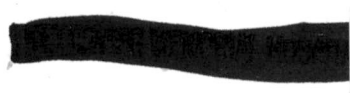

D1297985

## Sample Hospital Listing:

**ANYTOWN, Universal County**

⊠ **ANYTOWN HOSPITAL & CLINICS (777777)**, (Formerly Anytown Area Community Hospital and Clinic), 100 South Main Street, Zip 12345–6789; tel. 123/456–7890 **A**9 10  ]  ①

**F**10 12 23 24 29 30 31 37 39 49 51 55 57 64 65 66 68 70 71 72 77 78 83 87 88 91 96 97 106 107 110 111 113 124 **P**1 2 3 **S** Universal County Health System  ⑦ ② ③
Primary Contact: Ann M. Generic, Chief Executive Officer
COO: Ann M. Generic
CFO: Michael M. Generic
CMO: Peterl Van Generic, President Medical Staff  ④
CHR: Jerry Generic, Human Resources Director
Web address: www.website.org
**Control:** Other not–for–profit (including NFP Corporation) **Service:** General Medical and surgical  ⑤

**Staffed Beds:** 25 **Admissions:** 892 **Census:** 9 **Outpatient Visits:** 44014
**Births:** 51 **Total Expense ($000):** 19210 **Payroll Expense ($000):** 5864
**Personnel:** 182  ⑥

**ANYTOWN, Universal County**

⊠ **ANYTOWN HOSPITAL & CLINICS (777777)**, (Formerly Anytown Area Community Hospital and Clinic), 100 South Main Street, Zip 12345–6789; tel. 123/456–7890 **A**9 10

① = **Approval Codes**
② = **Physician Codes**
③ = **Health Care System Name**
④ = **Titles of Chief Administrators**
⑤ = **Control and Service Classifications**
⑥ = **Utilization Data**
⑦ = **Facility Codes**

---

**Hospital, Medicare Provider Number, Address, Telephone, Approval, Facility, and Physician Codes, Health Care System**

★ American Hospital Association (AHA) membership
□ The Joint Commission accreditation   ◇ DNV Healthcare Inc. accreditation
○ American Osteopathic Association (AOA) accreditation
△ Commission on Accreditation of Rehabilitation Facilities (CARF) accreditation

---

## ① Approval Codes

*Reported by the approving bodies specified, as of the dates noted.*

**1** Accreditation under the hospital program of The Joint Commission (May 2012).
**2** Cancer program approved by American College of Surgeons (March 2012).
†**3** Approval to participate in residency training, by the Accreditation Council for Graduate Medical Education (April 2012).
†**5** Medical school affiliation, reported to the American Medical Association (April 2012).
**6** Hospital–controlled professional nursing school, reported by National League for Nursing.
**7** Accreditation by Commission on Accreditation of Rehabilitation Facilities (March 2012).

**8** Member of Council of Teaching Hospitals of the Association of American Medical Colleges (February 2012).
**9** Hospitals contracting or participating in a Plan, reported by the Blue Cross and Blue Shield Association (April 2012).
**10** Certified for participation in the Health Insurance for the Aged (Medicare) Program by the Centers for Medicare and Medical Services (February 2012).
**11** Healthcare Facilities Accreditation Program *(formerly American Osteopathic Association accreditation)* (May 2012).

**12** Internship approved by American Osteopathic Association (April 2012).
**13** Residency approved by American Osteopathic Association (April 2012).
**18** Critical Access Hospitals (May 2012).
**19** Rural Referral Center (May 2012).
**20** Sole Community Provider (May 2012).
**21** Accreditation by DNV Healthcare Inc. (May 2012).

**Nonreporting** indicates that the 2011 Annual Survey questionnaire for the hospital was not received prior to publication.

---

## ② Physician Codes

*Actually available within, and reported by the institution; for definitions, see page A12.*

**(Alphabetical/Numerical Order)**

**1** Closed physician–hospital organization (PHO)
**2** Equity model
**3** Foundation

**4** Group practice without walls
**5** Independent practice association (IPA)
**6** Integrated salary model

**7** Management service organization (MSO)
**8** Open physician–hospital organization (PHO)

---

## ③ Health Care System Name

*The inclusion of the letter "S" (1) indicates that the hospital belongs to a health care system and (2) identifies the specific system to which the hospital belongs.*

---

## ④ Titles of Chief Administrators

## ⑤ Control and Service Classification

*For a list of control and service classifications, see page A13.*

**Control**–The type of organization that is responsible for establishing policy for overall operation of the hospital.

**Service**–The type of service the hospital provides to the majority of admissions.

---

## ⑥ Utilization Data

*Definitions are based on the American Hospital Association's Hospital Administration Terminology. In completing the survey, hospitals were requested to report data for a full year, in accord with their fiscal year, ending in 2011.*

**Beds**–Number of beds regularly maintained (set up and staffed for use) for inpatients as of the close of the reporting period. Excludes newborn bassinets.

**Admissions**–Number of patients accepted for inpatient service during a 12–month period; does not include newborn.

**Census**–Average number of inpatients receiving care each day during the 12–month reporting period; does not include newborn.

**Outpatient Visits**–A visit by a patient who is not lodged in the hospital while receiving medical, dental, or other services. Each appearance of an outpatient in each unit constitutes one visit regardless of the number of diagnostic and/or therapeutic treatments that a patient receives.

**Births**–Number of infants born in the hospital and accepted for service in a newborn infant bassinet during a 12–month period; excludes stillbirths.

**Expense:** Expense for a 12–month period; both total expense and payroll components are shown. Payroll expenses include all salaries and wages.

**Personnel:** Represents personnel situations as they existed at the end of the reporting period; includes full-time equivalents of part–time personnel. Full–time equivalents were calculated on the basis that two part–time persons equal one full–time person.

---

†Data from the Graduate Medical Education Database, Copyright 2012, American Medical Association, Chicago, Illinois.

## Sample Hospital Listing:

---

**Hospital, Medicare Provider Number, Address, Telephone, Approval, Facility, and Physician Codes, Health Care System**

★ American Hospital Association (AHA) membership    ○ American Osteopathic Association (AOA) accreditation
□ The Joint Commission accreditation    ◇ DNV Healthcare Inc. accreditation    △ Commission on Accreditation of Rehabilitation Facilities (CARF) accreditation

---

## ⑦ Facility Codes

*Provided directly by the hospital; for definitions, see page A6.*

### (Numerical Order)

1. Acute long-term care
2. Adult day care program
3. Airborne infection isolation room
4. Alcoholism-drug abuse or dependency inpatient unit
5. Alcoholism-drug abuse or dependency outpatient unit
6. Alzheimer center
7. Ambulance services
8. Ambulatory surgery center
9. Arthritis treatment center
10. Assisted living
11. Auxiliary
12. Bariatric/weight control services
13. Birthing room-LDR room-LDRP room
14. Blood donor center
15. Breast cancer screening/mammograms
16. Burn care services
17. Cardiac intensive care
18. Adult cardiology services
19. Pediatric cardiology services
20. Adult diagnostic catheterization
21. Pediatric diagnostic catheterization
22. Adult interventional cardiac catheterization
23. Pediatric diagnostic catheterization
24. Adult cardiac surgery
25. Pediatric cardiac surgery
26. Adult cardiac electrophysiology
27. Pediatric cardiac electrophysiology
28. Cardiac rehabilitation
29. Case management
30. Chaplaincy/pastoral care services
31. Chemotherapy
32. Children's wellness program
33. Chiropractic services
34. Community health education
35. Community outreach
36. Complementary and alternative medicine services
37. Computer assisted orthopedic surgery (CAOS)
38. Crisis prevention
39. Dental services
40. Emergency department
41. Pediatric emergency department
42. Satellite emergency department
43. Trauma center (certified)
44. Enabling services
45. Optical colonoscopy
46. Endoscopic ultrasound
47. Ablation of Barrett's esophagus
48. Esophageal impedance study

49. Endoscopic retrograde cholangiopancreatography (ERCP)
50. Enrollment assistance services
51. Extracorporeal shock wave lithotripter (ESWL)
52. Fertility clinic
53. Fitness center
54. Freestanding outpatient care center
55. Genetic testing/counseling
56. Geriatric services
57. Health fair
58. Health research
59. Health screenings
60. Hemodialysis
61. HIV–AIDS services
62. Home health services
63. Hospice program
64. Hospital–based outpatient care center services
65. Immunization program
66. Indigent care clinic
67. Intermediate nursing care
68. Linguistic/translation services
69. Meals on wheels
70. Medical surgical intensive care services
71. Mobile health services
72. Neonatal intensive care
73. Neonatal intermediate care
74. Neurological services
75. Nutrition programs
76. Obstetrics
77. Occupational health services
78. Oncology services
79. Orthopedic services
80. Other special care
81. Outpatient surgery
82. Pain management program
83. Inpatient palliative care unit
84. Palliative care program
85. Patient controlled analgesia (PCA)
86. Patient education center
87. Patient representative services
88. Pediatric intensive care services
89. Pediatric medical–surgical care
90. Physical rehabilitation inpatient services
91. Assistive technology center
92. Electrodiagnostic services
93. Physical rehabilitation outpatient services
94. Prosthetic and orthotic services
95. Robot-assisted walking therapy
96. Simulated rehabilitation environment
97. Primary care department
98. Psychiatric care
99. Psychiatric child–adolescent services
100. Psychiatric consultation–liaison services

101. Psychiatric education services
102. Psychiatric emergency services
103. Psychiatric geriatric services
104. Psychiatric outpatient services
105. Psychiatric partial hospitalization services
106. Psychiatric residential treatment
107. CT scanner
108. Diagnostic radioisotope facility
109. Electron beam computed tomography (EBCT)
110. Full–field digital mammography (FFDM)
111. Magnetic resonance imaging (MRI)
112. Intraoperative magnetic resonance imaging
113. Multi–slice spiral computed tomography (MSCT) (<64 slice CT)
114. Multi–slice spiral computed tomography (64 + slice CT)
115. Positron emission tomography (PET)
116. Positron emission tomography/CT (PET/CT)
117. Single photon emission computerized tomography (SPECT)
118. Ultrasound
119. Image–guided radiation therapy (IGRT)
120. Intensity–modulated radiation therapy (IMRT)
121. Proton beam therapy
122. Shaped beam radiation therapy
123. Stereotactic radiosurgery
124. Retirement housing
125. Robotic surgery
126. Rural health clinic
127. Skilled nursing care
128. Sleep center
129. Social work services
130. Sports medicine
131. Support groups
132. Swing bed services
133. Teen outreach services
134. Tobacco treatment/cessation program
135. Bone marrow transplant services
136. Heart transplant
137. Kidney transplant
138. Liver transplant
139. Lung transplant
140. Tissue transplant
141. Other transplant
142. Transportation to health services
143. Urgent care center
144. Virtual colonoscopy
145. Volunteer services department
146. Women's health center/services
147. Wound management services

# AHA Guide® to the Health Care Field

2013 Edition

AHA Guide® to the Health Care Field

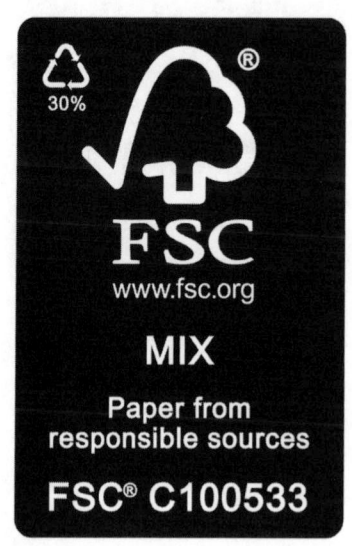

AHA Members $230
Nonmembers $350
AHA Item Number 010013
Telephone ORDERS 1–800–AHA–2626


ISSN 0094–8969
ISBN–13: 978–0–87258–906–3

# Contents

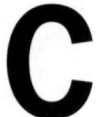

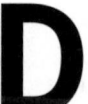

† List supplied by The Joint Commission

# Acknowledgements and Advisements

## Acknowledgements

The AHA Guide® to the Health Care Field is published annually by Health Forum LLC, an affiliate of the American Hospital Association. Contributions are made by Information Systems and Technology, Member Relations, Office of the President, Office of the Secretary, Printing Services Group, AHA Resource Center and the following participants:

| | |
|---|---|
| Stan Dziaba | Peter Kralovec |
| DeAnn Ellis | Andrea Liebig |
| Joan Finn | Denise Loggins |
| Deanna Frazier | Jennifer Pagan |
| Stella Hines | Steve Reczynski |
| Clisby Jackson | Christine Remedios |
| Danny Jackson | Elaine Singh |
| Kimberly Jackson | Judy Williams |

Health Forum LLC acknowledges the cooperation given by many professional groups and government agencies in the health care field, particularly the following: American College of Surgeons; American Medical Association; Blue Cross and Blue Shield Association; Council of Teaching Hospitals of the Association of American Medical Colleges; The Joint Commission; DNV Healthcare Inc.; National League for Nursing Accrediting Commission; Commission on Accreditation of Rehabilitation Facilities; American Osteopathic Association, Centers for Medicare & Medicaid Services; and various offices within the U.S. Department of Health and Human Services.

## Advisements

The data published here should be used with the following advisements: The data is based on replies to an annual survey that seeks a variety of information, not all of which is published in this book. The information gathered by the survey includes specific services, but not all of each hospital's services. Therefore, the data does not reflect an exhaustive list of all services offered by all hospitals. For information on the availability of additional data and products, please contact Health Forum LLC at 800/821–2039, or visit our web site.

Health Forum LLC does not assume responsibility for the accuracy of information voluntarily reported by the individual institutions surveyed. **The purpose of this publication is to provide basic data reflecting the delivery of health care in the United States and associated areas, and is not to serve as an official and all inclusive list of services offered by individual hospitals. The information reflected is based on data collected as of May 31, 2012.**

## An Introduction to *AHA Guide*®

Welcome, and thank you for purchasing the 2012 edition of *AHA Guide*®. This section is designed to aid you in using the book. While the primary focus of *AHA Guide* is on hospitals, it also contains information on other areas of the health care field, divided across its three major sections:

**A.** Hospitals
**B.** Health care systems, networks, and alliances
**C.** Health care organizations, agencies, and other health care providers

The information contained within this publication was compiled using AHA membership, and the AHA Annual Survey of Hospitals. *AHA Guide* is the leading hospital directory and represents hospitals with or without AHA membership.

Additional information contained in the front of AHA Guide includes:

- A section by section table of contents
- Recognition of the source of data in the *Acknowledgements and Advisements* section
- Information on AHA's history as well as a listing of our awards in *AHA Offices, Officers, Historical Data, and Awards*

## Getting Started: The AHA Guide Code Chart

Open the front cover and *AHA Guide* begins with the *2012 AHA Guide Code Chart*. This two page section (front and back) explains how to find and understand the most important elements of each hospital's listing. The chart is specially perforated and is meant to be extracted and used alongside Section A as a resource. The information found on these pages is repeated in the first section, so don't worry about removing the chart.

The *Code Chart* is a very useful tool to have when reading. It allows new users to become familiar with the data, and it aids returning users in understanding the new design and layout of *AHA Guide*. At the top of the chart, there is a sample listing. If you have used this publication before, you will notice the new columnar listing of all hospital entries by city. The city and county names are highlighted in gray, and all hospitals within the city follow. After the hospital name, you will find the address, telephone number, approval, facility and service codes, and health care systems to which the hospital belongs. Following this are the chief administrators and classifications for the hospital. Utilization data for the hospital is found in the box at the bottom of each hospital's entry in *AHA Guide*.

The chart further demonstrates how to understand these important elements:

1. **Approval codes** refer to certifications held by a hospital; they represent information supplied by various national approving and reporting bodies. For example, code A–3 indicates accreditation under one of the programs of the Accreditation Council for Graduate Medical Education, evidence that the hospital has been approved for participation in residency training.

2. **Physician codes** represent the different types of arrangements the hospital participates in with its physicians. In this section, code P-1 signifies a closed physician-hospital organization.

3. **Health Care System names** reference specific health care system headquarters to which the hospital belongs. The presence of a system name indicates that the hospital is a member. If no names are listed, the hospital does not belong to a system.

4. **Titles of Chief Administrators** including the Chief Executive Officer and, when available, other C-Suite officers such as the Chief Financial Officer, Chief Information Officer, Chief Medical Officer, Chief Operating Officer, and Chief Human Resources Officer.

5. **Classification** refers to two items in *AHA Guide*. **Control** classification indicates the organization that operates the hospital, and

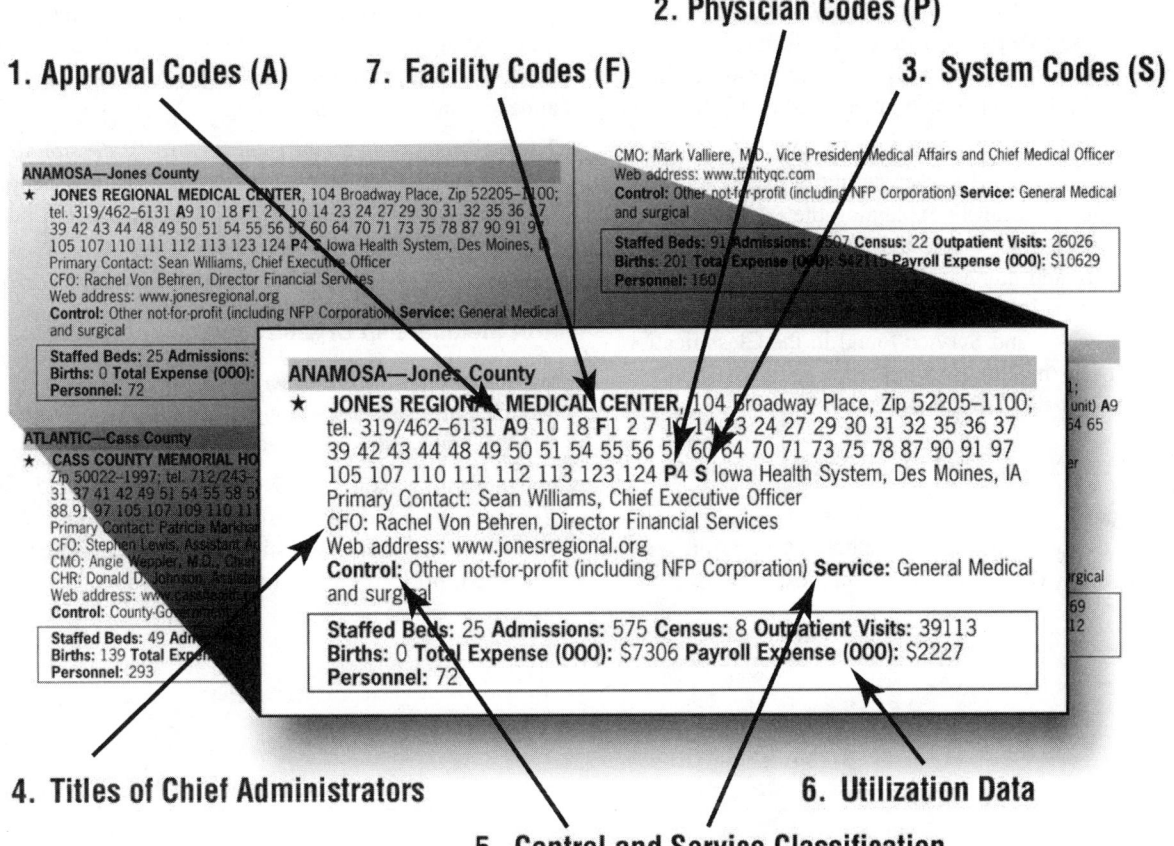

**1. Approval Codes (A)**

**7. Facility Codes (F)**

**2. Physician Codes (P)**

**3. System Codes (S)**

**4. Titles of Chief Administrators**

**5. Control and Service Classification**

**6. Utilization Data**

**Service** classification refers to the type of service the hospital offers. Previously, this section utilized numerical codes corresponding with a literal value, but the new design of *AHA Guide* bypasses the codes and instead displays the literal classifications for control and service.

- **Control:** In this section, organizations are divided among nonfederal government hospitals, nongovernment not-for-profit hospitals, investor owned for-profit hospitals, and federal government hospitals.
- **Service:** This section displays the primary type of service that a hospital offers. The most common value is general hospital. Among the other services listed in this section are specialties such as psychiatric hospitals or children's hospitals.

6. **Utilization Data** contains the statistics related to the day-to-day and cumulative operation of the hospital. The information included in this section consists of:
  - **Beds:** Number of beds regularly maintained.
  - **Admissions:** Amount of patients accepted for inpatient services over a 12-month period.

- **Census:** Average number of patients receiving care each day.
- **Outpatient Visits:** Amount of visits by patients not lodged in the hospital while receiving care.
- **Births:** Number of infants born in the hospital and accepted for service in a newborn infant bassinet.
- **Expense:** Includes all expenses (including payroll) that the hospital had over the 12-month period.
- **Personnel:** Represents personnel situations as they existed at the end of the reporting period. In this area, full time equivalency is calculated on the basis that two part-time persons equal one full-time person.

7. **Facility codes** provide a description of the specific services offered by a hospital. Code F-14, for instance, indicates that the hospital contains a Blood Donor Center.

### How To Use This Book

Section A begins with the *AHA Guide Hospital Listing Requirements*. This explains the requisite accreditations or characteristics a hospital must meet to be included in *AHA Guide*.

After this there is *An Explanation of the Hospital Listings*. These two pages review the information included in the Code Chart and are a vital resource in identifying the information, symbols, and codes for each hospital's listing.

Next up are the *Annual Survey* definitions, which go into even greater detail in explaining the facility and physician codes. Please note that these are arranged alphabetically and numerically to correspond with the code chart. Also included here are the definitions of the terms for Control and Service found in the Classification section. The listings of *Hospitals in the United States, by State* follow the definitions.

### Finding Hospitals & Health Care Professionals in Section A

There are two ways to locate hospitals in the print version of *AHA Guide*. One is by the hospital's geographic classification. In Section A, hospitals are arranged alphabetically by state and then by city. The second method is through the *Hospital Index* that appears directly after the listings.

There is also an *Index of Health Care Professionals* which begins after the first index that lists key people from hospitals and health systems. Look for fold out tabs and tabs on the sides of pages that mark the indices.

### AHA Membership Organizations

Section A ends with a description of the AHA Membership categories along with a listing of various AHA Membership organizations.

For more information on Systems, Networks, and Alliances, please read the introduction to Section B. Health organizations, agencies, and providers are described, prior to their listing, at the start of Section C.

# AHA Offices, Officers, and Historical Data

**Chicago:** 155 N. Wacker Drive, Chicago, IL 60606; tel. 312/422–3000

**Washington:** 325 Seventh Street, N.W., Suite 700, Washington, DC 20004; tel. 202/638–1100

## Past Presidents/Chairs†

| | | |
|---|---|---|
| 1899 ★James S. Knowles | 1938 ★Robert E. Neff | 1977 ★John M. Stagl |
| 1900 ★James S. Knowles | 1939 ★G. Harvey Agnew, M.D. | 1978 ★Samuel J. Tibbitts |
| 1901 ★Charles S. Howell | 1940 ★Fred G. Carter, M.D. | 1979 W. Daniel Barker |
| 1902 ★J. T. Duryea | 1941 ★B. W. Black, M.D. | 1980 ★Sister Irene Kraus |
| 1903 ★John Fehrenbatch | 1942 ★Basil C. MacLean, M.D. | 1981 ★Bernard J. Lachner |
| 1904 ★Daniel D. Test | 1943 ★James A. Hamilton | 1982 ★Stanley R. Nelson |
| 1905 ★George H. M. Rowe, M.D. | 1944 ★Frank J. Walter | 1983 Elbert E. Gilbertson |
| 1906 ★George P. Ludlam | 1945 ★Donald C. Smelzer, M.D. | 1984 Thomas R. Matherlee |
| 1907 ★Renwick R. Ross, M.D. | 1946 ★Peter D. Ward, M.D. | 1985 ★Jack A. Skarupa |
| 1908 ★Sigismund S. Goldwater, M.D. | 1947 ★John H. Hayes | 1986 Scott S. Parker |
| 1909 ★John M. Peters, M.D. | 1948 ★Graham L. Davis | 1987 Donald C. Wegmiller |
| 1910 ★H. B. Howard, M.D. | 1949 ★Joseph G. Norby | 1988 Eugene W. Arnett |
| 1911 ★W. L. Babcock, M.D. | 1950 ★John N. Hatfield | 1989 Edward J. Connors |
| 1912 ★Henry M. Hurd, M.D. | 1951 ★Charles F. Wilinsky, M.D. | 1990 David A. Reed |
| 1913 ★F. A. Washburn, M.D. | 1952 ★Anthony J. J. Rourke, M.D. | 1991 C. Thomas Smith |
| 1914 ★Thomas Howell, M.D. | 1953 ★Edwin L. Crosby, M.D. | 1992 D. Kirk Oglesby, Jr. |
| 1915 ★William O. Mann, M.D. | 1954 ★Ritz E. Heerman | 1993 Larry L. Mathis |
| 1916 ★Winford H. Smith, M.D. | 1955 ★Frank R. Bradley | 1994 Carolyn C. Roberts |
| 1917 ★Robert J. Wilson, M.D. | 1956 ★Ray E. Brown | 1995 Gail L. Warden |
| 1918 ★A. B. Ancker, M.D. | 1957 ★Albert W. Snoke, M.D. | 1996 Gordon M. Sprenger |
| 1919 ★A. R. Warner, M.D. | 1958 ★Tol Terrell | 1997 Reginald M. Ballantyne III |
| 1920 ★Joseph B. Howland, M.D. | 1959 ★Ray Amberg | 1998 John G. King |
| 1921 ★Louis B. Baldwin, M.D. | 1960 ★Russell A. Nelson, M.D. | 1999 Fred L. Brown |
| 1922 ★George O'Hanlon, M.D. | 1961 ★Frank S. Groner | 2000 ★Carolyn Boone Lewis |
| 1923 ★Asa S. Bacon | 1962 ★Jack Masur, M.D. | 2001 Gary A. Mecklenburg |
| 1924 ★Malcolm T. MacEachern, M.D. | 1963 ★T. Stewart Hamilton, M.D. | 2002 Sr. Mary Roch Rocklage, RSM |
| 1925 ★E. S. Gilmore | 1964 ★Stanley A. Ferguson | 2003 Dennis R. Barry |
| 1926 ★Arthur C. Bachmeyer, M.D. | 1965 ★Clarence E. Wonnacott | 2004 David L. Bernd |
| 1927 ★R. G. Brodrick, M.D. | 1966 ★Philip D. Bonnet, M.D. | 2005 George F. Lynn |
| 1928 ★Joseph C. Doane, M.D. | 1967 ★George E. Cartmill | **January–April 2006** Richard J. Umbdenstock |
| 1929 ★Louis H. Burlingham, M.D. | 1968 ★David B. Wilson, M.D. | **April–December 2006** George F. Lynn |
| 1930 ★Christopher G. Parnall, M.D. | 1969 ★George William Graham, M.D. | 2007 Kevin E. Lofton |
| 1931 ★Lewis A. Sexton, M.D. | 1970 ★Mark Berke | 2008 William D. Petasnick |
| 1932 ★Paul H. Fesler | 1971 ★Jack A. L. Hahn | 2009 Thomas M. Priselac |
| 1933 ★George F. Stephens, M.D. | 1972 ★Stephen M. Morris | 2010 Richard P. de Filippi |
| 1934 ★Nathaniel W. Faxon, M.D. | 1973 ★John W. Kauffman | 2011 John W. Bluford |
| 1935 ★Robert Jolly | 1974 ★Horace M. Cardwell | 2012 Teri G. Fontenot |
| 1936 ★Robin C. Buerki, M.D. | 1975 Wade Mountz | |
| 1937 ★Claude W. Munger, M.D. | 1976 H. Robert Cathcart | |

## Chief Executive Officers

| | | |
|---|---|---|
| 1917–18 ★William H. Walsh, M.D. | 1943–54 ★George Bugbee | 1986–91 Carol M. McCarthy, Ph.D., J.D. |
| 1919–24 ★Andrew Robert Warner, M.D. | 1954–72 ★Edwin L. Crosby, M.D. | 1991 Jack W. Owen (acting) |
| 1925–27 ★William H. Walsh, M.D. | 1972 Madison B. Brown, M.D. (acting) | 1991–2007 Richard J. Davidson |
| 1928–42 ★Bert W. Caldwell, M.D. | 1972–86 J. Alexander McMahon | 2007 Richard J. Umbdenstock (current) |

## Distinguished Service Award

The award recognizes significant lifetime contributions and service to health care institutions and associations.

| | | |
|---|---|---|
| 1934 Matthew O. Foley | 1964 Russell A. Nelson, M.D. | 1990 John W. Colloton |
| 1939 Malcolm T. MacEachern, M.D. | 1965 Albert W. Snoke, M.D. | 1991 Carol M. McCarthy, Ph.D., J.D. |
| 1940 Sigismund S. Goldwater, M.D. | 1966 Frank S. Groner | 1992 David H. Hitt |
| 1941 Frederic A. Washburn, M.D. | 1967 Rev. John J. Flanagan, S.J. | 1993 Edward J. Connors |
| 1942 Winford H. Smith, M.D. | 1968 Stanley W. Martin | Jack W. Owen |
| 1943 Arthur C. Bachmeyer, M.D. | 1969 T. Stewart Hamilton, M.D. | 1994 George Adams |
| 1944 Rt. Rev. Msgr. Maurice F. Griffin, LL.D. | 1970 Charles Patteson Cardwell, Jr. | 1995 Scott S. Parker |
| 1945 Asa S. Bacon | 1971 Mark Berke | 1996 John A. Russell |
| 1946 George F. Stephens, M.D. | 1972 Stanley A. Ferguson | 1997 D. Kirk Oglesby, Jr. |
| 1947 Robin C. Buerki, M.D. | 1973 Jack A. L. Hahn | 1998 Henry B. Betts, M.D. |
| 1948 James A. Hamilton | 1974 George William Graham, M.D. | 1999 Mitchell T. Rabkin, M.D. |
| 1949 Claude W. Munger, M.D. | 1975 George E. Cartmill | 2000 Gail L. Warden |
| 1950 Nathaniel W. Faxon, M.D. | 1976 D. O. McClusky, Jr. | 2001 Gordon M. Sprenger |
| 1951 Bert W. Caldwell, M.D. | 1977 Boone Powell | 2002 Carolyn Boone Lewis |
| 1952 Fred G. Carter, M.D. | 1978 Richard J. Stull | 2003 C. Thomas Smith |
| 1953 Basil C. MacLean, M.D. | 1979 Horace M. Cardwell | 2004 Michael C. Waters |
| 1954 George Bugbee | 1980 Donald W. Cordes | 2005 John G. King |
| 1955 Joseph G. Norby | 1981 Sister Mary Brigh Cassidy | 2006 Gary A. Mecklenburg |
| 1956 Charles F. Wilinsky, M.D. | 1982 R. Zach Thomas, Jr. | Sr. Mary Roch Rocklage, RSM |
| 1957 John H. Hayes | 1983 H. Robert Cathcart | 2007 Richard J. Davidson |
| 1958 John N. Hatfield | 1984 Matthew F. McNulty, Jr., Sc.D. | 2008 Fred L. Brown |
| 1959 Edwin L. Crosby, M.D. | 1985 J. Alexander McMahon | 2009 George F. Lynn |
| 1960 Oliver G. Pratt | 1986 Sister Irene Kraus | 2010 James J. Mongan, M.D. |
| 1961 E. M. Bluestone, M.D. | 1987 W. Daniel Barker | 2011 Thomas C. Royer, M.D. |
| 1962 Mother Loretto Bernard, S.C., R.N. | 1988 Elbert E. Gilbertson | 2012 Karen Davis, Ph.D. |
| 1963 Ray E. Brown | 1989 Donald G. Shropshire | |

★Deceased
†On June 3, 1972, the House of Delegates changed the title of the chief elected officer to chairman of the Board of Trustees, and the title of president was conferred on the chief executive officer of the Association.

# Award of Honor

Awarded to individuals, organizations, or groups to recognize an exemplary contribution to the health and well being of the people through leadership on a major health policy or social initiative.

| 1966 | Senator Lister Hill | 1996 | Stephen J. Hegarty | 2005 | Sr. Mary Jean Ryan |
|------|---------------------|------|--------------------|------|--------------------|
| 1967 | Emory W. Morris, D.D.S. | | Mothers Against Drunk Driving (MADD) | 2006 | Jordan J. Cohen, M.D. |
| 1971 | Special Committee on Provision of Health | 1997 | Paul B. Batalden, M.D. | | James W. Varnum |
| | Services (staff also) | | Habitat for Humanity International | 2007 | Edward A. Eckenhoff |
| 1982 | Walter J. McNemey | 1998 | John E. Curley, Jr. | | Stanley F. Hupfeld |
| 1989 | Ruth M. Rothstein | | National Civic League | 2008 | Regina M. Benjamin, MD, MBA |
| 1990 | Joyce C. Clifford, R.N. | 1999 | Joseph Cardinal Bernardin, Literacy | | Alfred G. Stubblefield |
| 1991 | Haynes Rice | | Volunteers of America | 2009 | The Center to Advance Palliative Care |
| 1992 | Donald W. Dunn | 2000 | Institute for Safe Medication Practices | | Paul B. Hofmann, Dr.PH |
| | Ira M. Lane, Jr. | 2001 | Dennis R. Barry | 2010 | Jack Bovender |
| 1993 | Elliott C. Roberts, Sr. | 2002 | Donald M. Berwick, M.D. | 2011 | Cary Medical Center, Caribou, ME |
| | William A. Spencer, M.D. | 2003 | Steven A. Schroeder, M.D. | 2012 | Ronald McDonald House Charities |
| 1994 | Robert A. Derzon | | Dan S. Wilford | | The Schwartz Center for Compassionate |
| 1995 | Russell G. Mawby, Ph.D. | 2004 | Ron J. Anderson, M.D. | | Healthcare |
| | John K. Springer | | Johnson & Johnson | | |

# Justin Ford Kimball Innovators Award

Recognition to individuals or organizations that have made outstanding, innovative contributions to health care financing and/or delivery that improves access or coordination of care.

| 1958 | E. A. van Steenwyk | 1973 | Herman M. Somers | 1994 | Donald A. Brennan |
|------|--------------------|------|------------------|------|-------------------|
| 1959 | George A. Newbury | 1974 | William H. Ford, Ph.D. | 1995 | E. George Middleton, Jr. |
| 1960 | C. Rufus Rorem, Ph.D. | 1975 | Earl H. Kammer | | Glenn R. Mitchell |
| 1961 | James E. Stuart | 1976 | J. Ed McConnell | 1997 | Harvey Pettry |
| 1962 | Frank Van Dyk | 1978 | Edwin R. Werner | | D. David Sniff |
| 1963 | William S. McNary | 1979 | Robert M. Cunningham, Jr. | 1998 | Montana Health Research and Education |
| 1964 | Frank S. Groner | 1981 | Maurice J. Norby | | Foundation |
| 1965 | J. Douglas Colman | 1982 | Robert E. Rinehimer | 1999 | Kenneth W. Kizer, M.D. |
| 1967 | Walter J. McNemey | 1983 | John B. Morgan, Jr. | 2002 | David M. Lawrence, M.D. |
| 1968 | John W. Paynter | 1984 | Joseph F. Duplinsky | 2003 | Lowell C. Kruse |
| 1970 | Edwin L. Crosby, M.D. | 1985 | David W. Stewart | 2006 | Spencer Foreman, M.D. |
| 1971 | H. Charles Abbott | 1988 | Ernest W. Saward, M.D. | 2009 | On Lok |
| 1972 | John R. Mannix | 1990 | James A. Vohs | 2012 | Thomas S. Nesbitt, M.D. |
| | | 1993 | John C. Lewin, M.D. | | |

# Board of Trustees Award

Individuals or groups who have made substantial and noteworthy contributions to the work of the American Hospital Association.

| 1959 | Joseph V. Friel | | Samuel J. Tibbitts | 1999 | Sister Carol Keehan |
|------|-----------------|------|--------------------|------|---------------------|
| | John H. Hayes | 1981 | Vernon A. Knutson | | C. Edward McCauley |
| 1960 | Duncan D. Sutphen, Jr. | | John E. Sullivan | | Stephen Rogness |
| 1963 | Eleanor C. Lambertsen, R.N., Ed.D. | 1982 | John Bigelow | 2000 | Dennis May |
| 1964 | John R. Mannix | | Robert W. O'Leary | 2001 | Spencer C. Johnson |
| 1965 | Albert G. Hahn | | Jack W. Owen | | Michael M. Mitchel |
| | Maurice J. Norby | 1984 | Howard J. Berman | 2002 | Victor L. Campbell |
| 1966 | Madison B. Brown, M.D. | | O. Ray Hurst | | Joseph A. Parker |
| | Kenneth Williamson | | James R. Neely | 2003 | J. Richard Gaintner, M.D. |
| 1967 | Alanson W. Wilcox | 1985 | James E. Ferguson | | Donald A. Wilson |
| 1968 | E. Dwight Barnett, M.D. | | Cleveland Rodgers | 2004 | Richard L. Clarke |
| 1969 | Vane M. Hoge, M.D. | 1986 | Rex N. Olsen | | Thelma Traut |
| | Joseph H. McNinch, M.D. | 1987 | Michael Lesparre | 2005 | Merrill Gappmayer |
| 1972 | David F. Drake, Ph.D. | 1988 | Barbara A. Donaho, R.N. | | Leo Greenawalt |
| | Paul W. Earle | 1989 | Walter H. MacDonald | 2006 | Robert L. Harman |
| | Michael Lesparre | | Donald R. Newkirk | | Kenneth G. Stella |
| | Andrew Pattullo | 1990 | William T. Robinson | 2007 | Deborah Freund, Ph.D. |
| 1973 | Tilden Cummings | 1992 | Jack C. Bills | | Michael D. Stephens |
| | Edmond J. Lanigan | | Anne Hall Davis | 2008 | James R. Castle |
| 1974 | James E. Hague | 1993 | Theodore C. Eickhoff, M.D. | 2009 | Richard M. Knapp, Ph.D. |
| | Sister Marybelle | | Stephen W. Gamble | 2010 | Fred Hessler |
| 1975 | Helen T. Yast | | Yoshi Honkawa | | John G. O'Brien |
| 1976 | Boynton P. Livingston | 1994 | Roger M. Busfield, Jr., Ph.D. | 2011 | Carolyn F. Scanlan |
| | James Ludlam | 1995 | Stephen E. Dorn | | Charlotte S. Yeh, MD |
| | Helen McGuire | | William L. Yates | 2012 | Larry S. Gage |
| 1979 | Newton J. Jacobson | 1996 | Leigh E. Morris | | Larry McAndrews |
| | Edward W. Weimer | | John Quigley | | |
| 1980 | Robert B. Hunter, M.D. | 1998 | John D. Leech | | |

# Citation for Meritorious Service

| 1968 | F. R. Knautz | | Gordon McLachlan | 1983 | David M. Kinzer |
|------|--------------|------|------------------|------|------------------|
| | Sister Conrad Mary, R.N. | 1977 | Theodore Cooper, M.D. | 1984 | Donald L. Custis, M.D. |
| 1971 | Hospital Council of Southern California | 1979 | Norman D. Burkett | 1985 | John A. D. Cooper, M.D. |
| 1972 | College of Misericordia, Dallas, PA | | John L. Quigley | | Imperial Council of the Ancient Arabic Order |
| 1973 | Madison B. Brown, M.D. | | William M. Whelan | | of the Nobles of the Mystic Shrine for |
| | Samuel J. Tibbitts | 1980 | Sister Grace Marie Hiltz | | North America |
| 1975 | Kenneth B. Babcock, M.D. | | Leo J. Gehrig, M.D. | 1986 | Howard F. Cook |
| | Sister Mary Maurita Sengelaube | 1981 | Richard Davi | 1987 | David H. Hitt |
| 1976 | Chaiker Abbis | | Pearl S. Fryar | | Lucile Packard |
| | Susan Jenkins | 1982 | Jorge Brull Nater | | |

This citation is no longer awarded

# AHA NOVA Awards

This award honors effective, collaborative programs focused on improving community health status.

## 1994

**Health Partners of Philadelphi (PA):** Albert Einstein Medical Center, Episcopal Hospital, Frankford Hospital, Medical College of Pennsylvania Hospital, St. Christopher's Hospital for Children, Temple University Hospital

**Decker Family Development Center:** Children's Hospital Medical Center of Akron (OH)

**Denver (CO) School–Based Clinics:** The Children's Hospital

**Basic Health Plan:** Dominican Network; Mount Carmel Hospital, Colville, WA; St. Joseph's

Hospital, Chewelah, WA; and Holy Family Hospital, Spokane, WA

**HealthLink:** Lakes Region General Hospital, Laconia, NH

## 1995

**Bladen Community Care Network:** Bladen County Hospital, Elizabethtown, NC

**Building a Healthier Community:** Community–Kimball Health Care System, Toms River, NJ

**Injury Prevention Program:** Harlem Hospital Center, New York City, NY

**The Community Ministries & Outreach Program:** Reaching Out to Our Vickery/Meadow

Neighborhood: Presbyterian Healthcare System, Dallas, TX

**"CHOICES":** Shriners Hospitals for Crippled Children, Tampa, FL

## 1996

**Lincoln and Sunnyslope:** John C. Lincoln Hospital and Health Center, Sunnyslope, AZ

**Growing into Life Task Force:** Aiken (SC) Regional Medical Centers

**People Caring for People:** Beatrice (NE) Community Hospital and Health Center

**Injury Prevention Center of the Greater Dayton (OH) Area:** The Children's Medical Center, Good

Samaritan Hospital and Health Center, Grandview Hospital, Kettering Memorial Hospital, Miami Valley Hospital, and St. Elizabeth Medical Center

**Family Road:** Hutzel Hospital, Detroit, MI

## 1997

**Health Promotion Schools of Excellence Program:** Alliant Health System and Kosair Children's Hospital, Louisville, KY

**Health, Outreach, Prevention, and Education (HOPE):** Health First Holmes Regional Medical Center, Melbourne, FL

**Healthy Community Initiative:** Roper Care Alliance, Charleston, SC

**Obstetrical Care and Prenatal Counseling Program:** St. Alexius Medical Center, Bismarck, ND

**HIV/AIDS Neighborhood Service Program:** Yale–New Haven Hospital, New Haven, CT

## 1998

**Partners for a Healthier Community:** Evergreen Community Health Care, Group Health Cooperative of Puget Sound, Overlake Hospital Medical Center, Providence Health System/Medalia HealthCare, Seattle, WA

**Glenwood–Lyndale Community Clinic:** Hennepin County Medical Center, Minneapolis, MN

**Greater Dallas (TX) Injury Prevention Center:** Parkland Health & Hospital System, Children's Medical Center of Dallas, Baylor Health Care System, Methodist Hospitals of Dallas, and Presbyterian Healthcare System

**Network of Trust:** Phoebe Putney Memorial Hospital, Albany, GA

**The Lauderdale Court: A Community Partnership:** St. Joseph Hospital and Health Centers, Memphis, TN

## 1999

**Making a Case for Community Health:** Middletown (OH) Regional Hospital

**The Family Resource Center:** Mount Carmel Medical Center, Pittsburgh, KS

**The Health Neighborhood Project:** St. Patrick Hospital, Missoula, MT

**Kids for Health:** Washington Regional Medical Center, Fayetteville, AR

**Children's Village:** Yakima Memorial Hospital, Yakima, WA

## 2000

**Community Healthcare Network:** Columbus (GA) Regional Healthcare System

**Pasadena County Asthma Project:** Huntington Memorial Hospital, Pasadena, CA

**Ashe County Health Council "Health Carolinias Task Force":** Ashe Memorial Hospital, Jefferson, NC

**Caritas–Connection Project:** St. Mary's Hospital, Passaic, NJ

**Correctional Health Care Program:** Baystate Health System, Springfield, MA

## 2001

**J.C. Lewis Health Center:** Memorial Health and St. Joseph's Candler Health System, Savannah, GA

**Project C.A.R.E.:** Mercy Medical Center, Canton, OH

**TeenHealthFX.com:** Atlantic Health System, Florham Park, NJ

**Vista ElderCARE:** Vista Health, Waukegan, IL

**Western Village Enterprise School:** INTEGRIS Health, Oklahoma City, OK

## 2002

**Chester Community Connections:** Crozer–Keystone Health System, Springfield, PA

**The Hope Street Family Center:** California Hospital Medical Center, Los Angeles, CA

**Mobile Health Outreach Ministry:** St. Vincent's Health System, Jacksonville, FL

**Operation Access:** Kaiser Foundation Hospitals, Oakland; Sutter Health, Sacramento; San Francisco General Hospital, San Francisco; St. Rose Hospital, Hayward; and Santa Rosa Memorial Hospital, Santa Rosa, CA

**Wilmington Health Access for Teens:** New Hanover Health Network, Wilmington, NC

## 2003

**C.O.A.C.H. for Kids:** Cedars–Sinai Medical Center, Los Angeles, CA

**Community Action Network:** Trinity Regional Medical Center, Fort Dodge, IA

**Hearts N' Health:** Glendale Adventist Medical Center, Glendale, CA

**Saint Joseph Health Center:** Saint Joseph Regional Medical Center, South Bend, IN

**St. Mary Medical Center Bensalem Ministries:** St. Mary Medical Center, Langhorne, PA

## 2004

**Better Beginnings:** Brockton Hospital, Brockton, MA

**Buffalo County Community Health Partners:** Good Samaritan Health Systems, Kearney, NE

**Quad City Health Initiative:** Genesis Health System, Davenport, IA and Trinity Regional Health System, Rock Island, IL

**Quality of Life in the Truckee Meadows:** Washoe Health System, Reno, NV

**Solano Coalition for Better Health, Inc.:** NorthBay Healthcare Group, Fairfield, CA; Sutter Solano Medical Center, Vallejo, CA; and Kaiser Permanente, Martinez, CA

## 2005

**Children's Health Connection:** McKay-Dee Hospital Center, Ogden, UT

**Palmetto Health's Vision Health Initiative:** Palmetto Health, Columbia, SC

**Project Dulce, Whittier Institute for Diabetes:** Scripps Health, San Diego, CA

**Toledo/Lucas County CareNet:** Mercy Health Partners, ProMedica Health System, and Medical

University of Ohio, all of Toledo, OH and St. Luke's Hospital, Maumee, OH

**Volunteer Health Advisor (VHA) Program:** Cambridge Health Alliance, Cambridge, MA

## 2006

**Healthy Learners, Columbia, SC:** Allendale County Hospital, Fairfax, SC; McLeod Medical Center–Dillon, Dillon, SC; Sisters of Charity Providence Hospitals, Columbia, SC; and Self Regional Healthcare, Greenwood, SC

**Primary Care Access Network (PCAN):** Health Central, Ocoee, FL; Florida Hospital, Winter Park, FL; and Orlando Regional Healthcare, Orlando, FL
**ProHealth Care Community Health Outreach Initiative:** ProHealth Care, Waukesha, WI

**St. Joseph Mobile Health Services:** Saint Joseph HealthCare Inc., Lexington, KY
**Yonkers Childhood Health Initiative:** St. John's Riverside, Yonkers, NY

## 2007

**Medical-Legal Partnership for Children:** Boston Medical Center, Boston, MA
**NOW (Nutritional Options for Wellness) Program:** Spectrum Health, Grand Rapids, MI

**Richland Care:** Palmetto Health, Columbia, SC
**Trauma Nurses Talk Tough:** Legacy Health System, Portland, OR

**UMass Memorial Medical Center Healthy Youth Development Initiative:** UMass Memorial Health Care, Worcester, MA
**Youth Health Partnership-Patee Market Youth Dental Clinic:** Heartland Health, St. Joseph, MO

## 2008

**Partnership for Community Health:** California Pacific Medical Center, San Francisco, CA
**Every Child Succeeds:** Cincinnati Children's Hospital Medical Center, Cincinnati, OH

**Memorial Hermann Health Centers for Schools:** Memorial Hermann, Houston, TX
**Nutrition Center of Maine:** Saint Mary's Health System, Lewiston, ME

*ENERGIZE!* **Pediatric Diabetes Intervention Program:** WakeMed Health & Hospitals, Raleigh, NC

## 2009

**Lighten Up 4 Life:** Mission Health System, Asheville, NC
**Project BRIEF:** Jacobi Medical Center and North Central Bronx Hospital, Bronx, NY

**Really Awesome Health (RAH) and Wholesome Routines:** Duke Raleigh Hospital, Raleigh, NC
**Student Success Jobs Program:** Brigham and Women's Hospital, Boston, MA

**Taos First Steps Program:** Holy Cross Hospital, Taos, NM

## 2010

**Community-Based Alternatives to the Emergency Room:** Lee Memorial Health System, Fort Meyers, FL
**Health-e-Access Telemedicine:** University of Rochester Medical Center, Rochester, NY

**Healthy Futures:** Munson Healthcare System, Traverse City, MI
**Healthy San Francisco:** San Francisco General Hospital, University of California Medical Center, Chinese Hospital, California Pacific Medical Center,

Saint Francis Memorial Hospital, St. Mary's Medical Center, and Kaiser Permanente, San Francisco, CA
**Pediatric Asthma Program:** Sinai Health System, Chicago, IL

## 2011

**Emergency Department Consistent Care Program:** Providence St. Peter Hospital, Olympia, WA
**Integrated Community Nursing Program at Parkview Health:** Parkview Health, Fort Wayne, IN

**Milwaukee Health Care Partnership:** Aurora Health Care, Children's Hospital & Health System, Inc., Columbia St. Mary's, and Froedtert Health, all of Milwaukee, WI, and Wheaton Franciscan Healthcare, Glendale, WI

**The Diabetes Collaborative:** Northwestern Memorial Hospital, Chicago, IL
**Rochester Youth Violence Partnership:** University of Rochester Medical Center and Rochester General Health System, Rochester, NY

## 2012

**The Beth Embraces Wellness: An Integrated Approach to Prevention in the Community:** Newark Beth Israel Medical Center and Children's Hospital of New Jersey, Newark, NJ

**CARE Network:** St. Joseph Health Queen of the Valley Medical Center, Napa, CA
**Fitness in the City:** Boston Children's Hospital, Boston, MA

**Puff City:** Henry Ford Health System, Detroit, MI
**Rural Health Initiative:** Shawano Medical Center of ThedaCare, Shawano, WI

# The Carolyn Boone Lewis Living the Vision Award

Organizations and individuals living AHA's vision of a society of healthy communities where all individuals reach their highest potential for health.

| | | | | | | |
|---|---|---|---|---|---|---|
| 1998 | Memorial Healthcare System, Hollywood, FL | | 2001 | Salina Regional Health Center, Salina, KS | 2005 | Fairbanks Memorial Hospital, Fairbanks, AK |
| 1999 | Baptist Health System, Montgomery, AL Robert A. DeVries, Battle Creek, MI | | 2002 | Health Improvement Collaborative of Greater Cincinnati, Cincinnati, OH | | Boston Medical Center, Boston, MA |
| 2000 | Memorial Health System, South Bend, IN Rockingham Memorial Hospital, Harrisonburg, VA | | 2003 | Franklin Memorial Hospital, Farmington, ME | 2010 | Lehigh Valley Health Network, Allentown, PA |
| | | | 2004 | Jamaica Hospital Medical Center, Jamaica, New York | 2011 | Alaska Native Tribal Health Consortium, Anchorage, AK |

# Circle of Life Award

This award celebrates innovation in palliative and end-of-life care.

## 2000

Improving Care through the End of Life, Franciscan Health System, Gig Harbor, WA

The Hospice of The Florida Suncoast, Largo, FL

Louisiana State Penitentiary Hospice Program, Angola, LA

## 2001

Department of Pain Medicine and Palliative Care, Beth Israel Medical Center, New York, NY

Palliative CareCenter & Hospice of the North Shore, Evanston , IL

St. Joseph's Manor, Trumbull, CT

## 2002

Children's Program of San Diego Hospice and Children's Hospital and Health Center of San Diego, San Diego, CA

Hospice of the Bluegrass, Lexington, KY
Project Safe Conduct, Hospice of the Western Reserve and Ireland Cancer Center, Cleveland, OH

**Special Circle of Life Award** Population–based Palliative Care Research Network (PoPCRN), Denver, CO

## 2003

Hospice & Palliative CareCenter, Winston–Salem, NC

Providence Health System, Portland, OR

University of California Davis Health System, Sacramento, CA

## 2004

Hope Hospice and Palliative Care, Fort Myers, FL

St. Mary's Healthcare System for Children, Bayside, NY

University of Texas M.D. Anderson Cancer Center Palliative Care, Houston, TX

## 2005

High Point Regional Health System, High Point, NC

Palliative and End-of-life Care Program, Hoag Memorial Hospital Presbyterian, Newport Beach, CA

Thomas Palliative Care Unit, VCU Massey Cancer Center, Richmond, VA

## 2006

Continuum Hospice Care, New York, NY

Mercy Supportive Care, St. Joseph Mercy Oakland, Pontiac, MI

Transitions and Life Choices, Fairview Health Services, Minneapolis, MN

| | | |
|---|---|---|
| **2007** | | |
| UCSF Palliative Care Program, San Francisco, CA | Covenant Hospice, Pensacola, FL | Woodwell: A Program of Presbyterian SeniorCare and Family Hospice and Palliative Care, Oakmont, PA |
| **2008** | | |
| Children's Hospitals and Clinics of Minnesota, Pain and Palliative Care Program, Minneapolis, MN | Haven Hospice, Gainesville, FL | The Pediatric Advanced Care Team, The Children's Hospital of Philadelphia, Philadelphia, PA |
| **2009** | | |
| Four Seasons, Flat Rock, NC | Oregon Health and Science University Palliative Medicine & Comfort Care Program, Portland, OR | Wishard Health Services Palliative Care Program, Indianapolis, IN |
| **2010** | | |
| Department of Veteran Affairs, VA New York/New Jersey Healthcare Network, Brooklyn, NY | Kansas City Hospice & Palliative Care, Kansas City, MO | Snohomish Palliative Partnership, Everett, WA |
| **2011** | | |
| The Center for Hospice & Palliative Care, Cheektowaga, NY | Gilchrist Hospice Care, Hunt Valley, MD | St. John Providence Health System, Detroit, MI |
| **2012** | | |
| Haslinger Family Pediatric Palliative Care Center, Akron Children's Hospital, Akron, OH | Calvary Hospital, Bronx, NY | Sharp HealthCare, San Diego, CA |

## The American Hospital Association–McKesson Quest for Quality Prize
Honoring Leadership and Innovation in Patient Care Quality, Safety, and Commitment

| | | |
|---|---|---|
| **2002** | | |
| Missouri Baptist Medical Center, St. Louis, MO | **Finalist:** Fairview Hospital, Greater, Barrington, MA | **Finalist:** Minnesota Children's Hospital and Clinics, Minneapolis, MN |
| **2003** | | |
| Abington Memorial Hospital, Abington, PA | **Finalist:** Beaumont Hospitals, Royal Oak, MI | **Finalist:** University of Wisconsin Hospital and Clinics, Madison, WI |
| **2004** | | |
| Sentara Norfolk General Hospital, Norfolk, VA | **Finalist:** The Johns Hopkins Hospital, Baltimore, MD | **Finalist:** Mary Lanning Memorial Hospital, Hastings, NE |
| **2005** | | |
| North Mississippi Medical Center, Tupelo, MS | **Finalist:** El Camino Hospital, Mountain View, CA | **Finalist:** NewYork-Presbyterian Hospital, New York, NY |
| **2006** | | |
| Cincinnati Children's Hospital Medical Center, Cincinnati, OH | | |
| **2007** | | |
| Columbus Regional Hospital, Columbus, IN | **Finalist:** Cedars-Sinai Medical Center, Los Angeles, CA | **Finalist:** INTEGRIS Baptist Medical Center, Oklahoma City, OK |
| **2008** | | |
| Munson Medical Center, Traverse City, MI | **Finalist:** University of Michigan Hospitals & Health Centers, Ann Arbor, MI | |
| **2009** | | |
| Bronson Methodist Hospital, Kalamazoo, MI | **Finalist:** Beth Israel Deaconess Medical Center, Boston, MA | |
| **2010** | | |
| McLeod Regional Medical Center, Florence, SC | **Finalist:** Henry Ford Hospital, Detroit, MI | |
| **2011** | | |
| Memorial Regional Hospital, Hollywood, FL | **Finalist:** AtlantiCare Regional Medical Center, Atlantic City, NJ | **Finalist:** Northwestern Memorial Hospital, Chicago, IL |
| **2012** | | |
| University Hospitals Case Medical Center, Cleveland, OH | **Finalist:** Lincoln Medical and Mental Health Center, Bronx, NY | **Finalist:** University of North Carolina Hospitals, Chapel Hill, NC and Life Choices, Fairview Health Services, Minneapolis, MN |

## Foster G. McGaw Prize
Honors health delivery organizations that have demonstrated exceptional commitment to community service.

| | | | | | |
|---|---|---|---|---|---|
| **1986** | Lutheran Medical Center, Brooklyn, NY | **1994** | Parkland Memorial Hospital, Dallas, TX | **2002** | John C. Lincoln Health Network, Phoenix, AZ |
| **1987** | Copley Hospital, Morrisville, VT | **1995** | Our Lady of Lourdes Medical Center, Camden, NJ | **2003** | Phoebe Putney Memorial Hospital, Albany, GA |
| | Mount Sinai Hospital, Hartford, CT | | | | |
| **1988** | MetroHealth System, Cleveland, OH | **1996** | St. Mary's Hospital, Rochester, NY | **2004** | Henry Ford Health System, Detroit, MI |
| **1989** | Greater Southeast Healthcare System, Washington, DC | **1997** | Bladen County Hospital Rural Health Network, Elizabethtown, NC | **2005** | Venice Family Clinic, Venice, CA |
| **1990** | Mount Zion Medical Center of The University of California-San Francisco, San Francisco, CA | **1998** | Allina Health System, Minneapolis, MN | **2006** | Memorial Healthcare System, Hollywood, FL |
| | | **1999** | LAC+USC Healthcare Network, Los Angeles, CA | **2007** | Harborview Medical Center, Seattle, WA |
| **1991** | Franklin Regional Hospital, Franklin, NH | | | **2008** | St. Mary's Health System, Lewiston, ME |
| **1992** | Mount Sinai Hospital Medical Center of Chicago, Chicago, IL | **2000** | Kaweah Delta Health Care District, Visalia, CA | **2009** | Heartland Health, St. Joseph, MO |
| | | | | **2010** | Allegiance Health, Jackson, MI |
| **1993** | The Cambridge Hospital, Cambridge, MA | **2001** | Memorial Hospital of South Bend, South Bend, IN | **2011** | Mt. Ascutney Hospital and Health Center, Windsor, VT |

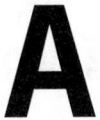
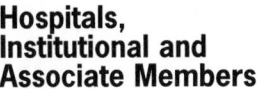

An institution may be listed by the American Hospital Association if it is accredited as a hospital by The Joint Commission, American Osteopathic Association, DNV Healthcare accredited, or Medicare certified as a provider of acute service under Title 18 of the Social Security Act. Membership in the American Hospital Association is not a prerequisite.

If none of the four conditions mentioned above are satisfied, an insititution licensed as a hospital by the appropriate state agency may be registered by AHA as a hospital by meeting the following alernative requirements:

**Function:** The primary function of the institution is to provide patient services, diagnostic and therapeutic, for particular or general medical conditions.

1. The institution shall maintain at least six inpatient beds, which shall be continuously available for the care of patients who are nonrelated and who stay on the average in excess of 24 hours per admission.

2. The institution shall be constructed, equipped, and maintained to ensure the health and safety of patients and to provide uncrowded, sanitary facilities for the treatment of patients.

3. There shall be an identifiable governing authority legally and morally responsible for the conduct of the hospital.

4. There shall be a chief executive to whom the governing authority delegates the continuous responsibility for the operation of the hospital in accordance with established policy.

5. There shall be an organized medical staff of fully licensed physicians* that may include other licensed individuals permitted by law and by the hospital to provide patient care services independently in the hospital. The medical staff shall be accountable to the governing authority for maintaining proper standards of medical care, and it shall be governed by bylaws adopted by said staff and approved by the governing authority.

6. Each patient shall be admitted on the authority of a member of the medical staff who has been granted the privilege to admit patients to inpatient services in accordance with state law and criteria for standards of medical care established by the individual medical staff. Each patient's general medical condition is the responsibility of a qualified physician member of the medical staff. When nonphysician members of the medical staff are granted privileges to admit patients, provision is made for prompt medical evaluation of these patients by a qualified physician. Any graduate of a foreign medical school who is permitted to assume responsibilities for patient care shall possess a valid license to practice medicine, or shall be certified by the Educational Commission for Foreign Medical Graduates, or shall have qualified for and have successfully completed an academic year of supervised clinical training under the direction of a medical school approved by the Liaison Committee on GAT Medical Education.

7. Registered nurse supervision and other nursing services are continuous.

8. A current and complete medical record shall be maintained by the institution for each patient and shall be available for reference.

9. Pharmacy service shall be maintained in the institution and shall be supervised by a registered pharmacist.

10. The institution shall provide patients with food service that meets their nutritional and therapeutic requirements; special diets shall also be available.

---

\* Physician–Term used to describe an individual with an M.D. or D.O. degree who is fully licensed to practice medicine in all its phases.

‡ The completed records in general shall contain at least the following: the patient's identifying data and consent forms, medical history, record of physical examination, physicians' progress notes, operative notes, nurses' notes, routine x–ray and laboratory reports, doctors' orders, and final diagnosis.

# Types of Hospitals

In addition to meeting these 10 general requirements, hospitals are listed as one of four types of hospitals: general, special, rehabilitation and chronic disease, or psychiatric. The following definitions of function by type of hospital and special requirements are:

## General

The primary function of the institution is to provide patient services, diagnostic and therapeutic, for a variety of medical conditions. A general hospital also shall provide:

- diagnostic x–ray services with facilities and staff for a variety of procedures
- clinical laboratory service with facilities and staff for a variety of procedures and with anatomical pathology services regularly and conveniently available
- operating room service with facilities and staff.

## Special

The primary function of the institution is to provide diagnostic and treatment services for patients who have specified medical conditions, both surgical and nonsurgical. A special hospital also shall provide:

- such diagnostic and treatment services as may be determined by the Executive Committee of the Board of Trustees of the American Hospital Association to

be appropriate for the specified medical conditions for which medical services are provided shall be maintained in the institution with suitable facilities and staff. If such conditions do not normally require diagnostic x–ray service, laboratory service, or operating room service, and if any such services are therefore not maintained in the institution, there shall be written arrangements to make them available to patients requiring them.

- clinical laboratory services capable of providing tissue diagnosis when offering pregancy termination services.

## Rehabilitation and Chronic Disease

The primary function of the institution is to provide diagnostic and treatment services to handicapped or disabled individuals requiring restorative and adjustive services. A rehabilitation and chronic disease hospital also shall provide:

- arrangements for diagnostic x–ray services, as required, on a regular and conveniently available basis
- arrangements for clinical laboratory service, as required on a regular and conveniently available basis
- arrangements for operating room service, as required, on a regular and conveniently available basis
- a physical therapy service with suitable facilities and staff in the institution
- an occupational therapy service with suitable facilities and staff in the institution

- arrangements for psychological and social work services on a regular and conveniently available basis
- arrangements for educational and vocational services on a regular and conveniently available basis
- written arrangements with a general hospital for the transfer of patients who require medical, obstetrical, or surgical services not available in the institution.

## Psychiatric

The primary function of the institution is to provide diagnostic and treatment services for patients who have psychiatric–related illnesses. A psychiatric hospital also shall provide:

- arrangements for clinical laboratory service, as required, on a regular and conveniently available basis
- arrangements for diagnostic x–ray services, as required on a regular and conveniently available basis
- psychiatric, psychological, and social work service with facilities and staff in the institution
- arrangements for electroencephalograph services, as required, on a regular and conveniently available basis.
- written arrangements with a general hospital for the transfer of patients who require medical, obstetrical, or surgical services not available in the institution.

The American Hospital Association may, at the sole discretion of the Executive Committee of the Board of Trustees, grant, deny, or withdraw the listing of an institution.

---

* Physician–Term used to describe an individual with an M.D. or D.O. degree who is fully licensed to practice medicine in all its phases.

‡ The completed records in general shall contain at least the following: the patient's identifying data and consent forms, medical history, record of physical examination, physicians' progress notes, operative notes, nurses' notes, routine x–ray and laboratory reports, doctors' orders, and final diagnosis.

# Explanation of Hospital Listings

## Sample Hospital Listing:

**ANYTOWN, Universal County**

✠ **ANYTOWN HOSPITAL & CLINICS (777777)**, (Formerly Anytown Area Community Hospital and Clinic), 100 South Main Street, Zip 12345–6789; tel. 123/456–7890 **A9** 10  ] ①

**F**10 12 23 24 29 30 31 37 39 49 51 55 57 64 65 66 68 70 71 72 77 78 83 87 88 91 96 97 106 107 110 111 113 124 **P**1 2 3 **S** Universal County Health System  ② ③  ⑦
Primary Contact: Ann M. Generic, Chief Executive Officer
COO: Ann M. Generic
CFO: Michael M. Generic
CMO: Peterl Van Generic, President Medical Staff  ④
CHR: Jerry Generic, Human Resources Director
Web address: www.website.org
**Control:** Other not–for–profit (including NFP Corporation) **Service:** General Medical and surgical  ⑤

**Staffed Beds:** 25 **Admissions:** 892 **Census:** 9 **Outpatient Visits:** 44014 **Births:** 51 **Total Expense ($000):** 19210 **Payroll Expense ($000):** 5864 **Personnel:** 182  ⑥

**ANYTOWN, Universal County**

✠ **ANYTOWN HOSPITAL & CLINICS (777777)**, (Formerly Anytown Area Community Hospital and Clinic), 100 South Main Street, Zip 12345–6789; tel. 123/456–7890 **A9** 10

① = Approval Codes
② = Physician Codes
③ = Health Care System Name
④ = Titles of Chief Administrators
⑤ = Control and Service Classifications
⑥ = Utilization Data
⑦ = Facility Codes

---

**Hospital, Medicare Provider Number, Address, Telephone, Approval, Facility, and Physician Codes, Health Care System**

★ American Hospital Association (AHA) membership
□ The Joint Commission accreditation
◇ DNV Healthcare Inc. accreditation
○ American Osteopathic Association (AOA) accreditation
△ Commission on Accreditation of Rehabilitation Facilities (CARF) accreditation

---

## ① Approval Codes

*Reported by the approving bodies specified, as of the dates noted.*

**1** Accreditation under the hospital program of The Joint Commission (May 2012).
**2** Cancer program approved by American College of Surgeons (March 2012).
**†3** Approval to participate in residency training, by the Accreditation Council for Graduate Medical Education (April 2012).
**†5** Medical school affiliation, reported to the American Medical Association (April 2012).
**6** Hospital–controlled professional nursing school, reported by National League for Nursing.
**7** Accreditation by Commission on Accreditation of Rehabilitation Facilities (March 2012).

**8** Member of Council of Teaching Hospitals of the Association of American Medical Colleges (February 2012).
**9** Hospitals contracting or participating in a Plan, reported by the Blue Cross and Blue Shield Association (April 2012).
**10** Certified for participation in the Health Insurance for the Aged (Medicare) Program by the Centers for Medicare and Medical Services (February 2012).
**11** Healthcare Facilities Accreditation Program *(formerly American Osteopathic Association accreditation)* (May 2012).

**12** Internship approved by American Osteopathic Association (April 2012).
**13** Residency approved by American Osteopathic Association (April 2012).
**18** Critical Access Hospitals (May 2012).
**19** Rural Referral Center (May 2012).
**20** Sole Community Provider (May 2012).
**21** Accreditation by DNV Healthcare Inc. (May 2012).

**Nonreporting** indicates that the 2011 Annual Survey questionnaire for the hospital was not received prior to publication.

## ② Physician Codes

*Actually available within, and reported by the institution; for definitions, see page A12.*

**(Alphabetical/Numerical Order)**

**1** Closed physician–hospital organization (PHO)
**2** Equity model
**3** Foundation

**4** Group practice without walls
**5** Independent practice association (IPA)
**6** Integrated salary model

**7** Management service organization (MSO)
**8** Open physician–hospital organization (PHO)

## ③ Health Care System Name

*The inclusion of the letter ''S'' (1) indicates that the hospital belongs to a health care system and (2) identifies the specific system to which the hospital belongs.*

## ④ Titles of Chief Administrators

## ⑤ Control and Service Classification

*For a list of control and service classifications, see page A13.*

**Control–**The type of organization that is responsible for establishing policy for overall operation of the hospital.

**Service–**The type of service the hospital provides to the majority of admissions.

## ⑥ Utilization Data

*Definitions are based on the American Hospital Association's Hospital Administration Terminology. In completing the survey, hospitals were requested to report data for a full year, in accord with their fiscal year, ending in 2011.*

**Beds–**Number of beds regularly maintained (set up and staffed for use) for inpatients as of the close of the reporting period. Excludes newborn bassinets.

**Admissions–**Number of patients accepted for inpatient service during a 12–month period; does not include newborn.

**Census–**Average number of inpatients receiving care each day during the 12–month reporting period; does not include newborn.

**Outpatient Visits–**A visit by a patient who is not lodged in the hospital while receiving medical, dental, or other services. Each appearance of an outpatient in each unit constitutes one visit regardless of the number of diagnostic and/or therapeutic treatments that a patient receives.

**Births–**Number of infants born in the hospital and accepted for service in a newborn infant bassinet during a 12–month period; excludes stillbirths.

**Expense:** Expense for a 12–month period; both total expense and payroll components are shown. Payroll expenses include all salaries and wages.

**Personnel:** Represents personnel situations as they existed at the end of the reporting period; includes full-time equivalents of part–time personnel. Full-time equivalents were calculated on the basis that two part–time persons equal one full–time person.

---

†Data from the Graduate Medical Education Database, Copyright 2012, American Medical Association, Chicago, Illinois.

## Sample Hospital Listing:

**ANYTOWN, Universal County**

✠ **ANYTOWN HOSPITAL & CLINICS (777777)**, (Formerly Anytown Area
Community Hospital and Clinic), 100 South Main Street, Zip 12345–6789;
tel. 123/456–7890 **A**9 10  ] ①

**F**10 12 23 24 29 30 31 37 39 49 51 55 57 64 65 66 68 70 71 72 77
78 83 87 88 91 96 97 106 107 110 111 113 124 **P**1 2 3 **S** Universal
County Health System
Primary Contact: Ann M. Generic, Chief Executive Officer
COO: Ann M. Generic
CFO: Michael M. Generic
CMO: Peterl Van Generic, President Medical Staff
CHR: Jerry Generic, Human Resources Director
Web address: www.website.org
**Control:** Other not–for–profit (including NFP Corporation) **Service:** General
Medical and surgical

**Staffed Beds:** 25 **Admissions:** 892 **Census:** 9 **Outpatient Visits:** 44014
**Births:** 51 **Total Expense ($000):** 19210 **Payroll Expense ($000):** 5864
**Personnel:** 182

**ANYTOWN, Universal County**

✠ **ANYTOWN HOSPITAL & CLINICS (777777)**, (Formerly Anytown Area
Community Hospital and Clinic), 100 South Main Street, Zip 12345–6789;
tel. 123/456–7890 **A**9 10

① = **Approval Codes**
② = **Physician Codes**
③ = **Health Care System Name**
④ = **Titles of Chief Administrators**
⑤ = **Control and Service Classifications**
⑥ = **Utilization Data**
⑦ = **Facility Codes**

---

**Hospital, Medicare Provider Number, Address, Telephone, Approval, Facility, and Physician Codes, Health Care System**

★ American Hospital Association (AHA) membership
☐ The Joint Commission accreditation
◇ DNV Healthcare Inc. accreditation
○ American Osteopathic Association (AOA) accreditation
△ Commission on Accreditation of Rehabilitation Facilities (CARF) accreditation

## ⑦ Facility Codes

*Provided directly by the hospital; for definitions, see page A6.*

### (Numerical Order)

1. Acute long-term care
2. Adult day care program
3. Airborne infection isolation room
4. Alcoholism-drug abuse or dependency inpatient unit
5. Alcoholism-drug abuse or dependency outpatient unit
6. Alzheimer center
7. Ambulance services
8. Ambulatory surgery center
9. Arthritis treatment center
10. Assisted living
11. Auxiliary
12. Bariatric/weight control services
13. Birthing room-LDR room-LDRP room
14. Blood donor center
15. Breast cancer screening/mammograms
16. Burn care services
17. Cardiac intensive care
18. Adult cardiology services
19. Pediatric cardiology services
20. Adult diagnostic catheterization
21. Pediatric diagnostic catheterization
22. Adult interventional cardiac catheterization
23. Pediatric diagnostic catheterization
24. Adult cardiac surgery
25. Pediatric cardiac surgery
26. Adult cardiac electrophysiology
27. Pediatric cardiac electrophysiology
28. Cardiac rehabilitation
29. Case management
30. Chaplaincy/pastoral care services
31. Chemotherapy
32. Children's wellness program
33. Chiropractic services
34. Community health education
35. Community outreach
36. Complementary and alternative medicine services
37. Computer assisted orthopedic surgery (CAOS)
38. Crisis prevention
39. Dental services
40. Emergency department
41. Pediatric emergency department
42. Satellite emergency department
43. Trauma center (certified)
44. Enabling services
45. Optical colonoscopy
46. Endoscopic ultrasound
47. Ablation of Barrett's esophagus
48. Esophageal impedance study
49. Endoscopic retrograde cholangiopancreatography (ERCP)
50. Enrollment assistance services
51. Extracorporeal shock wave lithotripter (ESWL)
52. Fertility clinic
53. Fitness center
54. Freestanding outpatient care center
55. Genetic testing/counseling
56. Geriatric services
57. Health fair
58. Health research
59. Health screenings
60. Hemodialysis
61. HIV–AIDS services
62. Home health services
63. Hospice program
64. Hospital–based outpatient care center services
65. Immunization program
66. Indigent care clinic
67. Intermediate nursing care
68. Linguistic/translation services
69. Meals on wheels
70. Medical surgical intensive care services
71. Mobile health services
72. Neonatal intensive care
73. Neonatal intermediate care
74. Neurological services
75. Nutrition programs
76. Obstetrics
77. Occupational health services
78. Oncology services
79. Orthopedic services
80. Other special care
81. Outpatient surgery
82. Pain management program
83. Inpatient palliative care unit
84. Palliative care program
85. Patient controlled analgesia (PCA)
86. Patient education center
87. Patient representative services
88. Pediatric intensive care services
89. Pediatric medical–surgical care
90. Physical rehabilitation inpatient services
91. Assistive technology center
92. Electrodiagnostic services
93. Physical rehabilitation outpatient services
94. Prosthetic and orthotic services
95. Robot-assisted walking therapy
96. Simulated rehabilitation environment
97. Primary care department
98. Psychiatric care
99. Psychiatric child–adolescent services
100. Psychiatric consultation–liaison services
101. Psychiatric education services
102. Psychiatric emergency services
103. Psychiatric geriatric services
104. Psychiatric outpatient services
105. Psychiatric partial hospitalization services
106. Psychiatric residential treatment
107. CT scanner
108. Diagnostic radioisotope facility
109. Electron beam computed tomography (EBCT)
110. Full–field digital mammography (FFDM)
111. Magnetic resonance imaging (MRI)
112. Intraoperative magnetic resonance imaging
113. Multi–slice spiral computed tomography (MSCT) (<64 slice CT)
114. Multi–slice spiral computed tomography (64 + slice CT)
115. Positron emission tomography (PET)
116. Positron emission tomography/CT (PET/CT)
117. Single photon emission computerized tomography (SPECT)
118. Ultrasound
119. Image–guided radiation therapy (IGRT)
120. Intensity–modulated radiation therapy (IMRT)
121. Proton beam therapy
122. Shaped beam radiation therapy
123. Stereotactic radiosurgery
124. Retirement housing
125. Robotic surgery
126. Rural health clinic
127. Skilled nursing care
128. Sleep center
129. Social work services
130. Sports medicine
131. Support groups
132. Swing bed services
133. Teen outreach services
134. Tobacco treatment/cessation program
135. Bone marrow transplant services
136. Heart transplant
137. Kidney transplant
138. Liver transplant
139. Lung transplant
140. Tissue transplant
141. Other transplant
142. Transportation to health services
143. Urgent care center
144. Virtual colonoscopy
145. Volunteer services department
146. Women's health center/services
147. Wound management services

# Annual Survey

Each year, an annual survey of hospitals is conducted by the American Hospital Association through its Health Forum affiliate.

The facilities and services found below are provided by the hospital. For data products reflecting the services provided by a hospital through its health care system, or network or through a formal arrangement with another provider contact Health Forum at 800/821–2039, or visit www.ahadata.com.

The AHA Guide to the Health Care Field does not include all data collected from the 2011 Annual Survey. Requests for purchasing other Annual Survey data should be directed to Health Forum LLC, an affiliate of the American Hospital Association, 155 N. Wacker Drive, Chicago, IL 60606, 800/821–2039.

## Definitions of Facility Codes

1. **Acute long–term care.** Provides specialized acute hospital care to medically complex patients who are critically ill, have multisystem complications and/or failure, and require hospitalization averaging 25 days, in a facility offering specialized treatment programs and therapeutic intervention on a 24–hour/7 day a week basis.

2. **Adult day care program.** Program providing supervision, medical and psychological care, and social activities for older adults who live at home or in another family setting, but cannot be alone or prefer to be with others during the day. May include intake assessment, health monitoring, occupational therapy, personal care, noon meal, and transportation services.

3. **Airborne infection isolation room.** A single–occupancy room for patient care where environmental factors are controlled in an effort to minimize the transmission of those infectious agents, usually spread person to person by droplet nuclei associated with coughing and inhalation. Such rooms typically have specific ventilation requirements for controlled ventilation, air pressure and filtration.

4. **Alcoholism–drug abuse or dependency inpatient unit.** Provides diagnosis and therapeutic services to patients with alcoholism or other drug dependencies. Includes care for inpatient/residential treatment for patients whose course of treatment involves more intensive care than provided in an outpatient setting or where patient requires supervised withdrawal.

5. **Alcoholism–drug abuse or dependency outpatient unit.** Organized hospital services that provide medical care and/or rehabilitative treatment services to outpatients for whom the primary diagnosis is alcoholism or other chemical dependency.

6. **Alzheimer center.** Facility that offers care to persons with Alzheimer's disease and their families through an integrated program of clinical services, research, and education.

7. **Ambulance services.** Provision of ambulance services to the ill and injured who require medical attention on a scheduled or unscheduled basis.

8. **Ambulatory surgery center.** Facility that provides care to patients requiring surgery who are admitted and discharged on the same day. Ambulatory surgery centers are distinct from same day surgical units within the hospital outpatient departments for purposes of Medicare payments.

9. **Arthritis treatment center.** Specifically equipped and staffed center for the diagnosis and treatment of arthritis and other joint disorders.

10. **Assisted living.** A special combination of housing, supportive services, personalized assistance and health care designed to respond to the individual needs of those who need help in activities of daily living and instrumental activities of daily living. Supportive services are available, 24 hours a day, to meet scheduled and unscheduled needs, in a way that promotes maximum independence and dignity for each resident and encourages the involvement of a resident's family, neighbor and friends.

11. **Auxiliary.** A volunteer community organization formed to assist the hospital in carrying out its purpose and to serve as a link between the institution and the community.

12. **Bariatric/weight control services.** Bariatrics is the medical practice of weight reduction.

13. **Birthing room–LDR room–LDRP room.** A single room–type of maternity care with a more homelike setting for families than the traditional three–room unit (labor/delivery/recovery) with a separate postpartum area. A birthing room combines labor and delivery in one room. An LDR room accommodates three stages in the birthing process— labor, delivery, and recovery. An LDRP room accommodates all four stages of the birth process—labor, delivery, recovery and postpartum.

14. **Blood donor center.** A facility that performs, or is responsible for the collection, processing, testing or distribution of blood and components.

15. **Breast cancer screening/mammograms.** Mammography screening–the use of breast x–ray to detect unsuspected breast cancer in asymptomatic women. Diagnostic mammography–the x–ray imaging of breast tissue in symptomatic women who are considered to have a substantial likelihood of having breast cancer already.

16. **Burn care services.** Provides care to severely burned patients. Severely burned patients are those with any of the following: 1. Second–degree burns of more than 25% total body surface area for adults or 20% total body surface area for children; 2. Third–degree burns of more than 10% total body surface area; 3. Any severe burns of the hands, face, eyes, ears or feet or; 4. All inhalation injuries, electrical burns, complicated burn injuries involving fractures and other major traumas, and all other poor risk factors.

17. **Cardiac intensive care.** Provides patient care of a more specialized

nature than the usual medical and surgical care, on the basis of physicians' orders and approved nursing care plans. The unit is staffed with specially trained nursing personnel and contains monitoring and specialized support or treatment equipment for patients who, because of heart seizure, open–heart surgery, or other life–threatening conditions, require intensified, comprehensive observation and care. May include myocardial infarction, pulmonary care, and heart transplant units.

18. **Adult cardiology services.** An organized clinical service offering diagnostic and interventional procedures to manage the full range of adult heart conditions.

19. **Pediatric cardiology services.**

20. **Adult diagnostic catheterization.** (also called coronary angiography or coronary arteriography) is used to assist in diagnosing complex heart conditions. Cardiac angiography involves the insertion of a tiny catheter up into the artery in the groin then carefully threading the catheter up into the aorta where the coronary arteries originate. Once the catheter is in place, a dye is injected which allows the cardiologist to see the size, shape and distribution of the coronary arteries. These images are used to diagnose heart disease and to determine, among other things, whether or not surgery is indicated.

21. **Pediatric diagnostic catheterization.** (also called coronary angiography or coronary arteriography) is used to assist in diagnosing complex heart conditions. Cardiac angiography involves the insertion of a tiny catheter up into the artery in the groin then carefully threading the catheter up into the aorta where the coronary arteries originate. Once the catheter is in place, a dye is injected which allows the cardiologist to see the size, shape and distribution of the coronary arteries. These images are used to diagnose heart disease and to determine, among other things, whether or not surgery is indicated.

22. **Adult interventional cardiac catheterization.** Nonsurgical procedure that utilizes the same basic principles as diagnostic cathereterization and then uses advanced the techniques to improve the heart's function. It can be less invasive alternative to heart surgery.

23. **Pediatric diagnostic catheterization.** Nonsurgical procedure that utilizes the same basic principles as diagnostic cathereterization and then uses advanced the techniques to improve the heart's function. It can be less invasive alternative to heart surgery.

24. **Adult cardiac surgery.** Includes minimally invasive procedures that include surgery done with only a small incision or no incision at all, such as through a laparoscope or an endoscope and more invasive major surgical procedures that include open chest and open heart surgery.

25. **Pediatric cardiac surgery.** Includes minimally invasive procedures that include surgery done with only a small incision or no incision at all, such as through a laparoscope or an endoscope and more invasive major surgical procedures that include open chest and open heart surgery defibrillator implantation and follow-up.

26. **Adult cardiac electrophysiology.** Evaluation and management of patients with complex rhythm or conduction abnormalities, including diagnostic testing, treatment of arrhythmias by catheter ablation or drug therapy, and pacemaker/defibrillator implantation and follow-up.

27. **Pediatric cardiac electrophysiology.**

28. **Cardiac rehabilitation.** A medically supervised program to help heart patients recover quickly and improve their overall physical and mental functioning. The goal is to reduce risk of another cardiac event or to keep an already present heart condition from getting worse. Cardiac rehabilitation programs include: counseling to patients, an exercise program, helping patients modify risk factors such as smoking and high blood pressure, providing vocational guidance to enable the patient to return to work, supplying information on physical limitations and lending emotional support.

29. **Case management.** A system of assessment, treatment planning, referral and follow–up that ensures the provision of comprehensive and continuous services and the coordination of payment and reimbursement for care.

30. **Chaplaincy/pastoral care services.** A service ministering religious activities and providing pastoral counseling to patients, their families,

and staff of a health care organization.

31. **Chemotherapy.** An organized program for the treatment of cancer by the use of drugs or chemicals.

32. **Children's wellness program.** A program that encourages improved health status and a healthful lifestyle of children through health education, exercise, nutrition and health promotion.

33. **Chiropractic services.** An organized clinical service including spinal manipulation or adjustment and related diagnostic and therapeutic services.

34. **Community health education.** Education that provides health information to individuals and populations as well as support for personal, family and community health decisions with the objective of improving health status.

35. **Community outreach.** A program that systematically interacts with the community to identify those in need of services, alerting persons and their families to the availability of services, locating needed services, and enabling persons to enter the service delivery system.

36. **Complementary and alternative medicine services.** Organized hospital services or formal arrangements to providers that provide care or treatment not based solely on traditional western allopathic medical teachings as instructed in most U.S. medical schools. Includes any of the following; acupuncture, chiropractic, homeopathy, osteopathy, diet and lifestyle changes, herbal medicine, massage therapy, etc.

37. **Computer assisted orthopedic surgery (CAOS).** Orthopedic surgery using computer technology, enabling three–dimensional graphic models to visualize a patient's anatomy.

38. **Crisis prevention** Services provided in order to promote physical and mental well being and the early identification of disease and ill health prior to the onset and recognition of symptoms so as to permit early treatment.

39. **Dental services.** An organized dental service, not necessarily involving special facilities, that provides dental or oral services to inpatients or outpatients.

40. **Emergency department.** Hospital facilities for the provision of

unscheduled outpatient services to patients whose conditions require immediate care. Must be staffed 24 hours a day.

**41. Pediatric emergency department.** Hospital facilities for the provision of unscheduled outpatient services to patients whose conditions require immediate care.

**42. Satellite emergency department.** A facility owned and operated by the hospital but physically separate from the hospital for the provision of unscheduled outpatient services to patients whose conditions require.

**43. Trauma center (certified).** A facility certified to provide emergency and specialized intensive care to critically ill and injured patients.

**44. Enabling services.** A program that is designed to help the patient access health care services by offering any of the following linguistic services, transportation services, and/or referrals to local social services agencies.

**45. Optical colonoscopy.** An examination of the interior of the colon using a long, flexible, lighted tube with a small built-in camera.

**46. Endoscopic ultrasound.** Specially designed endoscope that incorporates an ultrasound transducer used to obtain detailed images of organs in the chest and abdomen. The endoscope can be passed through the mouth or the anus. When combined with needle biopsy the procedure can assist in diagnosis and staging of cancer.

**47. Ablation of Barrett's esophagus.** Premalignant condition that can lead to adenocarcinoma of the esophagus. The non surgical ablation of the premalignant tissue in Barrett's esophagus by the application of thermal energy or light through an endoscope passed from the mouth into the esophagus.

**48. Esophageal impedance study.** A test in which a catheter is placed through the nose into the esophagus to measure whether gas or liquids are passing from the stomach into the esophagus and causing symptoms.

**49. Endoscopic retrograde cholangiopancreatography (ERCP).** A procedure in which a catheter is introduced through an endoscope into the bile ducts and pancreatic ducts. Injection of contrast materials permits detailed x–ray of these structures. The procedure is used diagnostically as

well as therapeutically to relieve obstruction or remove stones

**50. Enrollment assistance services.** A program that provides enrollment assistance for patients who are potentially eligible for public health insurance programs such as Medicaid, State Children's Health Insurance, or local/state indigent care programs. The specific services offered could include explanation of benefits, assist applicants in completing the application and locating all relevant documents, conduct eligibilty interviews, and/or forward applications and documentation to state/local social service or health agency.

**51. Extracorporeal shock wave lithotripter (ESWL).** A medical device used for treating stones in the kidney or urethra. The device disintegrates kidney stones noninvasively through the transmission of acoustic shock waves directed at the stones.

**52. Fertility clinic.** A specialized program set in an infertility center that provides counseling and education as well as advanced reproductive techniques such as: injectable therapy, reproductive surgeries, treatment for endometriosis, male factor infertility, tubal reversals, in vitro fertilization (IVF), donor eggs, and other such services to help patients achieve successful pregnancies.

**53. Fitness center.** Provides exercise, testing, or evaluation programs and fitness activities to the community and hospital employees.

**54. Freestanding outpatient care center.** A facility owned and operated by the hospital, but physically separate from the hospital, that provides various medical treatments on an outpatient basis only. In addition to treating minor illnesses or injuries, the center will stabilize seriously ill or injured patients before transporting them to a hospital. Laboratory and radiology services are usually available.

**55. Genetic testing/counseling** A service equipped with adequate laboratory facilities and directed by a qualified physician to advise parents and prospective parents on potential problems in cases of genetic defects. A genetic test is the analysis of human DNA, RNA, chromosomes, proteins, and certain metabolites in order to detect heritable disease–related genotypes, mutations,

phenotypes, or karyotypes for clinical purposes. Genetic tests can have diverse purposes, including the diagnosis of genetic diseases in newborns, children, and adults; the identification of future health risks; the prediction of drug responses; and the assessment of risks to future children.

**56. Geriatric services.** The branch of medicine dealing with the physiology of aging and the diagnosis and treatment of disease affecting the aged. Services could include: Adult day care program; Alzheimer's diagnostic–assessment services; Comprehensive geriatric assessment; Emergency response system; Geriatric acute care unit; and/or Geriatric clinics.

**57. Health fair.** Community health education events that focus on the prevention of disease and promotion of health through such activities as audiovisual exhibits and free diagnostic services.

**58. Health research.** Organized hospital research program in any of the following areas: basic research, clinical research, community health research, and/or research on innovative health care delivery.

**59. Health screenings.** A preliminary procedure, such as a test or examination to detect the most characteristic sign or signs of a disorder that may require further investigation.

**60. Hemodialysis.** Provision of equipment and personnel for the treatment of renal insufficiency on an inpatient or outpatient basis.

**61. HIV–AIDS services.** Services may include one or more of the following: HIV–AIDS unit (special unit or team designated and equipped specifically for diagnosis, treatment, continuing care planning, and counseling services for HIV–AIDS patients and their families.) General inpatient care for HIV–AIDS (inpatient diagnosis and treatment for human immunodeficiency virus and acquired immunodeficiency syndrome patients, but dedicated unit is not available.) Specialized outpatient program for HIV–AIDS (special outpatient program providing diagnostic, treatment, continuing care planning, and counseling for HIV–AIDS patients and their families.)

**62. Home health services.** Service providing nursing, therapy, and health–related homemaker or social services in the patient's home.

63. **Hospice program.** A program providing palliative care, chiefly medical relief of pain and supportive services, addressing the emotional, social, financial, and legal needs of terminally ill patients and their families. Care can be provided in a variety of settings, both inpatient and at home.

64. **Hospital–based outpatient care center services.** Organized hospital health care services offered by appointment on an ambulatory basis. Services may include outpatient surgery, examination, diagnosis, and treatment of a variety of medical conditions on a nonemergency basis, and laboratory and other diagnostic testing as ordered by staff or outside physician referral.

65. **Immunization program.** Program that plans, coordinates and conducts immunization services in the community.

66. **Indigent care clinic.** Health care services for uninsured and underinsured persons where care is free of charge or charged on a sliding scale. This would include "free clinics" staffed by volunteer practitioners, but could also be staffed by employees with sponsoring health care organizations subsidizing the cost of service.

67. **Intermediate nursing care.** Provides health–related services (skilled nursing care and social services) to residents with a variety of physical conditions or functional disabilities. These residents do not require the care provided by a hospital or skilled nursing facility, but do need supervision and support services.

68. **Linguistic/translation services.** Services provided by the hospital designed to make health care more accessible to non–English speaking patients and their physicians.

69. **Meals on wheels.** A hospital sponsored program which delivers meals to people, usually the elderly, who are unable to prepare their own meals. Low cost, nutritional meals are delivered to individuals' homes on a regular basis.

70. **Medical surgical intensive care services.** Provides patient care of a more intensive nature than the usual medical and surgical care, on the basis of physicians' orders and approved nursing care plans. These units are staffed with specially trained nursing personnel and contain monitoring and specialized support equipment of patients who, because of shock, trauma, or other life–threatening conditions, require intensified, comprehensive observation and care. Includes mixed intensive care units.

71. **Mobile health services.** Vans and other vehicles used to deliver primary care services.

72. **Neonatal intensive care.** A unit that must be separate from the newborn nursery providing intensive care to all sick infants including those with the very lowest birth weights (less that 1500 grams). NICU has potential for providing mechanical ventilation, neonatal surgery, and special care for the sickest infants born in the hospital or transferred from another institution. A full–time neonatologist serves as director of the NICU.

73. **Neonatal intermediate care.** A unit that must be separate from the normal newborn nursery and that provides intermediate and/or recovery care and some specialized services, including immediate resuscitation, intravenous therapy, and capacity for prolonged oxygen therapy and monitoring.

74. **Neurological services.** Services provided by the hospital dealing with the operative and nonoperative management of disorders of the central, peripheral, and autonomic nervous system.

75. **Nutrition programs.** Those services within a health care facility which are designed to provide inexpensive, nutritionally sound meals to patients.

76. **Obstetrics.** Levels should be designated: (1) unit provides services for uncomplicated maternity and newborn cases; (2) unit provides services for uncomplicated cases, the majority of complicated problems, and special neonatal services; and (3) unit provides services for all serious illnesses and abnormalities and is supervised by a full–time maternal/ fetal specialist.

77. **Occupational health services.** Includes services designed to protect the safety of employees from hazards in the work environment.

78. **Oncology services.** Inpatient and outpatient services for patients with cancer, including comprehensive care, support and guidance in addition to patient education and preventiion, chemotherapy, counseling, and other treatment methods.

79. **Orthopedic services.** Services provided for the prevention or correction of injuries or disorders of the skeletal system and associated muscles, joints, and ligaments.

80. **Other special care.** Provides care to patients requiring care more intensive than that provided in the acute area, yet not sufficiently intensive to require admission to an intensive care unit. Patients admitted to the area are usually transferred here from an intensive care unit once their condition has improved. These units are sometimes referred to as definitive observation, step–down, or progressive care units.

81. **Outpatient surgery.** Scheduled surgical services provided to patients who do not remain in the hospital overnight. The surgery may be performed in operating suites also used for inpatient surgery, specially designated surgical suites for outpatient surgery, or procedure rooms within an outpatient care facility.

82. **Pain management program.** A hospital wide formalized program that includes staff education for the management of chronic and acute pain based on guidelines and protocols like those developed by the agency for Health Care Policy Research, etc.

83. **Inpatient palliative care unit.** An inpatient palliative care ward is a physically discreet, inpatient nursing unit where the focus is palliative care. The patient care focus is on symptom relief for complex patients who may be continuing to undergo primary treatment. Care is delivered by palliative medicine specialists.

84. **Palliative care program.** An organized program providing specialized medical care, drugs or therapies for the management of acute or chronic pain and/or the control of symptoms adminstered by specially trained physicians and other clinicians; and supportive care services, such as counseling on advanced directives, spiritual care, and social services, to patients with advanced disease and their families.

85. **Patient controlled analgesia (PCA).** Patient Controlled Analgesia (PCA) is intravenously administered pain medicine under the patient's control. The patient has a button on the end of a cord than can be pushed at will, whenever more pain medicine is desired. This button will only deliver more pain medicine at pre–

determined intervals, as programmed by the doctor's order.

86. **Patient education center.** Written goals and objectives for the patient and/or family related to therapeutic regimens, medical procedures, and self care.

87. **Patient representative services.** Organized hospital services providing personnel through whom patients and staff can seek solutions to institutional problems affecting the delivery of high–quality care and services.

88. **Pediatric intensive care services.** Provides care to pediatric patients that is of a more intensive nature than that usually provided to pediatric patients. The unit is staffed with specially trained personnel and contains monitoring and specialized support equipment for treatment of patients who, because of shock, trauma, or other life–threatening conditions, require intensified, comprehensive observation and care.

89. **Pediatric medical–surgical care.** Provides acute care to pediatric patients on the basis of physicians' orders and approved nursing care plans.

90. **Physical rehabilitation inpatient services.** Provides care encompassing a comprehensive array of restoration services for the disabled and all support services necessary to help patients attain their maximum functional capacity.

91. **Assistive technology center.** A program providing access to specialized hardware and software with adaptations allowing individuals greater independence with mobility, dexterity, or increased communication options.

92. **Electrodiagnostic services.** Diagnostic testing services for nerve and muscle function including services such as nerve conduction studies and needle electromyography.

93. **Physical rehabilitation outpatient services.** Outpatient program providing medical, health–related, therapy, social, and/or vocational services to help disabled persons attain or retain their maximum functional capacity.

94. **Prosthetic and orthotic services.** Services providing comprehensive prosthetic and orthotic evaluation, fitting, and training.

95. **Robot-assisted walking therapy.** A form of physical therapy that uses a robotic device to assist patients who are relearning how to walk.

96. **Simulated rehabilitation environment.** Rehabilitation focused on retraining functional skills in a contextually appropriate environment (simulated home and community settings) or in a traditional setting (gymnasium) using motor learning principles.

97. **Primary care department.** A unit or clinic within the hospital that provides primary care services (e.g. general pediatric care, general internal medicine, family practice and gynecology) through hospital–salaried medical and or nursing staff, focusing on evaluating and diagnosing medical problems and providing medical treatment on an outpatient basis.

98. **Psychiatric care.** Provides acute or long–term care to emotionally disturbed patients, including patients admitted for diagnosis and those admitted for treatment of psychiatric problems, on the basis of physicians' orders and approved nursing care plans. Long–term care may include intensive supervision to the chronically mentally ill, mentally disordered, or other mentally incompetent persons.

99. **Psychiatric child–adolescent services.** Provides care to emotionally disturbed children and adolescents, including those admitted for diagnosis and those admitted for treatment.

100. **Psychiatric consultation–liaison services.** Provides organized psychiatric consultation/liaison services to nonpsychiatric hospital staff and/or department on psychological aspects of medical care that may be generic or specific to individual patients.

101. **Psychiatric education services.** Provides psychiatric educational services to community agencies and workers such as schools, police, courts, public health nurses, welfare agencies, clergy and so forth. The purpose is to expand the mental health knowledge and competence of personnel not working in the mental health field and to promote good mental health through improved understanding, attitudes, and behavioral patterns.

102. **Psychiatric emergency services.** Services or facilities available on a 24–hour basis to provide immediate unscheduled outpatient care, diagnosis, evaluation, crisis intervention, and assistance to persons suffering acute emotional or mental distress.

103. **Psychiatric geriatric services.** Provides care to emotionally disturbed elderly patients, including those admitted for diagnosis and those admitted for treatment.

104. **Psychiatric outpatient services.** Provides medical care, including diagnosis and treatment of psychiatric outpatients.

105. **Psychiatric partial hospitalization services.** Organized hospital services of intensive day/evening outpatient services of three hours or more duration, distinguished from other outpatient visits of one hour.

106. **Psychiatric residential treatment.**

107. **CT scanner.** Computed tomographic scanner for head and whole body scans.

108. **Diagnostic radioisotope facility.** The use of radioactive isotopes (Radiopharmaceutical) as tracers or indicators to detect an abnormal condition or disease.

109. **Electron beam computed tomography (EBCT).** A high tech computed tomography scan used to detect coronary artery disease by measuring coronary calcifications. This imaging procedure uses electron beams which are magnetically steered to produce a visual of the coronary artery and the images are produced faster than conventional CT scans.

110. **Full–field digital mammography (FFDM).** Combines the x–ray generators and tubes used in analog screen–film mammography (SFM) with a detector plate that converts the x–rays into a digital signal.

111. **Magnetic resonance imaging (MRI).** The use of a uniform magnetic field and radio frequencies to study tissue and structure of the body. This procedure enables the visualization of biochemical activity of the cell in vivo without the use of ionizing radiation, radioisotopic substances, or high–frequency sound.

112. **Intraoperative magnetic resonance imaging.** An integrated surgery system which provides an MRI system in an operating room. The system allows for immediate evaluation of the degree to tumor resection while the patient is undergoing a surgical resection. Intraoperative MRI exists when a MRI (low–field or high–field) is placed in the operating theater and is

used during surgical resection without moving the patient from the operating room to the diagnostic imaging suite.

113. **Multi–slice spiral computed tomography (MSCT) (<64 slice CT).** A specialized computed tomography procedure that provides three–dimensional processing and allows narrower and multiple slices with increased spatial resolution and faster scanning times as compared to a regular computed tomography scan.

114. **Multi–slice spiral computed tomography (64 + slice CT).** Involves the acquisition of volumetric tomographic x–ray absorption data expressed in Hounsfield units using multiple rows of detectors. 64+ systems reconstruct the equivalent of 64 or greater slices to cover the imaged volume.

115. **Positron emission tomography (PET).** A nuclear medicine imaging technology which uses radioactive (positron emitting) isotopes created in a cyclotron or generator and computers to produce composite pictures of the brain and heart at work. PET scanning produces sectional images depicting metabolic activity or blood flow rather than anatomy.

116. **Positron emission tomography/CT (PET/CT).** Provides metabolic functional information for the monitoring of chemotherapy, radiotherapy and surgical planning.

117. **Single photon emission computerized tomography (SPECT).** A nuclear medicine imaging technology that combines existing technology of gamma camera imaging with computed tomographic imaging technology to provide a more precise and clear image.

118. **Ultrasound.** The use of acoustic waves above the range of 20,000 cycles per second to visualize internal body structures.

119. **Image–guided radiation therapy (IGRT).** Automated system for image–guided radiation therapy that enables clinicians to obtain high–resolution x–ray images to pinpoint tumor sites, adjust patient positioning when necessary, and complete a treatment, all within the standard treatment time slot, allowing for more effective cancer treatments.

120. **Intensity–modulated radiation Therapy (IMRT).** A type of three–dimensional radiation therapy, which improves the targeting of treatment delivery in a way that is likely to decrease damage to normal tissues and allows varying intensities diagnosis of genetic diseases in newborns, children, and adults; the identification of future health risks; the prediction of drug responses; and the assessment of risks to future children.

121. **Proton beam therapy.** A form of radiation therapy which administers proton beams. While producing the same biologic effects as x–ray beams, the energy distribution of protons differs from conventional x–ray beams in that they can be more precisely focused in tissue volumes in a three–dimensional pattern resulting in less surrounding tissue damage than conventional radiation therapy permitting administration of higher doses.

122. **Shaped beam radiation therapy.** A precise, non–invasive treatment that involves targeting beams of radiation that mirror the exact size and shape of a tumor at a specific area of a tumor to shrink or destroy cancerous cells. This procedure delivers a therapeutic dose of radiation that conforms precisely to the shape of the tumor, thus minimizing the risk to nearby tissues.

123. **Stereotactic radiosurgery.** Stereotactic radiosurgery (SRS) is a radiotherapy modality that delivers a high dosage of radiation to a discrete treatment area in as few as one treatment session. Includes gamma knife, cyberknife, etc.

124. **Retirement housing.** A facility which provides social activities to senior citizens, usually retired persons, who do not require health care but some short–term skilled nursing care may be provided. A retirement center may furnish housing and may also have acute hospital and long–term care facilities, or it may arrange for acute and long term care through affiliated institutions.

125. **Robotic surgery.** The use of mechanical guidance devices to remotely manipulate surgical instrumentation.

126. **Rural health clinic.** A clinic located in a rural, medically under-served area in the United States that has a separate reimbursement structure from the standard medical office under the Medicare and Medicaid programs.

127. **Skilled nursing care.** Provides non–acute medical and skilled nursing care services, therapy, and social services under the supervision of a licensed registered nurse on a 24–hour basis.

128. **Sleep center.** Specially equipped and staffed center for the diagnosis and treatment of sleep disorders.

129. **Social work services.** Services may include one or more of the following: Organized social work services (services that are properly directed and sufficiently staffed by qualified individuals who provide assistance and counseling to patients and their families in dealing with social, emotional, and environmental problems associated with illness or disability, often in the context of financial or discharge planning coordination.) Outpatient social work services (social work services provided in ambulatory care areas.) Emergency department social work services (social work services provided to emergency department patients by social workers dedicated to the emergency department or on call.)

130. **Sports medicine.** Provision of diagnostic screening and assessment and clinical and rehabilitation services for the prevention and treatment of sports–related injuries.

131. **Support groups.** A hospital sponsored program which allows a group of individuals with the same or similar problems who meet periodically to share experiences, problems, and solutions, in order to support each other.

132. **Swing bed services.** A hospital bed that can be used to provide either acute or long–term care depending on community or patients needs. To be eligible a hospital must have a Medicare provider agreement in place, have fewer than 100 beds, be located in a rural area, not have a 24 hour nursing service waiver in effect, have not been terminated from the program in the prior two years, and meet various service conditions.

133. **Teen outreach services.** A program focusing on the teenager which encourages an improved health status and a healthful lifestyle including physical, emotional, mental, social, spiritual and economic health through education, exercise, nutrition and health promotion.

134. **Tobacco treatment/cessation program.** Organized hospital services with the purpose of ending tobacco-use habits of patients addicted to tobacco/nicotine.

**135.–141. Transplant services.** The branch of medicine that transfers an organ or tissue from one person to another or from one body part to another to replace a diseased structure or to restore function or to change appearance. Services could include: Bone marrow transplant program (**135. Bone marrow**); heart (**136. Heart transplant**), kidney (**137. Kidney transplant**), liver (**138. Liver transplant**) lung (**139. Lung transplant**), tissue (**140. Tissue transplant**). Please include heart/lung or other multi– transplant surgeries in other (**141. Other Transplant**).

**142. Transportation to health services.** A long–term care support service designed to assist the mobility of the elderly. Some programs offer improved financial access by offering reduced rates and barrier–free buses or vans with ramps and lifts to assist the elderly or handicapped; others offer subsidies for public transport systems or operate mini–bus services exclusively for use by senior citizens.

**143. Urgent care center.** A facility that provides care and treatment for problems that are not life–threatening but require attention over the short term. These units function like emergency rooms but are separate from hospitals with which they may have backup affiliation arrangements.

**144. Virtual colonoscopy.** Noninvasive screening procedure used to visualize, analyze and detect cancerous or potentially cancerous polyps in the colon.

**145. Volunteer services department.** An organized hospital department responsible for coordinating the services of volunteers working within the institution.

**146. Women's center.** An area set aside for coordinated education and treatment services specifically for and promoted by women as provided by this special unit. Services may or may not include obstetrics but include a range of services other than OB.

**147. Wound management services.** Services for patients with chronic wounds and non–healing wounds often resulting from diabetes, poor circulation, improper seating and immunocompromising conditions. The goals are to progress chronic wounds through stages of healing, reduce and eliminate infections, increase physical function to minimize complications from current wounds and prevent future chronic wounds. Wound management services are provided on an inpatient or outpatient basis, depending on the intensity of service needed.

# Definitions of Physician Codes

1. **Closed physician–hospital organization (PHO).** A PHO that restricts physician membership to those practitioners who meet criteria for cost effectiveness and/or high quality.

2. **Equity model.** Allows established practitioners to become shareholders in a professional corporation in exchange for tangible and intangible assets of their existing practices.

3. **Foundation.** A corporation, organized either as a hospital affiliate or subsidiary, which purchases both the tangible and intangible assets of one or more medical group practices. Physicians remain in a separate corporate entity but sign a professional services agreement with the foundation.

4. **Group practice without walls.** Hospital sponsors the formation of, or provides capital to physicians to establish, a 'quasi' group to share administrative expenses while remaining independent practitioners.

5. **Independent practice association (IPA).** A legal entity that hold managed care contracts. The IPA then contracts with physicians, usually in solo practice, to provide care either on a fee–for–services or capitated basis. The purpose of an IPA is to assist solo physicians in obtaining managed care contracts.

6. **Integrated salary model.** Physicians are salaried by the hospital or another entity of a health system to provide medical services for primary care and specialty care.

7. **Management services organization (MSO).** A corporation, owned by the hospital or a physician/hospital joint venture, that provides management services to one or more medical group practices. The MSO purchases the tangible assets of the practices and leases them back as part of a full–service management agreement, under which the MSO employs all non–physician staff and provides all supplies/administrative systems for a fee.

8. **Open physician–hospital organization (PHO).** A joint venture between the hospital and all members of the medical staff who wish to participate. The PHO can act as a unified agent in managed care contracting, own a managed care plan, own and operate ambulatory care centers or ancillary services projects, or provide administrative services to physician members.

# Control and Service Classifications

A13

## Control

### Government, nonfederal
State
County
City
City–county
Hospital district or authority

### Nongovernment not-for-profit
Church operated
Other

### Investor–owned (for–profit)
Individual
Partnership
Corporation

### Government, federal
Air Force
Army
Navy
Public Health Service other than 47
Veterans Affairs

Federal other than 41–45, 47–48
Public Health Service Indian Service
Department of Justice

### Osteopathic
Church operated
Other not–for–profit
Other
Individual for–profit
Partnership for–profit
Corporation for–profit

## Service

General medical and surgical
Hospital unit of an institution
 (prison hospital, college infirmary, etc.)
Hospital unit within an institution for the
 mentally retarded
Surgical
Psychiatric
Tuberculosis and other respiratory
 diseases
Cancer
Heart

Obstetrics and gynecology
Eye, ear, nose, and throat
Rehabilitation
Orthopedic
Chronic disease
Other specialty
Children's general
Children's hospital unit of an institution
Children's psychiatric
Children's tuberculosis and other
 respiratory diseases
Children's eye, ear, nose, and throat

Children's rehabilitation
Children's orthopedic
Children's chronic disease
Children's other specialty
Institution for mental retardation
Long–Term Acute Care
Alcoholism and other chemical
 dependency
Children's Long–Term Acute Care
Children's Cancer
Children's Heart

# Notes

# Notes

# Notes

# Notes

✠ **ST. VINCENT'S BIRMINGHAM (10056)**, 810 St. Vincent's Drive, Zip 35205–1695, Mailing Address: P.O. Box 12407, Zip 35202–2407; tel. 205/939–7000 **A**1 2 3 5 9 10 **F**3 11 13 15 17 18 20 22 24 26 28 29 30 31 34 35 36 37 40 43 45 50 53 54 57 58 59 60 62 65 66 68 70 72 74 75 76 77 78 79 81 82 84 85 86 87 93 97 107 108 110 111 113 114 118 119 120 122 125 128 129 130 134 145 146 147 **P**7 8 **S** Ascension Health, Saint Louis, MO
Primary Contact: Andy Davis, President
COO: Andy Davis, Chief Operating Officer
CFO: Wilma Newton, Executive Vice President and Chief Financial Officer
CMO: Gregory L. James, D.O., Chief Medical Officer
CIO: Timothy Stettheimer, Vice President and Chief Information Officer
CHR: Michelle Galipeau, Director Human Resources
Web address: www.stvhs.com
**Control:** Other not–for–profit (including NFP Corporation) **Service:** General Medical and Surgical

**Staffed Beds:** 439 **Admissions:** 20982 **Census:** 267 **Outpatient Visits:** 190529 **Births:** 2148 **Total Expense ($000):** 325743 **Payroll Expense ($000):** 94347 **Personnel:** 1875

✠ **ST. VINCENT'S EAST (10011)**, 50 Medical Park East Drive, Zip 35235–9987; tel. 205/838–3000 **A**1 2 3 5 9 10 **F**3 11 12 13 17 18 20 22 24 26 28 29 30 31 34 35 40 42 43 44 45 46 50 51 53 54 57 58 59 60 64 65 70 72 74 76 77 78 79 81 85 86 87 90 93 94 96 97 98 100 101 102 103 104 105 107 108 111 113 118 120 122 125 128 129 130 131 134 145 **P**7 8 **S** Ascension Health, Saint Louis, MO
Primary Contact: Sean Tinney, FACHE, President and Chief Operating Officer
CFO: Jan DiCesare, Vice President Financial Operations
CMO: Adeeb Thomas, M.D., Vice President Medical Affairs
CIO: Beverly Golightly, Director Information Technology
CHR: Carol Maietta, Vice President Human Resources and Chief Learning Officer
Web address: www.stvhs.com
**Control:** Other not–for–profit (including NFP Corporation) **Service:** General Medical and Surgical

**Staffed Beds:** 336 **Admissions:** 13277 **Census:** 178 **Outpatient Visits:** 135007 **Births:** 779 **Total Expense ($000):** 185901 **Payroll Expense ($000):** 62185 **Personnel:** 1046

✠ **THE CHILDREN'S HOSPITAL OF ALABAMA (13300)**, 1600 Seventh Avenue South, Zip 35233–1785; tel. 205/638–9100 **A**1 3 5 9 10 **F**3 7 8 11 12 16 19 29 30 31 32 34 35 38 39 40 41 43 46 48 49 50 54 55 57 58 60 61 64 65 68 72 74 75 77 78 79 80 81 82 84 85 86 87 88 89 92 93 94 97 98 99 100 101 102 104 107 111 113 114 117 118 128 129 130 131 133 134 135 141 142 143 145
Primary Contact: Wm. Michael Warren, Jr., Chief Executive Officer
COO: Tom Shufflebarger, Chief Operating Officer
CFO: Mike Burgess, Chief Financial Officer
CMO: Crayton A. Fargason, M.D., Medical Director
CIO: Mike McDevitt, Chief Information Officer
CHR: Douglas B. Dean, Chief Human Resources Officer
CNO: Deb Wesley, MSN, Chief Nursing Officer
Web address: www.childrensal.org
**Control:** Other not–for–profit (including NFP Corporation) **Service:** Children's general

**Staffed Beds:** 290 **Admissions:** 13357 **Census:** 218 **Outpatient Visits:** 634830 **Total Expense ($000):** 470597 **Payroll Expense ($000):** 189618 **Personnel:** 3322

✠ **TRINITY MEDICAL CENTER (10104)**, 800 Montclair Road, Zip 35213–1984; tel. 205/592–1000 **A**1 2 3 5 9 10 **F**3 12 13 15 17 18 20 22 24 26 28 29 30 31 34 35 40 43 45 46 47 48 49 50 51 53 54 57 58 59 64 70 72 73 74 75 76 77 78 79 81 82 85 90 93 96 98 99 102 103 106 107 108 109 110 111 113 114 116 117 118 119 121 123 125 128 129 130 131 145 146 147 **S** Community Health Systems, Inc., Franklin, TN
Primary Contact: Keith Granger, President and Chief Executive Officer
COO: Sean T. Dardeau, Chief Operating Officer
CFO: Julie Soekoro, Chief Financial Officer
CMO: Hugh O'Shields, M.D., President Medical Staff
CIO: Tim Townes, Director Information Systems
CHR: Joel R. Windham, Director Human Resources
CNO: Andy Romine, Chief Nursing Officer
Web address: www.bhsala.com
**Control:** Corporation, Investor–owned, for–profit **Service:** General Medical and Surgical

**Staffed Beds:** 379 **Admissions:** 13822 **Census:** 218 **Outpatient Visits:** 306029 **Births:** 601 **Total Expense ($000):** 222397 **Payroll Expense ($000):** 84204 **Personnel:** 1568

**UAB HIGHLANDS** See University of Alabama Hospital

✠ **UNIVERSITY OF ALABAMA HOSPITAL (10033)**, 619 19th Street South, Zip 35249; tel. 205/934–4011, (Includes UAB HIGHLANDS, 1201 11th Avenue South, Zip 35205–5299; tel. 205/930–7000; Anthony Patterson, Chief Operating Officer) **A**1 2 3 5 8 9 10 **F**3 4 5 6 8 9 11 12 13 15 16 17 18 19 20 21 22 23 24 25 26 27 28 29 30 31 33 34 35 37 38 39 40 43 44 45 46 47 49 50 52 53 54 55 56 57 58 59 60 61 62 64 65 66 68 70 71 72 73 74 75 76 77 78 79 81 82 83 84 85 86 87 90 91 92 93 94 95 96 97 98 99 100 101 102 103 104 107 108 110 111 113 114 115 116 117 118 119 120 122 123 125 128 129 130 131 134 135 136 137 138 139 140 141 142 143 144 145 146 147 **P**3 **S** UAB Health System, Birmingham, AL
Primary Contact: Michael Waldrum, M.D., Chief Executive Officer
CFO: Mary Beth Briscoe, Chief Financial Officer
CMO: Cynthia Brumfield, M.D., Chief of Staff
CIO: Joan Hicks, Chief Information Officer
CHR: Alesia Jones, Interim Chief Human Resources Officer
Web address: www.health.uab.edu
**Control:** State–Government, nonfederal **Service:** General Medical and Surgical

**Staffed Beds:** 1062 **Admissions:** 45936 **Census:** 812 **Outpatient Visits:** 420136 **Births:** 3994 **Total Expense ($000):** 1043685 **Payroll Expense ($000):** 378656 **Personnel:** 6838

✠ **VETERANS AFFAIRS MEDICAL CENTER**, 700 South 19th Street, Zip 35233–1927; tel. 205/933–8101 **A**1 2 3 5 8 **F**3 4 5 8 12 17 18 20 22 24 26 28 29 30 31 34 35 38 39 40 43 44 45 47 50 54 56 57 58 59 60 61 62 63 64 65 68 70 74 75 77 78 79 81 82 83 84 85 87 90 92 93 94 96 97 98 100 101 102 103 104 106 107 108 109 111 112 113 114 115 116 117 118 119 123 126 128 129 131 134 142 145 146 147 **S** Department of Veterans Affairs, Washington, DC
Primary Contact: Rica Lewis–Payton, Director
COO: Cynthia Cleveland, Ph.D., Acting Associate Director
COO: Phyllis Smith, Associate Director
CFO: Mary S. Mitchell, Chief Resource Management Services
CMO: Michael Thornsberry, M.D., Chief of Staff
CIO: Harald Carlisle, Acting Chief Information Officer
CIO: William Greer, Chief Information Officer
CHR: Jacqueline Caron, Chief Human Resources
CNO: Gregory S. Eagerton, Ph.D., Associate Director for Patient Care Services/Nurse Executive
Web address: www.va.gov/sta/guide/home.asp
**Control:** Veterans Affairs, Government, federal **Service:** General Medical and Surgical

**Staffed Beds:** 151 **Admissions:** 6212 **Census:** 102 **Outpatient Visits:** 705029 **Births:** 0 **Total Expense ($000):** 367459 **Payroll Expense ($000):** 146977 **Personnel:** 2022

**BOAZ—Marshall County**

✠ **MARSHALL MEDICAL CENTER SOUTH (10005)**, U.S. Highway 431 North, Zip 35957–0999, Mailing Address: P.O. Box 758, Zip 35957–0758; tel. 256/593–8310 **A**1 9 10 19 **F**3 7 8 11 12 13 15 18 20 22 26 28 29 32 34 37 40 43 45 46 50 53 54 57 59 64 68 70 74 75 76 78 79 81 85 86 87 93 100 107 108 110 111 113 116 118 120 122 128 129 130 131 134 140 144 145 146 147 **S** Marshall Health System, Guntersville, AL
Primary Contact: John D. Anderson, FACHE, Administrator
CFO: Kathy Nelson, Chief Financial Officer
Web address: www.mmcs.org
**Control:** Hospital district or authority, Government, nonfederal **Service:** General Medical and Surgical

**Staffed Beds:** 112 **Admissions:** 5322 **Census:** 52 **Outpatient Visits:** 192734 **Births:** 811 **Total Expense ($000):** 53045 **Payroll Expense ($000):** 29466 **Personnel:** 541

**BREWTON—Escambia County**

☐ **D. W. MCMILLAN MEMORIAL HOSPITAL (10099)**, 1301 Belleville Avenue, Zip 36426–1306, Mailing Address: P.O. Box 908, Zip 36427–0908; tel. 251/867–8061 **A**1 9 10 **F**3 7 11 13 15 31 34 35 40 45 57 59 62 64 70 75 76 78 79 81 85 86 89 93 100 107 108 111 113 118 126 128 129 130 131 132 134 142 145 **P**6
Primary Contact: Christopher B. Griffin, Chief Executive Officer
CFO: Richard Owens, Chief Financial Officer
CIO: Ian Vickery, Director Information Technology
CHR: Autherine Davis, Director Human Resources
CNO: Bob Ellis, Director of Nursing
Web address: www.dwmmh.org
**Control:** Hospital district or authority, Government, nonfederal **Service:** General Medical and Surgical

**Staffed Beds:** 49 **Admissions:** 2204 **Census:** 21 **Outpatient Visits:** 45168 **Births:** 278 **Total Expense ($000):** 19584 **Payroll Expense ($000):** 10344 **Personnel:** 229

---

**Hospital, Medicare Provider Number, Address, Telephone, Approval, Facility, and Physician Codes, Health Care System**

★ American Hospital Association (AHA) membership
☐ The Joint Commission accreditation
◇ DNV Healthcare Inc. accreditation
○ American Osteopathic Association (AOA) accreditation
△ Commission on Accreditation of Rehabilitation Facilities (CARF) accreditation

## CAMDEN—Wilcox County

**J. PAUL JONES HOSPITAL (10102)**, 317 McWilliams Avenue,
Zip 36726–1610; tel. 334/682–4131, (Nonreporting) **A**9 10 20
Primary Contact: Elizabeth M. Kennedy, Administrator
CMO: Willie White, M.D., Director Medical Staff
CIO: Jill Smith, Administrative Coordinator
CHR: Jill Smith, Administrative Coordinator
**Control:** City–County, Government, nonfederal **Service:** General Medical and
Surgical

**Staffed Beds:** 22

## CARROLLTON—Pickens County

**PICKENS COUNTY MEDICAL CENTER (10109)**, 241 Robert K. Wilson Drive,
Zip 35447, Mailing Address: P.O. Box 478, Zip 35447–0478;
tel. 205/367–8111, (Nonreporting) **A**9 10 20
Primary Contact: Wayne McElroy, Administrator
CFO: Janice Winters, Controller
CMO: William R. Brooke, M.D., President Medical Staff
CHR: Dottie Wilson, Director Human Resources
Web address: www.dchsystem.com
**Control:** County–Government, nonfederal **Service:** General Medical and Surgical

**Staffed Beds:** 52

## CENTRE—Cherokee County

✉ **CHEROKEE MEDICAL CENTER (10022)**, 400 Northwood Drive,
Zip 35960–1023; tel. 256/927–5531 **A**1 9 10 **F**3 11 15 29 30 35 40 43 45
48 57 59 64 70 81 87 107 108 111 113 118 126 128 129 130 132 145
**P**6 **S** Community Health Systems, Inc., Franklin, TN
Primary Contact: Patrick Trammell, Chief Executive Officer
CFO: Zac Allen, CPA, Chief Financial Officer
CHR: Marlene Benefield, Director Human Resources
Web address: www.cherokeemedicalcenter.com
**Control:** Corporation, Investor–owned, for–profit **Service:** General Medical and
Surgical

**Staffed Beds:** 45 **Admissions:** 991 **Census:** 12 **Outpatient Visits:** 20227
**Births:** 0 **Total Expense ($000):** 11392 **Payroll Expense ($000):** 5329
**Personnel:** 142

## CENTREVILLE—Bibb County

**BIBB MEDICAL CENTER (10058)**, 208 Pierson Avenue, Zip 35042–1199;
tel. 205/926–4881 **A**9 10 **F**3 11 15 29 35 40 50 57 59 62 64 81 93 107 118
124 126 129 132 143 145 **P**6
Primary Contact: Joseph Marchant, Administrator
CFO: Heather Desmond, Chief Financial Officer
CMO: John Meigs, Jr., M.D., Chief of Staff
CHR: Kim Hayes, Director Human Resources
Web address: www.bibbmedicalcenter.com
**Control:** County–Government, nonfederal **Service:** General Medical and Surgical

**Staffed Beds:** 20 **Admissions:** 250 **Census:** 2 **Outpatient Visits:** 39786
**Births:** 0 **Total Expense ($000):** 18224 **Payroll Expense ($000):** 7224
**Personnel:** 202

## CHATOM—Washington County

★ **WASHINGTON COUNTY HOSPITAL AND NURSING HOME (11300)**, 14600
St. Stephens Avenue, Zip 36518–9998, Mailing Address: P.O. Box 1299,
Zip 36518–1299; tel. 251/847–2223 **A**9 10 18 **F**15 29 34 40 59 64 89 107
113 118 127 132 147 **P**6
Primary Contact: Douglas Tanner, Chief Executive Officer
CFO: Alyson Overstreet, Chief Financial Officer
CMO: Steve Donald, M.D., Chief of Staff
CIO: Brady Wright, Information Technology Network Administrator
CHR: Linda Randolph, Director Personnel Services
CNO: Lamar Cooley, R.N., Director of Nursing
Web address: www.wchnh.org
**Control:** County–Government, nonfederal **Service:** General Medical and Surgical

**Staffed Beds:** 22 **Admissions:** 439 **Census:** 4 **Outpatient Visits:** 12263
**Births:** 0 **Total Expense ($000):** 5760 **Payroll Expense ($000):** 2346
**Personnel:** 72

## CLANTON—Chilton County

★ **CHILTON MEDICAL CENTER (10043)**, 1010 Lay Dam Road, Zip 35045–2306;
tel. 205/755–2500 **A**9 10 **F**3 11 15 29 34 35 40 41 45 57 59 64 68 71 75
79 81 82 85 86 87 97 98 107 108 113 117 118 129 132 134 144 145
Primary Contact: Ted G. Chapin, Chief Executive Officer
COO: David Pryor, Chief Operating Officer
CIO: Jimmy Smith, Coordinator Clinical Information Technology
CHR: Joann Turpen, Director Human Resources
Web address: www.chiltonmedicalcenter.net
**Control:** Corporation, Investor–owned, for–profit **Service:** General Medical and
Surgical

**Staffed Beds:** 20 **Admissions:** 629 **Census:** 5 **Outpatient Visits:** 33527
**Births:** 0 **Total Expense ($000):** 12268 **Payroll Expense ($000):** 5215
**Personnel:** 139

## CULLMAN—Cullman County

☐ **CULLMAN REGIONAL MEDICAL CENTER (10035)**, 1912 Alabama Highway
157, Zip 35055, Mailing Address: P.O. Box 1108, Zip 35056–1108;
tel. 256/737–2000 **A**1 9 10 19 **F**3 7 11 12 13 15 18 20 22 26 28 29 30 31
34 35 37 40 43 45 46 49 50 53 57 59 62 63 64 68 70 74 75 76 77 78 79
81 82 83 84 85 86 87 89 93 107 108 110 111 113 117 118 120 128 129
130 131 133 134 145 146 147
Primary Contact: James Weidner, President
COO: Jete Edmisson, Chief Operating Officer and Chief Financial Officer
CFO: Jete Edmisson, Chief Operating Officer and Chief Financial Officer
CMO: John Morris, M.D., Chief of Staff
CIO: Nancy Zavatchen, Director Information Technology
CHR: Toni Geddings, Director Human Resources
Web address: www.crmchospital.com
**Control:** Other not–for–profit (including NFP Corporation) **Service:** General
Medical and Surgical

**Staffed Beds:** 115 **Admissions:** 7195 **Census:** 79 **Outpatient Visits:** 105543
**Births:** 910 **Total Expense ($000):** 78181 **Payroll Expense ($000):** 39401
**Personnel:** 924

## DADEVILLE—Tallapoosa County

**LAKE MARTIN COMMUNITY HOSPITAL (10052)**, 201 Mariarden Road,
Zip 36853–6251, Mailing Address: P.O. Box 629, Zip 36853–0629;
tel. 256/825–7821, (Nonreporting) **A**9 10
Primary Contact: Michael D. Bruce, Chief Executive Officer
CHR: Karen Treadwell, Director Human Resources
Web address: www.lakemartincommunityhospital.com
**Control:** Partnership, Investor–owned, for–profit **Service:** General Medical and
Surgical

**Staffed Beds:** 28

## DECATUR—Morgan County

☐ **DECATUR GENERAL HOSPITAL (10085)**, 1201 Seventh Street S.E.,
Zip 35601–3303, Mailing Address: P.O. Box 2239, Zip 35609–2239;
tel. 256/341–2000, (Includes DECATUR GENERAL HOSPITAL–WEST, 2205
Beltline Road S.W., Zip 35601–3687, Mailing Address: P.O. Box 2240,
Zip 35609–2240; tel. 256/306–4000) **A**1 2 9 10 **F**3 6 11 13 15 18 20 28 29
30 31 34 35 38 40 41 43 45 49 50 53 55 56 57 59 60 61 65 68 70 73
74 75 76 77 78 79 81 85 86 87 89 91 92 93 97 98 99 100 101 102 103
104 107 108 110 111 113 118 119 120 122 125 128 129 130 131 133 134
144 145 146 147
Primary Contact: Dean A. Griffin, President and Chief Executive Officer
CFO: Kim Shrewsbury, Vice President and Chief Financial Officer
CMO: Allen J. Schmidt, M.D., President, Medical Staff
CIO: Mark Megehee, Vice President and Chief Information Officer
CNO: Anita Walden, Vice President and Chief Nursing Officer
Web address: www.decaturgeneral.org
**Control:** Hospital district or authority, Government, nonfederal **Service:** General
Medical and Surgical

**Staffed Beds:** 203 **Admissions:** 8298 **Census:** 106 **Outpatient Visits:**
128729 **Births:** 548 **Total Expense ($000):** 77144 **Payroll Expense ($000):**
41274 **Personnel:** 932

☐ **NORTH ALABAMA REGIONAL HOSPITAL (14009)**, 4218 Highway 31 South,
Zip 35603–5039; tel. 256/560–2200, (Nonreporting) **A**1 10
Primary Contact: J. Randall Phillips, FACHE, Chief Executive Officer
CFO: Roger Kalonick, Business Manager
CMO: Duard Bok, M.D., Clinical Director
CIO: Ronald J. Thomas, Coordinator Information Systems
CHR: Gregory Ethridge, Manager Personnel
Web address: www.narh.mh.alabama.gov
**Control:** State–Government, nonfederal **Service:** Psychiatric

**Staffed Beds:** 74

☐ **PARKWAY MEDICAL CENTER (10054)**, 1874 Beltline Road S.W.,
Zip 35601–5509, Mailing Address: P.O. Box 2211, Zip 35609–2211;
tel. 256/350–2211, (Nonreporting) **A**1 9 10 **S** Capella Healthcare, Franklin, TN
Primary Contact: Nathaniel Richardson, Jr., Interim President
COO: Wayne Bowman, Interim Chief Nursing Officer
CFO: Danny Crowe, Chief Financial Officer
CMO: Cara Hoffman, M.D., Chief of Staff
CIO: Doyle Haynes, Director Information Systems
CHR: Don Zamora, Director Human Resources
Web address: www.parkwaymedicalcenter.com
**Control:** Corporation, Investor–owned, for–profit **Service:** General Medical and
Surgical

**Staffed Beds:** 120

*Many Facility Codes have changed. Please refer to the AHA Guide Code Chart.*          © 2012 AHA Guide

## DEMOPOLIS—Marengo County

☐ **BRYAN W. WHITFIELD MEMORIAL HOSPITAL (10112)**, 105 U.S. Highway 80 East, Zip 36732–3616, Mailing Address: P.O. Box 890, Zip 36732–0890; tel. 334/289–4000, (Nonreporting) **A**1 9 10 20
Primary Contact: Michael D. Marshall, Administrator and Chief Executive Officer
CFO: Arthur D. Evans, Assistant Administrator
CHR: Danny Smith, Director Human Resources
Web address: www.bwwmh.com
**Control:** Hospital district or authority, Government, nonfederal **Service:** General Medical and Surgical

| Staffed Beds: 99 |
| --- |

## DOTHAN—Houston County

☒ **FLOWERS HOSPITAL (10055)**, 4370 West Main Street, Zip 36305–4000, Mailing Address: P.O. Box 6907, Zip 36302–6907; tel. 334/793–5000 **A**1 2 9 10 **F**1 3 4 12 13 15 16 17 18 20 22 24 26 28 29 31 34 35 40 46 48 49 50 51 56 57 59 60 61 64 67 68 70 74 75 76 77 78 79 80 81 82 85 86 87 89 90 92 93 97 98 107 108 110 111 113 114 115 116 117 118 125 127 128 129 131 133 134 145 146 147 **P**6 **S** Community Health Systems, Inc., Franklin, TN
Primary Contact: Suzanne Woods, President and Chief Executive Officer
CFO: Talana Bell, Chief Financial Officer
CHR: Scott H. Givens, Director Human Resources
CNO: Dan L. Cumbie, Chief Nursing Officer
Web address: www.flowershospital.com
**Control:** Corporation, Investor–owned, for–profit **Service:** General Medical and Surgical

| Staffed Beds: 235 Admissions: 11365 Census: 140 Outpatient Visits: 158145 Births: 1388 Total Expense ($000): 166914 Payroll Expense ($000): 59066 Personnel: 1197 |
| --- |

☒ **HEALTHSOUTH REHABILITATION HOSPITAL (13030)**, 1736 East Main Street, Zip 36301, Mailing Address: P.O. Box 6708, Zip 36302–6708; tel. 334/712–6333 **A**1 9 10 **F**28 29 34 35 56 57 59 64 74 75 77 79 90 91 93 95 96 129 131 **P**5 **S** HEALTHSOUTH Corporation, Birmingham, AL
Primary Contact: Margaret A. Futch, Chief Executive Officer
CFO: Heath Watson, Controller
CMO: Stephen L. Chastain, M.D., Medical Director
CHR: Lydia Christion, Director Human Resources
Web address: www.healthsouthdothan.com
**Control:** Corporation, Investor–owned, for–profit **Service:** Rehabilitation

| Staffed Beds: 39 Admissions: 1052 Census: 36 Outpatient Visits: 2546 Births: 0 Total Expense ($000): 8860 Payroll Expense ($000): 5019 Personnel: 127 |
| --- |

☐ **LAUREL OAKS BEHAVIORAL HEALTH CENTER (14013)**, 700 East Cottonwood Road, Zip 36301; tel. 334/794–7373 **A**1 9 10 **F**98 99 106 **S** Universal Health Services, Inc., King of Prussia, PA
Primary Contact: Derek Johnson, Chief Executive Officer
CMO: Nelson Handol, M.D., Medical Director
CHR: Lorrie Evans, Director Human Resources
Web address: www.laureloaksbhc.com
**Control:** Corporation, Investor–owned, for–profit **Service:** Children's hospital psychiatric

| Staffed Beds: 32 Admissions: 799 Census: 27 Outpatient Visits: 0 Births: 0 Total Expense ($000): 11008 Payroll Expense ($000): 6800 Personnel: 234 |
| --- |

☐ **NOLAND HOSPITAL DOTHAN (12010)**, 1108 Ross Clark Circle, 4th Floor, Zip 36302; tel. 334/699–4300, (Nonreporting) **A**1 9 10 **S** Noland Health Services, Inc., Birmingham, AL
Primary Contact: Kaye Burke, Administrator
Web address: www.nolandhealth.com
**Control:** Other not–for–profit (including NFP Corporation) **Service:** Long–Term Acute Care hospital

| Staffed Beds: 30 |
| --- |

☒ **SOUTHEAST ALABAMA MEDICAL CENTER (10001)**, 1108 Ross Clark Circle, Zip 36301–3024, Mailing Address: P.O. Box 6987, Zip 36302–6987; tel. 334/793–8111 **A**1 2 9 10 **F**3 8 12 13 15 18 20 22 24 26 28 29 30 31 32 34 35 37 40 43 44 45 49 50 51 53 56 57 59 60 62 63 64 68 70 71 74 75 76 77 78 79 81 82 85 86 87 89 93 94 98 100 101 102 103 104 105 107 108 110 111 113 114 115 116 117 118 119 120 122 123 125 128 129 131 134 145 146 147 **P**6
Primary Contact: Ronald S. Owen, FACHE, Chief Executive Officer
COO: Charles C. Brannen, Senior Vice President and Chief Operating Officer
CFO: Derek Miller, Senior Vice President and Chief Financial Officer
CMO: Charles Harkness, D.O., Vice President Medical Affairs
CHR: Peggy Sease, Vice President Human Resources
CNO: Diane Buntyn, MSN, Vice President Patient Care Services
Web address: www.samc.org
**Control:** Hospital district or authority, Government, nonfederal **Service:** General Medical and Surgical

| Staffed Beds: 420 Admissions: 18116 Census: 248 Outpatient Visits: 127085 Births: 2166 Total Expense ($000): 168660 Payroll Expense ($000): 109986 Personnel: 2191 |
| --- |

## ELBA—Coffee County

★ **ELBA GENERAL HOSPITAL (10027)**, 987 Drayton Street, Zip 36323–1494; tel. 334/897–2257, (Nonreporting) **A**9 10 **S** QHR, Brentwood, TN
Primary Contact: Ellen C. Briley, Administrator and Chief Executive Officer
COO: Ceina Spicer, R.N., Chief Operating Officer
CFO: Nicki Jinright, Chief Financial Officer
CMO: Lance K. Dyess, M.D., Chief Medical Officer
CIO: Mary Gray, R.N., Director Information Technology and Special Project
CHR: Judi Qualls, Director Human Resources
**Control:** Hospital district or authority, Government, nonfederal **Service:** General Medical and Surgical

| Staffed Beds: 20 |
| --- |

## ENTERPRISE—Coffee County

☒ **MEDICAL CENTER ENTERPRISE (10049)**, 400 North Edwards Street, Zip 36330; tel. 334/347–0584, (Nonreporting) **A**1 9 10 **S** Community Health Systems, Inc., Franklin, TN
Primary Contact: Jeffrey M. Brannon, Chief Executive Officer
CFO: Greg McGilvray, Chief Financial Officer
CHR: Toni Kaminski, Director Human Resources
Web address: www.mcehospital.com
**Control:** Corporation, Investor–owned, for–profit **Service:** General Medical and Surgical

| Staffed Beds: 117 |
| --- |

## EUFAULA—Barbour County

**MEDICAL CENTER BARBOUR (10069)**, 820 West Washington Street, Zip 36027–1899; tel. 334/688–7000 **A**9 10 20 **F**3 11 15 29 30 34 35 40 45 46 50 57 59 64 68 70 81 85 98 103 107 118 126 132 134 145
Primary Contact: Ralph H. Clark, Jr., FACHE, Chief Executive Officer
CFO: Debbie Norton, Chief Financial Officer
CHR: Cindy Griffin, Director Human Resources
CNO: Kathy Wilder, R.N., Chief Clinical Officer
Web address: www.medctrbarbour.org
**Control:** Hospital district or authority, Government, nonfederal **Service:** General Medical and Surgical

| Staffed Beds: 47 Admissions: 1612 Census: 19 Outpatient Visits: 29347 Total Expense ($000): 12382 Payroll Expense ($000): 6911 Personnel: 196 |
| --- |

## EUTAW—Greene County

★ **GREENE COUNTY HOSPITAL (10051)**, 509 Wilson Avenue, Zip 35462–1099; tel. 205/372–3388, (Nonreporting) **A**9 10
Primary Contact: Mark Chustz, Administrator
**Control:** County–Government, nonfederal **Service:** General Medical and Surgical

| Staffed Beds: 15 |
| --- |

---

**Hospital, Medicare Provider Number, Address, Telephone, Approval, Facility, and Physician Codes, Health Care System**

★ American Hospital Association (AHA) membership
☐ The Joint Commission accreditation
◇ DNV Healthcare Inc. accreditation
○ American Osteopathic Association (AOA) accreditation
△ Commission on Accreditation of Rehabilitation Facilities (CARF) accreditation

## EVERGREEN—Conecuh County

**EVERGREEN MEDICAL CENTER (10148)**, 101 Crestview Avenue,
Zip 36401–0706, Mailing Address: P.O. Box 706, Zip 36401–0706;
tel. 251/578–2480, (Nonreporting) **A**9 10 **S** Gilliard Health Services,
Montgomery, AL
Primary Contact: William G. McKenzie, Interim Administrator
CFO: Sharon Jones, Chief Financial Officer
CMO: William Farmer, M.D., Chief of Staff
Web address: www.evergreenmedical.org
**Control:** Corporation, Investor–owned, for–profit **Service:** General Medical and
Surgical

**Staffed Beds:** 44

## FAIRHOPE—Baldwin County

**THOMAS HOSPITAL (10100)**, 750 Morphy Avenue, Zip 36532–1812, Mailing
Address: P.O. Drawer 929, Zip 36533–0929; tel. 251/928–2375, (Nonreporting)
**A**5 9 10 19 **S** Infirmary Health System, Mobile, AL
Primary Contact: William J. McLaughlin, Administrator
COO: Douglas Garner, Vice President
CFO: Patrick Murphy, Vice President Finance
CMO: Michael McBrearty, M.D., Vice President Medical Affairs
Web address: www.thomashospital.com
**Control:** Hospital district or authority, Government, nonfederal **Service:** General
Medical and Surgical

**Staffed Beds:** 136

## FAYETTE—Fayette County

☐ **FAYETTE MEDICAL CENTER (10045)**, 1653 Temple Avenue North,
Zip 35555–1314, Mailing Address: P.O. Drawer 710, Zip 35555–0710;
tel. 205/932–5966, (Total facility includes 122 beds in nursing home–type unit)
**A**1 9 10 **F**3 11 15 28 29 31 34 40 59 64 70 78 81 107 111 118 129 132
145 **P**5 **S** DCH Health System, Tuscaloosa, AL
Primary Contact: Barry S. Cochran, FACHE, Administrator
CFO: Jeff Huff, Assistant Administrator Finance
CHR: Cindy Bohon, Director Human Resources
Web address: www.dchsystem.com
**Control:** Hospital district or authority, Government, nonfederal **Service:** General
Medical and Surgical

**Staffed Beds:** 167 **Admissions:** 1462 **Census:** 126 **Outpatient Visits:** 50485
**Births:** 0 **Total Expense ($000):** 20044 **Payroll Expense ($000):** 11651
**Personnel:** 327

## FLORALA—Covington County

**FLORALA MEMORIAL HOSPITAL (10066)**, 24273 Fifth Avenue, Zip 36442,
Mailing Address: P.O. Box 189, Zip 36442–0189; tel. 334/858–3287 **A**9 10 **F**40
107 108
Primary Contact: Mickey Rabuka, Administrator
Web address: www.floralahospital.org
**Control:** Corporation, Investor–owned, for–profit **Service:** General Medical and
Surgical

**Staffed Beds:** 23 **Admissions:** 377 **Census:** 3 **Outpatient Visits:** 5896
**Births:** 0 **Total Expense ($000):** 3329 **Payroll Expense ($000):** 1867

## FLORENCE—Lauderdale County

☐ **ELIZA COFFEE MEMORIAL HOSPITAL (10006)**, 205 Marengo Street,
Zip 35630–6033, Mailing Address: P.O. Box 818, Zip 35631–0818;
tel. 256/768–9191, (Nonreporting) **A**1 9 10 **S** RegionalCare Hospital Partners,
Brentwood, TN
Primary Contact: Russell Pigg, Chief Executive Officer
COO: Bryan Lee, Chief Operating Officer
Web address: www.chgroup.org
**Control:** Corporation, Investor–owned, for–profit **Service:** General Medical and
Surgical

**Staffed Beds:** 278

## FOLEY—Baldwin County

☒ **SOUTH BALDWIN REGIONAL MEDICAL CENTER (10083)**, 1613 North
McKenzie Street, Zip 36535–2299; tel. 251/949–3400, (Nonreporting) **A**1 9 10
19 **S** Community Health Systems, Inc., Franklin, TN
Primary Contact: Keith Newton, Chief Executive Officer
CMO: Karl Hakmiller, M.D., Chief Medical Officer
CIO: Jeannine O'Neill, Director Information Systems
CHR: Pam Brunson, Director Human Resources
Web address: www.southbaldwinrmc.com
**Control:** Corporation, Investor–owned, for–profit **Service:** General Medical and
Surgical

**Staffed Beds:** 110

## FORT PAYNE—Dekalb County

☒ **DEKALB REGIONAL MEDICAL CENTER (10012)**, 200 Medical Center Drive,
Zip 35968–3415, Mailing Address: P.O. Box 680778, Zip 35968–1608;
tel. 256/845–3150, (Nonreporting) **A**1 9 10 20 **S** Community Health Systems,
Inc., Franklin, TN
Primary Contact: Jeff G. Rains, Chief Executive Officer
COO: Jay Hinesley, Assistant Chief Executive Officer
CFO: Hugh Tobin, Chief Financial Officer
CMO: Jeff Thompson, M.D., Chief of Staff
CIO: Anthony Sherlin, Director Information Systems
CHR: Diane McMichen, Director Human Resources
CNO: Marquita Bailey, Chief Nursing Officer
Web address: www.dekalbregional.com
**Control:** Corporation, Investor–owned, for–profit **Service:** General Medical and
Surgical

**Staffed Beds:** 115

## GADSDEN—Etowah County

☒ **GADSDEN REGIONAL MEDICAL CENTER (10040)**, 1007 Goodyear Avenue,
Zip 35903–1195; tel. 256/494–4000 **A**1 2 9 10 **F**3 11 13 15 18 20 22 24 28
29 30 31 34 35 40 43 49 50 51 57 59 60 64 68 70 73 74 76 77 78 79 80
81 85 89 93 98 102 103 105 107 108 111 112 113 114 118 120 128 129
131 145 146 147 **S** Community Health Systems, Inc., Franklin, TN
Primary Contact: Stephen G. Pennington, Chief Executive Officer
COO: Paul Theriot, Chief Operating Officer
CFO: Michael Cotton, Chief Financial Officer
CMO: William Haller, III, M.D., Chief of Staff
CIO: Glenn Phillips, Director Information Systems
CHR: Gale H. Sanders, Director
CNO: Donna Nicholson, Chief Nursing Officer
Web address: www.gadsdenregional.com
**Control:** Corporation, Investor–owned, for–profit **Service:** General Medical and
Surgical

**Staffed Beds:** 299 **Admissions:** 11898 **Census:** 178 **Outpatient Visits:**
103215 **Births:** 1136 **Total Expense ($000):** 141061 **Payroll Expense
($000):** 48317 **Personnel:** 980

☒ **HEALTHSOUTH REHABILITATION OF GADSDEN (13032)**, 801 Goodyear
Avenue, Zip 35903; tel. 256/439–5000, (Nonreporting) **A**1 9 10
**S** HEALTHSOUTH Corporation, Birmingham, AL
Primary Contact: Michael W. Thompson, Chief Executive Officer
COO: Michael W. Thompson, Chief Executive Officer
CFO: Lori Norman, Chief Financial Officer
CMO: Catherine Harding, M.D., Medical Director
CIO: Lori Norman, Chief Financial Officer
CHR: Heather Blevins, Director Human Resources
Web address: www.healthsouth.com
**Control:** Corporation, Investor–owned, for–profit **Service:** Rehabilitation

**Staffed Beds:** 44

☐ **MOUNTAIN VIEW HOSPITAL (14006)**, 3001 Scenic Highway,
Zip 35901–9956, Mailing Address: P.O. Box 8406, Zip 35902–8406;
tel. 256/546–9265, (Nonreporting) **A**1 9 10
Primary Contact: G. Michael Shehi, M.D., Interim Chief Executive Officer
COO: Sara Romano, R.N., Vice President
CFO: Mary Jensen, Controller
CMO: G. Michael Shehi, M.D., Medical Director
CHR: Dave Jensen, Director Human Resources, Performance Improvement and
Risk Management
Web address: www.mtnviewhospital.com
**Control:** Corporation, Investor–owned, for–profit **Service:** Psychiatric

**Staffed Beds:** 68

☐ **RIVERVIEW REGIONAL MEDICAL CENTER (10046)**, 600 South Third Street,
Zip 35901–5399, Mailing Address: P.O. Box 268, Zip 35902;
tel. 256/543–5200, (Nonreporting) **A**1 9 10 **S** Health Management Associates,
Naples, FL
Primary Contact: Lloyd F. Ford, Jr., Ph.D., FACHE, Chief Executive Officer
COO: Bryan McCauley, Associate Executive Director
CFO: Gregory Pearson, Associate Executive Director Finance
CIO: Jay Terrell, Manager Management Information Systems
CHR: Dana Simpson, Manager Human Resources
Web address: www.riverviewregional.com
**Control:** Corporation, Investor–owned, for–profit **Service:** General Medical and
Surgical

**Staffed Beds:** 204

*Many Facility Codes have changed. Please refer to the AHA Guide Code Chart.*

© 2012 AHA Guide

## GENEVA—Geneva County

★ **WIREGRASS MEDICAL CENTER (10062)**, 1200 West Maple Avenue, Zip 36340–1694; tel. 334/684–3655, (Total facility includes 96 beds in nursing home–type unit) **A**9 10 **F**3 15 29 30 34 35 40 41 45 50 56 57 59 64 68 70 79 81 83 84 85 86 87 98 100 102 103 105 107 108 113 118 127 129 131 145 **P**5
Primary Contact: Charles A. Faulkner, FACHE, Chief Executive Officer
CFO: Gloria McGowan, Chief Financial Officer
CIO: Tom Garske, Director Information Systems
CHR: Pam Phillips, Chief Human Resource Officer
CNO: Craig Cassady, Director of Nursing
Web address: www.alaweb.com/~tgarske
**Control:** Hospital district or authority, Government, nonfederal **Service:** General Medical and Surgical

**Staffed Beds:** 167 **Admissions:** 1970 **Census:** 25 **Outpatient Visits:** 11517 **Births:** 0 **Total Expense ($000):** 21483 **Payroll Expense ($000):** 11622 **Personnel:** 300

## GEORGIANA—Butler County

**GEORGIANA HOSPITAL (10047)**, 515 Miranda Street, Zip 36033, Mailing Address: P.O. Box 548, Zip 36033–0548; tel. 334/376–2205, (Nonreporting) **A**9 10
Primary Contact: Harry Cole, Jr., Administrator
**Control:** Partnership, Investor–owned, for–profit **Service:** General Medical and Surgical

**Staffed Beds:** 22

## GREENSBORO—Hale County

**HALE COUNTY HOSPITAL (10095)**, 508 Green Street, Zip 36744–0017; tel. 334/624–3024, (Nonreporting) **A**9 10
Primary Contact: Thomas O. Lackey, Administrator
Web address: www.halecountyhospital.com
**Control:** County–Government, nonfederal **Service:** General Medical and Surgical

**Staffed Beds:** 28

## GREENVILLE—Butler County

⊞ **L. V. STABLER MEMORIAL HOSPITAL (10150)**, 29 L. V. Stabler Drive, Zip 36037–3800; tel. 334/382–2671, (Nonreporting) **A**1 9 10 **S** Community Health Systems, Inc., Franklin, TN
Primary Contact: Connie Nicholas, Interim Chief Executive Officer
COO: Connie Nicholas, Interim Chief Executive Officer
CFO: Vann Windham, Chief Financial Officer
CMO: Norman F. McGowin, III, M.D., Chief of Staff
CHR: Robert Foster, Director Human Resources
CNO: Kimberli Weaver, Chief Nursing Officer
Web address: www.lvstabler.com
**Control:** Corporation, Investor–owned, for–profit **Service:** General Medical and Surgical

**Staffed Beds:** 61

## GROVE HILL—Clarke County

★ **GROVE HILL MEMORIAL HOSPITAL (10091)**, 295 South Jackson Street, Zip 36451–0935, Mailing Address: P.O. Box 935, Zip 36451–0935; tel. 251/275–3191, (Nonreporting) **A**9 10
Primary Contact: Wes Nall, Administrator
CFO: Elaine Averett, Chief Financial Officer
CMO: David Hubbs, M.D., Chief Medical Staff
CHR: Emily Steadham, Administrative Assistant Human Resources and Public Relations
Web address: www.grovehillmemorial.org
**Control:** City–Government, nonfederal **Service:** General Medical and Surgical

**Staffed Beds:** 34

## GUNTERSVILLE—Marshall County

⊞ **MARSHALL MEDICAL CENTER NORTH (10010)**, 8000 Alabama Highway 69, Zip 35976; tel. 256/753–8000 **A**1 9 10 **F**3 7 8 11 12 15 26 28 29 32 34 35 37 38 40 43 45 49 50 51 53 54 57 59 64 68 70 74 75 76 79 81 82 85 86 87 93 99 100 102 103 104 107 108 110 111 113 118 129 130 131 132 134 140 145 146 **S** Marshall Health System, Guntersville, AL
Primary Contact: Cheryl M. Hays, FACHE, Administrator
COO: Cheryl M. Hays, FACHE, Administrator
CFO: Kathy Nelson, Chief Financial Officer
CIO: Kim Bunch, Director Information Technology
CHR: Jeff Stone, Director Human Resources
CNO: Kathy Woodruff, R.N., Chief Nursing Officer
Web address: www.mmcenters.com
**Control:** Hospital district or authority, Government, nonfederal **Service:** General Medical and Surgical

**Staffed Beds:** 90 **Admissions:** 4754 **Census:** 51 **Outpatient Visits:** 165270 **Births:** 296 **Total Expense ($000):** 40614 **Payroll Expense ($000):** 25369 **Personnel:** 368

## HALEYVILLE—Winston County

⊞ **LAKELAND COMMUNITY HOSPITAL (10125)**, Highway 195 East, Zip 35565–9536, Mailing Address: P.O. Box 780, Zip 35565–0780; tel. 205/486–5213, (Nonreporting) **A**1 9 10 20 **S** LifePoint Hospitals, Inc., Brentwood, TN
Primary Contact: James P. Jeansonne, Chief Executive Officer
CFO: Penny Westmoreland, Chief Financial Officer
Web address: www.lifepointhospitals.com
**Control:** Corporation, Investor–owned, for–profit **Service:** General Medical and Surgical

**Staffed Beds:** 42

## HAMILTON—Marion County

⊞ **NORTH MISSISSIPPI MEDICAL CENTER–HAMILTON (10044)**, 1256 Military Street South, Zip 35570–5001; tel. 205/921–6200, (Nonreporting) **A**1 9 10 **S** North Mississippi Health Services, Inc., Tupelo, MS
Primary Contact: Donald J. Jones, FACHE, Administrator
CMO: Jeff Hager, M.D., President Medical Staff
CHR: Anne Lawler, Director Human Resources
CNO: Tanya Brasher, Director of Nursing
Web address: www.nmhs.net
**Control:** Other not–for–profit (including NFP Corporation) **Service:** General Medical and Surgical

**Staffed Beds:** 36

## HUNTSVILLE—Madison County

⊞ **CRESTWOOD MEDICAL CENTER (10131)**, One Hospital Drive, Zip 35801–3403; tel. 256/429–4000 **A**1 9 10 **F**3 5 11 12 13 15 17 18 22 29 30 31 34 35 40 43 45 47 49 51 56 57 59 60 64 65 68 70 72 74 75 76 77 78 79 80 81 85 86 87 93 97 98 99 100 101 102 103 104 105 107 108 110 111 113 114 118 125 128 129 130 131 145 146 147 **S** Community Health Systems, Inc., Franklin, TN
Primary Contact: Pamela Hudson, M.D., Chief Executive Officer
COO: Bobby Ginn, Chief Operating Officer
CHR: Lynn Dingo, Director Human Resources
Web address: www.crestwoodmedcenter.com
**Control:** Corporation, Investor–owned, for–profit **Service:** General Medical and Surgical

**Staffed Beds:** 150 **Admissions:** 9101 **Census:** 98 **Outpatient Visits:** 112669 **Births:** 819 **Total Expense ($000):** 134558 **Payroll Expense ($000):** 46425 **Personnel:** 949

⊞ **HEALTHSOUTH REHABILITATION HOSPITAL OF NORTH ALABAMA (13029)**, 107 Governors Drive S.W., Zip 35801–4329; tel. 256/535–2300, (Nonreporting) **A**1 9 10 **S** HEALTHSOUTH Corporation, Birmingham, AL
Primary Contact: Douglas H. Beverly, Chief Executive Officer
Web address: www.healthsouthhuntsville.com
**Control:** Corporation, Investor–owned, for–profit **Service:** Rehabilitation

**Staffed Beds:** 70

---

**Hospital, Medicare Provider Number, Address, Telephone, Approval, Facility, and Physician Codes, Health Care System**

★ American Hospital Association (AHA) membership
☐ The Joint Commission accreditation
◇ DNV Healthcare Inc. accreditation

○ American Osteopathic Association (AOA) accreditation
△ Commission on Accreditation of Rehabilitation Facilities (CARF) accreditation

☐ **HUNTSVILLE HOSPITAL (10039)**, 101 Sivley Road, Zip 35801–4470;
tel. 256/265–1000, (Includes HUNTSVILLE HOSPITAL FOR WOMEN AND
CHILDREN, 911 Big Cove Road S.E., Zip 35801–3784; tel. 256/265–1000) **A**1 2
3 5 9 10 **F**5 7 8 12 13 14 15 17 18 19 20 21 22 23 24 25 26 28 29 30 31
35 37 38 39 40 41 43 48 49 50 51 53 54 56 57 59 60 64 68 70 71 72 73
74 76 78 79 80 81 82 88 89 93 96 98 99 100 101 102 103 104 105 107
108 109 110 111 113 114 115 116 117 118 125 128 129 130 141 143 144
145 146 147 **S** Huntsville Hospital Health System, Huntsville, AL
Primary Contact: David S. Spillers, Chief Executive Officer
COO: Jeff Samz, Chief Operating Officer
CFO: Lonnie D. Younger, Chief Financial Officer
CMO: Robert Chappell, M.D., Vice President and Chief Medical Officer
CIO: Rick Corn, Chief Information Officer
CHR: Andrea P. Rosler, Vice President Human Resources
Web address: www.huntsvillehospital.org
**Control:** Hospital district or authority, Government, nonfederal **Service:** General
Medical and Surgical

**Staffed Beds: 834 Admissions:** 43005 **Census:** 562 **Outpatient Visits:**
691267 **Births:** 5197 **Total Expense ($000):** 666468 **Payroll Expense
($000):** 259803 **Personnel:** 5690

**JACKSON—Clarke County**

**JACKSON MEDICAL CENTER (10128)**, 220 Hospital Drive, Zip 36545–2459,
Mailing Address: P.O. Box 428, Zip 36545–0428; tel. 251/246–9021,
(Nonreporting) **A**9 10 **S** Gilliard Health Services, Montgomery, AL
Primary Contact: Amy Gibson, Chief Executive Officer
COO: Jennifer M. Ryland, R.N., Chief Administrative Officer
CFO: Amy Gibson, Chief Executive Officer
CHR: Kathy Jones, Director Human Resources
Web address: www.jacksonmedicalcenter.org
**Control:** Corporation, Investor–owned, for–profit **Service:** General Medical and
Surgical

**Staffed Beds: 26**

**JACKSONVILLE—Calhoun County**

☐ **JACKSONVILLE MEDICAL CENTER (10146)**, 1701 Pelham Road South,
Zip 36265–3399, Mailing Address: P.O. Box 999, Zip 36265–0999;
tel. 256/435–4970 **A**1 9 10 **F**3 4 8 13 14 15 29 30 32 34 35 40 41 45 48 50
51 56 57 59 64 65 68 69 76 79 81 82 85 93 98 103 107 108 111 113 118
119 128 131 134 145 **P**6 **S** Capella Healthcare, Franklin, TN
Primary Contact: James H. Edmondson, Chief Executive Officer
COO: Jean Ann McMurray, R.N., Chief Nursing Officer
CFO: Tammy Cobb, Chief Financial Officer
CMO: James R. Yates, M.D., Chief of Staff
CIO: Richard Maust, Chief Information Officer
CHR: Doug Scott, Director Human Resources
Web address: www.jmchealth.com
**Control:** Corporation, Investor–owned, for–profit **Service:** General Medical and
Surgical

**Staffed Beds: 69 Admissions:** 2125 **Census:** 27 **Outpatient Visits:** 45919
**Births:** 354 **Total Expense ($000):** 28145 **Payroll Expense ($000):** 10242
**Personnel:** 202

**JASPER—Walker County**

☐ **WALKER BAPTIST MEDICAL CENTER (10089)**, 3400 Highway 78 East,
Zip 35501–8956, Mailing Address: P.O. Box 3547, Zip 35502–3547;
tel. 205/387–4000 **A**1 9 10 **F**3 8 11 13 15 18 20 22 26 29 30 31 34 35 40
41 43 45 47 49 50 56 57 59 64 67 68 70 76 77 78 79 81 85 87 93 94 96
97 98 100 103 104 107 108 110 111 113 114 116 118 125 129 131 145
146 147 **S** Baptist Health System, Birmingham, AL
Primary Contact: Robert Phillips, Administrator
CFO: John Langlois, Chief Financial Officer
CIO: Kenny Horton, Director Information Systems
CHR: Pat Morrow, Director Human Resources
CNO: Robbie Hindman, Vice President Patient Care Services and Chief Nursing
Officer
Web address: www.bhsala.com
**Control:** Church–operated, Nongovernment, not–for profit **Service:** General
Medical and Surgical

**Staffed Beds: 236 Admissions:** 7289 **Census:** 92 **Outpatient Visits:** 105831
**Births:** 753 **Total Expense ($000):** 82239 **Payroll Expense ($000):** 25873
**Personnel:** 546

**LUVERNE—Crenshaw County**

☐ **BEACON CHILDREN'S HOSPITAL (14015)**, 150 Hospital Drive,
Zip 36049–7350; tel. 334/335–5040, (Nonreporting) **A**1 9 10
Primary Contact: Carol Crowson, Administrator
Web address: www.beaconchildrenshospital.com
**Control:** Other not–for–profit (including NFP Corporation) **Service:** Psychiatric

**Staffed Beds: 24**

**CRENSHAW COMMUNITY HOSPITAL (10008)**, 101 Hospital Circle,
Zip 36049–7317; tel. 334/335–3374, (Nonreporting) **A**9 10
Primary Contact: Bradley Eisemann, Administrator
COO: Victoria Lawrenson, Chief Operating Officer
CMO: Charles Tompkins, M.D., Chief of Staff
CHR: Patricia Jarry, Manager Human Resources
**Control:** Corporation, Investor–owned, for–profit **Service:** General Medical and
Surgical

**Staffed Beds: 49**

**MADISON—Madison County**

**BRADFORD HEALTH SERVICES AT HUNTSVILLE**, 1600 Browns Ferry Road,
Zip 35758–9769, Mailing Address: P.O. Box 176, Zip 35758–0176;
tel. 256/461–7272, (Nonreporting) **S** Bradford Health Services, Birmingham, AL
Primary Contact: Bob Hinds, Executive Director
CFO: Bernard B. Stephens, Chief Financial Officer
CMO: Venkata S. Devabhaktuni, M.D., Medical Director
Web address: www.bradfordhealth.com
**Control:** Corporation, Investor–owned, for–profit **Service:** Alcoholism and other
chemical dependency

**Staffed Beds: 84**

**MADISON HOSPITAL**, 8375 Highway 72 West, Zip 35758–9573;
tel. 256/265–2012, (Nonreporting) **S** Huntsville Hospital Health System,
Huntsville, AL
Primary Contact: Mary Lynne Wright, R.N., President
Web address: www.madisonalhospital.org/
**Control:** Hospital district or authority, Government, nonfederal **Service:** General
Medical and Surgical

**Staffed Beds: 60**

**MOBILE—Mobile County**

**BAYPOINTE BEHAVIORAL HEALTH (14014)**, 5800 Southland Drive,
Zip 36693–3313; tel. 251/661–0153, (Nonreporting) **A**5 9 10
Primary Contact: Angela Ferrara, Administrator
Web address: www.altapointe.org/baypointe.asp
**Control:** Corporation, Investor–owned, for–profit **Service:** Psychiatric

**Staffed Beds: 60**

☐ **INFIRMARY LONG TERM ACUTE CARE HOSPITAL (12006)**, 5644 Girby
Road, Zip 36693–3320; tel. 251/660–5239, (Nonreporting) **A**1 9 10 **S** Infirmary
Health System, Mobile, AL
Primary Contact: Susanne Marmande, Administrator
Web address: www.theinfirmary.com/
**Control:** Other not–for–profit (including NFP Corporation) **Service:** Long–Term
Acute Care hospital

**Staffed Beds: 191**

☐ **INFIRMARY WEST (10152)**, 5600 Girby Road, Zip 36693–3398;
tel. 251/660–5120, (Nonreporting) **A**1 3 5 9 10 **S** Infirmary Health System,
Mobile, AL
Primary Contact: Alan R. Whaley, Administrator
COO: Joe Stough, Chief Operating Officer
CFO: Joe Denton, Chief Financial Officer
CMO: Kenneth Brewington, M.D., Vice President Administrator and Chief Marketing
Officer
CIO: Billy E. Stephens, Vice President Information Technology
CHR: Melissa Wheat, Manager Human Resources
Web address: www.southalabama.edu/usakph/index.html
**Control:** State–Government, nonfederal **Service:** General Medical and Surgical

**Staffed Beds: 63**

**INFIRMARY WEST AT KNOLLWOOD** See Infirmary West

☐ △ **MOBILE INFIRMARY MEDICAL CENTER (10113)**, 5 Mobile Infirmary Drive
North, Zip 36607–3513, Mailing Address: P.O. Box 2144, Zip 36652–2144;
tel. 251/435–2400, (Includes ROTARY REHABILITATION HOSPITAL, 5 Mobile
Infirmary Circle, Zip 36607, Mailing Address: P.O. Box 2144, Zip 36652;
tel. 334/431–3400), (Nonreporting) **A**1 2 3 5 7 9 10 **S** Infirmary Health System,
Mobile, AL
Primary Contact: Joe Strough, Administrator
CFO: Joe Denton, Executive Vice President and Chief Financial Officer
CIO: Eddy Stephens, Vice President Information Technology
CHR: Sheila C. Davidson, Vice President Human Resources
Web address: www.mobileinfirmary.org
**Control:** Other not–for–profit (including NFP Corporation) **Service:** General
Medical and Surgical

**Staffed Beds: 493**

★ **PROVIDENCE HOSPITAL (10090)**, 6801 Airport Boulevard, Zip 36608–3785, Mailing Address: P.O. Box 850429, Zip 36685–0429; tel. 251/633–1000 **A**2 3 5 9 10 **F**3 11 13 15 17 18 20 22 24 26 28 29 30 31 34 35 40 44 45 49 50 51 53 54 57 58 59 60 61 64 65 68 70 73 74 75 76 77 78 79 80 81 82 83 84 85 86 87 89 92 93 96 102 107 108 110 111 113 114 116 118 119 120 123 125 128 129 130 131 134 145 147 **P**6 **S** Ascension Health, Saint Louis, MO
Primary Contact: Clark P. Christianson, President and Chief Executive Officer
COO: Todd S. Kennedy, Executive Vice President and Chief Operating Officer
CFO: C. Susan Cornejo, Senior Vice President Finance and Chief Financial Officer
CMO: William M. Lightfoot, M.D., Vice President Medical Services
CHR: Kathy Ross, Chief Information Officer
CHR: H. Jaquita Tucker, Executive Director Human Resources
CNO: Susan E. Breslin, Vice President and Chief Nursing Officer
Web address: www.providencehospital.org
**Control:** Church–operated, Nongovernment, not–for profit **Service:** General Medical and Surgical

**Staffed Beds:** 349 **Admissions:** 14236 **Census:** 201 **Outpatient Visits:** 158868 **Births:** 1902 **Total Expense ($000):** 196914 **Payroll Expense ($000):** 68919 **Personnel:** 1392

**ROTARY REHABILITATION HOSPITAL** See Mobile Infirmary Medical Center

☐ **SPRINGHILL MEMORIAL HOSPITAL (10144)**, 3719 Dauphin Street, Zip 36608–1798, Mailing Address: P.O. Box 8246, Zip 36608–8246; tel. 251/344–9630 **A**1 3 5 9 10 **F**11 13 15 17 18 20 22 24 26 28 29 30 31 34 40 46 47 49 50 51 57 60 70 74 75 76 77 78 79 81 82 85 86 87 88 89 93 107 110 111 114 117 118 125 126 128 129 131 145 146 147
Primary Contact: Jeffery M. St. Clair, President and Chief Executive Officer
COO: Jeffery M. St Clair, President and Chief Executive Officer
CFO: Randy Sucher, Executive Vice President
CIO: Mark Kilborn, Director Information Systems
CHR: Daniela Batchelor, Director Human Resources
Web address: www.springhillmemorial.com
**Control:** Corporation, Investor–owned, for–profit **Service:** General Medical and Surgical

**Staffed Beds:** 203 **Admissions:** 7832 **Census:** 109 **Outpatient Visits:** 152612 **Births:** 671 **Total Expense ($000):** 128619 **Payroll Expense ($000):** 40043 **Personnel:** 1008

⊞ **UNIVERSITY OF SOUTH ALABAMA CHILDREN'S AND WOMEN'S HOSPITAL (13301)**, (Childrens and Womens), 1700 Center Street, Zip 36604–3301; tel. 251/415–1000 **A**1 3 5 9 10 **F**3 7 11 13 15 21 27 29 30 31 40 48 49 52 55 58 59 64 72 73 74 75 76 77 78 79 81 85 86 87 88 89 93 107 111 113 118 129 142 145 146 **S** University of South Alabama Hospitals, Mobile, AL
Primary Contact: Owen Bailey, Administrator
CFO: William B. Bush, CPA, Chief Financial Officer
CIO: David Blough, Chief Information Officer
CHR: Janice Rehm, Manager Human Resources
CNO: Carol Druckenmiller, R.N., Assistant Administrator and Chief Nursing Officer
Web address: www.usahealthsystem.com/usacwh
**Control:** State–Government, nonfederal **Service:** Other specialty

**Staffed Beds:** 198 **Admissions:** 8848 **Census:** 162 **Outpatient Visits:** 57551 **Births:** 2690 **Total Expense ($000):** 108604 **Payroll Expense ($000):** 46973 **Personnel:** 911

⊞ **UNIVERSITY OF SOUTH ALABAMA MEDICAL CENTER (10087)**, 2451 Fillingim Street, Zip 36617–2293; tel. 251/471–7000 **A**1 2 3 5 9 10 **F**3 11 16 17 18 20 22 24 26 29 31 34 40 43 46 49 57 58 59 60 61 64 70 74 78 79 81 85 87 107 108 111 113 114 118 129 145 147 **S** University of South Alabama Hospitals, Mobile, AL
Primary Contact: A. Elizabeth Anderson, Administrator
CFO: William B. Bush, CPA, Chief Financial Officer
CHR: Anita Shirah, Director Human Resources
Web address: www.usahospitals.org
**Control:** State–Government, nonfederal **Service:** General Medical and Surgical

**Staffed Beds:** 114 **Admissions:** 6345 **Census:** 111 **Outpatient Visits:** 42043 **Births:** 2 **Total Expense ($000):** 138364 **Payroll Expense ($000):** 68766 **Personnel:** 1369

**MONROEVILLE—Monroe County**

⊞ **MONROE COUNTY HOSPITAL (10120)**, 2016 South Alabama Avenue, Zip 36460, Mailing Address: P.O. Box 886, Zip 36461–0886; tel. 251/575–3111 **A**1 9 10 20 **F**3 11 13 15 29 30 31 34 35 40 45 57 59 62 64 70 75 76 81 93 107 109 111 118 128 131 147 **P**3
Primary Contact: Thomas J. Stone, FACHE, Chief Executive Officer
CFO: Michael Vaughn, Chief Financial Officer
CMO: Alexander Nettles, M.D., Chief of Staff
CIO: Lee Falkenberry, Director Information Systems
CHR: Tara Nowling, Director Human Resources
CNO: Barbara Harned, R.N., Chief Nursing Officer
Web address: www.mchcare.com
**Control:** Hospital district or authority, Government, nonfederal **Service:** General Medical and Surgical

**Staffed Beds:** 62 **Admissions:** 1658 **Census:** 13 **Outpatient Visits:** 28151 **Births:** 219

**MONTGOMERY—Montgomery County**

⊞ **BAPTIST MEDICAL CENTER EAST (10149)**, 400 Taylor Road, Zip 36117–3512, Mailing Address: P.O. Box 241267, Zip 36124–1267; tel. 334/277–8330 **A**1 9 10 **F**3 12 13 15 29 30 34 40 44 45 47 49 50 56 60 64 68 70 72 75 76 77 79 81 82 85 89 93 94 107 108 111 113 114 118 128 129 131 134 145 146 **S** Baptist Health, Montgomery, AL
Primary Contact: J. Peter Selman, Administrator and Chief Executive Officer
COO: Robin Barca, Chief Operating Officer
CFO: Katrina Belt, Chief Financial Officer
CIO: Wanda Sims, Chief Information Officer
CHR: Kay Bennett, Vice President Human Resources
Web address: www.baptistfirst.org
**Control:** Hospital district or authority, Government, nonfederal **Service:** General Medical and Surgical

**Staffed Beds:** 182 **Admissions:** 10672 **Census:** 118 **Outpatient Visits:** 83826 **Births:** 3387 **Total Expense ($000):** 93126 **Payroll Expense ($000):** 35119 **Personnel:** 804

⊞ **BAPTIST MEDICAL CENTER SOUTH (10023)**, 2105 East South Boulevard, Zip 36116–2498, Mailing Address: Box 11010, Zip 36111–0010; tel. 334/288–2100 **A**1 3 5 9 10 **F**3 5 11 12 13 15 17 18 19 20 22 24 26 28 29 30 31 35 40 44 45 49 50 56 61 63 64 68 70 72 74 75 76 78 79 81 82 84 85 87 89 93 98 100 101 102 103 104 105 107 108 110 111 113 114 117 118 128 129 130 131 145 147 **S** Baptist Health, Montgomery, AL
Primary Contact: Robin Barca, Chief Executive Officer
COO: Robin Barca, Chief Executive Officer
CFO: Lisa Goodlett, Chief Financial Officer
CMO: Donovan Kendrick, M.D., Chief of Staff
CIO: Wanda Sims, Chief Information Officer
CHR: Kay Bennett, System Director Human Resources
CNO: Teresa Parker, Vice President and Chief Nursing Officer
Web address: www.baptistfirst.org
**Control:** Hospital district or authority, Government, nonfederal **Service:** General Medical and Surgical

**Staffed Beds:** 386 **Admissions:** 17876 **Census:** 241 **Outpatient Visits:** 146357 **Births:** 832 **Total Expense ($000):** 248297 **Payroll Expense ($000):** 76905 **Personnel:** 1792

⊞ **CENTRAL ALABAMA VETERANS HEALTH CARE SYSTEM**, 215 Perry Hill Road, Zip 36109–3798; tel. 334/272–4670, (Includes MONTGOMERY DIVISION, 215 Perry Hill Road, tel. 334/272–4670; TUSKEGEE DIVISION, 2400 Hospital Road, Tuskegee, Zip 36083–5001; tel. 334/727–0550), (Nonreporting) **A**1 5 **S** Department of Veterans Affairs, Washington, DC
Primary Contact: Glen E. Struchtemeyer, Director
CFO: Brenda Schmitz, Manager Finance
CMO: N. Rao Chava, M.D., Director
CHR: Linda King, Chief Human Resources Management Service
Web address: www.centralalabama.va.gov/
**Control:** Veterans Affairs, Government, federal **Service:** General Medical and Surgical

**Staffed Beds:** 321

☐ **GREIL MEMORIAL PSYCHIATRIC HOSPITAL (14005)**, 2140 Upper Wetumpka Road, Zip 36107; tel. 334/262–0363, (Nonreporting) **A**1 10
Primary Contact: Susan Chambers, M.D., Administrator
**Control:** Corporation, Investor–owned, for–profit **Service:** Psychiatric

**Staffed Beds:** 25

**Hospital, Medicare Provider Number, Address, Telephone, Approval, Facility, and Physician Codes, Health Care System**

★ American Hospital Association (AHA) membership
☐ The Joint Commission accreditation
◇ DNV Healthcare Inc. accreditation
○ American Osteopathic Association (AOA) accreditation
△ Commission on Accreditation of Rehabilitation Facilities (CARF) accreditation

⊠ **HEALTHSOUTH REHABILITATION HOSPITAL OF MONTGOMERY (13028)**, 4465 Narrow Lane Road, Zip 36116–2900; tel. 334/284–7700 **A**1 9 10 **F**3 9 28 29 34 35 54 56 57 59 64 74 75 77 86 90 93 95 129 130 131 142 145 147 **P**5 **S** HEALTHSOUTH Corporation, Birmingham, AL
Primary Contact: Linda Wade, Chief Executive Officer
CFO: Heath Watson, Controller
CMO: Jeffrey Eng, M.D., Medical Director
CIO: Diane Davis, Manager Business Office
CHR: Kim McDaniel, Director Human Resources
Web address: www.healthsouthmontgomery.com
**Control:** Corporation, Investor–owned, for–profit **Service:** Rehabilitation

| | |
|---|---|
| **Staffed Beds:** 70 **Admissions:** 1438 **Census:** 53 **Outpatient Visits:** 5033 **Births:** 0 **Total Expense ($000):** 14914 **Payroll Expense ($000):** 8868 **Personnel:** 202 | |

⊠ **JACKSON HOSPITAL AND CLINIC (10024)**, 1725 Pine Street, Zip 36106–1117; tel. 334/293–8000 **A**1 9 10 **F**13 15 17 18 20 22 24 26 29 30 31 34 40 45 46 49 57 59 64 68 70 74 76 77 78 79 81 82 84 85 86 87 89 93 107 108 111 113 115 116 117 118 125 129 130 134 145 146 **P**6
Primary Contact: Joe B. Riley, President and Chief Executive Officer
CIO: Richard E. Caldwell, Vice President Support Services
Web address: www.jackson.org
**Control:** Other not–for–profit (including NFP Corporation) **Service:** General Medical and Surgical

| | |
|---|---|
| **Staffed Beds:** 251 **Admissions:** 13485 **Census:** 174 **Outpatient Visits:** 53245 **Births:** 1384 **Total Expense ($000):** 148285 **Payroll Expense ($000):** 58892 **Personnel:** 1322 | |

**LONG TERM CARE HOSPITAL** See Noland Hospital Montgomery

**MONTGOMERY DIVISION** See Central Alabama Veterans Health Care System

☐ **NOLAND HOSPITAL MONTGOMERY (12007)**, 1725 Pine Street, 5 North, Zip 36106–1109; tel. 334/240–0532, (Nonreporting) **A**1 9 10 **S** Noland Health Services, Inc., Birmingham, AL
Primary Contact: John Heffner, Interim Administrator
Web address: www.nolandhealth.com
**Control:** Other not–for–profit (including NFP Corporation) **Service:** Long–Term Acute Care hospital

| | |
|---|---|
| **Staffed Beds:** 36 | |

**MOULTON—Lawrence County**

**LAWRENCE MEDICAL CENTER (10059)**, 202 Hospital Street, Zip 35650, Mailing Address: P.O. Box 39, Zip 35650–0039; tel. 256/974–2200 **A**9 10 **F**3 15 28 29 30 34 35 40 45 46 47 50 54 56 57 59 62 64 65 66 68 70 75 81 85 86 87 93 97 107 108 111 113 117 118 126 129 131 134 145 146
Primary Contact: Cary J. Payne, Interim Chief Executive Officer
CFO: Jim Crawford, Chief Financial Officer
CIO: Jeremy Duncan, Director Information Systems
CHR: Diane K. Secor, Director Human Resources
Web address: www.attentushealthcare.com/lawrencemedicalcenter.htm
**Control:** County–Government, nonfederal **Service:** General Medical and Surgical

| | |
|---|---|
| **Staffed Beds:** 53 **Admissions:** 1387 **Census:** 19 **Outpatient Visits:** 35644 **Births:** 0 **Total Expense ($000):** 14670 **Payroll Expense ($000):** 8009 **Personnel:** 200 | |

**MOUNT VERNON—Mobile County**

☐ **SEARCY HOSPITAL (14008)**, 725 East Coy Smith Highway, Zip 36560–1090, Mailing Address: P.O. Box 1090, Zip 36560–1090; tel. 251/829–9411, (Nonreporting) **A**1 10
Primary Contact: Beatrice J. McLean, Director
CIO: Bobby McCarley, Director Information Management
**Control:** State–Government, nonfederal **Service:** Children's hospital psychiatric

| | |
|---|---|
| **Staffed Beds:** 467 | |

**MUSCLE SHOALS—Colbert County**

☐ **SHOALS HOSPITAL (10157)**, 201 Avalon Avenue, Zip 35661–2805, Mailing Address: P.O. Box 3359, Zip 35662–3359; tel. 256/386–1600, (Nonreporting) **A**1 9 10 **S** RegionalCare Hospital Partners, Brentwood, TN
Primary Contact: Ross Berry, Chief Executive Officer
Web address: www.chgroup.org
**Control:** Corporation, Investor–owned, for–profit **Service:** General Medical and Surgical

| | |
|---|---|
| **Staffed Beds:** 131 | |

**NORTHPORT—Tuscaloosa County**

☐ **NORTHPORT MEDICAL CENTER (10145)**, 2700 Hospital Drive, Zip 35476; tel. 205/333–4500 **A**1 9 10 **F**3 11 13 15 28 29 30 34 35 40 42 45 46 57 58 59 61 64 68 70 72 74 75 76 79 81 82 86 87 90 93 96 98 100 101 102 103 104 107 108 110 111 113 118 123 128 129 130 131 134 145 146 147 **P**7 8 **S** DCH Health System, Tuscaloosa, AL
Primary Contact: Luke Standeffer, Administrator
CFO: Jon Kramer, Controller and Assistant Administrator
CMO: David Rice, M.D., Vice President Medical Affairs
CIO: Kim Ligon, Director Information Services
CHR: Beth Francis, Vice President Human Resources
Web address: www.dchsystem.com
**Control:** Hospital district or authority, Government, nonfederal **Service:** General Medical and Surgical

| | |
|---|---|
| **Staffed Beds:** 196 **Admissions:** 8721 **Census:** 132 **Outpatient Visits:** 107937 **Births:** 1536 **Total Expense ($000):** 55132 **Payroll Expense ($000):** 40110 **Personnel:** 747 | |

**ONEONTA—Blount County**

⊠ **ST. VINCENT'S BLOUNT (10050)**, 150 Gilbreath, Zip 35121–2534, Mailing Address: P.O. Box 1000, Zip 35121–1000; tel. 205/274–3000 **A**1 9 10 **F**3 11 15 18 29 30 35 36 37 40 42 43 45 57 59 64 65 70 75 77 79 81 82 85 93 97 107 108 110 118 134 **P**7 8 **S** Ascension Health, Saint Louis, MO
Primary Contact: Kidada Hawkins, Interim President and Chief Operating Officer
COO: Kidada Hawkins, VP/COO Rural Hospital Operations
CFO: David Cauble, Chief Financial Officer
CMO: David R. Wilson, M.D., Chief of Staff
CIO: Timothy Stettheimer, Regional Chief Information Officer
CHR: Carol Maietta, Vice President and Talent Resource Officer Human Resources and Learning
CNO: Paula McCullough, VP Patient Care Services
Web address: www.stvhs.com
**Control:** Other not–for–profit (including NFP Corporation) **Service:** General Medical and Surgical

| | |
|---|---|
| **Staffed Beds:** 40 **Admissions:** 1367 **Census:** 14 **Outpatient Visits:** 37417 **Births:** 0 **Total Expense ($000):** 17716 **Payroll Expense ($000):** 6569 **Personnel:** 142 | |

**OPELIKA—Lee County**

⊠ **EAST ALABAMA MEDICAL CENTER (10029)**, 2000 Pepperell Parkway, Zip 36802–3201; tel. 334/749–3411, (Total facility includes 113 beds in nursing home–type unit) **A**1 2 9 10 19 **F**3 7 10 11 13 15 17 18 20 22 24 26 28 29 30 31 32 34 40 43 45 50 51 53 54 56 57 58 59 60 61 64 68 70 74 75 76 77 78 79 81 82 84 85 86 89 93 98 99 100 102 103 104 107 108 110 111 113 114 116 117 118 119 120 122 124 125 127 128 129 130 131 134 145 147 **P**6
Primary Contact: Terry W. Andrus, President
COO: Laura D. Grill, R.N., Executive Vice President and Administrator
CFO: Sam Price, Executive Vice President Finance/Chief Financial Officer
CMO: Michael Lisenby, M.D., Vice President and Chief Medical Officer
CIO: Tommy Chittom, Vice President Information Services
CHR: Susan Johnston, Director Human Resources
Web address: www.eamc.org
**Control:** Hospital district or authority, Government, nonfederal **Service:** General Medical and Surgical

| | |
|---|---|
| **Staffed Beds:** 377 **Admissions:** 14835 **Census:** 275 **Outpatient Visits:** 117475 **Births:** 1648 **Total Expense ($000):** 229364 **Payroll Expense ($000):** 87683 **Personnel:** 2382 | |

**OPP—Covington County**

★ **MIZELL MEMORIAL HOSPITAL (10007)**, 702 Main Street, Zip 36467–1626, Mailing Address: P.O. Box 1010, Zip 36467–1010; tel. 334/493–3541, (Nonreporting) **A**9 10
Primary Contact: Jana Wyatt, Chief Executive Officer
CFO: Amy Bess, Chief Financial Officer
CMO: Wheeler Gunnels, M.D., Medical Director
CIO: Elizabeth Cook, Chief Information Officer
CHR: Dianne Morrison, Director Human Resources
Web address: www.mizellmh.com
**Control:** Other not–for–profit (including NFP Corporation) **Service:** General Medical and Surgical

| | |
|---|---|
| **Staffed Beds:** 58 | |

**OZARK—Dale County**

**DALE MEDICAL CENTER (10021)**, 126 Hospital Avenue, Zip 36360–2080; tel. 334/774–2601, (Nonreporting) **A**9 10
Primary Contact: Vernon Johnson, Administrator
CFO: Brad Hull, Chief Financial Officer
CMO: Steve Brandt, M.D., Chief of Staff
CHR: Sheila Dunn, Assistant Administrator Human Resources
Web address: www.dalemedical.org
**Control:** County–Government, nonfederal **Service:** General Medical and Surgical

| | |
|---|---|
| **Staffed Beds:** 75 | |

*Many Facility Codes have changed. Please refer to the AHA Guide Code Chart.* © 2012 AHA Guide

**PELL CITY—St. Clair County**

★ **ST. VINCENT'S ST. CLAIR (10130)**, 2805 Doctor John Haynes Drive, Zip 35125–1499; tel. 205/338–3301 **A**9 10 **F**3 11 15 29 30 34 35 40 42 43 50 57 59 64 66 68 70 74 75 77 78 79 81 86 87 93 107 111 118 129 132 134 142 145 147 **P**7 8 **S** Ascension Health, Saint Louis, MO
Primary Contact: Kidada Hawkins, Interim President and Chief Operating Officer
COO: Kidada Hawkins, Vice President and Chief Operating Officer
CFO: Imelda Roberson, Director Finance
CMO: William McClanahan, M.D., Chief of Staff
CIO: Susan Evans, Director Health Information Services
CHR: Tamara Barr, Human Resources Generalist
Web address: www.stvhs.com
**Control:** Other not–for–profit (including NFP Corporation) **Service:** General Medical and Surgical

**Staffed Beds:** 36 **Admissions:** 1505 **Census:** 16 **Outpatient Visits:** 43495 **Births:** 0 **Total Expense ($000):** 19224 **Payroll Expense ($000):** 8105 **Personnel:** 168

**PHENIX CITY—Russell County**

**JACK HUGHSTON MEMORIAL HOSPITAL (10168)**, 4401 Riverchase Drive, Zip 36867; tel. 334/732–3000 **A**9 10 **F**3 40 45 70 79 81 107 113 114 118
Primary Contact: Mark A. Baker, Chief Executive Officer
COO: Divya Matai, Chief Operating Officer and Chief Financial Officer
CFO: Divya Matai, Chief Operating Officer and Chief Financial Officer
CMO: Lamar Carden, M.D., Chief Medical Officer
CHR: Lana Thomas–Folds, System Director Human Resources
Web address: www.jackhughstonmemorialhospital.com
**Control:** Corporation, Investor–owned, for–profit **Service:** General Medical and Surgical

**Staffed Beds:** 28 **Admissions:** 2403 **Census:** 23 **Outpatient Visits:** 20070 **Births:** 0 **Total Expense ($000):** 31732 **Payroll Expense ($000):** 11798 **Personnel:** 265

⊞ **REGIONAL REHABILITATION HOSPITAL (13033)**, 3715 Highway 280/431 North, Zip 36867; tel. 334/732–2200 **A**1 9 10 **F**3 29 30 90 93 95 131 **S** HEALTHSOUTH Corporation, Birmingham, AL
Primary Contact: Jill Jordan, Chief Executive Officer
CFO: Bobby Edmondson, Controller
CIO: Jacki Cuevas, Director Health Information Services
CHR: Cindy Glynn, Director Human Resources
CNO: Brandy Cook, Chief Nursing Officer
Web address: www.regionalrehabhospital.com
**Control:** Partnership, Investor–owned, for–profit **Service:** Rehabilitation

**Staffed Beds:** 48 **Admissions:** 1033 **Census:** 39 **Outpatient Visits:** 3854 **Births:** 0 **Total Expense ($000):** 12061 **Payroll Expense ($000):** 6515 **Personnel:** 137

**PRATTVILLE—Autauga County**

⊞ **PRATTVILLE BAPTIST HOSPITAL (10108)**, 124 South Memorial Drive, Zip 36067–3619, Mailing Address: P.O. Box 681630, Zip 36067–1638; tel. 334/365–0651 **A**1 9 10 **F**3 11 12 15 29 30 34 35 40 44 45 50 56 57 59 64 68 70 81 82 84 85 86 87 107 111 113 128 131 145 **S** Baptist Health, Montgomery, AL
Primary Contact: Ginger Henry, Chief Executive Officer
CFO: LaDonna McDaniel, Financial Manager
CIO: B. Blaine Brown, Vice President and General Counsel
CHR: Renee Drayton, Chief Human Resources
Web address: www.baptistfirst.org
**Control:** Hospital district or authority, Government, nonfederal **Service:** General Medical and Surgical

**Staffed Beds:** 56 **Admissions:** 2112 **Census:** 20 **Outpatient Visits:** 56807 **Births:** 0 **Total Expense ($000):** 28000 **Payroll Expense ($000):** 8955 **Personnel:** 175

**RED BAY—Franklin County**

**RED BAY HOSPITAL (11302)**, 211 Hospital Road, Zip 35582–0490, Mailing Address: P.O. Box 490, Zip 35582–0490; tel. 256/356–9532 **A**9 10 18 **F**15 29 30 34 39 40 50 53 56 57 59 64 65 75 81 86 93 107 111 118 127 129 132 134 143
Primary Contact: Glen M. Jones, Administrator
CFO: Samuel A. Strickland, Chief Financial Officer
CHR: Pam Bryant, Director Human Resources
Web address: www.redbayhospital.com
**Control:** Hospital district or authority, Government, nonfederal **Service:** General Medical and Surgical

**Staffed Beds:** 25 **Admissions:** 427 **Census:** 10 **Outpatient Visits:** 14168 **Total Expense ($000):** 7306 **Payroll Expense ($000):** 3535 **Personnel:** 81

**RUSSELLVILLE—Franklin County**

⊞ **RUSSELLVILLE HOSPITAL (10158)**, 15155 Highway 43, Zip 35653–1975, Mailing Address: P.O. Box 1089, Zip 35653–1089; tel. 256/332–1611, (Nonreporting) **A**1 9 10 **S** LifePoint Hospitals, Inc., Brentwood, TN
Primary Contact: Christine R. Stewart, FACHE, Chief Executive Officer
CFO: Penny Westmoreland, Chief Financial Officer
CHR: Stephen Proctor, Director of Human Resources/Risk
CNO: Belinda Johnson, R.N., Chief Nursing Officer/Chief Clinical Officer
Web address: www.russellvillehospital.com
**Control:** Corporation, Investor–owned, for–profit **Service:** General Medical and Surgical

**Staffed Beds:** 92

**SCOTTSBORO—Jackson County**

☐ **HIGHLANDS MEDICAL CENTER (10061)**, 380 Woods Cove Road, Zip 35768–2428, Mailing Address: P.O. Box 1050, Zip 35768–1050; tel. 256/259–4444, (Nonreporting) **A**1 9 10 20
Primary Contact: Kim Bryant, Chief Executive Officer
CFO: Dan Newell, Chief Financial Officer
CIO: Doug Newby, Chief Information Officer
CHR: Susanna S. Sivley, Chief Personnel Officer
Web address: www.highlandsmedcenter.com
**Control:** County–Government, nonfederal **Service:** General Medical and Surgical

**Staffed Beds:** 92

**SELMA—Dallas County**

⊞ **VAUGHAN REGIONAL MEDICAL CENTER (10118)**, 1015 Medical Center Parkway, Zip 36701–6352; tel. 334/418–4100 **A**1 3 5 9 10 20 **F**8 11 13 15 17 20 29 30 34 40 45 51 53 60 70 74 79 81 89 93 107 108 110 111 113 114 117 118 119 126 128 129 130 145 146 **S** LifePoint Hospitals, Inc., Brentwood, TN
Primary Contact: David R. Sirk, Chief Executive Officer
COO: Debbie Pace, Chief Operating Officer
CFO: Randy Rogers, Chief Financial Officer
CMO: Mark LeQuire, M.D., Chief of Staff
CHR: Dionne Williams, Director Human Resources
CNO: Verno Davidson, R.N., Chief Nursing Officer
Web address: www.vaughanregional.com
**Control:** Corporation, Investor–owned, for–profit **Service:** General Medical and Surgical

**Staffed Beds:** 149 **Admissions:** 7428 **Census:** 69 **Outpatient Visits:** 72010 **Births:** 692 **Total Expense ($000):** 64326 **Payroll Expense ($000):** 23755 **Personnel:** 469

**SHEFFIELD—Colbert County**

⊞ **HELEN KELLER HOSPITAL (10019)**, 1300 South Montgomery Avenue, Zip 35660–6334, Mailing Address: P.O. Box 610, Zip 35660–0610; tel. 256/386–4196 **A**1 9 10 **F**13 15 18 20 28 29 30 31 32 34 35 36 40 47 49 53 59 60 64 65 74 75 76 77 78 79 81 82 83 84 85 86 87 89 93 107 108 110 111 113 114 118 125 129 130 143 145 147
Primary Contact: Doug Arnold, President and Chief Executive Officer
COO: Steve Ezzell, Chief Information Officer
CFO: Morris S. Strickland, Chief Financial Officer
CHR: Pam Bryant, Director Human Resources
Web address: www.helenkeller.com
**Control:** Hospital district or authority, Government, nonfederal **Service:** General Medical and Surgical

**Staffed Beds:** 159 **Admissions:** 6620 **Census:** 70 **Outpatient Visits:** 96894 **Births:** 790 **Total Expense ($000):** 68102 **Payroll Expense ($000):** 27281 **Personnel:** 708

**SYLACAUGA—Talladega County**

☐ **COOSA VALLEY MEDICAL CENTER (10164)**, 315 West Hickory Street, Zip 35150–2996; tel. 256/401–4000, (Nonreporting) **A**1 9 10
Primary Contact: Glenn C. Sisk, President
CFO: Janice Brown, Chief Financial Officer
CIO: Sandra Murchison, Director Medical Records
CHR: Christy Knowles, Chief Human Resources Officer
Web address: www.cvhealth.net
**Control:** Other not–for–profit (including NFP Corporation) **Service:** General Medical and Surgical

**Staffed Beds:** 101

---

**Hospital, Medicare Provider Number, Address, Telephone, Approval, Facility, and Physician Codes, Health Care System**

★ American Hospital Association (AHA) membership
☐ The Joint Commission accreditation
◇ DNV Healthcare Inc. accreditation
○ American Osteopathic Association (AOA) accreditation
△ Commission on Accreditation of Rehabilitation Facilities (CARF) accreditation

### TALLADEGA—Talladega County

☐ **CITIZENS BAPTIST MEDICAL CENTER (10101)**, 604 Stone Avenue, Zip 35160–2217, Mailing Address: P.O. Box 978, Zip 35160–0978; tel. 256/362–8111 **A**1 9 10 19 **F**3 11 13 15 29 30 34 35 40 50 53 57 59 60 62 64 67 70 74 75 76 79 81 82 86 93 98 107 108 110 111 112 117 118 128 130 131 134 145 **S** Baptist Health System, Birmingham, AL
Primary Contact: Joel Taylor, Administrator
CFO: John Langlois, Vice President Finance
CHR: Sandra Willis, Manager Human Resources
Web address: www.bhsala.com
**Control:** Church–operated, Nongovernment, not–for profit **Service:** General Medical and Surgical

**Staffed Beds:** 116 **Admissions:** 3027 **Census:** 32 **Outpatient Visits:** 63797 **Births:** 306 **Total Expense ($000):** 32267 **Payroll Expense ($000):** 13999 **Personnel:** 306

### TALLASSEE—Elmore County

★ **COMMUNITY HOSPITAL (10034)**, 805 Friendship Road, Zip 36078–1234; tel. 334/283–6541, (Nonreporting) **A**9 10
Primary Contact: Jennie R. Rhinehart, Administrator and Chief Executive Officer
Web address: www.chal.org
**Control:** Other not–for–profit (including NFP Corporation) **Service:** General Medical and Surgical

**Staffed Beds:** 69

### TROY—Pike County

☐ **TROY REGIONAL MEDICAL CENTER (10126)**, 1330 Highway 231 South, Zip 36081–1224; tel. 334/670–5000, (Nonreporting) **A**1 9 10 **S** Gilliard Health Services, Montgomery, AL
Primary Contact: Teresa G. Grimes, Chief Executive Officer
CFO: Janet Smith, Chief Financial Officer
CIO: Brian Blackmon, Director Information Systems
CHR: Lori Austin, Director Human Resources
Web address: www.troymedicalcenter.com
**Control:** Corporation, Investor–owned, for–profit **Service:** General Medical and Surgical

**Staffed Beds:** 78

### TUSCALOOSA—Tuscaloosa County

☐ **BRYCE HOSPITAL (14007)**, 200 University Boulevard, Zip 35401–1294; tel. 205/759–0799, (Nonreporting) **A**1 10
Primary Contact: Roxanna Bender, Interim Administrator
CFO: Wendell Summerville, Chief Financial Officer
CMO: Cynthia Moore Sledge, M.D., Medical Director
CIO: Ronene Howell, Director Health Information Management
CHR: Jim Elliott, Director Human Resources
**Control:** State–Government, nonfederal **Service:** Psychiatric

**Staffed Beds:** 820

☐ **DCH REGIONAL MEDICAL CENTER (10092)**, 809 University Boulevard East, Zip 35401–9961; tel. 205/759–7111 **A**1 2 3 5 9 10 **F**3 11 12 13 15 17 18 20 22 24 26 29 30 31 35 38 40 43 45 48 49 50 51 57 59 60 61 62 64 66 68 70 72 74 75 76 77 78 79 81 82 86 87 88 89 94 107 108 110 111 113 114 115 116 117 118 120 125 128 129 131 145 146 147 **P**8 **S** DCH Health System, Tuscaloosa, AL
Primary Contact: William H. Cassels, Administrator
CFO: John W. Winfrey, Vice President Finance and Chief Financial Officer
CMO: Kenneth Aldridge, M.D., Vice President Medical Affairs
CIO: Kim Ligon, Director Information Services
CHR: Beth Francis, Vice President Human Resources
Web address: www.dchsystem.com
**Control:** Hospital district or authority, Government, nonfederal **Service:** General Medical and Surgical

**Staffed Beds:** 405 **Admissions:** 24099 **Census:** 320 **Outpatient Visits:** 352892 **Births:** 1657 **Total Expense ($000):** 276817 **Payroll Expense ($000):** 147230 **Personnel:** 2946

☐ **MARY S HARPER GERIATRIC PSYCHIATRY CENTER (14012)**, 200 University Boulevard, Zip 35401; tel. 205/759–0900, (Nonreporting) **A**1 10
Primary Contact: Beverly White, MS, Facility Director
CFO: Sarah Mitchell, Director Finance
CMO: Robin Barton Lariscy, M.D., Medical Director
CIO: Sarah Mitchell, Director Finance
CHR: Jim Elliott, Director Human Resources
Web address: www.mh.alabama.gov
**Control:** Corporation, Investor–owned, for–profit **Service:** Other specialty

**Staffed Beds:** 96

☐ **NOLAND HOSPITAL TUSCALOOSA (12012)**, 809 University Boulevard E, 4th Floor, Zip 35401; tel. 205/759–7241, (Nonreporting) **A**1 9 10 **S** Noland Health Services, Inc., Birmingham, AL
Primary Contact: Dale Jones, Administrator
Web address: www.nolandhealth.com
**Control:** Other not–for–profit (including NFP Corporation) **Service:** Long–Term Acute Care hospital

**Staffed Beds:** 27

☐ **TAYLOR HARDIN SECURE MEDICAL FACILITY (14011)**, 1301 Jack Warner Parkway, Zip 35404; tel. 205/556–7060, (Nonreporting) **A**1 3 5 10
Primary Contact: Shelia Taylor, Director
Web address: www.mh.alabama.gov/
**Control:** Corporation, Investor–owned, for–profit **Service:** Psychiatric

**Staffed Beds:** 114

⊠ △ **VETERANS AFFAIRS MEDICAL CENTER**, 3701 Loop Road, Zip 35404–5015; tel. 205/554–2000, (Nonreporting) **A**1 7 **S** Department of Veterans Affairs, Washington, DC
Primary Contact: Alan J. Tyler, MS, FACHE, Director
COO: Gary D. Trende, FACHE, Associate Director
CFO: Angelia Stevenson, Manager Finance
CMO: Mark Nissenbaum, M.D., Chief of Staff
CIO: Vicki Smallwood, Chief Information Officer
CHR: Janice Hardy, Chief Human Resources Management
Web address: www.tuscaloosa.va.gov
**Control:** Veterans Affairs, Government, federal **Service:** Psychiatric

**Staffed Beds:** 381

### TUSKEGEE—Macon County

**TUSKEGEE DIVISION** See Central Alabama Veterans Health Care System, Montgomery

### UNION SPRINGS—Bullock County

**BULLOCK COUNTY HOSPITAL (10110)**, 102 West Conecuh Avenue, Zip 36089–1303; tel. 334/738–2140, (Nonreporting) **A**9 10 20
Primary Contact: Jacques Jarry, Administrator
COO: Victoria Lawrenson, Chief Operating Officer
CFO: Allen J. Gamble, Comptroller
CMO: Maria Bernardo, M.D., Chief of Staff
CIO: Tony Lang, Chief Information Officer
**Control:** Corporation, Investor–owned, for–profit **Service:** General Medical and Surgical

**Staffed Beds:** 41

### VALLEY—Chambers County

☐ **LANIER HEALTH SERVICES (10025)**, 4800 48th Street, Zip 36854–3666; tel. 334/756–9180, (Total facility includes 103 beds in nursing home–type unit) **A**1 9 10 19 **F**3 11 13 15 18 20 22 28 29 30 34 40 41 43 45 46 47 48 49 57 59 62 64 68 70 74 76 77 78 79 81 85 86 87 89 93 100 102 107 108 110 111 117 118 123 127 128 129 131 132 134 145 146
Primary Contact: Doug Dewberry, Chief Executive Officer and Administrator
CFO: Tommy Lane, Chief Financial Officer
CMO: Krishna K. Reddy, M.D., President Medical Staff
CIO: Kurt Leroy, Manager Information Management
CHR: Clara Pitts, Director Human Resources
Web address: www.lanierhospital.com
**Control:** Other not–for–profit (including NFP Corporation) **Service:** General Medical and Surgical

**Staffed Beds:** 175 **Admissions:** 3070 **Census:** 136 **Outpatient Visits:** 50403 **Births:** 335 **Total Expense ($000):** 40640 **Payroll Expense ($000):** 17868 **Personnel:** 547

### WARRIOR—Jefferson County

**BRADFORD HEALTH SERVICES AT WARRIOR LODGE**, 1189 Allbritt Road, Zip 35180, Mailing Address: P.O. Box 129, Zip 35180–0129; tel. 205/647–1945, (Nonreporting) **S** Bradford Health Services, Birmingham, AL
Primary Contact: Roy M. Ramsey, Executive Director
Web address: www.bradfordhealth.com
**Control:** Corporation, Investor–owned, for–profit **Service:** Alcoholism and other chemical dependency

**Staffed Beds:** 100

### WEDOWEE—Randolph County

**WEDOWEE HOSPITAL (10032)**, 209 North Main Street, Zip 36278–5138, Mailing Address: P.O. Box 307, Zip 36278–0307; tel. 256/357–2111, (Nonreporting) **A**9 10
Primary Contact: Richard Daniel, Administrator
Web address: www.wedoweehospital.org/
**Control:** County–Government, nonfederal **Service:** General Medical and Surgical

**Staffed Beds:** 28

*Many Facility Codes have changed. Please refer to the AHA Guide Code Chart.* © 2012 AHA Guide

**WETUMPKA—Elmore County**

**ELMORE COMMUNITY HOSPITAL (10097)**, 500 Hospital Drive,
Zip 36092–1625, Mailing Address: P.O. Box 130, Zip 36092–0130;
tel. 334/567–4311, (Nonreporting) **A**9 10
Primary Contact: Gordon Faulk, Administrator
CFO: Mike Bruce, Chief Financial Officer
CHR: Cindy Futral, Director Human Resources
**Control:** Partnership, Investor–owned, for–profit **Service:** General Medical and
Surgical

| **Staffed Beds:** 49 |
| --- |

**WINFIELD—Marion County**

✖ **NORTHWEST MEDICAL CENTER (10086)**, 1530 U.S. Highway 43,
Zip 35594–5056; tel. 205/487–7000 **A**1 5 9 10 **F**3 8 15 28 29 34 35 40 45
53 57 59 62 64 68 70 75 77 79 81 86 87 90 93 97 98 103 107 108 110
111 113 115 116 117 118 123 128 130 132 146 147 **P**6 **S** LifePoint
Hospitals, Inc., Brentwood, TN
Primary Contact: Chuck Spann, Chief Executive Officer
CFO: James Gory, Chief Financial Officer
CMO: Gary Fowler, M.D., Chief of Staff Family Practice
CHR: Kelly Hagy, Director Human Resources and Professional Affairs
Web address: www.northwestmedcenter.com
**Control:** Corporation, Investor–owned, for–profit **Service:** General Medical and
Surgical

| **Staffed Beds:** 76 **Admissions:** 2375 **Census:** 31 **Outpatient Visits:** 43454 **Births:** 0 **Total Expense ($000):** 24640 **Payroll Expense ($000):** 9621 **Personnel:** 286 |
| --- |

**YORK—Sumter County**

**HILL HOSPITAL OF SUMTER COUNTY (10138)**, 751 Derby Drive, Zip 36925;
tel. 205/392–5263, (Nonreporting) **A**9 10
Primary Contact: Gerald Kidd, Administrator
CFO: Joyce Wedgeworth, Financial Clerk
CMO: Gary Walton, M.D., Chief Medical Officer
CHR: Annette Billingsley, Director Human Resources
**Control:** City–County, Government, nonfederal **Service:** General Medical and
Surgical

| **Staffed Beds:** 33 |
| --- |

---

**Hospital, Medicare Provider Number, Address, Telephone, Approval, Facility, and Physician Codes, Health Care System**

★ American Hospital Association (AHA) membership
☐ The Joint Commission accreditation    ◇ DNV Healthcare Inc. accreditation

○ American Osteopathic Association (AOA) accreditation
△ Commission on Accreditation of Rehabilitation Facilities (CARF) accreditation

# ALASKA

## ANCHORAGE—Anchorage Division

☒ **ALASKA NATIVE MEDICAL CENTER (20026)**, 4315 Diplomacy Drive,
Zip 99508; tel. 907/563–2662 **A**1 3 5 9 10 **F**3 7 11 13 15 29 30 31 34 35 40
41 43 45 46 47 49 50 51 55 57 58 59 61 64 65 68 70 72 73 74 75 76 77
78 79 81 85 86 87 88 89 93 94 102 107 108 111 113 114 118 128 129
131 134 141 142 145 146 147 **P**6
Primary Contact: Gary Shaw, Administrator
CFO: Gregory Burkel, Chief Financial Officer
CHR: Sonya Conant, Senior Director Human Resources
Web address: www.anmc.org
**Control:** Other not–for–profit (including NFP Corporation) **Service:** General
Medical and Surgical

**Staffed Beds:** 146 **Admissions:** 7316 **Census:** 99 **Outpatient Visits:** 411181
**Births:** 1550 **Total Expense ($000):** 150280 **Payroll Expense ($000):**
114229

☐ **ALASKA PSYCHIATRIC INSTITUTE (24002)**, 3700 Piper Street,
Zip 99508–4677; tel. 907/269–7100 **A**1 9 10 **F**29 59 75 87 98 99 100 101
129 131 134 **P**1
Primary Contact: Ronald M. Adler, Chief Executive Officer
COO: Ronald M. Adler, Chief Executive Officer
CFO: Tina Williams, Chief Financial Officer
CMO: Jenny Love, M.D., Medical Director
CIO: Stephen Schneider, Manager Information Services
CHR: Annalisa Haynie, Administrative Assistant III
Web address: www.hss.state.ak.us/dbh/API/
**Control:** State–Government, nonfederal **Service:** Psychiatric

**Staffed Beds:** 80 **Admissions:** 1325 **Census:** 71 **Outpatient Visits:** 0 **Births:**
0 **Total Expense ($000):** 31700 **Payroll Expense ($000):** 16100
**Personnel:** 246

☒ **ALASKA REGIONAL HOSPITAL (20017)**, 2801 Debarr Road, Zip 99508–2997,
Mailing Address: P.O. Box 143889, Zip 99514–3889; tel. 907/264–1754,
(Nonreporting) **A**1 2 9 10 **S** HCA, Nashville, TN
Primary Contact: Annie Holt, FACHE, Chief Executive Officer
CFO: Paul G. Morris, Chief Financial Officer
CMO: Norman Wilder, M.D., Vice President Medical Affairs
CIO: Michael Richardson, Director Information Services
CHR: Tammy Kaminski, Director Human Resources
Web address: www.alaskaregional.com
**Control:** Corporation, Investor–owned, for–profit **Service:** General Medical and
Surgical

**Staffed Beds:** 132

☒ **NORTH STAR BEHAVIORAL HEALTH SYSTEM (24001)**, 2530 DeBarr Road,
Zip 99508–2948; tel. 907/258–7575, (Includes NORTH STAR BEHAVIORAL
HEALTH, 1650 South Bragaw, Zip 99508–3467; tel. 907/258–7575) **A**1 5 9 10
**F**98 99 106 **P**8 **S** Universal Health Services, Inc., King of Prussia, PA
Primary Contact: Andrew Mayo, Chief Executive Officer and Managing Director
CFO: Michele Fissori, Chief Financial Officer
CMO: Ruth Dukoff, M.D., Medical Director
CIO: Terry Thompson, Director Information Services
CHR: Jana Durr, Director Human Resources
Web address: www.northstarbehavioral.com
**Control:** Corporation, Investor–owned, for–profit **Service:** Children's hospital
psychiatric

**Staffed Beds:** 200 **Admissions:** 1181 **Census:** 184 **Outpatient Visits:** 0
**Births:** 0 **Total Expense ($000):** 30958 **Payroll Expense ($000):** 16200
**Personnel:** 354

☒ **PROVIDENCE ALASKA MEDICAL CENTER (20001)**, 3200 Providence Drive,
Zip 99508–4615, Mailing Address: P.O. Box 196604, Zip 99519–6604;
tel. 907/562–2211, (Includes CHILDREN'S HOSPITAL AT PROVIDENCE, 3200
Providence Drive, Zip 99508; tel. 907/212–3130) **A**1 2 3 5 9 10 3 **F**3 5 11 12
13 15 16 17 18 19 20 21 22 23 24 26 27 28 29 30 31 34 37 38 40 45 46
49 50 51 53 55 57 58 59 60 62 63 64 65 68 70 72 73 74 75 76 77 78 79
80 81 82 84 85 86 87 88 89 90 91 92 93 98 99 100 101 102 103 104 107
108 111 113 114 117 118 120 122 123 125 128 129 130 131 134 144 145
147 **P**6 8 **S** Providence Health & Services, Renton, WA
Primary Contact: Bruce Lamoureux, Vice President and Chief Executive Officer
CFO: Anthony Dorsch, Chief Financial Officer
CMO: Roy Davis, M.D., Chief Medical Officer
CIO: Stephanie Morton, Chief Information Officer
CHR: Scott Jungwirth, Chief Human Resources Officer
Web address: www.providence.org/alaska/pamc/default.htm
**Control:** Church–operated, Nongovernment, not–for profit **Service:** General
Medical and Surgical

**Staffed Beds:** 371 **Admissions:** 16507 **Census:** 255 **Outpatient Visits:**
299896 **Births:** 2611 **Total Expense ($000):** 510098 **Payroll Expense**
**($000):** 185290 **Personnel:** 2392

☒ **ST. ELIAS SPECIALTY HOSPITAL (22001)**, 4800 Cordova Street, Zip 99503;
tel. 907/561–3333, (Nonreporting) **A**1 9 10
Primary Contact: Sharon H. Kurz, Ph.D., Chief Executive Officer
Web address: www.st–eliashospital.com
**Control:** Other not–for–profit (including NFP Corporation) **Service:** Long–Term
Acute Care hospital

**Staffed Beds:** 45

## BARROW—North Slope Division

☒ **SAMUEL SIMMONDS MEMORIAL HOSPITAL (21312)**, 1296 Agvik Street,
Zip 99723, Mailing Address: P.O. Box 29, Zip 99723; tel. 907/852–4611,
(Nonreporting) **A**1 10 18
Primary Contact: Donna Patterson, Administrator
Web address: www.arcticslope.org
**Control:** Other not–for–profit (including NFP Corporation) **Service:** General
Medical and Surgical

**Staffed Beds:** 14

## BETHEL—Bethel Division

☒ **YUKON–KUSKOKWIM DELTA REGIONAL HOSPITAL (20018)**, 700 Chief
Eddie Hoffman Highway, Zip 99559–3000, Mailing Address: P.O. Box 528,
Zip 99559–3000; tel. 907/543–6300, (Nonreporting) **A**1 10
Primary Contact: Gene Peltola, President and Chief Executive Officer
CFO: Vanetta Van Cleave, Chief Financial Officer
CIO: William Pearch, Chief Information Officer
CHR: Carla F. Romero–Erlanson, Director Human Resources
Web address: www.ykhc.org
**Control:** Other not–for–profit (including NFP Corporation) **Service:** General
Medical and Surgical

**Staffed Beds:** 37

## CORDOVA—Valdez–Cordova Division

★ **CORDOVA COMMUNITY MEDICAL CENTER (21307)**, 602 Chase Avenue,
Zip 99574, Mailing Address: P.O. Box 160, Zip 99574; tel. 907/424–8000,
(Nonreporting) **A**9 10 18
Primary Contact: Stephen Sundby, Interim Chief Executive Officer
CFO: Mary Staab, Director Finance
CMO: Murray Buttner, M.D., Medical Director
CIO: Kim Dunn, Attorney–at–Law
CHR: Mary Staab, Director Finance
Web address: www.cdvcmc.com
**Control:** City–Government, nonfederal **Service:** General Medical and Surgical

**Staffed Beds:** 23

## DILLINGHAM—Dillingham Division

☒ **BRISTOL BAY AREA HEALTH CORPORATION (21309)**, 6000 Kanakanak
Road, Zip 99576, Mailing Address: P.O. Box 130, Zip 99576; tel. 907/842–5201
**A**1 5 9 10 18 **F**3 4 5 13 15 29 32 34 35 39 40 43 45 50 57 58 59 64 65 66
68 85 93 99 100 101 102 104 107 110 118 129 132 134 **P**6
Primary Contact: Robert J. Clark, President and Chief Executive Officer
COO: Lorraine M. Jewett, Vice President and Chief Operating Officer
CFO: Tom Berner, Vice President and Chief Financial Officer
CMO: Arnold Loera, M.D., Vice President and Medical Director
Web address: www.bbahc.org
**Control:** Other not–for–profit (including NFP Corporation) **Service:** General
Medical and Surgical

**Staffed Beds:** 14 **Admissions:** 210 **Census:** 2 **Outpatient Visits:** 73564
**Births:** 45 **Total Expense ($000):** 50341 **Payroll Expense ($000):** 22548
**Personnel:** 340

## ELMENDORF AFB—Anchorage Division

☒ **U. S. AIR FORCE REGIONAL HOSPITAL**, 5955 Zeamer Avenue,
Zip 99506–3700; tel. 907/580–3006, (Nonreporting) **A**1 5 **S** Department of the
Air Force, Washington, DC
Primary Contact: Colonel Thomas Harrell, Commander
COO: Captain Jeffery Jones, Administrator
CFO: Shawn Bransky, Flight Commander Resources Management
CMO: Brian Affleck, M.D., Chief Medical Staff
CIO: Robert Traylor, Flight Commander Medical Information Systems
CHR: Mark Clark, Human Resources Liaison
Web address: www.elmendorf.af.mil/
**Control:** Air Force, Government, federal **Service:** General Medical and Surgical

**Staffed Beds:** 64

*Many Facility Codes have changed. Please refer to the AHA Guide Code Chart.*

## FAIRBANKS—Fairbanks North Star Division

✠ **FAIRBANKS MEMORIAL HOSPITAL (20012)**, 1650 Cowles Street,
Zip 99701–5998; tel. 907/452–8181, (Total facility includes 90 beds in nursing
home–type unit) **A**1 2 5 9 10 **F**11 13 15 18 20 22 28 29 30 31 34 35 40 45
50 51 62 64 67 70 76 79 81 82 85 86 87 89 93 98 102 107 108 110 111
113 114 118 120 127 128 129 131 145 146 147 **S** Banner Health,
Phoenix, AZ
Primary Contact: Michael K. Powers, FACHE, Chief Executive Officer
CFO: Jim Lynch, Chief Financial Officer
CMO: Randy McGregor, M.D., Medical Director
CIO: Carl J. Kegley, System Director Information Technology
Web address: www.bannerhealth.com
**Control:** Other not–for–profit (including NFP Corporation) **Service:** General
Medical and Surgical

**Staffed Beds:** 217 **Admissions:** 5668 **Census:** 135 **Outpatient Visits:**
302253 **Births:** 1101 **Total Expense ($000):** 213556 **Payroll Expense
($000):** 82702 **Personnel:** 1111

## FORT WAINWRIGHT—Fairbanks North Star Division

✠ **BASSETT ARMY COMMUNITY HOSPITAL**, 1060 Gaffney Road, Box 7400,
Zip 99703–7400, Mailing Address: 1060 Gaffney Road, Box 7440,
Zip 99703–7440; tel. 907/361–5172, (Nonreporting) **A**1 **S** Department of the
Army, Office of the Surgeon General, Falls Church, VA
Primary Contact: Colonel George Appenzeller, Commander
CFO: Major Doug Stratton, Chief Resource Management Division
CMO: Colonel Leo Bennett, M.D., Deputy Commander Clinical Services
CIO: Michele Krause, Chief Information Management Officer
CHR: Terri Morefield, Deputy Chief Human Resources Division
Web address: www.alaska.amedd.army.mil
**Control:** Army, Government, federal **Service:** General Medical and Surgical

**Staffed Beds:** 24

## HOMER—Kenai Peninsula Division

★ **SOUTH PENINSULA HOSPITAL (21313)**, 4300 Bartlett Street,
Zip 99603–7000; tel. 907/235–8101, (Total facility includes 28 beds in nursing
home–type unit) **A**9 10 18 **F**3 11 13 15 29 30 31 34 35 40 45 50 51 56 59 62
64 67 68 70 75 76 77 78 79 81 85 87 93 94 97 107 110 111 114 118 127
128 129 132 145 147 **P**8
Primary Contact: Robert F. Letson, Chief Executive Officer
CFO: Lori Meyer, Interim Chief Financial Officer
CMO: Kenneth Hahn, M.D., Chief of Staff
CIO: Jim Bartilson, Manager Information Systems
CHR: Cindy H. Brinkerhoff, Director Human Resources
CNO: Shara Sutherlin, R.N., Director Patient Care Services
Web address: www.sphosp.com
**Control:** Hospital district or authority, Government, nonfederal **Service:** General
Medical and Surgical

**Staffed Beds:** 50 **Admissions:** 862 **Census:** 34 **Outpatient Visits:** 27636
**Births:** 119 **Total Expense ($000):** 36640 **Payroll Expense ($000):** 15731
**Personnel:** 215

## JUNEAU—Juneau Division

✠ **BARTLETT REGIONAL HOSPITAL (20008)**, 3260 Hospital Drive,
Zip 99801–7808; tel. 907/796–8900 **A**1 9 10 20 **F**4 5 13 17 28 29 31 34 40
57 59 76 81 85 86 93 98 104 107 111 113 128 129 134 147 **S** QHR,
Brentwood, TN
Primary Contact: John H. Vowell, Interim Chief Executive Officer
CFO: Dennis Stillman, Interim Chief Financial Officer
CMO: Richard Welling, M.D., Chief of Staff
CIO: Doug Halstead, Manager Information Systems
CHR: Kyla Allred, Manager Human Resources
Web address: www.bartletthospital.org
**Control:** City–Government, nonfederal **Service:** General Medical and Surgical

**Staffed Beds:** 57 **Admissions:** 1475 **Census:** 29 **Births:** 400 **Total Expense
($000):** 79337 **Payroll Expense ($000):** 31774 **Personnel:** 430

## KETCHIKAN—Ketchikan Gateway Division

✠ **PEACEHEALTH KETCHIKAN MEDICAL CENTER (21311)**, 3100 Tongass
Avenue, Zip 99901–5746; tel. 907/225–5171 **A**1 9 10 18 **F**30 31 34 35 40 45
46 53 56 57 58 59 62 63 68 75 76 77 79 81 84 85 93 94 96 99 100 102
104 105 107 108 110 111 113 118 127 128 129 131 145 146 147
**S** PeaceHealth, Bellevue, WA
Primary Contact: Patrick J. Branco, Chief Executive Officer
CFO: Ken Tonjes, Chief Financial Officer
CMO: Peter Rice, M.D., Medical Director
CIO: Tim Walker, Manager Information Services
CHR: Lanetta Lundberg, Vice President Culture and People
CNO: Kendall Sawa, R.N., Vice President Patient Care Services
Web address: www.peacehealth.org
**Control:** Other not–for–profit (including NFP Corporation) **Service:** General
Medical and Surgical

**Staffed Beds:** 54 **Admissions:** 500 **Census:** 3 **Outpatient Visits:** 12000
**Births:** 350

## KODIAK—Kodiak Island Division

✠ **PROVIDENCE KODIAK ISLAND MEDICAL CENTER (21306)**, 1915 East
Rezanof Drive, Zip 99615–6602; tel. 907/486–3281, (Total facility includes 19
beds in nursing home–type unit) **A**1 9 10 18 **F**3 11 12 13 15 29 30 31 32 34
35 38 40 44 45 46 50 59 62 64 66 67 68 70 75 76 77 78 79 81 83 85 87
90 92 93 98 99 100 101 102 103 104 105 107 110 111 113 118 127 128
129 131 132 145 147 **S** Providence Health & Services, Renton, WA
Primary Contact: Donald J. Rush, Chief Executive Officer
CFO: Timothy Hocum, Chief Financial Officer
CMO: Paul Zimmer, M.D., Chief of Staff
CIO: Fritz Ferrante, Manager Information Services
CHR: Brenda Zawacki, Manager Human Resources
CNO: LeeAnn Horn, Chief Nurse Executive
Web address: www.providence.org
**Control:** Other not–for–profit (including NFP Corporation) **Service:** General
Medical and Surgical

**Staffed Beds:** 25 **Admissions:** 883 **Census:** 29 **Outpatient Visits:** 21036
**Births:** 163

## KOTZEBUE—Northwest Arctic Division

☐ **MANIILAQ HEALTH CENTER (21310)**, 436 5th Avenue, Zip 99752–0043,
Mailing Address: P.O. Box 43, Zip 99752–0043; tel. 907/442–7344,
(Nonreporting) **A**1 5 9 10 18
Primary Contact: Robert Ottone, Administrator
COO: Ian Erlich, President and Chief Executive Officer
CFO: Lucy Nelson, Director Finance
CMO: Ellen Elmore, M.D., Director Medical Services
CIO: Eugene Smith, Chief Information Officer
CHR: Deborah White, Director Human Resources
Web address: www.maniilaq.org
**Control:** Other not–for–profit (including NFP Corporation) **Service:** General
Medical and Surgical

**Staffed Beds:** 17

## NOME—Nome Division

✠ **NORTON SOUND REGIONAL HOSPITAL (21308)**, Bering Straits, Zip 99762,
Mailing Address: P.O. Box 966, Zip 99762–0966; tel. 907/443–3311,
(Nonreporting) **A**1 5 9 10 18
Primary Contact: Angela Gorn, Vice President
COO: Roy Agloinga, Chief Administrative Officer
CFO: Cynthia Brandt, Interim Chief Financial Officer
CMO: David Head, M.D., Chief Medical Staff
CIO: Dan Bailey, Director Information Systems
CHR: Tiffany Martinson, Director Human Resources
Web address: www.nortonsoundhealth.org
**Control:** Other not–for–profit (including NFP Corporation) **Service:** General
Medical and Surgical

**Staffed Beds:** 36

---

**Hospital, Medicare Provider Number, Address, Telephone, Approval, Facility, and Physician Codes, Health Care System**

★ American Hospital Association (AHA) membership
☐ The Joint Commission accreditation     ◇ DNV Healthcare Inc. accreditation
○ American Osteopathic Association (AOA) accreditation
△ Commission on Accreditation of Rehabilitation Facilities (CARF) accreditation

**AK**

## PALMER—Matanuska–Susitna Division

✠ **MAT–SU REGIONAL MEDICAL CENTER (20006)**, 2500 South Woodworth Loop, Zip 99645, Mailing Address: P.O. Box 1687, Zip 99645–1687; tel. 907/861–6000 **A**1 9 10 20 **F**3 8 13 15 18 19 20 22 26 28 29 30 34 35 40 45 51 54 57 64 65 68 70 74 75 76 79 81 85 86 87 93 97 107 108 110 111 113 114 118 125 127 128 129 131 132 134 143 145 147 **P**5
**S** Community Health Systems, Inc., Franklin, TN
Primary Contact: John R. Lee, Chief Executive Officer
CFO: Scott Bailey, Chief Financial Officer
CMO: Christopher Sahlstrom, M.D., Chief of Staff
CIO: Bryan Meurer, Director Information Systems
CHR: Cathy Babuscio, Director Human Resources
CNO: Emily Stevens, Chief Nursing Officer
Web address: www.matsuregional.com
**Control:** Partnership, Investor–owned, for–profit **Service:** General Medical and Surgical

**Staffed Beds:** 74 **Admissions:** 4552 **Census:** 41 **Outpatient Visits:** 99859 **Births:** 747 **Personnel:** 490

## PETERSBURG—Wrangell–Petersburg Division

★ **PETERSBURG MEDICAL CENTER (21304)**, 103 Fram Street, Zip 99833, Mailing Address: Box 589, Zip 99833–0589; tel. 907/772–4291, (Nonreporting) **A**9 10 18
Primary Contact: Elizabeth Woodyard, R.N., MSN, Chief Executive Officer
CFO: Leon Walsh, Chief Financial Officer
CHR: Cynthia Newman, Manager Human Resources
CNO: Jennifer Bryner, Chief Nursing Officer
Web address: www.pmc–health.com/
**Control:** City–Government, nonfederal **Service:** General Medical and Surgical

**Staffed Beds:** 27

## SEWARD—Kenai Peninsula Division

★ **PROVIDENCE SEWARD MEDICAL CENTER (21302)**, 417 First Avenue, Zip 99664, Mailing Address: P.O. Box 365, Zip 99664–0365; tel. 907/224–5205, (Nonreporting) **A**9 10 18 **S** Providence Health & Services, Renton, WA
Primary Contact: Christopher Bolton, Administrator
Web address: www.providence.org
**Control:** Church–operated, Nongovernment, not–for profit **Service:** General Medical and Surgical

**Staffed Beds:** 6

## SITKA—Sitka Division

✠ **SEARHC MT. EDGECUMBE HOSPITAL (20027)**, 222 Tongass Drive, Zip 99835–9416; tel. 907/966–2411 **A**1 9 10 **F**3 29 30 31 34 35 39 40 43 45 50 53 57 59 64 65 68 70 74 75 76 79 81 82 85 87 93 97 99 100 101 102 104 105 107 111 113 118 126 129 133 134 142 143 146
Primary Contact: Martin Grasmeder, M.D., Administrator
CFO: David Edwards, Chief Financial Officer
CMO: Martin Grasmeder, M.D., Medical Director
CIO: Bob Cita, Director Information Services
CHR: Melanie Millhorn, Director Human Resources
Web address: www.searhc.org
**Control:** Other not–for–profit (including NFP Corporation) **Service:** General Medical and Surgical

**Staffed Beds:** 27 **Admissions:** 983 **Census:** 13 **Outpatient Visits:** 79407 **Births:** 102

★ **SITKA COMMUNITY HOSPITAL (21303)**, 209 Moller Avenue, Zip 99835–7145; tel. 907/747–3241, (Nonreporting) **A**9 10 18
Primary Contact: Hugh R. Hallgren, Chief Executive Officer
CFO: Lee W. Bennett, Chief Financial Officer
CHR: Kelley Fink, Coordinator Human Resources
Web address: www.sitkahospital.org
**Control:** City–Government, nonfederal **Service:** General Medical and Surgical

**Staffed Beds:** 27

## SOLDOTNA—Kenai Peninsula Division

✠ **CENTRAL PENINSULA GENERAL HOSPITAL (20024)**, 250 Hospital Place, Zip 99669–6999; tel. 907/714–4404, (Total facility includes 58 beds in nursing home–type unit) **A**1 9 10 20 **F**3 4 5 11 13 15 28 29 30 31 34 35 36 38 40 49 53 57 59 68 70 74 75 76 77 78 79 81 82 84 85 86 87 93 100 104 105 106 107 108 111 113 117 118 127 128 129 130 132 133 134 144 145 146 147 **P**1
Primary Contact: Richard Davis, Chief Executive Officer
COO: Matt Dammeyer, Ph.D., Chief Operating Officer
CFO: Shaun Keef, Chief Financial Officer
CMO: Gregg Motonaga, M.D., Chief of Staff
CIO: Bryan Downs, Director Information Systems
CHR: John Dodd, Vice President Human Resources
Web address: www.cpgh.org
**Control:** Other not–for–profit (including NFP Corporation) **Service:** General Medical and Surgical

**Staffed Beds:** 117 **Admissions:** 2261 **Census:** 59 **Outpatient Visits:** 76474 **Births:** 448 **Total Expense ($000):** 96492 **Payroll Expense ($000):** 44177 **Personnel:** 642

## VALDEZ—Valdez–Cordova Division

★ **PROVIDENCE VALDEZ MEDICAL CENTER (21301)**, 911 Meals Avenue, Zip 99686–0550, Mailing Address: P.O. Box 550, Zip 99686–0550; tel. 907/835–2249, (Nonreporting) **A**9 10 18 **S** Providence Health & Services, Renton, WA
Primary Contact: Sean McCallister, Administrator
CFO: Jeremy O'Neil, Manager Finance
CMO: John Cullen, M.D., Chief of Staff and Medical Director Long Term Care
CHR: Maureen Radotich, Director Human Resources
Web address: www.providence.org/alaska
**Control:** City–Government, nonfederal **Service:** General Medical and Surgical

**Staffed Beds:** 21

## WRANGELL—Wrangell–Petersburg Division

★ **WRANGELL MEDICAL CENTER (21305)**, First Avenue & Bennett Street, Zip 99929, Mailing Address: P.O. Box 1081, Zip 99929; tel. 907/874–7000, (Nonreporting) **A**9 10 18
Primary Contact: Noel Rea, Chief Executive Officer
CFO: Olinda White, Chief Financial Officer
CIO: Cathy Gross, Director Health Information Management Systems
Web address: www.wrangellmedicalcenter.com
**Control:** City–Government, nonfederal **Service:** General Medical and Surgical

**Staffed Beds:** 22

*Many Facility Codes have changed. Please refer to the AHA Guide Code Chart.* © 2012 AHA Guide

# ARIZONA

## BENSON—Cochise County

**BENSON HOSPITAL (31301)**, 450 South Ocotillo Street, Zip 85602, Mailing Address: P.O. Box 2290, Zip 85602; tel. 520/586–2261, (Nonreporting) **A**9 10 18
Primary Contact: Ronald A. McKinnon, Chief Executive Officer
CFO: Denise Hurtado, Chief Financial Officer
Web address: www.bensonhospital.org
**Control:** Hospital district or authority, Government, nonfederal **Service:** General Medical and Surgical

| Staffed Beds: 22 |
| --- |

## BISBEE—Cochise County

★ **COPPER QUEEN COMMUNITY HOSPITAL (31312)**, 101 Cole Avenue, Zip 85603–1399; tel. 520/432–5383 **A**9 10 18 **F**11 15 18 40 43 45 46 62 75 77 81 85 93 107 110 113 118 126 129 132 134 146
Primary Contact: James J. Dickson, Administrator and Chief Executive Officer
COO: Lisa Cummings, Director Outpatient Services
CFO: Diane C. Moore, Chief Financial Officer
CMO: Jose Romo, M.D., Chief of Staff
CIO: David Chmura, Manager Management Information Systems
CHR: Virginia Martinez, Manager Human Resources
CNO: Linda Morin, Director of Nursing
Web address: www.cqch.org
**Control:** Other not–for–profit (including NFP Corporation) **Service:** General Medical and Surgical

| Staffed Beds: 14 **Admissions:** 471 **Census:** 3 **Outpatient Visits:** 115651 **Births:** 2 **Total Expense ($000):** 19531 **Payroll Expense ($000):** 10131 **Personnel:** 182 |
| --- |

## BULLHEAD CITY—Mohave County

⊞ **WESTERN ARIZONA REGIONAL MEDICAL CENTER (30101)**, 2735 Silver Creek Road, Zip 86442–8303; tel. 928/763–2273, (Nonreporting) **A**1 9 10 19 **S** Community Health Systems, Inc., Franklin, TN
Primary Contact: Barry S. Schneider, Chief Executive Officer
Web address: www.warmc.com
**Control:** Corporation, Investor–owned, for–profit **Service:** General Medical and Surgical

| Staffed Beds: 139 |
| --- |

## CASA GRANDE—Pinal County

⊞ **CASA GRANDE REGIONAL MEDICAL CENTER (30016)**, 1800 East Florence Boulevard, Zip 85222–5399; tel. 520/381–6300 **A**1 9 10 21 **F**11 13 15 18 20 22 28 29 30 31 34 40 45 46 49 50 57 59 60 68 70 74 75 76 78 79 81 85 87 89 93 98 103 107 108 110 111 112 114 115 116 117 118 128 129 131 143 145 146 147
Primary Contact: Rona Curphy, President and Chief Executive Officer
CFO: Karen Francis, Chief Financial Officer
CMO: Richard Stubbs, M.D., Vice President Medical Affairs
CIO: Walter Chisenski, Director Information Technology
CHR: Carol D'Souza, Director Human Resources
CNO: Cheryse Austin, Vice President Patient Care Services and Chief Nursing Officer
Web address: www.casagrandehospital.com
**Control:** Other not–for–profit (including NFP Corporation) **Service:** General Medical and Surgical

| Staffed Beds: 187 **Admissions:** 8399 **Census:** 93 **Outpatient Visits:** 108007 **Births:** 799 **Total Expense ($000):** 104216 **Payroll Expense ($000):** 47780 **Personnel:** 762 |
| --- |

## CHANDLER—Maricopa County

□ **ARIZONA ORTHOPEDIC SURGICAL HOSPITAL (30112)**, 2905 West Warner Road, Zip 85224; tel. 480/603–9000, (Nonreporting) **A**1 9 10 **S** United Surgical Partners International, Addison, TX
Primary Contact: Duane Scholer, Chief Executive Officer
Web address: www.azosh.com
**Control:** Corporation, Investor–owned, for–profit **Service:** Surgical

| Staffed Beds: 16 |
| --- |

⊞ **CHANDLER REGIONAL MEDICAL CENTER (30036)**, 1955 West Frye Road, Zip 85224–4230; tel. 480/728–3000 **A**1 9 10 **F**3 11 12 13 15 17 18 20 22 24 26 28 29 30 31 32 34 35 40 43 44 45 46 47 48 49 50 51 54 57 58 59 60 63 64 65 66 68 69 70 71 73 74 75 76 78 79 81 82 84 85 86 87 93 96 107 108 111 113 114 118 120 121 125 129 131 134 142 143 145 146 147 **P**6 **S** Dignity Health, San Francisco, CA
Primary Contact: Tim Bricker, President and Chief Executive Officer
COO: Peter Menor, Vice President Operations
CFO: Mark Kem, Vice President Finance and Chief Financial Officer
CMO: Terry J. Happel, M.D., Vice President and Chief Medical Officer
CHR: Renea Brunke, Vice President Human Resources
CNO: Peg Smith, Vice President and Chief Nursing Officer
Web address: www.chandlerregional.com
**Control:** Church–operated, Nongovernment, not–for profit **Service:** General Medical and Surgical

| Staffed Beds: 224 **Admissions:** 17886 **Census:** 201 **Outpatient Visits:** 116808 **Births:** 3674 **Total Expense ($000):** 280961 **Payroll Expense ($000):** 119969 **Personnel:** 1903 |
| --- |

## CHINLE—Apache County

⊞ **CHINLE COMPREHENSIVE HEALTH CARE FACILITY (30084)**, Highway 191, Zip 86503, Mailing Address: P.O. Drawer PH, Zip 86503; tel. 928/674–7011 **A**1 10 **F**5 15 29 34 35 38 39 40 45 46 47 48 50 53 57 59 62 64 65 68 70 75 76 77 81 82 85 86 87 89 90 93 97 98 99 100 101 102 103 104 107 108 110 118 126 129 130 131 132 143 144 145 146 147 **P**6 **S** U. S. Indian Health Service, Rockville, MD
Primary Contact: Ronald Tso, Chief Executive Officer
COO: Shirley Lewis
CFO: Philene Tyler, Chief Finance Officer
CMO: Kevin Rand, M.D., Clinical Director
CIO: Perry Francis, Supervisory Information Technology Specialist
CHR: Darlene J. Silverhatband, Supervisory Human Resource Specialist
CNO: Patricia Gorman, Chief Nurse Executive
Web address: www.ihs.gov
**Control:** PHS, Indian Service, Government, federal **Service:** General Medical and Surgical

| Staffed Beds: 60 **Admissions:** 2529 **Census:** 19 **Outpatient Visits:** 261986 **Births:** 525 **Total Expense ($000):** 182548 **Payroll Expense ($000):** 56584 **Personnel:** 873 |
| --- |

## COTTONWOOD—Yavapai County

★ **VERDE VALLEY MEDICAL CENTER (30007)**, 269 South Candy Lane, Zip 86326–4170; tel. 928/639–6000 **A**9 10 13 20 21 **F**3 8 11 13 15 18 20 22 28 29 30 31 32 34 35 36 40 44 46 47 48 49 50 53 57 59 60 64 68 70 74 75 76 77 78 79 81 82 85 86 87 89 93 98 100 101 103 106 107 108 110 111 113 114 116 117 118 119 120 122 128 129 130 131 134 142 144 145 146 147 **S** Northern Arizona Healthcare, Flagstaff, AZ
Primary Contact: James J. Bleicher, M.D., President and Chief Executive Officer
CFO: Gregory Kuzma, Vice President and Chief Financial Officer
CMO: Harry Alberti, M.D., Chief Medical Officer and Vice President Medical Affairs
CIO: Marilynn Black, Chief Information Officer
CHR: Lori L. Jackson, Director Human Resources
CNO: Jennifer Brewer, R.N., Chief Nursing Officer and Vice President Nursing Services
Web address: www.nahealth.com
**Control:** Other not–for–profit (including NFP Corporation) **Service:** General Medical and Surgical

| Staffed Beds: 110 **Admissions:** 4532 **Census:** 50 **Outpatient Visits:** 109135 **Births:** 542 **Total Expense ($000):** 139217 **Payroll Expense ($000):** 59240 **Personnel:** 720 |
| --- |

## DOUGLAS—Cochise County

**SOUTHEAST ARIZONA MEDICAL CENTER (31303)**, 2174 Oak Avenue, Zip 85607–9801; tel. 520/364–7931, (Nonreporting) **A**9 10 18
Primary Contact: Brian E. Bickel, President and Chief Executive Officer
COO: Annie Benson, Chief Operating Officer
CFO: Alvin Chilton, Chief Financial Officer
CMO: Christopher Spooner, M.D., Chief of Staff
CIO: Ann Bliss, Manager Computer Services
CHR: Roberta Berry, Manager Human Resources
Web address: www.samcdouglas.org
**Control:** Other not–for–profit (including NFP Corporation) **Service:** General Medical and Surgical

| Staffed Beds: 25 |
| --- |

| Hospital, Medicare Provider Number, Address, Telephone, Approval, Facility, and Physician Codes, Health Care System |
| --- |
| ★ American Hospital Association (AHA) membership  ○ American Osteopathic Association (AOA) accreditation |
| □ The Joint Commission accreditation  ◇ DNV Healthcare Inc. accreditation  △ Commission on Accreditation of Rehabilitation Facilities (CARF) accreditation |

**AZ**

## FLAGSTAFF—Coconino County

★ **FLAGSTAFF MEDICAL CENTER (30023)**, 1200 North Beaver Street, Zip 86001–3198; tel. 928/779–3366 **A**9 10 21 **F**3 5 7 11 12 13 15 17 18 20 22 24 28 29 30 31 32 34 35 36 37 40 43 45 49 50 53 54 57 58 59 60 61 64 68 70 72 74 75 76 77 78 79 81 82 84 85 86 87 88 89 90 93 98 99 100 101 102 103 104 105 107 108 111 113 114 115 116 117 118 119 120 122 125 129 130 131 134 144 145 146 147 **S** Northern Arizona Healthcare, Flagstaff, AZ
Primary Contact: William T. Bradel, President
COO: William T. Bradel, President
CFO: Gregory Kuzma, Vice President and Chief Financial Officer
CMO: Steven Lewis, M.D., Senior Vice President and Chief Medical Officer
CIO: John Schofield, Chief Information Officer
CHR: Patricia Crofford, Vice President Human Resources
Web address: www.flagstaffmedicalcenter.com
**Control:** Other not–for–profit (including NFP Corporation) **Service:** General Medical and Surgical

**Staffed Beds:** 267 **Admissions:** 13495 **Census:** 169 **Outpatient Visits:** 100427 **Births:** 1251 **Total Expense ($000):** 320994 **Payroll Expense ($000):** 121750 **Personnel:** 1594

## FLORENCE—Pinal County

**FLORENCE COMMUNITY HEALTHCARE (31316)**, 450 West Adamsville Road, Zip 85132–8582; tel. 520/868–3000, (Nonreporting) **A**9 10 21
Primary Contact: Gary Faulkner, Chief Executive Officer
Web address: www.florencecommunityhealthcare.com
**Control:** Corporation, Investor–owned, for–profit **Service:** General Medical and Surgical

**Staffed Beds:** 65

**FLORENCE HOSPITAL AT ANTHEM**, 4545 North Hunt Highway, Zip 85132; tel. 520/868–3333, (Nonreporting)
Primary Contact: David S. Wanger, Chief Executive Officer
Web address: www.florencehospital.org
**Control:** Partnership, Investor–owned, for–profit **Service:** General Medical and Surgical

**Staffed Beds:** 36

## FORT DEFIANCE—Apache County

★ **FORT DEFIANCE INDIAN HEALTH SERVICE HOSPITAL (30071)**, Zip 86504; tel. 928/729–8014, (Nonreporting) **A**10 **S** U. S. Indian Health Service, Rockville, MD
Primary Contact: Leland Leonard, M.D., Administrator
COO: Laverne Miles, Chief Operating Officer
CFO: Daniel E. Johnson, Chief Financial Officer
CMO: David Downing, M.D., Chief Medical Officer
CIO: Virgil Chavez, Chief Information Officer
CHR: Vivian Santistevan, Chief Human Resources
Web address: www.ihs.gov
**Control:** PHS, Indian Service, Government, federal **Service:** General Medical and Surgical

**Staffed Beds:** 39

## FORT MOHAVE—Mohave County

✠ **VALLEY VIEW MEDICAL CENTER (30117)**, 5330 South Highway 95, Zip 86426; tel. 928/788–2273, (Nonreporting) **A**1 9 10 **S** LifePoint Hospitals, Inc., Brentwood, TN
Primary Contact: Richard G. Carter, Chief Executive Officer
CFO: Meredith Nelson, Chief Financial Officer
CHR: Susan L. Scharles, Director Human Resources
CNO: Natasha Compton, Chief Nursing Officer
Web address: www.valleyviewmedicalcenter.net
**Control:** Corporation, Investor–owned, for–profit **Service:** Other specialty

**Staffed Beds:** 66

## GANADO—Apache County

✠ **SAGE MEMORIAL HOSPITAL (31309)**, Highway 264, Zip 86505, Mailing Address: P.O. Box 457, Zip 86505–0457; tel. 928/755–4500 **A**1 9 10 18 **F**1 5 7 11 18 29 32 34 35 39 40 50 53 54 57 59 62 64 65 68 75 100 101 104 107 118 126 132 133 143
Primary Contact: Ahmad Razaghi, Chief Executive Officer
COO: Tim Cousens, On–Site Administrator
CFO: Charity L. Askie, Director Finance
CMO: Sara Valladolid, M.D., Medical Director
CIO: Wayne White, Director Computer Services
CHR: Perphelia Fowler, Manager Human Resources
Web address: www.sagememorial.org
**Control:** Other not–for–profit (including NFP Corporation) **Service:** General Medical and Surgical

**Staffed Beds:** 25 **Admissions:** 460 **Census:** 6 **Outpatient Visits:** 18276 **Births:** 0 **Total Expense ($000):** 26349 **Payroll Expense ($000):** 8643 **Personnel:** 281

## GILBERT—Maricopa County

✠ **BANNER GATEWAY MEDICAL CENTER (30122)**, 1900 North Higley Road, Zip 85234; tel. 480/543–2000 **A**1 9 10 **F**3 8 12 13 21 29 30 31 34 40 45 46 47 48 49 50 54 57 59 60 64 68 70 73 74 75 76 77 78 79 81 85 86 87 107 108 109 111 112 113 118 125 129 145 147 **P**6 8 **S** Banner Health, Phoenix, AZ
Primary Contact: Todd S. Werner, Chief Executive Officer
CFO: Claire Agnew, Chief Financial Officer
CMO: David Edwards, M.D., Chief Medical Officer
CHR: Amber R. Kovacs, Chief Human Resources Officer
Web address: www.bannerhealth.com
**Control:** Other not–for–profit (including NFP Corporation) **Service:** General Medical and Surgical

**Staffed Beds:** 177 **Admissions:** 14039 **Census:** 117 **Outpatient Visits:** 115161 **Births:** 4172 **Total Expense ($000):** 177647 **Payroll Expense ($000):** 62252 **Personnel:** 1163

**GILBERT HOSPITAL (30120)**, 5656 South Power Road, Zip 85295; tel. 480/984–2000 **A**9 10 **F**3 29 34 40 41 45 49 50 59 70 79 81 82 87 107 108 111 114 118
Primary Contact: David S. Wanger, Chief Executive Officer
CFO: Randy Calvert, Chief Financial Officer
CMO: Timothy Johns, M.D., Chief Medical Officer and Board President
CIO: Michelle Cianfrani, Director Information Technology
CHR: David S. Wanger, Chief Executive Officer
Web address: www.gilberter.com
**Control:** Corporation, Investor–owned, for–profit **Service:** General Medical and Surgical

**Staffed Beds:** 19 **Admissions:** 1912 **Census:** 16 **Outpatient Visits:** 33476 **Total Expense ($000):** 38917 **Payroll Expense ($000):** 19239

✠ **MERCY GILBERT MEDICAL CENTER (30119)**, 3555 South Val Vista Road, Zip 85297; tel. 480/728–8000 **A**1 9 10 **F**3 11 12 13 15 20 22 26 29 30 31 32 34 35 39 40 43 44 45 49 50 51 57 58 59 60 63 64 65 68 70 73 74 75 76 79 81 82 83 84 85 86 87 89 107 108 110 111 113 114 118 128 129 131 134 142 143 145 147 **P**6 **S** Dignity Health, San Francisco, CA
Primary Contact: Tim Bricker, President and Chief Executive Officer
CFO: Mark Kem, Vice President Finance and Chief Financial Officer
CMO: Terry J. Happel, M.D., Vice President and Chief Medical Officer
CIO: Bob Campbell, Vice President Business Development and Chief Strategy Officer
CHR: Renea Brunke, Vice President Human Resources
Web address: www.mercygilbert.org
**Control:** Church–operated, Nongovernment, not–for profit **Service:** General Medical and Surgical

**Staffed Beds:** 212 **Admissions:** 14775 **Census:** 149 **Outpatient Visits:** 97841 **Births:** 2738 **Total Expense ($000):** 213241 **Payroll Expense ($000):** 84387 **Personnel:** 1249

## GLENDALE—Maricopa County

☐ **ARROWHEAD HOSPITAL (30094)**, 18701 North 67th Avenue, Zip 85308–5722; tel. 623/561–1000 **A**1 9 10 **F**3 11 13 15 17 18 20 22 24 26 28 29 30 31 34 35 37 40 41 42 45 46 47 48 49 57 59 64 70 72 74 75 76 77 78 79 81 85 87 107 108 110 111 113 117 118 129 145 147 **S** Vanguard Health System, Nashville, TN
Primary Contact: Frank L. Molinaro, Chief Executive Officer
CFO: Joel Snook, Chief Financial Officer
CMO: Patrick Smith, M.D., Chief Medical Officer
CHR: Sharon M. Chadwick, Director Human Resources
Web address: www.arrowheadhospital.com
**Control:** Corporation, Investor–owned, for–profit **Service:** General Medical and Surgical

**Staffed Beds:** 234 **Admissions:** 12610 **Census:** 122 **Outpatient Visits:** 70628 **Total Expense ($000):** 126848 **Payroll Expense ($000):** 58833 **Personnel:** 886

☐ **AURORA BEHAVIORAL HEALTH SYSTEM–GLENDALE (34024)**, 6015 West Peoria Avenue, Zip 85302–1201; tel. 623/344–4400, (Nonreporting) **A**1 9 10 **S** Aurora Behavioral Health Care, Corona, CA
Primary Contact: Bruce Waldo, Chief Executive Officer
CFO: Dino Quarante, Chief Financial Officer
CMO: Martin Newman, M.D., Chief Medical Officer
CHR: Vicki Thomsen, Director Human Resources
CNO: Ryan McKenzie, R.N., Director of Nursing
Web address: www.aurorabehavioral.com
**Control:** Corporation, Investor–owned, for–profit **Service:** Psychiatric

**Staffed Beds:** 80

*Many Facility Codes have changed. Please refer to the AHA Guide Code Chart.* © 2012 AHA Guide

★ **BANNER THUNDERBIRD MEDICAL CENTER (30089)**, 5555 West Thunderbird Road, Zip 85306–4696; tel. 602/865–5555, (Includes BANNER BEHAVIORAL HEALTH CENTER–THUNDERBIRD CAMPUS, 5555 West Thunderbird Road, Zip 85306; tel. 602/588–5555) **A**9 10 **F**3 13 15 17 18 20 22 24 26 28 29 30 31 34 35 36 37 38 40 43 45 46 47 49 51 55 57 58 59 60 64 67 68 70 72 74 75 76 77 78 79 81 82 85 86 87 88 89 93 98 99 102 103 104 107 108 109 110 111 113 114 116 118 119 120 122 123 125 128 129 131 133 134 142 145 146 147 **S** Banner Health, Phoenix, AZ
Primary Contact: Thomas C. Dickson, Chief Executive Officer
CFO: Richard Miller, Administrator Finance
CMO: Kathryn Perkins, M.D., Chief Medical Officer
CHR: Laura Witt, Administrator Human Resources
Web address: www.bannerhealth.com
**Control:** Other not–for–profit (including NFP Corporation) **Service:** General Medical and Surgical

**Staffed Beds:** 480 **Admissions:** 32792 **Census:** 362 **Outpatient Visits:** 304298 **Births:** 4765 **Total Expense ($000):** 389277 **Payroll Expense ($000):** 145858 **Personnel:** 2531

☒ **HEALTHSOUTH VALLEY OF THE SUN REHABILITATION HOSPITAL (33032)**, 13460 North 67th Avenue, Zip 85304–1042; tel. 623/878–8800, (Nonreporting) **A**1 9 10 **S** HEALTHSOUTH Corporation, Birmingham, AL
Primary Contact: Beth Bacher, Chief Executive Officer
CFO: Kathryn Haney, Chief Financial Officer
CFO: Kathryn Haney, Controller
CMO: Michael Kravetz, M.D., Medical Director
CHR: Danette Garcia, Director Human Resources
CNO: Beth Mooney, R.N., Chief Nursing Officer
Web address: www.healthsouthvalleyofthesun.com
**Control:** Corporation, Investor–owned, for–profit **Service:** Rehabilitation

**Staffed Beds:** 75

### GLOBE—Gila County

**COBRE VALLEY COMMUNITY HOSPITAL** See Cobre Valley Regional Medical Center

★ **COBRE VALLEY REGIONAL MEDICAL CENTER (31314)**, 5880 South Hospital Drive, Zip 85501–9454; tel. 928/425–3261 **A**9 10 18 **F**3 11 16 22 29 30 34 35 40 43 45 46 51 57 59 70 74 75 76 78 79 81 82 87 92 93 97 107 108 111 114 117 118 126 127 128 129 132 134 145 146 **P**5 **S** HealthTech Management Services, Franklin, TN
Primary Contact: Neal Jensen, Chief Executive Officer
CFO: James R. Childers, Chief Financial Officer
CIO: Sharon Bennett, Manager Information Systems
CHR: Rita Murphy, Director Human Resources
Web address: www.cvrmc.org
**Control:** Other not–for–profit (including NFP Corporation) **Service:** General Medical and Surgical

**Staffed Beds:** 25 **Admissions:** 1730 **Census:** 14 **Outpatient Visits:** 51879 **Births:** 332 **Total Expense ($000):** 35828 **Payroll Expense ($000):** 16303 **Personnel:** 200

### GOODYEAR—Maricopa County

☐ **WEST VALLEY HOSPITAL (30110)**, 13677 West McDowell Road, Zip 85338; tel. 623/882–1500, (Nonreporting) **A**1 9 10 **S** Vanguard Health System, Nashville, TN
Primary Contact: Jo Adkins, Chief Executive Officer
CFO: Richard Franco, Chief Financial Officer
CMO: Ron Kenneth, M.D., Chief Medical Officer
CHR: Deborah L. Rosenburg, Director Human Resources
Web address: www.wvhospital.com
**Control:** Corporation, Investor–owned, for–profit **Service:** General Medical and Surgical

**Staffed Beds:** 106

**WESTERN REGIONAL MEDICAL CENTER (30127)**, 14200 West Fillmore Street, Zip 85338–3005; tel. 623/207–3000, (Nonreporting) **A**10 **S** Cancer Treatment Centers of America, Schaumburg, IL
Primary Contact: David Veillette, President and Chief Executive Officer
Web address: www.cancercenter.com/western–hospital.cfm
**Control:** Corporation, Investor–owned, for–profit **Service:** Cancer

**Staffed Beds:** 24

### KEAMS CANYON—Navajo County

☒ **HOPI HEALTH CARE CENTER (31305)**, Zip 86034; Mailing Address: Polacca, tel. 928/737–6000 **A**1 10 18 **F**3 13 29 32 34 35 39 40 41 43 50 59 63 64 65 66 68 75 76 82 84 86 87 89 93 97 107 111 113 118 129 130 133 143 145 147 **P**4 6 **S** U. S. Indian Health Service, Rockville, MD
Primary Contact: De Alva Honahnie, Chief Executive Officer
CFO: Dorothy Sulu, Chief Financial Officer
CMO: Darren Vicenti, M.D., Clinical Director
CIO: Adrian Tom, Supervisor Management Information Systems
Web address: www.ihs.gov/index.asp
**Control:** PHS, Indian Service, Government, federal **Service:** General Medical and Surgical

**Staffed Beds:** 6 **Admissions:** 388 **Census:** 2 **Outpatient Visits:** 75137 **Births:** 39 **Payroll Expense ($000):** 12507 **Personnel:** 262

### KINGMAN—Mohave County

☒ **KINGMAN REGIONAL MEDICAL CENTER (30055)**, 3269 Stockton Hill Road, Zip 86409–3691; tel. 928/757–2101 **A**1 9 10 13 21 **F**3 11 13 15 17 18 22 24 28 29 30 31 34 35 40 42 43 49 51 53 57 59 60 62 63 64 70 74 75 76 77 78 79 81 82 84 85 86 87 89 90 93 97 104 105 107 108 110 111 113 114 115 116 117 118 120 122 126 128 129 131 134 142 143 145 146 147 **P**6 7
Primary Contact: Brian Turney, Chief Executive Officer
COO: Ryan Kennedy, Chief Operating Officer
CFO: Timothy D. Blanchard, Chief Financial Officer
CMO: Deborah Bennett, D.O., Chief Medical Officer
CIO: Robert (Bob) Sarnecki, Chief Information Officer
CHR: Heather N. Crowl, Chief Human Resources Officer
CNO: Kimberly Miyauchi, R.N., Chief Nursing Officer
Web address: www.azkrmc.com
**Control:** Hospital district or authority, Government, nonfederal **Service:** General Medical and Surgical

**Staffed Beds:** 180 **Admissions:** 8071 **Census:** 101 **Outpatient Visits:** 332758 **Births:** 641 **Total Expense ($000):** 196935 **Payroll Expense ($000):** 83986 **Personnel:** 1366

### LAKE HAVASU CITY—Mohave County

☒ **HAVASU REGIONAL MEDICAL CENTER (30069)**, 101 Civic Center Lane, Zip 86403–5683; tel. 928/855–8185, (Nonreporting) **A**1 9 10 **S** LifePoint Hospitals, Inc., Brentwood, TN
Primary Contact: Sandra C. Podley, Chief Executive Officer
CFO: Christopher Flores, Chief Financial Officer
CMO: Michael Rosen, M.D., Chief Medical Officer
CIO: Linda Toy, Director Information Systems
CHR: Sheena Benson, Director Human Resources
CNO: Julie Bowman, Chief Nursing Officer
Web address: www.havasuregional.com
**Control:** Corporation, Investor–owned, for–profit **Service:** General Medical and Surgical

**Staffed Beds:** 138

### MESA—Maricopa County

☐ **ARIZONA REGIONAL MEDICAL CENTER (30126)**, 515 North Mesa Drive, Zip 85201–5914; tel. 480/237–3200, (Includes APACHE JUNCTION HOSPITAL, 2050 West Southern Avenue, Apache Junction, Zip 85120–7305; tel. 480/223–3200), (Nonreporting) **A**1 9 10
Primary Contact: Brent A. Cope, Chief Executive Officer
Web address: www.myarmc.com
**Control:** Partnership, Investor–owned, for–profit **Service:** General Medical and Surgical

**Staffed Beds:** 103

☐ **ARIZONA SPINE AND JOINT HOSPITAL (30107)**, 4620 East Baseline Road, Zip 85206; tel. 480/832–4770, (Nonreporting) **A**1 9 10 **S** National Surgical Hospitals, Chicago, IL
Primary Contact: Kristi McShay, Chief Executive Officer
CFO: Brian Ebright, Chief Financial Officer
CHR: Lisa Garrett, Director Human Resources
Web address: www.azspineandjoint.com
**Control:** Corporation, Investor–owned, for–profit **Service:** Orthopedic

**Staffed Beds:** 23

---

**Hospital, Medicare Provider Number, Address, Telephone, Approval, Facility, and Physician Codes, Health Care System**

★ American Hospital Association (AHA) membership
☐ The Joint Commission accreditation
◇ DNV Healthcare Inc. accreditation
○ American Osteopathic Association (AOA) accreditation
△ Commission on Accreditation of Rehabilitation Facilities (CARF) accreditation

**AZ**

★ **BANNER BAYWOOD MEDICAL CENTER (30088)**, 6644 East Baywood Avenue, Zip 85206–1797; tel. 480/321–2000 **A**9 10 **F**3 11 13 15 29 30 31 34 36 37 40 45 46 49 51 54 56 57 58 59 60 61 64 68 70 74 75 76 77 78 79 80 81 85 86 87 90 91 92 100 102 104 107 108 110 111 113 114 115 118 125 128 129 131 134 145 146 147 **P**8 **S** Banner Health, Phoenix, AZ
Primary Contact: Laura Robertson, R.N., Chief Executive Officer
CFO: Stanley Adams, Chief Financial Officer
CMO: Larry Spratling, M.D., Chief Medical Officer
CHR: Justina M. Uzzell, Chief Human Resources Officer
Web address: www.bannerhealth.com
**Control:** Other not-for-profit (including NFP Corporation) **Service:** General Medical and Surgical

**Staffed Beds:** 340 **Admissions:** 21066 **Census:** 238 **Outpatient Visits:** 258040 **Births:** 803 **Total Expense ($000):** 239841 **Payroll Expense ($000):** 92237 **Personnel:** 1611

**BANNER CHILDREN'S HOSPITAL** See Cardon Children's Medical Center

⊞ **BANNER DESERT MEDICAL CENTER (30065)**, 1400 South Dobson Road, Zip 85202–9879; tel. 480/412–3000, (Includes CARDON CHILDREN'S MEDICAL CENTER, 1400 South Dobson Road, Zip 85202–4707; tel. 480/412–3000; Rhonda Anderson, R.N., FACHE, Chief Executive Officer; SAMARITAN BEHAVIORAL HEALTH CENTER–DESERT SAMARITAN MEDICAL CENTER, 2225 West Southern Avenue, Zip 85202; tel. 602/464–4000) **A**1 9 10 **F**3 5 11 13 15 18 20 22 24 26 28 29 30 31 32 35 36 38 40 43 44 45 46 47 48 49 51 57 58 59 60 61 64 68 70 72 74 75 76 77 78 79 81 82 84 85 86 87 88 89 92 93 96 107 108 109 111 113 115 116 117 118 120 121 122 125 128 129 131 134 142 143 145 146 147 **S** Banner Health, Phoenix, AZ
Primary Contact: Robert Gould, Chief Executive Officer
CFO: Clifford Loader, Chief Financial Officer
CMO: Marjorie Bessel, M.D., Chief Medical Officer
CIO: Stacey Hinkle, Director Information Technology
CHR: Kevin McVeigh, Chief Human Resources Officer
Web address: www.bannerhealth.com
**Control:** Other not-for-profit (including NFP Corporation) **Service:** General Medical and Surgical

**Staffed Beds:** 583 **Admissions:** 37639 **Census:** 406 **Outpatient Visits:** 337213 **Births:** 4916 **Total Expense ($000):** 481923 **Payroll Expense ($000):** 173910 **Personnel:** 2898

★ **BANNER HEART HOSPITAL (30105)**, 6750 East Baywood Avenue, Zip 85206; tel. 480/854–5000 **A**9 10 **F**3 17 18 20 22 24 26 28 29 30 58 75 81 86 87 107 118 125 129 131 134 145 146 147 **S** Banner Health, Phoenix, AZ
Primary Contact: Laura Robertson, R.N., Chief Executive Officer
CFO: Stanley Adams, Chief Financial Officer
CMO: Mark Starling, M.D., Chief Medical Officer
CIO: Michael S. Warden, Senior Vice President and Chief Information Officer
CHR: Justina M. Uzzell, Chief People Resources Officer
Web address: www.bannerhealth.com
**Control:** Other not-for-profit (including NFP Corporation) **Service:** Heart

**Staffed Beds:** 111 **Admissions:** 5874 **Census:** 61 **Outpatient Visits:** 41364 **Births:** 0 **Total Expense ($000):** 103988 **Payroll Expense ($000):** 28640 **Personnel:** 434

⊞ **HEALTHSOUTH EAST VALLEY REHABILITATION HOSPITAL (33037)**, 5652 East Baseline Road, Zip 85206–4713; tel. 480/567–0350, (Nonreporting) **A**1 9 10 **S** HEALTHSOUTH Corporation, Birmingham, AL
Primary Contact: Timothy T. Poore, Chief Executive Officer
Web address: www.healthsoesteastvalley.com
**Control:** Corporation, Investor–owned, for–profit **Service:** Rehabilitation

**Staffed Beds:** 40

**MOUNTAIN VISTA MEDICAL CENTER (30121)**, 1301 South Crismon Road, Zip 85208; tel. 480/358–6100, (Nonreporting) **A**9 10 21 **S** IASIS Healthcare, Franklin, TN
Primary Contact: Anthony Marinello, Chief Executive Officer
Web address: www.mvmedicalcenter.com
**Control:** Corporation, Investor–owned, for–profit **Service:** General Medical and Surgical

**Staffed Beds:** 172

**PROMISE HOSPITAL OF PHOENIX (32006)**, 433 East 6th Street, Zip 85203–7104; tel. 480/427–3000, (Nonreporting) **A**9 10 **S** Promise Healthcare, Boca Raton, FL
Primary Contact: Scott Floden, Chief Executive Officer
COO: Wendy Larson, Chief Clinical Officer
CFO: Theo Clark, Director Financial Services
CMO: Syed Shahryar, M.D., Medical Director
CHR: Christie Brea, Manager Human Resources
Web address: www.promise-phoenix.com
**Control:** Corporation, Investor–owned, for–profit **Service:** Long–Term Acute Care hospital

**Staffed Beds:** 40

**SAMARITAN BEHAVIORAL HEALTH CENTER–DESERT SAMARITAN MEDICAL CENTER** See Banner Desert Medical Center

**TRILLIUM SPECIALTY HOSPITAL–EAST VALLEY (32007)**, 215 South Power Road, Zip 85206–5235; tel. 480/985–6992, (Nonreporting) **A**10
**S** AcuityHealthcare, LP, Charlotte, NC
Primary Contact: Kevin Nicholson, Chief Executive Officer
Web address: www.trilliumhospital.net
**Control:** Corporation, Investor–owned, for–profit **Service:** Long–Term Acute Care hospital

**Staffed Beds:** 60

### NOGALES—Santa Cruz County

⊞ **CARONDELET HOLY CROSS HOSPITAL (31313)**, 1171 West Target Range Road, Zip 85621–2496; tel. 520/285–3000, (Total facility includes 31 beds in nursing home–type unit) **A**1 9 10 18 **F**11 13 29 30 32 35 40 50 51 56 57 59 60 63 64 68 70 75 76 77 79 81 84 86 87 89 93 102 107 111 118 127 129 131 132 133 134 145 **S** Ascension Health, Saint Louis, MO
Primary Contact: Debbie Knapheide, MSN, Site Administrator, Chief Nursing Officer and Chief Operating Officer
COO: Debbie Knapheide, MSN, Site Administrator, Chief Nursing Officer and Chief Operating Officer
CFO: Alan Strauss, Chief Financial Officer
CMO: Roy Farrell, M.D., Chief Medical Officer
CIO: Tony Fonze, Chief Information Officer
CHR: Daisy Jenkins, Vice President Human Resources
CNO: Debbie Knapheide, MSN, Site Administrator, Chief Nursing Officer and Chief Operating Officer
Web address: www.carondelet.org
**Control:** Church–operated, Nongovernment, not–for profit **Service:** General Medical and Surgical

**Staffed Beds:** 56 **Admissions:** 1481 **Census:** 39 **Outpatient Visits:** 37895 **Births:** 805 **Total Expense ($000):** 25631 **Payroll Expense ($000):** 10648 **Personnel:** 146

### ORO VALLEY—Pima County

⊞ **ORO VALLEY HOSPITAL (30114)**, 1551 East Tangerine Road, Zip 85737; tel. 520/901–3500 **A**1 9 10 **F**3 15 17 18 20 22 26 29 30 34 35 40 48 49 50 51 59 60 70 74 79 81 85 87 90 91 93 107 108 110 111 113 114 118 128 143 145 146 **S** Community Health Systems, Inc., Franklin, TN
Primary Contact: Jae Dale, Chief Executive Officer
COO: Kirkpatrick Conley, Assistant Chief Executive Officer
CFO: Mark Hoffman, Chief Financial Officer
CMO: Paul Bejarino, M.D., Chief of Staff
Web address: www.nmcorovalley.com
**Control:** Corporation, Investor–owned, for–profit **Service:** General Medical and Surgical

**Staffed Beds:** 144 **Admissions:** 4967 **Census:** 53 **Outpatient Visits:** 135984 **Births:** 0 **Total Expense ($000):** 69604 **Payroll Expense ($000):** 35016 **Personnel:** 446

### PAGE—Coconino County

⊞ **PAGE HOSPITAL (31304)**, 501 North Navajo Drive, Zip 86040, Mailing Address: P.O. Box 1447, Zip 86040–1447; tel. 928/645–2424 **A**1 9 10 18 **F**3 8 11 13 15 29 30 31 34 35 36 39 40 43 45 57 59 64 68 75 76 77 79 81 82 85 86 87 93 107 111 113 118 128 129 132 134 145 147 **S** Banner Health, Phoenix, AZ
Primary Contact: Sandy Haryasz, R.N., Chief Executive Officer
Web address: www.bannerhealth.com
**Control:** Other not-for-profit (including NFP Corporation) **Service:** General Medical and Surgical

**Staffed Beds:** 25 **Admissions:** 524 **Census:** 3 **Outpatient Visits:** 40150 **Births:** 232 **Total Expense ($000):** 14022 **Payroll Expense ($000):** 5916 **Personnel:** 108

### PARKER—La Paz County

○ **LA PAZ REGIONAL HOSPITAL (30067)**, 1200 West Mohave Road, Zip 85344–6349; tel. 928/669–9201 **A**9 10 11 20 **F**3 11 15 18 20 28 29 30 31 34 40 54 57 59 64 66 68 70 79 81 85 91 93 107 110 111 114 118 126 129 134 143 145 147
Primary Contact: M. Victoria Clark, Chief Executive Officer
CFO: James Ehasz, Chief Financial Officer
CMO: Melinda Astran, M.D., Chief of Staff
CHR: Regina M. Martinez, Director Human Resources
Web address: www.lapazhospital.org
**Control:** Other not-for-profit (including NFP Corporation) **Service:** General Medical and Surgical

**Staffed Beds:** 39 **Admissions:** 843 **Census:** 8 **Outpatient Visits:** 20356 **Births:** 0 **Total Expense ($000):** 18455 **Payroll Expense ($000):** 8233 **Personnel:** 169

⊠ **U. S. PUBLIC HEALTH SERVICE INDIAN HOSPITAL (31307)**, 12033 Agency Road, Zip 85344–7718; tel. 928/669–2137, (Nonreporting) **A**1 10 18 **S** U. S. Indian Health Service, Rockville, MD
Primary Contact: Dee Hutchison, Acting Chief Executive Officer
CFO: Robin Tahbo, Financial Management Officer
CMO: Laurence Norick, M.D., Clinical Director
CIO: JayLynn Saavedra, Chief Information Officer
Web address: www.ihs.gov
**Control:** Public Health Service, Government, federal **Service:** General Medical and Surgical

**Staffed Beds:** 20

### PAYSON—Gila County

⊠ **PAYSON REGIONAL MEDICAL CENTER (30033)**, 807 South Ponderosa Street, Zip 85541–5599; tel. 928/474–3222 **A**1 9 10 20 **F**13 15 18 29 30 35 37 40 51 70 75 76 77 78 79 81 82 85 86 87 91 93 96 97 107 110 111 113 118 131 145 146 147 **P**6 **S** Community Health Systems, Inc., Franklin, TN
Primary Contact: R. Chris Wolf, Chief Executive Officer
CFO: Peter Finelli, Chief Financial Officer
CMO: John Vandruff, M.D., Chief of Staff
CIO: Ross Skinner, Director Information Systems
CHR: Shawn M. Thomas, Director Human Resources
Web address: www.paysonhospital.com
**Control:** Corporation, Investor–owned, for–profit **Service:** General Medical and Surgical

**Staffed Beds:** 44 **Admissions:** 2467 **Census:** 18 **Births:** 162 **Total Expense ($000):** 39592 **Payroll Expense ($000):** 19167 **Personnel:** 297

### PEORIA—Maricopa County

**KINDRED HOSPITAL ARIZONA–NORTHWEST PHOENIX** See Kindred Hospital Arizona–Phoenix, Phoenix

### PHOENIX—Maricopa County

☐ **ARIZONA STATE HOSPITAL (34021)**, 2500 East Van Buren Street, Zip 85008–6079; tel. 602/244–1331 **A**1 10 **F**3 29 30 39 53 57 59 65 68 75 77 94 98 129 134 142 **P**6
Primary Contact: Ann M. Froio, Interim Chief Executive Officer
COO: Donna Noriega, Chief Operating Officer
CFO: Donna Noriega, Chief Operating Officer
CMO: Steve Dingle, M.D., Chief Medical Officer
CIO: Bruce Randolph, Chief Information Technology
CHR: Jeanine Decker, Manager Human Resources
Web address: www.hs.state.az.us
**Control:** State–Government, nonfederal **Service:** Psychiatric

**Staffed Beds:** 338 **Admissions:** 94 **Census:** 238 **Outpatient Visits:** 0 **Births:** 0 **Total Expense ($000):** 54776 **Payroll Expense ($000):** 27004 **Personnel:** 540

★ **BANNER ESTRELLA MEDICAL CENTER (30115)**, 9201 West Thomas Road, Zip 85037–3332; tel. 623/327–4000 **A**9 10 **F**3 17 18 20 22 24 26 28 29 30 31 36 40 43 46 48 49 51 60 68 70 72 76 78 79 81 85 92 107 108 111 113 114 117 118 125 129 144 145 147 **S** Banner Health, Phoenix, AZ
Primary Contact: Debra J. Krmpotic, R.N., Chief Executive Officer
COO: Gary Foster, R.N., Assistant Administrator
CFO: Patty Rhoden, Chief Financial Officer
CMO: Kenneth Welch, M.D., Chief Medical Officer
CHR: Dina Steinberg, Chief People Resources Officer
CNO: Nancy Adamson, R.N., Chief Nursing Officer
Web address: www.bannerhealth.com
**Control:** Other not–for–profit (including NFP Corporation) **Service:** General Medical and Surgical

**Staffed Beds:** 214 **Admissions:** 18739 **Census:** 176 **Outpatient Visits:** 191191 **Births:** 3725 **Total Expense ($000):** 202524 **Payroll Expense ($000):** 79471 **Personnel:** 1303

⊠ **BANNER GOOD SAMARITAN MEDICAL CENTER (30002)**, 1111 East McDowell Road, Zip 85006–2666, Mailing Address: P.O. Box 2989, Zip 85062–2989; tel. 602/239–2000 **A**1 2 3 5 8 9 10 **F**3 8 11 13 15 17 18 20 22 24 26 28 29 30 31 34 35 36 37 40 43 44 45 46 47 48 49 50 51 52 53 55 56 57 58 59 60 61 62 63 64 65 66 68 70 74 75 76 77 78 79 81 82 83 84 85 86 87 90 91 92 93 94 96 97 98 100 101 102 103 104 105 107 108 109 110 111 112 113 114 115 116 117 118 119 120 122 123 125 128 129 131 133 137 138 140 141 145 146 147 **S** Banner Health, Phoenix, AZ
Primary Contact: Larry E. Volkmar, Chief Executive Officer
CFO: Kathy Kotin, Chief Financial Officer
CMO: Paul Stander, M.D., Chief Medical Officer
CIO: Michael S. Warden, Senior Vice President Information Technology
CHR: Michael Fleming, Chief People Officer
Web address: www.bannerhealth.com
**Control:** Other not–for–profit (including NFP Corporation) **Service:** General Medical and Surgical

**Staffed Beds:** 640 **Admissions:** 38320 **Census:** 501 **Outpatient Visits:** 396121 **Births:** 5348 **Total Expense ($000):** 616553 **Payroll Expense ($000):** 240432 **Personnel:** 3882

**HAVEN SENIOR HORIZONS (34020)**, 1201 South 7th Avenue, Suite 200, Zip 85007–4076; tel. 623/236–2000, (Nonreporting) **S** Haven Behavioral Healthcare, Nashville, TN
Primary Contact: Kathy Shaw, Chief Executive Officer
CHR: Erin McEldowney, Manager Human Resources
CNO: Char Ralstin, Director of Nursing
Web address: www.havenbehavioral.com
**Control:** Corporation, Investor–owned, for–profit **Service:** Psychiatric

**Staffed Beds:** 30

★ ○ **JOHN C. LINCOLN DEER VALLEY HOSPITAL (30092)**, 19829 North 27th Avenue, Zip 85027–4002; tel. 623/879–6100 **A**9 10 11 **F**3 8 15 17 18 20 22 24 26 28 29 30 31 34 35 40 41 43 44 45 46 47 48 49 50 54 57 58 59 60 64 68 70 74 75 77 78 79 81 85 89 92 107 108 110 111 113 114 118 129 131 134 144 145 146 147 **S** John C. Lincoln Health Network, Phoenix, AZ
Primary Contact: Bruce Pearson, FACHE, Executive Vice President and Chief Executive Officer
CFO: David Lamparter, Senior Vice President and Chief Financial Officer
CMO: Mary Ann Turley, D.O., Medical Director
CHR: Frank L. Cummins, Vice President Human Resources
Web address: www.jcl.com
**Control:** Other not–for–profit (including NFP Corporation) **Service:** General Medical and Surgical

**Staffed Beds:** 204 **Admissions:** 12208 **Census:** 123 **Outpatient Visits:** 110116 **Births:** 0 **Total Expense ($000):** 173970 **Payroll Expense ($000):** 71413 **Personnel:** 1146

★ **JOHN C. LINCOLN NORTH MOUNTAIN HOSPITAL (30014)**, 250 East Dunlap Avenue, Zip 85020–2446; tel. 602/943–2381 **A**9 10 **F**2 3 11 15 17 18 20 22 24 26 28 29 30 31 34 35 36 37 40 43 44 45 46 47 48 49 50 53 54 56 57 58 59 60 64 68 70 74 75 76 77 78 79 81 85 89 92 97 103 107 108 111 113 114 118 125 129 131 134 143 144 145 146 147 **S** John C. Lincoln Health Network, Phoenix, AZ
Primary Contact: Bruce Pearson, FACHE, Executive Vice President and Chief Executive Officer
CFO: David Lamparter, Senior Vice President and Chief Financial Officer
CMO: Christopher Shearer, M.D., Chief Medical Officer
CIO: Robert Slepin, Vice President and Chief Information Officer
CHR: Frank L. Cummins, Vice President Human Resources
CNO: Maggi Griffin, Vice President and Chief Nursing Officer
Web address: www.jcl.com
**Control:** Other not–for–profit (including NFP Corporation) **Service:** General Medical and Surgical

**Staffed Beds:** 256 **Admissions:** 16152 **Census:** 191 **Outpatient Visits:** 101622 **Births:** 115 **Total Expense ($000):** 241935 **Payroll Expense ($000):** 98671 **Personnel:** 1867

⊠ **KINDRED HOSPITAL ARIZONA–PHOENIX (32000)**, 40 East Indianola Avenue, Zip 85012–2059; tel. 602/280–7000, (Includes KINDRED HOSPITAL ARIZONA–NORTHWEST PHOENIX, 13216 North Plaza Del Rio Boulevard, Peoria, Zip 85381–4907; tel. 623/974–5463; Karen Shammas, Chief Executive Officer; KINDRED HOSPITAL ARIZONA–SCOTTSDALE, 11250 North 92nd Street, Scottsdale, Zip 85260; tel. 480/391–4040; Heidi Miller, Market Chief Executive Officer), (Nonreporting) **A**1 9 10 **S** Kindred Healthcare, Louisville, KY
Primary Contact: Rachelle Spencer, Administrator
Web address: www.khphoenix.com/
**Control:** Corporation, Investor–owned, for–profit **Service:** Long–Term Acute Care hospital

**Staffed Beds:** 166

---

**Hospital, Medicare Provider Number, Address, Telephone, Approval, Facility, and Physician Codes, Health Care System**

★ American Hospital Association (AHA) membership
☐ The Joint Commission accreditation   ◇ DNV Healthcare Inc. accreditation
○ American Osteopathic Association (AOA) accreditation
△ Commission on Accreditation of Rehabilitation Facilities (CARF) accreditation

© 2012 AHA Guide    *Many Facility Codes have changed. Please refer to the AHA Guide Code Chart.*    Hospitals **A35**

**AZ**

**LOS NINOS HOSPITAL (33301)**, 2303 East Thomas Road, Zip 85016;
tel. 602/954–7311, (Nonreporting) **A**9 10
Primary Contact: William Timmons, Chief Executive Officer
Web address: www.losninoshospital.com
**Control:** Other not–for–profit (including NFP Corporation) **Service:** Other specialty

**Staffed Beds:** 15

★ **MARICOPA INTEGRATED HEALTH SYSTEM (30022)**, 2601 East Roosevelt
Street, Zip 85008–4956; tel. 602/344–5011, (Includes ARIZONA CHILDREN'S
CENTER, 2601 East Roosevelt Street, Zip 85008–4973; tel. 602/344–5051),
(Nonreporting) **A**3 5 8 9 10 21
Primary Contact: Betsey Bayless, President and Chief Executive Officer
COO: William F. Vanaskie, Executive Vice President and Chief Operating Officer
CMO: Robert Fromm, M.D., Senior Vice President and Chief Medical Officer
CIO: Dave Kempson, Chief Information Officer
CHR: Marshall Jones, Senior Vice President Human Resources
Web address: www.mihs.org
**Control:** County–Government, nonfederal **Service:** General Medical and Surgical

**Staffed Beds:** 578

☐ **MARYVALE HOSPITAL MEDICAL CENTER (30001)**, 5102 West Campbell
Avenue, Zip 85031–1799; tel. 623/848–5000 **A**1 9 10 **F**3 13 18 20 22 26 29
34 35 40 45 49 59 68 70 73 74 75 76 81 85 86 107 108 111 129 145
**S** Vanguard Health System, Nashville, TN
Primary Contact: Crystal Hamilton, R.N., Chief Executive Officer
CFO: Julie Hastings–Smith, Chief Financial Officer
CHR: Erin Gonzalez, Director Human Resources and Education
CNO: Scott Morey, Chief Nursing Officer
Web address: www.maryvalehospital.com
**Control:** Corporation, Investor–owned, for–profit **Service:** General Medical and
Surgical

**Staffed Beds:** 100 **Admissions:** 6072 **Census:** 55 **Outpatient Visits:** 53867
**Total Expense ($000):** 57661 **Payroll Expense ($000):** 30214 **Personnel:**
459

☒ **MAYO CLINIC HOSPITAL (30103)**, 5777 East Mayo Boulevard,
Zip 85054–4502; tel. 480/515–6296 **A**1 2 3 5 8 9 10 **F**3 6 8 9 12 15 17 18
20 22 24 26 28 29 30 31 34 35 36 37 39 40 45 46 47 48 49 50 51 54 55
56 58 59 60 61 64 68 70 74 75 77 78 79 80 81 82 84 85 86 87 90 92 93
96 97 100 103 104 107 108 110 111 112 113 114 115 116 117 118 119
120 122 123 125 128 129 130 131 134 135 136 137 138 140 141 144 145
146 147 **P**6 **S** Mayo Clinic Health System, Rochester, MN
Primary Contact: Ann M. Meyers, Chief Executive Officer
COO: Kevin Paige, Chief Operations Officer
CFO: Jeffrey R. Froisland, Chief Financial Officer
CMO: Jeff T. Mueller, M.D., Medical Director
CIO: John Cranmer, Chief Information Officer
CHR: Jamie Schmitgen, Chair Human Resources
CNO: Teresa Connolly, MSN, Chief Nursing Officer
Web address: www.mayoclinic.org/arizona/
**Control:** Other not–for–profit (including NFP Corporation) **Service:** General
Medical and Surgical

**Staffed Beds:** 244 **Admissions:** 12465 **Census:** 177 **Outpatient Visits:**
39386 **Births:** 0 **Total Expense ($000):** 350065 **Payroll Expense ($000):**
105703 **Personnel:** 3525

☐ **PARADISE VALLEY HOSPITAL (30083)**, 3929 East Bell Road,
Zip 85032–2196; tel. 602/923–5000, (Nonreporting) **A**1 9 10 **S** Vanguard Health
System, Nashville, TN
Primary Contact: Shawn G. Strash, Chief Executive Officer
COO: Sue Piarulli, Administrative Director Operations
CFO: Denise Chamberlain, Chief Financial Officer
CMO: David Tupponce, M.D., Chief Medical Officer
CHR: Michelle Wilkerson, Director Human Resources
CNO: Chris McConaughy, Chief Nursing Officer
Web address: www.paradisevalleyhospital.com
**Control:** Corporation, Investor–owned, for–profit **Service:** General Medical and
Surgical

**Staffed Beds:** 142

☒ **PHOENIX BAPTIST HOSPITAL (30030)**, 2000 West Bethany Home Road,
Zip 85015–2443; tel. 602/249–0212, (Includes ARIZONA HEART HOSPITAL,
1930 East Thomas Road, Zip 85016; tel. 602/532–1000; Jeffrey A. Ashin, Chief
Executive Officer), (Nonreporting) **A**1 3 5 9 10 **S** Vanguard Health System,
Nashville, TN
Primary Contact: Wayne Gillis, Interim Chief Executive Officer
COO: Wayne Gillis, Chief Operating Officer
CFO: Alan Germany, Chief Financial Officer
CMO: William Ellert, M.D., Chief Medical Officer
CHR: Julia Doucette, Director Human Resources
Web address: www.phoenixbaptisthospital.com
**Control:** Corporation, Investor–owned, for–profit **Service:** General Medical and
Surgical

**Staffed Beds:** 215

☒ **PHOENIX CHILDREN'S HOSPITAL (33302)**, 1919 East Thomas Road,
Zip 85016; tel. 602/546–1000 **A**1 3 5 8 9 10 **F**3 8 11 17 19 21 23 25 27 29
30 31 32 34 35 38 39 40 41 42 43 44 46 48 49 50 54 55 57 58 59 60 61
64 65 66 68 71 72 73 74 75 77 78 79 81 82 84 85 86 87 88 89 91 92 93
94 96 97 98 99 100 101 102 104 105 107 108 111 113 114 115 116 117
118 128 129 130 131 133 135 137 143 145 147 **P**6
Primary Contact: Robert L. Meyer, President and Chief Executive Officer
COO: Betsy Kuzas, Executive Vice President and Chief Operating Officer
CFO: Craig L. McKnight, Senior Vice President and Chief Financial Officer
CMO: Murray Pollack, M.D., Vice President and Chief Medical Officer
CIO: David Higginson, Senior Vice President and Chief Information Officer
CHR: Thomas Diederich, Senior Vice President Human Resources
CNO: Pam Carlson, Senior Vice President and Chief Nursing Officer
Web address: www.phoenixchildrens.com
**Control:** Other not–for–profit (including NFP Corporation) **Service:** Children's
general

**Staffed Beds:** 425 **Admissions:** 13404 **Census:** 224 **Outpatient Visits:**
178749 **Births:** 0 **Total Expense ($000):** 508968 **Payroll Expense ($000):**
217284 **Personnel:** 2884

☒ △ **PHOENIX VETERANS AFFAIRS HEALTH CARE SYSTEM**, 650 East Indian
School Road, Zip 85012–1892; tel. 602/277–5551, (Nonreporting) **A**1 2 5 7 9
**S** Department of Veterans Affairs, Washington, DC
Primary Contact: James Robbins, M.D., Director
CFO: Christine Hollingsworth, Chief Financial Officer
CMO: Raymond Chung, M.D., Chief of Staff
Web address: www.phoenix.med.va.gov
**Control:** Veterans Affairs, Government, federal **Service:** General Medical and
Surgical

**Staffed Beds:** 197

☒ **SELECT SPECIALTY HOSPITAL–PHOENIX (32001)**, 350 West Thomas Road,
Zip 85013; tel. 602/406–6802, (Nonreporting) **A**1 9 10 **S** Select Medical
Corporation, Mechanicsburg, PA
Primary Contact: Nancy L. Burton, Chief Executive Officer
Web address: www.selectmedicalcorp.com
**Control:** Corporation, Investor–owned, for–profit **Service:** Long–Term Acute Care
hospital

**Staffed Beds:** 48

**SELECT SPECIALTY HOSPITAL–PHOENIX DOWNTOWN** See Select Specialty
Hospital–Scottsdale, Scottsdale

☒ △ **ST. JOSEPH'S HOSPITAL AND MEDICAL CENTER (30024)**, 350 West
Thomas Road, Zip 85013–4496, Mailing Address: P.O. Box 2071,
Zip 85001–2071; tel. 602/406–3000, (Includes CHILDREN'S HEALTH CENTER,
350 West Thomas Road, Zip 85013–4409) **A**1 2 3 5 7 8 9 10 **F**3 6 11 13 15
17 18 19 20 21 22 24 25 26 27 28 29 30 31 34 35 39 40 41 43 45 46 47
48 49 51 53 55 56 57 58 59 64 66 68 70 71 72 73 74 75 76 77 78 79 81
82 84 85 86 87 88 89 90 91 92 93 96 97 100 102 103 104 107 108 110
111 112 113 114 116 117 118 120 122 123 125 129 130 131 133 134 136
139 140 145 146 147 **P**5 6 **S** Dignity Health, San Francisco, CA
Primary Contact: Linda A. Hunt, President
CFO: John Peters, Chief Financial Officer
CHR: Maureen Sterbach, Vice President Human Resources
Web address: www.stjosephs–phx.org
**Control:** Church–operated, Nongovernment, not–for profit **Service:** General
Medical and Surgical

**Staffed Beds:** 697 **Admissions:** 38257 **Census:** 500 **Outpatient Visits:**
470714 **Births:** 4592 **Total Expense ($000):** 884562 **Payroll Expense
($000):** 379592 **Personnel:** 4445

☐ **ST. LUKE'S BEHAVIORAL HEALTH CENTER (34013)**, 1800 East Van Buren,
Zip 85006–3742; tel. 602/251–8546, (Nonreporting) **A**1 9 10 21 **S** IASIS
Healthcare, Franklin, TN
Primary Contact: Gregory L. Jahn, R.N., Chief Executive Officer
CFO: Ruby Majhail, Chief Financial Officer
CMO: Mario Tafur, M.D., Chief of Staff
CIO: Chris Ulrey, Director Management Information Systems
CHR: Amy M. Howell, Director Human Resources
Web address: www.iasishealthcare.com
**Control:** Corporation, Investor–owned, for–profit **Service:** Psychiatric

**Staffed Beds:** 85

★ **ST. LUKE'S MEDICAL CENTER (30037)**, 1800 East Van Buren Street,
Zip 85006–3742; tel. 602/251–8100, (Includes TEMPE ST. LUKE'S HOSPITAL,
1500 South Mill Avenue, Tempe, Zip 85281–6699; tel. 480/784–5510; Dale
Larson, Administrator), (Nonreporting) **A**9 10 21 **S** IASIS Healthcare, Franklin, TN
Primary Contact: Edward W. Myers, Chief Executive Officer
CFO: Ken Walsh, Chief Financial Officer
CHR: Trinise Thompson, Director Human Resources
Web address: www.stlukesmedcenter.com
**Control:** Corporation, Investor–owned, for–profit **Service:** General Medical and
Surgical

**Staffed Beds:** 225

☐ **SURGICAL SPECIALTY HOSPITAL OF ARIZONA (30108)**, 6501 North 19th Avenue, Zip 85015; tel. 602/795–6020 **A**1 9 10 **F**12 29 45 49 70 79 81 107 111 113 **P**2
Primary Contact: Constance A. Harmsen, Ph.D., R.N., MS, FACHE, Chief Executive Officer
CFO: Greg Brink, Chief Financial Officer
CMO: Christopher A. Yeung, M.D., Chief of Staff
CHR: Deby Tooker, Director Human Resources
CNO: Karen Bonamase, R.N., Chief Nursing Officer
Web address: www.sshaz.com
**Control:** Corporation, Investor–owned, for–profit **Service:** Surgical

> **Staffed Beds:** 33 **Admissions:** 1578 **Census:** 7 **Outpatient Visits:** 1018 **Births:** 0 **Total Expense ($000):** 21714 **Payroll Expense ($000):** 6188 **Personnel:** 106

⊠ **U. S. PUBLIC HEALTH SERVICE PHOENIX INDIAN MEDICAL CENTER (30078)**, 4212 North 16th Street, Zip 85016–5389; tel. 602/263–1200, (Nonreporting) **A**1 5 9 10 **S** U. S. Indian Health Service, Rockville, MD
Primary Contact: John Molina, Chief Executive Officer
CFO: Geraldine Harney, Chief Financial Officer
CMO: Dave Civic, M.D., Associate Director Clinical Services
CIO: Vina Montour, Director Information Technology
CHR: Betty Weston, Chief Human Resources Officer
Web address: www.ihs.gov
**Control:** PHS, Indian Service, Government, federal **Service:** General Medical and Surgical

> **Staffed Beds:** 127

**VALLEY HOSPITAL PHOENIX (34026)**, 3550 East Pinchot Avenue, Zip 85018–7434; tel. 602/957–4000, (Nonreporting) **A**10 **S** Ascend Health Corporation, New York, NY
Primary Contact: Kim Whitelock, Chief Executive Officer
Web address: www.valleyhospital–phoenix.com
**Control:** Corporation, Investor–owned, for–profit **Service:** Psychiatric

> **Staffed Beds:** 122

### PRESCOTT—Yavapai County

⊠ **NORTHERN ARIZONA VA HEALTH CARE SYSTEM**, 500 Highway 89 North, Zip 86313–5000; tel. 928/445–4860 **A**1 9 **F**1 2 3 4 5 8 11 12 18 29 30 34 35 38 39 40 43 44 45 46 50 53 54 56 57 59 61 62 63 64 65 66 68 71 75 79 80 81 82 83 84 86 87 90 92 93 94 97 98 100 101 102 103 104 105 106 107 111 118 126 127 129 131 134 142 143 144 145 146 147 **S** Department of Veterans Affairs, Washington, DC
Primary Contact: Donna K. Jacobs, FACHE, Director
COO: James Belmont, Associate Director
CFO: Ame Callahan, Acting Manager Resource Management Service
CMO: A. Panneer Selvam, M.D., Chief of Staff
CIO: Scott McCrimmon, Manager Information Technology
CHR: Jane Lewerke, Manager Human Resources
CNO: Marianne Locke, R.N., Associate Director Patient Care Services
Web address: www.va.gov/sta/guide/home.asp
**Control:** Veterans Affairs, Government, federal **Service:** General Medical and Surgical

> **Staffed Beds:** 137 **Admissions:** 1575 **Census:** 19 **Outpatient Visits:** 276148 **Personnel:** 976

★ **YAVAPAI REGIONAL MEDICAL CENTER (30012)**, 1003 Willow Creek Road, Zip 86301–1668; tel. 928/445–2700 **A**9 10 **F**8 11 13 14 15 17 18 24 28 29 30 32 34 35 36 42 45 46 50 53 54 57 59 60 62 64 68 70 74 75 77 79 81 82 84 85 86 87 93 107 108 111 113 115 116 117 118 129 130 131 134 142 145 146 147 **P**5 7
Primary Contact: Timothy Barnett, President and Chief Executive Officer
COO: Larry P. Burns, Jr., Chief Operating Officer
CFO: Brian Hoefle, Chief Financial Officer
CMO: Joseph Goldberger, M.D., Chief Medical Officer
CIO: Randy Rahman, Chief Information Officer
CHR: Mark Timm, Director Human Resources
CNO: Diane Drexler, R.N., Chief Nursing Officer
Web address: www.yrmc.org
**Control:** Other not–for–profit (including NFP Corporation) **Service:** General Medical and Surgical

> **Staffed Beds:** 134 **Admissions:** 6916 **Census:** 67 **Outpatient Visits:** 83526 **Births:** 0 **Total Expense ($000):** 139068 **Payroll Expense ($000):** 60638 **Personnel:** 1002

### PRESCOTT VALLEY—Yavapai County

☐ **MOUNTAIN VALLEY REGIONAL REHABILITATION HOSPITAL (33036)**, 3700 North Windsong Drive, Zip 86314; tel. 928/759–8800, (Nonreporting) **A**1 9 10 **S** Ernest Health, Inc., Albuquerque, NM
Primary Contact: Jennifer Roel, Chief Executive Officer
Web address: www.mvrrh.ernesthealth.com
**Control:** Corporation, Investor–owned, for–profit **Service:** Rehabilitation

> **Staffed Beds:** 16

★ **YAVAPAI REGIONAL MEDICAL CENTER – EAST (30118)**, 7700 East Florentine Road, Zip 86314; tel. 928/445–2700 **A**9 10 **F**8 11 13 14 15 20 24 28 29 30 31 34 35 36 40 42 45 46 50 53 54 57 59 60 62 63 64 68 70 73 74 75 76 77 78 79 81 82 84 85 86 87 89 93 107 108 111 113 115 116 117 118 129 130 131 134 142 145 147 **P**7
Primary Contact: Timothy Barnett, Chief Executive Officer
COO: John Amos, COO East Campus
CFO: Brian Hoefle, Chief Financial Officer
CMO: Joseph Goldberger, M.D., Chief Medical Officer
CIO: Randy Rahman, Chief Information Officer
CHR: Mark Timm, Director Human Resources
CNO: Diane Drexler, R.N., Chief Nursing Officer
Web address: www.yrmc.org
**Control:** Other not–for–profit (including NFP Corporation) **Service:** General Medical and Surgical

> **Staffed Beds:** 72 **Admissions:** 4086 **Census:** 29 **Outpatient Visits:** 45215 **Births:** 993 **Total Expense ($000):** 42021 **Payroll Expense ($000):** 24025 **Personnel:** 400

### SACATON—Pinal County

⊠ **HUHUKAM MEMORIAL HOSPITAL (31308)**, 483 West Seed Farm Road, Zip 85147, Mailing Address: P.O. Box 38, Zip 85147–0001; tel. 602/528–1200 **A**1 9 10 18 **F**3 4 5 7 12 15 18 29 32 34 35 36 38 39 40 50 52 53 54 56 57 58 59 60 61 64 65 68 69 71 75 79 82 87 93 94 97 99 100 101 102 103 104 105 118 126 127 129 130 131 133 134 142 146 147
Primary Contact: Amish Purohit, Chief Executive Officer
COO: Pamela Thompson, Chief Operations Officer
CFO: Elisa Banigan, Chief Financial Officer
CMO: Noel Habib, M.D., Chief Medical Officer
CHR: Michael Freeman, Director Human Resources
Web address: www.grhc.org
**Control:** Other not–for–profit (including NFP Corporation) **Service:** General Medical and Surgical

> **Staffed Beds:** 15 **Admissions:** 58 **Census:** 1 **Outpatient Visits:** 365345 **Births:** 0 **Personnel:** 869

### SAFFORD—Graham County

★ **MT. GRAHAM REGIONAL MEDICAL CENTER (30068)**, 1600 20th Avenue, Zip 85546–4097; tel. 928/348–4000 **A**9 10 20 **F**3 11 13 15 29 31 34 35 40 45 46 53 54 57 58 59 62 63 64 65 68 70 75 76 78 79 81 83 84 85 87 93 107 108 110 111 114 115 118 128 129 131 132 133 134 140 145 **P**5
Primary Contact: Patrick Peters, Chief Executive Officer
CFO: Keith Bryce, Chief Financial Officer
CIO: Keith Bryce, Chief Financial Officer
CHR: Wick Lewis, Vice President Human Resources and Clinic Management
Web address: www.mtgraham.org
**Control:** Other not–for–profit (including NFP Corporation) **Service:** General Medical and Surgical

> **Staffed Beds:** 49 **Admissions:** 2088 **Census:** 20 **Outpatient Visits:** 91123 **Births:** 594 **Total Expense ($000):** 51626 **Payroll Expense ($000):** 23803

### SAN CARLOS—Gila County

⊠ **U. S. PUBLIC HEALTH SERVICE INDIAN HOSPITAL (30077)**, Zip 85550; tel. 928/475–2371, (Nonreporting) **A**1 10 **S** U. S. Indian Health Service, Rockville, MD
Primary Contact: Nella J. Ben, Chief Executive Officer
COO: Nella J. Ben, Chief Executive Officer
CFO: Vivie Hosteenez, Chief Financial Officer
CMO: Karen Health, M.D., Clinical Director
CIO: Lois Sprengeler Wesley, Director Quality Management
CHR: Shirley M. Boni, Administrative Officer
Web address: www.ihs.gov
**Control:** PHS, Indian Service, Government, federal **Service:** General Medical and Surgical

> **Staffed Beds:** 8

---

**Hospital, Medicare Provider Number, Address, Telephone, Approval, Facility, and Physician Codes, Health Care System**

★ American Hospital Association (AHA) membership
☐ The Joint Commission accreditation   ◇ DNV Healthcare Inc. accreditation
○ American Osteopathic Association (AOA) accreditation
△ Commission on Accreditation of Rehabilitation Facilities (CARF) accreditation

## SAN TAN VALLEY—Pinal County

✠ **BANNER IRONWOOD MEDICAL CENTER (30130)**, 37000 North Gantzel Road, Zip 85140–7303; tel. 480/394–4000, (Nonreporting) **A**1 9 10 **S** Banner Health, Phoenix, AZ
Primary Contact: Julie Nunley, R.N., Chief Executive Officer
CFO: Lori Linder, Chief Financial Officer
CMO: Michael O'Connor, M.D., Chief Medical Officer
CHR: Nancy M. English, Chief Human Resources Officer
CNO: Cathy Townsend, Chief Nursing Officer
Web address: www.bannerhealth.com
**Control:** Other not–for–profit (including NFP Corporation) **Service:** General Medical and Surgical

**Staffed Beds:** 36

## SCOTTSDALE—Maricopa County

✠ **BANNER BEHAVIORAL HEALTH HOSPITAL – SCOTTSDALE (34004)**, 7575 East Earll Drive, Zip 85251–6915; tel. 480/941–7500 **A**1 9 10 **F**4 5 29 30 34 35 38 50 56 64 65 68 75 86 87 98 99 100 101 103 104 105 129 131 133 134 142 145 **P**5 **S** Banner Health, Phoenix, AZ
Primary Contact: Cherie Martin, R.N., MSN, FACHE, Chief Executive Officer
CFO: Michael A. Cimino, Jr., Chief Financial Officer
CMO: Clifford Zeller, M.D., Chief Medical Officer
CHR: Kevin McVeigh, Interim Chief Human Resources Officer
CNO: Cherri Anderson, Chief Nursing Officer
Web address: www.bannerhealth.com
**Control:** Other not–for–profit (including NFP Corporation) **Service:** Psychiatric

**Staffed Beds:** 95 **Admissions:** 4069 **Census:** 83 **Outpatient Visits:** 27851
**Births:** 0 **Total Expense ($000):** 30147 **Payroll Expense ($000):** 16469
**Personnel:** 308

✠ **HEALTHSOUTH SCOTTSDALE REHABILITATION HOSPITAL (33025)**, 9630 East Shea Boulevard, Zip 85260; tel. 480/551–5400, (Nonreporting) **A**1 9 10 **S** HEALTHSOUTH Corporation, Birmingham, AL
Primary Contact: Richard Schulz, Chief Executive Officer
CFO: Lisa Barrick, Controller
CMO: Keith W. Cunningham, M.D., Medical Director
CHR: Mary Beth Giczi, Director Human Resources
CNO: Diane M. Caruso, MSN, Chief Nursing Officer
Web address: www.healthsouthscottsdale.com
**Control:** Corporation, Investor–owned, for–profit **Service:** Rehabilitation

**Staffed Beds:** 60

★ **SCOTTSDALE HEALTHCARE SHEA MEDICAL CENTER (30087)**, 9003 East Shea Boulevard, Zip 85260–6771; tel. 480/323–3000, (Nonreporting) **A**2 3 5 9 10 21 **S** Scottsdale Healthcare, Scottsdale, AZ
Primary Contact: Peggy J. Reiley, Ph.D., MS, R.N., Senior Vice President and Chief Clinical Officer
CFO: Todd La Porte, Senior Vice President and Chief Financial Officer
CMO: James Burke, M.D., Senior Vice President and Chief Medical Officer
CIO: James R. Cramer, Vice President and Chief Information Officer
CHR: Carol Henderson, Senior Vice President and Chief Talent Officer
Web address: www.shc.org
**Control:** Other not–for–profit (including NFP Corporation) **Service:** General Medical and Surgical

**Staffed Beds:** 409

★ **SCOTTSDALE HEALTHCARE THOMPSON PEAK HOSPITAL (30123)**, 7400 East Thompson Peak Parkway, Zip 85255; tel. 480/324–7000, (Nonreporting) **A**9 10 21 **S** Scottsdale Healthcare, Scottsdale, AZ
Primary Contact: Kimberly Post, R.N., Vice President and Administrator
CFO: Todd La Porte, Chief Financial Officer
CMO: James Burke, M.D., Senior Vice President and Chief Medical Officer
CIO: James R. Cramer, Chief Information Officer
CHR: Carol Henderson, Vice President Human Resources
Web address: www.shc.org
**Control:** Other not–for–profit (including NFP Corporation) **Service:** General Medical and Surgical

**Staffed Beds:** 64

★ **SCOTTSDALE HEALTHCARE–OSBORN MEDICAL CENTER (30038)**, 7400 East Osborn Road, Zip 85251–6403; tel. 480/882–4000, (Nonreporting) **A**2 3 5 8 9 10 21 **S** Scottsdale Healthcare, Scottsdale, AZ
Primary Contact: Gary E. Baker, Senior Vice President and Administrator
CFO: Todd La Porte, Senior Vice President and Chief Financial Officer
CMO: James Burke, M.D., Senior Vice President and Chief Medical Officer
CIO: James R. Cramer, Vice President and Chief Information Officer
CHR: Carol Henderson, Vice President Human Resources
Web address: www.shc.org
**Control:** Other not–for–profit (including NFP Corporation) **Service:** General Medical and Surgical

**Staffed Beds:** 347

✠ **SELECT SPECIALTY HOSPITAL–SCOTTSDALE (32005)**, 7400 East Osborn Road, 3 West, Zip 85251–6432; tel. 480/882–4360, (Includes SELECT SPECIALTY HOSPITAL–PHOENIX DOWNTOWN, 1012 East Wiletta Street, 4th Floor, Phoenix, Zip 85006; tel. 602/239–6134; Sharon Anthony, Market Administrator), (Nonreporting) **A**1 9 10 **S** Select Medical Corporation, Mechanicsburg, PA
Primary Contact: Nancy L. Burton, Chief Executive Officer
Web address: www.selectmedicalcorp.com
**Control:** Corporation, Investor–owned, for–profit **Service:** Long–Term Acute Care hospital

**Staffed Beds:** 62

## SELLS—Pima County

✠ **U. S. PUBLIC HEALTH SERVICE INDIAN HOSPITAL–SELLS (30074)**, Zip 85634; tel. 520/383–7251, (Nonreporting) **A**1 10 **S** U. S. Indian Health Service, Rockville, MD
Primary Contact: Priscilla Whitethorne, Chief Executive Officer
COO: Diane Shanley, Deputy Service Unit Director
CFO: Vivian Draper, Chief Financial Officer
CMO: Peter Ziegler, M.D., Acting Chief Medical Officer
CIO: Karen Wade, Chief Information Officer
CNO: Donna Hobbs, Nurse Executive
Web address: www.ihs.gov
**Control:** PHS, Indian Service, Government, federal **Service:** General Medical and Surgical

**Staffed Beds:** 12

## SHOW LOW—Navajo County

★ **SUMMIT HEALTHCARE REGIONAL MEDICAL CENTER (30062)**, 2200 East Show Low Lake Road, Zip 85901–7800; tel. 928/537–4375 **A**9 10 20 **F**3 11 13 15 18 20 22 28 29 30 31 32 34 35 36 38 40 41 43 45 46 47 53 54 57 59 62 64 65 68 70 71 73 75 76 77 78 79 81 82 92 93 107 108 110 111 113 114 118 120 126 128 129 130 131 134 145 **P**6
Primary Contact: Ronald L. McArthur, Chief Executive Officer
COO: Doug Gilchrist, Chief Operating Officer
CFO: Kurt Loveless, Chief Financial Officer
CMO: Jeffrey Northup, D.O., Chief Medical Officer
CIO: Kent McQuillan, Chief Information Officer
CHR: Connie Kakavas, Chief Human Resources Officer
CNO: Cynthia Ebert, R.N., Chief Nursing Officer
Web address: www.summithealthcare.net
**Control:** Other not–for–profit (including NFP Corporation) **Service:** General Medical and Surgical

**Staffed Beds:** 89 **Admissions:** 11477 **Census:** 99 **Outpatient Visits:** 52821
**Births:** 919 **Total Expense ($000):** 98218 **Payroll Expense ($000):** 41088
**Personnel:** 671

## SIERRA VISTA—Cochise County

✠ **SIERRA VISTA REGIONAL HEALTH CENTER (30043)**, 300 El Camino Real, Zip 85635–2899; tel. 520/417–3003 **A**1 9 10 13 20 **F**3 11 13 15 18 20 22 27 28 29 30 34 35 40 41 45 46 48 49 50 51 57 60 63 64 70 73 75 76 77 78 79 81 82 85 86 89 93 107 108 110 111 113 114 117 118 126 129 144 145 147
Primary Contact: Margaret Hepburn, MS, R.N., President and Chief Executive Officer
CFO: Bruce J. Norton, Senior Vice President and Chief Financial Officer
CMO: Jaya Maddur, M.D., Chief of Staff
CIO: Bruce J. Norton, Senior Vice President and Chief Financial Officer
CHR: Marie Wurth, Vice President Human Resources and Public Relations Officer
Web address: www.svrhc.org
**Control:** Other not–for–profit (including NFP Corporation) **Service:** General Medical and Surgical

**Staffed Beds:** 88 **Admissions:** 5540 **Census:** 46 **Outpatient Visits:** 90278
**Births:** 1178 **Total Expense ($000):** 88116 **Payroll Expense ($000):** 35735
**Personnel:** 715

## SPRINGERVILLE—Apache County

**WHITE MOUNTAIN REGIONAL MEDICAL CENTER (31315)**, 118 South Mountain Avenue, Zip 85938–5104; tel. 928/333–4368, (Nonreporting) **A**9 10 18
Primary Contact: Samuel Grant, Interim Chief Executive Officer
CFO: James Hamblin, Chief Financial Officer
CMO: Scott Hamblin, M.D., President Medical Staff
Web address: www.wmrmc.com
**Control:** Other not–for–profit (including NFP Corporation) **Service:** General Medical and Surgical

**Staffed Beds:** 20

*Many Facility Codes have changed. Please refer to the AHA Guide Code Chart.* © 2012 AHA Guide

## SUN CITY—Maricopa County

✠ **BANNER BOSWELL MEDICAL CENTER (30061)**, 10401 West Thunderbird Boulevard, Zip 85351–3004, Mailing Address: P.O. Box 1690, Zip 85372–1690; tel. 623/832–4000, (Total facility includes 71 beds in nursing home–type unit) **A**1 2 9 10 **F**3 11 15 17 22 24 28 29 30 31 37 40 47 49 53 54 56 58 60 64 65 69 70 74 75 77 78 79 81 82 85 87 90 93 107 108 109 111 112 113 114 115 116 117 118 125 127 129 144 145 146 147 **S** Banner Health, Phoenix, AZ
Primary Contact: David Cheney, Chief Executive Officer
CFO: Jeremy Williams, Chief Financial Officer
CMO: Terry Loftus, M.D., Chief Medical Officer
Web address: www.sunhealth.org
**Control:** Other not–for–profit (including NFP Corporation) **Service:** General Medical and Surgical

**Staffed Beds:** 489 **Admissions:** 24649 **Census:** 323 **Outpatient Visits:** 221227 **Births:** 0 **Total Expense ($000):** 282923 **Payroll Expense ($000):** 112778 **Personnel:** 1874

**TRILLIUM SPECIALTY HOSPITAL–WEST VALLEY (32008)**, 13818 North Thunderbird Boulevard, Zip 85351–2574; tel. 623/977–1325, (Nonreporting) **A**10 **S** AcuityHealthcare, LP, Charlotte, NC
Primary Contact: Rhonda Y. Williams, Chief Executive Officer
Web address: www.trilliumhospital.net
**Control:** Corporation, Investor–owned, for–profit **Service:** Long–Term Acute Care hospital

**Staffed Beds:** 120

## SUN CITY WEST—Maricopa County

★ **BANNER DEL E. WEBB MEDICAL CENTER (30093)**, 14502 West Meeker Boulevard, Zip 85375–5299, Mailing Address: P.O. Box 5169, Zip 85376–5169; tel. 623/214–4000 **A**9 10 **F**3 5 11 13 15 20 22 26 28 29 30 31 35 37 40 45 49 51 53 56 60 64 68 69 70 73 74 75 76 77 78 79 81 82 83 84 85 87 90 91 92 93 94 96 98 100 101 102 103 104 105 107 108 111 113 114 117 118 129 130 131 134 145 146 147 **P**1 8 **S** Banner Health, Phoenix, AZ
Primary Contact: Debbie Flores, Chief Executive Officer
CMO: Michel Dagher, D.O., Vice President and Chief Medical Officer
CIO: David Runt, Chief Information Officer
Web address: www.sunhealth.org
**Control:** Other not–for–profit (including NFP Corporation) **Service:** General Medical and Surgical

**Staffed Beds:** 373 **Admissions:** 19781 **Census:** 228 **Outpatient Visits:** 237132 **Births:** 1727 **Total Expense ($000):** 216243 **Payroll Expense ($000):** 91802 **Personnel:** 1541

## TUBA CITY—Coconino County

✠ **TUBA CITY REGIONAL HEALTH CARE CORPORATION (30073)**, 167 Main Street, Zip 86045–0611, Mailing Address: P.O. Box 600, Zip 86045–0600; tel. 928/283–2501 **A**1 5 9 10 **F**3 5 7 8 9 11 12 13 15 18 26 27 28 29 30 31 32 33 34 35 36 37 38 39 40 41 43 44 45 46 47 48 49 50 52 53 54 55 56 57 58 59 60 61 62 63 64 65 66 68 70 71 74 75 76 77 78 79 81 82 83 84 85 86 87 89 91 92 93 94 96 97 99 100 101 102 103 104 105 107 108 110 111 112 113 118 123 125 126 129 130 131 132 133 134 140 141 142 143 144 145 146 147 **P**6 7
Primary Contact: Joseph T. Engelken, Chief Executive Officer
COO: Lynette Bonar, Chief Support Services
CFO: Clifford Lee Olsson, Chief Financial Officer
CMO: Alan Spacone, M.D., Chief Medical Officer
CHR: John S. Pemberton, Director Human Resources
Web address: www.tchealth.org
**Control:** Other not–for–profit (including NFP Corporation) **Service:** General Medical and Surgical

**Staffed Beds:** 74 **Admissions:** 3874 **Census:** 39 **Outpatient Visits:** 495373 **Births:** 521 **Total Expense ($000):** 120215 **Payroll Expense ($000):** 64256 **Personnel:** 908

## TUCSON—Pima County

✠ **CARONDELET HEART & VASCULAR INSTITUTE (30100)**, 4888 North Stone Avenue, Zip 85704; tel. 520/696–2365 **A**1 9 10 **F**3 11 17 18 20 22 24 26 29 30 40 50 54 59 60 68 75 81 87 107 113 131 134 145 147 **S** Ascension Health, Saint Louis, MO
Primary Contact: Carol Erenberger, Site Administrator
CFO: Douglas B. Kell, Interim Chief Financial Officer
CMO: Michael Hecht, M.D., Chief Medical Officer
CIO: Tony Fonze, Vice President Information Services and Chief Information Officer
CHR: Daisy Jenkins, Vice President Human Resources
Web address: www.carondelet.org
**Control:** Church–operated, Nongovernment, not–for profit **Service:** General Medical and Surgical

**Staffed Beds:** 58 **Admissions:** 2827 **Census:** 28 **Outpatient Visits:** 14281 **Births:** 0 **Total Expense ($000):** 56675 **Payroll Expense ($000):** 18187 **Personnel:** 232

✠ **CARONDELET ST. JOSEPH'S HOSPITAL (30011)**, 350 North Wilmot Road, Zip 85711–2678; tel. 520/296–3211 **A**1 5 9 10 **F**3 5 11 12 13 15 17 18 20 22 24 28 29 30 34 38 40 44 45 46 47 49 50 57 59 60 61 63 64 68 69 70 72 74 75 76 77 78 79 81 82 83 84 87 90 93 98 100 101 102 103 104 105 107 108 110 111 113 114 117 118 125 128 129 130 131 132 134 144 145 146 147 **S** Ascension Health, Saint Louis, MO
Primary Contact: Mary Henrikson, Chief Executive Officer
CFO: Alan Strauss, Chief Financial Officer
CMO: Donald Denmark, M.D., Chief Medical Officer
CIO: Tony Fonze, Chief Information Officer, Carondelet Health Network
CHR: Daisy Jenkins, Chief Human Resources Officer
CNO: Debra A. Finch, Chief Operating Officer and Chief Nursing Officer
Web address: www.carondelet.org
**Control:** Church–operated, Nongovernment, not–for profit **Service:** General Medical and Surgical

**Staffed Beds:** 449 **Admissions:** 20073 **Census:** 265 **Outpatient Visits:** 153230 **Births:** 3111 **Total Expense ($000):** 262123 **Payroll Expense ($000):** 101275 **Personnel:** 1485

✠ **CARONDELET ST. MARY'S HOSPITAL (30010)**, 1601 West St. Mary's Road, Zip 85745–2682; tel. 520/872–3000 **A**1 5 9 10 **F**3 5 11 12 15 16 17 20 22 29 30 31 34 38 40 44 47 49 50 51 56 57 59 60 61 63 64 68 70 74 77 78 79 81 82 83 84 87 90 93 98 100 101 102 103 104 105 107 108 110 111 113 114 115 117 118 125 128 129 131 132 134 144 145 147 **S** Ascension Health, Saint Louis, MO
Primary Contact: Dorothy Sawyer, Chief Executive Officer
COO: Roberta B. Kaemmerling, MSN, Chief Operating Officer and Chief Nursing Officer
CFO: Deb Mohesky, Chief Financial Officer
CMO: Amy Beiter, M.D., Chief Medical Officer
CIO: Tony Fonze, Chief Information Officer
CHR: Daisy Jenkins, Vice President Human Resources
Web address: www.carondelet.org
**Control:** Church–operated, Nongovernment, not–for profit **Service:** General Medical and Surgical

**Staffed Beds:** 429 **Admissions:** 15557 **Census:** 224 **Outpatient Visits:** 196935 **Births:** 0 **Total Expense ($000):** 213260 **Payroll Expense ($000):** 85131 **Personnel:** 1186

☐ **CORNERSTONE HOSPITAL OF SOUTHEAST ARIZONA (32004)**, 7220 East Rosewood Drive, Zip 85710; tel. 520/546–4595, (Nonreporting) **A**1 10 **S** Cornerstone Healthcare Group, Dallas, TX
Primary Contact: Mindy S. Moore, Chief Executive Officer
CFO: Chad Deardorff, Group Chief Financial Officer
CMO: Paul Simon, M.D., Medical Director
CIO: Adam Davis, Director Information Technology
CHR: Isabel Dominguez, Director Human Resources and Payroll
Web address: www.chghospitals.com
**Control:** Corporation, Investor–owned, for–profit **Service:** Long–Term Acute Care hospital

**Staffed Beds:** 54

✠ **HEALTHSOUTH REHABILITATION HOSPITAL OF SOUTHERN ARIZONA (33029)**, 1921 West Hospital Drive, Zip 85704–7806; tel. 520/742–2800 **A**1 9 10 **F**3 29 34 59 64 69 90 93 95 96 129 130 131 142 147 **S** HEALTHSOUTH Corporation, Birmingham, AL
Primary Contact: Robin Conklin, R.N., Interim Chief Executive Officer
CFO: David Krogen, Controller
CMO: Susan Bulen, M.D., Medical Director
CHR: Maria Elena McElroy, Vice President Human Resources
Web address: www.healthsouthsouthernarizona.com
**Control:** Corporation, Investor–owned, for–profit **Service:** Rehabilitation

**Staffed Beds:** 60 **Admissions:** 1262 **Census:** 45 **Outpatient Visits:** 7132 **Births:** 0 **Total Expense ($000):** 19870 **Payroll Expense ($000):** 9127 **Personnel:** 168

---

**Hospital, Medicare Provider Number, Address, Telephone, Approval, Facility, and Physician Codes, Health Care System**

★ American Hospital Association (AHA) membership
☐ The Joint Commission accreditation
◇ DNV Healthcare Inc. accreditation
○ American Osteopathic Association (AOA) accreditation
△ Commission on Accreditation of Rehabilitation Facilities (CARF) accreditation

**AZ**

✠ **HEALTHSOUTH REHABILITATION INSTITUTE OF TUCSON (33028)**, 2650 North Wyatt Drive, Zip 85712–6108; tel. 520/325–1300, (Nonreporting) **A**1 9 10 **S** HEALTHSOUTH Corporation, Birmingham, AL
Primary Contact: Jeffrey Christensen, Chief Executive Officer
CFO: Mary Donovan, Controller
CMO: Jon Larson, M.D., Medical Director
CHR: Dawn Mosier, Director Human Resources
Web address: www.rehabinstituteoftucson.com
**Control:** Corporation, Investor–owned, for–profit **Service:** Rehabilitation

**Staffed Beds:** 80

✠ **KINDRED HOSPITAL–TUCSON (32002)**, 355 North Wilmot Road, Zip 85711–2635; tel. 520/584–4500, (Nonreporting) **A**1 9 10 **S** Kindred Healthcare, Louisville, KY
Primary Contact: Heidi Miller, Chief Executive Officer
COO: Kathleen D. Kobbes Adams, R.N., Chief Clinical Officer
CFO: M. Troy Carpenter, Chief Financial Officer
CMO: Sunil Natrajan, M.D., Medical Director
Web address: www.khtucson.com
**Control:** Corporation, Investor–owned, for–profit **Service:** General Medical and Surgical

**Staffed Beds:** 51

✠ **NORTHWEST MEDICAL CENTER (30085)**, 6200 North La Cholla Boulevard, Zip 85741–3599; tel. 520/742–9000 **A**1 3 5 9 10 **F**3 8 12 13 15 17 18 19 20 22 24 26 28 29 30 31 34 35 37 40 49 53 57 59 68 70 72 74 75 76 78 79 81 85 91 93 102 107 108 110 111 113 114 117 118 125 129 134 143 145 146 147 **P**6 **S** Community Health Systems, Inc., Franklin, TN
Primary Contact: Kevin Stockton, Chief Executive Officer
COO: Veronica Knudson, Chief Operating Officer
CFO: Ronald Patrick, Chief Financial Officer
CMO: Abram Aguilar, M.D., Chief Medical Officer
CIO: David Bullock, Director Information Services
CHR: John Zubiena, Director Human Resources
CNO: Karen Stubbs, Chief Nursing Officer
Web address: www.northwestmedicalcenter.com
**Control:** Corporation, Investor–owned, for–profit **Service:** General Medical and Surgical

**Staffed Beds:** 270 **Admissions:** 18302 **Census:** 173 **Outpatient Visits:** 186568 **Births:** 2778 **Total Expense ($000):** 222024 **Payroll Expense ($000):** 87944 **Personnel:** 1692

**PALO VERDE MENTAL HEALTH SERVICES** See TMC Healthcare

☐ **SONORA BEHAVIORAL HEALTH HOSPITAL (34022)**, 6050 North Corona Road, Zip 85704–1096; tel. 520/469–8700 **A**1 3 9 10 **F**5 98 99 100 103 104 142 **P**5 **S** Acadia Healthcare Company, Inc., Franklin, TN
Primary Contact: Brian Gill, Chief Executive Officer
**Control:** Corporation, Investor–owned, for–profit **Service:** Psychiatric

**Staffed Beds:** 56 **Admissions:** 2337 **Census:** 49 **Outpatient Visits:** 3278 **Births:** 0 **Total Expense ($000):** 12634 **Payroll Expense ($000):** 8365 **Personnel:** 152

✠ △ **SOUTHERN ARIZONA VETERANS AFFAIRS HEALTH CARE SYSTEM**, 3601 South 6th Avenue, Zip 85723–0002; tel. 520/792–1450, (Total facility includes 96 beds in nursing home–type unit) **A**1 3 5 7 8 9 **F**1 3 4 5 8 9 10 11 12 14 15 17 18 20 22 24 26 29 30 31 34 35 36 37 38 39 40 44 45 46 47 48 49 50 51 54 56 57 58 59 60 61 62 63 64 65 66 67 68 70 74 75 77 78 79 81 82 83 84 85 86 87 90 91 92 93 94 95 96 97 98 100 101 102 103 104 105 106 107 108 109 110 111 112 113 114 115 116 118 119 120 121 122 123 125 126 127 128 129 131 134 142 143 144 145 146 147 **S** Department of Veterans Affairs, Washington, DC
Primary Contact: Jonathan H. Gardner, Chief Executive Officer
COO: Joan M. Ricard, R.N., Chief Operating Officer
CFO: Larry Korn, Manager Finance
CMO: Jayendra H. Shah, M.D., Chief Medical Officer
CIO: John Walston, Chief Information Officer
CHR: Patrice Craig, Manager Human Resources
Web address: www.tucson.va.gov
**Control:** Veterans Affairs, Government, federal **Service:** General Medical and Surgical

**Staffed Beds:** 285 **Admissions:** 7767 **Census:** 108 **Outpatient Visits:** 720113 **Births:** 0 **Personnel:** 2394

★ **TMC HEALTHCARE (30006)**, 5301 East Grant Road, Zip 85712–2874; tel. 520/327–5461, (Includes PALO VERDE MENTAL HEALTH SERVICES, 2695 North Craycroft, Zip 85712–2244, Mailing Address: P.O. Box 40030, Zip 85717–0030; tel. 520/324–4340; TMC FOR CHILDREN, 5301 East Grant Road, Zip 85712–2805; tel. 520/327–5461) **A**3 5 8 9 10 **F**3 8 11 12 13 15 17 18 19 20 22 24 26 28 29 30 31 34 35 40 41 42 45 46 47 48 49 50 54 56 57 59 62 63 64 68 69 70 72 73 74 75 76 77 78 79 81 82 84 85 86 87 88 89 97 98 100 102 104 107 108 109 110 111 113 114 118 123 125 128 129 131 145 146 147 **P**4 7
Primary Contact: Judy F. Rich, President and Chief Executive Officer
COO: Linda Wojtowicz, R.N., Senior Vice President and Chief Operations Officer
CFO: Stephen Bush, Chief Financial Officer
CMO: Palmer Evans, M.D., Chief Medical Officer
CIO: Frank Marini, Vice President and Chief Information Officer
Web address: www.tmcaz.com
**Control:** Other not–for–profit (including NFP Corporation) **Service:** General Medical and Surgical

**Staffed Beds:** 553 **Admissions:** 32303 **Census:** 373 **Outpatient Visits:** 142436 **Births:** 5212 **Total Expense ($000):** 371407 **Payroll Expense ($000):** 163463 **Personnel:** 2763

**TUCSON HEART HOSPITAL** See Carondelet Heart & Vascular Institute

☐ **UNIVERSITY OF ARIZONA MEDICAL CENTER – UNIVERSITY CAMPUS (30111)**, 2800 East Ajo Way, Zip 85713–6289; tel. 520/874–2000 **A**1 9 10 **F**3 8 11 12 15 18 20 22 26 29 30 34 35 36 38 40 43 44 50 51 54 55 56 57 59 61 64 65 68 70 74 75 77 79 81 82 85 87 93 97 98 100 101 102 103 104 107 110 111 113 114 118 126 129 130 134 143 144 145 146 147 **P**4
Primary Contact: Diane Rafferty, Chief Executive Officer
COO: Sarah Frost, Associate Hospital Administrator
CFO: Timothy Kares, Chief Financial Officer
CMO: John Kettelle, M.D., Vice President Operations and Medical Director
CIO: Kevin Christiansen, Director Information Technology
CHR: Tere LeBarron, Vice President Planning and Integration
Web address: www.uph.org
**Control:** Other not–for–profit (including NFP Corporation) **Service:** General Medical and Surgical

**Staffed Beds:** 163 **Admissions:** 5965 **Census:** 95 **Outpatient Visits:** 183581 **Births:** 0 **Total Expense ($000):** 113407 **Payroll Expense ($000):** 45130 **Personnel:** 859

✠ **UNIVERSITY OF ARIZONA MEDICAL CENTER – UNIVERSITY CAMPUS (30064)**, 1501 North Campbell Avenue, Zip 85724–5128; tel. 520/694–0111 **A**1 3 5 8 9 10 **F**3 8 11 12 13 17 18 19 20 21 22 23 24 25 26 27 28 29 30 31 32 34 35 36 37 38 40 41 43 44 45 46 47 48 49 50 53 54 57 58 59 60 61 62 64 67 68 69 70 72 74 75 76 77 78 79 81 84 85 86 87 88 89 92 93 97 98 99 100 101 102 103 107 108 111 113 114 115 116 117 118 119 120 122 123 125 129 131 135 136 137 138 139 140 141 144 145 146 147 **P**4 6
Primary Contact: Jodi J. Mansfield, Interim President and Chief Executive Officer
CIO: Shirley Gabriel, Chief Information Officer
CHR: John Marques, Vice President Human Resources
Web address: www.umcarizona.org
**Control:** Other not–for–profit (including NFP Corporation) **Service:** General Medical and Surgical

**Staffed Beds:** 460 **Admissions:** 25270 **Census:** 358 **Outpatient Visits:** 435509 **Births:** 1871 **Total Expense ($000):** 574769 **Payroll Expense ($000):** 220836 **Personnel:** 3862

**WHITERIVER—Navajo County**

☐ **U. S. PUBLIC HEALTH SERVICE INDIAN HOSPITAL–WHITERIVER (30113)**, 200 West Hospital Drive, Zip 85941–0860, Mailing Address: State Route 73, Box 860, Zip 85941–0860; tel. 928/338–4911 **A**1 10 **F**3 8 13 29 31 32 34 35 36 38 39 40 44 45 46 50 53 54 56 57 59 61 64 65 66 75 78 79 81 82 84 85 86 87 89 91 93 94 97 100 101 104 107 111 113 118 129 130 131 134 143 145 146 147 **S** U. S. Indian Health Service, Rockville, MD
Primary Contact: Michelle Martinez, Interim Chief Executive Officer
CFO: Desdemona Leslie, Finance Officer
CMO: David Yost, M.D., Clinical Director
CIO: Russell Barker, Chief Information Officer
Web address: www.ihs.gov
**Control:** PHS, Indian Service, Government, federal **Service:** General Medical and Surgical

**Staffed Beds:** 35 **Admissions:** 1416 **Census:** 14 **Outpatient Visits:** 184078 **Births:** 352 **Personnel:** 502

*Many Facility Codes have changed. Please refer to the AHA Guide Code Chart.* © 2012 AHA Guide

**AZ**

### WICKENBURG—Maricopa County

★ **WICKENBURG COMMUNITY HOSPITAL (31300)**, 520 Rose Lane,
Zip 85390–1447; tel. 928/684–5421 **A**9 10 18 **F**11 15 34 40 53 57 59 63 93
107 110 111 114 116 118 132 147 **P**6
Primary Contact: James Tavary, Chief Executive Officer
CFO: Ron Smith, Chief Financial Officer
CMO: Dennis Barraco, D.O., Medical Director
CIO: Michael McKay, Manager Information Systems
CHR: Bill Horn, Director Human Resources
CNO: Linda Brockwell, R.N., Chief Nursing Officer
Web address: www.wickenburgcommunityhospital.com
**Control:** Other not–for–profit (including NFP Corporation) **Service:** General
Medical and Surgical

Staffed Beds: 19 Admissions: 564 Census: 7 Outpatient Visits: 25656
Births: 0 Total Expense ($000): 16861 Payroll Expense ($000): 7443
Personnel: 136

### WILLCOX—Cochise County

★ **NORTHERN COCHISE COMMUNITY HOSPITAL (31302)**, 901 West Rex Allen
Drive, Zip 85643–1009; tel. 520/384–3541, (Total facility includes 24 beds in
nursing home–type unit) **A**9 10 18 **F**19 29 34 40 56 57 59 65 68 77 90 93 98
101 103 104 107 110 111 113 118 127 129 132 142 145
Primary Contact: Roland Knox, Chief Executive Officer
COO: John Hilton, Operations Officer
CFO: Darcy Robertson, Financial Officer
CMO: Hisham Hamam, M.D., Chief of Staff
CHR: John Hilton, Director Human Resources
CNO: Laurel Kibler, Nursing Officer
Web address: www.ncch.com
**Control:** Hospital district or authority, Government, nonfederal **Service:** General
Medical and Surgical

Staffed Beds: 48 Admissions: 524 Census: 25 Outpatient Visits: 17637
Births: 0 Personnel: 107

### WINSLOW—Navajo County

★ **LITTLE COLORADO MEDICAL CENTER (31311)**, 1501 Williamson Avenue,
Zip 86047–2797; tel. 928/289–4691, (Nonreporting) **A**9 10 18
Primary Contact: Jeffrey J. Hamblen, Chief Executive Officer
CFO: Randy Glassman, Chief Financial Officer
CMO: Perry Mitchell, M.D., Chief of Staff
CHR: Nina L. Ferguson, Director Human Resources
Web address: www.lcmcwmh.org
**Control:** Other not–for–profit (including NFP Corporation) **Service:** General
Medical and Surgical

Staffed Beds: 25

### YUMA—Yuma County

★ **YUMA REGIONAL MEDICAL CENTER (30013)**, 2400 South Avenue A,
Zip 85364–7170; tel. 928/344–2000 **A**9 10 **F**3 8 11 12 13 14 15 17 18 20
22 24 26 28 29 30 31 32 34 35 38 39 40 41 45 46 47 48 49 50 54 56 57
58 59 64 65 68 70 72 73 74 75 76 77 78 79 81 82 83 84 85 86 87 89 94
97 100 102 107 108 110 111 113 114 115 116 117 118 123 129 131 132
145 146 147 **P**7
Primary Contact: Pat Walz, President and Chief Executive Officer
CFO: Tony Struck, Chief Financial Officer
CMO: Carl Myers, M.D., Vice President Medical Affairs and Chief Medical Officer
CIO: Gene Shaw, Chief Information Officer
CHR: Sharon R. Gardner, Vice President Human Resources
CNO: Brenda Hall, R.N., Vice President Patient Care Services
Web address: www.yumaregional.org
**Control:** Other not–for–profit (including NFP Corporation) **Service:** General
Medical and Surgical

Staffed Beds: 333 Admissions: 16272 Census: 181 Outpatient Visits:
165857 Births: 3473 Total Expense ($000): 271571 Payroll Expense
($000): 106608 Personnel: 1858

⌗ **YUMA REHABILITATION HOSPITAL (33034)**, 901 West 24th Street,
Zip 85364; tel. 928/726–5000, (Nonreporting) **A**1 9 10 **S** HEALTHSOUTH
Corporation, Birmingham, AL
Primary Contact: Larry Barclift, Interim Chief Executive Officer
CFO: Larry Barclift, Chief Financial Officer
CMO: Rinely Aguiar–Olsen, M.D., Medical Director
CHR: Linda Woen, Director Human Resources
Web address: www.yumarehabhospital.com
**Control:** Corporation, Investor–owned, for–profit **Service:** Rehabilitation

Staffed Beds: 41

---

**Hospital, Medicare Provider Number, Address, Telephone, Approval, Facility, and Physician Codes, Health Care System**

★ American Hospital Association (AHA) membership
□ The Joint Commission accreditation
◇ DNV Healthcare Inc. accreditation
○ American Osteopathic Association (AOA) accreditation
△ Commission on Accreditation of Rehabilitation Facilities (CARF) accreditation

## ARKANSAS

AR

**ARKADELPHIA—Clark County**

☒ **BAPTIST HEALTH MEDICAL CENTER–ARKADELPHIA (41321)**, 3050 Twin Rivers Drive, Zip 71923–4299; tel. 870/245–2622 **A**1 9 10 18 **F**3 7 11 13 15 28 29 30 40 43 57 59 61 62 63 65 68 69 70 76 81 93 107 110 111 113 118 128 129 132 134 145 **S** Baptist Health, Little Rock, AR
Primary Contact: Greg Stubblefield, Vice President and Administrator
COO: Greg Stubblefield, Vice President and Administrator
CFO: Robert C. Roberts, Vice President and Chief Financial Officer
CMO: Guy Gardner, M.D., Chief Medical Officer
CIO: David House, Vice President and Chief Information Officer
CHR: Anthony Kendall, Vice President Human Resources
Web address: www.baptist–health.org
**Control:** Other not–for–profit (including NFP Corporation) **Service:** General Medical and Surgical

**Staffed Beds:** 25 **Admissions:** 1206 **Census:** 12 **Outpatient Visits:** 24102 **Births:** 323 **Personnel:** 178

**ASHDOWN—Little River County**

★ **LITTLE RIVER MEMORIAL HOSPITAL (41320)**, 451 West Locke Street, Zip 71822–3398; tel. 870/898–5011, (Nonreporting) **A**9 10 18
Primary Contact: David Deaton, Administrator and Chief Executive Officer
CFO: Barbra Crow, Chief Financial Officer
CHR: Gina Strickland, Administrative Assistant and Director Human Resources
**Control:** County–Government, nonfederal **Service:** General Medical and Surgical

**Staffed Beds:** 25

**BARLING—Sebastian County**

☐ **VISTA HEALTH OF FORT SMITH (44006)**, 10301 Mayo Drive, Zip 72923; tel. 479/494–5700 **A**1 9 10 **F**29 34 35 38 57 59 64 68 86 87 98 99 100 101 102 104 105 106 129 133 **P**6
Primary Contact: Holli Baker, Chief Executive Officer
Web address: www.vistahealthservices.com
**Control:** Corporation, Investor–owned, for–profit **Service:** Psychiatric

**Staffed Beds:** 57 **Admissions:** 1506 **Census:** 50 **Outpatient Visits:** 32172 **Births:** 0 **Total Expense ($000):** 10961 **Payroll Expense ($000):** 7042 **Personnel:** 200

**BATESVILLE—Independence County**

★ △ **WHITE RIVER MEDICAL CENTER (40119)**, 1710 Harrison Street, Zip 72501–2197, Mailing Address: P.O. Box 2197, Zip 72503–2197; tel. 870/262–1200, (Total facility includes 12 beds in nursing home–type unit) **A**7 9 10 **F**3 8 11 12 13 15 17 18 20 22 28 29 30 31 34 35 38 40 43 44 50 51 56 57 59 60 64 68 70 72 74 75 76 77 78 79 81 82 85 86 87 90 93 98 99 100 101 103 104 107 108 110 111 113 114 116 118 120 125 126 127 128 129 130 131 134 143 145 146 147 **P**6 **S** White River Health System, Batesville, AR
Primary Contact: Gary Bebow, FACHE, Administrator and Chief Executive Officer
COO: Tammy Gavin, Assistant Administrator and Chief Operating Officer
CFO: Jana Richardson, Chief Financial Officer
CMO: Tom Cummins, M.D., Director Hospitalist Program
CIO: Gary Paxson, Chief Information Officer
CHR: Gary McDonald, Assistant Administrator Human Resources
CNO: Dede Strecker, Chief Nursing Officer
Web address: www.whiteriverhealthsystem.com
**Control:** Other not–for–profit (including NFP Corporation) **Service:** General Medical and Surgical

**Staffed Beds:** 171 **Admissions:** 9000 **Census:** 131 **Outpatient Visits:** 168516 **Births:** 704 **Total Expense ($000):** 125646 **Payroll Expense ($000):** 55412 **Personnel:** 1097

**BENTON—Saline County**

☐ **RIVENDELL BEHAVIORAL HEALTH SERVICES OF ARKANSAS (44007)**, 100 Rivendell Drive, Zip 72019–9100; tel. 501/316–1255 **A**1 9 10 **F**29 38 54 59 64 75 98 99 100 101 102 104 105 106 129 131 133 **P**5 **S** Universal Health Services, Inc., King of Prussia, PA
Primary Contact: Duane Runyan, Chief Executive Officer and Managing Director
CFO: Mike Rainbolt, Chief Financial Officer
Web address: www.rivendellofarkansas.com
**Control:** Corporation, Investor–owned, for–profit **Service:** Psychiatric

**Staffed Beds:** 77 **Admissions:** 2012 **Census:** 65 **Outpatient Visits:** 53933 **Births:** 0 **Total Expense ($000):** 19940 **Payroll Expense ($000):** 10904 **Personnel:** 225

★ **SALINE MEMORIAL HOSPITAL (40084)**, 1 Medical Park Drive, Zip 72015–3354; tel. 501/776–6000 **A**9 10 **F**3 7 11 13 15 17 18 20 22 29 30 34 35 40 41 45 57 59 62 63 64 70 74 75 76 77 79 81 85 87 89 90 93 96 98 107 108 110 111 114 117 118 128 129 131 134 147 **P**8
Primary Contact: Carla Robertson, Interim Chief Executive Officer
COO: Steve Henson, Vice President Operations
CFO: Larry Don Alford, Chief Financial Officer
CIO: Shawn Shuffield, Executive Director Information Services
CHR: Carol Matthews, Director Human Resources
Web address: www.salinememorial.org
**Control:** Other not–for–profit (including NFP Corporation) **Service:** General Medical and Surgical

**Staffed Beds:** 124 **Admissions:** 5455 **Census:** 70 **Outpatient Visits:** 73958 **Births:** 433 **Total Expense ($000):** 72088 **Payroll Expense ($000):** 33644 **Personnel:** 637

**BERRYVILLE—Carroll County**

☒ **MERCY HOSPITAL BERRYVILLE (41329)**, 214 Carter Street, Zip 72616–4303; tel. 870/423–3355 **A**1 9 10 18 **F**3 11 15 28 29 30 31 34 35 40 43 45 46 48 50 57 59 61 64 68 75 77 78 79 81 85 93 107 108 113 118 128 129 130 131 132 145 147 **P**6 8 **S** Mercy Health, Chesterfield, MO
Primary Contact: Kristy Estrem, FACHE, President
CFO: Sharon Ash, Vice President Finance
CFO: Sherry Clouse Day, Vice President Finance
CFO: Taya Flippo, Director
CHR: Taya James, Director
CNO: Michele Gann, Vice President Patient Services
Web address: www.mercy.net/berryvillear
**Control:** Church–operated, Nongovernment, not–for profit **Service:** General Medical and Surgical

**Staffed Beds:** 25 **Admissions:** 857 **Census:** 9 **Outpatient Visits:** 18649 **Births:** 0 **Total Expense ($000):** 15168 **Payroll Expense ($000):** 7521

**BLYTHEVILLE—Mississippi County**

☐ **GREAT RIVER MEDICAL CENTER (40069)**, 1520 North Division Street, Zip 72315–1448, Mailing Address: P.O. Box 108, Zip 72316–0108; tel. 870/838–7300 **A**1 9 10 **F**11 13 15 28 29 34 40 45 46 53 57 59 64 68 70 75 76 79 81 82 89 93 97 107 108 111 113 118 119 129 134 145 146 **P**7 **S** Mississippi County Hospital System, Blytheville, AR
Primary Contact: Ralph E. Beaty, Chief Executive Officer
COO: Chris Raymer, R.N., Chief Operating Officer and Chief Nursing Officer
CFO: Phil Norris, Chief Financial Officer
CMO: Jeffrey Hall, M.D., Chief of Staff
CHR: Cheri Blurton, Director Human Resources
**Control:** County–Government, nonfederal **Service:** General Medical and Surgical

**Staffed Beds:** 73 **Admissions:** 1632 **Census:** 12 **Outpatient Visits:** 27258 **Births:** 419 **Total Expense ($000):** 16979 **Payroll Expense ($000):** 8045 **Personnel:** 214

**BOONEVILLE—Logan County**

★ **BOONEVILLE COMMUNITY HOSPITAL (41318)**, 880 West Main Street, Zip 72927–3420, Mailing Address: P.O. Box 290, Zip 72927–0290; tel. 479/675–2800, (Nonreporting) **A**9 10 18
Primary Contact: Jerry Mitcham, Interim President and Chief Executive Officer
CMO: William Daniel, M.D., Chief Medical Officer
CIO: Aaron Albright, Chief Information Officer
CHR: Doris Whitaker, Vice President Human Resources
Web address: www.boonevillehospital.com
**Control:** Other not–for–profit (including NFP Corporation) **Service:** General Medical and Surgical

**Staffed Beds:** 25

**CALICO ROCK— County**

**COMMUNITY MEDICAL CENTER OF IZARD COUNTY (41306)**, 61 Grasse Street, Zip 72519, Mailing Address: P.O. Box 438, Zip 72519–0438; tel. 870/297–3726, (Nonreporting) **A**9 10 18
Primary Contact: Philip Hughes, Chief Executive Officer
CMO: Bethany Knight, M.D., Chief of Staff
Web address: www.cmcofic.org
**Control:** Other not–for–profit (including NFP Corporation) **Service:** General Medical and Surgical

**Staffed Beds:** 25

*Many Facility Codes have changed. Please refer to the AHA Guide Code Chart.* © 2012 AHA Guide

## CAMDEN—Ouachita County

✠ **OUACHITA COUNTY MEDICAL CENTER (40050)**, 638 California Avenue S.W., Zip 71701–4699, Mailing Address: P.O. Box 797, Zip 71711–0797; tel. 870/836–1000 **A**1 9 10 20 **F**3 4 5 7 8 11 13 15 29 31 34 40 41 43 46 48 49 56 57 59 62 63 64 65 68 69 70 75 76 77 78 81 85 87 89 93 98 100 102 103 107 108 111 113 114 118 126 128 129 131 132 134 145 147 **P**8
Primary Contact: James David Cicero, President and Chief Executive Officer
COO: Peggy Abbott, Vice President
CFO: Robert Anders, Chief Financial Officer
CIO: Walter Silliman, Chief Information Officer
CHR: Mary Bridges, Director Human Resources
CNO: Diane Isaacs, Director of Nursing
Web address: www.ouachitamedcenter.com
**Control:** Other not–for–profit (including NFP Corporation) **Service:** General Medical and Surgical

**Staffed Beds:** 65 **Admissions:** 2049 **Census:** 26 **Outpatient Visits:** 27144 **Births:** 252 **Total Expense ($000):** 30804 **Payroll Expense ($000):** 14214 **Personnel:** 437

**OUACHITA MEDICAL CENTER** See Ouachita County Medical Center

## CLARKSVILLE—Johnson County

★ **JOHNSON REGIONAL MEDICAL CENTER (40002)**, 1100 East Poplar Street, Zip 72830–4419, Mailing Address: P.O. Box 738, Zip 72830–0738; tel. 479/754–5454 **A**9 10 **F**3 7 11 13 15 29 34 35 40 43 45 50 56 57 59 62 64 68 70 75 76 77 79 81 85 90 91 92 93 96 98 103 104 107 108 110 111 113 117 118 128 129 131 146 147
Primary Contact: Larry Morse, Chief Executive Officer and Administrator
COO: Larry Morse, Chief Executive Officer and Administrator
CFO: Edward Anderson, Chief Financial Officer
CIO: Deb Bjorgum, Manager Data Processing
CHR: Maribel Baker, Director Human Resources
CNO: Terri Stumbaugh, R.N., Director Patient Care Services
Web address: www.jrmc.org
**Control:** Other not–for–profit (including NFP Corporation) **Service:** General Medical and Surgical

**Staffed Beds:** 80 **Admissions:** 3046 **Census:** 33 **Outpatient Visits:** 41889 **Births:** 497 **Total Expense ($000):** 30567 **Payroll Expense ($000):** 13719 **Personnel:** 344

## CLINTON—Van Buren County

★ **OZARK HEALTH MEDICAL CENTER (41313)**, Highway 65 South, Zip 72031–9045, Mailing Address: P.O. Box 206, Zip 72031–0206; tel. 501/745–7000, (Total facility includes 118 beds in nursing home–type unit) **A**9 10 18 **F**11 15 20 28 29 30 34 35 40 43 45 57 59 62 64 75 77 79 81 86 91 93 107 113 118 129 132 133 134 142 145
CFO: Rhonda Shipp, Chief Financial Officer
CMO: Steve Schoettle, M.D., Chief Medical Staff
CIO: Kathy Fugitt, Chief Information Officer
CHR: Lisa Swofford, Director Administrative Services
Web address: www.ozarkhealthinc.com
**Control:** Other not–for–profit (including NFP Corporation) **Service:** General Medical and Surgical

**Staffed Beds:** 143 **Admissions:** 840 **Census:** 95 **Outpatient Visits:** 20956 **Births:** 0 **Total Expense ($000):** 21438 **Payroll Expense ($000):** 9652 **Personnel:** 304

## CONWAY—Faulkner County

✠ **CONWAY REGIONAL MEDICAL CENTER (40029)**, 2302 College Avenue, Zip 72034–6297; tel. 501/329–3831 **A**1 2 9 10 **F**3 8 11 13 15 17 18 20 22 24 28 29 30 31 35 40 43 45 49 50 51 53 56 57 59 60 62 64 70 74 75 76 77 78 79 81 84 85 87 89 93 103 107 108 110 111 114 116 118 119 126 129 130 131 145 146 147 **P**8
Primary Contact: James M. Lambert, FACHE, President and Chief Executive Officer
COO: Alan Finley, Chief Operating Officer
CFO: Steven P. Rose, Chief Financial Officer
CMO: Keith Bell, M.D., Chief of Staff
CHR: Richard Tyler, Corporate Director Human Resources
CNO: Jacquelyn Wilkerson, R.N., Chief Nursing Officer
Web address: www.conwayregional.org
**Control:** Other not–for–profit (including NFP Corporation) **Service:** General Medical and Surgical

**Staffed Beds:** 146 **Admissions:** 7730 **Census:** 76 **Outpatient Visits:** 111228 **Births:** 1854 **Total Expense ($000):** 108493 **Payroll Expense ($000):** 47167 **Personnel:** 1020

**CONWAY REGIONAL REHAB HOSPITAL (43033)**, 2210 Robinson Street, Zip 72032; tel. 501/932–3500, (Nonreporting) **A**9 10
Primary Contact: Sherry Gann, Administrator
Web address: www.conwayregional.org
**Control:** Partnership, Investor–owned, for–profit **Service:** Rehabilitation

**Staffed Beds:** 24

## CROSSETT—Ashley County

★ **ASHLEY COUNTY MEDICAL CENTER (41323)**, 1015 Unity Road, Zip 71635–2930, Mailing Address: P.O. Box 400, Zip 71635–0400; tel. 870/364–4111 **A**9 10 18 **F**3 11 15 18 29 30 31 34 35 40 45 50 53 57 59 62 64 68 70 75 76 77 78 79 81 85 93 98 100 103 104 105 107 108 110 111 114 118 126 128 129 131 132 147
Primary Contact: Phillip K. Gilmore, FACHE, Chief Executive Officer
CFO: Bill Couch, Chief Financial Officer
CMO: Steve Lynn, M.D., Chief of Staff
CIO: Dan Austin, Manager Data Processing
CHR: Shirley White, Director Human Resources
CNO: Emily Bendinelli, Interim Director of Nurses
Web address: www.acmconline.org
**Control:** Other not–for–profit (including NFP Corporation) **Service:** General Medical and Surgical

**Staffed Beds:** 33 **Admissions:** 1166 **Census:** 15 **Outpatient Visits:** 70843 **Births:** 197 **Total Expense ($000):** 21656 **Payroll Expense ($000):** 10442 **Personnel:** 201

## DANVILLE—Yell County

★ **CHAMBERS MEMORIAL HOSPITAL (40011)**, Highway 10 at Detroit, Zip 72833, Mailing Address: P.O. Box 639, Zip 72833–0639; tel. 479/495–2241 **A**9 10 20 **F**3 11 29 35 40 43 57 62 81 107 113 118 127 129 132
Primary Contact: Michael Scott Peek, Chief Executive Officer
CMO: Philip Tippin, M.D., Chief of Staff
CIO: Amber Bottoms, Director Medical Records
CHR: Stacey Lane, Executive Assistant Human Resources
CNO: Joeann Bowerman, Director of Nursing Services
Web address: www.chambershospital.com
**Control:** Other not–for–profit (including NFP Corporation) **Service:** General Medical and Surgical

**Staffed Beds:** 41 **Admissions:** 2247 **Census:** 20 **Outpatient Visits:** 24788 **Births:** 0 **Total Expense ($000):** 16755 **Payroll Expense ($000):** 6964 **Personnel:** 166

## DARDANELLE—Yell County

**RIVER VALLEY MEDICAL CENTER (41302)**, 200 North Third Street, Zip 72834–3802, Mailing Address: P.O. Box 578, Zip 72834–0578; tel. 479/229–4677 **A**9 10 18 **F**3 29 40 45 56 57 59 64 65 68 75 81 93 98 103 107 127 128 132 147 **S** Allegiance Health Management, Shreveport, LA
Primary Contact: Jodi Love, R.N., Chief Executive Officer
CMO: William P. Scott, M.D., Chief of Staff
CHR: Kathy Hastin, Administrative Assistant Human Resources
**Control:** Corporation, Investor–owned, for–profit **Service:** General Medical and Surgical

**Staffed Beds:** 35 **Admissions:** 659 **Census:** 14 **Outpatient Visits:** 10890 **Births:** 0 **Personnel:** 117

## DE QUEEN—Sevier County

**DE QUEEN MEDICAL CENTER (41319)**, 1306 Collin Raye Drive, Zip 71832–2198; tel. 870/584–4111 **A**9 10 18 **F**3 11 15 29 40 42 57 59 75 77 90 93 107 113 118 128 132 145 147
Primary Contact: Jeremy Icenhower, Administrator and Chief Executive Officer
CMO: Darrin Green, M.D., Medical Director
CHR: Teresa Hodges, Assistant Administrator
Web address: www.dequeenhospital.com
**Control:** Corporation, Investor–owned, for–profit **Service:** General Medical and Surgical

**Staffed Beds:** 35 **Admissions:** 805 **Census:** 13 **Outpatient Visits:** 72528 **Births:** 0 **Total Expense ($000):** 6675 **Payroll Expense ($000):** 3764

---

**Hospital, Medicare Provider Number, Address, Telephone, Approval, Facility, and Physician Codes, Health Care System**

★ American Hospital Association (AHA) membership
☐ The Joint Commission accreditation
◇ DNV Healthcare Inc. accreditation
○ American Osteopathic Association (AOA) accreditation
△ Commission on Accreditation of Rehabilitation Facilities (CARF) accreditation

### DE WITT—Arkansas County

★ **DEWITT HOSPITAL (41314)**, Highway 1 and Madison Street, Zip 72042–9481, Mailing Address: P.O. Box 32, Zip 72042–0032; tel. 870/946–3571, (Total facility includes 59 beds in nursing home–type unit) **A**9 10 18 **F**3 7 29 33 34 35 40 57 62 64 75 107 118 126 127 132 142 144 **P**6
Primary Contact: Darren Caldwell, Chief Executive Officer
CMO: Stan Burleson, M.D., Chief Medical Staff
CIO: Jonathan Fuchs, Chief Information Officer
CHR: Hannah Hackney, Director Accounting and Human Resources
CNO: Rosie Killion, R.N., Chief Nursing Officer
Web address: www.dhnh.org
**Control:** Other not–for–profit (including NFP Corporation) **Service:** General Medical and Surgical

**Staffed Beds:** 85 **Admissions:** 913 **Census:** 55 **Outpatient Visits:** 5271
**Births:** 0 **Total Expense ($000):** 10560 **Payroll Expense ($000):** 5103
**Personnel:** 157

### DUMAS—Desha County

★ **DELTA MEMORIAL HOSPITAL (41326)**, 811 South Highway 65, Zip 71639, Mailing Address: P.O. Box 887, Zip 71639–0887; tel. 870/382–4303 **A**9 10 18 **F**3 11 13 15 29 34 35 40 43 45 50 55 57 59 62 76 81 93 94 95 96 97 107 113 118 119 126 129 132 134 147 **P**6
Primary Contact: Cris Bolin, Chief Executive Officer
CFO: Cris Bolin, Chief Executive Officer
CMO: Thomas Lewellen, D.O., Chief of Staff
CIO: Chris McTigrit, Manager Information Technology
CHR: Doris Fortenberry, Coordinator Human Resources
Web address: www.deltamem.org
**Control:** Other not–for–profit (including NFP Corporation) **Service:** General Medical and Surgical

**Staffed Beds:** 25 **Admissions:** 968 **Census:** 10 **Outpatient Visits:** 33807
**Births:** 111 **Total Expense ($000):** 14333 **Payroll Expense ($000):** 7012
**Personnel:** 142

### EL DORADO—Union County

⊞ **MEDICAL CENTER OF SOUTH ARKANSAS (40088)**, 700 West Grove Street, Zip 71730–4416, Mailing Address: P.O. Box 1998, Zip 71731–1998; tel. 870/863–2000 **A**1 9 10 **F**3 11 13 15 17 18 20 22 24 26 28 29 31 34 35 40 45 56 57 59 64 70 73 74 75 76 78 79 80 81 82 85 89 90 107 108 110 111 114 118 129 145 146 147 **P**7 8 **S** Community Health Systems, Inc., Franklin, TN
Primary Contact: Kyle Swift, Chief Executive Officer
COO: Kevin Decker, Assistant Chief Executive Officer
CFO: Mark Henke, Chief Financial Officer
CMO: Ken Gati, M.D., Chief of Staff
CIO: Rachel Scriber, Director of Marketing & Public Relations
CHR: LaKeitha Davis, Director Human Resources
CNO: Keitha Griffith, Chief Nursing Officer
Web address: www.themedcenter.net
**Control:** Corporation, Investor–owned, for–profit **Service:** General Medical and Surgical

**Staffed Beds:** 120 **Admissions:** 5432 **Census:** 54 **Outpatient Visits:** 62871
**Births:** 620 **Total Expense ($000):** 49626 **Payroll Expense ($000):** 28233
**Personnel:** 506

### EUREKA SPRINGS—Carroll County

★ **EUREKA SPRINGS HOSPITAL (41304)**, 24 Norris Street, Zip 72632–3541; tel. 479/253–7400 **A**9 10 18 **F**3 11 15 29 30 34 35 40 44 45 50 57 59 64 75 77 81 85 86 87 90 93 104 107 118 127 129 130 131 132 142 145 147
Primary Contact: Jodi Love, R.N., Chief Executive Officer
CFO: Sondra Wear, Director Financial Services
CMO: Gregory Kresse, M.D., Chairman Medical Staff
CHR: Jodi Smith, Administrative Assistant Human Resources
Web address: www.eurekaspringshospital.com
**Control:** Corporation, Investor–owned, for–profit **Service:** General Medical and Surgical

**Staffed Beds:** 15 **Admissions:** 353 **Census:** 4 **Outpatient Visits:** 5712
**Births:** 0 **Total Expense ($000):** 6490 **Payroll Expense ($000):** 2610
**Personnel:** 77

### FAYETTEVILLE—Washington County

⊞ **HEALTHSOUTH REHABILITATION HOSPITAL (43032)**, 153 East Monte Painter Drive, Zip 72703–4002; tel. 479/444–2200 **A**1 9 10 **F**3 29 34 57 59 64 75 77 79 90 91 92 93 94 95 96 **P**8 **S** HEALTHSOUTH Corporation, Birmingham, AL
Primary Contact: Jack C. Mitchell, FACHE, Chief Executive Officer
CFO: Robbi Hudson, Chief Financial Officer
CMO: Marty Hurlbut, M.D., Medical Director
CHR: Missy Cole, Director Human Resources
CNO: Miriam Irvin, CNO
Web address: www.healthsouthfayetteville.com
**Control:** Corporation, Investor–owned, for–profit **Service:** Rehabilitation

**Staffed Beds:** 60 **Admissions:** 1003 **Census:** 35 **Outpatient Visits:** 7123
**Births:** 0 **Total Expense ($000):** 12059 **Payroll Expense ($000):** 6089
**Personnel:** 129

○ **PHYSICIANS' SPECIALTY HOSPITAL (40152)**, 3875 North Parkview Drive, Zip 72703; tel. 479/571–7070 **A**9 10 11 **F**12 40 43 51 79 81 82 85 107 111 113 118 130 141
Primary Contact: Russ Greene, Chief Executive Officer
Web address: www.pshfay.com
**Control:** State–Government, nonfederal **Service:** Surgical

**Staffed Beds:** 21 **Admissions:** 857 **Census:** 6 **Outpatient Visits:** 9195
**Births:** 0 **Total Expense ($000):** 30321 **Payroll Expense ($000):** 8067
**Personnel:** 202

⊞ **REGENCY HOSPITAL OF NORTHWEST ARKANSAS (42009)**, 1125 North College, Zip 72703; tel. 479/713–7000, (Includes REGENCY HOSPITAL OF NORTHWEST ARKANSAS – SPRINGDALE, 609 West Maple Avenue, 6th Floor, Springdale, Zip 72764; tel. 479/757–2600) **A**1 9 10 **F**1 3 29 68 75 77 85 86 87 129 147 **P**5 8 **S** Select Medical Corporation, Mechanicsburg, PA
Primary Contact: Michael A. McLean, Chief Executive Officer
COO: Ruth Jones, Chief Operating Officer
CMO: Gary Templeton, M.D., Medical Director
CHR: Melissa Ross–Cole, Director Human Resources
Web address: www.regencyhospital.com
**Control:** Corporation, Investor–owned, for–profit **Service:** Long–Term Acute Care hospital

**Staffed Beds:** 50 **Admissions:** 487 **Census:** 37 **Outpatient Visits:** 0 **Births:** 0 **Total Expense ($000):** 20587 **Payroll Expense ($000):** 7014 **Personnel:** 126

☐ **SPRINGWOODS BEHAVIORAL HEALTH HOSPITAL (44019)**, 1955 West Truckers Drive, Zip 72704–5637; tel. 479/973–6000 **A**1 9 10 **F**98 99 100 101 102 103 104 105 129 **P**6
Primary Contact: Anthony Walters, Chief Executive Officer
Web address: www.springwoodsbehavioral.com
**Control:** Corporation, Investor–owned, for–profit **Service:** Psychiatric

**Staffed Beds:** 80 **Admissions:** 1620 **Census:** 41 **Outpatient Visits:** 1592
**Births:** 0 **Total Expense ($000):** 9341 **Payroll Expense ($000):** 4660
**Personnel:** 130

⊞ **VETERANS HEALTH CARE SYSTEM OF THE OZARKS**, 1100 North College Avenue, Zip 72703–6995; tel. 479/443–4301, (Nonreporting) **A**1 2 **S** Department of Veterans Affairs, Washington, DC
Primary Contact: John Henley, M.D., Interim Director
COO: Doris B. Cassidy, Associate Director
CMO: Bonnie Baker, M.D., Chief Medical Services
CIO: Michael Gracie, Chief Information Officer
CHR: Kathryn L. Barker, Chief Human Resources Management
Web address: www.va.gov/sta/guide/home.asp
**Control:** Veterans Affairs, Government, federal **Service:** General Medical and Surgical

**Staffed Beds:** 72

**VISTA HEALTH (44004)**, 4253 North Crossover Road, Zip 72703–4596; tel. 479/521–5731 **A**9 10 **F**87 98 99 100 101 102 103 104 106 129 131 **P**6
Primary Contact: Connie Borengasser, Chief Executive Officer
COO: Lee Christenson, Administrator
CFO: Johnny Lancaster, Chief Financial Officer
CMO: Norman Snyder, M.D., Medical Director
CIO: Margaret Brown, Director Medical Records
CHR: Sandy Stout, Director Human Resources
CNO: Angela Klinikowski, Director of Nursing
Web address: www.vistahealthservices.com
**Control:** Corporation, Investor–owned, for–profit **Service:** Psychiatric

**Staffed Beds:** 92 **Admissions:** 1788 **Census:** 78 **Outpatient Visits:** 97156
**Births:** 0 **Total Expense ($000):** 20411 **Payroll Expense ($000):** 12698
**Personnel:** 275

⊞ **WASHINGTON REGIONAL MEDICAL CENTER (40004)**, 3215 North Hills Boulevard, Zip 72703–1994; tel. 479/463–1000 **A**1 9 10 **F**3 9 11 13 14 17 18 20 22 24 26 28 29 30 31 32 34 35 40 43 45 46 47 48 49 50 51 53 54 56 57 58 59 60 61 62 63 64 68 70 72 73 74 75 76 77 78 79 81 82 83 84 85 86 87 89 93 97 100 102 107 108 110 111 113 114 117 118 124 125 128 129 130 131 134 145 146 147 **P**8
Primary Contact: William L. Bradley, President and Chief Executive Officer
CFO: Dan Eckels, Chief Financial Officer
CMO: David Ratcliff, M.D., Chief Medical Affairs
CIO: Becky Magee, Chief Information Officer
CHR: Steve Percival, Director Human Resources
CNO: Claudia Williams, R.N., CNO
Web address: www.wregional.com
**Control:** Other not–for–profit (including NFP Corporation) **Service:** General Medical and Surgical

**Staffed Beds:** 268 **Admissions:** 11540 **Census:** 126 **Outpatient Visits:** 152222 **Births:** 1004 **Total Expense ($000):** 155578 **Payroll Expense ($000):** 67790 **Personnel:** 1648

**FORDYCE—Dallas County**

★ **DALLAS COUNTY MEDICAL CENTER (41317)**, 201 Clifton Street,
Zip 71742–3099; tel. 870/352–6300 **A**9 10 18 **F**11 29 40 41 45 57 59 62 81
93 97 107 118 126 128 132 147
Primary Contact: Brian Miller, Administrator and Chief Executive Officer
CFO: Billie Launius, Director Business Finance
CMO: Michael Payne, M.D., Chief of Staff
CHR: Audrey Allen, Coordinator Benefits
Web address: www.dallascountymedicalcenter.com
**Control:** County–Government, nonfederal **Service:** General Medical and Surgical

**Staffed Beds:** 25 **Admissions:** 404 **Census:** 3 **Outpatient Visits:** 42489
**Births:** 0 **Total Expense ($000):** 8411 **Payroll Expense ($000):** 3286
**Personnel:** 97

**FORREST CITY—St. Francis County**

✠ **FORREST CITY MEDICAL CENTER (40019)**, 1601 Newcastle Road,
Zip 72335; tel. 870/261–0000 **A**1 9 10 20 **F**3 13 15 29 30 34 40 43 49 50
76 79 81 85 89 93 98 103 107 110 111 118 128 129 132 146 **S** Community
Health Systems, Inc., Franklin, TN
Primary Contact: Brett Kinman, Chief Executive Officer
CFO: Stephen Doherty, Chief Financial Officer
CMO: Brandy Davis, M.D., Chief of Staff
CIO: Scott Miller, Director Information Services
CHR: Sherry McLaughlin, Director Human Resources
CNO: Rhonda Nelson, Chief Nursing Officer
Web address: www.forrestcitymedicalcenter.com
**Control:** Corporation, Investor–owned, for–profit **Service:** General Medical and
Surgical

**Staffed Beds:** 70 **Admissions:** 2065 **Census:** 19 **Outpatient Visits:** 27143
**Births:** 688 **Total Expense ($000):** 18989 **Payroll Expense ($000):** 8324
**Personnel:** 174

**FORT SMITH—Sebastian County**

✠ **ADVANCE CARE HOSPITAL OF FORT SMITH (42008)**, 7301 Rogers Avenue,
4th Floor, Zip 72917; tel. 479/314–4900 **A**1 9 10 **F**1 3 29 30 68 75 77 82 84
85 91 129 147 **S** Dubuis Health System, Houston, TX
Primary Contact: Keith Rogers, Interim Administrator
CFO: Paul Veillon, CPA, Chief Financial Officer
Web address: www.dubuis.org
**Control:** Church–operated, Nongovernment, not–for profit **Service:** Long–Term
Acute Care hospital

**Staffed Beds:** 25 **Admissions:** 270 **Census:** 21 **Outpatient Visits:** 0 **Births:**
0 **Total Expense ($000):** 8716 **Payroll Expense ($000):** 3517 **Personnel:**
66

✠ **HEALTHSOUTH REHABILITATION HOSPITAL OF FORT SMITH (43028)**, 1401
South J Street, Zip 72901–5155; tel. 479/785–3300, (Nonreporting) **A**1 9 10
**S** HEALTHSOUTH Corporation, Birmingham, AL
Primary Contact: Ryan Cassedy, Chief Executive Officer
CFO: Brenda Forbes, Controller
CMO: Cygnet Schroeder, D.O., Medical Director
CIO: Donna England, Director Medical Records
CHR: S. Janette Daniels, Director Human Resources
CNO: Jacqueline Floyd, Chief Nursing Officer
Web address: www.healthsouthfortsmith.com
**Control:** Corporation, Investor–owned, for–profit **Service:** Rehabilitation

**Staffed Beds:** 80

✠ △ **MERCY HOSPITAL FORT SMITH (40062)**, 7301 Rogers Avenue,
Zip 72903–4189, Mailing Address: P.O. Box 17000, Zip 72917–7000;
tel. 479/314–6000 **A**1 2 7 9 10 **F**3 11 12 13 15 17 18 20 22 24 26 28 29 30
31 32 34 35 40 42 43 44 49 53 57 58 59 61 62 63 64 65 68 70 71 72 73
74 75 77 78 79 81 82 83 84 85 86 87 90 93 96 102 107 108 110 111 113
114 118 119 120 122 123 125 128 129 134 142 145 146 147 **P**6 8 **S** Mercy
Health, Chesterfield, MO
Primary Contact: Ryan Gehrig, President
COO: Steve Loveless, Chief Operating Officer
CFO: Greta Wilcher, Senior Vice President and Chief Financial Officer
CHR: Tim Murphy, Vice President, Human Resources
Web address: www.stedwardmercy.com
**Control:** Church–operated, Nongovernment, not–for profit **Service:** General
Medical and Surgical

**Staffed Beds:** 374 **Admissions:** 14412 **Census:** 206 **Outpatient Visits:**
130935 **Births:** 2228 **Total Expense ($000):** 203114 **Payroll Expense
($000):** 68706 **Personnel:** 1495

✠ **SELECT SPECIALTY HOSPITAL–FORT SMITH (42006)**, 1001 Towson Avenue,
Zip 72902–4921; tel. 479/441–3960 **A**1 9 10 **F**1 3 29 34 45 46 56 57 74 75
78 79 81 94 147 **S** Select Medical Corporation, Mechanicsburg, PA
Primary Contact: Cindy McLain, Chief Executive Officer
Web address: www.selectmedicalcorp.com
**Control:** Corporation, Investor–owned, for–profit **Service:** Long–Term Acute Care
hospital

**Staffed Beds:** 34 **Admissions:** 450 **Census:** 32 **Outpatient Visits:** 0 **Births:**
0 **Total Expense ($000):** 13444 **Payroll Expense ($000):** 4350 **Personnel:**
74

☐ **SPARKS REGIONAL MEDICAL CENTER (40055)**, 100 Towson Avenue,
Zip 72901–2632, Mailing Address: P.O. Box 17006, Zip 72917–7006;
tel. 479/441–4000 **A**1 2 9 10 **F**3 8 12 13 15 17 18 20 22 24 26 28 29 30 31
34 35 40 45 46 47 48 49 50 51 53 54 56 58 59 60 62 64 67 70 72 74 75
76 77 78 79 81 82 85 86 87 89 93 97 98 103 107 108 110 111 112 113
114 116 118 119 120 121 123 125 126 128 129 143 145 146 147 **P**8
**S** Health Management Associates, Naples, FL
Primary Contact: Melody Trimble, Chief Executive Officer
COO: Jeremy Drinkwitz, Chief Operating Officer
CFO: Richard Boone, Chief Financial Officer
CMO: Katherine Irish–Clardy, M.D., Chief Medical Officer
CIO: Tom Sallis, Director Information Systems
CHR: Robert Freeman, Director Human Resources
CNO: Cindy Slaydon, Chief Nursing Executive
Web address: www.sparks.org
**Control:** Individual, Investor–owned, for–profit **Service:** General Medical and
Surgical

**Staffed Beds:** 303 **Admissions:** 15432 **Census:** 208 **Outpatient Visits:**
149262 **Births:** 1230 **Total Expense ($000):** 194843 **Payroll Expense
($000):** 63422 **Personnel:** 1624

**GRAVETTE—Benton County**

**OZARKS COMMUNITY HOSPITAL (41331)**, 1101 Jackson Street S.W.,
Zip 72736–9121; tel. 479/787–5291 **A**9 10 18 **F**29 40 44 45 54 56 57 59 75
82 85 87 89 93 96 107 111 113 118 127 129 132 142 **P**6
Primary Contact: Paul Taylor, Administrator
Web address: www.ochonline.com/
**Control:** Individual, Investor–owned, for–profit **Service:** General Medical and
Surgical

**Staffed Beds:** 15 **Admissions:** 656 **Census:** 7 **Outpatient Visits:** 35972
**Births:** 1 **Total Expense ($000):** 13117 **Payroll Expense ($000):** 6676
**Personnel:** 170

**HARRISON—Boone County**

★ **NORTH ARKANSAS REGIONAL MEDICAL CENTER (40017)**, 620 North Main
Street, Zip 72601–2994; tel. 870/414–4000 **A**9 10 **F**3 7 8 11 13 15 17 18 28
29 31 34 35 39 40 48 50 51 57 59 62 63 64 65 68 70 75 76 77 78 79 81
85 86 87 92 93 97 107 108 110 111 113 114 117 118 119 120 122 126
127 128 129 131 145 146 147 **P**8
Primary Contact: Vincent Leist, President and Chief Executive Officer
COO: Richard McBryde, Senior Vice President and Chief Operating Officer
CFO: Debbie Henry, Vice President Financial Services
CIO: Kent Kimes, Director Information Systems
CHR: Linda Dickey Melton, Vice President Human Resources
Web address: www.narmc.com
**Control:** Other not–for–profit (including NFP Corporation) **Service:** General
Medical and Surgical

**Staffed Beds:** 125 **Admissions:** 4242 **Census:** 41 **Outpatient Visits:** 99389
**Births:** 732 **Total Expense ($000):** 59274 **Payroll Expense ($000):** 25213
**Personnel:** 568

**HEBER SPRINGS—Cleburne County**

✠ **BAPTIST HEALTH MEDICAL CENTER–HEBER SPRINGS (41312)**, 1800
Bypass Road, Zip 72543–9135; tel. 501/887–3000 **A**1 9 10 18 **F**3 8 11 15 28
29 30 31 34 35 36 40 43 45 48 57 59 62 64 68 74 75 77 78 79 81 85 93
102 107 110 111 114 115 116 118 126 128 130 131 132 133 134 142 145
**S** Baptist Health, Little Rock, AR
Primary Contact: Edward L. Lacy, FACHE, Vice President and Administrator
Web address: www.baptist–health.com
**Control:** Other not–for–profit (including NFP Corporation) **Service:** General
Medical and Surgical

**Staffed Beds:** 25 **Admissions:** 786 **Census:** 7 **Outpatient Visits:** 30847
**Births:** 0 **Total Expense ($000):** 13517 **Payroll Expense ($000):** 6771
**Personnel:** 155

AR

---

**Hospital, Medicare Provider Number, Address, Telephone, Approval, Facility, and Physician Codes, Health Care System**

★ American Hospital Association (AHA) membership
☐ The Joint Commission accreditation
◇ DNV Healthcare Inc. accreditation
○ American Osteopathic Association (AOA) accreditation
△ Commission on Accreditation of Rehabilitation Facilities (CARF) accreditation

**AR**

### HELENA—Phillips County

☒ **HELENA REGIONAL MEDICAL CENTER (40085)**, 1801 Martin Luther King Drive, Zip 72342, Mailing Address: P.O. Box 788, Zip 72342–0788; tel. 870/338–5800 **A**1 9 10 20 **F**3 13 15 28 29 34 35 40 43 59 60 62 64 70 75 76 77 79 81 86 87 90 91 93 97 107 108 111 118 129 131 132 134 144 145 146 147 **S** Community Health Systems, Inc., Franklin, TN
Primary Contact: James T. Sato, FACHE, Chief Executive Officer
CFO: Amy Rice, Chief Financial Officer
CIO: Robert White, Director Information Technology
CHR: Juril Fonzie, Director Human Resources
CNO: Shanna Pryor, R.N., Chief Nursing Officer
Web address: www.helenarmc.com
**Control:** Corporation, Investor–owned, for–profit **Service:** General Medical and Surgical

**Staffed Beds:** 100 **Admissions:** 2281 **Census:** 20 **Outpatient Visits:** 23857 **Births:** 238 **Total Expense ($000):** 22584 **Payroll Expense ($000):** 9010 **Personnel:** 154

### HOPE—Hempstead County

**MEDICAL PARK HOSPITAL (40091)**, 2001 South Main Street, Zip 71801–8194; tel. 870/777–2323, (Nonreporting) **A**9 10
Primary Contact: Teddy Cheek, Chief Executive Officer
COO: Faye Hughes, Chief Nursing Officer and Chief Operating Officer
CIO: Jeff Cook, Director Information Services
CHR: Vickie Barnhill–Keener, Director Human Resources
Web address: www.mphhope.com
**Control:** Corporation, Investor–owned, for–profit **Service:** General Medical and Surgical

**Staffed Beds:** 79

### HOT SPRINGS—Garland County

☐ △ **NATIONAL PARK MEDICAL CENTER (40078)**, 1910 Malvern Avenue, Zip 71901–7799; tel. 501/321–1000 **A**1 7 9 10 19 **F**3 11 13 15 17 18 20 22 24 28 29 30 31 34 35 40 45 46 47 49 56 57 59 62 64 70 73 74 75 76 78 79 81 85 87 89 90 93 107 108 110 111 113 118 123 127 128 129 130 131 142 145 146 147 **P**1 **S** Capella Healthcare, Franklin, TN
Primary Contact: Jerry D. Mabry, FACHE, Chief Executive Officer
COO: Brian Bell, Associate Administrator and Chief Operating Officer
CFO: Robbie Pettey, Chief Financial Officer
CMO: David Desoto, M.D., Chief of Staff
CIO: Thomas Elmore, Director Information System
CHR: Sandra Culliver, Director Human Resources
Web address: www.nationalparkmedical.com
**Control:** Corporation, Investor–owned, for–profit **Service:** General Medical and Surgical

**Staffed Beds:** 181 **Admissions:** 5810 **Census:** 87 **Outpatient Visits:** 45615 **Births:** 626 **Total Expense ($000):** 64527 **Payroll Expense ($000):** 24877 **Personnel:** 656

### HOT SPRINGS NATIONAL PARK—Garland County

☒ **ADVANCE CARE HOSPITAL (42004)**, 300 Werner Street, 3rd Floor East, Zip 71913; tel. 501/609–4300 **A**1 9 10 **F**1 3 29 30 45 68 77 79 85 87 117 129 134 147 **P**5 **S** Dubuis Health System, Houston, TX
Primary Contact: Keith Rogers, Administrator
CFO: Paul Veillon, CPA, Chief Financial Officer
CIO: David Cook, Manager Information Systems
CHR: Pearl Mohnkern, Vice President Human Resources
Web address: www.dubuis.org
**Control:** Church–operated, Nongovernment, not–for profit **Service:** Long–Term Acute Care hospital

**Staffed Beds:** 26 **Admissions:** 203 **Census:** 15 **Outpatient Visits:** 0 **Births:** 0 **Total Expense ($000):** 5962 **Payroll Expense ($000):** 2581 **Personnel:** 53

**HOT SPRINGS REHABILITATION CENTER (43027)**, 105 Reserve Avenue, Zip 71902, Mailing Address: P.O. Box 1358, Zip 71902; tel. 501/624–4411 **A**9 10 **F**12 29 30 38 39 44 64 68 75 79 87 90 91 93 97 99 100 101 104 129 131 142 147 **P**6
Primary Contact: Alan Phillips, M.D., Interim Administrator
CMO: Patricia Lang, M.D., Medical Director
CIO: Dean Ulmer, Manager Information Services
Web address: www.arsinfo.org/hsrehab.html
**Control:** State–Government, nonfederal **Service:** Rehabilitation

**Staffed Beds:** 24 **Admissions:** 21 **Census:** 1 **Outpatient Visits:** 4680 **Births:** 0 **Total Expense ($000):** 5536 **Payroll Expense ($000):** 3420 **Personnel:** 118

★ **LEVI HOSPITAL (40132)**, 300 Prospect Avenue, Zip 71901–4097; tel. 501/624–1281 **A**9 10 **F**40 57 59 64 93 98 102 103 104 129 130 131
Primary Contact: Patrick G. McCabe, Jr., FACHE, President and Chief Executive Officer
CFO: Charles Oswalt, Vice President and Chief Financial Officer
CMO: P. Ross Bandy, M.D., Chief Medical Officer and Chief of Staff
CIO: Charles Oswalt, Vice President, CFO and Compliance Officer
CHR: Susan Kramer, Director of Human Resources
CNO: Steven Boyd, R.N., Nurse Executive
Web address: www.levihospital.com
**Control:** Other not–for–profit (including NFP Corporation) **Service:** Psychiatric

**Staffed Beds:** 49 **Admissions:** 1443 **Census:** 26 **Outpatient Visits:** 17071 **Births:** 0 **Total Expense ($000):** 7382 **Payroll Expense ($000):** 4219 **Personnel:** 107

☒ **MERCY HOSPITAL HOT SPRINGS (40026)**, 300 Werner Street, Zip 71913–9937, Mailing Address: P.O. Box 29001, Zip 71913–9001; tel. 501/622–1000, (Includes HEALTHPARK HOSPITAL, 1636 Higdon Ferry Road, Zip 71913; tel. 501/520–2000) **A**1 2 9 10 **F**3 11 12 13 15 17 18 20 22 24 26 28 29 30 31 34 35 40 49 50 56 57 59 62 64 65 66 68 69 70 71 74 75 76 78 79 81 84 85 86 87 89 90 92 93 98 103 107 108 110 111 113 114 115 116 117 118 119 120 125 128 129 131 134 145 146 147 **P**6 **S** Mercy Health, Chesterfield, MO
Primary Contact: Timothy J. Johnsen, President and Chief Executive Officer
COO: Brenda Chase, Chief Operating Officer
CFO: Sarah Bradey, Vice President Finance
CIO: Bill Perry, Director Information Systems
CHR: Jed Liuzza, Vice President Human Resources
Web address: www.saintjosephs.com
**Control:** Church–operated, Nongovernment, not–for profit **Service:** General Medical and Surgical

**Staffed Beds:** 282 **Admissions:** 11567 **Census:** 167 **Outpatient Visits:** 169238 **Births:** 1019 **Total Expense ($000):** 169397 **Payroll Expense ($000):** 67531 **Personnel:** 1891

### JACKSONVILLE—Pulaski County

**ALLEGIANCE SPECIALTY HOSPITAL OF LITTLE ROCK (42010)**, 1400 Braden Street, Zip 72076–3721; tel. 501/985–7026 **A**9 10 **F**1 3 29 75 82 85 86 87 100 129 147 **P**5 **S** Allegiance Health Management, Shreveport, LA
Primary Contact: Cindy Stafford, Chief Executive Officer
CHR: Jennifer Rowen, Director Human Resources
CNO: Diane Cook, Chief Nursing Officer
Web address: www.allegiancespecialtyhospitaloflr.com
**Control:** Individual, Investor–owned, for–profit **Service:** Long–Term Acute Care hospital

**Staffed Beds:** 40 **Admissions:** 244 **Census:** 18 **Outpatient Visits:** 0 **Births:** 0 **Total Expense ($000):** 4588 **Payroll Expense ($000):** 1872 **Personnel:** 48

★ **NORTH METRO MEDICAL CENTER (40074)**, 1400 West Braden Street, Zip 72076–3788; tel. 501/985–7000 **A**9 10 **F**3 11 15 18 20 29 34 35 40 50 51 56 57 59 62 64 68 70 75 77 79 81 85 86 87 98 103 104 107 108 110 111 113 118 123 128 130 131 134 145 147 **P**1 3
Primary Contact: Jay Quebedeaux, Chief Executive Officer
CFO: Lynn Muller, Chief Financial Officer
CMO: Ann Layton, M.D., Chief of Staff
CHR: Jane Rockwell, Director Support Services
Web address: www.northmetromed.com
**Control:** Other not–for–profit (including NFP Corporation) **Service:** General Medical and Surgical

**Staffed Beds:** 76 **Admissions:** 1749 **Census:** 32 **Outpatient Visits:** 58293 **Births:** 0 **Total Expense ($000):** 28709 **Payroll Expense ($000):** 13589 **Personnel:** 301

### JONESBORO—Craighead County

☒ **HEALTHSOUTH REHABILITATION HOSPITAL OF JONESBORO (43029)**, 1201 Fleming Avenue, Zip 72401–4311, Mailing Address: P.O. Box 1680, Zip 72403–1680; tel. 870/932–0440, (Nonreporting) **A**1 9 10 **S** HEALTHSOUTH Corporation, Birmingham, AL
Primary Contact: Donna Harris, Chief Executive Officer
CFO: Allan Jones, Controller
CMO: Terence Braden, III, D.O., Medical Director
CHR: Tammy Barley, Director Human Resources
CHR: Tammy Barley, Manager Human Resources
Web address: www.healthsouthjonesboro.com
**Control:** Corporation, Investor–owned, for–profit **Service:** Rehabilitation

**Staffed Beds:** 67

⊞ **NEA BAPTIST MEMORIAL HOSPITAL (40118)**, 3024 Stadium Boulevard, Zip 72401-7493; tel. 870/972-7000 **A**1 9 10 **F**3 11 12 13 17 18 20 22 24 28 29 30 31 34 39 40 45 46 48 49 57 59 60 74 75 76 77 78 79 81 82 84 85 86 87 93 107 108 111 114 117 118 123 145 147 **P**8 **S** Baptist Memorial Health Care Corporation, Memphis, TN
Primary Contact: Brad Parsons, Administrator and Chief Executive Officer
CFO: David Webb, Chief Financial Officer
CMO: Stephen Woodruff, M.D., Chief Medical Officer
CHR: James Keller, Director Human Resources
Web address: www.neabaptist.com
**Control:** Other not-for-profit (including NFP Corporation) **Service:** General Medical and Surgical

**Staffed Beds:** 100 **Admissions:** 6787 **Census:** 71 **Outpatient Visits:** 43149 **Births:** 686 **Total Expense ($000):** 85998 **Payroll Expense ($000):** 27197 **Personnel:** 629

⊞ **ST. BERNARDS MEDICAL CENTER (40020)**, 225 East Jackson Avenue, Zip 72401; tel. 870/972-4429, (Total facility includes 27 beds in nursing home-type unit) **A**1 9 10 19 **F**2 3 11 17 18 20 22 24 26 28 29 30 31 32 34 35 37 38 40 43 45 46 48 49 50 51 53 54 55 56 57 58 59 60 61 62 63 64 68 69 70 71 74 75 76 77 78 79 81 82 84 85 86 87 89 92 93 96 98 99 100 101 102 103 104 105 107 108 110 111 113 114 115 116 118 119 120 122 123 125 127 128 129 130 131 134 135 140 143 144 145 146 147 **P**6 8
Primary Contact: Chris B. Barber, FACHE, President and Chief Executive Officer
COO: Michael K. Givens, FACHE, Administrator
CFO: Harry Hutchison, Vice President Fiscal Services
CMO: David Pyle, M.D., Vice President Medical Affairs
CIO: Charles Pigg, Chief Information Officer
CHR: Jacque Hurd, Vice President Human Resources
CNO: Brenda Million, R.N., Vice President and Chief Nursing Officer
Web address: www.stbernards.info
**Control:** Church-operated, Nongovernment, not-for profit **Service:** General Medical and Surgical

**Staffed Beds:** 375 **Admissions:** 18092 **Census:** 235 **Outpatient Visits:** 226832 **Births:** 1343 **Total Expense ($000):** 219673 **Payroll Expense ($000):** 78238 **Personnel:** 1835

**SURGICAL HOSPITAL OF JONESBORO**, 909 Enterprise Drive, Zip 72401; tel. 870/336-1100, (Nonreporting)
Primary Contact: Nate Miller, Chief Executive Officer
CFO: Carla Harral, Chief Financial Officer
CMO: Jason Brandt, M.D., Medical Director
CHR: Angie Stover, Administrative Assistant
Web address: www.tshj.com
**Control:** Corporation, Investor-owned, for-profit **Service:** Surgical

**Staffed Beds:** 12

★ **CHICOT MEMORIAL MEDICAL CENTER (41328)**, 2729 Highway 65 and 82 South, Zip 71653; tel. 870/265-5351 **A**9 10 18 **F**3 11 13 15 29 34 35 40 45 53 62 64 75 76 81 85 87 107 111 117 118 129 131 132 145 147
Primary Contact: Russ D. Sword, FACHE, Interim Chief Executive Officer
CFO: Vicki Allen, Chief Financial Officer
CMO: Michael Bradley Mayfield, M.D., Chief of Staff
CIO: David Andrews, Manager Information Systems
CHR: Bobbie Ivey, Director Human Resources
CNO: Eric Selby, R.N., Chief Nursing Officer
Web address: www.chicotmemorial.com
**Control:** Other not-for-profit (including NFP Corporation) **Service:** General Medical and Surgical

**Staffed Beds:** 25 **Admissions:** 1221 **Census:** 13 **Outpatient Visits:** 14572 **Births:** 109 **Total Expense ($000):** 13885 **Payroll Expense ($000):** 6585 **Personnel:** 149

**SOUTHEAST REHABILITATION HOSPITAL (43034)**, 2729-A Highway 65 and 82 South, Zip 71653; tel. 870/265-4333, (Nonreporting) **A**10
Primary Contact: Stacy Noble, Administrator
Web address: www.lakevillageclinic.com/SErehabhosp.html
**Control:** Partnership, Investor-owned, for-profit **Service:** Rehabilitation

**Staffed Beds:** 15

⊞ **ARKANSAS CHILDREN'S HOSPITAL (43300)**, 1 Children's Way, Zip 72202-3591; tel. 501/364-1100 **A**1 3 5 8 9 10 **F**3 7 8 9 11 12 16 17 19 21 23 25 27 28 29 30 31 32 34 35 38 39 40 41 43 45 46 48 50 53 55 57 58 59 60 61 64 68 71 72 74 75 77 78 79 81 82 84 85 86 87 88 89 91 93 94 97 99 100 102 107 113 114 115 116 117 118 125 128 129 130 131 134 135 136 137 142 145 **P**1
Primary Contact: Jonathan R. Bates, M.D., President and Chief Executive Officer
COO: David Berry, Senior Vice President and Chief Operating Officer
CFO: Gena Wingfield, Senior Vice President and Chief Financial Officer
CMO: W. Robert Morrow, M.D., Senior Vice President and Medical Director
CIO: Darrell Leonhardt, Senior Vice President Information Systems
CHR: Andree Trosclair, Vice President Human Resources
CNO: Lori J. Brown, MSN, Senior Vice President and Chief Nursing Officer
Web address: www.archildrens.org
**Control:** Other not-for-profit (including NFP Corporation) **Service:** Children's general

**Staffed Beds:** 312 **Admissions:** 14114 **Census:** 222 **Outpatient Visits:** 314937 **Births:** 0 **Total Expense ($000):** 447345 **Payroll Expense ($000):** 195364 **Personnel:** 3223

☐ **ARKANSAS HEART HOSPITAL (40134)**, 1701 South Shackleford Road, Zip 72211-4335; tel. 501/219-7000, (Nonreporting) **A**1 3 5 9 10
Primary Contact: Bruce Murphy, M.D., President and Chief Executive Officer
CHR: Brent Davis, Human Resources Team Leader
Web address: www.arheart.com
**Control:** Partnership, Investor-owned, for-profit **Service:** Heart

**Staffed Beds:** 112

☐ **ARKANSAS STATE HOSPITAL (44011)**, 305 South Palm Street, Zip 72205-5432; tel. 501/686-9000 **A**1 3 5 9 10 **F**98 99 101 106 **P**6
Primary Contact: Randall J. Fale, FACHE, Interim Chief Executive Officer
CFO: Jo Ann McDade, Assistant Administrator Finance
CMO: Albert Kittrell, M.D., Medical Director
CIO: Linda Jackson, Director Management Information Systems
CHR: Tracy Pearsall, Director Human Resources
Web address: www.state.ar.us/dhs/dmhs
**Control:** State-Government, nonfederal **Service:** Psychiatric

**Staffed Beds:** 220 **Admissions:** 954 **Census:** 217 **Outpatient Visits:** 0 **Births:** 0 **Total Expense ($000):** 44657 **Payroll Expense ($000):** 24074 **Personnel:** 724

★ **BAPTIST HEALTH EXTENDED CARE HOSPITAL (42012)**, 9601 Interstate 630, Exit 7, 10th Floor, Zip 72205-7202; tel. 501/202-1070 **A**9 10 **F**1 3 29 31 77 87 129 147 **S** Baptist Health, Little Rock, AR
Primary Contact: Mike Perkins, Administrator
CFO: Robert C. Roberts, Vice President
CIO: David House, Vice President
CHR: Anthony Kendall, Vice President Human Resources
CNO: Diane Smith, Chief Nursing Officer
Web address: www.baptist-health.com
**Control:** Other not-for-profit (including NFP Corporation) **Service:** Long-Term Acute Care hospital

**Staffed Beds:** 37 **Admissions:** 293 **Census:** 23 **Outpatient Visits:** 0 **Births:** 0 **Total Expense ($000):** 11045 **Payroll Expense ($000):** 4721 **Personnel:** 80

⊞ **BAPTIST HEALTH MEDICAL CENTER–LITTLE ROCK (40114)**, 9601 Interstate 630, Exit 7, Zip 72205-7299; tel. 501/202-2000 **A**1 5 6 9 10 **F**3 4 5 7 8 11 12 13 15 17 18 20 22 24 26 28 29 30 31 32 34 35 36 37 38 40 43 44 45 49 50 54 56 57 58 59 60 61 62 64 65 67 68 70 72 73 74 75 76 77 78 79 81 82 85 86 87 89 93 98 99 100 101 102 103 104 107 108 110 111 113 117 118 125 127 128 129 130 131 133 134 136 137 142 143 145 146 147 **S** Baptist Health, Little Rock, AR
Primary Contact: Steven Douglas Weeks, FACHE, Senior Vice President and Administrator
COO: Greg Stubblefield, Vice President and Administrator
CFO: Robert C. Roberts, Senior Vice President Financial Services
CMO: Anthony Bennett, M.D., Chief Clinical Affairs
CIO: David House, Vice President and Chief Information Officer
CHR: Anthony Kendall, Vice President Human Resources
CNO: Jill Massiet, R.N., Vice President Patient Care
Web address: www.baptist-health.org
**Control:** Other not-for-profit (including NFP Corporation) **Service:** General Medical and Surgical

**Staffed Beds:** 703 **Admissions:** 29486 **Census:** 435 **Outpatient Visits:** 88272 **Births:** 3367 **Total Expense ($000):** 377470 **Payroll Expense ($000):** 143846 **Personnel:** 2855

**AR**

---

**Hospital, Medicare Provider Number, Address, Telephone, Approval, Facility, and Physician Codes, Health Care System**

★ American Hospital Association (AHA) membership
☐ The Joint Commission accreditation
◇ DNV Healthcare Inc. accreditation
○ American Osteopathic Association (AOA) accreditation
△ Commission on Accreditation of Rehabilitation Facilities (CARF) accreditation

**AR**

⊠ △ **BAPTIST HEALTH REHABILITATION INSTITUTE (43026)**, 9601 Interstate 630, Exit 7, Zip 72205–7249; tel. 501/202–7000 **A**1 3 5 7 9 10 **F**11 29 30 35 50 53 64 75 79 87 90 93 95 96 129 131 142 145 **S** Baptist Health, Little Rock, AR
Primary Contact: Lee Gentry, FACHE, Vice President and Administrator
CFO: Robert C. Roberts, Senior Vice President
CIO: David House, Vice President and Chief Information Officer
CHR: Anthony Kendall, Vice President Human Resources
Web address: www.baptist–health.com
**Control:** Other not–for–profit (including NFP Corporation) **Service:** Rehabilitation

**Staffed Beds:** 100 **Admissions:** 1666 **Census:** 58 **Outpatient Visits:** 142912 **Births:** 0 **Total Expense ($000):** 28839 **Payroll Expense ($000):** 14146 **Personnel:** 270

⊠ △ **CENTRAL ARKANSAS VETERANS HEALTHCARE SYSTEM**, 4300 West Seventh Street, Zip 72205–5484; tel. 501/257–1000, (Includes NORTH LITTLE ROCK DIVISION, 2200 Fort Roots Drive, North Little Rock, Zip 72114–1706; tel. 501/661–1202), (Total facility includes 152 beds in nursing home–type unit) **A**1 2 3 5 7 8 **F**2 3 5 6 15 17 18 20 22 26 28 29 30 31 34 35 38 39 40 45 46 48 49 50 56 57 58 59 60 61 62 64 65 68 70 74 75 77 78 79 80 81 82 83 84 85 86 87 90 91 92 93 94 96 97 98 100 101 102 103 104 105 106 107 108 110 111 113 114 117 118 121 126 127 128 129 131 134 142 143 144 145 146 147 **P**1 6 **S** Department of Veterans Affairs, Washington, DC
Primary Contact: Michael R. Winn, Director
CFO: Debby Felton, Chief Financial Officer
CMO: Nicholas P. Lang, M.D., Chief of Staff
CIO: Jim Hall, Acting Chief Information Officer
CHR: Daniel Peterson, Chief Human Resource Management Service
Web address: www.va.gov/sta/guide/home.asp
**Control:** Veterans Affairs, Government, federal **Service:** General Medical and Surgical

**Staffed Beds:** 551 **Admissions:** 11750 **Census:** 430 **Outpatient Visits:** 822133 **Births:** 0 **Total Expense ($000):** 613800 **Payroll Expense ($000):** 235123 **Personnel:** 3333

☐ **PINNACLE POINTE HOSPITAL (44013)**, 11501 Financial Center Parkway, Zip 72211–3715; tel. 501/223–3322 **A**1 9 10 **F**29 34 98 99 100 101 102 104 106 129 **P**5 **S** Universal Health Services, Inc., King of Prussia, PA
Primary Contact: Lisa Evans, Chief Executive Officer
CMO: David Streett, M.D., Medical Director
CHR: James L. Howe, Chief Employee Relations
Web address: www.pinnaclepointehospital.com
**Control:** Corporation, Investor–owned, for–profit **Service:** Children's hospital psychiatric

**Staffed Beds:** 124 **Admissions:** 2619 **Census:** 108 **Outpatient Visits:** 275691 **Births:** 0 **Total Expense ($000):** 19971 **Payroll Expense ($000):** 12304 **Personnel:** 281

⊠ **SELECT SPECIALTY HOSPITAL–LITTLE ROCK (42000)**, 2 St. Vincent Circle, 6th Floor, Zip 72205; tel. 501/661–4198 **A**1 9 10 **F**1 3 29 74 75 77 78 79 82 85 86 91 97 100 129 147 **P**5 **S** Select Medical Corporation, Mechanicsburg, PA
Primary Contact: Barry Ewy, Chief Executive Officer
Web address: www.selectmedicalcorp.com
**Control:** Corporation, Investor–owned, for–profit **Service:** Long–Term Acute Care hospital

**Staffed Beds:** 43 **Admissions:** 409 **Census:** 32 **Outpatient Visits:** 0 **Births:** 0 **Total Expense ($000):** 15144 **Payroll Expense ($000):** 5454 **Personnel:** 132

⊠ **ST. VINCENT INFIRMARY MEDICAL CENTER (40007)**, Two St. Vincent Circle, Zip 72205–5499; tel. 501/552–3000, (Includes ST. VINCENT DOCTORS HOSPITAL, 6101 West Capitol, Zip 72205–5331; tel. 501/552–6000) **A**1 5 9 10 **F**3 11 13 17 18 20 22 24 26 28 29 30 31 34 35 37 40 43 44 45 50 51 53 54 56 57 59 60 61 62 64 70 72 74 75 76 77 78 79 81 82 84 85 86 87 91 92 93 97 98 107 108 109 110 111 113 114 115 116 117 118 123 125 128 129 131 134 142 145 146 147 **P**1 **S** Catholic Health Initiatives, Englewood, CO
Primary Contact: Peter D. Banko, FACHE, President and Chief Executive Officer
COO: Bob Lyons, Senior Vice President and Chief Operating Officer
CFO: Matthew Cox, Senior Vice President and Chief Financial Officer
CMO: James Tanner, M.D., Vice President and Chief Medical Officer
CIO: David Peterson, Regional Chief Information Officer
CHR: Darrick Paul, Vice President and Chief People Officer
Web address: www.stvincenthealth.com
**Control:** Church–operated, Nongovernment, not–for profit **Service:** General Medical and Surgical

**Staffed Beds:** 409 **Admissions:** 19621 **Census:** 271 **Outpatient Visits:** 107383 **Births:** 1763 **Total Expense ($000):** 274335 **Payroll Expense ($000):** 99875 **Personnel:** 1881

⊠ **UAMS MEDICAL CENTER (40016)**, 4301 West Markham Street, Zip 72205–7102; tel. 501/686–7000 **A**1 3 5 8 9 10 13 **F**3 11 12 13 14 15 17 18 20 22 24 26 29 30 31 40 43 44 45 46 47 49 50 53 55 56 58 59 60 61 64 68 70 72 73 74 75 76 77 78 79 80 81 82 84 85 86 87 91 92 93 94 96 97 98 99 100 101 102 103 104 107 108 110 111 113 114 117 118 125 129 130 131 135 137 138 140 145 146 **P**6
Primary Contact: Richard Pierson, Executive Director
COO: Melissa Fontaine, Chief Operating Officer
CFO: Daniel J. Riley, Chief Financial Officer
CMO: Nicholas P. Lang, M.D., Chief Medical Officer
CIO: David L. Miller, Chief Information Officer
CHR: Hosea Long, Director Human Resources
CNO: Mary Helen Forrest, R.N., Chief Nursing Officer
Web address: www.uams.edu/medcenter
**Control:** State–Government, nonfederal **Service:** General Medical and Surgical

**Staffed Beds:** 436 **Admissions:** 21304 **Census:** 368 **Outpatient Visits:** 446305 **Births:** 2662 **Total Expense ($000):** 526836 **Payroll Expense ($000):** 172171 **Personnel:** 3359

**MAGNOLIA—Columbia County**

★ **MAGNOLIA REGIONAL MEDICAL CENTER (40067)**, 101 Hospital Drive, Zip 71753–2416, Mailing Address: P.O. Box 629, Zip 71754–0629; tel. 870/235–3000 **A**9 10 20 **F**3 11 13 15 29 31 34 35 40 43 57 59 62 64 70 75 76 77 81 86 87 91 93 97 107 108 110 111 114 118 126 128 129 131 132 145 147 **S** CHRISTUS Health, Irving, TX
Primary Contact: Margaret M. West, MS, Chief Executive Officer
CMO: John Alexander, Jr., M.D., Chief of Staff
CHR: Shawnee Hicks, Director Human Resources
Web address: www.magnoliahospital.org
**Control:** City–Government, nonfederal **Service:** General Medical and Surgical

**Staffed Beds:** 49 **Admissions:** 1870 **Census:** 14 **Outpatient Visits:** 42794 **Births:** 235 **Total Expense ($000):** 22420 **Payroll Expense ($000):** 10446 **Personnel:** 241

**MALVERN—Hot Spring County**

★ **H.S.C. MEDICAL CENTER (40076)**, 1001 Schneider Drive, Zip 72104–4828; tel. 501/332–1000 **A**9 10 **F**3 8 11 15 17 29 30 34 35 40 50 57 59 62 64 70 75 77 81 87 98 101 102 103 107 111 113 118 128 129 131 144 145 147
Primary Contact: Sheila Williams, Chief Executive Officer
CHR: Kelli Hopkins, Director Human Resources
Web address: www.hscmc.org
**Control:** Other not–for–profit (including NFP Corporation) **Service:** General Medical and Surgical

**Staffed Beds:** 72 **Admissions:** 2217 **Census:** 25 **Outpatient Visits:** 26558 **Births:** 0 **Total Expense ($000):** 19287 **Payroll Expense ($000):** 9724 **Personnel:** 283

**MAUMELLE—Pulaski County**

☐ **METHODIST BEHAVIORAL HOSPITAL OF ARKANSAS (44017)**, 1601 Murphy Drive, Zip 72113; tel. 501/803–3388 **A**1 5 9 10 **F**30 32 38 50 54 64 75 86 87 98 99 104 106 **P**1
Primary Contact: Andy Alton, Chief Executive Officer
Web address: www.umch.org
**Control:** Other not–for–profit (including NFP Corporation) **Service:** Children's hospital psychiatric

**Staffed Beds:** 60 **Admissions:** 734 **Census:** 49 **Births:** 0 **Total Expense ($000):** 13115 **Payroll Expense ($000):** 6921 **Personnel:** 134

**MCGEHEE—Desha County**

★ **MCGEHEE–DESHA COUNTY HOSPITAL (41308)**, 900 South Third, Zip 71654–0351, Mailing Address: P.O. Box 351, Zip 71654–0351; tel. 870/222–5600 **A**9 10 18 **F**3 11 29 40 45 57 59 62 64 68 81 107 111 118 131 132 134 145 147
Primary Contact: John E. Heard, Chief Executive Officer
CFO: Teresa Morgan, Chief Financial Officer
CMO: James Young, M.D., Chief of Staff
CIO: Shaun Perry, Chief Information Officer
CHR: Judy A. Sass, Chief Human Resources Officer
CNO: Sarah Calvert, Chief Nursing Officer
**Control:** Other not–for–profit (including NFP Corporation) **Service:** General Medical and Surgical

**Staffed Beds:** 25 **Admissions:** 395 **Census:** 4 **Outpatient Visits:** 31705 **Births:** 0 **Total Expense ($000):** 9147 **Payroll Expense ($000):** 4155 **Personnel:** 96

**AR**

### MENA—Polk County

★ **MENA REGIONAL HEALTH SYSTEM (40015)**, 311 North Morrow Street, Zip 71953–2516; tel. 479/394–6100 **A**9 10 20 **F**3 11 13 15 29 30 31 32 34 35 40 43 45 49 50 54 56 57 59 64 68 70 75 76 77 78 79 81 86 87 90 91 93 96 98 100 101 103 104 107 108 111 113 114 117 118 128 129 130 132 143 145 146 **P**8
Primary Contact: Tim Bowen, Chief Executive Officer
COO: Richard A. Billingsley, MSN, Chief Operating Officer and Chief Nursing Officer
CFO: Paul Rogers, Chief Financial Officer
CMO: Patrick Fox, M.D., Chief of Staff
CIO: John Roberts, Director Information Systems
CHR: Mary Ellen Winters, Director Human Resources
Web address: www.menaregional.com
**Control:** City–Government, nonfederal **Service:** General Medical and Surgical

**Staffed Beds:** 35 **Admissions:** 1756 **Census:** 24 **Outpatient Visits:** 59284
**Births:** 375 **Total Expense ($000):** 24256 **Payroll Expense ($000):** 11904
**Personnel:** 274

### MONTICELLO—Drew County

★ **DREW MEMORIAL HOSPITAL (40051)**, 778 Scogin Drive, Zip 71655–5728; tel. 870/367–2411 **A**9 10 20 **F**3 13 17 34 35 40 45 50 57 59 62 64 68 70 76 81 85 86 89 97 104 107 108 110 111 114 118 132 142 147
Primary Contact: Michael G. Layfield, Chief Executive Officer
CFO: Shannon Clark, Chief Financial Officer
CMO: Jeffery Reinhart, M.D., Chief of Staff
CIO: Rusty Bryant, Director Information Technology
CHR: Keith Van Dee, Director Human Resources
CNO: Linda Orrell, Interim Chief Nursing Officer
Web address: www.drewmemorial.org
**Control:** County–Government, nonfederal **Service:** General Medical and Surgical

**Staffed Beds:** 49 **Admissions:** 2292 **Census:** 17 **Outpatient Visits:** 34538
**Births:** 347 **Total Expense ($000):** 18392 **Payroll Expense ($000):** 10247
**Personnel:** 341

### MORRILTON—Conway County

**ST. ANTHONY'S MEDICAL CENTER** See St. Vincent Morrilton

★ **ST. VINCENT MORRILTON (41324)**, 4 Hospital Drive, Zip 72110–4510; tel. 501/977–2300 **A**9 10 18 **F**2 3 11 17 28 29 30 34 35 40 50 56 57 59 62 64 77 79 81 85 87 93 107 111 113 118 126 129 130 131 132 134 142 145 **P**6 **S** Catholic Health Initiatives, Englewood, CO
Primary Contact: Thomas E. Fitz, Jr., FACHE, Interim Chief Executive Officer
COO: Bob Lyons, Chief Operating Officer
CFO: Amanda George, Assistant Controller
CMO: Charles Howard, M.D., Chief of Staff
CHR: Tammy Smith, Director Human Resources
Web address: www.stanthonysmorrilton.com/
**Control:** Church–operated, Nongovernment, not–for profit **Service:** General Medical and Surgical

**Staffed Beds:** 25 **Admissions:** 959 **Census:** 10 **Outpatient Visits:** 31519
**Births:** 60 **Total Expense ($000):** 15620 **Payroll Expense ($000):** 7098
**Personnel:** 159

### MOUNTAIN HOME—Baxter County

★ △ **BAXTER REGIONAL MEDICAL CENTER (40027)**, 624 Hospital Drive, Zip 72653–2955; tel. 870/508–1000 **A**7 9 10 **F**7 11 13 15 17 18 20 22 24 28 29 30 31 40 41 43 45 46 47 49 53 57 59 62 63 64 70 71 76 77 78 79 81 82 84 85 86 87 89 90 93 98 103 104 107 108 111 113 114 118 123 125 126 128 129 131 134 145 146 147 **P**6 8
Primary Contact: Ron Peterson, FACHE, President and Chief Executive Officer
COO: Rudy Darling, Chief Operating Officer
CFO: Ivan Holleman, Chief Financial Officer
CHR: Karen Adams, Director Human Resources
CNO: Cathleen Hamel, MS, Vice President and Chief Nursing Officer
Web address: www.baxterregional.org
**Control:** Other not–for–profit (including NFP Corporation) **Service:** General Medical and Surgical

**Staffed Beds:** 266 **Admissions:** 10397 **Census:** 117 **Outpatient Visits:** 97408 **Births:** 628 **Total Expense ($000):** 145555 **Payroll Expense ($000):** 56647 **Personnel:** 1241

### MOUNTAIN VIEW—Stone County

★ **STONE COUNTY MEDICAL CENTER (41310)**, 2106 East Main Street, Zip 72560, Mailing Address: P.O. Box 510, Zip 72560–0510; tel. 870/269–4361 **A**9 10 18 **F**11 15 29 34 40 43 50 57 59 64 68 75 77 79 81 91 93 107 111 113 118 132 134 145 146 **S** White River Health System, Batesville, AR
Primary Contact: Renie Taylor, Administrator
CFO: Gary L. Britten, Chief Financial Officer
CFO: Jana Richardson, Interim Chief Financial Officer
CIO: Ken Poole, Coordinator Information Systems
CHR: Gary McDonald, Assistant Administrator Human Resources
CNO: Diana Sheldon, CNO
Web address: www.whiteriverhealthsystem.com
**Control:** Other not–for–profit (including NFP Corporation) **Service:** General Medical and Surgical

**Staffed Beds:** 25 **Admissions:** 1010 **Census:** 11 **Outpatient Visits:** 21836
**Births:** 0 **Total Expense ($000):** 13699 **Payroll Expense ($000):** 6137
**Personnel:** 135

### NASHVILLE—Howard County

★ **HOWARD MEMORIAL HOSPITAL (41311)**, 130 Medical Circle, Zip 71852–8606; tel. 870/845–4400 **A**9 10 18 **F**3 11 15 29 30 34 35 39 40 43 45 50 57 64 65 70 77 81 85 87 93 102 107 108 110 118 132 145 **S** Mercy Health, Chesterfield, MO
Primary Contact: Debra J. Wright, R.N., Chief Executive Officer
CFO: William J. Craig, Chief Financial Officer
CMO: John Hearnsberger, M.D., Chief of Staff
CIO: Nathan Hale, Director Information Management
CHR: Gayla Lacefield, Director Human Resources
CNO: Angie Hanson, R.N., Chief Nursing Officer
Web address: www.howardmemorial.com
**Control:** Other not–for–profit (including NFP Corporation) **Service:** General Medical and Surgical

**Staffed Beds:** 20 **Admissions:** 781 **Census:** 9 **Outpatient Visits:** 26701
**Births:** 0 **Total Expense ($000):** 9700 **Payroll Expense ($000):** 5128
**Personnel:** 128

### NEWPORT—Jackson County

★ **HARRIS HOSPITAL (40080)**, 1205 McLain Street, Zip 72112–3533; tel. 870/523–8911 **A**9 10 20 **F**3 11 15 17 28 29 30 34 35 38 40 43 50 56 57 59 64 65 70 73 75 76 77 79 81 85 87 89 93 98 102 103 105 107 111 113 118 132 134 145 146 **S** Community Health Systems, Inc., Franklin, TN
Primary Contact: Robert Rupp, Chief Executive Officer
CFO: Misty Gates, Chief Financial Officer
CMO: Karen Jones, M.D., Chief of Staff
CHR: Margaret Gates, Chief Human Resources
CNO: Judy Haney, Chief Nursing Officer
Web address: www.harrishospital.com
**Control:** Corporation, Investor–owned, for–profit **Service:** General Medical and Surgical

**Staffed Beds:** 104 **Admissions:** 2483 **Census:** 27 **Outpatient Visits:** 30665
**Births:** 400 **Personnel:** 231

### NORTH LITTLE ROCK—Pulaski County

☐ **ARKANSAS SURGICAL HOSPITAL (40147)**, 5201 North Shore Drive, Zip 72118; tel. 501/748–8000 **A**1 9 10 **F**3 29 35 40 74 75 79 81 82 85 87 107 111 113 118 130 145
Primary Contact: Carrie Helm, Chief Executive Officer
CFO: Charles Powell, Chief Financial Officer
CMO: Kenneth A. Martin, M.D., Chief of Staff
CIO: Scott Davis, Manager Information Technology
CHR: Tina Albright, Vice President Human Resources and Consumer Advocacy
Web address: www.ArkSurgicalHospital.com
**Control:** Corporation, Investor–owned, for–profit **Service:** General Medical and Surgical

**Staffed Beds:** 51 **Admissions:** 3329 **Census:** 19 **Outpatient Visits:** 15813
**Births:** 0 **Total Expense ($000):** 44131 **Payroll Expense ($000):** 10465
**Personnel:** 204

---

**Hospital, Medicare Provider Number, Address, Telephone, Approval, Facility, and Physician Codes, Health Care System**

★ American Hospital Association (AHA) membership
☐ The Joint Commission accreditation
◇ DNV Healthcare Inc. accreditation
○ American Osteopathic Association (AOA) accreditation
△ Commission on Accreditation of Rehabilitation Facilities (CARF) accreditation

⊠ △ **BAPTIST HEALTH MEDICAL CENTER – NORTH LITTLE ROCK (40036)**, 3333 Springhill Drive, Zip 72117–2922; tel. 501/202–3000 **A**1 3 7 9 10 **F**3 8 11 13 15 17 18 20 22 24 26 28 29 30 31 37 38 40 43 45 46 47 49 50 53 54 56 59 60 64 65 68 70 74 75 76 77 78 79 81 85 86 87 89 90 93 94 97 107 108 111 115 116 118 123 125 128 129 131 134 142 143 145 146 147 **S** Baptist Health, Little Rock, AR
Primary Contact: Harrison M. Dean, FACHE, Senior Vice President and Administrator
CFO: Robert C. Roberts, Senior Vice President Financial Services
CMO: Guy Gardner, M.D., Chief Medical Affairs
CIO: David House, Vice President and Chief Information Officer
CHR: Anthony Kendall, Vice President Human Resources
Web address: www.baptist–health.org
**Control:** Other not–for–profit (including NFP Corporation) **Service:** General Medical and Surgical

**Staffed Beds: 220 Admissions: 11562 Census: 122 Outpatient Visits:** 111552 **Births:** 1501 **Total Expense ($000):** 129748 **Payroll Expense ($000):** 53794 **Personnel:** 1083

**NORTH LITTLE ROCK DIVISION** See Central Arkansas Veterans Healthcare System, Little Rock

☐ **THE BRIDGEWAY (44005)**, 21 Bridgeway Road, Zip 72113–9516; tel. 501/771–1500 **A**1 9 10 **F**4 5 98 99 104 105 106 **P**5 **S** Universal Health Services, Inc., King of Prussia, PA
Primary Contact: Barry Pipkin, Chief Executive Officer
COO: Jason Miller, Chief Operating Officer
CFO: Fred Woods, Chief Financial Officer
CMO: Philip L. Mizell, M.D., Medical Director
CHR: Neely Robison, Director Human Resources
CNO: Sherrie James, R.N., Director of Nursing
Web address: www.thebridgeway.com
**Control:** Corporation, Investor–owned, for–profit **Service:** Psychiatric

**Staffed Beds: 103 Admissions: 4102 Census: 86 Outpatient Visits:** 15180 **Births:** 0 **Total Expense ($000):** 16590 **Payroll Expense ($000):** 8200 **Personnel:** 153

**OSCEOLA—Mississippi County**

☐ **SOUTH MISSISSIPPI COUNTY REGIONAL MEDICAL CENTER (41316)**, 611 West Lee Avenue, Zip 72370–3001, Mailing Address: P.O. Box 607, Zip 72370–0607; tel. 870/563–7000 **A**1 9 10 18 **F**29 40 50 57 59 68 75 81 93 107 113 129 132 145 **S** Mississippi County Hospital System, Blytheville, AR
Primary Contact: Ralph E. Beaty, Chief Executive Officer
COO: Chris Raymer, R.N., Interim Chief Operating Officer
CFO: Paul Zuidema, Chief Financial Officer
CMO: Sherita Willis, M.D., Chief of Staff
Web address: www.mchealthsystem.com
**Control:** County–Government, nonfederal **Service:** General Medical and Surgical

**Staffed Beds: 25 Admissions: 822 Census: 8 Outpatient Visits:** 8384 **Births:** 0 **Total Expense ($000):** 8478 **Payroll Expense ($000):** 3746 **Personnel:** 73

**OZARK—Franklin County**

★ **MERCY HOSPITAL OZARK (41303)**, 801 West River Street, Zip 72949–3000; tel. 479/667–4138 **A**9 10 18 **F**3 8 28 34 35 40 42 57 59 64 68 81 85 107 118 132 145 **S** Mercy Health, Chesterfield, MO
Primary Contact: Michael K. Smith, Regional Administrator
CMO: John Lachowsky, M.D., Chief Medical Officer
CIO: Tiana Bolduc, Chief Information Officer
Web address: www.gravettehospital.org
**Control:** Church–operated, Nongovernment, not–for profit **Service:** General Medical and Surgical

**Staffed Beds: 25 Admissions: 537 Census: 6 Outpatient Visits:** 13033 **Births:** 0 **Total Expense ($000):** 8759 **Payroll Expense ($000):** 2078 **Personnel:** 53

**PARAGOULD—Greene County**

⊠ △ **ARKANSAS METHODIST MEDICAL CENTER (40039)**, 900 West Kingshighway, Zip 72450–5942, Mailing Address: P.O. Box 339, Zip 72451–0339; tel. 870/239–7000 **A**1 7 9 10 19 **F**3 7 10 11 13 15 18 20 22 28 29 31 32 34 35 39 40 43 45 49 50 51 53 54 57 59 62 64 68 70 75 76 78 79 81 85 86 87 89 90 93 107 108 111 113 118 124 128 129 130 131 132 134 145 146 147 **P**6 8
Primary Contact: Barry L. Davis, FACHE, President and Chief Executive Officer
CFO: Brad Bloemer, Vice President Finance and Chief Financial Officer
CMO: Frank Schefano, M.D., Chief of Staff
CIO: Mardy Holmes, Director Information Technology
CHR: Dennis Cooper, Director Human Resources
CNO: Debra Vassar, Chief Nursing Officer
Web address: www.arkansasmethodist.org
**Control:** Other not–for–profit (including NFP Corporation) **Service:** General Medical and Surgical

**Staffed Beds: 125 Admissions: 4535 Census: 59 Outpatient Visits:** 123924 **Births:** 533 **Total Expense ($000):** 61995 **Payroll Expense ($000):** 25450 **Personnel:** 575

**PARIS—Logan County**

★ **MERCY HOSPITAL PARIS (41300)**, 500 East Academy, Zip 72855–4099; tel. 479/963–6101 **A**9 10 18 **F**3 35 40 42 43 45 57 59 64 81 85 107 118 132 **S** Mercy Health, Chesterfield, MO
Primary Contact: Sharon Sorey, R.N., Regional Administrator
Web address: www.stedwardmercy.com
**Control:** Church–operated, Nongovernment, not–for profit **Service:** General Medical and Surgical

**Staffed Beds: 16 Admissions: 227 Census: 3 Outpatient Visits:** 12448 **Births:** 0 **Total Expense ($000):** 5647 **Payroll Expense ($000):** 1668 **Personnel:** 42

**PIGGOTT—Clay County**

★ **PIGGOTT COMMUNITY HOSPITAL (41330)**, 1206 Gordon Duckworth Drive, Zip 72454–1911; tel. 870/598–3881 **A**9 10 18 **F**7 15 18 29 34 35 40 43 57 59 62 64 77 93 107 111 113 118 126 128 129 132 142 145
Primary Contact: James L. Magee, Executive Director
CFO: Linda Ort, Chief Financial Officer
Web address: www.piggottcommunityhospital.com
**Control:** City–Government, nonfederal **Service:** General Medical and Surgical

**Staffed Beds: 25 Admissions: 804 Census: 12 Outpatient Visits:** 30796 **Births:** 0 **Total Expense ($000):** 12402 **Payroll Expense ($000):** 6822 **Personnel:** 179

**PINE BLUFF—Jefferson County**

**ARKANSAS DEPARTMENT OF CORRECTION HOSPITAL**, 7500 Correctional Circle, Zip 71603–1438; tel. 870/267–6999, (Nonreporting) **A**5
Primary Contact: Roland Anderson, M.D., Medical Director
**Control:** State–Government, nonfederal **Service:** Hospital unit of an institution (prison hospital, college infimary, etc.)

**Staffed Beds: 27**

⊠ △ **JEFFERSON REGIONAL MEDICAL CENTER (40071)**, 1600 West 40th Avenue, Zip 71603–7089; tel. 870/541–7100 **A**1 3 5 6 7 9 10 20 **F**3 11 13 15 17 18 20 22 24 28 29 30 31 34 35 40 43 45 46 48 49 50 51 53 54 56 57 59 60 61 64 65 70 72 73 74 75 76 77 78 79 81 85 86 87 89 90 96 97 98 100 101 102 103 107 108 110 111 113 114 115 117 118 123 127 129 130 131 134 142 143 144 145 146 147 **P**7
Primary Contact: Walter E. Johnson, Jr., President and Chief Executive Officer
COO: Brian N. Thomas, Senior Vice President and Chief Operating Officer
CFO: Bryan G. Jackson, Vice President and Chief Financial Officer
CMO: Doug Coleman, M.D., Chief of Staff
CIO: Patrick Neece, Chief Information Officer
CHR: M Daryl Scott, Assistant Vice President
CNO: Louise Hickman, R.N., Vice President of Patient Care Services
Web address: www.jrmc.org
**Control:** Other not–for–profit (including NFP Corporation) **Service:** General Medical and Surgical

**Staffed Beds: 333 Admissions: 10729 Census: 161 Outpatient Visits:** 174501 **Births:** 1039 **Total Expense ($000):** 173821 **Payroll Expense ($000):** 72837 **Personnel:** 1509

**POCAHONTAS—Randolph County**

**FIVE RIVERS MEDICAL CENTER (40047)**, 2801 Medical Center Drive, Zip 72455–9497; tel. 870/892–6000 **A**9 10 20 **F**3 11 15 29 40 43 45 47 57 59 62 70 81 85 93 98 103 104 107 111 113 118 129 132 145
Primary Contact: Luther J. Lewis, FACHE, Chief Executive Officer
CFO: Joey Radcliff, Chief Financial Officer
CHR: Alvin Taylor, Chief Human Resources
CNO: Mandy Dollins, R.N., Chief Nursing Officer
Web address: www.fiveriversmedicalcenter.com
**Control:** Other not–for–profit (including NFP Corporation) **Service:** General Medical and Surgical

**Staffed Beds: 46 Admissions: 1148 Census: 16 Outpatient Visits:** 16480 **Births:** 0 **Total Expense ($000):** 14832 **Payroll Expense ($000):** 8497 **Personnel:** 173

**ROGERS—Benton County**

⊠ **MERCY HOSPITAL ROGERS (40010)**, 2710 Rife Medical Lane, Zip 72758; tel. 479/338–8000 **A**1 9 10 **F**3 8 11 13 15 18 20 22 24 28 29 30 40 45 46 49 57 59 62 64 70 72 75 76 77 79 81 82 84 86 87 89 93 107 108 110 111 114 117 118 128 129 131 134 145 147 **P**6 **S** Mercy Health, Chesterfield, MO
Primary Contact: Scott Street, President and Chief Executive Officer
CFO: Benny Stover, Vice President Finance
CMO: Cynthia Wilson, M.D., Chief of Staff
CHR: Rick Barclay, Vice President Support Services
Web address: www.mercyhealthnwa.smhs.com
**Control:** Church–operated, Nongovernment, not–for profit **Service:** General Medical and Surgical

**Staffed Beds: 141 Admissions: 8779 Census: 85 Outpatient Visits:** 79375 **Births:** 1266 **Total Expense ($000):** 125938 **Payroll Expense ($000):** 36837 **Personnel:** 885

## RUSSELLVILLE—Pope County

☐ **SAINT MARY'S REGIONAL MEDICAL CENTER (40041)**, 1808 West Main Street, Zip 72801–2724; tel. 479/968–2841 **A**1 9 10 19 **F**3 11 13 15 18 20 22 29 31 34 35 40 43 45 50 51 53 54 56 57 59 62 64 68 70 74 75 76 78 79 81 85 86 87 89 90 93 98 107 108 109 110 111 113 117 118 120 122 126 128 129 130 131 145 146 147 **S** Capella Healthcare, Franklin, TN
Primary Contact: Donald J. Frederic, FACHE, Chief Executive Officer
COO: Mike McCoy, Chief Operating Officer
CFO: Wendell VanEs, Chief Financial Officer
CMO: Chris Horan, M.D., Chief of Staff
CHR: Connie Gragg, Director Human Resources
Web address: www.saintmarysregional.com
**Control:** Corporation, Investor–owned, for–profit **Service:** General Medical and Surgical

**Staffed Beds:** 137 **Admissions:** 5528 **Census:** 62 **Outpatient Visits:** 68716 **Births:** 904 **Total Expense ($000):** 62029 **Payroll Expense ($000):** 21355 **Personnel:** 500

## SALEM—Fulton County

**FULTON COUNTY HOSPITAL (41322)**, 679 North Main Street, Zip 72576–9122, Mailing Address: P.O. Box 517, Zip 72576–0517; tel. 870/895–2691 **A**9 10 18 **F**7 28 29 34 35 40 45 57 59 107 118 132 145
Primary Contact: Kim Thompson, Chief Executive Officer
Web address: www.fultoncountyhospital.org
**Control:** County–Government, nonfederal **Service:** General Medical and Surgical

**Staffed Beds:** 25 **Admissions:** 760 **Census:** 11 **Outpatient Visits:** 48204 **Births:** 0 **Total Expense ($000):** 10250 **Payroll Expense ($000):** 4936 **Personnel:** 152

## SEARCY—White County

**ADVANCED CARE HOSPITAL OF WHITE COUNTY (42011)**, 1200 South Main Street, Zip 72143; tel. 501/278–3155 **A**9 10 **F**1 3 29 31 60 68 75 91 100 129 134
Primary Contact: Terri L. Parsons, Administrator
Web address: www.achwc.org
**Control:** Other not–for–profit (including NFP Corporation) **Service:** Long–Term Acute Care hospital

**Staffed Beds:** 27 **Admissions:** 212 **Census:** 16 **Outpatient Visits:** 0 **Births:** 0 **Total Expense ($000):** 6803 **Payroll Expense ($000):** 2880 **Personnel:** 66

★ **WHITE COUNTY MEDICAL CENTER (40014)**, 3214 East Race Avenue, Zip 72143–4847; tel. 501/268–6121, (Includes CENTRAL ARKANSAS HOSPITAL, 1200 South Main Street, Zip 72143–7397; tel. 501/278–3100) **A**9 10 **F**1 3 10 11 12 13 17 18 20 22 24 28 29 30 31 34 35 39 40 43 45 51 54 57 59 61 62 64 68 70 74 75 76 77 78 79 81 86 87 89 90 93 98 100 102 103 105 107 108 111 114 118 124 128 129 130 131 133 134 144 145 146 147 **P**7
Primary Contact: Raymond W. Montgomery, II, FACHE, President and Chief Executive Officer
CFO: Stuart Hill, Vice President and Treasurer
CMO: Scott Dicus, M.D., Chief of Staff
CIO: Kevin Hoofman, Director Management Information
CHR: Pamela G. Williams, Director Human Resources
Web address: www.wcmc.org
**Control:** Other not–for–profit (including NFP Corporation) **Service:** General Medical and Surgical

**Staffed Beds:** 286 **Admissions:** 13027 **Census:** 152 **Outpatient Visits:** 87787 **Births:** 1202 **Total Expense ($000):** 152365 **Payroll Expense ($000):** 68909 **Personnel:** 1370

## SHERWOOD—Pulaski County

★ **ST. VINCENT MEDICAL CENTER–NORTH (40137)**, 2215 Wildwood Avenue, Zip 72120; tel. 501/552–7100 **A**9 10 **F**3 11 15 20 29 35 40 43 44 45 47 50 64 70 74 79 81 85 87 107 108 110 111 113 118 129 145 **S** Catholic Health Initiatives, Englewood, CO
Primary Contact: Tim Osterholm, Administrator and Chief Executive Officer
CMO: David Hall, M.D., Senior Vice President and Chief Medical Officer
CIO: Tommye Billing, Vice President and Chief Information Officer
CHR: Margaret Nixon, Director Human Resources
Web address: www.stvincenthealth.com
**Control:** Church–operated, Nongovernment, not–for profit **Service:** General Medical and Surgical

**Staffed Beds:** 58 **Admissions:** 2133 **Census:** 21 **Outpatient Visits:** 41555 **Births:** 0 **Total Expense ($000):** 26584 **Payroll Expense ($000):** 8463 **Personnel:** 175

⊠ **ST. VINCENT REHABILITATION HOSPITAL (43031)**, 2201 Wildwood Avenue, Zip 72120–5074, Mailing Address: P.O. Box 6930, Zip 72124–6930; tel. 501/834–1800 **A**1 9 10 **F**79 82 90 91 93 94 128 **S** HEALTHSOUTH Corporation, Birmingham, AL
Primary Contact: Lee Frazier, FACHE, Chief Executive Officer
CFO: Pat Robinson, Manager Accounting
CMO: Sean Foley, M.D., Medical Director
CHR: Sandra Pearson, Manager Human Resources
Web address: www.stvincenthealth.com/svrehabhospital/index.html
**Control:** Partnership, Investor–owned, for–profit **Service:** Rehabilitation

**Staffed Beds:** 71 **Admissions:** 1472 **Census:** 45 **Outpatient Visits:** 10967 **Births:** 0 **Total Expense ($000):** 14498 **Payroll Expense ($000):** 8817

## SILOAM SPRINGS—Benton County

⊠ **SILOAM SPRINGS MEMORIAL HOSPITAL (40001)**, 205 East Jefferson Street, Zip 72761–3697; tel. 479/524–4141, (Nonreporting) **A**1 9 10 **S** Community Health Systems, Inc., Franklin, TN
Primary Contact: Kevin J. Clement, Chief Executive Officer
CFO: James E. Little, Chief Financial Officer
CMO: Hunt Cooper, M.D., Chief of Staff
CHR: Carmen Burasco, Director Human Resources
Web address: www.ssmh.us
**Control:** City–Government, nonfederal **Service:** General Medical and Surgical

**Staffed Beds:** 43

## SPRINGDALE—Washington County

⊠ **NORTHWEST MEDICAL CENTER (40022)**, 609 West Maple Avenue, Zip 72764–5394, Mailing Address: P.O. Box 47, Zip 72765–0047; tel. 501/751–5711, (Includes NORTHWEST MEDICAL CENTER – BENTONVILLE, 3000 Medical Center Parkway, Bentonville, Zip 72712; tel. 479/553–1000; Tripp Smith, Chief Operating Officer; WILLOW CREEK WOMEN'S HOSPITAL, 4301 Greathouse Springs Road, Johnson, Zip 72741–0544, Mailing Address: P.O. Box 544, Zip 72741–0544; tel. 479/684–3000; Debbie A. Crandall, Administrative Director) **A**1 9 10 **F**3 8 11 12 13 14 15 17 18 20 22 24 26 28 29 30 31 35 36 40 43 45 46 47 48 49 50 51 56 57 59 60 64 68 70 71 72 74 75 76 77 78 79 81 85 86 87 88 89 90 93 97 98 102 107 108 110 111 112 113 114 117 118 125 128 129 130 131 134 143 145 146 147 **P**5 8
Primary Contact: Daniel E. McKay, Chief Executive Officer
CFO: Steve Flader, Chief Financial Officer
CMO: Robert Petrino, M.D., Chief of Staff
CIO: Paul DeMay, Chief Information Officer
Web address: www.northwesthealth.com
**Control:** Corporation, Investor–owned, for–profit **Service:** General Medical and Surgical

**Staffed Beds:** 358 **Admissions:** 18027 **Census:** 200 **Outpatient Visits:** 118442 **Births:** 3915 **Total Expense ($000):** 203974 **Payroll Expense ($000):** 76703 **Personnel:** 1516

## STUTTGART—Arkansas County

★ **BAPTIST HEALTH MEDICAL CENTER–STUTTGART (40072)**, North Buerkle Road, Zip 72160–3420, Mailing Address: P.O. Box 1905, Zip 72160–1905; tel. 870/673–3511 **A**9 10 **F**3 11 13 15 18 28 29 30 34 35 39 40 53 57 59 64 68 70 75 76 78 79 81 85 87 93 97 107 110 111 113 118 126 127 128 129 132 134 145 147 **S** Baptist Health, Little Rock, AR
Primary Contact: Steven B. Webb, FACHE, Administrator
CMO: Raymond Kirk Coker, M.D., Chief of Staff
CIO: Warren Horton, Information Technologist
Web address: www.baptist–health.org
**Control:** Other not–for–profit (including NFP Corporation) **Service:** General Medical and Surgical

**Staffed Beds:** 49 **Admissions:** 1711 **Census:** 16 **Outpatient Visits:** 36140 **Births:** 223 **Total Expense ($000):** 20723 **Payroll Expense ($000):** 8884 **Personnel:** 226

## TEXARKANA—Miller County

☐ **VISTA HEALTH TEXARKANA (44020)**, 701 Arkansas Boulevard, Zip 71854–2105; tel. 870/772–5028 **A**1 9 10 **F**54 56 98 99 100 101 102 103 104 106
Primary Contact: Michael S. Talmo, Chief Executive Officer
Web address: www.vistahealthservices.com
**Control:** Corporation, Investor–owned, for–profit **Service:** Psychiatric

**Staffed Beds:** 62 **Admissions:** 683 **Census:** 35 **Outpatient Visits:** 22630 **Births:** 0 **Total Expense ($000):** 10561 **Payroll Expense ($000):** 5785 **Personnel:** 94

---

**Hospital, Medicare Provider Number, Address, Telephone, Approval, Facility, and Physician Codes, Health Care System**

★ American Hospital Association (AHA) membership
☐ The Joint Commission accreditation
◇ DNV Healthcare Inc. accreditation
○ American Osteopathic Association (AOA) accreditation
△ Commission on Accreditation of Rehabilitation Facilities (CARF) accreditation

AR

### VAN BUREN—Crawford County

☐ **SUMMIT MEDICAL CENTER (40018)**, East Main and South 20th Streets, Zip 72956–5715, Mailing Address: P.O. Box 409, Zip 72957–0409; tel. 479/474–3401 **A**1 9 10 **F**3 11 15 29 30 34 40 43 45 50 51 56 57 59 64 65 68 70 74 75 77 78 79 81 82 85 86 87 93 100 107 108 110 111 113 118 129 130 131 134 145 147 **P**6 **S** Health Management Associates, Naples, FL
Primary Contact: Sue Conley, Chief Executive Officer
CHR: James Ford, Director Human Resources
CNO: Harlo McCall, Chief Nursing Officer
Web address: www.summitmedicalcenter.net
**Control:** Corporation, Investor–owned, for–profit **Service:** General Medical and Surgical

**Staffed Beds:** 103 **Admissions:** 1934 **Census:** 17 **Outpatient Visits:** 53563 **Births:** 0 **Personnel:** 182

### WALDRON—Scott County

★ **MERCY HOSPITAL WALDRON (41305)**, 1341 West 6th Street, Zip 72958–7001; tel. 479/637–4135 **A**9 10 18 **F**3 8 35 40 42 46 57 59 64 65 68 81 85 107 118 126 132 **S** Mercy Health, Chesterfield, MO
Primary Contact: Steve Loveless, Regional Administrator
CFO: Greta Wilcher, Senior Vice President and Chief Financial Officer
Web address: www.stedwardmercy.com
**Control:** Church–operated, Nongovernment, not–for profit **Service:** General Medical and Surgical

**Staffed Beds:** 24 **Admissions:** 528 **Census:** 6 **Outpatient Visits:** 26993 **Births:** 0 **Total Expense ($000):** 9238 **Payroll Expense ($000):** 2062 **Personnel:** 39

### WALNUT RIDGE—Lawrence County

✠ **LAWRENCE MEMORIAL HOSPITAL (41309)**, 1309 West Main, Zip 72476–1430, Mailing Address: P.O. Box 839, Zip 72476–0839; tel. 870/886–1200, (Includes LAWRENCE HALL NURSING HOME ), (Total facility includes 168 beds in nursing home–type unit) **A**1 9 10 18 **F**3 11 15 28 29 34 35 40 45 46 47 57 59 85 97 107 113 118 126 127 128 129 132
Primary Contact: Terry R. Lambert, FACHE, President
CFO: Vanessa Wagner, Chief Financial Officer
CHR: Sherri Brown, Director Human Resources
CNO: Rosalind Casillas, Director of Nursing
Web address: www.lawrencehealth.net
**Control:** County–Government, nonfederal **Service:** General Medical and Surgical

**Staffed Beds:** 194 **Admissions:** 1044 **Census:** 179 **Outpatient Visits:** 28876 **Births:** 0 **Total Expense ($000):** 17694 **Payroll Expense ($000):** 9601 **Personnel:** 285

### WARREN—Bradley County

★ **BRADLEY COUNTY MEDICAL CENTER (41327)**, 404 South Bradley Street, Zip 71671–3493; tel. 870/226–3731 **A**9 10 18 **F**3 11 13 15 29 31 40 57 62 63 76 81 93 98 103 104 107 111 113 117 118 127 128 129 131 132 134 **P**8
Primary Contact: Harold E. Mitchell, Jr., CPA, Administrator and Chief Executive Officer
CFO: Brandon Gorman, Controller
CMO: Joe H. Wharton, M.D., Chief of Staff
CHR: Debra Marshall, Director Human Resources
CNO: Paulette Tolefree, Chief Nursing Officer
Web address: www.bradleycountymedicalcenter.com
**Control:** Other not–for–profit (including NFP Corporation) **Service:** General Medical and Surgical

**Staffed Beds:** 35 **Admissions:** 1757 **Census:** 18 **Outpatient Visits:** 30288 **Births:** 181 **Total Expense ($000):** 17493 **Personnel:** 213

### WEST MEMPHIS—Crittenden County

☐ **CRITTENDEN REGIONAL HOSPITAL (40042)**, 200 Tyler Avenue, Zip 72301–4223, Mailing Address: P.O. Box 2248, Zip 72303–2248; tel. 870/735–1500 **A**1 9 10 **F**3 8 11 13 15 18 19 29 31 34 35 40 46 47 57 59 62 63 64 70 75 76 77 78 79 80 81 86 87 89 90 93 107 108 110 111 112 114 115 117 118 123 126 128 129 131 134 145 146 147 **P**6
Primary Contact: David G. Baytos, Interim Chief Executive Officer
COO: Justin Vernon, Chief Operating Officer
CFO: Paul Rogers, Chief Financial Officer
Web address: www.crittendenregional.org/
**Control:** Other not–for–profit (including NFP Corporation) **Service:** General Medical and Surgical

**Staffed Beds:** 142 **Admissions:** 3811 **Census:** 48 **Outpatient Visits:** 41434 **Births:** 731

### WYNNE—Cross County

✠ **CROSSRIDGE COMMUNITY HOSPITAL (41307)**, 310 South Falls Boulevard, Zip 72396–3013, Mailing Address: P.O. Box 590, Zip 72396–0590; tel. 870/238–3300 **A**1 9 10 18 **F**3 11 15 28 34 35 40 50 57 59 62 64 68 69 75 77 81 93 107 111 113 118 129 132 134 145
Primary Contact: Gary R. Sparks, Administrator
COO: Bryan Mattes, Associate Administrator
CFO: Janice Morris, Accountant
CIO: Gail Copeland, Director Management Information Systems
CHR: Bertha Ragle, Director Personnel
CNO: Amelia Davis, Director of Nursing
**Control:** Church–operated, Nongovernment, not–for profit **Service:** General Medical and Surgical

**Staffed Beds:** 15 **Admissions:** 661 **Census:** 7 **Outpatient Visits:** 16906 **Births:** 0 **Total Expense ($000):** 13057 **Payroll Expense ($000):** 5290 **Personnel:** 140

*Many Facility Codes have changed. Please refer to the AHA Guide Code Chart.* © 2012 AHA Guide

# CALIFORNIA

**CA**

## ALAMEDA—Alameda County

⊠ **ALAMEDA HOSPITAL (50211)**, 2070 Clinton Avenue, Zip 94501–4397;
tel. 510/522–3700, (Total facility includes 22 beds in nursing home–type unit) **A1**
9 10 **F3** 11 15 17 29 31 34 35 36 39 40 43 44 46 50 57 70 77 78 81 82 85
86 93 97 107 108 110 111 113 118 127 129 131 143 145 146 147
Primary Contact: Deborah E. Stebbins, FACHE, Chief Executive Officer
CFO: Robert C. Anderson, Interim Chief Financial Officer
CMO: Aika Sharma, M.D., President Medical Staff
CIO: Robert Lundy–Paine, Director Information Systems
CHR: Phyllis Weiss, Director Human Resources
Web address: www.alamedahospital.org
**Control:** Hospital district or authority, Government, nonfederal **Service:** General
Medical and Surgical

**Staffed Beds:** 126 **Admissions:** 2670 **Census:** 83 **Outpatient Visits:** 47255
**Births:** 0 **Total Expense ($000):** 59221 **Payroll Expense ($000):** 37619
**Personnel:** 390

## ALHAMBRA—Los Angeles County

☐ **ALHAMBRA HOSPITAL MEDICAL CENTER (50281)**, 100 South Raymond
Avenue, Zip 91801–3199, Mailing Address: P.O. Box 510, Zip 91802–0510;
tel. 626/570–1606, (Nonreporting) **A1** 9 10 **S** AHMC & Healthcare, Inc.,
Alhambra, CA
Primary Contact: Iris Lai, Chief Executive Officer
CFO: Linda Marsh, Vice President Financial Services and Chief Financial Officer
CIO: Johnson Legaspi, Director Information Systems
CHR: Elizabeth Sabandit, Director Human Resources
Web address: www.alhambrahospital.com
**Control:** Partnership, Investor–owned, for–profit **Service:** General Medical and
Surgical

**Staffed Beds:** 144

## ALTURAS—Modoc County

**MODOC MEDICAL CENTER (51330)**, 228 West Mcdowell Avenue,
Zip 96101–3934; tel. 530/233–5131, (Nonreporting) **A9** 10 18
Primary Contact: Monica Derner, Chief Executive Officer and Chief Financial
Officer
CFO: Monica Derner, Chief Executive Officer and Chief Financial Officer
CMO: Ed Richert, M.D., Chief of Staff
CHR: Diane Hagelthorn, Human Resources Generalist
Web address: www.modocmedicalcenter.com
**Control:** County–Government, nonfederal **Service:** General Medical and Surgical

**Staffed Beds:** 16

## ANAHEIM—Orange County

**ANAHEIM GENERAL HOSPITAL (50768)**, 3350 West Ball Road,
Zip 92804–3799; tel. 714/827–6700, (Nonreporting) **A10 S** Pacific Health
Corporation, Tustin, CA
Primary Contact: Michael O. Choo, Interim Chief Executive Officer
CFO: Mark Apodaca, Chief Financial Officer
CMO: Dilip Patel, M.D., President Medical Staff
**Control:** Individual, Investor–owned, for–profit **Service:** General Medical and
Surgical

**Staffed Beds:** 126

⊠ **ANAHEIM MEDICAL CENTER (50609)**, 441 North Lakeview Avenue,
Zip 92807–3089; tel. 714/279–4000, (Includes ORANGE COUNTY IRVINE
MEDICAL CENTER, 6640 Alton Parkway, Irvine, Zip 92618; tel. 949/932–5000)
**A1** 3 5 10 **F3** 13 14 15 17 18 19 20 29 30 31 35 37 40 44 45 46 47 48 49
50 59 61 62 63 64 65 68 70 72 74 75 76 78 79 80 81 82 84 85 87 89 92
93 100 107 108 111 113 118 129 134 142 145 147 **S** Kaiser Foundation
Hospitals, Oakland, CA
Primary Contact: Julie K. Miller–Phipps, Senior Vice President and Executive
Director
COO: Margie Harrier, Medical Center Chief Operations Officer
CFO: Melvin J. Benner, Assistant Administrator Finance
CMO: Nancy Gin, M.D., Area Associate Medical Director
CIO: Donald M. Carren, Information Technology Leader
CHR: Jocelyn A. Herrera, Director Human Resources
Web address: www.kp.org
**Control:** Other not–for–profit (including NFP Corporation) **Service:** General
Medical and Surgical

**Staffed Beds:** 326 **Admissions:** 21958 **Census:** 241 **Outpatient Visits:**
298439 **Births:** 4978 **Personnel:** 2127

☐ **ANAHEIM REGIONAL MEDICAL CENTER (50226)**, 1111 West La Palma
Avenue, Zip 92801–2881; tel. 714/774–1450, (Nonreporting) **A1** 2 9 10
**S** AHMC & Healthcare, Inc., Alhambra, CA
Primary Contact: Donald A. Lorack, Jr., Chief Executive Officer
COO: Deborah G. Webber, Chief Operating Officer
CFO: Frederick J. Drewette, Chief Financial Officer
CMO: Amitabh Prakash, M.D., Chief Medical Officer
CIO: Jeff DesRoches, Manager Information Systems
CHR: Kathy Doi, Executive Director Human Resources
CNO: Martha Dispoto, R.N., Chief Nursing Officer
Web address: www.anaheimregionalmc.com
**Control:** Other not–for–profit (including NFP Corporation) **Service:** General
Medical and Surgical

**Staffed Beds:** 223

☐ **WEST ANAHEIM MEDICAL CENTER (50426)**, 3033 West Orange Avenue,
Zip 92804–3184; tel. 714/827–3000, (Nonreporting) **A1** 5 10 **S** Prime
Healthcare Services, Ontario, CA
Primary Contact: Virgis Narbutas, Chief Executive Officer
CFO: Alan H. Smith, Chief Financial Officer
CMO: Hassan Alkhouli, M.D., Chief Medical Officer
CIO: Adam Morquecho, Director Information Technology
CHR: Stephanie Sioson, Director Human Resources
CNO: Virginia Edward, R.N., Administrator and Chief Nursing Officer
Web address: www.westanaheimmedctr.com
**Control:** Partnership, Investor–owned, for–profit **Service:** General Medical and
Surgical

**Staffed Beds:** 219

☐ **WESTERN MEDICAL CENTER ANAHEIM (50744)**, 1025 South Anaheim
Boulevard, Zip 92805–5806; tel. 714/533–6220, (Nonreporting) **A1** 9 10
**S** Integrated Healthcare, Santa Ana, CA
Primary Contact: Dennis M. Knox, Chief Executive Officer
CMO: Harmohinder Gogia, M.D., Chief Medical Officer
CIO: Nova Stewart, Chief Information Officer
Web address: www.westernmedanaheim.com
**Control:** Corporation, Investor–owned, for–profit **Service:** General Medical and
Surgical

**Staffed Beds:** 188

## ANTIOCH—Contra Costa County

⊠ **ANTIOCH MEDICAL CENTER (50760)**, 4501 Sand Creek Road, Zip 94531;
tel. 925/813–6500, (Nonreporting) **A1** 10 **S** Kaiser Foundation Hospitals,
Oakland, CA
Primary Contact: Tim F. Daly, Chief Operating Officer
CNO: Linda Krystof, Chief Nursing Officer
Web address: www.kaiserpermanente.org
**Control:** Other not–for–profit (including NFP Corporation) **Service:** General
Medical and Surgical

**Staffed Beds:** 150

⊠ **SUTTER DELTA MEDICAL CENTER (50523)**, 3901 Lone Tree Way,
Zip 94509–6253; tel. 925/779–7200 **A1** 9 10 **F8** 11 13 15 18 20 22 29 30
31 34 35 40 41 45 47 49 50 57 59 64 65 66 68 70 73 74 75 76 77 78 79
81 82 83 84 85 86 92 93 107 108 110 111 113 114 117 118 129 130 131
134 145 146 **S** Sutter Health, Sacramento, CA
Primary Contact: Gary D. Rapaport, Chief Executive Officer
COO: Susan C. Bumatay, R.N., Assistant Administrator
CFO: Julie Peterson, Chief Financial Officer
CMO: Bobby Glickman, M.D., Chief of Staff
CIO: Kathy Frederickson, Information Systems Site Lead
CHR: Christine Green, Administrative Director Human Resources
CNO: Dori Stevens, Chief Nursing Officer
Web address: www.sutterdelta.org
**Control:** Other not–for–profit (including NFP Corporation) **Service:** General
Medical and Surgical

**Staffed Beds:** 136 **Admissions:** 7754 **Census:** 84 **Outpatient Visits:** 83627
**Births:** 975 **Personnel:** 631

---

**Hospital, Medicare Provider Number, Address, Telephone, Approval, Facility, and Physician Codes, Health Care System**

★ American Hospital Association (AHA) membership
☐ The Joint Commission accreditation ◇ DNV Healthcare Inc. accreditation
○ American Osteopathic Association (AOA) accreditation
△ Commission on Accreditation of Rehabilitation Facilities (CARF) accreditation

**CA**

## APPLE VALLEY—San Bernardino County

★ ○ **ST. MARY MEDICAL CENTER (50300)**, 18300 Highway 18, Zip 92307–2206, Mailing Address: P.O. Box 7025, Zip 92307–0725; tel. 760/242–2311 **A**2 9 10 11 **F**8 11 13 15 18 20 22 24 26 28 29 30 34 35 40 45 46 50 57 59 60 64 65 68 70 71 72 75 76 77 78 79 81 82 83 84 85 86 87 89 93 107 108 111 114 118 125 126 129 131 134 142 145 147 **P**3 5 **S** St. Joseph Health, Orange, CA
Primary Contact: Alan H. Garrett, President and Chief Executive Officer
COO: David O'Brien, M.D., Senior Vice President, COO
CFO: Pitt Calkin, Interim Chief Financial Officer
CMO: James Kyle, M.D., Vice President Medical Affairs
CIO: Doug Kleine, IT Director
CHR: Stephen Eckberg, Vice President Human Resources
CNO: Marilyn Drone, R.N., Vice President, CNO
Web address: www.stmaryapplevalley.com/
**Control:** Church–operated, Nongovernment, not–for profit **Service:** General Medical and Surgical

**Staffed Beds:** 186 **Admissions:** 17773 **Census:** 192

## ARCADIA—Los Angeles County

✉ **METHODIST HOSPITAL OF SOUTHERN CALIFORNIA (50238)**, 300 West Huntington Drive, Zip 91007–3473, Mailing Address: P.O. Box 60016, Zip 91066–6016; tel. 626/898–8000 **A**1 2 9 10 **F**1 3 11 12 13 15 17 18 19 20 22 24 26 28 29 30 31 34 35 37 38 40 45 46 48 49 53 55 56 57 58 59 60 64 65 68 70 72 74 75 76 77 78 79 81 85 86 87 89 90 91 92 94 107 108 111 113 114 116 117 118 119 120 122 129 131 145 146 147
Primary Contact: Dan F. Ausman, President and Chief Executive Officer
COO: Steven A. Sisto, Senior Vice President and Chief Operating Officer
CFO: William E. Grigg, Senior Vice President and Chief Financial Officer
CHR: William Budzinski, Vice President Human Resources
Web address: www.methodisthospital.org
**Control:** Other not–for–profit (including NFP Corporation) **Service:** General Medical and Surgical

**Staffed Beds:** 394 **Admissions:** 16663 **Census:** 220 **Outpatient Visits:** 57123 **Births:** 1677 **Total Expense ($000):** 250563 **Payroll Expense ($000):** 117826 **Personnel:** 1601

## ARCATA—Humboldt County

○ **MAD RIVER COMMUNITY HOSPITAL (50028)**, 3800 Janes Road, Zip 95521–4788, Mailing Address: P.O. Box 1115, Zip 95518–1115; tel. 707/822–3621, (Nonreporting) **A**9 10 11
Primary Contact: Douglas A. Shaw, Chief Executive Officer
COO: Steve Engle, Chief Operations Officer
CFO: Michael Young, Chief Financial Officer
CMO: Gary Garcia, M.D., Chief of Staff
CIO: Steve Engle, Chief Operations Officer
CHR: Michele Bisgrove, Manager Human Resources
Web address: www.madriverhospital.com
**Control:** Corporation, Investor–owned, for–profit **Service:** General Medical and Surgical

**Staffed Beds:** 68

## ARROYO GRANDE—San Luis Obispo County

✉ **ARROYO GRANDE COMMUNITY HOSPITAL (50016)**, 345 South Halcyon Road, Zip 93420–3899; tel. 805/489–4261, (Total facility includes 14 beds in nursing home–type unit) **A**1 2 9 10 **F**8 11 15 29 30 34 35 37 39 40 50 51 54 57 59 64 68 70 75 77 78 79 81 84 87 90 93 94 96 100 107 108 109 110 111 113 116 117 118 128 129 131 145 147 **S** Dignity Health, San Francisco, CA
Primary Contact: Kenneth Dalebout, Chief Administrative Officer
CHR: Ami Padilla, Director Human Resources
Web address: www.arroyograndehospital.org
**Control:** Other not–for–profit (including NFP Corporation) **Service:** General Medical and Surgical

**Staffed Beds:** 67 **Admissions:** 2740 **Census:** 29 **Outpatient Visits:** 65717 **Births:** 0 **Total Expense ($000):** 55146 **Payroll Expense ($000):** 22698 **Personnel:** 286

## ATASCADERO—San Luis Obispo County

□ **ATASCADERO STATE HOSPITAL**, 10333 El Camino Real, Zip 93422–7001, Mailing Address: P.O. Box 7001, Zip 93423–7001; tel. 805/468–2000 **A**1 **F**34 39 53 57 59 75 77 82 86 87 98 103 129 131 143 145 **P**1
Primary Contact: Linda Persons, Executive Director
Web address: www.dmh.ca.gov/statehospitals/atascadero
**Control:** State–Government, nonfederal **Service:** Psychiatric

**Staffed Beds:** 1275 **Admissions:** 1153 **Census:** 1074 **Outpatient Visits:** 0 **Births:** 0 **Total Expense ($000):** 237862 **Payroll Expense ($000):** 142206 **Personnel:** 1941

## AUBURN—Placer County

✉ **SUTTER AUBURN FAITH HOSPITAL (50498)**, 11815 Education Street, Zip 95602–2410; tel. 530/888–4500 **A**1 2 9 10 **F**3 8 11 12 15 17 18 20 28 29 30 31 34 35 37 39 40 44 45 47 49 50 57 58 59 62 63 64 68 70 74 75 78 79 81 85 86 87 92 93 107 108 110 111 113 118 129 131 134 144 145 146 147 **P**5 **S** Sutter Health, Sacramento, CA
Primary Contact: Mitchell J. Hanna, Chief Executive Officer
CFO: Gary Hubschman, Administrative Director Finance
CMO: John Mesic, M.D., Chief Medical Officer
CIO: Tom Ream, Regional Chief Information Officer
CHR: Lynda Dasaro, Director Human Resources
CNO: Virgie Galindo, Chief Nurse Executive
Web address: www.sutterhealth.org
**Control:** Other not–for–profit (including NFP Corporation) **Service:** General Medical and Surgical

**Staffed Beds:** 78 **Admissions:** 4178 **Census:** 37 **Outpatient Visits:** 80561 **Births:** 195 **Total Expense ($000):** 97025 **Payroll Expense ($000):** 37607

## AVALON—Los Angeles County

**CATALINA ISLAND MEDICAL CENTER (51307)**, 100 Falls Canyon Road, Zip 90704, Mailing Address: P.O. Box 1563, Zip 90704–1563; tel. 310/510–0700, (Total facility includes 4 beds in nursing home–type unit) **A**9 10 18 **F**3 11 29 34 36 40 50 57 64 65 66 75 93 97 107 113 118 126 127 129 132 145
Primary Contact: Bryan M. Ballard, FACHE, Chief Executive Officer
CFO: John Lovrich, Chief Financial Officer
CMO: Monte Mellon, M.D., Chief of Staff
CIO: Richard Kleinman, R.N., Manager Medical Informatics
CHR: Krista Steuter, Director Human Resources
CNO: Nancy Mattis, Chief Patient Care Services
Web address: www.catalinaislandmedicalcenter.org
**Control:** Other not–for–profit (including NFP Corporation) **Service:** General Medical and Surgical

**Staffed Beds:** 12 **Admissions:** 24 **Census:** 7 **Outpatient Visits:** 11933 **Births:** 0 **Total Expense ($000):** 6311 **Payroll Expense ($000):** 2576 **Personnel:** 47

## BAKERSFIELD—Kern County

□ **BAKERSFIELD HEART HOSPITAL (50724)**, 3001 Sillect Avenue, Zip 93308–6337; tel. 661/316–6000, (Nonreporting) **A**1 10 **S** MedCath, Inc.
Primary Contact: Randall H. Rolfe, Chief Executive Officer
Web address: www.bakersfieldhearthospital.com
**Control:** Partnership, Investor–owned, for–profit **Service:** General Medical and Surgical

**Staffed Beds:** 47

✉ **BAKERSFIELD MEMORIAL HOSPITAL (50036)**, 420 34th Street, Zip 93301–2237; tel. 661/327–1792, (Nonreporting) **A**1 9 10 **S** Dignity Health, San Francisco, CA
Primary Contact: Jon Van Boening, President and Chief Executive Officer
COO: Bruce Peters, Vice President and Chief Operating Officer
CFO: Jesica Hanson, Vice President and Chief Financial Officer
CMO: Rodney Mark Root, D.O., Vice President Medical Affairs
CHR: Sheri Comaianni, Vice President Human Resources
Web address: www.bakersfieldmemorial.org
**Control:** Other not–for–profit (including NFP Corporation) **Service:** General Medical and Surgical

**Staffed Beds:** 255

□ **GOOD SAMARITAN HOSPITAL (50257)**, 901 Olive Drive, Zip 93308–4144, Mailing Address: P.O. Box 85002, Zip 93380–5002; tel. 661/399–4461 **A**1 9 10 **F**2 3 4 5 8 29 34 35 38 45 46 56 57 65 68 70 75 81 82 86 87 97 98 99 100 101 102 103 104 105 107 108 109 110 111 112 118 129 131 133 134 142 147
Primary Contact: S.A. Manohara, M.D., Chief Executive Officer
COO: Noel Cabezzas, Chief Operating Officer
CFO: Vicki Nguyen, Chief Financial Officer
CMO: Ronnie Claiborne, M.D., Chief Medical Officer
CIO: Anand Manohara, Associate Administrator
CHR: Milissa Newton, Supervisor Human Resources
**Control:** Partnership, Investor–owned, for–profit **Service:** Psychiatric

**Staffed Beds:** 120 **Admissions:** 3148 **Census:** 49 **Outpatient Visits:** 20032 **Births:** 0

✉ **HEALTHSOUTH BAKERSFIELD REHABILITATION HOSPITAL (53031)**, 5001 Commerce Drive, Zip 93309–0689; tel. 661/323–5500, (Nonreporting) **A**1 9 10 **S** HEALTHSOUTH Corporation, Birmingham, AL
Primary Contact: Sandra Hegland, Chief Executive Officer
CFO: Robert Mosesian, Controller
CMO: Chris Yoon, M.D., Medical Director
CIO: Tara DeMontgorency, Director Business Development
CHR: Tami Holden, Director Human Resources
Web address: www.healthsouthbakersfield.com
**Control:** Corporation, Investor–owned, for–profit **Service:** Rehabilitation

**Staffed Beds:** 60

☐ **KERN MEDICAL CENTER (50315)**, 1700 Mount Vernon Avenue, Zip 93306–4018; tel. 661/326–2000 **A**1 2 3 5 8 9 10 **F**2 3 11 15 20 29 31 34 40 43 44 45 49 50 51 54 57 59 61 62 64 66 68 70 72 73 74 75 76 78 79 81 85 87 89 92 93 94 97 98 106 107 108 111 113 114 118 129 145 146 **P**6
Primary Contact: Paul J. Hensler, Chief Executive Officer
CMO: Eugene Kercher, M.D., Chief Medical Officer
CIO: Bill Fawns, Interim Manager Information Systems
CHR: Steve O'Connor, Manager Human Resources
Web address: www.kernmedicalcenter.com
**Control:** County–Government, nonfederal **Service:** General Medical and Surgical

**Staffed Beds:** 172 **Admissions:** 14687 **Census:** 145 **Outpatient Visits:** 113881 **Births:** 3573 **Total Expense ($000):** 212923 **Payroll Expense ($000):** 117122 **Personnel:** 1614

☒ **MERCY HOSPITALS OF BAKERSFIELD (50295)**, 2215 Truxtun Avenue, Zip 93301–3698, Mailing Address: P.O. Box 119, Zip 93302–0119; tel. 661/632–5000, (Includes MERCY SOUTHWEST HOSPITAL, 400 Old River Road, Zip 93311; tel. 661/663–6000), (Nonreporting) **A**1 2 9 10 **S** Dignity Health, San Francisco, CA
Primary Contact: Russell V. Judd, President
COO: Jeremy Zoch, Chief Operating Officer
CFO: Rodney Winegarner, Chief Financial Officer
CIO: Jeff Vague, Regional Manager Information Systems
CHR: Jay King, Vice President Human Resources
Web address: www.mercybakersfield.org
**Control:** Church–operated, Nongovernment, not–for profit **Service:** General Medical and Surgical

**Staffed Beds:** 269

☒ **SAN JOAQUIN COMMUNITY HOSPITAL (50455)**, 2615 Chester Avenue, Zip 93301–2006, Mailing Address: P.O. Box 2615, Zip 93303–2615; tel. 661/395–3000 **A**1 9 10 **F**3 11 12 13 15 16 18 20 22 24 26 28 29 30 31 34 35 40 47 49 57 59 62 64 65 70 71 72 74 75 76 77 78 79 81 84 85 86 91 94 107 108 110 111 113 114 115 116 117 118 129 131 145 **P**7 **S** Adventist Health, Roseville, CA
Primary Contact: Robert J. Beehler, President and Chief Executive Officer
CFO: Brent Soper, Chief Financial Officer
CHR: Marlene Kreidler, Executive Director Human Resources
Web address: www.sanjoaquinhospital.org
**Control:** Church–operated, Nongovernment, not–for profit **Service:** General Medical and Surgical

**Staffed Beds:** 255 **Admissions:** 20815 **Census:** 216 **Outpatient Visits:** 80322 **Births:** 2652 **Total Expense ($000):** 286298 **Payroll Expense ($000):** 113329 **Personnel:** 1719

### BALDWIN PARK—Los Angeles County

☒ **BALDWIN PARK MEDICAL CENTER (50723)**, 1011 Baldwin Park Boulevard, Zip 91706–5806; tel. 626/851–1011 **A**1 10 **F**3 8 13 15 18 29 30 31 34 35 40 41 43 49 56 57 58 59 60 61 62 63 64 65 68 70 72 74 75 76 77 78 79 81 82 84 85 86 87 93 94 107 111 118 129 145 146 147 **S** Kaiser Foundation Hospitals, Oakland, CA
Primary Contact: Margaret H. Pierce, Executive Director
CFO: Rebecca Wheeler, Director Finance
CMO: John Bigley, M.D., Medical Director
CIO: Linda C. Salazar, Information Technology Leader
CHR: Leesa Malcom, Director Human Resources
Web address: www.kp.org
**Control:** Other not–for–profit (including NFP Corporation) **Service:** General Medical and Surgical

**Staffed Beds:** 254 **Admissions:** 14453 **Census:** 131 **Outpatient Visits:** 233126 **Births:** 2845

★ ○ **KINDRED HOSPITAL–BALDWIN PARK (52045)**, 14148 East Francisquito Avenue, Zip 91706; tel. 626/388–2700, (Nonreporting) **A**10 11 **S** Kindred Healthcare, Louisville, KY
Primary Contact: Swenda Moreh, Chief Executive Officer
COO: Dina Garrow, Chief Nursing Officer and Chief Operating Officer
CIO: Glenn P. Requierme, Director Information Technology
CHR: Antoinette Bibal, Director Human Resources
Web address: www.khbaldwinpark.com
**Control:** Corporation, Investor–owned, for–profit **Service:** Long–Term Acute Care hospital

**Staffed Beds:** 95

**VISTA SPECIALTY HOSPITAL OF SAN GABRIEL VALLEY** See Kindred Hospital–Baldwin Park

### BANNING—Riverside County

☒ **SAN GORGONIO MEMORIAL HOSPITAL (50054)**, 600 North Highland Springs Avenue, Zip 92220–3046; tel. 951/845–1121 **A**1 9 10 **F**3 5 8 11 13 15 18 28 29 30 34 35 40 45 49 56 57 64 70 76 79 81 82 85 87 93 104 107 108 110 114 118 127 129 145 146 147
Primary Contact: Mark S. Turner, Chief Executive Officer
CFO: David Recupero, Chief Financial Officer
CMO: Richard Sheldon, M.D., Vice President Medical Affairs
CIO: Linda Palmer, Coordinator Medical Records
CHR: Lynn M. Gomez, Executive Director Human Resources
CNO: Pat Brown, R.N., Chief Nursing Officer
Web address: www.sgmh.org
**Control:** Hospital district or authority, Government, nonfederal **Service:** General Medical and Surgical

**Staffed Beds:** 77 **Admissions:** 3002 **Census:** 34 **Outpatient Visits:** 40005 **Births:** 418 **Total Expense ($000):** 26750 **Payroll Expense ($000):** 19568 **Personnel:** 387

### BARSTOW—San Bernardino County

☒ **BARSTOW COMMUNITY HOSPITAL (50298)**, 555 South Seventh Avenue, Zip 92311–3043; tel. 760/256–1761, (Nonreporting) **A**1 9 10 20 **S** Community Health Systems, Inc., Franklin, TN
Primary Contact: S. Sean Fowler, Chief Executive Officer
CFO: Carrie Howell, Chief Financial Officer
CIO: Ian Riggall, Manager Data Processing
CHR: Vickie Hendricks, Director Human Resources
Web address: www.barstowhospital.com
**Control:** Corporation, Investor–owned, for–profit **Service:** General Medical and Surgical

**Staffed Beds:** 23

### BELLFLOWER—Los Angeles County

☐ **BELLFLOWER MEDICAL CENTER (50531)**, 9542 East Artesia Boulevard, Zip 90706–6511; tel. 562/925–8355, (Nonreporting) **A**1 3 5 9 10 **S** Pacific Health Corporation, Tustin, CA
Primary Contact: Michael O. Choo, President and Chief Executive Officer
COO: Lydia Rojas, Chief Operating Officer
CFO: Clara Blom, Chief Financial Officer
CMO: Virgilio Panganiban, M.D., Chief of Staff
CIO: Cesar Antangan, Director Information Systems
CHR: Liz Tran, Director Human Resources
Web address: www.bellflowermedicalctr.com
**Control:** Corporation, Investor–owned, for–profit **Service:** General Medical and Surgical

**Staffed Beds:** 110

### BERKELEY—Alameda County

☒ △ **ALTA BATES SUMMIT MEDICAL CENTER (50305)**, 2450 Ashby Avenue, Zip 94705–2067; tel. 510/204–4444, (Includes ALTA BATES MEDICAL CENTER–HERRICK CAMPUS, 2001 Dwight Way, Zip 94704; tel. 510/204–4444), (Nonreporting) **A**1 3 5 7 9 10 **S** Sutter Health, Sacramento, CA
Primary Contact: David Bradley, Chief Executive Officer
CFO: Robert Petrina, Chief Financial Officer
CMO: John Gentile, M.D., Vice President Medical Affairs
Web address: www.altabates.com
**Control:** Other not–for–profit (including NFP Corporation) **Service:** General Medical and Surgical

**Staffed Beds:** 527

### BIG BEAR LAKE—San Bernardino County

★ **BEAR VALLEY COMMUNITY HOSPITAL (50618)**, 41870 Garstin Drive, Zip 92315, Mailing Address: P.O. Box 1649, Zip 92315–1649; tel. 909/866–6501, (Nonreporting) **A**9 10 20
Primary Contact: Marc L. Hecksel, Chief Executive Officer
COO: Scott Rogers, Chief Operating Officer
CFO: Rudolph Shutta, Chief Financial Officer
CMO: Kurt Frauenpreis, M.D., Chief Medical Staff
CIO: Cindy Venuto, Public Information Officer
CHR: Karen Mathieu, Director Human Resources
CNO: Mary Norman, R.N., Chief Nursing Officer
Web address: www.bvchd.com
**Control:** Hospital district or authority, Government, nonfederal **Service:** General Medical and Surgical

**Staffed Beds:** 15

---

**Hospital, Medicare Provider Number, Address, Telephone, Approval, Facility, and Physician Codes, Health Care System**

★ American Hospital Association (AHA) membership
☐ The Joint Commission accreditation
◇ DNV Healthcare Inc. accreditation
○ American Osteopathic Association (AOA) accreditation
△ Commission on Accreditation of Rehabilitation Facilities (CARF) accreditation

**CA**

## BISHOP—Inyo County

☒ **NORTHERN INYO HOSPITAL (51324)**, 150 Pioneer Lane, Zip 93514–2599; tel. 760/873–5811, (Nonreporting) **A**1 9 10 18
Primary Contact: John Halfen, Administrator, Chief Executive Officer and Chief Financial Officer
CFO: John Halfen, Administrator, Chief Executive Officer and Chief Financial Officer
CMO: Charlotte Helvie, M.D., Chief of Staff
CIO: Adam Taylor, Manager Information Technology
CHR: Georgan L. Stottlemyre, Director Human Resources
Web address: www.nih.org
**Control:** Hospital district or authority, Government, nonfederal **Service:** General Medical and Surgical

**Staffed Beds:** 25

## BLYTHE—Riverside County

☐ **PALO VERDE HOSPITAL (50423)**, 250 North First Street, Zip 92225–1702; tel. 760/922–4115, (Nonreporting) **A**1 9 10 20
Primary Contact: Peter Klune, Chief Executive Officer
CFO: Dennis E. Rutherford, Chief Financial Officer
CMO: Mohommad Bahktavar, M.D., Chief of Staff
CIO: James C. Mayes, Manager Information Technology and Chief Security Officer
CHR: Rebecca Morse, Chief Human Resources Officer
CNO: Tara Barth, Chief Nursing Officer
Web address: www.paloverdehospital.org
**Control:** Hospital district or authority, Government, nonfederal **Service:** General Medical and Surgical

**Staffed Beds:** 20

## BRAWLEY—Imperial County

☐ **PIONEERS MEMORIAL HEALTHCARE DISTRICT (50342)**, 207 West Legion Road, Zip 92227–7780; tel. 760/351–3333 **A**1 9 10 **F**2 3 11 13 15 18 29 34 35 40 43 45 49 51 53 54 57 59 65 70 73 74 75 76 77 79 81 82 85 86 89 93 97 107 108 110 111 114 117 118 126 129 143 145 146 147
**S** HealthTech Management Services, Franklin, TN
Primary Contact: Greg Moore, CPA, Interim Chief Executive Officer
COO: Stephen J. Campbell, Chief Operating Officer
CFO: Daniel W. Smith, Chief Financial Officer
CMO: Travis Calvin, Jr., M.D., Chief of Staff
CIO: Doug Darby, Director Information Systems
CHR: Robert Honaker, Associate Administrator and Chief Human Resources Officer
Web address: www.pmhd.org
**Control:** Hospital district or authority, Government, nonfederal **Service:** General Medical and Surgical

**Staffed Beds:** 107 **Admissions:** 6831 **Census:** 61 **Outpatient Visits:** 104907 **Births:** 1844 **Total Expense ($000):** 77917 **Payroll Expense ($000):** 35297 **Personnel:** 668

## BREA—Orange County

☒ **KINDRED HOSPITAL–BREA (52039)**, 875 North Brea Boulevard, Zip 92821–2699; tel. 714/529–6842, (Nonreporting) **A**1 9 10 **S** Kindred Healthcare, Louisville, KY
Primary Contact: Joyce Winters, R.N., MSN, Administrator
COO: Denise Jenkins, Chief Clinical Officer
CFO: John Browne, Assistant Administrator Finance
CMO: Jyotika Wali, M.D., Chief of Staff
Web address: www.kindredhospitalbrea.com/
**Control:** Corporation, Investor–owned, for–profit **Service:** Long–Term Acute Care hospital

**Staffed Beds:** 48

## BURBANK—Los Angeles County

☒ △ **PROVIDENCE SAINT JOSEPH MEDICAL CENTER (50235)**, 501 South Buena Vista Street, Zip 91505–4866; tel. 818/843–5111 **A**1 2 7 9 10 **F**3 11 12 13 14 15 17 18 20 21 22 24 26 28 29 30 31 34 35 36 40 44 45 46 50 53 54 56 57 58 59 62 63 64 68 70 72 74 75 76 77 78 79 81 82 83 84 86 87 90 93 107 108 110 111 113 115 116 117 118 120 125 127 129 131 133 142 143 145 146 147 **S** Providence Health & Services, Renton, WA
Primary Contact: Kerry Carmody, Chief Executive Officer
CFO: Dave Mast, Chief Financial Officer
CMO: Myron Berdischewsky, M.D., Chief Medical Officer
CIO: Douglas Jones, Interim Chief Information Officer
CHR: John Saavedra, Service Area Director Human Resources
Web address: www.providence.org
**Control:** Church–operated, Nongovernment, not–for profit **Service:** General Medical and Surgical

**Staffed Beds:** 414 **Admissions:** 18228 **Census:** 239 **Outpatient Visits:** 371775 **Births:** 2524 **Total Expense ($000):** 408342 **Payroll Expense ($000):** 155577 **Personnel:** 1750

## BURLINGAME—San Mateo County

☒ **MILLS–PENINSULA HEALTH SERVICES (50007)**, 1501 Trousdale Drive, Zip 94010–3282; tel. 650/696–5400, (Includes MILLS HOSPITAL, 100 South San Mateo Drive, San Mateo, Zip 94401; tel. 415/696–4400; PENINSULA HOSPITAL, 1783 El Camino Real, Zip 94010–3205; tel. 650/696–5400), (Total facility includes 137 beds in nursing home–type unit) **A**1 2 9 10 **F**2 3 4 5 6 9 11 12 13 15 17 18 20 22 24 26 28 29 30 31 34 35 36 38 40 46 47 48 49 51 53 54 56 57 59 60 64 65 66 68 72 74 75 76 77 78 79 81 84 85 86 87 89 90 91 93 97 98 99 100 101 102 103 104 105 107 108 109 110 111 112 113 114 115 116 117 118 119 120 121 122 123 127 128 129 131 134 142 145 146 **P**5 **S** Sutter Health, Sacramento, CA
Primary Contact: Robert W. Merwin, Chief Executive Officer
CFO: Iftikhar Hussain, Chief Financial Officer
CMO: Michael K. Wood, M.D., Chief Medical Officer
CIO: Michael Reandeau, Chief Information Officer
CHR: Debbie Goodin, Vice President Human Resources
Web address: www.mills–peninsula.org
**Control:** Other not–for–profit (including NFP Corporation) **Service:** General Medical and Surgical

**Staffed Beds:** 393 **Admissions:** 14819 **Census:** 238 **Outpatient Visits:** 314738 **Births:** 1956 **Total Expense ($000):** 442285 **Payroll Expense ($000):** 182674 **Personnel:** 1757

## CAMARILLO—Ventura County

☒ **ST. JOHN'S PLEASANT VALLEY HOSPITAL (50616)**, 2309 Antonio Avenue, Zip 93010–1414; tel. 805/389–5800, (Nonreporting) **A**1 9 10 **S** Dignity Health, San Francisco, CA
Primary Contact: Laurie Eberst, R.N., President and Chief Executive Officer
COO: Kim A. Wilson, R.N., Chief Operating Officer
CFO: Robert D. Wardwell, Chief Financial Officer
CMO: Eugene Fussell, M.D., Chief Medical Officer
CIO: Jeff Perry, Director Information Technology
CHR: Ed Gonzales, Vice President Human Resources
CNO: Raye Burkhardt, Chief Nursing Officer
Web address: www.stjohnshealth.org
**Control:** Other not–for–profit (including NFP Corporation) **Service:** General Medical and Surgical

**Staffed Beds:** 127

## CAMP PENDLETON—San Diego County

☒ **NAVAL HOSPITAL**, Santa Margarita Road, Building H100, Zip 92055–5191, Mailing Address: P.O. Box 555191, Zip 92055–5191; tel. 760/725–1304, (Nonreporting) **A**1 3 5 **S** Bureau of Medicine and Surgery, Department of the Navy, Washington, DC
Primary Contact: Captain Kenneth J. Iverson, MC, USN, Commanding Officer
COO: Captain Jeff Plummer, Executive Officer
CFO: Commander Gordon Blighton, Director Resource Management
CMO: Lynn Bailey, M.D., Director Primary Care and Medical Services
CIO: Gabe Vallido, Chief Information Officer
CHR: Lieutenant Jet Ramos, Head Staff Administration
Web address: www.cpen.med.navy.mil
**Control:** Navy, Government, federal **Service:** General Medical and Surgical

**Staffed Beds:** 72

## CANOGA PARK—Los Angeles County, See Los Angeles

## CARMICHAEL—Sacramento County

☒ **MERCY SAN JUAN MEDICAL CENTER (50516)**, 6501 Coyle Avenue, Zip 95608–0306, Mailing Address: P.O. Box 479, Zip 95609–0479; tel. 916/537–5000 **A**1 2 9 10 **F**3 8 11 12 13 17 18 20 22 24 28 29 30 31 34 35 37 40 43 45 47 48 49 51 58 59 62 63 64 66 68 70 72 74 75 76 77 78 79 81 82 83 84 85 89 93 107 108 111 113 114 117 118 125 128 129 131 134 145 147 **S** Dignity Health, San Francisco, CA
Primary Contact: Brian K. Ivie, President
COO: Paul R. Luehrs, Chief Operating Officer
CFO: Robert Pascuzzi, Chief Financial Officer
CMO: Mark Owens, M.D., Vice President Medical Affairs
CHR: Donna Utley, Vice President Human Resources
Web address: www.mercysanjuan.org
**Control:** Church–operated, Nongovernment, not–for profit **Service:** General Medical and Surgical

**Staffed Beds:** 359 **Admissions:** 20700 **Census:** 264 **Outpatient Visits:** 140594 **Births:** 2617 **Total Expense ($000):** 468374 **Payroll Expense ($000):** 265302

## CASTRO VALLEY—Alameda County

☒ **EDEN MEDICAL CENTER (50488)**, 20103 Lake Chabot Road, Zip 94546–5341; tel. 510/537–1234, (Includes SAN LEANDRO HOSPITAL, 13855 East 14th Street, San Leandro, Zip 94578–2600; tel. 510/357–6500; Ronnie Bayduza, Administrator), (Nonreporting) **A**1 2 9 10 **S** Sutter Health, Sacramento, CA
Primary Contact: George Bischalaney, President and Chief Executive Officer
Web address: www.edenmedcenter.org
**Control:** Other not–for–profit (including NFP Corporation) **Service:** General Medical and Surgical

**Staffed Beds:** 271

*Many Facility Codes have changed. Please refer to the AHA Guide Code Chart.*  © 2012 AHA Guide

CA

## CEDARVILLE—Modoc County

**SURPRISE VALLEY HEALTHCARE DISTRICT (51308)**, 741 North Main Street, Zip 96104, Mailing Address: P.O. Box 246, Zip 96104–0246; tel. 530/279–6111, (Nonreporting) **A**9 10 18
Primary Contact: Wanda Grove, Chief Executive Officer
CFO: Renae Sweet, Chief Financial Officer
CMO: Chuck Colas, M.D., Medical Director
CHR: William Bostic, Administrative Assistant Human Resources
Web address: www.svhospital.org/
**Control:** Hospital district or authority, Government, nonfederal **Service:** General Medical and Surgical

**Staffed Beds:** 4

## CERRITOS—Los Angeles County

☐ **COLLEGE HOSPITAL (54055)**, 10802 College Place, Zip 90703–1579; tel. 562/924–9581, (Nonreporting) **A**1 9 10 **S** College Health Enterprises, Santa Fe Springs, CA
Primary Contact: Stephen Witt, President and Chief Executive Officer
CFO: Roderick Bell, Chief Financial Officer
CHR: Holly Risha, Administrative Director Human Resources
Web address: www.collegehospitals.com
**Control:** Corporation, Investor–owned, for–profit **Service:** Psychiatric

**Staffed Beds:** 157

## CHESTER—Plumas County

★ **SENECA HEALTHCARE DISTRICT (51327)**, 130 Brentwood Drive, Zip 96020–0737, Mailing Address: P.O. Box 737, Zip 96020–0737; tel. 530/258–2151, (Nonreporting) **A**9 10 18
Primary Contact: Linda S. Wagner, MSN, Interim Chief Executive Officer
CMO: Steen Jensen, M.D., Chief of Staff
CHR: Marie Stuersel, Director Human Resources
Web address: www.senecahospital.org
**Control:** Hospital district or authority, Government, nonfederal **Service:** General Medical and Surgical

**Staffed Beds:** 26

## CHICO—Butte County

⊞ **ENLOE MEDICAL CENTER (50039)**, 1531 Esplanade, Zip 95926–3386; tel. 530/332–7300, (Includes ENLOE MEDICAL CENTER–COHASSET, 560 Cohasset Road, Zip 95926; tel. 530/332–7300), (Nonreporting) **A**1 9 10
Primary Contact: Michael C. Wiltermood, President and Chief Executive Officer
CMO: Forrest Olson, M.D., Chief Medical Officer
CHR: Carol Linscheid, Vice President Human Resources
Web address: www.enloe.org
**Control:** Other not–for–profit (including NFP Corporation) **Service:** General Medical and Surgical

**Staffed Beds:** 263

## CHINO—San Bernardino County

○ **CANYON RIDGE HOSPITAL (54111)**, 5353 G Street, Zip 91710–5250; tel. 909/590–3700 **A**9 10 11 **F**3 4 5 29 35 98 99 100 101 102 104 105 129 131 **S** Universal Health Services, Inc., King of Prussia, PA
Primary Contact: Jeff McDonald, Chief Executive Officer
CFO: Burt Harris, Chief Financial Officer
CMO: Mir Ali–Khan, M.D., Medical Director
CIO: Maria Patterson, Manager Health Information Management
CHR: Ericca Lopez, Director Human Resources
Web address: www.canyonridgehospital.net
**Control:** Corporation, Investor–owned, for–profit **Service:** Psychiatric

**Staffed Beds:** 106 **Admissions:** 5108 **Census:** 83 **Outpatient Visits:** 11276 **Births:** 0

○ **CHINO VALLEY MEDICAL CENTER (50586)**, 5451 Walnut Avenue, Zip 91710–2672; tel. 909/464–8600, (Nonreporting) **A**10 11 12 13 **S** Prime Healthcare Services, Ontario, CA
Primary Contact: Lex Reddy, Chief Executive Officer
CFO: Gregory Brentano, Chief Financial Officer
CMO: James M. Lally, M.D., Chief Medical Officer
CIO: Vic Mahan, Chief Information Officer
CHR: Arti Dhuper, Regional Director Human Resources
Web address: www.cvmc.com
**Control:** Corporation, Investor–owned, for–profit **Service:** General Medical and Surgical

**Staffed Beds:** 112

## CHOWCHILLA—Madera County

**CHOWCHILLA DISTRICT MEMORIAL HOSPITAL**, 1104 Ventura Avenue, Zip 93610–2298; tel. 559/665–3781, (Nonreporting)
Primary Contact: Cathy Flores, R.N., Administrator
**Control:** Hospital district or authority, Government, nonfederal **Service:** General Medical and Surgical

**Staffed Beds:** 24

## CHULA VISTA—San Diego County

**BAYVIEW BEHAVIORAL HEALTH CAMPUS**, 330 Moss Street, Zip 91911–2005; tel. 619/426–6311, (Nonreporting)
Primary Contact: George Lewis, Executive Director
CFO: Robert Bourseau, Chief Financial Officer
Web address: www.bayviewhospital.com
**Control:** Corporation, Investor–owned, for–profit **Service:** Psychiatric

**Staffed Beds:** 64

**SCRIPPS MERCY HOSPITAL CHULA VISTA** See Scripps Mercy Hospital, San Diego

⊞ **SHARP CHULA VISTA MEDICAL CENTER (50222)**, 751 Medical Center Court, Zip 91911–6699, Mailing Address: P.O. Box 1297, Zip 91912–1297; tel. 619/482–5800, (Total facility includes 100 beds in nursing home–type unit) **A**1 2 9 10 **F**8 11 12 13 15 18 20 22 24 26 28 29 30 31 34 35 40 45 46 47 49 51 53 54 57 59 60 64 65 70 72 75 76 77 78 79 81 82 85 86 87 93 94 107 108 111 113 114 117 118 120 122 125 127 129 131 142 145 146 147 **P**5 **S** Sharp HealthCare, San Diego, CA
Primary Contact: Pablo Velez, Chief Executive Officer
CMO: Francisco Anguiano, M.D., Chief of Staff
CHR: Zoe Gardner, Manager Human Resources
Web address: www.sharp.com
**Control:** Other not–for–profit (including NFP Corporation) **Service:** General Medical and Surgical

**Staffed Beds:** 343 **Admissions:** 15131 **Census:** 275 **Outpatient Visits:** 104526 **Births:** 2948 **Total Expense ($000):** 279083 **Payroll Expense ($000):** 117814 **Personnel:** 1481

## CLEARLAKE—Lake County

⊞ **ST. HELENA HOSPITAL CLEARLAKE (51317)**, 15630 18th Avenue, Zip 95422–9339, Mailing Address: P.O. Box 6720, Zip 95422–6720; tel. 707/994–6486 **A**1 9 10 18 **F**18 29 30 34 35 40 45 50 57 59 62 70 76 81 87 93 97 107 108 110 111 113 116 118 126 129 132 133 142 143 **P**3 **S** Adventist Health, Roseville, CA
Primary Contact: Terry Newmyer, President and Chief Executive Officer
COO: David Santos, Chief Operating Officer (VP Operations)
CFO: Buck McDonald, Chief Financial Officer
CMO: Marc Shapiro, M.D., Chief Medical Officer
CIO: Joshua Cowan, Chief Information Officer
CHR: Wendi Fox, Human Resources Administrative Director
CNO: Joan Rogers, R.N., Chief Nursing Officer
Web address: www.adventisthealth.org
**Control:** Church–operated, Nongovernment, not–for profit **Service:** General Medical and Surgical

**Staffed Beds:** 25 **Admissions:** 1755 **Census:** 19 **Outpatient Visits:** 170438 **Births:** 193 **Total Expense ($000):** 56851 **Payroll Expense ($000):** 22453 **Personnel:** 394

## CLOVIS—Fresno County

☐ **CLOVIS COMMUNITY MEDICAL CENTER (50492)**, 2755 Herndon Avenue, Zip 93611–6800; tel. 559/324–4000, (Nonreporting) **A**1 9 10 **S** Community Medical Centers, Fresno, CA
Primary Contact: Craig Castro, Chief Executive Officer
COO: Craig Waggoner, Chief Operating Officer
CFO: Tracy Kiritani, Vice President and Chief Financial Officer
CIO: George Vasquez, Chief Technology Officer
CHR: Ginny Burdick, Senior Vice President and Chief Human Resources Officer
Web address: www.communitymedical.org
**Control:** Other not–for–profit (including NFP Corporation) **Service:** General Medical and Surgical

**Staffed Beds:** 109

## COALINGA—Fresno County

**COALINGA REGIONAL MEDICAL CENTER (50397)**, 1191 Phelps Avenue,
Zip 93210–9636; tel. 559/935–6400, (Nonreporting) **A**9 10 20
Primary Contact: Sharon A. Spurgeon, Chief Executive Officer
CFO: Sandra Earls, Chief Financial Officer
CMO: Lymar Bik, M.D., Medical Director
CIO: Rachael Diaz, Systems Operator
CHR: Amber Stiglianese, Manager Human Resources
CNO: Betty Hull, R.N., Director Patient Services
Web address: www.coalingamedicalcenter.com
**Control:** Hospital district or authority, Government, nonfederal **Service:** General
Medical and Surgical

**Staffed Beds: 138**

## COLTON—San Bernardino County

○ **ARROWHEAD REGIONAL MEDICAL CENTER (50245)**, 400 North Pepper
Avenue, Zip 92324–1819; tel. 909/580–1000 **A**2 3 5 10 11 12 13 **F**3 8 13 15
16 18 20 22 28 29 30 31 32 34 35 36 39 40 43 45 47 49 50 51 52 54 55
56 57 60 62 64 66 68 70 71 72 74 75 76 77 78 79 80 81 82 83 84 85 86
87 89 92 93 97 98 100 101 102 106 107 108 110 111 113 114 117 118
119 120 129 131 134 145 146 147 **P**5
Primary Contact: Patrick A. Petre, Chief Executive Officer
COO: Maureen A. Malone, Chief Operating Officer
CFO: Frank Arambula, Chief Financial Officer
CMO: Dev GnanaDev, M.D., Medical Director
CIO: Felix Ekpo, Interim Manager Information Systems
CHR: Victor Tordesillas, Director Human Resources
CNO: Michelle Sayre, R.N., Chief Nursing Officer
Web address: www.arrowheadmedcenter.org
**Control:** County–Government, nonfederal **Service:** General Medical and Surgical

**Staffed Beds: 373 Admissions:** 25170 **Census:** 301 **Outpatient Visits:**
382114 **Births:** 3193 **Total Expense ($000):** 474961 **Payroll Expense
($000):** 150789 **Personnel:** 2580

## COLUSA—Colusa County

⊠ **COLUSA REGIONAL MEDICAL CENTER (50434)**, 199 East Webster Street,
Zip 95932–2954, Mailing Address: P.O. Box 331, Zip 95932–0331;
tel. 530/458–5821, (Total facility includes 6 beds in nursing home–type unit) **A**1
9 10 20 **F**29 30 35 40 53 54 57 59 62 64 65 68 70 75 76 77 81 84 85 107
118 127 128 129 132 143 145
Primary Contact: Dale A. Kirby, Chief Executive Officer
CFO: Terry Deak, Chief Financial Officer
CMO: Samuel Medrano, M.D., Chief of Staff
CIO: Rachel Betke-Mena, Director Health Information Management
CHR: Dierdre Athenais, Director Human Resources
Web address: www.colusamedicalcenter.org
**Control:** Other not–for–profit (including NFP Corporation) **Service:** General
Medical and Surgical

**Staffed Beds: 30 Admissions:** 994 **Census:** 11 **Outpatient Visits:** 51756

## CONCORD—Contra Costa County

⊠ **JOHN MUIR BEHAVIORAL HEALTH CENTER (54131)**, 2740 Grant Street,
Zip 94520; tel. 925/674–4100, (Nonreporting) **A**1 9 10 **S** John Muir Health,
Walnut Creek, CA
Primary Contact: Elizabeth Stallings, Chief Operating Officer
COO: Elizabeth Stallings, Chief Operating Officer
CFO: Michael Moody, Senior Vice President and Chief Financial Officer
CMO: Nagui Achamallah, M.D., Chief of Staff
CIO: Eric Saff, Senior Vice President and Chief Information Officer
CHR: Alice A. Villanueva, Senior Vice President Human Resources
Web address: www.johnmuirhealth.com
**Control:** Other not–for–profit (including NFP Corporation) **Service:** Psychiatric

**Staffed Beds: 70**

⊠ **JOHN MUIR MEDICAL CENTER, CONCORD (50496)**, 2540 East Street,
Zip 94520; tel. 925/682–8200 **A**1 2 9 10 **F**3 12 15 17 18 20 22 24 26 28 29
30 31 34 37 39 40 44 46 47 48 49 50 54 56 57 58 59 64 70 74 75 78
79 80 81 82 84 85 86 87 93 107 108 110 111 113 114 117 118 119 120
122 123 125 129 131 134 140 142 145 147 **P**4 5 **S** John Muir Health, Walnut
Creek, CA
Primary Contact: Michael S. Thomas, President and Chief Administrative Officer
COO: Michael S. Thomas, President and Chief Administrative Officer
CFO: Michael Moody, Chief Financial Officer
CMO: Hartwell Lin, M.D., Chief of Staff
CIO: Jim Wesley, Interim Senior Vice President and Chief Information Officer
CHR: Alice A. Villanueva, Vice President Human Resources
CNO: Donna Brackley, Senior Vice President Patient Care Services
Web address: www.johnmuirhealth.com
**Control:** Other not–for–profit (including NFP Corporation) **Service:** General
Medical and Surgical

**Staffed Beds: 182 Admissions:** 9203 **Census:** 130 **Outpatient Visits:**
180937 **Births:** 0 **Total Expense ($000):** 354474 **Payroll Expense ($000):**
138435 **Personnel:** 1120

## CORCORAN—Kings County

★ **CORCORAN DISTRICT HOSPITAL (50349)**, 1310 Hanna Avenue,
Zip 93212–2395, Mailing Address: P.O. Box 758, Zip 93212–0758;
tel. 559/992–5051 **A**9 10 **F**29 40 45 49 50 51 57 64 66 68 79 81 85 93 107
113 118 126 129 132
Primary Contact: Jonathan Brenn, Chief Executive Officer
CIO: Eva Pierce, Chief Information Officer
CHR: Jose Romero, Director Human Resources
Web address: www.cdhosp.com
**Control:** Hospital district or authority, Government, nonfederal **Service:** General
Medical and Surgical

**Staffed Beds: 20 Admissions:** 499 **Census:** 4 **Outpatient Visits:** 35219
**Births:** 0 **Total Expense ($000):** 12075 **Personnel:** 93

## CORONA—Riverside County

□ **CORONA REGIONAL MEDICAL CENTER (50329)**, 800 South Main Street,
Zip 92882–3420; tel. 951/737–4343, (Includes CORONA REGIONAL MEDICAL
CENTER–REHABILITATION, 730 Magnolia Avenue, Zip 92879;
tel. 951/736–7200), (Nonreporting) **A**1 9 10 **S** Universal Health Services, Inc.,
King of Prussia, PA
Primary Contact: Kevan Metcalfe, Chief Executive Officer
CFO: Becky Cheng, Chief Financial Officer
CMO: Michael Molinari, M.D., Chief of Staff
CIO: Tura Heckler, Director Information Systems
CHR: Ruth Battles, Administrative Director Human Resources
Web address: www.coronaregional.com
**Control:** Other not–for–profit (including NFP Corporation) **Service:** General
Medical and Surgical

**Staffed Beds: 240**

## CORONADO—San Diego County

⊠ **SHARP CORONADO HOSPITAL AND HEALTHCARE CENTER (50234)**, 250
Prospect Place, Zip 92118–1999; tel. 619/522–3600, (Total facility includes 145
beds in nursing home–type unit) **A**1 9 10 **F**3 11 15 29 30 34 35 36 37 39 40
43 45 51 53 57 59 60 64 65 68 69 70 74 75 77 79 81 85 86 87 93 104
107 111 113 118 119 125 127 129 134 145 147 **S** Sharp HealthCare, San
Diego, CA
Primary Contact: Marcia K. Hall, Chief Executive Officer
COO: Tony Guerra, Chief Financial Officer and Chief Operating Officer
CFO: Tony Guerra, Chief Financial Officer and Chief Operating Officer
CHR: George Holtz, Manager Human Resources
Web address: www.sharp.com
**Control:** Other not–for–profit (including NFP Corporation) **Service:** General
Medical and Surgical

**Staffed Beds: 204 Admissions:** 3138 **Census:** 136 **Outpatient Visits:** 56622
**Births:** 0 **Total Expense ($000):** 77939 **Payroll Expense ($000):** 35321
**Personnel:** 496

## COSTA MESA—Orange County

□ **COLLEGE HOSPITAL COSTA MESA (50543)**, 301 Victoria Street,
Zip 92627–7131; tel. 949/642–2734, (Nonreporting) **A**1 9 10 **S** College Health
Enterprises, Santa Fe Springs, CA
Primary Contact: Susan L. Taylor, Chief Executive Officer
CFO: Dale Bracy, Chief Financial Officer
CMO: Craig A. Ross, M.D., Chief of Staff
CIO: Red Ladiana, Manager Information Systems
CHR: Sharon DuBruyne, Director Human Resources
Web address: www.collegehospitalcm.com
**Control:** Corporation, Investor–owned, for–profit **Service:** Psychiatric

**Staffed Beds: 122**

## COVINA—Los Angeles County

□ **AURORA CHARTER OAK HOSPITAL (54069)**, 1161 East Covina Boulevard,
Zip 91724–1599; tel. 626/966–1632, (Nonreporting) **A**1 9 10 **S** Aurora
Behavioral Health Care, Corona, CA
Primary Contact: Todd A. Smith, Chief Executive Officer
COO: Sheila Cordova, Director Clinical Services and Chief Operating Officer
CFO: Cory Delello, Chief Financial Officer
CMO: Adib Bitar, M.D., Medical Director
CHR: Christine de la Paz, Director Human Resources
Web address: www.aurorabehavioral.com
**Control:** Corporation, Investor–owned, for–profit **Service:** Psychiatric

**Staffed Beds: 95**

*Many Facility Codes have changed. Please refer to the AHA Guide Code Chart.* © 2012 AHA Guide

CA

**CITRUS VALLEY MEDICAL CENTER–INTER–COMMUNITY CAMPUS (50382)**, 210 West San Bernardino Road, Zip 91723–1901, Mailing Address: P.O. Box 6108, Zip 91722–5108; tel. 626/331–7331, (Nonreporting) **A**2 9 10 **S** Citrus Valley Health Partners, Covina, CA
Primary Contact: Robert H. Curry, President and Chief Executive Officer
COO: Elvia Foulke, Executive Vice President Healthcare Delivery and Chief Operating Officer
CFO: Lois Conyers, Senior Vice President and Chief Financial Officer
CMO: Richard Gisi, M.D., Chief Medical Officer
CIO: David McCobb, Chief Information Officer
CHR: Lisa Foust, Senior Vice President Human Resources
Web address: www.cvhp.org
**Control:** Other not–for–profit (including NFP Corporation) **Service:** General Medical and Surgical

**Staffed Beds:** 252

### CRESCENT CITY—Del Norte County

☒ **SUTTER COAST HOSPITAL (50417)**, 800 East Washington Boulevard, Zip 95531–8359; tel. 707/464–8511, (Nonreporting) **A**1 9 10 20 **S** Sutter Health, Sacramento, CA
Primary Contact: Eugene Suksi, Chief Executive Officer
CFO: Judi Swartout, Chief Financial Officer
Web address: www.sutterhealth.org
**Control:** Other not–for–profit (including NFP Corporation) **Service:** General Medical and Surgical

**Staffed Beds:** 59

### CULVER CITY—Los Angeles County

**BROTMAN MEDICAL CENTER (50752)**, 3828 Delmas Terrace, Zip 90232–6806; tel. 310/836–7000 **A**9 10 21 **F**4 17 18 20 22 24 26 29 40 41 45 49 51 57 60 70 74 78 79 81 90 98 107 108 111 113 117 118 142 **P**5
Primary Contact: Barbara Schneider, R.N., Chief Executive Officer
COO: Diane Rafferty, Chief Operating Officer
CFO: Vincent Rubin, Chief Financial Officer
CMO: Martha Sonnenberg, M.D., Chief of Staff
CIO: Carrie Bonar, Chief Information Officer
CHR: Betty J. Harris, Director Human Resources
Web address: www.brotmanmedicalcenter.com
**Control:** Corporation, Investor–owned, for–profit **Service:** General Medical and Surgical

**Staffed Beds:** 232 **Admissions:** 8460 **Census:** 164 **Outpatient Visits:** 26015 **Births:** 0 **Total Expense ($000):** 126255 **Payroll Expense ($000):** 49010 **Personnel:** 752

### DALY CITY—San Mateo County

☒ **SETON MEDICAL CENTER (50289)**, 1900 Sullivan Avenue, Zip 94015–2229; tel. 650/992–4000, (Nonreporting) **A**1 2 9 10 **S** Daughters of Charity Health System, Los Altos Hills, CA
Primary Contact: Lorraine P. Auerbach, President and Chief Executive Officer
COO: Stephanie Mearns, Vice President Patient Care Services and Chief Nurse Executive
CFO: Richard Wood, Chief Financial Officer
CMO: David Goldschmid, M.D., President Medical Staff
CIO: David Kerrins, Vice President Informatics, Information Technology and Chief Informatics Officer
CHR: Patricia White, Vice President Human Resources
Web address: www.setonmedicalcenter.org
**Control:** Church–operated, Nongovernment, not–for profit **Service:** General Medical and Surgical

**Staffed Beds:** 429

### DAVIS—Yolo County

☒ **SUTTER DAVIS HOSPITAL (50537)**, 2000 Sutter Place, Zip 95616–6201, Mailing Address: P.O. Box 1617, Zip 95617–1617; tel. 530/756–6440, (Nonreporting) **A**1 3 5 9 10 **S** Sutter Health, Sacramento, CA
Primary Contact: Janet Wagner, R.N., Chief Executive Officer
CFO: Richard SooHoo, Chief Financial Officer
CMO: Daniel Kennedy, M.D., Chief of Staff
CHR: Eva Hilliard, Director Human Resources
CNO: Tracy Needham, Director of Nursing
Web address: www.sutterhealth.org
**Control:** Other not–for–profit (including NFP Corporation) **Service:** General Medical and Surgical

**Staffed Beds:** 48

### DELANO—Kern County

○ **DELANO REGIONAL MEDICAL CENTER (50608)**, 1401 Garces Highway, Zip 93215–3690, Mailing Address: P.O. Box 460, Zip 93216–0460; tel. 661/725–4800, (Nonreporting) **A**9 10 11
Primary Contact: Bahram Ghaffari, Executive Director and Chief Financial Officer
CFO: Bahram Ghaffari, Executive Director and Chief Financial Officer
CIO: Sandy Bakich, Director Information Management
CHR: Del Garbanzos, Director Human Resources
Web address: www.drmc.com
**Control:** Other not–for–profit (including NFP Corporation) **Service:** General Medical and Surgical

**Staffed Beds:** 100

### DOWNEY—Los Angeles County

**DOWNEY REGIONAL MEDICAL CENTER (50393)**, 11500 Brookshire Avenue, Zip 90241; tel. 562/904–5000, (Nonreporting) **A**9 10 12 13
Primary Contact: Kenneth Strople, President and Chief Executive Officer
COO: Robert Fuller, Executive Vice President and Chief Operating Officer
CFO: Ed King, Chief Financial Officer
CIO: Nick Pappas, Chief Information Officer
CHR: Carole Everhart, Administrative Director Human Resources
CNO: Heather Conwell, Chief Nursing Officer
Web address: www.drmci.org
**Control:** Other not–for–profit (including NFP Corporation) **Service:** General Medical and Surgical

**Staffed Beds:** 181

★ **KAISER PERMANENTE DOWNEY MEDICAL CENTER (50139)**, 9333 Imperial Highway, Zip 90242–2812; tel. 562/657–9000, (Nonreporting) **A**10 21 **S** Kaiser Foundation Hospitals, Oakland, CA
Primary Contact: E. Jane Finley, Senior Vice President and Executive Director
COO: Jim Branchick, R.N., Chief Operating Officer
CNO: Patricia J. Clausen, R.N., Chief Nurse Executive
Web address: www.kaiserpermanente.org
**Control:** Other not–for–profit (including NFP Corporation) **Service:** General Medical and Surgical

**Staffed Beds:** 218

☐ △ **RANCHO LOS AMIGOS NATIONAL REHABILITATION CENTER (50717)**, 7601 East Imperial Highway, Zip 90242–3496; tel. 562/401–7022, (Nonreporting) **A**1 3 5 7 9 10 **S** Los Angeles County–Department of Health Services, Los Angeles, CA
Primary Contact: Jorge Orozco, Chief Executive Officer
COO: Benjamin Ovando, Chief Operations Officer
CFO: Robin Bayus, Chief Financial Officer
CMO: Mindy Aisen, M.D., Chief Medical Officer
CIO: Betty Romeo, Chief Information Officer
CHR: Melinda Fonseca, Associate Director Human Resources
CNO: Michelle Sterling, R.N., Acting Chief Nursing Officer
Web address: www.rancho.org
**Control:** County–Government, nonfederal **Service:** Rehabilitation

**Staffed Beds:** 207

### DUARTE—Los Angeles County

☒ **CITY OF HOPE'S HELFORD CLINICAL RESEARCH HOSPITAL (50146)**, 1500 East Duarte Road, Zip 91010–3012; tel. 626/256–4673 **A**1 2 3 5 8 9 10 **F**3 8 11 14 15 18 26 29 30 31 32 34 35 36 38 44 45 46 47 49 50 55 56 57 58 59 61 63 64 68 70 74 75 77 78 79 80 81 82 84 85 86 87 88 89 92 93 96 99 100 101 102 103 104 107 108 110 111 113 115 116 117 118 119 120 122 123 125 129 131 133 135 140 141 142 143 144 145 146 147 **P**3
Primary Contact: Michael A. Friedman, M.D., President and Chief Executive Officer
COO: Marty Sargeant, Chief Operating Officer
CFO: Gary F. Conner, Chief Financial Officer
CMO: Alexandra Levine, M.D., Chief Medical Officer
CIO: Paul Conocenti, Chief Information Officer
CHR: Stephanie Neuvirth, Chief Human Resource and Diversity Officer
CNO: Shirley Johnson, R.N., Chief Nursing and Patient Services Officer
Web address: www.cityofhope.org
**Control:** Other not–for–profit (including NFP Corporation) **Service:** General Medical and Surgical

**Staffed Beds:** 185 **Admissions:** 6020 **Census:** 150 **Outpatient Visits:** 171521 **Births:** 0 **Total Expense ($000):** 594770 **Payroll Expense ($000):** 202751 **Personnel:** 2787

---

**Hospital, Medicare Provider Number, Address, Telephone, Approval, Facility, and Physician Codes, Health Care System**

★ American Hospital Association (AHA) membership
☐ The Joint Commission accreditation
◇ DNV Healthcare Inc. accreditation
○ American Osteopathic Association (AOA) accreditation
△ Commission on Accreditation of Rehabilitation Facilities (CARF) accreditation

## EL CENTRO—Imperial County

☒ **EL CENTRO REGIONAL MEDICAL CENTER (50045)**, 1415 Ross Avenue, Zip 92243–4398; tel. 760/339–7100, (Nonreporting) **A**1 9 10
Primary Contact: David R. Green, Administrator and Chief Executive Officer
COO: Tomas Virgen, R.N., Chief Operating Officer
CFO: Kathleen Farmer, Assistant Administrator Finance and Chief Financial Officer
CIO: John Gaede, Director Information Systems
CHR: Bill Moore, Chief Human Resources
Web address: www.ecrmc.org
**Control:** City–Government, nonfederal **Service:** General Medical and Surgical

**Staffed Beds:** 165

## ELDRIDGE—Sonoma County

**SONOMA DEVELOPMENTAL CENTER (50547)**, 15000 Arnold Drive, Zip 95431, Mailing Address: P.O. Box 1493, Zip 95431–1493; tel. 707/938–6000, (Nonreporting) **A**10
Primary Contact: James E. Rogers, Executive Director
COO: Karen Clark, Director Administrative Services
CMO: Judith Bjorndal, M.D., Medical Director
CIO: Karen Litzenberg, Public Information Officer
CHR: Roy J. Johnson, Director Human Resources
Web address: www.dds.ca.gov/sonoma
**Control:** State–Government, nonfederal **Service:** Institution for mental retardation

**Staffed Beds:** 546

## ENCINITAS—San Diego County

☒ △ **SCRIPPS MEMORIAL HOSPITAL–ENCINITAS (50503)**, 354 Santa Fe Drive, Zip 92024–5182, Mailing Address: P.O. Box 230817, Zip 92023–0817; tel. 760/633–6501 **A**1 2 7 9 10 **F**3 8 11 13 14 15 18 20 26 28 29 30 31 34 35 40 44 49 54 57 58 59 64 65 68 70 74 75 76 77 78 79 81 82 84 85 86 87 90 91 92 93 94 96 102 107 108 111 113 114 118 129 131 145 147 **P**3 5 **S** Scripps Health, San Diego, CA
Primary Contact: Carl J. Etter, Senior Vice President and Chief Executive
COO: Rebecca Cofinas, Vice President and Chief Operating Executive Operations
CFO: Sharon Creal, Vice President Financial Operations
CHR: Cara Williams, Director Human Resources
Web address: www.scripps.org
**Control:** Other not–for–profit (including NFP Corporation) **Service:** General Medical and Surgical

**Staffed Beds:** 158 **Admissions:** 9623 **Census:** 117 **Outpatient Visits:** 72721 **Births:** 1648 **Total Expense ($000):** 194902 **Payroll Expense ($000):** 83893 **Personnel:** 1009

## ENCINO—Los Angeles County, See Los Angeles

## ESCONDIDO—San Diego County

☒ △ **PALOMAR MEDICAL CENTER (50115)**, 555 East Valley Parkway, Zip 92025–3084; tel. 760/739–3000, (Nonreporting) **A**1 7 9 10 **S** Palomar Health, San Diego, CA
Primary Contact: Gerald E. Bracht, Chief Administrative Officer
COO: Gerald E. Bracht, Chief Administrative Officer
CFO: Robert Hemker, Chief Financial Officer
CMO: Duane Buringrud, M.D., Chief Medical and Quality Officer
CIO: Paul Peabody, Chief Information Officer
CHR: Brenda C. Turner, Chief Human Resources Officer
Web address: www.pph.org
**Control:** Hospital district or authority, Government, nonfederal **Service:** General Medical and Surgical

**Staffed Beds:** 330

## EUREKA—Humboldt County

☒ **ST. JOSEPH HOSPITAL (50006)**, 2700 Dolbeer Street, Zip 95501–4799; tel. 707/445–8121, (Includes GENERAL HOSPITAL, 2200 Harrison Avenue, Zip 95501–3299; tel. 707/445–5111) **A**1 2 9 10 19 **F**3 8 11 12 13 15 17 18 20 22 24 26 28 29 30 31 35 40 45 46 47 48 49 53 54 62 63 64 68 70 72 75 76 77 78 79 81 82 84 85 86 87 89 90 93 96 107 108 110 111 113 114 116 117 118 119 120 122 123 128 129 143 145 147 **P**5 **S** St. Joseph Health, Orange, CA
Primary Contact: Joseph M. Mark, President and Chief Executive Officer
CFO: Andrew Rybolt, Chief Financial Officer
CMO: Scott Sageman, M.D., Vice President and Chief Medical Officer
CIO: Wendy Thorpe, Area Director Information Systems
CHR: Linda Cook, Vice President Human Resources
Web address: www.stjosepheureka.org
**Control:** Church–operated, Nongovernment, not–for profit **Service:** General Medical and Surgical

**Staffed Beds:** 128 **Admissions:** 6591 **Census:** 85 **Outpatient Visits:** 203231 **Births:** 646 **Total Expense ($000):** 181324 **Payroll Expense ($000):** 56032 **Personnel:** 983

## FAIRFIELD—Solano County

☒ **NORTHBAY MEDICAL CENTER (50367)**, 1200 B. Gale Wilson Boulevard, Zip 94533–3552; tel. 707/646–5000, (Includes NORTHBAY VACAVALLEY HOSPITAL, 1000 Nut Tree Road, Vacaville, Zip 95687–4100; tel. 707/624–7000) **A**1 2 9 10 **F**2 3 6 8 11 13 17 18 19 20 22 24 26 28 29 30 31 32 35 36 40 43 44 49 50 51 54 56 59 62 63 64 65 70 72 73 74 75 76 77 78 79 80 81 82 84 85 87 89 92 93 94 96 97 107 113 114 117 118 120 129 131 145 146 147 **P**6
Primary Contact: Deborah Sugiyama, President
CFO: Arthur E. DeNio, Vice President and Chief Financial Officer
CMO: Mitesh Patel, M.D., Vice President Medical Affairs
CIO: Paul Alcala, Vice President and Chief Information Officer
CHR: Ken McCollum, Vice President, Human Resources
Web address: www.northbay.org
**Control:** Other not–for–profit (including NFP Corporation) **Service:** General Medical and Surgical

**Staffed Beds:** 157 **Admissions:** 8205 **Census:** 92 **Outpatient Visits:** 229597 **Births:** 1431 **Total Expense ($000):** 304865 **Payroll Expense ($000):** 120875 **Personnel:** 1164

## FALL RIVER MILLS—Shasta County

★ **MAYERS MEMORIAL HOSPITAL DISTRICT (51305)**, 43563 Highway 299 East, Zip 96028–0459, Mailing Address: P.O. Box 459, Zip 96028–0459; tel. 530/336–5511, (Total facility includes 99 beds in nursing home–type unit) **A**9 10 18 **F**13 40 45 56 59 63 64 76 81 85 93 107 118 127 129 131 132 145
Primary Contact: Matthew Rees, Chief Executive Officer
CMO: Chris Camarata, M.D., Chief of Staff
CIO: Martha Lucero, Director Special Projects
CHR: Paul McCoy, Director Human Resources
CNO: Sherry Wilson, R.N., Chief Nursing Officer Long Term Care
Web address: www.mayersmemorial.com
**Control:** Hospital district or authority, Government, nonfederal **Service:** General Medical and Surgical

**Staffed Beds:** 121 **Admissions:** 494 **Census:** 81 **Outpatient Visits:** 16816 **Births:** 83 **Total Expense ($000):** 17680 **Payroll Expense ($000):** 7616 **Personnel:** 173

## FALLBROOK—San Diego County

☒ **FALLBROOK HOSPITAL (50435)**, 624 East Elder Street, Zip 92028–3099; tel. 760/728–1191, (Nonreporting) **A**1 9 10 20 **S** Community Health Systems, Inc., Franklin, TN
Primary Contact: Alex Villa, Chief Executive Officer
Web address: www.fallbrookhospital.com
**Control:** Hospital district or authority, Government, nonfederal **Service:** General Medical and Surgical

**Staffed Beds:** 86

## FOLSOM—Sacramento County

☒ **KINDRED HOSPITAL–SACRAMENTO (52033)**, 330 Montrose Drive, Zip 95630–2720; tel. 916/351–9151, (Nonreporting) **A**1 9 10 **S** Kindred Healthcare, Louisville, KY
Primary Contact: Janet Biedron, R.N., Chief Executive Officer
CFO: Bruce MacNeill, Chief Financial Officer
CMO: Alan Cubre, M.D., Medical Director
CHR: Michael G. Fanselau, District Director Human Resources
Web address: www.kindredsacramento.com/
**Control:** Corporation, Investor–owned, for–profit **Service:** Long–Term Acute Care hospital

**Staffed Beds:** 37

☒ **MERCY HOSPITAL OF FOLSOM (50414)**, 1650 Creekside Drive, Zip 95630–3405; tel. 916/983–7400 **A**1 5 9 10 **F**3 8 11 13 29 30 34 35 36 39 40 43 49 57 59 60 64 66 68 70 74 75 76 77 79 81 82 84 85 86 93 107 108 113 114 117 118 129 131 145 146 147 **P**4 5 **S** Dignity Health, San Francisco, CA
Primary Contact: Donald C. Hudson, President
CFO: Robin Rogness, Vice President and Chief Financial Officer
CHR: Amy Mantell, Vice President Human Resources
Web address: www.mercyfolsom.org
**Control:** Church–operated, Nongovernment, not–for profit **Service:** General Medical and Surgical

**Staffed Beds:** 106 **Admissions:** 5664 **Census:** 52 **Outpatient Visits:** 44557 **Births:** 973 **Total Expense ($000):** 127042 **Payroll Expense ($000):** 54210 **Personnel:** 505

*Many Facility Codes have changed. Please refer to the AHA Guide Code Chart.* © 2012 AHA Guide

## FONTANA—San Bernardino County

⊠ **FONTANA MEDICAL CENTER (50140)**, 9961 Sierra Avenue, Zip 92335–6720; tel. 909/427–5000 **A**1 3 5 10 **F**3 4 8 13 15 17 18 19 20 28 29 30 31 35 40 41 44 45 46 48 49 50 57 58 60 62 63 64 65 68 70 72 73 74 75 76 77 78 79 81 82 84 85 86 87 88 89 100 102 107 108 111 113 114 116 118 129 131 134 140 144 145 147 **S** Kaiser Foundation Hospitals, Oakland, CA
Primary Contact: Greg Christian, Executive Director
COO: Georgina R. Garcia, Chief Operating Officer
CFO: Donald P. Bernard, Chief Financial Officer
CMO: David Quam, M.D., Area Medical Director
CIO: Jennifer Resch–Silvestri, Director Public Affairs
CHR: Kimberly Labiaga, Human Resources Leader
Web address: www.kaiserpermanente.org
**Control:** Other not–for–profit (including NFP Corporation) **Service:** General Medical and Surgical

**Staffed Beds:** 390 **Admissions:** 25482 **Census:** 291 **Outpatient Visits:** 119649 **Births:** 4485 **Personnel:** 3819

## FORT BRAGG—Mendocino County

⊠ **MENDOCINO COAST DISTRICT HOSPITAL (51325)**, 700 River Drive, Zip 95437–5495; tel. 707/961–1234, (Nonreporting) **A**1 9 10 18
Primary Contact: Raymond T. Hino, Chief Executive Officer
COO: Raymond T. Hino, Chief Executive Officer
CFO: Wayne Allen, Chief Financial Officer
CMO: John Kermen, D.O., Chief Medical Staff
CIO: Jeff Edwards, Manager Information Services
CHR: Scott Kidd, Director Human Resources
CNO: Bonnie Kittner, R.N., Chief Nursing Officer
Web address: www.mcdh.org
**Control:** Hospital district or authority, Government, nonfederal **Service:** General Medical and Surgical

**Staffed Beds:** 25

## FORT IRWIN—San Bernardino County

⊠ **WEED ARMY COMMUNITY HOSPITAL**, Inner Loop Road and 4th Street, Building 166, Zip 92310–5065, Mailing Address: P.O. Box 105109, Zip 92310–5109; tel. 760/380–3108, (Nonreporting) **A**1 **S** Department of the Army, Office of the Surgeon General, Falls Church, VA
Primary Contact: Colonel Michael L. Kiefer, Commander
CFO: Bella R. Ibanez, Budget Officer
CMO: Lieutenant Colonel John Glorioso, M.D., Deputy Commander Clinical Services
CIO: Michael Haenelt, Chief Information Management
Web address: www.irwin.amedd.army.mil
**Control:** Army, Government, federal **Service:** General Medical and Surgical

**Staffed Beds:** 27

## FORTUNA—Humboldt County

⊠ **REDWOOD MEMORIAL HOSPITAL (51318)**, 3300 Renner Drive, Zip 95540–3198; tel. 707/725–3361 **A**1 2 9 10 18 **F**3 11 13 15 17 18 29 30 34 35 39 40 45 50 53 56 57 59 63 64 68 70 75 76 77 79 81 82 84 85 86 88 89 93 107 110 113 118 129 130 131 132 145 **P**5 **S** St. Joseph Health, Orange, CA
Primary Contact: Joseph M. Mark, Chief Executive Officer
COO: Joseph J. Rogers, Vice President and Chief Operating Officer
CFO: Andrew Rybolt, Vice President and Chief Financial Officer
CHR: Bob Sampson, Vice President Human Resources
Web address: www.stjosepheureka.org
**Control:** Church–operated, Nongovernment, not–for profit **Service:** General Medical and Surgical

**Staffed Beds:** 25 **Admissions:** 1593 **Census:** 15 **Outpatient Visits:** 42516 **Births:** 353 **Total Expense ($000):** 35266 **Payroll Expense ($000):** 13360 **Personnel:** 169

## FOUNTAIN VALLEY—Orange County

⊠ **FOUNTAIN VALLEY REGIONAL HOSPITAL AND MEDICAL CENTER (50570)**, 17100 Euclid Street, Zip 92708–4043; tel. 714/966–7200 **A**1 2 5 9 10 **F**3 12 13 15 17 18 20 22 24 26 29 30 31 34 35 40 44 49 50 51 57 58 59 60 64 65 68 70 72 74 75 76 77 78 79 81 82 85 86 87 88 89 107 108 110 111 113 114 118 129 131 145 146 147 **P**5 **S** TENET Healthcare Corporation, Dallas, TX
Primary Contact: Debbie Walsh, MSN, Chief Executive Officer
COO: Paul M. Czajka, Chief Operating Officer
CFO: Cari Welsh, Interim Chief Financial Officer
CFO: Jon Zilkow, Chief Financial Officer
CMO: Sara Myla, M.D., Chief of Staff
CIO: Edwin Del Los Santos, Director Information Systems
CHR: Tim Howard, Chief Human Resources Officer
CNO: Mary Botticella, R.N., Chief Nursing Officer
Web address: www.fountainvalleyhospital.com
**Control:** Corporation, Investor–owned, for–profit **Service:** General Medical and Surgical

**Staffed Beds:** 400 **Admissions:** 18042 **Census:** 236 **Outpatient Visits:** 71960 **Births:** 3145 **Total Expense ($000):** 260508 **Payroll Expense ($000):** 115263 **Personnel:** 1330

⊠ **ORANGE COAST MEMORIAL MEDICAL CENTER (50678)**, 9920 Talbert Avenue, Zip 92708–5153; tel. 714/378–7000 **A**1 2 9 10 **F**3 11 12 13 15 18 20 22 24 26 28 29 30 31 34 35 38 40 44 45 46 49 50 51 53 56 57 58 59 64 65 68 70 72 74 75 76 77 78 79 81 82 84 85 86 87 93 107 108 110 111 113 115 116 118 123 125 129 130 131 142 144 145 146 **P**3 5 **S** MemorialCare, Fountain Valley, CA
Primary Contact: Marcia Manker, Chief Executive Officer
COO: Emily Randle, Vice President Operations
CFO: Steve McNamara, Chief Financial Officer
CIO: Scott Raymond, Director Information Systems
CHR: Lorraine Booth, Executive Director Human Resources
Web address: www.memorialcare.org
**Control:** Other not–for–profit (including NFP Corporation) **Service:** General Medical and Surgical

**Staffed Beds:** 218 **Admissions:** 12299 **Census:** 124 **Outpatient Visits:** 63870 **Births:** 1645 **Total Expense ($000):** 222386 **Payroll Expense ($000):** 67095 **Personnel:** 989

## FREMONT—Alameda County

☐ **FREMONT HOSPITAL (54110)**, 39001 Sundale Drive, Zip 94538–2005; tel. 510/796–1100, (Nonreporting) **A**1 9 10 **S** Universal Health Services, Inc., King of Prussia, PA
Primary Contact: John C. Cooper, Chief Executive Officer
CMO: Travis Svensson, M.D., Medical Director
CHR: Mark Chatman, Director Human Resources
Web address: www.fremonthospital.com
**Control:** Corporation, Investor–owned, for–profit **Service:** Psychiatric

**Staffed Beds:** 96

⊠ **WASHINGTON HOSPITAL HEALTHCARE SYSTEM (50195)**, 2000 Mowry Avenue, Zip 94538–1746; tel. 510/797–1111, (Nonreporting) **A**1 2 9 10
Primary Contact: Nancy D. Farber, Chief Executive Officer
COO: Edward J. Fayen, Associate Administrator Operations and Support
CFO: Chris Henry, Associate Administrator and Chief Financial Officer
CMO: Albert Brooks, M.D., Chief Medical Staff Services
CIO: Robert Thorwald, Chief Information Officer
CHR: Bryant Welch, Chief Human Resources
CNO: Stephanie Williams, R.N., Chief Nursing Officer
Web address: www.whhs.com
**Control:** Hospital district or authority, Government, nonfederal **Service:** General Medical and Surgical

**Staffed Beds:** 323

## FRENCH CAMP—San Joaquin County

☐ **SAN JOAQUIN GENERAL HOSPITAL (50167)**, 500 West Hospital Road, Zip 95231, Mailing Address: P.O. Box 1020, Stockton, Zip 95201; tel. 209/468–6000, (Nonreporting) **A**1 3 5 9 10
Primary Contact: David K. Culberson, Chief Executive Officer
CMO: Jerry Royer, M.D., Chief Medical Officer
CIO: Don Johnston, Chief Information Officer
CHR: Patricia Wright, Personal Analyst
Web address: www.sjgeneralhospital.com/
**Control:** County–Government, nonfederal **Service:** General Medical and Surgical

**Staffed Beds:** 109

**CA**

---

**Hospital, Medicare Provider Number, Address, Telephone, Approval, Facility, and Physician Codes, Health Care System**

★ American Hospital Association (AHA) membership
☐ The Joint Commission accreditation  ◇ DNV Healthcare Inc. accreditation
○ American Osteopathic Association (AOA) accreditation
△ Commission on Accreditation of Rehabilitation Facilities (CARF) accreditation

CA

## FRESNO—Fresno County

**COMMUNITY BEHAVIORAL HEALTH CENTER**, 7171 North Cedar Avenue, Zip 93720–3311; tel. 559/449–8000, (Nonreporting) **S** Community Medical Centers, Fresno, CA
Primary Contact: Dawan Utecht, Chief Executive Officer
COO: Patrick W. Rafferty, Executive Vice President and Chief Operating Officer
CFO: Stephen Walter, Senior Vice President and Chief Financial Officer
CMO: Thomas Utecht, M.D., Senior Vice President and Chief Quality Officer
CIO: George Vasquez, Vice President Information Services
CHR: Ginny Burdick, Vice President Human Resources
Web address: www.communitymedical.org
**Control:** Corporation, Investor–owned, for–profit **Service:** Psychiatric

**Staffed Beds:** 60

☐ **COMMUNITY REGIONAL MEDICAL CENTER (50060)**, 2823 Fresno Street, Zip 93721–1324; tel. 559/459–6000, (Total facility includes 106 beds in nursing home–type unit) **A**1 2 5 8 9 10 **F**3 6 15 16 17 18 19 20 22 24 26 29 30 31 34 35 38 39 40 43 44 45 46 47 48 49 50 54 55 58 59 60 61 62 64 65 66 67 68 70 72 73 74 75 76 77 78 79 81 82 84 89 90 91 93 96 97 98 99 100 102 107 110 111 113 114 117 118 119 120 122 123 125 127 129 131 145 146 147 **S** Community Medical Centers, Fresno, CA
Primary Contact: John M. Chubb, Chief Executive Officer
COO: Patrick W. Rafferty, Executive Vice President and Chief Operating Officer
CFO: Stephen Walter, Senior Vice President and Chief Financial Officer
CMO: Thomas Utecht, M.D., Chief Quality Officer
CIO: Craig Castro, Chief Information Officer
CHR: Ginny Burdick, Vice President Human Resources
Web address: www.communitymedical.org
**Control:** Other not–for–profit (including NFP Corporation) **Service:** General Medical and Surgical

**Staffed Beds:** 677 **Admissions:** 37778 **Census:** 611 **Outpatient Visits:** 332661 **Births:** 6568 **Total Expense ($000):** 762474 **Payroll Expense ($000):** 276564 **Personnel:** 3758

☐ **FRESNO HEART AND SURGICAL HOSPITAL (50732)**, 15 East Audubon Drive, Zip 93720; tel. 559/433–8000, (Nonreporting) **A**1 9 10
Primary Contact: Wanda Holderman, Chief Executive Officer
CFO: Jon Edwards, Executive Director Finance
CMO: Keith Boone, M.D., Medical Director
CIO: Jonathon Anderson, Director Information Technology and Telecommunications
CHR: Lynn M. Horton, Executive Director Human Resources
Web address: www.fresnoheartandsurgical.org
**Control:** Corporation, Investor–owned, for–profit **Service:** Heart

**Staffed Beds:** 60

✠ **FRESNO MEDICAL CENTER (50710)**, 7300 North Fresno Street, Zip 93720–2941; tel. 559/448–4500 **A**1 10 **F**3 8 12 13 15 29 30 31 35 40 45 46 47 48 49 51 53 59 64 68 70 72 73 74 76 77 78 79 81 82 84 85 86 87 93 96 97 102 107 108 110 111 113 115 116 117 118 123 129 134 143 145 147 **S** Kaiser Foundation Hospitals, Oakland, CA
Primary Contact: Jeffrey A. Collins, Senior Vice President and Area Manager
CFO: Richard Alves, Chief Financial Officer
CMO: Varouj Altebarmakian, M.D., Physician in Chief
CIO: Brad Bain, Information Systems Leader
Web address: www.kaiserpermanente.org
**Control:** Other not–for–profit (including NFP Corporation) **Service:** General Medical and Surgical

**Staffed Beds:** 169 **Admissions:** 7398 **Census:** 77 **Outpatient Visits:** 720000 **Births:** 1132 **Personnel:** 1822

☐ **FRESNO SURGICAL HOSPITAL (50708)**, 6125 North Fresno Street, Zip 93710–5207; tel. 559/431–8000, (Nonreporting) **A**1 9 10
Primary Contact: Kristine Kassahn, Chief Executive Officer
CFO: Bruce Cecil, Chief Financial Officer
CMO: Bruce Witmer, M.D., Medical Director
CHR: Laura Patillo, Manager Human Resources
Web address: www.fresnosurgicalhospital.com
**Control:** Partnership, Investor–owned, for–profit **Service:** General Medical and Surgical

**Staffed Beds:** 16

✠ **SAINT AGNES MEDICAL CENTER (50093)**, 1303 East Herndon Avenue, Zip 93720–3309; tel. 559/450–3000 **A**1 2 9 10 **F**2 3 8 13 15 17 18 20 22 24 26 28 29 30 31 34 35 37 40 44 45 46 47 49 50 51 56 57 58 59 64 66 70 74 75 76 77 78 79 81 82 84 85 86 87 93 107 108 110 111 112 113 114 115 116 117 118 119 120 122 123 125 129 131 145 146 147 **S** Trinity Health, Novi, MI
Primary Contact: Nancy Hollingsworth, R.N., MSN, President and Chief Executive Officer
COO: Mark T. Bateman, Interim Chief Operating Officer
CFO: Christine Sarrico, Chief Financial Officer
CMO: Stephen Soldo, M.D., Chief Medical Officer
CIO: Irfan Ali, Director Information Services
CHR: Stacy Vaillancourt, Vice President Marketing, Communications, Advocacy and Human Resources
Web address: www.samc.com
**Control:** Church–operated, Nongovernment, not–for profit **Service:** General Medical and Surgical

**Staffed Beds:** 436 **Admissions:** 25995 **Census:** 291 **Outpatient Visits:** 311376 **Births:** 4130 **Total Expense ($000):** 461899 **Payroll Expense ($000):** 174222 **Personnel:** 2162

☐ △ **SAN JOAQUIN VALLEY REHABILITATION HOSPITAL (53032)**, 7173 North Sharon Avenue, Zip 93720–3329; tel. 559/436–3600, (Nonreporting) **A**1 7 9 10 **S** Vibra Healthcare, Mechanicsburg, PA
Primary Contact: Edward C. Palacios, Chief Executive Officer
CFO: Margaret Casarez, Chief Financial Officer
CMO: Michael Azevedo, M.D., Medical Director
CIO: Christi Rolff, Director Business Development
CHR: Jennifer Morrow, Director Human Resources
Web address: www.sjvrehab.com
**Control:** Corporation, Investor–owned, for–profit **Service:** Rehabilitation

**Staffed Beds:** 40

✠ **VETERANS AFFAIRS CENTRAL CALIFORNIA HEALTH CARE SYSTEM**, 2615 East Clinton Avenue, Zip 93703–2223; tel. 559/225–6100, (Nonreporting) **A**1 3 5 **S** Department of Veterans Affairs, Washington, DC
Primary Contact: Alan S. Perry, Director
CFO: Matthew Whetton, Chief Business Administration
CMO: Wessel Meyer, M.D., Chief of Staff
CIO: William Harris, Chief Information Resources Management
CHR: Sandra Stein, Chief Human Resources Management
Web address: www.va.gov/sta/guide/home.asp
**Control:** Veterans Affairs, Government, federal **Service:** General Medical and Surgical

**Staffed Beds:** 54

## FULLERTON—Orange County

✠ △ **ST. JUDE MEDICAL CENTER (50168)**, 101 East Valencia Mesa Drive, Zip 92835–3809; tel. 714/992–3000 **A**1 2 5 7 9 10 **F**2 3 8 9 11 13 15 18 20 22 24 26 28 29 30 31 32 34 35 36 39 40 43 44 45 46 47 48 49 50 51 53 54 55 56 57 58 59 60 61 62 63 64 65 66 68 70 71 72 74 75 76 77 78 79 81 82 83 84 85 86 87 89 90 91 92 93 95 96 97 100 107 108 109 110 111 113 114 115 116 117 118 119 120 122 123 125 127 128 129 130 131 133 134 142 143 145 146 147 **P**3 5 **S** St. Joseph Health, Orange, CA
Primary Contact: Lee Penrose, President and Chief Executive Officer
COO: Brian Helleland, Executive Vice President and Chief Operating Officer
CFO: Ed Salvador, Chief Financial Officer
CIO: Ryan Olsen, Vice President of Operations
CHR: Mark Jablonski, Senior Vice President Human Resources
CNO: Linda Jenkins, R.N., Vice President Patient Care Services
Web address: www.stjudemedicalcenter.org
**Control:** Church–operated, Nongovernment, not–for profit **Service:** General Medical and Surgical

**Staffed Beds:** 384 **Admissions:** 16244 **Census:** 225 **Outpatient Visits:** 371652 **Births:** 2145 **Total Expense ($000):** 426190 **Payroll Expense ($000):** 149349 **Personnel:** 2399

## GARBERVILLE—Humboldt County

**JEROLD PHELPS COMMUNITY HOSPITAL (51309)**, 733 Cedar Street, Zip 95542–3201; tel. 707/923–3921, (Nonreporting) **A**9 10 18
Primary Contact: Harry Jasper, Administrator
COO: Kent Scown, Director Operations and Information Services
CFO: Mike Nagle, Director Financial Services
CMO: Mark H. Phelps, M.D., Chief of Staff and Medical Director
CIO: Kent Scown, Director Operations and Information Services
CHR: Linda Feretto, Director Human Resources
Web address: www.shchd.org
**Control:** Hospital district or authority, Government, nonfederal **Service:** General Medical and Surgical

**Staffed Beds:** 16

*Many Facility Codes have changed. Please refer to the AHA Guide Code Chart.* © 2012 AHA Guide

## GARDEN GROVE—Orange County

☐ **GARDEN GROVE HOSPITAL AND MEDICAL CENTER (50230)**, 12601 Garden Grove Boulevard, Zip 92843–1908; tel. 714/537–5160, (Nonreporting) **A**1 9 10 **S** Prime Healthcare Services, Ontario, CA
Primary Contact: Virgis Narbutas, Chief Executive Officer
CFO: Alan H. Smith, Chief Financial Officer
CMO: Hassan Alkhouli, M.D., Chief Medical Officer
CIO: Adam Morquecho, Director Information Systems
CHR: Stephanie Sioson, Director Human Resources
CNO: Sofia Abrina, Administrator and Chief Nursing Officer
Web address: www.gardengrovehospital.com
**Control:** Corporation, Investor–owned, for–profit **Service:** General Medical and Surgical

**Staffed Beds:** 74

## GARDENA—Los Angeles County

★ ○ **KINDRED HOSPITAL OF SOUTH BAY (52050)**, 1246 West 155th Street, Zip 90247–4011; tel. 310/323–5330, (Nonreporting) **A**10 11 **S** Kindred Healthcare, Louisville, KY
Primary Contact: Kevin Chavez, Administrator
COO: Michael Grubb, Chief Operating Officer and Chief Financial Officer
CFO: Michael Grubb, Chief Operating Officer and Chief Financial Officer
CHR: Michelle Parra, Director Human Resources
Web address: www.khsouthbay.com/
**Control:** Corporation, Investor–owned, for–profit **Service:** Long–Term Acute Care hospital

**Staffed Beds:** 84

☐ **MEMORIAL HOSPITAL OF GARDENA (50468)**, 1145 West Redondo Beach Boulevard, Zip 90247–3528; tel. 310/532–4200, (Nonreporting) **A**1 9 10 **S** Avanti Hospitals, El Segundo, CA
Primary Contact: Araceli Lonergan, Chief Executive Officer
CFO: Daniel R. Heckathorne, Chief Financial Officer
CMO: Nosratian Farshao, M.D., Chief Medical Staff
CIO: Earle Johnson, Chief Information Officer
CHR: Matthew Kempiak, Director Human Resources and Administrative Services
CNO: Glenda Luce, Chief Nursing Officer
Web address: www.mhglax.com/
**Control:** Corporation, Investor–owned, for–profit **Service:** General Medical and Surgical

**Staffed Beds:** 172

**VISTA HOSPITAL OF SOUTH BAY** See Kindred Hospital of South Bay

## GILROY—Santa Clara County

⊠ **SAINT LOUISE REGIONAL HOSPITAL (50688)**, 9400 No Name Uno, Zip 95020–3528; tel. 408/848–2000 **A**1 9 10 **F**3 11 13 15 17 29 30 31 34 35 37 40 45 46 47 50 54 57 59 60 64 68 69 70 75 76 78 79 81 82 85 107 108 111 114 118 129 131 134 142 143 145 147 **S** Daughters of Charity Health System, Los Altos Hills, CA
Primary Contact: Joanne E. Allen, President and Chief Executive Officer
COO: Carol Furgurson, Chief Operating Officer
CFO: Nicole Thomson, Chief Financial Officer
CIO: Dick Hutsell, Vice President Information Technology Services
CHR: Lin Velasquez, Vice President Human Resources
CNO: Marilyn Gerrior, R.N., Chief Nursing Executive
Web address: www.dochs.org
**Control:** Church–operated, Nongovernment, not–for profit **Service:** General Medical and Surgical

**Staffed Beds:** 93 **Admissions:** 3536 **Census:** 35 **Outpatient Visits:** 58508 **Births:** 680 **Total Expense ($000):** 90463 **Payroll Expense ($000):** 38624 **Personnel:** 430

## GLENDALE—Los Angeles County

⊠ **GLENDALE ADVENTIST MEDICAL CENTER (50239)**, 1509 Wilson Terrace, Zip 91206–4098; tel. 818/409–8000 **A**1 2 3 5 9 10 **F**3 5 8 12 13 15 17 18 20 22 24 28 29 30 31 34 35 37 40 47 48 49 51 58 62 64 68 70 72 74 75 76 77 78 79 81 82 87 90 93 96 98 102 104 105 106 107 108 110 111 113 114 117 118 123 125 128 129 130 131 134 145 146 147 **S** Adventist Health, Roseville, CA
Primary Contact: Kevin A. Roberts, FACHE, President and Chief Executive Officer
COO: Warren Tetz, Senior Vice President and Chief Operating Officer
CFO: Kelly Turner, Senior Vice President Finance and Chief Financial Officer
CMO: Simon Keushkerian, M.D., Chief of Staff
CIO: Sharon Correa, Associate Vice President
CHR: Susan Crabtree, Director Human Resources
CNO: Judy Blair, Senior Vice President Clinical Services and Chief Nursing Officer
Web address: www.glendaleadventist.com
**Control:** Church–operated, Nongovernment, not–for profit **Service:** General Medical and Surgical

**Staffed Beds:** 414 **Admissions:** 19338 **Census:** 302 **Outpatient Visits:** 265122 **Births:** 2467 **Total Expense ($000):** 332561 **Payroll Expense ($000):** 136275 **Personnel:** 1994

⊠ **GLENDALE MEMORIAL HOSPITAL AND HEALTH CENTER (50058)**, 1420 South Central Avenue, Zip 91204–2508; tel. 818/502–1900, (Nonreporting) **A**1 9 10 **S** Dignity Health, San Francisco, CA
Primary Contact: Mark A. Meyers, President
COO: Matthew S. Gerlach, Vice President and Chief Operating Officer
CFO: Robert Allen, Vice President and Chief Financial Officer
CIO: David Gibbons, Chief Information Officer
CHR: Sandra Davis Houston, Vice President Human Resources and Organizational Development
CNO: Claire H. Hanks, R.N., Vice President and Chief Nursing Officer
Web address: www.glendalememorial.com
**Control:** Other not–for–profit (including NFP Corporation) **Service:** General Medical and Surgical

**Staffed Beds:** 334

**VERDUGO HILLS HOSPITAL (50124)**, 1812 Verdugo Boulevard, Zip 91208–1409; tel. 818/790–7100, (Nonreporting) **A**9 10 21
Primary Contact: Leonard LaBella, President and Chief Executive Officer
CFO: Cindy Trousdale, Chief Financial Officer
CHR: Paul Celuch, Vice President Human Resources and Support Services
Web address: www.verdugohillshospital.org
**Control:** Other not–for–profit (including NFP Corporation) **Service:** General Medical and Surgical

**Staffed Beds:** 114

## GLENDORA—Los Angeles County

○ **EAST VALLEY HOSPITAL MEDICAL CENTER (50205)**, 150 West Route 66, Zip 91740–6207; tel. 626/852–5000, (Nonreporting) **A**9 10 11
Primary Contact: C. Joseph Chang, President and Chief Executive Officer
CIO: Wayne Giddings, Manager Management Information Systems
CHR: Kim Bui, Director Human Resources
**Control:** Other not–for–profit (including NFP Corporation) **Service:** General Medical and Surgical

**Staffed Beds:** 118

⊠ **FOOTHILL PRESBYTERIAN HOSPITAL (50597)**, 250 South Grand Avenue, Zip 91741–4218; tel. 626/963–8411, (Nonreporting) **A**1 9 10 **S** Citrus Valley Health Partners, Covina, CA
Primary Contact: Diana Lugo–Zenner, R.N., Administrator
COO: Elvia Foulke, Executive Vice President and Chief Operating Officer
CFO: Lois Conyers, Senior Vice President and Chief Financial Officer
CMO: John DiMare, M.D., Medical Director
CIO: David McCobb, Chief Information Officer
CHR: Lisa Foust, Senior Vice President Human Resources
Web address: www.cvhp.org
**Control:** Church–operated, Nongovernment, not–for profit **Service:** General Medical and Surgical

**Staffed Beds:** 105

## GRANADA HILLS—Los Angeles County, See Los Angeles

**CA**

### GRASS VALLEY—Nevada County

⊠ **SIERRA NEVADA MEMORIAL HOSPITAL (50150)**, 155 Glasson Way, Zip 95945–5723, Mailing Address: P.O. Box 1029, Zip 95945–1029; tel. 530/274–6000 **A**1 2 9 10 19 **F**3 7 11 13 15 17 28 29 30 31 34 40 50 51 57 60 62 64 65 68 70 75 76 77 78 79 81 82 84 85 86 93 107 108 110 111 115 117 118 120 121 122 127 129 131 134 143 145 147 **P**5 **S** Dignity Health, San Francisco, CA
Primary Contact: Katherine Medeiros, President and Chief Executive Officer
COO: Mary L. Gish, R.N., Vice President and Chief Nursing Officer
CFO: Carolyn Canady, Chief Financial Officer
CMO: Frank Lang, Jr., M.D., Chief of Medicine
CHR: Annalise O'Connor, Director Human Resources
Web address: www.snmh.org
**Control:** Other not–for–profit (including NFP Corporation) **Service:** General Medical and Surgical

**Staffed Beds: 121 Admissions: 5464 Census: 62 Outpatient Visits: 204558 Births: 446 Total Expense ($000): 121496 Payroll Expense ($000): 58975 Personnel: 709**

### GREENBRAE—Marin County

⊠ **MARIN GENERAL HOSPITAL (50360)**, 250 Bon Air Road, Zip 94904–1784, Mailing Address: P.O. Box 8010, San Rafael, Zip 94912–8010; tel. 415/925–7000, (Nonreporting) **A**1 2 9 10
Primary Contact: Lee Domanico, Chief Executive Officer
CFO: David W. Cox, Chief Financial Officer
CMO: Joel Sklar, M.D., Chief Medical Officer
CIO: Somayaji Bulusu, Chief Information Officer
CHR: Theresa Gianfortune, Chief Human Resources Officer
CNO: Denise Perry, R.N., Vice President, Nursing Services
Web address: www.maringeneral.org
**Control:** Hospital district or authority, Government, nonfederal **Service:** General Medical and Surgical

**Staffed Beds: 235**

### GRIDLEY—Butte County

**BIGGS–GRIDLEY MEMORIAL HOSPITAL (51311)**, 240 Spruce Street, Zip 95948–2216, Mailing Address: P.O. Box 97, Zip 95948–0097; tel. 530/846–5671, (Total facility includes 21 beds in nursing home–type unit) **A**9 10 18 **F**11 15 18 29 30 34 35 36 40 45 49 50 54 59 64 65 68 70 71 75 77 79 81 93 97 107 110 111 113 118 127 129 132 145 147
Primary Contact: Tracy Atkins, Interim Chief Executive Officer
COO: Ryan Quist, Administrative Assistant
CFO: Kevin Woodward, Chief Financial Officer
CMO: Henry Starkes, M.D., Medical Director
CIO: Ryan Quist, Administrative Assistant
Web address: www.dmh.ca.gov/statehospitals/atascadero
**Control:** Other not–for–profit (including NFP Corporation) **Service:** General Medical and Surgical

**Staffed Beds: 45 Admissions: 920 Census: 29 Outpatient Visits: 39422 Total Expense ($000): 17116**

### HANFORD—Kings County

⊠ **CENTRAL VALLEY GENERAL HOSPITAL (50196)**, 1025 North Douty Street, Zip 93230–3722, Mailing Address: P.O. Box 480, Zip 93232–0480; tel. 559/583–2100, (Nonreporting) **A**1 9 10 **S** Adventist Health, Roseville, CA
Primary Contact: Wayne Ferch, President and Chief Executive Officer
Web address: www.hanfordhealth.com
**Control:** Corporation, Investor–owned, for–profit **Service:** General Medical and Surgical

**Staffed Beds: 30**

⊠ **HANFORD COMMUNITY MEDICAL CENTER (50121)**, 450 Greenfield Avenue, Zip 93230–3513; tel. 559/582–9000, (Includes ADVENTIST MEDICAL CENTER–SELMA, 1141 Rose Avenue, Selma, Zip 93662–3241; tel. 559/891–1000; Richard L. Rawson, President and Chief Executive Officer), (Nonreporting) **A**1 9 10 **S** Adventist Health, Roseville, CA
Primary Contact: Richard L. Rawson, President and Chief Executive Officer
CIO: Michael Aubry, Director Information Systems
**Control:** Church–operated, Nongovernment, not–for profit **Service:** General Medical and Surgical

**Staffed Beds: 94**

### HARBOR CITY—Los Angeles County, See Los Angeles

### HAWAIIAN GARDENS—Los Angeles County

**TRI–CITY REGIONAL MEDICAL CENTER (50575)**, 21530 South Pioneer Boulevard, Zip 90716; tel. 562/860–0401, (Nonreporting) **A**9 10 21
Primary Contact: Clifford Shiepe, President and Chief Executive Officer
COO: James Sherman, Executive Director Hospital Operations
CFO: Paul Brydon, Chief Financial Officer
CMO: Derek Dobalian, M.D., Chief of Staff
CIO: Anthony Carrasco, Director Information Systems
CHR: James Sherman, Executive Director Hospital Operations
CNO: Juliet Miranda, Chief Nursing Officer
Web address: www.tri–cityrmc.org
**Control:** Other not–for–profit (including NFP Corporation) **Service:** Other specialty

**Staffed Beds: 125**

### HAWTHORNE—Los Angeles County

**HAWTHORNE HOSPITAL** See Los Angeles Metropolitan Medical Center, Los Angeles

### HAYWARD—Alameda County

★ **HAYWARD MEDICAL CENTER (50512)**, 27400 Hesperian Boulevard, Zip 94545–4235; tel. 510/784–4000, (Includes FREMONT MEDICAL CENTER, 39400 Paseo Padre Parkway, Fremont, Zip 94538–2310; tel. 510/248–3000; Denise Vincenzi, Administrator), (Nonreporting) **A**3 5 10 **S** Kaiser Foundation Hospitals, Oakland, CA
Primary Contact: Colleen McKeown, Senior Vice President and Area Manager
Web address: www.kaiserpermanente.org
**Control:** Other not–for–profit (including NFP Corporation) **Service:** General Medical and Surgical

**Staffed Beds: 208**

☐ **ST. ROSE HOSPITAL (50002)**, 27200 Calaroga Avenue, Zip 94545–4383; tel. 510/264–4000, (Nonreporting) **A**1 2 9 10
Primary Contact: Michael P. Mahoney, President and Chief Executive Officer
CFO: Michael Taylor, Vice President Financial Services and Chief Financial Officer
CMO: Charles S. Feldstein, M.D., Vice President Medical Affairs
CHR: John Davini, Vice President
Web address: www.srhca.org
**Control:** Other not–for–profit (including NFP Corporation) **Service:** General Medical and Surgical

**Staffed Beds: 141**

### HEALDSBURG—Sonoma County

**HEALDSBURG DISTRICT HOSPITAL (51321)**, 1375 University Avenue, Zip 95448–3382; tel. 707/431–6500, (Nonreporting) **A**9 10 18
Primary Contact: Evan J. Rayner, Chief Executive Officer
COO: Janet Kiely, R.N., Chief Operating Officer and Chief Nursing Officer
CFO: Dan Hull, Chief Financial Officer
CMO: Paul Marguglio, M.D., Chief of Staff
CIO: Gary Crossan, Director Information Systems
CHR: George Protos, Director Human Resources
Web address: www.nschd.org
**Control:** Hospital district or authority, Government, nonfederal **Service:** General Medical and Surgical

**Staffed Beds: 24**

### HEMET—Riverside County

⊠ **HEMET VALLEY MEDICAL CENTER (50390)**, 1117 East Devonshire Avenue, Zip 92543–3083; tel. 951/652–2811, (Nonreporting) **A**1 9 10 **S** Physicians for Healthy Hospitals, Hemet, CA
Primary Contact: Joel Bergenfeld, Chief Executive Officer
CFO: John R. Collins, Chief Financial Officer
CHR: Michele Bird, Chief Human Resources Officer
CNO: Elizabeth C. Gardner, R.N., Chief Nursing Officer
Web address: www.valleyhealthsystem.com
**Control:** Hospital district or authority, Government, nonfederal **Service:** General Medical and Surgical

**Staffed Beds: 284**

### HOLLISTER—San Benito County

⊠ **HAZEL HAWKINS MEMORIAL HOSPITAL (50296)**, 911 Sunset Drive, Zip 95023–5695; tel. 831/637–5711, (Includes WILLIAM AND INEZ MABIE SKILLED NURSING FACILITY, 911 Sunset Drive, Zip 95023; tel. 408/637–5711), (Nonreporting) **A**1 9 10
Primary Contact: Ken Underwood, Chief Executive Officer
CFO: Mark Robinson, Associate Administrator and Chief Financial Officer
CIO: Julio Gil, Manager Information Services
CHR: Ysidro Gallardo, Associate Administrator Human Resources
Web address: www.hazelhawkins.com
**Control:** Hospital district or authority, Government, nonfederal **Service:** General Medical and Surgical

**Staffed Beds: 113**

**HOLLYWOOD—Los Angeles County, See Los Angeles**

**HUNTINGTON BEACH—Orange County**

☐ **HUNTINGTON BEACH HOSPITAL (50526)**, 17772 Beach Boulevard,
Zip 92647–6819; tel. 714/843–5000, (Nonreporting) **A**1 10 **S** Prime Healthcare
Services, Ontario, CA
Primary Contact: Virgis Narbutas, Chief Executive Officer
CFO: Alan H. Smith, Chief Financial Officer
CMO: Hassan Alkhouli, M.D., Medical Director
CIO: Adam Morquecho, Director Information Technology
CHR: Stephanie Sioson, Director Human Resources
CNO: Sofia Abrina, Administrator and Chief Nursing Officer
Web address: www.hbhospital.com
**Control:** Partnership, Investor–owned, for–profit **Service:** General Medical and
Surgical

| Staffed Beds: 130 |
|---|

**HUNTINGTON PARK—Los Angeles County**

**COMMUNITY AND MISSION HOSPITALS OF HUNTINGTON PARK** See
Community Hospital of Huntington Park

○ **COMMUNITY HOSPITAL OF HUNTINGTON PARK (50091)**, 2623 East
Slauson Avenue, Zip 90255–2900; tel. 323/583–1931, (Nonreporting) **A**10 11
**S** Avanti Hospitals, El Segundo, CA
Primary Contact: Hector Hernandez, Chief Administrative Officer
CFO: Steve K. Lopez, Chief Financial Officer
Web address: www.chhp.org
**Control:** Corporation, Investor–owned, for–profit **Service:** General Medical and
Surgical

| Staffed Beds: 157 |
|---|

**INDIO—Riverside County**

⌧ **JOHN F. KENNEDY MEMORIAL HOSPITAL (50534)**, 47111 Monroe Street,
Zip 92201; tel. 760/347–6191 **A**1 9 10 **F**3 8 13 18 20 29 30 31 34 35 37 40
46 47 48 49 50 54 56 57 59 68 70 72 74 76 77 78 79 81 85 87 89 97 107
108 111 117 118 125 129 130 132 134 145 147 **S** TENET Healthcare
Corporation, Dallas, TX
Primary Contact: Daniel Bowers, Chief Executive Officer
COO: Parrish Scarboro, Chief Operating Officer
CHR: Bill Peterson, Director Human Resources
Web address: www.jfkmemorialhosp.com
**Control:** Corporation, Investor–owned, for–profit **Service:** General Medical and
Surgical

| Staffed Beds: 126 Admissions: 8763 Census: 80 Outpatient Visits: 56060 |
|---|
| Births: 2417 Total Expense ($000): 103963 Payroll Expense ($000): 51004 Personnel: 581 |

**INGLEWOOD—Los Angeles County**

☐ **CENTINELA HOSPITAL MEDICAL CENTER (50739)**, 555 East Hardy Street,
Zip 90301–4011, Mailing Address: P.O. Box 720, Zip 90312–6720;
tel. 310/673–4660, (Nonreporting) **A**1 9 10 **S** Prime Healthcare Services,
Ontario, CA
Primary Contact: Linda Bradley, Chief Executive Officer
CFO: Mark Overeem, Chief Financial Officer
CMO: Etie Moghissi, M.D., Chief Medical Staff
CIO: Vicky Morgan, Director Information Services
CHR: Margaret Morgan, Director Human Resources
Web address: www.centinelamed.com
**Control:** Corporation, Investor–owned, for–profit **Service:** General Medical and
Surgical

| Staffed Beds: 369 |
|---|

**IRVINE—Orange County**

**HOAG HOSPITAL IRVINE (50769)**, 16200 Sand Canyon Avenue,
Zip 92618–3714; tel. 949/764–8240, (Nonreporting) **A**21
Primary Contact: Richard Afable, M.D., M.P.H., Chief Executive Officer
COO: Robert Braithwaite, Chief Operating Officer
CFO: Jennifer C. Mitzner, Chief Financial Officer
CMO: Jack Cox, M.D., Chief Quality Officer
CIO: Tim Moore, R.N., Chief Information Officer
CHR: Jan L. Blue, Senior Vice President Human Resources
CNO: Richard A. Martin, MSN, Chief Nursing Officer
Web address: www.hoag.org/locations/hospitals/hoag–hospital–irvine
**Control:** Other not–for–profit (including NFP Corporation) **Service:** General
Medical and Surgical

| Staffed Beds: 84 |
|---|

**ORANGE COUNTY IRVINE MEDICAL CENTER** See Anaheim Medical Center,
Anaheim

**JACKSON—Amador County**

⌧ **SUTTER AMADOR HOSPITAL (50014)**, 200 Mission Boulevard,
Zip 95642–2132; tel. 209/223–7500 **A**1 9 10 **F**29 34 35 40 46 47 49 54 59
64 65 70 75 76 77 78 79 81 84 85 87 93 102 107 108 110 111 114 118
126 128 129 131 145 146 147 **S** Sutter Health, Sacramento, CA
Primary Contact: Anne Platt, Chief Executive Officer
CFO: Brett Moore, CPA, Assistant Administrator Finance
CMO: Darrel K. Kerr, M.D., Chief of Staff
CIO: Tony Jackson, Director Information Technology
CHR: Beverly Revels, Director Human Resources
CNO: Nikki Allen, Patient Care Executive
Web address: www.sutteramador.org
**Control:** Other not–for–profit (including NFP Corporation) **Service:** General
Medical and Surgical

| Staffed Beds: 42 Admissions: 2199 Census: 21 Outpatient Visits: 54069 |
|---|
| Births: 327 Total Expense ($000): 64215 Payroll Expense ($000): 20500 Personnel: 285 |

**JOSHUA TREE—San Bernardino County**

⌧ **HI–DESERT MEDICAL CENTER (50279)**, 6601 White Feather Road,
Zip 92252–6601; tel. 760/366–3711, (Nonreporting) **A**1 9 10 20
Primary Contact: Lionel K. Chadwick, Chief Executive Officer
COO: Jackie Combs, Chief Operating and Nursing Officer
CFO: Thomas J. Duda, Chief Financial Officer
CMO: Andre Kasko, D.O., Chief Medical Staff
CIO: Dan McClure, Chief Information Officer
CHR: Barbara Staresinic, Director Human Resources
Web address: www.hdmc.org
**Control:** Hospital district or authority, Government, nonfederal **Service:** General
Medical and Surgical

| Staffed Beds: 70 |
|---|

**KENTFIELD—Marin County**

⌧ **KENTFIELD REHABILITATION AND SPECIALTY HOSPITAL (52043)**, 1125 Sir
Francis Drake Boulevard, Zip 94904–1455; tel. 415/456–9680, (Nonreporting)
**A**1 9 10 **S** Vibra Healthcare, Mechanicsburg, PA
Primary Contact: Ann Gors, Chief Executive Officer
CFO: Stephanie Lawrence, Chief Financial Officer
CMO: Curtis Roebken, M.D., Chief Medical Staff
CHR: Julene English, Director Human Resources
Web address: www.kentfieldrehab.com
**Control:** Corporation, Investor–owned, for–profit **Service:** Long–Term Acute Care
hospital

| Staffed Beds: 60 |
|---|

**KING CITY—Monterey County**

☐ **GEORGE L. MEE MEMORIAL HOSPITAL (50189)**, 300 Canal Street,
Zip 93930–3431; tel. 831/385–6000, (Nonreporting) **A**1 9 10 20
Primary Contact: Lex Smith, Chief Executive Officer
CFO: Gary L. Wangsmo, Chief Financial Officer
CMO: Schindelheim Roy, M.D., Chief of Staff
CIO: Mike McNamara, Chief Information Officer
CHR: Wendy Crawford, Director Human Resources
Web address: www.meememorial.com
**Control:** Other not–for–profit (including NFP Corporation) **Service:** General
Medical and Surgical

| Staffed Beds: 119 |
|---|

**LA JOLLA—San Diego County**

⌧ **SCRIPPS GREEN HOSPITAL (50424)**, 10666 North Torrey Pines Road,
Zip 92037–1093; tel. 858/455–9100 **A**1 2 8 9 10 **F**3 8 11 12 14 15 17 18 20
22 24 26 29 30 31 34 35 36 37 44 45 46 47 49 50 51 54 57 58 59 61 64
68 70 74 75 77 78 79 80 81 82 84 85 86 87 93 107 108 110 111 113 114
117 118 119 120 122 123 125 129 130 131 135 137 138 140 141 145 147
**P**3 5 **S** Scripps Health, San Diego, CA
Primary Contact: Robin Brown, Senior Vice President and Chief Executive
CMO: Brent Eastman, M.D., Chief Medical Officer
CHR: Victor Buzachero, Corporate Senior Vice President for Innovation, Human
Resources and Performance Management
Web address: www.scrippshealth.org
**Control:** Other not–for–profit (including NFP Corporation) **Service:** General
Medical and Surgical

| Staffed Beds: 173 Admissions: 11692 Census: 112 Outpatient Visits: 85252 Births: 0 Total Expense ($000): 290632 Payroll Expense ($000): 100659 Personnel: 1283 |
|---|

CA

**Hospital, Medicare Provider Number, Address, Telephone, Approval, Facility, and Physician Codes, Health Care System**

★ American Hospital Association (AHA) membership
☐ The Joint Commission accreditation　　◇ DNV Healthcare Inc. accreditation

○ American Osteopathic Association (AOA) accreditation
△ Commission on Accreditation of Rehabilitation Facilities (CARF) accreditation

☒ **SCRIPPS MEMORIAL HOSPITAL–LA JOLLA (50324)**, 9888 Genesee Avenue, Zip 92037–1200, Mailing Address: P.O. Box 28, Zip 92038–0028; tel. 858/626–4123 **A**1 2 3 5 9 10 **F**3 4 5 8 11 12 13 14 15 17 18 20 22 24 26 28 29 30 31 34 35 40 43 44 45 46 48 49 53 54 57 58 59 64 65 68 70 74 75 76 77 78 79 81 82 84 85 86 87 91 92 93 94 99 100 101 102 103 104 107 108 110 111 113 114 115 116 117 118 120 122 123 125 129 131 140 141 144 145 146 147 **P**5 **S** Scripps Health, San Diego, CA
Primary Contact: Gary G. Fybel, Senior Vice President and Chief Executive
COO: Cindy Steckel, Vice President Chief Nurse and Operations Executive
CFO: Linda Honaker, Vice President Financial Operations
CMO: Brent Eastman, M.D., Chief Medical Officer
CHR: Sandra Hughes, Executive Director Human Resources
CNO: Cindy Steckel, Vice President Chief Nurse and Operations Executive
Web address: www.scrippshealth.org
**Control:** Other not–for–profit (including NFP Corporation) **Service:** General Medical and Surgical

**Staffed Beds:** 351 **Admissions:** 17232 **Census:** 218 **Outpatient Visits:** 113102 **Births:** 3984 **Total Expense ($000):** 412238 **Payroll Expense ($000):** 154604 **Personnel:** 2032

### LA MESA—San Diego County

☒ △ **SHARP GROSSMONT HOSPITAL (50026)**, 5555 Grossmont Center Drive, Zip 91942–3019, Mailing Address: P.O. Box 158, Zip 91944–0158; tel. 619/740–6000, (Total facility includes 30 beds in nursing home–type unit) **A**1 2 7 9 10 **F**3 8 11 13 15 17 18 20 22 24 26 28 29 30 31 34 35 36 38 39 40 43 44 45 49 50 51 54 56 57 58 59 60 61 62 63 64 65 68 70 72 74 75 76 77 78 79 80 81 82 83 84 85 86 87 90 93 94 96 98 100 101 102 103 104 107 108 111 113 114 115 116 117 118 120 122 123 125 127 128 129 131 134 140 142 144 145 146 147 **P**5 **S** Sharp HealthCare, San Diego, CA
Primary Contact: Michele T. Tarbet, R.N., Chief Executive Officer
COO: Maryann Cone, Chief Operating Officer
CFO: Kari Cornicelli, Chief Financial Officer
CMO: Michael Murphy, M.D., Chief Medical Officer
CIO: William T. Spooner, Senior Vice President and Chief Information Officer
CHR: Ruth Shannon, Director Human Resources
CNO: Janet Hanley, Chief Nursing Officer
Web address: www.sharp.com
**Control:** Other not–for–profit (including NFP Corporation) **Service:** General Medical and Surgical

**Staffed Beds:** 521 **Admissions:** 28256 **Census:** 327 **Outpatient Visits:** 297373 **Births:** 3511 **Total Expense ($000):** 510773 **Payroll Expense ($000):** 211253 **Personnel:** 2805

### LA MIRADA—Los Angeles County

☒ **KINDRED HOSPITAL–LA MIRADA (52038)**, 14900 East Imperial Highway, Zip 90638; tel. 562/944–1900, (Includes KINDRED HOSPITAL SAN GABRIEL VALLEY, 845 North Lark Ellen Avenue, West Covina, Zip 91791–1069; tel. 626/339–5451; Harvey Ross, Administrator; KINDRED HOSPITAL SANTA ANA, 1901 North College Avenue, Santa Ana, Zip 92706–2334; tel. 714/564–7800; Brooke Saunders, Administrator), (Nonreporting) **A**1 9 10 **S** Kindred Healthcare, Louisville, KY
Primary Contact: April Myers, Administrator
COO: Jude Sullivan, Chief Clinical Officer
CFO: Nancy V. Wilson, Chief Financial Officer
CMO: Prakash Chandra Patel, M.D., Chief of Staff
CHR: Kristen Martinez, Coordinator Human Resources
Web address: www.kindredlamirada.com/
**Control:** Corporation, Investor–owned, for–profit **Service:** Long–Term Acute Care hospital

**Staffed Beds:** 216

### LA PALMA—Orange County

☐ **LA PALMA INTERCOMMUNITY HOSPITAL (50580)**, 7901 Walker Street, Zip 90623–1722; tel. 714/670–7400, (Nonreporting) **A**1 9 10 **S** Prime Healthcare Services, Ontario, CA
Primary Contact: Virgis Narbutas, Chief Executive Officer
CFO: Alan H. Smith, Chief Financial Officer
CMO: Sami Shoukair, M.D., Chief Medical Officer
CIO: Adam Morquecho, Director Information Technology
CHR: Stephanie Sioson, Director Human Resources
CNO: Margo Perusse, Administrator and Chief Nursing Officer
Web address: www.lapalmaintercommunityhospital.com
**Control:** Other not–for–profit (including NFP Corporation) **Service:** General Medical and Surgical

**Staffed Beds:** 141

### LAGUNA HILLS—Orange County

☒ **SADDLEBACK MEMORIAL MEDICAL CENTER (50603)**, 24451 Health Center Drive, Zip 92653–3689; tel. 949/837–4500, (Includes SADDLEBACK MEMORIAL MEDICAL CENTER – SAN CLEMENTE CAMPUS, 654 Camino De Los Mares, San Clemente, Zip 92673–2827; tel. 949/496–1122) **A**1 2 5 9 10 **F**3 11 12 13 14 15 18 20 22 24 26 28 29 30 31 34 35 36 38 40 44 45 49 50 51 53 54 55 56 57 58 59 62 63 64 65 68 70 72 74 75 76 77 78 79 81 82 84 85 86 87 90 93 94 96 100 107 108 110 111 113 114 117 118 119 120 122 125 129 131 134 140 141 142 144 145 146 147 **P**3 5 7 **S** MemorialCare, Fountain Valley, CA
Primary Contact: Steve Geidt, Chief Executive Officer
COO: Cheryl Jacob, Chief Operating Officer
CFO: Adolfo Chanez, Vice President Finance and Chief Financial Officer
CMO: Ronald Saltzman, M.D., Chief of Staff
CIO: J. Scott Joslyn, Senior Vice President and Chief Information Officer
CHR: Ron Salzberg, Executive Director Human Resources
Web address: www.memorialcare.org
**Control:** Other not–for–profit (including NFP Corporation) **Service:** General Medical and Surgical

**Staffed Beds:** 325 **Admissions:** 17018 **Census:** 188 **Outpatient Visits:** 288350 **Births:** 2629 **Total Expense ($000):** 299154 **Payroll Expense ($000):** 120280 **Personnel:** 1739

### LAKE ARROWHEAD—San Bernardino County

☒ **SAN BERNARDINO MOUNTAINS COMMUNITY HOSPITAL DISTRICT (51312)**, 29101 Hospital Road, Zip 92352, Mailing Address: P.O. Box 70, Zip 92352–0070; tel. 909/336–3651, (Nonreporting) **A**1 9 10 18
Primary Contact: Charles Harrison, Chief Executive Officer
COO: Susan Lowell, Chief Operating Officer and Chief Nursing Officer
CFO: Yvonne Waggener, Chief Financial Officer
CMO: Lawrence Walker, M.D., Chief of Staff
CIO: Trace Kateley, Manager Information Systems
CHR: Julie Atwood, Director Human Resources
Web address: www.mchcares.com
**Control:** Hospital district or authority, Government, nonfederal **Service:** General Medical and Surgical

**Staffed Beds:** 25

### LAKE ISABELLA—Kern County

**KERN VALLEY HEALTHCARE DISTRICT (51314)**, 6412 Laurel Avenue, Zip 93240–1628, Mailing Address: P.O. Box 1628, Zip 93240–1628; tel. 760/379–2681, (Nonreporting) **A**9 10 18
Primary Contact: Timothy McGlew, Chief Executive Officer
CFO: Chester Beedle, Chief Financial Officer
CMO: Gary A. Finstad, M.D., Chief of Staff
CIO: Dena Griffith, Manager Information Systems
CHR: Debra Hoffman, Manager Human Resources
Web address: www.kvhd.org
**Control:** Hospital district or authority, Government, nonfederal **Service:** General Medical and Surgical

**Staffed Beds:** 25

### LAKEPORT—Lake County

☒ **SUTTER LAKESIDE HOSPITAL (51329)**, 5176 Hill Road East, Zip 95453–6300; tel. 707/262–5000, (Nonreporting) **A**1 9 10 18 **S** Sutter Health, Sacramento, CA
Primary Contact: Siri Nelson, Chief Administrative Officer
CFO: Krista Touros, Assistant Administrator Finance
CMO: Diane Pege, M.D., Vice President Medical Affairs
CIO: Jack Buell, Director Information Services
CHR: Richard Abbate, Director Human Resources
CNO: Teresa L. Campbell, Chief Nurse Executive
Web address: www.sutterlakeside.org
**Control:** Other not–for–profit (including NFP Corporation) **Service:** General Medical and Surgical

**Staffed Beds:** 49

CA

**CA**

## LAKEWOOD—Los Angeles County

☒ **LAKEWOOD REGIONAL MEDICAL CENTER (50581)**, 3700 East South Street, Zip 90712–1498, Mailing Address: P.O. Box 6070, Zip 90714–6070; tel. 562/531–2550 **A**1 9 10 **F**3 11 15 17 18 20 22 24 26 29 30 34 35 38 40 45 49 50 51 57 59 64 68 70 74 75 77 81 85 87 90 93 107 108 109 111 114 117 118 119 129 131 142 145 147 **S** TENET Healthcare Corporation, Dallas, TX
Primary Contact: B. Joseph Badalian, President and Chief Executive Officer
COO: Nathaniel Malcolm, Chief Operating Officer
CFO: Mary Beth Formby, Chief Financial Officer
CMO: Ronald L. Kaufman, M.D., Chief Medical Officer
CIO: Pat Pierce, Director Information Systems
CHR: Mary Okuhara, Director Human Resources
CNO: Terri Newton, Chief Nursing Officer
Web address: www.lakewoodregional.com
**Control:** Corporation, Investor–owned, for–profit **Service:** General Medical and Surgical

**Staffed Beds:** 144 **Admissions:** 8032 **Census:** 101 **Outpatient Visits:** 54430 **Births:** 0 **Total Expense ($000):** 120270 **Payroll Expense ($000):** 58098 **Personnel:** 667

## LANCASTER—Los Angeles County

☒ **ANTELOPE VALLEY HOSPITAL (50056)**, 1600 West Avenue J, Zip 93534–2894; tel. 661/949–5000, (Nonreporting) **A**1 9 10
Primary Contact: Edward Mirzabegian, Chief Executive Officer
CFO: Cheryl Tong, Chief Financial Officer
CMO: Doddanna Krishna, M.D., Chief of Staff
CIO: Humberto Quintanar, Chief Information Officer
CHR: Marie Reed, Director Human Resources
CNO: Marcey Jorgenson, Chief Nursing Officer
Web address: www.avhospital.org
**Control:** Hospital district or authority, Government, nonfederal **Service:** General Medical and Surgical

**Staffed Beds:** 368

## LEMOORE—Kings County

☒ **NAVAL HOSPITAL**, 937 Franklin Avenue, Zip 93246–5004; tel. 559/998–4421, (Nonreporting) **A**1 **S** Bureau of Medicine and Surgery, Department of the Navy, Washington, DC
Primary Contact: Captain William J. Leonard, USN, Commanding Officer
CFO: Thomas M. Brui, Director Resource Management
CMO: Scott Cota, M.D., Director Medical Services
CIO: Victor Dela Torre, Command Legal Officer
CHR: Billy Newman, Department Head
Web address: www.lemoore.med.navy.mil
**Control:** Navy, Government, federal **Service:** General Medical and Surgical

**Staffed Beds:** 16

## LIVERMORE—Alameda County

**VALLEY MEMORIAL** See ValleyCare Medical Center, Pleasanton

**VETERANS AFFAIRS PALO ALTO HEALTH CARE SYSTEM, LIVERMORE DIVISION** See Veterans Affairs Palo Alto Health Care System, Palo Alto

## LODI—San Joaquin County

☒ **LODI MEMORIAL HOSPITAL (50336)**, 975 South Fairmont Avenue, Zip 95240–5179, Mailing Address: P.O. Box 3004, Zip 95241–1908; tel. 209/334–3411, (Includes LODI MEMORIAL HOSPITAL WEST, 800 South Lower Sacramento Road, Zip 95242; tel. 209/333–0211), (Nonreporting) **A**1 9 10
Primary Contact: Joseph P. Harrington, President and Chief Executive Officer
COO: Mark Sey, Vice President and Chief Administrative Officer
CFO: Ron Kreutner, Chief Financial Officer
CHR: Mark T. Wallace, Director Human Resources
Web address: www.lodihealth.org
**Control:** Other not–for–profit (including NFP Corporation) **Service:** General Medical and Surgical

**Staffed Beds:** 103

## LOMA LINDA—San Bernardino County

☒ △ **JERRY L. PETTIS MEMORIAL VETERANS MEDICAL CENTER**, 11201 Benton Street, Zip 92357; tel. 909/825–7084, (Nonreporting) **A**1 2 3 5 7 8 **S** Department of Veterans Affairs, Washington, DC
Primary Contact: Donald F. Moore, Director
COO: Shane Elliott, Associate Director Administration
CFO: Ron Pitts, Chief Financial Officer
CMO: Dwight Evans, M.D., Chief of Staff
CIO: Doug Wirthgen, Facility Chief Information Officer
CHR: Eugene Wylie, Chief Human Resources Officer
CNO: Anne Gillespie, R.N., Associate Director Patient Care and Nursing Services
Web address: www.lomalinda.va.gov
**Control:** Veterans Affairs, Government, federal **Service:** General Medical and Surgical

**Staffed Beds:** 97

**LOMA LINDA UNIVERSITY HEART & SURGICAL HOSPITAL** See Loma Linda University Medical Center

☒ △ **LOMA LINDA UNIVERSITY MEDICAL CENTER (50327)**, 11234 Anderson Street, Zip 92354–2870, Mailing Address: P.O. Box 2000, Zip 92354–0200; tel. 909/558–4000, (Includes LOMA LINDA UNIVERSITY CHILDREN'S HOSPITAL, 11234 Anderson Street, Zip 92354–2804; tel. 909/558–8000; LOMA LINDA UNIVERSITY EAST CAMPUS HOSPITAL, 25333 Barton Road, Zip 92354–3053; tel. 909/558–6000; LOMA LINDA UNIVERSITY HEART & SURGICAL HOSPITAL, 26780 Barton Road, Zip 92354; tel. 909/583–2900) **A**1 2 3 5 7 8 9 10 **F**2 3 8 11 12 13 15 17 18 19 20 21 22 23 24 25 26 27 28 29 30 31 32 34 35 37 40 41 43 45 46 47 48 49 50 54 57 59 60 62 64 65 68 72 74 75 76 77 78 79 81 82 84 85 87 88 89 90 91 92 93 94 107 108 110 111 112 113 114 115 116 117 118 119 120 121 122 123 125 128 129 131 133 135 136 137 138 140 141 142 143 145 146 147 **P**3 **S** Loma Linda University Adventist Health Sciences Center, Loma Linda, CA
Primary Contact: Ruthita J. Fike, Chief Executive Officer
COO: Ruthita J. Fike, Chief Executive Officer
CFO: Steve Mohr, Senior Vice President Finance and Chief Financial Officer
CMO: Daniel Giang, M.D., Vice President for Medical Administration
CIO: Mark Zirkelbach, Chief Information Officer
CHR: Lizette Norton, Associate Vice President Human Resources Management
Web address: www.llumc.edu
**Control:** Other not–for–profit (including NFP Corporation) **Service:** General Medical and Surgical

**Staffed Beds:** 815 **Admissions:** 28066 **Census:** 561 **Outpatient Visits:** 539253 **Births:** 2654 **Total Expense ($000):** 1024011 **Payroll Expense ($000):** 381512 **Personnel:** 6900

## LOMPOC—Santa Barbara County

☒ **LOMPOC VALLEY MEDICAL CENTER (50110)**, 1515 East Ocean Avenue, Zip 93436, Mailing Address: P.O. Box 1058, Zip 93438–1058; tel. 805/737–3300, (Nonreporting) **A**1 9 10
Primary Contact: James J. Raggio, Chief Executive Officer
COO: Naishadh Buch, Director Pharmacy and Chief Operating Officer
CFO: Robert M. Baden, Chief Financial Officer
CMO: Cecilia Ramos, M.D., Chief of Staff
CIO: Jim White, Chief Information Officer
CHR: Edwin R. Braxton, Director Human Resources
Web address: www.lompocvmc.com
**Control:** Hospital district or authority, Government, nonfederal **Service:** General Medical and Surgical

**Staffed Beds:** 60

## LONE PINE—Inyo County

★ **SOUTHERN INYO HEALTHCARE DISTRICT (51302)**, 501 East Locust Street, Zip 93545–1009, Mailing Address: P.O. Box 1009, Zip 93545–1009; tel. 760/876–5501, (Nonreporting) **A**9 10 18
Primary Contact: Lee Barron, Chief Executive Officer
CFO: Lee Barron, Chief Executive Officer
CIO: Patricia M. Murray, Information Officer
CHR: Ashley Williams, Manager Human Resources
Web address: www.sihd.org
**Control:** Hospital district or authority, Government, nonfederal **Service:** General Medical and Surgical

**Staffed Beds:** 4

---

**Hospital, Medicare Provider Number, Address, Telephone, Approval, Facility, and Physician Codes, Health Care System**

★ American Hospital Association (AHA) membership
□ The Joint Commission accreditation     ◇ DNV Healthcare Inc. accreditation
○ American Osteopathic Association (AOA) accreditation
△ Commission on Accreditation of Rehabilitation Facilities (CARF) accreditation

---

**LONG BEACH—Los Angeles County**

☐ **COMMUNITY HOSPITAL OF LONG BEACH (50727)**, 1720 Termino Avenue, Zip 90804–2180; tel. 562/498–1000 **A**1 9 10 **F**3 11 12 14 20 26 28 29 30 31 34 35 38 40 45 46 54 56 57 59 64 68 70 71 75 77 78 79 81 82 85 86 87 93 98 100 101 102 107 108 111 113 118 120 123 129 131 145 147 **P**3 5 **S** MemorialCare, Fountain Valley, CA
Primary Contact: Diana Hendel, PharmD, Chief Executive Officer
COO: Diane DeWalsche, R.N., Chief Operating Officer
CMO: Dennis Parmer, M.D., Chief Medical Staff
CIO: Rob Klingseis, Manager Information Systems
CHR: Valene J. Martin, Administrative Director Human Resources
Web address: www.chlb.org
**Control:** Other not–for–profit (including NFP Corporation) **Service:** General Medical and Surgical

**Staffed Beds:** 148 **Admissions:** 3824 **Census:** 50 **Outpatient Visits:** 26993 **Births:** 0 **Total Expense ($000):** 47468 **Payroll Expense ($000):** 21427 **Personnel:** 531

☒ △ **LONG BEACH MEMORIAL MEDICAL CENTER (50485)**, 2801 Atlantic Avenue, Zip 90806–1737, Mailing Address: P.O. Box 1428, Zip 90801–1428; tel. 562/933–2000 **A**1 2 3 5 7 8 9 10 **F**3 9 11 12 14 15 17 18 20 24 26 28 29 30 31 34 35 36 37 38 39 40 43 44 45 47 48 49 50 52 53 55 56 57 58 59 61 63 64 65 68 70 74 75 77 78 79 81 82 84 85 86 87 90 93 96 97 100 101 107 108 110 111 113 114 115 118 119 120 122 123 125 128 129 130 131 134 140 141 142 143 145 146 147 **P**3 4 5 **S** MemorialCare, Fountain Valley, CA
Primary Contact: Diana Hendel, PharmD, Chief Executive Officer
COO: Tamra Kaplan, Chief Operating Officer
CFO: John Bishop, Chief Financial Officer
CMO: Susan Melvin, D.O., Chief Medical Officer
CIO: Danny Asaoka, Executive Director Information Systems
CHR: Myra Gregorian, Vice President Human Resources
CNO: Judith A. Fix, R.N., Senior Vice President and Chief Nursing Officer
Web address: www.memorialcare.org/LongBeach
**Control:** Other not–for–profit (including NFP Corporation) **Service:** General Medical and Surgical

**Staffed Beds:** 420 **Admissions:** 21753 **Census:** 303 **Outpatient Visits:** 170154 **Births:** 0 **Total Expense ($000):** 435274 **Payroll Expense ($000):** 150987 **Personnel:** 3125

☐ **MILLER CHILDREN'S HOSPITAL (53309)**, 2801 Atlantic Avenue, Zip 90806; tel. 562/933–5437 **A**1 9 10 **F**3 11 12 13 14 19 21 23 25 27 29 30 31 32 34 35 36 37 38 40 41 43 44 45 47 48 50 52 53 54 55 57 58 59 61 64 65 66 68 72 74 75 76 77 78 79 81 84 85 86 87 88 89 93 96 97 99 100 101 102 107 108 111 113 114 115 116 118 119 120 122 123 125 128 129 131 133 134 140 141 142 143 145 146 147 **P**3 5 **S** MemorialCare, Fountain Valley, CA
Primary Contact: Diana Hendel, PharmD, Chief Executive Officer
Web address: www.memorialcare.org
**Control:** Other not–for–profit (including NFP Corporation) **Service:** Children's general

**Staffed Beds:** 383 **Admissions:** 15898 **Census:** 226 **Outpatient Visits:** 117739 **Births:** 5461 **Total Expense ($000):** 423579 **Payroll Expense ($000):** 130760 **Personnel:** 1225

☐ **PACIFIC HOSPITAL OF LONG BEACH (50277)**, 2776 Pacific Avenue, Zip 90806–2699, Mailing Address: P.O. Box 1268, Zip 90801; tel. 562/595–1911, (Nonreporting) **A**9 10 12 13 21
Primary Contact: Michael D. Drobot, Chief Executive Officer
COO: Jennifer Ensminger, Chief Operating Officer
CFO: Jim Canedo, Chief Financial Officer
CMO: Luke Watson, M.D., Chief of Staff
CIO: Rohan Corea, Director Healthcare Information Technology
CHR: Ann Mattia Schiller, Vice President Human Resources
CNO: Kathryn McLaughlin, Vice President and Chief Nursing Officer
Web address: www.phlb.org
**Control:** Other not–for–profit (including NFP Corporation) **Service:** General Medical and Surgical

**Staffed Beds:** 184

☐ **REDGATE MEMORIAL RECOVERY CENTER**, 1775 Chestnut Avenue, Zip 90813–1674; tel. 562/599–8444, (Nonreporting) **A**9
Primary Contact: Lawrence Gentile, President and Chief Executive Officer
Web address: www.bhs–inc.org/rmrc.html
**Control:** Other not–for–profit (including NFP Corporation) **Service:** Alcoholism and other chemical dependency

**Staffed Beds:** 63

☒ **ST. MARY MEDICAL CENTER (50191)**, 1050 Linden Avenue, Zip 90813, Mailing Address: P.O. Box 887, Zip 90801–0887; tel. 562/491–9000, (Nonreporting) **A**1 2 3 5 9 10 **S** Dignity Health, San Francisco, CA
Primary Contact: Thomas A. Salerno, President
COO: Gail Daly, Chief Operating Officer
CMO: Stanley Goldberg, M.D., Chief of Staff
CIO: Robert Erndt, Site Manager
CHR: Bob Bokern, Director Human Resources
Web address: www.stmarymedicalcenter.org
**Control:** Other not–for–profit (including NFP Corporation) **Service:** General Medical and Surgical

**Staffed Beds:** 165

☒ △ **VETERANS AFFAIRS LONG BEACH HEALTHCARE SYSTEM**, 5901 East 7th Street, Zip 90822–5201; tel. 562/826–8000, (Nonreporting) **A**1 2 3 5 7 8 **S** Department of Veterans Affairs, Washington, DC
Primary Contact: Isabel Duff, MS, Director
COO: Anthony DeFrancesco, Associate Director
CFO: Michael J. Rupert, Chief Financial Officer
CMO: Sandor Szabo, M.D., Chief of Staff
CIO: Rodney Sagmit, Chief Information Management
CHR: Mary E. McCartan, Manager Human Resources
Web address: www.va.gov/sta/guide/home.asp
**Control:** Veterans Affairs, Government, federal **Service:** General Medical and Surgical

**Staffed Beds:** 234

**LOS ALAMITOS—Orange County**

☒ **LOS ALAMITOS MEDICAL CENTER (50551)**, 3751 Katella Avenue, Zip 90720–3164; tel. 562/598–1311, (Nonreporting) **A**1 2 9 10 **S** TENET Healthcare Corporation, Dallas, TX
Primary Contact: Michele Finney, Chief Executive Officer
CFO: Dave Vickers, Chief Financial Officer
CIO: Sally Andrada, Chief Information Officer
CHR: Angie Driscoll, Director Human Resources
Web address: www.losalamitosmedctr.com
**Control:** Corporation, Investor–owned, for–profit **Service:** General Medical and Surgical

**Staffed Beds:** 120

**LOS ANGELES—Los Angeles County**

**(Mailing Addresses - Canoga Park, Encino, Granada Hills, Harbor City, Hollywood, Mission Hills, North Hollywood, Northridge, Panorama City, San Pedro, Sepulveda, Sherman Oaks, Sun Valley, Sylmar, Tarzana, Van Nuys, West Hills, West Los Angeles, Woodland Hills)**

☒ **BARLOW RESPIRATORY HOSPITAL (52031)**, 2000 Stadium Way, Zip 90026–2696; tel. 213/250–4200, (Nonreporting) **A**1 9 10
Primary Contact: Margaret W. Crane, Chief Executive Officer
COO: Mary B. Oelman, R.N., Chief Operating Officer and Chief Clinical Officer
CFO: Edward Engesser, Chief Financial Officer and Chief Information Officer
CMO: David Nelson, M.D., Medical Director
CIO: Edward Engesser, Chief Financial Officer and Chief Information Officer
CHR: Jeannine Coatsworth, Vice President Human Resources
Web address: www.barlow2000.com
**Control:** Other not–for–profit (including NFP Corporation) **Service:** Long–Term Acute Care hospital

**Staffed Beds:** 105

☒ **CALIFORNIA HOSPITAL MEDICAL CENTER (50149)**, 1401 South Grand Avenue, Zip 90015–3010; tel. 213/748–2411, (Total facility includes 31 beds in nursing home–type unit) **A**1 3 5 9 10 **F**3 11 17 29 30 31 34 35 40 43 45 49 51 53 57 59 64 70 72 76 78 79 81 84 89 102 107 108 111 113 118 120 127 129 142 145 146 **S** Dignity Health, San Francisco, CA
Primary Contact: Gerald B. Clute, President and Chief Executive Officer
CFO: Robert Allen, Chief Financial Officer
CMO: Bruce A. Greenfield, M.D., Chief of Staff
CIO: Rich Patla, Director Information Technology
CHR: Sandra Davis Houston, Vice President Human Resources
Web address: www.chmcla.org
**Control:** Other not–for–profit (including NFP Corporation) **Service:** General Medical and Surgical

**Staffed Beds:** 318 **Admissions:** 16149 **Census:** 176 **Outpatient Visits:** 115716 **Births:** 4660 **Total Expense ($000):** 296128 **Payroll Expense ($000):** 117674 **Personnel:** 1458

**CA**

⊠ △ **CEDARS–SINAI MEDICAL CENTER (50625)**, 8700 Beverly Boulevard, Zip 90048–1865, Mailing Address: Box 48750, Zip 90048–0750; tel. 310/423–5000 **A**1 2 3 5 7 8 9 10 **F**3 5 6 8 9 11 12 13 14 15 17 18 19 20 21 22 23 24 25 26 27 28 29 30 31 32 33 34 35 36 37 38 39 40 43 44 45 46 47 48 49 50 51 52 53 54 55 56 57 58 59 60 61 64 65 66 68 69 70 71 72 74 75 76 77 78 79 81 82 83 84 85 86 87 88 89 90 91 92 93 96 97 98 99 100 101 102 103 104 105 106 107 108 109 110 111 112 113 114 115 116 117 118 119 120 121 122 123 125 129 130 131 132 133 134 135 136 137 138 139 140 141 144 145 146 147 **P**3 5 8
Primary Contact: Thomas M. Priselac, President and Chief Executive Officer
COO: Mark R. Gavens, Senior Vice President Clinical Care Services and Chief Operating Officer
CFO: Edward M. Prunchunas, Senior Vice President and Chief Financial Officer
CMO: Michael L. Langberg, M.D., Senior Vice President Medical Affairs and Chief Medical Officer
CIO: Darren Dworkin, Senior Vice President and Chief Information Officer
CHR: Jeanne Flores, Senior Vice President Human Resources and Organizational Development
Web address: www.cedars–sinai.edu
**Control:** Other not–for–profit (including NFP Corporation) **Service:** General Medical and Surgical

**Staffed Beds:** 892 **Admissions:** 50453 **Census:** 765 **Outpatient Visits:** 681119 **Births:** 6678 **Total Expense ($000):** 2195635 **Payroll Expense ($000):** 849383 **Personnel:** 10742

⊠ **CHILDREN'S HOSPITAL LOS ANGELES (53302)**, 4650 Sunset Boulevard, Zip 90027–6062, Mailing Address: P.O. Box 27980, Zip 90027; tel. 323/660–2450 **A**1 3 5 9 10 **F**3 8 14 17 19 21 23 25 27 28 29 30 31 32 34 35 36 37 38 39 40 41 43 44 45 46 50 54 55 57 58 59 60 61 64 65 68 72 74 75 77 78 79 81 82 83 84 85 86 87 88 89 90 91 92 93 94 96 107 108 111 113 114 115 116 117 118 120 122 125 128 129 130 131 133 134 135 136 137 138 139 140 141 142 143 145 147
Primary Contact: Richard D. Cordova, President and Chief Executive Officer
COO: Rodney Hanners, Senior Vice President and Chief Operating Officer
CFO: Lannie Tonnu, Senior Vice President and Chief Financial Officer
CMO: Brent Polk, M.D., Chair Department of Pediatrics and Vice President Academic Affairs
CIO: Marty Miller, Vice President and Chief Information Officer
CHR: Hugo Santos, Vice President Human Resources
CNO: Mary Dee Hacker, R.N., Vice President, Patient Care Services and Chief Nursing Officer
Web address: www.chla.org
**Control:** Other not–for–profit (including NFP Corporation) **Service:** Children's general

**Staffed Beds:** 317 **Admissions:** 11866 **Census:** 243 **Births:** 0

☐ **EAST LOS ANGELES DOCTORS HOSPITAL (50641)**, 4060 East Whittier Boulevard, Zip 90023–2526; tel. 323/268–5514 **A**1 9 10 **F**1 3 7 8 13 17 29 30 35 40 41 76 80 89 107 118 129 **S** Avanti Hospitals, El Segundo, CA
Primary Contact: Hector Hernandez, Chief Executive Officer
CFO: Daniel R. Heckathorne, Regional Chief Financial Officer
CMO: Kamlesh Dhawan, M.D., Chief of Staff
CIO: Earle Johnson, Chief Information Officer
CHR: Rob Taylor, Corporate Director Human Resources
CNO: Carmelo James, Chief Nursing Officer
Web address: www.elalax.com
**Control:** Partnership, Investor–owned, for–profit **Service:** General Medical and Surgical

**Staffed Beds:** 127 **Admissions:** 4407 **Census:** 78 **Outpatient Visits:** 22088

☐ **ENCINO HOSPITAL MEDICAL CENTER (50158)**, 16237 Ventura Boulevard, Encino, Zip 91436–2201; tel. 818/995–5000, (Nonreporting) **A**1 10 **S** Prime Healthcare Services, Ontario, CA
Primary Contact: Robert C. Bills, Chief Executive Officer
CFO: Kanner Tillman, Chief Financial Officer
CMO: Muhammad Anwar, M.D., Chief Medical Officer
CIO: Edward Barrera, Director Communications
CHR: Barbara Back, Manager Human Resources
CNO: Vilma L. Dinham, R.N., Chief Nursing Officer
Web address: www.encinomed.com
**Control:** Corporation, Investor–owned, for–profit **Service:** General Medical and Surgical

**Staffed Beds:** 151

○ **GATEWAYS HOSPITAL AND MENTAL HEALTH CENTER (54028)**, 1891 Effie Street, Zip 90026–1711; tel. 323/644–2000 **A**10 11 **F**29 35 77 98 99 100 101 104 106 129 **P**6
Primary Contact: Mara Pelsman, Chief Executive Officer
COO: Jeff Emery, Chief Financial Officer and Chief Operating Officer
CFO: Jeff Emery, Chief Financial Officer and Chief Operating Officer
CMO: Mark Hantoot, M.D., Medical Director
CIO: Jeff Emery, Chief Financial Officer and Chief Operating Officer
CHR: Melanie Van Heusen, Director Human Resources
Web address: www.gatewayshospital.org
**Control:** Other not–for–profit (including NFP Corporation) **Service:** Psychiatric

**Staffed Beds:** 55 **Admissions:** 1035 **Census:** 35 **Outpatient Visits:** 115667 **Births:** 0 **Total Expense ($000):** 25785 **Payroll Expense ($000):** 13656 **Personnel:** 328

**GENERAL HOSPITAL** See LAC/University of Southern California Medical Center

☐ △ **GOOD SAMARITAN HOSPITAL (50471)**, 1225 Wilshire Boulevard, Zip 90017–1901; tel. 213/977–2121 **A**1 2 3 5 7 9 10 **F**3 7 8 9 11 13 14 15 17 18 20 22 24 26 28 29 30 31 34 35 36 37 40 43 45 46 47 48 49 50 51 53 56 57 58 59 60 61 64 65 68 70 72 74 76 77 78 79 81 85 86 87 93 107 108 110 111 113 114 116 117 118 119 120 122 123 125 129 131 142 143 144 145 147 **P**5 7
Primary Contact: Andrew B. Leeka, President and Chief Executive Officer
CFO: Alan Ino, Chief Financial Officer
CMO: Andrew Fishmann, M.D., Chairman, Medical Staff
CIO: Dean Campbell, Vice President Information Services and Chief Information Officer
CHR: Lexie Schuster, Vice President Human Resources
CNO: Margaret Pfeiffer, R.N., Vice President Patient Care Services
Web address: www.goodsam.org
**Control:** Other not–for–profit (including NFP Corporation) **Service:** General Medical and Surgical

**Staffed Beds:** 374 **Admissions:** 16547 **Census:** 209 **Outpatient Visits:** 92325 **Births:** 4801 **Total Expense ($000):** 272787 **Payroll Expense ($000):** 101225 **Personnel:** 1327

**HOLLYWOOD COMMUNITY HOSPITAL (50135)**, 6245 De Longpre Avenue, Zip 90028–9001; tel. 323/462–2271, (Includes HOLLYWOOD COMMUNITY HOSPITAL OF VAN NUYS, 14433 Emelita Street, Van Nuys, Zip 91401; tel. 818/787–1511), (Nonreporting) **A**10 **S** Alta Healthcare System, Los Angeles, CA
Primary Contact: Michael Sarian, Chief Executive Officer
Web address: www.hollywoodcommunityhospital.com
**Control:** Corporation, Investor–owned, for–profit **Service:** General Medical and Surgical

**Staffed Beds:** 45

**HOLLYWOOD COMMUNITY HOSPITAL OF VAN NUYS** See Hollywood Community Hospital

⊠ **HOLLYWOOD PRESBYTERIAN MEDICAL CENTER (50063)**, 1300 North Vermont Avenue, Zip 90027–6005; tel. 323/913–4800 **A**1 2 9 10 **F**3 7 15 17 18 20 22 24 26 29 30 31 34 35 39 40 45 46 49 55 57 58 59 61 64 65 68 70 72 74 75 76 77 78 79 80 81 82 84 85 87 89 90 92 93 96 107 108 111 113 118 119 129 131 145 147 **P**3 5 6
Primary Contact: Michael A. Rembis, FACHE, Chief Executive Officer
CFO: Allen Stefanek, Chief Financial Officer
CMO: Robert Chesne, M.D., Chief Medical Officer
CIO: Steve Giles, Chief Information Officer
CHR: Norma Braun, Vice President Human Resources
CNO: Kathy Wojno, R.N., Chief Nursing Officer
Web address: www.hollywoodpresbyterian.com
**Control:** Partnership, Investor–owned, for–profit **Service:** General Medical and Surgical

**Staffed Beds:** 434 **Admissions:** 15622 **Census:** 258 **Outpatient Visits:** 57808 **Births:** 4091 **Total Expense ($000):** 196374 **Payroll Expense ($000):** 98493 **Personnel:** 1163

**KAISER FOUNDATION MENTAL HEALTH CENTER** See Los Angeles Medical Center

---

**Hospital, Medicare Provider Number, Address, Telephone, Approval, Facility, and Physician Codes, Health Care System**

★ American Hospital Association (AHA) membership
☐ The Joint Commission accreditation          ◇ DNV Healthcare Inc. accreditation

○ American Osteopathic Association (AOA) accreditation
△ Commission on Accreditation of Rehabilitation Facilities (CARF) accreditation

⊠ **KECK HOSPITAL OF USC (50696)**, 1500 San Pablo Street, Zip 90033–4587; tel. 323/442–8500 **A**1 3 5 8 9 10 **F**3 6 12 15 17 18 20 22 24 26 29 30 34 35 39 44 45 46 47 48 49 50 51 53 54 55 56 57 58 59 60 61 64 65 68 70 74 75 77 78 79 81 82 83 84 85 86 87 91 92 93 94 96 97 98 100 101 103 104 105 106 107 108 110 111 112 113 114 115 116 117 118 119 120 122 123 125 128 129 130 131 135 136 137 138 139 140 141 144 145 146 147
Primary Contact: Scott Evans, PharmD, Chief Executive Officer
CFO: Jonathan Spees, Chief Financial Officer
CMO: Donald Larsen, M.D., Chief Medical Officer
CIO: Mark Amey, Chief Information Officer
CHR: Matthew McElrath, Chief Human Resources Officer
Web address: www.keckhospitalofusc.org
**Control:** Other not–for–profit (including NFP Corporation) **Service:** General Medical and Surgical

| Staffed Beds: 220 Admissions: 10138 Census: 207 Outpatient Visits: 95119 Births: 0 Total Expense ($000): 496136 Payroll Expense ($000): 175791 Personnel: 2076 |
| --- |

⊠ **KINDRED HOSPITAL–LOS ANGELES (52032)**, 5525 West Slauson Avenue, Zip 90056–1067; tel. 310/642–0325, (Nonreporting) **A**1 9 10 **S** Kindred Healthcare, Louisville, KY
Primary Contact: Luke Tharasri, Administrator
CFO: Dale Wagner, Chief Financial Officer
Web address: www.kindredhospitalalla.com/
**Control:** Corporation, Investor–owned, for–profit **Service:** General Medical and Surgical

| Staffed Beds: 81 |
| --- |

☐ **LAC–OLIVE VIEW–UCLA MEDICAL CENTER (50040)**, 14445 Olive View Drive, Sylmar, Zip 91342–1495; tel. 818/364–1555, (Nonreporting) **A**1 3 5 10 **S** Los Angeles County–Department of Health Services, Los Angeles, CA
Primary Contact: Carolyn F. Rhee, Chief Executive Officer
COO: Ernest Espinoza, Interim Chief Operating Officer
CFO: Anthony Gray, Chief Financial Officer
CMO: William Loos, M.D., Chief Medical Officer
CIO: Melvin Brewster, Chief Information Officer
CHR: Thomas Beggane, Manager Human Resources
Web address: www.ladhs.org
**Control:** County–Government, nonfederal **Service:** General Medical and Surgical

| Staffed Beds: 238 |
| --- |

☐ **LAC/UNIVERSITY OF SOUTHERN CALIFORNIA MEDICAL CENTER (50373)**, 1200 North State Street, Zip 90033–1029; tel. 323/226–2622, (Includes GENERAL HOSPITAL, 1200 North State Street, Zip 90033; WOMEN'S AND CHILDREN'S HOSPITAL, 1240 North Mission Road, Zip 90033), (Nonreporting) **A**1 2 3 5 8 9 10 **S** Los Angeles County–Department of Health Services, Los Angeles, CA
Primary Contact: Pete Delgado, Chief Executive Officer
COO: Henry Ornelas, Chief Operating Officer
CFO: Mark Corbet, Interim Chief Financial Officer
CMO: Stephanie Hall, M.D., Chief Medical Officer
CIO: Oscar Austelli, Chief Information Officer
Web address: www.lacusc.org
**Control:** County–Government, nonfederal **Service:** General Medical and Surgical

| Staffed Beds: 633 |
| --- |

☐ **LOS ANGELES COMMUNITY HOSPITAL (50663)**, 4081 East Olympic Boulevard, Zip 90023–3330; tel. 323/267–0477, (Includes LOS ANGELES COMMUNITY HOSPITAL OF NORWALK, 13222 Bloomfield Avenue, Norwalk, Zip 90650; tel. 562/863–4763), (Nonreporting) **A**1 10 21 **S** Alta Healthcare System, Los Angeles, CA
Primary Contact: Al Souza, Chief Executive Officer
CFO: Johnnette Chong, Chief Financial Officer
**Control:** Corporation, Investor–owned, for–profit **Service:** General Medical and Surgical

| Staffed Beds: 180 |
| --- |

**LOS ANGELES COUNTY CENTRAL JAIL HOSPITAL**, 441 Bauchet Street, Zip 90012–2994; tel. 213/473–6100, (Nonreporting)
Primary Contact: Tom Flaherty, Assistant Administrator
**Control:** County–Government, nonfederal **Service:** Hospital unit of an institution (prison hospital, college infimary, etc.)

| Staffed Beds: 190 |
| --- |

⊠ **LOS ANGELES MEDICAL CENTER (50138)**, 4867 Sunset Boulevard, Zip 90027–5969; tel. 323/783–4011, (Includes KAISER FOUNDATION MENTAL HEALTH CENTER, 765 West College Street, Zip 90012; tel. 213/580–7200) **A**1 3 5 10 **F**3 8 13 17 18 19 20 21 22 23 24 25 26 28 29 30 31 35 36 38 40 44 45 46 47 49 50 51 54 56 57 60 61 62 63 64 65 66 68 70 72 73 74 75 76 78 79 80 81 82 83 84 85 86 87 88 89 97 98 99 100 101 102 103 104 105 106 107 108 109 111 113 114 117 118 119 120 121 122 123 131 143 145 146 147 **P**6 **S** Kaiser Foundation Hospitals, Oakland, CA
Primary Contact: Mark E. Costa, Executive Director
COO: Alice H. Issai, Chief Operating Officer
CFO: Prasanna Mohanty, Assistant Administrator Finance
CMO: Donald H. Marcus, M.D., Medical Director
CHR: Paul J. Martin, Director Human Resources
Web address: www.kaiserpermanente.org
**Control:** Other not–for–profit (including NFP Corporation) **Service:** General Medical and Surgical

| Staffed Beds: 464 Admissions: 25663 Census: 328 Outpatient Visits: 2198712 Births: 2339 Personnel: 3018 |
| --- |

○ **LOS ANGELES METROPOLITAN MEDICAL CENTER (50644)**, 2231 South Western Avenue, Zip 90018–1302; tel. 323/730–7300, (Includes HAWTHORNE HOSPITAL, 13300 South Hawthorne Boulevard, Hawthorne, Zip 90250; tel. 310/679–3321) **A**10 11 **F**3 17 29 40 59 70 76 81 82 86 93 98 102 103 104 107 113 118 129 **S** Pacific Health Corporation, Tustin, CA
Primary Contact: Ron Stinnett, Chief Executive Officer
COO: Shannon Jones, Chief Operating Officer
CFO: Clara Blom, Chief Financial Officer
CMO: Fred Besharat, M.D., Chief of Staff
CIO: Maro Mercene, Chief Information Officer
CHR: Jacqueline Sanchez, Director Human Resources
Web address: www.lammc.com
**Control:** Partnership, Investor–owned, for–profit **Service:** General Medical and Surgical

| Staffed Beds: 213 Admissions: 5239 Census: 108 Outpatient Visits: 10378 Personnel: 536 |
| --- |

☐ **MIRACLE MILE MEDICAL CENTER (50751)**, 6000 San Vicente Boulevard, Zip 90036; tel. 323/930–1040, (Nonreporting) **A**1 10
Primary Contact: Jack Lahidjani, Chief Executive Officer
COO: Liz Cheever, Associate Administrator
CMO: Gil Tepper, M.D., Chief of Staff
CIO: Dipak Reddy, Director Information Technology
CHR: Liz Cheever, Associate Administrator
Web address: www.miraclemilemedicalcenter.com
**Control:** Corporation, Investor–owned, for–profit **Service:** General Medical and Surgical

| Staffed Beds: 17 |
| --- |

**MOTION PICTURE AND TELEVISION FUND HOSPITAL AND RESIDENTIAL SERVICES (50552)**, 23388 Mulholland Drive, Woodland Hills, Zip 91364–2733; tel. 818/876–1888, (Nonreporting) **A**9 10
Primary Contact: Bob Beitcher, Interim Chief Executive Officer
COO: Seth Ellis, Chief Operating Officer
CFO: Frank Guarrera, Executive Vice President and Chief Financial Officer
CHR: Jan Zlotowicz, Vice President Human Resources
Web address: www.mptvfund.org
**Control:** Other not–for–profit (including NFP Corporation) **Service:** General Medical and Surgical

| Staffed Beds: 250 |
| --- |

⊠ △ **NORTHRIDGE HOSPITAL MEDICAL CENTER–ROSCOE BOULEVARD CAMPUS (50116)**, 18300 Roscoe Boulevard, Northridge, Zip 91328–4167; tel. 818/885–8500 **A**1 2 3 5 7 8 9 10 **F**2 3 8 11 12 13 14 15 17 18 20 22 24 26 28 29 30 31 34 35 38 40 41 43 48 49 56 57 58 59 60 61 64 68 70 72 74 75 76 77 78 79 81 82 84 85 86 87 88 89 90 93 97 98 99 100 101 102 103 104 105 107 108 110 111 113 116 117 118 120 123 125 128 129 131 133 145 146 147 **S** Dignity Health, San Francisco, CA
Primary Contact: Michael L. Wall, President
COO: Saliba Salo, Chief Operating Officer
CHR: George Leisher, Vice President Human Resources
Web address: www.northridgehospital.org
**Control:** Other not–for–profit (including NFP Corporation) **Service:** General Medical and Surgical

| Staffed Beds: 371 Admissions: 18529 Census: 240 Outpatient Visits: 58901 Births: 2403 Total Expense ($000): 366885 Payroll Expense ($000): 156998 |
| --- |

**OLYMPIA MEDICAL CENTER (50742)**, 5900 West Olympic Boulevard, Zip 90036; tel. 310/657–5900 **A**9 10 21 **F**3 6 8 15 17 29 31 34 35 40 45 46 47 49 56 57 58 59 64 70 74 75 77 78 79 81 82 85 86 87 93 100 103 104 107 111 114 118 129 130 131 142 145
Primary Contact: John A. Calderone, Ph.D., Chief Executive Officer
CFO: Babur Ozkan, Chief Financial Officer
CMO: James Peace, M.D., Chief of Staff
CIO: Fritz Campbell, Director Information Systems
CHR: Judy Synder, Director Human Resources
CNO: Karen Knueven, Chief Nursing Officer
Web address: www.olympiamc.com
**Control:** Partnership, Investor–owned, for–profit **Service:** General Medical and Surgical

**Staffed Beds: 204 Admissions: 6424 Census: 92 Outpatient Visits: 37562 Births: 0 Total Expense ($000): 107309 Payroll Expense ($000): 49049 Personnel: 564**

☐ △ **PACIFIC ALLIANCE MEDICAL CENTER (50018)**, 531 West College Street, Zip 90012–2315; tel. 213/624–8411, (Nonreporting) **A**1 7 9 10
Primary Contact: John R. Edwards, Administrator and Chief Executive Officer
CFO: Allan Shubin, Chief Financial Officer
CIO: John D. Brown, Director Information Systems
Web address: www.pamc.net
**Control:** Partnership, Investor–owned, for–profit **Service:** General Medical and Surgical

**Staffed Beds: 138**

☐ **PACIFICA HOSPITAL OF THE VALLEY (50378)**, 9449 San Fernando Road, Sun Valley, Zip 91352–1421; tel. 818/767–3310, (Nonreporting) **A**1 9 10
Primary Contact: Ayman Mousa, R.N., Ph.D., Chief Executive Officer
CFO: Lawrence Tyrrell, Chief Financial Officer
CMO: Joseph Eipe, M.D., Chief Medical Officer
CIO: Mubashir Hashmi, Chief Information Officer
CHR: Patti Alonzo, Manager Human Resources
Web address: www.pacificahospital.com
**Control:** Corporation, Investor–owned, for–profit **Service:** General Medical and Surgical

**Staffed Beds: 231**

⊞ **PANORAMA CITY MEDICAL CENTER (50137)**, 13652 Cantara Street, Panorama City, Zip 91402–5497; tel. 818/375–2000, (Nonreporting) **A**1 3 5 10 **S** Kaiser Foundation Hospitals, Oakland, CA
Primary Contact: Dennis C. Benton, Administrator and Executive Director
COO: Barbara C. Zelinski, Chief Operating Officer
CFO: Mechi R. Caballero, Assistant Administrator
CMO: Mary L. Wilson, M.D., Area Medical Director
CHR: Carole L. Erken, Human Resources Leader
Web address: www.kaiserpermanente.org
**Control:** Other not–for–profit (including NFP Corporation) **Service:** General Medical and Surgical

**Staffed Beds: 218**

**PROMISE HOSPITAL OF EAST LOS ANGELES (52046)**, 443 South Soto Street, Zip 90033–4398; tel. 323/261–1181, (Nonreporting) **A**9 10 **S** Promise Healthcare, Boca Raton, FL
Primary Contact: Richard Luna, Chief Executive Officer
Web address: www.promiseeastla.com
**Control:** Corporation, Investor–owned, for–profit **Service:** Long–Term Acute Care hospital

**Staffed Beds: 36**

⊞ △ **PROVIDENCE HOLY CROSS MEDICAL CENTER (50278)**, 15031 Rinaldi Street, Mission Hills, Zip 91346–9600; tel. 818/365–8051, (Nonreporting) **A**1 2 7 9 10 **S** Providence Health & Services, Renton, WA
Primary Contact: Larry Bowe, Chief Executive
CFO: Dave Mast, Chief Financial Officer
CIO: Douglas Jones, Regional Chief Information Officer
CHR: Lori Curry, Regional Chief Human Resources Officer
Web address: www.providence.org/losangeles/facilities/providence_holy_cross/
**Control:** Church–operated, Nongovernment, not–for profit **Service:** General Medical and Surgical

**Staffed Beds: 254**

⊞ △ **PROVIDENCE LITTLE COMPANY OF MARY MEDICAL CENTER SAN PEDRO (50078)**, 1300 West Seventh Street, San Pedro, Zip 90732–3505; tel. 310/832–3311 **A**1 7 9 10 **F**2 3 4 5 11 13 14 15 18 29 30 31 32 34 35 40 44 45 49 50 51 57 59 60 66 68 70 71 74 75 76 77 78 79 81 82 85 86 87 90 92 93 94 96 98 100 101 102 103 104 105 107 108 110 111 113 118 119 122 127 129 131 132 134 144 145 **S** Providence Health & Services, Renton, WA
Primary Contact: Nancy Carlson, Chief Executive
COO: Carlos W. Priestley, Chief Operating Officer
CFO: Elizabeth Zuanich, Chief Financial Officer
CMO: Herbert Webb, M.D., Chief Medical Officer
CIO: Rachel Sanchez, Director Information Systems
CHR: Andreas Viggers, Director Human Resources
CNO: Mary Jane Jones, R.N., Chief Nursing Officer
Web address: www.https://california.providence.org/san–pedro
**Control:** Other not–for–profit (including NFP Corporation) **Service:** General Medical and Surgical

**Staffed Beds: 327 Admissions: 7254 Census: 173 Outpatient Visits: 71481 Births: 678 Total Expense ($000): 150764 Payroll Expense ($000): 66989 Personnel: 699**

⊞ **PROVIDENCE TARZANA MEDICAL CENTER (50761)**, 18321 Clark Street, Tarzana, Zip 91356–3521; tel. 818/881–0800 **A**1 9 10 **F**11 14 15 17 18 20 22 24 26 28 29 30 31 34 35 37 38 40 41 46 47 49 56 57 59 63 70 72 74 75 76 77 78 79 81 82 83 84 85 86 87 89 93 107 108 110 111 113 114 115 116 117 118 129 131 134 145 146 147 **S** Providence Health & Services, Renton, WA
Primary Contact: Dale Surowitz, Chief Executive
CFO: Nick Lymberopoulos, Chief Financial Officer
CMO: Glenn Irani, M.D., Chief Medical Officer
CIO: Craig Witmer, Chief Information Officer
CHR: Jo Lewis, Director Human Resources
Web address: www.providence.org/tarzana
**Control:** Other not–for–profit (including NFP Corporation) **Service:** General Medical and Surgical

**Staffed Beds: 245 Admissions: 14035 Census: 165 Outpatient Visits: 32262 Births: 1824**

⊞ **RONALD REAGAN UNIVERSITY OF CALIFORNIA LOS ANGELES MEDICAL CENTER (50262)**, 757 Westwood Plaza, Zip 90095–8358; tel. 310/825–9111, (Includes MATTEL CHILDREN'S HOSPITAL, 10833 Le Conte Avenue, Zip 90024; tel. 310/825–9111) **A**1 3 5 8 9 10 **F**3 6 7 8 9 11 12 13 14 15 17 18 19 20 21 22 23 24 25 26 27 28 29 30 31 32 34 35 36 40 41 43 44 45 46 47 48 49 50 51 52 54 55 56 57 58 59 61 62 64 65 66 68 70 71 72 74 75 76 77 78 79 81 82 83 84 85 86 87 88 89 90 92 93 94 96 97 102 107 108 110 111 112 113 114 115 116 117 118 119 120 122 123 125 128 129 130 131 135 136 137 138 139 140 141 142 144 145 146 147 **P**6 **S** University of California–Systemwide Administration, Oakland, CA
Primary Contact: David Feinberg, M.D., Chief Executive Officer
CFO: Paul Staton, Chief Financial Officer
CMO: J. Thomas Rosenthal, M.D., Chief Medical Officer
CIO: Virginia McFerran, Chief Information Officer
CHR: Mark Speare, Senior Associate Director Human Resources
Web address: www.uclahealth.org
**Control:** State–Government, nonfederal **Service:** General Medical and Surgical

**Staffed Beds: 466 Admissions: 23388 Census: 449 Outpatient Visits: 778173 Births: 2153 Total Expense ($000): 1155980 Payroll Expense ($000): 469570 Personnel: 6858**

○ **SHERMAN OAKS HOSPITAL (50755)**, 4929 Van Nuys Boulevard, Sherman Oaks, Zip 91403–1702; tel. 818/981–7111, (Nonreporting) **A**10 11 **S** Prime Healthcare Services, Ontario, CA
Primary Contact: Robert C. Bills, Chief Executive Officer
COO: Bockhi Park, Chief Operating Officer
CFO: Daniel Leon, Chief Financial Officer
CMO: Michael Malamed, M.D., Chief of Staff
Web address: www.shermanoakshospital.com
**Control:** Other not–for–profit (including NFP Corporation) **Service:** General Medical and Surgical

**Staffed Beds: 112**

**CA**

---

**Hospital, Medicare Provider Number, Address, Telephone, Approval, Facility, and Physician Codes, Health Care System**

★ American Hospital Association (AHA) membership
☐ The Joint Commission accreditation     ◇ DNV Healthcare Inc. accreditation
○ American Osteopathic Association (AOA) accreditation
△ Commission on Accreditation of Rehabilitation Facilities (CARF) accreditation

⊞ **SHRINERS HOSPITALS FOR CHILDREN, LOS ANGELES (53310)**, 3160 Geneva Street, Zip 90020–1199; tel. 213/388–3151 **A**1 3 5 10 **F**3 29 32 34 57 58 59 64 65 66 68 77 79 81 85 86 87 89 90 91 93 94 96 97 118 129 131 142 145 **S** Shriners Hospitals for Children, Tampa, FL
Primary Contact: Eugene Raynaud, Interim Chief Executive Officer and Administrator
CFO: David Burkitt, Director Fiscal Services
CMO: Hugh Watts, M.D., Chief of Staff
CIO: Mark Garrett, Chief Information Officer
CHR: Rashawn Woods, Director Human Resources
Web address: www.shrinershospitals.org
**Control:** Other not–for–profit (including NFP Corporation) **Service:** Children's general

**Staffed Beds:** 30 **Admissions:** 1120 **Census:** 8 **Outpatient Visits:** 19273 **Births:** 0

☐ **SILVER LAKE MEDICAL CENTER (50763)**, 1711 West Temple Street, Zip 90026–5421; tel. 213/989–6100, (Includes SILVER LAKE MEDICAL CENTER–INGLESIDE HOSPITAL, 7500 East Hellman Avenue, Rosemead, Zip 91770; tel. 626/288–1160), (Nonreporting) **A**1 10 **S** Success Healthcare, Boca Raton, FL
Primary Contact: Steve Popkin, Chief Executive Officer
CFO: John Cowles, Chief Financial Officer
CMO: Louis Acosta, M.D., Chief of Staff
CIO: Scott Musack, Chief Information Officer
CHR: Sylvia Cloud, Director Human Resources
Web address: www.silverlakemc.com
**Control:** Corporation, Investor–owned, for–profit **Service:** General Medical and Surgical

**Staffed Beds:** 150

⊞ **SOUTH BAY MEDICAL CENTER (50411)**, 25825 South Vermont Avenue, Harbor City, Zip 90710–3599; tel. 310/325–5111, (Nonreporting) **A**1 10 **S** Kaiser Foundation Hospitals, Oakland, CA
Primary Contact: Lesley A. Wille, Administrator and Executive Director
Web address: www.kaiserpermanente.org
**Control:** Other not–for–profit (including NFP Corporation) **Service:** General Medical and Surgical

**Staffed Beds:** 235

⊞ **ST. VINCENT MEDICAL CENTER (50502)**, 2131 West Third Street, Zip 90057–7992, Mailing Address: P.O. Box 57992, Zip 90057–7992; tel. 213/484–7111, (Total facility includes 27 beds in nursing home–type unit) **A**1 2 9 10 **F**3 11 15 17 18 20 22 24 26 29 30 31 34 35 36 40 47 49 50 54 57 58 59 60 63 64 65 68 69 70 71 74 75 77 78 79 80 81 82 85 87 90 91 93 96 107 108 110 111 117 118 119 120 124 127 128 135 137 141 142 145 147 **P**5 **S** Daughters of Charity Health System, Los Altos Hills, CA
Primary Contact: Catherine Fickes, R.N., President and Chief Executive Officer
COO: Douglas V. Kleam, Vice President and Chief Operating Officer
CFO: Michael Garko, Chief Financial Officer
CMO: Ronald Fishbach, M.D., Chief of Staff
CIO: Dan Robbins, Information Technology and Account Executive
CHR: Christine Carson, Vice President Human Resources
CNO: Kim Deese, R.N., Vice President/CNO
Web address: www.stvincentmedicalcenter.com
**Control:** Church–operated, Nongovernment, not–for profit **Service:** General Medical and Surgical

**Staffed Beds:** 271 **Admissions:** 8830 **Census:** 123 **Outpatient Visits:** 73079 **Births:** 0 **Total Expense ($000):** 220385 **Payroll Expense ($000):** 73129 **Personnel:** 1066

⊞ **STEWART & LYNDA RESNICK NEUROPSYCHIATRIC HOSPITAL AT UCLA (54009)**, 760 Westwood Plaza, Zip 90095–8353; tel. 310/825–9989 **A**1 3 5 9 10 **F**3 5 6 29 30 35 40 42 43 55 56 64 68 77 86 87 98 99 100 101 102 103 104 105 129 131 133 146 **P**1 **S** University of California–Systemwide Administration, Oakland, CA
Primary Contact: Thomas Strouse, M.D., Medical Director
COO: Ruth Irwin, Associate Director Clinical Operations
CHR: Cindy Cohen, Director Human Resources
Web address: www.semel.ucla.edu/resnick
**Control:** State–Government, nonfederal **Service:** Psychiatric

**Staffed Beds:** 74 **Admissions:** 1964 **Census:** 66 **Outpatient Visits:** 15722 **Births:** 0 **Total Expense ($000):** 44938 **Payroll Expense ($000):** 27276 **Personnel:** 295

☐ **TEMPLE COMMUNITY HOSPITAL (50111)**, 235 North Hoover Street, Zip 90004–3672; tel. 213/382–7252, (Nonreporting) **A**1 10
Primary Contact: Herbert G. Needman, President and Chief Executive Officer
CFO: John Skelton, Director Finance
CMO: Assa Weinberg, M.D., Chief of Staff
CIO: Diane Adams, Director Business Services
CHR: Leslie Beasley, Director Human Resources
Web address: www.templecommunityhospital.com
**Control:** Corporation, Investor–owned, for–profit **Service:** General Medical and Surgical

**Staffed Beds:** 130

☐ **UNIVERSITY OF SOUTHERN CALIFORNIA–NORRIS CANCER HOSPITAL (50660)**, 1441 Eastlake Avenue, Zip 90033–3804; tel. 323/865–3000, (Nonreporting) **A**1 2 3 5 9 10
Primary Contact: Scott Evans, PharmD, Chief Executive Officer
CMO: Alexandra Levine, M.D., Medical Director
CIO: David Wueste, Director Information Services
Web address: www.uscnorriscancerhospital.org
**Control:** Other not–for–profit (including NFP Corporation) **Service:** General Medical and Surgical

**Staffed Beds:** 60

**USC UNIVERSITY HOSPITAL** See Keck Hospital of USC

⊞ **VALLEY PRESBYTERIAN HOSPITAL (50126)**, 15107 Vanowen Street, Van Nuys, Zip 91405–4598; tel. 818/782–6600 **A**1 9 10 21 **F**3 13 18 20 22 24 28 29 31 34 35 40 44 45 46 49 50 53 57 59 64 65 70 72 74 75 76 77 78 79 81 85 86 87 88 89 90 96 107 108 109 113 114 118 121 122 129 144 145 146 147 **P**5
Primary Contact: Gustavo A. Valdespino, President and Chief Executive Officer
COO: Gayathri S. Jith, M.P.H., Vice President Operations
CFO: William Wilson, Interim Chief Financial Officer
CIO: Ray Moss, Vice President and Chief Information Officer
CHR: Norma Resneder, Senior Vice President Human Resources and Organizational Development
CNO: Michelle Ann Quigley, MS, Vice President and Chief Nursing Officer
Web address: www.valleypres.org
**Control:** Other not–for–profit (including NFP Corporation) **Service:** General Medical and Surgical

**Staffed Beds:** 350 **Admissions:** 16212 **Census:** 193 **Outpatient Visits:** 105077 **Births:** 4198 **Total Expense ($000):** 268137 **Payroll Expense ($000):** 103065 **Personnel:** 1543

★ △ **VETERANS AFFAIRS GREATER LOS ANGELES HEALTHCARE SYSTEM**, 11301 Wilshire Boulevard, Zip 90073–1003; tel. 310/478–3711, (Nonreporting) **A**2 5 7 8 **S** Department of Veterans Affairs, Washington, DC
Primary Contact: Donna M. Beiter, R.N., MSN, Director
COO: Lynn Carrier, Associate Director Administration and Support
CFO: Olivia Ortiz–Bitner, Acting Chief Financial Officer
CMO: Dennis Schaberg, M.D., Chief Medicine
CIO: Eugene Archey, Chief Information Technology
CHR: Harold Goings, Chief Human Resources
Web address: www.va.gov/sta/guide/home.asp
**Control:** Veterans Affairs, Government, federal **Service:** General Medical and Surgical

**Staffed Beds:** 1087

⊞ **WEST HILLS HOSPITAL AND MEDICAL CENTER (50481)**, 7300 Medical Center Drive, West Hills, Zip 91307–1910; tel. 818/676–4000 **A**1 9 10 **F**3 5 7 11 12 13 14 15 16 17 18 20 22 24 26 28 29 31 34 35 40 45 46 47 48 49 51 54 56 57 59 60 64 66 68 70 72 75 76 77 78 79 81 85 86 87 91 93 107 108 109 110 111 113 114 117 118 129 131 142 143 144 145 146 147 **S** HCA, Nashville, TN
Primary Contact: Beverly Gilmore, President and Chief Executive Officer
COO: Omar Chughtai, Vice President and Chief Operating Officer
CFO: Tony Lopez, Vice President and Chief Financial Officer
CMO: Ron Chitayat, M.D., Chief Medical Staff
CIO: Tony Lopez, Chief Financial Officer
CHR: Edward Battista, Vice President Human Resources
CNO: Janet Brooks, R.N., Vice President and Chief Nursing Officer
Web address: www.westhillshospital.com
**Control:** Corporation, Investor–owned, for–profit **Service:** General Medical and Surgical

**Staffed Beds:** 293 **Admissions:** 8100 **Census:** 116

⊞ **WEST LOS ANGELES MEDICAL CENTER (50561)**, 6041 Cadillac Avenue, Zip 90034–1702; tel. 323/857–2201, (Nonreporting) **A**1 3 5 10 **S** Kaiser Foundation Hospitals, Oakland, CA
Primary Contact: Gloria C. Blackburn, Executive Director
CFO: Alice H. Issai, Business Strategy and Finance Leader
CMO: Fred Alexander, M.D., Medical Director
CIO: Gregory M. Sincock, Information Technology Leader
Web address: www.kaiserpermanente.org
**Control:** Other not–for–profit (including NFP Corporation) **Service:** General Medical and Surgical

**Staffed Beds:** 172

☒ **WHITE MEMORIAL MEDICAL CENTER (50103)**, 1720 Cesar E Chavez Avenue, Zip 90033–2481; tel. 323/268–5000 **A**1 2 3 5 9 10 **F**3 8 11 13 15 17 18 19 20 22 24 26 27 28 29 30 31 34 35 40 45 46 47 48 49 50 51 53 56 57 58 59 64 68 70 72 74 75 76 78 79 81 82 84 85 86 87 88 89 90 91 92 93 96 98 100 102 103 107 108 109 110 111 113 114 115 116 117 118 119 120 122 127 129 130 131 142 145 146 147 **S** Adventist Health, Roseville, CA
Primary Contact: Beth D. Zachary, President and Chief Executive Officer
CFO: John Raffoul, Senior Vice President Finance
CIO: Ralf Weissenberger, Director Information Systems
CHR: Natasha Milatovich, Association Vice President Human Resources
Web address: www.whitememorial.com
**Control:** Church–operated, Nongovernment, not–for profit **Service:** General Medical and Surgical

**Staffed Beds:** 280 **Admissions:** 20017 **Census:** 255 **Total Expense ($000):** 294141

**WOMEN'S AND CHILDREN'S HOSPITAL** See LAC/University of Southern California Medical Center

☒ **WOODLAND HILLS MEDICAL CENTER (50677)**, 5601 DeSoto Avenue, Woodland Hills, Zip 91365–6701; tel. 818/719–2000 **A**1 3 5 10 **F**3 12 13 14 15 17 29 30 31 40 41 45 48 49 51 55 56 60 61 64 65 68 70 72 73 74 75 76 77 78 79 80 81 82 84 85 86 87 88 89 92 100 107 108 111 115 118 123 125 129 131 140 142 143 145 146 147 **P**6 **S** Kaiser Foundation Hospitals, Oakland, CA
Primary Contact: Catherine Casas, Executive Director
COO: Richard Trogman, FACHE, Chief Operating Officer
CFO: Marilou Cheung, Assistant Administrator Finance
CMO: Shirley Suda, M.D., Area Medical Director
CIO: David Snow, Area Information Officer
CHR: Cathy Cousineau, Director Human Resources
CNO: Nancy Tankel, R.N., Chief Nurse Executive
Web address: www.kaiserpermanente.org
**Control:** Other not–for–profit (including NFP Corporation) **Service:** General Medical and Surgical

**Staffed Beds:** 175 **Admissions:** 12084 **Census:** 138 **Outpatient Visits:** 44773 **Births:** 1541 **Personnel:** 1212

**LOS BANOS—Merced County**

☒ **MEMORIAL HOSPITAL LOS BANOS (50528)**, 520 West I Street, Zip 93635; tel. 209/826–0591, (Nonreporting) **A**1 9 10 20 **S** Sutter Health, Sacramento, CA
Primary Contact: Richard S. Liszewski, Chief Executive Officer
CFO: Timothy J. Noakes, Chief Financial Officer
CHR: Shawn Garcia, Manager Human Resources
CNO: Barbara Medeiros, R.N., Chief Nurse Executive
Web address: www.memoriallosbanos.org/
**Control:** Other not–for–profit (including NFP Corporation) **Service:** General Medical and Surgical

**Staffed Beds:** 46

**LYNWOOD—Los Angeles County**

☒ **ST. FRANCIS MEDICAL CENTER (50104)**, 3630 East Imperial Highway, Zip 90262–2636; tel. 310/900–8900, (Nonreporting) **A**1 9 10 **S** Daughters of Charity Health System, Los Altos Hills, CA
Primary Contact: Gerald T. Kozai, President
CFO: Jesse Guevara, Senior Vice President and Chief Financial Officer
CIO: Marsha Chan, PharmD, Chief Quality Officer
CHR: Laura Kato, Vice President Human Resources
Web address: www.dochs.org
**Control:** Church–operated, Nongovernment, not–for profit **Service:** General Medical and Surgical

**Staffed Beds:** 323

**MADERA—Madera County**

☐ △ **CHILDREN'S HOSPITAL CENTRAL CALIFORNIA (53300)**, 9300 Valley Children's Place, Zip 93636–8762; tel. 559/353–3000 **A**1 3 5 7 9 10 **F**3 8 9 11 19 21 23 25 27 28 29 30 31 32 34 35 36 38 39 40 41 44 46 48 50 54 55 57 58 59 60 61 62 64 65 68 72 73 74 75 77 78 79 81 82 84 85 86 87 88 89 90 93 94 97 107 108 111 113 114 118 126 128 129 130 131 142 145 146 147
Primary Contact: Todd Suntrapak, Interim Chief Executive Officer
COO: Todd Suntrapak, Executive Vice President and Chief Operating Officer
CFO: Michele Waldron, Vice President and Chief Financial Officer
CMO: David Christensen, M.D., Vice President Medical Affairs and Chief Medical Officer
CHR: Marta Boyer, Vice President Human Resources
Web address: www.childrenscentralcal.org
**Control:** Other not–for–profit (including NFP Corporation) **Service:** Children's general

**Staffed Beds:** 348 **Admissions:** 13265 **Census:** 231 **Outpatient Visits:** 201601 **Births:** 0 **Total Expense ($000):** 387368 **Payroll Expense ($000):** 156012 **Personnel:** 2337

○ **MADERA COMMUNITY HOSPITAL (50568)**, 1250 East Almond Avenue, Zip 93637–5696, Mailing Address: P.O. Box 1328, Zip 93639–1328; tel. 559/675–5501 **A**9 10 11 19 **F**3 13 29 30 31 34 35 40 45 46 47 48 49 54 62 63 64 70 75 76 77 78 79 81 82 93 107 108 110 111 113 118 126 131 145 146 147 **P**5
Primary Contact: John W. Frye, Jr., Chief Executive Officer
CFO: Mark Foote, Chief Financial Officer
CIO: Arthur Haggerty, Director Information Systems
CHR: Christine M. Watts–Johnson, Assistant Vice President
Web address: www.maderahospital.org
**Control:** Other not–for–profit (including NFP Corporation) **Service:** General Medical and Surgical

**Staffed Beds:** 106 **Admissions:** 5380 **Census:** 64 **Outpatient Visits:** 176806 **Births:** 1790 **Total Expense ($000):** 86498 **Payroll Expense ($000):** 36588 **Personnel:** 797

**MAMMOTH LAKES—Mono County**

**MAMMOTH HOSPITAL (51303)**, 85 Sierra Park Road, Zip 93546–0660, Mailing Address: P.O. Box 660, Zip 93546–0660; tel. 760/934–3311, (Nonreporting) **A**9 10 18
Primary Contact: Gary Boyd, M.P.H., Chief Executive Officer
COO: Glen Halverson, Chief Operating Officer
CFO: Melanie Van Winkle, Chief Financial Officer
CMO: Audrey Pauly, M.D., Chief of Staff
CIO: Mark Lind, Director Information Systems
CHR: Jeff Byberg, Manager Human Resources
CNO: Kathleen Alo, R.N., Chief Nursing Officer
Web address: www.mammothhospital.com
**Control:** Other not–for–profit (including NFP Corporation) **Service:** General Medical and Surgical

**Staffed Beds:** 17

**MANTECA—San Joaquin County**

☒ **DOCTORS HOSPITAL OF MANTECA (50118)**, 1205 East North Street, Zip 95336–4900; tel. 209/823–3111 **A**1 9 10 **F**3 11 13 15 29 31 34 35 40 45 49 50 51 75 76 78 79 81 85 102 107 108 110 111 114 115 117 118 129 145 146 147 **S** TENET Healthcare Corporation, Dallas, TX
Primary Contact: Mark P. Lisa, FACHE, Chief Executive Officer
COO: Carmen Silva, R.N., Chief Operating Officer
CFO: Tracy Roman, Chief Financial Officer
CHR: Traci Holzer, Director Human Resources
CNO: Patricia Pidge** Gooch, Chief Nursing Officer
Web address: www.doctorsmanteca.com
**Control:** Corporation, Investor–owned, for–profit **Service:** General Medical and Surgical

**Staffed Beds:** 73 **Admissions:** 3834 **Census:** 43 **Outpatient Visits:** 57426 **Births:** 720 **Total Expense ($000):** 61978 **Payroll Expense ($000):** 32002 **Personnel:** 370

---

⊠ **MANTECA MEDICAL CENTER (50748)**, 1777 West Yosemite Avenue, Zip 95337–5187; tel. 209/825–3500, (Includes MODESTO MEDICAL CENTER, 4601 Dale Road, Modesto, Zip 95356–9718; tel. 209/735–5000; Corwin N. Harper, Administrator), (Nonreporting) **A**1 10 **S** Kaiser Foundation Hospitals, Oakland, CA
Primary Contact: Corwin N. Harper, Senior Vice President and Area Manager
COO: Corwin N. Harper, Senior Vice President and Area Manager
CFO: Debra L. Brown, Area Financial Officer
CMO: Moses D. Elam, M.D., Physician–in–Chief
CIO: Tom J. Osteen, Director Area Technology
CHR: Pat McKeldin, Human Resource Business Partner
Web address: www.kaiserpermanente.org
**Control:** Church–operated, Nongovernment, not–for profit **Service:** General Medical and Surgical

| Staffed Beds: 146 |
| --- |

**MARINA DEL REY—Los Angeles County**

☐ **MARINA DEL REY HOSPITAL (50740)**, 4650 Lincoln Boulevard, Zip 90292–6360; tel. 310/823–8911 **A**1 9 10 **F**3 11 12 14 15 18 29 30 34 37 40 45 46 48 49 64 65 70 75 77 79 81 82 85 87 107 110 111 114 117 118 129 145 147
Primary Contact: Fred Hunter, Chief Executive Officer
COO: Phyllis Buchart, Chief Operating Officer
CFO: Stephen A. Hargett, Senior Vice President and Chief Financial Officer
Web address: www.marinahospital.com
**Control:** Corporation, Investor–owned, for–profit **Service:** General Medical and Surgical

| Staffed Beds: 90 Admissions: 4597 Census: 47 Outpatient Visits: 36643 Births: 0 Total Expense ($000): 88390 Payroll Expense ($000): 36365 Personnel: 504 |
| --- |

**MARIPOSA—Mariposa County**

★ **JOHN C. FREMONT HEALTHCARE DISTRICT (51304)**, 5189 Hospital Road, Zip 95338–9524, Mailing Address: P.O. Box 216, Zip 95338–0216; tel. 209/966–3631, (Nonreporting) **A**9 10 18
Primary Contact: David L. Hill, Chief Executive Officer
CFO: Tish Miller, Chief Financial Officer
CMO: Kenneth Smith, M.D., Chief of Staff
CIO: Joanne Eskra, Supervisor Data and Information Technology
CHR: Dawn Yesitis, Director Human Resources
CNO: Karen Gulbenkian, R.N., Director Patient Care Services
Web address: www.jcfhospital.com
**Control:** Hospital district or authority, Government, nonfederal **Service:** General Medical and Surgical

| Staffed Beds: 34 |
| --- |

**MARTINEZ—Contra Costa County**

☐ **CONTRA COSTA REGIONAL MEDICAL CENTER (50276)**, 2500 Alhambra Avenue, Zip 94553–3156; tel. 925/370–5000 **A**1 2 3 5 10 **F**3 11 13 15 30 31 36 39 40 50 52 54 56 59 61 62 64 65 66 68 70 71 72 73 74 76 77 78 79 81 85 86 87 93 97 98 100 102 103 104 107 108 111 113 118 129 131 142 145 146 147 **P**6
Primary Contact: Anna M. Roth, Chief Executive Officer
CFO: Patrick Godley, Chief Financial Officer
Web address: www.cchealth.org/medical_center/
**Control:** County–Government, nonfederal **Service:** General Medical and Surgical

| Staffed Beds: 112 Admissions: 9313 Census: 111 Outpatient Visits: 460250 Births: 2253 Total Expense ($000): 372829 Payroll Expense ($000): 139640 Personnel: 1715 |
| --- |

**KAISER FOUNDATION HOSPITAL** See Walnut Creek Medical Center, Walnut Creek

**MARYSVILLE—Yuba County**

⊠ **FREMONT–RIDEOUT HEALTH GROUP (50133)**, 726 Fourth Street, Zip 95901–5600; tel. 530/749–4300, (Includes FREMONT MEDICAL CENTER, 970 Plumas Street, Yuba City, Zip 95991–4087; tel. 530/751–4000) **A**1 2 9 10 **F**3 8 11 13 15 17 18 19 20 22 24 26 28 29 30 31 40 43 45 46 49 51 54 56 57 60 64 70 72 74 75 76 77 78 79 81 82 85 87 89 93 107 108 110 111 114 118 119 120 129 131 143 144 145 147 **P**7
Primary Contact: Theresa Hamilton, Chief Executive Officer
CMO: Robert Plass, M.D., Chief Medical Officer
CIO: Tarun Ghosh, Chief Information Officer
CHR: Tresha Moreland, Vice President Human Resources
Web address: www.frhg.org
**Control:** Other not–for–profit (including NFP Corporation) **Service:** General Medical and Surgical

| Staffed Beds: 212 Admissions: 11834 Census: 139 Outpatient Visits: 147992 Births: 2134 Total Expense ($000): 226881 Payroll Expense ($000): 70052 Personnel: 1516 |
| --- |

**MENLO PARK—San Mateo County**

⊠ **MENLO PARK SURGICAL HOSPITAL (50754)**, 570 Willow Road, Zip 94025–2617; tel. 650/324–8500, (Nonreporting) **A**1 5 9 10 **S** Sutter Health, Sacramento, CA
Primary Contact: Kathleen Palange, R.N., Chief Executive Officer
CMO: Andrew Gutow, M.D., Medical Director
Web address: www.pamf.org/mpsh
**Control:** Other not–for–profit (including NFP Corporation) **Service:** General Medical and Surgical

| Staffed Beds: 16 |
| --- |

**MERCED—Merced County**

⊠ **MERCY MEDICAL CENTER MERCED (50444)**, 333 Mercy Avenue, Zip 95340–8319; tel. 209/564–5000, (Includes MERCY MEDICAL CENTER MERCED–COMMUNITY CAMPUS, 301 East 13th Street, Zip 95340–6211; tel. 209/385–7000; MERCY MEDICAL CENTER MERCED–DOMINICAN CAMPUS, 2740 M Street, Zip 95340–2880; tel. 209/384–6444; David S. Dunham, President) **A**1 3 5 9 10 19 **F**3 8 13 15 18 20 28 29 30 33 34 35 40 45 46 50 57 62 64 66 68 70 74 75 76 77 78 79 81 84 85 86 87 91 92 93 97 107 108 109 110 111 113 118 120 122 129 131 145 147 **S** Dignity Health, San Francisco, CA
Primary Contact: David S. Dunham, President
CFO: Doreen Hartmann, Vice President and Chief Financial Officer
CMO: Robert Streeter, M.D., Vice President Medical Affairs
CIO: Noel Lee, Administrative Director and Chief Information Officer
CHR: Joe Lombardi, Vice President Human Resources
Web address: www.mercymercedcares.org
**Control:** Church–operated, Nongovernment, not–for profit **Service:** General Medical and Surgical

| Staffed Beds: 186 Admissions: 12029 Census: 140 Outpatient Visits: 137611 Births: 2811 Total Expense ($000): 235855 Payroll Expense ($000): 92831 Personnel: 1221 |
| --- |

**MISSION HILLS—Los Angeles County, See Los Angeles**

**MISSION VIEJO—Orange County**

☐ **CHILDREN'S HOSPITAL AT MISSION (53306)**, 27700 Medical Center Road, Zip 92691–6426; tel. 949/364–1400 **A**1 9 10 **F**3 11 36 72 74 79 81 85 88 89 145
Primary Contact: Kimberly C. Cripe, President and Chief Executive Officer
COO: Debra Mathias, Chief Operating Officer
CFO: Kerri Ruppert Schiller, Senior Vice President and Chief Financial Officer
CMO: Maria Minon, M.D., Vice President Medical Affairs and Chief Medical Officer
CIO: Mark Headland, Chief Information Officer
CHR: Susan M. Burrows, Vice President Human Resources
CNO: Louise White, R.N., Vice President Patient Care Services and Chief Nursing Officer
Web address: www.choc.org
**Control:** Other not–for–profit (including NFP Corporation) **Service:** Children's general

| Staffed Beds: 48 Admissions: 1923 Census: 25 Outpatient Visits: 26514 Births: 0 Total Expense ($000): 48522 Payroll Expense ($000): 8382 Personnel: 94 |
| --- |

⊠ △ **MISSION HOSPITAL (50567)**, 27700 Medical Center Road, Zip 92691–6426; tel. 949/364–1400, (Includes MISSION HOSPITAL LAGUNA BEACH, 31872 Coast Highway, Laguna Beach, Zip 92651–6775; tel. 949/499–1311) **A**1 2 7 9 10 **F**3 4 5 8 11 13 14 15 17 18 20 22 24 26 28 29 30 31 34 35 36 40 43 44 45 46 47 48 49 50 53 54 57 58 59 64 65 66 68 70 74 75 76 77 78 79 80 81 82 84 85 86 87 90 92 93 96 98 100 101 104 105 107 108 110 111 113 114 115 116 117 118 119 120 122 123 125 128 129 130 131 133 134 140 142 144 145 146 147 **P**3 5 **S** St. Joseph Health, Orange, CA
Primary Contact: Kenneth McFarland, President and Chief Executive Officer
COO: Markie Cowley, Executive Vice President and Chief Operating Officer
CMO: Dennis Haghighat, M.D., Vice President Medical Affairs
CIO: Cindy Emerson, Director Information Services
CHR: Shirley A. Barnes, Senior Vice President and Chief Human Resources Officer
Web address: www.mission4health.com
**Control:** Church–operated, Nongovernment, not–for profit **Service:** General Medical and Surgical

| Staffed Beds: 407 Admissions: 22225 Census: 259 Outpatient Visits: 175309 Births: 3094 Total Expense ($000): 436048 Payroll Expense ($000): 143313 Personnel: 1996 |
| --- |

*Many Facility Codes have changed. Please refer to the AHA Guide Code Chart.* © 2012 AHA Guide

CA

## MODESTO—Stanislaus County

⊠ **DOCTORS MEDICAL CENTER (50464)**, 1441 Florida Avenue, Zip 95350–4418, Mailing Address: P.O. Box 4138, Zip 95352–4138; tel. 209/578–1211 **A**1 2 9 10 **F**3 13 17 18 20 22 24 26 28 29 31 35 40 41 43 45 46 48 49 50 51 55 57 59 60 65 70 72 74 75 76 77 78 79 80 81 85 89 98 102 103 107 108 109 110 111 112 113 114 115 116 117 118 125 129 131 145 146 **P**4 **S** TENET Healthcare Corporation, Dallas, TX
Primary Contact: Warren J. Kirk, Chief Executive Officer
COO: Mike King, Chief Operating Officer
CFO: Greg Berry, Chief Financial Officer
CMO: Eric Ramos, M.D., Chief Medical Officer
CIO: Debbie Fuller, Director Health Information Systems and Chief Information Officer
CHR: Michele West, Director Human Resources
Web address: www.dmc-modesto.com
**Control:** Corporation, Investor–owned, for–profit **Service:** General Medical and Surgical

**Staffed Beds:** 441 **Admissions:** 21131 **Census:** 287 **Outpatient Visits:** 96719 **Births:** 3598 **Total Expense ($000):** 349815 **Payroll Expense ($000):** 177486 **Personnel:** 1829

⊠ **MEMORIAL MEDICAL CENTER (50557)**, 1700 Coffee Road, Zip 95355–2869, Mailing Address: P.O. Box 942, Zip 95353–0942; tel. 209/526–4500, (Includes MEMORIAL MEDICAL CENTER, 1700 Coffee Road, Zip 95355, Mailing Address: Box 942, Zip 95353; tel. 209/526–4500) **A**1 2 9 10 **F**8 11 12 13 15 18 20 22 24 28 29 30 31 34 35 40 43 57 59 60 62 70 73 74 75 76 77 78 79 81 82 85 86 89 107 108 111 113 114 117 118 119 120 123 129 145 147 **S** Sutter Health, Sacramento, CA
Primary Contact: James E. Conforti, Chief Executive Officer
COO: Steve Mitchell, Chief Operating Officer
CFO: Eric Dalton, Chief Financial Officer
CIO: Patrick Anderson, Chief Information Officer
CHR: Paula Rafala, Director, Human Resources
CNO: Sandra Proctor, R.N., Chief Nurse Executive
Web address: www.memorialmedicalcenter.org
**Control:** Other not–for–profit (including NFP Corporation) **Service:** General Medical and Surgical

**Staffed Beds:** 417 **Admissions:** 19954 **Census:** 264 **Outpatient Visits:** 110281 **Births:** 2005 **Total Expense ($000):** 479287 **Payroll Expense ($000):** 168433 **Personnel:** 2501

**MODESTO MEDICAL CENTER** See Manteca Medical Center, Manteca

**STANISLAUS SURGICAL HOSPITAL (50726)**, 1421 Oakdale Road, Zip 95355–3359; tel. 209/572–2700, (Nonreporting) **A**5 9 10
Primary Contact: Douglas V. Johnson, Chief Executive Officer
CMO: Harvey Palitz, M.D., Chief of Staff
CHR: Laura Boyles, Director Human Resources
Web address: www.stanislaussurgical.com
**Control:** Individual, Investor–owned, for–profit **Service:** General Medical and Surgical

**Staffed Beds:** 23

## MONROVIA—Los Angeles County

○ **MONROVIA MEMORIAL HOSPITAL (52054)**, 323 South Heliotrope Avenue, Zip 91016–2914; tel. 626/408–9800, (Nonreporting) **A**10 11
Primary Contact: Ron Kupferstein, Chief Executive Officer
Web address: www.monroviamemorial.com
**Control:** Partnership, Investor–owned, for–profit **Service:** Long–Term Acute Care hospital

**Staffed Beds:** 49

## MONTCLAIR—San Bernardino County

☐ **MONTCLAIR HOSPITAL MEDICAL CENTER (50758)**, 5000 San Bernardino Street, Zip 91763–2326; tel. 909/625–5411, (Nonreporting) **A**1 10 **S** Prime Healthcare Services, Ontario, CA
Primary Contact: Gregory Brentano, Chief Executive Officer
Web address: www.dhmcm.com
**Control:** Corporation, Investor–owned, for–profit **Service:** General Medical and Surgical

**Staffed Beds:** 102

## MONTEBELLO—Los Angeles County

**BEVERLY HOSPITAL (50350)**, 309 West Beverly Boulevard, Zip 90640–4308; tel. 323/726–1222, (Nonreporting) **A**9 10 21
Primary Contact: Gary V. Kiff, President and Chief Executive Officer
CFO: Narci Egan, Vice President and Chief Financial Officer
CIO: Ronnie O. Cobarrubias, Director Information Systems
Web address: www.beverly.org
**Control:** Other not–for–profit (including NFP Corporation) **Service:** General Medical and Surgical

**Staffed Beds:** 102

## MONTEREY—Monterey County

⊠ **COMMUNITY HOSPITAL OF THE MONTEREY PENINSULA (50145)**, 23625 Holman Highway, Zip 93962–6032, Mailing Address: Box 'HH', Zip 93942–6032; tel. 831/624–5311, (Total facility includes 28 beds in nursing home–type unit) **A**1 2 9 10 **F**3 5 11 12 13 14 15 17 18 20 22 24 26 28 29 30 31 34 35 37 40 44 45 46 47 48 49 50 51 53 54 57 58 59 60 61 62 63 64 68 70 73 74 75 76 77 78 79 81 82 84 85 86 87 89 91 92 93 94 96 98 99 100 101 102 103 104 105 107 108 109 110 111 113 114 115 116 117 118 119 120 122 123 127 128 129 131 133 134 144 145 147 **P**7
Primary Contact: Steven J. Packer, M.D., President and Chief Executive Officer
CFO: Laura Zehm, Vice President and Chief Financial Officer
CMO: Anthony D. Chavis, M.D., Vice President Medical Affairs and Patient Safety Officer
CIO: Tom McNamara, Director Information Technology
CHR: Joanne Webster, Director Human Resources
Web address: www.chomp.org
**Control:** Other not–for–profit (including NFP Corporation) **Service:** General Medical and Surgical

**Staffed Beds:** 235 **Admissions:** 12698 **Census:** 166 **Outpatient Visits:** 270477 **Births:** 1274 **Total Expense ($000):** 356879 **Payroll Expense ($000):** 140013 **Personnel:** 1587

## MONTEREY PARK—Los Angeles County

☐ **GARFIELD MEDICAL CENTER (50737)**, 525 North Garfield Avenue, Zip 91754–1205; tel. 626/573–2222 **A**1 9 10 12 13 **F**3 11 13 15 17 18 20 22 24 26 28 29 31 34 35 40 44 45 49 50 56 57 59 60 64 68 70 72 74 75 76 77 78 79 81 82 85 86 87 90 91 92 93 107 108 118 129 131 142 145 146 147 **P**5 **S** AHMC & Healthcare, Inc., Alhambra, CA
Primary Contact: David J. Batista, Chief Executive Officer
COO: David J. Batista, Chief Operating Officer
CFO: Steve Maekawa, Chief Financial Officer
CMO: Terry Lee, M.D., Chief of Staff
CIO: Ann Curnutt, Director Information Systems
CHR: Rebecca R. Ricartti, Interim Director Human Resources
CNO: Shirley Tang, R.N., Chief Nursing Officer
Web address: www.garfieldmedicalcenter.com
**Control:** Partnership, Investor–owned, for–profit **Service:** General Medical and Surgical

**Staffed Beds:** 210 **Admissions:** 12094 **Census:** 164 **Outpatient Visits:** 31061 **Births:** 3418 **Personnel:** 1070

☐ **MONTEREY PARK HOSPITAL (50736)**, 900 South Atlantic Boulevard, Zip 91754–4780; tel. 626/570–9000 **A**1 9 10 **F**3 15 29 34 35 40 49 50 57 59 60 70 75 76 81 86 87 89 107 113 118 129 141 142 145 **S** AHMC & Healthcare, Inc., Alhambra, CA
Primary Contact: Philip A. Cohen, Chief Executive Officer
COO: Ericka Smith, Chief Operating Officer
CFO: Daniel Song, Chief Financial Officer
CMO: Shawn Adhami, M.D., Chief of Staff
CIO: Ann Curnutt, Director Information Systems
CHR: Margaret Ettenheim, Director Human Resources
CNO: Evelyn Ku, Chief Nursing Officer
Web address: www.montereyparkhosp.com
**Control:** Partnership, Investor–owned, for–profit **Service:** General Medical and Surgical

**Staffed Beds:** 101 **Admissions:** 4916 **Census:** 45 **Outpatient Visits:** 19453 **Births:** 1667 **Total Expense ($000):** 67682 **Payroll Expense ($000):** 19493 **Personnel:** 306

## MORENO VALLEY—Riverside County

⊠ **MORENO VALLEY COMMUNITY HOSPITAL (50765)**, 27300 Iris Avenue, Zip 92555–4800; tel. 951/243–0811, (Nonreporting) **A**1 10 **S** Kaiser Foundation Hospitals, Oakland, CA
Primary Contact: Corey A. Seale, Administrator
CFO: Michael Garko, Chief Financial Officer
**Control:** Hospital district or authority, Government, nonfederal **Service:** General Medical and Surgical

**Staffed Beds:** 72

---

**Hospital, Medicare Provider Number, Address, Telephone, Approval, Facility, and Physician Codes, Health Care System**

★ American Hospital Association (AHA) membership
☐ The Joint Commission accreditation ◇ DNV Healthcare Inc. accreditation
○ American Osteopathic Association (AOA) accreditation
△ Commission on Accreditation of Rehabilitation Facilities (CARF) accreditation

**CA**

☒ **RIVERSIDE COUNTY REGIONAL MEDICAL CENTER (50292)**, 26520 Cactus Avenue, Zip 92555–3911; tel. 951/486–4000 **A**1 3 5 10 12 13 **F**3 8 11 13 15 29 30 31 32 35 39 40 43 44 47 49 50 56 57 58 59 60 64 65 66 68 70 71 72 74 75 77 78 79 81 82 85 87 88 93 97 98 100 107 108 111 113 117 118 129 134 142 145 146 147
Primary Contact: Douglas D. Bagley, Chief Executive Officer
COO: Ellie Bennett, Chief Operating Officer
CFO: David Runke, Chief Financial Officer
CMO: Arnold Tabuenca, M.D., Medical Director
Web address: www.rcrmc.org
**Control:** County–Government, nonfederal **Service:** General Medical and Surgical

**Staffed Beds:** 415 **Admissions:** 21443 **Census:** 324 **Outpatient Visits:** 263560 **Births:** 2539 **Total Expense ($000):** 389154 **Payroll Expense ($000):** 166331 **Personnel:** 2674

**MOUNT SHASTA—Siskiyou County**

☒ **MERCY MEDICAL CENTER MOUNT SHASTA (51319)**, 914 Pine Street, Zip 96067–2143; tel. 530/926–6111 **A**1 9 10 18 **F**3 11 13 15 29 30 31 35 40 43 50 53 56 57 59 62 63 64 68 70 72 75 76 77 79 81 82 84 93 107 108 111 113 117 118 120 126 129 130 131 132 142 145 147 **S** Dignity Health, San Francisco, CA
Primary Contact: Kenneth E. S. Platou, President
CFO: Tim Panks, Chief Financial Officer
CMO: Jill Schenk, M.D., Chief of Staff
CHR: Gary Blevins, Director Human Resources
Web address: www.mercymtshasta.org
**Control:** Other not–for–profit (including NFP Corporation) **Service:** General Medical and Surgical

**Staffed Beds:** 33 **Admissions:** 1224 **Census:** 9 **Outpatient Visits:** 45391 **Births:** 134 **Total Expense ($000):** 44790 **Payroll Expense ($000):** 19162 **Personnel:** 219

**MOUNTAIN VIEW—Santa Clara County**

☒ **EL CAMINO HOSPITAL (50308)**, 2500 Grant Road, Zip 94040, Mailing Address: P.O. Box 7025, Zip 94039–7025; tel. 650/940–7000, (Includes EL CAMINO HOSPITAL LOS GATOS, 815 Pollard Road, Los Gatos, Zip 95032–1438; tel. 408/378–6131) **A**1 9 10 **F**3 8 11 12 13 15 17 18 20 22 24 28 29 30 31 34 35 36 38 40 46 50 51 53 54 55 56 57 58 59 60 64 65 68 70 72 74 75 76 77 78 79 81 82 83 84 86 87 89 90 93 98 101 102 103 104 105 107 108 110 111 112 113 114 116 117 118 119 120 122 123 125 129 131 132 134 142 144 145 146
Primary Contact: Tomi S. Ryba, President and Chief Executive Officer
CFO: Michael King, Chief Financial Officer
CMO: Eric Pifer, M.D., Chief Medical Officer
CIO: Greg Walton, Chief Information Officer
CHR: Charlene Gliniecki, Vice President Human Resources
Web address: www.elcaminohospital.org
**Control:** Hospital district or authority, Government, nonfederal **Service:** General Medical and Surgical

**Staffed Beds:** 394 **Admissions:** 18927 **Census:** 224 **Outpatient Visits:** 789468 **Births:** 4877 **Total Expense ($000):** 523178 **Payroll Expense ($000):** 196381 **Personnel:** 1732

**MURRIETA—Riverside County**

**LOMA LINDA UNIVERSITY MEDICAL CENTER–MURRIETA (50770)**, 28062 Baxter Road, Zip 92563; tel. 951/290–4000, (Nonreporting) **S** Loma Linda University Adventist Health Sciences Center, Loma Linda, CA
Primary Contact: Richard L. Rawson, Chief Executive Officer
COO: Richard M. Tibbits, Vice President and Chief Operating Officer
CFO: Doug Loop, Vice President Finance and Chief Financial Officer
CMO: Jeff Conner, M.D., Chief Medical Staff
Web address: www.llumcmurrieta.org
**Control:** Other not–for–profit (including NFP Corporation) **Service:** General Medical and Surgical

**Staffed Beds:** 106

☐ **RANCHO SPRINGS MEDICAL CENTER (50701)**, 25500 Medical Center Drive, Zip 92562–5965; tel. 951/696–6000, (Nonreporting) **A**1 9 10 **S** Universal Health Services, Inc., King of Prussia, PA
Primary Contact: Kenneth I. Rivers, Chief Executive Officer
COO: Jared Giles, Chief Operating Officer
CFO: Diane Moon, Chief Financial Officer
CMO: Timothy Killeen, M.D., Chief of Staff
CIO: Tura Heckler, Director Information Services
CHR: Laura Culbertson, Director Human Resources
CNO: Anne Marie Watkins, R.N., Chief Nursing Officer
Web address: www.swhcs.com
**Control:** Corporation, Investor–owned, for–profit **Service:** General Medical and Surgical

**Staffed Beds:** 51

**NAPA—Napa County**

☐ **NAPA STATE HOSPITAL (54122)**, 2100 Napa–Vallejo Highway, Zip 94558–6293; tel. 707/253–5000 **A**1 3 5 10 **F**30 39 53 56 59 61 67 68 77 86 98 103 127 129 131 134 145 **P**6
Primary Contact: Dolly Matteucci, Interim Executive Director
COO: Dolly Matteucci, Interim Executive Director
Web address: www.dmh.ca.gov
**Control:** State–Government, nonfederal **Service:** Psychiatric

**Staffed Beds:** 1229 **Admissions:** 583 **Census:** 1149 **Outpatient Visits:** 0 **Births:** 0 **Total Expense ($000):** 255683 **Payroll Expense ($000):** 164517 **Personnel:** 2141

☒ **QUEEN OF THE VALLEY MEDICAL CENTER (50009)**, 1000 Trancas Street, Zip 94558–2906, Mailing Address: P.O. Box 2340, Zip 94558–2340; tel. 707/252–4411 **A**1 2 9 10 **F**3 8 11 13 15 17 18 20 22 24 26 28 29 30 31 32 34 35 39 40 43 44 45 46 47 48 49 50 51 53 57 59 60 61 64 68 70 72 75 76 77 78 79 81 82 84 85 86 87 89 90 91 92 93 97 102 107 108 110 111 113 114 115 116 117 118 119 120 122 123 125 129 131 134 142 145 147 **S** St. Joseph Health, Orange, CA
Primary Contact: Walt Mickens, President and Chief Executive Officer
CFO: Donald Miller, Vice President and Chief Financial Officer
CMO: Vincent Morgese, M.D., Vice President Medical Affairs
CHR: Ron Scott, Vice President Human Resources
Web address: www.thequeen.org
**Control:** Church–operated, Nongovernment, not–for profit **Service:** General Medical and Surgical

**Staffed Beds:** 174 **Admissions:** 7981 **Census:** 105 **Outpatient Visits:** 208114 **Births:** 867 **Total Expense ($000):** 246650 **Payroll Expense ($000):** 91772 **Personnel:** 1142

**NATIONAL CITY—San Diego County**

☐ △ **PARADISE VALLEY HOSPITAL (50024)**, 2400 East Fourth Street, Zip 91950–2099; tel. 619/470–4321, (Nonreporting) **A**1 7 10 **S** Prime Healthcare Services, Ontario, CA
Primary Contact: Luis Leon, Regional Chief Executive Officer
CFO: Janet L. Caceres, Chief Financial Officer
CMO: Genaro Fernandez, M.D., Chief of Staff
CIO: Amanda Kaems, Manager Information Systems
CHR: Lorraine Villegas, Manager Human Resources
Web address: www.paradisevalleyhospital.org
**Control:** Corporation, Investor–owned, for–profit **Service:** General Medical and Surgical

**Staffed Beds:** 205

**NEEDLES—San Bernardino County**

**COLORADO RIVER MEDICAL CENTER (51323)**, 1401 Bailey Avenue, Zip 92363–3103; tel. 760/326–4531, (Nonreporting) **A**9 10 18
Primary Contact: Mark H. Uffer, Chief Executive Officer
CIO: Ron Chieffo, Chief Information Officer
**Control:** Corporation, Investor–owned, for–profit **Service:** General Medical and Surgical

**Staffed Beds:** 25

**NEWPORT BEACH—Orange County**

★ **HOAG MEMORIAL HOSPITAL PRESBYTERIAN (50224)**, One Hoag Drive, Zip 92663–4120, Mailing Address: P.O. Box 6100, Zip 92658–6100; tel. 949/764–4624 **A**2 9 10 21 **F**3 4 5 11 13 14 15 17 18 20 22 24 26 28 29 30 31 34 35 36 37 40 44 45 46 47 48 49 50 51 54 55 57 58 59 60 64 68 70 71 72 74 75 76 77 78 79 81 82 84 85 86 87 92 93 96 100 102 103 107 108 110 111 113 114 115 116 117 118 119 120 122 123 125 128 129 131 134 140 142 144 145 146 147 **P**5
Primary Contact: Richard Afable, M.D., M.P.H., President and Chief Executive Officer
COO: Robert Braithwaite, Senior Vice President and Chief Operating Officer
CFO: Jennifer C. Mitzner, Senior Vice President Finance and Chief Financial Officer
CMO: Jack Cox, M.D., Senior Vice President and Chief Quality Officer
CIO: Tim Moore, R.N., Senior Vice President and Chief Information Officer
CHR: Jan L. Blue, Vice President Human Resources
CNO: Richard A. Martin, MSN, Senior Vice President and Chief Nursing Officer
Web address: www.hoaghospital.org
**Control:** Other not–for–profit (including NFP Corporation) **Service:** General Medical and Surgical

**Staffed Beds:** 451 **Admissions:** 26045 **Census:** 314 **Outpatient Visits:** 373732 **Births:** 6016 **Total Expense ($000):** 811538 **Payroll Expense ($000):** 269752 **Personnel:** 4120

**NEWPORT BAY HOSPITAL (54135)**, 1501 East 16th Street, Zip 92663–5924; tel. 949/650–9750, (Nonreporting) **A**10
Primary Contact: James E. Parkhurst, President and Chief Executive Officer
COO: Garry Hardwick, R.N., Chief Operating Officer
CFO: Rocky Gentner, Chief Financial Officer
CMO: Jason Kellogg, M.D., Chief of Staff
CIO: Nina Swenson, Director Business Services
CHR: Phyllis Parkhurst, Vice President Support Services
Web address: www.newportbayhospital.com
**Control:** Corporation, Investor–owned, for–profit **Service:** Psychiatric

**Staffed Beds:** 34

---

**NORTH HOLLYWOOD—Los Angeles County, See Los Angeles**

**NORTHRIDGE—Los Angeles County, See Los Angeles**

**NORWALK—Los Angeles County**

**COAST PLAZA DOCTORS HOSPITAL** See Coast Plaza Hospital

☐ ○ **COAST PLAZA HOSPITAL (50771)**, 13100 Studebaker Road, Zip 90650–2531; tel. 562/868–3751, (Nonreporting) **A**1 10 11 **S** Avanti Hospitals, El Segundo, CA
Primary Contact: John J. Ferrelli, Chief Executive Officer
CFO: Mihi Lee, Chief Financial Officer
CMO: Galal S. Gough, M.D., Chief of Staff
CIO: Linda K. Roman, Administrator
Web address: www.coastplaza.com
**Control:** Partnership, Investor–owned, for–profit **Service:** General Medical and Surgical

**Staffed Beds:** 123

**LOS ANGELES COMMUNITY HOSPITAL OF NORWALK** See Los Angeles Community Hospital, Los Angeles

☐ **METROPOLITAN STATE HOSPITAL (54133)**, 11401 Bloomfield Avenue, Zip 90650; tel. 562/863–7011, (Nonreporting) **A**1 10
Primary Contact: Sharon Smith–Nevins, Executive Director
CFO: Maybelle Manlagnit, Senior Accounting Officer
CMO: Michael Barsom, M.D., Medical Director
CIO: Paul Mello, Manager Data Processing
CHR: Eddie Park, Acting Director Human Resources
Web address: www.dmh.cahwnet.gov/statehospitals/metro
**Control:** State–Government, nonfederal **Service:** Psychiatric

**Staffed Beds:** 657

---

**NOVATO—Marin County**

★ **NOVATO COMMUNITY HOSPITAL (50131)**, 180 Rowland Way, Zip 94945–5009, Mailing Address: P.O. Box 1108, Zip 94948–1108; tel. 415/209–1300, (Nonreporting) **A**9 10 **S** Sutter Health, Sacramento, CA
Primary Contact: Anne L. Hosfeld, Chief Administrative Officer
CMO: Barbara Nylund, M.D., Chief of Staff
CIO: Kathryn Graham, Director Communications and Community Relations
CHR: Diana G. Johnson, Acting Chief Human Resources Officer
Web address: www.novatocommunity.sutterhealth.org
**Control:** Other not–for–profit (including NFP Corporation) **Service:** General Medical and Surgical

**Staffed Beds:** 47

---

**OAKDALE—Stanislaus County**

⊠ **OAK VALLEY HOSPITAL DISTRICT (50067)**, 350 South Oak Street, Zip 95361–3519; tel. 209/847–3011, (Nonreporting) **A**1 9 10 **S** Dignity Health, San Francisco, CA
Primary Contact: John P. Friel, Chief Executive Officer
CFO: John McCormick, Chief Financial Officer
CMO: Krystyna Belski, M.D., Chief of Staff
CIO: Sherry Peral, Manager Information Systems
CHR: Kim Bukhari, Manager Human Resources
Web address: www.oakvalleycares.org
**Control:** Church–operated, Nongovernment, not–for profit **Service:** General Medical and Surgical

**Staffed Beds:** 150

---

**OAKLAND—Alameda County**

⊠ **ALAMEDA COUNTY MEDICAL CENTER (50320)**, 1411 East 31st Street, Zip 94602–1018; tel. 510/437–4800, (Includes ALAMEDA COUNTY MEDICAL CENTER–FAIRMONT CAMPUS, 15400 Foothill Boulevard, San Leandro, Zip 94578–1009; tel. 510/895–4200) **A**1 3 5 10 **F**3 5 11 13 15 18 20 22 28 29 30 31 32 34 35 36 38 39 40 42 43 44 45 46 49 50 54 56 57 58 59 60 61 64 65 66 68 70 73 74 75 76 77 78 79 81 82 84 85 86 87 90 92 93 94 96 97 98 100 101 102 104 105 107 111 113 114 118 127 129 131 133 134 142 143 145 146 147 **P**6
Primary Contact: Wright L. Lassiter, III, Chief Executive Officer
COO: Bill Manns, Chief Operating Officer
CFO: Marion Schales, Chief Financial Officer
CMO: Sang–ick Chang, M.D., Chief Medical Officer
CIO: Mark Zielazinski, Chief Information Officer
CHR: Jeanette Louden–Corbett, Chief Human Resources Officer
Web address: www.acmedctr.org
**Control:** Hospital district or authority, Government, nonfederal **Service:** General Medical and Surgical

**Staffed Beds:** 387 **Admissions:** 13649 **Census:** 316 **Outpatient Visits:** 382406 **Births:** 1154 **Total Expense ($000):** 428486 **Payroll Expense ($000):** 231548 **Personnel:** 2423

⊠ **ALTA BATES SUMMIT MEDICAL CENTER – SUMMIT CAMPUS (50043)**, 350 Hawthorne Avenue, Zip 94609–3100; tel. 510/655–4000 **A**1 2 9 10 **F**3 8 11 12 15 17 18 20 22 24 26 29 30 31 34 35 36 40 46 47 49 56 57 58 59 60 61 64 68 70 74 75 77 78 79 81 82 84 85 86 87 97 107 108 113 118 119 120 121 122 125 127 129 131 134 145 147 **P**3 **S** Sutter Health, Sacramento, CA
Primary Contact: David Bradley, Chief Executive Officer
CFO: Robert Petrina, Chief Financial Officer
CMO: John Gentile, M.D., Vice President Medical Affairs
CHR: Mark Beiting, Vice President Human Resources
Web address: www.altabatessummit.com
**Control:** Other not–for–profit (including NFP Corporation) **Service:** General Medical and Surgical

**Staffed Beds:** 414 **Admissions:** 14102 **Census:** 219 **Outpatient Visits:** 140171 **Total Expense ($000):** 389345 **Payroll Expense ($000):** 178960

☐ **CHILDREN'S HOSPITAL AND RESEARCH CENTER AT OAKLAND (53301)**, 747 52nd Street, Zip 94609–1809; tel. 510/428–3000, (Nonreporting) **A**1 3 5 9 10
Primary Contact: Bertram Lubin, M.D., President and Chief Executive Officer
CFO: Doug Myers, Senior Vice President and Chief Financial Officer
CIO: Don Livsey, Vice President and Chief Information Officer
Web address: www.childrenshospitaloakland.org
**Control:** Other not–for–profit (including NFP Corporation) **Service:** Children's general

**Staffed Beds:** 190

⊠ **OAKLAND MEDICAL CENTER (50075)**, 280 West MacArthur Boulevard, Zip 94611–5693; tel. 510/752–1000, (Includes RICHMOND MEDICAL CENTER, 901 Nevin Avenue, Richmond, Zip 94801–2555; tel. 510/307–1500), (Nonreporting) **A**1 3 5 8 10 **S** Kaiser Foundation Hospitals, Oakland, CA
Primary Contact: Nathaniel L. Oubre, Jr., Senior Vice President and Area Manager
CFO: Dennis Morris, Area Finance Officer
CMO: John Loftus, M.D., Chief of Staff
CIO: Johnny Law, Area Information Officer
CHR: Rick Mead, Human Resources Leader
CNO: Charlene Boyer, Chief Nursing Officer
Web address: www.kaiserpermanente.org
**Control:** Other not–for–profit (including NFP Corporation) **Service:** General Medical and Surgical

**Staffed Beds:** 341

☐ **TELECARE HERITAGE PSYCHIATRIC HEALTH CENTER (54146)**, 2633 East 27th Street, Zip 94601–1912; tel. 510/535–5115, (Nonreporting) **A**1 9 10
Primary Contact: Linda Reese, Administrator
Web address: www.tbhcare.com/
**Control:** Partnership, Investor–owned, for–profit **Service:** Psychiatric

**Staffed Beds:** 26

---

**OCEANSIDE—San Diego County**

⊠ **TRI-CITY MEDICAL CENTER (50128)**, 4002 Vista Way, Zip 92056–4506; tel. 760/724–8411, (Nonreporting) **A**1 2 5 9 10
Primary Contact: Larry B. Anderson, Chief Executive Officer
COO: Casey Fatch, Chief Operating Officer
CFO: Alex Yu, Chief Financial Officer
CIO: Mark Facuri, Director Information Systems
Web address: www.tricitymed.org
**Control:** Hospital district or authority, Government, nonfederal **Service:** General Medical and Surgical

**Staffed Beds:** 330

---

**Hospital, Medicare Provider Number, Address, Telephone, Approval, Facility, and Physician Codes, Health Care System**

★ American Hospital Association (AHA) membership
☐ The Joint Commission accreditation
◇ DNV Healthcare Inc. accreditation
○ American Osteopathic Association (AOA) accreditation
△ Commission on Accreditation of Rehabilitation Facilities (CARF) accreditation

**CA**

### ONTARIO—San Bernardino County

☒ **KINDRED HOSPITAL–ONTARIO (52037)**, 550 North Monterey Avenue, Zip 91764–3399; tel. 909/391–0333, (Nonreporting) **A**1 9 10 **S** Kindred Healthcare, Louisville, KY
Primary Contact: Robin Rapp, MS, R.N., Chief Executive Officer
CFO: Omar Oregel, Controller
CMO: Marc Lynch, D.O., Chief of Staff
CHR: Laurel Scharber, Administrative Assistant and Coordinator Human Resources
CNO: Holly Ramos, R.N., Chief Clinical Officer
Web address: www.khontario.com/
**Control:** Corporation, Investor–owned, for–profit **Service:** General Medical and Surgical

**Staffed Beds: 91**

### ORANGE—Orange County

☐ **CHAPMAN MEDICAL CENTER (50745)**, 2601 East Chapman Avenue, Zip 92869–3206; tel. 714/633–0011, (Nonreporting) **A**1 9 10 **S** Integrated Healthcare, Santa Ana, CA
Primary Contact: Don Kreitz, Chief Executive Officer
COO: Ada Yeh, R.N., Chief Operating Officer and Chief Nursing Officer
CFO: Ray Rivas, Chief Financial Officer
CMO: Steven Duckor, M.D., Chief of Staff
CIO: Nova Stewart, Chief Information Officer
CHR: JoAnne Suehs, Manager Human Resources
Web address: www.chapmanmedicalcenter.com
**Control:** Corporation, Investor–owned, for–profit **Service:** General Medical and Surgical

**Staffed Beds: 100**

☐ **CHILDREN'S HOSPITAL OF ORANGE COUNTY (53304)**, 455 South Main Street, Zip 92868–3835, Mailing Address: PO Box 5700, Zip 92863–5700; tel. 714/997–3000 **A**1 3 5 9 10 **F**3 5 6 9 11 17 19 21 23 25 27 29 30 31 34 35 50 55 57 58 59 61 64 65 66 68 71 72 74 75 77 78 79 81 85 86 87 88 89 91 92 93 97 104 125 128 129 131 133 135 145 **P**5
Primary Contact: Kimberly C. Cripe, President and Chief Executive Officer
COO: Debra Mathias, Chief Operating Officer
CFO: Kerri Ruppert Schiller, Senior Vice President and Chief Financial Officer
CMO: Maria Minon, M.D., Vice President Medical Affairs and Chief Medical Officer
CIO: Mark Headland, Chief Information Officer
CHR: Susan M. Burrows, Vice President Human Resources
CNO: Louise White, R.N., Vice President Patient Care Services and Chief Nursing Officer
Web address: www.choc.org
**Control:** Other not–for–profit (including NFP Corporation) **Service:** Children's general

**Staffed Beds: 238 Admissions: 11810 Census: 163 Outpatient Visits: 212959 Total Expense ($000): 430536 Payroll Expense ($000): 120070 Personnel: 2066**

☐ **HEALTHBRIDGE CHILDRENS REHABILITATION HOSPITAL (53308)**, 393 South Tustin Street, Zip 92868; tel. 714/289–2400 **A**1 9 10 **F**64 65 75 77 90 93 127 129 131 145 **S** Nexus Health Systems, Houston, TX
Primary Contact: Ronell Myburgh, Administrator
Web address: www.nhsltd.com/HealthBridge–Orange/Default.htm
**Control:** Partnership, Investor–owned, for–profit **Service:** Children's general

**Staffed Beds: 27 Admissions: 330 Census: 26 Outpatient Visits: 0 Births: 0**

☒ **ST. JOSEPH HOSPITAL (50069)**, 1100 West Stewart Drive, Zip 92863–5600, Mailing Address: P.O. Box 5600, Zip 92863–5600; tel. 714/633–9111 **A**1 2 5 9 10 **F**3 5 8 11 12 13 14 15 17 18 19 20 21 22 23 24 25 26 27 28 29 30 31 34 35 39 40 41 45 46 47 49 50 51 54 57 58 59 60 64 65 66 68 69 70 71 74 75 76 77 78 79 80 81 82 84 85 86 87 91 92 93 98 100 102 103 104 105 106 107 108 110 111 113 114 115 116 117 118 120 122 123 125 128 129 130 131 134 137 140 145 146 147 **P**3 5 **S** St. Joseph Health, Orange, CA
Primary Contact: Steven C. Moreau, Chief Executive Officer
CFO: Tina Mycroft, Vice President and Chief Financial Officer
CMO: Raymond Casciari, M.D., Chief Medical Officer
CIO: Tina Mycroft, Vice President and Chief Financial Officer
CHR: Mary P. Leahy, Vice President Human Resources
Web address: www.sjo.org
**Control:** Other not–for–profit (including NFP Corporation) **Service:** General Medical and Surgical

**Staffed Beds: 379 Admissions: 20316 Census: 212 Outpatient Visits: 291875 Births: 5050 Total Expense ($000): 619759 Payroll Expense ($000): 198633 Personnel: 3255**

☒ **UNIVERSITY OF CALIFORNIA, IRVINE HEALTHCARE (50348)**, 101 The City Drive, Zip 92868–3298; tel. 714/456–6011 **A**1 2 3 5 8 9 10 **F**3 6 9 11 12 13 14 15 16 17 18 19 20 21 22 24 26 28 29 30 31 32 34 35 36 37 39 40 41 43 44 45 46 47 48 49 50 51 54 55 56 57 58 59 60 61 64 65 66 68 70 71 72 74 75 76 77 79 80 81 83 86 87 90 91 92 93 94 96 97 98 99 100 101 102 103 104 105 107 108 110 111 112 113 114 115 116 117 118 119 120 122 123 125 129 131 133 134 137 140 141 144 145 146 147 **S** University of California–Systemwide Administration, Oakland, CA
Primary Contact: Terry A. Belmont, Chief Executive Officer
COO: Alice H. Issai, Chief Operating Officer
CFO: Morris J. Frieling, Chief Financial Officer
CMO: Bill Barron, M.D., Chief Medical Officer
CIO: Jim Murry, Chief Information Officer
CHR: Julie Molleston, Executive Director Human Resources and Customer Services
CNO: Karen A. Grimley, R.N., Chief Nursing Officer
Web address: www.ucihealth.com
**Control:** State–Government, nonfederal **Service:** General Medical and Surgical

**Staffed Beds: 363 Admissions: 16365 Census: 281 Outpatient Visits: 510070 Births: 1135 Total Expense ($000): 611121 Payroll Expense ($000): 270017 Personnel: 3891**

### OROVILLE—Butte County

**OROVILLE HOSPITAL (50030)**, 2767 Olive Highway, Zip 95966–6118; tel. 530/533–8500, (Total facility includes 20 beds in nursing home–type unit) **A**9 10 **F**3 11 13 15 16 26 28 29 30 31 32 33 34 35 38 39 40 41 43 44 45 46 47 49 50 51 54 56 57 59 60 61 62 64 65 66 68 70 74 75 76 78 79 81 82 84 85 86 87 93 94 96 97 107 108 110 111 114 115 116 117 118 126 127 128 129 131 143 145 146 147
Primary Contact: Robert J. Wentz, President and Chief Executive Officer
COO: Scott Chapple, Chief Operating Officer
CFO: Ashok Khanchandani, Chief Financial Officer
CMO: Mark T. Heinrich, D.O., President Medical Staff
CIO: Denise LeFevre, Chief Information Officer
CHR: Scott Chapple, Chief Operating Officer
Web address: www.orovillehospital.com
**Control:** Other not–for–profit (including NFP Corporation) **Service:** General Medical and Surgical

**Staffed Beds: 133 Admissions: 9767 Census: 99 Outpatient Visits: 287635 Births: 440 Total Expense ($000): 133823 Payroll Expense ($000): 58906 Personnel: 1040**

### OXNARD—Ventura County

☒ **ST. JOHN'S REGIONAL MEDICAL CENTER (50082)**, 1600 North Rose Avenue, Zip 93030–3723; tel. 805/988–2500, (Nonreporting) **A**1 9 10 **S** Dignity Health, San Francisco, CA
Primary Contact: Laurie Eberst, R.N., President and Chief Executive Officer
COO: Kim A. Wilson, R.N., Chief Operating Officer
CFO: Robert D. Wardwell, Chief Financial Officer
CMO: Eugene Fussell, M.D., Chief Medical Officer
CIO: Jeff Perry, Director Information Technology
CHR: Ed Gonzales, Vice President Human Resources
CNO: Gudrun Moll, R.N., Chief Nursing Officer
Web address: www.stjohnshealth.org
**Control:** Other not–for–profit (including NFP Corporation) **Service:** General Medical and Surgical

**Staffed Beds: 266**

### PALM SPRINGS—Riverside County

☒ **DESERT REGIONAL MEDICAL CENTER (50243)**, 1150 North Indian Canyon Drive, Zip 92262–4872, Mailing Address: P.O. Box 2739, Zip 92263–2739; tel. 760/323–6511, (Total facility includes 30 beds in nursing home–type unit) **A**1 2 9 10 **F**3 12 13 14 15 17 18 20 22 24 26 28 29 30 31 34 35 40 43 45 46 47 48 49 51 52 53 54 55 57 58 59 60 61 62 63 64 65 68 70 72 74 75 76 77 78 79 81 82 83 84 85 86 87 89 90 92 93 94 100 102 107 108 109 110 111 113 114 115 116 118 119 123 125 127 129 130 131 145 146 147 **S** TENET Healthcare Corporation, Dallas, TX
Primary Contact: Karolee M. Sowle, R.N., MSN, FACHE, Chief Executive Officer
COO: Ken Wheat, Chief Operating Officer
CFO: Richard Phillips, Chief Financial Officer
Web address: www.desertmedctr.com
**Control:** Individual, Investor–owned, for–profit **Service:** General Medical and Surgical

**Staffed Beds: 387 Admissions: 17563 Census: 212 Outpatient Visits: 161057 Births: 3353 Personnel: 1497**

*Many Facility Codes have changed. Please refer to the AHA Guide Code Chart.* © 2012 AHA Guide

**PALMDALE—Los Angeles County**

☐ **PALMDALE REGIONAL MEDICAL CENTER (50204)**, 38600 Medical Center Drive, Zip 93551–4483; tel. 661/382–5000 **A**1 9 10 **F**3 8 11 12 18 20 24 26 29 30 40 45 46 47 49 50 51 64 68 70 77 79 81 85 87 93 107 108 111 113 114 118 129 140 145 147 **S** Universal Health Services, Inc., King of Prussia, PA
Primary Contact: Larry Coomes, Chief Executive Officer
COO: Karen Faulis, Chief Operating Officer
CFO: Kurt Broten, Chief Financial Officer
CIO: Roy Singleton, Director Computer Information Systems
CHR: Karen Hickling, Director Human Resources
CNO: Pat McClendon, MSN, Chief Nursing Officer
Web address: www.palmdaleregional.com
**Control:** Corporation, Investor–owned, for–profit **Service:** General Medical and Surgical

**Staffed Beds:** 157 **Admissions:** 7690 **Census:** 91 **Outpatient Visits:** 67214 **Births:** 0 **Total Expense ($000):** 118084 **Payroll Expense ($000):** 42792 **Personnel:** 588

**PALO ALTO—Santa Clara County**

☒ **LUCILE SALTER PACKARD CHILDREN'S HOSPITAL AT STANFORD (53305)**, 725 Welch Road, Zip 94304–1601; tel. 650/497–8000 **A**1 3 5 9 10 **F**3 11 12 13 17 19 25 27 28 29 30 31 32 34 35 36 38 44 45 46 47 48 49 50 54 55 57 58 59 60 61 64 65 66 68 71 72 73 74 75 76 77 78 79 80 81 82 84 85 86 87 88 89 91 92 93 96 97 99 100 104 107 111 114 118 125 128 129 130 131 133 135 136 137 138 139 140 141 143 144 145 147 **S** Stanford Health Care, Palo Alto, CA
Primary Contact: Christopher G. Dawes, President and Chief Executive Officer
COO: Susan Flanagan, Chief Operating Officer
CFO: Timothy W. Carmack, Chief Financial Officer
CMO: Kenneth Cox, M.D., Chief Medical Officer
CIO: James McCaughey, Chief Strategy Officer
CHR: Greg Souza, Vice President Human Resources
Web address: www.lpch.org
**Control:** Other not–for–profit (including NFP Corporation) **Service:** Children's general

**Staffed Beds:** 302 **Admissions:** 12799 **Census:** 222 **Outpatient Visits:** 143179 **Births:** 4373 **Total Expense ($000):** 698823 **Payroll Expense ($000):** 231001 **Personnel:** 2491

☒ **STANFORD HOSPITAL AND CLINICS (50441)**, 1520 Page Mill Road, Zip 94304–1125; tel. 650/723–4000 **A**1 2 3 5 8 9 10 **F**3 4 6 7 8 9 11 12 14 15 17 18 19 20 21 22 23 24 25 26 27 28 29 30 31 34 35 36 37 38 39 40 41 43 44 45 46 47 48 49 50 51 52 54 55 56 57 58 59 60 61 63 64 66 67 68 70 74 75 77 78 79 81 82 84 85 86 87 90 91 92 93 94 95 96 97 98 100 101 102 103 104 107 108 110 111 113 114 115 116 117 118 119 120 122 123 125 128 129 130 131 134 135 136 137 138 139 140 141 142 144 145 146 147 **P**6 **S** Stanford Health Care, Palo Alto, CA
Primary Contact: Amir Dan Rubin, President and Chief Executive Officer
COO: Margaret Vosburgh, Chief Operating Officer
CFO: Daniel Morrissette, Chief Financial Officer
CMO: Norman Rizk, M.D., Interim Chief Medical Officer
CIO: Carolyn Byerly, Chief Information Officer
CHR: Dale A. Spartz, Vice President Human Resources
CNO: Nancy Lee, R.N., Vice President Patient Care Services and Chief Nursing Officer
Web address: www.stanfordhospital.com/
**Control:** Other not–for–profit (including NFP Corporation) **Service:** General Medical and Surgical

**Staffed Beds:** 477 **Admissions:** 24970 **Census:** 377 **Outpatient Visits:** 902975 **Births:** 0 **Total Expense ($000):** 1921876 **Payroll Expense ($000):** 585042 **Personnel:** 6781

☒ △ **VETERANS AFFAIRS PALO ALTO HEALTH CARE SYSTEM**, 3801 Miranda Avenue, Zip 94304–1207; tel. 650/493–5000, (Includes PALO ALTO DIVISION, 3801 Miranda Avenue, tel. 650/493–5000; VETERANS AFFAIRS PALO ALTO HEALTH CARE SYSTEM, LIVERMORE DIVISION, 4951 Arroyo Road, tel. 510/447–2560) **A**1 2 3 5 7 8 **F**1 2 3 4 5 6 8 9 10 11 12 14 15 20 22 24 26 28 29 30 31 34 35 36 38 39 40 43 44 45 46 47 48 49 50 51 53 54 56 57 58 59 60 61 62 63 64 65 66 70 71 74 75 77 78 79 80 81 82 83 84 85 86 87 90 91 93 94 95 96 97 98 100 101 102 103 104 105 106 107 108 111 113 114 115 116 117 118 124 125 126 128 129 131 134 136 142 143 145 146 147 **P**6 **S** Department of Veterans Affairs, Washington, DC
Primary Contact: Elizabeth Joyce Freeman, Director
COO: Joanne Krumberger, Associate Director
CFO: Mel Niese, Chief Fiscal Service
CMO: Lawrence Leung, M.D., Chief of Staff
CIO: Doug Wirthgen, Chief Information Officer
CHR: Lori Peery, Chief Human Resource Management Services
Web address: www.va.gov/sta/guide/home.asp
**Control:** Veterans Affairs, Government, federal **Service:** General Medical and Surgical

**Staffed Beds:** 808 **Admissions:** 6502 **Census:** 606 **Outpatient Visits:** 958881 **Births:** 0

**PANORAMA CITY—Los Angeles County, See Los Angeles**

**PARADISE—Butte County**

☒ **FEATHER RIVER HOSPITAL (50225)**, 5974 Pentz Road, Zip 95969–5509; tel. 530/877–9361, (Nonreporting) **A**1 2 9 10 **S** Adventist Health, Roseville, CA
Primary Contact: Kevin R. Erich, President and Chief Executive Officer
CFO: Dan Gordon, Chief Financial Officer
CMO: Anthony Nasr, M.D., Chief Medical Staff
CIO: Dan Gordon, Chief Financial Officer
CHR: Denton Gruzensky, Director Human Resources
Web address: www.frhosp.org
**Control:** Church–operated, Nongovernment, not–for profit **Service:** General Medical and Surgical

**Staffed Beds:** 54

**PARAMOUNT—Los Angeles County**

☐ **PROMISE HOSPITAL OF EAST LOS ANGELES, SUBURBAN MEDICAL CENTER CAMPUS**, 16453 South Colorado Avenue, Zip 90723–5000; tel. 562/531–3110, (Nonreporting) **A**1 9 **S** Promise Healthcare, Boca Raton, FL
Primary Contact: Richard Luna, Chief Executive Officer
COO: Cynthia Duque, R.N., Chief Operating Officer
CMO: Mojtaba Sabahi, M.D., Chief of Staff
CIO: Jim Wilson, Vice President Information Technology
CHR: Sylvia Munoz, Director Human Resources
Web address: www.promiseeastla.com
**Control:** Corporation, Investor–owned, for–profit **Service:** General Medical and Surgical

**Staffed Beds:** 182

**PASADENA—Los Angeles County**

☐ **AURORA LAS ENCINAS HOSPITAL (54078)**, 2900 East Del Mar Boulevard, Zip 91107–4399; tel. 626/795–9901, (Nonreporting) **A**1 9 10 **S** Aurora Behavioral Health Care, Corona, CA
Primary Contact: Gerard Conway, Chief Executive Officer
COO: Steven Hytry, Chief Operating Officer
CFO: Tim Sides, Chief Financial Officer
CMO: Daniel Suzuki, M.D., Medical Director
CIO: Eric Kim, Chief Information Officer
CHR: Veronica Herrera, Director Human Resources
Web address: www.lasencinashospital.com
**Control:** Corporation, Investor–owned, for–profit **Service:** Psychiatric

**Staffed Beds:** 138

**CA**

---

**Hospital, Medicare Provider Number, Address, Telephone, Approval, Facility, and Physician Codes, Health Care System**

★ American Hospital Association (AHA) membership
☐ The Joint Commission accreditation
◇ DNV Healthcare Inc. accreditation
○ American Osteopathic Association (AOA) accreditation
△ Commission on Accreditation of Rehabilitation Facilities (CARF) accreditation

⌘ **HUNTINGTON MEMORIAL HOSPITAL (50438)**, 100 West California Boulevard, Zip 91105–3097, Mailing Address: P.O. Box 7013, Zip 91109–7013; tel. 626/397–5000 **A**1 2 3 5 9 10 **F**3 4 5 8 11 12 13 14 15 18 20 22 24 26 28 29 30 31 34 35 37 40 41 43 44 45 46 47 48 49 50 51 53 56 58 59 60 61 63 64 65 66 68 70 72 74 75 76 77 78 79 81 82 84 86 87 88 89 90 92 93 97 98 100 101 102 103 104 105 106 107 108 111 113 114 117 118 119 120 122 125 128 129 131 145 146 147 **P**3 5 7
Primary Contact: Stephen A. Ralph, President and Chief Executive Officer
CFO: James S. Noble, Senior Vice President Finance and Chief Financial Officer
CMO: Paula Verrette, M.D., Vice President Quality and Performance Improvement and Chief Medical Officer
CIO: Debbie Tafoya, Vice President and Chief Information Officer
CHR: Debbie Ortega, Chief Human Resource Officer and Vice President Administrative Services
CNO: Bonnie Kass, Chief Nursing Officer and Vice President Patient Care and Support Services
Web address: www.huntingtonhospital.com
**Control:** Other not–for–profit (including NFP Corporation) **Service:** General Medical and Surgical

**Staffed Beds: 540 Admissions: 27895 Census: 352 Outpatient Visits: 294681 Births: 3223 Total Expense ($000): 486674 Payroll Expense ($000): 187409 Personnel: 3604**

### PATTON—San Bernardino County

☐ **PATTON STATE HOSPITAL**, 3102 East Highland Avenue, Zip 92369; tel. 909/425–7000 **A**1 **F**3 29 30 39 53 57 58 59 61 65 74 75 77 86 87 98 100 101 103 129 131 134 142 145 **P**1
Primary Contact: Octavio C. Luna, Executive Director
CFO: Kathleen Gamble, Fiscal Officer
CMO: George Christison, M.D., Medical Director
CIO: Cindy Barrett, Administrative Assistant
CHR: Nancy Varela, Director Human Resources
Web address: www.dmh.cahwnet.gov/statehospitals/patton
**Control:** State–Government, nonfederal **Service:** Psychiatric

**Staffed Beds: 1517 Admissions: 986 Census: 1490 Births: 0 Total Expense ($000): 312355 Payroll Expense ($000): 199552**

### PERRIS—Riverside County

★ ○ **KINDRED HOSPITAL OF RIVERSIDE (52052)**, 2224 Medical Center Drive, Zip 92571; tel. 951/436–3535, (Nonreporting) **A**10 11 **S** Kindred Healthcare, Louisville, KY
Primary Contact: James Linhares, Administrator
COO: Bennie Montgomery, R.N., Chief Nursing Officer and Chief Operations Officer
CFO: Paul Smith, Chief Financial Officer
Web address: www.khriverside.com
**Control:** Corporation, Investor–owned, for–profit **Service:** Long–Term Acute Care hospital

**Staffed Beds: 40**

### PETALUMA—Sonoma County

⌘ **PETALUMA VALLEY HOSPITAL (50136)**, 400 North McDowell Boulevard, Zip 94954–2369; tel. 707/778–1111 **A**1 9 10 **F**3 11 13 15 29 30 34 35 40 44 45 46 49 50 51 57 60 63 64 68 69 70 75 76 77 78 79 81 82 84 85 86 87 93 97 107 108 111 114 118 129 145 147 **S** St. Joseph Health, Orange, CA
Primary Contact: Kevin Klockenga, President and Chief Executive Officer
CFO: Mich Riccioni, Chief Financial Officer
CMO: Gary Greensweig, D.O., Chief Medical Officer
CIO: Patrick Wylie, Director Information Systems
CHR: Debra Miller, Senior Vice President Human Resources
Web address: www.stjosephhealth.org/petalumavalley
**Control:** Other not–for–profit (including NFP Corporation) **Service:** General Medical and Surgical

**Staffed Beds: 29 Admissions: 2812 Census: 26 Outpatient Visits: 55892 Births: 464 Total Expense ($000): 76082 Payroll Expense ($000): 30289 Personnel: 329**

### PLACENTIA—Orange County

⌘ **PLACENTIA–LINDA HOSPITAL (50589)**, 1301 North Rose Drive, Zip 92870–3899; tel. 714/993–2000 **A**1 9 10 **F**3 11 12 15 17 29 30 31 34 40 45 46 47 48 49 57 59 65 70 75 79 81 82 85 87 93 107 108 111 117 118 129 130 131 134 144 145 **P**5 **S** TENET Healthcare Corporation, Dallas, TX
Primary Contact: Kent G. Clayton, President and Chief Executive Officer
COO: Pat Swaller, R.N., Chief Operating Officer
CFO: Kristi Liberatore, Chief Financial Officer
CMO: David Petreccia, M.D., Physician Advisor
CIO: Freddie T. Sanchez, Director Information Systems
CHR: Diane Worthington, Director Human Resources
CNO: Judy Chabot, R.N., Chief Nursing Officer
Web address: www.placentialinda.com
**Control:** Corporation, Investor–owned, for–profit **Service:** General Medical and Surgical

**Staffed Beds: 114 Admissions: 3788 Census: 33 Outpatient Visits: 49328 Births: 1 Total Expense ($000): 60168 Payroll Expense ($000): 28181 Personnel: 356**

### PLACERVILLE—El Dorado County

⌘ **MARSHALL MEDICAL CENTER (50254)**, 1100 Marshall Way, Zip 95667–6599; tel. 530/622–1441, (Nonreporting) **A**1 2 9 10
Primary Contact: James Whipple, Administrator and Chief Executive Officer
CFO: Laurie Eldridge, Chief Financial Officer
CMO: Rene Orona, M.D., Chief of Staff
CIO: Mike Jones, Director Information Services
CHR: Scott Comer, Director Administrative Services
Web address: www.marshallmedical.org
**Control:** Other not–for–profit (including NFP Corporation) **Service:** General Medical and Surgical

**Staffed Beds: 105**

### PLEASANTON—Alameda County

⌘ **VALLEYCARE MEDICAL CENTER (50283)**, 5555 West Las Positas Boulevard, Zip 94588–4000; tel. 925/847–3000, (Includes VALLEY MEMORIAL, 1111 East Stanley Boulevard, Livermore, Zip 94550–4115; tel. 925/447–7000), (Total facility includes 26 beds in nursing home–type unit) **A**1 2 9 10 **F**3 8 11 12 13 15 17 18 20 22 24 26 28 29 30 31 32 34 35 40 45 46 48 49 50 53 54 56 57 59 64 65 69 70 71 73 74 75 76 77 78 79 81 84 85 86 87 89 93 96 98 103 107 108 110 111 113 118 127 128 129 130 131 132 143 144 145 146 147 **P**3
Primary Contact: Marcy L. Feit, President and Chief Executive Officer
COO: Cindy Noonan, Chief Operating Officer
CFO: Ken Jensen, Chief Financial Officer
CMO: Dat Nguyen, M.D., Chief of Staff
CIO: Bob Woods, Chief Information Officer
CHR: Chris Faber, Human Resources Analyst
Web address: www.valleycare.com
**Control:** Other not–for–profit (including NFP Corporation) **Service:** General Medical and Surgical

**Staffed Beds: 207 Admissions: 7744 Census: 116 Outpatient Visits: 176133 Births: 1295 Total Expense ($000): 198237 Payroll Expense ($000): 100191 Personnel: 1138**

### POMONA—Los Angeles County

⌘ △ **CASA COLINA HOSPITAL FOR REHABILITATIVE MEDICINE (53027)**, 255 East Bonita Avenue, Zip 91767–1923, Mailing Address: P.O. Box 6001, Zip 91769–6001; tel. 909/596–7733 **A**1 7 9 10 **F**3 9 29 30 34 35 56 59 60 64 65 68 74 75 79 82 90 91 92 93 96 129 130 131 145 147
Primary Contact: Felice L. Loverso, Ph.D., President and Chief Executive Officer
CFO: David Morony, Chief Financial Officer
CMO: Christopher Chalian, M.D., Medical Director
CIO: Ross Lesins, Chief Information Officer
CHR: Karen Du Pont, Director Human Resources
CNO: Kathryn Johnson, Chief Nursing Officer
Web address: www.casacolina.org
**Control:** Other not–for–profit (including NFP Corporation) **Service:** Rehabilitation

**Staffed Beds: 68 Admissions: 1252 Census: 59 Outpatient Visits: 63184 Births: 0 Personnel: 359**

**LANTERMAN DEVELOPMENTAL CENTER (50545)**, 3530 Pomona Boulevard, Zip 91768–3238, Mailing Address: P.O. Box 100, Zip 91769–0100; tel. 909/444–7200, (Nonreporting) **A**10
Primary Contact: Cheryl Bright, Executive Director
COO: Ignacio Pina, Director Administrative Services
CFO: Rosie Flores–Ramirez, Director Fiscal Services
CMO: Hao Nguyen, M.D., Medical Director
CIO: George Oliva, Associate Information Systems Analyst
CHR: Mark Kaufman, Director Human Resources
Web address: www.dds.ca.gov
**Control:** State–Government, nonfederal **Service:** Hospital unit within an institution for the mentally retarded

**Staffed Beds: 481**

⌘ **POMONA VALLEY HOSPITAL MEDICAL CENTER (50231)**, 1798 North Garey Avenue, Zip 91767–2918; tel. 909/865–9500 **A**1 2 3 5 9 10 **F**3 11 13 15 17 18 20 22 24 26 28 29 30 31 34 35 40 45 47 49 50 51 53 54 55 57 58 59 60 61 63 64 66 68 69 70 72 74 75 76 77 78 79 81 84 85 89 92 93 107 108 110 111 113 114 115 116 117 118 119 120 122 123 125 127 128 129 130 131 134 143 144 145 146 147 **P**5
Primary Contact: Richard E. Yochum, President and Chief Executive Officer
COO: Kurt Weinmeister, Executive Vice President and Chief Operating Officer
CFO: Michael Nelson, Executive Vice President and Chief Financial Officer
CMO: Kenneth Nakamoto, M.D., Vice President Medical Affairs
CIO: Kent Hoyos, Chief Information Officer
CHR: Ray Inge, Vice President Human Resources
Web address: www.pvhmc.org
**Control:** Other not–for–profit (including NFP Corporation) **Service:** General Medical and Surgical

**Staffed Beds: 453 Admissions: 21688 Census: 271 Outpatient Visits: 439212 Births: 6869**

*Many Facility Codes have changed. Please refer to the AHA Guide Code Chart.* © 2012 AHA Guide

CA

## PORTERVILLE—Tulare County

**PORTERVILLE DEVELOPMENTAL CENTER (50546)**, 26501 Avenue 140, Zip 93257–9109, Mailing Address: P.O. Box 2000, Zip 93258–2000; tel. 559/782–2222, (Nonreporting) **A**10
Primary Contact: John Sawyer, Executive Director
COO: Larry Harris, Director Administrative Services
CFO: Karen Warren, Fiscal Officer
CMO: Rajachandran Srinivasan, M.D., Medical Director
CIO: Vincent Chandler, Director Information Services
CHR: Roger Wright, Director Human Resources
Web address: www.pdc.dds.ca.gov
**Control:** State–Government, nonfederal **Service:** Institution for mental retardation

**Staffed Beds:** 758

☐ **SIERRA VIEW DISTRICT HOSPITAL (50261)**, 465 West Putnam Avenue, Zip 93257–3320; tel. 559/784–1110, (Total facility includes 35 beds in nursing home–type unit) **A**1 9 10 **F**3 13 15 29 30 31 34 35 40 45 47 49 54 57 59 60 65 68 70 75 76 78 79 81 85 87 89 93 107 108 110 111 114 118 120 122 129 131 134 145 146 147
Primary Contact: Joseph A. Stewart, President and Chief Executive Officer
CFO: Douglas Dickson, Senior Vice President Finance
CIO: Kevin Shimamoto, Director Information Technology
CHR: Sharon Brown, Director Human Resources
Web address: www.sierra-view.com
**Control:** Hospital district or authority, Government, nonfederal **Service:** General Medical and Surgical

**Staffed Beds:** 151 **Admissions:** 7687 **Census:** 121 **Outpatient Visits:** 151372 **Births:** 1899 **Total Expense ($000):** 105759 **Payroll Expense ($000):** 47944 **Personnel:** 887

## PORTOLA—Plumas County

★ **EASTERN PLUMAS HEALTH CARE DISTRICT (51300)**, 500 First Avenue, Zip 96122–9406; tel. 530/832–6500, (Total facility includes 66 beds in nursing home–type unit) **A**9 10 18 **F**7 11 15 18 33 34 39 40 45 57 59 64 68 74 77 79 81 82 87 100 107 111 113 118 126 127 132 134
Primary Contact: Thomas P. Hayes, Chief Executive Officer
COO: Teresa L. Whitfield, MS, Director Quality and Outcomes
CFO: Jeri Nelson, Chief Financial Officer
CMO: Eric Bugna, M.D., Chief of Staff
CHR: Cathy Conant, Chief Human Resources and Personnel
Web address: www.ephc.org
**Control:** Hospital district or authority, Government, nonfederal **Service:** General Medical and Surgical

**Staffed Beds:** 75 **Admissions:** 537 **Census:** 58 **Outpatient Visits:** 42712 **Births:** 0 **Total Expense ($000):** 21243 **Payroll Expense ($000):** 9869 **Personnel:** 249

## POWAY—San Diego County

⊞ **POMERADO HOSPITAL (50636)**, 15615 Pomerado Road, Zip 92064–2460; tel. 858/613–4000, (Nonreporting) **A**1 9 10 **S** Palomar Health, San Diego, CA
Primary Contact: David A. Tam, M.D., FACHE, Chief Administrative Officer
CFO: Robert Hemker, Chief Financial Officer
CIO: Steven Tanaka, Chief Information Officer
CHR: Brenda C. Turner, Chief Human Resources Officer
Web address: www.pph.org
**Control:** Hospital district or authority, Government, nonfederal **Service:** General Medical and Surgical

**Staffed Beds:** 107

## QUINCY—Plumas County

☐ **PLUMAS DISTRICT HOSPITAL (51326)**, 1065 Bucks Lake Road, Zip 95971–9599; tel. 530/283–2121 **A**1 9 10 18 **F**3 7 13 15 18 19 30 32 39 40 45 57 61 64 68 75 79 81 82 85 107 111 113 118 126
Primary Contact: Douglas L. Lafferty, Chief Executive Officer
CMO: Vincent Frantz, M.D., Chief of Staff
CIO: Brenda Compton, Manager Information Technology
CHR: Denise Harding, Director Human Resources
Web address: www.pdh.org
**Control:** Hospital district or authority, Government, nonfederal **Service:** General Medical and Surgical

**Staffed Beds:** 25 **Admissions:** 488 **Census:** 4 **Outpatient Visits:** 99337 **Births:** 88 **Total Expense ($000):** 19843 **Payroll Expense ($000):** 9199 **Personnel:** 158

## RANCHO CUCAMONGA—San Bernardino County

★ ○ **KINDRED HOSPITAL RANCHO (52049)**, 10841 White Oak Avenue, Zip 91730–3811; tel. 909/581–6400, (Nonreporting) **A**9 10 11 **S** Kindred Healthcare, Louisville, KY
Primary Contact: Jody Knox, Administrator
Web address: www.khrancho.com
**Control:** Corporation, Investor–owned, for–profit **Service:** Long–Term Acute Care hospital

**Staffed Beds:** 55

## RANCHO MIRAGE—Riverside County

⊞ **EISENHOWER MEDICAL CENTER (50573)**, 39000 Bob Hope Drive, Zip 92270–3221; tel. 760/340–3911 **A**1 2 5 9 10 **F**2 3 9 11 12 15 17 18 20 22 24 26 28 29 30 31 34 35 37 40 41 45 47 49 50 53 54 56 57 59 60 61 64 65 68 70 74 75 77 78 79 81 82 85 86 87 89 90 93 96 97 98 100 101 102 103 107 108 109 110 111 112 113 114 115 116 118 119 120 122 123 125 128 129 130 131 134 143 144 145 146 147 **P**4 5 6
Primary Contact: G. Aubrey Serfling, President and Chief Executive Officer
COO: Martin Massiello, Senior Vice President and Chief Operating Officer
CFO: Kimberly Osborne, Vice President and Chief Financial Officer
CMO: Quinten VanderWerf, M.D., Chief Medical Officer
CIO: David Perez, Chief Information Officer
CHR: Liz Guignier, Vice President Human Resources
Web address: www.emc.org
**Control:** Other not–for–profit (including NFP Corporation) **Service:** General Medical and Surgical

**Staffed Beds:** 540 **Admissions:** 17922 **Census:** 210 **Outpatient Visits:** 72118 **Births:** 0 **Total Expense ($000):** 412071 **Payroll Expense ($000):** 148004 **Personnel:** 2206

## RED BLUFF—Tehama County

⊞ **ST. ELIZABETH COMMUNITY HOSPITAL (50042)**, 2550 Sister Mary Columba Drive, Zip 96080–4397; tel. 530/529–8000 **A**1 9 10 20 **F**3 7 11 13 15 29 30 32 35 40 43 45 51 54 57 62 63 64 68 70 75 76 81 82 84 85 89 93 107 108 110 111 113 118 129 130 131 132 144 145 147 **P**3 **S** Dignity Health, San Francisco, CA
Primary Contact: Jon W. Halfhide, President
CFO: Tim Panks, Chief Financial Officer
CMO: James DeSoto, M.D., Vice President Medical Affairs
CIO: Henry Niessink, Senior Manager Information Technology Systems
CHR: Dena Platz, Director Human Resources
Web address: www.mercy.org
**Control:** Church–operated, Nongovernment, not–for profit **Service:** General Medical and Surgical

**Staffed Beds:** 65 **Admissions:** 3283 **Census:** 25 **Outpatient Visits:** 61462 **Births:** 699 **Total Expense ($000):** 72910 **Payroll Expense ($000):** 32140 **Personnel:** 381

## REDDING—Shasta County

⊞ **MERCY MEDICAL CENTER REDDING (50280)**, 2175 Rosaline Avenue, Zip 96001–2509, Mailing Address: P.O. Box 496009, Zip 96049–6009; tel. 530/225–6000 **A**1 2 3 5 9 10 **F**2 3 7 11 13 15 17 18 20 22 24 28 29 30 31 34 35 37 40 43 45 46 47 48 49 50 54 57 59 61 62 63 64 66 68 70 72 75 76 77 78 79 81 82 84 85 89 91 97 107 108 111 113 114 117 118 129 131 134 142 143 144 145 146 147 **S** Dignity Health, San Francisco, CA
Primary Contact: Mark Korth, Chief Executive Officer
COO: Patrick Varga, Chief Operating Officer
CFO: Tim Panks, Regional Vice President Finance and Chief Financial Officer
CMO: James DeSoto, M.D., Vice President Medical Affairs
CIO: Henry Niessink, Regional Director Information Technology Services
CHR: Steve Hosler, Regional Vice President Human Resources
CNO: Andrea Kofl, Vice President Patient Care and Chief Nursing Executive
Web address: www.mercy.org
**Control:** Church–operated, Nongovernment, not–for profit **Service:** General Medical and Surgical

**Staffed Beds:** 261 **Admissions:** 14233 **Census:** 156 **Outpatient Visits:** 134074 **Births:** 2026 **Total Expense ($000):** 328454 **Payroll Expense ($000):** 122659 **Personnel:** 1378

---

**Hospital, Medicare Provider Number, Address, Telephone, Approval, Facility, and Physician Codes, Health Care System**

★ American Hospital Association (AHA) membership
☐ The Joint Commission accreditation   ◇ DNV Healthcare Inc. accreditation
○ American Osteopathic Association (AOA) accreditation
△ Commission on Accreditation of Rehabilitation Facilities (CARF) accreditation

**CA**

☐ **NORTHERN CALIFORNIA REHABILITATION HOSPITAL (52047)**, 2801 Eureka Way, Zip 96001; tel. 530/246–9000, (Nonreporting) **A**1 9 10 **S** Vibra Healthcare, Mechanicsburg, PA
Primary Contact: Chris Jones, Chief Executive Officer
COO: Lisa Stevens, Chief Clinical Officer and Chief Operating Officer
CFO: Rebecca Andrews, Chief Financial Officer
CMO: Nanda Kumar, M.D., Chief of Staff
CIO: Mark Cardenas, Director Plant Operations
CHR: Wendy Tempest, Director Human Resources
Web address: www.norcalrehab.com
**Control:** Corporation, Investor–owned, for–profit **Service:** Rehabilitation

**Staffed Beds:** 88

**PATIENTS' HOSPITAL OF REDDING (50697)**, 2900 Eureka Way, Zip 96001; tel. 530/225–8700 **A**9 10 **F**81 82 85
Primary Contact: Shari Lejsek, Administrator
CMO: James Tate, M.D., Chief of Staff
CIO: Kim Cameron, Manager Health Information Services
CHR: Traci Montgomery, Manager Human Resources
Web address: www.patientshospital.com
**Control:** Individual, Investor–owned, for–profit **Service:** General Medical and Surgical

**Staffed Beds:** 10 **Admissions:** 355 **Census:** 1 **Outpatient Visits:** 2333 **Births:** 0

**SHASTA REGIONAL MEDICAL CENTER (50764)**, 1100 Butte Street, Zip 96001–0853, Mailing Address: P.O. Box 496072, Zip 96049–6072; tel. 530/244–5400 **A**10 **F**3 11 17 18 20 22 24 26 28 29 30 34 35 40 43 45 49 50 51 59 65 70 74 75 77 79 81 84 85 86 107 108 111 114 118 131 145 147 **S** Prime Healthcare Services, Ontario, CA
Primary Contact: Randall Hempling, Chief Executive Officer
CFO: Sandra Bowen, Chief Financial Officer
CMO: Marcia McCampbell, M.D., Chief Medical Officer
CIO: Tony VanBoekel, Director Information Systems
CHR: Terry Jaqua, Director Human Resources
Web address: www.shastaregional.com
**Control:** Corporation, Investor–owned, for–profit **Service:** General Medical and Surgical

**Staffed Beds:** 135 **Admissions:** 8217 **Census:** 84 **Births:** 0 **Total Expense ($000):** 134610 **Payroll Expense ($000):** 39087 **Personnel:** 632

**REDLANDS—San Bernardino County**

☒ **LOMA LINDA UNIVERSITY BEHAVIORAL MEDICINE CENTER (54093)**, 1710 Barton Road, Zip 92373–5304; tel. 909/558–9200 **A**1 5 9 10 **F**4 5 29 30 34 35 57 87 98 99 100 101 102 103 104 105 129 131 **P**7 **S** Loma Linda University Adventist Health Sciences Center, Loma Linda, CA
Primary Contact: Ruthita J. Fike, Chief Executive Officer
COO: Ruthita J. Fike, Chief Executive Officer
CFO: Steve Mohr, Senior Vice President Finance and Chief Financial Officer
CMO: William Murdoch, M.D., Medical Director
CIO: Mark Zirkelback, Chief Information Officer
CHR: Mark Hubbard, Vice President Risk Management
Web address: www.llu.edu
**Control:** Other not–for–profit (including NFP Corporation) **Service:** Psychiatric

**Staffed Beds:** 89 **Admissions:** 4340 **Census:** 72 **Outpatient Visits:** 24495 **Births:** 0 **Total Expense ($000):** 28045 **Payroll Expense ($000):** 12506 **Personnel:** 233

☒ **REDLANDS COMMUNITY HOSPITAL (50272)**, 350 Terracina Boulevard, Zip 92373–4897, Mailing Address: P.O. Box 3391, Zip 92373–3391; tel. 909/335–5500, (Total facility includes 16 beds in nursing home–type unit) **A**1 9 10 **F**3 11 13 15 18 20 28 29 30 31 34 35 40 45 46 49 51 54 57 59 62 63 64 65 66 68 70 72 74 76 78 79 81 82 84 85 87 93 96 97 98 102 104 105 107 108 110 111 113 118 120 125 127 129 131 142 145 146 147 **P**5 7
Primary Contact: James R. Holmes, President and Chief Executive Officer
Web address: www.redlandshospital.org
**Control:** Other not–for–profit (including NFP Corporation) **Service:** General Medical and Surgical

**Staffed Beds:** 189 **Admissions:** 12486 **Census:** 145 **Outpatient Visits:** 147430 **Births:** 2582 **Total Expense ($000):** 231738 **Payroll Expense ($000):** 82662 **Personnel:** 1260

**REDWOOD CITY—San Mateo County**

☒ **REDWOOD CITY MEDICAL CENTER (50541)**, 1150 Veterans Boulevard, Zip 94063–2037; tel. 650/299–2000 **A**1 3 5 10 **F**2 3 5 13 15 18 20 22 26 28 29 30 31 32 34 35 36 40 45 49 50 51 54 55 56 57 58 59 64 65 68 70 73 74 75 76 77 78 79 80 81 82 84 85 86 87 91 92 93 94 95 96 97 99 100 101 103 104 107 108 110 111 113 114 118 123 128 129 130 131 133 134 145 146 147 **P**6 **S** Kaiser Foundation Hospitals, Oakland, CA
Primary Contact: Frank T. Beirne, Senior Vice President and Area Manager
COO: Maureen O'Brien, Chief Operating Officer
CIO: Angel Shew, Director Area Technology
CHR: Sharon Barncord, Business Partner Human Resources
Web address: www.kaiserpermanente.org
**Control:** Other not–for–profit (including NFP Corporation) **Service:** General Medical and Surgical

**Staffed Beds:** 213 **Admissions:** 7111 **Census:** 86 **Outpatient Visits:** 135629 **Births:** 1277 **Personnel:** 1486

☒ **SEQUOIA HOSPITAL (50197)**, 170 Alameda De Las Pulgas, Zip 94062–2799; tel. 650/369–5811 **A**1 9 10 **F**11 12 13 15 18 20 22 24 26 28 29 30 31 32 34 35 37 40 45 46 49 50 53 57 59 60 64 68 70 74 75 76 77 78 79 81 84 86 87 92 93 94 98 107 108 110 111 113 114 117 118 119 120 122 125 128 129 131 134 145 146 147 **P**3 **S** Dignity Health, San Francisco, CA
Primary Contact: Glenna L. Vaskelis, CPA, President and Administrator
CFO: Gratia Barton, Chief Financial Officer
CMO: Christopher Dunn, M.D., Vice President Medical Affairs
CIO: Gracie O'Brien, Chief Information Officer
CHR: Linde Cheema, Vice President Human Resources
Web address: www.sequoiahospital.org
**Control:** Other not–for–profit (including NFP Corporation) **Service:** General Medical and Surgical

**Staffed Beds:** 153 **Admissions:** 7599 **Census:** 84 **Outpatient Visits:** 116763 **Births:** 1605 **Total Expense ($000):** 219105 **Payroll Expense ($000):** 85088 **Personnel:** 793

**REEDLEY—Fresno County**

★ **ADVENTIST MEDICAL CENTER–REEDLEY (50192)**, 372 West Cypress Avenue, Zip 93654–2199; tel. 559/638–8155, (Nonreporting) **A**9 10 21 **S** Adventist Health, Roseville, CA
Primary Contact: Sandy Haskins, Interim Chief Executive Officer
CFO: Teresa Jacques, Interim Chief Financial Officer
CMO: Todd Spencer, M.D., Chief Medical Staff
CIO: Valerie Alvarez, Executive Assistant
CHR: Ramona Alvarado, Interim Manager Human Resources
Web address: www.skdh.org
**Control:** Hospital district or authority, Government, nonfederal **Service:** General Medical and Surgical

**Staffed Beds:** 44

**RICHMOND—Contra Costa County**

**RICHMOND MEDICAL CENTER** See Oakland Medical Center, Oakland

**RIDGECREST—Kern County**

★ **RIDGECREST REGIONAL HOSPITAL (50448)**, 1081 North China Lake Boulevard, Zip 93555–3130; tel. 760/446–3551 **A**9 10 20 21 **F**3 8 13 15 18 28 29 30 40 41 57 62 63 70 73 76 81 89 107 111 118 126 128 129 143 145 146 147
Primary Contact: James A. Suver, FACHE, Chief Executive Officer
CFO: Lois Johnson, Administrator Fiscal Services
CMO: Victoria Schauf, M.D., Chief of Staff
CIO: Randy Ferguson, Chief Information Officer
CHR: Dave Shary, Administrator Human Resources
Web address: www.rrh.org
**Control:** Other not–for–profit (including NFP Corporation) **Service:** General Medical and Surgical

**Staffed Beds:** 70 **Admissions:** 3207 **Census:** 27 **Total Expense ($000):** 69090 **Payroll Expense ($000):** 24612 **Personnel:** 467

**RIVERSIDE—Riverside County**

☐ **PARKVIEW COMMUNITY HOSPITAL MEDICAL CENTER (50102)**, 3865 Jackson Street, Zip 92503–3998; tel. 951/688–2211, (Nonreporting) **A**1 9 10
Primary Contact: Douglas Drumwright, Chief Executive Officer
CFO: Patti Lepe, Chief Financial Officer
CMO: Stephen Carney, M.D., Chief of Staff
CIO: John Ciccarelli, Chief Information Officer
CHR: Stacci Gary, Director Human Resources
CNO: Thomas Santos, R.N., Chief Nursing Officer and Director Quality Services
Web address: www.pchmc.org
**Control:** County–Government, nonfederal **Service:** General Medical and Surgical

**Staffed Beds:** 193

*Many Facility Codes have changed. Please refer to the AHA Guide Code Chart.* © 2012 AHA Guide

☐ **RIVERSIDE CENTER FOR BEHAVIORAL MEDICINE (54130)**, 5900 Brockton Avenue, Zip 92506; tel. 951/275–8400, (Nonreporting) **A1** 10
Primary Contact: Rence Leth, Administrator
Web address: www.rcbm.com/
**Control:** Other not–for–profit (including NFP Corporation) **Service:** Psychiatric

**Staffed Beds:** 68

☒ **RIVERSIDE COMMUNITY HOSPITAL (50022)**, 4445 Magnolia Avenue, Zip 92501–4199, Mailing Address: P.O. Box 1669, Zip 92502–1669; tel. 951/788–3000 **A1** 2 9 10 **F3** 11 12 13 15 17 18 20 22 24 26 28 29 30 31 34 35 40 43 53 57 59 60 64 68 70 72 74 75 76 77 78 79 81 84 85 86 89 93 107 108 110 111 114 118 120 121 122 123 125 129 131 137 141 145 146 147 **P5 S** HCA, Nashville, TN
Primary Contact: Patrick D. Brilliant, President and Chief Executive Officer
COO: C. Doug Long, Chief Operating Officer
CFO: Tracey Fernandez, Chief Financial Officer
CMO: Joseph Lee, M.D., President Medical Staff
CIO: Cae Swanger, Chief Information Officer
Web address: www.riversidecommunityhospital.com
**Control:** Corporation, Investor–owned, for–profit **Service:** General Medical and Surgical

**Staffed Beds:** 373 **Admissions:** 21648 **Census:** 281 **Outpatient Visits:** 119258 **Births:** 3861 **Total Expense ($000):** 315719 **Payroll Expense ($000):** 131661 **Personnel:** 1661

☒ **RIVERSIDE MEDICAL CENTER (50686)**, 10800 Magnolia Avenue, Zip 92505–3000; tel. 951/353–2000 **A1** 3 5 10 **F3** 13 15 17 29 30 31 35 40 45 46 47 49 60 64 65 68 70 72 74 75 76 77 78 79 81 82 84 85 87 89 97 100 102 107 108 111 113 114 116 117 118 129 145 146 147 **S** Kaiser Foundation Hospitals, Oakland, CA
Primary Contact: Vita M. Willett, Administrator and Executive Director
CFO: Lorna Curtis, Chief Financial Officer
CMO: Richard Rajatatnam, M.D., Area Medical Director
CIO: Alfred T. Velasquez, Area Information Officer
CHR: Wendy Sander, Director Human Resources
CNO: Kim E. Hadden, R.N., Chief Nurse Executive
Web address: www.kaiserpermanente.org
**Control:** Other not–for–profit (including NFP Corporation) **Service:** General Medical and Surgical

**Staffed Beds:** 215 **Admissions:** 15046 **Census:** 152 **Births:** 2072

### ROSEMEAD—Los Angeles County

☐ **BHC ALHAMBRA HOSPITAL (54032)**, 4619 North Rosemead Boulevard, Zip 91770–1478, Mailing Address: P.O. Box 369, Zip 91770–0369; tel. 626/286–1191, (Nonreporting) **A1** 9 10 **S** Universal Health Services, Inc., King of Prussia, PA
Primary Contact: Peggy Minnick, R.N., Chief Executive Officer
CFO: Michelle Jackson, Chief Financial Officer
CMO: Wakelin McNeel, M.D., Medical Director
CIO: Debbie Irvin, Director Health Information Management
CHR: Venus Taylor, Director Human Resources
Web address: www.bhcalhambra.com
**Control:** Corporation, Investor–owned, for–profit **Service:** Psychiatric

**Staffed Beds:** 85

**SILVER LAKE MEDICAL CENTER–INGLESIDE HOSPITAL** See Silver Lake Medical Center, Los Angeles

### ROSEVILLE—Placer County

☒ **ROSEVILLE MEDICAL CENTER (50772)**, 1600 Eureka Road, Zip 95661–3027; tel. 916/784–4000, (Nonreporting) **A1** 10 **S** Kaiser Foundation Hospitals, Oakland, CA
Primary Contact: Edward S. Glavis, Senior Vice President and Area Manager
Web address: www.kp.org
**Control:** Other not–for–profit (including NFP Corporation) **Service:** General Medical and Surgical

**Staffed Beds:** 340

☒ **SUTTER ROSEVILLE MEDICAL CENTER (50309)**, One Medical Plaza, Zip 95661–3037; tel. 916/781–1000, (Nonreporting) **A1** 2 5 9 10 **S** Sutter Health, Sacramento, CA
Primary Contact: Patrick R. Brady, Chief Executive Officer
COO: Dionne Miller, Chief Operating Officer
CFO: Gary Hubschman, Administrative Director Finance
CMO: Stuart Bostrom, M.D., Director Medical Affairs
CIO: Nancy Turner, Director Communications
CHR: Lynda Dasaro, Director Human Resources
CNO: Barbara J. Nelson, Ph.D., Chief Nursing Executive
Web address: www.sutterroseville.org
**Control:** Other not–for–profit (including NFP Corporation) **Service:** General Medical and Surgical

**Staffed Beds:** 313

### SACRAMENTO—Sacramento County

☐ **HERITAGE OAKS HOSPITAL (54104)**, 4250 Auburn Boulevard, Zip 95841–4164; tel. 916/489–3336, (Nonreporting) **A1** 5 9 10 **S** Universal Health Services, Inc., King of Prussia, PA
Primary Contact: Chris Diamond, Chief Executive Officer
CFO: Art Wong, Chief Financial Officer
CMO: Joseph Sison, M.D., Medical Director
CHR: Lisa Myers, Director Human Resources
Web address: www.heritageoakshospital.com
**Control:** Corporation, Investor–owned, for–profit **Service:** Psychiatric

**Staffed Beds:** 72

☒ △ **MERCY GENERAL HOSPITAL (50017)**, 4001 J Street, Zip 95819–3600; tel. 916/453–4545, (Total facility includes 38 beds in nursing home–type unit) **A1** 2 3 5 7 9 10 **F3** 8 11 13 15 17 18 20 22 24 26 28 29 30 31 34 37 39 40 42 43 45 46 49 50 51 53 56 57 58 59 63 64 66 68 70 74 75 76 77 78 79 81 82 83 84 85 87 90 93 94 96 99 107 108 111 113 114 117 118 125 127 129 130 131 134 142 144 145 146 147 **P3** 5 **S** Dignity Health, San Francisco, CA
Primary Contact: Phyllis Baltz, Interim President
COO: Patricia Monczewski, Chief Operating Officer
CFO: Ronald Kroll, Chief Financial Officer
CMO: Robert Wiebe, M.D., Chief Medical Officer
CHR: Cyndi Kirch, Vice President Human Resources
Web address: www.mercygeneral.org
**Control:** Church–operated, Nongovernment, not–for profit **Service:** General Medical and Surgical

**Staffed Beds:** 286 **Admissions:** 18810 **Census:** 245 **Outpatient Visits:** 149755 **Births:** 3172 **Total Expense ($000):** 458078 **Payroll Expense ($000):** 180415 **Personnel:** 1891

☒ **METHODIST HOSPITAL OF SACRAMENTO (50590)**, 7500 Hospital Drive, Zip 95823–5477; tel. 916/423–3000, (Total facility includes 171 beds in nursing home–type unit) **A1** 9 10 **F3** 11 12 17 29 30 35 37 39 40 41 47 49 50 56 59 60 61 64 68 70 72 74 75 76 77 79 81 84 85 86 87 89 93 96 97 107 108 111 115 116 117 118 125 127 129 130 131 142 145 146 147 **P5 S** Dignity Health, San Francisco, CA
Primary Contact: Eugene Bassett, Interim President and Chief Executive Officer
CHR: Christopher Joyce, Vice President Human Resources
Web address: www.methodistsacramento.org
**Control:** Other not–for–profit (including NFP Corporation) **Service:** General Medical and Surgical

**Staffed Beds:** 325 **Admissions:** 9136 **Census:** 246 **Outpatient Visits:** 62408 **Births:** 1188 **Total Expense ($000):** 216491 **Payroll Expense ($000):** 91435 **Personnel:** 961

★ **SACRAMENTO MEDICAL CENTER (50425)**, 2025 Morse Avenue, Zip 95825–2115; tel. 916/973–5000 **A3** 5 10 **F3** 8 15 17 18 20 29 31 35 40 45 46 48 49 50 56 60 64 68 70 74 75 77 78 79 81 82 84 85 107 108 111 113 114 118 129 145 147 **S** Kaiser Foundation Hospitals, Oakland, CA
Primary Contact: Ronald Groepper, Senior Vice President and Area Manager
CFO: Jim Eldridge, Area Financial Officer
CMO: Chris Palkowski, M.D., Physician in Chief
CIO: Philip Fasano, Chief Information Officer
CHR: Gay Westfall, Senior Vice President Human Resources
Web address: www.kp.org
**Control:** Other not–for–profit (including NFP Corporation) **Service:** General Medical and Surgical

**Staffed Beds:** 287 **Admissions:** 11314 **Census:** 137 **Outpatient Visits:** 217551 **Births:** 0

**CA**

---

**Hospital, Medicare Provider Number, Address, Telephone, Approval, Facility, and Physician Codes, Health Care System**

★ American Hospital Association (AHA) membership
☐ The Joint Commission accreditation      ◇ DNV Healthcare Inc. accreditation
○ American Osteopathic Association (AOA) accreditation
△ Commission on Accreditation of Rehabilitation Facilities (CARF) accreditation

□ **SHRINERS HOSPITALS FOR CHILDREN, NORTHERN CALIFORNIA (53310)**, 2425 Stockton Boulevard, Zip 95817–2215; tel. 916/453–2000, (Nonreporting) **A**1 3 5 10 **S** Shriners Hospitals for Children, Tampa, FL
Primary Contact: Margaret Bryan, Administrator
COO: Margaret Bryan, Administrator
CFO: William Dalby, Director Fiscal Services
CIO: John Bevel, Manager Information Systems
CHR: Deborah Rubens, Director Human Resources
Web address: www.shrinershq.org
**Control:** Other not–for–profit (including NFP Corporation) **Service:** Children's general

**Staffed Beds:** 70

□ **SIERRA VISTA HOSPITAL (54087)**, 8001 Bruceville Road, Zip 95823–2329; tel. 916/288–0300 **A**1 9 10 **F**5 29 35 38 98 99 100 101 103 104 105 129 131 **S** Universal Health Services, Inc., King of Prussia, PA
Primary Contact: Mike Zauner, Chief Executive Officer
COO: Barbara Roush, Chief Operating Officer
CFO: Irene McMillan, Chief Financial Officer
CMO: Okechukwu Nwangburuka, M.D., Medical Director
CIO: Mark Grip, Executive Director Business Development
CHR: David Lish, Director Human Resources
**Control:** Corporation, Investor–owned, for–profit **Service:** Psychiatric

**Staffed Beds:** 120 **Admissions:** 5130 **Census:** 93 **Outpatient Visits:** 2291 **Births:** 0 **Total Expense ($000):** 31231 **Payroll Expense ($000):** 12528 **Personnel:** 256

✠ **SOUTH SACRAMENTO MEDICAL CENTER (50674)**, 6600 Bruceville Road, Zip 95823–4671; tel. 916/688–2430 **A**1 3 5 10 **F**3 8 13 15 29 30 31 34 35 40 43 49 61 62 63 64 65 68 70 73 74 75 76 77 78 79 81 82 84 85 86 87 93 97 100 104 107 108 111 113 114 118 129 143 145 **S** Kaiser Foundation Hospitals, Oakland, CA
Primary Contact: Patricia Rodriguez, Senior Vice President and Area Manager
CIO: Kathleen McKenna, Public Affairs Leader
Web address: www.kp.org
**Control:** Other not–for–profit (including NFP Corporation) **Service:** General Medical and Surgical

**Staffed Beds:** 181 **Admissions:** 12546 **Census:** 119 **Outpatient Visits:** 86754 **Births:** 2414 **Personnel:** 1215

★ **SUTTER CENTER FOR PSYCHIATRY (54096)**, 7700 Folsom Boulevard, Zip 95826–2608; tel. 916/386–3000 **A**9 10 **F**29 30 44 68 98 99 100 101 102 103 104 105 129 131 132 142 **S** Sutter Health, Sacramento, CA
Primary Contact: John W. Boyd, PsyD, Chief Administrative Officer
CFO: Pamela Ansley, Director Finance
CMO: Cindy Thygeson, M.D., Director Medical Affairs
CHR: Kristin Daniels, Manager Human Resources
Web address: www.sutterpsychiatry.org
**Control:** Other not–for–profit (including NFP Corporation) **Service:** Psychiatric

**Staffed Beds:** 69 **Admissions:** 2279 **Census:** 45 **Births:** 0

✠ **SUTTER MEDICAL CENTER, SACRAMENTO (50108)**, 5151 F Street, Zip 95819–3295; tel. 916/454–3333, (Includes SUTTER CHILDREN'S CENTER, 5151 F. Street, Zip 95819–3223; tel. 800/478–8837; SUTTER GENERAL HOSPITAL, 2801 L Street, Zip 95816; tel. 916/454–2222), (Nonreporting) **A**1 2 3 5 9 10 **S** Sutter Health, Sacramento, CA
Primary Contact: Carrie Owen-Plietz, Chief Executive Officer
CFO: Richard SooHoo, Chief Financial Officer
CMO: Mark Leibenhaut, M.D., Chief of Staff
CIO: Julie Montera, Director Information Technology
CHR: Laurie Rose, Director Human Resources
Web address: www.sutterhealth.org
**Control:** Other not–for–profit (including NFP Corporation) **Service:** General Medical and Surgical

**Staffed Beds:** 654

✠ **UNIVERSITY OF CALIFORNIA, DAVIS MEDICAL CENTER (50599)**, 2315 Stockton Boulevard, Zip 95817–2282; tel. 916/734–2011, (Includes UNIVERSITY OF CALIFORNIA DAVIS CHILDREN'S HOSPITAL, 2315 Stockton Boulevard, Zip 95817–2201; tel. 800/282–3284) **A**1 2 3 5 8 9 10 **F**3 6 8 9 11 12 13 15 16 17 18 19 20 21 22 23 24 25 26 27 28 29 30 31 32 34 35 36 37 38 39 40 41 43 44 45 46 47 48 49 52 54 55 56 57 58 59 60 61 62 63 64 65 66 68 70 71 72 73 74 75 76 77 78 79 80 81 82 83 84 85 86 87 88 89 90 91 92 93 94 96 97 99 100 101 102 103 104 107 108 110 111 113 114 115 116 117 118 119 120 121 122 123 125 128 129 130 131 133 134 135 137 140 141 142 143 144 145 146 147 **P**6 **S** University of California–Systemwide Administration, Oakland, CA
Primary Contact: Ann Madden Rice, Chief Executive Officer
COO: Vincent Johnson, Chief Operating Officer
CFO: Timothy Maurice, Chief Financial Officer
CMO: Allan Siefkin, M.D., Chief Medical Officer
CIO: Michael N. Minear, Chief Information Officer
CHR: Stephen Chilcott, Associate Director Human Resources
Web address: www.ucdmc.ucdavis.edu
**Control:** State–Government, nonfederal **Service:** General Medical and Surgical

**Staffed Beds:** 567 **Admissions:** 31033 **Census:** 460 **Outpatient Visits:** 1131640 **Births:** 1954 **Total Expense ($000):** 1091556 **Payroll Expense ($000):** 538809 **Personnel:** 7762

✠ **ST. HELENA HOSPITAL (50013)**, 10 Woodland Road, Zip 94574; tel. 707/963–3611 **A**1 9 10 **F**3 4 5 8 15 17 18 20 22 24 26 28 29 30 31 34 35 36 37 39 40 45 47 50 51 53 54 57 58 59 60 62 64 65 70 74 75 76 77 78 79 81 82 84 85 86 87 92 97 98 99 100 101 102 104 105 107 108 110 111 114 116 118 119 120 125 128 129 130 134 145 146 147 **P**3 **S** Adventist Health, Roseville, CA
Primary Contact: Terry Newmyer, President and Chief Executive Officer
CFO: Edward A. McDonald, Senior Vice President and Chief Financial Officer
CIO: Mons Jensen, Information Systems Team Leader
CHR: Mark Fowler, Executive Director Human Resources
Web address: www.sthelenahospital.org
**Control:** Church–operated, Nongovernment, not–for profit **Service:** General Medical and Surgical

**Staffed Beds:** 116 **Admissions:** 6019 **Census:** 72 **Outpatient Visits:** 95728 **Births:** 256 **Total Expense ($000):** 165150 **Payroll Expense ($000):** 60153 **Personnel:** 874

✠ **NATIVIDAD MEDICAL CENTER (50248)**, 1441 Constitution Boulevard, Zip 93906–3100, Mailing Address: P.O. Box 81611, Zip 93912–1611; tel. 831/647–7611, (Nonreporting) **A**1 3 5 9 10
Primary Contact: Harry Weis, Chief Executive Officer
CMO: Gary Gray, D.O., Chief Medical Officer
CIO: Kirk Larson, Chief Information Officer
CHR: Janine Bouyea, Director Human Resources
Web address: www.natividad.com
**Control:** County–Government, nonfederal **Service:** General Medical and Surgical

**Staffed Beds:** 137

✠ **SALINAS VALLEY MEMORIAL HEALTHCARE SYSTEM (50334)**, 450 East Romie Lane, Zip 93901–4098; tel. 831/757–4333 **A**1 2 9 10 **F**3 13 15 17 18 20 22 24 26 29 31 34 35 40 42 44 45 46 47 48 49 50 55 57 58 59 60 61 63 68 70 72 74 75 76 77 78 79 81 82 83 84 85 86 87 89 93 94 107 108 110 111 112 113 114 115 116 117 118 123 125 128 129 131 132 133 145 146 147 **P**8
Primary Contact: Lowell W. Johnson, FACHE, Interim President and Chief Executive Officer
COO: James Griffith, Chief Operating Officer
CFO: Robert M. Dvorak, Interim Chief Financial Officer
CMO: Andrew Wilson, M.D., Interim Chief Medical Officer
CIO: Audrey Parks, Senior Administrative Director Information Technology
CHR: Michelle B. Childs, Executive Administrative Director Human Resources
CNO: Louella Freeman, Chief Nursing Officer
Web address: www.svmh.com
**Control:** Hospital district or authority, Government, nonfederal **Service:** General Medical and Surgical

**Staffed Beds:** 225 **Admissions:** 11000 **Census:** 121 **Outpatient Visits:** 82000 **Births:** 2000

✠ **MARK TWAIN ST. JOSEPH'S HOSPITAL (51332)**, 768 Mountain Ranch Road, Zip 95249–9707; tel. 209/754–3521, (Nonreporting) **A**1 9 10 18 **S** Dignity Health, San Francisco, CA
Primary Contact: Craig J. Marks, FACHE, President
CFO: Jacob Lewis, Chief Financial Officer
CHR: Nancy Vargas, Director Human Resources
Web address: www.marktwainhospital.com
**Control:** Other not–for–profit (including NFP Corporation) **Service:** General Medical and Surgical

**Staffed Beds:** 30

✠ **COMMUNITY HOSPITAL OF SAN BERNARDINO (50089)**, 1805 Medical Center Drive, Zip 92411–1214; tel. 909/887–6333, (Nonreporting) **A**1 9 10 **S** Dignity Health, San Francisco, CA
Primary Contact: June Collison, President
CFO: Ed Sorenson, Vice President Finance and Chief Financial Officer
CIO: Robert Redden, Site Director Information Technology
CHR: Denice C. Findlay, Director Human Resources
Web address: www.chsb.org
**Control:** Other not–for–profit (including NFP Corporation) **Service:** General Medical and Surgical

**Staffed Beds:** 321

□ △ **ROBERT H. BALLARD REHABILITATION HOSPITAL (53037)**, 1760 West 16th Street, Zip 92411; tel. 909/473–1200, (Nonreporting) **A**1 7 9 10 **S** Vibra Healthcare, Mechanicsburg, PA
Primary Contact: Edward C. Palacios, Chief Executive Officer
Web address: www.ballardhospital.com
**Control:** Corporation, Investor–owned, for–profit **Service:** Rehabilitation

**Staffed Beds:** 60

CA

★ **ST. BERNARDINE MEDICAL CENTER (50129)**, 2101 North Waterman Avenue, Zip 92404–4836; tel. 909/883–8711, (Nonreporting) **A**2 9 10 **S** Dignity Health, San Francisco, CA
Primary Contact: Steven R. Barron, President
COO: Jack Ivie, Chief Operating Officer
CFO: Darryl VandenBosch, Vice President and Chief Financial Officer
CMO: Betty Daniels, M.D., Chief of Staff
CIO: James Croker, Director Information Systems
CHR: Dee Webb, Vice President Human Resources
Web address: www.stbernardinemedicalcenter.com
**Control:** Other not–for–profit (including NFP Corporation) **Service:** General Medical and Surgical

| Staffed Beds: 250 |
| --- |

### SAN DIEGO—San Diego County

☐ **ALVARADO HOSPITAL (50757)**, 6655 Alvarado Road, Zip 92120–5208; tel. 619/287–3270, (Nonreporting) **A**1 2 9 10 **S** Prime Healthcare Services, Ontario, CA
Primary Contact: Robin Gomez, Administrator
CFO: Brian Kleven, Chief Financial Officer
CIO: Eric Logie, Director Information Systems
CNO: Peggy Bailey, Chief Nursing Officer
Web address: www.alvaradohospital.com
**Control:** Corporation, Investor–owned, for–profit **Service:** General Medical and Surgical

| Staffed Beds: 121 |
| --- |

☐ **AURORA BEHAVIORAL HEALTH CARE (54095)**, 11878 Avenue of Industry, Zip 92128–3423; tel. 858/487–3200, (Nonreporting) **A**1 9 10 **S** Aurora Behavioral Health Care, Corona, CA
Primary Contact: James S. Plummer, Chief Executive Officer
COO: Linda Achber, Director Clinical Services
CFO: Tim Sides, Chief Financial Officer
CMO: Thomas Flanagan, M.D., Medical Director
CIO: Alain Azcona, Director Business Development
CHR: Susan Haas, Human Resources
Web address: www.aurorasandiego.com
**Control:** Corporation, Investor–owned, for–profit **Service:** Psychiatric

| Staffed Beds: 80 |
| --- |

⊠ **KINDRED HOSPITAL–SAN DIEGO (52036)**, 1940 El Cajon Boulevard, Zip 92104–1096; tel. 619/543–4500, (Nonreporting) **A**1 9 10 **S** Kindred Healthcare, Louisville, KY
Primary Contact: Natalie Germuska, Chief Executive Officer
COO: Patricia Cavaness, Chief Clinical Officer
CFO: Gene Fantano, Controller
CMO: Davies Wong, M.D., Medical Director
CIO: Natalie Germuska, Chief Executive Officer
CHR: Jeffrey Sopko, District Director Human Resources
CNO: Maureen Bodme, Chief Clinical Officer
CNO: Catherine Rivera, Nurse Manager
Web address: www.kindredsandiego.com
**Control:** Corporation, Investor–owned, for–profit **Service:** General Medical and Surgical

| Staffed Beds: 70 |
| --- |

⊠ **NAVAL MEDICAL CENTER**, 34800 Bob Wilson Drive, Zip 92134–5000; tel. 619/532–6400, (Nonreporting) **A**1 2 3 5 **S** Bureau of Medicine and Surgery, Department of the Navy, Washington, DC
Primary Contact: Rear Admiral C. Forrest Faison, Commander
CFO: Captain O. G. Haugen, Director Resources
CIO: Lieutenant D. V. Gonzales, Head Information Technology Management
Web address: www.nmcsd.med.navy.mil
**Control:** Navy, Government, federal **Service:** General Medical and Surgical

| Staffed Beds: 285 |
| --- |

☐ **PROMISE HOSPITAL OF SAN DIEGO (52051)**, 5550 University Avenue, Zip 92105–2307; tel. 619/582–3800, (Nonreporting) **A**1 9 10 **S** Promise Healthcare, Boca Raton, FL
Primary Contact: Roy Rodriguez, Chief Executive Officer
COO: Tim Clark, Chief Operating Officer
CFO: Jim McCabe, Chief Financial Officer
CMO: Larry Emdur, M.D., Chief of Staff
CIO: Jim Wilson, Vice President Information Technology
CHR: Stacia Rasina, Director Human Resources
Web address: www.promisesandiego.com
**Control:** Partnership, Investor–owned, for–profit **Service:** Psychiatric

| Staffed Beds: 100 |
| --- |

⊠ **RADY CHILDREN'S HOSPITAL – SAN DIEGO (53303)**, 3020 Children's Way, Zip 92123–4282; tel. 858/576–1700, (Total facility includes 43 beds in nursing home–type unit) **A**1 3 5 9 10 **F**1 3 7 8 9 10 11 12 17 19 21 23 25 26 27 29 30 31 32 34 35 36 38 39 40 41 43 45 46 47 48 50 54 55 57 58 59 60 62 64 65 67 68 70 72 73 74 75 77 78 79 80 81 82 83 84 85 86 87 88 89 90 91 92 93 94 99 100 101 102 104 107 108 111 113 114 117 118 127 128 129 130 131 132 133 134 135 137 138 140 142 143 144 145 **P**3 5
Primary Contact: Kathleen Ann Sellick, President and Chief Executive Officer
COO: Meg Norton, Senior Vice President and Chief Operating Officer
CFO: Roger Roux, Senior Vice President Financial Affairs and Chief Financial Officer
CMO: Irvin A. Kaufman, M.D., Senior Vice President Health Affairs and Chief Medical Officer
CIO: Albert Oriol, Vice President Information Management and Chief Information Officer
CHR: Mamoon Syed, Vice President Human Resources
Web address: www.rchsd.org
**Control:** Other not–for–profit (including NFP Corporation) **Service:** Children's general

| Staffed Beds: 330 Admissions: 16341 Census: 255 Outpatient Visits: 317189 Births: 0 Total Expense ($000): 681364 Payroll Expense ($000): 232826 Personnel: 3030 |
| --- |

**RADY CHILDREN'S HOSPITAL AND HEALTH CENTER** See Rady Children's Hospital – San Diego

☐ **SAN DIEGO COUNTY PSYCHIATRIC HOSPITAL (54114)**, 3853 Rosecrans Street, Zip 92110–3115, Mailing Address: P.O. Box 85524, Zip 92186–5524; tel. 619/692–8211, (Nonreporting) **A**1 10
Primary Contact: Izabela Karmach, R.N., Administrator
COO: Izabela Karmach, R.N., Administrator
CFO: Raul J. Loyo–Rodriguez, Administrative Analyst III
CMO: Michael Krelstein, M.D., Medical Director
CIO: Linda Cannon, Chief Medical Records Services
CHR: Francisco Puentes, Human Resource Officer
Web address: www.sdcounty.ca.gov
**Control:** County–Government, nonfederal **Service:** Psychiatric

| Staffed Beds: 357 |
| --- |

★ **SAN DIEGO HOSPICE & THE INSTITUTE OF PALLIATIVE MEDICINE (50698)**, 4311 Third Avenue, Zip 92103–7499; tel. 619/688–1600, (Nonreporting) **A**10
Primary Contact: Kathleen Pacurar, President and Chief Executive Officer
COO: Kathleen Jones, Vice President Finance and Chief Financial Officer
CFO: Kathleen Jones, Vice President Finance and Chief Financial Officer
CMO: Steven Oppenheim, M.D., Vice President Medical Affairs
Web address: www.sdhospice.org
**Control:** Other not–for–profit (including NFP Corporation) **Service:** Other specialty

| Staffed Beds: 23 |
| --- |

⊠ **SAN DIEGO MEDICAL CENTER (50515)**, 4647 Zion Avenue, Zip 92120–2507; tel. 619/528–5000 **A**1 3 5 10 **F**3 8 13 14 15 29 30 31 34 40 41 44 45 46 47 48 49 50 51 54 55 56 57 58 59 60 61 62 63 64 65 68 70 71 72 74 75 76 77 78 79 81 82 83 84 85 86 87 89 93 97 100 102 103 104 107 108 111 113 114 116 117 118 129 130 131 132 142 143 145 147 **S** Kaiser Foundation Hospitals, Oakland, CA
Primary Contact: Mary Ann Barnes, Senior Vice President and Executive Director
COO: Joan Burritt, R.N., Chief Operating Officer
CFO: Lynette Seid, Area Chief Financial Officer
CMO: Paul E. Bernstein, M.D., Area Medical Director
CIO: Matthew T. Ebaugh, Area Information Officer
CHR: Cherie L. Sampson, Director Human Resources
CNO: Joan Burritt, R.N., Interim Chief Nurse Executive
Web address: www.kaiserpermanente.org
**Control:** Other not–for–profit (including NFP Corporation) **Service:** General Medical and Surgical

| Staffed Beds: 392 Admissions: 28733 Census: 297 Outpatient Visits: 225191 Births: 4312 Personnel: 2717 |
| --- |

CA

---

**Hospital, Medicare Provider Number, Address, Telephone, Approval, Facility, and Physician Codes, Health Care System**

★ American Hospital Association (AHA) membership
☐ The Joint Commission accreditation   ◇ DNV Healthcare Inc. accreditation

◯ American Osteopathic Association (AOA) accreditation
△ Commission on Accreditation of Rehabilitation Facilities (CARF) accreditation

**CA**

☒ **SCRIPPS MERCY HOSPITAL (50077)**, 4077 Fifth Avenue, Zip 92103–2105; tel. 619/294–8111, (Includes SCRIPPS MERCY HOSPITAL CHULA VISTA, 435 H Street, Chula Vista, Zip 91912–6617, Mailing Address: P.O. Box 1537, Zip 91910–1537; tel. 619/691–7000) **A**1 2 3 5 9 10 **F**3 8 11 12 13 14 15 17 18 20 22 24 26 28 29 30 31 32 34 35 39 40 43 44 45 46 49 50 51 54 56 57 58 59 61 64 65 66 68 70 73 74 75 76 77 78 79 81 82 83 84 85 86 87 92 93 97 98 100 101 102 103 104 105 107 108 110 111 113 114 117 118 125 128 129 131 133 134 140 145 146 147 **P**3 5 7 **S** Scripps Health, San Diego, CA
Primary Contact: Thomas A. Gammiere, Senior Vice President and Chief Executive
CFO: Edward Turk, Vice President Finance
CMO: Davis Cracroft, M.D., Senior Director Medical Affairs
CIO: Drexel DeFord, Chief Information Officer
Web address: www.scrippshealth.org
**Control:** Other not–for–profit (including NFP Corporation) **Service:** General Medical and Surgical

**Staffed Beds:** 439 **Admissions:** 33855 **Census:** 411 **Outpatient Visits:** 173877 **Births:** 4060 **Total Expense ($000):** 544732 **Payroll Expense ($000):** 238421 **Personnel:** 3108

☒ △ **SHARP MEMORIAL HOSPITAL (50100)**, 7901 Frost Street, Zip 92123–2701; tel. 858/939–3400 **A**1 2 7 9 10 **F**3 8 11 12 15 18 20 22 24 26 28 29 30 31 33 34 35 36 40 43 44 45 46 49 55 56 57 58 59 60 62 64 65 68 70 74 75 77 78 79 81 82 84 85 86 87 90 91 93 94 96 97 107 108 110 113 114 118 119 120 122 123 125 128 129 130 131 134 136 137 141 142 144 145 147 **P**3 5 **S** Sharp HealthCare, San Diego, CA
Primary Contact: Tim Smith, Chief Executive Officer
COO: Janie Kramer, Chief Operating Officer
CFO: Kevin Thompson, Chief Financial Officer
CMO: Ronald MacIntyre, M.D., Chief Medical Officer
CMO: Richard Santore, M.D., Chief Medical Officer
CIO: William T. Spooner, Senior Vice President and Chief Information Officer
CHR: Diane Delaney, Vice President Human Resources
CHR: Connie Duquette, Director Human Resources
CNO: Susan Stone, R.N., Chief Nursing Officer and VP of Patient Care Services
Web address: www.sharp.com
**Control:** Other not–for–profit (including NFP Corporation) **Service:** General Medical and Surgical

**Staffed Beds:** 400 **Admissions:** 19423 **Census:** 265 **Outpatient Visits:** 378607 **Births:** 0 **Total Expense ($000):** 568683 **Payroll Expense ($000):** 209681 **Personnel:** 2997

☒ **SHARP MESA VISTA HOSPITAL (54145)**, 7850 Vista Hill Avenue, Zip 92123–2717; tel. 858/278–4110, (Includes SHARP MCDONALD CENTER, 7989 Linda Vista Road, Zip 92111–5106; tel. 858/637–6920) **A**1 9 **F**4 5 29 35 40 43 56 58 64 87 98 99 100 101 102 103 104 105 129 131 142 **P**3 5 **S** Sharp HealthCare, San Diego, CA
Primary Contact: Kathi Lencioni, Chief Executive Officer
CFO: Kevin Thompson, Chief Financial Officer
CMO: Michael Plopper, M.D., Chief Medical Officer
CIO: William T. Spooner, Senior Vice President Information Systems
CHR: Carlisle Lewis, III, Senior Vice President Legal and Human Resources
CNO: Cheryl Odell, Chief Nursing Officer
Web address: www.sharp.com
**Control:** Other not–for–profit (including NFP Corporation) **Service:** Psychiatric

**Staffed Beds:** 149 **Admissions:** 5546 **Census:** 111 **Outpatient Visits:** 85836 **Births:** 0 **Total Expense ($000):** 59718 **Payroll Expense ($000):** 34849 **Personnel:** 506

☒ **UC SAN DIEGO HEALTH SYSTEM (50025)**, 200 West Arbor Drive, Zip 92103–8970; tel. 619/543–6222 **A**1 2 5 8 9 10 **F**3 6 9 11 12 13 15 16 17 18 20 22 24 26 29 30 31 34 36 37 40 43 44 45 46 47 48 49 50 51 55 56 57 58 59 60 61 64 65 66 68 70 72 74 75 76 77 78 79 80 81 82 84 85 86 87 92 93 97 98 99 100 101 102 103 107 109 110 111 113 114 116 117 118 119 120 122 123 125 128 129 130 131 135 136 137 138 139 140 141 143 144 145 146 147 **P**1 **S** University of California–Systemwide Administration, Oakland, CA
Primary Contact: Paul S. Viviano, Chief Executive Officer
COO: Margarita Baggett, MSN, Interim Chief Operating Officer
CFO: Lori Donaldson, Chief Financial Officer
CMO: Angela Scioscia, M.D., Chief Medical Officer
CIO: Ed Babakanian, Chief Information Officer
CHR: Paul A. Craig, R.N., Chief Human Resources and Risk Officer
CNO: Margarita Baggett, MSN, Chief Nursing Officer
Web address: www.health.ucsd.edu
**Control:** State–Government, nonfederal **Service:** General Medical and Surgical

**Staffed Beds:** 530 **Admissions:** 26722 **Census:** 384 **Outpatient Visits:** 633084 **Births:** 2609 **Total Expense ($000):** 883992 **Payroll Expense ($000):** 323782 **Personnel:** 4990

**UNIVERSITY OF CALIFORNIA SAN DIEGO MEDICAL CENTER** See UC San Diego Health System

☒ △ **VETERANS AFFAIRS SAN DIEGO HEALTHCARE SYSTEM**, 3350 LaJolla Village Drive, Zip 92161–0002; tel. 858/552–8585, (Total facility includes 39 beds in nursing home–type unit) **A**1 2 3 5 7 8 **F**3 5 8 12 15 18 20 22 24 26 29 30 31 34 35 36 38 39 40 44 45 46 47 48 49 54 55 56 58 59 60 61 62 63 64 68 70 71 74 75 77 78 79 81 82 83 84 85 86 87 91 92 93 94 96 97 98 100 101 102 103 104 107 108 110 111 113 114 115 116 117 118 125 126 127 128 129 130 131 132 134 142 144 145 146 147 **S** Department of Veterans Affairs, Washington, DC
Primary Contact: Robert M. Smith, M.D., Acting Director
COO: Cynthia Abair, Associate Director
CFO: Ronald Larson, Chief Financial Officer
CMO: Robert M. Smith, M.D., Chief of Staff
CIO: Ruey Keller, Acting Chief Information Officer
CHR: Stephanie Wright, Director Human Resources Management
Web address: www.sandiego.va.gov
**Control:** Veterans Affairs, Government, federal **Service:** General Medical and Surgical

**Staffed Beds:** 232 **Admissions:** 7607 **Census:** 149 **Outpatient Visits:** 767091 **Total Expense ($000):** 547196 **Payroll Expense ($000):** 231083 **Personnel:** 3210

☐ **VIBRA HOSPITAL OF SAN DIEGO (52044)**, 555 Washington Street, Zip 92103; tel. 619/260–8300, (Nonreporting) **A**1 9 10 **S** Vibra Healthcare, Mechanicsburg, PA
Primary Contact: Michael T. Phillips, FACHE, Chief Executive Officer
COO: Nancy Wiewiora, Chief Operating Officer
CMO: John Fox, M.D., Chief Medical Officer
CHR: Wes Burns, Director Human Resources
Web address: www.vhsandiego.com/
**Control:** Corporation, Investor–owned, for–profit **Service:** Long–Term Acute Care hospital

**Staffed Beds:** 57

**SAN DIMAS—Los Angeles County**

☐ **SAN DIMAS COMMUNITY HOSPITAL (50588)**, 1350 West Covina Boulevard, Zip 91773–3219; tel. 909/599–6811, (Nonreporting) **A**1 9 10 **S** Prime Healthcare Services, Ontario, CA
Primary Contact: Gregory Brentano, Chief Executive Officer
CFO: Dan Galles, Chief Financial Officer
CMO: Zuhair Yahya, M.D., Chief Medical Officer
CIO: Jason Beckett, Director Information Services
CHR: Arti Dhuper, Director Human Resources
Web address: www.sandimashospital.com
**Control:** Corporation, Investor–owned, for–profit **Service:** General Medical and Surgical

**Staffed Beds:** 64

**SAN FRANCISCO—San Francisco County**

☒ △ **CALIFORNIA PACIFIC MEDICAL CENTER (50047)**, 2333 Buchanan Street, Zip 94115–1925, Mailing Address: P.O. Box 7999, Zip 94120–7999; tel. 415/600–6000, (Includes CALIFORNIA PACIFIC MEDICAL CENTER–DAVIES CAMPUS, Castro and Duboce Streets, Zip 94114; tel. 415/565–6000), (Nonreporting) **A**1 2 3 5 7 8 9 10 **S** Sutter Health, Sacramento, CA
Primary Contact: Warren S. Browner, M.D., M.P.H., Chief Executive Officer
CFO: John Gates, Vice President Finance and Chief Financial Officer
CMO: Allan Pont, M.D., Vice President Medical Affairs
CIO: Craig Vercruysse, Chief Information Officer
Web address: www.cpmc.org
**Control:** Other not–for–profit (including NFP Corporation) **Service:** General Medical and Surgical

**Staffed Beds:** 967

☒ **CHINESE HOSPITAL (50407)**, 845 Jackson Street, Zip 94133–4899; tel. 415/982–2400 **A**1 9 10 **F**3 8 11 15 18 29 30 31 34 35 40 45 47 49 50 57 59 60 64 65 70 75 77 78 79 81 86 87 97 107 108 110 114 117 118 129 131 134 144 145 146 **P**5
Primary Contact: Brenda Yee, R.N., MSN, Chief Executive Officer
COO: Linda Schumacher, Chief Operating Officer
CFO: Thomas Bolger, Chief Financial Officer
CMO: James Yan, M.D., Chief of Staff
CIO: Helen Lee, Manager Information Systems
CHR: Karen Chow, Director Human Resources
CNO: Peggy Cmiel, R.N., Chief Nursing Officer
Web address: www.chinesehospital-sf.org
**Control:** Other not–for–profit (including NFP Corporation) **Service:** General Medical and Surgical

**Staffed Beds:** 54 **Admissions:** 1926 **Census:** 30 **Outpatient Visits:** 71490 **Births:** 0 **Total Expense ($000):** 90927 **Payroll Expense ($000):** 25669 **Personnel:** 298

*Many Facility Codes have changed. Please refer to the AHA Guide Code Chart.* © 2012 AHA Guide

★ **LAGUNA HONDA HOSPITAL AND REHABILITATION CENTER (50668)**, 375 Laguna Honda Boulevard, Zip 94116–1499; tel. 415/759–2300, (Total facility includes 765 beds in nursing home–type unit) **A**10 **F**3 29 30 53 56 61 63 64 65 74 75 77 83 84 90 92 93 94 100 103 104 127 129 131 134 145 147 **P**1
Primary Contact: Mivic Hirose, Executive Administrator
COO: Michael R. Llewellyn, Chief Operating Officer
CFO: Tess Navarro, Chief Financial Officer
CMO: Colleen Riley, M.D., Medical Director
CIO: Pat Skala, Chief Information Officer
CHR: Willie Ramirez, Manager Labor Relations
Web address: www.lagunahonda.org
**Control:** City–County, Government, nonfederal **Service:** Rehabilitation

**Staffed Beds:** 780 **Admissions:** 1131 **Census:** 749 **Outpatient Visits:** 24065 **Births:** 0 **Total Expense ($000):** 189821 **Payroll Expense ($000):** 104295 **Personnel:** 1379

☒ △ **SAINT FRANCIS MEMORIAL HOSPITAL (50152)**, 900 Hyde Street, Zip 94109–4899, Mailing Address: P.O. Box 7726, Zip 94120–7726; tel. 415/353–6000, (Nonreporting) **A**1 2 7 9 10 **S** Dignity Health, San Francisco, CA
Primary Contact: Thomas G. Hennessy, President and Chief Executive Officer
COO: James Jackson, Chief Operating Officer
CFO: Alan Fox, Chief Financial Officer
CHR: Richard Mead, Senior Director Human Resources
Web address: www.saintfrancismemorial.org
**Control:** Other not–for–profit (including NFP Corporation) **Service:** General Medical and Surgical

**Staffed Beds:** 239

☒ **SAN FRANCISCO GENERAL HOSPITAL MEDICAL CENTER (50228)**, 1001 Potrero Avenue, Zip 94110–3594; tel. 415/206–8000, (Nonreporting) **A**1 2 3 5 8 10
Primary Contact: Sue Currin, R.N., MS, Chief Executive Officer
COO: Sharon McCole–Wicher, R.N., Chief Nursing Officer
CFO: Valerie Inouye, Chief Financial Officer
CMO: John Luce, M.D., Chief Medical Officer
CIO: Pat Skala, Chief Information Officer
Web address: www.sfdph.org
**Control:** City–County, Government, nonfederal **Service:** General Medical and Surgical

**Staffed Beds:** 501

☒ **SAN FRANCISCO MEDICAL CENTER (50076)**, 2200 O'Farrell Street, Zip 94115–3358; tel. 415/833–2000 **A**1 3 5 10 **F**3 8 13 15 17 18 19 20 21 22 23 24 26 28 29 30 31 32 33 35 40 41 44 45 46 49 50 52 60 61 62 64 65 66 68 70 72 74 75 76 77 78 79 81 82 84 85 86 87 89 100 107 108 111 118 129 140 144 145 **P**3 **S** Kaiser Foundation Hospitals, Oakland, CA
Primary Contact: Christine Robisch, Senior Vice President and Area Manager
COO: Helen Archer–Duste, Chief Operating Officer
CFO: Alex Khoo, Interim Area Finance Officer
CMO: Robert Mithun, M.D., Physician in Chief
CIO: Peti Arunamata, Interim Area Director Information Technology
CHR: Diane J. Easterwood, Human Resources Business Partner
Web address: www.kaiserpermanente.org
**Control:** Other not–for–profit (including NFP Corporation) **Service:** General Medical and Surgical

**Staffed Beds:** 215 **Admissions:** 13864 **Census:** 167 **Outpatient Visits:** 68135 **Births:** 2752

★ **ST. LUKE'S HOSPITAL (50055)**, 3555 Cesar Chavez Street, Zip 94110–4490; tel. 415/600–6000, (Nonreporting) **A**5 10 **S** Sutter Health, Sacramento, CA
Primary Contact: Warren S. Browner, M.D., M.P.H., Chief Executive Officer
COO: Rick Stevens, Chief Administrative Officer
CFO: John Gates, Chief Financial Officer
CMO: Jerome Franz, M.D., Chief Medical Staff
CIO: Rob Seide, Manager Marketing and Communications
CHR: Linda Isaacs, Vice President Human Resources
CNO: Diana M. Karner, R.N., Chief Nursing Officer
Web address: www.stlukes–sf.org
**Control:** Other not–for–profit (including NFP Corporation) **Service:** General Medical and Surgical

**Staffed Beds:** 229

☒ **ST. MARY'S MEDICAL CENTER (50457)**, 450 Stanyan Street, Zip 94117–1079; tel. 415/668–1000, (Nonreporting) **A**1 3 5 9 10 **S** Dignity Health, San Francisco, CA
Primary Contact: Anna Cheung, President
COO: Deborah Kolhede, Vice President and Chief Operating Officer
CFO: Eric Brettner, Vice President and Chief Financial Officer
CMO: Francis Charlton, Jr., M.D., Chief Medical Staff
CHR: Barbara Morrissett, Vice President Human Resources
CNO: Barbara Eusebio, R.N., Vice President, Chief Nurse Executive
Web address: www.stmarysmedicalcenter.com
**Control:** Other not–for–profit (including NFP Corporation) **Service:** General Medical and Surgical

**Staffed Beds:** 232

☒ **UCSF MEDICAL CENTER (50454)**, 500 Parnassus Avenue, Zip 94143–0296, Mailing Address: 500 Parnassus Avenue, Box 0296, Zip 94143–0296; tel. 415/476–1000, (Includes UCSF BENIOFF CHILDREN'S HOSPITAL, 500 Parnassus Avenue, Zip 94143–2203, Mailing Address: 505 Parnassus Avenue, Zip 94143–2203; tel. 888/689–8273) **A**1 2 3 5 8 9 10 **F**3 6 7 8 9 11 12 13 14 15 17 18 19 20 21 22 23 24 25 26 27 29 30 31 32 33 34 35 36 37 39 40 44 45 46 47 48 49 50 51 52 53 54 55 56 57 58 59 60 61 62 63 64 65 66 68 70 72 74 75 76 77 78 79 81 82 83 84 85 86 87 88 89 93 94 95 96 97 99 100 101 102 103 104 105 107 108 109 110 111 112 113 114 115 116 117 118 119 120 122 123 125 128 129 130 131 133 134 135 136 137 138 139 140 141 143 144 145 146 147 **P**6 **S** University of California–Systemwide Administration, Oakland, CA
Primary Contact: Mark R. Laret, Chief Executive Officer
COO: Ken M. Jones, Interim Chief Operating Officer
CFO: Susan B. Moore, Interim Chief Financial Officer
CMO: Josh Adler, M.D., Interim Co–Chief Medical Officer
CIO: Larry Lotenero, Chief Information Officer
CHR: David Odato, Chief Administrative and Chief Human Resources Officer
Web address: www.ucsfhealth.org
**Control:** Other not–for–profit (including NFP Corporation) **Service:** General Medical and Surgical

**Staffed Beds:** 660 **Admissions:** 26935 **Census:** 500 **Outpatient Visits:** 1071433 **Births:** 1858 **Total Expense ($000):** 1750192 **Payroll Expense ($000):** 689451 **Personnel:** 7019

☒ **VETERANS AFFAIRS MEDICAL CENTER**, 4150 Clement Street, Zip 94121–1598; tel. 415/221–4810, (Total facility includes 120 beds in nursing home–type unit) **A**1 2 3 5 **F**5 8 12 17 18 20 22 24 26 28 29 30 31 34 35 37 38 39 40 45 46 47 48 49 50 54 56 57 58 59 60 61 62 63 64 65 70 74 75 77 78 79 81 82 83 84 86 87 92 93 94 97 98 100 101 102 103 104 105 106 107 108 109 111 112 113 114 115 116 117 118 125 126 127 128 129 131 134 142 143 145 146 147 **P**1 **S** Department of Veterans Affairs, Washington, DC
Primary Contact: Lawrence H. Carroll, Director
COO: Ezra R. Safdie, Associate Director
CFO: Brian Kelly, Acting Chief Fiscal Service
CMO: C. Diana Nicoll, M.D., Chief of Staff
CIO: Judith A. Ringler, Chief Information Resources Management
CHR: Terrence Vail, Acting Chief Human Resources Management Services
Web address: www.va.gov/sta/guide/home.asp
**Control:** Veterans Affairs, Government, federal **Service:** General Medical and Surgical

**Staffed Beds:** 244 **Admissions:** 5811 **Census:** 190 **Outpatient Visits:** 508081 **Births:** 0 **Total Expense ($000):** 516153 **Payroll Expense ($000):** 209580

**SAN GABRIEL—Los Angeles County**

☐ **SAN GABRIEL VALLEY MEDICAL CENTER (50132)**, 438 West Las Tunas Drive, Zip 91776–1216, Mailing Address: P.O. Box 1507, Zip 91778–1507; tel. 626/289–5454, (Nonreporting) **A**1 9 10 **S** AHMC & Healthcare, Inc., Alhambra, CA
Primary Contact: Michael Murray, Chief Executive Officer
COO: Harold Way, Chief Financial Officer and Chief Operating Officer
CFO: Harold Way, Chief Financial Officer and Chief Operating Officer
CIO: Bernie Sauer, Director Information Technology
CHR: Victor Voisard, Director Human Resources
Web address: www.sgvmc.org
**Control:** Other not–for–profit (including NFP Corporation) **Service:** General Medical and Surgical

**Staffed Beds:** 231

**CA**

---

**Hospital, Medicare Provider Number, Address, Telephone, Approval, Facility, and Physician Codes, Health Care System**

★ American Hospital Association (AHA) membership
☐ The Joint Commission accreditation
◇ DNV Healthcare Inc. accreditation
○ American Osteopathic Association (AOA) accreditation
△ Commission on Accreditation of Rehabilitation Facilities (CARF) accreditation

## SAN JOSE—Santa Clara County

☒ **GOOD SAMARITAN HOSPITAL (50380)**, 2425 Samaritan Drive, Zip 95124–3997, Mailing Address: P.O. Box 240002, Zip 95154–2402; tel. 408/559–2011 **A**1 2 9 10 **F**2 3 5 8 11 12 13 15 17 18 19 20 21 22 23 24 25 26 27 28 29 30 31 34 35 37 38 40 44 45 46 47 48 49 50 54 57 58 59 60 63 64 68 70 72 74 75 76 77 78 79 81 82 83 84 85 86 87 88 89 90 93 96 98 101 102 104 105 107 108 110 111 113 114 115 116 117 118 119 120 122 123 125 129 131 145 146 147 **S** HCA, Nashville, TN
Primary Contact: Paul Beaupre, M.D., Chief Executive Officer
COO: Robert Krieger, Interim Chief Operating Officer
CFO: Lana Aran, Chief Financial Officer
CMO: Arthur Douville, M.D., Chief Medical Officer
CIO: Darrell O'Dell, Director Information Services
CHR: John Omel, Interim Vice President Human Resources
CNO: Dian Adams, R.N., Chief Nursing Officer
Web address: www.goodsamsanjose.com
**Control:** Corporation, Investor–owned, for–profit **Service:** General Medical and Surgical

**Staffed Beds:** 349 **Admissions:** 16679 **Census:** 224 **Outpatient Visits:** 128595 **Births:** 3289 **Total Expense ($000):** 348958 **Payroll Expense ($000):** 173384 **Personnel:** 1429

☒ **O'CONNOR HOSPITAL (50153)**, 2105 Forest Avenue, Zip 95128–1471; tel. 408/947–2500, (Total facility includes 24 beds in nursing home–type unit) **A**1 2 9 10 **F**3 11 13 15 18 19 20 22 24 26 28 29 30 31 34 35 37 40 44 46 48 49 50 53 54 57 59 60 64 66 68 70 72 74 75 76 77 78 79 81 84 85 86 87 89 93 97 100 107 108 110 111 113 115 116 117 118 120 122 127 129 130 131 134 145 146 147 **S** Daughters of Charity Health System, Los Altos Hills, CA
Primary Contact: James F. Dover, FACHE, President and Chief Executive Officer
COO: Ronald J. Galonsky, Chief Operating Officer
CFO: David W. Carroll, Chief Financial Officer
CMO: George Block, M.D., Chief Medical Officer
CIO: Richard Hutsell, Vice President and Chief Information Officer
CHR: Julie Hatcher, Vice President Human Resources
CNO: Judy A. Watland, R.N., Chief Nursing Officer
Web address: www.oconnorhospital.org
**Control:** Other not–for–profit (including NFP Corporation) **Service:** General Medical and Surgical

**Staffed Beds:** 202 **Admissions:** 12746 **Census:** 144 **Outpatient Visits:** 155867 **Births:** 3341 **Total Expense ($000):** 317659 **Payroll Expense ($000):** 142646

☒ **REGIONAL MEDICAL CENTER OF SAN JOSE (50125)**, 225 North Jackson Avenue, Zip 95116–1691; tel. 408/259–5000, (Nonreporting) **A**1 9 10 **S** HCA, Nashville, TN
Primary Contact: Michael T. Johnson, Chief Executive Officer
COO: Brian J. Knecht, Chief Operating Officer
CFO: Raju Iyer, Chief Financial Officer
CMO: William Scott, M.D., Vice President Medical Affairs
CIO: Shirley Joyal, Director Information Systems
CHR: Nancy Clark, Vice President Human Resources
Web address: www.regionalmedicalsanjose.com
**Control:** Partnership, Investor–owned, for–profit **Service:** General Medical and Surgical

**Staffed Beds:** 193

☒ **SAN JOSE MEDICAL CENTER (50604)**, 250 Hospital Parkway, Zip 95119–1199; tel. 408/972–7000 **A**1 10 **F**3 8 13 17 18 20 22 29 30 31 35 40 46 49 51 56 68 70 73 74 76 78 79 81 82 84 85 87 104 107 110 111 113 114 118 129 134 140 145 147 **S** Kaiser Foundation Hospitals, Oakland, CA
Primary Contact: Irene Chavez, Senior Vice President and Area Manager
COO: Terry L. Austen, Senior Vice President and Area Manager
CFO: Stephen L. Kalsman, Area Finance Officer
CMO: Raj Bhandari, M.D., Physician–in–Chief
CIO: Ernie Japec, Area Information Officer
CHR: Susan Franzella, Human Resource Business Partner
Web address: www.kaiserpermanente.org
**Control:** Other not–for–profit (including NFP Corporation) **Service:** General Medical and Surgical

**Staffed Beds:** 217 **Admissions:** 11709 **Census:** 125 **Outpatient Visits:** 55998 **Births:** 1951 **Personnel:** 1282

☐ △ **SANTA CLARA VALLEY MEDICAL CENTER (50038)**, 751 South Bascom Avenue, Zip 95128–2604; tel. 408/885–5000 **A**1 3 5 7 9 10 **F**3 5 9 12 13 15 16 17 18 19 20 21 22 23 24 25 26 27 28 29 30 31 32 34 35 39 40 43 45 46 47 48 49 50 51 52 55 56 58 59 60 61 64 65 66 68 70 71 72 73 74 75 76 77 78 79 80 81 82 83 84 85 86 87 88 89 90 92 93 97 98 99 100 101 102 103 104 107 108 109 110 111 112 113 114 115 116 117 118 119 120 121 122 123 128 129 130 131 133 134 141 142 143 145 146 147 **P**6
Primary Contact: Linda Smith, FACHE, Chief Executive Officer
CFO: David S. McGrew, Chief Financial Officer
CMO: Alfonso F. Banuelos, Jr., M.D., Chief Medical Officer
CIO: Lee Herrmann, Chief Healthcare Technology Officer
CHR: David Manson, Manager Human Resources
CNO: Trudy Johnson, R.N., Chief Nursing Officer
Web address: www.scvmed.org
**Control:** County–Government, nonfederal **Service:** General Medical and Surgical

**Staffed Beds:** 554 **Admissions:** 22087 **Census:** 336 **Outpatient Visits:** 856486 **Births:** 4463 **Total Expense ($000):** 1022516 **Payroll Expense ($000):** 421154

## SAN LEANDRO—Alameda County

**ALAMEDA COUNTY MEDICAL CENTER–FAIRMONT CAMPUS** See Alameda County Medical Center, Oakland

☒ **KINDRED HOSPITAL–SAN FRANCISCO BAY AREA (52034)**, 2800 Benedict Drive, Zip 94577–6840; tel. 510/357–8300, (Nonreporting) **A**1 9 10 **S** Kindred Healthcare, Louisville, KY
Primary Contact: Kelli Cole, Chief Executive Officer
COO: Mary Schwind, R.N., Chief Clinical Officer
CFO: Ziba Aflak, Chief Financial Officer
CHR: Laurel Scharber, Coordinator Human Resources
Web address: www.kindredhospitalsfba.com
**Control:** Corporation, Investor–owned, for–profit **Service:** Long–Term Acute Care hospital

**Staffed Beds:** 99

## SAN LUIS OBISPO—San Luis Obispo County

**CALIFORNIA MENS COLONY HOSPITAL**, Highway 1, Zip 93409–8101, Mailing Address: P.O. Box 8101, Zip 93403–8101; tel. 805/547–7913, (Nonreporting)
Primary Contact: Galen Kirn, Administrator
CFO: William Cook, Associate Warden Business Service
CIO: Terry Knight, Public Information Officer and Administrative Assistant
Web address: www.yaca.ca.gov/visitors/fac_prison_cmc.html
**Control:** State–Government, nonfederal **Service:** Hospital unit of an institution (prison hospital, college infirmary, etc.)

**Staffed Beds:** 39

☒ **FRENCH HOSPITAL MEDICAL CENTER (50232)**, 1911 Johnson Avenue, Zip 93401–4131; tel. 805/543–5353 **A**1 9 10 **F**8 11 15 18 20 22 24 28 29 30 34 35 40 46 50 53 54 57 59 64 68 70 75 76 77 78 79 81 84 85 86 87 89 93 97 100 107 108 110 111 113 114 118 123 129 131 145 146 147 **S** Dignity Health, San Francisco, CA
Primary Contact: Alan Iftiniuk, Chief Executive Officer
CFO: Sue Andersen, Chief Financial Officer
CMO: J. Trees Ritter, D.O., Chief of Staff
CIO: Cyndi Lang, Director Information Services
CHR: Kristin Flynn, Manager Human Resources
CNO: Linda Riggle, R.N., Vice President Patient Care Services and Chief Nursing Executive
Web address: www.frenchmedicalcenter.org
**Control:** Other not–for–profit (including NFP Corporation) **Service:** General Medical and Surgical

**Staffed Beds:** 112 **Admissions:** 4750 **Census:** 46 **Outpatient Visits:** 103019 **Births:** 790 **Total Expense ($000):** 93303 **Payroll Expense ($000):** 36695 **Personnel:** 400

☒ **SIERRA VISTA REGIONAL MEDICAL CENTER (50506)**, 1010 Murray Avenue, Zip 93405–8800, Mailing Address: P.O. Box 1367, Zip 93406–1367; tel. 805/546–7600 **A**1 9 10 19 **F**3 4 11 13 15 16 17 18 20 29 31 34 35 38 39 40 45 46 49 50 51 57 64 65 67 70 72 73 74 75 76 77 78 79 80 81 84 85 86 88 89 90 98 107 108 110 114 118 125 127 129 130 131 144 145 146 147 **S** TENET Healthcare Corporation, Dallas, TX
Primary Contact: Candace L. Markwith, Chief Executive Officer
COO: Joseph DeSchryver, Chief Operating Officer
CFO: Rollie Pirkl, Chief Financial Officer
CIO: Robert Leonard, Director Information Services
CHR: Bill Peterson, Chief Human Resources Director
CNO: Christie Gonder, Chief Nursing Officer
Web address: www.sierravistaregional.com
**Control:** Corporation, Investor–owned, for–profit **Service:** General Medical and Surgical

**Staffed Beds:** 164 **Admissions:** 5839 **Census:** 72 **Outpatient Visits:** 55704 **Births:** 1299 **Total Expense ($000):** 107546 **Payroll Expense ($000):** 49862 **Personnel:** 655

*Many Facility Codes have changed. Please refer to the AHA Guide Code Chart.* © 2012 AHA Guide

## SAN MATEO—San Mateo County

**MILLS HOSPITAL** See Mills–Peninsula Health Services, Burlingame

☐ **SAN MATEO MEDICAL CENTER (50113)**, 222 West 39th Avenue, Zip 94403–4398; tel. 650/573–2222, (Total facility includes 257 beds in nursing home–type unit) **A**1 3 5 9 10 **F**1 3 15 18 19 29 30 31 32 39 40 45 47 49 51 54 56 59 60 61 64 65 66 68 69 70 71 74 75 78 79 81 82 83 84 87 89 90 93 97 98 100 101 102 103 104 105 107 114 118 127 129 133 142 143 145 146 147 **P**6 8
Primary Contact: Susan Ehrlich, M.D., Chief Executive Officer
COO: John Thomas, Chief Operating Officer
CFO: Philip Fortunato, Interim Chief Financial Officer
CMO: Chester Kunnappilly, M.D., Chief Medical Officer and Chief Quality Officer
CIO: Michael Aratow, M.D., Chief Information Officer
CHR: Sonya Siebe, Manager Human Resources
CNO: Liz Evans, Chief Nursing Officer
Web address: www.sanmateomedicalcenter.org
**Control:** County–Government, nonfederal **Service:** General Medical and Surgical

**Staffed Beds:** 307 **Admissions:** 4105 **Census:** 316 **Outpatient Visits:** 434616 **Births:** 0 **Total Expense ($000):** 233972 **Payroll Expense ($000):** 147573 **Personnel:** 1215

## SAN PABLO—Contra Costa County

☐ **DOCTORS MEDICAL CENTER–SAN PABLO CAMPUS (50079)**, 2000 Vale Road, Zip 94806–3808; tel. 510/970–5000 **A**1 2 9 10 **F**8 18 20 22 24 26 28 29 30 31 34 35 40 45 48 49 51 54 57 58 59 60 64 70 75 77 78 79 81 85 86 93 94 96 107 108 110 111 113 116 118 120 128 129 131 145 147
Primary Contact: Dawn M. Gideon, Interim Chief Executive Officer
COO: Kathy White, Interim Chief Operating Officer
CFO: James Boatman, Chief Financial Officer
CMO: Laurel Hodgson, M.D., President Medical Staff
CIO: Phyllis Moore, Director Information Systems and Data Center
CHR: John Hardy, Vice President Human Resources
CNO: Kathy White, Interim Chief Nursing Officer
Web address: www.doctorsmedicalcenter.org
**Control:** Hospital district or authority, Government, nonfederal **Service:** General Medical and Surgical

**Staffed Beds:** 140 **Admissions:** 6073 **Census:** 75 **Outpatient Visits:** 72791

## SAN PEDRO—Los Angeles County, See Los Angeles

## SAN RAFAEL—Marin County

☒ **SAN RAFAEL MEDICAL CENTER (50510)**, 99 Montecillo Road, Zip 94903–3308; tel. 415/444–2000, (Nonreporting) **A**1 10 **S** Kaiser Foundation Hospitals, Oakland, CA
Primary Contact: Judy Coffey, Senior Vice President and Area Manager
COO: Tony Fiorello, R.N., Chief Operating and Chief Nursing Officer
CFO: John Groesbeck, Area Finance Officer
CMO: Gary Mizono, M.D., Physician–in–Chief
CIO: Stanley Dobrawa, Area Technology Director
CHR: Rudy Collins, Human Resources Business Partner
CNO: Tony Fiorello, R.N., Chief Operating and Chief Nursing Officer
Web address: www.kaiserpermanente.org
**Control:** Other not–for–profit (including NFP Corporation) **Service:** General Medical and Surgical

**Staffed Beds:** 82

## SAN RAMON—Contra Costa County

☒ **SAN RAMON REGIONAL MEDICAL CENTER (50689)**, 6001 Norris Canyon Road, Zip 94583–5400; tel. 925/275–9200 **A**1 9 10 **F**3 8 13 15 17 18 20 22 24 26 28 29 30 31 34 35 37 40 45 46 47 48 49 53 57 59 70 72 76 78 79 81 85 86 87 89 93 107 108 110 113 117 118 125 129 130 131 145 146 147 **S** TENET Healthcare Corporation, Dallas, TX
Primary Contact: Gary Sloan, Chief Executive Officer
COO: Susan C. Micheletti, Chief Operating Officer
CFO: Beenu Chadha, Chief Financial Officer
CMO: Erik Gracer, M.D., Chief of Staff
CIO: Guy Tennyson, Director Information Systems and Telecommunications
CHR: Dennis Mills, Director Human Resources
CNO: Pam Pshea, R.N., Chief Nursing Officer
Web address: www.sanramonmedctr.com
**Control:** City–County, Government, nonfederal **Service:** General Medical and Surgical

**Staffed Beds:** 123 **Admissions:** 4744 **Census:** 52 **Outpatient Visits:** 70942 **Births:** 698 **Total Expense ($000):** 124475 **Payroll Expense ($000):** 69631 **Personnel:** 470

## SANTA ANA—Orange County

☐ **COASTAL COMMUNITIES HOSPITAL (50747)**, 2701 South Bristol Street, Zip 92704–6201; tel. 714/754–5454, (Nonreporting) **A**1 9 10 **S** Integrated Healthcare, Santa Ana, CA
Primary Contact: Craig G. Myers, Chief Executive Officer
CFO: Patricia Henry, Chief Financial Officer
CHR: Gretchen Lindeman, Director Human Resources
Web address: www.coastalcommhospital.com
**Control:** Corporation, Investor–owned, for–profit **Service:** General Medical and Surgical

**Staffed Beds:** 178

☐ **WESTERN MEDICAL CENTER–SANTA ANA (50746)**, 1001 North Tustin Avenue, Zip 92705–3577; tel. 714/835–3555, (Nonreporting) **A**1 3 5 9 10 **S** Integrated Healthcare, Santa Ana, CA
Primary Contact: Daniel Brothman, Chief Executive Officer
COO: Doug Norris, Administrator and Chief Operating Officer
CFO: Kathy Hammack, Chief Financial Officer
CMO: Seifolah Esfandiari, M.D., Chief of Staff
CIO: Nova Stewart, Chief Information Officer
CHR: Milas H. Kennington, Vice President, Human Resources
CNO: Patricia Rives, R.N., Chief Nursing Officer
Web address: www.westernmedicalcenter.com
**Control:** Corporation, Investor–owned, for–profit **Service:** General Medical and Surgical

**Staffed Beds:** 282

## SANTA BARBARA—Santa Barbara County

**COTTAGE REHABILITATION HOSPITAL** See Santa Barbara Cottage Hospital

☒ **GOLETA VALLEY COTTAGE HOSPITAL (50357)**, 351 South Patterson Avenue, Zip 93111–2496, Mailing Address: Box 6306, Zip 93160–6306; tel. 805/967–3411 **A**1 9 10 **F**8 11 12 15 29 40 65 68 70 79 81 107 110 113 118 123 147 **S** Cottage Health System, Santa Barbara, CA
Primary Contact: Ronald C. Werft, President and Chief Executive Officer
COO: Steven A. Fellows, Executive Vice President and Chief Operating Officer
CFO: Joan Bricher, Senior Vice President Finance and Chief Financial Officer
CMO: Edmund Wroblewski, M.D., Vice President Medical Affairs and Chief Medical Officer
CIO: Alberto Kywi, Chief Information Officer
CHR: Patrice Ryan, Vice President Human Resources
Web address: www.sbch.org
**Control:** Other not–for–profit (including NFP Corporation) **Service:** General Medical and Surgical

**Staffed Beds:** 78 **Admissions:** 1611 **Census:** 41 **Outpatient Visits:** 41729 **Births:** 0 **Total Expense ($000):** 54855 **Payroll Expense ($000):** 23866 **Personnel:** 296

☒ △ **SANTA BARBARA COTTAGE HOSPITAL (50396)**, 400 West Pueblo Street, Zip 93105–4390, Mailing Address: P.O. Box 689, Zip 93102–0689; tel. 805/682–7111, (Includes COTTAGE REHABILITATION HOSPITAL, 2415 De la Vina Street, Zip 93105–3819; tel. 805/687–7444; Melinda Staveley, President and Chief Executive Officer) **A**1 2 3 5 7 9 10 **F**3 4 5 8 11 12 13 15 17 18 20 22 24 26 28 29 30 31 34 35 40 43 46 50 53 54 57 59 60 64 68 70 72 74 75 76 78 79 81 84 86 88 89 90 91 92 93 96 98 100 102 103 104 106 107 110 111 113 114 118 125 129 131 134 145 147 **S** Cottage Health System, Santa Barbara, CA
Primary Contact: Ronald C. Werft, President and Chief Executive Officer
COO: Steven A. Fellows, Executive Vice President and Chief Operating Officer
CFO: Joan Bricher, Senior Vice President Finance and Chief Financial Officer
CMO: Edmund Wroblewski, M.D., Vice President Medical Affairs and Chief Medical Officer
CIO: Alberto Kywi, Chief Information Officer
CHR: Patrice Ryan, Vice President Human Resources
Web address: www.cottagehealthsystem.org
**Control:** Other not–for–profit (including NFP Corporation) **Service:** General Medical and Surgical

**Staffed Beds:** 345 **Admissions:** 18101 **Census:** 235 **Outpatient Visits:** 126938 **Births:** 2384 **Total Expense ($000):** 434903 **Payroll Expense ($000):** 174234 **Personnel:** 2378

---

**Hospital, Medicare Provider Number, Address, Telephone, Approval, Facility, and Physician Codes, Health Care System**

★ American Hospital Association (AHA) membership
☐ The Joint Commission accreditation ◇ DNV Healthcare Inc. accreditation
○ American Osteopathic Association (AOA) accreditation
△ Commission on Accreditation of Rehabilitation Facilities (CARF) accreditation

## SANTA CLARA—Santa Clara County

☒ **SANTA CLARA MEDICAL CENTER (50071)**, 700 Lawrence Expressway, Zip 95051–5173; tel. 408/851–1000 **A**1 3 5 10 **F**3 5 6 8 9 11 12 13 15 17 18 19 20 21 22 23 24 26 28 29 30 31 32 34 35 36 38 40 41 44 45 48 49 50 51 52 53 54 55 56 57 58 59 60 61 62 63 64 65 68 70 71 72 73 74 75 76 77 78 79 80 81 82 83 84 85 86 87 88 89 91 92 93 94 96 97 99 100 101 104 107 108 109 110 111 113 114 115 116 117 118 119 120 122 123 125 128 129 130 131 133 134 143 145 146 147 **P**3 **S** Kaiser Foundation Hospitals, Oakland, CA
Primary Contact: Christopher L. Boyd, Senior Vice President and Area Manager
COO: Susan G. Murphy, Chief Operating Officer
CFO: Carol Reeves, Interim Area Finance Officer
CMO: Susan Smarr, M.D., Physician–in–Chief
CIO: Scott May, Area Director Technology
CHR: Robert Hyde, Human Resources Business Partner
CNO: Anne M. Goldfisher, R.N., Chief Nursing Officer
Web address: www.kaiserpermanente.org
**Control:** Other not–for–profit (including NFP Corporation) **Service:** General Medical and Surgical

**Staffed Beds:** 327 **Admissions:** 23325 **Census:** 259 **Births:** 4156 **Personnel:** 4433

## SANTA CRUZ—Santa Cruz County

☒ **DOMINICAN HOSPITAL (50242)**, 1555 Soquel Drive, Zip 95065–1794; tel. 831/462–7700, (Nonreporting) **A**1 9 10 **S** Dignity Health, San Francisco, CA
Primary Contact: Nanette Mickiewicz, M.D., President and Chief Medical Officer
COO: Chris Wernke, Chief Operating Officer
CFO: Rick Harron, Chief Financial Officer
CMO: Nanette Mickiewicz, M.D., President and Chief Medical Officer
CIO: Lee Vanderpool, Vice President
CHR: Vicki Miranda, Vice President Human Resources
Web address: www.dominicanhospital.org
**Control:** Church–operated, Nongovernment, not–for profit **Service:** General Medical and Surgical

**Staffed Beds:** 276

☒ **SUTTER MATERNITY AND SURGERY CENTER OF SANTA CRUZ (50714)**, 2900 Chanticleer Avenue, Zip 95065–1816; tel. 831/477–2200, (Nonreporting) **A**1 9 10 **S** Sutter Health, Sacramento, CA
Primary Contact: Richard Nichols, Administrator
CFO: Iftikhar Hussain, Chief Financial Officer
CMO: Matthew Hansman, M.D., Chief of Staff
CIO: Michael Reandeau, Regional Chief Information Officer
CHR: Maynard Jenkins, Regional Vice President for Human Resources
CNO: Jacci Sterling, R.N., Chief Nursing Executive
Web address: www.suttermatsurg.org
**Control:** Other not–for–profit (including NFP Corporation) **Service:** Obstetrics and gynecology

**Staffed Beds:** 30

## SANTA MARIA—Santa Barbara County

☒ **MARIAN MEDICAL CENTER (50107)**, 1400 East Church Street, Zip 93454–5906; tel. 805/739–3000, (Total facility includes 95 beds in nursing home–type unit) **A**1 2 9 10 **F**3 8 11 13 15 17 18 20 22 24 28 29 30 31 34 35 36 39 40 46 49 50 53 54 56 57 58 59 60 62 63 64 65 66 68 69 72 74 75 76 77 78 79 81 82 84 85 86 87 89 93 97 100 107 108 110 111 113 117 118 125 126 127 129 131 133 134 142 143 145 146 147 **S** Dignity Health, San Francisco, CA
Primary Contact: Charles J. Cova, President and Chief Executive Officer
CFO: Sue Andersen, Chief Financial Officer
CMO: Chuck Merrill, M.D., Vice President Medical Affairs
CIO: Patricia Haase, Director Information Technology and Communications
CHR: Susan Winsell, Vice President Human Resources
Web address: www.marianmedicalcenter.org
**Control:** Church–operated, Nongovernment, not–for profit **Service:** General Medical and Surgical

**Staffed Beds:** 256 **Admissions:** 10527 **Census:** 181 **Outpatient Visits:** 181207 **Births:** 2745 **Total Expense ($000):** 210609 **Payroll Expense ($000):** 90661 **Personnel:** 1058

## SANTA MONICA—Los Angeles County

☒ **SAINT JOHN'S HEALTH CENTER (50290)**, 2121 Santa Monica Boulevard, Zip 90404; tel. 310/829–5511, (Nonreporting) **A**1 2 9 10 **S** Sisters of Charity of Leavenworth Health System, Denver, CO
Primary Contact: Lou Lazatin, President and Chief Executive Officer
COO: Eleanor Ramirez, R.N., Executive Vice President and Chief Operating Officer
CFO: Michelle Mok, Chief Financial Officer
CIO: Martha Ponce, Director Information Technologies and Telecommunications
CHR: Steven Sharrer, Vice President Human Resources
CNO: Dawna Hendel, R.N., Chief Nursing Officer and Vice President Patient Care Services
Web address: www.newstjohns.org
**Control:** Church–operated, Nongovernment, not–for profit **Service:** General Medical and Surgical

**Staffed Beds:** 223

☒ **SANTA MONICA–UCLA MEDICAL CENTER AND ORTHOPAEDIC HOSPITAL (50112)**, 1250 16th Street, Zip 90404; tel. 310/319–4000 **A**1 3 5 9 10 **F**3 8 9 11 12 13 15 18 20 22 24 26 27 29 30 31 34 35 37 40 41 45 46 47 48 49 50 52 54 55 56 57 58 59 64 65 68 70 72 74 75 76 78 79 81 82 84 85 86 87 89 93 96 97 102 107 108 110 111 113 114 115 116 117 118 129 130 142 144 145 146 **P**6 **S** University of California–Systemwide Administration, Oakland, CA
Primary Contact: Posie Carpenter, R.N., MSN, Chief Administrative Officer
COO: Posie Carpenter, R.N., Chief Administrative Officer
CFO: Paul Staton, Chief Financial Officer
CMO: James Atkinson, M.D., Medical Director
CIO: Virginia McFerran, Chief Information Officer
CHR: Mark Speare, Senior Associate Director Patient Relations and Human Resources
Web address: www.healthcare.ucla.edu
**Control:** State–Government, nonfederal **Service:** General Medical and Surgical

**Staffed Beds:** 316 **Admissions:** 14966 **Census:** 208 **Outpatient Visits:** 134695 **Births:** 1375 **Total Expense ($000):** 294340 **Payroll Expense ($000):** 127950 **Personnel:** 1511

## SANTA ROSA—Sonoma County

☒ **SANTA ROSA MEDICAL CENTER (50690)**, 401 Bicentennial Way, Zip 95403–2192; tel. 707/571–4000, (Nonreporting) **A**1 10 **S** Kaiser Foundation Hospitals, Oakland, CA
Primary Contact: Judy Coffey, Senior Vice President and Area Manager
COO: Susan Janvrin, R.N., Chief Operating and Chief Nursing Officer
CFO: John Groesbeck, Area Finance Officer
CMO: Kirk Pappas, M.D., Physician–in–Chief
CIO: Stanley Dobrawa, Area Technology Director
CHR: Rudy Collins, Human Resources Business Partner
CNO: Susan Janvrin, R.N., Chief Operating and Chief Nursing Officer
Web address: www.kaiserpermanente.org
**Control:** Other not–for–profit (including NFP Corporation) **Service:** General Medical and Surgical

**Staffed Beds:** 117

☒ **SANTA ROSA MEMORIAL HOSPITAL (50174)**, 1165 Montgomery Drive, Zip 95405–4897, Mailing Address: P.O. Box 522, Zip 95402–0522; tel. 707/546–3210 **A**1 2 9 10 **F**3 8 11 12 13 15 18 20 22 24 26 28 29 30 31 34 35 39 40 43 44 45 47 48 49 51 54 56 58 59 60 64 65 66 68 70 71 72 74 75 76 77 78 79 81 82 83 84 85 86 87 89 90 93 104 105 107 108 111 114 118 129 142 143 145 147 **S** St. Joseph Health, Orange, CA
Primary Contact: Kevin Klockenga, President and Chief Executive Officer
COO: Todd Salnas, Chief Operating Officer
CFO: Mich Riccioni, Chief Financial Officer
CMO: Gary Greensweig, D.O., Chief Medical Officer
CIO: Anna Shields, Executive Director Information Systems
CHR: Debra Miller, Vice President Human Resources
CNO: Rhonda Foster, Interim Chief Nursing Officer
Web address: www.stjosephhealth.org
**Control:** Other not–for–profit (including NFP Corporation) **Service:** General Medical and Surgical

**Staffed Beds:** 272 **Admissions:** 12781 **Census:** 156 **Outpatient Visits:** 164905 **Births:** 1005 **Total Expense ($000):** 329162 **Payroll Expense ($000):** 102146 **Personnel:** 1236

☒ **SUTTER MEDICAL CENTER OF SANTA ROSA, CHANATE CAMPUS (50291)**, 3325 Chanate Road, Zip 95404–1707; tel. 707/576–4000, (Includes WARRACK CAMPUS, 2449 Summerfield Road, Zip 95405–7815; tel. 707/576–4200), (Nonreporting) **A**1 3 5 9 10 **S** Sutter Health, Sacramento, CA
Primary Contact: Mike Purvis, Chief Administrative Officer
COO: F. Dana Ellerbe, Assistant Administrator
CFO: Avery Schlesenberg, Chief Financial Officer
CMO: Robert Heckey, M.D., Chief of Staff
CHR: Steve Morales, Director Human Resources
Web address: www.sutterhealth.org
**Control:** Other not–for–profit (including NFP Corporation) **Service:** General Medical and Surgical

**Staffed Beds:** 135

## SEBASTOPOL—Sonoma County

★ ○ **PALM DRIVE HOSPITAL (50385)**, 501 Petaluma Avenue, Zip 95472–4281; tel. 707/823–8511, (Nonreporting) **A**9 10 11
Primary Contact: Rick Reed, Interim Chief Executive Officer
CFO: David Glassburn, Interim Chief Financial Officer
CMO: Richard Powers, M.D., Chief of Staff
CIO: Bruce Espinosa, Manager Information Systems
CHR: Raoul McDuff, Director Human Resources
Web address: www.palmdrivehospital.org
**Control:** Other not–for–profit (including NFP Corporation) **Service:** General Medical and Surgical

**Staffed Beds:** 47

## SEPULVEDA—Los Angeles County, See Los Angeles

*Many Facility Codes have changed. Please refer to the AHA Guide Code Chart.* © 2012 AHA Guide

**SHERMAN OAKS—Los Angeles County, See Los Angeles**

**SIMI VALLEY—Ventura County**

⊞ **SIMI VALLEY HOSPITAL AND HEALTH CARE SERVICES (50236)**, 2975 North Sycamore Drive, Zip 93065–1201; tel. 805/955–6000, (Nonreporting) **A**1 2 9 10 **S** Adventist Health, Roseville, CA
Primary Contact: Caroline Esparza, Interim Chief Executive Officer
CFO: John Beaman, Senior Vice President and Chief Financial Officer
CFO: Jon Giese, Vice President and Chief Financial Officer
CMO: John Dingilian, M.D., Chief Medical Staff
CIO: Jeff Brown, Interim Director Information Systems
CHR: Sandy Werner, Director Human Resources
CNO: Caroline Esparza, Sr. VP to Patient Care Executive
Web address: www.simivalleyhospital.com
**Control:** Church–operated, Nongovernment, not–for profit **Service:** General Medical and Surgical

| Staffed Beds: 97 |
|---|

**SOLVANG—Santa Barbara County**

⊞ **SANTA YNEZ VALLEY COTTAGE HOSPITAL (51331)**, 2050 Viborg Road, Zip 93463–2295; tel. 805/688–6431 **A**1 9 10 18 **F**15 28 40 57 68 81 85 107 111 113 118 142 145 **S** Cottage Health System, Santa Barbara, CA
Primary Contact: Ronald C. Werft, President and Chief Executive Officer
COO: Steven A. Fellows, Executive Vice President and Chief Operating Officer
CFO: Joan Bricher, Senior Vice President Finance and Chief Financial Officer
CMO: Edmund Wroblewski, M.D., Vice President Medical Affairs and Chief Medical Officer
CIO: Alberto Kywi, Chief Information Officer
CHR: Patrice Ryan, Vice President Human Resources
Web address: www.cottagehealthsystem.org
**Control:** Other not–for–profit (including NFP Corporation) **Service:** General Medical and Surgical

| Staffed Beds: 10 Admissions: 302 Census: 3 Outpatient Visits: 28692 Births: 0 Personnel: 70 |
|---|

**SONOMA—Sonoma County**

⊞ **SONOMA VALLEY HOSPITAL (50090)**, 347 Andrieux Street, Zip 95476–6811, Mailing Address: P.O. Box 600, Zip 95476–0600; tel. 707/935–5000, (Total facility includes 27 beds in nursing home–type unit) **A**1 9 10 **F**11 12 13 15 18 28 29 35 40 49 70 75 76 77 79 80 81 93 107 108 110 111 114 117 118 127 129 145 147
Primary Contact: Kelly Mather, Chief Executive Officer
CFO: Richard Reid, Chief Financial Officer
CMO: Robert Cohen, M.D., Chief Medical Officer
CIO: Fe Sendaydiego, Director Information Systems
CHR: Paula M. Davis, Chief Human Resources Officer
CNO: Leslie Lovejoy, R.N., Chief Nursing and Quality Officer
Web address: www.svh.com
**Control:** Hospital district or authority, Government, nonfederal **Service:** General Medical and Surgical

| Staffed Beds: 65 Admissions: 2100 Census: 38 Outpatient Visits: 66357 Births: 180 Total Expense ($000): 45832 Payroll Expense ($000): 21922 Personnel: 242 |
|---|

**SONORA—Tuolumne County**

⊞ ○ **SONORA REGIONAL MEDICAL CENTER (50335)**, 1000 Greenley Road, Zip 95370–4819; tel. 209/536–5000, (Total facility includes 68 beds in nursing home–type unit) **A**1 9 10 11 **F**3 11 13 15 17 18 20 28 29 30 31 34 35 39 40 49 54 56 57 59 62 63 64 70 71 75 76 77 78 79 81 84 85 86 87 93 97 107 108 110 111 113 114 117 118 119 120 126 127 129 130 131 132 142 143 145 147 **P**6 **S** Adventist Health, Roseville, CA
Primary Contact: Jeff Eller, FACHE, President and Chief Executive Officer
CFO: Andrew Jahn, Vice President Finance
CMO: Ed Clinite, D.O., Chief of Staff
CIO: Bruce Chan, Director Business Planning and Marketing
CHR: Rick A. Dodds, Vice President Human Resources
CNO: Julie Kline, Senior Vice President Patient Services
Web address: www.sonorahospital.org
**Control:** Church–operated, Nongovernment, not–for profit **Service:** General Medical and Surgical

| Staffed Beds: 152 Admissions: 5094 Census: 121 Outpatient Visits: 289222 Births: 510 Total Expense ($000): 181025 Payroll Expense ($000): 67894 Personnel: 1067 |
|---|

**SOUTH EL MONTE—Los Angeles County**

☐ **GREATER EL MONTE COMMUNITY HOSPITAL (50738)**, 1701 Santa Anita Avenue, Zip 91733–3411; tel. 626/579–7777 **A**1 9 10 **F**3 13 17 18 19 29 34 35 40 49 56 57 59 65 68 70 76 81 87 89 93 107 118 127 129 142 145 **S** AHMC & Healthcare, Inc., Alhambra, CA
Primary Contact: Gale E. Gascho, Chief Executive Officer
COO: Jose Ortega, Administrator and Chief Operating Officer
CFO: Mary Anne Monje, Chief Financial Officer
CMO: Kamalakar Rambhatla, M.D., Chief of Staff
CIO: Jay Geldhof, Director Information Systems
CHR: Jason Jaquez, Director Human Resources
Web address: www.greaterelmonte.com
**Control:** Hospital district or authority, Government, nonfederal **Service:** General Medical and Surgical

| Staffed Beds: 46 Admissions: 4229 Census: 50 Births: 578 Total Expense ($000): 49368 Payroll Expense ($000): 19976 Personnel: 297 |
|---|

**SOUTH LAKE TAHOE—El Dorado County**

⊞ **BARTON HEALTHCARE SYSTEM (50352)**, 2170 South Avenue, Zip 96150–7026, Mailing Address: P.O. Box 9578, Zip 96158; tel. 530/541–3420, (Nonreporting) **A**1 9 10 20
Primary Contact: John G. Williams, President and Chief Executive Officer
COO: Kathy Cocking, R.N., Vice President Operations
CFO: Richard P. Derby, Vice President Finance
CMO: Clint Purvance, M.D., Chief Medical Officer
CIO: Rob Quadri, Director Management Information Systems
CHR: LeAnne Kankel, Vice President Human Relations
CNO: Mary J. Bittner, R.N., Vice President Nursing
Web address: www.bartonhealth.org
**Control:** Other not–for–profit (including NFP Corporation) **Service:** General Medical and Surgical

| Staffed Beds: 117 |
|---|

**SOUTH SAN FRANCISCO—San Mateo County**

⊞ **SOUTH SAN FRANCISCO MEDICAL CENTER (50070)**, 1200 El Camino Real, Zip 94080–3299; tel. 650/742–2000 **A**1 10 **F**3 5 8 12 15 18 29 30 31 32 34 35 36 40 45 46 47 48 49 50 51 54 56 57 58 59 62 63 64 65 68 70 74 75 77 78 79 81 82 84 85 86 87 91 92 93 94 95 97 99 100 101 103 104 107 108 110 111 113 114 117 118 119 120 122 123 128 129 130 131 134 145 146 147 **P**6 **S** Kaiser Foundation Hospitals, Oakland, CA
Primary Contact: Frank T. Beirne, Senior Vice President and Area Manager
CFO: Mark Okashima, Area Finance Officer
CMO: Michelle Caughey, M.D., Physician In Chief
CIO: Angel Shew, Director Area Technology
CHR: Sharon Barncord, Human Resource Business Partner
Web address: www.kaiserpermanente.org
**Control:** Other not–for–profit (including NFP Corporation) **Service:** General Medical and Surgical

| Staffed Beds: 120 Admissions: 5939 Census: 61 Outpatient Visits: 388294 Births: 0 Personnel: 882 |
|---|

**STOCKTON—San Joaquin County**

☐ **DAMERON HOSPITAL (50122)**, 525 West Acacia Street, Zip 95203–2484; tel. 209/944–5550, (Nonreporting) **A**1 9 10
Primary Contact: Christopher Arismendi, M.D., Chief Executive Officer
COO: Nicholas Arismendi, Chief Operating Officer
CFO: Cyrus E. Dah, Chief Financial Officer
CMO: Bradley Reinke, M.D., Chief of Staff
CIO: Glenn Whipple, Chief Information Officer
CHR: Maria Junez, Director Human Resources
CNO: Janine Hawkins, R.N., Chief Nursing Officer
Web address: www.dameronhospital.org
**Control:** Other not–for–profit (including NFP Corporation) **Service:** General Medical and Surgical

| Staffed Beds: 188 |
|---|

⊞ **ST. JOSEPH'S BEHAVIORAL HEALTH CENTER (54123)**, 2510 North California Street, Zip 95204–5502; tel. 209/461–2000 **A**1 9 10 **F**5 29 38 68 98 100 101 103 104 105 129 131 142 145 **S** Dignity Health, San Francisco, CA
Primary Contact: Paul Rains, R.N., MSN, President
CFO: Nikki Ochoa, Interim Chief Financial Officer
CMO: David Robinson, D.O., Medical Director
CHR: Nancy Vargas, Chief Human Resources
CNO: Alan Hall, Chief Nursing Officer
Web address: www.stjosephscanhelp.org
**Control:** Church–operated, Nongovernment, not–for profit **Service:** Psychiatric

| Staffed Beds: 35 Admissions: 1403 Census: 25 Outpatient Visits: 8656 Births: 0 Total Expense ($000): 12416 |
|---|

---

**Hospital, Medicare Provider Number, Address, Telephone, Approval, Facility, and Physician Codes, Health Care System**

★ American Hospital Association (AHA) membership
☐ The Joint Commission accreditation
◇ DNV Healthcare Inc. accreditation
○ American Osteopathic Association (AOA) accreditation
△ Commission on Accreditation of Rehabilitation Facilities (CARF) accreditation

⊠ **ST. JOSEPH'S MEDICAL CENTER (50084)**, 1800 North California Street, Zip 95204–6019, Mailing Address: P.O. Box 213008, Zip 95213–3008; tel. 209/943–2000, (Nonreporting) **A**1 2 9 10 **S** Dignity Health, San Francisco, CA
Primary Contact: Donald J. Wiley, President and Chief Executive Officer
COO: Michael Ricks, Chief Operating Officer
CFO: Nikki Ochoa, Interim Chief Financial Officer
CMO: Susan McDonald, M.D., Vice President
CIO: Randall Gamino, Director Perot Site
CHR: Nancy Vargas, Vice President Human Resources
Web address: www.stjosephsCARES.org
**Control:** Church–operated, Nongovernment, not–for profit **Service:** General Medical and Surgical

Staffed Beds: 273

**SUN CITY—Riverside County**

⊠ **MENIFEE VALLEY MEDICAL CENTER (50684)**, 28400 McCall Boulevard, Zip 92585–9537; tel. 951/679–8888, (Nonreporting) **A**1 9 10 **S** Physicians for Healthy Hospitals, Hemet, CA
Primary Contact: Joel Bergenfeld, Chief Executive Officer
CFO: Michael Garko, Chief Financial Officer
CHR: Michele Bird, Chief Human Resources Officer
Web address: www.valleyhealthsystem.com
**Control:** Hospital district or authority, Government, nonfederal **Service:** General Medical and Surgical

Staffed Beds: 82

**SUN VALLEY—Los Angeles County, See Los Angeles**

**SUSANVILLE—Lassen County**

⊠ **BANNER LASSEN MEDICAL CENTER (51320)**, 1800 Spring Ridge Drive, Zip 96130–4809; tel. 530/252–2000 **A**1 9 10 18 **F**3 11 13 15 29 31 34 35 40 45 50 56 57 59 64 68 75 76 77 78 79 81 85 87 92 107 108 110 111 113 118 128 145 147 **S** Banner Health, Phoenix, AZ
Primary Contact: Bob S. Edwards, Jr., FACHE, Chief Executive Officer
CFO: Shelby Diede, Chief Financial Officer
CMO: Hal Meadows, M.D., Chief Medical Officer
CHR: Melinda Moore, Chief Human Resources Officer
CNO: Catherine S. Harshbarger, R.N., Chief Nursing Officer
Web address: www.bannerhealth.com
**Control:** Other not–for–profit (including NFP Corporation) **Service:** General Medical and Surgical

Staffed Beds: 25 Admissions: 1352 Census: 11 Outpatient Visits: 52002 Births: 275 Total Expense ($000): 31645 Payroll Expense ($000): 12780 Personnel: 174

**SYLMAR—Los Angeles County, See Los Angeles**

**TARZANA—Los Angeles County, See Los Angeles**

**TEHACHAPI—Kern County**

★ **TEHACHAPI VALLEY HEALTHCARE DISTRICT (51301)**, 115 West E Street, Zip 93561, Mailing Address: P.O. Box 1900, Zip 93581–1900; tel. 661/823–3000, (Nonreporting) **A**9 10 18 21
Primary Contact: Alan J. Burgess, FACHE, Chief Executive Officer
CFO: William J. Van Noy, Chief Financial Officer
CMO: Susan Cribbs, D.O., Chief of Staff
CIO: Dusty Colvard, Manager Information Technology
CHR: Susan Nelson–Jones, Director Human Resources
CNO: Juliana Kay Kirby, R.N., Chief Nursing Officer and Director of Nursing
Web address: www.tvhd.org
**Control:** Hospital district or authority, Government, nonfederal **Service:** General Medical and Surgical

Staffed Beds: 24

**TEMPLETON—San Luis Obispo County**

⊠ **TWIN CITIES COMMUNITY HOSPITAL (50633)**, 1100 Las Tablas Road, Zip 93465–9704; tel. 805/434–3500 **A**1 9 10 **F**13 15 29 31 34 35 37 38 39 40 45 46 54 55 58 59 60 64 65 68 70 74 75 76 77 78 79 81 82 97 107 111 114 118 129 131 143 146 **S** TENET Healthcare Corporation, Dallas, TX
Primary Contact: Richard D. Lyons, Chief Executive Officer
COO: Nicholas Tejeda, Chief Operating Officer
CFO: Paul Posmoga, Chief Financial Officer
CMO: Paula Moore, R.N., Chief Nursing Officer
CIO: Scott Harrison, Director Information Systems
CHR: Eloise Rendon, Director Human Resources
Web address: www.twincitieshospital.com
**Control:** Corporation, Investor–owned, for–profit **Service:** General Medical and Surgical

Staffed Beds: 122 Admissions: 5982 Census: 64 Outpatient Visits: 43840 Births: 757 Total Expense ($000): 76777 Payroll Expense ($000): 32906 Personnel: 538

**THOUSAND OAKS—Ventura County**

⊠ **LOS ROBLES HOSPITAL AND MEDICAL CENTER (50549)**, 215 West Janss Road, Zip 91360–1847; tel. 805/497–2727, (Nonreporting) **A**1 2 9 10 **S** HCA, Nashville, TN
Primary Contact: Gregory R. Angle, President and Chief Executive Officer
CFO: Debra J. Herwaldt, Chief Financial Officer
CMO: Barry Thall, M.D., Medical Director
CIO: Dan Isozaki, Director Information Management
CHR: Dayle Dalton, Vice President Human Resources
Web address: www.losrobleshospital.com
**Control:** Corporation, Investor–owned, for–profit **Service:** General Medical and Surgical

Staffed Beds: 273

**THOUSAND OAKS SURGICAL HOSPITAL (50749)**, 401 East Rolling Oaks Drive, Zip 91361; tel. 805/777–7750, (Nonreporting) **A**9 10 21
Primary Contact: Robert C. Shaw, President and Chief Executive Officer
CFO: Craig Corley, Chief Financial Officer
CMO: Steven Bansbach, M.D., Medical Director
CIO: Michael Lashley, Network Administrator
CHR: Jean Callahan, Manager Human Resources
Web address: www.toshospital.com
**Control:** Partnership, Investor–owned, for–profit **Service:** General Medical and Surgical

Staffed Beds: 17

**TORRANCE—Los Angeles County**

☐ **DEL AMO HOSPITAL (54053)**, 23700 Camino Del Sol, Zip 90505–5000; tel. 310/530–1151, (Nonreporting) **A**1 9 10 **S** Universal Health Services, Inc., King of Prussia, PA
Primary Contact: Lisa K. Montes, Chief Executive Officer
Web address: www.delamohospital.com
**Control:** Corporation, Investor–owned, for–profit **Service:** Psychiatric

Staffed Beds: 70

☐ **LAC–HARBOR–UNIVERSITY OF CALIFORNIA AT LOS ANGELES MEDICAL CENTER (50376)**, 1000 West Carson Street, Zip 90502–2004; tel. 310/222–2345 **A**1 2 3 5 8 10 **F**3 11 12 13 14 15 17 18 19 20 22 24 25 26 29 30 31 32 34 35 39 40 41 43 44 45 46 47 48 49 52 54 55 56 57 59 60 61 64 66 68 70 72 74 76 77 78 79 81 82 85 87 88 89 93 97 98 100 101 102 107 108 114 118 128 129 130 131 133 134 137 143 145 146 147 **P**3 6 **S** Los Angeles County–Department of Health Services, Los Angeles, CA
Primary Contact: Delvecchio Finley, Chief Executive Officer
CFO: Jody Nakasuji, Chief Financial Officer
CMO: Gail Anderson, Jr., M.D., Chief Medical Officer
CIO: Sandy Mungovan, Chief Information Officer
CHR: Karyl Smith, Director Human Resources
Web address: www.humc.edu
**Control:** County–Government, nonfederal **Service:** General Medical and Surgical

Staffed Beds: 350 Admissions: 22064 Census: 347 Outpatient Visits: 418435 Births: 939 Total Expense ($000): 675671 Payroll Expense ($000): 281272 Personnel: 3660

⊠ **PROVIDENCE LITTLE COMPANY OF MARY MEDICAL CENTER (50353)**, 4101 Torrance Boulevard, Zip 90503–4698; tel. 310/540–7676, (Total facility includes 77 beds in nursing home–type unit) **A**1 2 9 10 **F**8 11 13 14 15 18 19 20 22 24 26 28 29 30 34 35 40 46 57 59 60 62 64 68 69 70 72 74 75 76 77 78 79 81 82 85 86 87 89 93 97 107 108 110 111 113 117 118 119 120 122 125 127 129 131 132 142 143 144 145 146 147 **S** Providence Health & Services, Renton, WA
Primary Contact: Elizabeth Dunne, Chief Executive Officer
CFO: Elizabeth Zuanich, Chief Financial Officer
CMO: Laurence Eason, M.D., Chief Medical Officer
CIO: Douglas Jones, Regional Chief Information Officer
Web address: www.lcmweb.org
**Control:** Other not–for–profit (including NFP Corporation) **Service:** General Medical and Surgical

Staffed Beds: 372 Admissions: 21380 Census: 259 Outpatient Visits: 220842 Births: 2754 Total Expense ($000): 331080 Payroll Expense ($000): 118979 Personnel: 1550

⊠ **TORRANCE MEMORIAL MEDICAL CENTER (50351)**, 3330 Lomita Boulevard, Zip 90505–5002; tel. 310/325–9110 **A**1 2 9 10 **F**3 5 8 11 12 13 14 15 16 17 18 20 22 24 26 28 29 30 31 34 35 37 40 46 49 50 51 54 57 58 59 60 62 63 64 70 72 74 75 76 77 78 79 81 82 83 84 85 86 87 89 91 93 96 107 108 109 110 111 113 114 115 116 117 118 119 120 122 125 127 128 129 131 133 134 142 143 144 145 146 147
Primary Contact: Craig Leach, President and Chief Executive Officer
CMO: David Rand, M.D., Chief of Staff
CIO: Robert Proto, Director Information Systems
CHR: Lois Michael, Vice President Human Resources
Web address: www.torrancememorial.org
**Control:** Other not–for–profit (including NFP Corporation) **Service:** General Medical and Surgical

Staffed Beds: 377 Admissions: 24765 Census: 276 Outpatient Visits: 257559 Births: 3318 Total Expense ($000): 418048 Payroll Expense ($000): 168126 Personnel: 2499

*Many Facility Codes have changed. Please refer to the AHA Guide Code Chart.* © 2012 AHA Guide

**TRACY—San Joaquin County**

☒ **SUTTER TRACY COMMUNITY HOSPITAL (50313)**, 1420 North Tracy Boulevard, Zip 95376–3497; tel. 209/835–1500 **A**1 9 10 **F**3 11 13 15 18 29 30 31 34 35 40 45 46 49 50 54 57 59 60 64 68 70 74 75 76 77 78 79 81 82 85 93 107 108 110 111 114 118 123 129 131 134 145 147 **S** Sutter Health, Sacramento, CA
Primary Contact: David M. Thompson, Chief Executive Officer
COO: Doug Archer, Assistant Administrator
CFO: Eric Dalton, Chief Financial Officer
CIO: Karen Mudd, Director Marketing and Public Affairs
CHR: Melanie Wallace, Manager Human Resources
Web address: www.suttertracy.org
**Control:** Other not–for–profit (including NFP Corporation) **Service:** General Medical and Surgical

**Staffed Beds:** 82 **Admissions:** 3975 **Census:** 40 **Outpatient Visits:** 86585 **Births:** 650 **Total Expense ($000):** 90670 **Payroll Expense ($000):** 32331 **Personnel:** 455

**TRAVIS AFB—Solano County**

☒ **DAVID GRANT MEDICAL CENTER**, 101 Bodin Circle, Zip 94535–1800; tel. 707/423–7300, (Nonreporting) **A**1 3 5 **S** Department of the Air Force, Washington, DC
Primary Contact: Colonel Brian T. Hayes, Commander
CFO: Major Jonathan Richards, Chief Financial Officer
CMO: Colonel Chris Scharenbrock, M.D., Chief Medical Staff
Web address: www.travis.af.mil/units/dgmc/index.asp
**Control:** Air Force, Government, federal **Service:** General Medical and Surgical

**Staffed Beds:** 110

**TRUCKEE—Nevada County**

**TAHOE FOREST HOSPITAL DISTRICT (51328)**, 10121 Pine Avenue, Zip 96161–4856, Mailing Address: P.O. Box 759, Zip 96160–0759; tel. 530/587–6011, (Nonreporting) **A**9 10 18 **S** Tahoe Forest Health System, Truckee, CA
Primary Contact: Robert A. Schapper, Chief Executive Officer
CFO: Crystal Betts, Chief Financial Officer
CMO: Richard Ganong, M.D., Chief of Staff
CIO: Mark Griffiths, Chief Systems Innovation Officer
CHR: Marcie Mortensson, Chief Human Resources Officer
Web address: www.tfhd.com
**Control:** Hospital district or authority, Government, nonfederal **Service:** General Medical and Surgical

**Staffed Beds:** 25

**TULARE—Tulare County**

☒ **TULARE REGIONAL MEDICAL CENTER (50359)**, 869 North Cherry Street, Zip 93274–2207; tel. 559/688–0821 **A**1 9 10 21 **F**3 11 13 15 18 20 26 29 31 34 35 40 45 46 47 48 49 50 53 56 57 59 60 62 65 68 70 71 73 74 75 76 77 78 79 81 85 86 89 92 93 97 107 108 110 111 113 118 125 126 128 129 130 131 145 146 147
Primary Contact: Shawn Bolouki, Chief Executive Officer
CFO: Michael Bernstein, Chief Financial Officer
CMO: Pradeep Kamboj, M.D., Chief Medical Staff
CIO: Jim Peelgren, Chief Information Officer
CHR: John Barbadian, Vice President Human Resources
CNO: Patricia Mathewson, Chief Nursing Officer
Web address: www.tulareregional.org
**Control:** Hospital district or authority, Government, nonfederal **Service:** General Medical and Surgical

**Staffed Beds:** 103 **Admissions:** 5884 **Census:** 61 **Outpatient Visits:** 85143 **Births:** 1218 **Total Expense ($000):** 81943 **Payroll Expense ($000):** 29560

**TURLOCK—Stanislaus County**

☒ **EMANUEL MEDICAL CENTER (50179)**, 825 Delbon Avenue, Zip 95382–2016, Mailing Address: P.O. Box 819005, Zip 95381–9005; tel. 209/667–4200, (Total facility includes 145 beds in nursing home–type unit) **A**1 2 9 10 **F**3 8 10 11 12 13 15 18 20 22 24 29 30 31 34 35 39 40 47 48 49 54 59 60 63 64 68 70 73 75 76 77 78 79 81 89 93 97 107 108 110 111 113 114 117 118 119 120 122 127 129 131 145 146
Primary Contact: John R. Sigsbury, President and Chief Executive Officer
COO: Michael T. Iltis, Vice President Professional Services
CFO: David Neapolitan, Chief Financial Officer
CMO: David Canton, D.O., Vice President Medical Affairs
CIO: Ken Hoach, Assistant Vice President and Chief Information Officer
CHR: Terry Gray, Vice President Human Resources
CNO: Constance Fairchilds, R.N., Vice President Patient Care Services
Web address: www.emanuelmed.org
**Control:** Church–operated, Nongovernment, not–for profit **Service:** General Medical and Surgical

**Staffed Beds:** 354 **Admissions:** 10600 **Census:** 250 **Outpatient Visits:** 83562 **Births:** 1383 **Total Expense ($000):** 190997 **Payroll Expense ($000):** 73369 **Personnel:** 1202

**TUSTIN—Orange County**

☒ **HEALTHSOUTH TUSTIN REHABILITATION HOSPITAL (53034)**, 14851 Yorba Street, Zip 92780–2925; tel. 714/832–9200, (Nonreporting) **A**1 9 10 **S** HEALTHSOUTH Corporation, Birmingham, AL
Primary Contact: Diana C. Hanyak, Chief Executive Officer
CFO: Paula Redmond, Controller
CMO: Rodric Bell, M.D., Medical Director
CHR: JoAnn Roiz, Director Human Resources
Web address: www.tustinrehab.com
**Control:** Corporation, Investor–owned, for–profit **Service:** Rehabilitation

**Staffed Beds:** 48

○ **NEWPORT SPECIALTY HOSPITAL (52053)**, 14662 Newport Avenue, Zip 92780–6064; tel. 714/838–9600, (Total facility includes 32 beds in nursing home–type unit) **A**10 11 **F**1 3 29 30 45 49 81 85 93 118 127 129 147 **S** Pacific Health Corporation, Tustin, CA
Primary Contact: Peter Friedman, President and Chief Executive Officer
COO: Kara Bourne, R.N., Chief Nursing Officer and Chief Operating Officer
CIO: Darla Kennedy, Chief Information Officer
CHR: Aprille Major, Director Human Resources
Web address: www.newportspecialtyhospital.com/
**Control:** Corporation, Investor–owned, for–profit **Service:** Long–Term Acute Care hospital

**Staffed Beds:** 155 **Admissions:** 405 **Census:** 53 **Outpatient Visits:** 646 **Births:** 0

**TWENTYNINE PALMS—San Bernardino County**

☒ **NAVAL HOSPITAL**, Zip 92278; tel. 760/830–2190 **A**1 **F**8 13 29 30 33 34 38 50 54 57 59 64 65 68 75 76 77 79 81 86 87 93 97 104 107 118 134 **S** Bureau of Medicine and Surgery, Department of the Navy, Washington, DC
Primary Contact: Captain Jay C. Sourbeer, Commanding Officer
COO: Captain Cynthia J. Gantt, Executive Officer
CFO: Lieutenant Commander Amy Sulog, Comptroller
CMO: Commander Michael E. Cardenas, M.D., Director Medical Services
CIO: Craig Palmer, Information Manager Officer
CHR: Virginia Ward, Human Resources Officer
CNO: Captain Sandra Mason, Director Nursing Services and Senior Nurse Executive
Web address: www.nhtp.med.navy.mil/nhtp
**Control:** Navy, Government, federal **Service:** General Medical and Surgical

**Staffed Beds:** 39 **Admissions:** 1447 **Census:** 7 **Outpatient Visits:** 142275 **Births:** 542 **Personnel:** 599

**UKIAH—Mendocino County**

☒ **UKIAH VALLEY MEDICAL CENTER (50301)**, 275 Hospital Drive, Zip 95482–4531; tel. 707/462–3111 **A**1 9 10 19 **F**3 11 12 13 15 18 29 30 31 32 34 35 38 40 43 44 45 46 48 49 50 51 54 57 59 60 64 65 68 70 72 75 76 77 78 79 81 82 84 85 86 87 93 97 107 108 110 111 113 114 115 116 117 118 126 129 130 131 134 143 145 146 147 **S** Adventist Health, Roseville, CA
Primary Contact: Gwen Matthews, R.N., MSN, Chief Executive Officer
CIO: David Eastman, Site Director
CHR: Rebecca Ryan, Interim Director Human Resources and Employee Health
Web address: www.adventisthealth.org
**Control:** Church–operated, Nongovernment, not–for profit **Service:** General Medical and Surgical

**Staffed Beds:** 62 **Admissions:** 4064 **Census:** 33 **Outpatient Visits:** 215661 **Births:** 846 **Total Expense ($000):** 95610 **Payroll Expense ($000):** 35249 **Personnel:** 645

CA

**Hospital, Medicare Provider Number, Address, Telephone, Approval, Facility, and Physician Codes, Health Care System**

★ American Hospital Association (AHA) membership
□ The Joint Commission accreditation
◇ DNV Healthcare Inc. accreditation
○ American Osteopathic Association (AOA) accreditation
△ Commission on Accreditation of Rehabilitation Facilities (CARF) accreditation

## UPLAND—San Bernardino County

☒ **SAN ANTONIO COMMUNITY HOSPITAL (50099)**, 999 San Bernardino Road, Zip 91786–4920, Mailing Address: Box 5001, Zip 91785–5001; tel. 909/985–2811 **A**1 2 9 10 **F**3 8 11 13 15 17 18 20 22 24 26 28 29 31 35 38 40 45 46 49 50 54 57 59 60 61 64 65 69 70 72 74 75 76 77 78 79 80 81 82 83 84 85 86 87 89 91 92 93 94 107 108 110 111 113 114 117 118 120 122 123 129 131 145 146 147
Primary Contact: Harris F. Koenig, President and Chief Executive Officer
CFO: Roger Parsons, Senior Vice President Finance
CMO: Thomas Easter, M.D., President Medical Staff
CIO: Perry Strength, Director Information Services
CHR: Lynn Kelly, Vice President Human Resources
Web address: www.sach.org
**Control:** Other not–for–profit (including NFP Corporation) **Service:** General Medical and Surgical

**Staffed Beds:** 279 **Admissions:** 15375 **Census:** 154 **Outpatient Visits:** 214883 **Births:** 2281 **Total Expense ($000):** 250733 **Payroll Expense ($000):** 109405 **Personnel:** 1638

## VACAVILLE—Solano County

**CALIFORNIA MEDICAL FACILITY**, 1600 California Drive, Zip 95696–2000; tel. 707/448–6841, (Nonreporting)
Primary Contact: Mary Lou Dunlap, Correctional Health Services Administrator
CMO: Raymond Andreasen, M.D., Chief Medical Officer–Inpatient
Web address: www.cya.ca.gov/visitors/fac_prison_cmf.html
**Control:** State–Government, nonfederal **Service:** Hospital unit of an institution (prison hospital, college infimary, etc.)

**Staffed Beds:** 215

**NORTHBAY VACAVALLEY HOSPITAL** See NorthBay Medical Center, Fairfield

☒ **VACAVILLE MEDICAL CENTER (50767)**, 1 Quality Drive, Zip 95688–9494; tel. 707/624–4000, (Nonreporting) **A**1 10 **S** Kaiser Foundation Hospitals, Oakland, CA
Primary Contact: Max Villalobos, Senior Vice President
Web address: www.kp.org
**Control:** Other not–for–profit (including NFP Corporation) **Service:** General Medical and Surgical

**Staffed Beds:** 64

## VALENCIA—Los Angeles County

☒ **HENRY MAYO NEWHALL MEMORIAL HOSPITAL (50624)**, 23845 McBean Parkway, Zip 91355–2083; tel. 661/253–8000 **A**1 2 9 10 **F**3 7 8 11 15 17 18 20 26 29 30 31 34 35 40 43 45 44 54 57 59 60 64 70 74 76 77 78 79 81 85 86 87 90 93 98 102 104 107 108 109 110 113 114 117 118 129 131 134 145 146 147 **P**5
Primary Contact: Roger E. Seaver, President and Chief Executive Officer
COO: John V. Schleif, Senior Vice President and Chief Operating Officer
CFO: C. R. Hudson, Senior Vice President and Chief Financial Officer
CMO: Richard Frankenstein, M.D., Vice President and Chief Medical Officer
CIO: Cindy Peterson, Vice President and Chief Information Officer
CHR: Mark Puleo, Vice President and Chief Human Resources Officer
CNO: Larry R. Kidd, R.N., Vice President and Chief Nursing Officer
Web address: www.henrymayo.com
**Control:** Other not–for–profit (including NFP Corporation) **Service:** General Medical and Surgical

**Staffed Beds:** 227 **Admissions:** 12066 **Census:** 154 **Outpatient Visits:** 86042 **Births:** 1248 **Total Expense ($000):** 194016 **Payroll Expense ($000):** 66500 **Personnel:** 1154

☐ **MISSION COMMUNITY HOSPITAL (50704)**, 14850 Roscoe Boulevard, Zip 91381; tel. 818/787–2222, (Nonreporting) **A**1 9 10
Primary Contact: James Theiring, Interim Chief Executive Officer
CFO: John Holder, Chief Financial Officer
CMO: Robert Thompson, M.D., Chief of Staff
CIO: Andre Henderson, Director Information Systems
CHR: Paul Williams, Director Human Resources
Web address: www.mchonline.org
**Control:** Other not–for–profit (including NFP Corporation) **Service:** General Medical and Surgical

**Staffed Beds:** 145

## VALLEJO—Solano County

☒ **ST. HELENA HOSPITAL–CENTER FOR BEHAVIORAL HEALTH (54074)**, 525 Oregon Street, Zip 94590–3201; tel. 707/648–2200, (Nonreporting) **A**1 9 10 **S** Adventist Health, Roseville, CA
Primary Contact: Terry Newmyer, President and Chief Executive Officer
CFO: Edward A. McDonald, Chief Financial Officer
Web address: www.sthelenahospital.org/Behavioral/
**Control:** Church–operated, Nongovernment, not–for profit **Service:** Psychiatric

**Staffed Beds:** 30

☒ **SUTTER SOLANO MEDICAL CENTER (50101)**, 300 Hospital Drive, Zip 94589–2517, Mailing Address: P.O. Box 3189, Zip 94590–0669; tel. 707/554–4444 **A**1 2 9 10 **F**3 8 11 13 15 18 26 29 30 31 34 35 40 45 49 50 51 55 57 58 59 64 68 70 74 75 76 77 78 79 81 84 85 86 87 89 90 100 107 108 110 111 113 117 118 119 120 122 129 131 145 **S** Sutter Health, Sacramento, CA
Primary Contact: Theresa Glubka, Chief Executive Officer
CFO: Cynthia van Hoff, Chief Financial Officer
CHR: Jean Willhite, Director Human Resources
Web address: www.suttersolano.org
**Control:** Other not–for–profit (including NFP Corporation) **Service:** General Medical and Surgical

**Staffed Beds:** 102 **Admissions:** 5155 **Census:** 53 **Outpatient Visits:** 67735 **Births:** 773 **Total Expense ($000):** 119448 **Payroll Expense ($000):** 42606 **Personnel:** 470

☒ △ **VALLEJO MEDICAL CENTER (50073)**, 975 Sereno Drive, Zip 94589–2441; tel. 707/651–1000, (Nonreporting) **A**1 7 10 **S** Kaiser Foundation Hospitals, Oakland, CA
Primary Contact: Max Villalobos, Senior Vice President and Area Manager
COO: Karen Grisnak, R.N., Chief Operating Officer and Assistant Administrator Quality Services
CFO: Joseph D'Angina, Area Finance Officer
CMO: Steven Stricker, M.D., Physician in Chief
CIO: Gale Austin–Moore, Director Area Technology
CHR: Sherri Stegge, Director Human Resources
Web address: www.kaiserpermanente.org
**Control:** Other not–for–profit (including NFP Corporation) **Service:** General Medical and Surgical

**Staffed Beds:** 287

## VAN NUYS—Los Angeles County, See Los Angeles

## VENTURA—Ventura County

☐ **AURORA VISTA DEL MAR HOSPITAL (54077)**, 801 Seneca Street, Zip 93001–1411; tel. 805/653–6434, (Nonreporting) **A**1 9 10 **S** Aurora Behavioral Health Care, Corona, CA
Primary Contact: Mayla Krebsbach, Chief Executive Officer
COO: Sherri Block, Chief Operating Officer
CFO: Cory Delello, Chief Financial Officer
CMO: Robert M. Carvalho, M.D., Medical Director
Web address: www.vistadelmarhospital.com
**Control:** Corporation, Investor–owned, for–profit **Service:** Psychiatric

**Staffed Beds:** 87

☒ **COMMUNITY MEMORIAL HEALTH SYSTEM (50394)**, 147 North Brent Street, Zip 93003–2854; tel. 805/652–5011, (Includes COMMUNITY MEMORIAL HOSPITAL, 147 North Brent Street, tel. 805/652–5011; OJAI VALLEY COMMUNITY HOSPITAL, 1306 Maricopa Highway, Ojai, Zip 93023–3163; tel. 805/646–1401; Haady Lashkari, Chief Administrative Officer), (Total facility includes 66 beds in nursing home–type unit) **A**1 2 9 10 21 **F**3 11 12 13 15 17 18 20 22 24 26 28 29 30 31 35 36 39 40 49 51 53 54 56 57 59 60 68 70 72 74 76 77 78 79 81 82 83 84 85 89 93 97 100 102 107 108 110 111 117 118 125 126 127 129 131 132 134 143 145 147 **P**7
Primary Contact: Gary Wilde, President and Chief Executive Officer
COO: Adam Thunell, Chief Operating Officer and Vice President Operations
CFO: David Glyer, Vice President Finance
CMO: Stanley Frochtzwajg, M.D., Chief Medical Officer
CIO: Ron Sandifer, Chief Information Officer
CHR: Diany Klein, Vice President Human Resources
Web address: www.cmhshealth.org
**Control:** Other not–for–profit (including NFP Corporation) **Service:** General Medical and Surgical

**Staffed Beds:** 345 **Admissions:** 13848 **Census:** 198 **Outpatient Visits:** 357939 **Births:** 2526 **Total Expense ($000):** 268436 **Payroll Expense ($000):** 100004 **Personnel:** 1787

☐ **VENTURA COUNTY MEDICAL CENTER (50159)**, 3291 Loma Vista Road, Zip 93003–3099; tel. 805/652–6000, (Nonreporting) **A**1 9 10
Primary Contact: Robert Gonzalez, M.D., Director
COO: Christina B. Thielst, Chief Operating Officer
CFO: Catherine Rodriguez, Chief Financial Officer
CIO: David Herzog, Chief Information Officer
CHR: Maria Teran, Personnel Officer
Web address: www.vchca.org
**Control:** County–Government, nonfederal **Service:** General Medical and Surgical

**Staffed Beds:** 160

## VICTORVILLE—San Bernardino County

★ ○ **DESERT VALLEY HOSPITAL (50709)**, 16850 Bear Valley Road, Zip 92395; tel. 760/241–8000 **A**10 11 **F**3 13 15 18 22 29 30 31 34 35 38 40 46 49 51 56 57 58 59 61 64 65 68 70 76 79 81 82 85 107 108 111 113 118 128 129 134 143 145 147 **S** Prime Healthcare Services, Ontario, CA
Primary Contact: Margaret R. Peterson, Ph.D., R.N., Chief Executive Officer
CFO: Roger Krissman, Chief Financial Officer
CIO: Sreekant Gotti, Director Information Systems
CHR: Arti Dhuper, Regional Director Human Resources
Web address: www.dvmc.com
**Control:** Corporation, Investor–owned, for–profit **Service:** General Medical and Surgical

**Staffed Beds: 75 Admissions:** 7134 **Census:** 65 **Outpatient Visits:** 62127 **Total Expense ($000):** 81053 **Personnel:** 565

★ ○ **VICTOR VALLEY COMMUNITY HOSPITAL (50517)**, 15248 Eleventh Street, Zip 92395; tel. 760/245–8691, (Nonreporting) **A**9 10 11 **S** Prime Healthcare Services, Ontario, CA
Primary Contact: Edward Matthews, Interim Chief Executive Officer
COO: Doreen Dann, R.N., Chief Operating Officer
CFO: Edward Matthews, Chief Financial Officer
CIO: Joe Archer, Chief Information Officer
CHR: Cesar Lugo, Director Human Resources
Web address: www.vvch.org
**Control:** Other not–for–profit (including NFP Corporation) **Service:** General Medical and Surgical

**Staffed Beds: 115**

## VISALIA—Tulare County

⊠ △ **KAWEAH DELTA MEDICAL CENTER (50057)**, 400 West Mineral King Boulevard, Zip 93291–6263; tel. 559/624–2000, (Includes SOUTH CAMPUS, 1633 South Court Street, Zip 93277; tel. 559/624–6090), (Total facility includes 63 beds in nursing home–type unit) **A**1 7 9 10 **F**3 5 13 15 17 18 20 22 24 26 28 29 30 31 34 35 40 41 43 45 49 50 51 53 54 56 57 59 60 62 63 64 65 68 70 73 74 75 76 77 78 79 81 82 84 85 86 87 89 90 93 97 98 99 100 101 102 103 104 107 108 110 111 113 115 116 117 118 122 123 125 126 127 128 129 130 131 133 134 143 145 146 147 **P**7
Primary Contact: Lindsay K. Mann, Chief Executive Officer
CFO: Gary Herbst, Senior Vice President and Chief Financial Officer
CMO: Mark Garfield, M.D., Vice President and Chief Medical Officer
CIO: Dave Gravender, Vice President and Chief Information Officer
CHR: Deb Wood, Vice President Human Resources
Web address: www.kaweahdelta.org
**Control:** Hospital district or authority, Government, nonfederal **Service:** General Medical and Surgical

**Staffed Beds: 429 Admissions:** 23960 **Census:** 389 **Outpatient Visits:** 535340 **Births:** 4343 **Total Expense ($000):** 401897 **Payroll Expense ($000):** 181155 **Personnel:** 2988

## WALNUT CREEK—Contra Costa County

⊠ **JOHN MUIR MEDICAL CENTER, WALNUT CREEK (50180)**, 1601 Ygnacio Valley Road, Zip 94598–3194; tel. 925/939–3000 **A**1 2 9 10 **F**3 11 13 15 17 18 20 22 24 26 28 29 30 31 34 35 37 39 40 43 44 45 46 47 49 50 54 56 57 58 59 60 62 64 65 68 70 72 74 75 76 77 78 79 80 81 82 84 85 86 87 89 90 93 96 100 102 107 108 110 111 113 114 117 118 119 120 122 123 125 129 130 131 134 140 144 145 146 147 **P**3 4 5 **S** John Muir Health, Walnut Creek, CA
Primary Contact: Jane Willemsen, Chief Administrative Officer
COO: Raymond Nassief, Senior Vice President Operations and Clinical Transformation
CFO: Michael Moody, Senior Vice President and Chief Financial Officer
CMO: Irving Pike, M.D., Chief Medical Officer
CIO: Jim Wesley, Interim Chief Information Officer
CHR: Alice A. Villanueva, Senior Vice President Human Resources
CNO: Debra Pendergast, Senior Vice President Patient Care Services and Chief Nursing Officer
Web address: www.jmmdhs.com/index.php/jmmdhs_jmmc.html
**Control:** Other not–for–profit (including NFP Corporation) **Service:** General Medical and Surgical

**Staffed Beds: 367 Admissions:** 17598 **Census:** 245 **Outpatient Visits:** 308536 **Births:** 2632 **Total Expense ($000):** 704449 **Payroll Expense ($000):** 267047 **Personnel:** 2501

⊠ **WALNUT CREEK MEDICAL CENTER (50072)**, 1425 South Main Street, Zip 94596–5300; tel. 925/295–4000, (Includes KAISER FOUNDATION HOSPITAL, 200 Muir Road, Martinez, Zip 94553–4696; tel. 510/372–1000), (Nonreporting) **A**1 3 5 10 **S** Kaiser Foundation Hospitals, Oakland, CA
Primary Contact: Ginger Campbell, Senior Vice President and Area Manager
CFO: Yakesun Wing, Business Strategy and Finance Leader
CIO: Kevin Wheeler, Information Technology Leader
Web address: www.kaiserpermanente.org
**Control:** Other not–for–profit (including NFP Corporation) **Service:** General Medical and Surgical

**Staffed Beds: 233**

## WATSONVILLE—Santa Cruz County

⊠ **WATSONVILLE COMMUNITY HOSPITAL (50194)**, 75 Nielson Street, Zip 95076–2468; tel. 831/724–4741, (Nonreporting) **A**1 9 10 **S** Community Health Systems, Inc., Franklin, TN
Primary Contact: Audra Earle, Chief Executive Officer
CFO: Dennis T. Bynum, Interim Chief Financial Officer
CMO: Robert Weber, M.D., Chief Medical Staff
CIO: Sergio Nell, Director Information Systems
CHR: Jeri Gilbert, Director Human Resources
CNO: Sherri Stout–Torres, Chief Nursing Officer
Web address: www.watsonvillehospital.com
**Control:** Other not–for–profit (including NFP Corporation) **Service:** General Medical and Surgical

**Staffed Beds: 106**

## WEAVERVILLE—Trinity County

**TRINITY HOSPITAL (51315)**, 60 Easter Avenue, Zip 96093, Mailing Address: P.O. Box 1229, Zip 96093–1229; tel. 530/623–5541, (Nonreporting) **A**9 10 18
Primary Contact: Thomas Pyper, Chief Executive Officer
COO: Thomas Pyper, Chief Executive Officer
CMO: Hank Edelstein, M.D., Chief of Staff
CIO: Jennifer Van Matre, Director Finance and Information Technology
CHR: Nanci Hankerd, Manager Human Resources
CNO: Veena Vangari, R.N., Director of Nursing
Web address: www.mcmedical.org
**Control:** Hospital district or authority, Government, nonfederal **Service:** General Medical and Surgical

**Staffed Beds: 51**

## WEST COVINA—Los Angeles County

☐ **CITRUS VALLEY MEDICAL CENTER–QUEEN OF THE VALLEY CAMPUS**, 1115 South Sunset Avenue, Zip 91790–3940, Mailing Address: P.O. Box 1980, Zip 91793–1980; tel. 626/962–4011, (Nonreporting) **A**1 9 **S** Citrus Valley Health Partners, Covina, CA
Primary Contact: Robert H. Curry, President and Chief Executive Officer
CFO: Roger Sharma, Chief Financial Officer
CMO: Pavel Bindra, M.D., Chief Information Officer and Chief Medical Officer
CIO: Pavel Bindra, M.D., Chief Medical Officer and Chief Information Officer
CHR: Lisa Foust, Senior Vice President Human Resources
CNO: Diana Lugo–Zenner, R.N., Chief Nursing Officer
Web address: www.cvhp.org
**Control:** Other not–for–profit (including NFP Corporation) **Service:** General Medical and Surgical

**Staffed Beds: 263**

☐ **DOCTORS HOSPITAL OF WEST COVINA (50096)**, 725 South Orange Avenue, Zip 91790–2614; tel. 626/338–8481, (Nonreporting) **A**1 9 10
Primary Contact: Gerald H. Wallman, Administrator
CFO: Kami Horvat, Chief Financial Officer
CMO: Nashat Ateia, M.D., Chief of Staff
CHR: Lourdes Meza, Coordinator Human Resources
CNO: Rita Lawrence, Director of Nursing
**Control:** Corporation, Investor–owned, for–profit **Service:** General Medical and Surgical

**Staffed Beds: 24**

## WEST HILLS—Los Angeles County, See Los Angeles

## WEST LOS ANGELES—Los Angeles County, See Los Angeles

---

**Hospital, Medicare Provider Number, Address, Telephone, Approval, Facility, and Physician Codes, Health Care System**

★ American Hospital Association (AHA) membership
☐ The Joint Commission accreditation    ◇ DNV Healthcare Inc. accreditation
○ American Osteopathic Association (AOA) accreditation
△ Commission on Accreditation of Rehabilitation Facilities (CARF) accreditation

CA

## WESTMINSTER—Orange County

⊠ **KINDRED HOSPITAL–WESTMINSTER (52035)**, 200 Hospital Circle,
Zip 92683–3910; tel. 714/893–4541, (Nonreporting) **A**1 9 10 **S** Kindred
Healthcare, Louisville, KY
Primary Contact: Adam Darvish, M.P.H., Chief Executive Officer
CFO: Dale Wagner, Chief Financial Officer
Web address: www.khwestminster.com/
**Control:** Corporation, Investor–owned, for–profit **Service:** Long–Term Acute Care
hospital

**Staffed Beds:** 109

## WHITTIER—Los Angeles County

⊠ **PRESBYTERIAN INTERCOMMUNITY HOSPITAL (50169)**, 12401 Washington
Boulevard, Zip 90602–1099; tel. 562/698–0811, (Total facility includes 35 beds
in nursing home–type unit) **A**1 2 9 10 **F**3 11 13 14 15 17 18 20 22 24 26 28
29 31 33 34 35 36 37 40 44 45 46 49 50 51 54 55 56 57 58 59 60 61 62
63 64 65 66 68 69 70 71 72 74 75 76 77 78 79 81 84 85 86 87 89 90 92
93 96 107 108 110 111 113 114 115 116 117 118 119 120 122 123 127
129 130 131 134 142 144 145 146 147 **P**3 5
Primary Contact: James R. West, President and Chief Executive Officer
CFO: Mitchell T. Thomas, Chief Financial Officer
CMO: Rosalio J. Lopez, M.D., Senior Vice President and Chief Medical Officer
CIO: Peggy Chulack, Chief Administrative Officer and Chief Information Officer
CHR: Lon Orey, Vice President Human Resources
Web address: www.whittierpres.com
**Control:** Other not–for–profit (including NFP Corporation) **Service:** General
Medical and Surgical

**Staffed Beds:** 444 **Admissions:** 19407 **Census:** 232 **Outpatient Visits:**
228619 **Births:** 3273 **Total Expense ($000):** 392771 **Payroll Expense
($000):** 150508 **Personnel:** 2549

☐ **WHITTIER HOSPITAL MEDICAL CENTER (50735)**, 9080 Colima Road,
Zip 90605–1600; tel. 562/945–3561, (Nonreporting) **A**1 9 10 **S** AHMC &
Healthcare, Inc., Alhambra, CA
Primary Contact: Lee Suyenaga, Chief Executive Officer
COO: Mary Anne Monje, Chief Financial Officer and Chief Operating Officer
CFO: Mary Anne Monje, Chief Financial Officer and Chief Operating Officer
CIO: Jay Geldhof, Director Information Systems
CHR: Tamera Jones, Director Human Resources
Web address: www.whittierhospital.com
**Control:** Corporation, Investor–owned, for–profit **Service:** General Medical and
Surgical

**Staffed Beds:** 81

## WILDOMAR—Riverside County

**INLAND VALLEY MEDICAL CENTER**, 36485 Inland Valley Drive,
Zip 92595–9700; tel. 951/677–1111 **A**9 **F**8 12 13 15 18 26 29 30 34 35 37
38 40 43 45 50 51 54 56 57 59 64 68 70 74 75 76 78 79 81 82 85 86 87
91 92 94 100 107 108 110 111 113 114 116 118 129 131 134 145 146
147 **S** Universal Health Services, Inc., King of Prussia, PA
Primary Contact: Kenneth I. Rivers, Chief Executive Officer
COO: Gino Patrizio, Chief Operating Officer
CFO: Diane Moon, Chief Financial Officer
CMO: Abayomi Odubela, M.D., Chief Medical Officer
CHR: Shannon Weidauer, Director Human Resources
Web address: www.swhealthcaresystem.com
**Control:** Corporation, Investor–owned, for–profit **Service:** General Medical and
Surgical

**Staffed Beds:** 252 **Admissions:** 17256 **Census:** 171 **Outpatient Visits:**
76613 **Births:** 3780 **Total Expense ($000):** 181682 **Payroll Expense
($000):** 109145 **Personnel:** 1259

## WILLITS—Mendocino County

⊠ **FRANK R. HOWARD MEMORIAL HOSPITAL (51310)**, One Madrone Street,
Zip 95490–4225; tel. 707/459–6801 **A**1 9 10 18 **F**11 15 29 30 34 35 40 57
59 68 70 75 79 81 93 107 110 111 114 118 130 131 132 134 145 146 147
**S** Adventist Health, Roseville, CA
Primary Contact: Rick Bockmann, Chief Executive Officer
CFO: Carlton Jacobson, Vice President Finance
Web address: www.howardhospital.com
**Control:** Church–operated, Nongovernment, not–for profit **Service:** General
Medical and Surgical

**Staffed Beds:** 25 **Admissions:** 1314 **Census:** 15 **Outpatient Visits:** 35135
**Births:** 0 **Total Expense ($000):** 40083 **Payroll Expense ($000):** 16459
**Personnel:** 222

## WILLOWS—Glenn County

**GLENN MEDICAL CENTER (51306)**, 1133 West Sycamore Street,
Zip 95988–2745; tel. 530/934–1800, (Nonreporting) **A**9 10 18
Primary Contact: Woody J. Laughnan, Jr., Administrator
CFO: Gary Pea, Chief Financial Officer
CMO: Mark Garrison, Chief of Staff
CHR: Deborah McMillan, Director Human Resources
Web address: www.glennmed.org
**Control:** Other not–for–profit (including NFP Corporation) **Service:** General
Medical and Surgical

**Staffed Beds:** 15

## WOODLAND—Yolo County

⊠ **WOODLAND HEALTHCARE (50127)**, 1325 Cottonwood Street,
Zip 95695–5199; tel. 530/662–3961, (Nonreporting) **A**1 5 9 10 **S** Dignity
Health, San Francisco, CA
Primary Contact: H. Kevin Vaziri, President
Web address: www.woodlandhealthcare.org
**Control:** Other not–for–profit (including NFP Corporation) **Service:** General
Medical and Surgical

**Staffed Beds:** 111

## WOODLAND HILLS—Los Angeles County, See Los Angeles

## YREKA—Siskiyou County

☐ **FAIRCHILD MEDICAL CENTER (51316)**, 444 Bruce Street, Zip 96097–3450;
tel. 530/842–4121 **A**1 9 10 18 **F**3 11 13 15 30 35 40 43 45 50 57 59 64 70
75 76 79 81 86 87 89 93 107 108 113 117 118 126 128 129 131 132
145 147
Primary Contact: Jonathon Andrus, Chief Executive Officer
CFO: Kelly Martin, Chief Financial Officer
CMO: David Della Lana, M.D., Chief of Staff
CIO: Joan Munson, Manager Information Systems
CHR: Joann Sarmento, Manager Human Resources
CNO: Kathy Shelvock, R.N., Assistant Administrator Patient Care Services
Web address: www.fairchildmed.org
**Control:** Other not–for–profit (including NFP Corporation) **Service:** General
Medical and Surgical

**Staffed Beds:** 25 **Admissions:** 1537 **Census:** 12 **Outpatient Visits:** 89658
**Births:** 212 **Personnel:** 349

## YUBA CITY—Sutter County

**FREMONT MEDICAL CENTER** See Fremont–Rideout Health Group, Marysville

☐ **SUTTER SURGICAL HOSPITAL – NORTH VALLEY (50766)**, 455 Plumas
Boulevard, Zip 95991–5074; tel. 530/749–5700, (Nonreporting) **A**1 10
Primary Contact: Toni Morris, Chief Executive Officer
COO: David Cooke, Chief Nursing Officer
CFO: Renee Schroyer, Chief Financial Officer
CHR: Cynthia Jeter, Director Human Resources
Web address: www.sshnv.org
**Control:** Partnership, Investor–owned, for–profit **Service:** Surgical

**Staffed Beds:** 14

**CA**

*Many Facility Codes have changed. Please refer to the AHA Guide Code Chart.* © 2012 AHA Guide

# COLORADO

## ALAMOSA—Alamosa County

★ **SAN LUIS VALLEY REGIONAL MEDICAL CENTER (60008)**, 106 Blanca Avenue, Zip 81101–2393; tel. 719/589–2511 **A**9 10 20 **F**3 7 11 13 15 29 30 31 33 40 43 53 70 75 76 77 78 79 81 85 93 104 107 111 113 118 128 129 130 145 146 147 **P**6
Primary Contact: Russell William Johnson, Chief Executive Officer
CFO: Shane Mortensen, Chief Financial Officer
CMO: Gregory McAuliffe, M.D., Chief Medical Officer
CIO: Patricia Allvin, Account Executive Information Technology
CHR: Mandy Lee Crockett, Director Human Resources
Web address: www.slvrmc.org
**Control:** Other not–for–profit (including NFP Corporation) **Service:** General Medical and Surgical

> **Staffed Beds:** 44 **Admissions:** 2313 **Census:** 20 **Outpatient Visits:** 112518 **Births:** 542 **Total Expense ($000):** 53202 **Payroll Expense ($000):** 25729 **Personnel:** 473

## ASPEN—Pitkin County

☒ **ASPEN VALLEY HOSPITAL DISTRICT (61324)**, 401 Castle Creek Road, Zip 81611–1159; tel. 970/925–1120 **A**1 9 10 18 **F**3 7 8 10 13 15 18 28 29 31 34 35 40 43 57 59 64 68 70 75 76 77 78 79 81 82 85 87 93 94 107 108 110 111 114 117 118 130 131 132 134 143 145 147
Primary Contact: David R. Ressler, Chief Executive Officer
CFO: Terry Collins, Chief Financial Officer
CMO: J. Christopher Beck, D.O., President Medical Staff
CIO: Ginny Dyche, Director Community Relations
CHR: Alicia Miller, Director Human Resources
CNO: Elaine Gerson, Chief Clinical Officer and General Counsel
Web address: www.avhaspen.org
**Control:** Hospital district or authority, Government, nonfederal **Service:** General Medical and Surgical

> **Staffed Beds:** 25 **Admissions:** 881 **Census:** 7 **Outpatient Visits:** 34612 **Births:** 260 **Total Expense ($000):** 55300 **Payroll Expense ($000):** 23953 **Personnel:** 300

## AURORA—Adams County

☒ **CHILDREN'S HOSPITAL COLORADO (63301)**, 13123 East 16th Avenue, Zip 80045; tel. 720/777–1234 **A**1 3 5 8 9 10 **F**3 11 12 13 14 17 19 21 23 25 27 29 30 31 32 34 35 36 38 39 40 41 42 43 44 45 46 48 49 50 53 54 55 58 59 60 61 63 64 65 66 68 71 72 74 75 77 78 79 81 82 84 85 86 87 88 89 91 92 93 95 96 97 98 99 100 101 102 104 105 107 108 111 113 114 115 116 118 125 128 129 130 131 133 135 136 137 138 140 143 144 145 146 147 **P**8
Primary Contact: James E. Shmerling, President and Chief Executive Officer
COO: Jena Hausmann, Executive Vice President and Chief Operating Officer
CFO: Len Dryer, Chief Financial Officer
CMO: Joan Bothner, M.D., Chief Medical Officer
CIO: Mary Ann Leach, Vice President and Chief Information Officer
CHR: Michael Wukitsch, Chief Human Resources Officer
Web address: www.thechildrenshospital.org
**Control:** Other not–for–profit (including NFP Corporation) **Service:** Children's general

> **Staffed Beds:** 301 **Admissions:** 13557 **Census:** 212 **Outpatient Visits:** 525952 **Births:** 6 **Total Expense ($000):** 595091 **Payroll Expense ($000):** 264605 **Personnel:** 3808

☒ **KINDRED HOSPITAL–AURORA (62013)**, 700 Potomac Street, Zip 80012; tel. 720/857–8333, (Nonreporting) **A**1 9 10 **S** Kindred Healthcare, Louisville, KY
Primary Contact: Linda A. W. McCaskill, Market Chief Executive Officer
Web address: www.khaurora.com/
**Control:** Corporation, Investor–owned, for–profit **Service:** Long–Term Acute Care hospital

> **Staffed Beds:** 37

☒ **MEDICAL CENTER OF AURORA (60100)**, 1501 South Potomac Street, Zip 80012–5499; tel. 303/695–2600, (Includes MEDICAL CENTER OF AURORA NORTH, 700 Potomac Street, Zip 80011–6792; tel. 303/363–7200; SOUTH CAMPUS, 1501 South Potomac, Zip 80012; tel. 303/695–2600) **A**1 2 9 10 **F**3 8 11 13 15 17 18 20 22 24 26 28 29 30 31 34 35 37 39 40 42 43 45 46 47 48 49 53 54 56 57 59 63 64 68 70 72 74 75 76 77 78 79 81 82 84 85 86 87 89 92 98 103 107 108 110 111 113 114 116 117 118 125 128 129 131 134 145 146 147 **P**6 8 **S** HCA, Nashville, TN
Primary Contact: Bill Voloch, Interim Chief Executive Officer
COO: Mary Berrigan, Chief Operating Officer
CFO: Bill Voloch, Chief Financial Officer
Web address: www.auroramed.com
**Control:** Corporation, Investor–owned, for–profit **Service:** General Medical and Surgical

> **Staffed Beds:** 303 **Admissions:** 13528 **Census:** 176 **Outpatient Visits:** 126319 **Births:** 1583 **Total Expense ($000):** 258722 **Payroll Expense ($000):** 103392 **Personnel:** 1179

☒ △ **SPALDING REHABILITATION HOSPITAL (63027)**, 900 Potomac Steet, Zip 80011–6716; tel. 303/367–1166, (Nonreporting) **A**1 7 10 **S** HCA, Nashville, TN
Primary Contact: Cynthia Kreutz, Chief Executive Officer
COO: Debbie Petersen, Chief Operating Officer and Chief Nursing Officer
CFO: Joyce Webber, Chief Financial Officer
CHR: Donna Greeley, Director Human Resources
CNO: Debbie Petersen, Chief Operating Officer and Chief Nursing Officer
Web address: www.spaldingrehab.com
**Control:** Partnership, Investor–owned, for–profit **Service:** Rehabilitation

> **Staffed Beds:** 40

☒ **UNIVERSITY OF COLORADO HOSPITAL (60024)**, 12605 East 16th Avenue, Zip 80045–2545; tel. 720/848–0000 **A**1 2 3 8 9 10 **F**3 4 5 6 8 9 11 12 13 15 16 17 18 20 22 24 26 28 29 30 31 33 34 35 36 37 38 39 40 43 44 45 46 47 48 49 50 52 53 54 55 56 57 58 59 60 61 64 65 68 70 72 74 75 76 77 78 79 81 82 84 85 86 87 90 92 93 94 96 97 99 100 101 102 103 104 107 108 110 111 113 114 116 117 118 119 120 122 123 125 129 130 131 133 134 135 136 137 138 139 140 141 145 146 147
Primary Contact: Bruce Schroffel, President and Chief Executive Officer
COO: John Harney, Chief Operating Officer
CFO: Anthony C. DeFurio, Vice President and Chief Financial Officer
CMO: Greg Stiegmann, M.D., Vice President Clinical Affairs
CIO: Steve Hess, Vice President Information Services and Chief Information Officer
CHR: Darryl Varnado, Vice President Human Resources
Web address: www.uch.edu
**Control:** Hospital district or authority, Government, nonfederal **Service:** General Medical and Surgical

> **Staffed Beds:** 467 **Admissions:** 22589 **Census:** 348 **Outpatient Visits:** 740640 **Births:** 3007 **Total Expense ($000):** 697786 **Payroll Expense ($000):** 269432 **Personnel:** 4199

## BOULDER—Boulder County

☒ △ **BOULDER COMMUNITY HOSPITAL (60027)**, 1100 Balsam Avenue, Zip 80304–3496, Mailing Address: P.O. Box 9019, Zip 80301–9019; tel. 303/440–2273, (Includes BOULDER COMMUNITY FOOTHILLS HOSPITAL, 4747 Arapahoe Avenue, Zip 80303–1133, Mailing Address: P.O. Box 9047, Zip 80301–9047; tel. 720/854–7000) **A**1 2 3 5 7 9 10 **F**8 13 15 18 20 22 24 26 28 29 30 34 37 40 43 46 50 53 54 57 59 60 61 62 64 68 70 72 74 75 76 77 78 79 81 82 87 90 97 98 102 104 107 111 115 118 123 125 128 129 130 143 145 146 147 **P**4 5
Primary Contact: David P. Gehant, President and Chief Executive Officer
CFO: Bill Munson, Vice President and Chief Financial Officer
Web address: www.bch.org
**Control:** Other not–for–profit (including NFP Corporation) **Service:** General Medical and Surgical

> **Staffed Beds:** 182 **Admissions:** 8730 **Census:** 104 **Outpatient Visits:** 418370 **Births:** 1198 **Total Expense ($000):** 262490 **Payroll Expense ($000):** 114116 **Personnel:** 2010

---

**Hospital, Medicare Provider Number, Address, Telephone, Approval, Facility, and Physician Codes, Health Care System**

★ American Hospital Association (AHA) membership
☐ The Joint Commission accreditation
◇ DNV Healthcare Inc. accreditation
○ American Osteopathic Association (AOA) accreditation
△ Commission on Accreditation of Rehabilitation Facilities (CARF) accreditation

**CO**

## BRIGHTON—Adams County

☒ **PLATTE VALLEY MEDICAL CENTER (60004)**, 1600 Prairie Center Parkway, Zip 80601–4006; tel. 303/498–1600 **A**1 5 9 10 **F**3 7 13 15 18 20 22 28 29 30 31 35 40 43 45 49 57 68 70 72 74 75 76 77 78 79 81 85 87 89 90 92 93 107 108 110 111 114 118 129 131 134 145 146 147
Primary Contact: John R. Hicks, President and Chief Executive Officer
COO: Kurt Gensert, R.N., Vice President Operations
CFO: Harold Dupper, Chief Financial Officer
CMO: Kirk Quackenbush, M.D., Chief of Staff
CIO: Darrell Messersmith, Director Information Systems
CHR: Jackie J. Dunkin, Director Human Resources
Web address: www.pvmc.org
**Control:** Other not–for–profit (including NFP Corporation) **Service:** General Medical and Surgical

**Staffed Beds:** 70 **Admissions:** 3157 **Census:** 26 **Outpatient Visits:** 64237 **Births:** 977 **Total Expense ($000):** 76752 **Payroll Expense ($000):** 27588 **Personnel:** 557

## BRUSH—Morgan County

★ **EAST MORGAN COUNTY HOSPITAL (61303)**, 2400 West Edison Street, Zip 80723–1640; tel. 970/842–6200 **A**9 10 18 **F**8 11 15 28 29 30 31 34 35 36 40 45 50 51 53 57 59 64 68 70 75 77 78 79 81 85 87 93 96 97 107 108 110 111 114 118 126 129 130 131 132 145 147 **P**6 **S** Banner Health, Phoenix, AZ
Primary Contact: Linda Thorpe, Chief Executive Officer
CFO: James Cussins, Chief Financial Officer
CMO: Jay Talluri, M.D., Chief Medical Officer
CIO: Michael S. Warden, Senior Vice President and Chief Information Officer
CHR: Jeannie Gallagher, Human Resource Generalist
CNO: Patience M. Samples, R.N., Chief Nursing Officer
Web address: www.emchbrush.com
**Control:** Other not–for–profit (including NFP Corporation) **Service:** General Medical and Surgical

**Staffed Beds:** 19 **Admissions:** 566 **Census:** 7 **Outpatient Visits:** 77086 **Births:** 0 **Total Expense ($000):** 22077 **Payroll Expense ($000):** 10833 **Personnel:** 155

## BURLINGTON—Kit Carson County

★ **KIT CARSON COUNTY MEMORIAL HOSPITAL (61313)**, 286 16th Street, Zip 80807–1697; tel. 719/346–5311, (Nonreporting) **A**9 10 18
Primary Contact: Joe Stratton, Chief Executive Officer
CFO: Mona Ebsen, Chief Financial Officer
CMO: James Perez, M.D., Chief Medical Officer
CIO: Arlan Tanner, Chief Information Officer
CHR: Robin Konecne, Manager Human Resources
Web address: www.kccmh.org
**Control:** Hospital district or authority, Government, nonfederal **Service:** General Medical and Surgical

**Staffed Beds:** 19

## CANON CITY—Fremont County

☒ **ST. THOMAS MORE HOSPITAL (60016)**, 1338 Phay Avenue, Zip 81212–2221; tel. 719/285–2000 **A**1 9 10 20 **F**3 8 11 12 13 14 15 29 30 34 35 40 43 51 53 57 59 64 66 69 70 75 76 77 79 81 82 85 86 87 89 93 97 107 108 110 111 118 126 127 128 130 131 132 134 145 146 147 **S** Catholic Health Initiatives, Englewood, CO
Primary Contact: Robert Ryder, Chief Executive Officer
COO: Rick Kamerzell, Vice President Operations
CFO: Sheri Trahern, Chief Administrative Officer and Chief Financial Officer
CMO: Victoria King, M.D., Chief Medical Officer
CIO: Jennifer Kemp, Director Marketing and Public Relations
CHR: Stan Miller, Executive Director Human Resources
Web address: www.stmhospital.org
**Control:** Other not–for–profit (including NFP Corporation) **Service:** General Medical and Surgical

**Staffed Beds:** 55 **Admissions:** 2040 **Census:** 21 **Outpatient Visits:** 33103 **Births:** 220 **Total Expense ($000):** 32962 **Payroll Expense ($000):** 15266 **Personnel:** 316

## CHEYENNE WELLS—Cheyenne County

★ **KEEFE MEMORIAL HOSPITAL (60043)**, 602 North 6th Street West, Zip 80810, Mailing Address: P.O. Box 578, Zip 80810–0578; tel. 719/767–5661 **A**9 10 20 **F**3 15 40 43 56 57 59 64 81 89 91 93 107 118 126 132 146 **P**6
Primary Contact: Jim Murphy, Interim Administrator
CFO: Kara Hoover, Controller and Director Human Resources
CMO: Christopher Williams, M.D., Chief of Staff
CHR: Kara Hoover, Controller and Director Human Resources
Web address: www.keefememorialhospital.org
**Control:** County–Government, nonfederal **Service:** General Medical and Surgical

**Staffed Beds:** 11 **Admissions:** 101 **Census:** 1 **Outpatient Visits:** 4932 **Births:** 0 **Total Expense ($000):** 4628 **Payroll Expense ($000):** 2975 **Personnel:** 66

## COLORADO SPRINGS—El Paso County

☐ **CEDAR SPRINGS BEHAVIORAL HEALTH SYSTEM (64009)**, 2135 Southgate Road, Zip 80906–2693; tel. 719/633–4114, (Nonreporting) **A**1 9 10 **S** Universal Health Services, Inc., King of Prussia, PA
Primary Contact: A. Elaine Crnkovic, Chief Executive Officer
CFO: Cynthia D. Deboer, Chief Financial Officer
CMO: Larry Shores, M.D., Executive Medical Director
CHR: Jessica McCoy, Director Human Resources
CNO: Jodi Mattson, Director of Nursing
Web address: www.cedarspringshospital.com
**Control:** Corporation, Investor–owned, for–profit **Service:** Psychiatric

**Staffed Beds:** 110

☒ **HEALTHSOUTH REHABILITATION HOSPITAL OF COLORADO SPRINGS (63030)**, 325 Parkside Drive, Zip 80910; tel. 719/630–8000, (Nonreporting) **A**1 10 **S** HEALTHSOUTH Corporation, Birmingham, AL
Primary Contact: Stephen Schaefer, Chief Executive Officer
CFO: Pat Penrod, Controller
CHR: Diana Crepeau, Director Human Resources
Web address: www.healthsouthcoloradosprings.com
**Control:** Corporation, Investor–owned, for–profit **Service:** Rehabilitation

**Staffed Beds:** 64

☒ △ **MEMORIAL HEALTH SYSTEM (60022)**, 1400 East Boulder Street, Zip 80909–5599, Mailing Address: P.O. Box 1326, Zip 80901–1326, (Includes MEMORIAL HOSPITAL FOR CHILDREN, 1400 East Boulder Street, Zip 80909–5533; tel. 719/365–5000) **A**1 2 7 9 10 **F**3 8 11 13 14 15 18 19 20 21 22 23 24 26 27 28 29 30 31 34 35 36 40 41 43 44 46 49 54 55 56 57 58 59 64 70 72 74 76 77 78 79 81 82 85 86 87 88 89 90 91 92 93 94 107 108 110 111 113 114 117 118 119 120 123 128 129 130 131 134 140 143 145 146 147 **P**6 8
Primary Contact: Lawrence R. McEvoy, M.D., Chief Executive Officer
CFO: Michael A. Scialdone, Chief Financial Officer
CMO: Lawrence R. McEvoy, M.D., Chief Executive Officer
Web address: www.memorialhealthsystem.com
**Control:** City–Government, nonfederal **Service:** General Medical and Surgical

**Staffed Beds:** 548 **Admissions:** 25663 **Census:** 326 **Outpatient Visits:** 520172 **Births:** 4596 **Total Expense ($000):** 561907 **Payroll Expense ($000):** 227381 **Personnel:** 3320

☐ **PEAK VIEW BEHAVIORAL HEALTH (64026)**, 7353 Sisters Grove, Zip 80923–2615; tel. 719/444–8484, (Nonreporting) **A**1 **S** Strategic Behavioral Health, LLC, Memphis, TN
Primary Contact: Gary Miller, Chief Executive Officer
Web address: www.strategicbh.com/peakview.html
**Control:** Corporation, Investor–owned, for–profit **Service:** Psychiatric

**Staffed Beds:** 24

☒ △ **PENROSE–ST. FRANCIS HEALTH SERVICES (60031)**, 2222 North Nevada Avenue, Zip 80907–6799, Mailing Address: P.O. Box 7021, Zip 80933–7021; tel. 719/776–5000, (Includes PENROSE HOSPITAL, 2215 North Cascade Avenue, Zip 80907, Mailing Address: P.O. Box 7021, Zip 80933–7021; tel. 719/776–5000; ST. FRANCIS MEDICAL CENTER, 6001 East Woodmen Road, Zip 80923–2601; tel. 719/776–5000) **A**1 2 7 9 10 **F**3 5 11 12 13 14 15 17 18 20 22 24 26 28 29 30 31 34 35 36 38 39 40 41 42 43 44 45 46 47 48 49 50 52 53 54 55 56 57 59 61 62 64 65 68 70 71 72 74 75 76 77 78 79 81 82 84 85 86 87 89 90 91 93 96 97 99 100 101 102 103 107 108 109 110 112 113 114 117 118 119 120 122 123 125 126 128 129 130 131 134 143 145 146 147 **S** Catholic Health Initiatives, Englewood, CO
Primary Contact: Margaret D. Sabin, President and Chief Executive Officer
COO: Andrea C. Coleman, Chief Operating Officer
CMO: Jeffrey C. Oram–Smith, M.D., Chief Medical Officer
CIO: Tanya Bell, Public Information Officer
CHR: James Humphrey, Director Human and Educational Resources
Web address: www.penrosestfrancis.org
**Control:** Church–operated, Nongovernment, not–for profit **Service:** General Medical and Surgical

**Staffed Beds:** 405 **Admissions:** 22296 **Census:** 247 **Outpatient Visits:** 300933 **Births:** 2611 **Total Expense ($000):** 465931 **Payroll Expense ($000):** 126240

☒ **SELECT LONG TERM CARE HOSPITAL – COLORADO SPRINGS (62016)**, 6001 East Woodmen Road, 6th Floor, Zip 80923–2601; tel. 719/571–6000, (Nonreporting) **A**1 10 **S** Select Medical Corporation, Mechanicsburg, PA
Primary Contact: James Elton, Chief Executive Officer
CMO: Dave Call, M.D., Medical Director
CHR: Lisa Gayler, Director Human Resources
CNO: Cathrine Viccellio, Chief Nursing Officer
Web address: www.selectmedical.com
**Control:** Corporation, Investor–owned, for–profit **Service:** Long–Term Acute Care hospital

**Staffed Beds:** 30

*Many Facility Codes have changed. Please refer to the AHA Guide Code Chart.* © 2012 AHA Guide

CO

## CORTEZ—Montezuma County

✠ **SOUTHWEST MEMORIAL HOSPITAL (61327)**, 1311 North Mildred Road, Zip 81321–2299; tel. 970/565–6666 **A**1 9 10 21 **F**3 7 11 13 15 28 29 34 40 50 59 62 64 70 75 76 79 81 93 97 107 108 110 111 114 118 126 128 129 132 147 **P**1
Primary Contact: Kent Helwig, Chief Executive Officer
CFO: John Nadone, Chief Financial Officer
CIO: David Cabana, Director Management Information Systems
CHR: Jim Bob Wynes, Director Human Resources
CNO: Liz Sellers, R.N., Chief Nursing Officer
Web address: www.swhealth.org
**Control:** Other not–for–profit (including NFP Corporation) **Service:** General Medical and Surgical

**Staffed Beds:** 25 **Admissions:** 1272 **Census:** 12 **Outpatient Visits:** 61244 **Births:** 174 **Total Expense ($000):** 39393 **Payroll Expense ($000):** 16365 **Personnel:** 325

## CRAIG—Moffat County

✠ **MEMORIAL HOSPITAL (61314)**, 750 Hospital Loop, Zip 81625–8750; tel. 970/824–9411 **A**1 9 10 18 **F**3 7 11 13 15 29 30 31 34 35 40 43 45 49 50 51 59 68 70 75 76 77 78 79 81 85 86 87 91 93 97 102 107 108 110 111 112 113 118 126 128 129 130 131 132 145 146 147 **S** QHR, Brentwood, TN
Primary Contact: George A. Rohrich, Chief Executive Officer
COO: Beka Warren, R.N., Interim Chief Clinical Officer
CFO: Bryan Chalmers, Chief Financial Officer
CMO: Larry Kipe, M.D., Chief of Staff
CIO: Samantha Johnston, Chief Organizational Excellence
CHR: Jade Wilhite, Manager Human Resource
Web address: www.thememorialhospital.com
**Control:** County–Government, nonfederal **Service:** General Medical and Surgical

**Staffed Beds:** 25 **Admissions:** 888 **Census:** 9

## DEL NORTE—Rio Grande County

★ **RIO GRANDE HOSPITAL (61301)**, 310 County Road 14, Zip 81132; tel. 719/657–2510 **A**9 10 18 **F**34 40 57 65 81 93 107 111 114 126 132 **P**6
Primary Contact: Arlene Harms, Chief Executive Officer
CFO: Greg Porter, Chief Financial Officer
CMO: Heidi E. Helgeson, M.D., Chief Medical Officer
CIO: Yael DeFaye, Director, Information Technology
CHR: Paula Warner–Pacheco, Chief Human Resources
CNO: Beverly Martinez, Director of Nursing
Web address: www.rio–grande–hospital.org/
**Control:** Other not–for–profit (including NFP Corporation) **Service:** General Medical and Surgical

**Staffed Beds:** 17 **Admissions:** 375 **Census:** 3 **Outpatient Visits:** 34817 **Births:** 0 **Total Expense ($000):** 11268 **Payroll Expense ($000):** 4970 **Personnel:** 111

## DELTA—Delta County

✠ **DELTA COUNTY MEMORIAL HOSPITAL (60071)**, 1501 East 3rd Street, Zip 81416–2297, Mailing Address: P.O. Box 10100, Zip 81416–5003; tel. 970/874–7681 **A**1 9 10 **F**3 11 13 15 28 30 31 34 40 43 57 62 70 75 76 78 79 81 85 87 93 107 110 111 113 114 118 123 128 145 147 **P**5 8
Primary Contact: John W. Mitchell, Administrator
CFO: Bev Carlson, Chief Financial Officer
CMO: John P. Knutson, M.D., Chief Medical Staff
CIO: Mitch Van Scoyk, Manager Information Systems
CHR: Larry Vincent, Director Human Resources
CNO: Jason Cleckler, Chief Clinical Officer
Web address: www.deltahospital.org
**Control:** Hospital district or authority, Government, nonfederal **Service:** General Medical and Surgical

**Staffed Beds:** 49 **Admissions:** 2659 **Census:** 22 **Outpatient Visits:** 91152 **Births:** 267 **Total Expense ($000):** 55733 **Payroll Expense ($000):** 24047 **Personnel:** 575

## DENVER—Denver, Adams and Arapaho Coun Counties

✠ **COLORADO ACUTE LONG TERM HOSPITAL (62012)**, 1690 Meade Street, Zip 80204; tel. 303/264–6900, (Nonreporting) **A**1 9 10 **S** LifeCare Management Services, Plano, TX
Primary Contact: Terry W. Kepler, Administrator
CFO: Nanette Pappas, Manager Business Office
Web address: www.lifecare–hospitals.com
**Control:** Corporation, Investor–owned, for–profit **Service:** Long–Term Acute Care hospital

**Staffed Beds:** 63

□ **COLORADO MENTAL HEALTH INSTITUTE AT FORT LOGAN (64003)**, 3520 West Oxford Avenue, Zip 80236–3197; tel. 303/761–0220, (Nonreporting) **A**1 3 5 10
Primary Contact: Elizabeth M. Stillman, Acting Director
CFO: Bob Fries, Director Fiscal Services
CIO: Billie Busby, Assistant Director
Web address: www.cdhs.state.co.us/cmhifl
**Control:** State–Government, nonfederal **Service:** Psychiatric

**Staffed Beds:** 297

□ **DENVER HEALTH MEDICAL CENTER (60011)**, 777 Bannock Street, Zip 80204–4507; tel. 303/436–6000 **A**1 3 5 9 10 **F**3 4 5 7 11 12 13 15 18 19 20 22 26 28 29 30 31 32 34 35 37 38 39 40 41 43 44 45 46 49 50 53 54 55 56 57 58 59 61 64 65 66 68 70 71 72 74 75 76 77 78 79 80 81 82 85 86 87 88 89 90 92 93 94 97 98 99 100 102 103 104 107 108 110 111 113 114 117 118 126 128 129 130 131 133 134 142 143 145 146 147 **P**6
Primary Contact: Patricia A. Gabow, M.D., Chief Executive Officer
COO: Stephanie Thomas, Chief Operating Officer
CFO: Peg Burnette, Chief Financial Officer
CMO: Philip Mehler, M.D., Chief Medical Officer
CIO: Gregory M. Veltri, Chief Information Officer
CHR: Greg Rossman, Chief Human Resource Officer
CNO: Kathy Boyle, R.N., Chief Nursing Officer
Web address: www.denverhealth.org
**Control:** Hospital district or authority, Government, nonfederal **Service:** General Medical and Surgical

**Staffed Beds:** 397 **Admissions:** 22847 **Census:** 282 **Outpatient Visits:** 530743 **Births:** 3190 **Total Expense ($000):** 621619 **Payroll Expense ($000):** 336114 **Personnel:** 5105

✠ **EXEMPLA SAINT JOSEPH HOSPITAL (60028)**, 1835 Franklin Street, Zip 80218–1191; tel. 303/837–7111 **A**1 3 5 9 10 **F**3 8 11 12 13 14 15 18 20 22 24 26 28 29 30 31 34 35 37 40 45 46 49 50 53 55 60 63 64 65 66 68 70 71 72 74 75 76 77 78 79 80 81 82 84 85 87 93 102 107 108 110 111 113 114 118 119 120 122 123 125 129 144 145 **P**6 **S** Exempla Healthcare, Inc., Denver, CO
Primary Contact: Bain J. Farris, President and Chief Executive Officer
COO: Barbara A. Jahn, Chief Operating Officer
CFO: Brad Ludford, Vice President Finance
CMO: Shawn Dufford, M.D., Vice President Medical Affairs and Chief Medical Officer
CNO: Mary Shepler, R.N., Vice President and Chief Nursing Officer
Web address: www.exempla.org
**Control:** Other not–for–profit (including NFP Corporation) **Service:** General Medical and Surgical

**Staffed Beds:** 371 **Admissions:** 20241 **Census:** 229 **Outpatient Visits:** 215015 **Births:** 4485 **Total Expense ($000):** 392716 **Payroll Expense ($000):** 156230 **Personnel:** 2232

✠ **KINDRED HOSPITAL–DENVER (62009)**, 1920 High Street, Zip 80218–1213; tel. 303/320–5871, (Nonreporting) **A**1 9 10 **S** Kindred Healthcare, Louisville, KY
Primary Contact: Linda A. W. McCaskill, Chief Executive Officer
CFO: Tim Stecker, Chief Financial Officer
CMO: Eric Yaeger, M.D., Medical Director
Web address: www.kh–denver.com
**Control:** Corporation, Investor–owned, for–profit **Service:** Long–Term Acute Care hospital

**Staffed Beds:** 68

✠ **NATIONAL JEWISH HEALTH (60107)**, (AllerCardioRespRheumIDGI), 1400 Jackson Street, Zip 80206–2762; tel. 303/388–4461 **A**1 3 5 9 10 **F**3 9 11 12 18 20 28 29 30 31 32 34 35 36 45 46 48 50 53 54 55 57 58 59 61 64 65 66 68 74 75 77 78 84 86 87 89 90 93 96 97 98 99 100 101 104 107 108 111 113 114 115 116 117 118 126 128 129 131 133 134 142 145 **P**6
Primary Contact: Michael Salem, M.D., President and Chief Executive Officer
COO: Ron Berge, Executive Vice President and Chief Operating Officer
CFO: Christine Forkner, Executive Vice President and Chief Financial Officer
CMO: Gary Cott, M.D., Executive Vice President Medical and Clinical Services
CIO: Lots Pook, Chief Information Officer
CHR: Susan Roll, Chief Human Resources
Web address: www.njhealth.org
**Control:** Other not–for–profit (including NFP Corporation) **Service:** Other specialty

**Staffed Beds:** 46 **Admissions:** 92 **Census:** 1 **Outpatient Visits:** 80811 **Births:** 0 **Total Expense ($000):** 202951 **Payroll Expense ($000):** 102759 **Personnel:** 1360

---

**Hospital, Medicare Provider Number, Address, Telephone, Approval, Facility, and Physician Codes, Health Care System**

★ American Hospital Association (AHA) membership
□ The Joint Commission accreditation
◇ DNV Healthcare Inc. accreditation
○ American Osteopathic Association (AOA) accreditation
△ Commission on Accreditation of Rehabilitation Facilities (CARF) accreditation

---

⊞ **PORTER ADVENTIST HOSPITAL (60064)**, 2525 South Downing Street, Zip 80210–5876; tel. 303/778–1955 **A**1 2 9 10 **F**3 5 8 11 15 18 20 22 24 26 28 29 30 31 34 35 36 37 38 40 45 46 47 48 49 53 54 55 56 57 58 59 60 64 65 68 70 74 75 77 78 79 81 82 84 85 86 87 90 91 92 93 96 97 98 100 101 102 103 104 105 106 107 108 109 110 111 112 113 114 115 116 117 118 119 120 121 122 123 125 128 129 131 134 136 137 138 139 140 141 145 146 147 **P**6 8 **S** Adventist Health System Sunbelt Health Care Corporation, Altamonte Springs, FL
Primary Contact: Randall L. Haffner, Ph.D., Chief Executive Officer
CFO: Andrew Gaasch, Chief Financial Officer
CMO: Diane McCallister, M.D., Chief Medical Officer
CHR: Oz Muller, Director Human Resources
CNO: Sharon H. Pappas, R.N., Chief Nursing Officer
Web address: www.centura.org
**Control:** Church–operated, Nongovernment, not–for profit **Service:** General Medical and Surgical

| | |
|---|---|
| **Staffed Beds:** 239 **Admissions:** 10322 **Census:** 137 **Outpatient Visits:** 65380 **Births:** 0 **Total Expense ($000):** 211824 **Payroll Expense ($000):** 70851 **Personnel:** 1272 | |

⊞ △ **PRESBYTERIAN–ST. LUKE'S MEDICAL CENTER (60014)**, 1719 East 19th Avenue, Zip 80218–1281; tel. 303/839–6000, (Includes ROCKY MOUNTAIN HOSPITAL FOR CHILDREN, 1719 East 19th Avenue, Zip 80218–1235; tel. 720/754–1000) **A**1 2 3 5 7 9 10 **F**3 8 9 11 12 13 14 15 18 19 20 21 22 23 24 25 26 28 29 30 31 34 35 37 38 40 41 43 44 45 46 47 48 49 50 51 54 56 57 58 59 60 61 63 64 65 66 68 70 72 73 74 75 76 78 79 80 81 82 83 84 85 86 87 88 89 97 99 100 101 102 103 107 108 110 111 112 113 114 115 116 118 119 120 122 125 126 128 129 130 131 134 135 137 144 145 147 **P**2 3 4 6 **S** HCA, Nashville, TN
Primary Contact: Madeleine Roberson, Chief Executive Officer
CMO: Reginald Washington, M.D., Chief Medical Officer
CIO: Jay Williams, Director Information Services
CHR: Shane Buer, Director Human Resources
Web address: www.pslmc.com
**Control:** Corporation, Investor–owned, for–profit **Service:** General Medical and Surgical

| | |
|---|---|
| **Staffed Beds:** 397 **Admissions:** 10296 **Census:** 200 **Outpatient Visits:** 85603 **Births:** 1341 **Personnel:** 1553 | |

⊞ **ROSE MEDICAL CENTER (60032)**, 4567 East Ninth Avenue, Zip 80220–3941; tel. 303/320–2121 **A**1 2 3 5 9 10 **F**3 8 11 12 13 15 18 20 22 24 26 28 29 30 31 34 35 40 44 45 49 50 53 54 55 58 59 60 61 64 68 70 72 74 75 76 77 78 79 81 82 84 85 86 87 89 92 93 94 97 102 107 108 110 111 112 113 114 115 116 117 118 119 120 121 122 125 128 129 130 131 134 142 145 146 147 **P**6 8 **S** HCA, Nashville, TN
Primary Contact: Kenneth H. Feiler, Chief Executive Officer
COO: Elizabeth Hunsicker, Chief Operating Officer
CFO: Jac Connelly, Chief Financial Officer
CIO: Dave Trevathan, Director Information Systems
CHR: Clarence McDavid, Vice President Human Resources
Web address: www.rosebabies.com
**Control:** Corporation, Investor–owned, for–profit **Service:** General Medical and Surgical

| | |
|---|---|
| **Staffed Beds:** 264 **Admissions:** 12674 **Census:** 138 **Outpatient Visits:** 95605 **Births:** 3711 **Total Expense ($000):** 190649 **Payroll Expense ($000):** 74779 **Personnel:** 958 | |

**SELECT SPECIALTY HOSPITAL DENVER SOUTH** See Select Specialty Hospital–Denver

⊞ **SELECT SPECIALTY HOSPITAL–DENVER (62015)**, 1719 East 19th Avenue, 5th Floor, Zip 80218; tel. 303/563–3700, (Includes SELECT SPECIALTY HOSPITAL DENVER SOUTH, 2525 South Downing Street, Zip 80210–5817; tel. 303/715–7373), (Nonreporting) **A**1 9 10 **S** Select Medical Corporation, Mechanicsburg, PA
Primary Contact: Deborah Dale, Chief Executive Officer
Web address: www.selectmedicalcorp.com
**Control:** Corporation, Investor–owned, for–profit **Service:** Long–Term Acute Care hospital

| | |
|---|---|
| **Staffed Beds:** 65 | |

⊞ △ **VETERANS AFFAIRS EASTERN COLORADO HEALTH CARE SYSTEM**, 1055 Clermont Street, Zip 80220–3877; tel. 303/399–8020, (Total facility includes 119 beds in nursing home–type unit) **A**1 3 5 7 8 **F**3 18 20 22 24 26 29 30 31 35 36 39 40 44 45 46 47 48 49 53 54 55 56 57 58 59 60 61 63 64 65 68 70 74 75 77 78 79 80 81 82 83 84 85 87 90 91 92 93 94 95 96 97 98 100 101 102 103 104 106 107 108 111 113 114 118 125 126 127 128 129 131 134 145 146 147 **S** Department of Veterans Affairs, Washington, DC
Primary Contact: Lynette A. Roff, Director
COO: Terry S. Atienza, Associate Director
CFO: Eliott R. Vanderstek, Chief Fiscal Service
CMO: Ellen Mangione, M.D., Chief of Staff
CIO: Don Huckaby, Chief Information Management Service
CHR: Lorene Connel, Chief Human Resources Management Service
Web address: www.va.gov/sta/guide/home.asp
**Control:** Veterans Affairs, Government, federal **Service:** General Medical and Surgical

| | |
|---|---|
| **Staffed Beds:** 252 **Admissions:** 5416 **Census:** 103 **Outpatient Visits:** 777900 **Births:** 0 **Total Expense ($000):** 475118 **Payroll Expense ($000):** 241594 **Personnel:** 2293 | |

**DURANGO—La Plata County**

⊞ **ANIMAS SURGICAL HOSPITAL (60117)**, 575 Rivergate Lane, Zip 81301; tel. 970/247–3537, (Nonreporting) **A**9 10
Primary Contact: Brett Gosney, Chief Executive Officer
Web address: www.animassurgical.com/index.htm
**Control:** Corporation, Investor–owned, for–profit **Service:** Surgical

| | |
|---|---|
| **Staffed Beds:** 12 | |

⊞ **MERCY REGIONAL MEDICAL CENTER (60013)**, 1010 Three Springs Boulevard, Zip 81301–5089; tel. 970/247–4311 **A**1 2 9 10 20 **F**11 13 15 17 18 20 22 24 26 27 28 29 30 31 35 36 40 42 43 50 59 60 61 66 70 72 73 76 79 81 84 85 89 94 96 107 111 114 118 126 128 129 130 131 132 134 145 146 147 **P**6 7 **S** Catholic Health Initiatives, Englewood, CO
Primary Contact: Kirk Dignum, Ph.D., Chief Executive Officer
CFO: Jane Strobel, Interim Chief Financial Officer
CMO: John A K Boyd, M.D., Vice President Mission and Medical Affairs and Chief Medical Officer
CIO: Neil Stock, Director Technology and Facilities
CHR: Cathy Roberts, Director Human Resources
CNO: Nancy Hoyt, R.N., Vice President Operations/Clinical and Chief Nursing Officer
Web address: www.mercydurango.org
**Control:** Church–operated, Nongovernment, not–for profit **Service:** General Medical and Surgical

| | |
|---|---|
| **Staffed Beds:** 82 **Admissions:** 4785 **Census:** 43 **Outpatient Visits:** 96356 **Births:** 906 **Total Expense ($000):** 114340 **Payroll Expense ($000):** 42991 **Personnel:** 653 | |

**EADS—Kiowa County**

★ **WEISBROD MEMORIAL COUNTY HOSPITAL (61300)**, 1208 Luther Street, Zip 81036, Mailing Address: P.O. Box 817, Zip 81036–0817; tel. 719/438–5401 **A**9 10 18 **F**7 11 34 40 59 62 67 80 93 126 129 132 145 **P**6
Primary Contact: Thomas Henton, Chief Executive Officer
CFO: Shannon Dixon, Manager Business Office
CMO: Jeff Waggoner, M.D., Chief of Staff
CHR: Shannon Dixon, Manager Business Office
Web address: www.weisbrod.org
**Control:** County–Government, nonfederal **Service:** General Medical and Surgical

| | |
|---|---|
| **Staffed Beds:** 42 **Admissions:** 78 **Census:** 1 **Outpatient Visits:** 9829 **Births:** 0 **Personnel:** 79 | |

**ENGLEWOOD—Arapahoe County**

⊞ **CRAIG HOSPITAL (62011)**, 3425 South Clarkson Street, Zip 80113–2899; tel. 303/789–8000 **A**1 3 5 9 10 **F**29 30 34 35 36 44 50 53 58 64 68 74 75 77 81 86 87 90 91 93 96 129 131 145 147
Primary Contact: Michael L. Fordyce, President and Chief Executive Officer
COO: Dana Polonsky, Vice President of Clinical Services
CFO: Julie Keegan, Vice President Finance
CMO: Thomas E. Balazy, M.D., Medical Director
CIO: Chris Watkins, Director of Information Technology
CHR: Stacy L. Abel, Director Human Resources
CNO: Diane Reinhard, R.N., Vice President of Patient Care Services
Web address: www.craighospital.org
**Control:** Other not–for–profit (including NFP Corporation) **Service:** Rehabilitation

| | |
|---|---|
| **Staffed Beds:** 78 **Admissions:** 468 **Census:** 71 **Outpatient Visits:** 5166 **Births:** 0 **Total Expense ($000):** 65292 **Payroll Expense ($000):** 31554 **Personnel:** 573 | |

⊞ **SWEDISH MEDICAL CENTER (60034)**, 501 East Hampden Avenue, Zip 80113; tel. 303/788–5000 **A**1 2 3 5 9 10 **F**3 7 8 11 12 13 15 18 20 22 24 26 29 30 31 34 35 38 39 40 42 43 44 45 47 48 49 50 53 55 57 58 59 60 64 66 68 70 72 73 74 75 76 77 78 79 81 82 84 85 86 87 88 90 92 97 102 107 108 109 111 113 114 115 116 117 118 119 120 121 122 123 125 128 129 130 131 145 146 147 **P**8 **S** HCA, Nashville, TN
Primary Contact: Mary M. White, Chief Executive Officer
COO: Daniel Miller, Chief Operating Officer
CFO: Kathy Ashenfelter, Chief Financial Officer
CMO: Patricia Howell, M.D., President Medical Staff
CIO: Robert Hollowell, Director Information Systems
CHR: Lisa Morris, Vice President Human Resources
CNO: Karleen Goerke, R.N., Chief Nursing Officer
Web address: www.swedishhospital.com
**Control:** Partnership, Investor–owned, for–profit **Service:** General Medical and Surgical

| | |
|---|---|
| **Staffed Beds:** 354 **Admissions:** 19115 **Census:** 248 **Outpatient Visits:** 112966 **Births:** 2115 **Personnel:** 1529 | |

## ESTES PARK—Larimer County

★ **ESTES PARK MEDICAL CENTER (61312)**, 555 Prospect Avenue, Zip 80517–2740, Mailing Address: P.O. Box 2740, Zip 80517–2740; tel. 970/586–2317, (Total facility includes 45 beds in nursing home–type unit) **A**9 10 18 **F**3 7 8 13 15 18 29 30 31 34 35 40 43 45 56 57 59 62 63 64 75 76 77 78 79 81 82 85 91 93 97 107 110 113 118 127 129 130 131 132 142 145 147
Primary Contact: Robert S. Austin, FACHE, Chief Executive Officer
CFO: Sam Radke, Vice President of Finance
CMO: Chris Daley, M.D., Chief of Staff
CIO: Gary Hall, Vice President of Information Technology
CHR: Robert Stansel, Vice President of Human Resources
CNO: Roberta Swenson, R.N., Vice President of Patient Services
Web address: www.epmedcenter.com
**Control:** Hospital district or authority, Government, nonfederal **Service:** General Medical and Surgical

**Staffed Beds:** 68 **Admissions:** 953 **Census:** 38 **Outpatient Visits:** 64863 **Births:** 76 **Total Expense ($000):** 29717 **Payroll Expense ($000):** 14391 **Personnel:** 243

## FORT CARSON—El Paso County

⊠ **EVANS U. S. ARMY COMMUNITY HOSPITAL**, 1650 Cochrane Circle, Building 7500, Zip 80913–5101; tel. 719/526–7200, (Nonreporting) **A**1 2 9 **S** Department of the Army, Office of the Surgeon General, Falls Church, VA
Primary Contact: Colonel Jimmie O. Keenan, Commander
CFO: Major Bradley Robinson, Chief Financial Officer
CMO: Colonel James Terrio, M.D., Chief Medical Officer
CHR: Lieutenant Colonel Lory Gurr, Chief Human Resources Division
Web address: www.evans.amedd.army.mil
**Control:** Army, Government, federal **Service:** General Medical and Surgical

**Staffed Beds:** 57

## FORT COLLINS—Larimer County

⊠ **POUDRE VALLEY HOSPITAL (60010)**, 1024 South Lemay Avenue, Zip 80524–3998; tel. 970/495–7000, (Includes MOUNTAIN CREST HOSPITAL, 4601 Corbett Drive, Zip 80525; tel. 970/270–4800) **A**1 2 9 10 **F**3 5 7 11 12 13 14 15 18 20 22 28 29 30 31 32 34 35 37 38 39 40 43 45 47 48 49 50 53 54 55 57 58 59 60 61 64 65 66 68 69 70 72 73 74 75 76 77 78 79 80 81 82 84 85 86 87 89 90 93 94 98 99 100 101 102 103 104 105 106 107 108 110 111 113 114 117 118 119 123 125 128 129 130 131 133 134 143 145 146 147 **P**5 6 **S** Poudre Valley Health System, Fort Collins, CO
Primary Contact: Kevin L. Unger, FACHE, President and Chief Executive Officer
COO: Dan Robinson, Vice President Operations
CFO: Stephanie Doughty, Chief Financial Officer
CMO: William Neff, M.D., Chief Medical Officer
CIO: Fernando Pedroza, Chief Information Officer
CHR: Patti Oakes, Interim Vice President Human Resources
Web address: www.pvhs.org
**Control:** Other not–for–profit (including NFP Corporation) **Service:** General Medical and Surgical

**Staffed Beds:** 238 **Admissions:** 15007 **Census:** 161 **Outpatient Visits:** 506067 **Births:** 2449 **Total Expense ($000):** 288792 **Payroll Expense ($000):** 124102 **Personnel:** 1759

## FORT MORGAN—Morgan County

⊠ **COLORADO PLAINS MEDICAL CENTER (60044)**, 1000 Lincoln Street, Zip 80701–3298; tel. 970/867–3391, (Nonreporting) **A**1 9 10 20 **S** LifePoint Hospitals, Inc., Brentwood, TN
Primary Contact: Michael N. Patterson, Chief Executive Officer
CFO: Christina Patton, Chief Financial Officer
CHR: Janet Brinkman, Director Human Resources
CNO: Sonya Bass, MS, Chief Nursing Officer
Web address: www.coloradoplainsmedicalcenter.com
**Control:** Corporation, Investor–owned, for–profit **Service:** General Medical and Surgical

**Staffed Beds:** 50

## FRISCO—Summit County

⊠ **ST. ANTHONY SUMMIT MEDICAL CENTER (60118)**, 340 Peak One Drive, Zip 80443, Mailing Address: P.O. Box 738, Zip 80443–0738; tel. 970/668–3300, (Includes ST. ANTHONY GRANBY MEDICAL CENTER, 480 East Agate, Granby, Zip 80446, Mailing Address: P.O. Box 397, Zip 80446; tel. 970/887–7400; Paul J. Chodkowski, Chief Executive Officer) **A**1 9 10 **F**3 34 40 42 43 45 57 59 68 70 75 76 77 79 81 82 84 85 97 107 110 111 113 118 128 129 131 143 145 146 **S** Catholic Health Initiatives, Englewood, CO
Primary Contact: Paul J. Chodkowski, Chief Executive Officer
CFO: David Thompson, Chief Financial Officer
CHR: Dana Laverdiere, Generalist
Web address: www.summitmedicalcenter.org
**Control:** Church–operated, Nongovernment, not–for–profit **Service:** General Medical and Surgical

**Staffed Beds:** 34 **Admissions:** 1451 **Census:** 11 **Outpatient Visits:** 18718 **Births:** 376 **Total Expense ($000):** 43579 **Payroll Expense ($000):** 13424 **Personnel:** 146

## FRUITA—Mesa County

★ **FAMILY HEALTH WEST (61302)**, 300 West Ottley Avenue, Zip 81521–2118, Mailing Address: P.O. Box 130, Zip 81521–0130; tel. 970/858–9871, (Nonreporting) **A**9 10 18
Primary Contact: Mark J. Francis, President Chief Executive Officer and Hospital Administrator
CFO: Jason McCormick, Vice President Finance and Chief Financial Officer
CMO: Michael Hughes, M.D., Medical Director
CIO: Camille Ficklin, Director Information Services
CHR: Kelly Murphy, Director Human Resources
Web address: www.familyhealthwest.org
**Control:** Other not–for–profit (including NFP Corporation) **Service:** General Medical and Surgical

**Staffed Beds:** 130

## GLENWOOD SPRINGS—Garfield County

⊠ **VALLEY VIEW HOSPITAL (60075)**, 1906 Blake Avenue, Zip 81601–4259; tel. 970/945–6535 **A**1 9 10 20 **F**3 11 12 13 14 15 18 20 22 28 29 30 31 34 35 36 38 40 43 45 49 50 51 55 57 59 64 65 68 69 70 74 75 76 77 78 79 80 81 82 85 86 87 93 97 104 107 110 111 114 116 117 118 128 129 130 131 134 144 145 146
Primary Contact: Gary L. Brewer, Chief Executive Officer
COO: Deb Wiepking, MSN, Chief Clinical Officer
CFO: Larry L. Dupper, Chief Financial Officer
CMO: Brian Murphy, M.D., Chief of Staff
CIO: Ron Hines, Director Information Technology
CHR: Daniel Biggs, Director Human Resources
Web address: www.vvh.org
**Control:** Other not–for–profit (including NFP Corporation) **Service:** General Medical and Surgical

**Staffed Beds:** 49 **Admissions:** 2706 **Census:** 29 **Outpatient Visits:** 70596 **Births:** 688 **Total Expense ($000):** 116434 **Payroll Expense ($000):** 50455 **Personnel:** 671

## GRANBY—Grand County

**ST. ANTHONY GRANBY MEDICAL CENTER** See St. Anthony Summit Medical Center, Frisco

## GRAND JUNCTION—Mesa County

**COLORADO WEST PSYCHIATRIC HOSPITAL (64023)**, 515 28 3/4 Road, Zip 81501–5016; tel. 970/263–4918, (Nonreporting)
Primary Contact: Kim Boe, Administrator
CNO: LaCinda Kelleher, Director of Nursing
Web address: www.cwrmhc.org/psychosp.htm
**Control:** Other not–for–profit (including NFP Corporation) **Service:** Psychiatric

**Staffed Beds:** 32

⊠ ○ **COMMUNITY HOSPITAL (60054)**, 2021 North 12th Street, Zip 81501–2999; tel. 970/242–0920 **A**1 9 10 11 **F**3 8 12 15 29 30 34 35 40 47 48 49 50 57 59 62 64 70 75 77 79 81 85 86 87 93 97 107 108 110 111 113 114 118 128 129 130 131 143 145 146 147 **S** QHR, Brentwood, TN
Primary Contact: Chris Thomas, FACHE, President and Chief Executive Officer
CFO: Wesley D. White, Chief Financial Officer
CMO: Donald Nicolay, M.D., Chief Medical Officer
CIO: Mike Kansgen, Director Information Services
CHR: Laurie K. Sinner, Director Human Resources
Web address: www.yourcommunityhospital.com
**Control:** Other not–for–profit (including NFP Corporation) **Service:** General Medical and Surgical

**Staffed Beds:** 44 **Admissions:** 1942 **Census:** 18 **Outpatient Visits:** 149931 **Births:** 0

---

**Hospital, Medicare Provider Number, Address, Telephone, Approval, Facility, and Physician Codes, Health Care System**

★ American Hospital Association (AHA) membership
☐ The Joint Commission accreditation ◇ DNV Healthcare Inc. accreditation
○ American Osteopathic Association (AOA) accreditation
△ Commission on Accreditation of Rehabilitation Facilities (CARF) accreditation

CO

⊞ **ST. MARY'S HOSPITAL AND MEDICAL CENTER (60023)**, 2635 North 7th Street, Zip 81501–8209, Mailing Address: P.O. Box 1628, Zip 81502–1628; tel. 970/298–2273 **A**1 2 9 10 **F**3 12 13 14 15 17 18 19 20 22 24 26 28 29 30 31 32 34 35 37 38 40 43 44 45 49 50 51 53 54 55 57 58 59 60 61 64 68 69 70 72 74 75 76 77 78 79 81 82 85 86 87 89 90 91 93 96 97 100 102 107 108 109 110 111 113 114 115 116 118 120 122 123 125 128 129 130 131 134 144 145 146 147 **P**6 **S** Sisters of Charity of Leavenworth Health System, Denver, CO
Primary Contact: Michael J. McBride, FACHE, President and Chief Executive Officer
COO: Reza Kaleel, Executive Vice President and Chief Operating Officer
CFO: Forest Binder, Vice President Finance
CMO: John C. Beeson, M.D., Vice President Medical Affairs
CIO: Jane Wild, Director Information Technology
CHR: Judy White House, Vice President Human Resources
CNO: Shelley Peterson, Vice President Patient Services and Chief Nursing Officer
Web address: www.stmarygj.com
**Control:** Church–operated, Nongovernment, not–for profit **Service:** General Medical and Surgical

**Staffed Beds:** 310 **Admissions:** 12496 **Census:** 149 **Outpatient Visits:** 367518 **Births:** 2190 **Total Expense ($000):** 319494 **Payroll Expense ($000):** 113776 **Personnel:** 1554

⊞ **VETERANS AFFAIRS MEDICAL CENTER**, 2121 North Avenue, Zip 81501–6499; tel. 970/242–0731, (Nonreporting) **A**1 **S** Department of Veterans Affairs, Washington, DC
Primary Contact: William R. Berryman, M.D., Acting Director
COO: Patricia A. Hitt, Associate Director
CFO: Laquita Gruver, Fiscal Officer
CMO: William R. Berryman, M.D., Chief of Staff
CIO: Craig Frerichs, Chief Information Technology Service
CHR: William Chester, Manager Human Resources
Web address: www.va.gov/sta/guide/home.asp
**Control:** Veterans Affairs, Government, federal **Service:** General Medical and Surgical

**Staffed Beds:** 23

### GREELEY—Weld County

⊞ **NORTH COLORADO MEDICAL CENTER (60001)**, 1801 16th Street, Zip 80634; tel. 970/352–4121 **A**1 2 9 10 **F**3 5 11 12 13 14 15 17 18 19 20 22 24 26 28 29 30 31 32 34 35 37 39 40 43 45 46 48 49 50 51 53 54 59 61 64 65 66 68 70 71 72 74 75 76 77 78 79 81 84 85 86 87 89 90 91 92 93 96 97 98 99 100 101 102 103 104 105 107 108 110 111 113 114 115 116 117 118 119 120 122 123 125 127 128 129 130 131 134 135 140 141 142 144 145 146 147 **P**1 8 **S** Banner Health, Phoenix, AZ
Primary Contact: Richard O. Sutton, Chief Executive Officer
CFO: Mary McCabe, Chief Financial Officer
CMO: Sheldon Stadnyk, M.D., Chief Medical Officer
CHR: Jimmy Duncan, Chief Human Resource Officer
Web address: www.ncmcgreeley.com
**Control:** Other not–for–profit (including NFP Corporation) **Service:** General Medical and Surgical

**Staffed Beds:** 258 **Admissions:** 15380 **Census:** 169 **Outpatient Visits:** 504456 **Births:** 2026 **Total Expense ($000):** 327581 **Payroll Expense ($000):** 119204 **Personnel:** 1928

### GUNNISON—Gunnison County

⊞ **GUNNISON VALLEY HOSPITAL (61320)**, 711 North Taylor Street, Zip 81230–2296; tel. 970/641–1456, (Nonreporting) **A**1 9 10 18
Primary Contact: M. Randell Phelps, Chief Executive Officer
COO: Betsy Bair, Chief Operating Officer
CFO: Tim Cashman, Chief Financial Officer
CMO: John S. Tarr, M.D., Chief Medical Officer
CIO: Trevor Smith, Chief Management Information Services
CHR: Elaine Crumpton, Director Human Resources
Web address: www.gvh–colorado.org
**Control:** County–Government, nonfederal **Service:** General Medical and Surgical

**Staffed Beds:** 24

### HAXTUN—Phillips County

★ **HAXTUN HOSPITAL DISTRICT (61304)**, 235 West Fletcher Street, Zip 80731–0308; tel. 970/774–6123 **A**9 10 18 **F**7 40 43 54 59 64 65 75 87 97 107 113 118 132 145
Primary Contact: Don Burris, Chief Executive Officer
CFO: Sandra Lambrecht, Chief Financial Officer
CMO: Lila Statz, M.D., Chief of Staff
CHR: Brenda Lechman, Director Human Resources
Web address: www.haxtunhealth.org
**Control:** Hospital district or authority, Government, nonfederal **Service:** General Medical and Surgical

**Staffed Beds:** 25 **Admissions:** 119 **Census:** 3 **Outpatient Visits:** 10234 **Births:** 0 **Total Expense ($000):** 6658 **Payroll Expense ($000):** 3441 **Personnel:** 87

### HOLYOKE—Phillips County

★ **MELISSA MEMORIAL HOSPITAL (61305)**, 1001 East Johnson Street, Zip 80734–1854; tel. 970/854–2241 **A**9 10 18 **F**3 7 11 15 28 29 31 32 34 35 40 43 45 50 53 57 59 64 65 67 68 75 81 84 85 87 89 93 97 107 113 118 126 127 128 129 132 145 147 **P**6
Primary Contact: John J. Ayoub, FACHE, Chief Executive Officer
CFO: Gregory J. Was, CPA, Chief Financial Officer
CMO: Dennis Jelden, M.D., Chief of Staff
CHR: Sharon Greenman, Director Human Resources
CNO: Claudia Powell, R.N., Director of Nursing
Web address: www.melissamemorial.org
**Control:** Hospital district or authority, Government, nonfederal **Service:** General Medical and Surgical

**Staffed Beds:** 15 **Admissions:** 323 **Census:** 4 **Outpatient Visits:** 9699 **Births:** 14 **Total Expense ($000):** 8627 **Payroll Expense ($000):** 3944 **Personnel:** 85

### HUGO—Lincoln County

**LINCOLN COMMUNITY HOSPITAL AND NURSING HOME (61306)**, 111 6th Street, Zip 80821–0248, Mailing Address: P.O. Box 248, Zip 80821–0248; tel. 719/743–2421, (Nonreporting) **A**9 10 18
Primary Contact: Herman Schreivogel, Chief Executive Officer
CFO: Herman Schreivogel, Chief Executive Officer
CMO: John E. Fox, M.D., Chief of Staff
Web address: www.lincolncommunityhospitalandnursinghome.com
**Control:** County–Government, nonfederal **Service:** General Medical and Surgical

**Staffed Beds:** 50

### JOHNSTOWN—Larimer County

☐ **NORTHERN COLORADO LONG TERM ACUTE HOSPITAL (62017)**, 4401A Union Street, Zip 80534; tel. 970/619–3663 **A**1 9 10 **F**3 28 29 34 70 75 85 86 87 91 96 129 131 142 147 **S** Ernest Health, Inc., Albuquerque, NM
Primary Contact: Joanne Fenton, MSN, FACHE, Chief Executive Officer
Web address: www.ncltah.ernesthealth.com/
**Control:** Partnership, Investor–owned, for–profit **Service:** Long–Term Acute Care hospital

**Staffed Beds:** 20 **Admissions:** 194 **Census:** 13 **Outpatient Visits:** 0 **Births:** 0 **Total Expense ($000):** 7848 **Payroll Expense ($000):** 3530 **Personnel:** 57

★ **NORTHERN COLORADO REHABILITATION HOSPITAL (63033)**, 4401 Union Street, Zip 80534; tel. 970/619–3400 **A**1 **F**29 34 35 50 57 59 64 75 79 82 90 93 96 129 131 142 147 **S** Ernest Health, Inc., Albuquerque, NM
Primary Contact: Sharon Scheller, Chief Executive Officer
CFO: Ken R. Derrington, Chief Financial Officer
CMO: Indria S. Lanig, M.D., Medical Director
CHR: Jill Scanlon, Director Human Resources
CNO: Rhonda Carolus, Director of Nursing Operations
Web address: www.ncrh.ernesthealth.com
**Control:** Corporation, Investor–owned, for–profit **Service:** Rehabilitation

**Staffed Beds:** 40 **Admissions:** 835 **Census:** 35 **Outpatient Visits:** 6282 **Births:** 0 **Total Expense ($000):** 12043 **Payroll Expense ($000):** 6419 **Personnel:** 172

### JULESBURG—Sedgwick County

**SEDGWICK COUNTY HEALTH CENTER (61310)**, 900 Cedar Street, Zip 80737–1199; tel. 970/474–3323, (Total facility includes 52 beds in nursing home–type unit) **A**9 10 18 **F**3 10 13 15 31 40 43 45 53 57 59 64 65 67 76 81 89 107 113 118 126 127 131 132 147 **P**6
Primary Contact: David Garnas, Chief Executive Officer
COO: David Garnas, Chief Executive Officer
CFO: Karla Dunker, Director Finance
CMO: Donald Regier, M.D., Chief Medical Officer
CHR: Sonja Bell, Coordinator Human Resources
**Control:** County–Government, nonfederal **Service:** General Medical and Surgical

**Staffed Beds:** 64 **Admissions:** 158 **Census:** 48 **Outpatient Visits:** 12662 **Births:** 22 **Total Expense ($000):** 7914 **Payroll Expense ($000):** 3842 **Personnel:** 92

### KREMMLING—Grand County

★ **KREMMLING MEMORIAL HOSPITAL (61318)**, 214 South Fourth Street, Zip 80459, Mailing Address: P.O. Box 399, Zip 80459–0399; tel. 970/724–3442, (Nonreporting) **A**9 10 18
Primary Contact: William Widener, Administrator and Chief Executive Officer
CFO: Cole White, Director Finance
CMO: Mark Paulsen, M.D., Medical Director
CIO: Eric Murray, Manager Public Relations
CHR: Marianne Hayes, Director Human Resources
Web address: www.kremmlinghospital.org
**Control:** Hospital district or authority, Government, nonfederal **Service:** General Medical and Surgical

**Staffed Beds:** 19

*Many Facility Codes have changed. Please refer to the AHA Guide Code Chart.* © 2012 AHA Guide

**CO**

**LA JARA—Conejos County**

★ **CONEJOS COUNTY HOSPITAL (61308)**, 19021 U.S. Highway 285, Zip 81140–0639, Mailing Address: P.O. Box 639, Zip 81140–0639; tel. 719/274–5121, (Nonreporting) **A**9 10 18
Primary Contact: Henry Garvin, Chief Executive Officer
CFO: Pat Cooper, Comptroller
CMO: Vaughn Jackson, M.D., Chief of Staff
CIO: Kathy Rogers, Vice President Marketing
CHR: Delilah Chavez, Human Resources Assistant
Web address: www.cchco.org
**Control:** Hospital district or authority, Government, nonfederal **Service:** General Medical and Surgical

**Staffed Beds:** 17

**LA JUNTA—Otero County**

⊞ **ARKANSAS VALLEY REGIONAL MEDICAL CENTER (60036)**, 1100 Carson Avenue, Zip 81050–2799; tel. 719/383–6000, (Total facility includes 99 beds in nursing home–type unit) **A**1 9 10 20 **F**3 8 11 13 15 29 31 34 35 40 43 45 57 59 64 67 68 70 75 76 77 78 79 81 84 85 86 87 89 93 97 107 108 110 111 114 117 118 127 128 129 131 144 146 147 **P**6 **S** QHR, Brentwood, TN
Primary Contact: Lynn Crowell, Chief Executive Officer
CFO: Janette Bender, Chief Financial Officer
CMO: Michael Martino, M.D., Chief of Staff
CIO: Rocky Ackelson, Director Information Services
CHR: Kerri Kimsey, Director Human Resources
Web address: www.avrmc.org
**Control:** Other not–for–profit (including NFP Corporation) **Service:** General Medical and Surgical

**Staffed Beds:** 163 **Admissions:** 2114 **Census:** 94 **Outpatient Visits:** 46450 **Births:** 254 **Total Expense ($000):** 35854 **Payroll Expense ($000):** 17728 **Personnel:** 378

**LAFAYETTE—Boulder County**

⊞ **EXEMPLA GOOD SAMARITAN MEDICAL CENTER (60116)**, 200 Exempla Circle, Zip 80026; tel. 303/689–4000 **A**1 9 10 **F**3 11 12 13 15 18 20 22 28 29 30 31 34 35 40 43 45 46 49 51 55 57 59 60 63 64 68 70 72 74 75 76 77 78 79 80 81 84 85 86 87 89 91 92 93 94 100 102 107 108 110 111 113 114 118 129 131 142 144 145 146 147 **P**6 **S** Exempla Healthcare, Inc., Denver, CO
Primary Contact: David Hamm, President and Chief Executive Officer
COO: Susan Kerschen, MSN, Vice President Chief Nursing Officer
CFO: John Higgins, Vice President Finance
CMO: Robert Billerbeck, M.D., Vice President and Chief Medical Officer
CHR: Amy Pacey, Vice President Human Resources
Web address: www.exempla.org
**Control:** Other not–for–profit (including NFP Corporation) **Service:** General Medical and Surgical

**Staffed Beds:** 192 **Admissions:** 13058 **Census:** 139 **Outpatient Visits:** 111071 **Births:** 2302 **Total Expense ($000):** 208540 **Payroll Expense ($000):** 83081 **Personnel:** 1226

**LAKEWOOD—Jefferson County**

**ORTHOCOLORADO HOSPITAL (60124)**, 11650 West 2nd Place, Zip 80228–1527; tel. 720/321–5000, (Nonreporting)
Primary Contact: Jude Torchia, Chief Executive Officer
Web address: www.orthocolorado.org
**Control:** Partnership, Investor–owned, for–profit **Service:** Orthopedic

**Staffed Beds:** 48

⊞ **ST. ANTHONY HOSPITAL (60015)**, 11600 West Second Place, Zip 80228–1527; tel. 720/321–0000 **A**1 2 3 5 9 10 **F**3 7 11 12 13 18 20 22 24 26 28 29 30 31 34 35 36 40 43 45 46 47 48 49 50 53 56 57 59 64 68 70 74 75 76 77 78 79 81 82 84 85 87 90 92 93 96 97 102 107 108 113 114 117 118 119 120 122 123 125 128 129 131 132 133 134 145 146 147 **S** Catholic Health Initiatives, Englewood, CO
Primary Contact: Jeffrey Brickman, FACHE, President and Chief Executive Officer
COO: Patrick Green, Chief Operating Officer
COO: Jay S. Weinstein, Chief Operating Officer
CFO: David Thompson, Chief Financial Officer
CMO: Jodi Chambers, M.D., Chief Medical Officer
CMO: Christopher Ott, M.D., Interim Chief Medical Officer
CIO: Dana Moore, Senior Vice President Information Services
CHR: Sheryl Blythe, Director Human Resources
CHR: Michelle Fornier–Johnson, Group Vice President Human Resources
Web address: www.stanthonyhosp.org
**Control:** Church–operated, Nongovernment, not–for profit **Service:** General Medical and Surgical

**Staffed Beds:** 222 **Admissions:** 11331 **Census:** 161 **Outpatient Visits:** 53367 **Births:** 392 **Total Expense ($000):** 251823 **Payroll Expense ($000):** 76929 **Personnel:** 1009

**LAMAR—Prowers County**

★ **PROWERS MEDICAL CENTER (61323)**, 401 Kendall Drive, Zip 81052–3993; tel. 719/336–4343 **A**9 10 18 **F**3 11 13 15 28 29 31 34 35 45 49 56 57 59 62 64 65 68 75 76 77 78 81 85 93 107 111 113 118 126 132 134 143 145 146 147 **P**3 6 **S** QHR, Brentwood, TN
Primary Contact: Craig Loveless, Interim Chief Executive Officer
COO: Karen Bryant, Chief Support Services Officer
CFO: Audrey Kane, Interim Chief Financial Officer
CMO: Barry Portner, M.D., Chief of Staff
CIO: Jason Spano, Manager Information Technology
CHR: Karen Bryant, Chief Support Services Officer
Web address: www.prowersmedical.com
**Control:** Hospital district or authority, Government, nonfederal **Service:** General Medical and Surgical

**Staffed Beds:** 25 **Admissions:** 984 **Census:** 9 **Outpatient Visits:** 6714 **Births:** 127 **Total Expense ($000):** 21755 **Payroll Expense ($000):** 10152 **Personnel:** 233

**LEADVILLE—Lake County**

**ST. VINCENT GENERAL HOSPITAL DISTRICT (61319)**, 822 West 4th Street, Zip 80461–3897; tel. 719/486–0230, (Total facility includes 13 beds in nursing home–type unit) **A**9 10 18 **F**3 7 15 29 40 45 62 81 93 107 118 126 132 **P**5 6
Primary Contact: Roger B. Oberg, Chief Executive Officer
CFO: Michael Choate, Interim Chief Financial Officer
CMO: William Bradshaw, M.D., Chief of Staff
CHR: Dawn Nelson, Director Human Resources
Web address: www.svghd.org
**Control:** Hospital district or authority, Government, nonfederal **Service:** General Medical and Surgical

**Staffed Beds:** 25 **Admissions:** 268 **Census:** 17 **Outpatient Visits:** 16582 **Births:** 2 **Total Expense ($000):** 11718 **Payroll Expense ($000):** 5718 **Personnel:** 92

**LITTLETON—Jefferson County**

**FEDERAL CORRECTIONAL INSTITUTE HOSPITAL**, 9595 West Quincy Street, Zip 80123; tel. 303/985–1566, (Nonreporting)
Primary Contact: Mark Ippolito, Administrator
**Control:** Department of Justice, Government, federal **Service:** Hospital unit of an institution (prison hospital, college infirmary, etc.)

**Staffed Beds:** 6

☐ **HIGHLANDS BEHAVIORAL HEALTH SYSTEM (64024)**, 8565 South Poplar Way, Zip 80130; tel. 720/348–2800, (Nonreporting) **A**1 9 10 **S** Universal Health Services, Inc., King of Prussia, PA
Primary Contact: David W. Morris, Chief Executive Officer
Web address: www.highlandsbhs.com
**Control:** Corporation, Investor–owned, for–profit **Service:** Psychiatric

**Staffed Beds:** 86

⊞ **LITTLETON ADVENTIST HOSPITAL (60113)**, 7700 South Broadway Street, Zip 80122–2628; tel. 303/730–8900 **A**1 9 10 **F**3 8 11 12 13 15 20 22 29 30 31 34 35 36 40 41 43 45 46 47 48 49 53 57 59 62 74 75 76 77 78 79 81 82 83 84 85 87 89 92 93 97 107 108 110 111 113 115 117 118 129 130 131 134 145 146 147 **P**6 **S** Adventist Health System Sunbelt Health Care Corporation, Altamonte Springs, FL
Primary Contact: Morre Dean, Interim Chief Executive Officer
COO: Geoff Lawton, Vice President Operations
CFO: Jeffrey Eitel, Chief Financial Officer
CMO: Lawrence Wood, M.D., Chief Medical Officer
CIO: Linda Hills, Director Information Technology
CHR: Rita K. Arthur, Director Human Resources
Web address: www.centura.org
**Control:** Church–operated, Nongovernment, not–for profit **Service:** General Medical and Surgical

**Staffed Beds:** 202 **Admissions:** 10169 **Census:** 113 **Outpatient Visits:** 71140 **Births:** 1566 **Total Expense ($000):** 153740 **Payroll Expense ($000):** 59030 **Personnel:** 947

---

**Hospital, Medicare Provider Number, Address, Telephone, Approval, Facility, and Physician Codes, Health Care System**

★ American Hospital Association (AHA) membership
☐ The Joint Commission accreditation
◇ DNV Healthcare Inc. accreditation
○ American Osteopathic Association (AOA) accreditation
△ Commission on Accreditation of Rehabilitation Facilities (CARF) accreditation

**CO**

## LONE TREE—Douglas County

☒ **SKY RIDGE MEDICAL CENTER (60112)**, 10101 Ridge Gate Parkway, Zip 80124; tel. 720/225–1000 **A**1 2 9 10 **F**3 5 8 11 12 13 15 18 20 22 24 28 29 30 31 34 35 36 39 40 43 45 46 47 48 49 56 57 59 61 64 70 72 74 75 76 77 78 79 81 82 84 85 86 87 89 93 97 107 108 111 113 114 117 118 120 122 125 128 129 130 134 145 146 147 **S** HCA, Nashville, TN
Primary Contact: Maureen Tarrant, Chief Executive Officer
COO: Susan Hicks, Chief Operating Officer
CFO: Craig Sammons, Chief Financial Officer
CMO: James Lingle, M.D., President Medical Staff
CIO: Ralph Crow, Director Information Technology and Systems
CHR: Linda Pruiett, Vice President Human Resources
Web address: www.skyridgemedcenter.com
**Control:** Corporation, Investor–owned, for–profit **Service:** General Medical and Surgical

**Staffed Beds:** 185 **Admissions:** 13118 **Census:** 129 **Outpatient Visits:** 95003 **Births:** 3056 **Payroll Expense ($000):** 60272 **Personnel:** 835

## LONGMONT—Boulder County

☒ **LONGMONT UNITED HOSPITAL (60003)**, 1950 West Mountain View Avenue, Zip 80501–3162, Mailing Address: P.O. Box 1659, Zip 80502–1659; tel. 303/651–5111, (Total facility includes 15 beds in nursing home–type unit) **A**1 2 9 10 **F**2 3 11 13 15 18 20 22 24 28 29 30 31 34 35 36 37 39 40 43 44 45 48 49 50 53 54 56 57 59 61 64 68 70 73 74 75 76 77 78 79 81 82 84 85 86 87 89 92 93 107 108 110 111 113 114 117 118 120 122 127 128 129 130 131 134 145 147 **P**6
Primary Contact: Mitchell C. Carson, President and Chief Executive Officer
CFO: Neil W. Bertrand, Chief Financial Officer
CMO: John Bradley, M.D., Chief of Staff
CMO: David Burnham, M.D., Chief of Staff
CIO: John Peterson, Vice President Information Systems
CHR: Warren Laughlin, Vice President Human Resources
CNO: Nancy Driscoll, R.N., Chief Nursing Officer
Web address: www.luhcares.org
**Control:** Other not–for–profit (including NFP Corporation) **Service:** General Medical and Surgical

**Staffed Beds:** 146 **Admissions:** 7865 **Census:** 90 **Outpatient Visits:** 116432 **Births:** 1083 **Total Expense ($000):** 158920 **Payroll Expense ($000):** 61511 **Personnel:** 1024

## LOUISVILLE—Boulder County

☒ **AVISTA ADVENTIST HOSPITAL (60103)**, 100 Health Park Drive, Zip 80027–9583; tel. 303/673–1000 **A**1 9 10 **F**3 8 11 13 15 17 18 20 22 29 30 31 34 40 44 45 47 48 49 50 59 60 62 63 64 68 70 72 73 74 75 76 77 79 80 81 82 85 86 87 89 93 107 108 110 111 113 114 118 128 129 130 131 134 145 146 147 **P**1 4 6 **S** Adventist Health System Sunbelt Health Care Corporation, Altamonte Springs, FL
Primary Contact: John Sackett, Chief Executive Officer
COO: David A. Smith, Vice President and Chief Operating Officer
CFO: Cheryl Curry, Vice President Finance
CMO: David Ehrenberger, M.D., Chief Medical Officer
CHR: Derek Morgan, Director Human Resources
Web address: www.avistahospital.org
**Control:** Church–operated, Nongovernment, not–for profit **Service:** General Medical and Surgical

**Staffed Beds:** 114 **Admissions:** 4324 **Census:** 38 **Outpatient Visits:** 44248 **Births:** 2090 **Total Expense ($000):** 72413 **Payroll Expense ($000):** 30093 **Personnel:** 495

☐ **CENTENNIAL PEAKS HOSPITAL (64007)**, 2255 South 88th Street, Zip 80027–9716; tel. 303/673–9990, (Nonreporting) **A**1 9 10 **S** Universal Health Services, Inc., King of Prussia, PA
Primary Contact: Elicia Bunch, Chief Executive Officer
CFO: Tim Ryan, Director Finance
CMO: Michael Zona, M.D., Medical Director
CHR: Tawnya Nordstrom, Director Human Resources
Web address: www.centennialpeaks.com
**Control:** Other not–for–profit (including NFP Corporation) **Service:** Psychiatric

**Staffed Beds:** 72

## LOVELAND—Larimer County

☒ **MCKEE MEDICAL CENTER (60030)**, 2000 Boise Avenue, Zip 80538–4281; tel. 970/669–4640 **A**1 2 9 10 **F**2 3 8 11 12 13 15 18 20 22 28 29 30 31 34 35 38 40 43 46 49 50 54 56 57 59 60 61 62 64 68 70 74 75 76 77 78 79 80 81 82 85 86 87 93 97 104 107 108 110 111 113 114 118 120 122 125 127 128 129 131 132 133 134 143 145 146 147 **P**1 6 **S** Banner Health, Phoenix, AZ
Primary Contact: Marilyn Schock, Chief Executive Officer
COO: Leslie Martin, Associate Administrator
CFO: Lori Sehrt, Chief Financial Officer
CMO: Bert Honea, M.D., Medical Director
CIO: Steve Rains, Director Information Services
CHR: Darlene Alvis, Chief Human Resources Officer
CNO: Debra Fox, Chief Nursing Officer
Web address: www.mckeeloveland.com
**Control:** Other not–for–profit (including NFP Corporation) **Service:** General Medical and Surgical

**Staffed Beds:** 121 **Admissions:** 6206 **Census:** 54 **Outpatient Visits:** 130818 **Births:** 833 **Total Expense ($000):** 120091 **Payroll Expense ($000):** 42669 **Personnel:** 733

☒ **MEDICAL CENTER OF THE ROCKIES (60119)**, 2500 Rocky Mountain Avenue, Zip 80538; tel. 970/624–2500 **A**1 9 10 **F**3 11 13 14 15 17 18 20 22 24 26 28 29 30 31 34 35 37 39 40 43 45 49 50 55 57 58 59 60 61 64 65 68 70 74 75 76 78 79 80 81 82 84 85 86 87 89 93 107 108 110 111 113 117 118 125 129 130 131 133 134 145 146 147 **P**5 6 **S** Poudre Valley Health System, Fort Collins, CO
Primary Contact: George E. Hayes, FACHE, President and Chief Executive Officer
CFO: Stephanie Doughty, Chief Financial Officer
CMO: William Neff, M.D., Chief Medical Officer
CIO: Steve Hess, Vice President & Chief Information Officer
CIO: Fernando Pedroza, Director Information Systems
CHR: Patti Oakes, Director Human Resources
CNO: Kay J. Miller, MS, Chief Nursing Officer
Web address: www.medctrrockies.org
**Control:** Other not–for–profit (including NFP Corporation) **Service:** General Medical and Surgical

**Staffed Beds:** 136 **Admissions:** 7143 **Census:** 75 **Outpatient Visits:** 138680 **Births:** 497 **Total Expense ($000):** 168512 **Payroll Expense ($000):** 57260 **Personnel:** 879

## MEEKER—Rio Blanco County

★ **PIONEERS MEDICAL CENTER (61325)**, 345 Cleveland Street, Zip 81641–3238; tel. 970/878–5047, (Includes WALBRIDGE MEMORIAL CONVALESCENT WING ), (Nonreporting) **A**9 10 18 **S** QHR, Brentwood, TN
Primary Contact: Kenneth Harman, Chief Executive Officer
COO: Drew Varland, Chief Nursing Officer and Chief Operating Officer
CFO: James W. Worrell, Chief Financial Officer
CMO: Albert Krueger, M.D., Chief of Staff
CIO: Curtis Cooper, Manager Information Systems
CHR: Twyla Jensen, Director Human Resources
Web address: www.pioneershospital.com
**Control:** County–Government, nonfederal **Service:** General Medical and Surgical

**Staffed Beds:** 50

## MONTROSE—Montrose County

☒ **MONTROSE MEMORIAL HOSPITAL (60006)**, 800 South Third Street, Zip 81401–4291; tel. 970/249–2211 **A**1 9 10 20 **F**3 12 13 15 17 18 20 22 28 29 30 31 34 35 40 43 45 46 51 57 66 70 73 74 75 76 78 79 80 81 85 88 89 90 93 107 108 110 111 113 118 125 126 128 129 130 145 **P**5 8 **S** QHR, Brentwood, TN
Primary Contact: David L. Hample, Chief Executive Officer
COO: Mary E. Snyder, Chief Operations Officer
CFO: Stephan A. Wilson, Chief Financial Officer
CMO: Richard Shannon, M.D., Chief of Staff
CIO: Carlos Lovera, Director Information Systems
CHR: Kathy McKie, Director Human Resources
Web address: www.montrosehospital.com
**Control:** Other not–for–profit (including NFP Corporation) **Service:** General Medical and Surgical

**Staffed Beds:** 69 **Admissions:** 3204 **Census:** 30 **Outpatient Visits:** 96535 **Births:** 457 **Total Expense ($000):** 73639 **Payroll Expense ($000):** 25818 **Personnel:** 502

## PAGOSA SPRINGS—Archuleta County

**PAGOSA SPRINGS MEDICAL CENTER (61328)**, 95 South Pagosa Boulevard, Zip 81147; tel. 970/731–3700, (Nonreporting) **A**9 10 18
Primary Contact: Bradley Cochennet, Chief Executive Officer
**Control:** Other not–for–profit (including NFP Corporation) **Service:** General Medical and Surgical

**Staffed Beds:** 11

**PARKER—Douglas County**

⊠ **PARKER ADVENTIST HOSPITAL (60114)**, 9395 Crown Crest Boulevard,
Zip 80138; tel. 303/269–4000 **A**1 9 10 **F**3 11 12 13 15 20 22 29 30 31 34
35 36 38 40 43 45 46 49 50 54 55 57 59 64 70 72 73 74 75 76 77 78 79
81 82 83 84 85 87 89 93 96 97 107 110 111 113 114 118 128 129 130
134 145 146 147 **P**6 **S** Adventist Health System Sunbelt Health Care
Corporation, Altamonte Springs, FL
Primary Contact: Morre Dean, Chief Executive Officer
CFO: Andrew Gaasch, Chief Financial Officer
CMO: Todd Mydler, M.D., Chief Medical Officer
Web address: www.parkerhospital.org
**Control:** Church–operated, Nongovernment, not–for profit **Service:** General
Medical and Surgical

> **Staffed Beds:** 142 **Admissions:** 6919 **Census:** 69 **Outpatient Visits:** 55413
> **Births:** 1531 **Total Expense ($000):** 111009 **Payroll Expense ($000):**
> 44005 **Personnel:** 708

**PUEBLO—Pueblo County**

☐ **COLORADO MENTAL HEALTH INSTITUTE AT PUEBLO (60115)**, 1600 West
24th Street, Zip 81003–1499; tel. 719/546–4000, (Nonreporting) **A**1 3 5 10
Primary Contact: John R. DeQuardo, M.D., Superintendent
CFO: Jim Duff, Chief Financial Officer
CMO: Al Singleton, M.D., Chief Psychiatry and Chief Medical Staff
CIO: Eunice Wolther, Public Information Officer
CHR: Mary Young, Director Human Resources
Web address: www.cdhs.state.co.us/cmhip
**Control:** State–Government, nonfederal **Service:** Psychiatric

> **Staffed Beds:** 514

**HAVEN BEHAVIORAL WAR HEROES HOSPITAL (64025)**, 1008 Minnequa
Avenue, Suite 6100, Zip 81004–3733; tel. 719/546–6000, (Nonreporting)
**S** Haven Behavioral Healthcare, Nashville, TN
Primary Contact: Carrin Harper, M.D., Chief Executive Officer
**Control:** Corporation, Investor–owned, for–profit **Service:** Psychiatric

> **Staffed Beds:** 20

⊠ △ **PARKVIEW MEDICAL CENTER (60020)**, 400 West 16th Street,
Zip 81003–2781; tel. 719/584–4000, (Total facility includes 20 beds in nursing
home–type unit) **A**1 7 9 10 **F**2 3 4 5 8 11 13 15 18 20 22 24 28 29 30 31 34
35 37 38 40 42 43 45 46 49 50 51 53 56 57 58 59 62 64 70 74 75 76 78
79 81 82 84 85 86 87 89 90 93 94 95 96 97 98 99 100 101 102 103 104
105 107 108 111 113 114 115 117 118 123 127 128 129 131 134 140 145
146 147 **P**6 8 **S** QHR, Brentwood, TN
Primary Contact: Michael T. Baxter, Chief Executive Officer
COO: Timothy Allen, Senior Vice President and Chief Operating Officer
CFO: William Patterson, Chief Financial Officer
CMO: Steve Nafziger, M.D., Vice President Medical Affairs
CIO: Steve Shirley, Chief Information Officer
CHR: Darrin Smith, Vice President Human Resources
Web address: www.parkviewmc.org
**Control:** Other not–for–profit (including NFP Corporation) **Service:** General
Medical and Surgical

> **Staffed Beds:** 370 **Admissions:** 14868 **Census:** 209 **Outpatient Visits:**
> 175395 **Births:** 1503 **Total Expense ($000):** 227733 **Payroll Expense**
> **($000):** 96363 **Personnel:** 1922

⊠ **ST. MARY–CORWIN MEDICAL CENTER (60012)**, 1008 Minnequa Avenue,
Zip 81004–3798; tel. 719/557–4000 **A**1 2 9 10 12 13 **F**3 13 15 18 20 22 26
28 29 30 31 34 35 40 43 45 47 48 49 50 51 53 55 57 58 59 64 68 70 72
73 75 76 78 79 81 82 84 85 86 87 89 90 107 108 110 111 113 114 116
118 119 120 122 123 125 128 129 130 131 134 145 146 147 **P**6 **S** Catholic
Health Initiatives, Englewood, CO
Primary Contact: Robert Ryder, Chief Executive Officer
COO: Michael Cafasso, Vice President Operations
CFO: Sheri Trahern, Chief Financial Officer
CMO: Stephen Brown, M.D., Chief Medical Officer
CHR: Rudy Krasovec, Director Human Resources
Web address: www.centura.org
**Control:** Church–operated, Nongovernment, not–for profit **Service:** General
Medical and Surgical

> **Staffed Beds:** 202 **Admissions:** 7390 **Census:** 93 **Outpatient Visits:** 87873
> **Births:** 558 **Total Expense ($000):** 136708 **Payroll Expense ($000):** 51471
> **Personnel:** 1013

**RANGELY—Rio Blanco County**

★ **RANGELY DISTRICT HOSPITAL (61307)**, 511 South White Avenue,
Zip 81648–2104; tel. 970/675–5011, (Nonreporting) **A**9 10 18
Primary Contact: Nick Goshe, Chief Executive Officer
CFO: Jim Dillon, Chief Financial Officer
CMO: Chris Adams, M.D., Physician
CHR: Kristin Beery, Executive Assistant and Director Human Resources
Web address: www.rangelyhospital.com
**Control:** Hospital district or authority, Government, nonfederal **Service:** General
Medical and Surgical

> **Staffed Beds:** 18

**RIFLE—Garfield County**

★ **GRAND RIVER HOSPITAL DISTRICT (61317)**, 501 Airport Road,
Zip 81650–2970, Mailing Address: P.O. Box 912, Zip 81650–0912;
tel. 970/625–1510, (Total facility includes 57 beds in nursing home–type unit) **A**9
10 18 **F**3 11 12 15 29 34 35 39 40 41 43 45 50 57 59 64 68 69 75 77 79
81 85 87 93 96 97 107 108 110 111 112 113 117 118 126 127 128 129
130 131 132 143 144 145 147 **P**6
Primary Contact: James Coombs, Chief Executive Officer
COO: Mary Desormeau, Chief Nursing Officer
CMO: Gary Meyer, M.D., Chief of Staff
CIO: Diana Murray, Director Information Systems
CHR: Michael Weerts, Director Human Resources
CNO: Mary Desormeau, Chief Nursing Officer
Web address: www.grhd.org
**Control:** Hospital district or authority, Government, nonfederal **Service:** General
Medical and Surgical

> **Staffed Beds:** 70 **Admissions:** 601 **Census:** 46 **Outpatient Visits:** 69836
> **Births:** 0 **Total Expense ($000):** 40808 **Payroll Expense ($000):** 19245
> **Personnel:** 300

**SALIDA—Chaffee County**

★ **HEART OF THE ROCKIES REGIONAL MEDICAL CENTER (61322)**, 1000 Rush
Drive, Zip 81201–0429, Mailing Address: P.O. Box 429, Zip 81201–0429;
tel. 719/530–2200 **A**9 10 18 **F**3 11 13 15 28 29 31 34 35 40 43 45 50 54
55 57 64 68 70 75 76 77 78 79 81 82 85 89 90 93 94 97 107 108 110 111
113 116 118 126 128 129 130 132 134 145 146 147
Primary Contact: Kenneth W. Leisher, Chief Executive Officer
CFO: Lesley Fagerberg, Vice President Fiscal Services
CMO: James Wigington, M.D., Chief of Staff
CIO: Andy Waldbart, Department Manager
CHR: Barbara J. Abel, Vice President Human Resources
CNO: Peg Arnett, Interim Vice President of Nursing
Web address: www.hrrmc.com
**Control:** Hospital district or authority, Government, nonfederal **Service:** General
Medical and Surgical

> **Staffed Beds:** 25 **Admissions:** 1130 **Census:** 11 **Outpatient Visits:** 37150
> **Births:** 147 **Total Expense ($000):** 30044 **Payroll Expense ($000):** 12065
> **Personnel:** 257

**SPRINGFIELD—Baca County**

★ **SOUTHEAST COLORADO HOSPITAL DISTRICT (61311)**, 373 East Tenth
Avenue, Zip 81073–1699; tel. 719/523–4501, (Total facility includes 56 beds in
nursing home–type unit) **A**9 10 18 **F**3 6 7 11 29 35 40 50 56 57 62 63 66 81
93 97 107 126 132 146 147
Primary Contact: Robert W. Omer, FACHE, Chief Executive Officer and
Administrator
CFO: James L. Forrest, Jr., Chief Financial Officer
CMO: Frank McDonald, D.O., Chief of Staff
CIO: Bobby L. Schaller, Chief Engineer
CHR: Sherrilyn Turner, Director Human Resources
Web address: www.sechosp.org
**Control:** Hospital district or authority, Government, nonfederal **Service:** General
Medical and Surgical

> **Staffed Beds:** 79 **Admissions:** 253 **Census:** 55 **Outpatient Visits:** 43505
> **Births:** 0 **Total Expense ($000):** 11511 **Payroll Expense ($000):** 5438
> **Personnel:** 182

**CO**

---

**Hospital, Medicare Provider Number, Address, Telephone, Approval, Facility, and Physician Codes, Health Care System**

★ American Hospital Association (AHA) membership
☐ The Joint Commission accreditation
◇ DNV Healthcare Inc. accreditation
○ American Osteopathic Association (AOA) accreditation
△ Commission on Accreditation of Rehabilitation Facilities (CARF) accreditation

## STEAMBOAT SPRINGS—Routt County

✠ **YAMPA VALLEY MEDICAL CENTER (60049)**, 1024 Central Park Drive,
Zip 80487–8813; tel. 970/879–1322, (Total facility includes 59 beds in nursing
home–type unit) **A**1 9 10 20 **F**3 11 13 15 18 28 29 30 31 34 35 36 40 43 45
46 49 50 51 57 64 68 70 73 75 76 77 78 79 81 82 85 86 87 93 107 111
114 118 127 128 129 130 131 132 134 142 145 146
Primary Contact: Frank May, Chief Executive Officer
CFO: Robert Flake, Chief Financial Officer
CMO: Larry Bookman, D.O., Chief Medical Officer
CIO: Mark Albright, Director of Information Services
CHR: Soniya Fidler, Senior Director Human Resources
CNO: Marie Timlin, R.N., Chief Nursing Officer
Web address: www.yvmc.org
**Control:** Other not–for–profit (including NFP Corporation) **Service:** General
Medical and Surgical

| | |
|---|---|
| **Staffed Beds:** 98 **Admissions:** 1816 **Census:** 66 **Outpatient Visits:** 66714 **Births:** 326 **Total Expense ($000):** 70017 **Payroll Expense ($000):** 25694 **Personnel:** 412 | |

## STERLING—Logan County

✠ **STERLING REGIONAL MEDCENTER (60076)**, 615 Fairhurst Street,
Zip 80751–0500; tel. 970/522–0122 **A**1 9 10 20 **F**3 13 15 18 19 28 29 30
31 32 34 40 41 43 44 45 50 51 57 59 60 64 68 69 70 75 76 77 78 79 81
82 85 86 87 93 97 107 108 110 111 113 117 118 126 128 129 130 142
145 147 **P**6 **S** Banner Health, Phoenix, AZ
Primary Contact: Julie Klein, Chief Executive Officer
CFO: Pamela Stieb, Chief Financial Officer
CMO: Thomas Soper, D.O., Medical Director
CHR: Randy Brigham, Chief Human Resource Officer
CNO: Karen A. Lund, R.N., Chief Nursing Officer
Web address: www.bannerhealth.com
**Control:** Other not–for–profit (including NFP Corporation) **Service:** General
Medical and Surgical

| | |
|---|---|
| **Staffed Beds:** 25 **Admissions:** 1386 **Census:** 13 **Outpatient Visits:** 147344 **Births:** 202 **Total Expense ($000):** 50300 **Payroll Expense ($000):** 19552 **Personnel:** 292 | |

## THORNTON—Adams County

**HAVEN BEHAVIORAL SENIOR CARE OF NORTH DENVER (64018)**, 8451
Pearl Street, Suite 100, Zip 80229–4804; tel. 303/288–7807, (Nonreporting)
**S** Haven Behavioral Healthcare, Nashville, TN
Primary Contact: Marc McComas, Executive Director
Web address: www.havenbehavioral.com/seniorcare/denver
**Control:** Corporation, Investor–owned, for–profit **Service:** Psychiatric

| | |
|---|---|
| **Staffed Beds:** 40 | |

✠ **NORTH SUBURBAN MEDICAL CENTER (60065)**, 9191 Grant Street,
Zip 80229–4341; tel. 303/451–7800 **A**1 9 10 **F**3 11 12 13 15 18 20 22 29
30 35 40 43 45 59 60 64 68 70 72 74 75 76 79 80 81 82 84 85 87 89 107
108 111 114 118 128 129 131 134 145 **P**2 **S** HCA, Nashville, TN
Primary Contact: Jennifer Alderfer, Chief Executive Officer
CFO: Deborah Hart, Chief Financial Officer
CIO: Jeff Schnoor, Director Information Technology and Systems
CHR: Suzanne Kelley, Director Human Resources
CNO: Erica Rossitto, R.N., Chief Nursing Officer
Web address: www.northsuburban.com
**Control:** Corporation, Investor–owned, for–profit **Service:** General Medical and
Surgical

| | |
|---|---|
| **Staffed Beds:** 136 **Admissions:** 6095 **Census:** 63 **Outpatient Visits:** 81805 **Births:** 1406 **Total Expense ($000):** 88101 **Payroll Expense ($000):** 37091 **Personnel:** 447 | |

☐ **VIBRA HOSPITAL OF DENVER (62014)**, 8451 Pearl Street, Zip 80229–4804;
tel. 303/288–3000, (Nonreporting) **A**1 9 10 **S** Vibra Healthcare,
Mechanicsburg, PA
Primary Contact: Dianne Chartier, R.N., Chief Executive Officer
CMO: Peter Cahill, M.D., President Medical Staff
CHR: Lorna Fulton, Director Human Resources
Web address: www.vhdenver.com
**Control:** Corporation, Investor–owned, for–profit **Service:** Long–Term Acute Care
hospital

| | |
|---|---|
| **Staffed Beds:** 71 | |

## TRINIDAD—Las Animas County

✠ **MT. SAN RAFAEL HOSPITAL (61321)**, 410 Benedicta Avenue,
Zip 81082–2093; tel. 719/846–9213 **A**1 9 10 18 **F**3 11 15 28 40 43 45 57
68 77 79 81 85 87 93 107 108 111 118 126 128 132 147 **S** QHR,
Brentwood, TN
Primary Contact: James Robertson, Chief Executive Officer
CFO: Woody Hathaway, Chief Financial Officer
CMO: Gerald Cichocki, M.D., Chief of Staff
CHR: Lori Silva, Director Human Resources
Web address: www.msrhc.org
**Control:** Other not–for–profit (including NFP Corporation) **Service:** General
Medical and Surgical

| | |
|---|---|
| **Staffed Beds:** 25 **Admissions:** 660 **Census:** 9 **Outpatient Visits:** 38813 **Births:** 0 **Total Expense ($000):** 23640 **Payroll Expense ($000):** 9199 **Personnel:** 168 | |

## VAIL—Eagle County

✠ **VAIL VALLEY MEDICAL CENTER (60096)**, 181 West Meadow Drive,
Zip 81657–5059, Mailing Address: P.O. Box 40000, Zip 81658;
tel. 970/476–2451, (Nonreporting) **A**1 2 9 10 20
Primary Contact: Doris Kirchner, Chief Executive Officer
COO: Tom Kyllo, Executive Vice President
CFO: Shaun J. Scanlon, Senior Vice President Finance and Chief Financial Officer
CMO: John Woodland, M.D., Medical Director
CIO: Dave Pluta, Chief Information Officer
CHR: David Blackwell, Vice President Human Resources
Web address: www.vvmc.com
**Control:** Other not–for–profit (including NFP Corporation) **Service:** General
Medical and Surgical

| | |
|---|---|
| **Staffed Beds:** 58 | |

## WALSENBURG—Huerfano County

★ **SPANISH PEAKS REGIONAL HEALTH CENTER (61316)**, 23500 U.S. Highway
160, Zip 81089–9524; tel. 719/738–5100 **A**9 10 18 **F**11 28 34 35 40 45 50
57 59 64 79 81 82 85 93 97 107 111 113 118 128 130 132 146 147 **P**6
Primary Contact: Todd Oberheu, Chief Executive Officer
CFO: Richard L. Corradino, Chief Financial Officer
CMO: Thomas Hoffeld, M.D., Chief of Staff
CHR: L. Anthony Marostica, Director Human Resources
CNO: Darlene Colt, R.N., Chief Nursing Officer
Web address: www.sprhc.org
**Control:** Hospital district or authority, Government, nonfederal **Service:** General
Medical and Surgical

| | |
|---|---|
| **Staffed Beds:** 25 **Admissions:** 365 **Census:** 5 **Outpatient Visits:** 32411 **Total Expense ($000):** 12300 **Payroll Expense ($000):** 7411 **Personnel:** 141 | |

## WESTMINSTER—Jefferson County

**CLEO WALLACE CENTERS HOSPITAL**, 8405 Church Ranch Boulevard,
Zip 80021–3918; tel. 303/466–7391, (Nonreporting) **A**9
Primary Contact: Michael J. Montgomery, President and Chief Executive Officer
CFO: Jonelle A. Roberts, Chief Financial Officer
Web address: www.devereux.org
**Control:** Other not–for–profit (including NFP Corporation) **Service:** Children's
hospital psychiatric

| | |
|---|---|
| **Staffed Beds:** 61 | |

✠ **ST. ANTHONY NORTH HOSPITAL (60104)**, 2551 West 84th Avenue,
Zip 80031; tel. 303/426–2151 **A**1 9 10 **F**3 11 13 15 18 20 22 26 28 29 30
31 34 35 36 40 43 45 46 49 54 57 60 63 64 65 68 70 72 74 75 76 77 78
79 81 85 87 92 93 97 102 107 108 110 113 114 118 128 129 145 146 147
**S** Catholic Health Initiatives, Englewood, CO
Primary Contact: Carole Peet, R.N., MSN, President and Chief Executive Officer
CFO: Alison Mizer, Chief Financial Officer
CMO: Patrick Sankovitz, M.D., Chief Medical Officer
CIO: Dana Moore, Senior Vice President Information Services
CHR: Robert Archibold, Director, Human Resources
CNO: Carol A. Butler, R.N., VP Patient Care Services & Operations
Web address: www.stanthonynorth.org
**Control:** Church–operated, Nongovernment, not–for profit **Service:** General
Medical and Surgical

| | |
|---|---|
| **Staffed Beds:** 138 **Admissions:** 6836 **Census:** 73 **Outpatient Visits:** 57222 **Births:** 926 **Total Expense ($000):** 99280 **Payroll Expense ($000):** 37465 **Personnel:** 645 | |

**CO**

## WHEAT RIDGE—Jefferson County

⊠ **EXEMPLA LUTHERAN MEDICAL CENTER (60009)**, 8300 West 38th Avenue, Zip 80033–6005; tel. 303/425–4500, (Includes EXEMPLA WEST PINES, 3400 Lutheran Parkway, Zip 80033; tel. 303/467–4000), (Total facility includes 113 beds in nursing home–type unit) **A**1 2 9 10 **F**3 4 5 10 11 13 15 18 20 22 24 26 28 29 30 31 33 34 35 36 40 43 45 47 48 49 50 54 55 58 59 60 62 63 64 67 68 70 72 74 75 76 77 78 79 81 84 85 86 87 94 98 100 101 102 103 104 105 107 108 110 111 113 114 118 119 120 122 123 124 125 127 128 129 131 145 146 147 **P**6 **S** Exempla Healthcare, Inc., Denver, CO
Primary Contact: Grant Wicklund, President and Chief Executive Officer
COO: Peggy Cain Price, Vice President and Chief Operating Officer
CFO: Karen Scremin, Vice President Finance
CMO: David Munch, M.D., Vice President and Chief Clinical and Quality Officer
CHR: Scott Day, Vice President Human Resources
Web address: www.exempla.org
**Control:** Other not–for–profit (including NFP Corporation) **Service:** General Medical and Surgical

**Staffed Beds:** 449 **Admissions:** 19632 **Census:** 363 **Outpatient Visits:** 180708 **Births:** 2717 **Total Expense ($000):** 325076 **Payroll Expense ($000):** 130138 **Personnel:** 1883

## WOODLAND PARK—Teller County

**PIKES PEAK REGIONAL HOSPITAL (61326)**, 16420 West Highway 24, Zip 80863; tel. 719/687–9999 **A**9 10 18 21 **F**3 15 29 30 34 40 43 45 50 59 64 68 77 79 81 82 85 86 87 93 107 110 111 113 118 132 134 145 147 **S** IASIS Healthcare, Franklin, TN
Primary Contact: Dolores A. Horvath, Chief Executive Officer
CFO: Kimberly Monvesky, Chief Financial Officer
CMO: Kurt Wever, M.D., Chief of Staff
CHR: Arianne Randolph, Director Human Resources
Web address: www.pprmc.org
**Control:** Corporation, Investor–owned, for–profit **Service:** General Medical and Surgical

**Staffed Beds:** 15 **Admissions:** 667 **Census:** 7

## WRAY—Yuma County

★ **WRAY COMMUNITY DISTRICT HOSPITAL (61309)**, 1017 West 7th Street, Zip 80758–1420; tel. 970/332–4811, (Nonreporting) **A**9 10 18
Primary Contact: Edward Finley, Administrator
CFO: Jennie Sullivan, Director Finance
CMO: Monte Uyemura, M.D., Chief of Staff
Web address: www.wcdh.org
**Control:** Hospital district or authority, Government, nonfederal **Service:** General Medical and Surgical

**Staffed Beds:** 16

## YUMA—Yuma County

★ **YUMA DISTRICT HOSPITAL (61315)**, 1000 West 8th Avenue, Zip 80759–2641; tel. 970/848–5405 **A**9 10 18 **F**3 11 13 15 28 30 31 34 35 36 40 43 44 50 53 57 59 62 64 65 68 74 75 76 77 78 79 81 82 87 93 97 99 101 102 103 104 107 111 114 118 126 129 132 147 **P**6
Primary Contact: John Gardner, Chief Executive Officer
COO: Lyndia Loppe, Chief Operating Officer
CFO: Cathy Wolff, Vice President Financial Services and Chief Financial Officer
CMO: John Wolz, M.D., Chief Medical Staff
CIO: Jason Hawley, Manager Information Services
CHR: Gini Adams, Director Employee and Public Relations
CNO: Beth Saxton, R.N., Vice President Patient Care Services
Web address: www.yumahospital.org
**Control:** Hospital district or authority, Government, nonfederal **Service:** General Medical and Surgical

**Staffed Beds:** 12 **Admissions:** 309 **Census:** 3 **Outpatient Visits:** 49230 **Births:** 11 **Total Expense ($000):** 18083 **Payroll Expense ($000):** 7706 **Personnel:** 131

CO

---

**Hospital, Medicare Provider Number, Address, Telephone, Approval, Facility, and Physician Codes, Health Care System**

★ American Hospital Association (AHA) membership
□ The Joint Commission accreditation     ◇ DNV Healthcare Inc. accreditation

○ American Osteopathic Association (AOA) accreditation
△ Commission on Accreditation of Rehabilitation Facilities (CARF) accreditation

# CONNECTICUT

**CT**

## BETHLEHEM—Litchfield County

**WELLSPRING FOUNDATION**, 21 Arch Bridge Road, Zip 06751–0370, Mailing Address: P.O. Box 370, Zip 06751–0370; tel. 203/266–7235, (Nonreporting) **A**9
Primary Contact: Richard E. Beauvais, Ph.D., Chief Executive Officer
CFO: Richard E. Beauvais, Ph.D., Chief Executive Officer
Web address: www.wellspring.org
**Control:** Other not–for–profit (including NFP Corporation) **Service:** Psychiatric

**Staffed Beds:** 36

## BRANFORD—New Haven County

☐ **THE CONNECTICUT HOSPICE (70038)**, 100 Double Beach Road,
Zip 06405–4909; tel. 203/315–7500, (Nonreporting) **A**1 10
Primary Contact: Rosemary Johnson Hurzeler, President and Chief Executive
Officer
Web address: www.hospice.com
**Control:** Other not–for–profit (including NFP Corporation) **Service:** Other specialty

**Staffed Beds:** 52

## BRIDGEPORT—Fairfield County

✠ **BRIDGEPORT HOSPITAL (70010)**, 267 Grant Street, Zip 06610–2805, Mailing
Address: P.O. Box 5000, Zip 06610–5000; tel. 203/384–3000 **A**1 2 3 5 6 8 9
10 **F**3 6 8 11 13 15 16 18 19 20 22 24 26 28 29 30 31 32 34 35 36 38 40
41 43 44 45 46 47 48 49 50 51 55 56 57 58 59 61 64 65 66 68 70 72 74
75 76 77 78 79 80 81 82 84 85 86 87 88 89 90 93 96 97 98 99 100 101
102 103 104 105 107 108 110 113 116 117 118 120 122 125 128 129 130
131 133 134 143 144 145 146 147 **P**6 **S** Yale New Haven Health System, New
Haven, CT
Primary Contact: William M. Jennings, President and Chief Executive Officer
COO: Norman G. Roth, Executive Vice President and Chief Operating Officer
CFO: Patrick McCabe, Senior Vice President Finance and Chief Financial Officer
CMO: Bruce M. McDonald, M.D., Senior Vice President Medical Affairs
CIO: Daniel Barchi, Senior Vice President, Technical Services and Chief
Information Officer
CHR: Melissa Turner, Senior Vice President Human Resources
CNO: MaryEllen Kosturko, R.N., Senior Vice President Patient Care Operations and
Chief Nursing Officer
Web address: www.bridgeporthospital.org
**Control:** Other not–for–profit (including NFP Corporation) **Service:** General
Medical and Surgical

**Staffed Beds:** 384 **Admissions:** 16996 **Census:** 272 **Outpatient Visits:**
271948 **Births:** 2241 **Total Expense ($000):** 370976 **Payroll Expense
($000):** 140185 **Personnel:** 1863

**SOUTHWEST CONNECTICUT MENTAL HEALTH SYSTEM (74012)**, 97 Middle
Street, Zip 6604; tel. 203/551–7400 **A**9 10 **F**29 35 38 50 98 100 102 104
129 131 **S** Connecticut Department of Mental Health and Addiction Services,
Hartford, CT
Primary Contact: James M. Pisciotta, Chief Executive Officer
CFO: Magnus Ezeji, Chief Financial Officer
CMO: Stephen R. Atkins, M.D., Medical Director
CIO: Paula Zwally, Director Quality Improvement Services and Compliance
CHR: Paula DeBarros, Director Human Resources
Web address: www.ct.gov/dmhas/cwp/view.asp?a=2946&q=378936
**Control:** State–Government, nonfederal **Service:** Psychiatric

**Staffed Beds:** 62 **Admissions:** 187 **Census:** 60 **Outpatient Visits:** 17489
**Births:** 0 **Personnel:** 381

✠ **ST. VINCENT'S MEDICAL CENTER (70028)**, 2800 Main Street,
Zip 06606–4292; tel. 203/576–5454, (Includes ST. VINCENT'S BEHAVIORAL
HEALTH, 47 Long Lots Road, Westport, Zip 06880–3800; tel. 203/221–8802;
James McCreath, Ph.D., President and Chief Executive Officer) **A**1 2 3 5 9 10 **F**3
4 5 8 12 13 15 17 18 20 22 24 26 28 29 30 31 34 35 36 38 40 43 44 45
46 47 49 50 53 54 55 56 57 58 59 60 61 63 64 65 66 68 70 71 72 73 74
75 76 77 78 79 80 81 82 84 85 86 87 90 91 92 93 96 97 98 99 100 101
102 103 104 105 106 107 108 110 111 113 114 116 117 118 119 120 122
123 125 129 131 133 142 143 144 145 146 147 **S** Ascension Health, Saint
Louis, MO
Primary Contact: Susan L. Davis, R.N., Ed.D., FACHE, President and Chief
Executive Officer
CFO: John Gleckler, Chief Financial Officer
CMO: Stuart Marcus, M.D., Senior Vice President and Chief Medical Officer
CIO: Betsy Thornquist, Chief Information Officer
CHR: Steven Younes, Vice President, Chief Human Resources Officer and
Employment Counsel
Web address: www.stvincents.org
**Control:** Other not–for–profit (including NFP Corporation) **Service:** General
Medical and Surgical

**Staffed Beds:** 396 **Admissions:** 21019 **Census:** 328 **Outpatient Visits:**
324127 **Births:** 1081 **Total Expense ($000):** 361247 **Payroll Expense
($000):** 165206 **Personnel:** 2231

## BRISTOL—Hartford County

✠ **BRISTOL HOSPITAL (70029)**, Brewster Road, Zip 6011, Mailing Address: P.O.
Box 977, Zip 06011–0977; tel. 860/585–3000 **A**1 2 5 9 10 **F**3 5 7 12 13 14
15 18 28 29 30 31 34 35 36 38 40 45 47 49 50 51 54 57 58 59 61 62 63
66 70 74 75 76 77 78 79 81 82 84 85 86 87 89 93 94 97 98 100 102 104
105 107 110 111 113 114 115 118 128 129 131 134 143 144 145 146
147 **P**3
Primary Contact: Kurt A. Barwis, FACHE, President and Chief Executive Officer
COO: Marc D. Edelman, Vice President Operations
CFO: Peter Freytag, Senior Vice President Finance and Chief Financial Officer
CMO: Leonard Banco, M.D., Senior Vice President and Chief Medical Officer
CIO: David Rackliffe, Assistant Vice President Information Services
CHR: Jeanine Reckdenwald, Assistant Vice President Human Resources
Web address: www.bristolhospital.org
**Control:** Other not–for–profit (including NFP Corporation) **Service:** General
Medical and Surgical

**Staffed Beds:** 134 **Admissions:** 6684 **Census:** 75 **Outpatient Visits:** 192283
**Births:** 622 **Total Expense ($000):** 122010 **Payroll Expense ($000):** 53092
**Personnel:** 916

## DANBURY—Fairfield County

✠ **DANBURY HOSPITAL (70033)**, 24 Hospital Avenue, Zip 06810–6099;
tel. 203/739–7000 **A**1 2 3 5 8 9 10 **F**3 4 5 8 9 12 13 14 15 17 18 20 22 24
26 28 29 30 31 32 33 34 35 36 37 38 39 40 43 44 45 46 47 48 49 50 51
54 55 56 57 58 59 60 61 64 65 66 68 70 72 73 74 75 76 77 78 79 80 81
82 83 84 85 86 87 89 90 93 94 96 97 98 99 100 101 102 103 104 105 107
108 109 110 111 112 113 114 115 116 117 118 119 120 122 123 125 128
129 130 131 133 134 143 144 145 146 147 **S** Western Connecticut
Healthcare, Inc., Danbury, CT
Primary Contact: John M. Murphy, M.D., President and Chief Executive Officer
COO: Michael Daglio, Chief Operating Officer
CFO: Steven Rosenberg, Chief Financial Officer
CMO: Matthew Miller, M.D., Vice President Medical Affairs
CIO: Kathleen DeMatteo, Chief Information Officer
CHR: Phyllis Zappala, Vice President Human Resources
CHR: Phyllis F. Zappala, Senior Vice President
CNO: Moreen Donahue, R.N., Chief Nursing Executive
Web address: www.danburyhospital.org
**Control:** Other not–for–profit (including NFP Corporation) **Service:** General
Medical and Surgical

**Staffed Beds:** 354 **Admissions:** 18887 **Census:** 250 **Outpatient Visits:**
386526 **Births:** 1994 **Total Expense ($000):** 479890 **Payroll Expense
($000):** 195165 **Personnel:** 2549

## DERBY—New Haven County

✠ **GRIFFIN HOSPITAL (70031)**, 130 Division Street, Zip 06418–1326;
tel. 203/735–7421 **A**1 2 9 10 **F**3 5 8 12 13 15 18 28 29 30 31 34 35 36 38
40 45 49 50 51 53 56 57 58 59 64 65 68 70 71 74 75 76 77 78 79 81 82
85 86 87 93 94 96 97 98 99 100 101 102 103 104 105 107 108 110 111
112 113 115 117 118 119 120 122 128 129 131 133 134 143 145 146 147
Primary Contact: Patrick Charmel, President and Chief Executive Officer
CMO: Kenneth V. Schwartz, M.D., Medical Director
CIO: George Tomas, Director Information Services
CHR: Steve Mordecai, Director Human Resources
CNO: Barbara J. Stumpo, R.N., Vice President Patient Care Services
Web address: www.griffinhealth.org
**Control:** Other not–for–profit (including NFP Corporation) **Service:** General
Medical and Surgical

**Staffed Beds:** 111 **Admissions:** 6850 **Census:** 81 **Outpatient Visits:** 191512
**Births:** 654 **Total Expense ($000):** 122819 **Payroll Expense ($000):** 53580
**Personnel:** 902

*Many Facility Codes have changed. Please refer to the AHA Guide Code Chart.*

**FARMINGTON—Hartford County**

✠ **UNIVERSITY OF CONNECTICUT HEALTH CENTER, JOHN DEMPSEY HOSPITAL (70036)**, 263 Farmington Avenue, Zip 06032–1941; tel. 860/679–2000 **A**1 2 3 5 8 9 10 12 13 19 **F**3 5 7 8 9 11 13 15 18 20 22 24 26 29 30 31 34 35 36 38 39 40 45 47 50 51 52 55 56 58 59 60 61 64 68 70 72 74 75 76 77 78 79 81 82 86 87 91 93 94 98 99 100 101 102 103 104 105 107 108 109 111 113 114 115 116 117 118 119 120 128 129 130 131 132 142 145 146 **P**6
Primary Contact: Mike H. Summerer, M.D., Chief Executive Officer
COO: Anne Diamond, JD, Chief Operating Officer
CFO: John Biancamano, Chief Financial Officer
CMO: Richard Simon, M.D., Chief of Staff
CIO: Sandra Armstrong, Chief Information Officer
CHR: Carolle Andrews, Interim Chief Human Resources Officer
CNO: Ellen Leone, R.N., Chief Nursing Officer
Web address: www.uchc.edu
**Control:** State–Government, nonfederal **Service:** General Medical and Surgical

**Staffed Beds:** 137 **Admissions:** 8653 **Census:** 139 **Outpatient Visits:** 271947 **Births:** 593 **Total Expense ($000):** 283069 **Payroll Expense ($000):** 95631 **Personnel:** 1329

**GREENWICH—Fairfield County**

✠ **GREENWICH HOSPITAL (70018)**, 5 Perryridge Road, Zip 06830–4697; tel. 203/863–3000 **A**1 2 3 5 9 10 **F**3 4 5 8 11 12 13 15 17 18 20 22 23 24 25 26 27 28 29 30 31 32 34 35 36 37 40 43 45 46 47 48 49 50 51 55 56 57 59 60 61 63 64 65 66 67 68 70 72 74 75 76 77 78 79 81 82 84 85 86 87 89 92 93 97 99 100 101 102 103 104 107 108 109 110 111 113 114 115 116 117 118 119 120 121 122 123 125 128 130 131 132 133 134 145 146 147 **P**6 **S** Yale New Haven Health System, New Haven, CT
Primary Contact: Frank A. Corvino, President and Chief Executive Officer
COO: Quinton J. Friesen, Executive Vice President and Chief Operating Officer
CFO: Eugene Colucci, Vice President Finance
CMO: A. Michael Marino, M.D., Senior Vice President Medical Administration
CIO: James Weeks, Chief Information Officer
Web address: www.greenhosp.org
**Control:** Other not–for–profit (including NFP Corporation) **Service:** General Medical and Surgical

**Staffed Beds:** 184 **Admissions:** 11234 **Census:** 123 **Outpatient Visits:** 413242 **Births:** 2245 **Total Expense ($000):** 296655 **Payroll Expense ($000):** 125959 **Personnel:** 1421

**HARTFORD—Hartford County**

✠ **CONNECTICUT CHILDREN'S MEDICAL CENTER (73300)**, 282 Washington Street, Zip 06106–3322; tel. 860/545–9000 **A**1 3 5 9 10 **F**3 8 11 19 21 23 25 27 29 30 31 32 34 35 36 41 44 45 46 47 48 55 57 58 59 60 61 64 65 68 72 74 75 77 78 79 81 82 85 86 87 88 89 91 92 93 94 95 96 97 107 111 113 118 119 125 128 129 130 131 133 134 137 143 145 147
Primary Contact: Martin J. Gavin, President and Chief Executive Officer
CFO: Gerald J. Boisvert, Executive Vice President and Chief Financial Officer
CMO: Paul Dworkin, M.D., Physician–in–Chief
CIO: Kelly R. Styles, Vice President and Chief Information Officer
CHR: Elizabeth Rudden, Vice President Human Resources
Web address: www.ccmckids.org
**Control:** Other not–for–profit (including NFP Corporation) **Service:** Children's general

**Staffed Beds:** 166 **Admissions:** 6096 **Census:** 104 **Outpatient Visits:** 131938 **Births:** 0 **Total Expense ($000):** 210162 **Payroll Expense ($000):** 89812 **Personnel:** 1786

✠ **HARTFORD HOSPITAL (70025)**, 80 Seymour Street, Zip 06102–5037, Mailing Address: P.O. Box 5037, Zip 06102–5037; tel. 860/545–5000, (Includes INSTITUTE OF LIVING, 400 Washington Street, Zip 06106–3392; tel. 860/545–7000) **A**1 2 3 5 8 9 10 **F**2 3 5 6 8 11 12 13 15 17 18 20 22 24 26 28 29 30 31 34 35 36 37 38 39 40 43 44 45 46 47 48 49 50 51 52 53 54 55 56 57 58 59 60 61 63 64 65 66 68 70 71 74 75 76 77 78 79 81 82 83 84 85 86 87 91 92 93 94 96 97 98 99 100 101 102 103 104 105 107 108 110 111 112 113 114 115 116 117 118 119 120 122 123 124 125 128 129 130 131 134 136 137 138 139 140 144 145 146 147 **S** Hartford Healthcare, Hartford, CT
Primary Contact: Jeffrey A. Flaks, President and Chief Executive Officer
CMO: Stuart Markowitz, M.D., Chief Medical Officer
CIO: Stephan O'Neill, Vice President Information Services
CHR: Richard McAloon, Vice President Human Resources
Web address: www.harthosp.org
**Control:** Other not–for–profit (including NFP Corporation) **Service:** General Medical and Surgical

**Staffed Beds:** 613 **Admissions:** 36841 **Census:** 587 **Outpatient Visits:** 204445 **Births:** 3760 **Total Expense ($000):** 951166 **Payroll Expense ($000):** 433339

✠ **MOUNT SINAI REHABILITATION HOSPITAL (73025)**, 490 Blue Hills Avenue, Zip 6112; tel. 860/714–3500 **A**1 10 **F**29 30 34 54 58 59 64 68 74 75 82 90 91 92 93 94 95 96 129 130 131 **P**6 8 **S** Saint Francis Care, Inc., Hartford, CT
Primary Contact: Christopher M. Dadlez, President and Chief Executive Officer
Web address: www.stfranciscare.org
**Control:** Other not–for–profit (including NFP Corporation) **Service:** Rehabilitation

**Staffed Beds:** 30 **Admissions:** 666 **Census:** 26 **Outpatient Visits:** 32304 **Births:** 0 **Total Expense ($000):** 20326 **Payroll Expense ($000):** 10665 **Personnel:** 136

✠ **SAINT FRANCIS HOSPITAL AND MEDICAL CENTER (70002)**, 114 Woodland Street, Zip 06105–1208; tel. 860/714–4000 **A**1 2 3 5 8 9 10 **F**3 8 11 12 13 15 17 18 20 22 24 26 28 29 30 31 34 35 36 38 39 40 43 46 47 48 49 50 53 54 55 56 57 58 59 61 64 65 66 68 70 72 74 75 76 77 78 79 81 82 84 85 87 92 93 94 95 96 97 98 99 100 101 102 103 104 107 111 114 116 117 118 119 120 122 123 125 128 129 130 131 133 134 143 144 145 146 147 **P**8 **S** Saint Francis Care, Inc., Hartford, CT
Primary Contact: Christopher M. Dadlez, President and Chief Executive Officer
COO: Kathleen M. Roche, R.N., Executive Vice President and Chief Operating Officer
CFO: John Giamalis, Senior Vice President and Chief Financial Officer
CMO: Rolf W. Knoll, M.D., Senior Vice President and Chief Medical Officer
CIO: Linda Shanley, Vice President and Chief Information Officer
CHR: Dawn L. Bryant, Senior Vice President and Chief Human Resource Officer
CNO: Rebecca Burke, R.N., Senior Vice President, Patient Care and Clinical Services and Chief Nursing Officer
Web address: www.saintfranciscare.com
**Control:** Church–operated, Nongovernment, not–for profit **Service:** General Medical and Surgical

**Staffed Beds:** 569 **Admissions:** 29113 **Census:** 414 **Outpatient Visits:** 297400 **Births:** 2990 **Total Expense ($000):** 631371 **Payroll Expense ($000):** 240078 **Personnel:** 4128

**MANCHESTER—Hartford County**

✠ **MANCHESTER MEMORIAL HOSPITAL (70027)**, 71 Haynes Street, Zip 06040–4188; tel. 860/646–1222 **A**1 2 5 9 10 **F**3 5 11 13 15 18 28 29 30 31 34 35 36 38 40 44 45 47 48 49 50 51 57 58 59 63 64 70 72 74 75 76 77 78 79 80 81 84 85 86 87 89 93 98 99 100 101 102 103 104 105 107 108 110 111 113 117 118 125 128 129 130 131 133 140 141 144 145 147 **P**1 5 6 **S** Eastern Connecticut Health Network, Manchester, CT
Primary Contact: Peter J. Karl, President and Chief Executive Officer
COO: Kathleen Sims, Vice President Operations
CFO: Kevin G. Murphy, Senior Vice President Finance and Chief Financial Officer
CMO: Joel R. Reich, M.D., Senior Vice President Medical Affairs
CIO: Charles Covin, Chief Information Officer
CHR: Deborah Gogliettino, Senior Vice President Human Resources
Web address: www.echn.org
**Control:** Other not–for–profit (including NFP Corporation) **Service:** General Medical and Surgical

**Staffed Beds:** 156 **Admissions:** 8079 **Census:** 110 **Outpatient Visits:** 368886 **Births:** 1222 **Total Expense ($000):** 167158 **Payroll Expense ($000):** 77582 **Personnel:** 1089

**MANSFIELD CENTER—Tolland County**

☐ **NATCHAUG HOSPITAL (74008)**, 189 Storrs Road, Zip 06250–0260; tel. 860/456–1311, (Nonreporting) **A**1 9 10 **S** Hartford Healthcare, Hartford, CT
Primary Contact: Stephen W. Larcen, Ph.D., President and Chief Executive Officer
COO: Sharon Hinton, Chief Nursing Officer
CFO: Paul V. Maloney, Chief Financial Officer
CMO: Deborah Weidner, M.D., Chief Medical Officer
CIO: Brian Jaworowski, Director Management Information Systems
CHR: Janet Keown, Director Human Resources
Web address: www.natchaug.org
**Control:** Other not–for–profit (including NFP Corporation) **Service:** Psychiatric

**Staffed Beds:** 57

CT

**MERIDEN—New Haven County**

☒ **MIDSTATE MEDICAL CENTER (70017)**, 435 Lewis Avenue, Zip 06451–2101;
tel. 203/694–8200 **A**1 2 9 10 **F**3 11 12 13 15 18 28 29 30 31 34 35 36 38
39 40 44 45 46 48 49 50 51 53 54 56 57 59 61 62 63 64 68 70 74 75 76
78 79 81 82 84 85 86 87 97 98 102 107 108 110 111 113 114 116 117
118 119 120 122 123 125 128 129 130 131 143 144 145 146 147 **P**5 7
**S** Hartford Healthcare, Hartford, CT
Primary Contact: Lucille A. Janatka, President and Chief Executive Officer
CFO: Ralph W. Becker, Chief Financial Officer
CMO: Kenneth R. Kurz, M.D., Chief of Staff
CIO: Jennifer Comerford, Manager Information Services
CHR: Ken Cesca, Vice President Human Resources
Web address: www.midstatemedical.org
**Control:** Other not–for–profit (including NFP Corporation) **Service:** General
Medical and Surgical

**Staffed Beds:** 134 **Admissions:** 9198 **Census:** 115 **Outpatient Visits:**
166901 **Births:** 1016 **Total Expense ($000):** 194874 **Payroll Expense
($000):** 73214 **Personnel:** 1080

**MIDDLETOWN—Middlesex County**

☐ **CONNECTICUT VALLEY HOSPITAL (74003)**, Eastern Drive, Zip 06457–3947,
Mailing Address: PO BOX 351, Zip 06457–7023; tel. 860/262–5000, (Includes
WHITING FORENSIC DIVISION OF CONNECTICUT VALLEY HOSPITAL, O'Brien Drive,
Zip 06457, Mailing Address: Box 70, Zip 06457–3942; tel. 203/344–2541),
(Nonreporting) **A**1 3 5 9 10 **S** Connecticut Department of Mental Health and
Addiction Services, Hartford, CT
Primary Contact: Helene M. Vartelas, Acting Chief Executive Officer
CFO: Paul Derdeyn, Director Fiscal Services and Plant Operations
CMO: Stuart Forman, M.D., Chief Professional Services
CHR: Shawn Kuhn, Facility Director Human Resources
**Control:** State–Government, nonfederal **Service:** Psychiatric

**Staffed Beds:** 537

☒ **MIDDLESEX HOSPITAL (70020)**, 28 Crescent Street, Zip 06457–3650;
tel. 860/358–6000 **A**1 2 3 5 9 10 **F**3 5 8 12 13 15 18 20 22 24 28 29 30 31
32 34 35 36 38 40 42 49 50 51 54 55 57 58 59 60 61 62 63 64 65 68 70
73 74 75 76 77 78 79 81 82 83 84 85 86 87 89 92 93 94 97 98 99 100
101 102 103 104 105 106 107 108 110 111 113 114 115 116 117 118 119
120 122 123 124 125 128 129 130 131 133 134 144 145 146 147 **P**6
Primary Contact: Vincent G. Capece, Jr., President and Chief Executive Officer
CFO: Susan Martin, Vice President Finance
CMO: Arthur V. McDowell, III, M.D., Vice President Clinical Affairs
CIO: Ludwig Johnson, Vice President Information Technology
CHR: Gregory B. Nokes, Vice President Human Resources
CNO: Jacquelyn Calamari, MSN, Vice President and Chief Nursing Officer
Web address: www.middlesexhospital.org
**Control:** Other not–for–profit (including NFP Corporation) **Service:** General
Medical and Surgical

**Staffed Beds:** 211 **Admissions:** 12762 **Census:** 156 **Outpatient Visits:**
1357744 **Births:** 1093 **Total Expense ($000):** 314945 **Payroll Expense
($000):** 155569 **Personnel:** 1837

☐ **RIVERVIEW HOSPITAL FOR CHILDREN AND YOUTH**, 915 River Road,
Zip 06457–2792, Mailing Address: P.O. Box 2792, Zip 06457–2792;
tel. 860/704–4000, (Nonreporting) **A**1 3 5
Primary Contact: Melodie J. Peet, Superintendent
CFO: Connie Tessarzik, Business Manager
CMO: Lesley Siegel, M.D., Medical Director
CIO: Andrew J A Kass, M.D., Assistant Superintendent
Web address: www.ct.gov/
**Control:** State–Government, nonfederal **Service:** Children's hospital psychiatric

**Staffed Beds:** 102

**WHITING FORENSIC DIVISION OF CONNECTICUT VALLEY HOSPITAL** See
Connecticut Valley Hospital

**MILFORD—New Haven County**

☒ **MILFORD HOSPITAL (70019)**, 300 Seaside Avenue, Zip 06460–4603;
tel. 203/876–4000, (Nonreporting) **A**1 9 10
Primary Contact: Joseph Pelaccia, President and Chief Executive Officer
COO: Lloyd Friedman, M.D., Vice President Medical Affairs and Chief Operating
Officer
CFO: Joseph Pelaccia, President and Chief Executive Officer
CMO: Lloyd Friedman, M.D., Vice President Medical Affairs and Chief Operating
Officer
CIO: Marilyn Christensen, Director Information Technology
CHR: Jeffrey Komornik, Director Human Resources
Web address: www.milfordhospital.org
**Control:** Other not–for–profit (including NFP Corporation) **Service:** General
Medical and Surgical

**Staffed Beds:** 87

**NEW BRITAIN—Hartford County**

☒ △ **HOSPITAL FOR SPECIAL CARE (72004)**, 2150 Corbin Avenue,
Zip 06053–2298; tel. 860/223–2761, (Nonreporting) **A**1 3 5 7 10
Primary Contact: David Crandall, FACHE, President and Chief Executive Officer
CFO: Laurie A. Whelan, Senior Vice President Finance and Chief Financial Officer
CMO: Paul Scalise, M.D., Chief Pulmonary Medicine and Internal Medicine
CIO: Stan Jankowski, Vice President and Chief Information Officer
CHR: Judi Trczinski, Vice President and Chief Human Resources Officer
Web address: www.hfsc.org
**Control:** Other not–for–profit (including NFP Corporation) **Service:** Long–Term
Acute Care hospital

**Staffed Beds:** 219

☒ **THE HOSPITAL OF CENTRAL CONNECTICUT (70035)**, 100 Grand Street,
Zip 06052–2017, Mailing Address: P.O. Box 100, Zip 06050–0100;
tel. 860/224–5011, (Includes BRADLEY MEMORIAL, 81 Meriden Avenue,
Southington, Zip 06489–3297; tel. 860/276–5000; NEW BRITAIN GENERAL, 100
Grand Street, Mailing Address: P.O. Box 100, Zip 06050–0100;
tel. 860/224–5011) **A**1 2 3 5 8 9 10 **F**2 3 4 11 12 13 15 17 18 20 22 27 28
29 30 31 34 35 38 40 44 45 49 50 51 52 53 54 57 58 59 60 61 62 64 65
66 68 70 72 74 75 76 77 78 79 81 84 85 86 87 89 93 97 98 99 100 101
102 103 104 105 107 108 110 111 113 114 115 116 117 118 119 120 122
123 125 128 129 130 131 134 141 142 143 145 146 147 **P**6 **S** Hartford
Healthcare, Hartford, CT
Primary Contact: Clarence J. Silvia, President and Chief Executive Officer
CFO: Brian Rogoz, Vice President Finance and Treasurer
CIO: Frank Pinto, Chief Information Officer
CHR: Elizabeth A. Lynch, Vice President Human Resources
Web address: www.thocc.org
**Control:** Other not–for–profit (including NFP Corporation) **Service:** General
Medical and Surgical

**Staffed Beds:** 249 **Admissions:** 18792 **Census:** 213 **Outpatient Visits:**
395964 **Births:** 1708 **Total Expense ($000):** 359374 **Payroll Expense
($000):** 173165 **Personnel:** 2157

**NEW CANAAN—Fairfield County**

☐ **SILVER HILL HOSPITAL (74014)**, 208 Valley Road, Zip 06840–3899;
tel. 203/966–3561, (Nonreporting) **A**1 9 10
Primary Contact: Sigurd H. Ackerman, M.D., President and Chief Executive Officer
COO: Elizabeth Moore, Chief Operating Officer
CFO: Ruurd Leegstra, Chief Financial Officer
CMO: Sigurd H. Ackerman, M.D., President and Chief Executive Officer
CIO: Maria Klinga, Director Management Information Systems
CHR: Rich Juliana, Director Human Resources
Web address: www.silverhillhospital.org
**Control:** Other not–for–profit (including NFP Corporation) **Service:** Psychiatric

**Staffed Beds:** 60

**NEW HAVEN—New Haven County**

☐ **CONNECTICUT MENTAL HEALTH CENTER (74011)**, 34 Park Street,
Zip 06508–1842, Mailing Address: P.O. Box 1842, Zip 06508–1842;
tel. 203/974–7144, (Nonreporting) **A**1 3 5 9 10 **S** Connecticut Department of
Mental Health and Addiction Services, Hartford, CT
Primary Contact: Michael Sernyak, M.D., Director
COO: Robert Cole, Chief Operating Officer
CFO: Robert Cole, Chief Operating Officer
CMO: Jeanne Steines, D.O., Medical Director
CIO: Paul Moore, Chief Information Officer
CHR: Carolyn Wallace, Director Human Resources
Web address: www.dmhas.state.ct.us/lmha.htm
**Control:** State–Government, nonfederal **Service:** Psychiatric

**Staffed Beds:** 39

☒ **HOSPITAL OF SAINT RAPHAEL (70001)**, 1450 Chapel Street,
Zip 06511–1450; tel. 203/789–3000, (Nonreporting) **A**1 2 3 5 8 9 10
Primary Contact: Christopher M. O'Connor, President and Chief Executive Officer
COO: Charles Hollander, M.D., Vice President and Chief Operating Officer
CIO: Gary Davidson, Vice President and Chief Information Officer
CHR: Elizabeth Conrad, Vice President Human Resources
Web address: www.srhs.org
**Control:** Church–operated, Nongovernment, not–for profit **Service:** General
Medical and Surgical

**Staffed Beds:** 406

✠ **YALE–NEW HAVEN HOSPITAL (70022)**, 20 York Street, Zip 06510–3202; tel. 203/688–4242, (Includes YALE–NEW HAVEN CHILDREN'S HOSPITAL, 1 Park Street, Zip 06504–8901; tel. 203/688–4242; YALE–NEW HAVEN PSYCHIATRIC HOSPITAL, 184 Liberty Street, Zip 06519–1625; tel. 203/688–9704; Paul Haeberle, Executive Director) **A**1 2 5 8 9 10 **F**3 5 6 8 11 12 13 14 15 17 18 19 20 21 22 23 24 25 26 27 28 29 30 31 32 34 35 36 37 38 39 40 41 42 43 44 45 46 47 48 49 50 51 52 54 55 56 57 58 59 61 64 65 66 68 70 71 72 73 74 75 76 77 78 79 80 81 82 84 85 86 87 88 89 91 92 93 96 97 98 99 100 101 102 103 104 105 107 108 109 110 111 112 113 114 115 116 117 118 119 120 122 123 125 128 129 130 131 132 133 134 135 136 137 138 140 141 142 143 144 145 146 147 **P**2 3 5 6 **S** Yale New Haven Health System, New Haven, CT
Primary Contact: Marna P. Borgstrom, President and Chief Executive Officer
COO: Richard D'Aquila, Executive Vice President and Chief Operating Officer
CFO: James Staten, Senior Vice President Finance
CMO: Peter N. Herbert, M.D., Senior Vice President Medical Affairs and Chief of Staff
CIO: Mark Andersen, Senior Vice President Information Systems and Chief Information Officer
CHR: Kevin A. Myatt, Senior Vice President Human Resources
Web address: www.ynhh.org
**Control:** Other not–for–profit (including NFP Corporation) **Service:** General Medical and Surgical

**Staffed Beds: 962 Admissions: 53032 Census: 752 Outpatient Visits: 634795 Births: 4419 Total Expense ($000): 1409417 Payroll Expense ($000): 537063 Personnel: 8741**

### NEW LONDON—New London County

✠ △ **LAWRENCE & MEMORIAL HOSPITAL (70007)**, 365 Montauk Avenue, Zip 06320–4769; tel. 860/442–0711, (Nonreporting) **A**1 2 3 7 9 10
Primary Contact: Bruce D. Cummings, President and Chief Executive Officer
COO: Daniel Rissi, M.D., Vice President, Chief Medical and Clinical Operations Officer
CFO: Lugene A. Inzana, Vice President and Chief Financial and Support Services Officer
CMO: Daniel Rissi, M.D., Chief Medical and Clinical Operations
CIO: Kimberly Kalajainen, Vice President and Chief Information Officer
CHR: Donna Epps, Vice President and Chief Human Resources Officer
CNO: Lauren Williams, R.N., Vice President of Professional Services and Chief Nursing Officer
Web address: www.lmhospital.org
**Control:** Other not–for–profit (including NFP Corporation) **Service:** General Medical and Surgical

**Staffed Beds: 252**

### NEW MILFORD—Litchfield County

✠ ○ **NEW MILFORD HOSPITAL (70015)**, 21 Elm Street, Zip 06776–2993; tel. 860/355–2611 **A**1 2 9 10 11 19 **F**3 8 13 14 15 17 18 28 29 30 31 32 34 35 36 38 39 40 45 46 47 48 49 50 51 53 55 56 57 58 59 61 62 63 64 65 68 70 74 75 76 77 78 79 81 82 84 85 86 87 89 99 100 101 102 107 108 109 110 111 114 115 116 118 119 120 121 122 123 128 129 131 132 133 134 144 145 146 147 **P**1 **S** Western Connecticut Healthcare, Inc., Danbury, CT
Primary Contact: John M. Murphy, M.D., Executive Director and Senior Vice President
COO: Deborah K. Weymouth, Executive Director and Senior Vice President
CFO: Steven Rosenberg, Senior Vice President, Chief Financial Officer and Treasurer
CMO: Fred Browne, M.D., Chief Medical Officer and Vice President Medical Affairs
CIO: Peter Courtway, Chief Information Officer
CHR: Phyllis Zappala, Senior Vice President Human Resources
CHR: Phyllis F. Zappala, Senior Vice President Human Resources
Web address: www.newmilfordhospital.org
**Control:** Other not–for–profit (including NFP Corporation) **Service:** General Medical and Surgical

**Staffed Beds: 62 Admissions: 2251 Census: 24 Outpatient Visits: 111624 Births: 264 Total Expense ($000): 91370 Payroll Expense ($000): 38861 Personnel: 403**

### NORWALK—Fairfield County

✠ △ **NORWALK HOSPITAL (70034)**, 34 Maple Street, Zip 06850–3894; tel. 203/852–2000 **A**1 2 3 5 7 9 10 **F**3 5 7 8 11 12 13 15 17 18 20 22 26 28 29 30 31 34 35 36 39 40 43 44 45 46 47 48 49 50 51 53 54 55 57 58 59 64 66 68 70 72 74 75 76 77 78 79 80 81 82 85 87 89 90 91 93 96 98 100 101 102 103 104 107 108 109 110 111 113 114 115 116 118 119 120 122 125 128 131 134 144 145 147 **P**6
Primary Contact: Daniel J. DeBarba, Jr., President and Chief Executive Officer
CFO: Michael Kruzick, Acting Chief Financial Officer
CMO: Michael Marks, M.D., Chief of Staff
CHR: Anthony Aceto, Vice President Human Resources
Web address: www.norwalkhospital.org
**Control:** Other not–for–profit (including NFP Corporation) **Service:** General Medical and Surgical

**Staffed Beds: 292 Admissions: 11223 Census: 182 Outpatient Visits: 159221 Births: 1629 Total Expense ($000): 297168 Payroll Expense ($000): 132292 Personnel: 1635**

### NORWICH—New London County

✠ **THE WILLIAM W. BACKUS HOSPITAL (70024)**, 326 Washington Street, Zip 06360–2733; tel. 860/889–8331 **A**1 2 9 10 **F**3 9 11 12 13 15 18 20 26 28 29 30 31 34 35 36 40 43 45 46 49 50 51 54 57 58 59 61 62 63 64 65 70 71 74 75 76 78 79 81 82 84 85 86 87 89 92 93 97 98 100 101 102 103 104 105 107 108 110 111 113 114 115 116 117 118 119 120 125 129 131 132 133 134 143 144 145 146 147 **P**6
Primary Contact: David Whitehead, President and Chief Executive Officer
CFO: Daniel E. Lohr, Senior Vice President and Chief Financial Officer
CMO: Peter H. Shea, M.D., Senior Vice President and Chief Medical Officer
CIO: Pamela M. Muccilli, Vice President and Chief Information Officer
CHR: Theresa L. Buss, Vice President, Human Resources and Organizational Development
Web address: www.backushospital.org
**Control:** Other not–for–profit (including NFP Corporation) **Service:** General Medical and Surgical

**Staffed Beds: 184 Admissions: 11050 Census: 130 Outpatient Visits: 435458 Births: 942 Total Expense ($000): 239963 Payroll Expense ($000): 110170 Personnel: 1371**

### PUTNAM—Windham County

✠ **DAY KIMBALL HOSPITAL (70003)**, 320 Pomfret Street, Zip 06260–0901, Mailing Address: P.O. Box 6001, Zip 06260–6001; tel. 860/928–6541 **A**1 9 10 **F**8 13 15 28 29 30 31 32 34 35 40 56 59 62 63 64 65 70 74 76 77 78 81 82 84 89 93 97 98 102 104 107 111 113 116 118 128 129 143 145 146 147
Primary Contact: Robert E. Smanik, FACHE, President and Chief Executive Officer
CFO: Christopher Ferraro, Chief Financial Officer
CMO: Douglas Waite, M.D., Vice President Medical Affairs
CIO: Marilyn Rath, Co–Director Management Information Systems and Chief Information Officer
CHR: Nancy Contillo, Director Human Resources
Web address: www.daykimball.org
**Control:** Other not–for–profit (including NFP Corporation) **Service:** General Medical and Surgical

**Staffed Beds: 63 Admissions: 4621 Census: 49 Outpatient Visits: 202995 Births: 547 Total Expense ($000): 104902 Payroll Expense ($000): 49631**

### ROCKY HILL—Hartford County

**VETERANS HOME AND HOSPITAL (72006)**, 287 West Street, Zip 06067–3501; tel. 860/529–2571, (Nonreporting) **A**10
Primary Contact: Margaret Concannon, Acting Administrator
CFO: Gregory J. Gioia, Chief Fiscal and Administrative Services
CMO: Michael M. Cebrik, M.D., Director Medical Staff
Web address: www.state.ct.us/ctva/
**Control:** State–Government, nonfederal **Service:** Long–Term Acute Care hospital

**Staffed Beds: 215**

### SHARON—Litchfield County

☐ **SHARON HOSPITAL (70004)**, 50 Hospital Hill Road, Zip 06069–0789, Mailing Address: P.O. Box 789, Zip 06069–0789; tel. 860/364–4000, (Nonreporting) **A**1 2 9 10 20 **S** RegionalCare Hospital Partners, Brentwood, TN
Primary Contact: Kim Lumia, Chief Executive Officer
CFO: Carolyn Allen, Chief Financial Officer
CMO: Michael Parker, M.D., Chief of Staff
CHR: Kathleen Berlinghoff, Director Human Resources
Web address: www.sharonhospital.com
**Control:** Corporation, Investor–owned, for–profit **Service:** General Medical and Surgical

**Staffed Beds: 78**

CT

## SOMERS—Tolland County

**CONNECTICUT DEPARTMENT OF CORRECTION'S HOSPITAL**, 100 Bilton Road, Zip 6071, Mailing Address: P.O. Box 100, Zip 06071–0100; tel. 860/749–8391, (Nonreporting)
Primary Contact: Edward A. Blanchette, M.D., Director
**Control:** State–Government, nonfederal **Service:** Hospital unit of an institution (prison hospital, college infimary, etc.)

**Staffed Beds:** 29

## SOUTHINGTON—Hartford County

**BRADLEY MEMORIAL** See The Hospital of Central Connecticut, New Britain

## STAFFORD SPRINGS—Tolland County

⊠ **JOHNSON MEMORIAL HOSPITAL (70008)**, 201 Chestnut Hill Road, Zip 06076–4005; tel. 860/684–4251 **A**1 9 10 **F**8 13 18 26 28 29 31 40 45 54 60 64 70 75 76 78 81 92 93 94 97 98 100 102 107 108 110 111 113 118 128 145
Primary Contact: David Morgan, Interim Chief Executive Officer
COO: David Morgan, Interim Chief Operating Officer
CFO: W. Frank Shiffer, Interim Chief Financial Officer
CIO: Andrew McFarlin, Director Information Services
CHR: Robert van Heiningen, Vice President Human Resources
Web address: www.johnsonhealthnetwork.com
**Control:** Other not–for–profit (including NFP Corporation) **Service:** General Medical and Surgical

**Staffed Beds:** 72 **Admissions:** 3035 **Census:** 41 **Outpatient Visits:** 80763 **Births:** 259 **Total Expense ($000):** 59565 **Payroll Expense ($000):** 26209 **Personnel:** 474

## STAMFORD—Fairfield County

⊠ **STAMFORD HOSPITAL (70006)**, 30 Shelburne Road, Zip 6902, Mailing Address: P.O. Box 9317, Zip 06904–9317; tel. 203/276–1000 **A**1 2 3 5 8 9 10 **F**3 8 11 12 13 15 17 18 20 22 24 26 28 29 30 31 32 34 35 36 38 40 43 44 45 46 49 50 52 53 54 55 57 58 59 60 61 64 65 66 68 70 71 72 73 74 75 76 78 79 81 82 84 85 86 87 89 90 93 96 97 98 100 101 102 103 104 107 108 110 111 113 114 117 118 119 120 122 123 125 128 129 130 131 134 143 144 145 146 147 **P**3 6
Primary Contact: Brian G. Grissler, President and Chief Executive Officer
COO: Kathleen A. Silard, R.N., Executive Vice President Operations and Chief Operating Officer
CFO: Kevin Gage, Chief Financial Officer
CMO: Sharon Kiely, M.D., Senior Vice President Medical Affairs and Chief Medical Officer
CIO: David Taylor, Vice President Information Systems and Chief Information Officer
CHR: Elaine Guglielmo, Vice President Human Resources and Organizational Development
CNO: Ellen M. Komar, R.N., Vice President Patient Care Services
Web address: www.stamhealth.org
**Control:** Other not–for–profit (including NFP Corporation) **Service:** General Medical and Surgical

**Staffed Beds:** 305 **Admissions:** 13431 **Census:** 193 **Outpatient Visits:** 385621 **Births:** 2155 **Total Expense ($000):** 414121 **Payroll Expense ($000):** 172458 **Personnel:** 1957

## TORRINGTON—Litchfield County

⊠ **THE CHARLOTTE HUNGERFORD HOSPITAL (70011)**, 540 Litchfield Street, Zip 06790–0988, Mailing Address: P.O. Box 988, Zip 06790–0988; tel. 860/496–6666 **A**1 2 9 10 **F**13 15 18 28 29 30 31 32 34 35 38 40 42 45 47 48 49 50 51 57 59 60 63 64 68 70 74 75 76 78 79 80 81 82 83 85 87 89 93 94 97 98 99 100 102 104 105 108 113 117 118 119 120 122 128 129 130 131 143 145 147 **P**6
Primary Contact: Daniel J. McIntyre, President and Chief Executive Officer
CFO: Susan Schapp, Vice President Finance and Treasurer
CMO: Mark Prete, M.D., Vice President Medical Affairs
CHR: R. James Elliott, Vice President Human Resources
Web address: www.charlottehungerford.org
**Control:** Other not–for–profit (including NFP Corporation) **Service:** General Medical and Surgical

**Staffed Beds:** 109 **Admissions:** 6145 **Census:** 73 **Outpatient Visits:** 237220 **Births:** 367 **Total Expense ($000):** 111751 **Payroll Expense ($000):** 53288 **Personnel:** 758

## VERNON ROCKVILLE—Tolland County

⊠ **ROCKVILLE GENERAL HOSPITAL (70012)**, 31 Union Street, Zip 06066–3160; tel. 860/872–0501 **A**1 9 10 **F**3 11 15 18 24 28 29 30 31 34 35 36 38 39 40 44 46 49 50 51 56 57 59 61 63 64 66 70 74 75 76 79 81 84 85 86 87 89 93 97 107 108 110 111 113 117 118 129 130 131 140 141 145 147 **P**1 5 6 **S** Eastern Connecticut Health Network, Manchester, CT
Primary Contact: Peter J. Karl, President and Chief Executive Officer
COO: Kathleen Sims, Vice President Operations
CFO: Kevin G. Murphy, Senior Vice President Finance and Chief Financial Officer
CMO: Joel R. Reich, M.D., Senior Vice President Medical Affairs
CIO: Charles Covin, Chief Information Officer
CHR: Deborah Gogliettino, Senior Vice President Human Resources
Web address: www.echn.org
**Control:** Other not–for–profit (including NFP Corporation) **Service:** General Medical and Surgical

**Staffed Beds:** 47 **Admissions:** 2461 **Census:** 34 **Outpatient Visits:** 87077 **Births:** 50 **Total Expense ($000):** 65092 **Payroll Expense ($000):** 29536 **Personnel:** 330

## WALLINGFORD—New Haven County

☐ △ **GAYLORD HOSPITAL (72003)**, Gaylord Farm Road, Zip 06492–7048, Mailing Address: P.O. Box 400, Zip 06492–0400; tel. 203/284–2800 **A**1 5 7 10 **F**1 3 29 30 34 54 56 64 75 85 91 92 93 94 96 107 118 128 129 131 134 147
Primary Contact: George M. Kyriacou, President and Chief Executive Officer
CFO: Janine L. Epright, Vice President and Chief Financial Officer
CMO: Luis Teba, M.D., Vice President and Chief Medical Officer
CIO: Brian Richard, Director Information Technology
CHR: Wally G. Harper, Vice President Human Resources
CNO: Charlotte Hyatt, MSN, Vice President Clinical Services
Web address: www.gaylord.org
**Control:** Other not–for–profit (including NFP Corporation) **Service:** Long–Term Acute Care hospital

**Staffed Beds:** 120 **Admissions:** 1383 **Census:** 110 **Outpatient Visits:** 52452 **Births:** 0 **Total Expense ($000):** 71006 **Payroll Expense ($000):** 37339 **Personnel:** 577

★ **MASONICARE HEALTH CENTER (70039)**, 22 Masonic Avenue, Zip 06492–3048, Mailing Address: P.O. Box 70, Zip 06492–7002; tel. 203/679–5900, (Nonreporting) **A**3 5 6 9 10
Primary Contact: William C. Piper, President
CFO: James F. Standish, Chief Financial Officer
CMO: Ronald Schwartz, M.D., Medical Director
CHR: Douglas T. Barrett, Senior Vice President Human Resources
Web address: www.masonicare.org
**Control:** Other not–for–profit (including NFP Corporation) **Service:** Other specialty

**Staffed Beds:** 65

## WATERBURY—New Haven County

⊠ **SAINT MARY'S HOSPITAL (70016)**, 56 Franklin Street, Zip 06706–1281; tel. 203/709–6000 **A**1 2 3 5 8 9 10 **F**3 5 8 11 12 13 15 17 18 20 22 24 28 29 30 31 32 34 35 36 37 39 40 41 43 45 49 50 53 54 57 59 64 70 72 74 75 76 77 78 79 80 81 85 87 93 96 98 100 102 104 105 107 108 110 112 113 114 117 118 125 128 129 131 134 145 146 **P**6
Primary Contact: Chad W. Wable, President and Chief Executive Officer
COO: Michael Novak, Vice President Operations
CFO: Chris Hayes, Interim Corporate Director of Finance
CMO: Steve Holland, M.D., Chief Medical Officer
CIO: Carolyn Orrell, Chief Information Officer
CHR: M. Clark Kearney, Vice President Human Resources
CNO: Elizabeth Bozzuto, R.N., Interim Chief Nursing Officer and Vice President Surgical Services
Web address: www.stmh.org
**Control:** Church–operated, Nongovernment, not–for profit **Service:** General Medical and Surgical

**Staffed Beds:** 168 **Admissions:** 12203 **Census:** 147 **Outpatient Visits:** 233213 **Births:** 1080 **Total Expense ($000):** 198097 **Payroll Expense ($000):** 77458 **Personnel:** 1154

⊠ **WATERBURY HOSPITAL (70005)**, 64 Robbins Street, Zip 06708–2600; tel. 203/573–6000, (Nonreporting) **A**1 2 3 5 9 10
Primary Contact: Darlene Stromstad, FACHE, President and Chief Executive Officer
CFO: Colleen M. Scott, Vice President Finance
CMO: David Puzzuto, M.D., Vice President Medical Affairs and Chief Medical Officer
CIO: Michael J. Cemeno, Chief Information Officer
CHR: Diane Woolley, Vice President Human Resources
CNO: Sandra Ladarola, Chief Nursing Officer
Web address: www.waterburyhospital.org
**Control:** Other not–for–profit (including NFP Corporation) **Service:** General Medical and Surgical

**Staffed Beds:** 214

## WEST HARTFORD—Hartford County

★ **THE HOSPITAL AT HEBREW HEALTH CARE (70040)**, 1 Abrahms Boulevard,
Zip 06117–1525; tel. 860/523–3800, (Nonreporting) **A**3 5 10
Primary Contact: Bonnie B. Gauthier, President and Chief Executive Officer
COO: Kathy Mon, Vice President Operations
CFO: David Houle, Executive Vice President and Chief Financial Officer
CMO: Henry Schneiderman, M.D., Vice President Medical Services and Physician
in Chief
CHR: Carmella Ross, Manager Human Resources
Web address: www.hebrewhealthcare.org
**Control:** Other not–for–profit (including NFP Corporation) **Service:** Long–Term
Acute Care hospital

| Staffed Beds: 332 |
| --- |

## WEST HAVEN—New Haven County

✶ △ **VETERANS AFFAIRS CONNECTICUT HEALTHCARE SYSTEM**, 950
Campbell Avenue, Zip 06516–2770; tel. 203/932–5711, (Includes WEST HAVEN
DIVISION, 950 Campbell Avenue, Zip 06516–2700; tel. 203/932–5711),
(Nonreporting) **A**1 2 3 5 7 8 9 **S** Department of Veterans Affairs, Washington, DC
Primary Contact: John Callahan, Acting Director
CFO: Joseph LaMadeleine, Chief Financial Officer
CMO: Michael Ebert, M.D., Chief of Staff
CIO: Joseph Erdos, M.D., Chief Information Officer
CHR: Mark Bain, Chief Human Resources
Web address: www.va.gov/sta/guide/home.asp
**Control:** Veterans Affairs, Government, federal **Service:** General Medical and
Surgical

| Staffed Beds: 160 |
| --- |

## WESTPORT—Fairfield County

**ST. VINCENT'S BEHAVIORAL HEALTH** See St. Vincent's Medical Center,
Bridgeport

## WILLIMANTIC—Windham County

**WINDHAM COMMUNITY MEMORIAL HOSPITAL** See Windham Hospital

✶ **WINDHAM HOSPITAL (70021)**, 112 Mansfield Avenue, Zip 06226–2040;
tel. 860/456–9116, (Nonreporting) **A**1 9 10 **S** Hartford Healthcare, Hartford, CT
Primary Contact: Stephen W. Larcen, Ph.D., President and Chief Executive Officer
COO: Cary Trantalis, R.N., Vice President Operations
CMO: Charles Shooks, M.D., Chief of Staff
CIO: Kevin Tupper, Director Information Technology
CHR: Marty Levine, Vice President Human Resources
CNO: Michael J. Dion, R.N., Vice President Patient Care Services
Web address: www.windhamhospital.org
**Control:** Other not–for–profit (including NFP Corporation) **Service:** General
Medical and Surgical

| Staffed Beds: 79 |
| --- |

CT

# DELAWARE

**DE**

## DOVER—Kent County

☒ △ **BAYHEALTH MEDICAL CENTER (80004)**, 640 South State Street, Zip 19901–3597; tel. 302/674–4700, (Includes BAYHEALTH MEDICAL CENTER AT KENT GENERAL, 640 South State Street; BAYHEALTH MEDICAL CENTER, MILFORD MEMORIAL HOSPITAL, 21 West Clarke Avenue, Milford, Zip 19963–1840, Mailing Address: P.O. Box 199, Zip 19963–0199; tel. 302/430–5738; Michael Ashton, Administrator) **A**1 2 7 9 10 **F**3 8 11 12 13 15 17 18 20 22 24 26 28 29 30 31 32 34 35 38 40 41 43 44 45 47 48 49 50 51 53 54 55 57 58 59 60 61 62 64 67 68 70 72 73 74 75 76 77 78 79 81 82 84 85 86 87 88 89 90 93 94 98 99 100 101 102 103 104 107 108 110 111 113 114 116 117 118 119 120 122 123 125 128 129 130 131 133 134 143 145 146 147
Primary Contact: Terry Murphy, President and Chief Executive Officer
COO: Deborah Watson, Senior Vice President and Chief Operating Officer
CFO: Earl P. Tanis, Senior Vice President Financial Operations
CMO: Gary M. Siegelman, M.D., Senior Vice President and Chief Medical Officer
CIO: Terry Feinour, Senior Vice President Corporate Services
CHR: Jon C. McDowell, Vice President Human Resources
Web address: www.bayhealth.org
**Control:** Other not–for–profit (including NFP Corporation) **Service:** General Medical and Surgical

**Staffed Beds:** 310 **Admissions:** 17524 **Census:** 248 **Outpatient Visits:** 463646 **Births:** 2322 **Total Expense ($000):** 369193 **Payroll Expense ($000):** 156981 **Personnel:** 2678

☐ **DOVER BEHAVIORAL HEALTH SYSTEM (84004)**, 725 Horsepond Road, Zip 19901; tel. 302/741–0140, (Nonreporting) **A**1 9 10 **S** Universal Health Services, Inc., King of Prussia, PA
Primary Contact: William Weaver, Chief Executive Officer
Web address: www.doverbehavioral.com
**Control:** Corporation, Investor–owned, for–profit **Service:** Psychiatric

**Staffed Beds:** 52

## LEWES—Sussex County

☒ **BEEBE MEDICAL CENTER (80007)**, 424 Savannah Road, Zip 19958–0226; tel. 302/645–3300 **A**1 2 6 9 10 19 **F**2 3 8 11 12 13 15 17 18 20 22 24 28 29 30 31 32 34 35 36 38 40 42 43 49 50 51 54 55 56 57 58 59 60 61 62 64 65 68 70 74 75 76 77 78 79 80 81 85 87 89 93 97 100 107 108 109 110 111 113 115 116 117 118 120 128 129 131 133 134 142 145 146 147
Primary Contact: Jeffrey M. Fried, FACHE, President and Chief Executive Officer
COO: Thomas Steiner, Chief Operating Officer
CFO: James W. Bartle, Vice President Finance
CMO: Andrejs Strauss, M.D., Interim Vice President Medical Affairs
CIO: Barbara P. Vugrinec, Vice President Information Systems
CHR: Catherine Halen, Vice President Human Resources
CNO: Paul E. Minnick, R.N., Vice President Patient Services
Web address: www.beebemed.org
**Control:** Other not–for–profit (including NFP Corporation) **Service:** General Medical and Surgical

**Staffed Beds:** 155 **Admissions:** 8794 **Census:** 101 **Outpatient Visits:** 466527 **Births:** 829 **Total Expense ($000):** 237911 **Payroll Expense ($000):** 86311 **Personnel:** 1594

## MILFORD—Sussex County

**BAYHEALTH MEDICAL CENTER, MILFORD MEMORIAL HOSPITAL** See Bayhealth Medical Center, Dover

## NEW CASTLE—New Castle County

☐ **DELAWARE PSYCHIATRIC CENTER (84001)**, 1901 North Dupont Highway, Zip 19720–1199; tel. 302/255–2700 **A**1 10 **F**30 34 39 58 59 65 68 75 86 87 98 100 101 103 106 129 131 134 142 145 **P**1
Primary Contact: Kevin Ann Huckshorn, R.N., MSN, Director
CIO: James Nau, Manager Computer and Applications Support
Web address: www.dhss.delaware.gov
**Control:** State–Government, nonfederal **Service:** Psychiatric

**Staffed Beds:** 189 **Admissions:** 566 **Census:** 164 **Outpatient Visits:** 0 **Births:** 0 **Total Expense ($000):** 42265 **Payroll Expense ($000):** 21010 **Personnel:** 443

☐ **MEADOW WOOD BEHAVIORAL HEALTH SYSTEM (84003)**, 575 South Dupont Highway, Zip 19720–4600; tel. 302/328–3330, (Nonreporting) **A**1 9 10 **S** Acadia Healthcare Company, Inc., Franklin, TN
Primary Contact: Bill A. Mason, Chief Executive Officer
CFO: John Greenly, Chief Financial Officer
Web address: www.meadowwoodhospital.com
**Control:** Corporation, Investor–owned, for–profit **Service:** Psychiatric

**Staffed Beds:** 53

## NEWARK—New Castle County

☒ △ **CHRISTIANA CARE HEALTH SYSTEM (80001)**, 4755 Ogletown–Stanton Road, Zip 19718–0002, Mailing Address: P.O. Box 6001, Zip 19726–6001; tel. 302/733–1000, (Includes CHRISTIANA HOSPITAL, 201 South Broom Street, Wilmington, Zip 19805, Mailing Address: P.O. Box 2653, Zip 19805; tel. 302/658–6711; WILMINGTON HOSPITAL, 501 West 14th Street, Wilmington, Zip 19801, Mailing Address: Box 1668, Zip 19899; tel. 302/733–1000) **A**1 2 3 5 7 8 9 10 12 13 **F**2 3 6 7 8 11 12 13 15 17 18 20 22 24 26 28 29 30 31 32 34 35 36 37 38 39 40 43 44 45 46 47 48 49 50 53 54 55 56 57 58 59 60 61 62 64 65 66 68 70 72 74 75 76 77 78 79 80 81 82 84 85 86 87 88 89 90 92 93 94 96 97 98 99 100 101 102 103 104 105 107 108 110 111 113 114 115 116 117 118 119 120 122 123 125 128 129 130 131 133 134 135 137 142 144 145 146 147 **P**6 **S** Christiana Care Health System, Wilmington, DE
Primary Contact: Robert J. Laskowski, M.D., President and Chief Executive Officer
COO: Gary W. Ferguson, Executive Vice President and Chief Operating Officer
CFO: Thomas L. Corrigan, Senior Vice President Finance, Managed Care and Chief Financial Officer
CMO: Janice E. Nevin, M.D., Chief Medical Officer
CIO: Randall Gaboriault, Chief Information Officer
CHR: Audrey C. Van Luven, Senior Vice President and Chief Human Resources Officer
Web address: www.christianacare.org
**Control:** Other not–for–profit (including NFP Corporation) **Service:** General Medical and Surgical

**Staffed Beds:** 988 **Admissions:** 52884 **Census:** 752 **Outpatient Visits:** 458291 **Births:** 6641 **Total Expense ($000):** 1238977 **Payroll Expense ($000):** 596451 **Personnel:** 8926

☐ **ROCKFORD CENTER (84002)**, 100 Rockford Drive, Zip 19713–2121; tel. 302/996–5480, (Nonreporting) **A**1 9 10 **S** Universal Health Services, Inc., King of Prussia, PA
Primary Contact: John F. McKenna, Chief Executive Officer and Managing Director
COO: Shawn Walsh, Chief Operating Officer
CFO: Kumar Purohit, Chief Financial Officer
CHR: Jessi Jeppi, Director Human Resources
Web address: www.rockfordcenter.com
**Control:** Corporation, Investor–owned, for–profit **Service:** Psychiatric

**Staffed Beds:** 94

## SEAFORD—Sussex County

☒ **NANTICOKE MEMORIAL HOSPITAL (80006)**, 801 Middleford Road, Zip 19973–3698; tel. 302/629–6611, (Total facility includes 110 beds in nursing home–type unit) **A**1 2 9 10 **F**3 11 13 15 17 18 20 22 28 29 30 31 32 34 35 40 43 47 48 49 50 51 57 59 65 68 70 74 75 76 77 79 81 85 86 87 89 93 107 108 109 110 111 113 114 120 122 123 127 128 129 131 134 145 146 147
Primary Contact: Steven A. Rose, R.N., Chief Executive Officer
COO: Tom Brown, Senior Vice President
CFO: Darr Hall, Chief Financial Officer
CIO: Susan Godesky, Director Information Technology
CHR: Barbara A. Hendricks, Vice President, Human Resources and Support Services
Web address: www.nanticoke.org
**Control:** Other not–for–profit (including NFP Corporation) **Service:** General Medical and Surgical

**Staffed Beds:** 249 **Admissions:** 5151 **Census:** 158 **Outpatient Visits:** 101219 **Births:** 862 **Total Expense ($000):** 112299 **Payroll Expense ($000):** 44324 **Personnel:** 773

## WILMINGTON—New Castle County

☒ △ **ALFRED I. DUPONT HOSPITAL FOR CHILDREN (83300)**, 1600 Rockland Road, Zip 19803–3616, Mailing Address: Box 269, Zip 19899–0269; tel. 302/651–4000 **A**1 3 5 7 9 10 **F**3 7 8 11 12 17 19 21 23 25 27 28 29 30 31 32 34 35 36 39 40 41 43 49 50 53 54 55 58 60 61 64 65 68 72 74 75 78 79 81 82 84 85 86 87 88 89 90 91 93 94 97 104 107 108 111 114 117 118 128 129 130 131 134 135 136 137 138 142 145 146 147
Primary Contact: Kevin B. Churchwell, M.D., Chief Executive Officer
COO: Paul D. Kempinski, Chief Operating Officer
CFO: William N. Britton, Associate Administrator Finance
CMO: Bernard J. Clark, III, M.D., Medical Director
CIO: Ann Altoe, Senior Director Information Systems and Security Officer
CHR: Terri Young, Vice President Human Resources
Web address: www.nemours.org
**Control:** Other not–for–profit (including NFP Corporation) **Service:** Children's general

**Staffed Beds:** 192 **Admissions:** 8845 **Census:** 131 **Outpatient Visits:** 179340 **Births:** 0 **Total Expense ($000):** 304204 **Payroll Expense ($000):** 104139

**CHRISTIANA HOSPITAL** See Christiana Care Health System, Newark

*Many Facility Codes have changed. Please refer to the AHA Guide Code Chart.* © 2012 AHA Guide

✠ **SELECT SPECIALTY HOSPITAL–WILMINGTON (82000)**, 7 Clayton Street, 5th Floor, Zip 19805; tel. 302/421–4545, (Nonreporting) **A**1 10 **S** Select Medical Corporation, Mechanicsburg, PA
Primary Contact: H. Frank Schneider, Chief Executive Officer
COO: Pam Lawson, Director Clinical Services
CFO: Melissa Smith, Vice President and Controller
CMO: John Chabalko, M.D., Medical Director
CHR: Shannon Oberman, Coordinator Human Resources
Web address: www.selectmedicalcorp.com
**Control:** Corporation, Investor–owned, for–profit **Service:** Long–Term Acute Care hospital

| Staffed Beds: 35 |
|---|

✠ **ST. FRANCIS HOSPITAL (80003)**, Seventh and Clayton Streets, Zip 19805–0500, Mailing Address: P.O. Box 2500, Zip 19805–0500; tel. 302/421–4100, (Nonreporting) **A**1 2 3 5 9 10 **S** Catholic Health East, Newtown Square, PA
Primary Contact: Julie A. Hester, President and Chief Executive Officer
COO: Ernest Baptiste, Executive Vice President and Chief Operating Officer
CIO: Paul W. Rowe, Director Information Technology
CHR: Charlene J. Wilson, Vice President Human Resources
Web address: www.stfrancishealthcare.org
**Control:** Other not–for–profit (including NFP Corporation) **Service:** General Medical and Surgical

| Staffed Beds: 214 |
|---|

✠ **VETERANS AFFAIRS MEDICAL CENTER**, 1601 Kirkwood Highway, Zip 19805–4989; tel. 302/994–2511, (Total facility includes 60 beds in nursing home–type unit) **A**1 2 3 5 8 9 **F**5 11 18 29 30 31 39 40 45 46 47 50 53 54 56 59 60 61 62 63 64 65 68 70 74 75 77 78 79 81 82 84 85 86 87 91 92 93 94 97 104 107 111 114 118 119 127 129 131 134 142 145 146 147 **S** Department of Veterans Affairs, Washington, DC
Primary Contact: Charles M. Dorman, FACHE, Director
CFO: Mary Ann Kozel, Chief Fiscal
CMO: Enrique Guttin, M.D., Chief of Staff
CIO: Scott Vlars, Chief Information Technology Services
CHR: Louis McCloskey, Chief Human Resources
Web address: www.va.gov/wilmington
**Control:** Veterans Affairs, Government, federal **Service:** General Medical and Surgical

| Staffed Beds: 120 **Admissions:** 1560 **Census:** 74 **Outpatient Visits:** 220946 **Births:** 0 |
|---|

**WILMINGTON HOSPITAL** See Christiana Care Health System, Newark

**DE**

---

**Hospital, Medicare Provider Number, Address, Telephone, Approval, Facility, and Physician Codes, Health Care System**

★ American Hospital Association (AHA) membership
☐ The Joint Commission accreditation
◇ DNV Healthcare Inc. accreditation
◯ American Osteopathic Association (AOA) accreditation
△ Commission on Accreditation of Rehabilitation Facilities (CARF) accreditation

# DISTRICT OF COLUMBIA

**WASHINGTON—District Of Columbia County**

☒ **CHILDREN'S NATIONAL MEDICAL CENTER (93300)**, 111 Michigan Avenue N.W., Zip 20010–2970; tel. 202/476–5000 **A**1 3 5 8 9 10 **F**3 5 7 8 11 12 14 17 18 19 20 21 22 23 25 27 28 29 30 31 32 34 35 38 39 40 41 42 43 44 48 50 54 55 57 58 59 60 61 64 65 66 68 71 72 74 75 77 78 79 81 82 83 84 85 86 87 88 89 93 97 98 99 100 101 102 104 107 108 111 112 113 118 128 129 130 131 132 133 134 135 136 141 142 143 145 147 **P**6
Primary Contact: Kurt Newman, M.D., President and Chief Executive Officer
COO: Douglas Myers, Executive Vice President, Chief Financial Officer and Interim Chief Operating Officer
CFO: Douglas Myers, Executive Vice President, Chief Financial Officer and Interim Chief Operating Officer
CMO: Mark L. Batshaw, M.D., Interim Chief Medical Officer and Chief Academic Officer
CIO: Cherie Pardue, Interim Chief Information Officer
CHR: Jack Gottschalk, Interim Vice President Human Resources
CNO: Nellie C. Robinson, R.N., Executive Vice President, Patient Services & Chief Nursing Officer
Web address: www.childrensnational.org
**Control:** Other not–for–profit (including NFP Corporation) **Service:** Children's general

> **Staffed Beds:** 283 **Admissions:** 14295 **Census:** 241 **Outpatient Visits:** 420882 **Births:** 0 **Total Expense ($000):** 610758 **Payroll Expense ($000):** 294200 **Personnel:** 5397

☒ △ **GEORGE WASHINGTON UNIVERSITY HOSPITAL (90001)**, 900 23rd Street N.W., Zip 20037–2377; tel. 202/715–4000 **A**1 2 3 5 7 8 9 10 **F**3 8 11 12 13 15 17 18 20 22 24 26 29 30 31 34 35 36 37 39 40 43 44 45 46 47 48 49 50 57 58 59 61 64 68 70 72 74 75 76 77 78 79 81 82 84 85 86 87 90 93 94 95 96 98 100 101 102 107 108 110 111 113 114 115 116 117 118 119 120 122 125 128 129 130 135 140 145 146 147 **S** Universal Health Services, Inc., King of Prussia, PA
Primary Contact: Barry A. Wolfman, Chief Executive Officer and Managing Director
COO: Kimberly Russo, Chief Operating Officer
CFO: Richard Davis, Chief Financial Officer
CMO: Gary Little, M.D., Medical Director
CIO: Louis Duhe, Senior Director Information Technology
CHR: Erin Fagan, Manager Human Resources
CNO: Jennifer Kirby, R.N., Chief Nursing Officer
Web address: www.gwhospital.com
**Control:** Partnership, Investor–owned, for–profit **Service:** General Medical and Surgical

> **Staffed Beds:** 367 **Admissions:** 18097 **Census:** 241 **Outpatient Visits:** 164282 **Births:** 1841 **Total Expense ($000):** 279993 **Payroll Expense ($000):** 121217 **Personnel:** 1671

**GEORGETOWN UNIVERSITY HOSPITAL** See Medstar Georgetown University Hospital

☒ **HOWARD UNIVERSITY HOSPITAL (90003)**, 2041 Georgia Avenue N.W., Zip 20060–0002; tel. 202/865–6100 **A**1 2 3 5 8 9 10 **F**3 6 8 11 12 13 15 17 18 24 26 28 29 30 31 32 34 35 36 38 39 40 41 43 44 45 46 50 53 54 55 56 57 58 59 60 61 64 65 66 68 70 71 72 73 74 75 76 77 78 79 81 82 84 85 86 87 89 93 97 98 99 100 101 102 103 104 107 108 110 111 113 114 117 118 122 123 128 129 130 131 133 134 142 143 145 146 147 **P**4
Primary Contact: Larry Warren, Chief Executive Officer
COO: Paul Mullings, Chief Operating Officer
CFO: John Grish, Assistant Executive Director and Chief Financial Officer
CMO: Thomas E. Gaiter, M.D., Chief Medical Officer
CIO: Bernie Galla, Interim Director Management Information Systems
CHR: Anthony Jacks, Director Human Resources
Web address: www.huhosp.org
**Control:** Other not–for–profit (including NFP Corporation) **Service:** General Medical and Surgical

> **Staffed Beds:** 266 **Admissions:** 12226 **Census:** 157 **Outpatient Visits:** 189142 **Births:** 753 **Total Expense ($000):** 383052 **Payroll Expense ($000):** 119267 **Personnel:** 2156

☒ **MEDSTAR GEORGETOWN UNIVERSITY HOSPITAL (90004)**, 3800 Reservoir Road N.W., Zip 20007–2197; tel. 202/444–2000 **A**1 2 3 5 8 9 10 **F**3 5 6 9 13 15 26 28 29 30 31 32 34 35 37 38 40 44 45 46 47 48 49 50 51 55 56 57 58 59 60 61 64 65 66 68 70 71 72 73 74 75 76 77 78 79 80 81 82 84 85 86 87 88 89 92 93 97 98 99 100 102 103 104 105 107 108 110 111 113 114 115 116 117 118 119 120 122 123 125 128 129 130 131 133 134 137 138 141 144 145 146 147 **P**6 **S** MedStar Health, Columbia, MD
Primary Contact: Richard L. Goldberg, M.D., President
COO: Michael Sachtleben, Chief Operating Officer
CFO: Paul Warda, Chief Financial Officer
CMO: Stephen Evans, M.D., Vice President Medical Affairs and Medical Director
CIO: Catherine Szenczy, Senior Vice President and Chief Information Officer
CHR: Mary Jo Schweickhardt, Vice President Human Resources
Web address: www.georgetownuniversityhospital.org
**Control:** Other not–for–profit (including NFP Corporation) **Service:** General Medical and Surgical

> **Staffed Beds:** 406 **Admissions:** 15069 **Census:** 294 **Outpatient Visits:** 670991 **Births:** 1033 **Total Expense ($000):** 728222 **Payroll Expense ($000):** 322389 **Personnel:** 4157

☒ △ **MEDSTAR NATIONAL REHABILITATION NETWORK (93025)**, 102 Irving Street N.W., Zip 20010–2949; tel. 202/877–1000, (Nonreporting) **A**1 3 5 7 9 10 **S** MedStar Health, Columbia, MD
Primary Contact: John D. Rockwood, President
CFO: Michael Boemmel, Vice President and Chief Financial Officer
CMO: Michael R. Yochelson, M.D., Vice President and Medical Director
CHR: Pamela Ashby, Vice President Human Resources
CNO: Rosemary C. Welch, R.N., Vice President and Chief Nursing Officer
Web address: www.medstarnrh.org
**Control:** Other not–for–profit (including NFP Corporation) **Service:** Rehabilitation

> **Staffed Beds:** 137

☒ **MEDSTAR WASHINGTON HOSPITAL CENTER (90011)**, 110 Irving Street N.W., Zip 20010–2975; tel. 202/877–7000 **A**1 2 3 5 8 9 10 **F**3 4 5 7 8 12 13 14 15 16 17 18 20 22 24 26 28 29 30 31 34 35 39 40 43 45 46 47 48 49 50 55 56 57 58 59 60 61 64 65 66 67 68 70 72 73 74 75 76 77 78 79 80 81 82 84 85 86 87 90 92 97 98 100 101 102 103 104 105 107 108 110 111 112 113 114 115 116 117 118 120 122 123 125 129 130 131 132 133 134 136 137 140 141 143 144 145 146 147 **P**1 6 7 **S** MedStar Health, Columbia, MD
Primary Contact: John Sullivan, President
COO: Catherine Monge, Senior Vice President Operations
CFO: Douglas A. Zehner, Senior Vice President and Chief Financial Officer
CMO: Janis M. Orlowski, M.D., Senior Vice President Medical Affairs and Chief Medical Officer
CIO: Joe Brothman, Vice President Information Systems
CHR: James P. Hill, Senior Vice President Human Resources
CNO: Susan Eckert, R.N., Senior Vice President and Chief Nursing Officer
Web address: www.whcenter.org
**Control:** Other not–for–profit (including NFP Corporation) **Service:** General Medical and Surgical

> **Staffed Beds:** 799 **Admissions:** 40192 **Census:** 614 **Outpatient Visits:** 411343 **Births:** 4079 **Total Expense ($000):** 1063416 **Payroll Expense ($000):** 498539 **Personnel:** 5626

**NATIONAL REHABILITATION HOSPITAL** See Medstar National Rehabilitation Network

☒ **PROVIDENCE HOSPITAL (90006)**, 1150 Varnum Street N.E., Zip 20017–2104; tel. 202/269–7000, (Nonreporting) **A**1 2 3 5 9 10 **S** Ascension Health, Saint Louis, MO
Primary Contact: Amy E. Freeman, President and Chief Executive Officer
CFO: Rick Talento, Senior Vice President and Chief Financial Officer
CMO: Raymond L. Cox, M.D., Chief Medical Officer
CIO: Alan Wyman, Chief Information Officer
CHR: Matt Lasecki, Interim Vice President Human Resources
CNO: Thedosia Munford, Senior Vice President and Chief Nursing Officer
Web address: www.provhosp.org
**Control:** Other not–for–profit (including NFP Corporation) **Service:** General Medical and Surgical

> **Staffed Beds:** 506

**DC**

☐ **PSYCHIATRIC INSTITUTE OF WASHINGTON (94004)**, 4228 Wisconsin Avenue N.W., Zip 20016–2138; tel. 202/885–5600 **A**1 5 9 10 **F**5 87 98 99 100 101 102 103 104 105 129 **P**6
Primary Contact: Kenneth F. Courage, Chief Executive Officer
COO: Carol Desjeunes, Chief Operating Officer
CFO: Charles J. Baumgardner, Vice President Corporate Operations
CMO: Howard Hoffman, M.D., Medical Director
CIO: Hector Benedi, Coordinator Information Systems
CHR: Randy Kellar, Director Human Resources
Web address: www.psychinstitute.com
**Control:** Corporation, Investor–owned, for–profit **Service:** Psychiatric

**Staffed Beds:** 114 **Admissions:** 3986 **Census:** 87 **Outpatient Visits:** 2510
**Births:** 0

☒ **SIBLEY MEMORIAL HOSPITAL (90005)**, 5255 Loughboro Road N.W., Zip 20016–2695; tel. 202/537–4000, (Total facility includes 45 beds in nursing home–type unit) **A**1 2 3 5 9 10 **F**3 6 8 10 12 13 14 15 17 20 22 29 30 31 34 35 40 46 47 48 51 53 55 56 57 59 60 62 64 65 68 70 73 74 75 76 77 78 79 81 82 84 85 86 87 92 93 96 98 100 102 103 105 107 108 109 110 111 113 114 116 117 118 119 120 122 123 125 127 128 129 130 131 134 140 144 145 146 147 **S** Johns Hopkins Health System, Baltimore, MD
Primary Contact: Richard O. Davis, Ph.D., President
COO: Stephen C. McDonnell, Senior Vice President, Chief Financial Officer and Chief Operating Officer
CFO: Stephen C. McDonnell, Senior Vice President, Chief Financial Officer and Chief Operating Officer
CMO: Peter E. Petrucci, M.D., Vice President Patient Safety, Quality and Medical Affairs
CIO: Kenda Tavakoli, Vice President Information Technology and Chief Information Officer
CHR: Queenie C. Plater, Vice President and Chief Human Resources Officer
Web address: www.sibley.org
**Control:** Other not–for–profit (including NFP Corporation) **Service:** General Medical and Surgical

**Staffed Beds:** 252 **Admissions:** 12470 **Census:** 170 **Outpatient Visits:** 87125 **Births:** 3521 **Total Expense ($000):** 209068 **Payroll Expense ($000):** 101748 **Personnel:** 1487

☐ **SPECIALTY HOSPITAL OF WASHINGTON (92002)**, 700 Constitution Avenue N.E., Zip 20002–6058; tel. 202/546–5700, (Nonreporting) **A**1 10 **S** Specialty Hospitals of America, LLC, Portsmouth, NH
Primary Contact: Susan P. Bailey, R.N., Chief Executive Officer
CFO: Ed Clark, Vice President Finance
CMO: Manisha Singal, M.D., Medical Director
CHR: Margaret A. Fisher, Executive Director Human Resources
Web address: www.specialtyhospitalofwashington.com
**Control:** Corporation, Investor–owned, for–profit **Service:** General Medical and Surgical

**Staffed Beds:** 177

☐ **SPECIALTY HOSPITAL OF WASHINGTON–HADLEY (92003)**, 4601 Martin Luther King Jr. Avenue, S.W., Zip 20032–1199; tel. 202/574–5700, (Nonreporting) **A**1 10 **S** Specialty Hospitals of America, LLC, Portsmouth, NH
Primary Contact: Peter Miller, FACHE, Chief Executive Officer
CFO: Ronald Davis, Chief Financial Officer
CMO: Samir Al–Khouri, M.D., Medical Director
CHR: Bing Lechoco, Director Human Resources
**Control:** Corporation, Investor–owned, for–profit **Service:** General Medical and Surgical

**Staffed Beds:** 82

★ **ST. ELIZABETHS HOSPITAL (94001)**, 1100 Alabama Avenue S.E., Zip 20032–4540; tel. 202/562–4000, (Nonreporting) **A**3 5 10
Primary Contact: Patrick J. Canavan, PsyD, Chief Executive Officer
COO: Anthea Seymour, Chief Operating Officer
CMO: Bernard Arons, M.D., Director Medical Affairs
CIO: Walter Vallierre, Chief Administrative Officer
CHR: James Gallo, Chief Human Resources Officer
Web address: www.dmh.dc.gov
**Control:** City–Government, nonfederal **Service:** Psychiatric

**Staffed Beds:** 292

☒ △ **THE HSC PEDIATRIC CENTER (93300)**, 1731 Bunker Hill Road N.E., Zip 20017–3096; tel. 202/832–4400 **A**1 7 9 10 **F**1 3 29 30 34 35 39 64 65 68 75 77 80 84 86 87 89 90 91 93 94 129 131 142 145 147 **P**6
Primary Contact: Bruce Goldman, Chief Operating Officer
COO: Bruce Goldman, Chief Operating Officer
CFO: Nancy J. Southers, Vice President and Chief Financial Officer
CMO: Michael Hauser, M.D., Chief Medical Officer
CIO: Eugene Greer, Chief Information Officer
CHR: Lynne Hostetter, Vice President Human Resources
Web address: www.hscpediatriccenter.org/
**Control:** Other not–for–profit (including NFP Corporation) **Service:** Children's chronic disease

**Staffed Beds:** 118 **Admissions:** 370 **Census:** 56 **Outpatient Visits:** 8404
**Births:** 0 **Total Expense ($000):** 39271 **Payroll Expense ($000):** 16526
**Personnel:** 336

☐ **UNITED MEDICAL CENTER (90008)**, 1310 Southern Avenue S.E., Zip 20032–4699; tel. 202/574–6000, (Total facility includes 120 beds in nursing home–type unit) **A**1 9 10 **F**3 13 15 18 29 30 35 40 41 45 46 50 60 61 64 65 70 74 75 76 77 79 81 85 87 93 94 96 97 98 100 102 107 108 111 113 118 129 145 146 147
Primary Contact: Frank G. DeLisi, III, Chief Executive Officer
CFO: Ronald P. Walker, Interim Chief Financial Officer
CMO: Cyril Allen, M.D., Chief Medical Officer
CIO: Janice Akintewe, Director Information Technology
CHR: Jackie Johnson, Vice President Human Resources
CNO: Jean C. Phaire, Executive Vice President Patient Care Services and Chief Nursing Executive
Web address: www.united–medicalcenter.com
**Control:** State–Government, nonfederal **Service:** General Medical and Surgical

**Staffed Beds:** 354 **Admissions:** 5207 **Census:** 166 **Outpatient Visits:** 67950
**Births:** 510 **Total Expense ($000):** 77389 **Payroll Expense ($000):** 50049
**Personnel:** 691

☒ △ **VETERANS AFFAIRS MEDICAL CENTER**, 50 Irving Street N.W., Zip 20422–0002; tel. 202/745–8100, (Nonreporting) **A**1 2 3 5 7 8 9 **S** Department of Veterans Affairs, Washington, DC
Primary Contact: Brian A. Hawkins, Director Medical Center
CFO: Frank Filosa, Fiscal Manager
CIO: Amanda Graves, Chief Information Systems
Web address: www.washingtondc.va.gov/
**Control:** Veterans Affairs, Government, federal **Service:** General Medical and Surgical

**Staffed Beds:** 291

**WASHINGTON HOSPITAL CENTER** See Medstar Washington Hospital Center

**DC**

---

**Hospital, Medicare Provider Number, Address, Telephone, Approval, Facility, and Physician Codes, Health Care System**

★ American Hospital Association (AHA) membership
☐ The Joint Commission accreditation
◇ DNV Healthcare Inc. accreditation
○ American Osteopathic Association (AOA) accreditation
△ Commission on Accreditation of Rehabilitation Facilities (CARF) accreditation

# FLORIDA

## ALTAMONTE SPRINGS—Seminole County

**FLORIDA HOSPITAL–ALTAMONTE** See Florida Hospital, Orlando

## APALACHICOLA—Franklin County

**GEORGE E. WEEMS MEMORIAL HOSPITAL (101305)**, 135 Avenue G.,
Zip 32320–1613, Mailing Address: P.O. Box 580, Zip 32329–0580;
tel. 850/653–8853, (Nonreporting) **A**9 10 18
Primary Contact: Cindy Drapal, Interim Chief Executive Officer
CFO: James Robinson, Chief Financial Officer
CIO: Dennis Peterson, Chief Information Officer
CHR: Ginny Grimer, Director Human Resources
CNO: Cindy Drapal, Chief Nursing Officer
Web address: www.weemsmemorial.com
**Control:** Partnership, Investor–owned, for–profit **Service:** General Medical and
Surgical

**Staffed Beds:** 25

## APOPKA—Orange County

**FLORIDA HOSPITAL–APOPKA** See Florida Hospital, Orlando

## ARCADIA—Desoto County

☐ **DESOTO MEMORIAL HOSPITAL (100175)**, 900 North Robert Avenue,
Zip 34266–8765, Mailing Address: P.O. Box 2180, Zip 34265–2180;
tel. 863/494–3535, (Nonreporting) **A**1 9 10 20
Primary Contact: Vincent A. Sica, President and Chief Executive Officer
CFO: Joe Amato, Interim Chief Financial Officer
CMO: Kayum Mohammadbhoy, M.D., Chief of Staff
CIO: Annie Curnow, Coordinator Medical Staff and Public Relations
CHR: Lois Hilton, Director Human Resources
Web address: www.dmh.org
**Control:** Other not–for–profit (including NFP Corporation) **Service:** General
Medical and Surgical

**Staffed Beds:** 49

## ATLANTIS—Palm Beach County

☒ **J. F. K. MEDICAL CENTER (100080)**, 5301 South Congress Avenue,
Zip 33462–1197; tel. 561/965–7300, (Nonreporting) **A**1 2 3 5 9 10 **S** HCA,
Nashville, TN
Primary Contact: Gina Melby, Chief Executive Officer
COO: Robbin M. Lee, Chief Operating Officer
CFO: Jim Leamon, Chief Financial Officer
CMO: Charles Posternack, M.D., Chief Medical Officer
CIO: Jane Stewart, Director Information Services
CHR: Trudy Bromley, Vice President Human Resources
Web address: www.jfkmc.com
**Control:** Corporation, Investor–owned, for–profit **Service:** General Medical and
Surgical

**Staffed Beds:** 424

## AVENTURA—Miami–Dade County

☒ **AVENTURA HOSPITAL AND MEDICAL CENTER (100131)**, 20900 Biscayne
Boulevard, Zip 33180–1407; tel. 305/682–7000, (Nonreporting) **A**1 2 10 **S** HCA,
Nashville, TN
Primary Contact: Heather J. Rohan, Chief Executive Officer
CFO: Alisa Bert, Chief Financial Officer
CMO: Charles Shenker, M.D., Chief of Staff
Web address: www.aventurahospital.com
**Control:** Corporation, Investor–owned, for–profit **Service:** General Medical and
Surgical

**Staffed Beds:** 359

## BARTOW—Polk County

☐ **BARTOW REGIONAL MEDICAL CENTER (100121)**, 2200 Osprey Boulevard,
Zip 33830–3308, Mailing Address: P.O. Box 1050, Zip 33831–1050;
tel. 863/533–8111, (Nonreporting) **A**1 9 10 **S** Health Management Associates,
Naples, FL
Primary Contact: Troy DeDecker, Chief Executive Officer
CFO: Brandon May, Chief Financial Officer
CMO: Stuart Patterson, M.D., Chief of Staff
CIO: Vilakon Champavannarath, Director Information Systems
CHR: Marie Horton, Director Associate Relations
Web address: www.bartowregional.com
**Control:** Corporation, Investor–owned, for–profit **Service:** General Medical and
Surgical

**Staffed Beds:** 72

## BAY PINES—Pinellas County

☒ △ **VETERANS AFFAIRS MEDICAL CENTER**, 10000 Bay Pines Boulevard,
Zip 33744, Mailing Address: P.O. Box 5005, Zip 33744–5005;
tel. 727/398–6661, (Nonreporting) **A**1 2 3 5 7 **S** Department of Veterans Affairs,
Washington, DC
Primary Contact: Suzanne M. Klinker, Director
COO: Kris Brown, Associate Director
CFO: Jeanine Ergle, Chief Financial Officer
CMO: George F. Van Buskirk, M.D., Chief of Staff
CIO: John Williams, Chief Information Officer
CHR: Paula Buchele, Chief Human Resources
Web address: www.baypines.va.gov/
**Control:** Veterans Affairs, Government, federal **Service:** General Medical and
Surgical

**Staffed Beds:** 291

## BELLE GLADE—Palm Beach County

**GLADES GENERAL HOSPITAL** See Lakeside Medical Center

☒ **LAKESIDE MEDICAL CENTER (100130)**, 39200 Hooker Highway,
Zip 33430–4911; tel. 561/996–6571 **A**1 9 10 **F**3 11 13 15 18 29 30 34 35
40 45 46 50 54 59 68 70 76 81 85 87 89 93 97 107 108 110 111 113 118
129 131 134 147
Primary Contact: Nancy L. O'Neal, Interim Administrator
COO: Nancy L. O'Neal, Director Operations
CFO: Larry Singleton, Chief Financial Officer
CMO: Ron Wiewora, M.D., Chief Medical Officer
CIO: Adam Levenson, Manager Information Systems
CHR: Matthew Morgan, Manager Human Resources
Web address: www.lakesidemedical.org
**Control:** Hospital district or authority, Government, nonfederal **Service:** General
Medical and Surgical

**Staffed Beds:** 70 **Admissions:** 6480 **Census:** 30 **Outpatient Visits:** 35939
**Births:** 616 **Total Expense ($000):** 27715 **Payroll Expense ($000):** 16772
**Personnel:** 270

## BLOUNTSTOWN—Calhoun County

★ **CALHOUN–LIBERTY HOSPITAL (101304)**, 20370 N.E. Burns Avenue,
Zip 32424–1097, Mailing Address: P.O. Box 419, Zip 32424–0419;
tel. 850/674–5411 **A**9 10 18 **F**3 7 34 40 45 50 54 57 59 66 107 110 113
118 132 134
Primary Contact: Phillip Hill, Interim Chief Executive Officer
CFO: Nathan Ebersole, Controller
CIO: Michael Flowers, Director Information Management
CHR: Lynn Pitts, Director Human Resources
Web address: www.calhoun–libertyhospital.com
**Control:** Other not–for–profit (including NFP Corporation) **Service:** General
Medical and Surgical

**Staffed Beds:** 25 **Admissions:** 632 **Census:** 14 **Outpatient Visits:** 20671
**Births:** 0 **Total Expense ($000):** 8173 **Payroll Expense ($000):** 4082
**Personnel:** 101

## BOCA RATON—Palm Beach County

**BOCA RATON COMMUNITY HOSPITAL** See Boca Raton Regional Hospital

☐ **BOCA RATON REGIONAL HOSPITAL (100168)**, 800 Meadows Road,
Zip 33486–2368; tel. 561/955–7100 **A**1 2 9 10 **F**3 8 11 13 15 17 18 20 22
24 26 28 29 30 31 34 35 40 44 45 46 47 48 49 50 51 53 54 55 56 57 58
59 60 62 64 68 70 71 72 74 75 76 77 78 79 81 82 84 85 86 87 91 92 93
94 96 97 100 102 103 107 108 110 111 113 114 115 116 117 118 119
120 122 123 125 129 130 131 134 143 144 145 146 147
Primary Contact: Jerry J. Fedele, President and Chief Executive Officer
COO: Karen Poole, Chief Operating Officer
CFO: Richard Jones, Vice President and Chief Financial Officer
CMO: M. Joseph Grennan, Jr., M.D., Vice President Medical Affairs
CIO: Robin Hildwein, Chief Information Officer
CHR: Mindy Raymond, Vice President Human Resources
Web address: www.brrh.com
**Control:** Other not–for–profit (including NFP Corporation) **Service:** General
Medical and Surgical

**Staffed Beds:** 394 **Admissions:** 16410 **Census:** 219 **Outpatient Visits:**
277652 **Births:** 1694 **Total Expense ($000):** 332951 **Payroll Expense
($000):** 120593 **Personnel:** 1883

*Many Facility Codes have changed. Please refer to the AHA Guide Code Chart.* © 2012 AHA Guide

☒ **WEST BOCA MEDICAL CENTER (100268)**, 21644 State Road 7, Zip 33428–1899; tel. 561/488–8000, (Nonreporting) **A**1 9 10 **S** TENET Healthcare Corporation, Dallas, TX
Primary Contact: Mitchell S. Feldman, Chief Executive Officer
COO: Laura A. Cillo, Chief Operating Officer
CFO: Brook Thomas, Chief Financial Officer
CMO: Jack L. Harari, M.D., Chief Medical Officer
CIO: Linda–Jean Long, Marketing Director
CHR: Stephanie Sherman, Chief Human Resources Officer
CNO: Ruth Schwarzkopf, R.N., Chief Nursing Officer
Web address: www.westbocamedctr.com
**Control:** Corporation, Investor–owned, for–profit **Service:** Other specialty

| Staffed Beds: 185 |
|---|

### BONIFAY—Holmes County

☐ **DOCTORS MEMORIAL HOSPITAL (101307)**, 2600 Hospital Drive, Zip 32425–3007, Mailing Address: P.O. Box 188, Zip 32425–0188; tel. 850/547–8000 **A**1 9 10 18 **F**3 11 15 29 30 40 45 57 59 64 70 77 81 90 93 107 110 113 118 130 132 145 147
Primary Contact: Joann Baker, Administrator
CFO: Haley Green, Chief Financial Officer
CMO: Leisa Bailey, M.D., Chief of Staff
CIO: Scott Scurlock, Chief Information Officer
CHR: Christy Booth, Chief Human Resources Officer
Web address: www.doctorsmemorialhospital.com
**Control:** Hospital district or authority, Government, nonfederal **Service:** General Medical and Surgical

| Staffed Beds: 20 Admissions: 1163 Census: 13 Outpatient Visits: 17002 Births: 0 Total Expense ($000): 11080 Payroll Expense ($000): 4918 Personnel: 137 |
|---|

### BOYNTON BEACH—Palm Beach County

☐ **BETHESDA MEMORIAL HOSPITAL (100002)**, 2815 South Seacrest Boulevard, Zip 33435–7995; tel. 561/737–7733 **A**1 2 9 10 **F**3 8 12 13 15 17 18 20 22 24 26 28 29 30 31 34 35 40 45 46 49 50 51 56 58 60 61 64 68 70 72 74 75 76 77 78 79 81 86 87 88 89 90 93 94 96 107 110 111 113 114 118 119 120 122 123 125 128 129 130 131 132 142 145 147
Primary Contact: Roger L. Kirk, President and Chief Executive Officer
CFO: Joanne Aquilina, Vice President Finance and Chief Financial Officer
CMO: Albert Biehl, M.D., Vice President Medical Affairs
CIO: Leslie Durham, Vice President Information Systems
CHR: Regina Crafa, Vice President Human Resources
Web address: www.bethesdaweb.com
**Control:** Other not–for–profit (including NFP Corporation) **Service:** General Medical and Surgical

| Staffed Beds: 401 Admissions: 20585 Census: 297 Outpatient Visits: 240631 Births: 2817 Total Expense ($000): 239882 Payroll Expense ($000): 91838 Personnel: 1570 |
|---|

### BRADENTON—Manatee County

☒ △ **BLAKE MEDICAL CENTER (100213)**, 2020 59th Street West, Zip 34209–4669; tel. 941/792–6611 **A**1 2 7 9 10 **F**3 8 11 15 17 18 20 22 24 26 28 29 30 31 34 35 37 40 45 46 48 49 56 57 59 64 70 74 75 77 78 79 80 81 82 85 86 87 90 92 93 96 97 102 107 108 110 111 113 114 117 118 123 128 129 130 131 134 144 145 **S** HCA, Nashville, TN
Primary Contact: Daniel J. Friedrich, III, Chief Executive Officer
COO: Justin Doss, Chief Operating Officer
CFO: Priscilla Parrish, Chief Financial Officer
CMO: Lawrence Lieberman, M.D., Medical Director
CIO: Shannon Piatkowski, Director Information Technology
CHR: Veronica Lequeux, Vice President Human Resources
Web address: www.blakemedicalcenter.com
**Control:** Corporation, Investor–owned, for–profit **Service:** General Medical and Surgical

| Staffed Beds: 294 Admissions: 13212 Census: 173 Outpatient Visits: 67649 Births: 0 Total Expense ($000): 130370 Payroll Expense ($000): 52102 Personnel: 860 |
|---|

☐ **LAKEWOOD RANCH MEDICAL CENTER (100299)**, 8330 Lakewood Ranch Boulevard, Zip 34202; tel. 941/782–2100, (Nonreporting) **A**1 9 10 **S** Universal Health Services, Inc., King of Prussia, PA
Primary Contact: James D. Wilson, Chief Executive Officer
COO: Linda S. Widra, FACHE, Chief Operating Officer
CFO: Gerald Christine, Chief Financial Officer
CHR: Trish Morales, Director Human Resources
Web address: www.lakewoodranchmedicalcenter.com
**Control:** Corporation, Investor–owned, for–profit **Service:** General Medical and Surgical

| Staffed Beds: 120 |
|---|

**MANATEE GLENS HOSPITAL AND ADDICTION CENTER (104040)**, 2020 26th Avenue East, Zip 34208, Mailing Address: P.O. Box 9478, Zip 34206–9478; tel. 941/782–4600, (Nonreporting) **A**9 10
Primary Contact: Mary Ruiz, Chief Executive Officer
COO: Deborah Kostroun, Chief Operating Officer
CFO: Don Biles, Chief Financial Officer
CMO: Jose Zaglul, M.D., Chief Medical Officer
CIO: Chris Mitchell, Director Information Systems
CHR: Chris McKenna, Director Human Resources
Web address: www.manateeglens.org
**Control:** Individual, Investor–owned, for–profit **Service:** Psychiatric

| Staffed Beds: 27 |
|---|

☐ **MANATEE MEMORIAL HOSPITAL (100035)**, 206 Second Street East, Zip 34208–1000; tel. 941/746–5111, (Nonreporting) **A**1 2 5 9 10 **S** Universal Health Services, Inc., King of Prussia, PA
Primary Contact: Kevin DiLallo, Chief Executive Officer
COO: Richard Fletcher, Chief Operating Officer
CFO: Mark A. Tierney, Chief Financial Officer
CMO: Waguih El Masry, M.D., Chief of Staff
CIO: Troy Beaubien, Director Information Services
CHR: Sheree Threewits, Director Human Resources
CNO: Darlette Tice, Chief Nursing Officer
Web address: www.manateememorial.com
**Control:** Corporation, Investor–owned, for–profit **Service:** General Medical and Surgical

| Staffed Beds: 319 |
|---|

**MANATEE PALMS YOUTH SERVICES**, 4480 51st Street West, Zip 34210; tel. 941/792–2222 **F**98 99 106 **S** Universal Health Services, Inc., King of Prussia, PA
Primary Contact: George Shopland, Chief Executive Officer
CFO: Linda Weymouth, Chief Financial Officer
CMO: Jaime Barker, M.D., Medical Director
Web address: www.mpys.com
**Control:** Corporation, Investor–owned, for–profit **Service:** Children's hospital psychiatric

| Staffed Beds: 60 Admissions: 157 Census: 57 Outpatient Visits: 0 Births: 0 Total Expense ($000): 7337 Payroll Expense ($000): 4406 Personnel: 146 |
|---|

### BRANDON—Hillsborough County

☒ **BRANDON REGIONAL HOSPITAL (100243)**, 119 Oakfield Drive, Zip 33511–5799; tel. 813/681–5551 **A**1 5 9 10 **F**3 11 12 13 15 17 18 20 22 24 26 28 29 31 40 41 45 46 47 48 49 51 57 59 60 64 68 70 72 73 74 75 76 77 78 79 81 82 85 89 97 98 100 102 103 107 108 111 113 117 118 125 131 145 146 147 **S** HCA, Nashville, TN
Primary Contact: Bland Eng, Chief Executive Officer
COO: Janice Balzano, Chief Operating Officer
COO: Alicia Schulhof, Chief Operating Officer
CFO: Michael T. Terrell, Chief Financial Officer
CMO: Craig Smestad, M.D., Chief Medical Officer
CIO: Shannon Piatkowski, Chief Information Officer
CHR: Patrick Kerrwood, Vice President Human Resources
CNO: Susan Laber, R.N., Chief Nursing Officer
Web address: www.brandonhospital.com
**Control:** Corporation, Investor–owned, for–profit **Service:** General Medical and Surgical

| Staffed Beds: 359 Admissions: 21774 Census: 235 Outpatient Visits: 117928 Births: 3240 Total Expense ($000): 204229 Payroll Expense ($000): 86085 Personnel: 1064 |
|---|

### BROOKSVILLE—Hernando County

☐ **BROOKSVILLE REGIONAL HOSPITAL (100071)**, 17240 Cortez Boulevard, Zip 34601, Mailing Address: P.O. Box 37, Zip 34605–0037; tel. 352/796–5111, (Nonreporting) **A**1 9 10 **S** Health Management Associates, Naples, FL
Primary Contact: Kenneth R. Wicker, Chief Executive Officer
COO: Scott Hartsell, Chief Operating Officer
CFO: Matthew Seagroves, Chief Financial Officer
CMO: Mohammad A. Joud, M.D., Chief of Staff
CIO: Lee Burch, Director Management Information Systems
CHR: Claudia L. Jack, Director Associate Relations
Web address: www.brooksvilleregionalhospital.org
**Control:** Corporation, Investor–owned, for–profit **Service:** General Medical and Surgical

| Staffed Beds: 91 |
|---|

---

**Hospital, Medicare Provider Number, Address, Telephone, Approval, Facility, and Physician Codes, Health Care System**

★ American Hospital Association (AHA) membership
☐ The Joint Commission accreditation
◇ DNV Healthcare Inc. accreditation
○ American Osteopathic Association (AOA) accreditation
△ Commission on Accreditation of Rehabilitation Facilities (CARF) accreditation

⊞ **HEALTHSOUTH REHABILITATION HOSPITAL OF SPRING HILL (103042)**, 12440 Cortez Boulevard, Zip 34613–2628; tel. 352/592–4250, (Nonreporting) **A**1 9 10 **S** HEALTHSOUTH Corporation, Birmingham, AL
Primary Contact: Lori Bedard, Chief Executive Officer
CFO: Debbie Punzirudu, Controller
CMO: Charles Dempsey, M.D., Medical Director
CIO: Myra Merillo, Supervisor Health Information Management
CHR: Ava McLellan, Coordinator Human Resources
Web address: www.healthsouthspringhill.com
**Control:** Corporation, Investor–owned, for–profit **Service:** Rehabilitation

**Staffed Beds:** 80

⊞ **OAK HILL HOSPITAL (100264)**, 11375 Cortez Boulevard, Zip 34613; tel. 352/596–6632, (Nonreporting) **A**1 2 9 10 **S** HCA, Nashville, TN
Primary Contact: Mickey Smith, Chief Executive Officer
COO: Sonia I. Gonzalez, R.N., Chief Operating Officer
CFO: Chance Phillips, Chief Financial Officer
CMO: Ganesh Chari, M.D., Chief of Staff
CIO: Cindy Peters, Chief Information Officer
CHR: Charles Snider, Vice President Human Resources
CNO: Melissa Bennett, R.N., Chief Nursing Officer
Web address: www.oakhillhospital.com
**Control:** Corporation, Investor–owned, for–profit **Service:** General Medical and Surgical

**Staffed Beds:** 214

☐ **SPRINGBROOK HOSPITAL (104057)**, 7007 Grove Road, Zip 34609–8610; tel. 352/596–4306, (Nonreporting) **A**1 9 10
Primary Contact: James E. O'Shea, Administrator
Web address: www.springbrookhospital.org/
**Control:** Other not–for–profit (including NFP Corporation) **Service:** Psychiatric

**Staffed Beds:** 50

**CAPE CORAL—Lee County**

★ **CAPE CORAL HOSPITAL (100244)**, 636 Del Prado Boulevard, Zip 33990–2695; tel. 239/424–2000 **A**9 10 21 **F**3 11 13 14 15 17 18 20 22 28 29 30 31 34 40 45 46 48 50 51 52 53 57 59 60 65 68 70 74 75 76 79 81 82 84 85 86 87 89 93 94 97 107 111 118 128 129 131 134 145 146 147 **S** Lee Memorial Health System, Fort Myers, FL
Primary Contact: James R. Nathan, President
COO: Lawrence Antonucci, M.D., Chief Operating Officer
CFO: Mike German, Chief Financial Officer
CMO: Mark Greenberg, M.D., Chief Medical Officer
CIO: Mike Smith, Chief Information Officer
CHR: Jon C. Cecil, Chief Human Resource Officer
Web address: www.leememorial.org
**Control:** Hospital district or authority, Government, nonfederal **Service:** General Medical and Surgical

**Staffed Beds:** 291 **Admissions:** 14886 **Census:** 180 **Outpatient Visits:** 220394 **Births:** 1368

**CELEBRATION—Osceola County**

**FLORIDA HOSPITAL CELEBRATION HEALTH** See Florida Hospital, Orlando

**CHATTAHOOCHEE—Gadsden County**

△ **FLORIDA STATE HOSPITAL (104000)**, U.S. Highway 90 East, Zip 32324–1000, Mailing Address: P.O. Box 1000, Zip 32324–1000; tel. 850/663–7536, (Nonreporting) **A**7 10
Primary Contact: Diane R. James, Administrator
CFO: Denise Smith, Director Financial Services
Web address: www.dcf.state.fl.us/institutions/fsh
**Control:** State–Government, nonfederal **Service:** Psychiatric

**Staffed Beds:** 987

**CHIPLEY—Washington County**

☐ **NORTHWEST FLORIDA COMMUNITY HOSPITAL (101308)**, 1360 Brickyard Road, Zip 32428–6303, Mailing Address: P.O. Box 889, Zip 32428–0889; tel. 850/638–1610, (Nonreporting) **A**1 9 10 18
Primary Contact: Patrick A. Schlenker, FACHE, President and Chief Executive Officer
COO: Janet Kinney, Chief Operating Officer
CFO: Marcey Black, Chief Financial Officer
CHR: Sue Byrd, Coordinator Human Resources
CNO: Joan Beard, Chief Nursing Officer
Web address: www.nfch.org
**Control:** Individual, Investor–owned, for–profit **Service:** General Medical and Surgical

**Staffed Beds:** 59

**CLEARWATER—Pinellas County**

⊞ **MORTON PLANT HOSPITAL (100127)**, 300 Pinellas Street, Zip 33756–3825, Mailing Address: P.O. Box 210, Zip 33757–0210; tel. 727/462–7000, (Nonreporting) **A**1 2 3 5 9 10 **S** Morton Plant Mease Health Care, Clearwater, FL
Primary Contact: Glenn D. Waters, FACHE, President
COO: N. Kristopher Hoce, Chief Operating Officer
CFO: Carl Tremonti, Chief Financial Officer
CMO: Donald Pocock, M.D., Chief Medical Officer
CHR: Sharon Collotta, Director Human Resources
CNO: Lisa Johnson, R.N., Chief Nursing Executive
Web address: www.mortonplant.com
**Control:** Other not–for–profit (including NFP Corporation) **Service:** General Medical and Surgical

**Staffed Beds:** 524

☐ **WINDMOOR HEALTHCARE OF CLEARWATER (104017)**, 11300 U.S. 19 North, Zip 33764; tel. 727/541–2646 **A**1 9 10 **F**4 5 29 34 35 38 75 98 100 101 102 103 105 129 131 142 **S** Universal Health Services, Inc., King of Prussia, PA
Primary Contact: Wendy Merson, Chief Executive Officer
Web address: www.windmoor–healthcare.com
**Control:** Corporation, Investor–owned, for–profit **Service:** Psychiatric

**Staffed Beds:** 120 **Admissions:** 2759 **Census:** 86 **Outpatient Visits:** 8040 **Births:** 0 **Total Expense ($000):** 14993 **Payroll Expense ($000):** 9092 **Personnel:** 178

**CLERMONT—Lake County**

☐ **SOUTH LAKE HOSPITAL (100051)**, 1900 Don Wickham Drive, Zip 34711–2787; tel. 352/394–4071 **A**1 9 10 **F**3 8 11 13 15 18 19 20 22 26 29 30 31 32 34 35 40 42 43 45 46 49 50 51 53 54 57 59 60 62 64 66 68 70 74 75 76 78 79 81 82 85 86 87 89 93 107 108 110 111 113 114 116 118 123 130 131 134 145 146 147 **P**6 **S** Orlando Health, Orlando, FL
Primary Contact: John Moore, Chief Executive Officer
CFO: Lance Sewell, Chief Financial Officer
CMO: Michael Goler, M.D., Chief Medical Officer
CHR: Sue Brown, Administrator Human Resources
Web address: www.southlakehospital.com
**Control:** Hospital district or authority, Government, nonfederal **Service:** General Medical and Surgical

**Staffed Beds:** 122 **Admissions:** 7122 **Census:** 86 **Outpatient Visits:** 83504 **Births:** 748 **Total Expense ($000):** 118270 **Payroll Expense ($000):** 46672 **Personnel:** 922

**CLEWISTON—Hendry County**

⊞ **HENDRY REGIONAL MEDICAL CENTER (101309)**, 524 West Sagamore Avenue, Zip 33440–3094; tel. 863/983–9121 **A**1 9 10 18 **F**3 11 15 18 29 34 35 40 45 50 57 59 64 65 68 70 71 75 77 81 82 85 93 97 107 110 111 113 118 126 128 132 134 145 147 **P**6 **S** QHR, Brentwood, TN
Primary Contact: Lynn W. Beasley, FACHE, Chief Executive Officer
CFO: William F. Stoltzfus, Interim Chief Financial Officer
CMO: Karim Kaki, M.D., Chief Medical Director
CIO: Leon Hoover, Director Information Systems
CHR: Lisa Miller, Director Human Resources
Web address: www.hendryregional.org
**Control:** Hospital district or authority, Government, nonfederal **Service:** General Medical and Surgical

**Staffed Beds:** 25 **Admissions:** 956 **Census:** 9 **Outpatient Visits:** 34397 **Births:** 0 **Total Expense ($000):** 17532 **Payroll Expense ($000):** 11602 **Personnel:** 199

**COCOA BEACH—Brevard County**

⊞ **CAPE CANAVERAL HOSPITAL (100177)**, 701 West Cocoa Beach Causeway, Zip 32931–5595, Mailing Address: P.O. Box 320069, Zip 32932–0069; tel. 321/799–7111 **A**1 2 9 10 **F**3 11 13 15 18 20 22 26 29 30 31 34 35 40 43 44 45 46 47 48 49 51 54 56 57 59 60 62 64 65 68 70 74 75 76 78 79 81 82 85 86 87 91 92 93 103 107 108 110 111 113 114 115 116 118 123 128 129 131 142 145 146 **P**6 7 **S** Health First, Inc., Rockledge, FL
Primary Contact: Roy Wright, FACHE, President and Chief Executive Officer
CFO: Robert Galloway, Senior Vice President Finance and Chief Financial Officer
CMO: Rodney Moore, M.D., Vice President Medical Affairs
CIO: Rich Rogers, Senior Vice President Support Services and Chief Information Officer
CHR: Robert W. Suttles, Vice President Human Resources
Web address: www.health–first.org
**Control:** Other not–for–profit (including NFP Corporation) **Service:** General Medical and Surgical

**Staffed Beds:** 145 **Admissions:** 6008 **Census:** 76 **Outpatient Visits:** 107327 **Births:** 638 **Total Expense ($000):** 104717 **Payroll Expense ($000):** 48318 **Personnel:** 548

FL

## COOPER CITY—Broward County

**FOCUS HEALTHCARE OF FLORIDA**, 5960 S.W. 106th Avenue, Zip 33328; tel. 954/680–2700, (Nonreporting)
Primary Contact: Manuel R. Llano, Chief Executive Officer
**Control:** Corporation, Investor–owned, for–profit **Service:** Alcoholism and other chemical dependency

**Staffed Beds:** 38

## CORAL GABLES—Miami–Dade County

✠ **BAPTIST HEALTH SOUTH FLORIDA, DOCTORS HOSPITAL (100296)**, 5000 University Drive, Zip 33146–2094; tel. 786/308–3000 **A**1 5 9 10 **F**3 11 18 29 30 31 34 35 37 40 45 47 49 53 57 60 63 64 68 70 74 75 77 78 79 81 82 84 85 86 87 93 94 100 102 107 108 111 113 114 118 123 125 129 130 131 134 142 145 147 **P**6 **S** Baptist Health South Florida, Coral Gables, FL
Primary Contact: Nelson Lazo, Chief Executive Officer
CFO: Maria J. Yanez, Chief Financial Officer
Web address: www.baptisthealth.net
**Control:** Other not–for–profit (including NFP Corporation) **Service:** General Medical and Surgical

**Staffed Beds:** 146 **Admissions:** 7136 **Census:** 108 **Outpatient Visits:** 62640 **Births:** 0 **Total Expense ($000):** 168297 **Payroll Expense ($000):** 57248 **Personnel:** 981

✠ **CORAL GABLES HOSPITAL (100183)**, 3100 Douglas Road, Zip 33134–6990; tel. 305/445–8461, (Nonreporting) **A**1 9 10 **S** TENET Healthcare Corporation, Dallas, TX
Primary Contact: Jay S. Miranda, Chief Executive Officer
COO: Caridad Nieves, Chief Nursing Officer and Chief Operating Officer
Web address: www.coralgableshospital.com
**Control:** Corporation, Investor–owned, for–profit **Service:** General Medical and Surgical

**Staffed Beds:** 256

## CORAL SPRINGS—Broward County

✠ **BROWARD HEALTH CORAL SPRINGS (100276)**, 3000 Coral Hills Drive, Zip 33065; tel. 954/344–3000 **A**1 9 10 **F**3 11 12 13 15 17 20 29 31 34 35 40 48 51 55 57 58 59 61 63 64 66 68 70 72 74 75 76 77 78 79 80 81 82 84 85 86 87 88 89 93 96 107 108 111 113 114 117 118 128 129 130 131 142 145 146 147 **S** Broward Health, Fort Lauderdale, FL
Primary Contact: Drew Grossman, Chief Executive Officer
COO: Kimberley Graham, R.N., Chief Nursing Officer and Chief Operating Officer
CFO: Arthur Wallace, Chief Financial Officer
CMO: Carrie Greenspan, M.D., Chief of Staff
CHR: Robert Diano, Director Human Resources
CNO: Kimberley Graham, R.N., Chief Nursing Officer and Chief Operating Officer
Web address: www.browardhealth.org
**Control:** Hospital district or authority, Government, nonfederal **Service:** General Medical and Surgical

**Staffed Beds:** 182 **Admissions:** 12831 **Census:** 139 **Outpatient Visits:** 125005 **Births:** 2316 **Total Expense ($000):** 135088 **Payroll Expense ($000):** 58609 **Personnel:** 845

## CRESTVIEW—Okaloosa County

✠ **NORTH OKALOOSA MEDICAL CENTER (100122)**, 151 Redstone Avenue S.E., Zip 32539–6026; tel. 850/689–8100, (Nonreporting) **A**1 9 10 **S** Community Health Systems, Inc., Franklin, TN
Primary Contact: David W. Fuller, Chief Executive Officer
COO: Heath Evans, Assistant Chief Executive Officer
CFO: Jim Andrews, Chief Financial Officer
CMO: Michael Foley, M.D., Chief Medical Officer
CIO: Jenny Zeitler, Network Administrator
CHR: Melody M. Miller–Collette, Director Human Resources
CNO: Nina Perez, R.N., Chief Nursing Officer
Web address: www.northokaloosa.com
**Control:** Corporation, Investor–owned, for–profit **Service:** General Medical and Surgical

**Staffed Beds:** 110

## CRYSTAL RIVER—Citrus County

☐ **SEVEN RIVERS REGIONAL MEDICAL CENTER (100249)**, 6201 North Suncoast Boulevard, Zip 34428–6712; tel. 352/795–6560, (Nonreporting) **A**1 9 10 19 **S** Health Management Associates, Naples, FL
Primary Contact: Joyce A. Brancato, Chief Executive Officer
COO: DeAnna Beverly, Chief Operating Officer
CFO: Steven Miller, Chief Financial Officer
CHR: Joann Mramor, Director Human Resources
CNO: Cynthia Heitzman, R.N., Chief Nursing Officer
Web address: www.srrmc.com
**Control:** Corporation, Investor–owned, for–profit **Service:** General Medical and Surgical

**Staffed Beds:** 128

## DADE CITY—Pasco County

☐ **PASCO REGIONAL MEDICAL CENTER (100211)**, 13100 Fort King Road, Zip 33525–5294; tel. 352/521–1100, (Nonreporting) **A**1 9 10 **S** Health Management Associates, Naples, FL
Primary Contact: Philip Minden, Chief Executive Officer
CFO: Linda Stockton, Chief Financial Officer
CMO: Petros Tsambiras, M.D., Chief of Staff
CIO: Cheryl Kaufman, Director Health Information Management
CHR: Tabatha Wallace, Director Human Resources
Web address: www.pascoregionalmc.com
**Control:** Corporation, Investor–owned, for–profit **Service:** General Medical and Surgical

**Staffed Beds:** 120

## DAVENPORT—Polk County

☐ **HEART OF FLORIDA REGIONAL MEDICAL CENTER (100137)**, 40100 Highway 27, Zip 33837–5906; tel. 863/422–4971, (Nonreporting) **A**1 9 10 **S** Health Management Associates, Naples, FL
Primary Contact: Donnie Breeding, Chief Executive Officer
COO: Brent Burish, Chief Operating Officer
CFO: Tonja Mosley, Chief Financial Officer
CMO: Mohamed Razak, M.D., Chief of Staff
CIO: Louis Jones, Director Management Information Systems
CHR: Joan Allard, Director Human Resources
CNO: Anne Carey, Chief Nursing Officer
Web address: www.heartofflorida.com
**Control:** Corporation, Investor–owned, for–profit **Service:** General Medical and Surgical

**Staffed Beds:** 194

## DAYTONA BEACH—Volusia County

✠ **FLORIDA HOSPITAL MEMORIAL MEDICAL CENTER (100068)**, 301 Memorial Medical Parkway, Zip 32117–5167; tel. 386/676–6000, (Includes FLORIDA HOSPITAL–OCEANSIDE, 264 South Atlantic Avenue, Ormond Beach, Zip 32176–8192; tel. 386/672–4161) **A**1 2 9 10 **F**2 3 11 12 13 15 17 18 20 22 24 26 28 29 30 31 32 34 35 40 42 45 46 47 54 57 58 59 68 70 74 75 76 77 78 79 81 82 86 87 90 91 92 93 97 100 107 108 109 110 111 112 113 115 116 118 119 120 122 123 129 130 131 134 143 145 146 147 **P**6 **S** Adventist Health System Sunbelt Health Care Corporation, Altamonte Springs, FL
Primary Contact: Daryl Tol, Chief Executive Officer
COO: Darlinda Copeland, Chief Operating Officer
CFO: Debora Thomas, Chief Financial Officer
CHR: Connie Schott, Administrative Assistant
Web address: www.floridahospitalmemorial.org
**Control:** Church–operated, Nongovernment, not–for profit **Service:** General Medical and Surgical

**Staffed Beds:** 396 **Admissions:** 13186 **Census:** 171 **Outpatient Visits:** 103194 **Births:** 1417 **Total Expense ($000):** 194437 **Payroll Expense ($000):** 75497

**FL**

---

**Hospital, Medicare Provider Number, Address, Telephone, Approval, Facility, and Physician Codes, Health Care System**

★ American Hospital Association (AHA) membership
☐ The Joint Commission accreditation
◇ DNV Healthcare Inc. accreditation
○ American Osteopathic Association (AOA) accreditation
△ Commission on Accreditation of Rehabilitation Facilities (CARF) accreditation

✠ **HALIFAX HEALTH MEDICAL CENTER OF DAYTONA BEACH (100017)**, 303 North Clyde Morris Boulevard, Zip 32114–2700; tel. 386/254–4000, (Includes HALIFAX BEHAVIORAL SERVICES, 841 Jimmy Ann Drive, Zip 32117–4599; tel. 904/274–5333; HALIFAX HEALTH MEDICAL CENTER OF PORT ORANGE, 1041 Dunlawton Avenue, Port Orange, Zip 32127; tel. 386/322–4700; Ann Martorano, Administrator) **A**1 2 3 5 9 10 **F**3 11 12 13 17 18 20 22 24 26 28 29 30 31 40 42 43 45 46 47 49 53 55 60 65 70 72 76 77 78 79 81 85 86 87 88 89 98 99 100 101 102 103 107 108 111 113 114 117 118 119 120 122 123 125 129 130 131 134 137 145 146 147
Primary Contact: Jeff Feasel, Chief Executive Officer
CFO: Eric Peburn, Chief Financial Officer
CMO: Donald Stoner, M.D., Chief Medical Officer
CIO: Lori Delone, Chief Technology Officer
CHR: Albert L. Alexander, Chief Human Resources Officer
Web address: www.halifax.org
**Control:** Hospital district or authority, Government, nonfederal **Service:** General Medical and Surgical

**Staffed Beds:** 582 **Admissions:** 23347 **Census:** 323 **Outpatient Visits:** 304758 **Births:** 1824 **Total Expense ($000):** 309465 **Payroll Expense ($000):** 172166 **Personnel:** 3156

### DEERFIELD BEACH—Broward County

✠ △ **BROWARD HEALTH NORTH (100086)**, 201 East Sample Road, Zip 33064–3502; tel. 954/941–8300 **A**1 2 7 9 10 **F**3 6 11 15 17 18 20 28 29 30 31 34 35 37 40 43 45 46 49 51 55 57 58 59 60 61 64 66 68 70 74 75 77 78 79 80 81 82 83 84 85 86 87 90 92 93 94 96 100 107 108 110 111 113 114 116 117 118 119 120 122 123 128 129 130 131 142 144 145 147 **S** Broward Health, Fort Lauderdale, FL
Primary Contact: Pauline Grant, FACHE, Chief Executive Officer
COO: Kevin Fusco, Chief Operating Officer
CFO: Robert Bugg, Chief Financial Officer
CMO: Douglas Ford, M.D., Chief of Staff
CIO: Doris Crain, Vice President and Chief Information Officer
CHR: Grace King, Regional Director Human Resources
CNO: Bettiann S. Ruditz, Chief Nursing Officer
Web address: www.browardhealth.org
**Control:** Hospital district or authority, Government, nonfederal **Service:** General Medical and Surgical

**Staffed Beds:** 360 **Admissions:** 13595 **Census:** 199 **Outpatient Visits:** 117485 **Births:** 0 **Total Expense ($000):** 200225 **Payroll Expense ($000):** 78581 **Personnel:** 1120

### DEFUNIAK SPRINGS—Walton County

**HEALTHMARK REGIONAL MEDICAL CENTER (100081)**, 4413 U.S. Highway 331 South, Zip 32435; tel. 850/951–4500, (Nonreporting) **A**9 10
Primary Contact: James H. Thompson, Ph.D., FACHE, Owner and Chief Executive Officer
COO: Gerald C. Beard, Chief Operating Officer
CFO: Jim Brewer, M.P.H., Chief Financial Officer
CMO: John H. Thomas, M.D., Chief of Staff
CIO: Nikki Galloway, Director Personnel and Administrative Secretary
CHR: Nikki Galloway, Director Personnel and Administrative Secretary
Web address: www.healthmarkregional.com
**Control:** Corporation, Investor–owned, for–profit **Service:** General Medical and Surgical

**Staffed Beds:** 50

### DELAND—Volusia County

✠ **FLORIDA HOSPITAL DELAND (100045)**, 701 West Plymouth Avenue, Zip 32720; tel. 386/943–4522 **A**1 9 10 **F**3 4 13 15 18 20 22 26 28 29 30 31 34 35 37 38 40 45 46 47 48 49 51 55 56 57 58 59 60 64 70 74 75 76 77 78 79 80 81 84 85 86 87 93 97 98 100 102 107 108 109 110 111 113 114 115 116 118 119 123 125 128 129 130 131 134 145 146 **S** Adventist Health System Sunbelt Health Care Corporation, Altamonte Springs, FL
Primary Contact: Mark LaRose, President and Chief Executive Officer
COO: Randy Surber, Chief Operating Officer
CFO: Nigel Hinds, Chief Financial Officer
CMO: Mark Hollmann, M.D., Chief of Staff
CIO: Kevin Piper, Director Information Systems
CHR: Opal R. Howard, Director Human Resources
CNO: Patricia Ann Stark, R.N., CNO
Web address: www.fhdeland.org
**Control:** Other not–for–profit (including NFP Corporation) **Service:** General Medical and Surgical

**Staffed Beds:** 156 **Admissions:** 8098 **Census:** 87 **Outpatient Visits:** 115852 **Births:** 851 **Total Expense ($000):** 110123 **Payroll Expense ($000):** 42064 **Personnel:** 757

### DELRAY BEACH—Palm Beach County

✠ **DELRAY MEDICAL CENTER (100258)**, 5352 Linton Boulevard, Zip 33484–6580; tel. 561/498–4440, (Includes FAIR OAKS PAVILION, 5440 Linton Boulevard, Zip 33484–6578; tel. 561/495–1000; PINECREST REHABILITATION HOSPITAL, 5360 Linton Boulevard, Zip 33484–6538; tel. 561/495–0400), (Nonreporting) **A**1 9 10 **S** TENET Healthcare Corporation, Dallas, TX
Primary Contact: Mark Bryan, Chief Executive Officer
COO: Jeffery L. Welch, Chief Operating Officer
CMO: Anthony Dardano, M.D., Chief Medical Officer
CIO: Robens Rosena, Director Information Systems
CHR: Shannon Wills, Director Human Resources
Web address: www.delraymedicalctr.com
**Control:** Corporation, Investor–owned, for–profit **Service:** General Medical and Surgical

**Staffed Beds:** 403

### DUNEDIN—Pinellas County

☐ **BAYCARE ALLIANT HOSPITAL (102021)**, 601 Main Street, Zip 34698–5848; tel. 727/736–9999 **A**1 9 10 **F**1 3 18 28 29 30 34 60 84 91 129 147
Primary Contact: Jacqueline Arocho, Administrator
CFO: John Proni, CPA, Manager Finance
CMO: Leonard Dunn, M.D., Chief Medical Officer
CHR: Darlene Shelton, Coordinator Team Resources
CNO: Karen Duffy, R.N., Director Patient Care Services
Web address: www.baycare.org
**Control:** Other not–for–profit (including NFP Corporation) **Service:** Long–Term Acute Care hospital

**Staffed Beds:** 38 **Admissions:** 385 **Census:** 29 **Outpatient Visits:** 0 **Births:** 0 **Total Expense ($000):** 15359 **Payroll Expense ($000):** 5342

☐ **MEASE HOSPITAL DUNEDIN (100043)**, 601 Main Street, Zip 34698–5891, Mailing Address: P.O. Box 760, Zip 34697–0760; tel. 727/733–1111, (Nonreporting) **A**1 9 10 **S** Morton Plant Mease Health Care, Clearwater, FL
Primary Contact: Glenn D. Waters, FACHE, President and Chief Executive Officer
COO: Lou Galdieri, R.N., Chief Operating Officer and Administrator
CFO: Carl Tremonti, Chief Financial Officer
CMO: Donald Pocock, M.D., Chief Medical Officer
CHR: Sharon Collotta, Director Human Resources
Web address: www.mpmhealth.com
**Control:** Other not–for–profit (including NFP Corporation) **Service:** General Medical and Surgical

**Staffed Beds:** 258

### EGLIN AFB—Okaloosa County

✠ **U. S. AIR FORCE REGIONAL HOSPITAL**, 307 Boatner Road, Suite 114, Zip 32542–1282; tel. 850/883–8221, (Nonreporting) **A**1 3 5 **S** Department of the Air Force, Washington, DC
Primary Contact: Colonel Gary Walker, Commander
Web address: www.eglin.af.mil
**Control:** Air Force, Government, federal **Service:** General Medical and Surgical

**Staffed Beds:** 57

### ENGLEWOOD—Sarasota County

✠ **ENGLEWOOD COMMUNITY HOSPITAL (100267)**, 700 Medical Boulevard, Zip 34223–3978; tel. 941/475–6571 **A**1 9 10 **F**3 15 18 20 29 30 34 35 40 45 48 49 50 51 56 57 59 60 61 64 65 70 74 75 77 78 79 81 85 87 91 92 93 107 108 110 111 113 118 128 129 130 131 132 142 145 146 147 **S** HCA, Nashville, TN
Primary Contact: Thomas J. Rice, FACHE, President and Chief Executive Officer
COO: Alex Chang, Chief Operating Officer
CFO: Michael Wyers, Chief Financial Officer
CMO: Eric Pressman, D.O., Chair Department of Medicine
CHR: Linda V. Smith, Director Human Resources
CHR: Tony Welch, VP Human Resources
CNO: Kathleen Pace, MSN, Chief Nursing Officer
Web address: www.englewoodcommunityhospital.com
**Control:** Corporation, Investor–owned, for–profit **Service:** General Medical and Surgical

**Staffed Beds:** 100 **Admissions:** 3072 **Census:** 31 **Outpatient Visits:** 36044 **Births:** 0 **Total Expense ($000):** 36722 **Payroll Expense ($000):** 15089 **Personnel:** 237

*Many Facility Codes have changed. Please refer to the AHA Guide Code Chart.* © 2012 AHA Guide

FL

## FERNANDINA BEACH—Nassau County

⊞ **BAPTIST MEDICAL CENTER NASSAU (100140)**, 1250 South 18th Street, Zip 32034–3098; tel. 904/321–3500 **A**1 9 10 **F**3 11 13 15 29 30 34 35 40 45 49 64 70 76 81 82 85 91 92 93 102 107 108 110 111 113 114 118 123 128 131 134 145 147 **S** Baptist Health, Jacksonville, FL
Primary Contact: Stephen Lee, President
COO: Patricia K. Hausauer, Director Finance
CFO: Patricia K. Hausauer, Director Finance
CHR: Katherine Howard, Director Human Resources
CNO: Barbara Gingher, R.N., Assistant Administrator for Patient Care Services
Web address: www.e–baptisthealth.com
**Control:** Other not–for–profit (including NFP Corporation) **Service:** General Medical and Surgical

**Staffed Beds:** 52 **Admissions:** 2981 **Census:** 27 **Outpatient Visits:** 60514 **Births:** 465 **Total Expense ($000):** 45670 **Payroll Expense ($000):** 16800

## FORT LAUDERDALE—Broward County

☐ **ATLANTIC SHORES HOSPITAL (104065)**, 4545 North Federal Highway, Zip 33308–5274; tel. 954/771–2711, (Nonreporting) **A**1 9 10 **S** Universal Health Services, Inc., King of Prussia, PA
Primary Contact: Manuel R. Llano, Chief Executive Officer
COO: Karin Carol, Chief Operating Officer
Web address: www.atlanticshoreshospital.com
**Control:** Individual, Investor–owned, for–profit **Service:** Psychiatric

**Staffed Beds:** 72

⊞ **BROWARD HEALTH IMPERIAL POINT (100200)**, 6401 North Federal Highway, Zip 33308–1495; tel. 954/776–8500 **A**1 9 10 **F**3 11 12 15 20 29 31 34 35 40 45 51 53 55 57 58 59 61 63 64 66 68 70 74 75 77 78 79 80 81 82 84 85 86 87 93 98 100 102 104 105 107 108 111 113 114 117 118 128 129 130 131 142 145 146 147 **S** Broward Health, Fort Lauderdale, FL
Primary Contact: Alice Taylor, R.N., MSN, Chief Executive Officer
CFO: Susan Newton, Chief Financial Officer
CHR: Melanie Hatcher, Region Director Human Resources
Web address: www.browardhealth.org
**Control:** Hospital district or authority, Government, nonfederal **Service:** General Medical and Surgical

**Staffed Beds:** 180 **Admissions:** 9340 **Census:** 111 **Outpatient Visits:** 84744 **Births:** 0 **Total Expense ($000):** 102600 **Payroll Expense ($000):** 41907 **Personnel:** 651

⊞ **BROWARD HEALTH MEDICAL CENTER (100039)**, 1600 South Andrews Avenue, Zip 33316–2510; tel. 954/355–4400, (Includes CHRIS EVERT CHILDRENS HOSPITAL, 1600 South Andrews Avenue, tel. 954/355–4400; Calvin E. Glidewell, Jr., Chief Executive Officer) **A**1 2 5 9 10 12 13 **F**3 11 13 15 17 18 20 22 24 26 28 29 30 31 34 35 40 43 45 48 49 51 53 57 59 60 61 62 63 64 65 66 68 70 71 72 73 74 75 76 77 78 79 80 81 82 83 84 85 87 88 89 93 94 98 100 102 105 107 108 110 111 113 114 115 116 118 119 120 128 129 138 145 **S** Broward Health, Fort Lauderdale, FL
Primary Contact: Calvin E. Glidewell, Jr., Chief Executive Officer
CFO: Mark Doyle, Chief Financial Officer
CMO: Rajiv Chokshi, M.D., Chief of Staff
CIO: Doris Crain, Vice President Information Services
CHR: Dionne Wong, Vice President and Chief Human Resources Officer
Web address: www.browardhealth.org
**Control:** Hospital district or authority, Government, nonfederal **Service:** General Medical and Surgical

**Staffed Beds:** 656 **Admissions:** 29613 **Census:** 426 **Outpatient Visits:** 271051 **Births:** 3173 **Total Expense ($000):** 428504 **Payroll Expense ($000):** 173345 **Personnel:** 2713

⊞ **FLORIDA MEDICAL CENTER (100210)**, 5000 West Oakland Park Boulevard, Zip 33313–1585; tel. 954/735–6000, (Nonreporting) **A**1 10 **S** TENET Healthcare Corporation, Dallas, TX
Primary Contact: Ben A. Rodriguez, Chief Executive Officer
Web address: www.floridamedicalctr.com
**Control:** Partnership, Investor–owned, for–profit **Service:** General Medical and Surgical

**Staffed Beds:** 459

☐ **FORT LAUDERDALE HOSPITAL (104026)**, 1601 East Las Olas Boulevard, Zip 33301–2393; tel. 954/463–4321, (Nonreporting) **A**1 9 10 **S** Universal Health Services, Inc., King of Prussia, PA
Primary Contact: Manuel R. Llano, Chief Executive Officer
CFO: Gina Lee, Chief Financial Officer
Web address: www.fortlauderdalehospital.org
**Control:** Corporation, Investor–owned, for–profit **Service:** Psychiatric

**Staffed Beds:** 100

⊞ **HEALTHSOUTH SUNRISE REHABILITATION HOSPITAL (103028)**, 4399 Nob Hill Road, Zip 33351–5899; tel. 954/749–0300 **A**1 9 10 **F**3 29 62 82 90 91 93 95 96 **S** HEALTHSOUTH Corporation, Birmingham, AL
Primary Contact: Kevin R. Conn, Chief Executive Officer
COO: Jay de los Reyes, Chief Operating Officer
CFO: Ruth Goodstein, Controller
CMO: Scott Tannenbaum, M.D., Medical Director
CIO: Angela Manning, Director Health Information Services
CHR: Barbara Dunkiel, Director Human Resources
CNO: Omaira D. Riano, Chief Nursing Officer
Web address: www.healthsouthsunrise.com
**Control:** Corporation, Investor–owned, for–profit **Service:** Rehabilitation

**Staffed Beds:** 126 **Admissions:** 2300 **Census:** 93 **Outpatient Visits:** 33175 **Births:** 0 **Total Expense ($000):** 31785 **Payroll Expense ($000):** 18085 **Personnel:** 372

⊞ **HOLY CROSS HOSPITAL (100073)**, 4725 North Federal Highway, Zip 33308–4668, Mailing Address: P.O. Box 23460, Zip 33307–3460; tel. 954/771–8000, (Nonreporting) **A**1 2 9 10 **S** Catholic Health East, Newtown Square, PA
Primary Contact: Patrick Taylor, M.D., President and Chief Executive Officer
COO: Luisa Gutman, Senior Vice President and Chief Operating Officer
CFO: Linda Wilford, CPA, Senior Vice President and Chief Financial Officer
CMO: Kenneth Homer, M.D., Chief Medical Officer
CIO: Jeff Smith, Chief Information Officer
CHR: Luisa Gutman, Vice President Human Resources
CNO: Margaret Scheaffel, R.N., Vice President and Chief Nursing Officer
Web address: www.holy–cross.com
**Control:** Church–operated, Nongovernment, not–for profit **Service:** General Medical and Surgical

**Staffed Beds:** 571

**IMPERIAL POINT MEDICAL CENTER** See Broward Health Imperial Point

⊞ **KINDRED HOSPITAL SOUTH FLORIDA–FORT LAUDERDALE (102010)**, 1516 East Las Olas Boulevard, Zip 33301–2399; tel. 954/764–8900, (Includes KINDRED HOSPITAL SOUTH FLORIDA–CORAL GABLES, 5190 S.W. Eighth Street, Coral Gables, Zip 33134–2495; tel. 305/445–1364; Charles Doten, Chief Executive Officer), (Nonreporting) **A**1 9 10 **S** Kindred Healthcare, Louisville, KY
Primary Contact: Theodore L. Welding, Administrator
CFO: Dean Card, Chief Financial Officer
Web address: www.khfortlauderdale.com/
**Control:** Corporation, Investor–owned, for–profit **Service:** Long–Term Acute Care hospital

**Staffed Beds:** 123

## FORT MYERS—Lee County

**CHILDREN'S HOSPITAL OF SOUTHWEST FLORIDA** See Lee Memorial Hospital

⊞ **GULF COAST MEDICAL CENTER (100220)**, 13681 Doctor's Way, Zip 33912–4300; tel. 239/343–1000 **A**1 2 9 10 21 **F**3 11 13 17 18 20 22 24 26 28 29 30 40 45 49 60 64 70 74 76 77 79 80 81 84 92 93 107 108 111 113 117 118 129 137 145 **S** Lee Memorial Health System, Fort Myers, FL
Primary Contact: James R. Nathan, President and Chief Executive Officer
COO: Lawrence Antonucci, M.D., Chief Operating Officer
CFO: Mike German, Chief Financial Officer
CMO: Mark Greenberg, M.D., Medical Director
CIO: Mike Smith, Chief Information Officer
CHR: Jon C. Cecil, Chief Human Resource Officer
CNO: Donna Giannuzzi, R.N., Chief Patient Care Officer
Web address: www.leememorial.org
**Control:** Hospital district or authority, Government, nonfederal **Service:** General Medical and Surgical

**Staffed Beds:** 349 **Admissions:** 22033 **Census:** 272 **Outpatient Visits:** 197329 **Births:** 1673

**FL**

★ △ **LEE MEMORIAL HOSPITAL (100012)**, 2776 Cleveland Avenue, Zip 33901–5855, Mailing Address: P.O. Box 2218, Zip 33902–2218; tel. 239/332–1111, (Includes CHILDREN'S HOSPITAL OF SOUTHWEST FLORIDA, 9981 South HealthPark Drive, Zip 33908; tel. 239/433–7799; HEALTHPARK MEDICAL CENTER, 9981 South HealthPark Drive, Zip 33908; tel. 239/433–7799; THE REHABILITATION HOSPITAL, 2776 Cleveland Avenue, Zip 33901; tel. 239/332–1111, (Total facility includes 112 beds in nursing home–type unit) **A**2 7 9 10 21 **F**3 11 13 14 15 17 18 19 20 21 22 24 26 28 29 30 31 32 34 35 38 40 43 45 48 50 51 56 57 58 59 64 65 68 70 72 73 74 75 76 77 78 79 80 81 82 84 85 86 87 88 89 90 93 94 97 98 102 103 106 107 108 110 113 114 118 125 127 128 129 131 134 145 146 147 **S** Lee Memorial Health System, Fort Myers, FL
Primary Contact: James R. Nathan, President
COO: Lawrence Antonucci, M.D., Chief Operating Officer
CMO: Chuck Krivenko, M.D., Chief Medical Officer, Clinical and Quality Services
CIO: Mike Smith, Chief Information Officer
CHR: Jon C. Cecil, Chief Human Resource Officer
Web address: www.leememorial.org
**Control:** Hospital district or authority, Government, nonfederal **Service:** General Medical and Surgical

| Staffed Beds: 835 Admissions: 38754 Census: 635 Outpatient Visits: 960632 Births: 3362 |
|---|

**FORT PIERCE—St. Lucie County**

✚ **LAWNWOOD REGIONAL MEDICAL CENTER (100246)**, 1700 South 23rd Street, Zip 34950–0188; tel. 772/461–4000, (Includes LAWNWOOD PAVILION, 1860 North Lawnwood Circle, Zip 34950, Mailing Address: P.O. Box 1540, Zip 34954–1540; tel. 361/466–1500), (Nonreporting) **A**1 9 10 **S** HCA, Nashville, TN
Primary Contact: Rodney R. Smith, Chief Executive Officer
COO: James R. Beatty, Chief Operating Officer
CFO: Robert Dunwoody, Chief Financial Officer
CIO: Eric Castle, Director Information Services
CHR: Pam Burchell, Director Human Resources
Web address: www.lawnwoodmed.com
**Control:** Corporation, Investor–owned, for–profit **Service:** General Medical and Surgical

| Staffed Beds: 331 |
|---|

**FORT WALTON BEACH—Okaloosa County**

✚ △ **FORT WALTON BEACH MEDICAL CENTER (100223)**, 1000 Mar–Walt Drive, Zip 32547–6795; tel. 850/862–1111, (Nonreporting) **A**1 2 7 9 10 **S** HCA, Nashville, TN
Primary Contact: John A. Deardorff, Chief Executive Officer
COO: Ellen Witterstaeter, Chief Operating Officer
CFO: Vincent N. Wyatt, Chief Financial Officer
CMO: Colonel Tama Van Decar, M.D., Chief Medical Officer
CIO: Lance Penton, Director Information Technology and Systems
CHR: Anna Garland, Director Human Resources
Web address: www.fwbmc.com
**Control:** Corporation, Investor–owned, for–profit **Service:** General Medical and Surgical

| Staffed Beds: 257 |
|---|

**GAINESVILLE—Alachua County**

✚ **MALCOM RANDALL VETERANS AFFAIRS MEDICAL CENTER**, 1601 S.W. Archer Road, Zip 32608–1197; tel. 352/376–1611, (Nonreporting) **A**1 3 5 8 **S** Department of Veterans Affairs, Washington, DC
Primary Contact: Nancy Reissener, Acting Director
COO: Thomas Sutton, Associate Director
CFO: Jim Taylor, Chief Business Office
CMO: Brad Bender, M.D., Chief of Staff
CIO: Deborah Michel–Ogborn, Chief Information Resource Management
CHR: Michelle Manderino, Chief Human Resources
Web address: www.northflorida.va.gov/
**Control:** Veterans Affairs, Government, federal **Service:** General Medical and Surgical

| Staffed Beds: 222 |
|---|

✚ **NORTH FLORIDA REGIONAL MEDICAL CENTER (100204)**, 6500 Newberry Road, Zip 32605–4392, Mailing Address: P.O. Box 147006, Zip 32614–7006; tel. 352/333–4000, (Nonreporting) **A**1 2 9 10 **S** HCA, Nashville, TN
Primary Contact: Ward Boston, III, Chief Executive Officer
COO: Matt Davis, Chief Operating Officer
CFO: Eric Lawson, Chief Financial Officer
CIO: Deborah Bush, Director Information Services
CHR: William Coorpender, Assistant Vice President Human Resources
Web address: www.nfrmc.com
**Control:** Corporation, Investor–owned, for–profit **Service:** General Medical and Surgical

| Staffed Beds: 278 |
|---|

✚ **SELECT SPECIALTY HOSPITAL–GAINESVILLE (102022)**, 2708 S.W. Archer Road, Zip 32608; tel. 352/337–3240, (Nonreporting) **A**1 9 10 **S** Select Medical Corporation, Mechanicsburg, PA
Primary Contact: Russell A. Test, Chief Executive Officer
Web address: www.selectspecialtyhospitals.com
**Control:** Corporation, Investor–owned, for–profit **Service:** Long–Term Acute Care hospital

| Staffed Beds: 44 |
|---|

✚ △ **SHANDS AT THE UNIVERSITY OF FLORIDA (100113)**, 1600 S.W. Archer Road, Zip 32610–0326, Mailing Address: P.O. Box 100326, Zip 32610–0326; tel. 352/265–0111, (Includes SHANDS AGH, 801 S.W. Second Avenue, Zip 32601–6289; tel. 352/733–0111; Francis A. Pommett, Jr., Administrator; SHANDS CHILDRENS HOSPITAL, 1600 S.W. Archer Road, Zip 32610–3003, Mailing Address: PO Box 100335, Zip 32610–0335; tel. 352/265–8000; SHANDS REHAB HOSPITAL, 4101 N.W. 89th Boulevard, Zip 32606–3813; tel. 352/265–5491; Marina T. Cecchini, Administrator) **A**1 2 3 5 7 8 9 10 **F**2 3 4 5 6 7 8 9 11 12 13 15 16 17 18 19 20 21 22 23 24 25 26 27 29 30 31 32 34 35 36 37 38 39 40 41 43 44 45 46 47 48 49 50 51 52 53 54 55 56 57 58 59 60 61 62 64 65 66 68 69 70 72 73 74 75 76 77 78 79 80 81 82 84 85 86 87 88 89 90 91 93 94 96 97 98 99 100 101 102 103 104 105 107 108 109 110 111 113 114 115 116 117 118 119 120 122 123 125 128 129 130 131 133 134 135 136 137 138 139 140 141 142 143 144 145 146 147 **P**6 **S** Shands HealthCare, Gainesville, FL
Primary Contact: Timothy M. Goldfarb, Chief Executive Officer
CFO: William J. Robinson, Senior Vice President and Treasurer
CMO: Timothy C. Flynn, M.D., Chief of Staff
CIO: Joan Hovhanesian, Vice President and Chief Information Officer
CHR: Janet L. Christie, Senior Vice President Human Resources
Web address: www.shands.org
**Control:** Other not–for–profit (including NFP Corporation) **Service:** General Medical and Surgical

| Staffed Beds: 939 Admissions: 39957 Census: 707 Outpatient Visits: 798775 Births: 2987 Total Expense ($000): 947723 Payroll Expense ($000): 364048 Personnel: 7207 |
|---|

**SHANDS REHAB HOSPITAL** See Shands at the University of Florida

**GRACEVILLE—Jackson County**

**CAMPBELLTON GRACEVILLE HOSPITAL (101302)**, 5429 College Drive, Zip 32440–1897; tel. 850/263–4431, (Nonreporting) **A**9 10 18
Primary Contact: Jimmy Rigsby, Chief Executive Officer
CFO: Dena Cooper, Chief Financial Officer
CMO: Steve Davis, M.D., Chief Medical Officer
CHR: Judy Austin, Director Human Resources
Web address: www.pahn.org/cgh.cfm
**Control:** Hospital district or authority, Government, nonfederal **Service:** General Medical and Surgical

| Staffed Beds: 25 |
|---|

**GREEN COVE SPRINGS—Clay County**

✚ **KINDRED HOSPITAL NORTH FLORIDA (102015)**, 801 Oak Street, Zip 32043–4317; tel. 904/284–9230 **A**1 9 10 **F**1 3 29 30 31 60 63 70 74 75 77 78 82 85 87 92 107 118 129 147 **S** Kindred Healthcare, Louisville, KY
Primary Contact: Hoyt Ross, Chief Executive Officer
CFO: Dean Cocchi, Chief Financial Officer
CFO: Steve Hart, Controller
CMO: Lionel J. Gatien, D.O., Chief of Staff
CIO: Rick Chapman, Chief Information Officer
CNO: Susan Drago, R.N., Chief Clinical Officer
Web address: www.khnorthflorida.com
**Control:** Corporation, Investor–owned, for–profit **Service:** Long–Term Acute Care hospital

| Staffed Beds: 80 Admissions: 671 Census: 51 Outpatient Visits: 0 Births: 0 Personnel: 229 |
|---|

**GULF BREEZE—Santa Rosa County**

✚ **GULF BREEZE HOSPITAL (100266)**, 1110 Gulf Breeze Parkway, Zip 32561; tel. 850/934–2000 **A**1 9 10 **F**3 8 11 15 29 30 31 40 44 45 46 50 54 57 59 64 68 70 74 75 78 79 81 85 86 93 107 108 111 113 118 119 120 122 129 130 131 142 145 146 **P**4 6 **S** Baptist Health Care Corporation, Pensacola, FL
Primary Contact: Robert Harriman, M.D., Administrator
CFO: Kerry Vermillion, Senior Vice President Finance and Chief Financial Officer
Web address: www.ebaptisthealthcare.org
**Control:** Other not–for–profit (including NFP Corporation) **Service:** General Medical and Surgical

| Staffed Beds: 77 Admissions: 4231 Census: 44 Outpatient Visits: 112169 Births: 0 Total Expense ($000): 67810 Payroll Expense ($000): 22588 Personnel: 428 |
|---|

FL

## HIALEAH—Miami–Dade County

☒ **HIALEAH HOSPITAL (100053)**, 651 East 25th Street, Zip 33013–3878; tel. 305/693–6100, (Nonreporting) **A**1 9 10 **S** TENET Healthcare Corporation, Dallas, TX
Primary Contact: Ralph A. Aleman, Chief Executive Officer
COO: Steven Burghart, Chief Operating Officer
CFO: Arthur West, Chief Financial Officer
CHR: Yamila Castro, Director Human Resources
Web address: www.hialeahhosp.com
**Control:** Corporation, Investor–owned, for–profit **Service:** General Medical and Surgical

**Staffed Beds:** 378

☐ **PALM SPRINGS GENERAL HOSPITAL (100050)**, 1475 West 49th Street, Zip 33012–3275, Mailing Address: P.O. Box 2804, Zip 33012–2804; tel. 305/558–2500, (Nonreporting) **A**1 10
Primary Contact: Tony Mazzorano, Chief Executive Officer
CFO: Tony Milian, Chief Financial Officer
CHR: Lourdes Anton, Director Human Resources
**Control:** Corporation, Investor–owned, for–profit **Service:** General Medical and Surgical

**Staffed Beds:** 190

☒ **PALMETTO GENERAL HOSPITAL (100187)**, 2001 West 68th Street, Zip 33016–1898; tel. 305/823–5000, (Nonreporting) **A**1 9 10 12 13 **S** TENET Healthcare Corporation, Dallas, TX
Primary Contact: Ana J. Mederos, Chief Executive Officer
COO: Georgina Diaz, Chief Operating Officer
CFO: Oscar Vicente, Chief Financial Officer
CMO: Eloy Roman, M.D., Chief of Staff
CHR: Ana Gonzalez–Fajardo, Human Resources Director
CNO: Jeanne Drouillard, R.N., Chief Nursing Officer
Web address: www.palmettogeneral.com
**Control:** Corporation, Investor–owned, for–profit **Service:** General Medical and Surgical

**Staffed Beds:** 360

**SOUTHERN WINDS HOSPITAL** See Westchester General Hospital, Miami

## HOLLYWOOD—Broward County

☐ **HOLLYWOOD PAVILION (104015)**, 1201 North 37th Avenue, Zip 33021–5498; tel. 954/962–1355, (Nonreporting) **A**1 9 10
Primary Contact: Karen Kallen–Zury, Chief Executive Officer
COO: Christopher Gabel, Chief Operating Officer
CFO: Rocky Davidson, Chief Financial Officer
CHR: Len Alpert, Director Human Resources
Web address: www.hollywoodpavilion.com
**Control:** Corporation, Investor–owned, for–profit **Service:** Psychiatric

**Staffed Beds:** 46

★ **KINDRED HOSPITAL SOUTH FLORIDA–HOLLYWOOD (102010)**, 1859 Van Buren Street, Zip 33020–5127; tel. 954/920–9000, (Nonreporting) **A**9 10 **S** Kindred Healthcare, Louisville, KY
Primary Contact: Christopher Clements, Administrator
COO: Carlene Nugent, Chief Clinical Officer
CFO: Donald Gemmel, Controller
CMO: James Stern, M.D., Senior Vice President Medical Staff
CIO: Linda McQuade, Director Information Management
Web address: www.khsfhollywood.com/
**Control:** Corporation, Investor–owned, for–profit **Service:** Long–Term Acute Care hospital

**Staffed Beds:** 118

☒ △ **MEMORIAL REGIONAL HOSPITAL (100038)**, 3501 Johnson Street, Zip 33021–5421; tel. 954/987–2000 **A**1 2 3 5 7 9 10 **F**3 4 5 7 8 11 12 13 15 16 17 18 19 20 21 22 23 24 25 26 27 28 29 30 31 34 35 36 37 38 39 40 41 42 43 44 45 46 47 49 50 51 53 54 55 56 57 58 59 60 61 62 64 65 66 67 68 70 71 72 73 74 75 76 77 78 79 80 81 82 84 85 87 88 90 93 96 97 98 99 100 101 102 103 104 105 107 108 110 111 113 114 117 118 119 120 122 129 130 131 133 134 135 136 144 145 146 147 **P**6 **S** Memorial Healthcare System, Hollywood, FL
Primary Contact: Zeff Ross, FACHE, Senior Vice President and Chief Executive Officer
COO: Angeline M. Marano, Chief Operating Officer
CFO: David Smith, Chief Financial Officer
CMO: Stanley Marks, M.D., Chief Medical Officer
CIO: Forest Blanton, Administrator Process Engineering
CHR: Ray Kendrick, Chief Human Resources Officer
CNO: Maggie Hansen, R.N., Chief Nursing Officer
Web address: www.mhs.net
**Control:** Hospital district or authority, Government, nonfederal **Service:** General Medical and Surgical

**Staffed Beds:** 713 **Admissions:** 33513 **Census:** 490 **Outpatient Visits:** 358854 **Births:** 4056 **Total Expense ($000):** 478221 **Payroll Expense ($000):** 258993 **Personnel:** 4003

★ △ **MEMORIAL REGIONAL HOSPITAL SOUTH (100225)**, 3600 Washington Street, Zip 33021–8216; tel. 954/966–4500, (Includes JOE DIMAGGIO CHILDREN'S HOSPITAL, 1000 Joe DiMaggio Drive, Zip 33021–5426; tel. 954/987–2000) **A**7 9 10 **F**3 8 15 17 18 29 30 34 40 45 50 51 56 57 59 60 64 70 77 79 81 84 85 86 90 95 96 107 108 110 111 112 113 114 118 128 129 131 134 145 146 147 **S** Memorial Healthcare System, Hollywood, FL
Primary Contact: Douglas Zaren, FACHE, Administrator
CFO: Veronica Bautista, Chief Financial Officer
CHR: Vivian Sandler, Director Human Resources
Web address: www.memorialregionalsouth.com
**Control:** Hospital district or authority, Government, nonfederal **Service:** General Medical and Surgical

**Staffed Beds:** 280 **Admissions:** 6442 **Census:** 78 **Outpatient Visits:** 23913 **Births:** 0 **Total Expense ($000):** 63245 **Payroll Expense ($000):** 34933 **Personnel:** 603

☐ **SOUTH FLORIDA STATE HOSPITAL (104001)**, 800 East Cypress Drive, Zip 33025–4543; tel. 954/392–3000, (Nonreporting) **A**1 10
Primary Contact: Sal A. Barbera, FACHE, Administrator
Web address: www.sfsh.org
**Control:** State–Government, nonfederal **Service:** Psychiatric

**Staffed Beds:** 355

## HOMESTEAD—Miami–Dade County

☒ **BAPTIST HEALTH SOUTH FLORIDA, HOMESTEAD HOSPITAL (100125)**, 975 Baptist Way, Zip 33033–7600; tel. 786/243–8000 **A**1 9 10 **F**3 11 13 15 18 29 30 31 34 35 40 41 45 47 49 50 51 53 57 59 60 61 63 64 68 70 74 75 76 78 79 81 82 84 85 86 87 89 93 102 107 108 110 111 113 114 118 128 129 130 131 133 134 144 145 146 147 **P**6 **S** Baptist Health South Florida, Coral Gables, FL
Primary Contact: Bill Duquette, Chief Executive Officer
COO: Kenneth R. Spell, Vice President Operations
CFO: Erik Long, Controller
CMO: Steven Fletcher, M.D., Chief of Staff
CIO: Mimi Taylor, Corporate Vice President Information Technology
CHR: Corey Heller, Corporate Vice President and Chief Human Resources Officer
CNO: Nancy Gail Gordon, R.N., CNO and VP of Nursing
Web address: www.baptisthealth.net
**Control:** Other not–for–profit (including NFP Corporation) **Service:** General Medical and Surgical

**Staffed Beds:** 142 **Admissions:** 10813 **Census:** 103 **Outpatient Visits:** 103587 **Births:** 1488 **Total Expense ($000):** 186679 **Payroll Expense ($000):** 68248 **Personnel:** 1122

## HUDSON—Pasco County

☒ **REGIONAL MEDICAL CENTER–BAYONET POINT (100256)**, 14000 Fivay Road, Zip 34667–7199; tel. 727/869–5400, (Nonreporting) **A**1 2 9 10 **S** HCA, Nashville, TN
Primary Contact: Shayne George, Chief Executive Officer
COO: Shalin Shah, Chief Operating Officer
CFO: Thomas Lawhorne, Chief Financial Officer
CMO: Ronald Gilberg, M.D., Chief of Staff
CIO: Stephen Goldstein, Director Information Systems
CHR: Patrick Kerrwood, Vice President Human Resources
Web address: www.rmchealth.com
**Control:** Corporation, Investor–owned, for–profit **Service:** General Medical and Surgical

**Staffed Beds:** 280

FL

---

**Hospital, Medicare Provider Number, Address, Telephone, Approval, Facility, and Physician Codes, Health Care System**

★ American Hospital Association (AHA) membership
☐ The Joint Commission accreditation
◇ DNV Healthcare Inc. accreditation
○ American Osteopathic Association (AOA) accreditation
△ Commission on Accreditation of Rehabilitation Facilities (CARF) accreditation

## INVERNESS—Citrus County

⊞ **CITRUS MEMORIAL HEALTH SYSTEM (100023)**, 502 West Highland Boulevard, Zip 34452–4754; tel. 352/726–1551 **A**1 9 10 19 **F**8 11 15 18 20 22 24 28 29 30 31 34 35 40 44 45 46 47 48 49 50 54 57 59 60 61 62 64 68 70 75 76 77 78 79 81 85 86 89 93 97 107 108 110 111 113 114 117 118 128 129 131 134 143 145 146 147 **P**6
Primary Contact: Ryan D. Beaty, President and Chief Executive Officer
COO: Jerrald Deloach, Chief Operating Officer
CFO: Mark Williams, Chief Financial Officer
CMO: Ralph Abadier, M.D., Chief of Staff
CIO: Tyler Whetstine, Director of Information Systems
CHR: Lee Glotzback, Director Human Resources
CNO: Linda M. McCarthy, R.N., VP/ Chief Nursing Officer
Web address: www.citrusmh.com
**Control:** Other not–for–profit (including NFP Corporation) **Service:** General Medical and Surgical

**Staffed Beds:** 198 **Admissions:** 10229 **Census:** 112 **Outpatient Visits:** 202183 **Births:** 581 **Total Expense ($000):** 157479 **Payroll Expense ($000):** 59198 **Personnel:** 997

## JACKSONVILLE—Duval County

⊞ **BAPTIST MEDICAL CENTER (100088)**, 800 Prudential Drive, Zip 32207–8203; tel. 904/202–2000, (Includes BAPTIST MEDICAL CENTER SOUTH, 14550 St. Augustine Road, Zip 32258–2160; tel. 904/821–6000; Ronald G. Robinson, Administrator; WOLFSON CHILDREN'S HOSPITAL, 800 Prudential Drive, Zip 32207; tel. 904/202–8000; Michael D. Aubin, President) **A**1 2 3 5 9 10 **F**3 5 8 11 12 13 15 17 18 19 20 21 22 23 24 25 26 27 28 29 30 31 32 34 35 36 37 38 39 40 41 44 45 46 47 48 49 50 51 53 54 55 56 57 58 59 60 61 62 64 68 70 72 73 74 75 76 78 79 80 81 82 85 86 87 88 89 92 93 94 98 99 100 101 102 103 104 105 107 108 109 110 111 113 114 115 116 117 118 119 120 122 123 125 128 129 130 131 133 134 135 140 144 145 146 147 **P**6 **S** Baptist Health, Jacksonville, FL
Primary Contact: Michael A. Mayo, FACHE, President
COO: John F. Wilbanks, FACHE, Chief Operating Officer
CFO: Mike Lukaszewski, Chief Financial Officer
CMO: Keith L. Stein, M.D., Senior Vice President Medical Affairs and Chief Medical Officer
CIO: Roland Garcia, Senior Vice President and Chief Information Officer
CHR: M. Beth Mehaffey, Vice President Human Resources
Web address: www.e–baptisthealth.com
**Control:** Other not–for–profit (including NFP Corporation) **Service:** General Medical and Surgical

**Staffed Beds:** 844 **Admissions:** 39596 **Census:** 540 **Outpatient Visits:** 398686 **Births:** 4303 **Total Expense ($000):** 696415 **Payroll Expense ($000):** 234973 **Personnel:** 5262

⊞ △ **BROOKS REHABILITATION HOSPITAL (103039)**, 3599 University Boulevard South, Zip 32216–0118; tel. 904/345–7600 **A**1 7 9 10 **F**29 30 54 62 64 90 91 93 95 96 129 131 145
Primary Contact: Douglas Baer, Chief Executive Officer
COO: Michael Spigel, Executive Vice President & Chief Operating Officer
CFO: Douglas Baer, Chief Executive Officer
CMO: Trevor Paris, M.D., Medical Director
CIO: Karen Green, Chief Information Officer
CHR: Karen Gallagher, Vice President Human Resources and Learning
CNO: Joanne Hoertz, Vice President of Nursing
Web address: www.brookshealth.org
**Control:** Other not–for–profit (including NFP Corporation) **Service:** Rehabilitation

**Staffed Beds:** 140 **Admissions:** 3010 **Census:** 124 **Outpatient Visits:** 133104 **Births:** 0 **Total Expense ($000):** 68489 **Payroll Expense ($000):** 27437 **Personnel:** 401

⊞ **MAYO CLINIC JACKSONVILLE (100151)**, 4500 San Pablo Road South, Zip 32224–1865; tel. 904/953–2000 **A**1 3 5 8 9 10 **F**3 9 12 14 15 17 18 20 22 24 26 28 29 30 31 34 35 36 37 40 45 46 47 48 49 50 51 54 55 56 58 59 60 64 65 68 70 74 75 77 78 79 81 82 84 85 86 87 92 93 96 97 100 107 108 110 111 112 113 114 115 116 117 118 119 120 122 123 125 128 129 130 131 134 135 136 137 138 139 140 141 144 145 146 147 **P**6 **S** Mayo Clinic Health System, Rochester, MN
Primary Contact: Hilary G. Mathews, MS, R.N., Administrator
COO: Hilary G. Mathews, MS, Administrator
CFO: Mary Hoffman, Chief Financial Officer
CMO: Nancy Dawson, M.D., Medical Director
CIO: Cheryl Croft, Chairman Information Services
CHR: Daniel Tomlinson, Chair Human Resources
CNO: Debra Harrison, MS, Chief Nursing Officer
Web address: www.mayoclinic.org
**Control:** Other not–for–profit (including NFP Corporation) **Service:** General Medical and Surgical

**Staffed Beds:** 214 **Admissions:** 12217 **Census:** 171 **Outpatient Visits:** 45051 **Births:** 0 **Total Expense ($000):** 328786 **Payroll Expense ($000):** 69302 **Personnel:** 1609

⊞ **MEMORIAL HOSPITAL JACKSONVILLE (100179)**, 3625 University Boulevard South, Zip 32216–4240, Mailing Address: P.O. Box 16325, Zip 32245–6325; tel. 904/399–6111, (Nonreporting) **A**1 2 9 10 **S** HCA, Nashville, TN
Primary Contact: James F. O'Loughlin, President and Chief Executive Officer
CFO: Ashley F. Johnson, Chief Financial Officer
CMO: Gary Winfield, M.D., Medical Director
CHR: Laura DeMotte, Vice President Human Resources
Web address: www.memorialhospitaljax.com
**Control:** Corporation, Investor–owned, for–profit **Service:** General Medical and Surgical

**Staffed Beds:** 425

⊞ **NAVAL HOSPITAL**, 2080 Child Street, Zip 32214–5000; tel. 904/542–7300 **A**1 3 5 **F**3 4 5 12 13 15 29 30 32 34 35 38 39 40 44 45 46 47 48 49 50 51 53 54 57 58 59 64 65 68 70 71 74 75 76 77 79 81 82 85 87 89 90 91 92 93 96 97 98 100 104 107 108 110 111 114 117 118 126 128 129 130 131 134 143 144 145 146 147 **P**6 **S** Bureau of Medicine and Surgery, Department of the Navy, Washington, DC
Primary Contact: Captain Lynn Welling, Commander
COO: Captain Mike Vernere, Executive Officer
CFO: Lieutenant Commander Michael Gregonis, Comptroller
CMO: Captain Christopher Quarles, M.D., Director Medical Services
CIO: Mike Haytaian, Head Director Information Resources Management
CHR: Commander Ruby Tennyson, Director Administration
Web address: www.navalhospitaljax.com
**Control:** Navy, Government, federal **Service:** General Medical and Surgical

**Staffed Beds:** 64 **Admissions:** 4070 **Census:** 25 **Outpatient Visits:** 492006 **Births:** 891 **Total Expense ($000):** 142000 **Personnel:** 1731

☐ **RIVER POINT BEHAVIORAL HEALTH (104016)**, 6300 Beach Boulevard, Zip 32216–2782; tel. 904/724–9202, (Nonreporting) **A**1 9 10 **S** Universal Health Services, Inc., King of Prussia, PA
Primary Contact: Gayle Eckerd, Chief Executive Officer
CFO: Jenni Stackhouse, Chief Financial Officer
CIO: Bill Willis, Director Information Technology
CHR: Cathy Calhoun, Director Human Resources
Web address: www.riverpointbehavioral.com
**Control:** Corporation, Investor–owned, for–profit **Service:** Psychiatric

**Staffed Beds:** 92

⊞ **SHANDS JACKSONVILLE MEDICAL CENTER (100001)**, 655 West Eighth Street, Zip 32209–6595; tel. 904/244–0411, (Total facility includes 56 beds in nursing home–type unit) **A**1 2 3 5 8 9 10 **F**3 5 6 7 8 11 12 13 15 17 18 19 20 22 24 25 26 28 29 30 31 32 33 34 35 38 39 40 41 43 47 48 49 50 51 53 49 50 51 52 53 54 56 57 58 59 60 61 62 64 65 66 68 70 71 72 73 74 75 76 77 78 79 80 81 82 84 85 86 87 88 89 92 93 94 96 97 98 99 100 101 102 103 104 105 107 108 109 110 111 113 114 115 116 117 118 119 120 122 123 125 127 128 129 130 131 133 134 140 143 144 145 146 147 **S** Shands HealthCare, Gainesville, FL
Primary Contact: James R. Burkhart, FACHE, President and Chief Executive Officer
COO: Greg Miller, Senior Vice President Operations
CFO: Mike Gleason, Vice President and Chief Financial Officer
CMO: David Vukich, M.D., Senior Vice President, Chief Medical Officer and Chief Quality Officer
CIO: Kari Cassel, Senior Vice President and Chief Information Officer
CHR: Lesli Ward, Vice President Human Resources
Web address: www.shandsjacksonville.org
**Control:** Other not–for–profit (including NFP Corporation) **Service:** General Medical and Surgical

**Staffed Beds:** 620 **Admissions:** 28644 **Census:** 476 **Outpatient Visits:** 378013 **Births:** 3107 **Total Expense ($000):** 437079 **Payroll Expense ($000):** 195182 **Personnel:** 3865

⊞ **SPECIALTY HOSPITAL JACKSONVILLE (102012)**, 4901 Richard Street, Zip 32207–7328; tel. 904/737–3120, (Nonreporting) **A**1 9 10 **S** HCA, Nashville, TN
Primary Contact: Barbara Walsh, Chief Executive Officer
CFO: Billy Wilcox, Chief Financial Officer
CMO: Wendell H. Williams, Jr., M.D., Medical Director
CIO: Liz Rhodes, Director Information Services
CHR: Lisa Ayala, R.N., Director Human Resources
Web address: www.specialtyhospitaljax.com
**Control:** Corporation, Investor–owned, for–profit **Service:** Long–Term Acute Care hospital

**Staffed Beds:** 62

*Many Facility Codes have changed. Please refer to the AHA Guide Code Chart.* © 2012 AHA Guide

FL

✠ **ST. VINCENT'S MEDICAL CENTER RIVERSIDE (100040)**, 1 Shircliff Way, Zip 32204–2982, Mailing Address: P.O. Box 2982, Zip 32203–2982; tel. 904/308–7300 **A**1 2 3 5 9 10 13 **F**3 7 12 13 15 17 18 20 22 24 26 28 29 30 31 34 35 38 40 43 45 48 49 50 51 53 54 56 57 58 59 60 61 64 65 66 68 70 71 72 74 75 76 78 79 81 84 85 86 87 93 94 96 97 107 108 110 111 113 114 116 117 118 119 120 122 123 125 128 129 130 131 132 134 142 145 146 147 **P**6 **S** Ascension Health, Saint Louis, MO
Primary Contact: Moody L. Chisholm, President & Chief Executive Officer
COO: Donnie Romine, Chief Operating Officer
CFO: Mark Doyle, Chief Financial Officer
CMO: Phil Perry, M.D., Chief Medical Officer
CIO: Ann Carey, Vice President and Chief Information Officer
CHR: Janice G. Lipsky, R.N., System Vice President Human Resources and Organizational Development
CNO: Rose Rivers, R.N., Chief Nursing Officer
Web address: www.jaxhealth.com
**Control:** Church–operated, Nongovernment, not–for profit **Service:** General Medical and Surgical

**Staffed Beds:** 501 **Admissions:** 27101 **Census:** 344 **Outpatient Visits:** 143637 **Births:** 1645 **Total Expense ($000):** 373404 **Payroll Expense ($000):** 121522 **Personnel:** 2480

✠ **ST. VINCENT'S MEDICAL CENTER SOUTHSIDE (100307)**, 4201 Belfort Road, Zip 32216; tel. 904/296–3700 **A**1 3 5 9 10 **F**3 12 13 15 18 20 22 26 29 30 31 34 35 37 40 44 45 47 49 51 57 59 60 64 65 70 72 74 75 76 78 79 81 82 85 86 87 93 96 107 108 110 111 113 118 127 128 129 130 131 142 145 146 **S** Ascension Health, Saint Louis, MO
Primary Contact: Moody L. Chisholm, President and Chief Executive Officer
COO: Donnie Romine, Chief Operating Officer
CFO: Mark Doyle, Chief Financial Officer
CMO: Phil Perry, M.D., Chief Medical Officer
CIO: Beth Fagin, Manager Information Systems
CHR: Edwina Coulliette, Manager Human Resources
CNO: Lorraine Keith, FACHE, Chief Nursing Officer
Web address: www.jaxhealth.com
**Control:** Church–operated, Nongovernment, not–for profit **Service:** General Medical and Surgical

**Staffed Beds:** 221 **Admissions:** 9332 **Census:** 124 **Outpatient Visits:** 36572 **Births:** 1336 **Total Expense ($000):** 129172 **Payroll Expense ($000):** 37699 **Personnel:** 672

**WEKIVA SPRINGS CENTER FOR WOMEN (104069)**, 3947 Salisbury Road, Zip 32216–6115; tel. 904/296–3533, (Nonreporting) **A**9 10 **S** Universal Health Services, Inc., King of Prussia, PA
Primary Contact: Gayle Eckerd, Chief Executive Officer
Web address: www.wekivacenter.com
**Control:** Other not–for–profit (including NFP Corporation) **Service:** Psychiatric

**Staffed Beds:** 60

**JACKSONVILLE BEACH—Duval County**

✠ **BAPTIST MEDICAL CENTER BEACHES (100117)**, 1350 13th Avenue South, Zip 32250–3205; tel. 904/627–2900 **A**1 9 10 **F**3 8 11 13 15 18 28 29 30 31 36 40 43 45 49 50 53 54 57 59 61 64 74 75 76 77 78 79 80 81 82 85 86 93 107 108 110 111 113 114 117 118 128 129 145 147 **S** Baptist Health, Jacksonville, FL
Primary Contact: Joseph M. Mitrick, FACHE, President
COO: John F. Wilbanks, FACHE, Chief Operating Officer
CFO: Mike Lukaszewski, Chief Financial Officer
CMO: Keith L. Stein, M.D., Chief Medical Officer
CIO: Roland Garcia, Senior Vice President and Chief Information Officer
CHR: Dana Voiselle, Director Human Resources
CNO: Diane Raines, R.N., Senior Vice President & CNO
Web address: www.e–baptisthealth.com
**Control:** Other not–for–profit (including NFP Corporation) **Service:** General Medical and Surgical

**Staffed Beds:** 136 **Admissions:** 7627 **Census:** 87 **Outpatient Visits:** 92510 **Births:** 1190 **Total Expense ($000):** 94026 **Payroll Expense ($000):** 33685 **Personnel:** 678

**JAY—Santa Rosa County**

★ **JAY HOSPITAL (100048)**, 14114 South Alabama Street, Zip 32565–1070; tel. 850/675–8000 **A**9 **F**11 15 18 29 30 34 35 40 45 46 48 49 50 57 59 64 75 77 81 82 85 93 107 111 113 118 129 131 132 134 145 146 **S** Baptist Health Care Corporation, Pensacola, FL
Primary Contact: Michael T. Hutchins, Administrator
CFO: Keith Strickling, Chief Accountant
CMO: Marian Stewart, M.D., Chief of Staff
CHR: Chanda Gay, Manager Human Resources
Web address: www.bhcpns.org/jayhospital/
**Control:** Other not–for–profit (including NFP Corporation) **Service:** General Medical and Surgical

**Staffed Beds:** 55 **Admissions:** 1043 **Census:** 20 **Outpatient Visits:** 24168 **Births:** 0 **Total Expense ($000):** 12478 **Payroll Expense ($000):** 5353 **Personnel:** 96

**JUPITER—Palm Beach County**

✠ **JUPITER MEDICAL CENTER (100253)**, 1210 South Old Dixie Highway, Zip 33458–7299; tel. 561/747–2234, (Total facility includes 120 beds in nursing home–type unit) **A**1 2 9 10 **F**3 8 11 12 13 15 18 20 26 28 29 30 31 34 35 40 47 48 49 50 53 54 55 57 58 59 66 70 74 75 76 77 78 79 80 81 82 84 85 86 87 92 93 107 108 109 110 111 113 114 115 116 117 118 119 120 122 125 127 128 129 131 134 142 145 146 147 **P**4
Primary Contact: John D. Couris, President and Chief Executive Officer
CFO: Stephen J. Grigsby, Chief Financial Officer
CIO: Mike Fehr, Vice President Operations and Chief Information Officer
CHR: John Wolf, Chief Human Resources Officer
Web address: www.jupitermed.com
**Control:** Other not–for–profit (including NFP Corporation) **Service:** General Medical and Surgical

**Staffed Beds:** 283 **Admissions:** 10853 **Census:** 221 **Outpatient Visits:** 118340 **Births:** 1116 **Total Expense ($000):** 180640 **Payroll Expense ($000):** 70331 **Personnel:** 1348

**KEY WEST—Monroe County**

☐ **LOWER KEYS MEDICAL CENTER (100150)**, 5900 College Road, Zip 33040–4396, Mailing Address: P.O. Box 9107, Zip 33041–9107; tel. 305/294–5531, (Includes DE POO HOSPITAL, 1200 Kennedy Drive, Zip 33041; tel. 305/294–4692), (Nonreporting) **A**1 9 10 **S** Health Management Associates, Naples, FL
Primary Contact: Nicki L. Will–Mowery, Ph.D., Chief Executive Officer
COO: Meylan Love–Watler, Chief Operating Officer
CFO: Dale Guffey, Chief Financial Officer
CMO: Jerome Covington, M.D., Chief Medical Officer
CIO: Les Jackson, Manager Information Systems
CHR: Donald Canalejo, Director Human Resources
Web address: www.lkmc.com
**Control:** Corporation, Investor–owned, for–profit **Service:** General Medical and Surgical

**Staffed Beds:** 90

**KISSIMMEE—Osceola County**

**FLORIDA HOSPITAL KISSIMMEE** See Florida Hospital, Orlando

✠ **OSCEOLA REGIONAL MEDICAL CENTER (100110)**, 700 West Oak Street, Zip 34741–4996; tel. 407/846–2266, (Nonreporting) **A**1 9 10 **S** HCA, Nashville, TN
Primary Contact: Kathryn Gillette, Chief Executive Officer
COO: David Cashwell, Chief Operating Officer
CFO: Glenn Romig, Chief Financial Officer
CMO: Aida Sanchez–Jimenez, M.D., Chief Medical Officer
CHR: Sylvia Lollis, Director Human Resources
CNO: Sonya Quintana, R.N., Chief Nursing Officer
Web address: www.osceolaregional.com
**Control:** Corporation, Investor–owned, for–profit **Service:** General Medical and Surgical

**Staffed Beds:** 235

**FL**

---

**Hospital, Medicare Provider Number, Address, Telephone, Approval, Facility, and Physician Codes, Health Care System**

★ American Hospital Association (AHA) membership
☐ The Joint Commission accreditation
◇ DNV Healthcare Inc. accreditation
○ American Osteopathic Association (AOA) accreditation
△ Commission on Accreditation of Rehabilitation Facilities (CARF) accreditation

## LAKE BUTLER—Union County

**LAKE BUTLER HOSPITAL HAND SURGERY CENTER (101303)**, 850 East Main Street, Zip 32054–1353, Mailing Address: P.O. Box 748, Zip 32054–0748; tel. 386/496–2323, (Nonreporting) **A**9 10 18
Primary Contact: Pamela B. Howard, R.N., Administrator
CFO: Paula Webb, Chief Financial Officer
CMO: Cynthia Larimer, M.D., Medical Director Emergency Room
CIO: Jennifer Thomas, Director Public Relations
CHR: Diane Cason, Supervisor Personnel and Payroll
CNO: Johnette Davis, Director of Nursing
Web address: www.lakebutlerhospital.com
**Control:** Corporation, Investor–owned, for–profit **Service:** General Medical and Surgical

**Staffed Beds:** 25

**RECEPTION AND MEDICAL CENTER**, State Road 231 South, Zip 32054, Mailing Address: P.O. Box 628, Zip 32054–0628; tel. 386/496–6000, (Nonreporting)
Primary Contact: Herbert L. Hall, Administrator
Web address: www.dc.state.fl.us
**Control:** State–Government, nonfederal **Service:** Hospital unit of an institution (prison hospital, college infirmary, etc.)

**Staffed Beds:** 133

## LAKE CITY—Columbia County

**LAKE CITY MEDICAL CENTER (100156)**, 340 N.W. Commerce Drive, Zip 32055–3718; tel. 386/719–9000, (Nonreporting) **A**1 9 10 **S** HCA, Nashville, TN
Primary Contact: Mark Robinson, FACHE, Chief Executive Officer
COO: Jennifer B. Adams, Chief Operating Officer and Chief Financial Officer
CFO: Jennifer B. Adams, Chief Operating Officer and Chief Financial Officer
CMO: Miguel Tepedino, M.D., Chief Medicine
CIO: Taylor Dickerson, Chief Information Officer
CHR: Steve Gordon, Director Human Resources
CNO: Barbara Kinder, R.N., Chief Nursing Officer
Web address: www.lakecitymedical.com
**Control:** Corporation, Investor–owned, for–profit **Service:** General Medical and Surgical

**Staffed Beds:** 67

**SHANDS LAKE SHORE (100102)**, 368 N.E. Franklin Street, Zip 32055–3047; tel. 386/292–8000, (Nonreporting) **A**1 9 10 **S** Health Management Associates, Naples, FL
Primary Contact: Rhonda Kay Sherrod, R.N., MSN, Administrator
CMO: Ricardo Rosato, M.D., President Medical Staff
CHR: Janice Jackson, Director Human Resources
Web address: www.shands.org
**Control:** Partnership, Investor–owned, for–profit **Service:** General Medical and Surgical

**Staffed Beds:** 85

★ △ **VETERANS AFFAIRS MEDICAL CENTER**, 619 South Marion Avenue, Zip 32025–5898; tel. 386/755–3016, (Nonreporting) **A**7 **S** Department of Veterans Affairs, Washington, DC
Primary Contact: Thomas A. Cappello, M.P.H., FACHE, Director
CIO: James Hudson, Assistant Chief Information Resource Management
Web address: www.va.gov/sta/guide/home.asp
**Control:** Veterans Affairs, Government, federal **Service:** General Medical and Surgical

**Staffed Beds:** 180

## LAKE WALES—Polk County

**LAKE WALES MEDICAL CENTER (100099)**, 410 South 11th Street, Zip 33853–4256; tel. 863/676–1433 **A**1 9 10 **F**3 11 15 18 20 29 30 34 35 40 45 46 49 50 57 59 64 70 74 75 79 81 82 85 86 87 89 91 92 93 94 96 107 108 110 111 113 114 118 123 128 130 131 145 146 147 **S** Community Health Systems, Inc., Franklin, TN
Primary Contact: Scott M. Smith, Chief Executive Officer
COO: Eric Lachance, Assistant Chief Executive Officer
CFO: Danny Warren, Chief Financial Officer
CMO: James Nelson, M.D., Chief Medical Staff
CMO: Sunil Nihalani, M.D., Chief Medical Staff
CIO: Erwin Jaropillo, Director Information Systems
CHR: Renee Latterner, Director Human Resources
CNO: Lee Clack, R.N., Chief Nursing Officer
Web address: www.lakewalesmedicalcenter.com
**Control:** Corporation, Investor–owned, for–profit **Service:** General Medical and Surgical

**Staffed Beds:** 131 **Admissions:** 5709 **Census:** 61 **Outpatient Visits:** 46364 **Births:** 0 **Total Expense ($000):** 52232 **Payroll Expense ($000):** 21044 **Personnel:** 453

## LAKE WORTH—Palm Beach County

**SELECT SPECIALTY HOSPITAL–PALM BEACH (102023)**, 3060 Melaleuca Lane, Zip 33461; tel. 561/357–7200, (Nonreporting) **A**1 9 10 **S** Select Medical Corporation, Mechanicsburg, PA
Primary Contact: Larry Melby, Chief Executive Officer
Web address: www.selectspecialtyhospitals.com
**Control:** Corporation, Investor–owned, for–profit **Service:** Long–Term Acute Care hospital

**Staffed Beds:** 60

## LAKELAND—Polk County

**LAKELAND REGIONAL MEDICAL CENTER (100157)**, 1324 Lakeland Hills Boulevard, Zip 33805–4543, Mailing Address: P.O. Box 95448, Zip 33804–5448; tel. 863/687–1100 **A**1 2 3 5 9 10 **F**3 4 11 13 17 18 20 22 24 26 28 29 30 31 34 37 38 40 41 43 44 45 46 47 49 51 55 56 57 58 59 60 61 64 65 70 71 72 74 75 76 77 78 79 80 81 82 83 84 85 86 87 88 89 93 98 99 100 101 102 103 104 105 107 108 109 110 111 113 114 117 118 119 120 122 123 125 129 131 134 142 143 145 146 147
Primary Contact: Elaine C. Thompson, Ph.D., President and Chief Executive Officer
CFO: Paul A. Powers, Vice President and Chief Financial Officer
CMO: Edwin Sammer, M.D., Vice President and Chief Medical Officer
CIO: Mary Ford, Vice President and Chief Information Officer
CHR: Jeffery L. Payne, Vice President Human Resources
Web address: www.lrmc.com
**Control:** Other not–for–profit (including NFP Corporation) **Service:** General Medical and Surgical

**Staffed Beds:** 788 **Admissions:** 37009 **Census:** 484 **Outpatient Visits:** 203364 **Births:** 3425 **Total Expense ($000):** 504090 **Payroll Expense ($000):** 206631 **Personnel:** 4348

## LAND O'LAKES—Pasco County

**FLORIDA HOSPITAL AT CONNERTON LONG TERM ACUTE CARE (102026)**, 9441 Health Center Drive, Zip 34637–5837; tel. 813/903–3701, (Nonreporting) **A**1 9 10 **S** Adventist Health System Sunbelt Health Care Corporation, Altamonte Springs, FL
Primary Contact: Debi Martoccio, R.N., Chief Operating Officer
COO: Debi Martoccio, R.N., Chief Operating Officer
CMO: Sharad Patel, M.D., Medical Director
CNO: Therese Murphy, Chief Nursing Officer
Web address: www.elevatinghealthcare.org
**Control:** Other not–for–profit (including NFP Corporation) **Service:** Long–Term Acute Care hospital

**Staffed Beds:** 8

## LARGO—Pinellas County

**HEALTHSOUTH REHABILITATION HOSPITAL (103037)**, 901 North Clearwater–Largo Road, Zip 33770–4126; tel. 727/586–2999, (Nonreporting) **A**1 9 10 **S** HEALTHSOUTH Corporation, Birmingham, AL
Primary Contact: Donald D. Evans, Chief Executive Officer
CFO: Judith Johnson, Controller
CMO: Richard A. Liles, M.D., Medical Director
CHR: Jackie Chalk, Director Human Resources
CNO: Pattie Brenner, R.N., Chief Nursing Officer
Web address: www.healthsouthlargo.com
**Control:** Corporation, Investor–owned, for–profit **Service:** Rehabilitation

**Staffed Beds:** 70

**LARGO MEDICAL CENTER (100248)**, 201 14th Street S.W., Zip 33770–3133, Mailing Address: P.O. Box 2905, Zip 33779–2905; tel. 727/588–5200, (Nonreporting) **A**1 2 5 9 10 12 13 **S** HCA, Nashville, TN
Primary Contact: Anthony M. Degina, President and Chief Executive Officer
COO: Timothy J. Cerullo, Chief Operating Officer
CFO: Robert E. Billings, Chief Financial Officer
CIO: Silvia Padro, Director Information Services
CHR: Eileen M. Corning, Director Human Resources
Web address: www.largomedical.com
**Control:** Corporation, Investor–owned, for–profit **Service:** General Medical and Surgical

**Staffed Beds:** 243

**SUN COAST HOSPITAL (100015)**, 2025 Indian Rocks Road, Zip 33774–1096, Mailing Address: P.O. Box 2025, Zip 33779–2025; tel. 727/581–9474, (Nonreporting)
Primary Contact: Darrell Lentz, Chief Executive Officer
COO: Nita Kasan, Chief Operating Officer and Chief Nursing Officer
Web address: www.suncoasthealthcare.com
**Control:** Other not–for–profit (including NFP Corporation) **Service:** General Medical and Surgical

**Staffed Beds:** 300

*Many Facility Codes have changed. Please refer to the AHA Guide Code Chart.*

FL

## LAUDERDALE LAKES—Broward County

☐ △ **ST. ANTHONY'S REHABILITATION HOSPITAL (103027)**, 3485 N.W. 30th Street, Zip 33311; tel. 954/739–6233 **A**1 7 9 10 **F**28 29 30 34 35 62 64 68 74 79 90 91 93 94 95 96 129 130 131 147
Primary Contact: Joe Catania, Chief Executive Officer
Web address: www.catholichealthservices.org
**Control:** Church–operated, Nongovernment, not–for profit **Service:** Rehabilitation

**Staffed Beds:** 26 **Admissions:** 530 **Census:** 20 **Outpatient Visits:** 2237 **Births:** 0 **Total Expense ($000):** 8130 **Payroll Expense ($000):** 2492 **Personnel:** 58

## LEESBURG—Lake County

☒ △ **LEESBURG REGIONAL MEDICAL CENTER (100084)**, 600 East Dixie Avenue, Zip 34748–5999; tel. 352/323–5762 **A**1 2 7 9 10 **F**3 8 11 13 15 17 18 20 22 24 26 28 29 30 31 34 35 40 45 53 54 57 59 60 64 66 68 70 74 75 76 77 78 79 81 82 85 87 89 90 93 96 107 110 111 113 118 129 131 143 145 147 **S** Central Florida Health Alliance, Leesburg, FL
Primary Contact: Donald G. Henderson, FACHE, President and Chief Executive Officer
CFO: Dale E. Hocking, Chief Financial Officer
CMO: Daniel Carlson, M.D., Senior Vice President and Chief Medical Officer
CIO: Nancy Vester, Vice President Information Technology
CNO: Cynde Gamache, R.N., Vice President and Chief Clinical Officer
Web address: www.cfhalliance.org
**Control:** Other not–for–profit (including NFP Corporation) **Service:** General Medical and Surgical

**Staffed Beds:** 316 **Admissions:** 17155 **Census:** 213 **Outpatient Visits:** 76612 **Births:** 1265 **Total Expense ($000):** 227293 **Payroll Expense ($000):** 83661 **Personnel:** 1653

## LEHIGH ACRES—Lee County

☐ **LEHIGH REGIONAL MEDICAL CENTER (100107)**, 1500 Lee Boulevard, Zip 33936–4897; tel. 239/369–2101, (Nonreporting) **A**1 10 **S** Health Management Associates, Naples, FL
Primary Contact: Joanie Jeannette, MSN, Chief Executive Officer
CFO: Bob Pulley, Interim Chief Financial Officer
CMO: Madhava Pally, M.D., Chief of Staff
CIO: Jeff Hampton, Director Information Systems
CHR: Carmen Bech de Garcia, Director Human Resources
Web address: www.lehighregional.com
**Control:** Corporation, Investor–owned, for–profit **Service:** General Medical and Surgical

**Staffed Beds:** 88

## LIVE OAK—Suwannee County

☒ **SHANDS LIVE OAK (101301)**, 1100 S.W. 11th Street, Zip 32060–3608; tel. 386/362–0800, (Nonreporting) **A**1 9 10 18 **S** Health Management Associates, Naples, FL
Primary Contact: Ricardo Diaz, Chief Executive Officer
Web address: www.shands.org
**Control:** Partnership, Investor–owned, for–profit **Service:** General Medical and Surgical

**Staffed Beds:** 15

## LONGWOOD—Seminole County

**ORLANDO REGIONAL SOUTH SEMINOLE HOSPITAL**, 555 West State Road 434, Zip 32750–4999; tel. 407/767–1200, (Nonreporting) **A**9 **S** Orlando Health, Orlando, FL
Primary Contact: Robert E. Snyder, Jr., President
CIO: Rick Schooler, Vice President Information Services
Web address: www.orhs.org
**Control:** Partnership, Investor–owned, for–profit **Service:** General Medical and Surgical

**Staffed Beds:** 206

## LOXAHATCHEE—Palm Beach County

☒ **PALMS WEST HOSPITAL (100269)**, 13001 Southern Boulevard, Zip 33470–1150; tel. 561/798–3300 **A**1 9 10 12 13 **F**3 8 11 13 15 17 18 19 20 22 29 30 31 34 35 39 40 41 45 46 47 49 50 51 56 57 58 59 60 61 64 70 74 75 76 77 78 79 81 82 84 85 87 88 89 93 107 108 110 111 113 118 125 129 130 131 145 146 147 **S** HCA, Nashville, TN
Primary Contact: Eric Goldman, Chief Executive Officer
COO: Laura Hilbert, Interim Chief Operating Officer
CFO: Joseph M. Paul, Chief Financial Officer
CIO: Fariba Borjian, Chief Information Officer
CHR: Marcy Mills–Mathews, Director Human Resources
Web address: www.palmswesthospital.com
**Control:** Corporation, Investor–owned, for–profit **Service:** General Medical and Surgical

**Staffed Beds:** 166 **Admissions:** 12403 **Census:** 129 **Outpatient Visits:** 74551 **Births:** 1015 **Total Expense ($000):** 111901 **Payroll Expense ($000):** 43806 **Personnel:** 644

## MACCLENNY—Baker County

**ED FRASER MEMORIAL HOSPITAL AND BAKER COMMUNITY HEALTH CENTER (100134)**, 159 North Third Street, Zip 32063–0484, Mailing Address: P.O. Box 484, Zip 32063–0484; tel. 904/259–3151, (Nonreporting) **A**9 10 20
Primary Contact: Dennis R. Markos, Chief Executive Officer
CFO: Maria Allen, Chief Financial Officer
CMO: Mark Hardin, M.D., Medical Director
CIO: Kelly Lowery, Director Health Information Management
CHR: Linda Fries, Director Personnel
Web address: www.bcmedsvcs.com
**Control:** Other not–for–profit (including NFP Corporation) **Service:** General Medical and Surgical

**Staffed Beds:** 68

## MADISON—Madison County

**MADISON COUNTY MEMORIAL HOSPITAL (101311)**, 309 N.E. Marion Street, Zip 32340–2561; tel. 850/973–2271, (Nonreporting) **A**9 10 18
Primary Contact: David Abercrombie, Chief Executive Officer
COO: Tammy Stevens, Chief Operating Officer
CFO: Patrick Halfhill, Chief Financial Officer
CMO: Brett Perkins, M.D., Chief Medical Staff
CIO: Patrick Stiff, Coordinator Information Technology
CHR: Cindi Burnett, Chief Human Resources Officer
Web address: www.mcmh.us/
**Control:** Other not–for–profit (including NFP Corporation) **Service:** General Medical and Surgical

**Staffed Beds:** 25

## MARATHON—Monroe County

☒ **FISHERMEN'S HOSPITAL (101312)**, 3301 Overseas Highway, Zip 33050–0068; tel. 305/743–5533, (Data for 182 days) **A**1 9 10 18 20 **F**3 8 11 15 17 18 29 30 34 35 40 45 50 51 53 57 59 68 70 75 77 79 81 82 85 91 93 107 108 111 113 118 123 140 145 **P**6 8 **S** QHR, Brentwood, TN
Primary Contact: Hal W. Leftwich, FACHE, Chief Executive Officer
CFO: Carmen Acker, Chief Financial Officer
CMO: Harlan Pettit, M.D., Chief of Staff
CIO: Joe Brake, Director Information Services
CHR: Michele Teller, Director Human Resources
Web address: www.fishermenshospital.com
**Control:** Other not–for–profit (including NFP Corporation) **Service:** General Medical and Surgical

**Staffed Beds:** 25 **Admissions:** 303 **Census:** 6 **Outpatient Visits:** 7927 **Births:** 0 **Total Expense ($000):** 8492 **Payroll Expense ($000):** 5192 **Personnel:** 186

## MARGATE—Broward County

☒ **NORTHWEST MEDICAL CENTER (100189)**, 2801 North State Road 7, Zip 33063; tel. 954/974–0400, (Nonreporting) **A**1 9 10 **S** HCA, Nashville, TN
Primary Contact: Dianne Goldenberg, Chief Executive Officer
COO: Stacy Modlin, Chief Operating Officer
CFO: Gary Mervak, Chief Financial Officer
CMO: Peter Gach, M.D., Chief of Staff
CHR: Scott Mazo, Vice President Human Resources
Web address: www.northwestmed.com
**Control:** Corporation, Investor–owned, for–profit **Service:** General Medical and Surgical

**Staffed Beds:** 215

FL

---

**Hospital, Medicare Provider Number, Address, Telephone, Approval, Facility, and Physician Codes, Health Care System**

★ American Hospital Association (AHA) membership
☐ The Joint Commission accreditation    ◇ DNV Healthcare Inc. accreditation
○ American Osteopathic Association (AOA) accreditation
△ Commission on Accreditation of Rehabilitation Facilities (CARF) accreditation

## MARIANNA—Jackson County

⊞ **JACKSON HOSPITAL (100142)**, 4250 Hospital Drive, Zip 32446–1939, Mailing Address: P.O. Box 1608, Zip 32447–1608; tel. 850/526–2200, (Nonreporting) **A**1 9 10 20 **S** QHR, Brentwood, TN
Primary Contact: Larry Meese, Chief Executive Officer
CFO: Kevin Rovito, Interim Chief Financial Officer
CMO: Doyle Bosse, M.D., Chief Medical Officer
CIO: Beth Medlock, Manager Information Technology
CHR: Brooke G. Donaldson, Assistant Administrator Human Resources
Web address: www.jacksonhosp.com
**Control:** Hospital district or authority, Government, nonfederal **Service:** General Medical and Surgical

**Staffed Beds: 65**

## MELBOURNE—Brevard County

☐ **CIRCLES OF CARE (104024)**, 400 East Sheridan Road, Zip 32901–3184; tel. 321/722–5200, (Nonreporting) **A**1 9 10
Primary Contact: James B. Whitaker, President
CFO: David L. Feldman, Executive Vice President and Treasurer
CMO: Jose Alvarez, M.D., Chief Medical Staff
CHR: Linda Brannon, Vice President Human Resources
Web address: www.circlesofcare.org
**Control:** Other not–for–profit (including NFP Corporation) **Service:** Psychiatric

**Staffed Beds: 134**

**DEVEREUX HOSPITAL AND CHILDREN'S CENTER OF FLORIDA**, 8000 Devereux Drive, Zip 32940–7907; tel. 321/242–9100, (Nonreporting) **A**9 **S** Devereux, Villanova, PA
Primary Contact: Steven Murphy, Executive Director
COO: Amy Blakely, Assistant Executive Director Operations
CFO: Pamela Griffith, Director Administrative Services
CMO: Emilio Roig, M.D., Network Medical Director
CIO: Rob Fensterer, Director Information Services
Web address: www.devereux.org
**Control:** Other not–for–profit (including NFP Corporation) **Service:** Children's hospital psychiatric

**Staffed Beds: 100**

⊞ **HEALTHSOUTH SEA PINES REHABILITATION HOSPITAL (103034)**, 101 East Florida Avenue, Zip 32901–9966; tel. 321/984–4600, (Nonreporting) **A**1 9 10 **S** HEALTHSOUTH Corporation, Birmingham, AL
Primary Contact: Denise B. McGrath, Chief Executive Officer
CFO: Dana Edwards, Chief Financial Officer
CMO: Stuart P. Miller, M.D., Medical Director
CHR: Donna C. Anderson, Director Human Resources
Web address: www.healthsouthseapines.com
**Control:** Corporation, Investor–owned, for–profit **Service:** Rehabilitation

**Staffed Beds: 90**

⊞ **HOLMES REGIONAL MEDICAL CENTER (100019)**, 1350 South Hickory Street, Zip 32901–3276; tel. 321/434–7000 **A**1 2 9 10 **F**3 7 11 13 15 17 18 20 22 24 26 29 30 31 34 35 40 43 45 46 47 48 49 56 57 59 60 65 68 70 72 73 74 75 76 77 78 79 81 82 83 84 85 87 89 91 92 93 100 107 108 110 111 113 114 115 116 117 118 123 125 128 129 131 145 146 147 **P**6 7 **S** Health First, Inc., Rockledge, FL
Primary Contact: Judy Killebrew, President
CFO: Robert Galloway, Senior Vice President Finance and Chief Financial Officer
CMO: Scott Gettings, M.D., Vice President and Chief Medical Officer
CIO: Rich Rogers, Senior Vice President Support Services and Chief Information Officer
CHR: Robert W. Suttles, Vice President Human Resources
Web address: www.health–first.org
**Control:** Other not–for–profit (including NFP Corporation) **Service:** General Medical and Surgical

**Staffed Beds: 514 Admissions: 25709 Census: 389 Outpatient Visits: 215455 Births: 2729 Total Expense ($000): 410521 Payroll Expense ($000): 174838 Personnel: 2061**

★ **KINDRED HOSPITAL MELBOURNE (100312)**, 765 West Nasa Boulevard, Zip 32901–1815; tel. 321/733–5725, (Nonreporting) **S** Kindred Healthcare, Louisville, KY
Primary Contact: Angelica Cotshott, Chief Executive Officer
Web address: www.khmelbourne.com
**Control:** Corporation, Investor–owned, for–profit **Service:** Long–Term Acute Care hospital

**Staffed Beds: 60**

**PALM BAY HOSPITAL (100316)**, 1425 Malabar Road N.E., Zip 32907; tel. 321/434–8000 **A**9 10 **F**3 11 15 18 20 29 30 34 40 45 49 51 57 59 60 65 68 70 74 75 79 81 84 85 87 91 92 93 107 108 110 111 113 114 117 118 129 131 142 144 145 **P**6 7 **S** Health First, Inc., Rockledge, FL
Primary Contact: Roy Wright, FACHE, President
COO: Stuart Mitchell, Executive Vice President and Chief Operating Officer
CFO: Joseph G. Felkner, Senior Vice President and Chief Financial Officer
CMO: Scott Gettings, M.D., Vice President Medical Affairs
CIO: Christi C. Rushnell, Vice President Information Technology
CHR: Robert W. Suttles, Vice President Human Resources
CNO: Suzanne Woods, R.N., Vice President Nursing and Chief Nursing Officer
Web address: www.health–first.org
**Control:** Other not–for–profit (including NFP Corporation) **Service:** General Medical and Surgical

**Staffed Beds: 119 Admissions: 5272 Census: 68 Outpatient Visits: 73964 Births: 0 Total Expense ($000): 76453 Payroll Expense ($000): 33900 Personnel: 373**

**VIERA HOSPITAL (100315)**, 8745 North Wickham Road, Zip 32940–5997; tel. 321/434–9164, (Data for 182 days) **A**9 10 **F**3 11 12 15 18 20 22 26 29 30 31 34 35 38 40 44 45 46 47 48 49 50 51 56 57 59 60 64 68 70 74 75 77 78 79 81 82 85 86 87 93 94 97 107 108 110 111 114 115 116 118 123 125 131 144 145 147 **P**6 **S** Health First, Inc., Rockledge, FL
Primary Contact: Christopher Kennedy, President
Web address: www.vierahospital.org
**Control:** Other not–for–profit (including NFP Corporation) **Service:** General Medical and Surgical

**Staffed Beds: 84 Admissions: 1119 Census: 24 Outpatient Visits: 14281 Total Expense ($000): 33498 Payroll Expense ($000): 14117 Personnel: 192**

☐ **WUESTHOFF MEDICAL CENTER – MELBOURNE (100291)**, 250 North Wickham Road, Zip 32935; tel. 321/752–1200 **A**1 9 10 **F**3 11 12 15 18 20 22 29 30 38 40 49 50 51 57 59 60 64 68 70 74 75 76 77 79 80 81 85 87 89 93 102 107 108 111 113 114 115 116 118 125 129 130 131 134 143 145 146 147 **S** Health Management Associates, Naples, FL
Primary Contact: Jeannette Skinner, R.N., FACHE, Chief Executive Officer
CFO: Steve Bender, Chief Financial Officer
Web address: www.wuesthoff.org
**Control:** Corporation, Investor–owned, for–profit **Service:** General Medical and Surgical

**Staffed Beds: 115 Admissions: 5798 Census: 70 Total Expense ($000): 49379 Personnel: 373**

## MIAMI—Miami–Dade County

⊞ △ **BAPTIST HEALTH SOUTH FLORIDA, BAPTIST HOSPITAL OF MIAMI (100008)**, 8900 North Kendall Drive, Zip 33176–2197; tel. 786/596–1960, (Includes BAPTIST CHILDREN'S HOSPITAL, 8900 North Kendall Drive, Zip 33176–2118; tel. 786/596–1960) **A**1 2 3 5 7 9 10 **F**3 8 11 13 15 17 18 19 20 22 24 26 28 29 30 31 32 34 35 40 41 45 46 47 49 50 51 53 54 55 56 57 58 59 60 61 62 63 64 66 68 70 72 73 74 75 76 77 78 79 81 82 84 85 86 87 88 89 90 91 92 93 96 100 102 107 108 109 110 111 113 114 115 116 117 118 119 120 122 123 125 128 129 131 134 143 144 145 146 147 **P**6 **S** Baptist Health South Florida, Coral Gables, FL
Primary Contact: Bo Boulenger, Chief Executive Officer
COO: Randall Lee, Vice President and Chief Operating Officer
CFO: Ralph E. Lawson, Executive Vice President and Chief Financial Officer
CMO: Mark J. Hauser, M.D., Chief Medical Officer
CIO: Mimi Taylor, Corporate Vice President Information Technology
CHR: Corey Heller, Corporate Vice President and Chief Human Resources Officer
Web address: www.baptisthealth.net
**Control:** Other not–for–profit (including NFP Corporation) **Service:** General Medical and Surgical

**Staffed Beds: 672 Admissions: 38016 Census: 517 Outpatient Visits: 349697 Births: 4426 Total Expense ($000): 741909 Payroll Expense ($000): 262375 Personnel: 4238**

⊞ **BAPTIST HEALTH SOUTH FLORIDA, SOUTH MIAMI HOSPITAL (100154)**, 6200 S.W. 73rd Street, Zip 33143–9990; tel. 786/662–4000 **A**1 2 9 10 **F**3 4 5 11 12 13 15 17 18 20 22 24 26 28 29 30 31 34 35 36 40 46 48 49 50 51 52 53 54 57 58 59 60 61 64 68 70 72 74 75 76 77 78 79 81 82 84 85 86 87 93 107 108 110 111 113 114 115 116 118 119 120 122 123 125 128 129 131 134 143 145 146 147 **P**6 **S** Baptist Health South Florida, Coral Gables, FL
Primary Contact: Lincoln S. Mendez, Chief Executive Officer
COO: Jeanette Stone, Vice President Operations
CFO: Berta Rufat, Controller
CMO: Yvonne Johnson, M.D., President Medical Staff
CIO: Mimi Taylor, Vice President Information Technology
CHR: Diana Montenegro, Director Human Resources
Web address: www.baptisthealth.net
**Control:** Other not–for–profit (including NFP Corporation) **Service:** General Medical and Surgical

**Staffed Beds: 357 Admissions: 16073 Census: 217 Outpatient Visits: 226675 Births: 4444 Total Expense ($000): 408504 Payroll Expense ($000): 140076 Personnel: 2331**

*Many Facility Codes have changed. Please refer to the AHA Guide Code Chart.* © 2012 AHA Guide

FL

★ **BAPTIST HEALTH SOUTH FLORIDA, WEST KENDALL BAPTIST HOSPITAL (100314)**, 9555 S.W. 162nd Avenue, Zip 33196; tel. 786/467-2000, (Data for 157 days) **A**10 **F**3 13 18 19 29 30 31 34 35 40 41 45 49 50 51 53 57 59 63 64 68 70 74 75 76 78 79 81 82 84 85 86 87 93 100 102 107 108 109 111 113 114 118 129 130 131 134 145 147 **P**6 **S** Baptist Health South Florida, Coral Gables, FL
Primary Contact: Javier Hernandez-Lichtl, Chief Executive Officer
CFO: Odalys Remigio, Assistant Vice President, Finance
CMO: Juan-Carlos Verdeja, M.D., President of Medical Staff
CHR: Hilde Zamora de Aguero, Human Resources Site Director
CNO: Denise H. Harris, R.N., Chief Nursing Officer
Web address: www.westkendallbaptist.com
**Control:** Other not-for-profit (including NFP Corporation) **Service:** General Medical and Surgical

**Staffed Beds:** 133 **Admissions:** 1993 **Census:** 49 **Outpatient Visits:** 15981 **Births:** 76 **Total Expense ($000):** 85533 **Payroll Expense ($000):** 28167 **Personnel:** 791

⊞ **BASCOM PALMER EYE INSTITUTE-ANNE BATES LEACH EYE HOSPITAL (100240)**, 900 N.W. 17th Street, Zip 33136-1199, Mailing Address: Box 016880, Zip 33101-6880; tel. 305/326-6000, (Nonreporting) **A**1 3 5 9 10
Primary Contact: Michael B. Gittelman, Administrator
COO: Charles Pappas, M.D., Chief Operating Officer
CFO: Harry Rohrer, Chief Financial Officer
CMO: Eduardo Alfonso, M.D., Chairman Ophthalmology
CHR: Paul Hudgins, Associate Vice President Human Resources
Web address: www.bascompalmer.org
**Control:** Other not-for-profit (including NFP Corporation) **Service:** Eye, ear, nose, and throat

**Staffed Beds:** 56

**HEALTHSOUTH REHABILITATION HOSPITAL** See HEALTHSOUTH Rehabilitation Hospital of Miami

⊞ **HEALTHSOUTH REHABILITATION HOSPITAL OF MIAMI (103038)**, 20601 Old Cutler Road, Zip 33189-2400; tel. 305/251-3800 **A**1 9 10 **F**3 29 57 67 77 86 87 90 91 94 95 96 129 131 147 **S** HEALTHSOUTH Corporation, Birmingham, AL
Primary Contact: Elizabeth L. Izquierdo, CPA, Chief Executive Officer
CFO: Reyna Hernandez, Chief Financial Officer
CHR: Susan Riley, Director Human Resources
Web address: www.healthsouthmiami.com
**Control:** Corporation, Investor-owned, for-profit **Service:** Rehabilitation

**Staffed Beds:** 60 **Admissions:** 1018 **Census:** 39 **Outpatient Visits:** 7004 **Births:** 0 **Total Expense ($000):** 14098 **Payroll Expense ($000):** 7781

**HIGHLAND PARK HOSPITAL** See Jackson Health System

⊞ △ **JACKSON HEALTH SYSTEM (100022)**, 1611 N.W. 12th Avenue, Zip 33136-1094, (Includes HIGHLAND PARK HOSPITAL, 1695 N.W. Ninth Avenue, Zip 33136; tel. 305/355-8234; HOLTZ CHILDREN'S HOSPITAL, 1611 N.W. 12th Avenue, Zip 33136-1005; tel. 305/585-5437; Daniel Armstrong, Chief Administrative Officer; JACKSON MEMORIAL HOSPITAL, 1611 N.W. 12th Avenue, Zip 33136; tel. 305/585-6661; Alex Contreras-Soto, Senior Vice President and Chief Administrative Officer; JACKSON NORTH MEDICAL CENTER, 160 N.W. 170th Street, North Miami Beach, Zip 33169-5576; tel. 305/651-1100; Sandy Sears, Senior Vice President and Chief Administrative Officer; JACKSON SOUTH COMMUNITY HOSPITAL, 9333 S.W. 152nd Street, Zip 33157-1780; tel. 305/251-2500; Martha Garcia, Senior Vice President and Chief Administrative Officer, (Total facility includes 310 beds in nursing home-type unit) **A**1 2 3 5 7 8 9 10 **F**1 3 4 5 9 11 12 13 15 16 17 18 19 20 21 22 23 24 25 26 27 28 29 30 31 34 35 36 38 39 40 41 43 44 45 46 47 48 49 50 51 54 56 57 58 59 60 61 63 64 65 66 68 70 71 72 73 74 75 76 77 78 79 80 81 82 83 84 85 86 87 88 89 90 91 92 93 94 96 97 98 99 100 101 102 103 104 105 106 107 108 110 111 113 114 116 117 118 119 120 122 125 127 128 129 130 131 133 134 135 136 137 138 139 140 141 143 144 145 146 147
Primary Contact: Carlos A. Migoya, President and Chief Executive Officer
COO: Don S. Steigman, Chief Operating Officer
CFO: Mark T. Knight, Executive Vice President and Chief Financial Officer
CMO: Michael K. Butler, M.D., Executive Vice President and Chief Medical Officer
CIO: Fernando Martinez, Vice President and Chief Information Officer
CHR: Trummell Valdera, Senior Vice President and Chief Human Resources Officer
Web address: www.um-jmh.org
**Control:** County-Government, nonfederal **Service:** General Medical and Surgical

**Staffed Beds:** 1637 **Admissions:** 64803 **Census:** 1155 **Outpatient Visits:** 320893 **Births:** 6884 **Total Expense ($000):** 1136299 **Payroll Expense ($000):** 735837 **Personnel:** 8570

**JACKSON SOUTH COMMUNITY HOSPITAL** See Jackson Health System

⊞ **KENDALL REGIONAL MEDICAL CENTER (100209)**, 11750 Bird Road, Zip 33175-3530; tel. 305/223-3000, (Nonreporting) **A**1 9 10 **S** HCA, Nashville, TN
Primary Contact: Scott A. Cihak, Chief Executive Officer
COO: Elizabeth Durrence, Chief Operating Officer
CFO: Ricardo Pavon, Chief Financial Officer
CIO: Ralph Ruiz, Director Information Technology and Services
CHR: Tom Nesbit, Director Human Resources
Web address: www.kendallmed.com
**Control:** Partnership, Investor-owned, for-profit **Service:** General Medical and Surgical

**Staffed Beds:** 300

☐ **METROPOLITAN HOSPITAL OF MIAMI (100076)**, 5959 N.W. Seventh Street, Zip 33126-3198; tel. 305/264-1000 **A**1 9 10 **F**3 15 26 29 31 40 43 45 49 56 57 60 61 64 68 70 74 75 77 78 79 81 83 84 85 87 93 107 108 111 112 113 118 129 134 140 142 145 147
Primary Contact: Ismael Roque-Velasco, M.D., Chief Executive Officer
CFO: Vivian Acevedo, Chief Financial Officer
CIO: Frank Canovaca, Director Management Information Systems
CHR: Mirelis Asper, Human Resources Generalist
Web address: www.mhmiami.com
**Control:** Corporation, Investor-owned, for-profit **Service:** General Medical and Surgical

**Staffed Beds:** 146 **Admissions:** 5016 **Census:** 67 **Outpatient Visits:** 31951 **Births:** 0

⊞ **MIAMI CHILDREN'S HOSPITAL (103301)**, 3100 S.W. 62nd Avenue, Zip 33155-3009; tel. 305/666-6511 **A**1 2 3 5 9 10 12 13 **F**1 3 4 7 8 9 16 17 19 20 21 22 23 25 27 29 30 31 32 34 35 36 38 39 40 42 43 44 45 46 50 53 54 55 57 58 59 60 61 64 65 66 67 68 70 71 72 73 74 75 77 78 79 80 81 82 85 86 87 88 89 90 93 97 98 99 100 101 102 104 105 106 107 108 111 113 115 116 117 118 126 127 128 129 130 131 133 135 143 145 **P**6
Primary Contact: M. Narendra Kini, M.D., President and Chief Executive Officer
COO: Kevin R. Hammeran, Executive Vice President and Chief Operating Officer
CFO: Pedro Alfaro, Vice President and Chief Financial Officer
CMO: Deise Granado-Villar, M.D., Chief Medical Officer and Senior Vice President Medical Affairs
CIO: Edward Martinez, Chief Information Officer
Web address: www.mch.com
**Control:** Other not-for-profit (including NFP Corporation) **Service:** Children's general

**Staffed Beds:** 272 **Admissions:** 12172 **Census:** 185 **Outpatient Visits:** 401926 **Births:** 0 **Total Expense ($000):** 442640 **Payroll Expense ($000):** 217031 **Personnel:** 3499

⊞ **MIAMI JEWISH HOME AND HOSPITAL FOR AGED (100277)**, 5200 N.E. Second Avenue, Zip 33137-2706; tel. 305/751-8626, (Nonreporting) **A**1 3 5 10
Primary Contact: Jeffrey P. Freimark, Chief Executive Officer
CFO: Lisa Jo Desmarteau, Chief Financial Officer
CMO: Brian Kiedrowski, M.D., Chief Medical Director
CHR: Larry McDonald, Director Human Resources
Web address: www.mjhha.org
**Control:** Other not-for-profit (including NFP Corporation) **Service:** General Medical and Surgical

**Staffed Beds:** 32

⊞ **NORTH SHORE MEDICAL CENTER (100029)**, 1100 N.W. 95th Street, Zip 33150-2098; tel. 305/835-6000, (Nonreporting) **A**1 2 9 10 **S** TENET Healthcare Corporation, Dallas, TX
Primary Contact: Manuel Linares, Chief Executive Officer
COO: Patricia Sechi, Chief Operating Officer
CFO: Alex Fernandez, Chief Financial Officer
CMO: Susan Baker, M.D., Chief of Staff
CIO: Luis Estrada, Director Multifacility Information Systems
CHR: Carmen Gomez, Director Human Resources
CNO: Rita Hess, R.N., Chief Nursing Officer
Web address: www.northshoremedical.com
**Control:** Corporation, Investor-owned, for-profit **Service:** General Medical and Surgical

**Staffed Beds:** 357

⊞ **SELECT SPECIALTY HOSPITAL-MIAMI (102001)**, 955 N.W. 3rd Street, Zip 33128; tel. 305/416-5700, (Nonreporting) **A**1 9 10 **S** Select Medical Corporation, Mechanicsburg, PA
Primary Contact: Dionisio Bencomo, Chief Executive Officer
Web address: www.selectmedicalcorp.com
**Control:** Corporation, Investor-owned, for-profit **Service:** Long-Term Acute Care hospital

**Staffed Beds:** 40

FL

☐ **SISTER EMMANUEL HOSPITAL (102016)**, 3663 South Miami Avenue, Zip 33133–4253; tel. 305/285–2939, (Nonreporting) **A**1 9 10
Primary Contact: Shed Boren, Administrator and Chief Executive Officer
CFO: Miguel Vasquez, Chief Financial Officer
CMO: Hugo Gonzalez, M.D., Chief Medical Officer
CIO: Macarena Restrepo, Manager Business Office
CHR: Kathy Mainieri, Human Resource Specialist
Web address: www.sisteremmanuelhospital.org/
**Control:** Church–operated, Nongovernment, not–for profit **Service:** Long–Term Acute Care hospital

**Staffed Beds:** 29

☒ **UNIVERSITY OF MIAMI HOSPITAL (100009)**, 1400 N.W. 12th Avenue, Zip 33136–1003; tel. 305/325–5511 **A**1 2 3 5 9 10 **F**3 11 12 15 17 18 20 22 24 26 29 30 31 34 35 36 39 40 44 45 47 48 49 50 51 56 57 58 59 60 61 63 64 68 70 74 75 77 78 79 80 81 82 84 85 86 87 93 96 97 98 102 103 107 108 111 113 114 140 134 140 145 147
Primary Contact: Daniel J. Snyder, Chief Executive Officer
COO: David Zambrana, R.N., Chief Operating Officer and Chief Nursing Officer
CFO: Darryl Caulton, Chief Financial Officer
CMO: Francisco Kerdel, M.D., President Medical Staff
CIO: Craig Scott, Interim Director Management Information Systems
CHR: Errol Douglas, Director Human Resources
Web address: www.umiamihospital.com
**Control:** Other not–for–profit (including NFP Corporation) **Service:** General Medical and Surgical

**Staffed Beds:** 525 **Admissions:** 19667 **Census:** 332 **Outpatient Visits:** 83627 **Births:** 0 **Total Expense ($000):** 318233 **Personnel:** 2033

☒ **UNIVERSITY OF MIAMI HOSPITAL AND CLINICS (100079)**, 1475 N.W. 12th Avenue, Zip 33136–1002; tel. 305/243–1000 **A**1 2 3 5 9 10 **F**3 9 11 15 29 30 31 34 35 36 38 44 45 46 47 48 49 54 56 57 58 59 60 61 64 68 70 74 75 77 78 79 81 82 84 85 86 87 97 99 100 101 102 103 104 107 108 110 111 113 114 116 117 118 119 120 122 123 129 131 134 140 145 146 **P**6
Primary Contact: Richard R. Ballard, Administrator
COO: Lazara Pagan, Chief Operating Officer
CFO: Harry Rohrer, Chief Financial Officer
CMO: W. Jarrad Goodwin, M.D., Director
CHR: Paul Hudgins, Associate Vice President Human Resources
Web address: www.uhealthsystem.com
**Control:** Other not–for–profit (including NFP Corporation) **Service:** General Medical and Surgical

**Staffed Beds:** 40 **Admissions:** 1143 **Census:** 17 **Outpatient Visits:** 305656 **Births:** 0 **Total Expense ($000):** 259195 **Payroll Expense ($000):** 55233 **Personnel:** 972

☒ △ **VETERANS AFFAIRS MEDICAL CENTER**, 1201 N.W. 16th Street, Zip 33125–1624; tel. 305/575–7000, (Nonreporting) **A**1 3 5 7 8 **S** Department of Veterans Affairs, Washington, DC
Primary Contact: Paul Russo, Director
COO: Paul D. Magalian, Associate Director
CFO: Rick Hunter, Chief Financial Officer
CMO: John Vara, M.D., Chief of Staff
CIO: Bill Tyson, Chief Information Officer
CHR: Larry Brinkman, Chief Human Resources
Web address: www.va.gov/miami
**Control:** Veterans Affairs, Government, federal **Service:** General Medical and Surgical

**Staffed Beds:** 281

☒ △ **WEST GABLES REHABILITATION HOSPITAL (103036)**, 2525 S.W. 75th Avenue, Zip 33155–2800; tel. 305/262–6800, (Nonreporting) **A**1 7 9 10 **S** Select Medical Corporation, Mechanicsburg, PA
Primary Contact: Walter Concepcion, Chief Executive Officer
CFO: Sara Reohr, Regional Controller
CMO: Jose L. Vargas, M.D., Medical Director
CHR: Barbara Etchason, HR Manager
CNO: Constance Hughes, Director of Nursing
Web address: www.westgablesrehabhospital.com/
**Control:** Corporation, Investor–owned, for–profit **Service:** Rehabilitation

**Staffed Beds:** 60

○ **WESTCHESTER GENERAL HOSPITAL (100284)**, 2500 S.W. 75th Avenue, Zip 33155–9947; tel. 305/264–5252, (Includes SOUTHERN WINDS HOSPITAL, 4225 West 20th Street, Hialeah, Zip 33012–5835; tel. 305/558–9700) **A**9 10 11 12 13 **F**3 15 18 29 31 40 45 49 56 65 70 74 75 77 78 79 81 85 87 98 99 100 102 103 107 108 110 113 114 118 129
Primary Contact: Gilda Baldwin, Chief Executive Officer
CFO: Henry Brown, Chief Financial Officer
CMO: Rogelio Zaldivar, M.D., Medical Director
CHR: Alicia Lund, Director Human Resources
Web address: www.westchesterhospital.com
**Control:** Corporation, Investor–owned, for–profit **Service:** General Medical and Surgical

**Staffed Beds:** 197 **Admissions:** 9021 **Census:** 149 **Outpatient Visits:** 31297 **Births:** 0 **Total Expense ($000):** 57004 **Payroll Expense ($000):** 30848 **Personnel:** 560

---

**MIAMI BEACH—Dade County**

**MIAMI HEART CAMPUS AT MOUNT SINAI MEDICAL CENTER** See Mount Sinai Medical Center

☐ △ **MOUNT SINAI MEDICAL CENTER (100034)**, 4300 Alton Road, Zip 33140–2800; tel. 305/674–2121, (Includes MIAMI HEART CAMPUS AT MOUNT SINAI MEDICAL CENTER, 4701 North Meridian Avenue, Zip 33140–2910; tel. 305/672–1111) **A**1 2 3 5 7 8 9 10 13 **F**3 6 8 13 14 15 17 18 20 22 24 26 28 29 30 31 34 35 37 39 40 42 43 44 45 46 47 48 49 50 51 53 54 55 56 57 58 59 60 61 62 64 65 66 70 71 72 73 74 75 76 77 78 79 81 82 83 84 85 86 87 90 91 92 93 96 97 98 100 101 102 103 104 107 108 109 110 111 113 114 115 116 117 118 119 120 121 122 123 125 127 128 129 130 131 134 136 142 144 145 146 147
Primary Contact: Steven D. Sonenreich, President and Chief Executive Officer
COO: Amy Perry, Senior Vice President and Chief Operating Officer
CFO: Alex A. Mendez, Senior Vice President and Chief Financial Officer
CMO: Robert Goldszer, M.D., Senior Vice President and Chief Medical Officer
CIO: Tom Gillette, Vice President and Chief Information Officer
CHR: Georgia McLean, Director Human Resources
Web address: www.msmc.com
**Control:** Other not–for–profit (including NFP Corporation) **Service:** General Medical and Surgical

**Staffed Beds:** 666 **Admissions:** 22926 **Census:** 391 **Outpatient Visits:** 183958 **Births:** 2748 **Total Expense ($000):** 450006 **Payroll Expense ($000):** 153841 **Personnel:** 3294

---

**MILTON—Santa Rosa County**

☐ **SANTA ROSA MEDICAL CENTER (100124)**, 1450 Berryhill Road, Zip 32570–4028, Mailing Address: P.O. Box 648, Zip 32572–0648; tel. 850/626–7762, (Nonreporting) **A**1 9 10 **S** Health Management Associates, Naples, FL
Primary Contact: Phillip L. Wright, FACHE, Chief Executive Officer
CFO: Kay Burns, Chief Financial Officer
CIO: Rick Payne, Director Information Systems
Web address: www.santarosamedicalcenter.org
**Control:** Corporation, Investor–owned, for–profit **Service:** General Medical and Surgical

**Staffed Beds:** 105

**WEST FLORIDA COMMUNITY CARE CENTER (104027)**, 5500 Stewart Street, Zip 32570–4304; tel. 850/983–5500, (Nonreporting) **A**10
Primary Contact: Carmen Paroby, Chief Executive Officer
**Control:** Other not–for–profit (including NFP Corporation) **Service:** Psychiatric

**Staffed Beds:** 100

---

**MIRAMAR—Broward County**

☒ **MEMORIAL HOSPITAL MIRAMAR (100285)**, 1901 S.W. 172nd Avenue, Zip 33029; tel. 954/538–5000 **A**1 9 10 **F**3 13 15 29 30 40 41 45 49 50 57 59 61 64 70 72 74 75 76 77 78 79 81 82 85 86 87 89 93 96 107 108 109 110 111 113 114 118 125 129 130 131 145 **S** Memorial Healthcare System, Hollywood, FL
Primary Contact: Leah A. Carpenter, Chief Executive Officer
CFO: Judy Sada, Chief Financial Officer
CMO: Stanley Marks, M.D., Chief Medical Officer
CIO: Forest Blanton, Senior VP and Chief Information Officer
CHR: Ray Kendrick, Chief Human Resources Officer
CNO: Denise Reynolds, Chief Nursing Officer
Web address: www.mhs.net
**Control:** Hospital district or authority, Government, nonfederal **Service:** General Medical and Surgical

**Staffed Beds:** 178 **Admissions:** 10512 **Census:** 104 **Outpatient Visits:** 117778 **Births:** 3350 **Total Expense ($000):** 131972 **Payroll Expense ($000):** 61810 **Personnel:** 803

---

**MIRAMAR BEACH—Walton County**

☒ **SACRED HEART HOSPITAL ON THE EMERALD COAST (100292)**, 7800 Highway 98 West, Zip 32550; tel. 850/278–3000 **A**1 9 10 **F**3 11 13 15 18 20 28 29 30 31 34 35 40 44 49 50 51 53 57 59 60 64 68 70 74 75 76 78 79 81 82 84 85 86 87 93 96 107 108 110 111 113 114 117 118 120 122 123 129 131 134 145 146 147 **S** Ascension Health, Saint Louis, MO
Primary Contact: Roger L. Hall, President
Web address: www.sacredheartemerald.org
**Control:** Other not–for–profit (including NFP Corporation) **Service:** General Medical and Surgical

**Staffed Beds:** 58 **Admissions:** 4101 **Census:** 36 **Outpatient Visits:** 222818 **Births:** 814 **Total Expense ($000):** 69936 **Payroll Expense ($000):** 23271 **Personnel:** 379

## NAPLES—Collier County

☒ △ **NCH DOWNTOWN NAPLES HOSPITAL (100018)**, 350 Seventh Street North, Zip 34102–4746, Mailing Address: P.O. Box 413029, Zip 34101–3029; tel. 239/436–5000, (Includes NCH NORTH NAPLES HOSPITAL, 11190 Health Park Boulevard, Zip 34110–5729, Mailing Address: 11190 Health Park Boulevard, Zip 34110–5729; tel. 239/552–7000) **A**1 2 7 9 10 **F**3 11 13 14 18 20 22 24 26 28 29 30 31 34 37 40 41 45 47 49 50 53 56 57 59 64 68 70 72 74 75 76 77 78 79 80 81 82 84 85 86 87 89 90 93 95 96 98 102 103 107 108 111 113 118 125 129 134 145 146
Primary Contact: Allen S. Weiss, M.D., President and Chief Executive Officer
COO: Phillip C. Dutcher, Chief Operating Officer
CFO: Vicki Hale, Chief Financial Officer
CMO: Aurora Estevez, M.D., Chief Medical Officer
CIO: Susan Wolff, Chief Information Officer
Web address: www.nchmd.org
**Control:** Other not–for–profit (including NFP Corporation) **Service:** General Medical and Surgical

**Staffed Beds:** 681 **Admissions:** 31974 **Census:** 399 **Outpatient Visits:** 289549 **Births:** 3033 **Total Expense ($000):** 358872 **Payroll Expense ($000):** 157998 **Personnel:** 2899

☐ **PHYSICIANS REGIONAL MEDICAL CENTER – PINE RIDGE (100286)**, 6101 Pine Ridge Road, Zip 34119; tel. 239/348–4000, (Includes PHYSICIANS REGIONAL MEDICAL CENTER, 8300 Collier Boulevard, Zip 34114; tel. 239/354–6000), (Nonreporting) **A**1 9 10 **S** Health Management Associates, Naples, FL
Primary Contact: Geoffrey D. Moebius, Chief Executive Officer
CIO: Lisa Gardiner, Director Marketing and Public Relations
CHR: Andrew Nottidge, Director Human Resources
Web address: www.physiciansregional.com
**Control:** Corporation, Investor–owned, for–profit **Service:** General Medical and Surgical

**Staffed Beds:** 70

☐ **WILLOUGH HEALTHCARE SYSTEM (104063)**, 9001 Tamiami Trail East, Zip 34113–3316; tel. 239/775–4500, (Nonreporting) **A**1 9 10
Primary Contact: James E. O'Shea, Administrator
CFO: Steve Baldwin, Vice President Finance
Web address: www.thewilloughatnaples.com/
**Control:** Corporation, Investor–owned, for–profit **Service:** Psychiatric

**Staffed Beds:** 80

## NEW PORT RICHEY—Pasco County

☒ △ **MORTON PLANT NORTH BAY HOSPITAL (100063)**, 6600 Madison Street, Zip 34652–1900; tel. 727/842–8468, (Nonreporting) **A**1 7 9 10 **S** Morton Plant Mease Health Care, Clearwater, FL
Primary Contact: Glenn D. Waters, FACHE, President
COO: Hal Ziecheck, Chief Operating Officer
CFO: Carl Tremonti, Chief Financial Officer
CMO: Donald Pocock, M.D., Chief Medical Officer
CHR: Sharon Collotta, Director Team Resources
CNO: Lisa Johnson, R.N., Chief Nursing Executive
Web address: www.mpmhealth.com
**Control:** Other not–for–profit (including NFP Corporation) **Service:** General Medical and Surgical

**Staffed Beds:** 122

## NEW SMYRNA BEACH—Volusia County

☒ **BERT FISH MEDICAL CENTER (100014)**, 401 Palmetto Street, Zip 32168–7399; tel. 386/424–5000, (Nonreporting) **A**1 9 10
Primary Contact: Steven W. Harrell, FACHE, Interim Chief Executive Officer
COO: Steven W. Harrell, FACHE, Chief Operating Officer
CFO: Al W. Allred, Chief Financial Officer
CMO: Rajesh Ailani, M.D., Chief Medical Staff
CIO: Debbie Burgess, Director Information Services
CHR: Nancy K. Evolga, Executive Director Human Resources
CNO: Linda Breum, R.N., Chief Nursing Officer
Web address: www.bertfish.com
**Control:** Hospital district or authority, Government, nonfederal **Service:** General Medical and Surgical

**Staffed Beds:** 112

## NICEVILLE—Okaloosa County

☒ **TWIN CITIES HOSPITAL (100054)**, 2190 Highway 85 North, Zip 32578–1045; tel. 850/678–4131, (Nonreporting) **A**1 9 10 **S** HCA, Nashville, TN
Primary Contact: David Whalen, Chief Executive Officer
CFO: Mark Day, Chief Financial Officer
CHR: Cyndi Ronca, Director Human Resources
Web address: www.tchealthcare.com
**Control:** Corporation, Investor–owned, for–profit **Service:** General Medical and Surgical

**Staffed Beds:** 65

## NORTH MIAMI—Miami–Dade County

☒ △ **ST. CATHERINE'S REHABILITATION HOSPITAL (103026)**, 1050 N.E. 125th Street, Zip 33161–5881; tel. 305/357–1735, (Nonreporting) **A**1 7 9 10
Primary Contact: Jaime Gonzalez, Administrator
COO: Jim Ball, Chief Operating Officer
CFO: Mary Jo Frick, Director Finance
CMO: Miriam Feliz, M.D., Medical Director
Web address: www.catholichealthservices.org
**Control:** Church–operated, Nongovernment, not–for profit **Service:** Rehabilitation

**Staffed Beds:** 60

## NORTH MIAMI BEACH—Dade County

**JACKSON NORTH MEDICAL CENTER** See Jackson Health System, Miami

## OCALA—Marion County

☒ **KINDRED HOSPITAL OCALA (102019)**, 1500 S.W. 1st Avenue, Zip 34474; tel. 352/369–0513, (Nonreporting) **A**1 10 **S** Kindred Healthcare, Louisville, KY
Primary Contact: Marc Lemon, Administrator
CFO: Joyce Caltrider, Chief Financial Officer
CFO: Dean Cocchi, Chief Financial Officer
CNO: Merlene Bhoorasingh, Chief Clinical Officer
Web address: www.kindredocala.com/
**Control:** Corporation, Investor–owned, for–profit **Service:** Other specialty

**Staffed Beds:** 31

**MARION–CITRUS MENTAL HEALTH CENTERS (104068)**, 5664 S.W. 60th Avenue, Zip 34474–5677; tel. 352/291–5500, (Nonreporting) **A**9 10
Primary Contact: Boswell Trowers, Director
Web address: www.marion–citrusmhc.org/
**Control:** Corporation, Investor–owned, for–profit **Service:** Other specialty

**Staffed Beds:** 40

☒ **MUNROE REGIONAL MEDICAL CENTER (100062)**, 1500 S.W. 1st Avenue, Zip 34471–4059, Mailing Address: P.O. Box 6000, Zip 34478–000; tel. 352/351–7200 **A**1 5 9 10 **F**3 11 12 13 15 17 18 20 22 24 26 28 29 30 34 35 36 37 40 41 42 45 46 47 48 49 51 53 56 57 58 59 60 64 65 67 70 71 74 75 76 77 79 81 83 84 85 86 87 89 93 96 107 111 113 114 118 119 123 125 129 130 131 133 134 145 146 147
Primary Contact: Stephen A. Purves, FACHE, President and Chief Executive Officer
COO: Paul Clark, Senior Vice President and Chief Operating Officer
CFO: Richard Mutarelli, Chief Financial Officer
CMO: Lon McPherson, M.D., Senior Vice President Medical Affairs and Chief Quality Officer
CIO: Carl Candullo, Chief Information Officer
CHR: Pamela W. Michell, R.N., Vice President and Chief Nursing Officer
CHR: Daniel O'Connor, Vice President Human Resources
CNO: Pamela W. Michell, R.N., Chief Nursing Officer
Web address: www.munroeregional.com
**Control:** Hospital district or authority, Government, nonfederal **Service:** General Medical and Surgical

**Staffed Beds:** 420 **Admissions:** 22494 **Census:** 278 **Outpatient Visits:** 155217 **Births:** 2668 **Total Expense ($000):** 252696 **Payroll Expense ($000):** 116862 **Personnel:** 2372

☒ **OCALA REGIONAL MEDICAL CENTER (100212)**, 1431 S.W. First Avenue, Zip 34474–4058, Mailing Address: P.O. Box 2200, Zip 34478–2200; tel. 352/401–1000, (Includes WEST MARION COMMUNITY HOSPITAL, 4600 S.W. 46th Court, Zip 34471; tel. 352/291–3000), (Nonreporting) **A**1 2 9 10 **S** HCA, Nashville, TN
Primary Contact: Randall McVay, Chief Executive Officer
COO: Brad Griffin, Chief Operating Officer
CMO: Art Osberg, M.D., Vice President and Chief Medical Officer
CIO: Taylor Dickerson, Director Information Services
CHR: Wayne Nielsen, Director Human Resources
Web address: www.ocalaregional.com
**Control:** Corporation, Investor–owned, for–profit **Service:** General Medical and Surgical

**Staffed Beds:** 270

FL

---

**Hospital, Medicare Provider Number, Address, Telephone, Approval, Facility, and Physician Codes, Health Care System**

★ American Hospital Association (AHA) membership
☐ The Joint Commission accreditation
◇ DNV Healthcare Inc. accreditation
○ American Osteopathic Association (AOA) accreditation
△ Commission on Accreditation of Rehabilitation Facilities (CARF) accreditation

**THE VINES (104071)**, 3130 S.W. 27th Avenue, Zip 34474; tel. 352/671-3130, (Nonreporting) **A**10 **S** Universal Health Services, Inc., King of Prussia, PA
Primary Contact: Michael McDonald, Chief Executive Officer
Web address: www.tenbroeckocala.com
**Control:** Corporation, Investor-owned, for-profit **Service:** Psychiatric

| Staffed Beds: 90 |
| --- |

### OCOEE—Orange County

**HEALTH CENTRAL (100030)**, 10000 West Colonial Drive, Zip 34761-3499; tel. 407/296-1000, (Total facility includes 228 beds in nursing home–type unit) **A**1 9 10 **F**3 8 11 12 13 15 17 18 20 22 26 28 29 30 34 35 37 40 45 49 50 51 57 59 60 64 70 73 74 75 76 77 79 81 82 85 86 87 89 92 93 97 107 108 110 111 113 114 117 118 127 128 129 131 143 145 146 147 **P**6 **S** Orlando Health, Orlando, FL
Primary Contact: Gregory P. Ohe, President and Chief Executive Officer
COO: Gregory P. Ohe, President and Chief Operating Officer
CFO: Michael E. Mueller, Chief Financial Officer
CMO: James Barton Rodier, M.D., Chief Quality Officer
CIO: John M. Sills, Chief Information Officer
CHR: John Sullivan, Vice President Human Resources
CNO: Susan E. Jackson, R.N., Senior Vice President
Web address: www.healthcentral.org
**Control:** Hospital district or authority, Government, nonfederal **Service:** General Medical and Surgical

| Staffed Beds: 399 Admissions: 11882 Census: 336 Outpatient Visits: 117326 Births: 1037 Total Expense ($000): 122831 Payroll Expense ($000): 72798 Personnel: 1257 |
| --- |

### OKEECHOBEE—Okeechobee County

**RAULERSON HOSPITAL (100252)**, 1796 Highway 441 North, Zip 34972-1918, Mailing Address: P.O. Box 1307, Zip 34973-1307; tel. 863/763-2151, (Nonreporting) **A**1 9 10 20 **S** HCA, Nashville, TN
Primary Contact: Robert H. Lee, President
CFO: Heather Garvey, Chief Financial Officer
CMO: Mohammad Riaz, M.D., Chief of Staff
CIO: Doug Schneider, Director Information Systems
CHR: Janis Stevens, Director Human Resources
Web address: www.raulersonhospital.com
**Control:** Corporation, Investor-owned, for-profit **Service:** General Medical and Surgical

| Staffed Beds: 100 |
| --- |

### ORANGE CITY—Volusia County

**FLORIDA HOSPITAL FISH MEMORIAL (100072)**, 1055 Saxon Boulevard, Zip 32763-8468; tel. 386/917-5000 **A**1 9 10 **F**3 11 15 20 28 29 30 31 34 35 37 40 45 48 49 59 64 70 74 75 77 78 79 81 82 85 87 91 92 93 100 104 107 108 110 111 113 114 115 116 117 118 119 120 128 129 131 134 143 145 146 147 **P**8 **S** Adventist Health System Sunbelt Health Care Corporation, Altamonte Springs, FL
Primary Contact: Ed Noseworthy, President and Chief Executive Officer
COO: Danielle Johnson, Chief Operating Officer
CFO: Eric Osterly, Chief Financial Officer
CIO: Trish Stebbins, Director Management Information Systems
CHR: Bonne S. Macpherson, Director Human Resources
CNO: Jennifer Shull, R.N., Chief Nursing Officer
Web address: www.fhfishmemorial.org
**Control:** Church-operated, Nongovernment, not-for profit **Service:** General Medical and Surgical

| Staffed Beds: 175 Admissions: 8394 Census: 101 Outpatient Visits: 99644 Births: 4 Total Expense ($000): 121284 Payroll Expense ($000): 46427 Personnel: 893 |
| --- |

### ORANGE PARK—Clay County

**ORANGE PARK MEDICAL CENTER (100226)**, 2001 Kingsley Avenue, Zip 32073-5156; tel. 904/276-8500, (Nonreporting) **A**1 2 9 10 **S** HCA, Nashville, TN
Primary Contact: Thomas R. Pentz, President and Chief Executive Officer
COO: Marsha A. Easley, Chief Operating Officer
CFO: Bryce DeHaven, Chief Financial Officer
CMO: Lawrence Coots, M.D., Chief Medical Officer
CIO: Karen Parish, Director Information Systems
CHR: Thomas R. Pentz, Chief Executive Officer
CNO: Kathy Hester, Chief Nursing Officer
Web address: www.opmedical.com
**Control:** Corporation, Investor-owned, for-profit **Service:** General Medical and Surgical

| Staffed Beds: 230 |
| --- |

### ORLANDO—Orange County

**ARNOLD PALMER CHILDREN'S HOSPITAL** See Orlando Regional Medical Center

**CENTRAL FLORIDA BEHAVIORAL HOSPITAL (104072)**, 6601 Central Florida Parkway, Zip 32821-8064; tel. 407/370-0111, (Nonreporting) **A**1 9 10 **S** Universal Health Services, Inc., King of Prussia, PA
Primary Contact: Vickie Lewis, Chief Executive Officer
Web address: www.centralfloridabehavioral.com
**Control:** Other not-for-profit (including NFP Corporation) **Service:** Psychiatric

| Staffed Beds: 120 |
| --- |

△ **FLORIDA HOSPITAL (100007)**, 601 East Rollins Street, Zip 32803-1489; tel. 407/303-6611, (Includes DISNEY CHILDREN'S HOSPITAL, 601 East Rollins Street, Zip 32803-1248; tel. 407/303-9732; FLORIDA HOSPITAL CELEBRATION HEALTH, 400 Clebration Place, Celebration, Zip 34747; tel. 407/303-4000; Monica Reed, M.D., Administrator; FLORIDA HOSPITAL EAST ORLANDO, 7727 Lake Underhill Drive, Zip 32822; tel. 407/277-8110; FLORIDA HOSPITAL KISSIMMEE, 2450 North Orange Blossom Trai, Kissimmee, Zip 34741; tel. 407/846-4343; William Haupt, Administrator; FLORIDA HOSPITAL-ALTAMONTE, 601 East Altamonte Drive, Altamonte Springs, Zip 32701; tel. 407/830-4321; Rob Fulbright, Administrator; FLORIDA HOSPITAL-APOPKA, 201 North Park Avenue, Apopka, Zip 32703; tel. 407/889-2566; Verbelee Neilsen Swanson, Administrator; WINTER PARK MEMORIAL HOSPITAL, 200 North Lakemont Avenue, Winter Park, Zip 32792-3273; tel. 407/646-7000; Ken Bradley, Administrator) **A**1 2 3 5 7 8 9 10 21 **F**3 7 9 11 12 13 14 15 17 18 19 20 21 22 24 26 28 29 30 31 32 34 35 36 37 38 39 40 41 44 45 46 47 48 49 50 51 53 54 56 57 58 59 60 61 62 64 65 66 68 70 72 73 74 75 76 77 78 79 80 81 82 84 85 86 87 88 89 90 91 92 93 94 96 97 98 100 101 102 103 104 107 108 110 111 112 113 114 115 116 117 118 119 120 122 123 125 128 129 130 131 133 134 135 136 137 138 140 141 144 145 146 147 **P**1 6 8 **S** Adventist Health System Sunbelt Health Care Corporation, Altamonte Springs, FL
Primary Contact: Lars D. Houmann, President
COO: Brian Paradis, Chief Operating Officer
CFO: Eddie Soler, Chief Financial Officer
CMO: David Moorhead, M.D., Chief Medical Officer
CIO: Andy Crowder, Chief Information Officer
CHR: Sheryl Dodds, Chief Clinical Officer
Web address: www.flhosp.org
**Control:** Other not-for-profit (including NFP Corporation) **Service:** General Medical and Surgical

| Staffed Beds: 2170 Admissions: 122729 Census: 1601 Outpatient Visits: 904759 Births: 9084 Total Expense ($000): 2691588 Payroll Expense ($000): 808071 Personnel: 16372 |
| --- |

**LAKESIDE BEHAVIORAL HEALTHCARE–PRINCETON PLAZA (104067)**, 1800 Mercy Drive, Zip 32808-5646; tel. 407/875-3700 **A**3 5 9 10 **F**98 102 104 **P**1
Primary Contact: Jerry Kassab, President and Chief Executive Officer
Web address: www.lakesidecares.org
**Control:** Other not-for-profit (including NFP Corporation) **Service:** Psychiatric

| Staffed Beds: 56 Admissions: 3250 Census: 49 Outpatient Visits: 33500 Births: 0 |
| --- |

**ORLANDO REGIONAL MEDICAL CENTER (100006)**, 1414 Kuhl Avenue, Zip 32806-2093; tel. 407/841-5111, (Includes ARNOLD PALMER CHILDREN'S HOSPITAL, 92 West Miller Street, Zip 32806; tel. 407/649-6960; John Bozard, President; ORLANDO REGIONAL–LUCERNE, 818 Main Lane, Zip 32801-3727; tel. 321/841-4200; Karen Frenier, Executive Director; WINNIE PALMER HOSPITAL FOR WOMEN AND BABIES, 83 West Miller Street, Zip 32806; tel. 321/843-2201; Kathy Swanson, President) **A**1 2 3 5 8 9 10 **F**3 5 7 8 11 12 13 15 16 17 18 19 20 21 22 23 24 25 26 27 28 29 30 31 34 35 36 37 40 41 43 44 45 46 48 49 50 51 53 54 55 57 58 59 60 61 62 64 65 68 70 71 72 73 74 75 76 77 78 79 80 81 82 84 85 86 87 88 89 90 91 92 93 94 96 97 98 99 100 101 102 103 104 107 108 110 111 113 114 115 116 117 118 119 120 122 123 125 128 129 130 131 133 134 145 146 147 **P**6 **S** Orlando Health, Orlando, FL
Primary Contact: Shannon Elswick, President
CFO: Paul Goldstein, Vice President Finance and Chief Financial Officer
CMO: Timothy Bullard, M.D., Chief of Staff
CIO: Rick Schooler, Vice President and Chief Information Officer
CHR: Nancy Dinon, Vice President Human Resources
Web address: www.orhs.org
**Control:** Other not-for-profit (including NFP Corporation) **Service:** General Medical and Surgical

| Staffed Beds: 1491 Admissions: 81666 Census: 1158 Outpatient Visits: 669168 Births: 12908 Total Expense ($000): 1441756 Payroll Expense ($000): 655462 Personnel: 13527 |
| --- |

**SELECT SPECIALTY HOSPITAL–ORLANDO (102003)**, 2250 Bedford Road, Zip 32803; tel. 407/303-7869, (Includes SELECT SPECIALTY HOSPITAL–ORLANDO SOUTH, 5579 South Orange Avenue, Zip 32809-3493; tel. 407/241-4800), (Nonreporting) **A**1 9 10 **S** Select Medical Corporation, Mechanicsburg, PA
Primary Contact: Nellie Castroman, Chief Executive Officer
Web address: www.selectmedicalcorp.com
**Control:** Corporation, Investor-owned, for-profit **Service:** Long-Term Acute Care hospital

| Staffed Beds: 75 |
| --- |

**SELECT SPECIALTY HOSPITAL–ORLANDO SOUTH** See Select Specialty Hospital–Orlando

**WINNIE PALMER HOSPITAL FOR WOMEN AND BABIES** See Orlando Regional Medical Center

*Many Facility Codes have changed. Please refer to the AHA Guide Code Chart.* © 2012 AHA Guide

FL

## PALATKA—Putnam County

**PUTNAM COMMUNITY MEDICAL CENTER (100232)**, Highway 20 West, Zip 32177–8118, Mailing Address: P.O. Box 778, Zip 32178–0778; tel. 386/328–5711 **A**1 9 10 19 **F**3 13 15 18 20 22 29 34 40 45 46 50 51 57 60 64 65 68 70 74 75 76 79 81 85 93 107 108 109 110 111 118 128 130 134 145 146 147 **S** LifePoint Hospitals, Inc., Brentwood, TN
Primary Contact: Jerry Christine, Chief Executive Officer
CFO: Debra Noyes, Chief Financial Officer
CMO: Joseph Stillword, Chief of Staff
CIO: Yvette A. Jones, HIM Director
CHR: John Schneider, Human Resources Director
CNO: Carol Negoshian, MSN, Chief Nursing Officer
Web address: www.pcmcfl.com
**Control:** Corporation, Investor–owned, for–profit **Service:** General Medical and Surgical

**Staffed Beds:** 99 **Admissions:** 5535 **Census:** 71 **Outpatient Visits:** 45305 **Births:** 442 **Total Expense ($000):** 51302 **Payroll Expense ($000):** 23823 **Personnel:** 476

## PALM BEACH GARDENS—Palm Beach County

**PALM BEACH GARDENS MEDICAL CENTER (100176)**, 3360 Burns Road, Zip 33410–4304; tel. 561/622–1411, (Nonreporting) **A**1 9 10 **S** TENET Healthcare Corporation, Dallas, TX
Primary Contact: Michael Cowling, Chief Executive Officer
CFO: Judi Stimson–Rusin, Chief Financial Officer
CIO: James Vega, Director Information Systems
CHR: Kevin Caracciolo, Chief Human Resources Officer
Web address: www.pbgmc.com
**Control:** Corporation, Investor–owned, for–profit **Service:** General Medical and Surgical

**Staffed Beds:** 199

## PALM COAST—Flagler County

**FLORIDA HOSPITAL–FLAGLER (100118)**, 60 Memorial Medical Parkway, Zip 32164; tel. 386/586–2000 **A**1 2 9 10 **F**11 15 20 28 29 30 31 34 40 45 46 49 50 51 57 59 60 62 63 64 68 70 74 75 77 78 79 81 85 86 87 93 107 108 110 111 113 115 116 117 118 119 120 123 125 131 134 145 146 **P**6 **S** Adventist Health System Sunbelt Health Care Corporation, Altamonte Springs, FL
Primary Contact: David Ottati, President and Chief Executive Officer
CFO: Valerie Ziesmer, Chief Financial Officer
CMO: John Walsh, M.D., Chief Medical Officer
CHR: Joshua I. Champion, Director
CHR: Alyson Parker, Director
CNO: Ellen R. Lenkevich, Chief Nursing Officer
Web address: www.fhms.com
**Control:** Church–operated, Nongovernment, not–for profit **Service:** General Medical and Surgical

**Staffed Beds:** 99 **Admissions:** 6270 **Census:** 69 **Outpatient Visits:** 144639 **Births:** 0 **Total Expense ($000):** 99031 **Payroll Expense ($000):** 35666

## PANAMA CITY—Bay County

**BAY MEDICAL CENTER (100026)**, 615 North Bonita Avenue, Zip 32401–3600, Mailing Address: P.O. Box 59515, Zip 32412–0515; tel. 850/769–1511 **A**1 2 9 10 **F**3 7 8 11 13 14 15 17 18 20 22 24 26 28 29 30 34 35 40 41 42 45 49 53 54 57 59 60 61 64 69 70 74 75 76 77 78 79 80 81 82 87 89 93 107 108 109 110 111 113 118 120 122 125 128 129 130 131 133 134 142 143 145 146 147 **S** LHP Hospital Group, Plano, TX
Primary Contact: Steven M. Johnson, President and Chief Executive Officer
COO: Daniel R. Morgan, Chief Operating Officer
CFO: Christopher Brooks, Vice President Finance
CMO: Ingrid Rachesky, M.D., President Medical Staff
CIO: Tom Bialorvcki, Chief Information Officer
CHR: Donna Baird, Vice President Corporate Services
Web address: www.baymedical.org
**Control:** Hospital district or authority, Government, nonfederal **Service:** General Medical and Surgical

**Staffed Beds:** 273 **Admissions:** 15975 **Census:** 205 **Outpatient Visits:** 194032 **Births:** 243 **Total Expense ($000):** 236194 **Payroll Expense ($000):** 88933 **Personnel:** 1516

**EMERALD COAST BEHAVIORAL HOSPITAL (104073)**, 1940 Harrison Avenue, Zip 32405–4542; tel. 850/763–0017, (Nonreporting) **A**1 10 **S** Universal Health Services, Inc., King of Prussia, PA
Primary Contact: Tim Bedford, Chief Executive Officer
Web address: www.emeraldcoastbehavioral.com
**Control:** Corporation, Investor–owned, for–profit **Service:** Psychiatric

**Staffed Beds:** 90

**GULF COAST MEDICAL CENTER (100242)**, 449 West 23rd Street, Zip 32405–4593, Mailing Address: P.O. Box 15309, Zip 32406–5309; tel. 850/769–8341 **A**1 2 9 10 **F**3 8 12 13 15 20 22 26 29 30 31 34 35 37 39 40 41 44 47 48 49 51 54 56 57 59 60 64 68 70 72 74 75 76 77 78 79 80 81 85 86 87 89 93 107 108 109 111 113 115 116 117 118 125 129 130 131 134 143 145 146 147 **S** HCA, Nashville, TN
Primary Contact: Carlton Ulmer, Chief Executive Officer
COO: Nancy Dodson, Chief Operating Officer
CFO: Laurie Haynes, Chief Financial Officer
CHR: Wanda Salley, Administrative Director Human Resources
Web address: www.egulfcoastmedical.com
**Control:** Corporation, Investor–owned, for–profit **Service:** General Medical and Surgical

**Staffed Beds:** 176 **Admissions:** 11036 **Census:** 111 **Outpatient Visits:** 111788 **Births:** 2282 **Total Expense ($000):** 113000 **Payroll Expense ($000):** 38000 **Personnel:** 588

**HEALTHSOUTH EMERALD COAST REHABILITATION HOSPITAL (103040)**, 1847 Florida Avenue, Zip 32405–4640; tel. 850/914–8600 **A**1 9 10 **F**3 28 29 34 57 59 64 68 75 77 85 86 87 90 91 93 95 96 128 129 130 131 145 147 **S** HEALTHSOUTH Corporation, Birmingham, AL
Primary Contact: Tony N. Bennett, Chief Executive Officer
CFO: Angela Eddins, Controller
CMO: Michael Hennigan, M.D., Medical Director
CHR: Traci Powell, Director Human Resources
Web address: www.healthsouthpanamacity.com
**Control:** Corporation, Investor–owned, for–profit **Service:** Rehabilitation

**Staffed Beds:** 75 **Admissions:** 1425 **Census:** 50 **Outpatient Visits:** 6316 **Births:** 0 **Total Expense ($000):** 18123 **Payroll Expense ($000):** 9301 **Personnel:** 208

**SELECT SPECIALTY HOSPITAL–PANAMA CITY (102017)**, 615 North Bonita Avenue, 3rd Floor, Zip 32401; tel. 850/767–3180, (Nonreporting) **A**1 9 10 **S** Select Medical Corporation, Mechanicsburg, PA
Primary Contact: Debra R. Gibson, Chief Executive Officer
CMO: Amir Manzoor, M.D., Medical Director
Web address: www.selectmedicalcorp.com
**Control:** Corporation, Investor–owned, for–profit **Service:** Long–Term Acute Care hospital

**Staffed Beds:** 30

## PEMBROKE PINES—Broward County

**MEMORIAL HOSPITAL PEMBROKE (100230)**, 7800 Sheridan Street, Zip 33024–2536; tel. 954/883–8482, (Nonreporting) **A**1 9 10 **S** Memorial Healthcare System, Hollywood, FL
Primary Contact: Chantal Leconte, Chief Executive Officer
CFO: Joseph Stuczynski, Assistant Administrator Finance and Support
CMO: Stanley Marks, M.D., Chief Medical Officer
CIO: Forest Blanton, Chief Information Officer
CHR: Margie Vargas, Director Human Resources
CNO: Judy Frum, R.N., Chief Nursing Officer
Web address: www.memorialpembroke.com/
**Control:** Hospital district or authority, Government, nonfederal **Service:** General Medical and Surgical

**Staffed Beds:** 149

**MEMORIAL HOSPITAL WEST (100281)**, 703 North Flamingo Road, Zip 33028–1014; tel. 954/436–5000 **A**1 2 9 10 **F**3 13 15 17 18 20 22 26 28 29 30 31 34 35 36 40 41 45 46 47 49 51 53 55 56 57 59 60 61 64 68 70 72 74 75 76 78 79 81 82 85 87 91 92 93 107 108 110 111 113 114 117 118 119 120 122 123 125 129 130 131 135 144 145 146 147 **S** Memorial Healthcare System, Hollywood, FL
Primary Contact: C. Kennon Hetlage, FACHE, Chief Executive Officer and Administrator
COO: Sue E. Bradford, R.N., Chief Nursing Officer
CFO: Walter Bussell, Chief Financial Officer
CMO: Eric Freling, M.D., Director Medical Staff Affairs
CMO: Miguel Venereo, M.D., Director Medical Staff
CIO: Forest Blanton, Chief Information Officer
CHR: Christopher Perry, Director Human Resources
CNO: Grisel Fernandez–Bravo, R.N., Chief Nursing Officer
Web address: www.mhs.net
**Control:** Hospital district or authority, Government, nonfederal **Service:** General Medical and Surgical

**Staffed Beds:** 304 **Admissions:** 22041 **Census:** 254 **Outpatient Visits:** 270329 **Births:** 4646 **Total Expense ($000):** 334074 **Payroll Expense ($000):** 135447 **Personnel:** 1870

FL

**Hospital, Medicare Provider Number, Address, Telephone, Approval, Facility, and Physician Codes, Health Care System**

★ American Hospital Association (AHA) membership
□ The Joint Commission accreditation
◇ DNV Healthcare Inc. accreditation
○ American Osteopathic Association (AOA) accreditation
△ Commission on Accreditation of Rehabilitation Facilities (CARF) accreditation

## PENSACOLA—Escambia County

☒ **BAPTIST HOSPITAL (100093)**, 1000 West Moreno, Zip 32501–2393, Mailing Address: P.O. Box 17500, Zip 32522–7500; tel. 850/434–4011 **A**1 2 9 10 **F**3 7 8 11 12 13 15 17 18 20 22 24 26 28 29 30 31 34 35 37 40 43 45 46 47 48 49 50 51 52 54 55 56 57 58 59 60 61 62 63 64 67 70 74 75 76 77 78 79 81 82 84 85 86 87 92 93 97 98 99 100 101 102 103 104 107 108 110 111 113 114 115 116 117 118 119 120 122 123 125 128 129 130 131 134 143 145 146 147 **P**4 6 **S** Baptist Health Care Corporation, Pensacola, FL
Primary Contact: David Wildebrandt, Administrator
CFO: Kerry Vermillion, Senior Vice President Finance and Chief Financial Officer
CMO: Coy Irvin, M.D., Vice President and Chief Medical Officer
CIO: Robert Johnson, Vice President and Chief Information Officer
CHR: Glenn Carnathan, Vice President Human Resources
Web address: www.ebaptisthealthcare.org
**Control:** Other not–for–profit (including NFP Corporation) **Service:** General Medical and Surgical

**Staffed Beds:** 339 **Admissions:** 16132 **Census:** 221 **Outpatient Visits:** 210516 **Births:** 1060 **Total Expense ($000):** 246171 **Payroll Expense ($000):** 84261 **Personnel:** 1383

☒ **NAVAL HOSPITAL**, 6000 West Highway 98, Zip 32512–0003; tel. 850/505–6413 **A**1 3 5 **F**3 5 13 15 18 29 30 32 33 34 35 38 39 40 45 49 50 51 53 54 55 57 58 59 64 65 68 70 74 75 76 77 79 81 85 86 87 92 93 97 100 101 102 104 107 108 110 111 113 114 117 118 123 128 129 130 134 145 146 147 **S** Bureau of Medicine and Surgery, Department of the Navy, Washington, DC
Primary Contact: Maureen Padden, Commander
COO: Commander Chris O'Donnell, Director for Administration
CFO: James L. Ayers, Director Resource Management
CMO: Commander Connie Stamateris, M.D., Director Medical Services
CIO: Lieutenant Russell Deason, Chief Information Officer
CHR: Commander Ron Martel, Director for Administration
Web address: www.psaweb.pcola.med.navy.mil
**Control:** Navy, Government, federal **Service:** General Medical and Surgical

**Staffed Beds:** 32 **Admissions:** 1861 **Census:** 14 **Outpatient Visits:** 528972 **Births:** 517 **Total Expense ($000):** 124829 **Payroll Expense ($000):** 37438 **Personnel:** 2270

**REHABILITATION INSTITUTE OF WEST FLORIDA** See West Florida Hospital

☒ **SACRED HEART HOSPITAL OF PENSACOLA (100025)**, 5151 North Ninth Avenue, Zip 32504–8795, Mailing Address: P.O. Box 2700, Zip 32513–2700; tel. 850/416–7000, (Nonreporting) **A**1 2 3 5 9 10 13 **S** Ascension Health, Saint Louis, MO
Primary Contact: Susan L. Davis, R.N., Ed.D., FACHE, President and Chief Executive Officer
COO: Carol Schmidt, Chief Operating Officer
CFO: Buddy Elmore, Chief Financial Officer
CMO: Paul T. Baroco, M.D., Chief Medical Officer
CMO: James Ward, M.D., Chief Medical Officer
CIO: Kathy Ross, Chief Information Officer
CHR: Carol Whittington, Chief Human Resources Officer
Web address: www.sacred–heart.org
**Control:** Church–operated, Nongovernment, not–for profit **Service:** General Medical and Surgical

**Staffed Beds:** 458

☒ **SELECT SPECIALTY HOSPITAL–PENSACOLA (102024)**, 7000 Cobble Creek Drive, Zip 32504; tel. 850/473–4800, (Nonreporting) **A**1 9 10 **S** Select Medical Corporation, Mechanicsburg, PA
Primary Contact: David Goodson, Chief Executive Officer
CMO: John Bray, M.D., Medical Director
Web address: www.selectmedicalcorp.com
**Control:** Corporation, Investor–owned, for–profit **Service:** Long–Term Acute Care hospital

**Staffed Beds:** 54

☒ **WEST FLORIDA HOSPITAL (100231)**, 8383 North Davis Highway, Zip 32514–6088; tel. 850/494–4000, (Includes REHABILITATION INSTITUTE OF WEST FLORIDA, 8383 North Davis Highway, Zip 32514, Mailing Address: P.O. Box 18900, Zip 32523; tel. 850/494–6000; THE PAVILION, 8383 North Davis Highway, Zip 32523, Mailing Address: P.O. Box 18900, Zip 32523; tel. 904/494–5000), (Nonreporting) **A**1 2 9 10 **S** HCA, Nashville, TN
Primary Contact: Brian Baumgardner, Chief Executive Officer
COO: Robert Peterson, Chief Operating Officer
CFO: Randy Butler, Chief Financial Officer
CIO: Jeff Amerson, Director Information System
CHR: Karen Oliver, Vice President Human Resources
Web address: www.westfloridahospital.com
**Control:** Corporation, Investor–owned, for–profit **Service:** General Medical and Surgical

**Staffed Beds:** 339

## PERRY—Taylor County

**DOCTOR'S MEMORIAL HOSPITAL (100106)**, 333 North Byron Butler Parkway, Zip 32347–2104; tel. 850/584–0800, (Nonreporting) **A**9 10 20
Primary Contact: Richard Huth, Chief Executive Officer
CFO: James L. Leis, Jr., Chief Financial Officer
CMO: Ron Emerick, M.D., Chief of Staff
CIO: Joseph Sprinkle, Chief Information Officer
CHR: Diana McRory, Director Human Resources
CNO: Michael Windham, Chief Nursing Officer
Web address: www.doctorsmemorial.com
**Control:** Other not–for–profit (including NFP Corporation) **Service:** General Medical and Surgical

**Staffed Beds:** 40

## PLANT CITY—Hillsborough County

☒ **SOUTH FLORIDA BAPTIST HOSPITAL (100132)**, 301 North Alexander Street, Zip 33563–9058, Mailing Address: Drawer H, Zip 33564–9058; tel. 813/757–1200, (Nonreporting) **A**1 9 10 **S** Catholic Health East, Newtown Square, PA
Primary Contact: Isaac Mallah, President and Chief Executive Officer
COO: Stephen Nierman, Chief Operating Officer
CFO: Cathy Yoder, Chief Financial Officer
CMO: Mark Vaaler, M.D., Chief Medical Officer
CHR: Juanita Radford, Coordinator Team Resource
Web address: www.sjbhealth.org
**Control:** Other not–for–profit (including NFP Corporation) **Service:** General Medical and Surgical

**Staffed Beds:** 147

## PLANTATION—Broward County

☒ **PLANTATION GENERAL HOSPITAL (100167)**, 401 N.W. 42nd Avenue, Zip 33317–2882; tel. 954/587–5010, (Includes MERCY HOSPITAL – A CAMPUS OF PLANTATION GENERAL HOSPITAL, 3663 South Miami Avenue, Miami, Zip 33133–4237; tel. 305/854–4400; Barbara Simmons, R.N., Chief Executive Officer), (Nonreporting) **A**1 9 10 **S** HCA, Nashville, TN
Primary Contact: Randy Gross, Chief Executive Officer
COO: Bryan Miller, Chief Operating Officer
CFO: Irfan Mirza, Chief Financial Officer
CIO: David Irizarri, Director Management Information Systems
CHR: Linda Bryan, Vice President Human Resources
CNO: Dolores Skaare, R.N., Chief Nursing Officer
Web address: www.plantationgeneral.com
**Control:** Corporation, Investor–owned, for–profit **Service:** General Medical and Surgical

**Staffed Beds:** 264

☒ **WESTSIDE REGIONAL MEDICAL CENTER (100228)**, 8201 West Broward Boulevard, Zip 33324–9937; tel. 954/473–6600 **A**1 2 9 10 **F**3 11 15 17 18 20 22 24 26 29 30 31 34 35 40 44 45 48 49 50 57 59 68 70 74 75 77 78 79 80 81 82 85 86 87 93 107 108 110 111 113 114 116 118 125 128 129 130 131 134 144 145 147 **S** HCA, Nashville, TN
Primary Contact: Lee B. Chaykin, Chief Executive Officer
COO: Shana Sappington–Crittenden, Chief Operating Officer
CFO: Kevin Corcoran, Chief Financial Officer
CMO: Brian Weinstein, M.D., Chief of Staff
CIO: Andres Blanco, Director Management Information Systems
CHR: Maria Rivera, Director Human Resources
Web address: www.westsideregional.com
**Control:** Corporation, Investor–owned, for–profit **Service:** General Medical and Surgical

**Staffed Beds:** 224 **Admissions:** 12480 **Census:** 146 **Outpatient Visits:** 56281 **Births:** 0 **Total Expense ($000):** 124453 **Payroll Expense ($000):** 48939 **Personnel:** 765

## PORT CHARLOTTE—Charlotte County

☒ △ **FAWCETT MEMORIAL HOSPITAL (100236)**, 21298 Olean Boulevard, Zip 33952–6765, Mailing Address: P.O. Box 494960, Punta Gorda, Zip 33949–4960; tel. 941/629–1181, (Nonreporting) **A**1 2 7 9 10 **S** HCA, Nashville, TN
Primary Contact: Thomas J. Rice, FACHE, President and Chief Executive Officer
COO: Alex Chang, Vice President and Chief Operating Officer
CFO: James P. Burns, Vice President and Chief Financial Officer
CHR: Tony Welch, Vice President Human Resources
Web address: www.fawcetthospital.com
**Control:** Corporation, Investor–owned, for–profit **Service:** General Medical and Surgical

**Staffed Beds:** 238

FL

*Many Facility Codes have changed. Please refer to the AHA Guide Code Chart.*           © 2012 AHA Guide

☐ **PEACE RIVER REGIONAL MEDICAL CENTER (100077)**, 2500 Harbor Boulevard, Zip 33952–5396; tel. 941/766–4122 **A**1 5 9 10 **F**3 11 12 13 15 17 18 20 22 24 26 28 29 30 31 34 35 36 37 38 40 44 45 46 49 50 51 54 56 57 58 59 60 61 62 64 65 68 70 72 74 75 76 77 79 81 84 85 86 87 89 93 100 107 108 110 111 113 114 117 118 125 130 134 145 146 **P**6 **S** Health Management Associates, Naples, FL
Primary Contact: Joseph T. Clancy, Chief Executive Officer
CFO: Robert Stiekes, Chief Financial Officer
CIO: Ted Bailey, Vice President Information Systems
Web address: www.peaceriverregional.com
**Control:** Corporation, Investor–owned, for–profit **Service:** General Medical and Surgical

**Staffed Beds:** 190 **Admissions:** 8766 **Census:** 112 **Outpatient Visits:** 45361 **Births:** 1143

### PORT ST. JOE—Gulf County

★ **SACRED HEART HOSPITAL ON THE GULF (100313)**, 3801 East Highway 98, Zip 32456–5318; tel. 850/229–5600, (Nonreporting) **A**9 10 **S** Ascension Health, Saint Louis, MO
Primary Contact: Roger L. Hall, President
Web address: www.sacred–heart.org/gulf/
**Control:** Other not–for–profit (including NFP Corporation) **Service:** General Medical and Surgical

**Staffed Beds:** 25

### PORT ST. LUCIE—St. Lucie County

**PORT ST. LUCIE HOSPITAL (104070)**, 2550 S.E. Walton Road, Zip 34952–7168; tel. 772/335–0500, (Nonreporting) **A**10
Primary Contact: Christopher Brooks, Chief Executive Officer
Web address: www.portstluciehospitalinc.com
**Control:** Other not–for–profit (including NFP Corporation) **Service:** Psychiatric

**Staffed Beds:** 75

⊞ **ST. LUCIE MEDICAL CENTER (100260)**, 1800 S.E. Tiffany Avenue, Zip 34952–7580; tel. 772/335–4000, (Nonreporting) **A**1 2 9 10 13 **S** HCA, Nashville, TN
Primary Contact: Gary Cantrell, President and Chief Executive Officer
COO: Calvin Thomas, IV, Chief Operating Officer
CFO: Kevin Keeling, Chief Financial Officer
Web address: www.stluciemed.com
**Control:** Corporation, Investor–owned, for–profit **Service:** General Medical and Surgical

**Staffed Beds:** 194

### PUNTA GORDA—Charlotte County

☐ **CHARLOTTE REGIONAL MEDICAL CENTER (100047)**, 809 East Marion Avenue, Zip 33950–3898, Mailing Address: P.O. Box 51–1328, Zip 33951–1328; tel. 941/639–3131 **A**1 9 10 **F**3 17 18 20 22 24 26 28 29 30 31 34 35 39 40 44 45 50 53 54 56 57 59 60 64 68 70 74 75 77 78 79 81 85 86 87 93 94 98 102 103 107 108 111 114 117 118 125 128 129 130 145 147 **S** Health Management Associates, Naples, FL
Primary Contact: Jose F. Morillo, Chief Executive Officer
CFO: Cheryl Tibbett, Chief Financial Officer
Web address: www.charlotteregional.com
**Control:** Corporation, Investor–owned, for–profit **Service:** General Medical and Surgical

**Staffed Beds:** 208 **Admissions:** 8800 **Census:** 134 **Births:** 0 **Personnel:** 679

### RIVIERA BEACH—Palm Beach County

⊞ **KINDRED HOSPITAL THE PALM BEACHES (102025)**, 5555 West Blue Heron Boulevard, Zip 33418–7813; tel. 561/840–0754, (Nonreporting) **A**1 9 10 **S** Kindred Healthcare, Louisville, KY
Primary Contact: Timothy Page, Chief Executive Officer
Web address: www.khthepalmbeaches.com/
**Control:** Corporation, Investor–owned, for–profit **Service:** Long–Term Acute Care hospital

**Staffed Beds:** 70

### ROCKLEDGE—Brevard County

☐ **WUESTHOFF MEDICAL CENTER – ROCKLEDGE (100092)**, 110 Longwood Avenue, Zip 32955–2887, Mailing Address: P.O. Box 565002, Mail Stop 1, Zip 32956–5002; tel. 321/636–2211, (Nonreporting) **A**1 2 9 10 **S** Health Management Associates, Naples, FL
Primary Contact: Devon Hyde, Chief Operating Officer
CFO: Richard Haun, Chief Financial Officer
CMO: Vinay Mehindru, M.D., Medical Director
CIO: David Barnhart, Director Information Systems
CHR: Marchita H. Marino, Vice President Human Resources
Web address: www.wuesthoff.org
**Control:** Corporation, Investor–owned, for–profit **Service:** General Medical and Surgical

**Staffed Beds:** 291

### SAFETY HARBOR—Pinellas County

☐ **MEASE COUNTRYSIDE HOSPITAL (100265)**, 3231 McMullen–Booth Road, Zip 34695–1098, Mailing Address: P.O. Box 1098, Zip 34695–1098; tel. 727/725–6222, (Nonreporting) **A**1 2 9 10 **S** Morton Plant Mease Health Care, Clearwater, FL
Primary Contact: Glenn D. Waters, FACHE, President
COO: Lou Galdieri, R.N., Chief Operating Officer and Administrator
CFO: Carl Tremonti, Chief Financial Officer
CMO: Donald Pocock, M.D., Chief Medical Officer
CHR: Sharon Collotta, Director Human Resources
Web address: www.mpmhealth.com
**Control:** Other not–for–profit (including NFP Corporation) **Service:** General Medical and Surgical

**Staffed Beds:** 100

### SAINT AUGUSTINE—St. Johns County

☐ **FLAGLER HOSPITAL (100090)**, 400 Health Park Boulevard, Zip 32086–5779; tel. 904/819–5155 **A**1 2 9 10 20 **F**3 11 12 13 15 18 20 22 24 28 29 30 31 34 35 40 46 49 51 53 54 57 59 64 65 66 68 70 72 74 75 76 77 78 79 81 82 85 86 87 89 93 97 100 101 102 103 107 108 111 113 118 128 129 131 134 145 147
Primary Contact: Joseph S. Gordy, President
COO: Jason P. Barrett, Chief Operating Officer
CFO: Lynda I. Kirker, Chief Financial Officer
CMO: Douglas Dew, M.D., President Medical Staff
CIO: Bill Rieger, Chief Information Officer
CHR: Jeff Hurley, Vice President Human Resources
Web address: www.flaglerhospital.org
**Control:** Other not–for–profit (including NFP Corporation) **Service:** General Medical and Surgical

**Staffed Beds:** 336 **Admissions:** 13816 **Census:** 188 **Outpatient Visits:** 172359 **Births:** 1129 **Total Expense ($000):** 184432 **Payroll Expense ($000):** 70605

### SAINT CLOUD—Osceola County

☐ **ST. CLOUD REGIONAL MEDICAL CENTER (100302)**, 2906 17th Street, Zip 34769–6099; tel. 407/892–2135 **A**1 9 10 **F**3 15 18 29 30 34 40 45 49 59 70 74 75 77 78 79 81 82 85 86 87 93 96 107 108 111 114 118 145 **S** Health Management Associates, Naples, FL
Primary Contact: Lindell W. Orr, Interim Chief Executive Officer
COO: Tom Patrias, Chief Operating Officer
CFO: Carmen Acker, Chief Financial Officer
CMO: Paul Thorne, M.D., Chief Medical Director
CIO: James Devlin, Director Information Systems
CHR: Daniel Avila, Director Human Resources
Web address: www.stcloudregional.com
**Control:** Corporation, Investor–owned, for–profit **Service:** General Medical and Surgical

**Staffed Beds:** 84 **Admissions:** 4940 **Census:** 56 **Births:** 0 **Total Expense ($000):** 45050 **Payroll Expense ($000):** 19372 **Personnel:** 383

FL

---

**Hospital, Medicare Provider Number, Address, Telephone, Approval, Facility, and Physician Codes, Health Care System**

★ American Hospital Association (AHA) membership
☐ The Joint Commission accreditation ◇ DNV Healthcare Inc. accreditation
○ American Osteopathic Association (AOA) accreditation
△ Commission on Accreditation of Rehabilitation Facilities (CARF) accreditation

## SAINT PETERSBURG—Pinellas County

⊞ **ALL CHILDREN'S HOSPITAL (103300)**, 501 6th Avenue South,
Zip 33701–4899; tel. 727/898–7451, (Data for 273 days) **A**1 3 5 8 9 10 **F**3 11
17 18 19 20 21 22 23 24 25 26 27 29 30 31 32 34 35 36 37 39 40 41 43
44 45 46 47 48 49 50 54 55 57 58 59 60 61 64 65 68 72 73 74 75 77 78
79 81 82 84 85 86 87 88 89 92 93 96 97 99 100 107 111 113 114 115 117
118 128 129 130 131 133 134 135 136 140 141 142 143 145 147 **P**6
**S** Johns Hopkins Health System, Baltimore, MD
Primary Contact: Arnold T. Stenberg, Jr., Executive Vice President and Chief
Administrative Officer
CFO: Nancy Templin, Vice President Finance and Chief Financial Officer
CMO: Michael Epstein, M.D., Senior Vice President Medical Affairs
CIO: Cal Popovich, Vice President Information Technology
CHR: Jay Kuhns, Vice President Human Resources
Web address: www.allkids.org
**Control:** Other not–for–profit (including NFP Corporation) **Service:** Children's
general

**Staffed Beds:** 259 **Admissions:** 7330 **Census:** 200 **Outpatient Visits:**
241349 **Births:** 0 **Total Expense ($000):** 252855 **Payroll Expense ($000):**
99807 **Personnel:** 2363

⊞ △ **BAYFRONT MEDICAL CENTER (100032)**, 701 Sixth Street South,
Zip 33701–4891; tel. 727/823–1234 **A**1 3 5 7 9 10 **F**3 8 11 13 15 17 18 20
22 24 26 27 28 29 30 31 34 35 36 38 40 41 43 45 46 49 50 53 56 57 58
59 61 64 65 68 70 74 75 76 77 78 79 81 82 84 85 86 87 90 93 96 97 107
108 109 110 111 113 114 117 118 120 122 123 125 126 128 129 130 131
134 145 146 147 **P**6
Primary Contact: Sue G. Brody, President and Chief Executive Officer
COO: Eric Feder, Exec. VP, Chief Operating Officer
CFO: Bob Thornton, Exec. VP, Chief Financial Officer
CMO: Paul McRae, M.D., Chief of Staff
CMO: David Weiland, M.D., VP Medical Affairs
CIO: Jennifer Greenman, Exec. Director, CIO
CHR: Deborah Menendez, VP Human Resources
CNO: Karen Long, R.N., VP Nursing
Web address: www.bayfront.org
**Control:** Other not–for–profit (including NFP Corporation) **Service:** General
Medical and Surgical

**Staffed Beds:** 395 **Admissions:** 17522 **Census:** 243 **Outpatient Visits:**
254254 **Births:** 3840 **Total Expense ($000):** 196692 **Payroll Expense
($000):** 96598 **Personnel:** 1988

⊞ **EDWARD WHITE HOSPITAL (100239)**, 2323 Ninth Avenue North,
Zip 33713–6898, Mailing Address: P.O. Box 12018, Zip 33733–2018;
tel. 727/323–1111, (Nonreporting) **A**1 9 10 **S** HCA, Nashville, TN
Primary Contact: Richard S. Frank, Interim Chief Executive Officer
COO: Richard S. Frank, Vice President Operations
CFO: Peggy Gatliff, Chief Financial Officer
CMO: Fadi Saba, M.D., Chief of Staff
CIO: Donna Leitenberger, Director Information Services
CHR: Bonnie O'Laskey, Vice President Human Resources
Web address: www.edwardwhitehospital.com
**Control:** Corporation, Investor–owned, for–profit **Service:** General Medical and
Surgical

**Staffed Beds:** 110

**KINDRED HOSPITAL–BAY AREA ST. PETERSBURG**, 3030 Sixth Street South,
Zip 33705–3720; tel. 727/894–8719, (Nonreporting) **A**9
Primary Contact: Kimberly Probus, Chief Executive Officer
CFO: John Miner, Chief Financial Officer
CNO: Niki Derrick, R.N., Chief Clinical Officer
Web address: www.kindredstpete.com
**Control:** Corporation, Investor–owned, for–profit **Service:** General Medical and
Surgical

**Staffed Beds:** 112

⊞ **NORTHSIDE HOSPITAL AND HEART INSTITUTE (100238)**, 6000 49th Street
North, Zip 33709–2145; tel. 727/521–4411 **A**1 9 10 12 13 **F**3 17 18 20 22 24
26 28 29 30 31 34 35 40 45 49 50 51 53 56 57 58 59 64 65 70 74 75 77
78 79 81 85 92 93 107 108 111 113 114 117 118 134 145 **S** HCA,
Nashville, TN
Primary Contact: Stephen J. Daugherty, Chief Executive Officer
COO: Betsy Bomar, Chief Operating Officer
CFO: Shalin Shah, Chief Financial Officer
CIO: Steve McDonald, Director Information Systems
CHR: Maggie Miklos, Director Human Resources
Web address: www.northsidehospital.com
**Control:** Corporation, Investor–owned, for–profit **Service:** General Medical and
Surgical

**Staffed Beds:** 227 **Admissions:** 9355 **Census:** 124 **Outpatient Visits:** 38750
**Births:** 0 **Total Expense ($000):** 112080 **Payroll Expense ($000):** 45211
**Personnel:** 656

△ **PALMS OF PASADENA HOSPITAL (100126)**, 1501 Pasadena Avenue South,
Zip 33707–3798; tel. 727/381–1000, (Nonreporting) **A**2 7 9 10 21 **S** IASIS
Healthcare, Franklin, TN
Primary Contact: Brian T. Flynn, Chief Executive Officer
CMO: David Long, M.D., Chief of Staff
CIO: Ron Truitt, Director Information Services
CHR: Karen Casteel, Director Human Resources
Web address: www.palmspasadena.com
**Control:** Corporation, Investor–owned, for–profit **Service:** General Medical and
Surgical

**Staffed Beds:** 307

⊞ **ST. ANTHONY'S HOSPITAL (100067)**, 1200 Seventh Avenue North,
Zip 33705–1388, Mailing Address: P.O. Box 12588, Zip 33733–2588;
tel. 727/825–1100, (Nonreporting) **A**1 2 9 10 **S** Catholic Health East, Newtown
Square, PA
Primary Contact: William G. Ulbricht, President
COO: Ronald J. Colaguori, Vice President Operations
CFO: Susan Olds, Chief Financial Officer
CMO: Teresa Bradley, M.D., Vice President Medical Affairs
CIO: Lindsey Jarrell, Vice President Information Services
CHR: Jim Bacon, Director Team Resources
Web address: www.stanthonys.com/
**Control:** Other not–for–profit (including NFP Corporation) **Service:** General
Medical and Surgical

**Staffed Beds:** 395

⊞ **ST. PETERSBURG GENERAL HOSPITAL (100180)**, 6500 38th Avenue North,
Zip 33710–1629; tel. 727/384–1414, (Nonreporting) **A**1 5 9 10 12 13 **S** HCA,
Nashville, TN
Primary Contact: Robert B. Conroy, Jr., Chief Executive Officer
COO: Stephanie McNulty, Chief Operating Officer
CFO: Andrew Smith, CFO
CHR: Guy Samuel, Director Human Resources
CNO: JoAnne Cattell, Chief Nursing Officer
Web address: www.stpetegeneral.com
**Control:** Corporation, Investor–owned, for–profit **Service:** General Medical and
Surgical

**Staffed Beds:** 219

## SANFORD—Seminole County

⊞ **CENTRAL FLORIDA REGIONAL HOSPITAL (100161)**, 1401 West Seminole
Boulevard, Zip 32771–6764; tel. 407/321–4500, (Nonreporting) **A**1 9 10 **S** HCA,
Nashville, TN
Primary Contact: Wendy H. Brandon, Chief Executive Officer
COO: Bobby McCullough, Chief Operating Officer
CFO: Russell T. Young, Chief Financial Officer
CIO: Nancy Ryerson, Director Information Systems
CHR: Karla Langlotz, Director Human Resources
Web address: www.centralfloridaregional.com
**Control:** Corporation, Investor–owned, for–profit **Service:** General Medical and
Surgical

**Staffed Beds:** 226

## SARASOTA—Sarasota County

⊞ **COMPLEX CARE HOSPITAL AT RIDGELAKE (102018)**, 6150 Edgelake Drive,
Zip 34240–8803; tel. 941/342–3000 **A**1 10 **F**1 29 129 147 **S** LifeCare
Management Services, Plano, TX
Primary Contact: Danny R. Edwards, Administrator
CFO: Leah Drabant, Director of Finance
CMO: Craig Harcup, M.D., Hospital Medical Director
CHR: Jennifer Sparks, Human Resources Generalist
CNO: Timothy Mitchell, R.N., Chief Nursing Officer
Web address: www.lifecare–hospitals.com/hospital.php?id=23
**Control:** Corporation, Investor–owned, for–profit **Service:** Long–Term Acute Care
hospital

**Staffed Beds:** 40 **Admissions:** 380 **Census:** 29 **Outpatient Visits:** 11 **Births:**
0 **Total Expense ($000):** 15478 **Payroll Expense ($000):** 7223 **Personnel:**
108

⊞ **DOCTORS HOSPITAL OF SARASOTA (100166)**, 5731 Bee Ridge Road,
Zip 34233–5056; tel. 941/342–1100, (Nonreporting) **A**1 9 10 **S** HCA,
Nashville, TN
Primary Contact: Robert C. Meade, Chief Executive Officer
COO: Valerie L. Powell–Stafford, Chief Operating Officer
CFO: Charles Schwaner, III, Chief Financial Officer
CHR: Theresa Levering, Director Human Resources
Web address: www.doctorsofsarasota.com
**Control:** Corporation, Investor–owned, for–profit **Service:** General Medical and
Surgical

**Staffed Beds:** 168

**FL**

⊠ △ **HEALTHSOUTH REHABILITATION HOSPITAL OF SARASOTA (103031)**, 6400 Edgelake Drive, Zip 34240–8813; tel. 941/921–8600, (Nonreporting) **A**1 7 9 10 **S** HEALTHSOUTH Corporation, Birmingham, AL
Primary Contact: Marcus Braz, Chief Executive Officer
CFO: Barbara Bierut, Chief Financial Officer
CMO: Alexander De Jesus, M.D., Medical Director
CHR: Brenda Benner, Director Human Resources
CHR: Marivee Jerome, Senior Human Resources Business Partner
CNO: Jacqueline Juenger, R.N., Chief Nursing Officer
Web address: www.healthsouthsarasota.com
**Control:** Corporation, Investor–owned, for–profit **Service:** Rehabilitation

**Staffed Beds:** 86

**HEALTHSOUTH RIDGELAKE HOSPITAL** See Complex Care Hospital at Ridgelake

☐ △ **SARASOTA MEMORIAL HOSPITAL (100087)**, 1700 South Tamiami Trail, Zip 34239–3555; tel. 941/917–9000 **A**1 2 3 5 7 9 10 **F**3 5 6 7 8 11 12 13 15 17 18 20 22 24 26 28 29 30 31 32 34 35 36 37 38 39 40 42 44 45 46 47 48 49 50 51 53 54 55 56 57 58 59 60 64 66 68 70 72 73 74 75 76 77 78 79 80 81 82 84 85 86 87 89 90 91 93 95 96 98 99 100 101 102 103 104 105 107 108 110 111 113 114 115 116 117 118 123 125 128 129 130 131 134 142 143 144 145 146 147
Primary Contact: Gwen MacKenzie, R.N., Chief Executive Officer
COO: Michael L. Harrington, Chief Operating Officer
CFO: Bill Woeltjen, Chief Financial Officer
CMO: Parlane Reid, M.D., Chief Medical Officer
CIO: Denis Baker, Chief Information Officer
CHR: Laurie Bennett, Director Human Resources
Web address: www.smh.com
**Control:** Hospital district or authority, Government, nonfederal **Service:** General Medical and Surgical

**Staffed Beds:** 628 **Admissions:** 24991 **Census:** 336 **Outpatient Visits:** 479309 **Births:** 3093 **Total Expense ($000):** 384518 **Payroll Expense ($000):** 166458 **Personnel:** 2685

**SEBASTIAN—Indian River County**

☐ **SEBASTIAN RIVER MEDICAL CENTER (100217)**, 13695 North U.S. Highway 1, Zip 32958–3230, Mailing Address: Box 780838, Zip 32978–0838; tel. 772/589–3186 **A**1 9 10 **F**3 12 15 18 20 22 28 29 31 34 40 41 45 46 49 50 51 57 59 60 62 63 64 68 70 74 75 77 78 79 81 82 83 84 85 86 87 89 91 92 93 95 107 110 111 113 114 115 118 125 128 129 131 144 145 147 **P**8 **S** Health Management Associates, Naples, FL
Primary Contact: Steven Salyer, Chief Executive Officer
CFO: John McEachern, Controller
CMO: Ralph Geiger, M.D., Chief of Staff
CHR: Kam Storey, Director Human Resources
Web address: www.sebastianrivermedical.com
**Control:** Corporation, Investor–owned, for–profit **Service:** General Medical and Surgical

**Staffed Beds:** 115 **Admissions:** 4930 **Census:** 58 **Outpatient Visits:** 28000 **Births:** 0 **Personnel:** 406

**SEBRING—Highlands County**

⊠ **FLORIDA HOSPITAL HEARTLAND MEDICAL CENTER (100109)**, 4200 Sun'n Lake Boulevard, Zip 33872–1986, Mailing Address: P.O. Box 9400, Zip 33871–9400; tel. 863/314–4466 **A**1 9 10 19 **F**8 11 13 15 18 20 22 24 28 29 30 34 35 37 40 44 45 49 50 51 53 54 57 59 60 62 64 70 75 76 79 81 82 86 87 89 98 100 101 103 104 107 108 110 111 113 117 118 126 128 129 131 132 133 145 146 147 **P**6 **S** Adventist Health System Sunbelt Health Care Corporation, Altamonte Springs, FL
Primary Contact: Timothy W. Cook, President and Chief Executive Officer
COO: Isaac Palmer, Chief Operating Officer
CFO: Dima Didenko, Vice President and Chief Financial Officer
CMO: Jorge F. Gonzalez, M.D., Chief Medical Officer
CHR: Anthony Stahl, Director Human Resources
Web address: www.fhheartland.org/
**Control:** Church–operated, Nongovernment, not–for profit **Service:** General Medical and Surgical

**Staffed Beds:** 222 **Admissions:** 12409 **Census:** 155 **Outpatient Visits:** 158354 **Births:** 804 **Total Expense ($000):** 165224 **Payroll Expense ($000):** 68089 **Personnel:** 1281

☐ **HIGHLANDS REGIONAL MEDICAL CENTER (100049)**, 3600 South Highlands Avenue, Zip 33870–5495, Mailing Address: Drawer 2066, Zip 33871–2066; tel. 863/471–5800, (Nonreporting) **A**1 9 10 19 **S** Health Management Associates, Naples, FL
Primary Contact: Brian Hess, Chief Executive Officer
COO: Kristen Kopinsky, Chief Operating Officer
CFO: Vicki DeRenzis, Chief Financial Officer
CMO: Robert Nudence, M.D., Chief of Staff
CIO: Felix Garcia, Director Health Information Services
CHR: Charlotte R. Lyda, Director Human Resources
CNO: Kari Bolin, R.N., Chief Nursing Officer
Web address: www.highlandsregional.com
**Control:** Corporation, Investor–owned, for–profit **Service:** General Medical and Surgical

**Staffed Beds:** 126

**SOUTH MIAMI—Miami–Dade County**

☐ **LARKIN COMMUNITY HOSPITAL (100181)**, 7031 S.W. 62nd Avenue, Zip 33143–4781; tel. 305/284–7500 **A**1 10 13 **F**3 12 18 29 30 31 35 40 45 46 49 51 59 62 70 74 75 78 79 81 82 85 87 98 102 103 105 107 108 111 115 116 118 129 134 142 147
Primary Contact: Sandra Sosa–Guerrero, Chief Executive Officer
COO: George J. Michel, Chief Operating Officer
CFO: Edgar Castillo, Chief Financial Officer
CMO: Jose David Suarez, M.D., Chief of Staff
CIO: Orlando Suarez, Manager Information Technology
CHR: Carlos R. Garcia, Vice President Clinical Services
CNO: Manuel Fernandez, Vice President Nursing
Web address: www.larkinhospital.com
**Control:** Individual, Investor–owned, for–profit **Service:** General Medical and Surgical

**Staffed Beds:** 146 **Admissions:** 5792 **Census:** 85 **Outpatient Visits:** 13512 **Births:** 0 **Total Expense ($000):** 55907 **Payroll Expense ($000):** 26864 **Personnel:** 469

**SPRING HILL—Hernando County**

**SPRING HILL REGIONAL HOSPITAL**, 10461 Quality Drive, Zip 34609–9634; tel. 352/688–8200, (Nonreporting) **A**9 **S** Health Management Associates, Naples, FL
Primary Contact: Patrick Maloney, Interim Chief Executive Officer
CMO: Mahmoud Bourghli, M.D., Chief of Staff
CIO: Deb Otis, Director Information Systems
CHR: Linda Campo, Director Human Resources
Web address: www.springhillregionalhospital.org
**Control:** Corporation, Investor–owned, for–profit **Service:** General Medical and Surgical

**Staffed Beds:** 75

**STARKE—Bradford County**

**SHANDS STARKE** See Shands Starke Regional Medical Center

⊠ **SHANDS STARKE REGIONAL MEDICAL CENTER (101310)**, 922 East Call Street, Zip 32091–3699; tel. 904/368–2300, (Nonreporting) **A**1 9 10 18 **S** Health Management Associates, Naples, FL
Primary Contact: Brent Burish, Chief Executive Officer
Web address: www.shands.org
**Control:** Partnership, Investor–owned, for–profit **Service:** General Medical and Surgical

**Staffed Beds:** 25

**STUART—Martin County**

⊠ **MARTIN HEALTH SYSTEM (100044)**, 200 S.E. Hospital Avenue, Zip 34994, Mailing Address: P.O. Box 9010, Zip 34995–9010; tel. 772/287–5200, (Includes MARTIN MEMORIAL HOSPITAL SOUTH, 2100 S.E. Salerno Road, Zip 34997; tel. 772/223–2300) **A**1 2 9 10 **F**3 8 11 12 13 15 17 18 20 22 24 26 28 29 30 31 35 36 37 40 42 45 46 47 49 50 51 53 55 60 64 68 70 72 74 75 76 77 78 79 81 82 85 86 87 89 91 93 94 95 107 108 110 111 113 114 116 117 118 119 120 122 123 125 128 129 131 142 143 145 **P**6
Primary Contact: Mark E. Robitaille, President and Chief Executive Officer
CFO: Mark Cocorullo, Senior Vice President and Chief Financial Officer
CMO: Howard M. Robbins, M.D., Senior Vice President and Chief Medical Officer
CIO: Edmund Collins, Chief Information Officer
CHR: Amy Barry, Vice President and Chief Human Resources Officer
Web address: www.mmhs.com
**Control:** Other not–for–profit (including NFP Corporation) **Service:** General Medical and Surgical

**Staffed Beds:** 316 **Admissions:** 16986 **Census:** 209 **Outpatient Visits:** 86211 **Births:** 1818 **Total Expense ($000):** 285970 **Payroll Expense ($000):** 116990 **Personnel:** 1412

FL

**Hospital, Medicare Provider Number, Address, Telephone, Approval, Facility, and Physician Codes, Health Care System**

★ American Hospital Association (AHA) membership
☐ The Joint Commission accreditation
◇ DNV Healthcare Inc. accreditation
○ American Osteopathic Association (AOA) accreditation
△ Commission on Accreditation of Rehabilitation Facilities (CARF) accreditation

## SUN CITY CENTER—Hillsborough County

☒ **SOUTH BAY HOSPITAL (100259)**, 4016 Sun City Center Boulevard, Zip 33573–5298; tel. 813/634–3301 **A**1 9 10 **F**3 15 18 29 30 31 34 35 40 45 49 50 51 57 59 64 68 70 74 75 77 78 79 81 85 86 87 93 107 108 110 111 113 117 118 130 131 145 147 **S** HCA, Nashville, TN
Primary Contact: Sharon L. Roush, Chief Executive Officer
COO: Gary Malaer, Chief Operating Officer
CFO: Shawn Gregory, Chief Financial Officer
CIO: Danny Waters, Director Information Technology and Systems
CHR: Dana Wheeler, Director Human Resources
CNO: Terrie Jefferson, R.N., Chief Nursing Officer
Web address: www.southbayhospital.com
**Control:** Corporation, Investor–owned, for–profit **Service:** General Medical and Surgical

Staffed Beds: 112 Admissions: 6890 Census: 87 Outpatient Visits: 37789 Births: 0 Total Expense ($000): 60145 Payroll Expense ($000): 22841 Personnel: 342

## TALLAHASSEE—Leon County

☒ **CAPITAL REGIONAL MEDICAL CENTER (100254)**, 2626 Capital Medical Boulevard, Zip 32308–4499; tel. 850/325–5000, (Nonreporting) **A**1 9 10 **S** HCA, Nashville, TN
Primary Contact: Brian Cook, FACHE, Chief Executive Officer
COO: Dale Neely, Chief Operating Officer
CFO: Michael Gordian, Chief Financial Officer
CMO: Steve West, M.D., Chief Medical Officer
CIO: Robert A. Steed, Director Information Systems
CHR: Louise Truitt, Vice President Human Resources
Web address: www.capitalregionalmedicalcenter.com
**Control:** Corporation, Investor–owned, for–profit **Service:** General Medical and Surgical

Staffed Beds: 198

**EASTSIDE PSYCHIATRIC HOSPITAL (104059)**, 2634 Capital Circle N.E., Zip 32308–4106; tel. 850/523–3333, (Nonreporting) **A**9 10
Primary Contact: Jay A. Reeve, President and Chief Executive Officer
COO: Sue Conger, Chief Operating Officer
CFO: Virginia Kelly, Chief Financial Officer
CMO: Ludmila de Faria, M.D., Chief Medical Officer
CIO: Thad Moorer, Chief Information Officer
CHR: Candy Landry, Chief Human Resource Officer
CNO: Judy Goreau, R.N., Director of Nursing
Web address: www.apalacheecenter.org
**Control:** Other not–for–profit (including NFP Corporation) **Service:** Psychiatric

Staffed Beds: 24

☒ **HEALTHSOUTH REHABILITATION HOSPITAL OF TALLAHASSEE (103033)**, 1675 Riggins Road, Zip 32308–5315; tel. 850/656–4800, (Nonreporting) **A**1 9 10 **S** HEALTHSOUTH Corporation, Birmingham, AL
Primary Contact: Heath Phillips, Chief Executive Officer
CFO: Jennifer Spooner, Controller
CMO: Robert Rowland, M.D., Medical Director
CIO: Charles O'Keefe, Director Health Information Services
CHR: Shelia Schiefelbein, Director Human Resources
Web address: www.healthsouthtallahassee.com
**Control:** Corporation, Investor–owned, for–profit **Service:** Rehabilitation

Staffed Beds: 76

☒ **SELECT SPECIALTY HOSPITAL–TALLAHASSEE (102020)**, 1554 Surgeons Drive, Zip 32308; tel. 850/219–6800, (Nonreporting) **A**1 9 10 **S** Select Medical Corporation, Mechanicsburg, PA
Primary Contact: Lora Davis, Chief Executive Officer
Web address: www.selectmedicalcorp.com
**Control:** Corporation, Investor–owned, for–profit **Service:** Long–Term Acute Care hospital

Staffed Beds: 29

☒ **TALLAHASSEE MEMORIAL HEALTHCARE (100135)**, 1300 Miccosukee Road, Zip 32308–5093; tel. 850/431–1155, (Total facility includes 42 beds in nursing home–type unit) **A**1 2 3 5 9 10 **F**2 3 5 6 8 11 12 15 16 17 18 20 22 24 26 29 30 31 34 35 37 40 43 45 46 47 48 49 50 51 53 54 55 56 57 58 59 60 61 62 64 65 68 70 72 73 74 75 76 77 78 79 80 81 82 84 85 86 87 88 89 91 93 96 97 98 99 100 102 103 104 107 108 110 113 114 116 117 118 119 120 122 123 125 126 127 128 129 130 131 134 142 143 145 146 147 **P**6
Primary Contact: G. Mark O'Bryant, President and Chief Executive Officer
COO: Jason H. Moore, Vice President and Chief Operating Officer
CFO: William A. Giudice, Vice President and Chief Financial Officer
CMO: Dean Watson, M.D., Chief Medical Officer
CIO: Don Lindsey, Vice President and Chief Information Officer
CHR: Steve W. Adriaanse, Vice President and Chief Human Resources Officer
Web address: www.tmh.org
**Control:** Other not–for–profit (including NFP Corporation) **Service:** General Medical and Surgical

Staffed Beds: 489 Admissions: 24721 Census: 356 Outpatient Visits: 400944 Births: 3704 Total Expense ($000): 394012 Payroll Expense ($000): 171011 Personnel: 3268

## TAMARAC—Broward County

☒ **UNIVERSITY HOSPITAL AND MEDICAL CENTER (100224)**, 7201 North University Drive, Zip 33321–2996; tel. 954/721–2200, (Includes UNIVERSITY PAVILION, 7425 North University Drive, Zip 33328; tel. 305/722–9933) **A**1 9 10 **F**3 15 29 30 31 34 35 40 45 46 49 50 51 57 58 59 60 64 68 70 74 75 77 78 79 81 82 85 86 87 91 93 98 99 100 101 102 103 105 107 108 110 111 116 118 123 128 129 131 134 145 146 147 **S** HCA, Nashville, TN
Primary Contact: Mark Rader, FACHE, Chief Executive Officer
CFO: Aurelio Gonzalez, Chief Financial Officer
CMO: Ran Abrahamy, M.D., Chief of Staff
CIO: Tom Scharff, Director Information Services
Web address: www.uhmchealth.com
**Control:** Corporation, Investor–owned, for–profit **Service:** General Medical and Surgical

Staffed Beds: 317 Admissions: 11056 Census: 139 Outpatient Visits: 48016 Births: 0 Total Expense ($000): 73848 Payroll Expense ($000): 38314 Personnel: 620

## TAMPA—Hillsborough County

☒ △ **FLORIDA HOSPITAL TAMPA (100173)**, 3100 East Fletcher Avenue, Zip 33613–4688; tel. 813/971–6000, (Nonreporting) **A**1 2 3 5 7 9 10 **S** Adventist Health System Sunbelt Health Care Corporation, Altamonte Springs, FL
Primary Contact: John R. Harding, Chief Executive Officer
COO: Jeffrey Oskin, Vice President Ancillary and Support Services
CFO: Marvin A. Kurtz, Senior Vice President Finance and Chief Financial Officer
CMO: Brad Bjornstad, M.D., Vice President and Chief Medical Officer
CIO: Brigitte W. Shaw, Chief Operating Officer, Pepin Heart Hospital
CHR: James Hackman, Corporate Vice President Human Resources
Web address: www.uch.org
**Control:** Other not–for–profit (including NFP Corporation) **Service:** General Medical and Surgical

Staffed Beds: 320

☒ **FLORIDA HOSPITAL–CARROLLWOOD (100069)**, 7171 North Dale Mabry Highway, Zip 33614–2699; tel. 813/932–2222 **A**1 9 10 **F**3 8 11 15 29 30 31 34 35 40 44 45 48 49 50 53 54 56 57 58 59 60 61 62 64 65 68 70 74 75 77 78 79 80 81 82 85 86 87 93 97 107 111 113 118 129 130 131 142 143 145 147 **S** Adventist Health System Sunbelt Health Care Corporation, Altamonte Springs, FL
Primary Contact: Brinsley B. Lewis, Chief Executive Officer
COO: Mary C. Whillock, R.N., Associate Nursing Officer and Chief Operating Officer
CFO: Marvin A. Kurtz, Chief Financial Officer
Web address: www.uch.org
**Control:** Church–operated, Nongovernment, not–for profit **Service:** General Medical and Surgical

Staffed Beds: 59 Admissions: 4769 Census: 51 Outpatient Visits: 48968 Births: 0 Total Expense ($000): 83413 Payroll Expense ($000): 26060 Personnel: 499

☒ **H. LEE MOFFITT CANCER CENTER AND RESEARCH INSTITUTE (100271)**, 12902 Magnolia Drive, Zip 33612–9497; tel. 813/972–4673 **A**1 2 3 5 8 9 10 **F**3 8 11 15 26 29 30 31 34 35 36 37 48 49 50 54 55 56 57 58 59 63 64 68 70 71 74 75 77 78 79 81 82 83 84 85 86 87 90 91 92 93 96 97 98 100 101 103 104 107 108 109 110 111 113 114 115 116 117 118 119 120 122 123 125 129 131 133 134 135 140 143 145 146 147 Primary Contact: William S. Dalton, Ph.D., M.D., President and Chief Executive Officer
COO: John A. Kolosky, Executive Vice President and Chief Operating Officer
CFO: Janene Culumber, Vice President and Chief Financial Officer
CMO: W. Michael Alberts, M.D., Vice President Medical Affairs
CIO: Mark Hulse, Vice President and Chief Information Officer
CHR: Yvette Tremonti, Vice President Human Resources
Web address: www.moffitt.org
**Control:** Other not–for–profit (including NFP Corporation) **Service:** Cancer

Staffed Beds: 206 Admissions: 8921 Census: 156 Outpatient Visits: 328311 Births: 0 Total Expense ($000): 734870 Payroll Expense ($000): 293426 Personnel: 4049

☒ △ **JAMES A. HALEY VETERANS HOSPITAL**, 13000 Bruce B. Downs Boulevard, Zip 33612–4798; tel. 813/972–2000, (Nonreporting) **A**1 3 5 7 8 **S** Department of Veterans Affairs, Washington, DC
Primary Contact: Nancy Reissener, Acting Director
COO: Michael C. Jorge, Ph.D., Associate Director
CFO: Rita Mercier, Manager Finance
CMO: Edward Cutolo, Jr., M.D., Chief of Staff
CIO: Jose Seymour, Chief Information Resource Management
CHR: Neal C. Hamilton, Chief Human Resources
Web address: www.va.gov/visn8/tampa
**Control:** Veterans Affairs, Government, federal **Service:** General Medical and Surgical

Staffed Beds: 93

FL

*Many Facility Codes have changed. Please refer to the AHA Guide Code Chart.* © 2012 AHA Guide

⊠ **KINDRED HOSPITAL BAY AREA–TAMPA (102009)**, 4555 South Manhattan Avenue, Zip 33611–2397; tel. 813/839–6341, (Nonreporting) **A**1 10 **S** Kindred Healthcare, Louisville, KY
Primary Contact: Julie Feasel, Chief Executive Officer
CFO: Frank Billy, Chief Financial Officer
CHR: Michael Grimes, Manager Human Resources
Web address: www.khtampa.com/
**Control:** Corporation, Investor–owned, for–profit **Service:** Long–Term Acute Care hospital

**Staffed Beds: 155**

⊠ **KINDRED HOSPITAL–CENTRAL TAMPA (102013)**, 4801 North Howard Avenue, Zip 33603–1484; tel. 813/874–7575, (Nonreporting) **A**1 9 10 **S** Kindred Healthcare, Louisville, KY
Primary Contact: Debra Plummer, Chief Executive Officer
CFO: John Miner, Chief Financial Officer
Web address: www.kindredcentraltampa.com/
**Control:** Corporation, Investor–owned, for–profit **Service:** Long–Term Acute Care hospital

**Staffed Beds: 102**

**MEMORIAL HOSPITAL OF TAMPA (100206)**, 2901 Swann Avenue, Zip 33609–4057; tel. 813/873–6400, (Nonreporting) **A**5 9 10 21 **S** IASIS Healthcare, Franklin, TN
Primary Contact: John J. Mainieri, Chief Executive Officer
CFO: Shelley V. Kolseth, Chief Financial Officer
CIO: John Riton, Director Information Services
Web address: www.memorialhospitaltampa.com
**Control:** Corporation, Investor–owned, for–profit **Service:** General Medical and Surgical

**Staffed Beds: 139**

☐ **SHRINERS HOSPITALS FOR CHILDREN, TAMPA (103303)**, 12502 USF Pine Drive, Zip 33612–9499; tel. 813/972–2250 **A**1 3 5 10 **F**3 34 35 50 57 64 68 74 77 79 81 85 89 91 93 94 107 130 145 **S** Shriners Hospitals for Children, Tampa, FL
Primary Contact: Alice Reed Lanford, R.N., MSN, FACHE, Administrator
CFO: Ruth Gregos, Director Finance
CMO: Dennis Grogan, M.D., Chief of Staff
Web address: www.shrinershq.org
**Control:** Other not–for–profit (including NFP Corporation) **Service:** Children's orthopedic

**Staffed Beds: 25 Admissions: 334 Census: 2 Outpatient Visits: 12000 Births: 0**

⊠ **ST. JOSEPH'S HOSPITAL (100075)**, 3001 West Martin Luther King Boulevard, Zip 33607–6387, Mailing Address: P.O. Box 4227, Zip 33677–4227; tel. 813/870–4000, (Includes ST. JOSEPH'S CHILDREN'S HOSPITAL OF TAMPA, 3001 Dr. Martin Luther King Jr. Boulevard, Zip 33607; tel. 813/554–8500; ST. JOSEPH'S WOMEN'S HOSPITAL – TAMPA, 3030 West Dr. Martin L. King Boulevard, Zip 33607–6394; tel. 813/872–2950; Kimberly Guy, Chief Operating Officer), (Nonreporting) **A**1 2 3 5 9 10 **S** Catholic Health East, Newtown Square, PA
Primary Contact: Isaac Mallah, President and Chief Executive Officer
COO: Lorraine Lutton, Chief Operating Officer
CFO: Cathy Yoder, Chief Financial Officer
CMO: Mark Vaaler, M.D., Vice President Medical Staff Affairs
CIO: Lindsey Jarrell, Vice President Information Services
CHR: Pat Teeuwen, Director Team Resources
Web address: www.sjbhealth.org
**Control:** Church–operated, Nongovernment, not–for profit **Service:** General Medical and Surgical

**Staffed Beds: 883**

⊠ △ **TAMPA GENERAL HOSPITAL (100128)**, 1 Tampa General Circle, Zip 33606–3508, Mailing Address: P.O. Box 1289, Zip 33601–1289; tel. 813/844–7000, (Includes TAMPA GENERAL HOSPITAL CHILDREN'S MEDICAL CENTER, 1 Tampa General Circle, Zip 33606–3571; tel. 813/844–7000) **A**1 3 5 7 8 9 10 **F**3 7 8 9 11 12 13 15 16 17 18 19 20 22 24 26 28 29 30 31 32 34 35 36 37 38 39 40 41 43 44 45 46 47 48 49 50 51 52 53 54 55 56 57 58 59 60 61 64 65 66 68 70 72 73 74 75 76 77 78 79 81 82 83 84 85 86 87 88 89 90 91 92 93 94 96 97 98 99 100 101 102 103 107 108 109 110 111 113 114 118 119 120 121 122 123 125 128 129 130 131 133 134 136 137 138 139 140 141 142 144 145 146 147 **P**6
Primary Contact: Ronald A. Hytoff, FACHE, President and Chief Executive Officer
COO: Deana Nelson, R.N., Executive Vice President and Chief Operating Officer
CFO: Steve Short, Executive Vice President Finance and Administration
CMO: Sally Houston, M.D., Senior Vice President and Chief Medical Officer
CIO: Elizabeth Lindsay-Wood, Vice President Information Systems
CHR: Chris Roederer, Vice President Human Resources
CNO: Janet Davis, R.N., Senior Vice President and Chief Nursing Officer
Web address: www.tgh.org
**Control:** Other not–for–profit (including NFP Corporation) **Service:** General Medical and Surgical

**Staffed Beds: 1018 Admissions: 39215 Census: 733 Outpatient Visits: 351315 Births: 5505 Total Expense ($000): 1008362 Payroll Expense ($000): 384692 Personnel: 6860**

**TOWN AND COUNTRY HOSPITAL (100255)**, 6001 Webb Road, Zip 33615–3291; tel. 813/888–7060, (Nonreporting) **A**5 9 10 21 **S** IASIS Healthcare, Franklin, TN
Primary Contact: Dale Johns, Administrator
CMO: Patrick Horan, M.D., Chief of Staff
CIO: Larry Mohammed, Director Information Systems
CHR: Judy Miller, Director Human Resources
Web address: www.townandcountryhospital.com
**Control:** Partnership, Investor–owned, for–profit **Service:** General Medical and Surgical

**Staffed Beds: 200**

## TARPON SPRINGS—Pinellas County

⊠ **FLORIDA HOSPITAL NORTH PINELLAS (100055)**, 1395 South Pinellas Avenue, Zip 34689–3721; tel. 727/942–5000, (Nonreporting) **A**1 9 10 **S** Adventist Health System Sunbelt Health Care Corporation, Altamonte Springs, FL
Primary Contact: Bruce Bergherm, Chief Executive Officer
COO: Karen Owensby, R.N., Chief Operating Officer and Chief Nursing Officer
COO: Amy Patterson, Chief Operating Officer and Chief Nursing Officer
CFO: Michael Mewhirter, Chief Financial Officer
CMO: Nicolas Pavouris, M.D., President Medical Staff
CMO: Nicolas Pavouris, M.D., Chief of Medical Staff
CIO: Francisco Manalo, Director of Information Services
CHR: Vernon Elarbee, Director of Human Resources
CNO: Karen Owensby, R.N., Chief Operating Officer and Chief Nursing Officer
Web address: www.hemh.com
**Control:** Other not–for–profit (including NFP Corporation) **Service:** General Medical and Surgical

**Staffed Beds: 150**

## TAVARES—Lake County

⊠ **FLORIDA HOSPITAL WATERMAN (100057)**, 1000 Waterman Way, Zip 32778–5266; tel. 352/253–3333, (Nonreporting) **A**1 2 9 10 **S** Adventist Health System Sunbelt Health Care Corporation, Altamonte Springs, FL
Primary Contact: Kenneth R. Mattison, President and Chief Executive Officer
COO: Carrie L. Fish, Senior Vice President and Chief Operating Officer
CFO: Frances H. Crunk, Vice President and Chief Financial Officer
CMO: Vinay Mehindru, M.D., Vice President/Chief Medical Officer
CHR: Madge Springer, Director Human Resources
CNO: Patricia R. Dolan, R.N., Vice President/ Chief Nursing Officer
Web address: www.fhwat.org
**Control:** Church–operated, Nongovernment, not–for profit **Service:** General Medical and Surgical

**Staffed Beds: 204**

FL

---

**Hospital, Medicare Provider Number, Address, Telephone, Approval, Facility, and Physician Codes, Health Care System**

★ American Hospital Association (AHA) membership
☐ The Joint Commission accreditation
◇ DNV Healthcare Inc. accreditation
○ American Osteopathic Association (AOA) accreditation
△ Commission on Accreditation of Rehabilitation Facilities (CARF) accreditation

## TAVERNIER—Monroe County

☒ **BAPTIST HEALTH SOUTH FLORIDA, MARINERS HOSPITAL (101313)**, 91500 Overseas Highway, Zip 33070–2547; tel. 305/434–3000 **A**1 9 10 18 20 **F**3 11 15 18 28 29 30 31 34 35 40 45 47 50 53 57 59 68 70 74 75 79 81 84 85 93 97 102 107 108 110 111 113 118 128 129 130 132 145 147 **P**6 8 **S** Baptist Health South Florida, Coral Gables, FL
Primary Contact: Rick Freeburg, Chief Executive Officer
CFO: Erik Long, Controller
CIO: Mimi Taylor, Vice President Information Technology
CHR: John Williamson, Human Resources Site Manager
Web address: www.baptisthealth.net
**Control:** Other not–for–profit (including NFP Corporation) **Service:** General Medical and Surgical

| | |
|---|---|
| **Staffed Beds:** 25 **Admissions:** 706 **Census:** 8 **Outpatient Visits:** 19843 **Births:** 0 **Total Expense ($000):** 39639 **Payroll Expense ($000):** 13612 **Personnel:** 206 | |

## THE VILLAGES—Sumter County

☒ **THE VILLAGES HEALTH SYSTEM (100290)**, 1451 El Camino Real, Zip 32159; tel. 352/751–8000 **A**1 9 10 **F**11 15 17 18 20 22 24 26 29 30 31 34 35 40 45 53 57 64 70 74 78 81 86 93 107 111 113 118 145 **S** Central Florida Health Alliance, Leesburg, FL
Primary Contact: Tim F. Hawkins, Chief Executive Officer
CFO: Dale E. Hocking, Senior Vice President and Chief Financial Officer
CMO: Daniel Carlson, M.D., Senior Vice President Medical Affairs and Chief Medical Officer
CIO: Nancy Vester, Vice President and Chief Information Officer
CHR: Darlene Stone, Senior Vice President Human Resources
CNO: Rosemary Reiner, MSN, Vice President and Chief Clinical Officer
Web address: www.cfhalliance.org
**Control:** Other not–for–profit (including NFP Corporation) **Service:** General Medical and Surgical

| | |
|---|---|
| **Staffed Beds:** 198 **Admissions:** 12212 **Census:** 138 **Outpatient Visits:** 50862 **Births:** 0 **Total Expense ($000):** 124848 **Payroll Expense ($000):** 44901 **Personnel:** 729 | |

**THE VILLAGES REGIONAL HOSPITAL** See The Villages Health System

## TITUSVILLE—Brevard County

☐ **PARRISH MEDICAL CENTER (100028)**, 951 North Washington Avenue, Zip 32796–2163; tel. 321/268–6111, (Nonreporting) **A**1 2 9 10
Primary Contact: George Mikitarian, Jr., Chief Executive Officer
CFO: Timothy K. Skeldon, Senior Vice President and Chief Financial Officer
CMO: Lisa Alexanda, M.D., Vice President Medical Affairs
CIO: William Moore, Chief Information Officer
CHR: Roberta Chaildin, Manager Human Resources
Web address: www.parrishmed.com
**Control:** Hospital district or authority, Government, nonfederal **Service:** General Medical and Surgical

| | |
|---|---|
| **Staffed Beds:** 210 | |

## TRINITY—Pasco County

☒ **MEDICAL CENTER OF TRINITY (100191)**, 9330 State Road 54, Zip 34655, Mailing Address: P.O. Box 996, New Port Richey, Zip 34656–0996; tel. 727/834–4900 **A**1 2 5 9 10 **F**8 11 18 20 22 26 29 30 31 34 35 38 40 45 46 47 48 49 57 59 60 67 68 70 74 75 76 77 78 79 80 81 82 84 85 86 87 93 94 97 98 102 103 107 108 110 111 118 125 129 131 134 145 146 147 **S** HCA, Nashville, TN
Primary Contact: Leigh Massengill, Chief Executive Officer
COO: Mary Ann Knight, Chief Operating Officer
COO: Thibaut vanMarcke, Chief Operating Officer
CFO: Alex Romanchik, Chief Financial Officer
CMO: Linda Badillo, M.D., Chief of Medical Staff
CIO: Kurt Hornung, Director
CHR: Christena Miano, Human Resources Director
CNO: Nancy Maysilles, R.N., Chief Nursing Officer
Web address: www.medicalcentertrinity.com
**Control:** Corporation, Investor–owned, for–profit **Service:** General Medical and Surgical

| | |
|---|---|
| **Staffed Beds:** 292 **Admissions:** 13443 **Census:** 168 **Outpatient Visits:** 64990 **Births:** 638 **Total Expense ($000):** 119529 **Payroll Expense ($000):** 49049 **Personnel:** 1080 | |

## VENICE—Sarasota County

☐ **VENICE REGIONAL MEDICAL CENTER (100070)**, 540 The Rialto, Zip 34285–2900; tel. 941/485–7711, (Nonreporting) **A**1 9 10 **S** Health Management Associates, Naples, FL
Primary Contact: Peter Wozniak, MS, R.N., Chief Executive Officer
CFO: Fred Ashworth, Chief Financial Officer
CHR: Dana Wheeler, Director Human Resources
Web address: www.veniceregional.com
**Control:** Corporation, Investor–owned, for–profit **Service:** General Medical and Surgical

| | |
|---|---|
| **Staffed Beds:** 220 | |

## VERO BEACH—Indian River County

☒ **HEALTHSOUTH TREASURE COAST REHABILITATION HOSPITAL (103032)**, 1600 37th Street, Zip 32960–6549; tel. 772/778–2100, (Nonreporting) **A**1 9 10 **S** HEALTHSOUTH Corporation, Birmingham, AL
Primary Contact: Kevin R. Conn, Interim Chief Executive Officer
CFO: Kevin Hardy, Chief Financial Officer
CMO: Jimmy Wayne Lockhart, M.D., Medical Director
CHR: Pearl Shisler, Director Human Resources
Web address: www.healthsouthtreasurecoast.com
**Control:** Corporation, Investor–owned, for–profit **Service:** Rehabilitation

| | |
|---|---|
| **Staffed Beds:** 90 | |

☒ **INDIAN RIVER MEDICAL CENTER (100105)**, 1000 36th Street, Zip 32960–6592; tel. 772/567–4311 **A**1 2 9 10 **F**3 11 12 13 17 18 20 22 24 26 28 29 30 31 34 35 37 40 44 49 50 51 57 58 59 60 61 64 70 74 75 76 77 78 79 80 81 82 83 84 85 86 87 89 92 93 96 97 98 99 100 101 102 103 104 107 108 111 113 114 117 118 119 120 122 128 129 130 131 134 143 145 146 147 **P**6
Primary Contact: Jeffrey L. Susi, President and Chief Executive Officer
CFO: Wael Fakhry, Senior Vice President and Chief Financial Officer
CHR: Barbara Horne, R.N., Vice President and Chief Human Resource Development Officer
Web address: www.irmc.cc
**Control:** Other not–for–profit (including NFP Corporation) **Service:** General Medical and Surgical

| | |
|---|---|
| **Staffed Beds:** 245 **Admissions:** 14522 **Census:** 170 **Outpatient Visits:** 156612 **Births:** 1140 **Total Expense ($000):** 183150 **Payroll Expense ($000):** 78542 **Personnel:** 1355 | |

## WAUCHULA—Hardee County

☒ **FLORIDA HOSPITAL WAUCHULA (101300)**, 533 West Carlton Street, Zip 33873; tel. 863/773–3101, (Nonreporting) **A**1 9 10 18 **S** Adventist Health System Sunbelt Health Care Corporation, Altamonte Springs, FL
Primary Contact: Linda Adler, Administrator
COO: Isaac Palmer, Chief Operating Officer
CFO: Dima Didenko, Vice President and Chief Financial Officer
CHR: Michelle F. Myers, Manager Human Resources
Web address: www.fhheartland.org
**Control:** Church–operated, Nongovernment, not–for profit **Service:** General Medical and Surgical

| | |
|---|---|
| **Staffed Beds:** 25 | |

## WEST PALM BEACH—Palm Beach County

☒ ○ **COLUMBIA HOSPITAL (100234)**, 2201 45th Street, Zip 33407–2069; tel. 561/842–6141, (Nonreporting) **A**1 9 10 11 12 13 **S** HCA, Nashville, TN
Primary Contact: Dana Oaks, Chief Executive Officer
COO: Patrick Connor, Chief Operating Officer
CFO: Oon Soo Ung, Chief Financial Officer
CMO: Paul Seltzer, M.D., Chief of Staff
CIO: Martha Stinson, Director
CHR: Donna Boyle, Director
Web address: www.columbiahospital.com
**Control:** Corporation, Investor–owned, for–profit **Service:** General Medical and Surgical

| | |
|---|---|
| **Staffed Beds:** 250 | |

☒ **GOOD SAMARITAN MEDICAL CENTER (100287)**, 1309 North Flagler Drive, Zip 33401–3499; tel. 561/655–5511, (Nonreporting) **A**1 2 9 10 **S** TENET Healthcare Corporation, Dallas, TX
Primary Contact: Mark Nosacka, Chief Executive Officer
CFO: Cynthia McCauley, Chief Financial Officer
CIO: Candace Helms, Director Information Services
CHR: Amy Linsin, Chief Human Resources Officer
Web address: www.goodsamaritanmc.com
**Control:** Corporation, Investor–owned, for–profit **Service:** General Medical and Surgical

| | |
|---|---|
| **Staffed Beds:** 174 | |

**JEROME GOLDEN CENTER FOR BEHAVIORAL HEALTH, INC. (104008)**, 1041 45th Street, Zip 33407–2494; tel. 561/383–8000, (Nonreporting) **A**9 10
Primary Contact: Linda De Piano, Ph.D., Chief Executive Officer
CFO: Pat Priola, Chief Financial Officer
CMO: Suresh Rajpara, M.D., Chief Medical Officer
CIO: Emiliano Fernandez, Director Information Services
CHR: Diane B. White, Director Human Resources
Web address: www.jeromegoldencenter.org
**Control:** Other not–for–profit (including NFP Corporation) **Service:** Psychiatric

| | |
|---|---|
| **Staffed Beds:** 44 | |

**PALM BEACH CHILDREN'S HOSPITAL** See St. Mary's Medical Center

FL

⊠ △ **ST. MARY'S MEDICAL CENTER (100288)**, 901 45th Street,
Zip 33407–2495; tel. 561/844–6300, (Includes PALM BEACH CHILDREN'S
HOSPITAL, 901 45th Street, Zip 33407; tel. 561/844–6300), (Nonreporting) **A**1
7 9 10 **S** TENET Healthcare Corporation, Dallas, TX
Primary Contact: Davide M. Carbone, FACHE, Chief Executive Officer
CFO: Tom Schlemmer, Chief Financial Officer
CMO: Jeffrey David, D.O., Chief Medical Officer
CIO: Rich Avato, Director
CHR: Sandy Wyant, Director Human Resources
Web address: www.stmarysmc.com
**Control:** Corporation, Investor–owned, for–profit **Service:** General Medical and
Surgical

**Staffed Beds:** 463

⊠ △ **VETERANS AFFAIRS MEDICAL CENTER**, 7305 North Military Trail,
Zip 33410–6400; tel. 561/422–8262, (Nonreporting) **A**1 3 5 7 **S** Department of
Veterans Affairs, Washington, DC
Primary Contact: Charleen R. Szabo, FACHE, Director
CFO: Lori Hancock, Chief Business Officer
CMO: Deepak Mandi, M.D., Chief of Staff
CIO: Karen Gabaldon, Chief Management Information Systems
CHR: David Green, Chief Human Resources
Web address: www.va.gov/sta/guide/home.asp
**Control:** Veterans Affairs, Government, federal **Service:** General Medical and
Surgical

**Staffed Beds:** 133

☐ **WELLINGTON REGIONAL MEDICAL CENTER (100275)**, 10101 Forest Hill
Boulevard, Zip 33414–6199; tel. 561/798–8500, (Nonreporting) **A**1 2 9 10 12
13 **S** Universal Health Services, Inc., King of Prussia, PA
Primary Contact: Jerel T. Humphrey, Chief Executive Officer
CFO: Woody White, Chief Financial Officer
CMO: Gordon Johnson, M.D., Chief of Staff
CIO: Pierre Bergeron, Director Information Services
CHR: Mary Jo Garski, Director Human Resources
CNO: Michelle Epps, R.N., Chief Nursing Officer
Web address: www.wellingtonregional.com
**Control:** Corporation, Investor–owned, for–profit **Service:** General Medical and
Surgical

**Staffed Beds:** 108

### WESTON—Broward County

⊠ **CLEVELAND CLINIC FLORIDA (100289)**, 3100 Weston Road,
Zip 33331–3602; tel. 954/659–6001 **A**1 2 3 5 9 10 **F**3 8 12 15 18 20 22 24
26 28 29 30 31 34 35 37 40 45 46 47 48 49 50 54 55 56 57 58 59 60 61
63 64 65 68 70 74 75 77 78 79 81 82 85 86 87 91 92 93 97 100 101 107
108 109 110 111 113 114 115 116 118 125 128 129 130 131 135 145 146
147 **P**6 **S** Cleveland Clinic Health System, Cleveland, OH
Primary Contact: Bernardo Fernandez, M.D., Chief Executive Officer
COO: Liz Matuk, Executive Director, Administrative and Clinical Services
COO: Marty Sargeant, Chief Operating Officer
CFO: Keith Nilsson, Chief Financial Officer
CMO: Juan Nogueras, M.D., Chief of Staff
CIO: John Santangelo, Director Information Technology
CHR: Paula Adamson, Manager Human Resources
CHR: Stuart Thompson, Director Human Resources
CNO: Kerry Major, R.N., Chief Nursing Officer
Web address: www.clevelandclinic.org/florida
**Control:** Other not–for–profit (including NFP Corporation) **Service:** General
Medical and Surgical

**Staffed Beds:** 155 **Admissions:** 10254 **Census:** 120 **Outpatient Visits:**
138243 **Births:** 0 **Total Expense ($000):** 136058 **Payroll Expense ($000):**
55406 **Personnel:** 2811

### WILLISTON—Levy County

**NATURE COAST REGIONAL HOSPITAL** See Tri–County Hospital – Williston

**TRI–COUNTY HOSPITAL – WILLISTON (100139)**, 125 S.W. Seventh Street,
Zip 32696–2403; tel. 352/528–2801, (Nonreporting) **A**9 10
Primary Contact: Jerry E. Gillman, Chief Executive Officer
CFO: Barbara Miller, Manager Business Office
CMO: Jeremie Young, M.D., Chief of Staff
CHR: Karla Dass, Director Human Resources
Web address: www.tricountyhosp.com/
**Control:** Partnership, Investor–owned, for–profit **Service:** Long–Term Acute Care
hospital

**Staffed Beds:** 20

### WINTER HAVEN—Polk County

⊠ △ **WINTER HAVEN HOSPITAL (100052)**, 200 Avenue F. N.E.,
Zip 33881–4193; tel. 863/293–1121 **A**1 7 9 10 **F**3 8 11 13 14 15 17 18 20
22 24 26 28 29 30 31 34 36 40 45 52 57 58 59 60 64 68 70 72 73 74 75
76 77 78 79 81 82 84 85 86 87 89 90 93 94 98 100 101 102 103 104 107
108 111 113 117 118 120 122 125 129 131 134 143 145 146 147 **P**6
Primary Contact: Lance W. Anastasio, President
COO: Mary Jo Schreiber, R.N., Vice President Patient Services
CFO: David MacDougall, Vice President Finance
CMO: Donald I. Gale, M.D., Vice President Medical Affairs
CIO: Pat Mongoven, Director Information Systems
Web address: www.winterhavenhospital.org
**Control:** Other not–for–profit (including NFP Corporation) **Service:** General
Medical and Surgical

**Staffed Beds:** 519 **Admissions:** 15319 **Census:** 188 **Outpatient Visits:**
281765 **Births:** 1654 **Total Expense ($000):** 234040 **Payroll Expense
($000):** 112185 **Personnel:** 2423

### WINTER PARK—Orange County

**WINTER PARK MEMORIAL HOSPITAL** See Florida Hospital, Orlando

### ZEPHYRHILLS—Pasco County

⊠ **FLORIDA HOSPITAL ZEPHYRHILLS (100046)**, 7050 Gall Boulevard,
Zip 33541–1399; tel. 813/788–0411, (Nonreporting) **A**1 5 9 10 **S** Adventist
Health System Sunbelt Health Care Corporation, Altamonte Springs, FL
Primary Contact: Douglas Duffield, President and Chief Executive Officer
COO: Donald E. Welch, Chief Operating Officer
CFO: Paul Ziegele, Chief Financial Officer
CIO: Kelley Sasser, Director Information Systems
CHR: Laura Asaftei, Administrative Director
CNO: Ruth Hemphill, R.N., Chief Nursing Officer
Web address: www.fhzeph.org
**Control:** Church–operated, Nongovernment, not–for profit **Service:** General
Medical and Surgical

**Staffed Beds:** 154

---

**Hospital, Medicare Provider Number, Address, Telephone, Approval, Facility, and Physician Codes, Health Care System**

★ American Hospital Association (AHA) membership
☐ The Joint Commission accreditation          ◇ DNV Healthcare Inc. accreditation

○ American Osteopathic Association (AOA) accreditation
△ Commission on Accreditation of Rehabilitation Facilities (CARF) accreditation

**FL**

# GEORGIA

### ADEL—Cook County

☐ **COOK MEDICAL CENTER–A CAMPUS OF TIFT REGIONAL MEDICAL CENTER (110101)**, 706 North Parrish Avenue, Zip 31620–0677; tel. 229/896–8000, (Total facility includes 95 beds in nursing home–type unit) **A**1 9 10 **F**11 13 15 29 30 34 35 40 46 56 57 59 64 70 75 76 81 86 87 93 97 107 110 111 117 118 129 132 134 145 146
Primary Contact: Michael L. Purvis, Chief Executive Officer
COO: Kim Wills, Chief Operating Officer
CIO: Barry Medley, Director Information Systems
CHR: Shirley Padgett, Director Human Resources
**Control:** Corporation, Investor–owned, for–profit **Service:** General Medical and Surgical

**Staffed Beds:** 155 **Admissions:** 1051 **Census:** 94 **Outpatient Visits:** 15896 **Births:** 112 **Total Expense ($000):** 13839 **Payroll Expense ($000):** 6171 **Personnel:** 226

### ALBANY—Dougherty County

⊠ **PHOEBE NORTH (110163)**, 2000 Palmyra Road, Zip 31702–1908, Mailing Address: P.O. Box 1908, Zip 31702–1908; tel. 229/434–2000 **A**1 9 10 **F**3 12 15 17 29 30 34 40 43 45 46 48 49 51 56 57 60 63 64 70 74 75 77 79 81 82 86 90 93 107 111 113 118 129 130 131 145 147 **P**5 **S** Phoebe Putney Health System, Albany, GA
Primary Contact: Hugh D. Wilson, Interim Chief Executive Officer
CFO: Karen Hayes, Chief Financial Officer
CHR: Tracy St. Amant, Director Human Resources
Web address: www.palmyramedicalcenters.com
**Control:** Hospital district or authority, Government, nonfederal **Service:** General Medical and Surgical

**Staffed Beds:** 102 **Admissions:** 3369 **Census:** 52 **Outpatient Visits:** 55696 **Births:** 0 **Total Expense ($000):** 62826 **Payroll Expense ($000):** 20993 **Personnel:** 360

⊠ **PHOEBE PUTNEY MEMORIAL HOSPITAL (110007)**, 417 Third Avenue, Zip 31701–1828, Mailing Address: P.O. Box 1828, Zip 31702–1828; tel. 229/883–1800 **A**1 2 3 5 9 10 **F**3 5 7 8 11 12 13 15 17 18 20 22 24 26 28 29 30 31 34 35 38 40 44 45 46 49 50 51 53 54 55 56 57 58 59 60 62 63 64 68 70 72 73 74 75 76 77 78 79 81 82 83 84 85 86 87 89 90 92 93 94 96 97 98 100 101 102 103 104 105 107 108 110 111 113 116 117 118 119 120 122 123 125 126 128 129 130 131 133 134 135 143 144 145 146 147 **P**1 7 **S** Phoebe Putney Health System, Albany, GA
Primary Contact: Joel Wernick, President and Chief Executive Officer
CFO: Kerry Loudermilk, Senior Vice President and Chief Financial Officer
CMO: Douglas Patten, M.D., Director Medical Affairs
CIO: Jesse Diaz, Chief Information Officer
CHR: David J. Baranski, Vice President Human Resources
Web address: www.phoebeputney.com
**Control:** Other not–for–profit (including NFP Corporation) **Service:** General Medical and Surgical

**Staffed Beds:** 440 **Admissions:** 18736 **Census:** 277 **Outpatient Visits:** 713484 **Births:** 2814 **Total Expense ($000):** 457431 **Payroll Expense ($000):** 138461 **Personnel:** 3233

### ALMA—Bacon County

⊠ **BACON COUNTY HOSPITAL AND HEALTH SYSTEM (111327)**, 302 South Wayne Street, Zip 31510–2997, Mailing Address: P.O. Drawer 1987, Zip 31510–1987; tel. 912/632–8961, (Nonreporting) **A**1 9 10 18
Primary Contact: Cindy R. Turner, Chief Executive Officer
COO: Cindy R. Turner, Chief Executive Officer
CFO: Kyle Kimmel, Chief Financial Officer
CMO: Lou Ellen Hutcheson, M.D., Chief of Staff
CHR: Jackie Lewis, Director Human Resources
CNO: Deanna Williams, R.N., Director of Nursing
Web address: www.baconcountyhospital.com
**Control:** Other not–for–profit (including NFP Corporation) **Service:** General Medical and Surgical

**Staffed Beds:** 113

### AMERICUS—Sumter County

⊠ **PHOEBE SUMTER MEDICAL CENTER (110044)**, 126 Highway 280 West, Zip 31719; tel. 229/924–6011, (Nonreporting) **A**1 9 10 **S** Phoebe Putney Health System, Albany, GA
Primary Contact: Keith J. Petersen, Chief Executive Officer
CFO: Laurie Hair, Chief Financial Officer
CMO: Andrew Carlson, M.D., Vice President Medical Staff Services
CIO: Becky Lightner, Director Information Systems
CHR: Deatrice Harris, Supervisor Human Resources and Employment
Web address: www.phoebesumter.org
**Control:** Other not–for–profit (including NFP Corporation) **Service:** General Medical and Surgical

**Staffed Beds:** 45

### ARLINGTON—Calhoun County

**CALHOUN MEMORIAL HOSPITAL (111309)**, 55 R.E. Jennings Avenue, Zip 39813–8722, Mailing Address: P.O. Box 496, Zip 39813–0496; tel. 229/725–4272, (Nonreporting) **A**9 10 18
Primary Contact: Earl S. Whiteley, Administrator
Web address: www.hacc–ga.com
**Control:** Hospital district or authority, Government, nonfederal **Service:** General Medical and Surgical

**Staffed Beds:** 25

### ATHENS—Clarke County

⊠ **ATHENS REGIONAL MEDICAL CENTER (110074)**, 1199 Prince Avenue, Zip 30606–2793; tel. 706/475–7000 **A**1 2 9 10 **F**3 8 11 13 15 17 18 20 22 24 26 28 29 30 31 34 35 36 40 43 45 46 47 48 51 54 56 57 59 60 62 68 70 72 73 74 76 77 78 79 80 81 83 84 85 86 87 89 92 93 94 96 107 108 110 111 115 116 118 119 120 122 123 128 129 130 131 134 144 145 146 147
Primary Contact: James G. Thaw, President and Chief Executive Officer
COO: Linda Della Torre, Senior Vice President and Chief Operating Officer
CFO: W. Larry Webb, Senior Vice President and Chief Financial Officer
CMO: Mark J. Costantino, M.D., Interim Chief Medical Officer
CIO: Steve W. Davis, Interim Chief Information Officer
CHR: Kevin Thigpen, Vice President Human Resources
Web address: www.armc.org
**Control:** Other not–for–profit (including NFP Corporation) **Service:** General Medical and Surgical

**Staffed Beds:** 359 **Admissions:** 17892 **Census:** 217 **Outpatient Visits:** 224152 **Births:** 2578 **Total Expense ($000):** 286177 **Payroll Expense ($000):** 136541 **Personnel:** 2538

☐ **LANDMARK HOSPITAL OF ATHENS (112017)**, 775 Sunset Drive, Zip 30606–2211; tel. 706/425–1500 **A**1 10 **F**1 3 29 30 45 118 129 147 **S** Landmark Hospitals, Cape Girardeau, MO
Primary Contact: Tommy Jackson, Chief Executive Officer
Web address: www.landmarkhospitals.com
**Control:** Individual, Investor–owned, for–profit **Service:** Long–Term Acute Care hospital

**Staffed Beds:** 42 **Admissions:** 458 **Census:** 32 **Outpatient Visits:** 0 **Births:** 0 **Personnel:** 122

⊠ △ **ST. MARY'S HEALTH CARE SYSTEM (110006)**, 1230 Baxter Street, Zip 30606–3791; tel. 706/389–3000 **A**1 7 9 10 **F**6 10 11 12 13 15 18 20 22 26 28 29 30 34 40 45 46 47 48 49 51 53 54 57 58 59 62 63 64 67 68 70 72 74 75 76 77 79 81 82 83 84 89 90 91 93 107 108 109 110 111 112 113 114 118 123 124 125 128 129 130 145 146 **S** Catholic Health East, Newtown Square, PA
Primary Contact: Donald McKenna, President and Chief Executive Officer
COO: Montez Carter, Vice President Operations
CFO: Marty Hutson, Chief Financial Officer
CMO: Bruce Middendorf, M.D., Chief Medical Officer
CIO: Kerry Vaughn, Chief Information Officer
CHR: Jeff English, Vice President Human Resources
CNO: Nina Evans, R.N., Vice President and Chief Nursing Officer
Web address: www.stmarysathens.com
**Control:** Church–operated, Nongovernment, not–for profit **Service:** General Medical and Surgical

**Staffed Beds:** 165 **Admissions:** 9386 **Census:** 114 **Outpatient Visits:** 118828 **Births:** 1420 **Total Expense ($000):** 155182 **Payroll Expense ($000):** 56815

*Many Facility Codes have changed. Please refer to the AHA Guide Code Chart.*   © 2012 AHA Guide

**ATLANTA—Fulton and De Kalb County**

**ANCHOR HOSPITAL (114032)**, 5454 Yorktowne Drive, Zip 30349–5305; tel. 770/991–6044, (Nonreporting) **A**10 **S** Universal Health Services, Inc., King of Prussia, PA
Primary Contact: Jennifer Morgan, Chief Executive Officer and Managing Director
COO: Jennifer Morgan, Chief Executive Officer and Managing Director
CMO: Joel Kirson, M.D., Medical Director
Web address: www.anchorhospital.com
**Control:** Corporation, Investor–owned, for–profit **Service:** Alcoholism and other chemical dependency

**Staffed Beds:** 111

⊞ **ATLANTA MEDICAL CENTER (110115)**, 303 Parkway Drive N.E., Zip 30312–1212; tel. 404/265–4000 **A**1 3 5 8 9 10 **F**11 12 13 15 17 18 20 22 24 26 28 29 30 31 34 35 36 37 38 40 43 44 45 46 50 51 53 54 56 57 59 60 61 64 65 66 68 70 72 73 74 75 76 77 78 79 81 84 85 86 87 90 93 96 97 98 100 101 102 103 104 107 108 111 113 117 118 128 129 131 133 145 146 147 **P**3 7 8 **S** TENET Healthcare Corporation, Dallas, TX
Primary Contact: William T. Moore, Chief Executive Officer
COO: Robert Russell, Chief Operating Officer
CFO: Lisa Napier, Chief Financial Officer
CMO: Pano Lamis, M.D., Medical Director
CIO: Maryland McCarty, Director Information Systems
CHR: Troy Bond, Chief Human Resources Officer
CNO: Jacqueline Herd, R.N., Chief Nursing Officer
Web address: www.atlantamedcenter.com
**Control:** Corporation, Investor–owned, for–profit **Service:** General Medical and Surgical

**Staffed Beds:** 403 **Admissions:** 14421 **Census:** 227 **Outpatient Visits:** 85153 **Births:** 3432 **Total Expense ($000):** 223522 **Payroll Expense ($000):** 81075 **Personnel:** 1423

☐ △ **CHILDREN'S HEALTHCARE OF ATLANTA (113300)**, 1600 Tullie Circle, N.E., Zip 30329–2303; tel. 404/325–6000, (Includes CHILDREN'S HEALTHCARE OF ATLANTA AT EGLESTON, 1600 Tullie Circle, Zip 30329; tel. 404/325–6000; CHILDREN'S HEALTHCARE OF ATLANTA AT SCOTTISH RITE, 1001 Johnson Ferry Road N.E., Zip 30342–1600; tel. 404/256–5252), (Nonreporting) **A**1 3 5 7 8 9 10
Primary Contact: Donna W. Hyland, President and Chief Executive Officer
COO: Carolyn Kenny, Executive Vice President Clinical Care
CFO: Ruth Fowler, Senior Vice President and Chief Financial Officer
CMO: Daniel Salinas, M.D., Senior Vice President and Chief Medical Officer
CIO: Praveen Chopra, Chief Information and Supply Chain Officer
CHR: Linda Matzigkeit, Senior Vice President Human Resources
Web address: www.choa.org
**Control:** Other not–for–profit (including NFP Corporation) **Service:** Children's general

**Staffed Beds:** 496

⊞ △ **EMORY UNIVERSITY HOSPITAL (110010)**, 1364 Clifton Road N.E., Zip 30322–1102; tel. 404/712–2000, (Includes EMORY UNIVERSITY ORTHOPAEDIC AND SPINE HOSPITAL, 1455 Montreal Road, Tucker, Zip 30084; tel. 404/251–3600; June Conner, R.N., Chief Operating Officer) **A**1 2 3 5 7 8 9 10 **F**3 9 11 12 14 15 17 18 20 22 24 26 28 29 30 31 34 35 37 38 40 44 45 46 47 49 50 55 57 58 59 60 61 64 65 68 70 74 75 77 78 79 81 82 83 84 85 86 87 90 93 98 99 100 101 102 103 104 107 108 110 111 113 114 115 116 117 118 119 120 122 123 125 129 130 131 134 135 136 137 138 139 140 141 144 145 146 147 **P**6 **S** Emory Healthcare, Atlanta, GA
Primary Contact: Robert J. Bachman, Chief Operating Officer
CMO: Ira Horowitz, M.D., Chief Medical Officer
CIO: Dedra Cantrell, Chief Information Officer
CHR: Margaret A. Bloomquist, Assistant Administrator Human Resources
Web address: www.emoryhealthcare.org
**Control:** Other not–for–profit (including NFP Corporation) **Service:** General Medical and Surgical

**Staffed Beds:** 579 **Admissions:** 25217 **Census:** 454 **Outpatient Visits:** 137921 **Births:** 0 **Total Expense ($000):** 681226 **Payroll Expense ($000):** 224592 **Personnel:** 3556

⊞ **EMORY UNIVERSITY HOSPITAL MIDTOWN (110078)**, 550 Peachtree Street N.E., Zip 30308; tel. 404/686–4411 **A**1 2 3 5 8 9 10 **F**3 11 12 13 15 17 18 20 22 24 26 28 29 30 31 34 35 38 40 44 46 50 51 52 55 57 58 59 60 61 64 65 68 70 72 73 74 75 76 77 78 79 80 81 82 83 84 85 86 87 93 100 102 104 107 108 110 111 113 114 115 116 117 118 119 120 122 123 125 129 130 131 134 145 146 147 **S** Emory Healthcare, Atlanta, GA
Primary Contact: Dane C. Peterson, Chief Operating Officer
COO: Dane C. Peterson, Chief Operating Officer
CFO: Greg E. Anderson, Chief Financial Officer
CMO: James P. Steinberg, M.D., Chief Medical Officer
CIO: Dedra Cantrell, Chief Information Officer
CHR: Dallis Howard–Crow, Chief Human Resources Officer
Web address: www.emoryhealthcare.org
**Control:** Other not–for–profit (including NFP Corporation) **Service:** General Medical and Surgical

**Staffed Beds:** 469 **Admissions:** 20959 **Census:** 301 **Outpatient Visits:** 162468 **Births:** 3576 **Total Expense ($000):** 472439 **Payroll Expense ($000):** 150918 **Personnel:** 2384

⊞ **GRADY MEMORIAL HOSPITAL (110079)**, 80 Jesse Hill Jr. Drive S.E., Zip 30303, Mailing Address: P.O. Box 26189, Zip 30303–3801; tel. 404/616–1000, (Total facility includes 261 beds in nursing home–type unit) **A**1 2 3 5 8 9 10 **F**3 5 7 8 13 15 16 17 18 20 22 24 26 29 30 31 34 35 39 40 43 44 45 50 51 52 53 54 56 57 59 60 61 62 64 65 66 68 70 72 73 74 75 76 77 78 79 80 81 82 84 85 86 87 93 97 98 99 100 101 102 103 104 105 106 107 108 109 110 111 113 114 115 116 117 118 119 120 127 129 131 133 134 135 136 137 138 139 140 141 142 143 145 146 147 **P**6
Primary Contact: John M. Haupert, FACHE, Chief Executive Officer
COO: Mark J. Chastang, FACHE, Chief Operating Officer
CFO: Sue McCarthy, Chief Financial Officer
CMO: Curtis Lewis, M.D., Chief of Staff
CIO: Deborah Cancilla, Chief Information Officer
CHR: Althea Williams, Senior Vice President Human Resources
Web address: www.gradyhealthsystem.org
**Control:** Other not–for–profit (including NFP Corporation) **Service:** General Medical and Surgical

**Staffed Beds:** 921 **Admissions:** 27570 **Census:** 680 **Outpatient Visits:** 540179 **Births:** 2971 **Total Expense ($000):** 377765 **Payroll Expense ($000):** 241977 **Personnel:** 4172

⊞ **KINDRED HOSPITAL–ATLANTA (112004)**, 705 Juniper Street N.E., Zip 30308; tel. 404/873–2871 **A**1 9 10 **F**1 3 29 30 57 60 63 75 82 86 87 92 96 119 129 131 147 **S** Kindred Healthcare, Louisville, KY
Primary Contact: Michael Schmitt, Chief Executive Officer
CFO: Phillip Johnson, CPA, Chief Financial Officer
CMO: David N. DeRuyter, M.D., President Medical Staff
CHR: Armetria Gibson, Human Resources Generalist
CNO: Annette Harrilson, Chief Clinical Officer
Web address: www.kindredatlanta.com/
**Control:** Partnership, Investor–owned, for–profit **Service:** Long–Term Acute Care hospital

**Staffed Beds:** 70 **Admissions:** 408 **Census:** 42 **Outpatient Visits:** 0 **Births:** 0 **Total Expense ($000):** 16630 **Payroll Expense ($000):** 8793 **Personnel:** 166

☐ **NORTHSIDE HOSPITAL (110161)**, 1000 Johnson Ferry Road N.E., Zip 30342–1611; tel. 404/851–8000 **A**1 2 9 10 **F**3 5 11 12 13 15 18 20 22 26 28 29 30 31 34 35 40 44 45 46 47 48 49 50 54 55 57 58 59 60 64 68 70 71 72 73 74 75 76 77 78 79 80 81 82 84 85 86 87 93 100 104 105 107 108 110 111 113 114 116 117 118 119 120 122 123 125 128 129 131 134 135 144 145 146 147 **S** Northside Healthcare System, Atlanta, GA
Primary Contact: Robert Quattrocchi, President and Chief Executive Officer
CFO: Debbie Mitcham, Chief Financial Officer
CIO: Tina Wakim, Vice President Information
CHR: Dwight Hill, Vice President Human Resources
Web address: www.northside.com
**Control:** Other not–for–profit (including NFP Corporation) **Service:** General Medical and Surgical

**Staffed Beds:** 571 **Admissions:** 32337 **Census:** 425 **Outpatient Visits:** 346012 **Births:** 14438 **Total Expense ($000):** 682741 **Payroll Expense ($000):** 266584 **Personnel:** 4436

☐ **PEACHFORD BEHAVIORAL HEALTH SYSTEM (114010)**, 2151 Peachford Road, Zip 30338–6599; tel. 770/455–3200, (Nonreporting) **A**1 9 10 **S** Universal Health Services, Inc., King of Prussia, PA
Primary Contact: Matthew Crouch, Chief Executive Officer and Managing Director
COO: Sharon Stackhouse, Assistant Administrator and Director Risk Management
CFO: April Hughes, Chief Financial Officer
CMO: Asaf Aleem, M.D., Medical Director
CHR: Clay Boyles, Director Human Resources
Web address: www.peachfordhospital.com
**Control:** Corporation, Investor–owned, for–profit **Service:** Psychiatric

**Staffed Beds:** 224

**GA**

**Hospital, Medicare Provider Number, Address, Telephone, Approval, Facility, and Physician Codes, Health Care System**

★ American Hospital Association (AHA) membership
☐ The Joint Commission accreditation
◇ DNV Healthcare Inc. accreditation
○ American Osteopathic Association (AOA) accreditation
△ Commission on Accreditation of Rehabilitation Facilities (CARF) accreditation

✠ **PIEDMONT HOSPITAL (110083)**, 1968 Peachtree Road N.W.,
Zip 30309–1231; tel. 404/605–5000 **A**1 2 3 5 9 10 **F**3 8 11 13 15 17 18 20
22 24 26 28 29 30 31 34 35 40 45 46 47 48 49 50 51 53 54 55 56 57 58
59 60 63 64 65 68 70 72 73 74 75 76 77 78 79 81 82 84 85 86 87 93 107
108 110 111 113 114 115 116 117 118 119 120 122 123 125 128 129 130
131 134 137 138 141 142 145 146 147 **S** Piedmont Healthcare, Atlanta, GA
Primary Contact: Leslie A. Donahue, President and Chief Executive Officer
COO: Denise Ray, Senior Vice President and Chief Operating Officer
CFO: Thomas Arnold, Chief Financial Officer
CMO: Matthew Schreiber, M.D., Chief Medical Officer
CIO: Mark Pasquale, Vice President Information Systems
CHR: Steve Karasick, Interim Vice President Human Resources
Web address: www.piedmonthospital.org
**Control:** Other not–for–profit (including NFP Corporation) **Service:** General
Medical and Surgical

**Staffed Beds:** 481 **Admissions:** 26260 **Census:** 365 **Outpatient Visits:**
346140 **Births:** 3453

✠ **SAINT JOSEPH'S HOSPITAL OF ATLANTA (110082)**, 5665 Peachtree
Dunwoody Road N.E., Zip 30342–1764; tel. 678/843–7001 **A**1 2 9 10 **F**3 11
15 17 18 20 22 24 26 28 29 30 31 34 35 37 40 44 45 46 47 48 49 50 54
55 57 58 59 60 64 68 70 71 74 75 78 79 81 82 84 85 87 93 107 108 110
111 113 114 115 116 117 118 119 120 122 123 125 129 131 134 136 144
145 146 **P**2 **S** Catholic Health East, Newtown Square, PA
Primary Contact: Scott Schmidly, Chief Executive Officer
CFO: Kevin Brenan, Chief Financial Officer
CMO: Paul Scheinberg, M.D., Chief of Staff
CIO: Scott Rattray, Vice President and Chief Information Officer
CHR: Audra Farish, Vice President Human Resources
Web address: www.stjosephsatlanta.org
**Control:** Other not–for–profit (including NFP Corporation) **Service:** General
Medical and Surgical

**Staffed Beds:** 258 **Admissions:** 14314 **Census:** 196 **Outpatient Visits:**
197757 **Births:** 0 **Total Expense ($000):** 318246 **Payroll Expense ($000):**
110588 **Personnel:** 1911

★ **SELECT SPECIALTY HOSPITAL–ATLANTA (112009)**, 550 Peachtree Street
N.E., Zip 30308; tel. 404/686–2270, (Nonreporting) **A**9 10 **S** Select Medical
Corporation, Mechanicsburg, PA
Primary Contact: Andrew Tatnall, Chief Executive Officer
Web address: www.selectmedical.com
**Control:** Corporation, Investor–owned, for–profit **Service:** Long–Term Acute Care
hospital

**Staffed Beds:** 30

☐ △ **SHEPHERD CENTER (112003)**, 2020 Peachtree Road N.W.,
Zip 30309–1465; tel. 404/352–2020, (Nonreporting) **A**1 3 5 7 9 10
Primary Contact: Gary R. Ulicny, Ph.D., President and Chief Executive Officer
COO: Sarah Morrison, Vice President Clinical Services
CFO: Stephen B. Holleman, Chief Financial Officer
CMO: Donald P. Leslie, M.D., Medical Director
CIO: Michael L. Jones, Ph.D., Chief Information Officer
CHR: Betsy Fox, Director Human Resources
CNO: Tamara King, R.N., Chief Nurse Executive
Web address: www.shepherd.org
**Control:** Other not–for–profit (including NFP Corporation) **Service:** Rehabilitation

**Staffed Beds:** 100

✠ **SOUTH FULTON MEDICAL CENTER (110219)**, 1170 Cleveland Avenue,
Zip 30344–3665; tel. 404/466–1170 **A**1 2 5 9 10 **F**3 11 13 15 17 18 20 22
29 30 31 40 48 49 53 57 59 60 61 64 66 72 74 75 76 77 78 79 81 93 94
98 101 102 107 108 110 111 113 114 118 128 129 146 147 **S** TENET
Healthcare Corporation, Dallas, TX
Primary Contact: James Clements, Chief Executive Officer
CFO: Jacob Spruit, Jr., Chief Financial Officer
CMO: Albert Barrocas, M.D., Chief Medical Officer
CHR: Detra Bickerstaff, Chief Human Resources Officer
Web address: www.southfultonmedicalcenter.com
**Control:** Corporation, Investor–owned, for–profit **Service:** General Medical and
Surgical

**Staffed Beds:** 210 **Admissions:** 7088 **Census:** 101 **Outpatient Visits:** 80887
**Births:** 1454 **Total Expense ($000):** 101357 **Payroll Expense ($000):**
50397 **Personnel:** 534

✠ **WESLEY WOODS GERIATRIC HOSPITAL OF EMORY UNIVERSITY (110203)**,
(Multi–Discrip Geri Hospital), 1821 Clifton Road N.E., Zip 30329–5102;
tel. 404/728–6200, (Total facility includes 250 beds in nursing home–type unit)
**A**1 3 5 9 10 **F**3 6 10 11 29 30 34 38 39 59 65 67 68 71 75 77 82 85 87
74 75 77 82 84 86 87 90 93 96 98 100 101 102 103 104 105 107 118 124
127 128 129 131 142 145 147 **S** Emory Healthcare, Atlanta, GA
Primary Contact: William Such, Chief Executive Officer
CFO: Greg E. Anderson, Chief Financial Officer
CMO: Frank Brown, M.D., Chief Medical Officer
CIO: Dedra Cantrell, Chief Information Officer
CHR: Dallis Howard–Crow, Chief Human Resources Officer
Web address: www.emoryhealthcare.org
**Control:** Other not–for–profit (including NFP Corporation) **Service:** Other specialty

**Staffed Beds:** 276 **Admissions:** 2532 **Census:** 213 **Outpatient Visits:** 15193
**Births:** 0 **Total Expense ($000):** 41902 **Payroll Expense ($000):** 27444
**Personnel:** 464

☐ **WESLEY WOODS LONG TERM CARE HOSPITAL (112005)**, 1821 Clifton Road
N.E., 2nd Floor, Zip 30329; tel. 404/728–6200 **A**1 10 **F**1 3 11 29 30 34 56 68
74 75 77 82 85 87 **S** Emory Healthcare, Atlanta, GA
Primary Contact: William Such, Chief Executive Officer
CFO: Theodore Saunders, Assistant Controller
CMO: Jeffrey Mikell, M.D., Chief Medical Officer
CIO: Vicky Goziah, Software Administrator
Web address: www.emoryhealthcare.org
**Control:** Other not–for–profit (including NFP Corporation) **Service:** Long–Term
Acute Care hospital

**Staffed Beds:** 18 **Admissions:** 218 **Census:** 16 **Outpatient Visits:** 0 **Births:**
0 **Total Expense ($000):** 8909 **Payroll Expense ($000):** 2679 **Personnel:**
42

**AUGUSTA—Richmond County**

✠ **DOCTORS HOSPITAL (110177)**, 3651 Wheeler Road, Zip 30909–6426;
tel. 706/651–3232 **A**1 2 5 9 10 **F**8 12 13 15 16 18 22 29 30 31 34 39 40 41
43 46 49 50 51 57 59 60 64 70 71 72 74 75 76 77 78 79 81 82 84 85 87
89 90 91 92 93 94 96 97 107 108 110 111 113 115 116 118 119 120 122
123 125 128 129 130 131 134 140 145 146 147 **P**1 **S** HCA, Nashville, TN
Primary Contact: Douglas Welch, Chief Executive Officer
CFO: Terence Van Arkel, Vice President and Chief Financial Officer
CIO: Dona Hornung, Director Information and Technology Services
Web address: www.doctors–hospital.net
**Control:** Corporation, Investor–owned, for–profit **Service:** General Medical and
Surgical

**Staffed Beds:** 287 **Admissions:** 12811 **Census:** 179 **Outpatient Visits:**
109485 **Births:** 1468 **Total Expense ($000):** 186131 **Payroll Expense**
**($000):** 60967 **Personnel:** 912

☐ **EAST CENTRAL REGIONAL HOSPITAL (114029)**, 3405 Mike Padgett
Highway, Zip 30906–3897; tel. 706/792–7000, (Includes EAST CENTRAL
REGIONAL HOSPITAL, 100 Myrtle Boulevard, Gracewood, Zip 30812–1299;
tel. 706/790–2011), (Total facility includes 391 beds in nursing home–type unit)
**A**1 3 5 9 10 **F**29 34 38 39 59 65 67 75 77 86 87 96 98 101 127 129
142 **P**6
Primary Contact: Nan M. Lewis, Administrator
CFO: Terry Tribble, Chief Financial Officer
Web address: www.augustareg.dhr.state.ga.us
**Control:** State–Government, nonfederal **Service:** Psychiatric

**Staffed Beds:** 552 **Admissions:** 1740 **Census:** 469 **Outpatient Visits:** 0
**Births:** 0 **Total Expense ($000):** 87977 **Payroll Expense ($000):** 35638
**Personnel:** 1627

✠ **GEORGIA HEALTH SCIENCES MEDICAL CENTER (110034)**, 1120 15th
Street, Zip 30912–5000; tel. 706/721–0211, (Includes MCG CHILDREN'S
MEDICAL CENTER, 1446 Harper Street, Zip 30912–0012; tel. 706/721–2273)
**A**1 2 3 5 8 9 10 13 **F**3 6 11 12 13 14 15 17 18 19 20 21 22 23 24 25 26 27
28 29 30 31 32 34 35 36 38 39 40 41 43 44 45 46 48 49 50 51 54 55 56
58 59 60 61 64 65 66 67 68 70 72 73 74 75 76 77 78 79 81 82 84 85 86
87 88 89 91 92 93 97 98 99 100 101 102 103 104 107 108 111 114 115
116 117 118 119 120 122 123 125 126 128 129 130 131 133 134 135 137
140 141 142 144 145 146 147 **P**3 7
Primary Contact: David S. Hefner, President and Chief Executive Officer
CFO: Dennis Roemer, Senior Vice President and Chief Financial Officer
CMO: William Kanto, M.D., Acting Senior Vice President and Chief Medical Officer
CIO: Richard R. Bias, Acting Vice President Information Systems and Chief
Information Officer
CHR: Derek Carissimi, Vice President Human Resources
Web address: www.mcghealth.org
**Control:** Other not–for–profit (including NFP Corporation) **Service:** General
Medical and Surgical

**Staffed Beds:** 503 **Admissions:** 19373 **Census:** 325 **Outpatient Visits:**
443463 **Births:** 775 **Total Expense ($000):** 472553 **Payroll Expense**
**($000):** 202094 **Personnel:** 3219

**MEDICAL COLLEGE OF GEORGIA HEALTH** See Georgia Health Sciences
Medical Center

**GA**

*Many Facility Codes have changed. Please refer to the AHA Guide Code Chart.* © 2012 AHA Guide

✠ **SELECT SPECIALTY HOSPITAL–AUGUSTA (112013)**, 1537 Walton Way, Zip 30904; tel. 706/731–1169 **A**1 9 10 **F**1 29 30 107 108 129 147 **S** Select Medical Corporation, Mechanicsburg, PA
Primary Contact: David L. Mork, Jr., FACHE, Chief Executive Officer
CHR: Terrie Richardson, Coordinator Human Resources
CNO: Kim Pippin, Chief Nursing Officer
Web address: www.selectmedical.com
**Control:** Corporation, Investor–owned, for–profit **Service:** Long–Term Acute Care hospital

**Staffed Beds:** 80 **Admissions:** 779 **Census:** 56 **Births:** 0

✠ **TRINITY HOSPITAL OF AUGUSTA (110039)**, 2260 Wrightsboro Road, Zip 30904–4726; tel. 706/481–7000, (Nonreporting) **A**1 5 9 10 **S** Community Health Systems, Inc., Franklin, TN
Primary Contact: James A. Cruickshank, Chief Executive Officer
CFO: Marc Nakagawa, Chief Financial Officer
CMO: Lawrence LaHatte, M.D., Chief of Staff
CIO: Charlotte Choate, Director Information Systems
CHR: Connie Martin, Director Human Resources
Web address: www.trinityofaugusta.com
**Control:** Corporation, Investor–owned, for–profit **Service:** General Medical and Surgical

**Staffed Beds:** 105

✠ **UNIVERSITY HEALTH CARE SYSTEM (110028)**, 1350 Walton Way, Zip 30901–2629; tel. 706/722–9011 **A**1 2 3 5 9 10 **F**3 13 15 17 18 20 22 24 26 28 29 30 31 34 35 37 38 40 41 44 48 49 50 53 54 56 57 59 60 62 64 68 70 72 73 74 75 76 77 78 79 80 81 82 83 84 85 86 87 89 93 97 100 107 108 111 113 114 115 117 118 125 128 129 131 133 134 143 145 146 147 **P**8
Primary Contact: James R. Davis, President and Chief Executive Officer
COO: Marilyn A. Bowcutt, R.N., Senior Vice President and Chief Operating Officer
CFO: David Belkoski, Executive Vice President and Chief Financial Officer
CMO: William L. Farr, M.D., Chief Medical Officer
CIO: Leslie Clonch, Vice President and Chief Information Officer
Web address: www.universityhealth.org
**Control:** Other not–for–profit (including NFP Corporation) **Service:** General Medical and Surgical

**Staffed Beds:** 510 **Admissions:** 21668 **Census:** 299 **Outpatient Visits:** 261821 **Births:** 3196 **Total Expense ($000):** 349714 **Payroll Expense ($000):** 130203 **Personnel:** 2332

✠ △ **VETERANS AFFAIRS MEDICAL CENTER**, 1 Freedom Way, Zip 30904–6285; tel. 706/733–0188, (Nonreporting) **A**1 2 3 5 7 8
**S** Department of Veterans Affairs, Washington, DC
Primary Contact: Patricia O. Pittman, Acting Director
COO: John S. Goldman, Associate Director
CFO: Earline Corder, Chief Fiscal
CMO: Thomas Kiernan, M.D., Chief of Staff
CIO: Susan Lloyd, Chief Health Information Management and Revenue Administration
CHR: Linda Dailey, Acting Chief Human Resources Officer
Web address: www.augusta.va.gov/
**Control:** Veterans Affairs, Government, federal **Service:** General Medical and Surgical

**Staffed Beds:** 338

☐ △ **WALTON REHABILITATION HOSPITAL (113026)**, 1355 Independence Drive, Zip 30901–1037; tel. 706/724–7746, (Nonreporting) **A**1 5 7 9 10
Primary Contact: Dennis B. Skelley, President and Chief Executive Officer
COO: Bob Orsini, Chief Operating Officer
CFO: Mike Harrell, Chief Financial Officer
CMO: Pamela Salazar, M.D., Chief of Staff
CIO: Ann Keller, Manager Health Information Management
CHR: Volante Henderson, Manager Human Resources
CNO: Leslie Baker, R.N., Chief Nursing Officer
Web address: www.wrh.org
**Control:** Other not–for–profit (including NFP Corporation) **Service:** Rehabilitation

**Staffed Beds:** 58

**AUSTELL—Cobb County**

✠ △ **WELLSTAR COBB HOSPITAL (110143)**, 3950 Austell Road, Zip 30106–1121; tel. 770/732–4000 **A**1 2 3 5 7 9 10 **F**3 4 11 13 15 16 17 18 20 22 26 28 29 30 31 37 38 40 41 44 45 48 49 50 53 54 58 61 62 63 64 66 68 70 72 73 74 75 76 77 78 79 80 81 82 84 85 86 87 90 93 94 96 98 100 101 102 103 106 107 108 110 111 113 114 117 118 125 129 140 145 146 147 **P**1 6 **S** WellStar Health System, Marietta, GA
Primary Contact: Kem Mullins, FACHE, Senior Vice President and Hospital President
COO: Ilona Wozniak, Vice President and Chief Operating Officer
CFO: Darold Etheridge, Vice President and Chief Financial Officer
CMO: Don Campbell, M.D., Senior Vice President and Chief Medical Officer
CMO: Thomas McNamara, D.O., Vice President Medical Management
CHR: Joseph W. Herzberg, Assistant Vice President Human Resources
CHR: Alma Stanfield, Director Human Resources
CNO: Lisa Person, MSN, Vice President and Chief Nursing Officer
Web address: www.wellstar.org
**Control:** Other not–for–profit (including NFP Corporation) **Service:** General Medical and Surgical

**Staffed Beds:** 370 **Admissions:** 22588 **Census:** 277 **Outpatient Visits:** 239034 **Births:** 4082 **Personnel:** 1941

**BAINBRIDGE—Decatur County**

✠ **MEMORIAL HOSPITAL AND MANOR (110132)**, 1500 East Shotwell Street, Zip 39819–4256; tel. 229/246–3500, (Nonreporting) **A**1 9 10
Primary Contact: William J. Walker, Jr., Chief Executive Officer
COO: Lee Harris, Assistant Administrator Support Services
CFO: Karen Faircloth, Chief Financial Officer
CMO: Shawn Surratt, M.D., Chief of Staff
CIO: Nelda Moore, Director Data Processing
CHR: Angel Sykes, Director Human Resources
CNO: Cynthia Vickers, R.N., Assistant Administrator for Nursing Services
Web address: www.mh–m.org
**Control:** Hospital district or authority, Government, nonfederal **Service:** General Medical and Surgical

**Staffed Beds:** 80

**BAXLEY—Appling County**

**APPLING HEALTHCARE SYSTEM (110071)**, 163 East Tollison Street, Zip 31513–2898; tel. 912/367–9841, (Total facility includes 101 beds in nursing home–type unit) **A**9 10 20 21 **F**1 7 8 11 13 15 29 30 31 35 40 47 56 60 68 70 75 76 78 80 81 93 98 103 107 111 115 118 126 131 132 142 145 146 147
Primary Contact: Dale Spell, Chief Executive Officer
COO: Dale Spell, Chief Executive Officer
CFO: Farell Turner, Chief Financial Officer
CIO: Brian Snow, Manager Information Systems
CHR: Carla McLendon, Director Human Resources
Web address: www.appling–hospital.org
**Control:** County–Government, nonfederal **Service:** General Medical and Surgical

**Staffed Beds:** 150 **Admissions:** 1580 **Census:** 117 **Outpatient Visits:** 34605 **Births:** 223 **Total Expense ($000):** 36526 **Payroll Expense ($000):** 16344 **Personnel:** 258

**BLAIRSVILLE—Union County**

✠ **UNION GENERAL HOSPITAL (110051)**, 35 Hospital Road, Zip 30512–3139; tel. 706/745–2111, (Nonreporting) **A**1 9 10 20
Primary Contact: Rebecca T. Dyer, Administrator
COO: Mike Gowder, Assistant Administrator
CFO: Tim Henry, Chief Financial Officer
CMO: Andre Schaeffer, M.D., Chief of Staff
CHR: Kathy Hood, Administrative Assistant
Web address: www.uniongeneralhospital.com
**Control:** Hospital district or authority, Government, nonfederal **Service:** General Medical and Surgical

**Staffed Beds:** 195

**BLAKELY—Early County**

✠ **PIONEER COMMUNITY HOSPITAL OF EARLY (111314)**, 11740 Columbia Street, Zip 39823–9604; tel. 229/723–4235, (Nonreporting) **A**1 9 10 18 21
**S** Pioneer Health Services, Magee, MS
Primary Contact: Adam Willmann, Administrator
CFO: Skip Hightower, Senior Vice President and Chief Financial Officer
Web address: www.pchearly.com
**Control:** Corporation, Investor–owned, for–profit **Service:** General Medical and Surgical

**Staffed Beds:** 25

**GA**

| Hospital, Medicare Provider Number, Address, Telephone, Approval, Facility, and Physician Codes, Health Care System |
|---|
| ★ American Hospital Association (AHA) membership      ○ American Osteopathic Association (AOA) accreditation |
| ☐ The Joint Commission accreditation      ◇ DNV Healthcare Inc. accreditation      △ Commission on Accreditation of Rehabilitation Facilities (CARF) accreditation |

## BLUE RIDGE—Fannin County

☒ **FANNIN REGIONAL HOSPITAL (110189)**, 2855 Old Highway 5,
Zip 30513–6248; tel. 706/632–3711 **A**1 9 10 **F**3 11 13 15 28 29 30 35 39
40 50 53 56 57 59 64 68 70 75 76 77 78 79 81 82 85 86 87 93 107 108
110 111 113 118 123 128 129 131 132 133 134 145 146 147 **S** Community
Health Systems, Inc., Franklin, TN
Primary Contact: David S. Sanders, Chief Executive Officer
CFO: Rodney Sisk, Chief Financial Officer
CIO: Timothy Snider, Manager Information Systems
CHR: Terrasina Ensley, Director Human Resources
CNO: Julia Barnett, Chief Nursing Officer
Web address: www.fanninregionalhospital.com
**Control:** Corporation, Investor–owned, for–profit **Service:** General Medical and
Surgical

**Staffed Beds:** 50 **Admissions:** 1912 **Census:** 15 **Outpatient Visits:** 27765
**Births:** 288 **Total Expense ($000):** 32021 **Payroll Expense ($000):** 11105
**Personnel:** 227

## BREMEN—Haralson County

☐ **HIGGINS GENERAL HOSPITAL (111320)**, 200 Allen Memorial Drive,
Zip 30110–2012, Mailing Address: P.O. Box 655, Zip 30110–0655;
tel. 770/537–5851, (Nonreporting) **A**1 9 10 18 **S** Tanner Health System,
Carrollton, GA
Primary Contact: Michael Alexander, Administrator
CIO: Dianne Reed, Director Information Systems
CHR: Vivian C. Barr, Director Human Resources
Web address: www.tanner.org
**Control:** Other not–for–profit (including NFP Corporation) **Service:** General
Medical and Surgical

**Staffed Beds:** 25

## BRUNSWICK—Glynn County

☒ **SOUTHEAST GEORGIA HEALTH SYSTEM BRUNSWICK CAMPUS (110025)**,
2415 Parkwood Drive, Zip 31520–4252, Mailing Address: P.O. Box 1518,
Zip 31521–1518; tel. 912/466–7000, (Total facility includes 250 beds in nursing
home–type unit) **A**1 2 9 10 **F**3 11 12 13 15 17 18 20 22 26 28 29 30 31 34
35 37 40 44 45 46 47 48 49 50 51 54 57 59 64 68 70 71 73 74 75 76 77
78 79 81 85 86 87 89 90 91 93 94 96 98 100 107 108 110 111 113 116
118 119 120 123 125 128 130 131 133 134 143 145 146 147 **P**5 **S** Southeast
Georgia Health System, Brunswick, GA
Primary Contact: Gary R. Colberg, FACHE, President and Chief Executive Officer
CFO: Michael D. Scherneck, Executive Vice President and Chief Financial Officer
CMO: Terry Reynolds, M.D., Chief of Staff
CIO: Chuck Bumgardner, Director Information Systems
CHR: Patrick Ebri, Ph.D., Vice President, Human Resources
Web address: www.sghs.org
**Control:** Hospital district or authority, Government, nonfederal **Service:** General
Medical and Surgical

**Staffed Beds:** 510 **Admissions:** 11848 **Census:** 351 **Outpatient Visits:**
181527 **Births:** 1322 **Total Expense ($000):** 236881 **Payroll Expense
($000):** 99787 **Personnel:** 1477

## CAIRO—Grady County

☒ **GRADY GENERAL HOSPITAL (110121)**, 1155 Fifth Street S.E.,
Zip 39828–0360, Mailing Address: P.O. Box 360, Zip 39828–0360;
tel. 229/377–1150 **A**1 9 10 **F**3 11 13 15 28 29 34 35 40 45 50 57 59 70 75
76 77 79 81 85 86 87 91 92 93 107 110 111 114 118 129 132 134 145 **P**6
**S** Archbold Medical Center, Thomasville, GA
Primary Contact: LaDon Toole, Chief Operating Officer and Administrator
COO: LaDon Toole, Chief Operating Officer and Administrator
CFO: Skip Hightower, Chief Financial Officer
CMO: Stephen Ruberdall, M.D., Chief Medical Officer
CIO: William Zimmermann, Chief Information Officer
CHR: Michelle Pledger, Coordinator Human Resources
Web address: www.archbold.org
**Control:** Hospital district or authority, Government, nonfederal **Service:** General
Medical and Surgical

**Staffed Beds:** 48 **Admissions:** 1362 **Census:** 16 **Outpatient Visits:** 39119
**Births:** 264 **Total Expense ($000):** 18222 **Payroll Expense ($000):** 7810
**Personnel:** 143

## CALHOUN—Gordon County

☒ ○ **GORDON HOSPITAL (110023)**, 1035 Red Bud Road, Zip 30701–2082,
Mailing Address: P.O. Box 12938, Zip 30703–7013; tel. 706/629–2895 **A**1 2 9
10 11 19 **F**3 7 11 13 15 18 20 29 30 31 34 35 37 40 46 57 59 62 64 70 71
75 76 77 78 79 81 82 85 86 87 93 107 108 111 113 115 118 128 129 134
143 145 146 147 **P**1 6 **S** Adventist Health System Sunbelt Health Care
Corporation, Altamonte Springs, FL
Primary Contact: Pete M. Weber, President and Chief Executive Officer
COO: Steve Hannah, Chief Operating Officer
CFO: Cory Reeves, Chief Financial Officer
CMO: Will Theus, M.D., Chief of Staff
CHR: Jeni Hasselbrack, Director Human Resources
Web address: www.gordonhospital.com
**Control:** Church–operated, Nongovernment, not–for profit **Service:** General
Medical and Surgical

**Staffed Beds:** 80 **Admissions:** 4492 **Census:** 51 **Outpatient Visits:** 130039
**Births:** 597 **Total Expense ($000):** 70777 **Payroll Expense ($000):** 31636
**Personnel:** 653

## CAMILLA—Mitchell County

☒ **MITCHELL COUNTY HOSPITAL (111331)**, 90 East Stephens Street,
Zip 31730–1836, Mailing Address: P.O. Box 639, Zip 31730–0639;
tel. 229/336–5284, (Total facility includes 156 beds in nursing home–type unit)
**A**1 9 10 18 **F**3 15 18 26 29 34 35 40 50 59 68 77 87 92 93 97 107 111
118 126 127 129 132 145 **P**6 **S** Archbold Medical Center, Thomasville, GA
Primary Contact: Mark E. Kimball, Administrator
COO: Kevin C. Taylor, Chief Operating Officer
CFO: Skip Hightower, Senior Vice President and Chief Financial Officer
CIO: William Zimmermann, Chief Information Officer
CHR: Vickie County–Teemer, Coordinator Human Resources
Web address: www.archbold.org
**Control:** Hospital district or authority, Government, nonfederal **Service:** General
Medical and Surgical

**Staffed Beds:** 181 **Admissions:** 517 **Census:** 166 **Outpatient Visits:** 29005
**Births:** 0 **Total Expense ($000):** 23763 **Payroll Expense ($000):** 10296
**Personnel:** 143

## CANTON—Cherokee County

☐ **NORTHSIDE HOSPITAL – CHEROKEE (110008)**, 201 Hospital Road,
Zip 30114–2408, Mailing Address: P.O. Box 906, Zip 30169; tel. 770/720–5100
**A**1 9 10 **F**3 8 11 12 13 15 18 20 22 26 28 29 30 31 34 35 40 44 45 50 54
57 59 60 64 68 70 73 74 76 78 79 81 82 85 86 87 93 107 108 110 111
113 118 119 120 122 125 128 129 131 145 146 147 **S** Northside Healthcare
System, Atlanta, GA
Primary Contact: William M. Hayes, Chief Executive Officer
COO: Mike Patterson, Director of Operations
CFO: Brian Jennette, Chief Financial Officer
CMO: Alexander Kessler, M.D., Chief of Staff
CIO: Bill Dunford, Manager
CHR: Roslyn Roberts, Manager
CNO: Jan Johnson, R.N., Chief Nursing Officer
Web address: www.northside.com
**Control:** Other not–for–profit (including NFP Corporation) **Service:** General
Medical and Surgical

**Staffed Beds:** 79 **Admissions:** 5005 **Census:** 58 **Outpatient Visits:** 82092
**Births:** 979 **Total Expense ($000):** 93093 **Payroll Expense ($000):** 36742
**Personnel:** 626

## CARROLLTON—Carroll County

☐ **TANNER MEDICAL CENTER (110011)**, 705 Dixie Street, Zip 30117–3818;
tel. 770/836–9666, (Nonreporting) **A**1 9 10 **S** Tanner Health System,
Carrollton, GA
Primary Contact: Loy M. Howard, President and Chief Executive Officer
CHR: Vivian C. Barr, Director Human Resources
Web address: www.tanner.org
**Control:** Other not–for–profit (including NFP Corporation) **Service:** General
Medical and Surgical

**Staffed Beds:** 176

## CARTERSVILLE—Bartow County

☒ **CARTERSVILLE MEDICAL CENTER (110030)**, 960 Joe Frank Harris Parkway,
Zip 30120–2129; tel. 770/382–1530, (Nonreporting) **A**1 2 9 10 **S** HCA,
Nashville, TN
Primary Contact: Keith Sandlin, Chief Executive Officer
Web address: www.cartersvillemedical.com
**Control:** Corporation, Investor–owned, for–profit **Service:** General Medical and
Surgical

**Staffed Beds:** 80

**GA**

## CEDARTOWN—Polk County

★ **POLK MEDICAL CENTER (111330)**, 424 North Main Street, Zip 30125–2698; tel. 770/748–2500, (Nonreporting) **A**9 10 18 **S** HCA, Nashville, TN
Primary Contact: Kim Scoggins, Administrator
CFO: Heath King, Controller
CHR: Jeanna Smith, Administrative Assistant and Human Resources Officer
Web address: www.polkmedicalcenter.com
**Control:** Corporation, Investor–owned, for–profit **Service:** General Medical and Surgical

**Staffed Beds:** 18

## CHATSWORTH—Murray County

☐ **MURRAY MEDICAL CENTER (110050)**, 707 Old Dalton Ellijay Road, Zip 30705–2060, Mailing Address: P.O. Box 1406, Zip 30705–1406; tel. 706/695–4564 **A**1 9 10 **F**7 15 29 34 40 45 57 59 81 107 110 111 113 118 145 **S** Hamilton Health Care System, Inc., Dalton, GA
Primary Contact: James C. Hazel, FACHE, Chief Executive Officer
CFO: Jana Briley, Director Financial Services
CMO: Michael A. Witt, M.D., Chief of Staff
CIO: Cynthia Austin, Manager Health Information Management
CHR: Jason Hopkins, Director Human Resources
Web address: www.hamiltonhealth.com/
**Control:** Hospital district or authority, Government, nonfederal **Service:** General Medical and Surgical

**Staffed Beds:** 19 **Admissions:** 679 **Census:** 6 **Outpatient Visits:** 27923 **Births:** 0 **Total Expense ($000):** 14976 **Payroll Expense ($000):** 7712

## CLAXTON—Evans County

⊠ **EVANS MEMORIAL HOSPITAL (110142)**, 200 North River Street, Zip 30417–1659, Mailing Address: P.O. Box 518, Zip 30417–0518; tel. 912/739–2611, (Total facility includes 120 beds in nursing home–type unit) **A**1 9 10 **F**3 15 34 40 45 53 57 59 68 81 93 97 107 108 110 111 114 118 126 127 129 134 145
Primary Contact: Martha F. Tatum, Chief Executive Officer
CFO: John Wiggins, Chief Financial Officer
CMO: Yelandra Daniels, M.D., Chief of Staff
CIO: Steve Schmidt, Director Information Systems
CHR: Gina Waters, Director Human Resources
CNO: Nikki NeSmith, Chief Nursing Officer
Web address: www.evansmemorialhospital.org
**Control:** Hospital district or authority, Government, nonfederal **Service:** General Medical and Surgical

**Staffed Beds:** 150 **Admissions:** 1111 **Census:** 119 **Outpatient Visits:** 31862 **Births:** 0 **Total Expense ($000):** 24386 **Payroll Expense ($000):** 10303 **Personnel:** 270

## CLAYTON—Rabun County

**MOUNTAIN LAKES MEDICAL CENTER (111336)**, 196 Ridgecrest Circle, Zip 30525–4111; tel. 706/782–4233, (Nonreporting) **A**9 10 18
Primary Contact: Kim Ingram, Chief Executive Officer
CFO: Jimmy Norman, Chief Financial Officer
CHR: Charles Harbaugh, Director Human Resources
Web address: www.mountainlakesmedicalcenter.com
**Control:** Hospital district or authority, Government, nonfederal **Service:** General Medical and Surgical

**Staffed Beds:** 24

## COCHRAN—Bleckley County

☐ **BLECKLEY MEMORIAL HOSPITAL (111302)**, 145 East Peacock Street, Zip 31014–1559, Mailing Address: P.O. Box 536, Zip 31014–0536; tel. 478/934–6211, (Nonreporting) **A**1 9 10 18
**Control:** Hospital district or authority, Government, nonfederal **Service:** General Medical and Surgical

**Staffed Beds:** 25

## COLQUITT—Miller County

**MILLER COUNTY HOSPITAL (111305)**, 209 North Cuthbert Street, Zip 39837, Mailing Address: P.O. Box 7, Zip 39837; tel. 229/758–3385, (Total facility includes 97 beds in nursing home–type unit) **A**9 10 18 **F**8 13 15 29 30 34 35 40 44 45 50 56 57 59 64 65 66 68 75 77 79 81 85 87 93 97 103 104 107 108 111 113 118 126 127 128 129 132 134 142 144 145 147
Primary Contact: Robin Rau, Chief Executive Officer
CFO: Jill Brown, Chief Financial Officer
CMO: Lamar Brand, M.D., Chief of Staff
CIO: Keith Lovering, Information Technician
CHR: Sharon Calhoun, R.N., Director Human Resources
CNO: Shawn Whittaker, Chief Nursing Officer
Web address: www.millercountyhospital.com
**Control:** Hospital district or authority, Government, nonfederal **Service:** General Medical and Surgical

**Staffed Beds:** 122 **Admissions:** 777 **Census:** 104 **Outpatient Visits:** 28164 **Births:** 0 **Total Expense ($000):** 14606 **Payroll Expense ($000):** 9859 **Personnel:** 252

## COLUMBUS—Muscogee County

**BRADLEY CENTER OF ST. FRANCIS** See St. Francis Hospital

⊠ **COLUMBUS SPECIALTY HOSPITAL (112012)**, 710 Center Street, 9th Floor, Zip 31901; tel. 706/321–6712 **A**1 9 10 **F**1 3 29 30 129 147
Primary Contact: Greg Thomsen, Ed.D., FACHE, Chief Executive Officer
CFO: William Eckstein, Chief Financial Officer
CHR: Melissa Lassiter, Coordinator Human Resources
CNO: Robert Saulnier, R.N., Chief Nurse Executive
Web address: www.columbusspecialtyhospital.net
**Control:** Other not–for–profit (including NFP Corporation) **Service:** Long–Term Acute Care hospital

**Staffed Beds:** 50 **Admissions:** 401 **Census:** 28 **Outpatient Visits:** 0 **Births:** 0 **Total Expense ($000):** 14486 **Payroll Expense ($000):** 5775 **Personnel:** 120

⊠ **DOCTORS HOSPITAL OF COLUMBUS (110186)**, 616 19th Street, Zip 31901–1528, Mailing Address: P.O. Box 2188, Zip 31902–2188; tel. 706/494–4262 **A**1 9 10 **F**3 11 13 29 40 45 50 61 70 74 75 76 77 78 79 81 82 85 87 107 111 113 118 128 129 131 145 146 147 **S** Columbus Regional Healthcare System, Columbus, GA
Primary Contact: Kevin Sass, FACHE, Senior Executive Officer
CMO: Thomas L. Theus, M.D., Chief of Medicine
CIO: Ryan Sanders, Director Information Services
Web address: www.doctorshospital.net
**Control:** Other not–for–profit (including NFP Corporation) **Service:** General Medical and Surgical

**Staffed Beds:** 171 **Admissions:** 5203 **Census:** 57 **Outpatient Visits:** 46701 **Births:** 1521 **Total Expense ($000):** 71344 **Payroll Expense ($000):** 25287 **Personnel:** 455

⊠ **HUGHSTON HOSPITAL (110200)**, 100 Frist Court, Zip 31908–7188, Mailing Address: P.O. Box 7188, Zip 31908–7188; tel. 706/576–2100, (Nonreporting) **A**1 9 10 **S** Columbus Regional Healthcare System, Columbus, GA
Primary Contact: Butch Wheeler, FACHE, Chief Executive Officer
COO: Michelle Breitfelder, Chief Operating Officer
CFO: Roland Thacker, Chief Financial Officer
CMO: Lyle Norwood, M.D., Chief of Staff
CIO: Douglas Colburn, Chief Information Officer
CHR: Becky Augustyniak, Director Human Resources
Web address: www.hughstonhospital.com
**Control:** Corporation, Investor–owned, for–profit **Service:** Orthopedic

**Staffed Beds:** 100

⊠ **ST. FRANCIS HOSPITAL (110129)**, 2122 Manchester Expressway, Zip 31904–6878, Mailing Address: P.O. Box 7000, Zip 31908–7000; tel. 706/596–4000, (Includes BRADLEY CENTER OF ST. FRANCIS, 2000 16th Avenue, Zip 31906–0308; tel. 706/320–3700) **A**1 9 10 **F**3 4 10 11 15 17 18 20 22 24 26 28 29 30 31 34 35 40 45 46 49 50 51 53 54 56 57 58 59 60 63 64 70 74 75 77 78 79 81 82 85 86 92 93 94 96 98 99 100 101 102 103 104 105 107 108 110 111 118 125 128 129 143 144 145 146 147 **P**6
Primary Contact: Robert P. Granger, President and Chief Executive Officer
CFO: Matthew Moore, Senior Vice President and Chief Financial Officer
CMO: Bobbi Farber, M.D., Chief Medical Officer
CIO: David Steele, Vice President and Chief Information Officer
CHR: E. Rick Lowe, FACHE, Senior Vice President and Chief Administrative Officer
Web address: www.sfhga.com
**Control:** Other not–for–profit (including NFP Corporation) **Service:** General Medical and Surgical

**Staffed Beds:** 313 **Admissions:** 12899 **Census:** 177 **Outpatient Visits:** 140046 **Births:** 0 **Total Expense ($000):** 184546 **Payroll Expense ($000):** 69187 **Personnel:** 1466

**GA**

**GA**

⊠ **THE MEDICAL CENTER (110064)**, 710 Center Street, Zip 31901–1527, Mailing Address: P.O. Box 951, Zip 31902–0951; tel. 706/571–1000, (Total facility includes 128 beds in nursing home–type unit) **A**1 2 3 5 9 10 12 13 **F**5 11 13 15 18 20 26 29 30 31 34 35 40 43 44 49 50 56 57 59 60 61 64 66 68 70 71 72 73 74 75 76 77 78 79 81 82 86 87 88 89 93 97 100 101 102 107 108 111 113 115 117 118 120 122 127 128 129 131 133 134 143 145 146 147 **S** Columbus Regional Healthcare System, Columbus, GA
Primary Contact: Ryan Chandler, President and Chief Executive Officer
CMO: Andrew P. Morley, Jr., M.D., Senior Vice President and Chief Medical Officer
CIO: Joseph T. Wood, Vice President and Chief Information Officer
CHR: Wayne Joiner, Vice President Human Resources
Web address: www.columbusregional.com
**Control:** Other not–for–profit (including NFP Corporation) **Service:** General Medical and Surgical

**Staffed Beds:** 497 **Admissions:** 12352 **Census:** 284 **Outpatient Visits:** 175327 **Births:** 2833 **Total Expense ($000):** 291569 **Payroll Expense ($000):** 108599 **Personnel:** 2013

☐ **WEST CENTRAL GEORGIA REGIONAL HOSPITAL (114013)**, 3000 Schatulga Road, Zip 31995–3117, Mailing Address: P.O. Box 12435, Zip 31917–2435; tel. 706/568–5000, (Nonreporting) **A**1 9 10
Primary Contact: John L. Robertson, Administrator
COO: Larmar Cunningham, Chief Operating Officer
CMO: Abiodun Famakinwa, M.D., Acting Clinical Director
CIO: Ron Buchanan, Director Information Services
CHR: Coreg Burns, Human Resources Lead
Web address: www.wcgrh.org
**Control:** State–Government, nonfederal **Service:** Psychiatric

**Staffed Beds:** 145

### COMMERCE—Jackson County

⊠ **NORTHRIDGE MEDICAL CENTER (110040)**, 70 Medical Center Drive, Zip 30529–9989; tel. 706/335–1000, (Total facility includes 167 beds in nursing home–type unit) **A**1 9 10 **F**3 11 15 17 29 30 33 40 45 46 50 53 70 79 81 89 93 98 107 111 118 127 128 129 132 145 147
Primary Contact: Bryan Dearing, Chief Executive Officer
CFO: Larry W. Ebert, Jr., Chief Financial Officer
CMO: Narasimhulu Neelagaru, M.D., Chief of Staff
CIO: Vince Jarnagin, Manager Information Technology
CHR: Robin Daniel, Director of Human Resources
CNO: Maura Cobb, R.N., Chief Nursing Officer
Web address: www.northridgemc.com
**Control:** Partnership, Investor–owned, for–profit **Service:** General Medical and Surgical

**Staffed Beds:** 257 **Admissions:** 1184 **Census:** 165 **Outpatient Visits:** 41186 **Births:** 0 **Total Expense ($000):** 18369 **Payroll Expense ($000):** 12201 **Personnel:** 284

### CONYERS—Rockdale County

⊠ **ROCKDALE MEDICAL CENTER (110091)**, 1412 Milstead Avenue N.E., Zip 30012; tel. 770/918–3000 **A**1 9 10 **F**3 11 13 15 18 20 28 29 30 31 34 35 36 40 45 46 47 49 57 59 62 64 68 70 73 74 75 76 78 79 81 82 85 86 87 92 93 107 108 110 111 113 114 117 118 125 129 130 131 134 144 145 146 147 **S** LifePoint Hospitals, Inc., Brentwood, TN
Primary Contact: Deborah Armstrong, Chief Executive Officer
COO: James Atkins, Chief Operating Officer
CFO: James Hughey, Chief Financial Officer
CMO: Lisa Gillespie, M.D., Chief Medical Officer
CIO: Gail Waldo, Director Information Technology
CHR: Marianne Freeman, Vice President Human Resources
CNO: Deborah Almauhy, R.N., Chief Nursing Officer
Web address: www.rockdalemedicalcenter.org
**Control:** Corporation, Investor–owned, for–profit **Service:** General Medical and Surgical

**Staffed Beds:** 146 **Admissions:** 8521 **Census:** 96 **Outpatient Visits:** 125878 **Births:** 2061 **Total Expense ($000):** 94514 **Payroll Expense ($000):** 44519 **Personnel:** 937

### CORDELE—Crisp County

⊠ **CRISP REGIONAL HOSPITAL (110104)**, 902 North Seventh Street, Zip 31015–5007; tel. 229/276–3100, (Total facility includes 143 beds in nursing home–type unit) **A**1 9 10 20 **F**3 10 11 13 15 28 29 30 31 34 35 40 44 45 48 50 51 54 56 57 58 59 60 61 62 63 64 65 68 70 75 76 77 78 81 84 85 86 87 89 90 93 96 97 107 108 110 111 114 117 124 126 127 128 131 132 134 143 145 146 147 **P**2 8
Primary Contact: Steven Gautney, Chief Executive Officer
COO: Mary Jim Montgomery, R.N., Chief Operating Officer
CFO: Jessica Y. Carter, Chief Financial Officer
CMO: David Kavtaradze, M.D., Chief of Staff
CHR: George M. Laurin, Interim Director Human Resources
CNO: Marsha L. Mulderig, R.N., Chief Nursing Officer
Web address: www.crispregional.com
**Control:** County–Government, nonfederal **Service:** General Medical and Surgical

**Staffed Beds:** 216 **Admissions:** 2797 **Census:** 136 **Outpatient Visits:** 100524 **Births:** 363 **Personnel:** 787

### COVINGTON—Newton County

⊠ **NEWTON MEDICAL CENTER (110018)**, 5126 Hospital Drive, Zip 30014–2567; tel. 770/786–7053 **A**1 9 10 **F**7 11 12 13 15 18 20 28 29 30 34 35 40 49 57 59 62 63 64 70 72 74 75 76 79 81 85 87 89 93 97 107 108 111 113 118 129 131 140 141 145 146 147
Primary Contact: James F. Weadick, Administrator and Chief Executive Officer
CFO: Troy Brooks, Assistant Administrator Fiscal Services
CMO: Mark C. Hanson, M.D., Chief of Staff
CIO: Steve Dickstein, Director
CHR: Greg Richardson, Director Human Resources
CNO: Patricia A. Waller, R.N., Assistant Administrator Patient Care Services
Web address: www.newtonmedical.com
**Control:** Other not–for–profit (including NFP Corporation) **Service:** General Medical and Surgical

**Staffed Beds:** 101 **Admissions:** 4986 **Census:** 50 **Outpatient Visits:** 249269 **Births:** 665 **Total Expense ($000):** 59390 **Payroll Expense ($000):** 34142 **Personnel:** 680

### CUMMING—Forsyth County

☐ **NORTHSIDE HOSPITAL FORSYTH (110005)**, 1200 Northside Forsyth Drive, Zip 30041–7659; tel. 770/844–3200 **A**1 9 10 **F**3 11 12 13 15 18 20 22 26 28 29 30 31 34 35 40 44 45 49 57 59 60 64 68 70 71 73 74 75 76 78 79 81 82 85 86 87 93 107 108 110 111 113 114 118 119 120 122 123 125 128 129 131 134 145 146 147 **S** Northside Healthcare System, Atlanta, GA
Primary Contact: Lynn Jackson, Administrator
CFO: Mitch Logan, Director Finance
Web address: www.northside.com
**Control:** Other not–for–profit (including NFP Corporation) **Service:** General Medical and Surgical

**Staffed Beds:** 187 **Admissions:** 11527 **Census:** 144 **Outpatient Visits:** 155449 **Births:** 2236 **Total Expense ($000):** 221844 **Payroll Expense ($000):** 72863 **Personnel:** 1371

### CUTHBERT—Randolph County

⊠ **SOUTHWEST GEORGIA REGIONAL MEDICAL CENTER (111300)**, 361 Randolph Street, Zip 39840–1338; tel. 229/732–2181, (Nonreporting) **A**1 9 10 18
Primary Contact: Derrick A. Frazier, Chief Executive Officer
CFO: Brent Rigsby, Chief Financial Officer
Web address: www.phoebeputney.com/
**Control:** Hospital district or authority, Government, nonfederal **Service:** General Medical and Surgical

**Staffed Beds:** 105

### DAHLONEGA—Lumpkin County

☐ **CHESTATEE REGIONAL HOSPITAL (110187)**, 227 Mountain Drive, Zip 30533–1606; tel. 706/864–6136 **A**1 9 10 **F**3 13 15 29 34 49 50 54 57 59 64 65 76 79 81 85 86 87 93 105 107 108 110 111 113 118 128 129 132 142 143 145 146 147 **P**8 **S** Sunlink Health Systems, Atlanta, GA
Primary Contact: Larry R. Jeter, Chief Executive Officer
CFO: Michael Deaton, Chief Financial Officer
CMO: Richard Wherry, M.D., Chief of Staff
CHR: Barbara Patrick, Director Human Resources
CNO: Barbara Arnau, R.N., Chief Nursing Officer
Web address: www.chestateeregionalhospital.com
**Control:** Corporation, Investor–owned, for–profit **Service:** General Medical and Surgical

**Staffed Beds:** 49 **Admissions:** 1651 **Census:** 14 **Outpatient Visits:** 24222 **Births:** 176 **Total Expense ($000):** 19572 **Payroll Expense ($000):** 7531 **Personnel:** 141

### DALLAS—Paulding County

⊠ **WELLSTAR PAULDING HOSPITAL (110042)**, 600 West Memorial Drive, Zip 30132–1335; tel. 770/445–4411, (Total facility includes 182 beds in nursing home–type unit) **A**1 2 9 10 **F**3 11 15 28 29 30 37 38 40 41 44 45 50 54 61 64 68 70 75 77 78 79 81 82 85 86 87 102 104 107 108 110 111 113 117 118 119 120 122 127 128 129 145 **P**1 6 **S** WellStar Health System, Marietta, GA
Primary Contact: Mark Haney, Senior Vice President and Administrator
CFO: Marsha Burke, Senior Vice President Financial Services
Web address: www.wellstar.org
**Control:** Other not–for–profit (including NFP Corporation) **Service:** General Medical and Surgical

**Staffed Beds:** 216 **Admissions:** 2299 **Census:** 192 **Outpatient Visits:** 85911 **Births:** 0 **Personnel:** 566

*Many Facility Codes have changed. Please refer to the AHA Guide Code Chart.* © 2012 AHA Guide

## DALTON—Whitfield County

☒ **HAMILTON MEDICAL CENTER (110001)**, 1200 Memorial Drive,
Zip 30720–2529, Mailing Address: P.O. Box 1168, Zip 30722–1168;
tel. 706/272–6000 **A**1 2 9 10 19 **F**3 4 5 8 11 12 13 15 18 20 22 26 28 29
30 31 34 35 40 43 44 49 50 51 53 54 57 59 60 62 63 64 68 70 72 74 75
76 77 78 79 81 82 83 84 85 86 87 89 93 96 97 98 99 100 101 102 103
104 105 107 108 110 111 113 114 116 118 119 120 122 125 128 129 130
131 134 143 145 146 147 **S** Hamilton Health Care System, Inc., Dalton, GA
Primary Contact: Jeffrey D. Myers, President and Chief Executive Officer
COO: Karen J. Wisdom, Executive Vice President and Chief Operating Officer
CFO: Gary L. Howard, Senior Vice President, Chief Financial Officer and Corporate
Compliance Officer
CMO: Carlton Lancaster, M.D., Medical Consultant
CIO: John M. Forrester, Director Information Services
CHR: Steven Pound, Vice President Human Resources
Web address: www.hamiltonhealth.com
**Control:** Other not–for–profit (including NFP Corporation) **Service:** General
Medical and Surgical

**Staffed Beds:** 230 **Admissions:** 9651 **Census:** 105 **Outpatient Visits:**
227237 **Births:** 1876 **Personnel:** 1160

## DECATUR—Dekalb County

☐ **DEKALB MEDICAL AT DOWNTOWN DECATUR (112006)**, 450 North Candler
Street, Zip 30030–2671; tel. 404/501–6700 **A**1 5 9 10 **F**1 3 29 30 50 60 74
75 77 79 87 118 129 147 **S** DeKalb Regional Health System, Decatur, GA
Primary Contact: John Shelton, President and Chief Executive Officer
COO: John Shelton, Executive Vice President and Chief Operating Officer
CMO: David Snyder, M.D., Chief of Staff
CHR: Tom Crawford, Vice President Human Resources
Web address: www.dekalbmedicalcenter.org
**Control:** Other not–for–profit (including NFP Corporation) **Service:** Long–Term
Acute Care hospital

**Staffed Beds:** 44 **Admissions:** 309 **Census:** 26 **Outpatient Visits:** 50 **Births:**
0 **Total Expense ($000):** 16476 **Payroll Expense ($000):** 6509 **Personnel:**
163

☒ **DEKALB MEDICAL AT NORTH DECATUR (110076)**, 2701 North Decatur
Road, Zip 30033–5995; tel. 404/501–1000 **A**1 2 3 9 10 **F**3 11 12 13 15 18
20 22 26 28 29 30 31 34 35 36 37 40 45 48 49 50 53 55 56 57 58 59 60
64 67 70 71 72 73 74 75 76 77 78 79 81 85 87 90 93 96 97 98 100 102
105 107 108 110 111 113 114 116 118 119 120 123 125 128 129 130 131
133 134 145 146 147 **P**1 **S** DeKalb Regional Health System, Decatur, GA
Primary Contact: John Shelton, President and Chief Executive Officer
COO: Dane Henry, Executive Vice President and Chief Operating Officer
CFO: Mal Underwood, Interim Sr. VP and Chief Financial Officer
CMO: Duane Barclay, D.O., Vice President Physician Support Services
CIO: Mark Trocino, Chief Information Officer
CHR: Joel Schuessler, Interim Vice President Human Resources
CNO: Cherie Kunik, R.N., Interim Vice President Patient Care Services & CNO
Web address: www.dekalbmedical.org
**Control:** Other not–for–profit (including NFP Corporation) **Service:** General
Medical and Surgical

**Staffed Beds:** 436 **Admissions:** 21510 **Census:** 279 **Outpatient Visits:**
182767 **Births:** 5230 **Total Expense ($000):** 285016 **Payroll Expense**
**($000):** 105368 **Personnel:** 2101

☐ **GEORGIA REGIONAL HOSPITAL AT ATLANTA (114019)**, 3073 Panthersville
Road, Zip 30034–3828; tel. 404/243–2100, (Total facility includes 24 beds in
nursing home–type unit) **A**1 3 5 9 10 **F**39 67 98 102 103 127 134 **P**6
Primary Contact: Susan Trueblood, Chief Executive Officer
COO: Sonny Slate, Chief Operating Officer
CFO: Reginald Jones, Business Manager
CMO: Emile Risby, M.D., Clinical Director
CIO: Elfie Early, Manager Data Services
CHR: Lorraine Farr, Manager Human Resources
Web address: www.atlantareg.dhr.state.ga.us
**Control:** State–Government, nonfederal **Service:** Psychiatric

**Staffed Beds:** 354 **Admissions:** 2069 **Census:** 175 **Outpatient Visits:** 146
**Births:** 0 **Total Expense ($000):** 47647 **Payroll Expense ($000):** 30775
**Personnel:** 1007

☒ △ **VETERANS AFFAIRS MEDICAL CENTER**, 1670 Clairmont Road,
Zip 30033–4004; tel. 404/321–6111, (Nonreporting) **A**1 2 3 5 7 8 9
**S** Department of Veterans Affairs, Washington, DC
Primary Contact: James A. Clark, M.P.H., Director
CFO: Pamela Watkins, Chief Financial Officer
CMO: David Bower, M.D., Chief of Staff
CIO: William Brock, Chief Information Officer
CHR: Zeta Ferguson, Chief Human Resources
CNO: Sandy Leake, MSN, Associate Director, Nursing and Patient Care Services
Web address: www.atlanta.va.gov/
**Control:** Veterans Affairs, Government, federal **Service:** General Medical and
Surgical

**Staffed Beds:** 239

## DEMOREST—Habersham County

☒ **HABERSHAM MEDICAL CENTER (110041)**, 541 Historic Highway 441,
Zip 30535–3118, Mailing Address: P.O. Box 37, Zip 30535–0037;
tel. 706/754–2161, (Total facility includes 84 beds in nursing home–type unit) **A**1
9 10 **F**3 7 11 13 15 28 29 30 35 38 40 45 53 54 57 59 62 64 68 70 77 79
81 82 85 86 87 93 107 108 111 113 115 116 118 123 127 128 129 130
131 132 145 146 **P**7 **S** QHR, Brentwood, TN
Primary Contact: C. Richard Dwozan, Chief Executive Officer
CFO: James Peterson, Senior Vice President Finance
CMO: James Hamilton, M.D., Chief of Staff
CIO: Roger Ivester, Manager Information Systems
CHR: Wanda Hardman, Director Human Resources
Web address: www.hcmcmed.org
**Control:** Hospital district or authority, Government, nonfederal **Service:** General
Medical and Surgical

**Staffed Beds:** 137 **Admissions:** 2580 **Census:** 104 **Outpatient Visits:** 90202
**Births:** 411 **Total Expense ($000):** 44943 **Payroll Expense ($000):** 19028
**Personnel:** 519

## DONALSONVILLE—Seminole County

☐ **DONALSONVILLE HOSPITAL (110194)**, 102 Hospital Circle, Zip 39845–1199;
tel. 229/524–5217, (Nonreporting) **A**1 9 10
Primary Contact: Charles H. Orrick, Administrator
CFO: James Moody, Chief Financial Officer
CMO: C. O. Walker, M.D., Chief of Staff
CHR: Jo Adams, Director Human Resources
**Control:** Other not–for–profit (including NFP Corporation) **Service:** General
Medical and Surgical

**Staffed Beds:** 140

## DOUGLAS—Coffee County

☒ **COFFEE REGIONAL MEDICAL CENTER (110089)**, 1101 Ocilla Road,
Zip 31533–3617, Mailing Address: P.O. Box 1287, Zip 31534–1287;
tel. 912/384–1900 **A**1 9 10 20 **F**3 7 8 11 13 15 28 29 31 32 34 35 40 47 50
51 53 54 56 57 59 61 65 68 70 75 76 78 79 81 82 85 86 87 89 97 107
108 110 111 113 114 118 126 129 130 131 134 142 143 145 146 147 **P**8
Primary Contact: George L. Heck, III, President and Chief Executive Officer
CFO: Donald C. Lewis, Jr., Vice President and Chief Financial Officer
CIO: George L. Heck, III, President and Chief Executive Officer
CHR: Laura Bloom, Director Human Resources
Web address: www.coffeeregional.org
**Control:** Other not–for–profit (including NFP Corporation) **Service:** General
Medical and Surgical

**Staffed Beds:** 88 **Admissions:** 5664 **Census:** 58 **Outpatient Visits:** 85000
**Births:** 595 **Total Expense ($000):** 76691 **Payroll Expense ($000):** 33859
**Personnel:** 668

## DOUGLASVILLE—Douglas County

☒ **WELLSTAR DOUGLAS HOSPITAL (110184)**, 8954 Hospital Drive,
Zip 30134–2282; tel. 770/949–1500 **A**1 2 9 10 **F**3 11 13 15 20 28 29 30 31
37 38 40 41 44 45 48 49 50 54 58 61 64 68 70 74 75 76 77 78 79 81 82
85 86 87 93 94 102 107 108 110 111 113 114 117 118 128 129 145 146
**P**1 6 **S** WellStar Health System, Marietta, GA
Primary Contact: Craig A. Owens, Senior Vice President and Administrator
CFO: Bradley Greene, Chief Financial Officer
CMO: Noel Holtz, M.D., Chief Medical Officer
CIO: Ronald Strachan, Chief Information Officer
CHR: Danyale Ziglor, Assistant Director Human Resources
Web address: www.wellstar.org
**Control:** Other not–for–profit (including NFP Corporation) **Service:** General
Medical and Surgical

**Staffed Beds:** 102 **Admissions:** 6696 **Census:** 74 **Outpatient Visits:** 127784
**Births:** 481 **Personnel:** 829

GA

---

**Hospital, Medicare Provider Number, Address, Telephone, Approval, Facility, and Physician Codes, Health Care System**

★ American Hospital Association (AHA) membership
☐ The Joint Commission accreditation   ◇ DNV Healthcare Inc. accreditation

○ American Osteopathic Association (AOA) accreditation
△ Commission on Accreditation of Rehabilitation Facilities (CARF) accreditation

**YOUTH VILLAGES INNER HARBOUR CAMPUS**, 4685 Dorsett Shoals Road, Zip 30135–4999; tel. 770/942–2391, (Nonreporting)
Primary Contact: Patrick Lawler, Chief Executive Officer
CFO: J. Steve Lewis, Director Finance
CIO: Laura Sellers, Director Information Systems
CHR: Sherry Kollmeyer, Vice President Human Resources
Web address: www.innerharbour.org
**Control:** Other not–for–profit (including NFP Corporation) **Service:** Children's hospital psychiatric

| Staffed Beds: 176 |
| --- |

### DUBLIN—Laurens County

☒ **CARL VINSON VETERANS AFFAIRS MEDICAL CENTER**, 1826 Veterans Boulevard, Zip 31021–3620; tel. 478/272–1210, (Nonreporting) **A**1
**S** Department of Veterans Affairs, Washington, DC
Primary Contact: J. Mark Anderson, Acting Director
CFO: Marcy Chambless, Manager Business Office
CMO: Eva Martin, M.D., Chief of Staff
CIO: Sandra Clem, Manager Information Management
CHR: Teresa L. Lindsey, Supervisor Human Resources
Web address: www.va.gov/sta/guide/home.asp
**Control:** Veterans Affairs, Government, federal **Service:** General Medical and Surgical

| Staffed Beds: 178 |
| --- |

☒ **FAIRVIEW PARK HOSPITAL (110125)**, 200 Industrial Boulevard, Zip 31021–2997, Mailing Address: P.O. Box 1408, Zip 31040–1408; tel. 478/275–2000, (Nonreporting) **A**1 9 10 19 **S** HCA, Nashville, TN
Primary Contact: Donald R. Avery, FACHE, President and Chief Executive Officer
COO: Michael Hoskins, Chief Operating Officer
CFO: Ted Short, Chief Financial Officer
CMO: David G. Shores, D.O., President Medical Staff
CIO: Marsha Morris, Manager Information Services
CHR: Jeff Bruton, Director Human Resources
Web address: www.fairviewparkhospital.com
**Control:** Corporation, Investor–owned, for–profit **Service:** General Medical and Surgical

| Staffed Beds: 168 |
| --- |

### DULUTH—De Kalb County

**GWINNETT MEDICAL CENTER–DULUTH** See Gwinnett Hospital System, Lawrenceville

### EAST POINT—Fulton County

☒ **REGENCY HOSPITAL OF SOUTH ATLANTA (112014)**, 1170 Cleveland Avenue, 4th Floor, Zip 30344; tel. 404/466–6250, (Nonreporting) **A**1 10
**S** Select Medical Corporation, Mechanicsburg, PA
Primary Contact: Alisa Jett, Chief Executive Officer
Web address: www.regencyhospital.com
**Control:** Corporation, Investor–owned, for–profit **Service:** Long–Term Acute Care hospital

| Staffed Beds: 37 |
| --- |

### EASTMAN—Dodge County

**DODGE COUNTY HOSPITAL (110092)**, 901 Griffin Avenue, Zip 31023–2223, Mailing Address: P.O. Box 4309, Zip 31023–4309; tel. 478/374–4000 **A**9 10 21 **F**3 11 13 15 29 30 31 40 45 53 57 59 64 69 70 75 76 79 81 85 86 107 108 111 113 118 129 145
Primary Contact: Kevin Bierschenk, Chief Executive Officer
CFO: Jan Hamrick, Chief Financial Officer
CIO: Victor Woodard, Manager Information Technology
CHR: Wendy Selph, Director Human Resources
CNO: Sandra M. Campbell, R.N., Chief Nursing Officer
Web address: www.dodgecountyhospital.com
**Control:** Hospital district or authority, Government, nonfederal **Service:** General Medical and Surgical

| Staffed Beds: 38 Admissions: 1814 Census: 19 Outpatient Visits: 38197 Births: 160 Total Expense ($000): 19558 Payroll Expense ($000): 8055 Personnel: 218 |
| --- |

### EATONTON—Putnam County

☐ **PUTNAM GENERAL HOSPITAL (111313)**, 101 Lake Oconee Parkway, Zip 31024; tel. 706/485–2711 **A**1 9 10 18 **F**3 11 15 28 29 34 35 40 50 57 59 64 68 75 79 81 93 97 107 110 111 113 118 128 132 145 **P**2
Primary Contact: Darrell M. Oglesby, Administrator
CFO: Brenda Jarrett, Chief Financial Officer
CMO: Omar Akhras, M.D., Chief of Staff
CIO: Steven Cason, Chief Information Officer
CHR: Ellen Ellard, Director Human Resources
Web address: www.putnamgeneral.com
**Control:** Hospital district or authority, Government, nonfederal **Service:** General Medical and Surgical

| Staffed Beds: 25 Admissions: 934 Census: 7 Outpatient Visits: 21720 Births: 0 Total Expense ($000): 10991 Payroll Expense ($000): 5481 Personnel: 138 |
| --- |

### ELBERTON—Elbert County

☒ **ELBERT MEMORIAL HOSPITAL (110026)**, 4 Medical Drive, Zip 30635–1897; tel. 706/283–3151, (Nonreporting) **A**1 9 10
Primary Contact: James Yarborough, FACHE, Interim Chief Executive Officer
CFO: Doug Faircloth, Interim Chief Financial Officer
CIO: Andy Chapin, Director Information Technology
CHR: Georgian Walton, Director Human Resources
Web address: www.emhcare.net
**Control:** Hospital district or authority, Government, nonfederal **Service:** General Medical and Surgical

| Staffed Beds: 42 |
| --- |

### ELLIJAY—Gilmer County

☐ **NORTH GEORGIA MEDICAL CENTER (110205)**, 1362 South Main Street, Zip 30540–0346, Mailing Address: P.O. Box 2239, Zip 30540–0346; tel. 706/276–4741, (Nonreporting) **A**1 9 10 **S** Sunlink Health Systems, Atlanta, GA
Primary Contact: Jeffrey Dunn, Chief Executive Officer
COO: Jeffrey Dunn, Chief Executive Officer
CFO: Debbie Self, Chief Financial Officer
CMO: Kelvin Haim, M.D., Chief of Staff
CHR: Mary Beth Ralston, Manager Human Resources
Web address: www.northgeorgiamedicalcenter.com
**Control:** Corporation, Investor–owned, for–profit **Service:** General Medical and Surgical

| Staffed Beds: 150 |
| --- |

### FAYETTEVILLE—Fayette County

☒ **PIEDMONT FAYETTE HOSPITAL (110215)**, 1255 Highway 54 West, Zip 30214; tel. 770/719–7000, (Nonreporting) **A**1 2 9 10 **S** Piedmont Healthcare, Atlanta, GA
Primary Contact: W. Darrell Cutts, President and Chief Executive Officer
COO: Michael Burnett, Chief Operating Officer
CFO: John Miles, Chief Financial Officer
CMO: Frederick Willms, M.D., Vice President Medical Affairs
CIO: Mark Pasquale, Vice President Information Services and Chief Information Officer
CHR: Catherine Crisler, Executive Director Human Resources
Web address: www.fayettehospital.org
**Control:** Other not–for–profit (including NFP Corporation) **Service:** General Medical and Surgical

| Staffed Beds: 148 |
| --- |

### FITZGERALD—Ben Hill County

☐ **DORMINY MEDICAL CENTER (110073)**, 200 Perry House Road, Zip 31750, Mailing Address: P.O. Box 1447, Zip 31750–1447; tel. 229/424–7100 **A**1 9 10 **F**3 11 13 15 29 30 34 35 40 50 57 59 60 63 64 68 70 75 76 81 82 84 87 89 90 93 107 111 118 126 128 129 131 132 147 **P**6
Primary Contact: Warren Manley, Administrator
COO: Debbie Thomas, Chief Operating Officer
CFO: Paige Wynn, Chief Financial Officer
CMO: Thomas Mann, M.D., Chief of Staff
CIO: Mike James, Director Management Information Systems
CHR: Denise Steverson, Director Human Resources
CNO: Staci Mims, Chief Nursing Officer
Web address: www.dorminymedical.org
**Control:** Hospital district or authority, Government, nonfederal **Service:** General Medical and Surgical

| Staffed Beds: 67 Admissions: 1541 Census: 14 Outpatient Visits: 25350 Births: 113 Total Expense ($000): 21969 Payroll Expense ($000): 10408 Personnel: 237 |
| --- |

### FOLKSTON—Charlton County

**CHARLTON MEMORIAL HOSPITAL (111315)**, 2449 Third Street, Zip 31537–1303, Mailing Address: P.O. Box 188, Zip 31537–0188; tel. 912/496–2531 **A**9 10 18 **F**3 7 15 29 30 35 40 45 50 57 59 61 64 81 107 108 111 117 118 126 128 132
Primary Contact: Farrell Turner, Interim Administrator
CFO: Kim Savage, Interim Controller
CMO: Albert Thompson, M.D., Chief of Staff
CHR: Darlene Tait, Director Human Resources
**Control:** Hospital district or authority, Government, nonfederal **Service:** General Medical and Surgical

| Staffed Beds: 22 Admissions: 356 Census: 3 Outpatient Visits: 9719 Births: 2 Total Expense ($000): 4920 Payroll Expense ($000): 4656 Personnel: 118 |
| --- |

**GA**

## FORSYTH—Monroe County

☐ **MONROE COUNTY HOSPITAL (111318)**, 88 Martin Luther King Jr. Drive, Zip 31029–1682, Mailing Address: P.O. Box 1068, Zip 31029–1068; tel. 478/994–2521 **A**1 9 10 18 **F**3 11 15 29 35 40 57 59 68 75 81 107 111 113 118 131 132 145 147 **P**1 2
Primary Contact: Kay A. Floyd, R.N., Chief Executive Officer
CFO: Marlene McLennan, Controller
CMO: Jeremy Goodwin, M.D., President, Medical Staff
CIO: Donna Hogg, Supervisor Medical Records
CHR: Deborah Flowers, Director Human Resources
CNO: Casey Fleckenstein, Medical and Surgical Nurse Manager
Web address: www.monroehospital.org
**Control:** Hospital district or authority, Government, nonfederal **Service:** General Medical and Surgical

**Staffed Beds:** 25 **Admissions:** 458 **Census:** 6 **Outpatient Visits:** 25301 **Births:** 0 **Total Expense ($000):** 7811 **Payroll Expense ($000):** 4346 **Personnel:** 123

## FORT BENNING—Muscogee County

☒ **MARTIN ARMY COMMUNITY HOSPITAL**, 7950 Martin Loop, Zip 31905–5648, Mailing Address: 7950 Martin Loop, B9200, Room 010, Zip 31905–5648; tel. 706/544–2516, (Nonreporting) **A**1 3 5 **S** Department of the Army, Office of the Surgeon General, Falls Church, VA
Primary Contact: Colonel Timothy E. Lamb, Commander
CFO: Major Sean Casperson, Chief Resource Management
CMO: Colonel Sonja Thompson, Deputy Commander Clinical Services
CIO: Major Tony Cromer, Chief Information Management
CHR: Major Bernita Hightower, Chief Human Resources
Web address: www.martin.amedd.army.mil
**Control:** Army, Government, federal **Service:** General Medical and Surgical

**Staffed Beds:** 57

## FORT GORDON—Richmond County

☒ **DWIGHT DAVID EISENHOWER ARMY MEDICAL CENTER**, Hospital Drive, Zip 30905–5650; tel. 706/787–5811 **A**1 2 3 5 **F**3 4 5 7 8 9 11 12 14 15 18 20 22 24 26 29 30 31 33 34 35 37 38 39 40 43 44 45 49 50 53 54 56 57 58 59 60 61 64 65 68 70 74 75 77 78 79 80 81 82 85 86 87 89 91 93 94 97 98 100 101 102 104 105 106 107 108 111 113 115 116 117 118 121 128 129 130 131 134 142 143 144 145 146 147 **P**6 **S** Department of the Army, Office of the Surgeon General, Falls Church, VA
Primary Contact: Commander Christopher M. Castle, Commander
CMO: Colonel James M. Baunchalk, Deputy Chief Clinical Services
CIO: Major Joseph A. Ponce, Chief Information Management
CHR: Elizabeth Shelt, Civilian Personnel Officer
Web address: www.ddeamc.amedd.army.mil
**Control:** Army, Government, federal **Service:** General Medical and Surgical

**Staffed Beds:** 125 **Admissions:** 4640 **Census:** 80 **Outpatient Visits:** 593335 **Births:** 698 **Personnel:** 2645

## FORT OGLETHORPE—Catoosa County

☐ **ERLANGER AT HUTCHESON (110004)**, 100 Gross Crescent Circle, Zip 30742–3669; tel. 706/858–2000, (Nonreporting) **A**1 9 10 **S** Erlanger Health System, Chattanooga, TN
Primary Contact: Roger Forgey, President and Chief Executive Officer
CFO: Denise Baker, Interim Chief Financial Officer
CMO: Maria Bowers, M.D., Chief of Staff
CIO: Ruth Wright, Director Information Services
CHR: Ella Cowden, Director Human Resources
Web address: www.hutcheson.org
**Control:** Hospital district or authority, Government, nonfederal **Service:** General Medical and Surgical

**Staffed Beds:** 185

## FORT VALLEY—Peach County

☒ **PEACH REGIONAL MEDICAL CENTER (111310)**, 601 Blue Bird Boulevard, Zip 31030–4599, Mailing Address: P.O. Box 1799, Zip 31030–1799; tel. 478/825–8691, (Nonreporting) **A**1 9 10 18
Primary Contact: Nancy Peed, Administrator and Chief Executive Officer
CFO: Lisa Urbistondo, Chief Financial Officer
CMO: Crystal Brown, M.D., Medical Director
CNO: Brenda Goodman, Chief Nursing Officer
Web address: www.peachregional.org
**Control:** Hospital district or authority, Government, nonfederal **Service:** General Medical and Surgical

**Staffed Beds:** 25

## GAINESVILLE—Hall County

☒ △ **NORTHEAST GEORGIA MEDICAL CENTER (110029)**, 743 Spring Street N.E., Zip 30501–3899; tel. 770/219–3553, (Nonreporting) **A**1 2 7 9 10 19 21
Primary Contact: Carol H. Burrell, President and Chief Executive Officer
CFO: Tony Herdener, Vice President Systems and Finance
CMO: Jim Bailey, M.D., Chief Medical Officer
CIO: Mark Jennings, Director Information Systems
Web address: www.nghs.com
**Control:** Other not–for–profit (including NFP Corporation) **Service:** General Medical and Surgical

**Staffed Beds:** 254

## GLENWOOD—Wheeler County

☐ **LOWER OCONEE COMMUNITY HOSPITAL (111321)**, 111 Third Street, Zip 30428–2301, Mailing Address: P.O. Box 398, Zip 30428–0398; tel. 912/523–5113, (Nonreporting) **A**1 9 10 18
Primary Contact: Peyton A. Smith, Chief Executive Officer
CFO: David R. Pike, Chief Financial Officer
CHR: Sheila Heaton, Chief Human Resources Officer
**Control:** Other not–for–profit (including NFP Corporation) **Service:** General Medical and Surgical

**Staffed Beds:** 25

## GRACEWOOD—Richmond County

**EAST CENTRAL REGIONAL HOSPITAL** See East Central Regional Hospital, Augusta

## GREENSBORO—Greene County

☒ **GOOD SAMARITAN HOSPITAL (111329)**, 1201 Siloam Highway, Zip 30642–2811; tel. 706/453–7331 **A**1 9 10 18 **F**3 11 15 18 29 30 34 35 40 50 56 57 59 64 65 75 79 81 86 87 89 93 107 111 114 118 127 128 132 134 147 **S** Catholic Health East, Newtown Square, PA
Primary Contact: Montez Carter, Interim President and Chief Executive Officer
CMO: Dave Ringer, M.D., Chief of Staff
CHR: Angela C. Adams, Director Human Resources
Web address: www.stmarysgoodsam.org
**Control:** Church–operated, Nongovernment, not–for profit **Service:** General Medical and Surgical

**Staffed Beds:** 25 **Admissions:** 415 **Census:** 5 **Outpatient Visits:** 16058 **Births:** 0 **Total Expense ($000):** 14362 **Payroll Expense ($000):** 6603 **Personnel:** 150

## GRIFFIN—Spalding County

☒ **SPALDING REGIONAL MEDICAL CENTER (110031)**, 601 South Eighth Street, Zip 30224–4294, Mailing Address: P.O. Drawer V, Zip 30224–1168; tel. 770/228–2721 **A**1 2 9 10 **F**3 7 11 13 15 18 19 20 22 29 30 31 34 35 40 50 51 53 54 57 59 64 70 73 74 75 76 77 78 79 81 85 89 93 107 108 111 113 114 115 118 123 128 129 130 134 142 143 145 146 147 **P**8 **S** TENET Healthcare Corporation, Dallas, TX
Primary Contact: John A. Quinn, Chief Executive Officer
COO: Christopher Locke, Chief Operating Officer
CFO: Tamara Ison, Chief Financial Officer
CIO: Steve Brown, Director Information Systems
CHR: Amanda Remington, Director Human Resources
CNO: Wadra McCullough, Chief Nursing Officer
Web address: www.spaldingregional.com
**Control:** Corporation, Investor–owned, for–profit **Service:** General Medical and Surgical

**Staffed Beds:** 160 **Admissions:** 8376 **Census:** 93 **Outpatient Visits:** 103402 **Births:** 879 **Total Expense ($000):** 86187 **Payroll Expense ($000):** 36693 **Personnel:** 689

## HARTWELL—Hart County

☒ **HART COUNTY HOSPITAL (110059)**, Gibson and Cade Streets, Zip 30643–0280, Mailing Address: P.O. Box 280, Zip 30643–0280; tel. 706/856–6100, (Total facility includes 92 beds in nursing home–type unit) **A**1 9 10 **F**3 11 29 30 34 35 40 45 50 57 59 64 70 75 79 81 85 87 93 96 107 108 113 118 127 129 130 132 **S** Ty Cobb Healthcare System, Inc., Royston, GA
Primary Contact: Jerry R. Wise, Administrator and Vice President
Web address: www.tycobbhealthcare.org
**Control:** Other not–for–profit (including NFP Corporation) **Service:** General Medical and Surgical

**Staffed Beds:** 120 **Admissions:** 784 **Census:** 95 **Outpatient Visits:** 22111 **Births:** 0 **Total Expense ($000):** 19599 **Payroll Expense ($000):** 7563 **Personnel:** 240

**GA**

---

**Hospital, Medicare Provider Number, Address, Telephone, Approval, Facility, and Physician Codes, Health Care System**

★ American Hospital Association (AHA) membership
☐ The Joint Commission accreditation
◇ DNV Healthcare Inc. accreditation
○ American Osteopathic Association (AOA) accreditation
△ Commission on Accreditation of Rehabilitation Facilities (CARF) accreditation

## HAWKINSVILLE—Pulaski County

☐ **TAYLOR REGIONAL HOSPITAL (110135)**, Macon Highway, Zip 31036, Mailing Address: P.O. Box 1297, Zip 31036–1297; tel. 478/783–0200, (Nonreporting) **A**1 9 10
Primary Contact: Dan S. Maddock, President
CFO: Lisa Halliday, Director Accounting Services
CMO: Al Baggett, M.D., Interim Chief of Staff
CIO: Dawn Warnock, Director Medical Records
Web address: www.taylorregional.org
**Control:** Other not–for–profit (including NFP Corporation) **Service:** General Medical and Surgical

| Staffed Beds: 55 |
| --- |

## HAZLEHURST—Jeff Davis County

☐ **JEFF DAVIS HOSPITAL (111333)**, 1215 South Tallahassee Street, Zip 31539–2921, Mailing Address: P.O. Box 1690, Zip 31539–1690; tel. 912/375–7781, (Nonreporting) **A**1 9 10 18
Primary Contact: Gerald A. Schoendienst, Chief Executive Officer
**Control:** Hospital district or authority, Government, nonfederal **Service:** General Medical and Surgical

| Staffed Beds: 25 |
| --- |

## HIAWASSEE—Towns County

**CHATUGE REGIONAL HOSPITAL AND NURSING HOME (111324)**, 110 Main Street, Zip 30546–2212, Mailing Address: P.O. Box 509, Zip 30546–0509; tel. 706/896–2222, (Nonreporting) **A**9 10 18
Primary Contact: R. Lewis Kelley, Administrator
CFO: Tim Henry, Accountant
CMO: Robert F. Stahlkuppe, M.D., Chief of Staff
CIO: Walt Stafford, Director Information Technology
CHR: Rita Bradshaw, Director Human Resources
Web address: www.chatugeregionalhospital.org
**Control:** County–Government, nonfederal **Service:** General Medical and Surgical

| Staffed Beds: 137 |
| --- |

## HINESVILLE—Liberty County

☐ **LIBERTY REGIONAL MEDICAL CENTER (111335)**, 462 Elma G. Miles Parkway, Zip 31313–4000, Mailing Address: P.O. Box 919, Zip 31310–0919; tel. 912/369–9400, (Total facility includes 108 beds in nursing home–type unit) **A**1 9 10 18 **F**3 6 7 8 13 15 18 26 28 29 34 35 40 45 46 50 57 59 65 68 77 79 81 82 87 89 91 93 97 107 108 110 111 113 118 123 127 130 132 134 142 145 146
Primary Contact: H. Scott Kroell, Jr., Chief Executive Officer
CFO: Sam Johnson, Chief Financial Officer
Web address: www.libertyregional.org
**Control:** Hospital district or authority, Government, nonfederal **Service:** General Medical and Surgical

| Staffed Beds: 133 Admissions: 2249 Census: 19 Outpatient Visits: 30000 Births: 400 Total Expense ($000): 40427 Payroll Expense ($000): 17795 Personnel: 462 |
| --- |

⊠ **WINN ARMY COMMUNITY HOSPITAL**, 1061 Harmon Avenue, Zip 31314–5674, Mailing Address: 1061 Harmon Avenue, Suite 2311B, Zip 31314–5674; tel. 912/435–6965, (Nonreporting) **A**1 5 **S** Department of the Army, Office of the Surgeon General, Falls Church, VA
Primary Contact: Colonel Ronald Place, M.D., Commander
COO: Jose A. Bonilla, Deputy Commander Administration
CFO: Captain Marcos Martinez, Chief Business Operations
CMO: Richard Malish, M.D., Deputy Commander Clinical Services
CIO: Arthur N. Kirshner, Chief Information Management
CHR: Major Yvette McCrea, Chief Human Resources
CNO: Colonel Sharon Brown, Deputy Commander Nursing
Web address: www.winn.amedd.army.mil/
**Control:** Army, Government, federal **Service:** General Medical and Surgical

| Staffed Beds: 79 |
| --- |

## HOMERVILLE—Clinch County

★ **CLINCH MEMORIAL HOSPITAL (111308)**, 1050 Valdosta Highway, Zip 31634–1507, Mailing Address: P.O. Box 516, Zip 31634–0516; tel. 912/487–5211 **A**9 10 18 **F**3 7 15 34 40 45 57 59 64 77 91 93 97 107 110 111 118 128 129 132 134 144 145
Primary Contact: Phillip Cook, Administrator
CFO: Sandra Hughes, Chief Financial Officer
CMO: Samuel Cobarrubias, M.D., Chief of Staff
CIO: Shelly Studebaker, Director Management Information Systems
CHR: Shelly Studebaker, Manager Human Resources
Web address: www.sgmc.org/healthsystem/clinchmemorial.htm
**Control:** County–Government, nonfederal **Service:** General Medical and Surgical

| Staffed Beds: 25 Admissions: 373 Census: 4 Outpatient Visits: 14607 Births: 0 Total Expense ($000): 9953 Payroll Expense ($000): 3619 Personnel: 118 |
| --- |

## JACKSON—Butts County

★ **SYLVAN GROVE HOSPITAL (111319)**, 1050 McDonough Road, Zip 30233–1599; tel. 770/775–7861 **A**9 10 18 **F**15 29 34 35 40 50 57 59 68 77 93 107 118 129 132 **S** TENET Healthcare Corporation, Dallas, TX
Primary Contact: Edward J. Whitehouse, Chief Executive Officer
CFO: Tamara Ison, Chief Financial Officer
CIO: Steve Brown, Chief Information Officer
CHR: Amanda Remington, Director Human Resources
Web address: www.sylvangrovehospital.com
**Control:** Corporation, Investor–owned, for–profit **Service:** General Medical and Surgical

| Staffed Beds: 23 Admissions: 473 Census: 13 Outpatient Visits: 17823 Births: 0 Total Expense ($000): 8421 Payroll Expense ($000): 4623 Personnel: 74 |
| --- |

## JASPER—Pickens County

⊠ **PIEDMONT MOUNTAINSIDE HOSPITAL (110225)**, 1266 Highway 515 South, Zip 30143; tel. 706/692–2441 **A**1 9 10 **F**3 13 15 20 29 34 40 46 47 49 57 64 70 76 77 79 81 85 107 108 110 111 118 128 129 132 134 147 **S** Piedmont Healthcare, Atlanta, GA
Primary Contact: Mike Robertson, President and Chief Executive Officer
CMO: Folsom Proctor, III, M.D., Vice President and Chief Medical Officer
CHR: Connie McLendon, Director Human Resources
Web address: www.piedmontmountainsidehospital.org
**Control:** Other not–for–profit (including NFP Corporation) **Service:** General Medical and Surgical

| Staffed Beds: 48 Admissions: 2962 Census: 33 Outpatient Visits: 36945 Births: 351 Personnel: 301 |
| --- |

## JESUP—Wayne County

⊠ **WAYNE MEMORIAL HOSPITAL (110124)**, 865 South First Street, Zip 31598–0210, Mailing Address: P.O. Box 410, Zip 31598–0410; tel. 912/427–6811, (Nonreporting) **A**1 9 10 20
Primary Contact: Joseph P. Ierardi, Chief Executive Officer
CFO: Greg Jones, Chief Financial Officer
CMO: Dan Collipp, M.D., Chief of Staff
CIO: Deborah Six, Coordinator Data Processing
CHR: John McIwain, Director Human Resources
Web address: www.wmhweb.com
**Control:** County–Government, nonfederal **Service:** General Medical and Surgical

| Staffed Beds: 84 |
| --- |

## JOHNS CREEK—Fulton County

⊠ **EMORY JOHNS CREEK HOSPITAL (110230)**, 6325 Hospital Parkway, Zip 30097; tel. 678/474–7000 **A**1 10 **F**3 11 12 13 15 18 20 22 26 29 30 31 34 35 40 46 47 49 51 57 59 64 70 72 74 75 76 77 78 79 81 82 93 107 110 111 114 118 125 128 129 131 145 147 **S** Emory Healthcare, Atlanta, GA
Primary Contact: Craig McCoy, Chief Executive Officer
COO: Laurie Hansen, Associate Administrator
CFO: JoAnn Manning, Chief Financial Officer
CMO: Alan Wang, M.D., Chief Medical Officer
CIO: Jose Diaz, Director Information Systems
CHR: Jennifer Elizabeth Garber, Vice President Human Resources
CNO: Marilyn Margolis, Chief Nursing Officer
Web address: www.emoryjohnscreek.com
**Control:** Other not–for–profit (including NFP Corporation) **Service:** General Medical and Surgical

| Staffed Beds: 84 Admissions: 5047 Census: 57 Outpatient Visits: 52834 Births: 926 Total Expense ($000): 94553 Payroll Expense ($000): 32257 Personnel: 565 |
| --- |

## KENNESAW—Cobb County

**DEVEREUX GEORGIA TREATMENT NETWORK**, 1291 Stanley Road N.W., Zip 30152–4359; tel. 770/427–0147, (Nonreporting) **S** Devereux, Villanova, PA
Primary Contact: Gwendolyn Skinner, Executive Director
COO: Mary H. Esposito, Assistant Executive Director
CFO: Kathy Goggin, Director Administrative Services
CMO: Yolanda Graham, M.D., Medical Director
CIO: Sam Maguta, Coordinator Information Systems
CHR: Rudie Delien, Director Human Resources
CNO: Amber Boyd, Nurse Practitioner and Director of Nursing
Web address: www.devereuxga.org
**Control:** Other not–for–profit (including NFP Corporation) **Service:** Children's hospital psychiatric

| Staffed Beds: 187 |
| --- |

**GA**

*Many Facility Codes have changed. Please refer to the AHA Guide Code Chart.* © 2012 AHA Guide

## LA GRANGE—Troup County

⊞ **WEST GEORGIA HEALTH (110016)**, 1514 Vernon Road, Zip 30240–4199; tel. 706/882–1411, (Total facility includes 260 beds in nursing home–type unit) **A**1 2 9 10 19 **F**2 3 8 11 12 13 15 18 20 22 26 28 29 30 31 34 35 40 47 48 49 50 51 54 56 57 58 59 60 62 63 64 66 68 70 73 74 75 76 77 78 79 80 81 82 85 86 89 92 93 96 102 107 108 110 113 114 118 119 120 122 127 128 129 131 134 145 146 **P**6
Primary Contact: Gerald N. Fulks, President and Chief Executive Officer
COO: Charis Acree, Senior Vice President
CFO: Paul R. Perrotti, CPA, Chief Financial Officer
CHR: Tommy Britt, Director Human Resources
Web address: www.wghealth.org/
**Control:** Other not–for–profit (including NFP Corporation) **Service:** General Medical and Surgical

**Staffed Beds:** 412 **Admissions:** 8129 **Census:** 315 **Outpatient Visits:** 128693 **Births:** 991 **Total Expense ($000):** 161421 **Payroll Expense ($000):** 60940 **Personnel:** 1307

## LAKELAND—Lanier County

⊞ **LOUIS SMITH MEMORIAL HOSPITAL (111326)**, (Sub–acute), 116 West Thigpen Avenue, Zip 31635–1099; tel. 229/482–3110, (Total facility includes 62 beds in nursing home–type unit) **A**1 9 10 18 **F**3 7 34 35 40 50 53 56 57 59 64 65 68 75 77 93 97 107 111 113 118 127 128 129 132 142 147 **P**6
Primary Contact: Neil W. Ginty, Administrator
CFO: Libby Flemming, Controller and Chief Information Officer
CMO: Bruce Herrington, M.D., Chief Medical Officer
CIO: Libby Flemming, Controller and Chief Information Officer
CHR: Vicki Dinkins, Director Human Resources
Web address: www.sgmc.org
**Control:** Other not–for–profit (including NFP Corporation) **Service:** Other specialty

**Staffed Beds:** 87 **Admissions:** 358 **Census:** 61 **Outpatient Visits:** 9930 **Births:** 0 **Total Expense ($000):** 9288 **Payroll Expense ($000):** 4139 **Personnel:** 193

## LAWRENCEVILLE—Gwinnett County

⊞ **GWINNETT HOSPITAL SYSTEM (110087)**, 1000 Medical Center Boulevard, Zip 30046–7694, Mailing Address: P.O. Box 348, Zip 30046; tel. 678/312–4321, (Includes GWINNETT MEDICAL CENTER, 1000 Medical Center Boulevard, Zip 30245, Mailing Address: Box 348, Zip 30246; tel. 770/995–4321; GWINNETT MEDICAL CENTER–DULUTH, 3620 Howell Ferry Road, Duluth, Zip 30096; tel. 678/312–6800), (Nonreporting) **A**1 2 9 10
Primary Contact: Philip R. Wolfe, President and Chief Executive Officer
COO: Jeffrey D. Nowlin, Executive Vice President and Chief Operating Officer
CFO: Thomas Y. McBride, III, Executive Vice President and Chief Financial Officer
CMO: Alan Bier, M.D., Executive Vice President and Chief Medical Officer
CIO: Ed Brown, Senior Vice President and Chief Information Officer
CHR: Steve Nadeau, Senior Vice President Human Resources
Web address: www.gwinnettmedicalcenter.org
**Control:** Other not–for–profit (including NFP Corporation) **Service:** General Medical and Surgical

**Staffed Beds:** 448

☐ **SUMMITRIDGE HOSPITAL (114004)**, 250 Scenic Highway, Zip 30046–5675; tel. 678/442–5800, (Nonreporting) **A**1 10
Primary Contact: Margaret P. Collier, Chief Executive Officer
Web address: www.summitridgehospital.net
**Control:** Other not–for–profit (including NFP Corporation) **Service:** Psychiatric

**Staffed Beds:** 25

## LITHONIA—Dekalb County

☐ **DEKALB MEDICAL AT HILLANDALE (110226)**, 2801 DeKalb Medical Parkway, Zip 30058; tel. 404/501–8700 **A**1 9 10 **F**3 11 12 15 18 29 30 35 40 45 49 50 60 70 74 75 77 79 81 85 87 93 107 108 110 111 113 118 129 145 **P**1 **S** DeKalb Regional Health System, Decatur, GA
Primary Contact: John Shelton, President and Chief Executive Officer
COO: John Shelton, Chief Operating Officer
CMO: Duane Barclay, D.O., Chief Medical Officer
CIO: Mark Trocino, Chief Information Officer
CHR: Tom Crawford, Vice President Human Resources
Web address: www.dekalbmedical.org
**Control:** Other not–for–profit (including NFP Corporation) **Service:** General Medical and Surgical

**Staffed Beds:** 100 **Admissions:** 4707 **Census:** 54 **Outpatient Visits:** 86547 **Births:** 0 **Total Expense ($000):** 58972 **Payroll Expense ($000):** 21822 **Personnel:** 368

## LOUISVILLE—Jefferson County

☐ **JEFFERSON HOSPITAL (110100)**, 1067 Peachtree Street, Zip 30434–1599; tel. 478/625–7000 **A**1 9 10 20 **F**11 15 30 34 40 45 53 54 57 59 63 64 65 66 79 81 85 89 93 97 107 109 113 118 126 128 132 134 **P**6
Primary Contact: Ralph X. Randall, FACHE, Chief Executive Officer
CFO: Michael J. Sombar, Jr., Chief Financial Officer
CIO: Ricky Wasden, Manager Information Technology
CHR: Catherine Hall, Manager Human Resources
Web address: www.jeffersonhosp.com
**Control:** City–County, Government, nonfederal **Service:** General Medical and Surgical

**Staffed Beds:** 37 **Admissions:** 669 **Census:** 8 **Outpatient Visits:** 74247 **Births:** 0 **Total Expense ($000):** 12662 **Payroll Expense ($000):** 6799 **Personnel:** 207

## MACON—Bibb County

⊞ **CENTRAL GEORGIA REHABILITATION HOSPITAL (113029)**, 3351 Northside Drive, Zip 31210–2591; tel. 478/201–6500, (Nonreporting) **A**1 9 10
Primary Contact: Elbert T. McQueen, President and Chief Executive Officer
CFO: Beverly Owens, Controller
CMO: Allison Scheetz, M.D., Medical Director
Web address: www.centralgarehab.com
**Control:** Other not–for–profit (including NFP Corporation) **Service:** Rehabilitation

**Staffed Beds:** 58

⊞ **COLISEUM MEDICAL CENTERS (110164)**, 350 Hospital Drive, Zip 31217–3871; tel. 478/765–7000, (Nonreporting) **A**1 2 9 10 **S** HCA, Nashville, TN
Primary Contact: Charles Briscoe, Chief Executive Officer
COO: David A. Portwood, Chief Operating Officer
CFO: Roger Simmons, Chief Financial Officer
CMO: Larry Grant, M.D., Chief Medical Officer
CIO: Joan Morstad, Director Information Systems
CHR: Pat Lattrell, Director Human Resources
Web address: www.coliseumhealthsystem.com
**Control:** Corporation, Investor–owned, for–profit **Service:** General Medical and Surgical

**Staffed Beds:** 227

⊞ **COLISEUM NORTHSIDE HOSPITAL (110201)**, 400 Charter Boulevard, Zip 31210–4853, Mailing Address: P.O. Box 4627, Zip 31208–4627; tel. 478/757–8200, (Nonreporting) **A**1 9 10 **S** HCA, Nashville, TN
Primary Contact: Mike Sherrod, Chief Executive Officer
CFO: Roger Simmons, Chief Financial Officer
CHR: Pat Luttrell, Director Human Resources
Web address: www.coliseumhealthsystem.com
**Control:** Corporation, Investor–owned, for–profit **Service:** General Medical and Surgical

**Staffed Beds:** 103

⊞ **COLISEUM PSYCHIATRIC CENTER (114015)**, 340 Hospital Drive, Zip 31217–8002; tel. 478/741–1355 **A**1 9 10 **F**4 5 29 30 35 38 56 75 98 100 101 102 103 104 105 129 131 **S** HCA, Nashville, TN
Primary Contact: James W. Eyler, FACHE, Chief Executive Officer
Web address: www.coliseumhealthsystem.com
**Control:** Corporation, Investor–owned, for–profit **Service:** Psychiatric

**Staffed Beds:** 34 **Admissions:** 1365 **Census:** 25 **Outpatient Visits:** 4125 **Births:** 0 **Personnel:** 85

⊞ **MEDICAL CENTER OF CENTRAL GEORGIA (110107)**, 777 Hemlock Street, Zip 31201–2155; tel. 478/633–1000, (Includes CHILDREN'S HOSPITAL, 777 Hemlock Street, tel. 478/633–1000) **A**1 2 3 5 8 9 10 **F**3 5 7 8 11 12 13 14 15 17 18 20 22 24 26 28 29 30 31 32 34 35 36 39 40 43 44 45 46 47 48 49 50 51 53 54 56 57 58 59 60 61 62 63 64 65 66 68 70 72 73 74 75 76 77 78 79 81 82 83 84 85 86 87 88 89 92 93 94 97 98 99 100 101 102 103 104 105 107 108 110 111 113 114 118 125 129 131 134 142 143 144 145 146 147 **P**1
Primary Contact: A. Donald Faulk, Jr., FACHE, President
COO: Joseph D. Lavelle, Executive Vice President and Chief Operating Officer
CFO: Rhonda Perry, Chief Financial Officer
CMO: James M. Cunningham, M.D., Vice President Medical Affairs
CIO: William Avenel, Assistant Vice President Information Services
CHR: Lori W. Cassidy, FACHE, Assistant Vice President
Web address: www.mccg.org
**Control:** Hospital district or authority, Government, nonfederal **Service:** General Medical and Surgical

**Staffed Beds:** 659 **Admissions:** 30963 **Census:** 473 **Outpatient Visits:** 350886 **Births:** 2666 **Total Expense ($000):** 586285 **Payroll Expense ($000):** 228790 **Personnel:** 4710

**GA**

GA

✠ **REGENCY HOSPITAL OF CENTRAL GEORGIA (112016)**, 535 Coliseum Drive, Zip 31217; tel. 478/803–7300, (Nonreporting) **A**1 10 **S** Select Medical Corporation, Mechanicsburg, PA
Primary Contact: Michael S. Boggs, Chief Executive Officer
Web address: www.regencyhospital.com
**Control:** Corporation, Investor–owned, for–profit **Service:** Long–Term Acute Care hospital

**Staffed Beds:** 34

### MADISON—Morgan County

☐ **MORGAN MEMORIAL HOSPITAL (111304)**, 1077 South Main Street, Zip 30650, Mailing Address: P.O. Box 860, Zip 30650–0860; tel. 706/342–1667 **A**1 9 10 18 **F**15 29 34 35 40 43 45 56 57 59 68 75 81 93 100 103 104 107 110 113 118 127 128 129 131 132 134 145
Primary Contact: Ralph Castillo, Chief Executive Officer
CFO: Courtney Moore, CPA, Chief Financial Officer
CMO: Eduardo M. Cossio, M.D., Chief of Staff
CIO: Patrick Cook, Vice President Support Services
CHR: Sarah Logan, Manager Human Resources
Web address: www.mmh.org
**Control:** Hospital district or authority, Government, nonfederal **Service:** General Medical and Surgical

**Staffed Beds:** 41 **Admissions:** 223 **Census:** 2 **Outpatient Visits:** 13027 **Births:** 0 **Total Expense ($000):** 11929 **Payroll Expense ($000):** 6553 **Personnel:** 158

### MARIETTA—Cobb County

✠ △ **WELLSTAR KENNESTONE HOSPITAL (110035)**, 677 Church Street, Zip 30060–1148; tel. 770/793–5000 **A**1 2 3 5 7 9 10 **F**3 10 11 12 13 15 17 18 20 22 24 26 28 29 30 31 37 38 40 41 44 45 48 49 50 53 54 58 61 64 66 68 70 72 73 74 75 76 77 78 79 80 81 82 84 85 86 87 90 93 94 96 100 102 107 108 110 111 113 114 116 117 118 120 122 123 124 125 129 140 145 146 147 **P**1 6 **S** WellStar Health System, Marietta, GA
Primary Contact: Candice Saunders, Senior Vice President and Administrator
COO: Michael L. Graue, Executive Vice President and Chief Operating Officer
CFO: A. James Budzinski, Vice President and Chief Financial Officer
CIO: Ronald Strachan, Senior Vice President and Chief Information Officer
CHR: David W. Anderson, Executive Vice President Human Resources and Chief Compliance Officer
Web address: www.wellstar.org
**Control:** Other not–for–profit (including NFP Corporation) **Service:** General Medical and Surgical

**Staffed Beds:** 580 **Admissions:** 37397 **Census:** 465 **Outpatient Visits:** 422124 **Births:** 5442 **Personnel:** 3465

✠ **WELLSTAR WINDY HILL HOSPITAL (112007)**, 2540 Windy Hill Road, Zip 30067–8632; tel. 770/644–1000 **A**1 2 9 10 **F**1 3 5 11 15 29 30 38 44 45 50 51 58 61 64 68 75 77 79 81 85 86 87 93 94 100 101 104 105 107 108 110 111 113 117 118 128 129 140 145 147 **P**1 6 **S** WellStar Health System, Marietta, GA
Primary Contact: Lou Little, Senior Vice President and Administrator
CFO: Marsha Burke, Senior Vice President and Chief Financial Officer
CMO: Larry Haldeman, M.D., Executive Vice President and Chief Medical Officer
CIO: Leigh Cox, Chief Information Officer
Web address: www.wellstar.org
**Control:** Other not–for–profit (including NFP Corporation) **Service:** General Medical and Surgical

**Staffed Beds:** 55 **Admissions:** 470 **Census:** 36 **Outpatient Visits:** 24022 **Births:** 0 **Personnel:** 256

### METTER—Candler County

☐ **CANDLER COUNTY HOSPITAL (111334)**, 400 Cedar Street, Zip 30439–3338, Mailing Address: P.O. Box 597, Zip 30439–0597; tel. 912/685–5741, (Nonreporting) **A**1 9 10 18
Primary Contact: Stephen C. Shepherd, Chief Executive Officer
Web address: www.candlercountyhospital.com
**Control:** Hospital district or authority, Government, nonfederal **Service:** General Medical and Surgical

**Staffed Beds:** 25

### MILLEDGEVILLE—Baldwin County

☐ **CENTRAL STATE HOSPITAL (114018)**, 620 Broad Street, Zip 31062–0001; tel. 478/445–4128, (Total facility includes 413 beds in nursing home–type unit) **A**1 9 10 **F**15 30 39 53 59 67 75 77 86 87 97 98 100 103 107 108 110 118 127 129 **P**6
Primary Contact: Randall Hines, Interim Administrator
COO: Terry McGee, Chief Operations Officer
CMO: Scott VanSant, M.D., Chief Medical Officer
CIO: Betsy Bradley, Coordinator Performance Improvement
CHR: Myra Holloway, Director Human Resources Management
Web address: www.centralstatehospital.org
**Control:** State–Government, nonfederal **Service:** Psychiatric

**Staffed Beds:** 597 **Admissions:** 111 **Census:** 496 **Outpatient Visits:** 0 **Births:** 0 **Total Expense ($000):** 111904 **Payroll Expense ($000):** 51173 **Personnel:** 1657

☐ **OCONEE REGIONAL MEDICAL CENTER (110150)**, 821 North Cobb Street, Zip 31061–2351, Mailing Address: P.O. Box 690, Zip 31059–0690; tel. 478/454–3500, (Total facility includes 15 beds in nursing home–type unit) **A**1 9 10 19 **F**3 11 13 15 28 29 30 31 34 35 37 40 45 46 49 50 53 57 59 64 68 70 75 76 78 79 80 81 82 85 86 87 89 107 108 111 113 115 116 118 119 120 122 127 131 134 142 145 146 147 **S** Oconee Regional Health Systems, Milledgeville, GA
Primary Contact: Jean Aycock, President and Chief Executive Officer
CFO: Brenda Qualls, Chief Financial Officer
Web address: www.oconeeregional.com
**Control:** Other not–for–profit (including NFP Corporation) **Service:** General Medical and Surgical

**Staffed Beds:** 89 **Admissions:** 3868 **Census:** 57 **Outpatient Visits:** 128258 **Births:** 642 **Total Expense ($000):** 74096 **Payroll Expense ($000):** 28192 **Personnel:** 602

### MILLEN—Jenkins County

**JENKINS COUNTY HOSPITAL (111311)**, 931 East Winthrope Avenue, Zip 30442–1839; tel. 478/982–4221, (Nonreporting) **A**9 10 18
Primary Contact: Brad Trower, Chief Executive Officer
**Control:** Hospital district or authority, Government, nonfederal **Service:** General Medical and Surgical

**Staffed Beds:** 25

### MONROE—Walton County

☐ **WALTON REGIONAL MEDICAL CENTER (110046)**, 330 Alcovy Street, Zip 30655–2140, Mailing Address: P.O. Box 1346, Zip 30655–1346; tel. 770/267–8461, (Nonreporting) **A**1 9 10 **S** Health Management Associates, Naples, FL
Primary Contact: J. T. Barnhart, Chief Executive Officer
COO: Jon–Paul Croom, Chief Operating Officer
CFO: Kevin Rinks, Chief Financial Officer
CMO: Terry Chongulia, M.D., Chief of Staff
CIO: Ed Stanley, Director Information Systems
CHR: Michele Monsrud, Director Human Resources
Web address: www.waltonregional.com
**Control:** Corporation, Investor–owned, for–profit **Service:** General Medical and Surgical

**Staffed Beds:** 115

### MONTEZUMA—Macon County

☐ **FLINT RIVER COMMUNITY HOSPITAL (110190)**, 509 Sumter Street, Zip 31063–0770, Mailing Address: P.O. Box 770, Zip 31063–0770; tel. 478/472–3100, (Nonreporting) **A**1 9 10
Primary Contact: Frank Schupp, Chief Executive Officer
CFO: Lara Busbee, Chief Financial Officer
CMO: Christopher Inhulsen, M.D., Chief of Staff
CIO: Shawn Reddick, Director Information Management
CHR: Tricia Johnson, Coordinator Human Resources
Web address: www.flintriverhospital.com/
**Control:** Corporation, Investor–owned, for–profit **Service:** General Medical and Surgical

**Staffed Beds:** 49

### MONTICELLO—Jasper County

**JASPER MEMORIAL HOSPITAL (111303)**, 898 College Street, Zip 31064–1298; tel. 706/468–6411, (Total facility includes 55 beds in nursing home–type unit) **A**9 10 18 **F**11 18 29 34 40 57 59 65 77 93 97 107 111 114 118 127 132 145 147 **P**6 **S** Oconee Regional Health Systems, Milledgeville, GA
Primary Contact: Jan Gaston, Administrator
CFO: Stuart Abney, Controller
CHR: Laura Hammonds, Assistant Administrator
CNO: Tammy Honeycutt, R.N., Director of Nursing
Web address: www.jaspermemorialhospital.org
**Control:** Other not–for–profit (including NFP Corporation) **Service:** General Medical and Surgical

**Staffed Beds:** 67 **Admissions:** 191 **Census:** 57 **Outpatient Visits:** 11658 **Births:** 0 **Total Expense ($000):** 8875 **Payroll Expense ($000):** 4575 **Personnel:** 116

## MOULTRIE—Colquitt County

☒ ○ **COLQUITT REGIONAL MEDICAL CENTER (110105)**, 3131 South Main Street, Zip 31768–6701, Mailing Address: P.O. Box 40, Zip 31776–0040; tel. 229/985–3420 **A**1 9 10 11 **F**3 7 11 12 13 15 17 20 29 30 31 32 34 35 39 40 45 47 48 49 56 57 59 60 61 62 63 65 68 70 74 75 76 77 78 79 81 82 85 86 87 89 91 93 97 107 108 110 111 114 118 126 128 129 130 131 134 142 143 145 146 147
Primary Contact: James L. Matney, President and Chief Executive Officer
CFO: W. Larry Sims, Chief Financial Officer and Vice President Financial Services
CMO: D. W. Adcock, M.D., Medical Director
CIO: Mitch Hiers, Director Information Services
CHR: Dawn Johns, Director Human Resources
Web address: www.colquittregional.com
**Control:** Hospital district or authority, Government, nonfederal **Service:** General Medical and Surgical

**Staffed Beds:** 73 **Admissions:** 3892 **Census:** 42 **Outpatient Visits:** 110741 **Births:** 665 **Total Expense ($000):** 72075 **Payroll Expense ($000):** 29551 **Personnel:** 656

**TURNING POINT HOSPITAL (110209)**, 3015 Veterans Parkway South, Zip 31788–6705, Mailing Address: P.O. Box 1177, Zip 31776–1177; tel. 229/985–4815 **A**9 10 **F**4 5 75 87 98 104 105 129 134 142 **P**6 **S** Universal Health Services, Inc., King of Prussia, PA
Primary Contact: Ben Marion, Chief Executive Officer and Managing Director
COO: Judy Payne, R.N., Chief Operating Officer
CFO: Edwin Bennett, Controller
CHR: Michelle Reddick, Director Human Resources
CNO: Faith Connell, Director of Nursing
Web address: www.turningpointcare.com
**Control:** Corporation, Investor–owned, for–profit **Service:** Alcoholism and other chemical dependency

**Staffed Beds:** 59 **Admissions:** 2468 **Census:** 30 **Outpatient Visits:** 17360 **Births:** 0 **Total Expense ($000):** 12948 **Payroll Expense ($000):** 5352 **Personnel:** 126

## NASHVILLE—Berrien County

☐ **BERRIEN COUNTY HOSPITAL (110112)**, 1221 East McPherson Avenue, Zip 31639–2326, Mailing Address: P.O. Box 665, Zip 31639–0665; tel. 229/543–7100, (Nonreporting) **A**1 9 10
Primary Contact: Stephanie Fletcher, Interim Chief Executive Officer
CFO: Stephanie Fletcher, Chief Financial Officer
Web address: www.berrienhospital.com
**Control:** Corporation, Investor–owned, for–profit **Service:** General Medical and Surgical

**Staffed Beds:** 63

## NEWNAN—Coweta County

☒ **PIEDMONT NEWNAN HOSPITAL (110229)**, 60 Hospital Road, Zip 30263–1210, Mailing Address: P.O. Box 997, Zip 30264–0997; tel. 770/253–1912 **A**1 9 10 **F**8 11 13 15 17 18 20 22 28 29 31 34 35 40 45 49 51 53 54 57 59 64 68 70 72 73 74 75 76 77 78 79 81 82 85 87 89 93 107 108 110 111 114 115 118 128 129 131 134 145 146 147 **S** Piedmont Healthcare, Atlanta, GA
Primary Contact: G. Michael Bass, President and Chief Executive Officer
COO: Nathan Nipper, Vice President and Chief Operating Officer
CFO: Courtney Reece, Chief Financial Officer
CMO: Jeffrey R. Folk, M.D., Vice President Medical Affairs and Chief Medical Officer
CIO: Sandra Romanow, Director Management Information Systems
CHR: Virginia H. Lyles, Vice President Human Resources
Web address: www.piedmontnewnan.org
**Control:** Other not–for–profit (including NFP Corporation) **Service:** General Medical and Surgical

**Staffed Beds:** 143 **Admissions:** 6008 **Census:** 74 **Outpatient Visits:** 74747 **Births:** 690 **Total Expense ($000):** 90649 **Payroll Expense ($000):** 40893 **Personnel:** 760

## OCILLA—Irwin County

☒ **IRWIN COUNTY HOSPITAL (110130)**, 710 North Irwin Avenue, Zip 31774–1098; tel. 229/468–3800, (Total facility includes 30 beds in nursing home–type unit) **A**1 9 10 **F**3 13 40 76 81 107 110 113 118 123 127 129
Primary Contact: Sue Spivey, Administrator
CFO: Tami Gray, Chief Financial Officer
CMO: Ashfaq Saiyed, M.D., Medical Director
CHR: Becky Edwards, Manager Human Resources
Web address: www.irwincntyhospital.com
**Control:** County–Government, nonfederal **Service:** General Medical and Surgical

**Staffed Beds:** 64 **Admissions:** 1244 **Census:** 33 **Outpatient Visits:** 11475 **Births:** 551 **Total Expense ($000):** 17246 **Payroll Expense ($000):** 7188 **Personnel:** 193

## PERRY—Houston County

☒ **PERRY HOSPITAL (110153)**, 1120 Morningside Drive, Zip 31069–2906; tel. 478/987–3600 **A**1 9 10 **F**3 11 15 29 30 34 35 39 40 45 48 49 50 51 56 57 58 59 61 68 70 75 79 81 82 85 86 87 89 100 107 110 113 114 118 128 129 130 131 132 133 134 145 146 147 **S** Houston Healthcare System, Warner Robins, GA
Primary Contact: David Campbell, Administrator
CFO: Sean Whilden, Chief Financial Officer
CMO: Jefferson Davis, M.D., Medical Director
CIO: Robert Rhodes, Director Information Systems
CHR: Michael O'Hara, Senior Executive Director
CNO: Melinda D. Hartley, R.N., Vice President Patient Care Services
Web address: www.hhc.org
**Control:** Other not–for–profit (including NFP Corporation) **Service:** General Medical and Surgical

**Staffed Beds:** 39 **Admissions:** 1511 **Census:** 18 **Outpatient Visits:** 37091 **Births:** 0 **Total Expense ($000):** 24067 **Payroll Expense ($000):** 9331 **Personnel:** 220

## QUITMAN—Brooks County

☒ **BROOKS COUNTY HOSPITAL (111332)**, 903 North Court Street, Zip 31643–1315, Mailing Address: P.O. Box 5000, Zip 31643–5000; tel. 229/263–4171 **A**1 9 10 18 **F**11 15 29 30 34 35 40 50 57 59 75 77 86 87 93 107 111 118 126 129 132 134 145 **P**6 **S** Archbold Medical Center, Thomasville, GA
Primary Contact: Kenneth D. Rhudy, Chief Executive Officer
COO: LaDon Toole, Administrator
CFO: LaDon Toole, Administrator
CMO: Michael Sopt, M.D., Chief of Staff
CHR: Janet Eldridge, Director Human Resources and Personnel
Web address: www.archbold.org
**Control:** Other not–for–profit (including NFP Corporation) **Service:** General Medical and Surgical

**Staffed Beds:** 25 **Admissions:** 525 **Census:** 14 **Outpatient Visits:** 19409 **Births:** 0 **Total Expense ($000):** 9787 **Payroll Expense ($000):** 5137 **Personnel:** 91

## REIDSVILLE—Tattnall County

★ **DOCTORS HOSPITAL OF TATTNALL (111323)**, 247 South Main Street, Zip 30453; tel. 912/557–1000, (Nonreporting) **A**9 10 18
Primary Contact: Jarrod G. Johnson, FACHE, President
Web address: www.tattnallhospital.com
**Control:** Partnership, Investor–owned, for–profit **Service:** Orthopedic

**Staffed Beds:** 25

## RICHLAND—Stewart County

**STEWART–WEBSTER HOSPITAL (111322)**, 580 Alston Street, Zip 31825–6012; tel. 229/887–3366 **A**9 10 18 **F**3 12 29 40 45 50 56 59 61 64 65 81 107 113 118 132 145
Primary Contact: Randy Stigleman, President and Chief Executive Officer
COO: Randy Stigleman, President and Chief Executive Officer
CFO: Randy Stigleman, President and Chief Executive Officer
CMO: Alliri Ragu, M.D., Chief of Staff
CHR: Merri Lynn Babb, Chief Human Resources
Web address: www.stewartcountyga.gov/stewartwebsterhospital.htm
**Control:** Corporation, Investor–owned, for–profit **Service:** General Medical and Surgical

**Staffed Beds:** 25 **Admissions:** 521 **Census:** 8 **Outpatient Visits:** 3526 **Births:** 0 **Total Expense ($000):** 4241 **Payroll Expense ($000):** 2086

## RIVERDALE—Clayton County

☐ **RIVERWOODS BEHAVIORAL HEALTH SYSTEM (114035)**, 233 Medical Center Drive, Zip 30274–2640; tel. 770/991–8500, (Nonreporting) **A**1 10
Primary Contact: Kirk Kureska, Chief Executive Officer
COO: Jenifer Harcourt, Chief Operating Officer
CFO: Tricia Nelson, Chief Financial Officer
CMO: Mahaveer Vakharia, M.D., Medical Director
CIO: Hema Patel, Director Medical Records
CHR: Tareka Beasley, Director Human Resources
Web address: www.riverwoodsbehavioral.com
**Control:** Corporation, Investor–owned, for–profit **Service:** Psychiatric

**Staffed Beds:** 75

**GA**

---

**Hospital, Medicare Provider Number, Address, Telephone, Approval, Facility, and Physician Codes, Health Care System**

★ American Hospital Association (AHA) membership
☐ The Joint Commission accreditation ◇ DNV Healthcare Inc. accreditation
○ American Osteopathic Association (AOA) accreditation
△ Commission on Accreditation of Rehabilitation Facilities (CARF) accreditation

✠ **SOUTHERN CRESCENT HOSPITAL FOR SPECIALTY CARE (112015)**, 11 Upper Riverdale Road S.W., 6th Floor, Zip 30274; tel. 770/897–7603 **A**1 10 **F**1 29 30 35 44 75 77 82 84 87 147 **P**8 **S** Dubuis Health System, Houston, TX
Primary Contact: Janice Hamilton–Crawford, Administrator
**Control:** Church–operated, Nongovernment, not–for profit **Service:** Long–Term Acute Care hospital

Staffed Beds: 30 Admissions: 301 Census: 22 Outpatient Visits: 0 Births: 0 Total Expense ($000): 11353 Payroll Expense ($000): 4265 Personnel: 75

☐ **SOUTHERN REGIONAL MEDICAL CENTER (110165)**, 11 Upper Riverdale Road S.W., Zip 30274–2615; tel. 770/991–8000, (Nonreporting) **A**1 2 3 5 9 10
Primary Contact: Stephen W. Mahan, President and Chief Executive Officer
COO: Therese O. Sucher, Senior Vice President Operations
CFO: Richard G. Stovall, Senior Vice President Fiscal Services and Chief Financial Officer
CMO: Willie Cochran, Jr., M.D., Chief of Staff
CIO: Karen Moore, Vice President Information Technology and Chief Information Officer
CHR: Norma Adams, Director Human Resources
Web address: www.southernregional.org
**Control:** Other not–for–profit (including NFP Corporation) **Service:** General Medical and Surgical

Staffed Beds: 274

### ROME—Floyd County

✠ **FLOYD MEDICAL CENTER (110054)**, 304 Turner McCall Boulevard, Zip 30165–2734, Mailing Address: P.O. Box 233, Zip 30162–0233; tel. 706/509–5000 **A**1 2 3 5 9 10 13 19 **F**3 4 5 6 7 8 9 11 12 13 15 17 18 20 22 26 28 29 30 31 32 34 35 36 37 38 39 40 43 44 45 46 48 49 50 51 53 54 56 57 58 59 61 63 64 65 66 68 70 71 72 74 75 76 77 78 79 81 82 84 85 86 87 88 89 90 93 96 97 98 100 101 102 103 104 105 107 108 110 111 113 114 117 118 128 129 130 131 133 134 142 143 145 146 147
Primary Contact: Kurt Stuenkel, FACHE, President and Chief Executive Officer
COO: Warren Alston Rigas, Executive Vice President and Chief Operating Officer
CFO: Rick Sheerin, Vice President Fiscal Services
CMO: Dee B. Russell, M.D., Vice President & Chief of Medical Affairs
CIO: Jeff Budda, Chief Information Officer
CHR: Beth Bradford, Director Human Resources
CNO: Sheila Bennett, R.N., Vice President & Chief Nursing Officer
Web address: www.floyd.org
**Control:** Other not–for–profit (including NFP Corporation) **Service:** General Medical and Surgical

Staffed Beds: 303 Admissions: 15130 Census: 199 Outpatient Visits: 237388 Births: 2374 Total Expense ($000): 292224 Payroll Expense ($000): 121172 Personnel: 2103

★ **KINDRED HOSPITAL ROME (112010)**, 304 Turner McCall Boulevard, Zip 30162; tel. 706/378–6800, (Nonreporting) **A**9 10 **S** Kindred Healthcare, Louisville, KY
Primary Contact: Susan M. Stovall, Chief Executive Officer
Web address: www.kindredrome.com
**Control:** Corporation, Investor–owned, for–profit **Service:** Long–Term Acute Care hospital

Staffed Beds: 45

✠ **REDMOND REGIONAL MEDICAL CENTER (110168)**, 501 Redmond Road, Zip 30165–7001, Mailing Address: P.O. Box 107001, Zip 30162–7001; tel. 706/291–0291, (Nonreporting) **A**1 2 9 10 19 **S** HCA, Nashville, TN
Primary Contact: John Quinlivan, Chief Executive Officer
COO: Carlton Ulmer, Chief Operating Officer
CFO: Danny Smith, Chief Financial Officer
CMO: Julie Coffman Barnes, M.D., Chief Medical Officer
CIO: Brad Treglown, Director Information Systems
CHR: Patsy Adams, Director Human Resources
CNO: Kay Rhodes, R.N., Chief Nursing Officer
Web address: www.redmondregional.com
**Control:** Corporation, Investor–owned, for–profit **Service:** General Medical and Surgical

Staffed Beds: 230

**SPECIALTY HOSPITAL** See Kindred Hospital Rome

### ROSWELL—Fulton County

✠ **NORTH FULTON REGIONAL HOSPITAL (110198)**, 3000 Hospital Boulevard, Zip 30076–3899; tel. 770/751–2500, (Nonreporting) **A**1 9 10 **S** TENET Healthcare Corporation, Dallas, TX
Primary Contact: Deborah C. Keel, Chief Executive Officer
CFO: Wesley James, Chief Financial Officer
CHR: Susan Brown, Chief Human Resources Officer
Web address: www.northfultonregional.com
**Control:** Corporation, Investor–owned, for–profit **Service:** General Medical and Surgical

Staffed Beds: 196

### ROYSTON—Franklin County

☐ **COBB MEMORIAL HOSPITAL (110027)**, 521 Franklin Springs Street, Zip 30662–3909, Mailing Address: P.O. Box 589, Zip 30662–0589; tel. 706/245–5071, (Includes BROWN MEMORIAL CONVALESCENT CENTER, COBB HEALTH CARE CENTER AND THE GABLES ), (Total facility includes 144 beds in nursing home–type unit) **A**1 9 10 **F**3 11 13 15 29 30 34 35 40 45 50 57 59 64 69 70 75 76 79 81 85 87 89 93 96 107 108 110 111 113 118 127 129 130 **S** Ty Cobb Healthcare System, Inc., Royston, GA
Primary Contact: David H. Seagraves, Chief Executive Officer
CFO: Kimberly Massey, Controller
Web address: www.tycobbhealthcare.org
**Control:** Other not–for–profit (including NFP Corporation) **Service:** General Medical and Surgical

Staffed Beds: 186 Admissions: 1348 Census: 153 Outpatient Visits: 33340 Births: 236 Total Expense ($000): 25804 Payroll Expense ($000): 10278 Personnel: 331

### SAINT MARYS—Camden County

✠ **SOUTHEAST GEORGIA HEALTH SYSTEM CAMDEN CAMPUS (110146)**, 2000 Dan Proctor Drive, Zip 31558–3810; tel. 912/576–6200 **A**1 9 10 20 **F**3 11 13 15 29 30 34 35 40 45 46 47 48 49 50 54 57 59 64 68 70 71 75 76 77 78 79 81 85 86 87 90 93 94 96 107 108 110 111 113 118 128 130 131 145 **P**5 **S** Southeast Georgia Health System, Brunswick, GA
Primary Contact: Howard W. Sepp, Jr., FACHE, Vice President and Administrator
CFO: Michael D. Scherneck, Executive Vice President
CMO: Robert Wilson, M.D., Chief of Staff
CHR: Patrick Ebri, Ph.D., Vice President Human Resources
Web address: www.sghs.org
**Control:** City–County, Government, nonfederal **Service:** General Medical and Surgical

Staffed Beds: 40 Admissions: 1811 Census: 21 Outpatient Visits: 77670 Births: 757 Total Expense ($000): 32057 Payroll Expense ($000): 13818 Personnel: 265

### SAINT SIMONS ISLAND—Glynn County

☐ **SAINT SIMONS BY–THE–SEA HOSPITAL (114016)**, 2927 Demere Road, Zip 31522–1620; tel. 912/638–1999, (Nonreporting) **A**1 9 10 **S** Universal Health Services, Inc., King of Prussia, PA
Primary Contact: Steve Glazier, Chief Executive Officer
CMO: Kim Masters, M.D., Medical Director
CIO: Chisty Mosely, Director Information Management
Web address: www.ssbythesea.com
**Control:** Corporation, Investor–owned, for–profit **Service:** Psychiatric

Staffed Beds: 101

### SANDERSVILLE—Washington County

☐ **WASHINGTON COUNTY REGIONAL MEDICAL CENTER (110086)**, 610 Sparta Road, Zip 31082–1362, Mailing Address: P.O. Box 636, Zip 31082–0636; tel. 478/240–2000, (Nonreporting) **A**1 9 10 20
Primary Contact: Jimmy Childre, Jr., Interim Chief Executive Officer
CFO: Cythia Parker, Fiscal Director
CMO: Robert Wright, M.D., Chief of Staff
CHR: Gayle Prince, Director Human Resources
Web address: www.wcrmc.com
**Control:** Hospital district or authority, Government, nonfederal **Service:** General Medical and Surgical

Staffed Beds: 116

### SAVANNAH—Chatham County

✠ △ **CANDLER HOSPITAL (110024)**, 5353 Reynolds Street, Zip 31405–6013; tel. 912/819–6000, (Total facility includes 11 beds in nursing home–type unit) **A**1 2 7 9 10 **F**2 3 11 13 15 18 20 28 29 30 31 32 34 35 36 37 38 39 40 41 44 45 46 47 48 49 50 53 54 57 58 59 60 61 64 65 68 70 71 73 74 75 76 77 78 80 81 82 84 85 86 87 89 90 93 94 96 107 108 110 113 115 116 117 118 119 120 122 123 127 128 129 130 131 134 145 146 147
Primary Contact: Paul P. Hinchey, President and Chief Executive Officer
CFO: Gregory J. Schaack, CPA, Vice President and Chief Financial Officer
CMO: James Scott, M.D., Vice President Medical Affairs
CIO: George Evans, Vice President and Chief Information Officer
CHR: Don Stubbs, Vice President Human Resources
Web address: www.sjchs.org
**Control:** Church–operated, Nongovernment, not–for profit **Service:** General Medical and Surgical

Staffed Beds: 285 Admissions: 11997 Census: 187 Outpatient Visits: 323806 Births: 2971 Total Expense ($000): 187168 Payroll Expense ($000): 73632 Personnel: 1487

**GA**

☐ **COASTAL HARBOR TREATMENT CENTER (114008)**, 1150 Cornell Avenue, Zip 31406–2797; tel. 912/354–3911 **A**1 9 10 **F**98 99 103 105 106 **S** Universal Health Services, Inc., King of Prussia, PA
Primary Contact: Ray Heckerman, Chief Executive Officer and Managing Director
COO: Ray Heckerman, Chief Executive Officer and Managing Director
CFO: Garry Ege, Chief Financial Officer
CMO: Ed Merves, M.D., Medical Director
CHR: Kellie Carlson, Director Human Resources
CNO: Jillisa Thornton, Director of Nursing
Web address: www.coastalharbor.com
**Control:** Corporation, Investor–owned, for–profit **Service:** Psychiatric

**Staffed Beds:** 195 **Admissions:** 2123 **Census:** 144 **Outpatient Visits:** 6277 **Births:** 0 **Total Expense ($000):** 24079 **Payroll Expense ($000):** 11009 **Personnel:** 301

**GEORGE AND MARIE BACKUS CHILDREN'S HOSPITAL** See Memorial Children's Hospital

☐ **GEORGIA REGIONAL HOSPITAL AT SAVANNAH (114028)**, 1915 Eisenhower Drive, Zip 31406–5098; tel. 912/356–2011, (Nonreporting) **A**1 9 10
Primary Contact: Charles Li, M.D., Regional Administrator
COO: Thomas F. Kurtz, Jr., Chief Operating Officer
CFO: Janet Edenfield, Director Financial Services
CMO: Donald Manning, M.D., Clinical Director
CHR: Jamekia Powers, Assistant Director Human Resources
Web address: www.garegionalsavannah.com
**Control:** State–Government, nonfederal **Service:** Psychiatric

**Staffed Beds:** 105

☒ △ **MEMORIAL HEALTH (110036)**, 4700 Waters Avenue, Zip 31404–6283, Mailing Address: P.O. Box 23089, Zip 31403–3089; tel. 912/350–8000, (Includes MEMORIAL CHILDREN'S HOSPITAL, 4700 Waters Avenue, Zip 31404–6220, Mailing Address: PO Box 23089, Zip 31403–3089; tel. 912/350–1543) **A**1 2 3 5 7 8 9 10 **F**3 8 11 12 13 14 15 17 18 19 20 22 24 26 28 29 30 31 32 34 35 36 37 39 40 41 43 44 45 46 49 50 52 53 54 55 56 57 58 59 60 61 64 65 66 68 70 71 72 73 74 75 76 77 78 79 80 81 82 83 84 85 86 87 88 89 90 92 93 96 97 98 100 101 102 103 104 107 108 110 111 113 114 116 117 118 119 120 122 123 125 128 129 130 131 134 142 143 145 146 147 **P**6
Primary Contact: Margaret Gill, Chief Executive Officer
CFO: Darcy Davis, Senior Vice President and Chief Financial Officer
CMO: Ramon V. Meguiar, M.D., Senior Vice President and Chief Medical Officer
CIO: Patricia A. Lavely, FACHE, Chief Information Officer
CHR: Richard J. Roche, Vice President Human Resources and Support Services
Web address: www.memorialhealth.com
**Control:** Other not–for–profit (including NFP Corporation) **Service:** General Medical and Surgical

**Staffed Beds:** 538 **Admissions:** 27169 **Census:** 396 **Outpatient Visits:** 271142 **Births:** 2688 **Total Expense ($000):** 442549 **Payroll Expense ($000):** 185550 **Personnel:** 3331

☒ **SELECT SPECIALTY HOSPITAL–SAVANNAH (112011)**, 5353 Reynolds Street, 4 South, Zip 31405; tel. 912/819–7972, (Nonreporting) **A**1 9 10 **S** Select Medical Corporation, Mechanicsburg, PA
Primary Contact: Coleen Zimmerman, Chief Executive Officer
Web address: www.selectmedicalcorp.com
**Control:** Corporation, Investor–owned, for–profit **Service:** Long–Term Acute Care hospital

**Staffed Beds:** 36

**ST. JOSEPH'S CANDLER HOSPITAL** See Candler Hospital

☐ △ **ST. JOSEPH'S HOSPITAL (110043)**, 11705 Mercy Boulevard, Zip 31419–1791; tel. 912/819–4100, (Total facility includes 11 beds in nursing home–type unit) **A**1 2 7 9 10 **F**3 11 15 17 18 20 22 24 26 28 29 30 34 35 36 37 38 39 40 41 44 45 49 50 54 56 57 58 59 60 61 65 68 70 74 75 77 79 80 81 82 84 85 86 87 90 93 94 96 107 108 110 111 113 114 117 118 122 123 125 127 129 130 131 134 145 147
Primary Contact: Paul P. Hinchey, President and Chief Executive Officer
CFO: Gregory J. Schaack, CPA, Vice President and Chief Financial Officer
CMO: James Jackson, M.D., Vice President Medical Affairs
CIO: John Adkins, Vice President and Chief Information Officer
CHR: Don Stubbs, Vice President Human Resources
Web address: www.sjchs.org
**Control:** Church–operated, Nongovernment, not–for profit **Service:** General Medical and Surgical

**Staffed Beds:** 236 **Admissions:** 10818 **Census:** 179 **Outpatient Visits:** 132027 **Births:** 0 **Total Expense ($000):** 178048 **Payroll Expense ($000):** 64228 **Personnel:** 1184

☒ **EMORY–ADVENTIST HOSPITAL (110183)**, 3949 South Cobb Drive S.E., Zip 30080–6300; tel. 770/434–0710 **A**1 9 10 **F**3 11 15 29 30 34 35 40 44 45 48 49 50 56 57 59 64 68 70 74 75 79 81 82 84 85 87 92 93 97 107 109 110 111 112 113 118 129 145 **S** Adventist Health System Sunbelt Health Care Corporation, Altamonte Springs, FL
Primary Contact: Dennis Kiley, President
COO: Ed Moyer, Chief Operating Officer
CFO: Carol Hazen, Vice President Finance
CHR: Shelli K. Johnson, Director Human Resources
Web address: www.emoryadventist.org
**Control:** Church–operated, Nongovernment, not–for profit **Service:** General Medical and Surgical

**Staffed Beds:** 52 **Admissions:** 1758 **Census:** 21 **Outpatient Visits:** 44255 **Births:** 0 **Total Expense ($000):** 46759 **Payroll Expense ($000):** 17080 **Personnel:** 388

☒ **RIDGEVIEW INSTITUTE (114012)**, 3995 South Cobb Drive S.E., Zip 30080–6397; tel. 770/434–4567 **A**1 5 9 10 **F**4 5 35 38 75 87 98 99 100 101 103 104 105 129 131 146 **P**8
Primary Contact: Paul Hackman, Chief Executive Officer
CFO: Jerry Magnison, Chief Financial Officer
CMO: Thomas Bradford Johns, M.D., Medical Director
CIO: Lynn Leger, Director Information Systems
CHR: Betty Sonderman, Manager Human Resources
Web address: www.ridgeviewinstitute.com
**Control:** Other not–for–profit (including NFP Corporation) **Service:** Psychiatric

**Staffed Beds:** 92 **Admissions:** 3815 **Census:** 66 **Outpatient Visits:** 39350 **Births:** 0 **Total Expense ($000):** 27561 **Payroll Expense ($000):** 15828 **Personnel:** 339

☒ **EASTSIDE MEDICAL CENTER (110192)**, 1700 Medical Way, Zip 30078–2195; tel. 770/979–0200 **A**1 2 9 10 **F**3 11 13 15 20 26 28 29 30 31 34 37 39 40 41 45 49 50 54 56 57 59 64 70 72 73 74 75 76 77 78 79 81 82 85 86 87 90 93 94 96 98 101 103 105 107 108 110 111 112 113 114 117 118 125 128 129 130 131 143 145 146 147 **S** HCA, Nashville, TN
Primary Contact: Kimberly Ryan, Chief Executive Officer
COO: Dustin Greene, Chief Operating Officer
CFO: Tom Jackson, Chief Financial Officer
CMO: Michael O'Neill, M.D., Chief Medical Officer
CIO: Pattie Page, Director Marketing and Public Relations
CHR: Nancy Dwyer, Vice President Human Resources
Web address: www.eastsidemedical.com
**Control:** Corporation, Investor–owned, for–profit **Service:** General Medical and Surgical

**Staffed Beds:** 247 **Admissions:** 10686 **Census:** 159 **Outpatient Visits:** 136872 **Births:** 1746 **Total Expense ($000):** 126372 **Payroll Expense ($000):** 55866 **Personnel:** 1030

☒ **EFFINGHAM HOSPITAL (111306)**, 459 Highway 119 South, Zip 31329–3021, Mailing Address: P.O. Box 386, Zip 31329–0386; tel. 912/754–6451, (Total facility includes 105 beds in nursing home–type unit) **A**1 9 10 18 **F**3 11 15 18 19 28 29 34 40 45 46 50 54 56 59 64 65 67 77 79 81 86 87 93 107 108 110 111 118 127 129 130 132 145 146 **P**6
Primary Contact: Norma J. Morgan, Chief Executive Officer
CFO: Ed Brown, Chief Financial Officer
CMO: George W. Brelsford, M.D., Chief Medical Staff
CIO: Bart Hunter, Manager Information Technology
CHR: Vicky Little, Director Human Resources
Web address: www.effinghamhospital.com
**Control:** Hospital district or authority, Government, nonfederal **Service:** General Medical and Surgical

**Staffed Beds:** 120 **Admissions:** 441 **Census:** 105 **Outpatient Visits:** 45037 **Births:** 0 **Total Expense ($000):** 20206 **Payroll Expense ($000):** 12035 **Personnel:** 300

**GA**

## STATESBORO—Bulloch County

☐ **EAST GEORGIA REGIONAL MEDICAL CENTER (110075)**, 1499 Fair Road, Zip 30458, Mailing Address: P.O. Box 1048, Zip 30459–1048; tel. 912/486–1000 **A**1 9 10 19 **F**3 11 13 15 18 20 22 29 30 31 35 40 46 48 49 57 59 60 67 68 70 74 75 76 77 78 79 81 82 85 87 89 93 103 107 108 111 112 113 114 115 116 117 118 128 131 145 146 147 **P**5 **S** Health Management Associates, Naples, FL
Primary Contact: Robert F. Bigley, President and Chief Executive Officer
COO: Cindi Butcher, Chief Operating Officer
CFO: Eric Smith, Chief Financial Officer
CMO: Benjamin Oldham, M.D., Chief of Staff
CIO: Marisa Smith, Director Information Services
CHR: Michael Black, Director Human Resources
CNO: Mary Anderson, R.N., Chief Nursing Officer
Web address: www.eastgeorgiaregional.com
**Control:** Corporation, Investor–owned, for–profit **Service:** General Medical and Surgical

**Staffed Beds:** 150 **Admissions:** 8562 **Census:** 85 **Outpatient Visits:** 126622 **Births:** 1544 **Personnel:** 629

**WILLINGWAY HOSPITAL**, 311 Jones Mill Road, Zip 30458–4765; tel. 912/764–6236, (Nonreporting) **A**9
Primary Contact: Jimmy Mooney, Chief Executive Officer
CFO: Barbara S. Reid, Chief Financial Officer
CMO: Robert W. Mooney, M.D., Medical Director
Web address: www.willingway.com
**Control:** Corporation, Investor–owned, for–profit **Service:** Alcoholism and other chemical dependency

**Staffed Beds:** 40

## STOCKBRIDGE—Henry County

⊠ **HENRY MEDICAL CENTER (110191)**, 1133 Eagle's Landing Parkway, Zip 30281–5099; tel. 678/604–1000, (Total facility includes 89 beds in nursing home–type unit) **A**1 2 9 10 **F**3 8 11 13 15 18 20 26 28 29 30 31 34 35 37 40 42 45 46 49 54 57 59 61 64 70 72 73 74 75 76 77 78 79 81 85 86 90 93 100 102 107 108 110 111 113 114 117 118 123 127 129 131 134 143 145 146 147 **S** Piedmont Healthcare, Atlanta, GA
Primary Contact: Charles F. Scott, President and Chief Executive Officer
CFO: Claude Carruth, Vice President and Chief Financial Officer
CMO: Jorge Spinolo, M.D., Chief of Staff
CIO: Terry Wilk, Chief Information Officer
CHR: Maribeth Ledford, Director Human Resources
Web address: www.henrymedical.com
**Control:** Hospital district or authority, Government, nonfederal **Service:** General Medical and Surgical

**Staffed Beds:** 289 **Admissions:** 12724 **Census:** 224 **Outpatient Visits:** 130933 **Births:** 2250 **Total Expense ($000):** 167469 **Payroll Expense ($000):** 65580 **Personnel:** 1193

## SWAINSBORO—Emanuel County

☐ **EMANUEL MEDICAL CENTER (110109)**, 117 Kite Road, Zip 30401–3231, Mailing Address: P.O. Box 879, Zip 30401–0879; tel. 478/289–1100, (Total facility includes 49 beds in nursing home–type unit) **A**1 9 10 20 **F**3 7 11 13 15 29 30 34 40 50 57 59 64 68 70 76 79 81 85 86 87 107 108 110 111 113 117 118 123 126 127 128 129 131 132 145 146
Primary Contact: Brian L. Riddle, Sr., FACHE, Chief Executive Officer
CFO: Rhonda Durden, Chief Financial Officer
CMO: Cedric Porter, M.D., President Medical Staff
CIO: Dave Flanders, Director Information Technology Systems
CHR: Ellen Boyd, Director Human Resources
Web address: www.emanuelmedical.org
**Control:** Hospital district or authority, Government, nonfederal **Service:** General Medical and Surgical

**Staffed Beds:** 91 **Admissions:** 1792 **Census:** 63 **Outpatient Visits:** 26360 **Births:** 89 **Total Expense ($000):** 14164 **Payroll Expense ($000):** 9259 **Personnel:** 314

## SYLVANIA—Screven County

★ **SCREVEN COUNTY HOSPITAL (111312)**, 215 Mims Road, Zip 30467–2097; tel. 912/564–7426, (Nonreporting) **A**9 10 18
Primary Contact: George H. St. George, FACHE, Chief Executive Officer
CFO: Marsha Carroll, Director Financial Services
**Control:** Hospital district or authority, Government, nonfederal **Service:** General Medical and Surgical

**Staffed Beds:** 25

## SYLVESTER—Worth County

⊠ **PHOEBE WORTH MEDICAL CENTER (111328)**, 807 South Isabella Street, Zip 31791–0545, Mailing Address: P.O. Box 545, Zip 31791–0545; tel. 229/776–6961 **A**1 9 10 18 **F**3 7 11 29 30 31 35 40 43 57 59 64 75 77 78 87 93 107 118 126 128 129 132 142 145 147 **P**6 **S** Phoebe Putney Health System, Albany, GA
Primary Contact: Kim Gilman, Chief Administrative Officer
CFO: John Graham, Chief Financial Officer
CMO: Natu M. Patel, M.D., Chief of Staff
CHR: Chris Foreman, Director
Web address: www.phobeputney.com
**Control:** Other not–for–profit (including NFP Corporation) **Service:** General Medical and Surgical

**Staffed Beds:** 25 **Admissions:** 294 **Census:** 3 **Outpatient Visits:** 16014 **Births:** 0 **Total Expense ($000):** 12604 **Payroll Expense ($000):** 6627 **Personnel:** 161

## THOMASTON—Upson County

⊠ **UPSON REGIONAL MEDICAL CENTER (110002)**, 801 West Gordon Street, Zip 30286–2831, Mailing Address: P.O. Box 1059, Zip 30286–1059; tel. 706/647–8111 **A**1 9 10 21 **F**3 11 13 15 28 29 30 31 34 35 40 45 46 49 50 53 57 59 61 64 70 75 76 78 79 80 81 82 85 86 89 107 108 110 111 113 114 117 118 123 129 131 132 134 147 **P**5 6 **S** HealthTech Management Services, Franklin, TN
Primary Contact: David L. Castleberry, Chief Executive Officer
CFO: John Williams, Chief Financial Officer
CIO: George Curtis, Director Information Technology Services
CHR: Rich Williams, Director Human Resources
Web address: www.urmc.org
**Control:** Other not–for–profit (including NFP Corporation) **Service:** General Medical and Surgical

**Staffed Beds:** 115 **Admissions:** 3920 **Census:** 40 **Outpatient Visits:** 77385 **Births:** 474 **Total Expense ($000):** 59668 **Payroll Expense ($000):** 23611 **Personnel:** 586

## THOMASVILLE—Thomas County

⊠ **JOHN D. ARCHBOLD MEMORIAL HOSPITAL (110038)**, 915 Gordon Avenue, Zip 31792–6614, Mailing Address: P.O. Box 1018, Zip 31799–1018; tel. 229/228–2000, (Total facility includes 64 beds in nursing home–type unit) **A**1 2 9 10 19 **F**1 3 4 5 8 11 12 13 15 17 18 20 22 26 28 29 30 31 34 35 36 38 40 43 45 46 48 49 50 51 54 56 57 58 59 60 61 64 65 67 68 70 74 75 76 77 78 79 81 82 85 86 87 89 90 93 98 99 100 101 102 103 104 105 107 108 110 111 113 114 115 116 117 118 120 122 123 125 127 128 129 130 131 133 134 142 143 145 146 147 **P**6 **S** Archbold Medical Center, Thomasville, GA
Primary Contact: J. Perry Mustian, President and Chief Executive Officer
COO: Kevin C. Taylor, Chief Operating Officer
CFO: Skip Hightower, Senior Vice President and Chief Financial Officer
CIO: William Zimmermann, Senior Vice President Information Services
CHR: Zach Wheeler, Senior Vice President Human Resources
Web address: www.archbold.org
**Control:** Other not–for–profit (including NFP Corporation) **Service:** General Medical and Surgical

**Staffed Beds:** 328 **Admissions:** 10546 **Census:** 220 **Outpatient Visits:** 287141 **Births:** 840 **Total Expense ($000):** 207644 **Payroll Expense ($000):** 78242 **Personnel:** 1564

☐ **SOUTHWESTERN STATE HOSPITAL (114021)**, Pine Tree Boulevard, Zip 31792, Mailing Address: P.O. Box 1378, Zip 31799–1378; tel. 229/227–2833, (Nonreporting) **A**1 9 10
Primary Contact: Hilary Hoo–You, Regional Administrator
COO: Susie Oates, Assistant Superintendent for Administration
CFO: Charles Barton, Business Manager
CMO: Joseph B. LeRoy, M.D., Clinical Director
CIO: Loma Owens, Data Manager
CHR: Clifton Mitchell, Manager Human Resources
Web address: www.swsh.org
**Control:** State–Government, nonfederal **Service:** Psychiatric

**Staffed Beds:** 236

## THOMSON—McDuffie County

★ **UNIVERSITY HOSPITAL MCDUFFIE (110111)**, 521 Hill Street S.W., Zip 30824–2199; tel. 706/595–1411 **A**9 10 21 **F**3 7 11 15 29 30 40 45 50 57 59 63 64 68 70 79 81 82 87 89 93 107 110 113 118 128 129 131 145 147
Primary Contact: Sandra I. McVicker, R.N., MSN, Chief Executive Officer
CFO: Pat Parris, Chief Financial Officer
CIO: Lisa Tucker, Chief Information Officer
CHR: Belinda H. Campbell, Director Human Resources, Legal Compliance and Risk Management
Web address: www.mrmc.org
**Control:** Hospital district or authority, Government, nonfederal **Service:** General Medical and Surgical

**Staffed Beds:** 25 **Admissions:** 768 **Census:** 8 **Outpatient Visits:** 32633 **Births:** 0 **Total Expense ($000):** 17809 **Payroll Expense ($000):** 6913 **Personnel:** 195

**GA**

*Many Facility Codes have changed. Please refer to the AHA Guide Code Chart.* © 2012 AHA Guide

## TIFTON—Tift County

☒ **TIFT REGIONAL MEDICAL CENTER (110095)**, 901 East 18th Street,
Zip 31794–3648, Mailing Address: Drawer 747, Zip 31793–0747;
tel. 229/382–7120, (Total facility includes 15 beds in nursing home–type unit) **A**1
2 9 10 19 **F**3 8 9 11 13 15 18 20 22 26 28 29 31 34 35 40 45 46 47 49 50
54 57 59 60 63 64 68 70 74 75 76 77 78 79 81 82 84 85 86 87 89 92 93
97 107 108 110 111 113 118 120 122 127 128 129 131 134 142 145 146
147 **P**6
Primary Contact: William T. Richardson, President and Chief Executive Officer
COO: Sarah Thompson, Vice President Operations
CFO: Dennis L. Crum, Vice President and Chief Financial Officer
CMO: Raymond Moreno, M.D., Vice President Medical Affairs
CIO: Guy McAllister, Assistant Vice President and Chief Information Officer
CHR: Ellen Eaton, Director Human Resources
Web address: www.tiftregional.com
**Control:** Hospital district or authority, Government, nonfederal **Service:** General
Medical and Surgical

> **Staffed Beds:** 191 **Admissions:** 11188 **Census:** 131 **Outpatient Visits:**
> 162195 **Births:** 1111 **Total Expense ($000):** 208712 **Payroll Expense**
> **($000):** 84094 **Personnel:** 1591

## TOCCOA—Stephens County

☒ **STEPHENS COUNTY HOSPITAL (110032)**, 163 Hospital Drive,
Zip 30577–9700; tel. 706/282–4200, (Total facility includes 92 beds in nursing
home–type unit) **A**1 9 10 **F**3 7 11 13 15 28 30 34 35 40 51 57 59 60 64 68
70 73 75 76 77 79 81 85 86 89 93 107 110 111 113 118 124 128 129
145 147
Primary Contact: Edward C. Gambrell, Jr., Administrator
CFO: Jeff Laird, Controller
CHR: Diane Hardeman, Director Personnel
Web address: www.stephenscountyhospital.com
**Control:** Hospital district or authority, Government, nonfederal **Service:** General
Medical and Surgical

> **Staffed Beds:** 188 **Admissions:** 3296 **Census:** 125 **Outpatient Visits:** 58314
> **Births:** 540 **Total Expense ($000):** 51360 **Payroll Expense ($000):** 24138
> **Personnel:** 578

## VALDOSTA—Lowndes County

☒ **SOUTH GEORGIA MEDICAL CENTER (110122)**, 2501 North Patterson Street,
Zip 31602–1735, Mailing Address: P.O. Box 1727, Zip 31603–1727;
tel. 229/333–1000, (Includes GREENLEAF CENTER, 2209 Pineview Drive,
Zip 31602–7316; tel. 229/247–4357; SMITH NORTHVIEW HOSPITAL, 4280
North Valdosta Road, Zip 31602, Mailing Address: P.O. Box 10010, Zip 31604;
tel. 229/671–2000; Sammie Dixon, M.D., Interim Chief Executive Officer) **A**1 2 9
10 19 **F**3 4 5 7 8 11 13 15 17 18 19 20 22 24 26 28 29 30 31 32 34 35 37
38 39 40 45 46 47 49 50 51 54 56 57 64 68 74 76 77
78 79 81 82 85 86 87 89 90 95 96 97 98 99 100 101 102 103 104 105 107
108 110 111 113 114 116 117 118 119 120 122 123 125 128 129 130 131
133 134 142 143 145 146 147 **P**6
Primary Contact: Randy Sauls, Chief Executive Officer and Administrator
CFO: Greg Hembree, Chief Financial Officer
CMO: Kimberly Megow, M.D., Chief Medical Officer
CIO: Bob Foster, Assistant Administrator Information Services
CHR: Charles Eidson, Assistant Administrator Human Resources
Web address: www.sgmc.org
**Control:** Hospital district or authority, Government, nonfederal **Service:** General
Medical and Surgical

> **Staffed Beds:** 380 **Admissions:** 13960 **Census:** 194 **Outpatient Visits:**
> 228134 **Births:** 1634 **Total Expense ($000):** 252864 **Payroll Expense**
> **($000):** 85516 **Personnel:** 2274

## VIDALIA—Toombs County

☒ **MEADOWS REGIONAL MEDICAL CENTER (110128)**, 1703 Meadows Lane,
Zip 30474–8915, Mailing Address: P.O. Box 1048, Zip 30475–1048;
tel. 912/535–5555 **A**1 9 10 20 **F**11 13 15 18 20 22 29 30 31 34 35 37 40
45 46 47 50 51 53 54 57 59 61 62 64 68 70 74 75 76 77 78 79 81 85 86
87 93 97 107 108 110 111 114 117 118 123 126 128 129 130 131 145
146 147 **P**6
Primary Contact: Alan Kent, Chief Executive Officer
COO: Shirley Hoskins, Chief Operating Officer
CFO: John Cornell, Vice President Finance
CIO: Charles Bondurant, Chief Information Officer
Web address: www.meadowsregional.org
**Control:** Other not–for–profit (including NFP Corporation) **Service:** General
Medical and Surgical

> **Staffed Beds:** 57 **Admissions:** 4783 **Census:** 35 **Outpatient Visits:** 56885
> **Births:** 717 **Total Expense ($000):** 64021 **Payroll Expense ($000):** 24707
> **Personnel:** 513

## VILLA RICA—Carroll County

☐ **TANNER MEDICAL CENTER–VILLA RICA (110015)**, 601 Dallas Road,
Zip 30180–1202, Mailing Address: P.O. Box 638, Zip 30180–0638;
tel. 770/456–3100, (Nonreporting) **A**1 9 10 **S** Tanner Health System,
Carrollton, GA
Primary Contact: Deborah Matthews, Administrator
Web address: www.tanner.org
**Control:** Other not–for–profit (including NFP Corporation) **Service:** General
Medical and Surgical

> **Staffed Beds:** 39

## WARM SPRINGS—Meriwether County

☐ **ROOSEVELT WARM SPRINGS INSTITUTE FOR REHABILITATION (113028)**,
6135 Roosevelt Highway, Zip 31830, Mailing Address: P.O. Box 1000,
Zip 31830–1000; tel. 706/655–5000, (Nonreporting) **A**1 9 10
Primary Contact: Greg Schmieg, Executive Director
CFO: David Cawthon, Director Financial Services
CMO: Burton McDaniel, M.D., Medical Director
CIO: Martin Harmon, Director Public Relations
CHR: Bill Bulloch, Director Human Resources
Web address: www.rooseveltrehab.org
**Control:** State–Government, nonfederal **Service:** Rehabilitation

> **Staffed Beds:** 52

**ROOSEVELT WARM SPRINGS LTAC HOSPITAL (112000)**, 6135 Roosevelt
Highway, Zip 31830; tel. 708/655–5000, (Nonreporting) **A**10
Primary Contact: Greg Schmieg, Executive Director
CFO: Ann Poston, Director Financial Services
CMO: W. Burton McDaniel, Jr., M.D., Physician Executive
CIO: Rufus Braddy, Director Management Information Systems
CHR: Kathy Albritton, Director Human Resources
Web address: www.rooseveltrehab.org/medical.php
**Control:** State–Government, nonfederal **Service:** Long–Term Acute Care hospital

> **Staffed Beds:** 30

☒ **WARM SPRINGS MEDICAL CENTER (111316)**, 5995 Spring Street,
Zip 31830–2149, Mailing Address: P.O. Box 8, Zip 31830–0008;
tel. 706/655–3331, (Total facility includes 79 beds in nursing home–type unit) **A**1
9 10 18 **F**3 11 15 29 30 40 45 54 57 64 67 68 79 81 90 93 107 111 113
118 127 129 132 145
Primary Contact: Richard Buchanan, Interim Chief Executive Officer
CFO: Karen Blanton, Chief Financial Officer
CMO: Alan Thompson, M.D., President Medical Staff
CIO: Milo Varnadoe, Director Information Systems
CHR: Barbara Nolan, Manager Human Resources
Web address: www.warmspringsmc.org
**Control:** Hospital district or authority, Government, nonfederal **Service:** General
Medical and Surgical

> **Staffed Beds:** 104 **Admissions:** 473 **Census:** 80 **Outpatient Visits:** 22403
> **Births:** 2 **Total Expense ($000):** 16652 **Payroll Expense ($000):** 8392
> **Personnel:** 145

## WARNER ROBINS—Houston County

☒ **HOUSTON MEDICAL CENTER (110069)**, 1601 Watson Boulevard,
Zip 31093–3431, Mailing Address: P.O. Box 2886, Zip 31099–2886;
tel. 478/922–4281 **A**1 9 10 **F**3 11 13 15 20 22 28 29 30 31 34 35 38 39 40
45 48 49 50 51 54 56 57 58 59 60 61 64 68 70 73 74 75 76 78 79 81 82
85 86 87 89 98 100 101 102 103 106 107 108 110 111 113 114 117 118
128 129 130 131 133 134 143 145 146 147 **P**6 **S** Houston Healthcare
System, Warner Robins, GA
Primary Contact: Cary Martin, Chief Executive Officer
CFO: Frank R. Powell, Chief Financial Officer
CFO: Sean Whilden, Chief Financial Officer
CIO: Robert Rhodes, Chief Information Officer
CHR: Michael O'Hara, Senior Executive Director Human Resources
Web address: www.hhc.org
**Control:** Other not–for–profit (including NFP Corporation) **Service:** General
Medical and Surgical

> **Staffed Beds:** 237 **Admissions:** 14344 **Census:** 179 **Outpatient Visits:**
> 230673 **Births:** 2183 **Total Expense ($000):** 187487 **Payroll Expense**
> **($000):** 78122 **Personnel:** 1891

**GA**

---

**Hospital, Medicare Provider Number, Address, Telephone, Approval, Facility, and Physician Codes, Health Care System**

★ American Hospital Association (AHA) membership
☐ The Joint Commission accreditation
◇ DNV Healthcare Inc. accreditation
○ American Osteopathic Association (AOA) accreditation
△ Commission on Accreditation of Rehabilitation Facilities (CARF) accreditation

## WASHINGTON—Wilkes County

☐ **WILLS MEMORIAL HOSPITAL (111325)**, 120 Gordon Street, Zip 30673–1602,
Mailing Address: P.O. Box 370, Zip 30673–0370; tel. 706/678–2151,
(Nonreporting) **A**1 9 10 18
Primary Contact: Jane Echols, Chief Executive Officer
CFO: Cliff Cooper, Chief Financial Officer
CHR: Tom Urban, Director Human Resources
Web address: www.willsmemorialhospital.com
**Control:** Hospital district or authority, Government, nonfederal **Service:** General
Medical and Surgical

**Staffed Beds:** 25

## WAYCROSS—Ware County

☒ **MAYO CLINIC HEALTH SYSTEM IN WAYCROSS (110003)**, 410 Darling
Avenue, Zip 31501–5246, Mailing Address: P.O. Box 139, Zip 31502–0139;
tel. 912/283–3030 **A**1 3 5 9 10 **F**3 13 15 17 18 20 22 28 29 30 34 35 40 45
49 51 57 59 60 70 73 74 75 76 77 78 79 80 81 85 87 89 90 92 93 98 107
108 111 113 114 115 116 117 118 128 129 131 134 145 **P**6 **S** Mayo Clinic
Health System, Rochester, MN
Primary Contact: Robert M. Trimm, Chief Administrative Officer
COO: Windell Smith, Chief Operating Officer
CFO: Katrina Wheeler, Chief Financial Officer
CMO: John Butler, M.D., Director Medical Staff
CIO: Barry Rudd, Chief Information Officer
Web address: www.satilla.org
**Control:** Other not–for–profit (including NFP Corporation) **Service:** General
Medical and Surgical

**Staffed Beds:** 200 **Admissions:** 7928 **Census:** 102 **Outpatient Visits:**
133224 **Births:** 469 **Total Expense ($000):** 115871 **Payroll Expense
($000):** 45602 **Personnel:** 1003

## WAYNESBORO—Burke County

☐ **BURKE MEDICAL CENTER (110113)**, 351 Liberty Street, Zip 30830–9686;
tel. 706/554–4435, (Nonreporting) **A**1 9 10
Primary Contact: Jennifer A. Royal, Administrator
CFO: Dianne Stewart, Controller
CHR: Danette Highsmith, Director Human Resources
Web address: www.burkemedical.net
**Control:** Hospital district or authority, Government, nonfederal **Service:** General
Medical and Surgical

**Staffed Beds:** 40

## WILDWOOD—Dade County

**WILDWOOD LIFESTYLE CENTER AND HOSPITAL**, 435 Lifestyle Lane,
Zip 30757–4128, Mailing Address: P.O. Box 129, Zip 30757–0129;
tel. 706/820–1493, (Nonreporting)
Primary Contact: Larry E. Clements, Administrator
Web address: www.wildwoodlsc.org
**Control:** Other not–for–profit (including NFP Corporation) **Service:** General
Medical and Surgical

**Staffed Beds:** 13

## WINDER—Barrow County

☐ **BARROW REGIONAL MEDICAL CENTER (110045)**, 316 North Broad Street,
Zip 30680–2150, Mailing Address: P.O. Box 688, Zip 30680–0688;
tel. 770/867–3400, (Nonreporting) **A**1 9 10 **S** Health Management Associates,
Naples, FL
Primary Contact: Todd Dixon, R.N., Chief Executive Officer
COO: Joshua Self, Chief Operating Officer
CFO: Jared Whipkey, Chief Financial Officer
CMO: William Lytollis, M.D., Chief of Staff
CIO: Ed Stanley, Director Information Systems
CHR: Tina Jackson, Director Human Resources
Web address: www.barrowregional.com
**Control:** Corporation, Investor–owned, for–profit **Service:** General Medical and
Surgical

**Staffed Beds:** 56

**GA**

# HAWAII

## AIEA—Honolulu County

✠ **PALI MOMI MEDICAL CENTER (120026)**, 98–1079 Moanalua Road, Zip 96701–4713; tel. 808/486–6000 **A**1 2 5 9 10 **F**3 8 12 15 18 20 22 26 29 30 31 34 35 40 46 47 49 50 57 59 64 67 70 74 75 77 78 79 81 82 85 86 107 108 110 111 113 114 118 129 131 134 141 145 146 147 **P**5 **S** Hawaii Pacific Health, Honolulu, HI
Primary Contact: Raymond Vara, Chief Executive Officer
COO: Jen Chahanovich, Chief Operating Officer
CFO: David Okabe, Executive Vice President, Chief Financial Officer and Treasurer
CMO: Mark Pitts, M.D., Chief of Staff
CIO: Steve Robertson, Senior Vice President
CHR: Gail Lerch, R.N., Vice President Human Resources
Web address: www.kapiolani.org
**Control:** Other not–for–profit (including NFP Corporation) **Service:** General Medical and Surgical

> **Staffed Beds:** 116 **Admissions:** 6316 **Census:** 108 **Outpatient Visits:** 115180 **Births:** 0 **Total Expense ($000):** 142134 **Payroll Expense ($000):** 55582 **Personnel:** 837

## EWA BEACH—Honolulu County

✠ **KAHI MOHALA BEHAVIORAL HEALTH (124001)**, 91–2301 Old Fort Weaver Road, Zip 96706–3602; tel. 808/671–8511 **A**1 9 10 **F**35 98 99 100 101 103 105 126 **P**6 **S** Sutter Health, Sacramento, CA
Primary Contact: Leonard Licina, Chief Executive Officer
CFO: Rose Choy, Chief Financial Officer
CMO: Steven Chaplin, M.D., Medical Director
CHR: Christina Enoka, Director Human Resources and Risk Management
Web address: www.kahi.org
**Control:** Other not–for–profit (including NFP Corporation) **Service:** Psychiatric

> **Staffed Beds:** 60 **Admissions:** 1462 **Census:** 58 **Outpatient Visits:** 2384 **Births:** 0 **Total Expense ($000):** 18621 **Payroll Expense ($000):** 11254 **Personnel:** 164

## HILO—Hawaii County

✠ **HILO MEDICAL CENTER (120005)**, 1190 Waianuenue Avenue, Zip 96720–2095; tel. 808/932–3000, (Total facility includes 112 beds in nursing home–type unit) **A**1 5 9 10 20 **F**1 3 17 18 20 29 30 31 34 40 49 50 51 57 59 62 67 70 74 75 76 77 78 81 85 86 87 93 98 100 101 102 103 107 111 113 120 122 127 129 134 145 147 **P**5 6 **S** Hawaii Health Systems Corporation, Honolulu, HI
Primary Contact: Howard N. Ainsley, Regional Chief Executive Officer
COO: Julie–Beth Ako, Director, Systems Services
CFO: Money Atwal, Chief Financial Officer
CMO: Ted Peskin, M.D., Acute Care Medical Director
CIO: Money Atwal, Chief Information Officer
CHR: Holly Ka'Akimaka, Director Human Resources
CNO: Dan Brinkman, Chief Nurse Executive
Web address: www.hmc.hhsc.org
**Control:** State–Government, nonfederal **Service:** General Medical and Surgical

> **Staffed Beds:** 276 **Admissions:** 7531 **Census:** 193 **Outpatient Visits:** 71004 **Births:** 1135 **Total Expense ($000):** 132951 **Payroll Expense ($000):** 50070 **Personnel:** 950

## HONOKAA—Hawaii County

★ **HALE HO'OLA HAMAKUA (121307)**, 45–547 Plumeria Street, Zip 96727–6902; tel. 808/775–7211, (Nonreporting) **A**5 9 10 18 **S** Hawaii Health Systems Corporation, Honolulu, HI
Primary Contact: Cathy Meyer–Uyehara, Administrator
CFO: Harlan Seo, Accountant
CMO: Gretchen Salmon, M.D., Medical Director
Web address: www.hhsc.org
**Control:** State–Government, nonfederal **Service:** General Medical and Surgical

> **Staffed Beds:** 52

## HONOLULU—Honolulu County

✠ **KAISER PERMANENTE MEDICAL CENTER (120011)**, 3288 Moanalua Road, Zip 96819–1469; tel. 808/432–0000, (Total facility includes 28 beds in nursing home–type unit) **A**1 3 5 10 **F**3 12 13 15 17 18 19 20 21 22 24 26 29 30 31 32 34 35 36 38 40 41 45 46 47 48 49 50 51 54 55 56 57 58 59 60 61 62 64 65 70 71 72 74 75 76 77 78 79 81 82 83 84 85 86 87 89 92 93 94 97 99 100 101 104 107 108 110 111 114 115 116 118 127 128 129 130 132 133 134 143 145 147 **P**1 **S** Kaiser Foundation Hospitals, Oakland, CA
Primary Contact: William F. Haug, FACHE, Administrator
CFO: Thomas Risse, Chief Financial Officer and Vice President Business Services
CMO: James Griffith, M.D., Associate Medical Director and Professional Chief of Staff
CIO: Brian Yoshii, Vice President Information Technology
CHR: Arlene F. Peasnall, Senior Vice President Human Resources
CNO: Linda Puu, Chief Nursing Officer
Web address: www.kaiserpermanente.org
**Control:** Other not–for–profit (including NFP Corporation) **Service:** General Medical and Surgical

> **Staffed Beds:** 235 **Admissions:** 11435 **Census:** 187 **Outpatient Visits:** 59377 **Births:** 1459 **Personnel:** 1788

☐ **KAPIOLANI MEDICAL CENTER FOR WOMEN & CHILDREN (123300)**, 1319 Punahou Street, Zip 96826–1032; tel. 808/983–6000, (Nonreporting) **A**1 2 3 5 9 10 **S** Hawaii Pacific Health, Honolulu, HI
Primary Contact: Raymond Vara, Chief Executive Officer
COO: Martha Smith, Chief Operating Officer
CFO: David Okabe, Senior Vice President, Chief Financial Officer and Treasurer
CIO: Steve Robertson, Vice President
CHR: Gail Lerch, R.N., Vice President
Web address: www.kapiolani.org
**Control:** Other not–for–profit (including NFP Corporation) **Service:** Children's general

> **Staffed Beds:** 225

✠ **KUAKINI MEDICAL CENTER (120007)**, 347 North Kuakini Street, Zip 96817–2381; tel. 808/536–2236 **A**1 2 3 5 9 10 **F**3 15 17 18 20 22 24 26 28 29 31 34 35 40 45 46 49 57 59 60 68 70 74 75 77 78 79 81 82 85 86 87 107 108 110 111 114 116 117 118 120 123 128 129 130 131 144 145 146 147 **P**1
Primary Contact: Gary K. Kajiwara, President and Chief Executive Officer
COO: Gregg Oishi, Senior Vice President and Chief Operating Officer
CFO: Quin Ogawa, Vice President and Chief Financial Officer
CMO: Nobuyuki Miki, M.D., Vice President Medical Affairs
CIO: Gary K. Kajiwara, President and Chief Executive Officer
CHR: Ann N. Choy, Manager Human Resources and Payroll
Web address: www.kuakini.org
**Control:** Other not–for–profit (including NFP Corporation) **Service:** General Medical and Surgical

> **Staffed Beds:** 92 **Admissions:** 5651 **Census:** 109 **Outpatient Visits:** 58762 **Births:** 0 **Total Expense ($000):** 132534 **Payroll Expense ($000):** 60629 **Personnel:** 897

★ **LEAHI HOSPITAL (122001)**, 3675 Kilauea Avenue, Zip 96816–2398; tel. 808/733–8000, (Nonreporting) **A**9 10 **S** Hawaii Health Systems Corporation, Honolulu, HI
Primary Contact: Vincent H. S. Lee, FACHE, Regional Chief Executive Officer
CFO: Edward Chu, Chief Financial Officer
CMO: Albert Yazawa, M.D., Regional Medical Director
CHR: Russel Higa, JD, Regional Director Human Resources
CNO: Amy Vasunaga, Chief Nurse Executive
Web address: www.hhsc.org
**Control:** State–Government, nonfederal **Service:** Other specialty

> **Staffed Beds:** 188

HI

---

| **Hospital, Medicare Provider Number, Address, Telephone, Approval, Facility, and Physician Codes, Health Care System** | |
|---|---|
| ★ American Hospital Association (AHA) membership | ○ American Osteopathic Association (AOA) accreditation |
| ☐ The Joint Commission accreditation   ◇ DNV Healthcare Inc. accreditation | △ Commission on Accreditation of Rehabilitation Facilities (CARF) accreditation |

⊠ **QUEEN'S MEDICAL CENTER (120001)**, 1301 Punchbowl Street, Zip 96813–2499; tel. 808/538–9011, (Total facility includes 28 beds in nursing home–type unit) **A**1 2 3 5 9 10 **F**3 5 11 12 13 15 17 18 20 22 24 26 28 29 31 34 35 37 38 39 40 43 44 45 46 47 48 49 50 51 55 56 57 59 60 61 62 63 64 66 68 70 73 74 75 76 77 78 79 81 82 84 85 86 87 93 96 97 98 99 100 101 102 103 104 105 107 108 110 111 113 114 116 118 119 120 123 125 127 128 129 130 131 134 135 142 145 146 147 **S** Queen's Health Systems, Honolulu, HI
Primary Contact: Arthur A. Ushijima, President
COO: Mark Yamakawa, Chief Operating Officer
CFO: Richard Keene, Chief Financial Officer
CMO: Gerard Akaka, M.D., Vice President Medical Affairs
CIO: Hunter Praywell, Vice President Information Technology and Chief Information Officer
CHR: Bert Kido, Vice President Human Resources
CNO: Cynthia Kamikawa, R.N., Vice President Nursing Emergency Department and Trauma and Chief Nursing Officer
Web address: www.queens.org
**Control:** Other not–for–profit (including NFP Corporation) **Service:** General Medical and Surgical

| | |
|---|---|
| **Staffed Beds:** 495 **Admissions:** 23040 **Census:** 389 **Outpatient Visits:** 322677 **Births:** 2411 **Personnel:** 3217 | |

⊠ **REHABILITATION HOSPITAL OF THE PACIFIC (123025)**, 226 North Kuakini Street, Zip 96817–9881; tel. 808/531–3511 **A**1 9 10 **F**3 11 29 54 64 74 75 77 79 90 91 93 94 95 96 129 130 131 142 145 146 147
Primary Contact: Timothy J. Roe, President and Chief Executive Officer
CFO: Ty Tomimoto, Acting Vice President Financial Affairs
CMO: Gary Okamoto, M.D., Senior Vice President and Chief Medical Executive
CIO: Dave Orme, Chief Information Officer
CHR: Faye Miyamoto, Vice President Human Resources
CNO: AMy Parungao, Director of Nursing
Web address: www.rehabhospital.org
**Control:** Other not–for–profit (including NFP Corporation) **Service:** Rehabilitation

| | |
|---|---|
| **Staffed Beds:** 69 **Admissions:** 1399 **Census:** 52 **Outpatient Visits:** 36811 **Births:** 0 **Total Expense ($000):** 33876 **Payroll Expense ($000):** 18128 **Personnel:** 265 | |

☐ **SHRINERS HOSPITALS FOR CHILDREN, HONOLULU (123301)**, 1310 Punahou Street, Zip 96826–1099; tel. 808/941–4466 **A**1 3 5 10 **F**29 35 39 58 75 77 79 81 85 89 93 94 118 129 131 145 147 **S** Shriners Hospitals for Children, Tampa, FL
Primary Contact: Stanley B. Berry, FACHE, Administrator
CFO: Patricia Miyasawa, CPA, Director Fiscal Service
CMO: Arabella Leet, M.D., Chief of Staff
CIO: Ross Imada, Director Information Systems
CHR: Derek Ito, Director Human Resources
CNO: Andrea Kubota, Director Patient Care Services
Web address: www.shrinershq.org
**Control:** Other not–for–profit (including NFP Corporation) **Service:** Children's orthopedic

| | |
|---|---|
| **Staffed Beds:** 16 **Admissions:** 305 **Census:** 4 **Outpatient Visits:** 10468 **Births:** 0 **Personnel:** 145 | |

☐ **STRAUB CLINIC & HOSPITAL (120022)**, 888 South King Street, Zip 96813–3009; tel. 808/522–4000 **A**1 2 3 5 9 10 **F**3 9 12 15 16 17 18 20 21 22 23 24 26 27 29 30 31 34 40 45 49 54 56 57 59 64 65 68 70 74 75 77 78 79 81 82 84 85 86 87 93 94 96 97 104 107 108 110 111 113 117 118 123 128 129 130 131 134 142 143 145 147 **P**6 **S** Hawaii Pacific Health, Honolulu, HI
Primary Contact: Raymond Vara, Chief Executive Officer
COO: Art Gladstone, R.N., Chief Operating Officer
CFO: David Okabe, Executive Vice President, Chief Financial Officer and Treasurer
CMO: Kenneth Robbins, M.D., Chief Medical Officer
CIO: Steve Robertson, Executive Vice President and Chief Information Officer
CHR: Gail Lerch, R.N., Executive Vice President Human Resources
Web address: www.straubhealth.org
**Control:** Other not–for–profit (including NFP Corporation) **Service:** General Medical and Surgical

| | |
|---|---|
| **Staffed Beds:** 107 **Admissions:** 6793 **Census:** 105 **Outpatient Visits:** 760875 **Births:** 0 **Total Expense ($000):** 207741 **Payroll Expense ($000):** 134036 **Personnel:** 1385 | |

⊠ **TRIPLER ARMY MEDICAL CENTER**, 1 Jarret White Road, Zip 96859–5000; tel. 808/433–6661, (Nonreporting) **A**1 2 3 5 **S** Department of the Army, Office of the Surgeon General, Falls Church, VA
Primary Contact: Brigadier General Keith W. Gallagher, FACHE, Commander
CMO: Captain David A. Lane, Deputy Commander Clinical Services
CIO: Major Donna E. Beed, Division Chief Information Management
CHR: Colonel Lisa P. Chisholm, Troop Commander
Web address: www.tamc.amedd.army.mil
**Control:** Army, Government, federal **Service:** General Medical and Surgical

| | |
|---|---|
| **Staffed Beds:** 198 | |

**KAHUKU MEDICAL CENTER (121304)**, 56–117 Pualalea Street, Zip 96731–2052; tel. 808/293–9221, (Nonreporting) **A**9 10 18
Primary Contact: Stephany Vaioleti, Administrator
CFO: Francis Daquioag, Controller
CMO: P. Douglas Nielson, M.D., Chief of Staff
Web address: www.hhsc.org/oahu/kahuku/index.html
**Control:** Other not–for–profit (including NFP Corporation) **Service:** General Medical and Surgical

| | |
|---|---|
| **Staffed Beds:** 11 | |

⊠ **CASTLE MEDICAL CENTER (120006)**, 640 Ulukahiki Street, Zip 96734–4498; tel. 808/263–5500 **A**1 9 10 **F**8 12 13 15 18 20 22 29 30 31 34 35 40 45 49 51 57 59 62 64 68 70 71 74 75 76 77 78 79 81 84 93 98 102 107 108 111 114 118 131 134 145 146 147 **P**8 **S** Adventist Health, Roseville, CA
Primary Contact: Kathryn A. Raethel, R.N., M.P.H., President and Chief Executive Officer
COO: A. John Monge, Vice President Operations
CFO: Dale Northrop, Vice President Finance
CMO: Alan Cheung, M.D., Vice President Medical Affairs
CIO: Brian Rothe, Site Director Information Systems
CHR: Adele Hoe, Director Human Resources
Web address: www.castlemed.org
**Control:** Church–operated, Nongovernment, not–for profit **Service:** General Medical and Surgical

| | |
|---|---|
| **Staffed Beds:** 160 **Admissions:** 7139 **Census:** 89 **Outpatient Visits:** 106854 **Births:** 853 **Total Expense ($000):** 117166 **Payroll Expense ($000):** 54175 **Personnel:** 755 | |

☐ **NORTH HAWAII COMMUNITY HOSPITAL (120028)**, 67–1125 Mamalahoa Highway, Zip 96743; tel. 808/885–4444, (Nonreporting) **A**1 5 9 10 20
Primary Contact: Ken Wood, President and Chief Executive Officer
CMO: Dana Lee, M.D., Chief of Staff
CHR: Bill Brown, Vice President Human Resources
Web address: www.northhawaiicommunityhospital.org
**Control:** Other not–for–profit (including NFP Corporation) **Service:** General Medical and Surgical

| | |
|---|---|
| **Staffed Beds:** 39 | |

☐ **HAWAII STATE HOSPITAL**, 45–710 Keaahala Road, Zip 96744–3597; tel. 808/236–8237 **A**1 3 5 **F**34 39 59 75 77 97 98 101 102 103 104 105 106 129 131 134 142 145
Primary Contact: Mark Fridovich, Ph.D., Administrator
COO: William T. Elliott, Associate Administrator Administrative and Support Services
CFO: Anthony Fraiola, Business Manager
CMO: James Westphal, M.D., Medical Director
CIO: John Jansen, Management Information Specialist
CHR: Karen Hara, Personnel Management Specialist
CNO: Leona Guest, Chief Nursing Unit
Web address: www.hshweb.health.state.hi.us
**Control:** State–Government, nonfederal **Service:** Psychiatric

| | |
|---|---|
| **Staffed Beds:** 178 **Admissions:** 219 **Census:** 185 **Outpatient Visits:** 0 **Births:** 0 **Total Expense ($000):** 36390 **Personnel:** 612 | |

★ **SAMUEL MAHELONA MEMORIAL HOSPITAL (121306)**, 4800 Kawaihau Road, Zip 96746–1998; tel. 808/822–4961, (Total facility includes 66 beds in nursing home–type unit) **A**9 10 18 **F**1 3 11 39 40 68 93 98 102 108 129 132 145 **P**6 **S** Hawaii Health Systems Corporation, Honolulu, HI
Primary Contact: Jerry Walker, Interim Regional Chief Executive Officer
CFO: Michael Perel, Regional Chief Financial Officer
CMO: Gerald Tomory, M.D., Regional Medical Director
CIO: Sandra McMaster, Regional Chief Information Officer
CHR: Lani Aranio, Regional Director Human Resources
Web address: www.smmh.hhsc.org
**Control:** State–Government, nonfederal **Service:** Long–Term Acute Care hospital

| | |
|---|---|
| **Staffed Beds:** 80 **Admissions:** 269 **Census:** 64 **Outpatient Visits:** 6070 **Births:** 0 **Total Expense ($000):** 15841 **Payroll Expense ($000):** 7481 | |

## KAUNAKAKAI—Maui County

⊞ **MOLOKAI GENERAL HOSPITAL (121303)**, Zip 96748–0408; tel. 808/553–5331, (Total facility includes 2 beds in nursing home–type unit) **A**1 5 9 10 18 **F**3 13 15 29 31 34 35 40 41 44 45 50 57 59 63 64 65 67 68 69 75 76 77 82 84 87 91 93 97 107 110 114 118 126 129 132 133 134 146 147 **P**6 **S** Queen's Health Systems, Honolulu, HI
Primary Contact: Janice Kalanihuia, President
CFO: Alyne Kikukawa, Accountant
CMO: William Thomas, Jr., M.D., Medical Director Clinical and Internal Affairs
CIO: Randy Lite, Vice President
CHR: Lei Mokiao, Coordinator Human Resources
Web address: www.queens.org
**Control:** Other not–for–profit (including NFP Corporation) **Service:** General Medical and Surgical

**Staffed Beds: 15 Admissions: 110 Census: 4 Outpatient Visits: 35594 Births: 38 Total Expense ($000): 11662 Payroll Expense ($000): 4483 Personnel: 84**

## KEALAKEKUA—Hawaii County

⊞ **KONA COMMUNITY HOSPITAL (120019)**, 79–1019 Haukapila Street, Zip 96750–7920; tel. 808/322–9311, (Nonreporting) **A**1 5 9 10 20 **S** Hawaii Health Systems Corporation, Honolulu, HI
Primary Contact: Jay E. Kreuzer, FACHE, Chief Executive Officer
CFO: Dean Herzog, Chief Financial Officer
CMO: Kathleen Rokavec, M.D., Medical Director
CHR: Kathryn Salomon, Director Human Resources
CNO: Patricia Kalua, Chief Nurse Executive
Web address: www.kch.hhsc.org
**Control:** Other not–for–profit (including NFP Corporation) **Service:** General Medical and Surgical

**Staffed Beds: 54**

## KOHALA—Hawaii County

★ **KOHALA HOSPITAL (121302)**, 54–383 Hospital Road, Zip 96755, Mailing Address: P.O. Box 10, Kapaau, Zip 96755–0010; tel. 808/889–6211, (Nonreporting) **A**9 10 18 **S** Hawaii Health Systems Corporation, Honolulu, HI
Primary Contact: Eugene Amar, Jr., Administrator
CMO: Silvia Sonnenschein, M.D., Chief of Staff
Web address: www.koh.hhsc.org
**Control:** State–Government, nonfederal **Service:** General Medical and Surgical

**Staffed Beds: 26**

## KULA—Maui County

★ **KULA HOSPITAL (121308)**, 100 Keokea Place, Zip 96790–7450; tel. 808/878–1221, (Nonreporting) **A**5 9 10 18 **S** Hawaii Health Systems Corporation, Honolulu, HI
Primary Contact: Paul Harper, Interim Administrator
CFO: Nerissa Garrity, Chief Financial Officer
CMO: Nicole Apoliona, M.D., Medical Director
Web address: www.hhsc.org
**Control:** State–Government, nonfederal **Service:** General Medical and Surgical

**Staffed Beds: 6**

## LANAI CITY—Maui County

★ **LANAI COMMUNITY HOSPITAL (121305)**, 628 Seventh Street, Zip 96763–0650, Mailing Address: P.O. Box 630650, Zip 96763–0650; tel. 808/565–8450, (Nonreporting) **A**9 10 18 **S** Hawaii Health Systems Corporation, Honolulu, HI
Primary Contact: Paul Harper, Interim Administrator
Web address: www.lch.hhsc.org
**Control:** Other not–for–profit (including NFP Corporation) **Service:** General Medical and Surgical

**Staffed Beds: 14**

## LIHUE—Kauai County

☐ **WILCOX MEMORIAL HOSPITAL (120014)**, 3–3420 Kuhio Highway, Zip 96766–1099; tel. 808/245–1100 **A**1 5 9 10 20 **F**3 11 13 15 29 30 31 37 40 43 59 60 61 64 68 70 75 76 77 81 84 85 93 107 108 110 111 113 118 129 132 134 145 146 147 **S** Hawaii Pacific Health, Honolulu, HI
Primary Contact: Kathleen Clark, President and Chief Executive Officer
CFO: David Okabe, Executive Vice President, Chief Financial Officer and Treasurer
CMO: Christopher Jordan, M.D., President Medical Staff
CIO: Steve Robertson, Executive Vice President Revenue Cycle Management and Chief Information Officer
CHR: Monica Reisner, Director Human Resources Operations
CNO: Nancy Wilson, Chief Nurse Executive
Web address: www.wilcoxhealth.org
**Control:** Other not–for–profit (including NFP Corporation) **Service:** General Medical and Surgical

**Staffed Beds: 64 Admissions: 3624 Census: 46 Outpatient Visits: 76747 Births: 552 Total Expense ($000): 79438 Payroll Expense ($000): 29424**

## PAHALA—Hawaii County

★ **KAU HOSPITAL (121301)**, 1 Kamani Street, Zip 96777, Mailing Address: P.O. Box 40, Zip 96777–0040; tel. 808/928–2050, (Nonreporting) **A**9 10 18 **S** Hawaii Health Systems Corporation, Honolulu, HI
Primary Contact: Merilyn Harris, Administrator
CFO: Susan Kingsley, Accountant
CMO: Clifford Field, M.D., Medical Director
Web address: www.hhsc.org
**Control:** State–Government, nonfederal **Service:** General Medical and Surgical

**Staffed Beds: 5**

## WAHIAWA—Honolulu County

⊞ **WAHIAWA GENERAL HOSPITAL (120004)**, 128 Lehua Street, Zip 96786–2036; tel. 808/621–8411, (Total facility includes 103 beds in nursing home–type unit) **A**1 3 5 9 10 **F**3 8 11 15 29 31 40 56 62 70 75 77 78 79 81 85 86 87 93 96 103 107 108 109 110 114 118 127 129 131 144 145 146 147 **P**8
Primary Contact: R. Don Olden, Chief Executive Officer
COO: R. Don Olden, Chief Executive Officer
CMO: Timothy Whiteside, M.D., Chief of Staff
CIO: Jason Fujinaka, Manager Information System
CHR: Richard Aea, Director Human Resources
Web address: www.wahiawageneral.org
**Control:** Other not–for–profit (including NFP Corporation) **Service:** General Medical and Surgical

**Staffed Beds: 160 Admissions: 1898 Census: 121 Outpatient Visits: 24321 Births: 0 Total Expense ($000): 49249 Payroll Expense ($000): 22478 Personnel: 331**

## WAILUKU—Maui County

⊞ **MAUI MEMORIAL MEDICAL CENTER (120002)**, 221 Mahalani Street, Zip 96793–2581; tel. 808/244–9056, (Nonreporting) **A**1 5 9 10 20 **S** Hawaii Health Systems Corporation, Honolulu, HI
Primary Contact: Wesley Lo, Regional Chief Executive Officer
CIO: Dana Mendoza, Chief Information Officer
Web address: www.mmmc.hhsc.org
**Control:** State–Government, nonfederal **Service:** General Medical and Surgical

**Staffed Beds: 213**

## WAIMEA—Kauai County

⊞ **KAUAI VETERANS MEMORIAL HOSPITAL (121300)**, Waimea Canyon Road, Zip 96796, Mailing Address: P.O. Box 337, Zip 96796–0337; tel. 808/338–9431, (Total facility includes 20 beds in nursing home–type unit) **A**1 9 10 18 **F**11 13 15 17 40 67 70 76 79 81 89 107 110 111 113 118 127 129 132 146 **S** Hawaii Health Systems Corporation, Honolulu, HI
Primary Contact: Jerry Walker, Interim Regional Chief Executive Officer
CFO: Michael Perel, Regional Chief Financial Officer
CMO: Gerald Tomory, M.D., Regional Medical Director
CIO: Sandra McMaster, Regional Chief Information Officer
CHR: Solette Perry, Regional Director Human Resources
Web address: www.kvmh.hhsc.org
**Control:** State–Government, nonfederal **Service:** General Medical and Surgical

**Staffed Beds: 45 Admissions: 983 Census: 27 Outpatient Visits: 10680 Births: 248 Total Expense ($000): 36567 Payroll Expense ($000): 20462**

**HI**

---

**Hospital, Medicare Provider Number, Address, Telephone, Approval, Facility, and Physician Codes, Health Care System**

★ American Hospital Association (AHA) membership
☐ The Joint Commission accreditation  ◇ DNV Healthcare Inc. accreditation
○ American Osteopathic Association (AOA) accreditation
△ Commission on Accreditation of Rehabilitation Facilities (CARF) accreditation

# IDAHO

## AMERICAN FALLS—Power County

★ **POWER COUNTY HOSPITAL DISTRICT (131304)**, 510 Roosevelt Road, Zip 83211–0420, Mailing Address: P.O. Box 420, Zip 83211–0420; tel. 208/226–3200, (Nonreporting) **A**9 10 18
Primary Contact: Dallas Clinger, Administrator
COO: Rock Roy, Professional Services Director
CFO: Shauna Croft, Chief Financial Officer
CMO: Bret Timmons, D.O., Chief Medical Staff
CIO: Mindy Earl, Health Information Manager
CHR: Norma Hartley, Director Human Resources
CNO: Daniel Kuta, R.N., Director of Nursing
Web address: www.pchd.net
**Control:** Hospital district or authority, Government, nonfederal **Service:** General Medical and Surgical

**Staffed Beds:** 10

## ARCO—Butte County

**LOST RIVERS DISTRICT HOSPITAL (131324)**, 551 Highland Drive, Zip 83213–9771, Mailing Address: P.O. Box 145, Zip 83213–0145; tel. 208/527–8206, (Nonreporting) **A**9 10 18
Primary Contact: Kim Dahlman, Administrator
COO: Kim Dahlman, Administrator
CFO: Kim Dahlman, Administrator
CMO: Jeffrey Haskell, M.D., Chief Medical Staff
CIO: Leann Wartchow, Assistant Chief Executive Officer and Certified Risk Manager
CHR: Leann Wartchow, Assistant Chief Executive Officer and Certified Risk Manager
Web address: www.lostrivershospital.com
**Control:** Hospital district or authority, Government, nonfederal **Service:** General Medical and Surgical

**Staffed Beds:** 43

## BLACKFOOT—Bingham County

★ **BINGHAM MEMORIAL HOSPITAL (131325)**, 98 Poplar Street, Zip 83221–1799; tel. 208/785–4100, (Total facility includes 70 beds in nursing home–type unit) **A**9 10 18 **F**2 3 12 13 15 29 34 35 37 39 40 45 47 50 55 56 57 64 68 70 74 76 77 79 81 82 85 86 87 93 97 107 108 109 110 111 114 118 126 127 128 129 130 131 132 133 134 143 145 146 147
Primary Contact: Louis D. Kraml, FACHE, Chief Executive Officer
COO: Dan Cochran, Chief Operating Officer
CFO: Jeff Daniels, Chief Financial Officer
CMO: Gary Call, M.D., Chief Medical Officer
CIO: Jack York, Director Information Systems
CHR: Dinah Karren, Director Human Resources
Web address: www.binghammemorial.org
**Control:** Other not–for–profit (including NFP Corporation) **Service:** General Medical and Surgical

**Staffed Beds:** 95 **Admissions:** 2038 **Census:** 62 **Outpatient Visits:** 46223 **Births:** 444 **Total Expense ($000):** 72364 **Payroll Expense ($000):** 32903 **Personnel:** 583

**MOUNTAIN RIVER BIRTHING AND SURGERY CENTER (130067)**, 350 North Meridian Street, Zip 83221; tel. 208/782–0300 **A**9 10 **F**3 12 68 79 81 85 86 87 107 129 134 147
Primary Contact: Louis D. Kraml, FACHE, Chief Executive Officer
**Control:** Corporation, Investor–owned, for–profit **Service:** Surgical

**Staffed Beds:** 8 **Admissions:** 127 **Census:** 1 **Outpatient Visits:** 6424 **Births:** 0 **Total Expense ($000):** 5769 **Payroll Expense ($000):** 712 **Personnel:** 21

☐ **STATE HOSPITAL SOUTH (134010)**, 700 East Alice Street, Zip 83221–0400, Mailing Address: P.O. Box 400, Zip 83221–0400; tel. 208/785–1200, (Nonreporting) **A**1 9 10
Primary Contact: Tracey Sessions, Administrator
COO: Greg Horton, Director Support Services
CFO: Eric Price, Financial Specialist, Senior
CMO: Kelly Palmer, M.D., Medical Director
CIO: Julie Sutton, Director Performance Improvement
CHR: Heidi Anderson, Human Resources Specialist
CNO: Randy Walker, Director Nursing Services
Web address: www.healthandwelfare.idaho.gov
**Control:** State–Government, nonfederal **Service:** Psychiatric

**Staffed Beds:** 77

## BOISE—Ada County

**BOISE BEHAVIORAL HEALTH HOSPITAL (134009)**, 8050 Northview Street, Zip 83704; tel. 208/327–0504 **A**5 9 10 **F**29 38 57 98 100 101 102 103 104 129 131 **P**1
Primary Contact: Phil Herink, Chief Executive Officer
CFO: Phil Herink, Chief Executive Officer
CMO: David Kent, M.D., Chief Medical Officer
CIO: Debra Alexander, Chief Information Officer
CHR: Kathy Cady, Coordinator Human Resources, Accounts Payable and Payroll
Web address: www.sunh.com
**Control:** Corporation, Investor–owned, for–profit **Service:** Psychiatric

**Staffed Beds:** 22 **Admissions:** 423 **Census:** 18 **Outpatient Visits:** 7560 **Births:** 0

★ △ **ELKS REHAB HOSPITAL (133025)**, 600 North Robbins Road, Zip 83702–4597, Mailing Address: P.O. Box 1100, Zip 83701–1100; tel. 208/489–4444, (Nonreporting) **A**5 7 10
Primary Contact: Joseph P. Caroselli, Chief Executive Officer
COO: Melissa Honsinger, Chief Operating Officer
CFO: Doug Lewis, Chief Financial Officer
CMO: Lee Kornfield, M.D., Medical Director
CIO: Scott Pyrah, Director Information Systems
CHR: Jim Atkins, Director Employee Services
Web address: www.idahoelksrehab.org
**Control:** Other not–for–profit (including NFP Corporation) **Service:** Rehabilitation

**Staffed Beds:** 31

**IDAHO ELKS REHABILITATION HOSPITAL** See Elks Rehab Hospital

☐ **INTERMOUNTAIN HOSPITAL (134002)**, 303 North Allumbaugh Street, Zip 83704–9266; tel. 208/377–8400, (Nonreporting) **A**1 9 10 **S** Universal Health Services, Inc., King of Prussia, PA
Primary Contact: Brent J. Bryson, Chief Executive Officer
CMO: Harry Silsby, M.D., Medical Director
CHR: Angela Billingsley, Director Human Resources
Web address: www.intermountainhospital.com
**Control:** Corporation, Investor–owned, for–profit **Service:** Psychiatric

**Staffed Beds:** 140

⊠ △ **SAINT ALPHONSUS REGIONAL MEDICAL CENTER (130007)**, 1055 North Curtis Road, Zip 83706–1370; tel. 208/367–2121 **A**1 2 3 5 7 9 10 **F**3 5 7 8 9 11 12 13 14 15 17 18 20 22 24 26 28 29 30 31 32 33 34 35 36 37 38 39 40 42 43 44 45 48 49 50 52 54 55 56 57 58 59 61 64 65 68 70 71 72 74 75 76 77 78 79 81 82 84 85 86 87 89 90 91 93 94 96 97 98 99 100 101 102 104 107 108 110 111 113 114 115 116 117 118 119 120 122 123 125 126 127 128 129 130 131 134 143 145 146 147 **P**6 8 **S** Trinity Health, Novi, MI
Primary Contact: Sally E. Jeffcoat, President and Chief Executive Officer
COO: Rodney D. Reider, Chief Operating Officer
CFO: Kenneth Fry, Chief Financial Officer
CMO: Steve Brown, M.D., Chief Quality Officer
CIO: Dwight Pond, TIS Boise
CHR: Susan Bundgard, Vice President Human Resources
CNO: Sherry Parks, R.N., Chief Nursing Officer
Web address: www.saintalphonsus.org
**Control:** Church–operated, Nongovernment, not–for profit **Service:** General Medical and Surgical

**Staffed Beds:** 399 **Admissions:** 17385 **Census:** 215 **Outpatient Visits:** 776155 **Births:** 1150 **Personnel:** 2975

☐ **SOUTHWEST IDAHO ADVANCED CARE HOSPITAL (132003)**, Franklin Road and Allumbaugh Street, Zip 83706; tel. 208/376–5700 **A**1 9 10 **F**1 18 20 29 34 50 75 107 129 147 **P**6 **S** Ernest Health, Inc., Albuquerque, NM
Primary Contact: Nolan Hoffer, Chief Executive Officer
Web address: www.siach.ernesthealth.com/
**Control:** Corporation, Investor–owned, for–profit **Service:** Long–Term Acute Care hospital

**Staffed Beds:** 40 **Admissions:** 270 **Census:** 22 **Outpatient Visits:** 0 **Births:** 0 **Total Expense ($000):** 13089 **Payroll Expense ($000):** 6922 **Personnel:** 134

**ID**

*Many Facility Codes have changed. Please refer to the AHA Guide Code Chart.*   © 2012 AHA Guide

☒ **ST. LUKE'S REGIONAL MEDICAL CENTER (130006)**, 190 East Bannock Street, Zip 83712–6298; tel. 208/381–2222, (Includes ST. LUKE'S CHILDREN'S HOSPITAL, 190 East Bannock Street, Zip 83712–6241; tel. 208/381–1200; ST. LUKE'S MERIDIAN MEDICAL CENTER, 520 South Eagle Road, Meridian, Zip 83642; tel. 208/706–5000) **A**1 2 3 5 9 10 **F**7 8 11 12 13 15 17 18 19 20 21 22 23 24 25 26 27 28 29 30 31 32 34 35 36 37 40 41 46 47 48 49 53 54 56 57 59 61 62 63 64 68 69 70 71 72 74 75 76 77 78 79 81 82 84 86 87 88 89 107 108 110 111 113 114 116 117 118 125 126 128 129 130 131 133 135 143 145 146 **P**5 6 8 **S** St. Luke's Health System, Boise, ID
Primary Contact: Chris Roth, Chief Executive Officer
COO: Kathy D. Moore, Chief Operating Officer
CFO: Jeff Taylor, Vice President Finance
CMO: Bart Hill, M.D., Vice President Medical Affairs
CHR: Maureen O'Keeffe, Vice President Human Resources
Web address: www.stlukesonline.org/boise
**Control:** Other not–for–profit (including NFP Corporation) **Service:** General Medical and Surgical

**Staffed Beds: 576 Admissions: 30640 Census: 293 Outpatient Visits:** 1179080 **Births: 5362 Total Expense ($000): 874703 Payroll Expense ($000): 380199 Personnel: 6474**

☐ **TREASURE VALLEY HOSPITAL (130063)**, 8800 West Emerald Street, Zip 83704; tel. 208/373–5000, (Nonreporting) **A**1 9 10
Primary Contact: Nick Genna, Administrator
CMO: Jeffrey Hessing, M.D., Medical Director
CHR: Kathleen Phelps, Director Human Resources
Web address: www.treasurevalleyhospital.com
**Control:** Corporation, Investor–owned, for–profit **Service:** General Medical and Surgical

**Staffed Beds: 9**

☒ △ **VETERANS AFFAIRS MEDICAL CENTER**, 500 West Fort Street, Zip 83702–4598; tel. 208/422–1000, (Total facility includes 24 beds in nursing home–type unit) **A**1 3 5 7 9 **F**1 2 3 4 5 8 9 10 12 16 29 30 31 34 35 38 39 40 45 46 47 50 53 54 56 57 58 59 60 61 62 63 64 65 66 67 68 71 74 75 77 78 79 80 81 82 83 84 85 86 87 90 91 92 93 94 96 97 98 100 101 102 103 104 105 106 107 108 111 112 118 119 120 121 122 123 126 127 128 129 131 132 134 142 143 144 145 146 147 **S** Department of Veterans Affairs, Washington, DC
Primary Contact: David Stockwell, Interim Director
CFO: Ron Blanton, Chief Fiscal Services
CMO: Paul Lambert, M.D., Chief of Staff
CHR: Randy Turner, Chief Human Resource Management Services
Web address: www.va.gov/directory/guide/home.asp
**Control:** Veterans Affairs, Government, federal **Service:** General Medical and Surgical

**Staffed Beds: 79 Admissions: 3053 Census: 56 Outpatient Visits: 332938 Births: 0 Total Expense ($000): 180000 Payroll Expense ($000): 105000 Personnel: 998**

★ **BOUNDARY COMMUNITY HOSPITAL (131301)**, 6640 Kaniksu Street, Zip 83805–7532; tel. 208/267–3141, (Includes BOUNDARY COUNTY NURSING HOME ), (Total facility includes 36 beds in nursing home–type unit) **A**9 10 18 **F**3 11 15 35 40 45 50 57 59 65 75 77 79 81 85 87 93 107 110 111 113 118 127 129 132 142 145 147
Primary Contact: Craig A. Johnson, Chief Executive Officer and Chief Financial Officer
COO: Jeffery Perkins, Chief Operating Officer
CFO: Craig A. Johnson, Chief Executive Officer and Chief Financial Officer
CHR: Ann Coughlin, Director Human Resources
CNO: Tari Yourzek, Chief Nursing Officer
Web address: www.boundaryhospital.org
**Control:** County–Government, nonfederal **Service:** General Medical and Surgical

**Staffed Beds: 56 Admissions: 263 Census: 32 Outpatient Visits: 19652 Births: 0 Total Expense ($000): 10801 Payroll Expense ($000): 5980 Personnel: 107**

☒ **CASSIA REGIONAL MEDICAL CENTER (131326)**, 1501 Hiland Avenue, Zip 83318–2648; tel. 208/678–4444 **A**1 9 10 18 **F**3 7 8 11 13 15 18 29 30 34 35 38 40 41 50 57 59 64 68 70 74 75 76 77 79 81 82 83 85 86 93 97 107 108 110 111 113 118 128 129 130 131 145 146 147 **P**6 **S** Intermountain Healthcare, Inc, Salt Lake City, UT
Primary Contact: Rod Barton, Administrator
CFO: Mark Christensen, Assistant Administrator Finance and Chief Financial Officer
CMO: Fred Wood, M.D., Medical Director
CIO: Carie Call, Director Computer Support
CHR: Keri Perrigot, Assistant Administrator Human Resources
CNO: Michele Pond–Bell, R.N., Administrator Nursing
Web address: www.cassiaregional.org
**Control:** Other not–for–profit (including NFP Corporation) **Service:** General Medical and Surgical

**Staffed Beds: 25 Admissions: 1727 Census: 14 Outpatient Visits: 83548 Births: 667 Total Expense ($000): 36144 Payroll Expense ($000): 16413 Personnel: 308**

☒ **WEST VALLEY MEDICAL CENTER (130014)**, 1717 Arlington, Zip 83605–4864; tel. 208/459–4641, (Nonreporting) **A**1 9 10 **S** HCA, Nashville, TN
Primary Contact: Julie Taylor, Chief Executive Officer
COO: Scott Davis, Chief Financial Officer and Chief Operating Officer
CFO: Scott Davis, Chief Financial Officer and Chief Operating Officer
CIO: Lance Christiansen, Chief Information Officer
CHR: Senta Cornelius, Director Human Resources
Web address: www.westvalleymedctr.com
**Control:** Corporation, Investor–owned, for–profit **Service:** General Medical and Surgical

**Staffed Beds: 122**

★ **CASCADE MEDICAL CENTER (131308)**, 402 Old State Highway, Zip 83611, Mailing Address: P.O. Box 1330, Zip 83611–1330; tel. 208/382–4242 **A**9 10 18 **F**11 29 32 34 40 45 53 57 59 64 65 67 89 93 97 102 107 113 126 127 129 130 132 134 146 147 **P**6
Primary Contact: William C. Behnke, Jr., Administrator
CMO: Douglas Hill, M.D., Medical Director
Web address: www.cascademedicalcenter.net
**Control:** Hospital district or authority, Government, nonfederal **Service:** General Medical and Surgical

**Staffed Beds: 10 Admissions: 14 Census: 1 Outpatient Visits: 3545 Births: 0 Total Expense ($000): 3174 Payroll Expense ($000): 1706 Personnel: 29**

☒ **KOOTENAI MEDICAL CENTER (130049)**, 2003 Kootenai Health Way, Zip 83814–2677; tel. 208/666–2000, (Includes NORTH IDAHO BEHAVIORAL HEALTH, DIVISION OF KOOTENAI MEDICAL CENTER, 2301 North Ironwood Place, Zip 83814–2650; tel. 208/765–4800) **A**1 2 9 10 19 **F**2 3 4 5 8 11 12 13 15 17 18 20 22 24 28 29 30 31 34 35 39 40 43 46 47 49 50 51 53 54 55 57 58 59 60 63 64 65 68 70 74 75 76 77 78 79 81 82 83 84 86 87 89 90 93 98 99 100 101 102 103 104 105 106 112 113 114 115 118 119 120 125 128 129 131 133 134 142 143 145 **P**7
Primary Contact: Jon Ness, Chief Executive Officer
CFO: Tom Legel, Vice President Finance and Information
CMO: Joseph Bujak, M.D., Vice President Medical Affairs
CIO: Tom Legel, Vice President and Chief Financial Officer
CHR: Daniel Klocko, Vice President Human Resources
Web address: www.kmc.org
**Control:** Hospital district or authority, Government, nonfederal **Service:** General Medical and Surgical

**Staffed Beds: 246 Admissions: 13408 Census: 159 Outpatient Visits: 70696 Births: 1510 Total Expense ($000): 225475 Payroll Expense ($000): 93782 Personnel: 1677**

**ID**

---

**Hospital, Medicare Provider Number, Address, Telephone, Approval, Facility, and Physician Codes, Health Care System**

★ American Hospital Association (AHA) membership
☐ The Joint Commission accreditation
◇ DNV Healthcare Inc. accreditation
○ American Osteopathic Association (AOA) accreditation
△ Commission on Accreditation of Rehabilitation Facilities (CARF) accreditation

© 2012 AHA Guide    *Many Facility Codes have changed. Please refer to the AHA Guide Code Chart.*    Hospitals **A167**

## COTTONWOOD—Idaho County

★ **ST. MARY'S HOSPITAL (131321)**, Lewiston and North Streets,
Zip 83522–9750, Mailing Address: P.O. Box 137, Zip 83522–0137;
tel. 208/962–3251, (Nonreporting) **A**9 10 18 **S** Essentia Health, Duluth, MN
Primary Contact: Casey Meza, Chief Executive Officer
COO: Larry Barker, Chief Operating Officer
CFO: Lenne Bonner, Chief Financial Officer
CHR: Debbie Schumacher, Manager Human Resource
Web address: www.stmaryshospital.net
**Control:** Other not–for–profit (including NFP Corporation) **Service:** General
Medical and Surgical

**Staffed Beds:** 28

## DRIGGS—Teton County

★ **TETON VALLEY HOSPITAL AND SURGICENTER (131313)**, 120 East Howard
Street, Zip 83422–5112; tel. 208/354–2383 **A**9 10 18 **F**3 7 8 15 30 31 32 34
35 40 50 57 59 64 65 68 75 77 79 81 82 87 93 97 107 110 113 118 126
130 132 145 147 **P**5
Primary Contact: Virgil Boss, Chief Executive Officer
CFO: Jason Hotchkiss, Controller
CMO: Chad Horrocks, M.D., Chief of Staff
CIO: Chuck Fischer, Director Information Technology Systems
CHR: Dory Harris, Manager Human Resource
CNO: Angela Booker, Director of Nursing Services
Web address: www.tvhcare.org
**Control:** County–Government, nonfederal **Service:** General Medical and Surgical

**Staffed Beds:** 13 **Admissions:** 152 **Census:** 2 **Outpatient Visits:** 27844
**Births:** 0 **Total Expense ($000):** 10615 **Payroll Expense ($000):** 6277
**Personnel:** 127

## EMMETT—Gem County

★ **WALTER KNOX MEMORIAL HOSPITAL (131318)**, 1202 East Locust Street,
Zip 83617–2715; tel. 208/365–3561 **A**9 10 18 **F**3 11 13 29 31 34 35 40 45
57 59 64 76 79 81 82 85 87 107 111 113 118 127 132 143 145
Primary Contact: John N. Olson, Chief Executive Officer
CFO: Larry Droppers, Chief Financial Officer
CHR: Susan Vahlberg, Director Employee and Community Relations
Web address: www.wkmh.org
**Control:** County–Government, nonfederal **Service:** General Medical and Surgical

**Staffed Beds:** 16 **Admissions:** 397 **Census:** 3 **Outpatient Visits:** 21589
**Births:** 73 **Total Expense ($000):** 7811 **Payroll Expense ($000):** 3725
**Personnel:** 86

## GOODING—Gooding County

★ **NORTH CANYON MEDICAL CENTER (131302)**, 267 North Canyon Drive,
Zip 83330; tel. 208/934–4433 **A**9 10 18 **F**3 11 15 29 34 35 40 44 45 46 47
48 50 53 57 59 64 68 75 77 81 82 85 86 87 93 107 110 113 118 128 129
132 134 145 **S** St. Luke's Health System, Boise, ID
Primary Contact: David Butler, Chief Executive Officer
CFO: Rod Larsen, Chief Financial Officer
CMO: Reid Lofgran, D.O., Chief of Staff
CIO: Paul Castronova, Chief Information Officer
CHR: Sara Otto, Director Human Resources
Web address: www.goodinghospital.org
**Control:** Other not–for–profit (including NFP Corporation) **Service:** General
Medical and Surgical

**Staffed Beds:** 15 **Admissions:** 653 **Census:** 5 **Outpatient Visits:** 20431
**Births:** 1 **Total Expense ($000):** 16130 **Payroll Expense ($000):** 4522
**Personnel:** 123

## GRANGEVILLE—Idaho County

★ **SYRINGA HOSPITAL AND CLINICS (131315)**, 607 West Main Street,
Zip 83530–1396; tel. 208/983–1700, (Nonreporting) **A**9 10 18
Primary Contact: Joseph Cladouhos, Chief Executive Officer
CFO: Betty A. Watson, Chief Financial Officer
CMO: Cheryl Mallory, M.D., Chief Medical Officer
CHR: Katy Eimers, Human Resources Officer
Web address: www.syringahospital.org
**Control:** Hospital district or authority, Government, nonfederal **Service:** General
Medical and Surgical

**Staffed Beds:** 15

## IDAHO FALLS—Bonneville County

⊞ **EASTERN IDAHO REGIONAL MEDICAL CENTER (130018)**, 3100 Channing
Way, Zip 83404–7533, Mailing Address: P.O. Box 2077, Zip 83403–2077;
tel. 208/529–6111, (Total facility includes 16 beds in nursing home–type unit) **A**1
2 9 10 **F**3 7 11 12 13 15 18 20 21 22 23 24 28 29 30 31 34 35 36 39 40
43 44 46 49 50 51 53 57 59 64 65 67 68 70 72 74 75 76 77 78 79 81 82
85 86 87 89 90 91 92 93 98 99 100 102 106 107 108 111 113 114 117
118 119 120 122 127 128 129 130 131 134 145 146 147 **P**5 **S** HCA,
Nashville, TN
Primary Contact: Douglas Crabtree, Chief Executive Officer
COO: Sandee Moore, Chief Operating Officer
CFO: Jeffrey D. Baiocco, Chief Financial Officer
CMO: Todd Williams, M.D., President Medical Staff
CHR: Wendy Andersen, Director Human Resources
CNO: Kathleen Nelson, R.N., Chief Nursing Officer
Web address: www.eirmc.com
**Control:** Corporation, Investor–owned, for–profit **Service:** General Medical and
Surgical

**Staffed Beds:** 309 **Admissions:** 10994 **Census:** 168 **Outpatient Visits:**
171002 **Births:** 1508 **Total Expense ($000):** 171610 **Payroll Expense
($000):** 63404 **Personnel:** 1143

**IDAHO FALLS RECOVERY CENTER (130062)**, 1957 East 17th Street,
Zip 83404–6429; tel. 208/529–5285, (Nonreporting) **A**9 10
Primary Contact: Lindee Hokanson, Administrator
COO: Lindee Hokanson, Administrator
Web address: www.ifrecoverycenter.com
**Control:** Other not–for–profit (including NFP Corporation) **Service:** General
Medical and Surgical

**Staffed Beds:** 10

**MOUNTAIN VIEW HOSPITAL (130065)**, 2325 Coronado Street, Zip 83404;
tel. 208/557–2700, (Nonreporting) **A**9 10
Primary Contact: James Adamson, Chief Executive Officer
COO: Peter Fabrick, Vice President Clinical Operations
CHR: Eilene Horne, Manager Human Resources
Web address: www.mountainviewhospital.org
**Control:** Corporation, Investor–owned, for–profit **Service:** General Medical and
Surgical

**Staffed Beds:** 22

## JEROME—Jerome County

**ST. LUKE'S JEROME FAMILY MEDICAL CENTER (131310)**, 709 North
Lincoln Street, Zip 83338–1851, Mailing Address: P.O. Box 586,
Zip 83338–0586; tel. 208/324–4301 **A**9 10 18 **F**7 13 15 29 30 32 34 39 40
56 57 59 64 65 68 77 79 81 86 87 97 107 111 118 126 132 145 146 **P**6
**S** Essentia Health, Duluth, MN
Primary Contact: James L. Angle, FACHE, Chief Executive Officer
COO: Curtis Maier, Assistant Administrator
CMO: H. Peter Doble, M.D., Director Medical Staff Affairs
CIO: Curtis Maier, Assistant Administrator
CHR: Dee Hartzell, Manager Human Resources
Web address: www.stbenshospital.org
**Control:** Other not–for–profit (including NFP Corporation) **Service:** General
Medical and Surgical

**Staffed Beds:** 25 **Admissions:** 635 **Census:** 5 **Outpatient Visits:** 34577
**Births:** 227 **Total Expense ($000):** 17794 **Payroll Expense ($000):** 9385
**Personnel:** 171

## KELLOGG—Shoshone County

**SHOSHONE MEDICAL CENTER (131314)**, 25 Jacobs Gulch, Zip 83837–2096;
tel. 208/784–1221, (Nonreporting) **A**9 10 18
Primary Contact: Gary Moore, Chief Executive Officer
CFO: Jerry Brantz, Chief Financial Officer
CMO: Berri Swasand, M.D., Chief of Staff
CIO: Russ Allred, Manager Information Systems
CHR: Joanna Radford, Chief Human Resources Officer
Web address: www.shoshonehealth.com
**Control:** Hospital district or authority, Government, nonfederal **Service:** General
Medical and Surgical

**Staffed Beds:** 25

## KETCHUM—Blaine County

⊞ **ST. LUKE'S WOOD RIVER MEDICAL CENTER (131323)**, 100 Hospital Drive,
Zip 83340, Mailing Address: P.O. Box 100, Zip 83340; tel. 208/727–8800 **A**1 9
10 18 **F**3 7 8 11 13 15 29 30 31 34 35 36 37 40 43 45 50 54 57 59 64 68
70 74 75 76 79 81 85 86 97 107 108 110 111 113 118 125 127 129 130
131 132 133 134 140 142 144 145 146 **P**6 8 **S** St. Luke's Health System,
Boise, ID
Primary Contact: Cody Langbehn, Chief Executive Officer
CFO: Carl Hollingsworth, Chief Financial Officer
Web address: www.slrmc.org
**Control:** Other not–for–profit (including NFP Corporation) **Service:** General
Medical and Surgical

**Staffed Beds:** 25 **Admissions:** 1311 **Census:** 8 **Births:** 221 **Total Expense
($000):** 46408 **Payroll Expense ($000):** 22821 **Personnel:** 309

ID

## LEWISTON—Nez Perce County

☒ **ST. JOSEPH REGIONAL MEDICAL CENTER (130003)**, 415 Sixth Street, Zip 83501–0816; tel. 208/743–2511, (Nonreporting) **A**1 2 9 10 **S** Ascension Health, Saint Louis, MO
Primary Contact: Timothy Sayler, President and Chief Executive Officer
CFO: Thomas Safley, Chief Financial Officer
CMO: Jay Hunter, M.D., Chief of Staff
CIO: Collin Lamb, Director Management Information Systems
CHR: Brenda J. Forge, Vice President Human Resources
Web address: www.sjrmc.org
**Control:** Church–operated, Nongovernment, not–for profit **Service:** General Medical and Surgical

**Staffed Beds:** 136

## MALAD CITY—Oneida County

**ONEIDA COUNTY HOSPITAL (131303)**, 150 North 200 West, Zip 83252–0126, Mailing Address: Box 126, Zip 83252–0126; tel. 208/766–2231, (Nonreporting) **A**9 10 18
Primary Contact: Todd V. Winder, Administrator and Chief Executive Officer
CFO: Cindy Howard, Director Financial Services
CHR: Kathy Hubbard, Manager Human Resources
Web address: www.oneidahospital.com
**Control:** County–Government, nonfederal **Service:** General Medical and Surgical

**Staffed Beds:** 11

## MCCALL—Valley County

★ **ST. LUKE'S MCCALL (131312)**, 1000 State Street, Zip 83638–3704; tel. 208/634–2221 **A**9 10 18 **F**3 8 9 11 15 30 32 34 35 36 38 40 45 46 50 57 59 64 68 70 76 79 81 85 86 87 93 97 107 114 118 129 131 132 133 134 145 **P**6 8 **S** St. Luke's Health System, Boise, ID
Primary Contact: Michael A. Fenello, Chief Executive Officer
CFO: Matt Groenig, Vice President Finance
CHR: Cindy E. Paget, Human Resources Manager
Web address: www.mccallhosp.org
**Control:** Other not–for–profit (including NFP Corporation) **Service:** General Medical and Surgical

**Staffed Beds:** 15 **Admissions:** 386 **Census:** 3 **Outpatient Visits:** 44863
**Births:** 81 **Total Expense ($000):** 19311 **Payroll Expense ($000):** 10169
**Personnel:** 174

## MERIDIAN—Ada County

☒ **COMPLEX CARE HOSPITAL OF IDAHO (132002)**, 2131 South Bonito Way, Zip 83642–1659; tel. 877/801–2244, (Nonreporting) **A**1 9 10 **S** LifeCare Management Services, Plano, TX
Primary Contact: Colin O'Sullivan, Administrator
Web address: www.lifecare–hospitals.com
**Control:** Corporation, Investor–owned, for–profit **Service:** Long–Term Acute Care hospital

**Staffed Beds:** 60

**ST. LUKE'S MERIDIAN MEDICAL CENTER** See St. Luke's Regional Medical Center, Boise

## MONTPELIER—Bear Lake County

★ **BEAR LAKE MEMORIAL HOSPITAL (131316)**, 164 South Fifth Street, Zip 83254–1597; tel. 208/847–1630, (Total facility includes 36 beds in nursing home–type unit) **A**9 10 18 **F**2 5 10 11 12 13 18 34 40 45 53 56 57 59 60 62 70 75 76 79 81 82 85 87 93 97 99 101 105 107 113 118 119 126 127 128 132 134 145
Primary Contact: Rodney D. Jacobson, Administrator
Web address: www.blmhospital.com
**Control:** County–Government, nonfederal **Service:** General Medical and Surgical

**Staffed Beds:** 57 **Admissions:** 452 **Census:** 40 **Outpatient Visits:** 4474
**Births:** 55 **Total Expense ($000):** 16097 **Payroll Expense ($000):** 7191
**Personnel:** 171

## MOSCOW—Latah County

☒ **GRITMAN MEDICAL CENTER (131327)**, 700 South Main Street, Zip 83843–3047; tel. 208/882–4511 **A**1 9 10 18 **F**2 3 8 11 13 15 19 28 29 34 35 36 37 40 46 49 51 53 54 56 57 59 60 63 64 65 70 75 76 77 79 81 82 84 85 86 87 89 93 96 107 108 111 113 118 126 128 129 130 131 134 142 145 146 147 **P**5 **S** QHR, Brentwood, TN
Primary Contact: Kara Besst, President and Chief Executive Officer
CFO: Lisa Mae Wood, Chief Financial Officer
CMO: John Visger, M.D., Chief Medical Staff
CIO: Kane Francetich, Chief Information Officer
CHR: Dennis Cockrell, Director Human Resources
CNO: Deena R. Rauch, R.N., Chief Nursing Officer
Web address: www.gritman.org
**Control:** Other not–for–profit (including NFP Corporation) **Service:** General Medical and Surgical

**Staffed Beds:** 25 **Admissions:** 1749 **Census:** 15 **Outpatient Visits:** 60158
**Births:** 374 **Total Expense ($000):** 39966 **Payroll Expense ($000):** 18316
**Personnel:** 367

## MOUNTAIN HOME—Elmore County

★ **ELMORE MEDICAL CENTER (131311)**, 895 North Sixth East Street, Zip 83647–2207, Mailing Address: P.O. Box 1270, Zip 83647–1270; tel. 208/587–8401, (Total facility includes 38 beds in nursing home–type unit) **A**9 10 18 **F**3 7 11 13 29 30 34 35 40 45 57 64 75 76 77 81 89 107 111 113 118 126 127 128 129 132 145 **S** St. Luke's Health System, Boise, ID
Primary Contact: Gregory L. Maurer, Administrator
COO: Betty Van Gheluwe, Chief Operating Officer
CFO: Tricia Senger, Chief Financial Officer
CNO: Debbie Plemmons, MSN, Chief Nursing Officer
Web address: www.elmoremedicalcenter.org
**Control:** Hospital district or authority, Government, nonfederal **Service:** General Medical and Surgical

**Staffed Beds:** 57 **Admissions:** 616 **Census:** 34 **Outpatient Visits:** 36960
**Births:** 108 **Total Expense ($000):** 21922 **Payroll Expense ($000):** 8378
**Personnel:** 245

## MOUNTAIN HOME AFB—Elmore County

☒ **U. S. AIR FORCE CLINIC**, 90 Hope Drive, Building 600, Zip 83648–5300; tel. 208/828–7610, (Nonreporting) **A**1 9 **S** Department of the Air Force, Washington, DC
Primary Contact: Lieutenant Colonel Gregory W. Carson, Administrator
CFO: Robert Magnuson, Business Operations Flight Chief
CIO: Richard Broemeling, Information Systems Flight Commander
**Control:** Air Force, Government, federal **Service:** General Medical and Surgical

**Staffed Beds:** 10

## NAMPA—Canyon County

**MERCY MEDICAL CENTER** See Saint Alphonsus Medical Center – Nampa

☒ **SAINT ALPHONSUS MEDICAL CENTER – NAMPA (130013)**, 1512 12th Avenue Road, Zip 83686–6008; tel. 208/463–5000 **A**1 9 10 **F**3 11 12 13 15 18 19 20 22 26 28 29 30 31 34 35 37 40 43 44 45 49 50 54 55 57 59 60 63 64 68 69 70 75 76 77 78 79 81 82 85 86 87 89 107 108 110 111 113 114 117 118 125 128 129 131 134 140 142 144 145 146 147 **S** Trinity Health, Novi, MI
Primary Contact: Karl Keeler, Chief Executive Officer
CFO: Richard Caffrey, Interim Assistant Chief Financial Officer
CIO: Daniel Wright, Director Information Technology
Web address: www.mercynampa.org
**Control:** Church–operated, Nongovernment, not–for profit **Service:** General Medical and Surgical

**Staffed Beds:** 118 **Admissions:** 5168 **Census:** 39 **Outpatient Visits:** 114417
**Births:** 1067 **Total Expense ($000):** 67120 **Payroll Expense ($000):** 25627
**Personnel:** 560

## OROFINO—Clearwater County

★ **CLEARWATER VALLEY HOSPITAL AND CLINICS (131320)**, 301 Cedar, Zip 83544–9029; tel. 208/476–4555, (Nonreporting) **A**9 10 18 **S** Essentia Health, Duluth, MN
Primary Contact: Casey Meza, Chief Executive Officer
COO: Larry Barker, Chief Operating Officer
CFO: Lenne Bonner, Chief Financial Officer
CHR: Debbie Schumacher, Chief Human Resources
Web address: www.smh–cvhc.org
**Control:** Other not–for–profit (including NFP Corporation) **Service:** General Medical and Surgical

**Staffed Beds:** 23

**ID**

---

**Hospital, Medicare Provider Number, Address, Telephone, Approval, Facility, and Physician Codes, Health Care System**

★ American Hospital Association (AHA) membership
☐ The Joint Commission accreditation
◇ DNV Healthcare Inc. accreditation
○ American Osteopathic Association (AOA) accreditation
△ Commission on Accreditation of Rehabilitation Facilities (CARF) accreditation

**STATE HOSPITAL NORTH**, 300 Hospital Drive, Zip 83544–9034;
tel. 208/476–4511, (Nonreporting) **A**9
Primary Contact: Debra Manfull, Interim Chief Executive Officer
CMO: Karla Eisele, M.D., Clinical Director
CIO: James Sarbacher, Chief Information Officer
CHR: Heather Vandenbark, Human Resources Specialist
Web address: www.healthandwelfare.idaho.gov
**Control:** State–Government, nonfederal **Service:** Psychiatric

Staffed Beds: 60

### POCATELLO—Bannock County

⊠ **PORTNEUF MEDICAL CENTER (130028)**, 777 Hospital Way,
Zip 83201–4004; tel. 208/239–1000 **A**1 2 3 5 9 10 20 **F**3 7 8 11 12 13 14
15 17 18 19 20 22 24 28 29 30 31 34 35 39 40 44 45 46 49 50 51 54 56
57 58 59 60 61 64 68 70 71 72 74 75 76 77 78 79 81 82 85 86 87 88 89
90 93 96 97 98 100 101 102 103 104 105 107 108 109 110 111 113 114
115 116 117 118 120 122 125 128 129 131 134 142 143 145 146 147 **P**4
6 **S** LHP Hospital Group, Plano, TX
Primary Contact: Norman F. Stephens, President and Chief Executive Officer
CFO: John Abreu, Vice President and Chief Financial Officer
CHR: Scott Lowe, Administrative Director Human Resources
CNO: Michael E. Zielaskiewicz, R.N., Vice President Patient Care Services and
Chief Nursing Officer
Web address: www.portmed.org
**Control:** Corporation, Investor–owned, for–profit **Service:** General Medical and
Surgical

Staffed Beds: 174 Admissions: 8188 Census: 81 Outpatient Visits: 166527
Births: 1562 Total Expense ($000): 146617 Payroll Expense ($000):
66218 Personnel: 952

**SAFE HAVEN HOSPITAL OF POCATELLO (134011)**, 1200 Hospital Way,
Zip 83201; tel. 208/232–2570, (Nonreporting) **A**9 10
Primary Contact: Josiah Dahlstrom, Administrator
Web address: www.safehavenhealthcare.org/safehaven_hospital/index.html
**Control:** Individual, Investor–owned, for–profit **Service:** Rehabilitation

Staffed Beds: 12

### POST FALLS—Kootenai County

☐ **NORTHERN IDAHO ADVANCED CARE HOSPITAL (132001)**, 600 North Cecil
Road, Zip 83854; tel. 208/262–2800, (Nonreporting) **A**1 9 10 **S** Ernest Health,
Inc., Albuquerque, NM
Primary Contact: Richard M. Richards, Chief Executive Officer
Web address: www.niach.ernesthealth.com
**Control:** Corporation, Investor–owned, for–profit **Service:** Long–Term Acute Care
hospital

Staffed Beds: 40

☐ **NORTHWEST SPECIALTY HOSPITAL (130066)**, 1593 East Polston Avenue,
Zip 83854; tel. 208/262–2300, (Nonreporting) **A**1 9 10 **S** National Surgical
Hospitals, Chicago, IL
Primary Contact: Ron Rock, Chief Executive Officer
Web address: www.northwestspecialtyhospital.com
**Control:** Corporation, Investor–owned, for–profit **Service:** Other specialty

Staffed Beds: 22

### PRESTON—Franklin County

★ **FRANKLIN COUNTY MEDICAL CENTER (131322)**, 44 North First East Street,
Zip 83263–1399; tel. 208/852–0137, (Nonreporting) **A**9 10 18
Primary Contact: Michael G. Andrus, Administrator and Chief Executive Officer
CFO: Paul Smart, CPA, Chief Financial Officer
CHR: Courtney Dursteler, Chief Human Resources Officer
CNO: LuAnn Nielsen, R.N., Chief Nursing Officer
Web address: www.fcmc.org
**Control:** County–Government, nonfederal **Service:** General Medical and Surgical

Staffed Beds: 65

### REXBURG—Madison County

★ **MADISON MEMORIAL HOSPITAL (130025)**, 450 East Main Street,
Zip 83440–2048, Mailing Address: P.O. Box 310, Zip 83440–0310;
tel. 208/359–6900 **A**9 10 21 **F**3 8 11 13 15 29 30 31 32 34 35 40 41 45 49
59 65 66 68 70 72 74 75 76 77 78 79 81 85 86 87 89 91 93 96 107 108
111 114 117 118 129 145 146 147
Primary Contact: Rachel Gonzales, MSN, R.N., Chief Executive Officer
CFO: Cecil Ricks, Interim Chief Financial Officer
CMO: Clay C. Prince, Chief Medical Officer
CNO: Terry Conrad, Interim CNO
Web address: www.madisonhospital.org
**Control:** County–Government, nonfederal **Service:** General Medical and Surgical

Staffed Beds: 69 Admissions: 4635 Census: 23 Outpatient Visits: 24263
Births: 1415 Total Expense ($000): 49478 Payroll Expense ($000): 17571
Personnel: 395

### RUPERT—Minidoka County

★ **MINIDOKA MEMORIAL HOSPITAL (131319)**, 1224 Eighth Street,
Zip 83350–1599; tel. 208/436–0481, (Total facility includes 59 beds in nursing
home–type unit) **A**9 10 18 **F**3 7 11 15 29 30 34 35 37 40 45 50 56 57 59 62
63 64 65 68 70 75 77 79 81 83 84 85 86 87 97 107 108 111 113 118 126
127 129 130 131 132 133 142 145 146 147 **P**1 3 5
Primary Contact: Carl Hanson, Administrator
COO: Joel Rogers, Chief Operating Officer
CFO: Jason Gibbons, Chief Financial Officer
CMO: Jeff Swenson, M.D., Chief of Staff
CHR: Tammy Hanks, Director Human Resources
Web address: www.minidokamemorial.com
**Control:** County–Government, nonfederal **Service:** General Medical and Surgical

Staffed Beds: 88 Admissions: 646 Census: 58 Outpatient Visits: 14764
Births: 0 Total Expense ($000): 19869 Payroll Expense ($000): 9496
Personnel: 206

**MINIDOKA MEMORIAL HOSPITAL AND EXTENDED CARE FACILITY** See
Minidoka Memorial Hospital

### SAINT MARIES—Benewah County

★ **BENEWAH COMMUNITY HOSPITAL (131317)**, 229 South Seventh Street,
Zip 83861–1803; tel. 208/245–5551 **A**9 10 18 **F**8 13 15 29 30 31 34 35 40
45 57 59 63 64 75 76 78 79 81 82 84 85 92 93 97 99 100 101 103 104
107 111 113 118 126 128 130 132 134 145 **P**6 **S** QHR, Brentwood, TN
Primary Contact: Brian Nall, Chief Executive Officer
COO: Debbie Kerns, Director Human Resources and Chief Operating Officer
CFO: Lori Stoltz, Chief Financial Officer
CMO: Richard Thurston, M.D., Chief of Staff
CHR: Debbie Kerns, Director Human Resources and Chief Operating Officer
CNO: Kim Wilson, Interim Director of Nursing
Web address: www.bchmed.org
**Control:** County–Government, nonfederal **Service:** General Medical and Surgical

Staffed Beds: 19 Admissions: 434 Census: 4 Outpatient Visits: 19946
Births: 50 Total Expense ($000): 13970 Payroll Expense ($000): 5953
Personnel: 124

### SALMON—Lemhi County

★ **STEELE MEMORIAL MEDICAL CENTER (131305)**, 203 South Daisy Street,
Zip 83467–4109; tel. 208/756–5600 **A**9 10 18 **F**3 11 13 15 28 29 31 34 35
40 45 55 57 59 64 65 66 68 75 76 77 78 79 81 82 85 87 90 93 97 104
107 114 118 126 128 130 131 132 134 144 145 147 **P**6 **S** QHR,
Brentwood, TN
Primary Contact: Jeff Hill, Chief Executive Officer
COO: Abner King, Chief Operating Officer
CFO: Gregory Hexum, Chief Financial Officer
CMO: Adam Deutchman, M.D., Chief of Staff
CNO: Stephanie Orr, R.N., Chief Nursing Officer
Web address: www.steelemh.org
**Control:** County–Government, nonfederal **Service:** General Medical and Surgical

Staffed Beds: 18 Admissions: 424 Census: 3 Outpatient Visits: 28007
Births: 39 Total Expense ($000): 14313 Payroll Expense ($000): 5807
Personnel: 131

### SANDPOINT—Bonner County

⊠ **BONNER GENERAL HOSPITAL (131328)**, 520 North Third Avenue,
Zip 83864–0877, Mailing Address: Box 1448, Zip 83864–0877;
tel. 208/263–1441 **A**1 9 10 18 **F**3 11 13 15 17 22 26 28 29 30 34 35 40 45
46 47 48 54 57 59 62 63 64 68 75 76 77 79 81 85 86 87 93 102 107 108
110 111 113 117 118 129 130 131 141 143 145 **P**8
Primary Contact: Sheryl Rickard, Chief Executive Officer
CFO: Norilina Harvel, Chief Financial Officer
CIO: Bob Hess, Chief Information Officer
CHR: Brad Waterbury, Director Human Resources
CNO: Linda Rammler, R.N., Chief Nursing Officer
Web address: www.bonnergen.org
**Control:** Other not–for–profit (including NFP Corporation) **Service:** General
Medical and Surgical

Staffed Beds: 25 Admissions: 2007 Census: 16 Outpatient Visits: 54536
Births: 321 Total Expense ($000): 40176 Payroll Expense ($000): 16343
Personnel: 284

### SODA SPRINGS—Caribou County

★ **CARIBOU MEMORIAL HOSPITAL AND LIVING CENTER (131309)**, 300 South
Third West, Zip 83276–1598; tel. 208/547–3341, (Total facility includes 30 beds
in nursing home–type unit) **A**9 10 18 **F**11 13 17 18 34 35 40 50 56 57 59 65
67 70 76 79 81 93 100 107 114 118 126 127 128 129 131 132 142 147
Primary Contact: John L. Hoopes, Chief Executive Officer
CFO: Leota Carver, Chief Financial Officer
CMO: John K. Franson, M.D., Chief Medical Staff
CIO: Kathey Peck, Manager Health Information
CHR: Michael D. Peck, Assistant Administrator
Web address: www.cariboumemorial.org
**Control:** County–Government, nonfederal **Service:** General Medical and Surgical

Staffed Beds: 55 Admissions: 403 Census: 28 Outpatient Visits: 11331
Births: 39 Total Expense ($000): 10412 Personnel: 152

**ID**

**TWIN FALLS—Twin Falls County**

⊞ **ST. LUKE'S MAGIC VALLEY MEDICAL CENTER (130002)**, 801 Pole Line Road West, Zip 83301, Mailing Address: P.O. Box 409, Zip 83303–0409; tel. 208/814–0000 **A**1 2 9 10 **F**3 4 5 7 8 11 13 15 18 20 22 29 30 31 35 40 57 62 63 68 70 72 76 77 78 79 81 85 87 89 90 93 96 98 107 110 111 113 118 129 145 **P**6 8 **S** St. Luke's Health System, Boise, ID
Primary Contact: James L. Angle, FACHE, Chief Executive Officer
Web address: www.stlukesonline.org
**Control:** Other not–for–profit (including NFP Corporation) **Service:** General Medical and Surgical

**Staffed Beds:** 201 **Admissions:** 9062 **Census:** 99 **Outpatient Visits:** 518567
**Births:** 1613 **Total Expense ($000):** 211655 **Payroll Expense ($000):** 79908 **Personnel:** 1762

**WEISER—Washington County**

★ **WEISER MEMORIAL HOSPITAL (131307)**, 645 East Fifth Street, Zip 83672–2202; tel. 208/549–0370, (Nonreporting) **A**9 10 18 21 **S** St. Luke's Health System, Boise, ID
Primary Contact: Tom Murphy, Chief Executive Officer
CFO: Nate Coburn, Chief Financial Officer
CMO: Suzanna D. Hubele, M.D., Chief of Staff
CHR: Terri Kautz, Manager Human Resources
CNO: Reuben J. DeKastle, Chief Nursing Officer
Web address: www.weisermemorialhospital.org
**Control:** Hospital district or authority, Government, nonfederal **Service:** General Medical and Surgical

**Staffed Beds:** 25

**ID**

---

**Hospital, Medicare Provider Number, Address, Telephone, Approval, Facility, and Physician Codes, Health Care System**

★ American Hospital Association (AHA) membership
☐ The Joint Commission accreditation
◇ DNV Healthcare Inc. accreditation
○ American Osteopathic Association (AOA) accreditation
△ Commission on Accreditation of Rehabilitation Facilities (CARF) accreditation

# ILLINOIS

## ALEDO—Mercer County

★ **MERCER COUNTY HOSPITAL (141304)**, 409 N.W. Ninth Avenue,
Zip 61231–1296; tel. 309/582–5301 **A**9 10 18 **F**3 11 15 29 30 34 35 40 45
54 56 57 59 62 63 64 69 77 79 81 85 87 93 97 107 108 113 118 126 127
129 130 132 145 146 **S** Genesis Health System, Davenport, IA
Primary Contact: Ted Rogalski, Chief Executive Officer
COO: Myron Higgins, Chief Operating Officer
CFO: Sandy Moore, Interim CFO
CMO: Dennis Palmer, D.O., Chief of Staff
CIO: Marcia Kelly, Manager, IT
CHR: Myron Higgins, Chief Operating Officer
CNO: Shelley Wiborg, MS, Chief Nursing Officer
Web address: www.mercerhospital.org
**Control:** County–Government, nonfederal **Service:** General Medical and Surgical

Staffed Beds: 22 Admissions: 346 Census: 4 Outpatient Visits: 36641
Births: 0 Total Expense ($000): 11808 Payroll Expense ($000): 5515
Personnel: 121

## ALTON—Madison County

⊠ **ALTON MEMORIAL HOSPITAL (140002)**, One Memorial Drive,
Zip 62002–6722; tel. 618/463–7311, (Total facility includes 88 beds in nursing
home–type unit) **A**1 2 9 10 **F**3 6 7 11 13 15 18 20 22 29 30 31 34 35 38 39
40 45 46 49 50 56 57 59 64 70 74 75 76 77 78 79 81 85 86 87 89 92 93
96 98 103 104 107 108 110 111 113 114 115 116 117 118 119 120 122
127 128 129 130 131 145 147 **S** BJC HealthCare, Saint Louis, MO
Primary Contact: David A. Braasch, President
COO: Doug Pytlinski, Vice President Administration
CFO: Brad Goacher, Director Finance
CMO: David Burnside, M.D., Chief Medical Officer
CIO: David Weiss, Vice President Information System
CHR: Tina Kristoff, Manager Human Resources
Web address: www.altonmemorialhospital.org
**Control:** Other not–for–profit (including NFP Corporation) **Service:** General Medical and Surgical

Staffed Beds: 253 Admissions: 6663 Census: 143 Outpatient Visits:
106490 Births: 581 Total Expense ($000): 114039 Payroll Expense
($000): 39639 Personnel: 724

☐ **ALTON MENTAL HEALTH CENTER (144016)**, 4500 College Avenue,
Zip 62002–5099; tel. 618/474–3800, (Nonreporting) **A**1 10 **S** Division of Mental
Health, Department of Human Services, Springfield, IL
Primary Contact: Brian E. Thomas, Administrator
CFO: Susan Shobe, Director Administration and Support Services
CMO: Claudia Kachigion, M.D., Medical Director
**Control:** State–Government, nonfederal **Service:** Psychiatric

Staffed Beds: 165

⊠ **SAINT ANTHONY'S HEALTH CENTER (140052)**, 1 Saint Anthony's Way,
Zip 62024–4579, Mailing Address: P.O. Box 340, Zip 62002–0340;
tel. 618/465–2571, (Includes SAINT CLARE'S HOSPITAL, 915 East Fifth Street,
Zip 62002–6434; tel. 618/463–5151), (Total facility includes 30 beds in nursing
home–type unit) **A**1 2 9 10 **F**2 3 10 11 13 15 18 20 22 26 29 30 31 32 34 35
38 39 40 41 44 45 46 47 49 50 51 54 56 57 58 59 61 62 63 64 65 67 70
74 75 76 78 79 81 82 84 85 86 87 89 90 91 92 93 94 95 96 99 100 101
102 103 104 107 108 110 111 113 114 117 118 119 120 122 127 128 129
130 131 133 134 145 146 147 **P**6
Primary Contact: Evert J. Kuiper, President and Chief Executive Officer
CFO: Mike Nelson, Chief Financial Officer
CMO: Larry Burch, M.D., Vice President Medical Affairs
CIO: Michael Russo, Chief Administrative Officer
CHR: Sister Mary Mikela, Vice President Mission Stewardship
Web address: www.sahc.org
**Control:** Church–operated, Nongovernment, not–for profit **Service:** General Medical and Surgical

Staffed Beds: 199 Admissions: 4043 Census: 66 Outpatient Visits: 131850
Births: 414 Total Expense ($000): 79869 Payroll Expense ($000): 30464
Personnel: 666

## ANNA—Union County

☐ **CHOATE MENTAL HEALTH CENTER (144038)**, 1000 North Main Street,
Zip 62906–1699; tel. 618/833–5161, (Nonreporting) **A**1 5 10 **S** Division of
Mental Health, Department of Human Services, Springfield, IL
Primary Contact: Elaine Ray, Administrator
COO: Elaine Ray, Administrator
CMO: John Larcas, M.D., Acting Medical Director
CIO: Cindy Flamm, Manager Quality
CHR: Tammy Tellor, Acting Director Human Resources
**Control:** State–Government, nonfederal **Service:** Psychiatric

Staffed Beds: 79

⊠ **UNION COUNTY HOSPITAL (141342)**, 517 North Main Street,
Zip 62906–1696; tel. 618/833–4511, (Total facility includes 22 beds in nursing
home–type unit) **A**1 9 10 18 **F**3 11 15 28 29 30 34 35 40 45 49 50 57 59 64
68 75 77 81 85 87 93 97 107 110 113 118 126 127 129 132 145 147 **P**6
**S** Community Health Systems, Inc., Franklin, TN
Primary Contact: James R. Farris, FACHE, Chief Executive Officer
COO: Jeanette L. Hook, R.N., Chief Nursing Officer
CFO: Terry Paligo, Chief Financial Officer
CMO: Christine Lucas, M.D., Chief of Staff
CIO: John Hegger, Director Information Systems
CHR: Tammy Samuels, Director Human Resources
Web address: www.unioncountyhospital.com
**Control:** Corporation, Investor–owned, for–profit **Service:** General Medical and Surgical

Staffed Beds: 47 Admissions: 840 Census: 30 Outpatient Visits: 38766
Births: 3 Total Expense ($000): 16390 Payroll Expense ($000): 7987
Personnel: 146

## ARLINGTON HEIGHTS—Cook County

⊠ **NORTHWEST COMMUNITY HOSPITAL (140252)**, 800 West Central Road,
Zip 60005–2392; tel. 847/618–1000 **A**1 2 9 10 **F**3 4 5 13 15 17 18 20 22 24
25 26 28 29 30 31 32 34 35 37 38 39 40 41 43 44 45 46 47 49 50 54 55
56 57 59 61 62 63 64 65 66 68 70 71 72 73 74 75 76 77 78 79 81 82 84
85 86 87 89 90 92 93 96 98 99 100 101 102 103 104 105 106 107 108
110 111 113 114 115 116 117 118 119 120 122 123 125 128 129 130 131
134 143 144 145 146 147 **P**5 8
Primary Contact: Bruce K. Crowther, President and Chief Executive Officer
COO: Michael B. Zenn, Executive Vice President, Chief Operating Officer and Chief Financial Officer
CFO: Michael B. Zenn, Executive Vice President, Chief Operating Officer and Chief Financial Officer
CMO: Leighton B. Smith, M.D., Vice President Medical Affairs
CIO: George Morris, Vice President Information Technology and Chief Information Officer
CHR: Mark Lusson, Vice President Human Resources
Web address: www.nch.org
**Control:** Other not–for–profit (including NFP Corporation) **Service:** General Medical and Surgical

Staffed Beds: 433 Admissions: 24225 Census: 273 Outpatient Visits:
357107 Births: 3135 Total Expense ($000): 397006 Payroll Expense
($000): 190404 Personnel: 3087

## AURORA—Du Page and Kane Counties

⊠ **PROVENA MERCY MEDICAL CENTER (140174)**, 1325 North Highland
Avenue, Zip 60506–1449; tel. 630/859–2222 **A**1 2 9 10 **F**3 5 11 12 13 15 18
20 22 24 26 28 29 30 31 34 35 36 38 40 43 46 49 56 57 59 61 65 68 70
73 75 76 77 78 79 81 82 85 86 87 93 97 98 99 100 101 102 103 104 105
107 111 113 114 118 129 131 134 143 145 146 **P**5 **S** Presence Health,
Chicago, IL
Primary Contact: Maureen A. Bryant, FACHE, President and Chief Executive Officer
COO: Mary Vonderau, Vice President Strategy and Operations
CHR: Diane Hargreaves, Vice President Human Resources
CNO: Suzette M. Mahneke, R.N., Chief Nursing Executive
Web address: www.provena.org/mercy/
**Control:** Other not–for–profit (including NFP Corporation) **Service:** General Medical and Surgical

Staffed Beds: 124 Admissions: 10015 Census: 124 Outpatient Visits:
189262 Births: 773 Total Expense ($000): 146479 Payroll Expense
($000): 54757 Personnel: 900

IL

⊠ △ **RUSH–COPLEY MEDICAL CENTER (140029)**, 2000 Ogden Avenue, Zip 60504–7222; tel. 630/978–6200 **A**1 2 3 5 7 9 10 **F**3 7 9 13 15 17 18 19 20 22 24 26 28 29 30 31 32 34 35 36 37 38 39 40 42 43 44 45 46 47 49 50 52 53 54 55 56 57 58 59 60 61 62 64 65 66 68 70 72 73 74 75 76 77 78 79 81 82 84 85 86 87 89 90 92 93 96 97 99 104 107 108 110 111 113 114 116 117 118 119 120 122 129 130 131 133 134 142 143 144 145 146 147 **P**6 **S** Rush University Medical Center, Chicago, IL
Primary Contact: Barry C. Finn, President and Chief Executive Officer
COO: John A. Diederich, Senior Vice President Operations and Chief Operating Officer
CFO: Brenda VanWyhe, Senior Vice President Finance and Chief Financial Officer
CMO: Steve B. Lowenthal, M.D., Senior Vice President Medical Affairs and Chief Medical Officer
CIO: Dennis DeMasie, Vice President Information Systems and Chief Information Officer
CHR: Darla Mullner, Director Human Resources
CNO: Mary Shilkaitis, Vice President Patient Care and Chief Nursing Officer
Web address: www.rushcopley.com
**Control:** Other not–for–profit (including NFP Corporation) **Service:** General Medical and Surgical

**Staffed Beds:** 210 **Admissions:** 13136 **Census:** 148 **Outpatient Visits:** 197103 **Births:** 3294 **Total Expense ($000):** 226276 **Payroll Expense ($000):** 89402 **Personnel:** 1393

### BARRINGTON—Lake County

⊠ **ADVOCATE GOOD SHEPHERD HOSPITAL (140291)**, 450 West Highway 22, Zip 60010–1901; tel. 847/381–0123 **A**1 2 9 10 **F**3 11 12 13 15 17 18 19 20 22 23 24 26 28 29 30 31 34 35 36 37 40 43 45 46 47 48 49 54 57 59 63 64 65 68 70 74 75 76 77 78 79 81 82 84 87 89 91 92 93 94 97 100 101 102 103 104 105 107 110 111 113 114 117 118 119 120 122 125 128 129 131 134 145 **P**8 **S** Advocate Health Care, Oak Brook, IL
Primary Contact: Karen A. Lambert, President
COO: Doug Ryder, Vice President Clinical Operations and Service Lines
CFO: George Teufel, Vice President Finance
CMO: Barry Rosen, M.D., Vice President Medical Management
CHR: Robert F. Scott, Vice President Human Resources
Web address: www.advocatehealth.com
**Control:** Church–operated, Nongovernment, not–for profit **Service:** General Medical and Surgical

**Staffed Beds:** 169 **Admissions:** 10817 **Census:** 112 **Outpatient Visits:** 209658 **Births:** 1469 **Total Expense ($000):** 220683 **Payroll Expense ($000):** 77744 **Personnel:** 800

### BELLEVILLE—St. Clair County

★ ○ **MEMORIAL HOSPITAL (140185)**, 4500 Memorial Drive, Zip 62226–5399; tel. 618/233–7750, (Total facility includes 70 beds in nursing home–type unit) **A**9 10 11 **F**3 11 13 15 18 20 22 24 26 28 29 30 31 34 39 40 45 46 49 51 53 54 57 59 60 62 64 70 71 74 75 76 77 79 81 82 84 85 86 87 89 92 93 94 96 107 108 110 111 112 113 114 117 118 127 128 129 130 131 134 144 145 146 147 **P**6 8
Primary Contact: Mark J. Turner, President and Chief Executive Officer
COO: Michael T. McManus, Chief Operating Officer
CFO: Amy Thomas, Vice President Finance
CMO: William Casperson, M.D., Vice President Medical Affairs
CIO: Jennifer Meinkoth, Chief Information Officer
CHR: John C. Ziegler, FACHE, Vice President Human Resources
CNO: Nancy R. Weston, R.N., Vice President Nursing Services
Web address: www.memhosp.com
**Control:** Other not–for–profit (including NFP Corporation) **Service:** General Medical and Surgical

**Staffed Beds:** 345 **Admissions:** 17300 **Census:** 245 **Outpatient Visits:** 316773 **Births:** 1533 **Total Expense ($000):** 234699 **Payroll Expense ($000):** 102658 **Personnel:** 1922

⊠ △ **ST. ELIZABETH'S HOSPITAL (140187)**, 211 South Third Street, Zip 62220–1998; tel. 618/234–2120 **A**1 3 5 7 9 10 **F**3 4 5 11 13 15 18 20 22 24 26 28 29 30 31 35 39 40 45 46 49 50 53 54 56 57 59 60 62 64 65 68 70 74 75 76 77 78 79 81 82 85 86 87 90 93 97 98 100 101 102 103 104 105 107 108 111 114 115 116 117 118 120 123 128 129 130 131 134 143 145 146 147 **P**6 8 **S** Hospital Sisters Health System, Springfield, IL
Primary Contact: Maryann Reese, R.N., FACHE, President and Chief Executive Officer
CFO: Leslie Eckert, Chief Financial Officer
CMO: Shelly Harkins, M.D., Chief Medical Officer
CIO: Dana Stephens, Director Information Technology
CHR: Margaret Dolan, Director People Services
CNO: Shelley Harris, MSN, Chief Nursing Officer
Web address: www.steliz.org
**Control:** Church–operated, Nongovernment, not–for profit **Service:** General Medical and Surgical

**Staffed Beds:** 260 **Admissions:** 11855 **Census:** 139 **Outpatient Visits:** 173488 **Births:** 1153 **Total Expense ($000):** 178022 **Payroll Expense ($000):** 60006 **Personnel:** 1105

### BENTON—Franklin County

★ **FRANKLIN HOSPITAL DISTRICT (141321)**, 201 Bailey Lane, Zip 62812–1969; tel. 618/439–3161 **A**9 10 18 **F**11 15 29 30 34 35 40 45 56 57 59 66 75 77 81 93 97 107 113 118 126 131 132 **P**6 **S** Alliant Management Services, Louisville, KY
Primary Contact: Hervey E. Davis, Chief Executive Officer
COO: Michael J. Budnick, FACHE, Chief Operating Officer and Clinic Manager
CFO: Howard Schou, Chief Financial Officer
CMO: David Hartman, M.D., Chief of Staff
CIO: David Williams, Director Information Technology
CHR: Nancy Seibert, Director Human Resources
CNO: Terri Hermann, R.N., Chief Nursing Officer
Web address: www.franklinhospital.net
**Control:** Hospital district or authority, Government, nonfederal **Service:** General Medical and Surgical

**Staffed Beds:** 25 **Admissions:** 345 **Census:** 3 **Outpatient Visits:** 21715 **Births:** 0 **Total Expense ($000):** 14825 **Payroll Expense ($000):** 7110 **Personnel:** 167

### BERWYN—Cook County

⊠ **MACNEAL HOSPITAL (140054)**, 3249 South Oak Park Avenue, Zip 60402–0715; tel. 708/783–9100 **A**1 2 3 5 8 9 10 13 **F**3 5 12 13 15 18 19 20 22 24 26 28 29 30 31 34 35 36 39 40 41 43 44 45 46 49 50 54 55 56 57 58 59 60 62 64 65 68 70 73 74 75 76 77 78 79 81 82 84 85 86 87 89 92 93 96 97 98 100 101 102 103 104 105 106 107 110 111 113 118 119 120 128 129 130 131 134 140 143 145 146 147 **P**5 8 **S** Vanguard Health System, Nashville, TN
Primary Contact: Brian J. Lemon, Chief Executive Officer
COO: J. Scott Steiner, Chief Operating Officer
CFO: Michael A. Lawrence, Chief Financial Officer
CMO: Charles Bareis, M.D., Medical Director
CIO: Nora Ellis, Market Chief Information Officer
CHR: Maggie Shontz, VP, Human Resources
CNO: Debra Albert, MSN, Chief Nursing Officer
Web address: www.macneal.com
**Control:** Corporation, Investor–owned, for–profit **Service:** General Medical and Surgical

**Staffed Beds:** 373 **Admissions:** 17096 **Census:** 225 **Outpatient Visits:** 197136 **Births:** 1891 **Total Expense ($000):** 232278 **Payroll Expense ($000):** 101751 **Personnel:** 2035

### BLOOMINGTON—Mclean County

⊠ **OSF ST. JOSEPH MEDICAL CENTER (140162)**, 2200 East Washington Street, Zip 61701–4323; tel. 309/662–3311, (Total facility includes 12 beds in nursing home–type unit) **A**1 2 9 10 **F**3 11 12 13 15 18 20 22 24 28 29 30 31 34 35 37 40 42 43 45 49 50 51 54 57 59 60 61 64 65 66 68 70 74 75 76 77 78 79 81 82 84 85 86 87 89 92 93 96 97 107 108 110 111 113 114 117 118 126 127 129 130 131 134 143 145 146 147 **P**6 **S** OSF Healthcare System, Peoria, IL
Primary Contact: Kenneth J. Natzke, President and Chief Executive Officer
COO: Lawrence E. Wills, Vice President Operations
CFO: John R. Zell, Chief Financial Officer
CMO: Paul E. Pedersen, M.D., Vice President and Chief Medical Officer
CHR: Sue A. Herriott, Director Human Resources
Web address: www.osfstjoseph.org
**Control:** Church–operated, Nongovernment, not–for profit **Service:** General Medical and Surgical

**Staffed Beds:** 149 **Admissions:** 6184 **Census:** 63 **Outpatient Visits:** 336541 **Births:** 786 **Total Expense ($000):** 137054 **Payroll Expense ($000):** 66905 **Personnel:** 875

IL

## BLUE ISLAND—Cook County

✠ **METROSOUTH MEDICAL CENTER (140118)**, 12935 South Gregory Street, Zip 60406–2470; tel. 708/597–2000 **A**1 9 10 **F**3 13 15 18 20 22 24 26 28 29 30 31 34 35 40 45 46 47 48 49 50 53 54 56 57 59 61 64 68 70 73 74 75 76 77 78 79 81 82 85 86 87 92 93 94 96 97 100 107 108 111 113 117 118 128 129 131 134 145 146 147 **S** Community Health Systems, Inc., Franklin, TN
Primary Contact: Enrique Beckmann, M.D., Ph.D., President and Chief Executive Officer
COO: Barbara Fideli, COO of Nonclinical
CFO: Pamela Cassara, Chief Financial Officer
CMO: Enrique Beckmann, M.D., President and Chief Executive Officer
CIO: Bashirat Hahn, Chief Information Officer
CHR: Jackie Montgomery, Director Human Resources
CNO: Linda M. St. Julien, R.N., CNO/COO of Clinical
Web address: www.metrosouthmedicalcenter.com
**Control:** Partnership, Investor–owned, for–profit **Service:** General Medical and Surgical

**Staffed Beds:** 180 **Admissions:** 10052 **Census:** 111 **Outpatient Visits:** 91886 **Births:** 1692 **Total Expense ($000):** 152256 **Payroll Expense ($000):** 63017 **Personnel:** 820

## BOLINGBROOK—Will County

★ **ADVENTIST BOLINGBROOK HOSPITAL (140304)**, 500 Remington Boulevard, Zip 60440; tel. 630/312–5000 **A**9 10 **F**3 11 12 13 15 18 20 22 28 29 30 31 33 34 35 36 37 39 40 43 45 46 47 49 50 51 52 54 56 57 58 59 60 61 64 65 68 70 73 74 75 76 78 79 81 82 85 86 87 92 93 96 107 108 110 111 113 114 118 128 129 130 131 144 145 146 **P**7 8 **S** Adventist Health System Sunbelt Health Care Corporation, Altamonte Springs, FL
Primary Contact: Rick Mace, Chief Executive Officer
CFO: Mike Murrill, Vice President and Chief Financial Officer
CMO: Richard Carroll, M.D., Chief Medical officer
CIO: John McLendon, Senior Vice President and Chief Information Officer
CHR: Shana Ross, Director Human Resources
CNO: Jolene Albaugh, R.N., Vice President and Chief Nursing Officer
Web address: www.keepingyouwell.com/abh/
**Control:** Church–operated, Nongovernment, not–for profit **Service:** General Medical and Surgical

**Staffed Beds:** 148 **Admissions:** 5590 **Census:** 53 **Outpatient Visits:** 80694 **Births:** 951 **Total Expense ($000):** 103669 **Payroll Expense ($000):** 33052 **Personnel:** 576

## BREESE—Clinton County

✠ **ST. JOSEPH'S HOSPITAL (140145)**, 9515 Holy Cross Lane, Zip 62230–0099; tel. 618/526–4511 **A**1 9 10 **F**3 11 13 15 28 29 30 32 34 35 40 43 50 53 56 57 59 68 70 76 79 81 85 89 93 103 107 108 110 111 114 117 118 126 128 129 130 131 133 134 143 145 147 **S** Hospital Sisters Health System, Springfield, IL
Primary Contact: Mark D. Klosterman, FACHE, President and Chief Executive Officer
CFO: John Jeffries, Chief Financial Officer
CHR: Kathryn Mines, Director Human Resources
Web address: www.stjoebreese.com
**Control:** Church–operated, Nongovernment, not–for profit **Service:** General Medical and Surgical

**Staffed Beds:** 47 **Admissions:** 1679 **Census:** 14 **Outpatient Visits:** 87474 **Births:** 463 **Total Expense ($000):** 42646 **Payroll Expense ($000):** 13982 **Personnel:** 293

## CANTON—Fulton County

✠ **GRAHAM HOSPITAL (140001)**, 210 West Walnut Street, Zip 61520–2497; tel. 309/647–5240, (Total facility includes 50 beds in nursing home–type unit) **A**1 6 9 10 20 **F**3 11 13 15 26 28 29 30 32 34 35 40 45 50 53 54 56 57 59 62 63 64 65 67 70 75 76 77 79 81 82 85 86 87 89 91 93 97 107 108 110 111 114 118 123 126 127 128 129 130 131 134 142 143 144 145 **P**3
Primary Contact: Robert G. Senneff, FACHE, President and Chief Executive Officer
CFO: Jim Stratton, Vice President Finance
Web address: www.grahamhospital.org
**Control:** Other not–for–profit (including NFP Corporation) **Service:** General Medical and Surgical

**Staffed Beds:** 99 **Admissions:** 2743 **Census:** 61 **Outpatient Visits:** 193107 **Births:** 262 **Total Expense ($000):** 67116 **Payroll Expense ($000):** 28008 **Personnel:** 585

## CARBONDALE—Jackson County

✠ **MEMORIAL HOSPITAL OF CARBONDALE (140164)**, 405 West Jackson Street, Zip 62901–1467, Mailing Address: P.O. Box 10000, Zip 62902–9000; tel. 618/549–0721 **A**1 2 3 5 9 10 13 19 **F**3 11 13 18 20 22 24 26 28 29 30 31 34 35 40 45 48 49 54 56 57 59 64 68 70 72 74 75 76 77 78 79 81 82 83 84 85 86 87 89 107 108 111 113 114 118 119 120 129 130 131 134 144 145 146 **S** Southern Illinois Hospital Services, Carbondale, IL
Primary Contact: Bart Millstead, Administrator
CMO: James D. Miller, M.D., Chief Medical Officer
CIO: Frank Sears, Vice President Information Services
Web address: www.sih.net
**Control:** Other not–for–profit (including NFP Corporation) **Service:** General Medical and Surgical

**Staffed Beds:** 153 **Admissions:** 10166 **Census:** 100 **Outpatient Visits:** 115481 **Births:** 2057 **Total Expense ($000):** 192134 **Payroll Expense ($000):** 53624 **Personnel:** 996

## CARLINVILLE—Macoupin County

★ **CARLINVILLE AREA HOSPITAL (141347)**, 20733 North Broad Street, Zip 62626–1499; tel. 217/854–3141 **A**9 10 18 **F**11 15 28 29 34 35 40 45 64 77 79 81 91 93 107 110 114 128 132 **P**6 **S** HealthTech Management Services, Franklin, TN
Primary Contact: Kenneth G. Reid, President and Chief Executive Officer
CFO: Greg Ward, Chief Financial Officer and Vice President Operations
CMO: Julie Fleischer, M.D., President Medical Staff
CIO: Jerod Cottingham, Director Information Systems
CHR: Tracy Koster, Director Human Resources
Web address: www.cahcare.com
**Control:** Other not–for–profit (including NFP Corporation) **Service:** General Medical and Surgical

**Staffed Beds:** 25 **Admissions:** 578 **Census:** 6 **Outpatient Visits:** 21349 **Births:** 0 **Total Expense ($000):** 19042 **Payroll Expense ($000):** 6354 **Personnel:** 138

## CARROLLTON—Greene County

**THOMAS H. BOYD MEMORIAL HOSPITAL (141300)**, 800 School Street, Zip 62016–1498; tel. 217/942–6946, (Includes REISCH MEMORIAL NURSING HOME ) **A**9 10 18 **F**3 7 11 15 34 40 53 57 77 89 93 97 107 118 126 129 132
Primary Contact: Deborah Campbell, Administrator
CHR: Lisa Eldridge, Human Resources Officer
**Control:** Other not–for–profit (including NFP Corporation) **Service:** General Medical and Surgical

**Staffed Beds:** 25 **Admissions:** 450 **Census:** 5 **Outpatient Visits:** 25625 **Births:** 0 **Total Expense ($000):** 9568 **Payroll Expense ($000):** 4856 **Personnel:** 137

## CARTHAGE—Hancock County

☐ **MEMORIAL HOSPITAL (141305)**, 1454 North County Road 2050, Zip 62321–1600, Mailing Address: P.O. Box 160, Zip 62321–0160; tel. 217/357–8500 **A**1 9 10 18 **F**3 11 13 15 28 29 30 31 34 35 36 40 45 56 57 59 64 75 76 80 81 82 85 103 107 108 110 114 118 124 126 128 129 131 132 143 145
Primary Contact: Ada Bair, Chief Executive Officer
CFO: Teresa Smith, Chief Financial Officer
CIO: Syndi Horn, Director Information Systems
CHR: Dan Smith, Director Human Resources
CNO: Florine Dixon, Vice President Clinical Services
Web address: www.mhtlc.org
**Control:** Other not–for–profit (including NFP Corporation) **Service:** General Medical and Surgical

**Staffed Beds:** 18 **Admissions:** 678 **Census:** 7 **Outpatient Visits:** 17713 **Births:** 102 **Total Expense ($000):** 18686 **Payroll Expense ($000):** 7858 **Personnel:** 164

## CENTRALIA—Marion County

✠ **ST. MARY'S HOSPITAL (140034)**, 400 North Pleasant Avenue, Zip 62801–3091; tel. 618/436–8000 **A**1 2 9 10 **F**3 5 11 13 15 18 20 26 28 29 30 31 32 34 35 38 40 44 45 50 51 54 57 59 61 64 68 70 73 74 75 76 77 78 79 80 81 82 84 85 86 87 89 92 93 94 98 99 100 101 102 103 104 105 107 108 110 111 113 117 118 119 120 128 129 130 131 134 145 146 147 **P**6 8 **S** SSM Health Care, Saint Louis, MO
Primary Contact: Bruce Merrell, FACHE, President
COO: Mark A. Clark, Vice President Operations
CFO: Kay Tinsley, Vice President Finance
CMO: Rajendra Shroff, M.D., Administrative Medical Director
CIO: Ralph Caudill, Director Information Systems
CHR: Thomas W. Blythe, Vice President Human Resources
Web address: www.smgsi.com
**Control:** Church–operated, Nongovernment, not–for profit **Service:** General Medical and Surgical

**Staffed Beds:** 104 **Admissions:** 6714 **Census:** 73 **Outpatient Visits:** 190186 **Births:** 351 **Total Expense ($000):** 97933 **Payroll Expense ($000):** 36792 **Personnel:** 877

*Many Facility Codes have changed. Please refer to the AHA Guide Code Chart.*

IL

## CENTREVILLE—St. Clair County

☐ **TOUCHETTE REGIONAL HOSPITALS (140077)**, 5900 Bond Avenue, Zip 62207–2326; tel. 618/332–3060 **A**1 9 10 **F**3 11 13 15 18 29 30 31 40 45 47 50 55 62 64 68 70 73 75 76 78 79 81 85 87 89 92 98 101 102 104 105 107 113 118 124 129 142 145 147 **P**6
Primary Contact: Larry W. McCulley, President and Chief Executive Officer
COO: Tom Mikkelson, M.D., Interim Chief Operating Officer
CFO: John Majchrzak, Chief Financial Officer
CMO: Tom Mikkelson, M.D., Vice President Medical Affairs
CIO: Michael Nichols, Corporate Vice President Information Technology
CHR: Wardell Sullivan, Director Human Resources
Web address: www.touchette.org
**Control:** Other not–for–profit (including NFP Corporation) **Service:** General Medical and Surgical

**Staffed Beds:** 96 **Admissions:** 2778 **Census:** 31 **Outpatient Visits:** 69666 **Births:** 338 **Total Expense ($000):** 59756 **Payroll Expense ($000):** 28772 **Personnel:** 460

## CHAMPAIGN—Champaign County

☐ **THE PAVILION (144029)**, 809 West Church Street, Zip 61820–3399; tel. 217/373–1700, (Nonreporting) **A**1 9 10 **S** Universal Health Services, Inc., King of Prussia, PA
Primary Contact: Joseph Sheehy, Chief Executive Officer and Managing Director
CFO: Edith Frasca, Controller and Chief Financial Officer
Web address: www.pavilionhospital.com
**Control:** Corporation, Investor–owned, for–profit **Service:** Psychiatric

**Staffed Beds:** 46

## CHESTER—Randolph County

☐ **CHESTER MENTAL HEALTH CENTER**, Chester Road, Zip 62233–0031, Mailing Address: Box 31, Zip 62233–0031; tel. 618/826–4571 **A**1 5 **F**29 30 39 86 98 106 129 **P**6 **S** Division of Mental Health, Department of Human Services, Springfield, IL
Primary Contact: Melissa Gross, Interim Administrator
**Control:** State–Government, nonfederal **Service:** Psychiatric

**Staffed Beds:** 245 **Admissions:** 252 **Census:** 240 **Outpatient Visits:** 0 **Births:** 0 **Total Expense ($000):** 35613 **Payroll Expense ($000):** 28565 **Personnel:** 449

☐ **MEMORIAL HOSPITAL (141338)**, 1900 State Street, Zip 62233–1116, Mailing Address: P.O. Box 609, Zip 62233–0609; tel. 618/826–4581, (Nonreporting) **A**1 9 10 18
Primary Contact: Steven A. Hayes, Administrator
CFO: Gail Miesner, Chief Financial Officer
CMO: Alan Liefer, M.D., President Medical Staff
CIO: Becky Bunselmeyer, Director Information Services
CHR: May Rose, Director Human Resources
Web address: www.mhchester.com
**Control:** Hospital district or authority, Government, nonfederal **Service:** General Medical and Surgical

**Staffed Beds:** 25

## CHICAGO—Cook County

**ADVOCATE BETHANY HOSPITAL** See RML Specialty Hospital

⊞ **ADVOCATE ILLINOIS MASONIC MEDICAL CENTER (140182)**, 836 West Wellington Avenue, Zip 60657–5193; tel. 773/975–1600 **A**1 2 3 5 8 9 10 12 13 **F**3 5 13 15 17 18 20 22 24 26 28 29 30 31 32 33 34 35 36 38 39 40 43 44 45 49 50 53 54 55 56 57 58 59 61 64 66 68 70 71 72 73 74 75 76 77 78 79 81 82 84 85 86 87 89 90 92 93 96 97 98 99 100 101 102 103 104 107 108 110 111 113 114 116 117 118 119 120 122 125 129 130 131 133 140 142 145 146 147 **P**6 8 **S** Advocate Health Care, Oak Brook, IL
Primary Contact: Susan Nordstrom Lopez, President
CFO: Jack Gilbert, Vice President Finance and Support Services
CMO: Robert Zadylak, M.D., Vice President Medical Management
CIO: Adem Arslani, Director Information Systems
CHR: Marc Senesac, Vice President Human Resources
CNO: Donna J. King, R.N., Vice President Clinical Operations and Chief Nursing Executive
Web address: www.advocatehealth.com/masonic
**Control:** Other not–for–profit (including NFP Corporation) **Service:** General Medical and Surgical

**Staffed Beds:** 335 **Admissions:** 16921 **Census:** 207 **Outpatient Visits:** 155438 **Births:** 2328 **Total Expense ($000):** 312421 **Payroll Expense ($000):** 134412 **Personnel:** 2252

⊞ **ADVOCATE TRINITY HOSPITAL (140048)**, 2320 East 93rd Street, Zip 60617–9984; tel. 773/967–2000 **A**1 9 10 **F**1 3 4 11 13 15 16 17 18 20 22 24 28 29 30 31 34 35 40 45 49 56 57 58 59 61 63 65 67 68 70 72 73 74 75 76 77 78 79 80 81 82 87 88 89 90 93 98 107 108 110 111 113 114 118 127 128 129 131 142 145 147 **P**5 8 **S** Advocate Health Care, Oak Brook, IL
Primary Contact: Jonathan R. Bruss, President
CFO: Maureen Morrison, Vice President Financial Services
CMO: Dianna Grant, M.D., Vice President Medical Management
CIO: Brenda Aranda, Director Communications and Government Relations
Web address: www.advocatehealth.com/trinity
**Control:** Other not–for–profit (including NFP Corporation) **Service:** General Medical and Surgical

**Staffed Beds:** 188 **Admissions:** 10905 **Census:** 115 **Outpatient Visits:** 86219 **Births:** 1309 **Total Expense ($000):** 152412 **Payroll Expense ($000):** 57887 **Personnel:** 964

⊞ **ANN & ROBERT H. LURIE CHILDREN'S HOSPITAL OF CHICAGO (143300)**, 225 East Chicago Avenue, Zip 60611–2605; tel. 312/227–4000 **A**1 2 3 5 8 9 10 **F**3 8 9 11 12 17 18 19 21 23 25 27 29 30 31 32 34 35 36 38 39 40 43 44 45 49 50 51 54 55 57 58 59 60 61 63 64 65 68 72 74 75 77 78 79 80 81 82 84 85 86 87 88 89 91 92 93 94 96 97 98 99 100 101 102 104 105 107 108 111 113 114 115 116 117 118 123 125 128 129 130 131 133 135 136 137 138 141 143 145 147
Primary Contact: Patrick M. Magoon, President and Chief Executive Officer
COO: Gordon B. Bass, Chief Operating Officer
CFO: Paula Noble, Chief Financial Officer and Treasurer
CMO: Edward S. Ogata, M.D., Chief Medical Officer
CIO: Stan Krok, Chief Information Officer
CHR: Barbara Bowman, Chief Human Resource Officer
Web address: www.luriechildrens.org
**Control:** Other not–for–profit (including NFP Corporation) **Service:** Children's general

**Staffed Beds:** 245 **Admissions:** 10897 **Census:** 180 **Outpatient Visits:** 486458 **Births:** 0 **Total Expense ($000):** 528536 **Payroll Expense ($000):** 229296 **Personnel:** 3385

☐ **AURORA CHICAGO LAKESHORE HOSPITAL (144005)**, 4840 North Marine Drive, Zip 60640–4296; tel. 773/878–9700, (Nonreporting) **A**1 3 5 9 10 **S** Aurora Behavioral Health Care, Corona, CA
Primary Contact: C. Alan Eaks, Chief Executive Officer
CFO: Carol Peart, Chief Financial Officer
CMO: Peter Nierman, M.D., Chief Medical Officer
CHR: Johanne Jeanty, Director Human Resources
Web address: www.chicagolakeshorehospital.com
**Control:** Corporation, Investor–owned, for–profit **Service:** Psychiatric

**Staffed Beds:** 108

**BERNARD MITCHELL HOSPITAL** See University of Chicago Medical Center

**CHICAGO LYING–IN HOSPITAL** See University of Chicago Medical Center

☐ **CHICAGO–READ MENTAL HEALTH CENTER (144010)**, 4200 North Oak Park Avenue, Zip 60634–1457; tel. 773/794–4000, (Nonreporting) **A**1 10 **S** Division of Mental Health, Department of Human Services, Springfield, IL
Primary Contact: Thomas Simpatico, M.D., Facility Director and Network System Manager
**Control:** State–Government, nonfederal **Service:** Psychiatric

**Staffed Beds:** 200

**CHILDREN'S MEMORIAL HOSPITAL** See Ann & Robert H. Lurie Children's Hospital of Chicago

⊞ **HARTGROVE HOSPITAL (144026)**, 5730 West Roosevelt Road, Zip 60644; tel. 773/413–1700, (Nonreporting) **A**1 9 10 **S** Universal Health Services, Inc., King of Prussia, PA
Primary Contact: Steven Airhart, Chief Executive Officer
CFO: Srbo Nikolic, Chief Financial Officer
CMO: Johnny Williamson, M.D., Chief Medical Officer
CHR: Anthony Rivera, Director Human Resources
CNO: Jody Bhambra, Chief Nursing Officer
Web address: www.uhsinc.com
**Control:** Corporation, Investor–owned, for–profit **Service:** Psychiatric

**Staffed Beds:** 128

---

**Hospital, Medicare Provider Number, Address, Telephone, Approval, Facility, and Physician Codes, Health Care System**

★ American Hospital Association (AHA) membership
☐ The Joint Commission accreditation
◇ DNV Healthcare Inc. accreditation
○ American Osteopathic Association (AOA) accreditation
△ Commission on Accreditation of Rehabilitation Facilities (CARF) accreditation

IL

★ ○ **HOLY CROSS HOSPITAL (140133)**, 2701 West 68th Street,
Zip 60629–1882; tel. 773/884–9000, (Nonreporting) **A**9 10 11
Primary Contact: Wayne M. Lerner, DPH, President and Chief Executive Officer
COO: Paul M. Teodo, Chief Operating Officer
CFO: Loren Chandler, Interim, Vice President and Chief Financial Officer
CMO: Catherine Kallal, M.D., Chief Medical Officer
CIO: Ken Slawkowski, Interim Director Information Systems
CHR: Doris Gutierrez, Director Human Resources
CNO: Katherine Loeb, R.N., Interim Vice President, Patient Care Services
Web address: www.holycrosshospital.org
**Control:** Corporation, Investor–owned, for–profit **Service:** General Medical and Surgical

| Staffed Beds: 160 |
| --- |

△ **JACKSON PARK HOSPITAL AND MEDICAL CENTER (140177)**, 7531 Stony Island Avenue, Zip 60649–3993; tel. 773/947–7500 **A**7 9 10 **F**3 5 18 19 29 30 31 34 38 40 56 57 59 61 63 64 65 66 68 70 75 76 77 78 79 81 82 84 85 87 89 92 93 97 98 100 101 102 103 104 105 107 108 109 110 114 118 129 131 134 143 147 **P**6
Primary Contact: Merritt J. Hasbrouck, President
COO: Randall Smith, Executive Vice President
CFO: Nelson Vasquez, Vice President Finance
CMO: Bangalore Murthy, M.D., Director Medical Staff
CIO: Thomas Pankow, Chief Information Officer
CHR: Tracey Jones, Director Human Resources
Web address: www.jacksonparkhospital.org
**Control:** Other not–for–profit (including NFP Corporation) **Service:** General Medical and Surgical

| Staffed Beds: 260 Admissions: 10429 Census: 117 Outpatient Visits: 53372 Births: 239 Total Expense ($000): 92201 Payroll Expense ($000): 38285 Personnel: 730 |
| --- |

☒ △ **JESSE BROWN VETERANS AFFAIRS CHICAGO HEALTH CARE SYSTEM**, 820 South Damen, Zip 60612–3776; tel. 312/569–8387 **A**1 3 5 7 8 9 **F**4 5 8 12 15 18 20 22 24 26 28 29 30 31 33 35 38 39 40 43 45 46 48 49 50 53 54 56 57 58 59 60 61 62 63 64 65 70 74 75 77 78 79 81 82 83 84 86 87 90 91 93 94 97 98 100 101 102 103 104 106 107 111 114 118 125 127 128 129 131 134 142 143 145 146 147 **P**6 **S** Department of Veterans Affairs, Washington, DC
Primary Contact: Michael A. Anaya, Sr., FACHE, Medical Center Director
COO: Michelle Blakely, Associate Director
CFO: Kalpana Mehta, Chief Fiscal Services
CMO: Wendy W. Brown, M.D., Chief of Staff
CIO: Howard Loewenstein, Chief Information Resource Management Services
CHR: Wayne Davis, Manager Human Resources
Web address: www.va.gov/sta/guide/home.asp
**Control:** Veterans Affairs, Government, federal **Service:** General Medical and Surgical

| Staffed Beds: 240 Admissions: 9819 Census: 240 Outpatient Visits: 897361 Births: 0 Total Expense ($000): 394717 Payroll Expense ($000): 250000 Personnel: 2437 |
| --- |

☒ **JOHN H. STROGER JR. HOSPITAL OF COOK COUNTY (140124)**, 1901 West Harrison Street, Zip 60612–3785; tel. 312/864–6000 **A**1 2 3 5 8 9 10 **F**3 5 11 13 15 16 17 18 19 20 22 24 28 29 30 31 35 36 38 39 40 41 42 43 44 45 46 47 48 49 52 54 55 56 58 60 61 64 65 68 70 72 74 75 76 77 78 79 81 82 84 85 86 87 88 89 91 92 93 94 97 99 100 101 102 103 104 107 110 111 113 114 117 118 120 128 129 131 133 134 145 146 147 **P**6 **S** Cook County Bureau of Health Services, Chicago, IL
Primary Contact: Carol L. Schneider, Chief Operating Officer
COO: Carol L. Schneider, Chief Operating Officer
CFO: John R. Morales, Chief Financial Officer
CMO: Claudia Fegan, M.D., Chief Medical Officer
CIO: Bala Hota, Interim Chief Information Officer
CHR: Paris I. Partee, Associate Administrator and Director Human Resources
CNO: Antoinette Williams, Chief Nursing Officer
Web address: www.cookcountyhealth.net
**Control:** County–Government, nonfederal **Service:** General Medical and Surgical

| Staffed Beds: 460 Admissions: 23133 Census: 317 Outpatient Visits: 724215 Births: 813 Payroll Expense ($000): 335904 Personnel: 4713 |
| --- |

**JOHNSTON R. BOWMAN HEALTH CENTER** See Rush University Medical Center

**KINDRED CHICAGO LAKESHORE** See Kindred Chicago–Central Hospital

★ **KINDRED CHICAGO–CENTRAL HOSPITAL (142009)**, 4058 West Melrose Street, Zip 60641–4797; tel. 773/736–7000, (Includes KINDRED CHICAGO LAKESHORE, 6130 North Sheridan Road, Zip 60660; tel. 773/381–1222; Diane Otteman, Chief Executive Officer; KINDRED HOSPITAL CHICAGO NORTH, 2544 West Montrose Avenue, Zip 60618–1589; tel. 773/267–2622; Larry Foster, R.N., MSN, Chief Executive Officer) **A**9 10 **F**1 3 29 82 129 147 **S** Kindred Healthcare, Louisville, KY
Primary Contact: Bruce Carey, Chief Executive Officer
COO: Joanne Garcia, Chief Operating Officer
CFO: Mary Treacy Shiff, Chief Financial Officer
Web address: www.khchicagocentral.com
**Control:** Corporation, Investor–owned, for–profit **Service:** Long–Term Acute Care hospital

| Staffed Beds: 54 Admissions: 701 Census: 47 Outpatient Visits: 0 Births: 0 Total Expense ($000): 25238 Payroll Expense ($000): 8189 Personnel: 129 |
| --- |

**KINDRED HOSPITAL CHICAGO NORTH** See Kindred Chicago–Central Hospital

☒ **LA RABIDA CHILDREN'S HOSPITAL (143301)**, East 65th Street at Lake Michigan, Zip 60649–1395; tel. 773/363–6700 **A**1 3 5 9 10 **F**3 12 28 29 30 32 34 35 38 40 41 50 57 58 59 64 65 74 75 77 79 82 85 86 87 89 91 93 96 97 99 100 102 104 129 131 133 142 143 145 147 **P**6
Primary Contact: Brenda J. Wolf, President and Chief Executive Officer
CFO: Mark Renfree, Chief Financial Officer
CMO: Dilek Bishku, M.D., Vice President Medical Affairs
CIO: Timothy Diamond, Chief Information Officer
CHR: Frances Lefkow, Director Human Resources
Web address: www.larabida.org
**Control:** Other not–for–profit (including NFP Corporation) **Service:** Children's chronic disease

| Staffed Beds: 49 Admissions: 852 Census: 28 Outpatient Visits: 31042 Births: 0 Total Expense ($000): 50808 Payroll Expense ($000): 23395 Personnel: 441 |
| --- |

☐ **LORETTO HOSPITAL (140083)**, 645 South Central Avenue, Zip 60644–9987; tel. 773/626–4300, (Nonreporting) **A**1 9 10
Primary Contact: Steven C. Drucker, President and Chief Executive Officer
CFO: John Valles, Senior Vice President and Chief Financial Officer
CMO: Amjad Khan, M.D., President Medical Staff
CIO: Ron Warren, Director Information Systems
CHR: Ruby Isom, Associate Vice President Human Resources
CNO: Marc Trznadel, Chief Nursing Officer
Web address: www.lorettohospital.org
**Control:** Other not–for–profit (including NFP Corporation) **Service:** General Medical and Surgical

| Staffed Beds: 187 |
| --- |

☒ **LOUIS A. WEISS MEMORIAL HOSPITAL (140082)**, 4646 North Marine Drive, Zip 60640–1501; tel. 773/878–8700 **A**1 2 3 5 9 10 **F**3 8 9 15 17 18 20 22 24 28 29 30 31 34 35 37 40 44 45 49 56 57 58 59 64 65 66 68 70 74 75 77 78 79 81 82 84 85 86 87 90 92 93 96 97 98 100 101 102 103 107 108 111 113 117 118 120 125 129 130 131 134 140 142 143 145 146 147 **P**6 **S** Vanguard Health System, Nashville, TN
Primary Contact: Jeffrey Steinberg, M.D., Chief Executive Officer
COO: James M. Renneker, MSN, Chief Operating Officer and Chief Nursing Officer
CFO: Jeffrey L. Meigs, Chief Financial Officer
CMO: Martin Siglin, M.D., Vice President Medical Affairs
CIO: Thomas Crawford, Chicago Market Chief Information Officer
CHR: Keoni Nader, Director Human Resources
Web address: www.weisshospital.com
**Control:** Corporation, Investor–owned, for–profit **Service:** General Medical and Surgical

| Staffed Beds: 184 Admissions: 7807 Census: 115 Outpatient Visits: 96075 Births: 0 Total Expense ($000): 138228 Payroll Expense ($000): 58515 Personnel: 804 |
| --- |

★ ○ **MERCY HOSPITAL AND MEDICAL CENTER (140158)**, 2525 South Michigan Avenue, Zip 60616–2477; tel. 312/567–2000 **A**2 3 5 9 10 11 **F**3 5 12 13 15 17 18 20 22 24 26 28 29 30 31 32 34 35 36 40 44 45 46 49 50 51 52 53 54 55 56 57 58 59 61 64 65 66 70 73 74 76 77 78 79 81 82 85 86 87 89 90 92 93 96 97 98 99 100 101 102 103 104 105 107 108 110 111 113 114 116 117 118 120 122 123 125 129 130 131 132 133 134 142 143 144 145 146 147 **P**5 **S** Trinity Health, Novi, MI
Primary Contact: Sister Sheila Lyne, President and Chief Executive Officer
COO: Richard Cerceo, Executive Vice President and Chief Operating Officer
CFO: Thomas J. Garvey, Chief Financial Officer
CMO: Warren Furey, M.D., Vice President Medical Affairs
CIO: Margaret Delaney, Chief Information Officer
CHR: Nancy L. Hill–Davis, Vice President Human Resources and Risk Management
CHR: Nancy L. Hill–Davis, Vice President Human Resources and Risk Management
Web address: www.mercy–chicago.org
**Control:** Other not–for–profit (including NFP Corporation) **Service:** General Medical and Surgical

| Staffed Beds: 291 Admissions: 16353 Census: 186 Outpatient Visits: 377168 Births: 2976 Total Expense ($000): 226441 Payroll Expense ($000): 95318 Personnel: 1578 |
| --- |

○ **METHODIST HOSPITAL OF CHICAGO (140197)**, 5025 North Paulina Street, Zip 60640–2797; tel. 773/271–9040, (Nonreporting) **A**9 10 11
Primary Contact: Steven H. Friedman, Ph.D., Executive Vice President
CFO: Harold Reisler, Controller
CIO: Bernie Ziegler, Manager Information Systems
Web address: www.bethanymethodist.org
**Control:** Other not–for–profit (including NFP Corporation) **Service:** General Medical and Surgical

| Staffed Beds: 189 |
| --- |

IL

*Many Facility Codes have changed. Please refer to the AHA Guide Code Chart.* © 2012 AHA Guide

⊠ △ **MOUNT SINAI HOSPITAL (140018)**, California Avenue at 15th Street, Zip 60608–1729; tel. 773/542–2000, (Includes SINAI CHILDREN'S HOSPITAL, California Avenue at 15th Street, Zip 60608; tel. 888/287–4624), (Nonreporting) **A**1 2 3 5 7 8 9 10 12 13 **S** Sinai Health System, Chicago, IL
Primary Contact: Alan H. Channing, President and Chief Executive Officer
COO: Karen Teitelbaum, Executive Vice President and Chief Operating Officer
CFO: Charles Weis, Chief Financial Officer
CMO: Jack Garon, M.D., Chief Medical Officer
CIO: Peter Ingram, Vice President and Chief Information Officer
CHR: Andrew Wissel, Director Human Resources
Web address: www.sinai.org
**Control:** Other not–for–profit (including NFP Corporation) **Service:** General Medical and Surgical

**Staffed Beds: 290**

⊠ **NORTHWESTERN MEMORIAL HOSPITAL (140281)**, 251 East Huron Street, Zip 60611–2908; tel. 312/926–2000, (Includes PRENTICE WOMEN'S HOSPITAL, 250 East Superior Street, Zip 60611; tel. 312/926–2000; STONE INSTITUTE OF PSYCHIATRY, 320 East Huron Street, Zip 60611; tel. 312/926–2000) **A**1 2 3 5 8 9 10 **F**3 4 5 6 8 9 11 12 13 14 15 17 18 20 22 24 26 28 29 30 31 32 33 34 35 36 37 38 39 40 43 44 45 46 47 48 49 50 51 52 53 54 55 56 57 58 59 60 61 62 63 64 65 66 68 70 72 73 74 75 76 77 78 79 80 81 82 83 84 85 86 87 92 93 97 98 99 100 101 102 103 104 105 106 107 108 110 111 113 114 115 116 117 118 119 120 122 123 125 128 129 130 131 133 134 135 136 137 138 140 141 142 143 144 145 146 147 **P**5 6 **S** Northwestern Memorial Healthcare, Chicago, IL
Primary Contact: Dean M. Harrison, President and Chief Executive Officer
COO: Dennis M. Murphy, Executive Vice President and Chief Operating Officer
CFO: Peter J. McCanna, Executive Vice President Administration and Chief Financial Officer
CMO: Michael G. Ankin, M.D., Vice President Medical Affairs & Chief Medical Officer
CIO: Timothy R. Zoph, Senior Vice President and Chief Information Officer
CHR: Dean Manheimer, Senior Vice President Human Resources
Web address: www.nmh.org
**Control:** Other not–for–profit (including NFP Corporation) **Service:** General Medical and Surgical

**Staffed Beds: 868 Admissions: 53626 Census: 700 Outpatient Visits: 604508 Births: 12241 Total Expense ($000): 1366947 Payroll Expense ($000): 460567 Personnel: 7104**

**NORWEGIAN AMERICAN HOSPITAL (140206)**, 1044 North Francisco Avenue, Zip 60622–2794; tel. 773/292–8200, (Nonreporting) **A**3 5 6 9 10
Primary Contact: Jose R. Sanchez, President and Chief Executive Officer
COO: Anthony Tedeschi, M.D., Chief Operating Officer
CFO: Duane Fitch, CPA, Chief Financial Officer
CMO: Mark Loafman, M.D., Vice President Medical Affairs
CIO: James Filkins, Chief Information Officer
CHR: Marcia Powers, Vice President Human Resources
Web address: www.nahospital.org
**Control:** Other not–for–profit (including NFP Corporation) **Service:** General Medical and Surgical

**Staffed Beds: 230**

★ ○ **OUR LADY OF THE RESURRECTION MEDICAL CENTER (140251)**, 5645 West Addison Street, Zip 60634–4403; tel. 773/282–7000, (Total facility includes 66 beds in nursing home–type unit) **A**9 10 11 **F**3 8 12 15 18 20 22 28 29 30 31 34 35 36 39 40 43 44 45 49 50 53 56 57 58 59 60 64 68 70 74 75 79 81 82 85 86 92 93 96 107 108 111 113 114 118 127 129 131 141 143 145 146 147 **P**5 8 **S** Presence Health, Chicago, IL
Primary Contact: Martin H. Judd, Executive Vice President and Chief Executive Officer
COO: Dennis FitzMaurice, Vice President, Professional Services
CFO: Donna Diblik, Chief Financial Officer
CMO: David Bordo, M.D., Vice President, Medical Affairs/Chief Medical Officer
CIO: George Chessum, Senior Vice President and Chief Information Officer
CHR: Ivy McKinley, Director Human Resources
CNO: Maryanne Bajgrowicz, Vice President, Patient Care Services/Chief Nursing Officer
Web address: www.reshealthcare.org
**Control:** Church–operated, Nongovernment, not–for profit **Service:** General Medical and Surgical

**Staffed Beds: 279 Admissions: 8600 Census: 133 Outpatient Visits: 106604 Births: 2 Total Expense ($000): 117372 Payroll Expense ($000): 44095 Personnel: 777**

**PRENTICE WOMEN'S HOSPITAL** See Northwestern Memorial Hospital

⊠ **PROVIDENT HOSPITAL OF COOK COUNTY (140300)**, 500 East 51st Street, Zip 60615–2494; tel. 312/572–2000 **A**1 3 5 9 10 **F**3 15 18 29 30 40 45 51 68 75 77 81 85 87 107 109 117 118 129 131 **S** Cook County Bureau of Health Services, Chicago, IL
Primary Contact: Robert Hamilton, Chief Operating Officer
COO: Michele T. Thompson, Deputy Chief Operating Officer
CFO: Barbara Patterson, Chief Financial Officer
CMO: Aaron Hamb, M.D., Chief Medical Officer
CIO: Donna Hart, Chief Information Officer
Web address: www.ccbhs.org/pages/ProvidentHospitalofCookCounty.htm
**Control:** County–Government, nonfederal **Service:** General Medical and Surgical

**Staffed Beds: 25 Admissions: 2198 Census: 20 Outpatient Visits: 43176 Total Expense ($000): 75972 Payroll Expense ($000): 40741 Personnel: 250**

⊠ **REHABILITATION INSTITUTE OF CHICAGO (143026)**, 345 East Superior Street, Zip 60611–4496; tel. 312/238–1000, (Nonreporting) **A**1 3 5 9 10
Primary Contact: Joanne C. Smith, M.D., President and Chief Executive Officer
COO: Peggy Kirk, Senior Vice President Clinical Operations
CFO: Ed Case, Executive Vice President and Chief Financial Officer
CMO: James Sliwa, M.D., Chief Medical Officer
CIO: Tim McKula, Vice President Information Systems and Chief Information Officer
CHR: Lois Huggins, Chief Human Resources Officer and Senior Vice President Human Resources
Web address: www.ric.org
**Control:** Other not–for–profit (including NFP Corporation) **Service:** Rehabilitation

**Staffed Beds: 182**

★ ○ △ **RESURRECTION MEDICAL CENTER (140117)**, 7435 West Talcott Avenue, Zip 60631–3746; tel. 773/774–8000, (Nonreporting) **A**2 3 5 7 9 10 11 13 **S** Presence Health, Chicago, IL
Primary Contact: John D. Baird, Chief Executive Officer
CFO: John Orsini, Executive Vice President Finance and Chief Financial Officer
CMO: Victor McKarry, M.D., President Medical Staff
CIO: George Chessum, Senior Vice President Information Systems and Chief Information Officer
CHR: Paul Skiem, Senior Vice President Human Resources
Web address: www.reshealthcare.org
**Control:** Church–operated, Nongovernment, not–for profit **Service:** General Medical and Surgical

**Staffed Beds: 402**

★ **RML SPECIALTY HOSPITAL (142012)**, 3435 West Van Buren Street, Zip 60624–3399; tel. 773/826–6300 **A**9 10 **F**1 3 29 30 31 40 50 58 74 85 87 107 113 118 129 131 145 147
Primary Contact: James R. Prister, President and Chief Executive Officer
COO: Ken Pawola, Chief Operating Officer
CFO: Tom Pater, Vice President Finance and Chief Financial Officer
CMO: Joseph Rosman, M.D., Chief Medical Director
CIO: Julie Ames, Chief Information Officer
CHR: John Landstrom, Vice President Human Resources and Operations
Web address: www.rmlspecialtyhospital.org
**Control:** Other not–for–profit (including NFP Corporation) **Service:** Long–Term Acute Care hospital

**Staffed Beds: 68 Admissions: 393 Census: 32 Outpatient Visits: 882 Births: 0 Total Expense ($000): 25004 Payroll Expense ($000): 12937 Personnel: 253**

○ **ROSELAND COMMUNITY HOSPITAL (140068)**, 45 West 111th Street, Zip 60628–4294; tel. 773/995–3000, (Nonreporting) **A**9 10 11
Primary Contact: Dian Powell, Chief Executive Officer
CMO: Rogelio Cave, M.D., Medical Director
CIO: William Spence, Director
CHR: Brenda Mitchell, Director Human Resources
Web address: www.roselandhospital.org
**Control:** Other not–for–profit (including NFP Corporation) **Service:** General Medical and Surgical

**Staffed Beds: 115**

IL

---

**Hospital, Medicare Provider Number, Address, Telephone, Approval, Facility, and Physician Codes, Health Care System**

★ American Hospital Association (AHA) membership
□ The Joint Commission accreditation
◇ DNV Healthcare Inc. accreditation
○ American Osteopathic Association (AOA) accreditation
△ Commission on Accreditation of Rehabilitation Facilities (CARF) accreditation

☒ △ **RUSH UNIVERSITY MEDICAL CENTER (140119)**, 1653 West Congress Parkway, Zip 60612–3833; tel. 312/942–5000, (Includes JOHNSTON R. BOWMAN HEALTH CENTER, 700 South Paulina, Zip 60612; tel. 312/942–7000) **A**1 2 3 5 7 8 9 10 **F**8 9 11 12 13 14 15 16 18 19 20 21 22 23 24 25 26 27 29 30 31 32 34 35 36 38 40 44 45 46 47 48 49 50 51 52 55 56 57 58 59 60 61 64 65 66 68 74 75 77 78 79 81 82 84 85 86 87 91 92 93 94 95 96 97 99 100 101 102 103 104 107 108 111 113 114 115 116 117 118 119 120 122 123 124 125 128 129 130 131 133 134 135 136 137 138 140 141 144 145 146 147 **S** Rush University Medical Center, Chicago, IL
Primary Contact: Peter W. Butler, President and Chief Operating Officer
CMO: David A. Ansell, M.D., Vice President and Chief Medical Officer
CIO: Lac Tran, Senior Vice President Information Services
CHR: Sheri L. Marker, Vice President Human Resources
CNO: Cynthia Barginere, MSN, Vice President Clinical Nursing and Chief Nursing Officer
Web address: www.rush.edu
**Control:** Other not–for–profit (including NFP Corporation) **Service:** General Medical and Surgical

| **Staffed Beds:** 664 **Admissions:** 30259 **Census:** 462 **Outpatient Visits:** 415508 **Births:** 2142 **Total Expense ($000):** 812159 **Payroll Expense ($000):** 274526 |

○ **SACRED HEART HOSPITAL (140151)**, 3240 West Franklin Boulevard, Zip 60624–1599; tel. 773/722–3020, (Nonreporting) **A**9 10 11
Primary Contact: Edward Novak, President and Chief Executive Officer
CFO: Roy Payawal, Executive Vice President Finance
Web address: www.sacredheartchicago.com/
**Control:** Corporation, Investor–owned, for–profit **Service:** General Medical and Surgical

| **Staffed Beds:** 96 |

☒ **SAINT ANTHONY HOSPITAL (140095)**, 2875 West 19th Street, Zip 60623–3596; tel. 773/484–1000 **A**1 5 9 10 **F**3 13 15 18 29 30 31 32 33 34 35 40 41 44 49 50 51 54 56 57 59 64 65 66 68 70 74 75 76 77 78 79 81 82 85 86 87 89 93 96 97 98 99 100 102 104 105 107 111 114 117 118 129 130 131 142 145 146 147 **P**1
Primary Contact: Guy A. Medaglia, President and Chief Executive Officer
CFO: Charles R. Brobst, Senior Vice President and Chief Financial Officer
CIO: Mark Jennings, Chief Information Officer
CHR: Michelle C. Morgan, Chief Human Resource Manager
CNO: Jill Stemmerman, R.N., Vice President Nursing
Web address: www.saintanthonyhospital.org
**Control:** Church–operated, Nongovernment, not–for profit **Service:** General Medical and Surgical

| **Staffed Beds:** 139 **Admissions:** 7039 **Census:** 84 **Outpatient Visits:** 94998 **Births:** 1797 **Total Expense ($000):** 93921 **Payroll Expense ($000):** 46271 **Personnel:** 818 |

★ ○ **SAINT JOSEPH HOSPITAL (140224)**, 2900 North Lake Shore Drive, Zip 60657–6274; tel. 773/665–3000, (Total facility includes 26 beds in nursing home–type unit) **A**2 3 5 9 10 11 **F**3 4 11 12 13 15 18 20 22 24 26 28 29 30 31 32 34 35 36 38 39 44 45 50 53 54 56 57 58 59 60 63 64 65 66 68 70 74 75 76 77 78 79 81 82 84 85 86 87 89 90 93 96 97 98 100 101 103 104 105 107 108 111 113 114 116 118 120 125 127 128 129 130 131 132 134 142 144 145 146 147 **S** Presence Health, Chicago, IL
Primary Contact: Roberta Luskin–Hawk, M.D., Chief Executive Officer
CFO: Stanley Kazmierczak, Controller
CMO: M. Todd Grendon, M.D., President Medical Staff
CIO: George Chessum, Senior Vice President Information Systems and Chief Information Officer
CHR: Denise Brown, Vice President Human Resources
Web address: www.reshealth.org
**Control:** Church–operated, Nongovernment, not–for profit **Service:** General Medical and Surgical

| **Staffed Beds:** 327 **Admissions:** 12724 **Census:** 187 **Outpatient Visits:** 180976 **Births:** 1689 **Total Expense ($000):** 187813 **Payroll Expense ($000):** 63437 **Personnel:** 1074 |

★ ○ **SAINTS MARY & ELIZABETH MEDICAL CENTER (140180)**, 2233 West Division Street, Zip 60622–3086; tel. 312/770–2000, (Includes SAINTS MARY & ELIZABETH MEDICAL CENTER, CLAREMONT AVENUE, 1431 North Claremont Avenue, Zip 60622–1791; tel. 773/278–2000; Margaret McDermott, Chief Executive Officer), (Total facility includes 26 beds in nursing home–type unit) **A**2 9 10 11 **F**3 4 5 13 15 17 18 19 20 22 24 26 28 29 30 31 32 34 35 36 40 45 47 49 50 51 57 58 59 60 64 65 66 68 70 72 74 75 76 77 78 79 81 82 85 86 87 89 90 92 93 96 97 98 99 100 101 102 103 104 105 106 107 108 110 111 113 114 117 118 120 122 127 128 129 131 134 142 145 146 147 **P**8 **S** Presence Health, Chicago, IL
Primary Contact: Margaret McDermott, Chief Executive Officer
CFO: Kenneth A. Kautzer, Senior Vice President Finance and Treasurer
CIO: Steven Smith, Chief Information Officer
Web address: www.stmaryofnazareth.org
**Control:** Church–operated, Nongovernment, not–for profit **Service:** General Medical and Surgical

| **Staffed Beds:** 495 **Admissions:** 22846 **Census:** 346 **Outpatient Visits:** 183041 **Births:** 1863 **Total Expense ($000):** 260998 **Payroll Expense ($000):** 96386 **Personnel:** 1569 |

☒ △ **SCHWAB REHABILITATION HOSPITAL (143025)**, 1401 South California Avenue, Zip 60608–1858; tel. 773/522–2010, (Nonreporting) **A**1 7 9 10 **S** Sinai Health System, Chicago, IL
Primary Contact: Alan H. Channing, President and Chief Executive Officer
COO: Karen Teitelbaum, Executive Vice President and Chief Operating Officer
CFO: Charles Weis, Chief Financial Officer
CMO: Susan Rayner, M.D., Executive Vice President
CIO: Peter Ingram, Vice President and Chief Information Officer
CHR: Andrew Wissel, Director Human Resources
Web address: www.schwabrehab.org
**Control:** Other not–for–profit (including NFP Corporation) **Service:** Rehabilitation

| **Staffed Beds:** 101 |

□ **SHRINERS HOSPITALS FOR CHILDREN–CHICAGO (143302)**, 2211 North Oak Park Avenue, Zip 60707–3392; tel. 773/622–5400, (Nonreporting) **A**1 3 5 10 **S** Shriners Hospitals for Children, Tampa, FL
Primary Contact: Terry Wheat, R.N., Acting Administrator
CFO: Philip Magid, Director Fiscal Services
CMO: Jeffrey D. Ackman, M.D., Chief of Staff
CIO: Robert Gilb, Director Information Services
CHR: James E. Pawlowicz, Director Human Resources
Web address: www.shrinershospitals.org
**Control:** Other not–for–profit (including NFP Corporation) **Service:** Children's orthopedic

| **Staffed Beds:** 36 |

□ **SOUTH SHORE HOSPITAL (140181)**, 8012 South Crandon Avenue, Zip 60617–1199; tel. 773/768–0810, (Nonreporting) **A**1 9 10
Primary Contact: Jesus M. Ong, President
CFO: Timothy Caveney, Chief Financial Officer
CMO: Abraham Jacob, M.D., President Medical Staff
CIO: Jim Ritchie, Director Management Information Systems
CHR: Roger Rak, Director Human Resources
Web address: www.southshorehospital.com
**Control:** Other not–for–profit (including NFP Corporation) **Service:** General Medical and Surgical

| **Staffed Beds:** 125 |

□ △ **ST. BERNARD HOSPITAL AND HEALTH CARE CENTER (140103)**, 326 West 64th Street, Zip 60621–3146; tel. 773/962–3900, (Nonreporting) **A**1 7 9 10
Primary Contact: Sister Elizabeth Van Straten, President and Chief Executive Officer
COO: Janet G. Nohos, Executive Vice President
CFO: Guy Alton, Chief Financial Officer
CIO: Guy Alton, Chief Financial Officer
CHR: Donna Dertz, Director Human Resources
Web address: www.stbernardhospital.com
**Control:** Church–operated, Nongovernment, not–for profit **Service:** General Medical and Surgical

| **Staffed Beds:** 194 |

★ ○ **SWEDISH COVENANT HOSPITAL (140114)**, 5145 North California Avenue, Zip 60625–3688; tel. 773/878–8200 **A**2 3 5 9 10 11 12 13 **F**3 12 13 15 18 19 20 22 24 26 28 29 30 31 32 34 35 36 38 39 40 43 45 46 47 49 50 53 56 57 58 59 60 62 64 68 70 74 75 76 78 79 81 82 84 85 86 87 89 90 92 93 96 97 98 100 101 102 103 104 105 107 108 110 111 113 114 116 117 118 120 122 125 127 128 129 130 131 133 134 142 145 146 147 **P**1 5 7
Primary Contact: Mark Newton, President and Chief Executive Officer
COO: Anthony Guaccio, Senior Vice President & Chief Operating Officer
CFO: Gary M. Krugel, Senior Vice President Operations and Chief Financial Officer
CIO: Karen Sheehan, Director Information Systems
CNO: Mary Shehan, R.N., Senior Vice President and Chief Nursing Officer
Web address: www.schosp.org
**Control:** Church–operated, Nongovernment, not–for profit **Service:** General Medical and Surgical

| **Staffed Beds:** 279 **Admissions:** 14064 **Census:** 195 **Outpatient Visits:** 249247 **Births:** 2199 **Total Expense ($000):** 246595 **Payroll Expense ($000):** 98359 **Personnel:** 1752 |

○ **THOREK MEMORIAL HOSPITAL (140115)**, 850 West Irving Park Road, Zip 60613–3077; tel. 773/525–6780, (Nonreporting) **A**2 9 10 11
Primary Contact: Edward Budd, President and Chief Executive Officer
COO: Peter N. Kamberos, Chief Operating Officer
CFO: Kevin J. Higdon, Chief Financial Officer
CMO: James Diesfeld, M.D., President Medical Staff
CIO: Eric Dodd, Chief Information Officer
CHR: Brett Wakefield, Director Human Resources
CNO: Mary McCahill, Chief Nursing Officer
Web address: www.thorek.org
**Control:** Other not–for–profit (including NFP Corporation) **Service:** General Medical and Surgical

| **Staffed Beds:** 134 |

**UNIVERSITY OF CHICAGO COMER CHILDREN'S HOSPITAL** See University of Chicago Medical Center

*Many Facility Codes have changed. Please refer to the AHA Guide Code Chart.* © 2012 AHA Guide

☒ **UNIVERSITY OF CHICAGO MEDICAL CENTER (140088)**, 5841 South Maryland Avenue, Zip 60637–1447; tel. 773/702–1000, (Includes BERNARD MITCHELL HOSPITAL, 950 East 59th Street, Zip 60637; CHICAGO LYING–IN HOSPITAL, 950 East 59th Street, Zip 60637; tel. 312/684–6100; UNIVERSITY OF CHICAGO COMER CHILDREN'S HOSPITAL, 5721 South Maryland Avenue, Zip 60637; tel. 312/702–6168) **A**1 2 3 5 8 9 10 **F**3 6 7 9 11 12 13 14 15 16 17 18 19 20 21 22 23 24 25 26 27 28 29 30 31 32 34 35 36 37 38 39 40 41 43 44 45 46 47 48 49 50 51 52 54 55 56 57 58 59 60 61 62 63 64 65 68 70 71 72 73 74 75 76 77 78 79 80 81 82 83 84 85 86 87 88 89 92 93 96 97 99 100 101 102 103 104 107 108 110 111 113 114 115 116 117 118 119 120 122 123 125 128 129 130 131 133 134 135 136 137 138 139 140 141 142 143 144 145 146 147 **P**1
Primary Contact: Kenneth Polonsky, M.D., Chief Executive Officer
CFO: Richard Miller, Vice President Finance
CMO: Harvey Golomb, M.D., Chief Medical Officer
CIO: Eric Yablonka, Vice President and Chief Information Officer
CHR: Larry Callahan, Interim Vice President and Chief Human Resources Officer
Web address: www.uchospitals.edu
**Control:** Other not–for–profit (including NFP Corporation) **Service:** General Medical and Surgical

**Staffed Beds:** 558 **Admissions:** 22797 **Census:** 391 **Outpatient Visits:** 629269 **Births:** 1487 **Total Expense ($000):** 1107586 **Payroll Expense ($000):** 362610 **Personnel:** 7010

☒ △ **UNIVERSITY OF ILLINOIS HOSPITAL & HEALTH SCIENCES SYSTEM (140150)**, 1740 West Taylor Street, Zip 60612–7236; tel. 312/996–7000 **A**1 2 3 5 7 8 9 10 **F**3 9 12 13 14 15 17 18 19 20 21 22 23 24 25 26 27 28 29 30 31 32 34 35 37 38 39 40 41 45 46 47 48 49 50 52 54 55 56 57 58 59 60 61 64 65 66 68 70 72 73 74 75 76 77 78 79 81 82 85 86 87 88 89 90 91 92 93 96 97 98 99 100 101 102 103 104 105 107 108 110 111 113 114 115 116 117 118 120 122 123 125 129 130 131 133 134 135 137 138 140 141 143 144 145 146 147 **P**4
Primary Contact: John J. DeNardo, Chief Executive Officer
COO: David Loffing, Chief Operating Officer
CFO: William Devoney, Chief Financial Officer
CMO: William Chamberlin, M.D., Chief Medical Officer
CIO: Rose Ann Laureto, Chief Information Officer
CHR: John R. Loya, Vice Chancellor Human Resources
Web address: www.hospital.uillinois.edu/
**Control:** State–Government, nonfederal **Service:** General Medical and Surgical

**Staffed Beds:** 483 **Admissions:** 17984 **Census:** 314 **Outpatient Visits:** 486828 **Births:** 2453 **Total Expense ($000):** 657243 **Payroll Expense ($000):** 267174 **Personnel:** 3887

**CHICAGO HEIGHTS—Cook County**

**ST. JAMES HOSPITAL AND HEALTH CENTERS – CHICAGO HEIGHTS CAMPUS** See Franciscan St. James Hospital and Health Centers, Olympia Fields

**CLINTON—De Witt County**

★ **DR. JOHN WARNER HOSPITAL (141303)**, 422 West White Street, Zip 61727–2199; tel. 217/935–9571 **A**9 10 18 **F**3 7 8 11 15 28 29 34 40 45 53 54 57 59 64 68 70 75 77 81 82 85 87 90 93 97 107 110 126 127 128 129 131 132 147 **P**6
Primary Contact: Earl N. Sheehy, Chief Executive Officer
CFO: Donna Wisner, Chief Financial Officer
CMO: Brit Williams, M.D., President Medical Staff
CIO: Larry Schleicher, Manager Information Services
CHR: Jennie Wernecke, Human Resources Manager
CNO: Heidi Cook, Chief Nursing Officer
Web address: www.djwhospital.org
**Control:** City–Government, nonfederal **Service:** General Medical and Surgical

**Staffed Beds:** 25 **Admissions:** 316 **Census:** 3 **Outpatient Visits:** 17486 **Births:** 0 **Total Expense ($000):** 15819 **Payroll Expense ($000):** 7501 **Personnel:** 163

**DANVILLE—Vermilion County**

☒ **PROVENA UNITED SAMARITANS MEDICAL CENTER (140093)**, 812 North Logan, Zip 61832–3788; tel. 217/443–5000 **A**1 2 9 10 19 **F**3 11 13 15 18 20 28 29 30 31 34 35 40 45 46 47 48 49 50 57 59 64 70 74 75 76 77 78 79 81 82 83 85 86 87 89 93 102 107 108 110 111 113 114 117 118 119 120 123 128 129 131 134 145 146 **S** Presence Health, Chicago, IL
Primary Contact: Michael L. Brown, President and Chief Executive Officer
COO: Jennifer Cord, Vice President of Operations
CFO: Deborah Schimerowski, Chief Financial Officer
CMO: Charles Canver, M.D., Chief Medical Officer
CIO: Paula Keele, Manager Information Systems
CIO: Jason Wheatley, Manager Information Systems
CHR: Janet S. Payne, Vice President Human Resources
CNO: Molly Nicholson, R.N., Vice President of Patient Care/Chief Nurse Executive
Web address: www.provena.org/usmc
**Control:** Church–operated, Nongovernment, not–for profit **Service:** General Medical and Surgical

**Staffed Beds:** 127 **Admissions:** 6421 **Census:** 63 **Outpatient Visits:** 197830 **Births:** 679 **Total Expense ($000):** 96560 **Payroll Expense ($000):** 34233 **Personnel:** 665

☒ △ **VETERANS AFFAIRS ILLIANA HEALTH CARE SYSTEM**, 1900 East Main Street, Zip 61832–5198; tel. 217/554–3000, (Total facility includes 186 beds in nursing home–type unit) **A**1 3 5 7 9 **F**1 3 5 6 8 12 29 30 33 34 35 36 38 39 40 44 45 46 50 51 53 54 56 57 59 61 62 63 64 65 66 74 75 77 79 81 82 83 84 85 86 87 92 93 94 96 97 98 100 101 102 103 104 106 107 108 111 118 126 127 128 129 131 134 143 145 146 147 **P**6 **S** Department of Veterans Affairs, Washington, DC
Primary Contact: Michael E. Hamilton, Director
COO: Diana Carranza, Associate Director
CFO: Becky Tissier, Chief Fiscal Service
CMO: Khiem Tran, M.D., Acting Chief of Staff
CIO: Sherry Boone, Chief Information Resource Management
CHR: Connie Ohl, Acting Chief Human Resources
Web address: www.va.gov/sta/guide/home.asp
**Control:** Veterans Affairs, Government, federal **Service:** General Medical and Surgical

**Staffed Beds:** 245 **Admissions:** 3369 **Census:** 187 **Outpatient Visits:** 324540 **Births:** 0 **Total Expense ($000):** 219882 **Payroll Expense ($000):** 117760 **Personnel:** 1479

**DECATUR—Macon County**

☒ △ **DECATUR MEMORIAL HOSPITAL (140135)**, 2300 North Edward Street, Zip 62526–4192; tel. 217/876–8121 **A**1 2 3 5 7 9 10 19 **F**3 11 12 13 14 15 17 18 20 22 24 26 28 29 30 31 34 40 45 46 47 48 49 51 53 54 56 57 58 59 60 61 62 63 64 65 69 70 73 74 75 76 77 78 79 81 82 86 87 89 91 92 93 94 96 107 108 110 111 112 113 114 115 116 117 118 119 120 122 125 127 128 129 130 131 132 142 143 144 145 146 147 **P**8
Primary Contact: Kenneth L. Smithmier, President and Chief Executive Officer
COO: Timothy D. Stone, Executive Vice President and Chief Operating Officer
CFO: Gary G. Peacock, Senior Vice President and Chief Financial Officer
CMO: Michael Zia, M.D., Vice President Quality Systems and Medical Affairs
CIO: James Blackwell, Director Information Systems
CHR: Kevin Horath, Director Human Resources
CNO: Linda L. Fahey, MS, Vice President and Chief Nurse Executive
Web address: www.dmhcares.org
**Control:** Other not–for–profit (including NFP Corporation) **Service:** General Medical and Surgical

**Staffed Beds:** 188 **Admissions:** 11941 **Census:** 130 **Outpatient Visits:** 305495 **Births:** 949 **Total Expense ($000):** 269338 **Payroll Expense ($000):** 110131 **Personnel:** 2089

☒ △ **ST. MARY'S HOSPITAL (140166)**, 1800 East Lake Shore Drive, Zip 62521–3883; tel. 217/464–2966, (Total facility includes 14 beds in nursing home–type unit) **A**1 3 5 7 9 10 **F**2 3 5 11 13 15 18 20 22 28 29 30 31 34 35 40 44 45 50 54 56 57 59 64 66 70 74 75 76 77 78 79 81 82 85 86 87 89 90 92 93 96 98 99 100 101 102 103 104 105 107 108 110 111 113 114 116 118 119 120 122 123 127 128 129 130 131 140 141 145 147 **P**7 **S** Hospital Sisters Health System, Springfield, IL
Primary Contact: Kevin F. Kast, President and Chief Executive Officer
COO: Theresa Rutherford, R.N., Chief Operating Officer
CFO: Rebecca Colker, Chief Financial Officer
CHR: Terri Kuhle, Director Human Resources
Web address: www.stmarys–hospital.com
**Control:** Church–operated, Nongovernment, not–for profit **Service:** General Medical and Surgical

**Staffed Beds:** 220 **Admissions:** 7145 **Census:** 93 **Outpatient Visits:** 156623 **Births:** 671 **Total Expense ($000):** 125564 **Payroll Expense ($000):** 41366 **Personnel:** 918

IL

**Hospital, Medicare Provider Number, Address, Telephone, Approval, Facility, and Physician Codes, Health Care System**

★ American Hospital Association (AHA) membership
□ The Joint Commission accreditation
◇ DNV Healthcare Inc. accreditation
○ American Osteopathic Association (AOA) accreditation
△ Commission on Accreditation of Rehabilitation Facilities (CARF) accreditation

## DEKALB—DeKalb County

⊞ **KISHWAUKEE COMMUNITY HOSPITAL (140286)**, 1 Kish Hospital Drive, Zip 60115–9602, Mailing Address: P.O. Box 707, Zip 60115–0707; tel. 815/756–1521 **A**1 2 9 10 **F**3 8 11 13 15 18 20 22 26 28 29 30 31 32 34 35 36 37 40 43 45 46 48 49 57 58 59 60 64 68 70 71 73 74 75 76 77 78 79 81 82 85 86 87 89 93 96 102 104 107 108 110 111 113 114 116 117 118 128 129 130 131 132 134 142 144 145 146 147 **P**8 **S** Kish Health System, De Kalb, IL
Primary Contact: Brad Copple, President
COO: Brad Copple, President
CFO: Loren Foelske, Vice President Finance
CMO: Michael Kulisz, D.O., Chief Medical Officer
CIO: Heath Bell, Chief Information Officer
CHR: Mark Thate, Vice President Human Resources
CNO: Pamela Duffy, Vice President Patient Care Services and Chief Nursing Officer
Web address: www.kishhospital.org
**Control:** Other not–for–profit (including NFP Corporation) **Service:** General Medical and Surgical

**Staffed Beds:** 94 **Admissions:** 6029 **Census:** 57 **Outpatient Visits:** 141944 **Births:** 893 **Total Expense ($000):** 137155 **Payroll Expense ($000):** 38580 **Personnel:** 741

## DES PLAINES—Cook County

★ ○ **HOLY FAMILY MEDICAL CENTER (142011)**, 100 North River Road, Zip 60016–1255; tel. 847/297–1800, (Nonreporting) **A**9 10 11 **S** Presence Health, Chicago, IL
Primary Contact: Pamela Bell, R.N., Chief Executive Officer
CFO: John Orsini, Executive Vice President and Chief Financial Officer
CMO: Manish Tanna, M.D., President Medical Staff
CIO: George Chessum, Senior Vice President Information Systems and Chief Information Officer
CHR: Paul Skiem, Senior Vice President Human Resources
CNO: Marti Edwards, MSN, Vice President Patient Care Services
Web address: www.reshealth.org
**Control:** Church–operated, Nongovernment, not–for profit **Service:** Long–Term Acute Care hospital

**Staffed Beds:** 118

☐ **MARYVILLE SCOTT NOLAN CENTER**, 555 Wilson Lane, Zip 60016; tel. 847/768–5430 **A**1 9 **F**29 98 99
Primary Contact: Randall Autry, Administrator
CFO: Timothy J. Morgan, Chief Financial Officer
CMO: Shiraz Butt, M.D., Medical Director
CIO: Richard Arceo, Director Information Technology
CHR: Betty Barnes, Director Human Resources
Web address: www.maryvilleacademy.org
**Control:** Church–operated, Nongovernment, not–for profit **Service:** Children's hospital psychiatric

**Staffed Beds:** 113 **Admissions:** 933 **Census:** 33 **Outpatient Visits:** 0 **Births:** 0 **Total Expense ($000):** 10756 **Payroll Expense ($000):** 5031 **Personnel:** 144

## DIXON—Lee County

★ **KATHERINE SHAW BETHEA HOSPITAL (140012)**, 403 East First Street, Zip 61021–3187; tel. 815/288–5531 **A**3 5 9 10 **F**3 5 11 13 15 18 20 22 28 29 30 31 32 33 34 35 36 38 40 43 44 45 46 47 49 50 52 54 56 57 59 62 63 64 65 66 68 69 70 71 74 75 77 78 79 81 84 85 86 87 89 91 93 94 97 98 99 100 101 102 103 104 105 107 108 110 111 114 117 118 128 129 130 131 133 134 143 144 145 146 **P**6
Primary Contact: David L. Schreiner, FACHE, President and Chief Executive Officer
CFO: Debra Didier, Vice President and Chief Financial Officer
CMO: Tim Appenheimer, M.D., Vice President and Chief Medical Officer
CIO: Timothy W. Broos, Vice President and Chief Information Officer
CHR: Suzanne M. Ravlin, Director Human Resources
CNO: Linda Clemen, R.N., Vice President and Chief Nursing Officer
Web address: www.ksbhospital.com
**Control:** Other not–for–profit (including NFP Corporation) **Service:** General Medical and Surgical

**Staffed Beds:** 80 **Admissions:** 4991 **Census:** 42 **Outpatient Visits:** 166337 **Births:** 341 **Total Expense ($000):** 110154 **Payroll Expense ($000):** 58437 **Personnel:** 829

## DOWNERS GROVE—Dupage County

⊞ **ADVOCATE GOOD SAMARITAN HOSPITAL (140288)**, 3815 Highland Avenue, Zip 60515–1590; tel. 630/275–5900 **A**1 2 3 5 9 10 **F**3 4 5 11 12 13 15 17 18 20 22 24 26 28 29 30 31 32 34 35 36 38 40 41 43 44 45 46 47 49 50 53 54 55 56 57 59 63 64 68 70 72 74 75 76 78 79 81 82 84 85 86 87 89 93 98 100 101 102 103 104 105 107 108 109 110 111 113 114 118 119 120 122 123 128 129 130 131 134 143 144 145 146 147 **P**8 **S** Advocate Health Care, Oak Brook, IL
Primary Contact: David S. Fox, President
COO: Marjorie A. Maurer, MSN, Vice President Operations and Chief Nursing Executive
CFO: Mary Treacy–Shiff, Vice President Finance
CMO: Charles Derus, M.D., Vice President Medical Management
CHR: Elizabeth Calby, Vice President Human Resources
Web address: www.advocatehealth.com/gsam
**Control:** Church–operated, Nongovernment, not–for profit **Service:** General Medical and Surgical

**Staffed Beds:** 326 **Admissions:** 19191 **Census:** 222 **Outpatient Visits:** 172855 **Births:** 1905 **Total Expense ($000):** 345762 **Payroll Expense ($000):** 131174 **Personnel:** 2151

## DU QUOIN—Perry County

⊞ **MARSHALL BROWNING HOSPITAL (141331)**, 900 North Washington Street, Zip 62832–1230, Mailing Address: P.O. Box 192, Zip 62832–0192; tel. 618/542–2146 **A**1 9 10 18 **F**3 11 15 28 29 35 40 59 69 81 85 93 107 108 113 118 124 126 128 132
Primary Contact: Edwin A. Gast, Chief Executive Officer
CFO: Brice Harsy, Chief Financial Officer
CHR: Sarah J. Dickey, Manager Personnel
Web address: www.marshallbrowninghospital.com
**Control:** Other not–for–profit (including NFP Corporation) **Service:** General Medical and Surgical

**Staffed Beds:** 25 **Admissions:** 587 **Census:** 8 **Outpatient Visits:** 30087 **Births:** 0 **Total Expense ($000):** 16086 **Payroll Expense ($000):** 6758 **Personnel:** 137

## EFFINGHAM—Effingham County

⊞ **ST. ANTHONY'S MEMORIAL HOSPITAL (140032)**, 503 North Maple Street, Zip 62401–2099; tel. 217/342–2121, (Total facility includes 13 beds in nursing home–type unit) **A**1 2 9 10 19 **F**3 8 11 13 15 18 19 20 28 29 30 31 34 37 40 45 57 59 60 62 64 65 68 70 76 79 81 82 85 89 93 107 108 110 111 113 114 117 118 127 128 129 131 145 146 147 **S** Hospital Sisters Health System, Springfield, IL
Primary Contact: Daniel J. Woods, President and Chief Executive Officer
COO: Robert W. Esker, Assistant Administrator
CFO: Dave Storm, Director Business Support
CHR: Kal Keitel, Manager Personnel Services
Web address: www.stanthonyshospital.org
**Control:** Church–operated, Nongovernment, not–for profit **Service:** General Medical and Surgical

**Staffed Beds:** 146 **Admissions:** 7042 **Census:** 73 **Outpatient Visits:** 248737 **Births:** 774 **Total Expense ($000):** 99830 **Payroll Expense ($000):** 31676 **Personnel:** 633

## ELDORADO—Saline County

**FERRELL HOSPITAL (141324)**, 1201 Pine Street, Zip 62930–1634; tel. 618/273–3361, (Nonreporting) **A**9 10 18 **S** Alliant Management Services, Louisville, KY
Primary Contact: Tom Barry, President and Chief Executive Officer
CFO: James Fraser, Chief Financial Officer
CIO: Doug Rash, Director Information Technology
CHR: Beth Anderton, Vice President Human Resources
Web address: www.ferrellhosp.org
**Control:** Other not–for–profit (including NFP Corporation) **Service:** General Medical and Surgical

**Staffed Beds:** 25

## ELGIN—Kane County

☐ **ELGIN MENTAL HEALTH CENTER (144037)**, 750 South State Street, Zip 60123–7692; tel. 847/742–1040, (Nonreporting) **A**1 5 10 **S** Division of Mental Health, Department of Human Services, Springfield, IL
Primary Contact: Amparo Lopez, Region Executive Director
CFO: Tajudeen Ibrahim, Interim Business Administrator
CMO: Malini Patel, M.D., Medical Director
CIO: Kelly Callahan, Public Information Officer
CHR: Darek Williams, Director Human Resources
Web address: www.dhs.state.il.us
**Control:** State–Government, nonfederal **Service:** Psychiatric

**Staffed Beds:** 500

⊠ △ **PROVENA SAINT JOSEPH HOSPITAL (140217)**, 77 North Airlite Street, Zip 60123–4912; tel. 847/695–3200 **A**1 2 5 7 9 10 **F**5 11 12 15 17 18 20 22 24 26 28 29 30 31 34 35 36 37 38 40 42 43 44 49 50 53 54 56 57 58 59 60 61 62 63 64 65 68 69 70 74 75 77 78 79 81 82 84 85 86 87 90 93 94 96 97 98 99 100 101 102 103 104 105 107 108 111 113 114 115 116 118 119 120 122 123 129 131 133 134 142 143 144 145 146 147 **P**5
**S** Presence Health, Chicago, IL
Primary Contact: Eugene J. McMahon, M.D., President and Chief Executive Officer
COO: Laurence Dry, Vice President, Support and Ambulatory Services
CFO: Paul E. Belter, Chief Financial Officer
CIO: Trevor O'Malley, Site Manager
CHR: Diane Hargreaves, Vice President Human Resources
Web address: www.provena.org
**Control:** Other not–for–profit (including NFP Corporation) **Service:** General Medical and Surgical

**Staffed Beds:** 119 **Admissions:** 7537 **Census:** 119 **Outpatient Visits:** 167884 **Births:** 0 **Total Expense ($000):** 144305 **Payroll Expense ($000):** 51501 **Personnel:** 880

⊠ **SHERMAN HOSPITAL (140030)**, 1425 North Randall Road, Zip 60123–2300; tel. 847/742–9800 **A**1 2 9 10 **F**3 11 13 15 18 19 20 22 24 26 27 28 29 30 31 34 35 38 40 43 45 46 47 48 49 50 55 57 59 64 65 68 70 74 75 76 77 78 79 81 82 85 87 89 93 100 107 108 110 111 113 114 117 118 119 120 125 128 129 131 134 143 145 146 147 **P**8
Primary Contact: Richard B. Floyd, President and Chief Executive Officer
COO: Linda Deering, R.N., Executive Vice President and Chief Operating Officer
CFO: Eric Krueger, Vice President, Finance and Chief Financial Officer
CMO: Ian V. Jones, M.D., Vice President Clinical Performance
CHR: Katie Bata, Vice President Human Resources
CNO: Judith Balcitis, MS, Vice President, Nursing and Chief Nursing Officer
Web address: www.shermanhealthsystems.com
**Control:** Other not–for–profit (including NFP Corporation) **Service:** General Medical and Surgical

**Staffed Beds:** 255 **Admissions:** 14603 **Census:** 151 **Outpatient Visits:** 319543 **Births:** 2949 **Total Expense ($000):** 256816 **Payroll Expense ($000):** 90170 **Personnel:** 1758

### ELK GROVE VILLAGE—Cook County

⊠ △ **ALEXIAN BROTHERS MEDICAL CENTER (140258)**, 800 Biesterfield Road, Zip 60007–3397; tel. 847/437–5500, (Includes ALEXIAN REHABILITATION HOSPITAL, 935 Beisner Road, Zip 60007; tel. 847/640–5600) **A**1 2 3 5 7 9 10 **F**3 12 13 15 17 18 20 22 24 26 28 29 30 31 34 35 36 37 39 40 41 43 45 46 47 48 49 50 54 56 57 58 59 60 62 63 64 66 68 70 74 75 76 78 79 81 82 84 85 86 87 90 91 92 93 95 96 107 108 110 111 113 114 115 116 118 119 120 122 123 125 128 129 131 134 142 144 145 146 147 **P**6
**S** Ascension Health, Saint Louis, MO
Primary Contact: John P. Werrbach, Chief Executive Officer
Web address: www.alexian.org
**Control:** Church–operated, Nongovernment, not–for profit **Service:** General Medical and Surgical

**Staffed Beds:** 370 **Admissions:** 20093 **Census:** 292 **Outpatient Visits:** 389861 **Births:** 2280 **Total Expense ($000):** 412712 **Payroll Expense ($000):** 138428 **Personnel:** 2378

### ELMHURST—Dupage County

⊠ **ELMHURST MEMORIAL HOSPITAL (140200)**, 155 East Brush Hill Road, Zip 60126–5658; tel. 331/221–1000, (Total facility includes 38 beds in nursing home–type unit) **A**1 2 9 10 **F**3 5 11 13 15 18 20 22 24 26 28 29 30 31 34 35 38 40 41 42 43 45 46 47 48 49 50 54 57 58 59 62 63 64 65 70 74 75 76 77 78 79 81 82 83 84 85 86 87 89 92 93 96 98 99 100 101 102 103 104 105 107 108 109 110 111 113 114 118 119 120 121 122 125 127 128 129 131 133 145 146 147 **P**8
Primary Contact: W. Peter Daniels, FACHE, President and Chief Executive Officer
CFO: James F. Doyle, Senior Vice President Finance and Chief Financial Officer
CMO: Michael Martirano, M.D., President Medical Staff
CIO: Charles Colander, Vice President Information Systems and Chief Information Officer
CHR: Lois Grubb, Vice President Human Resources
Web address: www.emhc.org
**Control:** Other not–for–profit (including NFP Corporation) **Service:** General Medical and Surgical

**Staffed Beds:** 315 **Admissions:** 14439 **Census:** 199 **Outpatient Visits:** 416878 **Births:** 1286 **Total Expense ($000):** 323007 **Payroll Expense ($000):** 121295 **Personnel:** 2246

### EUREKA—Woodford County

★ **ADVOCATE EUREKA HOSPITAL (141309)**, 101 South Major Street, Zip 61530; tel. 309/467–2371 **A**9 10 18 **F**3 15 28 29 30 31 34 35 39 40 44 45 57 59 64 65 67 68 74 75 77 78 79 81 82 85 86 87 89 90 93 107 108 110 111 113 118 127 128 129 131 132 145 **P**8 **S** Advocate Health Care, Oak Brook, IL
Primary Contact: Colleen Kannaday, FACHE, President
COO: Anna Laible, Administrator
CMO: Steven K. Jones, M.D., Medical Director
CIO: David Harper, Director, Site Information Systems
CHR: Tony Coletta, Vice President of Human Resources
CHR: Aron Klein, Vice President of Finance
CNO: Nancy Allen, R.N., Director, Patient Services/CNE
Web address: www.advocatehealth.com/bromenn
**Control:** Church–operated, Nongovernment, not–for profit **Service:** General Medical and Surgical

**Staffed Beds:** 18 **Admissions:** 496 **Census:** 5 **Outpatient Visits:** 40300 **Births:** 0 **Total Expense ($000):** 13901 **Payroll Expense ($000):** 5253 **Personnel:** 94

**EUREKA COMMUNITY HOSPITAL** See Advocate Eureka Hospital

### EVANSTON—Cook County

⊠ **NORTHSHORE UNIVERSITY HEALTH SYSTEM EVANSTON HOSPITAL (140010)**, 1301 Central Street, Zip 60201–1613; tel. 847/570–2000, (Includes NORTHSHORE GLENBROOK HOSPITAL, 2100 Pfingsten Road, Glenview, Zip 60025; tel. 847/657–5800; NORTHSHORE HIGHLAND PARK HOSPITAL, 718 Glenview Avenue, Highland Park, Zip 60035–2497; tel. 847/432–8000) **A**1 2 3 5 8 9 10 **F**2 3 5 8 9 11 12 13 14 15 18 19 20 22 24 26 28 29 30 31 32 34 35 36 37 38 39 40 43 44 45 46 47 48 49 50 54 55 56 57 58 59 60 61 62 63 64 66 68 70 72 74 75 76 77 78 79 81 82 83 84 85 86 87 89 90 92 93 96 97 98 99 100 101 102 103 104 105 107 108 109 110 111 113 114 115 116 117 118 119 120 122 123 125 128 129 130 131 133 134 135 144 145 146 147 **S** NorthShore University HealthSystem, Evanston, IL
Primary Contact: J. P. Gallagher, President
COO: Jeffrey H. Hillebrand, Chief Operating Officer
CFO: Gary Weiss, Chief Financial Officer
CIO: Thomas Smith, Chief Information Officer
CHR: Bill Luehrs, Chief Human Resources Officer
Web address: www.northshore.org
**Control:** Other not–for–profit (including NFP Corporation) **Service:** General Medical and Surgical

**Staffed Beds:** 755 **Admissions:** 42250 **Census:** 545 **Outpatient Visits:** 1797223 **Births:** 4633 **Total Expense ($000):** 1257866 **Payroll Expense ($000):** 416663 **Personnel:** 5971

★ ○ **SAINT FRANCIS HOSPITAL (140080)**, 355 Ridge Avenue, Zip 60202–3399; tel. 847/316–4000, (Nonreporting) **A**2 3 5 9 10 11 **S** Presence Health, Chicago, IL
Primary Contact: Jeffrey J. Murphy, Executive Vice President and Chief Executive Officer
CFO: John Orsini, Chief Financial Officer
CMO: David DiLoreto, M.D., Executive Vice President and Chief Medical Officer
CIO: George Chessum, Vice President Information Systems
CHR: Paul Skiem, Senior Vice President Human Resources
Web address: www.reshealth.org
**Control:** Church–operated, Nongovernment, not–for profit **Service:** General Medical and Surgical

**Staffed Beds:** 244

### EVERGREEN PARK—Cook County

□ **LITTLE COMPANY OF MARY HOSPITAL AND HEALTH CARE CENTERS (140179)**, 2800 West 95th Street, Zip 60805–2795; tel. 708/422–6200 **A**1 2 5 9 10 **F**2 3 5 11 12 13 15 17 18 20 22 23 29 30 31 34 35 40 45 46 48 49 54 57 59 60 62 63 64 70 71 72 75 76 78 79 81 82 83 84 85 86 87 89 92 93 94 98 101 102 103 104 105 107 108 111 113 118 119 120 125 128 129 131 134 143 145 146 147 **P**6 7 8 **S** American Province of Little Company of Mary Sisters, Evergreen Park, IL
Primary Contact: Dennis A. Reilly, President and Chief Executive Officer
COO: Mary Freyer, Chief Operating Officer
CFO: Randy Ruther, Vice President Finance and Chief Financial Officer
CMO: Dan Rowan, M.D., President Medical Staff
CIO: Darryl Mazzuca, Director Management Information Systems
CHR: Colleen Rohan, Director Human Resources
Web address: www.lcmh.org
**Control:** Other not–for–profit (including NFP Corporation) **Service:** General Medical and Surgical

**Staffed Beds:** 298 **Admissions:** 13590 **Census:** 175 **Outpatient Visits:** 175056 **Births:** 858 **Total Expense ($000):** 186733 **Payroll Expense ($000):** 80544 **Personnel:** 1511

IL

---

**Hospital, Medicare Provider Number, Address, Telephone, Approval, Facility, and Physician Codes, Health Care System**

★ American Hospital Association (AHA) membership
□ The Joint Commission accreditation ◇ DNV Healthcare Inc. accreditation
○ American Osteopathic Association (AOA) accreditation
△ Commission on Accreditation of Rehabilitation Facilities (CARF) accreditation

## FAIRFIELD—Wayne County

☒ **FAIRFIELD MEMORIAL HOSPITAL (141311)**, 303 N.W. 11th Street,
Zip 62837–1203; tel. 618/842–2611 **A**1 9 10 18 **F**3 11 15 18 28 30 31 34
38 40 41 56 57 59 62 64 69 70 75 78 81 87 93 103 104 107 108 111 115
118 126 127 128 129 131 134 144 145 **S** Alliant Management Services,
Louisville, KY
Primary Contact: Katherine Bunting, Chief Executive Officer
COO: Dana Shantel Taylor, Director of Organizational Development
CFO: Michael J. Brown, Chief Financial Officer
CMO: Michelle O'Neill, M.D., President Medical Staff
CIO: Bryan Mitchell, Director Information Systems
CHR: Kari Book, Director Human Resources
CNO: Ann Ignas, R.N., Chief Nurse Executive
Web address: www.fairfieldmemorial.org
**Control:** Other not–for–profit (including NFP Corporation) **Service:** General
Medical and Surgical

| |
|---|
| **Staffed Beds:** 55 **Admissions:** 893 **Census:** 26 **Outpatient Visits:** 38323 **Births:** 0 **Total Expense ($000):** 22591 **Payroll Expense ($000):** 9701 **Personnel:** 237 |

## FLORA—Clay County

☒ **CLAY COUNTY HOSPITAL (141351)**, 911 Stacy Burk Drive, Zip 62839–1823,
Mailing Address: P.O. Box 280, Zip 62839–0280; tel. 618/662–2131 **A**1 9 10
18 **F**3 7 15 28 29 30 32 40 41 43 56 57 59 64 75 77 81 85 93 103 107 110
113 118 126 132 147 **P**6 **S** BJC HealthCare, Saint Louis, MO
Primary Contact: Robert R. Sellers, President
CFO: Melissa Lucas, Chief Financial Officer
CMO: Michael Klingler, M.D., Chief of Staff
CHR: Darla Colwell, Director Human Resources and Marketing
Web address: www.claycountyhospital.org
**Control:** County–Government, nonfederal **Service:** General Medical and Surgical

| |
|---|
| **Staffed Beds:** 18 **Admissions:** 941 **Census:** 10 **Outpatient Visits:** 30687 **Births:** 0 **Total Expense ($000):** 18434 **Payroll Expense ($000):** 7533 **Personnel:** 185 |

## FOREST PARK—Cook County

☒ **RIVEREDGE HOSPITAL (144009)**, 8311 West Roosevelt Road,
Zip 60130–2500; tel. 708/771–7000, (Nonreporting) **A**1 5 9 10 **S** Universal
Health Services, Inc., King of Prussia, PA
Primary Contact: Carey Carlock, Chief Executive Officer
CFO: Michael E. Nelson, Chief Financial Officer
CMO: Lucyna M. Puszkarska, M.D., Medical Director
CIO: Kyle Heinze, Coordinator Information Technology
CHR: Joseph Baw, Director Human Resources
Web address: www.riveredgehospital.com
**Control:** Corporation, Investor–owned, for–profit **Service:** Psychiatric

| |
|---|
| **Staffed Beds:** 224 |

## FREEPORT—Stephenson County

★ **FHN MEMORIAL HOSPITAL (140160)**, 1045 West Stephenson Street,
Zip 61032–4899; tel. 815/599–6000 **A**9 10 **F**3 11 13 14 15 18 20 22 28 29
30 31 32 34 38 40 46 47 48 49 50 51 53 57 59 61 63 64 65 68 69 74 75
76 77 78 79 81 82 84 85 86 87 89 93 97 99 100 101 102 103 104 107 108
109 110 111 113 118 127 128 129 130 131 134 140 145 **P**6 8
Primary Contact: Michael R. Perry, M.D., President and Chief Executive Officer
COO: Sharon K. Summers, R.N., Executive Vice President and Chief Operating
Officer
CFO: Michael Clark, Vice President Finance
CMO: Robert D. Geller, M.D., Vice President Medical Affairs
CIO: Mike Willams, Chief Information Officer
CHR: Len Carter, Vice President Human Resources
CNO: Nancy Cutler, R.N., Vice President Patient Services/CNO
Web address: www.fhn.org
**Control:** Other not–for–profit (including NFP Corporation) **Service:** General
Medical and Surgical

| |
|---|
| **Staffed Beds:** 100 **Admissions:** 5038 **Census:** 58 **Outpatient Visits:** 102044 **Births:** 405 **Total Expense ($000):** 96931 **Payroll Expense ($000):** 30580 **Personnel:** 476 |

## GALENA—Jo Daviess County

★ **MIDWEST MEDICAL CENTER (141302)**, One Medical Center Drive,
Zip 61036–1697; tel. 815/777–1340, (Nonreporting) **A**9 10 18
Primary Contact: Tracy Bauer, Chief Executive Officer
COO: Steve Busch, Chief Operating Officer
CMO: Grant Westenfelder, M.D., Chief Medical Officer
CHR: Melissa Conley, Director Human Resources
Web address: www.midwestmedicalcenter.org
**Control:** Corporation, Investor–owned, for–profit **Service:** General Medical and
Surgical

| |
|---|
| **Staffed Beds:** 25 |

## GALESBURG—Knox County

☒ **GALESBURG COTTAGE HOSPITAL (140040)**, 695 North Kellogg Street,
Zip 61401–2885; tel. 309/343–8131, (Nonreporting) **A**1 9 10 **S** Community
Health Systems, Inc., Franklin, TN
Primary Contact: Earl J. Tamar, Chief Executive Officer
COO: Lance Porter, Assistant Chief Executive Officer
CFO: Rob Gasaway, Chief Financial Officer
CMO: Daniel Piper, M.D., President Medical Staff
CIO: Teresa Mach, Director Information Technology
CHR: Nancy Baird, Director Human Resources
CNO: Debra Rickard, R.N., Chief Nursing Officer
Web address: www.cottagehospital.com
**Control:** Other not–for–profit (including NFP Corporation) **Service:** General
Medical and Surgical

| |
|---|
| **Staffed Beds:** 119 |

★ **OSF ST. MARY MEDICAL CENTER (140064)**, 3333 North Seminary Street,
Zip 61401–1299; tel. 309/344–3161 **A**9 10 **F**3 11 13 15 18 20 26 28 29 30
31 34 40 41 43 45 49 51 53 56 57 58 59 61 62 63 68 70 74 75 76 77 78
79 81 82 84 85 86 87 89 93 94 97 107 110 111 113 114 116 118 128 129
131 134 144 145 146 **P**1 6 **S** OSF Healthcare System, Peoria, IL
Primary Contact: Richard S. Kowalski, FACHE, President and Chief Executive
Officer
CFO: Curt Lipe, Vice President, Chief Financial Officer
CMO: Mark Meeker, D.O., Medical Staff President
CIO: Becky Lynch, Manager Business Entity Management and Information Systems
CHR: Roxanna Crosser, Vice President, Operations
CNO: Alice Snyder, Vice President, Chief Nursing Officer
Web address: www.osfstmary.org
**Control:** Church–operated, Nongovernment, not–for profit **Service:** General
Medical and Surgical

| |
|---|
| **Staffed Beds:** 90 **Admissions:** 3704 **Census:** 40 **Outpatient Visits:** 144021 **Births:** 143 **Total Expense ($000):** 80876 **Payroll Expense ($000):** 38044 **Personnel:** 556 |

## GENESEO—Henry County

☒ **HAMMOND–HENRY HOSPITAL (141319)**, 600 North College Avenue,
Zip 61254–1099; tel. 309/944–4625, (Total facility includes 56 beds in nursing
home–type unit) **A**1 9 10 18 **F**3 8 11 12 13 15 17 18 28 29 34 35 40 43 44
45 57 59 62 67 70 75 76 78 79 81 87 88 89 93 107 111 113 118 127 128
129 130 131 132 134 143 145 **S** HealthTech Management Services,
Franklin, TN
Primary Contact: Bradley Solberg, FACHE, Chief Executive Officer
CFO: Jodie Criswell, Vice President Fiscal Services
CIO: Heather Henry, Manager Information Systems
CHR: Margaret Chavez, Manager Human Resources
Web address: www.hammondhenry.com
**Control:** Hospital district or authority, Government, nonfederal **Service:** General
Medical and Surgical

| |
|---|
| **Staffed Beds:** 79 **Admissions:** 1191 **Census:** 48 **Outpatient Visits:** 72641 **Births:** 196 **Total Expense ($000):** 28245 **Payroll Expense ($000):** 11562 **Personnel:** 279 |

## GENEVA—Kane County

☒ **DELNOR HOSPITAL (140211)**, 300 Randall Road, Zip 60134–4200;
tel. 630/208–3000, (Data for 303 days) **A**1 2 9 10 **F**3 11 13 15 18 20 22 26
28 29 30 31 32 34 35 36 39 40 43 44 49 50 53 55 57 59 60 64 65 68 70
74 75 76 77 78 79 81 82 85 86 87 89 93 94 96 102 104 107 108 110 111
113 114 117 118 119 120 125 128 129 130 131 134 142 143 144 145 146
147 **S** Cadence Health, Winfield, IL
Primary Contact: Robert Friedberg, President
COO: Robert Friedberg, President
CMO: Mark Daniels, M.D., Vice President Physician Enterprise
CIO: James Kearns, Chief Information Officer
Web address: www.delnor.com
**Control:** Other not–for–profit (including NFP Corporation) **Service:** General
Medical and Surgical

| |
|---|
| **Staffed Beds:** 159 **Admissions:** 7172 **Census:** 85 **Outpatient Visits:** 190529 **Births:** 1201 **Total Expense ($000):** 154590 **Payroll Expense ($000):** 58053 **Personnel:** 1058 |

IL

## GIBSON CITY—Ford County

✠ **GIBSON AREA HOSPITAL AND HEALTH SERVICES (141317)**, 1120 North Melvin Street, Zip 60936, Mailing Address: P.O. Box 429, Zip 60936–0429; tel. 217/784–4251, (Includes GIBSON COMMUNITY HOSPITAL NURSING HOME ), (Total facility includes 42 beds in nursing home–type unit) **A**1 9 10 18 **F**3 7 11 13 15 28 29 31 35 40 43 44 45 49 50 51 53 56 57 59 63 64 65 68 69 70 75 76 77 79 81 85 87 93 103 107 108 110 111 114 118 126 127 128 130 131 132 142 145 146 147 **P**1 6 7
Primary Contact: Robert C. Schmitt, II, Chief Executive Officer
COO: Robin Rose, R.N., Chief Nursing Officer
CFO: John Jacobson, Chief Financial Officer
CMO: David J. Hagan, M.D., Chief Medical Officer
CIO: Jim Edwards, Executive Director of Information Technology
CHR: Ty Royal, Executive Director of Support Services and Human Resources
CNO: Robin Rose, R.N., Chief Nursing Officer/Chief Operating Officer
Web address: www.gibsonhospital.org
**Control:** Other not–for–profit (including NFP Corporation) **Service:** General Medical and Surgical

**Staffed Beds:** 67 **Admissions:** 1036 **Census:** 49 **Outpatient Visits:** 114855
**Births:** 150 **Total Expense ($000):** 53448 **Payroll Expense ($000):** 24467
**Personnel:** 466

## GLENDALE HEIGHTS—Dupage County

✠ **ADVENTIST GLENOAKS HOSPITAL (140292)**, 701 Winthrop Avenue, Zip 60139–1403; tel. 630/545–8000 **A**1 9 10 **F**3 11 13 15 17 18 20 22 26 29 31 34 35 38 40 43 45 49 57 58 59 61 64 68 70 72 74 75 76 78 79 81 82 85 86 87 92 93 96 97 98 99 100 101 102 103 104 105 107 108 110 111 113 117 118 129 130 131 145 146 147 **P**7 8 **S** Adventist Health System Sunbelt Health Care Corporation, Altamonte Springs, FL
Primary Contact: Bruce C. Christian, Chief Executive Officer
CFO: Eric Moots, Vice President and Chief Financial Officer
CMO: Richard Carroll, M.D., Chief Medical Officer
CIO: Joe Granneman, Regional Chief Information Officer
CHR: Donald Russell, Vice President
Web address: www.keepingyouwell.com
**Control:** Church–operated, Nongovernment, not–for profit **Service:** General Medical and Surgical

**Staffed Beds:** 141 **Admissions:** 5448 **Census:** 85 **Outpatient Visits:** 37132
**Births:** 472 **Total Expense ($000):** 77423 **Payroll Expense ($000):** 32565
**Personnel:** 566

## GLENVIEW—Cook County

**NORTHSHORE GLENBROOK HOSPITAL** See NorthShore University Health System Evanston Hospital, Evanston

## GRANITE CITY—Madison County

✠ **GATEWAY REGIONAL MEDICAL CENTER (140125)**, 2100 Madison Avenue, Zip 62040–4799; tel. 618/798–3000 **A**1 9 10 **F**3 11 13 15 20 22 28 29 40 45 48 49 70 74 76 77 79 81 82 85 90 93 96 98 99 103 104 107 108 110 111 113 115 118 127 128 131 145 **S** Community Health Systems, Inc., Franklin, TN
Primary Contact: Mark Bethell, Chief Executive Officer
CFO: Ronald Leazer, Chief Financial Officer
CMO: Mike Adams, M.D., Chief Medical Officer
CIO: Dennis Kampwerth, Director Management Information Systems
CHR: J. Ronald Payton, Director Human Resources
Web address: www.gatewayregional.net
**Control:** Corporation, Investor–owned, for–profit **Service:** General Medical and Surgical

**Staffed Beds:** 337 **Admissions:** 7914 **Census:** 119 **Outpatient Visits:** 62244
**Births:** 264 **Total Expense ($000):** 89324 **Payroll Expense ($000):** 31087
**Personnel:** 768

## GREENVILLE—Bond County

★ ○ **GREENVILLE REGIONAL HOSPITAL (140137)**, 200 Healthcare Drive, Zip 62246–1156; tel. 618/664–1230, (Includes FAIR OAKS ), (Total facility includes 108 beds in nursing home–type unit) **A**9 10 11 **F**2 7 11 13 15 28 29 31 34 40 41 45 49 50 56 57 59 64 68 75 76 77 78 79 81 85 87 89 93 94 95 97 98 100 103 104 107 111 114 118 124 126 127 128 129 130 131 132 134 145 147 **P**6
Primary Contact: Morris L. Bond, Interim Chief Executive Officer
CFO: Sherry Koehler, Chief Financial Officer
CHR: Todd A. Ray, Director Human Resources
CNO: Tammy Lett, R.N., Chief Nursing Officer
Web address: www.greenvilleregionalhospital.com
**Control:** Other not–for–profit (including NFP Corporation) **Service:** General Medical and Surgical

**Staffed Beds:** 150 **Admissions:** 1538 **Census:** 80 **Outpatient Visits:** 40790
**Births:** 205 **Total Expense ($000):** 36183 **Payroll Expense ($000):** 16442
**Personnel:** 360

## HARRISBURG—Saline County

✠ **HARRISBURG MEDICAL CENTER (140210)**, 100 Drive Warren Tuttle Drive, Zip 62946, Mailing Address: P.O. Box 428, Zip 62946–0428; tel. 618/253–7671 **A**1 9 10 20 **F**3 8 11 15 28 29 30 31 34 40 50 56 57 59 61 62 64 75 77 78 81 85 87 89 91 93 97 98 99 100 101 102 103 104 105 107 108 110 113 117 118 126 128 129 130 132 145 147
Primary Contact: Vincent Ashley, Chief Executive Officer
CFO: John Riley, Chief Financial Officer
CIO: Rick Pyle, Director Information Systems
CHR: Rodney Smith, VP Support Services
CNO: Cindy Ford, R.N., Chief Nursing Officer
Web address: www.harrisburgmc.com
**Control:** Other not–for–profit (including NFP Corporation) **Service:** General Medical and Surgical

**Staffed Beds:** 74 **Admissions:** 2933 **Census:** 33 **Outpatient Visits:** 46767
**Births:** 0 **Total Expense ($000):** 37220 **Payroll Expense ($000):** 18964
**Personnel:** 324

## HARVARD—Mchenry County

✠ **MERCY HARVARD HOSPITAL (141335)**, 901 Grant Street, Zip 60033–1898, Mailing Address: P.O. Box 850, Zip 60033–0850; tel. 815/943–5431, (Total facility includes 34 beds in nursing home–type unit) **A**1 9 10 18 **F**3 11 12 15 28 29 30 35 40 45 46 53 57 59 64 69 70 75 77 79 81 82 85 87 93 94 96 97 107 108 109 113 118 127 128 129 131 142 145 **P**6 **S** Mercy Health System, Janesville, WI
Primary Contact: Jennifer Hallatt, Chief Operating Officer
CFO: John Cook, Chief Financial Officer
CHR: Heather Niles, Director Human Resources Operations
Web address: www.mercyhealthsystem.org
**Control:** Other not–for–profit (including NFP Corporation) **Service:** General Medical and Surgical

**Staffed Beds:** 54 **Admissions:** 743 **Census:** 31 **Outpatient Visits:** 73019
**Births:** 0 **Total Expense ($000):** 20809 **Payroll Expense ($000):** 8806
**Personnel:** 138

## HARVEY—Cook County

★ △ **INGALLS MEMORIAL HOSPITAL (140191)**, One Ingalls Drive, Zip 60426–3591; tel. 708/333–2300, (Nonreporting) **A**2 7 9 10 21
Primary Contact: Kurt E. Johnson, President and Chief Executive Officer
CFO: Andrew Stefo, Senior Vice President Finance and Chief Financial Officer
CHR: Aletha Ross, Vice President Human Resources
Web address: www.ingallshealthsystem.org
**Control:** Other not–for–profit (including NFP Corporation) **Service:** General Medical and Surgical

**Staffed Beds:** 419

## HAVANA—Mason County

✠ **MASON DISTRICT HOSPITAL (141313)**, 615 North Promenade Street, Zip 62644–0530, Mailing Address: P.O. Box 530, Zip 62644–0530; tel. 309/543–4431 **A**1 9 10 18 **F**7 8 11 15 18 28 29 30 34 35 40 42 45 49 50 53 54 56 57 59 62 64 65 68 69 75 79 81 93 97 103 107 108 113 117 118 126 128 129 131 132 142 145 **P**6
Primary Contact: Harry Wolin, Administrator and Chief Executive Officer
CFO: Robert J. Stolba, Chief Financial Officer
CMO: James T. Brown, M.D., President of Medical Staff
CIO: Aaron Coats, Information Technology Director
CHR: Anne Davis, Director Human Resources
CNO: Carman Wuebbels, R.N., Chief Nursing Officer
Web address: www.masondistricthospital.org
**Control:** Hospital district or authority, Government, nonfederal **Service:** General Medical and Surgical

**Staffed Beds:** 20 **Admissions:** 459 **Census:** 4 **Outpatient Visits:** 24338
**Births:** 0 **Total Expense ($000):** 19176 **Payroll Expense ($000):** 10389
**Personnel:** 222

**IL**

## HAZEL CREST—Cook County

☒ **ADVOCATE SOUTH SUBURBAN HOSPITAL (140250)**, 17800 South Kedzie Avenue, Zip 60429–0989; tel. 708/799–8000, (Total facility includes 37 beds in nursing home–type unit) **A**1 2 9 10 **F**3 11 13 15 18 20 22 24 26 28 29 30 31 34 35 36 40 45 46 47 49 50 51 53 57 59 60 63 64 68 70 75 76 78 79 81 82 85 87 107 108 110 111 113 114 117 118 125 127 128 129 131 144 145 146 147 **P**8 **S** Advocate Health Care, Oak Brook, IL
Primary Contact: Michael A. Engelhart, President
COO: Karen Clark, MS, Vice President Operations
CFO: Brian Kelly, Vice President Finance
CIO: Beth Turek, Site Manager Information Systems
Web address: www.advocatehealth.com/ssub/
**Control:** Church–operated, Nongovernment, not–for profit **Service:** General Medical and Surgical

**Staffed Beds: 225 Admissions: 12168 Census: 143 Outpatient Visits: 112814 Births: 950**

## HERRIN—Williamson County

☐ **HERRIN HOSPITAL (140011)**, 201 South 14th Street, Zip 62948–3631; tel. 618/942–2171 **A**1 5 9 10 **F**3 11 12 18 28 29 30 34 35 40 45 47 49 54 56 57 59 60 64 68 70 74 75 78 79 81 82 84 85 86 87 90 93 100 107 108 111 113 114 118 129 130 131 134 142 145 147 **S** Southern Illinois Hospital Services, Carbondale, IL
Primary Contact: Terence Farrell, Administrator
CFO: Michael Kasser, Chief Financial Officer
CMO: Michelle Jenkins, M.D., President Medical Staff
CIO: David Holland, Chief Information Officer
CHR: Teresa A. Lovellette, Manager Human Resources
Web address: www.sih.net
**Control:** Other not–for–profit (including NFP Corporation) **Service:** General Medical and Surgical

**Staffed Beds: 104 Admissions: 5258 Census: 77 Outpatient Visits: 96113 Births: 0 Total Expense ($000): 95444 Payroll Expense ($000): 31420 Personnel: 630**

## HIGHLAND—Madison County

☒ **ST. JOSEPH'S HOSPITAL (141336)**, 1515 Main Street, Zip 62249–1656; tel. 618/654–7421, (Nonreporting) **A**1 9 10 18 **S** Hospital Sisters Health System, Springfield, IL
Primary Contact: Peggy A. Sebastian, MSN, R.N., President and Chief Executive Officer
CFO: James Johnson, Chief Financial Officer
CMO: A. Greg Miranda, D.O., President Medical Staff
Web address: www.stjosephshighland.com
**Control:** Church–operated, Nongovernment, not–for profit **Service:** General Medical and Surgical

**Staffed Beds: 25**

## HIGHLAND PARK—Lake County

**NORTHSHORE HIGHLAND PARK HOSPITAL** See NorthShore University Health System Evanston Hospital, Evanston

## HILLSBORO—Montgomery County

☒ **HILLSBORO AREA HOSPITAL (141332)**, 1200 East Tremont Street, Zip 62049–1900; tel. 217/532–6111 **A**1 9 10 18 **F**10 15 28 29 30 34 35 40 56 57 59 64 65 75 77 79 81 85 86 87 89 92 93 97 107 110 114 124 128 129 130 132 134 145 147 **S** HealthTech Management Services, Franklin, TN
Primary Contact: Rex H. Brown, Chief Executive Officer
CFO: Terri L. Carroll, Vice President Financial Services
CHR: Sharon Clark, Director Human Resources
Web address: www.hillsborohealth.org
**Control:** Other not–for–profit (including NFP Corporation) **Service:** General Medical and Surgical

**Staffed Beds: 25 Admissions: 576 Census: 8 Outpatient Visits: 21906 Births: 0 Total Expense ($000): 16490 Payroll Expense ($000): 6055 Personnel: 155**

## HINES—Cook County

☐ **JOHN J. MADDEN MENTAL HEALTH CENTER (144028)**, 1200 South First Avenue, Zip 60141; tel. 708/338–7202, (Nonreporting) **A**1 3 5 10 **S** Division of Mental Health, Department of Human Services, Springfield, IL
Primary Contact: Edith Newman, Interim Administrator
CFO: Janice Evans, Chief Financial Officer
**Control:** State–Government, nonfederal **Service:** Psychiatric

**Staffed Beds: 150**

☒ △ **VETERANS AFFAIRS EDWARD HINES, JR. HOSPITAL**, Fifth Avenue & Roosevelt Road, Zip 60141–5000, Mailing Address: P.O. Box 5000, Zip 60141–5000; tel. 708/202–8387 **A**1 2 3 5 7 8 9 **F**3 4 5 8 12 17 18 20 22 24 26 28 30 31 34 35 38 39 40 43 46 47 48 49 50 54 56 57 58 59 60 61 62 63 64 65 68 70 74 75 77 78 79 81 82 83 84 85 86 87 90 92 93 94 95 96 97 98 100 101 102 103 104 105 106 107 111 114 115 116 117 118 119 120 122 125 126 127 128 129 131 134 140 142 143 145 146 147 **S** Department of Veterans Affairs, Washington, DC
Primary Contact: Nathan L. Geraths, Director
COO: Nathan L. Geraths, Director
CFO: Raleigh Beard, Chief Fiscal Services
CMO: Barbara Temeck, M.D., Chief of Staff
CIO: Gordon Brown, Chief Information Resources Management
CHR: Clare Hadjuk, Director Human Resources
Web address: www.va.gov/sta/guide/home.asp
**Control:** Veterans Affairs, Government, federal **Service:** General Medical and Surgical

**Staffed Beds: 385 Admissions: 9445 Census: 325 Outpatient Visits: 700000 Births: 0**

## HINSDALE—Dupage County

☒ △ **ADVENTIST HINSDALE HOSPITAL (140122)**, 120 North Oak Street, Zip 60521–3890; tel. 630/856–9000 **A**1 2 3 5 7 9 10 13 **F**3 5 8 11 12 13 14 15 17 18 20 22 24 26 27 28 29 30 31 34 35 37 38 39 40 43 44 45 48 49 52 54 55 56 57 58 59 61 62 63 64 68 70 72 73 74 75 76 78 79 81 82 84 85 86 87 88 89 90 92 96 97 98 99 100 101 102 103 104 105 107 108 110 111 113 114 117 118 119 120 122 123 125 128 129 130 131 135 140 145 146 147 **P**7 8 **S** Adventist Health System Sunbelt Health Care Corporation, Altamonte Springs, FL
Primary Contact: Michael Goebel, Chief Executive Officer
CFO: Rebecca Mathis, Vice President and Chief Financial Officer
CMO: Gary Lipinski, M.D., Regional Vice President and Chief Medical Officer
CIO: Joe Granneman, Chief Information Officer
CHR: Donald Russell, Regional Vice President Human Resources
CNO: Shawn O. Tyrrell, R.N., VP/Chief Nursing Officer
Web address: www.keepingyouwell.com
**Control:** Church–operated, Nongovernment, not–for profit **Service:** General Medical and Surgical

**Staffed Beds: 271 Admissions: 12842 Census: 159 Outpatient Visits: 267898 Births: 1762 Total Expense ($000): 280234 Payroll Expense ($000): 100708 Personnel: 1885**

☒ **R M L SPECIALTY HOSPITAL (142010)**, 5601 South County Line Road, Zip 60521–8900; tel. 630/286–4000 **A**1 5 9 10 **F**1 3 29 30 31 40 50 58 74 85 87 107 113 118 129 131 145 147
Primary Contact: James R. Prister, President and Chief Executive Officer
COO: Ken Pawola, Chief Operating Officer
CFO: Tom Pater, Chief Financial Officer
CMO: John Brofman, M.D., Medical Director
CIO: Julie Ames, Chief Information Officer
CHR: John Landstrom, Director Human Resources
CNO: Maura Hopkins, R.N., Chief Nursing Officer
Web address: www.rmlspecialtyhospital.org
**Control:** Other not–for–profit (including NFP Corporation) **Service:** Long–Term Acute Care hospital

**Staffed Beds: 87 Admissions: 759 Census: 68 Outpatient Visits: 0 Births: 0 Total Expense ($000): 45408 Payroll Expense ($000): 22567 Personnel: 357**

## HOFFMAN ESTATES—Cook County

☒ **ALEXIAN BROTHERS BEHAVIORAL HEALTH HOSPITAL (144031)**, 1650 Moon Lake Boulevard, Zip 60194–5000; tel. 847/882–1600 **A**1 5 9 10 **F**4 5 29 30 34 35 44 50 56 58 59 65 68 75 77 87 98 99 100 101 102 103 104 105 129 131 **P**4 **S** Ascension Health, Saint Louis, MO
Primary Contact: Clayton Ciha, President and Chief Executive Officer
COO: Christopher Novak, Chief Operating Officer
CFO: David Jones, Chief Financial Officer
CMO: Gregory Teas, M.D., Chief Medical Officer
CIO: Sherrie Russell, Vice President and Chief Information Officer
CHR: James Lewandowski, Vice President Corporate Human Resources
CNO: Christine Quinlan, MS, Chief Nursing Officer
Web address: www.abbhh.org
**Control:** Church–operated, Nongovernment, not–for profit **Service:** Psychiatric

**Staffed Beds: 141 Admissions: 6120 Census: 129 Outpatient Visits: 139988 Births: 0 Total Expense ($000): 59413 Payroll Expense ($000): 32719 Personnel: 461**

IL

⊠ **ST. ALEXIUS MEDICAL CENTER (140290)**, 1555 Barrington Road,
Zip 60169–1019; tel. 847/843–2000 **A**1 2 3 5 9 10 **F**3 8 12 13 15 17 18 19
20 21 22 23 26 29 30 31 32 33 34 35 36 37 39 40 41 42 43 45 46 47 48
49 50 54 55 56 57 59 60 64 65 70 72 73 74 75 76 77 78 79 81 82 84 85
86 87 88 89 93 96 97 107 108 110 111 113 114 117 118 119 120 125 129
130 131 144 145 146 147 **S** Ascension Health, Saint Louis, MO
Primary Contact: Edward M. Goldberg, President and Chief Executive Officer
CFO: Sherril Vincent, Vice President Finance/CFO, Alexian Brothers Acute Care
Ministries
CMO: Scott Neeley, M.D., Chief Medical Officer
CIO: Sherrie Russell, Chief Information Officer
CHR: Linda Baker, Director Human Resources
CNO: Chris Budzinsky, R.N., Vice President Nursing/CNO Alexian Brothers Acute
Care Ministries
Web address: www.stalexius.org
**Control:** Church–operated, Nongovernment, not–for profit **Service:** General
Medical and Surgical

**Staffed Beds: 305 Admissions: 18032 Census: 207 Outpatient Visits:**
266763 **Births: 3138 Total Expense ($000): 297960 Payroll Expense**
**($000): 105245 Personnel: 1623**

### HOOPESTON—Vermilion County

⊠ **HOOPESTON REGIONAL HEALTH CENTER (141316)**, 701 East Orange
Street, Zip 60942–1871; tel. 217/283–5531, (Total facility includes 75 beds in
nursing home–type unit) **A**1 9 10 18 **F**1 4 7 15 16 17 34 40 51 59 67 70 72
73 79 80 81 85 88 89 90 93 98 103 107 110 111 114 118 124 126 127
129 132 142 **S** QHR, Brentwood, TN
Primary Contact: Harry Brockus, Chief Executive Officer
COO: Jacqueline Johnson, Chief Clinical Officer
CIO: Bernie McCarty, Director Facilities
CHR: Betsy Morgenroth, Director Human Resources
Web address: www.hoopestonhospital.org
**Control:** Other not–for–profit (including NFP Corporation) **Service:** General
Medical and Surgical

**Staffed Beds: 99 Admissions: 871 Census: 79 Outpatient Visits: 24580**
**Births: 0 Total Expense ($000): 22073 Payroll Expense ($000): 9159**
**Personnel: 228**

### HOPEDALE—Tazewell County

**HOPEDALE MEDICAL COMPLEX (141330)**, 107 Tremont Street, Zip 61747;
tel. 309/449–3321, (Nonreporting) **A**9 10 18
Primary Contact: Alfred N. Rossi, M.D., Chief Executive Officer
COO: Mark F. Rossi, Chief Operating Officer and General Counsel
CFO: Larry Kloc, Chief Financial Officer
CHR: Ann Wilson, Acting Director Human Resources
Web address: www.hopedalemc.com
**Control:** Other not–for–profit (including NFP Corporation) **Service:** General
Medical and Surgical

**Staffed Beds: 25**

### JACKSONVILLE—Morgan County

⊠ **PASSAVANT AREA HOSPITAL (140058)**, 1600 West Walnut Street,
Zip 62650–1136; tel. 217/245–9541, (Total facility includes 15 beds in nursing
home–type unit) **A**1 9 10 **F**1 3 4 8 11 12 13 15 16 17 28 29 30 34 35 38 40
45 47 50 51 56 57 59 64 67 68 69 70 72 73 75 76 77 79 80 81 82 85 86
87 88 89 90 93 96 98 100 104 107 108 111 114 118 127 128 129 130 131
145 147 **P**4 6
Primary Contact: Chester A. Wynn, President and Chief Executive Officer
CFO: David Bolen, Vice President and Chief Financial Officer
CMO: Tara Ramsey, M.D., President Medical Staff
CIO: Marc E. Steinberg, Vice President Community Relations and Physician
Recruitment
CHR: Rick A. Mogler, Director Human Resources
Web address: www.passavanthospital.com
**Control:** Other not–for–profit (including NFP Corporation) **Service:** General
Medical and Surgical

**Staffed Beds: 112 Admissions: 3770 Census: 47 Outpatient Visits: 90346**
**Births: 305 Total Expense ($000): 74974 Payroll Expense ($000): 31813**
**Personnel: 755**

### JERSEYVILLE—Jersey County

⊠ **JERSEY COMMUNITY HOSPITAL (140059)**, 400 Maple Summit Road,
Zip 62052–2028, Mailing Address: P.O. Box 426, Zip 62052–0426;
tel. 618/498–6402 **A**1 9 10 **F**3 7 8 11 12 13 15 28 29 31 32 34 35 36 40 45
51 53 56 57 59 64 65 68 69 70 74 75 76 78 79 81 85 86 89 93 107 108
110 111 114 118 128 129 130 131 132 133 134 145 146 147
Primary Contact: Lawrence P. Bear, Administrator and Chief Executive Officer
COO: Lawrence P. Bear, Administrator and Chief Executive Officer
CFO: David Kennett, Chief Financial Officer
CMO: Julie Smith, R.N., Director of Nursing
CIO: Bob Bray, Chief Information Officer
CHR: Sharon K. Sanford, Director Human Resources
Web address: www.jch.org
**Control:** Hospital district or authority, Government, nonfederal **Service:** General
Medical and Surgical

**Staffed Beds: 65 Admissions: 1396 Census: 11 Outpatient Visits: 61503**
**Births: 165 Total Expense ($000): 27836 Payroll Expense ($000): 11171**
**Personnel: 255**

### JOLIET—Will County

⊠ △ **PROVENA SAINT JOSEPH MEDICAL CENTER (140007)**, 333 North
Madison Street, Zip 60435–6595; tel. 815/725–7133 **A**1 2 5 7 9 10 **F**3 5 8 11
12 13 15 17 18 20 22 24 26 28 29 30 31 32 34 35 36 37 38 39 40 41 43
44 45 46 49 50 53 54 56 57 58 59 60 61 64 65 68 70 71 72 74 75 76 77
78 79 80 81 82 84 85 86 87 88 89 90 92 93 96 97 98 99 100 101 102 103
105 107 108 110 111 113 114 117 118 119 120 122 123 125 128 129 130
131 133 134 142 143 144 145 146 **P**8 **S** Presence Health, Chicago, IL
Primary Contact: Beth Hughes, President and Chief Executive Officer
COO: Amy Dirks Stevens, Chief Operating Officer
CFO: Gary Gasbarra, Regional Chief Financial Officer
CMO: Gary Plundo, D.O., Chief Medical Officer
CIO: Russell Soliman, System Manager Client Services and Management
Information Services
CHR: Terry S. Solem, System Vice President Human Resources
Web address: www.provena.org/stjoes
**Control:** Church–operated, Nongovernment, not–for profit **Service:** General
Medical and Surgical

**Staffed Beds: 457 Admissions: 24508 Census: 297 Outpatient Visits:**
500601 **Births: 1617 Total Expense ($000): 358982 Payroll Expense**
**($000): 130765 Personnel: 2089**

### KANKAKEE—Kankakee County

⊠ **PROVENA ST. MARY'S HOSPITAL (140155)**, 500 West Court Street,
Zip 60901–3661; tel. 815/937–2400 **A**1 2 9 10 **F**3 5 11 12 13 15 18 20 22
26 28 29 30 31 32 34 35 36 38 39 40 43 45 48 49 50 53 54 56 57 58 59
60 61 64 65 68 70 74 75 76 77 78 79 81 82 83 84 85 86 87 89 92 93 97
98 99 100 101 102 103 104 105 106 107 108 110 111 113 114 115 118
128 129 130 131 134 142 145 146 147 **S** Presence Health, Chicago, IL
Primary Contact: Amy LaFine, R.N., MSN, President and Chief Executive Officer
CFO: Frank McHugh, Chief Financial Officer
CIO: Russell Soliman, Director Information Services
CNO: Barbara Decker, R.N., Chief Nursing Officer
Web address: www.provena.org/stmarys/
**Control:** Church–operated, Nongovernment, not–for profit **Service:** General
Medical and Surgical

**Staffed Beds: 143 Admissions: 7281 Census: 83 Outpatient Visits: 215848**
**Births: 418 Total Expense ($000): 122435 Payroll Expense ($000): 40791**
**Personnel: 759**

⊠ **RIVERSIDE MEDICAL CENTER (140186)**, 350 North Wall Street,
Zip 60901–0749; tel. 815/933–1671 **A**1 2 5 9 10 13 **F**3 4 5 6 7 8 9 11 12 13
15 17 18 19 20 22 24 26 28 29 30 31 32 34 35 36 38 39 40 41 43 44 45
46 47 48 49 50 51 54 55 56 57 58 59 61 62 64 65 66 68 70 71 74 75 76
77 78 79 81 82 84 85 86 87 89 90 92 93 96 97 98 99 100 101 102 103
104 105 107 108 110 111 113 114 117 118 119 120 122 125 126 128 129
130 131 133 134 140 142 144 145 146 147
Primary Contact: Phillip M. Kambic, Chief Executive Officer
COO: David Duda, Senior Vice President and Chief Operating Officer
CFO: Bill Douglas, Senior Vice President and Chief Financial Officer
CMO: John Jurica, M.D., Vice President Medical Affairs
CIO: Kyle Hansen, Corporate Director Information Systems
CHR: Becky Hinrichs, Vice President Human Resources
CNO: Allen Kelly, R.N., Vice President Procedural Services & CNO
Web address: www.riversidehealthcare.org
**Control:** Other not–for–profit (including NFP Corporation) **Service:** General
Medical and Surgical

**Staffed Beds: 325 Admissions: 11816 Census: 156 Outpatient Visits:**
331142 **Births: 1013 Total Expense ($000): 216414 Payroll Expense**
**($000): 87257 Personnel: 1487**

**IL**

**Hospital, Medicare Provider Number, Address, Telephone, Approval, Facility, and Physician Codes, Health Care System**

★ American Hospital Association (AHA) membership
□ The Joint Commission accreditation
◇ DNV Healthcare Inc. accreditation
○ American Osteopathic Association (AOA) accreditation
△ Commission on Accreditation of Rehabilitation Facilities (CARF) accreditation

## KEWANEE—Henry County

★ **KEWANEE HOSPITAL (141325)**, 1051 West South Street, Zip 61443–2711, Mailing Address: P.O. Box 747, Zip 61443–0747; tel. 309/852–7500 **A**9 10 18 **F**3 11 15 18 29 31 32 34 35 36 38 40 45 50 57 59 64 65 66 68 70 75 77 78 79 81 82 85 86 87 92 93 96 97 107 108 110 114 118 126 128 130 131 132 134 145 147 **P**6
Primary Contact: Lynn Fulton, Chief Executive Officer
CFO: Preston Becker, Chief Financial Officer
CIO: Jeremy Johnson, Director of Information Technology
CHR: Renee A. Salisbury, Director Human Resources
CNO: Jennifer Junis, Chief Nursing Officer
Web address: www.kewaneehospital.com
**Control:** Other not–for–profit (including NFP Corporation) **Service:** General Medical and Surgical

**Staffed Beds:** 25 **Admissions:** 704 **Census:** 6 **Outpatient Visits:** 33061 **Births:** 0 **Total Expense ($000):** 26027 **Payroll Expense ($000):** 9266 **Personnel:** 204

## LA GRANGE—Cook County

✠ **ADVENTIST LA GRANGE MEMORIAL HOSPITAL (140065)**, 5101 South Willow Spring Road, Zip 60525–2680; tel. 708/245–9000 **A**1 2 3 5 9 10 13 **F**3 12 13 15 17 18 20 22 24 26 28 29 30 31 34 35 37 39 40 43 44 45 49 50 56 57 58 59 60 61 64 68 70 73 74 75 76 78 79 81 82 85 86 87 93 96 97 100 107 108 110 111 113 114 117 118 119 120 122 128 129 130 131 145 146 147 **P**7 8 **S** Adventist Health System Sunbelt Health Care Corporation, Altamonte Springs, FL
Primary Contact: Lary Davis, President and Chief Executive Officer
COO: Edward Gervain, Chief Operating Officer
CFO: Keith Richardson, Chief Financial Officer
CMO: Gary Lipinski, M.D., Regional Vice President and Chief Medical Officer
CIO: Russ Solimon, Chief Information Officer
CHR: Patty Sanchez, Site Manager Human Resources
Web address: www.keepingyouwell.com
**Control:** Church–operated, Nongovernment, not–for profit **Service:** General Medical and Surgical

**Staffed Beds:** 179 **Admissions:** 8626 **Census:** 110 **Outpatient Visits:** 116275 **Births:** 583 **Total Expense ($000):** 151529 **Payroll Expense ($000):** 55034 **Personnel:** 982

## LAKE FOREST—Lake County

**LAKE FOREST HOSPITAL** See Northwestern Lake Forest Hospital

✠ **NORTHWESTERN LAKE FOREST HOSPITAL (140130)**, 660 North Westmoreland Road, Zip 60045–1696; tel. 847/234–5600, (Total facility includes 72 beds in nursing home–type unit) **A**1 2 9 10 **F**2 3 8 9 11 13 15 18 19 20 22 26 28 29 30 31 32 34 35 36 38 40 42 43 44 45 46 48 49 50 51 53 54 56 57 58 59 62 64 65 70 73 74 75 76 77 78 79 81 82 85 86 87 89 92 93 96 97 107 108 110 111 113 114 115 116 118 119 120 122 127 128 129 130 131 134 145 146 147 **P**6 8 **S** Northwestern Memorial Healthcare, Chicago, IL
Primary Contact: Thomas J. McAfee, President
CFO: Matthew J. Flynn, Senior Vice President and Chief Financial Officer
CMO: Michael G. Ankin, M.D., Vice President Medical Affairs & Chief Medical Officer
CIO: Timothy R. Zoph, Senior Vice President and Chief Information Officer
CHR: Marsha Oberrieder, Vice President Operations
CNO: Kimberly Nagy, R.N., Vice President Operations and Chief Nurse Executive
Web address: www.lfh.org
**Control:** Other not–for–profit (including NFP Corporation) **Service:** General Medical and Surgical

**Staffed Beds:** 205 **Admissions:** 9024 **Census:** 127 **Outpatient Visits:** 203209 **Births:** 1718 **Total Expense ($000):** 226422 **Payroll Expense ($000):** 88760 **Personnel:** 1315

## LAWRENCEVILLE—Lawrence County

★ **LAWRENCE COUNTY MEMORIAL HOSPITAL (141344)**, 2200 West State Street, Zip 62439–1853; tel. 618/943–1000 **A**9 10 18 **F**3 11 15 28 30 40 75 81 93 107 113 126 129 132 142 **S** QHR, Brentwood, TN
Primary Contact: Doug Florkowski, Chief Executive Officer
CFO: Jerry Klein, Chief Financial Officer
CHR: Kim Kendall, Director Human Resources
Web address: www.lcmhosp.org
**Control:** Other not–for–profit (including NFP Corporation) **Service:** General Medical and Surgical

**Staffed Beds:** 25 **Admissions:** 894 **Census:** 9 **Outpatient Visits:** 29850 **Births:** 0 **Total Expense ($000):** 12369 **Payroll Expense ($000):** 4514 **Personnel:** 127

## LIBERTYVILLE—Lake County

✠ **ADVOCATE CONDELL MEDICAL CENTER (140202)**, 801 South Milwaukee Avenue, Zip 60048–3199; tel. 847/362–2900 **A**1 2 9 10 **F**2 3 11 12 13 15 18 19 20 22 24 26 28 29 30 31 32 34 35 36 40 41 43 45 46 48 49 50 51 53 54 56 57 59 60 64 65 68 70 73 74 75 76 77 78 79 81 82 85 86 87 89 92 93 95 96 107 108 110 111 113 114 116 117 118 120 122 125 128 129 130 131 134 143 144 145 146 147 **P**8 **S** Advocate Health Care, Oak Brook, IL
Primary Contact: Dominica Tallarico, President
CFO: David A. Cartwright, Vice President Finance
CMO: Joan Boomsma, M.D., Vice President Medical Management
CIO: Eileen Matzek, Director Information Technology
CHR: Gwenn Leschke, Vice President Human Resources
Web address: www.advocatehealth.com/condell/
**Control:** Other not–for–profit (including NFP Corporation) **Service:** General Medical and Surgical

**Staffed Beds:** 269 **Admissions:** 17386 **Census:** 186 **Outpatient Visits:** 205370 **Births:** 2312 **Total Expense ($000):** 273652 **Payroll Expense ($000):** 91705

## LINCOLN—Logan County

✠ **ABRAHAM LINCOLN MEMORIAL HOSPITAL (141322)**, 200 Stahlhut Drive, Zip 62656–2698; tel. 217/732–2161 **A**1 5 9 10 18 **F**13 15 28 29 30 35 40 57 59 64 71 75 76 77 78 81 82 93 107 108 111 118 128 129 130 131 132 143 145 **P**5 **S** Memorial Health System, Springfield, IL
Primary Contact: Dolan Dalpoas, President and Chief Executive Officer
COO: Kathleen Vipond, Assistant Administrator and Director
CFO: Andrew Costic, Regional Chief Financial Officer
CMO: Tracy Mizeur, M.D., President Medical Staff
CIO: Darrell Oller, Director Information Systems
CHR: Kaylee Tanner, Human Resources Business Partner
Web address: www.almh.org
**Control:** Other not–for–profit (including NFP Corporation) **Service:** General Medical and Surgical

**Staffed Beds:** 25 **Admissions:** 1046 **Census:** 9 **Outpatient Visits:** 54828 **Births:** 228 **Total Expense ($000):** 35889 **Payroll Expense ($000):** 13239 **Personnel:** 346

## LITCHFIELD—Montgomery County

✠ **ST. FRANCIS HOSPITAL (141350)**, 1215 Franciscan Drive, Zip 62056–1799, Mailing Address: P.O. Box 1215, Zip 62056–1215; tel. 217/324–2191 **A**1 9 10 18 **F**11 12 13 15 18 19 28 29 30 34 35 36 40 44 45 46 50 56 57 59 64 68 70 74 75 76 77 78 79 81 82 85 86 87 92 93 107 111 113 117 118 128 130 131 132 133 134 145 146 **S** Hospital Sisters Health System, Springfield, IL
Primary Contact: Daniel L. Perryman, President and Chief Executive Officer
COO: Carol Jaco, R.N., Chief Operating Officer and Chief Nursing Officer
CFO: Diane Lindsay, Chief Financial Officer
Web address: www.stfrancis–litchfield.org
**Control:** Church–operated, Nongovernment, not–for profit **Service:** General Medical and Surgical

**Staffed Beds:** 25 **Admissions:** 1508 **Census:** 15 **Outpatient Visits:** 52323 **Births:** 320 **Total Expense ($000):** 32519 **Payroll Expense ($000):** 11144 **Personnel:** 232

## MACOMB—Mcdonough County

✠ **MCDONOUGH DISTRICT HOSPITAL (140089)**, 525 East Grant Street, Zip 61455–3318; tel. 309/833–4101, (Total facility includes 16 beds in nursing home–type unit) **A**1 2 9 10 20 **F**2 3 5 7 8 11 12 13 15 18 19 26 27 28 31 34 35 37 38 40 41 43 45 48 51 56 57 59 62 63 64 68 70 74 75 76 77 78 79 81 82 84 85 86 89 91 93 94 96 97 99 100 101 102 103 104 107 108 110 111 113 114 115 118 123 127 128 129 130 131 134 140 145 147 **P**8
Primary Contact: Kenneth Boyd, Jr., President and Chief Executive Officer
COO: Lori Moon, R.N., Vice President Clinical Operations/ Business Development
CFO: Linda Dace, Vice President Finance
CMO: Christopher Stortzum, M.D., President Medical Staff
CIO: Harlan T. Baker, Department Leader Information Systems
CHR: Sue Dexter, Administrative Department Leader Human Resources
CNO: Wanda Foster, R.N., Vice President Nursing
Web address: www.mdh.org
**Control:** Hospital district or authority, Government, nonfederal **Service:** General Medical and Surgical

**Staffed Beds:** 95 **Admissions:** 2214 **Census:** 25 **Outpatient Visits:** 105813 **Births:** 321 **Total Expense ($000):** 52045 **Payroll Expense ($000):** 27110 **Personnel:** 506

## MARION—Williamson County

✠ **HEARTLAND REGIONAL MEDICAL CENTER (140184)**, 3333 West DeYoung, Zip 62959; tel. 618/998–7000, (Nonreporting) **A**1 9 10 **S** Community Health Systems, Inc., Franklin, TN
Primary Contact: Stephen Lunn, Chief Executive Officer
CFO: Loren Rials, Chief Financial Officer
CHR: Ed Daech, Director Human Resources
Web address: www.heartlandregional.com
**Control:** Corporation, Investor–owned, for–profit **Service:** General Medical and Surgical

**Staffed Beds:** 92

IL

*Many Facility Codes have changed. Please refer to the AHA Guide Code Chart.* © 2012 AHA Guide

⊞ **VETERANS AFFAIRS MEDICAL CENTER**, 2401 West Main Street, Zip 62959–1194; tel. 618/997–5311, (Nonreporting) **A**1 3 5 **S** Department of Veterans Affairs, Washington, DC
Primary Contact: Paul Bockelman, Director
COO: Frank Kehus, Associate Director for Operations
CFO: Wayne Morris, Chief Financial Officer
CMO: Farhana Hasan, M.D., Chief of Staff
CIO: Clint Bishop, Program Manager
CHR: Tonya L. Searby, Chief Human Resources
CNO: Barbara Southworth, R.N., Associate Director for Patient Care Services
Web address: www.marion.va.gov
**Control:** Veterans Affairs, Government, federal **Service:** General Medical and Surgical

**Staffed Beds:** 55

### MARYVILLE—Madison County

⊞ △ **ANDERSON HOSPITAL (140289)**, 6800 State Route 162, Zip 62062–8500; tel. 618/288–5711 **A**1 7 9 10 **F**3 11 13 15 18 20 22 28 29 30 34 35 40 49 51 57 59 62 63 70 74 75 76 78 79 81 82 85 90 93 107 108 110 111 114 117 118 119 123 125 128 129 131 143 145 146 147
Primary Contact: Keith Allen Page, President and Chief Executive Officer
CFO: Michael Marshall, Vice President Finance and Chief Financial Officer
CMO: Michael Mulligan, M.D., President Medical Staff
CIO: Michael Ward, Director Information Services
CHR: Robin Steinmann, Administrative Director Human Resources
CNO: Lisa Klaustermeier, R.N., Chief Nursing Officer
Web address: www.andersonhospital.org
**Control:** Other not–for–profit (including NFP Corporation) **Service:** General Medical and Surgical

**Staffed Beds:** 151 **Admissions:** 7578 **Census:** 80 **Outpatient Visits:** 169977 **Births:** 1843 **Total Expense ($000):** 104523 **Payroll Expense ($000):** 44990 **Personnel:** 915

### MATTOON—Coles County

⊞ **SARAH BUSH LINCOLN HEALTH CENTER (140189)**, 1000 Health Center Drive, Zip 61938–0372, Mailing Address: P.O. Box 372, Zip 61938–0372; tel. 217/258–2525, (Nonreporting) **A**1 9 10 20
Primary Contact: Timothy A. Ols, FACHE, President and Chief Executive Officer
COO: Dennis Pluard, Vice President Operations
CFO: Craig Sheagren, Vice President Finance
CMO: James Hildebrandt, D.O., President Medical Staff
CIO: Mike DeLuca, Vice President Information Systems
CHR: Eric Benson, Vice President Human Resources
CNO: Mary Lou Wild, Vice President Patient Care Services
Web address: www.sarahbush.org
**Control:** Other not–for–profit (including NFP Corporation) **Service:** General Medical and Surgical

**Staffed Beds:** 143

### MAYWOOD—Cook County

⊞ △ **LOYOLA UNIVERSITY MEDICAL CENTER (140276)**, 2160 South First Avenue, Zip 60153–5585; tel. 708/216–9000 **A**1 2 3 5 7 8 9 10 **F**3 4 5 6 7 8 9 11 12 13 14 15 16 17 18 19 20 21 22 23 24 25 26 27 28 29 30 31 32 34 35 36 37 38 39 40 43 44 45 46 47 48 49 50 51 53 54 55 56 57 58 59 60 61 62 63 64 65 66 68 70 71 72 73 74 75 77 78 79 80 81 82 84 85 86 87 88 89 90 92 93 94 96 97 98 99 100 101 102 103 104 107 108 110 111 113 114 115 116 117 118 119 120 122 123 125 128 129 130 131 133 134 135 136 137 138 139 140 141 143 144 145 146 147 **P**6 **S** Trinity Health, Novi, MI
Primary Contact: Patricia Cassidy, Interim President and Chief Executive Officer
CFO: Thomas Honan, Interim Chief Financial Officer
CMO: Robert Cherry, M.D., Chief Medical Officer
CIO: Arthur J. Krumrey, Chief Information Officer
CHR: Vicky Piper, Vice President Human Resources
Web address: www.loyolamedicine.org/Medical_Services/index.cfm
**Control:** Other not–for–profit (including NFP Corporation) **Service:** General Medical and Surgical

**Staffed Beds:** 535 **Admissions:** 24496 **Census:** 354 **Outpatient Visits:** 1261113 **Births:** 874 **Total Expense ($000):** 669814 **Payroll Expense ($000):** 423416 **Personnel:** 5854

### MCHENRY—Mchenry County

⊞ **CENTEGRA HOSPITAL – MCHENRY (140116)**, 4201 Medical Center Drive, Zip 60050–9506; tel. 815/344–5000 **A**1 2 5 9 10 **F**3 4 11 13 15 18 20 22 24 26 28 29 30 31 34 35 37 38 39 40 43 44 49 50 54 57 58 59 62 64 68 69 70 74 75 76 78 79 81 85 86 87 90 92 93 96 100 102 107 108 110 111 113 114 115 116 117 118 119 120 122 128 129 130 131 142 145 146 147 **P**5 **S** Centegra Health System, Crystal Lake, IL
Primary Contact: Michael S. Eesley, Chief Executive Officer
COO: Jason Sciarro, President and Chief Operating Officer
CFO: Robert Rosenberger, Executive Vice President and Chief Financial Officer
CMO: Ted Lorenc, M.D., Vice President Medical Affairs
CIO: David Tomlinson, Senior Vice President, Chief Information Officer
CHR: Bernadette S. Szczepanski, Vice President, Human Resources Development
CNO: Neil W. Murphy, R.N., Senior Vice President and Chief Nursing Officer
Web address: www.centegra.org
**Control:** Other not–for–profit (including NFP Corporation) **Service:** General Medical and Surgical

**Staffed Beds:** 173 **Admissions:** 10369 **Census:** 121 **Outpatient Visits:** 157065 **Births:** 831 **Total Expense ($000):** 203014 **Payroll Expense ($000):** 83918 **Personnel:** 1081

### MCLEANSBORO—Hamilton County

**HAMILTON MEMORIAL HOSPITAL DISTRICT (141326)**, 611 South Marshall Avenue, Zip 62859–0429, Mailing Address: P.O. Box 429, Mc Leansboro, Zip 62859–0429; tel. 618/643–2361 **A**9 10 18 **F**3 11 15 28 29 40 43 57 81 93 107 108 113 118 126 128 129 132
Primary Contact: Randall W. Dauby, Chief Executive Officer
COO: Bradley Futrell, Chief Operating Officer
CFO: Kent Mitchell, Chief Financial Officer
CIO: Don Darnell, Chief Information Officer
CNO: Patty Blazier, Chief Nursing Officer
Web address: www.hmhospital.org
**Control:** Hospital district or authority, Government, nonfederal **Service:** General Medical and Surgical

**Staffed Beds:** 25 **Admissions:** 1078 **Census:** 9 **Outpatient Visits:** 37119 **Births:** 0 **Total Expense ($000):** 12841 **Payroll Expense ($000):** 5289 **Personnel:** 129

### MELROSE PARK—Cook County

⊞ **GOTTLIEB MEMORIAL HOSPITAL (140008)**, 701 West North Avenue, Zip 60160–1692; tel. 708/681–3200, (Nonreporting) **A**1 3 5 9 10 **S** Trinity Health, Novi, MI
Primary Contact: Patricia Cassidy, President
COO: Ken Fishbain, Chief Operating Officer
CFO: Ellyn Chin, Vice President Finance
CMO: Gerald Luger, M.D., President Medical Staff
CIO: Maurita Adler, Director Information Services
CHR: Brett Wakefield, Vice President Human Resources
Web address: www.gottliebhospital.org
**Control:** Other not–for–profit (including NFP Corporation) **Service:** General Medical and Surgical

**Staffed Beds:** 268

○ **WESTLAKE HOSPITAL (140240)**, 1225 Lake Street, Zip 60160–4000; tel. 708/681–3000, (Nonreporting) **A**3 5 9 10 11 **S** Vanguard Health System, Nashville, TN
Primary Contact: William A. Brown, FACHE, Chief Executive Officer
COO: Patrick Durkin, Vice President Professional Services
CFO: John Orsini, Chief Financial Officer
CMO: Glenn Kushner, M.D., President Medical Staff
CIO: George Chessum, Chief Information Officer
CHR: Robert Mueller, Director Human Resources
Web address: www.wlhospital.com/Home.aspx
**Control:** Corporation, Investor–owned, for–profit **Service:** General Medical and Surgical

**Staffed Beds:** 181

**IL**

---

**Hospital, Medicare Provider Number, Address, Telephone, Approval, Facility, and Physician Codes, Health Care System**

★ American Hospital Association (AHA) membership
□ The Joint Commission accreditation
◇ DNV Healthcare Inc. accreditation
○ American Osteopathic Association (AOA) accreditation
△ Commission on Accreditation of Rehabilitation Facilities (CARF) accreditation

© 2012 AHA Guide    *Many Facility Codes have changed. Please refer to the AHA Guide Code Chart.*    Hospitals **A187**

**MENDOTA—Lasalle County**

★ **MENDOTA COMMUNITY HOSPITAL (141310)**, 1401 East 12th Street, Zip 61342–9216; tel. 815/539–7461 **A**9 10 18 **F**3 11 15 28 29 31 34 40 45 49 59 62 69 70 75 77 79 81 85 93 107 110 113 128 129 130 131 132 144 145 **P**6
Primary Contact: Lynn E. Klein, Administrator
CFO: Larry Peach, Assistant Administrator and Chief Financial Officer
CMO: William Schuler, M.D., President Medical Staff
CIO: Gilbert Hermosillo, Manager Information Services
CHR: Kimberly Kennedy, Manager Human Resources
Web address: www.mendotahospital.org
**Control:** Other not–for–profit (including NFP Corporation) **Service:** General Medical and Surgical

| | |
|---|---|
| **Staffed Beds:** 25 **Admissions:** 877 **Census:** 10 **Outpatient Visits:** 50910 **Births:** 0 **Total Expense ($000):** 30343 **Payroll Expense ($000):** 13197 **Personnel:** 234 | |

**METROPOLIS—Massac County**

★ **MASSAC MEMORIAL HOSPITAL (141323)**, 28 Chick Street, Zip 62960, Mailing Address: P.O. Box 850, Zip 62960–0850; tel. 618/524–2176, (Nonreporting) **A**9 10 18
Primary Contact: David G. Fuqua, Chief Executive Officer
CFO: Chelle Keplinger, Chief Financial Officer
CHR: Joel Foster, Director Human Resources
CNO: Janet Barrett, R.N., Chief Nurse Executive
Web address: www.massachealth.org
**Control:** Hospital district or authority, Government, nonfederal **Service:** General Medical and Surgical

| | |
|---|---|
| **Staffed Beds:** 25 | |

**MOLINE—Rock Island County**

**TRINITY MOLINE** See Trinity Rock Island, Rock Island

**MONMOUTH—Warren County**

★ **OSF HOLY FAMILY MEDICAL CENTER (141318)**, 1000 West Harlem Avenue, Zip 61462–1099; tel. 309/734–3141 **A**9 10 18 **F**11 15 28 29 30 34 40 45 46 50 57 59 64 65 68 75 77 81 85 87 93 97 107 110 111 114 117 118 126 128 129 131 132 134 144 145 147 **P**6 **S** OSF Healthcare System, Peoria, IL
Primary Contact: Patricia A. Luker, Chief Executive Officer
CFO: Theresa Springer, Chief Financial Officer
CMO: Ruben Medrano, M.D., President Medical Staff
CIO: Lew McCann, Director Management Information Systems
CHR: Irene Kress, Director Human Resources
Web address: www.osfholyfamily.org
**Control:** Church–operated, Nongovernment, not–for profit **Service:** General Medical and Surgical

| | |
|---|---|
| **Staffed Beds:** 23 **Admissions:** 483 **Census:** 5 **Outpatient Visits:** 74944 **Births:** 0 **Total Expense ($000):** 23370 **Payroll Expense ($000):** 10774 **Personnel:** 198 | |

**MONTICELLO—Piatt County**

⊞ **KIRBY MEDICAL CENTER (141301)**, 1000 Medical Center Drive, Zip 61856–1116; tel. 217/762–2115, (Nonreporting) **A**1 9 10 18
Primary Contact: Steven Tenhouse, Chief Executive Officer
CFO: C. David Harms, Chief Financial Officer
CMO: Narain Mandhan, M.D., President Medical Staff
CIO: Kyle Willams, Chief Information Officer
Web address: www.kirbyhealth.org
**Control:** Other not–for–profit (including NFP Corporation) **Service:** General Medical and Surgical

| | |
|---|---|
| **Staffed Beds:** 16 | |

**MORRIS—Grundy County**

★ **MORRIS HOSPITAL & HEALTHCARE CENTERS (140101)**, 150 West High Street, Zip 60450–1497; tel. 815/942–2932 **A**2 9 10 **F**3 11 13 15 18 19 20 22 26 28 29 34 35 40 43 47 49 50 54 57 59 64 66 69 70 74 75 76 77 78 79 81 82 85 86 87 89 93 97 99 102 107 108 110 111 113 114 117 118 119 120 122 129 131 132 134 142 143 145 **P**6
Primary Contact: Mark B. Steadham, President and Chief Executive Officer
COO: Patrick O'Connor, Chief Operating Officer
CFO: Thomas Meyer, Vice President Finance
CIO: Dean M. Marketti, Chief Information Officer
CHR: Erin Murphy–Frobish, Vice President Human Resources
CNO: Carol Havel, R.N., Vice President Patient Care Services
Web address: www.morrishospital.org
**Control:** Other not–for–profit (including NFP Corporation) **Service:** General Medical and Surgical

| | |
|---|---|
| **Staffed Beds:** 89 **Admissions:** 4147 **Census:** 42 **Outpatient Visits:** 219161 **Births:** 612 **Total Expense ($000):** 102579 **Payroll Expense ($000):** 45838 **Personnel:** 688 | |

**MORRISON—Whiteside County**

★ **MORRISON COMMUNITY HOSPITAL (141329)**, 303 North Jackson Street, Zip 61270–3042; tel. 815/772–4003, (Nonreporting) **A**9 10 18 **S** Trinity Health, Novi, MI
Primary Contact: Kent Jorgensen, Chief Executive Officer
COO: Pam Pfister, Associate Administrator
CFO: Cami Megli, Controller
CMO: Duncan Dinkha, M.D., Chief of Staff
CIO: Pam Pfister, Associate Administrator
CHR: Kathy Pennock, Director Human Resources
Web address: www.morrisonhospital.com
**Control:** Hospital district or authority, Government, nonfederal **Service:** General Medical and Surgical

| | |
|---|---|
| **Staffed Beds:** 60 | |

**MOUNT CARMEL—Wabash County**

⊞ **WABASH GENERAL HOSPITAL (141327)**, 1418 College Drive, Zip 62863–2638; tel. 618/262–8621 **A**1 9 10 18 **F**3 7 11 28 29 31 34 40 45 46 50 59 64 75 77 78 79 81 91 92 94 107 110 111 113 118 126 128 129 130 132 134 142 143 **S** Alliant Management Services, Louisville, KY
Primary Contact: Jay Purvis, Administrator
CFO: Steve McGill, Chief Financial Officer
Web address: www.wabashgeneral.com
**Control:** County–Government, nonfederal **Service:** General Medical and Surgical

| | |
|---|---|
| **Staffed Beds:** 25 **Admissions:** 716 **Census:** 7 **Outpatient Visits:** 40945 **Births:** 0 **Total Expense ($000):** 29166 **Payroll Expense ($000):** 11682 **Personnel:** 234 | |

**MOUNT VERNON—Jefferson County**

⊞ **CROSSROADS COMMUNITY HOSPITAL (140294)**, 8 Doctors Park Road, Zip 62864–6224; tel. 618/244–5500, (Nonreporting) **A**1 9 10 **S** Community Health Systems, Inc., Franklin, TN
Primary Contact: M. Edward Cunningham, Chief Executive Officer
CMO: Norman Cohen, M.D., Chief Medical Officer
CIO: Regina Garrett, Director Health Information Management
CHR: Reva Weems, Director Human Resources
Web address: www.crossroadscommunityhospital.com
**Control:** Corporation, Investor–owned, for–profit **Service:** General Medical and Surgical

| | |
|---|---|
| **Staffed Beds:** 41 | |

⊞ **GOOD SAMARITAN REGIONAL HEALTH CENTER (140046)**, 605 North 12th Street, Zip 62864–2899; tel. 618/242–4600 **A**1 2 9 10 19 **F**3 11 13 15 18 20 22 24 26 28 29 30 31 34 35 38 40 44 45 50 51 54 57 59 61 64 68 70 74 75 76 77 78 79 80 81 82 84 85 86 87 89 90 93 94 107 108 109 110 111 113 114 117 118 125 129 131 134 144 145 146 147 **P**6 8 **S** SSM Health Care, Saint Louis, MO
Primary Contact: Michael D. Warren, President
COO: Chris Adams, Vice President Operations
CFO: Kay Tinsley, Vice President Fiscal Services
CMO: Daniel Hoffman, M.D., Administrative Medical Director
CIO: Steve Murphy, Director Networks
CHR: Thomas W. Blythe, Vice President Human Resources
Web address: www.smgsi.com
**Control:** Church–operated, Nongovernment, not–for profit **Service:** General Medical and Surgical

| | |
|---|---|
| **Staffed Beds:** 148 **Admissions:** 6581 **Census:** 69 **Outpatient Visits:** 199141 **Births:** 845 **Total Expense ($000):** 113821 **Payroll Expense ($000):** 42126 **Personnel:** 1009 | |

**MURPHYSBORO—Jackson County**

★ **ST. JOSEPH MEMORIAL HOSPITAL (141334)**, 2 South Hospital Drive, Zip 62966–3333; tel. 618/684–3156 **A**9 10 18 **F**3 11 18 28 29 30 34 35 40 45 56 57 59 64 74 75 77 78 79 81 85 93 107 113 118 128 129 131 134 145 147 **S** Southern Illinois Hospital Services, Carbondale, IL
Primary Contact: Scott Seaborn, Administrator
CMO: Gerald McClallen, President Medical Staff
CIO: David Holland, Vice President Information Services
CHR: Kelly Stevens, Manager Human Resources
Web address: www.sih.net
**Control:** Other not–for–profit (including NFP Corporation) **Service:** General Medical and Surgical

| | |
|---|---|
| **Staffed Beds:** 25 **Admissions:** 875 **Census:** 8 **Outpatient Visits:** 57764 **Births:** 0 **Total Expense ($000):** 34140 **Payroll Expense ($000):** 12215 **Personnel:** 223 | |

IL

*Many Facility Codes have changed. Please refer to the AHA Guide Code Chart.*   © 2012 AHA Guide

## NAPERVILLE—Dupage County

⊠ **EDWARD HOSPITAL (140231)**, 801 South Washington Street,
Zip 60540–7499; tel. 630/527–3000 **A**1 2 9 10 **F**3 13 15 17 18 20 22 24 26
28 29 30 31 32 34 35 37 38 40 41 42 43 45 47 49 50 54 55 57 58 59 61
64 68 70 72 73 74 75 76 77 78 79 80 81 82 84 85 86 87 88 89 93 96 97
102 107 108 109 110 111 113 114 115 116 117 118 119 120 122 123 125
128 129 130 131 134 143 145 146 147 **P**1 6 7
Primary Contact: Pamela M. Davis, President and Chief Executive Officer
COO: Marianne Spencer, R.N., Vice President Operations and Chief Operating
Officer
CFO: Vincent Pryor, Senior Vice President Finance and Chief Financial Officer
CMO: Brent Smith, M.D., Chief Medical Officer and Vice President Clinical
Integration
CIO: Bobbie Byrne, M.D., Vice President Chief Information Officer
CHR: Dennise Vaughn, Vice President Corporate Resources
CNO: Patti Ludwig–Beymer, Ph.D., Chief Nursing Officer
Web address: www.edward.org
**Control:** Other not–for–profit (including NFP Corporation) **Service:** General
Medical and Surgical

**Staffed Beds:** 330 **Admissions:** 20254 **Census:** 213 **Outpatient Visits:**
505001 **Births:** 3427 **Total Expense ($000):** 440079 **Payroll Expense
($000):** 148833 **Personnel:** 2339

⊠ **LINDEN OAKS HOSPITAL AT EDWARD (144035)**, 852 West Street,
Zip 60540–6400; tel. 630/305–5500 **A**1 5 9 10 **F**4 5 29 30 34 35 38 56 57
59 64 68 75 87 98 99 100 101 103 104 105 106 129 131 133 **P**1 6 7
Primary Contact: Mary Lou Mastro, President
COO: Gina Sharp, Executive Director
CFO: Gina Sharp, Executive Director
CMO: Barry Rabin, M.D., Medical Director
CIO: Hugh Siddiqui, Senior Applications Analyst
CHR: Dennise Vaughn, Vice President Corporate Resources
CNO: Beth Jelesky, Director Quality, Risk Management, CNO
Web address: www.edward.org
**Control:** Other not–for–profit (including NFP Corporation) **Service:** Psychiatric

**Staffed Beds:** 94 **Admissions:** 3893 **Census:** 76 **Outpatient Visits:** 40709
**Births:** 0 **Total Expense ($000):** 31483 **Payroll Expense ($000):** 16442
**Personnel:** 315

## NASHVILLE—Washington County

⊠ **WASHINGTON COUNTY HOSPITAL (141308)**, 705 South Grand Avenue,
Zip 62263–1534; tel. 618/327–8236, (Total facility includes 28 beds in nursing
home–type unit) **A**1 9 10 18 **F**11 15 28 29 31 34 40 49 57 65 66 78 81 85 93
104 107 113 118 126 132 144 145 147
Primary Contact: Nancy M. Newby, R.N., Ph.D., FACHE, President and Chief
Executive Officer
CFO: Elaine Matzenbacher, Chief Financial Officer
CMO: Alfonso Urdaneta, M.D., President Medical Staff
CIO: Kim Larkin, Chief Information Officer
CHR: Alanna Barker, Director Human Resources
CNO: Tammy Amizich, Chief Nursing Executive
Web address: www.washingtoncountyhospital.org
**Control:** Hospital district or authority, Government, nonfederal **Service:** General
Medical and Surgical

**Staffed Beds:** 50 **Admissions:** 343 **Census:** 33 **Outpatient Visits:** 35933
**Births:** 0 **Total Expense ($000):** 14977 **Payroll Expense ($000):** 6811
**Personnel:** 148

## NEW LENOX—Will County

⊠ △ **SILVER CROSS HOSPITAL (140213)**, 1900 Silver Cross Boulevard,
Zip 60451–9509; tel. 815/300–1100 **A**1 2 7 9 10 **F**3 5 7 11 12 13 15 18 20
22 26 28 29 30 31 32 34 35 37 38 40 42 43 44 45 46 47 48 49 50 53 54
57 59 60 62 64 68 70 74 75 76 77 78 79 81 82 85 89 90 92 93 96 98 100
101 102 103 104 105 107 108 110 111 113 114 117 118 129 130 131 133
134 145 146 147 **P**1 5 8
Primary Contact: Paul Pawlak, President and Chief Executive Officer
COO: Mary Bakken, Executive Vice President and Chief Operating Officer
CFO: William R. Brownlow, Senior Vice President Finance
CMO: Alexander Sosenko, M.D., Chief of Staff
CIO: Kevin Lane, Vice President Information Systems
CHR: Mark Jepson, Vice President
CNO: Peggy Gricus, R.N., Vice President, Patient Care Services/CNO
Web address: www.silvercross.org
**Control:** Other not–for–profit (including NFP Corporation) **Service:** General
Medical and Surgical

**Staffed Beds:** 246 **Admissions:** 14902 **Census:** 162 **Outpatient Visits:**
208952 **Births:** 1715 **Total Expense ($000):** 218619 **Payroll Expense
($000):** 83629 **Personnel:** 1312

## NORMAL—Mclean County

⊠ **ADVOCATE BROMENN MEDICAL CENTER (140127)**, 1304 Franklin Avenue,
Zip 61761, Mailing Address: P.O. Box 2850, Bloomington, Zip 61702–2850;
tel. 309/454–1400, (Includes BROMENN REGIONAL MEDICAL CENTER, Virginia
and Franklin Streets, Mailing Address: P.O. Box 2850, Bloomington,
Zip 61702–2850; tel. 309/454–1400) **A**1 2 10 12 13 **F**2 3 4 12 13 15 18 20
22 24 26 28 29 30 31 32 34 35 38 39 40 43 44 45 49 57 59 64 65 66 68
70 74 75 76 77 78 79 81 82 83 84 85 86 87 89 90 93 96 97 98 100 101
102 103 107 108 110 111 113 114 117 118 125 129 130 131 134 140 143
145 146 147 **P**8 **S** Advocate Health Care, Oak Brook, IL
Primary Contact: Colleen Kannaday, FACHE, President
COO: Gary Hagens, Chief Operating Officer and Vice President Medical Affairs
CMO: Gary Hagens, Chief Operating Officer and Vice President Medical Affairs
CIO: Vincent Vitali, Vice President and Chief Information Officer
CHR: Alex Horvath, Vice President Human Resources
Web address: www.bromenn.org
**Control:** Church–operated, Nongovernment, not–for profit **Service:** General
Medical and Surgical

**Staffed Beds:** 200 **Admissions:** 9942 **Census:** 100 **Outpatient Visits:**
165402 **Births:** 1489 **Total Expense ($000):** 164729 **Payroll Expense
($000):** 56706 **Personnel:** 1122

**ADVOCATE BROMENN REGIONAL MEDICAL CENTER** See Advocate BroMenn
Medical Center

## NORTH CHICAGO—Lake County

⊠ **CAPTAIN JAMES A. LOVELL FEDERAL HEALTH CARE CENTER**, 3001 Green
Bay Road, Zip 60064–3049; tel. 847/688–1900, (Nonreporting) **A**1 3 5 9
**S** Department of Veterans Affairs, Washington, DC
Primary Contact: Patrick L. Sullivan, FACHE, Director
COO: Marianne Semrad, Associate Director Administrative Services
CFO: Barbara Meadows, Chief Financial Manager
CMO: Tariq Hassan, M.D., Associate Director of Patient Care
CIO: Jonathan Friedman, Public Affairs Officer
CHR: Amy Sanders, Chief Human Resources
CNO: Sarah Fouse, Associate Director of Patient Services
Web address: www.lovell.fhcc.va.gov
**Control:** Veterans Affairs, Government, federal **Service:** Other specialty

**Staffed Beds:** 103

## NORTHLAKE—Cook County

⊠ **KINDRED HOSPITAL CHICAGO–NORTHLAKE (142008)**, 365 East North
Avenue, Zip 60164–2628; tel. 708/345–8100 **A**1 9 10 **F**1 3 29 45 77 80 85
91 107 118 129 147 **S** Kindred Healthcare, Louisville, KY
Primary Contact: Beverly Foster, Chief Executive Officer
COO: Sandra Buckhoy, Chief Clinical Officer
CFO: Jay Schweikart, Chief Financial Officer
CMO: Maher Najjar, M.D., Medical Director
Web address: www.kindrednorthlake.com/
**Control:** Corporation, Investor–owned, for–profit **Service:** Long–Term Acute Care
hospital

**Staffed Beds:** 94 **Admissions:** 573 **Census:** 56 **Outpatient Visits:** 0 **Births:**
0 **Total Expense ($000):** 30351 **Payroll Expense ($000):** 10037
**Personnel:** 133

## OAK LAWN—Cook County

⊠ △ **ADVOCATE CHRIST MEDICAL CENTER (140208)**, 4440 West 95th
Street, Zip 60453–2699; tel. 708/684–8000, (Includes ADVOCATE HOPE
CHILDREN'S HOSPITAL, 4440 West 95th Street, Zip 60453–2600;
tel. 708/684–8000) **A**1 2 3 5 7 8 9 10 13 **F**3 5 6 11 13 15 17 18 19 20 21
22 23 24 25 26 27 28 29 30 31 32 34 35 37 38 39 40 41 43 44 45 46 48
49 50 51 52 54 55 56 57 58 59 60 61 62 64 65 66 68 69 70 71 72 74
75 76 77 78 79 81 82 84 85 86 87 88 89 90 93 96 97 98 99 100 101 102
103 104 105 107 108 109 110 111 113 114 117 118 119 120 122 123 125
128 129 130 131 133 134 136 137 142 144 145 146 147 **P**8 **S** Advocate
Health Care, Oak Brook, IL
Primary Contact: Kenneth W. Lukhard, President
COO: Dominica Tallarico, Chief Operating Officer
CFO: Robert Pekofske, Vice President Finance
CMO: Robert Stein, M.D., Vice President Medical Management
CIO: Brian Banbury, Director Site Information Systems
Web address: www.advocatehealth.com/christ
**Control:** Other not–for–profit (including NFP Corporation) **Service:** General
Medical and Surgical

**Staffed Beds:** 672 **Admissions:** 40767 **Census:** 575 **Outpatient Visits:**
318341 **Births:** 4012 **Total Expense ($000):** 812548 **Payroll Expense
($000):** 315074 **Personnel:** 4200

IL

**Hospital, Medicare Provider Number, Address, Telephone, Approval, Facility, and Physician Codes, Health Care System**

★ American Hospital Association (AHA) membership
□ The Joint Commission accreditation
◇ DNV Healthcare Inc. accreditation
○ American Osteopathic Association (AOA) accreditation
△ Commission on Accreditation of Rehabilitation Facilities (CARF) accreditation

© 2012 AHA Guide    *Many Facility Codes have changed. Please refer to the AHA Guide Code Chart.*    Hospitals **A189**

## OAK PARK—Cook County

☒ △ **RUSH OAK PARK HOSPITAL (140063)**, 520 South Maple Avenue,
Zip 60304–1097; tel. 708/383–9300, (Total facility includes 20 beds in nursing
home–type unit) **A**1 3 5 7 9 10 **F**3 11 15 18 20 22 29 30 34 35 40 45 47 49
50 56 57 59 64 68 70 74 75 77 79 81 82 85 87 90 92 93 94 96 107 108
111 113 114 118 127 129 144 145 147 **P**8 **S** Wheaton Franciscan Healthcare,
Wheaton, IL
Primary Contact: Bruce M. Elegant, President and Chief Executive Officer
COO: James Kaese, Vice President Administration
CFO: Deborah Wilberding, Controller
CMO: Michael R. Silver, M.D., Vice President Medical Affairs
CIO: Dewey Gosnell, Manager
CHR: Cristina Diaz, Director
CNO: Karen Mayer, VP Patient Care Services
Web address: www.roph.org
**Control:** Church–operated, Nongovernment, not–for profit **Service:** General
Medical and Surgical

**Staffed Beds:** 114 **Admissions:** 4383 **Census:** 68 **Outpatient Visits:** 94386
**Births:** 0 **Total Expense ($000):** 97474 **Payroll Expense ($000):** 45138
**Personnel:** 777

○ **WEST SUBURBAN MEDICAL CENTER (140049)**, 3 Erie Court,
Zip 60302–2599; tel. 708/383–6200, (Nonreporting) **A**2 3 5 9 10 11 13
**S** Vanguard Health System, Nashville, TN
Primary Contact: John J. Cleary, Chief Executive Officer
COO: Joan Ormsby, Vice President
CFO: John Orsini, Chief Financial Officer
CMO: Michael DeHaan, M.D., President Medical Staff
CIO: George Chessum, Chief Information Officer
CHR: Robert Mueller, Director Human Resources
Web address: www.westsuburbanmc.com/Home.aspx
**Control:** Corporation, Investor–owned, for–profit **Service:** General Medical and
Surgical

**Staffed Beds:** 172

## OLNEY—Richland County

★ ○ **RICHLAND MEMORIAL HOSPITAL (140147)**, 800 East Locust Street,
Zip 62450–2553; tel. 618/395–2131, (Total facility includes 34 beds in nursing
home–type unit) **A**9 10 11 **F**3 7 11 13 15 28 29 31 34 35 40 51 57 59 61 62
63 64 68 69 70 75 76 78 79 81 85 87 89 93 97 98 100 102 103 104 107
108 110 111 114 118 127 128 129 130 131 132 134 142 145 146 **P**6
Primary Contact: David B. Allen, Chief Executive Officer
CFO: Mike Stoverink, Chief Financial Officer
CMO: Robert Nash, M.D., Chief of Staff
CIO: Tim Gillespie, Manager Information Systems
CHR: Jill Van Hyning, Director Human Resources
CNO: Cindy Bailey, R.N., Chief Nursing Officer
Web address: www.richlandmemorial.com
**Control:** Other not–for–profit (including NFP Corporation) **Service:** General
Medical and Surgical

**Staffed Beds:** 90 **Admissions:** 2989 **Census:** 54 **Outpatient Visits:** 50257
**Births:** 347 **Personnel:** 378

## OLYMPIA FIELDS—Cook County

○ **FRANCISCAN ST. JAMES HOSPITAL AND HEALTH CENTERS (140172)**,
20201 South Crawford Avenue, Zip 60461–1080; tel. 708/747–4000, (Includes
ST. JAMES HOSPITAL AND HEALTH CENTERS – CHICAGO HEIGHTS CAMPUS,
1423 Chicago Road, Chicago Heights, Zip 60411–3483; tel. 708/756–1000; ST.
JAMES HOSPITALS AND HEALTH CENTERS – OLYMPIA FIELDS CAMPUS, 20201
Crawford Avenue, Zip 60461–1010; tel. 708/747–4000), (Nonreporting) **A**2 9 10
11 12 13 **S** Franciscan Alliance, Mishawaka, IN
Primary Contact: Seth C. R. Warren, President
CIO: Stephen Maes, Director Information Systems
Web address: www.stjameshhc.org
**Control:** Other not–for–profit (including NFP Corporation) **Service:** General
Medical and Surgical

**Staffed Beds:** 402

**ST. JAMES HOSPITAL AND HEALTH CENTERS** See Franciscan St. James
Hospital and Health Centers

## OTTAWA—Lasalle County

☒ **OTTAWA REGIONAL HOSPITAL AND HEALTHCARE CENTER (140110)**,
1100 East Norris Drive, Zip 61350–1687; tel. 815/433–3100 **A**1 9 10 **F**3 11
13 15 18 28 30 31 34 35 40 43 45 47 48 49 53 56 57 59 62 63 68 70 75
76 77 79 81 82 84 85 86 87 93 94 98 101 102 103 104 105 107 108 110
111 113 114 117 118 129 130 131 134 142 143 145 146 147
Primary Contact: Robert A. Chaffin, President and Chief Executive Officer
COO: Judy A. Christiansen, R.N., Chief Operating Officer
CFO: Dawn Trompeter, Vice President Finance
CMO: David O. Manigold, M.D., President Medical Staff
CIO: John Maynard, Director Information Systems
CHR: Robert Gibson, Senior Director Operating Services
Web address: www.ottawaregional.org
**Control:** Other not–for–profit (including NFP Corporation) **Service:** General
Medical and Surgical

**Staffed Beds:** 91 **Admissions:** 3693 **Census:** 35 **Outpatient Visits:** 194031
**Births:** 357 **Total Expense ($000):** 70661 **Payroll Expense ($000):** 29934
**Personnel:** 541

## PALOS HEIGHTS—Cook County

☒ **PALOS COMMUNITY HOSPITAL (140062)**, 12251 South 80th Avenue,
Zip 60463–0930; tel. 708/923–4000 **A**1 2 9 10 **F**3 4 5 13 15 17 18 20 22 24
26 28 29 30 31 32 34 35 36 38 40 49 50 54 56 57 59 61 62 63 64 69 70
74 75 76 78 79 81 84 85 87 89 93 98 99 100 102 103 104 105 107 108
110 111 113 114 116 117 118 129 131 134 143 145 146 147 **P**6
Primary Contact: Sister Margaret Wright, President
CFO: Hugh Rose, Vice President Fiscal Management
CIO: Peggy Carroll, Chief Information Officer
CHR: Mary Denisienko, Vice President Human Resources
Web address: www.paloscommunityhospital.org
**Control:** Other not–for–profit (including NFP Corporation) **Service:** General
Medical and Surgical

**Staffed Beds:** 377 **Admissions:** 19968 **Census:** 244 **Outpatient Visits:**
405000 **Births:** 1169 **Total Expense ($000):** 318749 **Payroll Expense
($000):** 163715 **Personnel:** 2286

## PANA—Christian County

★ ○ **PANA COMMUNITY HOSPITAL (141341)**, 101 East Ninth Street,
Zip 62557–1785; tel. 217/562–2131 **A**9 10 11 18 **F**3 11 15 28 30 31 34 35
40 53 57 59 62 63 69 75 78 79 81 87 93 94 100 104 110 113 126 129
130 132
Primary Contact: Roland R. Carlson, President and Chief Executive Officer
CFO: Trina Casner, Chief Financial Officer and Chief Operating Officer
CMO: Alan Frigy, M.D., President Medical Staff
CIO: Dianne Bailey, Coordinator Information Systems
CHR: Luann Funk, Administrative Assistant and Manager Human Resources
Web address: www.panahospital.com
**Control:** Other not–for–profit (including NFP Corporation) **Service:** General
Medical and Surgical

**Staffed Beds:** 22 **Admissions:** 527 **Census:** 4 **Outpatient Visits:** 48926
**Births:** 0 **Total Expense ($000):** 16088 **Payroll Expense ($000):** 7241
**Personnel:** 146

## PARIS—Edgar County

☒ **PARIS COMMUNITY HOSPITAL (141320)**, 721 East Court Street, Zip 61944;
tel. 217/465–4141 **A**1 9 10 18 **F**3 15 28 29 30 31 34 35 40 45 57 59 64 65
67 69 74 75 77 78 79 81 82 85 86 87 89 90 93 107 108 110 111 113 118
126 127 129 130 131 132 134 143 145 147 **P**6 **S** Alliant Management
Services, Louisville, KY
Primary Contact: Randy Simmons, President and Chief Executive Officer
CFO: Terry Brinkley, Vice President Finance
CIO: Gary Taylor, Manager Information Services
CHR: Ollie Smith, Vice President Human Resources
Web address: www.pariscommunityhospital.com
**Control:** Other not–for–profit (including NFP Corporation) **Service:** General
Medical and Surgical

**Staffed Beds:** 25 **Admissions:** 511 **Census:** 5 **Outpatient Visits:** 91527
**Births:** 0 **Total Expense ($000):** 30506 **Payroll Expense ($000):** 14372
**Personnel:** 219

*Many Facility Codes have changed. Please refer to the AHA Guide Code Chart.* © 2012 AHA Guide

## PARK RIDGE—Cook County

⊞ △ **ADVOCATE LUTHERAN GENERAL HOSPITAL (140223)**, 1775 Dempster Street, Zip 60068–1174; tel. 847/723–2210 **A**1 2 3 5 7 8 9 10 13 **F**2 3 5 6 8 9 11 13 15 17 18 19 20 21 22 23 24 25 26 27 28 29 30 31 32 34 35 37 38 39 40 41 43 44 45 46 47 48 49 50 53 55 56 57 58 59 60 61 63 64 65 66 68 69 70 72 74 75 76 78 79 80 81 82 84 85 86 87 88 89 90 92 93 94 97 98 99 100 101 102 103 104 105 106 107 108 110 111 112 113 114 115 116 117 118 119 120 122 123 125 128 129 130 131 133 134 135 140 142 145 146 147 **P**6 8 **S** Advocate Health Care, Oak Brook, IL
Primary Contact: Anthony A. Armada, President
COO: Barbara Weber, Chief Operating Officer
CFO: Jim Kelley, Vice President Finance and Support Services
CMO: Michael McKenna, M.D., Vice President Medical Management
CIO: Mark Beitzel, Director Information Systems
CHR: Penny Pilarczyk, Vice President Human Resources
Web address: www.advocatehealth.com
**Control:** Other not–for–profit (including NFP Corporation) **Service:** General Medical and Surgical

**Staffed Beds:** 624 **Admissions:** 29586 **Census:** 409 **Outpatient Visits:** 296251 **Births:** 3911 **Total Expense ($000):** 588678 **Payroll Expense ($000):** 222275 **Personnel:** 3378

## PEKIN—Tazewell County

⊞ **PEKIN HOSPITAL (140120)**, 600 South 13th Street, Zip 61554–5098; tel. 309/347–1151 **A**1 9 10 **F**3 8 11 13 15 18 20 22 28 29 30 31 34 35 40 42 45 46 47 48 49 50 51 53 57 59 60 62 64 68 69 70 74 75 76 78 79 81 82 85 86 87 89 97 107 108 110 111 114 118 127 128 129 131 134 143 144 145 146 147 **P**1 **S** QHR, Brentwood, TN
Primary Contact: Gary L. Jepson, Chief Executive Officer
CFO: Steve Hall, Chief Financial Officer
CMO: Kathryn Kramer, M.D., President Medical Staff
CHR: Anne Dierker, Vice President Hospital Services
Web address: www.pekinhospital.org
**Control:** Other not–for–profit (including NFP Corporation) **Service:** General Medical and Surgical

**Staffed Beds:** 125 **Admissions:** 4016 **Census:** 48 **Outpatient Visits:** 100955 **Births:** 430 **Total Expense ($000):** 63790 **Payroll Expense ($000):** 27362 **Personnel:** 643

## PEORIA—Peoria County

**GREATER PEORIA SPECIALTY HOSPITAL** See Kindred Hospital Peoria

⊞ **KINDRED HOSPITAL PEORIA (142013)**, 500 West Romeo B. Garrett Avenue, Zip 61605; tel. 309/680–1500, (Nonreporting) **A**1 10 **S** Kindred Healthcare, Louisville, KY
Primary Contact: Adam Novak, Chief Executive Officer
Web address: www.khpeoria.com/
**Control:** Partnership, Investor–owned, for–profit **Service:** Long–Term Acute Care hospital

**Staffed Beds:** 50

⊞ △ **METHODIST MEDICAL CENTER OF ILLINOIS (140209)**, 221 N.E. Glen Oak Avenue, Zip 61636–4310; tel. 309/672–5522 **A**1 2 3 5 7 9 10 **F**3 8 9 11 12 13 15 17 18 20 22 24 26 28 29 30 31 32 34 35 36 38 40 43 44 45 46 47 48 49 50 53 54 56 57 58 59 60 62 63 64 68 70 74 75 76 77 78 79 81 82 84 85 86 87 89 90 92 93 96 98 99 100 101 102 103 104 105 107 108 110 111 113 114 115 116 117 118 120 125 126 128 129 130 131 133 134 135 142 143 144 145 146 147 **P**8 **S** Iowa Health System, Des Moines, IA
Primary Contact: Deborah R. Simon, R.N., President and Chief Executive Officer
CFO: Calvin R. MacKay, Chief Financial Officer
CMO: Rick Anderson, M.D., Senior Vice President Medical Affairs and Chief Medical Officer
CIO: Steven Riney, Vice President Information Technology and Chief Information Officer
CHR: Joy Ledbetter, Director Human Resources
Web address: www.mymethodist.net
**Control:** Other not–for–profit (including NFP Corporation) **Service:** General Medical and Surgical

**Staffed Beds:** 282 **Admissions:** 15638 **Census:** 210 **Outpatient Visits:** 539927 **Births:** 1750 **Total Expense ($000):** 353585 **Payroll Expense ($000):** 138086 **Personnel:** 2124

⊞ △ **OSF SAINT FRANCIS MEDICAL CENTER (140067)**, 530 N.E. Glen Oak Avenue, Zip 61637–0001; tel. 309/655–2000, (Includes CHILDREN'S HOSPITAL OF ILLINOIS, 530 N.E. Glen Oak Avenue, tel. 309/655–7171), (Nonreporting) **A**1 2 3 5 7 8 9 10 **S** OSF Healthcare System, Peoria, IL
Primary Contact: Keith E. Steffen, President and Chief Executive Officer
COO: Susan C. Wozniak, R.N., Senior Vice President and Chief Operating Officer
CFO: Ken Harbaugh, Vice President and Chief Financial Officer
CMO: Tim C. Miller, M.D., Vice President, Chief Medical Officer and Director Academy Affairs
CIO: Michael B. Nauman, Senior Vice President and Chief Information Officer
CHR: Lynn J. Gillespie, Vice President Human Resources and Organizational Development
Web address: www.osfsaintfrancis.org
**Control:** Church–operated, Nongovernment, not–for profit **Service:** General Medical and Surgical

**Staffed Beds:** 574

☐ **PROCTOR HOSPITAL (140013)**, 5409 North Knoxville Avenue, Zip 61614–5094; tel. 309/691–1000, (Total facility includes 20 beds in nursing home–type unit) **A**1 9 10 **F**3 4 5 11 13 15 18 20 22 24 28 29 30 34 40 45 49 51 53 57 59 62 64 65 70 74 75 76 79 81 85 86 87 89 107 108 110 111 114 117 118 127 128 129 134 144 145 147
Primary Contact: Paul E. Macek, President and Chief Executive Officer
CFO: Roger Armstrong, Vice President Finance and Chief Financial Officer
CHR: Linda K. Buck, Vice President Human Resources
Web address: www.proctor.org
**Control:** Other not–for–profit (including NFP Corporation) **Service:** General Medical and Surgical

**Staffed Beds:** 163 **Admissions:** 6544 **Census:** 82 **Outpatient Visits:** 179510 **Births:** 635 **Total Expense ($000):** 107120 **Payroll Expense ($000):** 39083 **Personnel:** 1021

## PERU—Lasalle County

★ **ILLINOIS VALLEY COMMUNITY HOSPITAL (140234)**, 925 West Street, Zip 61354–2757; tel. 815/223–3300 **A**9 10 **F**2 3 11 13 15 28 29 30 31 34 35 38 40 45 49 50 51 54 56 57 59 64 65 68 69 70 74 75 76 77 79 81 82 84 85 86 87 89 91 93 94 96 104 107 110 111 114 117 118 128 129 130 131 132 134 142 143 145 146 147 **P**8
Primary Contact: Tommy Hobbs, Chief Executive Officer
COO: Bobby Smith, Vice President Physician Services and Quality
CFO: Stephen Davis, Chief Financial Officer
CMO: Mario Cote, M.D., Chief of Staff and President Medical Staff
CIO: Nancy McDonnell, Manager Information Systems
CHR: Mary Beth Herron, Director of Human Resources
CNO: Wilma Hart–Flynn, Vice President Patient Care Services/CNO
Web address: www.ivch.org
**Control:** Other not–for–profit (including NFP Corporation) **Service:** General Medical and Surgical

**Staffed Beds:** 72 **Admissions:** 2733 **Census:** 26 **Outpatient Visits:** 103707 **Births:** 398 **Total Expense ($000):** 60240 **Payroll Expense ($000):** 19753 **Personnel:** 444

## PINCKNEYVILLE—Perry County

★ **PINCKNEYVILLE COMMUNITY HOSPITAL (141307)**, 101 North Walnut Street, Zip 62274–1099; tel. 618/357–5901 **A**9 10 18 **F**3 15 29 31 40 43 45 50 53 57 78 81 85 93 107 108 118 126 129 132 147 **P**6
Primary Contact: Thomas J. Hudgins, FACHE, Administrator and Chief Executive Officer
CFO: Kara Jo Carson, Chief Financial Officer
CIO: Tina Grafton, Director Information Technology
CHR: Christie Gajewski, Director Human Resources
CNO: Eva Hopp, Chief Nurse Executive
Web address: www.pvillehosp.org/
**Control:** Hospital district or authority, Government, nonfederal **Service:** General Medical and Surgical

**Staffed Beds:** 25 **Admissions:** 564 **Census:** 6 **Outpatient Visits:** 46216 **Births:** 0 **Total Expense ($000):** 18378 **Payroll Expense ($000):** 8100 **Personnel:** 175

**IL**

---

**Hospital, Medicare Provider Number, Address, Telephone, Approval, Facility, and Physician Codes, Health Care System**

★ American Hospital Association (AHA) membership
☐ The Joint Commission accreditation
◇ DNV Healthcare Inc. accreditation
○ American Osteopathic Association (AOA) accreditation
△ Commission on Accreditation of Rehabilitation Facilities (CARF) accreditation

## PITTSFIELD—Pike County

★ ○ **ILLINI COMMUNITY HOSPITAL (141315)**, 640 West Washington Street, Zip 62363–1397; tel. 217/285–2113 **A**9 10 11 18 **F**3 15 18 19 28 30 31 34 40 46 50 53 59 64 65 68 70 75 78 81 82 85 87 89 93 97 107 110 114 118 126 128 129 130 132 145
Primary Contact: Kathy Hull, President and Chief Executive Officer
CFO: Sandra Purcell, Administrative Director Business and Financial Services
CMO: Paul Hibbert, D.O., President Medical Staff
CHR: Becky Myers, Human Resources Specialist
Web address: www.illinihospital.org
**Control:** Other not–for–profit (including NFP Corporation) **Service:** General Medical and Surgical

**Staffed Beds:** 21 **Admissions:** 640 **Census:** 7 **Outpatient Visits:** 7840 **Births:** 0 **Total Expense ($000):** 18404 **Payroll Expense ($000):** 7334 **Personnel:** 171

## PONTIAC—Livingston County

⊞ **OSF SAINT JAMES – JOHN W. ALBRECHT MEDICAL CENTER (140161)**, 2500 West Reynolds, Zip 61764–2194; tel. 815/842–2828 **A**1 9 10 20 **F**3 8 11 13 15 18 28 29 30 32 34 35 40 45 50 56 57 59 64 68 70 75 76 77 79 81 82 84 85 86 87 89 90 91 93 96 97 107 110 111 114 116 117 118 126 127 129 130 131 132 134 143 145 146 **P**7 **S** OSF Healthcare System, Peoria, IL
Primary Contact: David T. Ochs, President and Chief Executive Officer
CFO: Paula Corrigan, Vice President and Chief Financial Officer
CHR: Kenneth Beutke, Vice President Organization Development and Planning
Web address: www.osfsaintjames.org
**Control:** Church–operated, Nongovernment, not–for profit **Service:** General Medical and Surgical

**Staffed Beds:** 42 **Admissions:** 1545 **Census:** 13 **Outpatient Visits:** 154905 **Births:** 201 **Total Expense ($000):** 62081 **Payroll Expense ($000):** 23637 **Personnel:** 331

## PRINCETON—Bureau County

**PERRY MEMORIAL HOSPITAL (141337)**, 530 Park Avenue East, Zip 61356–2598; tel. 815/875–2811 **A**9 10 18 **F**11 13 15 28 29 30 31 34 35 40 45 47 48 49 56 57 59 64 70 75 76 77 78 79 81 82 85 86 87 93 107 108 110 111 114 115 116 118 128 129 130 131 132 145 146 **P**8
Primary Contact: Rex D. Conger, FACHE, President and Chief Executive Officer
CFO: Patricia Ellison, Chief Financial Officer
CMO: Robert E. Mestan, M.D., Chief of Staff
CIO: Karen Behrens, Director Technology Services
CHR: Karen Russell, Director Human Resources
Web address: www.perry–memorial.org
**Control:** City–Government, nonfederal **Service:** General Medical and Surgical

**Staffed Beds:** 25 **Admissions:** 1452 **Census:** 14 **Outpatient Visits:** 62516 **Births:** 116 **Total Expense ($000):** 34656 **Payroll Expense ($000):** 14670 **Personnel:** 270

## QUINCY—Adams County

⊞ △ **BLESSING HOSPITAL (140015)**, Broadway at 11th Street, Zip 62305–7005, Mailing Address: P.O. Box 7005, Zip 62305–7005; tel. 217/223–1200, (Includes BLESSING HOSPITAL, Broadway & 14th Street, Zip 62301, Mailing Address: P.O. Box 7005, Zip 62305–7005; tel. 217/223–1200), (Total facility includes 20 beds in nursing home–type unit) **A**1 2 3 5 7 9 10 13 **F**3 5 8 11 13 15 17 18 20 22 24 28 29 30 31 32 34 35 40 43 44 48 49 50 53 56 61 62 63 64 66 68 70 73 74 75 76 77 78 79 81 82 84 85 86 87 89 90 93 94 96 98 99 100 101 102 103 104 107 108 110 111 113 114 117 118 119 120 122 123 125 126 127 128 129 130 131 134 143 145 146 147 **P**8
Primary Contact: Maureen A. Kahn, R.N., President and Chief Executive Officer
COO: Tim Moore, Chief Accounting Officer and Vice President Ancillary Services
CFO: Patrick M. Gerveler, Vice President Finance and Chief Financial Officer
Web address: www.blessinghospital.org
**Control:** Other not–for–profit (including NFP Corporation) **Service:** General Medical and Surgical

**Staffed Beds:** 340 **Admissions:** 13872 **Census:** 176 **Outpatient Visits:** 380031 **Births:** 1151 **Total Expense ($000):** 251506 **Payroll Expense ($000):** 100378 **Personnel:** 2039

## RED BUD—Randolph County

⊞ **RED BUD REGIONAL HOSPITAL (141348)**, 325 Spring Street, Zip 62278–1194; tel. 618/282–3831, (Total facility includes 115 beds in nursing home–type unit) **A**1 9 10 18 **F**3 15 29 34 40 56 57 59 64 79 81 85 86 89 91 93 107 108 110 111 113 118 126 127 128 131 132 134 144 145 147 **P**6 **S** Community Health Systems, Inc., Franklin, TN
Primary Contact: Shane Watson, Chief Executive Officer
CFO: David L. Jones, Chief Financial Officer
CMO: Pamella S. Gronemeyer, M.D., President Medical Staff
CIO: Casey Baldridge, Supervisor Information Technology
CHR: Lori Brooks, Director Human Resources
Web address: www.redbudhospital.com
**Control:** Corporation, Investor–owned, for–profit **Service:** General Medical and Surgical

**Staffed Beds:** 140 **Admissions:** 1352 **Census:** 106 **Outpatient Visits:** 27547 **Births:** 0 **Total Expense ($000):** 19914 **Payroll Expense ($000):** 8062 **Personnel:** 196

## ROBINSON—Crawford County

⊞ **CRAWFORD MEMORIAL HOSPITAL (141343)**, 1000 North Allen Street, Zip 62454–1167; tel. 618/544–3131, (Nonreporting) **A**1 9 10 18 **S** QHR, Brentwood, TN
Primary Contact: Donald E. Annis, Chief Executive Officer
CFO: Richard Carlson, Chief Financial Officer
CMO: Gary Tennison, D.O., Chief of Staff
CIO: Tim Richard, IT Coordinator
CHR: Kristi Zane, Chief Human Resources Officer
CNO: Sandra Burtron, MS, Chief Nursing Officer
Web address: www.crawfordmh.org
**Control:** Hospital district or authority, Government, nonfederal **Service:** General Medical and Surgical

**Staffed Beds:** 63

## ROCHELLE—Ogle County

⊞ **ROCHELLE COMMUNITY HOSPITAL (141312)**, 900 North Second Street, Zip 61068–0330; tel. 815/562–2181 **A**1 9 10 18 **F**3 8 15 29 30 31 34 35 40 41 50 53 57 59 64 68 70 74 75 77 78 81 82 85 86 87 93 97 107 110 114 129 131 132 134 143 145 **P**6
Primary Contact: Mark Batty, Chief Executive Officer
CFO: Lori Gutierrez, Chief Financial Officer
CFO: John M. Ross, Vice President Finance and Chief Financial Officer
CMO: Jason Popp, Chief of Medical Staff
CIO: Scott Stewart, Manager Information Services
CHR: Robert Johns, Senior Vice President Administration
CNO: Jennifer Montgomery, Chief Nursing Officer
Web address: www.rcha.net
**Control:** Other not–for–profit (including NFP Corporation) **Service:** General Medical and Surgical

**Staffed Beds:** 16 **Admissions:** 541 **Census:** 4 **Outpatient Visits:** 9621 **Births:** 0 **Total Expense ($000):** 22795 **Payroll Expense ($000):** 8691 **Personnel:** 214

## ROCK ISLAND—Rock Island County

⊞ △ **TRINITY ROCK ISLAND (140280)**, 2701 17th Street, Zip 61201–5393; tel. 309/779–5000, (Includes TRINITY MOLINE, 500 John Deere Road, Moline, Zip 61265; tel. 309/779–5000), (Total facility includes 29 beds in nursing home–type unit) **A**1 2 7 9 10 **F**3 5 7 11 12 13 15 18 20 22 24 26 28 29 30 31 34 35 37 38 40 43 44 45 49 50 51 57 58 59 64 70 74 75 76 78 79 81 82 85 86 87 89 90 93 96 97 98 99 100 101 102 103 104 105 106 107 108 110 111 113 114 118 119 120 122 125 127 128 129 131 133 134 142 143 145 146 147 **P**6 **S** Iowa Health System, Des Moines, IA
Primary Contact: Richard A. Seidler, FACHE, President and Chief Executive Officer
COO: Michael J. Patterson, Vice President Operations
CFO: Greg Pagliuzza, Chief Financial Officer
CMO: Paul McLoone, M.D., Chief Medical Officer
CHR: Jeffery Stolze, Vice President Human Resources
Web address: www.trinityqc.com
**Control:** Other not–for–profit (including NFP Corporation) **Service:** General Medical and Surgical

**Staffed Beds:** 317 **Admissions:** 16488 **Census:** 212 **Outpatient Visits:** 391357 **Births:** 1496 **Total Expense ($000):** 258595 **Payroll Expense ($000):** 93862 **Personnel:** 1697

## ROCKFORD—Winnebago County

☐ **H. DOUGLAS SINGER MENTAL HEALTH AND DEVELOPMENTAL CENTER (144023)**, 4402 North Main Street, Zip 61103–1278; tel. 815/987–7096, (Nonreporting) **A**1 10 **S** Division of Mental Health, Department of Human Services, Springfield, IL
Primary Contact: Gail Tennant, Director
**Control:** State–Government, nonfederal **Service:** Psychiatric

**Staffed Beds:** 162

⊞ **OSF SAINT ANTHONY MEDICAL CENTER (140233)**, 5666 East State Street, Zip 61108–2425; tel. 815/226–2000 **A**1 2 5 9 10 **F**3 11 12 13 15 16 17 18 20 22 24 26 28 29 30 31 32 34 35 36 37 38 39 40 41 43 44 45 49 50 51 53 55 56 57 58 59 64 66 70 73 74 75 76 77 78 79 81 82 84 85 86 87 89 92 93 107 108 110 111 113 114 115 116 117 118 119 120 122 123 128 129 130 131 134 144 145 146 147 **P**6 **S** OSF Healthcare System, Peoria, IL
Primary Contact: David A. Schertz, President and Chief Executive Officer
CFO: David Stenerson, Vice President Fiscal Services and Chief Financial Officer
CMO: Eric Benink, M.D., Vice President and Chief Medical Officer
CIO: Kathy Peterson, Director Information Services
CHR: Karen C. Brown, Vice President Strategic Human Resources
Web address: www.osfhealth.com
**Control:** Church–operated, Nongovernment, not–for–profit **Service:** General Medical and Surgical

**Staffed Beds:** 235 **Admissions:** 10418 **Census:** 134 **Outpatient Visits:** 405232 **Births:** 456 **Total Expense ($000):** 315364 **Payroll Expense ($000):** 131697 **Personnel:** 1811

⊞ **ROCKFORD MEMORIAL HOSPITAL (140239)**, 2400 North Rockton Avenue, Zip 61103–3692; tel. 815/971–5000 **A**1 2 5 9 10 **F**3 11 13 18 19 20 22 24 25 26 27 28 29 30 31 32 34 35 39 40 41 43 44 45 48 49 50 54 55 57 59 63 64 65 68 70 71 72 74 75 76 77 78 79 80 81 82 84 85 86 87 88 89 93 97 98 99 100 101 102 103 107 108 111 113 114 117 118 120 122 125 128 129 131 134 144 145 146 147 **P**6
Primary Contact: Gary E. Kaatz, President and Chief Executive Officer
COO: Daniel A. Parod, Senior Vice President Hospital and Administrative Affairs
CFO: Henry Seybold, Senior Vice President and Chief Financial Officer
CMO: Milton G. Schmitt, Jr., M.D., Chief Medical Officer
CIO: Dennis P. L'Heureux, Chief Information Officer
CHR: Daniel A. Parod, Senior Vice President Hospital and Administrative Affairs
CNO: Susan Schreier, R.N., Chief Nursing Executive
Web address: www.rhsnet.org
**Control:** Other not–for–profit (including NFP Corporation) **Service:** General Medical and Surgical

**Staffed Beds:** 292 **Admissions:** 13719 **Census:** 194 **Outpatient Visits:** 431421 **Births:** 1608 **Total Expense ($000):** 277546 **Payroll Expense ($000):** 107842 **Personnel:** 2000

⊞ **SWEDISHAMERICAN HOSPITAL (140228)**, 1401 East State Street, Zip 61104–2315; tel. 815/968–4400 **A**1 2 3 5 9 10 **F**3 13 15 17 18 20 22 24 26 28 29 30 31 34 35 36 37 38 39 40 43 44 45 46 49 50 56 57 58 59 61 64 65 68 70 72 74 75 76 77 78 79 81 82 84 85 86 87 89 92 93 98 99 100 101 102 103 104 105 107 108 110 111 113 114 116 117 118 120 122 128 129 131 145 146 147 **P**6
Primary Contact: William R. Gorski, M.D., President and Chief Executive Officer
COO: Richard Walsh, Executive Vice President and Chief Operating Officer
CFO: Don Haring, Vice President Finance and Treasurer
CMO: Kathleen Kelly, M.D., Chief Medical Officer and Chief Quality Officer
CIO: Phil Wasson, Chief Information Officer
CHR: Jerry Guinane, Vice President Human Resources
Web address: www.swedishamerican.org
**Control:** Other not–for–profit (including NFP Corporation) **Service:** General Medical and Surgical

**Staffed Beds:** 326 **Admissions:** 17691 **Census:** 214 **Outpatient Visits:** 271048 **Births:** 2449 **Total Expense ($000):** 293101 **Payroll Expense ($000):** 113393 **Personnel:** 2083

⊞ △ **VAN MATRE HEALTHSOUTH REHABILITATION HOSPITAL (143028)**, 950 South Mulford Road, Zip 61108; tel. 815/381–8500 **A**1 7 9 10 **F**29 64 68 74 75 86 90 91 93 95 96 129 130 131 147 **S** HEALTHSOUTH Corporation, Birmingham, AL
Primary Contact: Ken Bowman, Chief Executive Officer
CFO: Mark Lundvall, Controller
CMO: Scott Craig, M.D., Medical Director
CIO: Dianne Miller, Director Health Information Management
CHR: Lisa Vitale, Director Human Resources
CNO: Nancy Miller, R.N., Chief Nursing Officer
Web address: www.healthsouth.com
**Control:** Partnership, Investor–owned, for–profit **Service:** Rehabilitation

**Staffed Beds:** 50 **Admissions:** 1209 **Census:** 44 **Outpatient Visits:** 7272 **Births:** 0 **Total Expense ($000):** 16260 **Payroll Expense ($000):** 9131 **Personnel:** 124

**ROSICLARE—Hardin County**

★ **HARDIN COUNTY GENERAL HOSPITAL (141328)**, 6 Ferrell Road, Zip 62982, Mailing Address: PO BOX 2467, Zip 62982–2467; tel. 618/285–6634 **A**9 10 18 **F**15 29 34 40 59 64 65 75 77 93 97 107 113 118 126 128 129 132
Primary Contact: Roby D. Williams, Administrator
CFO: Janie Parker, Chief Financial Officer
CMO: Marcos N. Sunga, M.D., Chief of Staff
CHR: Joyce Shelby, Manager Human Resources
Web address: www.ilhcgh.org
**Control:** Other not–for–profit (including NFP Corporation) **Service:** General Medical and Surgical

**Staffed Beds:** 25 **Admissions:** 606 **Census:** 8 **Outpatient Visits:** 16180 **Births:** 0 **Total Expense ($000):** 9485 **Payroll Expense ($000):** 5440 **Personnel:** 134

**RUSHVILLE—Schuyler County**

★ **SARAH D. CULBERTSON MEMORIAL HOSPITAL (141333)**, 238 South Congress Street, Zip 62681–1472; tel. 217/322–4321, (Total facility includes 24 beds in nursing home–type unit) **A**9 10 18 **F**11 15 18 28 31 34 40 45 57 59 69 77 78 79 81 82 93 107 110 113 118 124 126 128 131 132 145 147
Primary Contact: Lynn E. Stambaugh, R.N., Chief Executive Officer
CFO: Alan Palo, Chief Financial Officer
CMO: S. K. Kanthilal, M.D., President Medical Staff
Web address: www.cmhospital.com
**Control:** Hospital district or authority, Government, nonfederal **Service:** General Medical and Surgical

**Staffed Beds:** 46 **Admissions:** 375 **Census:** 26 **Outpatient Visits:** 38064 **Births:** 0 **Total Expense ($000):** 18622 **Payroll Expense ($000):** 7949 **Personnel:** 158

**SALEM—Marion County**

★ ○ **SALEM TOWNSHIP HOSPITAL (141345)**, 1201 Ricker Drive, Zip 62881–6250; tel. 618/548–3194, (Nonreporting) **A**9 10 11 18
Primary Contact: Stephanie Hilton–Siebert, President and Chief Executive Officer
CFO: Teresa Stroud, Chief Financial Officer
CMO: Gautam Jha, M.D., Chief of Staff
CIO: Steve Turner, Director Information Technology
CHR: Diane Boswell, Director Human Resources and Marketing
CNO: Kendra Taylor, Director Inpatient Nursing
Web address: www.sthcares.org
**Control:** City–Government, nonfederal **Service:** General Medical and Surgical

**Staffed Beds:** 25

**SANDWICH—Dekalb County**

⊞ **VALLEY WEST COMMUNITY HOSPITAL (141340)**, 11 East Pleasant Avenue, Zip 60548–0901; tel. 815/786–8484 **A**1 9 10 18 **F**11 13 15 18 28 29 30 31 32 34 35 40 45 46 49 51 57 58 59 64 68 70 71 75 76 77 78 79 81 82 85 87 93 102 104 107 110 114 118 128 129 130 131 134 145 146 **S** Kish Health System, De Kalb, IL
Primary Contact: Brad Copple, President
COO: David R. Proulx, Assistant Vice President Operations
CFO: Loren Foelske, Vice President Finance
CMO: Michael Kulisz, D.O., Chief Medical Officer
CIO: Heath Bell, Chief Information Officer
CHR: Mark Thate, Vice President Human Resources
CNO: Pamela Duffy, Vice President Patient Services and CNO
Web address: www.vwch.org
**Control:** Other not–for–profit (including NFP Corporation) **Service:** General Medical and Surgical

**Staffed Beds:** 25 **Admissions:** 1194 **Census:** 9 **Outpatient Visits:** 36779 **Births:** 252 **Total Expense ($000):** 38701 **Payroll Expense ($000):** 10555 **Personnel:** 182

**SHELBYVILLE—Shelby County**

★ **SHELBY MEMORIAL HOSPITAL (140019)**, 200 South Cedar Street, Zip 62565–1899; tel. 217/774–3961, (Nonreporting) **A**9 10 20
Primary Contact: Marilyn Sears, President and Chief Executive Officer
CFO: Phil Miller, Chief Financial Officer
CMO: Arnold Agapito, M.D., President Medical Staff
CHR: Amy Koehler, Director Human Resources
Web address: www.mysmh.org
**Control:** Other not–for–profit (including NFP Corporation) **Service:** General Medical and Surgical

**Staffed Beds:** 45

**SILVIS—Rock Island County**

★ **GENESIS MEDICAL CENTER, ILLINI CAMPUS (140275)**, 801 Illini Drive, Zip 61282–1893; tel. 309/281–4000 **A**9 10 **F**3 7 11 13 15 18 20 26 28 29 30 31 34 35 38 40 43 44 46 47 48 50 53 54 57 59 63 64 68 70 74 75 76 77 78 79 81 82 84 85 86 87 89 97 107 108 110 111 113 118 128 129 130 131 134 145 146 **S** Genesis Health System, Davenport, IA
Primary Contact: Florence Spyrow, President
CFO: Mark G. Rogers, Interim Vice President Finance and Chief Financial Officer
CMO: Peter Metcalf, M.D., President Medical Staff
CIO: Robert Frieden, Vice President Information Systems
CHR: Heidi Kahly–McMahon, Vice President Human Resources
Web address: www.genesishealth.com
**Control:** Other not–for–profit (including NFP Corporation) **Service:** General Medical and Surgical

**Staffed Beds:** 101 **Admissions:** 4585 **Census:** 40 **Outpatient Visits:** 101408 **Births:** 608 **Total Expense ($000):** 76460 **Payroll Expense ($000):** 25156 **Personnel:** 535

IL

**Hospital, Medicare Provider Number, Address, Telephone, Approval, Facility, and Physician Codes, Health Care System**

★ American Hospital Association (AHA) membership
□ The Joint Commission accreditation ◇ DNV Healthcare Inc. accreditation
○ American Osteopathic Association (AOA) accreditation
△ Commission on Accreditation of Rehabilitation Facilities (CARF) accreditation

## SKOKIE—Cook County

⊠ **NORTHSHORE UNIVERSITY HEALTH SYSTEM SKOKIE HOSPITAL (140051)**, 9600 Gross Point Road, Zip 60076–1257; tel. 847/677–9600, (Nonreporting) **A**1 3 5 9 10 **S** NorthShore University HealthSystem, Evanston, IL
Primary Contact: Kristen Murtos, FACHE, President
COO: Anthony Di Lorenzo, Vice President Operations
CMO: Michael Raymond, M.D., Chief Medical Officer
CIO: Kerry Kerlin, Vice President Information Technology
CHR: Richard J. Casey, Assistant Vice President Operations
Web address: www.northshore.org
**Control:** Other not–for–profit (including NFP Corporation) **Service:** General Medical and Surgical

| Staffed Beds: 234 |
| --- |

## SPARTA—Randolph County

○ **SPARTA COMMUNITY HOSPITAL (141349)**, 818 East Broadway Street, Zip 62286–0297, Mailing Address: P.O. Box 297, Zip 62286–0297; tel. 618/443–2177 **A**9 10 11 18 **F**3 11 15 28 34 35 40 41 53 54 57 59 62 64 77 81 89 93 97 107 113 118 126 128 129 131 132 142 145 146 **P**5
Primary Contact: Joann Emge, Chief Executive Officer
COO: Joann Emge, Chief Executive Officer
CFO: Steven A. Bricker, Chief Financial Officer
CMO: Franklin James, Jr., M.D., Chief Medical Staff
CIO: Susan Gutjahr, Reimbursement Specialist
CHR: Darla Shawgo, Director Human Resources
CNO: Lori Clinton, Chief Nursing Officer
Web address: www.spartahospital.com
**Control:** Hospital district or authority, Government, nonfederal **Service:** General Medical and Surgical

| Staffed Beds: 25 Admissions: 985 Census: 9 Outpatient Visits: 42700 Births: 0 Total Expense ($000): 18820 Payroll Expense ($000): 11543 Personnel: 268 |
| --- |

## SPRING VALLEY—Bureau County

**ST. MARGARET'S HOSPITAL (140143)**, 600 East First Street, Zip 61362–2034; tel. 815/664–5311, (Nonreporting) **A**9 10 **S** Sisters of Mary of the Presentation Health System, Fargo, ND
Primary Contact: Tim Muntz, President and Chief Executive Officer
CFO: Kim D. Santman, Vice President Finance
CIO: John Sabotta, Director Information Systems
CHR: Cheri D. Adrian, Director Human Resources
Web address: www.aboutsmh.org
**Control:** Church–operated, Nongovernment, not–for profit **Service:** General Medical and Surgical

| Staffed Beds: 86 |
| --- |

## SPRINGFIELD—Sangamon County

□ **ANDREW MCFARLAND MENTAL HEALTH CENTER (144021)**, 901 East Southwind Road, Zip 62703–5125; tel. 217/786–6994, (Nonreporting) **A**1 3 5 10
Primary Contact: Karen Schweighart, R.N., MS, Administrator
CFO: Jeff Frey, Business Administrator
CIO: Josh Kates, Information Technology Analyst
CHR: Robert Braasch, Administrator Human Resources
**Control:** State–Government, nonfederal **Service:** Psychiatric

| Staffed Beds: 118 |
| --- |

⊠ **KINDRED HOSPITAL SPRINGFIELD (142014)**, 701 North Walnut Street, Zip 62702–4913; tel. 217/528–1217, (Nonreporting) **A**1 10 **S** Kindred Healthcare, Louisville, KY
Primary Contact: Sherry L. Hendricksen, R.N., MSN, Chief Executive Officer
Web address: www.kindredspringfield.com/
**Control:** Corporation, Investor–owned, for–profit **Service:** Long–Term Acute Care hospital

| Staffed Beds: 50 |
| --- |

□ **LINCOLN PRAIRIE BEHAVIORAL HEALTH CENTER**, 5230 South Sixth Street, Zip 62703; tel. 217/585–1180 **A**1 3 5 9 **F**35 38 98 99 100 101 104 **S** Universal Health Services, Inc., King of Prussia, PA
Primary Contact: Mark Littrell, Chief Executive Officer
Web address: www.lincolnprairiebhc.com/
**Control:** Corporation, Investor–owned, for–profit **Service:** Children's hospital psychiatric

| Staffed Beds: 88 Admissions: 1460 Census: 52 Outpatient Visits: 5260 Births: 0 Total Expense ($000): 11530 Payroll Expense ($000): 6368 Personnel: 206 |
| --- |

⊠ △ **MEMORIAL MEDICAL CENTER (140148)**, 701 North First Street, Zip 62781–0001; tel. 217/788–3000 **A**1 2 3 5 7 8 9 10 **F**3 8 11 12 13 14 15 16 17 18 20 22 24 26 28 29 30 31 32 34 35 36 37 40 43 44 45 46 47 48 49 50 51 54 57 58 59 60 61 63 64 68 69 70 74 75 76 77 78 79 81 82 84 85 86 87 89 90 92 93 96 97 98 100 101 102 103 104 105 107 108 110 111 113 114 115 116 117 118 119 120 123 125 128 129 130 131 133 134 137 140 141 143 144 145 146 147 **P**3 5 **S** Memorial Health System, Springfield, IL
Primary Contact: Edgar J. Curtis, President and Chief Executive Officer
COO: Douglas L. Rahn, Senior Vice President and Chief Operating Officer
CFO: Robert W. Kay, Senior Vice President and Chief Financial Officer
CMO: Rajesh G. Govindaiah, M.D., Chief Medical Officer
CIO: David B. Graham, M.D., Senior Vice President and Chief Information Officer
CHR: Bradley J. Warren, Senior Vice President and Chief People Officer
CNO: Marsha A. Prater, Ph.D., Senior Vice President and Chief Nursing Officer
Web address: www.memorialmedical.com
**Control:** Other not–for–profit (including NFP Corporation) **Service:** General Medical and Surgical

| Staffed Beds: 471 Admissions: 24496 Census: 336 Outpatient Visits: 493859 Births: 1756 Total Expense ($000): 541953 Payroll Expense ($000): 174877 Personnel: 3784 |
| --- |

⊠ **ST. JOHN'S HOSPITAL (140053)**, 800 East Carpenter Street, Zip 62769–0002; tel. 217/544–6464, (Includes ST. JOHN'S CHILDREN'S HOSPITAL, 800 East Carpenter Street, Zip 62769; tel. 217/544–6464), (Total facility includes 37 beds in nursing home–type unit) **A**1 2 3 5 8 9 10 **F**2 3 11 12 13 15 17 18 19 20 22 24 26 28 29 30 31 32 34 35 36 39 40 41 43 44 45 46 47 48 49 50 51 53 54 56 57 58 59 60 61 62 63 64 66 68 70 72 74 75 76 77 78 79 81 82 84 85 86 87 88 89 92 93 94 98 100 101 102 103 104 107 108 110 111 113 114 116 117 118 119 120 121 122 123 125 127 128 129 130 131 134 144 145 146 147 **S** Hospital Sisters Health System, Springfield, IL
Primary Contact: Robert P. Ritz, Chief Executive Officer
CFO: Larry Ragel, Chief Financial Officer
CMO: Craig Backs, M.D., Medical Director
CIO: Kirk Mahlen, Chief Information Officer
CHR: Joseph W. Bretz, Director Human Resources
Web address: www.st–johns.org
**Control:** Church–operated, Nongovernment, not–for profit **Service:** General Medical and Surgical

| Staffed Beds: 430 Admissions: 19486 Census: 280 Outpatient Visits: 240615 Births: 1856 Total Expense ($000): 430647 Payroll Expense ($000): 134673 Personnel: 2527 |
| --- |

## STAUNTON—Macoupin County

**COMMUNITY MEMORIAL HOSPITAL (141306)**, 400 Caldwell Street, Zip 62088–1499; tel. 618/635–2200 **A**9 10 18 **F**3 11 15 28 29 30 34 35 40 45 56 57 59 63 64 70 77 78 79 81 82 85 86 87 97 103 107 108 110 114 118 129 131 132 134 145 **P**6
Primary Contact: Susie Campbell, Chief Executive Officer
CFO: Donald Brunnworth, Chief Financial Officer
CMO: Bryan Siegfried, M.D., President Medical Staff
CIO: Cheryl Horner, Supervisor Data Processing
CHR: Marilyn Herbeck, Coordinator Human Resources
Web address: www.stauntonhospital.org
**Control:** Other not–for–profit (including NFP Corporation) **Service:** General Medical and Surgical

| Staffed Beds: 25 Admissions: 354 Census: 4 Outpatient Visits: 27960 Births: 0 Total Expense ($000): 12672 Payroll Expense ($000): 5040 Personnel: 133 |
| --- |

## STERLING—Whiteside County

⊠ **CGH MEDICAL CENTER (140043)**, 100 East LeFevre Road, Zip 61081–1279; tel. 815/625–0400 **A**1 9 10 **F**3 7 8 11 13 15 18 20 22 28 29 30 31 34 35 40 45 47 49 50 51 57 59 62 64 68 70 74 76 78 79 81 85 86 87 89 93 97 107 108 110 111 113 114 117 118 123 128 129 131 132 134 144 145 147 **P**6
Primary Contact: Edward Andersen, President and Chief Executive Officer
COO: Norm Deets, Vice President and Chief Operating Officer
CFO: Ben Schaab, VP Fiscal Services/ Chief Financial Officer
CMO: Mark Schmelzel, M.D., Vice President and Medical Director
CIO: Raymond Sharp, Vice President and Chief Information Officer
CHR: Thomas J. McCawley, Manager Human Resources
CNO: Kristie A. Geil, VP, Chief Nursing Officer
Web address: www.cghmc.com
**Control:** City–Government, nonfederal **Service:** General Medical and Surgical

| Staffed Beds: 99 Admissions: 5710 Census: 49 Outpatient Visits: 129416 Births: 562 Total Expense ($000): 105299 Payroll Expense ($000): 43458 Personnel: 1219 |
| --- |

**IL**

*Many Facility Codes have changed. Please refer to the AHA Guide Code Chart.*

## STREAMWOOD—Cook County

☐ **STREAMWOOD BEHAVIORAL HEALTH CENTER (144034)**, 1400 East Irving Park Road, Zip 60107–3203; tel. 630/837–9000, (Nonreporting) **A**1 9 10 **S** Universal Health Services, Inc., King of Prussia, PA
Primary Contact: Roxane Harcourt, Chief Executive Officer
COO: Ron Weglarz, Chief Operating Officer
CFO: Karen Williams, Chief Financial Officer
CMO: Joseph McNally, M.D., Medical Director
CHR: Michael Isaacs, Director Human Resources
CNO: Olieth Lightbourne, Chief Nursing Officer
Web address: www.streamwoodhospital.com
**Control:** Corporation, Investor–owned, for–profit **Service:** Children's hospital psychiatric

**Staffed Beds:** 177

## STREATOR—Lasalle County

☒ **ST. MARY'S HOSPITAL (140026)**, 111 Spring Street, Zip 61364–3399; tel. 815/673–2311, (Total facility includes 30 beds in nursing home–type unit) **A**1 9 10 **F**2 3 11 13 15 18 28 29 30 31 34 35 40 41 45 47 50 54 56 57 59 62 70 75 76 77 78 79 81 82 84 85 87 89 93 107 108 110 111 114 117 118 127 129 130 131 142 145 146 147 **P**8 **S** Hospital Sisters Health System, Springfield, IL
Primary Contact: Brian E. Dietz, FACHE, Interim President and Chief Executive Officer
CFO: Karen S. Clark, Chief Financial Officer
CMO: Larry Jones, M.D., Chief Medical Officer
CIO: Georgene Lansford, Director Information Systems
Web address: www.stmaryshospital.org
**Control:** Church–operated, Nongovernment, not–for profit **Service:** General Medical and Surgical

**Staffed Beds:** 98 **Admissions:** 2860 **Census:** 41 **Outpatient Visits:** 88381 **Births:** 238 **Total Expense ($000):** 61143 **Payroll Expense ($000):** 20826 **Personnel:** 431

## SYCAMORE—Dekalb County

☒ **KINDRED HOSPITAL–SYCAMORE (142006)**, 225 Edward Street, Zip 60178–2197; tel. 815/895–2144 **A**1 10 **F**1 3 29 30 45 46 60 63 68 74 80 82 84 85 129 147 **S** Kindred Healthcare, Louisville, KY
Primary Contact: Cindy Smith, Chief Executive Officer
CFO: Jay Schweikart, Chief Financial Officer
CMO: Thomas Liske, M.D., Chief Medical Officer
CHR: Eileen Strachan, Coordinator Human Resources
Web address: www.kindredhospitalsyc.com/
**Control:** Corporation, Investor–owned, for–profit **Service:** Long–Term Acute Care hospital

**Staffed Beds:** 69 **Admissions:** 509 **Census:** 40 **Outpatient Visits:** 0 **Births:** 0 **Total Expense ($000):** 17506 **Payroll Expense ($000):** 6554 **Personnel:** 123

## TAYLORVILLE—Christian County

★ **TAYLORVILLE MEMORIAL HOSPITAL (141339)**, 201 East Pleasant Street, Zip 62568–1597; tel. 217/824–3331, (Nonreporting) **A**9 10 18 **S** Memorial Health System, Springfield, IL
Primary Contact: Daniel J. Raab, President and Chief Executive Officer
CFO: Sue Hill, Director Finance
CHR: Jackie Broaddus, Business Partner
Web address: www.taylorvillememorial.org
**Control:** Church–operated, Nongovernment, not–for profit **Service:** General Medical and Surgical

**Staffed Beds:** 45

## URBANA—Champaign County

☒ △ **CARLE FOUNDATION HOSPITAL (140091)**, 611 West Park Street, Zip 61801–2595; tel. 217/383–3311 **A**1 2 3 5 7 9 10 13 **F**3 7 8 11 12 13 15 17 20 22 24 26 29 30 34 35 40 43 44 45 46 47 48 49 50 51 53 56 57 58 59 60 61 62 63 64 65 68 70 72 74 75 76 78 79 80 81 84 85 86 87 89 90 91 93 94 96 107 108 110 111 113 114 115 116 118 125 128 129 130 131 134 144 145 147
Primary Contact: James C. Leonard, M.D., President and Chief Executive Officer
COO: John Snyder, Executive Vice President and Chief Operating Officer
CFO: Dennis Hesch, Executive Vice President Finance and Chief Financial Officer
CMO: Kirk Moberg, M.D., Executive Vice President and Chief Medical Officer
CIO: Rick Rinehart, Chief Information Officer
CHR: Philip L. Kubow, Senior Vice President Human Resources
Web address: www.carle.com/hospital
**Control:** Other not–for–profit (including NFP Corporation) **Service:** General Medical and Surgical

**Staffed Beds:** 313 **Admissions:** 18421 **Census:** 244 **Outpatient Visits:** 255805 **Births:** 2563 **Total Expense ($000):** 291376 **Payroll Expense ($000):** 96227 **Personnel:** 1841

☒ △ **PROVENA COVENANT MEDICAL CENTER (140113)**, 1400 West Park Street, Zip 61801–2396; tel. 217/337–2000 **A**1 3 5 7 9 10 **F**3 7 13 15 18 20 22 24 26 28 29 30 31 34 35 38 40 49 50 56 57 59 61 63 64 65 68 70 74 75 76 78 79 81 82 83 84 85 89 90 93 98 100 101 102 103 107 108 110 111 113 114 118 125 129 131 134 145 146 147 **S** Presence Health, Chicago, IL
Primary Contact: Michael L. Brown, President and Chief Executive Officer
COO: Eric Rhodes, Assistant Vice President of Operations
CFO: Deborah Schimerowski, Vice President Finance and Chief Financial Officer
CMO: Jared Rogers, M.D., Chief Medical Officer
CIO: Jason Wheatley, Manager Information Systems
CHR: Janet S. Payne, Vice President Human Resources
Web address: www.provenacovenant.org
**Control:** Church–operated, Nongovernment, not–for profit **Service:** General Medical and Surgical

**Staffed Beds:** 181 **Admissions:** 7949 **Census:** 85 **Outpatient Visits:** 250012 **Births:** 874 **Total Expense ($000):** 137239 **Payroll Expense ($000):** 42249 **Personnel:** 784

## VANDALIA—Fayette County

☒ **FAYETTE COUNTY HOSPITAL (141346)**, 650 West Taylor Street, Zip 62471–1296; tel. 618/283–1231, (Total facility includes 85 beds in nursing home–type unit) **A**1 9 10 18 **F**3 7 11 15 28 29 30 34 35 40 44 45 49 57 59 80 81 86 93 107 110 111 112 113 115 116 118 126 127 128 129 131 132 144 145 147 **P**5 **S** Alliant Management Services, Louisville, KY
Primary Contact: Gregory D. Starnes, Chief Executive Officer
CFO: Shelley Bay, Chief Financial Officer
CMO: Raymond Ryan, M.D., Chief of Staff
CIO: Susan Crawford, Manager Human Resources
Web address: www.fayettecountyhospital.org
**Control:** Corporation, Investor–owned, for–profit **Service:** General Medical and Surgical

**Staffed Beds:** 110 **Admissions:** 1557 **Census:** 68 **Outpatient Visits:** 30589 **Births:** 0 **Total Expense ($000):** 21262 **Payroll Expense ($000):** 7893 **Personnel:** 230

## WATSEKA—Iroquois County

☒ **IROQUOIS MEMORIAL HOSPITAL AND RESIDENT HOME (140167)**, 200 Fairman Avenue, Zip 60970–1644; tel. 815/432–5841, (Total facility includes 35 beds in nursing home–type unit) **A**1 9 10 20 **F**3 7 11 13 15 18 20 22 28 29 30 31 34 35 40 43 45 47 51 53 54 56 57 59 62 63 64 65 66 68 70 75 76 77 78 79 80 81 82 84 85 87 93 97 107 108 110 111 114 118 124 126 127 128 129 130 131 132 134 142 145 146 **P**4 **S** QHR, Brentwood, TN
Primary Contact: Michael J. Stenger, Interim President and Chief Executive Officer
CFO: Joseph A. Swab, Chief Financial Officer
CMO: Mohammed Razvi, M.D., Chief of Staff
CIO: Tim Smith, Director Information Systems
CHR: Jamie Neumann, Director Human Resources
Web address: www.iroquoismemorial.com
**Control:** Other not–for–profit (including NFP Corporation) **Service:** General Medical and Surgical

**Staffed Beds:** 84 **Admissions:** 1654 **Census:** 39 **Outpatient Visits:** 48649 **Births:** 121 **Total Expense ($000):** 36253 **Payroll Expense ($000):** 16576 **Personnel:** 287

IL

---

**Hospital, Medicare Provider Number, Address, Telephone, Approval, Facility, and Physician Codes, Health Care System**

★ American Hospital Association (AHA) membership
☐ The Joint Commission accreditation
◇ DNV Healthcare Inc. accreditation
◯ American Osteopathic Association (AOA) accreditation
△ Commission on Accreditation of Rehabilitation Facilities (CARF) accreditation

## WAUKEGAN—Lake County

★ **VISTA MEDICAL CENTER EAST (140084)**, 1324 North Sheridan Road, Zip 60085–2181; tel. 847/360–3000 **A**2 9 10 **F**3 12 13 15 18 20 22 24 26 28 29 30 31 34 35 38 40 42 43 44 45 46 47 48 49 50 57 59 68 70 73 74 76 78 79 81 82 85 87 89 93 100 102 107 110 111 112 113 114 118 125 128 129 131 145 146 147 **P**5 6 **S** Community Health Systems, Inc., Franklin, TN
Primary Contact: Barbara J. Martin, R.N., President and Chief Executive Officer
COO: Kim Needham, Assistant Chief Executive Officer
CFO: Pamela German Hill, Chief Financial Officer
CMO: Michael Scheer, M.D., President Medical Staff
CIO: Cathy Adler–Marks, Director Information Technology
CHR: Nancy Alonso, Vice President Human Resources
Web address: www.vistahealth.com
**Control:** Corporation, Investor–owned, for–profit **Service:** General Medical and Surgical

**Staffed Beds:** 192 **Admissions:** 11481 **Census:** 121 **Outpatient Visits:** 117024 **Births:** 1286 **Total Expense ($000):** 143122 **Payroll Expense ($000):** 51726 **Personnel:** 747

★ △ **VISTA MEDICAL CENTER WEST (140033)**, 2615 Washington Street, Zip 60085–4988; tel. 847/249–3900 **A**7 9 10 **F**29 30 34 35 38 40 50 56 57 59 64 68 77 87 90 98 99 101 102 103 104 105 107 113 118 129 131 134 **P**5 6 **S** Community Health Systems, Inc., Franklin, TN
Primary Contact: Barbara J. Martin, R.N., President and Chief Executive Officer
COO: Kim Needham, Assistant Chief Executive Officer
CFO: Pamela German Hill, Chief Financial Officer
CMO: Wendy Lotts, M.D., President Medical Staff
CIO: Cathy Adler–Marks, Director Information Technology
CHR: Robyn Matsil, Human Resources Director
CNO: Rosetta Speights, R.N., Chief Nursing Officer
Web address: www.vistahealth.com
**Control:** Corporation, Investor–owned, for–profit **Service:** Psychiatric

**Staffed Beds:** 67 **Admissions:** 1807 **Census:** 40 **Outpatient Visits:** 24145 **Births:** 0 **Total Expense ($000):** 17283 **Payroll Expense ($000):** 7702 **Personnel:** 106

## WHEATON—Du Page County

⊞ △ **MARIANJOY REHABILITATION HOSPITAL (143027)**, 26 West 171 Roosevelt Road, Zip 60187–0795, Mailing Address: P.O. Box 795, Zip 60187–0795; tel. 630/909–8000, (Total facility includes 20 beds in nursing home–type unit) **A**1 3 5 7 9 10 **F**11 29 30 34 35 36 56 64 68 75 86 87 90 91 93 94 127 131 142 145 147 **P**6 **S** Wheaton Franciscan Healthcare, Wheaton, IL
Primary Contact: Kathleen C. Yosko, President and Chief Executive Officer
COO: John Brady, Vice President Physician Services and Organizational Planning
CFO: Michael Hedderman, Senior Vice President Finance and Chief Financial Officer
CMO: Noel Rao, M.D., Medical Director
CIO: Pat Orrison, Director Information Services
CHR: Teresa Chapman, Vice President Human Resources
Web address: www.marianjoy.org
**Control:** Church–operated, Nongovernment, not–for profit **Service:** Rehabilitation

**Staffed Beds:** 128 **Admissions:** 2991 **Census:** 115 **Outpatient Visits:** 48837 **Births:** 0 **Total Expense ($000):** 68041 **Payroll Expense ($000):** 35189 **Personnel:** 711

## WINFIELD—DuPage County

⊞ **CENTRAL DUPAGE HOSPITAL (140242)**, 25 North Winfield Road, Zip 60190; tel. 630/933–1600, (Includes BEHAVIORAL HEALTH CENTER, 27 West 350 High Lake Road, tel. 630/653–4000) **A**1 2 5 9 10 **F**3 4 5 8 11 12 13 14 15 17 18 19 20 22 24 26 28 29 30 31 34 35 36 37 39 40 41 42 43 44 45 46 47 48 49 50 54 55 57 58 59 60 64 68 70 72 73 74 75 76 78 79 81 82 84 85 86 87 88 89 91 92 93 94 96 98 99 100 101 102 103 104 105 106 107 108 110 111 112 113 114 115 116 117 118 119 120 121 122 123 125 128 129 131 134 140 141 142 143 144 145 146 147 **S** Cadence Health, Winfield, IL
Primary Contact: Michael Vivoda, President
CFO: James Spear, Executive Vice President and Chief Financial Officer
CMO: Kevin Most, D.O., Vice President Medical Affairs
CIO: David Printz, Vice President and Chief Information Officer
Web address: www.cdh.org
**Control:** Other not–for–profit (including NFP Corporation) **Service:** General Medical and Surgical

**Staffed Beds:** 344 **Admissions:** 22691 **Census:** 240 **Outpatient Visits:** 686970 **Births:** 3087 **Total Expense ($000):** 486597 **Payroll Expense ($000):** 174402 **Personnel:** 3083

## WOODSTOCK—Mchenry County

⊞ **CENTEGRA HOSPITAL – WOODSTOCK (140176)**, 3701 Doty Road, Zip 60098–7509, Mailing Address: P.O. Box 1990, Zip 60098–1990; tel. 815/338–2500, (Total facility includes 25 beds in nursing home–type unit) **A**1 2 9 10 **F**3 4 5 11 12 13 15 18 28 29 30 31 34 35 37 38 39 40 43 44 49 50 54 57 58 59 64 68 69 70 74 75 76 78 79 81 85 86 87 92 93 98 100 101 102 103 105 107 108 110 111 113 114 117 118 127 128 129 130 131 142 145 146 147 **P**5 **S** Centegra Health System, Crystal Lake, IL
Primary Contact: Michael S. Eesley, Chief Executive Officer
COO: Jason Sciarro, Chief Operating Officer
CFO: Robert Rosenberger, Executive Vice President, Chief Financial Officer
CMO: Ted Lorenc, M.D., Chief Medical Officer
CIO: Paul Solverson, Interim Chief Information Officer
CIO: David Tomlinson, Senior Vice President, Chief Information Officer
CHR: Barbara Jo Johnson, R.N., Senior Vice President Human Resources Development
CHR: Bernadette S. Szczepanski, Vice President Human Resources Development
CNO: Neil W. Murphy, R.N., Senior Vice President, Chief Nursing Officer
Web address: www.centegra.org
**Control:** Other not–for–profit (including NFP Corporation) **Service:** General Medical and Surgical

**Staffed Beds:** 135 **Admissions:** 8292 **Census:** 103 **Outpatient Visits:** 121476 **Births:** 918 **Total Expense ($000):** 135360 **Payroll Expense ($000):** 58787 **Personnel:** 794

## ZION—Lake County

☐ **MIDWESTERN REGIONAL MEDICAL CENTER (140100)**, 2520 Elisha Avenue, Zip 60099–2587; tel. 847/872–4561, (Nonreporting) **A**1 2 3 5 9 10 **S** Cancer Treatment Centers of America, Schaumburg, IL
Primary Contact: Anne Meisner, MSN, President and Chief Executive Officer
COO: Scott Jones, Chief Operating Officer
CFO: Cecilia Taylor, Chief Financial Officer
CMO: Edgar Staren, M.D., Senior Vice President Medical Affairs
CIO: Chad Eckes, Chief Information Officer
CHR: Scott Gallo, Assistant Vice President Talent
Web address: www.cancercenter.com
**Control:** Corporation, Investor–owned, for–profit **Service:** General Medical and Surgical

**Staffed Beds:** 73

IL

*Many Facility Codes have changed. Please refer to the AHA Guide Code Chart.* © 2012 AHA Guide

# INDIANA

## ANDERSON—Madison County

☐ **COMMUNITY HOSPITAL OF ANDERSON AND MADISON COUNTY (150113)**, 1515 North Madison Avenue, Zip 46011–3453; tel. 765/298–4242, (Nonreporting) **A**1 2 9 10 **S** Community Health Network, Indianapolis, IN
Primary Contact: William C. Vanness, II, M.D., President
Web address: www.communityanderson.com
**Control:** Other not–for–profit (including NFP Corporation) **Service:** General Medical and Surgical

**Staffed Beds:** 173

⊠ ◯ **SAINT JOHN'S HEALTH SYSTEM (150088)**, 2015 Jackson Street, Zip 46016–4339; tel. 765/649–2511 **A**1 2 9 10 11 **F**3 4 5 8 11 13 14 15 18 20 22 28 29 30 31 32 34 35 38 40 44 45 49 50 51 54 56 57 58 59 60 61 62 63 64 65 66 68 70 74 75 76 77 78 79 81 82 84 85 86 87 89 90 92 93 94 96 98 99 100 101 102 103 104 105 106 107 108 110 111 113 115 116 117 118 119 120 122 128 129 131 133 134 143 144 145 146 147 **P**6 **S** Ascension Health, Saint Louis, MO
Primary Contact: Thomas J. VanOsdol, President
COO: David Maxwell, Vice President Operations
CFO: Donald L. Apple, Chief Financial Officer
CMO: Gary Brazel, M.D., Chief Medical Officer
CIO: Robert Pope, Information Technology Director and Ministry Liaison
CHR: Glenn Fields, Vice President Human Resources
CNO: Nancy Pitcock, Vice President of Nursing and Chief Nursing Officer
Web address: www.saintjohns.stvincent.org
**Control:** Church–operated, Nongovernment, not–for profit **Service:** General Medical and Surgical

**Staffed Beds:** 185 **Admissions:** 7465 **Census:** 110 **Outpatient Visits:** 256383 **Births:** 465 **Total Expense ($000):** 180777 **Payroll Expense ($000):** 70054 **Personnel:** 1298

## ANGOLA—Steuben County

★ △ **CAMERON MEMORIAL COMMUNITY HOSPITAL (151315)**, 416 East Maumee Street, Zip 46703–2015; tel. 260/665–2141 **A**7 9 10 18 **F**3 5 10 11 13 15 28 29 30 34 45 54 57 59 62 63 68 76 77 81 82 84 85 87 93 107 108 111 113 115 116 117 118 131 132 143 145
Primary Contact: Gregory T. Burns, President and Chief Executive Officer
COO: Ellen Bisson, Chief Operating Officer
CFO: Darryl Faye, Chief Financial Officer
CMO: Berry Miller, M.D., Chief Medical Officer
CHR: Nancy Covell, Director Human Resources
Web address: www.cameronmch.com
**Control:** Other not–for–profit (including NFP Corporation) **Service:** General Medical and Surgical

**Staffed Beds:** 25 **Admissions:** 927 **Census:** 8 **Outpatient Visits:** 102394 **Births:** 160 **Total Expense ($000):** 35357 **Payroll Expense ($000):** 14340 **Personnel:** 339

## AUBURN—Dekalb County

★ **DEKALB HEALTH (150045)**, 1316 East Seventh Street, Zip 46706–2515, Mailing Address: P.O. Box 542, Zip 46706–0542; tel. 260/925–4600 **A**9 10 **F**3 7 11 13 15 28 29 32 34 35 36 40 45 53 56 57 59 62 63 64 70 73 75 76 77 79 81 82 84 85 86 87 89 93 97 107 108 110 111 113 114 117 118 128 129 131 134 145 146 147 **P**6 8
Primary Contact: Kirk M. Ray, Chief Executive Officer
CFO: Amy Crouch, Chief Financial Officer
CMO: Emilio Vazquez, M.D., Chief Medical Officer
CIO: Ed Hobbs, Director Information Services
CHR: Deb Arend Sinclair, Vice President Human Resources
CNO: Donna S. Freund, MSN, Chief Nursing Officer
Web address: www.dekalbhealth.com
**Control:** Other not–for–profit (including NFP Corporation) **Service:** General Medical and Surgical

**Staffed Beds:** 53 **Admissions:** 1840 **Census:** 15 **Outpatient Visits:** 73339 **Births:** 445 **Total Expense ($000):** 43635 **Payroll Expense ($000):** 19282 **Personnel:** 401

## AVON—Hendricks County

**CLARIAN WEST MEDICAL CENTER** See Indiana University Health West Hospital

⊠ **INDIANA UNIVERSITY HEALTH WEST HOSPITAL (150158)**, 1111 North Ronald Reagan Parkway, Zip 46123; tel. 317/217–3000 **A**1 2 5 9 10 **F**3 8 13 15 18 20 22 26 28 29 30 34 35 40 45 47 48 49 51 57 59 64 70 73 74 75 76 77 78 79 81 85 87 89 93 100 107 110 111 113 114 118 119 120 128 129 131 134 145 146 **S** Indiana University Health, Indianapolis, IN
Primary Contact: Matthew D. Bailey, FACHE, President and Chief Executive Officer
CMO: James Fesenmeier, M.D., Chief of Staff
CHR: Lana Funkhouser, Vice President Human Resources
Web address: www.iuhealth.org
**Control:** Other not–for–profit (including NFP Corporation) **Service:** General Medical and Surgical

**Staffed Beds:** 127 **Admissions:** 7489 **Census:** 83 **Outpatient Visits:** 117982 **Births:** 1189 **Total Expense ($000):** 128561 **Payroll Expense ($000):** 45666 **Personnel:** 760

## BATESVILLE—Franklin County

⊠ **MARGARET MARY COMMUNITY HOSPITAL (151329)**, 321 Mitchell Avenue, Zip 47006–0226, Mailing Address: P.O. Box 226, Zip 47006–0226; tel. 812/934–6624, (Nonreporting) **A**1 2 9 10 18
Primary Contact: Timothy L. Putnam, FACHE, President and Chief Executive Officer
CFO: Brian Daeger, Vice President Financial Services
CMO: Andrew Poltrack, M.D., Chief of Staff
CIO: Donna Nobbe, Director Information Systems
CHR: Kimberly Inscho, Vice President Community Relations and Human Resources
Web address: www.mmch.org
**Control:** Other not–for–profit (including NFP Corporation) **Service:** General Medical and Surgical

**Staffed Beds:** 25

## BEDFORD—Lawrence County

**BEDFORD REGIONAL MEDICAL CENTER** See Indiana University Health Bedford Hospital

**DUNN MEMORIAL HOSPITAL** See St. Vincent Dunn Hospital

⊠ **INDIANA UNIVERSITY HEALTH BEDFORD HOSPITAL (151328)**, 2900 West 16th Street, Zip 47421–3583; tel. 812/275–1200 **A**1 2 9 10 18 **F**3 7 11 15 18 28 29 30 31 34 35 36 37 38 39 40 41 44 45 46 49 50 53 57 59 62 64 65 68 70 71 74 75 77 78 79 81 82 84 85 86 87 90 91 92 93 94 97 102 107 108 110 111 114 117 118 128 129 130 131 132 133 134 143 144 145 146 147 **P**6 **S** Indiana University Health, Indianapolis, IN
Primary Contact: Bradford W. Dykes, President and Chief Executive Officer
CFO: Charles L. Shetler, CPA, Chief Financial Officer
CHR: Cindy Smale, Director Human Resources
CNO: Brenda Davis, R.N., Vice President of Patient Services
Web address: www.iuhealth.com
**Control:** Other not–for–profit (including NFP Corporation) **Service:** General Medical and Surgical

**Staffed Beds:** 25 **Admissions:** 1312 **Census:** 14 **Outpatient Visits:** 88519 **Births:** 0 **Total Expense ($000):** 50330 **Payroll Expense ($000):** 25615 **Personnel:** 453

⊠ **ST. VINCENT DUNN HOSPITAL (151335)**, 1600 23rd Street, Zip 47421–4704; tel. 812/275–3331 **A**1 9 10 18 **F**3 11 13 14 15 18 20 22 26 28 29 30 32 34 35 40 48 49 53 54 56 57 59 64 68 70 71 75 76 77 79 81 93 107 108 111 113 115 116 118 130 134 145 146 147 **S** Ascension Health, Saint Louis, MO
Primary Contact: Deborah Bruner, Chief Executive Officer
CFO: Crystal Plano, Controller
CMO: Deborah W. Craton, M.D., Chief Medical Officer
CIO: Chad Damon, Chief Information Officer
CHR: Darci Medlock, Manager Human Resources
Web address: www.stvincent.org/st–vincent–dunn
**Control:** Other not–for–profit (including NFP Corporation) **Service:** General Medical and Surgical

**Staffed Beds:** 25 **Admissions:** 1428 **Census:** 13 **Outpatient Visits:** 47898 **Births:** 321 **Total Expense ($000):** 28508 **Payroll Expense ($000):** 12875 **Personnel:** 289

IN

---

**Hospital, Medicare Provider Number, Address, Telephone, Approval, Facility, and Physician Codes, Health Care System**

★ American Hospital Association (AHA) membership
☐ The Joint Commission accreditation
◇ DNV Healthcare Inc. accreditation
◯ American Osteopathic Association (AOA) accreditation
△ Commission on Accreditation of Rehabilitation Facilities (CARF) accreditation

## BEECH GROVE—Marion County

✉ **SELECT SPECIALTY HOSPITAL–BEECH GROVE (152013)**, 1600 Albany Street, Suite 200, Zip 46107; tel. 317/783–8913, (Nonreporting) **A**1 10 **S** Select Medical Corporation, Mechanicsburg, PA
Primary Contact: Cheryl G. Gentry, Chief Executive Officer
CHR: Kelly Becker, Administrative Coordinator Human Resources
Web address: www.selectmedicalcorp.com
**Control:** Corporation, Investor–owned, for–profit **Service:** Long–Term Acute Care hospital

| | |
|---|---|
| **Staffed Beds:** 45 | |

**ST. FRANCIS HOSPITAL AND HEALTH CENTERS – NORTH CAMPUS** See Franciscan St. Francis Health – Beech Grove

## BLOOMINGTON—Monroe County

**BLOOMINGTON HOSPITAL** See Indiana University Health Bloomington Hospital

☐ **BLOOMINGTON MEADOWS HOSPITAL (154041)**, 3600 North Prow Road, Zip 47404; tel. 812/331–8000 **A**1 9 10 **F**4 98 99 101 102 104 105 106 **S** Universal Health Services, Inc., King of Prussia, PA
Primary Contact: Jean Scallon, Chief Executive Officer
CFO: Becky T. Nyberg, Chief Financial Officer
CMO: Jonathan Bevers, M.D., Medical Director
CHR: Amanda Shettlesworth, Director Human Resources
CNO: Susan Calabrese, Director of Nursing
Web address: www.bloomingtonmeadows.com
**Control:** Corporation, Investor–owned, for–profit **Service:** Psychiatric

| | |
|---|---|
| **Staffed Beds:** 67 **Admissions:** 1235 **Census:** 48 **Outpatient Visits:** 5976 **Births:** 0 **Total Expense ($000):** 7613 **Payroll Expense ($000):** 5194 **Personnel:** 112 | |

✉ **INDIANA UNIVERSITY HEALTH BLOOMINGTON HOSPITAL (150051)**, 709 W. 1st Street, Zip 47402, Mailing Address: P.O. Box 1149, Zip 47402–1149; tel. 812/336–6821 **A**1 2 5 9 10 19 **F**3 7 8 11 12 13 15 17 18 20 22 24 26 28 29 30 31 32 34 35 38 40 43 45 46 47 48 49 50 53 54 55 57 58 59 60 61 62 63 64 65 68 70 71 74 75 76 77 78 79 81 82 84 85 86 87 89 90 91 92 93 96 97 98 100 101 102 103 104 105 107 108 111 113 114 117 118 119 120 122 125 128 129 130 131 134 142 143 145 146 147 **P**6 **S** Indiana University Health, Indianapolis, IN
Primary Contact: Mark E. Moore, President and Chief Executive Officer
CFO: Jim Myers, Chief Financial Officer
CMO: Ken Marshall, M.D., Chief Medical Officer
CIO: Mark W. McMath, Chief Information Officer
CHR: Steven Deckard, Vice President Human Resources
Web address: www.iuhealth.org
**Control:** Other not–for–profit (including NFP Corporation) **Service:** General Medical and Surgical

| | |
|---|---|
| **Staffed Beds:** 293 **Admissions:** 13148 **Census:** 155 **Outpatient Visits:** 244429 **Births:** 1953 **Total Expense ($000):** 283404 **Payroll Expense ($000):** 121409 **Personnel:** 2324 | |

✉ **MONROE HOSPITAL (150164)**, 4011 South Monroe Medical Park Boulevard, Zip 47403–8000; tel. 812/825–1111, (Nonreporting) **A**1 9 10
Primary Contact: Theodore M. Lewis, Interim Chief Executive Officer
CFO: Dan Urban, Vice President of Finance
CMO: Brian Murphy, M.D., Chief of Staff
CHR: Pamela S. Hoffman, Director of Human Resources
CNO: Mary Jane Fleener, Director of Clinical Services
Web address: www.monroehospital.com
**Control:** Corporation, Investor–owned, for–profit **Service:** General Medical and Surgical

| | |
|---|---|
| **Staffed Beds:** 32 | |

## BLUFFTON—Wells County

✉ **BLUFFTON REGIONAL MEDICAL CENTER (150075)**, 303 South Main Street, Zip 46714–2529; tel. 260/824–3210, (Total facility includes 13 beds in nursing home–type unit) **A**1 9 10 **F**3 13 15 18 28 29 30 31 34 35 40 46 48 57 59 65 68 70 71 75 76 77 79 81 82 85 89 93 107 110 111 113 118 127 128 129 134 145 146 147 **S** Community Health Systems, Inc., Franklin, TN
Primary Contact: Brandon Haushalter, Chief Executive Officer
CFO: Larry DeBolt, Chief Financial Officer
CMO: Kay Johnson, M.D., Chief of Staff
Web address: www.blufftonregional.com
**Control:** Corporation, Investor–owned, for–profit **Service:** General Medical and Surgical

| | |
|---|---|
| **Staffed Beds:** 79 **Admissions:** 2267 **Census:** 23 **Outpatient Visits:** 66975 **Births:** 269 **Total Expense ($000):** 29582 **Payroll Expense ($000):** 13919 **Personnel:** 347 | |

## BOONVILLE—Warrick County

✉ **ST. MARY'S WARRICK HOSPITAL (151325)**, 1116 Millis Avenue, Zip 47601–0629; tel. 812/897–4800 **A**1 9 10 18 **F**3 11 15 28 29 30 40 42 45 50 53 56 57 59 61 64 68 74 79 81 87 89 93 97 98 103 107 111 113 118 127 129 131 132 134 145 **S** Ascension Health, Saint Louis, MO
Primary Contact: Carol Godsey, Administrator
COO: Jared Richey, Chief Operating Officer
CFO: Cheryl Richey, Director of Finance
CMO: Peter Rosario, M.D., Chief Medical Officer
CHR: Dorothy Gehlhausen, Manager Human Resources
CNO: Karen Waters, Chief Nursing Officer
Web address: www.stmarys.org/warrick
**Control:** Other not–for–profit (including NFP Corporation) **Service:** General Medical and Surgical

| | |
|---|---|
| **Staffed Beds:** 35 **Admissions:** 1004 **Census:** 21 **Outpatient Visits:** 22949 **Births:** 0 **Total Expense ($000):** 14417 **Payroll Expense ($000):** 7083 **Personnel:** 161 | |

## BRAZIL—Clay County

✉ ○ **ST. VINCENT CLAY HOSPITAL (151309)**, 1206 East National Avenue, Zip 47834–2797, Mailing Address: P.O. Box 489, Zip 47834–0489; tel. 812/442–2500 **A**1 9 10 11 18 **F**3 11 15 18 29 30 34 35 40 45 50 57 59 65 67 68 75 77 79 81 82 85 86 87 107 108 111 113 118 129 130 131 132 134 145 **S** Ascension Health, Saint Louis, MO
Primary Contact: Jerry Laue, Administrator
CFO: Wayne Knight, Director Finance
CMO: Craig Johnson, D.O., Medical Director
CHR: Jennifer French, Director Organizational Quality
Web address: www.stvincent.org
**Control:** Church–operated, Nongovernment, not–for profit **Service:** General Medical and Surgical

| | |
|---|---|
| **Staffed Beds:** 25 **Admissions:** 602 **Census:** 8 **Outpatient Visits:** 37732 **Births:** 0 **Total Expense ($000):** 18482 **Payroll Expense ($000):** 7101 **Personnel:** 131 | |

## BREMEN—Marshall County

✉ **COMMUNITY HOSPITAL OF BREMEN (151300)**, 1020 High Road, Zip 46506, Mailing Address: P.O. Box 8, Zip 46506–0008; tel. 574/546–2211 **A**1 9 10 18 **F**3 11 13 15 29 34 35 40 45 50 57 59 64 69 75 76 77 79 81 82 85 89 93 107 110 111 113 118 128 129 131 132 134 145
Primary Contact: Scott R. Graybill, President and Chief Executive Officer
CFO: Debra Kipfer, Chief Financial Officer
CMO: Michael McClaid, M.D., President Medical Staff
CIO: Linda Barrett, Vice President of Information Services
CHR: Patricia Board, Vice President Human Resources
CNO: Andrea Koontz, R.N., Vice President of Nursing Services
Web address: www.bremenhospital.com
**Control:** Other not–for–profit (including NFP Corporation) **Service:** General Medical and Surgical

| | |
|---|---|
| **Staffed Beds:** 24 **Admissions:** 485 **Census:** 4 **Outpatient Visits:** 28459 **Births:** 80 **Total Expense ($000):** 14287 **Payroll Expense ($000):** 5972 **Personnel:** 120 | |

**DOCTOR'S HOSPITAL AND NEUROMUSCULAR CENTER (153040)**, 411 South Whitlock Street, Zip 46506, Mailing Address: P.O. Box 36, Zip 46506–0036; tel. 574/546–3830, (Nonreporting) **A**9 10 **S** Physicians Hospital System, Mishawaka, IN
Primary Contact: DeWayne Long, Chief Executive Officer
COO: John M. Day, Chief Operating Officer
CFO: Bernie Hebert, Jr., Chief Financial Officer
CMO: Steven Posar, M.D., Chief of Medicine
CHR: Emyle Kruyer–Collins, Director Human Resources
Web address: www.physicianshospitalsystem.net
**Control:** Partnership, Investor–owned, for–profit **Service:** Rehabilitation

| | |
|---|---|
| **Staffed Beds:** 20 | |

## CARMEL—Hamilton County

**CLARIAN NORTH MEDICAL CENTER** See Indiana University Health North Hospital

**FRANCISCAN ST. FRANCIS HEALTH–CARMEL**, 12188B North Meridian Street, Zip 46032; tel. 317/705–4500, (Nonreporting) **S** Franciscan Alliance, Mishawaka, IN
**Control:** Other not–for–profit (including NFP Corporation) **Service:** General Medical and Surgical

| | |
|---|---|
| **Staffed Beds:** 6 | |

*Many Facility Codes have changed. Please refer to the AHA Guide Code Chart.* © 2012 AHA Guide

IN

✠ **INDIANA UNIVERSITY HEALTH NORTH HOSPITAL (150161)**, 11700 North Meridian Avenue, Zip 46032; tel. 317/688–2000 **A**1 5 9 10 **F**3 13 15 18 19 20 22 25 29 30 31 34 35 36 37 40 45 47 49 52 53 55 57 59 60 64 68 70 72 74 75 76 78 79 81 85 87 88 89 93 107 108 110 111 114 118 123 125 128 129 131 134 145 146 147 **S** Indiana University Health, Indianapolis, IN
Primary Contact: Jonathan R. Goble, FACHE, President and Chief Executive Officer
COO: Randall C. Yust, Chief Operating Officer and Chief Financial Officer
CFO: Randall C. Yust, Chief Operating Officer and Chief Financial Officer
CMO: Lynda Ann Smirz, M.D., Chief Medical Officer
CIO: Terrence Baker, Manager Information Services
CHR: Angela S. Thompson, Vice President Human Resources and Support Services
CNO: Suzanne DelBoccio, Chief Nursing Officer and Vice President Patient Care Services
Web address: www.iuhealth.org
**Control:** Other not–for–profit (including NFP Corporation) **Service:** General Medical and Surgical

**Staffed Beds: 161 Admissions: 9136 Census: 92 Outpatient Visits: 106945 Births: 2578 Total Expense ($000): 194362 Payroll Expense ($000): 64355 Personnel: 1079**

✠ ○ **ST. VINCENT CARMEL HOSPITAL (150157)**, 13500 North Meridian Street, Zip 46032; tel. 317/582–7000, (Nonreporting) **A**1 9 10 11 **S** Ascension Health, Saint Louis, MO
Primary Contact: Michael D. Chittenden, President
COO: Daniel LaReau, Executive Director Operations and Information
CFO: Robert A. Bates, Executive Director Finance and Chief Financial Officer
CMO: Steven L. Priddy, M.D., Vice President Physician Affairs and Chief Medical Officer
CIO: Daniel LaReau, Executive Director Operations and Information
CHR: Charles Jeffras, Executive Director Human Resources
CNO: Gwynn Perlich, Vice President of Patient Services and Chief Nursing Officer
Web address: www.stvincent.org
**Control:** Church–operated, Nongovernment, not–for profit **Service:** General Medical and Surgical

**Staffed Beds: 104**

### CHARLESTOWN—Clark County

☐ **SAINT CATHERINE REGIONAL HOSPITAL (150163)**, 2200 Market Street, Zip 47111–0009, Mailing Address: P.O. Box 9, Zip 47111–0009; tel. 812/256–3301, (Nonreporting) **A**1 9 10 **S** Saint Catherine Healthcare, LLC, Ashland, PA
Primary Contact: Daniel A. Colon, President and Chief Executive Officer
CMO: William Garner, M.D., Chief Medical Officer
CIO: Kevin McLaughlin, Director Information Systems
Web address: www.saintcatherinehospital.com
**Control:** Corporation, Investor–owned, for–profit **Service:** General Medical and Surgical

**Staffed Beds: 64**

### CLARKSVILLE—Clark County

○ **KENTUCKIANA MEDICAL CENTER (150176)**, 4601 Medical Plaza Way, Zip 47130; tel. 812/284–6100, (Nonreporting) **A**9 10 11
Primary Contact: Paul Newsom, Chief Operating Officer
Web address: www.kentuckianamedcen.com/
**Control:** Corporation, Investor–owned, for–profit **Service:** General Medical and Surgical

**Staffed Beds: 40**

### CLINTON—Vermillion County

○ **UNION HOSPITAL CLINTON (151326)**, 801 South Main Street, Zip 47842–0349; tel. 765/832–2451 **A**9 10 11 18 **F**3 11 15 18 29 30 34 35 40 45 46 50 57 59 64 68 70 75 77 79 81 85 86 87 93 97 107 108 110 113 118 129 130 132 145 146 147 **P**6
Primary Contact: Terri L. Hill, Vice President and Administrator
COO: Scott L. Teffeteller, President and Chief Executive Officer
CFO: Wayne Hutson, Chief Financial Officer
CIO: Kym Pfrank, Vice President Information Systems
CHR: Sally Zuel, Vice President Human Resources
CNO: Rhonda E. Smith, R.N., Chief Nursing Officer
Web address: www.uhhg.org/wcch/index.html
**Control:** Other not–for–profit (including NFP Corporation) **Service:** General Medical and Surgical

**Staffed Beds: 25 Admissions: 1343 Census: 10 Outpatient Visits: 49473 Births: 0 Total Expense ($000): 21482 Payroll Expense ($000): 9545 Personnel: 151**

### COLUMBIA CITY—Whitley County

✠ **PARKVIEW WHITLEY HOSPITAL (150101)**, 1260 East State Road 205, Zip 46725–9492; tel. 260/248–9000, (Total facility includes 67 beds in nursing home–type unit) **A**1 9 10 **F**3 7 8 13 15 28 29 34 35 38 40 45 50 54 57 59 64 69 70 75 76 79 81 82 85 89 91 93 96 102 107 108 111 113 118 124 127 128 131 134 142 143 145 147 **S** Parkview Health, Fort Wayne, IN
Primary Contact: Scott F. Gabriel, Senior Vice President and Chief Operating Officer
COO: Scott F. Gabriel, Senior Vice President and Chief Operating Officer
CFO: Lisa Peppler, Financial Operations Analyst
CMO: Jeffrey Brookes, M.D., Medical Director
CHR: Stephen P. Gagle, Manager Human Resources
CNO: Bridget Dolohanty–Johnson, R.N., Vice President Patient Care Services
Web address: www.parkview.com
**Control:** Other not–for–profit (including NFP Corporation) **Service:** General Medical and Surgical

**Staffed Beds: 97 Admissions: 1605 Census: 65 Outpatient Visits: 39380 Births: 188 Total Expense ($000): 36275 Payroll Expense ($000): 12221 Personnel: 256**

### COLUMBUS—Bartholomew County

★ ○ **COLUMBUS REGIONAL HOSPITAL (150112)**, 2400 East 17th Street, Zip 47201–5360; tel. 812/379–4441 **A**2 9 10 11 19 **F**3 7 8 11 12 13 15 18 20 22 24 26 28 29 30 31 34 35 36 38 39 40 46 49 50 51 53 57 58 59 64 66 68 70 73 74 75 76 77 78 79 81 84 85 86 87 89 90 93 98 100 101 102 103 107 108 110 111 113 116 117 118 119 120 122 128 129 130 131 134 142 143 145 146 147
Primary Contact: James Bickel, Chief Executive Officer
CFO: Marlene Weatherwax, Vice President and Chief Financial Officer
CMO: Thomas Sonderman, M.D., Vice President and Chief Medical Officer
CIO: Diana Boyer, Chief Information Officer
CHR: Joseph Turco, Director Human Resources
Web address: www.crh.org
**Control:** County–Government, nonfederal **Service:** General Medical and Surgical

**Staffed Beds: 198 Admissions: 8990 Census: 99 Outpatient Visits: 234514 Births: 1158 Total Expense ($000): 189972 Payroll Expense ($000): 69850 Personnel: 1258**

### CONNERSVILLE—Fayette County

○ **FAYETTE REGIONAL HEALTH SYSTEM (150064)**, 1941 Virginia Avenue, Zip 47331–9990; tel. 765/825–5131, (Nonreporting) **A**9 10 11
Primary Contact: Randall White, Chief Executive Officer
CMO: Steven Johnson, D.O., Chief of Staff
CIO: Roy Cupp, Director Management Information Systems
CHR: Rhonda McPherson, Vice President Human Resources
Web address: www.fayetteregional.org
**Control:** Other not–for–profit (including NFP Corporation) **Service:** General Medical and Surgical

**Staffed Beds: 118**

### CORYDON—Harrison County

★ ○ **HARRISON COUNTY HOSPITAL (151331)**, 1141 Hospital Drive North W., Zip 47112–1774; tel. 812/738–4251, (Nonreporting) **A**9 10 11 18
Primary Contact: Steven L. Taylor, Chief Executive Officer
CFO: Jeff Davis, Chief Financial Officer
CIO: Chuck Wiley, Manager Information Systems
CHR: Angie Phelps Sells, Manager Human Resources
Web address: www.hchin.org
**Control:** County–Government, nonfederal **Service:** General Medical and Surgical

**Staffed Beds: 25**

### CRAWFORDSVILLE—Montgomery County

○ **FRANCISCAN ST. ELIZABETH HEALTH – CRAWFORDSVILLE (150022)**, 1710 Lafayette Road, Zip 47933–1099; tel. 765/362–2800, (Nonreporting) **A**9 10 11 **S** Franciscan Alliance, Mishawaka, IN
Primary Contact: Thomas R. Peck, Chief Executive Officer
COO: Nancy Sennett, R.N., Vice President Nursing Services
CFO: Keith Lauter, Vice President Finance
Web address: www.stclaremedical.org
**Control:** Other not–for–profit (including NFP Corporation) **Service:** General Medical and Surgical

**Staffed Beds: 76**

**ST. CLARE MEDICAL CENTER** See Franciscan St. Elizabeth Health – Crawfordsville

IN

---

**Hospital, Medicare Provider Number, Address, Telephone, Approval, Facility, and Physician Codes, Health Care System**

★ American Hospital Association (AHA) membership
☐ The Joint Commission accreditation
◇ DNV Healthcare Inc. accreditation
○ American Osteopathic Association (AOA) accreditation
△ Commission on Accreditation of Rehabilitation Facilities (CARF) accreditation

## CROWN POINT—Lake County

○ **FRANCISCAN ST. ANTHONY HEALTH – CROWN POINT (150126)**, 1201 South Main Street, Zip 46307–8483; tel. 219/738–2100, (Nonreporting) **A**2 5 9 10 11 **S** Franciscan Alliance, Mishawaka, IN
Primary Contact: David Ruskowski, President
CFO: Larry Stazinski, Vice President Finance
CMO: John T. King, M.D., Vice President Medical Staff Affairs
CIO: Nader Eskander, Director
CHR: Donna Wimmer, Director Human Resources
Web address: www.stanthonymedicalcenter.com
**Control:** Church–operated, Nongovernment, not–for profit **Service:** General Medical and Surgical

**Staffed Beds:** 254

**PINNACLE HOSPITAL (150166)**, 9301 Connecticut Drive, Zip 46307; tel. 219/756–2100, (Nonreporting) **A**9 10
Primary Contact: Haroon Naz, Chief Executive Officer
Web address: www.pinnaclehealthcare.net
**Control:** Partnership, Investor–owned, for–profit **Service:** General Medical and Surgical

**Staffed Beds:** 18

**ST. ANTHONY MEDICAL CENTER** See Franciscan St. Anthony Health – Crown Point

**VIBRA HOSPITAL OF NORTHWESTERN INDIANA (152028)**, 9509 Georgia Street, Zip 46307–6518; tel. 219/472–2200, (Nonreporting) **S** Vibra Healthcare, Mechanicsburg, PA
Primary Contact: Mark Senko, Chief Executive Officer
Web address: www.vhnwindiana.com/
**Control:** Corporation, Investor–owned, for–profit **Service:** Long–Term Acute Care hospital

**Staffed Beds:** 40

## DANVILLE—Hendricks County

★ ○ **HENDRICKS REGIONAL HEALTH (150005)**, 1000 East Main Street, Zip 46122–0409, Mailing Address: P.O. Box 409, Zip 46122–0409; tel. 317/745–4451 **A**2 5 9 10 11 **F**3 8 11 13 15 20 28 29 30 31 32 34 35 40 54 55 56 57 59 60 61 64 66 69 70 74 75 76 77 78 79 81 85 86 87 89 93 96 97 107 108 109 110 111 114 116 117 118 119 120 122 128 129 130 131 134 143 145 146 147 **P**6
Primary Contact: John Sparzo, M.D., Interim Chief Executive Officer
CFO: John Komenda, Chief Financial Officer
CMO: John Sparzo, M.D., Vice President Medical Affairs
CIO: Lowell Nicodemus, Director Information Systems
CHR: Gary Lenard, Director Human Resources
Web address: www.hendrickshospital.org
**Control:** County–Government, nonfederal **Service:** General Medical and Surgical

**Staffed Beds:** 121 **Admissions:** 5554 **Census:** 57 **Outpatient Visits:** 315983 **Births:** 1026 **Total Expense ($000):** 158661 **Payroll Expense ($000):** 75101 **Personnel:** 1295

## DECATUR—Adams County

★ ○ **ADAMS MEMORIAL HOSPITAL (151330)**, 1100 Mercer Avenue, Zip 46733–2311, Mailing Address: P.O. Box 151, Zip 46733–0151; tel. 260/724–2145, (Total facility includes 194 beds in nursing home–type unit) **A**9 10 11 18 **F**2 3 5 7 10 11 13 15 29 31 34 35 38 40 45 47 50 53 56 57 59 64 65 66 67 68 70 71 75 76 77 79 81 82 84 85 86 87 92 93 94 96 97 98 99 100 101 102 103 104 105 107 108 110 111 113 118 124 127 128 129 130 131 132 133 134 142 143 144 145 146 147 **P**6
Primary Contact: Thomas Joseph Nordwick, Executive Director
COO: JoEllen Eidam, Chief Operating Officer
CFO: Dane Wheeler, Chief Financial Officer
CMO: Scott Smith, M.D., Chief of Staff
CIO: Nick Nelson, Director Support Services
CHR: Alison Kukelhan, Manager Human Resources
CNO: Jo McIntire, Chief Nursing Officer
Web address: www.adamshospital.com
**Control:** County–Government, nonfederal **Service:** General Medical and Surgical

**Staffed Beds:** 229 **Admissions:** 2470 **Census:** 209 **Outpatient Visits:** 90556 **Births:** 191 **Total Expense ($000):** 46518 **Payroll Expense ($000):** 25462 **Personnel:** 524

## DYER—Lake County

**FRANCISCAN ST. MARGARET HEALTH – DYER** See Franciscan St. Margaret Health – Hammond, Hammond

**SAINT MARGARET MERCY HEALTHCARE CENTERS–SOUTH CAMPUS** See Franciscan St. Margaret Health – Dyer

## EAST CHICAGO—Lake County

⊠ **REGENCY HOSPITAL OF NORTHWEST INDIANA (152024)**, 4321 Fir Street, 4th Floor, Zip 46312; tel. 219/392–7790, (Includes REGENCY HOSPITAL OF PORTER COUNTY, 3630 Willow Creek Road, Portage, Zip 46368; tel. 219/364–3800), (Nonreporting) **A**1 10 **S** Select Medical Corporation, Mechanicsburg, PA
Primary Contact: Victor J. Galfano, FACHE, Chief Executive Officer
Web address: www.regencyhospital.com
**Control:** Corporation, Investor–owned, for–profit **Service:** Long–Term Acute Care hospital

**Staffed Beds:** 25

△ **ST. CATHERINE HOSPITAL (150008)**, 4321 Fir Street, Zip 46312–3097; tel. 219/392–1700 **A**5 7 9 10 **F**1 3 5 11 13 15 17 18 20 22 24 26 28 29 30 31 34 35 40 49 50 54 57 58 59 60 61 62 64 68 74 75 76 77 78 79 80 81 82 85 86 87 89 92 93 98 99 100 101 102 103 104 107 108 110 111 113 118 119 128 129 131 134 145 146 147 **P**1 **S** Community Healthcare System, Hammond, IN
Primary Contact: JoAnn Birdzell, Chief Executive Officer and Administrator
COO: Craig Bolda, Chief Operating Officer
CFO: Luis Molina, Chief Financial Officer
CMO: John Griep, M.D., Chief Medical Director
CIO: Gary Weiner, Chief Information Officer
CNO: Paula C. Swenson, R.N., Vice President and Chief Nursing Officer
Web address: www.stcatherinehospital.org
**Control:** Other not–for–profit (including NFP Corporation) **Service:** General Medical and Surgical

**Staffed Beds:** 189 **Admissions:** 8674 **Census:** 114 **Outpatient Visits:** 151903 **Births:** 630 **Total Expense ($000):** 158300 **Payroll Expense ($000):** 57422 **Personnel:** 981

## ELKHART—Elkhart County

★ ○ △ **ELKHART GENERAL HEALTHCARE SYSTEM (150018)**, 600 East Boulevard, Zip 46514–2499, Mailing Address: P.O. Box 1329, Zip 46515–1329; tel. 574/294–2621 **A**2 5 7 9 10 11 **F**3 11 12 13 15 17 18 20 22 24 26 28 29 30 31 34 35 36 40 45 46 49 50 57 59 62 64 68 69 70 72 74 75 76 77 78 79 81 82 85 86 87 89 90 92 93 98 99 100 102 104 105 107 108 110 111 113 114 117 118 119 120 122 128 129 131 133 134 145 146 147 **P**4
Primary Contact: Greg Losasso, President
CMO: Karl W. Schultz, M.D., Chief of Staff
CIO: David Vick, Chief Information Officer
CHR: Kurt A. Meyer, Vice President Human Resources
Web address: www.egh.org
**Control:** Other not–for–profit (including NFP Corporation) **Service:** General Medical and Surgical

**Staffed Beds:** 305 **Admissions:** 12543 **Census:** 141 **Outpatient Visits:** 430580 **Births:** 1551 **Total Expense ($000):** 223815 **Payroll Expense ($000):** 82421 **Personnel:** 1135

## ELWOOD—Madison County

⊠ ○ **ST. VINCENT MERCY HOSPITAL (151308)**, 1331 South A Street, Zip 46036–1942; tel. 765/552–4600 **A**1 2 9 10 11 18 **F**3 5 8 11 15 18 28 29 30 31 32 34 35 40 43 44 45 46 47 50 53 54 57 59 64 67 74 75 78 79 81 82 85 86 87 89 93 96 107 108 111 113 118 127 128 129 130 131 132 133 134 140 145 147 **P**6 **S** Ascension Health, Saint Louis, MO
Primary Contact: Deborah Y. Rasper, FACHE, Administrator
CFO: Joseph Kubala, Chief Financial Officer
CMO: Stephen Berghofer, M.D., Chief Medical Officer
CHR: Barbara Whitenack, Manager Human Resources
CNO: Ann C. Yates, R.N., Director Patient Care and Clinical Services
Web address: www.stvincent.org
**Control:** Church–operated, Nongovernment, not–for profit **Service:** General Medical and Surgical

**Staffed Beds:** 25 **Admissions:** 615 **Census:** 8 **Outpatient Visits:** 34207 **Births:** 0 **Total Expense ($000):** 23486 **Payroll Expense ($000):** 10646 **Personnel:** 143

## EVANSVILLE—Vanderburgh County

★ ○ **DEACONESS HOSPITAL (150082)**, 600 Mary Street, Zip 47747–0001; tel. 812/450–5000, (Includes DEACONESS CROSS POINTE CENTER, 7200 East Indiana Street, Zip 47715; tel. 812/476–7200; Cheryl Rietman, Chief Administrative Officer) **A**2 3 5 9 10 11 **F**3 5 9 11 12 15 17 18 19 20 22 24 26 29 30 31 34 35 36 38 39 40 43 44 45 46 49 50 53 54 56 57 58 59 60 61 62 63 64 65 66 68 70 71 74 75 77 78 79 81 82 84 85 86 87 88 89 94 96 97 98 99 100 101 102 104 105 107 108 110 111 113 114 115 116 117 118 119 120 122 125 128 129 131 133 134 142 143 144 145 147 **P**6 **S** Deaconess Health System, Evansville, IN
Primary Contact: Shawn W. McCoy, Chief Administrative Officer
CFO: Cheryl Wathen, Interim Chief Financial Officer
CMO: James Porter, M.D., Vice President Medical Affairs
CHR: Larry Pile, Director Human Resources
Web address: www.deaconess.com
**Control:** Other not–for–profit (including NFP Corporation) **Service:** General Medical and Surgical

**Staffed Beds:** 541 **Admissions:** 25141 **Census:** 341 **Outpatient Visits:** 554261 **Births:** 0 **Total Expense ($000):** 476501 **Payroll Expense ($000):** 188011 **Personnel:** 3225

**EVANSVILLE PSYCHIATRIC CHILDREN CENTER**, 3300 East Morgan Avenue, Zip 47715–2232; tel. 812/477–6436, (Nonreporting)
Primary Contact: Lottie Cook, Superintendent
Web address: www.khrh.org
**Control:** State–Government, nonfederal **Service:** Children's hospital psychiatric

**Staffed Beds:** 28

□ **EVANSVILLE STATE HOSPITAL**, 3400 Lincoln Avenue, Zip 47714–0146; tel. 812/469–6800 **A**1 **F**30 98 129 131 134 145
Primary Contact: Cathe Fulcher, Superintendent
CFO: Janet Kelsey, Director Business
CMO: Melba Briones, M.D., Medical Director
CHR: Cheryl Lutey, Director Human Resources
**Control:** State–Government, nonfederal **Service:** Psychiatric

**Staffed Beds:** 168 **Admissions:** 61 **Census:** 155 **Outpatient Visits:** 0 **Births:** 0 **Total Expense ($000):** 59418 **Payroll Expense ($000):** 13686 **Personnel:** 390

⊞ **HEALTHSOUTH DEACONESS REHABILITATION HOSPITAL (153025)**, 4100 Covert Avenue, Zip 47714–5567, Mailing Address: P.O. Box 5349, Zip 47716–5349; tel. 812/476–9983 **A**1 9 10 **F**28 29 64 68 75 87 90 91 93 94 95 96 129 131 142 147 **S** HEALTHSOUTH Corporation, Birmingham, AL
Primary Contact: Barbara Butler, Chief Executive Officer
CFO: Diane Riley, Controller
CMO: Ashok Dhingra, M.D., Executive Medical Director
CHR: Blake Bunner, Director Human Resources
Web address: www.healthsouthdeaconess.com
**Control:** Corporation, Investor–owned, for–profit **Service:** Rehabilitation

**Staffed Beds:** 80 **Admissions:** 1482 **Census:** 60 **Outpatient Visits:** 7150 **Births:** 0 **Total Expense ($000):** 19538 **Payroll Expense ($000):** 9622 **Personnel:** 236

⊞ **SELECT SPECIALTY HOSPITAL–EVANSVILLE (152014)**, 400 S.E. 4th Street, Zip 47713; tel. 812/421–2500, (Nonreporting) **A**1 10 **S** Select Medical Corporation, Mechanicsburg, PA
Primary Contact: Tracy Conroy, Chief Executive Officer
Web address: www.selectmedicalcorp.com
**Control:** Corporation, Investor–owned, for–profit **Service:** Long–Term Acute Care hospital

**Staffed Beds:** 60

⊞ △ **ST. MARY'S MEDICAL CENTER OF EVANSVILLE (150100)**, 3700 Washington Avenue, Zip 47750–0002; tel. 812/485–4000 **A**1 2 5 7 9 10 **F**3 8 11 12 13 15 17 18 19 20 22 24 26 28 29 30 31 32 34 35 36 37 39 40 43 45 46 47 48 49 50 51 53 54 55 56 59 60 61 64 65 66 70 71 72 73 74 75 76 77 78 79 80 81 84 85 86 87 88 89 90 92 93 96 97 98 100 101 102 103 107 108 110 111 113 114 116 117 118 125 128 129 130 131 134 142 143 145 146 147 **P**4 6 **S** Ascension Health, Saint Louis, MO
Primary Contact: Timothy A. Flesch, President and Chief Executive Officer
CFO: Kimberly Hodgkinson, Senior Vice President and Chief Financial Officer
CMO: John Gallagher, M.D., Chief Medical Officer
CIO: Cynthia Hyde, Interim Chief Information Officer
CHR: Claudia Richardt, Director Human Resources and Organization Development
CNO: Darcy Ellison, R.N., Senior Vice President, Chief Nursing Officer and Inpatient Flow
Web address: www.stmarys.org
**Control:** Church–operated, Nongovernment, not–for profit **Service:** General Medical and Surgical

**Staffed Beds:** 430 **Admissions:** 18133 **Census:** 243 **Outpatient Visits:** 348794 **Births:** 1643 **Total Expense ($000):** 358297 **Payroll Expense ($000):** 118088 **Personnel:** 2198

## FORT WAYNE—Allen County

⊞ **DUPONT HOSPITAL (150150)**, 2520 East Dupont Road, Zip 46825; tel. 260/416–3000 **A**1 9 10 **F**3 13 15 20 22 26 29 30 34 35 40 45 49 51 56 57 59 64 65 68 70 72 73 74 75 79 81 82 85 86 87 107 108 111 112 113 114 118 123 125 128 130 131 134 140 144 145 146 147 **P**1 5 **S** Community Health Systems, Inc., Franklin, TN
Primary Contact: Chad Towner, Chief Executive Officer
COO: Bonnie Hanson, Chief Operating Officer
CFO: Brian Schneider, Chief Financial Officer
CMO: Theresa Herman, M.D., Chief Medical Officer and Chief Quality Officer
CIO: Keith A. Neuman, Chief Information Officer
CNO: Karra Heggen, R.N., Chief Nursing Officer
Web address: www.thedupontdifference.com
**Control:** Partnership, Investor–owned, for–profit **Service:** General Medical and Surgical

**Staffed Beds:** 131 **Admissions:** 5119 **Census:** 54 **Outpatient Visits:** 103920 **Births:** 2264 **Total Expense ($000):** 72105 **Payroll Expense ($000):** 29100 **Personnel:** 447

⊞ **LUTHERAN HOSPITAL OF INDIANA (150017)**, 7950 West Jefferson Boulevard, Zip 46804–1677; tel. 260/435–7001 **A**1 2 3 5 9 10 **F**17 70 72 76 80 88 89 98 **S** Community Health Systems, Inc., Franklin, TN
Primary Contact: Brian Bauer, Chief Executive Officer
COO: Erica Wehrmeister, Chief Operating Officer
CFO: Michael McCullough, Chief Financial Officer
CMO: Geoffrey Randolph, M.D., Chief Medical Officer
CIO: Randy Cox, Chief Information Officer
CHR: Bruce Hamilton, Vice President Human Resources
Web address: www.lutheranhospital.com
**Control:** Corporation, Investor–owned, for–profit **Service:** General Medical and Surgical

**Staffed Beds:** 396 **Admissions:** 18347 **Census:** 254 **Outpatient Visits:** 423424 **Births:** 1209 **Total Expense ($000):** 286106 **Payroll Expense ($000):** 103206

⊞ **ORTHOPAEDIC HOSPITAL OF LUTHERAN HEALTH (150168)**, 7952 West Jefferson Boulevard, Zip 46804–4140; tel. 260/435–2999 **A**1 9 10 **F**29 34 35 37 64 77 79 80 81 82 93 94 96 111 130 **P**8 **S** Community Health Systems, Inc., Franklin, TN
Primary Contact: Shelly Miller, R.N., Chief Executive Officer
CFO: Michael McCullough, Chief Financial Officer
CMO: Steven Fisher, M.D., President Medical Staff
CHR: Bruce Hamilton, Director Human Resources
Web address: www.theorthohospital.com
**Control:** Corporation, Investor–owned, for–profit **Service:** Orthopedic

**Staffed Beds:** 44 **Admissions:** 2029 **Census:** 14 **Outpatient Visits:** 39193 **Births:** 0 **Total Expense ($000):** 39981 **Payroll Expense ($000):** 9683 **Personnel:** 158

⊞ △ **PARKVIEW HOSPITAL (150021)**, 2200 Randallia Drive, Zip 46805–4699; tel. 260/373–4000, (Includes PARKVIEW NORTH HOSPITAL, 11115 Parkview Plaza Drive, Zip 46845; tel. 260/672–4000), (Total facility includes 28 beds in nursing home–type unit) **A**1 2 3 5 7 9 10 **F**3 5 7 11 13 14 15 18 20 22 24 26 28 29 30 31 32 34 35 40 43 44 45 46 49 50 51 53 54 55 57 58 59 60 61 62 63 64 65 68 69 70 72 74 75 76 78 79 81 82 84 85 86 87 88 89 90 92 93 96 98 99 100 101 102 103 104 105 107 108 109 111 113 114 117 118 119 120 122 123 125 127 128 129 130 131 134 140 145 146 147 **S** Parkview Health, Fort Wayne, IN
Primary Contact: Sue Ehinger, Ph.D., Executive Vice President and Chief Operating Officer
COO: Sue Ehinger, Ph.D., Executive Vice President and Chief Operating Officer
CMO: Michael Grabowski, M.D., President Medical Staff
CIO: Ron Double, Chief Information Officer
CHR: Debra Williams, Senior Vice President Human Resources
Web address: www.parkview.com
**Control:** Other not–for–profit (including NFP Corporation) **Service:** General Medical and Surgical

**Staffed Beds:** 620 **Admissions:** 27139 **Census:** 399 **Outpatient Visits:** 240727 **Births:** 2696 **Total Expense ($000):** 500867 **Payroll Expense ($000):** 149711 **Personnel:** 2820

**PARKVIEW ORTHO HOSPITAL**, 11130 Parkview Circle Drive, Zip 46845–1735; tel. 260/672–5000 **S** Parkview Health, Fort Wayne, IN
Primary Contact: Julie Fleck, Chief Operating Officer
Web address: www.parkview.com
**Control:** Corporation, Investor–owned, for–profit **Service:** Orthopedic

**Staffed Beds:** 30

---

**Hospital, Medicare Provider Number, Address, Telephone, Approval, Facility, and Physician Codes, Health Care System**

★ American Hospital Association (AHA) membership
□ The Joint Commission accreditation
◇ DNV Healthcare Inc. accreditation
○ American Osteopathic Association (AOA) accreditation
△ Commission on Accreditation of Rehabilitation Facilities (CARF) accreditation

☒ △ **REHABILITATION HOSPITAL OF FORT WAYNE (153030)**, 7970 West Jefferson Boulevard, Zip 46804–4140; tel. 260/435–6100 **A**1 7 9 10 **F**29 30 90 93 96 129 131 145 **P**5 **S** Community Health Systems, Inc., Franklin, TN
Primary Contact: Ted Scholten, Chief Operating Officer
COO: Ted Scholten, Chief Operating Officer
CFO: Michael McCullough, Chief Financial Officer
CMO: Thomas Banas, Chief Medical Officer
CIO: Keith A. Neuman, Chief Information Officer
CHR: Deborah Giardina, Director Human Resources and Medical Staff Services
CNO: Shelley Boxell, R.N., Chief Nursing Officer and Quality Coordinator
Web address: www.rehabhospital.com
**Control:** Corporation, Investor–owned, for–profit **Service:** Rehabilitation

**Staffed Beds:** 36 **Admissions:** 543 **Census:** 18 **Outpatient Visits:** 68 **Births:** 0 **Total Expense ($000):** 8102 **Payroll Expense ($000):** 4671 **Personnel:** 88

☒ **SELECT SPECIALTY HOSPITAL–FORT WAYNE (152016)**, 700 Broadway, 7th Floor, Zip 46802; tel. 260/425–3810, (Nonreporting) **A**1 10 **S** Select Medical Corporation, Mechanicsburg, PA
Primary Contact: Lea Ann Klarner, Chief Executive Officer
CMO: Yogesh Amin, M.D., Medical Director
CNO: Marielle Lael, R.N., Chief Nursing Officer
Web address: www.selectmedicalcorp.com
**Control:** Corporation, Investor–owned, for–profit **Service:** Long–Term Acute Care hospital

**Staffed Beds:** 32

☒ **ST. JOSEPH HOSPITAL (150047)**, 700 Broadway, Zip 46802–1493; tel. 260/425–3000, (Total facility includes 21 beds in nursing home–type unit) **A**1 3 5 9 10 **F**1 3 4 5 13 15 16 17 18 20 22 24 26 28 29 30 31 34 35 40 43 44 45 46 47 49 50 53 56 57 68 69 70 71 72 73 74 75 76 77 79 80 81 82 85 86 87 88 89 90 93 96 97 98 100 101 102 103 104 105 107 108 110 111 114 117 118 127 129 131 140 145 147 **P**6 **S** Community Health Systems, Inc., Franklin, TN
Primary Contact: Eric N. Looper, Chief Executive Officer
CFO: Pamela Hess, Chief Financial Officer
CIO: Randy Cox, Chief Information Officer
CHR: Steve Heggen, Administrative Director Human Resources
Web address: www.stjoehospital.com
**Control:** Corporation, Investor–owned, for–profit **Service:** General Medical and Surgical

**Staffed Beds:** 191 **Admissions:** 5560 **Census:** 94 **Outpatient Visits:** 112544 **Births:** 473 **Total Expense ($000):** 74093 **Payroll Expense ($000):** 33055 **Personnel:** 576

☒ **VETERANS AFFAIRS NORTHERN INDIANA HEALTH CARE SYSTEM**, 2121 Lake Avenue, Zip 46805–5347; tel. 260/460–1310, (Includes VETERANS AFFAIRS NORTHERN INDIANA HEALTH CARE SYSTEM–MARION CAMPUS, 1700 East 38th Street, Marion, Zip 46953–4589; tel. 765/674–3321), (Nonreporting) **A**1 **S** Department of Veterans Affairs, Washington, DC
Primary Contact: Daniel D. Hendee, Director
COO: Helen Rhodes, R.N., Associate Director Operations
CFO: Jay H. Vandermark, Chief Financial Officer
CMO: Mark D. Wooten, M.D., Chief of Staff
CIO: David Troyer, Chief Information Officer
CHR: Brian Flynn, Chief Human Resources Officer
Web address: www.va.gov/sta/guide/home.asp
**Control:** Veterans Affairs, Government, federal **Service:** General Medical and Surgical

**Staffed Beds:** 105

☐ **VIBRA HOSPITAL OF FORT WAYNE (152027)**, 2626 Fairfield Avenue, Zip 46807–1215; tel. 260/399–2900, (Nonreporting) **A**1 **S** Vibra Healthcare, Mechanicsburg, PA
Primary Contact: Robert P. Gerick, Interim Chief Executive Officer
Web address: www.vhfortwayne.com
**Control:** Corporation, Investor–owned, for–profit **Service:** Long–Term Acute Care hospital

**Staffed Beds:** 50

**FRANKFORT—Clinton County**

☒ ○ **ST. VINCENT FRANKFORT HOSPITAL (151316)**, 1300 South Jackson Street, Zip 46041–3394, Mailing Address: P.O. Box 669, Zip 46041–0669; tel. 765/656–3000 **A**1 9 10 11 18 **F**3 8 13 15 28 29 30 31 34 35 40 45 50 53 57 59 64 68 75 76 78 79 81 82 85 86 87 89 90 93 107 110 111 113 118 129 131 132 134 145 **S** Ascension Health, Saint Louis, MO
Primary Contact: Thomas Crawford, Administrator
CFO: Jerry Marks, Chief Financial Officer
CMO: Stephen Tharp, M.D., Medical Director
CHR: Krista Wright, Director Human Resources
Web address: www.stvincent.org
**Control:** Church–operated, Nongovernment, not–for profit **Service:** General Medical and Surgical

**Staffed Beds:** 25 **Admissions:** 997 **Census:** 11 **Outpatient Visits:** 32344 **Births:** 231 **Total Expense ($000):** 22095 **Payroll Expense ($000):** 8530 **Personnel:** 98

**FRANKLIN—Johnson County**

★ ○ **JOHNSON MEMORIAL HOSPITAL (150001)**, 1125 West Jefferson Street, Zip 46131–2140, Mailing Address: P.O. Box 549, Zip 46131–0549; tel. 317/736–3300 **A**2 5 9 10 11 **F**12 13 15 18 20 28 29 30 31 34 35 36 40 44 45 49 50 54 57 59 62 64 68 70 74 75 76 77 78 79 81 82 85 87 90 93 97 107 111 113 117 118 120 128 129 130 131 133 134 143 145 146 147 **P**8
Primary Contact: Larry Heydon, President and Chief Executive Officer
COO: Steve Wohlford, Chief Operating Officer–Hospital Services
CFO: Andrew Walker, Chief Financial Officer
CMO: John Norris, M.D., Chief Medical Officer
CIO: Scott Krodel, Director Information Systems
CHR: Judy Ware, Director Human Resources
CNO: Anita M. Trackwell, R.N., Chief Nursing Officer
Web address: www.johnsonmemorial.org
**Control:** County–Government, nonfederal **Service:** General Medical and Surgical

**Staffed Beds:** 101 **Admissions:** 2666 **Census:** 32 **Outpatient Visits:** 160740 **Births:** 494 **Total Expense ($000):** 76802 **Payroll Expense ($000):** 33995 **Personnel:** 580

**GARY—Lake County**

☐ ○ △ **METHODIST HOSPITALS (150002)**, 600 Grant Street, Zip 46402–6099; tel. 219/886–4000, (Includes SOUTHLAKE CAMPUS, 8701 Broadway, Merrillville, Zip 46410; tel. 219/738–5500) **A**1 2 3 5 7 9 10 11 **F**3 8 10 11 12 13 15 20 22 24 28 29 30 31 32 34 35 40 45 47 48 49 50 51 54 55 57 59 62 64 68 70 72 73 74 75 76 77 78 79 81 82 85 86 87 89 90 93 97 98 99 100 101 102 104 105 107 108 110 111 113 114 116 118 119 120 122 123 129 131 132 145 146 147 **P**6
Primary Contact: Ian McFadden, President and Chief Executive Officer
CMO: Charles O. Davidson, M.D., Vice President Medical Affairs
CIO: Shaw Collins, Director Information Technology
CHR: Joyce McGlory, Vice President Human Resources
Web address: www.methodisthospitals.org
**Control:** Other not–for–profit (including NFP Corporation) **Service:** General Medical and Surgical

**Staffed Beds:** 505 **Admissions:** 17447 **Census:** 285 **Outpatient Visits:** 206525 **Births:** 1438 **Total Expense ($000):** 273596 **Payroll Expense ($000):** 106863 **Personnel:** 1753

**GOSHEN—Elkhart County**

**GOSHEN GENERAL HOSPITAL** See Indiana University Health Goshen Hospital

☒ **INDIANA UNIVERSITY HEALTH GOSHEN HOSPITAL (150026)**, 200 High Park Avenue, Zip 46526–4899, Mailing Address: P.O. Box 139, Zip 46527–0139; tel. 574/533–2141, (Nonreporting) **A**1 2 9 10 **S** Indiana University Health, Indianapolis, IN
Primary Contact: James O. Dague, President and Chief Executive Officer
COO: Paulette Brown, Chief Operating Officer
CFO: Randal Christophel, Executive Vice President and Chief Financial Officer
CMO: Randall Cammenga, M.D., Vice President Medical Affairs
CIO: Dolph Voelker, Director Information Services
CHR: Alan Weldy, Vice President Human Resources, Compliance and Legal Services
Web address: www.iuhealth.org
**Control:** Other not–for–profit (including NFP Corporation) **Service:** General Medical and Surgical

**Staffed Beds:** 122

**OAKLAWN PSYCHIATRIC CENTER (154031)**, 330 Lakeview Drive, Zip 46528–9365, Mailing Address: P.O. Box 809, Zip 46527–0809; tel. 574/533–1234 **A**9 10 **F**4 5 29 30 35 38 54 56 98 99 100 101 103 104 106 126 129 145 **P**6
Primary Contact: Laurie N. Nafziger, President and Chief Executive Officer
CFO: Lynn J. Miller, Vice President Financial Services
CMO: Daniel Kinsey, M.D., Medical Director
CIO: Gloria Holub, Manager Communications
CHR: Jill Seifer, Vice President Human Resources
CNO: Elaine G. Miller, Director of Nursing
Web address: www.oaklawn.org
**Control:** Other not–for–profit (including NFP Corporation) **Service:** Psychiatric

**Staffed Beds:** 16 **Admissions:** 811 **Census:** 13 **Outpatient Visits:** 227373 **Births:** 0 **Total Expense ($000):** 33131 **Payroll Expense ($000):** 18502 **Personnel:** 387

**GREENCASTLE—Putnam County**

○ **PUTNAM COUNTY HOSPITAL (151333)**, 1542 Bloomington Street, Zip 46135–2297; tel. 765/653–5121, (Nonreporting) **A**2 9 10 11 18
Primary Contact: Dennis Weatherford, Chief Executive Officer
CFO: Kevin Fowler, Director Finance
Web address: www.pchosp.org/
**Control:** County–Government, nonfederal **Service:** General Medical and Surgical

**Staffed Beds:** 25

**IN**

## GREENFIELD—Hancock County

★ ○ **HANCOCK REGIONAL HOSPITAL (150037)**, 801 North State Street, Zip 46140–1270, Mailing Address: P.O. Box 827, Zip 46140–0827; tel. 317/462–5544 **A**5 9 10 11 **F**3 11 12 13 15 17 18 20 22 28 29 30 31 32 34 35 36 38 40 44 45 47 48 49 50 53 54 56 57 59 62 63 64 66 68 69 70 74 75 76 78 79 81 82 83 84 85 86 87 89 90 93 96 98 103 107 110 111 113 114 118 126 128 129 130 131 133 134 143 145 146 147 **P**2 8
Primary Contact: Robert C. Keen, Ph.D., FACHE, President and Chief Executive Officer
CFO: Rick Edwards, Vice President Finance Services
CMO: Michael Fletcher, M.D., President Medical Staff
CIO: Jon Miller, Team Leader Accounting and Information Services
CHR: Laura L. Nichols, Team Leader Human Resources
CNO: Sherry Gehring, R.N., Vice President Nursing, Inpatient Care and Chief Nursing Officer
Web address: www.hancockregional.org
**Control:** County–Government, nonfederal **Service:** General Medical and Surgical

**Staffed Beds:** 85 **Admissions:** 3469 **Census:** 39 **Outpatient Visits:** 168908 **Births:** 390 **Total Expense ($000):** 77019 **Payroll Expense ($000):** 37074 **Personnel:** 697

## GREENSBURG—Decatur County

⊞ **DECATUR COUNTY MEMORIAL HOSPITAL (151332)**, 720 North Lincoln Street, Zip 47240–1398; tel. 812/663–4331 **A**1 2 9 10 18 21 **F**3 7 8 11 13 15 18 28 29 31 32 34 35 40 45 50 54 56 57 59 62 64 65 68 69 75 76 77 78 79 80 81 82 85 86 87 89 92 93 94 96 97 107 108 110 111 113 114 116 117 118 127 128 129 130 131 132 134 144 145 146 147 **P**6
Primary Contact: Linda V. Simmons, President and Chief Executive Officer
CFO: Michael R. Ruckel, Vice President Finance
CIO: Michael R. Ruckel, Vice President Finance
CHR: Robin Meyer, Vice President Support Services
CNO: Diane McKinney, R.N., Vice President Patient Care Service
Web address: www.dcmh.net
**Control:** County–Government, nonfederal **Service:** General Medical and Surgical

**Staffed Beds:** 25 **Admissions:** 1159 **Census:** 9 **Outpatient Visits:** 109099 **Births:** 263 **Total Expense ($000):** 41865 **Payroll Expense ($000):** 20745 **Personnel:** 358

## GREENWOOD—Johnson County

★ **KINDRED HOSPITAL INDIANAPOLIS SOUTH (152008)**, 607 Greenwood Springs Drive, Zip 46143–1400; tel. 317/888–8155, (Nonreporting) **A**10 **S** Kindred Healthcare, Louisville, KY
Primary Contact: Mona Euler, Chief Executive Officer
COO: Michelle Estes, Chief Clinical Officer
CFO: William Brenner, Chief Financial Officer
CMO: Steven Samuels, M.D., Medical Director
Web address: www.khindysouth.com/
**Control:** Corporation, Investor–owned, for–profit **Service:** Long–Term Acute Care hospital

**Staffed Beds:** 60

☐ **VALLE VISTA HOSPITAL (154024)**, 898 East Main Street, Zip 46143–1400; tel. 317/887–1348 **A**1 9 10 **F**4 5 35 64 98 99 100 101 104 105 106 **P**6 **S** Universal Health Services, Inc., King of Prussia, PA
Primary Contact: Sherri R. Jewett, Chief Executive Officer
CFO: Anne Knapp, Chief Financial Officer
CMO: Jennifer Comer, M.D., Medical Director
CIO: Karen Hayden, Director Health Information Services, Performance Improvement and Risk Management
CHR: Ismael Santos, Director Human Resources
Web address: www.vallevistahospital.com
**Control:** Corporation, Investor–owned, for–profit **Service:** Psychiatric

**Staffed Beds:** 102 **Admissions:** 2001 **Census:** 53 **Outpatient Visits:** 9889 **Births:** 0 **Total Expense ($000):** 11277 **Payroll Expense ($000):** 5993 **Personnel:** 160

## HAMMOND—Lake County

○ △ **FRANCISCAN ST. MARGARET HEALTH – HAMMOND (150004)**, 5454 Hohman Avenue, Zip 46320–1999; tel. 219/933–2074, (Includes FRANCISCAN ST. MARGARET HEALTH – DYER, 24 Joliet Street, Dyer, Zip 46311–1799; tel. 219/865–2141; SAINT MARGARET MERCY HEALTHCARE CENTERS–NORTH CAMPUS, 5454 Hohman Avenue, Zip 46320; tel. 219/932–2300), (Nonreporting) **A**2 5 7 9 10 11 **S** Franciscan Alliance, Mishawaka, IN
Primary Contact: Thomas J. Gryzbek, President
CFO: Jim Lipinski, Chief Financial Officer
Web address: www.smmhc.com
**Control:** Church–operated, Nongovernment, not–for profit **Service:** General Medical and Surgical

**Staffed Beds:** 500

⊞ **KINDRED HOSPITAL NORTHWEST INDIANA (152012)**, 5454 Hohman Avenue, 5th Floor, Zip 46320; tel. 219/937–9900, (Nonreporting) **A**1 10 **S** Kindred Healthcare, Louisville, KY
Primary Contact: Jeff Cellucci, Interim Chief Executive Officer
Web address: www.khnwindiana.com
**Control:** Corporation, Investor–owned, for–profit **Service:** Long–Term Acute Care hospital

**Staffed Beds:** 70

**SAINT MARGARET MERCY HEALTHCARE CENTERS** See Franciscan St. Margaret Health – Hammond

**TRIUMPH HOSPITAL NORTHWEST INDIANA** See Kindred Hospital Northwest Indiana

## HARTFORD CITY—Blackford County

**BLACKFORD COMMUNITY HOSPITAL** See Indiana University Health Blackford Hospital

⊞ **INDIANA UNIVERSITY HEALTH BLACKFORD HOSPITAL (151302)**, 410 Pilgrim Boulevard, Zip 47348–1897; tel. 765/348–0300 **A**1 9 10 18 **F**3 7 11 15 28 29 34 35 40 44 45 50 57 59 64 75 81 85 86 93 107 110 113 118 128 131 132 134 142 **S** Indiana University Health, Indianapolis, IN
Primary Contact: Steven J. West, Chief Executive Officer
CIO: Robert McKelvey, Chief Information Officer
CHR: John Crosbie, Director Support Services
Web address: www.iuhealth.org
**Control:** Other not–for–profit (including NFP Corporation) **Service:** General Medical and Surgical

**Staffed Beds:** 15 **Admissions:** 498 **Census:** 5 **Outpatient Visits:** 25630 **Births:** 0 **Total Expense ($000):** 15467 **Payroll Expense ($000):** 7180 **Personnel:** 127

## HOBART—Lake County

**HIND GENERAL HOSPITAL**, 101 West 61st Avenue, Zip 46342; tel. 219/947–3030 **F**3 75 79 81 82 87
Primary Contact: Raghu Nayak, Chief Executive Officer
**Control:** Partnership, Investor–owned, for–profit **Service:** Surgical

**Staffed Beds:** 8 **Admissions:** 113 **Census:** 1 **Outpatient Visits:** 519 **Births:** 0 **Personnel:** 34

☐ △ **ST. MARY MEDICAL CENTER (150034)**, 1500 South Lake Park Avenue, Zip 46342–6699; tel. 219/942–0551 **A**1 7 9 10 **F**3 8 11 12 13 15 18 20 22 24 26 28 29 30 31 34 35 36 38 39 40 45 46 47 49 50 51 54 57 58 59 60 62 64 65 67 68 70 74 75 76 77 78 79 81 82 85 86 87 89 90 93 107 108 110 111 113 115 117 118 120 122 128 129 131 133 134 145 146 147 **P**6 8 **S** Community Healthcare System, Hammond, IN
Primary Contact: Janice L. Ryba, JD, Chief Executive Officer
CFO: Mary Sudicky, Chief Financial Officer
CIO: Gary Weiner, Vice President Information Technology and Chief Information Officer
CHR: Tony Ferracane, Vice President Human Resources
Web address: www.comhs.org
**Control:** Other not–for–profit (including NFP Corporation) **Service:** General Medical and Surgical

**Staffed Beds:** 190 **Admissions:** 10499 **Census:** 152 **Outpatient Visits:** 178939 **Births:** 733 **Total Expense ($000):** 180218 **Payroll Expense ($000):** 63509 **Personnel:** 1045

## HUNTINGTON—Huntington County

⊞ **PARKVIEW HUNTINGTON HOSPITAL (150091)**, 2001 Stults Road, Zip 46750–3696; tel. 260/355–3000 **A**1 9 10 **F**3 7 8 13 15 28 29 30 31 32 34 35 36 38 39 40 44 45 46 50 53 56 57 59 64 68 69 70 75 76 77 78 79 81 85 86 87 93 96 97 107 108 111 118 129 130 131 133 134 145 147 **S** Parkview Health, Fort Wayne, IN
Primary Contact: Darlene Garrett, Chief Operating Officer
COO: Darlene Garrett, Chief Operating Officer
Web address: www.parkview.com
**Control:** Other not–for–profit (including NFP Corporation) **Service:** General Medical and Surgical

**Staffed Beds:** 36 **Admissions:** 1906 **Census:** 16 **Outpatient Visits:** 41174 **Births:** 374 **Total Expense ($000):** 35370 **Payroll Expense ($000):** 11025 **Personnel:** 225

## INDIANAPOLIS—Marion County

**CLARIAN HEALTH PARTNERS** See Indiana University Health University Hospital

**IN**

---

**Hospital, Medicare Provider Number, Address, Telephone, Approval, Facility, and Physician Codes, Health Care System**

★ American Hospital Association (AHA) membership
☐ The Joint Commission accreditation
◇ DNV Healthcare Inc. accreditation
○ American Osteopathic Association (AOA) accreditation
△ Commission on Accreditation of Rehabilitation Facilities (CARF) accreditation

☐ △ **COMMUNITY HOSPITAL EAST (150074)**, 1500 North Ritter Avenue, Zip 46219–3095; tel. 317/355–1411, (Nonreporting) **A**1 2 3 5 7 9 10 **S** Community Health Network, Indianapolis, IN
Primary Contact: Robin Ledyard, M.D., M.P.H., President
Web address: www.ecommunity.org
**Control:** Other not–for–profit (including NFP Corporation) **Service:** General Medical and Surgical

**Staffed Beds: 233**

☐ **COMMUNITY HOSPITAL NORTH (150169)**, 7150 Clearvista Drive, Zip 46256; tel. 317/621–6262, (Nonreporting) **A**1 9 10 **S** Community Health Network, Indianapolis, IN
Primary Contact: Barbara Summers, President
COO: Mike Blanchet, President, CHI
CFO: Jeff Kirkham, Chief Financial Officer
CMO: Clif Knight, M.D., Vice President Medical and Academic Affairs
CIO: Edward Koschka, Network Vice President Information Technology and Chief Information Officer
CHR: Jill Parris, Network Vice President Human Resources
Web address: www.ecommunity.com
**Control:** Other not–for–profit (including NFP Corporation) **Service:** General Medical and Surgical

**Staffed Beds: 389**

☐ **COMMUNITY HOSPITAL SOUTH (150128)**, 1402 East County Line Road South, Zip 46227; tel. 317/887–7000, (Nonreporting) **A**1 9 10 **S** Community Health Network, Indianapolis, IN
Primary Contact: Anthony B. Lennen, President
Web address: www.ecommunity.com
**Control:** Other not–for–profit (including NFP Corporation) **Service:** General Medical and Surgical

**Staffed Beds: 108**

○ **COMMUNITY WESTVIEW HOSPITAL (150129)**, 3630 Guion Road, Zip 46222–1699; tel. 317/924–6661, (Nonreporting) **A**3 5 9 10 11 12 13 **S** Community Health Network, Indianapolis, IN
Primary Contact: Jon P. Anderson, CPA, Chief Executive Officer
CMO: James M. Williams, D.O., Vice President Medical Affairs
CHR: Emily Rogers, Manager Human Resources
CNO: Deborah Lee, Chief Nursing Officer
Web address: www.westviewhospital.org
**Control:** Hospital district or authority, Government, nonfederal **Service:** General Medical and Surgical

**Staffed Beds: 68**

**FAIRBANKS (154034)**, 8102 Clearvista Parkway, Zip 46256–4698; tel. 317/849–8222 **A**9 10 **F**4 5 29 30 35 36 75 87 100 105 129 131 134 145 **P**8
Primary Contact: Helene M. Cross, President and Chief Executive Officer
COO: Cindy Leigh, Chief Operating Officer
CFO: Barb Elliott, Chief Financial Officer
CMO: Timothy J. Kelly, M.D., Medical Director
CIO: Randy Walls, Manager Information Services
CHR: Sharon Baker, Director Support Services
Web address: www.fairbankscd.org
**Control:** Other not–for–profit (including NFP Corporation) **Service:** Alcoholism and other chemical dependency

**Staffed Beds: 86 Admissions: 3238 Census: 56 Outpatient Visits: 24620 Births: 0 Total Expense ($000): 17942 Payroll Expense ($000): 9643 Personnel: 223**

○ **FRANCISCAN ST. FRANCIS HEALTH – INDIANAPOLIS (150162)**, 8111 South Emerson Avenue, Zip 46217; tel. 317/528–5000 **A**9 10 11 **F**8 11 12 13 15 17 18 22 24 28 29 30 31 32 34 35 36 40 46 47 49 50 55 56 57 60 61 62 63 64 65 66 68 72 74 75 76 77 78 79 80 81 82 84 85 86 87 89 93 97 107 108 109 110 111 114 115 116 117 118 119 120 122 123 125 128 129 130 131 134 143 145 146 147 **P**7 8 **S** Franciscan Alliance, Mishawaka, IN
Primary Contact: Robert J. Brody, President and Chief Executive Officer
COO: D. Keith Jewell, Senior Vice President and Chief Operating Officer
CFO: Jay R. Brehm, Executive Vice President and Chief Financial Officer
CMO: Christopher Doehring, M.D., Vice President Medical Affairs
CIO: Barbara Coulter, Director Information Systems
CHR: Karen S. Sagar, Vice President Human Resources
CNO: Susan McRoberts, R.N., Vice President and Chief Nursing Officer
Web address: www.stfrancishospitals.org
**Control:** Church–operated, Nongovernment, not–for profit **Service:** General Medical and Surgical

**Staffed Beds: 234 Admissions: 9993 Census: 116 Outpatient Visits: 369218 Births: 2566 Total Expense ($000): 188167 Payroll Expense ($000): 51835 Personnel: 1061**

☐ **INDIANA HEART HOSPITAL (150154)**, 8075 North Shadeland Avenue, Zip 46250; tel. 317/621–8000, (Nonreporting) **A**1 9 10 **S** Community Health Network, Indianapolis, IN
Primary Contact: Thomas A. Malasto, Chief Executive Officer
COO: Susan Holbrook–Preston, Chief Operating Officer and Chief Nursing Officer
CFO: W. Kevin Fowler, Chief Financial Officer
CMO: Robert Shoemaker, M.D., Chief of Staff Community Heart and Vascular
CIO: Ed Koschka, Network Vice President Information Technology and Chief Information Officer
CHR: Sharon McCullough, Director Human Resources
Web address: www.hearthospital.com
**Control:** Other not–for–profit (including NFP Corporation) **Service:** General Medical and Surgical

**Staffed Beds: 56**

○ **INDIANA ORTHOPAEDIC HOSPITAL (150160)**, 8400 Northwest Boulevard, Zip 46278; tel. 317/956–1000, (Nonreporting) **A**9 10 11
Primary Contact: Jane Keller, R.N., Chief Executive Officer
COO: Stacie Vance, Vice President Clinical Services
CFO: Anthony Gioia, Chief Financial Officer
CMO: Jeffrey J. Soldatis, M.D., Chairman Medical Executive Committee
CIO: Paul Frey, Director Information Technology Applications
CHR: Amanda Gleason, Director Human Resources
Web address: www.orthoindy.com
**Control:** Corporation, Investor–owned, for–profit **Service:** Orthopedic

**Staffed Beds: 37**

**INDIANA UNIVERSITY HEALTH METHODIST HOSPITAL** See Indiana University Health University Hospital

★ **INDIANA UNIVERSITY HEALTH UNIVERSITY HOSPITAL (150056)**, 550 University Boulevard, Zip 46202–5149, Mailing Address: P.O. Box 1367, Zip 46206–1367; tel. 317/962–2000, (Includes INDIANA UNIVERSITY HEALTH METHODIST HOSPITAL, 1701 North Senate Boulevard, Zip 46202, Mailing Address: 1701 North Senate Bouleverd, Zip 46202; tel. 317/962–2000; INDIANA UNIVERSITY HOSPITAL, 550 North University Boulevard, Zip 46202–5262; tel. 317/274–5000; RILEY HOSPITAL FOR CHILDREN AT INDIANA UNIVERSITY HEALTH, 702 Barnhill Drive, Zip 46202–5225; tel. 317/274–5000; Jeff Sperring, M.D., President and Chief Executive Officer) **A**2 3 5 8 9 10 **F**3 4 5 6 7 8 9 11 12 13 15 16 17 18 19 20 21 22 23 24 25 26 27 28 29 30 31 32 34 35 36 37 38 39 40 43 44 45 46 47 48 49 50 51 52 53 54 55 56 57 58 59 60 61 62 63 64 65 68 69 70 71 72 73 74 75 76 77 78 79 81 82 83 84 85 86 87 88 89 91 92 93 94 96 97 98 99 100 101 102 103 104 105 107 108 109 110 111 112 113 114 115 116 117 118 119 120 121 122 123 125 128 129 130 131 133 134 135 136 137 138 139 140 143 144 145 146 147 **P**6 **S** Indiana University Health, Indianapolis, IN
Primary Contact: Daniel F. Evans, Jr., JD, President and Chief Executive Officer
CMO: Richard Graffis, M.D., Executive Vice President and Chief Medical Officer
CIO: Richard F. Johnson, Senior Vice President and Chief Information Officer
CHR: Steve Wantz, Senior Vice President Human Resources and Administration
Web address: www.iuhealth.org
**Control:** Other not–for–profit (including NFP Corporation) **Service:** General Medical and Surgical

**Staffed Beds: 1407 Admissions: 57167 Census: 1005 Outpatient Visits: 1035175 Births: 3849 Total Expense ($000): 2243080 Payroll Expense ($000): 790184 Personnel: 12247**

**INDIANA UNIVERSITY HOSPITAL** See Indiana University Health University Hospital

⊠ **KINDRED HOSPITAL–INDIANAPOLIS (152007)**, 1700 West 10th Street, Zip 46222–3802; tel. 317/636–4400, (Nonreporting) **A**1 10 **S** Kindred Healthcare, Louisville, KY
Primary Contact: Kristy Walden, R.N., Interim Administrator
CFO: William Brenner, Chief Financial Officer
CHR: Linda Russell, Director Human Resources
Web address: www.kindredhospitalindy.com/
**Control:** Corporation, Investor–owned, for–profit **Service:** Long–Term Acute Care hospital

**Staffed Beds: 59**

☐ **LARUE D. CARTER MEMORIAL HOSPITAL (154008)**, 2601 Cold Spring Road, Zip 46222–2273; tel. 317/941–4000, (Nonreporting) **A**1 3 5 10
Primary Contact: Lawrence D. Lisak, Superintendent
CFO: Michael Logar, Assistant Superintendent
CMO: Beth Pfau, M.D., Chief Medical Officer
CIO: Denton Gross, Director Information Services
CHR: Rebecca Dutton, Director Human Resources
CNO: Todd Rittman, Director of Nursing
**Control:** State–Government, nonfederal **Service:** Psychiatric

**Staffed Beds: 159**

**METHODIST HOSPITAL** See Indiana University Health Methodist Hospital

**IN**

☐ △ **REHABILITATION HOSPITAL OF INDIANA (153028)**, 4141 Shore Drive, Zip 46254–2607; tel. 317/329–2000, (Nonreporting) **A**1 3 5 7 9 10
Primary Contact: Daniel B. Woloszyn, Chief Executive Officer
COO: Monte Spence, Chief Operating Officer
CFO: Marjorie Basey, Chief Financial Officer
CMO: Flora Hammond, M.D., Chief Medical Affairs
CHR: Joni Brown, Director Human Resources
Web address: www.rhin.com
**Control:** Other not–for–profit (including NFP Corporation) **Service:** Rehabilitation

**Staffed Beds:** 80

☒ △ **RICHARD L. ROUDEBUSH VETERANS AFFAIRS MEDICAL CENTER**, 1481 West Tenth Street, Zip 46202–2884; tel. 317/554–0000 **A**1 2 3 5 7 8 **F**2 3 5 8 18 20 22 24 26 28 29 30 31 34 35 36 38 39 40 45 46 49 50 53 54 56 57 58 59 60 61 62 63 64 65 67 70 74 75 77 78 79 80 81 82 83 84 85 86 87 90 91 92 93 94 97 98 100 101 102 103 104 105 107 111 114 116 118 119 120 126 128 129 130 131 134 142 143 145 146 147 **S** Department of Veterans Affairs, Washington, DC
Primary Contact: Thomas Mattice, Director
COO: Major Jeff Nechanicky, Assistant Director
CFO: Paul Pessagno, Chief Financial Officer
CMO: Ken Klotz, M.D., Chief of Staff
CIO: Steve Stoner, Chief Information Officer
CHR: Corey Baute, Chief Human Resources Management Services
Web address: www.indianapolis.va.gov
**Control:** Veterans Affairs, Government, federal **Service:** General Medical and Surgical

**Staffed Beds:** 209 **Admissions:** 8322 **Census:** 166 **Outpatient Visits:** 584432 **Births:** 0 **Total Expense ($000):** 409703 **Payroll Expense ($000):** 149171 **Personnel:** 2117

**RILEY HOSPITAL FOR CHILDREN** See Riley Hospital for Children at Indiana University Health

**RILEY HOSPITAL FOR CHILDREN AT INDIANA UNIVERSITY HEALTH** See Indiana University Health University Hospital

**ST. FRANCIS HOSPITAL AND HEALTH CENTERS – SOUTH CAMPUS** See Franciscan St. Francis Health – Indianapolis

★ ○ **ST. VINCENT HEART CENTER OF INDIANA (150153)**, 10580 North Meridian Street, Zip 46290; tel. 317/583–5000 **A**9 10 11 **F**3 18 20 22 24 26 28 29 30 34 35 40 45 46 57 58 59 75 81 85 86 87 107 111 114 118 128 129 134 147 **P**2 **S** Ascension Health, Saint Louis, MO
Primary Contact: Blake A. Dye, President
COO: Mike Schroyer, Chief Operating Officer
CFO: Becky Jacobson, Vice President Finance
CMO: William Storer, M.D., Medical Director
CIO: Roger Strange, Chief Information Officer
CHR: Jane Richardson, Vice President Human Resources
Web address: www.theheartcenter.com
**Control:** Partnership, Investor–owned, for–profit **Service:** Heart

**Staffed Beds:** 107 **Admissions:** 5220 **Census:** 54 **Outpatient Visits:** 11871 **Births:** 0 **Total Expense ($000):** 104576 **Payroll Expense ($000):** 28595 **Personnel:** 301

☒ ○ **ST. VINCENT INDIANAPOLIS HOSPITAL (150084)**, 2001 West 86th Street, Zip 46260–1991, Mailing Address: P.O. Box 40970, Zip 46240–0970; tel. 317/338–2345, (Includes PEYTON MANNING CHILDREN'S HOSPITAL, 1707 West 86th Street, Zip 46240, Mailing Address: P.O. Box 40407, Zip 46240; tel. 317/415–5500; Anne Coleman, Administrator; PEYTON MANNING CHILDREN'S HOSPITAL AT ST. VINCENT, 2001 West 86th Street, Zip 46260, Mailing Address: P.O. Box 40970, Zip 46240–0970; tel. 317/415–8111; Anne Coleman, Administrator; ST. VINCENT STRESS CENTER, 8401 Harcourt Road, Zip 46260, Mailing Address: P.O. Box 80160, Zip 46280; tel. 317/338–4600; Sheila Mishler, Chief Executive Officer; ST. VINCENT WOMEN'S HOSPITAL, 8111 Township Line Road, Zip 46260–8043; tel. 317/415–8111; Anne Coleman, Administrator) **A**1 2 3 5 8 9 10 11 **F**2 3 4 5 9 11 13 15 17 18 19 20 21 22 23 24 25 26 27 28 29 30 31 32 34 35 37 38 39 40 41 42 43 44 45 46 47 48 49 50 51 53 54 55 56 57 58 59 61 62 63 64 66 68 70 71 72 73 74 75 76 78 79 80 81 82 84 85 86 87 88 89 90 91 93 94 96 97 98 99 100 101 102 103 104 105 107 108 110 111 113 114 115 116 117 118 119 120 122 123 125 128 129 130 131 133 134 135 136 137 142 143 145 146 147 **P**6 **S** Ascension Health, Saint Louis, MO
Primary Contact: Kyle De Fur, FACHE, President
COO: Darcy Burthay, MSN, Chief Nursing Officer and Chief Operating Officer
CFO: Thomas M. Cook, CPA, Chief Financial Officer
CMO: Daniel LeGrand, M.D., Chief Medical Officer
CIO: Brian Peters, Chief Information Officer
CHR: Marty Du Rall, Executive Director Human Resources
Web address: www.stvincent.org
**Control:** Church–operated, Nongovernment, not–for profit **Service:** General Medical and Surgical

**Staffed Beds:** 873 **Admissions:** 34270 **Census:** 524 **Outpatient Visits:** 893832 **Births:** 3757 **Total Expense ($000):** 929240 **Payroll Expense ($000):** 347056 **Personnel:** 4903

☒ **ST. VINCENT SETON SPECIALTY HOSPITAL (152020)**, 8050 Township Line Road, Zip 46260; tel. 317/415–8353, (Nonreporting) **A**1 9 10 **S** Ascension Health, Saint Louis, MO
Primary Contact: Peter H. Alexander, Administrator
COO: Troy T. Reiff, Corporate Director Operations
CFO: David M. Girten, Corporate Director Financial Services
CMO: Ronald Reisman, M.D., Chief Medical Director
CHR: Terry A. Wignall, Director Human Resources
Web address: www.stvincent.org/
**Control:** Church–operated, Nongovernment, not–for profit **Service:** Long–Term Acute Care hospital

**Staffed Beds:** 74

**WESTVIEW HOSPITAL** See Community Westview Hospital

☐ **WISHARD HEALTH SERVICES (150024)**, 1001 West 10th Street, Zip 46202–2879; tel. 317/630–7033 **A**1 3 5 8 9 10 **F**3 5 7 10 12 13 14 15 16 18 19 20 21 22 28 29 30 31 32 34 35 36 38 39 40 43 44 47 48 50 54 55 56 57 59 61 62 64 65 66 68 70 71 72 74 75 76 77 78 79 81 82 84 85 86 87 93 96 97 98 99 100 101 102 103 104 105 106 107 110 111 115 116 117 118 129 131 133 134 142 143 144 145 146 147
Primary Contact: Lisa E. Harris, M.D., Chief Executive Officer and Medical Director
CFO: Lee Livin, Chief Financial Officer
CMO: Lisa E. Harris, M.D., Chief Executive Officer and Medical Director
CIO: David Shaw, Vice President Information Systems
CHR: Nancy Foster, Vice President Human Resources
Web address: www.wishard.edu
**Control:** County–Government, nonfederal **Service:** General Medical and Surgical

**Staffed Beds:** 293 **Admissions:** 16650 **Census:** 250 **Outpatient Visits:** 990165 **Births:** 2195 **Total Expense ($000):** 501017 **Payroll Expense ($000):** 203386 **Personnel:** 3813

### JASPER—Dubois County

☒ **MEMORIAL HOSPITAL AND HEALTH CARE CENTER (150115)**, 800 West Ninth Street, Zip 47546–2516; tel. 812/996–2345, (Nonreporting) **A**1 2 9 10 19 **S** American Province of Little Company of Mary Sisters, Evergreen Park, IL
Primary Contact: Raymond W. Snowden, President and Chief Executive Officer
CFO: E. Kyle Bennett, Executive Vice President
CMO: Stan Tretter, M.D., President Medical Staff
CIO: Todd Mehringer, Director Information Systems
CHR: Richard Pea, Director Human Resources
CNO: Tonya Heim, R.N., Vice President Patient Services and Chief Nursing Officer
Web address: www.mhhcc.org
**Control:** Church–operated, Nongovernment, not–for profit **Service:** General Medical and Surgical

**Staffed Beds:** 135

### JEFFERSONVILLE—Clark County

☒ **CLARK MEMORIAL HOSPITAL (150009)**, 1220 Missouri Avenue, Zip 47130–3743, Mailing Address: P.O. Box 69, Zip 47131–0069; tel. 812/282–6631 **A**1 2 5 9 10 **F**3 5 8 11 12 13 15 17 18 20 22 26 28 29 30 31 34 35 38 40 45 46 49 50 53 54 56 57 59 64 65 70 74 75 76 77 78 79 81 82 85 86 87 91 92 97 98 100 101 102 103 104 105 107 108 110 111 113 114 118 123 129 131 134 143 144 145 146 147 **P**6
Primary Contact: Martin Padgett, President and Chief Executive Officer
CFO: Kirk Strack, Vice President and Chief Financial Officer
CMO: William Templeton, III, M.D., Medical Director
CIO: Larry Reverman, Director Information Systems
CHR: Fred J. Horlander, Vice President
Web address: www.clarkmemorial.org
**Control:** County–Government, nonfederal **Service:** General Medical and Surgical

**Staffed Beds:** 172 **Admissions:** 14322 **Census:** 162 **Outpatient Visits:** 155853 **Births:** 1561 **Total Expense ($000):** 95854 **Payroll Expense ($000):** 57170 **Personnel:** 1363

☐ **WELLSTONE REGIONAL HOSPITAL (154051)**, 2700 Vissing Park Road, Zip 47130; tel. 812/284–8000 **A**1 9 10 **F**4 5 29 33 34 56 59 71 75 87 98 99 101 103 104 105 129 131 **P**5 **S** Universal Health Services, Inc., King of Prussia, PA
Primary Contact: Thomas Stormanns, Chief Executive Officer
CFO: Gracia Winsett, Chief Financial Officer
CMO: Asad Ismail, M.D., Medical Director
CHR: Tiffany Smith, Director Human Resources
Web address: www.wellstonehospital.com
**Control:** Corporation, Investor–owned, for–profit **Service:** Psychiatric

**Staffed Beds:** 100 **Admissions:** 3126 **Census:** 82 **Outpatient Visits:** 7101 **Births:** 0 **Total Expense ($000):** 14227 **Payroll Expense ($000):** 8724 **Personnel:** 211

IN

**KENDALLVILLE—Noble County**

✠ **PARKVIEW NOBLE HOSPITAL (150146)**, 401 Sawyer Road, Zip 46755–0728; tel. 260/347–8700 **A**1 9 10 **F**3 7 11 12 13 15 28 29 34 35 40 45 46 47 50 54 57 59 64 70 74 75 76 79 81 82 85 87 93 97 107 108 110 111 113 117 118 128 129 131 134 142 144 145 **P**4 **S** Parkview Health, Fort Wayne, IN
Primary Contact: David C. Hunter, Chief Operating Officer
COO: David C. Hunter, Chief Operating Officer
CFO: Michael P. Browning, Chief Financial Officer
CMO: Phil Corbin, M.D., Chief Medical Officer
CIO: Ron Double, Chief Information Officer
CHR: Rebecca Gonzalez, Manager Human Resources
Web address: www.parkview.com
**Control:** Other not–for–profit (including NFP Corporation) **Service:** General Medical and Surgical

Staffed Beds: 31 **Admissions:** 1860 **Census:** 16 **Outpatient Visits:** 48756 **Births:** 306 **Total Expense ($000):** 35609 **Payroll Expense ($000):** 11251 **Personnel:** 201

**KNOX—Starke County**

✠ **INDIANA UNIVERSITY HEALTH STARKE HOSPITAL (150102)**, 102 East Culver Road, Zip 46534–2299, Mailing Address: P.O. Box 339, Zip 46534–0339; tel. 574/772–6231 **A**1 9 10 **F**3 15 18 28 29 30 34 35 36 40 45 47 50 57 59 68 74 75 77 79 81 85 89 93 94 107 108 110 111 113 115 116 118 129 132 134 145 147 **S** Indiana University Health, Indianapolis, IN
Primary Contact: David W. Hyatt, Interim Chief Executive Officer
COO: David W. Hyatt, Vice President Operations
CFO: Rosemarie Heise, Vice President Finance
CMO: A. N. Damodaran, M.D., President Medical Staff
CIO: Ashley Norem, Chief Information Systems
CHR: Doug Jesch, Director Human Resources
Web address: www.iuhealth.org
**Control:** Other not–for–profit (including NFP Corporation) **Service:** General Medical and Surgical

Staffed Beds: 20 **Admissions:** 853 **Census:** 7 **Outpatient Visits:** 27101 **Births:** 0 **Total Expense ($000):** 14090 **Payroll Expense ($000):** 7768 **Personnel:** 150

**STARKE MEMORIAL HOSPITAL** See Indiana University Health Starke Hospital

**KOKOMO—Howard County**

✠ **COMMUNITY HOWARD REGIONAL HOSPITAL (150007)**, 3500 South Lafountain Street, Zip 46904–9011, Mailing Address: P.O. Box 9011, Zip 46904–9011; tel. 765/453–0702, (Nonreporting) **A**1 2 9 10 **S** Community Health Network, Indianapolis, IN
Primary Contact: James P. Alender, President and Chief Executive Officer
COO: Theodore Brown, Chief Operating Officer
CFO: Alan W. Biggs, Vice President Financial Services
CIO: Sharon Miller, Chief Information Officer
CHR: Michael L. Williams, FACHE, Vice President Human Resources
CHR: Michael L. Williams, Vice President Human Resources
Web address: www.howardregional.org
**Control:** Other not–for–profit (including NFP Corporation) **Service:** General Medical and Surgical

Staffed Beds: 152

✠ **COMMUNITY HOWARD SPECIALTY HOSPITAL (153039)**, 829 North Dixon Road, Zip 46901–7709; tel. 765/452–6700 **A**1 9 10 **F**29 30 68 87 90 93 128 131 142 **S** Community Health Network, Indianapolis, IN
Primary Contact: Michelle L. Russell, Administrator
CFO: Julie Pena, Director Finance
CMO: Brad Vossberg, M.D., Chief Rehabilitation
CHR: Kathy Leonard, Manager Human Resources
Web address: www.howardregional.org
**Control:** Corporation, Investor–owned, for–profit **Service:** Rehabilitation

Staffed Beds: 30 **Admissions:** 650 **Census:** 18 **Outpatient Visits:** 32974 **Births:** 0 **Total Expense ($000):** 13173 **Payroll Expense ($000):** 7118 **Personnel:** 162

**HOWARD REGIONAL HEALTH SYSTEM** See Community Howard Regional Hospital

**HOWARD REGIONAL HEALTH SYSTEM WEST CAMPUS SPECIALTY HOSPITAL** See Community Howard Specialty Hospital

✠ ○ **ST. JOSEPH HOSPITAL AND HEALTH CENTER (150010)**, 1907 West Sycamore Street, Zip 46901–4197, Mailing Address: P.O. Box 9010, Zip 46904–9010; tel. 765/452–5611 **A**1 9 10 11 **F**3 4 5 7 8 13 15 18 20 28 29 30 34 35 36 40 44 45 49 50 51 55 57 59 64 66 68 69 70 73 74 75 76 77 78 79 81 82 84 85 86 87 89 90 93 96 97 98 99 100 101 102 103 104 105 107 108 110 111 113 117 118 119 120 122 128 129 130 131 134 142 143 144 145 146 **P**6 **S** Ascension Health, Saint Louis, MO
Primary Contact: Kathlene A. Young, MS, FACHE, President and Chief Executive Officer
CFO: Dennis Ressler, Chief Financial Officer
CMO: David L. Williams, M.D., Chief Medical Officer
CIO: Jeffrey Scott, Chief Information Officer
CHR: Cindy Babb, Executive Director Human Resources and Organizational Effectiveness
CNO: Kathleen K. Peoples, R.N., Vice President and Nursing
Web address: www.stjoseph.stvincent.org
**Control:** Church–operated, Nongovernment, not–for profit **Service:** General Medical and Surgical

Staffed Beds: 137 **Admissions:** 5440 **Census:** 73 **Outpatient Visits:** 150077 **Births:** 595 **Total Expense ($000):** 97573 **Payroll Expense ($000):** 41605 **Personnel:** 814

**LA PORTE—Laporte County**

✠ **INDIANA UNIVERSITY HEALTH LA PORTE HOSPITAL (150006)**, 1007 Lincolnway, Zip 46350–3201, Mailing Address: P.O. Box 250, Zip 46352–0250; tel. 219/326–1234, (Total facility includes 55 beds in nursing home–type unit) **A**1 2 5 9 10 19 **F**3 8 11 13 15 17 18 20 22 24 26 28 29 30 31 32 34 35 36 38 39 40 45 46 47 48 49 50 51 53 54 56 57 58 59 60 62 63 64 65 66 67 68 70 71 74 75 76 77 78 79 81 82 84 85 86 87 89 90 93 96 98 100 101 102 103 107 108 110 111 113 114 117 118 125 127 128 129 130 131 134 143 144 145 146 147 **S** Indiana University Health, Indianapolis, IN
Primary Contact: G. Thor Thordarson, President and Chief Executive Officer
COO: Linda L. Satkoski, R.N., Chief Operating Officer
CFO: Mark Rafalski, CPA, Chief Financial Officer
CMO: William J. Houston, M.D., Medical Director
CIO: Earl Adams, Chief Information Officer
CHR: Connie Ford, Vice President Human Resources
CNO: Pauline Arnold, MSN, Chief Nursing and Quality Officer
Web address: www.iuhealth.org
**Control:** Other not–for–profit (including NFP Corporation) **Service:** General Medical and Surgical

Staffed Beds: 204 **Admissions:** 6244 **Census:** 109 **Outpatient Visits:** 107137 **Births:** 690 **Total Expense ($000):** 149684 **Payroll Expense ($000):** 57859 **Personnel:** 1382

**LA PORTE REGIONAL HEALTH SYSTEM** See Indiana University Health La Porte Hospital

**LAFAYETTE—Tippecanoe County**

**CLARIAN ARNETT HOSPITAL** See Indiana University Health Arnett Hospital

○ **FRANCISCAN ST. ELIZABETH HEALTH – LAFAYETTE CENTRAL (150003)**, 1501 Hartford Street, Zip 47904–2134; tel. 765/423–6011, (Includes LAFAYETTE HOME HOSPITAL, 2400 South Street, Zip 47904–3052; tel. 765/447–6811; ST. ELIZABETH MEDICAL CENTER, 1501 Hartford Street, Zip 47904–2126; tel. 765/423–6011), (Nonreporting) **A**2 6 9 10 11 **S** Franciscan Alliance, Mishawaka, IN
Primary Contact: Terrance E. Wilson, President and Chief Executive Officer
CFO: Keith Lauter, Chief Financial Officer
CMO: Donald B. Edelen, M.D., Vice President Medical Services and Quality Initiatives
CIO: Lisa K. Decker, Director Public Relations and Marketing
CHR: Jan Garvin, Vice President Human Resources
Web address: www.ste.org
**Control:** Other not–for–profit (including NFP Corporation) **Service:** General Medical and Surgical

Staffed Beds: 302

★ ○ **INDIANA UNIVERSITY HEALTH ARNETT HOSPITAL (150173)**, 5165 McCarty Lane, Zip 47905–8764, Mailing Address: P.O. Box 5545, Zip 47903–5545; tel. 765/448–8000 **A**9 10 11 **F**3 8 11 13 15 17 18 19 20 22 24 26 27 28 29 30 31 34 35 40 45 49 50 54 57 59 60 64 65 68 69 70 72 74 75 76 77 78 79 81 82 84 85 87 89 93 97 107 108 111 113 114 115 117 118 120 128 129 130 **P**6 **S** Indiana University Health, Indianapolis, IN
Primary Contact: Alfonso W. Gatmaitan, Chief Executive Officer
COO: Brian T. Shockney, FACHE, Chief Operating Officer
CMO: Jim Bien, M.D., Vice President Quality and Patient Safety
CIO: John Rich, System Director Information Technology
CHR: Koreen H. Kyhnell, Vice President Human Resources
Web address: www.iuhealth.org
**Control:** Other not–for–profit (including NFP Corporation) **Service:** General Medical and Surgical

Staffed Beds: 141 **Admissions:** 8735 **Census:** 103 **Outpatient Visits:** 65729 **Births:** 1110 **Total Expense ($000):** 319166 **Payroll Expense ($000):** 137251 **Personnel:** 1714

**ST. ELIZABETH CENTRAL** See Franciscan St. Elizabeth Health – Lafayette Central

*Many Facility Codes have changed. Please refer to the AHA Guide Code Chart.* © 2012 AHA Guide

**ST. ELIZABETH EAST (150109)**, 1701 South Creasy Lane, Zip 47905–4972; tel. 765/502–4000, (Nonreporting) **S** Franciscan Alliance, Mishawaka, IN
Primary Contact: Terrance E. Wilson, President and Chief Executive Officer
Web address: www.ste.org
**Control:** Other not–for–profit (including NFP Corporation) **Service:** General Medical and Surgical

**Staffed Beds: 140**

✉ ○ **ST. VINCENT SETON SPECIALTY HOSPITAL (152021)**, 1501 Hartford Street, Zip 47904; tel. 765/236–8900, (Nonreporting) **A**1 9 10 11 **S** Ascension Health, Saint Louis, MO
Primary Contact: Peter H. Alexander, Administrator
COO: Troy T. Reiff, Corporate Director Operations
CFO: David M. Girten, Corporate Director Financial Services
CMO: Ronald Reisman, M.D., rireisma@stvincent.org
CHR: Terry A. Wignall, Director Human Resources
Web address: www.stvincent.org
**Control:** Church–operated, Nongovernment, not–for profit **Service:** Long–Term Acute Care hospital

**Staffed Beds: 30**

### LAGRANGE—Lagrange County

✉ **PARKVIEW LAGRANGE HOSPITAL (151323)**, 207 North Townline Road, Zip 46761–1325; tel. 260/463–2143 **A**1 9 10 18 **F**3 7 13 15 17 26 29 30 34 35 40 45 50 51 57 59 63 64 70 75 76 79 81 82 83 84 85 86 87 89 90 93 96 107 108 109 111 113 118 127 128 129 132 142 145 147 **S** Parkview Health, Fort Wayne, IN
Primary Contact: Robert T. Myers, Chief Operating Officer
COO: Robert T. Myers, Chief Operating Officer
CFO: Vickie Stanski, Financial Analyst
CMO: Jeffrey Brookes, M.D., Chief Medical Officer
CHR: Rebecca Gonzalez, Director Human Resources
Web address: www.parkview.com
**Control:** Other not–for–profit (including NFP Corporation) **Service:** General Medical and Surgical

**Staffed Beds: 25 Admissions: 1200 Census: 12 Outpatient Visits: 20267 Births: 308 Total Expense ($000): 24475 Payroll Expense ($000): 7632 Personnel: 155**

### LAWRENCEBURG—Dearborn County

**COMMUNITY MENTAL HEALTH CENTER (154011)**, 285 Bielby Road, Zip 47025–1055; tel. 812/537–1302 **A**9 10 **F**4 98 99 100 101 102 103 104 105 106 129 134 **P**5
Primary Contact: Tom Talbot, Chief Executive Officer
Web address: www.cmhcinc.org
**Control:** Other not–for–profit (including NFP Corporation) **Service:** Psychiatric

**Staffed Beds: 14 Admissions: 510 Census: 9 Outpatient Visits: 26876 Births: 0 Total Expense ($000): 1710 Payroll Expense ($000): 1064**

★ ○ **DEARBORN COUNTY HOSPITAL (150086)**, 600 Wilson Creek Road, Zip 47025–1199; tel. 812/537–1010 **A**9 10 11 **F**3 11 13 15 20 28 30 31 34 35 37 40 43 44 45 46 47 49 50 57 59 62 63 64 70 75 76 77 78 79 81 84 85 86 87 92 93 107 108 110 111 113 115 116 117 118 129 130 131 145 147 **P**6
Primary Contact: Roger Howard, President and Chief Executive Officer
CFO: Philip A. Meyer, Director Finance
CHR: Pat Sutton, Director Human Resources
Web address: www.dch.org
**Control:** County–Government, nonfederal **Service:** General Medical and Surgical

**Staffed Beds: 78 Admissions: 4275 Census: 46 Outpatient Visits: 137790 Births: 531 Total Expense ($000): 68133 Payroll Expense ($000): 32628 Personnel: 663**

### LEBANON—Boone County

✉ **WITHAM MEMORIAL HOSPITAL (150104)**, 2605 North Lebanon Street, Zip 46052, Mailing Address: P.O. Box 1200, Zip 46052–3005; tel. 765/485–8000, (Total facility includes 1 beds in nursing home–type unit) **A**1 9 10 **F**3 7 8 13 15 18 20 22 28 29 30 31 34 40 42 45 50 54 56 57 59 60 64 65 68 69 70 75 76 77 79 81 82 83 85 86 87 93 94 97 98 103 107 108 110 111 114 116 117 118 128 129 131 134 140 145 146 147 **P**1
Primary Contact: Raymond V. Ingham, M.D., Ph.D., President and Chief Executive Officer
COO: Diane Feder, MSN, Senior Vice President and Chief Operating Officer
CFO: George Pogas, CPA, Senior Vice President and Chief Financial Officer
CMO: Thomas Cartwright, M.D., Chief of Staff
CMO: C. Layton Elliott, M.D., Chief of Staff
CIO: George Pogas, CPA, Senior Vice President and Chief Financial Officer
CHR: Gary A. Deater, Vice President Administration, Human Resources and Risk Management
CNO: Diane Feder, MSN, Senior Vice President and Chief Operating Officer
Web address: www.witham.org
**Control:** County–Government, nonfederal **Service:** General Medical and Surgical

**Staffed Beds: 52 Admissions: 2607 Census: 25 Outpatient Visits: 123883 Births: 419 Total Expense ($000): 83453 Payroll Expense ($000): 32611 Personnel: 548**

### LINTON—Greene County

✉ **GREENE COUNTY GENERAL HOSPITAL (151317)**, 1185 North 1000 W., Zip 47441; tel. 812/847–2281 **A**1 9 10 18 **F**13 18 30 31 34 45 57 59 64 65 70 74 76 77 78 81 85 89 93 107 108 110 113 118 129 132 134 147
Primary Contact: Jonas S. Uland, Executive Director
COO: Brenda Reetz, R.N., Chief Operating Officer
CFO: Timothy Norris, Chief Financial Officer
CMO: Owen A. Batterton, M.D., Chief of Staff
CIO: Steve Phillips, Information Officer
CHR: Timothy Norris, Chief Financial Officer
CNO: Lea Ann Camp, R.N., Chief Nursing Officer
Web address: www.greenecountyhospital.com
**Control:** County–Government, nonfederal **Service:** General Medical and Surgical

**Staffed Beds: 25 Admissions: 911 Census: 8 Outpatient Visits: 536110 Births: 86 Total Expense ($000): 24507 Payroll Expense ($000): 10311 Personnel: 212**

### LOGANSPORT—Cass County

★ ○ **LOGANSPORT MEMORIAL HOSPITAL (150072)**, 1101 Michigan Avenue, Zip 46947–7013, Mailing Address: P.O. Box 7013, Zip 46947–7013; tel. 574/753–7541 **A**9 10 11 20 **F**3 7 11 13 15 28 29 30 32 34 35 36 40 44 45 48 49 50 51 57 59 64 65 68 69 70 75 76 77 78 79 81 85 86 87 93 97 107 108 110 111 113 118 123 128 129 131 132 134 145 146 **P**6
Primary Contact: David J. Ameen, President and Chief Executive Officer
CFO: Julia L. Berndt, Chief Financial Officer
CMO: Charles Montgomery, M.D., Medical Director
CIO: Beth Jump, Chief Information Officer
CHR: Lynda J. Murphy, Vice President Human Resources
Web address: www.logansportmemorial.org
**Control:** County–Government, nonfederal **Service:** General Medical and Surgical

**Staffed Beds: 83 Admissions: 1922 Census: 17 Outpatient Visits: 97759 Births: 518 Total Expense ($000): 54851 Payroll Expense ($000): 27120 Personnel: 540**

□ **LOGANSPORT STATE HOSPITAL**, 1098 South State Road 25, Zip 46947–9699; tel. 574/737–3633, (Nonreporting) **A**1
Primary Contact: Mark E. Schutter, Ph.D., Superintendent and Chief Executive Officer
COO: Robert Clover, Assistant Superintendent
CFO: Misty Moss, Director Business Administration
CMO: Danny Meadows, M.D., Medical Director
CIO: Joe McIntosh, Director Management Information Systems
CHR: Dianne Renner, Director Human Resources
Web address: www.lshonline.org
**Control:** State–Government, nonfederal **Service:** Psychiatric

**Staffed Beds: 396**

IN

---

**Hospital, Medicare Provider Number, Address, Telephone, Approval, Facility, and Physician Codes, Health Care System**

★ American Hospital Association (AHA) membership
□ The Joint Commission accreditation  ◇ DNV Healthcare Inc. accreditation
○ American Osteopathic Association (AOA) accreditation
△ Commission on Accreditation of Rehabilitation Facilities (CARF) accreditation

## MADISON—Jefferson County

★ ○ **KING'S DAUGHTERS' HOSPITAL AND HEALTH SERVICES (150069)**, One King's Daughters' Drive, Zip 47250–3357, Mailing Address: P.O. Box 447, Zip 47250–0447; tel. 812/265–5211 **A**2 9 10 11 **F**3 7 8 13 15 20 28 29 30 31 32 34 35 40 45 48 49 50 56 57 59 62 63 64 65 68 70 74 75 76 77 78 79 81 82 84 85 86 89 91 94 97 107 108 111 113 114 118 119 120 122 128 129 130 131 133 134 143 144 145 146 147 **P**6
Primary Contact: Roger J. Allman, Chief Executive Officer
CFO: Steve Meacham, Vice President Finance
CMO: Judy Kuehler, M.D., President Medical Staff
CIO: Linda Darnell, Director Management Information Systems
CHR: Susan Poling, Director Human Resources
Web address: www.kdhhs.org
**Control:** Other not–for–profit (including NFP Corporation) **Service:** General Medical and Surgical

| **Staffed Beds:** 82 **Admissions:** 3143 **Census:** 31 **Outpatient Visits:** 160066 **Births:** 348 **Total Expense ($000):** 92877 **Payroll Expense ($000):** 48317 **Personnel:** 782 |

☐ **MADISON STATE HOSPITAL (154019)**, 711 Green Road, Zip 47250–2199; tel. 812/265–2611, (Nonreporting) **A**1 10
Primary Contact: Peggy Stephens, M.D., Superintendent and Medical Director
COO: Peggy Stephens, M.D., Superintendent and Medical Director
CFO: Carolyn Copeland, Business Administrator
CMO: Peggy Stephens, M.D., Superintendent and Medical Director
CIO: Ric Martin, Information Specialist
Web address: www.in.gov/fssa/msh
**Control:** State–Government, nonfederal **Service:** Psychiatric

| **Staffed Beds:** 150 |

## MARION—Grant County

☐ **GRANT–BLACKFORD MENTAL HEALTH CENTER (154021)**, 505 North Wabash Avenue, Zip 46952–2608; tel. 765/662–3971, (Nonreporting) **A**1 10
Primary Contact: Paul Kuczora, Chief Executive Officer
Web address: www.cornerstone.org/
**Control:** Other not–for–profit (including NFP Corporation) **Service:** Psychiatric

| **Staffed Beds:** 16 |

★ ○ **MARION GENERAL HOSPITAL (150011)**, 441 North Wabash Avenue, Zip 46952–2690; tel. 765/660–6000 **A**2 9 10 11 **F**3 7 8 11 13 15 18 20 22 26 28 29 30 31 34 35 40 41 45 50 57 58 59 64 65 66 68 70 74 75 76 77 78 79 81 82 85 86 87 89 90 91 92 93 96 97 107 108 110 111 113 114 117 118 128 129 131 134 142 144 145 146 147 **P**6
Primary Contact: Paul L. Usher, President and Chief Executive Officer
COO: Bernadine L. Wallace, MSN, Chief Nursing Officer and Chief Operating Officer
CFO: Robyn L. Powell, Chief Financial Officer
CMO: Edward L. Keppler, M.D., Chief Medical Officer
CIO: Emmanuel Ndow, Chief Information Officer
CHR: Karen Jones, Administrative Director Human Resources
Web address: www.mgh.net
**Control:** Other not–for–profit (including NFP Corporation) **Service:** General Medical and Surgical

| **Staffed Beds:** 115 **Admissions:** 5168 **Census:** 56 **Outpatient Visits:** 203812 **Births:** 691 **Total Expense ($000):** 119614 **Payroll Expense ($000):** 42807 **Personnel:** 861 |

**VETERANS AFFAIRS NORTHERN INDIANA HEALTH CARE SYSTEM–MARION CAMPUS** See Veterans Affairs Northern Indiana Health Care System, Fort Wayne

## MARTINSVILLE—Morgan County

⊞ **INDIANA UNIVERSITY HEALTH MORGAN HOSPITAL (150038)**, 2209 John R. Wooden Drive, Zip 46151–1840, Mailing Address: P.O. Box 1717, Zip 46151–1717; tel. 765/342–8441 **A**1 2 9 10 **F**3 8 11 13 15 28 29 30 31 32 34 35 40 45 50 55 56 57 59 64 69 70 73 75 76 77 78 79 81 82 84 85 86 90 93 97 98 103 107 108 110 111 113 118 119 120 122 128 129 131 143 145 146 147 **P**1 6 **S** Indiana University Health, Indianapolis, IN
Primary Contact: Doug Puckett, President and Chief Executive Officer
CFO: Scott Andritsch, Vice President and Chief Financial Officer
CMO: Warren L. Gray, M.D., Chief of Staff
CHR: Charlene Hall, Vice President Human Resources and Guest Support Services
Web address: www.iuhealth.org/morgan/
**Control:** Other not–for–profit (including NFP Corporation) **Service:** General Medical and Surgical

| **Staffed Beds:** 92 **Admissions:** 1717 **Census:** 21 **Outpatient Visits:** 70267 **Births:** 199 **Total Expense ($000):** 40082 **Payroll Expense ($000):** 16145 **Personnel:** 316 |

## MERRILLVILLE—Lake County

**REGIONAL MENTAL HEALTH CENTER (154020)**, 8555 Taft Street, Zip 46410–6123; tel. 219/769–4005, (Nonreporting) **A**9 10
Primary Contact: Robert D. Krumwied, President and Chief Executive Officer
Web address: www.regionalmentalhealth.org/
**Control:** Corporation, Investor–owned, for–profit **Service:** Psychiatric

| **Staffed Beds:** 16 |

**SOUTHLAKE CAMPUS** See Methodist Hospitals, Gary

## MICHIGAN CITY—Laporte County

○ **FRANCISCAN ST. ANTHONY HEALTH – MICHIGAN CITY (150015)**, 301 West Homer Street, Zip 46360–4358; tel. 219/879–8511, (Nonreporting) **A**2 9 10 11 19 **S** Franciscan Alliance, Mishawaka, IN
Primary Contact: James Callaghan, III, M.D., President
CFO: Jim Lipinski, Regional Chief Financial Officer
CIO: Terry Veith, Director Management Information Systems
CHR: Susan King–Schreiber, Vice President Human Resources
Web address: www.saintanthonymemorial.org
**Control:** Church–operated, Nongovernment, not–for profit **Service:** General Medical and Surgical

| **Staffed Beds:** 171 |

**SAINT ANTHONY MEMORIAL** See Franciscan St. Anthony Health – Michigan City

## MISHAWAKA—St. Joseph County

⊞ **KINDRED HOSPITAL OF NORTHERN INDIANA (152018)**, 215 West Fourth Street, Suite 200, Zip 46544–1917; tel. 574/252–2000, (Nonreporting) **A**1 9 10 **S** Kindred Healthcare, Louisville, KY
Primary Contact: Christine T. Voorde, Chief Executive Officer
CFO: Christy Henrich, Controller
CMO: Shaya Mokfi, M.D., Medical Director and President Medical Staff
CHR: Brenda Schweizer, Coordinator Human Resources
CNO: Jane G. Mason, Chief Clinical Officer
Web address: www.khnorthernindiana.com/
**Control:** Corporation, Investor–owned, for–profit **Service:** Long–Term Acute Care hospital

| **Staffed Beds:** 32 |

○ **RIVERCREST SPECIALTY HOSPITAL (152026)**, 1625 East Jefferson Boulevard, Zip 46545; tel. 574/255–1400, (Nonreporting) **A**10 11 **S** Physicians Hospital System, Mishawaka, IN
Primary Contact: Ronni Banks, Administrator
Web address: www.physicianshospitalsystem.net/
**Control:** Partnership, Investor–owned, for–profit **Service:** Long–Term Acute Care hospital

| **Staffed Beds:** 30 |

⊞ **SAINT JOSEPH REGIONAL MEDICAL CENTER (150012)**, 5215 Holy Cross Parkway, Zip 46545–1469; tel. 574/335–5000, (Nonreporting) **A**1 2 9 10 13 **S** Trinity Health, Novi, MI
Primary Contact: Albert Gutierrez, FACHE, President and Chief Executive Officer
CFO: Terry Heck, Vice President Finance and Chief Financial Officer
CIO: Gary L. Miller, Regional Director Information Systems
CHR: Aaron Austin, Vice President Human Resources
Web address: www.sjmed.com
**Control:** Church–operated, Nongovernment, not–for profit **Service:** General Medical and Surgical

| **Staffed Beds:** 258 |

**TRIUMPH OUR LADY OF PEACE HOSPITAL** See Kindred Hospital of Northern Indiana

○ **UNITY MEDICAL & SURGICAL HOSPITAL (150177)**, 4455 Edison Lakes Parkway, Zip 46545–1442; tel. 574/968–0867, (Nonreporting) **A**9 10 11 **S** Physicians Hospital System, Mishawaka, IN
Primary Contact: John M. Day, Chief Executive Officer
CFO: Bernie Hebert, Jr., Chief Financial Officer
CMO: Viraj Patel, M.D., Chief Medical Officer
CIO: Tim Morningstar, Blue Star
CHR: Emyle Kruyer–Collins, Vice President Human Resources
Web address: www.physicianshospitalsystem.net
**Control:** Corporation, Investor–owned, for–profit **Service:** General Medical and Surgical

| **Staffed Beds:** 15 |

## MONTICELLO—White County

★ ○ **INDIANA UNIVERSITY HEALTH WHITE MEMORIAL HOSPITAL (151312)**, 720 South Sixth Street, Zip 47960–8182; tel. 574/583–7111 **A**9 10 11 18 **F**3 8 11 13 15 29 30 31 34 35 40 45 50 57 59 62 64 75 76 77 78 80 81 85 91 93 107 108 110 111 113 118 128 132 134 145 146 **S** Indiana University Health, Indianapolis, IN
Primary Contact: Stephanie Long, Chief Executive Officer
COO: Mary Minier, Vice President Operations
CMO: Adel Khdour, M.D., Chief Medical Officer
CIO: Michelle Baker, Director Information Systems
CHR: JoEllyn Brockmeyer, Director Human Resources
CNO: Robin S. Smith, Chief Nursing Officer
Web address: www.iuhealth.org/white–memorial
**Control:** Other not–for–profit (including NFP Corporation) **Service:** General Medical and Surgical

| **Staffed Beds:** 25 **Admissions:** 1189 **Census:** 13 **Outpatient Visits:** 69571 **Births:** 216 **Total Expense ($000):** 25698 **Payroll Expense ($000):** 8640 **Personnel:** 216 |

**IN**

*Many Facility Codes have changed. Please refer to the AHA Guide Code Chart.* © 2012 AHA Guide

## MOORESVILLE—Morgan County

○ **FRANCISCAN ST. FRANCIS HEALTH – MOORESVILLE (150057)**, 1201 Hadley Road, Zip 46158–1789; tel. 317/831–1160 **A**9 10 11 **F**8 12 13 15 29 30 31 35 37 46 47 49 50 57 58 59 64 70 75 76 77 78 79 81 87 91 107 108 109 110 111 115 116 118 119 120 122 123 128 129 143 144 145 146 **P**7 8 **S** Franciscan Alliance, Mishawaka, IN
Primary Contact: Jared Stark, Executive Director
COO: D. Keith Jewell, Senior Vice President and Chief Operating Officer
CMO: Donald Kerner, M.D., Vice President Medical Affairs
CIO: Barbara Coulter, Director Information Systems
CHR: John Ross, Vice President
Web address: www.stfrancishospitals.org
**Control:** Church–operated, Nongovernment, not–for profit **Service:** General Medical and Surgical

**Staffed Beds:** 92 **Admissions:** 3733 **Census:** 32 **Outpatient Visits:** 131816 **Births:** 433 **Total Expense ($000):** 73898 **Payroll Expense ($000):** 23156 **Personnel:** 363

**ST. FRANCIS HOSPITAL–MOORESVILLE** See Franciscan St. Francis Health – Mooresville

## MUNCIE—Delaware County

**BALL MEMORIAL HOSPITAL** See Indiana University Health Ball Memorial Hospital

⊠ △ **INDIANA UNIVERSITY HEALTH BALL MEMORIAL HOSPITAL (150089)**, 2401 University Avenue, Zip 47303–3499; tel. 765/747–3111, (Total facility includes 30 beds in nursing home–type unit) **A**1 2 3 5 7 8 9 10 19 **F**3 11 12 13 15 17 18 20 22 24 26 28 29 30 31 34 35 39 40 45 46 49 50 51 52 53 54 55 57 58 59 64 65 69 70 72 73 74 75 76 77 78 79 80 81 82 85 86 87 89 90 91 92 93 94 97 98 100 102 107 110 111 113 114 116 117 118 119 120 122 123 125 126 127 128 129 130 131 145 146 147 **P**6 8 **S** Indiana University Health, Indianapolis, IN
Primary Contact: Michael E. Haley, President and Chief Executive Officer
COO: Harold Berfiend, Chief Operating Officer
CFO: Carol Seals, Chief Financial Officer
CMO: Jeffrey C. Bird, M.D., Chief Medical Officer
CIO: Robert McKelvey, Director Information System, Mergers and Integrations
CHR: Ann M. McGuire, Vice President Human Resources
Web address: www.iuhealth.org
**Control:** Other not–for–profit (including NFP Corporation) **Service:** General Medical and Surgical

**Staffed Beds:** 347 **Admissions:** 18425 **Census:** 232 **Outpatient Visits:** 306231 **Births:** 1726 **Total Expense ($000):** 299831 **Payroll Expense ($000):** 97660 **Personnel:** 2288

○ **INTEGRA SPECIALTY HOSPITAL (152025)**, 2401 West University Avenue, 8th Floor, Zip 47303–3428; tel. 765/282–5822, (Nonreporting) **A**10 11
Primary Contact: Ryan Ott, Chief Executive Officer
Web address: www.integraspecialty.com/
**Control:** Corporation, Investor–owned, for–profit **Service:** Long–Term Acute Care hospital

**Staffed Beds:** 32

**RENAISSANCE SPECIALTY HOSPITAL OF CENTRAL INDIANA** See Integra Specialty Hospital

## MUNSTER—Lake County

☐ △ **COMMUNITY HOSPITAL (150125)**, 901 MacArthur Boulevard, Zip 46321–2959; tel. 219/836–1600 **A**1 2 5 7 9 10 **F**3 8 11 13 15 17 18 20 22 24 26 28 29 31 34 35 40 45 49 50 51 53 54 57 58 59 60 62 64 68 70 72 73 74 75 76 78 79 80 81 82 85 86 87 89 90 92 93 94 96 107 108 110 111 113 114 116 118 119 120 122 123 125 128 129 131 134 143 145 146 147 **P**6 **S** Community Healthcare System, Hammond, IN
Primary Contact: Donald P. Fesko, Chief Executive Officer and Administrator
CFO: Luis Molina, Vice President Finance and Chief Financial Officer
CMO: Don Henry, M.D., President Medical and Dental Staff
CIO: Gary Weiner, Vice President Information Technology, Chief Information Officer
CHR: Michael Graham, Director Human Resources
CNO: Ronda McKay, MSN, Vice President Patient Care Services, Chief Nursing Officer
Web address: www.comhs.org
**Control:** Other not–for–profit (including NFP Corporation) **Service:** General Medical and Surgical

**Staffed Beds:** 449 **Admissions:** 21563 **Census:** 314 **Outpatient Visits:** 359245 **Births:** 2267 **Total Expense ($000):** 396243 **Payroll Expense ($000):** 160696 **Personnel:** 2554

○ **FRANCISCAN PHYSICIANS HOSPITAL (150165)**, 701 Superior Avenue, Zip 46321–4029; tel. 219/924–1300, (Nonreporting) **A**9 10 11 **S** Franciscan Alliance, Mishawaka, IN
Primary Contact: Barbara M. Greene, President
CFO: Harold E. Collins, JD, Chief Financial Officer
CMO: Vijay D. Gupta, M.D., President and Chief Executive Officer
CIO: Steven Krause, Manager Information Technology
Web address: www.heartlandmemorial.org
**Control:** Church–operated, Nongovernment, not–for profit **Service:** General Medical and Surgical

**Staffed Beds:** 32

## NEW ALBANY—Floyd County

★ ○ **FLOYD MEMORIAL HOSPITAL AND HEALTH SERVICES (150044)**, 1850 State Street, Zip 47150–4997; tel. 812/949–5500 **A**2 3 5 9 10 11 **F**8 11 12 13 15 17 18 20 22 24 28 29 30 31 34 35 40 43 49 50 56 57 59 62 64 70 71 74 75 76 77 78 79 80 81 82 85 86 87 89 93 100 107 108 110 111 113 114 117 118 119 120 122 128 129 130 131 134 143 145 146 147
Primary Contact: Mark D. Shugarman, President and Chief Executive Officer
COO: Mark Truman, Vice President of Operations
CFO: Ted Miller, Chief Financial Officer
CMO: Daniel J. Eichenberger, M.D., Medical Director
CIO: Brian Cox, Director Information Systems
CHR: Mike Ford, Vice President Human Resources
Web address: www.floydmemorial.com
**Control:** County–Government, nonfederal **Service:** General Medical and Surgical

**Staffed Beds:** 211 **Admissions:** 14611 **Census:** 166 **Outpatient Visits:** 368727 **Births:** 931 **Total Expense ($000):** 191168 **Payroll Expense ($000):** 91343 **Personnel:** 1760

☐ **PHYSICIANS' MEDICAL CENTER (150172)**, 4023 Reas Lane, Zip 47150; tel. 812/206–7660, (Nonreporting) **A**1 9 10
Primary Contact: Dennis Medley, Administrator
CMO: John Rademaker, M.D., Medical Director
CNO: Rob Jones, Chief Nursing Officer
Web address: www.pmcindiana.com
**Control:** Individual, Investor–owned, for–profit **Service:** General Medical and Surgical

**Staffed Beds:** 12

⊠ △ **SOUTHERN INDIANA REHABILITATION HOSPITAL (153037)**, 3104 Blackiston Boulevard, Zip 47150–9579; tel. 812/941–8300, (Total facility includes 26 beds in nursing home–type unit) **A**1 7 9 10 **F**29 34 35 57 59 74 75 77 79 86 87 90 91 93 96 127 129 131 134 142 145 **S** Jewish Hospital & St. Mary's HealthCare, Louisville, KY
Primary Contact: Randy L. Napier, President and Chief Executive Officer
CFO: Robert Steltenpohl, Controller
CMO: John C. Shaw, M.D., Medical Director
CHR: Lisa Burris, Director Human Resources
CNO: Suzann Byers, Director of Nursing
Web address: www.sirh.org
**Control:** Other not–for–profit (including NFP Corporation) **Service:** Rehabilitation

**Staffed Beds:** 60 **Admissions:** 1275 **Census:** 45 **Outpatient Visits:** 25431 **Births:** 0 **Total Expense ($000):** 17397 **Payroll Expense ($000):** 9225 **Personnel:** 200

## NEW CASTLE—Henry County

★ ○ **HENRY COUNTY HOSPITAL (150030)**, 1000 North 16th Street, Zip 47362–4319, Mailing Address: P.O. Box 490, Zip 47362–0490; tel. 765/521–0890 **A**9 10 11 **F**3 8 11 13 15 18 28 29 30 34 35 40 45 46 50 51 53 57 59 62 63 64 68 70 74 75 76 77 79 81 82 85 87 89 91 92 93 94 97 107 110 111 113 117 118 126 128 129 130 131 134 143 145 146 147 **P**1
Primary Contact: Paul Janssen, President and Chief Executive Officer
COO: Brian K. Ring, Chief Operating Officer
CMO: Wylie McGlothlin, M.D., Chief Medical Officer
CIO: Mike Spencer, Chief Information Officer
CHR: Deanna Malott, Director Human Resources
CNO: Carrie Williams, R.N., Chief Nursing Officer
Web address: www.hcmhcares.org
**Control:** County–Government, nonfederal **Service:** General Medical and Surgical

**Staffed Beds:** 90 **Admissions:** 2822 **Census:** 29 **Outpatient Visits:** 136444 **Births:** 354 **Total Expense ($000):** 58185 **Payroll Expense ($000):** 23612 **Personnel:** 611

IN

**Hospital, Medicare Provider Number, Address, Telephone, Approval, Facility, and Physician Codes, Health Care System**

★ American Hospital Association (AHA) membership
☐ The Joint Commission accreditation  ◇ DNV Healthcare Inc. accreditation
○ American Osteopathic Association (AOA) accreditation
△ Commission on Accreditation of Rehabilitation Facilities (CARF) accreditation

## NEWBURGH—Warrick County

○ **THE HEART HOSPITAL AT DEACONESS GATEWAY (150175)**, 4007 Gateway Boulevard, Zip 47630–8947; tel. 812/842–4784 **A**9 10 11 **F**17 18 20 22 24 26 28 29 30 34 35 57 58 59 60 62 63 64 68 81 83 84 85 86 87 107 108 109 111 113 114 115 116 117 118 129 131 **S** Deaconess Health System, Evansville, IN
Primary Contact: Rebecca Malotte, Executive Director and Chief Nursing Officer
Web address: www.deaconess.com/
**Control:** Partnership, Investor–owned, for–profit **Service:** Heart

**Staffed Beds:** 24 **Admissions:** 1630 **Census:** 17 **Outpatient Visits:** 5841 **Births:** 0 **Total Expense ($000):** 36647 **Payroll Expense ($000):** 6300 **Personnel:** 117

★ ○ **THE WOMEN'S HOSPITAL (150149)**, 4199 Gateway Boulevard, Zip 47630; tel. 812/842–4200 **A**9 10 11 **F**3 7 13 29 30 34 44 50 52 53 55 57 59 63 65 72 73 75 76 77 81 84 85 86 87 93 118 125 129 131 133 134 145 146 **P**6 **S** Deaconess Health System, Evansville, IN
Primary Contact: Christina M. Ryan, R.N., Chief Executive Officer
CFO: Tina Cady, Controller
CIO: Liz Adams, Manager Informatics
CHR: Jerri Sue Traylor, Manager Human Resources
CNO: Christina M. Ryan, R.N., Chief Executive Officer and Chief Nursing Officer
Web address: www.deaconess.com
**Control:** Partnership, Investor–owned, for–profit **Service:** Obstetrics and gynecology

**Staffed Beds:** 74 **Admissions:** 3211 **Census:** 39 **Outpatient Visits:** 16218 **Births:** 2904 **Total Expense ($000):** 47081 **Payroll Expense ($000):** 18790 **Personnel:** 355

## NOBLESVILLE—Hamilton County

○ △ **RIVERVIEW HOSPITAL (150059)**, 395 Westfield Road, Zip 46060–1425, Mailing Address: P.O. Box 220, Zip 46061–0220; tel. 317/773–0760, (Nonreporting) **A**5 7 9 10 11
Primary Contact: Patricia K. Fox, President and Chief Executive Officer
COO: Lawrence Christman, Chief Financial Officer and Chief Operating Officer
CFO: Lawrence Christman, Chief Financial Officer and Chief Operating Officer
CMO: John Paris, M.D., Chief Medical Officer
CIO: Michael Mover, Chief Information Officer
Web address: www.riverview.org
**Control:** County–Government, nonfederal **Service:** General Medical and Surgical

**Staffed Beds:** 162

## NORTH VERNON—Jennings County

⊞ ○ **ST. VINCENT JENNINGS HOSPITAL (151303)**, 301 Henry Street, Zip 47265–1097; tel. 812/352–4200 **A**1 9 10 11 18 **F**3 15 29 30 32 34 35 36 40 44 46 47 50 56 57 59 64 65 66 74 77 79 81 85 93 97 107 111 113 118 123 131 132 134 143 145 147 **P**5 **S** Ascension Health, Saint Louis, MO
Primary Contact: Carl W. Risk, II, Administrator
CFO: John Lines, Chief Financial Officer
CMO: Jennifer Stanley, M.D., President Medical Staff
CHR: Kathryn Johnson, Manager Human Resources, Marketing and Public Relations
CNO: Karen Shaw, Chief Nursing Officer and Director of Clinical Services
Web address: www.stvincent.org
**Control:** Other not–for–profit (including NFP Corporation) **Service:** General Medical and Surgical

**Staffed Beds:** 25 **Admissions:** 376 **Census:** 5 **Outpatient Visits:** 35526 **Births:** 0 **Total Expense ($000):** 17450 **Payroll Expense ($000):** 6277 **Personnel:** 130

## PAOLI—Orange County

**BLOOMINGTON HOSPITAL OF ORANGE COUNTY** See Indiana University Health Paoli Hospital

⊞ **INDIANA UNIVERSITY HEALTH PAOLI HOSPITAL (151306)**, 642 West Hospital Road, Zip 47454–0499, Mailing Address: P.O. Box 499, Zip 47454–0499; tel. 812/723–2811 **A**1 9 10 18 **F**3 7 13 15 29 30 35 40 45 50 57 59 64 76 77 81 84 85 89 93 107 110 111 113 118 128 131 132 134 145 147 **S** Indiana University Health, Indianapolis, IN
Primary Contact: Larry Bailey, Chief Executive Officer
COO: Candace Isom, Chief Operating Officer
CFO: Sue Brock, Chief Financial Officer
CMO: Dan O'Brien, D.O., Medical Director
CHR: Jessica Fortner, Director Human Resources
Web address: www.bhhs.org
**Control:** Other not–for–profit (including NFP Corporation) **Service:** General Medical and Surgical

**Staffed Beds:** 24 **Admissions:** 559 **Census:** 4 **Outpatient Visits:** 28713 **Births:** 129 **Total Expense ($000):** 22014 **Payroll Expense ($000):** 10613 **Personnel:** 203

## PERU—Miami County

⊞ **DUKES MEMORIAL HOSPITAL (151318)**, 275 West 12th Street, Zip 46970–1698; tel. 765/472–8000 **A**1 9 10 18 **F**3 7 13 15 28 29 30 40 50 51 56 57 59 64 68 69 70 75 76 77 79 81 82 85 87 90 93 107 108 110 111 113 117 118 128 129 132 134 143 145 146 147 **P**6 **S** Community Health Systems, Inc., Franklin, TN
Primary Contact: Debra Close, Chief Executive Officer
CMO: Neil Stalker, M.D., Chief of Staff
CHR: Kim Black, Manager Human Resources
Web address: www.dukesmemorialhosp.com
**Control:** Corporation, Investor–owned, for–profit **Service:** General Medical and Surgical

**Staffed Beds:** 25 **Admissions:** 1478 **Census:** 14 **Outpatient Visits:** 46366 **Births:** 227 **Total Expense ($000):** 28601 **Payroll Expense ($000):** 15087 **Personnel:** 260

## PLYMOUTH—Marshall County

□ **MICHIANA BEHAVIORAL HEALTH CENTER (154047)**, 1800 North Oak Drive, Zip 46563–3492; tel. 574/936–3784, (Nonreporting) **A**1 9 10 **S** Universal Health Services, Inc., King of Prussia, PA
Primary Contact: Bryan W. Lett, Chief Executive Officer
CFO: Jeff Calvin, Chief Financial Officer
CMO: Robert Raster, M.D., Medical Director
CIO: Bob Kedalis, Director Business Development
CHR: Becky Nowicki, Director Human Resources
Web address: www.michianabhc.com
**Control:** Corporation, Investor–owned, for–profit **Service:** Psychiatric

**Staffed Beds:** 76

⊞ **SAINT JOSEPH REGIONAL MEDICAL CENTER–PLYMOUTH CAMPUS (150076)**, 1915 Lake Avenue, Zip 46563–9905, Mailing Address: P.O. Box 670, Zip 46563–9905; tel. 574/936–3181, (Nonreporting) **A**1 9 10 **S** Trinity Health, Novi, MI
Primary Contact: Lori Price, President
CFO: Terry Heck, Vice President Finance and Chief Financial Officer
CIO: Gary L. Miller, Regional Director Information Systems
CHR: Aaron Austin, Vice President Human Resources
Web address: www.sjmed.com
**Control:** Church–operated, Nongovernment, not–for profit **Service:** General Medical and Surgical

**Staffed Beds:** 45

## PORTLAND—Jay County

⊞ **JAY COUNTY HOSPITAL (151320)**, 500 West Votaw Street, Zip 47371–1322; tel. 260/726–7131 **A**1 9 10 18 **F**3 8 11 13 15 28 29 30 32 34 35 40 45 50 57 59 68 70 75 76 77 81 85 86 87 103 107 108 110 111 113 118 128 129 131 132 134 143 145 **P**6 **S** Indiana University Health, Indianapolis, IN
Primary Contact: Joe Johnston, Chief Executive Officer
CFO: Don Michael, Chief Financial Officer
CIO: Jeff Horn, Coordinator Information Systems
CHR: Jerry Bozell, Administrative Director Human Resources
CNO: Lisa Craiger, Chief Nursing Officer
Web address: www.jaycountyhospital.com
**Control:** County–Government, nonfederal **Service:** General Medical and Surgical

**Staffed Beds:** 35 **Admissions:** 1169 **Census:** 17 **Outpatient Visits:** 47227 **Births:** 74 **Total Expense ($000):** 25847 **Payroll Expense ($000):** 13801 **Personnel:** 273

## PRINCETON—Gibson County

⊞ **GIBSON GENERAL HOSPITAL (151319)**, 1808 Sherman Drive, Zip 47670–1043; tel. 812/385–3401, (Total facility includes 45 beds in nursing home–type unit) **A**1 9 10 18 **F**3 5 11 15 28 29 30 34 35 38 40 45 54 56 57 59 62 64 68 70 75 77 79 81 89 93 97 99 100 101 102 103 104 107 110 111 114 118 127 128 129 130 131 132 145 147 **P**6 **S** Alliant Management Services, Louisville, KY
Primary Contact: Emmett C. Schuster, President and Chief Executive Officer
CFO: Ron Harrington, Vice President and Chief Financial Officer
CMO: Thomas Joseph, M.D., Chief of Staff
CIO: Patricia Ping, Director Information Services
CHR: D. Deann Hunt, Director Human Resources
CNO: Lori Phillips, Vice President and Chief Nursing Officer
Web address: www.gibsongeneral.com
**Control:** Other not–for–profit (including NFP Corporation) **Service:** General Medical and Surgical

**Staffed Beds:** 70 **Admissions:** 753 **Census:** 45 **Outpatient Visits:** 32273 **Births:** 0 **Total Expense ($000):** 24438 **Payroll Expense ($000):** 10148 **Personnel:** 132

IN

## RENSSELAER—Jasper County

★ **JASPER COUNTY HOSPITAL (151324)**, 1104 East Grace Street, Zip 47978–3296; tel. 219/866–5141, (Nonreporting) **A**9 10 18
Primary Contact: Timothy M. Schreeg, President and Chief Executive Officer
CFO: Jeffrey D. Webb, CPA, Chief Financial Officer
CIO: Kirby Reed, Director Information Systems
CHR: Deana Brown, Director Administrative Services
Web address: www.jchh.com
**Control:** County–Government, nonfederal **Service:** General Medical and Surgical

**Staffed Beds:** 42

## RICHMOND—Wayne County

★ ○ **REID HOSPITAL AND HEALTH CARE SERVICES (150048)**, 1100 Reid Parkway, Zip 47374; tel. 765/983–3000 **A**2 5 9 10 11 **F**3 11 13 15 18 20 22 24 26 27 28 29 30 31 32 34 35 36 39 40 43 44 45 47 49 50 51 54 56 57 59 61 63 64 70 74 75 76 77 78 79 81 82 83 84 85 86 87 89 90 93 96 97 98 100 101 102 103 104 107 108 110 111 113 114 115 116 117 118 119 120 122 125 128 129 130 131 134 143 145 146 147 **P**6 7 8
Primary Contact: Craig C. Kinyon, President
CFO: James Puffenberger, Vice President and Chief Financial Officer
CMO: Thomas Huth, M.D., Vice President Medical Affairs
CIO: Tim Love, Director Information Services
CHR: Scott C. Rauch, Vice President Human Resources
CNO: Kay B. Cartwright, R.N., Vice President and Chief Nursing Officer
Web address: www.reidhosp.com
**Control:** Other not–for–profit (including NFP Corporation) **Service:** General Medical and Surgical

**Staffed Beds:** 207 **Admissions:** 11520 **Census:** 145 **Outpatient Visits:** 146524 **Births:** 700 **Total Expense ($000):** 315848 **Payroll Expense ($000):** 113520 **Personnel:** 1656

□ **RICHMOND STATE HOSPITAL (154018)**, 498 N.W. 18th Street, Zip 47374–2898; tel. 765/966–0511 **A**1 10 **F**29 30 39 68 75 77 87 98 100 101 103 129 131 134 145 **P**6
Primary Contact: Jeffrey Butler, Superintendent
CFO: Dave Shelford, Assistant Superintendent
CMO: Donald Graber, M.D., Medical Director
CIO: Robert Boatman, Director Information Technology
CHR: Sarah Witt, Director Human Resources
Web address: www.richmondstatehospital.org
**Control:** State–Government, nonfederal **Service:** Psychiatric

**Staffed Beds:** 234 **Admissions:** 310 **Census:** 234 **Outpatient Visits:** 0 **Births:** 0 **Total Expense ($000):** 38589 **Payroll Expense ($000):** 19378 **Personnel:** 490

## ROCHESTER—Fulton County

★ ○ **WOODLAWN HOSPITAL (151313)**, 1400 East Ninth Street, Zip 46975–8937; tel. 574/223–3141 **A**9 10 11 18 **F**3 11 13 15 29 30 31 40 46 56 57 59 63 65 68 69 75 76 77 78 79 81 82 87 93 97 107 108 111 114 115 118 128 129 131 132 134 142 145 147 **P**6
Primary Contact: John L. Alley, Chief Executive Officer
CFO: Dave Cholger, Chief Financial Officer
CHR: Deb Lemasters, Director Human Resources
Web address: www.woodlawnhospital.com
**Control:** County–Government, nonfederal **Service:** General Medical and Surgical

**Staffed Beds:** 25 **Admissions:** 935 **Census:** 10 **Outpatient Visits:** 85207 **Births:** 174 **Total Expense ($000):** 38203 **Payroll Expense ($000):** 17758 **Personnel:** 304

## RUSHVILLE—Rush County

★ **RUSH MEMORIAL HOSPITAL (151304)**, 1300 North Main Street, Zip 46173–1198, Mailing Address: P.O. Box 608, Zip 46173–0608; tel. 765/932–4111 **A**9 10 18 **F**3 7 11 15 18 24 28 29 31 35 36 40 46 51 52 57 59 64 65 74 75 77 78 79 81 85 93 97 107 111 113 116 119 120 121 128 129 130 131 132 134 145 146 147 **P**6
Primary Contact: Bradley Smith, President and Chief Executive Officer
COO: Debbie Jones–Browning, Vice President Operations and Physician Services and Chief Operating Officer
CFO: Karen Meyer, Vice President Finance and Chief Financial Officer
CMO: Daniel Stahl, D.O., Chief of Staff
CIO: Jim Boyer, Vice President Information Technology and Chief Information Officer
CNO: Gretchen Smith, Vice President Nursing and Compliance and Risk
Web address: www.rushmemorial.com
**Control:** County–Government, nonfederal **Service:** General Medical and Surgical

**Staffed Beds:** 25 **Admissions:** 479 **Census:** 4 **Outpatient Visits:** 35469 **Births:** 0 **Total Expense ($000):** 21328 **Payroll Expense ($000):** 10676 **Personnel:** 219

## SALEM—Washington County

⊞ **ST. VINCENT SALEM HOSPITAL (151314)**, 911 North Shelby Street, Zip 47167–1694; tel. 812/883–5881 **A**1 9 10 18 **F**3 11 15 28 29 30 34 40 45 47 49 57 59 75 79 81 82 85 89 93 104 107 111 113 118 128 129 131 132 **P**6 **S** Ascension Health, Saint Louis, MO
Primary Contact: Lee Jaeger, FACHE, Chief Executive Officer
CFO: John Lines, Director Financial and Support Services
CMO: S. E. Kemker, M.D., President Medical Staff
CIO: Scott Cox, Manager Information Systems
CHR: Val Potter, Director Human Resources
Web address: www.wcmhospital.org
**Control:** Other not–for–profit (including NFP Corporation) **Service:** General Medical and Surgical

**Staffed Beds:** 25 **Admissions:** 439 **Census:** 5 **Outpatient Visits:** 29125 **Births:** 0 **Total Expense ($000):** 16742 **Payroll Expense ($000):** 7539 **Personnel:** 126

## SCOTTSBURG—Scott County

⊞ **SCOTT MEMORIAL HOSPITAL (151334)**, 1415 North Gardner Street, Zip 47170–0430, Mailing Address: Box 430, Zip 47170–0430; tel. 812/752–3456 **A**1 9 10 18 **F**3 11 13 15 28 29 30 34 35 40 57 59 64 68 70 74 76 79 81 85 86 107 108 111 113 128 131 134 145 146 **P**6 **S** Jewish Hospital & St. Mary's HealthCare, Louisville, KY
Primary Contact: Clifford D. Nay, Executive Director
CFO: Angela Doan, Chief Financial Officer
Web address: www.scottmemorial.com
**Control:** County–Government, nonfederal **Service:** General Medical and Surgical

**Staffed Beds:** 25 **Admissions:** 1095 **Census:** 12 **Outpatient Visits:** 37994 **Births:** 176 **Total Expense ($000):** 22308 **Payroll Expense ($000):** 10057 **Personnel:** 235

## SEYMOUR—Jackson County

⊞ **SCHNECK MEDICAL CENTER (150065)**, 411 West Tipton Street, Zip 47274–5000, Mailing Address: P.O. Box 2349, Zip 47274–2349; tel. 812/522–2349 **A**1 2 9 10 **F**3 8 12 13 15 18 28 29 30 31 34 35 36 40 45 50 51 56 57 58 59 60 61 62 63 64 68 69 70 74 75 76 77 78 79 81 82 83 84 85 86 87 89 93 104 107 110 111 114 115 117 118 119 120 122 123 125 128 129 130 131 132 134 143 145 146 147 **P**8
Primary Contact: Gary A. Meyer, President and Chief Executive Officer
CFO: Warren Forgey, Executive Vice President Fiscal Services and Business Development
CIO: Craig Rice, Director Information
CHR: William Lewis, Vice President Human Resources
Web address: www.schneckmed.org
**Control:** County–Government, nonfederal **Service:** General Medical and Surgical

**Staffed Beds:** 93 **Admissions:** 3727 **Census:** 40 **Outpatient Visits:** 149950 **Births:** 675 **Total Expense ($000):** 96788 **Payroll Expense ($000):** 40961 **Personnel:** 751

## SHELBYVILLE—Shelby County

★ ○ **MAJOR HOSPITAL (150097)**, 150 West Washington Street, Zip 46176–1236; tel. 317/392–3211 **A**9 10 11 **F**3 12 13 15 28 29 30 31 34 35 40 50 57 59 62 63 68 70 73 75 76 77 78 80 81 82 85 89 93 97 107 108 110 111 113 117 118 119 120 122 128 129 131 134 145 146 147 **P**6
Primary Contact: John M. Horner, President and Chief Executive Officer
CFO: Ralph Mercuri, Vice President and Chief Financial Officer
CHR: Nicki Sparling, Manager Human Resources
Web address: www.majorhospital.org
**Control:** City–County, Government, nonfederal **Service:** General Medical and Surgical

**Staffed Beds:** 73 **Admissions:** 2666 **Census:** 25 **Outpatient Visits:** 138902 **Births:** 403 **Total Expense ($000):** 72187 **Payroll Expense ($000):** 29960 **Personnel:** 547

## SOUTH BEND—St. Joseph County

**MADISON CENTER AND HOSPITAL (154040)**, 403 East Madison Street, Zip 46617; tel. 574/234–0061, (Nonreporting) **A**9 10
Primary Contact: Kenneth A. Davis, Interim Chief Executive Officer
COO: Sharon DeVinney, Interim Chief Operating Officer
CMO: John Zwerneman, M.D., Chief Medical Officer
CIO: Jim Shelley, Manager Operations
Web address: www.madison.org
**Control:** Corporation, Investor–owned, for–profit **Service:** Psychiatric

**Staffed Beds:** 91

IN

---

**Hospital, Medicare Provider Number, Address, Telephone, Approval, Facility, and Physician Codes, Health Care System**

★ American Hospital Association (AHA) membership
□ The Joint Commission accreditation
◇ DNV Healthcare Inc. accreditation
○ American Osteopathic Association (AOA) accreditation
△ Commission on Accreditation of Rehabilitation Facilities (CARF) accreditation

⊠ △ **MEMORIAL HOSPITAL OF SOUTH BEND (150058)**, 615 North Michigan Street, Zip 46601–9986; tel. 574/647–1000, (Includes MEMORIAL CHILDREN'S HOSPITAL, 615 North Michigan Street, Zip 46601, Mailing Address: 516 North Michigan Street, Zip 46601; tel. 574/647–1000) **A**1 2 3 5 7 9 10 **F**7 8 9 12 13 15 17 18 19 20 22 24 26 29 30 31 35 38 40 43 46 49 50 53 56 59 60 61 64 67 68 70 72 74 75 76 77 78 79 81 82 84 85 86 87 88 89 90 92 93 98 99 102 103 107 108 113 114 115 116 118 120 123 125 128 129 130 131 133 134 145 146 147 **P**8
Primary Contact: Kreg Gruber, President
CFO: Jeff Costello, Chief Financial Officer
CMO: Cheryl Wibbens, M.D., Vice President Medical Staff Affairs
CIO: Steve Huffman, Chief Information Officer
Web address: www.qualityoflife.org
**Control:** Other not–for–profit (including NFP Corporation) **Service:** General Medical and Surgical

**Staffed Beds: 464 Admissions:** 19821 **Census:** 231 **Outpatient Visits:** 178192 **Births:** 2916 **Total Expense ($000):** 289137 **Payroll Expense ($000):** 117969 **Personnel:** 2117

**RIVERSIDE HOSPITAL (154049)**, 533 North Niles Avenue, Zip 46617; tel. 574/283–1104, (Nonreporting) **A**9 10
Primary Contact: Kenneth A. Davis, Interim Chief Executive Officer
CFO: Andrew J. Poole, Chief Financial Officer
CMO: John Zwerneman, M.D., Chief Medical Officer
Web address: www.madison.com
**Control:** Corporation, Investor–owned, for–profit **Service:** Psychiatric

**Staffed Beds:** 16

### SULLIVAN—Sullivan County

★ ○ **SULLIVAN COUNTY COMMUNITY HOSPITAL (151327)**, 2200 North Section Street, Zip 47882, Mailing Address: P.O. Box 10, Zip 47882–0010; tel. 812/268–4311 **A**9 10 11 18 **F**3 8 13 15 28 29 32 34 35 40 44 45 47 48 53 56 57 59 61 62 69 70 75 76 77 78 79 81 86 87 93 97 107 110 111 113 128 129 130 132 145 146 147 **P**8 **S** QHR, Brentwood, TN
Primary Contact: Michelle Sly–Smith, Chief Executive Officer
CFO: Alan J. Montella, Assistant Administrator Finance
CMO: Gene Bourgasser, M.D., Chief of Staff
CIO: Hap Beckes, Director Information Systems
CHR: Denise Hart, Director Human Resources
Web address: www.schosp.com
**Control:** County–Government, nonfederal **Service:** General Medical and Surgical

**Staffed Beds: 25 Admissions:** 987 **Census:** 8 **Outpatient Visits:** 66638 **Births:** 143 **Total Expense ($000):** 22946 **Payroll Expense ($000):** 9278 **Personnel:** 206

### TELL CITY—Perry County

★ ○ **PERRY COUNTY MEMORIAL HOSPITAL (151322)**, 1 Hospital Road, Zip 47586–0362; tel. 812/547–7011 **A**9 10 11 18 **F**3 7 11 13 15 28 29 30 31 34 35 38 40 50 56 57 59 62 64 68 70 74 75 76 77 78 79 81 86 87 93 102 107 108 110 111 113 117 118 128 129 131 132 134 145 146 **S** Alliant Management Services, Louisville, KY
Primary Contact: Joseph A. Stuber, President and Chief Executive Officer
COO: Becky Elder, Vice President Clinical Services
CFO: Kathy Clayton, Chief Financial Officer
CMO: Anastacia Lagunzad, M.D., Chief of Staff
CIO: Debbie Kleeman, Manager Information Systems
CHR: Sheila Gaynor, Director Human Resources
Web address: www.pchospital.org
**Control:** County–Government, nonfederal **Service:** General Medical and Surgical

**Staffed Beds: 25 Admissions:** 1367 **Census:** 14 **Outpatient Visits:** 66663 **Births:** 83 **Total Expense ($000):** 27679 **Payroll Expense ($000):** 9580 **Personnel:** 260

### TERRE HAUTE—Vigo County

**HAMILTON CENTER (154009)**, 620 Eighth Avenue, Zip 47804–0323; tel. 812/231–8323, (Nonreporting) **A**9 10
Primary Contact: Galen Goode, Chief Executive Officer
COO: Robb Johnson, Director Operations
CFO: Susie Thompson, Executive Director Fiscal Services
CMO: David Hilton, M.D., Medical Director
CIO: Mel Burks, Executive Director Administrative Services
CHR: Mel Burks, Executive Director Administrative Services
Web address: www.hamiltoncenter.org
**Control:** Other not–for–profit (including NFP Corporation) **Service:** Psychiatric

**Staffed Beds:** 16

**HARSHA BEHAVIORAL CENTER (154054)**, 1420 East Crossing Boulevard, Zip 47802–5316; tel. 866/644–8880, (Nonreporting) **A**9 10
Primary Contact: Roopam Harshawat, Chief Executive Officer
Web address: www.harshacenter.com
**Control:** Corporation, Investor–owned, for–profit **Service:** Psychiatric

**Staffed Beds:** 36

⊠ **TERRE HAUTE REGIONAL HOSPITAL (150046)**, 3901 South Seventh Street, Zip 47802–5709; tel. 812/232–0021, (Nonreporting) **A**1 2 5 9 10 **S** HCA, Nashville, TN
Primary Contact: Mary Ann Conroy, Chief Executive Officer
CMO: Francis Tapia, M.D., President Medical Staff
CIO: Mike Kuckewich, Director Information Systems
CHR: Aaron Garofola, Director Human Resources
Web address: www.regionalhospital.com
**Control:** Corporation, Investor–owned, for–profit **Service:** General Medical and Surgical

**Staffed Beds:** 231

★ ○ △ **UNION HOSPITAL (150023)**, 1606 North Seventh Street, Zip 47804–2780; tel. 812/238–7000 **A**2 3 5 7 9 10 11 19 **F**3 8 13 15 18 20 22 24 26 28 29 30 31 34 35 36 39 40 46 49 50 53 54 57 59 64 68 70 72 73 74 75 76 77 78 79 81 82 85 86 87 89 90 92 93 94 97 107 108 110 111 112 113 114 115 116 117 118 119 120 122 125 126 129 130 131 134 145 146 147 **P**6
Primary Contact: Scott L. Teffeteller, President and Chief Executive Officer
CFO: Wayne Hutson, Chief Financial Officer
CMO: John Bolinger, M.D., Vice President Medical Affairs
CIO: Kym Pfrank, Senior Vice President and Chief Information Officer
CHR: Sally Zuel, Vice President Human Resources and Education
CNO: Rhonda E. Smith, R.N., Vice President Patient Care Services and Chief Nursing Officer
Web address: www.uhhg.org
**Control:** Other not–for–profit (including NFP Corporation) **Service:** General Medical and Surgical

**Staffed Beds: 318 Admissions:** 17370 **Census:** 215 **Outpatient Visits:** 363242 **Births:** 1556 **Total Expense ($000):** 353106 **Payroll Expense ($000):** 107582 **Personnel:** 1910

### TIPTON—Tipton County

⊠ **INDIANA UNIVERSITY HEALTH TIPTON HOSPITAL (151311)**, 1000 South Main Street, Zip 46072–9799; tel. 765/675–8500 **A**1 2 9 10 18 **F**3 11 15 18 28 29 31 34 35 40 45 46 47 48 53 57 58 59 68 70 74 75 77 78 79 81 82 85 86 87 93 94 107 108 110 111 114 118 124 128 129 130 131 132 133 134 145 146 147 **P**8 **S** Indiana University Health, Indianapolis, IN
Primary Contact: Michael Harlowe, President and Chief Executive Officer
CFO: Vern J. Schmaltz, Vice President Finance
Web address: www.iuhealth.org
**Control:** Other not–for–profit (including NFP Corporation) **Service:** General Medical and Surgical

**Staffed Beds: 25 Admissions:** 1373 **Census:** 16 **Outpatient Visits:** 45653 **Births:** 0 **Total Expense ($000):** 37540 **Payroll Expense ($000):** 17805 **Personnel:** 298

**TIPTON HOSPITAL** See Indiana University Health Tipton Hospital

### VALPARAISO—Porter County

⊠ **PORTER–VALPARAISO HOSPITAL CAMPUS (150035)**, 814 La Porte Avenue, Zip 46383–5898; tel. 219/263–4600, (Nonreporting) **A**1 9 10 **S** Community Health Systems, Inc., Franklin, TN
Primary Contact: Jonathan Nalli, Chief Executive Officer
COO: Brian Sinotte, Chief Operating Officer
CMO: Ramireddy K. Tummuru, M.D., Chief Medical Officer
CHR: Angie Hampton, Director Human Resources
Web address: www.porterhealth.org
**Control:** Corporation, Investor–owned, for–profit **Service:** General Medical and Surgical

**Staffed Beds:** 276

### VINCENNES—Knox County

⊠ △ **GOOD SAMARITAN HOSPITAL (150042)**, 520 South Seventh Street, Zip 47591–1098; tel. 812/882–5220 **A**1 2 7 9 10 19 **F**3 5 8 11 13 15 17 18 20 22 24 28 29 30 31 32 34 35 38 39 40 45 48 49 51 53 57 59 60 63 66 67 68 70 74 75 76 77 78 79 81 85 87 89 90 92 93 96 97 98 99 100 101 102 103 104 106 107 108 110 111 114 117 118 120 128 129 130 131 133 134 143 144 145 146 147 **P**6
Primary Contact: Robert D. McLin, President and Chief Executive Officer
COO: Gerald E. Waldroup, Senior Vice President
CFO: Jerry Stump, Chief Financial Officer
CMO: Charles C. Hedde, M.D., Vice President Medical Affairs
CIO: Charles Christian, Chief Information Officer and Director Information Systems
CHR: Dean Wagoner, Director Human Resources
Web address: www.gshvin.org/goodsamaritan
**Control:** County–Government, nonfederal **Service:** General Medical and Surgical

**Staffed Beds: 176 Admissions:** 7653 **Census:** 95 **Outpatient Visits:** 318609 **Births:** 502 **Total Expense ($000):** 170766 **Payroll Expense ($000):** 75363 **Personnel:** 1630

IN

## WABASH—Wabash County

☒ **WABASH COUNTY HOSPITAL (151310)**, 710 North East Street,
Zip 46992–1924, Mailing Address: P.O. Box 548, Zip 46992–0548;
tel. 260/563–3131, (Total facility includes 25 beds in nursing home–type unit) **A**1
2 9 10 18 **F**3 11 15 17 32 34 35 53 57 58 59 62 63 64 65 68 69 70 75 77
81 85 86 87 89 93 97 107 108 111 118 127 129 130 131 132 145 146
**S** Alliant Management Services, Louisville, KY
Primary Contact: Marilyn J. Custer–Mitchell, President and Chief Executive Officer
CFO: Jane Bissel, Chief Financial Officer
CMO: Dean Gifford, M.D., Chief of Staff
CIO: David Brinson, Director Information Technology
CHR: Kimberly R. Shininger, Director Human Resources
CNO: Sonia R. Strevy, Chief Nursing Officer
Web address: www.wchospital.com
**Control:** County–Government, nonfederal **Service:** General Medical and Surgical

**Staffed Beds:** 50 **Admissions:** 829 **Census:** 22 **Outpatient Visits:** 45805
**Births:** 0 **Total Expense ($000):** 34561 **Payroll Expense ($000):** 14935
**Personnel:** 317

## WARSAW—Kosciusko County

☒ **KOSCIUSKO COMMUNITY HOSPITAL (150133)**, 2101 East Dubois Drive,
Zip 46580–3288; tel. 574/267–3200 **A**1 2 9 10 19 **F**3 12 13 15 28 29 30 31
32 34 35 40 42 44 50 51 53 57 58 59 64 65 68 70 74 75 76 77 78 79 81
82 85 86 89 92 93 98 107 108 110 111 114 115 116 117 118 119 120 128
129 130 131 143 145 146 147 **P**6 **S** Community Health Systems, Inc.,
Franklin, TN
Primary Contact: Stephen R. Miller, Chief Executive Officer
CFO: Douglas J. BeMent, Chief Financial Officer
CFO: Finny Mathew, Chief Operating Officer
CMO: Patrick Silveus, M.D., Medical Director
CIO: Tammy Lukens, Director Information
CHR: Joe Jarboe, Director Human Resources
CNO: Kim Finch, Chief Nursing Officer
Web address: www.kch.com
**Control:** Corporation, Investor–owned, for–profit **Service:** General Medical and
Surgical

**Staffed Beds:** 72 **Admissions:** 3958 **Census:** 34 **Outpatient Visits:** 105777
**Births:** 718 **Total Expense ($000):** 56022 **Payroll Expense ($000):** 22964
**Personnel:** 467

**OTIS R BOWEN CENTER FOR HUMAN SERVICES (154014)**, 850 North
Harrison Street, Zip 46580–3163; tel. 574/267–7169 **A**9 10 **F**4 5 29 34 35 38
50 86 98 99 100 102 103 104 106 126 129 131 133 134 142 **P**1
Primary Contact: Kurt Carlson, Chief Executive Officer
Web address: www.bowencenter.org
**Control:** Other not–for–profit (including NFP Corporation) **Service:** Psychiatric

**Staffed Beds:** 16 **Admissions:** 929 **Census:** 12 **Outpatient Visits:** 391644
**Births:** 0 **Total Expense ($000):** 29181 **Payroll Expense ($000):** 17950
**Personnel:** 578

## WASHINGTON—Daviess County

☒ △ **DAVIESS COMMUNITY HOSPITAL (150061)**, 1314 East Walnut Street,
Zip 47501–2198, Mailing Address: P.O. Box 760, Zip 47501–0760;
tel. 812/254–2760, (Nonreporting) **A**1 7 9 10 **S** QHR, Brentwood, TN
Primary Contact: David Bixler, Chief Executive Officer
CMO: Michael Baker, D.O., Chief of Staff
CIO: Richard Meinhart, Manager Information Systems
CHR: Marilyn Richard, Director Human Resources
CNO: Brenda L. Sturm, MSN, Vice President of Nursing
Web address: www.dchosp.org
**Control:** County–Government, nonfederal **Service:** General Medical and Surgical

**Staffed Beds:** 48

## WEST LAFAYETTE—Tippecanoe County

★ **RIVER BEND HOSPITAL (154005)**, 2900 North River Road, Zip 47906–3766;
tel. 765/463–2555, (Nonreporting) **A**9 10
Primary Contact: John R. Walling, President
COO: Tom Gillian, Chief Operating Officer
CFO: Jeff Nagy, Chief Financial Officer
CMO: Richard Rahdert, M.D., Medical Director
CIO: Craig Anderson, Director Management Information Systems
CHR: Jan Shaw, Director Personnel
CNO: Megan Gibson, Nurse Manager
Web address: www.nchsi.com/riverbendhospital.cfm
**Control:** Other not–for–profit (including NFP Corporation) **Service:** Psychiatric

**Staffed Beds:** 16

**WABASH VALLEY HOSPITAL** See River Bend Hospital

## WILLIAMSPORT—Warren County

☒ ○ **ST. VINCENT WILLIAMSPORT HOSPITAL (151307)**, 412 North Monroe
Street, Zip 47993–0215; tel. 765/762–4000 **A**1 9 10 11 18 **F**3 7 15 29 30 34
35 40 45 50 51 57 59 64 75 77 79 81 85 86 87 93 97 107 111 113 118
126 130 131 132 134 142 145 **P**6 **S** Ascension Health, Saint Louis, MO
Primary Contact: Jane Craigin, Chief Executive Officer
CFO: Janet Merritt, Chief Financial Officer
Web address: www.stvincent.org
**Control:** Other not–for–profit (including NFP Corporation) **Service:** General
Medical and Surgical

**Staffed Beds:** 16 **Admissions:** 862 **Census:** 8 **Outpatient Visits:** 97007
**Births:** 0 **Total Expense ($000):** 19363 **Payroll Expense ($000):** 9844
**Personnel:** 149

## WINAMAC—Pulaski County

★ ○ **PULASKI MEMORIAL HOSPITAL (151305)**, 616 East 13th Street,
Zip 46996–1117, Mailing Address: P.O. Box 279, Zip 46996–0279;
tel. 574/946–2100 **A**9 10 11 18 **F**1 4 11 13 15 18 28 29 30 31 34 35 40 43
45 50 53 57 59 62 63 64 65 67 68 73 75 76 77 78 79 80 81 82 85 86 87
89 90 91 93 96 98 107 110 113 118 127 129 130 131 132 134 145 **P**6
Primary Contact: Richard H. Mynark, Chief Executive Officer
CFO: Gregg Malott, Chief Financial Officer
CMO: Rex Allman, M.D., President Medical Staff
CIO: Jeff Boer, Director Information Technology
CHR: Mark Fenn, Director Human Resources
CNO: Linda Webb, R.N., Chief Nursing Executive
Web address: www.pulaskimemorial.com
**Control:** County–Government, nonfederal **Service:** General Medical and Surgical

**Staffed Beds:** 25 **Admissions:** 613 **Census:** 6 **Outpatient Visits:** 24755
**Births:** 112 **Total Expense ($000):** 17343 **Payroll Expense ($000):** 8344
**Personnel:** 180

## WINCHESTER—Randolph County

☒ ○ **ST. VINCENT RANDOLPH HOSPITAL (151301)**, 473 Greenville Avenue,
Zip 47394–2235, Mailing Address: P.O. Box 407, Zip 47394–0407;
tel. 765/584–0004 **A**1 9 10 11 18 **F**3 11 13 15 28 29 30 34 35 40 45 48 50
57 59 62 63 68 75 76 77 79 81 85 86 87 89 93 107 111 113 118 123 128
129 130 131 132 134 145 146 147 **S** Ascension Health, Saint Louis, MO
Primary Contact: Francis G. Albarano, Administrator
CFO: John Arthur, Chief Financial Officer
CMO: Daniel Wegg, M.D., Medical Director
CHR: Ross Brodhead, Human Resource Assistant
CNO: Carla Fouse, Chief Nursing Officer
Web address: www.stvincent.org
**Control:** Other not–for–profit (including NFP Corporation) **Service:** General
Medical and Surgical

**Staffed Beds:** 25 **Admissions:** 1234 **Census:** 11 **Outpatient Visits:** 51588
**Births:** 219 **Total Expense ($000):** 24993 **Payroll Expense ($000):** 10868
**Personnel:** 198

**IN**

---

# IOWA

## ALBIA—Monroe County

★ **MONROE COUNTY HOSPITAL (161342)**, 6580 165th Street,
Zip 52531–8793; tel. 641/932–2134 **A**9 10 18 **F**1 4 7 8 11 15 16 17 28 29
31 35 40 45 57 59 63 64 67 70 72 73 80 81 85 88 89 90 93 98 107 114
118 126 127 132 134 **P**6
Primary Contact: Gregory A. Paris, FACHE, Chief Executive Officer
Web address: www.mchalbia.com
**Control:** County–Government, nonfederal **Service:** General Medical and Surgical

**Staffed Beds:** 25 **Admissions:** 438 **Census:** 8 **Outpatient Visits:** 48571
**Births:** 0 **Total Expense ($000):** 14281 **Payroll Expense ($000):** 6730
**Personnel:** 143

## ALGONA—Kossuth County

★ **KOSSUTH REGIONAL HEALTH CENTER (161353)**, 1515 South Phillips Street,
Zip 50511–3649; tel. 515/295–2451 **A**9 10 18 **F**11 13 15 17 28 29 30 31 32
34 35 36 40 41 43 50 56 57 59 62 63 64 65 67 68 70 75 76 77 78 81 82
84 86 87 89 90 92 93 97 104 107 113 118 126 127 128 129 130 131 132
134 145 146 **P**8 **S** Trinity Health, Novi, MI
Primary Contact: Scott A. Curtis, Administrator and Chief Executive Officer
CFO: Dan Myers, Controller
CMO: Michael Lampe, M.D., Chief of Staff
CIO: Nancy Erickson, Administrator Information Systems
CHR: Paula Seely, Manager Human Resources
CNO: Darlene M. Elbert, R.N., Assistant Administrator and Chief Nursing Officer
Web address: www.krhc.com
**Control:** County–Government, nonfederal **Service:** General Medical and Surgical

**Staffed Beds:** 22 **Admissions:** 770 **Census:** 10 **Outpatient Visits:** 28142
**Births:** 107 **Total Expense ($000):** 27118 **Payroll Expense ($000):** 9075
**Personnel:** 175

## AMES—Story County

⊞ **MARY GREELEY MEDICAL CENTER (160030)**, 1111 Duff Avenue,
Zip 50010–5745; tel. 515/239–2011, (Total facility includes 11 beds in nursing
home–type unit) **A**1 2 9 10 19 **F**3 7 8 11 12 13 15 17 18 20 22 26 28 29 30
31 34 35 36 37 38 39 40 43 45 46 49 50 53 55 56 57 58 59 61 62 63 64
65 68 69 70 72 74 75 76 77 78 79 81 82 85 86 89 90 92 93 96 98 99 100
101 102 103 104 107 108 110 111 113 114 117 118 120 122 123 125 127
128 129 130 131 134 144 145 147
Primary Contact: Brian Dieter, President and Chief Executive Officer
CFO: Mike Tretina, Vice President and Chief Financial Officer
CIO: JaNelle Anderson, Director
CHR: Betsy V. Schoeller, Director Human Resources and Education
Web address: www.mgmc.org
**Control:** City–Government, nonfederal **Service:** General Medical and Surgical

**Staffed Beds:** 197 **Admissions:** 9782 **Census:** 114 **Outpatient Visits:**
150574 **Births:** 1164 **Total Expense ($000):** 146293 **Payroll Expense
($000):** 56693 **Personnel:** 1062

## ANAMOSA—Jones County

★ **JONES REGIONAL MEDICAL CENTER (161306)**, 1795 Highway 64 East,
Zip 52205–2112; tel. 319/462–6131 **A**9 10 18 **F**1 3 7 11 12 15 28 29 31 34
35 38 40 43 45 50 56 57 59 64 67 68 71 75 81 82 84 85 87 90 91 93 96
97 99 100 101 102 103 104 107 110 111 113 117 118 127 129 131 132
134 144 145 147 **P**4 **S** Iowa Health System, Des Moines, IA
Primary Contact: Eric Briesemeister, Chief Executive Officer
CFO: Rachel Von Behren, Director Financial Services
CMO: Victor Salas, M.D., President Medical Staff
CHR: Donna Condry, Director Human Resources
Web address: www.jonesregional.org
**Control:** Other not–for–profit (including NFP Corporation) **Service:** General
Medical and Surgical

**Staffed Beds:** 22 **Admissions:** 612 **Census:** 8 **Outpatient Visits:** 55536
**Births:** 1 **Total Expense ($000):** 14717 **Payroll Expense ($000):** 5442
**Personnel:** 125

## ATLANTIC—Cass County

★ **CASS COUNTY MEMORIAL HOSPITAL (161376)**, 1501 East Tenth Street,
Zip 50022–1997; tel. 712/243–3250 **A**9 10 18 **F**11 13 15 28 29 40 57 59 64
69 70 75 76 77 78 81 82 93 98 99 101 102 103 104 105 107 108 111 118
123 126 128 129 131 132 134 146 147 **P**8
Primary Contact: Patricia A. Markham, Administrator and Chief Executive Officer
CFO: Stephen Lewis, Assistant Administrator and Chief Financial Officer
CMO: Chad McCance, M.D., Chief of Staff
CIO: Steve Stark, Chief Information Officer
CHR: Donald D. Johnson, Assistant Administrator Human Resources
CNO: Linda Hemminger, MSN, Assistant Administrator Clinical Services
Web address: www.casshealth.org
**Control:** County–Government, nonfederal **Service:** General Medical and Surgical

**Staffed Beds:** 33 **Admissions:** 1090 **Census:** 12 **Outpatient Visits:** 92817
**Births:** 134 **Total Expense ($000):** 31017 **Payroll Expense ($000):** 14010
**Personnel:** 333

## AUDUBON—Audubon County

**AUDUBON COUNTY MEMORIAL HOSPITAL (161330)**, 515 Pacific Street,
Zip 50025–1052; tel. 712/563–2611 **A**9 10 18 **F**3 11 15 28 31 40 43 45 53
59 64 67 78 79 81 85 90 93 98 104 110 118 126 127 132 134
Primary Contact: Thomas G. Smith, Administrator and Chief Executive Officer
CFO: Karen McGuire, Chief Financial Officer
CMO: James Brokke, M.D., Chief of Staff
CIO: Kelli Burgin, Director Information Technology
Web address: www.acmhhosp.org
**Control:** County–Government, nonfederal **Service:** General Medical and Surgical

**Staffed Beds:** 25 **Admissions:** 197 **Census:** 2 **Outpatient Visits:** 15562
**Births:** 0 **Total Expense ($000):** 9528 **Payroll Expense ($000):** 3691
**Personnel:** 86

## BELMOND—Wright County

★ **IOWA SPECIALTY HOSPITAL–BELMOND (161301)**, 403 First Street S.E.,
Zip 50421–1201; tel. 641/444–3223 **A**9 10 18 **F**7 11 15 26 28 29 32 34 35
40 43 45 46 50 53 56 57 59 62 63 64 65 67 68 75 77 79 81 82 85 87 89
92 93 97 107 110 111 118 127 128 130 132 134 145 147 **P**6
Primary Contact: Nancy Gabrielson, Administrator and Chief Executive Officer
CFO: Greg Polzin, Chief Financial Officer
CMO: Charles B. Brindle, M.D., Chief Medical Staff
CHR: Reagan Swisher, Director Human Resources
Web address: www.belmondmedicalcenter.com
**Control:** City–Government, nonfederal **Service:** General Medical and Surgical

**Staffed Beds:** 22 **Admissions:** 370 **Census:** 5 **Outpatient Visits:** 24776
**Births:** 0 **Total Expense ($000):** 11609 **Payroll Expense ($000):** 3546
**Personnel:** 101

## BETTENDORF—Scott County

⊞ **TRINITY BETTENDORF (160104)**, 4500 Utica Ridge Road, Zip 52722–1626;
tel. 563/742–5000 **A**1 9 10 13 **F**3 11 13 15 18 20 22 26 29 30 34 35 37 40
44 45 46 57 58 59 64 65 70 74 75 76 79 81 82 85 86 87 93 96 97 107
108 110 113 118 128 129 131 134 145 146 147 **P**6 **S** Iowa Health System,
Des Moines, IA
Primary Contact: Richard A. Seidler, FACHE, President and Chief Executive Officer
COO: Mykl Garrett, Executive Vice President and Chief Operating Officer
CFO: Greg Pagliuzza, Chief Financial Officer
CMO: Paul McLoone, M.D., Chief Medical Officer
CHR: Jeffery Stolze, Vice President Human Resources
Web address: www.trinityqc.com
**Control:** Other not–for–profit (including NFP Corporation) **Service:** General
Medical and Surgical

**Staffed Beds:** 59 **Admissions:** 3618 **Census:** 31 **Outpatient Visits:** 41952
**Births:** 538 **Total Expense ($000):** 56549 **Payroll Expense ($000):** 17569
**Personnel:** 222

IA

## BLOOMFIELD—Davis County

★ **DAVIS COUNTY HOSPITAL (161327)**, 509 North Madison Street,
Zip 52537–1271; tel. 641/664–2145, (Total facility includes 32 beds in nursing
home–type unit) **A**9 10 18 **F**3 7 11 13 15 29 34 35 40 44 45 50 57 59 61 62
63 64 65 67 68 69 75 76 78 79 81 85 86 87 97 107 111 118 129 131 132
145 **P**6
Primary Contact: Deborah L. Herzberg, R.N., MS, FACHE, Chief Executive Officer
COO: Debbie Scott, Chief Operating Officer
CFO: William Giles, Chief Financial Officer
CMO: Sean Brodale, D.O., Chief Medical Staff
CIO: William Giles, Chief Financial Officer
CHR: Pam Young, Human Resources Leader
CNO: Ronda Reimer, R.N., Chief Nursing Officer
Web address: www.daviscountyhospital.org
**Control:** County–Government, nonfederal **Service:** General Medical and Surgical

**Staffed Beds:** 57 **Admissions:** 532 **Census:** 38 **Outpatient Visits:** 20191
**Births:** 35 **Total Expense ($000):** 19262 **Payroll Expense ($000):** 7775
**Personnel:** 162

## BOONE—Boone County

★ **BOONE COUNTY HOSPITAL (161372)**, 1015 Union Street, Zip 50036–4821;
tel. 515/432–3140 **A**9 10 18 **F**2 7 11 13 15 28 30 31 34 35 40 43 50 57 59
62 64 65 69 70 75 76 77 78 79 81 86 91 93 97 107 111 113 118 127 131
132 144 145 146 147 **P**6 **S** QHR, Brentwood, TN
Primary Contact: Joseph S. Smith, Chief Executive Officer
CFO: David Mellett, Chief Financial Officer
CMO: Scott Thiel, M.D., Chief of Staff
CIO: Matthew Sabus, Director Information Systems
CHR: Kim K. Schwartz, Director Human Resources and Physician Clinics
Web address: www.boonehospital.com
**Control:** County–Government, nonfederal **Service:** General Medical and Surgical

**Staffed Beds:** 25 **Admissions:** 1409 **Census:** 16 **Outpatient Visits:** 69000
**Births:** 176 **Total Expense ($000):** 38534 **Payroll Expense ($000):** 15735
**Personnel:** 314

## BRITT—Hancock County

★ **HANCOCK COUNTY MEMORIAL HOSPITAL (161307)**, 532 First Street N.W.,
Zip 50423; tel. 641/843–5000 **A**9 10 18 **F**11 15 28 29 31 34 35 36 40 43 45
46 53 56 57 59 64 65 75 77 78 81 82 85 93 97 107 113 118 128 129 130
131 132 145 147 **P**1 **S** Trinity Health, Novi, MI
Primary Contact: Vance Jackson, FACHE, Administrator and Chief Executive
Officer
CFO: Julie Damm, Chief Financial Officer
CMO: Catherine Butler, M.D., Chief Medical Staff
CIO: Julie Damm, Chief Financial Officer
CHR: Denise Jakoubeck, Director Human Resources
Web address: www.hancockmemhospital.com
**Control:** County–Government, nonfederal **Service:** General Medical and Surgical

**Staffed Beds:** 25 **Admissions:** 565 **Census:** 9 **Outpatient Visits:** 18142
**Births:** 0 **Total Expense ($000):** 13530 **Payroll Expense ($000):** 4811
**Personnel:** 128

## CARROLL—Carroll County

★ **ST. ANTHONY REGIONAL HOSPITAL (160005)**, 311 South Clark Street,
Zip 51401–3038, Mailing Address: P.O. Box 628, Zip 51401–0628;
tel. 712/792–3581, (Total facility includes 79 beds in nursing home–type unit) **A**9
10 19 20 **F**6 11 13 15 28 29 30 31 34 35 37 38 39 40 43 44 45 46 50 51
56 57 59 60 61 62 63 64 65 67 68 69 70 74 75 76 77 78 79 81 82 84 85
86 87 89 93 97 98 99 100 101 102 103 104 107 108 110 111 113 117 118
124 126 128 129 130 131 132 133 134 144 145 146 147 **P**6
Primary Contact: Edward H. Smith, Jr., Interim Chief Executive Officer
CFO: John Munson, Vice President and Chief Financial Officer
CMO: Tracey Wellendorf, M.D., Chief of Staff
CIO: Randy Eischeid, Director Information Systems
CHR: Gina Ramaekers, Director Human Resources
Web address: www.stanthonyhospital.org
**Control:** Church–operated, Nongovernment, not–for profit **Service:** General
Medical and Surgical

**Staffed Beds:** 155 **Admissions:** 2290 **Census:** 107 **Outpatient Visits:** 92669
**Births:** 359 **Total Expense ($000):** 53791 **Payroll Expense ($000):** 22392
**Personnel:** 500

## CEDAR FALLS—Black Hawk County

⊞ **SARTORI MEMORIAL HOSPITAL (160040)**, 515 College Street,
Zip 50613–2500; tel. 319/268–3000 **A**1 9 10 **F**3 7 8 11 12 15 29 30 35 40
43 44 46 53 57 59 64 68 70 75 77 79 81 91 93 97 98 103 107 111 118
129 130 131 145 **P**1 6 **S** Wheaton Franciscan Healthcare, Wheaton, IL
Primary Contact: Rose Fowler, MS, Administrator
CFO: Michele Panicucci, Chief Financial Officer
CMO: Paul Franke, M.D., Vice President Medical Affairs
CHR: Vicki L. Parsons, Regional Vice President Human Resources
Web address: www.wheatoniowa.org
**Control:** Church–operated, Nongovernment, not–for profit **Service:** General
Medical and Surgical

**Staffed Beds:** 50 **Admissions:** 1389 **Census:** 21 **Outpatient Visits:** 53379
**Births:** 0 **Total Expense ($000):** 28389 **Payroll Expense ($000):** 10217
**Personnel:** 181

## CEDAR RAPIDS—Linn County

☐ **CONTINUING CARE HOSPITAL AT ST. LUKE'S (162002)**, 1026 A Avenue
N.E., 6th Floor, Zip 52402; tel. 319/369–8142 **A**1 10 **F**1 3 18 29 30 34 60 68
74 75 78 79 82 84 85 87 100 107 111 113 114 118 142 147 **S** Dubuis
Health System, Houston, TX
Primary Contact: Elly Steffen, Chief Executive Officer and Administrator
CNO: Mary Beth Keuter, Director Patient Care
Web address: www.stlukescr.org
**Control:** Church–operated, Nongovernment, not–for profit **Service:** Long–Term
Acute Care hospital

**Staffed Beds:** 17 **Admissions:** 172 **Census:** 12 **Outpatient Visits:** 0 **Births:**
0 **Total Expense ($000):** 6844 **Payroll Expense ($000):** 2235 **Personnel:**
46

⊞ **MERCY MEDICAL CENTER (160079)**, 701 Tenth Street S.E.,
Zip 52403–1292; tel. 319/398–6011, (Total facility includes 76 beds in nursing
home–type unit) **A**1 2 3 5 9 10 **F**3 5 6 10 12 15 16 17 19 20 22 26 28 29 30 33
32 34 35 38 40 43 44 49 50 53 54 55 56 57 58 59 60 61 62 63 64 65 67
68 70 71 72 74 75 76 77 78 79 81 82 84 85 86 87 88 89 90 91 92 93 94
98 99 100 101 102 103 104 107 108 109 110 113 114 115 116 117 118
119 120 122 123 125 127 129 130 131 134 142 144 145 146 147 **P**7 8
Primary Contact: Timothy L. Charles, President and Chief Executive Officer
COO: Michael D. Trachta, FACHE, Executive Vice President and Chief Operating
Officer
CFO: Philip Peterson, Executive Vice President and Chief Financial Officer
CMO: Mark Valliere, M.D., Senior Vice President Medical Affairs and Chief Medical
Officer
CIO: Jeff Cash, Senior Vice President and Chief Information Officer
Web address: www.mercycare.org
**Control:** Church–operated, Nongovernment, not–for profit **Service:** General
Medical and Surgical

**Staffed Beds:** 314 **Admissions:** 11196 **Census:** 187 **Outpatient Visits:**
229185 **Births:** 754 **Total Expense ($000):** 237308 **Payroll Expense
($000):** 89956 **Personnel:** 1872

⊞ △ **ST. LUKE'S HOSPITAL (160045)**, 1026 A Avenue N.E., Zip 52402–3026,
Mailing Address: P.O. Box 3026, Zip 52406–3026; tel. 319/369–7211 **A**1 2 3 5
7 9 10 **F**3 5 8 11 12 13 14 15 17 18 19 20 22 24 26 28 29 30 31 32 34 35
36 37 39 40 43 45 46 49 50 54 55 56 57 59 60 61 63 64 65 66 70 72 74
75 76 77 78 79 81 82 84 85 86 87 88 89 90 92 93 96 98 99 100 101 103
104 105 107 108 110 111 113 114 117 118 125 129 130 131 133 134 144
145 146 147 **P**4 6 **S** Iowa Health System, Des Moines, IA
Primary Contact: Theodore E. Townsend, FACHE, President and Chief Executive
Officer
COO: John C. Sheehan, FACHE, Executive Vice President and Chief Operating
Officer
CFO: Milton E. Aunan, II, CPA, Vice President and Chief Financial Officer
CMO: Charles W. Schauberger, M.D., Vice President and Chief Medical Officer
CHR: Sue Slattery, Director Human Resources
Web address: www.crstlukes.org
**Control:** Other not–for–profit (including NFP Corporation) **Service:** General
Medical and Surgical

**Staffed Beds:** 363 **Admissions:** 16560 **Census:** 217 **Outpatient Visits:**
480480 **Births:** 2602 **Total Expense ($000):** 275487 **Payroll Expense
($000):** 111697 **Personnel:** 2529

**IA**

---

**Hospital, Medicare Provider Number, Address, Telephone, Approval, Facility, and Physician Codes, Health Care System**

★ American Hospital Association (AHA) membership
☐ The Joint Commission accreditation
◇ DNV Healthcare Inc. accreditation
○ American Osteopathic Association (AOA) accreditation
△ Commission on Accreditation of Rehabilitation Facilities (CARF) accreditation

---

## CENTERVILLE—Appanoose County

★ **MERCY MEDICAL CENTER–CENTERVILLE (161377)**, 1 St. Joseph's Drive, Zip 52544–8055; tel. 641/437–4111, (Total facility includes 20 beds in nursing home–type unit) **A**9 10 18 **F**1 3 4 7 8 11 13 15 16 17 28 29 30 31 34 40 45 46 50 51 54 57 59 60 62 63 64 67 70 72 73 75 76 77 78 79 80 81 85 86 87 88 89 90 93 97 98 107 111 114 116 118 126 127 128 129 131 132 134 **P**6 **S** Catholic Health Initiatives, Englewood, CO
Primary Contact: Clinton J. Christianson, FACHE, President and Chief Executive Officer
COO: Lori Rathbun, Vice President Operations
CFO: Lori Rathbun, Vice President Operations
CIO: Ann Young, Vice President Community and Staff Relations
CHR: Tonya Clawson, Manager Human Resources
CNO: Sherri L. Doggett, Vice President Patient Services
Web address: www.mercycenterville.org
**Control:** Church–operated, Nongovernment, not–for profit **Service:** General Medical and Surgical

**Staffed Beds:** 45 **Admissions:** 1055 **Census:** 31 **Outpatient Visits:** 86086 **Births:** 86 **Total Expense ($000):** 22420 **Payroll Expense ($000):** 10023 **Personnel:** 194

## CHARITON—Lucas County

★ **LUCAS COUNTY HEALTH CENTER (161341)**, 1200 North Seventh Street, Zip 50049–1258; tel. 641/774–3000 **A**9 10 18 **F**3 5 7 13 15 28 29 31 34 38 40 41 43 44 45 47 50 59 64 68 70 75 76 77 81 86 87 89 93 107 114 118 126 127 129 130 131 132 142 144 145 147
Primary Contact: Veronica Fuhs, Chief Executive Officer
CFO: Larry Brown, Chief Financial Officer
CMO: Philip Sundquist, M.D., Chief Medical Staff
CIO: Brett Grinde, Network Manager
CHR: Lana Kuball, Director Administrative Services
CNO: JoBeth Lawless, Director of Nursing, Nursing Services and Director Emergency Management Services
Web address: www.lchcia.com
**Control:** County–Government, nonfederal **Service:** General Medical and Surgical

**Staffed Beds:** 25 **Admissions:** 525 **Census:** 5 **Outpatient Visits:** 18986 **Births:** 72 **Total Expense ($000):** 14965 **Payroll Expense ($000):** 6571 **Personnel:** 180

## CHARLES CITY—Floyd County

**FLOYD COUNTY MEDICAL CENTER (161347)**, 800 Eleventh Street, Zip 50616–3499; tel. 641/228–6830 **A**9 10 18 **F**3 11 13 15 28 29 31 34 35 40 45 48 57 59 64 69 75 76 79 81 85 89 91 93 97 107 114 118 126 129 131 132 145 147 **S** Mayo Clinic Health System, Rochester, MN
Primary Contact: Bill D. Faust, Administrator
CFO: Ron James, Chief Financial Officer
CHR: Don Nosbisch, Director Human Resources
Web address: www.fcmc.us.com/
**Control:** County–Government, nonfederal **Service:** General Medical and Surgical

**Staffed Beds:** 25 **Admissions:** 984 **Census:** 11 **Outpatient Visits:** 50912 **Births:** 95 **Total Expense ($000):** 21294 **Payroll Expense ($000):** 7940 **Personnel:** 173

## CHEROKEE—Cherokee County

★ **CHEROKEE REGIONAL MEDICAL CENTER (161362)**, 300 Sioux Valley Drive, Zip 51012–1205; tel. 712/225–5101 **A**9 10 18 **F**7 11 13 15 17 28 29 34 35 40 43 45 53 56 57 59 62 63 64 65 67 68 69 75 76 77 78 81 84 86 87 89 93 96 97 107 111 113 116 118 124 126 127 128 129 130 131 132 134 145 146 147 **P**6
Primary Contact: John M. Comstock, Chief Executive Officer
CFO: Joan Bierman, Vice President Finance
Web address: www.cherokeermc.org
**Control:** Other not–for–profit (including NFP Corporation) **Service:** General Medical and Surgical

**Staffed Beds:** 25 **Admissions:** 1226 **Census:** 12 **Outpatient Visits:** 43321 **Births:** 135 **Total Expense ($000):** 18517 **Payroll Expense ($000):** 8098 **Personnel:** 175

☐ **MENTAL HEALTH INSTITUTE (164002)**, 1251 West Cedar Loop, Zip 51012–1599; tel. 712/225–2594 **A**1 9 10 **F**3 98 99 100 101 102 104 129 **P**6
Primary Contact: Daniel Gillette, M.D., Clinical Director
CFO: Tony Morris, Business Manager
CMO: Daniel Gillette, M.D., Clinical Director
CHR: Mary Ann Hanson, Director Personnel
Web address: www.dhs.state.ia.us
**Control:** State–Government, nonfederal **Service:** Psychiatric

**Staffed Beds:** 37 **Admissions:** 429 **Census:** 27 **Outpatient Visits:** 26 **Births:** 0 **Total Expense ($000):** 12158 **Payroll Expense ($000):** 8063 **Personnel:** 167

## CLARINDA—Page County

★ **CLARINDA REGIONAL HEALTH CENTER (161352)**, 823 South 17th Street, Zip 51632, Mailing Address: P.O. Box 217, Zip 51632–0217; tel. 712/542–2176 **A**9 10 18 **F**3 7 11 15 28 29 31 34 36 40 43 50 57 59 64 65 66 69 74 75 77 78 79 81 82 85 86 87 93 97 107 110 111 113 117 118 123 126 127 128 129 131 132 134 142 145 147 **P**6
Primary Contact: Christopher R. Stipe, FACHE, Chief Executive Officer
COO: Elaine Otte, Chief Operating Officer
CFO: Melissa Walter, Chief Financial Officer
CHR: Tammie Driftmier, Director Human Resources
Web address: www.clarindahealth.com
**Control:** City–Government, nonfederal **Service:** General Medical and Surgical

**Staffed Beds:** 25 **Admissions:** 447 **Census:** 3 **Outpatient Visits:** 55022 **Births:** 0 **Total Expense ($000):** 19426 **Payroll Expense ($000):** 8463 **Personnel:** 186

**MENTAL HEALTH INSTITUTE (164005)**, 1800 North 16Th Street, Zip 51632–1101; tel. 712/542–2161, (Total facility includes 20 beds in nursing home–type unit) **A**9 10 **F**67 98 101 103 129 145 **P**6
Primary Contact: Mark Lund, Superintendent
COO: Mark Lund, Superintendent
CFO: Roger Stirle, Business Manager
CMO: Teresa Rosales, M.D., Clinical Director
CIO: Jeri Nielsen, Compliance Officer
CHR: Anna Fengel, Personnel Assistant
Web address: www.dhs.state.ia.us/
**Control:** State–Government, nonfederal **Service:** Psychiatric

**Staffed Beds:** 35 **Admissions:** 175 **Census:** 35 **Outpatient Visits:** 0 **Births:** 0 **Personnel:** 91

## CLARION—Wright County

★ **IOWA SPECIALTY HOSPITAL–CLARION (161302)**, 1316 South Main Street, Zip 50525–2019; tel. 515/532–2811 **A**9 10 18 **F**11 13 15 28 29 31 32 34 35 40 43 45 46 50 56 57 59 63 64 65 68 69 75 76 77 79 81 82 85 87 92 93 97 107 110 111 113 118 124 126 128 130 131 132 133 134 145 147 **P**6
Primary Contact: Steven J. Simonin, Chief Executive Officer
CFO: Amy McDaniel, Chief Financial Officer
CMO: Jon Ahrendsen, M.D., Chief of Staff
CHR: Holly Martin, Human Resources Leader
Web address: www.wrightmed.com
**Control:** City–Government, nonfederal **Service:** General Medical and Surgical

**Staffed Beds:** 25 **Admissions:** 1443 **Census:** 10 **Outpatient Visits:** 101782 **Births:** 207 **Total Expense ($000):** 42769 **Payroll Expense ($000):** 17131 **Personnel:** 279

## CLINTON—Clinton County

⊠ **MERCY MEDICAL CENTER–CLINTON (160080)**, 1410 North Fourth Street, Zip 52732–2940; tel. 563/244–5555, (Includes MERCY SERVICES FOR AGING, 600 14th Avenue North, Zip 52732; tel. 563/244–3888), (Total facility includes 183 beds in nursing home–type unit) **A**1 9 10 **F**3 11 13 15 18 20 22 28 29 30 31 34 35 36 38 40 44 45 47 49 50 53 56 57 59 60 61 62 63 64 68 70 74 75 76 77 78 79 80 81 82 84 85 87 89 90 93 98 99 100 101 102 103 107 108 110 114 117 118 120 122 127 128 129 131 145 147 **S** Trinity Health, Novi, MI
Primary Contact: Sean J. Williams, President and Chief Financial Officer
CFO: Paul Mangin, Vice President Finance
Web address: www.mercyclinton.com
**Control:** Church–operated, Nongovernment, not–for profit **Service:** General Medical and Surgical

**Staffed Beds:** 341 **Admissions:** 6359 **Census:** 192 **Outpatient Visits:** 50963 **Births:** 531 **Total Expense ($000):** 84152 **Payroll Expense ($000):** 34358 **Personnel:** 754

**IA**

*Many Facility Codes have changed. Please refer to the AHA Guide Code Chart.* © 2012 AHA Guide

## CORNING—Adams County

★ **ALEGENT HEALTH MERCY HOSPITAL (161304)**, 603 Rosary Drive,
Zip 50841–1685; tel. 641/322–3121 **A**9 10 18 **F**3 11 15 28 30 31 34 40 43
50 53 56 57 59 62 64 67 69 74 75 81 85 107 118 126 127 128 129 132
134 145 146 147 **S** Alegent Health, Omaha, NE
Primary Contact: Debra Goldsmith, Chief Executive Officer
CMO: Maen Haddadin, M.D., President Medical Staff
CHR: Sandra Lammers, Coordinator Human Resources and Finance
Web address: www.alegent.com
**Control:** Church–operated, Nongovernment, not–for profit **Service:** General
Medical and Surgical

**Staffed Beds:** 22 **Admissions:** 309 **Census:** 4 **Outpatient Visits:** 49868
**Births:** 0 **Total Expense ($000):** 14894 **Payroll Expense ($000):** 4578
**Personnel:** 118

## CORYDON—Wayne County

★ **WAYNE COUNTY HOSPITAL (161358)**, 417 South East Street,
Zip 50060–1860, Mailing Address: P.O. Box 305, Zip 50060–0305;
tel. 641/872–2260 **A**9 10 18 **F**7 10 11 13 15 30 34 35 36 39 40 43 51 56
57 59 60 69 70 75 76 77 79 81 85 87 89 91 92 93 97 107 110 113 118
124 126 129 130 131 132 **P**6
Primary Contact: Daren Relph, Chief Executive Officer
COO: Michael Thomas, Associate Administrator
CFO: Diane Hook, Chief Financial Officer
CMO: Joel Baker, D.O., Chief Medical Officer
CIO: Laurie Ehrich, Chief Communications Officer
CHR: Dave Carlyle, Director Human Resources
CNO: Sheila Mattly, Chief Nursing Officer
Web address: www.waynecountyhospital.org
**Control:** County–Government, nonfederal **Service:** General Medical and Surgical

**Staffed Beds:** 25 **Admissions:** 713 **Census:** 5 **Outpatient Visits:** 15050
**Births:** 118 **Total Expense ($000):** 16698 **Payroll Expense ($000):** 7556
**Personnel:** 192

## COUNCIL BLUFFS—Pottawattamie County

⊠ **ALEGENT HEALTH–MERCY HOSPITAL (160028)**, 800 Mercy Drive,
Zip 51503–3128, Mailing Address: P.O. Box 1C, Zip 51502–3001;
tel. 712/328–5000 **A**1 2 9 10 **F**3 5 11 12 13 15 18 20 22 28 29 30 31 34 35
38 39 40 43 44 47 48 49 50 56 57 59 60 62 64 65 68 70 74 75 76 77 78
79 81 82 84 85 87 89 93 97 98 99 100 101 102 103 104 105 107 108 110
111 113 114 118 128 129 131 133 134 142 145 146 147 **P**6 8 **S** Alegent
Health, Omaha, NE
Primary Contact: Marie E. Knedler, R.N., Vice President and Chief Operating
Officer
COO: Marie E. Knedler, R.N., Vice President and Chief Operating Officer
CFO: Amy Knott, Chief Financial Officer
CMO: Joseph Hoagbin, M.D., Chief Quality Officer
CIO: Kenneth Lawonn, Senior Vice President and Chief Information Officer
CHR: Nancy Wallace, Senior Vice President Human Resources
CNO: Jane Carmody, R.N., Chief Nursing Officer
Web address: www.alegent.com/mercy
**Control:** Church–operated, Nongovernment, not–for profit **Service:** General
Medical and Surgical

**Staffed Beds:** 163 **Admissions:** 7890 **Census:** 87 **Outpatient Visits:** 72630
**Births:** 602 **Total Expense ($000):** 96037 **Payroll Expense ($000):** 32614
**Personnel:** 658

⊠ **JENNIE EDMUNDSON HOSPITAL (160047)**, 933 East Pierce Street,
Zip 51503–4652, Mailing Address: P.O. Box 2C, Zip 51502–3002;
tel. 712/396–6000 **A**1 2 5 9 10 **F**3 11 13 15 18 20 22 26 28 29 30 31 34 35
39 40 43 45 49 50 57 58 59 61 64 68 70 74 75 76 78 79 81 82 85 86 87
89 92 93 98 100 101 102 103 107 108 110 111 113 115 117 118 120 122
128 129 130 131 134 142 144 145 146 147 **S** Nebraska Methodist Health
System, Inc., Omaha, NE
Primary Contact: Steven P. Baumert, President and Chief Executive Officer
CFO: Linda K. Burt, Corporate Vice President Finance
CMO: Michael A. Romano, M.D., Vice President Medical Affairs
CIO: Roger Hertz, Vice President
CHR: Holly Huerter, Vice President Human Resources
CNO: Peggy Helget, R.N., Vice President Patient Services and Chief Nursing
Officer
Web address: www.bestcare.org
**Control:** Other not–for–profit (including NFP Corporation) **Service:** General
Medical and Surgical

**Staffed Beds:** 114 **Admissions:** 5614 **Census:** 65 **Outpatient Visits:** 106256
**Births:** 331 **Total Expense ($000):** 85138 **Payroll Expense ($000):** 34488
**Personnel:** 588

## CRESCO—Howard County

★ **REGIONAL HEALTH SERVICES OF HOWARD COUNTY (161328)**, 235 Eighth
Avenue West, Zip 52136–1098; tel. 563/547–2101 **A**9 10 18 **F**1 4 7 11 13 15
16 17 18 28 29 31 34 40 43 44 47 58 59 62 63 64 65 67 68 70 72 73 75
76 77 79 80 81 85 86 87 88 89 90 93 98 107 110 113 127 129 131 132
145 147 **P**8 **S** Trinity Health, Novi, MI
Primary Contact: Vance Jackson, FACHE, Interim Chief Executive Officer
CFO: Brenda Moser, Vice President Finance
CMO: Paul Jensen, M.D., Chief of Staff
CIO: Brenda Moser, Chief Information Officer
CHR: Connie Kuennen, Director Human Resources and Community Relations
CNO: Staci Urzak, Director Patient Care Services
Web address: www.rhshc.com
**Control:** County–Government, nonfederal **Service:** General Medical and Surgical

**Staffed Beds:** 20 **Admissions:** 364 **Census:** 4 **Outpatient Visits:** 21569
**Births:** 70 **Total Expense ($000):** 13099 **Payroll Expense ($000):** 5427
**Personnel:** 136

## CRESTON—Union County

★ **GREATER REGIONAL MEDICAL CENTER (161365)**, 1700 West Townline,
Zip 50801–1099; tel. 641/782–7091 **A**9 10 18 **F**3 7 11 13 15 28 29 31 34
35 40 43 45 56 57 59 62 63 64 65 68 70 75 76 77 78 79 81 82 84 86 93
96 97 107 108 110 111 113 118 119 120 123 124 126 128 129 130 131
132 134 145 147 **P**6 **S** Iowa Health System, Des Moines, IA
Primary Contact: Monte Neitzel, Chief Executive Officer
CFO: Matt McCutchan, Chief Financial Officer
CMO: Steve Reeves, M.D., Chief Medical Officer
CIO: Karla Winn, Chief Information Officer
CHR: Lisa Ross, Human Resources Officer
Web address: www.greaterregional.org
**Control:** County–Government, nonfederal **Service:** General Medical and Surgical

**Staffed Beds:** 25 **Admissions:** 891 **Census:** 9 **Outpatient Visits:** 70377
**Births:** 186 **Total Expense ($000):** 36201 **Payroll Expense ($000):** 15903
**Personnel:** 292

## DAVENPORT—Scott County

⊠ △ **GENESIS MEDICAL CENTER–DAVENPORT (160033)**, 1227 East
Rusholme Street, Zip 52803–2498; tel. 563/421–1000, (Includes GENESIS
MEDICAL CENTER–EAST CAMPUS, 1227 East Rusholme Street, Zip 52803;
tel. 563/421–1000; GENESIS MEDICAL CENTER–WEST CAMPUS, 1401 West
Central Park, Zip 52804–1769; tel. 563/421–1000) **A**1 2 3 5 7 9 10 **F**3 7 11
12 13 15 18 20 22 24 26 28 29 30 31 34 35 37 38 40 43 44 46 49 50 53
54 57 58 59 60 63 64 68 70 72 74 75 76 77 78 79 80 81 82 84 85 86 87
89 90 91 92 93 94 96 97 98 100 102 107 110 111 113 115 117 118 119
120 122 123 125 128 129 130 131 134 145 146 147 **S** Genesis Health
System, Davenport, IA
Primary Contact: Wayne A. Diewald, President
CFO: Mark G. Rogers, Interim Vice President Finance and Chief Financial Officer
CMO: Frank Claudy, M.D., Vice President Medical Staff Affairs
CIO: Robert Frieden, Vice President Information Systems
CHR: Heidi Kahly–McMahon, Interim Vice President Human Resources
Web address: www.genesishealth.com
**Control:** Other not–for–profit (including NFP Corporation) **Service:** General
Medical and Surgical

**Staffed Beds:** 380 **Admissions:** 19053 **Census:** 220 **Outpatient Visits:**
179279 **Births:** 2294 **Total Expense ($000):** 293895 **Payroll Expense
($000):** 88984 **Personnel:** 1723

⊠ **SELECT SPECIALTY HOSPITAL–QUAD CITIES (162001)**, 1111 West Kimberly
Road, Zip 52806–5711; tel. 563/468–2000 **A**1 10 **F**1 3 29 75 77 85 100 118
129 147 **S** Select Medical Corporation, Mechanicsburg, PA
Primary Contact: Austin B. Cleveland, Chief Executive Officer
Web address: www.selectmedicalcorp.com
**Control:** Corporation, Investor–owned, for–profit **Service:** Long–Term Acute Care
hospital

**Staffed Beds:** 50 **Admissions:** 347 **Census:** 24 **Outpatient Visits:** 0 **Births:**
0 **Total Expense ($000):** 14213 **Payroll Expense ($000):** 4896 **Personnel:**
120

**IA**

---

**Hospital, Medicare Provider Number, Address, Telephone, Approval, Facility, and Physician Codes, Health Care System**

★ American Hospital Association (AHA) membership
☐ The Joint Commission accreditation ◇ DNV Healthcare Inc. accreditation

○ American Osteopathic Association (AOA) accreditation
△ Commission on Accreditation of Rehabilitation Facilities (CARF) accreditation

**DE WITT—Clinton County**

✠ **GENESIS MEDICAL CENTER, DEWITT (161313)**, 1118 11th Street, Zip 52742–1296; tel. 563/659–4200, (Total facility includes 75 beds in nursing home–type unit) **A**1 9 10 18 **F**7 11 15 29 30 31 34 35 38 40 43 44 50 53 57 59 64 74 75 77 78 79 81 85 86 87 97 102 107 110 111 113 118 128 129 130 131 132 134 **S** Genesis Health System, Davenport, IA
Primary Contact: Jeffrey M. Cooper, President
CMO: Steven Fowler, M.D., President Medical Staff
CHR: Kristin Nicholson, Coordinator Human Resources
CNO: Wanda Haack, MSN, Chief Nursing Officer
Web address: www.genesishealth.com
**Control:** Other not–for–profit (including NFP Corporation) **Service:** General Medical and Surgical

| | |
|---|---|
| **Staffed Beds:** 86 **Admissions:** 345 **Census:** 65 **Outpatient Visits:** 18240 **Births:** 0 **Total Expense ($000):** 15266 **Payroll Expense ($000):** 6335 **Personnel:** 110 | |

**DECORAH—Winneshiek County**

✠ **WINNESHIEK MEDICAL CENTER (161371)**, 901 Montgomery Street, Zip 52101–2325; tel. 563/382–2911 **A**1 9 10 18 **F**3 7 11 13 15 17 28 29 31 34 35 38 40 43 50 57 59 61 62 63 64 68 69 70 75 76 77 78 79 81 86 93 97 102 107 111 113 118 127 128 129 130 131 132 134 143 145 146 **S** Mayo Clinic Health System, Rochester, MN
Primary Contact: Gretchen M. Dahlen, FACHE, Chief Executive Officer
COO: David B. Jordahl, FACHE, Chief Operating Officer
CFO: Lynn Luloff, Chief Financial Officer
CMO: Susan Halter, M.D., Chief Medical Officer
CHR: Laurie Bulman, Director Human Resources
Web address: www.winmedical.org
**Control:** County–Government, nonfederal **Service:** General Medical and Surgical

| | |
|---|---|
| **Staffed Beds:** 25 **Admissions:** 1153 **Census:** 11 **Outpatient Visits:** 57555 **Births:** 180 **Total Expense ($000):** 42128 **Payroll Expense ($000):** 15154 **Personnel:** 363 | |

**DENISON—Crawford County**

★ **CRAWFORD COUNTY MEMORIAL HOSPITAL (161369)**, 100 Medical Parkway, Zip 51442–2210; tel. 712/265–2500 **A**9 10 18 **F**3 7 8 11 13 15 17 28 29 31 35 39 40 45 56 57 59 64 67 68 70 75 76 77 78 79 81 85 89 93 97 107 113 118 126 127 132 134 147 **P**6
Primary Contact: Bill Bruce, FACHE, Chief Executive Officer
CFO: Nancy Carlson, Chief Financial Officer
CIO: Angie Anderson, Director Information Technology
CNO: Diane Arkfeld, R.N., Director of Nursing
Web address: www.ccmhia.com
**Control:** County–Government, nonfederal **Service:** General Medical and Surgical

| | |
|---|---|
| **Staffed Beds:** 25 **Admissions:** 763 **Census:** 6 **Outpatient Visits:** 38940 **Births:** 119 **Total Expense ($000):** 21135 **Payroll Expense ($000):** 11362 **Personnel:** 197 | |

**DES MOINES—Polk County**

✠ **BROADLAWNS MEDICAL CENTER (160101)**, 1801 Hickman Road, Zip 50314–1597; tel. 515/282–2200 **A**1 3 5 9 10 15 18 29 30 31 32 34 35 38 39 40 42 43 44 45 48 50 52 53 56 57 58 59 64 65 66 68 70 74 75 76 77 78 79 81 82 85 86 87 92 93 94 97 98 99 100 101 102 103 104 105 106 107 111 113 118 129 130 131 134 143 145 146 147 **P**6
Primary Contact: Jody J. Jenner, President and Chief Executive Officer
CFO: Al White, CPA, Senior Vice President Business Services
CMO: Vincent Mandracchia, DPM, Chief Medical Officer
CNO: Susan N. Kirstein, R.N., Chief Nursing Officer
Web address: www.broadlawns.org
**Control:** County–Government, nonfederal **Service:** General Medical and Surgical

| | |
|---|---|
| **Staffed Beds:** 91 **Admissions:** 3591 **Census:** 44 **Outpatient Visits:** 182760 **Births:** 265 **Total Expense ($000):** 99746 **Payroll Expense ($000):** 47631 **Personnel:** 810 | |

**DES MOINES DIVISION** See Veterans Affairs Central Iowa Health Care System

★ **IOWA LUTHERAN HOSPITAL (160024)**, 700 East University Avenue, Zip 50316–2392; tel. 515/263–5612, (Total facility includes 16 beds in nursing home–type unit) **A**3 5 9 10 21 **F**3 4 5 8 11 13 15 17 18 20 22 24 26 28 29 30 34 35 38 39 40 43 44 45 49 50 51 53 56 57 58 59 60 61 64 65 66 68 70 71 74 75 76 79 81 82 84 85 86 87 93 97 98 99 100 101 102 103 104 105 107 108 110 111 113 114 117 118 127 129 131 133 134 141 145 146 147 **P**6 **S** Iowa Health System, Des Moines, IA
Primary Contact: Eric T. Crowell, President and Chief Executive Officer
COO: Eric L. Lothe, Vice President and Administrator
CFO: Joe Corfits, Chief Financial Officer
CMO: Mark Purtle, M.D., Vice President Medical Affairs
CHR: Joyce McDanel, Vice President Human Resources and Education
Web address: www.iowahealth.org
**Control:** Other not–for–profit (including NFP Corporation) **Service:** General Medical and Surgical

| | |
|---|---|
| **Staffed Beds:** 187 **Admissions:** 8151 **Census:** 117 **Outpatient Visits:** 97562 **Births:** 456 **Total Expense ($000):** 117747 **Payroll Expense ($000):** 58884 **Personnel:** 894 | |

★ △ **IOWA METHODIST MEDICAL CENTER (160082)**, 1200 Pleasant Street, Zip 50309–9976; tel. 515/241–6212, (Includes BLANK CHILDREN'S HOSPITAL, 1200 Pleasant Street, Zip 50309–1406; tel. 515/241–5437; JOHN STODDARD CANCER CENTER, 1221 Pleasant Street, Zip 50309–1423; tel. 515/241–6212; METHODIST WEST HOSPITAL, 1660 60th Street, West Des Moines, Zip 50266–7700; tel. 515/343–1000; Eric T. Crowell, Chief Executive Officer; POWELL CONVALESCENT CENTER, 1200 Pleasant, Zip 50309; RAYMOND BLANK MEMORIAL HOSPITAL FOR CHILDREN, Zip 50308; YOUNKER MEMORIAL REHABILITATION CENTER, 1200 Pleasant Road, Zip 50308) **A**2 7 8 9 10 21 **F**3 7 8 11 12 13 17 18 20 22 24 26 29 30 31 32 34 35 39 40 41 43 45 46 49 50 53 54 55 56 57 58 59 60 61 64 65 68 70 71 72 74 75 76 77 78 79 81 82 84 85 86 87 88 89 90 91 92 93 94 96 97 100 107 108 111 114 115 116 117 118 119 120 122 123 125 128 129 130 131 133 134 137 141 145 146 147 **P**6 **S** Iowa Health System, Des Moines, IA
Primary Contact: Eric T. Crowell, President and Chief Executive Officer
COO: Steve R. Stephenson, M.D., Executive Vice President and Chief Operating Officer
CFO: Joe Corfits, Senior Vice President Finance
CMO: Mark Purtle, M.D., Vice President Medical Affairs
CHR: Joyce McDanel, Vice President Human Resources
Web address: www.iowahealth.org
**Control:** Other not–for–profit (including NFP Corporation) **Service:** General Medical and Surgical

| | |
|---|---|
| **Staffed Beds:** 415 **Admissions:** 19950 **Census:** 303 **Outpatient Visits:** 254596 **Births:** 3197 **Total Expense ($000):** 399249 **Payroll Expense ($000):** 180605 **Personnel:** 3228 | |

✠ △ **MERCY MEDICAL CENTER–DES MOINES (160083)**, 1111 6th Avenue, Zip 50314–2611; tel. 515/247–3121, (Includes MERCY FRANKLIN CENTER, 1818 48th Street, Zip 50310; tel. 515/271–6000) **A**1 2 3 5 7 9 10 13 **F**3 4 5 6 7 8 9 10 11 13 15 16 17 18 19 20 21 22 23 24 25 26 27 28 29 30 31 32 34 35 36 38 39 40 41 43 44 46 48 49 50 51 53 54 55 57 58 59 60 61 62 63 64 65 66 68 70 72 73 74 75 76 77 78 79 81 82 84 85 86 87 88 89 90 91 92 93 94 96 97 98 99 100 101 102 103 104 105 106 107 108 109 110 111 113 114 115 116 117 118 119 120 122 123 124 125 128 129 130 131 133 134 137 140 141 142 143 144 145 146 147 **P**6 **S** Catholic Health Initiatives, Englewood, CO
Primary Contact: David H. Vellinga, FACHE, President and Chief Executive Officer
COO: Jackie Frost–Kunnen, Senior Vice President Operations
CFO: Steven F. Kukla, Senior Vice President and Chief Financial Officer
CMO: Dale Andres, D.O., Senior Vice President Medical Affairs
CIO: Cristina Thomas, Vice President and Chief Information Officer
CHR: Robyn Wilkinson, Senior Vice President Human Resources
Web address: www.mercydesmoines.org
**Control:** Church–operated, Nongovernment, not–for profit **Service:** General Medical and Surgical

| | |
|---|---|
| **Staffed Beds:** 567 **Admissions:** 29824 **Census:** 407 **Outpatient Visits:** 250702 **Births:** 4833 **Total Expense ($000):** 569392 **Payroll Expense ($000):** 238399 **Personnel:** 4141 | |

✠ △ **VETERANS AFFAIRS CENTRAL IOWA HEALTH CARE SYSTEM**, 3600 30th Street, Zip 50310–5774; tel. 515/699–5999, (Includes DES MOINES DIVISION, 3600 30th Street, tel. 515/699–5999; KNOXVILLE DIVISION, 1515 West Pleasant, Knoxville, Zip 50138–3399; tel. 515/842–3101), (Total facility includes 140 beds in nursing home–type unit) **A**1 3 5 7 9 **F**2 3 5 11 15 18 20 22 28 29 30 31 33 34 35 36 38 39 40 44 46 50 56 57 59 61 62 64 65 66 70 71 74 75 77 78 79 80 81 82 83 84 85 86 87 93 94 97 98 100 101 102 103 104 105 106 107 108 111 113 114 117 118 127 128 129 131 134 145 146 147 **S** Department of Veterans Affairs, Washington, DC
Primary Contact: Donald C. Cooper, Director
CMO: Fredrick Bahls, M.D., Chief of Staff
CIO: James Danuser, Chief Information Officer
CHR: Sabrina Owen, Human Resources Officer
Web address: www.va.centra/iowa.va.gov
**Control:** Veterans Affairs, Government, federal **Service:** General Medical and Surgical

| | |
|---|---|
| **Staffed Beds:** 255 **Admissions:** 4831 **Census:** 214 **Outpatient Visits:** 307464 **Births:** 0 **Total Expense ($000):** 215000 **Payroll Expense ($000):** 121818 **Personnel:** 1392 | |

IA

*Many Facility Codes have changed. Please refer to the AHA Guide Code Chart.* © 2012 AHA Guide

## DUBUQUE—Dubuque County

✠ △ **FINLEY HOSPITAL (160117)**, 350 North Grandview Avenue,
Zip 52001–6392; tel. 563/582–1881 **A**1 2 7 9 10 **F**3 11 12 13 15 18 26 28
29 30 31 34 35 39 40 43 44 45 46 48 49 50 53 56 57 58 59 60 61 62 64
65 69 70 72 74 75 76 77 78 79 81 82 84 85 86 90 93 96 97 98 103 107
108 111 114 115 116 117 118 119 120 122 123 128 129 130 131 134 143
145 146 147 **P**1 5 **S** Iowa Health System, Des Moines, IA
Primary Contact: David R. Brandon, President and Chief Executive Officer
COO: Chad Wolbers, Chief Operating Officer
CFO: Dan Carpenter, Chief Financial Officer
CMO: Bryan Pechous, M.D., Vice President Medical Affairs
CIO: Tim Loeffelholz, Account Executive Information Technology
CHR: Karla Waldbillig, Director Human Resources
CNO: Diana Batchelor, Chief Nursing Officer
Web address: www.finleyhospital.org
**Control:** Other not–for–profit (including NFP Corporation) **Service:** General
Medical and Surgical

> **Staffed Beds:** 119 **Admissions:** 4669 **Census:** 54 **Outpatient Visits:** 94506
> **Births:** 684 **Total Expense ($000):** 88953 **Payroll Expense ($000):** 32205
> **Personnel:** 654

✠ △ **MERCY MEDICAL CENTER–DUBUQUE (160069)**, 250 Mercy Drive,
Zip 52001–7360; tel. 563/589–8000, (Total facility includes 40 beds in nursing
home–type unit) **A**1 7 9 10 **F**3 4 5 8 11 13 15 18 20 22 24 26 28 29 30 31
32 34 35 36 38 39 40 43 44 49 50 51 53 56 57 58 59 61 62 64 65 67 68
70 72 74 75 76 77 78 79 80 81 85 86 87 89 90 91 93 97 98 99 100 101
102 103 104 107 108 111 113 115 118 127 128 129 130 131 133 134 142
143 145 146 147 **P**8 **S** Trinity Health, Novi, MI
Primary Contact: Russell M. Knight, President and Chief Executive Officer
CFO: Robert Shafer, Vice President Finance
CIO: Matt Trimmer, Director Information Services
CNO: Kay Takes, R.N., Vice President Patient Care Services and Chief Nursing
Officer
Web address: www.mercydubuque.com
**Control:** Church–operated, Nongovernment, not–for profit **Service:** General
Medical and Surgical

> **Staffed Beds:** 272 **Admissions:** 8864 **Census:** 141 **Outpatient Visits:** 41524
> **Births:** 864 **Total Expense ($000):** 61621 **Payroll Expense ($000):** 42991
> **Personnel:** 979

## DYERSVILLE—Dubuque County

★ **MERCY MEDICAL CENTER–DYERSVILLE (161378)**, 1111 Third Street S.W.,
Zip 52040; tel. 563/875–7101 **A**9 10 18 **F**11 15 34 35 36 39 40 44 50 56 57
59 64 65 68 75 79 81 85 86 93 118 129 130 131 132 133 134 145 146 **P**8
**S** Trinity Health, Novi, MI
Primary Contact: Russell M. Knight, President and Chief Executive Officer
CFO: Robert Shafer, Vice President Finance
Web address: www.mercydubuque.com/dyersville
**Control:** Church–operated, Nongovernment, not–for profit **Service:** General
Medical and Surgical

> **Staffed Beds:** 25 **Admissions:** 92 **Census:** 3 **Outpatient Visits:** 3958 **Births:**
> 0 **Total Expense ($000):** 4806 **Payroll Expense ($000):** 2230 **Personnel:**
> 47

## ELKADER—Clayton County

★ **CENTRAL COMMUNITY HOSPITAL (161319)**, 901 Davidson Street N.W.,
Zip 52043–9015; tel. 563/245–7000 **A**9 10 18 **F**7 11 15 18 28 34 35 40 43
50 56 57 59 64 65 67 68 70 75 81 85 86 87 89 102 107 113 127 129 131
132 133 134 142 147 **S** Trinity Health, Novi, MI
Primary Contact: Frances J. Zichal, Chief Executive Officer
CFO: Patricia Borel, Chief Financial Officer
CIO: Nathan Baker, Manager Information Technology
CHR: Angie Gerndt, Human Resources Generalist
CNO: Mary Walters, Chief Nursing Officer
Web address: www.centralcommunityhospital.com
**Control:** Other not–for–profit (including NFP Corporation) **Service:** General
Medical and Surgical

> **Staffed Beds:** 16 **Admissions:** 201 **Census:** 3 **Outpatient Visits:** 14842
> **Births:** 0 **Total Expense ($000):** 5718 **Payroll Expense ($000):** 1836
> **Personnel:** 57

## EMMETSBURG—Palo Alto County

★ **PALO ALTO COUNTY HEALTH SYSTEM (161357)**, 3201 First Street,
Zip 50536; tel. 712/852–5500, (Total facility includes 22 beds in nursing home–
type unit) **A**9 10 18 **F**3 7 11 13 15 28 31 34 35 40 45 50 57 59 62 63 64 65
67 68 69 70 75 76 77 79 81 85 86 87 93 96 107 110 114 118 124 126 129
131 132 134 142 145 **P**6 **S** Trinity Health, Novi, MI
Primary Contact: Vance Jackson, FACHE, Interim Administrator
CFO: Renay Hauswirth, Chief Financial Officer
CMO: Frank Veltri, M.D., President Medical Staff
CIO: Randy Beaver, Chief Information Officer
CHR: Kelly Bond, Director Human Resources
Web address: www.pachs.com
**Control:** County–Government, nonfederal **Service:** General Medical and Surgical

> **Staffed Beds:** 47 **Admissions:** 597 **Census:** 28 **Outpatient Visits:** 26844
> **Births:** 108 **Total Expense ($000):** 20667 **Payroll Expense ($000):** 7953
> **Personnel:** 172

## ESTHERVILLE—Emmet County

★ **AVERA HOLY FAMILY HOSPITAL (161351)**, 826 North Eighth Street,
Zip 51334–1598; tel. 712/362–2631 **A**9 10 18 **F**3 11 13 15 28 29 30 31 34
35 40 45 59 62 63 64 68 69 70 75 76 77 78 79 81 85 87 93 107 113 118
129 131 132 145 **P**4 **S** Avera Health, Sioux Falls, SD
Primary Contact: Michael L. Hall, Chief Executive Officer
CMO: James Creech, M.D., Chief of Staff
CHR: Janette Jensen, Manager Human Resources
Web address: www.avera–holyfamily.org
**Control:** Church–operated, Nongovernment, not–for profit **Service:** General
Medical and Surgical

> **Staffed Beds:** 25 **Admissions:** 720 **Census:** 7 **Outpatient Visits:** 65169
> **Births:** 0 **Total Expense ($000):** 20385 **Payroll Expense ($000):** 7076
> **Personnel:** 175

## FAIRFIELD—Jefferson County

★ **JEFFERSON COUNTY HEALTH CENTER (161364)**, 2000 South Main,
Zip 52556–9572, Mailing Address: P.O. Box 588, Zip 52556–0588;
tel. 641/472–4111 **A**9 10 18 **F**11 15 28 30 31 34 35 36 40 43 45 57 59 67
68 70 75 77 78 79 81 85 89 93 96 102 107 110 113 118 127 128 132 134
142 145 147
Primary Contact: Deborah Cardin, R.N., FACHE, MS, Chief Executive Officer
CFO: Gene Irwin, Chief Financial Officer
CHR: Nanette Everly, Manager Human Resources and Administrative Assistant
Web address: www.jeffersoncountyhealthcenter.org
**Control:** County–Government, nonfederal **Service:** General Medical and Surgical

> **Staffed Beds:** 25 **Admissions:** 788 **Census:** 12 **Outpatient Visits:** 42512
> **Births:** 0 **Total Expense ($000):** 21076 **Payroll Expense ($000):** 7414
> **Personnel:** 165

## FORT DODGE—Webster County

★ **TRINITY REGIONAL MEDICAL CENTER (160016)**, 802 Kenyon Road,
Zip 50501–5795; tel. 515/573–3101 **A**2 9 10 21 **F**3 7 8 11 13 15 18 20 22
24 28 29 30 31 32 34 35 36 40 43 45 49 50 53 57 59 60 64 68 70 73
75 76 77 78 79 81 82 84 86 87 89 93 107 108 111 114 117 118 128 129
130 131 134 145 147 **P**6 **S** Iowa Health System, Des Moines, IA
Primary Contact: Susan K. Thompson, President and Chief Executive Officer
COO: Troy Martens, Chief Operating Officer
CFO: Mike Dewerff, Chief Financial Officer
CHR: Ted W. Vaughn, Director Human Resources
CNO: Debra Shriver, R.N., Chief Nurse Executive
Web address: www.trmc.org
**Control:** Other not–for–profit (including NFP Corporation) **Service:** General
Medical and Surgical

> **Staffed Beds:** 132 **Admissions:** 4725 **Census:** 44 **Outpatient Visits:** 101038
> **Births:** 492 **Total Expense ($000):** 99188 **Payroll Expense ($000):** 44069
> **Personnel:** 720

**IA**

---

**Hospital, Medicare Provider Number, Address, Telephone, Approval, Facility, and Physician Codes, Health Care System**

★ American Hospital Association (AHA) membership
☐ The Joint Commission accreditation
◇ DNV Healthcare Inc. accreditation
○ American Osteopathic Association (AOA) accreditation
△ Commission on Accreditation of Rehabilitation Facilities (CARF) accreditation

## FORT MADISON—Lee County

✠ **FORT MADISON COMMUNITY HOSPITAL (160122)**, 5445 Avenue O,
Zip 52627–0174, Mailing Address: P.O. Box 174, Zip 52627–0174;
tel. 319/372–6530 **A**1 9 10 **F**3 11 13 15 28 29 31 34 40 43 45 50 51 53 57
59 62 64 67 68 70 74 75 76 77 78 79 81 85 86 87 90 91 93 94 96 97 99
100 101 102 103 104 107 108 110 111 113 116 117 118 127 128 129 130
131 132 142 143 145 146 147 **P**6 **S** QHR, Brentwood, TN
Primary Contact: C. James Platt, Chief Executive Officer
CFO: Bradley J. Kokjohn, Chief Financial Officer
CMO: David Wenger–Keller, M.D., Chief of Staff
CIO: Shane Tapper, Director Management Information Systems
CHR: Vicki Kokjohn, Director Employee Relations
Web address: www.fmchosp.com
**Control:** Other not–for–profit (including NFP Corporation) **Service:** General
Medical and Surgical

**Staffed Beds:** 50 **Admissions:** 2220 **Census:** 22 **Outpatient Visits:** 73562
**Births:** 286 **Total Expense ($000):** 46487 **Payroll Expense ($000):** 23246
**Personnel:** 421

## GREENFIELD—Adair County

**ADAIR COUNTY MEMORIAL HOSPITAL (161310)**, 609 S.E. Kent Street,
Zip 50849–9454; tel. 641/743–2123 **A**9 10 18 **F**3 7 11 15 18 28 29 31 34
35 36 40 43 45 48 57 59 62 64 65 69 70 75 77 79 81 89 91 93 97 107
108 110 111 113 115 117 118 126 127 128 129 132 145 147 **P**6
Primary Contact: Angela Mortoza, Administrator
CFO: Lisa Blazek, Chief Financial Officer
CMO: Melissa Thompson, M.D., Chief Medical Officer
CIO: Andy Christie, Chief Information Technology
CHR: Angie Shatava, Director Human Resources
Web address: www.adaircountyhealthsystem.org
**Control:** County–Government, nonfederal **Service:** General Medical and Surgical

**Staffed Beds:** 18 **Admissions:** 175 **Census:** 2 **Outpatient Visits:** 11957
**Births:** 0 **Total Expense ($000):** 10262 **Payroll Expense ($000):** 4020
**Personnel:** 97

## GRINNELL—Poweshiek County

★ **GRINNELL REGIONAL MEDICAL CENTER (160147)**, 210 Fourth Avenue,
Zip 50112–1833; tel. 641/236–7511 **A**9 10 **F**3 11 12 13 15 28 29 30 31 32
34 35 36 37 38 40 43 44 45 46 47 50 53 54 56 57 59 61 62 63 64 65 66
70 75 76 77 78 81 84 85 86 87 89 93 97 107 108 110 111 113 117 118
126 128 129 130 131 132 133 134 145 146 147 **P**6 7
Primary Contact: Todd C. Linden, President and Chief Executive Officer
COO: Suzanne Cooner, R.N., Vice President Operations
CFO: Jack Fritts, Vice President Finance and Chief Financial Officer
CMO: David C. Cranston, M.D., Vice President Medical Staff Affairs
CIO: David L. Ness, Vice President Operations
CHR: Debra S. Nowachek, Director Human Resources
Web address: www.grmc.us
**Control:** Other not–for–profit (including NFP Corporation) **Service:** General
Medical and Surgical

**Staffed Beds:** 49 **Admissions:** 1518 **Census:** 14 **Outpatient Visits:** 50707
**Births:** 181 **Total Expense ($000):** 40357 **Payroll Expense ($000):** 19167
**Personnel:** 380

## GRUNDY CENTER—Grundy County

★ **GRUNDY COUNTY MEMORIAL HOSPITAL (161303)**, 201 East J Avenue,
Zip 50638–2096; tel. 319/824–5421, (Total facility includes 55 beds in nursing
home–type unit) **A**9 10 18 **F**15 28 29 34 35 40 43 57 59 63 67 75 78 79 81
82 86 87 93 107 110 111 113 118 127 128 129 130 131 132 134 145 147
**S** Iowa Health System, Des Moines, IA
Primary Contact: Pamela K. Delagardelle, Chief Executive Officer
COO: Ryan Bingman, Director Operations
CFO: Lisa Zinkula, Chief Financial Officer
CMO: Douglas Cooper, M.D., Chief Medical Officer
CIO: Nicholas Betts, Director Management Information Technology
CHR: Nicole Larson, Manager Human Resources
Web address: www.grundycountyhospital.com
**Control:** County–Government, nonfederal **Service:** General Medical and Surgical

**Staffed Beds:** 80 **Admissions:** 390 **Census:** 57 **Outpatient Visits:** 30526
**Births:** 0 **Total Expense ($000):** 16216 **Payroll Expense ($000):** 6879
**Personnel:** 109

## GUTHRIE CENTER—Guthrie County

★ **GUTHRIE COUNTY HOSPITAL (161314)**, 710 North 12th Street,
Zip 50115–1544; tel. 641/332–2201 **A**9 10 18 **F**11 15 18 28 29 31 34 35 40
43 45 53 56 57 59 64 69 75 77 79 81 85 93 107 110 118 127 129 131 132
142 **P**5 **S** Iowa Health System, Des Moines, IA
Primary Contact: Gerald D. Neal, Chief Executive Officer and Administrator
CFO: Melinda Alt, Chief Financial Officer
CMO: Steven Bascom, M.D., Chief Medical Officer
CIO: Jeff Cobb, Information Technologist
CHR: Kimberly Myers, Director Human Resources
CNO: Danielle Navarro, R.N., Chief Nursing Officer
Web address: www.guthriecountyhospital.org
**Control:** County–Government, nonfederal **Service:** General Medical and Surgical

**Staffed Beds:** 25 **Admissions:** 591 **Census:** 6 **Outpatient Visits:** 34368
**Births:** 0 **Total Expense ($000):** 12586 **Payroll Expense ($000):** 5939
**Personnel:** 112

## GUTTENBERG—Clayton County

✠ **GUTTENBERG MUNICIPAL HOSPITAL (161312)**, 200 Main Street,
Zip 52052–0550, Mailing Address: P.O. Box 550, Zip 52052–0550;
tel. 563/252–1121 **A**1 9 10 18 **F**3 7 8 11 13 15 28 34 35 40 43 45 50 53 57
59 64 68 76 81 82 85 89 93 102 107 110 111 113 118 127 129 131 132
**P**5 6 **S** Iowa Health System, Des Moines, IA
Primary Contact: Kimberley A. Gau, FACHE, Chief Executive Officer
CMO: Andrew Smith, M.D., Chief Medical Staff
CIO: Ken Kaiser, Director Information Technology
CHR: Leigh Ann Judge, Manager Human Resources
CNO: Laura Beyer, Director Patient Care
Web address: www.guttenberghospital.org
**Control:** City–Government, nonfederal **Service:** General Medical and Surgical

**Staffed Beds:** 20 **Admissions:** 504 **Census:** 5 **Outpatient Visits:** 20547
**Births:** 28 **Total Expense ($000):** 9144 **Payroll Expense ($000):** 3444
**Personnel:** 79

## HAMBURG—Fremont County

**GEORGE C GRAPE COMMUNITY HOSPITAL (161324)**, 2959 U.S. Highway
275, Zip 51640–5067; tel. 712/382–1515, (Total facility includes 6 beds in
nursing home–type unit) **A**9 10 18 **F**11 15 18 28 31 34 40 43 45 49 50 53 57
59 62 64 65 68 69 74 75 77 78 79 81 82 91 93 107 113 118 127 128 129
130 132 134 147
Primary Contact: Michael O'Neal, Administrator and Chief Executive Officer
CFO: Hilary Christiansen, Chief Financial Officer
CMO: Kelli Woltemath, D.O., Chief Medical Staff
CIO: Nancy Tiemeyer, Director Health Information Management
CHR: Jackie Wertz, Director Human Resources
Web address: www.grapehospital.com
**Control:** Other not–for–profit (including NFP Corporation) **Service:** General
Medical and Surgical

**Staffed Beds:** 25 **Admissions:** 301 **Census:** 8 **Outpatient Visits:** 16283
**Births:** 0 **Total Expense ($000):** 9244 **Payroll Expense ($000):** 3970
**Personnel:** 100

## HAMPTON—Franklin County

★ **FRANKLIN GENERAL HOSPITAL (161308)**, 1720 Central Avenue East,
Zip 50441–1859; tel. 641/456–5000, (Total facility includes 52 beds in nursing
home–type unit) **A**9 10 18 **F**7 10 11 15 28 30 31 34 40 43 57 59 63 64 65 67
68 75 77 81 82 85 86 89 90 93 107 111 113 118 126 127 128 129 131
132 134 145 **P**8 **S** Trinity Health, Novi, MI
Primary Contact: Kim Price, Chief Executive Officer
CFO: Michelle Craighton, Manager Finance
CHR: Victoria Kruse, Manager Human Resources
Web address: www.franklingeneral.org
**Control:** County–Government, nonfederal **Service:** General Medical and Surgical

**Staffed Beds:** 77 **Admissions:** 321 **Census:** 55 **Outpatient Visits:** 17504
**Births:** 0 **Total Expense ($000):** 15371 **Payroll Expense ($000):** 6009
**Personnel:** 137

## HARLAN—Shelby County

★ **MYRTUE MEDICAL CENTER (161374)**, 1213 Garfield Avenue,
Zip 51537–2057; tel. 712/755–5161 **A**9 10 18 **F**3 11 13 15 28 29 31 34 35
38 40 43 45 46 50 53 56 57 59 62 63 64 65 68 75 76 77 78 81 85 87 92
93 97 99 101 102 103 104 107 110 113 118 126 128 129 130 131 132
134 145 147 **P**6 8
Primary Contact: Barry Jacobsen, Chief Executive Officer
CFO: Sue Blake, Chief Financial Officer
CMO: Sarah Devine, M.D., Chief of Staff
CIO: David Sirek, Chief Information Officer
CHR: Donna Christensen–Mores, Director Human Resources
CNO: Karen Buman, Chief Nurse Executive
Web address: www.myrtuemedical.org
**Control:** County–Government, nonfederal **Service:** General Medical and Surgical

**Staffed Beds:** 25 **Admissions:** 1190 **Census:** 13 **Outpatient Visits:** 71586
**Births:** 81 **Total Expense ($000):** 28461 **Payroll Expense ($000):** 12179
**Personnel:** 351

**IA**

**HAWARDEN—Sioux County**

★ **HAWARDEN COMMUNITY HOSPITAL (161311)**, 1111 11th Street,
Zip 51023–1999; tel. 712/551–3100 **A**9 10 18 **F**11 15 28 29 31 34 35 40 43
53 56 57 59 64 67 69 75 77 80 81 89 90 93 107 108 118 127 131 132 145
147 **P**3 7 **S** Trinity Health, Novi, MI
Primary Contact: Jayson Pullman, Chief Executive Officer
CFO: Kathy Ranniger, Director Finance
CHR: Amy A. Miller, Human Resources Assistant
Web address: www.hawardencommunityhospital.org
**Control:** City–Government, nonfederal **Service:** General Medical and Surgical

**Staffed Beds:** 18 **Admissions:** 141 **Census:** 2 **Outpatient Visits:** 16717
**Births:** 0 **Total Expense ($000):** 6094 **Payroll Expense ($000):** 2102
**Personnel:** 47

**HUMBOLDT—Humboldt County**

★ **HUMBOLDT COUNTY MEMORIAL HOSPITAL (161334)**, 1000 North 15th
Street, Zip 50548–1008; tel. 515/332–4200, (Total facility includes 28 beds in
nursing home–type unit) **A**9 10 18 **F**7 8 10 11 12 14 15 28 29 31 32 34 35 40
41 43 45 47 50 51 59 65 69 75 77 78 79 81 82 85 87 89 90 93 102 107
110 111 113 118 124 127 129 132 133 **S** Iowa Health System, Des Moines, IA
Primary Contact: James Atty, Chief Executive Officer
CFO: Betty Etherington, Chief Financial Officer
CHR: Mary Moritz, Administrator Human Resources
Web address: www.humboldthospital.org
**Control:** County–Government, nonfederal **Service:** General Medical and Surgical

**Staffed Beds:** 49 **Admissions:** 277 **Census:** 30 **Outpatient Visits:** 38401
**Births:** 0 **Total Expense ($000):** 11708 **Payroll Expense ($000):** 4711
**Personnel:** 117

**IDA GROVE—Ida County**

★ **HORN MEMORIAL HOSPITAL (161354)**, 701 East Second Street,
Zip 51445–1699; tel. 712/364–3311 **A**9 10 18 **F**11 13 15 28 29 31 34 40 45
57 59 62 63 64 65 66 68 69 71 75 76 77 78 79 81 85 89 93 97 104 107
108 111 113 118 126 128 131 132 134 145 147 **P**6
Primary Contact: Marc Augsburger, President and Chief Executive Officer
CFO: Marcia Fehring, Chief Financial Officer
CIO: Robbie Todd, Director Information Technology
CHR: Lorraine Davis, Vice President Human Resources
CNO: Sharon A. Wellendorf, Chief Nursing Officer
Web address: www.hornmemorialhospital.org
**Control:** Other not–for–profit (including NFP Corporation) **Service:** General
Medical and Surgical

**Staffed Beds:** 25 **Admissions:** 593 **Census:** 8 **Outpatient Visits:** 23039
**Births:** 46 **Total Expense ($000):** 16307 **Payroll Expense ($000):** 6609
**Personnel:** 150

**INDEPENDENCE—Buchanan County**

★ **BUCHANAN COUNTY HEALTH CENTER (161335)**, 1600 First Street East,
Zip 50644–3155; tel. 319/332–0999, (Total facility includes 39 beds in nursing
home–type unit) **A**9 10 18 **F**3 11 15 28 29 32 34 35 40 43 45 53 56 57 59 64
65 67 70 75 77 79 81 82 86 87 89 93 107 110 113 118 124 128 129 130
131 132 134 145
Primary Contact: Danielle Gearhart, Chief Executive Officer
CFO: Ronald Timpe, Associate Administrator
CHR: Shelbie Medina, Chief People Officer
Web address: www.bchealth.info
**Control:** County–Government, nonfederal **Service:** General Medical and Surgical

**Staffed Beds:** 64 **Admissions:** 364 **Census:** 33 **Outpatient Visits:** 44401
**Births:** 0 **Total Expense ($000):** 14923 **Payroll Expense ($000):** 6684
**Personnel:** 178

☐ **MENTAL HEALTH INSTITUTE (164003)**, 2277 Iowa Avenue, Zip 50644–9106;
tel. 319/334–2583 **A**1 9 10 **F**65 98 99 101 102 106 129 142 145 **P**6
Primary Contact: Bhasker J. Dave, M.D., Superintendent
CFO: Kevin Jimmerson, Business Manager
CMO: Bhasker J. Dave, M.D., Superintendent
Web address: www.dhs.state.ia.us
**Control:** State–Government, nonfederal **Service:** Psychiatric

**Staffed Beds:** 75 **Admissions:** 239 **Census:** 59 **Outpatient Visits:** 3 **Births:**
0 **Total Expense ($000):** 20400 **Payroll Expense ($000):** 11544
**Personnel:** 235

**IOWA CITY—Johnson County**

⊞ **IOWA CITY VETERANS AFFAIRS HEALTH CARE SYSTEM**, 601 Highway 6
West, Zip 52246–2208; tel. 319/339–7100 **A**1 3 5 8 9 **F**1 3 4 5 7 8 15 16 17
18 20 22 26 29 30 31 35 39 40 44 45 47 54 56 57 58 59 60 61 62 63
64 65 67 70 72 73 74 75 76 77 78 79 80 81 82 83 84 85 86 87 88 89 90
91 92 93 94 97 98 100 101 102 103 104 107 108 111 113 114 116 117
118 126 127 128 129 131 134 137 142 143 145 146 147 **S** Department of
Veterans Affairs, Washington, DC
Primary Contact: Barry Sharp, Director
COO: Timothy McMurry, Associate Director Operations
CFO: Kevin Kosek, Chief Financial Officer
CMO: Mark H. Smith, M.D., Chief of Staff
CIO: Dwight Schuessler, Chief Information Officer
CHR: Dan Helle, Human Resources Officer
CNO: Dawn Oxley, R.N., Associate Director Patient Care Services and Nurse
Executive
Web address: www.iowacity.va.gov/
**Control:** Veterans Affairs, Government, federal **Service:** General Medical and
Surgical

**Staffed Beds:** 83 **Admissions:** 3384 **Census:** 47 **Outpatient Visits:** 400972
**Births:** 0 **Total Expense ($000):** 257111 **Payroll Expense ($000):** 99451
**Personnel:** 1546

⊞ **MERCY IOWA CITY (160029)**, 500 East Market Street, Zip 52245–2689;
tel. 319/339–0300, (Total facility includes 16 beds in nursing home–type unit) **A**1
2 9 10 **F**3 11 13 15 18 20 22 24 26 28 29 30 31 34 35 36 37 38 40 41 42
43 44 45 48 49 50 51 56 57 58 59 62 63 64 65 70 72 73 74 75 76 77 78
79 81 82 85 86 87 89 97 98 100 101 102 103 107 108 110 111 113 114
117 118 125 127 129 131 134 143 144 145 147 **P**8
Primary Contact: Ronald R. Reed, President and Chief Executive Officer
CFO: Michael G. Heinrich, Executive Vice President and Chief Financial Officer
CMO: Martin Izakovic, M.D., Vice President Medical Staff Affairs and Chief Medical
Officer
CIO: Paul Foelsch, Vice President Information Services and Chief Information
Officer
CHR: Marie Peeters, Director Human Resources
CNO: Cindy L. Penney, R.N., Vice President Nursing
Web address: www.mercyiowacity.org
**Control:** Church–operated, Nongovernment, not–for profit **Service:** General
Medical and Surgical

**Staffed Beds:** 234 **Admissions:** 8334 **Census:** 96 **Outpatient Visits:** 338076
**Births:** 1130 **Total Expense ($000):** 137038 **Payroll Expense ($000):**
56044 **Personnel:** 985

**UNIVERSITY HOSPITAL SCHOOL** See Center for Disabilities and Development

⊞ **UNIVERSITY OF IOWA HOSPITALS AND CLINICS (160058)**, 200 Hawkins
Drive, Zip 52242–1009; tel. 319/356–1616, (Includes CENTER FOR DISABILITIES
AND DEVELOPMENT, 200 Hawkins Drive, Zip 52242; tel. 319/353–6456;
CHEMICAL DEPENDENCY CENTER, 200 Hawkins Drive, Oakdale,
Zip 52242–1007; tel. 319/384–8765; STATE PSYCHIATRIC HOSPITAL, 200
Hawkins Drive, Zip 52242; tel. 319/356–4658; UNIVERSITY OF IOWA CHILDREN'S
HOSPITAL, 200 Hawkins Drive, tel. 319/384–8442) **A**1 2 3 5 8 9 10 **F**3 5 6 7 8
9 11 12 13 14 15 16 17 18 19 20 21 22 23 24 25 26 27 28 29 30 31 32 34
35 36 37 38 39 40 43 44 45 46 47 48 49 50 51 52 53 54 55 56 57 58 59
60 61 62 63 64 65 66 68 70 72 73 74 75 76 77 78 79 80 81 82 83 84 85
86 87 88 89 90 91 92 93 94 97 98 99 100 101 102 103 104 105 107 108
109 110 111 113 114 115 116 117 118 119 120 122 123 125 126 128 129
130 131 134 135 136 137 138 139 140 141 142 143 144 145 146 147
**P**1 7
Primary Contact: Kenneth P. Kates, Chief Executive Officer
COO: John H. Staley, Ph.D., Senior Associate Director and Interim Chief Operating
Officer
CFO: Kenneth Fisher, Associate Vice President Finance and Chief Financial Officer
CMO: Theresa Brennan, M.D., Chief Medical Officer
CIO: Lee Carmen, Associate Vice President Health Care Information Systems
CHR: Jana Wessels, Associate Vice President Human Resources
Web address: www.uihealthcare.com
**Control:** State–Government, nonfederal **Service:** General Medical and Surgical

**Staffed Beds:** 692 **Admissions:** 29949 **Census:** 538 **Outpatient Visits:**
1065371 **Births:** 1951 **Total Expense ($000):** 955520 **Payroll Expense
($000):** 360959 **Personnel:** 6675

**IA**

---

**Hospital, Medicare Provider Number, Address, Telephone, Approval, Facility, and Physician Codes, Health Care System**

★ American Hospital Association (AHA) membership
☐ The Joint Commission accreditation          ◇ DNV Healthcare Inc. accreditation

○ American Osteopathic Association (AOA) accreditation
△ Commission on Accreditation of Rehabilitation Facilities (CARF) accreditation

## IOWA FALLS—Hardin County

★ **ELLSWORTH MUNICIPAL HOSPITAL (161380)**, 110 Rocksylvania Avenue, Zip 50126–2400; tel. 641/648–4631 **A**9 10 18 **F**11 13 15 28 29 34 35 40 43 45 50 53 57 59 64 65 75 76 77 81 85 86 87 93 97 100 101 102 104 107 110 113 118 129 131 132 **P**6 **S** Trinity Health, Novi, MI
Primary Contact: Cherelle Montanye, Chief Executive Officer
CFO: Betty Riley, Chief Financial Officer
CMO: Kathleen Haverkamp, M.D., Chief Medical Officer
CHR: Cheri Geitz, Director Human Resources
Web address: www.emhia.com
**Control:** City–Government, nonfederal **Service:** General Medical and Surgical

**Staffed Beds: 25 Admissions: 1031 Census: 11 Outpatient Visits: 30844 Births: 79 Total Expense ($000): 18169 Payroll Expense ($000): 8360 Personnel: 203**

## JEFFERSON—Greene County

★ **GREENE COUNTY MEDICAL CENTER (161325)**, 1000 West Lincolnway, Zip 50129–1697; tel. 515/386–2114, (Total facility includes 65 beds in nursing home–type unit) **A**9 10 18 **F**11 13 15 28 29 35 36 40 46 56 57 59 62 63 64 65 67 68 75 76 78 79 81 83 93 107 113 118 124 127 129 130 131 132 146 **P**5 6 **S** Iowa Health System, Des Moines, IA
Primary Contact: Carl P. Behne, Administrator and Chief Executive Officer
CFO: William Steussy, Chief Financial Officer
CMO: Steven Karber, M.D., Medical Director
CIO: Roger Overby, Executive Director Information Systems
CHR: Tammy Ford, Executive Director Human Resources
CNO: Cynthia Kail, Chief Nursing Officer and Executive Director Public Health
Web address: www.gcmchealth.com
**Control:** County–Government, nonfederal **Service:** General Medical and Surgical

**Staffed Beds: 90 Admissions: 608 Census: 62 Outpatient Visits: 26236 Births: 42 Total Expense ($000): 19748 Payroll Expense ($000): 9523 Personnel: 225**

## KEOKUK—Lee County

☒ **KEOKUK AREA HOSPITAL (160008)**, 1600 Morgan Street, Zip 52632–3456; tel. 319/524–7150 **A**1 9 10 **F**3 13 15 28 31 34 35 40 43 45 46 57 59 62 64 68 70 76 79 81 85 86 87 89 93 96 98 100 101 102 107 108 113 114 117 118 128 129 130 131 132 145 147 **P**6
Primary Contact: Walter Winkler, Chief Executive Officer
CFO: Walter Winkler, Chief Executive Officer
CMO: Kiran Khanolkar, M.D., Chief of Staff
CIO: Linda Schaffner, Chief Information Officer
CHR: Rhonda Schreck, Director Human Resources
CNO: Susan Pankey, Vice President Clinical Services
Web address: www.keokukhealthsystems.org
**Control:** Other not–for–profit (including NFP Corporation) **Service:** General Medical and Surgical

**Staffed Beds: 75 Admissions: 1947 Census: 22 Outpatient Visits: 37423 Births: 189 Total Expense ($000): 28831 Payroll Expense ($000): 13230 Personnel: 349**

## KEOSAUQUA—Van Buren County

★ **VAN BUREN COUNTY HOSPITAL (161337)**, 304 Franklin Street, Zip 52565; tel. 319/293–3171 **A**9 10 18 **F**3 7 10 11 13 15 28 29 32 34 35 40 43 45 46 50 57 59 64 65 70 75 76 77 81 85 86 87 89 93 97 102 107 110 111 113 118 124 126 127 129 131 132 134 145 146 147 **P**6
Primary Contact: Lisa W. Schnedler, FACHE, Chief Executive Officer and Administrator
CFO: Kara McEntee, Chief Financial Officer
CIO: Chris McEntee, Network Specialist
Web address: www.vbch.org
**Control:** County–Government, nonfederal **Service:** General Medical and Surgical

**Staffed Beds: 25 Admissions: 560 Census: 7 Outpatient Visits: 15859 Births: 32 Total Expense ($000): 13367 Payroll Expense ($000): 6086 Personnel: 150**

## KNOXVILLE—Marion County

**KNOXVILLE DIVISION** See Veterans Affairs Central Iowa Health Care System, Des Moines

## KNOXVILLE HOSPITAL & CLINICS (161355), 1002 South Lincoln Street,

★ **KNOXVILLE HOSPITAL & CLINICS (161355)**, 1002 South Lincoln Street, Zip 50138–3155; tel. 641/842–2151 **A**9 10 18 21 **F**3 8 11 13 15 28 29 31 34 40 43 45 47 48 49 50 54 57 59 64 65 68 75 76 77 79 81 85 86 93 97 102 107 108 110 111 113 117 118 128 129 131 132 134 145 146 147 **P**6
Primary Contact: Kevin Kincaid, Chief Executive Officer
COO: Christine Buttell, Chief Operating Officer
CFO: Maggie Hamilton–Beyer, Chief Financial Officer
CMO: Bryon Schaeffer, M.D., Chief of Medical Staff
CIO: Thom Richards, Director Information Technology
CHR: Brian Sims, Director Administrative Services
CNO: Mary Jane Applegate, Chief Nursing Officer
Web address: www.knoxvillehospital.org
**Control:** Other not–for–profit (including NFP Corporation) **Service:** General Medical and Surgical

**Staffed Beds: 25 Admissions: 665 Census: 10 Outpatient Visits: 24801 Births: 40 Total Expense ($000): 22808 Payroll Expense ($000): 10484 Personnel: 203**

## LAKE CITY—Calhoun County

★ **STEWART MEMORIAL COMMUNITY HOSPITAL (161350)**, 1301 West Main, Zip 51449–1585; tel. 712/464–3171 **A**9 10 18 **F**7 11 12 13 15 28 29 30 31 34 40 43 59 62 63 64 65 69 70 75 76 77 78 79 81 82 86 93 94 107 110 118 126 129 132 134 146 **P**5 6
Primary Contact: Leah Marxen, Administrator and Chief Executive Officer
CFO: Jim Henkenius, Chief Financial Officer
CHR: Bill Albright, Director Human Resources
Web address: www.stewartmemorial.org
**Control:** Other not–for–profit (including NFP Corporation) **Service:** General Medical and Surgical

**Staffed Beds: 25 Admissions: 627 Census: 7 Outpatient Visits: 46275 Births: 70 Total Expense ($000): 28543 Payroll Expense ($000): 12075 Personnel: 212**

## LE MARS—Plymouth County

★ **FLOYD VALLEY HOSPITAL (161368)**, 714 Lincoln Street N.E., Zip 51031–3314; tel. 712/546–7871 **A**9 10 18 **F**3 10 11 13 15 28 29 31 32 34 35 40 43 45 53 57 59 62 64 65 67 76 78 79 80 81 85 86 87 89 107 113 118 127 129 131 132 134 145 147 **S** Avera Health, Sioux Falls, SD
Primary Contact: Michael T. Donlin, FACHE, Administrator
CFO: Daryl Friedenbach, Director Fiscal Services
CMO: Shahid Naqvi, M.D., President Medical Staff
CHR: Mary Helen Gibson, Director Human Resources
Web address: www.floydvalleyhospital.org
**Control:** City–Government, nonfederal **Service:** General Medical and Surgical

**Staffed Beds: 25 Admissions: 1030 Census: 10 Outpatient Visits: 49775 Births: 106 Total Expense ($000): 28978 Payroll Expense ($000): 10203 Personnel: 242**

## LEON—Decatur County

★ **DECATUR COUNTY HOSPITAL (161340)**, 1405 N.W. Church Street, Zip 50144–1299; tel. 641/446–4871 **A**9 10 18 **F**7 11 15 28 29 31 40 57 59 64 67 68 75 78 79 81 85 89 93 107 111 113 118 127 129 132
Primary Contact: Lynn Milnes, Chief Executive Officer
CFO: Tara Spidle, Controller
CMO: Larry Richard, M.D., Chief Medical Staff
CHR: Jo Beth Smith, Director Support Services and Human Resources
Web address: www.decaturcountyhospital.org
**Control:** County–Government, nonfederal **Service:** General Medical and Surgical

**Staffed Beds: 25 Admissions: 332 Census: 5 Outpatient Visits: 12406 Births: 0 Total Expense ($000): 8654 Payroll Expense ($000): 3393 Personnel: 91**

## MANCHESTER—Delaware County

★ **REGIONAL MEDICAL CENTER (161343)**, 709 West Main Street, Zip 52057–0359, Mailing Address: P.O. Box 359, Zip 52057–0359; tel. 563/927–3232 **A**9 10 18 **F**3 7 11 13 15 17 28 29 34 35 36 38 40 43 44 50 53 57 59 61 62 63 64 65 66 68 70 75 76 77 79 81 82 85 86 89 93 94 97 104 107 108 110 111 113 118 126 127 128 129 130 131 132 133 145 147 **P**6
Primary Contact: Lon D. Butikofer, R.N., Ph.D., Chief Executive Officer
CFO: Danette Kramer, Chief Financial Officer
CIO: Amy Mensen, Chief Administrative Officer
CHR: Amy Mensen, Chief Administrative Officer
CNO: Patricia S. Doyle, R.N., Chief Nursing Officer
Web address: www.regmedctr.org
**Control:** County–Government, nonfederal **Service:** General Medical and Surgical

**Staffed Beds: 25 Admissions: 903 Census: 8 Outpatient Visits: 144410 Births: 164 Total Expense ($000): 31300 Payroll Expense ($000): 15617 Personnel: 305**

IA

## MANNING—Carroll County

★ **MANNING REGIONAL HEALTHCARE CENTER (161332)**, 410 Main Street, Zip 51455–1093; tel. 712/655–2072, (Total facility includes 56 beds in nursing home–type unit) **A**9 10 18 **F**3 4 5 11 13 15 34 35 38 40 43 45 46 50 51 56 57 59 61 64 68 71 74 75 76 77 78 79 81 82 84 85 87 89 92 93 107 108 113 118 127 129 131 132 145 147 **P**5
Primary Contact: John O'Brien, Chief Executive Officer
CFO: Abbey Stangl, Chief Financial Officer
CMO: Tracy Kahl, M.D., Chief Medical Officer
CIO: Kim C. Jahn, Director Support Services
CHR: Shelli Lorenzen, Director Human Resources
CNO: Amy S. Dawson, Chief Clinical Officer
Web address: www.mrhcia.com
**Control:** Other not–for–profit (including NFP Corporation) **Service:** General Medical and Surgical

**Staffed Beds:** 73 **Admissions:** 351 **Census:** 50 **Outpatient Visits:** 8061
**Births:** 31 **Total Expense ($000):** 11152 **Payroll Expense ($000):** 5017
**Personnel:** 156

## MAQUOKETA—Jackson County

✉ **JACKSON COUNTY REGIONAL HEALTH CENTER (161329)**, 700 West Grove Street, Zip 52060–0910; tel. 563/652–2474 **A**1 9 10 18 **F**3 7 11 15 28 34 40 43 45 53 59 62 64 65 70 75 76 77 81 87 89 93 107 113 118 128 129 131 132 145 **S** Genesis Health System, Davenport, IA
Primary Contact: Curt Coleman, FACHE, Chief Executive Officer
CFO: Donna Roeder, Chief Financial Officer
CHR: Shannon Langenberg, Director Human Resources
Web address: www.jcrhc.org
**Control:** County–Government, nonfederal **Service:** General Medical and Surgical

**Staffed Beds:** 25 **Admissions:** 277 **Census:** 3 **Outpatient Visits:** 19830
**Births:** 0 **Total Expense ($000):** 12623 **Payroll Expense ($000):** 5206
**Personnel:** 113

## MARENGO—Iowa County

★ **MARENGO MEMORIAL HOSPITAL (161317)**, 300 West May Street, Zip 52301–1261, Mailing Address: P.O. Box 228, Zip 52301–0228; tel. 319/642–5543 **A**9 10 18 **F**3 7 28 29 34 35 38 40 43 44 45 50 57 59 60 64 68 69 75 77 81 82 85 87 96 97 107 113 129 132 142 145 **P**6
Primary Contact: Barry Goettsch, Chief Executive Officer
COO: Mikaela Kienitz, Assistant Administrator
CFO: Nancy Kohrt, Chief Financial Officer
CHR: Lesa Waddell, Director Human Resources
Web address: www.marengohospital.org
**Control:** City–Government, nonfederal **Service:** General Medical and Surgical

**Staffed Beds:** 25 **Admissions:** 302 **Census:** 12 **Outpatient Visits:** 17583
**Births:** 0 **Total Expense ($000):** 13821 **Payroll Expense ($000):** 6279
**Personnel:** 138

## MARSHALLTOWN—Marshall County

★ **MARSHALLTOWN MEDICAL & SURGICAL CENTER (160001)**, 3 South Fourth Avenue, Zip 50158–2998; tel. 641/754–5151, (Total facility includes 26 beds in nursing home–type unit) **A**9 10 **F**3 7 11 13 15 18 20 22 26 28 29 30 35 40 41 42 43 44 45 46 48 50 53 54 57 59 62 64 65 67 68 70 71 74 75 76 77 79 81 82 85 86 87 89 91 92 93 94 97 107 108 110 111 114 118 126 127 128 129 130 131 134 145 146 147
Primary Contact: Brian D. Burnside, FACHE, Chief Executive Officer
CFO: Robert Downey, Chief Financial Officer
CMO: Milt Van Gundy, M.D., President Medical Staff
CIO: Robert Downey, Chief Financial Officer
CHR: Jill Petermeier, Senior Executive Human Resources
Web address: www.everydaychampions.org
**Control:** Other not–for–profit (including NFP Corporation) **Service:** General Medical and Surgical

**Staffed Beds:** 105 **Admissions:** 3311 **Census:** 32 **Outpatient Visits:** 205371
**Births:** 528 **Total Expense ($000):** 54272 **Payroll Expense ($000):** 27815
**Personnel:** 513

## MASON CITY—Cerro Gordo County

✠ **MERCY MEDICAL CENTER–NORTH IOWA (160064)**, 1000 Fourth Street S.W., Zip 50401–2800; tel. 641/428–7000 **A**1 2 3 5 9 10 13 **F**3 11 12 13 15 17 18 20 22 24 26 28 29 30 31 32 34 35 36 37 38 39 40 43 44 45 46 47 48 49 50 54 56 57 59 60 61 62 63 64 65 66 68 70 71 72 74 75 76 77 78 79 81 82 84 85 86 87 89 90 92 93 96 97 98 99 100 101 102 103 104 105 107 108 110 111 113 114 116 117 118 119 120 122 124 125 127 128 129 130 131 133 134 143 145 146 147 **P**1 6 **S** Trinity Health, Novi, MI
Primary Contact: Rod G. Schlader, Interim President and Chief Executive Officer
COO: Diane Fischels, Senior Vice President and Chief Operating Officer
CFO: Moni Haxtom, Interim Chief Financial Officer
CMO: Paul Manternach, M.D., Senior Vice President Physician Integration
CIO: Randy Haskins, Director Information Systems
CHR: Jackie Luecht, Chief Human Resources Officer
CNO: Kim Chamberlin, Vice President Patient Services and Chief Nursing Officer
Web address: www.mercynorthiowa.com
**Control:** Church–operated, Nongovernment, not–for profit **Service:** General Medical and Surgical

**Staffed Beds:** 240 **Admissions:** 13479 **Census:** 143 **Outpatient Visits:** 423897 **Births:** 923 **Total Expense ($000):** 292787 **Payroll Expense ($000):** 122914 **Personnel:** 1994

## MISSOURI VALLEY—Harrison County

★ **ALEGENT HEALTH–COMMUNITY MEMORIAL HOSPITAL (161309)**, 631 North Eighth Street, Zip 51555–1199; tel. 712/642–2784 **A**9 10 18 **F**3 11 15 18 28 29 30 31 35 39 40 43 45 50 54 59 64 71 75 77 78 79 81 82 85 93 99 100 102 103 104 107 110 113 118 126 128 132 134 143 145 **P**8 **S** Alegent Health, Omaha, NE
Primary Contact: Robert A. Valentine, Regional Administrator
CFO: Matthew Smith, Operations Director Finance and Support Services
CMO: Daniel Richter, M.D., Chief of Staff
CHR: Julie Brown, Human Resources Specialist
CNO: Darcy Behrendt, R.N., Chief Nurse Executive
Web address: www.alegent.org
**Control:** Other not–for–profit (including NFP Corporation) **Service:** General Medical and Surgical

**Staffed Beds:** 16 **Admissions:** 559 **Census:** 6 **Outpatient Visits:** 60680
**Births:** 1 **Total Expense ($000):** 21191 **Payroll Expense ($000):** 7001
**Personnel:** 158

## MOUNT AYR—Ringgold County

**RINGGOLD COUNTY HOSPITAL (161373)**, 504 North Cleveland Street, Zip 50854–2201; tel. 641/464–3226 **A**9 10 18 **F**3 7 11 15 28 29 31 35 38 40 43 56 57 59 60 64 65 81 93 107 111 113 118 132 147 **P**6
Primary Contact: Gordon W. Winkler, Administrator and Chief Executive Officer
CFO: Teresa Roberts, Chief Financial Officer
CIO: Jan Lyons, Regional Director Health Improvement Management
CHR: Mitzi Hymbaugh, Chief Personnel
Web address: www.rchmtayr.org
**Control:** County–Government, nonfederal **Service:** General Medical and Surgical

**Staffed Beds:** 16 **Admissions:** 327 **Census:** 3 **Outpatient Visits:** 24287
**Births:** 0 **Total Expense ($000):** 15286 **Payroll Expense ($000):** 6108
**Personnel:** 117

## MOUNT PLEASANT—Henry County

★ **HENRY COUNTY HEALTH CENTER (161356)**, 407 South White Street, Zip 52641–2299; tel. 319/385–3141, (Total facility includes 49 beds in nursing home–type unit) **A**9 10 18 **F**3 7 11 13 15 28 29 31 32 34 35 40 41 43 45 50 57 59 64 67 68 70 75 76 77 78 79 81 85 86 87 89 93 102 107 108 110 114 117 118 127 128 129 130 131 132 134 142 144 145 147 **P**6
Primary Contact: Robb Gardner, Chief Executive Officer
CFO: David Muhs, Chief Financial Officer
CMO: Steve Davis, M.D., Chief of Staff
CIO: Steve Stewart, Director Information Technology
CHR: Jim Carson, Director Human Resources
CNO: Jodi Geerts, Chief Nursing Officer
Web address: www.hchc.org
**Control:** County–Government, nonfederal **Service:** General Medical and Surgical

**Staffed Beds:** 74 **Admissions:** 767 **Census:** 51 **Outpatient Visits:** 168983
**Births:** 138 **Total Expense ($000):** 29373 **Payroll Expense ($000):** 12518
**Personnel:** 253

**IA**

---

**Hospital, Medicare Provider Number, Address, Telephone, Approval, Facility, and Physician Codes, Health Care System**

★ American Hospital Association (AHA) membership
☐ The Joint Commission accreditation ◇ DNV Healthcare Inc. accreditation
○ American Osteopathic Association (AOA) accreditation
△ Commission on Accreditation of Rehabilitation Facilities (CARF) accreditation

**MENTAL HEALTH INSTITUTE (164004)**, 1200 East Washington Street, Zip 52641–1898; tel. 319/385–7231 **A**9 10 **F**4 5 29 75 86 98 100 101 103 129 131 134
Primary Contact: Ron Mullen, Superintendent
CFO: Barb Wheeler, Business Manager
CHR: Janice Creighton, Human Resources Associate
Web address: www.dhs.state.ia.us
**Control:** State–Government, nonfederal **Service:** Alcoholism and other chemical dependency

**Staffed Beds:** 79 **Admissions:** 768 **Census:** 61 **Outpatient Visits:** 35 **Births:** 0 **Total Expense ($000):** 8408 **Payroll Expense ($000):** 4729 **Personnel:** 82

### MUSCATINE—Muscatine County

✠ **TRINITY MUSCATINE (160013)**, 1518 Mulberry Avenue, Zip 52761–3499; tel. 563/264–9100 **A**1 9 10 20 **F**3 11 13 15 28 31 40 43 46 50 56 57 59 61 64 68 69 70 75 76 79 81 83 85 87 89 102 107 108 110 113 118 128 129 132 147 **S** Iowa Health System, Des Moines, IA
Primary Contact: James M. Hayes, Chief Executive Officer
CFO: Greg Pagliuzza, Chief Financial Officer
CMO: Manasi Nadkarni, M.D., Vice President Medical Affairs
CIO: Richard E. Maere, Account Executive Information Technology
CHR: Karla Blaser, Director Human Resources
CNO: Pam Askew, R.N., Vice President Patient Care Services
Web address: www.trinitymuscatine.org
**Control:** Other not–for–profit (including NFP Corporation) **Service:** General Medical and Surgical

**Staffed Beds:** 56 **Admissions:** 1523 **Census:** 14 **Outpatient Visits:** 86917 **Births:** 317 **Total Expense ($000):** 37599 **Payroll Expense ($000):** 15702 **Personnel:** 334

### NEVADA—Story County

★ **STORY COUNTY MEDICAL CENTER (161333)**, 640 South 19th Street, Zip 50201–2266; tel. 515/382–2111, (Total facility includes 60 beds in nursing home–type unit) **A**9 10 18 **F**3 7 11 28 29 31 32 35 36 40 43 50 53 57 59 64 68 75 77 79 81 85 93 97 107 113 126 129 130 131 132 134 142 145 147 **P**6
Primary Contact: Todd Willert, Administrator
COO: Julie Schreitmueller, Chief Operating Officer
CFO: Jane Ramthun, Chief Financial Officer
CHR: Kaylee Siebrecht, Director Human Resources
Web address: www.storymedical.org
**Control:** County–Government, nonfederal **Service:** General Medical and Surgical

**Staffed Beds:** 77 **Admissions:** 440 **Census:** 67 **Outpatient Visits:** 27516 **Births:** 0 **Total Expense ($000):** 17358 **Payroll Expense ($000):** 8287 **Personnel:** 168

### NEW HAMPTON—Chickasaw County

★ **MERCY MEDICAL CENTER–NEW HAMPTON (161331)**, 308 North Maple Avenue, Zip 50659–1142; tel. 641/394–4121 **A**9 10 18 **F**3 11 13 15 28 29 34 35 40 43 45 48 56 57 59 64 65 68 74 76 77 79 81 85 93 97 107 108 110 113 118 130 132 145 147 **P**1 **S** Trinity Health, Novi, MI
Primary Contact: Bruce E. Roesler, FACHE, President and Chief Executive Officer
CFO: Jennifer Rapenske, Manager Financial Services
CMO: D. Paul McQuillen, D.O., Chief of Staff
CIO: Randy Haskins, Director Information Systems
CHR: Lisa Heller, Manager Human Resources
CNO: Sherrie L. Laubenthal, R.N., Chief Nursing Officer
Web address: www.mercynewhampton.com
**Control:** Church–operated, Nongovernment, not–for profit **Service:** General Medical and Surgical

**Staffed Beds:** 18 **Admissions:** 454 **Census:** 5 **Outpatient Visits:** 17825 **Births:** 15 **Total Expense ($000):** 14137 **Payroll Expense ($000):** 5042 **Personnel:** 86

### NEWTON—Jasper County

★ ○ **SKIFF MEDICAL CENTER (160032)**, 204 Fourth Avenue East, Zip 50208–3100, Mailing Address: P.O. Box 1006, Zip 50208–1006; tel. 641/792–1273 **A**9 10 11 **F**3 11 13 15 17 28 29 30 31 32 34 35 36 40 43 44 45 57 59 62 63 64 65 70 75 76 77 78 79 81 84 85 93 96 102 107 108 110 111 114 117 118 123 129 130 131 132 134 145 147 **P**6
Primary Contact: Steve Long, FACHE, President and Chief Executive Officer
COO: Brett Altman, Clinical Operations Officer
CFO: Mike Anderson, Chief Financial Officer
CIO: Janice Bilmer, Director, Information Services
CHR: Ellen Graber, Director, Human Resources
CNO: Mary Swoboda, R.N., Chief Nursing Officer
Web address: www.skiffmed.com
**Control:** City–Government, nonfederal **Service:** General Medical and Surgical

**Staffed Beds:** 48 **Admissions:** 1888 **Census:** 19 **Outpatient Visits:** 71969 **Births:** 165 **Total Expense ($000):** 32241 **Payroll Expense ($000):** 16694 **Personnel:** 295

### OAKDALE—Johnson County

**IOWA MEDICAL AND CLASSIFICATION CENTER**, Highway 965, Zip 52319, Mailing Address: IMCC, Box A, Zip 52319; tel. 319/626–2391 **F**29 38 39 59 75 98 101 102 103 105 129 131 142
Primary Contact: Daniel Craig, Warden
Web address: www.oakdaleprison.com/
**Control:** State–Government, nonfederal **Service:** Psychiatric

**Staffed Beds:** 27 **Admissions:** 42 **Census:** 25 **Outpatient Visits:** 5 **Births:** 0 **Personnel:** 26

### OELWEIN—Fayette County

★ **MERCY HOSPITAL OF FRANCISCAN SISTERS (161338)**, 201 Eighth Avenue S.E., Zip 50662–2447; tel. 319/283–6000, (Total facility includes 39 beds in nursing home–type unit) **A**9 10 18 **F**7 11 15 29 30 34 35 46 56 57 59 69 75 79 81 97 107 111 118 126 127 129 131 132 145 **P**1 **S** Wheaton Franciscan Healthcare, Wheaton, IL
Primary Contact: Terri Derflinger, Administrator
CFO: Timothy Huber, Manager Financial Support
CIO: Todd Richardson, Regional Vice President Information Services
CHR: Vicki L. Parsons, Regional Vice President Human Resources
Web address: www.covhealth.com
**Control:** Church–operated, Nongovernment, not–for profit **Service:** General Medical and Surgical

**Staffed Beds:** 64 **Admissions:** 461 **Census:** 36 **Outpatient Visits:** 31632 **Births:** 0 **Total Expense ($000):** 13376 **Payroll Expense ($000):** 5693 **Personnel:** 105

### ONAWA—Monona County

★ **BURGESS HEALTH CENTER (161359)**, 1600 Diamond Street, Zip 51040–1548; tel. 712/423–2311 **A**9 10 18 **F**3 7 11 13 15 28 29 31 32 34 35 40 56 57 59 62 63 64 65 70 75 76 77 78 79 81 82 85 89 93 97 99 100 101 103 104 107 113 118 126 129 131 132 134 145 147 **P**6
Primary Contact: Francis G. Tramp, President
CFO: Shawn Gosch, Chief Financial Officer
CMO: John Garred, Sr., M.D., Chief Medical Officer
CIO: Kim Norby, Chief Information Officer
CHR: Denise Trukenmiller, Director Human Resources
Web address: www.burgesshc.org
**Control:** Other not–for–profit (including NFP Corporation) **Service:** General Medical and Surgical

**Staffed Beds:** 25 **Admissions:** 827 **Census:** 10 **Outpatient Visits:** 70429 **Births:** 27 **Total Expense ($000):** 23359 **Payroll Expense ($000):** 9737 **Personnel:** 232

### ORANGE CITY—Sioux County

★ **ORANGE CITY AREA HEALTH SYSTEM (161360)**, 1000 Lincoln Circle S.E., Zip 51041–1398; tel. 712/737–4984, (Total facility includes 79 beds in nursing home–type unit) **A**9 10 18 **F**7 10 11 13 15 18 28 29 31 34 35 40 45 50 53 56 57 59 60 62 63 64 67 68 69 70 75 76 77 78 79 81 82 85 86 87 89 93 97 107 110 111 113 116 119 124 126 129 130 131 132 145 146 147 **P**6 **S** Sanford Health, Sioux Falls, SD
Primary Contact: Martin W. Guthmiller, Chief Executive Officer
COO: Daniel P. McCarty, Chief Operating Officer
CFO: Dina Baas, Director Financial Services
CHR: Shari Baker, Director Human Resources
Web address: www.ochealthsystem.org
**Control:** City–Government, nonfederal **Service:** General Medical and Surgical

**Staffed Beds:** 104 **Admissions:** 956 **Census:** 85 **Outpatient Visits:** 70180 **Births:** 186 **Total Expense ($000):** 35123 **Payroll Expense ($000):** 15383 **Personnel:** 375

**IA**

## OSAGE—Mitchell County

★ **MITCHELL COUNTY REGIONAL HEALTH CENTER (161323)**, 616 North
Eighth Street, Zip 50461–1498; tel. 641/732–6000 **A**9 10 18 **F**7 8 11 15 18
28 29 34 35 40 50 57 59 63 64 65 75 81 85 87 91 93 107 110 113 118
126 129 131 132 143 145 **P**8 **S** Trinity Health, Novi, MI
Primary Contact: Desiree Einsweiler, Interim Chief Executive Officer
CFO: Alan W. Streeter, Chief Financial Officer
CMO: Kelly Ross, M.D., Chief of Staff
CHR: Tom Nelson, Director Human Resources
Web address: www.mitchellcohospital–clinics.com
**Control:** County–Government, nonfederal **Service:** General Medical and Surgical

**Staffed Beds:** 25 **Admissions:** 490 **Census:** 6 **Outpatient Visits:** 57292
**Births:** 0 **Total Expense ($000):** 16065 **Payroll Expense ($000):** 5617
**Personnel:** 134

## OSCEOLA—Clarke County

★ **CLARKE COUNTY HOSPITAL (161348)**, 800 South Fillmore Street,
Zip 50213–1619; tel. 641/342–2184 **A**9 10 18 **F**7 11 15 18 28 29 31 34 35
40 45 53 57 59 64 67 68 75 81 89 90 93 94 96 107 111 114 115 116 117
118 127 128 129 132 134 143 **S** Iowa Health System, Des Moines, IA
Primary Contact: Brian G. Evans, FACHE, Chief Executive Officer
CFO: Michael Thilges, Chief Financial Officer
CMO: George Fotiadis, M.D., Chief of Staff
CIO: Dennis Blazek, Chief Information Officer
CHR: Kate Emanuel, Director Human Resources
Web address: www.clarkehosp.org
**Control:** County–Government, nonfederal **Service:** General Medical and Surgical

**Staffed Beds:** 25 **Admissions:** 377 **Census:** 14 **Outpatient Visits:** 20760
**Births:** 0 **Total Expense ($000):** 16567 **Payroll Expense ($000):** 5450
**Personnel:** 143

## OSKALOOSA—Mahaska County

⊠ **MAHASKA HEALTH PARTNERSHIP (161379)**, 1229 C Avenue East,
Zip 52577–4298; tel. 641/672–3100 **A**1 9 10 18 **F**5 7 11 13 15 28 29 30 31
34 35 40 43 45 47 50 54 56 57 59 62 63 64 68 69 70 75 76 77 78 79 81
87 93 97 98 99 100 101 102 103 104 107 110 111 113 118 128 129 132
134 145 147 **P**6
Primary Contact: Jay Christensen, FACHE, Administrator
CFO: Susan Horras, Chief Financial Officer
CMO: Sreedhar Somisetty, M.D., Chief Medical Officer
CHR: Jacky Bresnahan, Director Human Resources
Web address: www.mahaskahealth.com
**Control:** County–Government, nonfederal **Service:** General Medical and Surgical

**Staffed Beds:** 33 **Admissions:** 1748 **Census:** 20 **Outpatient Visits:** 91506
**Births:** 195 **Total Expense ($000):** 33196 **Payroll Expense ($000):** 18162
**Personnel:** 316

## OTTUMWA—Wapello County

☐ △ **OTTUMWA REGIONAL HEALTH CENTER (160089)**, 1001 Pennsylvania
Avenue, Zip 52501–2186; tel. 641/684–2300 **A**1 2 7 9 10 **F**3 7 11 13 15 20
22 26 28 29 30 31 34 35 40 43 46 47 48 51 54 56 57 59 62 64 68 70 72
73 75 76 77 78 79 81 82 85 86 87 89 90 93 100 102 107 108 110 111 112
118 124 125 128 129 131 134 144 145 146 147 **P**6 **S** RegionalCare Hospital
Partners, Brentwood, TN
Primary Contact: Philip G. Dionne, Chief Executive Officer
CFO: Dan Porter, Vice President and Chief Financial Officer
CMO: Kenneth Wayne, M.D., Chief Medical Officer
CHR: JoEllen Randall, Administrative Director Human Resources
Web address: www.orhc.com
**Control:** Corporation, Investor–owned, for–profit **Service:** General Medical and
Surgical

**Staffed Beds:** 88 **Admissions:** 3398 **Census:** 40 **Outpatient Visits:** 123658
**Births:** 605 **Total Expense ($000):** 69939 **Payroll Expense ($000):** 25016
**Personnel:** 588

## PELLA—Marion County

⊠ **PELLA REGIONAL HEALTH CENTER (161367)**, 404 Jefferson Street,
Zip 50219–1257; tel. 641/628–3150, (Total facility includes 63 beds in nursing
home–type unit) **A**1 9 10 18 **F**3 11 13 15 28 29 30 31 34 35 40 43 48 50 59
60 62 63 64 65 67 70 75 76 77 78 79 81 85 86 87 93 97 107 108 110 111
114 118 125 126 127 128 129 130 131 132 140 143 145 146 147 **P**6
Primary Contact: Robert D. Kroese, FACHE, Chief Executive Officer
COO: Robert D. Kroese, FACHE, Chief Executive Officer
CFO: Ron Wauters, Chief Financial Officer
CIO: Tait Smock, Manager Information Systems
CHR: Teri Lickteig, HR Director
CNO: Yvonne M. O'Brien, MS, Chief of Nursing
Web address: www.pellahealth.org
**Control:** Other not–for–profit (including NFP Corporation) **Service:** General
Medical and Surgical

**Staffed Beds:** 88 **Admissions:** 1713 **Census:** 66 **Outpatient Visits:** 141678
**Births:** 375 **Total Expense ($000):** 47600 **Payroll Expense ($000):** 20076
**Personnel:** 552

## PERRY—Dallas County

★ **DALLAS COUNTY HOSPITAL (161322)**, 610 10th Street, Zip 50220–2221;
tel. 515/465–3547 **A**9 10 18 **F**11 15 28 29 31 34 35 40 43 57 59 68 75 78
79 81 82 85 89 107 110 111 115 118 127 128 131 132 145 147
Primary Contact: Matt Wille, Chief Executive Officer
CFO: Sandra Christensen, Chief Financial Officer
CMO: Steven Sohn, M.D., President Medical Staff
CHR: Sherry Smith, Manager Human Resources
Web address: www.dallascohospital.org
**Control:** County–Government, nonfederal **Service:** General Medical and Surgical

**Staffed Beds:** 18 **Admissions:** 310 **Census:** 4 **Outpatient Visits:** 27681
**Births:** 0 **Total Expense ($000):** 13966 **Payroll Expense ($000):** 4417
**Personnel:** 90

## POCAHONTAS—Pocahontas County

★ **POCAHONTAS COMMUNITY HOSPITAL (161305)**, 606 N.W. Seventh,
Zip 50574–1099; tel. 712/335–3501 **A**9 10 18 **F**7 11 15 17 28 29 31 35 40
43 45 59 62 63 64 70 75 76 77 78 79 81 84 89 93 107 110 118 127 129
131 132 134 145 147 **P**6 **S** Iowa Health System, Des Moines, IA
Primary Contact: James D. Roetman, President and Chief Executive Officer
CFO: Lynn Raveling, Chief Financial Officer
Web address: www.pocahontashospital.org
**Control:** City–Government, nonfederal **Service:** General Medical and Surgical

**Staffed Beds:** 20 **Admissions:** 307 **Census:** 3 **Outpatient Visits:** 32064
**Births:** 0 **Total Expense ($000):** 8348 **Payroll Expense ($000):** 2885
**Personnel:** 83

## PRIMGHAR—O'brien County

★ **BAUM HARMON MERCY HOSPITAL (161300)**, 255 North Welch Avenue,
Zip 51245–1034, Mailing Address: P.O. Box 528, Zip 51245–0528;
tel. 712/957–2300 **A**9 10 18 **F**11 15 28 29 30 31 32 34 35 40 45 53 57 59
64 67 70 75 77 78 81 89 118 126 127 131 132 **P**6 **S** Trinity Health, Novi, MI
Primary Contact: David Liebsack, Chief Executive Officer
CFO: Sue E. McCauley, Director Finance
CMO: Shailesh Desai, M.D., Chief of Staff
Web address: www.baumharmon.org
**Control:** Church–operated, Nongovernment, not–for profit **Service:** General
Medical and Surgical

**Staffed Beds:** 13 **Admissions:** 156 **Census:** 1 **Outpatient Visits:** 23299
**Births:** 0 **Total Expense ($000):** 7095 **Payroll Expense ($000):** 3387
**Personnel:** 61

## RED OAK—Montgomery County

★ **MONTGOMERY COUNTY MEMORIAL HOSPITAL (161363)**, 2301 Eastern
Avenue, Zip 51566–1300, Mailing Address: P.O. Box 498, Zip 51566–0498;
tel. 712/623–7000 **A**9 10 18 **F**11 13 15 28 29 31 34 35 40 44 45 50 53 57
59 62 63 64 68 69 70 75 76 77 78 79 81 82 85 86 87 89 93 107 110 111
113 117 118 128 129 132 134 145 146 147
Primary Contact: Allen E. Pohren, Administrator
CFO: Rick Leinen, Chief Financial Officer
CMO: William Artherholt, M.D., Chief of Staff
CIO: Ron Kloewer, Chief Information Officer
Web address: www.mcmh.org
**Control:** County–Government, nonfederal **Service:** General Medical and Surgical

**Staffed Beds:** 25 **Admissions:** 1156 **Census:** 15 **Outpatient Visits:** 46503
**Births:** 78 **Total Expense ($000):** 26746 **Payroll Expense ($000):** 12517
**Personnel:** 247

**IA**

**Hospital, Medicare Provider Number, Address, Telephone, Approval, Facility, and Physician Codes, Health Care System**

★ American Hospital Association (AHA) membership
☐ The Joint Commission accreditation ◇ DNV Healthcare Inc. accreditation
○ American Osteopathic Association (AOA) accreditation
△ Commission on Accreditation of Rehabilitation Facilities (CARF) accreditation

© 2012 AHA Guide *Many Facility Codes have changed. Please refer to the AHA Guide Code Chart.* Hospitals **A225**

## ROCK RAPIDS—Lyon County

★ **SANFORD MEDICAL CENTER ROCK RAPIDS (161321)**, 801 South Greene Street, Zip 51246–1998; tel. 712/472–2591 **A**9 10 18 **F**11 28 31 34 40 41 45 53 57 59 77 81 87 89 97 107 118 126 129 130 132 134 145 **P**6 **S** Sanford Health, Sioux Falls, SD
Primary Contact: Tammy Loosbrock, Chief Executive Officer
CFO: Stanley Knobloch, Chief Financial Officer
CMO: David Springer, M.D., President Medical Staff
CHR: Rachel K. Ask, Supervisor Human Resources
Web address: www.sanfordmerrill.org
**Control:** Other not–for–profit (including NFP Corporation) **Service:** General Medical and Surgical

**Staffed Beds:** 16 **Admissions:** 290 **Census:** 3 **Outpatient Visits:** 17614
**Births:** 0 **Total Expense ($000):** 7663 **Payroll Expense ($000):** 3500
**Personnel:** 66

**SANFORD MERRILL MEDICAL CENTER** See Sanford Medical Center Rock Rapids

## ROCK VALLEY—Sioux County

★ **HEGG MEMORIAL HEALTH CENTER AVERA (161336)**, 1202 21st Avenue, Zip 51247–1497; tel. 712/476–8000, (Total facility includes 60 beds in nursing home–type unit) **A**9 10 18 **F**3 11 13 15 28 29 31 34 35 36 40 41 43 45 53 57 59 62 64 67 68 70 75 76 77 78 79 81 85 89 93 97 107 110 111 113 118 127 129 130 131 132 134 143 146 147 **S** Avera Health, Sioux Falls, SD
Primary Contact: Glenn Zevenbergen, Chief Executive Officer
CFO: Kari Timmer, Chief Financial Officer
CMO: Kevin Post, D.O., Chief Medical Officer
CHR: Tammy Faber, Director Human Resources
CNO: Sherri Kerr, Director of Nursing
Web address: www.hegghc.org
**Control:** Other not–for–profit (including NFP Corporation) **Service:** General Medical and Surgical

**Staffed Beds:** 85 **Admissions:** 366 **Census:** 63 **Outpatient Visits:** 33289
**Births:** 82 **Total Expense ($000):** 14374 **Payroll Expense ($000):** 6981
**Personnel:** 193

## SAC CITY—Sac County

★ **LORING HOSPITAL (161370)**, 211 Highland Avenue, Zip 50583–0217; tel. 712/662–7105 **A**9 10 18 **F**3 11 15 28 29 30 31 34 35 40 45 57 59 62 63 64 68 75 78 79 81 86 87 93 107 110 114 118 124 128 129 131 132 145 **S** Iowa Health System, Des Moines, IA
Primary Contact: Michael S. Ketcham, President and Chief Executive Officer
CFO: Angie Fischer, Chief Financial Officer
CMO: Les Marczewski, M.D., Chief Medical Officer
CIO: Kathy Veit, Director Health Information Services
CHR: Becky Pontious, Human Resources/Accounting
CNO: Lori Forneris, R.N., Chief Clinical Officer
Web address: www.loringhospital.org
**Control:** Other not–for–profit (including NFP Corporation) **Service:** General Medical and Surgical

**Staffed Beds:** 25 **Admissions:** 991 **Census:** 9 **Outpatient Visits:** 26128
**Births:** 0 **Total Expense ($000):** 11522 **Payroll Expense ($000):** 4253
**Personnel:** 109

## SHELDON—O'brien County

★ **SANFORD SHELDON MEDICAL CENTER (161381)**, 118 North Seventh Avenue, Zip 51201–1235, Mailing Address: P.O. Box 250, Zip 51201–0250; tel. 712/324–5041, (Total facility includes 70 beds in nursing home–type unit) **A**9 10 18 **F**11 13 15 28 29 31 34 35 38 40 45 50 53 56 57 59 62 63 64 65 67 68 74 75 76 77 78 79 81 82 84 86 87 91 93 96 107 110 113 114 118 126 128 129 130 131 132 134 145 147 **P**6 **S** Sanford Health, Sioux Falls, SD
Primary Contact: Richard E. Nordahl, Chief Executive Officer
CFO: Deb Rosburg, Chief Financial Officer
CMO: Shane Smith, M.D., Physician
CIO: Scott Moffitt, Director Information Systems
CHR: Dianne Wolthuizen, Director Human Resources
CNO: Joni DeKok, Chief Nursing Officer
Web address: www.sanfordsheldon.org
**Control:** Other not–for–profit (including NFP Corporation) **Service:** General Medical and Surgical

**Staffed Beds:** 95 **Admissions:** 863 **Census:** 72 **Outpatient Visits:** 81118
**Births:** 124 **Total Expense ($000):** 24850 **Payroll Expense ($000):** 12040
**Personnel:** 280

## SHENANDOAH—Page County

★ **SHENANDOAH MEDICAL CENTER (161366)**, 300 Pershing Avenue, Zip 51601–2397; tel. 712/246–1230, (Total facility includes 53 beds in nursing home–type unit) **A**9 10 18 **F**3 10 11 13 15 18 28 31 34 36 40 43 45 50 53 56 57 59 62 63 64 67 68 69 70 75 76 77 78 79 81 85 87 93 99 104 107 108 111 113 116 117 118 128 129 131 132 134 145 146 147 **P**6
Primary Contact: Karen S. Cole, MS, FACHE, Chief Executive Officer
CFO: Sandra Chesshire, Chief Financial Officer
CMO: Jerry Schaaf, M.D., Chief Medical Officer
CIO: John Eckmann, Director Information Systems
CHR: Keli Royal, Director Human Resources
CNO: Victor Bycroft, R.N., Chief Nursing Officer
Web address: www.shenandoahmedcenter.com
**Control:** Other not–for–profit (including NFP Corporation) **Service:** General Medical and Surgical

**Staffed Beds:** 78 **Admissions:** 784 **Census:** 54 **Outpatient Visits:** 171721
**Births:** 115 **Total Expense ($000):** 24116 **Payroll Expense ($000):** 11129
**Personnel:** 199

## SIBLEY—Osceola County

★ **OSCEOLA COMMUNITY HOSPITAL (161345)**, Ninth Avenue North, Zip 51249–0258, Mailing Address: P.O. Box 258, Zip 51249–0258; tel. 712/754–2574, (Data for 273 days) **A**9 10 18 **F**3 8 9 10 11 13 15 17 18 26 28 29 31 32 34 35 36 40 43 45 49 53 56 57 59 61 62 64 65 67 68 70 75 76 77 78 79 81 82 83 84 85 86 87 89 93 107 108 110 113 118 124 127 128 129 130 131 132 134 142 143 144 145 146 147 **P**5 **S** Avera Health, Sioux Falls, SD
Primary Contact: Janet H. Dykstra, Chief Executive Officer
CFO: Jerri Palsrok, Manager Business Office
CMO: Gregory J. Kosters, D.O., Chief Medical Officer
CIO: Sherry McElroy, Director Health Information Management
Web address: www.osceolacommunityhospital.org
**Control:** Other not–for–profit (including NFP Corporation) **Service:** General Medical and Surgical

**Staffed Beds:** 25 **Admissions:** 291 **Census:** 4 **Outpatient Visits:** 14825
**Births:** 21 **Total Expense ($000):** 7669 **Payroll Expense ($000):** 2455
**Personnel:** 79

## SIGOURNEY—Keokuk County

**KEOKUK COUNTY HEALTH CENTER (161315)**, 23019 Highway 149, Zip 52591; tel. 641/622–2720 **A**9 10 18 **F**1 3 7 11 12 28 29 30 34 35 38 40 43 45 46 50 56 57 59 63 64 65 67 75 77 82 84 86 87 90 91 93 97 107 113 127 129 130 131 132 133 134 143 145 147 **P**5 6
Primary Contact: Matthew Ives, Interim Chief Executive Officer and Chief Financial Officer
CFO: Matthew Ives, Interim Chief Executive Officer and Chief Financial Officer
Web address: www.kchc.net
**Control:** County–Government, nonfederal **Service:** General Medical and Surgical

**Staffed Beds:** 14 **Admissions:** 100 **Census:** 7 **Outpatient Visits:** 6578
**Births:** 0 **Total Expense ($000):** 7418 **Payroll Expense ($000):** 3304
**Personnel:** 83

## SIOUX CENTER—Sioux County

★ **SIOUX CENTER COMMUNITY HOSPITAL AND HEALTH CENTER AVERA (161346)**, 605 South Main Avenue, Zip 51250–1398; tel. 712/722–1271, (Total facility includes 69 beds in nursing home–type unit) **A**9 10 18 **F**3 8 10 13 15 17 18 28 29 30 31 34 35 40 41 43 45 56 57 59 62 63 64 67 68 74 75 76 77 78 79 81 82 83 84 85 86 89 93 97 107 111 113 118 124 127 129 130 131 132 134 143 145 146 147 **P**6 **S** Avera Health, Sioux Falls, SD
Primary Contact: Kayleen R. Lee, Chief Executive Officer
COO: Marla Toering, Chief Operating Officer
CFO: Jackson Schuiteman, Chief Financial Officer
CHR: Gail Vonk, Director Human Resources and Marketing
Web address: www.schospital.org
**Control:** Other not–for–profit (including NFP Corporation) **Service:** General Medical and Surgical

**Staffed Beds:** 90 **Admissions:** 617 **Census:** 75 **Outpatient Visits:** 47316
**Births:** 196 **Total Expense ($000):** 26602 **Payroll Expense ($000):** 12784
**Personnel:** 302

IA

## SIOUX CITY—Woodbury County

✠ **MERCY MEDICAL CENTER–SIOUX CITY (160153)**, 801 Fifth Street, Zip 51101–1326, Mailing Address: P.O. Box 3168, Zip 51102–3168; tel. 712/279–2010 **A**1 2 3 5 9 10 **F**3 5 11 13 15 17 18 20 22 24 26 28 29 30 32 34 35 36 37 38 40 43 44 45 48 49 50 51 55 56 57 59 61 64 65 68 70 71 74 75 76 77 78 79 81 82 84 85 86 87 89 90 92 93 94 96 97 98 99 100 101 102 103 104 105 107 108 110 111 113 114 117 118 123 125 128 129 131 134 143 145 146 147 **P**6 7 8 **S** Trinity Health, Novi, MI
Primary Contact: Robert J. Peebles, President and Chief Executive Officer
COO: Mari Kaptain–Dahlen, Chief Operating Officer
CFO: J. Steven Eavenson, Interim Vice President and Chief Financial Officer
CMO: Larry W. Sellers, M.D., Chief Medical Officer
CIO: Steve Larson, M.D., Director Information Systems
CHR: Julie Anfinson, Director Human Resources
Web address: www.mercysiouxcity.com
**Control:** Church–operated, Nongovernment, not–for profit **Service:** General Medical and Surgical

**Staffed Beds:** 238 **Admissions:** 11261 **Census:** 152 **Outpatient Visits:** 270361 **Births:** 390 **Total Expense ($000):** 195319 **Payroll Expense ($000):** 78969 **Personnel:** 1288

★ **ST. LUKE'S REGIONAL MEDICAL CENTER (160146)**, 2720 Stone Park Boulevard, Zip 51104–2000; tel. 712/279–3500 **A**3 5 9 10 21 **F**3 11 13 15 17 18 20 22 26 28 29 30 32 34 35 39 40 45 49 50 51 54 57 59 60 63 64 68 70 72 73 74 75 76 77 78 79 81 82 84 86 88 89 90 92 93 96 97 98 102 105 107 108 111 113 117 118 128 129 130 131 134 141 144 145 146 **P**6 **S** Iowa Health System, Des Moines, IA
Primary Contact: Peter W. Thoreen, FACHE, President and Chief Executive Officer
COO: Lynn Wold, Chief Operation Officer
CFO: James Gobell, Chief Financial Officer
CMO: Richard D. Hildebrand, M.D., Vice President Medical Affairs and Chief Medical Officer
CIO: James Gobell, Chief Financial Officer
CHR: Gary Johnson, Director Human Resources
CNO: Priscilla Stokes, MS, Vice President Patient Care and Chief Nursing Officer
Web address: www.stlukes.org
**Control:** Other not–for–profit (including NFP Corporation) **Service:** General Medical and Surgical

**Staffed Beds:** 160 **Admissions:** 9412 **Census:** 107 **Outpatient Visits:** 65731 **Births:** 2079 **Total Expense ($000):** 118294 **Payroll Expense ($000):** 48993 **Personnel:** 1036

## SPENCER—Clay County

★ **SPENCER HOSPITAL (160112)**, 1200 First Avenue East, Zip 51301; tel. 712/264–6111 **A**9 10 **F**3 7 8 11 13 15 28 29 30 31 34 35 39 40 43 50 53 56 57 59 60 62 63 64 65 69 70 75 76 77 78 79 81 82 84 85 86 87 93 97 98 99 100 101 102 103 104 105 107 108 109 111 114 117 118 119 120 122 126 128 129 130 131 132 134 145 146 147 **P**5
Primary Contact: William J. Bumgarner, President
COO: Susan Zulk, Vice President Marketing and Fund Development
CFO: Mark Gaworski, Vice President Finance, Chief Financial Officer
CMO: Brian Wilson, D.O., Medical Staff President
CIO: Brenda Marie Tiefenthaler BSN, MSN, MHA, R.N., Vice President Patient Care and Informatics
CHR: Stephen Duetsch, Vice President Operations and Support
CNO: Brenda Marie Tiefenthaler BSN, MSN, MHA, R.N., Vice President Patient Care and Informatics
Web address: www.spencerhospital.org
**Control:** City–Government, nonfederal **Service:** General Medical and Surgical

**Staffed Beds:** 80 **Admissions:** 3111 **Census:** 35 **Outpatient Visits:** 98609 **Births:** 274 **Total Expense ($000):** 60805 **Payroll Expense ($000):** 21001 **Personnel:** 467

## SPIRIT LAKE—Dickinson County

**LAKES REGIONAL HEALTHCARE (160124)**, Highway 71 South, Zip 51360–6810, Mailing Address: P.O. Box AB, Zip 51360–6810; tel. 712/336–1230 **A**9 10 **F**7 11 13 15 28 30 31 34 35 40 41 43 45 57 59 62 63 64 65 69 70 75 76 77 78 79 81 85 93 107 111 113 118 128 129 131 132 142 145 147
Primary Contact: Jason Harrington, President and Chief Executive Officer
CFO: Steve Alger, Senior Vice President and Chief Financial Officer
Web address: www.lakeshealth.org
**Control:** County–Government, nonfederal **Service:** General Medical and Surgical

**Staffed Beds:** 28 **Admissions:** 1058 **Census:** 11 **Outpatient Visits:** 32996 **Births:** 140 **Total Expense ($000):** 26385 **Payroll Expense ($000):** 10463 **Personnel:** 197

## STORM LAKE—Buena Vista County

✠ **BUENA VISTA REGIONAL MEDICAL CENTER (161375)**, 1525 West Fifth Street, Zip 50588–0309, Mailing Address: P.O. Box 309, Zip 50588–0309; tel. 712/732–4030 **A**1 9 10 18 **F**3 7 8 11 13 15 18 28 29 30 31 34 40 45 53 57 59 62 63 64 68 70 74 75 76 77 78 79 81 82 84 85 86 87 93 96 98 103 107 108 110 111 113 116 117 118 128 129 130 131 132 134 145 146 147 **S** Iowa Health System, Des Moines, IA
Primary Contact: Steven Colerick, Chief Executive Officer
CFO: Krista Ketcham, Chief Financial Officer
CMO: Jason Huisenga, D.O., Chief Medical Staff
CIO: Brian Granville, Director Information Technology
CHR: Carrie Turnquist, Director Human Resources
CNO: Dawn M. Bach, MS, Chief Clinical Officer
Web address: www.bvrmc.org
**Control:** County–Government, nonfederal **Service:** General Medical and Surgical

**Staffed Beds:** 35 **Admissions:** 1621 **Census:** 22 **Outpatient Visits:** 73830 **Births:** 299 **Total Expense ($000):** 37628 **Payroll Expense ($000):** 16116 **Personnel:** 354

## SUMNER—Bremer County

★ **COMMUNITY MEMORIAL HOSPITAL (161320)**, 909 West First Street, Zip 50674–1203, Mailing Address: P.O. Box 148, Zip 50674–0148; tel. 563/578–3275 **A**9 10 18 **F**3 11 15 28 29 34 40 45 57 59 64 81 85 86 97 107 113 126 127 128 130 132 134 147 **P**5 6 **S** Iowa Health System, Des Moines, IA
Primary Contact: Mary S. Wells, R.N., Chief Executive Officer
CFO: Sara Trainor, Chief Financial Officer
CMO: Troy Buchholz, M.D., Chief Medical Staff
CHR: Robin Elliott, Personnel Officer
CNO: Lynne Niemann, Director Nurses and Patient Care
Web address: www.cmhsumner.org
**Control:** Other not–for–profit (including NFP Corporation) **Service:** General Medical and Surgical

**Staffed Beds:** 16 **Admissions:** 301 **Census:** 4 **Outpatient Visits:** 10707 **Births:** 0 **Total Expense ($000):** 9143 **Payroll Expense ($000):** 3799 **Personnel:** 81

## VINTON—Benton County

★ **VIRGINIA GAY HOSPITAL (161349)**, 502 North Ninth Avenue, Zip 52349–2299; tel. 319/472–6200, (Total facility includes 47 beds in nursing home–type unit) **A**9 10 18 **F**28 34 35 40 42 43 45 59 62 65 67 75 77 81 85 86 87 96 97 107 111 112 113 118 124 126 128 129 130 131 132 142 **P**6
Primary Contact: Michael J. Riege, Chief Executive Officer
COO: Tedd Kipper, Chief Operating Officer
CFO: Julia Meadows, Chief Financial Officer
CMO: Brian Meeker, D.O., President Medical Staff
CHR: Kim Frank, Chief Human Resources Officer
Web address: www.vghinc.com
**Control:** Other not–for–profit (including NFP Corporation) **Service:** General Medical and Surgical

**Staffed Beds:** 72 **Admissions:** 492 **Census:** 42 **Outpatient Visits:** 90923 **Births:** 0 **Total Expense ($000):** 19390 **Payroll Expense ($000):** 9468 **Personnel:** 188

IA

**Hospital, Medicare Provider Number, Address, Telephone, Approval, Facility, and Physician Codes, Health Care System**

★ American Hospital Association (AHA) membership
☐ The Joint Commission accreditation ◇ DNV Healthcare Inc. accreditation
○ American Osteopathic Association (AOA) accreditation
△ Commission on Accreditation of Rehabilitation Facilities (CARF) accreditation

## WASHINGTON—Washington County

★ **WASHINGTON COUNTY HOSPITAL AND CLINICS (161344)**, 400 East Polk Street, Zip 52353, Mailing Address: P.O. Box 909, Zip 52353–0909; tel. 319/653–5481, (Total facility includes 43 beds in nursing home–type unit) **A**9 10 18 **F**3 13 15 28 29 34 40 43 45 53 55 57 59 64 67 68 69 75 76 81 82 84 85 86 93 97 107 110 113 118 129 132 145 146 147 **P**6
Primary Contact: Dennis Hunger, Chief Executive Officer
CFO: Steve Sanders, Chief Financial Officer
CMO: Donald Miller, M.D., Chief of Staff
CIO: Jennifer Durst, Director Information Services
CHR: Tracy Ousey, Director Human Resources
CNO: Barbara Griswold, Chief Nursing Officer
Web address: www.wchc.org
**Control:** County–Government, nonfederal **Service:** General Medical and Surgical

**Staffed Beds:** 68 **Admissions:** 1720 **Census:** 54 **Outpatient Visits:** 44262 **Births:** 134 **Total Expense ($000):** 21676 **Payroll Expense ($000):** 10681 **Personnel:** 231

## WATERLOO—Black Hawk County

✠ **ALLEN MEMORIAL HOSPITAL (160110)**, 1825 Logan Avenue, Zip 50703–1916; tel. 319/235–3941 **A**1 3 5 9 10 **F**3 8 11 13 15 17 18 20 22 24 26 28 29 30 31 34 35 39 40 43 45 46 48 49 50 51 52 54 56 57 59 63 64 66 68 70 72 74 75 76 77 78 79 81 82 84 85 86 87 88 89 90 91 92 93 96 97 98 99 100 101 102 103 104 107 108 110 111 113 114 117 118 125 126 128 129 131 134 145 146 147 **S** Iowa Health System, Des Moines, IA
Primary Contact: Thomas Tibbitts, Interim Chief Executive Officer
CFO: Renee Rasmussen, Senior Vice President and Chief Financial Officer
CMO: Jeff Crandall, M.D., Chief Medical Officer
Web address: www.allenhospital.org
**Control:** Other not–for–profit (including NFP Corporation) **Service:** General Medical and Surgical

**Staffed Beds:** 201 **Admissions:** 10777 **Census:** 109 **Outpatient Visits:** 294073 **Births:** 929 **Total Expense ($000):** 188053 **Payroll Expense ($000):** 65721 **Personnel:** 1245

✠ △ **COVENANT MEDICAL CENTER (160067)**, 3421 West Ninth Street, Zip 50702–5499; tel. 319/272–8000, (Includes KIMBALL–RIDGE CENTER, 2101 Kimball Avenue, Zip 50702; tel. 319/291–3131) **A**1 2 3 5 7 9 10 **F**3 4 5 7 11 13 15 18 19 20 22 26 28 29 30 31 33 34 35 39 40 43 44 46 49 51 53 57 58 59 60 61 62 64 68 70 71 72 74 75 76 77 78 79 81 82 89 90 93 97 98 99 100 104 105 107 108 111 113 114 117 118 119 126 128 129 130 131 134 142 143 145 146 147 **P**1 6 **S** Wheaton Franciscan Healthcare, Wheaton, IL
Primary Contact: Jack Dusenbery, President and Chief Executive Officer
CFO: Michele Panicucci, Senior Vice President and Chief Financial Officer ·
CMO: Paul Franke, M.D., Vice President Medical Affairs
CIO: Gregory Smith, Chief Information Officer
CHR: Vicki L. Parsons, Regional Vice President Human Resources
Web address: www.wheatoniowa.org
**Control:** Church–operated, Nongovernment, not–for profit **Service:** General Medical and Surgical

**Staffed Beds:** 243 **Admissions:** 8500 **Census:** 98 **Outpatient Visits:** 645595 **Births:** 1416 **Total Expense ($000):** 230911 **Payroll Expense ($000):** 106666 **Personnel:** 1647

## WAUKON—Allamakee County

★ **VETERANS MEMORIAL HOSPITAL (161318)**, 40 First Street S.E., Zip 52172–2099; tel. 563/568–3411 **A**9 10 18 **F**7 11 13 15 28 31 34 35 40 45 57 59 62 64 65 75 76 78 81 107 118 130 131 132 133 143 145
Primary Contact: Michael D. Myers, Chief Executive Officer
CFO: Scott Knode, Chief Financial Officer
CHR: Erin Berns, Director Human Resources
Web address: www.vmhospital.com
**Control:** City–Government, nonfederal **Service:** General Medical and Surgical

**Staffed Beds:** 25 **Admissions:** 741 **Census:** 7 **Outpatient Visits:** 43395 **Births:** 109 **Total Expense ($000):** 12446 **Payroll Expense ($000):** 5788 **Personnel:** 142

## WAVERLY—Bremer County

✠ **WAVERLY HEALTH CENTER (161339)**, 312 Ninth Street S.W., Zip 50677–2999; tel. 319/352–4120 **A**1 9 10 18 **F**3 7 8 11 13 15 28 34 35 36 40 43 45 57 59 63 64 68 75 76 77 79 81 85 86 97 107 110 111 113 118 126 129 131 132 133 134 143 145 146 **P**6
Primary Contact: Kyle Richards, Chief Executive Officer
CFO: Lisa Bennett, Chief Financial Officer
CMO: Clay Dahlquist, M.D., Chief Medical Officer
CIO: Jerry Tiedt, Director Information Systems
CHR: Angie Tye, Director Human Resources
CNO: Rhonda DeBuhr, R.N., Chief Clinical and Nursing Officer
Web address: www.waverlyhealthcenter.org
**Control:** City–Government, nonfederal **Service:** General Medical and Surgical

**Staffed Beds:** 25 **Admissions:** 1041 **Census:** 10 **Outpatient Visits:** 94306 **Births:** 229 **Total Expense ($000):** 44447 **Payroll Expense ($000):** 20550 **Personnel:** 327

## WEBSTER CITY—Hamilton County

**HAMILTON HOSPITAL** See Van Diest Medical Center

★ **VAN DIEST MEDICAL CENTER (161361)**, 2350 Hospital Drive, Zip 50595–2824, Mailing Address: P.O. Box 430, Zip 50595–0430; tel. 515/832–9400 **A**9 10 18 **F**3 7 11 13 15 28 29 35 38 40 43 44 45 59 64 75 76 77 79 81 82 85 86 87 89 93 107 111 118 128 129 131 132 134 145 146 **P**6
Primary Contact: Palmer Schneider, Administrator
COO: Janet Naset–Payne, R.N., Chief Operating Officer
CFO: Alice Heinrichs, CPA, Chief Financial Officer
CMO: Mark Andrew, M.D., Chief of Staff
CIO: Dave Dawson, Director Information Services
Web address: www.hamiltonhospital.com
**Control:** County–Government, nonfederal **Service:** General Medical and Surgical

**Staffed Beds:** 25 **Admissions:** 1296 **Census:** 13 **Outpatient Visits:** 20493 **Births:** 114 **Total Expense ($000):** 21861 **Payroll Expense ($000):** 8489 **Personnel:** 182

## WEST BURLINGTON—Des Moines County

✠ △ **GREAT RIVER MEDICAL CENTER (160057)**, 1221 South Gear Avenue, Zip 52655–1681; tel. 319/768–1000, (Total facility includes 165 beds in nursing home–type unit) **A**1 7 9 10 19 **F**3 4 5 7 11 13 15 18 20 22 28 29 30 31 32 34 35 36 38 40 43 48 50 53 57 59 60 62 63 64 67 68 69 70 73 75 76 77 78 79 81 82 84 85 86 87 89 90 91 92 93 96 98 99 100 101 102 103 104 107 108 110 111 113 114 117 118 120 122 127 128 129 130 131 142 145 146 147 **P**6
Primary Contact: Mark D. Richardson, FACHE, President and Chief Executive Officer
CFO: Todd J. Sladky, Chief Financial Officer
CMO: William Daws, M.D., Chief of Staff
CIO: Gary Davis, Director Information Systems
CHR: Ron Halligan, Vice President Support Services
CHR: James M. Kammerer, Vice President Support Services
CNO: Teresa Colgan, VP of Nursing
Web address: www.greatrivermedical.org
**Control:** Other not–for–profit (including NFP Corporation) **Service:** General Medical and Surgical

**Staffed Beds:** 378 **Admissions:** 7423 **Census:** 191 **Outpatient Visits:** 245000 **Births:** 533 **Total Expense ($000):** 148789 **Payroll Expense ($000):** 61064 **Personnel:** 1200

## WEST DES MOINES—Dallas County

★ **MERCY MEDICAL CENTER – WEST LAKES**, 1755 59th Place, Zip 50266–7736; tel. 515/358–8000 **A**9 **F**3 7 11 12 13 15 18 20 22 26 29 30 40 41 43 44 50 56 61 62 64 65 68 70 75 76 77 78 79 81 85 86 87 93 96 107 108 111 113 117 118 129 131 134 142 145 **S** Catholic Health Initiatives, Englewood, CO
Primary Contact: Laurie A. Conner, FACHE, Vice President and Administrator
COO: Sheryl L. Barnes, MSN, Senior Director Clinical Services
Web address: www.mercywestlakes.org/
**Control:** Church–operated, Nongovernment, not–for profit **Service:** General Medical and Surgical

**Staffed Beds:** 82 **Admissions:** 3619 **Census:** 35 **Outpatient Visits:** 18870 **Births:** 186 **Total Expense ($000):** 45182 **Payroll Expense ($000):** 14461 **Personnel:** 273

## WEST UNION—Fayette County

★ **PALMER LUTHERAN HEALTH CENTER (161316)**, 112 Jefferson Street, Zip 52175–1022; tel. 563/422–3811 **A**9 10 18 **F**3 8 11 13 15 28 29 30 31 34 40 43 56 57 59 62 63 64 65 68 70 76 77 78 79 81 82 85 86 93 96 107 111 113 118 127 128 129 132 133 134 143 145 147
Primary Contact: Debrah Chensvold, FACHE, President and Chief Executive Officer
CFO: Joni Gisleson, Director Finance
CMO: Chaudri Rasool, D.O., Chief of Staff
CIO: Kurt Chicken, Director Support Services
CHR: Cheryl Meyer, Director Human Resources
CNO: Kathy Begalske, Chief Nursing Officer
Web address: www.palmerlutheran.org
**Control:** Other not–for–profit (including NFP Corporation) **Service:** General Medical and Surgical

**Staffed Beds:** 25 **Admissions:** 480 **Census:** 6 **Outpatient Visits:** 65001 **Births:** 103 **Total Expense ($000):** 21880 **Payroll Expense ($000):** 8492 **Personnel:** 188

IA

**WINTERSET—Madison County**

★ **MADISON COUNTY HEALTH CARE SYSTEM (161326)**, 300 Hutchings Street,
Zip 50273–2109; tel. 515/462–2373 **A**9 10 18 **F**3 4 15 18 28 31 35 37 40
43 45 57 59 63 70 78 79 81 89 93 97 107 110 111 113 118 126 127 128
129 130 131 132 134 145 **P**6
Primary Contact: Marcia Hendricks, R.N., Chief Executive Officer
COO: Terry E. Simmons, Chief Nursing Officer
CFO: Rebekah Mitchell, Chief Financial Officer
CMO: Jonathan Suddarth, D.O., Chief of Staff
CIO: Gary Mullen, Chief Information Officer
CHR: Jennifer Hannon, Director Human Resources
Web address: www.madisonhealth.com
**Control:** County–Government, nonfederal **Service:** General Medical and Surgical

**Staffed Beds:** 21 **Admissions:** 540 **Census:** 7 **Outpatient Visits:** 61136
**Births:** 0 **Total Expense ($000):** 16157 **Payroll Expense ($000):** 7171
**Personnel:** 134

**Hospital, Medicare Provider Number, Address, Telephone, Approval, Facility, and Physician Codes, Health Care System**

★ American Hospital Association (AHA) membership    ○ American Osteopathic Association (AOA) accreditation
□ The Joint Commission accreditation    ◇ DNV Healthcare Inc. accreditation    △ Commission on Accreditation of Rehabilitation Facilities (CARF) accreditation

# KANSAS

### ABILENE—Dickinson County

★ **MEMORIAL HEALTH SYSTEM (171381)**, 511 N.E. Tenth Street,
Zip 67410–2153; tel. 785/263–2100, (Total facility includes 75 beds in nursing
home–type unit) **A**9 10 18 **F**3 13 15 18 28 29 31 34 36 40 45 53 57 59 62 63
64 68 69 71 75 77 78 79 81 82 85 87 93 98 103 107 108 111 113 116 118
126 127 129 130 131 132 134 142 145 147 **P**6
Primary Contact: Mark A. Miller, FACHE, Chief Executive Officer
COO: Robert Brazil, Chief Operating Officer
CFO: Elgin Glanzer, Chief Financial Officer
CMO: W. L. Short, M.D., Chief Medical Officer
CIO: Blaine Cappel, Director Information Systems
CHR: Robert Brazil, Chief Operating Officer
Web address: www.mhsks.org
**Control:** Hospital district or authority, Government, nonfederal **Service:** General
Medical and Surgical

> **Staffed Beds:** 110 **Admissions:** 973 **Census:** 84 **Outpatient Visits:** 45359
> **Births:** 59 **Total Expense ($000):** 22398 **Payroll Expense ($000):** 11824
> **Personnel:** 306

### ANDOVER—Butler County

**KANSAS MEDICAL CENTER (170197)**, 1124 West 21st Street, Zip 67002;
tel. 316/300–4000 **A**9 10 **F**3 17 18 20 22 24 29 30 40 49 51 60 64 68 70
75 77 79 81 82 85 87 102 107 108 114 118 129 130 145 147
Primary Contact: Badr Idbeis, M.D., Chief Executive Officer
COO: Daryl W. Thornton, Chief Operating Officer
CFO: Steven N. Hadley, Chief Financial Officer
Web address: www.ksmedcenter.com/
**Control:** Corporation, Investor–owned, for–profit **Service:** General Medical and
Surgical

> **Staffed Beds:** 58 **Admissions:** 2644 **Census:** 28 **Outpatient Visits:** 8655
> **Births:** 0 **Personnel:** 233

### ANTHONY—Harper County

★ **ANTHONY MEDICAL CENTER (171346)**, 1101 East Spring Street,
Zip 67003–2122; tel. 620/842–5111 **A**9 10 18 **F**40 48 53 57 64 67 81 93 97
107 118 126 127 132 **P**6
Primary Contact: J. Bryant Anderson, Administrator and Chief Executive Officer
CFO: Lori Allen, Chief Financial Officer
CHR: Kim Barwick, Vice President Human Resources
**Control:** Hospital district or authority, Government, nonfederal **Service:** General
Medical and Surgical

> **Staffed Beds:** 25 **Admissions:** 217 **Census:** 9 **Outpatient Visits:** 19233
> **Births:** 0 **Total Expense ($000):** 6210 **Payroll Expense ($000):** 3453
> **Personnel:** 79

### ARKANSAS CITY—Cowley County

★ **SOUTH CENTRAL KANSAS MEDICAL CENTER (170150)**, 6401 Patterson
Parkway, Zip 67005, Mailing Address: P.O. Box 1107, Zip 67005–1107;
tel. 620/442–2500 **A**9 10 **F**11 12 13 15 29 30 34 35 39 40 45 50 59 64 68
70 75 76 77 79 81 82 85 87 93 107 108 110 111 112 114 118 128 131
132 147
Primary Contact: Steven J. Perkins, Chief Executive Officer
CFO: Holly Beaty, Chief Financial Officer
CMO: David Schmeidler, M.D., Chief Medical Staff
CMO: Kamran Shahzada, M.D., Chief Medical Staff
CHR: Clayton Pappan, Director Human Resources and Marketing
CNO: Patricia Davis, Chief Nursing Officer
Web address: www.sckrmc.org
**Control:** City–Government, nonfederal **Service:** General Medical and Surgical

> **Staffed Beds:** 37 **Admissions:** 1134 **Census:** 12 **Outpatient Visits:** 16395
> **Births:** 115 **Total Expense ($000):** 13424 **Payroll Expense ($000):** 7559
> **Personnel:** 197

### ASHLAND—Clark County

★ **ASHLAND HEALTH CENTER (171304)**, 709 Oak Street, Zip 67831–0188,
Mailing Address: P.O. Box 188, Zip 67831–0188; tel. 620/635–2241, (Total
facility includes 21 beds in nursing home–type unit) **A**9 10 18 **F**2 30 34 40 53
59 62 64 67 68 85 87 93 107 126 127 132 142 **P**6 **S** Great Plains Health
Alliance, Inc., Phillipsburg, KS
Primary Contact: Benjamin Anderson, Chief Executive Officer
CFO: Debbie Filson, Chief Financial Officer
CMO: Daniel Shuman, D.O., Chief Medical Officer
CIO: Alan Romans, Director Information Technology
CHR: Debbie Filson, Chief Financial Officer
CNO: Patty Young, R.N., Hospital Director of Nursing
Web address: www.ashlandhc.org
**Control:** Hospital district or authority, Government, nonfederal **Service:** General
Medical and Surgical

> **Staffed Beds:** 45 **Admissions:** 115 **Census:** 25 **Outpatient Visits:** 6443
> **Births:** 0 **Total Expense ($000):** 5057 **Payroll Expense ($000):** 2306
> **Personnel:** 69

### ATCHISON—Atchison County

★ ○ **ATCHISON HOSPITAL (171382)**, 800 Raven Hill Drive, Zip 66002;
tel. 913/367–2131 **A**9 10 11 18 **F**3 7 8 11 12 13 15 28 29 30 31 34 35 40
45 49 50 57 59 62 63 64 68 70 75 76 77 79 81 82 85 87 89 92 93 97 107
108 110 111 113 117 118 126 128 129 130 131 132 134 145 146 **P**6
Primary Contact: John L. Jacobson, Chief Executive Officer
CFO: Gary R. Foll, Chief Financial Officer
CMO: Michael Jones, M.D., Chief of Staff
CIO: Michael Gaul, Manager Information Systems
CHR: Pamela K. Sweger, Director Human Resources
Web address: www.atchisonhospital.org
**Control:** Other not–for–profit (including NFP Corporation) **Service:** General
Medical and Surgical

> **Staffed Beds:** 25 **Admissions:** 1042 **Census:** 10 **Outpatient Visits:** 49581
> **Births:** 182 **Total Expense ($000):** 31261 **Payroll Expense ($000):** 13829
> **Personnel:** 255

### ATWOOD—Rawlins County

★ **RAWLINS COUNTY HEALTH CENTER (171307)**, 707 Grant Street,
Zip 67730–4700, Mailing Address: P.O. Box 47, Zip 67730–4700;
tel. 785/626–3211 **A**9 10 18 **F**3 28 30 40 45 57 64 75 81 85 93 107 114
124 126 127 129 132 134 145 147 **P**6 **S** Great Plains Health Alliance, Inc.,
Phillipsburg, KS
Primary Contact: Deanna Freeman, Administrator and Chief Executive Officer
CFO: Heather Prideaux, Director Finance
Web address: www.rchc.us
**Control:** County–Government, nonfederal **Service:** General Medical and Surgical

> **Staffed Beds:** 24 **Admissions:** 311 **Census:** 4 **Outpatient Visits:** 17915
> **Births:** 0 **Total Expense ($000):** 5791 **Payroll Expense ($000):** 2697
> **Personnel:** 69

### BELLEVILLE—Republic County

▣ **REPUBLIC COUNTY HOSPITAL (171361)**, 2420 G Street, Zip 66935–2400;
tel. 785/527–2254, (Total facility includes 38 beds in nursing home–type unit) **A**1
9 10 18 **F**3 13 15 28 29 30 31 35 39 40 45 56 57 64 67 68 75 76 77 78 79
81 85 86 87 89 93 107 108 113 118 127 129 130 132 **S** Great Plains Health
Alliance, Inc., Phillipsburg, KS
Primary Contact: Blaine K. Miller, Administrator
CFO: Barry Bottger, Chief Financial Officer
Web address: www.rphospital.org
**Control:** Other not–for–profit (including NFP Corporation) **Service:** General
Medical and Surgical

> **Staffed Beds:** 63 **Admissions:** 1188 **Census:** 41 **Outpatient Visits:** 15171
> **Births:** 54 **Total Expense ($000):** 13550 **Payroll Expense ($000):** 6529
> **Personnel:** 155

**KS**

*Many Facility Codes have changed. Please refer to the AHA Guide Code Chart.* © 2012 AHA Guide

## BELOIT—Mitchell County

★ **MITCHELL COUNTY HOSPITAL HEALTH SYSTEMS (171375)**, 400 West Eighth, Zip 67420–1605, Mailing Address: P.O. Box 399, Zip 67420–0399; tel. 785/738–2266, (Total facility includes 40 beds in nursing home–type unit) **A**9 10 18 **F**11 13 15 28 29 31 34 40 45 48 50 56 59 62 63 64 68 69 74 76 77 81 82 84 86 87 93 98 103 106 107 111 113 118 127 128 129 131 132 134 147
Primary Contact: David Dick, Chief Executive Officer
CFO: Eldon Koepke, Chief Financial Officer
CIO: Nate Richards, Director Information Technology
CHR: Phyllis Oetting, Director Human Resources
CNO: Jan Kemmerer, Director of Nursing
Web address: www.mchks.com
**Control:** County–Government, nonfederal **Service:** General Medical and Surgical

> **Staffed Beds:** 75 **Admissions:** 1321 **Census:** 51 **Outpatient Visits:** 16243 **Births:** 102 **Total Expense ($000):** 22976 **Payroll Expense ($000):** 10588 **Personnel:** 266

## BURLINGTON—Coffey County

★ **COFFEY COUNTY HOSPITAL (170094)**, 801 North Fourth Street, Zip 66839–0189, Mailing Address: P.O. Box 189, Zip 66839–0189; tel. 620/364–2121, (Total facility includes 42 beds in nursing home–type unit) **A**9 10 20 **F**3 7 10 11 13 15 17 29 30 31 34 40 45 50 57 59 62 64 65 67 68 70 75 76 77 78 79 81 82 85 87 93 107 110 111 113 118 124 126 127 129 132 145 **P**6
Primary Contact: Karen Smith, Interim Chief Executive Officer
CFO: James H. Garner, Chief Financial Officer
CHR: Larry V. Gales, Director Human Resources
Web address: www.coffeyhealth.org
**Control:** County–Government, nonfederal **Service:** General Medical and Surgical

> **Staffed Beds:** 78 **Admissions:** 943 **Census:** 44 **Outpatient Visits:** 20606 **Births:** 79 **Total Expense ($000):** 18695 **Payroll Expense ($000):** 11031 **Personnel:** 144

## CALDWELL—Sumner County

★ **SUMNER COUNTY HOSPITAL DISTRICT ONE (171329)**, 601 South Osage Street, Zip 67022–1654; tel. 620/845–6492 **A**9 10 18 **F**1 4 7 11 16 17 40 57 62 67 70 72 73 75 76 80 81 88 89 90 93 98 107 111 118 127 128 132 **P**5
Primary Contact: Virgil Watson, Administrator
CFO: Jennifer Marcrum, Chief Financial Officer
CMO: Jim Blunk, D.O., Chief Medical Officer
CIO: Trey Watson, Network Administrator
Web address: www.schd1.com
**Control:** Hospital district or authority, Government, nonfederal **Service:** General Medical and Surgical

> **Staffed Beds:** 15 **Admissions:** 173 **Census:** 2 **Outpatient Visits:** 4609 **Births:** 0 **Total Expense ($000):** 4130 **Payroll Expense ($000):** 1793 **Personnel:** 57

## CHANUTE—Neosho County

★ **NEOSHO MEMORIAL REGIONAL MEDICAL CENTER (171380)**, 629 South Plummer, Zip 66720–0426, Mailing Address: P.O. Box 426, Zip 66720–0426; tel. 620/431–4000 **A**5 9 10 18 **F**3 7 11 13 15 29 30 40 53 57 62 63 76 77 79 81 82 89 93 107 108 111 113 118 127 128 129 132 134 142 145 146 **P**8 **S** QHR, Brentwood, TN
Primary Contact: Dennis Franks, FACHE, Chief Executive Officer
CFO: Nancy Woodyard, Chief Financial Officer
CMO: Brian Kueser, M.D., Chief Medical Officer
CIO: Wanda W. Thomas, Director Health Information
CHR: R. C. Rowan, Director Human Resources
Web address: www.nmrmc.com
**Control:** County–Government, nonfederal **Service:** General Medical and Surgical

> **Staffed Beds:** 25 **Admissions:** 2013 **Census:** 19 **Outpatient Visits:** 33232 **Births:** 316 **Total Expense ($000):** 33761 **Payroll Expense ($000):** 15960 **Personnel:** 293

## CLAY CENTER—Clay County

★ **CLAY COUNTY MEDICAL CENTER (171371)**, 617 Liberty Street, Zip 67432–0512, Mailing Address: P.O. Box 512, Zip 67432–0512; tel. 785/632–2144 **A**9 10 18 **F**13 15 18 19 28 30 31 40 50 51 53 55 59 63 64 67 68 70 74 75 76 77 78 79 81 82 84 85 86 87 88 89 93 96 108 110 111 113 116 118 127 129 131 132 147
Primary Contact: Ron Bender, Chief Executive Officer
COO: Tyce Young, Patient Services Officer
CFO: Jim Brinkman, Chief Financial Officer
CIO: Jim Seley, Chief Information Officer
CHR: Cindy Rush, Director Human Resources
Web address: www.ccmcks.org
**Control:** County–Government, nonfederal **Service:** General Medical and Surgical

> **Staffed Beds:** 25 **Admissions:** 800 **Census:** 10 **Outpatient Visits:** 42627 **Births:** 65 **Total Expense ($000):** 14447 **Payroll Expense ($000):** 7213 **Personnel:** 179

## COFFEYVILLE—Montgomery County

⊠ **COFFEYVILLE REGIONAL MEDICAL CENTER (170145)**, 1400 West Fourth, Zip 67337–0856; tel. 620/251–1200, (Total facility includes 20 beds in nursing home–type unit) **A**1 2 9 10 **F**3 7 11 13 15 28 29 30 31 34 40 45 46 50 57 59 62 64 68 70 75 76 77 78 79 81 82 85 90 93 94 96 97 107 108 110 113 114 118 127 131 134 144 146 **P**8 **S** QHR, Brentwood, TN
Primary Contact: John Smith, Chief Executive Officer
CIO: Chris Crist, Director Information Systems
CHR: Becky McCune, Director Human Resources, Community Relations and Education
CNO: Lori Rexwinkle, Chief Nursing Officer
Web address: www.crmcinc.com
**Control:** Other not–for–profit (including NFP Corporation) **Service:** General Medical and Surgical

> **Staffed Beds:** 88 **Admissions:** 2568 **Census:** 32 **Outpatient Visits:** 49410 **Births:** 200 **Total Expense ($000):** 36775 **Payroll Expense ($000):** 15359 **Personnel:** 331

## COLBY—Thomas County

**CITIZENS MEDICAL CENTER (171362)**, 100 East College Drive, Zip 67701–3799; tel. 785/462–7511, (Total facility includes 68 beds in nursing home–type unit) **A**9 10 18 **F**3 11 13 15 28 30 31 34 40 64 67 74 76 78 79 81 85 86 87 93 97 107 108 110 111 113 118 126 129 132 145 **P**6
Primary Contact: Kevan Trenkle, Chief Executive Officer
CFO: Patsy Evans, Chief Financial Officer
CMO: Brewster Kellogg, D.O., Chief Medical Staff
CIO: Rod Williams, Manager Information Systems
CHR: Margaret Kummer, Vice President Human Resources
CNO: Victoria Duffey, Director of Nursing
Web address: www.nwkshealthcare.com
**Control:** Other not–for–profit (including NFP Corporation) **Service:** General Medical and Surgical

> **Staffed Beds:** 93 **Admissions:** 647 **Census:** 63 **Outpatient Visits:** 11218 **Births:** 116 **Total Expense ($000):** 20796 **Payroll Expense ($000):** 10150 **Personnel:** 232

## COLDWATER—Comanche County

★ **COMANCHE COUNTY HOSPITAL (171312)**, 202 South Frisco Street, Zip 67029, Mailing Address: HC 65, Box 8A, Zip 67029; tel. 620/582–2144 **A**9 10 18 **F**11 30 31 40 53 59 61 62 68 75 77 78 93 102 127 132 **P**6 **S** Great Plains Health Alliance, Inc., Phillipsburg, KS
Primary Contact: Nancy Zimmerman, R.N., Administrator
CFO: Lisa Brooks, Chief Financial Officer
CMO: Daniel Schowengerdt, M.D., Chief of Staff
CIO: LaNell Wagnon, Director Medical Records
CHR: Lisa Brooks, Chief Financial Officer
CNO: Sandra Dobrinski, Director of Nursing
Web address: www.gpha.com
**Control:** County–Government, nonfederal **Service:** General Medical and Surgical

> **Staffed Beds:** 12 **Admissions:** 95 **Census:** 2 **Outpatient Visits:** 11976 **Births:** 0 **Total Expense ($000):** 4235 **Payroll Expense ($000):** 2083 **Personnel:** 49

---

**Hospital, Medicare Provider Number, Address, Telephone, Approval, Facility, and Physician Codes, Health Care System**

★ American Hospital Association (AHA) membership
☐ The Joint Commission accreditation
◇ DNV Healthcare Inc. accreditation
○ American Osteopathic Association (AOA) accreditation
△ Commission on Accreditation of Rehabilitation Facilities (CARF) accreditation

**KS**

## COLUMBUS—Cherokee County

★ **MERCY HOSPITAL COLUMBUS (171308)**, 220 North Pennsylvania Street,
Zip 66725–1110; tel. 620/429–2545 **A**9 10 18 **F**11 15 39 40 45 57 59 77 81
93 118 132 144 **S** Mercy Health, Chesterfield, MO
Primary Contact: Cindy Neely, Administrator
CMO: Darcy Selenke, M.D., Chief of Staff
Web address: www.mercy.ne
**Control:** Church–operated, Nongovernment, not–for profit **Service:** General
Medical and Surgical

**Staffed Beds:** 18 **Admissions:** 110 **Census:** 2 **Outpatient Visits:** 9025
**Births:** 0 **Total Expense ($000):** 3355 **Payroll Expense ($000):** 1989
**Personnel:** 45

## CONCORDIA—Cloud County

**CLOUD COUNTY HEALTH CENTER (171349)**, 1100 Highland Drive,
Zip 66901–3923; tel. 785/243–1234 **A**9 10 18 **F**3 11 13 15 20 28 31 34 35
40 41 45 56 57 59 64 65 70 74 75 76 77 79 81 82 85 86 87 89 93 96 97
102 107 108 113 117 118 126 129 131 132 134 145 147 **P**6
Primary Contact: James E. Wahlmeier, President and Chief Executive Officer
CMO: Justin Poore, D.O., Chief Medical Staff
CIO: Mitch Wing, Network Administrator
CHR: Nicole Nelson, Director Human Resources
Web address: www.cchc.org
**Control:** Other not–for–profit (including NFP Corporation) **Service:** General
Medical and Surgical

**Staffed Beds:** 25 **Admissions:** 775 **Census:** 9 **Outpatient Visits:** 23319
**Births:** 29 **Total Expense ($000):** 12766 **Payroll Expense ($000):** 7208
**Personnel:** 157

## COUNCIL GROVE—Morris County

★ **MORRIS COUNTY HOSPITAL (171379)**, 600 North Washington Street,
Zip 66846–1422; tel. 620/767–6811 **A**9 10 18 **F**7 11 13 15 18 28 31 35 40
45 59 64 65 70 76 77 81 87 93 94 96 107 110 129 131 132 145 147 **P**5
Primary Contact: James H. Reagan, Jr., Ph.D., Chief Executive Officer
CFO: Ron Christenson, Chief Financial Officer
CMO: Joel Hornuug, M.D., Chief Medical Officer
CIO: Bill Lauer, Chief Information Officer
CHR: Don Zimmerman, Director Human Resources
CNO: Stephanne Wolf, Chief Nursing Officer
Web address: www.mrcohosp.com
**Control:** County–Government, nonfederal **Service:** General Medical and Surgical

**Staffed Beds:** 25 **Admissions:** 519 **Census:** 6 **Outpatient Visits:** 14677
**Births:** 41 **Total Expense ($000):** 8426 **Payroll Expense ($000):** 3005
**Personnel:** 88

## DIGHTON—Lane County

★ **LANE COUNTY HOSPITAL (171303)**, 235 West Vine, Zip 67839–0969, Mailing
Address: P.O. Box 969, Zip 67839–0969; tel. 620/397–5321, (Total facility
includes 14 beds in nursing home–type unit) **A**9 10 18 **F**30 40 56 67 77 85 93
97 126 127 130 132 **P**6 **S** Great Plains Health Alliance, Inc., Phillipsburg, KS
Primary Contact: Donna McGowan, Administrator
CFO: Marcia Gabel, Chief Financial Officer
CMO: Paul Chinburg, M.D., Medical Director
CHR: Dina Casey, Human Resources Officer
Web address: www.lchospital.com
**Control:** County–Government, nonfederal **Service:** General Medical and Surgical

**Staffed Beds:** 31 **Admissions:** 107 **Census:** 18 **Outpatient Visits:** 13247
**Births:** 0 **Total Expense ($000):** 4486 **Payroll Expense ($000):** 2160
**Personnel:** 52

## DODGE CITY—Ford County

⊞ **WESTERN PLAINS MEDICAL COMPLEX (170175)**, 3001 Avenue A,
Zip 67801–6508, Mailing Address: P.O. Box 1478, Zip 67801–1478;
tel. 620/225–8400 **A**1 3 5 9 10 20 **F**3 8 11 13 15 17 18 20 22 28 29 30 35
40 43 50 51 59 60 70 72 73 74 75 76 77 79 81 85 86 87 88 89 93 107
108 111 114 118 128 129 132 145 **S** LifePoint Hospitals, Inc., Brentwood, TN
Primary Contact: Michael R. Burroughs, FACHE, Chief Executive Officer
CFO: Scott Hankinson, Chief Financial Officer
CMO: Aye Mya Win, M.D., Chief Medical Staff
CIO: Shawna Culver, Director Information Systems
Web address: www.westernplainsmc.com
**Control:** Corporation, Investor–owned, for–profit **Service:** General Medical and
Surgical

**Staffed Beds:** 89 **Admissions:** 2634 **Census:** 22 **Outpatient Visits:** 32054
**Births:** 755 **Personnel:** 252

## EL DORADO—Butler County

⊞ **SUSAN B. ALLEN MEMORIAL HOSPITAL (170017)**, 720 West Central Avenue,
Zip 67042–2112; tel. 316/321–3300 **A**1 5 9 10 **F**3 11 13 15 28 30 40 45 59
60 62 68 69 70 76 79 81 85 92 93 96 97 98 103 107 108 110 111 114 118
120 122 129 132 145 147
Primary Contact: Gayle Arnett, President and Chief Executive Officer
COO: David Shaw, Vice President and Chief Operating Officer
CFO: Robin Crawford, Vice President and Chief Financial Officer
CIO: Mark Rooker, Director Information Systems
CHR: Gay Kimble, Director Human Resources
Web address: www.sbamh.com
**Control:** Other not–for–profit (including NFP Corporation) **Service:** General
Medical and Surgical

**Staffed Beds:** 52 **Admissions:** 1877 **Census:** 20 **Outpatient Visits:** 78597
**Births:** 294 **Total Expense ($000):** 41943 **Payroll Expense ($000):** 17664
**Personnel:** 345

## ELKHART—Morton County

★ **MORTON COUNTY HEALTH SYSTEM (170166)**, 445 Hilltop Street,
Zip 67950–0937, Mailing Address: P.O. Box 937, Zip 67950–0937;
tel. 620/697–2141, (Total facility includes 80 beds in nursing home–type unit) **A**9
10 20 **F**10 11 15 18 28 29 31 34 40 45 54 56 57 59 64 67 68 70 75 77 79
81 86 87 93 94 96 97 98 99 100 101 102 103 104 107 111 113 118 129
130 131 132 134 142 145 146 147 **P**5 6
Primary Contact: Leonard Hernandez, Chief Executive Officer
CFO: Jeff Weaver, Chief Financial Officer
CHR: Sonja May, Director Human Resources
Web address: www.mchswecare.com
**Control:** County–Government, nonfederal **Service:** General Medical and Surgical

**Staffed Beds:** 120 **Admissions:** 729 **Census:** 80 **Outpatient Visits:** 23851
**Births:** 0 **Total Expense ($000):** 15911 **Payroll Expense ($000):** 9729
**Personnel:** 199

## ELLINWOOD—Barton County

★ **ELLINWOOD DISTRICT HOSPITAL (171301)**, 605 North Main Street,
Zip 67526–1440; tel. 620/564–2548 **A**9 10 18 **F**11 40 64 65 93 107 126 127
132 **P**6 **S** Great Plains Health Alliance, Inc., Phillipsburg, KS
Primary Contact: Joyce Schulte, Chief Executive Officer
CFO: Penny Stephenson, Chief Financial Officer
CMO: Charles Joslin, M.D., Chief of Staff
CIO: Becky L. Burns, Manager Health Information Management
CHR: Penny Stephenson, Chief Financial Officer
CNO: Aletha Budig, R.N., Director of Nursing
Web address: www.ellinwood.org
**Control:** Other not–for–profit (including NFP Corporation) **Service:** General
Medical and Surgical

**Staffed Beds:** 25 **Admissions:** 234 **Census:** 10 **Outpatient Visits:** 14514
**Births:** 0 **Total Expense ($000):** 5965 **Payroll Expense ($000):** 2811
**Personnel:** 63

## ELLSWORTH—Ellsworth County

★ **ELLSWORTH COUNTY MEDICAL CENTER (171327)**, 1604 Aylward Street,
Zip 67439–0087, Mailing Address: P.O. Box 87, Zip 67439–0087;
tel. 785/472–3111 **A**9 10 18 **F**3 11 28 29 34 35 40 45 47 53 57 59 62 64
67 77 85 86 87 93 97 107 113 118 126 127 129 132 134 145
Primary Contact: Roger A. Masse, FACHE, Chief Executive Officer
CFO: Preston Sauers, Chief Financial Officer
CIO: Lynette Dick, Director of Support Services
CHR: Sandy Wedel, Director Human Resources
CNO: Laura Stofferson, Director of Nursing
Web address: www.ewmed.com
**Control:** County–Government, nonfederal **Service:** General Medical and Surgical

**Staffed Beds:** 20 **Admissions:** 790 **Census:** 9 **Outpatient Visits:** 17258
**Births:** 0 **Total Expense ($000):** 13270 **Payroll Expense ($000):** 6629
**Personnel:** 143

## EMPORIA—Lyon County

★ ○ **NEWMAN REGIONAL HEALTH (170001)**, 1201 West 12th Avenue,
Zip 66801–2597; tel. 620/343–6800 **A**5 9 10 11 20 **F**3 11 13 28 29 31 39
40 41 45 51 53 59 61 63 64 65 68 70 76 77 78 79 81 82 84 85 86 87 89
90 93 96 100 102 107 108 111 113 117 118 128 129 130 131 132 134
145 146 147 **P**6 **S** QHR, Brentwood, TN
Primary Contact: John Rossfeld, Interim Chief Executive Officer
CFO: Holly French, Chief Financial Officer
CMO: Cy Anderson, M.D., Chief of Staff
CIO: Donald Cope, Director Information Systems
CHR: Kathy Orear, Director Human Resources
CNO: Julia Pyle, R.N., Chief Nursing Officer
Web address: www.newmanrh.org
**Control:** County–Government, nonfederal **Service:** General Medical and Surgical

**Staffed Beds:** 59 **Admissions:** 2698 **Census:** 32 **Outpatient Visits:** 88234
**Births:** 404 **Total Expense ($000):** 50003 **Payroll Expense ($000):** 22026
**Personnel:** 449

### EUREKA—Greenwood County

**GREENWOOD COUNTY HOSPITAL (171339)**, 100 West 16th Street, Zip 67045–1064; tel. 620/583–7451 **A**9 10 18 **F**3 40 53 62 64 81 93 107 118 126 132 **P**6
Primary Contact: Edward E. Riley, Chief Executive Officer
CFO: Lisa Ramsey, Chief Financial Officer
CIO: Filiberto J. Ojeda, Director Quality Improvement, Risk Management and Information System
CHR: Janel M. Palmer, Director Human Resources
Web address: www.gwch.org
**Control:** County–Government, nonfederal **Service:** General Medical and Surgical

**Staffed Beds:** 25 **Admissions:** 583 **Census:** 5 **Outpatient Visits:** 17378 **Births:** 0 **Total Expense ($000):** 12744 **Payroll Expense ($000):** 6183 **Personnel:** 139

### FORT SCOTT—Bourbon County

⊠ **MERCY HOSPITAL FORT SCOTT (170058)**, 401 Woodland Hills Boulevard, Zip 66701–8797; tel. 620/223–2200 **A**1 5 9 10 **F**3 7 11 13 15 28 30 34 35 40 53 57 59 62 65 70 72 75 76 77 79 81 82 84 85 90 93 97 107 108 110 111 113 117 118 126 128 129 130 131 132 142 143 144 145 147 **P**6
**S** Mercy Health, Chesterfield, MO
Primary Contact: Reta K. Baker, President
CFO: Terri Del Chiaro, Chief Financial Officer
CMO: Robert R. Nichols, M.D., Vice President Medical Affairs
CIO: Rose Ludeke, Site Administrator Management Information Systems
CHR: Linda Noll, Executive Director Human Resources
Web address: www.mercykansas.com
**Control:** Church–operated, Nongovernment, not–for profit **Service:** General Medical and Surgical

**Staffed Beds:** 61 **Admissions:** 1788 **Census:** 19 **Outpatient Visits:** 82600 **Births:** 231 **Total Expense ($000):** 30370 **Payroll Expense ($000):** 14340 **Personnel:** 284

### FREDONIA—Wilson County

★ **FREDONIA REGIONAL HOSPITAL (171374)**, 1527 Madison Street, Zip 66736–1751, Mailing Address: P.O. Box 579, Zip 66736–0579; tel. 620/378–2121 **A**9 10 18 **F**3 7 11 15 30 40 81 82 85 93 98 103 107 110 113 118 127 132 **S** Great Plains Health Alliance, Inc., Phillipsburg, KS
Primary Contact: Terry Deschaine, Chief Executive Officer
CFO: Wendy Barton, Manager Business Office
CHR: Debbie Marr, Administrative Assistant and Director Human Resources
Web address: www.fredoniaregionalhospital.org
**Control:** City–Government, nonfederal **Service:** General Medical and Surgical

**Staffed Beds:** 34 **Admissions:** 777 **Census:** 13 **Outpatient Visits:** 18061 **Births:** 0 **Total Expense ($000):** 12432 **Payroll Expense ($000):** 4279 **Personnel:** 117

### GARDEN CITY—Finney County

⊠ **ST. CATHERINE HOSPITAL (170023)**, 401 East Spuce Street, Zip 67846–5679; tel. 620/272–2561 **A**1 9 10 20 **F**3 13 15 18 20 22 24 29 30 31 34 35 40 45 51 57 59 60 63 64 65 69 70 73 75 76 77 78 79 81 85 87 89 93 97 98 100 102 107 108 109 111 114 115 117 118 119 120 121 122 123 128 129 131 134 145 146 147 **P**5 6 **S** Catholic Health Initiatives, Englewood, CO
Primary Contact: Scott J. Taylor, President and Chief Executive Officer
COO: John Yox, Senior Vice President and Chief Operating Officer
CFO: Amanda Vaughan, Chief Financial Officer
CIO: Lance Kellenbarger, Site Director Information Systems
CHR: Kathy E. Morrison, Executive Director Human Resources
CNO: Carol Schmekel, R.N., Senior Vice President Patient Services
Web address: www.stcath–hosp.org
**Control:** Church–operated, Nongovernment, not–for profit **Service:** General Medical and Surgical

**Staffed Beds:** 110 **Admissions:** 3531 **Census:** 43 **Outpatient Visits:** 128286 **Births:** 859 **Total Expense ($000):** 78528 **Payroll Expense ($000):** 28872 **Personnel:** 525

### GARDNER—Johnson County

★ △ **MEADOWBROOK REHABILITATION HOSPITAL (170180)**, 427 West Main Street, Zip 66030–1183; tel. 913/856–8747, (Total facility includes 42 beds in nursing home–type unit) **A**7 9 10 **F**90 127 129 131 142 145 147
Primary Contact: Mark LeNeave, Administrator
CFO: Renee Morrow, Business Manager
CMO: Magdy Tadros, M.D., Medical Director
CHR: Carrie Moore, Director Human Resources
Web address: www.meadowbrookrehab.com
**Control:** Partnership, Investor–owned, for–profit **Service:** Rehabilitation

**Staffed Beds:** 96 **Admissions:** 375 **Census:** 58 **Outpatient Visits:** 925 **Births:** 0 **Total Expense ($000):** 11654 **Payroll Expense ($000):** 4960 **Personnel:** 138

### GARNETT—Anderson County

**ANDERSON COUNTY HOSPITAL (171316)**, 421 South Maple, Zip 66032–1334, Mailing Address: P.O. Box 309, Zip 66032–0309; tel. 785/448–3131, (Total facility includes 30 beds in nursing home–type unit) **A**9 10 18 **F**3 7 11 15 34 40 57 59 64 67 75 81 93 97 107 108 113 126 129 132 **P**6 **S** Saint Luke's Health System, Kansas City, MO
Primary Contact: Dennis A. Hachenberg, FACHE, Chief Executive Officer
CFO: Vicki L. Mills, Chief Financial Officer
CMO: George A. Pagels, M.D., Senior Vice President and Chief Medical Officer
CHR: Karen Gillespie, Director Human Resources
CNO: Margo L. Williams, R.N., Chief Nursing Officer
Web address: www.saint–lukes.org
**Control:** Other not–for–profit (including NFP Corporation) **Service:** General Medical and Surgical

**Staffed Beds:** 41 **Admissions:** 168 **Census:** 30 **Outpatient Visits:** 38613 **Births:** 0 **Total Expense ($000):** 14938 **Payroll Expense ($000):** 6805 **Personnel:** 137

### GIRARD—Crawford County

★ **GIRARD MEDICAL CENTER (171376)**, 302 North Hospital Drive, Zip 66743–2000; tel. 620/724–8291 **A**9 10 18 **F**3 11 12 15 28 34 35 40 47 49 50 53 56 57 59 62 64 65 70 75 77 79 81 87 93 98 100 101 102 103 104 105 106 107 108 118 126 129 131 132 145 146 147 **P**6
Primary Contact: Michael E. Payne, Administrator
CFO: Holly Koch, Chief Financial Officer
CIO: Jeff Barnes, Director of Information Technology
CHR: Mary Ann Holloway, Manager Human Resources
CNO: Patty Ridings, Director of Nursing
Web address: www.girardmedicalcenter.com
**Control:** Hospital district or authority, Government, nonfederal **Service:** General Medical and Surgical

**Staffed Beds:** 35 **Admissions:** 1205 **Census:** 20 **Outpatient Visits:** 27154 **Births:** 0 **Total Expense ($000):** 19774 **Payroll Expense ($000):** 8747 **Personnel:** 193

### GOODLAND—Sherman County

**GOODLAND REGIONAL MEDICAL CENTER (171370)**, 220 West Second Street, Zip 67735–1602; tel. 785/890–3625 **A**9 10 18 **F**3 7 11 13 15 28 31 34 40 44 45 57 59 64 65 67 69 75 76 79 81 82 85 87 89 93 97 107 113 118 126 127 129 131 132 **P**6
Primary Contact: Jay P. Jolly, Chief Executive Officer
CFO: James Precht, Chief Financial Officer
CIO: Kevin Sanderson, Director Information Systems
CHR: Dale Schields, Director Human Resources
Web address: www.goodlandregional.com
**Control:** County–Government, nonfederal **Service:** General Medical and Surgical

**Staffed Beds:** 25 **Admissions:** 389 **Census:** 4 **Outpatient Visits:** 42686 **Births:** 57 **Total Expense ($000):** 13780 **Payroll Expense ($000):** 5940 **Personnel:** 124

### GREAT BEND—Barton County

**GREAT BEND REGIONAL HOSPITAL (170191)**, 514 Cleveland Street, Zip 67530; tel. 620/792–8833 **A**9 10 **F**3 13 29 30 34 40 57 59 64 68 69 70 75 76 79 81 82 89 107 111 113 118 126 129 146 **P**5
Primary Contact: Pamela Chambers, Chief Executive Officer
CFO: Larry T. Fore, Controller
CMO: Adina Gregory, Chief Nursing Officer
CIO: Susan Read, Director Information Technology Support
CHR: Ruth Bealer, Director Human Resources
Web address: www.greatbendsurgical.com
**Control:** Partnership, Investor–owned, for–profit **Service:** General Medical and Surgical

**Staffed Beds:** 33 **Admissions:** 1451 **Census:** 13 **Outpatient Visits:** 19061 **Births:** 180 **Total Expense ($000):** 27371 **Payroll Expense ($000):** 9055 **Personnel:** 181

---

**Hospital, Medicare Provider Number, Address, Telephone, Approval, Facility, and Physician Codes, Health Care System**

★ American Hospital Association (AHA) membership
□ The Joint Commission accreditation ◇ DNV Healthcare Inc. accreditation
○ American Osteopathic Association (AOA) accreditation
△ Commission on Accreditation of Rehabilitation Facilities (CARF) accreditation

**KS**

## GREENSBURG—Kiowa County

★ **KIOWA COUNTY MEMORIAL HOSPITAL (171332)**, 721 West Kansas Avenue, Zip 67054–1951; tel. 620/723–3341 **A**9 10 18 **F**3 7 11 40 50 53 59 64 68 107 114 126 127 132 **P**6 **S** Great Plains Health Alliance, Inc., Phillipsburg, KS
Primary Contact: Mary Sweet, Administrator
CFO: Ron Tucker, Business Office Manager
CMO: Nizar Kibar, M.D., Chief Medical Staff
CIO: Jeremy Hoover, Chief Information Officer
CHR: Cathy McFall, Human Resources Manager
CNO: Vanessa Kirk, Director of Nursing
Web address: www.kcmh.net
**Control:** County–Government, nonfederal **Service:** General Medical and Surgical

> **Staffed Beds:** 15 **Admissions:** 122 **Census:** 3 **Outpatient Visits:** 12029 **Births:** 0 **Total Expense ($000):** 7885 **Payroll Expense ($000):** 2733 **Personnel:** 68

## HANOVER—Washington County

★ **HANOVER HOSPITAL (171365)**, (Critical Access Hospital), 205 South Hanover, Zip 66945–0038, Mailing Address: P.O. Box 38, Zip 66945–0038; tel. 785/337–2214 **A**9 10 18 **F**7 40 53 64 69 81 132 **P**5
Primary Contact: Roger D. Warren, M.D., Administrator
CFO: Sheryl Adam, Chief Financial Officer
CMO: Roger D. Warren, M.D., Administrator
**Control:** Hospital district or authority, Government, nonfederal **Service:** General Medical and Surgical

> **Staffed Beds:** 25 **Admissions:** 1493 **Census:** 19 **Outpatient Visits:** 2169 **Births:** 10 **Total Expense ($000):** 3242 **Payroll Expense ($000):** 1700 **Personnel:** 51

## HARPER—Harper County

★ **HARPER HOSPITAL DISTRICT FIVE (171366)**, 700 West 13th Street, Zip 67058–1401; tel. 620/896–7324 **A**9 10 18 **F**3 10 12 29 32 34 35 40 43 45 46 50 53 57 59 62 64 65 67 68 69 75 77 79 81 84 87 93 97 107 111 113 118 124 126 127 128 129 132 134 145 146 147
Primary Contact: Kim Cinelli, Administrator and Chief Executive Officer
CFO: Sandra Owen, Director Fiscal and Accounting
CMO: Ralph Imlay, M.D., Chief of Staff
CIO: Cindi Beadman, Director Medical Records
CHR: Vicki Longbine, Director Human Resources
CNO: Karen Aldis, Director of Nursing
Web address: www.hhd5.com
**Control:** Hospital district or authority, Government, nonfederal **Service:** General Medical and Surgical

> **Staffed Beds:** 25 **Admissions:** 334 **Census:** 10 **Outpatient Visits:** 81515 **Births:** 0 **Total Expense ($000):** 7043 **Payroll Expense ($000):** 3752 **Personnel:** 99

## HAYS—Ellis County

★ **HAYS MEDICAL CENTER (170013)**, 2220 Canterbury Drive, Zip 67601–2370, Mailing Address: P.O. Box 8100, Zip 67601–8100; tel. 785/623–5000 **A**2 5 9 10 21 **F**3 11 12 13 15 17 18 20 22 24 26 28 29 30 31 32 34 35 36 37 38 39 40 43 45 46 49 53 55 56 57 59 60 63 64 65 66 68 69 70 71 72 74 75 76 77 78 79 80 81 82 84 85 86 87 89 90 92 93 97 98 100 101 102 103 104 107 108 110 111 114 117 118 119 120 126 128 129 130 131 134 145 146 147 **P**6
Primary Contact: John H. Jeter, M.D., President and Chief Executive Officer
COO: Bryce A. Young, Chief Operating Officer
CFO: Bill Overbey, Chief Financial Officer and Chief Information Officer
CMO: Larry Watts, Chief Medical Officer
CIO: Bill Overbey, Chief Financial Officer and Chief Information Officer
CHR: Bruce Whittington, Vice President Human Resources
CNO: Terry Siek, MSN, Chief Nursing Officer
Web address: www.haysmed.com
**Control:** Other not–for–profit (including NFP Corporation) **Service:** General Medical and Surgical

> **Staffed Beds:** 172 **Admissions:** 5165 **Census:** 70 **Outpatient Visits:** 313857 **Births:** 703 **Total Expense ($000):** 172262 **Payroll Expense ($000):** 73249 **Personnel:** 1196

## HERINGTON—Dickinson County

**HERINGTON MUNICIPAL HOSPITAL (171340)**, 100 East Helen Street, Zip 67449–1606; tel. 785/258–2207 **A**9 10 18 **F**15 28 29 40 45 57 64 77 81 93 97 107 118 126 132 147
Primary Contact: Michael J. Ryan, Chief Executive Officer
CFO: Patricia M. Moyer, Chief Financial Officer
CMO: John Mosier, D.O., Chief of Staff
CHR: Debbie Stewart, Human Resources Officer
CNO: Kathy Kershner, Director of Nursing
Web address: www.heringtonhospital.org
**Control:** City–Government, nonfederal **Service:** General Medical and Surgical

> **Staffed Beds:** 25 **Admissions:** 427 **Census:** 6 **Outpatient Visits:** 14050 **Births:** 0 **Total Expense ($000):** 6286 **Payroll Expense ($000):** 3061 **Personnel:** 74

## HIAWATHA—Brown County

★ **HIAWATHA COMMUNITY HOSPITAL (171341)**, 300 Utah Street, Zip 66434–2314; tel. 785/742–2131 **A**9 10 18 **F**8 13 15 28 40 45 62 67 69 70 76 81 85 107 113 118 126 127 129 132 145 **P**6
Primary Contact: John Moore, Administrator
CFO: Jenny Knudson, Controller
CMO: Bryon Bigham, M.D., Chief of Staff
CIO: Cheryl Wenger, Manager Health Information and Quality Assurance
CHR: Katie Sisk, Director Human Resources
CNO: Lisa Thompson, MSN, Director of Nursing
Web address: www.hch-ks.org
**Control:** Other not-for-profit (including NFP Corporation) **Service:** General Medical and Surgical

> **Staffed Beds:** 25 **Admissions:** 1039 **Census:** 12 **Outpatient Visits:** 26766 **Births:** 106 **Total Expense ($000):** 18226 **Payroll Expense ($000):** 7846 **Personnel:** 218

## HILL CITY—Graham County

★ **GRAHAM COUNTY HOSPITAL (171325)**, 304 West Prout Street, Zip 67642–1435; tel. 785/421–2121 **A**9 10 18 **F**3 8 11 28 29 30 31 34 35 40 45 50 53 57 59 63 64 69 81 84 93 97 107 126 127 129 132 145 147 **P**6
Primary Contact: Melissa Atkins, CPA, Chief Executive Officer
CHR: Donella Belleau, Director Human Resources
Web address: www.grahamcountyhospital.org
**Control:** County–Government, nonfederal **Service:** General Medical and Surgical

> **Staffed Beds:** 25 **Admissions:** 621 **Census:** 7 **Outpatient Visits:** 966 **Births:** 0 **Total Expense ($000):** 7764 **Payroll Expense ($000):** 3929 **Personnel:** 94

## HILLSBORO—Marion County

★ **HILLSBORO COMMUNITY HOSPITAL (171357)**, 701 South Main Street, Zip 67063–1595; tel. 620/947–3114 **A**9 10 18 **F**3 11 29 30 34 35 40 45 47 50 57 59 64 65 75 77 81 85 86 87 93 107 113 126 129 131 132 145 147 **P**5 6 **S** HMC/CAH Consolidated, Inc., Kansas City, MO
Primary Contact: Marion Regier, Chief Executive Officer
COO: Johna Magnuson, Director Nursing
CIO: Marsha Setzkorn–Meyer, Director Public Relations and Marketing
CHR: Wendy McCarty, Director Human Resources
Web address: www.hchks.com
**Control:** Corporation, Investor–owned, for–profit **Service:** General Medical and Surgical

> **Staffed Beds:** 16 **Admissions:** 163 **Census:** 2 **Outpatient Visits:** 6061 **Births:** 0 **Total Expense ($000):** 3655 **Payroll Expense ($000):** 1582 **Personnel:** 32

## HOISINGTON—Barton County

★ **CLARA BARTON HOSPITAL (171333)**, 250 West Ninth Street, Zip 67544–1706; tel. 620/653–2114 **A**9 10 18 **F**11 15 28 40 51 56 57 59 64 69 77 81 85 93 97 107 113 118 126 127 132 147 **P**3
Primary Contact: Curt Colson, President and Chief Executive Officer
CFO: James Blackwell, Vice President and Chief Financial Officer
CMO: Josh Durham, D.O., Chief of Staff
CHR: John Moshier, Director Human Resources
CNO: Jane Schepmann, Vice President and Chief Nursing Officer
Web address: www.clarabartonhospital.org
**Control:** Other not–for–profit (including NFP Corporation) **Service:** General Medical and Surgical

> **Staffed Beds:** 23 **Admissions:** 555 **Census:** 8 **Outpatient Visits:** 48226 **Births:** 0 **Total Expense ($000):** 15649 **Payroll Expense ($000):** 6885 **Personnel:** 147

## HOLTON—Jackson County

★ **HOLTON COMMUNITY HOSPITAL (171319)**, 1110 Columbine Drive, Zip 66436–1545; tel. 785/364–2116 **A**9 10 18 **F**3 11 13 15 18 28 34 40 45 62 63 64 65 75 76 77 81 82 89 90 93 97 107 113 118 126 127 129 130 131 132 134 145 146 147
Primary Contact: Carrie L. Saia, R.N., Interim Chief Executive Officer
CFO: Marlene Kranz, Controller
CMO: Lee Schnee, M.D., Chief Medical Staff
CIO: Sarah Larison, Director Health Information Management
CHR: Gretchen Snavely, Director Human Resources
Web address: www.holtonhospital.com
**Control:** Other not–for–profit (including NFP Corporation) **Service:** General Medical and Surgical

> **Staffed Beds:** 12 **Admissions:** 389 **Census:** 5 **Outpatient Visits:** 49135 **Births:** 35 **Total Expense ($000):** 9976 **Payroll Expense ($000):** 5092 **Personnel:** 116

*Many Facility Codes have changed. Please refer to the AHA Guide Code Chart.* © 2012 AHA Guide

## HORTON—Brown County

★ **HORTON COMMUNITY HOSPITAL (171320)**, 240 West 18th Street, Zip 66439–1245; tel. 785/486–2642 **A**9 10 18 **F**7 15 18 28 29 31 40 45 46 64 81 93 107 113 118 126 127 132 **P**6 **S** HMC/CAH Consolidated, Inc., Kansas City, MO
Primary Contact: Terry Nichols, Interim Chief Executive Officer
CFO: Sue Kidd, Chief Financial Officer
CMO: Galen Seymour, M.D., Chief of Staff
CHR: Ty Compton, Chief Nursing Executive
**Control:** Corporation, Investor–owned, for–profit **Service:** General Medical and Surgical

**Staffed Beds:** 25 **Admissions:** 269 **Census:** 2 **Outpatient Visits:** 1996
**Births:** 0 **Total Expense ($000):** 5978 **Payroll Expense ($000):** 2989
**Personnel:** 60

## HOXIE—Sheridan County

**SHERIDAN COUNTY HEALTH COMPLEX (171347)**, 826 18th Street, Zip 67740–0167, Mailing Address: P.O. Box 167, Zip 67740–0167; tel. 785/675–3281, (Total facility includes 35 beds in nursing home–type unit) **A**9 10 18 **F**2 3 10 11 29 30 34 40 45 49 50 53 57 59 64 68 69 75 81 85 86 93 97 107 113 118 126 127 129 133 134 143 145 146 147
Primary Contact: Steven L. Granzow, Chief Executive Officer
CFO: Christine Niblock, Chief Financial Officer
CMO: Thomas R. Plumeri, Chief of Staff
CNO: Maria Zimmerman, R.N., Chief Nursing Officer
Web address: www.sheridancountyhospital.com
**Control:** County–Government, nonfederal **Service:** General Medical and Surgical

**Staffed Beds:** 53 **Admissions:** 151 **Census:** 28 **Outpatient Visits:** 7689
**Births:** 0 **Total Expense ($000):** 6356 **Payroll Expense ($000):** 3381
**Personnel:** 98

## HUGOTON—Stevens County

**STEVENS COUNTY HOSPITAL (171335)**, 1006 South Jackson Street, Zip 67951–2842, Mailing Address: P.O. Box 10, Zip 67951–0010; tel. 620/544–8511, (Total facility includes 58 beds in nursing home–type unit) **A**9 10 18 **F**3 6 11 15 28 29 34 40 45 57 59 62 67 68 81 97 107 118 126 127 129 131 132 134 145
Primary Contact: Linda Stalcup, Chief Executive Officer
CMO: Samer Al–hashmi, M.D., Chief Medical Staff
Web address: www.healthcarefor the heartland.org
**Control:** County–Government, nonfederal **Service:** General Medical and Surgical

**Staffed Beds:** 75 **Admissions:** 267 **Census:** 54 **Outpatient Visits:** 11764
**Births:** 0 **Total Expense ($000):** 14485 **Payroll Expense ($000):** 6938
**Personnel:** 89

## HUTCHINSON—Reno County

★ **HUTCHINSON REGIONAL MEDICAL CENTER (170020)**, 1701 East 23rd Avenue, Zip 67502–1191; tel. 620/665–2000, (Total facility includes 70 beds in nursing home–type unit) **A**3 5 9 10 **F**3 7 10 11 13 18 20 22 24 28 29 30 31 40 48 49 50 51 60 62 63 64 67 68 70 74 75 76 77 78 79 81 82 83 84 85 89 90 93 98 102 103 106 107 108 111 113 114 118 119 120 122 124 125 127 128 129 145 147
Primary Contact: Kevin J. Miller, FACHE, President and Chief Executive Officer
COO: James McComas, Vice President Operations
CFO: David A. Busatti, Vice President Finance
CMO: Verlin Janzen, M.D., Chief of Staff
CIO: David Mendenhall, Chief Information Officer
CHR: Janet Hamons, Vice President Human Resources
Web address: www.promiseregional.com
**Control:** Other not–for–profit (including NFP Corporation) **Service:** General Medical and Surgical

**Staffed Beds:** 209 **Admissions:** 7635 **Census:** 188 **Outpatient Visits:** 134168 **Births:** 667 **Total Expense ($000):** 140112 **Payroll Expense ($000):** 53817 **Personnel:** 1063

**SUMMIT SURGICAL, LLC (170198)**, 1818 East 23rd Avenue, Zip 67502; tel. 620/663–4800 **A**9 10 **F**3 29 45 50 64 79 81 82 85 **P**2
Primary Contact: Gordon Funk, Chief Executive Officer
CFO: Kevin Crunkleton, Chief Financial Officer
CMO: Ann Hentzen Page, M.D., Medical Director
CIO: Monty Moore, Director Information Services
CHR: Jonathan D. Funk, Director Human Resources and Marketing
Web address: www.summitks.com/
**Control:** Partnership, Investor–owned, for–profit **Service:** Surgical

**Staffed Beds:** 10 **Admissions:** 246 **Census:** 1 **Outpatient Visits:** 1181
**Births:** 0 **Total Expense ($000):** 3655 **Payroll Expense ($000):** 1041
**Personnel:** 18

## INDEPENDENCE—Montgomery County

⊠ **MERCY HOSPITAL INDEPENDENCE (170010)**, 800 West Myrtle Street, Zip 67301–9980, Mailing Address: P.O. Box 388, Zip 67301–0388; tel. 620/331–2200 **A**1 9 10 **F**1 3 4 11 13 15 16 17 18 28 30 34 40 45 53 57 59 62 65 67 70 72 73 76 77 79 80 81 84 88 89 90 91 93 97 98 107 108 110 111 113 117 118 126 127 128 129 130 132 134 142 143 145 **P**3 6 **S** Mercy Health, Chesterfield, MO
Primary Contact: Eric Ammons, President and Chief Executive Officer
CFO: Terri Del Chiaro, Vice President and Chief Financial Officer
CMO: Chris Lewis, M.D., Vice President Medical Affairs
CHR: Linda Noll, Executive Director Human Resources
Web address: www.mercykansas.com
**Control:** Church–operated, Nongovernment, not–for profit **Service:** General Medical and Surgical

**Staffed Beds:** 40 **Admissions:** 1129 **Census:** 11 **Outpatient Visits:** 46890
**Births:** 229 **Total Expense ($000):** 20306 **Payroll Expense ($000):** 9192
**Personnel:** 183

## IOLA—Allen County

⊠ **ALLEN COUNTY HOSPITAL (171373)**, 101 South First Street, Zip 66749–3505, Mailing Address: P.O. Box 540, Zip 66749–0540; tel. 620/365–1000, (Nonreporting) **A**1 9 10 18 **S** HCA, Nashville, TN
Primary Contact: Cristina Rivera, Chief Executive Officer
CFO: Larry Peterson, Chief Financial Officer
CMO: Tim Spears, D.O., Chief of Staff
CHR: Paula Sell, Director Human Resources
CNO: Patty McGuffin, R.N., Chief Nursing Officer
Web address: www.allencountyhospital.com
**Control:** Corporation, Investor–owned, for–profit **Service:** General Medical and Surgical

**Staffed Beds:** 25

## JETMORE—Hodgeman County

★ **HODGEMAN COUNTY HEALTH CENTER (171369)**, 809 Bramley Street, Zip 67854–9320, Mailing Address: P.O. Box 310, Zip 67854–0310; tel. 620/357–8361, (Total facility includes 25 beds in nursing home–type unit) **A**9 10 18 **F**3 40 53 67 70 81 107 113 124 126 129 132 142 **P**4
Primary Contact: Teresa L. Deuel, Chief Executive Officer
Web address: www.hchconline.org
**Control:** County–Government, nonfederal **Service:** General Medical and Surgical

**Staffed Beds:** 38 **Admissions:** 341 **Census:** 26 **Outpatient Visits:** 5794
**Births:** 0 **Total Expense ($000):** 6027 **Payroll Expense ($000):** 2643
**Personnel:** 99

## JOHNSON—Stanton County

**STANTON COUNTY HOSPITAL (171343)**, 404 North Chestnut Street, Zip 67855–0779, Mailing Address: P.O. Box 779, Zip 67855–0779; tel. 620/492–6250, (Total facility includes 17 beds in nursing home–type unit) **A**9 10 18 **F**3 13 34 40 41 45 50 57 59 64 68 76 81 86 87 89 93 97 107 127 129 131 132 142 145 **P**6
Primary Contact: Jay Tusten, Chief Executive Officer
CFO: Barbara Anderson, Chief Financial Officer
CMO: Charles Weintz, D.O., Chief of Staff
CIO: Marco Medina, Chief Information Officer
CHR: Camille Davidson, Director Human Resources
CNO: Marianne Mills, R.N., Chairperson
Web address: www.stantoncountyhospital.com
**Control:** County–Government, nonfederal **Service:** General Medical and Surgical

**Staffed Beds:** 26 **Admissions:** 105 **Census:** 16 **Outpatient Visits:** 9932
**Births:** 19 **Total Expense ($000):** 5081 **Payroll Expense ($000):** 2680
**Personnel:** 72

## JUNCTION CITY—Geary County

⊠ **GEARY COMMUNITY HOSPITAL (170074)**, 1102 St. Mary's Road, Zip 66441–4196, Mailing Address: P.O. Box 490, Zip 66441–0490; tel. 785/238–4131 **A**1 3 5 9 10 **F**3 8 11 12 13 16 18 28 29 30 34 35 40 50 56 57 59 61 62 63 64 65 68 70 75 76 77 79 81 85 86 87 89 90 97 98 103 107 108 109 110 111 113 114 117 118 126 128 129 130 131 132 134 142 143 144 145 146 147
Primary Contact: David K. Bradley, FACHE, Chief Executive Officer
COO: Alice J. Jensen, Chief Operating Officer
CFO: Darren K. Rumford, Chief Financial Officer
CHR: Teto E. Henderson, Director Human Resources
Web address: www.gchks.org
**Control:** County–Government, nonfederal **Service:** General Medical and Surgical

**Staffed Beds:** 65 **Admissions:** 1783 **Census:** 18 **Outpatient Visits:** 57104
**Births:** 356 **Total Expense ($000):** 37849 **Payroll Expense ($000):** 19343
**Personnel:** 377

⊞ **IRWIN ARMY COMMUNITY HOSPITAL**, 600 Caisson Hill Road,
Zip 66442–5037; tel. 785/239–7000, (Nonreporting) **A**1 2 5 **S** Department of
the Army, Office of the Surgeon General, Falls Church, VA
Primary Contact: Colonel Barry R. Pockrandt, Commander
COO: Lieutenant Colonel Daniel G. Bonnichsen, Deputy Commander for
Administration
CFO: Lieutenant Colonel Daniel G. Bonnichsen, Deputy Commander for
Administration
CMO: Colonel Craig R. Webb, M.D., Deputy Commander for Clinical Services
CIO: David Dougherty, Chief Information Management Officer
CHR: Dianna Kallenberger, Chief Manpower Branch
CNO: Colonel Robert E. Dettmer, Deputy Commander for Health Services
Web address: www.iach.amedd.army.mil/
**Control:** Army, Government, federal **Service:** General Medical and Surgical

| Staffed Beds: 44 |
| --- |

### KANSAS CITY—Wyandotte County

☐ **KVC PSYCHIATRIC HOSPITAL**, 4300 Brenner Drive, Zip 66104;
tel. 913/334–0294 **A**1 3 5 9 **F**98 99 **P**5
Primary Contact: B. Wayne Sims, President and Chief Executive Officer
Web address: www.kvc.org
**Control:** Other not–for–profit (including NFP Corporation) **Service:** Children's
hospital psychiatric

| Staffed Beds: 57 Admissions: 1643 Census: 37 Outpatient Visits: 0 Births: 0 Total Expense ($000): 7480 Payroll Expense ($000): 3386 Personnel: 96 |
| --- |

⊞ **PROVIDENCE MEDICAL CENTER (170146)**, 8929 Parallel Parkway,
Zip 66112–1636; tel. 913/596–4000 **A**1 2 9 10 **F**3 13 15 17 18 20 22 24 28
29 30 31 34 35 40 44 46 56 57 59 61 62 64 68 70 73 74 75 76 77 78 79
80 81 82 84 85 86 89 93 97 107 108 111 113 114 117 118 119 120 122
123 128 129 130 131 134 145 146 147 **P**6 **S** Sisters of Charity of
Leavenworth Health System, Denver, CO
Primary Contact: Randall G. Nyp, FACHE, President and Chief Executive Officer
CFO: Joe Jeans, Vice President Finance
CIO: Kevin Mapes, Regional Information Technology Director
CHR: Winifred Williams, Vice President Human Resources
CNO: Barbara Wertz, Vice President Patient Care Services
Web address: www.providence–health.org
**Control:** Church–operated, Nongovernment, not–for profit **Service:** General
Medical and Surgical

| Staffed Beds: 196 Admissions: 7421 Census: 91 Outpatient Visits: 114424 Births: 908 Total Expense ($000): 146768 Payroll Expense ($000): 59978 Personnel: 844 |
| --- |

☐ **RAINBOW MENTAL HEALTH FACILITY (174010)**, 2205 West 36th Avenue,
Zip 66103–2107; tel. 913/755–7000 **A**1 10 **F**11 30 50 86 87 98 101 103 129
134 145 **P**6
Primary Contact: Gregory Valentine, Superintendent
CFO: Donna Dean, Chief Financial Officer
CMO: Maria Gustilo, M.D., Medical Director
CHR: Marilyn Williamson, Chief Human Resources Officer
Web address: www.srskansas.org/osh/osh–rmhf_main.html
**Control:** State–Government, nonfederal **Service:** Psychiatric

| Staffed Beds: 36 Admissions: 704 Census: 36 Outpatient Visits: 0 Births: 0 Total Expense ($000): 8727 Payroll Expense ($000): 4973 Personnel: 106 |
| --- |

⊞ **SELECT SPECIALTY HOSPITAL–KANSAS CITY (172005)**, 8929 Parallel
Parkway, 4th Floor, Zip 66112; tel. 913/596–7220 **A**1 9 10 **F**1 3 18 29 82 85
91 129 147 **P**5 **S** Select Medical Corporation, Mechanicsburg, PA
Primary Contact: Matthew H. Blevins, Chief Executive Officer
Web address: www.selectmedicalcorp.com
**Control:** Corporation, Investor–owned, for–profit **Service:** Long–Term Acute Care
hospital

| Staffed Beds: 40 Admissions: 385 Census: 26 Outpatient Visits: 0 Births: 0 Total Expense ($000): 14943 Payroll Expense ($000): 5774 Personnel: 115 |
| --- |

⊞ △ **THE UNIVERSITY OF KANSAS HOSPITAL (170040)**, 3901 Rainbow
Boulevard, Zip 66160–7200; tel. 913/588–5000 **A**1 2 3 5 7 8 9 10 **F**3 8 11 12
13 14 15 16 17 18 20 21 22 24 25 26 27 28 29 30 31 32 33 34 35 36 38
39 40 41 43 44 45 46 47 48 49 50 51 52 54 55 56 57 58 59 60 61 63 64
65 68 70 72 74 75 76 77 78 79 80 81 82 83 84 85 86 87 88 89 90 92 93
96 97 98 99 100 101 102 103 104 107 108 110 111 113 114 115 116 117
118 119 120 122 123 125 128 129 130 131 134 135 137 138 140 141 143
144 145 146 147 **P**6
Primary Contact: Bob Page, Chief Executive Officer
COO: Tammy Peterman, R.N., Executive Vice President, Chief Operating Officer
and Chief Nursing Officer
CFO: Bill Marting, Senior Vice President and Chief Financial Officer
CMO: H. William Barkman, M.D., Chief of Staff
CIO: Chris Hansen, Senior Vice President Ambulatory Services and Chief
Information Officer
CHR: Dwight Kasperbauer, Vice President Human Resources
CNO: Tammy Peterman, R.N., Executive Vice President, Chief Operating Officer
and Chief Nursing Officer
Web address: www.kumed.com
**Control:** Hospital district or authority, Government, nonfederal **Service:** General
Medical and Surgical

| Staffed Beds: 600 Admissions: 26033 Census: 422 Outpatient Visits: 365223 Births: 1539 Total Expense ($000): 832481 Payroll Expense ($000): 300357 Personnel: 5222 |
| --- |

### KINGMAN—Kingman County

★ **NINNESCAH VALLEY HEALTH SYSTEM (171378)**, 750 Avenue D West,
Zip 67068–0376, Mailing Address: P.O. Box 376, Zip 67068–0376;
tel. 620/532–3147 **A**9 10 18 **F**3 11 15 17 28 29 31 34 35 40 56 57 59 62
64 67 69 70 75 77 78 81 86 87 89 90 93 97 107 113 118 127 129 131 132
144 145 147
Primary Contact: Gary L. Tiller, Chief Executive Officer
CFO: Kent Hudson, Chief Financial Officer
CIO: Jay Gehring, Director Information Systems
CHR: Nancy Stucky, Director Human Resources and Public Relations
CNO: Nita McFarland, Director of Nursing
Web address: www.nvhsinc.com
**Control:** Other not–for–profit (including NFP Corporation) **Service:** General
Medical and Surgical

| Staffed Beds: 25 Admissions: 609 Census: 10 Outpatient Visits: 29437 Births: 0 Total Expense ($000): 9932 Payroll Expense ($000): 4776 Personnel: 126 |
| --- |

### KINSLEY—Edwards County

★ **EDWARDS COUNTY HOSPITAL AND HEALTHCARE CENTER (171317)**, 620
West Eighth Street, Zip 67547–2329, Mailing Address: P.O. Box 99,
Zip 67547–0099; tel. 620/659–3621 **A**9 10 18 **F**3 7 11 15 18 19 28 29 30
34 35 39 40 53 56 57 59 64 65 67 68 77 79 81 93 97 98 103 107 110 111
118 126 127 129 132 147
Primary Contact: Robert Krickbaum, Chief Executive Officer
CFO: Jennifer L. Jones, Chief Financial Officer
CMO: Robert Wray, D.O., Chief Medical Staff
CHR: Cheryl Gross, Director Human Resources
Web address: www.edwardscohospital.com
**Control:** County–Government, nonfederal **Service:** General Medical and Surgical

| Staffed Beds: 22 Admissions: 408 Census: 14 Outpatient Visits: 9552 Births: 0 Total Expense ($000): 7633 Payroll Expense ($000): 2946 Personnel: 61 |
| --- |

### KIOWA—Barber County

★ **KIOWA DISTRICT HOSPITAL AND MANOR (171331)**, 810 Drumm Street,
Zip 67070–1626; tel. 620/825–4131, (Total facility includes 34 beds in nursing
home–type unit) **A**9 10 18 **F**2 29 40 45 64 67 81 85 92 93 97 107 111 118
126 129 132 **P**6
Primary Contact: Alden M. Vandeveer, Jr., FACHE, Chief Executive Officer
CFO: Robin Lewis, Chief Financial Officer
CMO: Paul Wilhelm, M.D., Chief of Staff
CHR: Tara Girty, Director Human Resources
**Control:** Hospital district or authority, Government, nonfederal **Service:** General
Medical and Surgical

| Staffed Beds: 58 Admissions: 185 Census: 27 Outpatient Visits: 6202 Births: 0 Total Expense ($000): 3208 Payroll Expense ($000): 1821 Personnel: 77 |
| --- |

*Many Facility Codes have changed. Please refer to the AHA Guide Code Chart.* © 2012 AHA Guide

## LA CROSSE—Rush County

★ **RUSH COUNTY MEMORIAL HOSPITAL (171342)**, 801 Locust Street, Zip 67548–9673, Mailing Address: P.O. Box 520, Zip 67548–0520; tel. 785/222–2545, (Total facility includes 20 beds in nursing home–type unit) **A**9 10 18 **F**40 45 53 63 64 68 77 81 93 97 107 111 113 118 126 132 **P**6
Primary Contact: Jonathan Owens, Chief Executive Officer
CFO: Duane Fields, Chief Financial Officer
CMO: J. Scott Appling, M.D., Chief of Staff
CHR: Pam Seltman, Director Human Resources
Web address: www.rushcounty.org/
**Control:** County–Government, nonfederal **Service:** General Medical and Surgical

**Staffed Beds: 36 Admissions: 123 Census: 22 Outpatient Visits: 6900 Births: 0 Total Expense ($000): 5191 Payroll Expense ($000): 2040 Personnel: 63**

## LAKIN—Kearny County

**KEARNY COUNTY HOSPITAL (171313)**, 500 Thorpe Street, Zip 67860; tel. 620/355–7111, (Total facility includes 75 beds in nursing home–type unit) **A**9 10 18 **F**2 3 6 10 13 28 34 35 40 45 50 56 59 62 64 67 68 75 76 81 85 86 89 93 97 107 118 124 127 130 131 132 142 **P**6
Primary Contact: John Loebl, Chief Executive Officer
CFO: ReChelle Kennedy, Chief Financial Officer
CMO: Arlo Reimer, M.D., Chief of Staff
CIO: Scott Good, Manager Information Services
CHR: Donna Winright, Director Human Resources and Senior Services
Web address: www.kearnycountyhospital.com
**Control:** County–Government, nonfederal **Service:** General Medical and Surgical

**Staffed Beds: 100 Admissions: 539 Census: 67 Outpatient Visits: 33993 Births: 148 Total Expense ($000): 14794 Payroll Expense ($000): 7973 Personnel: 200**

## LARNED—Pawnee County

☐ **LARNED STATE HOSPITAL (174006)**, 1301 Kansas Highway 264, Zip 67550; tel. 620/285–2131 **A**1 10 **F**30 50 53 57 61 68 75 77 86 87 98 99 101 103 106 129 131 134 142 145
Primary Contact: Robert Connell, PsyD, Superintendent
CFO: Mary Odom, Accountant
CMO: Geoffrey Hammond, M.D., Medical Director
CIO: Sid Smith, Director Information Resources
CHR: Adele Dunn, Director Human Resources
Web address: www.larnedstatehospital.org
**Control:** State–Government, nonfederal **Service:** Psychiatric

**Staffed Beds: 468 Admissions: 1543 Census: 468 Outpatient Visits: 0 Births: 0 Total Expense ($000): 57150 Payroll Expense ($000): 44042 Personnel: 709**

★ **PAWNEE VALLEY COMMUNITY HOSPITAL (171345)**, 923 Carroll Avenue, Zip 67550; tel. 620/285–3161 **A**9 10 18 **F**3 11 28 29 30 34 40 45 46 57 68 77 81 84 87 93 102 107 113 118 129 130 132 134 147
Primary Contact: Matt Heyn, Administrator
COO: Bryce A. Young, Chief Operating Officer
CFO: Bill Overbey, Chief Financial Officer
CMO: David Sanger, M.D., Chief Medical Officer
CHR: Bruce Whittington, Vice President Human Resources
Web address: www.pawneevalleyhospital.com
**Control:** County–Government, nonfederal **Service:** General Medical and Surgical

**Staffed Beds: 25 Admissions: 382 Census: 8 Outpatient Visits: 39407 Births: 0 Total Expense ($000): 8989 Payroll Expense ($000): 3777 Personnel: 74**

## LAWRENCE—Douglas County

☒ △ **LAWRENCE MEMORIAL HOSPITAL (170137)**, 325 Maine Street, Zip 66044–1389; tel. 785/505–5000, (Total facility includes 12 beds in nursing home–type unit) **A**1 3 5 7 9 10 20 **F**3 11 13 15 18 20 22 26 28 29 30 31 34 36 38 40 44 45 50 51 54 55 57 59 61 64 68 70 74 75 76 77 78 79 81 82 84 85 86 87 89 90 91 93 94 96 100 102 107 108 110 111 113 114 115 116 117 118 121 127 128 129 133 134 144 145 146 147 **P**6 8
Primary Contact: Eugene W. Meyer, President and Chief Executive Officer
COO: Karen J. Shumate, R.N., Chief Operating Officer
CFO: Joe Pedley, CPA, Vice President and Chief Financial Officer
CIO: Jane Maskus, Vice President and Chief Information Officer
CNO: Dana R. Hale, R.N., Vice President Nursing
Web address: www.lmh.org
**Control:** City–Government, nonfederal **Service:** General Medical and Surgical

**Staffed Beds: 152 Admissions: 6655 Census: 63 Outpatient Visits: 193499 Births: 1086 Total Expense ($000): 157168 Payroll Expense ($000): 64988 Personnel: 1139**

## LEAVENWORTH—Leavenworth County

☐ **CUSHING MEMORIAL HOSPITAL (170133)**, 711 Marshall Street, Zip 66048–3235; tel. 913/684–1100 **A**1 5 9 10 **F**11 13 15 18 28 29 31 34 40 45 50 51 57 59 64 70 74 75 76 77 79 81 82 85 87 93 94 98 100 101 102 103 108 110 111 113 118 128 129 130 131 145 147 **P**6 **S** Saint Luke's Health System, Kansas City, MO
Primary Contact: N. Gary Wages, FACHE, Interim Chief Executive Officer
CFO: Sally Border, Chief Financial Officer
CMO: Kathleen McBratney, M.D., President
CHR: Bertt Matthews, Director Human Resources
Web address: www.cushinghospital.org
**Control:** Other not–for–profit (including NFP Corporation) **Service:** General Medical and Surgical

**Staffed Beds: 53 Admissions: 1968 Census: 20 Outpatient Visits: 32875 Births: 138 Total Expense ($000): 31668 Payroll Expense ($000): 13558 Personnel: 263**

**DWIGHT D. EISENHOWER VETERANS AFFAIRS MEDICAL CENTER** See Veterans Affairs Eastern Kansas Health Care System, Topeka

☒ **SAINT JOHN HOSPITAL (170009)**, 3500 South Fourth Street, Zip 66048–5043; tel. 913/680–6000 **A**1 9 10 **F**3 8 13 15 18 29 30 34 35 40 44 46 54 56 57 59 61 64 65 70 74 75 76 77 78 79 81 82 84 85 93 98 103 105 107 113 117 118 129 131 132 134 145 146 147 **P**6 **S** Sisters of Charity of Leavenworth Health System, Denver, CO
Primary Contact: Randall G. Nyp, FACHE, President and Chief Executive Officer
CFO: Joe Jeans, Chief Financial Officer
CIO: Kevin Mapes, Regional Information Technology Director
CHR: Winifred Williams, Vice President Human Resources
CNO: Barbara Wertz, Vice President Patient Care Services
Web address: www.providence–health.org/sjh
**Control:** Church–operated, Nongovernment, not–for profit **Service:** General Medical and Surgical

**Staffed Beds: 56 Admissions: 1944 Census: 30 Outpatient Visits: 44217 Births: 128 Total Expense ($000): 33101 Payroll Expense ($000): 14912 Personnel: 233**

## LEAWOOD—Johnson County

☐ **DOCTOR'S HOSPITAL (170194)**, 4901 College Boulevard, Zip 66211; tel. 913/529–1801 **A**1 10 **F**79 81 82 111 **P**5
Primary Contact: Phil Harness, Chief Executive Officer
Web address: www.dshospital.net
**Control:** Partnership, Investor–owned, for–profit **Service:** General Medical and Surgical

**Staffed Beds: 10 Admissions: 243 Census: 1 Outpatient Visits: 10987 Births: 0 Total Expense ($000): 14301 Payroll Expense ($000): 2086 Personnel: 27**

**KANSAS CITY ORTHOPAEDIC INSTITUTE (170188)**, 3651 College Boulevard, Zip 66211; tel. 913/338–4100 **A**3 5 9 10 **F**29 77 79 81 82 93 111
Primary Contact: Charles E. Rhoades, M.D., Chief Executive Officer
CIO: Jim Leveling, Director Information Technology
CHR: Laura Sinclair, Director Human Resources
Web address: www.kcoi.com
**Control:** Partnership, Investor–owned, for–profit **Service:** Orthopedic

**Staffed Beds: 9 Admissions: 711 Census: 6 Outpatient Visits: 32245 Births: 0 Personnel: 96**

## LENEXA—Johnson County

☐ **MINIMALLY INVASIVE SURGERY CENTER (170199)**, 11217 Lakeview Avenue, Zip 66219; tel. 913/322–7401 **A**1 9 **F**12 81 107 118
Primary Contact: Parajeet Sabharrwal, Administrator
Web address: www.laplose.com/
**Control:** Hospital district or authority, Government, nonfederal **Service:** Surgical

**Staffed Beds: 9 Admissions: 97 Census: 1 Outpatient Visits: 720 Births: 0 Personnel: 16**

## LEOTI—Wichita County

★ **WICHITA COUNTY HEALTH CENTER (171306)**, 211 East Earl Street,
Zip 67861–9620; tel. 620/375–2233, (Total facility includes 12 beds in nursing
home–type unit) **A**9 10 18 **F**2 3 11 29 34 35 40 41 45 50 56 57 59 64 67 69
75 77 86 87 89 93 97 107 126 127 129 132 134 145 **P**6
Primary Contact: Victoria J. Hahn, Administrator and Chief Executive Officer
CFO: Janice Campas, Chief Financial Officer
CMO: Jeffrey Alpert, M.D., Medical Director
CHR: Patti Whalen, Manager Human Resources
CNO: Teresa Clark, Director of Nursing
Web address: www.wichitacountyhealthcenter.com
**Control:** County–Government, nonfederal **Service:** General Medical and Surgical

**Staffed Beds:** 37 **Admissions:** 218 **Census:** 15 **Outpatient Visits:** 22601
**Births:** 0 **Total Expense ($000):** 6379 **Payroll Expense ($000):** 3064
**Personnel:** 67

## LIBERAL—Seward County

⊠ **SOUTHWEST MEDICAL CENTER (170068)**, 315 West 15th Street,
Zip 67901–1340, Mailing Address: Box 1340, Zip 67905–1340;
tel. 620/624–1651, (Total facility includes 18 beds in nursing home–type unit) **A**1
5 9 10 **F**3 11 13 15 29 31 34 40 45 48 49 57 59 68 70 73 75 76 77 79 81
85 87 89 93 96 98 103 104 107 108 110 111 113 117 118 127 128
129 144
Primary Contact: Bill Ermann, Interim Chief Executive Officer
COO: Michele Gillespie, Vice President of Operations
CFO: Bill Ermann, Vice President and Chief Financial Officer
CIO: Shelley Mayes, Director of Medical Information Services
CHR: Lisa L. Mathes, Director of Human Resources
CNO: Jo L. Harrison, Vice President of Patient Care Services
Web address: www.swmedcenter.com
**Control:** County–Government, nonfederal **Service:** General Medical and Surgical

**Staffed Beds:** 101 **Admissions:** 1865 **Census:** 20 **Outpatient Visits:** 57583
**Births:** 697 **Total Expense ($000):** 39432 **Payroll Expense ($000):** 16773
**Personnel:** 344

## LINCOLN—Lincoln County

**LINCOLN COUNTY HOSPITAL (171360)**, 624 North Second Street,
Zip 67455–1738, Mailing Address: P.O. Box 406, Zip 67455–0406;
tel. 785/524–4403 **A**9 10 18 **F**11 40 69 107 118 126 132 **P**6
Primary Contact: Greg R. McNeil, Chief Executive Officer
**Control:** County–Government, nonfederal **Service:** General Medical and Surgical

**Staffed Beds:** 14 **Admissions:** 188 **Census:** 2 **Outpatient Visits:** 4552
**Births:** 0 **Total Expense ($000):** 5876 **Payroll Expense ($000):** 2762
**Personnel:** 76

## LINDSBORG—Mcpherson County

★ **LINDSBORG COMMUNITY HOSPITAL (171358)**, 605 West Lincoln Street,
Zip 67456–2328; tel. 785/227–3308 **A**9 10 18 **F**3 28 29 40 53 59 62 67 75
77 81 93 107 113 118 127 129 132 **P**6
Primary Contact: Larry VanDerWege, Administrator and Chief Executive Officer
CFO: Laraine Gengler, Chief Financial Officer
CMO: Craig Nickel, M.D., Chief of Staff
CIO: Betty Nelson, Director of Marketing and Development
CHR: Brad Malm, Director Human Resources and Education
CNO: Beth Hedberg, R.N., Director of Nursing
Web address: www.lindsborghospital.org
**Control:** Other not–for–profit (including NFP Corporation) **Service:** General
Medical and Surgical

**Staffed Beds:** 25 **Admissions:** 337 **Census:** 5 **Outpatient Visits:** 20847
**Births:** 0 **Total Expense ($000):** 5771 **Payroll Expense ($000):** 2746
**Personnel:** 70

## LYONS—Rice County

★ **RICE COUNTY DISTRICT HOSPITAL (171330)**, 619 South Clark Street,
Zip 67554–0828, Mailing Address: P.O. Box 828, Zip 67554–0828;
tel. 620/257–5173 **A**9 10 18 **F**1 3 10 13 29 30 34 35 40 45 47 57 67 70 75
76 77 81 89 93 107 124 126 127 129 131 132 142
Primary Contact: George M. Stover, Chief Executive Officer
CFO: Terry Pound, Chief Financial Officer
Web address: www.ricecountyhospital.com
**Control:** Hospital district or authority, Government, nonfederal **Service:** General
Medical and Surgical

**Staffed Beds:** 25 **Admissions:** 303 **Census:** 15 **Outpatient Visits:** 8829
**Births:** 41 **Total Expense ($000):** 10314 **Payroll Expense ($000):** 5133
**Personnel:** 108

## MANHATTAN—Riley County

**MANHATTAN SURGICAL CENTER (170190)**, 1829 College Avenue,
Zip 66502; tel. 785/776–5100 **A**9 10 **F**45 48 51 81 82 129
Primary Contact: Scott Chapman, Administrator
Web address: www.manhattansurgical.com
**Control:** Corporation, Investor–owned, for–profit **Service:** Surgical

**Staffed Beds:** 13 **Admissions:** 429 **Census:** 2 **Outpatient Visits:** 9268
**Births:** 0 **Personnel:** 73

★ ○ **MERCY REGIONAL HEALTH CENTER (170142)**, 1823 College Avenue,
Zip 66502, Mailing Address: P.O. Box 1289, Zip 66505–1289;
tel. 785/776–3322 **A**5 9 10 11 19 **F**3 5 11 12 13 15 18 20 22 28 29 30 31
34 35 37 40 44 45 46 49 56 60 64 70 74 75 76 77 78 79 80 81 82 84 85
86 87 89 90 93 96 102 103 104 107 108 110 111 113 114 118 128 129
131 132 142 145 146 147 **S** Via Christi Health, Wichita, KS
Primary Contact: John R. Broberg, FACHE, President and Chief Executive Officer
COO: Carla J. Yost, R.N., Chief Operating Officer
CFO: Susan Morgan, Chief Financial Officer
CMO: Joseph Philipp, M.D., Chief Medical Officer
CIO: Andy Gagnon, Director Information Systems
CHR: Floyd Chasse, Vice President Human Resources
Web address: www.mercyregional.org
**Control:** Other not–for–profit (including NFP Corporation) **Service:** General
Medical and Surgical

**Staffed Beds:** 111 **Admissions:** 5143 **Census:** 49 **Outpatient Visits:** 121811
**Births:** 1076 **Total Expense ($000):** 84916 **Payroll Expense ($000):** 34600
**Personnel:** 669

## MANKATO—Jewell County

**JEWELL COUNTY HOSPITAL (171309)**, 100 Crestvue Avenue,
Zip 66956–2407, Mailing Address: P.O. Box 327, Zip 66956–0327;
tel. 785/378–3137, (Total facility includes 19 beds in nursing home–type unit) **A**9
10 18 **F**28 29 32 40 50 64 75 81 93 107 126 132
Primary Contact: Doyle L. McKimmy, FACHE, Chief Executive Officer
COO: Eric Borden, Chief Operating Officer and Chief Financial Officer
CFO: Eric Borden, Chief Operating Officer and Chief Financial Officer
**Control:** County–Government, nonfederal **Service:** General Medical and Surgical

**Staffed Beds:** 41 **Admissions:** 107 **Census:** 27 **Outpatient Visits:** 5119
**Births:** 0 **Total Expense ($000):** 3975 **Payroll Expense ($000):** 2174
**Personnel:** 72

## MARION—Marion County

★ **ST. LUKE HOSPITAL AND LIVING CENTER (171356)**, 535 South Freeborn,
Zip 66861–1299; tel. 620/382–2177, (Total facility includes 32 beds in nursing
home–type unit) **A**9 10 18 **F**3 11 15 28 29 34 40 45 62 64 81 97 107 108
113 126 127 132 **P**6 **S** QHR, Brentwood, TN
Primary Contact: Jeremy Armstrong, FACHE, Chief Executive Officer
CFO: Bev Reid, Chief Financial Officer
CMO: Don Hodson, M.D., Chief Medical Officer
CIO: Jeff Methvin, Manager Information Technology
CHR: Sharon Zogelman, Director Human Resources
Web address: www.slhmarion.org
**Control:** Hospital district or authority, Government, nonfederal **Service:** General
Medical and Surgical

**Staffed Beds:** 37 **Admissions:** 151 **Census:** 32 **Outpatient Visits:** 20675
**Births:** 0 **Total Expense ($000):** 7570 **Payroll Expense ($000):** 3170
**Personnel:** 94

## MARYSVILLE—Marshall County

★ **COMMUNITY MEMORIAL HEALTHCARE (171363)**, 708 North 18th Street,
Zip 66508–1338; tel. 785/562–2311 **A**9 10 18 **F**3 13 15 28 29 30 31 34 35
40 45 50 57 59 62 64 68 69 75 76 77 78 79 81 87 91 93 94 97 107 108
113 126 127 128 129 130 131 132 134 145 146 147 **P**6
Primary Contact: Curtis R. Hawkinson, Chief Executive Officer
CFO: William H. Storck, Chief Financial Officer
CMO: Michelle Stone, D.O., Chief Medical Staff
CHR: Jessie Schneider, Director Human Resources
Web address: www.cmhcare.org
**Control:** Other not–for–profit (including NFP Corporation) **Service:** General
Medical and Surgical

**Staffed Beds:** 25 **Admissions:** 811 **Census:** 10 **Outpatient Visits:** 28195
**Births:** 77 **Total Expense ($000):** 19384 **Payroll Expense ($000):** 9077
**Personnel:** 194

## MCPHERSON—Mcpherson County

★ **MCPHERSON HOSPITAL (170105)**, 1000 Hospital Drive, Zip 67460–2321;
tel. 620/241–2250 **A**5 9 10 **F**3 7 11 13 15 28 34 35 40 45 53 57 59 64 65
70 75 76 77 79 81 82 85 97 107 108 113 118 132 145 **P**6
Primary Contact: Robert Monical, President and Chief Executive Officer
COO: Terri Gehring, Vice President Operations
CHR: Jill Wenger, Vice President Human Resources
Web address: www.mcphersonmemorial.org
**Control:** Other not–for–profit (including NFP Corporation) **Service:** General
Medical and Surgical

**Staffed Beds:** 41 **Admissions:** 1208 **Census:** 13 **Outpatient Visits:** 40690
**Births:** 177 **Total Expense ($000):** 23408 **Payroll Expense ($000):** 10892
**Personnel:** 290

**MEMORIAL HOSPITAL** See McPherson Hospital

*Many Facility Codes have changed. Please refer to the AHA Guide Code Chart.*

## MEADE—Meade County

★ **MEADE DISTRICT HOSPITAL (171321)**, 510 East Carthage Street,
Zip 67864–0820, Mailing Address: P.O. Box 820, Zip 67864–0820;
tel. 620/873–2141, (Total facility includes 60 beds in nursing home–type unit) **A**9
10 18 **F**3 15 28 29 34 35 40 45 53 56 57 59 62 64 79 81 82 85 87 93 107
108 113 118 126 127 129 130 132 142 147 **P**6
Primary Contact: Michael P. Thomas, Administrator
CFO: Lori Smith, Chief Financial Officer
CIO: Leighton Miller, Chief Information Officer
Web address: www.meadehospital.com
**Control:** Hospital district or authority, Government, nonfederal **Service:** General
Medical and Surgical

| | | |
|---|---|---|
| **Staffed Beds:** 80 **Admissions:** 397 **Census:** 51 **Outpatient Visits:** 10734 | | |
| **Births:** 0 **Total Expense ($000):** 14181 **Payroll Expense ($000):** 7142 | | |
| **Personnel:** 178 | | |

## MEDICINE LODGE—Barber County

★ **MEDICINE LODGE MEMORIAL HOSPITAL (171334)**, 710 North Walnut Street,
Zip 67104–1019; tel. 620/886–3771 **A**9 10 18 **F**7 11 40 44 45 53 56 64 81
93 107 118 126 127 132 147 **P**6 **S** Great Plains Health Alliance, Inc.,
Phillipsburg, KS
Primary Contact: Kevin A. White, Administrator
CFO: Thomas G. Lee, Chief Financial Officer
CHR: Johnnie Davis, Director Human Resources
CNO: Kathryn I. Burns, R.N., Director of Nursing
Web address: www.mlmh.net/
**Control:** Hospital district or authority, Government, nonfederal **Service:** General
Medical and Surgical

| | | |
|---|---|---|
| **Staffed Beds:** 25 **Admissions:** 339 **Census:** 16 **Outpatient Visits:** 24577 | | |
| **Births:** 0 **Total Expense ($000):** 8650 **Payroll Expense ($000):** 4763 | | |
| **Personnel:** 96 | | |

## MINNEAPOLIS—Ottawa County

★ **OTTAWA COUNTY HEALTH CENTER (171328)**, 215 East Eighth,
Zip 67467–1999, Mailing Address: P.O. Box 290, Zip 67467–0290;
tel. 785/392–2122, (Total facility includes 17 beds in nursing home–type unit) **A**9
10 18 **F**10 28 35 40 53 56 62 64 67 69 85 86 93 127 129 132 142 **S** Great
Plains Health Alliance, Inc., Phillipsburg, KS
Primary Contact: Joy Johnson, R.N., Interim Chief Executive Officer
CFO: Cheryl Lanoue, Chief Financial Officer
CIO: Linda Wright, Director Information
CHR: Jenny Johnson, Chief Human Resource Officer
Web address: www.ottawacountyhealthcenter.com
**Control:** Other not–for–profit (including NFP Corporation) **Service:** General
Medical and Surgical

| | | |
|---|---|---|
| **Staffed Beds:** 42 **Admissions:** 376 **Census:** 35 **Outpatient Visits:** 9883 | | |
| **Births:** 0 **Total Expense ($000):** 5492 **Payroll Expense ($000):** 2836 | | |
| **Personnel:** 82 | | |

## MINNEOLA—Ford County

★ **MINNEOLA DISTRICT HOSPITAL (171368)**, 212 Main Street,
Zip 67865–0127, Mailing Address: P.O. Box 127, Zip 67865–0127;
tel. 620/885–4264, (Total facility includes 36 beds in nursing home–type unit) **A**9
10 18 **F**13 29 40 45 46 56 57 64 65 67 81 83 93 102 107 126 127 129 132
147 **P**6 **S** Great Plains Health Alliance, Inc., Phillipsburg, KS
Primary Contact: Brian Roland, Administrator and Chief Executive Officer
CFO: Marion Blanton, Chief Financial Officer
CMO: Tony Luna, M.D., Chief of Staff
CHR: Vena Harris, Director Human Resources
Web address: www.minneolahealthcare.com
**Control:** Hospital district or authority, Government, nonfederal **Service:** General
Medical and Surgical

| | | |
|---|---|---|
| **Staffed Beds:** 54 **Admissions:** 603 **Census:** 40 **Outpatient Visits:** 22270 | | |
| **Births:** 50 **Total Expense ($000):** 10064 **Payroll Expense ($000):** 5105 | | |
| **Personnel:** 127 | | |

## MOUNDRIDGE—Mcpherson County

★ **MERCY HOSPITAL (170075)**, 218 East Pack Street, Zip 67107–0180, Mailing
Address: P.O. Box 180, Zip 67107–0180; tel. 620/345–6391 **A**9 10 **F**40 56 76
81 89 129 132
Primary Contact: Doyle K. Johnson, Administrator
CFO: Royce Holdeman, Chief Financial Officer
Web address: www.mercyh.org/
**Control:** Church–operated, Nongovernment, not–for profit **Service:** General
Medical and Surgical

| | | |
|---|---|---|
| **Staffed Beds:** 21 **Admissions:** 330 **Census:** 5 **Outpatient Visits:** 8371 | | |
| **Births:** 35 **Total Expense ($000):** 2586 **Payroll Expense ($000):** 1188 | | |
| **Personnel:** 42 | | |

## NEODESHA—Wilson County

★ **WILSON MEDICAL CENTER (171344)**, 2600 Ottawa Road, Zip 66757–1817,
Mailing Address: P.O. Box 360, Zip 66757–0360; tel. 620/325–2611 **A**9 10 18
**F**3 11 29 34 40 45 53 57 59 64 81 85 89 93 107 108 114 118 127 132 147
**S** QHR, Brentwood, TN
Primary Contact: Dennis R. Shelby, Chief Executive Officer
CFO: John Gutschenritter, Chief Financial Officer
CIO: Julie Quanstrom, Director Information Systems and Reimbursement Specialist
CHR: Laura Dean, Director Human Resources
CNO: Michelle Bohannon, Director of Nursing Operations and Risk, Compliance,
Quality and Safety
Web address: www.wilsonmedical.org
**Control:** County–Government, nonfederal **Service:** General Medical and Surgical

| | | |
|---|---|---|
| **Staffed Beds:** 15 **Admissions:** 360 **Census:** 6 **Outpatient Visits:** 11670 | | |
| **Births:** 0 **Total Expense ($000):** 11177 **Payroll Expense ($000):** 4462 | | |
| **Personnel:** 106 | | |

## NESS CITY—Ness County

★ **NESS COUNTY HOSPITAL (171336)**, 312 Custer Street, Zip 67560–1654;
tel. 785/798–2291, (Total facility includes 43 beds in nursing home–type unit) **A**9
10 18 **F**3 7 15 28 32 40 45 59 62 65 67 93 107 111 118 124 126 127
132 **P**6
Primary Contact: Curt Thomas, Administrator
CFO: Debra Frank, Chief Financial Officer
CMO: Mikhail Imseis, M.D., Chief of Staff
CIO: Vicki Howe, Chief Information Officer
CHR: Lori Hensley, Chief Human Resources Officer
CNO: Brenda Dinges, Director of Nursing
Web address: www.nesscountyhospital.com/
**Control:** Hospital district or authority, Government, nonfederal **Service:** General
Medical and Surgical

| | | |
|---|---|---|
| **Staffed Beds:** 63 **Admissions:** 204 **Census:** 44 **Outpatient Visits:** 10724 | | |
| **Births:** 0 **Total Expense ($000):** 8190 **Payroll Expense ($000):** 3786 | | |
| **Personnel:** 108 | | |

## NEWTON—Harvey County

★ ○ **NEWTON MEDICAL CENTER (170103)**, 600 Medical Center Drive,
Zip 67114–0308, Mailing Address: P.O. Box 308, Zip 67114–0308;
tel. 316/283–2700 **A**5 9 10 11 **F**3 8 13 15 20 22 28 29 30 40 45 49 51 59
64 68 70 73 75 76 81 85 86 90 107 108 110 111 113 117 118 125 129
132 145 146 147 **P**6
Primary Contact: Steven G. Kelly, President and Chief Executive Officer
COO: J. Michael Keller, Vice President Operations
CFO: Paul Lavender, Vice President Finance
CIO: Prableen Singh, Chief Information Officer
CHR: Todd Tangeman, Director Human Resources
Web address: www.newtonmedicalcenter.com
**Control:** Other not–for–profit (including NFP Corporation) **Service:** General
Medical and Surgical

| | | |
|---|---|---|
| **Staffed Beds:** 103 **Admissions:** 3262 **Census:** 41 **Outpatient Visits:** 65219 | | |
| **Births:** 554 **Total Expense ($000):** 57281 **Payroll Expense ($000):** 24821 | | |
| **Personnel:** 530 | | |

☐ **PRAIRIE VIEW (174016)**, 1901 East First Street, Zip 67114–0467, Mailing
Address: P.O. Box 467, Zip 67114–0467; tel. 316/284–6400, (Nonreporting) **A**1
9 10
Primary Contact: Jessie Kaye, Chief Executive Officer
CFO: Dan Evans, Vice President Business and Finance
CIO: Merle Enns, Director Information Services
CHR: Joy Robb, Vice President Human Resources
Web address: www.prairieview.org
**Control:** Other not–for–profit (including NFP Corporation) **Service:** Psychiatric

| | | |
|---|---|---|
| **Staffed Beds:** 38 | | |

## NORTON—Norton County

★ **NORTON COUNTY HOSPITAL (171348)**, 102 East Holme, Zip 67654–0250,
Mailing Address: P.O. Box 250, Zip 67654–0250; tel. 785/877–3351 **A**9 10 18
**F**3 13 15 28 31 34 40 41 45 50 57 59 64 67 69 76 78 81 89 93 97 107 110
113 118 126 127 129 132 134 **P**6
Primary Contact: Richard Miller, Administrator and Chief Executive Officer
CFO: Ryan Stover, Chief Financial Officer
CHR: Shannan Hempler, Director Human Resources
Web address: www.ntcohosp.com
**Control:** City–County, Government, nonfederal **Service:** General Medical and
Surgical

| | | |
|---|---|---|
| **Staffed Beds:** 25 **Admissions:** 657 **Census:** 5 **Outpatient Visits:** 46887 | | |
| **Births:** 54 **Total Expense ($000):** 10075 **Payroll Expense ($000):** 4985 | | |
| **Personnel:** 117 | | |

---

**KS**

## OAKLEY—Logan County

**LOGAN COUNTY HOSPITAL (171326)**, 211 Cherry Street, Zip 67748–1201; tel. 785/672–3211, (Total facility includes 46 beds in nursing home–type unit) **A**9 10 18 **F**26 27 28 40 45 50 64 67 69 81 93 107 126 129 132 142 147 **P**5 6
Primary Contact: Darcy Howard, Chief Executive Officer and Chief Financial Officer
CFO: Darcy Howard, Chief Executive Officer and Chief Financial Officer
CMO: Celeste Rains, D.O., Chief of Staff
CIO: Mike Jacobs, Director Information Technology
CHR: Steve Allison, Director Human Resources
Web address: www.logancountyhospital.org
**Control:** County–Government, nonfederal **Service:** General Medical and Surgical

**Staffed Beds:** 71 **Admissions:** 464 **Census:** 50 **Outpatient Visits:** 16919
**Births:** 0 **Total Expense ($000):** 9892 **Payroll Expense ($000):** 5088
**Personnel:** 130

## OBERLIN—Decatur County

★ **DECATUR COUNTY HOSPITAL AND CEDAR LIVING CENTER (171352)**, 810 West Columbia Street, Zip 67749–2450, Mailing Address: P.O. Box 268, Zip 67749–0268; tel. 785/475–2208, (Total facility includes 37 beds in nursing home–type unit) **A**9 10 18 **F**3 13 15 28 29 31 34 35 40 45 53 56 57 62 64 69 75 76 78 80 81 84 85 86 93 107 113 126 129 132 134 **P**6
Primary Contact: Lynn Doeden, Chief Executive Officer
CFO: Amanda Fortin, Manager Finance
CMO: Elizabeth Sliter, M.D., Chairman Medical Staff
CIO: Natasha Weishapl, Manager Business Office and Human Resources
CHR: Natasha Weishapl, Manager Business Office and Human Resources
Web address: www.decaturhealthsystems.org
**Control:** Other not–for–profit (including NFP Corporation) **Service:** General Medical and Surgical

**Staffed Beds:** 61 **Admissions:** 344 **Census:** 29 **Outpatient Visits:** 8483
**Births:** 0 **Total Expense ($000):** 5885 **Payroll Expense ($000):** 3085
**Personnel:** 98

## OLATHE—Johnson County

☐ **OLATHE MEDICAL CENTER (170049)**, 20333 West 151st Street, Zip 66061–5350; tel. 913/791–4200 **A**1 2 5 9 10 **F**3 8 11 12 13 15 18 20 22 24 26 28 29 30 31 34 35 39 40 41 46 49 56 57 58 59 61 62 63 64 65 68 70 74 75 76 77 78 79 81 82 84 85 86 87 89 93 107 108 110 111 113 114 117 118 128 129 130 131 134 143 144 145 146 147
Primary Contact: Frank H. Devocelle, President and Chief Executive Officer
CFO: Tierney Grasser, Senior Vice President Finance
CIO: Georeg Dix, Chief Information Officer
CHR: David Klimek, Chief Human Resources Officer
CNO: Elaine Patton, Vice President Nursing
Web address: www.ohsi.com
**Control:** Other not–for–profit (including NFP Corporation) **Service:** General Medical and Surgical

**Staffed Beds:** 230 **Admissions:** 10839 **Census:** 115 **Outpatient Visits:** 296580 **Births:** 1301 **Personnel:** 1443

## ONAGA—Pottawatomie County

★ **COMMUNITY HEALTH CARE SYSTEM (171354)**, 120 West Eighth Street, Zip 66521–0120; tel. 785/889–4272, (Total facility includes 78 beds in nursing home–type unit) **A**9 10 18 **F**2 3 5 6 10 11 12 13 15 29 31 32 34 35 36 40 43 45 50 53 56 57 59 62 64 65 67 70 74 75 76 77 78 79 81 82 84 85 86 87 89 93 97 99 100 101 102 103 104 105 106 107 113 118 124 126 127 129 130 131 132 133 134 142 143 144 145 146 147 **P**6
Primary Contact: Greg Unruh, Chief Executive Officer
COO: Marcia S. Walsh, M.P.H., Chief Operating Officer
CFO: Monica Holthaus, Chief Financial Officer
CMO: Nancy Zidek, M.D., Chief of Staff
CIO: Paul Zidek, Chief Information Officer
CHR: Terry Bernatis, Manager Human Resources
CNO: Rosalind Lewis, R.N., Chief Nursing Officer
Web address: www.chcsks.org
**Control:** Other not–for–profit (including NFP Corporation) **Service:** General Medical and Surgical

**Staffed Beds:** 159 **Admissions:** 1106 **Census:** 74 **Outpatient Visits:** 95643
**Births:** 114 **Total Expense ($000):** 23323 **Payroll Expense ($000):** 14531
**Personnel:** 254

## OSAWATOMIE—Miami County

☐ **OSAWATOMIE STATE HOSPITAL (174004)**, 500 State Hospital Drive, Zip 66064–0500, Mailing Address: P.O. Box 500, Zip 66064–0500; tel. 913/755–7000 **A**1 10 **F**11 30 50 75 86 87 98 101 103 129 131 134 145 **P**6
Primary Contact: Gregory Valentine, Superintendent
CFO: Donna Dean, Chief Financial Officer
CMO: Maria Gustilo, M.D., Medical Director
CIO: Lester Vohs, Chief Information Management
CHR: Marilyn Williamson, Director Human Resources
Web address: www.srskansas.org/osh/osh-rmhf_info.html
**Control:** State–Government, nonfederal **Service:** Psychiatric

**Staffed Beds:** 176 **Admissions:** 2288 **Census:** 176 **Outpatient Visits:** 0
**Births:** 0 **Total Expense ($000):** 29295 **Payroll Expense ($000):** 17155
**Personnel:** 323

## OSBORNE—Osborne County

★ **OSBORNE COUNTY MEMORIAL HOSPITAL (171364)**, 424 West New Hampshire Street, Zip 67473–0070, Mailing Address: P.O. Box 70, Zip 67473–0070; tel. 785/346–2121 **A**9 10 18 **F**3 11 13 40 45 64 69 76 81 107 127 132 **P**6 **S** Great Plains Health Alliance, Inc., Phillipsburg, KS
Primary Contact: Kiley Floyd, Administrator
CFO: Linda Murphy, Chief Financial Officer
CMO: Barbara Brown, D.O., Chief of Staff
CIO: Kiley Floyd, Administrator
Web address: www.ocmh.org
**Control:** County–Government, nonfederal **Service:** General Medical and Surgical

**Staffed Beds:** 25 **Admissions:** 306 **Census:** 4 **Outpatient Visits:** 9830
**Births:** 16 **Total Expense ($000):** 4975 **Payroll Expense ($000):** 2411
**Personnel:** 58

## OSWEGO—Labette County

★ **OSWEGO COMMUNITY HOSPITAL (171302)**, 800 Barker Drive, Zip 67356–9033; tel. 620/795–2921 **A**9 10 18 **F**3 9 12 30 32 33 40 57 59 64 65 77 93 97 126 128 129 131 132 134 142 145 146 147 **P**5 **S** HMC/CAH Consolidated, Inc., Kansas City, MO
Primary Contact: Daniel Hiben, Chief Executive Officer
CFO: Christina Schlatter, Chief Financial Officer
CMO: Gordon Kern, M.D., Medical Director
CHR: Christina Schlatter, Chief Financial Officer
Web address: www.oswegocommunityhospital.com
**Control:** Corporation, Investor–owned, for–profit **Service:** General Medical and Surgical

**Staffed Beds:** 12 **Admissions:** 114 **Census:** 5 **Outpatient Visits:** 9044
**Births:** 0 **Total Expense ($000):** 4168 **Payroll Expense ($000):** 2044
**Personnel:** 43

## OTTAWA—Franklin County

⊠ **RANSOM MEMORIAL HOSPITAL (170014)**, 1301 South Main Street, Zip 66067–3598; tel. 785/229–8200 **A**1 9 10 **F**3 11 13 15 28 30 34 35 36 40 45 46 49 53 56 57 59 64 70 75 76 77 79 81 82 85 86 92 93 96 97 107 108 110 111 114 117 118 128 129 130 131 132 133 134 143 145 146 147 **P**8
Primary Contact: Larry A. Felix, FACHE, Chief Executive Officer
CFO: Dean Ohmart, Assistant Administrator and Chief Financial Officer
Web address: www.ransom.org
**Control:** County–Government, nonfederal **Service:** General Medical and Surgical

**Staffed Beds:** 44 **Admissions:** 1539 **Census:** 14 **Outpatient Visits:** 100525
**Births:** 150 **Total Expense ($000):** 26880 **Payroll Expense ($000):** 15949
**Personnel:** 285

## OVERLAND PARK—Johnson County

**CHILDREN'S MERCY SOUTH (173300)**, 5808 West 110th Street, Zip 66211; tel. 913/696–8000 **A**9 10 **F**3 9 29 30 32 35 36 44 48 50 59 62 64 68 75 77 79 81 82 85 87 89 93 94 100 101 104 107 111 113 118 128 129 130 131 133 143 145 147 **P**6 8
Primary Contact: Randall L. O'Donnell, Ph.D., President and Chief Executive Officer
CFO: Sandra A J Lawrence, Executive Vice President and Chief Financial Officer
CMO: Charles Roberts, M.D., Medical Director
CIO: Jean Ann Breedlove, Chief Information Officer
CHR: Dan Wright, Vice President Human Resources
Web address: www.childrens-mercy.org
**Control:** Other not–for–profit (including NFP Corporation) **Service:** Children's general

**Staffed Beds:** 45 **Admissions:** 2541 **Census:** 15 **Outpatient Visits:** 105522
**Births:** 0 **Total Expense ($000):** 81166 **Payroll Expense ($000):** 44699
**Personnel:** 630

**HEARTLAND SPINE & SPECIALTY HOSPITAL** See Heartland Surgical Specialty Hospital

☐ **HEARTLAND SURGICAL SPECIALTY HOSPITAL (170195)**, 10720 Nall Avenue, Zip 66211; tel. 913/754–5000 **A**1 9 10 **F**3 12 29 45 51 64 77 79 81 82 85 89 90 96 97 107 111 114 118 130 131 **P**5
Primary Contact: Don Burman, Chief Executive Officer
CFO: Jesse Saucedo, Chief Financial Officer
CMO: David Anderson, M.D., Medical Director
CIO: Matt Czugala, Manager Information Systems
CHR: Jan Mathieu, Director Human Resources
Web address: www.hssh.org
**Control:** Partnership, Investor–owned, for–profit **Service:** General Medical and Surgical

**Staffed Beds:** 48 **Admissions:** 619 **Census:** 4 **Outpatient Visits:** 9427
**Births:** 0 **Total Expense ($000):** 28141 **Payroll Expense ($000):** 7612
**Personnel:** 128

*Many Facility Codes have changed. Please refer to the AHA Guide Code Chart.* © 2012 AHA Guide

⊞ **MENORAH MEDICAL CENTER (170182)**, 5721 West 119th Street, Zip 66209–3722; tel. 913/498–6000 **A**1 2 9 10 **F**3 12 13 15 18 20 22 24 26 28 29 30 31 34 35 38 40 45 46 47 49 55 57 58 59 60 64 65 68 70 72 74 75 76 77 78 79 81 82 85 86 87 90 93 97 102 107 108 110 111 113 114 116 118 120 123 125 128 129 130 131 134 143 144 145 146 147 **P**5 **S** HCA, Nashville, TN
Primary Contact: Steven D. Wilkinson, President and Chief Executive Officer
CFO: Deborah Gafford, Chief Financial Officer
Web address: www.menorahmedicalcenter.com
**Control:** Corporation, Investor–owned, for–profit **Service:** General Medical and Surgical

**Staffed Beds:** 158 **Admissions:** 7063 **Census:** 82 **Outpatient Visits:** 69475 **Births:** 1033 **Total Expense ($000):** 143835 **Payroll Expense ($000):** 41915 **Personnel:** 725

⊞ **OVERLAND PARK REGIONAL MEDICAL CENTER (170176)**, 10500 Quivira Road, Zip 66215–2306, Mailing Address: P.O. Box 15959, Zip 66215–5959; tel. 913/541–5000 **A**1 5 9 10 **F**3 13 15 18 20 22 24 26 28 29 30 31 34 35 37 40 43 45 49 50 56 57 59 60 61 64 65 67 70 72 73 74 75 76 77 78 79 81 82 83 84 85 86 87 91 92 93 107 108 110 111 113 118 125 128 129 130 134 144 145 146 147 **S** HCA, Nashville, TN
Primary Contact: Damond Boatwright, Chief Executive Officer
COO: Dean Carucci, Chief Operating Officer
CFO: Shari Collier, Chief Financial Officer
CMO: John A. Romito, M.D., Chief Medical Officer
CHR: Connie Miller, Vice President Human Resources
Web address: www.oprmc.com
**Control:** Corporation, Investor–owned, for–profit **Service:** General Medical and Surgical

**Staffed Beds:** 276 **Admissions:** 10306 **Census:** 142 **Outpatient Visits:** 65721 **Births:** 3077 **Total Expense ($000):** 163676 **Payroll Expense ($000):** 52173 **Personnel:** 819

⊞ **SAINT LUKE'S SOUTH HOSPITAL (170185)**, 12300 Metcalf Avenue, Zip 66213; tel. 913/317–7000 **A**1 9 10 **F**3 8 12 13 15 18 20 22 26 28 29 30 31 34 38 40 45 47 49 55 57 58 59 64 65 70 72 74 75 76 77 78 79 81 82 84 85 87 90 93 94 107 108 110 111 113 116 117 118 128 129 130 131 145 147 **S** Saint Luke's Health System, Kansas City, MO
Primary Contact: Kathy A. Howell, R.N., Chief Executive Officer
CFO: Shelby Frigon, Chief Financial Officer
CMO: Wendell Clarkston, M.D., President Medical Staff
CIO: Deborah Gash, Chief Information Officer
CHR: Donna Kunz, Manager Human Resources
CNO: Julia Woods, MSN, Vice President and Chief Nursing Officer
Web address: www.saint–lukes.org
**Control:** Church–operated, Nongovernment, not–for profit **Service:** General Medical and Surgical

**Staffed Beds:** 110 **Admissions:** 5316 **Census:** 54 **Outpatient Visits:** 79051 **Births:** 1148 **Total Expense ($000):** 94044 **Payroll Expense ($000):** 34141 **Personnel:** 526

☐ **SPECIALTY HOSPITAL OF MID–AMERICA (172004)**, 6509 West 103rd Street, Zip 66212–1728; tel. 913/649–3701, (Total facility includes 52 beds in nursing home–type unit) **A**1 9 10 **F**1 29 60 127 142 **S** Fundamental Long Term Care Holdings, LLC, Sparks Glencoe, MD
Primary Contact: Karen Leverich, Chief Executive Officer
CFO: William Scott, Chief Financial Officer
CHR: Darren Enochs, Director Human Resources
Web address: www.thicare.com/SpecHospOfMidAmerica/
**Control:** Corporation, Investor–owned, for–profit **Service:** Long–Term Acute Care hospital

**Staffed Beds:** 104 **Admissions:** 318 **Census:** 61 **Outpatient Visits:** 0 **Births:** 0 **Total Expense ($000):** 4420 **Payroll Expense ($000):** 3236 **Personnel:** 119

**PAOLA—Miami County**

☐ **MIAMI COUNTY MEDICAL CENTER (170109)**, 2100 Baptiste Drive, Zip 66071–0365, Mailing Address: P.O. Box 365, Zip 66071–0365; tel. 913/294–2327 **A**1 9 10 **F**3 11 15 30 40 59 61 64 68 75 77 78 79 81 82 85 87 89 90 93 102 107 108 110 111 113 118 126 128 129 130 145 147
Primary Contact: Gerald Wiesner, Administrator
Web address: www.olathehealth.org
**Control:** Other not–for–profit (including NFP Corporation) **Service:** General Medical and Surgical

**Staffed Beds:** 18 **Admissions:** 484 **Census:** 3 **Outpatient Visits:** 33820 **Births:** 0 **Personnel:** 147

**PARSONS—Labette County**

★ ○ **LABETTE HEALTH (170120)**, 1902 South U.S. Highway 59, Zip 67357–7404; tel. 620/421–4880 **A**9 10 11 **F**3 7 11 13 15 29 30 40 43 53 57 59 62 64 70 75 76 77 79 81 82 85 86 90 93 107 111 117 118 126 128 129 130 131 142 145 146 147 **P**6 7
Primary Contact: Jodi A. Schmidt, President and Chief Executive Officer
CFO: Thomas Macaronas, Chief Financial Officer
CHR: Christina Sykes, Director Human Resources
Web address: www.labettehealth.com
**Control:** County–Government, nonfederal **Service:** General Medical and Surgical

**Staffed Beds:** 62 **Admissions:** 2723 **Census:** 26 **Outpatient Visits:** 71684 **Births:** 230 **Total Expense ($000):** 50376 **Payroll Expense ($000):** 22179 **Personnel:** 466

**PARSONS STATE HOSPITAL AND TRAINING CENTER**, 2601 Gabriel Avenue, Zip 67357–0738, Mailing Address: P.O. Box 738, Zip 67357–0738; tel. 620/421–6550 **F**35 39 67 129 145
Primary Contact: Jerry A. Rea, Ph.D., Superintendent
CFO: John Spare, Accountant
CMO: Rema Menon, M.D., Clinical Director
CIO: Ron Malmstrom, Information Research Specialist
CHR: Tim B. Posch, Business Manager and Director Personnel
Web address: www.pshtc.org
**Control:** State–Government, nonfederal **Service:** Institution for mental retardation

**Staffed Beds:** 188 **Admissions:** 17 **Census:** 185 **Outpatient Visits:** 0 **Births:** 0 **Total Expense ($000):** 25373 **Payroll Expense ($000):** 16249 **Personnel:** 453

**PHILLIPSBURG—Phillips County**

★ **PHILLIPS COUNTY HOSPITAL (171353)**, 1150 State Street, Zip 67661–1799, Mailing Address: P.O. Box 607, Zip 67661–0607; tel. 785/543–5226 **A**9 10 18 **F**3 11 13 15 28 30 31 40 45 59 64 68 75 76 77 78 81 86 87 93 107 113 118 126 127 129 131 132 144 145 147 **P**6 **S** Great Plains Health Alliance, Inc., Phillipsburg, KS
Primary Contact: David Engel, Chief Executive Officer
CFO: Dennis Fredrickson, Chief Financial Officer
CMO: Ben Stephenson, M.D., Chief of Staff
CIO: Steven Seems, Director of Information Technology
CNO: Diane Jarvis, R.N., Director of Nursing
Web address: www.phillipshospital.org
**Control:** Other not–for–profit (including NFP Corporation) **Service:** General Medical and Surgical

**Staffed Beds:** 25 **Admissions:** 350 **Census:** 6 **Outpatient Visits:** 20606 **Births:** 0 **Total Expense ($000):** 8573 **Payroll Expense ($000):** 3658 **Personnel:** 91

**PITTSBURG—Crawford County**

⊞ **VIA CHRISTI HOSPITAL (170006)**, 1 Mt. Carmel Way, Zip 66762–6643; tel. 620/232–0109 **A**1 2 5 9 10 **F**3 5 11 12 13 15 18 20 22 26 28 29 30 31 34 35 40 42 43 45 47 48 50 51 53 54 55 56 57 58 59 62 64 68 69 70 71 73 75 76 77 78 79 80 81 82 84 85 86 89 90 93 99 100 101 103 104 107 108 109 110 111 112 113 114 117 118 119 120 121 122 128 129 130 131 132 134 142 143 144 145 146 147 **P**8 **S** Via Christi Health, Wichita, KS
Primary Contact: Randall R. Cason, FACHE, President and Chief Executive Officer
COO: Drew Talbott, Vice President Operations
CFO: Deb Bainbridge, Chief Financial Officer
CIO: Troy Mascher, Director Information Systems
CHR: Connie McCune, Vice President Human Resources
Web address: www.viachristi.org
**Control:** Church–operated, Nongovernment, not–for profit **Service:** General Medical and Surgical

**Staffed Beds:** 111 **Admissions:** 4316 **Census:** 55 **Outpatient Visits:** 114422 **Births:** 556 **Total Expense ($000):** 80643 **Payroll Expense ($000):** 36496 **Personnel:** 648

KS

**Hospital, Medicare Provider Number, Address, Telephone, Approval, Facility, and Physician Codes, Health Care System**

★ American Hospital Association (AHA) membership
☐ The Joint Commission accreditation
◇ DNV Healthcare Inc. accreditation
○ American Osteopathic Association (AOA) accreditation
△ Commission on Accreditation of Rehabilitation Facilities (CARF) accreditation

## PLAINVILLE—Rooks County

★ **ROOKS COUNTY HEALTH CENTER (171311)**, 1210 North Washington Street, Zip 67663-1632, Mailing Address: P.O. Box 389, Zip 67663-0389; tel. 785/434-4553 **A**9 10 18 **F**3 11 13 15 28 34 40 45 50 57 59 64 65 75 76 77 81 87 91 93 107 110 113 118 124 132 142 143 145 147 **P**5
Primary Contact: Michael Sinclair, Chief Executive Officer
COO: William D. Stahl, Chief Operating Officer
CFO: Julie Price, Chief Financial Officer
CMO: Lynn Fisher, M.D., Chief of Staff
CIO: Kathy Ramsay, R.N., Director Communications and Development
CHR: Cindi Knipp, Director Human Resources
Web address: www.rookscountyhealthcenter.com
**Control:** Hospital district or authority, Government, nonfederal **Service:** General Medical and Surgical

**Staffed Beds:** 20 **Admissions:** 318 **Census:** 6 **Outpatient Visits:** 16160 **Births:** 26 **Total Expense ($000):** 10721 **Payroll Expense ($000):** 4025 **Personnel:** 105

## PRATT—Pratt County

★ **PRATT REGIONAL MEDICAL CENTER (170027)**, 200 Commodore Street, Zip 67124-2903; tel. 620/672-7451, (Total facility includes 47 beds in nursing home-type unit) **A**5 9 10 20 **F**3 11 13 15 30 31 34 40 45 49 56 57 59 61 62 64 68 69 70 75 76 77 79 81 82 85 86 87 89 90 93 107 108 113 117 118 123 126 127 129 130 132 144 145 146 147 **P**6
Primary Contact: Susan M. Page, President and Chief Executive Officer
CFO: Hilary Dolbee, Vice President and Chief Financial Officer
CIO: Stacy Glennie, Director Health Information Services
CHR: Ken Brown, Vice President and Chief Human Resource Officer
CNO: Sherry L. Besser, R.N., Vice President Quality, Risk Management and Chief Nursing Officer
Web address: www.prmc.org
**Control:** Other not-for-profit (including NFP Corporation) **Service:** General Medical and Surgical

**Staffed Beds:** 85 **Admissions:** 1674 **Census:** 53 **Outpatient Visits:** 95711 **Births:** 282 **Total Expense ($000):** 34982 **Payroll Expense ($000):** 19148 **Personnel:** 351

## QUINTER—Gove County

**GOVE COUNTY MEDICAL CENTER (171367)**, 520 West Fifth Street, Zip 67752-0129, Mailing Address: P.O. Box 129, Zip 67752-0129; tel. 785/754-3341, (Total facility includes 49 beds in nursing home-type unit) **A**9 10 18 **F**3 11 13 28 29 31 34 40 45 57 62 67 75 81 93 107 118 124 132 134 142 147
Primary Contact: Richard Q. Bergling, Chief Executive Officer
CFO: Joy Bretz, Chief Financial Officer
CHR: Valerie Schneider, Director Human Resources
CNO: Tammy Hutchison, R.N., Director of Nursing
Web address: www.gcmc.ws
**Control:** County-Government, nonfederal **Service:** General Medical and Surgical

**Staffed Beds:** 70 **Admissions:** 790 **Census:** 55 **Outpatient Visits:** 9648 **Births:** 72 **Total Expense ($000):** 11882 **Payroll Expense ($000):** 5617 **Personnel:** 172

## RANSOM—Ness County

★ **GRISELL MEMORIAL HOSPITAL DISTRICT ONE (171300)**, 210 South Vermont Avenue, Zip 67572; tel. 785/731-2231, (Total facility includes 34 beds in nursing home-type unit) **A**9 10 18 **F**3 40 56 67 69 85 93 97 126 127 132 **P**6 **S** Great Plains Health Alliance, Inc., Phillipsburg, KS
Primary Contact: Kristine Ochs, R.N., Administrator
CFO: Tammy Schweitzer, Chief Financial Officer
CMO: Allen McLain, M.D., Chief of Staff
CNO: Joni Pfaff, Chief Nursing Officer
Web address: www.grisellmemorialhospital.org
**Control:** Hospital district or authority, Government, nonfederal **Service:** General Medical and Surgical

**Staffed Beds:** 46 **Admissions:** 54 **Census:** 34 **Outpatient Visits:** 7107 **Births:** 0 **Total Expense ($000):** 4453 **Payroll Expense ($000):** 2319 **Personnel:** 70

## RUSSELL—Russell County

★ **RUSSELL REGIONAL HOSPITAL (171350)**, 200 South Main Street, Zip 67665-2997; tel. 785/483-3131, (Total facility includes 29 beds in nursing home-type unit) **A**9 10 18 **F**7 11 15 29 30 32 34 35 40 50 53 57 59 64 65 66 67 69 75 83 85 87 93 107 110 113 118 126 127 129 130 132 134 144 145 146 147 **P**6
Primary Contact: Shelley Boden, Administrator and Chief Executive Officer
CFO: Janel Burch, Chief Financial Officer
CMO: Earl Merkel, M.D., Chief of Staff
CIO: David Schraeder, Director Information Systems
CHR: Sharon Collins, Director Human Resources and Executive Administrative Assistant
Web address: www.russellhospital.org
**Control:** Other not-for-profit (including NFP Corporation) **Service:** General Medical and Surgical

**Staffed Beds:** 52 **Admissions:** 400 **Census:** 27 **Outpatient Visits:** 35040 **Births:** 0 **Total Expense ($000):** 12449 **Payroll Expense ($000):** 7602 **Personnel:** 157

## SABETHA—Nemaha County

★ **SABETHA COMMUNITY HOSPITAL (171338)**, 14th and Oregon Streets, Zip 66534-0229, Mailing Address: P.O. Box 229, Zip 66534-0229; tel. 785/284-2121 **A**9 10 18 **F**3 11 13 15 28 34 35 40 45 50 56 57 59 62 63 64 68 75 76 77 78 79 81 82 84 86 93 107 113 118 127 129 132 145 147 **P**6 **S** Great Plains Health Alliance, Inc., Phillipsburg, KS
Primary Contact: Lora Key, Chief Executive Officer
CFO: Lori Lackey, Chief Financial Officer
CMO: Kevin Kennally, M.D., Chief of Medical Staff
CIO: Holli Dieckmann, Director Health Information
CHR: Julie K. Holthaus, Director Human Resources
CNO: Stacy Scott, Director of Nursing
Web address: www.sabethahospital.com
**Control:** Other not-for-profit (including NFP Corporation) **Service:** General Medical and Surgical

**Staffed Beds:** 25 **Admissions:** 390 **Census:** 7 **Outpatient Visits:** 42080 **Births:** 47 **Total Expense ($000):** 10110 **Payroll Expense ($000):** 4750 **Personnel:** 105

## SAINT FRANCIS—Cheyenne County

★ **CHEYENNE COUNTY HOSPITAL (171310)**, 210 West First Street, Zip 67756-0547, Mailing Address: P.O. Box 547, Zip 67756-0547; tel. 785/332-2104 **A**9 10 18 **F**3 8 11 13 28 31 40 57 59 65 66 69 76 78 81 85 89 93 97 107 118 126 127 132 **P**6 **S** Great Plains Health Alliance, Inc., Phillipsburg, KS
Primary Contact: Leslie Lacy, Administrator
CFO: Heidi Tice, Chief Financial Officer
CMO: Rebecca Allard, M.D., Chief of Staff
CHR: Tabetha Ketzner, Director Human Resources
Web address: www.cheyennecountyhospital.com
**Control:** Other not-for-profit (including NFP Corporation) **Service:** General Medical and Surgical

**Staffed Beds:** 16 **Admissions:** 385 **Census:** 4 **Outpatient Visits:** 20179 **Births:** 22 **Total Expense ($000):** 7854 **Payroll Expense ($000):** 3590 **Personnel:** 80

## SALINA—Saline County

★ ○ **SALINA REGIONAL HEALTH CENTER (170012)**, 400 South Santa Fe Avenue, Zip 67401-4198, Mailing Address: P.O. Box 5080, Zip 67402-5080; tel. 785/452-7000, (Includes SALINA REGIONAL HEALTH CENTER- PENN CAMPUS, 139 North Penn Street, Zip 67401, Mailing Address: P.O. Box 5080, Zip 67402-5080; tel. 913/452-7000; SALINA REGIONAL HEALTH CENTER-SANTA FE CAMPUS, 400 South Santa Fe Avenue, Zip 67401, Mailing Address: Box 5080, Zip 67402-5080; tel. 913/452-7000) **A**2 3 5 9 10 11 **F**3 13 15 20 22 24 26 28 29 30 31 35 40 46 47 48 49 51 53 64 70 71 72 73 74 76 77 78 79 81 85 86 87 89 90 91 92 93 94 98 100 102 103 104 105 107 108 110 111 113 115 116 117 118 119 120 121 122 128 129 142 143 144 145 146 147
Primary Contact: Micheal Terry, President and Chief Executive Officer
COO: Joel Phelps, Chief Operating Officer
CFO: Joe Tallon, Vice President Finance
CIO: Larry Barnes, Vice President Information Technology
CHR: David Moody, Vice President Human Resources
Web address: www.srhc.com
**Control:** Other not-for-profit (including NFP Corporation) **Service:** General Medical and Surgical

**Staffed Beds:** 204 **Admissions:** 8356 **Census:** 100 **Outpatient Visits:** 163782 **Births:** 1126 **Total Expense ($000):** 138019 **Payroll Expense ($000):** 57764 **Personnel:** 1035

**SALINA SURGICAL HOSPITAL (170187)**, 401 South Sante Fe,
Zip 67401–2697; tel. 785/827–0610 **A**9 10 **F**29 45 48 49 51 74 77 79 81
85 130
Primary Contact: LuAnn Puvogel, R.N., Administrator
CFO: Geri Leibham, Manager Business Office
CMO: Michael Johnson, M.D., Medical Director
CIO: Rex Harrell, Information Technologist
CHR: Geri Leibham, Manager Business Office
Web address: www.salinasurgical.com/
**Control:** Partnership, Investor–owned, for–profit **Service:** Surgical

**Staffed Beds:** 16 **Admissions:** 552 **Census:** 4 **Outpatient Visits:** 7086
**Births:** 0 **Total Expense ($000):** 12764 **Payroll Expense ($000):** 4561
**Personnel:** 78

### SATANTA—Haskell County

★ **SATANTA DISTRICT HOSPITAL (171324)**, 401 South Cheyenne Street,
Zip 67870–0159, Mailing Address: P.O. Box 159, Zip 67870–0159;
tel. 620/649–2761, (Total facility includes 44 beds in nursing home–type unit) **A**9
10 18 **F**3 11 40 45 57 64 67 68 75 81 82 87 93 104 107 118 126 127 129
132 **P**4 **S** Great Plains Health Alliance, Inc., Phillipsburg, KS
Primary Contact: Ron Baker, Administrator
CFO: Libby Anderson, Chief Financial Officer
CMO: Virgilio Taduran, M.D., Chief Medical Officer
CIO: Ben Leppke, Chief Information Officer
CHR: Sam Hett, Manager Human Resources
CNO: Tina Pendergraft, Chief Nursing Officer
Web address: www.satantahospital.org
**Control:** Hospital district or authority, Government, nonfederal **Service:** General
Medical and Surgical

**Staffed Beds:** 57 **Admissions:** 199 **Census:** 36 **Outpatient Visits:** 27820
**Births:** 0 **Total Expense ($000):** 12087 **Payroll Expense ($000):** 5164
**Personnel:** 128

### SCOTT CITY—Scott County

★ **SCOTT COUNTY HOSPITAL (171372)**, 310 East Third Street,
Zip 67871–1203; tel. 620/872–5811 **A**9 10 18 **F**3 7 11 13 15 28 29 30 31
35 40 45 57 59 62 64 68 69 75 76 77 78 79 81 85 93 107 118 126 127
129 132 147 **P**6
Primary Contact: Mark Burnett, President and Chief Executive Officer
COO: Karma Huck, Chief Operating Officer
CFO: Joe S. Meyer, Chief Financial Officer
CMO: Elizabeth Hineman, M.D., Chief Medical Staff
CHR: Pam Wheeler, Manager Human Resources
Web address: www.scotthospital.net
**Control:** Other not–for–profit (including NFP Corporation) **Service:** General
Medical and Surgical

**Staffed Beds:** 23 **Admissions:** 558 **Census:** 8 **Outpatient Visits:** 14798
**Births:** 64 **Total Expense ($000):** 12240 **Payroll Expense ($000):** 6514
**Personnel:** 166

### SEDAN—Chautauqua County

**SEDAN CITY HOSPITAL (171318)**, 300 North Street, Zip 67361–0427, Mailing
Address: P.O. Box C, Zip 67361–0427; tel. 620/725–3115 **A**9 10 18 **F**29 34
40 53 57 64 107 127 129 132 147
Primary Contact: Michelle Williams, Administrator
CFO: Jennifer Seever, Regional Chief Financial Officer
CMO: James McDermott, M.D., Chief of Staff
**Control:** City–Government, nonfederal **Service:** General Medical and Surgical

**Staffed Beds:** 25 **Admissions:** 238 **Census:** 2 **Outpatient Visits:** 5109 **Total
Expense ($000):** 2984 **Payroll Expense ($000):** 1577 **Personnel:** 41

### SENECA—Nemaha County

★ **NEMAHA VALLEY COMMUNITY HOSPITAL (171315)**, 1600 Community Drive,
Zip 66538–9739; tel. 785/336–6181 **A**9 10 18 **F**11 12 13 15 28 31 40 56 57
59 64 75 76 77 78 79 81 84 85 89 93 107 111 113 116 118 126 128 129
130 131 132 **P**6
Primary Contact: Stan Regehr, President and Chief Executive Officer
CFO: Connie Ingwerson, Chief Financial Officer
CHR: Jan Lueb, Coordinator Human Resources
Web address: www.nemvch.org
**Control:** Other not–for–profit (including NFP Corporation) **Service:** General
Medical and Surgical

**Staffed Beds:** 24 **Admissions:** 342 **Census:** 4 **Outpatient Visits:** 19012
**Births:** 46 **Total Expense ($000):** 10241 **Payroll Expense ($000):** 4844
**Personnel:** 111

### SHAWNEE MISSION—Johnson County

⊠ **MID–AMERICA REHABILITATION HOSPITAL (173026)**, 5701 West 110th
Street, Zip 66211–2503; tel. 913/491–2400 **A**1 **F**29 35 56 64 86 90 93 131
142 147 **S** HEALTHSOUTH Corporation, Birmingham, AL
Primary Contact: Kristen De Hart, Chief Executive Officer
CFO: Richard Lane, Chief Financial Officer
CMO: Cielo Dehning, M.D., Medical Director
CHR: Holly Ray, Director Human Resources
Web address: www.midamericarehabhospital.com
**Control:** Corporation, Investor–owned, for–profit **Service:** Rehabilitation

**Staffed Beds:** 98 **Admissions:** 2079 **Census:** 80 **Outpatient Visits:** 9594
**Births:** 0 **Total Expense ($000):** 24333 **Payroll Expense ($000):** 12614
**Personnel:** 212

⊠ **SHAWNEE MISSION MEDICAL CENTER (170104)**, 9100 West 74th Street,
Zip 66204–4004, Mailing Address: Box 2923, Zip 66201–1323;
tel. 913/676–2000 **A**1 2 3 5 9 10 **F**3 4 5 8 11 12 13 15 17 18 20 22 24 28
29 30 31 32 34 35 36 40 42 45 47 48 49 52 54 55 56 57 59 60 61 62 64
70 72 74 75 76 77 78 79 81 82 84 85 86 87 89 93 96 98 100 101 102 103
104 105 107 108 110 111 113 114 117 118 125 128 129 130 131 134 143
145 146 147 **P**6 **S** Adventist Health System Sunbelt Health Care Corporation,
Altamonte Springs, FL
Primary Contact: Ken J. Bacon, President and Chief Executive Officer
CFO: Jack W. Wagner, Executive Vice President and Chief Financial Officer
CMO: Leah Ridgway, M.D., President Medical Staff
CIO: Mike Allen, Director Information Services
CHR: Brad Hoffman, Administrative Director Human Resources
Web address: www.shawneemission.org
**Control:** Church–operated, Nongovernment, not–for profit **Service:** General
Medical and Surgical

**Staffed Beds:** 374 **Admissions:** 20520 **Census:** 213 **Outpatient Visits:**
509170 **Births:** 3914 **Total Expense ($000):** 324294 **Payroll Expense
($000):** 128251 **Personnel:** 2158

### SMITH CENTER—Smith County

★ **SMITH COUNTY MEMORIAL HOSPITAL (171377)**, 614 South Main Street,
Zip 66967–0349; tel. 785/282–6845, (Total facility includes 28 beds in nursing
home–type unit) **A**9 10 18 **F**2 13 15 28 30 31 40 45 53 64 67 68 69 75 76 81
93 107 118 126 127 132 **P**6 **S** Great Plains Health Alliance, Inc.,
Phillipsburg, KS
Primary Contact: Carolyn K. Hess, R.N., Administrator
CFO: Julie Williams, Chief Financial Officer
CIO: Tammy Gaston, Chief Information Officer
CHR: Jody Maxwell, Manager Business Office
CNO: Sarah Ragsdale, R.N., Chief Nursing Officer
Web address: www.gpha.com
**Control:** Other not–for–profit (including NFP Corporation) **Service:** General
Medical and Surgical

**Staffed Beds:** 53 **Admissions:** 412 **Census:** 27 **Outpatient Visits:** 25294
**Births:** 34 **Total Expense ($000):** 10045 **Payroll Expense ($000):** 4619
**Personnel:** 119

### STAFFORD—Stafford County

★ **STAFFORD COUNTY HOSPITAL (171323)**, 502 South Buckeye Street,
Zip 67578–2035, Mailing Address: P.O. Box 190, Zip 67578–0190;
tel. 620/234–5221 **A**9 10 18 **F**3 29 30 35 40 59 62 64 67 77 87 93 107 126
127 129 132 **P**5
Primary Contact: Todd Taylor, Chief Executive Officer
CFO: Janell Goodno, Chief Financial Officer
Web address: www.staffordcountyhospital.org
**Control:** County–Government, nonfederal **Service:** General Medical and Surgical

**Staffed Beds:** 25 **Admissions:** 149 **Census:** 8 **Outpatient Visits:** 44845
**Births:** 0 **Total Expense ($000):** 3298 **Payroll Expense ($000):** 2132
**Personnel:** 56

### SYRACUSE—Hamilton County

**HAMILTON COUNTY HOSPITAL (171322)**, East Avenue G & Huser Street,
Zip 67878–0948, Mailing Address: P.O. Box 948, Zip 67878–0948;
tel. 620/384–7461, (Total facility includes 44 beds in nursing home–type unit) **A**9
10 18 **F**3 40 50 64 81 93 107 126 132 147
Primary Contact: Jeremy Clingenpeel, Administrator and Chief Executive Officer
CFO: Phyllis Horning, Chief Financial Officer
CHR: Angela Talbot, Manager Human Resources
Web address: www.phn.org
**Control:** County–Government, nonfederal **Service:** General Medical and Surgical

**Staffed Beds:** 69 **Admissions:** 285 **Census:** 36 **Outpatient Visits:** 5739
**Births:** 0 **Total Expense ($000):** 6083 **Payroll Expense ($000):** 3183
**Personnel:** 81

---

**Hospital, Medicare Provider Number, Address, Telephone, Approval, Facility, and Physician Codes, Health Care System**

★ American Hospital Association (AHA) membership
☐ The Joint Commission accreditation
◇ DNV Healthcare Inc. accreditation
○ American Osteopathic Association (AOA) accreditation
△ Commission on Accreditation of Rehabilitation Facilities (CARF) accreditation

**KS**

## TOPEKA—Shawnee County

**COLMERY–O'NEIL VETERANS AFFAIRS MEDICAL CENTER** See Veterans Affairs Eastern Kansas Health Care System

**KANSAS NEUROLOGICAL INSTITUTE**, 3107 West 21st Street, Zip 66604–3298; tel. 785/296–5301 **F**29 30 35 39 67 91 97 129 142 145 **P**6
Primary Contact: Barney Hubert, Superintendent
COO: Barney Hubert, Superintendent
CFO: Sara Mock, Director Administrative Services
CMO: Kimberley Scott, Director Health Care Services
CIO: Cheryl Fuller, Director Information Resources
CHR: Shawna Mercer, Director Human Resources
Web address: www.srsnet.srs.ks.gov/hospitals/kni/
**Control:** State–Government, nonfederal **Service:** Institution for mental retardation

**Staffed Beds:** 156 **Admissions:** 2 **Census:** 156 **Outpatient Visits:** 0 **Births:** 0 **Total Expense ($000):** 26985 **Payroll Expense ($000):** 17345 **Personnel:** 539

**KANSAS REHABILITATION HOSPITAL (173025)**, 1504 S.W. Eighth Avenue, Zip 66606–1632; tel. 785/235–6600 **A**1 9 10 **F**3 29 53 62 64 68 75 90 91 93 96 129 131 147 **S** HEALTHSOUTH Corporation, Birmingham, AL
Primary Contact: Marty Dernier, Chief Financial Officer and Administrator
CFO: Marty Dernier, Chief Financial Officer
CMO: Joseph Sankoorikal, M.D., Chief Medical Staff
CHR: Dina Cox, Director Human Resources
CNO: Carol Swanger, Chief Nursing Officer
Web address: www.kansasrehabhospital.com
**Control:** Corporation, Investor–owned, for–profit **Service:** Rehabilitation

**Staffed Beds:** 59 **Admissions:** 1245 **Census:** 40 **Outpatient Visits:** 18343 **Births:** 0 **Total Expense ($000):** 15154 **Payroll Expense ($000):** 7744 **Personnel:** 169

**SELECT SPECIALTY HOSPITAL–TOPEKA (172006)**, 1700 S.W. Seventh Street, Suite 840, Zip 66606–1660; tel. 785/295–5551 **A**1 9 10 **F**1 3 29 75 77 85 87 129 147 **S** Select Medical Corporation, Mechanicsburg, PA
Primary Contact: Jon W. Scott, Chief Executive Officer
CMO: Jed McKee, M.D., Medical Director
CNO: Sarah Herrmann, R.N., Chief Nursing Officer
Web address: www.selectmedical.com
**Control:** Corporation, Investor–owned, for–profit **Service:** Long–Term Acute Care hospital

**Staffed Beds:** 34 **Admissions:** 295 **Census:** 21 **Outpatient Visits:** 0 **Births:** 0 **Total Expense ($000):** 10326 **Payroll Expense ($000):** 4479 **Personnel:** 76

△ **ST. FRANCIS HEALTH CENTER (170016)**, 1700 S.W. 7th Street, Zip 66606–1690; tel. 785/295–8000 **A**1 2 7 9 10 **F**3 5 12 13 15 18 19 20 22 24 26 28 29 30 31 34 35 37 39 40 45 47 48 49 50 51 53 57 58 59 61 62 64 68 70 74 75 76 77 78 79 80 81 82 84 85 86 87 89 90 91 92 93 94 95 96 97 107 108 110 111 113 114 115 116 117 118 119 120 122 125 129 130 131 133 134 145 146 147 **P**8 **S** Sisters of Charity of Leavenworth Health System, Denver, CO
Primary Contact: Robert J. Erickson, Chief Executive Officer
COO: Dan Fieker, D.O., Chief Medical Officer and Chief Operating Officer
CFO: Gary Zmrhal, Interim Vice President Finance
CMO: Dan Fieker, D.O., Chief Medical Officer and Chief Operating Officer
CIO: Kevin Mapes, Director Kansas Division System and Technology Service Center
CHR: Byron Waldy, Director Human Resources
CNO: Scott E. Wells, MSN, Chief Nursing Officer
Web address: www.stfrancistopeka.org
**Control:** Church–operated, Nongovernment, not–for profit **Service:** General Medical and Surgical

**Staffed Beds:** 291 **Admissions:** 9675 **Census:** 119 **Outpatient Visits:** 514441 **Births:** 953 **Total Expense ($000):** 225300 **Payroll Expense ($000):** 96472 **Personnel:** 1372

**STORMONT–VAIL HEALTHCARE (170086)**, 1500 S.W. Tenth Avenue, Zip 66604–1353; tel. 785/354–6000 **A**1 2 5 9 10 **F**3 11 12 13 15 17 18 19 20 22 24 26 28 29 30 31 34 35 37 40 43 45 47 49 51 53 55 56 57 58 59 60 61 64 65 68 69 70 71 72 74 75 76 77 78 79 81 82 83 84 85 86 87 88 89 91 93 94 97 98 99 101 102 103 104 105 107 108 110 111 112 113 114 116 118 119 120 122 128 129 130 131 134 142 143 144 145 146 147 **P**6
Primary Contact: Randall Peterson, President and Chief Executive Officer
COO: Janet Stanek, Executive Vice President
CFO: Kevin Han, Vice President and Chief Financial Officer
CMO: Kent Palmberg, M.D., Senior Vice President and Chief Medical Officer
CIO: Judy Corzine, Administrative Director and Chief Information Officer
CHR: Bernard H. Becker, Vice President and Chief Human Resources Officer
CNO: Carol Perry, R.N., Vice President and Chief Nursing Officer
Web address: www.stormontvail.org
**Control:** Other not–for–profit (including NFP Corporation) **Service:** General Medical and Surgical

**Staffed Beds:** 359 **Admissions:** 20136 **Census:** 231 **Outpatient Visits:** 120158 **Births:** 2069 **Total Expense ($000):** 463603 **Payroll Expense ($000):** 236226 **Personnel:** 3485

△ **VETERANS AFFAIRS EASTERN KANSAS HEALTH CARE SYSTEM**, 2200 Gage Boulevard, Zip 66622–0002; tel. 785/350–3111, (Includes COLMERY–O'NEIL VETERANS AFFAIRS MEDICAL CENTER, 2200 Gage Boulevard, tel. 785/350–3111; DWIGHT D. EISENHOWER VETERANS AFFAIRS MEDICAL CENTER, 4101 S. 4th Street Trafficway, Leavenworth, Zip 66048–5055; tel. 913/682–2000), (Nonreporting) **A**1 3 5 7 **S** Department of Veterans Affairs, Washington, DC
Primary Contact: John Moon, Associate Director
COO: Karen Glotzbach, Acting Associate Director
CMO: Rajeev Trehan, M.D., Chief of Staff
CIO: Joni Davin, Director Information and Business Management Service Line
Web address: www.va.gov/sta/guide/home.asp
**Control:** Veterans Affairs, Government, federal **Service:** General Medical and Surgical

**Staffed Beds:** 213

## TRIBUNE—Greeley County

★ **GREELEY COUNTY HEALTH SERVICES (171359)**, 506 Third Street, Zip 67879–0338, Mailing Address: P.O. Box 338, Zip 67879–0338; tel. 620/376–4221, (Total facility includes 32 beds in nursing home–type unit) **A**9 10 18 **F**28 31 40 45 46 59 64 65 66 69 81 82 93 97 126 132 146 **S** QHR, Brentwood, TN
Primary Contact: Deborah Lehner, Administrator
CFO: James L. Smith, Chief Financial Officer
CMO: Wendel Ellis, D.O., Chief Medical Staff
CIO: Shanon Schneider, Chief Information Officer
CHR: Tiffany Kleymann, Manager Human Resources
CNO: Stephanie Wineinger, Director of Nursing
Web address: www.phn.org
**Control:** Other not–for–profit (including NFP Corporation) **Service:** General Medical and Surgical

**Staffed Beds:** 50 **Admissions:** 251 **Census:** 27 **Outpatient Visits:** 12110 **Births:** 2 **Total Expense ($000):** 9143 **Payroll Expense ($000):** 4583 **Personnel:** 112

## ULYSSES—Grant County

★ **BOB WILSON MEMORIAL GRANT COUNTY HOSPITAL (170110)**, 415 North Main Street, Zip 67880–2133; tel. 620/356–1266 **A**9 10 20 **F**3 11 13 15 29 30 34 35 40 45 50 57 59 62 64 68 75 76 79 81 82 85 86 87 91 93 96 97 107 118 126 129 132 145 147 **P**6
Primary Contact: Arthur H. Frable, Chief Executive Officer
CFO: Robert Jacobi, Chief Financial Officer
CIO: Chris Moffet, Director Information Services
CHR: Tammy Oxford, Director Human Resources
Web address: www.bwmgch.com
**Control:** County–Government, nonfederal **Service:** General Medical and Surgical

**Staffed Beds:** 26 **Admissions:** 366 **Census:** 4 **Outpatient Visits:** 10655 **Births:** 104 **Total Expense ($000):** 13649 **Payroll Expense ($000):** 6301 **Personnel:** 131

## WAKEENEY—Trego County

★ **TREGO COUNTY–LEMKE MEMORIAL HOSPITAL (171355)**, 320 North 13th Street, Zip 67672–2099; tel. 785/743–2182, (Total facility includes 37 beds in nursing home–type unit) **A**9 10 18 **F**3 8 10 11 15 28 29 34 40 45 57 59 62 67 69 81 86 89 93 107 110 113 126 127 129 132 142 145 147 **P**6 **S** Great Plains Health Alliance, Inc., Phillipsburg, KS
Primary Contact: Harold Courtois, Administrator and Chief Executive Officer
CFO: Gail Jensen, Chief Financial Officer
CMO: Gordon Lang, M.D., Chief of Staff
CIO: Jolene Schuster, Director Information Technology
CHR: Cindy Meiar, Human Resources and Payroll Coordinator
CNO: Sandy Purinton, Chief Nursing Officer
Web address: www.tclmh.org
**Control:** County–Government, nonfederal **Service:** General Medical and Surgical

**Staffed Beds:** 62 **Admissions:** 1049 **Census:** 51 **Outpatient Visits:** 32929 **Births:** 0 **Total Expense ($000):** 14913 **Payroll Expense ($000):** 6831 **Personnel:** 167

## WAMEGO—Pottawatomie County

★ **WAMEGO CITY HOSPITAL (171337)**, 711 Genn Drive, Zip 66547–1179; tel. 785/456–2295 **A**9 10 18 **F**3 11 15 29 32 34 35 40 45 56 59 75 77 81 93 97 107 113 118 126 129 131 132 141 142 145 146 147
Primary Contact: Shannan Flach, Chief Executive Officer
COO: Brian Smith, Chief Operating Officer
CFO: Keith Zachariasen, Chief Financial Officer
CMO: Roland Darey, M.D., Medical Director
CIO: Wes Janzen, Chief Information Officer
CHR: Marcie Holsteen, Human Resources Officer
CNO: Tresha Flanary, R.N., Chief Clinical Services Officer
Web address: www.wamegocityhospital.com
**Control:** Other not–for–profit (including NFP Corporation) **Service:** General Medical and Surgical

**Staffed Beds:** 18 **Admissions:** 272 **Census:** 3 **Outpatient Visits:** 26349 **Births:** 0 **Total Expense ($000):** 8378 **Payroll Expense ($000):** 4274 **Personnel:** 66

*Many Facility Codes have changed. Please refer to the AHA Guide Code Chart.* © 2012 AHA Guide

## WASHINGTON—Washington County

**WASHINGTON COUNTY HOSPITAL (171351)**, 304 East Third Street, Zip 66968–2033; tel. 785/325–2211 **A**9 10 18 **F**2 3 11 13 15 28 29 30 31 35 40 45 53 57 64 67 70 76 81 85 89 93 107 113 127 129 132 147 **P**5
Primary Contact: Doyle L. McKimmy, FACHE, Chief Executive Officer
CFO: Linda Rettig, Director Financial Services
Web address: www.washingtoncountyhospital.com
**Control:** County–Government, nonfederal **Service:** General Medical and Surgical

**Staffed Beds:** 25 **Admissions:** 168 **Census:** 6 **Outpatient Visits:** 4620 **Births:** 10 **Total Expense ($000):** 4078 **Payroll Expense ($000):** 1736 **Personnel:** 44

## WELLINGTON—Sumner County

**SUMNER REGIONAL MEDICAL CENTER (170039)**, 1323 North A Street, Zip 67152–4350; tel. 620/326–7451, (Total facility includes 9 beds in nursing home–type unit) **A**9 10 **F**10 11 13 15 31 34 35 40 45 56 57 59 76 79 81 82 85 98 103 107 108 110 111 118 127 128 129 147 **P**6
Primary Contact: Robert H. Bean, Ph.D., President and Chief Executive Officer
CFO: Kim Weaver, CPA, Chief Financial Officer
CIO: Lori Young, Manager Health Information Management
CHR: Allen Keller, Director Human Resources
CNO: Darlene Cooney, Director Nursing
Web address: www.srmcks.org
**Control:** City–Government, nonfederal **Service:** General Medical and Surgical

**Staffed Beds:** 57 **Admissions:** 709 **Census:** 15 **Outpatient Visits:** 26712 **Births:** 152 **Total Expense ($000):** 13664 **Payroll Expense ($000):** 5507 **Personnel:** 134

## WICHITA—Sedgwick County

**KANSAS HEART HOSPITAL (170186)**, 3601 North Webb Road, Zip 67226; tel. 316/630–5000 **A**9 10 **F**3 17 18 20 22 24 29 30 64 81 86 107 108 114 118 129
Primary Contact: Thomas L. Ashcom, M.D., Ph.D., Chief Executive Officer
COO: I. Lynn Jeane, Chief Operating Officer
CFO: Steve Smith, Chief Financial Officer
CHR: Teresa E. Wolfe, Manager Human Resources
Web address: www.kansasheart.com
**Control:** Corporation, Investor–owned, for–profit **Service:** Heart

**Staffed Beds:** 54 **Admissions:** 2288 **Census:** 28 **Outpatient Visits:** 9599 **Births:** 0 **Personnel:** 211

**KANSAS SPINE HOSPITAL (170196)**, 3333 North Webb Road, Zip 67226; tel. 316/462–5000 **A**9 10 **F**3 29 79 81 82 85 87 107 111 113
Primary Contact: Thomas M. Schmitt, Chief Executive Officer
CFO: Kevin P. Vaughn, Chief Financial Officer
CIO: Michael Knocke, Chief Information Officer
CHR: Jean–Marie Jimeson, Coordinator Human Resources
Web address: www.ksspine.com
**Control:** Corporation, Investor–owned, for–profit **Service:** General Medical and Surgical

**Staffed Beds:** 38 **Admissions:** 1668 **Census:** 10 **Outpatient Visits:** 4580 **Births:** 0 **Personnel:** 82

**KANSAS SURGERY AND RECOVERY CENTER (170183)**, 2770 North Webb Road, Zip 67226–8112; tel. 316/634–0090 **A**9 10 **F**51 64 68 81 85 87 107 111 113 118 **S** Via Christi Health, Wichita, KS
Primary Contact: Ely Bartal, M.D., Chief Executive Officer
CFO: Ashley Simon, Chief Financial Officer
CMO: Ely Bartal, M.D., Chief Executive Officer and Medical Director
CIO: Jonathan Wells, Supervisor Information Technology
CNO: Becky Bailey, R.N., Director of Nursing
Web address: www.ksrc.org
**Control:** Partnership, Investor–owned, for–profit **Service:** General Medical and Surgical

**Staffed Beds:** 32 **Admissions:** 1562 **Census:** 12 **Outpatient Visits:** 7979 **Births:** 0 **Total Expense ($000):** 24429 **Payroll Expense ($000):** 6370 **Personnel:** 135

☐ **LTAC OF WICHITA (172003)**, 8080 East Pawnee Street, Zip 67207–5475; tel. 316/682–0004 **A**1 9 10 **F**1 29 30 77 100 142 147 **S** AMG Integrated Healthcare Management, Lafayette, LA
Primary Contact: William Wild, Chief Executive Officer
CFO: Myra Dick, Manager Business Office
CIO: Michelle Bradley, Director Health Information Management
CHR: Adrienne Burkholder, Director Human Resources
**Control:** Corporation, Investor–owned, for–profit **Service:** Long–Term Acute Care hospital

**Staffed Beds:** 26 **Admissions:** 192 **Census:** 15 **Outpatient Visits:** 0 **Births:** 0 **Personnel:** 42

⊠ **ROBERT J. DOLE VETERANS AFFAIRS MEDICAL CENTER**, 5500 East Kellogg, Zip 67218; tel. 316/685–2221, (Nonreporting) **A**1 5 **S** Department of Veterans Affairs, Washington, DC
Primary Contact: Thomas J. Sanders, FACHE, Director
COO: Thomas J. Sanders, FACHE, Director
CFO: Ronald Dreher, Finance Officer
CMO: Kent Murray, M.D., Chief of Staff
CIO: Sharon Williamson, Chief Information Technology
CHR: Nancy Gerstner, Manager Human Resources
Web address: www.va.gov/sta/guide/home.asp
**Control:** Veterans Affairs, Government, federal **Service:** General Medical and Surgical

**Staffed Beds:** 41

⊠ **SELECT SPECIALTY HOSPITAL–WICHITA (172007)**, 929 North St. Francis Street, Zip 67214; tel. 316/261–8303 **A**1 9 10 **F**1 3 12 18 29 50 56 60 61 75 82 84 85 86 87 129 147 **S** Select Medical Corporation, Mechanicsburg, PA
Primary Contact: Peggy Cliffe, Chief Executive Officer
Web address: www.selectmedicalcorp.com
**Control:** Corporation, Investor–owned, for–profit **Service:** Long–Term Acute Care hospital

**Staffed Beds:** 58 **Admissions:** 466 **Census:** 35 **Outpatient Visits:** 0 **Births:** 0 **Total Expense ($000):** 16221 **Payroll Expense ($000):** 5896 **Personnel:** 116

⊠ **VIA CHRISTI HOSPITAL (170200)**, 14800 West St. Teresa, Zip 67235–9602; tel. 316/796–7000 **A**1 10 **F**3 8 13 18 20 22 26 29 30 34 35 40 45 50 64 68 70 75 76 79 81 85 87 107 108 111 113 117 118 129 145 146 147 **S** Via Christi Health, Wichita, KS
Primary Contact: Kevin Strecker, President
Web address: www.via–christi.org
**Control:** Church–operated, Nongovernment, not–for profit **Service:** General Medical and Surgical

**Staffed Beds:** 68 **Admissions:** 1719 **Census:** 14 **Outpatient Visits:** 16152 **Births:** 249 **Total Expense ($000):** 40881 **Payroll Expense ($000):** 14634 **Personnel:** 192

⊠ **VIA CHRISTI HOSPITALS WICHITA (170122)**, 929 North St. Francis Street, Zip 67214–3882; tel. 316/268–5000, (Includes GOOD SHEPHERD CAMPUS, 8901 East Orme, Zip 67207; tel. 316/858–0333; ST. FRANCIS CAMPUS, 929 North St. Francis Street, tel. 316/268–5000; Sherry Hausmann, President; ST. JOSEPH CAMPUS, 3600 East Harry Street, Zip 67218–3713; tel. 316/685–1111; Claudio J. Ferraro, President) **A**1 2 3 5 9 10 13 **F**3 5 7 11 12 13 15 16 17 18 19 20 21 22 23 24 26 27 28 29 30 31 32 34 35 38 40 43 44 45 49 50 51 54 56 57 58 59 60 61 64 68 70 72 74 75 76 77 78 79 81 82 84 85 86 87 88 89 92 93 97 98 99 100 101 102 103 104 105 107 108 110 111 113 114 115 116 117 118 119 120 122 123 125 129 130 131 134 135 137 140 141 142 145 146 147 **P**3 6 7 **S** Via Christi Health, Wichita, KS
Primary Contact: Sherry Hausmann, President
COO: Laurie Labarca, Executive Vice President and Chief Operating Officer
CFO: Mike Wegner, Chief Financial Officer
CMO: Steven Nesbit, D.O., Chief Medical Officer
CIO: Diana Hilburn, Vice President Information Technology and Chief Information Officer
CHR: Sherrie String, Vice President Human Resources
Web address: www.via–christi.org
**Control:** Church–operated, Nongovernment, not–for profit **Service:** General Medical and Surgical

**Staffed Beds:** 801 **Admissions:** 33638 **Census:** 442 **Outpatient Visits:** 296348 **Births:** 2393 **Total Expense ($000):** 458612 **Payroll Expense ($000):** 209430 **Personnel:** 3777

**VIA CHRISTI REGIONAL MEDICAL CENTER** See Via Christi Hospitals Wichita

⊠ △ **VIA CHRISTI REHABILITATION CENTER (173028)**, 1151 North Rock Road, Zip 67206–1262; tel. 316/634–3400 **A**1 7 9 10 **F**11 29 30 34 44 50 54 57 58 59 64 77 86 87 90 92 93 96 118 128 129 130 131 142 145 147 **S** Via Christi Health, Wichita, KS
Primary Contact: Cindy LaFleur, President
CMO: Kevin Rieg, M.D., President Medical Staff
Web address: www.via–christi.org
**Control:** Church–operated, Nongovernment, not–for profit **Service:** Rehabilitation

**Staffed Beds:** 58 **Admissions:** 826 **Census:** 29 **Outpatient Visits:** 94020 **Births:** 0 **Total Expense ($000):** 22265 **Payroll Expense ($000):** 11614 **Personnel:** 249

---

**Hospital, Medicare Provider Number, Address, Telephone, Approval, Facility, and Physician Codes, Health Care System**

★ American Hospital Association (AHA) membership
☐ The Joint Commission accreditation ◇ DNV Healthcare Inc. accreditation
○ American Osteopathic Association (AOA) accreditation
△ Commission on Accreditation of Rehabilitation Facilities (CARF) accreditation

**KS**

✠ **WESLEY MEDICAL CENTER (170123)**, 550 North Hillside, Zip 67214–4976; tel. 316/962–2000, (Includes GALICHIA HEART HOSPITAL, 2610 North Woodlawn, Zip 67220; tel. 316/858–2610; Stephen J. Harris, Chief Executive Officer) **A**1 3 5 9 10 **F**3 7 11 12 13 15 17 18 19 20 22 24 26 28 29 30 31 34 35 39 40 42 43 44 45 46 48 49 50 51 54 55 56 57 58 59 60 64 65 68 70 72 73 74 76 78 79 81 85 86 87 88 89 92 93 94 97 100 102 107 108 111 113 114 118 120 122 123 125 128 129 130 131 133 134 145 146 147 **P**6 **S** HCA, Nashville, TN
Primary Contact: Hugh C. Tappan, President and Chief Executive Officer
COO: G. B. Serrill, Chief Operating Officer
CFO: Matt Leary, Chief Financial Officer
CMO: Francie H. Ekengren, M.D., Chief Medical Officer
CIO: Larry Forsyth, Director Information System
CHR: Don Morris, Vice President Human Resources
Web address: www.wesleymc.com
**Control:** Corporation, Investor–owned, for–profit **Service:** General Medical and Surgical

**Staffed Beds:** 524 **Admissions:** 23424 **Census:** 313 **Outpatient Visits:** 293625 **Births:** 6399 **Total Expense ($000):** 333247 **Payroll Expense ($000):** 128309 **Personnel:** 2127

✠ **WESLEY REHABILITATION HOSPITAL (173027)**, 8338 West 13th Street North, Zip 67212–2984; tel. 316/729–9999 **A**1 9 10 **F**29 34 35 62 64 90 91 93 95 96 131 146 147 **S** HEALTHSOUTH Corporation, Birmingham, AL
Primary Contact: Bob Peck, Interim Chief Executive Officer
CFO: Bob Peck, Chief Financial Officer
CMO: Kevin F. Brown, D.O., Medical Director
CIO: Debbie Patterson, Director Health Information Management
CHR: Betty Shuman, Director Human Resources
Web address: www.wesleyrehabhospital.com
**Control:** Corporation, Investor–owned, for–profit **Service:** Rehabilitation

**Staffed Beds:** 65 **Admissions:** 975 **Census:** 34 **Outpatient Visits:** 22456 **Births:** 0 **Total Expense ($000):** 15438 **Payroll Expense ($000):** 7359 **Personnel:** 165

**WICHITA SPECIALTY HOSPITAL** See LTAC of Wichita

**WINCHESTER—Jefferson County**

★ **F. W. HUSTON MEDICAL CENTER (171314)**, 408 Delaware Street, Zip 66097–4003; tel. 913/774–4340, (Total facility includes 43 beds in nursing home–type unit) **A**9 10 18 **F**3 10 34 40 44 50 56 57 59 64 65 67 69 75 87 93 97 103 104 107 124 127 129 131 132 134 142 143 **P**6 8
Primary Contact: LaMont Cook, Administrator
CFO: Shelly Ludwig, Controller
CHR: Lois Wheeler, Manager Human Resources
Web address: www.jcmhospital.org
**Control:** Other not–for–profit (including NFP Corporation) **Service:** General Medical and Surgical

**Staffed Beds:** 74 **Admissions:** 86 **Census:** 31 **Outpatient Visits:** 4740 **Births:** 0 **Total Expense ($000):** 4537 **Payroll Expense ($000):** 2793 **Personnel:** 83

**JEFFERSON COUNTY MEMORIAL HOSPITAL** See F. W. Huston Medical Center

**WINFIELD—Cowley County**

★ **WILLIAM NEWTON HOSPITAL (171383)**, 1300 East Fifth Street, Zip 67156–2407; tel. 620/221–2300 **A**9 10 18 **F**3 11 13 15 18 28 29 32 34 35 38 39 40 44 45 47 51 57 59 62 64 65 68 70 74 75 76 77 78 79 81 82 85 86 87 93 102 107 108 111 113 117 118 120 122 126 128 129 130 131 132 134 145 146 147
Primary Contact: Richard H. Vaught, Administrator
COO: Tom Embers, Assistant Administrator and Chief Operating Officer
CFO: Debbie Hockenbury, Assistant Administrator and Chief Financial Officer
CMO: Wade Turner, M.D., Chief of Staff
CIO: Randy Mayo, Director Information Technology
CHR: Cathy McClurg, Director Human Resources
CNO: Kristie Ball, Director of Nursing
Web address: www.wnmh.org
**Control:** City–Government, nonfederal **Service:** General Medical and Surgical

**Staffed Beds:** 25 **Admissions:** 1006 **Census:** 8 **Outpatient Visits:** 60056 **Births:** 257 **Total Expense ($000):** 25741 **Payroll Expense ($000):** 11236 **Personnel:** 251

**KS**

# KENTUCKY

## ALBANY—Clinton County

**CLINTON COUNTY HOSPITAL (180106)**, 723 Burkesville Road,
Zip 42602–1654; tel. 606/387–6421, (Nonreporting) **A**9 10
Primary Contact: John David Mullins, Jr., Administrator
CHR: Pat Beard, Director Human Resources
Web address: www.clintoncountyhospital.com
**Control:** Other not–for–profit (including NFP Corporation) **Service:** General
Medical and Surgical

**Staffed Beds:** 42

## ASHLAND—Boyd County

☐ △ **KING'S DAUGHTERS MEDICAL CENTER (180009)**, 2201 Lexington
Avenue, Zip 41101–2874, Mailing Address: P.O. Box 151, Zip 41105–0151;
tel. 606/408–4000, (Total facility includes 147 beds in nursing home–type unit)
**A**1 2 7 9 10 **F**3 7 8 9 10 11 12 13 15 17 18 20 22 24 26 28 29 30 31 34 35
37 38 40 44 45 46 47 48 49 50 51 54 55 56 57 58 59 60 61 62 64 65 70
71 72 74 75 76 77 78 79 81 82 84 85 86 87 89 90 91 92 93 96 97 98 100
101 102 103 107 108 110 111 113 114 115 116 117 118 125 127 128 129
130 131 133 134 142 143 144 145 146 147 **P**8
Primary Contact: Fred L. Jackson, FACHE, Chief Executive Officer
COO: Bob Lucas, Vice President Operations
CFO: Paul L. McDowell, Vice President Finance and Chief Financial Officer
CMO: Phil Fioret, M.D., Vice President Medical Affairs
CIO: David Oliver, Director Information Systems
CHR: Larry Higgins, Vice President Human Resources
Web address: www.kdmc.com
**Control:** Other not–for–profit (including NFP Corporation) **Service:** General
Medical and Surgical

**Staffed Beds:** 612 **Admissions:** 23447 **Census:** 423 **Outpatient Visits:**
683974 **Births:** 1524 **Total Expense ($000):** 474693 **Payroll Expense
($000):** 175995 **Personnel:** 3289

☒ **OUR LADY OF BELLEFONTE HOSPITAL (180036)**, St. Christopher Drive,
Zip 41101, Mailing Address: P.O. Box 789, Zip 41105–0789; tel. 606/833–3333
**A**1 2 9 10 12 13 **F**3 4 5 8 11 12 15 18 19 20 28 29 30 31 34 35 37 39 40
44 45 49 50 53 54 55 57 58 59 62 64 65 66 69 70 71 74 75 77 78 79 81
82 84 85 86 87 89 93 96 97 98 100 101 102 103 106 107 108 110 111
113 114 117 118 128 129 130 131 134 142 143 144 145 146 147 **P**7 8
**S** Bon Secours Health System, Inc., Marriottsville, MD
Primary Contact: Kevin Halter, Chief Executive Officer
CFO: Joe Buchheit, Chief Financial Officer
CIO: Mike Gomez, Site Manager Medical Information Systems
CHR: Judy Daniels, Vice President Human Resources
Web address: www.olbh.com
**Control:** Church–operated, Nongovernment, not–for profit **Service:** General
Medical and Surgical

**Staffed Beds:** 151 **Admissions:** 7398 **Census:** 77 **Outpatient Visits:** 220286
**Births:** 0 **Total Expense ($000):** 129954 **Payroll Expense ($000):** 42924
**Personnel:** 1170

## BARBOURVILLE—Knox County

☐ **KNOX COUNTY HOSPITAL (181328)**, 80 Hospital Drive, Zip 40906–1317,
Mailing Address: P.O. Box 10, Zip 40906–0160; tel. 606/546–4175,
(Nonreporting) **A**1 9 10 18 **S** Pacer Health Corporation, Miami Lakes, FL
Primary Contact: Craig Morgan, Chief Executive Officer
CFO: Amanda Ellis, Chief Financial Officer
CMO: Kamran Hasni, M.D., Chief of Medical Staff
CIO: Evan Davis, Director Technology and Environmental Services
CHR: Janet Wilder, Coordinator Human Resources
CNO: Brenda Graham, Chief Nursing Officer
Web address: www.knoxcohospital.com
**Control:** Corporation, Investor–owned, for–profit **Service:** General Medical and
Surgical

**Staffed Beds:** 25

## BARDSTOWN—Nelson County

☒ **FLAGET MEMORIAL HOSPITAL (180025)**, 4305 New Shepherdsville Road,
Zip 40004; tel. 502/350–5000, (Total facility includes 12 beds in nursing home–
type unit) **A**1 9 10 **F**11 12 13 15 18 28 29 30 31 34 35 37 40 45 49 59 62
63 64 70 76 78 79 81 82 84 85 96 107 111 115 118 126 127 128 129 131
143 145 146 147 **P**3 **S** Catholic Health Initiatives, Englewood, CO
Primary Contact: Sue Downs, R.N., MSN, President
COO: Norma Goss, R.N., COO/CNO
CFO: John Bradford, Vice President Finance
CMO: Mark Abramovich, M.D., Chief of Staff
CHR: Deborah Cowles, Vice President Human Resources
CNO: Norma Goss, R.N., COO/CNO
Web address: www.flaget.com
**Control:** Other not–for–profit (including NFP Corporation) **Service:** General
Medical and Surgical

**Staffed Beds:** 40 **Admissions:** 2525 **Census:** 24 **Outpatient Visits:** 63377
**Births:** 228 **Total Expense ($000):** 54786 **Payroll Expense ($000):** 19605
**Personnel:** 413

## BENTON—Marshall County

☐ **MARSHALL COUNTY HOSPITAL (181327)**, 615 Old Symsonia Road,
Zip 42025–5042, Mailing Address: P.O. Box 630, Zip 42025–0630;
tel. 270/527–4800 **A**1 9 10 18 **F**3 7 11 15 18 28 29 30 34 35 40 51 53 57
59 62 77 79 81 85 89 90 93 107 108 118 127 131 132 134 **P**6
Primary Contact: Kathy Long, Chief Executive Officer
CFO: Janice Kelley, Chief Financial Officer
CMO: Glen Van Loon, M.D., Chief of Staff
CIO: Patrick Waters, Director Information Technology
CHR: Jeannie Lee, Director Human Resources
Web address: www.marshallcountyhospital.org
**Control:** Hospital district or authority, Government, nonfederal **Service:** General
Medical and Surgical

**Staffed Beds:** 25 **Admissions:** 931 **Census:** 8 **Outpatient Visits:** 26503
**Births:** 0 **Total Expense ($000):** 19269 **Payroll Expense ($000):** 7563
**Personnel:** 190

## BEREA—Madison County

☒ **SAINT JOSEPH BEREA (181329)**, 305 Estill Street, Zip 40403–1909;
tel. 859/986–3151, (Nonreporting) **A**1 5 9 10 18 **S** Catholic Health Initiatives,
Englewood, CO
Primary Contact: Greg D. Gerard, President
CMO: Patrick Kelleher, M.D., Chief Medical Staff
CIO: Katie Heckman, Director Community Relations
CHR: Renee Bullock, Vice President Human Resources
Web address: www.saintjosephberea.org
**Control:** Other not–for–profit (including NFP Corporation) **Service:** General
Medical and Surgical

**Staffed Beds:** 25

## BOWLING GREEN—Warren County

**COMMONWEALTH REGIONAL SPECIALTY HOSPITAL (182005)**, 250 Park
Drive, 6th Floor, Zip 42101, Mailing Address: P.O. Box 90010, Zip 42101;
tel. 270/796–6200 **A**9 10 **F**1 3 29 30 129 **S** Commonwealth Health
Corporation, Bowling Green, KY
Primary Contact: Emily Howard Martin, Administrator
CFO: Ronald G. Sowell, Executive Vice President
CMO: Doug Thomson, M.D., Chief Medical Officer
CIO: Jean Cherry, Executive Vice President
CHR: Lynn Williams, Vice President
Web address: www.commonwealthregionalspecialtyhospital.org
**Control:** Other not–for–profit (including NFP Corporation) **Service:** General
Medical and Surgical

**Staffed Beds:** 28 **Admissions:** 251 **Census:** 18 **Outpatient Visits:** 0 **Births:**
0 **Personnel:** 57

**Hospital, Medicare Provider Number, Address, Telephone, Approval, Facility, and Physician Codes, Health Care System**

★ American Hospital Association (AHA) membership
☐ The Joint Commission accreditation   ◇ DNV Healthcare Inc. accreditation
○ American Osteopathic Association (AOA) accreditation
△ Commission on Accreditation of Rehabilitation Facilities (CARF) accreditation

⌧ **GREENVIEW REGIONAL HOSPITAL (180124)**, 1801 Ashley Circle,
Zip 42104–3362; tel. 270/793–1000 **A**1 2 9 10 19 **F**3 8 11 15 18 20 22 29
30 31 34 35 37 40 45 46 48 49 50 51 57 59 64 65 68 70 74 75 77 78 79
81 82 85 86 87 107 108 110 111 113 117 118 123 127 128 129 130 131
132 134 144 145 **S** HCA, Nashville, TN
Primary Contact: Mark A. Marsh, Chief Executive Officer
CFO: Richard Patterson, Chief Financial Officer
CMO: Tim Long, M.D., Chief of Staff
CIO: Cyndi Talley, Director Information Systems
CHR: Judy Fulkerson, Director Human Resources
Web address: www.greenviewhospital.com
**Control:** Corporation, Investor–owned, for–profit **Service:** General Medical and
Surgical

> **Staffed Beds:** 167 **Admissions:** 4224 **Census:** 58 **Outpatient Visits:** 46888
> **Births:** 0 **Total Expense ($000):** 60655 **Payroll Expense ($000):** 20166
> **Personnel:** 450

☐ **MEDICAL CENTER AT BOWLING GREEN (180013)**, 250 Park Street,
Zip 42101–1795, Mailing Address: P.O. Box 90010, Zip 42102–9010;
tel. 270/745–1000 **A**1 2 9 10 19 **F**1 3 7 13 15 17 18 20 22 24 26 28 29 30
31 32 34 35 37 39 40 46 50 51 56 57 59 60 62 64 68 70 72 74 75 76 78
79 80 81 82 84 85 86 87 89 91 93 98 100 102 103 104 105 107 108 110
111 113 115 116 118 120 122 128 129 131 134 144 145 146 147
**S** Commonwealth Health Corporation, Bowling Green, KY
Primary Contact: Connie Smith, Chief Executive Officer
CFO: Ronald G. Sowell, Executive Vice President
CIO: Jean Cherry, Executive Vice President and Chief Information Officer
CHR: Lynn Williams, Vice President Human Resources
Web address: www.themedicalcenter.org
**Control:** Other not–for–profit (including NFP Corporation) **Service:** General
Medical and Surgical

> **Staffed Beds:** 337 **Admissions:** 16346 **Census:** 212 **Outpatient Visits:**
> 107431 **Births:** 2324 **Personnel:** 1550

☐ **RIVENDELL BEHAVIORAL HEALTH (184017)**, 1035 Porter Pike, Zip 42103;
tel. 270/843–1199, (Nonreporting) **A**1 9 10 **S** Universal Health Services, Inc.,
King of Prussia, PA
Primary Contact: Janice Richardson, Chief Executive Officer and Managing
Director
CFO: Tim Gore, Chief Financial Officer
Web address: www.rivendellbehavioral.com
**Control:** Corporation, Investor–owned, for–profit **Service:** Psychiatric

> **Staffed Beds:** 125

☐ △ **SOUTHERN KENTUCKY REHABILITATION HOSPITAL (183029)**, 1300
Campbell Lane, Zip 42104–4162; tel. 270/782–6900, (Nonreporting) **A**1 7 9 10
**S** Vibra Healthcare, Mechanicsburg, PA
Primary Contact: Stuart Locke, Interim Chief Executive Officer
COO: Dana Lewis, Director Clinical Services
CFO: Stuart Locke, Chief Financial Officer
CMO: Jim Farrage, M.D., Medical Director
CHR: Suzanne Cornett, Director Human Resources
Web address: www.skyrehab.com
**Control:** Corporation, Investor–owned, for–profit **Service:** Rehabilitation

> **Staffed Beds:** 60

### BURKESVILLE—Cumberland County

**CUMBERLAND COUNTY HOSPITAL (181317)**, 299 Glasgow Road,
Zip 42717–9696, Mailing Address: P.O. Box 280, Zip 42717–0280;
tel. 270/864–2511, (Nonreporting) **A**9 10 18
Primary Contact: Richard Neikirk, Chief Executive Officer
CFO: Rick Capps, Chief Financial Officer
CMO: Christian Konsavage, M.D., Chief of Staff
CHR: Martha Young, Director Human Resources
Web address: www.cchospital.org
**Control:** Other not–for–profit (including NFP Corporation) **Service:** General
Medical and Surgical

> **Staffed Beds:** 25

### CADIZ—Trigg County

★ **TRIGG COUNTY HOSPITAL (181304)**, 254 Main Street, Zip 42211–9153,
Mailing Address: P.O. Box 312, Zip 42211–0312; tel. 270/522–3215 **A**9 10 18
**F**3 7 8 11 15 29 34 40 50 54 57 59 68 74 75 77 81 87 93 97 100 101 103
104 107 111 113 118 126 132 134 142 **P**3 6
Primary Contact: Alisa Coleman, Chief Executive Officer
CFO: Liz Snodgrass, Chief Financial Officer
CMO: Stuart Harris, M.D., Chief of Staff
CHR: Janet James, Director Human Resources
Web address: www.trigghospital.org
**Control:** County–Government, nonfederal **Service:** General Medical and Surgical

> **Staffed Beds:** 25 **Admissions:** 600 **Census:** 9 **Outpatient Visits:** 27310
> **Births:** 0 **Total Expense ($000):** 10279 **Payroll Expense ($000):** 5215
> **Personnel:** 138

### CAMPBELLSVILLE—Taylor County

★ **TAYLOR REGIONAL HOSPITAL (180087)**, 1700 Old Lebanon Road,
Zip 42718–9600; tel. 270/465–3561 **A**2 9 10 **F**3 8 11 13 15 18 20 28 29 30
31 34 35 36 39 40 43 44 45 46 48 49 50 51 54 56 57 59 60 64 65 68 70
75 76 77 78 79 81 83 84 85 86 93 97 100 107 108 110 111 113 114 117
118 121 126 128 129 131 134 140 142 143 145 146 147 **S** Jewish
Hospital & St. Mary's HealthCare, Louisville, KY
Primary Contact: Jane Wheatley, Chief Executive Officer
CFO: David Massengale, Chief Financial Officer
CIO: Gary Neat, Director Information Management Systems
CHR: Andrea Settle, Director Human Resources
Web address: www.trhosp.org
**Control:** Hospital district or authority, Government, nonfederal **Service:** General
Medical and Surgical

> **Staffed Beds:** 90 **Admissions:** 3059 **Census:** 34 **Outpatient Visits:** 86133
> **Births:** 290 **Total Expense ($000):** 62761 **Payroll Expense ($000):** 28394
> **Personnel:** 562

### CARLISLE—Nicholas County

☐ **NICHOLAS COUNTY HOSPITAL (181303)**, 2323 Concrete Road,
Zip 40311–9721, Mailing Address: P.O. Box 232, Zip 40311–0232;
tel. 859/289–7181, (Includes JOHNSON–MATHERS NURSING HOME ) **A**1 9 10
18 **F**3 11 15 40 57 59 77 81 90 107 113 118 126 132 134 145 **P**1
Primary Contact: Barry A. Papania, Administrator
CFO: Wesley Berry, Chief Financial Officer
CMO: Osias Villaflor, M.D., Chief Medical Staff
CHR: Wendy Price, Manager Human Resources
Web address: www.johnsonmathers.org
**Control:** Other not–for–profit (including NFP Corporation) **Service:** General
Medical and Surgical

> **Staffed Beds:** 16 **Admissions:** 424 **Census:** 4 **Outpatient Visits:** 10318
> **Births:** 0 **Total Expense ($000):** 5881 **Payroll Expense ($000):** 2601
> **Personnel:** 78

### CARROLLTON—Carroll County

★ **CARROLL COUNTY MEMORIAL HOSPITAL (181310)**, 309 11th Street,
Zip 41008–1400; tel. 502/732–4321, (Nonreporting) **A**9 10 18 **S** Alliant
Management Services, Louisville, KY
Primary Contact: Kanute Rarey, Chief Executive Officer
CFO: Steve Eigel, Chief Financial Officer
CMO: Kathy Short, D.O., Family Practice
CHR: Kimberly Puckett, Manager Human Resources
CNO: Lisa Penick, R.N., Chief Nursing Officer
Web address: www.ccmhosp.com
**Control:** County–Government, nonfederal **Service:** General Medical and Surgical

> **Staffed Beds:** 25

### COLUMBIA—Adair County

☐ **WESTLAKE REGIONAL HOSPITAL (180149)**, 901 Westlake Drive,
Zip 42728–1149, Mailing Address: P.O. Box 1269, Zip 42728–1269;
tel. 270/384–4753 **A**1 9 10 **F**3 11 15 18 28 29 35 45 57 59 79 81 87 93 98
107 113 118 126 129 147 **P**6
Primary Contact: Timothy P. Menton, Interim Chief Executive Officer
CFO: Ken Doran, Interim Chief Financial Officer
CMO: Gary Partin, M.D., President Medical Staff
CHR: Nanette Kenyon, Director Human Resources
Web address: www.westlake–healthcare.org
**Control:** Hospital district or authority, Government, nonfederal **Service:** General
Medical and Surgical

> **Staffed Beds:** 77 **Admissions:** 1840 **Census:** 18 **Outpatient Visits:** 18926
> **Births:** 0 **Total Expense ($000):** 15720 **Payroll Expense ($000):** 7541
> **Personnel:** 234

### CORBIN—Whitley County

★ **BAPTIST REGIONAL MEDICAL CENTER (180080)**, 1 Trillium Way,
Zip 40701–8420; tel. 606/528–1212 **A**9 10 19 21 **F**1 3 4 5 11 12 13 15 18
20 29 30 31 32 34 35 38 40 45 47 48 49 53 54 57 59 64 68 70 73 76 78
79 81 85 86 89 90 93 98 99 100 101 102 103 104 105 107 108 110 111
113 114 117 118 125 129 131 132 134 144 145 146 147 **S** Baptist
Healthcare System, Louisville, KY
Primary Contact: Larry Gray, President and Chief Executive Officer
CIO: Jeff Thurmond, Vice President Information Systems
CHR: Tim Perry, Director Human Resources
CNO: Anthony Powers, Vice President Patient Care Services
Web address: www.baptistregional.com
**Control:** Other not–for–profit (including NFP Corporation) **Service:** General
Medical and Surgical

> **Staffed Beds:** 273 **Admissions:** 10185 **Census:** 140 **Outpatient Visits:**
> 94520 **Births:** 824 **Total Expense ($000):** 117074 **Payroll Expense ($000):**
> 50276 **Personnel:** 1021

**OAK TREE HOSPITAL (182006)**, One Trillium Way, Lower Level, Zip 40701;
tel. 606/523–5150 **A**9 10 21 **F**1 3 29 30 39 50 60 70 80 129 147
Primary Contact: R. Alan Coppock, FACHE, President and Chief Executive Officer
CFO: Jeff Hamlin, Director Finance
CMO: Bill Durham, M.D., Chief Medical Officer
CIO: Jackie Lucas, Vice President
CHR: Janice Caldwell, Director Human Resources
Web address: www.oaktreecorbin.com
**Control:** Other not–for–profit (including NFP Corporation) **Service:** Long–Term
Acute Care hospital

**Staffed Beds:** 32 **Admissions:** 372 **Census:** 26 **Outpatient Visits:** 0 **Births:**
0 **Total Expense ($000):** 11764 **Payroll Expense ($000):** 4353 **Personnel:**
83

### COVINGTON—Kenton County

**NORTHKEY COMMUNITY CARE (184006)**, 502 Farrell Drive,
Zip 41011–3799, Mailing Address: P.O. Box 2680, Zip 41012–2680;
tel. 859/578–3200, (Nonreporting) **A**9 10
Primary Contact: Owen Nichols, PsyD, President and Chief Executive Officer
CFO: John Metzger, Controller
Web address: www.northkey.org
**Control:** Other not–for–profit (including NFP Corporation) **Service:** Children's
hospital psychiatric

**Staffed Beds:** 25

**ST. ELIZABETH MEDICAL CENTER–NORTH** See St. Elizabeth Covington

### CYNTHIANA—Harrison County

**HARRISON MEMORIAL HOSPITAL (180079)**, 1210 KY Highway 36E,
Zip 41031–7498; tel. 859/234–2300 **A**1 9 10 **F**3 11 13 15 18 20 28 29 30
31 34 35 36 39 40 44 45 47 49 50 53 57 59 61 64 68 69 70 74 75 76 77
78 79 81 82 85 86 87 89 93 97 107 108 111 114 117 118 128 129 130
131 132 134 145 146 147 **P**6
Primary Contact: Sheila Currans, Chief Executive Officer
CFO: James Spears, Chief Financial Officer
CIO: Martha Sullivan, Chief Information Officer
CHR: Rebecca Jenkins, Director Human Resources Management
CNO: Wendy Reeder, R.N., Chief Nursing Officer
Web address: www.harrisonmemhosp.com
**Control:** Other not–for–profit (including NFP Corporation) **Service:** General
Medical and Surgical

**Staffed Beds:** 49 **Admissions:** 1849 **Census:** 17 **Outpatient Visits:** 51005
**Births:** 253 **Total Expense ($000):** 29545 **Payroll Expense ($000):** 14252
**Personnel:** 279

### DANVILLE—Boyle County

**EPHRAIM MCDOWELL REGIONAL MEDICAL CENTER (180048)**, 217 South
Third Street, Zip 40422–9983; tel. 859/239–1000, (Total facility includes 18
beds in nursing home–type unit) **A**1 5 9 10 19 **F**3 8 10 11 13 15 17 18 20 22
29 30 31 32 34 35 40 43 45 49 51 53 56 57 59 60 64 65 66 70 73 75
76 77 78 79 81 82 85 87 89 93 96 97 98 100 101 102 103 107 108 110
111 113 116 117 118 124 126 127 128 129 131 143 145 146 147 **P**5
Primary Contact: Vicki A. Darnell, President and Chief Executive Officer
CFO: William R. Snapp, III, Vice President Finance and Chief Financial Officer
CMO: Gary Ahnquist, M.D., President Medical Staff
CIO: Allen Levi, Director Information Services
CHR: Carl Metz, Vice President Human Resources
CNO: Sally Davenport, Vice President of Patient Care Services & CNO
Web address: www.emrmc.org
**Control:** Other not–for–profit (including NFP Corporation) **Service:** General
Medical and Surgical

**Staffed Beds:** 153 **Admissions:** 7490 **Census:** 99 **Outpatient Visits:** 122067
**Births:** 668 **Total Expense ($000):** 111150 **Payroll Expense ($000):** 45313
**Personnel:** 983

### EDGEWOOD—Kenton County

**HEALTHSOUTH NORTHERN KENTUCKY REHABILITATION HOSPITAL
(183027)**, 201 Medical Village Drive, Zip 41017–3407; tel. 859/341–2044 **A**1
9 10 **F**64 79 82 93 94 **P**6 **S** HEALTHSOUTH Corporation, Birmingham, AL
Primary Contact: Richard R. Evens, Chief Executive Officer
CFO: Lisa McGue, Controller
CMO: Neal Moser, M.D., Medical Director
CHR: Bridgette Keith, Director Human Resources
CNO: Scott Toney, R.N., Chief Nursing Officer
Web address: www.healthsouthkentucky.com
**Control:** Partnership, Investor–owned, for–profit **Service:** Rehabilitation

**Staffed Beds:** 40 **Admissions:** 996 **Census:** 32 **Outpatient Visits:** 4948
**Births:** 0

**ST. ELIZABETH EDGEWOOD (180035)**, 1 Medical Village Drive,
Zip 41017–3403; tel. 859/301–2000, (Includes ST. ELIZABETH COVINGTON,
1500 James Simpson Jr. Way, Covington, Zip 41014–1585; tel. 859/655–8800)
**A**1 2 3 5 9 10 **F**3 5 8 11 12 13 14 15 17 18 20 22 24 26 28 29 30 31 34 35
36 38 40 44 45 46 47 48 49 50 55 57 58 59 60 63 64 68 70 71 73 74 75
76 77 78 79 80 81 82 83 84 85 86 89 92 93 97 98 102 103 104 107 108
109 110 111 112 113 114 118 119 120 121 122 123 125 128
129 130 131 134 144 145 146 147 **P**6 7 **S** St. Elizabeth Healthcare,
Edgewood, KY
Primary Contact: John S. Dubis, FACHE, President and Chief Executive Officer
COO: John S. Dubis, FACHE, President and Chief Executive Officer
CFO: Garren Colvin, Senior Vice President and Chief Financial Officer
CMO: Karl Schmitt, M.D., Chief of Staff
CIO: Alex Rodriguez, Vice President and Chief Information Officer
CHR: Martin Oscadal, Vice President Human Resources
Web address: www.stelizabeth.com
**Control:** Church–operated, Nongovernment, not–for profit **Service:** General
Medical and Surgical

**Staffed Beds:** 510 **Admissions:** 29308 **Census:** 358 **Outpatient Visits:**
810013 **Births:** 3987 **Total Expense ($000):** 566612 **Payroll Expense
($000):** 230087 **Personnel:** 3635

**ST. ELIZABETH HEALTHCARE–EDGEWOOD** See St. Elizabeth Edgewood

### ELIZABETHTOWN—Hardin County

**HARDIN MEMORIAL HOSPITAL (180012)**, 913 North Dixie Avenue, Zip 42701;
tel. 270/737–1212, (Total facility includes 15 beds in nursing home–type unit) **A**1
2 5 9 10 19 **F**3 8 11 12 13 15 17 18 20 22 24 28 29 30 31 32 34 35 37 39
40 44 45 48 49 50 51 52 54 57 58 59 64 68 70 71 73 74 75 76 77 78 79
80 81 82 84 85 86 87 89 93 94 96 98 102 107 108 110 111 113 114 116
117 118 119 120 123 125 127 128 129 130 131 133 134 143 145 146 147
**S** Baptist Healthcare System, Louisville, KY
Primary Contact: Dennis B. Johnson, Chief Executive Officer
COO: Diane Logsdon, Vice President Planning and Development
CFO: Elmer Cummings, Vice President and Chief Financial Officer
CMO: Stephen Toadvine, M.D., Chief Medical Officer
CIO: Mark Brookman, Director Information Technology
CHR: Ann Kelley, Director Human Resources
Web address: www.hmh.net
**Control:** County–Government, nonfederal **Service:** General Medical and Surgical

**Staffed Beds:** 268 **Admissions:** 13025 **Census:** 160 **Outpatient Visits:**
289484 **Births:** 1551 **Total Expense ($000):** 182493 **Payroll Expense
($000):** 74525 **Personnel:** 1577

**HEALTHSOUTH LAKEVIEW REHABILITATION HOSPITAL (183028)**, 134
Heartland Drive, Zip 42701–2778; tel. 270/769–3100, (Nonreporting) **A**1 9 10
**S** HEALTHSOUTH Corporation, Birmingham, AL
Primary Contact: Lori Jarboe, Chief Executive Officer
CFO: Scott Hart, Controller
CMO: Vickie Lowe, M.D., Medical Director
CHR: Janet Morris, Director Human Resources
Web address: www.healthsouthlakeview.com
**Control:** Corporation, Investor–owned, for–profit **Service:** Rehabilitation

**Staffed Beds:** 40

### FLEMINGSBURG—Fleming County

**FLEMING COUNTY HOSPITAL (180053)**, 55 Foundation Drive,
Zip 41041–9815, Mailing Address: P.O. Box 388, Zip 41041–0388;
tel. 606/849–5000 **A**1 9 10 **F**15 29 31 34 35 67 68 70 79 81 87 93
107 108 110 111 113 117 118 128 129 132 134 145 **P**6 **S** QHR,
Brentwood, TN
Primary Contact: David M. Faulkner, Chief Executive Officer
CFO: David Pike, Interim Chief Financial Officer
CMO: William Bacon, M.D., Chief of Staff
CIO: Don Daugherty, Director Information Systems
CHR: Marsha Mitchell, Director Human Resources
CNO: Lynda Skaggs, Chief Nursing Officer
Web address: www.flemingcountyhospital.org
**Control:** Other not–for–profit (including NFP Corporation) **Service:** General
Medical and Surgical

**Staffed Beds:** 52 **Admissions:** 1473 **Census:** 18 **Outpatient Visits:** 27276
**Births:** 0 **Total Expense ($000):** 21393 **Payroll Expense ($000):** 10121
**Personnel:** 196

### FLORENCE—Boone County

**GATEWAY REHABILITATION HOSPITAL (183030)**, 5940 Merchant Street,
Zip 41042; tel. 859/426–2400, (Nonreporting) **A**1 9 10
Primary Contact: Jim Burcham, Chief Executive Officer
Web address: www.gatewayflorence.com/
**Control:** Corporation, Investor–owned, for–profit **Service:** Rehabilitation

**Staffed Beds:** 40

---

**Hospital, Medicare Provider Number, Address, Telephone, Approval, Facility, and Physician Codes, Health Care System**

★ American Hospital Association (AHA) membership
□ The Joint Commission accreditation
◇ DNV Healthcare Inc. accreditation
○ American Osteopathic Association (AOA) accreditation
△ Commission on Accreditation of Rehabilitation Facilities (CARF) accreditation

☐ **ST. ELIZABETH FLORENCE (180045)**, 4900 Houston Road, Zip 41042–4824; tel. 859/212–5200, (Total facility includes 16 beds in nursing home–type unit) **A**1 10 **F**3 11 12 13 15 18 20 28 29 30 31 32 34 35 36 40 44 45 47 48 49 50 55 56 57 59 60 64 68 71 73 74 75 76 77 78 79 80 81 82 85 86 87 92 93 97 98 102 107 110 111 113 114 117 118 127 128 129 131 134 143 145 146 **P**6 7 **S** St. Elizabeth Healthcare, Edgewood, KY
Primary Contact: Chris Carle, Senior Vice President and Chief Operating Officer
COO: Chris Carle, Senior Vice President and Chief Operating Officer
CFO: Garren Colvin, Senior Vice President Finance and Chief Financial Officer
CMO: George Hall, M.D., Vice President Medical Affairs
CIO: Alex Rodriguez, Vice President and Chief Information Officer
CHR: Martin Oscadal, Senior Vice President Human Resources
Web address: www.stelizabeth.com
**Control:** Church–operated, Nongovernment, not–for profit **Service:** General Medical and Surgical

**Staffed Beds:** 170 **Admissions:** 9125 **Census:** 114 **Outpatient Visits:** 161716 **Births:** 473 **Total Expense ($000):** 98324 **Payroll Expense ($000):** 45824 **Personnel:** 674

**ST. ELIZABETH HEALTHCARE FLORENCE** See St. Elizabeth Florence

### FORT CAMPBELL—Montgomery County

⊠ **COLONEL FLORENCE A. BLANCHFIELD ARMY COMMUNITY HOSPITAL**, 650 Joel Drive, Zip 42223; tel. 270/798–8040, (Nonreporting) **A**1 3 5 **S** Department of the Army, Office of the Surgeon General, Falls Church, VA
Primary Contact: Colonel Paul Cordts, Commander
CMO: Lieutenant Colonel Michael Place, M.D., Deputy Commander Clinical Services
CIO: Gloria K. Davis, Chief Information Management
CHR: Major Travis Burchett, Troop Commander Human Resources
Web address: www.campbell.amedd.army.mil/
**Control:** Army, Government, federal **Service:** General Medical and Surgical

**Staffed Beds:** 66

### FORT KNOX—Hardin County

⊠ **IRELAND ARMY COMMUNITY HOSPITAL**, 289 Ireland Avenue, Zip 40121–5111; tel. 502/624–9333, (Nonreporting) **A**1 5 9 **S** Department of the Army, Office of the Surgeon General, Falls Church, VA
Primary Contact: Colonel Cornelius C. Maher, Commander
Web address: www.iach.knox.amedd.army.mil/
**Control:** Army, Government, federal **Service:** General Medical and Surgical

**Staffed Beds:** 33

### FORT THOMAS—Campbell County

☐ **CARDINAL HILL SPECIALTY HOSPITAL (182004)**, 85 North Grand Avenue, Zip 41075; tel. 859/572–3880, (Nonreporting) **A**1 9 10 **S** Cardinal Hill Healthcare System, Lexington, KY
Primary Contact: Janice Bauer, Administrator
**Control:** Other not–for–profit (including NFP Corporation) **Service:** Long–Term Acute Care hospital

**Staffed Beds:** 32

☐ **ST. ELIZABETH FORT THOMAS (180001)**, 85 North Grand Avenue, Zip 41075–1796; tel. 859/572–3100, (Total facility includes 26 beds in nursing home–type unit) **A**1 2 10 **F**3 4 11 12 15 17 18 20 28 29 30 31 34 35 36 40 44 45 47 48 49 50 55 56 57 59 60 61 64 68 70 71 74 75 77 78 79 80 81 82 85 86 87 92 93 97 107 108 110 111 113 114 117 118 120 122 123 125 127 128 129 131 134 145 146 **P**6 7 **S** St. Elizabeth Healthcare, Edgewood, KY
Primary Contact: Thomas Saalfeld, Senior Vice President and Chief Operating Officer
COO: Thomas Saalfeld, Senior Vice President and Chief Operating Officer
CFO: Garren Colvin, Senior Vice President and Chief Financial Officer
CMO: George Hall, M.D., Vice President Medical Affairs
CIO: Alex Rodriguez, Vice President and Chief Information Officer
CHR: Martin Oscadal, Senior Vice President Human Resources
Web address: www.stelizabeth.com
**Control:** Church–operated, Nongovernment, not–for profit **Service:** General Medical and Surgical

**Staffed Beds:** 194 **Admissions:** 7612 **Census:** 107 **Outpatient Visits:** 124331 **Births:** 0 **Total Expense ($000):** 85495 **Payroll Expense ($000):** 40744 **Personnel:** 626

**ST. ELIZABETH HEALTHCARE FORT THOMAS** See St. Elizabeth Fort Thomas

### FRANKFORT—Franklin County

⊠ **FRANKFORT REGIONAL MEDICAL CENTER (180127)**, 299 King's Daughters Drive, Zip 40601–4186; tel. 502/875–5240 **A**1 9 10 19 **F**3 13 15 17 18 20 22 28 29 30 34 40 45 57 70 72 73 75 76 77 81 82 89 93 107 111 118 123 125 128 129 132 144 145 146 147 **S** HCA, Nashville, TN
Primary Contact: Chip Peal, Chief Executive Officer
CFO: Osman Gruhonjic, Chief Financial Officer
CMO: Willis P. McKee, Jr., M.D., Chief Medical Officer
CIO: Craig Willard, Director Information Technology and Systems
CHR: Bev Young, Director Human Resources
Web address: www.frankfortregional.com
**Control:** Corporation, Investor–owned, for–profit **Service:** Long–Term Acute Care hospital

**Staffed Beds:** 134 **Admissions:** 4418 **Census:** 46 **Outpatient Visits:** 84786 **Births:** 761 **Total Expense ($000):** 58812 **Payroll Expense ($000):** 26531 **Personnel:** 419

### FRANKLIN—Simpson County

☐ **MEDICAL CENTER AT FRANKLIN (181318)**, 1100 Brookhaven Road, Zip 42134–2746; tel. 270/598–4800 **A**1 9 10 18 **F**3 15 28 29 30 32 34 35 40 46 57 59 64 68 75 77 81 86 87 93 107 111 113 118 126 129 132 134 145 147 **S** Commonwealth Health Corporation, Bowling Green, KY
Primary Contact: Clara M. Sumner, Senior Vice President and Chief Executive Officer
CFO: Ronald G. Sowell, Executive Vice President
CIO: Jean Cherry, Executive Vice President
Web address: www.themedicalcenterfranklin.org
**Control:** Other not–for–profit (including NFP Corporation) **Service:** General Medical and Surgical

**Staffed Beds:** 25 **Admissions:** 1158 **Census:** 16 **Outpatient Visits:** 19197 **Births:** 0 **Personnel:** 116

### FULTON—Fulton County

⊠ **PARKWAY REGIONAL HOSPITAL (180117)**, 2000 Holiday Lane, Zip 42041–8468; tel. 270/472–2522, (Nonreporting) **A**1 9 10 **S** Community Health Systems, Inc., Franklin, TN
Primary Contact: Dana Lawrence, Interim Chief Executive Officer
CFO: Dana Lawrence, Chief Financial Officer
CMO: F. Gregory Cox, M.D., Chief of Staff
CHR: Janice Bone, Director Human Resources
Web address: www.parkwayregionalhospital.com
**Control:** Corporation, Investor–owned, for–profit **Service:** General Medical and Surgical

**Staffed Beds:** 70

### GEORGETOWN—Scott County

⊠ **GEORGETOWN COMMUNITY HOSPITAL (180101)**, 1140 Lexington Road, Zip 40324–9362; tel. 502/868–1100 **A**1 5 9 10 **F**3 12 13 15 18 28 29 30 31 34 35 40 50 56 57 59 66 70 74 75 76 77 78 79 81 85 93 107 108 109 110 111 113 114 118 128 129 130 131 132 134 144 145 146 **S** LifePoint Hospitals, Inc., Brentwood, TN
Primary Contact: Jerry C. Dooley, Chief Executive Officer
CFO: Patrick C. Bolander, Chief Financial Officer
CMO: Brian Allen, M.D., President Medical Staff
CHR: Marianne Slonina, Director Human Resources
Web address: www.georgetowncommunityhospital.com
**Control:** Corporation, Investor–owned, for–profit **Service:** General Medical and Surgical

**Staffed Beds:** 58 **Admissions:** 2024 **Census:** 17 **Outpatient Visits:** 59184 **Births:** 130 **Total Expense ($000):** 34771 **Payroll Expense ($000):** 13698 **Personnel:** 265

### GLASGOW—Barren County

⊠ **T. J. SAMSON COMMUNITY HOSPITAL (180017)**, 1301 North Race Street, Zip 42141–3483; tel. 270/651–4444, (Total facility includes 16 beds in nursing home–type unit) **A**1 3 5 9 10 19 **F**2 3 11 13 15 18 20 22 24 28 29 30 31 34 40 45 57 59 60 62 63 64 70 71 72 74 75 77 78 79 81 82 85 86 87 93 97 107 110 111 112 113 118 123 127 128 129 131 134 145 147 **P**5
Primary Contact: Bill Kindred, Chief Executive Officer
COO: Larry Morgan, Controller
CFO: Anthony G. Sudduth, CPA, Chief Financial Officer
CMO: Michael Shadowen, M.D., Chief of Staff
CIO: Debbie Caudel–Logsdon, Director Information System
CHR: LaDonna Rogers, Director Human Resources
Web address: www.tjsamson.org
**Control:** Other not–for–profit (including NFP Corporation) **Service:** General Medical and Surgical

**Staffed Beds:** 196 **Admissions:** 6403 **Census:** 62 **Outpatient Visits:** 103265 **Births:** 1072 **Total Expense ($000):** 107596 **Payroll Expense ($000):** 46851 **Personnel:** 927

## GREENSBURG—Green County

**JANE TODD CRAWFORD HOSPITAL (181325)**, 202–206 Milby Street, Zip 42743–1100, Mailing Address: P.O. Box 220, Zip 42743–0220; tel. 270/932–4211, (Nonreporting) **A**9 10 18
Primary Contact: Rex A. Tungate, Administrator
CMO: James G. Bland, M.D., Chief of Staff
**Control:** County–Government, nonfederal **Service:** General Medical and Surgical

**Staffed Beds:** 45

## GREENVILLE—Muhlenberg County

✖ **MUHLENBERG COMMUNITY HOSPITAL (180004)**, 440 Hopkinsville Street, Zip 42345–1172, Mailing Address: P.O. Box 387, Zip 42345–0387; tel. 270/338–8000, (Total facility includes 45 beds in nursing home–type unit) **A**1 9 10 **F**3 7 8 11 13 15 28 29 30 34 35 40 50 56 57 59 62 64 65 68 70 75 76 77 79 81 82 85 86 87 89 93 94 107 110 111 113 118 127 128 129 130 134 145 147 **P**6 **S** Alliant Management Services, Louisville, KY
Primary Contact: John Countzler, Chief Executive Officer
CFO: Joseph Swab, Chief Financial Officer
CMO: Vincent P. Genovese, M.D., President Medical Staff
CIO: Alan Trail, Director Information Systems
CHR: Lisa R. Hope, Director Human Resources
CNO: Kathy Mitchell, Chief Nursing Officer
Web address: www.mchky.org
**Control:** Other not–for–profit (including NFP Corporation) **Service:** General Medical and Surgical

**Staffed Beds:** 105 **Admissions:** 2328 **Census:** 57 **Outpatient Visits:** 63635 **Births:** 169 **Total Expense ($000):** 32301 **Payroll Expense ($000):** 14661 **Personnel:** 420

## HARDINSBURG—Breckinridge County

✖ **BRECKINRIDGE MEMORIAL HOSPITAL (181319)**, 1011 Old Highway 60, Zip 40143–2597; tel. 270/756–7000, (Total facility includes 18 beds in nursing home–type unit) **A**1 9 10 18 **F**3 11 15 18 28 29 30 34 35 40 48 49 50 53 56 57 59 62 63 64 65 68 75 77 79 81 82 85 87 93 100 107 110 111 118 126 128 129 131 132 133 134 142 145 **P**6 **S** Alliant Management Services, Louisville, KY
Primary Contact: Michael W. Cooper, Chief Executive Officer
CMO: Brian O'Donoghue, M.D., Chief Medical Officer
CIO: Virginia D. Bradley, Chief Information Officer
CHR: Clara Cordelia Hall, Chief Human Resources Officer
Web address: www.breckhealth.org
**Control:** Other not–for–profit (including NFP Corporation) **Service:** General Medical and Surgical

**Staffed Beds:** 43 **Admissions:** 1169 **Census:** 33 **Outpatient Visits:** 33956 **Total Expense ($000):** 17138 **Payroll Expense ($000):** 7036 **Personnel:** 201

## HARLAN—Harlan County

☐ **HARLAN ARH HOSPITAL (180050)**, 81 Ball Park Road, Zip 40831–1792; tel. 606/573–8100 **A**1 9 10 19 **F**3 11 13 15 29 30 32 34 35 40 50 54 57 59 62 64 70 75 76 77 78 79 81 82 85 86 87 89 90 93 97 98 102 103 107 108 111 114 117 118 126 128 129 131 145 146 **S** Appalachian Regional Healthcare, Inc., Lexington, KY
Primary Contact: Dan Stone, Community Chief Executive Officer
CFO: Brad Burkhart, Assistant Administrator
CHR: Sabra Howard, Manager Human Resources
Web address: www.arh.org
**Control:** Other not–for–profit (including NFP Corporation) **Service:** General Medical and Surgical

**Staffed Beds:** 137 **Admissions:** 5350 **Census:** 69 **Outpatient Visits:** 66889 **Births:** 271 **Total Expense ($000):** 50513 **Payroll Expense ($000):** 17457

## HARRODSBURG—Mercer County

✖ **JAMES B. HAGGIN MEMORIAL HOSPITAL (181302)**, 464 Linden Avenue, Zip 40330–1862; tel. 859/734–5441, (Nonreporting) **A**1 5 9 10 18 **S** Alliant Management Services, Louisville, KY
Primary Contact: Victoria L. Reed, R.N., FACHE, Chief Executive Officer
CFO: Tony Patterson, Chief Financial Officer
Web address: www.hagginhosp.org
**Control:** Other not–for–profit (including NFP Corporation) **Service:** General Medical and Surgical

**Staffed Beds:** 25

## HARTFORD—Ohio County

✖ **OHIO COUNTY HOSPITAL (181323)**, 1211 Main Street, Zip 42347–1619; tel. 270/298–7411, (Nonreporting) **A**1 9 10 18 **S** QHR, Brentwood, TN
Primary Contact: Blaine Pieper, Chief Executive Officer
CFO: John Tichenor, Chief Financial Officer
CMO: Janna Pathi, M.D., Chief Medical Officer
CHR: Sue Wydick, Director Human Resources
Web address: www.ohiocountyhospital.com
**Control:** Other not–for–profit (including NFP Corporation) **Service:** General Medical and Surgical

**Staffed Beds:** 25

## HAZARD—Perry County

☐ **HAZARD ARH REGIONAL MEDICAL CENTER (180029)**, 100 Medical Center Drive, Zip 41701–1000; tel. 606/439–6600, (Nonreporting) **A**1 2 3 5 9 10 19 **S** Appalachian Regional Healthcare, Inc., Lexington, KY
Primary Contact: Donald R. Fields, Senior Community Chief Executive Officer
COO: Donald R. Fields, Senior Community Chief Executive Officer
CMO: J. D. Miller, M.D., Chief Medical Officer
CIO: Jeff Brady, Director Information Systems
CHR: Sheila Cornett, Manager Human Resources
Web address: www.arh.org
**Control:** Other not–for–profit (including NFP Corporation) **Service:** General Medical and Surgical

**Staffed Beds:** 308

## HENDERSON—Henderson County

☐ **METHODIST HOSPITAL (180056)**, 1305 North Elm Street, Zip 42420–2775, Mailing Address: P.O. Box 48, Zip 42420–0048; tel. 270/827–7700 **A**1 9 10 13 **F**3 7 11 13 15 18 20 29 30 31 34 35 40 45 46 47 49 50 51 53 54 57 58 59 64 66 68 70 72 74 75 76 77 78 79 81 82 85 86 87 92 93 98 102 107 108 110 111 113 115 118 125 126 128 131 134 145 146 147 **P**8
Primary Contact: Bruce D. Begley, Executive Director
COO: Wayne Meriwether, Chief Operating Officer
CFO: Gregory P. Hebbeler, Chief Financial Officer
CMO: Gerald Rightmyer, M.D., Chief of Staff
CIO: Gregory P. Hebbeler, Chief Financial Officer
CHR: Marty Mattingly, Vice President Human Resources
Web address: www.methodisthospital.net
**Control:** Church–operated, Nongovernment, not–for profit **Service:** General Medical and Surgical

**Staffed Beds:** 192 **Admissions:** 5435 **Census:** 72 **Outpatient Visits:** 254883 **Births:** 675 **Total Expense ($000):** 91889 **Payroll Expense ($000):** 36336 **Personnel:** 1009

## HOPKINSVILLE—Christian County

☐ **CUMBERLAND HALL HOSPITAL (184014)**, 210 West 17th Street, Zip 42240–1912; tel. 270/886–1919 **A**1 9 10 **F**98 106 142 **S** Universal Health Services, Inc., King of Prussia, PA
Primary Contact: James Spruyt, Chief Executive Officer
COO: Lance Folske, Chief Operating Officer
CFO: Chris Jagoditz, Chief Financial Officer
CMO: Deepak Patel, M.D., Medical Director
CIO: Patricia Gray, Director Health Information Management
CHR: Tracy Thomas, Director Human Resources
CNO: Jackie Wurth, Director of Nursing
Web address: www.cumberlandhallhospital.com
**Control:** Corporation, Investor–owned, for–profit **Service:** Psychiatric

**Staffed Beds:** 64 **Admissions:** 1127 **Census:** 59 **Outpatient Visits:** 0 **Births:** 0 **Total Expense ($000):** 5842 **Payroll Expense ($000):** 4338 **Personnel:** 124

✖ **JENNIE STUART MEDICAL CENTER (180051)**, 320 West 18th Street, Zip 42241–2400, Mailing Address: P.O. Box 2400, Zip 42241–2400; tel. 270/887–0100, (Nonreporting) **A**1 9 10 **S** QHR, Brentwood, TN
Primary Contact: Eric A. Lee, President and Chief Executive Officer
CFO: Samuel L. Brown, CPA, Vice President Financial Services
CMO: Casey Covington, M.D., President Elect, Medical Staff
CIO: Jerry Houston, Director Information Systems
CHR: Austin Moss, Vice President Human Resources
Web address: www.jsmc.org
**Control:** Other not–for–profit (including NFP Corporation) **Service:** General Medical and Surgical

**Staffed Beds:** 139

---

**Hospital, Medicare Provider Number, Address, Telephone, Approval, Facility, and Physician Codes, Health Care System**

★ American Hospital Association (AHA) membership
☐ The Joint Commission accreditation
◇ DNV Healthcare Inc. accreditation
○ American Osteopathic Association (AOA) accreditation
△ Commission on Accreditation of Rehabilitation Facilities (CARF) accreditation

☐ **WESTERN STATE HOSPITAL (184002)**, Russellville Road, Zip 42240–3017, Mailing Address: P.O. Box 2200, Zip 42241–2200; tel. 270/889–6025 **A**1 10 **F**98 103 129 **P**5
Primary Contact: Stephen P. Wiggins, Director
CFO: Jessica Cates, Fiscal Manager
CMO: Nayyar Iqbal, M.D., Director Medical Staff
CIO: Valerie Majors, Director Information Services
CHR: James L. Hayes, Director Human Resources
**Control:** State–Government, nonfederal **Service:** Psychiatric

**Staffed Beds:** 207 **Admissions:** 1946 **Census:** 101 **Outpatient Visits:** 0
**Births:** 0 **Total Expense ($000):** 13943 **Payroll Expense ($000):** 9066
**Personnel:** 595

### HORSE CAVE—Hart County

★ **CAVERNA MEMORIAL HOSPITAL (181314)**, 1501 South Dixie Street, Zip 42749–1477; tel. 270/786–2191 **A**9 10 18 **F**3 15 34 40 57 59 64 70 81 85 89 107 111 113 118 126 127 132 134 **P**6 **S** Alliant Management Services, Louisville, KY
Primary Contact: Alan B. Alexander, Chief Executive Officer
CFO: Debra Riggs, Chief Financial Officer
CMO: Swaranjik K. Chani, M.D., Chief of Staff
CIO: Brad Lowe, Director Information Systems
CHR: Cathy Szabo, Director Human Resources
CNO: Vanessa Burd, R.N., Chief Nursing Officer
Web address: www.cavernahospital.com
**Control:** Other not–for–profit (including NFP Corporation) **Service:** General Medical and Surgical

**Staffed Beds:** 25 **Admissions:** 535 **Census:** 6 **Outpatient Visits:** 20305
**Births:** 0 **Total Expense ($000):** 10379 **Payroll Expense ($000):** 4829
**Personnel:** 117

### HYDEN—Leslie County

**MARY BRECKINRIDGE ARH HOSPITAL (181316)**, 130 Kate Ireland Drive, Zip 41749–0000, Mailing Address: P.O. Box 447–A, Zip 41749–0000; tel. 606/672–2901 **A**9 10 18 **F**3 11 15 29 40 42 45 46 47 49 57 62 64 65 66 81 83 90 91 93 107 113 114 118 126 129 132 134 145 146 **S** Appalachian Regional Healthcare, Inc., Lexington, KY
Primary Contact: Mallie S. Noble, Administrator
COO: Nathan W. Lee, Chief Executive Officer
CFO: Robert Besten, Chief Financial Officer
CMO: Roy Varghese, M.D., Chief of Staff
CIO: Frank Baker, Chief Information Officer
CHR: Beulah Couch, Director Human Resources
Web address: www.frontiernursing.org
**Control:** Other not–for–profit (including NFP Corporation) **Service:** General Medical and Surgical

**Staffed Beds:** 25 **Admissions:** 1029 **Census:** 10 **Outpatient Visits:** 11609
**Births:** 67 **Personnel:** 122

### IRVINE—Estill County

★ **MARCUM AND WALLACE MEMORIAL HOSPITAL (181301)**, 60 Mercy Court, Zip 40336–1331; tel. 606/723–2115 **A**9 10 18 **F**3 11 15 29 30 34 40 43 57 59 75 81 87 97 107 110 114 117 118 126 128 132 146 **P**6 **S** Catholic Health Partners, Cincinnati, OH
Primary Contact: Susan Starling, President and Chief Executive Officer
CFO: Della Deerfield, Vice President Finance
CMO: Mark Rukavina, M.D., Chief Medical Staff
CIO: Tracy Bryant, Coordinator Information Technology
CHR: Dana Stepp, Human Resources Officer
Web address: www.marcumandwallace.org
**Control:** Church–operated, Nongovernment, not–for profit **Service:** General Medical and Surgical

**Staffed Beds:** 25 **Admissions:** 842 **Census:** 8 **Outpatient Visits:** 63109
**Births:** 0 **Total Expense ($000):** 11876 **Payroll Expense ($000):** 6373
**Personnel:** 170

### JACKSON—Breathitt County

☒ **KENTUCKY RIVER MEDICAL CENTER (180139)**, 540 Jett Drive, Zip 41339–9620; tel. 606/666–6000, (Nonreporting) **A**1 9 10 20 **S** Community Health Systems, Inc., Franklin, TN
Primary Contact: William Chad French, Chief Executive Officer
CFO: Michael Ackley, Chief Financial Officer
CMO: Eunice Johnson, M.D., Chief Medical Staff
CIO: Diana Tyra, Director Health Information
CHR: Naomi Mitchell, Director Human Resources
Web address: www.kentuckyrivermc.com
**Control:** Corporation, Investor–owned, for–profit **Service:** General Medical and Surgical

**Staffed Beds:** 54

### LA GRANGE—Oldham County

★ ○ **BAPTIST HOSPITAL NORTHEAST (180138)**, 1025 New Moody Lane, Zip 40031–0559; tel. 502/222–5388, (Total facility includes 30 beds in nursing home–type unit) **A**3 5 9 10 11 **F**3 11 13 15 18 28 29 30 34 35 36 40 43 45 46 49 50 54 56 57 59 64 68 70 74 75 76 77 78 79 81 82 85 86 87 93 97 107 108 110 111 113 118 127 128 129 130 131 132 134 145 146 147 **P**6 **S** Baptist Healthcare System, Louisville, KY
Primary Contact: Chris Roty, President
CFO: Susanne Haynes, Executive Director Finance
CMO: Matt McDanald, M.D., Chief Medical Officer
CIO: Jackie Lucas, Vice President Information Systems
CHR: Jean Harden, Executive Director Human Resources
Web address: www.baptistnortheast.com
**Control:** Other not–for–profit (including NFP Corporation) **Service:** General Medical and Surgical

**Staffed Beds:** 108 **Admissions:** 3228 **Census:** 33 **Outpatient Visits:** 59110
**Births:** 539 **Total Expense ($000):** 46642 **Payroll Expense ($000):** 21380
**Personnel:** 301

### LEBANON—Marion County

☒ **SPRING VIEW HOSPITAL (180024)**, 320 Loretto Road, Zip 40033–1300; tel. 270/692–3161 **A**1 9 10 **F**3 11 13 15 28 29 30 34 35 40 45 48 49 50 51 57 59 64 68 70 75 76 77 79 81 85 86 87 90 92 93 107 108 110 111 113 117 118 129 130 132 134 145 146 147 **S** LifePoint Hospitals, Inc., Brentwood, TN
Primary Contact: Ruth A. McDaniel, Chief Executive Officer
CFO: Denise Thomas, Chief Financial Officer
CIO: Douglas Bland, Manager Information Services
CHR: Ann Dabney, Manager Human Resources
CNO: Kathleen Ferriell, Chief Nursing Officer
Web address: www.springviewhospital.com
**Control:** Corporation, Investor–owned, for–profit **Service:** General Medical and Surgical

**Staffed Beds:** 60 **Admissions:** 1734 **Census:** 16 **Outpatient Visits:** 42120
**Births:** 361 **Total Expense ($000):** 22860 **Payroll Expense ($000):** 9572
**Personnel:** 232

### LEITCHFIELD—Grayson County

☒ **TWIN LAKES REGIONAL MEDICAL CENTER (180070)**, 910 Wallace Avenue, Zip 42754–1499; tel. 270/259–9400 **A**1 9 10 **F**3 11 13 15 28 29 30 31 34 40 53 57 59 68 70 76 78 79 81 82 85 86 87 89 93 107 108 110 111 114 117 118 128 129 130 131 132 134 143 145 147 **P**6 **S** Alliant Management Services, Louisville, KY
Primary Contact: Stephen L. Meredith, Chief Executive Officer
COO: Deneace Clemons, Chief Operating Officer
CFO: Scott Arndell, Chief Financial Officer
CMO: John Evans, M.D., Chief Medical Officer
CIO: Mandy Bryant, Chief Information Officer
CHR: Mandi Filburn, Director Human Resources
Web address: www.tlrmc.com
**Control:** Other not–for–profit (including NFP Corporation) **Service:** General Medical and Surgical

**Staffed Beds:** 75 **Admissions:** 2432 **Census:** 26 **Outpatient Visits:** 72611
**Births:** 340 **Total Expense ($000):** 31548 **Payroll Expense ($000):** 12000
**Personnel:** 314

### LEXINGTON—Fayette County

★ △ **CARDINAL HILL REHABILITATION HOSPITAL (183026)**, 2050 Versailles Road, Zip 40504–1405; tel. 859/254–5701 **A**3 5 7 9 10 **F**2 3 9 11 29 30 32 34 35 38 50 53 56 57 58 59 62 64 65 68 74 75 79 82 86 87 90 91 92 93 94 95 96 127 129 130 131 133 134 142 145 146 147 **S** Cardinal Hill Healthcare System, Lexington, KY
Primary Contact: Gary Payne, Chief Executive Officer
COO: Beth Monarch, Executive Vice President and Chief Operating Officer
CFO: Marty Lautner, Vice President Finance and Chief Financial Officer
CMO: William Lester, M.D., Vice President Medical Affairs
CIO: LouAnn Hydor, Director Information Integrity Management
CHR: Tracy Murford, Director Human Resources
Web address: www.cardinalhill.org
**Control:** Other not–for–profit (including NFP Corporation) **Service:** Rehabilitation

**Staffed Beds:** 108 **Admissions:** 2088 **Census:** 86 **Outpatient Visits:** 54163
**Births:** 0 **Total Expense ($000):** 50425 **Payroll Expense ($000):** 29419
**Personnel:** 557

⊞ **CENTRAL BAPTIST HOSPITAL (180103)**, 1740 Nicholasville Road, Zip 40503–1499; tel. 859/260–6100 **A**1 2 9 10 **F**3 11 12 13 15 17 18 20 22 24 26 28 29 30 31 34 35 36 40 44 45 49 53 54 55 57 58 59 60 62 63 64 68 70 72 74 75 76 77 78 79 81 83 84 85 86 87 89 93 97 107 108 110 111 112 113 114 116 117 118 119 120 123 125 128 129 130 131 134 143 145 146 147 **P**5 **S** Baptist Healthcare System, Louisville, KY
Primary Contact: William G. Sisson, President
COO: Karen S. Hill, R.N., Chief Operating Officer and Chief Nursing Officer
CFO: Bobbie L. Prather, Chief Financial Officer
CMO: Preston Nunelley, M.D., Chief Medical Officer
CIO: Lisa Fluty, Director Information Services
CHR: Lynette Walker, R.N., Executive Director Human Resources
Web address: www.centralbap.com
**Control:** Other not–for–profit (including NFP Corporation) **Service:** General Medical and Surgical

**Staffed Beds:** 344 **Admissions:** 18198 **Census:** 228 **Outpatient Visits:** 218928 **Births:** 3804 **Total Expense ($000):** 352835 **Payroll Expense ($000):** 128143 **Personnel:** 1983

★ **CONTINUING CARE HOSPITAL (182002)**, 150 North Eagle Creek Drive, 5th Floor, Zip 40509; tel. 859/967–5744, (Nonreporting) **A**9 10 **S** Catholic Health Initiatives, Englewood, CO
Primary Contact: Tonja Williams, MSN, R.N., President and Chief Executive Officer
CMO: Michael Miedler, M.D., Chief Medical Officer
CNO: Regina Masters, R.N., Director of Nursing
**Control:** Church–operated, Nongovernment, not–for profit **Service:** Long–Term Acute Care hospital

**Staffed Beds:** 45

☐ **EASTERN STATE HOSPITAL (184004)**, 627 West Fourth Street, Zip 40508–1294; tel. 859/246–7000, (Nonreporting) **A**1 5 9 10
Primary Contact: Shannon Ware, President and Chief Executive Officer
COO: Susan M. Griffith, Chief Operations Officer
CFO: Tambara Nalle, Chief Financial Officer
CMO: Scott A. Haas, M.D., Chief Medical Officer
CIO: Bud Stone, Director Information Systems
CHR: Jerry Kersey, Director Employee Relations
CNO: Kristan Mowder, Director Administration and Patient Care Services
Web address: www.bluegrass.org
**Control:** State–Government, nonfederal **Service:** Psychiatric

**Staffed Beds:** 197

**FEDERAL MEDICAL CENTER**, 3301 Leestown Road, Zip 40511–8799; tel. 859/255–6812, (Nonreporting)
Primary Contact: Stephen DeWalt, Warden
CFO: Mike Kinsel, Controller
CMO: Michael Growse, M.D., Clinical Director
**Control:** Department of Justice, Government, federal **Service:** Hospital unit of an institution (prison hospital, college infimary, etc.)

**Staffed Beds:** 22

☐ **RIDGE BEHAVIORAL HEALTH SYSTEM (184009)**, 3050 Rio Dosa Drive, Zip 40509–9990; tel. 859/269–2325, (Nonreporting) **A**1 3 5 9 10 **S** Universal Health Services, Inc., King of Prussia, PA
Primary Contact: Nina W. Eisner, Chief Executive Officer and Managing Director
CFO: Richard McDowell, Chief Financial Officer
CMO: Michael Rieser, M.D., Medical Director
CHR: Samantha Castle, Director Human Resources and Performance Improvement
CNO: Georgia Swank, Chief Nursing Officer
Web address: www.ridgebhs.com
**Control:** Corporation, Investor–owned, for–profit **Service:** Psychiatric

**Staffed Beds:** 110

⊞ **SAINT JOSEPH EAST (180143)**, 150 North Eagle Creek Drive, Zip 40509–1807; tel. 859/967–5000, (Nonreporting) **A**1 5 9 10 **S** Catholic Health Initiatives, Englewood, CO
Primary Contact: Eric Gilliam, Administrator
COO: Christine Mays, R.N., Chief Operating Officer and Chief Nurse Executive
CFO: Melinda S. Evans, Vice President Finance
CIO: Janie Fergus, Director and Chief Information Officer
CHR: Edward Carthew, Chief Human Resources Officer
Web address: www.sjhlex.org
**Control:** Church–operated, Nongovernment, not–for profit **Service:** General Medical and Surgical

**Staffed Beds:** 144

⊞ **SAINT JOSEPH HOSPITAL (180010)**, One St. Joseph Drive, Zip 40504–3754; tel. 859/278–3436, (Nonreporting) **A**1 2 3 5 9 10 **S** Catholic Health Initiatives, Englewood, CO
Primary Contact: Ken D. Haynes, President
COO: Christine Mays, R.N., Chief Operating Officer and Chief Nurse Executive
CFO: Melinda S. Evans, Vice President Finance
CIO: Janie Fergus, Director and Chief Information Officer
CHR: Edward Carthew, Chief Human Resources Officer
Web address: www.sjhlex.org
**Control:** Church–operated, Nongovernment, not–for profit **Service:** General Medical and Surgical

**Staffed Beds:** 366

⊞ **SELECT SPECIALTY HOSPITAL–LEXINGTON (182003)**, 310 South Limestone Street, 3rd Floor, Zip 40508; tel. 859/226–7096, (Nonreporting) **A**1 9 10 **S** Select Medical Corporation, Mechanicsburg, PA
Primary Contact: Mary Lou Guinle, FACHE, Chief Executive Officer
Web address: www.selectmedicalcorp.com
**Control:** Corporation, Investor–owned, for–profit **Service:** Long–Term Acute Care hospital

**Staffed Beds:** 41

☐ **SHRINERS HOSPITALS FOR CHILDREN–LEXINGTON (183300)**, 1900 Richmond Road, Zip 40502–1298; tel. 859/266–2101, (Nonreporting) **A**1 3 5 10 **S** Shriners Hospitals for Children, Tampa, FL
Primary Contact: Tony Lewgood, Administrator
CFO: Robert Montgomery, Chief Financial Officer
CMO: Chester Tylkowski, M.D., Chief of Staff
CIO: David Brian, Director Information Services
Web address: www.shrinershq.com
**Control:** Other not–for–profit (including NFP Corporation) **Service:** Children's orthopedic

**Staffed Beds:** 50

★ **UK HEALTHCARE GOOD SAMARITAN HOSPITAL (180007)**, 310 South Limestone Street, Zip 40508–3008; tel. 859/226–7000 **A**5 9 10 **F**3 28 29 30 40 45 46 49 51 57 59 64 68 70 79 81 82 85 97 98 99 100 101 102 103 107 111 113 118 128 129 145 146 147 **P**6 **S** UK HealthCare, Lexington, KY
Primary Contact: Willem de Villiers, M.D., Chief Administrative Officer
COO: Mark Armstrong, Chief Operating Officer
CFO: Sergio L. Melgar, Vice President Health Affairs and Chief Financial Officer
CMO: Paul Duane DePriest, M.D., Chief Medical Officer
CIO: Zed Day, Associate Vice President Information Technology
CHR: Kimberly P. Wilson, Associate Vice President
Web address: www.ukhealthcare.uky.edu/samaritan
**Control:** State–Government, nonfederal **Service:** General Medical and Surgical

**Staffed Beds:** 158 **Admissions:** 7976 **Census:** 102 **Outpatient Visits:** 60463 **Births:** 0 **Total Expense ($000):** 101920 **Payroll Expense ($000):** 33127 **Personnel:** 702

⊞ **UNIVERSITY OF KENTUCKY ALBERT B. CHANDLER HOSPITAL (180067)**, 800 Rose Street, N100, Zip 40536–0293; tel. 859/323–5000, (Includes KENTUCKY CHILDREN'S HOSPITAL, N–100 – 800 Rose Street, tel. 859/257–1000) **A**1 2 3 5 8 9 10 **F**3 5 6 7 9 11 12 13 15 16 17 18 19 20 21 22 23 24 25 26 27 28 29 30 31 32 34 35 36 37 38 39 40 41 42 43 44 45 46 47 48 49 50 52 55 56 57 58 59 60 61 64 65 66 68 70 71 72 73 74 75 76 77 78 79 81 82 84 85 86 87 88 89 92 93 94 95 96 97 100 104 107 108 110 111 113 114 117 118 119 120 122 123 125 129 130 131 133 134 135 136 137 138 139 140 141 145 146 147 **P**6 **S** UK HealthCare, Lexington, KY
Primary Contact: Richard P. Lofgren, M.D., Vice President Health Care Operations
CFO: Jay Sial, Chief Financial Officer
CMO: Paul Duane DePriest, M.D., Chief Medical Officer
CIO: Tim Tarnowski, Chief Information Officer
CHR: Kimberly P. Wilson, Director Human Resources
Web address: www.ukhealthcare.uky.edu
**Control:** State–Government, nonfederal **Service:** General Medical and Surgical

**Staffed Beds:** 524 **Admissions:** 24562 **Census:** 427 **Outpatient Visits:** 590627 **Births:** 1760 **Total Expense ($000):** 698801 **Payroll Expense ($000):** 217321 **Personnel:** 4925

**UNIVERSITY OF KENTUCKY HOSPITAL** See University of Kentucky Albert B. Chandler Hospital

---

**Hospital, Medicare Provider Number, Address, Telephone, Approval, Facility, and Physician Codes, Health Care System**

★ American Hospital Association (AHA) membership
☐ The Joint Commission accreditation
◇ DNV Healthcare Inc. accreditation
○ American Osteopathic Association (AOA) accreditation
△ Commission on Accreditation of Rehabilitation Facilities (CARF) accreditation

⊞ **VETERANS AFFAIRS MEDICAL CENTER–LEXINGTON**, 1101 Veterans Drive, Zip 40502; tel. 859/233–4511, (Nonreporting) **A**1 2 3 5 8 **S** Department of Veterans Affairs, Washington, DC
Primary Contact: DeWayne Hamlin, Director
CFO: Patricia Swisshelm, Acting Chief Fiscal Service
CMO: Joseph Pellecchia, M.D., Chief of Staff
CIO: Michael Gross, Chief Information Officer
CHR: Laura Faulkner, Chief Human Resource Management Service
Web address: www.va.gov/sta/guide/home.asp
**Control:** Veterans Affairs, Government, federal **Service:** General Medical and Surgical

| Staffed Beds: 138 |
|---|

### LIBERTY—Casey County

☐ **CASEY COUNTY HOSPITAL (181309)**, 187 Wolford Avenue, Zip 42539; tel. 606/787–6275, (Nonreporting) **A**1 9 10 18
Primary Contact: Rex A. Tungate, Administrator
**Control:** County–Government, nonfederal **Service:** General Medical and Surgical

| Staffed Beds: 24 |
|---|

### LONDON—Laurel County

⊞ **SAINT JOSEPH – LONDON (180011)**, 310 East Ninth Street, Zip 40741–1299; tel. 606/330–6000, (Nonreporting) **A**1 9 10 19 **S** Catholic Health Initiatives, Englewood, CO
Primary Contact: Virginia B. Dempsey, President
COO: Peggy Green, Chief Operating Officer and Chief Nursing Officer
CFO: Robert Brock, Vice President Finance and Business Development
CMO: John Abe, M.D., Chief of Staff
CIO: Debbie Mullins, Director
CHR: Kevin P. Richie, Senior Human Resources Business Partner
Web address: www.saintjosephhealthsystem.org
**Control:** Church–operated, Nongovernment, not–for profit **Service:** General Medical and Surgical

| Staffed Beds: 89 |
|---|

### LOUISA—Lawrence County

⊞ **THREE RIVERS MEDICAL CENTER (180128)**, Highway 644, Zip 41230–9632, Mailing Address: P.O. Box 769, Zip 41230–0769; tel. 606/638–9451 **A**1 9 10 20 **F**3 12 13 15 17 18 29 34 40 45 49 50 51 57 59 70 76 77 79 81 85 86 87 93 97 98 102 103 104 107 111 114 118 129 131 132 145 147 **S** Community Health Systems, Inc., Franklin, TN
Primary Contact: Greg Kiser, Chief Executive Officer
CFO: Adam Cruse, Chief Financial Officer
CHR: Pat Hart, Director Human Resources
Web address: www.threeriversmedicalcenter.com
**Control:** Corporation, Investor–owned, for–profit **Service:** General Medical and Surgical

| Staffed Beds: 80 Admissions: 3436 Census: 36 Outpatient Visits: 39532 Births: 183 Total Expense ($000): 25219 Personnel: 345 |
|---|

### LOUISVILLE—Jefferson County

⊞ △ **BAPTIST HOSPITAL EAST (180130)**, 4000 Kresge Way, Zip 40207–4676; tel. 502/897–8100 **A**1 2 3 5 7 9 10 **F**3 5 8 11 12 13 15 17 18 20 22 24 26 28 29 30 31 33 34 36 37 38 40 41 44 45 46 47 48 49 50 51 53 54 56 57 58 59 60 61 62 64 68 70 72 74 75 76 78 79 81 82 83 84 85 86 87 89 90 93 97 98 100 101 102 103 104 105 107 108 110 111 113 114 115 116 117 118 119 120 122 123 125 128 129 130 131 133 134 144 145 146 147 **S** Baptist Healthcare System, Louisville, KY
Primary Contact: David L. Gray, FACHE, President
CFO: Jim Morris, Vice President Finance
CIO: Shari Price, Director Information Services
CHR: Steven Rudolf, Vice President Human Resources
Web address: www.baptisteast.com
**Control:** Other not–for–profit (including NFP Corporation) **Service:** General Medical and Surgical

| Staffed Beds: 519 Admissions: 29405 Census: 385 Outpatient Visits: 220726 Births: 3037 Total Expense ($000): 433398 Payroll Expense ($000): 164040 Personnel: 2873 |
|---|

☐ **CENTRAL STATE HOSPITAL (184015)**, 10510 LaGrange Road, Zip 40223–1228; tel. 502/253–7000, (Nonreporting) **A**1 3 5 10
Primary Contact: Vital Shah, M.D., Director
CFO: Mark Reynolds, Controller
CMO: Vital Shah, M.D., Director
**Control:** State–Government, nonfederal **Service:** Psychiatric

| Staffed Beds: 116 |
|---|

★ △ **FRAZIER REHAB INSTITUTE**, 220 Abraham Flexner Way, Zip 40202–1887; tel. 502/582–7400 **A**3 5 7 9 **F**28 29 30 34 35 42 44 50 54 56 57 58 59 60 64 68 74 75 77 78 79 82 84 85 86 87 90 91 93 95 96 100 129 130 131 145 147 **P**6 **S** Jewish Hospital & St. Mary's HealthCare, Louisville, KY
Primary Contact: Douglas Howell, Interim President and Chief Executive Officer
COO: Randy L. Napier, Administrator
CFO: Ronald Farr, Senior Vice President and Chief Financial Officer
CMO: William P. Williamson, M.D., Medical Director
CHR: Lisa Burris, Manager Human Resources
Web address: www.frazierrehab.org
**Control:** Other not–for–profit (including NFP Corporation) **Service:** Rehabilitation

| Staffed Beds: 79 Admissions: 1653 Census: 69 Outpatient Visits: 10669 Births: 0 Total Expense ($000): 51189 Payroll Expense ($000): 19988 Personnel: 445 |
|---|

⊞ **JEWISH HOSPITAL (180040)**, 200 Abraham Flexner Way, Zip 40202–1886; tel. 502/587–4011 **A**1 2 3 5 9 10 **F**1 3 8 11 14 15 17 18 20 22 24 26 28 29 30 31 34 35 37 39 40 42 43 44 45 46 48 49 50 54 55 56 57 58 59 60 61 63 64 68 70 71 74 75 77 78 79 80 81 82 84 85 86 87 92 97 98 100 103 107 108 110 111 113 114 115 116 117 118 119 120 123 125 128 129 130 131 134 136 137 138 139 140 141 144 145 146 147 **P**6 **S** Jewish Hospital & St. Mary's HealthCare, Louisville, KY
Primary Contact: Douglas Howell, Interim President and Chief Executive Officer
CFO: Ronald Farr, Chief Financial Officer
CMO: James P. Ketterhagen, M.D., Senior Vice President and Chief Medical Officer
CIO: Thomas Wittman, Chief Information Officer
CHR: Julie McGregor, Vice President and Chief People Officer
CNO: Cheryl Fugatte, Vice President and Chief Nursing Officer
Web address: www.jewishhospital.org
**Control:** Other not–for–profit (including NFP Corporation) **Service:** General Medical and Surgical

| Staffed Beds: 462 Admissions: 18744 Census: 275 Outpatient Visits: 167470 Births: 0 Total Expense ($000): 449598 Payroll Expense ($000): 121248 Personnel: 2113 |
|---|

**KINDRED HOSPITAL LOUISVILLE AT JEWISH HOSPITAL** See Kindred Hospital–Louisville

⊞ **KINDRED HOSPITAL–LOUISVILLE (182001)**, 1313 Saint Anthony Place, Zip 40204–1740; tel. 502/587–7001, (Includes KINDRED HOSPITAL LOUISVILLE AT JEWISH HOSPITAL, 200 Abraham Flexner Way, 2nd Floor, Zip 40202; tel. 502/587–3999; David Johnson, Chief Executive Officer), (Total facility includes 47 beds in nursing home–type unit) **A**1 3 5 9 10 **F**1 3 29 45 50 64 70 81 107 118 127 129 147 **S** Kindred Healthcare, Louisville, KY
Primary Contact: Michael L. Moody, Market Chief Executive Officer
CFO: Debra Michalek, Chief Financial Officer
Web address: www.kindredlouisville.com/
**Control:** Corporation, Investor–owned, for–profit **Service:** Long–Term Acute Care hospital

| Staffed Beds: 164 Admissions: 1096 Census: 133 Outpatient Visits: 59 Births: 0 Total Expense ($000): 52030 Payroll Expense ($000): 19734 Personnel: 459 |
|---|

★ **KOSAIR CHILDREN'S HOSPITAL (189801)**, 231 East Chestnut Street, Zip 40202; tel. 502/629–6000 **A**2 3 5 9 **F**3 8 11 19 21 23 25 27 29 30 31 32 34 35 38 39 40 41 42 43 44 50 54 57 58 59 64 68 72 74 75 77 78 79 81 82 84 85 86 87 88 89 92 93 96 98 99 100 101 102 107 108 111 112 113 118 128 129 131 133 135 136 137 142 145 **S** Norton Healthcare, Louisville, KY
Primary Contact: Thomas D. Kmetz, President
Web address: www.nortonhealthcare.org
**Control:** Other not–for–profit (including NFP Corporation) **Service:** Children's general

| Staffed Beds: 263 Admissions: 9988 Census: 197 Outpatient Visits: 132428 Births: 0 Total Expense ($000): 275931 Payroll Expense ($000): 91919 Personnel: 1540 |
|---|

★ **NORTON AUDUBON HOSPITAL**, One Audubon Plaza Drive, Zip 40217–1397, Mailing Address: P.O. Box 17550, Zip 40217–0550; tel. 502/636–7111 **A**2 3 5 9 10 **F**3 11 15 17 18 20 22 24 26 29 30 31 34 35 37 40 43 45 46 47 48 49 50 56 57 59 64 68 70 74 75 77 78 79 81 82 85 86 87 107 108 110 111 112 113 114 117 118 128 129 131 145 146 147 **S** Norton Healthcare, Louisville, KY
Primary Contact: Steven MacLauchlan, President
CFO: Jonathan Presser, Vice President Finance and Operations
Web address: www.nortonhealthcare.org
**Control:** Other not–for–profit (including NFP Corporation) **Service:** General Medical and Surgical

| Staffed Beds: 262 Admissions: 13993 Census: 201 Outpatient Visits: 119937 Births: 0 Total Expense ($000): 220959 Payroll Expense ($000): 73246 Personnel: 1298 |
|---|

★ **NORTON BROWNSBORO HOSPITAL**, 4960 Norton Healthcare Boulevard, Zip 40141; tel. 502/446–8000 **A**9 10 **F**3 11 12 15 18 20 29 30 31 34 35 37 40 43 44 45 46 47 48 49 56 57 59 64 68 70 74 75 77 78 79 81 82 85 86 87 92 107 108 110 111 112 113 114 118 128 129 130 131 142 143 145 147 **S** Norton Healthcare, Louisville, KY
Primary Contact: Doug Winkelhake, President
CFO: Andy Strausbaugh, Vice President Finance and Operations
Web address: www.nortonhealthcare.org
**Control:** Other not–for–profit (including NFP Corporation) **Service:** General Medical and Surgical

**Staffed Beds:** 98 **Admissions:** 5286 **Census:** 52 **Outpatient Visits:** 46742 **Births:** 0 **Total Expense ($000):** 104361 **Payroll Expense ($000):** 31274 **Personnel:** 586

**NORTON HEALTHCARE PAVILION** See Norton Hospital

☒ **NORTON HOSPITAL (180088)**, 200 East Chestnut Street, Zip 40202–1800, Mailing Address: P.O. Box 35070, Zip 40232–5070; tel. 502/629–8000, (Includes NORTON HEALTHCARE PAVILION, 315 East Broadway, Zip 40202–1703; tel. 502/629–2000) **A**1 2 3 5 9 10 **F**1 3 4 11 12 13 15 16 17 18 20 22 24 26 28 29 30 31 34 35 36 38 39 40 43 44 45 46 49 50 51 53 55 56 57 59 64 67 68 70 72 73 74 75 76 78 79 80 81 82 84 85 86 87 88 90 92 93 96 98 100 101 102 107 108 110 111 112 113 115 116 117 118 125 127 129 131 142 145 146 147 **S** Norton Healthcare, Louisville, KY
Primary Contact: Kevin S. Wardell, President
CFO: Carl Amorose, Vice President Finance
Web address: www.nortonhealthcare.org
**Control:** Other not–for–profit (including NFP Corporation) **Service:** General Medical and Surgical

**Staffed Beds:** 340 **Admissions:** 16789 **Census:** 245 **Outpatient Visits:** 234982 **Births:** 2943 **Total Expense ($000):** 313941 **Payroll Expense ($000):** 97367 **Personnel:** 1651

★ **NORTON SUBURBAN HOSPITAL**, 4001 Dutchmans Lane, Zip 40207–4799; tel. 502/893–1000 **A**2 5 9 10 **F**3 11 12 13 15 18 20 29 30 31 34 35 40 43 44 45 47 49 50 56 57 59 64 68 70 72 73 74 75 76 78 79 81 82 85 86 87 107 108 110 111 113 114 117 118 119 120 122 123 125 129 131 145 146 **S** Norton Healthcare, Louisville, KY
Primary Contact: Charlotte Ipsan, President
CFO: Mark Kircher, Associate Vice President Finance
CMO: Steven Hester, M.D., Vice President Medical Affairs
CIO: Joseph DeVenuto, Vice President and Chief Information Officer
Web address: www.nortonhealthcare.com
**Control:** Other not–for–profit (including NFP Corporation) **Service:** General Medical and Surgical

**Staffed Beds:** 364 **Admissions:** 15772 **Census:** 198 **Outpatient Visits:** 105675 **Births:** 5387 **Total Expense ($000):** 206462 **Payroll Expense ($000):** 71582 **Personnel:** 1268

★ **OUR LADY OF PEACE**, 2020 Newburg Road, Zip 40205–1879; tel. 502/479–4500 **A**9 **F**2 9 20 30 34 35 53 59 68 98 99 100 101 104 105 106 129 131 142 145 **S** Jewish Hospital & St. Mary's HealthCare, Louisville, KY
Primary Contact: Jennifer Nolan, President and Chief Executive Officer
COO: Martha Mathers, COO/VP
CFO: Beckie Kistler, Controller
CHR: Jan Ostbloom, Human Resources Consultant
CNO: Brad Lincks, R.N., Chief Nursing Officer/ Vice President
Web address: www.hopehasaplace.org
**Control:** Other not–for–profit (including NFP Corporation) **Service:** Psychiatric

**Staffed Beds:** 261 **Admissions:** 4301 **Census:** 213 **Outpatient Visits:** 18958 **Births:** 0 **Total Expense ($000):** 54969 **Payroll Expense ($000):** 26658 **Personnel:** 603

★ **STS. MARY & ELIZABETH HOSPITAL**, 1850 Bluegrass Avenue, Zip 40215–1199; tel. 502/361–6000 **A**3 5 9 **F**3 8 11 12 15 18 20 22 29 30 31 34 35 39 40 42 43 44 45 47 49 50 53 54 59 60 64 68 69 70 74 75 78 79 81 82 84 85 86 87 107 108 110 111 113 114 117 118 128 129 131 134 145 146 147 **P**6 **S** Jewish Hospital & St. Mary's HealthCare, Louisville, KY
Primary Contact: James Parobek, President
COO: Kenneth Johnson, Vice President
CFO: Elaine Hayes, Controller
CMO: Val Slayton, M.D., Vice President Medical Affairs
CHR: Julie McGregor, Director Human Resources
Web address: www.jhsmh.org
**Control:** Other not–for–profit (including NFP Corporation) **Service:** General Medical and Surgical

**Staffed Beds:** 163 **Admissions:** 10366 **Census:** 123 **Outpatient Visits:** 156224 **Births:** 0 **Total Expense ($000):** 136833 **Payroll Expense ($000):** 48108 **Personnel:** 873

**TEN BROECK DUPONT** See The Brook at Dupont

☐ **THE BROOK AT DUPONT (184007)**, 1405 Browns Lane, Zip 40207; tel. 502/896–0495, (Nonreporting) **A**1 10 **S** Universal Health Services, Inc., King of Prussia, PA
Primary Contact: Paul Andrews, Chief Executive Officer
Web address: www.thebrookhospitals.com/
**Control:** Corporation, Investor–owned, for–profit **Service:** Psychiatric

**Staffed Beds:** 66

☐ **THE BROOK HOSPITAL – KMI (184008)**, 8521 Old Lagrange Road, Zip 40223; tel. 502/426–6380 **A**1 5 9 10 **F**4 5 64 98 99 100 101 102 103 104 105 106 129 **S** Universal Health Services, Inc., King of Prussia, PA
Primary Contact: Paul Andrews, Chief Executive Officer
COO: Kim Peabody, Chief Operating Officer
CFO: Dennis Collins, Chief Financial Officer
CMO: Timothy Burke, M.D., Medical Director
CIO: Joel Roy, Manager Information Systems
CHR: Christina Taylor, Director Human Resources
Web address: www.thebrookhospitals.com
**Control:** Corporation, Investor–owned, for–profit **Service:** Psychiatric

**Staffed Beds:** 110 **Admissions:** 1973 **Census:** 98 **Outpatient Visits:** 16089 **Births:** 0 **Total Expense ($000):** 17159 **Payroll Expense ($000):** 7696 **Personnel:** 160

☒ **UNIVERSITY OF LOUISVILLE HOSPITAL (180141)**, 530 South Jackson Street, Zip 40202–3611; tel. 502/562–3000 **A**1 2 3 5 8 9 10 **F**3 13 15 16 17 18 20 22 24 26 29 30 31 34 35 39 40 43 45 47 49 50 51 54 55 56 57 58 59 60 61 64 65 66 68 70 71 72 73 74 75 76 78 79 80 81 82 84 85 86 87 92 93 94 98 100 102 103 104 107 108 110 111 113 114 116 117 118 119 120 122 123 125 128 129 131 134 135 143 145 147
Primary Contact: James H. Taylor, FACHE, President and Chief Executive Officer
COO: Kenneth P. Marshall, Senior Vice President and Chief Operating Officer
CFO: Robert P. Barbier, Senior Vice President and Chief Financial Officer
CMO: Mark P. Pfeifer, M.D., Senior Vice President and Chief Medical Officer
CIO: Troy May, Chief Information Officer
CHR: Gary Bensing, Vice President Human Resources
CNO: Mary Jane Adams, R.N., Senior Vice President and Chief Nursing Officer
Web address: www.ulh.org
**Control:** Other not–for–profit (including NFP Corporation) **Service:** General Medical and Surgical

**Staffed Beds:** 329 **Admissions:** 17401 **Census:** 262 **Outpatient Visits:** 213002 **Births:** 1753 **Total Expense ($000):** 442527 **Payroll Expense ($000):** 140992 **Personnel:** 2528

☒ **VETERANS AFFAIRS MEDICAL CENTER–LOUISVILLE**, 800 Zorn Avenue, Zip 40206–1499; tel. 502/287–5500, (Nonreporting) **A**1 2 3 5 8 **S** Department of Veterans Affairs, Washington, DC
Primary Contact: Wayne L. Pfeffer, FACHE, Director
CFO: Barbara Roberts, Chief Financial Officer
CMO: Marylee Rothschild, M.D., Chief of Staff
CIO: Augustine Bittner, Chief Information Officer
CHR: Angela Dutton, Chief Human Resources Management Service
Web address: www.louisville.va.gov
**Control:** Veterans Affairs, Government, federal **Service:** General Medical and Surgical

**Staffed Beds:** 116

**MADISONVILLE—Hopkins County**

☒ **REGIONAL MEDICAL CENTER OF HOPKINS COUNTY (180093)**, 900 Hospital Drive, Zip 42431–1694; tel. 270/825–5100, (Total facility includes 20 beds in nursing home–type unit) **A**1 2 3 5 9 10 **F**3 8 11 13 14 18 20 22 24 26 28 29 30 31 34 35 40 44 49 51 53 57 58 59 60 62 63 64 68 70 73 76 78 79 81 85 87 88 89 90 93 96 107 108 111 113 116 117 118 119 120 122 127 128 129 130 131 145 147
Primary Contact: E. Berton Whitaker, FACHE, Chief Executive Officer
CFO: C. Thomas Moore, Chief Financial Officer
CIO: Sheila Bruce, Director Information System
CHR: David Lang, Vice President Human Resources
Web address: www.troverfoundation.org
**Control:** Other not–for–profit (including NFP Corporation) **Service:** General Medical and Surgical

**Staffed Beds:** 197 **Admissions:** 8249 **Census:** 101 **Outpatient Visits:** 207974 **Births:** 849 **Total Expense ($000):** 123982 **Payroll Expense ($000):** 56027 **Personnel:** 1210

---

**Hospital, Medicare Provider Number, Address, Telephone, Approval, Facility, and Physician Codes, Health Care System**

★ American Hospital Association (AHA) membership
☐ The Joint Commission accreditation
◇ DNV Healthcare Inc. accreditation
○ American Osteopathic Association (AOA) accreditation
△ Commission on Accreditation of Rehabilitation Facilities (CARF) accreditation

## MANCHESTER—Clay County

⊠ ○ **MANCHESTER MEMORIAL HOSPITAL (180043)**, 210 Marie Langdon Drive, Zip 40962–9156; tel. 606/598–5104 **A**1 9 10 11 **F**1 3 4 13 15 16 17 29 30 34 35 40 45 50 57 59 62 65 67 68 70 71 72 73 75 76 77 80 81 85 86 87 88 89 90 93 97 98 107 108 110 111 118 126 127 129 130 134 145 146 **S** Adventist Health System Sunbelt Health Care Corporation, Altamonte Springs, FL
Primary Contact: Erika Skula, President and Chief Executive Officer
CFO: Daniel T. Walker, Vice President Finance and Chief Financial Officer
CMO: Neeraj Mahboob, M.D., Chief Medical Officer
CHR: Joe Skula, Director Human Resources
Web address: www.manchestermemorial.org
**Control:** Church–operated, Nongovernment, not–for profit **Service:** General Medical and Surgical

**Staffed Beds:** 63 **Admissions:** 4469 **Census:** 32 **Outpatient Visits:** 45048 **Births:** 114

## MARION—Crittenden County

⊠ **CRITTENDEN COUNTY HOSPITAL (180095)**, 520 West Gum Street, Zip 42064–6201, Mailing Address: P.O. Box 386, Zip 42064–0386; tel. 270/965–5281 **A**1 9 10 20 **F**3 7 11 15 17 28 29 30 34 35 40 45 50 57 59 62 64 68 75 77 81 85 86 87 93 97 107 108 111 118 126 128 129 132 145 **P**6
Primary Contact: Jim Christensen, Chief Executive Officer
COO: Robin Curnel, Chief Operating Officer and Chief Nursing Officer
CFO: Tom Hales, CPA, Chief Financial Officer
CMO: Steven Burkhart, M.D., Chief Medical Officer
CIO: Reese Baker, Director Information Systems
CHR: Jan Gregory, Chief of Human Resources
CNO: Robin Curnel, Chief Operating Officer and Chief Nursing Officer
Web address: www.crittenden–health.org
**Control:** Other not–for–profit (including NFP Corporation) **Service:** General Medical and Surgical

**Staffed Beds:** 48 **Admissions:** 1543 **Census:** 18 **Outpatient Visits:** 14965 **Births:** 0 **Total Expense ($000):** 14324 **Payroll Expense ($000):** 8064 **Personnel:** 198

## MARTIN—Floyd County

⊠ **SAINT JOSEPH – MARTIN (181305)**, 11203 Main Street, Zip 41649–0910; tel. 606/285–6400, (Nonreporting) **A**1 9 10 18 **S** Catholic Health Initiatives, Englewood, CO
Primary Contact: Kathy Stumbo, President
CFO: Robert Brock, Vice President Finance
CMO: John Triplett, D.O., President Medical Staff
CIO: Chris Dye, Director Information Systems
Web address: www.saintjosephmartin.org
**Control:** Church–operated, Nongovernment, not–for profit **Service:** General Medical and Surgical

**Staffed Beds:** 25

## MAYFIELD—Graves County

⊠ **JACKSON PURCHASE MEDICAL CENTER (180116)**, 1099 Medical Center Circle, Zip 42066–1179; tel. 270/251–4100 **A**1 9 10 19 **F**3 11 12 13 15 18 22 28 29 30 31 34 35 37 40 43 46 47 48 49 51 57 59 64 68 74 75 76 77 79 80 81 85 87 93 97 107 110 111 114 116 118 128 130 131 132 134 142 145 146 147 **P**7 **S** LifePoint Hospitals, Inc., Brentwood, TN
Primary Contact: Fred L. Pelle, FACHE, Chief Executive Officer
COO: Matt Tavenner, Assistant Administrator
CFO: Greg Cook, Chief Financial Officer
CMO: David Zetter, M.D., Chief of Staff
CIO: Tracy Watt, Director Information Systems
CHR: Tressa B. Hargrove, Director Human Resources
Web address: www.jacksonpurchase.com
**Control:** Corporation, Investor–owned, for–profit **Service:** General Medical and Surgical

**Staffed Beds:** 106 **Admissions:** 4068 **Census:** 50 **Outpatient Visits:** 85919 **Births:** 398 **Total Expense ($000):** 47923 **Payroll Expense ($000):** 21387 **Personnel:** 520

## MAYSVILLE—Mason County

⊠ **MEADOWVIEW REGIONAL MEDICAL CENTER (180019)**, 989 Medical Park Drive, Zip 41056–8750; tel. 606/759–5311, (Nonreporting) **A**1 9 10 **S** LifePoint Hospitals, Inc., Brentwood, TN
Primary Contact: Robert Parker, Chief Executive Officer
CFO: Clayton Kolodziejczyk, Chief Financial Officer
CMO: Eric Lohman, M.D., Chief of Staff
CHR: Diana Kennedy, Director Human Resources
Web address: www.meadowviewregional.com
**Control:** Corporation, Investor–owned, for–profit **Service:** General Medical and Surgical

**Staffed Beds:** 101

## MCDOWELL—Floyd County

☐ **MCDOWELL ARH HOSPITAL (181331)**, Route 122, Zip 41647, Mailing Address: P.O. Box 247, Zip 41647–0247; tel. 606/377–3400, (Nonreporting) **A**1 9 10 18 **S** Appalachian Regional Healthcare, Inc., Lexington, KY
Primary Contact: Russell Barker, Community Chief Executive Officer
COO: Russell Barker, Community Chief Executive Officer
CFO: Joseph Grossman, Chief Financial Officer
CMO: Mary A. Hall, Chief Medical Staff
CIO: Jeff Brady, Director Information Systems
CHR: Stephanie Owens, Manager Human Resources
Web address: www.arh.org
**Control:** Other not–for–profit (including NFP Corporation) **Service:** General Medical and Surgical

**Staffed Beds:** 25

## MIDDLESBORO—Bell County

☐ **MIDDLESBORO ARH HOSPITAL (180020)**, 3600 West Cumberland Avenue, Zip 40965–2614, Mailing Address: P.O. Box 340, Zip 40965–0340; tel. 606/242–1100, (Nonreporting) **A**1 9 10 **S** Appalachian Regional Healthcare, Inc., Lexington, KY
Primary Contact: Michael Slusher, Community Chief Executive Officer
CFO: Jeremy Hall, Assistant Administrator and Chief Financial Officer
CMO: Rogelio Uy, M.D., Chief of Staff
CIO: Lisa Dooley, Health Information Officer
CHR: Ashley Kelly, Manager Human Resources
Web address: www.arh.org/middlesboro
**Control:** Other not–for–profit (including NFP Corporation) **Service:** General Medical and Surgical

**Staffed Beds:** 96

## MONTICELLO—Wayne County

○ **WAYNE COUNTY HOSPITAL (181321)**, 166 Hospital Street, Zip 42633–2416; tel. 606/348–9343 **A**9 10 11 18 **F**3 15 29 30 40 63 64 81 107 108 110 113 118 126 132 134 145
Primary Contact: Joseph Murrell, Chief Executive Officer
CFO: Anne Sawyer, Chief Financial Officer
CMO: Cory Ryan, M.D., Chief of Staff
CIO: Angela Griffin, Privacy Officer
CHR: Mollie Dick, Coordinator Human Resources
Web address: www.waynehospital.org
**Control:** County–Government, nonfederal **Service:** General Medical and Surgical

**Staffed Beds:** 25 **Admissions:** 891 **Census:** 12 **Outpatient Visits:** 24846 **Births:** 0 **Total Expense ($000):** 13753 **Payroll Expense ($000):** 5292 **Personnel:** 154

## MOREHEAD—Rowan County

⊠ **ST. CLAIRE REGIONAL MEDICAL CENTER (180018)**, 222 Medical Circle, Zip 40351–1180; tel. 606/783–6500, (Total facility includes 10 beds in nursing home–type unit) **A**1 2 3 5 9 10 **F**3 5 11 13 15 18 20 22 28 29 30 31 34 35 38 39 40 45 48 49 50 51 54 56 57 58 59 60 61 62 63 64 65 68 70 74 75 76 77 78 79 81 82 84 85 86 87 89 90 93 97 98 99 100 101 102 103 104 107 108 111 114 117 118 127 128 129 131 134 145 146 147 **P**6
Primary Contact: Mark J. Neff, FACHE, President and Chief Executive Officer
CFO: G.R. Sonny Jones, Vice President Finance and Chief Financial Officer
CMO: Will L. Melahn, M.D., Vice President Medical Affairs and Chief Medical Officer
CIO: Randy McCleese, Vice President Information Services and Chief Information Officer
CHR: Travis A. Bailey, Vice President Administration
CNO: Lerae Wilson, R.N., Vice President Patient Services and Chief Nursing Officer
Web address: www.st–claire.org
**Control:** Church–operated, Nongovernment, not–for profit **Service:** General Medical and Surgical

**Staffed Beds:** 133 **Admissions:** 5239 **Census:** 49 **Outpatient Visits:** 213579 **Births:** 422 **Total Expense ($000):** 118314 **Payroll Expense ($000):** 58798 **Personnel:** 1234

## MORGANFIELD—Union County

⊠ **METHODIST HOSPITAL UNION COUNTY (181306)**, 4604 Highway 60 West, Zip 42437–9570; tel. 270/389–5000 **A**1 9 10 18 **F**3 7 11 15 29 30 34 40 45 53 57 64 75 77 81 85 93 107 118 129 132 134 145
Primary Contact: Patrick Donahue, Administrator
CFO: Gregory P. Hebbeler, Chief Financial Officer
CMO: John Holeman, M.D., Chief of Staff
CNO: Peggy F. Creighton, R.N., Director of Nursing Services
Web address: www.methodisthospitaluc.net
**Control:** Church–operated, Nongovernment, not–for profit **Service:** General Medical and Surgical

**Staffed Beds:** 25 **Admissions:** 804 **Census:** 15 **Outpatient Visits:** 22280 **Births:** 0 **Total Expense ($000):** 12355 **Payroll Expense ($000):** 5189 **Personnel:** 136

*Many Facility Codes have changed. Please refer to the AHA Guide Code Chart.*

© 2012 AHA Guide

## MOUNT STERLING—Montgomery County

✠ **SAINT JOSEPH MOUNT STERLING (180064)**, 50 Sterling Avenue, Zip 40353–1158, Mailing Address: P.O. Box 7, Zip 40353–0007; tel. 859/497–6000, (Nonreporting) **A**1 5 9 10 **S** Catholic Health Initiatives, Englewood, CO
Primary Contact: Benny Nolen, President
CFO: Janelle Pugh, Vice President Finance and Operations
CMO: James Rollins, M.D., President Medical Staff
CIO: Jeff Ryder, Director Information Systems
CHR: Cindy Clark, Human Resource Consultant
Web address: www.sjhlex.org
**Control:** Other not–for–profit (including NFP Corporation) **Service:** General Medical and Surgical

**Staffed Beds:** 56

## MOUNT VERNON—Rockcastle County

✠ **ROCKCASTLE REGIONAL HOSPITAL AND RESPIRATORY CARE CENTER (180115)**, 145 Newcomb Avenue, Zip 40456–2733, Mailing Address: P.O. Box 1310, Zip 40456–1310; tel. 606/256–2195, (Total facility includes 93 beds in nursing home–type unit) **A**1 9 10 **F**3 12 15 28 29 31 34 35 40 45 53 57 59 62 64 68 75 81 86 87 93 107 111 114 117 118 126 127 129 131 132 134 145 146 **P**8
Primary Contact: Stephen A. Estes, Chief Executive Officer
CFO: Charles Black, Jr., Chief Financial Officer
CMO: Jon A. Arvin, M.D., Chief Medical Officer
CIO: Maleigha Amyx, Chief Information Officer
CHR: Carmen Poynter, Director Human Resources
CNO: Cynthia Burton, R.N., Chief Nursing Officer
Web address: www.rockcastleregional.org
**Control:** Other not–for–profit (including NFP Corporation) **Service:** General Medical and Surgical

**Staffed Beds:** 119 **Admissions:** 1158 **Census:** 97 **Outpatient Visits:** 43147 **Births:** 0 **Total Expense ($000):** 34479 **Payroll Expense ($000):** 20101

## MURRAY—Calloway County

✠ **MURRAY–CALLOWAY COUNTY HOSPITAL (180027)**, 803 Poplar Street, Zip 42071–2432; tel. 270/762–1100, (Nonreporting) **A**1 2 9 10 19
Primary Contact: Colonel Jerome Penner, Chief Executive Officer
CFO: Vicki Parks, Vice President
CMO: Robert Tucker, M.D., Chief Medical Officer
CIO: Regina Davison, Director Information Systems
CHR: John R. Wilson, Vice President, Human Resources
CNO: Lisa Ray, R.N., Vice President, Patient Care Services
Web address: www.murrayhospital.org
**Control:** City–County, Government, nonfederal **Service:** General Medical and Surgical

**Staffed Beds:** 335

## OWENSBORO—Daviess County

✠ △ **OWENSBORO MEDICAL HEALTH SYSTEM (180038)**, 811 East Parrish Avenue, Zip 42303, Mailing Address: P.O. Box 20007, Zip 42304–0007; tel. 270/688–2000, (Includes HEALTHPARK, 1006 Ford Avenue, Zip 42301, Mailing Address: P.O. Box 2839, Zip 42302; tel. 270/688–5433), (Total facility includes 30 beds in nursing home–type unit) **A**1 2 5 7 9 10 **F**3 5 11 12 13 15 17 18 20 22 24 26 28 29 30 31 32 34 35 40 45 46 49 53 54 56 57 58 59 61 62 63 64 65 66 70 72 74 75 76 77 78 79 81 82 84 85 86 87 89 90 91 92 93 97 98 100 101 102 103 104 105 107 108 110 111 113 114 115 116 117 118 119 120 122 123 125 127 128 129 130 131 134 143 144 145 146 147 **P**6 8
Primary Contact: Jeffrey B. Barber, Dr.PH, FACHE, President and Chief Executive Officer
COO: Greg Strahan, Chief Operating Officer
CFO: John Hackbarth, CPA, Senior Vice President Finance and Chief Financial Officer
CMO: Wathen Medley, M.D., Chief Medical Officer
CHR: Mia Suter, Senior Vice President Organizational Development
Web address: www.omhs.org
**Control:** Other not–for–profit (including NFP Corporation) **Service:** General Medical and Surgical

**Staffed Beds:** 372 **Admissions:** 18349 **Census:** 236 **Outpatient Visits:** 539642 **Births:** 1805 **Total Expense ($000):** 314898 **Payroll Expense ($000):** 115923 **Personnel:** 2555

**RIVERVALLEY BEHAVIORAL HEALTH HOSPITAL (184013)**, 1000 Industrial Drive, Zip 42301–8715; tel. 270/689–6500 **A**9 10 **F**29 98 99 100 101 102 104 106 129 **P**6
Primary Contact: Gayle DiCesare, President and Chief Executive Officer
COO: Michelle Parks, Administrator
CFO: J. Michael Mountain, Chief Financial Officer
CMO: David Harmon, D.O., Vice President Medical Services
CIO: Travis Taggart, Director Information Technology
CHR: Cathryn Gaddis, Director Human Resources
Web address: www.rvbh.com
**Control:** Other not–for–profit (including NFP Corporation) **Service:** Children's hospital psychiatric

**Staffed Beds:** 80 **Admissions:** 612 **Census:** 40 **Outpatient Visits:** 0 **Births:** 0 **Total Expense ($000):** 7943 **Payroll Expense ($000):** 4031 **Personnel:** 85

## OWENTON—Owen County

★ ○ **NEW HORIZONS HEALTH SYSTEMS (181312)**, 330 Roland Avenue, Zip 40359–1502; tel. 502/484–3663, (Nonreporting) **A**9 10 11 18
Primary Contact: Bernard T. Poe, Administrator
COO: Bernard T. Poe, Administrator
CFO: Roger Williams, Chief Financial Officer
CMO: Larry C. Johnson, M.D., Medical Director Rural Health Clinic
CIO: Edward Seale, Chief Information Officer
CHR: Kelly Perkins, Director Human Resources
Web address: www.newhorizonsmedicalcenter.com
**Control:** Other not–for–profit (including NFP Corporation) **Service:** General Medical and Surgical

**Staffed Beds:** 25

## PADUCAH—Mccracken County

✠ △ **LOURDES HOSPITAL (180102)**, 1530 Lone Oak Road, Zip 42003–7900, Mailing Address: P.O. Box 7100, Zip 42002–7100; tel. 270/444–2444, (Total facility includes 20 beds in nursing home–type unit) **A**1 7 9 10 19 **F**7 8 11 12 13 15 17 18 20 22 24 26 28 29 30 31 32 34 35 40 42 45 46 54 57 59 60 62 63 64 66 68 70 74 75 76 77 78 79 81 82 83 84 85 87 90 93 96 97 98 100 101 102 103 105 107 110 111 113 114 116 118 126 127 128 129 134 135 140 142 145 146 147 **P**3 6 **S** Catholic Health Partners, Cincinnati, OH
Primary Contact: Steven Grinnell, President and Chief Executive Officer
COO: Nicholas P. Lewis, Chief Operating Officer
CFO: Mark Thompson, Vice President Finance and Chief Financial Officer
CHR: Kim Lindsey, Chief Human Resources Officer
Web address: www.lourdes–pad.org
**Control:** Church–operated, Nongovernment, not–for profit **Service:** General Medical and Surgical

**Staffed Beds:** 277 **Admissions:** 11365 **Census:** 151 **Outpatient Visits:** 232849 **Births:** 253 **Total Expense ($000):** 160760 **Payroll Expense ($000):** 77203

✠ **WESTERN BAPTIST HOSPITAL (180104)**, 2501 Kentucky Avenue, Zip 42003–3200; tel. 270/575–2100, (Total facility includes 24 beds in nursing home–type unit) **A**1 2 9 10 19 **F**11 13 15 17 18 20 22 24 28 29 30 31 34 35 40 45 46 57 58 59 64 70 72 73 74 75 76 77 78 79 81 84 85 86 87 89 93 97 107 108 110 111 113 114 116 118 120 125 127 128 129 130 131 134 142 144 145 146 **P**6 8 **S** Baptist Healthcare System, Louisville, KY
Primary Contact: Larry O. Barton, FACHE, President
COO: Scott T. Ware, Chief Operating Officer
CFO: Jim Carmain, Vice President Financial and Information Services
CMO: Pat Withrow, M.D., Vice President Medical Affairs
CIO: Mike Cromika, Director Information Services
CHR: Donald L. Brown, Director Human Resources
Web address: www.westernbaptist.com
**Control:** Other not–for–profit (including NFP Corporation) **Service:** General Medical and Surgical

**Staffed Beds:** 320 **Admissions:** 15390 **Census:** 198 **Outpatient Visits:** 153248 **Births:** 1385 **Total Expense ($000):** 219969 **Payroll Expense ($000):** 77725 **Personnel:** 1624

## PAINTSVILLE—Johnson County

☐ **PAUL B. HALL REGIONAL MEDICAL CENTER (180078)**, 625 James S. Trimble Boulevard, Zip 41240–0000; tel. 606/789–3511, (Nonreporting) **A**1 9 10 **S** Health Management Associates, Naples, FL
Primary Contact: Deborah Trimble, R.N., Chief Executive Officer
CFO: Pattie Major, Chief Financial Officer
CMO: F. K. Belhasen, M.D., Medical Director
CHR: Carla J. Stapleton, Director Human Resources
Web address: www.pbhrmc.com
**Control:** Corporation, Investor–owned, for–profit **Service:** General Medical and Surgical

**Staffed Beds:** 72

---

**Hospital, Medicare Provider Number, Address, Telephone, Approval, Facility, and Physician Codes, Health Care System**

★ American Hospital Association (AHA) membership
☐ The Joint Commission accreditation
◇ DNV Healthcare Inc. accreditation
○ American Osteopathic Association (AOA) accreditation
△ Commission on Accreditation of Rehabilitation Facilities (CARF) accreditation

**PARIS—Bourbon County**

☒ **BOURBON COMMUNITY HOSPITAL (180046)**, 9 Linville Drive,
Zip 40361–2196; tel. 859/987–3600 **A**1 9 10 **F**3 15 29 34 35 38 39 40 44
45 49 50 51 56 57 59 64 68 70 74 75 79 81 86 87 93 98 99 100 101 102
103 107 108 110 111 113 118 128 129 132 145 147 **S** LifePoint Hospitals,
Inc., Brentwood, TN
Primary Contact: Joseph G. Koch, Chief Executive Officer
COO: Donna Davis, Chief Nursing Officer
CFO: Michael Snedegar, Chief Financial Officer
CMO: Hunter Housman, M.D., Chief Medical Officer
CIO: Phil Osborne, Director Information Technology
CHR: Roger K. Davis, Director Human Resources
CNO: Brian Springate, Chief Nursing Officer
Web address: www.bourbonhospital.com
**Control:** Corporation, Investor–owned, for–profit **Service:** General Medical and
Surgical

**Staffed Beds:** 58 **Admissions:** 1904 **Census:** 26 **Outpatient Visits:** 28971
**Births:** 0 **Total Expense ($000):** 18834 **Payroll Expense ($000):** 10005
**Personnel:** 190

**PIKEVILLE—Pike County**

☐ **PIKEVILLE MEDICAL CENTER (180044)**, 911 Bypass Road, Zip 41501–1595;
tel. 606/218–3500 **A**1 2 9 10 13 **F**3 11 12 13 15 18 20 22 24 26 29 30
31 34 35 39 40 45 49 50 51 57 59 60 61 62 64 66 68 69 70 72 74 75 76
77 78 79 81 82 84 85 86 87 89 90 93 95 96 97 107 108 110 111 114 115
116 117 118 120 122 123 126 128 129 130 131 134 145 146 147 **P**6
Primary Contact: Walter E. May, President and Chief Executive Officer
COO: Juanita Deskins, Chief Operating Officer
CFO: Michael Hagy, Chief Financial Officer
CMO: William Johnson, M.D., Chief Medical Director
CIO: Bernie Galla, Director Information Services
CHR: Melissa Coleman, Assistant Vice President Human Resources
CNO: Estella Clark, Chief Nursing Officer
Web address: www.pikevillehospital.org
**Control:** Other not–for–profit (including NFP Corporation) **Service:** General
Medical and Surgical

**Staffed Beds:** 228 **Admissions:** 10830 **Census:** 150 **Outpatient Visits:**
357087 **Births:** 888 **Total Expense ($000):** 288989 **Payroll Expense**
**($000):** 120541 **Personnel:** 2012

**PINEVILLE—Bell County**

**PINEVILLE COMMUNITY HOSPITAL ASSOCIATION (180021)**, 850 Riverview
Avenue, Zip 40977–0850; tel. 606/337–3051, (Nonreporting) **A**9 10
Primary Contact: J. Milton Brooks, III, Administrator
CFO: Colan Kelly, Chief Financial Officer
CIO: David Hall, Chief Information Officer
CHR: Greg Nunnelley, Director Human Resources
Web address: www.pinevillehospital.com
**Control:** Other not–for–profit (including NFP Corporation) **Service:** General
Medical and Surgical

**Staffed Beds:** 150

**PRESTONSBURG—Floyd County**

☒ **HIGHLANDS REGIONAL MEDICAL CENTER (180005)**, 5000 Kentucky Route
321, Zip 41653–1273, Mailing Address: P.O. Box 668, Zip 41653–0668;
tel. 606/886–8511, (Nonreporting) **A**1 2 5 9 10 19 21
Primary Contact: Harold C. Warman, Jr., FACHE, President and Chief Executive
Officer
COO: Chris Hoffman, Chief Operating Officer
CFO: Jack Blackwell, Chief Financial Officer
CIO: J. D. Jackson, Chief Information Officer
CHR: Susan Ellis, R.N., Vice President of Human Resources
CNO: Terresa O. Booher, Vice President of Patient Care Services
Web address: www.hrmc.org
**Control:** Other not–for–profit (including NFP Corporation) **Service:** General
Medical and Surgical

**Staffed Beds:** 145

**PRINCETON—Caldwell County**

☒ **CALDWELL MEDICAL CENTER (181322)**, 100 Medical Center Drive,
Zip 42445–2430, Mailing Address: P.O. Box 410, Zip 42445–0410;
tel. 270/365–0300 **A**1 9 10 18 **F**11 15 28 29 34 35 40 57 59 62 68 77 81
85 107 108 111 117 118 128 132 134 145 **S** QHR, Brentwood, TN
Primary Contact: Charles D. Lovell, Jr., FACHE, President and Chief Executive
Officer
CFO: Shane Whittington, Chief Financial Officer
CHR: Chad A. Walker, Director Human Resources
CNO: Douglas James, Chief Nursing Officer
Web address: www.caldwellhosp.org
**Control:** Other not–for–profit (including NFP Corporation) **Service:** General
Medical and Surgical

**Staffed Beds:** 25 **Admissions:** 667 **Census:** 6 **Outpatient Visits:** 30438
**Births:** 0 **Total Expense ($000):** 18676 **Payroll Expense ($000):** 6150
**Personnel:** 174

**RADCLIFF—Hardin County**

☐ **LINCOLN TRAIL BEHAVIORAL HEALTH SYSTEM (184012)**, 3909 South
Wilson Road, Zip 40160–9714, Mailing Address: P.O. Box 369, Zip 40159–0369;
tel. 270/351–9444, (Nonreporting) **A**1 9 10 **S** Universal Health Services, Inc.,
King of Prussia, PA
Primary Contact: Charles L. Webb, Jr., Administrator
CFO: Debbie Ditto, CPA, Controller
CMO: Muhammad W. Sajid, M.D., Medical Director
CHR: Charlotte C. Davis, Director Human Resources
Web address: www.lincolnbehavioral.com
**Control:** Corporation, Investor–owned, for–profit **Service:** Psychiatric

**Staffed Beds:** 67

**RICHMOND—Madison County**

★ ○ **PATTIE A. CLAY REGIONAL MEDICAL CENTER (180049)**, 801 Eastern
Bypass, Zip 40475–2405, Mailing Address: P.O. Box 1600, Zip 40476–2603;
tel. 859/623–3131 **A**9 10 11 19 **F**3 11 13 18 20 28 29 30 34 35 40 46 48
49 50 51 57 59 64 68 70 75 76 77 79 81 84 85 87 89 91 92 93 107 108
110 111 113 117 118 123 128 129 131 132 143 145 146 147 **S** Baptist
Healthcare System, Louisville, KY
Primary Contact: Todd Jones, President and Chief Executive Officer
CFO: Chris McClurg, Chief Financial Officer
CMO: Tom Cervoni, M.D., Chief of Staff
CHR: Joy M. Benedict, Director Human Resources
Web address: www.pattieaclay.org
**Control:** Other not–for–profit (including NFP Corporation) **Service:** General
Medical and Surgical

**Staffed Beds:** 66 **Admissions:** 3439 **Census:** 36 **Outpatient Visits:** 96770
**Births:** 791 **Total Expense ($000):** 64265 **Payroll Expense ($000):** 25249
**Personnel:** 542

**RUSSELL SPRINGS—Russell County**

★ **RUSSELL COUNTY HOSPITAL (181330)**, 153 Dowell Road, Zip 42642–4236,
Mailing Address: P.O. Box 1610, Zip 42642–1610; tel. 270/866–4141,
(Nonreporting) **A**9 10 18 **S** Alliant Management Services, Louisville, KY
Primary Contact: David D. Rasmussen, Chief Executive Officer
CFO: Ken Kimsal, Chief Financial Officer
CMO: Miles Gibson, M.D., Chief of Staff
CIO: Monte Monsanto, Chief Information Systems
CHR: Jennifer Dykes, Director Human Resources
Web address: www.russellcohospital.org
**Control:** County–Government, nonfederal **Service:** General Medical and Surgical

**Staffed Beds:** 25

**RUSSELLVILLE—Logan County**

☒ **LOGAN MEMORIAL HOSPITAL (180066)**, 1625 South Nashville Road,
Zip 42276–8834, Mailing Address: P.O. Box 10, Zip 42276–0010;
tel. 270/726–4011, (Nonreporting) **A**1 9 10 **S** LifePoint Hospitals, Inc.,
Brentwood, TN
Primary Contact: William Haugh, Chief Executive Officer
COO: Julia Murphy, Chief Nursing Officer
CFO: Jason Schmiedt, Chief Financial Officer
CMO: Patrick Hayden, M.D., Chief of Staff
CIO: Mike Katz, Director Information Systems
CHR: Courtney Jackson, Director Human Resources
CNO: Julia Murphy, Chief Nursing Officer
Web address: www.loganmemorial.com
**Control:** Corporation, Investor–owned, for–profit **Service:** General Medical and
Surgical

**Staffed Beds:** 52

**SALEM—Livingston County**

★ **LIVINGSTON HOSPITAL AND HEALTHCARE SERVICES (181320)**, 131
Hospital Drive, Zip 42078–8043; tel. 270/988–2299 **A**9 10 18 **F**3 15 29 30 34
35 40 46 50 56 57 59 62 64 70 75 77 81 87 103 107 111 113 114 118 126
127 129 131 132 134 144 145 146 147 **S** Alliant Management Services,
Louisville, KY
Primary Contact: Mark A. Edwards, Chief Executive Officer
CFO: John Hubbell, Chief Financial Officer
CMO: William Guyette, M.D., President Medical Staff
CIO: Shannan Landreth, Information Systems
CHR: Carla Wiggins, Director Human Resources
CNO: Joanna Stone, Chief Nursing Officer
Web address: www.lhhs.org
**Control:** Other not–for–profit (including NFP Corporation) **Service:** General
Medical and Surgical

**Staffed Beds:** 25 **Admissions:** 1146 **Census:** 13 **Outpatient Visits:** 12669
**Births:** 0 **Total Expense ($000):** 12330 **Payroll Expense ($000):** 5545
**Personnel:** 153

*Many Facility Codes have changed. Please refer to the AHA Guide Code Chart.* © 2012 AHA Guide

## SCOTTSVILLE—Allen County

**MEDICAL CENTER AT SCOTTSVILLE (181324)**, 456 Burnley Road,
Zip 42164–6355; tel. 270/622–2800, (Total facility includes 110 beds in nursing home–type unit) **A**9 10 18 **F**3 15 28 29 30 40 56 57 59 64 68 71 74 75 79 81 85 86 87 90 93 97 102 104 107 111 113 118 126 127 129 131 132 142 145 147 **S** Commonwealth Health Corporation, Bowling Green, KY
Primary Contact: Eric Hagan, R.N., Vice President
COO: Connie Smith, Chief Executive Officer and Chief Operating Officer
CFO: Ronald G. Sowell, Chief Financial Officer
CIO: Jean Cherry, Chief Information Officer
CHR: Lynn Williams, Vice President Human Resources
Web address: www.mcbg.org/scottsville
**Control:** Other not–for–profit (including NFP Corporation) **Service:** General Medical and Surgical

**Staffed Beds:** 135 **Admissions:** 818 **Census:** 120 **Outpatient Visits:** 20099 **Births:** 0 **Personnel:** 185

## SHELBYVILLE—Shelby County

**JEWISH HOSPITAL–SHELBYVILLE (180016)**, 727 Hospital Drive,
Zip 40065–1699; tel. 502/647–4000 **A**1 9 10 **F**3 11 15 18 28 29 30 34 35 39 40 44 45 46 50 57 59 64 68 70 75 79 81 82 84 85 87 93 107 108 110 111 113 118 128 131 134 145 146 147 **P**6 **S** Jewish Hospital & St. Mary's HealthCare, Louisville, KY
Primary Contact: Michael L. Collins, President and Chief Executive Officer
CFO: Erika McGimsey, Controller
CMO: Tony Perez, M.D., President Medical Staff
CHR: Cindy Stewart Rattray, Director Human Resources
Web address: www.jhsmh.org
**Control:** Other not–for–profit (including NFP Corporation) **Service:** General Medical and Surgical

**Staffed Beds:** 41 **Admissions:** 1750 **Census:** 19 **Outpatient Visits:** 46322 **Births:** 0 **Total Expense ($000):** 32853 **Payroll Expense ($000):** 11459 **Personnel:** 214

## SOMERSET—Pulaski County

**LAKE CUMBERLAND REGIONAL HOSPITAL (180132)**, 305 Langdon Street,
Zip 42501–2750, Mailing Address: P.O. Box 620, Zip 42502–2750; tel. 606/679–7441, (Total facility includes 12 beds in nursing home–type unit) **A**1 2 9 10 **F**3 8 11 12 13 15 17 18 20 22 24 26 28 29 30 31 34 35 40 45 47 49 50 54 56 57 59 61 64 65 68 70 73 74 75 76 77 78 79 81 82 85 86 87 89 90 93 97 98 102 103 107 108 109 110 111 113 114 118 120 123 126 127 128 129 131 134 145 146 147 **P**5 **S** LifePoint Hospitals, Inc., Brentwood, TN
Primary Contact: Mark T. Brenzel, Chief Executive Officer
CFO: Steve Sloan, Chief Financial Officer
CMO: Michael Citak, M.D., Chief Medical Officer
CIO: Thomas Gilbert, Director Information Technology Services
CHR: James Hughes, Director Human Resources
Web address: www.lakecumberlandhospital.com
**Control:** Corporation, Investor–owned, for–profit **Service:** General Medical and Surgical

**Staffed Beds:** 295 **Admissions:** 12844 **Census:** 165 **Outpatient Visits:** 120726 **Births:** 1430 **Total Expense ($000):** 124608 **Payroll Expense ($000):** 50900 **Personnel:** 1138

## SOUTH WILLIAMSON—Pike County

**WILLIAMSON ARH HOSPITAL (180069)**, 260 Hospital Drive, Zip 41503–4072; tel. 606/237–1710, (Nonreporting) **A**1 9 10 **S** Appalachian Regional Healthcare, Inc., Lexington, KY
Primary Contact: Timothy A. Hatfield, Community Chief Executive Officer
CMO: J. D. Miller, M.D., Vice President Medical Affairs
CIO: Jeff Brady, Chief Information Officer
Web address: www.arh.org
**Control:** Other not–for–profit (including NFP Corporation) **Service:** General Medical and Surgical

**Staffed Beds:** 123

## STANFORD—Lincoln County

★ **EPHRAIM MCDOWELL FORT LOGAN HOSPITAL (181315)**, 110 Metker Trail, Zip 40484–1020; tel. 606/365–4600 **A**9 10 18 **F**3 11 13 15 29 30 34 35 40 57 59 64 76 81 87 89 107 110 111 118 129 132 134 145 **P**5
Primary Contact: Mike Jackson, President and Chief Executive Officer
CFO: William R. Snapp, III, Vice President and Chief Financial Officer
CMO: Naren James, M.D., Chief of Staff
CIO: Sharon McWhorter, Director Information Systems
Web address: www.fortloganhospital.org
**Control:** Other not–for–profit (including NFP Corporation) **Service:** General Medical and Surgical

**Staffed Beds:** 22 **Admissions:** 874 **Census:** 7 **Outpatient Visits:** 42300 **Births:** 286 **Total Expense ($000):** 11698 **Payroll Expense ($000):** 6815 **Personnel:** 155

## TOMPKINSVILLE—Monroe County

**MONROE COUNTY MEDICAL CENTER (180105)**, 529 Capp Harlan Road, Zip 42167–1840; tel. 270/487–9231 **A**1 9 10 **F**2 3 7 15 29 30 40 45 57 62 64 85 93 110 111 113 118 131 **P**8 **S** QHR, Brentwood, TN
Primary Contact: Vicky McFall, Chief Executive Officer
CFO: Rickie F. Brown, Chief Financial Officer
CIO: Paul McKiddy, Director Information Technology
CHR: Sue Page, Director Human Resources
Web address: www.mcmccares.com
**Control:** Other not–for–profit (including NFP Corporation) **Service:** General Medical and Surgical

**Staffed Beds:** 49 **Admissions:** 2117 **Census:** 27 **Outpatient Visits:** 50175 **Births:** 0 **Total Expense ($000):** 17601 **Payroll Expense ($000):** 8895 **Personnel:** 230

## VERSAILLES—Woodford County

★ **BLUEGRASS COMMUNITY HOSPITAL (181308)**, 360 Amsden Avenue, Zip 40383–1286; tel. 859/873–3111, (Nonreporting) **A**9 10 18 **S** LifePoint Hospitals, Inc., Brentwood, TN
Primary Contact: Tommy Haggard, Chief Executive Officer
CFO: Shellie Shouse, Chief Financial Officer
CMO: Jon Sanchez, M.D., Chief of Staff
CHR: Marcia Carter, Director Human Resources
CNO: Kathy Russell, R.N., Chief Nursing Officer
Web address: www.bluegrasscommunityhospital.com
**Control:** Other not–for–profit (including NFP Corporation) **Service:** General Medical and Surgical

**Staffed Beds:** 25

## WEST LIBERTY—Morgan County

**MORGAN COUNTY ARH HOSPITAL (181307)**, 476 Liberty Road, Zip 41472–2049, Mailing Address: P.O. Box 579, Zip 41472–0579; tel. 606/743–3186, (Nonreporting) **A**1 9 10 18 **S** Appalachian Regional Healthcare, Inc., Lexington, KY
Primary Contact: Stephen M. Gavalchik, FACHE, Community Chief Executive Officer
COO: Paul V. Miles, Chief Operating Officer
CMO: J. D. Miller, M.D., Vice President Medical Affairs
CIO: Jeff Brady, Director Information Systems
CHR: Lisa Redding, Manager Human Resources
Web address: www.arh.org
**Control:** Other not–for–profit (including NFP Corporation) **Service:** General Medical and Surgical

**Staffed Beds:** 25

## WHITESBURG—Letcher County

**WHITESBURG ARH HOSPITAL (180002)**, 240 Hospital Road, Zip 41858–1254; tel. 606/633–3600, (Nonreporting) **A**1 9 10 **S** Appalachian Regional Healthcare, Inc., Lexington, KY
Primary Contact: Dena C. Sparkman, FACHE, Community Chief Executive Officer
COO: Paul V. Miles, Vice President Administration
CFO: Joseph Grossman, Vice President Fiscal Affairs
CMO: Ricky M. Collins, M.D., Chief of Staff
CIO: Brent Styer, Director Information Technology
CHR: Daniel Fitzpatrick, Director Human Resources
Web address: www.arh.org/whitesburg
**Control:** Other not–for–profit (including NFP Corporation) **Service:** General Medical and Surgical

**Staffed Beds:** 82

## WILLIAMSTOWN—Grant County

**ST. ELIZABETH GRANT (181311)**, 238 Barnes Road, Zip 41097–9460;
tel. 859/824–8240 **A**9 10 18 **F**3 11 15 29 30 31 34 35 38 40 42 44 46 50
57 59 63 64 68 74 75 78 79 82 84 87 93 97 107 108 110 111 113 118 128
129 130 131 134 145 147 **P**6 7 **S** St. Elizabeth Healthcare, Edgewood, KY
Primary Contact: Paula Roe, Assistant Vice President Operations
Web address: www.stelizabeth.com
**Control:** Church–operated, Nongovernment, not–for profit **Service:** General
Medical and Surgical

**Staffed Beds:** 16 **Admissions:** 490 **Census:** 4 **Outpatient Visits:** 41127
**Births:** 0 **Total Expense ($000):** 16933 **Payroll Expense ($000):** 6298
**Personnel:** 97

**ST. ELIZABETH MEDICAL CENTER–GRANT COUNTY** See St. Elizabeth Grant

## WINCHESTER—Clark County

★ ○ **CLARK REGIONAL MEDICAL CENTER (180092)**, 175 Hospital Drive,
Zip 40391–9591; tel. 859/745–3500, (Nonreporting) **A**5 9 10 11 **S** LifePoint
Hospitals, Inc., Brentwood, TN
Primary Contact: Katherine S. Love, Chief Executive Officer
CMO: Freddie Terrell, M.D., Chief of Staff
CHR: Barry K. Lindeman, Director Human Resources
Web address: www.clarkregional.org
**Control:** Corporation, Investor–owned, for–profit **Service:** General Medical and
Surgical

**Staffed Beds:** 100

# LOUISIANA

## ABBEVILLE—Vermilion Parish

☒ **ABBEVILLE GENERAL HOSPITAL (190034)**, 118 North Hospital Drive, Zip 70510–4077, Mailing Address: P.O. Box 580, Zip 70511–0580; tel. 337/893–5466 **A**1 9 10 **F**11 13 15 29 30 40 45 50 54 59 60 64 66 70 75 76 79 81 82 85 86 87 89 97 98 103 105 107 108 111 113 118 126 127 129 132 145 **P**6
Primary Contact: Ray A. Landry, Chief Executive Officer
CFO: Troy Hair, Chief Financial Officer
CIO: Kelly Cousins, Director Information Technology
Web address: www.abbgen.net
**Control:** Hospital district or authority, Government, nonfederal **Service:** General Medical and Surgical

**Staffed Beds:** 60 **Admissions:** 2142 **Census:** 35 **Outpatient Visits:** 58986 **Births:** 138

## ALEXANDRIA—Rapides Parish

**CENTRAL LOUISIANA SURGICAL HOSPITAL (190298)**, 651 North Bolton Avenue, Zip 71301–7449, Mailing Address: P.O. Box 8646, Zip 71306–1646; tel. 318/443–3511, (Nonreporting) **A**9 10 21
Primary Contact: Louise Barker, R.N., Chief Executive Officer
CFO: Michael Fuselier, FACHE, Chief Financial Officer
CMO: Renick Webb, M.D., Chief Medical Director
CHR: Debbie Norman, Director Human Resources
CNO: Carol Wells, R.N., Chief Nursing Officer
Web address: www.clshospital.com
**Control:** Other not–for–profit (including NFP Corporation) **Service:** Surgical

**Staffed Beds:** 13

☒ **CHRISTUS ST. FRANCES CABRINI HOSPITAL (190019)**, 3330 Masonic Drive, Zip 71301–3899; tel. 318/487–1122 **A**1 2 9 10 **F**11 12 13 15 18 20 22 24 26 28 29 30 31 32 34 35 37 40 43 44 45 46 47 48 49 50 51 53 54 57 58 59 60 63 64 68 70 71 72 74 75 76 77 78 79 81 82 84 85 86 87 89 90 93 94 96 107 108 110 111 113 114 116 118 119 120 125 128 129 130 131 134 142 143 144 145 146 147 **P**6 **S** CHRISTUS Health, Irving, TX
Primary Contact: Stephen F. Wright, President and Chief Executive Officer
COO: Lisa R. Lauve, R.N., Regional Chief Nursing Executive and Chief Operating Officer
CFO: Debbie White, Chief Financial Officer
CIO: Ron Dekeyzer, Regional Management Information Officer
CHR: Wendy White, Regional Vice President Human Resources
Web address: www.christushealth.org/sfcabrini
**Control:** Church–operated, Nongovernment, not–for profit **Service:** General Medical and Surgical

**Staffed Beds:** 281 **Admissions:** 12339 **Census:** 173 **Outpatient Visits:** 193780 **Births:** 986 **Total Expense ($000):** 194393 **Payroll Expense ($000):** 65099 **Personnel:** 1354

☐ **CROSSROADS REGIONAL HOSPITAL (194022)**, 110 John Eskew Drive, Zip 71303; tel. 318/445–5111, (Nonreporting) **A**1 9 10
Primary Contact: Brian Brunson, Chief Executive Officer
Web address: www.crossroadshospital.com
**Control:** Corporation, Investor–owned, for–profit **Service:** Psychiatric

**Staffed Beds:** 70

☒ **DUBUIS HOSPITAL OF ALEXANDRIA (192012)**, 3330 Masonic Drive, 4th Floor, Zip 71301; tel. 318/448–6505 **A**1 10 **F**1 3 29 77 84 85 147 **S** Dubuis Health System, Houston, TX
Primary Contact: Stephen D. Peters, Administrator
Web address: www.dubuis.org
**Control:** Church–operated, Nongovernment, not–for profit **Service:** General Medical and Surgical

**Staffed Beds:** 33 **Admissions:** 336 **Census:** 20 **Outpatient Visits:** 0 **Births:** 0 **Personnel:** 86

☒ **HEALTHSOUTH REHABILITATION HOSPITAL OF ALEXANDRIA (193031)**, 104 North Third Street, Zip 71301–8581; tel. 318/449–1370, (Nonreporting) **A**1 10 **S** HEALTHSOUTH Corporation, Birmingham, AL
Primary Contact: William Bush, Chief Executive Officer
CFO: Bobby Bouillion, Chief Financial Officer
CMO: Vasudeva Dhulipala, M.D., Medical Director
CHR: Suzie Wagner, Director Human Resources
Web address: www.healthsouthalexandria.com
**Control:** Partnership, Investor–owned, for–profit **Service:** Rehabilitation

**Staffed Beds:** 47

☐ **OCEANS BEHAVIORAL HOSPITAL OF ALEXANDRIA (194096)**, 2621 North Bolton Avenue, Zip 71303–4506; tel. 318/448–8473 **A**1 9 10 **F**29 98 100 101 103 104 **S** Oceans Healthcare, Lake Charles, LA
Primary Contact: Gene Amons, Administrator
Web address: www.obha.info/
**Control:** Corporation, Investor–owned, for–profit **Service:** Psychiatric

**Staffed Beds:** 24 **Admissions:** 390 **Census:** 16 **Outpatient Visits:** 1872 **Births:** 0 **Total Expense ($000):** 4039 **Payroll Expense ($000):** 1716 **Personnel:** 48

☒ **RAPIDES REGIONAL MEDICAL CENTER (190026)**, 211 Fourth Street, Zip 71301; tel. 318/473–3000 **A**1 2 3 5 9 10 **F**3 11 13 15 17 18 19 20 22 24 26 28 29 30 31 32 34 35 36 38 40 41 43 44 45 46 47 48 49 50 51 52 54 55 57 59 60 61 64 65 68 70 72 74 75 76 77 78 79 81 82 84 85 86 87 88 89 97 107 108 110 111 113 114 117 118 119 120 122 123 128 129 130 131 134 145 146 147 **P**8 **S** HCA, Nashville, TN
Primary Contact: David R. Williams, President and Chief Executive Officer
COO: Cheryl A. Wilson, Chief Operating Officer
CFO: Daniel E. Davis, Chief Financial Officer
CMO: Francis Brian, M.D., Senior Vice President Medical Affairs
CHR: Allen Crain, Director Human Resources
Web address: www.rapidesregional.com
**Control:** Partnership, Investor–owned, for–profit **Service:** General Medical and Surgical

**Staffed Beds:** 349 **Admissions:** 16409 **Census:** 243 **Outpatient Visits:** 126107 **Births:** 1588 **Total Expense ($000):** 195503 **Payroll Expense ($000):** 74122 **Personnel:** 1350

☐ **RIVERSIDE HOSPITAL OF LOUISIANA (192043)**, 211 Fourth Street, 5th Floor, Zip 71301; tel. 318/767–2900, (Nonreporting) **A**1 10
Primary Contact: Christopher Kemp Wright, Chief Executive Officer
**Control:** Corporation, Investor–owned, for–profit **Service:** Long–Term Acute Care hospital

**Staffed Beds:** 27

## AMITE—Tangipahoa Parish

★ **HOOD MEMORIAL HOSPITAL (191309)**, 301 West Walnut Street, Zip 70422–2098; tel. 985/748–9485, (Nonreporting) **A**9 10 18
Primary Contact: John C. Neal, Chief Executive Officer
CHR: Cynthia Rutherford, Manager Business Office
**Control:** Hospital district or authority, Government, nonfederal **Service:** General Medical and Surgical

**Staffed Beds:** 17

## ARCADIA—Bienville Parish

**BIENVILLE MEDICAL CENTER (191320)**, 1175 Pine Street, Suite 200, Zip 71001; tel. 318/263–4700, (Nonreporting) **A**9 10 18
Primary Contact: Richard T. Merk, Chief Executive Officer
**Control:** Other not–for–profit (including NFP Corporation) **Service:** General Medical and Surgical

**Staffed Beds:** 21

---

**Hospital, Medicare Provider Number, Address, Telephone, Approval, Facility, and Physician Codes, Health Care System**

★ American Hospital Association (AHA) membership
☐ The Joint Commission accreditation
◇ DNV Healthcare Inc. accreditation
○ American Osteopathic Association (AOA) accreditation
△ Commission on Accreditation of Rehabilitation Facilities (CARF) accreditation

**LA**

### BASTROP—Morehouse Parish

**BASTROP REHABILITATION HOSPITAL (193058)**, 323 West Walnut Street, Zip 71220, Mailing Address: P.O. Box 1531, Zip 71221–1531; tel. 318/556–1191, (Nonreporting) **A**10
Primary Contact: William H. Means, Jr., Administrator
COO: Tena Hughes, R.N., Program Director and Director Nursing
CFO: William H. Means, Jr., Administrator
CMO: James M. Smith, M.D., Medical Director
CIO: Debbie Chunn, Director Medical Records
CHR: Renee Walker, Director Human Resources
**Control:** Corporation, Investor–owned, for–profit **Service:** Rehabilitation

**Staffed Beds:** 15

☐ **LIBERTY HEALTHCARE SYSTEMS (194083)**, 4673 Eugene Ware Boulevard, Zip 71220–1425; tel. 318/281–2448, (Nonreporting) **A**1 9 10
Primary Contact: William W. Bing, Chief Executive Officer
Web address: www.libertybh.com/
**Control:** Corporation, Investor–owned, for–profit **Service:** Psychiatric

**Staffed Beds:** 60

★ **MOREHOUSE GENERAL HOSPITAL (190116)**, 323 West Walnut Avenue, Zip 71220–4521, Mailing Address: P.O. Box 1060, Zip 71221–1060; tel. 318/283–3600, (Nonreporting) **A**9 10
Primary Contact: Stephen R. Pitts, Chief Executive Officer
CFO: James Allbritton, Chief Financial Officer
CMO: John Coats, M.D., Chief Medical Staff
CIO: B. J. Vail, Director Information Systems
CHR: Debbie Spann, Director Human Resources
CNO: Melinda Jones, R.N., Chief Nursing Officer
Web address: www.mghospital.com
**Control:** Hospital district or authority, Government, nonfederal **Service:** General Medical and Surgical

**Staffed Beds:** 40

### BATON ROUGE—East Baton Rouge Parish

☐ **BATON ROUGE GENERAL MEDICAL CENTER (190065)**, 3600 Florida Street, Zip 70806–3889, Mailing Address: P.O. Box 2511, Zip 70821–2511; tel. 225/387–7000, (Includes BATON ROUGE GENERAL MEDICAL CENTER–BLUEBONNET, 8585 Picardy Avenue, Zip 70809–3679, Mailing Address: P.O. Box 84330, Zip 70884–4330; tel. 225/763–4000) **A**1 2 3 5 6 8 9 10 **F**3 8 11 12 13 15 16 17 18 19 20 22 24 26 28 29 30 31 34 35 38 40 44 45 46 47 49 50 53 56 57 58 59 60 61 64 65 68 70 72 74 75 76 77 78 79 81 82 84 86 87 88 89 90 93 96 97 98 101 102 103 104 107 108 110 111 113 114 116 117 118 119 120 122 123 125 126 127 128 129 130 131 134 142 143 145 146 147 **P**4 6
Primary Contact: William R. Holman, FACHE, President and Chief Executive Officer
COO: Edgardo Tenreiro, Chief Operating Officer
CFO: Kendall Johnson, Chief Financial Officer
CMO: Floyd Roberts, M.D., Chief Medical Officer
CIO: David Hastings, Director Information Technology
CHR: Paul Douglas, Vice President Human Resources
Web address: www.brgeneral.org
**Control:** Other not–for–profit (including NFP Corporation) **Service:** General Medical and Surgical

**Staffed Beds:** 404 **Admissions:** 19314 **Census:** 280 **Outpatient Visits:** 216459 **Births:** 872 **Total Expense ($000):** 293042 **Payroll Expense ($000):** 107326 **Personnel:** 2416

☒ **BATON ROUGE REHABILITATION HOSPITAL (193028)**, 8595 United Plaza Boulevard, Zip 70809–2251; tel. 225/927–0567, (Nonreporting) **A**1 10
Primary Contact: Jacque Shadle, Chief Executive Officer
CFO: Nicholas Hluchy, Business Analyst, Support Services Manager
CMO: Sundararama R. Vatsavai, M.D., Medical Director
CIO: Roxane Bingham, Director Marketing
CHR: Michelle Smith, Coordinator Human Resources
CNO: Derrick Landreneau, Director of Nursing
Web address: www.brrehab.com
**Control:** Corporation, Investor–owned, for–profit **Service:** Rehabilitation

**Staffed Beds:** 80

**BECK BEHAVIORAL HOSPITAL (194071)**, 4363 Convention Street, Suite A., Zip 70806; tel. 225/336–8940, (Nonreporting) **A**10
Primary Contact: Kenneth O'Rourke, Administrator
Web address: www.beckhospital.com
**Control:** Partnership, Investor–owned, for–profit **Service:** Psychiatric

**Staffed Beds:** 30

○ **BEHAVIORAL HOSPITAL OF SOUTHEAST LOUISIANA (194101)**, 7414 Sumrall Drive, Zip 70812; tel. 225/364–2715, (Nonreporting) **A**10 11
Primary Contact: Reuben Patel, Administrator
Web address: www.bhsela.com
**Control:** Other not–for–profit (including NFP Corporation) **Service:** Psychiatric

**Staffed Beds:** 10

**BETHESDA REHABILITATION HOSPITAL (193092)**, 7414 Sumrall Drive, Zip 70812–1240, Mailing Address: 8225 Summa Avenue, Suite B., Zip 70809–3422; tel. 225/767–2034, (Nonreporting) **A**10
Primary Contact: Monica Nix, Administrator
**Control:** Corporation, Investor–owned, for–profit **Service:** Rehabilitation

**Staffed Beds:** 18

**CYPRESS PSYCHIATRIC HOSPITAL** See Beck Behavioral Hospital

☐ **EARL K. LONG MEDICAL CENTER (190122)**, 5825 Airline Highway, Zip 70805–2498; tel. 225/358–1000 **A**1 3 5 9 10 **F**3 8 14 15 18 29 31 32 40 45 48 49 50 59 60 61 64 66 68 70 72 73 75 76 77 78 79 81 85 87 93 97 102 107 108 110 111 113 114 116 118 129 130 134 146 147 **P**6 **S** LSU Health Care Services Division, Baton Rouge, LA
Primary Contact: Roxane A. Townsend, M.D., Chief Executive Officer
CFO: Sue Tolbert, Chief Financial Officer
CIO: Kevin Bolds, Director Information Technology
Web address: www.lsuhsc.edu
**Control:** State–Government, nonfederal **Service:** General Medical and Surgical

**Staffed Beds:** 103 **Admissions:** 4975 **Census:** 52 **Outpatient Visits:** 241273 **Births:** 516 **Total Expense ($000):** 156561 **Payroll Expense ($000):** 55297 **Personnel:** 1595

**GREATER BATON ROUGE SURGICAL HOSPITAL (190273)**, 7855 Howell Place Boulevard, Zip 70807; tel. 225/358–4900, (Nonreporting) **A**9 10
Primary Contact: Laura Broadhurst, R.N., Chief Executive Officer
Web address: www.gbrsh.com
**Control:** Corporation, Investor–owned, for–profit **Service:** Surgical

**Staffed Beds:** 10

**HEALTHSOUTH REHABILITATION HOSPITAL OF BATON ROUGE** See Baton Rouge Rehabilitation Hospital

**NEUROMEDICAL CENTER REHABILITATION HOSPITAL (193090)**, 10101 Park Rowe Avenue, Suite 500, Zip 70810; tel. 225/906–2999, (Nonreporting) **A**10 **S** AMG Integrated Healthcare Management, Lafayette, LA
Primary Contact: Jay Ivy, R.N., Chief Executive Officer
Web address: www.theneuromedicalcenter.com
**Control:** Corporation, Investor–owned, for–profit **Service:** Rehabilitation

**Staffed Beds:** 23

**OCEANS BEHAVIORAL HOSPITAL OF BATON ROUGE (194086)**, 11135 Florida Boulevard, Zip 70815–2013; tel. 225/356–7030, (Nonreporting) **A**10 **S** Oceans Healthcare, Lake Charles, LA
Primary Contact: Gene Amos, Administrator
Web address: www.obhbr.info/
**Control:** Corporation, Investor–owned, for–profit **Service:** Psychiatric

**Staffed Beds:** 20

★ **OCHSNER MEDICAL CENTER–BATON ROUGE (190202)**, 17000 Medical Center Drive, Zip 70816–3224; tel. 225/752–2470, (Nonreporting) **A**9 10 **S** Ochsner Health System, New Orleans, LA
Primary Contact: Eric McMillen, Interim Chief Executive Officer
CFO: Barry M. Chambers, CPA, Chief Financial Officer
CMO: F. Ralph Dauterive, M.D., Vice President Medical Affairs
CHR: Chris Atkinson, Director of Human Resources
Web address: www.ochsner.org/page.cfm?id=103
**Control:** Corporation, Investor–owned, for–profit **Service:** General Medical and Surgical

**Staffed Beds:** 115

☒ **OUR LADY OF THE LAKE REGIONAL MEDICAL CENTER (190064)**, 5000 Hennessy Boulevard, Zip 70808–4375; tel. 225/765–6565, (Includes OUR LADY OF THE LAKE CHILDREN'S HOSPITAL, 5000 Hennessy Boulevard, tel. 225/765–8886), (Total facility includes 390 beds in nursing home–type unit) **A**1 2 3 5 8 9 10 **F**3 4 5 10 11 12 14 15 17 18 19 20 21 22 23 24 25 26 28 29 30 31 34 35 37 38 39 40 41 45 46 49 50 53 54 55 56 57 58 59 61 64 68 70 71 74 75 77 78 79 81 82 84 85 86 87 88 89 90 93 96 97 98 99 100 101 102 103 104 105 107 108 110 111 113 114 117 118 124 125 126 127 128 129 130 131 134 140 141 142 145 147 **P**6 **S** Franciscan Missionaries of Our Lady Health System, Inc., Baton Rouge, LA
Primary Contact: K. Scott Wester, FACHE, President and Chief Executive Officer
COO: Terrie Sterling, R.N., Chief Operating Officer
CFO: Jeff Limbocker, Chief Financial Officer
CMO: Richard Vath, M.D., Vice President Medical Affairs
CIO: Stephanie Mills, Vice President Information and Materials Systems
CHR: Cora Ford, Assistant Vice President Human Resources
Web address: www.ololrmc.com
**Control:** Church–operated, Nongovernment, not–for profit **Service:** General Medical and Surgical

**Staffed Beds:** 1049 **Admissions:** 35337 **Census:** 758 **Outpatient Visits:** 363751 **Births:** 0 **Total Expense ($000):** 655528 **Payroll Expense ($000):** 255119 **Personnel:** 4421

*Many Facility Codes have changed. Please refer to the AHA Guide Code Chart.*
© 2012 AHA Guide

**PROMISE HOSPITAL BATON ROUGE (192045)**, 5130 Mancuso Lane, Zip 70809–3583; tel. 225/621–1248 **A**9 10 **F**1 3 18 28 29 35 50 56 75 91 92 96 104 129 147 **P**5 **S** Promise Healthcare, Boca Raton, FL
Primary Contact: Richard Knowland, Area Chief Executive Officer
COO: Christopher A. Stegall, Regional Chief Financial Officer and Chief Operating Officer
CFO: Christopher A. Stegall, Regional Chief Financial Officer and Chief Operating Officer
CMO: Peter J. Monteyne, M.D., Chief Medical Staff
CHR: Wendy Cobbs, Director Human Resources
Web address: www.promisehealthcare.com
**Control:** Corporation, Investor–owned, for–profit **Service:** Long–Term Acute Care hospital

**Staffed Beds:** 50 **Admissions:** 550 **Census:** 42 **Outpatient Visits:** 2600 **Births:** 0 **Total Expense ($000):** 14782 **Payroll Expense ($000):** 7852 **Personnel:** 151

**PROMISE HOSPITAL OF BATON ROUGE (192004)**, 3600 Florida Boulevard, 4th Floor, Zip 70806; tel. 225/387–7770 **A**10 **F**1 3 18 28 29 50 56 75 82 96 129 147 **P**5 **S** Promise Healthcare, Boca Raton, FL
Primary Contact: Richard Knowland, Area Chief Executive Officer
COO: Michael J. Nolan, Area Chief Operating Officer and Safety
CMO: Venkat Banda, M.D., President of the Medical Staff
CMO: Subhaker Gummadi, M.D., President Medical Staff
Web address: www.promise–batonrouge.com
**Control:** Corporation, Investor–owned, for–profit **Service:** Long–Term Acute Care hospital

**Staffed Beds:** 28 **Admissions:** 348 **Census:** 26 **Outpatient Visits:** 0 **Births:** 0 **Total Expense ($000):** 11055 **Payroll Expense ($000):** 4382 **Personnel:** 75

☐ **PROMISE HOSPITAL OF BATON ROUGE (192049)**, 17000 Medical Center Drive, 3rd Floor, Zip 70816; tel. 225/236–5440 **A**1 10 **F**1 3 18 28 29 56 75 96 104 129 147 **P**5 **S** Promise Healthcare, Boca Raton, FL
Primary Contact: Richard Knowland, Area Chief Executive Officer
COO: Michael J. Nolan, Area Safety Director
CMO: Venkat Banda, M.D., President Medical Staff
CHR: Wendy Cobbs, Director of Human Resources
Web address: www.promise–batonrouge.com
**Control:** Corporation, Investor–owned, for–profit **Service:** Long–Term Acute Care hospital

**Staffed Beds:** 22 **Admissions:** 180 **Census:** 13 **Outpatient Visits:** 1680 **Births:** 0 **Total Expense ($000):** 5367 **Payroll Expense ($000):** 2257 **Personnel:** 42

**SAGE REHABILITATION HOSPITAL (193078)**, 8000 Summa Avenue, Zip 70809, Mailing Address: P.O. Box 82681, Zip 70884; tel. 225/819–0703, (Nonreporting) **A**10
Primary Contact: Theresa Brinkhaus, Chief Financial Officer and Compliance
CFO: Theresa Brinkhaus, Chief Financial Officer
CMO: Christopher Belleau, M.D., Medical Director
CIO: Garon Leblanc, Chief Plant Operations
CHR: Kathy Ringe, Director Human Resources
Web address: www.aboutseniorhealthcare.com/sage/
**Control:** Individual, Investor–owned, for–profit **Service:** Rehabilitation

**Staffed Beds:** 22

☐ **SURGICAL SPECIALTY CENTER OF BATON ROUGE (190251)**, 8080 Bluebonnet Boulevard, Zip 70810; tel. 225/408–8080, (Nonreporting) **A**1 9 10
Primary Contact: Craig P. Hume, Chief Executive Officer
Web address: www.sscbr.com
**Control:** Corporation, Investor–owned, for–profit **Service:** Surgical

**Staffed Beds:** 14

**THE NEUROMEDICAL CENTER SURGICAL HOSPITAL (190266)**, 10105 Park Rowe Avenue, Suite 250, Zip 70810; tel. 225/763–9900, (Nonreporting) **A**9 10
Primary Contact: Robert D. Blair, Chief Executive Officer
CFO: Allison Doherty, Chief Financial Officer
CMO: Shawn Dunn, M.D., Medical Director
CHR: Shannon Juge, Human Resources Representative
Web address: www.theneuromedicalcenter.com
**Control:** Corporation, Investor–owned, for–profit **Service:** Surgical

**Staffed Beds:** 23

☒ **WOMAN'S HOSPITAL (190128)**, 100 Woman's Way, Zip 70817, Mailing Address: P.O. Box 95009, Zip 70895–5009; tel. 225/927–1300 **A**1 2 9 10 **F**3 11 12 13 15 31 32 34 35 36 38 45 50 53 54 57 58 59 61 62 64 65 68 70 71 72 73 74 75 76 77 78 79 81 84 85 86 87 89 93 107 110 111 113 118 125 128 129 131 133 134 145 146 **P**6
Primary Contact: Teri G. Fontenot, FACHE, President and Chief Executive Officer
COO: Jamie Haeuser, Senior Vice President Operations
CFO: Stephanie Anderson, Senior Vice President, Finance and Administration
CMO: Kenneth Brown, M.D., Medical Director
CIO: Paul Kirk, Vice President
CHR: Donna L. Bodin, Vice President
CNO: Patricia R. Johnson, R.N., Senior Vice President
Web address: www.womans.org
**Control:** Other not–for–profit (including NFP Corporation) **Service:** Obstetrics and gynecology

**Staffed Beds:** 226 **Admissions:** 12483 **Census:** 134 **Outpatient Visits:** 117264 **Births:** 7953 **Total Expense ($000):** 188378 **Payroll Expense ($000):** 98487 **Personnel:** 1548

## BERNICE—Union Parish

**REEVES MEMORIAL MEDICAL CENTER (191326)**, 409 First Street, Zip 71222–0697, Mailing Address: P.O. Box 697, Zip 71222–0697; tel. 318/285–9066, (Nonreporting) **A**9 10 18
Primary Contact: Landon Tooke, Chief Executive Officer
COO: Beth Jones, Chief Operating Officer
CFO: Charlotte Thompson, Chief Financial Officer
CMO: R. Brian Harris, M.D., Chief of Staff
CHR: Robin Adams, Director Human Resources
Web address: www.reevesmemorial.com/
**Control:** Hospital district or authority, Government, nonfederal **Service:** General Medical and Surgical

**Staffed Beds:** 11

**TRI–WARD GENERAL HOSPITAL** See Reeves Memorial Medical Center

## BOGALUSA—Washington Parish

☐ **LSU BOGALUSA MEDICAL CENTER (190095)**, 433 Plaza Street, Zip 70427–3793; tel. 985/730–6700, (Includes AMG SPECIALTY HOSPITAL BOGALUSA, 621 Columbia Street, Zip 70427–0040; tel. 985/735–1322; BOGALUSA COMMUNITY MEDICAL CENTER, 433 Plaza Street, tel. 985/730–6700) **A**1 3 9 10 **F**3 11 13 15 18 28 29 34 35 38 40 41 45 49 50 51 56 57 58 59 60 61 64 66 68 70 74 75 76 81 85 86 87 89 93 97 98 104 107 108 111 113 118 129 131 134 140 145 146 147 **P**6 **S** LSU Health Care Services Division, Baton Rouge, LA
Primary Contact: Kurt M. Scott, FACHE, Administrator
CFO: Brooke Cummings, Chief Financial Officer
CMO: Lee Roy Joyner, M.D., Medical Director
CIO: Betina Owens, Chief Information Officer
CHR: Christi Brown, Director Human Resources
Web address: www.lsuhospitals.org
**Control:** State–Government, nonfederal **Service:** General Medical and Surgical

**Staffed Beds:** 74 **Admissions:** 3403 **Census:** 42 **Outpatient Visits:** 151067 **Births:** 167 **Total Expense ($000):** 68203 **Payroll Expense ($000):** 30357 **Personnel:** 574

## BOSSIER CITY—Bossier Parish

**CHRISTUS SCHUMPERT BOSSIER** See CHRISTUS Health Shreveport–Bossier, Shreveport

☐ **CORNERSTONE HOSPITAL OF BOSSIER CITY (192006)**, 4900 Medical Drive, Zip 71112–4596; tel. 318/747–9500, (Nonreporting) **A**1 9 10 **S** Cornerstone Healthcare Group, Dallas, TX
Primary Contact: Sheri Burnette, R.N., Chief Executive Officer and Administrator
CFO: Chad Deardorff, Chief Financial Officer
CMO: James Jackson, M.D., Chief of Staff
Web address: www.chghospitals.com/
**Control:** Corporation, Investor–owned, for–profit **Service:** Long–Term Acute Care hospital

**Staffed Beds:** 54

**PATHWAY REHABILITATION HOSPITAL (193094)**, 4900 Medical Drive, Zip 71112–4521, (Nonreporting)
**Control:** Corporation, Investor–owned, for–profit **Service:** Rehabilitation

**Staffed Beds:** 24

---

**Hospital, Medicare Provider Number, Address, Telephone, Approval, Facility, and Physician Codes, Health Care System**

★ American Hospital Association (AHA) membership
☐ The Joint Commission accreditation
◇ DNV Healthcare Inc. accreditation
○ American Osteopathic Association (AOA) accreditation
△ Commission on Accreditation of Rehabilitation Facilities (CARF) accreditation

**LA**

**PROMISE HOSPITAL OF BOSSIER CITY**, 2525 Viking Drive, Zip 71111; tel. 318/841–2525, (Nonreporting) **S** Promise Healthcare, Boca Raton, FL
Primary Contact: Rick Stockton, Chief Executive Officer
Web address: www.promise–bossiercity.com
**Control:** Corporation, Investor–owned, for–profit **Service:** Long–Term Acute Care hospital

| Staffed Beds: 50 |
| --- |

**RED RIVER BEHAVIORAL CENTER (194079)**, 2800 Melrose Avenue, Zip 71111; tel. 318/549–2033, (Nonreporting) **A**9 10
Primary Contact: Susan Kottenbrook, Chief Executive Officer
Web address: www.redriverbehavioral.com/
**Control:** State–Government, nonfederal **Service:** Psychiatric

| Staffed Beds: 20 |
| --- |

**WILLIS–KNIGHTON BOSSIER HEALTH CENTER** See WK Bossier Health Center

⊠ △ **WK BOSSIER HEALTH CENTER (190236)**, 2400 Hospital Drive, Zip 71111; tel. 318/212–7000 **A**1 7 9 10 **F**3 8 11 12 13 15 18 20 22 24 28 29 30 34 35 38 40 44 45 46 47 48 49 50 53 54 56 57 59 60 61 64 65 68 70 74 75 76 77 78 79 80 81 82 84 85 86 87 89 93 96 97 100 101 102 103 107 108 109 110 111 113 117 118 126 128 129 130 131 134 143 145 146 147 **P**6 7 **S** Willis–Knighton Health System, Shreveport, LA
Primary Contact: Clifford M. Broussard, FACHE, Administrator
COO: Charles D. Daigle, Chief Operating Officer
CFO: Robert D. Huie, Chief Financial Officer
CMO: Charles Powers, M.D., Administrative Medical Director
CIO: Charles Laster, Director Information Management
CHR: Debbie Fortson, Director Human Resources
CNO: Sharon Hudnell, R.N., Chief Nursing Officer
Web address: www.wkhs.com/wkb/
**Control:** Other not–for–profit (including NFP Corporation) **Service:** General Medical and Surgical

| Staffed Beds: 134 **Admissions:** 10391 **Census:** 93 **Outpatient Visits:** 120791 **Births:** 913 **Personnel:** 938 |
| --- |

**BREAUX BRIDGE—St. Martin Parish**

**GENESIS BEHAVIORAL HOSPITAL (194089)**, 606 Latiolais Drive, Zip 70517–4231; tel. 337/442–6084, (Nonreporting) **A**9 10
Primary Contact: Will Alredge, Administrator
**Control:** Other not–for–profit (including NFP Corporation) **Service:** Psychiatric

| Staffed Beds: 12 |
| --- |

**ST. MARTIN HOSPITAL (191302)**, 210 Champagne Boulevard, Zip 70517–3852, Mailing Address: P.O. Box 357, Zip 70517–0357; tel. 337/332–2178 **A**9 10 18 **F**3 29 40 56 77 93 110 118 **P**8
Primary Contact: Katherine D. Hebert, Chief Executive Officer
CFO: Shadelle Huval, Director Finance
CHR: Rena B. Mouisset, Director Human Resources and Contract Compliance
Web address: www.stmartinhospital.org
**Control:** Other not–for–profit (including NFP Corporation) **Service:** General Medical and Surgical

| Staffed Beds: 25 **Admissions:** 333 **Census:** 39 **Outpatient Visits:** 13535 **Births:** 0 **Total Expense ($000):** 11384 **Payroll Expense ($000):** 4458 |
| --- |

**BROUSSARD—Lafayette Parish**

☐ **OCEANS BEHAVIORAL HOSPITAL OF BROUSSARD (194073)**, 418 Albertson Parkway, Zip 70518; tel. 337/237–6444, (Nonreporting) **A**1 9 10 **S** Oceans Healthcare, Lake Charles, LA
Primary Contact: Marlene Lucas, Administrator
Web address: www.obhb.info/
**Control:** Corporation, Investor–owned, for–profit **Service:** Psychiatric

| Staffed Beds: 38 |
| --- |

**BUNKIE—Avoyelles Parish**

★ **BUNKIE GENERAL HOSPITAL (191311)**, 427 Evergreen Highway, Zip 71322–3901, Mailing Address: P.O. Box 380, Zip 71322–0380; tel. 318/346–6681, (Nonreporting) **A**9 10 18
Primary Contact: Linda F. Deville, Chief Executive Officer
COO: Lonnie L. Dufour, Chief Operating Officer, Chief Information Officer and Director Human Resources
CFO: Terry Willett, Chief Financial Officer
CMO: Mohit Srivastava, M.D., Chief of Staff
CIO: Lonnie L. Dufour, Chief Operating Officer, Chief Information Officer and Director Human Resources
CHR: Lonnie L. Dufour, Chief Operating Officer, Chief Information Officer and Director Human Resource
Web address: www.bunkiegeneral.com
**Control:** Hospital district or authority, Government, nonfederal **Service:** General Medical and Surgical

| Staffed Beds: 18 |
| --- |

**CAMERON—Cameron Parish**

**SOUTH CAMERON MEMORIAL HOSPITAL (190307)**, 5360 West Creole Highway, Zip 70631–5127; tel. 337/542–4111, (Nonreporting) **A**20 21
Primary Contact: David Byrns, Chief Executive Officer
**Control:** Hospital district or authority, Government, nonfederal **Service:** General Medical and Surgical

| Staffed Beds: 49 |
| --- |

**CHURCH POINT—Acadia Parish**

**ACADIA–ST. LANDRY HOSPITAL (191319)**, 810 South Broadway Street, Zip 70525–4497; tel. 337/684–5435, (Nonreporting) **A**9 10 18
Primary Contact: F. Peter Savoy, III, Chief Executive Officer
CFO: Judy Young, Chief Financial Officer
CMO: Ty Hargroder, M.D., Chief of Staff
CHR: Judy Young, Chief Financial Officer
Web address: www.aslh.org
**Control:** Other not–for–profit (including NFP Corporation) **Service:** General Medical and Surgical

| Staffed Beds: 25 |
| --- |

**CLINTON—East Feliciana Parish**

**AMG SPECIALTY HOSPITAL–FELICIANA (192041)**, 9725 Grace Lane, Zip 70722; tel. 225/683–1600, (Nonreporting) **A**10 **S** AMG Integrated Healthcare Management, Lafayette, LA
Primary Contact: Karen Crayton, Chief Executive Officer
Web address: www.amgihm.com/ltac_of_feliciana
**Control:** Corporation, Investor–owned, for–profit **Service:** Long–Term Acute Care hospital

| Staffed Beds: 16 |
| --- |

**COLUMBIA—Caldwell Parish**

**CALDWELL MEMORIAL HOSPITAL (190190)**, 411 Main Street, Zip 71418, Mailing Address: P.O. Box 899, Zip 71418–0899; tel. 318/649–6111, (Nonreporting) **A**9 10
Primary Contact: Heather Clark, Chief Executive Officer
COO: Lisa Patrick, Chief Operating Officer
**Control:** Corporation, Investor–owned, for–profit **Service:** Long–Term Acute Care hospital

| Staffed Beds: 25 |
| --- |

**CITIZENS MEDICAL CENTER (190184)**, 7939 U.S. Highway 165, Zip 71418–1079, Mailing Address: P.O. Box 1079, Zip 71418–1079; tel. 318/649–6106, (Nonreporting) **A**9 10
Primary Contact: Steve Barbo, R.N., Administrator
**Control:** Hospital district or authority, Government, nonfederal **Service:** General Medical and Surgical

| Staffed Beds: 40 |
| --- |

**COUSHATTA—Red River Parish**

⊠ **CHRISTUS COUSHATTA HEALTH CARE CENTER (191312)**, 1635 Marvel Street, Zip 71019–9022, Mailing Address: P.O. Box 589, Zip 71019–0589; tel. 318/932–2000, (Nonreporting) **A**1 9 10 18 **S** CHRISTUS Health, Irving, TX
Primary Contact: Nancy R. Hellyer, Interim Chief Executive Officer
CFO: Scott Merryman, Chief Financial Officer
CMO: Jonathan Weisul, M.D., Vice President Medical Affairs and Chief Medical Officer
CIO: Bruce Honea, Director Information Services
CHR: Donnette Craig, Director Human Resources
Web address: www.christuscoushatta.org
**Control:** Church–operated, Nongovernment, not–for profit **Service:** General Medical and Surgical

| Staffed Beds: 25 |
| --- |

**SPECIALTY REHABILITATION HOSPITAL (193080)**, 1110 Ringgold Avenue Suite B., Zip 71019–9073; tel. 318/932–1770, (Nonreporting) **A**10 **S** Specialty Healthcare, LLC, Leesville, LA
Primary Contact: Craig Ball, Chief Executive Officer
COO: Charlie Ball, Chief Operating Officer
CFO: Connie Ball, Chief Financial Officer
CMO: Jalal Joudeh, M.D., Chief Medical Officer
CHR: Denise Logan, Director Human Resources
Web address: www.specialtyhealthcare.com
**Control:** Individual, Investor–owned, for–profit **Service:** Rehabilitation

| Staffed Beds: 12 |
| --- |

## COVINGTON—St. Tammany Parish

**FAIRWAY MEDICAL CENTER (190267)**, 67252 Industry Lane,
Zip 70433–8704; tel. 985/809–9888, (Nonreporting) **A**9 10 21
Primary Contact: David J. Guzan, Chief Executive Officer
CFO: Sandy Badinger, Chief Financial Officer
CMO: William Preau, M.D., Medical Director
CIO: Skip Federico, Director Information Systems
CHR: Pam Collins, Director Human Resources
Web address: www.fairwaymedical.com
**Control:** Corporation, Investor–owned, for–profit **Service:** General Medical and
Surgical

**Staffed Beds: 21**

**GREENBRIER HOSPITAL (194069)**, 201 Greenbrier Boulevard, Zip 70433;
tel. 985/893–2970, (Nonreporting) **A**10
Primary Contact: Kristie Overstreet, Administrator
CMO: Jason Coe, M.D., Medical Director
**Control:** Corporation, Investor–owned, for–profit **Service:** Psychiatric

**Staffed Beds: 58**

**GULF STATES LONG TERM ACUTE CARE OF COVINGTON** See Northshore
Specialty Hospital

⊠ **LAKEVIEW REGIONAL MEDICAL CENTER (190177)**, 95 Judge Tanner
Boulevard, Zip 70433–7507; tel. 985/867–3800 **A**1 9 10 **F**11 12 13 15 18 20
22 24 26 27 28 29 34 35 40 49 57 59 64 68 70 75 76 77 78 81 85 89 91
92 93 98 102 103 106 107 108 110 111 113 114 118 129 131 142 143
145 146 **S** HCA, Nashville, TN
Primary Contact: Jason E. Cobb, FACHE, Chief Executive Officer
COO: Stephen Robinson, Chief Operating Officer
CFO: Tim Breslin, Chief Financial Officer
CMO: George Barnes, M.D., Medical Director
CIO: Debra Hasling, Director Medical Records
CHR: Lyle Theriot, Director Human Resources
CNO: Bonnie Pratt, R.N., Chief Nursing Officer
Web address: www.lakeviewregional.com
**Control:** Corporation, Investor–owned, for–profit **Service:** General Medical and
Surgical

**Staffed Beds: 172 Admissions: 6886 Census: 98 Outpatient Visits: 39077
Births: 866 Total Expense ($000): 91519 Payroll Expense ($000): 34480
Personnel: 636**

☐ **NORTHSHORE SPECIALTY HOSPITAL (192048)**, 20050 Crestwood
Boulevard, Zip 70433; tel. 985/875–7525, (Nonreporting) **A**1 10 **S** Post Acute
Medical, LLC, Camp Hill, PA
Primary Contact: Douglas L. Johnson, FACHE, Chief Executive Officer
Web address: www.northshoreltach.com
**Control:** Corporation, Investor–owned, for–profit **Service:** Long–Term Acute Care
hospital

**Staffed Beds: 58**

⊠ **REGENCY HOSPITAL OF COVINGTON (192051)**, 195 Highland Park Entrance,
Zip 70433; tel. 985/867–3977, (Nonreporting) **A**1 10 **S** Select Medical
Corporation, Mechanicsburg, PA
Primary Contact: Keith Carruth, Chief Executive Officer
CMO: Merrill Laurent, M.D., Medical Director
CHR: Beth Sayler, Director Human Resources
Web address: www.regencyhospital.com
**Control:** Corporation, Investor–owned, for–profit **Service:** Long–Term Acute Care
hospital

**Staffed Beds: 38**

☐ **ST. TAMMANY PARISH HOSPITAL (190045)**, 1202 South Tyler Street,
Zip 70433–2330; tel. 985/898–4000, (Nonreporting) **A**1 2 9 10
Primary Contact: Patti M. Ellish, President and Chief Executive Officer
COO: Sharon A. Toups, Senior Vice President and Chief Operating Officer
CMO: Robert Capitelli, M.D., Senior Vice President and Chief Medical Officer
CHR: Judy Gracia, Vice President Human Resources
Web address: www.stph.org
**Control:** Hospital district or authority, Government, nonfederal **Service:** General
Medical and Surgical

**Staffed Beds: 218**

## CROWLEY—Acadia Parish

★ **AMERICAN LEGION HOSPITAL (190044)**, 1305 Crowley Rayne Highway,
Zip 70526–8202; tel. 337/783–3222, (Nonreporting) **A**9 10
Primary Contact: Terry W. Osborne, CPA, Chief Executive Officer
CFO: Charmaine Vidrine, CPA, Chief Financial Officer
CMO: Neal J. Duhon, M.D., Chief of Staff
**Control:** Other not–for–profit (including NFP Corporation) **Service:** General
Medical and Surgical

**Staffed Beds: 178**

**COMPASS BEHAVIORAL CENTER OF CROWLEY (194085)**, 1526 North
Avenue I., Zip 70526–2434; tel. 337/788–3380 **A**9 10 **F**64 98 100 101 103
104 105 **P**8
Primary Contact: Aimee Monaghan, Administrator
Web address: www.compashealthcare.com
**Control:** Corporation, Investor–owned, for–profit **Service:** Psychiatric

**Staffed Beds: 18 Admissions: 297 Census: 9 Births: 0**

**CROWLEY REHABILITATION HOSPITAL (192050)**, 713 North Avenue L.,
Zip 70526–3832; tel. 337/783–2859 **A**10 **F**1 3 29
Primary Contact: Gil Pinac, Chief Executive Officer
**Control:** Corporation, Investor–owned, for–profit **Service:** Long–Term Acute Care
hospital

**Staffed Beds: 15 Admissions: 113 Census: 8 Outpatient Visits: 0 Births: 0
Personnel: 31**

## CUT OFF—Lafourche Parish

★ **LADY OF THE SEA GENERAL HOSPITAL (191325)**, 200 West 134th Place,
Zip 70345–4143; tel. 985/632–6401, (Nonreporting) **A**9 10 18 21
Primary Contact: Don Werner, Chief Executive Officer
CFO: Randy Tabor, Chief Financial Officer
CHR: Bennie Smith, Director Human Resources and Risk Management
Web address: www.losgh.org
**Control:** Hospital district or authority, Government, nonfederal **Service:** General
Medical and Surgical

**Staffed Beds: 25**

## DE RIDDER—Beauregard Parish

⊠ **BEAUREGARD MEMORIAL HOSPITAL (190050)**, 600 South Pine Street,
Zip 70634–4998, Mailing Address: P.O. Box 730, Zip 70634–0730;
tel. 337/462–7100 **A**1 9 10 **F**3 11 13 15 18 20 26 28 29 30 31 34 35 39 40
45 46 50 53 57 64 70 75 76 78 79 81 85 89 91 93 96 107 108 110 111
113 118 129 132 145 147 **P**6
Primary Contact: Theodore J. Badger, Jr., FACHE, Chief Executive Officer
CFO: Darrell L. Kingham, CPA, Vice President Finance
CMO: Chris Granger, M.D., President Medical Staff
CIO: Meg Jackson, Director Biomedical and Management Information Systems
CHR: Hope Leedom, Director Human Resources
CNO: Jackie Reviel, R.N., Vice President Patient Care Services
Web address: www.beauregard.org
**Control:** Hospital district or authority, Government, nonfederal **Service:** General
Medical and Surgical

**Staffed Beds: 60 Admissions: 2593 Census: 27 Outpatient Visits: 42560
Births: 323 Total Expense ($000): 32236 Payroll Expense ($000): 15448
Personnel: 332**

## DELHI—Richland Parish

**RICHLAND PARISH HOSPITAL (191323)**, 407 Cincinnati Street,
Zip 71232–3009; tel. 318/878–5171, (Nonreporting) **A**9 10 18
Primary Contact: Michael W. Carroll, Administrator
CIO: Barbra Hutchison, Director Medical Records
CHR: Patsy Stout, Director Personnel
Web address: www.delhihospital.com
**Control:** Hospital district or authority, Government, nonfederal **Service:** General
Medical and Surgical

**Staffed Beds: 25**

## DENHAM SPRINGS—Livingston Parish

**AMG SPECIALTY HOSPITAL–DENHAM SPRINGS (192008)**, 8375 Florida
Boulevard, Zip 70726; tel. 225/665–2664, (Nonreporting) **A**9 10 **S** AMG
Integrated Healthcare Management, Lafayette, LA
Primary Contact: Ricky Robeson, Administrator
Web address: www.amgihm.com/ltac_of_denham_springs
**Control:** Corporation, Investor–owned, for–profit **Service:** Long–Term Acute Care
hospital

**Staffed Beds: 117**

---

**Hospital, Medicare Provider Number, Address, Telephone, Approval, Facility, and Physician Codes, Health Care System**

★ American Hospital Association (AHA) membership
☐ The Joint Commission accreditation      ◇ DNV Healthcare Inc. accreditation
○ American Osteopathic Association (AOA) accreditation
△ Commission on Accreditation of Rehabilitation Facilities (CARF) accreditation

**LA**

## DEQUINCY—Calcasieu Parish

☐ **DEQUINCY MEMORIAL HOSPITAL (191307)**, 110 West Fourth Street, Zip 70633–3508, Mailing Address: P.O. Box 1166, Zip 70633–1166; tel. 337/786–1200, (Nonreporting) **A**1 9 10 18
Primary Contact: Michael Ashford, Administrator
CFO: Brandy Maddox, Chief Financial Officer
CMO: Jalal Joudeh, M.D., Chief of Staff
Web address: www.dequincyhospital.com
**Control:** City–Government, nonfederal **Service:** General Medical and Surgical

**Staffed Beds:** 19

**REHABILITATION HOSPITAL OF DEQUINCY**, 110 West Fourth Street, Zip 70633; tel. 337/786–6100, (Nonreporting)
Primary Contact: Heath Hairgrove, Administrator
Web address: www.triparishrehab.com
**Control:** Corporation, Investor–owned, for–profit **Service:** Rehabilitation

**Staffed Beds:** 13

## DERIDDER—Beauregard Parish

☐ **OCEANS BEHAVIORAL HOSPITAL OF DE RIDDER (194081)**, 1420 Blankenship Drive, Zip 70634–4604; tel. 337/460–9472 **A**1 9 10 **F**29 56 64 98 103 104 129 **P**5 **S** Oceans Healthcare, Lake Charles, LA
Primary Contact: Ronald E. Hand, Administrator
Web address: www.obhd.info/
**Control:** Corporation, Investor–owned, for–profit **Service:** Psychiatric

**Staffed Beds:** 20 **Admissions:** 345 **Census:** 16 **Outpatient Visits:** 0 **Births:** 0

## DONALDSONVILLE—Ascension Parish

☒ **PREVOST MEMORIAL HOSPITAL (191308)**, 301 Memorial Drive, Zip 70346–4376; tel. 225/473–7931, (Nonreporting) **A**1 9 10 18
Primary Contact: Vincent A. Cataldo, Administrator
CFO: Jane Arboneaux, Chief Financial Officer
CMO: Michel Y. Hirsch, M.D., Chief Medical Staff
CHR: Linda Cataldo, Human Resources Secretary
Web address: www.prevosthospital.net
**Control:** Hospital district or authority, Government, nonfederal **Service:** General Medical and Surgical

**Staffed Beds:** 25

## EUNICE—St. Landry Parish

**EUNICE EXTENDED CARE HOSPITAL**, 1879 Highway 190, Zip 70535; tel. 337/546–0024, (Nonreporting)
Primary Contact: Cayle P. Guillory, Administrator
**Control:** Other not–for–profit (including NFP Corporation) **Service:** Long–Term Acute Care hospital

**Staffed Beds:** 18

## FARMERVILLE—Union Parish

**LIBERTY HEALTHCARE SYSTEMS** See Serenity Springs Specialty Hospital

**SERENITY SPRINGS SPECIALTY HOSPITAL (194074)**, 309 North Main Street, Zip 71241; tel. 318/368–0110, (Nonreporting) **A**9 10
Primary Contact: Kendall Corkern, Administrator
Web address: www.serenityhospital.com
**Control:** Corporation, Investor–owned, for–profit **Service:** Psychiatric

**Staffed Beds:** 18

**UNION GENERAL HOSPITAL (191301)**, 901 James Avenue, Zip 71241–0398, Mailing Address: P.O. Box 398, Zip 71241–0398; tel. 318/368–9751 **A**9 10 18 **F**15 32 35 40 45 56 93 104 107 118 126 127 132 142
Primary Contact: Evalyn Ormond, Chief Executive Officer
CFO: William Adcock, Chief Financial Officer
CHR: Sheri Cooper, Director Human Resources
Web address: www.uniongen.com
**Control:** Other not–for–profit (including NFP Corporation) **Service:** General Medical and Surgical

**Staffed Beds:** 25 **Admissions:** 588 **Census:** 8 **Outpatient Visits:** 25934 **Total Expense ($000):** 10966 **Payroll Expense ($000):** 4309 **Personnel:** 104

## FERRIDAY—Concordia Parish

**RIVERLAND MEDICAL CENTER (191318)**, 1700 N.E. Wallace Boulevard, Zip 71334–0111, Mailing Address: P.O. Box 111, Zip 71334–0111; tel. 318/757–6551, (Nonreporting) **A**9 10 18
Primary Contact: Lana Stamper, Chief Executive Officer
CFO: Lynda Jones, Financial Officer
CFO: Lynda Jones, Financial Officer
CMO: J. Kevin Ingram, M.D., Chief of Staff
CIO: Nekisha Smith, Director Medical Records
CHR: Norma Jean Price, Manager Personnel
Web address: www.riverlandmedcenter.com/
**Control:** Church–operated, Nongovernment, not–for profit **Service:** General Medical and Surgical

**Staffed Beds:** 25

## FORT POLK—Vernon Parish

☒ **BAYNE–JONES ARMY COMMUNITY HOSPITAL**, 1585 3rd Street, Zip 71459–5102; tel. 337/531–3928 **A**1 9 **F**3 8 11 13 15 18 29 30 32 33 34 35 38 39 40 44 45 46 50 54 57 59 64 65 68 75 76 77 79 81 82 87 92 97 99 100 101 104 107 110 111 114 118 129 130 131 134 142 143 145 146 147 **S** Department of the Army, Office of the Surgeon General, Falls Church, VA
Primary Contact: Colonel David Dunning, Commander
COO: Lieutenant Colonel Jeffrey Hillard, FACHE, Deputy Commander for Administration
CFO: Captain Wayne Schintisen, Chief Resource Management Division
CMO: Colonel Glynda Lucas, M.D., Deputy Commander Clinical Services
CIO: Thomas Baker, Chief Information Management Division
CHR: Captain Lucinda Duncan, Chief Human Resources
Web address: www.polk.amedd.army.mil
**Control:** Army, Government, federal **Service:** General Medical and Surgical

**Staffed Beds:** 22 **Admissions:** 1135 **Census:** 7 **Outpatient Visits:** 195615 **Births:** 564 **Payroll Expense ($000):** 37376 **Personnel:** 719

## FRANKLIN—St. Mary Parish

☒ **FRANKLIN FOUNDATION HOSPITAL (191310)**, 1097 Northwest Boulevard, Zip 70538–3724, Mailing Address: P.O. Box 577, Zip 70538–0577; tel. 337/828–0760 **A**1 9 10 18 **F**3 11 13 15 18 28 29 34 40 45 50 57 59 68 70 74 75 76 77 79 81 85 93 107 110 111 113 118 132 134 145 146 147 **P**6 **S** QHR, Brentwood, TN
Primary Contact: Parker Templeton, FACHE, Chief Executive Officer
CFO: Ron Bailey, Chief Financial Officer
CMO: Jesus Chua, M.D., Chief of Staff
CMO: Sharad Gunda, M.D., Chief of Staff
CIO: Hal Goree, Chief Information Officer
CIO: John Spradlin, Information Systems Director
CHR: Elmo Vinas, Director Human Resources
CNO: Jennifer Wise, Chief Nursing Officer
Web address: www.franklinfoundation.org
**Control:** Hospital district or authority, Government, nonfederal **Service:** General Medical and Surgical

**Staffed Beds:** 22 **Admissions:** 991 **Census:** 14 **Outpatient Visits:** 22206 **Births:** 95 **Total Expense ($000):** 21097 **Payroll Expense ($000):** 9369 **Personnel:** 158

## FRANKLINTON—Washington Parish

☒ **RIVERSIDE MEDICAL CENTER (191313)**, 1900 Main Street, Zip 70438–3688; tel. 985/839–4431, (Nonreporting) **A**1 9 10 18
Primary Contact: Calvin Green, Chief Executive Officer
CFO: Patricia A. Mizell, Chief Financial Officer
CMO: Mark James, M.D., Chief of Staff
CIO: Herman Ingram, Director
CHR: John Seal, Director Human Resources
Web address: www.rmchospital.com
**Control:** Hospital district or authority, Government, nonfederal **Service:** General Medical and Surgical

**Staffed Beds:** 25

## GONZALES—Ascension Parish

☐ **ASCENSION GONZALES REHABILITATION HOSPITAL (193089)**, 333 East Worthy Road, Zip 70737; tel. 225/450–2231, (Nonreporting) **A**1 10
Primary Contact: Bruce Walker, MSN, R.N., Chief Executive Officer
COO: Shawanza L. Alston, Administrator
CMO: Rosiland Cropper, M.D., Medical Director
Web address: www.agrehab.com
**Control:** Corporation, Investor–owned, for–profit **Service:** Rehabilitation

**Staffed Beds:** 12

**SOUTH BATON ROUGE REHABILITATION HOSPITAL** See Ascension Gonzales Rehabilitation Hospital

*Many Facility Codes have changed. Please refer to the AHA Guide Code Chart.* © 2012 AHA Guide

★ **ST. ELIZABETH HOSPITAL (190242)**, 1125 West Highway 30, Zip 70737–5004; tel. 225/647–5000 **A**9 10 **F**3 8 11 12 15 29 30 34 35 40 43 45 46 47 48 49 51 57 59 66 70 74 75 79 80 81 82 85 107 108 110 111 113 114 118 129 132 145 **P**6 **S** Franciscan Missionaries of Our Lady Health System, Inc., Baton Rouge, LA
Primary Contact: Dolores N. LeJeune, R.N., President and Chief Executive Officer
COO: Sue Knight, CPA, Chief Operating Officer
CFO: Scott Richard, Vice President Finance and Chief Financial Officer
CMO: Craig Vitrano, M.D., Medical Director
CIO: Joe Bumpus, Director Information Technology
CHR: Victor Vidaurre, Assistant Vice President Human Resources
Web address: www.steh.com
**Control:** Church–operated, Nongovernment, not–for profit **Service:** General Medical and Surgical

| | |
|---|---|
| **Staffed Beds:** 48 **Admissions:** 2876 **Census:** 29 **Outpatient Visits:** 266403 **Births:** 0 **Total Expense ($000):** 81023 **Payroll Expense ($000):** 37995 **Personnel:** 687 | |

**ST. JAMES BEHAVIORAL HEALTH HOSPITAL (194088)**, 3136 South Saint Landry Road, Zip 70737–5801; tel. 225/647–7524, (Nonreporting) **A**10
Primary Contact: Rick Bennett, Administrator
COO: Wendell Smith, Chief Operating Officer
CFO: Gopinath Gopalam, Chief Financial Officer
CMO: Lance Bullock, M.D., Medical Director
CHR: Charla Burchfield, Manager Human Resources
Web address: www.sjbhh.com/
**Control:** Corporation, Investor–owned, for–profit **Service:** Psychiatric

**Staffed Beds:** 10

**GREENSBURG—St. Helena Parish**

**ST. HELENA PARISH HOSPITAL (191300)**, 16874 Highway 43, Zip 70441–4834; tel. 225/222–6111, (Nonreporting) **A**9 10 18
Primary Contact: Naveed Awan, FACHE, Chief Executive Officer
CFO: Ken Cox, Chief Financial Officer
CMO: Anjanette Varnado, M.D., Chief Medical Officer
CHR: Lorraine L. Ballard, Director Human Resources
Web address: www.sthelenaparishhospital.com
**Control:** Other not–for–profit (including NFP Corporation) **Service:** General Medical and Surgical

**Staffed Beds:** 25

**GRETNA—Jefferson Parish**

**MEADOWCREST SPECIALTY HOSPITAL** See Oceans Specialty Hospital of Gretna

**OCEANS SPECIALTY HOSPITAL OF GRETNA (192014)**, 535 Commerce Street, Suite B., Zip 70056–7316; tel. 504/391–1500, (Nonreporting) **A**10
**S** Oceans Healthcare, Lake Charles, LA
Primary Contact: Michael Rabalais, Chief Executive Officer
Web address: www.oshla.info
**Control:** Corporation, Investor–owned, for–profit **Service:** Long–Term Acute Care hospital

**Staffed Beds:** 27

**UNITED MEDICAL HEALTHWEST–NEW ORLEANS (193074)**, 3201 Wall Boulevard, Suite B., Zip 70056; tel. 504/433–5551, (Nonreporting) **A**10
Primary Contact: Hugh Cassidy, Administrator
**Control:** Individual, Investor–owned, for–profit **Service:** Rehabilitation

**Staffed Beds:** 15

**HAMMOND—Tangipahoa Parish**

**CYPRESS POINTE SURGICAL HOSPITAL (190303)**, 42570 South Airport Road, Zip 70403–0946; tel. 985/510–6200, (Nonreporting) **A**10 21
Primary Contact: Don Trexler, Chief Executive Officer
Web address: www.cypresspointsurgical.com
**Control:** Other not–for–profit (including NFP Corporation) **Service:** Surgical

**Staffed Beds:** 24

⊠ △ **NORTH OAKS MEDICAL CENTER (190015)**, 15790 Paul Vega, M. D. Drive, Zip 70403–1436, Mailing Address: PO Box 2668, Zip 70404–2668; tel. 985/345–2700 **A**1 7 9 10 19 **F**3 13 15 18 20 22 24 26 28 29 30 31 32 34 40 45 50 54 56 57 58 59 63 64 68 70 72 73 74 75 76 77 78 79 81 82 84 85 86 87 89 93 94 96 102 103 107 108 110 111 113 114 117 118 125 128 129 130 131 134 142 143 145 146 147 **P**6 **S** North Oaks Health System, Hammond, LA
Primary Contact: James E. Cathey, Jr., President and Chief Executive Officer
COO: Michele K. Sutton, Executive Vice President and Chief Operating Officer
CFO: Shirley Hsing, Senior Vice President and Chief Financial Officer
CMO: Robert Peltier, M.D., Senior Vice President and Chief Medical Officer
CIO: Chris Smith, Vice President Information Technology
CHR: Carolyn Adema, Senior Vice President Human Resources
CNO: Shelly Welch, R.N., Senior Vice President and Chief Nursing Officer
Web address: www.northoaks.org
**Control:** Hospital district or authority, Government, nonfederal **Service:** General Medical and Surgical

| | |
|---|---|
| **Staffed Beds:** 255 **Admissions:** 12953 **Census:** 187 **Outpatient Visits:** 350829 **Births:** 1495 **Total Expense ($000):** 237063 **Payroll Expense ($000):** 124276 **Personnel:** 2225 | |

☐ **NORTH OAKS REHABILITATION HOSPITAL (193044)**, 1900 South Morrison Boulevard, Zip 70403; tel. 504/230–5700 **A**1 9 10 **F**29 56 75 86 87 90 103 129 131 142 **P**6 **S** North Oaks Health System, Hammond, LA
Primary Contact: Sybil K. Paulson, R.N., Administrator
Web address: www.northoaks.org
**Control:** Hospital district or authority, Government, nonfederal **Service:** Rehabilitation

| | |
|---|---|
| **Staffed Beds:** 27 **Admissions:** 519 **Census:** 17 **Outpatient Visits:** 0 **Births:** 0 **Total Expense ($000):** 13445 **Payroll Expense ($000):** 3176 **Personnel:** 69 | |

☐ **SPECIALTY LONG TERM ACUTE CARE HOSPITAL OF HAMMOND (192036)**, 42074 Veterans Avenue, Zip 70403; tel. 985/902–8148, (Nonreporting) **A**1 10 **S** Specialty Healthcare, LLC, Leesville, LA
Primary Contact: Charles Ball, Administrator
Web address: www.specialtyltchhammond.com
**Control:** Corporation, Investor–owned, for–profit **Service:** Long–Term Acute Care hospital

**Staffed Beds:** 20

**UNITED MEDICAL REHABILITATION HOSPITAL (193079)**, 15717 Belle Drive, Zip 70403; tel. 985/340–5998, (Nonreporting) **A**10
Primary Contact: Cyrillia Bonds, Administrator
CFO: Warren Swenson, Chief Financial Officer
CMO: Luis Franco, M.D., Medical Director
CHR: Mark Gros, Director Human Resources
Web address: www.umrhospital.com
**Control:** Corporation, Investor–owned, for–profit **Service:** Rehabilitation

**Staffed Beds:** 20

**HOMER—Claiborne Parish**

**HOMER MEMORIAL HOSPITAL (190114)**, 620 East College Street, Zip 71040–3202; tel. 318/927–2024 **A**9 10 **F**3 13 15 29 35 38 40 45 56 57 64 65 70 75 76 81 85 86 89 98 101 103 107 108 113 118 127 129 131 132 134 142 147
Primary Contact: Scott G. Barrilleaux, FACHE, Chief Executive Officer
CFO: Michael Randle, Chief Financial Officer
CMO: Mark Haynes, M.D., Chief of Staff
CIO: Vance Robinson, Chief Information Officer
CHR: William Colvin, Human Resources Officer
Web address: www.homerhospital.com
**Control:** City–Government, nonfederal **Service:** General Medical and Surgical

| | |
|---|---|
| **Staffed Beds:** 60 **Admissions:** 1994 **Census:** 32 **Outpatient Visits:** 18344 **Births:** 11 **Total Expense ($000):** 11381 **Payroll Expense ($000):** 7661 **Personnel:** 202 | |

**HOUMA—Terrebonne Parish**

**AMG SPECIALTY HOSPITAL–HOUMA (192037)**, 629 Dunn Street, Zip 70360–4707; tel. 985/274–0001, (Nonreporting) **A**10 **S** AMG Integrated Healthcare Management, Lafayette, LA
Primary Contact: Ricky Robeson, Chief Executive Officer
**Control:** Corporation, Investor–owned, for–profit **Service:** Long–Term Acute Care hospital

**Staffed Beds:** 40

---

| Hospital, Medicare Provider Number, Address, Telephone, Approval, Facility, and Physician Codes, Health Care System | |
|---|---|
| ★ American Hospital Association (AHA) membership | ○ American Osteopathic Association (AOA) accreditation |
| ☐ The Joint Commission accreditation ◇ DNV Healthcare Inc. accreditation | △ Commission on Accreditation of Rehabilitation Facilities (CARF) accreditation |

☐ **LEONARD J. CHABERT MEDICAL CENTER (190183)**, 1978 Industrial Boulevard, Zip 70363–7094; tel. 985/873–2200 **A**1 3 5 9 10 **F**3 13 15 18 20 29 30 31 32 39 40 45 48 49 50 58 59 60 61 64 65 66 70 72 73 74 75 76 77 78 79 81 82 84 85 86 87 89 93 97 98 107 108 111 114 118 129 134 145 146 147 **P**4 **S** LSU Health Care Services Division, Baton Rouge, LA
Primary Contact: Rhonda G. Green, Administrator
CFO: Elizabeth Callais, Chief Fiscal Officer
CMO: Michael Garcia, M.D., Medical Director
CIO: Susan Arceneaux, R.N., Coordinator Information Technology
CHR: Bain Manning, Director Human Resources
Web address: www.lsuhsc.edu/hcsd/ljc
**Control:** State–Government, nonfederal **Service:** General Medical and Surgical

**Staffed Beds:** 87 **Admissions:** 4837 **Census:** 66 **Outpatient Visits:** 217353 **Births:** 426 **Total Expense ($000):** 108446 **Payroll Expense ($000):** 40074 **Personnel:** 964

**PHYSICIANS ALLIANCE HOSPITAL OF HOUMA** See AMG Specialty Hospital–Houma

**PHYSICIANS MEDICAL CENTER (190241)**, 218 Corporate Drive, Zip 70360–2764; tel. 985/853–1390, (Nonreporting) **A**9 10
Primary Contact: Connie Martin, Administrator
**Control:** Corporation, Investor–owned, for–profit **Service:** Other specialty

**Staffed Beds:** 10

⊞ △ **TERREBONNE GENERAL MEDICAL CENTER (190008)**, 8166 Main Street, Zip 70360–3498, Mailing Address: P.O. Box 6037, Zip 70361–6037; tel. 985/873–4141, (Total facility includes 8 beds in nursing home–type unit) **A**1 2 7 9 10 **F**8 11 13 14 15 17 18 20 22 24 26 29 30 31 34 35 40 44 49 50 57 58 59 64 65 68 70 72 74 75 76 77 78 79 81 82 84 85 86 87 89 90 92 93 107 108 109 110 111 113 114 116 117 118 120 122 123 127 129 131 133 134 145 146 147 **P**3 6
Primary Contact: Phyllis Peoples, MSN, R.N., President and Chief Executive Officer
COO: Diane Yeates, Chief Operating Officer
CFO: Dean Verret, Vice President Financial Services
CMO: Richard Abben, M.D., Chief of Staff
CHR: Mickie Rousseau, Director Human Resources
CNO: Teresita McNabb, R.N., Vice President Nursing Services
Web address: www.tgmc.com
**Control:** Hospital district or authority, Government, nonfederal **Service:** General Medical and Surgical

**Staffed Beds:** 218 **Admissions:** 9881 **Census:** 132 **Outpatient Visits:** 114195 **Births:** 1860 **Total Expense ($000):** 165256 **Payroll Expense ($000):** 63505 **Personnel:** 1213

### INDEPENDENCE—Tangipahoa Parish

☐ **LALLIE KEMP MEDICAL CENTER (191321)**, 52579 Highway 51 South, Zip 70443–2231; tel. 985/878–9421 **A**1 3 5 9 10 18 **F**3 15 18 29 31 34 35 40 45 50 56 59 61 64 65 66 70 75 78 79 81 85 86 87 97 107 108 113 118 127 129 131 132 134 145 146 **P**6 **S** LSU Health Care Services Division, Baton Rouge, LA
Primary Contact: Sherre Pack–Hookfin, Administrator
COO: Lisa G. Bruhl, Chief Operating Officer
CFO: Chad Thompson, Chief Financial Officer
CMO: Kathy Willis, M.D., Medical Director
CIO: Charles Tate, Director Information Technology
CHR: Diane Farnham, Acting Director Human Resources
Web address: www.lsuhospitals.org
**Control:** State–Government, nonfederal **Service:** General Medical and Surgical

**Staffed Beds:** 25 **Admissions:** 1173 **Census:** 12 **Outpatient Visits:** 110715 **Births:** 0 **Total Expense ($000):** 44201 **Payroll Expense ($000):** 19210 **Personnel:** 400

### JACKSON—East Feliciana Parish

☐ **EASTERN LOUISIANA MENTAL HEALTH SYSTEM (194008)**, 4502 Highway 951, Zip 70748–5842, Mailing Address: P.O. Box 498, Zip 70748–0498; tel. 225/634–0100, (Nonreporting) **A**1 10 **S** Louisiana State Hospitals, Baton Rouge, LA
Primary Contact: Patricia Gonzales, Chief Executive Officer
COO: Hampton P S Lea, Chief Operating Officer
CFO: Janet O'Dell, Administrative Director
CMO: John W. Thompson, M.D., Chief of Staff
CIO: Deborah Brandon, Director Total Quality Management
CHR: Evelyn Perkins, Director Human Resources
Web address: www.dhh.louisiana.gov/offices/locations.asp?ID=62&Detail=126
**Control:** State–Government, nonfederal **Service:** Psychiatric

**Staffed Beds:** 593

**VILLA FELICIANA MEDICAL COMPLEX (190199)**, 5002 Highway 10, Zip 70748–3627, Mailing Address: P.O. Box 438, Zip 70748–0438; tel. 225/634–4017, (Nonreporting) **A**10
Primary Contact: Michael C. Crump, Administrator
CFO: Kim Jelks, Fiscal Officer
CMO: John F. Piker, M.D., Medical Director
CIO: Michael James, Information Technology Technical Support Specialist 1
CHR: Sandra Delatte, Director Human Resources
CNO: Linda Williams, Director of Nursing
Web address: www.dhh.state.la.us/
**Control:** State–Government, nonfederal **Service:** Other specialty

**Staffed Beds:** 10

### JENA—La Salle Parish

★ **LASALLE GENERAL HOSPITAL (190145)**, 187 Ninth Street, Zip 71342–2780, Mailing Address: P.O. Box 2780, Zip 71342–2780; tel. 318/992–9200 **A**9 10 **F**7 11 15 24 29 40 45 53 57 59 62 64 71 81 89 93 107 108 110 113 117 118 126 129 132 **P**6
Primary Contact: Douglas A. Newman, Chief Executive Officer
CHR: Allyson Fannin, Director Human Resources
Web address: www.lasallegeneralhospital.com
**Control:** Hospital district or authority, Government, nonfederal **Service:** General Medical and Surgical

**Staffed Beds:** 49 **Admissions:** 968 **Census:** 12 **Outpatient Visits:** 26127 **Births:** 0 **Total Expense ($000):** 16532 **Payroll Expense ($000):** 9261 **Personnel:** 249

### JENNINGS—Jefferson Davis Parish

☐ **JENNINGS AMERICAN LEGION HOSPITAL (190053)**, 1634 Elton Road, Zip 70546–3614; tel. 337/616–7000, (Nonreporting) **A**1 9 10
Primary Contact: Dana D. Williams, Chief Executive Officer
COO: Keith J. Simpson, Chief Operating Officer
CFO: Pam Primeaux, Chief Financial Officer
CIO: Gary Courrege, Chief Information Officer
CHR: Ruth Carnes, Manager Human Resources
Web address: www.jalh.com
**Control:** Other not–for–profit (including NFP Corporation) **Service:** General Medical and Surgical

**Staffed Beds:** 60

**JENNINGS SENIOR CARE HOSPITAL (194082)**, 1 Hospital Drive, Suite 201, Zip 70546–3641; tel. 337/785–8003, (Nonreporting) **A**9 10
Primary Contact: April Bearb, Administrator
**Control:** Corporation, Investor–owned, for–profit **Service:** General Medical and Surgical

**Staffed Beds:** 18

**REHABILITATION HOSPITAL OF JENNINGS (193067)**, 1 Hospital Drive. Suite 101, Zip 70546–3641; tel. 337/821–5353 **A**10 **F**29 34 56 62 75 77 90 129 147
Primary Contact: Michael Holland, M.D., Chief Executive Officer
**Control:** State–Government, nonfederal **Service:** Rehabilitation

**Staffed Beds:** 16 **Admissions:** 228 **Census:** 8 **Outpatient Visits:** 0 **Births:** 0 **Total Expense ($000):** 1783 **Payroll Expense ($000):** 1234 **Personnel:** 49

**WESTEND HOSPITAL (194075)**, 1530 Highway 90 West, Zip 70546; tel. 337/616–8122, (Nonreporting) **A**10
CFO: Ronnie Callais, Chief Financial Officer
CMO: Charles Bramliet, M.D., Medical Director
CHR: Gloria Conner, Director Human Resources
Web address: www.westendhospital.com
**Control:** Corporation, Investor–owned, for–profit **Service:** Psychiatric

**Staffed Beds:** 20

### JONESBORO—Jackson Parish

**JACKSON PARISH HOSPITAL (191317)**, 165 Beech Springs Road, Zip 71251–2059; tel. 318/259–4435, (Nonreporting) **A**9 10 18
Primary Contact: Lloyd Monger, Chief Executive Officer
CFO: David Sanders, Chief Financial Officer
CHR: Elizabeth Cheatwood, Human Resource Director and Administrative Assistant
Web address: www.jacksonparishhospital.com
**Control:** Hospital district or authority, Government, nonfederal **Service:** General Medical and Surgical

**Staffed Beds:** 25

*Many Facility Codes have changed. Please refer to the AHA Guide Code Chart.* © 2012 AHA Guide

## KAPLAN—Vermilion Parish

**ABROM KAPLAN MEMORIAL HOSPITAL (191322)**, 1310 West Seventh Street, Zip 70548–2998; tel. 337/643–8300, (Nonreporting) **A**9 10 18
Primary Contact: Lyman Trahan, Chief Executive Officer
CFO: Mary Melancon, Chief Financial Officer
CMO: Scott Bergeaux, M.D., Chief Medical Staff
Web address: www.lafayettegeneral.com
**Control:** Hospital district or authority, Government, nonfederal **Service:** General Medical and Surgical

**Staffed Beds:** 35

## KENNER—Jefferson Parish

**LOUISIANA EXTENDED CARE HOSPITAL OF KENNER** See Ochsner Extended Care Hospital of Kenner

**OCEANS BEHAVIORAL HOSPITAL OF GREATER NEW ORLEANS (194098)**, 716 Village Road, Zip 70065–2751; tel. 504/464–8895, (Nonreporting) **A**9 10 **S** Oceans Healthcare, Lake Charles, LA
Primary Contact: Deborah Spier, Administrator
Web address: www.obhgno.info/
**Control:** Corporation, Investor–owned, for–profit **Service:** Psychiatric

**Staffed Beds:** 18

☐ **OCHSNER EXTENDED CARE HOSPITAL OF KENNER (192015)**, 180 West Esplanade Avenue, 5th Floor, Zip 70065–2467; tel. 504/464–8590, (Nonreporting) **A**1 10 **S** LHC Group, Lafayette, LA
Primary Contact: Fritz Nelson, Administrator
Web address: www.lhcgroup.com/
**Control:** Corporation, Investor–owned, for–profit **Service:** Long–Term Acute Care hospital

**Staffed Beds:** 34

⌧ **OCHSNER MEDICAL CENTER – KENNER (190274)**, 180 West Esplanade Avenue, Zip 70065–6001; tel. 504/468–8600 **A**1 3 5 8 9 10 **F**3 13 15 18 20 22 24 26 28 29 30 34 35 37 40 43 45 46 47 49 54 56 57 58 59 60 63 64 65 68 70 72 74 75 76 77 78 79 81 84 85 87 93 97 102 107 108 110 111 114 118 119 123 128 129 130 131 134 145 146 147 **S** Ochsner Health System, New Orleans, LA
Primary Contact: Paolo Zambito, Chief Executive Officer
COO: Eddy Ramirez, Vice President Operations
CFO: Mark Eckert, Vice President Finance
CMO: James Tebbe, M.D., Vice President Medical Affairs
CIO: Dere Krummel, Director Information Systems
CHR: Wendy L. Willis, Assistant Vice President Human Resources
Web address: www.ochsner.org/locations/ochsner_health_center_kenner_w_esplanade_ave/
**Control:** Other not–for–profit (including NFP Corporation) **Service:** General Medical and Surgical

**Staffed Beds:** 119 **Admissions:** 5456 **Census:** 56 **Outpatient Visits:** 101542 **Births:** 1234 **Total Expense ($000):** 89546 **Payroll Expense ($000):** 32168 **Personnel:** 606

## KENTWOOD—Tangipahoa Parish

**OCEANS BEHAVIORAL HOSPITAL OF KENTWOOD (194091)**, 921 Avenue G., Zip 70444–2636; tel. 985/229–0717, (Nonreporting) **A**9 10 **S** Oceans Healthcare, Lake Charles, LA
Primary Contact: Robert Pound, Administrator
Web address: www.obhk.info/
**Control:** Corporation, Investor–owned, for–profit **Service:** Psychiatric

**Staffed Beds:** 18

**SOUTHEAST REGIONAL MEDICAL CENTER (192040)**, 719 Avenue G., Zip 70444–2601; tel. 985/229–9193, (Nonreporting) **A**10
Primary Contact: Lionel Murphy, Chief Executive Officer
**Control:** Corporation, Investor–owned, for–profit **Service:** Long–Term Acute Care hospital

**Staffed Beds:** 14

## KINDER—Allen Parish

★ **ALLEN PARISH HOSPITAL (190133)**, 108 Sixth Avenue, Zip 70648–3519, Mailing Address: P.O. Box 1670, Zip 70648–1670; tel. 337/738–2527 **A**9 10 **F**3 29 34 40 45 50 57 59 62 80 89 93 98 107 111 118 126 127 129 132 **P**6
Primary Contact: Terry Willet, Chief Executive Officer
CFO: Suzette Fatula, Chief Financial Officer
CMO: Ejiro Ughouwa, M.D., Chief of Staff
CIO: Bill Marcantel, Chief Information Systems
CHR: Amand Lambert, Director Human Resources
Web address: www.allenparishhospital.com
**Control:** Hospital district or authority, Government, nonfederal **Service:** General Medical and Surgical

**Staffed Beds:** 49 **Admissions:** 1169 **Census:** 23 **Outpatient Visits:** 33831 **Births:** 0 **Total Expense ($000):** 9643 **Payroll Expense ($000):** 5842 **Personnel:** 162

## LA PLACE—St. John The Baptist Parish

⌧ **RIVER PARISHES HOSPITAL (190175)**, 500 Rue De Sante, Zip 70068–5418; tel. 985/652–7000, (Nonreporting) **A**1 9 10 **S** LifePoint Hospitals, Inc., Brentwood, TN
Primary Contact: Gerald A. Fornoff, Interim Chief Executive Officer
CFO: Thomas Ramsey, Chief Financial Officer
CMO: Andrew St. Martin, M.D., Chief of Staff
CHR: Katherine Trepagnier, Director Human Resources
CNO: Joyce Neville, Chief Nursing Officer
Web address: www.riverparisheshospital.com
**Control:** Corporation, Investor–owned, for–profit **Service:** General Medical and Surgical

**Staffed Beds:** 106

## LACOMBE—St. Tammany Parish

☐ **LOUISIANA MEDICAL CENTER AND HEART HOSPITAL (190250)**, 64030 Highway 434, Zip 70445–3456; tel. 985/690–7500, (Nonreporting) **A**1 9 10
Primary Contact: Charles D. Nasem, FACHE, President and Chief Executive Officer
CFO: Christopher W. Daniel, Chief Financial Officer
CMO: Vasanth Bethala, M.D., Medical Director
CIO: Alan Chapman, Director Information Systems
CHR: Alana Roche, Director Human Resources
CNO: Glenda Dobson, Vice President Clinical Services
Web address: www.louisianaheart.com
**Control:** Corporation, Investor–owned, for–profit **Service:** Heart

**Staffed Beds:** 58

**MAGNOLIA BEHAVIORAL HEALTHCARE (194080)**, 64026 Highway 434, Suite 300, Zip 70445–5412; tel. 985/882–0226, (Nonreporting) **A**9 10
Primary Contact: Gerry Morris, Administrator
Web address: www.magnoliabehavioralhealth.com
**Control:** Corporation, Investor–owned, for–profit **Service:** Psychiatric

**Staffed Beds:** 15

## LAFAYETTE—Lafayette Parish

**ACADIA VERMILION HOSPITAL (194044)**, 2520 North University Avenue, Zip 70507–5306; tel. 337/234–5614 **A**9 10 **F**29 64 98 99 101 103 104 105 129 **P**5 **S** Acadia Healthcare Company, Inc., Franklin, TN
Primary Contact: Joseph Rodriguez, Chief Executive Officer
CFO: Doug Lahasky, Chief Financial Officer
CMO: Bob Winston, M.D., Medical Director
CHR: Claire Rowland, Director Human Resources
Web address: www.vermilionhospital.com
**Control:** Corporation, Investor–owned, for–profit **Service:** Psychiatric

**Staffed Beds:** 54 **Admissions:** 2156 **Census:** 44 **Outpatient Visits:** 4343 **Births:** 0 **Total Expense ($000):** 10197 **Payroll Expense ($000):** 5265 **Personnel:** 59

**AMG SPECIALTY HOSPITAL – LAFAYETTE (192029)**, 310 Youngsville Highway, Zip 70508; tel. 337/839–9880 **A**10 **F**1 3 29 30 34 35 50 56 60 75 77 79 91 118 129 134 142 147 **P**5 **S** AMG Integrated Healthcare Management, Lafayette, LA
Primary Contact: Jason Branson, Chief Executive Officer
CFO: Jessica McGee, Chief Financial Officer
CMO: Bradley Blappert, M.D., Chief Medical Officer
CHR: Heather Lamarche, Manager Human Resources
CNO: Mary Bollich, Director of Nurses
Web address: www.amglafayette.com
**Control:** Corporation, Investor–owned, for–profit **Service:** General Medical and Surgical

**Staffed Beds:** 58 **Admissions:** 425 **Census:** 27 **Outpatient Visits:** 0 **Births:** 0 **Personnel:** 85

---

**Hospital, Medicare Provider Number, Address, Telephone, Approval, Facility, and Physician Codes, Health Care System**

★ American Hospital Association (AHA) membership
☐ The Joint Commission accreditation
◇ DNV Healthcare Inc. accreditation
○ American Osteopathic Association (AOA) accreditation
△ Commission on Accreditation of Rehabilitation Facilities (CARF) accreditation

**LA**

✠ **AMG SPECIALTY HOSPITAL–LAFAYETTE REGIONAL CAMPUS (190205)**, 2810 Ambassador Caffery Parkway, Zip 70506–5906; tel. 337/981–2949, (Includes WOMEN'S AND CHILDREN'S HOSPITAL, 4600 Ambassador Caffery Parkway, Zip 70508–6923, Mailing Address: P.O. Box 88030, Zip 70598–8030; tel. 337/521–9100; Kathy J. Bobbs, FACHE, Chief Executive Officer), (Nonreporting) **A**1 9 10 **S** HCA, Nashville, TN
Primary Contact: Kathy J. Bobbs, FACHE, Interim Chief Executive Officer
COO: Mario J. Garner, FACHE, Chief Operating Officer
CFO: James Miller, CPA, Chief Financial Officer
CMO: Charles Wyatt, M.D., Medical Director
CHR: Jane Fuller, Director Human Resources
Web address: www.medicalcenterofacadiana.com
**Control:** Corporation, Investor–owned, for–profit **Service:** General Medical and Surgical

**Staffed Beds:** 142

**COMMUNITY SPECIALTY HOSPITAL (192020)**, 408 S.E. Evangeline Thruway, Zip 70501–7129; tel. 337/234–4031, (Nonreporting) **A**10
Primary Contact: Mark Goff, Owner and Administrator
COO: John E. Jumonville, III, Chief Operating Officer
CFO: Carolyn Guidry, Business Manager
CMO: John Charles Dugal, M.D., Medical Director
**Control:** Corporation, Investor–owned, for–profit **Service:** Rehabilitation

**Staffed Beds:** 22

✠ **HEART HOSPITAL OF LAFAYETTE (190263)**, 1105 Kaliste Saloom, Zip 70508; tel. 337/521–1000 **A**1 9 10 **F**3 17 18 20 22 24 26 28 29 30 34 35 40 46 50 57 59 64 68 74 75 81 85 87 107 108 114 134
Primary Contact: Donna Landry, Interim Administrator
CFO: James P. Barbuat, Chief Financial Officer
CHR: Thomas Duhon, Director Human Resources
Web address: www.hearthospitallafayette.com
**Control:** Partnership, Investor–owned, for–profit **Service:** Heart

**Staffed Beds:** 32 **Admissions:** 2012 **Census:** 18 **Outpatient Visits:** 20405 **Births:** 0 **Total Expense ($000):** 33438 **Payroll Expense ($000):** 10327 **Personnel:** 164

✠ **KINDRED HOSPITAL LAFAYETTE (192033)**, 204 Energy Parkway, Zip 70508–3816; tel. 337/232–1905 **A**1 10 **F**1 3 29 30 34 35 56 57 59 74 75 77 78 79 85 86 87 91 96 107 134 142 147 **S** Kindred Healthcare, Louisville, KY
Primary Contact: Sharon Black, Chief Executive Officer
CFO: Eva De La Paz, Regional Controller
CMO: Vitalis C. Okechukwu, M.D., President Medical Staff
CHR: Donna Stelly, Human Resources Coordinator
CNO: Major Stephanie Rossyion, Chief Clinical Officer
Web address: www.khlafayette.com
**Control:** Corporation, Investor–owned, for–profit **Service:** Long–Term Acute Care hospital

**Staffed Beds:** 50 **Admissions:** 452 **Census:** 31 **Outpatient Visits:** 0 **Births:** 0 **Total Expense ($000):** 13082 **Payroll Expense ($000):** 6877 **Personnel:** 151

✠ **LAFAYETTE GENERAL MEDICAL CENTER (190002)**, 1214 Coolidge Avenue, Zip 70503–2696, Mailing Address: P.O. Box 52009 OCS, Zip 70505–2009; tel. 337/289–7991 **A**1 2 9 10 **F**3 5 8 10 11 12 13 15 18 19 20 21 22 23 24 26 28 29 30 31 35 40 45 47 48 49 50 53 54 56 57 59 64 65 70 72 74 75 76 77 78 79 81 84 85 87 88 89 90 100 102 103 107 108 110 111 113 116 117 118 119 120 122 123 125 129 131 134 143 145 146 147 **P**8
Primary Contact: David L. Callecod, FACHE, President and Chief Executive Officer
COO: Patrick W. Gandy, Chief Operating Officer
CFO: Roger Mattke, Chief Financial Officer
CMO: Ziad Ashkar, M.D., Chief Medical Officer
CIO: Edwina Mallery, Vice President Information Systems
CHR: Sheena Mitchell, Director Human Resources
CNO: Rebecca Benoit, R.N., Chief Nursing Officer
Web address: www.lafayettegeneral.org
**Control:** Other not–for–profit (including NFP Corporation) **Service:** General Medical and Surgical

**Staffed Beds:** 319 **Admissions:** 14069 **Census:** 193 **Outpatient Visits:** 170327 **Births:** 1914 **Total Expense ($000):** 204220 **Payroll Expense ($000):** 82247 **Personnel:** 1837

**LAFAYETTE GENERAL SURGICAL HOSPITAL (190268)**, 1000 West Pinhook Road, Zip 70503; tel. 337/289–8088 **A**9 10 **F**3 29 51 68 81 140 **P**2
Primary Contact: Carrie E. Templeton, FACHE, Chief Executive Officer
CFO: Sandi Hernandez, Controller
CNO: Susan Woollen, R.N., Director of Nursing
Web address: www.lgsh.us
**Control:** Partnership, Investor–owned, for–profit **Service:** General Medical and Surgical

**Staffed Beds:** 10 **Admissions:** 44 **Census:** 1 **Outpatient Visits:** 7151 **Births:** 0 **Personnel:** 49

**LAFAYETTE PHYSICAL REHABILITATION HOSPITAL (193093)**, 307 Polly Lane, Zip 70508–4960; tel. 337/314–1111, (Nonreporting) **A**10 **S** AMG Integrated Healthcare Management, Lafayette, LA
Primary Contact: Jonathan Landreth, Chief Executive Officer
**Control:** Corporation, Investor–owned, for–profit **Service:** Rehabilitation

**Staffed Beds:** 32

☐ **LAFAYETTE SURGICAL SPECIALTY HOSPITAL (190259)**, 1101 Kaliste Saloom Road, Zip 70508; tel. 337/769–4100, (Nonreporting) **A**1 9 10 **S** National Surgical Hospitals, Chicago, IL
Primary Contact: Buffy Domingue, Chief Executive Officer
Web address: www.lafayettesurgical.com
**Control:** Corporation, Investor–owned, for–profit **Service:** Surgical

**Staffed Beds:** 20

**LONG TERM ACUTE CARE OF ACADIANA** See AMG Specialty Hospital – Lafayette

**LOUISIANA EXTENDED CARE HOSPITAL OF LAFAYETTE (192032)**, 1214 Coolidge Boulevard, 8th Floor, Zip 70503–2621; tel. 337/289–8180, (Nonreporting) **A**10 **S** LHC Group, Lafayette, LA
Primary Contact: Kevin Frank, Administrator
Web address: www.lhcgroup.com
**Control:** Other not–for–profit (including NFP Corporation) **Service:** Long–Term Acute Care hospital

**Staffed Beds:** 42

**MEADOWBROOK SPECIALTY HOSPITAL OF LAFAYETTE** See Kindred Hospital Lafayette

**OPTIMA SPECIALTY HOSPITAL (194078)**, 1131 Rue De Belier, Zip 70506–6532; tel. 337/991–0571, (Nonreporting) **A**10
Primary Contact: Michael E. Geissler, Chief Executive Officer
Web address: www.optimaspecialtyhospital.com/
**Control:** Corporation, Investor–owned, for–profit **Service:** General Medical and Surgical

**Staffed Beds:** 24

✠ **OUR LADY OF LOURDES REGIONAL MEDICAL CENTER (190102)**, 611 St. Landry Street, Zip 70506–4627, Mailing Address: P.O. Box 4027, Zip 70502–4027; tel. 337/289–2000 **A**1 2 9 10 **F**3 9 11 12 15 16 17 18 20 22 24 26 28 29 30 31 32 34 35 38 40 42 43 45 46 47 48 49 50 51 53 54 57 58 59 60 64 65 66 67 68 70 71 74 75 77 78 79 81 82 84 85 86 87 90 93 96 107 108 110 111 113 114 115 116 117 118 125 126 128 129 131 133 134 142 143 144 145 146 147 **P**6 **S** Franciscan Missionaries of Our Lady Health System, Inc., Baton Rouge, LA
Primary Contact: William F. Barrow, II, President and Chief Executive Officer
COO: Robert Davis, III, M.D., Chief Operating Officer
CFO: Kim Hebert, Chief Financial Officer
CMO: Andy Blalock, M.D., Physician Executive
CIO: Nona Mire, Director Information Systems
CHR: Kevin Domingue, Director Human Resources and Medical Affairs
Web address: www.lourdes.net
**Control:** Church–operated, Nongovernment, not–for profit **Service:** General Medical and Surgical

**Staffed Beds:** 218 **Admissions:** 10092 **Census:** 132 **Outpatient Visits:** 85901 **Births:** 0 **Total Expense ($000):** 204202 **Payroll Expense ($000):** 65666 **Personnel:** 1165

**PARK PLACE SURGICAL HOSPITAL (190255)**, 901 Wilson Street, Zip 70503; tel. 337/237–8119, (Nonreporting) **A**9 10
Primary Contact: Brandon Moore, Administrator and Chief Executive Officer
Web address: www.parkplacesurgery.com/
**Control:** Corporation, Investor–owned, for–profit **Service:** Other specialty

**Staffed Beds:** 10

☐ **UNIVERSITY MEDICAL CENTER (190006)**, 2390 West Congress Street, Zip 70506–4298, Mailing Address: P.O. Box 69300, Zip 70596–9300; tel. 337/261–6001 **A**1 2 3 5 9 10 **F**3 4 15 17 18 20 29 30 31 32 34 40 49 50 56 57 58 59 61 64 65 66 70 72 75 76 77 78 79 81 85 87 89 97 98 100 102 103 107 108 110 111 113 114 118 128 129 131 134 141 143 147 **P**1 **S** LSU Health Care Services Division, Baton Rouge, LA
Primary Contact: Lawrence T. Dorsey, Administrator
COO: Glenn L. Craig, Chief Operating Officer
CFO: Karen Gardiner, Director Fiscal Services
CMO: James B. Falterman, Jr., M.D., Medical Director
CIO: J. Barry Daigle, Manager Information Systems
CHR: Jennifer Simms, Director Human Resources
Web address: www.lsuhospitals.org
**Control:** State–Government, nonfederal **Service:** General Medical and Surgical

**Staffed Beds:** 100 **Admissions:** 4672 **Census:** 65 **Outpatient Visits:** 182256 **Births:** 238 **Total Expense ($000):** 118190 **Payroll Expense ($000):** 45773 **Personnel:** 853

*Many Facility Codes have changed. Please refer to the AHA Guide Code Chart.* © 2012 AHA Guide

**UNIVERSITY MEDICAL CENTER–PSYCHIATRIC UNIT**, 302 Dulles Drive, Zip 70506–3008; tel. 337/262–4190, (Nonreporting)
Primary Contact: Joyce M. Ben, Regional Manager
Web address: www.lsuhospitals.org/
**Control:** State–Government, nonfederal **Service:** Psychiatric

**Staffed Beds: 20**

## LAKE CHARLES—Calcasieu Parish

**CALCASIEU OAKS GERIATRIC PSYCHIATRIC HOSPITAL**, 2837 Ernest Street, Zip 70601; tel. 337/439–8111, (Nonreporting) **S** Pacer Health Corporation, Miami Lakes, FL
Primary Contact: Charles Getwood, Assistant Chief Executive Officer
**Control:** Corporation, Investor–owned, for–profit **Service:** Psychiatric

**Staffed Beds: 24**

⊠ △ **CHRISTUS ST. PATRICK HOSPITAL OF LAKE CHARLES (190027)**, 524 Dr. Michael Debakey Drive, Zip 70601–5799, Mailing Address: P.O. Box 3401, Zip 70602–3401; tel. 337/436–2511 **A**1 2 7 9 10 **F**2 3 11 12 15 17 18 20 22 24 26 28 29 30 31 32 34 35 38 40 44 45 46 47 48 49 50 56 57 59 61 64 65 68 70 74 75 78 79 81 84 85 86 87 89 90 93 98 100 101 102 103 104 105 107 108 110 117 118 119 120 121 122 123 125 129 130 131 133 134 145 146 147 **P**8 **S** CHRISTUS Health, Irving, TX
Primary Contact: Stephen F. Wright, President and Chief Executive Officer
COO: Dianne P. Teal, MSN, Vice President Clinical Operations
CFO: Debbie White, Chief Financial Officer
CMO: David Engleking, M.D., Vice President Medical Affairs
CIO: Allen Abshire, Director Information Services
CHR: Wendy White, Assistant Administrator Human Resources
Web address: www.stpatrickhospital.org
**Control:** Church–operated, Nongovernment, not–for profit **Service:** General Medical and Surgical

**Staffed Beds: 228 Admissions: 7445 Census: 115 Outpatient Visits: 74499 Births: 0 Total Expense ($000): 129654 Payroll Expense ($000): 41677 Personnel: 695**

⊠ **DUBUIS HOSPITAL OF LAKE CHARLES (192024)**, 524 Dr. Michael DeBakey Drive, 5th Floor, Zip 70601–5725; tel. 337/491–7752 **A**1 10 **F**1 3 29 30 35 75 147 **S** Dubuis Health System, Houston, TX
Primary Contact: William L. Willis, Administrator
CMO: Ron Lewis, M.D., Medical Director
Web address: www.dubuis.com
**Control:** Church–operated, Nongovernment, not–for profit **Service:** Long–Term Acute Care hospital

**Staffed Beds: 23 Admissions: 228 Census: 15 Outpatient Visits: 0 Births: 0 Total Expense ($000): 7558 Payroll Expense ($000): 2685 Personnel: 59**

**EXTENDED CARE OF SOUTHWEST LOUISIANA (192019)**, 2837 Ernest Street, Building B., Zip 70601; tel. 337/436–6111, (Nonreporting) **A**10
Primary Contact: Ronald Hunt, Chief Executive Officer
Web address: www.lcmh.com/extcare.htm
**Control:** Other not–for–profit (including NFP Corporation) **Service:** Long–Term Acute Care hospital

**Staffed Beds: 28**

⊠ **LAKE CHARLES MEMORIAL HOSPITAL (190060)**, 1701 Oak Park Boulevard, Zip 70601–8911; tel. 337/494–3000 **A**1 2 3 5 9 10 **F**3 8 11 13 14 15 17 18 20 22 24 25 26 28 29 30 31 34 37 40 43 45 49 50 51 53 56 57 58 60 62 64 66 68 70 71 72 73 74 75 76 77 78 79 81 85 86 87 88 89 90 93 98 99 102 103 107 108 110 111 113 114 118 119 120 122 123 126 128 129 130 131 134 142 143 145 146 147 **P**1 6 7
Primary Contact: Larry M. Graham, FACHE, President and Chief Executive Officer
COO: Timothy O. Coffey, Senior Vice President Operations
CFO: Charles P. Whitson, CPA, Senior Vice President Finance
CMO: Kevin Mocklin, M.D., Director Medical Staff
CIO: Belinda Sommers, Chief Information Officer
CHR: Ginger Consigney, Vice President Human Resources
Web address: www.lcmh.com
**Control:** Other not–for–profit (including NFP Corporation) **Service:** General Medical and Surgical

**Staffed Beds: 306 Admissions: 10777 Census: 148 Outpatient Visits: 140299 Births: 1679 Total Expense ($000): 149896 Payroll Expense ($000): 54854 Personnel: 1440**

**LAKE CHARLES MEMORIAL HOSPITAL FOR WOMEN**, 1900 West Gauthier Road, Zip 70605–7170; tel. 337/480–7000, (Nonreporting) **A**9
Primary Contact: Marilyn McSwain, R.N., MSN, Administrator
Web address: www.lcmh.com/womens–hospital
**Control:** Corporation, Investor–owned, for–profit **Service:** Other specialty

**Staffed Beds: 38**

**OCEANS BEHAVIORAL HOSPITAL OF LAKE CHARLES (194090)**, 302 West Mcneese Street, Zip 70605–5604; tel. 337/474–7581, (Nonreporting) **A**9 10 **S** Oceans Healthcare, Lake Charles, LA
Primary Contact: Nicholas D. Guillory, MSN, Administrator
Web address: www.obhlc.info/
**Control:** Corporation, Investor–owned, for–profit **Service:** Psychiatric

**Staffed Beds: 20**

☐ **WALTER OLIN MOSS REGIONAL MEDICAL CENTER (190161)**, 1000 Walters Street, Zip 70607–4647; tel. 337/475–8100 **A**1 9 10 **F**3 8 9 11 15 29 31 34 39 40 45 50 57 58 59 61 64 66 68 70 75 78 81 85 86 87 97 98 100 102 103 107 110 113 118 129 134 145 146 147 **P**4 **S** LSU Health Care Services Division, Baton Rouge, LA
Primary Contact: Jimmy Pottorff, Interim Administrator
CFO: Ranelda Benoit, Administrative Manager and Fiscal Officer
CMO: Mohammed Sarwar, M.D., Medical Director
CIO: Steve Demourelle, Chief Information Officer
CHR: Sharon Powell, Director Human Resources
Web address: www.lsuhospitals.org/Hospitals/WOM/WOM.htm
**Control:** State–Government, nonfederal **Service:** General Medical and Surgical

**Staffed Beds: 36 Admissions: 1278 Census: 23 Outpatient Visits: 123192 Births: 0 Total Expense ($000): 33891 Payroll Expense ($000): 18502 Personnel: 384**

⊠ **WOMEN AND CHILDREN'S HOSPITAL (190201)**, 4200 Nelson Road, Zip 70605–4118; tel. 337/474–6370 **A**1 9 10 **F**12 13 15 29 40 45 46 47 48 49 50 57 70 72 75 76 77 79 81 85 89 91 93 107 110 113 118 129 131 145 146 **S** Community Health Systems, Inc., Franklin, TN
Primary Contact: Bryan S. Bateman, Chief Executive Officer
CFO: Dawn Johnson–Hatcher, Chief Financial Officer
CMO: Floyd Guidry, M.D., Medical Director
CIO: Aaron Cook, Director Information Services
CHR: Charles Buchert, Director Human Resources
CNO: Robbin Odom, R.N., Chief Nursing Officer
Web address: www.women–childrens.com
**Control:** Corporation, Investor–owned, for–profit **Service:** General Medical and Surgical

**Staffed Beds: 88 Admissions: 3282 Census: 33 Outpatient Visits: 43276 Births: 1342 Total Expense ($000): 38848 Payroll Expense ($000): 18307 Personnel: 355**

## LAKE PROVIDENCE—East Carroll Parish

**EAST CARROLL PARISH HOSPITAL (190208)**, 336 North Hood Street, Zip 71254–2194; tel. 318/559–4023, (Nonreporting) **A**9 10
Primary Contact: Ladonna Englerth, Administrator
**Control:** Hospital district or authority, Government, nonfederal **Service:** Other specialty

**Staffed Beds: 11**

## LEESVILLE—Vernon Parish

⊠ **BYRD REGIONAL HOSPITAL (190164)**, 1020 West Fertitta Boulevard, Zip 71446–4645; tel. 337/239–9041 **A**1 9 10 **F**3 8 13 15 18 20 29 34 37 40 45 48 50 54 57 65 70 76 79 81 87 107 110 111 114 118 132 **P**7 **S** Community Health Systems, Inc., Franklin, TN
Primary Contact: Roger C. LeDoux, Chief Executive Officer
CFO: Wendell Wilkes, Chief Financial Officer
CMO: Hanna Lubbos, M.D., Chief of Staff
CHR: Karolyne Christian, Director Human Resources
Web address: www.byrdregional.com
**Control:** Corporation, Investor–owned, for–profit **Service:** General Medical and Surgical

**Staffed Beds: 60 Admissions: 3921 Census: 37 Outpatient Visits: 29287 Births: 426 Total Expense ($000): 32114 Payroll Expense ($000): 14054 Personnel: 329**

**DOCTOR'S HOSPITAL OF DEER CREEK (190297)**, 815 South 10th Street, Zip 71446–4611, Mailing Address: P.O. Box 1391, Zip 71496–1391; tel. 337/392–5088 **A**9 10 **F**3 29 45 56 75 79 81 82 85 87 89 107 113 147
Primary Contact: Robert R. Bash, FACHE, Chief Executive Officer and Administrator
CHR: Annette Hillman, Director Human Resources
CNO: Elizabeth Bennett, Director of Nursing
Web address: www.dhdc.md
**Control:** Corporation, Investor–owned, for–profit **Service:** General Medical and Surgical

**Staffed Beds: 10 Admissions: 588 Census: 5 Outpatient Visits: 1962 Births: 0 Total Expense ($000): 6362 Payroll Expense ($000): 2137 Personnel: 54**

---

**Hospital, Medicare Provider Number, Address, Telephone, Approval, Facility, and Physician Codes, Health Care System**

★ American Hospital Association (AHA) membership
☐ The Joint Commission accreditation
◇ DNV Healthcare Inc. accreditation
○ American Osteopathic Association (AOA) accreditation
△ Commission on Accreditation of Rehabilitation Facilities (CARF) accreditation

**LA**

☐ **LEESVILLE REHABILITATION HOSPITAL (193086)**, 900 South 6th Street, Zip 71446–4723; tel. 337/392–8118, (Nonreporting) **A**1 10
Primary Contact: Jason Carroll, Administrator and Chief Executive Officer
CMO: Gregory D. Lord, M.D., Chief Medical Officer
CHR: Jackie Rubar, Administrative Assistant and Director Human Resources
Web address: www.leesvillerehab.com
**Control:** Corporation, Investor–owned, for–profit **Service:** Rehabilitation

Staffed Beds: 16

☐ **TRI PARISH REHABILITATION HOSPITAL (193050)**, 8088 Hawks Road, Zip 71446–6649; tel. 337/462–8880, (Nonreporting) **A**1 10
Primary Contact: Heath Hairgrove, Administrator
Web address: www.triparishrehab.com
**Control:** Corporation, Investor–owned, for–profit **Service:** Rehabilitation

Staffed Beds: 33

**LULING—St. Charles Parish**

☐ **SPECIALTY REHABILITATION HOSPITAL OF LULING (193064)**, 1125 Paul Maillard Road, Zip 70070–4351; tel. 985/785–5233, (Nonreporting) **A**1 10 **S** Specialty Healthcare, LLC, Leesville, LA
Primary Contact: Lisa Miller, Administrator
Web address: www.specialtyrehabluling.com
**Control:** Corporation, Investor–owned, for–profit **Service:** Rehabilitation

Staffed Beds: 21

☐ **ST. CHARLES PARISH HOSPITAL (190079)**, 1057 Paul Maillard Road, Zip 70070–4349, Mailing Address: P.O. Box 87, Zip 70070–0087; tel. 985/785–6242 **A**1 9 10 **F**3 7 11 15 18 28 29 30 31 34 35 40 45 56 57 59 60 64 65 70 74 75 77 78 79 81 82 86 93 96 98 100 101 102 103 107 110 111 113 118 129 130 131 145 147 **P**5
Primary Contact: Fred Martinez, Jr., Chief Executive Officer
COO: Karen Guillot, R.N., Chief Operating Officer
CMO: Chemmele Jayakrishnan, M.D., Chief Medical Staff
CIO: Angela Duet, Director Information Technology
CHR: Carolyn Faucheaux, Director Human Resources
Web address: www.stch.net
**Control:** Hospital district or authority, Government, nonfederal **Service:** General Medical and Surgical

Staffed Beds: 59 Admissions: 1759 Census: 35 Outpatient Visits: 35144 Births: 0 Total Expense ($000): 35451 Payroll Expense ($000): 15668 Personnel: 390

**ST. CHARLES SPECIALTY REHABILITATION HOSPITAL (193060)**, 1057 Paul Maillard Road, Zip 70070, Mailing Address: P.O. Box 243, Zip 70070–0243; tel. 985/331–2281, (Nonreporting) **A**10
Primary Contact: Juanita Ann Bates, Administrator
Web address: www.lulingrehab.com
**Control:** County–Government, nonfederal **Service:** Rehabilitation

Staffed Beds: 16

**LUTCHER—St. James Parish**

⊞ **ST. JAMES PARISH HOSPITAL (191305)**, 1645 Lutcher Avenue, Zip 70071–5150; tel. 225/869–5512 **A**1 9 10 18 **F**3 15 29 30 34 35 40 57 59 64 75 77 81 107 111 113 118 127 131 132
Primary Contact: Mary Ellen Pratt, FACHE, Chief Executive Officer
CFO: Tracy L. George, Chief Financial Officer
CIO: Susan Duhon, Director Medical Records
CHR: Lisa Faucheux, Director Human Resources
Web address: www.sjph.org
**Control:** Hospital district or authority, Government, nonfederal **Service:** General Medical and Surgical

Staffed Beds: 20 Admissions: 706 Census: 11

**MAMOU—Evangeline Parish**

**EVANGELINE EXTENDED CARE HOSPITAL–MAMOU**, 801 Poinciana Avenue, Zip 70554; tel. 337/468–4203, (Nonreporting)
Primary Contact: Biff David, Administrator
Web address: www.lhcgroup.com
**Control:** Corporation, Investor–owned, for–profit **Service:** Long–Term Acute Care hospital

Staffed Beds: 18

⊞ **SAVOY MEDICAL CENTER (190025)**, 801 Poinciana Avenue, Zip 70554–2298; tel. 337/468–5261, (Nonreporting) **A**1 9 10
Primary Contact: Ted Smith, Chief Executive Officer
COO: Gerald Fuselier, Chief Operating Officer
CMO: Greg Savoy, M.D., Chief Medical Officer
CIO: Daniel Lahaye, Manager
CHR: Annette Thibodeaux, Director Human Resources
Web address: www.savoymedicalcenter.com
**Control:** Corporation, Investor–owned, for–profit **Service:** General Medical and Surgical

Staffed Beds: 180

**MANDEVILLE—St. Tammany Parish**

☐ **SOUTHEAST LOUISIANA HOSPITAL (194007)**, 23515 Highway 190, Zip 70448–5612, Mailing Address: P.O. Box 3850, Zip 70470–3850; tel. 985/626–6300, (Nonreporting) **A**1 3 5 10 **S** Louisiana State Hospitals, Baton Rouge, LA
Primary Contact: Richard Kramer, Interim Chief Executive Officer
COO: Richard Kramer, Chief Operating Officer
CFO: Denise Businelle, Account Administrator
CMO: Girishkumar Shah, M.D., Clinical Director
CIO: Mike Ziemba, Information Technology Project Lead
CHR: Daphne Stewart, Director Human Resources
Web address: www.selh.org
**Control:** State–Government, nonfederal **Service:** Psychiatric

Staffed Beds: 153

**MANSFIELD—De Soto Parish**

**DE SOTO REGIONAL HEALTH SYSTEM (190118)**, 207 Jefferson Street, Zip 71052–2603, Mailing Address: P.O. Box 1636, Zip 71052–2603; tel. 318/871–3100, (Nonreporting) **A**9 10 20 **S** HealthTech Management Services, Franklin, TN
Primary Contact: Douglas P. Efferson, FACHE, Chief Executive Officer
CMO: Leigh Dillard, M.D., Chief of Staff
CHR: Rhonda Potter, Director Human Resources
Web address: www.desotoregional.com
**Control:** Other not–for–profit (including NFP Corporation) **Service:** General Medical and Surgical

Staffed Beds: 37

**MANY—Sabine Parish**

**SABINE MEDICAL CENTER (190218)**, 240 Highland Drive, Zip 71449–3718; tel. 318/256–5691 **A**9 10 20 **F**3 15 29 34 40 41 45 50 57 59 64 81 89 104 107 111 114 118 126 127 129 132
Primary Contact: Chris Beddoe, Chief Executive Officer
CFO: Frances F. Hopkins, Chief Financial Officer
Web address: www.sabinemedicalcenter.net
**Control:** Individual, Investor–owned, for–profit **Service:** General Medical and Surgical

Staffed Beds: 44 Admissions: 1139 Census: 9 Outpatient Visits: 53964 Births: 0 Total Expense ($000): 14188 Personnel: 135

**MARKSVILLE—Avoyelles Parish**

☐ **AVOYELLES HOSPITAL (190099)**, 4231 Highway 1192, Zip 71351, Mailing Address: P.O. Box 249, Zip 71351–0249; tel. 318/253–8611 **A**1 9 10 **F**3 15 29 34 40 45 59 64 67 70 81 85 89 107 110 118 127 132 134 145
Primary Contact: David M. Mitchel, Chief Executive Officer
CMO: Fernando Garcia, M.D., Chief of Staff
CIO: Billy Tingle, Director Information Systems and Respiratory Therapy
CHR: Allison Ferguson, Director Human Resources
Web address: www.avoyelleshospital.com
**Control:** Corporation, Investor–owned, for–profit **Service:** General Medical and Surgical

Staffed Beds: 35 Admissions: 1608 Census: 17 Outpatient Visits: 43151 Births: 0 Payroll Expense ($000): 6502 Personnel: 193

**MARRERO—Jefferson Parish**

★ **KINDRED HOSPITAL WEST–JEFFERSON (192007)**, 1111 Medical Center Boulevard, Suite S–550, Zip 70072; tel. 504/349–2470, (Nonreporting) **A**10 **S** Kindred Healthcare, Louisville, KY
Primary Contact: Paul R. Newhouse, Chief Executive Officer
Web address: www.khwestjefferson.com/
**Control:** Corporation, Investor–owned, for–profit **Service:** Long–Term Acute Care hospital

Staffed Beds: 56

⊞ △ **WEST JEFFERSON MEDICAL CENTER (190039)**, 1101 Medical Center Boulevard, Zip 70072–3191; tel. 504/347–5511 **A**1 2 3 5 7 9 10 **F**3 6 7 11 12 13 15 17 18 20 22 24 26 28 29 30 31 34 35 37 38 39 40 41 43 45 46 47 49 50 51 53 56 57 59 60 61 64 65 68 70 72 74 75 76 78 79 81 82 85 86 87 89 90 91 93 96 97 98 100 101 102 104 105 107 108 110 111 113 114 116 117 118 119 120 123 125 126 128 129 131 134 145 146 147 **P**6
Primary Contact: Nancy R. Cassagne, FACHE, Chief Executive Officer
COO: Angela Greener, Chief Administrative Officer
CMO: Mark Workman, M.D., Chief Medical Officer
CIO: Nicholas Thimis, Chief Information Officer
CHR: Frank Martinez, Vice President Human Resources
CNO: Adonna F. Lowe, R.N., Chief Nursing Officer
Web address: www.wjmc.org
**Control:** Hospital district or authority, Government, nonfederal **Service:** General Medical and Surgical

Staffed Beds: 327 Admissions: 13356 Census: 197 Outpatient Visits: 212049 Births: 1212 Total Expense ($000): 217824 Payroll Expense ($000): 88431

*Many Facility Codes have changed. Please refer to the AHA Guide Code Chart.* © 2012 AHA Guide

## METAIRIE—Jefferson Parish

☒ △ **EAST JEFFERSON GENERAL HOSPITAL (190146)**, 4200 Houma Boulevard, Zip 70006–2996; tel. 504/454–4000, (Includes DOCTORS HOSPITAL OF JEFFERSON, 4320 Houma Boulevard, Zip 70006–2973; tel. 504/849–4000) **A**1 2 3 5 7 9 10 **F**3 7 8 11 13 14 15 17 18 20 22 24 28 29 30 31 34 35 40 43 45 46 47 48 49 50 51 53 56 57 59 60 64 68 70 72 73 74 75 76 77 78 79 81 82 84 85 86 87 90 91 93 94 96 98 100 101 102 103 104 107 108 109 110 111 112 114 115 116 117 118 119 120 121 122 123 125 127 128 129 130 131 134 142 144 145 146 147 **P**4 6 8
Primary Contact: Mark J. Peters, M.D., President and Chief Executive Officer
COO: Janice Kishner, Chief Operating Officer and Nurse Executive
CFO: Ted Shaw, Interim Chief Financial Officer
CMO: Raymond P. DeCorte, M.D., Chief Medical Officer
CIO: Bernie Clement, Chief Information Officer
CHR: Donna Ammons, Director Human Resources
Web address: www.ejgh.org
**Control:** Hospital district or authority, Government, nonfederal **Service:** General Medical and Surgical

**Staffed Beds:** 420 **Admissions:** 18934 **Census:** 295 **Outpatient Visits:** 198265 **Births:** 1578 **Total Expense ($000):** 323463 **Payroll Expense ($000):** 122916 **Personnel:** 2327

**OMEGA HOSPITAL (190302)**, 2525 Severn Avenue, Zip 70002; tel. 504/832–4200, (Nonreporting) **A**10 21
Primary Contact: Debbie Schenck, Administrator
Web address: www.omega–institute.com
**Control:** Individual, Investor–owned, for–profit **Service:** Surgical

**Staffed Beds:** 10

☐ **ST. THERESA SPECIALTY HOSPITAL (192030)**, 4200 Houma Boulevard, Zip 70006; tel. 504/780–3041, (Nonreporting) **A**1 10
Primary Contact: Glynda Troyo, Chief Executive Officer
Web address: www.stmck.com
**Control:** Corporation, Investor–owned, for–profit **Service:** Long–Term Acute Care hospital

**Staffed Beds:** 31

★ **TULANE–LAKESIDE HOSPITAL**, 4700 South I. 10 Service Road West, Zip 70001–1269; tel. 504/780–4200, (Nonreporting) **A**9 **S** HCA, Nashville, TN
Primary Contact: Robert Lynch, M.D., Chief Executive Officer
COO: Andre duPlessis, Chief Operating Officer
Web address: www.tuhc.com
**Control:** Corporation, Investor–owned, for–profit **Service:** General Medical and Surgical

**Staffed Beds:** 116

## MINDEN—Webster Parish

☒ **MINDEN MEDICAL CENTER (190144)**, 1 Medical Plaza, Zip 71055–3330, Mailing Address: P.O. Box 5003, Zip 71058–5003; tel. 318/377–2321 **A**1 9 10 19 **F**11 13 15 18 20 22 29 30 34 40 45 46 56 57 59 62 64 70 75 76 77 79 81 82 87 89 90 93 98 103 107 111 114 118 128 129 131 145 146 147 **S** LifePoint Hospitals, Inc., Brentwood, TN
Primary Contact: George E. French, III, FACHE, Chief Executive Officer
CFO: Jim Williams, Chief Financial Officer
CMO: G. Max Stell, M.D., Medical Director
CIO: Mace Morgan, Director Information Systems
CHR: Mary Winget, Director Human Resources
CNO: Donna Carter, MSN, Chief Nursing Officer
Web address: www.mindenmedicalcenter.com
**Control:** Corporation, Investor–owned, for–profit **Service:** General Medical and Surgical

**Staffed Beds:** 161 **Admissions:** 5125 **Census:** 54 **Outpatient Visits:** 39678 **Births:** 749 **Total Expense ($000):** 43909 **Payroll Expense ($000):** 20911 **Personnel:** 366

## MONROE—Ouachita Parish

☐ **E. A. CONWAY MEDICAL CENTER (190011)**, 4864 Jackson Street, Zip 71202–6497, Mailing Address: P.O. Box 1881, Zip 71210–8005; tel. 318/330–7000 **A**1 3 5 9 10 **F**11 13 15 29 30 31 35 40 43 49 50 54 57 58 59 61 64 65 66 70 72 74 75 76 77 78 79 81 85 87 89 92 93 97 98 100 102 107 108 110 111 113 118 129 134 145 **P**1
Primary Contact: H. Aryon McGuire, Administrator
CFO: Linda Lochbrunner, Chief Financial Officer
CMO: LaDonna Ford, M.D., Medical Director
CHR: Kaye Clark, Assistant Director Human Resources Management
Web address: www.conway.lsuhsc.edu
**Control:** State–Government, nonfederal **Service:** General Medical and Surgical

**Staffed Beds:** 158 **Admissions:** 5770 **Census:** 94 **Outpatient Visits:** 143807 **Births:** 946 **Total Expense ($000):** 78876 **Payroll Expense ($000):** 35229 **Personnel:** 813

☐ **MONROE SURGICAL HOSPITAL (190245)**, 2408 Broadmoor Boulevard, Zip 71201, Mailing Address: P.O. Box 4887, Zip 71211–4887; tel. 318/410–0002 **A**1 9 10 **F**3 15 29 51 64 68 79 81 85 107 108 110 111 113 118 130 **P**5
Primary Contact: Scooter Chriceol, Chief Executive Officer
Web address: www.monroesurgical.com
**Control:** Corporation, Investor–owned, for–profit **Service:** General Medical and Surgical

**Staffed Beds:** 10 **Admissions:** 296 **Census:** 2 **Outpatient Visits:** 14823 **Births:** 0 **Total Expense ($000):** 13752 **Payroll Expense ($000):** 4402 **Personnel:** 98

★ **P & S SURGICAL HOSPITAL (190246)**, 312 Grammont Street Suite 101, Zip 71201–7403; tel. 318/388–4040, (Nonreporting) **A**9 10
Primary Contact: Linda S. Holyfield, R.N., MSN, President and Chief Executive Officer
COO: Terri Hicks, Chief Operating Officer and Chief Financial Officer
CFO: Terri Hicks, Chief Operating Officer and Chief Financial Officer
CMO: Mark Napoli, M.D., Chief of Staff
CIO: Joseph Vicknair, Chief Information Officer
CHR: Joseph Vicknair, Director Human Resources
CNO: Debbie W. Austin, R.N., Vice President Patient Care Services
Web address: www.pssurgery.com
**Control:** Partnership, Investor–owned, for–profit **Service:** General Medical and Surgical

**Staffed Beds:** 22

**SPECIALTY EXTENDED CARE OF MONROE (192016)**, 309 Jackson Street, Zip 71210, Mailing Address: P.O. Box 1532, Zip 71210–1532; tel. 318/327–4000, (Nonreporting) **A**9 10
Primary Contact: Cleta Munholland, Administrator
Web address: www.specialtyhospital.com
**Control:** Church–operated, Nongovernment, not–for profit **Service:** General Medical and Surgical

**Staffed Beds:** 32

☒ **ST. FRANCIS MEDICAL CENTER (190125)**, 309 Jackson Street, Zip 71201–7407, Mailing Address: P.O. Box 1901, Zip 71210–1901; tel. 318/966–4000, (Includes ST. FRANCIS NORTH HOSPITAL, 3421 Medical Park Drive, Zip 71203–2399; tel. 318/388–1946; Cindy J. Rogers, FACHE, Administrator) **A**1 2 9 10 **F**2 3 12 13 15 17 18 19 20 21 22 23 24 26 27 28 29 30 31 32 34 35 37 39 40 44 45 46 49 50 54 55 56 57 59 64 65 68 69 70 72 74 75 76 77 78 79 81 85 87 88 89 90 92 93 96 97 98 102 103 104 105 107 108 110 111 113 114 115 116 117 118 123 127 128 129 130 131 133 134 143 145 146 147 **P**8 **S** Franciscan Missionaries of Our Lady Health System, Inc., Baton Rouge, LA
Primary Contact: Louis H. Bremer, Jr., President and Chief Executive Officer
CFO: Ronald E. Hogan, Senior Vice President and Chief Financial Officer
CMO: R. Louis Gavioli, M.D., Vice President Medical Affairs
CIO: Thomas H. Hammond, Chief Information Officer
CHR: James Novak, Vice President, Human Resources
CNO: Darline Smith, R.N., Vice President Patient Care Services and Chief Nursing Officer
Web address: www.stfran.com
**Control:** Church–operated, Nongovernment, not–for profit **Service:** General Medical and Surgical

**Staffed Beds:** 343 **Admissions:** 16088 **Census:** 242 **Outpatient Visits:** 227248 **Births:** 1760 **Total Expense ($000):** 240740 **Payroll Expense ($000):** 92078 **Personnel:** 1844

**ST. FRANCIS SPECIALTY HOSPITAL** See Specialty Extended Care of Monroe

## MORGAN CITY—St. Mary Parish

☒ **TECHE REGIONAL MEDICAL CENTER (190014)**, 1125 Marguerite Street, Zip 70380–1855, Mailing Address: P.O. Box 2308, Zip 70381–2308; tel. 985/384–2200 **A**1 9 10 20 **F**3 13 15 18 20 22 29 30 31 34 40 45 50 57 60 70 76 79 81 85 89 90 93 98 102 104 105 107 108 110 111 114 118 129 140 145 146 **S** LifePoint Hospitals, Inc., Brentwood, TN
Primary Contact: James P. Frazier, III, Chief Executive Officer
CFO: Michael Mayeux, Chief Financial Officer
CMO: Kimberly Thorguson, M.D., Chief of Staff
CIO: Cheryl Lipari, Manager Information Systems
CHR: Timothy Hebert, Director Human Resources
Web address: www.techeregional.com
**Control:** Corporation, Investor–owned, for–profit **Service:** General Medical and Surgical

**Staffed Beds:** 165 **Admissions:** 3583 **Census:** 48 **Outpatient Visits:** 51295 **Births:** 409 **Total Expense ($000):** 40072 **Payroll Expense ($000):** 14551 **Personnel:** 284

---

**Hospital, Medicare Provider Number, Address, Telephone, Approval, Facility, and Physician Codes, Health Care System**

★ American Hospital Association (AHA) membership
☐ The Joint Commission accreditation
◇ DNV Healthcare Inc. accreditation
○ American Osteopathic Association (AOA) accreditation
△ Commission on Accreditation of Rehabilitation Facilities (CARF) accreditation

**LA**

## NAPOLEONVILLE—Assumption Parish

★ **ASSUMPTION COMMUNITY HOSPITAL (191303)**, 135 Highway 402,
Zip 70390–2217; tel. 985/369–3600, (Nonreporting) **A**9 10 18 **S** Franciscan
Missionaries of Our Lady Health System, Inc., Baton Rouge, LA
Primary Contact: Wayne M. Arboneaux, Chief Executive Officer
CHR: Letonia Pierre, Coordinator Human Resources
CNO: Donna Mullings, Director of Nursing
Web address: www.ololrmc.com
**Control:** Other not–for–profit (including NFP Corporation) **Service:** General
Medical and Surgical

**Staffed Beds:** 6

## NATCHITOCHES—Natchitoches Parish

**LOUISIANA EXTENDED CARE HOSPITAL OF NATCHITOCHES (192035)**, 501
Keyser Avenue, Zip 71457; tel. 318/354–2044, (Nonreporting) **A**10 **S** LHC
Group, Lafayette, LA
Primary Contact: Kermit Simmons, Administrator
Web address: www.lhcgroup.com
**Control:** Corporation, Investor–owned, for–profit **Service:** Long–Term Acute Care
hospital

**Staffed Beds:** 21

⊠ **NATCHITOCHES REGIONAL MEDICAL CENTER (190007)**, 501 Keyser
Avenue, Zip 71457–6036, Mailing Address: P.O. Box 2009, Zip 71457–2009;
tel. 318/214–4200, (Nonreporting) **A**1 9 10 20 **S** CHRISTUS Health, Irving, TX
Primary Contact: Mark E. Marley, FACHE, Chief Executive Officer
CFO: Billy Page, Chief Financial Officer
CIO: Steve Crowder, Manager Information Technology
CHR: Ernie Scott, Director Human Resources
CNO: Dawna DeBlieux, Chief Nurse Executive
Web address: www.natchitocheshospital.org
**Control:** Hospital district or authority, Government, nonfederal **Service:** General
Medical and Surgical

**Staffed Beds:** 78

## NEW IBERIA—Iberia Parish

⊠ ○ **DAUTERIVE HOSPITAL (190003)**, 600 North Lewis Street, Zip 70563;
tel. 337/365–7311 **A**1 9 10 11 19 **F**13 15 17 18 28 29 40 56 57 70 76 81
86 87 89 90 93 98 103 107 111 118 129 131 145 **S** HCA, Nashville, TN
Primary Contact: Alan J. Fabian, Chief Executive Officer
CFO: Laura Allen, Chief Financial Officer
CMO: Mike Alvarez, M.D., Chief Medical Officer
CIO: Terry Stewart, Director Information Systems
CHR: Candice Ardoin, Director Human Resources
Web address: www.dauterivehospital.com
**Control:** Corporation, Investor–owned, for–profit **Service:** General Medical and
Surgical

**Staffed Beds:** 103 **Admissions:** 2974 **Census:** 38 **Outpatient Visits:** 21220
**Births:** 428 **Total Expense ($000):** 53634 **Payroll Expense ($000):** 17420
**Personnel:** 318

**IBERIA EXTENDED CARE HOSPITAL**, 2315 East Main Street, 3rd Floor,
Zip 70560; tel. 337/369–1100, (Nonreporting)
Primary Contact: Kevin Frank, Administrator
**Control:** Corporation, Investor–owned, for–profit **Service:** Long–Term Acute Care
hospital

**Staffed Beds:** 16

☐ **IBERIA MEDICAL CENTER (190054)**, 2315 East Main Street,
Zip 70560–4031, Mailing Address: P.O. Box 13338, Zip 70562–3338;
tel. 337/364–0441 **A**1 9 10 **F**3 11 13 15 18 20 22 28 29 30 31 34 39 40 45
46 47 48 49 57 62 64 65 68 70 72 74 75 76 77 78 79 81 85 86 87 89 93
97 107 108 113 114 118 126 129 145 147 **P**6 **S** HealthTech Management
Services, Franklin, TN
Primary Contact: John A. Tucker, Chief Executive Officer
COO: Shane P. Myers, Chief Operating Officer
CFO: Wally Piekarczyk, Chief Financial Officer
CMO: Ellen Mullen, M.D., Chief of Staff
CIO: Ross Leleux, Chief Information Officer
CHR: Lori Spann, Director Human Resources
Web address: www.iberiamedicalcenter.com
**Control:** Hospital district or authority, Government, nonfederal **Service:** General
Medical and Surgical

**Staffed Beds:** 83 **Admissions:** 4228 **Census:** 39 **Outpatient Visits:** 86967
**Births:** 451 **Total Expense ($000):** 41300 **Payroll Expense ($000):** 24180
**Personnel:** 467

☐ **IBERIA REHABILITATION HOSPITAL (190304)**, 532 Jefferson Terrace,
Zip 70560–4948; tel. 337/364–6923, (Nonreporting) **A**1 10
Primary Contact: Athan Oliver, Administrator and Chief Executive Officer
Web address: www.iberiarehab.net/
**Control:** Corporation, Investor–owned, for–profit **Service:** Rehabilitation

**Staffed Beds:** 24

## NEW ORLEANS—Orleans Parish

**BEACON BEHAVIORAL HOSPITAL – NEW ORLEANS (194084)**, 14500 Hayne
Boulevard, Suite 200, Zip 70128–1751; tel. 504/210–0460, (Nonreporting)
**A**9 10
Primary Contact: Mandy Henry, Administrator
**Control:** Corporation, Investor–owned, for–profit **Service:** Psychiatric

**Staffed Beds:** 24

☐ **CHILDREN'S HOSPITAL (193300)**, 200 Henry Clay Avenue, Zip 70118–5720;
tel. 504/899–9511 **A**1 2 3 5 9 10 **F**3 8 9 11 16 17 19 21 23 25 27 29 30 31
32 34 35 36 39 40 41 43 50 54 55 57 58 59 60 61 64 65 66 71 72 74 75
78 79 80 81 82 84 85 86 87 88 89 90 93 97 98 99 100 102 104 107 108
111 114 118 128 129 130 131 135 137 140 143 145 147 **P**4 8
Primary Contact: Steve Worley, President and Chief Executive Officer
CFO: Greg Feirn, Senior Vice President and Chief Financial Officer
CMO: Alan M. Robson, M.D., Senior Vice President and Medical Director
CIO: Tammy Reites, Vice President Patient Financial Services
CHR: Doug Mittelstaedt, Vice President Human Resources
CNO: Diane Michel, Vice President Nursing
Web address: www.chnola.org
**Control:** Other not–for–profit (including NFP Corporation) **Service:** Children's
general

**Staffed Beds:** 200 **Admissions:** 8655 **Census:** 144 **Outpatient Visits:**
410709 **Births:** 0 **Personnel:** 1649

☐ **COMMUNITY CARE HOSPITAL (194056)**, 1421 General Taylor Street,
Zip 70115; tel. 504/899–2500, (Nonreporting) **A**1 9 10
Primary Contact: Paul B. Kavanaugh, President and Chief Executive Officer
Web address: www.communitycarehospital.com
**Control:** State–Government, nonfederal **Service:** Psychiatric

**Staffed Beds:** 36

**INTERIM LSU PUBLIC HOSPITAL (190005)**, 2021 Perdido Street,
Zip 70112–1396; tel. 504/903–3000 **A**2 5 8 9 10 **F**3 4 8 11 12 15 18 20 22
24 26 29 30 31 34 35 39 40 43 44 45 46 48 49 50 51 54 55 58 59 60
61 64 65 66 68 70 74 75 77 78 79 81 82 84 85 86 87 92 93 94 97 98 100
101 102 107 108 110 111 113 114 116 117 118 128 129 131 134 141 143
145 146 147 **P**1 **S** LSU Health Care Services Division, Baton Rouge, LA
Primary Contact: Roxane A. Townsend, M.D., Chief Executive Officer
COO: Adler Voltaire, Chief Administrative Officer
CFO: Ed Burke, Chief Financial Officer
CMO: Cathi E. Fontenot, M.D., Medical Director
CIO: Mitch Perlin, Chief Information Officer
CHR: Ronald Broadus, Assistant Administrator Human Resources
Web address: www.lsuhospitals.org/hospitals/mclno/mclno–directory.htm
**Control:** State–Government, nonfederal **Service:** General Medical and Surgical

**Staffed Beds:** 255 **Admissions:** 12116 **Census:** 193 **Outpatient Visits:**
279945 **Births:** 42 **Total Expense ($000):** 398803 **Payroll Expense ($000):**
128960 **Personnel:** 2251

⊠ **KINDRED HOSPITAL–NEW ORLEANS (192009)**, 3601 Coliseum Street,
Zip 70115–3606; tel. 504/899–1555 **A**1 10 **F**1 3 28 29 30 31 40 46 56 57
60 74 75 77 78 85 86 87 90 96 98 100 103 105 118 147 **P**8 **S** Kindred
Healthcare, Louisville, KY
Primary Contact: Thomas G. Alexander, Chief Executive Officer
CFO: Mary Kay Nations, Chief Financial Officer
CMO: Juzar Ali, M.D., Chief of Staff
Web address: www.kindredhospitalnola.com
**Control:** Individual, Investor–owned, for–profit **Service:** General Medical and
Surgical

**Staffed Beds:** 80 **Admissions:** 545 **Census:** 43 **Outpatient Visits:** 0 **Births:**
0 **Total Expense ($000):** 21932 **Payroll Expense ($000):** 8703 **Personnel:**
167

**MEDICAL CENTER OF LOUISIANA AT NEW ORLEANS** See Interim LSU Public
Hospital

⊠ **OCHSNER BAPTIST MEDICAL CENTER (190135)**, 2700 Napoleon Avenue,
Zip 70115–6914; tel. 504/899–9311 **A**1 9 10 **F**3 15 20 22 29 30 34 37 40
41 45 46 47 48 49 50 53 54 57 59 60 64 70 74 75 77 79 81 82 107 109
110 111 113 114 118 128 129 134 **P**8 **S** Ochsner Health System, New
Orleans, LA
Primary Contact: Bradley R. Goodson, Chief Executive Officer
COO: Ava Jo Collins, Vice President Operations
CFO: Christy Migaud, Controller
CMO: Allen Brown, M.D., Vice President Medical Affairs
CHR: Bill Ramsey, Director Human Resources
CNO: Donna Martin, R.N., Chief Nursing Officer
Web address: www.ochsner.org
**Control:** Other not–for–profit (including NFP Corporation) **Service:** General
Medical and Surgical

**Staffed Beds:** 55 **Admissions:** 3426 **Census:** 36 **Outpatient Visits:** 41287
**Births:** 0 **Total Expense ($000):** 63261 **Payroll Expense ($000):** 20653
**Personnel:** 393

☒ △ **OCHSNER MEDICAL CENTER (190036)**, 1514 Jefferson Highway, Zip 70121–2429; tel. 504/842–3000, (Includes OCHSNER MEDICAL CENTER – WEST BANK, 2500 Belle Chasse Highway, Gretna, Zip 70056–7127; tel. 504/392–3131; Travis Capers, Chief Executive Officer), (Total facility includes 32 beds in nursing home–type unit) **A**1 2 3 5 7 8 9 10 **F**2 3 5 8 9 11 12 13 14 15 17 18 19 20 21 22 23 24 25 26 27 28 29 30 31 32 34 37 38 40 41 43 44 45 46 47 48 49 50 51 54 55 56 57 58 59 60 61 64 65 68 70 72 74 75 76 77 78 79 81 84 85 86 87 88 89 90 93 94 96 98 99 100 101 102 103 104 105 107 108 110 111 113 114 116 117 118 119 120 122 123 125 127 128 129 130 131 132 133 134 135 136 137 138 139 140 141 144 145 146 147 **P**6 **S** Ochsner Health System, New Orleans, LA
Primary Contact: Michael Hulefeld, Chief Executive Officer
COO: Warner L. Thomas, FACHE, System President and Chief Operating Officer
CFO: Scott J. Posecai, Executive Vice President and Chief Financial Officer
CMO: Patrick J. Quinlan, M.D., Chief Executive Officer
CIO: Lynn Witherspoon, Vice President and Chief Information Officer
CHR: Joan Mollohan, Vice President Human Resources
Web address: www.ochsner.org
**Control:** Other not–for–profit (including NFP Corporation) **Service:** General Medical and Surgical

**Staffed Beds:** 771 **Admissions:** 34179 **Census:** 495 **Outpatient Visits:** 378942 **Births:** 3464 **Total Expense ($000):** 773119 **Payroll Expense ($000):** 289600 **Personnel:** 4042

**PSYCHIATRIC PAVILION NEW ORLEANS** See Beacon Behavioral Hospital – New Orleans

☐ **RIVER OAKS HOSPITAL (194031)**, 1525 River Oaks Road West, Zip 70123–2162; tel. 504/734–1740, (Includes RIVER OAKS CHILD AND ADOLESCENT HOSPITAL, 1525 River Oaks Road West, tel. 504/734–1740) **A**1 9 10 **F**4 5 29 40 98 99 102 105 129 **S** Universal Health Services, Inc., King of Prussia, PA
Primary Contact: Evelyn Nolting, Chief Executive Officer and Managing Director
CFO: James Todd, Chief Financial Officer
CMO: Lincoln Paine, M.D., Medical Director
CIO: Vincent Chastelain, Director Business Development
CIO: Kim Epperson, Director Business Development
CHR: Wanda Hoffmann, Director Human Resources
Web address: www.riveroakshospital.com
**Control:** Corporation, Investor–owned, for–profit **Service:** Psychiatric

**Staffed Beds:** 126 **Admissions:** 2957 **Census:** 77 **Births:** 0

**ST. CATHERINE MEMORIAL HOSPITAL (192023)**, 14500 Hayne Boulevard, Zip 70128–1751; tel. 504/210–3000, (Nonreporting) **A**10
Primary Contact: Wayne Landry, Administrator and Chief Executive Officer
Web address: www.stcatherine–hospital.com
**Control:** Corporation, Investor–owned, for–profit **Service:** Long–Term Acute Care hospital

**Staffed Beds:** 21

**ST. CHARLES SURGICAL HOSPITAL (190300)**, 1717 Saint Charles Avenue, Zip 70130–5223; tel. 504/529–6600, (Nonreporting) **A**10 21
Primary Contact: Cheri Saltaformaggio, Chief Executive Officer
Web address: www.scsh.com
**Control:** Other not–for–profit (including NFP Corporation) **Service:** Surgical

**Staffed Beds:** 17

☒ △ **TOURO INFIRMARY (190046)**, 1401 Foucher Street, Zip 70115–3593; tel. 504/897–7011, (Includes TOURO REHABILITATION CENTER, 1401 Foucher Street, Zip 70115–3515; tel. 504/897–8560) **A**1 2 3 5 7 8 9 10 **F**3 8 10 11 13 15 18 20 22 24 28 29 30 31 34 35 36 37 39 40 43 44 45 50 53 54 57 59 60 61 62 63 64 68 70 72 74 75 76 77 78 79 81 83 84 85 86 87 90 93 96 97 107 108 109 110 111 113 114 115 116 117 118 119 120 122 123 124 127 129 130 131 134 142 145 146 147 **P**8
Primary Contact: James T. Montgomery, FACHE, President
COO: Susan Pitoscia, MSN, Chief Operating Officer
CIO: Jeff Lott, Director Information Services
CHR: Chad Courrege, Vice President Human Resources
Web address: www.touro.com
**Control:** Other not–for–profit (including NFP Corporation) **Service:** General Medical and Surgical

**Staffed Beds:** 380 **Admissions:** 14165 **Census:** 210 **Outpatient Visits:** 243373 **Births:** 2938 **Total Expense ($000):** 213367 **Payroll Expense ($000):** 79498 **Personnel:** 1471

☒ **TULANE MEDICAL CENTER (190176)**, 1415 Tulane Avenue, Zip 70112–2600; tel. 504/988–5263, (Nonreporting) **A**1 2 5 8 9 10 **S** HCA, Nashville, TN
Primary Contact: Robert Lynch, M.D., Chief Executive Officer
COO: Jennifer Eslinger, Chief Operating Officer
CFO: Robert Hatcher, Chief Financial Officer
CMO: John Pigott, M.D., Chief Medical Officer
CIO: Sue Rachuig, Director Information Services
CHR: Beth Babin, Vice President Human Resources
CNO: Danita S. Sullivan, R.N., Chief Nursing Officer
Web address: www.tuhc.com
**Control:** Corporation, Investor–owned, for–profit **Service:** General Medical and Surgical

**Staffed Beds:** 327

### NEW ROADS—Pointe Coupee Parish

★ **POINTE COUPEE GENERAL HOSPITAL (191316)**, 2202 False River Drive, Zip 70760–2614; tel. 225/638–6331, (Nonreporting) **A**9 10 18
Primary Contact: Chad E. Olinde, Administrator and Chief Executive Officer
CFO: John Cazayoux, Chief Financial Officer
CMO: Carol Smothers, M.D., Chief of Staff
CHR: Lisa Patterson, Director Human Resources
Web address: www.pcgh.org
**Control:** Hospital district or authority, Government, nonfederal **Service:** General Medical and Surgical

**Staffed Beds:** 25

### OAK GROVE—West Carroll Parish

**WEST CARROLL MEMORIAL HOSPITAL (190081)**, 706 Ross Street, Zip 71263; tel. 318/428–3237, (Nonreporting) **A**9 10
Primary Contact: R. Randall Morris, Administrator
**Control:** Other not–for–profit (including NFP Corporation) **Service:** General Medical and Surgical

**Staffed Beds:** 21

### OAKDALE—Allen Parish

☐ **OAKDALE COMMUNITY HOSPITAL (190106)**, 130 North Hospital Drive, Zip 71463, Mailing Address: P.O. Box 629, Zip 71463–0629; tel. 318/335–3700, (Nonreporting) **A**1 9 10
Primary Contact: D. Kirk Soileau, Chief Executive Officer
CFO: Michael Fontenot, Interim Chief Financial Officer
CMO: Tommy Davis, M.D., Chief of Staff
CIO: Melissa Welch, Director Health Information Management
CHR: Dana Blood, Director Human Resources
Web address: www.oakdalecommunityhospital.com/
**Control:** Partnership, Investor–owned, for–profit **Service:** General Medical and Surgical

**Staffed Beds:** 27

### OLLA—Caldwell Parish

**HARDTNER MEDICAL CENTER (191315)**, 1102 North Pine Road, Zip 71465; tel. 318/495–3131, (Nonreporting) **A**9 10 18
Primary Contact: Paul G. Mathews, CPA, Administrator
CIO: Destini Bubrig, Director Health Information Management
Web address: www.hardtnermedical.com
**Control:** Hospital district or authority, Government, nonfederal **Service:** General Medical and Surgical

**Staffed Beds:** 35

### OPELOUSAS—St. Landry Parish

☐ **OCEANS BEHAVIORAL HOSPITAL OF OPELOUSAS (194095)**, 1310 Heather Drive, Zip 70570–7714; tel. 337/948–8820, (Nonreporting) **A**1 9 10 **S** Oceans Healthcare, Lake Charles, LA
Primary Contact: Remi Savoy, Administrator
Web address: www.obho.info/
**Control:** Corporation, Investor–owned, for–profit **Service:** Psychiatric

**Staffed Beds:** 20

---

**Hospital, Medicare Provider Number, Address, Telephone, Approval, Facility, and Physician Codes, Health Care System**

★ American Hospital Association (AHA) membership
☐ The Joint Commission accreditation
◇ DNV Healthcare Inc. accreditation
◯ American Osteopathic Association (AOA) accreditation
△ Commission on Accreditation of Rehabilitation Facilities (CARF) accreditation

**LA**

⊞ **OPELOUSAS GENERAL HEALTH SYSTEM (190017)**, 539 East Prudhomme Street, Zip 70570, Mailing Address: P.O. Box 1389, Zip 70571–1389; tel. 337/948–3011, (Includes OPELOUSAS GENERAL HEALTH SYSTEM–SOUTH CAMPUS, 3983 I–49 South Service Road, Zip 70570–8975; tel. 337/948–2100) **A**1 2 9 10 19 **F**3 13 15 18 20 22 28 29 30 31 34 35 38 40 49 51 57 59 61 70 74 75 77 78 79 80 81 86 87 89 90 93 98 103 104 107 108 110 111 113 116 117 118 120 128 129 131 134 145 146 **S** QHR, Brentwood, TN
Primary Contact: Gary I. Keller, President and Chief Executive Officer
COO: Bob Hardy, Chief Operating Officer
CFO: James B. Juneau, Chief Financial Officer
CMO: Derek Metoyer, M.D., Chief of Staff
CIO: Jared Lormand, Vice President Information Technology
CHR: Suzanne Kidder, Director Human Resources
CNO: Karen Gremillion, R.N., Chief Nursing Officer
Web address: www.opelousasgeneral.com
**Control:** Hospital district or authority, Government, nonfederal **Service:** General Medical and Surgical

**Staffed Beds:** 201 **Admissions:** 9618 **Census:** 124 **Outpatient Visits:** 121374 **Births:** 1129 **Total Expense ($000):** 108571 **Payroll Expense ($000):** 45582 **Personnel:** 984

**ST. LANDRY EXTENDED CARE HOSPITAL (192034)**, 3983 I–49 South Service Road, 2nd Floor, Zip 70570; tel. 337/948–5184, (Nonreporting) **A**10
Primary Contact: Biff David, Administrator
Web address: www.lhcgroup.com
**Control:** Corporation, Investor–owned, for–profit **Service:** Long–Term Acute Care hospital

**Staffed Beds:** 23

### PINEVILLE—Rapides Parish

☐ **CENTRAL LOUISIANA STATE HOSPITAL (194025)**, 242 West Shamrock Avenue, Zip 71360, Mailing Address: P.O. Box 5031, Zip 71361–5031; tel. 318/484–6200, (Nonreporting) **A**1 10 **S** Louisiana State Hospitals, Baton Rouge, LA
Primary Contact: Wayne Hallford, Chief Executive Officer
COO: Paul Benoit, Associate Administrator
CFO: Tina Darbonne, Chief Financial Officer
CMO: L. Lee Tynes, Jr., M.D., Medical Director
CIO: William Haynes, Director Information Technology
CHR: Tom Crout, MS, Director Human Resources
Web address: www.dhh.la.gov/omh/inpatient–serv/clsh.htm
**Control:** State–Government, nonfederal **Service:** Psychiatric

**Staffed Beds:** 128

☐ **HUEY P. LONG MEDICAL CENTER (190009)**, 352 Hospital Boulevard, Zip 71360, Mailing Address: P.O. Box 5352, Zip 71361–5352; tel. 318/448–0811 **A**1 3 5 9 10 **F**3 8 11 13 15 18 29 30 31 32 35 38 40 43 46 49 50 54 57 59 61 64 65 66 70 75 77 78 79 81 85 86 87 89 93 97 98 102 107 113 118 129 131 134 145 146 147 **P**6
Primary Contact: Gary L. Crockett, Administrator
CFO: Beldia Bebee, Acting Chief Financial Officer
CMO: David Barnard, M.D., Medical Director
CIO: Mickey Roberts, Director Information Systems
CHR: Marsha Crittle, Director Human Resources
Web address: www.lsuhscshreveport.edu/index.php?src=gendocs&ref=HP–Long&submenu=HP–Long
**Control:** State–Government, nonfederal **Service:** General Medical and Surgical

**Staffed Beds:** 60 **Admissions:** 2297 **Census:** 37 **Outpatient Visits:** 86073 **Births:** 43 **Personnel:** 487

⊞ **VETERANS AFFAIRS MEDICAL CENTER – ALEXANDRIA**, 2495 Shreveport Highway, 71 N., Zip 71360, Mailing Address: P.O. Box 69004, Alexandria, Zip 71306–9004; tel. 318/466–2205, (Nonreporting) **A**1 2 5 **S** Department of Veterans Affairs, Washington, DC
Primary Contact: Gracie Specks, MS, Director
CFO: Denise Morton, Chief Financial Officer
CMO: Hollis Reed, M.D., Chief of Staff
CIO: David Thurmond, Chief Information Resource Management Service
CHR: Cindy Twilligear, Manager Human Resources
Web address: www.va.gov/sta/guide/home.asp
**Control:** Veterans Affairs, Government, federal **Service:** General Medical and Surgical

**Staffed Beds:** 143

### PLAQUEMINE—Iberville Parish

**MMO REHABILITATION AND WELLNESS CENTER (193070)**, 59213 Riverwest Drive, Zip 70764; tel. 225/687–8100, (Nonreporting) **A**10
Primary Contact: Bridget Suire, Acting Administrator
Web address: www.mmoinc.com
**Control:** Other not–for–profit (including NFP Corporation) **Service:** Rehabilitation

**Staffed Beds:** 8

### RACELAND—Lafourche Parish

⊞ **OCHSNER ST. ANNE GENERAL HOSPITAL (191324)**, 4608 Highway 1, Zip 70394–2623; tel. 985/537–6841, (Nonreporting) **A**1 9 10 18 **S** Ochsner Health System, New Orleans, LA
Primary Contact: Milton D. Bourgeois, Jr., Chief Executive Officer
CHR: Ann Ritchie, Director Human Resources
Web address: www.ochsnerstanne.org
**Control:** Hospital district or authority, Government, nonfederal **Service:** General Medical and Surgical

**Staffed Beds:** 35

### RAYNE—Acadia Parish

☐ **PHOENIX BEHAVIORAL HOSPITAL (194097)**, 2021 Crowley Rayne Highway, Zip 70578–4027; tel. 337/788–0091, (Nonreporting) **A**1 9 10
Primary Contact: Nancy Bourque, Administrator
**Control:** Other not–for–profit (including NFP Corporation) **Service:** Psychiatric

**Staffed Beds:** 18

### RAYVILLE—Richland Parish

★ **RICHARDSON MEDICAL CENTER (190151)**, 254 Highway 3048 Christian Drive, Zip 71269–0388, Mailing Address: P.O. Box 388, Zip 71269–0388; tel. 318/728–4181, (Nonreporting) **A**9 10
Primary Contact: James W. Barrett, Jr., Chief Executive Officer
CFO: Shawnia Taylor, Chief Financial Officer
CMO: David Thompson, M.D., Chief of Staff
CHR: Rita Brown, Director Human Resources
Web address: www.richardsonmed.org
**Control:** Hospital district or authority, Government, nonfederal **Service:** General Medical and Surgical

**Staffed Beds:** 38

### RUSTON—Lincoln Parish

**ALLEGIANCE HEALTH CENTER OF RUSTON (194087)**, 1401 Ezelle Street, Zip 71270–7218; tel. 318/226–8202, (Nonreporting) **A**9 10
Primary Contact: Donna K. Thompson, Chief Executive Officer
**Control:** Corporation, Investor–owned, for–profit **Service:** Psychiatric

**Staffed Beds:** 14

**GREEN CLINIC SURGICAL HOSPITAL (190257)**, 1118 Farmerville Street, Zip 71270; tel. 318/232–7700, (Nonreporting) **A**9 10
Primary Contact: Chad Conner, Interim Administrator
Web address: www.green–clinic.com
**Control:** Corporation, Investor–owned, for–profit **Service:** Other specialty

**Staffed Beds:** 13

⊞ **LIFECARE SPECIALTY HOSPITAL OF NORTH LOUISIANA (192022)**, 1401 Ezell Street, Zip 71270–7221; tel. 318/251–3126, (Nonreporting) **A**1 10 **S** LifeCare Management Services, Plano, TX
Primary Contact: Brent Martin, Chief Executive Officer
Web address: www.lifecare–hospitals.com/hospital.php?id=19
**Control:** Corporation, Investor–owned, for–profit **Service:** Long–Term Acute Care hospital

**Staffed Beds:** 90

⊞ **NORTHERN LOUISIANA MEDICAL CENTER (190086)**, 401 East Vaughn Avenue, Zip 71270–5950; tel. 318/254–2100, (Nonreporting) **A**1 9 10 19 **S** Community Health Systems, Inc., Franklin, TN
Primary Contact: Brady Dubois, Interim Chief Executive Officer
COO: James W. McClung, Assistant Chief Executive Officer
CFO: Frank Malek, Chief Financial Officer
CMO: Derek McClusky, M.D., Chief of Staff
CIO: Heather Nolan, Director Information Services
CHR: Tonya Duggan, Director Human Resources
Web address: www.northernlouisianamedicalcenter.com
**Control:** Other not–for–profit (including NFP Corporation) **Service:** General Medical and Surgical

**Staffed Beds:** 91

### SAINT FRANCISVILLE—West Feliciana Parish

⊞ **WEST FELICIANA PARISH HOSPITAL (191306)**, 5266 Commerce Street, Zip 70775–0368, Mailing Address: P.O. Box 368, Zip 70775–0368; tel. 225/635–3811 **A**1 9 10 18 **F**34 35 40 57 58 81 107 118 127 129 132 134 142
Primary Contact: Lee Chastant, M.D., Chief Executive Officer
CFO: Linda Harvey, Chief Financial Officer
CHR: Neta F. Leake, Administrative Assistant Human Resources
Web address: www.wfph.org
**Control:** Hospital district or authority, Government, nonfederal **Service:** General Medical and Surgical

**Staffed Beds:** 22 **Admissions:** 143 **Census:** 1 **Outpatient Visits:** 21986 **Births:** 0 **Total Expense ($000):** 11860 **Payroll Expense ($000):** 4618 **Personnel:** 90

**SHREVEPORT—Caddo Parish**

☐ **BRENTWOOD HOSPITAL (194020)**, 1006 Highland Avenue, Zip 71101–4103; tel. 318/678–7500, (Nonreporting) **A**1 9 10 **S** Universal Health Services, Inc., King of Prussia, PA
Primary Contact: James Duff, Chief Executive Officer
CFO: Kisha Scruggs, Chief Financial Officer
Web address: www.brentwoodbehavioral.com
**Control:** Corporation, Investor–owned, for–profit **Service:** Psychiatric

Staffed Beds: 160

⊠ **CHRISTUS HEALTH SHREVEPORT–BOSSIER (190041)**, One St. Mary Place, Zip 71101–4399; tel. 318/681–4500, (Includes CHRISTUS HIGHLAND MEDICAL CENTER, 1453 East Bert Kouns Industrial Loop, Zip 71105–6050; tel. 318/681–5000; CHRISTUS SCHUMPERT BOSSIER, 2105 Airline Drive, Bossier City, Zip 71111–3190; tel. 318/848–8000; CHRISTUS SCHUMPERT MEDICAL CENTER, One St. Mary Place, tel. 318/681–4500; CHRISTUS SCHUMPERT SUTTON CHILDREN'S MEDICAL CENTER, One Saint Mary Place, Zip 71101; tel. 318/424–5437) **A**1 2 3 5 9 10 **F**3 7 11 12 13 15 17 18 20 22 24 26 29 30 31 32 34 35 40 41 43 45 46 47 48 49 53 54 56 57 58 59 60 61 64 70 72 74 75 76 77 78 79 81 82 85 86 87 88 89 90 93 96 97 102 107 108 110 111 113 114 118 119 120 122 123 125 129 130 131 133 134 142 145 146 147 **S** CHRISTUS Health, Irving, TX
Primary Contact: Stephen F. Wright, President and Chief Executive Officer
COO: William Lunn, M.D., Chief Operating Officer
CFO: Frank Canova, Jr., Chief Financial Officer
CMO: Deirdre Barfield, M.D., Vice President Medical Affairs and Chief Medical Officer
CIO: Jeff Davis, Market Information Officer
CHR: Wendy White, Vice President Human Resources
Web address: www.christusschumpert.org
**Control:** Church–operated, Nongovernment, not–for profit **Service:** General Medical and Surgical

Staffed Beds: 302 Admissions: 14433 Census: 185 Outpatient Visits: 204600 Births: 1152 Total Expense ($000): 215147 Payroll Expense ($000): 82565 Personnel: 1207

⊠ **DUBUIS HOSPITAL OF SHREVEPORT (192025)**, One St. Mary Place, 6th Floor, Zip 71101; tel. 318/221–3802, (Nonreporting) **A**1 10 **S** Dubuis Health System, Houston, TX
Primary Contact: Holly Powell, Interim Administrator
Web address: www.dubuis.org
**Control:** Church–operated, Nongovernment, not–for profit **Service:** General Medical and Surgical

Staffed Beds: 36

⊠ **LIFECARE HOSPITALS OF SHREVEPORT (192011)**, 9320 Linwood Avenue, Zip 71106–7003; tel. 318/688–8504, (Includes LIFECARE HOSPITALS OF SHREVEPORT–WILLIS KNIGHTON, 8001 Youree Drive, Zip 71115–2302; Keith Cox, Chief Executive Officer and Administrator; LIFECARE HOSPITALS OF SOUTH SHREVEPORT–WILLIS KNIGHTON NORTH, 2550 Kings Highway, Zip 71103–3922; Keith Cox, Chief Executive Officer and Administrator), (Nonreporting) **A**1 9 10 **S** LifeCare Management Services, Plano, TX
Primary Contact: Keith Cox, Administrator
Web address: www.lifecare–hospitals.com
**Control:** Corporation, Investor–owned, for–profit **Service:** Long–Term Acute Care hospital

Staffed Beds: 119

☐ **LSU MEDICAL CENTER–UNIVERSITY HOSPITAL (190098)**, 1501 Kings Highway, Zip 71130–4299, Mailing Address: P.O. Box 33932, Zip 71130–3932; tel. 318/675–5000, (Includes CHILDREN'S HOSPITAL OF SHREVEPORT, 1501 Kings Highway, Zip 71103–4228, Mailing Address: PO Box 33932, Zip 71130–3932; tel. 318/675–5000) **A**1 2 3 5 9 10 **F**3 8 11 13 14 15 16 18 19 20 21 22 23 24 26 27 29 30 31 33 43 47 49 50 51 54 55 59 60 61 64 66 68 70 72 74 75 76 77 78 79 80 81 82 85 88 89 93 97 98 99 100 101 102 103 104 107 108 110 111 113 114 117 118 119 120 122 123 128 129 134 135 145 146 147 **P**1 4 5 8
Primary Contact: Joseph M. Miciotto, Administrator
COO: Betty Johnson, Associate Administrator
CFO: Harold White, Vice Chancellor
CMO: Kevin Sittig, M.D., Senior Associate Dean and Chief Medical Officer
CIO: Marcus Hobgood, Director Information Services
CHR: David Fuqua, Director Human Resources Management
Web address: www.lsuhscshreveport.edu
**Control:** State–Government, nonfederal **Service:** General Medical and Surgical

Staffed Beds: 502 Admissions: 20602 Census: 349 Outpatient Visits: 449072 Births: 1502 Total Expense ($000): 328817 Payroll Expense ($000): 176258 Personnel: 3402

⊠ **OVERTON BROOKS VETERANS AFFAIRS MEDICAL CENTER**, 510 East Stoner Avenue, Zip 71101–4295; tel. 318/221–8411, (Nonreporting) **A**1 2 3 5 8 9 **S** Department of Veterans Affairs, Washington, DC
Primary Contact: Shirley Bealer, Director
CFO: Kim Lane, Chief Fiscal Service
CIO: Janey Taylor, Chief Information and Technology
CHR: Michael L. Palmier, Chief Human Resources Management
Web address: www.va.gov/sta/guide/home.asp
**Control:** Veterans Affairs, Government, federal **Service:** General Medical and Surgical

Staffed Beds: 119

**PHYSICIANS BEHAVIORAL HOSPITAL (194094)**, 2025 Desoto Street, Zip 71103–4717; tel. 337/223–4165, (Nonreporting) **A**10
Primary Contact: Debbie Priebe, Administrator
**Control:** Corporation, Investor–owned, for–profit **Service:** Psychiatric

Staffed Beds: 12

☐ **PROMISE HOSPITAL OF LOUISIANA – SHREVEPORT CAMPUS (192010)**, 1800 Irving Place, Zip 71101–4608; tel. 318/425–4096, (Nonreporting) **A**1 9 10 **S** Promise Healthcare, Boca Raton, FL
Primary Contact: Rick Stockton, Chief Executive Officer
Web address: www.promise–shreveport.com
**Control:** Corporation, Investor–owned, for–profit **Service:** Long–Term Acute Care hospital

Staffed Beds: 146

**PROMISE SPECIALTY HOSPITAL OF SHREVEPORT** See Promise Hospital of Louisiana – Shreveport Campus

☐ **SHRINERS HOSPITALS FOR CHILDREN, SHREVEPORT (193301)**, 3100 Samford Avenue, Zip 71103–4289; tel. 318/222–5704, (Nonreporting) **A**1 3 5 10 **S** Shriners Hospitals for Children, Tampa, FL
Primary Contact: Garry Kim Green, FACHE, Administrator
CFO: Lori Lucas, Director Fiscal Services
CMO: Philip E. Gates, M.D., Chief of Staff
CIO: Kim Crockett, Director Management Information Systems
CHR: Rena Arbuthnot, Director Human Resources
CNO: Gail Rains, R.N., Director Patient Care Services
Web address: www.shriners.com
**Control:** Other not–for–profit (including NFP Corporation) **Service:** Children's other specialty

Staffed Beds: 45

**SPECIALISTS HOSPITAL – SHREVEPORT (190278)**, 1500 Line Avenue, Zip 71101–4639; tel. 318/213–3800, (Nonreporting) **A**9 10
Primary Contact: Kandi Moore, Administrator
Web address: www.specialistshospitalshreveport.com/
**Control:** Corporation, Investor–owned, for–profit **Service:** General Medical and Surgical

Staffed Beds: 15

⊠ △ **WILLIS–KNIGHTON MEDICAL CENTER (190111)**, 2600 Greenwood Road, Zip 71103–2600, Mailing Address: P.O. Box 32600, Zip 71130–2600; tel. 318/212–4600, (Includes WILLIS–KNIGHTON PIERREMONT HEALTH CENTER, 8001 Youree Drive, Zip 71115; tel. 318/212–3000; WILLIS–KNIGHTON SOUTH – THE CENTER FOR WOMEN'S HEALTH, 2510 Bert Kouns Industrial Loop, Zip 71118; tel. 318/212–5000; Keri Elrod, Administrator) **A**1 2 3 5 7 9 10 **F**3 7 8 9 10 11 12 13 15 17 18 20 22 24 26 28 29 30 31 34 35 38 40 44 45 47 48 49 50 51 52 53 54 55 56 57 58 59 60 61 62 63 64 65 66 68 70 72 74 75 76 77 78 79 80 81 82 84 85 86 87 88 89 90 93 96 97 98 100 101 102 103 104 106 107 108 109 110 111 112 113 114 117 118 119 120 122 123 124 125 126 127 128 129 130 131 133 134 136 137 138 141 143 144 145 146 147 **P**6 7 **S** Willis–Knighton Health System, Shreveport, LA
Primary Contact: Jaf Fielder, Vice President and Administrator
COO: Charles D. Daigle, Senior Vice President and Chief Operating Officer
CFO: Robert D. Huie, Executive Vice President and Chief Financial Officer
CMO: Frederick Kinder, M.D., Chief of Staff
CIO: Charles Laster, Director Information Management
CHR: Jaf Fielder, Vice President and Administrator
Web address: www.wkhs.com
**Control:** Other not–for–profit (including NFP Corporation) **Service:** General Medical and Surgical

Staffed Beds: 902 Admissions: 37175 Census: 452 Outpatient Visits: 367849 Births: 3049 Personnel: 4321

---

**Hospital, Medicare Provider Number, Address, Telephone, Approval, Facility, and Physician Codes, Health Care System**

★ American Hospital Association (AHA) membership
☐ The Joint Commission accreditation
◇ DNV Healthcare Inc. accreditation
○ American Osteopathic Association (AOA) accreditation
△ Commission on Accreditation of Rehabilitation Facilities (CARF) accreditation

LA

## SLIDELL—St. Tammany Parish

**AMG SPECIALTY HOSPITAL–SLIDELL (192046)**, 1400 Lindberg Drive, Zip 70458–8056; tel. 985/326–0440, (Nonreporting) **A**10 **S** AMG Integrated Healthcare Management, Lafayette, LA
Primary Contact: Richard Daughdrill, R.N., Chief Executive Officer
COO: Gene Smith, Senior Vice President Operations
CFO: Jessica McGee, Chief Financial Officer
CMO: Marie Mahoney, M.D., Chief Medical Officer
CHR: Kim Hernandez, Director Human Resources
Web address: www.acadianamanagementgroup.com
**Control:** Partnership, Investor–owned, for–profit **Service:** Long–Term Acute Care hospital

**Staffed Beds:** 40

**CYPRESS POINTE HOSPITAL EAST (190256)**, 989 Robert Boulevard, Zip 70458–2009; tel. 985/690–8200 **A**10 **F**29 81 107 118
Primary Contact: Sarah C. Garvin, Chief Executive Officer
**Control:** Corporation, Investor–owned, for–profit **Service:** Surgical

**Staffed Beds:** 10 **Admissions:** 43 **Census:** 1 **Outpatient Visits:** 1166 **Births:** 0 **Personnel:** 44

**NORTHSHORE REGIONAL MEDICAL CENTER** See Ochsner Medical Center – North Shore

☒ **OCHSNER MEDICAL CENTER – NORTH SHORE (190204)**, 100 Medical Center Drive, Zip 70461–5520; tel. 985/646–5000 **A**1 9 10 **F**8 11 13 15 18 19 20 24 29 30 31 40 43 45 49 50 51 54 60 72 76 77 81 82 87 88 89 90 93 95 96 107 108 110 111 118 128 131 145 146 147 **S** Ochsner Health System, New Orleans, LA
Primary Contact: Polly J. Davenport, R.N., Chief Executive Officer
COO: Alan Hodges, Chief Operating Officer
CFO: Forrest Whichard, Chief Financial Officer
CMO: James Newcomb, M.D., Vice President Medical
CHR: Terri Joseph–Taylor, Chief Human Resource Manager
CNO: Cheryl Woods, Chief Nursing Officer
Web address: www.ochsner.org/locations/northshore
**Control:** Other not–for–profit (including NFP Corporation) **Service:** General Medical and Surgical

**Staffed Beds:** 110 **Admissions:** 5148 **Census:** 61 **Outpatient Visits:** 51168 **Births:** 487 **Total Expense ($000):** 66767 **Payroll Expense ($000):** 31064

☒ **SLIDELL MEMORIAL HOSPITAL (190040)**, 1001 Gause Boulevard, Zip 70458–2987; tel. 985/643–2200 **A**1 2 3 5 9 10 **F**3 11 13 15 17 18 19 20 21 22 23 24 25 26 28 29 31 32 34 35 40 45 46 49 54 56 57 59 64 70 72 74 75 76 78 79 81 82 85 86 87 89 90 93 96 97 107 108 109 110 111 113 114 116 117 118 119 120 122 123 128 129 131 134 144 145 146 147 **P**6
Primary Contact: John William Davis, Chief Executive Officer and Chief Financial Officer
CFO: John William Davis, Chief Executive Officer and Chief Financial Officer
Web address: www.slidellmemorial.org
**Control:** Hospital district or authority, Government, nonfederal **Service:** General Medical and Surgical

**Staffed Beds:** 170 **Admissions:** 6500 **Census:** 88 **Outpatient Visits:** 120283 **Births:** 784 **Total Expense ($000):** 113573 **Payroll Expense ($000):** 50933

☐ **SOUTHERN SURGICAL HOSPITAL (190270)**, 1700 Lindberg Drive, Zip 70458–8062; tel. 985/641–0600, (Nonreporting) **A**1 9 10
Primary Contact: Michael J. Pisciotta, Chief Executive Officer
CFO: Michael J. Maurin, Chief Financial Officer
CMO: J. Gosey, M.D., Medical Director
CIO: Buddy Graves, Chief Information Officer
CHR: Lorrie Alfred, Director Human Resources
Web address: www.sshla.com/
**Control:** Corporation, Investor–owned, for–profit **Service:** Surgical

**Staffed Beds:** 39

## SPRINGHILL—Webster Parish

☐ **SPRINGHILL MEDICAL CENTER (190088)**, 2001 Doctors Drive, Zip 71075–4526, Mailing Address: P.O. Box 920, Zip 71075–0920; tel. 318/539–1000, (Nonreporting) **A**1 9 10
Primary Contact: Todd Eppler, Chief Executive Officer
CFO: Layla Chase, Chief Financial Officer
CMO: Michelle Pardue, M.D., Chief Medical Staff
CIO: Brian Griffin, Director Information Services
CHR: Derek Melancon, Director Human Resources and Marketing
CNO: Dana Jones, R.N., Chief Nursing Officer
Web address: www.smccare.com
**Control:** Other not–for–profit (including NFP Corporation) **Service:** General Medical and Surgical

**Staffed Beds:** 35

## STERLINGTON—Ouachita Parish

**STERLINGTON REHABILITATION HOSPITAL (193069)**, 111 Highway 2, Zip 71280, Mailing Address: P.O. Box 627, Zip 71280–0627; tel. 318/665–9950, (Nonreporting) **A**10
Primary Contact: Cathy Martin, Administrator
Web address: www.www.sterlingtonrehab.com
**Control:** Corporation, Investor–owned, for–profit **Service:** Rehabilitation

**Staffed Beds:** 19

## STONEWALL—De Soto Parish

**STONEWALL HOSPITAL (194093)**, 960 Highway 171 South, Zip 71078–9594; tel. 318/925–6660, (Nonreporting) **A**9 10
Primary Contact: Del Humphrey, Administrator and Chief Executive Officer
**Control:** Corporation, Investor–owned, for–profit **Service:** Psychiatric

**Staffed Beds:** 22

## SULPHUR—Calcasieu Parish

☐ **CORNERSTONE HOSPITAL OF SOUTHWEST LOUISIANA (192013)**, 703 Cypress Street, Zip 70663; tel. 337/527–1102, (Nonreporting) **A**1 9 10 **S** Cornerstone Healthcare Group, Dallas, TX
Primary Contact: Robert R. Lafleur, Chief Executive Officer
CFO: Amy Bryant, Chief Financial Officer
Web address: www.cornerstonehealthcaregroup.com
**Control:** Partnership, Investor–owned, for–profit **Service:** Long–Term Acute Care hospital

**Staffed Beds:** 30

☐ **WEST CALCASIEU CAMERON HOSPITAL (190013)**, 701 Cypress Street, Zip 70663–5000, Mailing Address: P.O. Box 2509, Zip 70664–2509; tel. 337/527–4240 **A**1 9 10 **F**3 7 11 13 15 18 20 22 26 28 29 30 31 32 34 35 37 38 40 44 45 46 50 53 54 57 59 62 64 65 68 70 75 76 77 78 79 81 85 86 89 93 94 107 108 109 110 111 114 117 118 126 129 133 144 145 147
Primary Contact: J. William Hankins, FACHE, Chief Executive Officer
COO: Janie Fruge, Chief Operating Officer and Chief Nursing Officer
CFO: Tammy Broussard, Chief Financial Officer
CIO: Trey Rion, Chief Information Officer
CHR: Christi Kingsley, Director Human Resources
CNO: Janie Fruge, Chief Operating Officer and Chief Nursing Officer
Web address: www.wcch.com
**Control:** Hospital district or authority, Government, nonfederal **Service:** General Medical and Surgical

**Staffed Beds:** 76 **Admissions:** 3362 **Census:** 36 **Outpatient Visits:** 74937 **Births:** 200 **Total Expense ($000):** 51364 **Payroll Expense ($000):** 22976 **Personnel:** 548

## TALLULAH—Madison Parish

**MADISON PARISH HOSPITAL (191314)**, 900 Johnson Street, Zip 71282–4537, Mailing Address: P.O. Box 1559, Zip 71284–1559; tel. 318/574–2374, (Nonreporting) **A**9 10 18
Primary Contact: Wendell Alford, Administrator
CIO: Charles Whitaker, Director Information Technology
CHR: Chasity Whitaker, Administrative Assistant
Web address: www.madisonparishhospital.com
**Control:** Other not–for–profit (including NFP Corporation) **Service:** General Medical and Surgical

**Staffed Beds:** 25

## THIBODAUX—Lafourche Parish

☒ △ **THIBODAUX REGIONAL MEDICAL CENTER (190004)**, 602 North Acadia Road, Zip 70301–4847, Mailing Address: P.O. Box 1118, Zip 70302–1118; tel. 985/447–5500 **A**1 2 7 9 10 **F**3 8 11 12 13 15 18 19 20 22 24 28 29 30 31 32 34 40 46 49 57 59 62 64 70 73 74 75 76 77 78 79 81 85 86 87 90 92 93 96 97 104 105 107 108 110 111 114 115 116 118 119 120 122 123 125 126 128 129 130 131 145 146 147
Primary Contact: Greg K. Stock, Chief Executive Officer
COO: Kim Keene, Vice President Professional Services
CFO: Steve C. Gaubert, Chief Financial Officer
CMO: Greg Chaisson, M.D., Chief Medical Staff
CIO: Terry Evans, Chief Information Officer
CHR: Eric Degravelle, Director Human Resources
Web address: www.thibodaux.com
**Control:** Hospital district or authority, Government, nonfederal **Service:** General Medical and Surgical

**Staffed Beds:** 140 **Admissions:** 7991 **Census:** 95 **Outpatient Visits:** 137588 **Births:** 736 **Total Expense ($000):** 124778 **Payroll Expense ($000):** 48121 **Personnel:** 856

*Many Facility Codes have changed. Please refer to the AHA Guide Code Chart.*  © 2012 AHA Guide

## VIDALIA—Concordia Parish

☐ **PROMISE HOSPITAL OF MISS LOU (192028)**, 209 Front Street, Zip 71373–2837; tel. 318/336–6500, (Data for 325 days) **A**1 9 **F**1 3 29 60 75 93 104 129 147 **S** Promise Healthcare, Boca Raton, FL
Primary Contact: Benny Costello, Chief Executive Officer
COO: Howard B. Koslow, President and Chief Executive Officer
CFO: Larry Leder, Chief Financial Officer
CMO: Barry Tillman, M.D., Chief Medical Staff
CIO: Elizabeth Carpenter, Director Quality Assurance and Quality Improvement and Assistant Administrator
CHR: Roxan Houghton, Director Human Resources
Web address: www.promise–misslou.com
**Control:** Corporation, Investor–owned, for–profit **Service:** Long–Term Acute Care hospital

**Staffed Beds: 40 Admissions: 316 Census: 26 Outpatient Visits: 11314 Births: 0**

## VILLE PLATTE—Evangeline Parish

★ **MERCY REGIONAL MEDICAL CENTER (190167)**, 800 East Main Street, Zip 70586, Mailing Address: P.O. Box 349, Zip 70586–0349; tel. 337/363–5684, (Includes ACADIAN MEDICAL CENTER, 3501 Highway 190, Eunice, Zip 70535–5129; tel. 337/580–7500) **A**9 10 **F**3 8 11 13 15 29 30 31 34 35 38 40 45 51 53 55 57 59 64 65 70 75 76 77 78 79 81 82 83 84 85 86 87 89 90 91 92 93 94 96 97 107 108 111 113 118 129 130 131 132 134 145 146 147 **S** LifePoint Hospitals, Inc., Brentwood, TN
Primary Contact: Robert Alan Daugherty, Chief Executive Officer
COO: Sandy Morein, Chief Operating Officer
CFO: Lori Petrie, Chief Financial Officer
CMO: Brandon Fontenot, M.D., Chief of Staff
CIO: Courtney Bieber, Director Information Systems
CHR: Sue Thomas, Director Human Resources
Web address: www.mercyregionalmedicalcenter.com
**Control:** Corporation, Investor–owned, for–profit **Service:** General Medical and Surgical

**Staffed Beds: 70 Admissions: 5200 Census: 54 Outpatient Visits: 45832 Births: 499 Total Expense ($000): 58610 Payroll Expense ($000): 21681 Personnel: 460**

## VIVIAN—Caddo Parish

**NORTH CADDO MEDICAL CENTER (191304)**, 1000 South Spruce Street, Zip 71082–3232, Mailing Address: P.O. Box 792, Zip 71082–0792; tel. 318/375–3235, (Nonreporting) **A**9 10 18
Primary Contact: David C. Jones, Administrator
CFO: Carol Reisz, Chief Financial Officer
CMO: John H. Haynes, Jr., M.D., Chief of Medical Staff
CIO: Allyson Allums, Director Medical Records
CHR: Lanell Audirsch, Administrative Assistant
Web address: www.northcaddomedicalcenter.com
**Control:** Hospital district or authority, Government, nonfederal **Service:** General Medical and Surgical

**Staffed Beds: 25**

## WEST MONROE—Ouachita Parish

☐ **CORNERSTONE HOSPITAL–WEST MONROE (192031)**, 6198 Cypress Street, Zip 71291–9010; tel. 318/396–5600, (Nonreporting) **A**1 9 10 **S** Cornerstone Healthcare Group, Dallas, TX
Primary Contact: Chris Simpson, Chief Executive Officer
COO: Jay Quintana, Vice President Operations
CFO: Laura Nowell, Chief Financial Officer
CMO: Khaled Shafici, M.D., President Medical Staff
CIO: Adam Davis, Chief Information Officer
CHR: Dan Perkins, Corporate Director Human Resources
Web address: www.cornerstonehealthcaregroup.com
**Control:** Corporation, Investor–owned, for–profit **Service:** Long–Term Acute Care hospital

**Staffed Beds: 40**

**GLENWOOD REGIONAL MEDICAL CENTER (190160)**, 503 McMillan Road, Zip 71291–5327; tel. 318/329–4200, (Nonreporting) **A**2 9 10 21 **S** IASIS Healthcare, Franklin, TN
Primary Contact: Ronald J. Elder, Chief Executive Officer
COO: Larry D. Walker, Chief Operating Officer
CFO: John DeSantis, Chief Financial Officer
CMO: John Maxwell, M.D., Chief of Staff
CIO: Ronnie Maxwell, Director Information Systems
CHR: Jan Walker, Director Human Resources
CNO: Sharon Lewis, Chief Nursing Officer
Web address: www.grmc.com
**Control:** Other not–for–profit (including NFP Corporation) **Service:** General Medical and Surgical

**Staffed Beds: 247**

**LOUISIANA EXTENDED CARE HOSPITAL WEST MONROE (192055)**, 503 McMillan Road, 3rd Floor, Zip 71291; tel. 318/329–4300, (Nonreporting) **A**10 **S** LHC Group, Lafayette, LA
Primary Contact: Cleta Munholland, Administrator
**Control:** Corporation, Investor–owned, for–profit **Service:** Long–Term Acute Care hospital

**Staffed Beds: 18**

**OUACHITA COMMUNITY HOSPITAL (190261)**, 1275 Glenwood Drive, Zip 71291; tel. 318/322–1339 **A**9 10 21 **F**3 12 34 35 45 57 65 79 81 82 85 131
Primary Contact: Robert L. Colvin, Administrator
CFO: John DeSantis, Chief Financial Officer
CMO: H. Jerrel Fontenot, M.D., Medical Director
CMO: Brenda Wallace, R.N., Chief Nursing Officer
Web address: www.ouachitacommunityhospital.com
**Control:** Partnership, Investor–owned, for–profit **Service:** Surgical

**Staffed Beds: 10 Admissions: 49 Census: 1 Outpatient Visits: 2906 Births: 0 Total Expense ($000): 4951 Payroll Expense ($000): 1823 Personnel: 27**

## WINNFIELD—Winn Parish

☐ **SPECIALTY HOSPITAL OF WINNFIELD (192052)**, 915 First Street, Zip 71483–2945; tel. 318/648–0212, (Nonreporting) **A**1 10
Primary Contact: Christopher Kemp Wright, Chief Executive Officer
CFO: Charlie Jurek, Business Office Manager
CIO: Shamada Venzant, Manager Health Information
**Control:** Corporation, Investor–owned, for–profit **Service:** Long–Term Acute Care hospital

**Staffed Beds: 20**

**WINN PARISH MEDICAL CENTER (190090)**, 301 West Boundary Street, Zip 71483–3427, Mailing Address: P.O. Box 152, Zip 71483–0152; tel. 318/648–3000, (Nonreporting) **A**9 10
Primary Contact: Bryan Bogle, Interim Chief Executive Officer
CFO: Leah Lashley, Chief Financial Officer
CMO: Julio Iglesias, M.D., Chief of Staff
CHR: Kimberly Ingles, Director Human Resources
Web address: www.winnparishmedical.com
**Control:** Corporation, Investor–owned, for–profit **Service:** General Medical and Surgical

**Staffed Beds: 60**

**WOODLANDS BEHAVIORAL CENTER (194076)**, 1400 West Court Street, Zip 71483–1338, Mailing Address: P.O. Box 138, Zip 71483–1338; tel. 318/628–5445, (Nonreporting) **A**9 10
Primary Contact: Bobby G. Jordan, Administrator
Web address: www.woodlandsbehavioral.com/
**Control:** Corporation, Investor–owned, for–profit **Service:** Psychiatric

**Staffed Beds: 19**

## WINNSBORO—Franklin Parish

★ **FRANKLIN MEDICAL CENTER (190140)**, 2106 Loop Road, Zip 71295–3398, Mailing Address: P.O. Box 1300, Zip 71295–1300; tel. 318/435–9411, (Nonreporting) **A**9 10
Primary Contact: Blake Kramer, Chief Executive Officer
CMO: Jay Busby, M.D., President Medical Staff
CIO: Judy Ogden, Director Information Technology
Web address: www.fmc–cares.com
**Control:** Hospital district or authority, Government, nonfederal **Service:** General Medical and Surgical

**Staffed Beds: 43**

---

**Hospital, Medicare Provider Number, Address, Telephone, Approval, Facility, and Physician Codes, Health Care System**

★ American Hospital Association (AHA) membership
☐ The Joint Commission accreditation
◇ DNV Healthcare Inc. accreditation
○ American Osteopathic Association (AOA) accreditation
△ Commission on Accreditation of Rehabilitation Facilities (CARF) accreditation

**LA**

✠ **LANE REGIONAL MEDICAL CENTER (190020)**, 6300 Main Street, Zip 70791–4037; tel. 225/658–4000, (Nonreporting) **A**1 9 10
Primary Contact: Randall M. Olson, Chief Executive Officer
CFO: Mark Anderson, Chief Financial Officer
CMO: David Rabalais, M.D., Chief Medical Staff
CIO: Scarlet Collier, Chief Information Officer
CHR: David Beck, Chief Operating Officer and Director Human Resources
CNO: Jennifer Johnson, R.N., Chief Nursing Officer
Web address: www.lanermc.org
**Control:** Hospital district or authority, Government, nonfederal **Service:** General Medical and Surgical

**Staffed Beds:** 176

*Many Facility Codes have changed. Please refer to the AHA Guide Code Chart.*
© 2012 AHA Guide

# MAINE

## AUGUSTA—Kennebec County

**MAINEGENERAL MEDICAL CENTER–AUGUSTA CAMPUS** See MaineGeneral Medical Center–Waterville Campus, Waterville

☐ **RIVERVIEW PSYCHIATRIC CENTER (204007)**, 250 Arsenal Street, 11 State House Station, Zip 4330, Mailing Address: P.O. Box 724, Zip 04332–0724; tel. 207/624–3900 **A**1 9 10 **F**29 30 39 64 75 86 87 97 98 100 101 103 104 129 131 134 **P**6
Primary Contact: Mary Louise McEwen, Superintendent
CFO: Jenny Boyden, Chief Financial Officer
CMO: William Nelson, M.D., Medical Director
CHR: Kristine Albert, Personnel Officer
CNO: Tami Cooper, Acting Director of Nursing
Web address: www.state.me.us/dhhs/riverview
**Control:** State–Government, nonfederal **Service:** Psychiatric

**Staffed Beds:** 92 **Admissions:** 295 **Census:** 80 **Outpatient Visits:** 7197
**Births:** 0 **Total Expense ($000):** 34832 **Payroll Expense ($000):** 13192
**Personnel:** 291

## BANGOR—Penobscot County

☐ **DOROTHEA DIX PSYCHIATRIC CENTER (204004)**, 656 State Street, Zip 4401, Mailing Address: P.O. Box 926, Zip 04402–0926; tel. 207/941–4000 **A**1 9 10 **F**39 98 101 104 129 **P**6
Primary Contact: Linda O. Abernethy, MSN, R.N., Superintendent
COO: Sharon Sprague, Director Therapeutic Services
CFO: Steven Thebarge, Chief Operating Officer and Chief Financial Officer
CMO: Marjorie Snyder, M.D., Clinical Director
CIO: Larry Larson, Management Analyst
CHR: Ruth Mullaney, Personnel Officer
Web address: www.maine.gov/dhhs/ddpc/index.shtml
**Control:** State–Government, nonfederal **Service:** Psychiatric

**Staffed Beds:** 51 **Admissions:** 308 **Census:** 55 **Outpatient Visits:** 2200
**Births:** 0 **Total Expense ($000):** 27143 **Payroll Expense ($000):** 12856
**Personnel:** 246

⊞ **EASTERN MAINE MEDICAL CENTER (200033)**, 489 State Street, Zip 04401–6674, Mailing Address: P.O. Box 404, Zip 04402–0404; tel. 207/973–7000, (Includes ROSS SKILLED NURSING FACILITY ), (Data for 364 days) **A**1 2 3 5 9 10 13 **F**3 11 12 13 15 17 18 19 20 22 24 26 28 29 30 31 34 36 37 39 40 43 44 45 46 47 48 49 50 51 53 54 55 57 58 59 60 61 64 70 72 74 75 76 77 78 79 81 82 84 85 86 87 88 89 90 92 93 94 96 97 102 107 108 110 111 113 114 116 117 118 119 120 122 123 125 128 129 130 131 143 144 145 146 147 **P**6 **S** Eastern Maine Healthcare Systems, Brewer, ME
Primary Contact: Deborah Carey Johnson, R.N., President and Chief Executive Officer
CFO: Elmer Doucette, Vice President and Chief Financial Officer
CMO: James Raczek, M.D., Sr. Vice President of Operations and Chief Medical Officer
CIO: Catherine Bruno, FACHE, Chief Information Officer
CHR: Greg Howat, Vice President Human Resources
CNO: Jodi Galli, Chief Nursing Officer
Web address: www.emh.org
**Control:** Other not–for–profit (including NFP Corporation) **Service:** General Medical and Surgical

**Staffed Beds:** 349 **Admissions:** 19302 **Census:** 271 **Outpatient Visits:** 412756 **Births:** 1619 **Total Expense ($000):** 556299 **Payroll Expense ($000):** 226663 **Personnel:** 3191

⊞ **ST. JOSEPH HOSPITAL (200001)**, 360 Broadway, Zip 04401–3897, Mailing Address: P.O. Box 403, Zip 04402–0403; tel. 207/262–1000 **A**1 9 10 **F**8 15 18 28 29 30 31 35 40 45 48 49 51 55 56 57 62 63 64 70 74 75 78 79 81 82 84 86 87 107 108 110 114 118 128 129 131 134 145 146 147 **S** Covenant Health Systems, Inc., Tewksbury, MA
Primary Contact: Mary Prybylo, President and Chief Executive Officer
CFO: Wayne Woodford, Executive Vice President and Chief Financial Officer
CMO: David Renedo, M.D., Chief of Staff
CIO: Karen Bowling, Chief Information Officer
CHR: Patricia Brezovsky, Director Human Resources
Web address: www.sjhhealth.com
**Control:** Church–operated, Nongovernment, not–for profit **Service:** General Medical and Surgical

**Staffed Beds:** 84 **Admissions:** 5858 **Census:** 55 **Outpatient Visits:** 103102
**Births:** 0 **Total Expense ($000):** 82348 **Payroll Expense ($000):** 34267
**Personnel:** 624

⊞ **THE ACADIA HOSPITAL (204006)**, 268 Stillwater Avenue, Zip 04401–3945, Mailing Address: P.O. Box 422, Zip 04402–0422; tel. 207/973–6100 **A**1 9 10 **F**5 29 30 50 57 66 68 75 77 87 98 99 100 101 103 104 105 129 131 **P**6 **S** Eastern Maine Healthcare Systems, Brewer, ME
Primary Contact: Daniel B. Coffey, President and Chief Executive Officer
CFO: Marie Suitter, Chief Financial Officer
CMO: Anthony Ng, M.D., Vice President and Chief Medical Officer
CIO: Jeanne Paradis, Director Information Services
CHR: Ted Helberg, Vice President, Human Resources
CNO: Karen Clements, R.N., Vice President, Chief Nursing Officer
Web address: www.acadiahospital.org
**Control:** Other not–for–profit (including NFP Corporation) **Service:** Psychiatric

**Staffed Beds:** 72 **Admissions:** 1691 **Census:** 59 **Outpatient Visits:** 94619
**Births:** 0 **Total Expense ($000):** 47664 **Payroll Expense ($000):** 25038
**Personnel:** 439

## BAR HARBOR—Hancock County

★ **MOUNT DESERT ISLAND HOSPITAL (201304)**, 10 Wayman Lane, Zip 04609–0008, Mailing Address: P.O. Box 8, Zip 04609–0008; tel. 207/288–5081 **A**9 10 18 **F**3 5 6 10 11 13 15 28 29 31 34 35 36 40 54 56 57 59 64 65 70 74 75 76 77 78 79 81 82 84 85 87 91 92 93 97 99 100 101 104 107 108 113 118 124 126 129 130 131 132 134 144 145 146 **P**6 7
Primary Contact: Arthur J. Blank, President and Chief Executive Officer
CFO: Christina Harding, Vice President Finance
CMO: Julian Kuffler, M.D., President Medical Staff
CIO: Mark White, Director Information Services
CHR: Joanne Harris, Director Human Resources
CNO: Barbara A. Hannon, MSN, VP Nursing
Web address: www.mdihospital.org
**Control:** Other not–for–profit (including NFP Corporation) **Service:** General Medical and Surgical

**Staffed Beds:** 25 **Admissions:** 1010 **Census:** 10 **Outpatient Visits:** 171948
**Births:** 119 **Total Expense ($000):** 48342 **Payroll Expense ($000):** 22786
**Personnel:** 353

## BELFAST—Waldo County

**WALDO COUNTY GENERAL HOSPITAL (201312)**, 118 Northport Avenue, Zip 04915–6072, Mailing Address: P.O. Box 287, Zip 04915–0287; tel. 207/338–2500 **A**9 10 18 **F**3 11 13 15 18 19 28 29 31 34 40 45 46 51 57 59 62 63 64 65 70 74 75 76 78 79 81 83 85 93 97 107 108 110 111 113 116 117 118 126 128 129 131 132 134 144 145 146 147 **P**8 **S** MaineHealth, Portland, ME
Primary Contact: Mark A. Biscone, Executive Director
COO: Dan Bennett, Director Operations
CFO: Linda Drinkwater, Chief Financial Officer
CMO: Kent Clark, M.D., Chief Medical Affairs and Quality
CIO: David Felton, Manager Information Systems
CHR: Karen Littlefield, Manager Human Resources
CNO: Teri R. Young–Hise, Director of Nursing
Web address: www.wchi.com
**Control:** Other not–for–profit (including NFP Corporation) **Service:** General Medical and Surgical

**Staffed Beds:** 25 **Admissions:** 1625 **Census:** 16 **Outpatient Visits:** 125663
**Births:** 169 **Total Expense ($000):** 64964 **Payroll Expense ($000):** 32891
**Personnel:** 480

---

**Hospital, Medicare Provider Number, Address, Telephone, Approval, Facility, and Physician Codes, Health Care System**

★ American Hospital Association (AHA) membership
☐ The Joint Commission accreditation
◇ DNV Healthcare Inc. accreditation
○ American Osteopathic Association (AOA) accreditation
△ Commission on Accreditation of Rehabilitation Facilities (CARF) accreditation

**ME**

## BIDDEFORD—York County

✠ **SOUTHERN MAINE MEDICAL CENTER (200019)**, One Medical Center Drive, Zip 04005–9496, Mailing Address: P.O. Box 626, Zip 04005–0626; tel. 207/283–7000 **A**1 2 9 10 **F**3 5 8 11 12 13 15 18 20 22 24 28 29 30 34 35 36 38 40 44 45 46 47 48 49 50 51 54 57 58 59 62 65 66 68 70 74 75 76 77 79 81 85 86 87 89 93 98 99 100 101 102 103 105 107 108 110 111 113 114 117 118 128 129 131 145 146 147 **P**6 **S** MaineHealth, Portland, ME
Primary Contact: Edward J. McGeachey, President and Chief Executive Officer
COO: Frank Lavoie, M.D., Executive Vice President and Chief Operating Officer
CFO: Norman Belair, Chief Financial Officer and Vice President Finance
CMO: Robert Fernandez, M.D., Chief Medical Staff
CIO: Mary Jane Kamps, Chief Information Officer
CHR: Lorraine Bouchard, Vice President Human Resources
CNO: Patricia M. Camire, MS, Chief Nursing Officer
Web address: www.smmc.org
**Control:** Other not–for–profit (including NFP Corporation) **Service:** General Medical and Surgical

**Staffed Beds:** 110 **Admissions:** 5888 **Census:** 68 **Outpatient Visits:** 277635 **Births:** 519 **Total Expense ($000):** 160839 **Payroll Expense ($000):** 79161 **Personnel:** 1154

## BLUE HILL—Hancock County

★ **BLUE HILL MEMORIAL HOSPITAL (201300)**, 57 Water Street, Zip 04614–0823, Mailing Address: P.O. Box 1029, Zip 04614–1029; tel. 207/374–3400, (Nonreporting) **A**9 10 18 **S** Eastern Maine Healthcare Systems, Brewer, ME
Primary Contact: Gregory E. Roraff, President and Chief Executive Officer
CFO: Scott Oxley, Interim Chief Financial Officer
CMO: Kathleen Ober, M.D., Chief Medical Officer
CHR: David Wheaton, Director Human Resources
Web address: www.bhmh.org
**Control:** Other not–for–profit (including NFP Corporation) **Service:** General Medical and Surgical

**Staffed Beds:** 25

## BOOTHBAY HARBOR—Lincoln County

★ **ST. ANDREWS HOSPITAL AND HEALTHCARE CENTER (201302)**, 6 St. Andrews Lane, Zip 04538–1732, Mailing Address: P.O. Box 417, Zip 04538–0417; tel. 207/633–2121, (Total facility includes 54 beds in nursing home–type unit) **A**9 10 18 **F**3 6 10 11 15 29 30 34 35 40 43 44 45 50 56 57 59 64 65 67 75 79 81 85 87 93 96 97 107 110 113 118 124 126 127 129 131 132 134 142 145 147 **P**6 **S** MaineHealth, Portland, ME
Primary Contact: James W. Donovan, President and Chief Executive Officer
COO: Cynthia Leavitt, R.N., Senior Vice President, Hospital Operations
CFO: Wayne Printy, Chief Financial Officer and Senior Vice President Finance
CMO: Russell Mack, M.D., Chief Medical Officer
CIO: Brooks Betts, Vice President and Chief Information Officer
CHR: Lisa McIlwain, Vice President Human Resources
Web address: www.lincolncountyhealthcare.org
**Control:** Other not–for–profit (including NFP Corporation) **Service:** General Medical and Surgical

**Staffed Beds:** 73 **Admissions:** 356 **Census:** 63 **Outpatient Visits:** 24535 **Births:** 0 **Total Expense ($000):** 18371 **Payroll Expense ($000):** 6443 **Personnel:** 157

## BRIDGTON—Cumberland County

★ **BRIDGTON HOSPITAL (201310)**, 10 Hospital Drive, Zip 4009; tel. 207/647–6000 **A**9 10 18 **F**3 11 13 15 29 30 31 35 40 53 54 57 59 70 75 76 78 79 81 85 86 97 107 108 110 113 118 129 130 131 132 134 142 145 146 147 **P**4 8
Primary Contact: R. David Frum, President
COO: John A. Ludwig, R.N., Vice President Administration
CFO: Philip Morissette, Chief Financial Officer
CMO: Suzanne Dater, M.D., President Medical Staff
CHR: Joyce McPhetres, Vice President Human Resources
Web address: www.bridgtonhospital.org
**Control:** Other not–for–profit (including NFP Corporation) **Service:** General Medical and Surgical

**Staffed Beds:** 22 **Admissions:** 1204 **Census:** 12 **Outpatient Visits:** 103961 **Births:** 98 **Total Expense ($000):** 38157 **Payroll Expense ($000):** 14758 **Personnel:** 239

## BRUNSWICK—Cumberland County

✠ **MID COAST HOSPITAL (200021)**, 123 Medical Center Drive, Zip 4011; tel. 207/729–0181 **A**1 9 10 **F**3 5 11 12 13 15 18 20 28 29 30 31 32 34 35 36 40 41 44 45 46 47 48 49 51 53 54 57 58 59 61 64 66 68 70 74 75 76 77 78 79 81 82 84 85 86 87 89 92 93 97 98 103 105 107 108 110 111 114 117 118 128 129 130 131 133 134 143 145 146 147 **P**6
Primary Contact: Lois N. Skillings, R.N., MSN, President and Chief Executive Officer
COO: Philip A. Ortolani, Vice President Operations
CFO: Robert N. McCue, Vice President Finance
CMO: Scott Mills, M.D., Vice President Medical Staff Administration and Chief Medical Officer
CIO: Gale Stoy, Manager Information Systems
Web address: www.midcoasthealth.com
**Control:** Other not–for–profit (including NFP Corporation) **Service:** General Medical and Surgical

**Staffed Beds:** 92 **Admissions:** 4791 **Census:** 56 **Outpatient Visits:** 168404 **Births:** 563 **Total Expense ($000):** 109350 **Payroll Expense ($000):** 49414 **Personnel:** 825

★ **PARKVIEW ADVENTIST MEDICAL CENTER (200025)**, 329 Maine Street, Zip 04011–3398; tel. 207/373–2000 **A**9 10 **F**11 15 29 30 31 34 35 36 37 38 40 45 50 56 59 61 64 65 66 68 70 75 77 78 79 81 82 85 86 87 89 90 93 107 108 110 111 113 115 116 118 128 129 131 134 144 145 146 **P**8
Primary Contact: Randee Reynolds, Interim President
CFO: Scott Heatley, Controller
CMO: Ramesh Gaindh, M.D., President Medical Staff
CIO: Bill McQuaid, Assistant Vice President and Chief Information Officer
CHR: Robin White, Assistant Vice President Human Resources
Web address: www.parkviewamc.org
**Control:** Church–operated, Nongovernment, not–for profit **Service:** General Medical and Surgical

**Staffed Beds:** 55 **Admissions:** 1037 **Census:** 11 **Outpatient Visits:** 66498 **Births:** 0 **Total Expense ($000):** 32700 **Payroll Expense ($000):** 11242 **Personnel:** 182

## CALAIS—Washington County

★ **CALAIS REGIONAL HOSPITAL (201305)**, 24 Hospital Lane, Zip 04619–1398; tel. 207/454–7521 **A**9 10 18 **F**1 3 11 13 15 28 29 31 32 34 35 36 40 45 50 57 59 62 64 65 67 68 70 75 76 77 78 79 81 83 84 85 86 87 89 90 93 97 98 107 108 111 113 118 126 127 128 129 131 132 134 145 146 147 **P**6 **S** QHR, Brentwood, TN
Primary Contact: Michael K. Lally, Chief Executive Officer
CFO: Nancy Glidden, Chief Financial Officer
CMO: Robert Chagrasulis, M.D., Chief of Staff
CIO: Dee Dee Travis, Director Community Relations
CHR: Kristi K. Saunders, Director and Compliance Officer
CNO: Cheryl Zwingman–Bagley, R.N., Chief Nursing Officer
Web address: www.calaishospital.com
**Control:** Other not–for–profit (including NFP Corporation) **Service:** General Medical and Surgical

**Staffed Beds:** 25 **Admissions:** 985 **Census:** 8 **Outpatient Visits:** 34480 **Births:** 61 **Total Expense ($000):** 33388 **Payroll Expense ($000):** 10624 **Personnel:** 240

## CARIBOU—Aroostook County

✠ **CARY MEDICAL CENTER (200031)**, 163 Van Buren Road, Suite 1, Zip 04736–2599; tel. 207/498–3111, (Total facility includes 9 beds in nursing home–type unit) **A**1 9 10 **F**3 8 11 13 15 28 29 31 32 34 35 36 38 40 43 44 51 53 54 56 57 59 61 64 67 68 70 75 76 77 78 79 81 82 84 85 86 87 89 90 93 97 107 108 111 114 117 118 120 129 130 131 134 143 145 146 147 **S** QHR, Brentwood, TN
Primary Contact: Kris A. Doody, R.N., Chief Executive Officer
COO: Shawn Anderson, Chief Operating Officer
CFO: Galen Dickinson, Chief Financial Officer
CMO: Beth Collamore, M.D., Chief of Staff
CIO: Dave Silsbee, Chief Information Officer
CHR: Paula A. Parent, R.N., Director Human Resources and Nursing Administration
Web address: www.carymedicalcenter.org
**Control:** City–Government, nonfederal **Service:** General Medical and Surgical

**Staffed Beds:** 49 **Admissions:** 1726 **Census:** 30 **Outpatient Visits:** 80652 **Births:** 182 **Total Expense ($000):** 42548 **Payroll Expense ($000):** 18515 **Personnel:** 387

*Many Facility Codes have changed. Please refer to the AHA Guide Code Chart.* © 2012 AHA Guide

**DAMARISCOTTA—Lincoln County**

★ **MILES MEMORIAL HOSPITAL (200002)**, 35 Miles Street, Zip 04543–9767;
tel. 207/563–1234 **A**9 10 20 **F**3 11 13 15 29 30 32 34 35 40 43 44 45 50
57 59 64 65 70 75 76 79 81 85 86 87 93 96 97 107 108 110 111 113 117
118 126 129 131 132 134 145 146 147 **P**6 **S** MaineHealth, Portland, ME
Primary Contact: James W. Donovan, President and Chief Executive Officer
COO: Cynthia Leavitt, R.N., Senior Vice President, Hospital Operations
CFO: Wayne Printy, Chief Financial Officer and Senior Vice President Finance
CMO: Russell Mack, M.D., Chief Medical Officer
CIO: Brooks Betts, Vice President and Chief Information Officer
CHR: Lisa McIlwain, Vice President Human Resources
Web address: www.lchcare.org
**Control:** Other not–for–profit (including NFP Corporation) **Service:** General
Medical and Surgical

| | |
|---|---|
| **Staffed Beds:** 38 **Admissions:** 1646 **Census:** 18 **Outpatient Visits:** 86475 **Births:** 171 **Total Expense ($000):** 53220 **Payroll Expense ($000):** 14307 **Personnel:** 338 | |

**DOVER–FOXCROFT—Piscataquis County**

★ **MAYO REGIONAL HOSPITAL (201309)**, 897 West Main Street,
Zip 04426–1099; tel. 207/564–8401 **A**9 10 18 **F**3 5 7 8 11 13 15 29 30 31
34 35 38 40 45 50 57 59 64 65 70 75 76 77 78 79 81 85 86 87 93 94 97
99 100 104 107 110 111 113 117 118 126 127 128 129 132 145 146 147
Primary Contact: Ralph Gabarro, Chief Executive Officer
CFO: Jeff Provenzano, Chief Financial Officer
CMO: Richard Evans, M.D., President Medical Staff
CHR: Ken Proctor, Director Human Resources
Web address: www.mayohospital.com
**Control:** Hospital district or authority, Government, nonfederal **Service:** General
Medical and Surgical

| | |
|---|---|
| **Staffed Beds:** 25 **Admissions:** 1117 **Census:** 11 **Outpatient Visits:** 108129 **Births:** 144 **Total Expense ($000):** 44167 **Payroll Expense ($000):** 23340 **Personnel:** 443 | |

**ELLSWORTH—Hancock County**

⊠ **MAINE COAST MEMORIAL HOSPITAL (200050)**, 50 Union Street,
Zip 04605–1599; tel. 207/664–5311 **A**1 9 10 **F**13 15 18 28 29 31 34 35 40
45 51 55 57 59 61 64 65 68 70 74 75 76 77 78 79 81 84 85 93 97 99 107
108 111 114 118 128 129 131 132 143 145 146 147
Primary Contact: Charles D. Therrien, Chief Executive Officer
COO: Barbara Hocking, R.N., Chief Operating Officer
CFO: Michael Hendrix, Chief Financial Officer
CMO: Sheena Whittaker, M.D., President Medical Staff
CIO: Mary Jo MacLaughlin, Director Information Systems
CHR: Karen Dickson, Director, Human Resources
CNO: Barbara Hocking, R.N., Chief Nursing Officer
Web address: www.mainehospital.org
**Control:** Other not–for–profit (including NFP Corporation) **Service:** General
Medical and Surgical

| | |
|---|---|
| **Staffed Beds:** 48 **Admissions:** 3010 **Census:** 28 **Outpatient Visits:** 104127 **Births:** 307 **Total Expense ($000):** 81029 **Payroll Expense ($000):** 41630 **Personnel:** 583 | |

**FARMINGTON—Franklin County**

⊠ **FRANKLIN MEMORIAL HOSPITAL (200037)**, 111 Franklin Health Commons,
Zip 04938–9990; tel. 207/778–6031 **A**1 9 10 20 **F**3 5 7 8 11 13 15 18 28 29
30 31 32 34 35 36 40 41 45 46 50 51 54 56 59 61 64 65 70 75 76 77 78
79 81 82 83 84 85 86 87 89 93 97 99 100 101 102 103 104 107 108 110
111 114 117 118 128 129 130 131 134 145 146 147 **P**6 8
Primary Contact: Rebecca L. Ryder, R.N., President and Chief Executive Officer
COO: Gerald Cayer, Executive Vice President and Chief Operating Officer
CFO: Wayne Bennett, Chief Financial Officer
CMO: Michael Rowland, M.D., Vice President Medical Affairs
CIO: Ralph Johnson, Chief Information Officer
CHR: Joline Hart, Vice President Human Resources
CNO: Pam Ernest, R.N., CNO/ VP Patient Care Services
Web address: www.fchn.org
**Control:** Other not–for–profit (including NFP Corporation) **Service:** General
Medical and Surgical

| | |
|---|---|
| **Staffed Beds:** 43 **Admissions:** 2854 **Census:** 25 **Outpatient Visits:** 134958 **Births:** 296 **Total Expense ($000):** 83646 **Payroll Expense ($000):** 41037 **Personnel:** 702 | |

**FORT FAIRFIELD—Aroostook County**

**COMMUNITY GENERAL HEALTH CENTER** See The Aroostook Medical Center,
Presque Isle

**FORT KENT—Aroostook County**

⊠ **NORTHERN MAINE MEDICAL CENTER (200052)**, 194 East Main Street,
Zip 04743–1497; tel. 207/834–3155, (Total facility includes 45 beds in nursing
home–type unit) **A**1 9 10 20 **F**13 15 28 29 31 34 40 45 53 54 57 59 62 64 67
68 69 70 75 76 77 78 79 81 82 86 87 93 98 99 100 101 102 103 104 107
108 111 118 126 127 129 130 131 134 145 146 147 **P**6
Primary Contact: Peter Sirois, Interim Chief Executive Officer
COO: Joanne Fortin, R.N., Director of Clinical Services
COO: Peter Sirois, Associate Administrator
CFO: Roger Lagasse, Chief Financial Officer
CMO: Michael Sullivan, M.D., Chief Medical Officer
CIO: Adam Landry, Coordinator Computer Systems
CHR: Robin Damboise, Director Human Resources
CNO: Cheryl Daigle, R.N., Director of Nursing
Web address: www.nmmc.org
**Control:** Other not–for–profit (including NFP Corporation) **Service:** General
Medical and Surgical

| | |
|---|---|
| **Staffed Beds:** 81 **Admissions:** 1642 **Census:** 64 **Outpatient Visits:** 50504 **Births:** 75 **Total Expense ($000):** 44914 **Payroll Expense ($000):** 24389 **Personnel:** 405 | |

**GREENVILLE—Piscataquis County**

★ **CHARLES A. DEAN MEMORIAL HOSPITAL (201301)**, 364 Pritham Avenue,
Zip 04441–1395, Mailing Address: P.O. Box 1129, Zip 04441–1129;
tel. 207/695–5200, (Nonreporting) **A**9 10 18 **S** Eastern Maine Healthcare
Systems, Brewer, ME
Primary Contact: Geno Murray, President and Chief Executive Officer
CFO: Edward Olivier, Chief Financial Officer
CMO: Darin Peck, M.D., Chief of Staff
Web address: www.cadean.org
**Control:** Other not–for–profit (including NFP Corporation) **Service:** General
Medical and Surgical

| | |
|---|---|
| **Staffed Beds:** 36 | |

**HOULTON—Aroostook County**

★ **HOULTON REGIONAL HOSPITAL (201308)**, 20 Hartford Street,
Zip 04730–9998; tel. 207/532–9471, (Total facility includes 26 beds in nursing
home–type unit) **A**9 10 18 **F**1 3 4 11 13 15 16 17 28 29 30 34 40 43 51 59
65 67 70 72 73 75 76 79 80 81 85 86 87 88 89 90 93 97 98 107 108 110
111 113 118 126 127 129 131 134 145 147 **P**5 6
Primary Contact: Thomas J. Moakler, Chief Executive Officer
CFO: Cindy Daigle, Chief Financial Officer
CHR: Vicky Moody, Director Human Resources
Web address: www.houlton.net/hrh
**Control:** Other not–for–profit (including NFP Corporation) **Service:** General
Medical and Surgical

| | |
|---|---|
| **Staffed Beds:** 51 **Admissions:** 1503 **Census:** 32 **Outpatient Visits:** 95440 **Births:** 170 **Total Expense ($000):** 45321 **Payroll Expense ($000):** 21101 **Personnel:** 400 | |

**LEWISTON—Androscoggin County**

⊠ **CENTRAL MAINE MEDICAL CENTER (200024)**, 300 Main Street,
Zip 04240–0305; tel. 207/795–0111 **A**1 2 3 5 9 10 13 **F**3 11 12 13 15 18 19
20 22 24 26 28 29 30 31 32 34 35 36 40 43 44 45 46 47 48 49 50 51
52 53 55 57 58 59 61 64 65 66 67 68 70 71 73 74 75 76 77 78 79 81 82
84 85 86 87 89 90 91 92 93 97 102 107 108 110 113 114 117 118 119
120 122 123 128 129 130 131 134 142 143 145 146 147 **P**4 5 6 8
Primary Contact: Laird P. Covey, President
CFO: Matthew Cox, Chief Financial Officer
CMO: Edmund Claxton, M.D., President, Medical Staff
CIO: Denis Tanguay, Chief Information Officer
CHR: Kirk Miklavic, Director, Human Resources
CNO: Sharron Sieleman, R.N., VP, Nursing
Web address: www.cmmc.org
**Control:** Other not–for–profit (including NFP Corporation) **Service:** General
Medical and Surgical

| | |
|---|---|
| **Staffed Beds:** 190 **Admissions:** 9854 **Census:** 115 **Outpatient Visits:** 768907 **Births:** 772 **Total Expense ($000):** 299268 **Payroll Expense ($000):** 136153 **Personnel:** 1859 | |

ME

⊠ **ST. MARY'S REGIONAL MEDICAL CENTER (200034)**, 330 Sabattus Street, Zip 4240, Mailing Address: P.O. Box 291, Zip 04243–0291; tel. 207/777–8100 **A**1 2 9 10 **F**3 4 5 7 11 13 15 17 18 20 28 29 30 31 34 35 40 44 45 46 49 50 51 53 54 57 58 59 60 61 64 65 68 70 74 75 76 77 78 79 80 81 82 84 85 86 87 89 91 93 96 97 98 99 100 101 102 103 104 105 107 108 110 111 113 115 116 117 118 128 129 131 133 134 143 145 146 147 **P**1 6 **S** Covenant Health Systems, Inc., Tewksbury, MA
Primary Contact: Lee T. Myles, Chief Executive Officer
COO: Susan Keiler, Chief Operating Officer
CFO: Carolyn Kasabian, Chief Financial Officer
CMO: Ira Shapiro, M.D., Chief Medical Officer
CIO: Rene Dumont, CIO/ Vice President Strategic Growth
CHR: Kevin Healey, Vice President Human Resources
Web address: www.stmarysmaine.com
**Control:** Other not–for–profit (including NFP Corporation) **Service:** General Medical and Surgical

**Staffed Beds:** 171 **Admissions:** 6507 **Census:** 89 **Outpatient Visits:** 357666 **Births:** 655 **Total Expense ($000):** 146076 **Payroll Expense ($000):** 68121 **Personnel:** 1621

### LINCOLN—Penobscot County

★ **PENOBSCOT VALLEY HOSPITAL (201303)**, 7 Transalpine Road, Zip 04457–0368, Mailing Address: P.O. Box 368, Zip 04457–0368; tel. 207/794–3321 **A**9 10 18 **F**3 7 8 11 13 15 28 29 30 34 40 41 45 50 57 59 64 65 68 70 76 77 79 81 84 85 89 90 93 107 108 113 118 126 127 129 131 132 134 145 146 147 **P**6 **S** QHR, Brentwood, TN
Primary Contact: David A. Shannon, Chief Executive Officer
CFO: Ann Marie Rush, Chief Financial Officer
CHR: Sarah Loman, Director Human Resources
Web address: www.pvhme.org
**Control:** Other not–for–profit (including NFP Corporation) **Service:** General Medical and Surgical

**Staffed Beds:** 25 **Admissions:** 979 **Census:** 9 **Outpatient Visits:** 38504 **Births:** 77 **Total Expense ($000):** 24711 **Payroll Expense ($000):** 9733 **Personnel:** 184

### MACHIAS—Washington County

★ **DOWN EAST COMMUNITY HOSPITAL (201311)**, 11 Hospital Drive, Zip 04654–3325; tel. 207/255–3356, (Total facility includes 28 beds in nursing home–type unit) **A**9 10 18 **F**3 4 13 15 28 29 30 34 35 40 42 43 45 46 56 57 59 63 64 65 68 75 76 77 79 81 82 84 85 86 89 93 97 107 108 110 111 118 126 127 128 129 131 145 146 147 **P**6
Primary Contact: Douglas T. Jones, President and Chief Executive Officer
CFO: Lynnette Parr, Chief Financial Officer
CMO: Kara Dwight, Chief of Staff
CIO: Lynnette Parr, Chief Financial Officer
CHR: Ernestine O. Reisman, Vice President Human Resources
Web address: www.dech.org
**Control:** Other not–for–profit (including NFP Corporation) **Service:** General Medical and Surgical

**Staffed Beds:** 53 **Admissions:** 942 **Census:** 32 **Outpatient Visits:** 32635 **Births:** 113 **Total Expense ($000):** 38761 **Payroll Expense ($000):** 17771 **Personnel:** 211

### MARS HILL—Aroostook County

**AROOSTOOK HEALTH CENTER** See The Aroostook Medical Center, Presque Isle

### MILLINOCKET—Penobscot County

★ **MILLINOCKET REGIONAL HOSPITAL (201307)**, 200 Somerset Street, Zip 04462–1298; tel. 207/723–5161 **A**9 10 18 **F**3 8 11 15 28 29 30 31 34 35 37 40 43 45 47 48 50 53 55 59 64 65 75 79 81 84 85 86 87 89 93 97 107 108 127 129 132 134 146 **P**6
Primary Contact: Marie E. Vienneau, R.N., Chief Executive Officer
CFO: Christine McLaughlin, Chief Financial Officer
CMO: Daniel Herbert, M.D., Medical Administrative Officer
CIO: Tom Folsom, Manager Information Systems
CHR: Lisa Arsenault, Director Human Resources
Web address: www.mrhme.org
**Control:** Other not–for–profit (including NFP Corporation) **Service:** General Medical and Surgical

**Staffed Beds:** 25 **Admissions:** 989 **Census:** 10 **Outpatient Visits:** 34213 **Births:** 0 **Total Expense ($000):** 26391 **Payroll Expense ($000):** 13305 **Personnel:** 179

### NORWAY—Oxford County

★ **STEPHENS MEMORIAL HOSPITAL (201315)**, 181 Main Street, Zip 04268–1297; tel. 207/743–5933 **A**2 9 10 18 **F**3 7 8 13 15 28 29 30 31 34 35 40 43 45 57 59 61 64 65 68 70 75 76 78 79 81 84 85 86 89 93 96 102 107 108 111 114 118 129 131 145 147 **S** MaineHealth, Portland, ME
Primary Contact: Timothy A. Churchill, President
CMO: Gregory Hardy, M.D., President Medical Staff
CHR: Roberta Metivier, Vice President Human Resources and Administrator, Western Main Nursing Home
Web address: www.wmhcc.com
**Control:** Other not–for–profit (including NFP Corporation) **Service:** General Medical and Surgical

**Staffed Beds:** 25 **Admissions:** 1715 **Census:** 15 **Outpatient Visits:** 105067 **Births:** 172 **Total Expense ($000):** 43823 **Payroll Expense ($000):** 19680 **Personnel:** 389

### PITTSFIELD—Somerset County

⊠ **SEBASTICOOK VALLEY HEALTH (201313)**, 447 North Main Street, Zip 04967–1199; tel. 207/487–4000 **A**1 9 10 18 **F**7 11 15 28 29 35 40 45 50 51 57 59 64 65 70 75 78 79 81 85 87 93 96 97 107 108 111 114 117 118 126 128 129 131 132 134 142 145 146 147 **P**6 **S** Eastern Maine Healthcare Systems, Brewer, ME
Primary Contact: Victoria Alexander–Lane, President and Chief Executive Officer
COO: Terri Vieira, Vice President Operations
CFO: Randal Clark, Vice President Finance
CMO: Howard Margolskee, M.D., Chief of Staff
CIO: Michael Peterson, Vice President Ancillary and Support Services and Chief Information Officer
CHR: Liisa H. Janelle, Vice President Human Resources
Web address: www.sebasticookvalleyhealth.org
**Control:** Other not–for–profit (including NFP Corporation) **Service:** General Medical and Surgical

**Staffed Beds:** 25 **Admissions:** 912 **Census:** 12 **Outpatient Visits:** 103541 **Births:** 0 **Total Expense ($000):** 31937 **Payroll Expense ($000):** 15018 **Personnel:** 291

### PORTLAND—Cumberland County

⊠ △ **MAINE MEDICAL CENTER (200009)**, 22 Bramhall Street, Zip 04102–3175; tel. 207/662–0111, (Includes BARBARA BUSH CHILDREN'S HOSPITAL, 22 Bramhall Street, Zip 04102–3134; tel. 207/662–0111; MAINE MEDICAL CENTER, BRIGHTON CAMPUS, 335 Brighton Avenue, Zip 04102–9735, Mailing Address: P.O. Box 9735, Zip 04102–9735; tel. 207/879–8000) **A**1 2 3 5 7 8 9 10 **F**3 5 8 11 12 13 15 16 17 18 19 20 21 22 23 24 25 26 27 28 29 30 31 32 34 35 36 37 38 40 41 42 43 45 46 47 48 49 50 51 54 55 56 57 58 59 60 61 64 65 66 68 70 72 73 74 75 76 77 78 79 81 82 83 84 85 86 87 88 89 92 93 94 97 98 100 101 102 103 104 105 107 108 110 111 113 114 117 118 119 120 122 123 125 128 129 130 131 133 134 135 137 141 142 143 144 145 146 147 **P**4 6 8 **S** MaineHealth, Portland, ME
Primary Contact: Richard W. Petersen, President and Chief Executive Officer
COO: Jeff Sanders, Chief Operating Officer
CFO: John E. Heye, Chief Financial Officer
CMO: Peter Bates, M.D., Vice President Medical Affairs and Chief Medical Officer
CIO: Barry Blumenfeld, M.D., Chief Information Officer
CHR: Judy West, Vice President Human Resources
Web address: www.mmc.org
**Control:** Other not–for–profit (including NFP Corporation) **Service:** General Medical and Surgical

**Staffed Beds:** 637 **Admissions:** 28451 **Census:** 417 **Outpatient Visits:** 351479 **Births:** 2647 **Total Expense ($000):** 780846 **Payroll Expense ($000):** 325890 **Personnel:** 5546

⊠ **MERCY HOSPITAL OF PORTLAND (200008)**, 144 State Street, Zip 04101–3795; tel. 207/879–3000 **A**1 2 9 10 **F**4 5 11 13 15 18 20 26 29 30 31 34 35 36 40 44 45 48 49 50 51 54 56 57 58 59 61 64 68 70 74 75 76 77 78 79 81 82 84 86 87 93 97 100 102 104 105 107 108 110 111 114 118 129 131 134 142 143 145 146 147 **P**6 **S** Catholic Health East, Newtown Square, PA
Primary Contact: Eileen F. Skinner, FACHE, President and Chief Executive Officer
COO: Robert Nutter, COO, Vice President of Human Resources and Support Services
CFO: Anthony Marple, Vice President of Strategy
CMO: Scott Rusk, M.D., Vice President Medical Administration
CIO: Don Huff, Interim Chief Information Officer
CHR: Elizabeth B. Christensen, Director, Human Resources
CNO: Bette Neville, R.N., Interim CNO and Director of Nursing
Web address: www.mercyhospital.org
**Control:** Church–operated, Nongovernment, not–for profit **Service:** General Medical and Surgical

**Staffed Beds:** 168 **Admissions:** 7714 **Census:** 81 **Outpatient Visits:** 341511 **Births:** 787 **Total Expense ($000):** 207097 **Payroll Expense ($000):** 89403 **Personnel:** 1022

*Many Facility Codes have changed. Please refer to the AHA Guide Code Chart.* © 2012 AHA Guide

⊠ **NEW ENGLAND REHABILITATION HOSPITAL OF PORTLAND (203025)**, 335 Brighton Avenue, Zip 04102–9735; tel. 207/775–4000 **A**1 10 **F**29 34 35 60 68 75 79 82 90 93 95 96 129 130 131 134 142 145 **S** HEALTHSOUTH Corporation, Birmingham, AL
Primary Contact: Jeanine Chesley, Chief Executive Officer
CMO: Elissa Charbonneau, D.O., Medical Director
CHR: Leigh Baade, Director Human Resources
Web address: www.nerhp.org
**Control:** Partnership, Investor–owned, for–profit **Service:** Rehabilitation

**Staffed Beds:** 90 **Admissions:** 1917 **Census:** 72 **Outpatient Visits:** 15003 **Births:** 0 **Total Expense ($000):** 21412 **Payroll Expense ($000):** 13398 **Personnel:** 248

### PRESQUE ISLE—Aroostook County

⊠ **THE AROOSTOOK MEDICAL CENTER (200018)**, 140 Academy Street, Zip 04769–3171, Mailing Address: P.O. Box 151, Zip 04769–0151; tel. 207/768–4000, (Includes AROOSTOOK HEALTH CENTER, 15 Highland Avenue, Mars Hill, Zip 04758; tel. 207/768–4900; ARTHUR R. GOULD MEMORIAL HOSPITAL, 140 Academy Street, Zip 04769, Mailing Address: P.O. Box 151, Zip 04769; tel. 207/768–4000; COMMUNITY GENERAL HEALTH CENTER, 3 Green Street, Fort Fairfield, Zip 04742; tel. 207/768–4700), (Total facility includes 64 beds in nursing home–type unit) **A**1 9 10 **F**3 7 8 12 13 15 18 20 28 29 30 31 32 34 35 36 38 40 43 45 46 50 51 52 53 54 56 57 59 60 61 63 64 65 67 68 69 70 74 75 76 77 78 79 80 81 82 84 85 86 87 89 90 91 93 96 97 99 104 107 108 110 111 113 114 117 118 120 122 127 128 129 130 131 133 134 142 145 146 147 **P**6 **S** Eastern Maine Healthcare Systems, Brewer, ME
Primary Contact: Sylvia Getman, President and Chief Executive Officer
COO: Jay Reynolds, M.D., Chief Operating Officer and Chief Medical Officer
CFO: C. Bruce Sandstrom, Vice President and Chief Financial Officer
CMO: Jay Reynolds, M.D., Vice President Medical Affairs and Chief Operating Officer
CIO: Catherine Bruno, FACHE, Chief Information Officer
CHR: Thomas Umphrey, Senior Vice President Human Resources
Web address: www.tamc.org
**Control:** Other not–for–profit (including NFP Corporation) **Service:** General Medical and Surgical

**Staffed Beds:** 122 **Admissions:** 2229 **Census:** 85 **Outpatient Visits:** 176080 **Births:** 208 **Total Expense ($000):** 96507 **Payroll Expense ($000):** 51232 **Personnel:** 935

### ROCKPORT—Knox County

⊠ **PEN BAY MEDICAL CENTER (200063)**, 6 Glen Cove Drive, Zip 04856–4240; tel. 207/596–8000, (Total facility includes 84 beds in nursing home–type unit) **A**1 2 9 10 20 **F**3 4 5 6 13 15 17 18 28 29 30 31 32 34 35 40 43 45 51 58 59 61 64 65 67 70 74 75 76 77 78 79 81 82 83 85 86 87 89 93 97 98 100 107 113 117 118 127 128 129 130 131 133 134 143 145 146 147 **P**1 **S** MaineHealth, Portland, ME
Primary Contact: Wade C. Johnson, MS, FACHE, Chief Executive Officer
COO: Eric Waters, Vice President Operations
CFO: Maura Kelly, Vice President Fiscal Services
CMO: Dana L. Goldsmith, M.D., Vice President Medical Affairs
CIO: Brooks Betts, Director Information Systems and Chief Information Officer
CHR: Thomas Girard, Vice President Human Resources
Web address: www.penbayhealthcare.org
**Control:** Other not–for–profit (including NFP Corporation) **Service:** General Medical and Surgical

**Staffed Beds:** 165 **Admissions:** 4443 **Census:** 132 **Outpatient Visits:** 348512 **Births:** 323 **Total Expense ($000):** 114657 **Payroll Expense ($000):** 55924 **Personnel:** 824

**PENOBSCOT BAY MEDICAL CENTER** See Pen Bay Medical Center

### RUMFORD—Oxford County

★ **RUMFORD HOSPITAL (201306)**, 420 Franklin Street, Zip 04276–2145; tel. 207/369–1000 **A**9 10 18 **F**3 8 11 13 15 18 28 29 31 34 35 38 40 50 53 57 59 64 70 75 76 77 78 79 81 82 84 85 87 93 94 97 107 111 113 118 126 127 129 131 132 145 147 **P**6 8
Primary Contact: R. David Frum, President
Web address: www.rumfordhospital.org
**Control:** Other not–for–profit (including NFP Corporation) **Service:** General Medical and Surgical

**Staffed Beds:** 21 **Admissions:** 1171 **Census:** 15 **Outpatient Visits:** 81865 **Births:** 79 **Total Expense ($000):** 32810 **Payroll Expense ($000):** 13062 **Personnel:** 234

### SANFORD—York County

⊠ **HENRIETTA D. GOODALL HOSPITAL (200040)**, 25 June Street, Zip 04073–2645; tel. 207/324–4310, (Total facility includes 112 beds in nursing home–type unit) **A**1 2 9 10 **F**1 2 3 6 10 13 15 18 26 27 28 29 30 31 32 34 35 40 45 47 50 53 59 64 65 67 70 73 75 76 77 79 81 82 85 89 90 93 97 107 108 111 113 117 118 124 127 128 129 130 133 134 144 145 146 **P**6
Primary Contact: Patricia Aprile, Chief Executive Officer
CFO: Dan Forgues, Chief Financial Officer
CMO: Mukesh Bhargava, M.D., Vice President Medical Affairs
CIO: Charles Caruso, Chief Information Officer
CHR: Carolyn Burgess, Director Human Resources
Web address: www.goodallhospital.org
**Control:** Other not–for–profit (including NFP Corporation) **Service:** General Medical and Surgical

**Staffed Beds:** 157 **Admissions:** 2142 **Census:** 128 **Outpatient Visits:** 201394 **Births:** 190 **Total Expense ($000):** 72854 **Payroll Expense ($000):** 39649 **Personnel:** 587

### SKOWHEGAN—Somerset County

★ **REDINGTON–FAIRVIEW GENERAL HOSPITAL (201314)**, Fairview Avenue, Zip 4976, Mailing Address: P.O. Box 468, Zip 04976–0468; tel. 207/474–5121 **A**2 9 10 18 **F**3 7 11 13 15 18 28 29 30 31 34 35 40 50 53 56 57 59 65 68 70 74 75 76 77 78 79 81 82 85 92 93 97 107 108 110 113 114 117 118 129 130 131 133 134 145 146 **P**6
Primary Contact: Richard Willett, Chief Executive Officer
CFO: Dana Kempton, Associate Director and Chief Financial Officer
CMO: Michael Lambke, M.D., Medical Director
CHR: Deborah Buckingham, R.N., Director Human Resources
CNO: Sherry L. Rogers, MS, Chief Nursing Officer
Web address: www.rfgh.net
**Control:** Other not–for–profit (including NFP Corporation) **Service:** General Medical and Surgical

**Staffed Beds:** 25 **Admissions:** 1616 **Census:** 22 **Outpatient Visits:** 78941 **Births:** 139 **Total Expense ($000):** 67259 **Payroll Expense ($000):** 27105 **Personnel:** 489

### TOGUS—Kennebec County

⊠ **VETERANS AFFAIRS MEDICAL CENTER**, 1 VA Center, Zip 4330; tel. 207/623–8411, (Nonreporting) **A**1 **S** Department of Veterans Affairs, Washington, DC
Primary Contact: Brian Stiller, Director
CFO: Daniel Howard, Chief Financial Officer
CMO: Timothy J. Richardson, M.D., Chief of Staff
CIO: Richard McNaughton, Chief Information Management Service
CHR: Christine Miller, Chief Human Resources Management Services
Web address: www.visn1.med.va.gov/togus/
**Control:** Veterans Affairs, Government, federal **Service:** General Medical and Surgical

**Staffed Beds:** 167

### WATERVILLE—Kennebec County

★ ○ **INLAND HOSPITAL (200041)**, 200 Kennedy Memorial Drive, Zip 04901–4595; tel. 207/861–3000 **A**9 10 11 **F**3 13 15 18 28 29 30 34 35 36 40 45 48 50 54 57 59 65 66 68 70 74 75 76 77 79 81 82 85 86 89 93 97 107 108 110 111 114 117 118 126 128 131 134 143 145 146 147 **S** Eastern Maine Healthcare Systems, Brewer, ME
Primary Contact: John Dalton, President and Chief Executive Officer
COO: Daniel Booth, Vice President Operations and Chief Human Resources Officer
CFO: Dean Bither, Chief Financial Officer
CIO: Kevin Dieterich, Director Information Services
CHR: Daniel Booth, Vice President Operations and Chief Human Resources Officer
Web address: www.inlandhospital.org
**Control:** Other not–for–profit (including NFP Corporation) **Service:** General Medical and Surgical

**Staffed Beds:** 46 **Admissions:** 1491 **Census:** 15 **Outpatient Visits:** 87179 **Births:** 322 **Total Expense ($000):** 64847 **Payroll Expense ($000):** 31244 **Personnel:** 535

---

**Hospital, Medicare Provider Number, Address, Telephone, Approval, Facility, and Physician Codes, Health Care System**

★ American Hospital Association (AHA) membership
□ The Joint Commission accreditation
◇ DNV Healthcare Inc. accreditation
○ American Osteopathic Association (AOA) accreditation
△ Commission on Accreditation of Rehabilitation Facilities (CARF) accreditation

☒ **MAINEGENERAL MEDICAL CENTER–WATERVILLE CAMPUS (200039)**, 149 North Street, Zip 04901–4974; tel. 207/872–1000, (Includes MAINEGENERAL MEDICAL CENTER–AUGUSTA CAMPUS, 6 East Chestnut Street, Augusta, Zip 04330–9988; tel. 207/626–1000; Chuck Hays, President), (Nonreporting) **A**1 2 9 10
Primary Contact: Chuck Hays, President
CMO: Steve Diaz, M.D., Chief Medical Officer
CIO: Daniel Burgess, Chief Information Officer
CHR: Rebecca Lamey, Vice President Human Resources
Web address: www.mainegeneral.org
**Control:** Other not–for–profit (including NFP Corporation) **Service:** General Medical and Surgical

**Staffed Beds:** 264

### WESTBROOK—Cumberland County

☒ **SPRING HARBOR HOSPITAL (204005)**, 123 Andover Road, Zip 04092–3850; tel. 207/761–2200, (Nonreporting) **A**1 9 10 **S** MaineHealth, Portland, ME
Primary Contact: Dennis P. King, Chief Executive Officer
COO: Richard Hanley, Chief Operating Officer
CFO: Gregory Bowers, Chief Financial Officer
CMO: Girard Robinson, M.D., Chief Medical Officer
CIO: Chris Simons, Director Health Information Management and Utilization Review
Web address: www.springharbor.org
**Control:** Other not–for–profit (including NFP Corporation) **Service:** Psychiatric

**Staffed Beds:** 88

### YORK—York County

★ **YORK HOSPITAL (200020)**, 15 Hospital Drive, Zip 03909–1099; tel. 207/363–4321 **A**2 9 10 **F**3 4 5 8 11 13 15 17 18 20 22 26 28 29 30 31 32 34 35 36 40 42 43 45 48 49 50 53 54 56 57 59 62 64 65 69 70 71 74 75 76 77 78 79 81 82 85 87 89 90 93 96 97 98 100 104 107 108 110 111 112 113 114 117 118 128 129 130 131 134 142 143 145 146 147 **P**6
Primary Contact: Jud Knox, President
COO: Stephen Pelletier, Leader Guest Services
CFO: Robin LaBonte, Leader Financial Care
CMO: Lawrence Petrovich, M.D., Chief Medical Officer
CIO: Robin LaBonte, Leader Financial Care
CHR: Olivia Chayer, Lead Human Resources
CNO: Kathy Lane, Leader–ICU, Home Care, MedSurg
Web address: www.yorkhospital.com
**Control:** Other not–for–profit (including NFP Corporation) **Service:** General Medical and Surgical

**Staffed Beds:** 79 **Admissions:** 3721 **Census:** 39 **Outpatient Visits:** 300525 **Births:** 332 **Total Expense ($000):** 143762 **Payroll Expense ($000):** 66228 **Personnel:** 880

# MARYLAND

## ANNAPOLIS—Anne Arundel County

✠ **ANNE ARUNDEL MEDICAL CENTER (210023)**, 2001 Medical Parkway, Zip 21401–3019; tel. 443/481–1000, (Total facility includes 40 beds in nursing home–type unit) **A**1 2 5 9 10 **F**3 4 5 9 11 13 14 15 18 20 22 26 28 29 30 31 32 34 35 36 37 38 39 40 41 44 45 46 49 50 51 53 54 55 56 57 58 59 60 61 63 64 66 68 70 72 74 75 76 77 78 79 81 82 84 85 86 87 89 91 92 93 94 96 97 100 102 107 108 110 111 113 114 115 116 117 118 119 120 122 123 125 128 129 130 131 133 134 144 145 146 147
Primary Contact: Victoria Bayless, President and Chief Executive Officer
COO: Sherry Perkins, Ph.D., Chief Operating Officer and Chief Nursing Officer
CFO: Robert Reilly, Vice President and Chief Financial Officer
CMO: Joseph Moser, M.D., Vice President Medical Staff Affairs
CIO: Douglas A. Abel, Chief Information Officer
CHR: Nancy Luttrell, Vice President Human Resources
Web address: www.aahs.org
**Control:** Other not–for–profit (including NFP Corporation) **Service:** General Medical and Surgical

**Staffed Beds:** 401 **Admissions:** 25751 **Census:** 269 **Outpatient Visits:** 515791 **Births:** 5112 **Total Expense ($000):** 422534 **Payroll Expense ($000):** 163617 **Personnel:** 3064

## BALTIMORE—Baltimore City County

✠ **BON SECOURS BALTIMORE HEALTH SYSTEM (210013)**, 2000 West Baltimore Street, Zip 21223–1597; tel. 410/362–3000 **A**1 9 10 **F**3 11 15 18 20 26 29 30 31 40 44 49 59 60 64 66 70 78 79 81 84 85 98 99 100 101 102 103 104 105 107 108 110 111 114 118 129 142 145 147 **P**6 **S** Bon Secours Health System, Inc., Marriottsville, MD
Primary Contact: Samuel Lee Ross, M.D., MS, Chief Executive Officer
CFO: Richard Jones, Chief Financial Officer
CMO: Sidney Mir, M.D., Vice President Medical Affairs and Chief Medical Officer
CIO: Sanjay Purushotham, Executive Director Information Systems
CHR: Michelle Wiles, Vice President Human Resources
CNO: Lesia Douglas, R.N., Vice President Patient Care Services and Chief Nurse Executive
Web address: www.bonsecoursbaltimore.com
**Control:** Church–operated, Nongovernment, not–for profit **Service:** General Medical and Surgical

**Staffed Beds:** 89 **Admissions:** 7390 **Census:** 88 **Outpatient Visits:** 198947 **Births:** 0 **Total Expense ($000):** 124271 **Payroll Expense ($000):** 49853 **Personnel:** 883

**FRANKLIN SQUARE HOSPITAL CENTER** See Medstar Franklin Square Medical Center

**GOOD SAMARITAN HOSPITAL OF MARYLAND** See Medstar Good Samaritan Hospital

✠ **GREATER BALTIMORE MEDICAL CENTER (210044)**, 6701 North Charles Street, Zip 21204–6892; tel. 443/849–2000, (Total facility includes 23 beds in nursing home–type unit) **A**1 2 3 5 9 10 **F**3 8 11 12 13 18 20 22 26 29 30 31 34 35 40 44 45 46 47 48 49 50 51 54 55 56 57 58 59 60 61 63 64 68 70 72 73 74 75 76 77 78 79 80 81 82 84 85 86 87 89 92 96 97 102 107 108 113 114 118 119 120 122 123 125 127 128 129 131 134 143 144 145 146 147 **P**4
Primary Contact: John B. Chessare, M.D., M.P.H., FACHE, President and Chief Executive Officer
COO: Keith R. Poisson, Executive Vice President and Chief Operating Officer
CFO: Eric L. Melchior, Executive Vice President and Chief Financial Officer
CMO: John R. Saunders, M.D., Senior Vice President Medical Affairs and Chief Medical Officer
CIO: Tressa Springmann, Chief Information Officer
CHR: Delois Simpson–Tuggle, Vice President Human Resources and Organizational Development and Chief Human Resources Officer
CNO: Jody Porter, R.N., Senior Vice President Patient Care Services and Chief Nursing Officer
Web address: www.gbmc.org
**Control:** Other not–for–profit (including NFP Corporation) **Service:** General Medical and Surgical

**Staffed Beds:** 249 **Admissions:** 24276 **Census:** 251 **Outpatient Visits:** 127603 **Births:** 4372 **Total Expense ($000):** 383165 **Payroll Expense ($000):** 167484 **Personnel:** 3116

**HARBOR HOSPITAL** See Medstar Harbor Hospital

✠ **JOHNS HOPKINS BAYVIEW MEDICAL CENTER (210029)**, 4940 Eastern Avenue, Zip 21224–2780; tel. 410/550–0100, (Total facility includes 158 beds in nursing home–type unit) **A**1 2 3 5 8 9 10 **F**2 3 4 5 6 8 9 10 11 12 13 15 16 17 18 20 22 26 28 29 30 31 32 34 35 36 38 39 40 43 44 45 47 48 49 50 51 54 55 56 57 58 59 60 61 64 65 66 68 70 71 72 74 75 76 77 78 79 80 81 82 84 85 86 87 89 90 92 93 94 97 98 99 100 101 102 103 104 105 107 111 113 114 115 117 118 119 125 127 128 129 130 131 133 134 140 142 144 145 146 147 **S** Johns Hopkins Health System, Baltimore, MD
Primary Contact: Richard G. Bennett, M.D., President
COO: Charlie Reuland, Sc.D., Executive Vice President and Chief Operating Officer
CFO: Carl H. Francioli, Vice President Finance
CIO: Sandy Reckert, Director Communications and Public Affairs
CHR: Craig Brodian, Vice President Human Resources
Web address: www.hopkinsbayview.org
**Control:** Other not–for–profit (including NFP Corporation) **Service:** General Medical and Surgical

**Staffed Beds:** 518 **Admissions:** 22252 **Census:** 387 **Outpatient Visits:** 428715 **Births:** 1646 **Total Expense ($000):** 378376 **Payroll Expense ($000):** 140680 **Personnel:** 3148

✠ △ **JOHNS HOPKINS HOSPITAL (210009)**, 600 North Wolfe Street, Zip 21287–2182; tel. 410/955–5000, (Includes JOHNS HOPKINS CHILDREN'S CENTER, 600 North Wolfe Street, Zip 21287–0005; tel. 410/955–5000) **A**1 2 3 5 7 8 9 10 **F**3 5 6 7 8 9 11 13 14 15 16 17 18 19 20 21 22 23 24 25 26 27 28 29 30 31 32 34 35 36 38 39 40 41 43 44 45 46 47 48 49 50 52 54 55 56 57 58 59 60 61 63 64 65 66 68 70 72 74 75 76 77 78 79 80 81 82 84 85 86 87 88 89 90 92 93 94 96 97 98 99 100 101 102 103 104 105 107 108 110 111 112 113 114 115 116 117 118 119 120 122 123 125 128 129 130 131 133 134 135 136 137 138 139 140 141 142 144 145 146 147 **S** Johns Hopkins Health System, Baltimore, MD
Primary Contact: Ronald R. Peterson, President
COO: Judy A. Reitz, Sc.D., Executive Vice President and Chief Operating Officer
CFO: Ronald J. Werthman, Vice President Finance, Chief Financial Officer and Treasurer
CMO: Redonda Miller, M.D., Vice President Medical Affairs
CIO: Stephanie L. Reel, Vice President Information Services
CHR: Pamela Paulk, Vice President Human Resources
Web address: www.hopkinsmedicine.org
**Control:** Other not–for–profit (including NFP Corporation) **Service:** General Medical and Surgical

**Staffed Beds:** 912 **Admissions:** 46573 **Census:** 764 **Outpatient Visits:** 510814 **Births:** 1929 **Total Expense ($000):** 1605701 **Payroll Expense ($000):** 504564 **Personnel:** 8686

☐ △ **KENNEDY KRIEGER INSTITUTE (213301)**, 707 North Broadway, Zip 21205–1890; tel. 443/923–9200, (Nonreporting) **A**1 3 5 7 9 10
Primary Contact: Gary W. Goldstein, M.D., President and Chief Executive Officer
COO: James M. Anders, Jr., Administrator and Chief Operating Officer
CFO: Michael J. Neuman, Vice President Finance
CMO: Michael V. Johnston, M.D., Chief Medical Officer and Senior Vice President Medical Programs
CIO: Kenneth Davis, Assistant Vice President Information Systems
CHR: Michael Loughran, Vice President Human Resources
Web address: www.kennedykrieger.org
**Control:** Other not–for–profit (including NFP Corporation) **Service:** Children's other specialty

**Staffed Beds:** 70

✠ △ **KERNAN ORTHOPAEDICS AND REHABILITATION (210058)**, 2200 Kernan Drive, Zip 21207–6697; tel. 410/448–2500 **A**1 3 5 7 9 10 **F**1 8 11 29 39 70 74 77 79 81 82 90 93 95 96 107 114 130 131 145 147 **S** University of Maryland Medical System, Baltimore, MD
Primary Contact: Michael Jablonover, M.D., President and Chief Executive Officer
COO: Juanita D. Robbins, Chief Operating and Development Officer
CFO: W. Walter Augustin, III, CPA, Vice President Financial Services and Chief Financial Officer
CMO: John P. Straumanis, M.D., Vice President Medical Affairs and Chief Medical Officer
CIO: Linda Hines, Vice President Information Technology and Information Systems
CHR: David Swift, Vice President Human Resources, Volunteer and Community Services
Web address: www.kernan.org
**Control:** Other not–for–profit (including NFP Corporation) **Service:** Rehabilitation

**Staffed Beds:** 104 **Admissions:** 3286 **Census:** 104 **Outpatient Visits:** 74417 **Births:** 0 **Total Expense ($000):** 90594 **Payroll Expense ($000):** 37184 **Personnel:** 572

---

**Hospital, Medicare Provider Number, Address, Telephone, Approval, Facility, and Physician Codes, Health Care System**

★ American Hospital Association (AHA) membership
☐ The Joint Commission accreditation
◇ DNV Healthcare Inc. accreditation
○ American Osteopathic Association (AOA) accreditation
△ Commission on Accreditation of Rehabilitation Facilities (CARF) accreditation

**MD**

⊞ △ **LEVINDALE HEBREW GERIATRIC CENTER AND HOSPITAL (212005)**, 2434 West Belvedere Avenue, Zip 21215–5299; tel. 410/466–8700, (Total facility includes 323 beds in nursing home–type unit) **A**1 7 9 10 **F**2 11 29 30 50 56 60 63 68 69 82 84 87 93 103 104 105 127 129 131 145 147 **P**6 **S** LifeBridge Health, Baltimore, MD
Primary Contact: Aric Spitulnik, President and Chief Operating Officer
CFO: David Krajewski, Vice President Finance
CMO: Susan M. Levy, M.D., Vice President Medical Affairs
CIO: Karen Barker, Vice President and Chief Information Officer
CHR: Cheryl T. Boyer, Vice President Human Resources
CNO: Cathy M. Gallo, Vice President and Chief Nursing Officer
Web address: www.sinai–balt.com
**Control:** Other not–for–profit (including NFP Corporation) **Service:** Long–Term Acute Care hospital

> **Staffed Beds: 443 Admissions: 1616 Census: 407 Outpatient Visits:** 24141 **Births:** 0 **Total Expense ($000):** 86659 **Payroll Expense ($000):** 39922 **Personnel:** 776

⊞ △ **MARYLAND GENERAL HOSPITAL (210038)**, 827 Linden Avenue, Zip 21201–4681; tel. 410/225–8000 **A**1 3 5 7 9 10 **F**5 11 13 15 18 20 29 30 31 34 35 40 44 45 49 50 51 56 57 59 60 61 64 65 66 68 70 74 75 76 77 78 79 81 82 85 87 90 93 94 96 97 98 100 101 102 103 104 106 107 108 111 113 114 117 118 128 129 142 146 147 **S** University of Maryland Medical System, Baltimore, MD
Primary Contact: Sylvia Smith Johnson, President and Chief Executive Officer
COO: Donald Ray, Vice President of Operations
CFO: Brian Bailey, Chief Administrative and Financial Officer
CMO: W. Eugene Egerton, M.D., Chief Medical Officer
CIO: Jon P. Burns, Senior Vice President and Chief Information Officer
CHR: David Swift, Vice President Human Resources
CNO: Edward Streyle, MS, Senior Vice President and Chief Nursing Officer
Web address: www.marylandgeneral.org
**Control:** Other not–for–profit (including NFP Corporation) **Service:** General Medical and Surgical

> **Staffed Beds: 212 Admissions: 9692 Census: 128 Outpatient Visits:** 115034 **Births:** 749 **Total Expense ($000):** 160526 **Payroll Expense ($000):** 66159 **Personnel:** 1117

⊞ **MEDSTAR FRANKLIN SQUARE MEDICAL CENTER (210015)**, 9000 Franklin Square Drive, Zip 21237–2998; tel. 443/777–7000 **A**1 2 3 5 8 9 10 **F**3 5 8 10 11 12 13 14 15 18 20 22 26 28 29 30 31 32 34 35 36 37 38 39 40 42 44 45 46 47 48 49 50 51 52 55 56 57 58 59 60 61 64 65 66 70 71 72 74 75 76 77 78 79 81 82 84 85 86 87 89 91 92 93 94 97 98 99 100 101 102 103 104 105 107 111 113 114 117 118 128 129 130 131 133 134 143 144 145 146 147 **P**6 **S** MedStar Health, Columbia, MD
Primary Contact: Samuel E. Moskowitz, President
CFO: Robert P. Lally, Jr., Vice President Finance
CMO: Tony Sclama, M.D., Vice President Medical Affairs
CIO: Stephen Mannion, Assistant Vice President Information Systems Customer Service
CHR: Karen Robertson–Keck, Vice President Human Resources
CNO: Lawrence F. Strassner III, R.N., Vice President, Patient Care Services and Chief Nursing Officer
Web address: www.medstarfranklin.org
**Control:** Other not–for–profit (including NFP Corporation) **Service:** General Medical and Surgical

> **Staffed Beds: 368 Admissions: 21711 Census: 244 Outpatient Visits:** 271800 **Births:** 2549 **Total Expense ($000):** 417428 **Payroll Expense ($000):** 177352 **Personnel:** 2860

⊞ △ **MEDSTAR GOOD SAMARITAN HOSPITAL (210056)**, 5601 Loch Raven Boulevard, Zip 21239–2995; tel. 443/444–8000, (Total facility includes 30 beds in nursing home–type unit) **A**1 2 3 5 7 9 10 **F**3 9 11 14 15 17 18 20 26 28 29 30 31 34 35 36 37 38 40 44 45 50 51 53 56 57 58 59 60 61 64 65 66 67 68 70 74 75 77 78 79 80 81 82 84 85 86 87 90 91 93 96 97 99 100 101 102 103 104 107 108 111 113 117 118 120 127 128 129 130 131 134 142 145 147 **P**6 **S** MedStar Health, Columbia, MD
Primary Contact: Jeffrey A. Matton, President and Chief Executive Officer
CFO: Deana Stout, Vice President Financial Services
Web address: www.goodsam–md.org
**Control:** Other not–for–profit (including NFP Corporation) **Service:** General Medical and Surgical

> **Staffed Beds: 310 Admissions: 16060 Census: 225 Outpatient Visits:** 149345 **Births:** 0 **Total Expense ($000):** 299519 **Payroll Expense ($000):** 123118 **Personnel:** 2110

⊞ **MEDSTAR HARBOR HOSPITAL (210034)**, 3001 South Hanover Street, Zip 21225–1290; tel. 410/350–3200 **A**1 2 3 5 9 10 **F**3 9 11 13 14 15 17 18 20 26 29 30 31 34 35 36 40 44 45 46 48 49 50 51 53 55 56 57 58 59 60 61 64 65 66 68 70 72 73 74 76 77 78 79 81 82 84 85 86 87 89 92 93 94 97 102 103 107 108 110 111 113 118 119 120 128 129 130 131 134 145 146 **P**6 **S** MedStar Health, Columbia, MD
Primary Contact: Dennis W. Pullin, Chief Executive Officer
CFO: David R. Pitman, Vice President Finance
CMO: Allan Birenberg, Vice President Medical Affairs
CIO: David B. Smith, Assistant Vice President Information Services
CHR: Pamela S. Williams, Vice President Human Resources
Web address: www.harborhospital.org
**Control:** Other not–for–profit (including NFP Corporation) **Service:** General Medical and Surgical

> **Staffed Beds: 187 Admissions: 10677 Census: 127 Outpatient Visits:** 86649 **Births:** 1555 **Total Expense ($000):** 183462 **Payroll Expense ($000):** 79260 **Personnel:** 1267

★ △ **MEDSTAR UNION MEMORIAL HOSPITAL (210024)**, 201 East University Parkway, Zip 21218–2895; tel. 410/554–2000 **A**2 3 5 7 9 10 **F**3 5 8 9 11 14 15 17 18 20 22 24 26 28 29 30 31 34 35 37 38 39 40 43 44 45 46 47 48 49 50 51 52 53 54 55 56 57 58 59 60 61 63 64 65 66 68 70 74 75 77 78 79 80 81 82 84 85 86 87 89 90 91 92 93 94 96 97 98 100 101 102 103 104 105 107 108 110 111 113 114 117 118 119 120 122 128 129 130 131 134 141 142 145 147 **P**6 **S** MedStar Health, Columbia, MD
Primary Contact: Bradley Chambers, President
COO: Neil MacDonald, Vice President Operations
CFO: Joseph B. Smith, Vice President Finance
CMO: Stuart Bell, M.D., Vice President Medical Affairs
CIO: Catherine Szenczy, Senior Vice President and Chief Information Officer
CHR: Holly Phipps–Adams, Vice President Human Resources
CNO: Sharon A. Bottcher, R.N., Vice President Patient Care Services
Web address: www.unionmemorial.org
**Control:** Other not–for–profit (including NFP Corporation) **Service:** General Medical and Surgical

> **Staffed Beds: 271 Admissions: 14979 Census: 170 Outpatient Visits:** 164499 **Births:** 0 **Total Expense ($000):** 395227 **Payroll Expense ($000):** 153035 **Personnel:** 2185

⊞ **MERCY MEDICAL CENTER (210008)**, 301 St. Paul Place, Zip 21202–2165; tel. 410/332–9000 **A**1 2 3 5 8 9 10 **F**3 4 8 11 13 14 15 17 18 20 29 30 31 34 35 39 40 41 44 45 46 47 49 50 51 55 57 58 59 64 65 66 68 70 72 74 75 76 77 78 79 81 82 85 86 87 89 92 93 94 100 102 107 108 110 111 113 114 115 117 118 120 122 125 127 128 129 131 134 140 141 142 143 144 145 146 147 **P**6
Primary Contact: Thomas R. Mullen, President and Chief Executive Officer
COO: Christopher G. Thomaskutty, Vice President Corporate Affairs
CFO: John E. Topper, Senior Vice President and Chief Financial Officer
CMO: Scott A. Spier, M.D., Senior Vice President Medical Affairs
CIO: Kathleen Perry, Vice President and Chief Information Officer
CHR: Tammy Janus, Vice President Human Resources
CNO: Susan D. Finlayson, R.N., Senior Vice President and Chief Nursing Officer
Web address: www.mdmercy.com
**Control:** Church–operated, Nongovernment, not–for profit **Service:** General Medical and Surgical

> **Staffed Beds: 299 Admissions: 18313 Census: 197 Outpatient Visits:** 334300 **Births:** 2704 **Total Expense ($000):** 350633 **Payroll Expense ($000):** 143816 **Personnel:** 3207

⊞ △ **MT. WASHINGTON PEDIATRIC HOSPITAL (213300)**, 1708 West Rogers Avenue, Zip 21209–4537; tel. 410/578–8600, (Nonreporting) **A**1 3 5 7 9 10 **S** University of Maryland Medical System, Baltimore, MD
Primary Contact: Sheldon J. Stein, President and Chief Executive Officer
CFO: Mary Miller, Vice President Finance and Business Development
CMO: Richard Katz, M.D., Vice President Medical Affairs
CIO: Tim Brady, Director Information Systems
CHR: Thomas J. Ellis, Vice President Human Resources
Web address: www.mwph.org
**Control:** Other not–for–profit (including NFP Corporation) **Service:** Children's other specialty

> **Staffed Beds:** 70

⊞ **SAINT AGNES HOSPITAL (210011)**, 900 Caton Avenue, Zip 21229–5299; tel. 410/368–6000 **A**1 2 3 5 9 10 **F**3 8 11 12 13 14 15 17 18 20 22 26 28 29 30 31 32 34 35 40 41 44 45 46 51 53 54 55 56 57 58 59 60 61 65 68 70 72 74 75 76 77 78 79 81 82 84 85 86 87 88 89 92 93 96 97 102 103 107 108 110 111 113 114 116 117 118 119 120 122 123 128 129 130 131 133 134 143 145 146 147 **P**6 **S** Ascension Health, Saint Louis, MO
Primary Contact: Bonnie Phipps, President and Chief Executive Officer
CFO: Scott Furniss, Senior Vice President and Chief Financial Officer
CMO: Adrian Long, M.D., Executive Vice President and Chief Medical Officer
CIO: William Greskovich, Chief Information Officer
CHR: James Bobbitt, Vice President Human Resources
Web address: www.stagnes.org
**Control:** Church–operated, Nongovernment, not–for profit **Service:** General Medical and Surgical

> **Staffed Beds: 372 Admissions: 19602 Census: 219 Outpatient Visits:** 468885 **Births:** 1952 **Total Expense ($000):** 362160 **Payroll Expense ($000):** 183514 **Personnel:** 2599

*Many Facility Codes have changed. Please refer to the AHA Guide Code Chart.* © 2012 AHA Guide

☐ **SHEPPARD AND ENOCH PRATT HOSPITAL (214000)**, 6501 North Charles Street, Zip 21285, Mailing Address: P.O. Box 6815, Zip 21285–6815; tel. 410/938–3000 **A**1 3 5 9 10 **F**10 30 35 38 56 58 64 75 87 98 99 101 103 104 105 106 129 131 142 145 **P**4
Primary Contact: Steven S. Sharfstein, M.D., President and Chief Executive Officer
CFO: Patricia Pinkerton, Vice President and Chief Financial Officer
CMO: Robert Roca, M.D., Vice President Medical Affairs
CIO: Greg Merkle, Director Information Systems
CHR: Cathy Doughty, Vice President Human Resources
CNO: Ernestine Cosby, Vice President Clinical Services and Chief Nursing Officer
Web address: www.sheppardpratt.org
**Control:** Other not–for–profit (including NFP Corporation) **Service:** Psychiatric

**Staffed Beds: 336 Admissions: 8289 Census: 261 Outpatient Visits: 34579 Births: 0 Total Expense ($000): 177384 Payroll Expense ($000): 87690 Personnel: 1844**

☒ △ **SINAI HOSPITAL OF BALTIMORE (210012)**, 2401 West Belvedere Avenue, Zip 21215–5271; tel. 410/601–9000 **A**1 2 3 5 7 9 10 **F**3 5 6 8 9 11 12 13 15 17 18 20 22 24 26 28 29 30 31 32 34 35 36 37 38 39 40 41 43 44 45 46 47 48 49 50 55 57 58 59 60 61 64 65 66 68 70 72 73 74 75 76 77 78 79 81 82 85 86 87 88 89 90 92 93 94 96 97 98 100 101 102 103 104 105 107 108 110 111 113 114 116 118 120 122 123 125 128 129 131 133 134 142 145 146 **P**6 **S** LifeBridge Health, Baltimore, MD
Primary Contact: Neil M. Meltzer, President and Chief Operating Officer
COO: Neil M. Meltzer, President and Chief Operating Officer
CFO: Charles Orlando, Senior Vice President and Chief Financial Officer
CMO: Daniel C. Silverman, M.D., Vice President and Chief Medical Officer
CIO: Karen Barker, Vice President and Chief Information Officer
CHR: Taylor Foss, Vice President Human Resources
Web address: www.lifebridgehealth.org
**Control:** Other not–for–profit (including NFP Corporation) **Service:** General Medical and Surgical

**Staffed Beds: 456 Admissions: 26157 Census: 343 Outpatient Visits: 163906 Births: 2239 Total Expense ($000): 626814 Payroll Expense ($000): 277867 Personnel: 4121**

☐ **SPRING GROVE HOSPITAL CENTER (214018)**, 55 Wade Avenue, Zip 21228–4689; tel. 410/402–6000, (Nonreporting) **A**1 5 9 10
Primary Contact: David S. Helsel, M.D., Chief Executive Officer
CFO: Edward Swartz, Chief Financial Officer
CMO: Devika Krishnan, M.D., Clinical Director and Chief of Staff
Web address: www.springgrove.com
**Control:** State–Government, nonfederal **Service:** Psychiatric

**Staffed Beds: 425**

**UNION MEMORIAL HOSPITAL** See Medstar Union Memorial Hospital

☒ **UNIVERSITY OF MARYLAND MEDICAL CENTER (210002)**, 22 South Greene Street, Zip 21201–1595; tel. 410/328–8667, (Includes UNIVERSITY OF MARYLAND HOSPITAL FOR CHILDREN, 22 South Greene Street, Zip 21201–1544; tel. 800/492–5538) **A**1 2 3 5 8 9 10 **F**3 5 6 7 9 11 12 13 14 15 17 18 19 20 21 22 23 24 25 26 27 28 29 30 31 32 34 35 36 38 39 40 41 43 44 45 46 47 48 49 50 51 52 54 55 56 57 58 59 60 61 64 65 66 68 70 71 72 74 75 76 77 78 79 80 81 82 84 85 86 87 88 89 91 92 93 94 97 98 99 100 101 102 103 104 105 107 108 109 110 111 113 114 115 116 117 118 119 120 122 123 125 128 129 130 131 133 134 135 136 137 138 139 140 141 142 143 144 145 146 147 **P**6 **S** University of Maryland Medical System, Baltimore, MD
Primary Contact: Jeffrey A. Rivest, FACHE, President and Chief Executive Officer
COO: Herbert Buchanan, Senior Vice President and Chief Operating Officer
CFO: Keith D. Persinger, Senior Vice President Finance and Chief Financial Officer
CMO: Jonathan Gottlieb, M.D., Senior Vice President and Chief Medical Officer
CIO: Jon P. Burns, Chief Information Officer
CHR: R. Keith Allen, Senior Vice President Human Resources
Web address: www.umm.edu
**Control:** Other not–for–profit (including NFP Corporation) **Service:** General Medical and Surgical

**Staffed Beds: 819 Admissions: 38627 Census: 597 Outpatient Visits: 270198 Births: 1376 Total Expense ($000): 1147922 Payroll Expense ($000): 452989 Personnel: 8676**

☒ △ **VETERANS AFFAIRS MARYLAND HEALTH CARE SYSTEM–BALTIMORE DIVISION**, 10 North Greene Street, Zip 21201–1524; tel. 410/605–7001, (Includes VETERANS AFFAIRS MARYLAND HEALTH CARE SYSTEM–PERRY POINT DIVISION, Circle Drive, Perry Point, Zip 21902; tel. 410/642–2411; Dennis H. Smith, Director), (Nonreporting) **A**1 2 3 5 7 8 9 **S** Department of Veterans Affairs, Washington, DC
Primary Contact: Dennis H. Smith, Director
CFO: Major Tom Scheffler, Chief Fiscal Officer
CMO: Dorothy Snow, M.D., Chief of Staff
CIO: Sharon Zielinski, Chief Information Resource Officer
CHR: Jeff Craig, Chief Human Resource Management
Web address: www.va.gov/sta/guide/home.asp
**Control:** Veterans Affairs, Government, federal **Service:** General Medical and Surgical

**Staffed Beds: 452**

**MD**

### BEL AIR—Harford County

☐ **UPPER CHESAPEAKE MEDICAL CENTER (210049)**, 500 Upper Chesapeake Drive, Zip 21014–4324; tel. 443/643–1000 **A**1 2 9 10 **F**3 11 13 15 18 20 22 26 28 29 30 31 34 35 36 38 40 41 42 45 46 49 50 51 54 57 59 60 64 65 68 70 71 74 75 76 77 78 79 81 82 84 85 86 87 89 92 93 96 107 108 110 111 113 114 117 118 129 130 131 142 145 146 **S** Upper Chesapeake Health System, Bel Air, MD
Primary Contact: Lyle Ernest Sheldon, FACHE, President and Chief Executive Officer
CFO: Joseph E. Hoffman, III, Senior Vice President and Chief Financial Officer
CMO: Peggy Vaughan, M.D., Senior Vice President Medical Affairs
CIO: Rick Casteel, Vice President Management Information Systems and Chief Information Officer
CHR: Toni Shivery, Vice President Human Resources
Web address: www.uchs.org
**Control:** Other not–for–profit (including NFP Corporation) **Service:** General Medical and Surgical

**Staffed Beds: 175 Admissions: 13486 Census: 131 Outpatient Visits: 176716 Births: 1416 Total Expense ($000): 198754 Payroll Expense ($000): 77300 Personnel: 1592**

### BERLIN—Worcester County

☒ **ATLANTIC GENERAL HOSPITAL (210061)**, 9733 Healthway Drive, Zip 21811–1155; tel. 410/641–1100 **A**1 9 10 **F**3 8 11 12 15 17 18 29 30 31 34 35 38 40 45 50 54 57 58 59 64 65 66 70 74 75 77 78 79 81 83 84 85 87 92 97 104 107 108 110 111 113 118 128 131 134 143 145 146 147 **P**7
Primary Contact: Michael A. Franklin, FACHE, President and Chief Executive Officer
COO: Kim Justice, Vice President Planning and Operations
CFO: Cheryl Nottingham, Chief Financial Officer
CMO: Stephen F. Waters, M.D., Medical Director
CIO: Barbara Riddell, Vice President Information Services
CHR: Jim Brannon, Vice President Human Resources
CNO: Colleen Wareing, Vice President Patient Care Services
Web address: www.atlanticgeneral.org
**Control:** Other not–for–profit (including NFP Corporation) **Service:** General Medical and Surgical

**Staffed Beds: 58 Admissions: 4011 Census: 37 Outpatient Visits: 107725 Births: 0 Total Expense ($000): 82890 Payroll Expense ($000): 37563 Personnel: 697**

### BETHESDA—Montgomery County

☒ **NATIONAL INSTITUTES OF HEALTH CLINICAL CENTER**, (Biomedical Research), 9000 Rockville Pike, Building 10, Room 6–2551, Zip 20892–1504; tel. 301/496–4000, (Includes CHILDREN'S INN AT NIH, 7 West Drive, Zip 20814–1509; tel. 301/496–5672) **A**1 3 5 8 **F**3 4 5 8 14 15 20 22 26 30 31 36 39 45 52 53 55 58 59 60 61 64 65 68 70 74 75 77 78 79 81 82 84 85 86 87 89 91 92 93 94 95 96 98 99 100 101 104 105 107 108 110 111 112 113 114 115 116 117 118 119 120 123 125 128 129 131 134 135 140 141 144 145 147 **S** U. S. Indian Health Service, Rockville, MD
Primary Contact: John I. Gallin, M.D., Director
COO: Maureen E. Gormley, R.N., Chief Operating Officer
CFO: Maria Joyce, Chief Financial Officer
CMO: David K. Henderson, M.D., Deputy Director Clinical Care
CIO: Jon W. McKeeby, Chief Information Officer
CHR: Bonnie Tuma, Human Resources Team Lead
Web address: www.clinicalcenter.nih.gov
**Control:** Public Health Service, Government, federal **Service:** Other specialty

**Staffed Beds: 161 Admissions: 6082 Census: 155 Outpatient Visits: 106134 Births: 0 Total Expense ($000): 391534 Payroll Expense ($000): 174684 Personnel: 1896**

**NATIONAL NAVAL MEDICAL CENTER** See Walter Reed National Military Medical Center

---

**Hospital, Medicare Provider Number, Address, Telephone, Approval, Facility, and Physician Codes, Health Care System**

★ American Hospital Association (AHA) membership
☐ The Joint Commission accreditation
◇ DNV Healthcare Inc. accreditation
○ American Osteopathic Association (AOA) accreditation
△ Commission on Accreditation of Rehabilitation Facilities (CARF) accreditation

✠ **SUBURBAN HOSPITAL (210022)**, 8600 Old Georgetown Road,
Zip 20814–1497; tel. 301/896–3100 **A**1 2 3 5 9 10 **F**3 4 5 8 11 15 17 18 20
22 24 26 28 29 30 31 34 35 36 37 38 39 40 43 44 45 46 49 50 51 53 54
56 57 58 59 60 64 70 71 74 75 77 78 79 80 81 82 84 85 86 87 89 92 93
98 99 100 101 102 103 104 105 107 108 110 111 113 114 116 117 118
119 120 122 125 128 129 131 133 134 145 146 147 **P**6 **S** Johns Hopkins
Health System, Baltimore, MD
Primary Contact: Brian A. Gragnolati, FACHE, President and Chief Executive
Officer
COO: Jacky Schultz, R.N., Executive Vice President and Chief Operating Officer
CFO: Marty Basso, Senior Vice President Finance
CMO: Robert Rothstein, M.D., Vice President Medical Affairs
CIO: Christopher T. Timbers, Vice President and Chief Information Officer
CHR: Dennis Parnell, Senior Vice President Human Resources
CNO: Barbara Stewart Jacobs, MSN, Suburban Hospital Nursing and Patient Care
Administrator
Web address: www.suburbanhospital.org
**Control:** Other not–for–profit (including NFP Corporation) **Service:** General
Medical and Surgical

**Staffed Beds:** 234 **Admissions:** 14217 **Census:** 166 **Outpatient Visits:**
129718 **Births:** 0 **Total Expense ($000):** 228738 **Payroll Expense ($000):**
94880 **Personnel:** 1283

✠ **WALTER REED NATIONAL MILITARY MEDICAL CENTER**, 8901 Wisconsin
Avenue, Zip 20889–5600; tel. 301/295–4611, (Nonreporting) **A**1 2 3 5 9
**S** Bureau of Medicine and Surgery, Department of the Navy, Washington, DC
Primary Contact: Rear Admiral Alton Stocks, Commander
CFO: Commander Joseph Pickel, Director Resource Management
CMO: Paul Florentino, M.D., Director Medical Services
CIO: Commander Cayetano Thornton, Chief Information Officer
CHR: Captain Jaime Carroll, Department Head
Web address: www.bethesda.med.navy.mil
**Control:** Navy, Government, federal **Service:** General Medical and Surgical

**Staffed Beds:** 240

### CAMBRIDGE—Dorchester County

✠ **DORCHESTER GENERAL HOSPITAL**, 300 Byrn Street, Zip 21613–1908;
tel. 410/228–5511 **A**1 9 **F**3 11 15 18 19 20 22 28 29 30 31 39 40 45 57 59
64 68 70 74 75 77 78 79 81 82 85 87 91 93 98 99 100 102 103 104 107
108 111 113 117 118 129 131 **S** University of Maryland Medical System,
Baltimore, MD
Primary Contact: Kenneth D. Kozel, FACHE, President and Chief Executive Officer
COO: Gerard M. Walsh, Senior Vice President and Chief Operating Officer
CFO: Walter Zajac, Senior Vice President and Chief Financial Officer
CMO: Michael Tooke, M.D., Vice President Medical Affairs
CIO: Elizabeth Fish, Chief Information Officer
CHR: Michael Zimmerman, Vice President Human Resources
Web address: www.shorehealth.org
**Control:** Other not–for–profit (including NFP Corporation) **Service:** General
Medical and Surgical

**Staffed Beds:** 44 **Admissions:** 3447 **Census:** 36 **Outpatient Visits:** 109185
**Births:** 0 **Total Expense ($000):** 44051 **Payroll Expense ($000):** 20234
**Personnel:** 270

☐ **EASTERN SHORE HOSPITAL CENTER (214002)**, 5262 Woods Road,
Zip 21613, Mailing Address: P.O. Box 800, Zip 21613–0800;
tel. 410/221–2525, (Nonreporting) **A**1 9 10
Primary Contact: Mary Kay Noren, Chief Executive Officer
COO: Randy L. Bradford, Assistant Superintendent
CFO: Ida Bundick, Chief Financial Officer
CMO: David Pytlewski, M.D., Clinical Director
CHR: Cassandra Stanley, Director Personnel
Web address: www.dhmh.state.md.us/eshc
**Control:** State–Government, nonfederal **Service:** Psychiatric

**Staffed Beds:** 76

### CHESTERTOWN—Kent County

✠ **CHESTER RIVER HEALTH SYSTEM (210030)**, 100 Brown Street,
Zip 21620–1499; tel. 410/778–3300 **A**1 9 10 **F**3 11 13 15 18 20 24 28 29
30 31 34 35 39 40 41 42 45 46 47 50 53 55 56 57 59 60 62 63 64 65 68
70 75 76 78 79 80 81 82 85 87 89 97 102 107 110 111 114 118 128 129
131 145 146 **S** University of Maryland Medical System, Baltimore, MD
Primary Contact: James E. Ross, FACHE, President and Chief Executive Officer
COO: Scott D. Burleson, Executive Vice President
CFO: Samuel Marinelli, Vice President Finance and Chief Financial Officer
CMO: Stanley Minken, M.D., Chief Medical Officer
CIO: Elizabeth Fish, Senior Director Site Executive and Information Technology
CHR: Patricia Kuhl, Vice President Human Resources
CNO: Mary Jo Keefe, R.N., Vice President Patient Care Services and Chief Nursing
Officer
Web address: www.chesterriverhealth.org
**Control:** Other not–for–profit (including NFP Corporation) **Service:** General
Medical and Surgical

**Staffed Beds:** 47 **Admissions:** 2789 **Census:** 32 **Outpatient Visits:** 56389
**Births:** 183 **Total Expense ($000):** 53037 **Payroll Expense ($000):** 22795
**Personnel:** 384

**CHESTER RIVER HOSPITAL CENTER** See Chester River Health System

### CHEVERLY—Prince George's County

**GLADYS SPELLMAN SPECIALTY HOSPITAL AND NURSING CENTER**, 2900
Mercy Lane, Zip 20785–1157; tel. 301/618–2010, (Nonreporting)
Primary Contact: Stewart R. Seitz, Chief Executive Officer
CFO: Ketty Taboado, Chief Financial Officer
CMO: Paul A. Devore, M.D., Medical Director
CIO: Dennis Lilik, Chief Information Officer
CHR: Michael Jacobs, Vice President Human Resources
Web address: www.dimensionshealth.org
**Control:** Corporation, Investor–owned, for–profit **Service:** Chronic disease

**Staffed Beds:** 30

☐ **PRINCE GEORGE'S HOSPITAL CENTER (210003)**, 3001 Hospital Drive,
Zip 20785–1189; tel. 301/618–2000, (Total facility includes 107 beds in nursing
home–type unit) **A**1 3 5 9 10 **F**1 3 11 13 15 17 18 20 22 24 26 28 29 31 34
35 38 40 42 43 45 46 47 48 49 50 54 55 56 57 59 60 61 63 64 65 66 68
69 70 72 74 75 76 77 78 79 81 82 84 85 86 87 89 92 93 97 98 100 101
102 103 104 105 107 108 110 111 113 114 117 118 127 129 130 131 133
134 141 143 145 147 **P**6 **S** Dimensions Healthcare System, Cheverly, MD
Primary Contact: John A. O'Brien, FACHE, President
CFO: Neil J. Moore, Chief Financial Officer
CMO: David Goldman, M.D., Vice President Medical Affairs and Education
CIO: Dennis Lilik, Chief Information Officer
CHR: Michael Jacobs, Vice President Human Resources
Web address: www.princegeorgeshospital.org
**Control:** Other not–for–profit (including NFP Corporation) **Service:** General
Medical and Surgical

**Staffed Beds:** 411 **Admissions:** 13086 **Census:** 238 **Outpatient Visits:**
89591 **Births:** 2307 **Total Expense ($000):** 236027 **Payroll Expense
($000):** 107844 **Personnel:** 1754

### CLINTON—Prince George's County

✠ **SOUTHERN MARYLAND HOSPITAL CENTER (210054)**, 7503 Surratts Road,
Zip 20735–3397; tel. 301/868–8000, (Nonreporting) **A**1 2 9 10
Primary Contact: Michael J. Chiaramonte, Chief Executive Officer
COO: Patricia Christensen, MSN, Chief Operating Officer
CFO: Charles R. Stewart, Vice President Business, Finance and Corporate
Compliance
CMO: J. Andrew Sumner, M.D., Vice President Medical Affairs
CIO: Lou Mavromatis, Vice President Data Processing
CHR: Paul Zeller, Vice President Human Resources
Web address: www.smhchealth.org
**Control:** Corporation, Investor–owned, for–profit **Service:** General Medical and
Surgical

**Staffed Beds:** 294

### COLUMBIA—Howard County

✠ **HOWARD COUNTY GENERAL HOSPITAL (210048)**, 5755 Cedar Lane,
Zip 21044–2999; tel. 410/740–7890 **A**1 2 5 9 10 **F**3 8 11 13 15 18 20 22 26
28 29 30 31 32 34 35 36 39 40 41 44 45 46 47 49 50 51 55 56 57 58 59
61 64 65 68 70 72 74 75 76 77 78 79 81 82 85 86 87 89 91 92 93 94 96
98 100 101 102 103 107 108 110 111 113 114 118 129 130 131 133 134
145 146 147 **S** Johns Hopkins Health System, Baltimore, MD
Primary Contact: Victor A. Broccolino, President and Chief Executive Officer
COO: Jay H. Blackman, Senior Vice President and Chief Operating Officer
CFO: James Young, Senior Vice President Finance and Chief Financial Officer
CIO: Rick Edwards, Director Information Systems
CHR: Dorothy Brillantes, Senior Vice President Human Resources
Web address: www.hcgh.org
**Control:** Other not–for–profit (including NFP Corporation) **Service:** General
Medical and Surgical

**Staffed Beds:** 256 **Admissions:** 16068 **Census:** 178 **Outpatient Visits:**
148272 **Births:** 3229 **Total Expense ($000):** 214459 **Payroll Expense
($000):** 83979 **Personnel:** 1351

### CRISFIELD—Somerset County

☐ **MCCREADY HEALTH SERVICES FOUNDATION (210045)**, 201 Hall Highway,
Zip 21817–1299; tel. 410/968–1200, (Nonreporting) **A**1 9 10
Primary Contact: Robert Jones, Chief Executive Officer
CFO: Gary W. Broadwater, Chief Financial Officer
Web address: www.mccreadyfoundation.org
**Control:** Other not–for–profit (including NFP Corporation) **Service:** General
Medical and Surgical

**Staffed Beds:** 89

*Many Facility Codes have changed. Please refer to the AHA Guide Code Chart.* © 2012 AHA Guide

## CUMBERLAND—Allegany County

☐ **THOMAS B. FINAN CENTER (214012)**, 10102 Country Club Road S.E., Zip 21502–8339, Mailing Address: P.O. Box 1722, Zip 21501–1722; tel. 301/777–2240, (Nonreporting) **A**1 9 10
Primary Contact: Judith Hott, Chief Executive Officer
COO: John Cullen, Assistant Superintendent
CFO: Craig Alexander, Fiscal Specialist
CMO: Linda de Hoyos, M.D., Clinical Director
CHR: Chris Loney, Director Personnel
CNO: Gayle Walter, Director of Nursing
Web address: www.dhmh.state.md.us
**Control:** State–Government, nonfederal **Service:** Psychiatric

**Staffed Beds:** 80

⊠ △ **WESTERN MARYLAND REGIONAL MEDICAL CENTER (210027)**, 12500 Willowbrook Road, Zip 21502–6393, Mailing Address: P.O. Box 539, Zip 21501–0539; tel. 240/964–7000, (Total facility includes 88 beds in nursing home–type unit) **A**1 2 7 9 10 **F**3 5 11 13 14 15 17 18 20 22 24 26 28 29 30 31 32 34 35 38 40 43 44 45 50 51 54 56 57 59 60 62 63 64 68 69 70 73 74 75 76 77 78 79 80 81 82 84 85 86 87 89 90 93 94 96 97 98 100 102 103 104 107 108 110 111 113 114 115 116 117 118 119 120 122 127 128 129 131 134 143 145 147 **P**6
Primary Contact: Barry P. Ronan, President and Chief Executive Officer
COO: Thomas C. Dowdell, FACHE, Senior Vice President and Chief Operating Officer
CFO: Kimberly S. Repac, Senior Vice President and Chief Financial Officer
CMO: George Garrow, M.D., Senior Vice President and Chief Medical Officer
CIO: William Byers, Vice President and Chief Information Officer
CHR: Mark J. Sullivan, Vice President Human Resources
CNO: Nancy D. Adams, R.N., Senior Vice President and Chief Nurse Executive
Web address: www.wmhs.com
**Control:** Other not–for–profit (including NFP Corporation) **Service:** General Medical and Surgical

**Staffed Beds:** 373 **Admissions:** 15626 **Census:** 269 **Outpatient Visits:** 503866 **Births:** 1011 **Total Expense ($000):** 288558 **Payroll Expense ($000):** 100384 **Personnel:** 1837

## EAST NEW MARKET—Dorchester County

**WARWICK MANOR BEHAVIORAL HEALTH**, 3680 Warwick Road, Zip 21631–1420; tel. 410/943–8108, (Nonreporting) **A**9
Primary Contact: Marie McBee, Chief Executive Officer
Web address: www.warwickmanor.org/
**Control:** Corporation, Investor–owned, for–profit **Service:** Alcoholism and other chemical dependency

**Staffed Beds:** 42

## EASTON—Talbot County

⊠ △ **MEMORIAL HOSPITAL AT EASTON MARYLAND (210037)**, 219 South Washington Street, Zip 21601–2996; tel. 410/822–1000 **A**1 2 7 9 10 **F**3 8 11 13 15 18 20 22 28 29 30 31 34 37 39 40 42 45 49 51 54 57 58 59 60 62 63 64 65 70 74 76 78 79 81 82 83 84 85 86 89 90 91 93 95 100 102 107 108 111 113 115 116 117 118 119 120 122 123 125 128 129 131 143 146 147 **P**3 **S** University of Maryland Medical System, Baltimore, MD
Primary Contact: Kenneth D. Kozel, FACHE, President and Chief Executive Officer
COO: Gerard M. Walsh, Senior Vice President and Chief Operating Officer
CFO: Walter Zajac, Senior Vice President and Chief Financial Officer
CMO: Michael Tooke, M.D., Chief Medical Officer
CIO: Elizabeth Fish, Chief Information Officer
CHR: Michael Zimmerman, Vice President Human Resources
CNO: Christopher J. Parker, R.N., Chief Nursing Officer
Web address: www.shorehealth.org
**Control:** Other not–for–profit (including NFP Corporation) **Service:** General Medical and Surgical

**Staffed Beds:** 107 **Admissions:** 9435 **Census:** 97 **Outpatient Visits:** 300906 **Births:** 1082 **Total Expense ($000):** 159613 **Payroll Expense ($000):** 59450 **Personnel:** 1125

## ELKTON—Cecil County

⊠ △ **UNION HOSPITAL (210032)**, 106 Bow Street, Zip 21921–5596; tel. 410/398–4000 **A**1 2 3 5 7 9 10 **F**2 3 11 13 15 18 26 29 30 31 34 35 40 44 45 46 49 50 51 54 57 59 61 63 64 69 70 74 75 76 77 78 79 81 82 84 85 86 87 89 92 97 98 100 102 104 105 107 108 110 111 113 117 118 128 129 130 131 134 145 146 147 **P**6
Primary Contact: Kenneth S. Lewis, M.D., JD, President and Chief Executive Officer
COO: David N. Gipson, Senior Vice President and Chief Clinical Operations Officer
CFO: Laurie Beyer, Senior Vice President and Chief Financial Officer
CMO: Jose Ma, M.D., Vice President Medical Affairs
CIO: Mary Jane Kamps, Chief Information Officer
CHR: Peter Gloggner, Vice President Human Resources
Web address: www.uhcc.com
**Control:** Other not–for–profit (including NFP Corporation) **Service:** General Medical and Surgical

**Staffed Beds:** 119 **Admissions:** 7032 **Census:** 72 **Outpatient Visits:** 166709 **Births:** 668 **Total Expense ($000):** 126875 **Payroll Expense ($000):** 53622 **Personnel:** 890

## EMMITSBURG—Frederick County

**MOUNTAIN MANOR TREATMENT CENTER**, Route 15, Zip 21727, Mailing Address: Box 136, Zip 21727; tel. 301/447–2361, (Nonreporting)
Primary Contact: William J. Roby, Executive Vice President
CFO: Susan Liedlich, Director Finance
CHR: Craig Cutter, Corporate Director Human Resources
Web address: www.mountainmanor.org
**Control:** Corporation, Investor–owned, for–profit **Service:** Alcoholism and other chemical dependency

**Staffed Beds:** 140

## FORT WASHINGTON—Prince George's County

⊠ **FORT WASHINGTON MEDICAL CENTER (210060)**, 11711 Livingston Road, Zip 20744–5164; tel. 301/292–7000 **A**1 9 10 **F**3 15 29 34 40 49 70 75 77 79 80 81 85 87 90 107 108 118 129
Primary Contact: Verna Meacham, Chief Executive Officer
CFO: Joseph B. Tucker, Senior Vice President and Chief Financial Officer
CMO: Elias Debbas, M.D., President Medical Staff
CIO: Fred Ashby, Director Information Technology
CHR: Alexander Morris, Corporate Director Human Resources
CNO: Marjorie Quint–Bouzid, Chief Nursing Officer and Vice President Patient Care Services
Web address: www.fortwashingtonmc.org
**Control:** Other not–for–profit (including NFP Corporation) **Service:** General Medical and Surgical

**Staffed Beds:** 37 **Admissions:** 2393 **Census:** 24 **Outpatient Visits:** 50264 **Births:** 0 **Total Expense ($000):** 38479 **Payroll Expense ($000):** 18408 **Personnel:** 289

## FREDERICK—Frederick County

⊠ **FREDERICK MEMORIAL HOSPITAL (210005)**, 400 West Seventh Street, Zip 21701–4593; tel. 240/566–3300, (Total facility includes 20 beds in nursing home–type unit) **A**1 2 5 9 10 **F**3 8 11 13 15 18 20 22 26 28 29 30 31 32 34 35 36 37 38 39 40 41 44 45 46 48 49 50 51 53 54 57 58 59 60 61 62 63 64 66 68 70 71 72 74 75 76 77 78 79 81 82 83 84 85 86 87 89 93 94 96 97 98 100 101 102 103 104 105 107 108 109 110 111 113 114 115 116 117 118 119 120 123 125 127 128 129 130 131 134 142 143 144 145 146 147 **P**6 7
Primary Contact: Thomas A. Kleinhanzl, President and Chief Executive Officer
COO: John R. Verbus, Senior Vice President and Chief Operating Officer
CFO: Michelle K. Mahan, Senior Vice President and Chief Financial Officer
CMO: Manuel Casiano, M.D., Vice President Medical Affairs
CIO: David Quirke, Vice President Information Services
CHR: Terry O'Malley, Vice President Human Resources
Web address: www.fmh.org
**Control:** Other not–for–profit (including NFP Corporation) **Service:** General Medical and Surgical

**Staffed Beds:** 308 **Admissions:** 20413 **Census:** 247 **Outpatient Visits:** 434576 **Births:** 2382 **Total Expense ($000):** 325811 **Payroll Expense ($000):** 140081 **Personnel:** 2324

---

**Hospital, Medicare Provider Number, Address, Telephone, Approval, Facility, and Physician Codes, Health Care System**

★ American Hospital Association (AHA) membership
☐ The Joint Commission accreditation
◇ DNV Healthcare Inc. accreditation
○ American Osteopathic Association (AOA) accreditation
△ Commission on Accreditation of Rehabilitation Facilities (CARF) accreditation

**MD**

## GLEN BURNIE—Anne Arundel County

☒ **BALTIMORE WASHINGTON MEDICAL CENTER (210043)**, 301 Hospital Drive, Zip 21061–5899; tel. 410/787–4000 **A**1 2 9 10 **F**3 8 10 11 13 14 18 20 22 26 28 29 30 31 34 35 40 44 45 46 48 49 50 54 55 56 57 58 59 60 64 68 70 74 75 76 77 78 79 81 82 84 85 87 89 93 94 98 100 102 105 107 108 111 113 114 115 116 117 118 119 120 122 125 128 129 130 131 134 145 146 147 **P**6 **S** University of Maryland Medical System, Baltimore, MD
Primary Contact: Karen E. Olscamp, Chief Executive Officer
COO: Ronald J. Andro, Senior Vice President and Chief Operating Officer
CFO: Al Pietsch, CPA, Senior Vice President and Chief Financial Officer
CMO: Lawrence Linder, M.D., Senior Vice President and Chief Medical Officer
CIO: Linda Hines, Vice President and Site Executive
CHR: Frank Venuto, Vice President Human Resources
Web address: www.bwmc.umms.org
**Control:** Other not–for–profit (including NFP Corporation) **Service:** General Medical and Surgical

**Staffed Beds:** 321 **Admissions:** 19776 **Census:** 225 **Outpatient Visits:** 137166 **Births:** 753 **Total Expense ($000):** 291450 **Payroll Expense ($000):** 119651 **Personnel:** 2166

## HAGERSTOWN—Washington County

☐ **BROOK LANE HEALTH SERVICES (214003)**, 13218 Brook Lane Drive, Zip 21742–1945, Mailing Address: P.O. Box 1945, Zip 21742–1945; tel. 301/733–0330 **A**1 9 10 **F**5 26 27 30 56 68 98 99 100 101 103 104 105 129 142 145 **P**4 6
Primary Contact: R. Lynn Rushing, Chief Executive Officer
CFO: Floyd Klauka, Chief Financial Officer
CIO: Sharon Gladfelter, Health Information Officer
CHR: Patricia Bourdeau, Director Human Resources
Web address: www.brooklane.org
**Control:** Other not–for–profit (including NFP Corporation) **Service:** Psychiatric

**Staffed Beds:** 44 **Admissions:** 1694 **Census:** 30 **Outpatient Visits:** 42488 **Births:** 0 **Total Expense ($000):** 17699 **Payroll Expense ($000):** 10824 **Personnel:** 259

☒ △ **MERITUS MEDICAL CENTER (210001)**, 11116 Medical Campus Road, Zip 21742–6710; tel. 301/790–8000 **A**1 2 7 9 10 **F**3 5 11 12 13 15 17 18 20 22 26 28 29 30 31 34 35 38 40 43 44 49 51 52 54 56 57 58 59 60 61 62 64 65 70 74 75 76 77 78 79 81 82 83 84 85 86 87 89 90 93 94 96 97 98 99 100 101 102 103 104 105 107 108 111 113 114 117 118 119 120 122 129 130 131 134 142 143 144 145 146 147 **P**6 8
Primary Contact: Joseph P. Ross, President and Chief Executive Officer
COO: Deborah Addo–Samuels, Senior Vice President and Chief Operating Officer
CFO: Raymond A. Grahe, Senior Vice President Strategic Ventures and Chief Financial Officer
CMO: Robert L. Brooks, M.D., Vice President Medical Affairs
CMO: Heather Lorenzo, M.D., Vice President and Chief Medical Officer
CIO: Jake Dorst, Vice President and Chief Information Officer
CIO: Carey O. Leverett, Vice President Information Services
CHR: Kelly Corbi, Chief Administrative Officer and Vice President Human Resources and Development
CNO: Jesus Cepero, R.N., Vice President Nursing and Chief Nursing Officer
Web address: www.meritushealth.com
**Control:** Other not–for–profit (including NFP Corporation) **Service:** General Medical and Surgical

**Staffed Beds:** 278 **Admissions:** 16206 **Census:** 192 **Outpatient Visits:** 198508 **Births:** 1948 **Total Expense ($000):** 257607 **Payroll Expense ($000):** 111849 **Personnel:** 1836

**WASHINGTON COUNTY HEALTH SYSTEM** See Meritus Medical Center

☐ **WESTERN MARYLAND HOSPITAL CENTER (212002)**, 1500 Pennsylvania Avenue, Zip 21742–3194; tel. 301/791–4400, (Nonreporting) **A**1 9 10
Primary Contact: Cynthia Miller Pellegrino, Chief Executive Officer
COO: David Davis, Chief Operating Officer
CFO: Kelly Edmonds, Chief Financial Officer
CMO: Monica Stallworth, M.D., Chief of Staff
CIO: Ron Keplinger, Chief Information Officer
CHR: David Davis, Chief Operating Officer
Web address: www.wmhc.us
**Control:** State–Government, nonfederal **Service:** Long–Term Acute Care hospital

**Staffed Beds:** 120

## HAVRE DE GRACE—Harford County

☐ **HARFORD MEMORIAL HOSPITAL (210006)**, 501 South Union Avenue, Zip 21078–3493; tel. 443/843–5000 **A**1 2 9 10 **F**3 11 12 15 28 29 30 31 34 35 36 38 40 42 46 49 50 51 57 59 60 64 65 66 68 70 71 74 75 77 78 79 81 82 84 85 86 87 92 93 96 98 102 103 104 107 108 110 111 113 114 117 118 128 129 130 131 134 145 147 **S** Upper Chesapeake Health System, Bel Air, MD
Primary Contact: Lyle Ernest Sheldon, FACHE, President and Chief Executive Officer
CFO: Joseph E. Hoffman, III, Senior Vice President and Chief Financial Officer
CMO: Peggy Vaughan, M.D., Senior Vice President Medical Affairs
CIO: Rick Casteel, Vice President Management Information Systems and Chief Information Officer
CHR: Toni Shivery, Vice President Human Resources
Web address: www.uchs.org
**Control:** Other not–for–profit (including NFP Corporation) **Service:** General Medical and Surgical

**Staffed Beds:** 105 **Admissions:** 5566 **Census:** 65 **Outpatient Visits:** 88999 **Births:** 0 **Total Expense ($000):** 80375 **Payroll Expense ($000):** 35955 **Personnel:** 673

## JESSUP—Howard County

☐ **CLIFTON T. PERKINS HOSPITAL CENTER**, 8450 Dorsey Run Road, Zip 20794–9414; tel. 410/724–3000, (Nonreporting) **A**1 3 5
Primary Contact: Sheilah Davenport, JD, MS, R.N., Chief Executive Officer and Superintendent
COO: Steve Mason, Assistant Superintendent and Chief Operating Officer
CFO: George Parnel, Chief Financial Officer
CMO: Muhammed Ajanah, M.D., Clinical Director
CIO: Chanda Hamilton, Chief Information Officer
CHR: Beverly Stacie, Director Human Resources
Web address: www.dhmh.state.md.us/perkins/
**Control:** State–Government, nonfederal **Service:** Psychiatric

**Staffed Beds:** 218

## LA PLATA—Charles County

☒ **CIVISTA HEALTH (210035)**, 5 Garrett Avenue, Zip 20646–1070, Mailing Address: P.O. Box 1070, Zip 20646–1070; tel. 301/609–4000 **A**1 2 9 10 **F**3 8 11 13 15 18 20 26 28 29 30 31 34 35 36 40 45 46 50 51 54 57 59 60 61 64 70 74 76 77 78 79 81 82 85 86 87 89 93 97 107 108 109 111 113 114 117 118 128 129 131 144 145 146 147 **S** University of Maryland Medical System, Baltimore, MD
Primary Contact: Noel A. Cervino, President and Chief Executive Officer
COO: Gary J. Herbek, Chief Operating Officer
CFO: Erik Boas, Vice President Finance
CMO: Sanjeeb Mishra, M.D., Chief of Staff
CIO: Kevin Burbules, Chief Information Officer
CHR: Stacey Cook, Director Human Resources
Web address: www.civista.org
**Control:** Other not–for–profit (including NFP Corporation) **Service:** General Medical and Surgical

**Staffed Beds:** 124 **Admissions:** 7850 **Census:** 86 **Outpatient Visits:** 55229 **Births:** 828 **Total Expense ($000):** 94882 **Payroll Expense ($000):** 41138 **Personnel:** 689

## LANHAM—Prince George's County

☒ **DOCTORS COMMUNITY HOSPITAL (210051)**, 8118 Good Luck Road, Zip 20706–3596; tel. 301/552–8118 **A**1 9 10 **F**3 8 11 12 14 15 17 20 28 29 30 31 34 35 40 45 50 51 57 59 60 61 68 70 74 75 77 78 79 81 82 84 85 86 91 92 93 102 107 108 109 110 111 113 114 115 116 117 118 123 125 128 129 130 131 143 145 146 147 **P**2
Primary Contact: Philip B. Down, President and Chief Executive Officer
COO: Paul Grenaldo, Executive Vice President and Chief Operating Officer
CFO: Dennis P. Scanlon, Vice President Finance
CMO: Gabriel Jaffe, M.D., Vice President Medical Affairs
CIO: Alan Johnson, Chief Information Officer
CHR: Charlene B. Lundgren, Vice President
Web address: www.dchweb.org
**Control:** Other not–for–profit (including NFP Corporation) **Service:** General Medical and Surgical

**Staffed Beds:** 150 **Admissions:** 13147 **Census:** 163 **Outpatient Visits:** 78944 **Births:** 0 **Total Expense ($000):** 180056 **Payroll Expense ($000):** 76457 **Personnel:** 1204

*Many Facility Codes have changed. Please refer to the AHA Guide Code Chart.* © 2012 AHA Guide

## LAUREL—Prince George's County

☐ △ **LAUREL REGIONAL HOSPITAL (210055)**, 7300 Van Dusen Road, Zip 20707–9266; tel. 301/725–4300 **A**1 7 9 10 **F**3 11 13 15 18 20 29 30 31 34 35 40 46 49 50 51 57 59 60 61 63 64 65 66 68 69 70 74 75 76 77 78 79 80 81 82 84 85 87 90 92 93 98 100 102 103 104 105 107 108 110 111 113 114 117 118 128 129 131 145 147 **S** Dimensions Healthcare System, Cheverly, MD
Primary Contact: Gloria Ceballos, R.N., MS, Interim President
COO: John A. O'Brien, FACHE, Chief Operating Officer
CFO: Neil J. Moore, Chief Financial Officer
CMO: Gita Shah, M.D., Vice President Medical Affairs
CIO: Dennis Lilik, Chief Information Officer
CHR: Michael Jacobs, Vice President Human Resources
Web address: www.laurelregionalhospital.org
**Control:** Other not–for–profit (including NFP Corporation) **Service:** General Medical and Surgical

**Staffed Beds:** 124 **Admissions:** 5663 **Census:** 64 **Outpatient Visits:** 40285 **Births:** 901 **Total Expense ($000):** 92738 **Payroll Expense ($000):** 40854 **Personnel:** 688

## LEONARDTOWN—St. Mary's County

⊠ **MEDSTAR ST. MARY'S HOSPITAL (210028)**, 25500 Point Lookout Road, Zip 20650–0527, Mailing Address: P.O. Box 527, Zip 20650–0527; tel. 301/475–6001 **A**1 2 9 10 **F**2 3 5 8 11 13 15 18 28 29 30 31 32 34 35 36 39 40 44 45 50 51 53 54 56 57 59 60 63 64 65 66 68 70 71 74 75 76 77 78 79 81 82 84 85 86 87 89 93 98 102 104 105 107 108 110 111 113 114 115 117 118 126 128 129 131 134 143 145 146 147 **P**1 6 **S** MedStar Health, Columbia, MD
Primary Contact: Christine R. Wray, President
CFO: Richard Braam, Vice President Finance
CMO: Avani D. Shah, M.D., Chief of Medical Staff
CIO: Donald Sirk, Director Information Systems
CHR: Evelyn Campos–Diaz, Director Human Resources
CNO: Mary Lou Watson, MS, Vice President Nursing
Web address: www.medstarstmarys.org
**Control:** Other not–for–profit (including NFP Corporation) **Service:** General Medical and Surgical

**Staffed Beds:** 115 **Admissions:** 7857 **Census:** 64 **Outpatient Visits:** 277008 **Births:** 1191 **Total Expense ($000):** 113805 **Payroll Expense ($000):** 49148 **Personnel:** 883

## OAKLAND—Garrett County

⊠ **GARRETT COUNTY MEMORIAL HOSPITAL (210017)**, 251 North Fourth Street, Zip 21550–1398; tel. 301/533–4000, (Total facility includes 10 beds in nursing home–type unit) **A**1 9 10 **F**3 11 13 28 29 30 31 32 34 35 38 40 45 56 57 59 65 70 74 75 76 78 79 81 82 85 87 89 102 107 108 109 113 117 118 127 129 134 145 146 147 **P**6 7
Primary Contact: Donald P. Battista, President and Chief Executive Officer
COO: Denise R. Liston, R.N., Vice President Clinical and Support Services
CFO: Tracy Lipscomb, Vice President Financial Services and Chief Financial Officer
CIO: Stephen Peterson, Director Information Systems
CHR: Annette Livengood, Vice President Human Resources
Web address: www.gcmh.com
**Control:** Other not–for–profit (including NFP Corporation) **Service:** General Medical and Surgical

**Staffed Beds:** 55 **Admissions:** 2451 **Census:** 22 **Outpatient Visits:** 74070 **Births:** 274 **Total Expense ($000):** 33330 **Payroll Expense ($000):** 15609 **Personnel:** 306

## OLNEY—Montgomery County

⊠ **MEDSTAR MONTGOMERY MEDICAL CENTER (210018)**, 18101 Prince Philip Drive, Zip 20832–1512; tel. 301/774–8882 **A**1 2 9 10 **F**3 5 11 13 18 20 26 28 29 30 31 34 35 37 38 40 41 45 46 48 49 50 51 55 56 57 59 62 65 70 74 75 76 77 78 79 80 81 84 85 86 89 92 93 98 99 100 102 103 104 105 107 108 113 114 117 118 125 128 129 131 133 134 142 145 **S** MedStar Health, Columbia, MD
Primary Contact: Peter W. Monge, President
CFO: David A. Havrilla, Chief Financial Officer
CMO: Roger Leonard, M.D., Vice President Medical Affairs
CHR: Kevin Mell, Vice President Operations
Web address: www.montgomerygeneral.com
**Control:** Other not–for–profit (including NFP Corporation) **Service:** General Medical and Surgical

**Staffed Beds:** 158 **Admissions:** 9877 **Census:** 109 **Outpatient Visits:** 65610 **Births:** 735 **Total Expense ($000):** 133010 **Payroll Expense ($000):** 56134 **Personnel:** 830

## PERRY POINT—Cecil County

**VETERANS AFFAIRS MARYLAND HEALTH CARE SYSTEM–PERRY POINT DIVISION** See Veterans Affairs Maryland Health Care System–Baltimore Division, Baltimore

## PRINCE FREDERICK—Calvert County

⊠ **CALVERT MEMORIAL HOSPITAL (210039)**, 100 Hospital Road, Zip 20678–9675; tel. 410/535–4000, (Total facility includes 18 beds in nursing home–type unit) **A**1 2 9 10 **F**3 8 11 13 15 18 28 29 30 31 32 33 34 35 36 38 40 49 50 54 57 59 62 68 70 75 76 77 78 79 81 82 84 85 86 87 89 98 99 101 102 105 107 108 111 113 117 118 128 129 130 131 133 134 143 145 146 147 **P**4
Primary Contact: James J. Xinis, President and Chief Executive Officer
COO: Dean Teague, Chief Operating Officer
CFO: Robert Kertis, Vice President Finance
CMO: Barbara Estes, M.D., Chief of Staff
CIO: Ed Grogan, Vice President Information Services and Chief Information Officer
CHR: Anthony M. Bladen, Vice President Human Resources
CNO: Robert McWhirt, Vice President Patient Care Services and Chief Nursing Executive
Web address: www.calverthospital.com
**Control:** Other not–for–profit (including NFP Corporation) **Service:** General Medical and Surgical

**Staffed Beds:** 116 **Admissions:** 7918 **Census:** 80 **Outpatient Visits:** 135040 **Births:** 896 **Total Expense ($000):** 124479 **Payroll Expense ($000):** 54431 **Personnel:** 896

## RANDALLSTOWN—Baltimore County

⊠ **NORTHWEST HOSPITAL (210040)**, 5401 Old Court Road, Zip 21133–5185; tel. 410/521–2200, (Total facility includes 29 beds in nursing home–type unit) **A**1 2 9 10 **F**3 8 11 12 15 18 20 26 28 29 30 31 34 35 36 37 38 40 49 50 56 57 59 60 64 65 68 70 74 75 77 78 79 80 81 82 83 85 87 92 93 97 98 100 102 107 110 111 113 114 118 125 127 128 129 130 131 134 145 146 147 **S** LifeBridge Health, Baltimore, MD
Primary Contact: Brian M. White, President and Chief Operating Officer
CFO: David Krajewski, Vice President Finance
CMO: Ronald L. Ginsberg, M.D., Vice President Medical Affairs
CIO: Karen Barker, Vice President and Chief Information Officer
CHR: Valerie Brandenburg, Director Human Resources
Web address: www.lifebridgehealth.org
**Control:** Other not–for–profit (including NFP Corporation) **Service:** General Medical and Surgical

**Staffed Beds:** 230 **Admissions:** 14262 **Census:** 186 **Outpatient Visits:** 93521 **Births:** 0 **Total Expense ($000):** 189502 **Payroll Expense ($000):** 80063 **Personnel:** 1339

## ROCKVILLE—Montgomery County

⊠ **ADVENTIST BEHAVIORAL HEALTH ROCKVILLE (214013)**, 14901 Broschart Road, Zip 20850–3395; tel. 301/251–4500, (Nonreporting) **A**1 9 10 **S** Adventist HealthCare, Rockville, MD
Primary Contact: Kevin Young, FACHE, President and Chief Executive Officer
CFO: Randy Reimer, Chief Financial Officer
CMO: Peter H. Levine, M.D., Executive Medical Director Behavioral Health Services
CIO: Kathleen Dyer, Vice President and Chief Information Officer
CHR: Mary Cloutier, Director Human Resources
Web address: www.adventistbehavioralhealth.com
**Control:** Other not–for–profit (including NFP Corporation) **Service:** Psychiatric

**Staffed Beds:** 283

⊠ △ **ADVENTIST REHABILITATION HOSPITAL OF MARYLAND (213029)**, 9909 Medical Center Drive, Zip 20850; tel. 240/864–6000, (Nonreporting) **A**1 7 9 10 **S** Adventist HealthCare, Rockville, MD
Primary Contact: Brent Reitz, Vice President and Administrator
CFO: Val C. Daniels, Chief Financial Officer
CMO: Terrence P. Sheehan, M.D., Medical Director
CHR: Ana S. Doll, Manager Human Resources
Web address: www.adventistrehab.com
**Control:** Other not–for–profit (including NFP Corporation) **Service:** Rehabilitation

**Staffed Beds:** 77

**POTOMAC RIDGE BEHAVIORAL HEALTH** See Adventist Behavioral Health Rockville

---

**Hospital, Medicare Provider Number, Address, Telephone, Approval, Facility, and Physician Codes, Health Care System**

★ American Hospital Association (AHA) membership
☐ The Joint Commission accreditation
◇ DNV Healthcare Inc. accreditation
○ American Osteopathic Association (AOA) accreditation
△ Commission on Accreditation of Rehabilitation Facilities (CARF) accreditation

**MD**

☒ **SHADY GROVE ADVENTIST HOSPITAL (210057)**, 9901 Medical Center Drive, Zip 20850–3395; tel. 240/826–6000, (Nonreporting) **A**1 2 9 10 **S** Adventist HealthCare, Rockville, MD
Primary Contact: Dennis Hansen, President
COO: Dennis Hansen, President
CFO: Daniel Cochran, Vice President and Chief Financial Officer
CMO: Stephen Lakner, M.D., President Medical and Affiliate Staff
CIO: Kathleen Dyer, Vice President and Chief Information Officer
CHR: Eric Brown, Senior Business Partner
CNO: Skip Margot, Vice President Patient Care Services and Chief Nurse Executive
Web address: www.adventisthealthcare.com
**Control:** Church–operated, Nongovernment, not–for profit **Service:** General Medical and Surgical

**Staffed Beds:** 327

### SALISBURY—Wicomico County

☐ **DEER'S HEAD HOSPITAL CENTER (212003)**, 351 Deer's Head Hospital Road, Zip 21801, Mailing Address: P.O. Box 2018, Zip 21802–2018; tel. 410/543–4000, (Total facility includes 57 beds in nursing home–type unit) **A**1 10 **F**1 3 11 28 29 30 44 50 56 57 59 60 61 65 68 75 77 82 84 85 86 87 90 91 93 94 96 127 129 131 134 145 147 **P**6
Primary Contact: Sandra K. Smith, Chief Executive Officer
CFO: Kenneth Waller, Fiscal Administrator
CMO: Thomas F. Kelly, M.D., Medical Director
CIO: Mac Beattie, Computer Network Specialist
CHR: Michael Dollinger, Personnel Administrator
Web address: www.deershead.org
**Control:** State–Government, nonfederal **Service:** Chronic disease

**Staffed Beds:** 81 **Admissions:** 149 **Census:** 75 **Outpatient Visits:** 15470 **Births:** 0 **Total Expense ($000):** 21589 **Payroll Expense ($000):** 9620 **Personnel:** 228

☒ △ **HEALTHSOUTH CHESAPEAKE REHABILITATION HOSPITAL (213028)**, 220 Tilghman Road, Zip 21804–1921; tel. 410/546–4600 **A**1 7 10 **F**29 30 57 59 62 64 90 93 130 131 **S** HEALTHSOUTH Corporation, Birmingham, AL
Primary Contact: Steven Walas, Chief Executive Officer
CFO: Karen Rounsley, Controller
CHR: Belinda Thompson, Coordinator Human Resources
Web address: www.healthsouthchesapeake.com
**Control:** Corporation, Investor–owned, for–profit **Service:** Rehabilitation

**Staffed Beds:** 54 **Admissions:** 1191 **Census:** 45 **Births:** 0

☒ **PENINSULA REGIONAL HEALTH SYSTEM (210019)**, 100 East Carroll Street, Zip 21801–5422; tel. 410/546–6400, (Total facility includes 30 beds in nursing home–type unit) **A**1 2 9 10 **F**3 12 13 15 17 18 20 22 24 26 28 29 30 31 34 35 40 43 45 46 47 48 49 50 51 53 54 57 58 59 60 61 62 64 68 70 71 72 74 75 76 77 78 79 81 82 84 85 87 89 93 96 97 98 100 102 107 108 110 111 113 114 115 116 117 118 119 120 122 123 125 127 129 142 143 144 145 146 147 **P**5 8
Primary Contact: Peggy Naleppa, President and Chief Executive Officer
COO: Cindy Lunsford, Executive Vice President and Chief Operating Officer
CFO: Bruce Ritchie, Vice President of Finance and Chief Financial Officer
CMO: Charles B. Silvia, M.D., Chief Medical Officer and Vice President Medical Affairs
CIO: Raymond Adkins, Chief Information Officer
CHR: Scott Peterson, Vice President of People and Organizational Development
CNO: Karen C. Poisker, MSN, Vice President Patient Care Services and Chief Nursing Officer
Web address: www.peninsula.org
**Control:** Other not–for–profit (including NFP Corporation) **Service:** General Medical and Surgical

**Staffed Beds:** 403 **Admissions:** 22037 **Census:** 275 **Outpatient Visits:** 479937 **Births:** 2035 **Total Expense ($000):** 356637 **Payroll Expense ($000):** 138742 **Personnel:** 2516

### SILVER SPRING—Montgomery County

☒ **HOLY CROSS HOSPITAL (210004)**, 1500 Forest Glen Road, Zip 20910–1487; tel. 301/754–7000 **A**1 2 3 5 8 9 10 **F**2 3 11 12 13 15 17 18 19 20 22 26 29 30 31 32 34 35 36 37 40 41 45 46 49 50 54 55 56 57 58 59 60 64 66 68 70 72 74 75 76 77 78 79 81 82 84 85 86 87 89 93 97 100 107 108 110 111 113 114 118 119 120 122 123 125 128 129 130 131 133 134 143 145 146 **S** Trinity Health, Novi, MI
Primary Contact: Kevin J. Sexton, President and Chief Executive Officer
COO: Judith Rogers, R.N., Senior Vice President Operations
CFO: Anne Gillis, Chief Financial Officer
CMO: Blair Eig, M.D., Senior Vice President Medical Affairs
CIO: Heather Smith, Director Information Services
CHR: J. Manuel Ocasio, Vice President Human Resources
CNO: Celia Guarino, R.N., Vice President and Chief Nursing Officer
Web address: www.holycrosshealth.org
**Control:** Church–operated, Nongovernment, not–for profit **Service:** General Medical and Surgical

**Staffed Beds:** 425 **Admissions:** 33210 **Census:** 356 **Outpatient Visits:** 170317 **Births:** 8539 **Total Expense ($000):** 369945 **Payroll Expense ($000):** 162163 **Personnel:** 2194

**SAINT LUKE INSTITUTE**, 8901 New Hampshire Avenue, Zip 20903–3611; tel. 301/445–7970, (Nonreporting)
Primary Contact: Father Stephen J. Rossetti, Ph.D., President and Chief Executive Officer
COO: Sister Danile Lynch, Chief Operating Officer
Web address: www.sli.org
**Control:** Other not–for–profit (including NFP Corporation) **Service:** Psychiatric

**Staffed Beds:** 24

### SYKESVILLE—Carroll County

☐ **SPRINGFIELD HOSPITAL CENTER (214004)**, 6655 Sykesville Road, Zip 21784–7966; tel. 410/970–7000 **A**1 9 10 **F**10 11 35 39 44 53 56 57 68 75 77 86 87 98 101 103 106 129 131 134 145 **P**6
Primary Contact: Paula A. Langmead, Chief Executive Officer
COO: Barry Stabile, Chief Operating Officer
CFO: Dallas Snyder, Chief Financial Officer
CMO: Jonathan D. Book, M.D., Clinical Director
CMO: Gloria Merek, Director of Nursing
CIO: Denise Maskell, Chief Information Officer
CHR: Sherry L. Miller, Director Human Resources
Web address: www.dhmh.state.md.us/springfield
**Control:** State–Government, nonfederal **Service:** Psychiatric

**Staffed Beds:** 285 **Admissions:** 391 **Census:** 265 **Outpatient Visits:** 0 **Births:** 0 **Total Expense ($000):** 70067 **Payroll Expense ($000):** 39268 **Personnel:** 809

### TAKOMA PARK—Montgomery County

☒ △ **WASHINGTON ADVENTIST HOSPITAL (210016)**, 7600 Carroll Avenue, Zip 20912–6392; tel. 301/891–7600, (Nonreporting) **A**1 2 3 5 7 9 10 **S** Adventist HealthCare, Rockville, MD
Primary Contact: Joyce Newmyer, President
Web address: www.adventisthealthcare.com
**Control:** Other not–for–profit (including NFP Corporation) **Service:** General Medical and Surgical

**Staffed Beds:** 204

### TOWSON—Baltimore County

☒ **ST. JOSEPH MEDICAL CENTER (210007)**, 7601 Osler Drive, Zip 21204–7582; tel. 410/337–1000 **A**1 2 9 10 **F**3 11 12 13 17 18 19 20 21 22 23 24 26 28 29 30 31 34 35 36 37 40 41 44 45 46 47 48 49 50 55 56 57 58 59 60 61 64 65 66 68 70 71 72 74 75 76 77 78 79 81 82 85 86 87 89 91 92 93 97 98 99 100 101 102 103 104 105 107 108 110 113 114 117 118 119 120 121 122 123 125 128 129 130 131 133 134 143 145 146 147 **P**6 **S** Catholic Health Initiatives, Englewood, CO
Primary Contact: Charles W. Neumann, President and Chief Executive Officer
COO: Craig Carmichael, Vice President, Operations
CFO: Richard Imbimbo, Chief Financial Officer
CMO: Gail Cunningham, Interim Chief Medical Officer
CIO: Sean Shuffield, Regional Chief Information Officer
CHR: Dianne Wassall, Director Human Resources
CNO: Pamela Jamieson, Vice President Patient Care Services and Chief Nursing Officer
Web address: www.sjmcmd.org
**Control:** Church–operated, Nongovernment, not–for profit **Service:** General Medical and Surgical

**Staffed Beds:** 320 **Admissions:** 16740 **Census:** 185 **Outpatient Visits:** 159724 **Births:** 2095 **Total Expense ($000):** 347676 **Payroll Expense ($000):** 126162 **Personnel:** 1693

### WESTMINSTER—Carroll County

☒ **CARROLL HOSPITAL CENTER (210033)**, 200 Memorial Avenue, Zip 21157–5799; tel. 410/848–3000 **A**1 2 9 10 **F**3 5 11 13 15 18 19 20 22 26 28 29 30 31 32 34 35 36 37 38 39 40 44 45 49 50 51 55 56 57 59 62 63 64 65 70 75 76 77 78 79 81 82 83 84 85 86 87 89 93 94 98 99 100 101 102 103 104 105 107 108 109 111 113 114 117 118 119 120 128 129 131 134 144 145 146 147 **P**5 6
Primary Contact: John M. Sernulka, President and Chief Executive Officer
COO: Leslie Simmons, Executive Vice President and Chief Operating Officer
CFO: Kevin Kelbly, Senior Vice President Finance and Corporate Fiscal Affairs
CMO: Kevin Smothers, M.D., Senior Vice President Medical Affairs and Chief Medical and Quality Officer
CIO: Kim Moreau, Assistant Vice President Information Systems
CHR: Tracey Ellison, Vice President Human Resources
CNO: Stephanie Reid, R.N., Vice President of Quality and Chief Nursing Officer
Web address: www.carrollhospitalcenter.org
**Control:** Other not–for–profit (including NFP Corporation) **Service:** General Medical and Surgical

**Staffed Beds:** 195 **Admissions:** 14339 **Census:** 129 **Outpatient Visits:** 157590 **Births:** 1119 **Total Expense ($000):** 235383 **Payroll Expense ($000):** 103350 **Personnel:** 1417

*Many Facility Codes have changed. Please refer to the AHA Guide Code Chart.* © 2012 AHA Guide

# MASSACHUSETTS

## ANDOVER—Essex County

**ISHAM HEALTH CENTER**, 180 Main Street, Zip 01810–4161;
tel. 978/749–4455, (Nonreporting)
Primary Contact: Catherine Golas, Administrator
Web address: www.andover.edu
**Control:** Other not–for–profit (including NFP Corporation) **Service:** Children's other specialty

**Staffed Beds:** 20

## ATHOL—Worcester County

☐ **ATHOL MEMORIAL HOSPITAL (221303)**, 2033 Main Street, Zip 01331–3598;
tel. 978/249–3511, (Nonreporting) **A**1 9 10 18
Primary Contact: Steven Penka, President and Chief Executive Officer
COO: Lucille Songer, Acting Chief Operating Officer
CFO: Dean Fleming, Chief Financial Officer
CMO: Donald Mruk, M.D., President Medical Staff
CIO: Lorrie Bernard, Manager Patient Accounts and Information Systems
CHR: John G. Kelleher, Manager Human Resources
CNO: Lucille Songer, Chief Nursing Officer
Web address: www.atholhospital.org
**Control:** Other not–for–profit (including NFP Corporation) **Service:** General Medical and Surgical

**Staffed Beds:** 12

## ATTLEBORO—Bristol County

☐ **ARBOUR–FULLER HOSPITAL (224021)**, 200 May Street, Zip 02703–5520;
tel. 508/761–8500, (Nonreporting) **A**1 9 10 **S** Universal Health Services, Inc., King of Prussia, PA
Primary Contact: Lisa Pappone, Chief Executive Officer
CFO: James Rollins, Chief Financial Officer
CMO: Aminadav Zakai, M.D., Medical Director
CHR: Brian Jenkins, Director Human Resources
Web address: www.arbourhealth.com
**Control:** Corporation, Investor–owned, for–profit **Service:** Psychiatric

**Staffed Beds:** 46

☒ **STURDY MEMORIAL HOSPITAL (220008)**, 211 Park Street, Zip 02703–3137,
Mailing Address: PO Box 2963, Zip 02703–0963; tel. 508/222–5200 **A**1 2 9 10
**F**3 8 13 15 18 20 28 29 30 31 32 34 35 36 39 40 44 45 49 50 54 56 57 58 59 61 64 70 74 75 76 77 78 79 81 82 85 86 87 89 93 97 107 108 110 111 114 117 118 128 129 130 131 133 143 145 146 147 **P**6
Primary Contact: Linda Shyavitz, President and Chief Executive Officer
CFO: Joseph Casey, Chief Financial Officer
CMO: Daniel Pietro, M.D., Medical Director
CHR: Cheryl Barrows, Vice President Human Resources
Web address: www.sturdymemorial.org
**Control:** Other not–for–profit (including NFP Corporation) **Service:** General Medical and Surgical

**Staffed Beds:** 128 **Admissions:** 7262 **Census:** 78 **Outpatient Visits:** 218300 **Births:** 798 **Total Expense ($000):** 141750 **Payroll Expense ($000):** 72875 **Personnel:** 978

## AYER—Middlesex County

☐ **NASHOBA VALLEY MEDICAL CENTER (220098)**, 200 Groton Road,
Zip 01432–3300; tel. 978/784–9000, (Nonreporting) **A**1 9 10 **S** Steward Health Care System, LLC, Boston, MA
Primary Contact: Steven P. Roach, Chief Executive Officer
CFO: Ben Moll, Assistant Chief Financial Officer
CMO: Michael Older, M.D., President Medical Staff
CIO: Armen Arakelian, Chief Information Officer
Web address: www.nashobamed.com
**Control:** Corporation, Investor–owned, for–profit **Service:** General Medical and Surgical

**Staffed Beds:** 42

## BEDFORD—Middlesex County

☒ △ **EDITH NOURSE ROGERS MEMORIAL VETERANS HOSPITAL**, 200
Springs Road, Zip 01730–1198; tel. 781/687–2000, (Nonreporting) **A**1 3 5 7
**S** Department of Veterans Affairs, Washington, DC
Primary Contact: Christine Croteau, Acting Director
CFO: Warren Berger, Chief Fiscal Service
CIO: Joseph Calabresi, Chief Information Service
Web address: www.va.gov/sta/guide/home.asp
**Control:** Veterans Affairs, Government, federal **Service:** Psychiatric

**Staffed Beds:** 147

## BELMONT—Middlesex County

☒ **MCLEAN HOSPITAL (224007)**, 115 Mill Street, Zip 02478–9106;
tel. 617/855–2000 **A**1 3 5 9 10 **F**4 5 11 29 50 53 56 58 59 64 68 74 75 77 86 98 99 101 103 104 105 106 111 118 129 145 **P**6 **S** Partners HealthCare System, Inc., Boston, MA
Primary Contact: Scott L. Rauch, M.D., President
COO: Michele L. Gougeon, Executive Vice President and Chief Operating Officer
CFO: David A. Lagasse, Senior Vice President Fiscal Affairs
CMO: Joseph Gold, M.D., Chief Medical Officer
CIO: Andrew Laband, Chief Information Officer
CHR: Jean Mansfield, Director Human Resources
CNO: Linda Flaherty, R.N., Senior Vice President, Patient Care Services
Web address: www.mclean.harvard.edu
**Control:** Other not–for–profit (including NFP Corporation) **Service:** Psychiatric

**Staffed Beds:** 177 **Admissions:** 6074 **Census:** 157 **Outpatient Visits:** 112822 **Births:** 0 **Total Expense ($000):** 164612 **Payroll Expense ($000):** 69831 **Personnel:** 1433

## BEVERLY—Essex County

☒ **BEVERLY HOSPITAL (220033)**, 85 Herrick Street, Zip 01915–1777;
tel. 978/922–3000, (Includes ADDISON GILBERT HOSPITAL, 298 Washington Street, Gloucester, Zip 01930–4887; tel. 978/283–4000) **A**1 2 5 9 10 **F**3 5 8 9 11 12 13 15 18 20 22 24 26 28 29 30 31 32 34 35 40 44 45 48 49 50 51 52 53 54 56 57 59 60 63 64 65 68 70 71 73 74 75 76 77 78 79 81 82 83 84 85 86 87 89 93 96 97 98 100 102 103 104 105 107 108 110 111 113 114 118 126 128 129 130 131 133 134 144 145 146 147 **P**1 6
Primary Contact: Kenneth Hanover, President and Chief Executive Officer
COO: Pauline Pike, Chief Operating Officer
CFO: Denis Conroy, Chief Financial Officer
CMO: Peter H. Short, M.D., Senior Vice President Medical Affairs
CIO: Robert Laramie, Chief Information Officer
CHR: Althea C. Lyons, Vice President Human Resources
Web address: www.nhshealth.org
**Control:** Other not–for–profit (including NFP Corporation) **Service:** General Medical and Surgical

**Staffed Beds:** 348 **Admissions:** 16172 **Census:** 183 **Outpatient Visits:** 464314 **Births:** 2140 **Total Expense ($000):** 318599 **Payroll Expense ($000):** 166831 **Personnel:** 2030

## BOSTON—Suffolk County

☐ **ARBOUR HOSPITAL (224013)**, 49 Robinwood Avenue, Zip 02130–2156;
tel. 617/522–4400, (Nonreporting) **A**1 9 10 **S** Universal Health Services, Inc., King of Prussia, PA
Primary Contact: Joseph Murphy, Chief Executive Officer
Web address: www.arbourhealth.com
**Control:** Other not–for–profit (including NFP Corporation) **Service:** Psychiatric

**Staffed Beds:** 118

---

**Hospital, Medicare Provider Number, Address, Telephone, Approval, Facility, and Physician Codes, Health Care System**

★ American Hospital Association (AHA) membership
☐ The Joint Commission accreditation
◇ DNV Healthcare Inc. accreditation
○ American Osteopathic Association (AOA) accreditation
△ Commission on Accreditation of Rehabilitation Facilities (CARF) accreditation

**MA**

✠ **BETH ISRAEL DEACONESS MEDICAL CENTER (220086)**, 330 Brookline Avenue, Zip 02215–5491; tel. 617/667–7000, (Includes BETH ISRAEL DEACONESS HOSPITAL–NEEDHAM CAMPUS, 148 Chestnut Street, Needham, Zip 02492; tel. 781/453–3000; John M. Fogarty, President and Chief Executive Officer) **A**1 2 3 5 8 9 10 **F**3 6 9 11 12 13 14 15 17 18 20 22 24 26 28 29 30 31 34 35 36 38 40 43 44 45 46 47 48 49 50 51 53 54 56 57 58 59 60 61 63 64 65 66 68 70 72 73 74 75 76 77 78 79 81 82 84 85 86 87 91 92 93 94 97 98 100 101 102 103 104 107 108 109 110 111 113 114 115 116 117 118 119 120 122 123 125 126 129 130 131 133 134 135 137 138 141 142 144 145 146 147 **P**5 7
Primary Contact: Kevin Tabb, M.D., President and Chief Executive Officer
COO: Marsha L. Maurer, R.N., Interim Chief Operating Officer
CFO: Steven P. Fischer, Chief Financial Officer
CIO: John Halamka, M.D., Chief Information Officer
CHR: Lisa Zankman, Senior Vice President Human Resources
Web address: www.bidmc.harvard.edu
**Control:** Other not–for–profit (including NFP Corporation) **Service:** General Medical and Surgical

**Staffed Beds:** 642 **Admissions:** 37308 **Census:** 518 **Outpatient Visits:** 595228 **Births:** 4748 **Total Expense ($000):** 1297568 **Payroll Expense ($000):** 529971 **Personnel:** 7324

✠ △ **BOSTON MEDICAL CENTER (220031)**, 1 Boston Medical Center Place, Zip 02118–2908; tel. 617/638–8000 **A**1 2 3 5 7 8 9 10 **F**3 5 8 9 12 13 15 17 18 20 22 24 26 28 29 30 31 32 34 35 36 38 40 41 43 44 45 46 47 48 49 50 51 54 55 56 57 58 59 60 61 64 65 66 68 70 72 73 74 75 76 77 78 79 81 82 84 85 86 87 88 89 90 93 97 99 100 101 102 103 104 107 108 110 111 113 115 116 117 118 119 120 122 123 125 128 129 130 131 133 134 135 137 141 142 143 144 145 146 147 **P**7
Primary Contact: Kate Walsh, President and Chief Executive Officer
CFO: Ronald E. Bartlett, Chief Financial Officer
CMO: Ravin Davidoff, M.D., Chief Medical Officer
CHR: Stephanie Lovell, Vice President and General Counsel
Web address: www.bmc.org
**Control:** Other not–for–profit (including NFP Corporation) **Service:** General Medical and Surgical

**Staffed Beds:** 474 **Admissions:** 26874 **Census:** 340 **Outpatient Visits:** 944454 **Births:** 2410 **Total Expense ($000):** 971990 **Payroll Expense ($000):** 349530 **Personnel:** 4919

✠ **BRIGHAM AND WOMEN'S HOSPITAL (220110)**, 75 Francis Street, Zip 02115–6110; tel. 617/732–5500 **A**1 3 5 8 9 10 **F**3 5 6 8 9 11 12 13 14 15 16 17 18 20 22 24 26 28 29 30 31 32 33 34 35 36 37 38 39 40 43 44 45 46 47 48 49 50 51 52 54 55 56 57 58 59 60 61 63 64 65 66 68 70 71 72 74 75 76 77 78 79 81 82 83 84 85 86 87 92 93 97 99 100 101 102 103 104 105 107 108 110 111 112 113 114 115 116 117 118 119 120 122 123 125 128 129 130 131 132 133 134 135 136 137 139 140 141 142 143 144 145 146 147 **P**6 **S** Partners HealthCare System, Inc., Boston, MA
Primary Contact: Elizabeth Nabel, M.D., President
COO: Mairead Hickey, Ph.D., Executive Vice President and Chief Operating Officer
CFO: Michael Reney, Chief Financial Officer
CMO: Stanley Ashley, M.D., Chief Medical Officer
CIO: Sue Schade, Chief Information Officer
CHR: Julie Celano, Vice President Human Resources
CNO: Jacqueline G. Somerville, R.N., Senior Vice President for Patient Care Services and Chief Nursing Officer
Web address: www.brighamandwomens.org
**Control:** Other not–for–profit (including NFP Corporation) **Service:** General Medical and Surgical

**Staffed Beds:** 779 **Admissions:** 46498 **Census:** 706 **Outpatient Visits:** 786122 **Births:** 7883 **Total Expense ($000):** 2176141 **Payroll Expense ($000):** 653939 **Personnel:** 12497

☐ **CARNEY HOSPITAL (220017)**, 2100 Dorchester Avenue, Zip 02124–5615; tel. 617/296–4000, (Nonreporting) **A**1 2 3 5 10 **S** Steward Health Care System, LLC, Boston, MA
Primary Contact: Margaret Hanson, R.N., Interim President
CFO: Nancy Hoffmann, Vice President Finance
CMO: Greg McSweeney, M.D., Vice President Medical Affairs
CIO: Nancy Hoffmann, Vice President Finance
CHR: Mary Orlandi, Manager Human Resources
Web address: www.carneyhospital.org
**Control:** Corporation, Investor–owned, for–profit **Service:** General Medical and Surgical

**Staffed Beds:** 133

✠ **CHILDREN'S HOSPITAL BOSTON (223302)**, 300 Longwood Avenue, Zip 02115–5737; tel. 617/355–6000 **A**1 3 5 8 9 10 **F**3 5 8 11 12 14 18 19 20 21 22 23 24 25 26 27 28 29 30 31 32 34 35 36 37 38 39 40 41 43 44 45 46 48 50 54 55 57 58 59 60 61 62 63 64 65 68 72 74 75 77 78 79 80 81 82 83 84 85 86 87 88 89 92 93 94 97 98 99 100 101 102 104 107 108 109 111 112 113 114 115 116 117 118 119 120 122 123 125 128 129 130 131 133 134 135 136 137 138 139 140 141 142 143 145 146 147 **P**3 5
Primary Contact: James Mandell, M.D., President and Chief Executive Officer
COO: Sandra Fenwick, Chief Operating Officer
CFO: David Kirshner, Senior Vice President and Chief Financial Officer
CIO: Daniel Nigrin, M.D., Vice President Information Services and Chief Information Officer
CHR: Inez Stewart, Vice President
Web address: www.childrenshospital.org/
**Control:** Other not–for–profit (including NFP Corporation) **Service:** Children's general

**Staffed Beds:** 395 **Admissions:** 17173 **Census:** 317 **Outpatient Visits:** 635899 **Births:** 0 **Total Expense ($000):** 1242547 **Payroll Expense ($000):** 442571 **Personnel:** 8210

✠ **DANA–FARBER CANCER INSTITUTE (220162)**, 44 Binney Street, Zip 02115–6084; tel. 617/632–3000 **A**1 3 5 9 10 **F**3 11 14 15 29 30 31 34 35 36 44 50 54 55 57 58 59 64 65 66 68 71 75 77 78 82 83 84 85 86 87 99 100 101 104 107 108 110 111 113 114 116 118 119 120 122 123 129 131 133 134 135 145 146 147 **P**6
Primary Contact: Edward J. Benz, Jr., M.D., President and Chief Executive Officer
COO: Janet E. Porter, Ph.D., Executive Vice President and Chief Operating Officer
CFO: Dorothy E. Puhy, Executive Vice President and Chief Financial Officer
CMO: Lawrence N. Shulman, M.D., Senior Vice President Medical Affairs and Chief Medical Officer
CIO: Jeffrey R. Kessler, Vice President Information Services
CHR: Emily Barclay, Vice President Human Resources
Web address: www.dana–farber.org
**Control:** Other not–for–profit (including NFP Corporation) **Service:** General Medical and Surgical

**Staffed Beds:** 30 **Admissions:** 1073 **Census:** 26 **Outpatient Visits:** 320849 **Births:** 0 **Total Expense ($000):** 955382 **Payroll Expense ($000):** 288413 **Personnel:** 4090

**DR. SOLOMON CARTER FULLER MENTAL HEALTH CENTER (224040)**, 85 East Newton Street, Zip 02118–2340; tel. 617/626–8700, (Nonreporting) **A**10
Primary Contact: Mary–Louise White, M.D., Chief Executive Officer
**Control:** Other not–for–profit (including NFP Corporation) **Service:** Psychiatric

**Staffed Beds:** 32

✠ **FAULKNER HOSPITAL (220119)**, 1153 Centre Street, Zip 02130–3400; tel. 617/983–7000 **A**1 2 3 5 8 9 10 **F**3 4 5 11 15 18 28 29 30 34 35 40 45 46 48 50 51 56 57 59 60 65 68 70 74 75 77 79 81 82 85 86 87 93 94 98 100 101 102 103 104 105 107 108 110 111 113 114 118 123 125 128 129 130 131 134 144 145 146 **S** Partners HealthCare System, Inc., Boston, MA
Primary Contact: Elizabeth Nabel, M.D., President
COO: Michael Gustafson, M.D., Chief Operating Officer
CFO: Vincent McDermott, Executive Director Finance
CMO: Stephen C. Wright, M.D., Chief Medical Officer
CIO: Jim Anzeveno, Chief Information Officer
CHR: Rebecca Blair, Vice President Human Resources and Service Excellence
Web address: www.faulknerhospital.org
**Control:** Other not–for–profit (including NFP Corporation) **Service:** General Medical and Surgical

**Staffed Beds:** 93 **Admissions:** 7573 **Census:** 94 **Outpatient Visits:** 195131 **Births:** 0 **Total Expense ($000):** 172598 **Payroll Expense ($000):** 83846 **Personnel:** 1117

✠ **FRANCISCAN HOSPITAL FOR CHILDREN (223300)**, 30 Warren Street, Zip 02135–3680; tel. 617/254–3800, (Nonreporting) **A**1 3 5 9 10
Primary Contact: John D. Nash, President and Chief Executive Officer
COO: Donna Polselli, Chief Operating Officer
CFO: Alex Denucci, Chief Financial Officer
CMO: Jane E. O'Brien, M.D., Medical Director
CHR: Steven Snyder, Vice President Human Resources
Web address: www.franciscanhospital.org
**Control:** Other not–for–profit (including NFP Corporation) **Service:** Children's rehabilitation

**Staffed Beds:** 52

*Many Facility Codes have changed. Please refer to the AHA Guide Code Chart.* © 2012 AHA Guide

△ **HEBREW REHABILITATION CENTER (222007)**, 1200 Centre Street, Zip 02131–1097; tel. 617/323–8000, (Total facility includes 50 beds in nursing home–type unit) **A**7 10 **F**1 2 18 29 30 34 39 50 53 56 58 59 60 64 65 68 69 75 77 82 93 100 103 104 118 127 129 142 145 147 **P**6
Primary Contact: Louis J. Woolf, President
COO: Mary K. Moscato, Chief Operating Officer–Hebrew Rehabilitation Center and Hebrew Senior Life Health Care Services
CFO: James Hart, Chief Financial Officer
CMO: Rob Schreiber, M.D., Chief Medical Officer
CIO: Fran Hinckley, Chief Information Officer
CHR: Alessandra de Vaca, Chief Administrative Officer
CNO: Tammy B. Retalic, R.N., Vice President Nursing and Patient and Family Centered Care
Web address: www.hebrewseniorlife.org
**Control:** Other not–for–profit (including NFP Corporation) **Service:** Long–Term Acute Care hospital

**Staffed Beds: 725 Admissions: 1492 Census: 679 Births: 0 Total Expense ($000): 121091 Payroll Expense ($000): 71326**

☐ **MASSACHUSETTS EYE AND EAR INFIRMARY (220075)**, 243 Charles Street, Zip 02114–3002; tel. 617/523–7900 **A**1 3 5 9 10 **F**3 7 8 11 29 30 31 34 35 36 40 41 44 50 54 55 56 57 58 59 64 65 66 68 74 75 77 78 81 82 85 86 87 89 107 111 113 118 129 131 140 142 143 145 147 **P**6
Primary Contact: John R. Fernandez, President and Chief Executive Officer
CFO: Peter J. Chinetti, Chief Financial Officer
CIO: Alec Cheloff, Chief Information Officer
CHR: Christine Regan, Vice President Human Resources
Web address: www.masseyeandear.org
**Control:** Other not–for–profit (including NFP Corporation) **Service:** Eye, ear, nose, and throat

**Staffed Beds: 41 Admissions: 1475 Census: 15 Outpatient Visits: 306328 Births: 0 Total Expense ($000): 197530 Payroll Expense ($000): 57857 Personnel: 1572**

⊠ **MASSACHUSETTS GENERAL HOSPITAL (220071)**, 55 Fruit Street, Zip 02114–2696; tel. 617/726–2000, (Includes MASSGENERAL HOSPITAL FOR CHILDREN, 55 Fruit Street, Zip 02114–2621; tel. 888/644–3248) **A**1 3 5 8 9 10 **F**2 3 5 6 8 9 11 12 13 14 15 16 17 18 19 20 22 24 25 26 27 28 29 30 31 32 33 34 35 36 37 38 39 40 41 43 44 45 46 47 48 49 50 51 52 53 54 55 56 57 58 59 60 61 62 63 64 65 66 70 72 73 74 75 76 77 78 79 80 81 82 84 85 86 87 88 89 91 92 93 94 95 96 97 98 99 100 101 102 103 104 107 108 110 111 112 113 114 115 116 117 118 119 120 121 122 123 125 128 129 130 131 133 134 135 136 137 138 139 140 141 142 143 144 145 146 147 **P**6 7 **S** Partners HealthCare System, Inc., Boston, MA
Primary Contact: Peter L. Slavin, M.D., President
CFO: Sally Mason Boemer, Senior Vice President Finance
CMO: Britain Nicholson, M.D., Chief Medical Officer
CIO: James W. Noga, Chief Information Officer
CHR: Jeff Davis, Senior Vice President Human Resources
Web address: www.massgeneral.org
**Control:** Other not–for–profit (including NFP Corporation) **Service:** General Medical and Surgical

**Staffed Beds: 945 Admissions: 47118 Census: 760 Outpatient Visits: 933412 Births: 3657 Total Expense ($000): 2748389 Payroll Expense ($000): 880274 Personnel: 15611**

⊠ **NEW ENGLAND BAPTIST HOSPITAL (220088)**, 125 Parker Hill Avenue, Zip 02120–2847; tel. 617/754–5800 **A**1 3 5 9 10 **F**3 8 9 11 14 18 20 29 30 34 35 36 37 44 45 50 51 54 57 58 59 60 64 65 68 70 74 75 77 79 81 82 85 86 87 91 92 93 96 97 100 107 108 111 118 129 130 131 140 142 143 145 147 **P**8
Primary Contact: Trish Hannon, FACHE, President and Chief Executive Officer
CFO: Thomas Gheringhelli, Chief Financial Officer
CHR: Linda Thompson, Vice President Human Resources
Web address: www.nebh.org
**Control:** Other not–for–profit (including NFP Corporation) **Service:** Orthopedic

**Staffed Beds: 122 Admissions: 7088 Census: 69 Outpatient Visits: 141190 Births: 0 Total Expense ($000): 194077 Payroll Expense ($000): 70159 Personnel: 1009**

⊠ **RADIUS SPECIALTY HOSPITAL BOSTON (222010)**, 59 Townsend Street, Zip 02119–1318; tel. 617/442–8760 **A**1 10 **F**1 3 28 29 30 60 82 118 129 147
Primary Contact: Christine Bassett, Chief Executive Officer
COO: Dan Mitchell, Chief Operating Officer
CMO: Raul Octaviani, M.D., Chief Medical Officer
CHR: Christine Bresnahan, Manager Human Resources
Web address: www.radiushospital.com
**Control:** Corporation, Investor–owned, for–profit **Service:** Long–Term Acute Care hospital

**Staffed Beds: 98 Admissions: 1046 Census: 91 Outpatient Visits: 0 Births: 0**

☐ **SHRINERS HOSPITALS FOR CHILDREN–BOSTON (223304)**, (Pediatric Burns, Orthopaedics), 51 Blossom Street, Zip 02114–2601; tel. 617/722–3000 **A**1 3 5 10 **F**3 16 29 30 34 35 57 64 75 77 79 81 85 86 87 93 99 104 129 131 140 142 145 147 **S** Shriners Hospitals for Children, Tampa, FL
Primary Contact: C. Thomas D'Esmond, FACHE, Administrator
CFO: Maria Chung, CPA, Director Fiscal Services
CMO: Ronald G. Tompkins, M.D., Chief of Staff and Director Research
CIO: Kenneth Ward, Regional Director Information Services
CHR: Sharyn D. Gazit, Director Human Resources
Web address: www.shrinershospitals.org
**Control:** Other not–for–profit (including NFP Corporation) **Service:** Children's other specialty

**Staffed Beds: 30 Admissions: 579 Census: 9 Outpatient Visits: 5730 Births: 0 Personnel: 205**

⊠ △ **SPAULDING REHABILITATION HOSPITAL (223034)**, 125 Nashua Street, Zip 02114–1198; tel. 617/573–7000 **A**1 3 5 7 10 **F**3 7 29 30 34 35 36 39 50 57 58 59 60 64 74 75 77 82 85 86 87 90 91 92 93 94 95 96 100 104 118 128 129 130 131 142 145 147 **P**8 **S** Partners HealthCare System, Inc., Boston, MA
Primary Contact: David E. Storto, President
COO: Maureen Banks, R.N., Chief Operating Officer
CFO: Mary Shaughnessy, Vice President Finance
CMO: David Lowell, M.D., Medical Director
CMO: Ross Zafonte, D.O., Chief, Physical Medicine and Rehabilitation and Vice President Medical Affairs, Research and Education
CIO: John Campbell, Director Management Information Systems
CHR: Russell Averna, Director Human Resources
Web address: www.spauldingrehab.org
**Control:** Other not–for–profit (including NFP Corporation) **Service:** Rehabilitation

**Staffed Beds: 196 Admissions: 2327 Census: 147 Outpatient Visits: 154749 Births: 0 Total Expense ($000): 102816 Payroll Expense ($000): 53235 Personnel: 872**

⊠ **TUFTS MEDICAL CENTER (220116)**, 800 Washington Street, Zip 02111–1552; tel. 617/636–5000 **A**1 2 3 5 8 9 10 **F**3 12 13 14 15 17 18 19 20 21 22 23 24 25 26 27 28 29 30 31 32 34 35 39 40 43 44 45 47 49 50 51 55 57 58 59 61 64 65 68 70 71 72 74 75 76 77 78 79 81 82 85 86 87 88 89 93 97 98 99 100 102 104 107 108 111 113 114 115 116 117 118 119 120 122 123 125 128 129 130 131 133 134 135 136 137 142 145 146 **P**3
Primary Contact: Eric J. Beyer, President and Chief Executive Officer
CFO: C. Okey Agba, Senior Vice President, Chief Financial Officer and Treasurer
CMO: David Fairchild, M.D., Chief Medical Officer
CIO: William Shickolovich, Chief Information Officer
Web address: www.tuftsmedicalcenter.org
**Control:** Other not–for–profit (including NFP Corporation) **Service:** General Medical and Surgical

**Staffed Beds: 284 Admissions: 20452 Census: 273 Outpatient Visits: 400062 Births: 1093 Total Expense ($000): 588504 Payroll Expense ($000): 244563 Personnel: 4111**

★ △ **VETERANS AFFAIRS BOSTON HEALTHCARE SYSTEM**, 1400 VFW Parkway, Zip 2132; tel. 617/232–9500, (Nonreporting) **A**2 3 5 7 8 **S** Department of Veterans Affairs, Washington, DC
Primary Contact: Michael E. Lawson, Director
COO: Susan A. MacKenzie, Ph.D., Associate Director
CFO: Joe Costa, Chief Financial Officer
CMO: Brian Hoffman, M.D., Chief Medical Services
CIO: David M. Goodman, Ph.D., Chief Information Officer
CHR: William Warfield, Chief Human Resources Management
Web address: www.va.gov/sta/guide/home.asp
**Control:** Veterans Affairs, Government, federal **Service:** General Medical and Surgical

**Staffed Beds: 361**

**VETERANS AFFAIRS MEDICAL CENTER** See Brockton Veterans Affairs Medical Center, Brockton

### BRADFORD—Essex County

⊠ △ **WHITTIER REHABILITATION HOSPITAL (222047)**, 145 Ward Hill Avenue, Zip 1835; tel. 978/372–8000, (Nonreporting) **A**1 7 9 10 **S** Whittier Health Network, Haverhill, MA
Primary Contact: Alfred J. Arcidi, M.D., Senior Vice President
Web address: www.whittierhealth.com
**Control:** Partnership, Investor–owned, for–profit **Service:** Rehabilitation

**Staffed Beds: 60**

**MA**

---

**Hospital, Medicare Provider Number, Address, Telephone, Approval, Facility, and Physician Codes, Health Care System**

★ American Hospital Association (AHA) membership
☐ The Joint Commission accreditation
◇ DNV Healthcare Inc. accreditation
○ American Osteopathic Association (AOA) accreditation
△ Commission on Accreditation of Rehabilitation Facilities (CARF) accreditation

**BRAINTREE—Norfolk County**

☐ **BRAINTREE REHABILITATION HOSPITAL (223027)**, 250 Pond Street, Zip 02184–5351; tel. 781/348–2500 **A**1 5 10 **F**29 34 35 54 57 59 64 74 75 77 78 79 86 87 90 91 92 93 94 95 101 108 118 129 130 131 145 147 **P**5 **S** Five Star Quality Care, Newton, MA
Primary Contact: Randy Doherty, Administrator
CFO: Thomas Whalen, Chief Financial Officer
CMO: Arthur Williams, M.D., Medical Director
CHR: Tara Spellacy, Director Human Resources
Web address: www.braintreerehabhospital.com
**Control:** Corporation, Investor–owned, for–profit **Service:** Rehabilitation

| |
|---|
| **Staffed Beds:** 187 **Admissions:** 2233 **Census:** 98 **Outpatient Visits:** 111032 **Births:** 0 **Total Expense ($000):** 51246 **Payroll Expense ($000):** 32139 **Personnel:** 601 |

**BRIDGEWATER—Plymouth County**

☐ **BRIDGEWATER STATE HOSPITAL**, 20 Administration Road, Zip 02324–3201; tel. 508/279–4521, (Nonreporting) **A**3 5
Primary Contact: Kenneth W. Nelson, Superintendent
CFO: Diane Wholley, Director Fiscal Services
**Control:** State–Government, nonfederal **Service:** Psychiatric

| |
|---|
| **Staffed Beds:** 350 |

**BRIGHTON—Suffolk County**

**CARITAS ST. ELIZABETH'S MEDICAL CENTER** See St. Elizabeth's Medical Center

⊞ **KINDRED HOSPITAL–BOSTON (222045)**, 1515 Commonwealth Avenue, Zip 02135–3617; tel. 617/254–1100, (Nonreporting) **A**1 10 **S** Kindred Healthcare, Louisville, KY
Primary Contact: Susan Downey, Chief Executive Officer
CFO: Lawrence J. Toye, Chief Financial Officer
CMO: Mark Rohrer, M.D., Chief Medical Officer
CHR: Kristen Ward, Coordinator Human Resources
Web address: www.kindredbos.com/
**Control:** Corporation, Investor–owned, for–profit **Service:** General Medical and Surgical

| |
|---|
| **Staffed Beds:** 59 |

☐ **ST. ELIZABETH'S MEDICAL CENTER (220036)**, 736 Cambridge Street, Zip 02135–2997; tel. 617/789–3000, (Nonreporting) **A**1 2 3 5 8 9 10 **S** Steward Health Care System, LLC, Boston, MA
Primary Contact: John Polanowicz, President
COO: Nathan Howell, Chief Operating Officer
CFO: Jeffrey P. Dion, Vice President Finance
CIO: Joseph Schmitt, Chief Information Officer
CHR: Claudia Henderson, Chief Human Resources
CNO: Suzanne G. McLaughlin, R.N., Chief Nursing Officer and Vice President Patient Care
Web address: www.stewardhealth.org/St_Elizabeths
**Control:** Corporation, Investor–owned, for–profit **Service:** General Medical and Surgical

| |
|---|
| **Staffed Beds:** 338 |

**BROCKTON—Plymouth County**

⊞ △ **BROCKTON VETERANS AFFAIRS MEDICAL CENTER**, 940 Belmont Street, Zip 02401–5596; tel. 508/583–4500, (Includes VETERANS AFFAIRS MEDICAL CENTER, 1400 VFW Parkway, West Roxbury, Boston, Zip 02132, Mailing Address: 1400 VVF Parkway, West Roxbury, Zip 02132; tel. 617/323–7700; William H. Kelleher, Director), (Nonreporting) **A**1 3 5 7 8 **S** Department of Veterans Affairs, Washington, DC
Primary Contact: Michael E. Lawson, Director
CFO: Joe Costa, Acting Chief Fiscal Officer
Web address: www.va.gov/sta/guide/home.asp
**Control:** Veterans Affairs, Government, federal **Service:** General Medical and Surgical

| |
|---|
| **Staffed Beds:** 375 |

**CARITAS GOOD SAMARITAN MEDICAL CENTER** See Good Samaritan Medical Center

☐ **GOOD SAMARITAN MEDICAL CENTER (220111)**, 235 North Pearl Street, Zip 02301–1794; tel. 508/427–3000, (Includes GOOD SAMARITAN MEDICAL CENTER – CUSHING CAMPUS, 235 North Pearl Street, Zip 02401–1794; tel. 508/427–3000), (Nonreporting) **A**1 2 3 5 9 10 **S** Steward Health Care System, LLC, Boston, MA
Primary Contact: Jeffrey H. Liebman, President
COO: Donna Rubinate, R.N., Chief Operating Officer
CFO: Thomas Whalen, Vice President Finance
CMO: Scott Stewart, M.D., Vice President Medical Management
CIO: Lori Caswell, Director Information Technology
CHR: David J. Cronin, Regional Vice President Human Resources
Web address: www.stewardhealth.org/Good–Samaritan
**Control:** Corporation, Investor–owned, for–profit **Service:** General Medical and Surgical

| |
|---|
| **Staffed Beds:** 190 |

⊞ **SIGNATURE HEALTHCARE BROCKTON HOSPITAL (220052)**, 680 Centre Street, Zip 02302–3395; tel. 508/941–7000, (Total facility includes 29 beds in nursing home–type unit) **A**1 2 6 10 **F**11 12 13 15 17 18 20 22 24 28 29 30 31 32 34 35 38 40 45 46 47 48 49 50 51 52 54 55 56 57 58 59 60 61 64 65 66 68 70 73 74 75 76 77 78 79 81 82 84 85 87 89 93 97 98 100 101 102 103 104 105 107 108 111 113 114 116 117 118 119 120 122 127 129 130 131 134 142 143 145 146 147 **P**6 8
Primary Contact: Kim Norton Hollon, FACHE, Chief Executive Officer
CFO: James Papadakos, Chief Financial Officer
CIO: Paul J. Pettinato, M.D., Chief Information Officer
CHR: David Fisher, Vice President Human Resources
CNO: Kim Walsh, Chief Nursing Officer
Web address: www.signature–healthcare.org
**Control:** Other not–for–profit (including NFP Corporation) **Service:** General Medical and Surgical

| |
|---|
| **Staffed Beds:** 253 **Admissions:** 13177 **Census:** 157 **Outpatient Visits:** 87895 **Births:** 1010 **Total Expense ($000):** 189911 **Payroll Expense ($000):** 85582 **Personnel:** 1319 |

**BROOKLINE—Norfolk County**

☐ **ARBOUR H. R. I. HOSPITAL (224018)**, 227 Babcock Street, Zip 02146–6799; tel. 617/731–3200, (Nonreporting) **A**1 9 10 **S** Universal Health Services, Inc., King of Prussia, PA
Primary Contact: Patrick Moallemian, Chief Executive Officer and Managing Director
CFO: James Rollins, Chief Financial Officer
CMO: Anthony Raynes, M.D., Psychiatrist in Chief
CHR: Kris Munson, Director Human Resources
Web address: www.arbourhealth.com
**Control:** Corporation, Investor–owned, for–profit **Service:** Psychiatric

| |
|---|
| **Staffed Beds:** 68 |

☐ **BOURNEWOOD HEALTH SYSTEMS (224022)**, 300 South Street, Zip 02467–3658; tel. 617/469–0300 **A**1 5 9 10 **F**4 5 98 99 104 105 129 131 **P**1
Primary Contact: Nasir A. Khan, M.D., Chief Executive Officer
CFO: Michael Gale, Chief Financial Officer
CMO: Carmel Heinsohn, M.D., Medical Director
CHR: Paula Berardi, Manager Human Resources
Web address: www.bournewood.com
**Control:** Corporation, Investor–owned, for–profit **Service:** Psychiatric

| |
|---|
| **Staffed Beds:** 81 **Admissions:** 3593 **Census:** 75 **Outpatient Visits:** 10813 **Births:** 0 **Total Expense ($000):** 18193 **Payroll Expense ($000):** 11522 **Personnel:** 178 |

**BURLINGTON—Middlesex County**

⊞ **LAHEY CLINIC HOSPITAL (220171)**, 41 Mall Road, Zip 01805–0001; tel. 781/744–5100 **A**1 2 3 5 8 9 10 **F**3 5 6 8 9 11 12 14 15 17 18 20 22 24 26 28 29 30 31 34 35 36 37 38 40 41 42 43 44 45 46 47 48 49 50 51 52 53 54 55 56 57 58 59 61 63 64 65 66 68 70 74 75 77 78 79 81 82 83 84 85 86 87 91 92 93 94 96 97 99 100 101 102 103 104 107 108 110 111 113 114 115 116 117 118 119 120 122 123 125 128 129 130 131 134 135 137 138 140 141 142 143 144 145 146 147 **P**6
Primary Contact: Howard R. Grant, JD, M.D., President and Chief Executive Officer
COO: Donald F. Snell, Executive Vice President and Chief Operating Officer
CFO: Timothy O'Connor, Executive Vice President and Chief Financial Officer
CMO: Richard W. Nesto, M.D., Executive Vice President and Chief Medical Officer
CIO: Bruce Metz, Ph.D., Chief Information Officer
CHR: Joan M. Robbio, Senior Vice President and Chief Human Resources Officer
CNO: Kathleen S. Jose, MSN, Chief Nursing Officer
Web address: www.lahey.org
**Control:** Other not–for–profit (including NFP Corporation) **Service:** General Medical and Surgical

| |
|---|
| **Staffed Beds:** 327 **Admissions:** 22190 **Census:** 285 **Outpatient Visits:** 1100684 **Births:** 0 **Total Expense ($000):** 681917 **Payroll Expense ($000):** 241301 **Personnel:** 5074 |

*Many Facility Codes have changed. Please refer to the AHA Guide Code Chart.* © 2012 AHA Guide

MA

**CAMBRIDGE—Middlesex County**

✠ **CAMBRIDGE HEALTH ALLIANCE (220011)**, 1493 Cambridge Street, Zip 02139–1099; tel. 617/665–1000, (Includes CAMBRIDGE HOSPITAL, 1493 Cambridge Street, tel. 617/498–1000; SOMERVILLE HOSPITAL, 230 Highland Avenue, Somerville, Zip 02143; tel. 617/666–4400; WHIDDEN MEMORIAL HOSPITAL, 103 Garland Street, Everett, Zip 02149–5095; tel. 617/389–6270) **A**1 2 3 5 8 9 10 **F**5 11 13 15 29 30 31 32 34 35 36 38 39 40 44 45 46 47 48 49 50 51 52 56 57 58 59 61 64 65 66 68 70 75 76 77 78 79 81 82 86 87 93 97 98 99 100 101 102 103 104 107 108 110 111 113 114 118 128 129 130 131 133 134 142 145 146 147 **P**6
Primary Contact: Patrick R. Wardell, Chief Executive Officer
COO: Allison Bayer, Executive Vice President and Chief Operating Officer
CFO: Gordon Boudrow, Chief Financial Officer
CMO: David Bor, M.D., Chief of Medicine
CIO: Judith S. Klickstein, Chief Information Officer
CHR: Joan Bennett, Senior Vice President Human Resources
Web address: www.challiance.org
**Control:** Hospital district or authority, Government, nonfederal **Service:** General Medical and Surgical

**Staffed Beds:** 229 **Admissions:** 11582 **Census:** 167 **Outpatient Visits:** 637328 **Births:** 1245 **Total Expense ($000):** 489653 **Payroll Expense ($000):** 283995 **Personnel:** 3197

✠ **MOUNT AUBURN HOSPITAL (220002)**, 330 Mount Auburn Street, Zip 02138–5597; tel. 617/492–3500 **A**1 2 3 5 8 9 10 **F**3 5 11 12 13 14 15 17 18 20 22 24 26 29 30 31 34 35 37 40 45 49 50 51 52 55 56 57 58 59 60 61 62 64 65 68 70 73 74 75 76 77 78 79 81 86 87 93 97 98 100 101 102 103 104 107 108 110 111 113 114 116 117 118 119 120 122 123 125 128 129 130 131 134 143 144 145 146 **P**5 6 7
Primary Contact: Jeanette G. Clough, President and Chief Executive Officer
COO: Nicholas T. Dileso, R.N., Chief Operating Officer
CFO: William Sullivan, Chief Financial Officer
CMO: A. Kim Saal, M.D., President Medical Staff
CIO: Bob Todd, Director Information Systems
CHR: Tom Fabiano, Director Human Resources
Web address: www.mountauburnhospital.org
**Control:** Other not–for–profit (including NFP Corporation) **Service:** General Medical and Surgical

**Staffed Beds:** 209 **Admissions:** 11919 **Census:** 150 **Outpatient Visits:** 180957 **Births:** 2340 **Total Expense ($000):** 285240 **Payroll Expense ($000):** 134651 **Personnel:** 2773

**SPAULDING HOSPITAL CAMBRIDGE** See Spaulding Hospital for Continuing Medical Care Cambridge

✠ **SPAULDING HOSPITAL FOR CONTINUING MEDICAL CARE CAMBRIDGE (222000)**, 1575 Cambridge Street, Zip 02138–4308; tel. 617/876–4344, (Nonreporting) **A**1 10 **S** Partners HealthCare System, Inc., Boston, MA
Primary Contact: Maureen Banks, R.N., MS, President
COO: Timothy Lynch, Vice President Operations
CFO: Michael J. Keller, Vice President Financial Affairs and Chief Financial Officer
CMO: Jonathon Schwartz, M.D., Medical Director and Chief Medical Officer
CIO: John Wilder, Director Information Systems
CHR: Jack Carroll, Senior Director Human Resources
Web address: www.spauldingrehab.org/OurLocations/HospitalCambridge
**Control:** Other not–for–profit (including NFP Corporation) **Service:** Long–Term Acute Care hospital

**Staffed Beds:** 180

**CANTON—Norfolk County**

✠ **MASSACHUSETTS HOSPITAL SCHOOL (222025)**, 3 Randolph Street, Zip 02021–2397; tel. 781/828–2440 **A**1 5 10 **F**1 19 29 34 39 44 50 54 59 61 64 65 75 77 79 85 86 87 90 91 93 97 107 118 129 133 142 145 **S** Massachusetts Department of Public Health, Boston, MA
Primary Contact: Katherine Ann Chmiel, R.N., MS, Chief Executive Officer
COO: Brian V. Devin, Chief Operating Officer
CFO: Sharon Porter, Chief Financial Officer
CMO: Aruna Sachdev, M.D., Medical Director
CIO: Robert Lima, Director Information Systems
CHR: Trish Scully, Manager Employment Services
Web address: www.mhsf.us/
**Control:** State–Government, nonfederal **Service:** Children's general

**Staffed Beds:** 93 **Admissions:** 32 **Census:** 72 **Outpatient Visits:** 0 **Births:** 0 **Total Expense ($000):** 17444 **Payroll Expense ($000):** 11315 **Personnel:** 218

**CLINTON—Worcester County**

★ **CLINTON HOSPITAL (220058)**, 201 Highland Street, Zip 01510–1096; tel. 978/368–3000, (Nonreporting) **A**3 5 9 10 21 **S** UMass Memorial Health Care, Inc., Worcester, MA
Primary Contact: Sheila Daly, President and Chief Executive Officer
CFO: Steven McCue, Chief Financial Officer
CHR: Martha Chiarchiaro, Vice President Human Resources
CNO: Charlene Elie, Vice President Patient Care Services
Web address: www.clintonhospital.org
**Control:** Other not–for–profit (including NFP Corporation) **Service:** General Medical and Surgical

**Staffed Beds:** 41

**CONCORD—Middlesex County**

✠ **EMERSON HOSPITAL (220084)**, 133 Old Road to Nine Acre Corner, Zip 01742–9120; tel. 978/369–1400 **A**1 2 5 9 10 **F**3 7 8 11 12 13 14 15 17 18 28 29 30 31 32 34 35 36 37 38 40 45 48 49 50 51 54 57 59 60 62 64 65 68 74 75 76 77 78 79 81 85 86 87 89 93 98 100 101 102 103 104 105 107 110 111 113 114 118 120 127 128 129 130 131 140 144 145 147 **P**5 8
Primary Contact: Christine C. Schuster, President and Chief Executive Officer
CFO: John O. Wilhelm, Jr., Senior Vice President and Chief Financial Officer
CMO: C. Gregory Martin, M.D., Chief Medical Officer
CIO: John O. Wilhelm, Jr., Senior Vice President and Chief Financial Officer
CHR: Eric Stastny, Vice President Human Resources
Web address: www.emersonhospital.org
**Control:** Other not–for–profit (including NFP Corporation) **Service:** General Medical and Surgical

**Staffed Beds:** 170 **Admissions:** 8499 **Census:** 113 **Outpatient Visits:** 278843 **Births:** 1162 **Total Expense ($000):** 172070 **Payroll Expense ($000):** 80984 **Personnel:** 1233

**EAST SANDWICH—Barnstable County**

✠ **SPAULDING REHABILITATION HOSPITAL CAPE COD (223032)**, 311 Service Road, Zip 02537–1370; tel. 508/833–4000 **A**1 10 **F**3 74 75 79 82 90 92 93 94 96 100 129 130 131 145 146 147 **S** Partners HealthCare System, Inc., Boston, MA
Primary Contact: Maureen Banks, R.N., MS, President and Chief Executive Officer
COO: Stephanie Nadolny, Vice President Clinical Services
CFO: Mary Shaughnessy, Vice President Finance
CMO: David Lowell, M.D., Medical Director
CIO: John Campbell, Chief Information Officer
CHR: Del Pontremoli, Director Human Resources
Web address: www.rhci.org
**Control:** Other not–for–profit (including NFP Corporation) **Service:** Rehabilitation

**Staffed Beds:** 60 **Admissions:** 1024 **Census:** 38 **Outpatient Visits:** 85158 **Births:** 0 **Total Expense ($000):** 30592 **Payroll Expense ($000):** 16678 **Personnel:** 342

**EVERETT—Middlesex County**

**WHIDDEN MEMORIAL HOSPITAL** See Cambridge Health Alliance, Cambridge

**FALL RIVER—Bristol County**

**CHARLTON MEMORIAL HOSPITAL** See Southcoast Hospitals Group

**DR. J. CORRIGAN MENTAL HEALTH CENTER (224028)**, 49 Hillside Street, Zip 02720–5266; tel. 508/235–7200, (Nonreporting) **A**10 **S** Massachusetts Department of Mental Health, Boston, MA
Primary Contact: Steve Figueiredo, Director
**Control:** State–Government, nonfederal **Service:** Psychiatric

**Staffed Beds:** 16

☐ **SAINT ANNE'S HOSPITAL (220020)**, 795 Middle Street, Zip 02721–1798; tel. 508/674–5741, (Nonreporting) **A**1 2 9 10 **S** Steward Health Care System, LLC, Boston, MA
Primary Contact: Craig A. Jesiolowski, FACHE, President
CFO: Michael Bushell, Vice President Finance, Business Development and Support Services
CMO: Harvey Kowaloff, M.D., Vice President Medical Affairs
CHR: Lisa Berry, Director
CNO: Carole Billington, R.N., Vice President Patient Care Services
Web address: www.saintanneshospital.org
**Control:** Corporation, Investor–owned, for–profit **Service:** General Medical and Surgical

**Staffed Beds:** 92

| Hospital, Medicare Provider Number, Address, Telephone, Approval, Facility, and Physician Codes, Health Care System |
|---|
| ★ American Hospital Association (AHA) membership      ○ American Osteopathic Association (AOA) accreditation |
| ☐ The Joint Commission accreditation    ◇ DNV Healthcare Inc. accreditation      △ Commission on Accreditation of Rehabilitation Facilities (CARF) accreditation |

MA

**MA**

✠ **SOUTHCOAST HOSPITALS GROUP (220074)**, 363 Highland Avenue, Zip 02720–3703; tel. 508/679–3131, (Includes CHARLTON MEMORIAL HOSPITAL, 363 Highland Avenue, tel. 508/679–3131; ST. LUKE'S HOSPITAL, 101 Page Street, New Bedford, Zip 02740; tel. 508/997–1515; TOBEY HOSPITAL, 43 High Street, Wareham, Zip 02571; tel. 508/295–0880) **A**1 2 9 10 **F**3 8 11 12 13 14 15 17 18 20 22 24 26 28 29 30 31 32 34 35 36 37 40 44 45 47 48 49 50 51 54 56 57 59 60 61 62 63 64 68 70 71 73 74 75 76 77 78 79 81 83 84 85 86 87 89 90 91 92 93 98 101 102 103 104 107 108 110 111 113 114 116 117 118 119 120 122 123 125 129 130 131 133 143 145 146 147 **P**5
Primary Contact: Keith A. Hovan, President and Chief Executive Officer
COO: Linda Bodenmann, Chief Operating Officer
CIO: Christopher Baldwin, Vice President Information Systems
CHR: David DeJesus, Vice President Human Resources
Web address: www.southcoast.org
**Control:** Other not–for–profit (including NFP Corporation) **Service:** General Medical and Surgical

**Staffed Beds:** 742 **Admissions:** 41443 **Census:** 556 **Outpatient Visits:** 975171 **Births:** 3406 **Total Expense ($000):** 629534 **Payroll Expense ($000):** 301082 **Personnel:** 4315

**FALMOUTH—Barnstable County**

✠ **FALMOUTH HOSPITAL (220135)**, 100 Ter Heun Drive, Zip 02540–2599; tel. 508/548–5300 **A**1 2 9 10 **F**3 11 13 15 18 20 22 28 29 30 34 35 37 38 40 45 50 51 54 57 59 60 61 64 68 70 75 76 77 79 81 82 87 89 93 94 100 102 107 108 110 111 113 117 118 128 129 130 131 142 145 146 147 **P**5 6 8 **S** Cape Cod Healthcare, Inc., Hyannis, MA
Primary Contact: Susan M. Wing, R.N., Chief Operating Officer
COO: Susan M. Wing, R.N., Chief Operating Officer
CFO: Michael Connors, Senior Vice President and Chief Financial Officer
CMO: Herb Gray, M.D., Chief Medical Officer
CIO: Sheryl Crowley, Chief Information Officer
CHR: David Ryan, Vice President Human Resources
Web address: www.capecodhealth.org
**Control:** Other not–for–profit (including NFP Corporation) **Service:** General Medical and Surgical

**Staffed Beds:** 95 **Admissions:** 6171 **Census:** 68 **Outpatient Visits:** 160535 **Births:** 501 **Total Expense ($000):** 131017 **Payroll Expense ($000):** 56694 **Personnel:** 538

**FRAMINGHAM—Middlesex County**

✠ **METROWEST MEDICAL CENTER (220175)**, 115 Lincoln Street, Zip 01702–6342; tel. 508/383–1000, (Includes FRAMINGHAM UNION HOSPITAL, 115 Lincoln Street, Zip 01702; tel. 508/383–1000; LEONARD MORSE HOSPITAL, 67 Union Street, Natick, Zip 01760; tel. 508/650–7000) **A**1 2 3 5 9 10 **F**3 5 12 13 14 15 18 20 22 26 28 29 30 31 32 34 35 36 40 44 45 49 50 54 56 57 59 61 62 63 64 65 68 70 72 74 75 76 77 78 79 81 82 85 86 87 89 93 97 98 99 100 102 103 104 105 107 108 110 113 114 117 118 119 120 128 129 130 131 133 134 142 143 145 146 147 **S** Vanguard Health System, Nashville, TN
Primary Contact: Andrei Soran, Chief Executive Officer
CFO: Roger D. Wiseman, Chief Financial Officer
CMO: Michael Gottlieb, M.D., Chief Medical Officer
CIO: Michael Hebert, Director Technology
CHR: Rebecca Heffernan, Director Human Resources
Web address: www.mwmc.com
**Control:** Corporation, Investor–owned, for–profit **Service:** General Medical and Surgical

**Staffed Beds:** 160 **Admissions:** 14625 **Census:** 165 **Outpatient Visits:** 392276 **Births:** 1187 **Total Expense ($000):** 246639 **Payroll Expense ($000):** 122360 **Personnel:** 1845

**GARDNER—Worcester County**

✠ **HEYWOOD HOSPITAL (220095)**, 242 Green Street, Zip 01440–1373; tel. 978/632–3420, (Nonreporting) **A**1 5 9 10
Primary Contact: Winfield S. Brown, President and Chief Executive Officer
CFO: Robert Crosby, Senior Vice President and Chief Financial Officer
CHR: Thomas Cady, Vice President Human Resources
Web address: www.heywood.org
**Control:** Other not–for–profit (including NFP Corporation) **Service:** General Medical and Surgical

**Staffed Beds:** 128

**GLOUCESTER—Essex County**

**ADDISON GILBERT HOSPITAL** See Beverly Hospital, Beverly

**GREAT BARRINGTON—Berkshire County**

✠ **FAIRVIEW HOSPITAL (221302)**, 29 Lewis Avenue, Zip 01230–1713; tel. 413/528–0790 **A**1 9 10 18 **F**3 11 13 15 18 26 29 30 34 35 40 45 46 49 50 54 57 59 64 65 68 70 75 79 81 85 86 87 93 94 97 107 108 110 113 118 129 130 131 132 134 145 146 **P**6 **S** Berkshire Health Systems, Inc., Pittsfield, MA
Primary Contact: Eugene A. Dellea, President
COO: Doreen M. Sylvia–Hutchinson, Vice President Operations and Chief Nurse Executive
CFO: Anthony Rinaldi, Executive Vice President
CMO: Brian Burke, M.D., President Medical Staff
CHR: Laura Farkas, Director Human Resources
Web address: www.berkshirehealthsystems.com
**Control:** Other not–for–profit (including NFP Corporation) **Service:** General Medical and Surgical

**Staffed Beds:** 24 **Admissions:** 1092 **Census:** 11 **Outpatient Visits:** 62662 **Births:** 174 **Total Expense ($000):** 40170 **Payroll Expense ($000):** 17377 **Personnel:** 209

**GREENFIELD—Franklin County**

✠ **BAYSTATE FRANKLIN MEDICAL CENTER (220016)**, 164 High Street, Zip 01301–2613; tel. 413/773–0211 **A**1 2 9 10 **F**3 7 11 12 13 14 15 18 24 28 29 30 31 34 36 40 45 46 47 48 49 50 51 55 57 59 60 64 68 70 74 75 76 77 78 79 81 82 85 86 87 89 93 98 105 107 108 110 111 114 117 118 128 129 130 131 145 146 **S** Baystate Health, Inc., Springfield, MA
Primary Contact: Charles Gijanto, President, Baystate Northern Region
CFO: Andrea Nathanson, Director Finance
CMO: Jacques Blanchet, M.D., Director Medical Affairs
CHR: Jill Wyman, Interim Director Human Resources
Web address: www.baystatehealth.com
**Control:** Other not–for–profit (including NFP Corporation) **Service:** General Medical and Surgical

**Staffed Beds:** 90 **Admissions:** 3621 **Census:** 48 **Outpatient Visits:** 122747 **Births:** 479 **Total Expense ($000):** 77664 **Payroll Expense ($000):** 33669 **Personnel:** 421

**HAVERHILL—Essex County**

**BALDPATE HOSPITAL (224033)**, 83 Baldpate Road, Zip 01833–2399; tel. 978/352–2131, (Nonreporting) **A**9 10
Primary Contact: Lucille M. Batal, Administrator
Web address: www.baldpateh.com
**Control:** Corporation, Investor–owned, for–profit **Service:** Psychiatric

**Staffed Beds:** 59

☐ **MERRIMACK VALLEY HOSPITAL (220174)**, 140 Lincoln Avenue, Zip 01830–6798; tel. 978/374–2000, (Nonreporting) **A**1 9 10 **S** Steward Health Care System, LLC, Boston, MA
Primary Contact: Michael F. Collins, Chief Executive Officer
COO: Diane Lovallo, R.N., Chief Nursing Officer
CMO: George Kwass, M.D., Chief of Staff
CIO: Mark Nightingale, Senior Administrator
CHR: Gina Lagana, Director Human Resources
Web address: www.merrimackvalleyhospital.com
**Control:** Corporation, Investor–owned, for–profit **Service:** General Medical and Surgical

**Staffed Beds:** 90

**HOLYOKE—Hampden County**

✠ **HOLYOKE MEDICAL CENTER (220024)**, 575 Beech Street, Zip 01040–2223; tel. 413/534–2500 **A**1 2 5 9 10 **F**3 5 9 11 13 14 15 17 18 28 29 31 34 35 38 40 44 45 46 49 50 51 57 59 60 64 65 68 70 74 75 76 77 78 79 81 82 85 86 87 89 91 92 93 96 98 100 101 102 104 105 107 108 110 111 113 117 118 119 120 122 128 129 131 134 142 144 145 146 147 **P**8
Primary Contact: Hank J. Porten, FACHE, President and Chief Executive Officer
CFO: Antonio Correia, Chief Financial Officer
CMO: Karen Ferroni, M.D., Medical Director
CIO: Carl Cameron, Director Information Systems
CHR: Mary Kelleher, Vice President Human Resources
Web address: www.holyokehealth.com
**Control:** Other not–for–profit (including NFP Corporation) **Service:** General Medical and Surgical

**Staffed Beds:** 203 **Admissions:** 5949 **Census:** 80 **Outpatient Visits:** 285015 **Births:** 487 **Total Expense ($000):** 112141 **Payroll Expense ($000):** 62546 **Personnel:** 885

*Many Facility Codes have changed. Please refer to the AHA Guide Code Chart.* © 2012 AHA Guide

**SOLDIERS' HOME IN HOLYOKE (220153)**, 110 Cherry Street, Zip 01040–2829; tel. 413/532–9475, (Nonreporting) **A**10
Primary Contact: Paul Barabani, Superintendent
COO: Lee Anne St Martin, Director Operations
CFO: Anthony Di Stefano, Director Finance
CMO: David Clinton, M.D., Medical Director
CIO: Anthony Di Stefano, Coordinator Management Information Systems
CHR: James M. Black, Director Administration
CNO: Pamela Quirk, Director of Nursing
Web address: www.mass.gov/hly
**Control:** State–Government, nonfederal **Service:** General Medical and Surgical

**Staffed Beds:** 308

### HYANNIS—Barnstable County

**CAPE COD HOSPITAL (220012)**, 27 Park Street, Zip 02601–5230;
tel. 508/771–1800 **A**1 2 5 9 10 20 **F**3 5 11 13 14 15 17 18 20 22 24 26 29 30 31 34 35 37 38 40 44 45 49 50 51 54 55 57 58 59 60 61 64 65 68 70 74 75 76 77 78 79 81 82 86 87 89 93 94 97 98 99 100 101 102 103 104 105 107 108 110 111 113 114 116 118 119 120 122 123 125 129 130 131 134 142 145 146 **P**5 6 8 **S** Cape Cod Healthcare, Inc., Hyannis, MA
Primary Contact: Jason M. Adams, Chief Operating Officer
CFO: Michael Connors, Senior Vice President and Chief Financial Officer
CMO: James D. Butterick, M.D., Chief Medical Officer
CIO: John E. Kilroy, Vice President and Chief Information Officer
Web address: www.capecodhealth.org
**Control:** Other not–for–profit (including NFP Corporation) **Service:** General Medical and Surgical

**Staffed Beds:** 259 **Admissions:** 16096 **Census:** 180 **Outpatient Visits:** 661361 **Births:** 804 **Total Expense ($000):** 369979 **Payroll Expense ($000):** 143077 **Personnel:** 1435

### JAMAICA PLAIN—Suffolk County

**LEMUEL SHATTUCK HOSPITAL (222006)**, 170 Morton Street, Zip 02130–3735; tel. 617/522–8110, (Nonreporting) **A**1 3 10 **S** Massachusetts Department of Public Health, Boston, MA
Primary Contact: Paul Romary, Chief Executive Officer
CFO: Mike Donovan, Chief Financial Officer
CMO: Kenneth Freedman, M.D., Chief Medical Officer
CIO: Kathryn Noonan, Director Information Management
CHR: Jill Sampson, Director Human Resources
Web address: www.mass.gov/shattuckhospital.org
**Control:** State–Government, nonfederal **Service:** General Medical and Surgical

**Staffed Beds:** 260

### LAWRENCE—Essex County

**LAWRENCE GENERAL HOSPITAL (220010)**, 1 General Street, Zip 01842–0389, Mailing Address: P.O. Box 189, Zip 01842–0389; tel. 978/683–4000, (Nonreporting) **A**1 2 9 10
Primary Contact: Dianne J. Anderson, MS, R.N., President and Chief Executive Officer
COO: Denise S. Palumbo, MSN, Executive Vice President and Chief Operating Officer
CFO: Deborah J. Wilson, Senior Vice President and Chief Financial Officer
CMO: Neil S. Meehan, D.O., Chief Medical Officer and Chief Medical Information Officer
CIO: Jeffrey L. Brown, Director Information Systems
CHR: Cynthia Phelan, Vice President Human Resources
CNO: Elizabeth Hale, R.N., Vice President Patient Services and Chief Nursing Officer
Web address: www.lawrencegeneral.org
**Control:** Other not–for–profit (including NFP Corporation) **Service:** General Medical and Surgical

**Staffed Beds:** 189

### LEEDS—Hampshire County

**VETERANS AFFAIRS MEDICAL CENTER**, 421 North Main Street, Zip 01053–9764; tel. 413/582–3000, (Total facility includes 66 beds in nursing home–type unit) **A**1 **F**5 18 29 30 35 38 39 50 54 56 59 61 62 64 65 68 74 75 77 82 83 84 86 87 93 94 97 98 101 102 103 104 106 107 118 129 131 134 142 143 145 146 147 **S** Department of Veterans Affairs, Washington, DC
Primary Contact: Roger L. Johnson, Director
COO: Richard Tremaine, Associate Director
CFO: David Cichocki, Chief Fiscal Officer
CMO: Neil Nusbaum, M.D., Chief of Staff
CIO: Michael Marley, Chief Information Officer
CHR: Michelle Krause, Manager Human Resources
Web address: www.va.gov/sta/guide/home.asp
**Control:** Veterans Affairs, Government, federal **Service:** Psychiatric

**Staffed Beds:** 167 **Admissions:** 933 **Census:** 121 **Outpatient Visits:** 202464 **Births:** 0 **Total Expense ($000):** 126122 **Payroll Expense ($000):** 47197 **Personnel:** 649

### LEOMINSTER—Worcester County

**HEALTH ALLIANCE HOSPITALS (220001)**, 60 Hospital Road, Zip 01453–8004; tel. 978/466–2000 **A**1 2 5 7 9 10 13 **F**3 13 15 28 29 30 31 34 35 36 40 46 47 49 50 51 59 62 63 64 68 70 74 75 76 77 78 81 82 84 85 86 87 89 92 93 96 97 100 105 107 108 110 113 117 118 129 130 131 134 143 145 146 **P**6 **S** UMass Memorial Health Care, Inc., Worcester, MA
Primary Contact: Patrick L. Muldoon, FACHE, President and Chief Executive Officer
CFO: Michael Cofone, Chief Financial Officer
CMO: Lisa Colombo, R.N., Vice President Patient Care Services and Chief Nursing Officer
CMO: Daniel H. O'Leary, M.D., Chief Medical Officer
CIO: Margaret Campbell, Vice President, Associate Chief Information Officer
CHR: Cynthia Ring, Vice President Human Resources
Web address: www.healthalliance.com
**Control:** Other not–for–profit (including NFP Corporation) **Service:** General Medical and Surgical

**Staffed Beds:** 83 **Admissions:** 6949 **Census:** 65 **Outpatient Visits:** 254701 **Births:** 1042 **Total Expense ($000):** 150565 **Payroll Expense ($000):** 65685 **Personnel:** 912

### LOWELL—Middlesex County

**LOWELL GENERAL HOSPITAL (220063)**, 295 Varnum Avenue, Zip 01854–2134; tel. 978/937–6000 **A**1 2 9 10 **F**3 8 11 12 13 15 18 20 22 26 28 29 30 31 32 34 35 36 38 40 43 44 49 50 51 54 55 56 57 58 59 61 62 63 64 66 68 70 73 74 75 76 77 78 79 81 82 84 85 86 87 89 92 93 97 107 108 110 111 113 114 117 118 120 122 123 125 128 129 130 131 133 134 143 145 146 **P**6 8
Primary Contact: Normand E. Deschene, FACHE, President and Chief Executive Officer
COO: Jody White, Executive Vice President and Chief Operating Officer
CFO: Susan Green, Chief Financial Officer
CMO: Wayne Pasanen, M.D., Vice President Medical Affairs
CIO: Maureen Belley, Director Information Services
CHR: Peter Zarrilla, Vice President and Chief Human Resources Officer
Web address: www.lowellgeneral.org
**Control:** Other not–for–profit (including NFP Corporation) **Service:** General Medical and Surgical

**Staffed Beds:** 189 **Admissions:** 14163 **Census:** 133 **Outpatient Visits:** 287675 **Births:** 2403 **Total Expense ($000):** 238148 **Payroll Expense ($000):** 96338 **Personnel:** 1595

**SAINTS MEDICAL CENTER (220082)**, 1 Hospital Drive, Zip 01852–1311; tel. 978/458–1411 **A**1 2 9 10 **F**3 7 8 14 15 18 20 22 28 29 30 31 34 35 40 45 46 48 49 50 51 54 55 57 59 60 64 65 67 68 70 75 77 78 79 81 82 84 85 86 87 89 93 97 107 108 110 113 114 117 118 119 120 122 128 129 130 131 134 143 144 145 146 147 **P**5
Primary Contact: Stephen J. Guimond, President and Chief Executive Officer
COO: Judith Casagrande, Chief Operating Officer
CFO: Stephen J. Guimond, President and Chief Executive Officer
CIO: Paul Englund, Chief Information Officer
CHR: Ann–Marie E. Driscoll, Director Human Resources
Web address: www.saintsmedicalcenter.com
**Control:** Church–operated, Nongovernment, not–for profit **Service:** General Medical and Surgical

**Staffed Beds:** 102 **Admissions:** 6531 **Census:** 70 **Outpatient Visits:** 215326 **Births:** 0 **Total Expense ($000):** 138906 **Payroll Expense ($000):** 56000 **Personnel:** 851

---

**Hospital, Medicare Provider Number, Address, Telephone, Approval, Facility, and Physician Codes, Health Care System**

★ American Hospital Association (AHA) membership
□ The Joint Commission accreditation
◇ DNV Healthcare Inc. accreditation
○ American Osteopathic Association (AOA) accreditation
△ Commission on Accreditation of Rehabilitation Facilities (CARF) accreditation

MA

## LUDLOW—Hampden County

⊠ **HEALTHSOUTH REHABILITATION HOSPITAL OF WESTERN MASSACHUSETTS (223030)**, 14 Chestnut Place, Zip 01056–3476; tel. 413/589–7581, (Nonreporting) **A**1 10 **S** HEALTHSOUTH Corporation, Birmingham, AL
Primary Contact: Scott R. Keen, Chief Executive Officer
CFO: Victoria Healy, Controller
CMO: Adnan Dahdul, M.D., Medical Director
CHR: Mary Mazza, Director Human Resources
CNO: Deborah Cabanas, R.N., Chief Nursing Officer
Web address: www.healthsouthrehab.com
**Control:** Corporation, Investor–owned, for–profit **Service:** Rehabilitation

**Staffed Beds:** 53

## LYNN—Essex County

**UNION CAMPUS** See North Shore Medical Center, Salem

**UNION HOSPITAL** See Union Campus

## MARLBOROUGH—Bristol County

⊠ **UMASS MEMORIAL–MARLBOROUGH HOSPITAL (220049)**, 157 Union Street, Zip 01752–1297; tel. 508/481–5000 **A**1 5 9 10 **F**3 11 15 18 28 29 30 31 34 35 40 49 50 57 68 70 75 77 78 79 81 85 93 98 100 101 105 107 113 118 131 140 145 146 **S** UMass Memorial Health Care, Inc., Worcester, MA
Primary Contact: Karen O. Moore, MS, R.N., President and Chief Executive Officer
COO: Candra Szymanski, Chief Operating Officer
CFO: Jeff Dion, Chief Financial Officer
CFO: Steven McCue, Chief Financial Officer
CMO: Lalita Matta, M.D., Chief Medical Officer and Vice President Medical Affairs
CHR: Suzanne Parsons, Vice President Human Resources
CNO: Mary Brown, Chief Nursing Officer
Web address: www.marlboroughhospital.org
**Control:** Other not–for–profit (including NFP Corporation) **Service:** General Medical and Surgical

**Staffed Beds:** 67 **Admissions:** 4272 **Census:** 51 **Outpatient Visits:** 103706 **Births:** 0 **Total Expense ($000):** 71934 **Payroll Expense ($000):** 29794 **Personnel:** 427

## MEDFORD—Middlesex County

**LAWRENCE MEMORIAL HOSPITAL OF MEDFORD** See Hallmark Health System, Melrose

## MELROSE—Middlesex County

★ **HALLMARK HEALTH SYSTEM (220070)**, 585 Lebanon Street, Zip 2176; tel. 781/979–3000, (Includes LAWRENCE MEMORIAL HOSPITAL OF MEDFORD, 170 Governors Avenue, Medford, Zip 02155–1643; tel. 781/306–6000; MELROSE–WAKEFIELD HOSPITAL, 585 Lebanon Street, Zip 02176; tel. 781/979–3000; Michael V. Sack, Chief Executive Officer) **A**2 5 10 **F**2 3 11 12 13 15 18 20 22 26 28 29 30 31 34 35 38 40 45 46 47 49 50 51 54 55 56 57 58 59 60 61 62 63 64 65 68 70 72 74 75 76 77 78 79 81 82 84 85 86 87 93 97 98 100 101 102 103 104 105 107 108 110 111 113 114 118 119 120 122 129 130 131 134 140 142 143 145 146 **P**5 6
Primary Contact: Michael V. Sack, President and Chief Executive Officer
CFO: James A. Nania, System Vice President and Chief Financial Officer
CIO: Richard A. Pozniak, Director Marketing and Communications
CHR: Richard Kenny, Vice President Human Resources
Web address: www.hallmarkhealth.org
**Control:** Other not–for–profit (including NFP Corporation) **Service:** General Medical and Surgical

**Staffed Beds:** 297 **Admissions:** 14949 **Census:** 202 **Outpatient Visits:** 563154 **Births:** 1082 **Total Expense ($000):** 258959 **Payroll Expense ($000):** 131924 **Personnel:** 1548

## METHUEN—Essex County

☐ **HOLY FAMILY HOSPITAL AND MEDICAL CENTER (220080)**, 70 East Street, Zip 01844–4597; tel. 978/687–0151, (Nonreporting) **A**1 2 5 9 10 **S** Steward Health Care System, LLC, Boston, MA
Primary Contact: Lester P. Schindel, President and Chief Executive Officer
COO: Martha M. McDrury, R.N., Chief Operating Officer and Chief Nursing Officer
CFO: Kevin Kilday, Vice President Finance
CMO: Paul Allen, M.D., Vice President Medical Affairs
CHR: Deborah Bradshaw, Director Human Resources
CNO: Martha M. McDrury, R.N., Chief Operating Officer and Chief Nursing Officer
Web address: www.stewardhealth.org/Holy–Family–Hospital
**Control:** Corporation, Investor–owned, for–profit **Service:** General Medical and Surgical

**Staffed Beds:** 239

## MILFORD—Worcester County

⊠ **MILFORD REGIONAL MEDICAL CENTER (220090)**, 14 Prospect Street, Zip 01757–3003; tel. 508/473–1190, (Includes WHITINSVILLE MEDICAL CENTER, 18 Granite Street, Whitinsville, Zip 01588; tel. 508/234–6311) **A**1 2 5 9 10 **F**3 11 13 15 18 20 28 29 30 31 32 34 35 40 41 49 50 51 52 57 59 62 63 64 65 68 70 74 75 76 77 78 79 80 81 82 85 86 87 89 93 107 108 110 113 114 117 118 123 129 130 131 133 134 145 146 147 **P**6
Primary Contact: Francis M. Saba, Chief Executive Officer
CFO: Edward Kelly, President
CMO: William Muller, M.D., Vice President Medical Affairs
CIO: Larry Fraize, Director Management Information Systems
CHR: Linda Greasom, Vice President Human Resources
Web address: www.milfordregional.org
**Control:** Other not–for–profit (including NFP Corporation) **Service:** General Medical and Surgical

**Staffed Beds:** 121 **Admissions:** 7825 **Census:** 84 **Outpatient Visits:** 414411 **Births:** 968 **Total Expense ($000):** 175556 **Payroll Expense ($000):** 81148 **Personnel:** 1522

## MILTON—Norfolk County

☐ **MILTON HOSPITAL (220108)**, 199 Reedsdale Road, Zip 02186–3926; tel. 617/696–4600, (Nonreporting) **A**1 9 10
Primary Contact: Joseph V. Morrissey, President
CFO: Jason Radzevich, Vice President Finance
CIO: Jean Fernandez, Chief Information Officer
CHR: Kathleen Harrington, Vice President Human Resources
Web address: www.miltonhospital.org
**Control:** Other not–for–profit (including NFP Corporation) **Service:** General Medical and Surgical

**Staffed Beds:** 82

## NANTUCKET—Nantucket County

⊠ **NANTUCKET COTTAGE HOSPITAL (220177)**, 57 Prospect Street, Zip 02554–2799; tel. 508/825–8100, (Nonreporting) **A**1 9 10 **S** Partners HealthCare System, Inc., Boston, MA
Primary Contact: Margot Hartmann, M.D., Ph.D., President and Chief Executive Officer
CFO: David J. Burke, Director Finance and Chief Financial Officer
CMO: Timothy J. Lepore, FACS, Medical Director
CIO: Terry Hughes, Manager Management Information Systems
CHR: Grace Hull, Director Human Resources
Web address: www.nantuckethospital.org
**Control:** Other not–for–profit (including NFP Corporation) **Service:** General Medical and Surgical

**Staffed Beds:** 19

## NATICK—Middlesex County

**LEONARD MORSE HOSPITAL** See MetroWest Medical Center, Framingham

## NEEDHAM—Norfolk County

**BETH ISRAEL DEACONESS HOSPITAL–NEEDHAM CAMPUS** See Beth Israel Deaconess Medical Center, Boston

## NEW BEDFORD—Bristol County

☐ **NEW BEDFORD REHABILITATION HOSPITAL (222043)**, 4499 Acushnet Avenue, Zip 2745; tel. 508/995–6900, (Nonreporting) **A**1 10 **S** Vibra Healthcare, Mechanicsburg, PA
Primary Contact: Edward B. Leary, Chief Executive Officer
CFO: Cheryl Perry, Chief Financial Officer
CMO: Albert Loerinc, M.D., Medical Director
CHR: Ilene Mirabella, Director Human Resources
Web address: www.newbedfordrehab.com
**Control:** Corporation, Investor–owned, for–profit **Service:** Rehabilitation

**Staffed Beds:** 90

**ST. LUKE'S HOSPITAL** See Southcoast Hospitals Group, Fall River

## NEWBURYPORT—Essex County

★ **ANNA JAQUES HOSPITAL (220029)**, 25 Highland Avenue, Zip 01950–3894; tel. 978/463–1000 **A**9 10 **F**13 14 15 18 28 29 31 34 35 38 40 43 45 57 64 70 75 76 77 78 79 81 82 85 86 87 89 93 97 98 102 105 107 108 110 111 114 117 118 128 129 134 145 **P**8
Primary Contact: Delia O'Connor, Chief Executive Officer
CFO: Mark L. Goldstein, Chief Financial Officer
CMO: Gail Fayre, M.D., Medical Director
CIO: Robert Buchanan, Chief Information Officer
CHR: Stephen Salvo, Vice President Human Resources
CNO: Richard Maki, R.N., Vice President Nursing and Chief Nursing Officer
Web address: www.ajh.org
**Control:** Other not–for–profit (including NFP Corporation) **Service:** General Medical and Surgical

**Staffed Beds:** 127 **Admissions:** 7113 **Census:** 83 **Outpatient Visits:** 233198 **Births:** 595 **Total Expense ($000):** 102921 **Payroll Expense ($000):** 49780 **Personnel:** 688

MA

**NEWTON LOWER FALLS—Middlesex County**

⊞ **NEWTON–WELLESLEY HOSPITAL (220101)**, 2014 Washington Street, Zip 02462–1699; tel. 617/243–6000, (Includes MASSGENERAL FOR CHILDREN AT NEWTON–WELLESLEY HOSPITAL, 2000 Washington Street, Newton, Zip 02462–1650; tel. 617/243–6585) **A**1 2 3 5 9 10 **F**3 8 11 12 13 15 18 28 29 30 31 32 34 35 38 40 41 44 45 46 49 50 51 52 53 54 55 56 57 58 59 60 61 63 64 65 68 70 72 74 75 76 77 78 79 81 82 84 85 86 87 89 93 94 97 98 100 101 102 107 108 110 111 113 114 115 116 117 118 128 129 130 131 134 142 143 145 146 147 **P**1 6 **S** Partners HealthCare System, Inc., Boston, MA
Primary Contact: Michael Jellinek, M.D., President
COO: Patrick Jordan, Senior Vice President Administration
CFO: Daniel Gross, Senior Vice President Finance and Chief Financial Officer
CMO: Leslie Selbovitz, M.D., Senior Vice President Medical Affairs
CIO: Scott T. MacLean, Chief Information Officer
CHR: Beth Taylor, Director Human Resources
Web address: www.nwh.org
**Control:** Other not–for–profit (including NFP Corporation) **Service:** General Medical and Surgical

**Staffed Beds:** 232 **Admissions:** 17402 **Census:** 185 **Outpatient Visits:** 569150 **Births:** 3968 **Total Expense ($000):** 358226 **Payroll Expense ($000):** 167993 **Personnel:** 2280

**NORTH ADAMS—Berkshire County**

⊞ **NORTH ADAMS REGIONAL HOSPITAL (220051)**, 71 Hospital Avenue, Zip 01247–2584; tel. 413/664–5000 **A**1 2 9 10 **F**3 8 13 15 18 29 30 32 34 35 40 43 45 50 51 57 59 61 64 68 70 75 76 77 79 81 85 87 89 93 96 98 100 101 103 107 108 111 114 118 129 131 134 145 146 147 **P**6
Primary Contact: William Frado, Jr., President and Chief Executive Officer
COO: Arthur B. Scott, Vice President Operations
CFO: Christopher Hickey, Chief Financial Officer
CMO: Jeffrey Bath, M.D., President Medical Staff
CIO: Charles Groh, Interim Chief Information Officer
CHR: Paul Kulp, Director Human Resources
Web address: www.nbhealth.org
**Control:** Other not–for–profit (including NFP Corporation) **Service:** General Medical and Surgical

**Staffed Beds:** 36 **Admissions:** 2602 **Census:** 28 **Outpatient Visits:** 125606 **Births:** 281 **Total Expense ($000):** 61330 **Payroll Expense ($000):** 24622

**NORTHAMPTON—Hampshire County**

⊞ **COOLEY DICKINSON HOSPITAL (220015)**, 30 Locust Street, Zip 01060–2093, Mailing Address: P.O. Box 5001, Zip 01061–5001; tel. 413/582–2000 **A**1 2 9 10 **F**3 11 12 13 14 15 18 20 26 28 29 30 31 34 35 36 38 39 40 49 50 51 54 56 57 59 60 61 64 68 70 74 75 76 78 79 81 82 86 87 89 92 93 94 96 98 100 107 108 110 111 113 116 118 119 120 122 125 129 130 131 133 134 143 145 146 147 **P**8
Primary Contact: Craig N. Melin, President and Chief Executive Officer
CFO: Edith S. Peter, Chief Financial Officer and Vice President Finance
CIO: Wayne Freeberg, Chief Information Officer
CHR: Wilmont Davis, Vice President Human Resources
Web address: www.cooley–dickinson.org
**Control:** Other not–for–profit (including NFP Corporation) **Service:** General Medical and Surgical

**Staffed Beds:** 101 **Admissions:** 8177 **Census:** 82 **Outpatient Visits:** 211603 **Births:** 860 **Total Expense ($000):** 147940 **Payroll Expense ($000):** 64973 **Personnel:** 865

**NORWOOD—Norfolk County**

⊞ **NORWOOD HOSPITAL (220126)**, 800 Washington Street, Zip 02062–3487; tel. 781/769–4000, (Nonreporting) **A**1 2 5 9 10 **S** Steward Health Care System, LLC, Boston, MA
Primary Contact: Emily L. Holliman, President
COO: William P. Fleming, Chief Operating Officer
CFO: Victoria Lobban, Interim Vice President Finance
CHR: Kimberly Brosnan, Director Human Resources
CNO: Kathleen Davidson, Vice President, Patient Care Services and Chief Nursing Officer
CNO: Matthew Lowry, M.D., Vice President of Medical Affairs
Web address: www.stewardhealth.org/Norwood–Hospital
**Control:** Corporation, Investor–owned, for–profit **Service:** General Medical and Surgical

**Staffed Beds:** 205

**OAK BLUFFS—Dukes County**

⊞ **MARTHA'S VINEYARD HOSPITAL (221300)**, One Hospital Road, Zip 2557, Mailing Address: P.O. Box 1477, Zip 02557–1477; tel. 508/693–0410, (Nonreporting) **A**1 9 10 18 **S** Partners HealthCare System, Inc., Boston, MA
Primary Contact: Timothy J. Walsh, Chief Executive Officer
CFO: Thomas Lenkowski, Chief Financial Officer
CMO: Pieter Pil, M.D., Chief Medical Staff
CHR: Ken Chisholm, Director Human Resources
CNO: Carol A. Bardwell, R.N., Chief Nurse Executive
Web address: www.marthasvineyardhospital.org
**Control:** Other not–for–profit (including NFP Corporation) **Service:** General Medical and Surgical

**Staffed Beds:** 25

**PALMER—Hampden County**

⊞ **WING MEMORIAL HOSPITAL AND MEDICAL CENTERS (220030)**, 40 Wright Street, Zip 01069–1138; tel. 413/283–7651 **A**1 5 9 10 **F**3 5 11 12 15 18 29 30 31 33 34 36 37 40 49 50 51 56 57 59 61 62 63 64 65 68 70 74 75 77 78 79 81 82 85 89 92 93 97 98 99 100 101 102 103 104 107 108 110 114 117 118 128 129 130 131 145 146 147 **P**6 **S** UMass Memorial Health Care, Inc., Worcester, MA
Primary Contact: Charles E. Cavagnaro, III, M.D., President and Chief Executive Officer
CFO: Keary T. Allicon, Vice President Finance and Chief Financial Officer
CMO: David L. Maguire, M.D., Vice President Medical Affairs
CIO: Kenneth Riley, Director Information Systems
CHR: Thomas Guilfoil, Director Human Resources
Web address: www.winghealth.org
**Control:** Other not–for–profit (including NFP Corporation) **Service:** General Medical and Surgical

**Staffed Beds:** 74 **Admissions:** 3734 **Census:** 54 **Outpatient Visits:** 244798 **Births:** 0 **Total Expense ($000):** 90000 **Payroll Expense ($000):** 40056 **Personnel:** 565

**PEABODY—Essex County**

⊞ **KINDRED HOSPITAL BOSTON–NORTH SHORE (222044)**, 15 King Street, Zip 01960–4379; tel. 978/531–2900, (Nonreporting) **A**1 10 **S** Kindred Healthcare, Louisville, KY
Primary Contact: Yolande Wilson, Chief Executive Officer
CFO: John Couillard, Chief Financial Officer
CMO: M. Akbarian, M.D., Medical Director
CHR: Jan Pray, Coordinator Payroll and Benefits
Web address: www.kindredbns.com
**Control:** Corporation, Investor–owned, for–profit **Service:** General Medical and Surgical

**Staffed Beds:** 50

**PEMBROKE—Plymouth County**

**PEMBROKE HOSPITAL**, 199 Oak Street, Zip 02359–1953; tel. 781/829–7000, (Nonreporting) **A**9 **S** Universal Health Services, Inc., King of Prussia, PA
Primary Contact: Thomas P. Hickey, Chief Executive Officer and Managing Director
CFO: Diane Airosus, Chief Financial Officer
CMO: Gary Jacobson, M.D., Chief Medical Officer
Web address: www.arbourhealth.com/pembroke.htm
**Control:** Partnership, Investor–owned, for–profit **Service:** Psychiatric

**Staffed Beds:** 80

**PITTSFIELD—Berkshire County**

⊞ **BERKSHIRE MEDICAL CENTER (220046)**, 725 North Street, Zip 01201–4124; tel. 413/447–2000, (Includes HILLCREST HOSPITAL, 165 Tor Court, Zip 01201–3099, Mailing Address: Box 1155, Zip 01202–1155; tel. 413/443–4761) **A**1 2 3 5 8 9 10 12 13 **F**3 4 5 8 12 13 14 15 17 18 20 26 28 29 30 31 32 34 35 38 39 40 43 44 49 50 51 53 54 55 56 57 58 59 60 61 62 64 65 68 70 71 74 75 76 77 78 79 81 82 84 85 86 87 89 90 93 96 98 99 100 101 102 103 104 105 107 108 110 111 112 113 114 117 118 119 120 122 123 125 128 129 130 131 133 134 143 144 145 146 147 **P**6 **S** Berkshire Health Systems, Inc., Pittsfield, MA
Primary Contact: Diane Kelly, R.N., Chief Operating Officer
CFO: Darlene Rodowicz, Chief Financial Officer
CMO: Robert Cella, M.D., Vice President Medical Affairs
CHR: Arthur D. Milano, Vice President Human Resources
Web address: www.berkshirehealthsystems.com
**Control:** Other not–for–profit (including NFP Corporation) **Service:** General Medical and Surgical

**Staffed Beds:** 278 **Admissions:** 11883 **Census:** 171 **Outpatient Visits:** 432065 **Births:** 655 **Total Expense ($000):** 307689 **Payroll Expense ($000):** 149352 **Personnel:** 2037

MA

---

**Hospital, Medicare Provider Number, Address, Telephone, Approval, Facility, and Physician Codes, Health Care System**

★ American Hospital Association (AHA) membership
☐ The Joint Commission accreditation
◇ DNV Healthcare Inc. accreditation
○ American Osteopathic Association (AOA) accreditation
△ Commission on Accreditation of Rehabilitation Facilities (CARF) accreditation

**MA**

## PLYMOUTH—Plymouth County

⊞ **JORDAN HOSPITAL (220060)**, 275 Sandwich Street, Zip 02360–2196;
tel. 508/746–2000 **A**1 2 9 10 **F**3 13 15 17 18 20 28 29 30 31 34 35 36 37
40 44 45 51 57 58 59 61 62 64 68 70 73 74 75 76 77 78 79 81 82 85 86
87 89 93 96 98 100 102 103 104 107 108 109 110 111 114 116 117 118
119 120 122 128 129 130 131 133 134 142 143 145 146 147 **P**6
Primary Contact: Peter J. Holden, President and Chief Executive Officer
COO: James E. Fanale, M.D., Senior Vice President System Development
CFO: Joseph Iannoni, Vice President Finance
CIO: James Albert, Chief Information Officer
CNO: Donna Doherty, R.N., Vice President of Nursing and Chief Nursing Officer
Web address: www.jordanhospital.org
**Control:** Other not–for–profit (including NFP Corporation) **Service:** General
Medical and Surgical

Staffed Beds: 155 Admissions: 10567 Census: 122 Outpatient Visits:
274808 Births: 590 Total Expense ($000): 190046 Payroll Expense
($000): 82308 Personnel: 862

## POCASSET—Barnstable County

**CAPE COD & ISLAND COMMUNITY MENTAL HEALTH CENTER (224031)**,
830 County Road, Zip 02559–2110; tel. 508/564–9600, (Nonreporting) **A**10
Primary Contact: Steven Jochim, Administrator
**Control:** Other not–for–profit (including NFP Corporation) **Service:** Psychiatric

Staffed Beds: 24

## QUINCY—Norfolk County

☐ **QUINCY MEDICAL CENTER (220067)**, 114 Whitwell Street, Zip 02169–1899;
tel. 617/773–6100, (Nonreporting) **A**1 2 3 5 9 10 **S** Steward Health Care
System, LLC, Boston, MA
Primary Contact: Daniel J. Knell, MSN, President
CMO: Apurv Gupta, M.D., Chief Medical Officer
CHR: Victor Munger, Vice President Human Resources
Web address: www.quincymc.org
**Control:** Corporation, Investor–owned, for–profit **Service:** General Medical and
Surgical

Staffed Beds: 116

## ROCHDALE—Worcester County

**KINDRED HOSPITAL PARK VIEW–CENTRAL MASSACHUSETTS** See Kindred
Hospital Park View, Springfield

## SALEM—Essex County

**NORTH SHORE CHILDREN'S HOSPITAL** See MassGeneral for Children at North
Shore Medical Center

⊞ **NORTH SHORE MEDICAL CENTER (220035)**, 81 Highland Avenue,
Zip 01970–2714; tel. 978/741–1200, (Includes MASSGENERAL FOR CHILDREN
AT NORTH SHORE MEDICAL CENTER, 57 Highland Avenue, Zip 01970–6508;
tel. 978/745–2100; SALEM CAMPUS, 81 Highland Avenue, Zip 01970;
tel. 978/741–1200; UNION CAMPUS, 500 Lynnfield Street, Lynn,
Zip 01904–1487; tel. 781/581–9200) **A**1 3 5 9 10 **F**5 12 13 15 17 18 20 22
24 26 28 29 30 31 32 34 35 36 38 40 43 45 46 49 50 51 55 57 59 61 63
64 68 70 73 74 75 76 77 78 79 81 82 84 85 86 87 89 93 98 99 100 101
102 103 104 105 107 108 111 113 115 117 118 120 122 128 129 130 131
134 142 145 146 147 **P**6 8 **S** Partners HealthCare System, Inc., Boston, MA
Primary Contact: Robert G. Norton, President and Chief Executive Officer
CFO: Sally Mason Boemer, Chief Financial Officer
CMO: Mitchell S. Rein, M.D., Chief Medical Officer
CIO: Patricia George, Chief Information Officer
CHR: Arthur Bowes, Senior Vice President Human Resources
Web address: www.nsmc.partners.org
**Control:** Other not–for–profit (including NFP Corporation) **Service:** General
Medical and Surgical

Staffed Beds: 395 Admissions: 19467 Census: 255 Outpatient Visits:
634987 Births: 1549 Total Expense ($000): 412082 Payroll Expense
($000): 193917 Personnel: 2466

**SALEM HOSPITAL** See Salem Campus

⊞ △ **SPAULDING HOSPITAL FOR CONTINUING MEDICAL CARE NORTH
SHORE (222026)**, 1 Dove Avenue, Zip 01970–2999; tel. 978/825–8900,
(Nonreporting) **A**1 7 10 **S** Partners HealthCare System, Inc., Boston, MA
Primary Contact: Maureen Banks, R.N., MS, President
COO: Joanne Fucile, R.N., Vice President Patient Care Services
CFO: Virginia Mirisola, Fiscal Director
CIO: Robert Sawyer, Senior Project Specialist
CHR: Colleen M. Moran, Director Human Resources
Web address: www.shaughnessy–kaplan.org
**Control:** Other not–for–profit (including NFP Corporation) **Service:** General
Medical and Surgical

Staffed Beds: 160

## SOMERVILLE—Middlesex County

**SOMERVILLE HOSPITAL** See Cambridge Health Alliance, Cambridge

## SOUTH WEYMOUTH—Norfolk County

⊞ **SOUTH SHORE HOSPITAL (220100)**, 55 Fogg Road, Zip 02190–2432;
tel. 781/624–8000 **A**1 2 3 5 9 10 **F**3 7 11 13 15 17 18 20 22 24 26 28 29
30 31 32 34 35 36 37 40 41 43 44 45 46 49 50 51 53 54 55 57 58 59 60
62 63 64 65 68 70 72 73 74 75 76 78 79 81 82 84 85 86 87 89 91 92 93
107 108 110 111 113 114 117 118 123 125 128 129 131 133 134 142 145
146 147 **P**1
Primary Contact: Richard H. Aubut, R.N., President and Chief Executive Officer
COO: Joseph Cahill, Executive Vice President and Chief Operating Officer
CFO: Michael Cullen, Senior Vice President and Chief Financial Officer
CMO: John Stevenson, M.D., Senior Vice President and Chief Medical Officer
CIO: Del Dixon, Chief Information Officer
CHR: Robert Wheeler, Vice President Human Resources
Web address: www.southshorehospital.org
**Control:** Other not–for–profit (including NFP Corporation) **Service:** General
Medical and Surgical

Staffed Beds: 327 Admissions: 23070 Census: 256 Outpatient Visits:
508729 Births: 3639 Total Expense ($000): 417772 Payroll Expense
($000): 205608 Personnel: 3092

## SOUTHBRIDGE—Worcester County

⊞ **HARRINGTON MEMORIAL HOSPITAL (220019)**, 100 South Street,
Zip 01550–4051; tel. 508/765–9771 **A**1 5 9 10 **F**3 5 8 11 13 15 17 18 19 28
29 30 31 32 34 35 38 39 40 42 45 49 50 51 54 57 59 61 64 65 68 70
71 74 75 76 77 78 79 81 82 85 86 87 89 92 93 94 96 98 99 100 101 102
103 104 107 108 110 111 113 114 116 117 118 119 120 122 123 128 129
130 131 133 134 145 146 147 **P**8
Primary Contact: Edward H. Moore, President and Chief Executive Officer
COO: Douglas Crapser, Executive Vice President
CFO: Thomas Sullivan, Vice President Fiscal Services
CMO: Arthur Russo, M.D., Director Medical Affairs
CIO: Hadley Zabinsky, Chief Information Officer
CHR: Charlene Richard, Director Human Resources
Web address: www.harringtonhospital.org
**Control:** Other not–for–profit (including NFP Corporation) **Service:** General
Medical and Surgical

Staffed Beds: 114 Admissions: 4488 Census: 54 Outpatient Visits: 306567
Births: 309 Total Expense ($000): 103731 Payroll Expense ($000): 48852
Personnel: 669

## SPRINGFIELD—Hampden County

⊞ **BAYSTATE MEDICAL CENTER (220077)**, 759 Chestnut Street,
Zip 01199–0001; tel. 413/794–0000, (Includes BAYSTATE CHILDREN'S
HOSPITAL, 759 Chestnut Street, Zip 01199–1001; tel. 413/794–0000) **A**1 2 3 5
8 9 10 **F**3 5 8 12 13 14 15 17 18 19 20 22 24 26 28 29 30 31 32 34 35 38
40 41 43 44 45 46 47 48 49 50 51 52 53 54 55 56 57 58 59 60 61 64 65
66 68 70 72 74 75 76 77 78 79 81 82 85 86 87 88 89 91 92 93 97 98 99
100 101 102 103 104 105 107 108 110 111 113 114 117 118 119 120 122
123 125 128 129 130 131 137 140 142 144 145 146 147 **P**5 8 **S** Baystate
Health, Inc., Springfield, MA
Primary Contact: Mark R. Tolosky, JD, FACHE, President and Chief Executive
Officer
COO: Gregory A. Harb, FACHE, Executive Vice President and Chief Operating
Officer
CFO: Keith C McLean Shinaman, Senior Vice President Finance
CMO: Loring S. Flint, Jr., M.D., Senior Vice President Medical Affairs
CIO: Mark Gorrell, Vice President Information Services
CHR: Paula C. Squires, Senior Vice President Human Resources
Web address: www.baystatehealth.org
**Control:** Other not–for–profit (including NFP Corporation) **Service:** General
Medical and Surgical

Staffed Beds: 659 Admissions: 32716 Census: 461 Outpatient Visits:
729430 Births: 4264 Total Expense ($000): 825845 Payroll Expense
($000): 336434 Personnel: 8492

★ **KINDRED HOSPITAL PARK VIEW (222046)**, 1400 State Street,
Zip 01109–2550; tel. 413/726–6700, (Includes KINDRED HOSPITAL PARK
VIEW–CENTRAL MASSACHUSETTS, 111 Huntoon Memorial Highway, Rochdale,
Zip 01542; tel. 508/892–6000; Scott MacLean, Administrator), (Nonreporting)
**A**10 **S** Kindred Healthcare, Louisville, KY
Primary Contact: Jake Socha, Chief Executive Officer
CFO: Anna Dyrkacz, Chief Financial Officer
CHR: Donna Ciarefella, Director Human Resources
Web address: www.khparkview.com/
**Control:** Corporation, Investor–owned, for–profit **Service:** Long–Term Acute Care
hospital

Staffed Beds: 202

⊠ △ **MERCY MEDICAL CENTER (220066)**, 271 Carew Street, Zip 01104–2398, Mailing Address: P.O. Box 9012, Zip 01102–9012; tel. 413/748–9000, (Nonreporting) **A**1 2 7 9 10 **S** Catholic Health East, Newtown Square, PA
Primary Contact: Daniel P. Moen, President and Chief Executive Officer
COO: William Bithoney, M.D., Chief Operating Officer
CFO: Michael Hammond, Chief Financial Officer
CMO: William Bithoney, M.D., Chief Operating Officer
CIO: Joan Methe, Chief Information Officer
CHR: Leonard F. Pansa, Senior Vice President Human Resources
Web address: www.mercycares.com
**Control:** Other not–for–profit (including NFP Corporation) **Service:** General Medical and Surgical

**Staffed Beds:** 221

☐ **SHRINERS HOSPITALS FOR CHILDREN, SPRINGFIELD (223303)**, 516 Carew Street, Zip 01104–2396; tel. 413/787–2000 **A**1 3 5 10 **F**34 35 37 39 44 50 58 59 62 64 68 74 75 77 79 81 85 86 87 89 91 92 93 94 96 108 118 129 145 147 **P**6 **S** Shriners Hospitals for Children, Tampa, FL
Primary Contact: Charles Walczak, FACHE, Administrator
COO: Charles Walczak, FACHE, Administrator
CFO: Richard Fulkerson, Director Fiscal Services
CMO: David M. Drvaric, M.D., Chief of Staff
CIO: Kenneth Ward, Director Information Services
CHR: Kathleen Bachetti, Director Human Resources
Web address: www.shrinershq.org
**Control:** Other not–for–profit (including NFP Corporation) **Service:** Children's orthopedic

**Staffed Beds:** 20 **Admissions:** 359 **Census:** 4 **Outpatient Visits:** 14685 **Births:** 0 **Total Expense ($000):** 23190 **Payroll Expense ($000):** 11177 **Personnel:** 176

**STOCKBRIDGE—Berkshire County**

⊠ **AUSTEN RIGGS CENTER**, 25 Main Street, Zip 01262–0962, Mailing Address: P.O. Box 962, Zip 01262–0962; tel. 413/298–5511 **A**1 3 **F**98 105 106
Primary Contact: Chauncey Collins, Director Operations
COO: Edward R. Shapiro, M.D., Medical Director and Chief Executive Officer
CFO: Chauncey Collins, Director Operations
CMO: Edward R. Shapiro, M.D., Medical Director and Chief Executive Officer
CIO: Ave Schwartz, Chief Information Officer
CHR: Bertha Connelley, Director Human Resources
Web address: www.austenriggs.org
**Control:** Other not–for–profit (including NFP Corporation) **Service:** Psychiatric

**Staffed Beds:** 74 **Admissions:** 92 **Census:** 58 **Outpatient Visits:** 0 **Births:** 0 **Total Expense ($000):** 16317 **Payroll Expense ($000):** 8507 **Personnel:** 141

**STOUGHTON—Norfolk County**

⊠ **KINDRED HOSPITAL NORTHEAST–STOUGHTON (222002)**, 909 Sumner Street, 1st Floor, Zip 2072; tel. 781/297–8200, (Nonreporting) **A**1 10 **S** Kindred Healthcare, Louisville, KY
Primary Contact: Robert A. Gundersen, Market Chief Executive Officer
Web address: www.khstoughton.com
**Control:** Corporation, Investor–owned, for–profit **Service:** Long–Term Acute Care hospital

**Staffed Beds:** 170

⊠ △ **NEW ENGLAND SINAI HOSPITAL AND REHABILITATION CENTER (222027)**, 150 York Street, Zip 02072–1881; tel. 781/344–0600 **A**1 3 5 7 10 **F**1 2 3 6 29 30 34 50 56 57 58 59 60 61 64 65 68 75 77 78 82 83 84 85 86 87 90 91 92 93 94 96 128 129 130 131 134 145 147 **P**6
Primary Contact: Judith C. Waterston, R.N., MS, President and Chief Executive Officer
CFO: Kevin Leonard, Vice President for Finance and Chief Financial Officer
CMO: Lawrence S. Hotes, M.D., Chief Medical Officer
CIO: Francine Sousa, Director Management Information Service
CHR: Nanette Smith Callihan, Vice President Human Resources
CNO: Janet M. Madigan, MS, Vice President for Patient Care Services
Web address: www.newenglandsinai.org
**Control:** Other not–for–profit (including NFP Corporation) **Service:** Long–Term Acute Care hospital

**Staffed Beds:** 212 **Admissions:** 1650 **Census:** 158 **Outpatient Visits:** 31426 **Births:** 0 **Total Expense ($000):** 79229 **Payroll Expense ($000):** 44945 **Personnel:** 669

**TAUNTON—Bristol County**

⊠ **MORTON HOSPITAL AND MEDICAL CENTER (220073)**, 88 Washington Street, Zip 02780–2465; tel. 508/828–7000, (Nonreporting) **A**1 2 9 10 **S** Steward Health Care System, LLC, Boston, MA
Primary Contact: Michael J. Schwartz, Interim President
CFO: Richard Jeffcote, Chief Financial Officer
CIO: Harry Lemieux, Chief Information and Innovation Officer
CHR: Cara Hart, Director Human Resources
Web address: www.mortonhospital.org
**Control:** Corporation, Investor–owned, for–profit **Service:** General Medical and Surgical

**Staffed Beds:** 153

☐ **TAUNTON STATE HOSPITAL (224001)**, 60 Hodges Avenue Extension, Zip 02780–3034, Mailing Address: PO Box 4007, Zip 02780–0997; tel. 508/977–3000, (Nonreporting) **A**1 10 **S** Massachusetts Department of Mental Health, Boston, MA
Primary Contact: Roberta H. Guez, Chief Operating Officer
COO: Roberta H. Guez, Chief Operating Officer
CMO: Whitney Wolff, M.D., Medical Director
CHR: Trish Scully, Director Human Resources
**Control:** State–Government, nonfederal **Service:** Psychiatric

**Staffed Beds:** 185

**TEWKSBURY—Middlesex County**

☐ **TEWKSBURY HOSPITAL (222003)**, 365 East Street, Zip 01876–1998; tel. 978/851–7321, (Nonreporting) **A**1 10 **S** Massachusetts Department of Public Health, Boston, MA
Primary Contact: Debra Tosti, Interim Chief Executive Officer
COO: Debra Tosti, Chief Operating Officer
CFO: Maureen DiPalma, Director Finance
Web address: www.state.ma.us/dph/hosp/th.htm
**Control:** State–Government, nonfederal **Service:** Long–Term Acute Care hospital

**Staffed Beds:** 720

**WALTHAM—Middlesex County**

☐ **WALDEN PSYCHIATRIC CARE (224038)**, 9 Hope Avenue, Zip 02453–2741; tel. 781/647–6700, (Nonreporting) **A**1 9 10
Primary Contact: Stuart Koman, Ph.D., President and Chief Executive Officer
Web address: www.waldenbehavioralcare.com/
**Control:** Other not–for–profit (including NFP Corporation) **Service:** Psychiatric

**Staffed Beds:** 45

**WARE—Hampshire County**

⊠ **BAYSTATE MARY LANE HOSPITAL (220050)**, 85 South Street, Zip 01082–1697; tel. 413/967–6211, (Nonreporting) **A**1 9 10 **S** Baystate Health, Inc., Springfield, MA
Primary Contact: Charles Gijanto, President
COO: Gregory A. Harb, FACHE, Executive Vice President and Chief Operating Officer
CFO: Curtis Davis, Director Finance
CMO: Mohammed Shafeeq Ahmed, M.D., Chief Operating Officer and Chief Medical Officer
CIO: Joel L. Vengco, MS, Vice President and Chief Information Officer, Baystate Health
CHR: Donna Arsenault, Director Human Resources
CNO: Lisa Beaudry, M.P.H., Director, Patient Care
Web address: www.baystatehealth.com
**Control:** Other not–for–profit (including NFP Corporation) **Service:** General Medical and Surgical

**Staffed Beds:** 31

**WAREHAM—Plymouth County**

**TOBEY HOSPITAL** See Southcoast Hospitals Group, Fall River

**WESTBOROUGH—Worcester County**

☐ **WHITTIER REHABILITATION HOSPITAL (222048)**, 150 Flanders Road, Zip 1581; tel. 508/871–2000, (Nonreporting) **A**1 10 **S** Whittier Health Network, Haverhill, MA
Primary Contact: Alfred J. Arcidi, M.D., Senior Vice President
Web address: www.whittierhealth.com
**Control:** Partnership, Investor–owned, for–profit **Service:** Long–Term Acute Care hospital

**Staffed Beds:** 74

---

**Hospital, Medicare Provider Number, Address, Telephone, Approval, Facility, and Physician Codes, Health Care System**

★ American Hospital Association (AHA) membership
☐ The Joint Commission accreditation
◇ DNV Healthcare Inc. accreditation
○ American Osteopathic Association (AOA) accreditation
△ Commission on Accreditation of Rehabilitation Facilities (CARF) accreditation

## WESTFIELD—Hampden County

✠ **NOBLE HOSPITAL (220065)**, 115 West Silver Street, Zip 01086–1634;
tel. 413/568–2811 **A**1 2 5 9 10 **F**8 14 15 18 29 30 31 34 35 40 57 59 68 70
75 77 78 79 80 81 86 87 89 90 93 98 100 101 102 103 104 105 107 108
110 111 114 115 116 118 129 131 145 146 147 **P**8
Primary Contact: Ron Bryant, President and Chief Executive Officer
CFO: John Shaver, Chief Financial Officer
CMO: Stanley Strzempko, M.D., Vice President Medical Affairs and Chief Medical Officer
CIO: Steven Cummings, Chief Operating Officer and Chief Information Officer
CHR: Joanne Ollson, Vice President Human Resources
CNO: Diane Brunelle, MSN, Vice President of Patient Care Services and Chief Nursing Officer
Web address: www.noblehealth.org
**Control:** Other not–for–profit (including NFP Corporation) **Service:** General Medical and Surgical

**Staffed Beds:** 97 **Admissions:** 3454 **Census:** 54 **Outpatient Visits:** 118241 **Births:** 0 **Total Expense ($000):** 52035 **Payroll Expense ($000):** 24516 **Personnel:** 327

☐ **WESTERN MASSACHUSETTS HOSPITAL (222023)**, 91 East Mountain Road,
Zip 1085; tel. 413/562–4131, (Nonreporting) **A**1 10 **S** Massachusetts
Department of Public Health, Boston, MA
Primary Contact: Derrick Tallman, Chief Executive Officer
CMO: Chabilal Neergheen, M.D., Medical Director
CHR: James E. Duggan, Director Human Resources
Web address: www.mass.gov/dph/hosp/wmh.htm
**Control:** State–Government, nonfederal **Service:** General Medical and Surgical

**Staffed Beds:** 70

## WESTWOOD—Norfolk County

☐ **WESTWOOD LODGE HOSPITAL (224023)**, 45 Clapboardtree Street,
Zip 02090–2930; tel. 781/762–7764 **A**1 9 10 **F**29 98 99 105 **S** Universal
Health Services, Inc., King of Prussia, PA
Primary Contact: Gregory Brownstein, Chief Executive Officer
CFO: Charles Denno, Chief Financial Officer
Web address: www.arbourhealth.com
**Control:** Corporation, Investor–owned, for–profit **Service:** Psychiatric

**Staffed Beds:** 130 **Admissions:** 3681 **Census:** 105 **Outpatient Visits:** 0 **Births:** 0

## WHITINSVILLE—Worcester County

**WHITINSVILLE MEDICAL CENTER** See Milford Regional Medical Center, Milford

## WINCHESTER—Middlesex County

✠ **WINCHESTER HOSPITAL (220105)**, 41 Highland Avenue, Zip 01890–1496;
tel. 781/729–9000 **A**1 2 3 5 9 10 **F**12 13 15 18 28 29 30 31 32 34 35 36 38
40 41 42 46 48 49 50 51 56 57 59 62 64 68 70 72 74 75 76 77 78 79 81
82 85 86 87 89 93 107 108 110 111 113 114 116 117 118 125 128 129
131 134 143 144 145 146 147 **P**2 5 6 7
Primary Contact: Kevin F. Smith, President and Chief Executive Officer
CFO: Matthew Woods, Executive Vice President Finance and Chief Financial Officer
CMO: Richard Iseke, M.D., Vice President Medical Affairs
CHR: Anne Lang, Vice President Human Resources and Compliance and Privacy Officer
CNO: Kathy Schuler, R.N., Vice President of Patient Care Services
Web address: www.winchesterhospital.org
**Control:** Other not–for–profit (including NFP Corporation) **Service:** General Medical and Surgical

**Staffed Beds:** 200 **Admissions:** 13429 **Census:** 141 **Outpatient Visits:** 584930 **Births:** 2100 **Total Expense ($000):** 253384 **Payroll Expense ($000):** 119979 **Personnel:** 1737

## WOBURN—Middlesex County

☐ **NEW ENGLAND REHABILITATION HOSPITAL (223026)**, Two Rehabilitation
Way, Zip 01801–6098; tel. 781/935–5050, (Nonreporting) **A**1 10 **S** Five Star
Quality Care, Newton, MA
Primary Contact: Joel Rudin, Chief Executive Officer
CFO: Lester Felege, Controller
CMO: A. Deniz Ozel, M.D., Medical Director
CHR: Annamarie Cronin, Director Human Resources
Web address: www.newenglandrehab.com
**Control:** Corporation, Investor–owned, for–profit **Service:** Rehabilitation

**Staffed Beds:** 210

## WORCESTER—Worcester County

**ADCARE HOSPITAL OF WORCESTER (220062)**, 107 Lincoln Street,
Zip 01605–2499; tel. 508/799–9000, (Nonreporting) **A**5 9 10
Primary Contact: David W. Hillis, President and Chief Executive Officer
COO: Jeffrey W. Hillis, Chief Operating Officer
CFO: Christine Judycki–Crepeault, Chief Financial Officer
CMO: Ronald F. Pike, M.D., Medical Director
CHR: Joan L. Bertrand, Vice President Human Resources
Web address: www.adcare.com
**Control:** Other not–for–profit (including NFP Corporation) **Service:** Alcoholism and other chemical dependency

**Staffed Beds:** 114

★ **FAIRLAWN REHABILITATION HOSPITAL (223029)**, 189 May Street,
Zip 01602–4339; tel. 508/791–6351 **A**3 5 10 **F**28 29 34 35 56 57 59 64 74
75 77 79 82 86 87 90 91 93 95 96 129 131 134 145 147 **P**8
**S** HEALTHSOUTH Corporation, Birmingham, AL
Primary Contact: R. David Richer, Chief Executive Officer
CFO: John Flaherty, Controller
CMO: Peter Bagley, M.D., Medical Director
CIO: Elizabeth Hemingway, Director Health Information
CHR: Rosalie Lawless, Director Human Resources
Web address: www.fairlawnrehab.org
**Control:** Corporation, Investor–owned, for–profit **Service:** Rehabilitation

**Staffed Beds:** 110 **Admissions:** 2121 **Census:** 80 **Outpatient Visits:** 8953 **Births:** 0 **Total Expense ($000):** 26160 **Payroll Expense ($000):** 14570 **Personnel:** 277

✠ **SAINT VINCENT HOSPITAL (220176)**, 123 Summer Street, Zip 1608;
tel. 508/363–5000 **A**1 2 3 5 9 10 12 **F**12 13 15 17 18 20 22 24 26 28 29 30
31 35 38 40 45 46 47 48 49 50 57 59 60 63 64 68 70 74 75 76 77 78 79
81 82 84 85 86 87 89 92 93 97 98 100 101 102 107 108 110 111 113 114
116 117 118 119 120 122 123 125 128 129 130 131 134 145 **S** Vanguard
Health System, Nashville, TN
Primary Contact: Erik G. Wexler, President and Chief Executive Officer
COO: Deborah Bitsoli, Chief Operating Officer
CFO: Stephen Gilmore, Chief Financial Officer
CMO: Octavio Diaz, M.D., Chief Medical Officer
CIO: Tara Jones, Director Information Services
CHR: Jan Peters, Vice President Human Resources
Web address: www.stvincenthospital.com
**Control:** Corporation, Investor–owned, for–profit **Service:** General Medical and Surgical

**Staffed Beds:** 297 **Admissions:** 17609 **Census:** 179 **Outpatient Visits:** 238755 **Births:** 1910 **Total Expense ($000):** 283873 **Payroll Expense ($000):** 127695 **Personnel:** 1378

✠ **UMASS MEMORIAL MEDICAL CENTER (220163)**, 119 Belmont Street,
Zip 01605–2982; tel. 508/334–1000, (Includes HAHNEMANN CAMPUS, 281
Lincoln Street, Zip 01605; tel. 508/334–1000; MEMORIAL CAMPUS, 119
Belmont Street, Zip 01605; tel. 508/334–1000; UMASS MEMORIAL CHILDREN'S
MEDICAL CENTER, 55 Lake Avenue North, Zip 01655–0002; tel. 508/334–1000;
UNIVERSITY CAMPUS, 55 Lake Avenue North, Zip 01655–0002;
tel. 508/334–1000) **A**1 2 3 5 8 9 10 **F**3 5 7 8 9 12 13 14 15 16 17 18 19 20
22 24 25 26 28 29 30 31 32 38 40 41 43 45 46 47 48 49 50 51 52 54 55
56 60 61 62 63 64 65 68 70 71 72 73 74 75 76 78 79 81 82 83 84 85 87
88 89 91 92 93 97 98 99 100 101 102 103 104 107 108 110 113 114 117
118 119 120 122 123 125 126 128 129 130 131 132 133 134 135 137 138
141 143 144 145 146 147 **P**1 8 **S** UMass Memorial Health Care, Inc.,
Worcester, MA
Primary Contact: John G. O'Brien, President and Chief Executive Officer
COO: Andrew Sussman, M.D., Chief Operating Officer
CFO: Therese Day, Chief Financial Officer
CMO: Stephen Tosi, M.D., Chief Medical Officer
CIO: George Brenkle, Chief Information Officer
CHR: Patricia G. Webb, Senior Vice President Human Resources
Web address: www.umassmemorial.org
**Control:** Other not–for–profit (including NFP Corporation) **Service:** General Medical and Surgical

**Staffed Beds:** 682 **Admissions:** 42727 **Census:** 589 **Outpatient Visits:** 1029928 **Births:** 4115 **Total Expense ($000):** 1288816 **Payroll Expense ($000):** 464122 **Personnel:** 8871

☐ **WORCESTER STATE HOSPITAL (224032)**, 305 Belmont Street,
Zip 01604–1695; tel. 508/368–3300, (Nonreporting) **A**1 3 5 10
**S** Massachusetts Department of Mental Health, Boston, MA
Primary Contact: Anthony Riccitelli, Chief Operating Officer
COO: Anthony Riccitelli, Chief Operating Officer
CMO: Kathleen Whitley, M.D., Director Clinical and Professional Service
CIO: Ron Medciros, Director Applied Information Technology
**Control:** State–Government, nonfederal **Service:** Psychiatric

**Staffed Beds:** 126

MA

*Many Facility Codes have changed. Please refer to the AHA Guide Code Chart.* © 2012 AHA Guide

# MICHIGAN

## ADRIAN—Lenawee County

★ ○ **PROMEDICA BIXBY HOSPITAL (230005)**, 818 Riverside Avenue, Zip 49221–1496; tel. 517/265–0900 **A**2 9 10 11 **F**3 11 13 15 18 20 28 29 31 34 40 45 50 51 57 59 60 64 65 68 70 74 75 76 77 78 79 81 82 85 92 93 100 102 103 104 107 108 110 111 113 116 117 118 119 120 129 130 131 134 144 145 147 **P**6 7 8 **S** ProMedica Health System, Toledo, OH
Primary Contact: Timothy Jakacki, President
CFO: Bernie Nawrocki, Administrative Director Finance
CMO: Julie Yaroch, D.O., Vice President Medical Affairs
CIO: Carol Boyce, Administrative Director Support Services
CHR: Cathy J. Davis, Director Human Resources
CNO: Kathryn M. Greenlee, R.N., Vice President, Clinical Services/CNO
Web address: www.promedica.org
**Control:** Other not–for–profit (including NFP Corporation) **Service:** General Medical and Surgical

**Staffed Beds:** 66 **Admissions:** 4217 **Census:** 41 **Outpatient Visits:** 150867 **Births:** 776 **Total Expense ($000):** 72814 **Payroll Expense ($000):** 24320 **Personnel:** 515

## ALLEGAN—Allegan County

★ △ **ALLEGAN GENERAL HOSPITAL (231328)**, 555 Linn Street, Zip 49010–1524; tel. 269/673–8424 **A**7 9 10 18 **F**3 12 15 28 29 31 32 34 35 40 45 47 48 50 57 59 62 64 65 68 70 75 77 78 79 81 85 86 87 93 96 99 100 101 104 107 108 110 113 118 126 128 129 130 131 134 144 145 **S** QHR, Brentwood, TN
Primary Contact: Gerald J. Barbini, President and Chief Executive Officer
CFO: Richard Harning, Vice President Finance and Chief Financial Officer
CMO: Nabil Nouna, M.D., Chief of Staff
CIO: David Federinko, Chief Information Officer
CHR: Denise A. Eberth, Director Human Resources
Web address: www.aghosp.org
**Control:** Other not–for–profit (including NFP Corporation) **Service:** General Medical and Surgical

**Staffed Beds:** 25 **Admissions:** 879 **Census:** 9 **Outpatient Visits:** 81007 **Births:** 0 **Total Expense ($000):** 39451 **Payroll Expense ($000):** 16529 **Personnel:** 281

## ALMA—Gratiot County

**GRATIOT MEDICAL CENTER** See MidMichigan Medical Center–Gratiot

⊞ △ **MIDMICHIGAN MEDICAL CENTER–GRATIOT (230030)**, 300 East Warwick Drive, Zip 48801–1014; tel. 989/463–1101, (Nonreporting) **A**1 7 9 10 19 **S** MidMichigan Health, Midland, MI
Primary Contact: Mark A. Santamaria, President
CFO: Victor Morgan, Chief Financial Officer
CIO: Michael Larson, Chief Information Officer
Web address: www.midmichigan.org/gratiot
**Control:** Other not–for–profit (including NFP Corporation) **Service:** General Medical and Surgical

**Staffed Beds:** 136

## ALPENA—Alpena County

⊞ **ALPENA REGIONAL MEDICAL CENTER (230036)**, 1501 West Chisholm Street, Zip 49707–1401; tel. 989/356–7390 **A**1 2 9 10 **F**3 5 11 13 14 15 20 22 28 29 31 34 35 40 43 44 45 46 47 48 49 50 59 62 64 65 70 71 73 74 75 76 77 78 79 81 82 85 86 87 90 93 96 97 98 99 100 101 102 103 104 106 107 108 110 111 113 114 117 118 128 129 130 131 134 145 146 147 **P**6
Primary Contact: Karmon T. Bjella, Chief Executive Officer
COO: Aldean J. Moe, Chief Operating Officer
CFO: George J. Smart, VP Finance & IT
CHR: Diane Shields, Chief Human Resources Officer
CNO: Gayle Bruski, R.N., Chief Nursing Officer
Web address: www.agh.org
**Control:** County–Government, nonfederal **Service:** General Medical and Surgical

**Staffed Beds:** 125 **Admissions:** 4902 **Census:** 63 **Outpatient Visits:** 188851 **Births:** 397 **Total Expense ($000):** 119566 **Payroll Expense ($000):** 47242 **Personnel:** 802

## ANN ARBOR—Washtenaw County

⊞ **UNIVERSITY OF MICHIGAN HOSPITALS AND HEALTH CENTERS (230046)**, 1500 East Medical Center Drive, Zip 48109–5000; tel. 734/936–4000, (Includes C.S. MOTT CHILDREN'S HOSPITAL, 1500 East Medical Center Drive, Zip 48109–5475; tel. 734/936–4000) **A**1 2 3 5 8 9 10 **F**3 5 6 8 9 11 12 13 15 16 17 18 19 20 21 22 23 24 25 26 27 28 29 30 31 32 34 35 36 37 38 39 40 41 43 44 45 46 47 48 49 50 51 52 53 54 55 56 57 58 59 60 61 62 64 65 66 68 69 70 72 74 75 76 77 78 79 80 81 82 84 85 86 87 88 89 90 91 92 93 94 95 97 98 99 100 101 102 103 104 107 108 110 111 113 114 115 116 117 118 119 120 122 123 125 126 128 129 130 131 133 134 135 136 137 138 139 140 141 144 145 146 147 **P**6
Primary Contact: Douglas Strong, Chief Executive Officer
COO: Tony Denton, JD, Chief Operating Officer
CFO: Paul Castillo, Chief Financial Officer
CMO: Darrell Campbell, M.D., Chief Clinical Affairs
CIO: Jocelyn DeWitt, Chief Information Officer
CHR: Deborah Childs, Chief Human Resources Officer
Web address: www.med.umich.edu
**Control:** Other not–for–profit (including NFP Corporation) **Service:** General Medical and Surgical

**Staffed Beds:** 919 **Admissions:** 45137 **Census:** 752 **Outpatient Visits:** 1719649 **Births:** 3738 **Total Expense ($000):** 1957168 **Payroll Expense ($000):** 785953 **Personnel:** 12853

⊞ △ **VETERANS AFFAIRS ANN ARBOR HEALTHCARE SYSTEM**, 2215 Fuller Road, Zip 48105–2399; tel. 734/769–7100, (Total facility includes 40 beds in nursing home–type unit) **A**1 2 3 5 7 8 9 **F**3 5 12 18 20 22 24 26 28 29 30 31 34 35 36 38 39 40 45 46 49 50 54 56 57 58 59 60 61 62 63 64 65 68 70 71 74 75 77 78 79 80 81 82 83 84 85 86 87 91 92 93 94 96 97 98 100 101 102 103 104 105 107 108 111 113 115 116 118 120 122 127 128 129 131 134 142 143 145 146 147 **P**6 **S** Department of Veterans Affairs, Washington, DC
Primary Contact: Robert P. McDivitt, FACHE, Director
COO: Randall Ritter, Associate Director
CFO: Walter Zawisza, Chief Financial Officer
CMO: Eric Young, M.D., Chief of Staff
CIO: Rob Whitehurst, Chief, Office of Information and Technology
CHR: James S. Lodge, Chief Human Resources
CNO: Stacey Breedveld, R.N., Associate Director for Patient Care
Web address: www.annarbor.va.gov
**Control:** Veterans Affairs, Government, federal **Service:** General Medical and Surgical

**Staffed Beds:** 105 **Admissions:** 5674 **Census:** 83 **Outpatient Visits:** 466235 **Births:** 0 **Personnel:** 1971

## AUBURN HILLS—Oakland County

☐ **HAVENWYCK HOSPITAL (234023)**, 1525 University Drive, Zip 48326–2673; tel. 248/373–9200 **A**1 9 10 **F**98 99 102 105 129 **P**8 **S** Universal Health Services, Inc., King of Prussia, PA
Primary Contact: David C. Bell, Chief Executive Officer
CFO: Mirhee Chun, Chief Financial Officer
Web address: www.havenwyckhospital.com
**Control:** Corporation, Investor–owned, for–profit **Service:** Psychiatric

**Staffed Beds:** 242 **Admissions:** 5567 **Census:** 189 **Outpatient Visits:** 4291 **Births:** 0 **Total Expense ($000):** 33476 **Payroll Expense ($000):** 13688 **Personnel:** 315

## BAD AXE—Huron County

★ **HURON MEDICAL CENTER (230118)**, 1100 South Van Dyke Road, Zip 48413–9615; tel. 989/269–9521 **A**9 10 20 **F**3 11 13 14 15 18 20 28 29 31 32 34 35 40 45 53 56 57 59 64 70 74 75 76 77 78 79 81 85 93 97 107 108 113 118 126 129 131 133 134 143 145 **P**6
Primary Contact: Janet Sternberg, President and Chief Executive Officer
CFO: Jeffery Longbrake, Chief Financial Officer
CMO: Jerome Yaklic, M.D., Chief of Staff
CHR: Nancy Bouck, Director Human Resources
Web address: www.huronmedicalcenter.org
**Control:** Other not–for–profit (including NFP Corporation) **Service:** General Medical and Surgical

**Staffed Beds:** 37 **Admissions:** 1592 **Census:** 12 **Outpatient Visits:** 52689 **Births:** 359 **Total Expense ($000):** 34109 **Payroll Expense ($000):** 13823 **Personnel:** 421

---

**Hospital, Medicare Provider Number, Address, Telephone, Approval, Facility, and Physician Codes, Health Care System**

★ American Hospital Association (AHA) membership
☐ The Joint Commission accreditation
◇ DNV Healthcare Inc. accreditation
○ American Osteopathic Association (AOA) accreditation
△ Commission on Accreditation of Rehabilitation Facilities (CARF) accreditation

## BATTLE CREEK—Calhoun County

☒ **BRONSON BATTLE CREEK (230075)**, 300 North Avenue, Zip 49017-3307; tel. 269/966-8000, (Includes FIELDSTONE CENTER, 165 North Washington Avenue, Zip 49037; tel. 616/964-7121; MAIN CAMPUS, 300 North Avenue, Zip 49017; tel. 616/966-8000) **A**1 2 9 10 **F**3 13 15 18 20 26 28 29 30 31 35 40 43 49 50 58 59 60 64 65 68 70 71 74 75 76 77 78 79 81 84 85 86 87 92 93 97 98 100 101 102 103 104 107 108 110 111 113 114 117 118 119 120 122 125 128 129 130 131 134 142 143 145 146 147 **P**6 8 **S** Bronson Healthcare Group, Inc., Kalamazoo, MI
Primary Contact: Denise Brooks–Williams, President and Chief Executive Officer
CFO: Anne Regling, Interim Chief Financial Officer
CMO: Thomas Ignaczak, M.D., Interim Vice President Medical Affairs
CIO: Jim Keller, Director Information Services
CHR: Cathy Edwards, Director Organization and Talent Effectiveness
Web address: www.bchealth.com
**Control:** Other not–for–profit (including NFP Corporation) **Service:** General Medical and Surgical

**Staffed Beds:** 218 **Admissions:** 10361 **Census:** 119 **Outpatient Visits:** 198976 **Births:** 921 **Total Expense ($000):** 219665 **Payroll Expense ($000):** 77944 **Personnel:** 1203

☒ **SELECT SPECIALTY HOSPITAL–BATTLE CREEK (232035)**, 300 North Avenue, Zip 49017-3307; tel. 269/964-9075, (Nonreporting) **A**1 9 10 **S** Select Medical Corporation, Mechanicsburg, PA
Primary Contact: Gerrie Baarson, Chief Executive Officer
Web address: www.selectmedicalcorp.com
**Control:** Corporation, Investor–owned, for–profit **Service:** Long–Term Acute Care hospital

**Staffed Beds:** 25

☐ **SOUTHWEST REGIONAL REHABILITATION CENTER (233025)**, 393 East Roosevelt Avenue, Zip 49017-3333; tel. 269/965-3206, (Nonreporting) **A**1 9 10
Primary Contact: Stan Tooley, President and Chief Executive Officer
CFO: Stephen Jessup, Chief Financial Officer
CMO: Mehmet Yilmaz, M.D., Medical Director
CIO: Rick Albaugh, Manager Information Services
CHR: Karol A. Jenney, Director Business Operations
Web address: www.sw–rehab.org
**Control:** Other not–for–profit (including NFP Corporation) **Service:** Rehabilitation

**Staffed Beds:** 26

☒ △ **VETERANS AFFAIRS MEDICAL CENTER**, 5500 Armstrong Road, Zip 49037; tel. 269/966-5600, (Nonreporting) **A**1 7 9 **S** Department of Veterans Affairs, Washington, DC
Primary Contact: Denise Deitzen, Acting Director
COO: Edward G. Dornoff, Associate Director
CFO: James M. Rupert, Chief Fiscal Services
CMO: Wilfredo Rodriguez, M.D., Chief of Staff
CIO: Scott Hershberger, Acting Chief Information Management Services
CHR: Palma Simkins, Chief Human Resources Management Services
CNO: Kay Bower, Associate Director for Patient Care Services
Web address: www.battlecreek.va.gov/
**Control:** Veterans Affairs, Government, federal **Service:** Psychiatric

**Staffed Beds:** 313

## BAY CITY—Bay County

☒ △ **MCLAREN BAY REGION (230041)**, 1900 Columbus Avenue, Zip 48708-6831; tel. 989/894-3000, (Includes BAY REGIONAL MEDICAL CENTER–WEST CAMPUS, 3250 East Midland Road, Zip 48706; tel. 989/667-6750) **A**1 2 7 9 10 12 13 **F**3 7 11 13 15 17 18 20 22 24 26 28 29 30 31 32 34 35 36 38 40 44 49 50 57 58 59 64 65 68 70 73 74 75 76 78 79 81 82 85 86 87 89 90 92 93 96 97 98 100 102 103 107 108 110 111 113 114 118 119 120 122 123 128 129 130 131 134 140 142 145 146 147 **P**6 **S** McLaren Health Care Corporation, Flint, MI
Primary Contact: Alice M. Gerard, President and Chief Executive Officer
CFO: Brian Kay, Chief Financial Officer
CMO: Ashok Vashishta, M.D., Vice President Medical Affairs
CIO: Curt Valley, Customer Site Manager
CHR: Joseph A. Lyons, Vice President Human Resources
Web address: www.bayregional.org
**Control:** Other not–for–profit (including NFP Corporation) **Service:** General Medical and Surgical

**Staffed Beds:** 338 **Admissions:** 16647 **Census:** 216 **Outpatient Visits:** 363195 **Births:** 937 **Total Expense ($000):** 239164 **Payroll Expense ($000):** 106449 **Personnel:** 1760

☒ **MCLAREN BAY SPECIAL CARE (232020)**, 3250 East Midland Road, Suite 1, Zip 48706-2835; tel. 989/667-6802 **A**1 10 **F**1 3 29 30 31 79 87 96 147 **S** McLaren Health Care Corporation, Flint, MI
Primary Contact: Cheryl A. Burzynski, President
CFO: Brian Kay, Chief Financial Officer
CMO: Janet Sutton, M.D., Medical Director
CIO: Darren Frye, Manager
CHR: Greg Purtell, Vice President Human Resources
Web address: www.bayspecialcare.org
**Control:** Other not–for–profit (including NFP Corporation) **Service:** Long–Term Acute Care hospital

**Staffed Beds:** 26 **Admissions:** 339 **Census:** 25 **Outpatient Visits:** 0 **Births:** 0 **Total Expense ($000):** 7467 **Payroll Expense ($000):** 3833 **Personnel:** 74

## BERRIEN CENTER—Berrien County

☐ **LAKELAND SPECIALTY HOSPITAL–BERRIEN CENTER (232025)**, 6418 Deans Hill Road, Zip 49102-9750; tel. 269/473-3003, (Nonreporting) **A**1 9 10 **S** Lakeland Healthcare, Saint Joseph, MI
Primary Contact: Loren Hamel, M.D., President and Chief Executive Officer
Web address: www.lakelandhealth.org
**Control:** Other not–for–profit (including NFP Corporation) **Service:** Long–Term Acute Care hospital

**Staffed Beds:** 26

## BIG RAPIDS—Mecosta County

☒ **MECOSTA COUNTY MEDICAL CENTER (230093)**, 605 Oak Street, Zip 49307-2099; tel. 231/796-8691 **A**1 9 10 20 **F**3 11 13 15 17 28 29 34 40 43 45 59 62 64 65 75 76 77 79 81 85 86 87 89 90 93 107 108 110 111 114 118 123 126 128 129 131 134 145 147 **P**1
Primary Contact: Thomas E. Daugherty, Administrator
CFO: Joseph W. Hohenberger, Chief Financial Officer
Web address: www.mcmcbr.com
**Control:** County–Government, nonfederal **Service:** General Medical and Surgical

**Staffed Beds:** 49 **Admissions:** 2324 **Census:** 19 **Outpatient Visits:** 129175 **Births:** 656 **Total Expense ($000):** 50004 **Payroll Expense ($000):** 22388 **Personnel:** 418

## BRIGHTON—Livingston County

★ **BRIGHTON CENTER FOR RECOVERY (230279)**, 12851 Grand River Road, Zip 48116-8506; tel. 810/227-1211 **A**10 **F**4 5 35 58 68 75 104 129 131 **P**6 **S** Ascension Health, Saint Louis, MO
Primary Contact: Ken Van Elsander, Director
COO: Ken Van Elsander, Director
CFO: Jackie Hill, Chief Financial Officer
CMO: Jeffrey Berger, M.D., Chief Medical Officer
CIO: Melissa Whelan, Director Health Information
CHR: Carol Tucker, Worklife Services Consultant
CNO: Barbara Shaw, Nursing Manager/ Chief Nursing Officer
Web address: www.brightonhospital.org
**Control:** Other not–for–profit (including NFP Corporation) **Service:** Alcoholism and other chemical dependency

**Staffed Beds:** 99 **Admissions:** 3161 **Census:** 69 **Outpatient Visits:** 43791 **Births:** 0 **Total Expense ($000):** 18213 **Payroll Expense ($000):** 9073 **Personnel:** 145

## CADILLAC—Wexford County

☒ **MERCY HOSPITAL CADILLAC (230081)**, 400 Hobart Street, Zip 49601-2331; tel. 231/876-7200 **A**1 9 10 20 **F**3 11 13 15 18 28 29 30 34 35 40 44 45 50 51 59 64 68 70 75 76 77 78 79 81 82 85 87 89 93 97 107 108 111 113 115 118 128 129 131 145 146 147 **P**6 8 **S** Trinity Health, Novi, MI
Primary Contact: John L. MacLeod, President and Chief Executive Officer
COO: Mary L. Neff, R.N., Chief Operating Officer and Chief Nursing Officer
CMO: Gerald Dudek, M.D., Chief of Staff
CIO: Randi Oehlers, Site Director Management Information Systems
CHR: Michael Stebbins, Director Organization and Talent Effectiveness
CNO: Mary L. Neff, R.N., Chief Nursing Officer
Web address: www.munsonhealthcare.org
**Control:** Church–operated, Nongovernment, not–for profit **Service:** General Medical and Surgical

**Staffed Beds:** 65 **Admissions:** 4044 **Census:** 35 **Outpatient Visits:** 80986 **Births:** 392 **Total Expense ($000):** 63216 **Payroll Expense ($000):** 22114 **Personnel:** 492

## CARO—Tuscola County

☐ **CARO CENTER (234025)**, 2000 Chambers Road, Zip 48723-9296; tel. 989/673-3191, (Nonreporting) **A**1 9 10
Primary Contact: Rose Laskowski, R.N., Director
COO: Rose Laskowski, R.N., Director
CFO: Mary Jo Drzewiecki–Burger, Administrative Manager
CMO: William Clark, M.D., Chief Clinical Affairs
CIO: Michele Wills, Registered Health Information Administrator
CHR: Barbara Frank, Human Resource Specialist
**Control:** State–Government, nonfederal **Service:** Psychiatric

**Staffed Beds:** 193

*Many Facility Codes have changed. Please refer to the AHA Guide Code Chart.*

© 2012 AHA Guide

MI

★ **CARO COMMUNITY HOSPITAL (231329)**, 401 North Hooper Street,
Zip 48723–1476, Mailing Address: P.O. Box 435, Zip 48723–0435;
tel. 989/673–3141 **A**9 10 18 **F**3 11 15 18 29 31 40 45 50 57 59 75 79 81
85 87 92 93 97 107 108 110 113 117 118 128 129 134 **P**6
Primary Contact: William P. Miller, President and Chief Executive Officer
CFO: Ron Srebinski, Chief Financial Officer
Web address: www.cch–mi.org
**Control:** Other not–for–profit (including NFP Corporation) **Service:** General
Medical and Surgical

**Staffed Beds:** 25 **Admissions:** 183 **Census:** 1 **Outpatient Visits:** 30800
**Births:** 0 **Total Expense ($000):** 13049 **Payroll Expense ($000):** 5309
**Personnel:** 120

### CARSON CITY—Montcalm County

★ ○ **CARSON CITY HOSPITAL (230208)**, 406 East Elm Street,
Zip 48811–0879, Mailing Address: P.O. Box 879, Zip 48811–0879;
tel. 989/584–3131 **A**9 10 11 19 **F**11 13 15 29 30 31 34 35 37 40 45 46 57
59 62 65 68 70 74 75 76 77 78 79 81 82 93 97 98 100 101 102 104 107
108 110 111 114 118 125 126 129 131 134 145 146 147 **P**8
Primary Contact: Matthew J. Thompson, Chief Executive Officer
CFO: Duane Miller, Senior Vice President Finance
CMO: Robert Seals, D.O., Medical Director
CIO: Richard Terry, Vice President & Chief Information Officer
CHR: Georgette Russell, Vice President of Talent & Organizational Effectiveness
CNO: Nancy Weaver, Vice President of Nursing, Chief Nursing Officer
Web address: www.carsoncityhospital.com
**Control:** Other not–for–profit (including NFP Corporation) **Service:** General
Medical and Surgical

**Staffed Beds:** 62 **Admissions:** 1874 **Census:** 18 **Outpatient Visits:** 67245
**Births:** 319 **Total Expense ($000):** 55301 **Payroll Expense ($000):** 27807
**Personnel:** 505

### CASS CITY—Tuscola County

★ ○ **HILLS & DALES GENERAL HOSPITAL (231316)**, 4675 Hill Street,
Zip 48726–1099; tel. 989/872–2121 **A**9 10 11 18 **F**3 11 15 29 30 31 32 34
35 40 46 53 56 57 59 61 64 74 75 77 79 81 85 86 87 93 97 107 108 109
110 114 117 118 126 128 129 130 131 134 143 145 146 147 **P**5 6
Primary Contact: Michael J. Falatko, FACHE, President and Chief Executive Officer
COO: Jean Anthony, Chief Operating Officer and Vice President Patient Services
CFO: Kenneth Baranski, Chief Financial Officer
CMO: Nancy Wade, M.D., Chief of Staff
CHR: Tom Bardwell, Vice President Human Resources
CNO: Jennifer TerBush, Director of Nursing
Web address: www.hdghmi.org
**Control:** Other not–for–profit (including NFP Corporation) **Service:** General
Medical and Surgical

**Staffed Beds:** 25 **Admissions:** 503 **Census:** 4 **Outpatient Visits:** 41175
**Births:** 0 **Total Expense ($000):** 18564 **Payroll Expense ($000):** 8268
**Personnel:** 167

### CHARLEVOIX—Charlevoix County

⊞ **CHARLEVOIX AREA HOSPITAL (231322)**, 14700 Lake Shore Drive,
Zip 49720–1931; tel. 231/547–4024 **A**1 9 10 18 **F**11 13 15 28 40 57 59 70
76 77 78 79 81 89 93 107 108 111 118 128 129 130 132 134 143 145
Primary Contact: Lyn Jenks, President
COO: Christine Wilhelm, Vice President Operations
CFO: Joseph Schodde, Vice President Financial Services
CIO: David Priest, Director Information Systems
CHR: Patty Fitzgerald, Staff Services
Web address: www.cah.org
**Control:** Other not–for–profit (including NFP Corporation) **Service:** General
Medical and Surgical

**Staffed Beds:** 25 **Admissions:** 1018 **Census:** 9 **Outpatient Visits:** 30870
**Births:** 221 **Total Expense ($000):** 33475 **Payroll Expense ($000):** 15310
**Personnel:** 286

### CHARLOTTE—Eaton County

⊞ △ **HAYES GREEN BEACH MEMORIAL HOSPITAL (231327)**, 321 East Harris
Street, Zip 48813–1629; tel. 517/543–1050 **A**1 7 9 10 18 **F**3 7 11 15 18 26
28 29 34 35 36 40 45 46 50 53 57 59 62 64 65 68 69 75 77 79 81 82 85
87 89 92 93 97 107 108 110 111 113 117 118 128 129 130 131 134 142
143 145 147 **P**6 **S** QHR, Brentwood, TN
Primary Contact: Matthew Rush, President and Chief Executive Officer
CFO: Kim Capps, Chief Financial Officer
CMO: Robert Leeser, M.D., Chief Medical Officer
CIO: Kim Capps, Chief Financial Officer
CHR: Jennifer Bucienski, Director Human Resources
Web address: www.hgbhealth.com
**Control:** Other not–for–profit (including NFP Corporation) **Service:** General
Medical and Surgical

**Staffed Beds:** 25 **Admissions:** 654 **Census:** 5 **Outpatient Visits:** 145515
**Births:** 0 **Total Expense ($000):** 44099 **Payroll Expense ($000):** 19227
**Personnel:** 364

### CHELSEA—Washtenaw County

⊞ **CHELSEA COMMUNITY HOSPITAL (230259)**, 775 South Main Street,
Zip 48118–1383; tel. 734/475–1311 **A**1 3 5 9 10 **F**3 5 8 9 11 15 28 29 30
31 34 35 36 40 45 51 53 59 62 64 65 68 70 75 77 78 79 81 82 85 86 87
90 91 93 97 98 99 100 101 104 107 110 111 113 114 118 128 129 130
131 133 134 145 146 147 **S** Trinity Health, Novi, MI
Primary Contact: Nancy Kay Graebner, President and Chief Executive Officer
CFO: James Birchler, Vice President Finance
CMO: Larry Handelsman, M.D., Vice President Medical Affairs
CIO: Sherry Brown, Director Information Services
CHR: Cindy Harrison, Vice President Human Resources
Web address: www.cch.org
**Control:** Other not–for–profit (including NFP Corporation) **Service:** General
Medical and Surgical

**Staffed Beds:** 102 **Admissions:** 3835 **Census:** 53 **Outpatient Visits:** 159282
**Births:** 0 **Total Expense ($000):** 98261 **Payroll Expense ($000):** 45528
**Personnel:** 676

### CLARE—Clare County

⊞ **MIDMICHIGAN MEDICAL CENTER–CLARE (230180)**, 703 North Mcewan
Street, Zip 48617–1440; tel. 989/802–5000 **A**1 9 10 **F**3 11 15 18 28 30 31
34 35 40 45 53 57 59 61 64 70 74 75 77 79 81 85 87 89 93 107 108 110
113 117 118 126 128 129 131 134 143 145 147 **S** MidMichigan Health,
Midland, MI
Primary Contact: Raymond Stover, President
CFO: Josh Wiggins, Vice President Controller
CMO: David Bremer, D.O., Chief of Staff
CIO: Michael Larson, Vice President Chief Information Officer
CHR: Lynn Bruchhof, Vice President Human Resources
CNO: Glenn King, Vice President, Chief Nursing Officer
Web address: www.midmichigan.org
**Control:** Other not–for–profit (including NFP Corporation) **Service:** General
Medical and Surgical

**Staffed Beds:** 49 **Admissions:** 1608 **Census:** 14 **Outpatient Visits:** 109437
**Births:** 0 **Total Expense ($000):** 42560 **Payroll Expense ($000):** 15091
**Personnel:** 275

### CLINTON TOWNSHIP—Macomb County

⊞ △ **HENRY FORD MACOMB HOSPITALS (230047)**, 15855 19 Mile Road,
Zip 48038–6324; tel. 586/263–2300, (Includes HENRY FORD MACOMB
HOSPITAL – MOUNT CLEMENS CAMPUS, 215 North Avenue, Mount Clemens,
Zip 48043; tel. 586/466–9300; ST. JOSEPH'S MERCY HOSPITAL–WEST, 15855
19 Mile Road, Zip 48038; tel. 586/263–2707; ST. JOSEPH'S MERCY–NORTH,
80650 North Van Dyke, Romeo, Zip 48065; tel. 810/798–3551) **A**1 2 7 9 10 12
13 **F**3 7 11 13 15 18 19 20 22 24 26 28 29 30 31 32 34 35 36 38 40 44 45
46 47 49 50 51 54 56 57 58 59 60 61 64 65 66 68 70 74 75 76 77 78 79
81 82 84 85 86 87 89 90 92 93 94 96 97 98 99 100 101 102 103 104 105
107 108 110 111 113 114 116 117 118 119 120 123 125 128 129 130 131
133 143 145 146 147 **P**6 8 **S** Henry Ford Health System, Detroit, MI
Primary Contact: Barbara Rossmann, President and Chief Executive Officer
COO: Gary Beaulac, Chief Operating Officer
CFO: Terry Goodbalian, Vice President Finance and Chief Financial Officer
CMO: Charles Kelly, D.O., Vice President Medical Affairs and Chief Medical Officer
CIO: Cathy Geiger, Director Information Systems
CHR: Joel Gibson, Vice President Human Resources
Web address: www.henryfordmacomb.com
**Control:** Other not–for–profit (including NFP Corporation) **Service:** General
Medical and Surgical

**Staffed Beds:** 421 **Admissions:** 23651 **Census:** 334 **Outpatient Visits:**
374212 **Births:** 1695 **Total Expense ($000):** 374419 **Payroll Expense
($000):** 154887 **Personnel:** 2603

MI

---

**Hospital, Medicare Provider Number, Address, Telephone, Approval, Facility, and Physician Codes, Health Care System**

★ American Hospital Association (AHA) membership
□ The Joint Commission accreditation
◇ DNV Healthcare Inc. accreditation
○ American Osteopathic Association (AOA) accreditation
△ Commission on Accreditation of Rehabilitation Facilities (CARF) accreditation

## COLDWATER—Branch County

⊞ **COMMUNITY HEALTH CENTER OF BRANCH COUNTY (230022)**, 274 East Chicago Street, Zip 49036–2041; tel. 517/279–5400 **A**1 9 10 13 19 **F**3 5 8 11 12 13 15 28 29 30 31 34 37 40 43 45 46 57 59 61 62 63 64 65 66 70 74 75 76 78 79 81 84 85 87 89 91 92 93 96 97 98 100 101 102 103 104 107 108 110 111 114 115 116 117 118 126 128 129 131 134 145 147 **P**6 8
Primary Contact: Randy DeGroot, President and Chief Executive Officer
COO: Mary R. Rose, R.N., Chief Clinical Officer
CFO: Steve Anderson, Chief Financial Officer
CMO: Joudat Daoud, M.D., Chief of Staff
CIO: Joel Lederman, Director Information Systems
CHR: Amy Jensen, Director Human Resources
Web address: www.chcbc.com
**Control:** County–Government, nonfederal **Service:** General Medical and Surgical

**Staffed Beds: 96 Admissions: 3508 Census: 38 Outpatient Visits:** 147120 **Births: 239 Total Expense ($000):** 65052 **Payroll Expense ($000):** 27503 **Personnel: 543**

## COMMERCE TOWNSHIP—Oakland County

⊞ **HURON VALLEY–SINAI HOSPITAL (230277)**, 1 William Carls Drive, Zip 48382–2201; tel. 248/937–3300 **A**1 3 5 9 10 12 13 **F**3 11 12 13 15 18 20 22 26 28 29 30 31 34 35 39 40 42 43 44 45 46 47 48 49 50 51 56 57 58 59 60 61 64 65 68 70 74 75 76 77 78 79 80 81 84 85 87 89 92 107 108 110 111 113 114 116 118 119 120 122 125 128 129 130 131 133 134 140 145 146 147 **P**8 **S** Vanguard Health System, Nashville, TN
Primary Contact: Lynn M. Torossian, President
COO: Karen Fordham, Vice President Chief Operating Officer
CFO: William Lantzy, Vice President Finance
CMO: Marc Bocknek, D.O., Vice President Medical Affairs
CHR: Ayanna Weber, Director Human Resources
CNO: Cathy Grant, R.N., Associate Vice President, Patient Services
Web address: www.hvsh.org
**Control:** Corporation, Investor–owned, for–profit **Service:** General Medical and Surgical

**Staffed Beds: 153 Admissions: 9136 Census: 109 Outpatient Visits:** 91529 **Births: 1300 Total Expense ($000):** 143026 **Payroll Expense ($000):** 55884 **Personnel: 981**

## DEARBORN—Wayne County

⊞ **OAKWOOD HOSPITAL & MEDICAL CENTER–DEARBORN (230020)**, 18101 Oakwood Boulevard, Zip 48124–4089, Mailing Address: P.O. Box 2500, Zip 48123–2500; tel. 313/593–7000 **A**1 2 3 5 8 9 10 **F**3 11 12 13 15 17 18 20 22 24 26 28 29 30 31 32 34 35 37 38 39 40 43 44 46 47 49 50 52 55 56 57 58 59 60 61 64 65 68 70 72 74 75 76 77 78 79 80 81 82 84 85 86 87 89 92 93 96 97 100 102 107 108 110 111 113 114 117 118 119 120 122 123 125 129 130 131 134 145 146 147 **P**5 8 **S** Oakwood Healthcare, Inc., Dearborn, MI
Primary Contact: Michael Geheb, M.D., Division President
CFO: Douglas D. Welday, Executive Vice President and Chief Financial Officer
CMO: Malcolm S. Henoch, M.D., Chief Medical Officer
CIO: Paula Smith, Leader Information Services and Chief Information Officer
CHR: John Paul Conway, Executive Vice President Human Resources
Web address: www.oakwood.org
**Control:** Other not–for–profit (including NFP Corporation) **Service:** General Medical and Surgical

**Staffed Beds: 553 Admissions: 31762 Census: 439 Outpatient Visits:** 186894 **Births: 4104 Total Expense ($000):** 564333 **Payroll Expense ($000):** 206019 **Personnel: 3153**

## DECKERVILLE—Sanilac County

**DECKERVILLE COMMUNITY HOSPITAL (231311)**, 3559 Pine Street, Zip 48427–7703, Mailing Address: P.O. Box 126, Zip 48427–0126; tel. 810/376–2835, (Nonreporting) **A**9 10 18
Primary Contact: Ethan Lipkind, President and Chief Executive Officer
COO: David West, Chief Operating Officer
CFO: Michael Beeman, Chief Financial Officer
CMO: Levi Guerrero, M.D., Chief of Staff
Web address: www.deckervillehosp.org
**Control:** Other not–for–profit (including NFP Corporation) **Service:** General Medical and Surgical

**Staffed Beds: 15**

## DETROIT—Wayne County

☐ **BCA STONECREST HOSPITAL (234038)**, 15000 Gratiot Avenue, Zip 48205–1973; tel. 313/245–0600, (Nonreporting) **A**1 10 **S** Behavioral Centers of America, Nashville, TN
Primary Contact: Steve Savage, Chief Operating Officer
Web address: www.bcastonecrestcenter.com
**Control:** Corporation, Investor–owned, for–profit **Service:** Psychiatric

**Staffed Beds: 90**

⊞ △ **CHILDREN'S HOSPITAL OF MICHIGAN (233300)**, 3901 Beaubien Street, Zip 48201–2119; tel. 313/745–5437 **A**1 3 5 7 9 10 **F**3 7 8 11 16 17 18 19 20 21 22 23 24 25 26 27 29 30 31 32 34 35 36 38 39 40 41 43 44 45 48 49 50 51 54 55 57 58 59 60 61 63 64 65 68 71 72 74 75 77 78 79 80 81 82 84 85 86 87 88 89 90 91 92 93 94 95 96 97 99 100 101 102 104 107 108 111 113 114 115 116 117 118 119 120 122 123 128 129 130 131 133 135 136 137 138 140 143 145 147 **P**6 8 **S** Vanguard Health System, Nashville, TN
Primary Contact: Herman B. Gray, M.D., President
CFO: Joseph Scallen, Jr., Chief Financial Officer
CMO: Charles Barone, M.D., Vice President Medical Affairs
CIO: Srinivasan Suresh, M.D., Chief Medical Information Officer
CHR: Tarry Paylor, Director Human Resources
Web address: www.chmkids.org
**Control:** Corporation, Investor–owned, for–profit **Service:** Children's general

**Staffed Beds: 222 Admissions: 11333 Census: 144 Outpatient Visits:** 254818 **Births: 0 Total Expense ($000):** 320891 **Payroll Expense ($000):** 122058 **Personnel: 1933**

⊞ △ **DETROIT RECEIVING HOSPITAL/UNIVERSITY HEALTH CENTER (230273)**, 4201 Saint Antoine Street, Zip 48201–2153; tel. 313/745–3000 **A**1 3 5 7 9 10 **F**3 16 17 18 29 30 34 35 38 40 42 43 44 50 56 57 59 64 65 66 68 70 74 75 77 79 81 82 84 85 87 97 98 99 100 102 103 104 107 113 114 118 128 129 130 131 134 140 142 143 145 147 **P**1 6 **S** Vanguard Health System, Nashville, TN
Primary Contact: Iris Taylor, Ph.D., R.N., President
COO: Jeff Dawkins, Chief Operating Officer
CFO: Gloria Larkins, Vice President Finance
CMO: Safwan Badr, M.D., Executive Vice President and Chief Medical Officer
CIO: Michael LeRoy, Senior Vice President and Chief Information Officer
CHR: Paulette Griffin, Vice President Human Resources
Web address: www.dmc.org
**Control:** Corporation, Investor–owned, for–profit **Service:** General Medical and Surgical

**Staffed Beds: 268 Admissions: 12977 Census: 186 Outpatient Visits:** 174004 **Births: 0 Total Expense ($000):** 186446 **Payroll Expense ($000):** 97268 **Personnel: 1681**

**HARPER UNIVERSITY HOSPITAL** See Harper University Hospital/Hutzel Women's Hospital

⊞ **HARPER UNIVERSITY HOSPITAL/HUTZEL WOMEN'S HOSPITAL (230104)**, 3990 John R Street, Zip 48201–2018; tel. 313/745–8040, (Includes DMC SURGERY HOSPITAL, 30671 Stephenson Highway, Madison Heights, Zip 48071–1678; tel. 248/733–2200; Frank P. Iacobell, President; HUTZEL HOSPITAL, 4707 St. Antoine Boulevard, Zip 48201–0154; tel. 313/745–6211) **A**1 3 5 9 10 **F**3 8 9 11 12 13 15 17 18 20 22 24 26 28 29 30 34 35 36 39 40 42 43 44 45 46 47 48 49 50 52 54 55 56 57 58 59 60 61 63 64 65 66 68 70 72 73 74 75 76 78 79 80 81 82 83 84 85 86 87 92 94 97 98 100 107 108 109 111 112 113 114 118 123 125 129 130 131 133 134 135 137 140 142 145 146 147 **P**6 8 **S** Vanguard Health System, Nashville, TN
Primary Contact: Thomas Malone, M.D., President
COO: Valerie Gibson, Chief Operating Officer
CFO: Tina Wood, Vice President Finance
CMO: Reginald J. Eadie, M.D., Vice President Medical Affairs
CIO: Michael LeRoy, Senior Vice President and Chief Information Officer
CHR: Deloris Hunt, Corporate Vice President Human Resources
Web address: www.harperhospital.org
**Control:** Corporation, Investor–owned, for–profit **Service:** General Medical and Surgical

**Staffed Beds: 535 Admissions: 21547 Census: 285 Outpatient Visits:** 211861 **Births: 5323 Total Expense ($000):** 499880 **Payroll Expense ($000):** 168228 **Personnel: 2909**

⊞ **HENRY FORD HOSPITAL (230053)**, 2799 West Grand Boulevard, Zip 48202–2608; tel. 313/916–2600 **A**1 2 3 5 8 9 10 **F**3 5 6 8 9 11 12 15 17 18 19 20 22 24 26 27 28 29 30 31 32 33 34 35 36 38 39 40 42 43 44 45 46 47 48 49 50 51 52 53 54 55 56 57 58 59 60 61 64 65 66 68 70 71 72 73 74 75 76 77 78 79 80 81 82 83 84 85 86 87 89 91 92 93 94 96 97 99 100 101 102 103 104 105 107 108 110 111 112 113 114 115 116 117 118 119 120 122 125 128 129 130 131 133 134 135 136 137 138 139 140 141 143 144 145 146 147 **P**6 **S** Henry Ford Health System, Detroit, MI
Primary Contact: John Popovich, M.D., President and Chief Executive Officer
COO: Veronica Hall, R.N., Chief Operating Officer
CFO: Joseph Schmitt, III, Senior Vice President Finance and Chief Financial Officer
CMO: Mark A. Kelley, M.D., Executive Vice President and Chief Medical Officer
CIO: Mary Alice Annecharico, Chief Information Officer
CHR: Kathy Oswald, Senior Vice President and Chief Human Resources Officer
CNO: Gwen Gnam, R.N., Chief Nursing Officer
Web address: www.henryfordhealth.org
**Control:** Other not–for–profit (including NFP Corporation) **Service:** General Medical and Surgical

**Staffed Beds: 759 Admissions: 41056 Census: 603 Outpatient Visits:** 2027001 **Births: 1583 Total Expense ($000):** 1598629 **Payroll Expense ($000):** 801021 **Personnel: 9924**

*Many Facility Codes have changed. Please refer to the AHA Guide Code Chart.* © 2012 AHA Guide

⊠ △ **JOHN D. DINGELL VETERANS AFFAIRS MEDICAL CENTER**, 4646 John R Street, Zip 48201–1932; tel. 313/576–1000, (Total facility includes 84 beds in nursing home–type unit) **A**1 2 3 5 7 8 9 **F**3 4 5 8 9 11 12 17 18 20 26 28 29 30 31 34 35 36 38 39 40 44 45 49 50 54 56 57 58 59 60 61 62 63 64 65 66 67 68 70 74 75 77 78 79 80 81 82 83 84 85 86 87 90 93 94 97 98 99 100 101 102 103 104 105 107 108 111 113 114 117 118 120 122 126 127 128 129 131 134 142 143 144 145 146 147 **P**6 **S** Department of Veterans Affairs, Washington, DC
Primary Contact: Pamela Reeves, M.D., Director
COO: Brent Thelen, Associate Director
CFO: Sherry Kilgore, Chief Financial Management Service
CMO: Scott Gruber, M.D., Chief of Staff
CIO: Jonathan Small, Chief Operations Information and Technology
CHR: Kathleen Osinski, Chief Human Resources Service
CNO: Ann Herm, Associate Director Patient Care Services
Web address: www.va.gov/sta/guide/home.asp
**Control:** Veterans Affairs, Government, federal **Service:** General Medical and Surgical

**Staffed Beds:** 188 **Admissions:** 4452 **Census:** 120 **Outpatient Visits:** 445281 **Births:** 0 **Total Expense ($000):** 303441 **Payroll Expense ($000):** 179630 **Personnel:** 1786

⊠ **KARMANOS CANCER CENTER (230297)**, 4100 John R Street, Zip 48201–2013; tel. 313/576–8670 **A**1 2 3 5 9 10 **F**3 8 15 29 31 34 35 36 39 44 50 54 55 56 57 58 59 63 64 65 68 74 75 78 79 82 83 84 85 86 87 107 108 109 110 111 113 114 115 116 117 118 119 120 122 123 125 129 131 132 134 135 145 146 147 **P**6
Primary Contact: Gerold Bepler, M.D., Ph.D., President and Chief Executive Officer
COO: Gary Morrison, Chief Operating Officer
CFO: Michael Grisdela, Chief Financial Officer
CMO: George Yoo, M.D., Chief Medical Officer
CIO: Scott McCarter, Chief Information Officer
CHR: David Jansen, Vice President Human Resources
Web address: www.karmanos.org
**Control:** Other not–for–profit (including NFP Corporation) **Service:** Cancer

**Staffed Beds:** 84 **Admissions:** 4104 **Census:** 74 **Outpatient Visits:** 159295 **Births:** 0 **Total Expense ($000):** 227749 **Payroll Expense ($000):** 53761 **Personnel:** 1077

⊠ **KINDRED HOSPITAL DETROIT (232027)**, 4777 East Outer Drive, Zip 48234–3241; tel. 313/369–5800, (Nonreporting) **A**1 9 10 **S** Kindred Healthcare, Louisville, KY
Primary Contact: Andrew G. Escamilla, MS, R.N., Chief Executive Officer
CFO: Steven Smith, Chief Financial Officer
CMO: Christopher Hughes, M.D., Medical Director
CHR: John Lucido, Director Human Resources
Web address: www.kindreddetroit.com/
**Control:** Corporation, Investor–owned, for–profit **Service:** Long–Term Acute Care hospital

**Staffed Beds:** 77

⊠ △ **REHABILITATION INSTITUTE OF MICHIGAN (233027)**, 261 Mack Boulevard, Zip 48201–2495; tel. 313/745–1203 **A**1 3 5 7 9 10 **F**28 29 30 34 35 36 43 44 50 53 58 64 68 86 87 90 91 92 93 94 95 96 118 129 130 131 133 145 147 **P**6 8 **S** Vanguard Health System, Nashville, TN
Primary Contact: William H. Restum, Ph.D., President
COO: Patty Jobbitt, Vice President Operations
CFO: Kevin Smith, Vice President Finance and Support Services
CMO: Ali Bitar, M.D., Vice President Medical Affairs
CHR: Paul Sturgis, Vice President Human Resources
CNO: Julia Libcke, R.N., VP Patient Care Services
Web address: www.rimrehab.org
**Control:** Corporation, Investor–owned, for–profit **Service:** Rehabilitation

**Staffed Beds:** 74 **Admissions:** 1267 **Census:** 61 **Outpatient Visits:** 241825 **Births:** 0 **Total Expense ($000):** 76097 **Payroll Expense ($000):** 38424 **Personnel:** 655

⊠ **SELECT SPECIALTY HOSPITAL–NORTHWEST DETROIT (232032)**, 6071 West Outer Drrive, Zip 48235–2624; tel. 313/966–4747, (Nonreporting) **A**1 9 10 **S** Select Medical Corporation, Mechanicsburg, PA
Primary Contact: Sandra Baumchen, Chief Executive Officer
Web address: www.selectmedicalcorp.com
**Control:** Corporation, Investor–owned, for–profit **Service:** Long–Term Acute Care hospital

**Staffed Beds:** 36

⊠ **SINAI–GRACE HOSPITAL (230024)**, 6071 West Outer Drive, Zip 48235–2679; tel. 313/966–3300 **A**1 3 5 8 9 10 13 **F**3 5 7 8 11 13 15 17 18 20 22 24 26 28 29 30 31 32 34 35 37 38 39 40 42 43 44 45 47 49 50 51 52 54 55 56 57 58 59 60 61 63 64 65 66 68 70 72 74 75 76 77 78 79 80 81 82 83 84 85 86 87 93 94 96 97 98 100 101 102 103 104 107 108 110 111 113 114 116 117 118 119 120 122 125 128 129 130 131 133 134 142 143 145 146 147 **P**6 8 **S** Vanguard Health System, Nashville, TN
Primary Contact: Reginald J. Eadie, M.D., President
CFO: Michael Prusatis, Vice President Finance
CMO: Matthew Griffin, M.D., Vice President Medical Affairs
CHR: Paulette Griffin, Director Human Resources
Web address: www.sinaigrace.org
**Control:** Corporation, Investor–owned, for–profit **Service:** General Medical and Surgical

**Staffed Beds:** 337 **Admissions:** 18414 **Census:** 272 **Outpatient Visits:** 213897 **Births:** 1512 **Total Expense ($000):** 300952 **Payroll Expense ($000):** 130905 **Personnel:** 2388

⊠ **ST. JOHN HOSPITAL AND MEDICAL CENTER (230165)**, 22101 Moross Road, Zip 48236–2172; tel. 313/343–4000 **A**1 2 3 5 8 9 10 **F**3 8 9 11 12 13 14 15 17 18 20 22 24 26 28 29 30 31 32 34 35 36 37 38 39 40 41 42 43 44 45 46 47 48 49 50 51 54 55 56 57 58 59 60 61 63 64 65 66 68 70 72 73 74 75 76 77 78 79 80 81 82 84 85 86 87 88 89 90 91 92 93 95 96 97 98 100 101 102 103 107 108 110 111 113 114 115 116 117 118 119 120 122 123 125 129 130 131 134 137 140 141 142 143 145 146 147 **P**6 8 **S** Ascension Health, Saint Louis, MO
Primary Contact: Frank W. Poma, Interim President
CFO: Tomasine Marx, Chief Financial Officer
CMO: Michael Haynes, M.D., Chief Medical Officer
CIO: Claudia Allen, Chief Information Officer
CHR: Mary Naber, Senior Vice President Worklife Services
Web address: www.stjohn.org
**Control:** Church–operated, Nongovernment, not–for profit **Service:** General Medical and Surgical

**Staffed Beds:** 680 **Admissions:** 34376 **Census:** 476 **Outpatient Visits:** 777537 **Births:** 3354 **Total Expense ($000):** 661269 **Payroll Expense ($000):** 259695 **Personnel:** 4392

**TRIUMPH HOSPITAL DETROIT** See Kindred Hospital Detroit

## DOWAGIAC—Cass County

⊠ **BORGESS–LEE MEMORIAL HOSPITAL (231315)**, 420 West High Street, Zip 49047–1943; tel. 269/782–8681 **A**1 9 10 18 **F**3 11 15 18 29 30 31 34 35 40 41 50 54 57 59 64 65 66 68 70 75 77 78 79 81 85 86 87 93 97 100 104 107 108 113 118 126 127 129 131 132 134 145 147 **P**6 **S** Ascension Health, Saint Louis, MO
Primary Contact: John Ryder, Interim Chief Executive Officer
CFO: Ken Holst, Chief Financial Officer
CMO: James L. Wierman, M.D., Chief of Staff
CHR: Pete Krueger, Director Human Resources
Web address: www.borgess.com
**Control:** Church–operated, Nongovernment, not–for profit **Service:** General Medical and Surgical

**Staffed Beds:** 25 **Admissions:** 830 **Census:** 8 **Outpatient Visits:** 108145 **Births:** 0 **Total Expense ($000):** 28937 **Payroll Expense ($000):** 13692 **Personnel:** 223

## EAST CHINA—St. Clair County

⊠ **ST. JOHN RIVER DISTRICT HOSPITAL (230241)**, 4100 River Road, Zip 48054–2909; tel. 810/329–7111 **A**1 9 10 **F**3 7 11 13 15 18 20 29 31 34 35 36 40 44 49 50 55 56 59 60 63 64 65 68 70 74 75 76 77 78 79 81 82 84 85 87 89 92 93 97 102 107 108 110 111 114 115 116 118 128 129 131 145 146 147 **P**7 8 **S** Ascension Health, Saint Louis, MO
Primary Contact: Frank W. Poma, President
CFO: Tomasine Marx, Chief Financial Officer
CMO: H. Lee Bacheldor, D.O., Medical Director
CIO: Linda Osterland, Director Information Services
CHR: Dawn Beindit, Director Work Life Services
Web address: www.stjohn.org
**Control:** Church–operated, Nongovernment, not–for profit **Service:** General Medical and Surgical

**Staffed Beds:** 68 **Admissions:** 1888 **Census:** 21 **Outpatient Visits:** 62978 **Births:** 266 **Total Expense ($000):** 43389 **Payroll Expense ($000):** 17478 **Personnel:** 336

MI

**Hospital, Medicare Provider Number, Address, Telephone, Approval, Facility, and Physician Codes, Health Care System**

★ American Hospital Association (AHA) membership
□ The Joint Commission accreditation          ◇ DNV Healthcare Inc. accreditation
○ American Osteopathic Association (AOA) accreditation
△ Commission on Accreditation of Rehabilitation Facilities (CARF) accreditation

## EATON RAPIDS—Eaton County

⊞ **EATON RAPIDS MEDICAL CENTER (231324)**, 1500 South Main Street, Zip 48827–0130, Mailing Address: P.O. Box 130, Zip 48827–0130; tel. 517/663–2671 **A**1 9 10 18 **F**3 11 15 18 29 30 34 35 40 45 53 54 57 59 64 68 75 77 79 81 82 85 86 87 89 90 93 95 96 107 113 118 126 129 131 132 134 143 145
Primary Contact: Timothy Johnson, President and Chief Executive Officer
CFO: Shari Glynn, Vice President Finance and Chief Financial Officer
CMO: Ashok K. Gupta, M.D., Chief of Staff
CIO: Mark Rodge, Director Information Systems
CHR: Laurie Field, Director Human Resources
Web address: www.eatonrapidsmedicalcenter.org
**Control:** Other not–for–profit (including NFP Corporation) **Service:** General Medical and Surgical

**Staffed Beds:** 20 **Admissions:** 368 **Census:** 3 **Outpatient Visits:** 14599 **Births:** 0 **Total Expense ($000):** 19385 **Payroll Expense ($000):** 7903 **Personnel:** 142

## ESCANABA—Delta County

⊞ **OSF ST. FRANCIS HOSPITAL (230101)**, 3401 Ludington Street, Zip 49829–1377; tel. 906/786–3311 **A**1 9 10 20 **F**3 11 13 15 28 29 30 34 35 40 45 46 56 57 59 62 63 64 65 66 68 70 74 75 76 77 78 79 81 83 84 85 86 93 96 97 107 108 110 111 114 118 126 128 129 130 131 132 143 144 145 146 147 **P**6 **S** OSF Healthcare System, Peoria, IL
Primary Contact: Peter G. Jennings, President and Chief Executive Officer
CFO: Jim Wayne, Chief Financial Officer
CMO: Mark Povich, D.O., Medical Director
CIO: Mark Irving, Manager Management Information Systems
CHR: Elizabeth Zorza, Assistant Administrator
Web address: www.osfstfrancis.org
**Control:** Church–operated, Nongovernment, not–for profit **Service:** General Medical and Surgical

**Staffed Beds:** 48 **Admissions:** 2042 **Census:** 20 **Outpatient Visits:** 190432 **Births:** 256 **Total Expense ($000):** 71674 **Payroll Expense ($000):** 29277 **Personnel:** 433

## FARMINGTON HILLS—Oakland County

★ ○ **BOTSFORD HOSPITAL (230151)**, 28050 Grand River Avenue, Zip 48336–5933; tel. 248/471–8000 **A**9 10 11 12 13 **F**3 8 9 11 12 13 15 17 18 20 22 26 28 29 30 31 32 34 35 36 38 39 40 41 43 44 45 46 47 48 49 50 51 53 54 56 57 58 59 60 61 63 64 65 68 70 74 75 76 77 78 79 80 81 82 83 84 85 86 87 89 90 92 93 94 96 97 98 100 101 102 103 107 108 109 110 111 113 114 117 118 119 120 122 123 125 128 129 130 131 133 134 143 145 146 147 **P**1 5 6
Primary Contact: Paul E. LaCasse, D.O., President and Chief Executive Officer
CFO: David Marcellino, Executive Vice President and Chief Financial Officer
CMO: David Walters, D.O., Vice President and Chief Medical Officer
CIO: John Czahor, Chief Information Officer
CHR: Barbara Palmer, Corporate Vice President Human Resources
Web address: www.botsford.org
**Control:** Other not–for–profit (including NFP Corporation) **Service:** General Medical and Surgical

**Staffed Beds:** 306 **Admissions:** 16364 **Census:** 214 **Outpatient Visits:** 442950 **Births:** 829 **Total Expense ($000):** 271601 **Payroll Expense ($000):** 132415 **Personnel:** 2101

## FERNDALE—Oakland County

★ **HENRY FORD KINGSWOOD HOSPITAL (234011)**, 10300 West Eight Mile Road, Zip 48220–2100; tel. 248/398–3200 **A**9 10 **F**4 29 30 32 34 35 44 50 56 57 59 68 75 77 82 86 87 98 99 101 103 129 133 134 **P**6 **S** Henry Ford Health System, Detroit, MI
Primary Contact: C. Edward Coffey, M.D., Chief Executive Officer and Director Behavioral Health Services
CFO: Tony Gaglio, Chief Financial Officer
CMO: Taft Parson, M.D., Medical Director
CNO: Cheryl Taylor, R.N., Director of Nursing
Web address: www.henryford.com
**Control:** Other not–for–profit (including NFP Corporation) **Service:** Psychiatric

**Staffed Beds:** 100 **Admissions:** 3306 **Census:** 58 **Outpatient Visits:** 0 **Births:** 0 **Total Expense ($000):** 15830 **Payroll Expense ($000):** 9417 **Personnel:** 171

## FLINT—Genesee County

⊞ **HURLEY MEDICAL CENTER (230132)**, One Hurley Plaza, Zip 48503–5993; tel. 810/262–6887 **A**1 2 3 5 8 9 10 **F**3 5 11 12 13 15 16 17 18 19 20 22 26 28 29 30 31 32 35 39 40 41 43 45 46 49 50 52 53 54 55 56 57 58 59 61 64 66 70 72 74 75 76 77 78 79 80 81 82 84 85 86 87 88 89 90 93 96 97 98 100 101 102 103 104 107 108 110 111 113 114 117 118 119 120 122 123 128 129 130 131 134 140 142 145 146 147
Primary Contact: Melany Gavulic, President & Chief Executive Officer
COO: Melany Gavulic, Senior Vice President Operations & COO
CFO: Cass Wisniewski, Interim Chief Financial Officer
CMO: Michael Jaggi, D.O., Vice President and Chief Medical Officer
CIO: Gary Townsend, Chief Information Officer
CHR: Beth Brophy, Interim VP for Human Resources
CNO: Teresa Bourque, Sr. Administrator for Nursing/Chief Nurse
Web address: www.hurleymc.com
**Control:** City–Government, nonfederal **Service:** General Medical and Surgical

**Staffed Beds:** 418 **Admissions:** 17988 **Census:** 293 **Outpatient Visits:** 396160 **Births:** 2614 **Total Expense ($000):** 350226 **Payroll Expense ($000):** 150174 **Personnel:** 2291

⊞ **MCLAREN FLINT (230141)**, 401 South Ballenger Highway, Zip 48532–3685; tel. 810/342–2000 **A**1 2 3 5 8 9 10 **F**3 5 11 12 13 15 17 18 20 22 24 26 28 29 30 31 32 34 35 36 38 39 40 43 44 45 46 49 50 52 53 54 55 56 57 58 59 60 61 64 68 70 74 75 76 77 78 79 81 82 85 86 87 89 90 93 96 97 98 99 100 101 102 103 104 105 107 108 113 114 117 118 119 120 122 123 125 128 129 130 131 134 140 143 145 146 147 **P**6 7 **S** McLaren Health Care Corporation, Flint, MI
Primary Contact: Donald C. Kooy, President and Chief Executive Officer
COO: Brent Wheeler, Vice President Ancillary and Support Services
CFO: Rick Wyles, Chief Financial Officer
CIO: Gayle Consiglio, Chief Information Officer
CHR: Timothy G. Srock, Vice President Human Resources
Web address: www.mclarenregional.org
**Control:** Other not–for–profit (including NFP Corporation) **Service:** General Medical and Surgical

**Staffed Beds:** 336 **Admissions:** 21520 **Census:** 256 **Outpatient Visits:** 422477 **Births:** 549 **Total Expense ($000):** 361377 **Payroll Expense ($000):** 152364 **Personnel:** 2415

⊞ **SELECT SPECIALTY HOSPITAL–FLINT (232012)**, 401 South Ballenger Highway, 5th Floor, Zip 48532–3638; tel. 810/342–4500, (Nonreporting) **A**1 9 10 **S** Select Medical Corporation, Mechanicsburg, PA
Primary Contact: Lorie Powell, Chief Executive Officer
CMO: Jitendra P. Katneni, M.D., Medical Director
CHR: Gayle Barthel, Coordinator Human Resources
CNO: Nicole McLean, Chief Nursing Officer
Web address: www.selectmedicalcorp.com
**Control:** Corporation, Investor–owned, for–profit **Service:** Long–Term Acute Care hospital

**Staffed Beds:** 26

## FRANKFORT—Benzie County

★ **PAUL OLIVER MEMORIAL HOSPITAL (231300)**, 224 Park Avenue, Zip 49635–9658; tel. 231/352–2200, (Total facility includes 39 beds in nursing home–type unit) **A**9 10 18 **F**11 15 28 30 34 35 40 45 46 50 53 57 59 64 75 77 81 86 93 107 110 111 113 118 128 129 131 132 145 147 **S** Munson Healthcare, Traverse City, MI
Primary Contact: James D. Austin, FACHE, Administrator
COO: Peter Marinoff, Director Operations
CMO: Gerard Mahoney, M.D., Chief of Staff
CHR: Julie Banktson, Manager Human Resources
Web address: www.munsonhealthcare.org
**Control:** Other not–for–profit (including NFP Corporation) **Service:** General Medical and Surgical

**Staffed Beds:** 47 **Admissions:** 77 **Census:** 36 **Outpatient Visits:** 40817 **Births:** 0 **Total Expense ($000):** 14156 **Payroll Expense ($000):** 4829 **Personnel:** 110

## FREMONT—Newaygo County

⊞ **SPECTRUM HEALTH GERBER MEMORIAL (230106)**, 212 South Sullivan Avenue, Zip 49412–1548; tel. 231/924–3300 **A**1 9 10 **F**3 11 15 28 29 31 32 34 35 36 40 43 45 48 53 56 59 62 64 68 70 75 76 77 78 79 81 86 87 93 96 107 108 110 111 114 117 118 126 128 129 130 131 134 145 146 **S** Spectrum Health, Grand Rapids, MI
Primary Contact: Randall Stasik, President and Chief Executive Officer
COO: Janice Stone, Vice President Clinical Integration
CFO: John Sella, Chief Financial Officer
CMO: Mark Byland, M.D., Chief of Staff
CIO: Patrick Whiteside, Director Information Systems
CHR: Christine Schurkamp, Human Resources Director
CNO: Patti Wethington, R.N., Chief Nursing Officer
Web address: www.gerberhospital.org
**Control:** Other not–for–profit (including NFP Corporation) **Service:** General Medical and Surgical

**Staffed Beds:** 40 **Admissions:** 2571 **Census:** 20 **Outpatient Visits:** 116793 **Births:** 478 **Total Expense ($000):** 64106 **Payroll Expense ($000):** 27219 **Personnel:** 505

*Many Facility Codes have changed. Please refer to the AHA Guide Code Chart.* © 2012 AHA Guide

MI

## GARDEN CITY—Wayne County

★ ○ **GARDEN CITY HOSPITAL (230244)**, 6245 North Inkster Road, Zip 48135–4001; tel. 734/421–3300 **A**9 10 11 12 13 **F**3 4 11 13 15 17 18 20 22 26 28 29 31 34 35 36 40 43 44 46 47 49 50 51 57 59 62 64 65 68 70 74 75 76 77 78 79 80 81 82 85 87 89 90 91 92 93 96 97 107 111 112 113 114 118 128 129 130 131 134 142 145 147 **P**5 6
Primary Contact: Gary R. Ley, President and Chief Executive Officer
CFO: Timothy Jodway, Chief Financial Officer
CMO: Kirsten Waarala, D.O., Vice President Medical Services
CIO: Albert Fadool, Director Information Systems
CHR: Steven Solomon, Vice President Human Resources
CNO: Bette Fitz, Chief Nursing Officer
Web address: www.gchosp.org
**Control:** Other not–for–profit (including NFP Corporation) **Service:** General Medical and Surgical

**Staffed Beds:** 220 **Admissions:** 9480 **Census:** 118 **Outpatient Visits:** 138332 **Births:** 712 **Total Expense ($000):** 132110 **Payroll Expense ($000):** 55337 **Personnel:** 1033

## GAYLORD—Otsego County

⊠ **OTSEGO MEMORIAL HOSPITAL (230133)**, 825 North Center Avenue, Zip 49735–1592; tel. 989/731–2100, (Includes MCREYNOLDS HALL ), (Total facility includes 34 beds in nursing home–type unit) **A**1 9 10 20 **F**3 13 15 28 29 31 32 34 35 36 37 40 43 44 45 46 49 50 51 54 56 57 59 60 64 65 70 74 75 76 77 78 79 81 82 85 86 87 93 96 97 107 108 110 111 114 117 118 123 126 127 128 129 130 131 133 134 143 145 146 147 **P**6 7
Primary Contact: Thomas R. Lemon, Chief Executive Officer
COO: James D. Flickema, VP, Professional & Ancillary Services
CFO: Robert Courtois, Vice President Finance
CMO: Peter Handley, M.D., Chief of Staff
CIO: Timothy Hella, Chief Information Officer
CHR: Terra Deming, Director Human Resources
CNO: Diane Fisher, R.N., VP, Patient Care Services
Web address: www.myomh.org
**Control:** Other not–for–profit (including NFP Corporation) **Service:** General Medical and Surgical

**Staffed Beds:** 80 **Admissions:** 1584 **Census:** 47 **Outpatient Visits:** 178828 **Births:** 264 **Total Expense ($000):** 66746 **Payroll Expense ($000):** 30155 **Personnel:** 479

## GLADWIN—Gladwin County

⊠ **MIDMICHIGAN MEDICAL CENTER–GLADWIN (231325)**, 515 South Quarter Street, Zip 48624–1959; tel. 989/426–9286 **A**1 9 10 18 **F**3 11 15 18 28 29 30 31 34 40 53 74 77 81 85 86 89 93 97 107 108 110 111 113 117 118 126 128 129 131 134 142 145 **S** MidMichigan Health, Midland, MI
Primary Contact: Raymond Stover, President and Chief Executive Officer
CFO: Josh Wiggins, Vice President and Controller
CMO: Marcelino Barreto, M.D., Chief Medical Staff
CIO: Michael Larson, Vice President and Chief Information Officer
CHR: Lynn Bruchhof, Vice President
CNO: Glenn King, Vice President and Chief Nursing Officer
Web address: www.midmichigan.org
**Control:** Other not–for–profit (including NFP Corporation) **Service:** General Medical and Surgical

**Staffed Beds:** 25 **Admissions:** 592 **Census:** 5 **Outpatient Visits:** 58960 **Births:** 0 **Total Expense ($000):** 22647 **Payroll Expense ($000):** 8042 **Personnel:** 146

## GRAND BLANC—Genesee County

⊠ ○ △ **GENESYS REGIONAL MEDICAL CENTER (230197)**, One Genesys Parkway, Zip 48439–8066; tel. 810/606–5000 **A**1 2 3 5 7 9 10 11 12 13 **F**3 11 13 15 17 18 20 22 24 26 28 29 30 31 34 35 37 40 43 44 45 46 47 48 49 50 51 54 58 59 60 61 64 70 74 75 76 77 78 79 81 82 84 85 86 87 89 90 92 93 96 97 102 107 108 110 111 113 114 116 117 118 128 129 131 134 144 145 146 147 **P**6 **S** Ascension Health, Saint Louis, MO
Primary Contact: Elizabeth Aderholdt, President
COO: Christopher Palazzolo, Senior Vice President and Chief Operating Officer
CFO: Nancy Haywood, Chief Financial Officer
CMO: James C. Bonnette, M.D., Chief Clinical Officer
CIO: Daniel Stross, Chief Information Officer
CNO: Polly Gates, Senior Vice President and Chief Nursing Officer
Web address: www.genesys.org
**Control:** Church–operated, Nongovernment, not–for profit **Service:** General Medical and Surgical

**Staffed Beds:** 410 **Admissions:** 22057 **Census:** 289 **Outpatient Visits:** 645885 **Births:** 2385 **Total Expense ($000):** 413287 **Payroll Expense ($000):** 180694 **Personnel:** 2697

## GRAND HAVEN—Ottawa County

⊠ **NORTH OTTAWA COMMUNITY HOSPITAL (230174)**, 1309 Sheldon Road, Zip 49417–2488; tel. 616/842–3600, (Nonreporting) **A**1 9 10 21
Primary Contact: Shelleye Yaklin, President and Chief Executive Officer
CFO: Donald J. Longpre, Vice President Finance and Chief Financial Officer
CMO: Haney Assaad, Chief of Staff
CHR: Carla Wallis, Director Human Resources
CNO: Cindy Van Kampen, Chief Nursing Officer
Web address: www.noch.org
**Control:** Other not–for–profit (including NFP Corporation) **Service:** General Medical and Surgical

**Staffed Beds:** 39

## GRAND RAPIDS—Kent County

☐ **FOREST VIEW PSYCHIATRIC HOSPITAL (234030)**, 1055 Medical Park Drive S.E., Zip 49546–3607; tel. 616/942–9610 **A**1 9 10 **F**75 87 98 99 100 101 102 104 105 129 131 **S** Universal Health Services, Inc., King of Prussia, PA
Primary Contact: Andrew Hotaling, Chief Executive Officer
CFO: Gabrielle Gale, Chief Financial Officer
CMO: James VanHaren, M.D., Medical Director
CHR: Mike Henderson, Director Human Resources
Web address: www.forestviewhospital.com
**Control:** Corporation, Investor–owned, for–profit **Service:** Psychiatric

**Staffed Beds:** 82 **Admissions:** 2286 **Census:** 67 **Outpatient Visits:** 3766 **Births:** 0 **Personnel:** 126

⊠ **GREAT LAKES SPECIALTY HOSPITAL–OAK CAMPUS (232026)**, 200 Jefferson Avenue S.E., 5th Floor, Zip 49503–4502; tel. 616/965–8701, (Nonreporting) **A**1 9 10 **S** Select Medical Corporation, Mechanicsburg, PA
Primary Contact: Brian Pangle, Chief Executive Officer
COO: Jennifer Groeneweg, R.N., Chief Clinical Officer
CMO: Mark J. Ivey, M.D., Medical Director
CNO: Tracie Peterson, R.N., Chief Nursing Officer
Web address: www.selectmedicalcorp.com
**Control:** Corporation, Investor–owned, for–profit **Service:** Long–Term Acute Care hospital

**Staffed Beds:** 20

⊠ △ **MARY FREE BED REHABILITATION HOSPITAL (233026)**, 235 Wealthy Street S.E., Zip 49503–5247; tel. 616/242–0300 **A**1 7 9 10 **F**30 34 54 64 68 75 77 82 86 90 91 93 94 100 104 129 130 131 142 145 **P**6
Primary Contact: Kent Riddle, Interim President
COO: Bruce A. Brasser, R.N., VP of Inpatient and Network Operations
CFO: Randall DeNeff, Vice President Finance
CMO: John Butzer, M.D., Medical Director
CIO: Jeff Burns, Manager of Information Technology
CHR: Kelli Miller, Vice President Human Resources
CNO: Connie A. Brown–Olds, R.N., Chief Nursing Officer
Web address: www.maryfreebed.com
**Control:** Other not–for–profit (including NFP Corporation) **Service:** Rehabilitation

**Staffed Beds:** 80 **Admissions:** 863 **Census:** 43 **Outpatient Visits:** 56272 **Births:** 0 **Total Expense ($000):** 44258 **Payroll Expense ($000):** 25191 **Personnel:** 507

⊠ **PINE REST CHRISTIAN MENTAL HEALTH SERVICES (234006)**, 300 68th Street S.E., Zip 49501–0165, Mailing Address: P.O. Box 165, Zip 49501–0165; tel. 616/455–5000 **A**1 5 9 10 **F**2 4 5 6 29 30 32 34 35 38 55 56 58 59 66 68 75 77 82 86 87 91 98 99 100 101 103 104 105 106 129 131 133 134 145 **P**6
Primary Contact: Mark C. Eastburg, Ph.D., President and Chief Executive Officer
COO: Robert Nykamp, Vice President and Chief Operating Officer
CFO: Paul H. Karsten, Vice President Finance and Chief Financial Officer
CMO: Alan Armstrong, M.D., Chief Medical Officer
Web address: www.pinerest.org
**Control:** Other not–for–profit (including NFP Corporation) **Service:** Psychiatric

**Staffed Beds:** 450 **Admissions:** 5403 **Census:** 142 **Outpatient Visits:** 265011 **Births:** 0 **Total Expense ($000):** 91997 **Payroll Expense ($000):** 53400 **Personnel:** 1133

---

**Hospital, Medicare Provider Number, Address, Telephone, Approval, Facility, and Physician Codes, Health Care System**

★ American Hospital Association (AHA) membership
☐ The Joint Commission accreditation
◇ DNV Healthcare Inc. accreditation
○ American Osteopathic Association (AOA) accreditation
△ Commission on Accreditation of Rehabilitation Facilities (CARF) accreditation

✠ **SAINT MARY'S HEALTH CARE (230059)**, 200 Jefferson Avenue S.E., Zip 49503–4598; tel. 616/685–5000 **A**1 2 3 5 9 10 **F**3 8 13 15 18 20 22 26 28 29 30 31 34 35 36 37 40 43 44 45 46 48 49 50 53 54 56 57 58 59 60 61 64 66 68 70 72 74 75 76 77 78 79 80 81 82 83 84 85 86 87 97 98 99 100 102 105 107 108 110 111 113 114 115 116 117 118 119 120 122 123 125 128 129 130 131 134 137 143 145 146 147 **P**1 6 **S** Trinity Health, Novi, MI
Primary Contact: Philip H. McCorkle, Jr., President and Chief Executive Officer
COO: Randall J. Wagner, Chief Operating Officer
CFO: Steve Pirog, Vice President Finance
CMO: David Baumgartner, M.D., Vice President Medical Affairs
CMO: Rolland Mambourg, M.D., Vice President Medical Affairs
CIO: Jim Keller, Site Director Information Services
CHR: Thomas Karel, Vice President Organization and Talent Effectiveness
CNO: Elizabeth A. Murphy, R.N., Vice President for Patient Care Services
Web address: www.mercyhealthsaintmarys.org
**Control:** Church–operated, Nongovernment, not–for profit **Service:** General Medical and Surgical

> **Staffed Beds:** 344 **Admissions:** 19919 **Census:** 259 **Outpatient Visits:** 750205 **Births:** 2135 **Total Expense ($000):** 397001 **Payroll Expense ($000):** 123012 **Personnel:** 2098

✠ **SPECTRUM HEALTH BUTTERWORTH HOSPITAL (230038)**, 100 Michigan Street N.E., Zip 49503–2560; tel. 616/774–7444, (Includes HELEN DEVOS CHILDREN'S HOSPITAL, 100 Michigan Street N.E., tel. 616/391–9000; SPECTRUM HEALTH, 100 Michigan Street N.E., Zip 49503–2551; tel. 616/391–1774; SPECTRUM HEALTH – BLODGETT CAMPUS, 1840 Wealthy Street S.E., Zip 49506–2921; tel. 616/774–7444) **A**1 2 3 5 8 9 10 **F**3 7 8 9 11 12 13 15 16 17 18 19 20 21 22 23 24 25 26 27 28 29 30 31 32 34 35 36 37 38 40 41 43 44 49 50 51 52 54 55 56 57 58 59 60 61 64 65 66 68 70 71 72 73 74 75 76 77 78 79 80 81 82 84 85 86 87 88 89 93 107 108 110 111 113 114 116 117 118 119 120 122 123 125 128 129 130 131 133 134 135 136 137 142 143 144 145 146 147 **P**5 6 **S** Spectrum Health, Grand Rapids, MI
Primary Contact: Matthew Van Vranken, President, Spectrum Health Hospital Group
COO: Marc Chircop, Senior Vice President
CMO: Lowell Bursch, M.D., Executive Vice President Medical Affairs
CHR: Tanja Oquendo, Vice President Human Resources
Web address: www.spectrum–health.org
**Control:** Other not–for–profit (including NFP Corporation) **Service:** General Medical and Surgical

> **Staffed Beds:** 1066 **Admissions:** 57057 **Census:** 709 **Outpatient Visits:** 1217905 **Births:** 7302 **Total Expense ($000):** 1276634 **Payroll Expense ($000):** 465612 **Personnel:** 7752

✠ **SPECTRUM HEALTH SPECIAL CARE HOSPITAL (232029)**, 750 Fuller Avenue N.E., Zip 49503–1995; tel. 616/486–3000, (Nonreporting) **A**1 10 **S** Spectrum Health, Grand Rapids, MI
Primary Contact: Charles Tozer, Chief Executive Officer
CFO: Larry Oberst, Vice President Finance
CIO: Mary Nader, Director Applications
CHR: Lori Gibson, Chief Human Resources Officer
Web address: www.spectrum–health.org
**Control:** Other not–for–profit (including NFP Corporation) **Service:** Long–Term Acute Care hospital

> **Staffed Beds:** 36

**GRAYLING—Crawford County**

✠ **MERCY HOSPITAL GRAYLING (230058)**, 1100 East Michigan Avenue, Zip 49738–1312; tel. 989/348–5461, (Total facility includes 39 beds in nursing home–type unit) **A**1 9 10 20 **F**3 11 13 15 28 29 30 32 34 35 36 38 40 44 45 50 51 54 56 57 58 59 64 65 66 70 75 76 77 79 81 85 86 87 93 97 107 108 111 114 118 126 128 129 130 134 145 146 147 **P**6 8 **S** Trinity Health, Novi, MI
Primary Contact: Stephanie J. Riemer–Matuzak, Chief Executive Officer
COO: Kirsten Korth–White, Vice President Operations
CFO: David Boyer, Chief Financial Officer
CHR: Kirsten Korth–White, Vice President Operations
Web address: www.mercygrayling.munsonhealthcare.org/
**Control:** Church–operated, Nongovernment, not–for profit **Service:** General Medical and Surgical

> **Staffed Beds:** 94 **Admissions:** 3761 **Census:** 63 **Outpatient Visits:** 136690 **Births:** 292 **Total Expense ($000):** 68597 **Payroll Expense ($000):** 26048 **Personnel:** 416

**GREENVILLE—Montcalm County**

✠ **SPECTRUM HEALTH UNITED HOSPITAL (230035)**, 615 South Bower Street, Zip 48838–2614; tel. 616/754–4691, (Includes SPECTRUM HEALTH KELSEY HOSPITAL, 418 Washington Avenue, Lakeview, Zip 48850; tel. 989/352–7211), (Total facility includes 71 beds in nursing home–type unit) **A**1 9 10 **F**3 8 11 13 15 18 29 31 32 40 41 43 44 45 50 64 65 70 76 77 78 79 81 85 86 87 89 97 107 108 110 111 113 118 123 126 127 128 129 130 131 132 134 145 146 147 **P**8 **S** Spectrum Health, Grand Rapids, MI
Primary Contact: Christina Freese–Decker, President
COO: Priscillia Mahar, Chief Clinical and Compliance Officer
CFO: David J. Oehring, Chief Financial Officer
CMO: Bennett Walstatler, M.D., President
CIO: David Dutmers, Team Leader Information and Technology Management
CHR: Vicki Jensen, Chief Human Resources Officer
Web address: www.spectrum–health.org/
**Control:** Other not–for–profit (including NFP Corporation) **Service:** General Medical and Surgical

> **Staffed Beds:** 117 **Admissions:** 3069 **Census:** 90 **Outpatient Visits:** 148612 **Births:** 424 **Total Expense ($000):** 66445 **Payroll Expense ($000):** 26928 **Personnel:** 626

**GROSSE POINTE—Wayne County**

✠ **BEAUMONT HOSPITAL GROSSE POINTE (230089)**, 468 Cadieux Road, Zip 48230–1507; tel. 313/473–1000 **A**1 9 10 **F**3 11 12 13 15 18 20 26 28 29 30 31 34 35 39 40 44 45 46 49 50 51 53 54 57 58 59 60 61 63 64 65 66 68 69 70 71 74 75 76 77 78 79 80 81 82 84 85 86 87 89 92 93 94 96 97 100 107 108 110 111 113 114 116 118 123 125 129 130 131 134 145 146 147 **P**6 **S** Beaumont Health System, Royal Oak, MI
Primary Contact: Richard P. Swaine, President
COO: Chris Stesney–Ridenour, Vice President Operations
CFO: Nickolas A. Vitale, Senior Vice President and Chief Financial Officer
CMO: Donna Hoban, M.D., Senior Vice President and Physician–in–Chief
CIO: Subra Sripada, Senior Vice President and Chief Information Officer
CHR: Jay T. Holden, Vice President, Human Resources
CNO: Phyllis Reynolds, R.N., VP, Nursing
Web address: www.beaumont.edu
**Control:** Other not–for–profit (including NFP Corporation) **Service:** General Medical and Surgical

> **Staffed Beds:** 250 **Admissions:** 10301 **Census:** 114 **Outpatient Visits:** 254792 **Births:** 632 **Total Expense ($000):** 148811 **Payroll Expense ($000):** 47689 **Personnel:** 990

**GROSSE POINTE FARMS—Wayne County**

✠ **SELECT SPECIALTY HOSPITAL–GROSSE POINTE (232038)**, 468 Cadieux Road, Zip 48230–1507; tel. 313/473–6131, (Nonreporting) **A**1 9 10 **S** Select Medical Corporation, Mechanicsburg, PA
Primary Contact: Miriam Deemer, Chief Executive Officer
Web address: www.selectmedicalcorp.com
**Control:** Corporation, Investor–owned, for–profit **Service:** Long–Term Acute Care hospital

> **Staffed Beds:** 30

**HANCOCK—Houghton County**

✠ **PORTAGE HEALTH (230108)**, 500 Campus Drive, Zip 49930–1569; tel. 906/483–1000, (Total facility includes 60 beds in nursing home–type unit) **A**1 9 10 20 **F**3 7 8 11 13 15 28 29 30 31 34 35 40 43 46 50 53 54 56 57 59 60 62 63 64 65 67 68 69 70 75 76 77 78 79 81 82 84 85 86 87 89 90 93 94 97 107 108 110 111 114 117 118 126 128 129 130 131 132 134 142 143 144 145 146 147 **P**6
Primary Contact: James Bogan, FACHE, President and Chief Executive Officer
CFO: Brian Donahue, Chief Financial Officer
CMO: Kirk Lufkin, M.D., Chief Medical Officer
CIO: John Steenport, Director Information Technology
CHR: Robbyn Lucier, Chief Human Resources Officer
Web address: www.portagehealth.org
**Control:** Other not–for–profit (including NFP Corporation) **Service:** General Medical and Surgical

> **Staffed Beds:** 96 **Admissions:** 1730 **Census:** 73 **Outpatient Visits:** 106925 **Births:** 389 **Total Expense ($000):** 70108 **Payroll Expense ($000):** 33781 **Personnel:** 569

MI

MI

## HARBOR BEACH—Huron County

**HARBOR BEACH COMMUNITY HOSPITAL (231313)**, 210 South First Street, Zip 48441–1236; tel. 989/479–3201, (Total facility includes 39 beds in nursing home–type unit) **A**9 10 18 **F**2 3 15 29 35 40 56 57 59 64 75 81 86 93 107 108 113 117 118 126 127 129 131 132 145 146 147 **P**6
Primary Contact: Edward L. Gamache, President and Chief Executive Officer
CFO: Jill Wehner, Vice President Financial Services
CMO: Richard Lloyd, D.O., Chief of Staff
CIO: Tami Nickrand, Director Information Technology
CHR: Tina Osantoski, Director Human Resources
Web address: www.hbch.org
**Control:** Other not–for–profit (including NFP Corporation) **Service:** General Medical and Surgical

**Staffed Beds:** 54 **Admissions:** 137 **Census:** 38 **Outpatient Visits:** 9921
**Births:** 0 **Total Expense ($000):** 10807 **Payroll Expense ($000):** 4705
**Personnel:** 130

## HASTINGS—Barry County

⊠ **PENNOCK HOSPITAL (230040)**, 1009 West Green Street, Zip 49058–1790; tel. 269/945–3451 **A**1 9 10 **F**3 11 13 15 29 30 32 34 35 36 39 40 44 45 50 53 54 56 57 59 62 63 64 65 68 70 74 75 76 77 78 79 81 82 84 85 86 87 89 91 93 96 97 107 108 110 111 114 118 124 128 129 130 131 134 143 145 146 147 **P**6 8
Primary Contact: Sheryl Lewis Blake, FACHE, Chief Executive Officer
COO: Carla Wilson–Neil, Chief Operating Officer
CFO: Connie Downs, Chief Financial Officer
CHR: Anita Henderson, Director Human Resources
Web address: www.pennockhealth.com
**Control:** Other not–for–profit (including NFP Corporation) **Service:** General Medical and Surgical

**Staffed Beds:** 58 **Admissions:** 2673 **Census:** 28 **Outpatient Visits:** 457023
**Births:** 347 **Total Expense ($000):** 52019 **Payroll Expense ($000):** 22556
**Personnel:** 473

## HILLSDALE—Hillsdale County

★ ○ **HILLSDALE COMMUNITY HEALTH CENTER (230037)**, 168 South Howell Street, Zip 49242–2081; tel. 517/437–4451, (Total facility includes 21 beds in nursing home–type unit) **A**9 10 11 12 13 19 **F**3 11 12 13 15 28 29 31 34 35 37 38 40 45 48 50 59 62 70 75 76 78 79 81 87 89 93 97 98 102 104 107 110 111 114 118 126 127 129 130 131 134 145 146 147 **P**6 8
Primary Contact: Duke Anderson, President and Chief Executive Officer
CFO: Valerie Fetters, Chief Financial Officer
CMO: Barry Collins, D.O., Chief of Staff
CIO: Steve Rausch, Manager Information Technology
CHR: Mike Pacheco, Human Resources Manager
CNO: Julie Walters, Chief Nursing Officer
Web address: www.hchc.com
**Control:** Other not–for–profit (including NFP Corporation) **Service:** General Medical and Surgical

**Staffed Beds:** 84 **Admissions:** 3564 **Census:** 53 **Outpatient Visits:** 127863
**Births:** 355 **Total Expense ($000):** 54463 **Payroll Expense ($000):** 19941
**Personnel:** 397

## HOLLAND—Ottawa County

★ **HOLLAND HOSPITAL (230072)**, 602 Michigan Avenue, Zip 49423–4999; tel. 616/392–5141, (Nonreporting) **A**9 10 21
Primary Contact: Dale Sowders, President and Chief Executive Officer
CFO: Terry L. Steele, Vice President Finance and Chief Financial Officer
CMO: William Vandervliet, M.D., Vice President Medical Affairs
CIO: Randy J. Paruch, Director, Information Systems
CHR: Chuck Kohlruss, Vice President Human Resources and Operations Support
CNO: Patti J. VanDort, MSN, Vice President Nursing/Chief Nursing Officer
Web address: www.hollandhospital.org
**Control:** Other not–for–profit (including NFP Corporation) **Service:** General Medical and Surgical

**Staffed Beds:** 130

## HOWELL—Livingston County

⊠ **ST. JOSEPH MERCY LIVINGSTON HOSPITAL (230069)**, 620 Byron Road, Zip 48843–1093; tel. 517/545–6000 **A**1 3 5 9 10 13 **F**3 5 8 11 13 15 18 28 29 30 31 34 35 40 41 42 45 51 54 56 57 59 62 63 64 65 68 70 74 75 76 77 78 79 81 82 83 84 85 86 87 93 97 100 104 107 108 110 111 113 114 115 118 119 125 128 129 130 131 134 143 144 145 146 147 **S** Trinity Health, Novi, MI
Primary Contact: Robert F. Casalou, President and Chief Executive Officer
COO: Michael J. Markel, MSN, Executive Director of Operations
CFO: Charles Hoffman, Vice President Financial Services and Chief Financial Officer
CMO: Mark Baumeier, M.D., Chief of Staff
CIO: Frank Rademacher, Director, Information Systems
CHR: Kenneth Antczak, Vice President Human Resources
CNO: Joyce Young, R.N., VP, Patient Services & Chief Nursing Officer
Web address: www.sjmh.com/who/mcphersn.shtml
**Control:** Church–operated, Nongovernment, not–for profit **Service:** General Medical and Surgical

**Staffed Beds:** 55 **Admissions:** 3481 **Census:** 31 **Outpatient Visits:** 341622
**Births:** 187 **Total Expense ($000):** 108185 **Payroll Expense ($000):** 39903
**Personnel:** 680

## IONIA—Ionia County

⊠ **SPARROW IONIA HOSPITAL (231331)**, 479 Lafayette Street, Zip 48846–1834, Mailing Address: Box 1001, Zip 48846–1899; tel. 616/523–1400 **A**1 9 10 18 **F**3 12 15 29 31 34 35 40 45 50 54 57 59 64 65 68 70 74 75 77 78 79 81 85 89 93 107 108 114 118 126 128 129 130 145 147 **S** Sparrow Health System, Lansing, MI
Primary Contact: William Roeser, President and Chief Executive Officer
COO: George W. Rutherford, Vice President and Chief Operating Officer
CFO: Mark Brisboe, Vice President and Chief Financial Officer
CMO: Amy Jentz, M.D., Chief of Staff
CIO: Bob Neal, Director Information Technology
CHR: Jolene Jacobs, Director Human Resources
Web address: www.ioniahospital.org
**Control:** Other not–for–profit (including NFP Corporation) **Service:** General Medical and Surgical

**Staffed Beds:** 25 **Admissions:** 501 **Census:** 4 **Outpatient Visits:** 55170
**Births:** 0 **Total Expense ($000):** 22520 **Payroll Expense ($000):** 12649
**Personnel:** 227

## IRON MOUNTAIN—Dickinson County

⊠ **DICKINSON COUNTY HEALTHCARE SYSTEM (230055)**, 1721 South Stephenson Avenue, Zip 49801–3637; tel. 906/774–1313 **A**1 9 10 20 **F**3 11 13 15 17 18 28 29 30 31 34 35 40 45 46 51 53 56 57 59 61 62 64 67 68 70 74 75 76 77 79 81 85 86 87 89 91 93 94 96 97 107 108 110 111 113 114 118 120 122 126 128 129 130 131 132 134 144 145 **P**6
Primary Contact: John Schon, Administrator and Chief Executive Officer
COO: Jeff Gussert, Director Operations
CFO: Eileen Sparpana, Director Finance
CMO: Don Kube, M.D., Chief of Staff
CIO: Dean Decremer, Chief Information Officer
CHR: Paula Swartout, HR Manager
CNO: Susan Hadley, R.N., Director of Nursing
Web address: www.dchs.org
**Control:** County–Government, nonfederal **Service:** General Medical and Surgical

**Staffed Beds:** 96 **Admissions:** 3397 **Census:** 34 **Outpatient Visits:** 231777
**Births:** 472 **Total Expense ($000):** 73156 **Payroll Expense ($000):** 36815
**Personnel:** 596

⊠ **VETERANS AFFAIRS MEDICAL CENTER**, 325 East H Street, Zip 49801–4792; tel. 906/774–3300, (Nonreporting) **A**1 9 **S** Department of Veterans Affairs, Washington, DC
Primary Contact: James W. Rice, Director
Web address: www.va.gov/sta/guide/home.asp
**Control:** Veterans Affairs, Government, federal **Service:** General Medical and Surgical

**Staffed Beds:** 17

---

**Hospital, Medicare Provider Number, Address, Telephone, Approval, Facility, and Physician Codes, Health Care System**

★ American Hospital Association (AHA) membership
□ The Joint Commission accreditation ◇ DNV Healthcare Inc. accreditation
○ American Osteopathic Association (AOA) accreditation
△ Commission on Accreditation of Rehabilitation Facilities (CARF) accreditation

---

## IRON RIVER—Iron County

⊞ **NORTHSTAR HEALTH SYSTEM (231318)**, 1400 West Ice Lake Road, Zip 49935–9526; tel. 906/265–6121 **A**1 9 10 18 **F**7 11 15 28 29 31 32 33 34 35 40 43 50 53 54 56 57 59 60 62 63 64 70 75 77 78 79 81 86 87 89 93 97 104 107 111 114 118 127 129 130 131 132 134 143 144 145 146 147
Primary Contact: Bruce E. Rampage, Chief Executive Officer
COO: Connie L. Koutouzos, R.N., COO/Vice President of Patient Care Services
COO: Robert Lindberg, R.N., Chief Operating Officer and Chief Nursing Officer
CFO: Glenn E. Dobson, Chief Financial Officer
CMO: Ronald Dalton, M.D., Chief Medical Officer
CMO: Kim Mahler, M.D., Chief Medical Officer
CHR: Carol Bastianello, Director Employee Services
Web address: www.northstarhs.org
**Control:** Other not–for–profit (including NFP Corporation) **Service:** General Medical and Surgical

**Staffed Beds:** 25 **Admissions:** 906 **Census:** 9 **Outpatient Visits:** 65235 **Births:** 0 **Total Expense ($000):** 36214 **Payroll Expense ($000):** 14517 **Personnel:** 275

## IRONWOOD—Gogebic County

⊞ **ASPIRUS GRAND VIEW HOSPITAL (231333)**, N10561 Grand View Lane, Zip 49938–9622; tel. 906/932–2525 **A**1 9 10 18 **F**3 11 13 15 28 29 31 34 35 40 44 45 50 56 57 59 62 63 64 65 66 70 75 76 77 81 85 86 87 89 97 100 101 102 103 104 105 107 108 110 113 118 119 120 128 129 131 132 143 145 146 147 **P**6
Primary Contact: Carol Goffnett, Chief Executive Officer
CFO: Charmaine Chiantello, Chief Financial Officer
CMO: Jeffrey Edwards, M.D., Chief Medical Staff
CIO: Ron Eyer, Manager Information Services
CHR: Keri Kartheiser, Manager Human Resources
Web address: www.gvhs.org
**Control:** Other not–for–profit (including NFP Corporation) **Service:** General Medical and Surgical

**Staffed Beds:** 25 **Admissions:** 496 **Census:** 4 **Outpatient Visits:** 29116 **Births:** 76 **Total Expense ($000):** 14218 **Payroll Expense ($000):** 5293 **Personnel:** 248

## ISHPEMING—Marquette County

★ **BELL HOSPITAL (231321)**, 901 Lakeshore Drive, Zip 49849–1367; tel. 906/486–4431 **A**9 10 18 **F**3 7 10 11 13 15 29 30 32 34 35 40 51 53 57 59 70 75 76 77 79 81 85 87 89 92 93 96 97 107 108 110 118 128 130 132 142 143 145 146 **P**6
Primary Contact: Barbara Larson, Interim Chief Executive Officer
COO: Barbara Larson, Chief Operating Officer
CFO: Darin Sizemore, Controller
CMO: Shahar Madjar, M.D., Chief of Staff
CHR: Ruth Solinski, Vice President Organizational Development
Web address: www.bellmemorial.org
**Control:** Other not–for–profit (including NFP Corporation) **Service:** General Medical and Surgical

**Staffed Beds:** 25 **Admissions:** 1396 **Census:** 9 **Outpatient Visits:** 82186 **Births:** 257 **Total Expense ($000):** 38108 **Payroll Expense ($000):** 16611 **Personnel:** 259

## JACKSON—Jackson County

⊞ **ALLEGIANCE HEALTH (230092)**, 205 North East Avenue, Zip 49201–1753; tel. 517/788–4800, (Total facility includes 20 beds in nursing home–type unit) **A**1 2 9 10 **F**3 4 5 8 9 11 13 15 17 18 20 22 24 26 28 29 30 31 34 35 38 40 44 45 46 47 48 49 50 51 53 54 56 57 58 59 61 62 63 64 65 68 69 70 73 74 75 76 77 78 79 81 82 84 85 87 89 92 93 96 98 99 100 101 102 103 104 105 106 107 108 110 111 112 113 114 117 118 120 125 127 128 129 130 131 133 134 145 146 147 **P**6
Primary Contact: Georgia R. Fojtasek, President and Chief Executive Officer
COO: Karen Chaprnka, Senior Vice President and Chief Operating Officer
CFO: Jeanne Wickens, Chief Financial Officer
CMO: Ray King, M.D., Senior Vice President and Chief Medical Officer
CIO: Richard Warren, Vice President Health Information Systems
CHR: Cheryl Lamborn, Vice President Human Resources
CNO: Jacalyn A. Liebowitz, Senior Vice President Patient Care Continuum & CNO
Web address: www.allegiancehealth.org
**Control:** Other not–for–profit (including NFP Corporation) **Service:** General Medical and Surgical

**Staffed Beds:** 305 **Admissions:** 20280 **Census:** 218 **Outpatient Visits:** 512185 **Births:** 1740 **Total Expense ($000):** 378112 **Payroll Expense ($000):** 178842 **Personnel:** 3128

⊞ **CARELINK OF JACKSON (232036)**, 110 North Elm Avenue, Zip 49202–3595; tel. 517/787–1440 **A**1 9 10 **F**1 3 29 30 31 50 57 60 77 85 87 129 145 147
Primary Contact: J. Mark Fall, Chief Executive Officer
COO: Nancy D. Fitzgerald, Chief Operating Officer
CFO: Dale L. Friesen, Chief Financial Officer
CMO: Gregg Patten, M.D., Chief Medical Officer
Web address: www.carelinkofjackson.org
**Control:** Other not–for–profit (including NFP Corporation) **Service:** Long–Term Acute Care hospital

**Staffed Beds:** 44 **Admissions:** 442 **Census:** 35 **Outpatient Visits:** 0 **Births:** 0 **Total Expense ($000):** 14585 **Payroll Expense ($000):** 5160 **Personnel:** 127

**DUANE L. WATERS HOSPITAL**, 3857 Cooper Street, Zip 49201–7521; tel. 517/780–5600, (Nonreporting)
Primary Contact: Gerald De Voss, Acting Administrator
**Control:** State–Government, nonfederal **Service:** Hospital unit of an institution (prison hospital, college infirmary, etc.)

**Staffed Beds:** 150

## KALAMAZOO—Kalamazoo County

⊞ △ **BORGESS MEDICAL CENTER (230117)**, 1521 Gull Road, Zip 49048–1640; tel. 269/226–7000 **A**1 3 5 7 9 10 **F**1 3 7 8 9 11 12 13 15 17 18 20 22 24 26 28 29 30 31 32 33 34 35 36 37 38 39 40 43 44 45 46 49 50 53 54 56 57 58 59 60 61 64 68 70 74 75 76 77 78 79 81 82 84 85 86 87 90 91 92 93 94 96 97 98 99 100 101 102 103 104 105 107 108 110 113 114 117 118 125 128 129 130 131 134 143 145 146 147 **P**1 3 6
**S** Ascension Health, Saint Louis, MO
Primary Contact: Paul A. Spaude, FACHE, President and Chief Executive Officer
COO: Mark Anthony, Executive Vice President and Chief Operating Officer
CFO: Richard Felbinger, Senior Vice President and Chief Financial Officer
CMO: Anthony F. Oliva, D.O., Sr. Vice President & Chief Medical Officer
CIO: Donna Roach, Chief Information Officer
CHR: Laura Lentenbrink, Vice President, Human Resources
CNO: Lois J. Van Donselaar, R.N., Vice President & Chief Nursing Officer
Web address: www.borgess.com
**Control:** Church–operated, Nongovernment, not–for profit **Service:** General Medical and Surgical

**Staffed Beds:** 387 **Admissions:** 19607 **Census:** 248 **Outpatient Visits:** 471622 **Births:** 1341 **Total Expense ($000):** 453242 **Payroll Expense ($000):** 170713 **Personnel:** 2208

⊞ **BRONSON METHODIST HOSPITAL (230017)**, 601 John Street, Zip 49007–5346; tel. 269/341–6000, (Includes BRONSON VICKSBURG HOSPITAL, 13326 North Boulevard, Vicksburg, Zip 49097–1099; tel. 269/649–2321; Frank J. Sardone, President and Chief Executive Officer; CHILDREN'S HOSPITAL AT BRONSON, 601 John Street, Zip 49007–5341; tel. 269/341–7654) **A**1 3 5 8 9 10 **F**3 11 12 13 15 16 17 18 19 20 22 24 26 28 29 30 31 32 34 35 37 39 40 43 45 46 47 49 50 55 56 57 58 59 61 62 64 65 68 70 72 73 74 75 76 77 78 79 81 82 84 85 86 87 88 89 90 92 93 97 102 107 108 110 111 113 114 117 118 125 129 130 131 133 134 140 144 145 146 147 **P**6 **S** Bronson Healthcare Group, Inc., Kalamazoo, MI
Primary Contact: Frank J. Sardone, President and Chief Executive Officer
COO: Kenneth L. Taft, Executive Vice President and Chief Operating Officer
CFO: Mary Meitz, Vice President Finance
CMO: Scott Larson, M.D., Vice President Medical Affairs and Chief Medical Officer
CHR: John Hayden, Vice President and Chief Human Resources Officer
Web address: www.bronsonhealth.com
**Control:** Other not–for–profit (including NFP Corporation) **Service:** General Medical and Surgical

**Staffed Beds:** 368 **Admissions:** 22681 **Census:** 272 **Outpatient Visits:** 536191 **Births:** 3363 **Total Expense ($000):** 505112 **Payroll Expense ($000):** 218005 **Personnel:** 3046

☐ **KALAMAZOO PSYCHIATRIC HOSPITAL (234026)**, 1312 Oakland Drive, Zip 49008–1205; tel. 269/337–3000 **A**1 9 10 12 13 **F**3 39 50 53 56 65 75 77 86 87 97 98 101 103 129 131 134 142 145 **P**6
Primary Contact: James J. Coleman, Ed.D., Director
COO: James J. Coleman, Ed.D., Director
CFO: Sue Glenn, Director Administrative Services
CMO: N. Gajare, M.D., Chief Clinical Affairs
CIO: Gerry Wood, Information Technologist
CHR: Kerry Bloom, Director Human Resources
**Control:** State–Government, nonfederal **Service:** Psychiatric

**Staffed Beds:** 205 **Admissions:** 516 **Census:** 169 **Outpatient Visits:** 0 **Births:** 0 **Total Expense ($000):** 40400 **Payroll Expense ($000):** 25170 **Personnel:** 479

*Many Facility Codes have changed. Please refer to the AHA Guide Code Chart.* © 2012 AHA Guide

MI

## KALKASKA—Kalkaska County

★ **KALKASKA MEMORIAL HEALTH CENTER (231301)**, 419 South Coral Street, Zip 49646–2503; tel. 231/258–7500, (Total facility includes 88 beds in nursing home–type unit) **A**9 10 18 **F**2 7 10 15 28 34 35 40 44 45 50 56 57 59 60 64 65 66 78 81 84 87 93 97 107 110 118 126 127 128 129 131 133 142 143 145 146 147 **S** Munson Healthcare, Traverse City, MI
Primary Contact: James D. Austin, FACHE, Administrator
COO: Sheila Atwood, R.N., Chief Operating Officer
CMO: Jeremy Holmes, D.O., Chief of Staff
CHR: Kimberly Babcock, Administrator Human Resources
CNO: Christine Bissonette, R.N., Chief Nursing Officer
Web address: www.munsonhealthcare.org
**Control:** Hospital district or authority, Government, nonfederal **Service:** General Medical and Surgical

**Staffed Beds:** 96 **Admissions:** 183 **Census:** 82 **Outpatient Visits:** 57104 **Births:** 0 **Total Expense ($000):** 27731 **Payroll Expense ($000):** 10472 **Personnel:** 235

## L'ANSE—L'Anse County

☐ **BARAGA COUNTY MEMORIAL HOSPITAL (231307)**, 18341 U.S. Highway 41, Zip 49946–8024; tel. 906/524–3300 **A**1 9 10 18 **F**3 8 11 15 28 31 40 45 53 59 62 63 64 74 78 79 81 82 84 89 93 107 108 110 113 117 118 129 131 132 145 **P**6
Primary Contact: Tim E. Zwickey, Chief Executive Officer
CFO: Gail Jestila–Peltola, Chief Financial Officer
CMO: Todd Ingram, M.D., Chief of Staff
CIO: Taylor Makela, Director Information Technology
CHR: Carol Seppanen, Director Human Resources
CNO: Becky D'Agostino, R.N., Director of Nursing
Web address: www.bcmh.org
**Control:** County–Government, nonfederal **Service:** General Medical and Surgical

**Staffed Beds:** 15 **Admissions:** 558 **Census:** 4 **Outpatient Visits:** 34673 **Total Expense ($000):** 20781 **Payroll Expense ($000):** 7491 **Personnel:** 105

## LAKEVIEW—Montcalm County

**SPECTRUM HEALTH KELSEY HOSPITAL** See Spectrum Health United Hospital, Greenville

## LANSING—Ingham County

★ ○ **MCLAREN GREATER LANSING (230167)**, 401 West Greenlawn Avenue, Zip 48910–2819; tel. 517/975–6000, (Includes INGHAM REGIONAL MEDICAL CENTER, GREENLAWN CAMPUS, 401 West Greenlawn Avenue, tel. 517/334–2121; MCLAREN ORTHOPEDIC HOSPITAL, 2727 South Pennsylvania Avenue, Zip 48910–3490; tel. 517/975–6000; Rick Wright, President and Chief Executive Officer) **A**2 3 5 8 9 10 11 12 13 **F**3 5 8 10 11 13 15 17 18 19 20 22 24 26 28 29 30 31 34 35 37 40 44 45 49 50 51 55 56 57 58 59 60 61 63 64 65 66 70 74 75 76 77 78 79 81 82 83 84 85 86 87 89 90 93 97 98 100 101 102 103 104 105 107 108 110 111 113 114 115 116 117 118 119 120 123 125 128 129 130 131 134 145 146 147 **S** McLaren Health Care Corporation, Flint, MI
Primary Contact: Rick Wright, President and Chief Executive Officer
CFO: Kevin Lanciotti, Chief Financial Officer
CMO: Thomas Petroff, D.O., Vice President Medical Affairs
CHR: Laurie Brewis, Vice President Human Resources
Web address: www.irmc.org
**Control:** Other not–for–profit (including NFP Corporation) **Service:** General Medical and Surgical

**Staffed Beds:** 318 **Admissions:** 15927 **Census:** 188 **Outpatient Visits:** 386291 **Births:** 1269 **Total Expense ($000):** 300237 **Payroll Expense ($000):** 117952 **Personnel:** 1723

☒ ○ △ **SPARROW HOSPITAL (230230)**, 1215 East Michigan Avenue, Zip 48912–1811, Mailing Address: P.O. Box 30480, Zip 48909–7980; tel. 517/364–1000, (Includes SPARROW REGIONAL CHILDREN'S CENTER, 1215 East Michigan Avenue, tel. 517/364–1000) **A**1 2 3 5 7 9 10 11 12 13 **F**2 3 4 5 11 12 13 15 17 18 20 22 24 26 28 29 30 33 34 35 36 38 40 41 43 44 45 46 49 50 51 54 55 56 57 58 59 60 63 64 65 66 68 70 72 74 75 76 77 78 79 81 82 84 85 86 87 88 89 90 92 93 96 97 98 99 100 101 102 103 104 105 107 108 109 110 113 114 116 117 118 119 120 122 123 125 127 128 129 130 131 134 142 143 145 146 147 **P**1 6 **S** Sparrow Health System, Lansing, MI
Primary Contact: Dennis A. Swan, President and Chief Executive Officer
COO: Joseph Ruth, Executive Vice President and Chief Operating Officer
CFO: Scott Wilkerson, Interim Senior Vice President and Chief Financial Officer
CMO: Larry Rawsthorne, M.D., Senior Vice President Medical Affairs
CIO: Thomas Bres, Vice President and Chief Information Officer
CHR: Thomas Ostrander, Vice President Human Resources
Web address: www.sparrow.org
**Control:** Other not–for–profit (including NFP Corporation) **Service:** General Medical and Surgical

**Staffed Beds:** 638 **Admissions:** 32611 **Census:** 440 **Outpatient Visits:** 629702 **Births:** 4196 **Total Expense ($000):** 720003 **Payroll Expense ($000):** 336090 **Personnel:** 5038

★ ○ **SPARROW SPECIALTY HOSPITAL (232037)**, 1210 West Saginaw Street, Zip 48915–1927, Mailing Address: P.O. Box 85201, Zip 48915; tel. 517/364–6800 **A**9 10 11 **F**1 3 29 30 36 60 68 85 100 101 118 129 147 **S** Sparrow Health System, Lansing, MI
Primary Contact: Kira Carter–Robertson, Chief Executive Officer
CFO: David Przybylski, Interim Controller
CMO: Paul Entler, D.O., Medical Director
CHR: LaChelle Flowers, Administrative Assistant Human Resources
CNO: Tina Gross, Director of Clinical Services
Web address: www.sparrowspecialty.org
**Control:** Other not–for–profit (including NFP Corporation) **Service:** Long–Term Acute Care hospital

**Staffed Beds:** 36 **Admissions:** 325 **Census:** 26 **Outpatient Visits:** 0 **Births:** 0 **Total Expense ($000):** 11904 **Payroll Expense ($000):** 5992 **Personnel:** 129

## LAPEER—Lapeer County

★ ○ **MCLAREN LAPEER REGION (230193)**, 1375 North Main Street, Zip 48446–1350; tel. 810/667–5500, (Total facility includes 19 beds in nursing home–type unit) **A**2 9 10 11 **F**3 11 13 15 18 20 28 29 30 31 34 40 45 46 49 50 51 54 56 57 59 64 68 70 74 75 76 77 78 79 81 82 83 85 86 87 92 93 97 98 102 107 108 111 113 114 118 122 123 127 128 129 130 131 145 147 **S** McLaren Health Care Corporation, Flint, MI
Primary Contact: Barton Buxton, Ed.D., President and Chief Executive Officer
COO: Thomas Mee, R.N., Vice President Operations
CFO: Mary Beth Callahan, Chief Financial Officer
CMO: Gary Salem, M.D., Vice President Medical Affairs
CIO: Gayle Consiglio, Chief Information Officer
CHR: Amy Dorr, Vice President Human Resources
Web address: www.lapeerregional.org
**Control:** Other not–for–profit (including NFP Corporation) **Service:** General Medical and Surgical

**Staffed Beds:** 157 **Admissions:** 6914 **Census:** 84 **Outpatient Visits:** 131584 **Births:** 606 **Total Expense ($000):** 89131 **Payroll Expense ($000):** 35849 **Personnel:** 610

## LAURIUM—Houghton County

☒ **ASPIRUS KEWEENAW HOSPITAL (231319)**, 205 Osceola Street, Zip 49913–2134; tel. 906/337–6500 **A**1 9 10 18 **F**3 7 11 13 15 17 18 28 29 30 31 35 40 45 52 53 56 57 59 61 62 63 70 76 78 79 81 87 89 93 107 108 110 114 118 126 128 129 130 131 132 134 144 145 146 **P**6 **S** Aspirus, Inc., Wausau, WI
Primary Contact: Charles Nelson, Chief Executive Officer
COO: Michael Hauswirth, Chief Operating Officer
CFO: Shane Jacques, Chief Financial Officer
CMO: Glenn Kauppila, D.O., Chief of Staff
CIO: Dave Olsson, Director of Marketing
CHR: Chad D. Rowe, Director Human Resources
CNO: Grace Tousignant, R.N., Chief Nursing Officer
Web address: www.aspiruskeweenaw.org
**Control:** Other not–for–profit (including NFP Corporation) **Service:** General Medical and Surgical

**Staffed Beds:** 25 **Admissions:** 1097 **Census:** 9 **Outpatient Visits:** 37086 **Births:** 77 **Total Expense ($000):** 33285 **Payroll Expense ($000):** 15809 **Personnel:** 302

MI

## LINCOLN PARK—Wayne County

☐ **VIBRA HOSPITAL OF SOUTHEASTERN MICHIGAN (232019)**, 26400 West Outer Drive, Zip 48146–2088; tel. 313/386–2000, (Nonreporting) **A**1 9 10 **S** Vibra Healthcare, Mechanicsburg, PA
Primary Contact: Jonathan Cohee, Chief Executive Officer
COO: Cindy Brassinger, Chief Operating Officer
CFO: Douglas Morris, Chief Financial Officer
CHR: Karen D. Gray, Director Human Resources
Web address: www.vhsemichigan.com/
**Control:** Corporation, Investor–owned, for–profit **Service:** Long–Term Acute Care hospital

**Staffed Beds:** 140

## LIVONIA—Wayne County

✉ **ST. MARY MERCY HOSPITAL (230002)**, 36475 West Five Mile Road, Zip 48154–1988; tel. 734/655–4800 **A**1 2 9 10 **F**3 4 5 12 13 15 17 18 20 22 26 29 30 31 34 35 38 40 45 46 47 49 50 51 56 57 58 59 64 68 70 74 75 76 78 79 81 83 84 85 87 90 93 98 100 101 102 103 104 107 108 110 111 113 114 115 116 117 118 119 120 125 128 129 131 134 142 144 145 146 147 **P**5 6 **S** Trinity Health, Novi, MI
Primary Contact: David A. Spivey, President and Chief Executive Officer
COO: C. W. Lauderbach, Jr., Vice President Clinical Services
CFO: Mike Samyn, Vice President, Finance and Chief Financial Officer
CIO: Janet Yim, Director Information Services
CHR: Kenneth Antczak, Vice President Human Resources
Web address: www.stmarymercy.org
**Control:** Church–operated, Nongovernment, not–for profit **Service:** General Medical and Surgical

**Staffed Beds:** 289 **Admissions:** 16877 **Census:** 225 **Outpatient Visits:** 191479 **Births:** 687 **Total Expense ($000):** 208167 **Payroll Expense ($000):** 84876 **Personnel:** 1253

## LUDINGTON—Mason County

**MEMORIAL MEDICAL CENTER OF WEST MICHIGAN (230110)**, One Atkinson Drive, Zip 49431–1906; tel. 231/843–2591 **A**9 10 20 21 **F**8 11 13 15 17 28 29 34 35 40 45 49 51 57 59 62 68 75 76 77 79 81 82 85 92 93 98 100 102 103 107 108 110 111 113 117 118 128 129 130 131 134 145 146
Primary Contact: Mark Vipperman, President and Chief Executive Officer
COO: Timothy Heinrich, Senior Vice President and Chief Operating Officer
CFO: Kerri Nelson, Chief Financial Officer
CMO: Stanley Seuferer, D.O., Chief of Staff
CIO: Daryl Crowley, Director Information Services
CHR: James Wood, Director Human Resources
Web address: www.mmcwm.com
**Control:** Other not–for–profit (including NFP Corporation) **Service:** General Medical and Surgical

**Staffed Beds:** 80 **Admissions:** 2379 **Census:** 30 **Outpatient Visits:** 94934 **Births:** 311 **Total Expense ($000):** 49098 **Payroll Expense ($000):** 21174 **Personnel:** 446

## MADISON HEIGHTS—Oakland County

**DMC SURGERY HOSPITAL** See Harper University Hospital/Hutzel Women's Hospital, Detroit

★ **ST. JOHN MACOMB–OAKLAND HOSPITAL, OAKLAND CENTER (230195)**, 27351 Dequindre, Zip 48071–3499; tel. 248/967–7000 **A**9 10 **F**3 11 12 15 18 20 28 29 30 31 34 35 36 38 39 40 41 44 45 46 49 50 51 57 59 60 61 63 64 65 68 70 74 75 77 78 79 81 82 84 85 86 87 91 92 93 96 97 98 100 101 102 103 104 105 107 108 113 114 118 128 129 131 134 142 145 147 **P**8 **S** Ascension Health, Saint Louis, MO
Primary Contact: Diane M. Radloff, President and Chief Executive Officer
COO: Deborah A. Condino, Site Administrator
CFO: Tomasine Marx, Chief Financial Officer
CFO: Tomasine Marx, Chief Financial Officer
CMO: Gary L. Berg, D.O., Chief Medical Officer
CIO: Karen McCormick, Director Client Services
CHR: Joanne E. Tuscany, Director Work life Services
Web address: www.stjohnprovidence.org/oakland
**Control:** Church–operated, Nongovernment, not–for profit **Service:** General Medical and Surgical

**Staffed Beds:** 157 **Admissions:** 7425 **Census:** 99 **Outpatient Visits:** 136960 **Births:** 0 **Total Expense ($000):** 96430 **Payroll Expense ($000):** 42744 **Personnel:** 822

## MANISTEE—Manistee County

**WEST SHORE MEDICAL CENTER (231335)**, 1465 East Parkdale Avenue, Zip 49660–9709; tel. 231/398–1000 **A**9 10 18 **F**3 7 11 13 15 17 28 29 32 34 39 40 46 53 54 57 59 74 75 76 77 79 81 85 86 93 107 108 110 111 114 117 118 126 128 131 134 145 146 147 **P**6
Primary Contact: James Barker, President
COO: Donn J. Lemmer, Vice President Finance
CFO: Donn J. Lemmer, Vice President Finance
Web address: www.westshoremedcenter.org
**Control:** County–Government, nonfederal **Service:** General Medical and Surgical

**Staffed Beds:** 34 **Admissions:** 1666 **Census:** 17 **Outpatient Visits:** 90386 **Births:** 170 **Total Expense ($000):** 42240 **Payroll Expense ($000):** 20340 **Personnel:** 304

## MANISTIQUE—Schoolcraft County

★ **SCHOOLCRAFT MEMORIAL HOSPITAL (231303)**, 500 Main Street, Zip 49854–1522; tel. 906/341–3200 **A**9 10 18 **F**3 10 11 15 28 29 30 31 32 34 35 40 41 44 45 50 53 56 57 59 62 63 64 65 70 75 77 78 79 81 84 85 86 87 89 93 97 107 108 110 113 118 126 127 128 129 131 132 134 143 145 146 147 **P**6
Primary Contact: George H. Montgomery, Chief Executive Officer
CFO: Tanya Hoar, Chief Financial Officer
CMO: Randy Olli, M.D., Chief Medical Officer
CIO: Kent La Croix, IT Supervisor
CHR: Gina Lindquist, Director Human Resources
CNO: Cindy Olli, R.N., Chief Nursing Officer
Web address: www.scmh.org
**Control:** County–Government, nonfederal **Service:** General Medical and Surgical

**Staffed Beds:** 18 **Admissions:** 336 **Census:** 3 **Outpatient Visits:** 35939 **Births:** 0 **Total Expense ($000):** 21205 **Payroll Expense ($000):** 11377 **Personnel:** 179

## MARLETTE—Sanilac County

✉ **MARLETTE REGIONAL HOSPITAL (231330)**, 2770 Main Street, Zip 48453–0307, Mailing Address: P.O. Box 307, Zip 48453–0307; tel. 989/635–4000, (Nonreporting) **A**1 9 10 18
Primary Contact: Daniel Babcock, Chief Executive Officer
CFO: James L. Singles, Chief Financial Officer
CMO: William Starbird, M.D., Chief of Staff
CIO: Rod Livingston, Manager Information Technology
CHR: Connie Kennedy, Director Human Resources
Web address: www.marlettecommunityhospital.com
**Control:** Other not–for–profit (including NFP Corporation) **Service:** General Medical and Surgical

**Staffed Beds:** 74

## MARQUETTE—Marquette County

✉ **MARQUETTE GENERAL HEALTH SYSTEM (230054)**, 580 West College Avenue, Zip 49855–2705; tel. 906/228–9440 **A**1 2 3 5 9 10 13 **F**3 4 5 7 8 11 12 13 14 15 17 18 20 22 24 26 28 29 30 31 32 34 35 37 38 40 43 45 46 48 49 50 51 55 56 57 58 59 60 62 63 64 65 68 70 72 74 75 76 77 78 79 81 82 85 86 87 89 90 93 94 98 99 100 101 102 103 104 107 108 110 111 113 114 115 116 117 118 119 120 121 122 123 126 128 129 130 131 134 142 144 145 146 147 **P**6
Primary Contact: A. Gary Muller, FACHE, President and Chief Executive Officer
COO: David Graser, Chief Information Officer
CFO: Jerry L. Worden, Chief Financial Officer
CMO: Tom Noren, M.D., Chief Medical Officer
CIO: David Graser, Chief Information Officer
CHR: David Smith, Senior Director Human Resources
CNO: Dagmar Ann Raica, R.N., Chief Nursing Officer
Web address: www.mgh.org
**Control:** Other not–for–profit (including NFP Corporation) **Service:** General Medical and Surgical

**Staffed Beds:** 276 **Admissions:** 10535 **Census:** 152 **Outpatient Visits:** 268307 **Births:** 672 **Total Expense ($000):** 294204 **Payroll Expense ($000):** 126539 **Personnel:** 1954

## MARSHALL—Calhoun County

★ **OAKLAWN HOSPITAL (230217)**, 200 North Madison Street, Zip 49068–1199; tel. 269/781–4271 **A**9 10 21 **F**3 11 13 15 18 19 26 28 29 30 31 32 34 35 36 37 38 40 44 45 46 48 50 53 54 57 58 59 60 62 63 64 65 68 69 70 74 75 76 77 78 79 81 82 85 86 87 89 93 94 97 98 99 100 101 102 103 104 105 106 107 108 110 111 113 114 116 117 118 125 128 129 130 131 134 145 146 147 **P**1 6
Primary Contact: Rob Covert, President and Chief Executive Officer
CFO: Colleen Koppenhaver, Chief Financial Officer
CMO: Ginger Williams, M.D., Chief Medical Officer
CIO: Natalie Spivak, Director Information Services
CHR: Jan Sinclair, Director Personnel
Web address: www.oaklawnhospital.org
**Control:** Other not–for–profit (including NFP Corporation) **Service:** General Medical and Surgical

**Staffed Beds:** 78 **Admissions:** 3805 **Census:** 41 **Outpatient Visits:** 162707 **Births:** 686 **Total Expense ($000):** 99910 **Payroll Expense ($000):** 48081 **Personnel:** 825

MI

*Many Facility Codes have changed. Please refer to the AHA Guide Code Chart.* © 2012 AHA Guide

## MIDLAND—Midland County

⊠ **MIDMICHIGAN MEDICAL CENTER–MIDLAND (230222)**, 4000 Wellness Drive, Zip 48670–0001; tel. 989/839–3000 **A**1 2 3 5 9 10 20 **F**3 7 11 12 13 15 18 20 22 24 26 28 29 30 31 34 40 45 46 48 49 50 53 54 55 57 58 59 64 65 68 70 74 75 76 77 78 79 81 85 86 87 89 92 93 96 97 98 100 101 102 104 107 108 110 111 113 114 117 118 119 120 122 123 125 128 129 130 131 132 134 142 144 145 146 147 **S** MidMichigan Health, Midland, MI
Primary Contact: Gregory H. Rogers, President
CFO: Scott D. Currie, Vice President and Chief Financial Officer
CMO: James Bicknell, M.D., Medical Director
CIO: C. Harlan Goodrich, Vice President and Chief Information Officer
CHR: Lynn Bruchhof, Vice President
Web address: www.midmichigan.org
**Control:** Other not–for–profit (including NFP Corporation) **Service:** General Medical and Surgical

**Staffed Beds:** 250 **Admissions:** 11133 **Census:** 116 **Outpatient Visits:** 295445 **Births:** 1188 **Total Expense ($000):** 274074 **Payroll Expense ($000):** 92376 **Personnel:** 1935

## MONROE—Monroe County

⊠ **MERCY MEMORIAL HOSPITAL SYSTEM (230099)**, 718 North Macomb Street, Zip 48162–7815; tel. 734/240–8400, (Total facility includes 70 beds in nursing home–type unit) **A**1 2 9 10 **F**3 5 8 11 13 15 18 28 29 30 34 35 38 40 44 45 46 49 50 51 54 56 57 59 62 63 64 65 69 70 71 74 75 76 77 79 81 84 85 86 87 89 92 93 97 98 100 101 102 103 104 107 108 109 110 111 113 114 115 116 117 118 125 128 129 130 131 134 143 144 145 146 147 **P**6
Primary Contact: Annette S. Phillips, President and Chief Executive Officer
CFO: Thomas Schilling, Chief Financial Officer and Senior Vice President Finance
CMO: Mark Sherrard, D.O., Chief Medical Officer and Senior Vice President Medical Affairs
CIO: Bruce Kelly, Chief Information Officer
CHR: Maureen Henson, Vice President Human Resources
CNO: Pamela A. Urbanski, R.N., Chief Nursing Officer, Senior Vice President, Patient Care Services
Web address: www.mercymemorial.org
**Control:** Other not–for–profit (including NFP Corporation) **Service:** General Medical and Surgical

**Staffed Beds:** 169 **Admissions:** 9605 **Census:** 108 **Outpatient Visits:** 176432 **Births:** 794 **Total Expense ($000):** 151512 **Payroll Expense ($000):** 65803 **Personnel:** 1386

## MOUNT CLEMENS—Macomb County

**HENRY FORD MACOMB HOSPITAL – MOUNT CLEMENS CAMPUS** See Henry Ford Macomb Hospitals, Clinton Township

★ ○ **MCLAREN MACOMB (230227)**, 1000 Harrington Boulevard, Zip 48043–2920; tel. 586/493–8000 **A**2 9 10 11 12 13 **F**3 7 8 13 15 17 18 20 22 24 26 28 29 30 31 34 35 36 37 39 40 42 43 45 47 48 49 50 51 52 54 57 58 59 60 61 62 63 64 65 66 68 70 71 74 75 76 77 78 79 81 82 85 86 87 89 90 92 93 97 100 102 107 108 109 110 111 112 113 114 115 116 117 118 119 120 123 125 128 129 131 134 144 145 146 147 **P**8 **S** McLaren Health Care Corporation, Flint, MI
Primary Contact: Mark S. O'Halla, President and Chief Executive Officer
COO: Sue Durst, R.N., Vice President Plant Operations
CMO: Michael K. Smith, D.O., Vice President Medical Affairs
CNO: Patricia Rosenberg, R.N., Vice President Patient Care Services and Chief Nursing Officer
Web address: www.mcrmc.org
**Control:** Other not–for–profit (including NFP Corporation) **Service:** General Medical and Surgical

**Staffed Beds:** 288 **Admissions:** 14941 **Census:** 164 **Outpatient Visits:** 155148 **Births:** 926 **Total Expense ($000):** 255132 **Payroll Expense ($000):** 104448 **Personnel:** 1537

⊠ **SELECT SPECIALTY HOSPITAL–MACOMB COUNTY (232023)**, 215 North Avenue, Zip 48043–1716; tel. 586/307–9000 **A**1 9 10 **F**1 3 17 18 29 30 70 77 80 90 91 **P**8 **S** Select Medical Corporation, Mechanicsburg, PA
Primary Contact: Jon P. O'Malley, Chief Executive Officer
Web address: www.selectmedicalcorp.com
**Control:** Individual, Investor–owned, for–profit **Service:** Children's Long–Term Acute Care

**Staffed Beds:** 30 **Admissions:** 36 **Census:** 30 **Outpatient Visits:** 0 **Births:** 0 **Total Expense ($000):** 13900 **Payroll Expense ($000):** 6700 **Personnel:** 161

## MOUNT PLEASANT—Isabella County

★ ○ **MCLAREN CENTRAL MICHIGAN (230080)**, 1221 South Drive, Zip 48858–3234; tel. 989/772–6700 **A**9 10 11 **F**3 12 13 15 18 20 22 26 28 29 30 31 34 35 40 44 45 48 49 50 54 57 59 62 64 65 68 70 74 75 76 77 78 79 81 82 85 86 87 89 96 97 107 108 110 111 113 116 117 118 119 120 122 123 128 129 130 131 143 144 145 146 **P**1 **S** McLaren Health Care Corporation, Flint, MI
Primary Contact: William P. Lawrence, President and Chief Executive Officer
CFO: Gregg Beeg, Chief Financial Officer
CMO: Ashok Vashishta, M.D., Vice President Medical Affairs
CIO: Nicolette Zalud, Customer Site Manager
CHR: Carolyn Potter, Director Human Resources
CNO: Sheri Myers, Vice President Patient Care Services
Web address: www.cmch.org
**Control:** Other not–for–profit (including NFP Corporation) **Service:** General Medical and Surgical

**Staffed Beds:** 78 **Admissions:** 3813 **Census:** 33 **Outpatient Visits:** 221934 **Births:** 595 **Total Expense ($000):** 78379 **Payroll Expense ($000):** 34855 **Personnel:** 562

## MUNISING—Alger County

**MUNISING MEMORIAL HOSPITAL (231308)**, 1500 Sand Point Road, Zip 49862–1406; tel. 906/387–4110, (Nonreporting) **A**9 10 18
Primary Contact: Kevin P. Calhoun, Chief Executive Officer
CFO: Barb Trombley, Director Financial Services
CMO: Christine Krueger, M.D., Chief of Staff
CHR: Melissa Hall, Human Resources
Web address: www.munisingmemorial.org
**Control:** Other not–for–profit (including NFP Corporation) **Service:** General Medical and Surgical

**Staffed Beds:** 25

## MUSKEGON—Muskegon County

⊠ **GREAT LAKES SPECIALTY HOSPITAL–HACKLEY CAMPUS (232021)**, 1700 Clinton Street, S2, Zip 49442–5502; tel. 231/728–5811, (Nonreporting) **A**1 9 10 **S** Select Medical Corporation, Mechanicsburg, PA
Primary Contact: Brian Pangle, Chief Executive Officer
Web address: www.selectmedical.com
**Control:** Corporation, Investor–owned, for–profit **Service:** Long–Term Acute Care hospital

**Staffed Beds:** 31

⊠ **MERCY HEALTH PARTNERS, HACKLEY CAMPUS (230066)**, 1700 Clinton Street, Zip 49442–5502, Mailing Address: P.O. Box 3302, Zip 49443–3302; tel. 231/726–3511 **A**1 2 9 10 **F**3 11 12 13 15 18 20 26 29 30 35 39 40 45 49 50 51 53 54 57 59 61 64 68 70 74 76 77 79 81 82 84 85 87 89 90 93 96 97 98 99 100 101 102 103 104 105 106 107 108 109 111 113 114 115 116 117 118 126 143 145 146 147 **P**6 8 **S** Trinity Health, Novi, MI
Primary Contact: Roger Spoelman, President and Chief Executive Officer
COO: Greg Loomis, Chief Operating Officer
CFO: Gary Allore, Chief Financial Officer
CMO: F. Remington Sprague, M.D., Chief Medical Officer
CIO: William Stefl, Director Information Systems
Web address: www.hackley.org
**Control:** Other not–for–profit (including NFP Corporation) **Service:** General Medical and Surgical

**Staffed Beds:** 213 **Admissions:** 8902 **Census:** 92 **Outpatient Visits:** 283052 **Births:** 1753 **Total Expense ($000):** 152838 **Payroll Expense ($000):** 58021 **Personnel:** 1052

⊠ ○ **MERCY HEALTH PARTNERS, MERCY CAMPUS (230004)**, 1500 East Sherman Boulevard, Zip 49444–1849; tel. 231/672–2000, (Includes MERCY HEALTH PARTNERS–MUSKEGON GENERAL CAMPUS, 1700 Oak Avenue, Zip 49442; tel. 231/672–3311) **A**1 2 9 10 11 12 13 **F**3 11 12 15 18 20 22 24 26 28 29 30 31 34 35 40 44 50 51 53 54 56 57 58 59 64 68 70 74 75 76 77 78 79 81 82 84 85 86 87 91 93 94 96 97 107 108 111 113 114 115 116 117 118 119 120 121 122 123 128 129 130 131 134 143 145 146 147 **P**6 8 **S** Trinity Health, Novi, MI
Primary Contact: Roger Spoelman, President and Chief Executive Officer
COO: Greg Loomis, Chief Operation Officer
CFO: Gary Allore, Chief Financial Officer
CMO: F. Remington Sprague, M.D., Chief Medical Officer
Web address: www.mghp.org
**Control:** Other not–for–profit (including NFP Corporation) **Service:** General Medical and Surgical

**Staffed Beds:** 188 **Admissions:** 10170 **Census:** 110 **Outpatient Visits:** 592613 **Births:** 427 **Total Expense ($000):** 288404 **Payroll Expense ($000):** 119213 **Personnel:** 1804

**SELECT SPECIALTY HOSPITAL–WESTERN MICHIGAN** See Great Lakes Specialty Hospital–Hackley Campus

**MI**

---

### NEW BALTIMORE—Macomb County

**HARBOR OAKS HOSPITAL (234021)**, 35031 23 Mile Road, Zip 48047–3649;
tel. 586/725–5777, (Nonreporting) **A**9 10 **S** Acadia Healthcare Company, Inc.,
Franklin, TN
Primary Contact: Sari Abromovich, Chief Executive Officer
CFO: Michael Ferguson, Chief Financial Officer
CMO: James D. Adamo, M.D., Medical Director
CHR: DeShawna Boden, Director Human Resources
Web address: www.harboroaks.com
**Control:** Corporation, Investor–owned, for–profit **Service:** Psychiatric

Staffed Beds: 45

### NEWBERRY—Luce County

**HELEN NEWBERRY JOY HOSPITAL (231304)**, 502 West Harrie Street,
Zip 49868–1209; tel. 906/293–9200, (Includes HELEN NEWBERRY JOY
HOSPITAL ANNEX ), (Total facility includes 48 beds in nursing home–type unit) **A**1
9 10 18 21 **F**1 4 15 16 17 28 29 30 31 32 34 35 36 38 40 44 45 53 57 59
63 64 65 67 70 72 73 75 78 80 81 85 86 87 88 89 90 93 97 98 107 108
113 117 118 126 127 128 129 130 131 132 133 134 142 143 145 147 **P**6
Primary Contact: Scott Pillion, Chief Executive Officer
CMO: Raghu Rao, M.D., Chief of Staff
CIO: Michelle Sears, Director Information Systems
CHR: Roger Bergh, Director Human Resources
Web address: www.hnjh.org
**Control:** County–Government, nonfederal **Service:** General Medical and Surgical

Staffed Beds: 73 **Admissions:** 504 **Census:** 44 **Outpatient Visits:** 64319
**Births:** 0 **Total Expense ($000):** 29012 **Payroll Expense ($000):** 12928
**Personnel:** 262

### NORTHVILLE—Wayne County

**HAWTHORN CENTER**, 18471 Haggerty Road, Zip 48167–9575;
tel. 248/735–6771, (Nonreporting) **A**1 3 5 9
Primary Contact: Roy Kelly, Facility Director
CIO: Robert W. Bailey, Chief Information Officer
**Control:** State–Government, nonfederal **Service:** Children's hospital psychiatric

Staffed Beds: 69

### ONTONAGON—Ontonagon County

**ASPIRUS ONTONAGON HOSPITAL (231309)**, 601 South Seventh Street,
Zip 49953–1448; tel. 906/884–8000, (Nonreporting) **A**1 9 10 18 **S** Aspirus,
Inc., Wausau, WI
Primary Contact: Michael Hauswirth, Chief Operating Officer
CMO: John Austin, M.D., Director Medical Staff
CHR: Gina Linna, Manager Human Resources
CNO: Deanna Wilson, VP Patient Care Services/Site Manager
Web address: www.aspirus–ontonagon.org
**Control:** City–Government, nonfederal **Service:** General Medical and Surgical

Staffed Beds: 18

### OWOSSO—Shiawassee County

**MEMORIAL HEALTHCARE (230121)**, 826 West King Street, Zip 48867–2120;
tel. 989/723–5211, (Total facility includes 17 beds in nursing home–type unit) **A**1
2 5 9 10 **F**11 12 13 15 28 29 30 31 32 34 35 36 40 45 46 47 49 50 51 56
57 58 59 62 63 64 65 69 70 74 75 76 78 79 81 82 85 87 89 93 98 100
101 102 103 107 108 111 114 118 126 127 128 129 130 131 142 143 145
147 **P**6 7
Primary Contact: James M. Full, FACHE, President and Chief Executive Officer
CFO: Brian Long, Vice President Finance
CMO: Wael Salman, M.D., Vice President Medical Affairs
CIO: Frank Fear, Chief Information Officer
CHR: Ruthann Liagre, Vice President Human Resources
CNO: Dawn Blackwell, R.N., VP of Patient Care Services
Web address: www.memorialhealthcare.org
**Control:** Other not–for–profit (including NFP Corporation) **Service:** General
Medical and Surgical

Staffed Beds: 134 **Admissions:** 4039 **Census:** 63 **Outpatient Visits:** 248288
**Births:** 457 **Total Expense ($000):** 94823 **Payroll Expense ($000):** 42007
**Personnel:** 860

### PAW PAW—Van Buren County

**BRONSON LAKEVIEW HOSPITAL (231332)**, 408 Hazen Street,
Zip 49079–1019, Mailing Address: P.O. Box 209, Zip 49079–0209;
tel. 269/657–3141 **A**1 9 10 18 **F**3 11 15 29 30 34 35 40 56 57 59 64 65 68
74 75 77 79 81 82 85 86 87 89 93 98 100 101 102 103 104 107 110 113
118 126 129 145 146 147 **P**6 **S** Bronson Healthcare Group, Inc., Kalamazoo, MI
Primary Contact: Frank J. Sardone, President and Chief Executive Officer
COO: Sally L. Berglin, Vice President
CMO: Ravinder P. Mediratta, M.D., Chief of Staff
CHR: John Hayden, Senior Vice President and Chief Human Resources Officer
Web address: www.bronsonhealth.com/lakeview
**Control:** Other not–for–profit (including NFP Corporation) **Service:** General
Medical and Surgical

Staffed Beds: 35 **Admissions:** 1007 **Census:** 14 **Outpatient Visits:** 95742
**Births:** 0 **Total Expense ($000):** 38047 **Payroll Expense ($000):** 12451
**Personnel:** 361

### PETOSKEY—Emmet County

**MCLAREN NORTHERN MICHIGAN (230105)**, 416 Connable Avenue,
Zip 49770–2297; tel. 231/487–4000 **A**1 2 9 10 **F**3 12 13 15 17 18 20 22 24
26 28 29 30 31 32 34 35 36 38 40 43 44 45 49 50 51 53 57 58 59 60 64
68 70 74 75 76 77 78 79 81 82 85 86 87 89 90 91 93 94 96 107 108 110
111 113 114 118 119 120 122 123 128 129 131 134 145 147 **S** McLaren
Health Care Corporation, Flint, MI
Primary Contact: Reezie DeVet, R.N., Ph.D., President and Chief Executive Officer
COO: Mary–Anne D. Ponti, R.N., Chief Operating Officer and Chief Nurse Executive
CFO: Stephen J. Scannell, Chief Financial Officer
CMO: Kirk Lufkin, M.D., VPMA
CIO: Mark Gray, Chief Information Officer
CHR: Gene Kaminski, Vice President Human Resources
CNO: Jennifer Woods, R.N., Chief Nursing Officer
Web address: www.northernhealth.org
**Control:** Other not–for–profit (including NFP Corporation) **Service:** General
Medical and Surgical

Staffed Beds: 178 **Admissions:** 8803 **Census:** 94 **Outpatient Visits:** 127516
**Births:** 766 **Total Expense ($000):** 161812 **Payroll Expense ($000):** 58945
**Personnel:** 1169

### PIGEON—Huron County

**SCHEURER HOSPITAL (231310)**, 170 North Caseville Road, Zip 48755–9704;
tel. 989/453–3223, (Total facility includes 19 beds in nursing home–type unit) **A**1
9 10 18 **F**3 7 10 11 15 28 29 30 31 34 36 40 44 45 50 53 54 56 57 59 64
68 69 75 77 78 79 81 85 86 87 91 92 93 97 107 108 110 113 118 124 126
129 130 131 132 142 145 **P**6
Primary Contact: Dwight Gascho, President and Chief Executive Officer
CFO: Terry Lutz, Chief Financial Officer
CMO: Scott Reiter, D.O., Chief of Staff
CIO: Suzanne LeMaire, Manager Health Information Management Services and
Corporate Compliance Officer
CHR: Greg Foy, Human Resources System Leader
CNO: Sue Lathrom, Director of Nursing/Patient Care System Leader
Web address: www.scheurer.org
**Control:** Other not–for–profit (including NFP Corporation) **Service:** General
Medical and Surgical

Staffed Beds: 44 **Admissions:** 555 **Census:** 23 **Outpatient Visits:** 47370
**Births:** 0 **Total Expense ($000):** 30405 **Payroll Expense ($000):** 14716
**Personnel:** 316

### PLAINWELL—Allegan County

**BORGESS–PIPP HOSPITAL (232034)**, 411 Naomi Street, Zip 49080–1222;
tel. 269/685–6811, (Nonreporting) **A**1 9 10 **S** Ascension Health, Saint Louis, MO
Primary Contact: John Ryder, Administrator and Chief Executive Officer
Web address: www.borgess.com
**Control:** Other not–for–profit (including NFP Corporation) **Service:** Long–Term
Acute Care hospital

Staffed Beds: 43

### PONTIAC—Oakland County

**DOCTORS' HOSPITAL OF MICHIGAN (230013)**, 461 West Huron Street,
Zip 48341–1601; tel. 248/857–7200, (Nonreporting) **A**9 10
Primary Contact: Sam Gizzi, President and Chief Executive Officer
COO: Dennis Franks, Vice President Operations
CFO: Dennis Franks, Interim Chief Financial Officer
CMO: Ray Breitenbach, M.D., Chief of Staff
CIO: Albert Sinisi, Director Information Systems
Web address: www.dhofm.com
**Control:** Other not–for–profit (including NFP Corporation) **Service:** General
Medical and Surgical

Staffed Beds: 106

*Many Facility Codes have changed. Please refer to the AHA Guide Code Chart.* © 2012 AHA Guide

★ ○ **MCLAREN OAKLAND (230207)**, 50 North Perry Street, Zip 48342–2253; tel. 248/338–5000, (Total facility includes 120 beds in nursing home–type unit) **A**9 10 11 12 13 **F**3 4 7 8 11 12 14 15 18 20 24 26 28 29 30 31 32 33 34 35 36 40 42 43 44 45 50 53 54 57 59 62 63 64 65 66 68 70 74 75 77 78 79 81 82 90 92 93 94 98 103 107 108 111 113 117 118 123 127 129 130 131 134 135 136 137 138 139 140 141 142 143 145 147 **P**4 8 **S** McLaren Health Care Corporation, Flint, MI
Primary Contact: Clarence Sevillian, President and Chief Executive Officer
CFO: Fred Korte, Chief Financial Officer
CMO: Steven Calkin, D.O., Vice President Medical Affairs
CIO: Teresa Rodges, Executive Director Marketing and Public Relations
CHR: Laura Gibbard, Vice President Human Resources
Web address: www.pohmedical.org
**Control:** Other not–for–profit (including NFP Corporation) **Service:** General Medical and Surgical

**Staffed Beds:** 288 **Admissions:** 6160 **Census:** 209 **Outpatient Visits:** 149723 **Births:** 0 **Total Expense ($000):** 129920 **Payroll Expense ($000):** 51180 **Personnel:** 1067

⊞ **SELECT SPECIALTY HOSPITAL–PONTIAC (232030)**, 44405 Woodward Avenue, 8th Floor, Zip 48341–5023; tel. 248/452–5252, (Nonreporting) **A**1 9 10 **S** Select Medical Corporation, Mechanicsburg, PA
Primary Contact: Peggy Kingston, Chief Executive Officer
CMO: Fadi Salloum, M.D., Medical Director
CNO: Catherine Folson, MSN, Chief Nursing Officer
Web address: www.https://www.selectmedicalcorp.com
**Control:** Corporation, Investor–owned, for–profit **Service:** Long–Term Acute Care hospital

**Staffed Beds:** 30

⊞ **ST. JOSEPH MERCY OAKLAND (230029)**, 44405 Woodward Avenue, Zip 48341–5023; tel. 248/858–3000 **A**1 2 3 5 9 10 12 13 **F**3 8 12 13 15 17 18 20 22 24 26 28 29 30 31 32 34 35 36 37 38 39 40 43 44 45 46 48 49 50 51 54 55 56 57 58 59 61 64 65 66 68 70 72 74 75 76 77 78 79 81 82 84 85 86 87 89 90 92 93 96 97 98 100 101 102 103 105 107 108 110 111 113 114 118 125 128 129 130 131 134 143 145 146 **P**6 **S** Trinity Health, Novi, MI
Primary Contact: Jack Weiner, President and Chief Executive Officer
COO: Barbara Hertzler, Chief Operating Officer
CFO: Michael Gusho, Chief Financial Officer
CMO: Donald Bignotti, M.D., Vice President Medical Affairs
CIO: Robert Jones, Director Management Information Systems
CHR: Martha Murphy, Vice President Human Resources
CNO: Ann McDonald–Upton, Chief Nursing Officer
Web address: www.stjoesoakland.com
**Control:** Church–operated, Nongovernment, not–for profit **Service:** General Medical and Surgical

**Staffed Beds:** 409 **Admissions:** 19385 **Census:** 268 **Outpatient Visits:** 325194 **Births:** 1969 **Total Expense ($000):** 369990 **Payroll Expense ($000):** 143437 **Personnel:** 2555

**PORT HURON—St. Clair County**

⊞ **PORT HURON HOSPITAL (230216)**, 1221 Pine Grove Avenue, Zip 48060–3511; tel. 810/987–5000 **A**1 2 9 10 **F**3 5 11 12 13 15 17 18 20 22 24 26 29 30 31 32 34 35 36 39 40 43 44 45 46 48 49 50 51 54 56 57 58 59 61 64 65 66 68 70 72 74 75 76 78 79 81 82 84 85 86 87 89 92 93 96 97 98 99 100 101 102 103 104 107 108 110 113 114 115 116 117 118 128 129 130 131 133 134 143 144 145 146 147 **P**6 **S** Blue Water Health Services Corporation, Port Huron, MI
Primary Contact: Thomas D. DeFauw, FACHE, President and Chief Executive Officer
COO: David S. McEwen, Vice President Operations
CFO: John Liston, Chief Financial Officer
CMO: Michael W. Tawney, D.O., Vice President Medical Affairs
CIO: John Kaiser, Director Information Systems
CHR: Doris A. Seidl, Vice President Human Resources
CNO: Jennifer Montgomery, Vice President, Nursing
Web address: www.porthuronhospital.org
**Control:** Other not–for–profit (including NFP Corporation) **Service:** General Medical and Surgical

**Staffed Beds:** 186 **Admissions:** 12017 **Census:** 143 **Outpatient Visits:** 170821 **Births:** 1326 **Total Expense ($000):** 156651 **Payroll Expense ($000):** 64264

⊞ **ST. JOSEPH MERCY PORT HURON (230031)**, 2601 Electric Avenue, Zip 48060–6518; tel. 810/985–1500 **A**1 2 9 10 **F**3 11 15 18 20 29 30 31 34 35 40 43 45 49 50 54 57 58 59 61 62 63 64 66 68 70 74 75 77 78 79 81 82 83 84 85 86 87 89 90 93 96 97 107 108 110 113 115 116 117 118 119 120 122 125 128 129 130 131 145 146 147 **P**6 8 **S** Trinity Health, Novi, MI
Primary Contact: Rebecca Smith, Chief Executive Officer
CFO: Deborah Armstrong, Chief Financial Officer
CMO: Philip Matich, M.D., Vice President Medical Affairs
CIO: Cathy Geiger, Director Information Services
CHR: Robert Gunn, Vice President Human Resources
Web address: www.mercyporthuron.com
**Control:** Church–operated, Nongovernment, not–for profit **Service:** General Medical and Surgical

**Staffed Beds:** 119 **Admissions:** 4196 **Census:** 51 **Outpatient Visits:** 123248 **Births:** 0 **Total Expense ($000):** 79665 **Payroll Expense ($000):** 27857 **Personnel:** 632

**REED CITY—Osceola County**

⊞ **SPECTRUM HEALTH REED CITY HOSPITAL (231323)**, 300 North Patterson Road, Zip 49677–0075, Mailing Address: P.O. Box 75, Zip 49677–0075; tel. 231/832–3271, (Total facility includes 54 beds in nursing home–type unit) **A**1 9 10 18 **F**3 15 29 30 31 34 35 40 45 50 53 54 57 59 64 65 70 75 77 78 79 81 84 85 86 87 93 97 107 108 110 111 113 117 118 119 120 122 123 126 127 128 129 130 132 145 **P**6 **S** Spectrum Health, Grand Rapids, MI
Primary Contact: Sam Daugherty, Ed.D., President
COO: Linda Rubin, Chief Operating Officer
CFO: Thomas Knoerl, Chief Financial Officer
CMO: Alan Grillo, M.D., Chief of Staff
CHR: Kris Miller, Director Human Resources
Web address: www.reedcity.spectrum–health.org
**Control:** Other not–for–profit (including NFP Corporation) **Service:** General Medical and Surgical

**Staffed Beds:** 74 **Admissions:** 858 **Census:** 56 **Outpatient Visits:** 116067 **Births:** 0 **Total Expense ($000):** 43592 **Payroll Expense ($000):** 16316 **Personnel:** 377

**ROCHESTER—Oakland County**

☐ △ **CRITTENTON HOSPITAL MEDICAL CENTER (230254)**, 1101 West University Drive, Zip 48307–1831; tel. 248/652–5000 **A**1 2 3 5 7 9 10 **F**3 11 12 13 15 17 18 20 22 24 26 28 29 30 31 32 34 35 36 37 39 40 44 45 46 47 48 49 50 51 53 54 55 57 58 59 60 62 63 64 65 68 70 73 74 75 76 77 78 79 81 82 84 85 86 87 89 90 92 93 94 96 97 98 100 101 102 107 108 110 113 114 117 118 125 128 129 130 131 133 134 142 143 145 146 147 **P**6
Primary Contact: Frank Sottile, M.D., Interim Chief Executive Officer
COO: Gregory A. Partamian, Chief Operating Officer
CFO: Donna Kopinski, Chief Financial Officer
CMO: Frank Sottile, M.D., Chief Medical Officer
CIO: Tom Ventameglia, Director Information Systems
Web address: www.crittenton.com
**Control:** Other not–for–profit (including NFP Corporation) **Service:** General Medical and Surgical

**Staffed Beds:** 254 **Admissions:** 12921 **Census:** 174 **Outpatient Visits:** 238097 **Births:** 1287 **Personnel:** 1133

**ROGERS CITY—Presque Isle County**

☐ **ROGERS CITY REHABILITATION HOSPITAL (233029)**, 555 North Bradley Highway, Suite C., Zip 49779–1539; tel. 989/734–7545, (Nonreporting) **A**1 9 10
Primary Contact: Joyal Pavey, Executive Director
CFO: Dylan Moore, Controller
CMO: Diana Hernandez Drozdowicz, M.D., Medical Director
Web address: www.rogerscityrehab.com
**Control:** Corporation, Investor–owned, for–profit **Service:** Rehabilitation

**Staffed Beds:** 15

**ROMEO—Macomb County**

**ST. JOSEPH'S MERCY–NORTH** See Henry Ford Macomb Hospitals, Clinton Township

MI

---

**Hospital, Medicare Provider Number, Address, Telephone, Approval, Facility, and Physician Codes, Health Care System**

★ American Hospital Association (AHA) membership
☐ The Joint Commission accreditation  ◇ DNV Healthcare Inc. accreditation
○ American Osteopathic Association (AOA) accreditation
△ Commission on Accreditation of Rehabilitation Facilities (CARF) accreditation

## ROYAL OAK—Oakland County

✠ **BEAUMONT HOSPITAL – ROYAL OAK (230130)**, 3601 West Thirteen Mile Road, Zip 48073–6712; tel. 248/898–5000, (Includes BEAUMONT CHILDREN'S HOSPITAL, 3601 West 13 Mile Road, tel. 248/898–5000) **A**1 2 3 5 8 9 10 13 **F**3 5 6 11 12 13 14 15 17 18 19 20 22 24 26 28 29 30 31 32 34 35 36 37 38 39 40 41 43 44 45 46 47 48 49 50 51 54 55 56 57 58 59 60 61 62 63 64 65 66 68 70 71 72 74 75 76 77 78 79 80 81 82 83 84 85 86 87 88 89 90 91 92 93 94 95 96 97 98 99 100 101 102 103 104 105 107 108 109 110 111 113 114 115 116 117 118 119 120 122 123 125 128 129 130 131 133 134 137 138 140 141 142 143 144 145 146 147 **P**6 **S** Beaumont Health System, Royal Oak, MI
Primary Contact: Shane Cerone, President
COO: Gene Michalski, Executive Vice President and Chief Operating Officer
CFO: Nickolas A. Vitale, Executive Vice President and Chief Financial Officer
CMO: Ananias C. Diokno, M.D., Executive Vice President and Chief Medical Officer
CIO: Subra Sripada, Senior Vice President and Chief Information Officer
Web address: www.beaumonthospitals.com
**Control:** Other not–for–profit (including NFP Corporation) **Service:** General Medical and Surgical

**Staffed Beds:** 1070 **Admissions:** 55689 **Census:** 837 **Outpatient Visits:** 1298056 **Births:** 5088 **Total Expense ($000):** 1086657 **Payroll Expense ($000):** 355050 **Personnel:** 7602

## SAGINAW—Saginaw County

✠ **ALEDA E. LUTZ VETERANS AFFAIRS MEDICAL CENTER**, 1500 Weiss Street, Zip 48602–5298; tel. 989/497–2500, (Total facility includes 81 beds in nursing home–type unit) **A**1 9 **F**3 5 6 11 15 18 29 30 31 34 35 36 38 39 40 44 45 50 53 54 56 57 58 59 61 63 64 68 74 75 77 78 81 82 83 84 85 86 87 93 94 97 100 101 102 103 104 107 108 118 126 127 129 130 131 132 134 135 136 137 138 139 140 141 142 143 145 146 147 **P**6 **S** Department of Veterans Affairs, Washington, DC
Primary Contact: Denise Deitzen, Director
CFO: Jeff Drew, Fiscal Officer
CMO: Nicholas Haddad, M.D., Acting Chief Medical Service
CIO: Stephanie Young, Chief Information Technology
CHR: Kathy Seymour, Acting Chief Human Resources Management Service
Web address: www.saginaw.va.gov/
**Control:** Veterans Affairs, Government, federal **Service:** General Medical and Surgical

**Staffed Beds:** 100 **Admissions:** 1348 **Census:** 55 **Outpatient Visits:** 291507 **Births:** 0 **Total Expense ($000):** 165268 **Payroll Expense ($000):** 64471 **Personnel:** 894

★ ○ △ **COVENANT MEDICAL CENTER (230070)**, 1447 North Harrison Street, Zip 48602–4727; tel. 989/583–0000, (Includes COVENANT MEDICAL CENTER–COOPER, 700 Cooper Avenue, Zip 48602–5399; tel. 517/583–0000; COVENANT MEDICAL CENTER–HARRISON, 1447 North Harrison Street, Zip 48602–4785; tel. 517/583–0000), (Nonreporting) **A**2 3 5 7 9 10 11
Primary Contact: Spencer Maidlow, President and Chief Executive Officer
COO: Edward Bruff, Executive Vice President and Chief Operating Officer
CFO: Mark E. Gronda, Vice President and Chief Financial Officer
CMO: John Kosanovich, M.D., Vice President Medical Affairs
CIO: Keith Grantham, Director Information Technology
CHR: Al Van Arsdal, Director Human Resources
Web address: www.covenanthealthcare.com
**Control:** Other not–for–profit (including NFP Corporation) **Service:** General Medical and Surgical

**Staffed Beds:** 533

☐ **HEALTHSOURCE SAGINAW (230275)**, (LTC Rehab Psych Chem Dependenc), 3340 Hospital Road, Zip 48603–9622, Mailing Address: P.O. Box 6280, Zip 48608–6280; tel. 989/790–7700, (Total facility includes 213 beds in nursing home–type unit) **A**1 9 10 **F**4 5 11 56 57 61 64 75 77 82 86 87 90 91 93 94 95 98 99 100 101 103 104 127 129 131 134 142 145 147 **P**6
Primary Contact: Lester Heyboer, Jr., President and Chief Executive Officer
CFO: Lisa Lapham, Chief Financial Officer
CMO: Daniel Duffy, D.O., Chief Medical Director
CIO: Randall Sanborn, Director Information Technology
CHR: Rebecca Oster, Director Human Resources
Web address: www.healthsourcesaginaw.org
**Control:** Other not–for–profit (including NFP Corporation) **Service:** Other specialty

**Staffed Beds:** 319 **Admissions:** 3131 **Census:** 263 **Outpatient Visits:** 3256 **Births:** 0 **Total Expense ($000):** 39128 **Payroll Expense ($000):** 18463 **Personnel:** 484

✠ **SELECT SPECIALTY HOSPITAL–SAGINAW (232033)**, 1447 North Harrison Street, Zip 48602–4727; tel. 989/583–4235, (Nonreporting) **A**1 9 10 **S** Select Medical Corporation, Mechanicsburg, PA
Primary Contact: Dawn Frisbie, Chief Executive Officer
Web address: www.selectmedicalcorp.com
**Control:** Corporation, Investor–owned, for–profit **Service:** Long–Term Acute Care hospital

**Staffed Beds:** 32

✠ **ST. MARY'S OF MICHIGAN (230077)**, 800 South Washington Avenue, Zip 48601–2551; tel. 989/907–8000 **A**1 2 3 5 9 10 **F**2 3 11 15 17 18 20 22 24 26 28 29 30 31 34 35 36 40 42 43 44 45 49 50 51 54 57 58 59 64 66 68 70 74 75 77 78 79 80 81 82 84 85 86 87 92 93 96 100 102 107 108 110 111 113 114 117 118 119 120 122 123 125 128 129 131 145 146 **P**6 7 8 **S** Ascension Health, Saint Louis, MO
Primary Contact: John R. Graham, President and Chief Executive Officer
COO: Rick L. Ohle, Chief Operating Officer
CFO: Gina Butcher, Chief Financial Officer
CIO: David Wanner, Chief Information Officer
CHR: Ron Haase, Vice President Human Resources
Web address: www.stmarysofmichigan.org
**Control:** Church–operated, Nongovernment, not–for profit **Service:** General Medical and Surgical

**Staffed Beds:** 228 **Admissions:** 11149 **Census:** 175 **Outpatient Visits:** 157728 **Births:** 0 **Total Expense ($000):** 243231 **Payroll Expense ($000):** 93316 **Personnel:** 1738

## SAINT IGNACE—Mackinac County

★ **MACKINAC STRAITS HEALTH SYSTEM (231306)**, 1140 North State Street, Zip 49781–1013; tel. 906/643–8585, (Total facility includes 48 beds in nursing home–type unit) **A**9 10 18 **F**11 15 28 31 32 40 42 54 56 59 60 64 65 77 78 91 93 97 104 107 111 113 118 126 127 129 131 132 145 146 **P**6
Primary Contact: Rodney M. Nelson, Chief Executive Officer
CFO: Jason Anderson, Chief Financial Officer
CMO: John Stephenson, M.D., Chief of Staff
CHR: Karen Cheeseman, Director Human Resources
Web address: www.mshosp.org
**Control:** Other not–for–profit (including NFP Corporation) **Service:** General Medical and Surgical

**Staffed Beds:** 63 **Admissions:** 320 **Census:** 52 **Outpatient Visits:** 28783 **Births:** 0 **Total Expense ($000):** 29409 **Payroll Expense ($000):** 10671 **Personnel:** 187

## SAINT JOHNS—Clinton County

✠ **SPARROW CLINTON HOSPITAL (231326)**, 805 South Oakland Street, Zip 48879–2253; tel. 989/227–3400 **A**1 9 10 18 **F**8 11 15 18 19 31 32 34 35 40 45 53 57 59 64 70 75 77 78 79 81 85 93 107 110 111 113 118 128 129 130 132 144 145 147 **P**6 **S** Sparrow Health System, Lansing, MI
Primary Contact: Edward Bruun, President and Chief Executive Officer
COO: Kevin A. Price, Vice President and Chief Operating Officer
CFO: Mark Brisboe, Vice President & CFO
CMO: Gregory Holzhei, D.O., Chief of Staff
CHR: Lucy M. Vail, Director Human Resources & Partner Relations
Web address: www.clintonmemorial.org
**Control:** Other not–for–profit (including NFP Corporation) **Service:** General Medical and Surgical

**Staffed Beds:** 25 **Admissions:** 769 **Census:** 7 **Outpatient Visits:** 54280 **Births:** 0 **Total Expense ($000):** 37853 **Payroll Expense ($000):** 13511 **Personnel:** 211

## SAINT JOSEPH—Berrien County

☐ **LAKELAND REGIONAL MEDICAL CENTER–ST. JOSEPH (230021)**, 1234 Napier Avenue, Zip 49085–2112; tel. 269/983–8300 **A**1 2 9 10 13 **F**3 11 12 13 15 18 20 22 24 26 28 29 30 31 32 34 35 36 37 38 40 45 46 49 50 51 54 56 57 59 60 61 62 63 64 68 70 74 75 76 77 78 79 81 85 86 89 90 91 92 93 96 98 101 102 103 107 110 111 113 114 117 118 119 120 122 123 125 128 129 130 131 133 134 144 145 146 **P**8 **S** Lakeland Healthcare, Saint Joseph, MI
Primary Contact: Loren Hamel, M.D., President and Chief Executive Officer
CFO: Timothy Calhoun, Vice President Finance and Chief Financial Officer
CMO: Stephen Hempel, M.D., President Medical Staff
CIO: Emily Gallay, Vice President and Chief Information Officer
CHR: Gerard Guinane, Vice President Human Resources and Diversity Management
Web address: www.lakelandhealth.org
**Control:** Other not–for–profit (including NFP Corporation) **Service:** General Medical and Surgical

**Staffed Beds:** 250 **Admissions:** 16105 **Census:** 188 **Outpatient Visits:** 302967 **Births:** 1845 **Total Expense ($000):** 286942 **Payroll Expense ($000):** 110707 **Personnel:** 2678

## SANDUSKY—Sanilac County

**MCKENZIE HEALTH SYSTEM (231314)**, 120 Delaware Street, Zip 48471–1087; tel. 810/648–3770, (Nonreporting) **A**9 10 18
Primary Contact: Steve Barnett, MS, President and Chief Executive Officer
COO: Janet Herbert, R.N., Chief Operating Officer
CFO: Amy Ruedisueli, Chief Financial Officer
CMO: Mark E. English, M.D., Chief of Staff
CHR: Carrie Krampits, Director Human Resources
CNO: Tammy Cliff, R.N., Director Nursing Services
Web address: www.mckenziehealth.org
**Control:** Other not–for–profit (including NFP Corporation) **Service:** General Medical and Surgical

**Staffed Beds:** 25

**MI**

## SAULT SAINTE MARIE—Chippewa County

✠ **WAR MEMORIAL HOSPITAL (230239)**, 500 Osborn Boulevard,
Zip 49783–1822; tel. 906/635–4460, (Total facility includes 51 beds in nursing
home–type unit) **A**1 9 10 20 21 **F**3 11 12 13 15 18 28 29 30 31 34 35 36 38
40 43 44 45 50 53 54 56 57 59 60 61 62 64 65 66 68 70 74 75 76 77 78
79 81 82 84 85 87 91 92 93 94 96 97 98 100 101 103 104 107 110 111
114 118 126 127 128 129 130 131 132 134 142 143 145 146 147
Primary Contact: David B. Jahn, President and Chief Executive Officer
COO: Marla Bunker, Vice President of Operations
CFO: Kevin Kalchik, Chief Financial Officer
CMO: Ted Ludwig, Chief Medical Officer
CIO: Steve Pietrangelo, Director Information Services
CHR: Susan Sliger, Director Human Resources
CNO: Sue Tetzlaff, Vice President of Nursing
Web address: www.warmemorialhospital.org
**Control:** Other not–for–profit (including NFP Corporation) **Service:** General
Medical and Surgical

**Staffed Beds: 139 Admissions: 3316 Census: 91 Outpatient Visits: 149006
Births: 339 Total Expense ($000): 83631 Payroll Expense ($000): 32871
Personnel: 767**

## SHELBY—Oceana County

✠ **MERCY HEALTH PARTNERS, LAKESHORE CAMPUS (231320)**, 72 South
State Street, Zip 49455–1299; tel. 231/861–2156 **A**1 9 10 18 **F**3 11 15 29 30
34 35 40 57 59 68 81 85 87 89 97 107 111 114 118 126 128 131 145
**S** Trinity Health, Novi, MI
Primary Contact: Jay Bryan, President and Chief Executive Officer
CFO: Mark Gross, Senior Business Director Finance
Web address: www.mercyhealthpartners.org
**Control:** Other not–for–profit (including NFP Corporation) **Service:** General
Medical and Surgical

**Staffed Beds: 24 Admissions: 488 Census: 4 Outpatient Visits: 16909
Births: 47 Total Expense ($000): 20428 Payroll Expense ($000): 10141
Personnel: 149**

## SHERIDAN—Montcalm County

★ ○ **SHERIDAN COMMUNITY HOSPITAL (231312)**, 301 North Main Street,
Zip 48884–9235, Mailing Address: P.O. Box 279, Zip 48884–0279;
tel. 989/291–3261 **A**9 10 11 18 **F**3 15 34 35 40 42 45 54 57 59 64 74 81
85 93 97 107 110 113 118 126 128 132 143 145 **P**8
Primary Contact: Kevin J. Cawley, Chief Executive Officer
COO: Steve Scott, Chief Operating Officer
CFO: Kevin J. Cawley, Chief Executive Officer
CMO: Maria Charlotte Alvarez, M.D., Chief of Staff
CIO: David Bussler, Chief Information Officer
CHR: Sharon Bowers, R.N., Manager of Community, Public and Employee
Relations
CNO: Elizabeth Edwards, R.N., Director, Nursing Services
Web address: www.sheridanhospital.com
**Control:** Other not–for–profit (including NFP Corporation) **Service:** General
Medical and Surgical

**Staffed Beds: 22 Admissions: 276 Census: 3 Outpatient Visits: 28566
Births: 0 Total Expense ($000): 12836 Payroll Expense ($000): 6823
Personnel: 140**

## SOUTH HAVEN—Van Buren County

**SOUTH HAVEN COMMUNITY HOSPITAL** See South Haven Health System

✠ **SOUTH HAVEN HEALTH SYSTEM (230085)**, 955 South Bailey Avenue,
Zip 49090–9701; tel. 269/637–5271 **A**1 9 10 **F**3 11 13 15 28 29 30 31 34
35 36 40 41 53 57 59 62 64 65 68 75 76 77 78 79 81 85 87 89 93 95 96
97 107 108 110 112 114 117 118 126 128 129 131 134 145 146 147 **P**4
Primary Contact: Joanne Urbanski, President and Chief Executive Officer
CFO: Jim Wheeler, Executive Vice President and Chief Financial Officer
CMO: Maura Buckingham, D.O., Chief of Staff
CIO: Dennis Sorenson, Supervisor Information Technology
CHR: Bill Wood, Director Human Resources
Web address: www.shch.org
**Control:** Hospital district or authority, Government, nonfederal **Service:** General
Medical and Surgical

**Staffed Beds: 33 Admissions: 1135 Census: 8 Outpatient Visits: 125816
Births: 427 Total Expense ($000): 32631 Payroll Expense ($000): 17955
Personnel: 316**

## SOUTHFIELD—Oakland County

★ ○ **OAKLAND REGIONAL HOSPITAL (230301)**, 22401 Foster Winter Drive,
Zip 48075–3724; tel. 248/423–5100, (Total facility includes 26 beds in nursing
home–type unit) **A**9 10 11 **F**29 45 79 81 82 85 90 93 111 127
Primary Contact: Daniel R. Babb, Chief Executive Officer
COO: Amelia Jones, Chief Operating Officer
CMO: Robert Barbosa, D.O., Chief Medical Officer
CIO: Bill Moncrief, ORH IT Client Executive
CHR: Gordon Meyer, Director Human Resources
Web address: www.oaklandregionalhospital.com
**Control:** Corporation, Investor–owned, for–profit **Service:** General Medical and
Surgical

**Staffed Beds: 71 Admissions: 323 Census: 20 Outpatient Visits: 11387
Births: 0 Total Expense ($000): 25169 Payroll Expense ($000): 8262
Personnel: 130**

✠ **PROVIDENCE HOSPITAL (230019)**, 16001 West Nine Mile Road,
Zip 48075–4818, Mailing Address: P.O. Box 2043, Zip 48037–2043;
tel. 248/424–3000, (Includes PROVIDENCE PARK HOSPITAL, 47601 Grand River
Avebue, Novi, Zip 48374–1233; tel. 248/465–4100; Peter Karadjoff, President)
**A**1 2 3 5 9 10 **F**3 5 8 9 11 12 13 15 17 18 20 22 24 26 28 29 30 31 34 35
36 38 39 40 44 45 46 47 48 49 50 54 55 57 58 59 60 61 63 64 65 66
68 70 72 74 75 76 77 78 79 80 81 82 84 85 86 87 90 92 93 97 98 99 100
101 102 103 104 105 107 108 110 111 113 114 115 116 117 118 119 120
122 125 129 130 131 134 140 142 145 146 147 **P**6 8 **S** Ascension Health,
Saint Louis, MO
Primary Contact: Michael Wiemann, M.D., President
CFO: Douglas Winner, Chief Financial Officer
CMO: Tammy S. Lundstrom, M.D., Chief Medical Officer
CHR: Sue Gronbach, Director Human Resources
Web address: www.providence-stjohnhealth.org
**Control:** Church–operated, Nongovernment, not–for profit **Service:** General
Medical and Surgical

**Staffed Beds: 430 Admissions: 20728 Census: 297 Outpatient Visits:
192504 Births: 1856 Total Expense ($000): 392948 Payroll Expense
($000): 161383 Personnel: 2568**

✠ **STRAITH HOSPITAL FOR SPECIAL SURGERY (230071)**, 23901 Lahser Road,
Zip 48033–6035; tel. 248/357–3360 **A**1 9 10 **F**29 81 129 140 147 **P**5
Primary Contact: Gregory R. Hoose, Chief Executive Officer
CFO: H. Roger Jones, Chief Financial Officer
Web address: www.straith.org/
**Control:** Other not–for–profit (including NFP Corporation) **Service:** General
Medical and Surgical

**Staffed Beds: 24 Admissions: 611 Census: 13 Outpatient Visits: 1882
Births: 0 Total Expense ($000): 11325 Payroll Expense ($000): 4545
Personnel: 98**

## STANDISH—Arenac County

✠ **ST. MARY'S OF MICHIGAN STANDISH HOSPITAL (231305)**, 805 West Cedar
Street, Zip 48658–9526; tel. 989/846–4521, (Nonreporting) **A**1 9 10 18
**S** Ascension Health, Saint Louis, MO
Primary Contact: Sheri Leaman–Case, Administrator and Chief Executive Officer
CFO: Tony Doud, Controller
CMO: Jaya Sankaran, M.D., Chief of Staff
CIO: Tammy Copes, Director Information Systems
CHR: Renee Reetz, Director Human Resources
Web address: www.stmarysofmichigan.org/standish
**Control:** Other not–for–profit (including NFP Corporation) **Service:** General
Medical and Surgical

**Staffed Beds: 68**

## STURGIS—St. Joseph County

★ **STURGIS HOSPITAL (230096)**, 916 Myrtle Street, Zip 49091–2326;
tel. 269/651–7824 **A**9 10 21 **F**3 11 13 15 28 29 30 31 34 35 40 42 45 46
49 50 57 59 62 63 64 65 68 70 75 76 77 78 79 81 85 87 89 93 97 102
107 108 114 117 118 126 128 129 131 143 145 146 147 **P**6 **S** QHR,
Brentwood, TN
Primary Contact: Robert J. LaBarge, Chief Executive Officer
CFO: David Miller, Chief Financial Officer
CMO: Keyar Patel, M.D., President Medical Staff
CIO: Rita Denison, Manager Information Systems
CHR: Mary Kay Schultz, Director Human Resources
CNO: Charlotte J. Pavilanis, R.N., Director of Patient Care Services
Web address: www.sturgishospital.com
**Control:** Other not–for–profit (including NFP Corporation) **Service:** General
Medical and Surgical

**Staffed Beds: 49 Admissions: 1625 Census: 14 Outpatient Visits: 92090
Births: 428 Total Expense ($000): 40169 Payroll Expense ($000): 17476
Personnel: 251**

MI

---

**Hospital, Medicare Provider Number, Address, Telephone, Approval, Facility, and Physician Codes, Health Care System**

★ American Hospital Association (AHA) membership
☐ The Joint Commission accreditation
◇ DNV Healthcare Inc. accreditation
○ American Osteopathic Association (AOA) accreditation
△ Commission on Accreditation of Rehabilitation Facilities (CARF) accreditation

**MI**

### TAWAS CITY—Iosco County

⊠ **ST. JOSEPH HEALTH SYSTEM (230100)**, 200 Hemlock Street, Zip 48763–9237, Mailing Address: P.O. Box 659, Zip 48764–0659; tel. 989/362–3411, (Nonreporting) **A**1 9 10 20 **S** Ascension Health, Saint Louis, MO
Primary Contact: Ann M. Balfour, R.N., Administrator
CFO: Linda Stancill, Vice President and Chief Financial Officer
CHR: Nancy Bodenner, Director Human Resources
Web address: www.sjhsys.org
**Control:** Other not–for–profit (including NFP Corporation) **Service:** General Medical and Surgical

**Staffed Beds: 20**

### TAYLOR—Wayne County

⊠ **OAKWOOD HERITAGE HOSPITAL (230270)**, 10000 Telegraph Road, Zip 48180–3330; tel. 313/295–5000 **A**1 3 5 9 10 **F**3 11 15 29 30 34 37 38 39 40 44 49 50 56 57 59 60 61 64 65 68 70 74 75 78 79 80 81 82 84 85 86 87 90 92 93 96 98 100 101 102 103 105 107 108 111 113 114 117 118 127 129 130 131 134 145 147 **P**5 8 **S** Oakwood Healthcare, Inc., Dearborn, MI
Primary Contact: Michael Geheb, M.D., Division President
COO: Kelly C. Smith, Chief Operating Officer
CFO: Mark Deming, Controller
CMO: Vijay Khanna, M.D., Chief of Staff
CIO: Paula Smith, Chief Information Officer
CHR: Sherry Huffman, Administrator Human Resources
Web address: www.oakwood.org
**Control:** Other not–for–profit (including NFP Corporation) **Service:** General Medical and Surgical

**Staffed Beds: 183 Admissions: 8029 Census: 127 Outpatient Visits: 62375 Births: 0 Total Expense ($000): 118085 Payroll Expense ($000): 47929 Personnel: 759**

⊠ **SELECT SPECIALTY HOSPITAL–DOWNRIVER (232031)**, 10000 Telegraph Road, 2nd Floor, Zip 48180–3330; tel. 313/375–7075, (Nonreporting) **A**1 9 10 **S** Select Medical Corporation, Mechanicsburg, PA
Primary Contact: Robert Padalino, Chief Executive Officer
CMO: Roderick Boyer, M.D., Medical Director
CHR: Barb Wierzbicki, Manager Human Resources
Web address: www.selectmedicalcorp.com
**Control:** Corporation, Investor–owned, for–profit **Service:** Long–Term Acute Care hospital

**Staffed Beds: 40**

### TECUMSEH—Lenawee County

★ ○ **PROMEDICA HERRICK HOSPITAL (231334)**, 500 East Pottawatamie Street, Zip 49286–2097; tel. 517/424–3000, (Total facility includes 25 beds in nursing home–type unit) **A**9 10 11 18 **F**3 11 15 18 29 34 40 45 50 53 57 59 60 64 68 74 75 77 79 81 85 92 93 98 100 101 102 104 107 108 110 113 118 123 127 128 129 130 131 134 144 145 146 **P**6 7 8 **S** ProMedica Health System, Toledo, OH
Primary Contact: Timothy Jakacki, President
CFO: Bernie Nawrocki, Administrative Director Finance
CMO: Julie Yaroch, D.O., Vice President Medical Affairs
CIO: Carol Boyce, Administrative Director Support Services
CHR: Cathy J. Davis, Director Human Resources
CNO: Kathryn M. Greenlee, R.N., Vice President, Clinical Services/CNO
Web address: www.promedica.org
**Control:** Other not–for–profit (including NFP Corporation) **Service:** General Medical and Surgical

**Staffed Beds: 60 Admissions: 1640 Census: 38 Outpatient Visits: 46264 Births: 0 Total Expense ($000): 35515 Payroll Expense ($000): 11505 Personnel: 161**

### THREE RIVERS—St. Joseph County

⊠ **THREE RIVERS HEALTH (230015)**, 701 South Houthealth Parkway, Zip 49093–8352; tel. 269/278–1145, (Nonreporting) **A**1 9 10 **S** QHR, Brentwood, TN
Primary Contact: William B. Russell, Chief Executive Officer
COO: Laurie Herbert, Vice President Operations
CFO: Steve Andrews, Chief Financial Officer
CIO: Dave Parks, Chief Information Officer
Web address: www.threerivershealth.org
**Control:** Hospital district or authority, Government, nonfederal **Service:** General Medical and Surgical

**Staffed Beds: 35**

### TRAVERSE CITY—Grand Traverse County

⊠ △ **MUNSON MEDICAL CENTER (230097)**, 1105 Sixth Street, Zip 49684–2345; tel. 231/935–5000 **A**1 2 3 5 7 9 10 12 13 **F**3 4 5 6 11 12 13 15 17 18 20 22 24 26 28 29 30 31 32 34 35 36 38 39 40 43 44 45 46 48 49 50 53 54 55 56 57 58 59 60 61 62 63 64 65 68 70 71 72 74 75 76 77 78 79 81 82 84 85 86 87 89 90 92 93 94 96 97 98 100 101 102 103 104 105 107 108 110 111 113 114 115 116 117 118 119 120 122 123 125 128 129 130 131 133 134 140 141 142 143 144 145 146 147 **P**6 **S** Munson Healthcare, Traverse City, MI
Primary Contact: Edwin Ness, President and Chief Executive Officer
COO: Kathleen A. McManus, Executive Vice President/Chief Operating Officer
CFO: Mark A. Helper, Vice President, Chief Financial Officer
CMO: David S. McGreaham, M.D., Vice President Medical Affairs
CIO: Christopher J. Podges, Vice President and Chief Information Officer
CHR: Sue Peters, Vice President Human Resources
CNO: James Fischer, R.N., Vice President Patient Care Services/Chief Nursing Officer
Web address: www.munsonhealthcare.org
**Control:** Other not–for–profit (including NFP Corporation) **Service:** General Medical and Surgical

**Staffed Beds: 391 Admissions: 23392 Census: 299 Outpatient Visits: 474066 Births: 1764 Total Expense ($000): 435006 Payroll Expense ($000): 173681 Personnel: 2965**

### TRENTON—Wayne County

⊠ ○ **OAKWOOD SOUTHSHORE MEDICAL CENTER (230176)**, 5450 Fort Street, Zip 48183–4625; tel. 734/671–3800 **A**1 9 10 11 12 13 **F**3 8 11 13 15 17 18 20 22 26 28 29 30 31 34 35 38 39 40 43 44 46 47 49 50 56 57 59 60 61 64 65 68 70 74 75 76 78 79 80 81 82 85 86 87 92 93 96 100 102 107 108 110 111 114 117 118 129 130 131 134 145 146 147 **P**5 8 **S** Oakwood Healthcare, Inc., Dearborn, MI
Primary Contact: Edith M. Hughes, President
COO: J. Joseph Diederich, Executive Vice President and Chief Operating Officer
CFO: Patricia Vannoy, Controller
CMO: Iqbal Nasir, M.D., Chief of Staff
CIO: Paula Smith, Vice President Information Services and Chief Information Officer
CHR: Juliet Hafford, Director Human Resources
Web address: www.oakwood.org
**Control:** Other not–for–profit (including NFP Corporation) **Service:** General Medical and Surgical

**Staffed Beds: 144 Admissions: 8334 Census: 102 Outpatient Visits: 62957 Births: 678 Total Expense ($000): 129543 Payroll Expense ($000): 45930 Personnel: 642**

### TROY—Oakland County

⊠ **BEAUMONT HOSPITAL – TROY (230269)**, 44201 Dequindre Road, Zip 48085–1117; tel. 248/964–5000 **A**1 2 9 10 **F**3 11 12 13 14 15 17 18 20 22 24 26 28 29 30 31 32 34 35 36 39 40 44 45 46 47 48 49 50 51 52 54 56 57 58 59 60 61 62 63 64 65 66 68 70 71 72 74 75 76 77 78 79 80 81 82 84 85 86 87 89 91 92 93 94 96 97 100 102 103 107 108 109 110 111 113 114 115 116 117 118 119 120 122 125 128 129 130 131 134 140 141 142 143 144 145 146 147 **P**6 **S** Beaumont Health System, Royal Oak, MI
Primary Contact: Nancy Susick, MSN, President
CFO: Mark Leonard, Vice President Finance
CMO: Roger Howard, M.D., Senior Vice President and Medical Director
CIO: Subra Sripada, Senior Vice President and Chief Information Officer
CHR: Lisa Ouelette, Director Human Resources
Web address: www.beaumonthospitals.com
**Control:** Other not–for–profit (including NFP Corporation) **Service:** General Medical and Surgical

**Staffed Beds: 394 Admissions: 28966 Census: 311 Outpatient Visits: 659117 Births: 3331 Total Expense ($000): 327720 Payroll Expense ($000): 179960 Personnel: 2620**

### VICKSBURG—Kalamazoo County

**BRONSON VICKSBURG HOSPITAL** See Bronson Methodist Hospital, Kalamazoo

### WARREN—Macomb County

**BEHAVIORAL CENTER OF MICHIGAN (234039)**, 4050 East 12 Mile Road, Zip 48092–2534; tel. 586/261–2266, (Nonreporting) **A**9 10
Primary Contact: Ryan Gunabalan, Chief Executive Officer
COO: Efren Lusterio, Director of Nursing
CFO: Mark Corey, Chief Financial Officer
CMO: Eleanor Medina, M.D., Chief Medical Officer
CIO: Kashmira Khade, Coordinator Non–Clinical Services
CHR: Erin R. Youngblood, Chief Human Resources Officer
Web address: www.behavioralcenter.com
**Control:** Corporation, Investor–owned, for–profit **Service:** Psychiatric

**Staffed Beds: 42**

☐ **SOUTHEAST MICHIGAN SURGICAL HOSPITAL (230264)**, 21230 Dequindre, Zip 48091–2287; tel. 586/427–1000, (Nonreporting) **A**1 9 10 **S** National Surgical Hospitals, Chicago, IL
Primary Contact: John Kolozsvary, Chief Executive Officer
CMO: Benjamin Paolucci, D.O., Chief of Staff
CHR: Dawn Meiers, Coordinator Medical Staff and Personnel Services
Web address: www.nshinc.com
**Control:** Corporation, Investor–owned, for–profit **Service:** General Medical and Surgical

| Staffed Beds: 13 |
| --- |

⊞ ○ **ST. JOHN MACOMB–OAKLAND HOSPITAL, MACOMB CENTER (230195)**, 11800 East Twelve Mile Road, Zip 48093–3494; tel. 586/573–5000 **A**1 2 9 10 11 12 13 **F**3 11 13 15 17 18 20 22 24 26 28 29 30 31 34 35 36 38 39 40 41 44 45 46 48 49 50 51 56 57 58 59 60 61 63 64 65 68 70 74 75 76 78 79 80 81 82 84 85 86 87 90 91 92 93 96 97 98 100 101 102 103 104 105 107 108 110 113 114 115 116 118 120 122 125 129 130 131 134 140 142 145 146 147 **P**8 **S** Ascension Health, Saint Louis, MO
Primary Contact: Terry Hamilton, President
CFO: Tomasine Marx, Chief Financial Officer
CMO: Gary L. Berg, D.O., Chief Medical Officer
CIO: Mary Kay LaChance, Director Information Systems
CHR: Joanne E. Tuscany, Director Worklife Services
Web address: www.stjohnprovidence.org/macomb
**Control:** Church–operated, Nongovernment, not–for profit **Service:** General Medical and Surgical

| Staffed Beds: 336 Admissions: 20029 Census: 281 Outpatient Visits: 301449 Births: 1234 Total Expense ($000): 281935 Payroll Expense ($000): 117807 Personnel: 2006 |
| --- |

## WATERVLIET—Berrien County

**COMMUNITY HOSPITAL** See Lakeland Community Hospital Watervliet

⊞ △ **LAKELAND COMMUNITY HOSPITAL WATERVLIET (230078)**, 400 Medical Park Drive, Zip 49098–9225; tel. 269/463–3111 **A**1 7 9 10 **F**3 11 15 29 30 34 35 38 40 45 50 54 57 59 68 70 75 77 79 81 85 86 87 90 93 97 107 118 126 129 130 131 134 143 145 **S** Lakeland Healthcare, Saint Joseph, MI
Primary Contact: Ray Cruse, Chief Executive Officer
CFO: Chris Kuhlmann, Chief Financial Officer
CHR: Heather West, Director Human Resources
Web address: www.communityhospitalwatervliet.com
**Control:** Other not–for–profit (including NFP Corporation) **Service:** General Medical and Surgical

| Staffed Beds: 38 Admissions: 834 Census: 10 Outpatient Visits: 55571 Births: 0 Total Expense ($000): 25839 Payroll Expense ($000): 11247 Personnel: 194 |
| --- |

## WAYNE—Wayne County

⊞ **OAKWOOD ANNAPOLIS HOSPITAL (230142)**, 33155 Annapolis Street, Zip 48184–2405; tel. 734/467–4000 **A**1 9 10 13 **F**3 11 13 15 18 20 22 26 28 29 30 31 34 35 38 40 44 47 49 50 51 64 65 68 70 74 75 76 78 79 80 81 82 84 85 86 87 92 93 96 100 102 107 108 111 113 114 117 118 129 130 131 134 145 146 147 **P**5 8 **S** Oakwood Healthcare, Inc., Dearborn, MI
Primary Contact: Eric W. Widner, President
COO: J. Joseph Diederich, Executive Vice President and Chief Operating Officer
CFO: Roy Birmingham, Controller
CMO: Ashok Jain, M.D., Chief of Staff
CIO: Paula Smith, Senior Vice President Chief Information Officer
CHR: Robert L. James, Director Human Resources
CNO: Diane L. Hartley, R.N., Director of Patient Care Services
Web address: www.oakwood.org
**Control:** Other not–for–profit (including NFP Corporation) **Service:** General Medical and Surgical

| Staffed Beds: 211 Admissions: 8748 Census: 105 Outpatient Visits: 84326 Births: 906 Total Expense ($000): 130686 Payroll Expense ($000): 53925 Personnel: 807 |
| --- |

## WEST BLOOMFIELD—Oakland County

★ **HENRY FORD WEST BLOOMFIELD HOSPITAL (230302)**, 6777 West Maple Road, Zip 48322–3013; tel. 248/661–4100 **A**2 9 10 21 **F**3 11 12 13 15 18 20 26 28 29 30 31 32 33 34 35 36 38 40 44 45 46 47 49 50 51 53 55 56 57 58 59 60 61 64 65 68 70 74 75 76 77 78 79 81 82 84 85 86 87 89 97 100 102 103 107 108 110 111 113 114 115 116 117 118 119 120 122 123 125 128 129 130 131 134 145 146 147 **P**6 **S** Henry Ford Health System, Detroit, MI
Primary Contact: Gerard van Grinsven, President and Chief Executive Officer
COO: Christine Zambrini, Chief Operating Officer and Chief Nursing Officer
Web address: www.henryford.com
**Control:** Other not–for–profit (including NFP Corporation) **Service:** General Medical and Surgical

| Staffed Beds: 191 Admissions: 12553 Census: 133 Outpatient Visits: 344361 Births: 1487 Total Expense ($000): 238808 Payroll Expense ($000): 95926 Personnel: 1559 |
| --- |

## WEST BRANCH—Ogemaw County

★ ○ **WEST BRANCH REGIONAL MEDICAL CENTER (230095)**, 2463 South M–30, Zip 48661–1199; tel. 989/345–3660 **A**9 10 11 20 **F**3 11 15 17 20 28 29 30 34 35 40 45 50 57 59 63 64 75 77 79 81 84 93 107 111 113 114 116 118 129 145 **P**6
Primary Contact: Edward A. Napierala, Chief Executive Officer
CFO: Robert McGrail, Chief Financial Officer
CMO: Patrick Morse, M.D., President Medical Staff
CIO: Doug Danitz, Director Information Technology
CHR: Dane J. Turner, Director Human Resources
CNO: Noreen B. Connolly, MS, Chief Nurse Executive
Web address: www.wbrmc.com
**Control:** City–Government, nonfederal **Service:** General Medical and Surgical

| Staffed Beds: 78 Admissions: 2330 Census: 28 Outpatient Visits: 81401 Births: 41 Total Expense ($000): 37441 Payroll Expense ($000): 13008 Personnel: 291 |
| --- |

## WESTLAND—Wayne County

☐ **WALTER P. REUTHER PSYCHIATRIC HOSPITAL (234035)**, 30901 Palmer Road, Zip 48186–5389; tel. 734/367–8400, (Nonreporting) **A**1 9 10
Primary Contact: Ron Denstedt, Acting Director
CMO: Venkata Lingam, M.D., Chief Clinical Affairs
CHR: Gerald Gibson, Director Human Resources
Web address: www.mhweb.org/wayne/reuther.htm
**Control:** State–Government, nonfederal **Service:** Psychiatric

| Staffed Beds: 239 |
| --- |

## WYANDOTTE—Wayne County

★ ○ △ **HENRY FORD WYANDOTTE HOSPITAL (230146)**, 2333 Biddle Avenue, Zip 48192–4668; tel. 734/246–6000 **A**7 9 10 11 12 13 21 **F**3 8 11 12 13 15 17 18 20 22 26 28 29 30 31 32 34 35 36 38 40 42 44 45 46 47 49 50 51 54 56 57 58 59 60 63 64 65 66 68 69 70 74 75 76 77 78 79 80 81 82 83 84 85 86 87 90 92 93 94 96 98 100 101 102 103 107 108 110 111 113 114 115 116 117 118 125 128 129 130 131 134 145 146 147 **P**6 **S** Henry Ford Health System, Detroit, MI
Primary Contact: James J. Sexton, FACHE, President and Chief Executive Officer
COO: Rand O'Leary, Senior Vice President and Chief Operating Officer
CFO: James J. Miller, Vice President and Chief Financial Officer
CMO: Dennis R. Lemanski, D.O., Senior Vice President Medical Affairs and Medical Education/CMO
CMO: Mohinder S. Singh–Sandhu, M.D., President Medical Staff
CIO: Mary Alice Annecharico, Senior VP and CIO, Henry Ford Health System
CIO: Arthur K. Gross, FACHE, Executive Vice President and Chief Information Officer
CHR: Aline S. Lafferty, Vice President Human Resources
CNO: Josephine Sclafani Wahl, R.N., VP, Patient Care Services & CNO
Web address: www.henryfordhealth.org
**Control:** Other not–for–profit (including NFP Corporation) **Service:** General Medical and Surgical

| Staffed Beds: 348 Admissions: 19648 Census: 266 Outpatient Visits: 301804 Births: 1460 Total Expense ($000): 262894 Payroll Expense ($000): 111088 Personnel: 1952 |
| --- |

| **Hospital, Medicare Provider Number, Address, Telephone, Approval, Facility, and Physician Codes, Health Care System** |
| --- |
| ★ American Hospital Association (AHA) membership      ○ American Osteopathic Association (AOA) accreditation <br> ☐ The Joint Commission accreditation      ◇ DNV Healthcare Inc. accreditation      △ Commission on Accreditation of Rehabilitation Facilities (CARF) accreditation |

## WYOMING—Kent County

★ ○ **METRO HEALTH HOSPITAL (230236)**, 5900 Byron Center Avenue S.W.,
Zip 49519–9606, Mailing Address: P.O. Box 916, Zip 49509–0916;
tel. 616/252–7200 **A**9 10 11 12 13 **F**1 3 12 13 15 18 20 22 24 26 29 30 31
34 35 40 44 45 49 50 51 54 57 58 59 64 65 67 70 71 74 75 76 77 78 79
81 82 85 86 90 91 92 93 94 96 97 107 108 110 111 113 114 116 118 125
128 129 130 131 134 145 146 147 **P**8
Primary Contact: Michael D. Faas, President and Chief Executive Officer
COO: Jamal Ghani, Chief Operating Officer
CFO: Tim Susterich, Chief Financial Officer
CMO: William Cunningham, D.O., Chief Medical Officer
CIO: William Lewkowski, Executive Vice President Information Services and Chief
Information Officer
CHR: Floyd Wilson, Jr., Executive Vice President Human Resources
Web address: www.metrohealth.net
**Control:** Other not–for–profit (including NFP Corporation) **Service:** General
Medical and Surgical

| |
|---|
| **Staffed Beds:** 208 **Admissions:** 10147 **Census:** 143 **Outpatient Visits:** 384198 **Births:** 1686 **Total Expense ($000):** 245458 **Payroll Expense ($000):** 87682 **Personnel:** 1739 |

## YPSILANTI—Washtenaw County

☐ **FOREST HEALTH MEDICAL CENTER (230144)**, 135 South Prospect Street,
Zip 48198–7914; tel. 734/547–4700 **A**1 9 10 **F**12 30 46 64 75 79 81 85 118
129 131
Primary Contact: Trevor J. Dyksterhouse, President
COO: Trevor J. Dyksterhouse, President
CFO: Dan Miller, Vice President Finance
CMO: Steven Poplawski, M.D., Medical Director
CIO: Steve Jerant, Vice President Information Technology
CHR: Karen Pinto, Coordinator Human Resources
Web address: www.barixclinics.com
**Control:** Corporation, Investor–owned, for–profit **Service:** General Medical and
Surgical

| |
|---|
| **Staffed Beds:** 24 **Admissions:** 1463 **Census:** 5 **Outpatient Visits:** 2083 **Births:** 0 **Personnel:** 43 |

✠ **SELECT SPECIALTY HOSPITAL–ANN ARBOR (232024)**, 5301 East Huron
River Drive, 5th Floor, Zip 48197–1051; tel. 734/712–0111, (Nonreporting) **A**1
10 **S** Select Medical Corporation, Mechanicsburg, PA
Primary Contact: John O'Malley, FACHE, Chief Executive Officer
CMO: Jim Hayner, M.D., Medical Director
CHR: Cambrea Baker, Coordinator Human Resources
Web address: www.selectspecialtyhospitals.com
**Control:** Corporation, Investor–owned, for–profit **Service:** Long–Term Acute Care
hospital

| |
|---|
| **Staffed Beds:** 36 |

✠ **ST. JOSEPH MERCY HOSPITAL (230156)**, 5301 McAuley Drive, Zip 48197,
Mailing Address: P.O. Box 995, Ann Arbor, Zip 48106–0995; tel. 734/712–3456
**A**1 2 3 5 8 9 10 **F**3 4 5 6 8 9 11 12 13 15 17 18 20 22 24 26 28 29 30 31
32 33 34 35 36 37 38 40 41 42 43 44 45 46 50 51 53 54 56 57 58 59 60
61 62 63 64 65 66 67 68 70 71 72 73 74 75 76 77 78 79 81 82 83 84 85
86 87 89 90 91 92 93 94 97 98 99 100 101 102 103 104 105 107 108 109
110 111 113 114 115 116 117 118 119 120 122 123 124 125 127 128 129
130 131 132 133 134 142 143 144 145 146 147 **P**1 **S** Trinity Health, Novi, MI
Primary Contact: Robert F. Casalou, President and Chief Executive Officer
CFO: Kathy O'Connor, Vice President, Finance and Chief Financial Officer
CMO: Rolland Mambourg, M.D., Vice President Physician Services
CIO: Joan Hurray, Regional Director Information Services
CHR: Kathleen Rhine, Vice President Administrative Services and Chief Operating
Officer
Web address: www.sjmercyhealth.org
**Control:** Church–operated, Nongovernment, not–for profit **Service:** General
Medical and Surgical

| |
|---|
| **Staffed Beds:** 530 **Admissions:** 31956 **Census:** 387 **Outpatient Visits:** 1129843 **Births:** 3577 **Total Expense ($000):** 674510 **Payroll Expense ($000):** 244810 **Personnel:** 5485 |

## ZEELAND—Ottawa County

✠ **SPECTRUM HEALTH ZEELAND COMMUNITY HOSPITAL (230003)**, 8333
Felch Street, Zip 49464–2608; tel. 616/772–4644 **A**1 9 10 **F**3 12 13 15 17 18
29 34 35 40 45 54 57 59 63 64 65 68 69 70 75 76 79 81 85 89 93 97 107
110 111 114 118 128 129 131 134 143 145
Primary Contact: Henry A. Veenstra, President
CFO: Ryan Powers, Chief Financial Officer
CMO: Dale Terpstra, D.O., Medical Director
CIO: George J. Smart, Vice President Finance and System Services
CHR: Jane Czerew, Vice President Clinical Services, Quality Systems, Human
Resources and Volunteer Services
Web address: www.zch.org
**Control:** Other not–for–profit (including NFP Corporation) **Service:** General
Medical and Surgical

| |
|---|
| **Staffed Beds:** 57 **Admissions:** 1590 **Census:** 15 **Outpatient Visits:** 57915 **Births:** 386 **Total Expense ($000):** 36842 **Payroll Expense ($000):** 16019 **Personnel:** 325 |

**ZEELAND COMMUNITY HOSPITAL** See Spectrum Health Zeeland Community
Hospital

# MINNESOTA

## ADA—Norman County

**BRIDGES MEDICAL CENTER** See Essentia Health Ada

★ **ESSENTIA HEALTH ADA (241313)**, 201 9th Street West, Zip 56510–1243; tel. 218/784–5000, (Nonreporting) **A**9 10 18 **S** Essentia Health, Duluth, MN
Primary Contact: Ryan Hill, Interim Chief Executive Officer
CFO: Ryan Hill, Chief Financial Officer
CMO: Jeff Peterson, M.D., Chief of Staff
CHR: Shayla Hennenberg, Director Human Resources
Web address: www.essentiahealth.org
**Control:** Other not–for–profit (including NFP Corporation) **Service:** General Medical and Surgical

**Staffed Beds:** 14

## AITKIN—Crow Wing County

★ **RIVERWOOD HEALTHCARE CENTER (241305)**, 200 Bunker Hill Drive, Zip 56431–1844; tel. 218/927–2121 **A**9 10 18 **F**3 8 11 13 15 28 29 31 32 34 35 40 43 45 54 56 57 59 64 65 70 75 76 77 78 79 81 82 86 87 93 97 104 107 110 111 113 118 126 128 129 130 131 132 134 143 144 145 146 147 **P**6
Primary Contact: Michael Hagen, Chief Executive Officer
CFO: Kent Dumonseau, Chief Financial Officer
CMO: Mark Heggem, M.D., Chief Medical Officer
CIO: Daryl Kallevig, Chief Information Officer
CHR: Cindi Hills, Director Human Resources
CNO: Kristine Layne, R.N., Chief Nursing Officer
Web address: www.riverwoodhealthcare.com
**Control:** Other not–for–profit (including NFP Corporation) **Service:** General Medical and Surgical

**Staffed Beds:** 24 **Admissions:** 1081 **Census:** 9 **Outpatient Visits:** 69146 **Births:** 63 **Total Expense ($000):** 42825 **Payroll Expense ($000):** 17931 **Personnel:** 280

## ALBANY—Stearns County

★ **ALBANY AREA HOSPITAL AND MEDICAL CENTER (241331)**, 300 Third Avenue, Zip 56307–9363; tel. 320/845–2121 **A**9 10 18 **F**13 15 30 34 35 40 45 50 59 64 65 76 77 79 81 93 107 113 118 126 128 129 131 132 134 145 **P**6 **S** Catholic Health Initiatives, Englewood, CO
Primary Contact: Sandra Day, Administrator, Chief Nursing Officer
CFO: Steve Smith, Chief Financial Officer
CMO: Aaron Gersch, M.D., Chief of Staff
CHR: Bernie Cekalla, Manager Human Resources
CNO: Sandra Day, Administrator, Chief Nursing Officer
Web address: www.albanyareahospital.com
**Control:** Church–operated, Nongovernment, not–for profit **Service:** General Medical and Surgical

**Staffed Beds:** 17 **Admissions:** 288 **Census:** 3 **Outpatient Visits:** 28286 **Births:** 57 **Total Expense ($000):** 10468 **Payroll Expense ($000):** 4580 **Personnel:** 81

## ALBERT LEA—Freeborn County

☐ **MAYO CLINIC HEALTH SYSTEM IN ALBERT LEA (240043)**, 404 West Fountain Street, Zip 56007–2473; tel. 507/373–2384, (Nonreporting) **A**1 5 9 10 **S** Mayo Clinic Health System, Rochester, MN
Primary Contact: Mark Ciota, M.D., Chief Executive Officer
CFO: Dave Pilot, Chief Financial Officer
CMO: John Grzybowski, M.D., Medical Director
CHR: Monica Fleegel, Director Human Resources
Web address: www.almedcenter.org
**Control:** Other not–for–profit (including NFP Corporation) **Service:** General Medical and Surgical

**Staffed Beds:** 129

## ALEXANDRIA—Sherburne County

☐ **COMMUNITY BEHAVIORAL HEALTH HOSPITAL – ALEXANDRIA (244012)**, 1610 8th Avenue East, Zip 55308; tel. 320/335–6201, (Nonreporting) **A**1 9 10 **S** Minnesota Department of Human Services, Saint Paul, MN
Primary Contact: John A. Cosco, Ph.D., FACHE, Administrator
CFO: Shirley Jacobson, Chief Financial Officer
Web address: www.health.state.mn.us
**Control:** State–Government, nonfederal **Service:** Psychiatric

**Staffed Beds:** 16

★ ○ **DOUGLAS COUNTY HOSPITAL (240030)**, 111 17th Avenue East, Zip 56308–3798; tel. 320/762–1511 **A**9 10 11 **F**3 8 11 13 15 28 30 31 34 36 40 43 45 57 61 64 68 69 70 76 77 78 79 81 85 86 89 93 107 108 111 114 116 118 128 129 130 131 134 145
Primary Contact: Carl P. Vaagenes, Chief Executive Officer
CFO: Nate Meyer, Director Finance
CHR: Sister Patrice Kiefer, Director Human Resources
Web address: www.dchospital.com
**Control:** County–Government, nonfederal **Service:** General Medical and Surgical

**Staffed Beds:** 99 **Admissions:** 3931 **Census:** 39 **Outpatient Visits:** 48700 **Births:** 623 **Personnel:** 463

## ANNANDALE—Wright County

☐ **COMMUNITY BEHAVIORAL HEALTH HOSPITAL – ANNANDALE (244011)**, 400 Annandale Boulevard, Zip 55302–3141; tel. 651/259–3850, (Nonreporting) **A**1 9 10 **S** Minnesota Department of Human Services, Saint Paul, MN
Primary Contact: Pamela R. Bajari, R.N., Interim Administrator
Web address: www.health.state.mn.us
**Control:** State–Government, nonfederal **Service:** Psychiatric

**Staffed Beds:** 16

## ANOKA—Anoka County

**ANOKA–METROPOLITAN REGIONAL TREATMENT CENTER (244002)**, 3301 Seventh Avenue, Zip 55303–1119; tel. 763/712–4000 **A**10 **F**29 30 38 39 50 53 68 75 86 87 91 97 98 100 101 103 104 106 129 131 **S** Minnesota Department of Human Services, Saint Paul, MN
Primary Contact: David Hartford, Administrator
Web address: www.health.state.mn.us
**Control:** State–Government, nonfederal **Service:** Psychiatric

**Staffed Beds:** 112 **Admissions:** 450 **Census:** 110 **Outpatient Visits:** 0 **Births:** 0 **Personnel:** 309

## APPLETON—Swift County

★ **APPLETON AREA HEALTH SERVICES (241341)**, 30 South Behl Street, Zip 56208–1699; tel. 320/289–2422, (Total facility includes 53 beds in nursing home–type unit) **A**9 10 18 **F**2 7 8 15 18 34 35 40 43 45 56 57 62 63 64 65 69 71 75 81 85 93 107 110 111 118 127 129 132 145 147 **P**6
Primary Contact: Kathy Johnson, Chief Executive Officer
CFO: Anne Kells, Interim Chief Financial Officer
Web address: www.appletonareahealth.com
**Control:** City–Government, nonfederal **Service:** General Medical and Surgical

**Staffed Beds:** 68 **Admissions:** 286 **Census:** 57 **Outpatient Visits:** 1408 **Births:** 0 **Total Expense ($000):** 10500 **Payroll Expense ($000):** 4622 **Personnel:** 104

## ARLINGTON—Sibley County

★ **SIBLEY MEDICAL CENTER (241311)**, 601 West Chandler Street, Zip 55307–4500; tel. 507/964–2271, (Nonreporting) **A**9 10 18
Primary Contact: Todd Sandberg, Chief Executive Officer
CFO: Darla Anderson, Chief Financial Officer
CMO: Ehtaisham Mohammed, M.D., Chief Medical Officer
CIO: Chris Bulau, Manager Information Technology
CHR: Sara Christiansen, Interim Director Human Resources
CNO: Sandy Domeier, Director Patient Care Services
Web address: www.sibleymedical.org
**Control:** City–Government, nonfederal **Service:** General Medical and Surgical

**Staffed Beds:** 17

---

**Hospital, Medicare Provider Number, Address, Telephone, Approval, Facility, and Physician Codes, Health Care System**

★ American Hospital Association (AHA) membership
☐ The Joint Commission accreditation
◇ DNV Healthcare Inc. accreditation
○ American Osteopathic Association (AOA) accreditation
△ Commission on Accreditation of Rehabilitation Facilities (CARF) accreditation

**MN**

## AURORA—St. Louis County

★ **ESSENTIA HEALTH NORTHERN PINES (241340)**, 5211 Highway 110,
Zip 55705–1599; tel. 218/229–2211, (Total facility includes 50 beds in nursing
home–type unit) **A**9 10 18 **F**3 28 29 34 40 56 59 64 65 75 77 81 91 93 102
107 127 129 130 132 134 147 **P**8 **S** Essentia Health, Duluth, MN
Primary Contact: Laura Ackman, Administrator
CFO: Barbara Johnson, Chief Financial Officer
CMO: Michelle Oman, D.O., Chief Medical Officer
CHR: Kim Carlson, Director Human Resources
CNO: Cindy Loe, Director of Nursing
Web address: www.essentiahealth.org
**Control:** Other not–for–profit (including NFP Corporation) **Service:** General
Medical and Surgical

**Staffed Beds:** 58 **Admissions:** 219 **Census:** 58 **Outpatient Visits:** 4422
**Births:** 0 **Total Expense ($000):** 7389 **Payroll Expense ($000):** 3469
**Personnel:** 48

**WHITE COMMUNITY HOSPITAL** See Essentia Health Northern Pines

## AUSTIN—Mower County

☐ **MAYO CLINIC HEALTH SYSTEM IN AUSTIN (240117)**, 1000 First Drive N.W.,
Zip 55912–2904; tel. 507/433–7351, (Nonreporting) **A**1 5 9 10 **S** Mayo Clinic
Health System, Rochester, MN
Primary Contact: David Agerter, President and Chief Executive Officer
COO: Adam Rees, Executive Vice President and Chief Administrative Officer
CFO: Sheri Dankert, Vice President Finance
CMO: Cynthia Dube, M.D., Medical Director
CIO: Tammy Kritzer, Vice President Clinic Operations
CHR: Rodney Nording, Vice President Organizational Support
Web address: www.austinmedicalcenter.org
**Control:** Other not–for–profit (including NFP Corporation) **Service:** General
Medical and Surgical

**Staffed Beds:** 82

## BAGLEY—Clearwater County

★ **SANFORD BAGLEY MEDICAL CENTER (241328)**, 203 Fourth Street N.W.,
Zip 56621–8307; tel. 218/694–6501, (Nonreporting) **A**9 10 18 **S** Sanford
Health, Sioux Falls, SD
Primary Contact: Kirby Johnson, Administrator
CFO: Rachel Rosenbush, Account Manager
CMO: Esther Potti, M.D., Chief Medical Staff
Web address: www.clearwaterhealthservices.com
**Control:** County–Government, nonfederal **Service:** General Medical and Surgical

**Staffed Beds:** 95

## BAUDETTE—Lake Of The Woods County

★ **LAKEWOOD HEALTH CENTER (241301)**, 600 Main Avenue South,
Zip 56623–2855; tel. 218/634–2120, (Total facility includes 44 beds in nursing
home–type unit) **A**9 10 18 **F**3 7 10 15 28 30 31 34 35 40 45 50 53 57 64 66
68 79 81 85 89 107 118 127 129 132 133 **P**6 **S** Catholic Health Initiatives,
Englewood, CO
Primary Contact: Jason Breuer, Administrator
CFO: Lynn Ellis, Chief Financial Officer
CIO: Darlene Bushaw, Information Technology Systems Site Lead
CHR: Lois Slick, Director Human Resources
Web address: www.lakewoodhealthcenter.org
**Control:** Church–operated, Nongovernment, not–for profit **Service:** General
Medical and Surgical

**Staffed Beds:** 59 **Admissions:** 246 **Census:** 43 **Outpatient Visits:** 21378
**Births:** 0 **Total Expense ($000):** 13965 **Payroll Expense ($000):** 6247
**Personnel:** 127

## BAXTER—Crow Wing County

☐ **COMMUNITY BEHAVIORAL HEALTH HOSPITAL – BAXTER (244015)**, 14241
Grand Oaks Drive, Zip 56425; tel. 218/316–3101, (Nonreporting) **A**1 9 10
**S** Minnesota Department of Human Services, Saint Paul, MN
Primary Contact: Richard G. Slieter, Jr., Administrator
**Control:** State–Government, nonfederal **Service:** Psychiatric

**Staffed Beds:** 16

## BEMIDJI—Beltrami County

☐ **COMMUNITY BEHAVIORAL HEALTH HOSPITAL – BEMIDJI (244014)**, 800
Bemidji Avenue North, Zip 56601–3054; tel. 218/308–2400, (Nonreporting) **A**1
10 **S** Minnesota Department of Human Services, Saint Paul, MN
Primary Contact: Theresa Vander Eyck, Administrator
**Control:** State–Government, nonfederal **Service:** Psychiatric

**Staffed Beds:** 16

**NORTH COUNTRY REGIONAL HOSPITAL** See Sanford Bemidji Medical Center

★ **SANFORD BEMIDJI MEDICAL CENTER (240100)**, 1300 Anne Street N.W.,
Zip 56601; tel. 218/751–5430, (Total facility includes 78 beds in nursing home–
type unit) **A**9 10 **F**3 6 8 10 11 13 15 20 22 28 29 30 31 34 35 40 45 46 50
51 53 59 62 63 64 70 74 75 76 77 78 79 81 82 85 86 87 90 93 97 103
107 108 110 111 113 114 116 118 119 120 122 123 124 126 127 128 129
130 131 134 143 144 145 147 **P**6 **S** Sanford Health, Sioux Falls, SD
Primary Contact: Paul A. Hanson, Chief Executive Officer
CFO: Craig Boyer, Vice President Finance
CMO: Daniel DeKrey, M.D., Chief of Staff
CIO: Dan Moffatt, Chief Information Officer
Web address: www.nchs.org
**Control:** Other not–for–profit (including NFP Corporation) **Service:** General
Medical and Surgical

**Staffed Beds:** 196 **Admissions:** 6499 **Census:** 141 **Outpatient Visits:**
113954 **Births:** 999 **Total Expense ($000):** 95565 **Payroll Expense ($000):**
38102 **Personnel:** 673

## BENSON—Swift County

★ **SWIFT COUNTY–BENSON HOSPITAL (241365)**, 1815 Wisconsin Avenue,
Zip 56215–1653; tel. 320/843–1311 **A**9 10 18 **F**7 11 15 17 18 28 29 31 34
38 40 46 50 57 62 68 69 70 75 77 78 79 81 82 83 84 85 91 93 104 110
126 127 131 132 147
Primary Contact: Frank Lawatsch, Chief Financial Officer
CFO: Jayne Thielke, Chief Financial Officer
CMO: Roger Bauer, M.D., Chief Medical Officer
CIO: Jayne Thielke, Chief Financial Officer
CHR: Stella Kalthoff, Administrative Assistant, Manager Human Resources and
Coordinator Quality Improvement
Web address: www.scbh.org
**Control:** Hospital district or authority, Government, nonfederal **Service:** General
Medical and Surgical

**Staffed Beds:** 18 **Admissions:** 334 **Census:** 3 **Outpatient Visits:** 20577
**Births:** 0 **Total Expense ($000):** 12295 **Payroll Expense ($000):** 4412
**Personnel:** 93

## BIGFORK—Itasca County

★ **BIGFORK VALLEY HOSPITAL (241316)**, 258 Pine Tree Drive, Zip 56628,
Mailing Address: P.O. Box 258, Zip 56628–0258; tel. 218/743–3177,
(Nonreporting) **A**9 10 18
Primary Contact: Daniel D. Odegaard, Chief Executive Officer
CFO: Karen M. Campbell, Director Finance
CMO: George Rounds, M.D., Chief of Staff
CIO: Sally Sedgwick, Manager Public Relations and Marketing
CHR: Jennifer Drotts, Manager Human Resources
Web address: www.bigforkvalley.org
**Control:** Hospital district or authority, Government, nonfederal **Service:** General
Medical and Surgical

**Staffed Beds:** 60

## BLUE EARTH—Faribault County

⊞ **UNITED HOSPITAL DISTRICT (241369)**, 515 South Moore Street,
Zip 56013–2158, Mailing Address: P.O. Box 160, Zip 56013–0160;
tel. 507/526–3273, (Nonreporting) **A**1 9 10 18
Primary Contact: Jeffrey M. Lang, Chief Executive Officer
CFO: Larry Lee, Chief Financial Officer
Web address: www.uhd.org
**Control:** Hospital district or authority, Government, nonfederal **Service:** General
Medical and Surgical

**Staffed Beds:** 41

## BRAINERD—Crow Wing County

**BRAINERD REGIONAL HUMAN SERVICES CENTER**, 11800 State Highway 18,
Zip 56401–7300; tel. 218/828–2201, (Nonreporting) **A**9
Primary Contact: Bill Peters, Acting Director of Psychiatry
**Control:** State–Government, nonfederal **Service:** Psychiatric

**Staffed Beds:** 16

☐ **ESSENTIA HEALTH ST. JOSEPH'S MEDICAL CENTER (240075)**, 523 North
Third Street, Zip 56401–3098; tel. 218/829–2861 **A**1 2 9 10 **F**3 4 5 11 12 13
15 18 26 28 29 30 31 34 35 40 43 44 45 48 49 52 56 57 59 64 65 70 74
75 76 77 78 79 81 85 86 87 89 90 92 93 94 95 96 98 100 101 102 103
104 105 107 108 111 114 118 125 126 128 129 130 131 143 145 146 147
**P**2 **S** Essentia Health, Duluth, MN
Primary Contact: Jani M. Wiebolt, President and Chief Executive Officer
CFO: James Winch, Vice President Finance
CMO: David Boran, M.D., Chief Medical Officer
CHR: Dale Benson, Vice President Human Resources
Web address: www.sjmcmn.org
**Control:** Church–operated, Nongovernment, not–for profit **Service:** General
Medical and Surgical

**Staffed Beds:** 162 **Admissions:** 6522 **Census:** 61 **Outpatient Visits:** 146554
**Births:** 459 **Total Expense ($000):** 158261 **Payroll Expense ($000):** 75983
**Personnel:** 1078

☐ **MINNESOTA NEUROREHABILITATION HOSPITAL (243025)**, 11615 State Avenue, Zip 56401–7306; tel. 218/828–2458, (Nonreporting) **A**1
Primary Contact: Dawn Barnard, Administrator
**Control:** State–Government, nonfederal **Service:** Rehabilitation

> **Staffed Beds:** 15

**ST. JOSEPH'S MEDICAL CENTER** See Essentia Health St. Joseph's Medical Center

**BRECKENRIDGE—Wilkin County**

★ **ST. FRANCIS HEALTHCARE CAMPUS (241377)**, 2400 St. Francis Drive, Zip 56520–1298; tel. 218/643–3000, (Total facility includes 120 beds in nursing home–type unit) **A**5 9 10 18 **F**3 5 8 11 13 15 17 28 29 30 32 34 35 38 39 40 43 45 46 50 53 56 57 59 64 70 75 76 77 79 81 87 89 93 96 97 99 100 101 102 103 104 107 110 111 114 118 124 126 127 128 129 130 131 132 142 145 **P**6 **S** Catholic Health Initiatives, Englewood, CO
Primary Contact: David A. Nelson, President and Chief Executive Officer
CFO: Nancy Whitney, Chief Financial Officer
Web address: www.sfcare.org
**Control:** Church–operated, Nongovernment, not–for profit **Service:** General Medical and Surgical

> **Staffed Beds:** 145 **Admissions:** 1229 **Census:** 127 **Outpatient Visits:** 20543
> **Births:** 179 **Total Expense ($000):** 28685 **Payroll Expense ($000):** 12382
> **Personnel:** 265

**BUFFALO—Wright County**

⊞ **BUFFALO HOSPITAL (240076)**, 303 Catlin Street, Zip 55313–1947; tel. 763/682–1212 **A**1 9 10 **F**3 11 13 15 17 28 29 31 35 40 44 57 59 70 75 76 78 79 81 84 85 86 87 89 93 107 111 113 118 128 129 130 143 145 **S** Allina Health, Minneapolis, MN
Primary Contact: Jennifer Myster, President
COO: Laura Jenkins, Director Operations Finance and Business Development
CFO: Sandra Matrella, Manager Finance
CMO: Corey Martin, M.D., Director Medical Affairs
CIO: Lois Nevinski, Manager Information Services
CHR: Nikki Mills, Director Human Resources and Operations
CNO: Gretchen A. Frederick, R.N., Director Patient Care Services
Web address: www.buffalohospital.org
**Control:** Other not–for–profit (including NFP Corporation) **Service:** General Medical and Surgical

> **Staffed Beds:** 44 **Admissions:** 2582 **Census:** 16 **Outpatient Visits:** 69743
> **Births:** 626 **Total Expense ($000):** 53948 **Payroll Expense ($000):** 22968
> **Personnel:** 312

**BURNSVILLE—Dakota County**

⊞ **FAIRVIEW RIDGES HOSPITAL (240207)**, 201 East Nicollet Boulevard, Zip 55337–5799; tel. 952/892–2000 **A**1 2 9 10 **F**3 11 13 15 18 20 28 29 30 31 34 35 36 40 43 44 45 49 50 51 55 57 64 68 70 72 74 75 76 77 78 79 81 82 84 85 87 89 93 100 107 108 109 110 110 111 113 117 118 129 131 145 **S** Fairview Health Services, Minneapolis, MN
Primary Contact: Beth Krehbiel, President and Chief Executive Officer
COO: Brian A. Knapp, Vice President Operations
CFO: Alan Lem, Vice President Finance
CMO: Lizbeth Thomas, M.D., Vice President Medical Affairs
CHR: Mary Kaphings, Director Human Resources
CNO: Carol Koeppel–Olsen, R.N., Vice President Patient Care Services
Web address: www.fairview.org
**Control:** Other not–for–profit (including NFP Corporation) **Service:** General Medical and Surgical

> **Staffed Beds:** 165 **Admissions:** 11531 **Census:** 103 **Outpatient Visits:** 100783 **Births:** 2649 **Total Expense ($000):** 154271 **Payroll Expense ($000):** 77445 **Personnel:** 911

**CAMBRIDGE—Isanti County**

⊞ **CAMBRIDGE MEDICAL CENTER (240020)**, 701 South Dellwood Street, Zip 55008–1920; tel. 763/689–7700 **A**1 9 10 **F**3 4 5 11 13 14 15 18 28 29 30 31 32 34 35 38 40 43 45 50 56 57 59 61 64 65 69 70 74 75 76 77 78 79 81 82 85 86 87 89 93 97 98 99 100 101 102 103 104 107 108 111 113 118 124 128 129 130 131 133 134 143 144 145 146 147 **P**5 6 **S** Allina Health, Minneapolis, MN
Primary Contact: Dennis J. Doran, President
CFO: Nancy Treacy, Director Finance
CHR: Diane Rasmussen, Director Human Resources
CNO: Mari J. Holt, R.N., Director Patient Care Services
Web address: www.allina.com/ahs/cambridge.nsf
**Control:** Other not–for–profit (including NFP Corporation) **Service:** General Medical and Surgical

> **Staffed Beds:** 78 **Admissions:** 3963 **Census:** 39 **Outpatient Visits:** 101909
> **Births:** 481 **Total Expense ($000):** 71913 **Payroll Expense ($000):** 29160
> **Personnel:** 649

**CANBY—Yellow Medicine County**

★ **SANFORD MEDICAL CENTER CANBY (241347)**, 112 St. Olaf Avenue South, Zip 56220–1433; tel. 507/223–7277, (Includes SENIOR HAVEN CONVALESCENT NURSING CENTER ), (Total facility includes 75 beds in nursing–type units) **A**9 10 18 **F**2 3 7 10 11 13 15 28 29 31 35 39 40 45 46 49 53 56 59 60 62 64 65 70 71 75 76 79 81 89 93 107 110 118 127 129 131 132 142 143 **P**6 **S** Sanford Health, Sioux Falls, SD
Primary Contact: Robert J. Salmon, Chief Executive Officer
CFO: Allison Nelson, Chief Financial Officer
CMO: Maritza Lopez, M.D., Chief of Staff
CIO: Cheryl L. Ferguson, Associate Administrator
CNO: Lori Sisk, R.N., Chief Nursing Officer
Web address: www.sanfordcanby.org
**Control:** Other not–for–profit (including NFP Corporation) **Service:** General Medical and Surgical

> **Staffed Beds:** 100 **Admissions:** 443 **Census:** 76 **Outpatient Visits:** 29591
> **Births:** 32 **Total Expense ($000):** 20710 **Payroll Expense ($000):** 10283
> **Personnel:** 226

**CANNON FALLS—Goodhue County**

⊞ **MAYO CLINIC HEALTH SYSTEM IN CANNON FALLS (241346)**, 1116 West Mill Street, Zip 55009–1898; tel. 507/263–4221, (Nonreporting) **A**1 9 10 18 **S** Mayo Clinic Health System, Rochester, MN
Primary Contact: Thomas J. Witt, M.D., President and Chief Executive Officer
COO: Glenn Christian, Administrator
CFO: Edward A. Tusa, Chief Financial Officer
CMO: Tarlochan Turna, M.D., Medical Director
CHR: Mary Garlets, Director Human Resources
Web address: www.cannonhealth.org/
**Control:** Hospital district or authority, Government, nonfederal **Service:** General Medical and Surgical

> **Staffed Beds:** 21

**CASS LAKE—Cass County**

★ **U. S. PUBLIC HEALTH SERVICE INDIAN HOSPITAL (241358)**, 7th Street & Grant Utley Avenue N.W., Zip 56633, Mailing Address: Rural Route 3, Box 211, Zip 56633; tel. 218/335–3200, (Nonreporting) **A**5 9 10 18 **S** U. S. Indian Health Service, Rockville, MD
Primary Contact: Norine Smith, Chief Executive Officer
CFO: Randall Jordan, Budget Analyst
Web address: www.ihs.gov
**Control:** PHS, Indian Service, Government, federal **Service:** General Medical and Surgical

> **Staffed Beds:** 11

**CLOQUET—Carlton County**

★ **COMMUNITY MEMORIAL HOSPITAL (241364)**, 512 Skyline Boulevard, Zip 55720–1199; tel. 218/879–4641, (Nonreporting) **A**9 10 18
Primary Contact: Rick Breuer, Chief Executive Officer and Administrator
CFO: Brad Anderson, Chief Financial Officer
CIO: Jason Stoeke, Director Management Information Systems
CHR: Cory Glad, Director Human Resources
Web address: www.cloquethospital.com
**Control:** Other not–for–profit (including NFP Corporation) **Service:** General Medical and Surgical

> **Staffed Beds:** 113

**COOK—St. Louis County**

★ **COOK HOSPITAL AND CONVALESCENT NURSING CARE UNIT (241312)**, 10 Fifth Street S.E., Zip 55723–9745; tel. 218/666–5945, (Total facility includes 28 beds in nursing home–type unit) **A**9 10 18 **F**2 3 11 15 28 29 35 40 53 56 57 64 77 81 93 96 107 110 111 118 127 132 147
Primary Contact: Allen J. Vogt, Chief Executive Officer
CFO: Kaylee S. Hoard, Chief Financial Officer
Web address: www.cookhospital.org
**Control:** Hospital district or authority, Government, nonfederal **Service:** General Medical and Surgical

> **Staffed Beds:** 42 **Admissions:** 372 **Census:** 31 **Outpatient Visits:** 15147
> **Births:** 0 **Total Expense ($000):** 10753 **Payroll Expense ($000):** 4911
> **Personnel:** 99

**Hospital, Medicare Provider Number, Address, Telephone, Approval, Facility, and Physician Codes, Health Care System**

★ American Hospital Association (AHA) membership
☐ The Joint Commission accreditation   ◇ DNV Healthcare Inc. accreditation
○ American Osteopathic Association (AOA) accreditation
△ Commission on Accreditation of Rehabilitation Facilities (CARF) accreditation

## COON RAPIDS—Anoka County

⊠ **MERCY HOSPITAL (240115)**, 4050 Coon Rapids Boulevard, Zip 55433–2586; tel. 763/236–6000 **A**1 2 5 9 10 **F**3 8 11 13 17 18 20 22 24 26 28 29 30 31 34 35 36 37 38 40 43 45 49 53 55 59 63 64 65 68 69 70 72 73 74 75 76 77 78 79 81 82 85 87 89 93 97 98 99 100 101 102 103 104 105 107 108 111 114 118 125 128 129 131 134 145 146 147 **P**4 5 6 **S** Allina Health, Minneapolis, MN
Primary Contact: Sara J. Criger, President
COO: Brandi Lunneborg, Vice President Operations
CFO: Earl Beitzel, Vice President Finance
CMO: Ryan Else, M.D., Interim Vice President Medical Affairs
CIO: Susan Heichert, Chief Information Officer
CHR: Nancy Watson, Director Human Resources
CNO: MariBeth Olson, R.N., Vice President Patient Care Services
Web address: www.allinamercy.org
**Control:** Other not–for–profit (including NFP Corporation) **Service:** General Medical and Surgical

**Staffed Beds:** 251 **Admissions:** 21062 **Census:** 196 **Outpatient Visits:** 131128 **Births:** 2048 **Total Expense ($000):** 340914 **Payroll Expense ($000):** 126042 **Personnel:** 1498

## CROOKSTON—Polk County

★ **RIVERVIEW HEALTH (241320)**, 323 South Minnesota Street, Zip 56716–1600; tel. 218/281–9200, (Nonreporting) **A**5 9 10 18
Primary Contact: Ross A. Matlack, FACHE, Chief Executive Officer
CFO: William Bennett, Chief Financial Officer
CMO: Mirza Baig, M.D., Chief of Staff
CIO: Chris Bruggeman, Chief Information Officer
CHR: Jean Tate, Manager Human Resources
Web address: www.riverviewhealth.org
**Control:** Other not–for–profit (including NFP Corporation) **Service:** General Medical and Surgical

**Staffed Beds:** 52

## CROSBY—Crow Wing County

⊠ **CUYUNA REGIONAL MEDICAL CENTER (241353)**, 320 East Main Street, Zip 56441–1690; tel. 218/546–7000, (Total facility includes 120 beds in nursing home–type unit) **A**1 9 10 18 **F**3 7 12 13 15 18 28 29 31 34 35 40 43 45 46 47 48 49 50 51 56 57 59 62 63 64 65 68 70 75 76 77 78 79 81 82 84 85 86 87 91 92 93 94 97 99 100 101 103 104 107 110 111 114 115 116 118 123 126 127 129 130 131 132 142 143 145 146 147 **P**6
Primary Contact: John H. Solheim, Chief Executive Officer
COO: Theresa Sullivan, Chief Operating Officer
CFO: Kyle Bauer, Chief Financial Officer
CMO: George Kuhlmann, M.D., Chief of Staff
CHR: Rebecca A. Thiesfeld, Executive Director Human Resources
Web address: www.cuyunamed.org
**Control:** Hospital district or authority, Government, nonfederal **Service:** General Medical and Surgical

**Staffed Beds:** 145 **Admissions:** 2409 **Census:** 131 **Outpatient Visits:** 36819 **Births:** 261 **Total Expense ($000):** 62210 **Payroll Expense ($000):** 25188 **Personnel:** 465

## DAWSON—Lac Qui Parle County

**JOHNSON MEMORIAL HEALTH SERVICES (241314)**, 1282 Walnut Street, Zip 56232–2333; tel. 320/769–4323, (Total facility includes 56 beds in nursing home–type unit) **A**9 10 18 **F**3 7 8 11 13 15 28 34 40 56 57 62 64 65 68 71 76 77 81 85 93 107 110 111 118 126 127 129 132 134 144 145 **P**6
Primary Contact: Kathy Johnson, Administrator
CFO: Stacey Lee, Chief Financial Officer
CMO: Ralph Gerbig, M.D., Chief of Staff
CIO: Derrick Ochsendorf, Manager Information Technology and Systems
CHR: Ellen Alberg, Director Human Resources
Web address: www.jmhsdawson.com
**Control:** Hospital district or authority, Government, nonfederal **Service:** General Medical and Surgical

**Staffed Beds:** 79 **Admissions:** 357 **Census:** 57 **Outpatient Visits:** 1937 **Births:** 11 **Total Expense ($000):** 12292 **Payroll Expense ($000):** 6706 **Personnel:** 137

## DEER RIVER—Itasca County

★ **DEER RIVER HEALTHCARE CENTER (241360)**, 115 10th Avenue N.E., Zip 56636–9700; tel. 218/246–2900, (Total facility includes 32 beds in nursing home–type unit) **A**9 10 18 **F**2 7 10 11 12 13 15 18 29 31 34 35 36 37 40 43 56 57 59 62 64 75 77 78 79 80 81 82 90 93 96 107 110 111 115 116 117 118 123 124 127 128 129 131 132 134 141 142 144 145 147 **P**6
Primary Contact: Jeffry Stampohar, Chief Executive Officer
CMO: David Goodall, M.D., Chief Medical Staff
CHR: Brittany Mohler, Director Human Resources
Web address: www.drhc.org
**Control:** Other not–for–profit (including NFP Corporation) **Service:** General Medical and Surgical

**Staffed Beds:** 52 **Admissions:** 546 **Census:** 33 **Outpatient Visits:** 16292 **Births:** 99 **Total Expense ($000):** 21096 **Payroll Expense ($000):** 7972 **Personnel:** 122

## DETROIT LAKES—Becker County

⊠ **ESSENTIA HEALTH ST. MARY'S HOSPITAL – DETROIT LAKES (240101)**, 1027 Washington Avenue, Zip 56501–3598; tel. 218/847–5611, (Nonreporting) **A**1 5 9 10 **S** Essentia Health, Duluth, MN
Primary Contact: Peter Jacobson, President
CFO: Ryan Hill, Chief Financial Officer
CMO: Rich Vetter, M.D., Associate Chief
CIO: Ken Gilles, Associate Chief Information Officer
CHR: Diane Sundrud, Human Resource Service Partner
CNO: Diana Johnson, R.N., Chief Nursing Officer
Web address: www.trustedcareforlife.org
**Control:** Church–operated, Nongovernment, not–for profit **Service:** General Medical and Surgical

**Staffed Beds:** 58

**ST. MARY'S INNOVIS HEALTH** See Essentia Health St. Mary's Hospital – Detroit Lakes

## DULUTH—St. Louis County

⊠ △ **ESSENTIA HEALTH DULUTH (240019)**, 502 East Second Street, Zip 55805–1982; tel. 218/727–8762 **A**1 2 3 5 7 9 10 **F**3 5 11 12 15 16 19 29 30 31 32 34 35 45 46 47 49 50 51 52 54 55 56 57 58 59 61 64 65 70 74 75 77 78 79 81 82 84 85 86 87 90 92 93 95 96 97 98 99 100 101 103 104 105 107 108 110 111 113 114 115 116 117 118 119 120 122 123 128 129 130 131 133 134 140 143 145 146 147 **P**6 **S** Essentia Health, Duluth, MN
Primary Contact: Mike Metcalf, Chief Administrative Officer
CFO: Barbara Johnson, Chief Financial Officer
CMO: Hugh Renier, M.D., Vice President Medical Affairs
CIO: Dennis Dassenko, Chief Information Officer
CHR: Diane Davidson, Senior Vice President Human Resources
Web address: www.smdcmedicalcenter.org
**Control:** Other not–for–profit (including NFP Corporation) **Service:** General Medical and Surgical

**Staffed Beds:** 154 **Admissions:** 4537 **Census:** 77 **Outpatient Visits:** 38951 **Births:** 20 **Total Expense ($000):** 344714 **Payroll Expense ($000):** 200186 **Personnel:** 2790

⊠ **ESSENTIA HEALTH ST. MARY'S MEDICAL CENTER (240002)**, 407 East Third Street, Zip 55805–1984; tel. 218/786–4000, (Includes ST. MARY'S CHILDREN'S HOSPITAL, 407 East Third Street, Zip 55805–1950; tel. 218/786–5437) **A**1 2 3 5 9 10 **F**3 11 12 13 17 18 20 22 24 26 28 29 30 34 35 37 40 43 46 48 49 50 57 59 61 63 64 65 67 70 72 74 76 78 79 81 83 84 85 86 87 88 89 107 108 111 114 118 125 128 129 131 140 145 **P**6 **S** Essentia Health, Duluth, MN
Primary Contact: Daniel B. McGinty, Administrator
CMO: Hugh Renier, M.D., Vice President Medical Affairs
CIO: Tess Jettergren, Director Clinical Informatics
CHR: Glen Porter, Vice President Human Resources
Web address: www.smdc.org
**Control:** Other not–for–profit (including NFP Corporation) **Service:** General Medical and Surgical

**Staffed Beds:** 316 **Admissions:** 17147 **Census:** 196 **Outpatient Visits:** 112491 **Births:** 1461 **Total Expense ($000):** 301473 **Payroll Expense ($000):** 128727 **Personnel:** 1952

**SMDC MEDICAL CENTER** See Essentia Health Duluth

⊠ △ **ST. LUKE'S HOSPITAL (240047)**, 915 East First Street, Zip 55805–2193; tel. 218/249–5555 **A**1 2 3 5 7 9 10 **F**3 8 9 11 12 13 15 17 18 20 22 24 26 28 29 30 31 34 35 39 40 43 46 47 48 49 51 53 54 57 58 59 60 61 62 63 64 65 70 74 75 76 77 78 79 81 82 83 84 85 86 87 89 90 92 93 97 98 100 101 102 103 104 107 108 110 111 113 114 115 117 118 119 120 122 123 125 128 129 130 131 143 145 147 **P**6
Primary Contact: John Strange, President and Chief Executive Officer
CMO: Gary Peterson, M.D., Vice President Medical Affairs and Medical Director
CIO: Clark Averill, Director Information Technology
CHR: Marla Halvorson, Director Human Resources
CNO: Susan Hamel, Chief Nursing Officer
Web address: www.slhduluth.com
**Control:** Other not–for–profit (including NFP Corporation) **Service:** General Medical and Surgical

**Staffed Beds:** 267 **Admissions:** 11424 **Census:** 134 **Outpatient Visits:** 157420 **Births:** 956 **Total Expense ($000):** 316391 **Payroll Expense ($000):** 156719 **Personnel:** 1878

**ST. MARY'S MEDICAL CENTER** See Essentia Health St. Mary's Medical Center

*Many Facility Codes have changed. Please refer to the AHA Guide Code Chart.* © 2012 AHA Guide

## EDINA—Hennepin County

✠ **FAIRVIEW SOUTHDALE HOSPITAL (240078)**, 6401 France Avenue South, Zip 55435–2199; tel. 952/924–5000 **A**1 2 3 5 9 10 **F**3 5 8 11 12 13 15 17 18 20 22 24 26 28 29 30 31 34 35 38 40 43 49 50 51 55 57 59 60 64 65 69 70 73 74 75 76 78 79 81 82 84 87 92 93 94 98 100 102 107 108 109 110 111 113 114 115 118 120 123 125 128 129 130 131 133 134 145 146 147 **P**6 **S** Fairview Health Services, Minneapolis, MN
Primary Contact: Bradley Beard, President
CFO: Alan Lem, Vice President Finance
CHR: Rich Lutz, Director Human Resources
CNO: Judith Pechacek, R.N., Vice President Patient Care
Web address: www.fairview.org
**Control:** Other not–for–profit (including NFP Corporation) **Service:** General Medical and Surgical

**Staffed Beds:** 335 **Admissions:** 18417 **Census:** 203 **Outpatient Visits:** 133666 **Births:** 3052 **Total Expense ($000):** 371117 **Payroll Expense ($000):** 145657 **Personnel:** 1621

## ELBOW LAKE—Grant County

**ELEAH MEDICAL CENTER** See Prairie Ridge Hospital and Health Services

★ **PRAIRIE RIDGE HOSPITAL AND HEALTH SERVICES (241379)**, 930 First Street N.E., Zip 56531–4611; tel. 218/685–4461 **A**9 10 18 **F**7 15 28 31 40 43 45 46 47 48 53 59 64 65 67 90 93 107 127 132 147 **P**5
Primary Contact: Thomas Kooiman, Chief Executive Officer
CFO: Claude Priest, Chief Financial Officer
CMO: Larry Rapp, M.D., Chief Medical Officer
Web address: www.eleahmed.org
**Control:** Other not–for–profit (including NFP Corporation) **Service:** General Medical and Surgical

**Staffed Beds:** 20 **Admissions:** 256 **Census:** 3 **Outpatient Visits:** 26774 **Births:** 0 **Total Expense ($000):** 11973 **Payroll Expense ($000):** 3481 **Personnel:** 113

## ELY—St. Louis County

★ **ELY–BLOOMENSON COMMUNITY HOSPITAL (241318)**, 328 West Conan Street, Zip 55731–1198; tel. 218/365–3271, (Nonreporting) **A**9 10 18
Primary Contact: John Fossum, Chief Executive Officer and Administrator
CFO: Scott Kellerman, Chief Financial Officer
CHR: Richard Rand, Director Human Resources
Web address: www.ebch.org
**Control:** Other not–for–profit (including NFP Corporation) **Service:** General Medical and Surgical

**Staffed Beds:** 84

## FAIRMONT—Martin County

✠ **MAYO CLINIC HEALTH SYSTEM IN FAIRMONT (240166)**, 800 Medical Center Drive, Zip 56031–0800; tel. 507/238–8100, (Includes LUTZ WING CONVALESCENT AND NURSING CARE UNIT ), (Total facility includes 40 beds in nursing home–type unit) **A**1 9 10 20 **F**3 8 11 13 15 17 28 29 30 31 34 40 43 47 48 59 64 65 68 75 76 77 78 79 81 82 84 85 86 87 92 93 97 99 100 101 103 104 107 108 110 111 114 117 118 127 128 129 131 132 143 145 **P**6 **S** Mayo Clinic Health System, Rochester, MN
Primary Contact: Robert Bartingale, Chief Administrative Officer
COO: Gayle B. Hansen, R.N., Chief Operating Officer
CFO: Brian Suter, Chief Financial Officer
CMO: Rufus Rodriguez, M.D., Medical Director
Web address: www.fairmontmedicalcenter.org
**Control:** Other not–for–profit (including NFP Corporation) **Service:** General Medical and Surgical

**Staffed Beds:** 96 **Admissions:** 2299 **Census:** 61 **Outpatient Visits:** 133656 **Births:** 272 **Total Expense ($000):** 76476 **Payroll Expense ($000):** 38124 **Personnel:** 572

## FARIBAULT—Rice County

★ **DISTRICT ONE HOSPITAL (240071)**, 200 State Avenue, Zip 55021–6345; tel. 507/334–6451, (Nonreporting) **A**9 10
Primary Contact: Stephen J. Pribyl, FACHE, Chief Executive Officer
COO: Joan Boysen, Chief Operating Officer
CFO: Rick Miller, Chief Financial Officer
CMO: Brant Barr, M.D., Chief Medical Officer
CIO: Glenn Gregersen, Director Information Technology
CHR: Lucy G. Dupree, Director Human Resources
CNO: Lynette Dickson, Director Clinical Operations and Director of Nursing
Web address: www.districtonehospital.com
**Control:** Hospital district or authority, Government, nonfederal **Service:** General Medical and Surgical

**Staffed Beds:** 42

## FERGUS FALLS—Otter Tail County

☐ **COMMUNITY BEHAVIORAL HEALTH HOSPITAL – FERGUS FALLS (244013)**, 1801 West Alcott Avenue, Zip 56538–0478, Mailing Address: P.O. Box 478, Zip 56538–0478; tel. 218/332–5001, (Nonreporting) **A**1 9 10 **S** Minnesota Department of Human Services, Saint Paul, MN
Primary Contact: Derrick A. Jones, Administrator
**Control:** State–Government, nonfederal **Service:** Psychiatric

**Staffed Beds:** 16

✠ △ **LAKE REGION HEALTHCARE CORPORATION (240052)**, 712 South Cascade Street, Zip 56537–2900, Mailing Address: P.O. Box 728, Zip 56538–0728; tel. 218/736–8000 **A**1 7 9 10 20 **F**3 10 11 13 15 17 28 29 30 31 32 33 34 35 36 40 41 43 44 45 50 51 53 54 56 57 59 61 64 65 68 70 74 75 76 77 78 79 81 82 84 85 86 87 89 90 92 93 94 96 98 100 101 102 103 104 107 108 110 111 114 116 117 118 119 120 122 129 130 131 134 143 145 146 147
Primary Contact: Larry A. Schulz, Chief Executive Officer
CFO: Edward A. Strand, CPA, Chief Financial Officer
CMO: Wade Swenson, M.D., Chief of Staff
CIO: Wade A. Jurkas, Director Computer Information Systems
CHR: Cheryl Buck, Vice President Human Resources
CNO: Lucia E. Anderson, Senior Vice President Nursing and Chief Nurse Executive
Web address: www.lrhc.org
**Control:** Other not–for–profit (including NFP Corporation) **Service:** General Medical and Surgical

**Staffed Beds:** 108 **Admissions:** 3086 **Census:** 33 **Outpatient Visits:** 53841 **Births:** 301 **Total Expense ($000):** 97633 **Payroll Expense ($000):** 34486 **Personnel:** 694

## FOSSTON—Polk County

★ **ESSENTIA HEALTH FOSSTON (241357)**, 900 Hilligoss Boulevard S.E., Zip 56542–1599; tel. 218/435–1133, (Total facility includes 50 beds in nursing home–type unit) **A**9 10 18 **F**2 3 7 10 11 13 28 29 31 34 35 36 40 43 45 48 53 54 56 57 59 62 63 64 65 68 75 76 77 80 81 82 84 85 87 89 90 93 97 107 118 124 126 127 129 130 131 132 134 142 144 145 147 **P**6 **S** Essentia Health, Duluth, MN
Primary Contact: Patricia Wangler, Chief Executive Officer
CFO: Kim Bodensteiner, Chief Financial Officer
CIO: Abe Deusterman, Manager Information Technology
CHR: Diane Sundrud, Director Human Resources
Web address: www.firstcare.org
**Control:** Other not–for–profit (including NFP Corporation) **Service:** General Medical and Surgical

**Staffed Beds:** 75 **Admissions:** 590 **Census:** 55 **Outpatient Visits:** 67275 **Births:** 70 **Total Expense ($000):** 18891 **Payroll Expense ($000):** 10444 **Personnel:** 207

**FIRST CARE MEDICAL SERVICES** See Essentia Health Fosston

## FRIDLEY—Anoka County

✠ **UNITY HOSPITAL (240132)**, 550 Osborne Road N.E., Zip 55432–2799; tel. 763/236–5000 **A**1 2 5 9 10 **F**3 4 5 11 12 13 15 18 20 22 24 26 28 29 30 31 34 35 36 40 43 45 49 50 55 56 57 59 63 64 65 69 70 73 75 76 77 78 79 81 82 85 86 87 89 93 97 98 99 100 101 102 103 104 107 108 111 113 114 118 128 129 131 134 144 145 146 147 **S** Allina Health, Minneapolis, MN
Primary Contact: Lori Wightman, R.N., MSN, FACHE, President
COO: Patrick Belland, Vice President Operations
CFO: Lisa K. Anderson, Vice President Finance
CMO: Paul Kettler, M.D., Vice President Medical Affairs
CIO: Susan Heichert, Chief Information Officer
CHR: Kenneth E. Auer, Director Human Resources
CNO: Julianne Lapensky, MS, Vice President Patient Care Services
Web address: www.allina.com
**Control:** Other not–for–profit (including NFP Corporation) **Service:** General Medical and Surgical

**Staffed Beds:** 220 **Admissions:** 13001 **Census:** 131 **Outpatient Visits:** 91668 **Births:** 1377 **Total Expense ($000):** 180555 **Payroll Expense ($000):** 73074 **Personnel:** 888

**MN**

---

**Hospital, Medicare Provider Number, Address, Telephone, Approval, Facility, and Physician Codes, Health Care System**

★ American Hospital Association (AHA) membership
☐ The Joint Commission accreditation ◇ DNV Healthcare Inc. accreditation
○ American Osteopathic Association (AOA) accreditation
△ Commission on Accreditation of Rehabilitation Facilities (CARF) accreditation

## GLENCOE—Mcleod County

★ **GLENCOE REGIONAL HEALTH SERVICES (241355)**, 1805 Hennepin Avenue North, Zip 55336–1416; tel. 320/864–3121, (Total facility includes 110 beds in nursing home–type unit) **A**9 10 18 **F**3 7 11 13 15 17 28 29 31 34 40 43 56 64 68 70 75 76 77 81 86 87 89 93 97 107 110 113 118 124 127 129 131 132 134 144 145 **P**6 **S** Park Nicollet Health Services, Saint Louis Park, MN
Primary Contact: Jon D. Braband, FACHE, President and Chief Executive Officer
CFO: John C. Doidge, Vice President Finance
CMO: John H. Bergseng, D.O., Vice President Medical Affairs
CIO: Tony Alsleben, Director Information Technology
CHR: Jill Hatlestad, Vice President Human Resources and Organizational Support
CNO: Gayle Sturgis, Vice President Nursing
Web address: www.grhsonline.org
**Control:** Other not–for–profit (including NFP Corporation) **Service:** General Medical and Surgical

**Staffed Beds:** 135 **Admissions:** 1087 **Census:** 111 **Outpatient Visits:** 24033
**Births:** 163 **Total Expense ($000):** 46022 **Payroll Expense ($000):** 23066
**Personnel:** 384

## GLENWOOD—Pope County

★ **GLACIAL RIDGE HEALTH SYSTEM (241376)**, 10 Fourth Avenue S.E., Zip 56334–1898; tel. 320/634–4521 **A**9 10 18 **F**7 11 12 13 15 17 28 31 34 35 40 41 43 53 59 62 63 64 75 76 81 107 110 113 118 126 129 132 145 147 **P**6
Primary Contact: Kirk A. Stensrud, Chief Executive Officer
CFO: Kyle Chase, Chief Financial Officer
CMO: Robert Montenegro, M.D., Chief of Staff
CIO: Heidi Engle, Manager Information Technology
CHR: Gordon Paulson, Manager Personnel
Web address: www.glacialridge.org
**Control:** Hospital district or authority, Government, nonfederal **Service:** General Medical and Surgical

**Staffed Beds:** 19 **Admissions:** 677 **Census:** 6 **Outpatient Visits:** 12656
**Births:** 33 **Total Expense ($000):** 19867 **Payroll Expense ($000):** 9439
**Personnel:** 166

## GOLDEN VALLEY—Hennepin County

⊞ **REGENCY HOSPITAL OF MINNEAPOLIS (242005)**, 1300 Hidden Lakes Parkway, Zip 55422–4299; tel. 763/588–2750, (Nonreporting) **A**1 10 **S** Select Medical Corporation, Mechanicsburg, PA
Primary Contact: John Allen, Chief Executive Officer
COO: Jan Cwynar, Vice President Operations
CMO: Norm Yunis, M.D., Medical Director
Web address: www.regencyhospital.com
**Control:** Corporation, Investor–owned, for–profit **Service:** General Medical and Surgical

**Staffed Beds:** 54

## GRACEVILLE—Big Stone County

**ESSENTIA HEALTH–HOLY TRINITY HOSPITAL (241321)**, 115 West Second Street, Zip 56240–0157, Mailing Address: P.O. Box 157, Zip 56240–0157; tel. 320/748–7223, (Total facility includes 50 beds in nursing home–type unit) **A**9 10 18 **F**3 8 15 28 30 34 35 40 41 43 57 59 62 63 64 71 77 81 85 91 93 107 111 113 118 127 131 132 **S** Essentia Health, Duluth, MN
Primary Contact: Kevin Gish, Chief Executive Officer
CFO: John Campion, Chief Financial Officer
CMO: Arthur Van Vranken, M.D., Chief Medical Officer
CIO: Brad Tostenson, Chief Information Officer
CHR: Jenny Lee, Human Resources Generalist
CNO: Jill Johnsrud, Director of Nursing
Web address: www.essentiahealth.org/HolyTrinityHospital/FindaClinic/Essentia–HealthHoly–Trinity–Hospital–96.aspx
**Control:** Other not–for–profit (including NFP Corporation) **Service:** General Medical and Surgical

**Staffed Beds:** 65 **Admissions:** 276 **Census:** 49 **Outpatient Visits:** 9172
**Births:** 0

**GRACEVILLE HEALTH CENTER** See Essentia Health–Holy Trinity Hospital

## GRAND MARAIS—Cook County

**COOK COUNTY NORTH SHORE HOSPITAL (241317)**, 515 5th Avenue West, Zip 55604–9716; tel. 218/387–3040, (Total facility includes 37 beds in nursing home–type unit) **A**9 10 18 **F**7 11 13 15 18 28 31 40 43 45 56 59 62 64 76 77 84 85 89 93 107 110 111 113 118 127 129 132
Primary Contact: Kimber L. Wraalstad, FACHE, Administrator and Chief Executive Officer
CFO: Yvonne Gennrich, Controller
CHR: Shelly Starkey, Personnel Coordinator
CNO: Bridget Sobieck, Director of Nursing
Web address: www.nshorehospital.com
**Control:** Hospital district or authority, Government, nonfederal **Service:** General Medical and Surgical

**Staffed Beds:** 53 **Admissions:** 153 **Census:** 40 **Outpatient Visits:** 9523
**Births:** 14 **Total Expense ($000):** 11757 **Payroll Expense ($000):** 5664
**Personnel:** 123

## GRAND RAPIDS—Itasca County

⊞ **GRAND ITASCA CLINIC AND HOSPITAL (240064)**, 1601 Golf Course Road, Zip 55744–3698; tel. 218/326–5000, (Nonreporting) **A**1 9 10 20
Primary Contact: Michael Youso, Chief Executive Officer
CFO: Bruce Lorenz, Senior Vice President Finance and Chief Financial Officer
CHR: Robert Cocker, Vice President Organizational Effectiveness
Web address: www.granditasca.org
**Control:** Other not–for–profit (including NFP Corporation) **Service:** General Medical and Surgical

**Staffed Beds:** 64

## GRANITE FALLS—Yellow Medicine County

★ **GRANITE FALLS MUNICIPAL HOSPITAL AND MANOR (241343)**, 345 Tenth Avenue, Zip 56241–1499; tel. 320/564–3111, (Total facility includes 57 beds in nursing home–type unit) **A**9 10 18 **F**3 7 13 15 28 34 40 43 45 56 57 59 62 64 69 71 76 79 81 84 85 93 107 127 128 129 132 142
Primary Contact: George Gerlach, Chief Executive Officer
CFO: Val Hoffman, Chief Financial Officer
CIO: Kris Wilke, Manager Health Information
CHR: Sue Tollefson, Coordinator Payroll Personnel
CNO: Patty Massman, Director of Nursing
Web address: www.granitefallshealthcare.com
**Control:** City–Government, nonfederal **Service:** General Medical and Surgical

**Staffed Beds:** 82 **Admissions:** 673 **Census:** 55 **Outpatient Visits:** 28493
**Births:** 40 **Total Expense ($000):** 16637 **Payroll Expense ($000):** 8081
**Personnel:** 145

## HALLOCK—Kittson County

★ **KITTSON MEMORIAL HEALTHCARE CENTER (241336)**, 1010 South Birch Street, Zip 56728–0700, Mailing Address: P.O. Box 700, Zip 56728–0700; tel. 218/843–3612, (Total facility includes 70 beds in nursing home–type unit) **A**9 10 18 **F**7 10 11 15 34 40 45 53 59 62 63 81 126 127 132
Primary Contact: Richard J. Failing, Chief Executive Officer
CFO: Jeni Schwenzfeier, Chief Financial Officer
CMO: Thomas Lohstreter, M.D., Chief of Staff
CIO: Holly Knutson, Manager Information Technology
CHR: Carlene Cole, Manager Human Resources
Web address: www.kmhc.net
**Control:** Other not–for–profit (including NFP Corporation) **Service:** General Medical and Surgical

**Staffed Beds:** 85 **Admissions:** 181 **Census:** 70 **Outpatient Visits:** 9800
**Births:** 0 **Total Expense ($000):** 11813 **Payroll Expense ($000):** 5700
**Personnel:** 135

## HASTINGS—Dakota County

☐ **REGINA MEDICAL CENTER (240059)**, 1175 Nininger Road, Zip 55033–1098; tel. 651/480–4100, (Total facility includes 61 beds in nursing home–type unit) **A**1 9 10 **F**3 8 10 11 13 15 29 30 34 40 43 46 49 50 57 59 63 68 69 70 75 76 77 81 83 87 93 107 111 113 118 124 127 128 129 131 142 145
Primary Contact: Ty W. Erickson, Chief Executive Officer
CFO: Greg Kopp, Chief Financial Officer
CMO: James Noreen, M.D., Chief Medical Officer
CHR: Kirstin D. Swenson, Director Human Resources
Web address: www.reginamedical.org
**Control:** Other not–for–profit (including NFP Corporation) **Service:** General Medical and Surgical

**Staffed Beds:** 115 **Admissions:** 1712 **Census:** 54 **Outpatient Visits:** 43146
**Births:** 425 **Total Expense ($000):** 49272 **Payroll Expense ($000):** 19922
**Personnel:** 521

## HENDRICKS—Lincoln County

★ **HENDRICKS COMMUNITY HOSPITAL (241339)**, 503 East Lincoln Street, Zip 56136–0106, Mailing Address: P.O. Box 106, Zip 56136–0106; tel. 507/275–3134, (Total facility includes 58 beds in nursing home–type unit) **A**9 10 18 **F**2 3 7 10 11 15 17 28 29 31 34 35 40 59 62 63 70 81 89 93 124 126 127 129 131 132 145
Primary Contact: Jeffrey Gollaher, Chief Executive Officer
CMO: Tabb McCluskey, M.D., Chief Medical Officer
CHR: Lynn R. Olson, Director Human Resources
Web address: www.hendrickshosp.org
**Control:** Other not–for–profit (including NFP Corporation) **Service:** General Medical and Surgical

**Staffed Beds:** 70 **Admissions:** 240 **Census:** 54 **Outpatient Visits:** 12837
**Births:** 0 **Total Expense ($000):** 11178 **Payroll Expense ($000):** 4394
**Personnel:** 112

MN

**HIBBING—St. Louis County**

⊠ **RANGE REGIONAL HEALTH SERVICES (240040)**, 750 East 34th Street, Zip 55746–4600; tel. 218/262–4881 **A**1 2 10 **F**3 6 11 13 15 28 29 30 31 34 35 40 43 45 48 49 57 59 62 63 64 65 70 75 76 77 78 81 82 85 86 87 89 93 97 98 102 107 108 110 114 115 118 119 120 128 129 134 143 144 145 146 147 **S** Fairview Health Services, Minneapolis, MN
Primary Contact: Debra K. Boardman, FACHE, President and Chief Executive Officer
COO: Vicky Korynta, Senior Vice President and Chief Operating Officer
CFO: John D. Kritz, Senior Vice President and Chief Financial Officer
CMO: Jim Hartert, M.D., Senior Vice President and Medical Director
CIO: Jessica Valento, Director Information Systems
CHR: Mitch Vincent, Vice President Organizational Support
CNO: Connie Harle, Chief Nursing Officer
Web address: www.range.fairview.org
**Control:** Other not–for–profit (including NFP Corporation) **Service:** General Medical and Surgical

**Staffed Beds:** 76 **Admissions:** 3277 **Census:** 36 **Outpatient Visits:** 13505 **Births:** 379 **Total Expense ($000):** 93543 **Payroll Expense ($000):** 45858 **Personnel:** 685

**HUTCHINSON—Mcleod County**

⊠ **HUTCHINSON AREA HEALTH CARE (240187)**, 1095 Highway 15 South, Zip 55350–3182; tel. 320/234–5000, (Total facility includes 120 beds in nursing home–type unit) **A**1 9 10 20 **F**2 3 5 7 11 13 15 28 29 31 34 35 36 38 40 43 45 56 57 59 64 69 70 75 76 77 78 79 81 82 85 87 93 98 99 100 101 102 103 104 107 110 111 113 118 126 127 128 129 130 131 145 146 147 **S** Allina Health, Minneapolis, MN
Primary Contact: Steven Mulder, M.D., President and Chief Executive Officer
CFO: Pamela Larson, Division Director Financial Services
CIO: Pamela Larson, Division Director Financial Services
CHR: Rebecca Streich, Manager Human Resources and Education Manager
Web address: www.hahc–hmc.com
**Control:** Other not–for–profit (including NFP Corporation) **Service:** General Medical and Surgical

**Staffed Beds:** 177 **Admissions:** 2776 **Census:** 128 **Outpatient Visits:** 90126 **Births:** 274 **Total Expense ($000):** 65457 **Payroll Expense ($000):** 23691 **Personnel:** 342

**INTERNATIONAL FALLS—Koochiching County**

⊠ **RAINY LAKE MEDICAL CENTER (241322)**, 1400 Highway 71, Zip 56649–2189; tel. 218/283–4481 **A**1 9 10 18 **F**11 13 15 28 29 31 34 40 43 59 76 77 81 85 89 93 99 100 101 102 103 104 107 113 114 118 132 143 **S** QHR, Brentwood, TN
Primary Contact: Bob Haley, Interim Chief Executive Officer
CMO: Douglas A. Johnson, M.D., Chief of Staff
CIO: Michael Blesi, Director Information Technology
Web address: www.rainylakemedical.com
**Control:** Other not–for–profit (including NFP Corporation) **Service:** General Medical and Surgical

**Staffed Beds:** 25 **Admissions:** 581 **Census:** 5 **Outpatient Visits:** 29810 **Births:** 88 **Total Expense ($000):** 24354 **Payroll Expense ($000):** 8097 **Personnel:** 149

**JACKSON—Jackson County**

★ **SANFORD JACKSON MEDICAL CENTER (241315)**, 1430 North Highway, Zip 56143–1098; tel. 507/847–2420 **A**9 10 18 **F**1 3 15 18 28 29 31 34 35 40 43 45 46 50 56 57 59 64 65 67 68 75 77 78 79 81 82 85 86 87 89 90 93 97 107 108 110 111 113 117 118 126 127 128 130 131 132 147 **P**6 **S** Sanford Health, Sioux Falls, SD
Primary Contact: Mary J. Ruyter, Chief Executive Officer
CFO: Gail Eike, Chief Financial Officer
CMO: Sister Marie Paul Lockerd, M.D., Chief Medical Officer
CNO: Dawn Schnell, Chief Nursing Officer
Web address: www.sanfordjackson.org
**Control:** Other not–for–profit (including NFP Corporation) **Service:** General Medical and Surgical

**Staffed Beds:** 20 **Admissions:** 171 **Census:** 2 **Outpatient Visits:** 24685 **Births:** 0 **Total Expense ($000):** 6698 **Payroll Expense ($000):** 2525 **Personnel:** 60

**LAKE CITY—Goodhue County**

⊠ **MAYO CLINIC HEALTH SYSTEM IN LAKE CITY (241338)**, 500 West Grant Street, Zip 55041–1143; tel. 651/345–3321, (Nonreporting) **A**1 9 10 18 **S** Mayo Clinic Health System, Rochester, MN
Primary Contact: Thomas J. Witt, M.D., President and Chief Executive Officer
COO: Cheri Kramer, Chief Administrative Officer
CFO: David Biren, Chief Financial Officer
CMO: Dennis Spano, M.D., Medical Director
CHR: Jacqueline Ryan, Director Human Resources
Web address: www.lakecitymedicalcenter.org
**Control:** Other not–for–profit (including NFP Corporation) **Service:** General Medical and Surgical

**Staffed Beds:** 108

**LE SUEUR—Le Sueur County**

**MINNESOTA VALLEY HEALTH CENTER (241375)**, 621 South Fourth Street, Zip 56058–2298; tel. 507/665–3375, (Includes GARDENVIEW NURSING HOME ), (Nonreporting) **A**9 10 18 **S** Essentia Health, Duluth, MN
Primary Contact: Patricia J. Townsdin–Woodruff, President and Chief Executive Officer
CFO: Patricia Schlegel, Executive Director Finance
CMO: Carolyn Stelter, M.D., Chief of Staff
CHR: Bonnie Barnhardt, Executive Director Human Resources
Web address: www.mvhc.org
**Control:** Other not–for–profit (including NFP Corporation) **Service:** General Medical and Surgical

**Staffed Beds:** 110

**LITCHFIELD—Meeker County**

★ **MEEKER MEMORIAL HOSPITAL (241366)**, 612 South Sibley Avenue, Zip 55355–3398; tel. 320/693–3242 **A**9 10 18 **F**11 13 15 28 29 31 34 40 43 56 57 59 68 70 75 76 77 78 81 89 90 93 103 107 111 118 129 131 132 145 147
Primary Contact: Kyle Rasmussen, Chief Executive Officer
CFO: Stephen Plaisance, Chief Financial Officer
CMO: Tim Peterson, M.D., Chief of Staff
CIO: Connie Liimatta, Director Medical Records and Business Office
CHR: Cindi Twardy, Manager Human Resources
CNO: Ann Lien, R.N., Chief Nursing Officer
Web address: www.meekermemorial.com
**Control:** County–Government, nonfederal **Service:** General Medical and Surgical

**Staffed Beds:** 39 **Admissions:** 1095 **Census:** 15 **Outpatient Visits:** 27318 **Births:** 166 **Total Expense ($000):** 24269 **Payroll Expense ($000):** 8667 **Personnel:** 144

**LITTLE FALLS—Morrison County**

★ **ST. GABRIEL'S HOSPITAL (241370)**, 815 Second Street S.E., Zip 56345–3596; tel. 320/632–5441 **A**9 10 18 **F**3 11 13 15 26 28 29 30 31 34 40 43 45 59 62 63 64 65 68 70 75 76 77 79 81 82 84 85 86 87 93 107 108 110 111 114 118 127 129 130 131 132 145 **P**6 **S** Catholic Health Initiatives, Englewood, CO
Primary Contact: Chad D. Cooper, President and Chief Executive Officer
CMO: Thomas Stoy, M.D., Chief of Staff
CHR: Barb Miller, Director Human Resources
Web address: www.stgabriels.com
**Control:** Church–operated, Nongovernment, not–for profit **Service:** General Medical and Surgical

**Staffed Beds:** 25 **Admissions:** 1419 **Census:** 12 **Outpatient Visits:** 134528 **Births:** 189 **Total Expense ($000):** 55909 **Payroll Expense ($000):** 25549 **Personnel:** 356

**LONG PRAIRIE—Todd County**

★ **CENTRACARE HEALTH SYSTEM – LONG PRAIRIE (241326)**, 20 Ninth Street S.E., Zip 56347–1404; tel. 320/732–2141, (Nonreporting) **A**9 10 18 **S** CentraCare Health System, Saint Cloud, MN
Primary Contact: Daniel J. Swenson, Chief Executive Officer
CFO: Larry Knutson, Director Finance
CMO: Rene Eldidy, M.D., Chief of Staff
Web address: www.centracare.com
**Control:** Other not–for–profit (including NFP Corporation) **Service:** General Medical and Surgical

**Staffed Beds:** 20

**LONG PRAIRIE MEMORIAL HOSPITAL AND HOME** See CentraCare Health System – Long Prairie

---

**Hospital, Medicare Provider Number, Address, Telephone, Approval, Facility, and Physician Codes, Health Care System**

★ American Hospital Association (AHA) membership
□ The Joint Commission accreditation
◇ DNV Healthcare Inc. accreditation
○ American Osteopathic Association (AOA) accreditation
△ Commission on Accreditation of Rehabilitation Facilities (CARF) accreditation

## LUVERNE—Rock County

★ **SANFORD LUVERNE MEDICAL CENTER (241371)**, 1600 North Kniss Avenue, Zip 56156–1067; tel. 507/283–2321 **A**9 10 18 **F**3 4 5 7 8 11 13 15 18 19 28 29 31 32 34 35 40 45 56 57 59 63 64 65 68 75 76 77 78 81 82 83 84 85 86 87 90 93 96 97 107 113 114 117 118 128 130 131 132 134 145 146 147 **P**6 **S** Sanford Health, Sioux Falls, SD
Primary Contact: Tammy Loosbrock, Chief Executive Officer
CFO: Stanley Knobloch, Chief Financial Officer
CMO: Richard P. Morgan, M.D., Chief of Staff
Web address: www.sanfordluverne.org
**Control:** Other not–for–profit (including NFP Corporation) **Service:** General Medical and Surgical

**Staffed Beds:** 25 **Admissions:** 672 **Census:** 7 **Outpatient Visits:** 35840 **Births:** 112 **Total Expense ($000):** 18439 **Payroll Expense ($000):** 7579 **Personnel:** 171

## MADELIA—Watonwan County

⊠ **MADELIA COMMUNITY HOSPITAL (241323)**, 121 Drew Avenue S.E., Zip 56062–1899; tel. 507/642–3255 **A**1 3 5 9 10 18 **F**11 13 15 34 35 40 57 59 62 64 68 69 75 76 77 81 84 85 86 93 102 107 110 113 127 129 131 132 143 144 **P**6
Primary Contact: Candace Fenske, Chief Executive Officer
CFO: Donna M. Klinkner, Chief Financial Officer
CMO: Timothy Bachenberg, M.D., Chief Medical Officer
CIO: Marie Schneeberger, Director of Health
CHR: Donna M. Klinkner, Chief Financial Officer
CNO: Deidre Hruby, Director of Patient Care
Web address: www.mchospital.org
**Control:** Other not–for–profit (including NFP Corporation) **Service:** General Medical and Surgical

**Staffed Beds:** 21 **Admissions:** 277 **Census:** 4 **Outpatient Visits:** 5085 **Births:** 31 **Total Expense ($000):** 8611 **Payroll Expense ($000):** 3267 **Personnel:** 70

## MADISON—Lac Qui Parle County

★ **MADISON HOSPITAL (241372)**, 900 Second Avenue, Zip 56256–1006; tel. 320/598–7556, (Nonreporting) **A**9 10 18
Primary Contact: Scott C. Larson, Chief Executive Officer
CFO: Carol Borgerson, Business Office Manager and Chief Financial Officer
CIO: Jerry Harberts, Information Technologist
CHR: Bridget Sabin, Director Human Resources
Web address: www.madisonlutheranhome.com
**Control:** Other not–for–profit (including NFP Corporation) **Service:** General Medical and Surgical

**Staffed Beds:** 12

## MAHNOMEN—Mahnomen County

★ **MAHNOMEN HEALTH CENTER (241300)**, 414 West Jefferson Avenue, Zip 56557–4912, Mailing Address: P.O. Box 396, Zip 56557–0396; tel. 218/935–2511, (Nonreporting) **A**9 10 18 **S** Sanford Health, Sioux Falls, SD
Primary Contact: Susan K. Klassen, Chief Executive Officer and Administrator
CFO: Mary Pazdernik, Chief Financial Officer
CMO: Anju Gurung, M.D., Chief Medical Officer
CHR: Kristi Stall, Chief Human Resources Officer
Web address: www.mahnomenhealthcenter.com
**Control:** City–County, Government, nonfederal **Service:** General Medical and Surgical

**Staffed Beds:** 18

## MANKATO—Blue Earth County

⊠ **MAYO CLINIC HEALTH SYSTEM IN MANKATO (240093)**, 1025 Marsh Street, Zip 56002–8673, Mailing Address: P.O. Box 8673, Zip 56002–8673; tel. 507/625–4031 **A**1 3 5 9 10 **F**3 5 11 13 15 18 20 22 26 27 28 29 30 31 33 35 36 38 39 40 41 43 45 49 53 54 57 58 59 60 61 62 63 64 65 66 68 70 74 75 76 77 78 79 81 82 83 84 85 86 87 89 91 92 93 97 98 99 100 102 103 104 107 108 110 111 113 114 115 117 118 119 120 122 126 128 129 131 134 143 145 146 147 **P**6 **S** Mayo Clinic Health System, Rochester, MN
Primary Contact: Gregory Kutcher, M.D., President and Chief Executive Officer
CFO: Stanley Marczak, Chief Financial Officer
CMO: Brian Whited, M.D., Medical Director
CIO: Thomas Borowski, Chief Information Officer
CHR: Julie Oliver, Chief Human Resources Officer
Web address: www.isj–mhs.org
**Control:** Other not–for–profit (including NFP Corporation) **Service:** General Medical and Surgical

**Staffed Beds:** 166 **Admissions:** 10626 **Census:** 111 **Outpatient Visits:** 360639 **Births:** 1580 **Total Expense ($000):** 252801 **Payroll Expense ($000):** 132079 **Personnel:** 1720

## MAPLE GROVE—Hennepin County

⊠ **MAPLE GROVE HOSPITAL (240214)**, 9875 Hospital Drive, Zip 55369–4648; tel. 763/581–1000 **A**1 9 10 **F**3 13 15 18 29 30 40 43 45 60 68 70 73 76 77 79 81 84 85 89 90 100 102 107 108 111 114 117 118 129 145 147 **P**8
Primary Contact: Andrew S. Cochrane, Chief Executive Officer
CFO: Jason Weaver, Finance Manager
CHR: Kate J. Law, Director Human Resources
Web address: www.maplegrovehospital.org
**Control:** Other not–for–profit (including NFP Corporation) **Service:** General Medical and Surgical

**Staffed Beds:** 90 **Admissions:** 5952 **Census:** 42 **Births:** 3026

## MARSHALL—Lyon County

⊠ **AVERA MARSHALL REGIONAL MEDICAL CENTER (241359)**, 300 South Bruce Street, Zip 56258–3900; tel. 507/532–9661, (Nonreporting) **A**1 9 10 18 **S** Avera Health, Sioux Falls, SD
Primary Contact: Mary B. Maertens, FACHE, President and Chief Executive Officer
CFO: Sharon Williams, Vice President Finance and Information Technology
CMO: Steven Meister, M.D., Chief of Staff
CIO: Sharon Williams, Vice President Finance and Information Technology
CHR: Amber Crowley, Vice President Human Resources
Web address: www.averamarshall.org
**Control:** City–Government, nonfederal **Service:** General Medical and Surgical

**Staffed Beds:** 25

## MELROSE—Stearns County

★ **CENTRACARE HEALTH SYSTEM – MELROSE (241330)**, 525 Main Street West, Zip 56352–1098; tel. 320/256–4231, (Total facility includes 75 beds in nursing home–type unit) **A**9 10 18 **F**2 7 10 13 15 28 30 34 35 40 46 56 57 59 70 75 77 78 79 81 82 83 85 93 99 103 107 110 113 118 120 121 124 127 128 129 131 132 145 147 **S** CentraCare Health System, Saint Cloud, MN
Primary Contact: Gerry Gilbertson, FACHE, Administrator
COO: Gerry Gilbertson, FACHE, Administrator
CFO: Adam Paulson, Director Finance
CMO: Dante Beretta, M.D., Chief of Staff
CIO: Janet Kruzel, Health Information Manager
CHR: Joyce Chan, Chief Human Resources Officer
CNO: Keri Wimmer, R.N., Patient Care Director
Web address: www.centracare.com
**Control:** Other not–for–profit (including NFP Corporation) **Service:** General Medical and Surgical

**Staffed Beds:** 93 **Admissions:** 520 **Census:** 79 **Outpatient Visits:** 22179 **Births:** 92 **Total Expense ($000):** 21725 **Payroll Expense ($000):** 9979 **Personnel:** 204

## MINNEAPOLIS—Hennepin County

⊠ **ABBOTT NORTHWESTERN HOSPITAL (240057)**, 800 East 28th Street, Zip 55407–3799; tel. 612/863–4000, (Includes SISTER KENNY REHABILITATION INSTITUTE, 810 East 27th Street, Zip 55407; tel. 612/874–4000) **A**1 2 3 5 8 9 10 **F**3 8 9 12 13 15 17 18 20 22 24 26 28 29 30 31 34 35 36 37 38 39 40 43 44 45 46 47 48 49 50 51 52 53 54 57 58 59 60 61 63 64 65 66 68 70 71 74 75 76 77 78 79 81 82 84 85 86 87 90 91 92 93 94 95 96 97 98 99 100 101 102 103 104 105 107 108 109 110 111 112 113 114 115 116 117 118 119 120 122 123 125 128 129 130 131 134 135 136 137 140 142 144 145 146 147 **P**6 **S** Allina Health, Minneapolis, MN
Primary Contact: Ben Bache–Wiig, M.D., President
CFO: Brian Weinreis, Vice President Operations and Finance
CHR: Margaret Butler, Vice President Human Resources
Web address: www.abbottnorthwestern.com
**Control:** Other not–for–profit (including NFP Corporation) **Service:** General Medical and Surgical

**Staffed Beds:** 649 **Admissions:** 37555 **Census:** 463 **Outpatient Visits:** 392581 **Births:** 3908 **Total Expense ($000):** 890327 **Payroll Expense ($000):** 361343 **Personnel:** 3726

☐ **CHILDREN'S HOSPITALS AND CLINICS OF MINNESOTA (243302)**, 2525 Chicago Avenue South, Zip 55404–9976; tel. 612/813–6100 **A**1 3 5 9 10 **F**3 8 9 11 12 17 18 19 20 21 22 23 24 25 26 27 28 29 30 31 32 34 35 36 38 39 40 41 43 44 48 49 50 51 54 55 57 58 59 60 61 62 63 64 65 66 68 72 73 74 75 77 78 79 80 81 82 84 85 86 87 88 89 92 93 97 99 100 101 102 104 107 108 109 111 112 113 114 117 118 128 129 130 131 133 134 135 142 144 145 146 147 **P**6 8 **S** Children's Hospitals and Clinics of Minnesota, Minneapolis, MN
Primary Contact: Alan L. Goldbloom, M.D., President and Chief Executive Officer
COO: David S. Overman, Chief Operating Officer
CFO: Jerry Massmann, Chief Financial Officer
CMO: Phillip M. Kibort, M.D., Chief Medical Officer
CMO: Phillip M. Kibort, M.D., Vice President Medical Affairs and Chief Medical Officer
CIO: Jeffrey D. Young, Chief Information Officer
CHR: David Brumbaugh, Vice President Human Resources
Web address: www.childrensmn.org
**Control:** Other not–for–profit (including NFP Corporation) **Service:** Children's general

> **Staffed Beds:** 347 **Admissions:** 12209 **Census:** 218 **Outpatient Visits:** 321191 **Births:** 0 **Total Expense ($000):** 571461 **Payroll Expense ($000):** 266178 **Personnel:** 3113

**FAIRVIEW RIVERSIDE HOSPITAL** See University of Minnesota Medical Center, Fairview

☐ △ **HENNEPIN COUNTY MEDICAL CENTER (240004)**, 701 Park Avenue South, Zip 55415–1829; tel. 612/873–3000, (Includes HCMC DEPARTMENT OF PEDIATRICS, 701 Park Avenue, Zip 55415–1623; tel. 612/873–2064) **A**1 2 3 5 7 8 9 10 **F**3 5 7 11 12 13 15 16 17 18 20 22 24 26 28 29 30 31 32 34 35 38 39 40 41 43 44 45 46 47 49 50 51 52 53 54 55 56 57 58 59 61 64 65 66 68 70 72 74 75 76 77 78 79 81 82 84 85 86 87 88 89 90 92 93 96 97 98 99 100 101 102 104 105 107 108 110 111 112 113 114 115 116 117 118 120 122 128 129 130 131 133 134 137 143 145 146 147
Primary Contact: Arthur A. Gonzalez, Dr.PH, FACHE, Chief Executive Officer
COO: Timothy Harlin, Chief Operating Officer
CFO: Larry Kryzaniak, Chief Financial Officer
CMO: Michael Belzer, M.D., Medical Director
CIO: Joanne Sunquist, Chief Information Officer
CHR: Hilary Marden–Resnik, Vice President Human Resources
Web address: www.hcmc.org
**Control:** County–Government, nonfederal **Service:** General Medical and Surgical

> **Staffed Beds:** 462 **Admissions:** 21315 **Census:** 324 **Outpatient Visits:** 480768 **Births:** 2327 **Total Expense ($000):** 552098 **Payroll Expense ($000):** 260683 **Personnel:** 3785

☒ △ **MINNEAPOLIS VETERANS AFFAIRS HEALTH CARE SYSTEM**, One Veterans Drive, Zip 55417–2399; tel. 612/725–2000, (Total facility includes 80 beds in nursing home–type unit) **A**1 2 3 5 7 8 **F**2 3 5 6 8 12 17 18 20 22 24 26 28 29 30 31 34 35 36 38 39 40 44 46 47 49 50 51 53 55 56 57 58 59 60 61 62 63 64 65 67 70 74 75 77 78 79 80 81 82 83 84 85 86 87 89 91 92 93 94 95 96 97 98 100 101 102 103 104 105 107 108 111 114 115 116 117 118 119 120 122 126 127 128 129 130 131 134 143 145 146 147
**S** Department of Veterans Affairs, Washington, DC
Primary Contact: Barry Sharp, Acting Director
COO: Kurt Thielen, Manager Business Office
CFO: LeAnn Stomberg, Chief Financial Officer
CMO: Kent Crossley, M.D., Acting Chief of Staff
CIO: Karl Reid, Chief Information Officer
CHR: Kevin Upham, Chief Human Resources Officer
CNO: Helen Pearlman, Nurse Executive
Web address: www.minneapolis.va.gov
**Control:** Veterans Affairs, Government, federal **Service:** General Medical and Surgical

> **Staffed Beds:** 305 **Admissions:** 7817 **Census:** 144 **Outpatient Visits:** 791146 **Births:** 0 **Personnel:** 3413

☒ **PHILLIPS EYE INSTITUTE (240196)**, 2215 Park Avenue, Zip 55404–3756; tel. 612/775–8800 **A**1 9 10 **F**81 **S** Allina Health, Minneapolis, MN
Primary Contact: Joan M. Arbach, Interim President
CFO: Chris Verdon, Director Finance
CMO: Emmett Carpel, M.D., Medical Director and Chief of Staff
CNO: Margaret Watry, Director of Patient Care Services and Nurse Executive
Web address: www.allina.com
**Control:** Other not–for–profit (including NFP Corporation) **Service:** Eye, ear, nose, and throat

> **Staffed Beds:** 8 **Admissions:** 191 **Census:** 1 **Outpatient Visits:** 14440 **Births:** 0 **Total Expense ($000):** 28803 **Payroll Expense ($000):** 9008 **Personnel:** 103

☐ **SHRINERS HOSPITALS FOR CHILDREN, TWIN CITIES (243303)**, 2025 East River Parkway, Zip 55414–3696; tel. 612/596–6100 **A**1 10 **F**3 11 29 34 35 57 58 59 64 68 75 77 79 80 81 82 85 86 87 89 93 94 118 129 133 **P**6 **S** Shriners Hospitals for Children, Tampa, FL
Primary Contact: Charles C. Lobeck, Administrator
CMO: Kenneth Guidera, M.D., Chief of Staff
CHR: Karen Frigen, Director Human Resources
Web address: www.shrinershq.org
**Control:** Other not–for–profit (including NFP Corporation) **Service:** Children's orthopedic

> **Staffed Beds:** 40 **Admissions:** 385 **Census:** 4 **Outpatient Visits:** 7775 **Births:** 0

**SISTER KENNY REHABILITATION INSTITUTE** See Abbott Northwestern Hospital

**ST. MARY'S HOSPITAL AND REHABILITATION CENTER** See University of Minnesota Medical Center, Fairview

**UNIVERSITY OF MINNESOTA HOSPITAL AND CLINIC** See University of Minnesota Medical Center, Fairview

☒ **UNIVERSITY OF MINNESOTA MEDICAL CENTER, FAIRVIEW (240080)**, 2450 Riverside Avenue, Zip 55454–1400; tel. 612/672–6000, (Includes FAIRVIEW RIVERSIDE HOSPITAL, 2312 South Sixth Street, Zip 55454; tel. 612/371–6300; ST. MARY'S HOSPITAL AND REHABILITATION CENTER, 2414 South Seventh Street, Zip 55454; tel. 612/338–2229; UNIVERSITY OF MINNESOTA CHILDREN'S HOSPITAL, FAIRVIEW, 420 Delaware Street, S.E., Zip 55455–0341; tel. 888/543–7866; UNIVERSITY OF MINNESOTA HOSPITAL AND CLINIC, 420 S.E. Delaware Street, Zip 55455–0392; tel. 612/626–3000), (Total facility includes 36 beds in nursing home–type unit) **A**1 3 5 8 9 10 **F**2 3 4 5 6 8 9 11 12 13 14 15 17 18 19 20 21 22 23 24 25 26 27 28 29 30 31 32 33 34 35 36 37 38 39 40 41 43 44 45 46 47 48 49 50 51 52 54 55 56 57 58 59 60 61 62 63 64 65 66 67 68 69 70 71 72 74 75 76 77 78 79 80 81 82 83 84 85 86 87 88 89 90 91 92 93 94 96 97 98 99 100 101 102 103 104 105 106 107 108 110 111 112 113 114 115 116 117 118 119 120 122 123 125 126 127 128 129 130 131 132 133 134 135 136 137 138 139 140 141 142 144 145 146 147 **P**5 **S** Fairview Health Services, Minneapolis, MN
Primary Contact: Carolyn Wilson, President
CFO: Steven Hill, Vice President Finance
CHR: Charles McIntosh, Senior Director Human Resources
Web address: www.fairview.org
**Control:** Other not–for–profit (including NFP Corporation) **Service:** General Medical and Surgical

> **Staffed Beds:** 814 **Admissions:** 32212 **Census:** 546 **Outpatient Visits:** 668104 **Births:** 2334 **Total Expense ($000):** 1147262 **Payroll Expense ($000):** 420358 **Personnel:** 5954

**VETERANS AFFAIRS MEDICAL CENTER** See Minneapolis Veterans Affairs Health Care System

### MONTEVIDEO—Chippewa County

★ **CHIPPEWA COUNTY–MONTEVIDEO HOSPITAL (241325)**, 824 North 11th Street, Zip 56265–1683; tel. 320/269–8877, (Nonreporting) **A**9 10 18
Primary Contact: Mark E. Paulson, Chief Executive Officer
CFO: Darlene Boike, Chief Financial Officer
CIO: Jane Myhre, MS, Director Health Information
CNO: Linda M. Nelson, R.N., Director of Nursing Services
Web address: www.montevideomedical.com
**Control:** City–County, Government, nonfederal **Service:** General Medical and Surgical

> **Staffed Beds:** 25

### MONTICELLO—Wright County

☒ **NEW RIVER MEDICAL CENTER (241362)**, 1013 Hart Boulevard, Zip 55362–8230; tel. 763/295–2945, (Nonreporting) **A**1 5 9 10 18
Primary Contact: Marshall E. Smith, FACHE, Chief Executive Officer
CFO: Nancy Friesen, Chief Financial Officer
CMO: Mark Dietz, Chief Medical Officer
CIO: Ruth Kremer, Director Information Services
CHR: Kathy Voss, Director Human Resources
CNO: Euretta Sorenson, R.N., Chief Nursing Officer
Web address: www.newrivermedical.com
**Control:** Hospital district or authority, Government, nonfederal **Service:** General Medical and Surgical

> **Staffed Beds:** 25

MN

---

**Hospital, Medicare Provider Number, Address, Telephone, Approval, Facility, and Physician Codes, Health Care System**

★ American Hospital Association (AHA) membership
☐ The Joint Commission accreditation   ◇ DNV Healthcare Inc. accreditation

○ American Osteopathic Association (AOA) accreditation
△ Commission on Accreditation of Rehabilitation Facilities (CARF) accreditation

## MOOSE LAKE—Carlton County

★ **MERCY HOSPITAL (241350)**, 710 South Kenwood Avenue, Zip 55767–9405; tel. 218/485–4481 **A**9 10 18 **F**3 7 8 11 13 15 28 29 31 34 35 40 43 45 46 53 57 59 62 64 68 70 75 76 77 79 81 85 86 87 89 93 107 111 113 118 129 131 132 134 142 143 145 147 **P**5
Primary Contact: Jason T. Douglas, Chief Executive Officer
CFO: Gregg Chartrand, Chief Financial Officer
CHR: Sonya Towle, Director Human Resources
CNO: Donita Korpela, R.N., Director of Patient Care Services
Web address: www.mercymooselake.org
**Control:** Hospital district or authority, Government, nonfederal **Service:** General Medical and Surgical

**Staffed Beds:** 25 **Admissions:** 951 **Census:** 8 **Outpatient Visits:** 26543
**Births:** 162 **Total Expense ($000):** 28488 **Payroll Expense ($000):** 12598
**Personnel:** 205

## MORA—Kanabec County

☒ **FIRSTLIGHT HEALTH SYSTEM (241367)**, 301 South Highway 65, Zip 55051; tel. 320/679–1212 **A**1 9 10 18 **F**3 7 11 13 15 28 30 31 34 35 40 43 51 53 57 63 70 75 76 77 78 79 81 85 87 93 94 107 108 110 111 114 117 118 129 131 132 134 145 147
Primary Contact: Randy Ulseth, Chief Executive Officer
COO: Christine M. Kimbler, R.N., Chief Operating Officer
CFO: David H. Amundson, Chief Financial Officer
CMO: Scott Lagaard, M.D., Chief of Staff
CHR: Kim Carlson, Manager Human Resources
Web address: www.firstlighthealthsystem.org
**Control:** County–Government, nonfederal **Service:** General Medical and Surgical

**Staffed Beds:** 25 **Admissions:** 1018 **Census:** 7 **Outpatient Visits:** 31302
**Total Expense ($000):** 41865 **Payroll Expense ($000):** 15968 **Personnel:** 300

## MORRIS—Stevens County

★ **STEVENS COMMUNITY MEDICAL CENTER (241363)**, 400 East First Street, Zip 56267–0660, Mailing Address: P.O. Box 660, Zip 56267–0660; tel. 320/589–1313 **A**9 10 18 **F**3 11 12 13 15 28 29 31 34 35 40 44 45 50 57 59 64 70 76 79 81 85 86 87 89 97 107 111 113 118 129 130 131 132 134 144 145 147 **P**6
Primary Contact: John Rau, President and Chief Executive Officer
CFO: Kerrie McEvilly, Director Finance and Information Systems
CIO: Kerrie McEvilly, Director Finance and Information Systems
CHR: Karla Larson, Director Human Resources
Web address: www.scmcinc.org
**Control:** Other not–for–profit (including NFP Corporation) **Service:** General Medical and Surgical

**Staffed Beds:** 25 **Admissions:** 1307 **Census:** 12 **Outpatient Visits:** 71451
**Births:** 90 **Total Expense ($000):** 35814 **Payroll Expense ($000):** 17673
**Personnel:** 258

## NEW PRAGUE—Scott County

☒ **MAYO CLINIC HEALTH SYSTEM IN NEW PRAGUE (241361)**, 301 Second Street N.E., Zip 56071–1799; tel. 952/758–4431 **A**1 9 10 18 **F**8 11 13 15 17 28 29 30 31 34 35 36 39 40 43 46 53 57 59 62 63 64 68 70 74 75 76 77 78 79 81 82 85 87 89 90 93 97 107 108 111 113 116 118 124 128 129 130 131 132 134 145 146 **P**6 **S** Mayo Clinic Health System, Rochester, MN
Primary Contact: Mary J. Klimp, Chief Administrative Officer
COO: Anna L. Herrmann, JD, Assistant Administrator
CMO: Marty Herrmann, M.D., Medical Director
CNO: Laura Hopkins, Director of Nursing
Web address: www.mayoclinichealthsystem.org/locations/new-prague
**Control:** Other not–for–profit (including NFP Corporation) **Service:** General Medical and Surgical

**Staffed Beds:** 25 **Admissions:** 1211 **Census:** 10 **Outpatient Visits:** 31376
**Births:** 172 **Total Expense ($000):** 29782 **Payroll Expense ($000):** 13995
**Personnel:** 217

## NEW ULM—Brown County

☒ **NEW ULM MEDICAL CENTER (241378)**, 1324 Fifth Street North, Zip 56073–1553; tel. 507/217–5000 **A**1 9 10 18 **F**3 4 5 7 8 11 13 15 28 29 31 32 34 40 45 54 55 56 57 59 62 63 64 68 70 75 76 77 78 79 81 82 84 85 89 93 97 98 99 100 101 102 103 104 105 106 107 111 113 118 119 120 121 122 123 128 129 130 131 134 143 145 147 **S** Allina Health, Minneapolis, MN
Primary Contact: Toby Freier, President
CFO: Toby Freier, President
CMO: Joan Krikava, M.D., Director Medical Affairs
CIO: Toby Freier, President
CHR: Anne Makepeace, Director Human Resources
Web address: www.newulmmedicalcenter.com
**Control:** Other not–for–profit (including NFP Corporation) **Service:** General Medical and Surgical

**Staffed Beds:** 45 **Admissions:** 2307 **Census:** 19 **Outpatient Visits:** 102226
**Births:** 329 **Total Expense ($000):** 64498 **Payroll Expense ($000):** 22415
**Personnel:** 329

## NORTHFIELD—Dakota County

★ **NORTHFIELD HOSPITAL (240014)**, 2000 North Avenue, Zip 55057–1498; tel. 507/646–1000, (Includes LONG TERM CARE CENTER ), (Total facility includes 40 beds in nursing home–type unit) **A**9 10 **F**3 7 11 15 29 30 31 34 35 43 45 46 47 48 49 57 59 62 63 64 68 69 70 75 76 77 78 79 81 85 86 87 93 94 97 107 110 111 114 116 118 119 127 128 129 130 131 132 145 146 **P**6
Primary Contact: Mark Henke, President and Chief Executive Officer
CFO: Timothy L. Gronseth, Vice President and Chief Financial Officer
CMO: Jeff Meland, M.D., Vice President, Chief Medical Officer
CHR: Kirsten Budin, Director Human Resources
Web address: www.northfieldhospital.org
**Control:** City–Government, nonfederal **Service:** General Medical and Surgical

**Staffed Beds:** 77 **Admissions:** 2039 **Census:** 52 **Outpatient Visits:** 115780
**Births:** 488 **Total Expense ($000):** 65254 **Payroll Expense ($000):** 28028
**Personnel:** 464

## OLIVIA—Renville County

**RC HOSPITAL AND CLINICS (241306)**, 611 East Fairview Avenue, Zip 56277–0800; tel. 320/523–1261, (Nonreporting) **A**9 10 18
Primary Contact: Glenn Haugo, Chief Executive Officer
CFO: Nate Blad, Chief Financial Officer
CIO: Cherry Weigel, Director Health Information Management
Web address: www.renvillecountyhospital.org
**Control:** County–Government, nonfederal **Service:** General Medical and Surgical

**Staffed Beds:** 25

## ONAMIA—Mille Lacs County

★ **MILLE LACS HEALTH SYSTEM (241356)**, 200 North Elm Street, Zip 56359–7978; tel. 320/532–3154, (Total facility includes 57 beds in nursing home–type unit) **A**9 10 18 **F**7 11 13 15 28 29 30 31 33 34 40 43 45 59 62 63 64 75 76 77 81 85 93 98 103 107 110 113 126 128 129 131 132 134 143 **P**6
Primary Contact: Bill Nelson, Chief Executive Officer
COO: Kim Kucera, Chief Operating Officer
CFO: John Unzen, Chief Financial Officer
CMO: Thomas H. Bracken, M.D., Vice President Medical Affairs
CIO: Robert Litke, Chief Information Officer
CHR: Fern Gershone, Vice President Human Resources
Web address: www.mlhealth.org
**Control:** Other not–for–profit (including NFP Corporation) **Service:** General Medical and Surgical

**Staffed Beds:** 85 **Admissions:** 980 **Census:** 69 **Outpatient Visits:** 21164
**Births:** 73 **Total Expense ($000):** 33190 **Payroll Expense ($000):** 15920
**Personnel:** 359

## ORTONVILLE—Big Stone County

★ **ORTONVILLE AREA HEALTH SERVICES (241342)**, 450 Eastvold Avenue, Zip 56278–1133; tel. 320/839–2502, (Total facility includes 64 beds in nursing home–type unit) **A**5 9 10 18 **F**2 3 11 13 15 18 19 28 30 31 34 35 40 44 45 49 50 56 57 59 62 63 64 65 68 69 74 75 76 77 78 79 81 82 84 85 86 87 89 92 93 107 111 113 116 118 127 129 130 132 134 145 **P**4 **S** Sanford Health, Sioux Falls, SD
Primary Contact: Richard M. Ash, Chief Executive Officer
CFO: James Foster, Chief Financial Officer and Assistant Administrator
CMO: Robert Ross, M.D., Chief of Staff
CIO: Barbara Voecks, Chief Information Officer
CHR: Kim McCrea, Chief Human Resources Officer
CNO: Jennifer Wiik, Chief Nursing Officer
Web address: www.oahs.us
**Control:** City–Government, nonfederal **Service:** General Medical and Surgical

**Staffed Beds:** 89 **Admissions:** 624 **Census:** 65 **Outpatient Visits:** 21050
**Births:** 65 **Total Expense ($000):** 20289 **Payroll Expense ($000):** 7042
**Personnel:** 96

## OWATONNA—Steele County

☒ **OWATONNA HOSPITAL (240069)**, 2250 N.W. 26th Street, Zip 55060–5503; tel. 507/451–3850 **A**1 9 10 **F**11 13 28 29 34 35 40 57 76 77 79 80 81 89 93 98 100 101 102 103 107 108 118 128 129 130 144 **S** Allina Health, Minneapolis, MN
Primary Contact: David L. Albrecht, President
CFO: Mark T. Gillen, Director Finance and Operations
CHR: Mark Sevenich, Director Human Resources
Web address: www.owatonnahospital.com
**Control:** Other not–for–profit (including NFP Corporation) **Service:** General Medical and Surgical

**Staffed Beds:** 43 **Admissions:** 2853 **Census:** 25 **Outpatient Visits:** 33055
**Births:** 526 **Total Expense ($000):** 46558 **Payroll Expense ($000):** 16319
**Personnel:** 216

*Many Facility Codes have changed. Please refer to the AHA Guide Code Chart.*

MN

## PARK RAPIDS—Hubbard County

✠ **ST. JOSEPH'S AREA HEALTH SERVICES (241380)**, 600 Pleasant Avenue, Zip 56470–1432; tel. 218/732–3311 **A**1 5 9 10 18 **F**3 11 12 13 15 28 29 30 32 34 35 39 40 43 45 47 57 59 62 63 64 65 70 75 76 77 79 81 82 84 85 93 107 108 110 111 113 117 118 128 129 130 131 132 133 145 **S** Catholic Health Initiatives, Englewood, CO
Primary Contact: Benjamin Koppelman, President and Chief Executive Officer
CFO: Jay Ross, Chief Financial Officer
CFO: Brent Schmidt, Chief Financial Officer
CMO: Darryl Beehler, D.O., Chief of Staff
CHR: John Tormanen, Director Mission and Human Resources
CNO: Deb Haagenson, R.N., Vice President of Patient Care
Web address: www.sjahs.org
**Control:** Church-operated, Nongovernment, not–for profit **Service:** General Medical and Surgical

**Staffed Beds:** 25 **Admissions:** 1761 **Census:** 15 **Outpatient Visits:** 36195
**Births:** 156 **Total Expense ($000):** 40263 **Payroll Expense ($000):** 16512
**Personnel:** 281

## PAYNESVILLE—Stearns County

**PAYNESVILLE AREA HEALTH CARE SYSTEM (241349)**, 200 West 1st Street, Zip 56362–1496; tel. 320/243–3767, (Total facility includes 102 beds in nursing home–type unit) **A**9 10 18 **F**7 10 11 13 15 17 28 31 40 56 64 75 76 81 107 114 118 124 126 127 129 131 132 142 144 145 147 **P**8
Primary Contact: Ronald A. Ommen, Interim Chief Executive Officer
COO: Greg Wilson, Chief Operating Officer and Chief Financial Officer
CFO: Greg Wilson, Chief Operating Officer and Chief Financial Officer
CIO: Gary Smith, Manager Information Technology
CHR: Paulette Hagen, Director Human Resources
Web address: www.pahcs.org
**Control:** Hospital district or authority, Government, nonfederal **Service:** General Medical and Surgical

**Staffed Beds:** 127 **Admissions:** 617 **Census:** 99 **Outpatient Visits:** 18306
**Births:** 83 **Total Expense ($000):** 27359 **Payroll Expense ($000):** 11934
**Personnel:** 282

## PERHAM—Otter Tail County

✠ **PERHAM HEALTH (241373)**, 1000 Coney Street West, Zip 56573–1199; tel. 218/347–4500, (Nonreporting) **A**1 9 10 18 **S** Sanford Health, Sioux Falls, SD
Primary Contact: Chuck Hofius, Chief Executive Officer
CFO: Brad D. Wurgler, Chief Financial Officer
CMO: Corey Nyhus, M.D., President Medical Staff
CIO: Jim Rieber, Director Information Systems
CHR: Kathy Johnson, Director Human Resources
CNO: Bonnie Johnson, R.N., Vice President of Patient Services
Web address: www.perhamhealth.org
**Control:** Hospital district or authority, Government, nonfederal **Service:** General Medical and Surgical

**Staffed Beds:** 19

## PINE CITY—Pine County

**LAKESIDE MEDICAL CENTER (240211)**, 129 East Sixth Avenue, Zip 55063; tel. 320/629–2542, (Nonreporting) **A**9 10
Primary Contact: Max Blaufuss, Administrator and Chief Executive Officer
Web address: www.lmc–pcac.com
**Control:** Corporation, Investor–owned, for–profit **Service:** Other specialty

**Staffed Beds:** 10

## PIPESTONE—Pipestone County

★ **PIPESTONE COUNTY MEDICAL CENTER AVERA (241374)**, 916 4th Avenue S.W., Zip 56164–0370; tel. 507/825–5811, (Nonreporting) **A**9 10 18 **S** Avera Health, Sioux Falls, SD
Primary Contact: Bradley D. Burris, Chief Executive Officer
CFO: Dave Keeler, Chief Financial Officer
CHR: Judy Raschke, Director Human Resources
Web address: www.pcmchealth.org
**Control:** County–Government, nonfederal **Service:** General Medical and Surgical

**Staffed Beds:** 25

## PRINCETON—Sherburne County

✠ **FAIRVIEW NORTHLAND MEDICAL CENTER (240141)**, 911 Northland Drive, Zip 55371–2173; tel. 763/389–1313 **A**1 5 9 10 **F**3 11 13 15 18 19 20 28 29 30 31 32 34 35 40 45 46 50 57 59 64 70 75 76 77 81 85 87 89 91 93 107 110 111 113 114 118 129 131 145 **P**6 **S** Fairview Health Services, Minneapolis, MN
Primary Contact: John W. Herman, Chief Executive Officer
CFO: Kim Ericson, Vice President Finance
CMO: Greg Schoen, M.D., Regional Medical Director
Web address: www.northland.fairview.org
**Control:** Other not–for–profit (including NFP Corporation) **Service:** General Medical and Surgical

**Staffed Beds:** 31 **Admissions:** 1959 **Census:** 14 **Outpatient Visits:** 48301
**Births:** 460 **Total Expense ($000):** 48386 **Payroll Expense ($000):** 23609
**Personnel:** 254

## RED WING—Goodhue County

✠ **MAYO CLINIC HEALTH SYSTEM IN RED WING (240018)**, 701 Fairview Boulevard, Zip 55066–2848, Mailing Address: P.O. Box 95, Zip 55066–0095; tel. 651/267–5000, (Total facility includes 84 beds in nursing home–type unit) **A**1 9 10 **F**3 8 11 13 15 18 19 28 29 30 31 34 35 36 38 40 43 45 49 50 54 56 57 59 62 63 64 68 69 70 75 76 77 78 79 81 83 84 85 86 87 93 96 97 99 104 107 108 110 111 113 117 118 124 127 128 129 130 131 134 143 145 146 147 **P**6 **S** Mayo Clinic Health System, Rochester, MN
Primary Contact: Thomas J. Witt, M.D., President and Chief Executive Officer
CFO: Mike Larson, Chief Financial Officer
CMO: Jack Alexander, M.D., Chief Medical Officer
CIO: Kendra Shaw, Manager Information Services
CHR: Kim Trittin, Manager Human Resources
Web address: www.mayoclinichealthsystem.org/locations/red–wing
**Control:** Other not–for–profit (including NFP Corporation) **Service:** General Medical and Surgical

**Staffed Beds:** 134 **Admissions:** 2075 **Census:** 80 **Outpatient Visits:** 60101
**Births:** 356 **Total Expense ($000):** 98921 **Payroll Expense ($000):** 47090
**Personnel:** 560

## REDLAKE—Beltrami County

✠ **U.S. PUBLIC HEALTH SERVICE INDIAN HOSPITAL (240206)**, Highway 1, Zip 56671, Mailing Address: P.O. Box 497, Zip 56671–0497; tel. 218/679–3912, (Nonreporting) **A**1 9 10 **S** U. S. Indian Health Service, Rockville, MD
Primary Contact: Mark Karzon, Chief Executive Officer
CMO: John Robinson, M.D., Clinical Director
Web address: www.ihs.gov
**Control:** PHS, Indian Service, Government, federal **Service:** General Medical and Surgical

**Staffed Beds:** 19

## REDWOOD FALLS—Redwood County

★ **REDWOOD AREA HOSPITAL (241351)**, 100 Fallwood Road, Zip 56283–1828; tel. 507/637–4500, (Nonreporting) **A**9 10 18
Primary Contact: James E. Schulte, Chief Executive Officer
CFO: John Peyerl, Chief Financial Officer
CIO: Tom Balko, Manager Information Systems
CHR: Jody Rindfleisch, Manager Human Resources
CNO: Dawn Allen, R.N., Chief Clinical Officer
Web address: www.redwoodareahospital.org
**Control:** City–Government, nonfederal **Service:** General Medical and Surgical

**Staffed Beds:** 25

**MN**

---

**Hospital, Medicare Provider Number, Address, Telephone, Approval, Facility, and Physician Codes, Health Care System**

★ American Hospital Association (AHA) membership
□ The Joint Commission accreditation   ◇ DNV Healthcare Inc. accreditation
○ American Osteopathic Association (AOA) accreditation
△ Commission on Accreditation of Rehabilitation Facilities (CARF) accreditation

## ROBBINSDALE—Hennepin County

✠ △ **NORTH MEMORIAL HEALTH CARE (240001)**, 3300 Oakdale Avenue North, Zip 55422–2926; tel. 763/520–5200 **A**1 2 3 5 7 9 10 **F**3 7 11 13 15 17 18 20 22 24 26 28 29 30 31 32 34 35 38 40 43 44 45 46 49 50 53 54 55 56 57 58 59 60 62 63 64 68 70 72 73 74 75 76 77 78 79 81 82 83 84 85 86 87 89 90 91 92 93 96 97 98 100 102 103 107 108 110 111 113 114 116 117 118 123 125 128 129 131 132 134 142 143 145 146 147 **P**6 8
Primary Contact: Loren L. Taylor, Chief Executive Officer
COO: Andrew S. Cochrane, President Hospital Operations
CFO: Patrick Boran, Chief Financial Officer
CMO: J. Kevin Croston, M.D., Chief Medical Officer
CIO: Patrick Taffe, Vice President Information Services
CHR: David Abrams, Vice President Human Resources
CNO: Ginger L. Malone, MSN, Chief Nursing Officer
Web address: www.northmemorial.com
**Control:** Other not–for–profit (including NFP Corporation) **Service:** General Medical and Surgical

**Staffed Beds:** 353 **Admissions:** 22760 **Census:** 254 **Outpatient Visits:** 431050 **Births:** 1525 **Total Expense ($000):** 613390 **Payroll Expense ($000):** 297092 **Personnel:** 4538

## ROCHESTER—Olmsted County

☐ **COMMUNITY BEHAVIORAL HEALTH HOSPITAL – ROCHESTER**, 251 Wood Lake Drive S.E., Zip 55904; tel. 507/206–2561, (Nonreporting) **A**1 9
**S** Minnesota Department of Human Services, Saint Paul, MN
Primary Contact: Mark S. Lancet, Administrator
Web address: www.health.state.mn.us
**Control:** State–Government, nonfederal **Service:** Psychiatric

**Staffed Beds:** 16

✠ **MAYO CLINIC – METHODIST HOSPITAL (240061)**, 201 West Center Street, Zip 55902–3084; tel. 507/266–7890, (Nonreporting) **A**1 3 5 9 10 **S** Mayo Clinic Health System, Rochester, MN
Primary Contact: Lynn Frederick, Administrator
COO: Shirley Weis, Chief Administrative Officer
CFO: Brad Schmidt, Chief Financial Officer
CMO: Michael Rock, M.D., Chief Medical Officer
CIO: Jessica Grosset, Director Information Technology
CHR: Ken Schneider, Chair Human Resources
CNO: Pamela O. Johnson, MS, Chief Nursing Officer
Web address: www.mayoclinic.org
**Control:** Other not–for–profit (including NFP Corporation) **Service:** General Medical and Surgical

**Staffed Beds:** 335

✠ △ **MAYO CLINIC – SAINT MARYS HOSPITAL (240010)**, 1216 Second Street S.W., Zip 55902–1970; tel. 507/255–5123, (Includes MAYO EUGENIO LITTA CHILDREN'S HOSPITAL, 200 First Street, S.W., Zip 55905–0001; tel. 507/255–5123), (Nonreporting) **A**1 3 5 7 8 9 10 **S** Mayo Clinic Health System, Rochester, MN
Primary Contact: Lynn Frederick, Administrator
COO: Shirley Weis, Chief Administrative Officer
CFO: Brad Schmidt, Chief Financial Officer
CMO: Michael Rock, M.D., Chief Medical Officer
CIO: Jessica Grosset, Director Information Technology
CHR: Ken Schneider, Chair Human Resources
Web address: www.mayoclinic.org
**Control:** Other not–for–profit (including NFP Corporation) **Service:** General Medical and Surgical

**Staffed Beds:** 797

★ **OLMSTED MEDICAL CENTER (240006)**, 1650 Fourth Street S.E., Zip 55904–4717, Mailing Address: 210 Ninth Street S.E., Zip 55904–4717; tel. 507/288–3443, (Nonreporting) **A**9 10
Primary Contact: Roy A. Yawn, M.D., President and Chief Executive Officer
CFO: Kevin A. Higgins, Chief Financial Officer
CMO: David E. Westgard, M.D., Chief Medical Officer
CIO: Susan M. Schuett, Chief Information Officer
CHR: David P. Johnson, Director Human Resources
Web address: www.olmmed.org
**Control:** Other not–for–profit (including NFP Corporation) **Service:** General Medical and Surgical

**Staffed Beds:** 37

## ROSEAU—Roseau County

✠ **LIFECARE MEDICAL CENTER (241344)**, 715 Delmore Avenue, Zip 56751–1599; tel. 218/463–2500, (Total facility includes 104 beds in nursing home–type unit) **A**1 5 9 10 18 **F**3 7 10 11 13 15 28 29 30 31 32 34 35 36 40 43 45 53 56 57 59 62 63 64 65 68 75 76 77 81 82 84 85 86 93 104 107 110 111 113 114 117 118 127 128 129 131 132 134 143 145 146 147 **P**6
Primary Contact: Keith Okeson, President and Chief Executive Officer
COO: Susan C. Lisell, Vice President of Clinical Services
CFO: Cathy Huss, Chief Financial Officer
CIO: Kevin Schumacher, Director of Information Services
CHR: Carol Klotz, Director Human Resources
CNO: Roxanne Fabian, Director of Nursing–Acute Care
Web address: www.lifecaremedicalcenter.org
**Control:** Other not–for–profit (including NFP Corporation) **Service:** General Medical and Surgical

**Staffed Beds:** 129 **Admissions:** 873 **Census:** 107 **Outpatient Visits:** 42834 **Births:** 193 **Total Expense ($000):** 33739 **Payroll Expense ($000):** 15423 **Personnel:** 300

## SAINT CLOUD—Stearns County

✠ △ **ST. CLOUD HOSPITAL (240036)**, 1406 Sixth Avenue North, Zip 56303–1901; tel. 320/251–2700 **A**1 2 3 5 7 9 10 13 20 **F**3 5 11 12 13 14 15 17 18 19 20 22 24 26 27 28 29 30 31 32 34 35 36 37 38 39 40 43 44 45 46 47 48 49 50 51 54 56 57 58 59 60 61 62 63 64 66 68 69 70 72 74 75 76 77 78 79 80 81 82 84 85 86 87 88 89 90 92 93 94 96 97 98 99 100 101 102 103 104 105 106 107 108 110 111 113 114 116 117 118 119 120 122 123 125 128 129 130 131 133 134 140 144 145 146 147 **P**6
**S** CentraCare Health System, Saint Cloud, MN
Primary Contact: Craig J. Broman, FACHE, President, St. Cloud Hospital
COO: Linda Chmielewski, R.N., Vice President Operations
CFO: Greg Klugherz, Vice President Corporate Services and Chief Financial Officer
CMO: Mark Matthias, M.D., Vice President of Medical Affairs
CIO: Amy Porwoll, Vice President of Information Systems
CHR: Duane Rasmusson, Vice President Human Resources
CNO: Linda Chmielewski, R.N., Vice President Operations
Web address: www.centracare.com
**Control:** Other not–for–profit (including NFP Corporation) **Service:** General Medical and Surgical

**Staffed Beds:** 467 **Admissions:** 26321 **Census:** 300 **Outpatient Visits:** 421846 **Births:** 2569 **Total Expense ($000):** 538535 **Payroll Expense ($000):** 223021 **Personnel:** 4023

✠ △ **ST. CLOUD VETERANS AFFAIRS HEALTH CARE SYSTEM**, 4801 Veterans Drive, Zip 56303–2099; tel. 320/252–1670, (Total facility includes 225 beds in nursing home–type unit) **A**1 7 **F**2 3 4 5 11 12 15 18 28 29 30 31 35 39 46 47 50 53 54 56 58 59 61 63 64 65 68 75 77 78 79 81 82 83 84 87 93 94 97 98 100 102 103 104 105 106 107 114 118 127 129 131 134 142 143 145 146 147 **P**6 **S** Department of Veterans Affairs, Washington, DC
Primary Contact: Barry I. Bahl, Director
COO: Barry I. Bahl, Director
CFO: Joseph Schmitz, Chief Financial Officer
CMO: Susan Markstrom, M.D., Chief of Staff
CIO: Denise Hanson, Information Technology Specialist
CHR: Lisa Rosendahl, Director Human Resources
CNO: Meri Hauge, R.N., Associate Director of Patient Care Services and Nurse Executive
Web address: www.stcloud.va.gov
**Control:** Veterans Affairs, Government, federal **Service:** General Medical and Surgical

**Staffed Beds:** 388 **Admissions:** 2510 **Census:** 351 **Outpatient Visits:** 283401 **Births:** 0 **Total Expense ($000):** 212226 **Payroll Expense ($000):** 122052 **Personnel:** 1443

**VETERANS AFFAIRS MEDICAL CENTER** See St. Cloud Veterans Affairs Health Care System

## SAINT JAMES—Watonwan County

✠ **MAYO CLINIC HEALTH SYSTEM IN SAINT JAMES (241333)**, 1101 Moulton and Parsons Drive, Zip 56081; tel. 507/375–3261 **A**1 9 10 18 **F**3 15 18 28 34 35 40 43 53 57 59 75 77 79 81 86 87 97 107 110 113 118 126 127 129 131 132 134 143 145 147 **P**6 **S** Mayo Clinic Health System, Rochester, MN
Primary Contact: Ryan J. Smith, Administrator
COO: Mark Fratzke, R.N., Chief Nursing Officer and Chief Operating Officer
CFO: James Tarasovich, Chief Financial Officer
CMO: Jennifer Langbehn, Medical Director
CIO: Thomas Borowski, Chief Information Officer
CHR: Gayle B. Hansen, R.N., Chief Integration Officer
CNO: Mark Fratzke, R.N., Chief Nursing Officer and Chief Operating Officer
Web address: www.mayoclinichealthsystem.org/locations/st-james
**Control:** Other not–for–profit (including NFP Corporation) **Service:** General Medical and Surgical

**Staffed Beds:** 13 **Admissions:** 287 **Census:** 4 **Outpatient Visits:** 30479 **Births:** 0 **Total Expense ($000):** 13853 **Payroll Expense ($000):** 5114 **Personnel:** 64

*Many Facility Codes have changed. Please refer to the AHA Guide Code Chart.*  © 2012 AHA Guide

MN

## SAINT LOUIS PARK—Hennepin County

⊠ △ **PARK NICOLLET METHODIST HOSPITAL (240053)**, 6500 Excelsior Boulevard, Zip 55426–4702; Mailing Address: Minneapolis, tel. 952/993–5000, (Nonreporting) **A**1 2 3 5 7 9 10 **S** Park Nicollet Health Services, Saint Louis Park, MN
Primary Contact: David Abelson, M.D., President and Chief Executive Officer
COO: Michael Kaupa, Executive Vice President and Chief Operating Officer
CFO: Sheila McMillan, Chief Financial Officer
CMO: Steven Connelly, M.D., Chief Medical Officer
CIO: Julie Flaschenriem, Chief Information Officer
CHR: Paul Dominski, Vice President Human Resources
CNO: Roxanna L. Gapstur, Ph.D., Chief Nursing Officer
Web address: www.parknicollet.com
**Control:** Other not–for–profit (including NFP Corporation) **Service:** General Medical and Surgical

**Staffed Beds:** 426

## SAINT PAUL—Ramsey County

⊠ **CHILDREN'S HOSPITALS AND CLINICS OF MINNESOTA (243301)**, 345 North Smith Avenue, Zip 55102–2392; tel. 651/220–6000, (Nonreporting) **A**1 3 5 9 10 **S** Children's Hospitals and Clinics of Minnesota, Minneapolis, MN
Primary Contact: Alan L. Goldbloom, M.D., President and Chief Executive Officer
COO: David S. Overman, Chief Operating Officer
CFO: Jerry Massmann, Chief Financial Officer
CMO: Phillip M. Kibort, M.D., Vice President Medical Affairs and Chief Medical Officer
CIO: Jeffrey D. Young, Chief Information Officer
CHR: David Brumbaugh, Vice President Human Resources
Web address: www.childrensmn.org
**Control:** Other not–for–profit (including NFP Corporation) **Service:** Children's general

**Staffed Beds:** 133

☐ △ **GILLETTE CHILDREN'S SPECIALTY HEALTHCARE (243300)**, (Pediatric Specialty Hospital), 200 East University Avenue, Zip 55101–2598; tel. 651/291–2848 **A**1 3 5 7 9 10 **F**3 29 30 35 36 39 50 54 64 68 71 74 79 81 82 84 85 88 89 90 91 92 93 94 107 111 114 118 128 129 145 **P**6
Primary Contact: Margaret E. Perryman, President and Chief Executive Officer
CFO: James Haddican, Vice President Finance
CMO: Steven Koop, M.D., Medical Director
CIQ: Jennifer Fall, Chief Information Officer
CHR: Betty Rivard, Vice President Human Resources
Web address: www.gillettechildrens.org
**Control:** Other not–for–profit (including NFP Corporation) **Service:** Children's other specialty

**Staffed Beds:** 60 **Admissions:** 2275 **Census:** 31 **Outpatient Visits:** 128257 **Births:** 0 **Total Expense ($000):** 163117 **Payroll Expense ($000):** 77325 **Personnel:** 989

⊠ △ **HEALTHEAST BETHESDA HOSPITAL (242004)**, 559 Capitol Boulevard, Zip 55103–2101; tel. 651/232–2000 **A**1 2 5 7 9 10 **F**1 3 6 11 29 30 38 44 45 50 53 56 60 61 64 68 74 75 77 79 85 86 87 91 93 100 101 103 104 105 107 111 113 118 129 131 145 **P**8 **S** HealthEast Care System, Saint Paul, MN
Primary Contact: Catherine Barr, President
CFO: Lea Jilek, Director Finance
CMO: Stephen J. Kolar, M.D., Vice President Medical Affairs
CIO: Mac McClurkan, Chief Information Officer
Web address: www.healtheast.org
**Control:** Other not–for–profit (including NFP Corporation) **Service:** Long–Term Acute Care hospital

**Staffed Beds:** 126 **Admissions:** 1077 **Census:** 92 **Outpatient Visits:** 10357 **Births:** 0 **Total Expense ($000):** 70140 **Payroll Expense ($000):** 32148 **Personnel:** 491

☐ △ **REGIONS HOSPITAL (240106)**, 640 Jackson Street, Zip 55101–2595; tel. 651/254–3456, (Nonreporting) **A**1 2 3 5 7 8 9 10 **S** HealthPartners, Bloomington, MN
Primary Contact: Brock D. Nelson, President and Chief Executive Officer
CFO: Heidi Conrad, Vice President and Chief Financial Officer
CMO: George J. Isham, M.D., Chief Health Officer and Medical Director Health Plan
CIO: Kim LaReau, Vice President and Chief Information Officer
Web address: www.regionshospital.com
**Control:** Other not–for–profit (including NFP Corporation) **Service:** General Medical and Surgical

**Staffed Beds:** 424

⊠ **ST. JOHN'S HOSPITAL (240210)**, 1575 Beam Avenue, Zip 55109–1126; tel. 651/232–7000 **A**1 2 10 **F**3 13 15 28 29 30 31 34 35 36 37 38 40 43 44 50 54 55 57 59 60 61 63 64 68 70 72 74 75 76 77 78 79 81 85 86 87 89 93 96 97 100 102 104 107 108 110 111 113 114 116 117 118 120 122 125 129 130 131 145 146 147 **P**8 **S** HealthEast Care System, Saint Paul, MN
Primary Contact: Scott L. North, FACHE, Chief Executive Officer
CFO: Mike Nass, Vice President and Chief Financial Officer
CMO: John Kvasnicka, M.D., Medical Director
CIO: Mac McClurkan, Chief Information Officer
CHR: Mary Arnold, Interim Vice President Human Resources
Web address: www.stjohnshospital–mn.org
**Control:** Other not–for–profit (including NFP Corporation) **Service:** General Medical and Surgical

**Staffed Beds:** 192 **Admissions:** 14437 **Census:** 126 **Outpatient Visits:** 210321 **Births:** 2788 **Total Expense ($000):** 224909 **Payroll Expense ($000):** 83039 **Personnel:** 1139

⊠ **ST. JOSEPH'S HOSPITAL (240063)**, 45 West 10th Street, Zip 55102–1053; tel. 651/232–3000 **A**1 2 3 5 9 10 **F**3 4 5 11 12 13 15 17 18 20 22 24 26 28 29 30 31 34 35 36 37 38 40 43 44 46 49 50 56 57 58 59 60 61 63 64 68 70 74 75 76 77 78 79 81 83 84 85 87 92 93 96 98 100 101 102 103 104 105 107 108 111 113 118 119 120 123 129 131 145 146 147 **P**8 **S** HealthEast Care System, Saint Paul, MN
Primary Contact: Scott L. North, FACHE, Chief Executive Officer
CFO: Mike Nass, Vice President and Chief Financial Officer
CMO: Stephen J. Kolar, M.D., Vice President Medical Affairs
Web address: www.healtheast.org
**Control:** Other not–for–profit (including NFP Corporation) **Service:** General Medical and Surgical

**Staffed Beds:** 232 **Admissions:** 13539 **Census:** 178 **Outpatient Visits:** 118918 **Births:** 1222 **Total Expense ($000):** 243489 **Payroll Expense ($000):** 91551 **Personnel:** 1403

⊠ △ **UNITED HOSPITAL (240038)**, 333 North Smith Avenue, Zip 55102–2389; tel. 651/241–8000, (Nonreporting) **A**1 2 3 5 7 9 10 **S** Allina Health, Minneapolis, MN
Primary Contact: Thomas O'Connor, President
CFO: John Bien, Vice President Finance
CMO: Daniel Foley, M.D., Vice President Medical Affairs
CHR: James McGlade, Director Human Resources
Web address: www.allina.com
**Control:** Other not–for–profit (including NFP Corporation) **Service:** General Medical and Surgical

**Staffed Beds:** 398

## SAINT PETER—Nicollet County

☐ **COMMUNITY BEHAVIORAL HEALTH HOSPITAL – ST. PETER (244010)**, 2000 Klein Street, Zip 56082–5800; tel. 507/933–5001, (Nonreporting) **A**1 5 9 10 **S** Minnesota Department of Human Services, Saint Paul, MN
Primary Contact: Carol Olson, Administrator
CFO: Shirley Jacobson, Chief Financial Officer
Web address: www.health.state.mn.us
**Control:** State–Government, nonfederal **Service:** Psychiatric

**Staffed Beds:** 16

★ **RIVER'S EDGE HOSPITAL AND CLINIC (241334)**, 1900 North Sunrise Drive, Zip 56082–1327; tel. 507/931–2200, (Nonreporting) **A**5 9 10 18 21
Primary Contact: Colleen A. Spike, Chief Executive Officer
CFO: Curt Savstrom, Chief Financial Officer and Chief Information Officer
CMO: Michael Sparacino, M.D., Chief Medical Staff
CIO: Curt Savstrom, Chief Financial Officer and Chief Information Officer
CHR: Tammie Hudspith, Director Human Resources
Web address: www.riversedgehealth.org
**Control:** City–Government, nonfederal **Service:** General Medical and Surgical

**Staffed Beds:** 17

## SANDSTONE—Pine County

★ **ESSENTIA HEALTH SANDSTONE (241309)**, 109 Court Avenue South, Zip 55072–5120; tel. 320/245–2212, (Total facility includes 60 beds in nursing home–type unit) **A**9 10 18 **F**7 11 15 28 29 30 34 35 40 43 51 57 64 75 77 80 81 93 107 113 127 129 132 143 **P**5 **S** Essentia Health, Duluth, MN
Primary Contact: Michael D. Hedrix, Interim Chief Executive Officer
CFO: Chris Johnson, Assistant Administrator and Chief Financial Officer
CMO: Sarah Aldredge, M.D., Chief Medical Officer
Web address: www.pinemedicalcenter.org
**Control:** Hospital district or authority, Government, nonfederal **Service:** General Medical and Surgical

**Staffed Beds:** 85 **Admissions:** 413 **Census:** 61 **Outpatient Visits:** 20443 **Births:** 0 **Total Expense ($000):** 18344 **Payroll Expense ($000):** 7525 **Personnel:** 175

MN

---

**Hospital, Medicare Provider Number, Address, Telephone, Approval, Facility, and Physician Codes, Health Care System**

★ American Hospital Association (AHA) membership
☐ The Joint Commission accreditation
◇ DNV Healthcare Inc. accreditation
○ American Osteopathic Association (AOA) accreditation
△ Commission on Accreditation of Rehabilitation Facilities (CARF) accreditation

---

## SAUK CENTRE—Stearns County

★ **ST. MICHAEL'S HOSPITAL AND NURSING HOME (241368)**, 425 North Elm Street, Zip 56378–1010; tel. 320/352–2221, (Nonreporting) **A**9 10 18
Primary Contact: Delano Christianson, Administrator
CFO: Delano Christianson, Administrator
Web address: www.stmichaelshospital.org
**Control:** City–Government, nonfederal **Service:** General Medical and Surgical

> **Staffed Beds:** 85

## SHAKOPEE—Scott County

⊠ **ST. FRANCIS REGIONAL MEDICAL CENTER (240104)**, 1455 St. Francis Avenue, Zip 55379–3380; tel. 952/428–3000 **A**1 2 5 9 10 **F**3 11 13 14 15 29 30 31 34 35 38 40 45 46 50 53 57 59 68 70 73 75 76 77 78 79 81 82 84 86 87 89 93 107 108 110 111 114 118 119 124 128 129 130 131 134 142 143 145 146 **P**3 **S** Allina Health, Minneapolis, MN
Primary Contact: Michael A. Baumgartner, President
CFO: Cynthia Vincent, Vice President Finance
CMO: Brian Prokosch, M.D., Vice President Medical Affairs
CIO: Joe Delveaux, Manager Information Services
CHR: Ann Glaves, Vice President Human Resources
CNO: Debora Ryan, R.N., Vice President Patient Care
Web address: www.stfrancis–shakopee.com
**Control:** Other not–for–profit (including NFP Corporation) **Service:** General Medical and Surgical

> **Staffed Beds:** 86 **Admissions:** 5799 **Census:** 43 **Outpatient Visits:** 110169 **Births:** 1164 **Total Expense ($000):** 109136 **Payroll Expense ($000):** 40704 **Personnel:** 486

## SLAYTON—Murray County

★ **MURRAY COUNTY MEDICAL CENTER (241319)**, 2042 Juniper Avenue, Zip 56172–1016; tel. 507/836–6111 **A**9 10 18 **F**3 7 8 11 28 29 31 32 34 35 40 43 45 53 56 57 59 64 65 70 75 79 81 85 86 87 93 97 107 118 126 128 129 130 131 132 134 145 147 **P**5 **S** Sanford Health, Sioux Falls, SD
Primary Contact: Meldon L. Snow, Chief Executive Officer
CFO: Renee Logan, Chief Financial Officer
CMO: Joyce Tarbet, M.D., Chief Medical Officer
CIO: Justin Keller, Director Information Technology
CHR: Nancy Andert, Director Human Resources
CNO: Shari Achterhoff, R.N., Chief Nursing Officer
Web address: www.murraycountymed.org
**Control:** County–Government, nonfederal **Service:** General Medical and Surgical

> **Staffed Beds:** 18 **Admissions:** 410 **Census:** 4 **Outpatient Visits:** 15710 **Births:** 0 **Total Expense ($000):** 15161 **Payroll Expense ($000):** 6418 **Personnel:** 104

## SLEEPY EYE—Brown County

**SLEEPY EYE MEDICAL CENTER (241327)**, 400 Fourth Avenue N.W., Zip 56085–1109, Mailing Address: P.O. Box 323, Zip 56085–0323; tel. 507/794–3571 **A**9 10 18 **F**13 15 28 34 40 43 45 59 68 76 77 81 91 93 107 113 118 126 128 129 132 **P**6
Primary Contact: Kevin Sellheim, Chief Executive Officer
CHR: Connie Dahlberg, Director Business and Employee
CNO: Sue Schweiss, Director of Nursing
Web address: www.semedicalcenter.org
**Control:** City–Government, nonfederal **Service:** General Medical and Surgical

> **Staffed Beds:** 17 **Admissions:** 392 **Census:** 4 **Outpatient Visits:** 11505 **Births:** 23 **Total Expense ($000):** 9249 **Payroll Expense ($000):** 4367 **Personnel:** 97

## SPRINGFIELD—Brown County

☐ **MAYO CLINIC HEALTH SYSTEM IN SPRINGFIELD (241352)**, 625 North Jackson Avenue, Zip 56087–1714, Mailing Address: P.O. Box 146, Zip 56087–0146; tel. 507/723–6201 **A**1 9 10 18 **F**3 13 15 28 32 34 39 40 45 57 59 65 75 76 81 85 89 93 97 107 110 113 127 129 131 132 134 147 **P**6 **S** Mayo Clinic Health System, Rochester, MN
Primary Contact: Scott D. Thoreson, FACHE, Administrator
COO: Scott D. Thoreson, FACHE, Administrator
CFO: James Tarasovich, Chief Financial Officer
CMO: Annette Schmit–Cline, M.D., Medical Director
CIO: Margo Woodford, Assistant Administrator
CHR: Marian Schoper, Manager Human Resources
Web address: www.smc–mhs.org
**Control:** Other not–for–profit (including NFP Corporation) **Service:** General Medical and Surgical

> **Staffed Beds:** 24 **Admissions:** 573 **Census:** 5 **Outpatient Visits:** 30142 **Births:** 38 **Total Expense ($000):** 14763 **Payroll Expense ($000):** 7164 **Personnel:** 73

## STAPLES—Wadena County

**LAKEWOOD HEALTH SYSTEM (241329)**, 49725 County 83, Zip 56479–5280; tel. 218/894–1515, (Total facility includes 100 beds in nursing home–type unit) **A**9 10 18 **F**3 6 7 8 10 11 12 13 15 28 29 30 31 34 35 36 39 40 43 50 52 53 56 57 59 62 63 64 65 68 75 77 78 79 81 82 84 85 86 87 93 98 99 100 101 102 103 104 105 107 110 113 118 124 126 127 128 129 130 131 132 134 142 145 146 147 **P**7
Primary Contact: Tim Rice, President and Chief Executive Officer
CFO: Jim Dregney, Chief Financial Officer
CMO: John Halfen, M.D., Medical Director
CIO: Jeff Osegard, Chief Information Officer
CHR: Janet Jacobson, Director Human Resources
Web address: www.lakewoodhealthsystem.com
**Control:** Other not–for–profit (including NFP Corporation) **Service:** General Medical and Surgical

> **Staffed Beds:** 135 **Admissions:** 1512 **Census:** 103 **Outpatient Visits:** 240131 **Births:** 393 **Total Expense ($000):** 77634 **Payroll Expense ($000):** 32655 **Personnel:** 725

## STILLWATER—Washington County

⊠ **LAKEVIEW HOSPITAL (240066)**, 927 Churchill Street West, Zip 55082–5930; tel. 651/439–5330, (Nonreporting) **A**1 5 9 10 **S** HealthPartners, Bloomington, MN
Primary Contact: Curt Geissler, President
CFO: Doug Johnson, Chief Financial Officer
CMO: Charles Bransford, M.D., Medical Director
CIO: Carol Lundstrom, Interim Director Information Systems
CHR: Angy Duchesneau, Senior Director Human Resources
CNO: Jo Sittlow, Senior Director of Patient Care and Chief Nursing Officer
Web address: www.lakeview.org
**Control:** Other not–for–profit (including NFP Corporation) **Service:** General Medical and Surgical

> **Staffed Beds:** 66

## THIEF RIVER FALLS—Pennington County

**MERITCARE THIEF RIVER FALLS NORTHWEST MEDICAL CENTER** See Sanford Medical Center Thief River Falls

★ **SANFORD MEDICAL CENTER THIEF RIVER FALLS (241381)**, 120 LaBree Avenue South, Zip 56701–2840; tel. 218/681–4240 **A**9 10 18 **F**3 8 11 13 15 28 29 31 33 34 40 43 45 50 53 54 57 64 68 70 76 77 78 79 81 85 86 87 93 94 96 98 99 100 101 102 104 106 107 110 111 113 118 128 131 132 134 143 145 146 147 **P**6 **S** Sanford Health, Sioux Falls, SD
Primary Contact: Christine K. Harff, Chief Executive Officer
COO: Rob Lovejoy, Chief Operating Officer
CFO: Casey R. Johnson, Chief Financial Officer
CMO: Janell Hudson, M.D., Chief Clinical Officer
CHR: Rob Lovejoy, Chief Operating Officer
Web address: www.sanfordhealth.org
**Control:** Other not–for–profit (including NFP Corporation) **Service:** General Medical and Surgical

> **Staffed Beds:** 35 **Admissions:** 1917 **Census:** 19 **Outpatient Visits:** 43102 **Births:** 291 **Total Expense ($000):** 58474 **Payroll Expense ($000):** 21379 **Personnel:** 331

## TRACY—Lyon County

★ **SANFORD TRACY MEDICAL CENTER (241303)**, 251 Fifth Street East, Zip 56175–1536; tel. 507/629–3200 **A**9 10 18 **F**3 11 28 31 32 34 40 41 56 57 59 62 64 68 71 77 81 85 87 89 93 97 107 108 111 124 128 129 130 131 132 134 142 **S** Sanford Health, Sioux Falls, SD
Primary Contact: Stacy Barstad, Chief Executive Officer
CFO: Jerry Thompson, Chief Financial Officer
CMO: Louisa Paul, M.D., Chief Medical Officer
CIO: Janet Theisen, Chief Information Officer
CHR: Becky Foster, Manager Human Resources
Web address: www.sanfordtracy.org
**Control:** Other not–for–profit (including NFP Corporation) **Service:** General Medical and Surgical

> **Staffed Beds:** 25 **Admissions:** 168 **Census:** 2 **Outpatient Visits:** 18434 **Births:** 0 **Total Expense ($000):** 9875 **Payroll Expense ($000):** 4313 **Personnel:** 106

## TWO HARBORS—Lake County

**LAKE VIEW MEMORIAL HOSPITAL (241308)**, 325 11th Avenue, Zip 55616–1360; tel. 218/834–7300 **A**9 10 18 **F**5 10 15 17 28 35 40 43 53 59 63 64 75 77 81 82 84 93 111 113 118 129 132 143 147
Primary Contact: Brian J. Carlson, FACHE, President and Chief Executive Officer
Web address: www.lvmhospital.com
**Control:** Other not–for–profit (including NFP Corporation) **Service:** General Medical and Surgical

> **Staffed Beds:** 17 **Admissions:** 226 **Census:** 6 **Outpatient Visits:** 31906 **Births:** 0 **Total Expense ($000):** 12422 **Payroll Expense ($000):** 5122 **Personnel:** 93

MN

## TYLER—Lincoln County

**TYLER HEALTHCARE CENTER AVERA (241348)**, 240 Willow Street, Zip 56178–0280, Mailing Address: P.O. Box 280, Zip 56178–0280; tel. 507/247–5521, (Total facility includes 38 beds in nursing home–type unit) **A**9 10 18 **F**2 7 12 15 28 31 34 40 43 45 53 57 59 62 63 64 65 67 69 77 78 79 81 90 93 107 126 127 129 131 132 **P**3 **S** Avera Health, Sioux Falls, SD
Primary Contact: Dale K. Kruger, Chief Executive Officer and Chief Financial Officer
CFO: Dale K. Kruger, Chief Executive Officer and Chief Financial Officer
Web address: www.averamckennan.org/amck/regionalfacilities/tyler/
**Control:** Other not–for–profit (including NFP Corporation) **Service:** General Medical and Surgical

**Staffed Beds:** 56 **Admissions:** 197 **Census:** 36 **Outpatient Visits:** 2744 **Births:** 0 **Total Expense ($000):** 10280 **Payroll Expense ($000):** 5516 **Personnel:** 68

## VIRGINIA—St. Louis County

✠ △ **VIRGINIA REGIONAL MEDICAL CENTER (240084)**, 901 Ninth Street North, Zip 55792–2398; tel. 218/741–3340, (Total facility includes 90 beds in nursing home–type unit) **A**1 7 9 10 **F**1 3 8 11 13 15 17 18 28 29 30 34 35 40 43 51 56 57 59 64 70 74 75 76 79 80 81 83 87 89 90 97 107 108 111 114 118 126 127 128 129 145 146 147 **P**6
Primary Contact: William R. Smith, Chief Executive Officer and Director Human Resources
CFO: Steven Feltman, CPA, Interim Chief Financial Officer
CIO: Brenda Skorich, Manager Business and Medical Records
CHR: William R. Smith, Chief Executive Officer and Director Human Resources
CNO: Michelle Fleming, Chief Nursing Officer
Web address: www.vrmc.org
**Control:** City–Government, nonfederal **Service:** General Medical and Surgical

**Staffed Beds:** 173 **Admissions:** 2202 **Census:** 104 **Outpatient Visits:** 53353 **Births:** 261 **Total Expense ($000):** 52608 **Payroll Expense ($000):** 22945

## WABASHA—Wabasha County

★ **SAINT ELIZABETH'S MEDICAL CENTER (241335)**, 1200 Grant Boulevard West, Zip 55981–1042; tel. 651/565–4531, (Total facility includes 148 beds in nursing home–type unit) **A**9 10 18 **F**1 2 4 6 10 11 12 13 15 16 17 28 29 30 34 35 40 43 45 46 49 50 53 56 59 62 65 67 70 72 73 75 76 77 80 81 85 88 89 90 93 94 98 100 103 104 107 110 113 118 124 127 129 132 134 142 143 144 145 147 **P**6 **S** Marian Health System, Tulsa, OK
Primary Contact: Thomas Crowley, President and Chief Executive Officer
CFO: John Wolfe, Chief Financial Officer
CMO: Brian E. Kelly, M.D., President Medical Staff
CHR: Jim Root, Vice President Human Resources
CNO: Kathy Lueders, R.N., Director of Nursing–Acute Care
Web address: www.stelizabethswabasha.org
**Control:** Church–operated, Nongovernment, not–for profit **Service:** General Medical and Surgical

**Staffed Beds:** 168 **Admissions:** 614 **Census:** 146 **Outpatient Visits:** 25976 **Births:** 85 **Total Expense ($000):** 22740 **Payroll Expense ($000):** 10798 **Personnel:** 354

## WACONIA—Carver County

★ **RIDGEVIEW MEDICAL CENTER (240056)**, 500 South Maple Street, Zip 55387–1791; tel. 952/442–2191 **A**2 9 10 21 **F**3 7 8 12 13 15 18 20 22 28 29 30 31 32 34 35 36 38 40 42 43 45 48 49 54 57 58 59 62 63 64 65 66 70 73 74 75 76 77 78 79 81 84 85 86 87 89 93 96 107 108 110 113 114 117 118 125 128 129 130 131 134 143 145 146 147 **P**6
Primary Contact: Robert Stevens, President and Chief Executive Officer
CFO: Gordon Gablenz, Vice President Finance
CIO: Tamara Korbel, Director Management Information Systems
CHR: Sarah M. Hastings, Vice President Human Resources
Web address: www.ridgeviewmedical.org
**Control:** Other not–for–profit (including NFP Corporation) **Service:** General Medical and Surgical

**Staffed Beds:** 105 **Admissions:** 5181 **Census:** 45 **Outpatient Visits:** 141208 **Births:** 1249 **Total Expense ($000):** 160916 **Payroll Expense ($000):** 78692 **Personnel:** 1073

## WADENA—Wadena County

☐ **TRI–COUNTY HOSPITAL (241354)**, 415 Jefferson Street North, Zip 56482–1297; tel. 218/631–3510 **A**1 9 10 18 **F**3 7 11 13 15 17 28 31 34 35 40 50 54 57 59 64 65 70 75 76 77 81 85 86 89 93 99 104 107 110 111 113 117 118 126 128 129 130 131 132 134 145 147 **P**6
Primary Contact: Joel Beiswenger, Chief Executive Officer
CFO: Kim Aagard, Chief Financial Officer
CMO: John Pate, M.D., Chief Medical Officer
CIO: Bill Blaha, Manager Information Technology
CHR: Lisa Reddick, Director Organizational Resources
CNO: Kathy Kleen, Chief Nursing Officer
Web address: www.tricountyhospital.org
**Control:** Other not–for–profit (including NFP Corporation) **Service:** General Medical and Surgical

**Staffed Beds:** 25 **Admissions:** 1137 **Census:** 11 **Outpatient Visits:** 70889 **Births:** 172 **Total Expense ($000):** 42656 **Payroll Expense ($000):** 15805 **Personnel:** 311

## WARREN—Marshall County

★ **NORTH VALLEY HEALTH CENTER (241337)**, 109 South Minnesota Street, Zip 56762–1499; tel. 218/745–4211, (Nonreporting) **A**9 10 18
Primary Contact: Ashley King, Chief Executive Officer
CFO: Mitchell Kotrba, Chief Financial Officer
Web address: www.nvhc.net
**Control:** Other not–for–profit (including NFP Corporation) **Service:** General Medical and Surgical

**Staffed Beds:** 20

## WASECA—Waseca County

✠ **MAYO CLINIC HEALTH SYSTEM IN WASECA (241345)**, 501 North State Street, Zip 56093–2811; tel. 507/835–1210 **A**1 5 9 10 18 **F**3 7 11 13 15 18 28 29 30 31 32 34 35 40 45 50 53 56 57 59 63 64 65 68 74 75 77 79 81 87 90 93 97 103 104 107 110 111 113 118 127 129 130 131 132 142 143 145 146 147 **P**6 **S** Mayo Clinic Health System, Rochester, MN
Primary Contact: Jeffrey Carlson, Chief Executive Officer
CMO: Daniel Stahl, M.D., Medical Director
Web address: www.mayoclinichealthsystem.org
**Control:** Other not–for–profit (including NFP Corporation) **Service:** General Medical and Surgical

**Staffed Beds:** 25 **Admissions:** 412 **Census:** 6 **Outpatient Visits:** 50681 **Births:** 0 **Total Expense ($000):** 18105 **Payroll Expense ($000):** 8243 **Personnel:** 114

## WESTBROOK—Cottonwood County

★ **SANFORD WESTBROOK MEDICAL CENTER (241302)**, 920 Bell Avenue, Zip 56183–0188, Mailing Address: P.O. Box 188, Zip 56183–0188; tel. 507/274–6121 **A**9 10 18 **F**3 31 34 40 56 57 59 62 64 68 71 75 77 81 85 89 91 93 97 99 100 101 102 103 104 107 108 111 124 129 130 131 132 134 142 **P**6 **S** Sanford Health, Sioux Falls, SD
Primary Contact: Stacy Barstad, Chief Executive Officer
COO: Gordon Kopperud, Director Operations
CFO: Jerry Thompson, Chief Financial Officer
CIO: Janet Theisen, Chief Information Officer
CHR: Becky Foster, Manager Human Resources
Web address: www.sanfordwestbrook.org
**Control:** Other not–for–profit (including NFP Corporation) **Service:** General Medical and Surgical

**Staffed Beds:** 6 **Admissions:** 89 **Census:** 1 **Outpatient Visits:** 9646 **Births:** 0 **Total Expense ($000):** 5573 **Payroll Expense ($000):** 2379 **Personnel:** 44

## WHEATON—Traverse County

★ **SANFORD WHEATON MEDICAL CENTER (241304)**, 401 12th Street North, Zip 56296–1099; tel. 320/563–8226, (Nonreporting) **A**9 10 18 **S** Sanford Health, Sioux Falls, SD
Primary Contact: JoAnn M. Foltz, R.N., Chief Executive Officer
CFO: Shane Ayres, Chief Financial Officer
CHR: Brenda Petersen, Director Human Resources
Web address: www.wheatonhealthcare.org
**Control:** City–Government, nonfederal **Service:** General Medical and Surgical

**Staffed Beds:** 15

**MN**

---

**Hospital, Medicare Provider Number, Address, Telephone, Approval, Facility, and Physician Codes, Health Care System**

★ American Hospital Association (AHA) membership
☐ The Joint Commission accreditation
◇ DNV Healthcare Inc. accreditation
○ American Osteopathic Association (AOA) accreditation
△ Commission on Accreditation of Rehabilitation Facilities (CARF) accreditation

## WILLMAR—Kandiyohi County

✠ **RICE MEMORIAL HOSPITAL (240088)**, 301 Becker Avenue S.W.,
Zip 56201–3395; tel. 320/235–4543, (Total facility includes 77 beds in nursing
home–type unit) **A**1 2 9 10 **F**7 11 12 13 15 18 28 29 30 31 34 35 36 39 40
43 45 47 48 49 57 59 60 63 64 68 70 73 75 76 77 78 79 81 82 84 86 87
89 90 93 98 100 101 102 103 104 105 107 108 111 113 117 118 120 127
128 129 130 131 134 142 145 146 147
Primary Contact: Michael Schramm, Chief Executive Officer
CIO: Teri Beyer, Chief Information Officer
CHR: Dale Hustedt, Associate Administrator Administrative Services
Web address: www.ricehospital.com
**Control:** City–Government, nonfederal **Service:** General Medical and Surgical

> **Staffed Beds:** 187 **Admissions:** 3990 **Census:** 103 **Outpatient Visits:** 88927
> **Births:** 820 **Total Expense ($000):** 97336 **Payroll Expense ($000):** 42619
> **Personnel:** 561

## WINDOM—Cottonwood County

★ **WINDOM AREA HOSPITAL (241332)**, 2150 Hospital Drive, Zip 56101–0339,
Mailing Address: P.O. Box 339, Zip 56101–0339; tel. 507/831–2400 **A**9 10 18
**F**11 13 15 28 31 34 35 40 45 53 57 59 76 77 81 93 107 113 118 129 132
**S** Sanford Health, Sioux Falls, SD
Primary Contact: Geraldine F. Burmeister, FACHE, Chief Executive Officer
CFO: Kim Armstrong, Chief Financial Officer
CIO: Lori Ling, Information Technician
CHR: Katie Slette, Director Human Resources and Marketing
CNO: Kari Witte, Director of Patient Care
Web address: www.windomareahospital.com
**Control:** City–Government, nonfederal **Service:** General Medical and Surgical

> **Staffed Beds:** 25 **Admissions:** 472 **Census:** 4 **Outpatient Visits:** 20579
> **Births:** 119 **Total Expense ($000):** 12493 **Payroll Expense ($000):** 5253
> **Personnel:** 100

## WINONA—Winona County

★ **WINONA HEALTH (240044)**, 855 Mankato Avenue, Zip 55987–5377, Mailing
Address: P.O. Box 5600, Zip 55987–0600; tel. 507/454–3650 **A**9 10 20 **F**11
13 15 28 29 30 31 32 34 35 36 38 40 43 48 50 53 56 57 59 60 61 64 68
70 74 75 76 77 78 79 81 82 84 85 86 87 89 93 97 98 99 100 101 102 103
104 107 108 110 111 114 117 118 126 128 129 130 131 134 143 145 146
147 **P**6
Primary Contact: Rachelle H. Schultz, President and Chief Executive Officer
CFO: Michael Allen, Chief Financial Officer
CMO: Charles Shepard, M.D., Medical Director
CHR: Bill Gould, Chief People Resource Officer
Web address: www.winonahealth.org
**Control:** Other not–for–profit (including NFP Corporation) **Service:** General
Medical and Surgical

> **Staffed Beds:** 68 **Admissions:** 2840 **Census:** 28 **Outpatient Visits:** 235780
> **Births:** 335 **Total Expense ($000):** 99209 **Payroll Expense ($000):** 42291
> **Personnel:** 895

## WOODBURY—Washington County

✠ **WOODWINDS HEALTH CAMPUS (240213)**, 1925 Woodwinds Drive,
Zip 55125–4445; tel. 651/232–0228 **A**1 2 5 9 10 **F**3 13 15 28 29 30 31 34
35 36 37 38 40 43 44 49 50 57 58 59 61 63 64 68 70 74 75 76 77 78 79
81 85 86 87 93 107 108 111 113 118 128 129 131 134 145 **P**8 **S** HealthEast
Care System, Saint Paul, MN
Primary Contact: Scott L. North, FACHE, Chief Executive Officer
CFO: Robert D. Gill, Chief Financial Officer
CMO: Lynne Lillie, M.D., Medical Director
CIO: Mac McClurkan, Chief Information Officer
CHR: Tammy Arrigoni, Human Resources Lead
Web address: www.woodwinds.org
**Control:** Other not–for–profit (including NFP Corporation) **Service:** General
Medical and Surgical

> **Staffed Beds:** 86 **Admissions:** 7192 **Census:** 57 **Outpatient Visits:** 80543
> **Births:** 1641 **Total Expense ($000):** 113512 **Payroll Expense ($000):**
> 41844 **Personnel:** 575

## WORTHINGTON—Nobles County

**SANFORD REGIONAL HOSPITAL WORTHINGTON** See Sanford Worthington
Medical Center

★ **SANFORD WORTHINGTON MEDICAL CENTER (240022)**, 1018 Sixth Avenue,
Zip 56187–2202, Mailing Address: P.O. Box 997, Zip 56187–0997;
tel. 507/372–2941 **A**9 10 **F**8 17 34 40 43 45 50 57 59 60 62 64 68 69 70
75 76 81 85 86 87 89 90 93 107 110 111 113 118 119 120 127 128 129
130 131 132 134 143 145 146 147 **S** Sanford Health, Sioux Falls, SD
Primary Contact: Michael Hammer, Chief Executive Officer
COO: Jeffrey J. Rotert, Chief Operating Officer
CFO: Linda Wagner, Chief Financial Officer
CMO: James D. Harris, M.D., Chief of Staff
CHR: Jeffrey J. Rotert, Chief Operating Officer
CNO: Jennifer Weg, R.N., Chief Nursing Officer
Web address: www.sanfordregionalworthington.org
**Control:** Other not–for–profit (including NFP Corporation) **Service:** General
Medical and Surgical

> **Staffed Beds:** 48 **Admissions:** 1172 **Census:** 9 **Outpatient Visits:** 49974
> **Total Expense ($000):** 25846 **Payroll Expense ($000):** 11609 **Personnel:**
> 273

## WYOMING—Chisago County

✠ **FAIRVIEW LAKES HEALTH SERVICES (240050)**, 5200 Fairview Boulevard,
Zip 55092–8013; tel. 651/982–7000 **A**1 9 10 **F**3 11 13 15 28 29 30 31 32
34 35 37 40 43 45 51 52 53 54 56 57 59 62 63 64 65 68 70 75 76 77 78
79 81 82 83 84 85 86 87 89 90 93 97 107 110 111 113 114 118 128 129 130
131 133 142 143 145 146 147 **P**6 **S** Fairview Health Services, Minneapolis, MN
Primary Contact: Steven C. Housh, President
CFO: Kim Ericson, Vice President Finance
CMO: David Milbrandt, M.D., Vice President Medical Affairs
CHR: Don Moschkau, Director Human Resources
CNO: Mary Jo Brueggeman, R.N., Vice President Patient Care
Web address: www.fairview.org/
**Control:** Other not–for–profit (including NFP Corporation) **Service:** General
Medical and Surgical

> **Staffed Beds:** 47 **Admissions:** 3743 **Census:** 28 **Outpatient Visits:** 96515
> **Births:** 740 **Personnel:** 495

**MN**

# MISSISSIPPI

## ABERDEEN—Monroe County

★ **PIONEER COMMUNITY HOSPITAL OF ABERDEEN (251302)**, 400 South Chestnut Street, Zip 39730–3335, Mailing Address: P.O. Box 548, Zip 39730–0747; tel. 662/369–2455 **A**9 10 18 21 **F**29 35 40 43 53 70 75 81 82 86 87 89 90 93 97 98 103 107 118 129 130 132 145 **S** Pioneer Health Services, Magee, MS
Primary Contact: John Tompkins, Administrator
CFO: Julie Gieger, Chief Financial Officer
CMO: Kevin Hayes, M.D., Chief of Staff
CHR: Lee Rob, Director Human Resources
Web address: www.pchaberdeen.com
**Control:** Corporation, Investor–owned, for–profit **Service:** General Medical and Surgical

**Staffed Beds:** 35 **Admissions:** 444 **Census:** 7 **Outpatient Visits:** 3893
**Births:** 0 **Personnel:** 183

## ACKERMAN—Choctaw County

★ **PIONEER COMMUNITY HOSPITAL OF CHOCTAW (251310)**, 311 West Cherry Street, Zip 39735–8708; tel. 662/285–6235, (Nonreporting) **A**9 10 18 21 **S** Pioneer Health Services, Magee, MS
Primary Contact: Sean Johnson, Chief Executive Officer
Web address: www.pchchoctaw.com
**Control:** Corporation, Investor–owned, for–profit **Service:** General Medical and Surgical

**Staffed Beds:** 20

## AMORY—Monroe County

☐ **GILMORE MEMORIAL REGIONAL MEDICAL CENTER (250025)**, 1105 Earl Frye Boulevard, Zip 38821–5500, Mailing Address: P.O. Box 459, Zip 38821–0459; tel. 662/256–7111 **A**1 9 10 **F**13 15 17 29 35 40 43 53 70 72 73 75 76 77 81 86 87 88 89 90 93 107 108 111 118 129 145 146 **P**6 **S** Health Management Associates, Naples, FL
Primary Contact: L. Dwayne Blaylock, Chief Executive Officer
CFO: Jimmy Young, Chief Financial Officer
CMO: William Rogers, Chief Medical Officer
CIO: Jeff Wideman, Director Information Systems
CHR: Angie L. Weaver, Director Human Resources
Web address: www.gilmorehealth.com
**Control:** Corporation, Investor–owned, for–profit **Service:** General Medical and Surgical

**Staffed Beds:** 95 **Admissions:** 3736 **Census:** 38 **Outpatient Visits:** 41809
**Births:** 498 **Personnel:** 296

## BATESVILLE—Panola County

**BATESVILLE SPECIALTY HOSPITAL (252011)**, 303 Medical Center Drive, Zip 38606; tel. 662/712–2484, (Nonreporting) **A**10
Primary Contact: Candace Eldib, Administrator
**Control:** Other not–for–profit (including NFP Corporation) **Service:** Long–Term Acute Care hospital

**Staffed Beds:** 12

**TRI–LAKES MEDICAL CENTER (250128)**, 303 Medical Center Drive, Zip 38606–8608; tel. 662/563–5611 **A**9 10 **F**3 4 5 11 12 13 15 29 30 31 32 34 35 38 40 43 45 50 56 57 59 64 65 68 70 74 76 77 81 85 87 89 97 98 100 101 102 103 104 107 108 113 118 126 128 129 131 134 142 145 146 147 **P**3 **S** Health Management Associates, Naples, FL
Primary Contact: Wes Sigler, Chief Executive Officer
COO: Vince Brummett, Director Administrative Services
CMO: Michael R. Hovens, M.D., Chief Medical Officer
CIO: Will Morris, Director Information Technology
Web address: www.trilakesmc.com
**Control:** Corporation, Investor–owned, for–profit **Service:** General Medical and Surgical

**Staffed Beds:** 112 **Admissions:** 3048 **Census:** 46 **Outpatient Visits:** 19140
**Births:** 174 **Total Expense ($000):** 30360 **Payroll Expense ($000):** 13196
**Personnel:** 357

## BAY SAINT LOUIS—Hancock County

⊠ **HANCOCK MEDICAL CENTER (250162)**, 149 Drinkwater Boulevard, Zip 39521–2790, Mailing Address: P.O. Box 2790, Zip 39521–2790; tel. 228/467–8600 **A**1 9 10 **F**3 11 13 15 17 18 28 29 31 32 34 35 40 43 45 51 57 59 64 65 68 70 75 76 77 79 81 82 85 86 87 89 90 93 97 107 108 110 111 113 114 117 118 126 128 129 130 134 143 144 145 146 147 **S** QHR, Brentwood, TN
Primary Contact: Robert A. Pascasio, FACHE, Chief Executive Officer
CHR: Audrey L. Dunn, Director Human Resources
CNO: Angela Gambino, R.N., Chief Nursing Officer
Web address: www.hmc.org
**Control:** County–Government, nonfederal **Service:** General Medical and Surgical

**Staffed Beds:** 47 **Admissions:** 1907 **Census:** 18 **Outpatient Visits:** 49755
**Births:** 190 **Total Expense ($000):** 39981 **Payroll Expense ($000):** 18781
**Personnel:** 356

## BAY SPRINGS—Jasper County

★ **JASPER GENERAL HOSPITAL (250018)**, 15 A South Sixth Street, Zip 39422–9738, Mailing Address: P.O. Box 527, Zip 39422–0527; tel. 601/764–2101, (Includes JASPER COUNTY NURSING HOME ), (Total facility includes 110 beds in nursing home–type unit) **A**9 10 **F**10 62 127 129 132
Primary Contact: M. Kenneth Posey, FACHE, Administrator
CFO: Steve Green, Comptroller
CMO: A. K. Lay, Sr., M.D., Chief Medical Officer
CHR: JoAnn Boyd, Administrative Assistant
**Control:** County–Government, nonfederal **Service:** General Medical and Surgical

**Staffed Beds:** 126 **Admissions:** 40 **Census:** 108 **Outpatient Visits:** 0 **Births:** 0 **Personnel:** 46

## BELZONI—Humphreys County

**PATIENT'S CHOICE MEDICAL CENTER (251311)**, 500 CCC Road, Zip 39038–3806, Mailing Address: P.O. Box 510, Zip 39038–0510; tel. 662/247–3831 **A**9 10 18 **F**3 13 29 40 43 70 76 89 90 93 97 98 103 126 129 132
Primary Contact: Paula Lang, Chief Executive Officer
CHR: Ruth Hayes, Director Human Resources
**Control:** Corporation, Investor–owned, for–profit **Service:** General Medical and Surgical

**Staffed Beds:** 34 **Admissions:** 694 **Census:** 11 **Outpatient Visits:** 6219
**Births:** 0 **Total Expense ($000):** 7173 **Payroll Expense ($000):** 3500
**Personnel:** 96

## BILOXI—Harrison County

☐ **BILOXI REGIONAL MEDICAL CENTER (250007)**, 150 Reynoir Street, Zip 39530–4199, Mailing Address: P.O. Box 128, Zip 39533–0128; tel. 228/432–1571 **A**1 9 10 **F**3 11 12 13 15 17 18 20 29 31 32 34 35 37 40 43 45 46 47 48 49 50 54 59 61 64 65 68 70 73 74 75 76 77 78 79 81 82 85 86 87 89 90 93 97 98 100 102 103 104 107 108 110 111 112 113 114 116 118 125 129 134 142 145 146 147 **S** Health Management Associates, Naples, FL
Primary Contact: Monte J. Bostwick, Chief Executive Officer
CFO: Mark Wack, Chief Financial Officer
CMO: David Harris, M.D., President Medical Affairs
CHR: Brian Stanford, Director Human Resources
Web address: www.hmamississippi.com
**Control:** Corporation, Investor–owned, for–profit **Service:** General Medical and Surgical

**Staffed Beds:** 198 **Admissions:** 7627 **Census:** 102 **Outpatient Visits:** 88008
**Births:** 791 **Total Expense ($000):** 85925 **Payroll Expense ($000):** 30666
**Personnel:** 708

---

**Hospital, Medicare Provider Number, Address, Telephone, Approval, Facility, and Physician Codes, Health Care System**

★ American Hospital Association (AHA) membership
☐ The Joint Commission accreditation ◇ DNV Healthcare Inc. accreditation
○ American Osteopathic Association (AOA) accreditation
△ Commission on Accreditation of Rehabilitation Facilities (CARF) accreditation

⊠ △ **VETERANS AFFAIRS GULF COAST VETERANS HEALTH CARE SYSTEM**, 400 Veterans Avenue, Zip 39531–2410; tel. 228/523–5000, (Nonreporting) **A**1 3 5 7 **S** Department of Veterans Affairs, Washington, DC
Primary Contact: Thomas Wisnieski, Director
COO: Deborah M. Johnson, Associate Director
CFO: Teresa Pisarich, Acting Chief Financial Officer
CMO: Barry–Lewis Harris, II, M.D., Chief of Staff
CIO: David D. Wagner, Chief Information Management Service
CHR: Johnnie M. Jones, Acting Chief Human Resource Management and Workforce Development Service
Web address: www.va.gov/biloxi
**Control:** Veterans Affairs, Government, federal **Service:** General Medical and Surgical

> **Staffed Beds:** 392

### BOONEVILLE—Prentiss County

⊠ **BAPTIST MEMORIAL HOSPITAL–BOONEVILLE (250044)**, 100 Hospital Street, Zip 38829–3359; tel. 662/720–5000 **A**1 9 10 **F**3 11 15 17 28 29 30 40 43 70 75 81 87 89 98 103 107 108 111 117 118 129 131 132 **P**3 **S** Baptist Memorial Health Care Corporation, Memphis, TN
Primary Contact: James Grantham, Administrator
CFO: Donavan Leonard, Chief Financial Officer
CMO: Nathan Baldwin, M.D., President Medical Staff
CIO: Linda Chaffin, Director Medical Review
CHR: Shannon Bolen, Director Human Resources
Web address: www.bmhcc.org
**Control:** Other not–for–profit (including NFP Corporation) **Service:** General Medical and Surgical

> **Staffed Beds:** 114 **Admissions:** 1353 **Census:** 21 **Outpatient Visits:** 29587 **Births:** 0 **Total Expense ($000):** 20640 **Payroll Expense ($000):** 8349 **Personnel:** 225

### BRANDON—Rankin County

☐ **CROSSGATES RIVER OAKS HOSPITAL (250096)**, 350 Crossgates Boulevard, Zip 39042–2698; tel. 601/825–2811 **A**1 9 10 **F**16 17 40 43 70 77 78 81 87 89 90 93 97 98 103 107 108 111 115 117 118 129 145 **P**8 **S** Health Management Associates, Naples, FL
Primary Contact: J. Allen Tyra, Chief Executive Officer
COO: Brandon Downey, Chief Operating Officer
CFO: Brad Sinclair, Chief Financial Officer
CMO: Edward Rigdon, M.D., Chief Medical Officer
CIO: Christy Murphy, Director Health Information Systems
CHR: Mark Cook, Director Human Resources
Web address: www.crossgatesriveroaks.com
**Control:** Corporation, Investor–owned, for–profit **Service:** General Medical and Surgical

> **Staffed Beds:** 134 **Admissions:** 5165 **Census:** 74 **Outpatient Visits:** 73542 **Births:** 0 **Personnel:** 410

### BROOKHAVEN—Lincoln County

⊠ **KING'S DAUGHTERS MEDICAL CENTER (250057)**, 427 Highway 51 North, Zip 39601–2600, Mailing Address: P.O. Box 948, Zip 39602–0948; tel. 601/833–6011 **A**1 9 10 20 **F**3 7 11 13 15 17 19 28 29 30 34 35 39 40 41 42 43 46 53 57 59 60 61 63 64 70 73 75 76 77 79 80 81 86 88 89 92 93 96 97 107 108 110 111 113 114 117 118 123 128 129 130 131 134 145 146 147 **S** QHR, Brentwood, TN
Primary Contact: Alvin Hoover, FACHE, Chief Executive Officer
COO: Phil Campbell, Chief Operating Officer
CFO: Randy B. Pirtle, Chief Financial Officer
CMO: Leigh Cher Gray, M.D., Chief of Staff
CIO: Carl Smith, Director Information Systems
CHR: Celine Craig, Director Human Resources
CNO: Cheri Walker, R.N., Chief Nursing Officer
Web address: www.kdmc.org
**Control:** Other not–for–profit (including NFP Corporation) **Service:** General Medical and Surgical

> **Staffed Beds:** 91 **Admissions:** 3430 **Census:** 32 **Outpatient Visits:** 80508 **Births:** 641 **Total Expense ($000):** 57956 **Payroll Expense ($000):** 24377 **Personnel:** 470

### CALHOUN CITY—Calhoun County

★ **CALHOUN HEALTH SERVICES (251331)**, 140 Burke–Calhoun City Road, Zip 38916–9690; tel. 662/628–6611, (Total facility includes 120 beds in nursing home–type unit) **A**9 10 **F**7 40 43 68 70 87 89 90 98 103 107 113 118 127 129 132 **S** North Mississippi Health Services, Inc., Tupelo, MS
Primary Contact: James P. Franklin, Administrator
CFO: Mandy Suber, Controller
CMO: Guy Farmer, M.D., President Medical Staff
Web address: www.nmhs.net/calhoun_city
**Control:** City–County, Government, nonfederal **Service:** General Medical and Surgical

> **Staffed Beds:** 150 **Admissions:** 537 **Census:** 113 **Outpatient Visits:** 6537 **Births:** 0 **Total Expense ($000):** 15929 **Payroll Expense ($000):** 7642 **Personnel:** 278

### CANTON—Madison County

**MADISON RIVER OAKS MEDICAL CENTER (250038)**, Highway 16 East, Zip 39046–8823, Mailing Address: P.O. Box 1607, Zip 39046–1607; tel. 601/859–1331 **A**9 10 **F**3 8 13 15 29 40 43 45 57 70 76 79 81 85 87 89 107 108 110 113 118 125 129 **S** Health Management Associates, Naples, FL
Primary Contact: Glen Silverman, Chief Executive Officer
CFO: Ken Warriner, Chief Financial Officer
CMO: Robert Tatum, M.D., Chief of Staff
CIO: Michelle Hughes, Director Health Information Management
CHR: Jackie Williams, Director Human Resources
CHR: Jackie Williams, Director Human Resources
Web address: www.madisonriveroaks.com
**Control:** Partnership, Investor–owned, for–profit **Service:** General Medical and Surgical

> **Staffed Beds:** 67 **Admissions:** 1576 **Census:** 12 **Outpatient Visits:** 28615 **Births:** 266 **Total Expense ($000):** 16521 **Payroll Expense ($000):** 6834 **Personnel:** 204

### CARTHAGE—Leake County

★ **BAPTIST MEDICAL CENTER LEAKE (251315)**, 310 Ellis Street, Zip 39051–3809, Mailing Address: P.O. Box 909, Zip 39051–0909; tel. 601/267–1100, (Total facility includes 44 beds in nursing home–type unit) **A**9 10 18 **F**29 40 43 70 87 107 118 127 129 132 **P**6 **S** Mississippi Baptist Health System, Jackson, MS
Primary Contact: Wayne Walters, Chief Executive Officer
COO: Jerry Cotton, Interim COO
CFO: David Jackson, Chief Financial Officer
CMO: Doug Perry, M.D., Chief of Staff
Web address: www.leakemh.org
**Control:** Other not–for–profit (including NFP Corporation) **Service:** General Medical and Surgical

> **Staffed Beds:** 69 **Admissions:** 738 **Census:** 49 **Outpatient Visits:** 19450 **Births:** 5 **Personnel:** 192

### CENTREVILLE—Wilkinson County

⊠ **FIELD MEMORIAL COMMUNITY HOSPITAL (251309)**, 270 West Main Street, Zip 39631, Mailing Address: P.O. Box 639, Zip 39631–0639; tel. 601/645–5221 **A**1 9 10 18 **F**15 29 39 40 43 45 50 57 61 64 68 70 75 77 79 81 89 90 93 107 108 113 118 126 129 132 145
Primary Contact: Chad Netterville, Administrator
CFO: Jacquelyn Richoux, Chief Financial Officer
CHR: Debbie Willingham, Administrative Assistant
Web address: www.fmch.org
**Control:** County–Government, nonfederal **Service:** General Medical and Surgical

> **Staffed Beds:** 25 **Admissions:** 638 **Census:** 7 **Outpatient Visits:** 14306 **Births:** 0 **Total Expense ($000):** 13189 **Payroll Expense ($000):** 7895 **Personnel:** 172

### CHARLESTON—Tallahatchie County

**TALLAHATCHIE GENERAL HOSPITAL (251304)**, 201 South Market, Zip 38921–2236, Mailing Address: P.O. Box 230, Zip 38921–0230; tel. 662/647–5535, (Total facility includes 98 beds in nursing home–type unit) **A**9 10 18 **F**29 39 40 70 87 107 127 129 132 **P**6
Primary Contact: Jim Blackwood, Chief Executive Officer
CFO: Sammie Bell, Jr., Chief Financial Officer
**Control:** County–Government, nonfederal **Service:** General Medical and Surgical

> **Staffed Beds:** 107 **Admissions:** 344 **Census:** 74 **Outpatient Visits:** 3536 **Births:** 0 **Personnel:** 229

### CLARKSDALE—Coahoma County

☐ **NORTHWEST MISSISSIPPI REGIONAL MEDICAL CENTER (250042)**, 1970 Hospital Drive, Zip 38614–7204, Mailing Address: P.O. Box 1218, Zip 38614–1218; tel. 662/627–3211 **A**1 9 10 19 **F**3 13 15 17 18 20 29 30 34 35 40 43 45 47 49 57 59 64 70 74 76 79 81 86 87 89 90 93 107 108 110 111 114 117 118 123 125 128 129 131 134 144 147 **S** Health Management Associates, Naples, FL
Primary Contact: Joan Strayham, R.N., Interim Chief Executive Officer
COO: Joseph Webb, Chief Operating Officer
CFO: Steve Marinelli, Chief Financial Officer
CMO: Rodney Baine, M.D., Chief of Staff
CIO: Kayla Carpenter, Health Information Management Systems Officer
CHR: Sarah Dale Shaffer, Director Human Resources
Web address: www.northwestregional.org
**Control:** Corporation, Investor–owned, for–profit **Service:** General Medical and Surgical

> **Staffed Beds:** 195 **Admissions:** 5857 **Census:** 64 **Outpatient Visits:** 49940 **Births:** 887 **Total Expense ($000):** 58371 **Payroll Expense ($000):** 23071 **Personnel:** 477

MS

## CLEVELAND—Bolivar County

☒ **BOLIVAR MEDICAL CENTER (250093)**, 901 East Sunflower Road, Zip 38732–9722, Mailing Address: P.O. Box 1380, Zip 38732–1380; tel. 662/846–0061, (Total facility includes 35 beds in nursing home–type unit) **A**1 9 10 20 **F**3 11 13 15 17 18 26 29 30 35 39 40 43 45 46 56 59 60 70 73 74 76 79 81 82 85 87 88 89 93 103 107 108 110 111 112 114 115 117 118 119 127 129 131 132 145 **S** LifePoint Hospitals, Inc., Brentwood, TN
Primary Contact: Scott M. Smith, Chief Executive Officer
CFO: Chad Miller, Chief Financial Officer
CMO: Michael Portner, M.D., Chief Medical Staff
CIO: Dusty Griffith, Director Information Systems
CHR: David Kent, Director Human Resources
Web address: www.bolivarmedical.com
**Control:** Corporation, Investor–owned, for–profit **Service:** General Medical and Surgical

**Staffed Beds:** 127 **Admissions:** 3822 **Census:** 75 **Outpatient Visits:** 51156 **Births:** 443 **Total Expense ($000):** 41129 **Payroll Expense ($000):** 16870 **Personnel:** 324

## COLLINS—Covington County

☒ **COVINGTON COUNTY HOSPITAL (251325)**, Gerald McRaney Street, Zip 39428–3899, Mailing Address: P.O. Box 1149, Zip 39428–1149; tel. 601/765–6711, (Total facility includes 60 beds in nursing home–type unit) **A**1 9 10 18 **F**3 7 40 43 45 57 70 81 89 93 103 105 107 118 126 127 129 132 143
Primary Contact: Jamie Rodgers, Chief Executive Officer
CFO: Kirstie Evans, Chief Financial Officer
CHR: Lee Robb, Director Human Resources
Web address: www.covingtoncountyhospital.com
**Control:** County–Government, nonfederal **Service:** General Medical and Surgical

**Staffed Beds:** 95 **Admissions:** 561 **Census:** 43 **Outpatient Visits:** 25817 **Births:** 0 **Total Expense ($000):** 18701 **Payroll Expense ($000):** 8386 **Personnel:** 250

## COLUMBIA—Marion County

**MARION GENERAL HOSPITAL (250085)**, 1560 Sumrall Road, Zip 39429–2654, Mailing Address: P.O. Box 630, Zip 39429–0630; tel. 601/736–6303 **A**9 10 **F**29 35 39 40 43 61 62 70 75 81 87 89 90 93 97 107 108 111 118 129 130 132 143 145
Primary Contact: Bryan K. Maxie, Administrator
CFO: Randall Pigott, Chief Financial Officer
CMO: Jeff Johnson, M.D., Chief Medical Staff
CIO: Donny Bracey, Director Information Services
**Control:** County–Government, nonfederal **Service:** General Medical and Surgical

**Staffed Beds:** 49 **Admissions:** 663 **Census:** 8 **Outpatient Visits:** 30429 **Births:** 1 **Personnel:** 190

## COLUMBUS—Lowndes County

☒ **BAPTIST MEMORIAL HOSPITAL–GOLDEN TRIANGLE (250100)**, 2520 Fifth Street North, Zip 39705–2095, Mailing Address: P.O. Box 1307, Zip 39703–1307; tel. 662/244–1000 **A**1 9 10 19 **F**3 4 5 7 11 13 15 17 18 20 22 24 28 29 30 31 34 38 39 40 42 43 49 51 57 59 61 64 70 73 75 76 77 78 79 80 81 84 85 87 88 89 91 93 94 98 100 102 104 105 107 108 109 110 111 113 114 115 116 117 118 119 120 122 123 125 128 131 133 145 146 **P**3 6 **S** Baptist Memorial Health Care Corporation, Memphis, TN
Primary Contact: Paul Cade, Administrator and Chief Executive Officer
CFO: Jimmy Robertson, Chief Financial Officer
CMO: John E. Reed, M.D., Medical Director
CIO: Sheila Bardwell, Director Information Systems
CHR: Bob McCallister, Director Human Resources
CNO: Mary Ellen Sumrall, Chief Nursing Officer
Web address: www.bmhcc.org
**Control:** Other not–for–profit (including NFP Corporation) **Service:** General Medical and Surgical

**Staffed Beds:** 249 **Admissions:** 7153 **Census:** 95 **Outpatient Visits:** 97828 **Births:** 899 **Total Expense ($000):** 115428 **Payroll Expense ($000):** 40259 **Personnel:** 921

## CORINTH—Alcorn County

☐ **MAGNOLIA REGIONAL HEALTH CENTER (250009)**, 611 Alcorn Drive, Zip 38834–9321; tel. 662/293–1000 **A**1 9 10 13 19 **F**13 15 17 29 35 39 40 43 51 53 62 63 70 75 76 77 78 81 82 86 87 89 93 98 100 101 102 103 107 108 111 115 117 118 129 130 131 142 145 146 **P**7 8
Primary Contact: Rick D. Napper, President and Chief Executive Officer
COO: Ronny Humes, Chief Operating Officer
CFO: Jeff Taylor, Senior Vice President Finance
CMO: Felton Combest, M.D., Vice President Medical Affairs
CIO: Hershell Foster, Vice President Information Technology
CHR: Regenia Brown, Vice President Human Resources
Web address: www.mrhc.org
**Control:** City–County, Government, nonfederal **Service:** General Medical and Surgical

**Staffed Beds:** 164 **Admissions:** 7787 **Census:** 102 **Outpatient Visits:** 133547 **Births:** 524 **Personnel:** 1129

## DE KALB—Kemper County

★ **JOHN C. STENNIS MEMORIAL HOSPITAL (251335)**, 14365 Highway 16 West, Zip 39328–7974; tel. 769/486–1000, (Data for 204 days) **A**10 21 **F**29 40 70 75 107 132 **P**6 7 **S** Rush Health Systems, Meridian, MS
Primary Contact: Jason Payne, Administrator
Web address: www.rushhealthsystems.org/stennis/
**Control:** Other not–for–profit (including NFP Corporation) **Service:** General Medical and Surgical

**Staffed Beds:** 25 **Admissions:** 103 **Census:** 2 **Outpatient Visits:** 2296 **Births:** 0 **Personnel:** 90

## EUPORA—Webster County

☒ **NORTH MISSISSIPPI MEDICAL CENTER–EUPORA (250020)**, 70 Medical Plaza, Zip 39744–4018; tel. 662/258–6221, (Total facility includes 35 beds in nursing home–type unit) **A**1 9 10 **F**35 40 43 53 70 86 87 89 98 107 118 127 129 132 **S** North Mississippi Health Services, Inc., Tupelo, MS
Primary Contact: John R. Jones, Administrator
CFO: Adonna Mitchell, Director Fiscal Services
CMO: Charles Ozborn, M.D., Chief of Staff
CIO: Shirley Griffin, Director Health Information
CHR: Dorothy Castle, Director Human Resources
Web address: www.nmhs.net/eupora
**Control:** Other not–for–profit (including NFP Corporation) **Service:** General Medical and Surgical

**Staffed Beds:** 73 **Admissions:** 1267 **Census:** 52 **Outpatient Visits:** 17840 **Births:** 0 **Personnel:** 217

## FAYETTE—Jefferson County

**JEFFERSON COUNTY HOSPITAL (250060)**, 870 South Main Street, Zip 39069, Mailing Address: P.O. Box 577, Zip 39069–0577; tel. 601/786–3401, (Nonreporting) **A**9 10
Primary Contact: Jerry Kennedy, Administrator
CFO: Jerry Kennedy, Administrator
CMO: Khar Omolara, M.D., Chief Medical Staff
CHR: Patricia Selmon, Director Public Relations and Chief Human Resources
**Control:** County–Government, nonfederal **Service:** General Medical and Surgical

**Staffed Beds:** 30

## FLOWOOD—Rankin County

☒ **RIVER OAKS HOSPITAL (250138)**, 1030 River Oaks Drive, Zip 39232–9553, Mailing Address: P.O. Box 5100, Jackson, Zip 39296–5100; tel. 601/932–1030 **A**1 9 10 **F**3 12 13 15 17 18 29 30 31 34 35 37 39 40 43 49 51 57 59 61 70 72 73 74 76 78 79 81 82 85 87 93 108 111 114 125 129 145 146 **S** Health Management Associates, Naples, FL
Primary Contact: Dennis R. Bruns, Chief Executive Officer
COO: Paul V. Peiffer, Executive Vice President and Chief Operating Officer
CFO: Jeff Bedford, Executive Vice President and Chief Financial Officer
CMO: C. Ron Cannon, M.D., Medical Director
CIO: Pat Jones, Director Information Systems
CHR: Warren Weed, Director Human Resources
Web address: www.riveroakshosp.org
**Control:** Corporation, Investor–owned, for–profit **Service:** General Medical and Surgical

**Staffed Beds:** 158 **Admissions:** 7136 **Census:** 72 **Outpatient Visits:** 59069 **Births:** 1916 **Personnel:** 703

**MS**

---

**Hospital, Medicare Provider Number, Address, Telephone, Approval, Facility, and Physician Codes, Health Care System**

★ American Hospital Association (AHA) membership
☐ The Joint Commission accreditation
◇ DNV Healthcare Inc. accreditation
○ American Osteopathic Association (AOA) accreditation
△ Commission on Accreditation of Rehabilitation Facilities (CARF) accreditation

☐ **WOMAN'S HOSPITAL (250136)**, 1026 North Flowood Drive, Zip 39232–9532, Mailing Address: P.O. Box 4546, Jackson, Zip 39296–4546; tel. 601/932–1000 **A**1 10 **F**13 15 30 34 35 39 57 59 70 72 73 76 81 85 108 125 129 146 **S** Health Management Associates, Naples, FL
Primary Contact: Sherry J. Pitts, Chief Executive Officer
COO: Paul V. Peiffer, Chief Operating Officer
CFO: Jeff Bedford, Executive Vice President and Chief Financial Officer
CMO: Edra Kimmel, M.D., Chief of Staff
CHR: Warren Weed, Director Associate Relations
Web address: www.womanshospitalms.com
**Control:** Corporation, Investor–owned, for–profit **Service:** Obstetrics and gynecology

**Staffed Beds:** 60 **Admissions:** 2135 **Census:** 20 **Outpatient Visits:** 16443 **Births:** 1392 **Total Expense ($000):** 25332 **Payroll Expense ($000):** 11395 **Personnel:** 202

### FOREST—Scott County

★ **S. E. LACKEY MEMORIAL HOSPITAL (251300)**, 330 Broad Street, Zip 39074–0428, Mailing Address: P.O. Box 428, Zip 39074–0428; tel. 601/469–4151, (Total facility includes 20 beds in nursing home–type unit) **A**9 10 18 21 **F**3 15 18 29 34 35 39 42 43 45 56 65 70 79 81 86 89 98 103 107 108 111 118 125 126 127 129 132 **P**5 6 **S** Pioneer Health Services, Magee, MS
Primary Contact: Donna Riser, Administrator
CFO: Julie Gieger, Chief Financial Officer
CMO: John Paul Lee, M.D., Chief of Staff
CIO: Eddie Pope, Chief Information Officer
CHR: Donn Paul, Chief Human Resources
Web address: www.selackey.com
**Control:** Other not–for–profit (including NFP Corporation) **Service:** General Medical and Surgical

**Staffed Beds:** 55 **Admissions:** 1644 **Census:** 34 **Outpatient Visits:** 32057 **Births:** 0 **Personnel:** 221

### GREENVILLE—Washington County

✚ **DELTA REGIONAL MEDICAL CENTER (250082)**, 1400 East Union Street, Zip 38703; tel. 662/378–3783, (Includes THE KING'S DAUGHTERS HOSPITAL, 300 Washington Avenue, Zip 38701–3614, Mailing Address: P.O. Box 1857, Zip 38702–1857; tel. 662/378–2020) **A**1 9 10 19 **F**3 4 7 11 13 15 17 18 20 22 24 28 29 34 35 40 42 43 49 51 57 59 62 63 70 72 73 76 78 79 81 82 89 90 93 94 96 97 98 103 104 107 108 110 111 113 114 115 116 117 118 126 128 130 131 133 134 145 146 147 **P**6 8
Primary Contact: Stansel Harvey, FACHE, Chief Executive Officer
CFO: Courtney Phillips, Chief Financial Officer
CIO: Shane Coleman, Director Information Services
CHR: Alphe Wells, Vice President Human Resources and Support Services
Web address: www.deltaregional.com
**Control:** County–Government, nonfederal **Service:** General Medical and Surgical

**Staffed Beds:** 217 **Admissions:** 8219 **Census:** 120 **Outpatient Visits:** 90061 **Births:** 837 **Total Expense ($000):** 101111 **Payroll Expense ($000):** 42573 **Personnel:** 850

### GREENWOOD—Leflore County

☐ △ **GREENWOOD LEFLORE HOSPITAL (250099)**, 1401 River Road, Zip 38930, Mailing Address: Drawer 1410, Zip 38935–1410; tel. 662/459–7000 **A**1 7 9 10 19 **F**3 13 15 18 20 26 27 28 29 31 32 35 39 40 43 45 47 50 53 56 57 59 61 65 68 70 74 75 76 79 81 82 84 85 86 87 89 90 92 93 96 98 103 107 108 110 111 113 116 117 118 123 126 128 129 131 134 145 146 147 **P**6 8
Primary Contact: James H. Jackson, Jr., Executive Director
COO: Jeff Curtis, Chief Operating Officer
CMO: A. Randle White, M.D., Chief Medical Staff
CIO: Mark S. Hutson, Chief Information Officer
CHR: Key Britt, Associate Director
Web address: www.glh.org
**Control:** City–County, Government, nonfederal **Service:** General Medical and Surgical

**Staffed Beds:** 196 **Admissions:** 7839 **Census:** 105 **Outpatient Visits:** 142915 **Births:** 700 **Total Expense ($000):** 123040 **Payroll Expense ($000):** 53745 **Personnel:** 957

**LTAC HOSPITAL OF GREENWOOD (252010)**, 1401 River Road Floor 2, Zip 38930–4030; tel. 662/459–2681 **A**9 10 **F**57 108 129 147 **S** AMG Integrated Healthcare Management, Lafayette, LA
Primary Contact: Tommy Strohe, Interim Chief Executive Officer
COO: Jason Nassif, Chief Operating Officer
CMO: Gutti Rao, M.D., Medical Director
CIO: Larry Bramlett, Chief Information Officer
CHR: Shelia Brown, Director Human Resources
Web address: www.amgihm.com/ltac_of_greenwood
**Control:** Partnership, Investor–owned, for–profit **Service:** Long–Term Acute Care hospital

**Staffed Beds:** 40 **Admissions:** 372 **Census:** 25 **Outpatient Visits:** 0 **Births:** 0 **Total Expense ($000):** 9407 **Payroll Expense ($000):** 3750 **Personnel:** 9

### GRENADA—Grenada County

★ **GRENADA LAKE MEDICAL CENTER (250015)**, 960 Avent Drive, Zip 38901–5230; tel. 662/227–7000 **A**9 10 20 21 **F**3 8 11 13 14 15 17 29 30 35 39 40 43 49 53 57 60 62 64 70 73 76 77 79 80 81 83 86 89 90 93 94 96 97 107 108 111 113 117 118 126 127 129 142 145 146
Primary Contact: Charles L. Denton, Chief Executive Officer
CFO: Keith Heartsill, Chief Financial Officer
CMO: David Simmons, M.D., Chief of Staff
CIO: Sarah Longest, Chief Information Officer
CHR: Ken Baker, Administrative Director Human Resources
Web address: www.glmc.net
**Control:** County–Government, nonfederal **Service:** General Medical and Surgical

**Staffed Beds:** 141 **Admissions:** 2914 **Census:** 36 **Outpatient Visits:** 47580 **Births:** 482 **Personnel:** 431

### GULFPORT—Harrison County

✚ **GARDEN PARK MEDICAL CENTER (250123)**, 15200 Community Road, Zip 39503–3085, Mailing Address: P.O. Box 1240, Zip 39502–1240; tel. 228/575–7000 **A**1 9 10 **F**3 12 13 15 18 19 29 31 34 35 45 49 57 59 70 73 74 76 78 79 81 85 86 87 89 90 93 97 98 103 107 108 110 111 113 117 118 125 128 129 145 146 147 **S** HCA, Nashville, TN
Primary Contact: Brenda M. Waltz, FACHE, Chief Executive Officer
COO: Daphne David, Chief Operating Officer
CFO: Regina Ramazani, Chief Financial Officer
CIO: Jackson Balch, IT Director
CHR: Krystyna Varnado, Director Human Resources
CNO: Cheryl Thompson, Chief Nursing Officer
Web address: www.gpmedical.com
**Control:** Corporation, Investor–owned, for–profit **Service:** General Medical and Surgical

**Staffed Beds:** 130 **Admissions:** 3806 **Census:** 45 **Outpatient Visits:** 62289 **Births:** 464 **Total Expense ($000):** 54173 **Payroll Expense ($000):** 22562 **Personnel:** 420

✚ △ **MEMORIAL HOSPITAL AT GULFPORT (250019)**, 4500 13th Street, Zip 39501–2569, Mailing Address: P.O. Box 1810, Zip 39502–1810; tel. 228/867–4000, (Includes MEMORIAL BEHAVIORAL HEALTH, 11150 Highway 49 North, Zip 39503–4110; tel. 228/831–1700; Michael A. Zieman, Administrator) **A**1 2 7 9 10 **F**3 4 5 8 11 13 15 17 18 20 22 24 26 28 29 30 31 34 35 40 42 43 45 46 47 48 49 50 51 53 54 57 58 59 64 65 70 71 72 73 74 76 77 78 79 80 81 85 87 89 90 91 92 93 95 96 98 99 100 101 102 104 105 107 108 110 111 113 114 115 116 117 118 119 120 122 123 125 129 131 134 145 147 **P**3 8
Primary Contact: Gary G. Marchand, President and Chief Executive Officer
CFO: Jeffrey T. Steiner, Vice President Finance
CMO: Nancy Downs, M.D., Vice President Medical Affairs
CIO: Richard Ferrans, M.D., Vice President and Medical Information Officer
CHR: Cathy Wood, Director Human Resources
Web address: www.gulfportmemorial.com
**Control:** City–County, Government, nonfederal **Service:** General Medical and Surgical

**Staffed Beds:** 445 **Admissions:** 15684 **Census:** 231 **Outpatient Visits:** 450399 **Births:** 1415 **Total Expense ($000):** 229036 **Payroll Expense ($000):** 154131 **Personnel:** 2541

✚ **SELECT SPECIALTY HOSPITAL–GULF COAST (252005)**, 1520 Broad Avenue, Suite 300, Zip 39501; tel. 228/575–7500 **A**1 10 **F**70 80 82 87 90 129 **S** Select Medical Corporation, Mechanicsburg, PA
Primary Contact: John O'Keefe, Chief Executive Officer
Web address: www.selectmedicalcorp.com
**Control:** Corporation, Investor–owned, for–profit **Service:** Long–Term Acute Care hospital

**Staffed Beds:** 61 **Admissions:** 290 **Census:** 20 **Outpatient Visits:** 0 **Births:** 0 **Personnel:** 104

### HATTIESBURG—Forrest County

★ △ **FORREST GENERAL HOSPITAL (250078)**, 6051 U.S. Highway 49, Zip 39401–7243, Mailing Address: P.O. Box 16389, Zip 39404–6389; tel. 601/288–7000 **A**2 3 5 7 9 10 19 21 **F**3 4 5 8 13 15 17 18 20 22 24 26 28 29 30 31 32 34 35 37 40 43 45 46 48 49 50 53 54 57 58 59 60 62 63 64 68 70 72 73 74 76 77 78 79 81 84 85 86 87 89 90 92 93 94 95 96 98 99 100 102 103 104 107 108 111 113 114 117 118 119 120 122 129 130 131 134 145 146 147 **P**8
Primary Contact: Evan S. Dillard, M.P.H., FACHE, President and Chief Executive Officer
CFO: Andy Woodward, Chief Financial Officer
CMO: Steven E. Farrell, M.D., Chief Medical Officer
CIO: G. Edward Tucker, Jr., Vice President Corporate Services
Web address: www.forrestgeneral.com
**Control:** County–Government, nonfederal **Service:** General Medical and Surgical

**Staffed Beds:** 512 **Admissions:** 26657 **Census:** 340 **Outpatient Visits:** 128447 **Births:** 2368 **Total Expense ($000):** 311006 **Payroll Expense ($000):** 132145 **Personnel:** 2546

*Many Facility Codes have changed. Please refer to the AHA Guide Code Chart.*  © 2012 AHA Guide

MS

⊠ **REGENCY HOSPITAL OF HATTIESBURG (252009)**, 220 South 27th Avenue, Zip 39401; tel. 601/288–8510 **A**1 10 **F**40 70 **S** Select Medical Corporation, Mechanicsburg, PA
Primary Contact: Robert J. Trautman, Chief Executive Officer
CMO: Ralph Kahler, M.D., Medical Director
CHR: Jared Burns, Coordinator Human Resources
Web address: www.regencyhospital.com/hattiesburg
**Control:** Corporation, Investor–owned, for–profit **Service:** Long–Term Acute Care hospital

**Staffed Beds:** 33 **Admissions:** 385 **Census:** 28 **Outpatient Visits:** 0 **Births:** 0 **Personnel:** 88

⊠ **WESLEY MEDICAL CENTER (250094)**, 5001 Hardy Street, Zip 39402–1366, Mailing Address: P.O. Box 16509, Zip 39404–6509; tel. 601/268–8000 **A**1 9 10 19 **F**13 15 17 29 35 39 40 53 56 60 61 70 72 73 75 76 77 78 81 87 89 90 93 97 107 108 111 117 118 129 131 145 **P**6 7 **S** Community Health Systems, Inc., Franklin, TN
Primary Contact: Michael Neuendorf, Chief Executive Officer
COO: Travis Sisson, Chief Operating Officer
CFO: Randy Humphrey, Chief Financial Officer
CMO: William Reno, III, M.D., President Medical Staff
CIO: William Toon, Director Information Technology
CHR: Terry Trigg, Director Human Resources
Web address: www.wesley.com
**Control:** Corporation, Investor–owned, for–profit **Service:** General Medical and Surgical

**Staffed Beds:** 211 **Admissions:** 9121 **Census:** 123 **Outpatient Visits:** 87344 **Births:** 1481 **Personnel:** 943

**HAZLEHURST—Copiah County**

★ **HARDY WILSON MEMORIAL HOSPITAL (251327)**, 233 Magnolia Street, Zip 39083–2229, Mailing Address: P.O. Box 889, Zip 39083–0889; tel. 601/894–4541 **A**9 10 18 **F**3 7 15 34 35 40 45 56 57 59 64 70 81 91 93 98 107 111 113 116 118 129 132 147
Primary Contact: Larry Joe Walker, Administrator and Chief Executive Officer
Web address: www.hardywilsonhospital.com
**Control:** County–Government, nonfederal **Service:** General Medical and Surgical

**Staffed Beds:** 25 **Admissions:** 688 **Census:** 12 **Outpatient Visits:** 10147 **Births:** 0 **Payroll Expense ($000):** 8753 **Personnel:** 190

**HOLLY SPRINGS—Marshall County**

**ALLIANCE HEALTHCARE SYSTEM (250012)**, 1430 Highway 4 East, Zip 38635, Mailing Address: P.O. Box 6000, Zip 38634–6000; tel. 662/252–1212 **A**9 10 20 **F**15 29 35 40 43 57 70 75 81 84 87 89 98 103 104 107 118 129 131 132 142
Primary Contact: Perry E. Williams, Sr., Administrator and Chief Executive Officer
COO: Cecelia Bost, Chief Operating Officer
CFO: William F. Magee, Chief Financial Officer
CMO: Subbu Rayudu, M.D., Chief of Staff
CIO: Saul Mbenga, Manager Information Technology
CHR: Judy Eggers, Manager Human Resources
Web address: www.alliancehealth.us
**Control:** Corporation, Investor–owned, for–profit **Service:** General Medical and Surgical

**Staffed Beds:** 40 **Admissions:** 794 **Census:** 10 **Outpatient Visits:** 10006 **Births:** 0 **Personnel:** 92

**HOUSTON—Chickasaw County**

**TRACE REGIONAL HOSPITAL (250017)**, Highway 8 East, Zip 38851–9396, Mailing Address: P.O. Box 626, Zip 38851–0626; tel. 662/456–3700 **A**9 10 **F**3 15 34 35 40 42 45 57 59 61 64 66 70 75 89 90 91 93 98 103 107 111 118 126 127 129 132 134 145 **P**6 **S** Sunlink Health Systems, Atlanta, GA
Primary Contact: Gary L. Staten, Chief Executive Officer
CFO: Pamela W. Cook, Chief Financial Officer
CMO: J. Ronald Staten, M.D., Chief of Staff
CHR: Carol Colbert, Director Human Resources
Web address: www.traceregional.com
**Control:** Corporation, Investor–owned, for–profit **Service:** General Medical and Surgical

**Staffed Beds:** 61 **Admissions:** 900 **Census:** 12 **Outpatient Visits:** 19814 **Births:** 0 **Personnel:** 220

**INDIANOLA—Sunflower County**

★ **SOUTH SUNFLOWER COUNTY HOSPITAL (250095)**, 121 East Baker Street, Zip 38751–2498; tel. 662/887–5235 **A**9 10 20 **F**13 15 40 43 70 76 81 85 107 111 118 126 129 **P**8
Primary Contact: Harold J. Blessitt, Administrator
COO: Barbara Prichard, Assistant Administrator
CFO: Meredith Taylor, Comptroller
CMO: Wade Dowell, M.D., Chief of Staff
CIO: Julie Sterling, Manager Information System
**Control:** County–Government, nonfederal **Service:** General Medical and Surgical

**Staffed Beds:** 49 **Admissions:** 1669 **Census:** 14 **Outpatient Visits:** 12366 **Births:** 256 **Total Expense ($000):** 15265 **Payroll Expense ($000):** 9195 **Personnel:** 130

**IUKA—Tishomingo County**

⊠ **NORTH MISSISSIPPI MEDICAL CENTER–IUKA (250002)**, 1777 Curtis Drive, Zip 38852–1001, Mailing Address: P.O. Box 860, Zip 38852–0860; tel. 662/423–6051 **A**1 9 10 **F**17 29 35 40 43 53 70 75 82 86 87 89 90 93 107 108 111 118 129 131 132 133 **S** North Mississippi Health Services, Inc., Tupelo, MS
Primary Contact: Fred A. Truesdale, Jr., Administrator
CFO: Betty Moore, Business Manager
CMO: Margaret Glynn, M.D., Chief Medical Officer
CIO: Fred A. Truesdale, Jr., Administrator
CHR: Jane Chamblee, Manager Human Resources
Web address: www.nmhs.net
**Control:** Other not–for–profit (including NFP Corporation) **Service:** General Medical and Surgical

**Staffed Beds:** 48 **Admissions:** 820 **Census:** 8 **Outpatient Visits:** 12755 **Births:** 0 **Personnel:** 159

**JACKSON—Hinds County**

☐ **BRENTWOOD BEHAVIORAL HEALTHCARE OF MISSISSIPPI (254007)**, 3531 East Lakeland Drive, Zip 39296–9794; tel. 601/936–2024 **A**1 9 10 **F**98 99 101 102 104 **S** Universal Health Services, Inc., King of Prussia, PA
Primary Contact: Michael J. Carney, Chief Executive Officer
Web address: www.brentwoodjackson.com
**Control:** Corporation, Investor–owned, for–profit **Service:** Psychiatric

**Staffed Beds:** 105 **Admissions:** 2693 **Census:** 81 **Outpatient Visits:** 0 **Births:** 0 **Total Expense ($000):** 12174 **Payroll Expense ($000):** 7188 **Personnel:** 243

☐ **CENTRAL MISSISSIPPI MEDICAL CENTER (250072)**, 1850 Chadwick Drive, Zip 39204–3479, Mailing Address: P.O. Box 59001, Zip 39204–9001; tel. 601/376–1000 **A**1 2 10 **F**13 15 17 29 35 40 43 51 61 70 72 73 75 76 77 78 80 81 82 86 87 89 90 93 97 98 100 102 103 107 108 111 115 117 118 129 131 145 146 **S** Health Management Associates, Naples, FL
Primary Contact: Charlotte W. Dupre', Chief Executive Officer
CHR: Kevin Korner, Director Human Resources
Web address: www.centralmississippimedicalcenter.com
**Control:** Corporation, Investor–owned, for–profit **Service:** General Medical and Surgical

**Staffed Beds:** 377 **Admissions:** 9778 **Census:** 138 **Outpatient Visits:** 45737 **Births:** 1036 **Personnel:** 895

⊠ △ **G.V. MONTGOMERY VETERANS AFFAIRS MEDICAL CENTER**, 1500 East Woodrow Wilson Drive, Zip 39216–5199; tel. 601/364–1201, (Nonreporting) **A**1 2 3 5 7 8 **S** Department of Veterans Affairs, Washington, DC
Primary Contact: Linda Watson, Director
COO: Jed Fillingim, Acting Chief Operating Officer and Associate Director
CFO: Joy Willis, Acting Chief Fiscal Service
CMO: Kent Kirchner, M.D., Chief of Staff
CIO: Robert Wolak, Chief Information Resource Management Service
CHR: Sam Evans, Chief Human Resources Management
Web address: www.va.gov
**Control:** Veterans Affairs, Government, federal **Service:** General Medical and Surgical

**Staffed Beds:** 323

**MS**

---

**Hospital, Medicare Provider Number, Address, Telephone, Approval, Facility, and Physician Codes, Health Care System**

★ American Hospital Association (AHA) membership
☐ The Joint Commission accreditation          ◇ DNV Healthcare Inc. accreditation
○ American Osteopathic Association (AOA) accreditation
△ Commission on Accreditation of Rehabilitation Facilities (CARF) accreditation

☒ △ **METHODIST REHABILITATION CENTER (250152)**, 1350 Woodrow Wilson Drive, Zip 39216–5198; tel. 601/981–2611, (Total facility includes 60 beds in nursing home–type unit) **A**1 5 7 8 9 10 **F**29 35 70 77 81 82 86 87 90 93 118 127 129 131 142 145
Primary Contact: Mark A. Adams, President and Chief Executive Officer
COO: Joseph M. Morette, Executive Vice President
CFO: Gary Armstrong, Executive Vice President
CIO: Gary Armstrong, Executive Vice President
CHR: Steve Hope, Vice President Corporate Services
Web address: www.methodistrehab.org
**Control:** Other not–for–profit (including NFP Corporation) **Service:** Rehabilitation

**Staffed Beds:** 184 **Admissions:** 1177 **Census:** 107 **Outpatient Visits:** 36314 **Births:** 0 **Personnel:** 434

☒ **MISSISSIPPI BAPTIST MEDICAL CENTER (250102)**, 1225 North State Street, Zip 39202–2002; tel. 601/968–1000 **A**1 2 3 5 9 10 **F**4 5 13 15 17 29 35 39 40 51 61 70 72 73 75 76 78 80 81 82 86 89 90 93 98 100 103 104 105 107 108 111 115 117 118 129 131 143 145 146 **S** Mississippi Baptist Health System, Jackson, MS
Primary Contact: Kerry R. Tirman, JD, FACHE, President
CFO: Russell W. York, Chief Financial Officer
CMO: Eric A. McVey, M.D., Vice President and Chief Medical Officer
CIO: Steve M. Stanic, Vice President and Chief Information Officer
CHR: Lee Ann Foreman, Vice President Human Resources
CNO: Bobbie K. Ware, R.N., Vice President/Patient Care/Chief Nursing Officer
Web address: www.mbhs.org
**Control:** Other not–for–profit (including NFP Corporation) **Service:** General Medical and Surgical

**Staffed Beds:** 638 **Admissions:** 19025 **Census:** 284 **Outpatient Visits:** 141319 **Births:** 1232 **Personnel:** 2684

☒ **MISSISSIPPI HOSPITAL FOR RESTORATIVE CARE (252003)**, 1225 North State Street, Zip 39202–2097, Mailing Address: P.O. Box 23695, Zip 39225–3695; tel. 601/968–1000 **A**1 10 **F**29 39 56 61 65 70 74 79 80 82 85 129 **P**7 **S** Mississippi Baptist Health System, Jackson, MS
Primary Contact: Bobbie K. Ware, R.N., FACHE, Chief Executive Officer and Chief Nursing Officer
CFO: Russell W. York, Vice President and Chief Financial Officer
CMO: Holland M. Addison, M.D., Medical Director
CIO: Steve M. Stanic, Vice President and Chief Information Officer
CHR: Lee Ann Foreman, Vice President Human Resources
Web address: www.mbhs.org
**Control:** Other not–for–profit (including NFP Corporation) **Service:** Long–Term Acute Care hospital

**Staffed Beds:** 25 **Admissions:** 244 **Census:** 19 **Outpatient Visits:** 0 **Births:** 0 **Total Expense ($000):** 12064 **Payroll Expense ($000):** 3800 **Personnel:** 58

☒ **REGENCY HOSPITAL OF JACKSON (252012)**, 971 Lakeland Drive, Zip 39216; tel. 601/364–6200 **A**1 9 10 **F**3 18 29 74 79 129 147 **S** Select Medical Corporation, Mechanicsburg, PA
Primary Contact: Michael L. Moore, Chief Executive Officer
Web address: www.regencyhospital.com
**Control:** Corporation, Investor–owned, for–profit **Service:** Long–Term Acute Care hospital

**Staffed Beds:** 36 **Admissions:** 384 **Census:** 28 **Outpatient Visits:** 0 **Births:** 0 **Personnel:** 93

☒ **SELECT SPECIALTY HOSPITAL–JACKSON (252007)**, 5903 Ridgewood Road, Zip 39211; tel. 601/899–3800 **A**1 10 **F**82 93 **S** Select Medical Corporation, Mechanicsburg, PA
Primary Contact: R. Shannon Canard, Chief Executive Officer
CFO: Melissa Smith, Controller
CMO: Greg Oden, M.D., Medical Director and Chief of Staff
CIO: Jacqueline Barnes, Manager Health Information
CHR: Vicki Watson, Manager Human Resources
Web address: www.selectmedicalcorp.com
**Control:** Corporation, Investor–owned, for–profit **Service:** Long–Term Acute Care hospital

**Staffed Beds:** 53 **Admissions:** 670 **Census:** 46 **Outpatient Visits:** 0 **Births:** 0 **Personnel:** 208

☒ **ST. DOMINIC–JACKSON MEMORIAL HOSPITAL (250048)**, 969 Lakeland Drive, Zip 39216–4606; tel. 601/200–2000 **A**1 2 3 5 9 10 **F**3 4 5 11 12 13 15 17 18 20 22 24 26 28 29 30 31 34 35 36 37 38 39 40 43 47 49 51 53 58 60 61 64 65 68 70 72 73 74 75 76 77 78 79 80 81 82 84 85 86 89 90 92 93 97 98 100 101 102 103 107 108 109 110 111 113 114 115 116 117 118 119 120 122 123 125 129 130 145 146 147 **P**8
Primary Contact: Lester K. Diamond, President
CFO: Jennifer Sinclair, Vice President Finance
CMO: Robert L. Mobley, M.D., Executive Vice President Medical Affairs and Quality
CIO: Keith Van Camp, Vice President Information Services
CHR: Lorraine Washington, Vice President Human Resources
Web address: www.stdom.com
**Control:** Other not–for–profit (including NFP Corporation) **Service:** General Medical and Surgical

**Staffed Beds:** 477 **Admissions:** 29937 **Census:** 342 **Outpatient Visits:** 103160 **Births:** 1282 **Total Expense ($000):** 338775 **Payroll Expense ($000):** 133379 **Personnel:** 2592

☒ △ **UNIVERSITY HOSPITALS AND HEALTH SYSTEM, UNIVERSITY OF MISSISSIPPI MEDICAL CENTER (250001)**, 2500 North State Street, Zip 39216–4505; tel. 601/984–1000, (Includes BLAIR E. BATSON HOSPITAL FOR CHILDREN, 2500 North State State Room W019, Zip 39216–4500; tel. 601/984–1000) **A**1 2 3 5 7 8 9 10 **F**3 6 7 11 12 13 15 17 18 19 20 21 22 23 24 25 26 27 28 29 30 31 32 33 34 35 36 37 38 39 40 42 43 44 45 46 48 49 50 52 53 54 55 56 57 58 59 60 61 64 65 68 70 72 73 74 75 76 77 78 79 80 81 82 83 84 85 86 87 88 89 90 91 92 93 94 95 96 97 98 99 100 101 102 103 104 107 108 109 110 111 112 113 114 115 116 118 119 120 121 122 123 124 125 128 129 130 131 133 134 135 136 137 140 141 142 143 144 145 146 147 **P**6
Primary Contact: Janet Y. Harris, R.N., MSN, Chief Executive Officer and Chief Nursing Officer
CFO: Dan Janicak, Chief Financial Officer
CMO: William H. Cleland, M.D., Chief Medical Officer
CIO: Charles Enicks, Chief Information Officer
CHR: Michael Estes, Director Human Resources
Web address: www.umc.edu
**Control:** State–Government, nonfederal **Service:** General Medical and Surgical

**Staffed Beds:** 623 **Admissions:** 27368 **Census:** 488 **Outpatient Visits:** 213226 **Births:** 2330 **Total Expense ($000):** 561949 **Payroll Expense ($000):** 322536 **Personnel:** 5461

## KEESLER AFB—Harrison County

☒ **U. S. AIR FORCE MEDICAL CENTER KEESLER**, 301 Fisher Street, Room 1A132, Zip 39534–2519; tel. 228/376–2550, (Nonreporting) **A**1 2 3 5 **S** Department of the Air Force, Washington, DC
Primary Contact: Colonel Robert Cothron, USAF, MSC, Administrator
COO: Brigadier General James Dougherty, Commander
CFO: Major Brenda Yi, Director Medical Resource Management and Chief Financial Officer
CMO: Colonel James Gasque, M.D., Chief Hospital Services
CIO: Major Samuel Silverthorne, Chief Information Officer
CHR: Major Brenda Yi, Director Medical Resource Management and Chief Financial Officer
Web address: www.keesler.af.mil
**Control:** Air Force, Government, federal **Service:** General Medical and Surgical

**Staffed Beds:** 56

## KILMICHAEL—Montgomery County

★ **KILMICHAEL HOSPITAL (250051)**, 301 Lamar Avenue, Zip 39747–0188, Mailing Address: P.O. Box 188, Zip 39747–0188; tel. 662/262–4311 **A**9 10 **F**70 89 132 **P**8
Primary Contact: Calvin D. Johnson, Administrator
**Control:** County–Government, nonfederal **Service:** General Medical and Surgical

**Staffed Beds:** 19 **Admissions:** 251 **Census:** 2 **Outpatient Visits:** 0 **Births:** 0 **Personnel:** 44

## KOSCIUSKO—Attala County

**MONTFORT JONES MEMORIAL HOSPITAL (250059)**, 220 Highway 12 West, Zip 39090–3209, Mailing Address: P.O. Box 887, Zip 39090–0887; tel. 662/289–4311 **A**9 10 **F**3 15 17 35 39 40 42 43 45 56 64 65 70 81 89 90 103 107 108 114 117 118 129 132 144 147
Primary Contact: John Dawson, Chief Executive Officer
CFO: James Thomas, Chief Financial Officer
CIO: Jimmy Chesteen, Director Information Technology
CHR: Linnie Pearson, Coordinator Human Resources and Benefits
CNO: Allison Schuler, R.N., Chief Nursing Officer
Web address: www.montfortjones.com
**Control:** County–Government, nonfederal **Service:** General Medical and Surgical

**Staffed Beds:** 71 **Admissions:** 1898 **Census:** 22 **Outpatient Visits:** 17680 **Births:** 0 **Total Expense ($000):** 14329 **Payroll Expense ($000):** 5252 **Personnel:** 150

## LAUREL—Jones County

★ **SOUTH CENTRAL REGIONAL MEDICAL CENTER (250058)**, 1220 Jefferson Street, Zip 39440–4374, Mailing Address: P.O. Box 607, Zip 39441–0607; tel. 601/426–4000, (Total facility includes 244 beds in nursing home–type unit) **A**9 10 21 **F**3 4 7 10 13 15 17 18 20 28 29 30 31 34 35 37 40 43 48 49 51 53 56 57 59 62 63 64 68 70 73 74 75 76 77 78 79 81 84 85 86 87 89 90 92 93 100 102 103 105 108 110 111 113 116 117 118 126 127 129 130 131 133 142 143 145 146 **P**6
Primary Contact: G. Douglas Higginbotham, Executive Director
CFO: Tom Canizaro, Vice President and Chief Financial Officer
CMO: James Holston, M.D., Vice President and Chief Quality Officer
CIO: Linda Gavin, Associate Executive Director Marketing and Physician Recruitment
CHR: Janet Staples, Vice President Human Resources
CNO: Beth W. Endom, R.N., Vice President and Chief Nursing Officer
Web address: www.scrmc.com
**Control:** County–Government, nonfederal **Service:** General Medical and Surgical

**Staffed Beds:** 412 **Admissions:** 7939 **Census:** 320 **Outpatient Visits:** 73062 **Births:** 827 **Total Expense ($000):** 115535 **Payroll Expense ($000):** 66087 **Personnel:** 1572

**MS**

*Many Facility Codes have changed. Please refer to the AHA Guide Code Chart.* © 2012 AHA Guide

## LEAKESVILLE—Greene County

**GREENE COUNTY HOSPITAL (251329)**, 1017 Jackson Avenue,
Zip 39451–9105; tel. 601/394–4139 **A**10 18 **F**40 43 70 107 132
Primary Contact: Deborah Berry, Director of Operations
CFO: Debbie Brannan, Chief Financial Officer
CMO: Larry Henderson, M.D., Medical Director
CHR: Carla Shows, Payroll Clerk
Web address: www.georgeregional.com
**Control:** County–Government, nonfederal **Service:** General Medical and Surgical

**Staffed Beds:** 3 **Admissions:** 29 **Census:** 1 **Outpatient Visits:** 3177 **Births:** 0 **Personnel:** 52

## LEXINGTON—Holmes County

⊠ **HOLMES COUNTY HOSPITAL AND CLINICS (251319)**, 239 Bowling Green
Road, Zip 39095–5167; tel. 662/834–1321 **A**1 10 18 **F**3 11 15 29 34 35 40
43 45 50 56 57 59 64 65 70 86 87 89 93 103 107 108 113 118 126 129
132 134 145 **P**6
Primary Contact: Phillip L. Grady, Administrator
COO: Dewery Montgomery, Chief Operating Officer
CFO: Dan Janicak, Chief Financial Officer
CMO: Mark Smothers, M.D., Chief Medical Staff
CIO: Paula Pepper, Lan Administrator
CHR: Gloria Bordelon, Human Resources Generalist
**Control:** State–Government, nonfederal **Service:** General Medical and Surgical

**Staffed Beds:** 25 **Admissions:** 383 **Census:** 3 **Outpatient Visits:** 16057
**Births:** 0 **Total Expense ($000):** 8617 **Payroll Expense ($000):** 6437
**Personnel:** 111

## LOUISVILLE—Winston County

**DIAMOND GROVE CENTER FOR CHILDREN AND ADOLESCENTS**, 2311
Highway 15 South, Zip 39339, Mailing Address: P.O. Box 848, Zip 39339;
tel. 662/779–0119, (Total facility includes 30 beds in nursing home–type unit) **A**9
**F**35 38 86 87 98 99 100 101 102 129 145 **P**6 **S** Universal Health Services,
Inc., King of Prussia, PA
Primary Contact: Patrick R. Swoopes, Administrator
Web address: www.ccs.state.ms.us
**Control:** Corporation, Investor–owned, for–profit **Service:** Children's hospital
psychiatric

**Staffed Beds:** 55 **Admissions:** 424 **Census:** 51 **Outpatient Visits:** 0 **Births:** 0 **Total Expense ($000):** 6347 **Payroll Expense ($000):** 3615 **Personnel:** 75

**WINSTON MEDICAL CENTER (250027)**, 562 East Main Street,
Zip 39339–2742, Mailing Address: P.O. Box 967, Zip 39339–0967;
tel. 662/773–6211, (Total facility includes 120 beds in nursing home–type unit)
**A**9 10 20 **F**15 29 34 35 40 43 45 46 57 59 64 65 68 70 81 89 93 103 107
110 113 118 127 129 132 134 145 147
Primary Contact: Lee McCall, Administrator
Web address: www.winstonmedical.org
**Control:** Other not–for–profit (including NFP Corporation) **Service:** General
Medical and Surgical

**Staffed Beds:** 150 **Admissions:** 711 **Census:** 120 **Outpatient Visits:** 22171
**Births:** 0 **Total Expense ($000):** 10502 **Payroll Expense ($000):** 3415
**Personnel:** 193

## LUCEDALE—Jackson County

**GEORGE COUNTY HOSPITAL (250036)**, 859 Winter Street, Zip 39452–6603,
Mailing Address: P.O. Box 607, Zip 39452–0607; tel. 601/947–3161 **A**9 10 20
**F**13 15 17 35 40 43 53 70 76 81 86 87 93 107 108 111 118 129 132
145 **P**8
Primary Contact: Paul A. Gardner, CPA, Administrator
CFO: Debbie Brannan, Chief Financial Officer
CMO: Seth Scott, M.D., Chief of Staff
CHR: Carla Shows, Payroll Clerk
Web address: www.georgeregional.com
**Control:** County–Government, nonfederal **Service:** General Medical and Surgical

**Staffed Beds:** 48 **Admissions:** 1394 **Census:** 13 **Outpatient Visits:** 38465
**Births:** 17 **Personnel:** 346

## MACON—Noxubee County

**NOXUBEE GENERAL HOSPITAL (251307)**, 606 North Jefferson Street,
Zip 39341–2236, Mailing Address: P.O. Box 480, Zip 39341–0480;
tel. 662/726–4231, (Total facility includes 60 beds in nursing home–type unit) **A**9
10 18 **F**40 43 70 89 107 127 129 132
Primary Contact: Danny H. McKay, Administrator
Web address: www.noxubeemedical.com
**Control:** County–Government, nonfederal **Service:** General Medical and Surgical

**Staffed Beds:** 85 **Admissions:** 755 **Census:** 61 **Outpatient Visits:** 3859
**Births:** 0 **Personnel:** 177

## MAGEE—Simpson County

**MAGEE GENERAL HOSPITAL (250124)**, 300 Third Avenue, S.E.,
Zip 39111–3698; tel. 601/849–5070 **A**9 10 **F**13 15 40 43 70 76 81 89 93
107 108 111 118 129 132 145
Primary Contact: Althea H. Crumpton, Administrator
CFO: Melissa Bruntlett, Chief Financial Officer
CMO: Kelli Smith, M.D., Chief of Staff
CIO: Kirby Craft, Chief Information Officer
CHR: Steve Beckham, Director Human Resources
CNO: Cindy McIntyre, R.N., Administrative Director Clinical Services
Web address: www.mghosp.org
**Control:** Other not–for–profit (including NFP Corporation) **Service:** General
Medical and Surgical

**Staffed Beds:** 61 **Admissions:** 1640 **Census:** 18 **Outpatient Visits:** 76153
**Births:** 224 **Personnel:** 302

## MAGNOLIA—Pike County

★ **BEACHAM MEMORIAL HOSPITAL (250049)**, 205 North Cherry Street,
Zip 39652–2819, Mailing Address: P.O. Box 351, Zip 39652–0351;
tel. 601/783–2351 **A**9 10 **F**3 34 35 59 65 68 70 107 113 126 129 132 145
Primary Contact: Guy Geller, Administrator and Chief Executive Officer
CMO: Lucius Lampton, M.D., Medical Director
CHR: Jackie McKenzie, Director Administrative Services
Web address: www.beachammemhos.com
**Control:** Other not–for–profit (including NFP Corporation) **Service:** General
Medical and Surgical

**Staffed Beds:** 37 **Admissions:** 954 **Census:** 15 **Outpatient Visits:** 0 **Births:** 0 **Total Expense ($000):** 6468 **Payroll Expense ($000):** 3148 **Personnel:** 106

## MARKS—Quitman County

**QUITMAN COUNTY HOSPITAL (251314)**, 340 Getwell Drive, Zip 38646–9785;
tel. 662/326–8031 **A**9 10 18 **F**40 43 56 70 89 107 118 132
Primary Contact: Stephen Nichols, Chief Executive Officer
CFO: Jane Moore, Director, Fiscal Services
CMO: James E. Warrington, Sr., M.D., Chief of Staff
CHR: Sandra Biffle, Personnel Clerk
CNO: Dana Hall, Director of Nursing
**Control:** Corporation, Investor–owned, for–profit **Service:** General Medical and
Surgical

**Staffed Beds:** 33 **Admissions:** 716 **Census:** 10 **Outpatient Visits:** 8307
**Births:** 0 **Personnel:** 88

## MCCOMB—Pike County

★ **SOUTHWEST MISSISSIPPI REGIONAL MEDICAL CENTER (250097)**, 215
Marion Avenue, Zip 39648–2798, Mailing Address: P.O. Box 1307,
Zip 39649–1307; tel. 601/249–5500 **A**9 10 19 21 **F**3 13 15 17 18 20 22 24
28 29 30 31 34 38 39 40 41 42 43 45 47 48 49 51 53 57 59 64 65 68 70
72 73 74 75 76 77 78 79 81 85 86 87 89 91 93 96 107 108 109 110 111
112 113 114 117 118 119 120 126 128 129 130 131 134 144 145 **P**6
**S** Southwest Health Systems, Mccomb, MS
Primary Contact: Norman M. Price, FACHE, Chief Executive Officer
COO: Richard Williams, Chief Operating Officer
CFO: Reece Nunnery, Chief Financial Officer
CMO: Kevin Richardson, M.D., Chief of Staff
CIO: Mike Moak, Chief Information Officer
CHR: Don Haskins, Administrative Director Human Resources
CNO: Katie McKinley, Assistant Administrator/Nursing
Web address: www.smrmc.com
**Control:** Hospital district or authority, Government, nonfederal **Service:** General
Medical and Surgical

**Staffed Beds:** 143 **Admissions:** 7061 **Census:** 65 **Outpatient Visits:** 63297
**Births:** 938 **Total Expense ($000):** 64247 **Payroll Expense ($000):** 48969
**Personnel:** 970

**MS**

---

**Hospital, Medicare Provider Number, Address, Telephone, Approval, Facility, and Physician Codes, Health Care System**

★ American Hospital Association (AHA) membership
□ The Joint Commission accreditation  ◇ DNV Healthcare Inc. accreditation
○ American Osteopathic Association (AOA) accreditation
△ Commission on Accreditation of Rehabilitation Facilities (CARF) accreditation

---

## MEADVILLE—Franklin County

**FRANKLIN COUNTY MEMORIAL HOSPITAL (251330)**, 40 Union Church Road,
Zip 39653–8336, Mailing Address: P.O. Box 636, Zip 39653–0636;
tel. 601/384–5801 **A**9 10 **F**29 35 40 43 56 70 81 86 89 93 98 103 107 118
129 132 142 **P**6
Primary Contact: W. P. Dickey, Jr., Chief Executive Officer
Web address: www.fcmh.net
**Control:** County–Government, nonfederal **Service:** General Medical and Surgical

**Staffed Beds:** 34 **Admissions:** 571 **Census:** 10 **Outpatient Visits:** 25054
**Births:** 0 **Personnel:** 206

## MENDENHALL—Simpson County

★ **SIMPSON GENERAL HOSPITAL (251317)**, 1842 Simpson Highway 149,
Zip 39114–3592; tel. 601/847–2221 **A**9 10 18 **F**35 40 53 56 61 70 81 86 87
90 98 103 106 107 118 129 131 132 133 145 **P**5 7
Primary Contact: Randall Neely, Chief Executive Officer
COO: Al Gary, COO
CFO: Al Gary, COO
CMO: Chip Holbrook, M.D., Chief of Staff
CIO: David Welch, Director Information Technology
CHR: Randall Neely, CEO
CNO: Sharon Burnham, Director of Nursing
Web address: www.simpsongeneralhospital.com
**Control:** Other not–for–profit (including NFP Corporation) **Service:** General
Medical and Surgical

**Staffed Beds:** 35 **Admissions:** 756 **Census:** 10 **Outpatient Visits:** 9540
**Births:** 0 **Personnel:** 85

## MERIDIAN—Lauderdale County

☐ **ALLIANCE HEALTH CENTER (250151)**, 5000 Highway 39 North,
Zip 39301–1021; tel. 601/483–6211 **A**1 9 10 **F**4 35 70 86 87 98 99 100 101
103 **P**6 **S** Universal Health Services, Inc., King of Prussia, PA
Primary Contact: William M. Patterson, Chief Executive Officer
CFO: Robert Jackson, Chief Financial Officer
CMO: Terry Jordan, M.D., Chief of Staff
CIO: Brenda Smith, Director Financial Services
CHR: Shrea Johnson, Director Human Resources
Web address: www.alliancehealthcenter.com
**Control:** Corporation, Investor–owned, for–profit **Service:** Psychiatric

**Staffed Beds:** 134 **Admissions:** 2443 **Census:** 78 **Outpatient Visits:** 0
**Births:** 0 **Personnel:** 286

⊞ **ANDERSON REGIONAL MEDICAL CENTER (250104)**, 2124 14th Street,
Zip 39301–4040; tel. 601/553–6000 **A**1 2 9 10 19 **F**13 15 17 35 39 40 43
53 70 72 73 75 76 77 78 80 81 86 87 88 89 90 93 98 107 108 115 117
118 129 130 131 145 **P**7 8
Primary Contact: L. Ray Humphreys, Chief Executive Officer
CFO: Anthony C. Rispoli, Vice President Finance
CHR: Irby Lang, Vice President Human Resources
Web address: www.jarmc.org
**Control:** Other not–for–profit (including NFP Corporation) **Service:** General
Medical and Surgical

**Staffed Beds:** 260 **Admissions:** 9453 **Census:** 136 **Outpatient Visits:** 99677
**Births:** 1327 **Personnel:** 1183

☐ △ **ANDERSON REGIONAL MEDICAL CENTER–SOUTH CAMPUS (250081)**,
1102 Constitution Avenue, Zip 39301–4001; tel. 601/693–2511, (Data for 273
days) **A**1 7 9 10 **F**4 15 17 29 35 60 61 70 75 77 78 81 82 86 87 90 93 97
98 107 108 117 118 129 131 143 145 146 **P**7 8
Primary Contact: Ray Humphreys, Chief Executive Officer
CFO: Anthony C. Rispoli, Vice President Finance
CMO: Bradley Boone, M.D., Chief Medical Staff
CHR: Jamie Shuster, Director Associate Relations
Web address: www.jarmc.org
**Control:** Other not–for–profit (including NFP Corporation) **Service:** General
Medical and Surgical

**Staffed Beds:** 140 **Admissions:** 1664 **Census:** 36 **Outpatient Visits:** 27917
**Births:** 101 **Personnel:** 339

**EAST MISSISSIPPI STATE HOSPITAL**, 4555 Highland Park Drive,
Zip 39307–5498, Mailing Address: Box 4128, West Station, Zip 39304–4128;
tel. 601/482–6186 **F**4 10 11 29 30 32 38 44 50 56 59 87 98 99 101 103
127 129 145 **S** Mississippi State Department of Mental Health, Jackson, MS
Primary Contact: Charles Carlisle, Director
CFO: Geri Rutledge, Director Business
CMO: Gloria Gomez, M.D., Medical Director
CIO: Susie Broadhead, Director Public Information
CHR: Shearmaine Calaway, Director Human Resources
Web address: www.emsh.state.ms.us
**Control:** State–Government, nonfederal **Service:** Psychiatric

**Staffed Beds:** 327 **Admissions:** 1095 **Census:** 311 **Outpatient Visits:** 0
**Births:** 0 **Personnel:** 1075

⊞ **REGENCY HOSPITAL OF MERIDIAN (252006)**, 1102 Constitution Avenue, 2nd
Floor, Zip 39301–4001; tel. 601/484–7900 **A**1 10 **F**40 70 **S** Select Medical
Corporation, Mechanicsburg, PA
Primary Contact: Clifton Quinn, Chief Executive Officer
Web address: www.regencyhospital.com
**Control:** Corporation, Investor–owned, for–profit **Service:** Long–Term Acute Care
hospital

**Staffed Beds:** 40 **Admissions:** 402 **Census:** 29 **Outpatient Visits:** 0 **Births:**
0 **Personnel:** 106

**RILEY HOSPITAL** See Anderson Regional Medical Center–South Campus

★ **RUSH FOUNDATION HOSPITAL (250069)**, 1314 19th Avenue,
Zip 39301–4195; tel. 601/483–0011 **A**9 10 19 21 **F**13 15 17 29 35 39 40 43
70 72 73 76 77 81 82 86 89 90 93 97 107 108 117 118 129 130 145 146
**P**3 8 **S** Rush Health Systems, Meridian, MS
Primary Contact: Christopher Rush, Vice President and Administrator
COO: Morris A. Reece, Executive Vice President and Chief Operating Officer
CMO: W. Scot Bell, M.D., Chief Medical Officer
CIO: Angela Sherrill, Corporate Director Information System
CHR: Donnie Smith, Director Human Resources
Web address: www.rushhealthsystems.org
**Control:** Other not–for–profit (including NFP Corporation) **Service:** General
Medical and Surgical

**Staffed Beds:** 182 **Admissions:** 5817 **Census:** 74 **Outpatient Visits:** 22524
**Births:** 790 **Personnel:** 820

★ **SPECIALTY HOSPITAL OF MERIDIAN (252004)**, 1314 19th Avenue,
Zip 39301–4116; tel. 601/703–4211 **A**10 **F**70 78 87 132 143 **S** Rush Health
Systems, Meridian, MS
Primary Contact: Elizabeth C. Mitchell, Vice President and Administrator
CFO: Lexie Fuller, Controller
CMO: Richmond Alexander, M.D., President Medical Staff
CIO: Angela Sherrill, Corporate Director Information System
Web address: www.rushhealthsystems.org
**Control:** Other not–for–profit (including NFP Corporation) **Service:** Long–Term
Acute Care hospital

**Staffed Beds:** 49 **Admissions:** 473 **Census:** 48 **Outpatient Visits:** 0 **Births:**
0 **Personnel:** 300

## MONTICELLO—Lawrence County

**LAWRENCE COUNTY HOSPITAL (251305)**, Highway 84 East,
Zip 39654–0788, Mailing Address: P.O. Box 788, Zip 39654–0788;
tel. 601/587–4051 **A**10 18 **F**3 34 39 40 43 57 59 64 70 87 107 113 126
129 132 134 **S** Southwest Health Systems, Mccomb, MS
Primary Contact: Semmes Ross, Jr., Administrator
CFO: Jennifer Moak, Business Office Manager
Web address: www.smrmc.com
**Control:** County–Government, nonfederal **Service:** General Medical and Surgical

**Staffed Beds:** 25 **Admissions:** 299 **Census:** 3 **Outpatient Visits:** 10220
**Births:** 0 **Total Expense ($000):** 4504 **Payroll Expense ($000):** 4426
**Personnel:** 123

## MORTON—Scott County

★ **SCOTT REGIONAL HOSPITAL (251323)**, 317 Highway 13 South,
Zip 39117–3353, Mailing Address: P.O. Box 259, Zip 39117–0259;
tel. 601/732–6301 **A**9 10 18 **F**3 30 34 35 40 42 43 45 57 68 70 77 81 89
93 107 111 118 128 129 132 134 **S** Rush Health Systems, Meridian, MS
Primary Contact: Michael R. Edwards, Chief Executive Officer
CFO: Paul S. Black, Chief Financial Officer
CHR: Amy Sugg, Director Human Resources
Web address: www.rushhealthsystems.org
**Control:** Other not–for–profit (including NFP Corporation) **Service:** General
Medical and Surgical

**Staffed Beds:** 25 **Admissions:** 911 **Census:** 9 **Outpatient Visits:** 13920
**Births:** 0 **Total Expense ($000):** 11097 **Payroll Expense ($000):** 4167
**Personnel:** 102

## NATCHEZ—Adams County

☐ **NATCHEZ COMMUNITY HOSPITAL (250122)**, 129 Jefferson Davis Boulevard,
Zip 39120–5100, Mailing Address: P.O. Box 1203, Zip 39121–1203;
tel. 601/445–6200 **A**1 9 10 **F**13 17 29 35 40 43 51 60 61 70 73 76 78 81
82 87 89 93 107 108 118 129 145 **P**6 **S** Health Management Associates,
Naples, FL
Primary Contact: Donald Rentfro, Chief Executive Officer
CFO: Warren Ladner, Chief Financial Officer
CHR: Hal Harrington, Director Human Resources
Web address: www.natchezcommunityhospital.com/default.aspx
**Control:** Partnership, Investor–owned, for–profit **Service:** General Medical and
Surgical

**Staffed Beds:** 101 **Admissions:** 4325 **Census:** 48 **Outpatient Visits:** 34948
**Births:** 506 **Personnel:** 277

*Many Facility Codes have changed. Please refer to the AHA Guide Code Chart.*

△ **NATCHEZ REGIONAL MEDICAL CENTER (250084)**, 54 Seargent S Prentiss Drive, Zip 39120–4726; tel. 601/443–2100 **A**7 9 10 **F**13 15 17 29 35 40 43 60 70 73 75 76 77 78 81 82 86 87 88 89 90 93 103 107 108 111 115 118 129 130 131 133 145 146 **P**3
Primary Contact: William R. Heburn, Chief Executive Officer
CFO: Charles Mack, Vice President Finance and Chief Financial Officer
CMO: John O'Brien, M.D., Chief of Staff
CIO: Walt Roddy, Director Information Management Systems
CHR: Sherri L. Clifton–LeMay, Director Human Resources
Web address: www.natchezregional.com
**Control:** County–Government, nonfederal **Service:** General Medical and Surgical

**Staffed Beds:** 155 **Admissions:** 3350 **Census:** 41 **Outpatient Visits:** 26879 **Births:** 472 **Personnel:** 297

**NEW ALBANY—Union County**

⊞ **BAPTIST MEMORIAL HOSPITAL–UNION COUNTY (250006)**, 200 State Highway 30 West, Zip 38652–3112; tel. 662/538–7631 **A**1 9 10 **F**13 15 17 29 35 39 40 51 53 70 75 76 77 81 86 87 89 90 93 107 108 111 118 129 131 132 145 146 **S** Baptist Memorial Health Care Corporation, Memphis, TN
Primary Contact: Walter Grace, Chief Executive Officer and Administrator
CFO: Kim High, Chief Financial Officer
CMO: Justin Lohmeier, M.D., Chief of Staff
CIO: Missy Coltharp, Director
CHR: Lori Goode, Director Human Resources
CNO: Randy White, Chief Nursing Officer
Web address: www.bmhcc.org
**Control:** Other not–for–profit (including NFP Corporation) **Service:** General Medical and Surgical

**Staffed Beds:** 153 **Admissions:** 4077 **Census:** 37 **Outpatient Visits:** 44906 **Births:** 1124 **Personnel:** 443

**NEWTON—Newton County**

**NEWTON REGIONAL HOSPITAL** See Pioneer Community Hospital of Newton

★ **PIONEER COMMUNITY HOSPITAL OF NEWTON (251332)**, 9421 Eastside Drive, Zip 39345–0299; tel. 601/683–2031 **A**9 10 18 21 **F**3 8 11 29 30 34 35 39 40 42 43 53 54 57 59 64 65 70 77 81 90 93 98 103 107 111 113 118 126 129 132 134 145 **P**6 **S** Pioneer Health Services, Magee, MS
Primary Contact: Mark Norman, Administrator
CFO: Julie Gieger, Chief Financial Officer
CMO: Sohaib Arair, M.D., Chairman of Medical Staff
CIO: Eric Two Bears, Chief Information Officer
CHR: Tracy Rushing, Executive Assistant Human Resources and Payroll
CNO: Christie Malbrough, Director of Nursing
Web address: www.pchnewton.com
**Control:** Corporation, Investor–owned, for–profit **Service:** General Medical and Surgical

**Staffed Beds:** 30 **Admissions:** 790 **Census:** 10 **Outpatient Visits:** 10893 **Births:** 0 **Total Expense ($000):** 10886 **Payroll Expense ($000):** 5271 **Personnel:** 99

**OCEAN SPRINGS—Jackson County**

**OCEAN SPRINGS HOSPITAL** See Singing River Health System, Pascagoula

**OLIVE BRANCH—Desoto County**

☐ **PARKWOOD BEHAVIORAL HEALTH SYSTEM (254005)**, 8135 Goodman Road, Zip 38654–2103; tel. 662/895–4900, (Total facility includes 40 beds in nursing home–type unit) **A**1 9 10 **F**4 5 29 34 35 38 42 54 57 65 75 82 86 87 98 99 100 101 102 104 105 129 **P**5 **S** Universal Health Services, Inc., King of Prussia, PA
Primary Contact: Ethan Permenter, Chief Executive Officer
CFO: Sandra Wallace, Chief Financial Officer
CMO: Paul King, M.D., Medical Director
CHR: Audrey Johnson, Director Human Resources
CNO: Alicia Plunkett, Director of Nursing
Web address: www.parkwoodbhs.com
**Control:** Corporation, Investor–owned, for–profit **Service:** Psychiatric

**Staffed Beds:** 128 **Admissions:** 2200 **Census:** 91 **Outpatient Visits:** 0 **Births:** 0 **Total Expense ($000):** 15803 **Payroll Expense ($000):** 7814 **Personnel:** 202

**OXFORD—Lafayette County**

⊞ △ **BAPTIST MEMORIAL HOSPITAL–NORTH MISSISSIPPI (250034)**, 2301 South Lamar Boulevard, Zip 38655–5373, Mailing Address: P.O. Box 946, Zip 38655–6002; tel. 662/232–8100 **A**1 2 7 9 10 19 **F**13 15 17 29 35 39 40 43 53 70 73 76 78 81 86 87 89 90 107 108 111 115 117 118 129 130 131 145 146 **S** Baptist Memorial Health Care Corporation, Memphis, TN
Primary Contact: Donald Hutson, Administrator and Chief Executive Officer
CFO: Dana Williams, Assistant Administrator and Chief Financial Officer
CMO: Brett Lampton, M.D., Chief of Staff
CIO: Linda Britt, Director Information Systems
CHR: Dennis Fisher, Director Human Resources
Web address: www.bmhcc.org
**Control:** Other not–for–profit (including NFP Corporation) **Service:** General Medical and Surgical

**Staffed Beds:** 217 **Admissions:** 7950 **Census:** 106 **Outpatient Visits:** 66225 **Births:** 900 **Personnel:** 981

**PASCAGOULA—Jackson County**

⊞ △ **SINGING RIVER HEALTH SYSTEM (250040)**, 2809 Denny Avenue, Zip 39581–5301; tel. 228/809–5000, (Includes OCEAN SPRINGS HOSPITAL, 3109 Bienville Boulevard, Ocean Springs, Zip 39564–4361; tel. 228/818–1111; Heath Thompson, R.N., Administrator; SINGING RIVER HOSPITAL, 2809 Denny Avenue, tel. 228/809–5000; Davis Walton, Administrator) **A**1 2 7 9 10 **F**13 15 17 30 39 40 43 53 61 70 73 76 78 80 81 82 86 87 89 90 98 100 101 102 103 104 107 108 111 117 118
Primary Contact: Chris Anderson, Chief Executive Officer
COO: Kevin Holland, Chief Operating Officer
CFO: Michael E. Crews, Chief Financial Officer
CMO: Larry D. Shoemaker, M.D., Chief Medical Officer
CIO: Chris Oubre, Director Information Systems
CHR: Nebo Carter, Chief Human Resources Officer
Web address: www.mysrhs.com
**Control:** County–Government, nonfederal **Service:** General Medical and Surgical

**Staffed Beds:** 381 **Admissions:** 18824 **Census:** 220 **Outpatient Visits:** 445371 **Births:** 1628 **Personnel:** 2559

**PHILADELPHIA—Neshoba County**

☐ **CHOCTAW HEALTH CENTER (250127)**, 210 Hospital Circle, Zip 39350–6781; tel. 601/656–2211 **A**1 9 10 **F**35 40 70 77 107 118 129 132
Primary Contact: Gary Ben, Administrator
CFO: Donita Stephens, Director Financial Services
CMO: Chandrashekhar V. Joshi, M.D., Chief of Staff
CIO: Charlene Sam, Manager Health Information
CHR: Linda McMillan, Human Resources Specialist
Web address: www.choctaw.org
**Control:** Corporation, Investor–owned, for–profit **Service:** General Medical and Surgical

**Staffed Beds:** 25 **Admissions:** 122 **Census:** 1 **Outpatient Visits:** 7320 **Births:** 0 **Personnel:** 130

**NESHOBA COUNTY GENERAL HOSPITAL (250043)**, 1001 Holland Avenue, Zip 39350–2161, Mailing Address: P.O. Box 648, Zip 39350–0648; tel. 601/663–1200, (Total facility includes 160 beds in nursing home–type unit) **A**9 10 20 **F**3 6 7 11 15 29 34 35 40 43 45 57 59 64 70 77 81 85 87 89 90 93 103 107 108 111 113 118 126 127 129 131 132 142 143 145
Primary Contact: Lawrence Graeber, Chief Executive Officer
CFO: Calvin J. Brummund, Interim Chief Financial Officer
CMO: Walt Willis, M.D., Medical Director
CHR: Hedda Stewart, Director Human Resources
Web address: www.neshobageneral.com
**Control:** County–Government, nonfederal **Service:** General Medical and Surgical

**Staffed Beds:** 208 **Admissions:** 1133 **Census:** 175 **Outpatient Visits:** 65114 **Births:** 0 **Total Expense ($000):** 27500 **Payroll Expense ($000):** 20717 **Personnel:** 457

**PICAYUNE—Pearl River County**

**HIGHLAND COMMUNITY HOSPITAL (250117)**, 801 Goodyear Boulevard, Zip 39466–3221, Mailing Address: P.O. Box 909, Zip 39466–0909; tel. 601/798–4711 **A**9 10 **F**12 13 15 18 29 40 43 45 70 74 75 76 81 86 87 89 93 107 108 111 113 118 129 130 134 145 146
Primary Contact: Mark Stockstill, R.N., Administrator
CFO: Bryan N. Stevens, Chief Financial Officer
CHR: Josh Lowery, Director Human Resources
CNO: MaryBeth Cooper, R.N., Chief Nursing Officer
Web address: www.highlandch.com
**Control:** County–Government, nonfederal **Service:** General Medical and Surgical

**Staffed Beds:** 55 **Admissions:** 2095 **Census:** 16 **Outpatient Visits:** 39297 **Births:** 262 **Total Expense ($000):** 20816 **Payroll Expense ($000):** 13245 **Personnel:** 257

**MS**

**Hospital, Medicare Provider Number, Address, Telephone, Approval, Facility, and Physician Codes, Health Care System**

★ American Hospital Association (AHA) membership
☐ The Joint Commission accreditation ◇ DNV Healthcare Inc. accreditation

○ American Osteopathic Association (AOA) accreditation
△ Commission on Accreditation of Rehabilitation Facilities (CARF) accreditation

**PONTOTOC—Pontotoc County**

⊠ **NORTH MISSISSIPPI MEDICAL CENTER–PONTOTOC HOSPITAL AND NURSING HOME (251308)**, 176 South Main Street, Zip 38863–3311, Mailing Address: P.O. Box 790, Zip 38863–0790; tel. 662/488–7640, (Total facility includes 44 beds in nursing home–type unit) **A**1 9 10 18 **F**35 40 43 70 82 86 87 90 107 118 127 129 132 145 **S** North Mississippi Health Services, Inc., Tupelo, MS
Primary Contact: Fred B. Hood, FACHE, Administrator
CFO: M. Denise Heard, Director Business Services
CHR: P. Marie Barnes, Director, Human Resources
CNO: Cathy Waldrop, Director, Hospital Nursing Services
Web address: www.nmhs.net
**Control:** Other not-for-profit (including NFP Corporation) **Service:** General Medical and Surgical

**Staffed Beds:** 69 **Admissions:** 523 **Census:** 49 **Outpatient Visits:** 17551 **Births:** 0 **Personnel:** 161

**POPLARVILLE—Pearl River County**

**PEARL RIVER COUNTY HOSPITAL (251333)**, 305 West Moody Street, Zip 39470–7242, Mailing Address: P.O. Box 392, Zip 39470–0392; tel. 601/795–4543, (Total facility includes 126 beds in nursing home–type unit) **A**9 10 **F**35 40 43 70 107 118 127 129 132 142 145
Primary Contact: Mike Boleware, Administrator
**Control:** County–Government, nonfederal **Service:** General Medical and Surgical

**Staffed Beds:** 150 **Admissions:** 239 **Census:** 90 **Outpatient Visits:** 0 **Births:** 0 **Personnel:** 290

**PORT GIBSON—Claiborne County**

☐ **PATIENT'S CHOICE MEDICAL CENTER OF CLAIBORNE COUNTY (251320)**, 123 McComb Avenue, Zip 39150–2915, Mailing Address: P.O. Box 1004, Zip 39150–1004; tel. 601/437–5141 **A**1 9 10 18 **F**3 34 40 42 43 64 70 89 90 98 103 118 126 129 132
Primary Contact: William Cockrell, Administrator and Chief Executive Officer
CFO: Linda Caho–Mooney, Chief Financial Officer
CIO: Ada Ratliff, Chief Information Officer
Web address: www.claibornehospital.net/
**Control:** Corporation, Investor–owned, for–profit **Service:** General Medical and Surgical

**Staffed Beds:** 32 **Admissions:** 761 **Census:** 11 **Outpatient Visits:** 5082 **Births:** 0 **Total Expense ($000):** 6505 **Payroll Expense ($000):** 3942 **Personnel:** 171

**PRENTISS—Jefferson Davis County**

**JEFFERSON DAVIS COMMUNITY HOSPITAL (251326)**, 1102 Rose Street, Zip 39474, Mailing Address: P.O. Box 1288, Zip 39474; tel. 601/792–4276, (Total facility includes 60 beds in nursing home–type unit) **A**9 10 18 **F**35 40 43 53 56 70 86 87 89 90 93 98 103 107 111 118 127 129 131 132
Primary Contact: Charles Phillips, Chief Executive Officer
CFO: Paul S. Black, Chief Financial Officer
CHR: Diane Daughdrill, Director Human Resources
Web address: www.jdchospital.com
**Control:** County–Government, nonfederal **Service:** General Medical and Surgical

**Staffed Beds:** 95 **Admissions:** 522 **Census:** 67 **Outpatient Visits:** 11553 **Births:** 0 **Total Expense ($000):** 11384 **Payroll Expense ($000):** 4663 **Personnel:** 118

**PURVIS—Lamar County**

☐ **SOUTH MISSISSIPPI STATE HOSPITAL (254008)**, 823 Highway 589, Zip 39475–4194; tel. 601/794–0100 **A**1 10 **F**98 129 145 **S** Mississippi State Department of Mental Health, Jackson, MS
Primary Contact: Clint Ashley, Director
Web address: www.smsh.state.ms.us
**Control:** State–Government, nonfederal **Service:** Psychiatric

**Staffed Beds:** 50 **Admissions:** 546 **Census:** 44 **Outpatient Visits:** 0 **Births:** 0 **Personnel:** 94

**QUITMAN—Clarke County**

★ **H. C. WATKINS MEMORIAL HOSPITAL (251316)**, 605 South Archusa Avenue, Zip 39355–2331; tel. 601/776–6925 **A**9 10 18 **F**29 40 43 70 80 81 89 107 111 127 132 **S** Rush Health Systems, Meridian, MS
Primary Contact: Clinton Eaves, Administrator
CFO: Paul S. Black, Controller
CMO: O. Wayne Byrd, M.D., Chief of Staff
CIO: Melinda Smith, Chief Information Systems
CHR: Leigh Moore, Administrative Assistant Human Resources
Web address: www.rushhealthsystems.org/hcw/
**Control:** Other not-for-profit (including NFP Corporation) **Service:** General Medical and Surgical

**Staffed Beds:** 25 **Admissions:** 456 **Census:** 5 **Outpatient Visits:** 6707 **Births:** 0 **Personnel:** 118

**RICHTON—Perry County**

**PERRY COUNTY GENERAL HOSPITAL (251306)**, 206 Bay Avenue, Zip 39476; tel. 601/788–6316 **A**9 10 18 **F**40 43 70 75 107 118 132
Primary Contact: David Paris, Chief Executive Officer
Web address: www.pcghospital.com/
**Control:** Partnership, Investor–owned, for–profit **Service:** General Medical and Surgical

**Staffed Beds:** 22 **Admissions:** 180 **Census:** 2 **Outpatient Visits:** 2700 **Births:** 0 **Personnel:** 61

**RIPLEY—Tippah County**

⊠ **TIPPAH COUNTY HOSPITAL (250010)**, 1005 City Avenue North, Zip 38663–0499, Mailing Address: P.O. Box 499, Zip 38663–0499; tel. 601/837–9221, (Total facility includes 40 beds in nursing home–type unit) **A**1 9 10 20 **F**15 29 40 43 53 56 70 81 93 107 118 127 129 132 **P**1 **S** QHR, Brentwood, TN
Primary Contact: Tom Hood, Administrator
CFO: Charles Knight, Chief Financial Officer
CMO: Charles M. Elliott, M.D., Chief of Staff
CHR: Margaret Weeks, Manager Personnel
Web address: www.tippahcounty.ripley.ms/hospital.html
**Control:** County–Government, nonfederal **Service:** General Medical and Surgical

**Staffed Beds:** 85 **Admissions:** 968 **Census:** 50 **Outpatient Visits:** 16159 **Births:** 0 **Personnel:** 192

**ROLLING FORK—Sharkey County**

**SHARKEY–ISSAQUENA COMMUNITY HOSPITAL (250079)**, 108 South Fourth Street, Zip 39159–2612, Mailing Address: P.O. Box 339, Zip 39159–0339; tel. 662/873–4396 **A**9 10 **F**40 53 56 70 89 103 107 111 118 132
Primary Contact: Jerry Keever, Administrator
**Control:** County–Government, nonfederal **Service:** General Medical and Surgical

**Staffed Beds:** 29 **Admissions:** 431 **Census:** 6 **Outpatient Visits:** 2527 **Births:** 0 **Personnel:** 70

**RULEVILLE—Sunflower County**

★ **NORTH SUNFLOWER MEDICAL CENTER (251318)**, 840 North Oak Avenue, Zip 38771–0369, Mailing Address: P.O. Box 369, Zip 38771–0369; tel. 662/756–2711, (Total facility includes 60 beds in nursing home–type unit) **A**9 10 18 **F**3 8 15 29 30 32 34 35 39 40 42 43 45 53 56 57 59 62 64 70 75 77 81 82 87 90 93 97 103 107 108 113 117 118 126 127 128 129 131 132 133 134 142 147 **P**6
Primary Contact: Billy Marlow, Administrator/CEO
COO: Sam Miller, Chief Operating Officer
CFO: Charlotte Sherwood, Chief Financial Officer
CMO: Vicente Luciano, M.D., Chief of Staff
CIO: Roger Goss, Director, Information Services
CHR: Robbie Taylor, Director Human Resources
CNO: Lisa Miller, R.N., Director of Nursing
Web address: www.northsunflower.com
**Control:** County–Government, nonfederal **Service:** General Medical and Surgical

**Staffed Beds:** 95 **Admissions:** 897 **Census:** 73 **Outpatient Visits:** 20553 **Births:** 0 **Total Expense ($000):** 29718 **Payroll Expense ($000):** 16505 **Personnel:** 336

**SENATOBIA—Tate County**

☐ **NORTH OAK REGIONAL MEDICAL CENTER (250126)**, 401 Getwell Drive, Zip 38668–2213, Mailing Address: P.O. Box 648, Zip 38668–0648; tel. 662/562–3100 **A**1 9 10 **F**3 29 34 35 40 43 45 56 57 64 70 81 86 89 98 103 107 113 118 129
Primary Contact: Sonja Graham, Chief Executive Officer
CMO: Pravinchandra Patel, M.D., Chief Medical Officer
CHR: Vickie Barksdale, Manager Human Resources
Web address: www.normc.org
**Control:** Corporation, Investor–owned, for–profit **Service:** General Medical and Surgical

**Staffed Beds:** 55 **Admissions:** 1266 **Census:** 17 **Outpatient Visits:** 12247 **Births:** 0 **Total Expense ($000):** 12392 **Payroll Expense ($000):** 5256 **Personnel:** 111

**SOUTHAVEN—Desoto County**

⊠ △ **BAPTIST MEMORIAL HOSPITAL–DESOTO (250141)**, 7601 Southcrest Parkway, Zip 38671–4742; tel. 662/772–4000 **A**1 7 9 10 **F**13 15 17 29 35 40 43 51 63 61 70 73 75 76 77 78 80 81 82 86 87 90 93 107 108 111 115 117 118 129 130 131 142 143 145 146 **S** Baptist Memorial Health Care Corporation, Memphis, TN
Primary Contact: James Huffman, Chief Executive Officer and Administrator
CFO: Kimberly Young, Chief Financial Officer
CHR: Walter Banks, Director Human Resources
Web address: www.bmhcc.org
**Control:** Other not-for-profit (including NFP Corporation) **Service:** General Medical and Surgical

**Staffed Beds:** 249 **Admissions:** 16386 **Census:** 204 **Outpatient Visits:** 102411 **Births:** 2043 **Personnel:** 1650

*Many Facility Codes have changed. Please refer to the AHA Guide Code Chart.* © 2012 AHA Guide

**MS**

**STARKVILLE—Oktibbeha County**

★ **OCH REGIONAL MEDICAL CENTER (250050)**, 400 Hospital Road, Zip 39759–2163, Mailing Address: P.O. Box 1506, Zip 39760–1506; tel. 662/323–4320 **A**9 10 21 **F**3 7 11 13 15 17 28 29 32 34 35 39 40 42 43 45 48 51 53 57 59 61 64 65 66 70 73 74 75 76 77 79 81 82 85 86 88 89 90 93 97 98 107 108 110 111 112 113 114 117 118 126 128 129 130 131 132 133 134 145 147 **P**6
Primary Contact: Arthur C. Kelly, Administrator and Chief Executive Officer
COO: Mike Andrews, Assistant Administrator and Chief Operating Officer
CFO: Richard G. Hilton, Associate Administrator and Chief Financial Officer
CIO: Chamath Wijewardane, Director Information Technology
CHR: Mike Andrews, Assistant Administrator and Chief Operating Officer
Web address: www.och.org
**Control:** County–Government, nonfederal **Service:** General Medical and Surgical

**Staffed Beds:** 96 **Admissions:** 3101 **Census:** 32 **Outpatient Visits:** 198224 **Births:** 952 **Total Expense ($000):** 51321 **Payroll Expense ($000):** 30866 **Personnel:** 580

**TUPELO—Lee County**

✖ △ **NORTH MISSISSIPPI MEDICAL CENTER – TUPELO (250004)**, 830 South Gloster Street, Zip 38801–4934; tel. 662/377–3000, (Total facility includes 107 beds in nursing home–type unit) **A**1 2 3 5 7 9 10 19 **F**4 5 13 15 17 29 35 40 43 51 53 56 61 62 63 69 70 72 73 75 76 77 78 80 81 86 87 88 89 90 93 97 98 100 101 103 104 107 108 111 115 117 118 127 129 130 131 133 145 146 **S** North Mississippi Health Services, Inc., Tupelo, MS
Primary Contact: Steve Altmiller, President and Chief Executive Officer
CIO: Tom Bozeman, Chief Information Officer
CHR: Rodger Brown, Vice President Human Resources
Web address: www.nmhs.net
**Control:** Other not–for–profit (including NFP Corporation) **Service:** General Medical and Surgical

**Staffed Beds:** 757 **Admissions:** 24812 **Census:** 454 **Outpatient Visits:** 221683 **Births:** 2073 **Personnel:** 3876

☐ **NORTH MISSISSIPPI STATE HOSPITAL (254009)**, 1937 Briar Ridge Road, Zip 38804; tel. 662/690–4200 **A**1 10 **F**3 29 87 98 101 129 131 142 145 **S** Mississippi State Department of Mental Health, Jackson, MS
Primary Contact: Paul A. Callens, Ph.D., Director
CFO: Joe Rials, Director Fiscal Services
CMO: Ken Lippincott, M.D., Chief of Staff
CIO: James Wilhite, Director Systems Information
Web address: www.nmsh.state.ms.us
**Control:** State–Government, nonfederal **Service:** Psychiatric

**Staffed Beds:** 50 **Admissions:** 546 **Census:** 48 **Outpatient Visits:** 0 **Births:** 0 **Total Expense ($000):** 8345 **Payroll Expense ($000):** 4106 **Personnel:** 112

**TYLERTOWN—Walthall County**

★ **WALTHALL COUNTY GENERAL HOSPITAL (251324)**, 100 Hospital Drive, Zip 39667–2099; tel. 601/876–2122 **A**9 10 18 **F**40 43 70 81 89 93 107 118 129 132 145
Primary Contact: Jimmy Graves, Administrator
Web address: www.wcghospital.datastar.net/
**Control:** County–Government, nonfederal **Service:** General Medical and Surgical

**Staffed Beds:** 25 **Admissions:** 397 **Census:** 4 **Outpatient Visits:** 16153 **Births:** 0 **Personnel:** 121

**UNION—Newton County**

★ **LAIRD HOSPITAL (251322)**, 25117 Highway 15, Zip 39365–9099; tel. 601/774–8214 **A**9 10 18 **F**15 29 35 40 43 70 81 87 89 93 107 118 129 131 132 145 **S** Rush Health Systems, Meridian, MS
Primary Contact: Thomas G. Bartlett, III, M.D., Administrator
COO: Morris A. Reece, EVP/COO
CFO: Jennifer Flint, Chief Financial Officer
CMO: John Mutziger, M.D., Chief Medical Officer
CIO: Angela Sherrill, Chief Information Officer
CHR: Donnie Smith, Chief Human Resources Officer
CNO: Pam Rigdon, Director Nursing
Web address: www.rushhealthsystems.org/laird/
**Control:** Other not–for–profit (including NFP Corporation) **Service:** General Medical and Surgical

**Staffed Beds:** 25 **Admissions:** 634 **Census:** 6 **Outpatient Visits:** 18059 **Births:** 0 **Personnel:** 176

**VICKSBURG—Warren County**

**PROMISE HOSPITAL OF VICKSBURG (252008)**, 1111 North Frontage Road, 2nd Floor, Zip 39180–5102; tel. 601/619–3526 **A**10 **F**3 11 70 90 147
**S** Promise Healthcare, Boca Raton, FL
Primary Contact: Lee Huckaby, Chief Executive Officer
COO: Dawn Posey, Chief Operating Officer
CFO: Christopher A. Stegall, Regional Chief Financial Officer and Chief Operating Officer
CMO: Daniel Edney, M.D., Chief of Staff
CIO: Barbara Whiting, Director Health Information Management
CHR: Debbie Carson, Director Human Resources
Web address: www.promise–vicksburg.com
**Control:** Corporation, Investor–owned, for–profit **Service:** Long–Term Acute Care hospital

**Staffed Beds:** 33 **Admissions:** 362 **Census:** 26 **Outpatient Visits:** 0 **Births:** 0 **Total Expense ($000):** 5415 **Payroll Expense ($000):** 4721 **Personnel:** 75

✖ **RIVER REGION MEDICAL CENTER (250031)**, 2100 Highway 61 North, Zip 39183, Mailing Address: P.O. Box 590, Zip 39181–0590; tel. 601/883–5000, (Includes RIVER REGION WEST CAMPUS, 1111 North Frontage Road, Zip 39180–5102; tel. 601/883–5000) **A**1 2 10 **F**4 13 15 17 29 35 39 40 43 51 56 60 70 73 75 76 77 78 81 82 87 89 90 93 97 98 100 101 102 103 108 111 117 118 129 130 131 145 146 **S** Community Health Systems, Inc., Franklin, TN
Primary Contact: Doug Sills, Chief Executive Officer
CFO: John Milazzo, Chief Financial Officer
CMO: W. Briggs Hopson, M.D., Clinical Medical Director
CIO: J. B. White, Director Information Systems
CHR: Rebecca Columbus, Vice President Human Resources
Web address: www.riverregion.com
**Control:** Corporation, Investor–owned, for–profit **Service:** General Medical and Surgical

**Staffed Beds:** 297 **Admissions:** 10079 **Census:** 152 **Outpatient Visits:** 126122 **Births:** 723 **Personnel:** 891

**WATER VALLEY—Yalobusha County**

**YALOBUSHA GENERAL HOSPITAL (250061)**, 630 South Main, Zip 38965, Mailing Address: P.O. Box 728, Zip 38965–0728; tel. 662/473–1411, (Total facility includes 122 beds in nursing home–type unit) **A**9 10 **F**7 29 32 33 57 59 66 70 107 113 118 126 127 129 132 142 145 **P**6
Primary Contact: Terry Varner, Administrator
COO: Ashlee Langdon, Controller
CHR: Katie Rotenberry–Baggett, Administrative Assistant and Human Resources
Web address: www.yalobushageneral.com/
**Control:** County–Government, nonfederal **Service:** General Medical and Surgical

**Staffed Beds:** 148 **Admissions:** 619 **Census:** 122 **Outpatient Visits:** 3208 **Births:** 0 **Total Expense ($000):** 14439 **Payroll Expense ($000):** 10346 **Personnel:** 235

**WAYNESBORO—Wayne County**

☐ **WAYNE GENERAL HOSPITAL (250077)**, 950 Matthew Drive, Zip 39367–2590, Mailing Address: P.O. Box 1249, Zip 39367–1249; tel. 601/735–5151 **A**1 9 10 20 **F**13 15 35 39 40 43 53 61 62 63 70 75 76 81 86 88 89 90 93 107 108 111 118 129 131 132 145
Primary Contact: Donald Hemeter, Administrator
Web address: www.waynegeneralhospital.org
**Control:** County–Government, nonfederal **Service:** General Medical and Surgical

**Staffed Beds:** 80 **Admissions:** 2158 **Census:** 27 **Outpatient Visits:** 32297 **Births:** 221 **Personnel:** 343

**WEST POINT—Clay County**

✖ **NORTH MISSISSIPPI MEDICAL CENTER–WEST POINT (250067)**, 835 Medical Center Drive, Zip 39773–9320; tel. 662/495–2300 **A**1 9 10 **F**3 7 8 11 13 15 17 28 29 30 31 32 34 35 39 40 42 43 45 48 53 57 59 64 65 70 73 75 76 78 79 80 81 85 86 87 89 90 97 107 108 109 110 111 113 118 119 128 129 131 132 134 142 144 145 146 147 **S** North Mississippi Health Services, Inc., Tupelo, MS
Primary Contact: James W. Hahn, Administrator
CFO: Kay Lawler, Business Office Manager
CMO: Timothy E. Whittle, M.D., Chief Medical Staff
CHR: Brenda Johnson, Director Human Resources
CNO: Jane Windle, R.N., Director of Nurses
Web address: www.nmhs.net/westpoint
**Control:** Other not–for–profit (including NFP Corporation) **Service:** General Medical and Surgical

**Staffed Beds:** 60 **Admissions:** 2000 **Census:** 19 **Outpatient Visits:** 44081 **Births:** 396 **Total Expense ($000):** 27105 **Payroll Expense ($000):** 12465 **Personnel:** 266

## WHITFIELD—Rankin County

☒ **MISSISSIPPI STATE HOSPITAL (254010)**, 3550 Highway 468 West,
Zip 39193, Mailing Address: P.O. Box 157–A, Zip 39193–0157;
tel. 601/351–8000, (Includes WHITFIELD MEDICAL SURGICAL HOSPITAL, Oak
Circle, tel. 601/351–8023), (Total facility includes 423 beds in nursing home–
type unit) **A**1 9 10 **F**4 29 30 39 70 75 82 87 89 98 99 100 101 102 104 106
107 108 118 127 129 142 145 **P**1 **S** Mississippi State Department of Mental
Health, Jackson, MS
Primary Contact: James G. Chastain, FACHE, Director
COO: Kelly R. Breland, CPA, Director Support Services
CFO: Warren Williams, CPA, Director Fiscal Services
CMO: Duncan Stone, D.D.S., Chief Medical Staff
CIO: James Dunaway, Director Information Management
CHR: Katie Storr, Director Personnel
Web address: www.msh.state.ms.us
**Control:** State–Government, nonfederal **Service:** Psychiatric

**Staffed Beds:** 938 **Admissions:** 2503 **Census:** 836 **Outpatient Visits:** 5784
**Births:** 0 **Total Expense ($000):** 115957 **Payroll Expense ($000):** 56218
**Personnel:** 1153

## WIGGINS—Stone County

**STONE COUNTY HOSPITAL (251303)**, 1434 East Central Avenue, Zip 39577;
tel. 601/928–6600 **A**9 10 18 **F**3 7 19 27 29 34 40 43 45 47 50 55 57 59 65
68 70 77 79 81 85 89 90 92 96 97 107 111 114 118 126 128 129 132 144
147 **P**6
Primary Contact: Julie Cain, Administrator
Web address: www.schospital.net/
**Control:** Corporation, Investor–owned, for–profit **Service:** General Medical and
Surgical

**Staffed Beds:** 25 **Admissions:** 369 **Census:** 3 **Outpatient Visits:** 7368
**Births:** 0 **Total Expense ($000):** 18663 **Payroll Expense ($000):** 7265
**Personnel:** 168

## WINONA—Montgomery County

**TYLER HOLMES MEMORIAL HOSPITAL (251312)**, 409 Tyler Holmes Drive,
Zip 38967–1599; tel. 662/283–4114 **A**9 10 18 **F**11 35 40 43 57 64 66 70 87
107 113 118 129 132 134 **P**8
Primary Contact: Rosamond M. Tyler, Administrator
CFO: Cori Bailey, Accountant
CHR: Becky Corley, Director Human Resources
**Control:** County–Government, nonfederal **Service:** General Medical and Surgical

**Staffed Beds:** 25 **Admissions:** 573 **Census:** 5 **Outpatient Visits:** 13563
**Births:** 0 **Total Expense ($000):** 8419 **Payroll Expense ($000):** 4193
**Personnel:** 138

## YAZOO CITY—Yazoo County

★ **KING'S DAUGHTERS HOSPITAL (251313)**, 823 Grand Avenue,
Zip 39194–3233; tel. 662/746–2261 **A**9 10 18 **F**15 29 40 53 56 70 81 89 93
103 107 108 111 117 118 132
Primary Contact: Daryl W. Weaver, Chief Executive Officer
COO: Marsha Jones, R.N., Director Nursing
CFO: Robert E. Harper, Chief Financial Officer
CMO: Heath Scott, M.D., Chief of Staff
CHR: Stephanie Washington, Director Community Relations and Human Resources
Web address: www.kdhyazoo.com
**Control:** Other not–for–profit (including NFP Corporation) **Service:** General
Medical and Surgical

**Staffed Beds:** 35 **Admissions:** 1073 **Census:** 15 **Outpatient Visits:** 23044
**Births:** 12 **Personnel:** 164

**MS**

# MISSOURI

## ALBANY—Gentry County

★ **NORTHWEST MEDICAL CENTER (261328)**, (Critical Access Hospital), 705
North College Street, Zip 64402–1433; tel. 660/726–3941 **A**9 10 18 **F**3 11 15
28 29 34 35 39 40 44 45 50 56 57 59 62 64 68 75 81 85 86 87 90 93 97
107 108 110 111 113 116 117 118 126 127 129 130 132 134 147 **P**6
Primary Contact: Jon D. Doolittle, President and Chief Executive Officer
COO: Jon D. Doolittle, President and Chief Executive Officer
CMO: Jackie Miller, D.O., Chief of Staff
CIO: James Crouch, Vice President Technical Services
CHR: Vickie Cline, Director Human Resources
Web address: www.northwestmedicalcenter.org
**Control:** Other not–for–profit (including NFP Corporation) **Service:** General
Medical and Surgical

| | |
|---|---|
| **Staffed Beds:** 25 **Admissions:** 763 **Census:** 10 **Outpatient Visits:** 40084 **Births:** 0 **Total Expense ($000):** 13766 **Payroll Expense ($000):** 6567 **Personnel:** 160 | |

## APPLETON CITY—St. Clair County

★ **ELLETT MEMORIAL HOSPITAL (261301)**, 610 North Ohio Avenue,
Zip 64724–1609, Mailing Address: P.O. Box 6, Zip 64724–0006;
tel. 660/476–2111 **A**9 10 18 **F**3 7 11 18 34 40 45 59 64 65 68 77 79 81 90
93 107 111 113 118 126 127 128 129 132 142 **P**6
Primary Contact: Raymond M. Magers, Chief Executive Officer
CFO: Tom Hollis, Chief Financial Officer
CMO: James Wirkkula, M.D., Chief Medical Officer
Web address: www.ellettmemorial.com
**Control:** Hospital district or authority, Government, nonfederal **Service:** General
Medical and Surgical

| | |
|---|---|
| **Staffed Beds:** 12 **Admissions:** 287 **Census:** 4 **Outpatient Visits:** 18506 **Births:** 0 **Total Expense ($000):** 9074 **Payroll Expense ($000):** 3921 **Personnel:** 80 | |

## AURORA—Lawrence County

✠ **MERCY HOSPITAL AURORA (261316)**, 500 Porter Street, Zip 65605–2365;
tel. 417/678–2122 **A**1 9 10 18 **F**3 11 13 15 28 29 30 34 35 40 41 45 50 57
59 64 65 75 76 77 80 81 85 86 87 89 92 93 94 96 107 108 110 111 113
118 128 129 131 132 134 147 **P**6 **S** Mercy Health, Chesterfield, MO
Primary Contact: Douglas M. Stroemel, President
COO: David Steinmann, VP/COO
CFO: Sherry Clouse Day, CPA, VP Finance/ Regional Chief Financial Officer
CMO: Christie Hurt, M.D., Chief of Staff and Medical Director
CHR: George Roden, Vice President Human Resources
CNO: Nicki Gamet, R.N., VP/Chief Nursing Officer
Web address: www.stjohns.com/aboutus/aurora.aspx
**Control:** Church–operated, Nongovernment, not–for profit **Service:** General
Medical and Surgical

| | |
|---|---|
| **Staffed Beds:** 25 **Admissions:** 746 **Census:** 6 **Outpatient Visits:** 27733 **Births:** 232 **Total Expense ($000):** 16875 **Payroll Expense ($000):** 8661 **Personnel:** 177 | |

## BELTON—Cass County

✠ **BELTON REGIONAL MEDICAL CENTER (260214)**, 17065 South 71 Highway,
Zip 64012–4631; tel. 816/348–1200 **A**1 9 10 **F**3 15 18 29 30 31 34 35 37
40 43 45 57 59 64 65 68 70 74 75 77 78 79 81 82 85 87 90 93 107 108
110 111 117 118 128 129 130 131 145 **P**5 **S** HCA, Nashville, TN
Primary Contact: Todd Krass, R.N., Chief Executive Officer
COO: Nicole Smith Hendricks, Vice President Operations
CFO: Susan Shreeve, Chief Financial Officer
CMO: Douglas Bradley, M.D., Vice President Medical Affairs
CIO: Sarah Bloom, Director Information Systems
CHR: Yvonne Brewington, Director Human Resources
CNO: Karen Lee, MSN, Chief Nursing Officer
Web address: www.beltonregionalmedicalcenter.com
**Control:** Corporation, Investor–owned, for–profit **Service:** General Medical and
Surgical

| | |
|---|---|
| **Staffed Beds:** 38 **Admissions:** 1651 **Census:** 15 **Outpatient Visits:** 88582 **Births:** 0 **Total Expense ($000):** 32975 **Payroll Expense ($000):** 11523 **Personnel:** 174 | |

**RESEARCH BELTON HOSPITAL** See Belton Regional Medical Center

## BETHANY—Harrison County

★ **HARRISON COUNTY COMMUNITY HOSPITAL (261312)**, 2600 Miller Street,
Zip 64424–2701, Mailing Address: P.O. Box 428, Zip 64424–0428;
tel. 660/425–2211 **A**5 9 10 18 **F**3 11 15 28 29 34 40 44 45 53 54 57 59 62
64 65 66 67 68 75 77 79 81 82 87 89 90 93 96 107 108 110 111 113 118
126 127 128 129 132 142 144 145 146 147 **P**5
Primary Contact: Richard C. Hamilton, Administrator
CFO: Christina Gillespie, Chief Financial Officer
CIO: Brenda Siemer, Director of Information Technology
CHR: Brenda Gabriel, Director Human Resources
CNO: Crystal Hicks, R.N., Chief Nursing Officer
Web address: www.hcchospital.org
**Control:** Hospital district or authority, Government, nonfederal **Service:** General
Medical and Surgical

| | |
|---|---|
| **Staffed Beds:** 20 **Admissions:** 358 **Census:** 5 **Outpatient Visits:** 35452 **Births:** 0 **Total Expense ($000):** 13861 **Payroll Expense ($000):** 6162 **Personnel:** 159 | |

## BLUE SPRINGS—Jackson County

✠ **ST. MARY'S MEDICAL CENTER (260193)**, 201 West R. D. Mize Road,
Zip 64014–2518; tel. 816/228–5900 **A**1 9 10 13 **F**3 8 11 13 15 18 20 22 28
29 30 31 34 35 40 49 50 53 56 57 59 60 64 68 70 72 74 75 76 77 78 79
81 82 84 85 86 87 90 93 96 107 108 110 111 117 118 120 122 128 129
131 134 142 145 146 147 **S** Ascension Health, Saint Louis, MO
Primary Contact: Annette Small, R.N., Chief Executive Officer
CFO: Steven R. Cleary, Vice President Finance
CMO: Stephens Stoops, M.D., Chief Medical Officer
Web address: www.carondelethealth.org
**Control:** Other not–for–profit (including NFP Corporation) **Service:** General
Medical and Surgical

| | |
|---|---|
| **Staffed Beds:** 131 **Admissions:** 4997 **Census:** 59 **Outpatient Visits:** 88289 **Births:** 898 **Total Expense ($000):** 76864 **Payroll Expense ($000):** 27123 **Personnel:** 458 | |

## BOLIVAR—Polk County

✠ **CITIZENS MEMORIAL HOSPITAL (260195)**, 1500 North Oakland Avenue,
Zip 65613–3011; tel. 417/326–6000 **A**1 9 10 20 **F**3 7 11 13 15 18 20 22 26
28 29 31 34 35 36 39 40 43 45 46 50 51 56 57 59 62 63 64 66 68 70 74
75 76 77 78 79 80 81 82 83 84 85 86 87 89 90 93 94 96 98 100 102 103
104 107 108 110 111 114 116 117 118 123 126 127 128 129 130 131 132
134 142 145 146 147 **P**6
Primary Contact: Donald J. Babb, Chief Executive Officer
COO: Jeff Miller, Chief Operating Officer
CFO: Gary D. Fullbright, Comptroller
CMO: Steven Butcher, D.O., Director Medical Affairs
CIO: Denni McColm, Chief Information Officer
CHR: Jeremy MacLaughlin, Director Human Resources
CNO: Pamela A. Reese, FACHE, Chief Clinical Officer
Web address: www.citizensmemorial.com
**Control:** Hospital district or authority, Government, nonfederal **Service:** General
Medical and Surgical

| | |
|---|---|
| **Staffed Beds:** 62 **Admissions:** 3072 **Census:** 32 **Outpatient Visits:** 292530 **Births:** 496 **Total Expense ($000):** 94197 **Payroll Expense ($000):** 42994 **Personnel:** 842 | |

## BONNE TERRE—St. Francois County

✠ **PARKLAND HEALTH CENTER–BONNE TERRE (261315)**, 7245 Raider Road,
Zip 63628–3767; tel. 573/358–1400, (Nonreporting) **A**1 9 10 18 **S** BJC
HealthCare, Saint Louis, MO
Primary Contact: Thomas P. Karl, President
CFO: Cheri L. Goldsmith, Director Financial Services
CMO: Brett M. Dickinson, M.D., Chief of Staff
CHR: Sheri S. Graham, Director Human Resources and Administrative Services
Web address: www.parklandhealthcenter.org
**Control:** Other not–for–profit (including NFP Corporation) **Service:** General
Medical and Surgical

| | |
|---|---|
| **Staffed Beds:** 6 | |

MO

## BOONVILLE—Cooper County

★ **COOPER COUNTY MEMORIAL HOSPITAL (260004)**, 17651 B Highway,
Zip 65233–2839, Mailing Address: P.O. Box 88, Zip 65233–0088;
tel. 660/882–7461, (Total facility includes 14 beds in nursing home–type unit) **A**5
9 10 20 **F**3 7 11 28 29 34 35 40 45 53 57 59 62 64 67 68 75 79 81 85 89
93 94 100 107 111 113 118 126 127 129 130 131 132 134 145 147
**S** University of Missouri Health Care, Columbia, MO
Primary Contact: Allen J. Waldo, FACHE, CPA, Chief Executive Officer
CFO: Patricia Nowlin, Director of Accounting
CMO: Robert Koch, M.D., Chief Medical Staff
CIO: Steve Weekley, Director Information Technology
CHR: Kim Ashcraft, Director Human Resources
CNO: Nancy Fredrich, R.N., Chief Clinical Officer
Web address: www.coopercmh.com
**Control:** County–Government, nonfederal **Service:** General Medical and Surgical

**Staffed Beds:** 32 **Admissions:** 387 **Census:** 13 **Outpatient Visits:** 38214
**Births:** 0 **Payroll Expense ($000):** 5522 **Personnel:** 155

## BRANSON—Taney County

☒ △ **SKAGGS REGIONAL MEDICAL CENTER (260094)**, 251 Skaggs Road,
Zip 65616–2035, Mailing Address: P.O. Box 650, Zip 65615–0650;
tel. 417/335–7000 **A**1 5 7 9 10 **F**3 8 11 13 15 17 18 20 22 26 28 29 31 32
34 35 40 41 44 45 46 47 50 51 53 56 57 59 60 61 62 63 64 65 68 70 74
75 76 77 78 79 80 81 82 84 85 86 87 89 90 93 97 98 100 103 106 107
108 110 111 113 116 117 118 120 122 123 126 128 129 130 131 134 142
143 145 146 147 **P**3 6 8
Primary Contact: William K. Mahoney, President and Chief Executive Officer
CFO: David Strong, Chief Financial Officer/Vice President Finance
CIO: Michael Elley, Chief Information Officer
CHR: Carol Murrow, Vice President Business Development
CNO: Sheryl Tilus, R.N., Vice President Clinical Services/Chief Nursing Officer
Web address: www.skaggs.net
**Control:** Other not–for–profit (including NFP Corporation) **Service:** General
Medical and Surgical

**Staffed Beds:** 128 **Admissions:** 7106 **Census:** 74 **Outpatient Visits:** 274355
**Births:** 603 **Total Expense ($000):** 151596 **Payroll Expense ($000):** 56839
**Personnel:** 1074

## BRIDGETON—St. Louis County

☒ **SSM DEPAUL HEALTH CENTER (260104)**, 12303 De Paul Drive,
Zip 63044–2512; tel. 314/344–6000 **A**1 2 9 10 **F**3 5 11 12 13 15 17 18 20
22 24 28 29 30 31 34 35 36 40 43 44 50 51 53 55 56 57 59 60 61 64
68 69 70 73 74 75 76 78 79 81 82 84 85 86 87 89 98 99 100 101 102 103
104 105 107 108 111 113 114 116 118 119 120 123 125 127 129 131 134
142 145 146 147 **P**6 8 **S** SSM Health Care, Saint Louis, MO
Primary Contact: Sean Hogan, President
COO: Tina Garrison, Vice President, Operations
CFO: Hal Holder, Director Finance
CMO: Andrew Karanas, M.D., Vice President Medical Affairs
CMO: Jay Moore, M.D., Vice President, Medical Affairs
CIO: Matt Woodall, Director Information Management
CHR: Patricia Campbell, Director Employee Relations
CNO: Kathleen Bonser, R.N., Vice President, Nursing/CNO
Web address: www.ssmdepaul.com
**Control:** Church–operated, Nongovernment, not–for profit **Service:** General
Medical and Surgical

**Staffed Beds:** 476 **Admissions:** 22190 **Census:** 345 **Outpatient Visits:**
193510 **Births:** 1148 **Total Expense ($000):** 302178 **Payroll Expense**
**($000):** 106468 **Personnel:** 1874

**SSM REHABILITATION HOSPITAL**, 12380 De Paul Drive, Zip 63044–2511;
tel. 314/447–9705, (Nonreporting)
**Control:** Partnership, Investor–owned, for–profit **Service:** Rehabilitation

**Staffed Beds:** 60

## BROOKFIELD—Linn County

**GENERAL JOHN J. PERSHING MEMORIAL HOSPITAL (261307)**, 130 East
Lockling Avenue, Zip 64628–0130, Mailing Address: P.O. Box 408,
Zip 64628–0408; tel. 660/258–2222 **A**9 10 18 **F**11 15 28 29 36 40 44 54 57
59 62 63 64 75 81 87 93 97 107 111 113 118 126 129 132 145 **P**6
Primary Contact: Phil Hamilton, R.N., Chief Executive Officer
CFO: Gary R. Tandy, Chief Financial Officer
CMO: B. K. Knowles, D.O., Chief of Staff
CIO: Elaine Sutton, Chief Information Officer
CHR: Amy Sayre, Director Human Resources
Web address: www.pershinghealthsystem.com
**Control:** Other not–for–profit (including NFP Corporation) **Service:** General
Medical and Surgical

**Staffed Beds:** 25 **Admissions:** 579 **Census:** 7 **Outpatient Visits:** 62130
**Births:** 0 **Total Expense ($000):** 15244 **Payroll Expense ($000):** 5787
**Personnel:** 132

## BUTLER—Bates County

**BATES COUNTY MEMORIAL HOSPITAL (260034)**, 615 West Nursery Street,
Zip 64730–0370, Mailing Address: P.O. Box 370, Zip 64730–0370;
tel. 660/200–7000 **A**9 10 20 **F**3 7 11 15 28 29 30 31 34 40 50 57 59 62 64
68 70 77 79 81 87 90 93 107 108 109 110 111 114 117 118 126 128 129
131 132 142 **P**6
Primary Contact: Wendell R. Harris, CPA, Ph.D., Chief Executive Officer
CFO: Wendell R. Harris, CPA, Chief Executive Officer
CMO: Joseph Brewster, M.D., Chief of Staff
CIO: Marcia Cook, Director Information Technology
CHR: Melinda Jackson, Director Human Resources
Web address: www.bcmhospital.com
**Control:** County–Government, nonfederal **Service:** General Medical and Surgical

**Staffed Beds:** 49 **Admissions:** 1131 **Census:** 13 **Outpatient Visits:** 61935
**Births:** 0 **Total Expense ($000):** 37059 **Payroll Expense ($000):** 14361
**Personnel:** 293

## CAMERON—Clinton County

**CAMERON REGIONAL MEDICAL CENTER (260057)**, 1600 East Evergreen,
Zip 64429–1498, Mailing Address: P.O. Box 557, Zip 64429–0557;
tel. 816/632–2101 **A**9 10 **F**3 11 13 15 17 18 28 29 30 31 34 35 39 40 46
47 49 56 57 59 61 62 63 64 67 70 74 75 76 77 78 79 81 82 84 85 86 87
89 90 98 100 104 107 110 111 114 118 127 128 129 130 132 142 145
146 147 **P**6
Primary Contact: Joseph F. Abrutz, Jr., Administrator
CFO: Rosa Patti, Chief Financial Officer
CIO: Bill Walser, Coordinator Technology
CHR: Pat Bestgen, Manager Human Resources
Web address: www.cameronregional.org
**Control:** Other not–for–profit (including NFP Corporation) **Service:** General
Medical and Surgical

**Staffed Beds:** 58 **Admissions:** 2040 **Census:** 33 **Outpatient Visits:** 336782
**Births:** 153 **Total Expense ($000):** 42193 **Payroll Expense ($000):** 18920
**Personnel:** 334

## CAPE GIRARDEAU—Cape Girardeau County

☐ **LANDMARK HOSPITAL (262015)**, 3255 Independence Street,
Zip 63701–4904; tel. 573/335–1091 **A**1 9 10 **F**1 29 75 118 129 147
**S** Landmark Hospitals, Cape Girardeau, MO
Primary Contact: Rodney Brown, Chief Executive Officer
COO: Michael L. Norman, Executive Vice President and Chief Operating Officer
CFO: Richard H. Hogan, CPA, Chief Financial Officer
CMO: William Fritsch, M.D., Medical Director
CIO: Renee Hesselrode, Director Health Information Management
CHR: Angela Kisner, Director Human Resources and Coordinator Medical Staff
Web address: www.landmarkhospitals.com
**Control:** Partnership, Investor–owned, for–profit **Service:** Long–Term Acute Care
hospital

**Staffed Beds:** 30 **Admissions:** 337 **Census:** 26 **Outpatient Visits:** 0 **Births:**
0 **Total Expense ($000):** 13744 **Payroll Expense ($000):** 4405 **Personnel:**
125

☒ **SAINT FRANCIS MEDICAL CENTER (260183)**, 211 St. Francis Drive,
Zip 63703–5049; tel. 573/331–3000 **A**1 2 5 9 10 19 **F**3 9 11 12 13 15 17 18
20 22 24 26 28 29 30 31 32 34 35 39 40 43 44 45 46 47 48 49 50 53 54
56 57 58 59 60 61 62 64 65 70 72 73 74 75 76 77 78 79 80 81 82 84 85
86 87 89 90 91 92 93 97 107 108 110 111 113 114 116 117 118 119 120
122 123 125 128 129 130 131 134 140 141 142 143 144 145 146 147 **P**6
Primary Contact: Steven C. Bjelich, President and Chief Executive Officer
COO: Marilyn K. Curtis, Vice President, Professional Services
CFO: Tony Balsano, Vice President Finance
CMO: James Schell, M.D., Vice President Medical Affairs
CIO: Diane Gammon, Director Information Systems
CHR: Teri Kreitzer, Director Human Resources
CNO: Jeannie Fadler, R.N., Vice President, Patient Care Services
Web address: www.sfmc.net
**Control:** Church–operated, Nongovernment, not–for profit **Service:** General
Medical and Surgical

**Staffed Beds:** 261 **Admissions:** 11122 **Census:** 160 **Outpatient Visits:**
270536 **Births:** 920 **Total Expense ($000):** 332415 **Payroll Expense**
**($000):** 128805 **Personnel:** 1933

*Many Facility Codes have changed. Please refer to the AHA Guide Code Chart.* © 2012 AHA Guide

**MO**

⊠ **SOUTHEAST HOSPITAL (260110)**, 1701 Lacey Street, Zip 63701–5230; tel. 573/334–4822 **A**1 2 5 9 10 19 **F**3 11 12 13 15 17 18 20 22 24 26 28 29 30 31 32 34 40 45 46 49 50 51 53 54 57 58 59 60 61 62 63 64 65 68 70 72 73 74 75 76 77 78 79 80 81 82 85 86 87 88 89 90 92 93 96 97 98 100 102 103 107 108 110 111 113 114 116 118 119 120 122 123 125 126 128 129 130 131 143 145 146 147 **P**6 **S** SoutheastHEALTH, Cape Girardeau, MO
Primary Contact: Wayne Smith, Interim President and Chief Executive Officer
CFO: David Strong, Vice President and Chief Financial Officer
CMO: Lee Taylor, M.D., Vice President and Chief Medical Officer
CIO: Jay McGuire, Director Information Systems
Web address: www.southeastmissourihospital.com
**Control:** Other not–for–profit (including NFP Corporation) **Service:** General Medical and Surgical

**Staffed Beds:** 227 **Admissions:** 10344 **Census:** 125 **Outpatient Visits:** 280960 **Births:** 841 **Total Expense ($000):** 300950 **Payroll Expense ($000):** 108306 **Personnel:** 1816

### CARROLLTON—Carroll County

**CARROLL COUNTY MEMORIAL HOSPITAL (261332)**, 1502 North Jefferson Street, Zip 64633–1948; tel. 660/542–1695 **A**5 9 10 18 **F**3 11 15 28 29 30 34 35 38 40 45 53 56 57 59 62 64 65 75 77 79 86 87 90 91 93 107 108 111 113 116 118 124 127 128 129 130 131 132 145 **P**6
Primary Contact: Jeff A. Tindle, Chief Executive Officer
CMO: Timothy Reid, M.D., Chief Medical Staff
CHR: Karen Pfaff, Director Human Resources
Web address: www.carrollcountyhospital.org
**Control:** Other not–for–profit (including NFP Corporation) **Service:** General Medical and Surgical

**Staffed Beds:** 25 **Admissions:** 500 **Census:** 5 **Outpatient Visits:** 39778 **Births:** 0 **Total Expense ($000):** 12114 **Payroll Expense ($000):** 5692 **Personnel:** 131

### CARTHAGE—Jasper County

★ **MERCY MCCUNE–BROOKS HOSPITAL (261326)**, 3125 Drive Russell Smith Way, Zip 64836–7402; tel. 417/358–8121 **A**9 10 18 **F**3 7 11 13 15 28 29 30 34 35 40 45 50 53 57 59 62 64 68 69 70 75 76 79 81 89 90 98 104 107 111 113 118 128 129 130 131 132 134 145 146 **P**6 **S** Mercy Health, Chesterfield, MO
Primary Contact: Robert Y. Copeland, Jr., FACHE, Chief Executive Officer
CFO: Tony Wright, Chief Financial Officer
CIO: Ken Masters, Director Information Systems
CHR: Tracy G. Lemmons, Director Human Resources
Web address: www.mccune–brooks.org
**Control:** City–Government, nonfederal **Service:** Surgical

**Staffed Beds:** 35 **Admissions:** 1617 **Census:** 13 **Outpatient Visits:** 61640 **Births:** 184 **Total Expense ($000):** 45352 **Payroll Expense ($000):** 15343 **Personnel:** 332

### CASSVILLE—Barry County

⊠ **MERCY HOSPITAL CASSVILLE (261317)**, 94 Main Street, Zip 65625–1610; tel. 417/847–6000 **A**1 9 10 18 **F**3 11 15 28 29 30 34 40 41 45 50 53 57 59 64 65 75 77 81 85 86 87 89 92 93 94 96 107 110 111 113 118 131 132 134 147 **P**6 **S** Mercy Health, Chesterfield, MO
Primary Contact: Douglas M. Stroemel, President
COO: David Steinmann, Chief Operating Officer
CFO: Sherry Clouse Day, CPA, Chief Financial Officer
CMO: Jamie Zengotita, M.D., Chief Medical Staff
CHR: George Roden, Vice President Human Resources
CNO: Nicki Gamet, R.N., Chief Nursing Officer
Web address: www.southbarrycountyhospital.com
**Control:** Church–operated, Nongovernment, not–for profit **Service:** General Medical and Surgical

**Staffed Beds:** 18 **Admissions:** 306 **Census:** 3 **Outpatient Visits:** 21184 **Births:** 0 **Total Expense ($000):** 12471 **Payroll Expense ($000):** 6248 **Personnel:** 116

### CHESTERFIELD—St. Louis County

**DUBUIS HOSPITAL OF ST. LOUIS** See Mercy Continuing Care Hospital

⊠ **MERCY CONTINUING CARE HOSPITAL (262012)**, 13190 South Outer Forty Road, Zip 63017–5917; tel. 314/392–6380 **A**1 9 10 **F**1 3 29 30 147 **S** Dubuis Health System, Houston, TX
Primary Contact: Matthew B. Schweigert, Administrator
CFO: Paul Veillon, CPA, Chief Financial Officer
CMO: Rekha Lakshmanan, M.D., Medical Director
CNO: Jennifer Ryder, Director of Nursing
Web address: www.dubuis.org
**Control:** Other not–for–profit (including NFP Corporation) **Service:** Long–Term Acute Care hospital

**Staffed Beds:** 54 **Admissions:** 313 **Census:** 25 **Outpatient Visits:** 0 **Births:** 0 **Total Expense ($000):** 14435 **Payroll Expense ($000):** 6759 **Personnel:** 92

⊠ △ **MERCY REHABILITATION HOSPITAL (263029)**, 14561 North Outer Forty Road, Zip 63017; tel. 314/881–4000 **A**1 7 9 10 **F**16 29 30 75 90 91 93 129 130 131 142 147 **S** Mercy Health, Chesterfield, MO
Primary Contact: Donna M. Flannery, Chief Executive Officer
CFO: Jerry Wise, Controller
CMO: Siresha Samudrala, M.D., Medical Director
Web address: www.stjohnsmercyrehab.com
**Control:** Partnership, Investor–owned, for–profit **Service:** Rehabilitation

**Staffed Beds:** 68 **Admissions:** 1306 **Census:** 54 **Outpatient Visits:** 21192 **Births:** 0 **Total Expense ($000):** 24863 **Payroll Expense ($000):** 10994 **Personnel:** 204

⊠ **ST. LUKE'S HOSPITAL (260179)**, 232 South Woods Mill Road, Zip 63017–3417; tel. 314/434–1500, (Total facility includes 140 beds in nursing home–type unit) **A**1 2 3 5 9 10 **F**3 10 11 12 13 15 17 18 20 22 24 26 28 29 30 31 32 34 35 36 39 40 41 42 44 45 46 49 50 52 53 54 55 56 57 58 59 60 61 62 63 64 65 66 68 69 70 71 73 74 75 76 77 78 79 81 82 83 84 85 86 87 89 90 93 97 107 108 110 111 113 114 117 118 119 120 122 123 125 127 128 129 130 131 134 143 144 145 146 147 **P**6 8
Primary Contact: Gary R. Olson, President and Chief Executive Officer
CFO: Scott Johnson, Vice President Finance
CIO: William Meyers, Chief Information Officer
CHR: Janette Taaffe, Administrator Human Resources
Web address: www.stlukes–stl.com
**Control:** Church–operated, Nongovernment, not–for profit **Service:** General Medical and Surgical

**Staffed Beds:** 580 **Admissions:** 17639 **Census:** 323 **Outpatient Visits:** 756430 **Births:** 1972 **Total Expense ($000):** 414570 **Payroll Expense ($000):** 187271 **Personnel:** 3130

⊠ **ST. LUKE'S REHABILITATION HOSPITAL (263030)**, 14709 Olive Boulevard, Zip 63017–2221; tel. 314/317–5700 **A**1 9 10 **F**3 12 28 29 34 54 75 79 90 93 94 96 100 118 129 131 147 **P**8 **S** Kindred Healthcare, Louisville, KY
Primary Contact: Della Abboud, Chief Executive Officer
Web address: www.khrehabstluke.com
**Control:** Partnership, Investor–owned, for–profit **Service:** Rehabilitation

**Staffed Beds:** 35 **Admissions:** 683 **Census:** 25 **Outpatient Visits:** 22606 **Births:** 0 **Total Expense ($000):** 11566 **Payroll Expense ($000):** 4119 **Personnel:** 72

### CHILLICOTHE—Livingston County

☐ **HEDRICK MEDICAL CENTER (261321)**, 100 Central Avenue, Zip 64601–1554; tel. 660/646–1480 **A**1 5 9 10 18 **F**3 11 13 15 18 28 29 30 31 34 35 40 41 44 50 57 59 62 63 64 65 68 69 70 74 75 76 77 78 79 81 82 85 86 87 89 90 92 93 96 97 100 102 104 107 108 111 114 117 118 126 127 128 129 130 132 134 145 146 147 **P**6 **S** Saint Luke's Health System, Kansas City, MO
Primary Contact: Matthew J. Wenzel, Chief Executive Officer
CFO: Dana Hoover, Chief Financial Officer
CMO: George A. Pagels, M.D., President and Chief Executive Officer
CHR: Lisa Hecker, Director Human Resources
Web address: www.saintlukeshealthsystem.org
**Control:** Other not–for–profit (including NFP Corporation) **Service:** General Medical and Surgical

**Staffed Beds:** 25 **Admissions:** 987 **Census:** 11 **Outpatient Visits:** 79041 **Births:** 151 **Total Expense ($000):** 31588 **Payroll Expense ($000):** 14003 **Personnel:** 260

**MO**

---

**Hospital, Medicare Provider Number, Address, Telephone, Approval, Facility, and Physician Codes, Health Care System**

★ American Hospital Association (AHA) membership
☐ The Joint Commission accreditation ◇ DNV Healthcare Inc. accreditation
○ American Osteopathic Association (AOA) accreditation
△ Commission on Accreditation of Rehabilitation Facilities (CARF) accreditation

## CLINTON—Henry County

✠ **GOLDEN VALLEY MEMORIAL HEALTHCARE (260175)**, 1600 North Second Street, Zip 64735–1192; tel. 660/885–5511 **A**1 9 10 **F**3 7 11 13 15 18 28 29 30 31 34 35 40 45 47 48 53 57 59 61 62 64 68 70 74 75 76 77 78 79 81 85 86 87 90 93 96 107 108 111 114 116 117 118 126 127 128 129 130 131 134 142 145 146 147
Primary Contact: Randy S. Wertz, Chief Executive Officer
CFO: Gordon Glass, Chief Financial Officer
CIO: James Begin, Director Information Technology
CHR: Roger Cook, Director Human Resources
CNO: Mark D. Mattes, R.N., Assistant Administrator/Patient Care Services
Web address: www.gvmh.org
**Control:** Hospital district or authority, Government, nonfederal **Service:** General Medical and Surgical

**Staffed Beds:** 56 **Admissions:** 2959 **Census:** 31 **Outpatient Visits:** 218832 **Births:** 360 **Total Expense ($000):** 56852 **Payroll Expense ($000):** 29027 **Personnel:** 593

## COLUMBIA—Boone County

✠ **BOONE HOSPITAL CENTER (260068)**, 1600 East Broadway, Zip 65201–5844; tel. 573/815–8000 **A**1 2 3 5 9 10 **F**3 7 11 12 13 15 17 18 20 22 24 26 28 29 30 31 34 35 36 40 45 46 47 48 49 50 51 53 56 57 59 60 61 64 65 68 70 72 73 74 75 76 77 78 79 80 81 82 84 85 86 87 89 90 93 96 97 107 108 110 111 113 114 116 117 118 125 128 129 130 131 134 144 145 146 147 **S** BJC HealthCare, Saint Louis, MO
Primary Contact: Daniel J. Rothery, President
COO: Randy Morrow, Vice President and Chief Operating Officer
CFO: Randy Morrow, Vice President and Chief Operating Officer
CMO: Jerry Kennett, M.D., Chief Medical Officer
CHR: Michelle Zvanut, Vice President Human Resources
Web address: www.boone.org
**Control:** Other not–for–profit (including NFP Corporation) **Service:** General Medical and Surgical

**Staffed Beds:** 360 **Admissions:** 17347 **Census:** 209 **Outpatient Visits:** 157623 **Births:** 2208 **Total Expense ($000):** 292202 **Payroll Expense ($000):** 75895 **Personnel:** 1668

**ELLIS FISCHEL CANCER CENTER** See University of Missouri Hospitals and Clinics

✠ △ **HARRY S. TRUMAN MEMORIAL VETERANS HOSPITAL**, 800 Hospital Drive, Zip 65201–5275; tel. 573/814–6000, (Total facility includes 41 beds in nursing home–type unit) **A**1 3 5 7 **F**3 4 5 17 18 20 22 24 26 28 29 30 31 34 35 39 40 44 49 54 56 58 59 61 62 63 64 67 70 74 75 78 79 81 82 83 84 85 86 87 90 92 93 94 97 98 100 101 102 103 104 105 106 107 108 111 114 115 117 118 126 127 128 129 131 134 145 146 **P**6 **S** Department of Veterans Affairs, Washington, DC
Primary Contact: Sallie Houser–Hanfelder, FACHE, Director
COO: Robert G. Ritter, Associate Director
CFO: Paul Hopkins, Chief Financial Officer
CMO: Lana Zerrer, M.D., Chief of Staff
CIO: Donna Krause, Chief Information Officer
CHR: Jimmy Powell, Manager Human Resources
Web address: www.columbiamo.va.gov
**Control:** Veterans Affairs, Government, federal **Service:** General Medical and Surgical

**Staffed Beds:** 126 **Admissions:** 4053 **Census:** 88 **Outpatient Visits:** 633414 **Births:** 0 **Total Expense ($000):** 255071 **Payroll Expense ($000):** 90060 **Personnel:** 1311

✠ **HOWARD A. RUSK REHABILITATION CENTER (263027)**, 315 Business Loop 70 West, Zip 65203–3248; tel. 573/817–2703 **A**1 3 5 9 10 **F**29 34 59 90 93 96 131 142 147 **S** HEALTHSOUTH Corporation, Birmingham, AL
Primary Contact: Bruce Eady, Chief Executive Officer
CFO: Ted Weatherford, Chief Financial Officer
CMO: Gregory Worsowicz, M.D., Medical Director
CHR: Robin Prater, Chief Nursing Officer
CNO: Mary Schnell, R.N., Chief Nursing Officer
Web address: www.ruskrehab.com
**Control:** Partnership, Investor–owned, for–profit **Service:** Rehabilitation

**Staffed Beds:** 60 **Admissions:** 1075 **Census:** 47 **Outpatient Visits:** 8616 **Births:** 0 **Total Expense ($000):** 18368 **Payroll Expense ($000):** 8475 **Personnel:** 192

**LANDMARK HOSPITAL OF COLUMBIA (262020)**, 604 Old 63 North, Zip 65201–6308; tel. 573/499–6600 **A**9 10 **F**1 29 75 147 **S** Landmark Hospitals, Cape Girardeau, MO
Primary Contact: Deborah Sabella, R.N., Chief Executive Officer
Web address: www.landmarkhospitals.com
**Control:** Partnership, Investor–owned, for–profit **Service:** Long–Term Acute Care hospital

**Staffed Beds:** 42 **Admissions:** 447 **Census:** 32 **Outpatient Visits:** 0 **Births:** 0 **Total Expense ($000):** 15414 **Payroll Expense ($000):** 5398 **Personnel:** 117

✠ **UNIVERSITY OF MISSOURI HOSPITALS AND CLINICS (260141)**, One Hospital Drive, Zip 65212–0001; tel. 573/882–4141, (Includes ELLIS FISCHEL CANCER CENTER, 115 Business Loop 70 West, Zip 65203; tel. 573/882–5460) **A**1 2 3 5 8 9 10 **F**3 4 7 9 11 12 13 15 16 17 18 19 20 22 24 26 28 29 30 31 32 34 35 37 38 39 40 41 43 44 45 46 47 48 49 50 51 52 53 54 55 56 57 58 59 60 61 64 65 68 70 71 72 73 74 75 76 77 78 79 81 82 84 85 86 87 88 89 92 93 97 98 99 100 101 102 104 107 108 110 111 113 114 116 117 118 119 120 122 123 125 128 129 130 131 133 134 137 140 141 143 145 146 147 **P**1 6 **S** University of Missouri Health Care, Columbia, MO
Primary Contact: James H. Ross, Chief Executive Officer
COO: Anita Larsen, R.N., Interim Chief Operating Officer
CFO: Kevin Necas, Chief Financial Officer
CMO: Les Hall, M.D., Chief Medical Officer
CHR: Sue Kopfle, Chief Human Resources Officer
Web address: www.muhealth.org
**Control:** State–Government, nonfederal **Service:** General Medical and Surgical

**Staffed Beds:** 477 **Admissions:** 21698 **Census:** 298 **Outpatient Visits:** 732030 **Births:** 1714 **Total Expense ($000):** 587619 **Payroll Expense ($000):** 209273 **Personnel:** 4692

★ **WOMEN'S AND CHILDREN'S HOSPITAL (260178)**, 404 Keene Street, Zip 65201–6626; tel. 573/875–9000, (Nonreporting) **A**9 10 **S** University of Missouri Health Care, Columbia, MO
Primary Contact: Keri Simon, Executive Director
COO: Mitchell L. Wasden, Ed.D., Chief Operating Officer
CFO: Kevin Necas, Chief Financial Officer
CMO: Les Hall, M.D., Chief of Staff
CIO: Joanne Burns, Chief Information Officer
CHR: Sue Kopfle, Chief Human Resources Officer
CNO: Anita Larsen, R.N., Chief Nursing Officer
Web address: www.muchildrenshospital.org
**Control:** State–Government, nonfederal **Service:** Children's general

**Staffed Beds:** 108

## CRYSTAL CITY—Jefferson County

○ △ **JEFFERSON REGIONAL MEDICAL CENTER (260023)**, Highway 61 South, Zip 63019, Mailing Address: P.O. Box 350, Zip 63019–0350; tel. 636/933–1000 **A**7 9 10 11 **F**3 4 5 7 8 11 12 13 15 18 20 22 24 26 28 29 30 34 35 37 40 44 45 49 50 51 53 54 57 59 62 63 64 70 74 75 76 77 79 81 82 84 85 86 87 89 90 92 93 94 96 97 98 99 100 101 102 103 104 105 107 110 111 113 114 115 116 117 118 128 129 130 131 134 142 143 145 146 147 **P**6
Primary Contact: Jeffrey W. Buck, Interim Chief Executive Officer
CMO: Mark Briete, M.D., Vice President Medical Affairs
CIO: Jan Poneta, Director Information Services
CHR: Saundra G. Turner, Director Human Resources
Web address: www.jhsmo.com
**Control:** Other not–for–profit (including NFP Corporation) **Service:** General Medical and Surgical

**Staffed Beds:** 219 **Admissions:** 12453 **Census:** 127 **Outpatient Visits:** 112110 **Births:** 207 **Total Expense ($000):** 116247 **Payroll Expense ($000):** 49926 **Personnel:** 1153

## DEXTER—Stoddard County

**MISSOURI SOUTHERN HEALTHCARE (260160)**, 1200 North One Mile Road, Zip 63841–1000; tel. 573/624–5566 **A**9 10 **F**3 11 15 29 34 39 40 57 59 62 65 70 75 77 80 81 85 89 90 93 97 107 108 113 118 126 127 129 132 134 **P**6 **S** Sunlink Health Systems, Atlanta, GA
Primary Contact: Amy Akers, Chief Executive Officer
CHR: Judy Bowling, Director Human Resources
Web address: www.msh–hospital.com
**Control:** Corporation, Investor–owned, for–profit **Service:** General Medical and Surgical

**Staffed Beds:** 45 **Admissions:** 1078 **Census:** 9 **Outpatient Visits:** 93324 **Births:** 0 **Total Expense ($000):** 12049 **Payroll Expense ($000):** 5433 **Personnel:** 157

## DONIPHAN—Ripley County

★ **SOUTHEAST HEALTH CENTER OF RIPLEY COUNTY (260080)**, 109 Plum Street, Zip 63935–1299; tel. 573/996–2141 **A**9 10 **F**11 29 40 59 62 65 87 93 107 114 118 126 129 134 **S** SoutheastHEALTH, Cape Girardeau, MO
Primary Contact: Robert E. Garrison, Chief Executive Officer
CFO: Rickie Maples, Interim Chief Financial Officer
CMO: Ureej Mansoor, M.D., Chief of Staff
CIO: Riley March, Manager Information Technology
CHR: Peggy Teasdale, Director Human Resources
Web address: www.rcmhospital.net
**Control:** County–Government, nonfederal **Service:** General Medical and Surgical

**Staffed Beds:** 27 **Admissions:** 331 **Census:** 3 **Outpatient Visits:** 25287 **Births:** 0 **Total Expense ($000):** 8961 **Payroll Expense ($000):** 4770 **Personnel:** 125

MO

## EL DORADO SPRINGS—Cedar County

**CEDAR COUNTY MEMORIAL HOSPITAL (261323)**, 1401 South Park Street, Zip 64744–2037; tel. 417/876–2511 **A**9 10 18 **F**11 13 15 18 28 29 30 34 35 40 45 53 56 57 59 62 64 65 68 74 75 76 77 81 85 89 93 102 107 110 111 113 118 126 127 128 129 132 145 146 147 **P**6
Primary Contact: Jana Witt, Chief Executive Officer
CFO: Carla Gilbert, Controller
CMO: George Methven, M.D., Chief Medical Staff
CIO: Lois Willmore, Supervisor Health Information Management
CHR: Diana Pyle, Director Human Resources
Web address: www.cedarcountyhospital.org
**Control:** County–Government, nonfederal **Service:** General Medical and Surgical

**Staffed Beds: 25 Admissions: 559 Census: 6 Outpatient Visits:** 37184
**Births: 65 Total Expense ($000):** 10696 **Payroll Expense ($000):** 5263
**Personnel:** 123

**SOUTHWEST MISSOURI PSYCHIATRIC REHABILITATION CENTER (264027)**, 1301 Industrial Parkway East, Zip 64744–6263; tel. 417/876–1000 **A**10 **F**98 101 102
Primary Contact: Denise Norbury, Regional Executive Officer
CFO: Ronald Chandler, Accountant II
CMO: Ronald Lacey, M.D., Medical Director
CHR: James Stacy, Director Human Resources
**Control:** State–Government, nonfederal **Service:** Psychiatric

**Staffed Beds: 16 Admissions: 106 Census: 14 Outpatient Visits: 0 Births:**
0 **Total Expense ($000):** 3397 **Payroll Expense ($000):** 2865 **Personnel:** 6

## ELLINGTON—Reynolds County

**ADVANCED HEALTHCARE MEDICAL CENTER (261304)**, 100 Highway 21 South, Zip 63638–7427, Mailing Address: Rural Route 4, Box 4269, Zip 63638–9409; tel. 573/663–2511 **A**9 10 18 **F**3 40 62 64 87 107 111 113 118 126 129 132 **P**6
Primary Contact: Paula Harris, Chief Executive Officer
COO: Steve Myers, Assistant Administrator
CFO: Katie Caudel, Controller
CIO: Thomas Barker, Director Information
**Control:** Partnership, Investor–owned, for–profit **Service:** General Medical and Surgical

**Staffed Beds: 12 Admissions: 381 Census: 4 Outpatient Visits: 0 Births:** 1
**Total Expense ($000):** 12854 **Payroll Expense ($000):** 6529 **Personnel:** 19

## EXCELSIOR SPRINGS—Clay County

✠ **EXCELSIOR SPRINGS HOSPITAL (261322)**, 1700 Rainbow Boulevard, Zip 64024–1190; tel. 816/630–6081, (Total facility includes 80 beds in nursing home–type unit) **A**1 9 10 18 **F**3 10 11 15 18 29 30 31 32 34 35 39 40 45 49 56 57 59 62 63 64 67 68 70 75 77 78 79 81 82 84 85 86 89 90 93 102 107 108 110 111 113 115 116 117 118 124 127 128 129 131 132 134 142 145 146
Primary Contact: Sally S. Nance, Chief Executive Officer
CFO: Dennis Hartman, Chief Financial Officer
CMO: Manoch Kuangparichat, M.D., President Medical Staff
CIO: Alicia Harrison, Data Management Officer
CHR: Joni Schwan, Director Human Resources
Web address: www.esmc.org
**Control:** City–Government, nonfederal **Service:** General Medical and Surgical

**Staffed Beds: 105 Admissions: 512 Census: 76 Outpatient Visits:** 13665
**Births: 0 Total Expense ($000):** 22382 **Payroll Expense ($000):** 9333
**Personnel:** 225

## FAIRFAX—Atchison County

**COMMUNITY HOSPITAL ASSOCIATION** See Community Hospital–Fairfax

★ **COMMUNITY HOSPITAL–FAIRFAX (261303)**, 26136 U.S. Highway 59, Zip 64446–9105, Mailing Address: P.O. Box 107, Zip 64446–0107; tel. 660/686–2211 **A**5 9 10 18 **F**3 11 13 15 28 30 34 40 45 57 59 62 64 67 76 79 81 85 87 89 93 107 113 118 127 132
Primary Contact: Myra L. Evans, Chief Executive Officer
COO: Rhonda Evans, R.N., Chief Operating Officer
CFO: Suzanne Southard, Director Finance
CMO: Aron Burke, M.D., Chief Medical Officer
CIO: Michelle Oswald, Director of Information Systems
CHR: Deanna Lamb, Director of Human Resources
Web address: www.fairfaxmed.com
**Control:** Other not–for–profit (including NFP Corporation) **Service:** General Medical and Surgical

**Staffed Beds: 18 Admissions: 620 Census: 6 Outpatient Visits:** 16371
**Births: 46 Total Expense ($000):** 10622 **Payroll Expense ($000):** 3889
**Personnel:** 92

## FARMINGTON—St. Francois County

○ **MINERAL AREA REGIONAL MEDICAL CENTER (260116)**, 1212 Weber Road, Zip 63640–3325; tel. 573/756–4581 **A**9 10 11 19 **F**3 12 13 15 28 29 30 34 40 45 50 51 57 59 60 62 64 68 70 76 77 79 81 85 89 90 93 98 100 102 103 107 111 113 118 128 129 131 132 145 146 **S** Capella Healthcare, Franklin, TN
Primary Contact: David P. Steitz, Interim Chief Executive Officer
CFO: Paul Rogers, Chief Financial Officer
CMO: Richard Secor, Jr., M.D., Chief of Staff
CIO: Jim Smith, Director Information Systems
CHR: Regina K. Sons, Administrative Director Human Resources and Volunteer Services Associate Ethics and Compliance Officer
Web address: www.marmc.net
**Control:** Corporation, Investor–owned, for–profit **Service:** General Medical and Surgical

**Staffed Beds: 98 Admissions: 3519 Census: 40 Outpatient Visits:** 78083
**Births: 344 Total Expense ($000):** 35714 **Payroll Expense ($000):** 15561
**Personnel:** 385

✠ **PARKLAND HEALTH CENTER (260163)**, 1101 West Liberty Street, Zip 63640–1921; tel. 573/756–6451 **A**1 5 9 10 **F**3 11 13 15 28 29 30 34 35 39 40 44 45 46 49 50 51 53 57 59 60 61 64 65 68 69 70 74 75 76 77 79 81 85 86 87 89 93 98 103 107 108 111 114 117 118 129 130 131 134 145 146 147 **P**6 **S** BJC HealthCare, Saint Louis, MO
Primary Contact: Thomas P. Karl, President
CFO: Cheri L. Goldsmith, Director Financial Services
CMO: Brett M. Dickinson, M.D., Chief of Staff
CHR: Sheri S. Graham, Director Human Resources and Administrative Services
Web address: www.parklandhealthcenter.org
**Control:** Other not–for–profit (including NFP Corporation) **Service:** General Medical and Surgical

**Staffed Beds: 98 Admissions: 3935 Census: 35 Outpatient Visits:** 81288
**Births: 531 Total Expense ($000):** 71188 **Payroll Expense ($000):** 23341
**Personnel:** 470

□ **SOUTHEAST MISSOURI MENTAL HEALTH CENTER (264005)**, 1010 West Columbia Street, Zip 63640–2997; tel. 573/218–6792 **A**1 9 10 **F**4 30 39 40 53 65 75 77 86 87 93 97 98 101 102 103 106 129 131 134 142 145
Primary Contact: Julie Inman, Regional Executive Officer
COO: Melissa Ring, Ph.D., Chief Operating Officer
CMO: Jay Englehart, M.D., Medical Director
CHR: Mark Remspecher, Director Human Resources
Web address: www.dmh.missouri.gov/southeast/
**Control:** State–Government, nonfederal **Service:** Psychiatric

**Staffed Beds: 298 Admissions: 280 Census: 283 Outpatient Visits:** 157
**Births: 0 Total Expense ($000):** 49464 **Payroll Expense ($000):** 28339
**Personnel:** 762

## FENTON—St. Louis County

✠ **SSM ST. CLARE HEALTH CENTER (260081)**, 1015 Bowles Avenue, Zip 63026–2394; tel. 636/496–2000 **A**1 9 10 **F**3 11 12 13 15 18 20 22 24 28 29 30 31 34 35 40 44 45 49 50 51 53 54 56 57 59 61 64 65 70 73 74 75 76 78 79 81 82 85 86 87 100 102 103 107 108 110 111 113 114 116 117 118 119 120 129 131 134 142 145 146 147 **P**6 8 **S** SSM Health Care, Saint Louis, MO
Primary Contact: R. William Hoefer, FACHE, President
COO: Kelly Pearce, Vice President of Operations
CFO: Karen Rewerts, Vice President Finance and Chief Financial Officer
CMO: Timothy J. Pratt, M.D., Vice President of Medical Affairs/Chief Medical Officer
CIO: Leighton Wassilak, Manager, Information Systems/ Telecommunications
CHR: Patricia Campbell, Vice President Human Resources
CNO: Mary Brobst, R.N., Vice President of Nursing
Web address: www.ssmstclare.com
**Control:** Church–operated, Nongovernment, not–for profit **Service:** General Medical and Surgical

**Staffed Beds: 184 Admissions: 12414 Census: 129 Outpatient Visits:** 100461 **Births: 1415 Total Expense ($000):** 169923 **Payroll Expense ($000):** 56244 **Personnel:** 937

**MO**

---

**Hospital, Medicare Provider Number, Address, Telephone, Approval, Facility, and Physician Codes, Health Care System**

★ American Hospital Association (AHA) membership
□ The Joint Commission accreditation      ◇ DNV Healthcare Inc. accreditation

○ American Osteopathic Association (AOA) accreditation
△ Commission on Accreditation of Rehabilitation Facilities (CARF) accreditation

## FORT LEONARD WOOD—Pulaski County

✠ **GENERAL LEONARD WOOD ARMY COMMUNITY HOSPITAL**, 126 Missouri Avenue, Zip 65473–8952; tel. 573/596–0414 **A**1 5 **F**3 4 7 13 14 15 18 29 30 33 34 35 39 45 50 54 57 59 64 65 68 70 74 75 76 77 79 81 85 86 87 89 90 93 94 97 98 99 100 102 104 107 110 111 113 131 134 145 146 **S** Department of the Army, Office of the Surgeon General, Falls Church, VA
Primary Contact: Colonel Marie Dominguez, Commander
CFO: Major Michael Hogan, Chief Resource Management
CMO: Lieutenant Colonel John Lowery, M.D., Deputy Commander Clinical Services
CHR: Major Sandra Roper, Chief Human Resources
Web address: www.amedd.army.mil
**Control:** Army, Government, federal **Service:** General Medical and Surgical

> **Staffed Beds:** 54 **Admissions:** 1625 **Census:** 22 **Outpatient Visits:** 565199
> **Births:** 600 **Personnel:** 1278

## FREDERICKTOWN—Madison County

**MADISON MEDICAL CENTER (261302)**, 611 West Main Street, Zip 63645–1111; tel. 573/783–3341, (Total facility includes 80 beds in nursing home–type unit) **A**9 10 18 **F**6 11 15 35 40 59 62 64 67 70 77 79 81 87 93 97 103 107 111 118 126 127 129 132 145
Primary Contact: Lisa Twidwell, Administrator
CMO: P. A. George, M.D., Chief of Staff
CHR: Jennifer Penuel, Director Human Resources
Web address: www.madisonmedicalcenter.net
**Control:** County–Government, nonfederal **Service:** General Medical and Surgical

> **Staffed Beds:** 97 **Admissions:** 530 **Census:** 76 **Outpatient Visits:** 54707
> **Births:** 0 **Total Expense ($000):** 15996 **Payroll Expense ($000):** 8191
> **Personnel:** 243

## FULTON—Callaway County

☐ **CALLAWAY COMMUNITY HOSPITAL (260209)**, 10 South Hospital Drive, Zip 65251–2510; tel. 573/642–3376 **A**1 3 5 9 10 **F**3 11 13 15 29 30 34 35 40 45 50 57 59 67 76 81 85 89 97 107 108 111 113 118 126 127 132 **S** Sunlink Health Systems, Atlanta, GA
Primary Contact: Allen D. AufderHeide, Chief Executive Officer
COO: Chuck Baker, R.N., Chief Operating Officer and Chief Nursing Officer
CHR: Martie Jeney, Director Human Resources
Web address: www.mycallaway.org
**Control:** Corporation, Investor–owned, for–profit **Service:** General Medical and Surgical

> **Staffed Beds:** 31 **Admissions:** 655 **Census:** 4 **Outpatient Visits:** 36269
> **Births:** 95 **Total Expense ($000):** 18370 **Payroll Expense ($000):** 7356
> **Personnel:** 122

☐ **FULTON STATE HOSPITAL (264004)**, 600 East Fifth Street, Zip 65251–1753; tel. 573/592–4100 **A**1 3 5 10 **F**3 4 11 29 30 39 44 50 53 56 57 58 59 65 75 77 82 86 87 98 100 101 102 103 129 131 134 142 145 **P**6
Primary Contact: Robert Reitz, Ph.D., Regional Executive Officer
COO: Marty Ann Martin–Forman, Chief Operating Officer
CFO: J. Kenneth Lyle, Jr., Chief Financial Officer
CMO: Bruce Harry, M.D., Clinical Director
CIO: Robert Smith, Chief Information Officer
CHR: Lori Hollinger, Manager Human Resources
Web address: www.dmh.missouri.gov/fulton
**Control:** State–Government, nonfederal **Service:** Psychiatric

> **Staffed Beds:** 356 **Admissions:** 169 **Census:** 356 **Outpatient Visits:** 0
> **Births:** 0 **Total Expense ($000):** 84746 **Payroll Expense ($000):** 42699
> **Personnel:** 1018

## HANNIBAL—Marion County

✠ **HANNIBAL REGIONAL HOSPITAL (260025)**, 6000 Hospital Drive, Zip 63401–6749, Mailing Address: P.O. Box 551, Zip 63401–0551; tel. 573/248–1300 **A**1 2 5 9 10 **F**3 11 13 15 18 20 22 26 28 30 31 35 39 40 45 47 49 51 57 59 60 62 64 68 70 74 75 76 77 78 79 81 82 85 86 87 89 90 92 93 96 97 98 100 102 104 107 108 110 111 114 116 117 118 119 120 122 123 126 128 129 130 131 143 144 145 147 **P**1
Primary Contact: Lynn W. Olson, President and Chief Executive Officer
CFO: Roger J. Dix, Senior Vice President and Chief Financial Officer
CMO: Roderick Bartlett, M.D., President Medical Staff
CIO: Jeff W. Evans, Vice President Information and Technology
CHR: Penny Nunley, Vice President Human Resources
Web address: www.hrhonline.org
**Control:** Other not–for–profit (including NFP Corporation) **Service:** General Medical and Surgical

> **Staffed Beds:** 105 **Admissions:** 5392 **Census:** 57 **Outpatient Visits:** 114992
> **Births:** 602 **Total Expense ($000):** 106580 **Payroll Expense ($000):** 49363
> **Personnel:** 867

## HARRISONVILLE—Cass County

✠ **CASS REGIONAL MEDICAL CENTER (261324)**, 2800 East Rock Haven Road, Zip 64701–4411; tel. 816/380–3474 **A**1 9 10 18 **F**3 11 15 18 28 29 30 31 32 34 35 39 40 45 48 50 54 56 57 59 64 65 66 68 70 74 75 77 78 79 81 85 86 87 89 92 93 96 97 98 107 110 111 113 114 118 126 128 129 130 131 132 134 145 146 147 **P**6
Primary Contact: John Christopher Lang, Chief Executive Officer
CFO: Brent Probasco, Chief Financial Officer
CIO: Cynthia Miltenberger, Director Organizational Effectiveness
CHR: Carla Wallen, Manager Human Resources
Web address: www.cassregional.org
**Control:** County–Government, nonfederal **Service:** General Medical and Surgical

> **Staffed Beds:** 35 **Admissions:** 1690 **Census:** 20 **Outpatient Visits:** 101686
> **Births:** 0 **Total Expense ($000):** 54002 **Payroll Expense ($000):** 20945
> **Personnel:** 397

## HAYTI—Pemiscot County

**PEMISCOT MEMORIAL HEALTH SYSTEM (260070)**, 946 East Road, Zip 63851–1245, Mailing Address: P.O. Box 489, Zip 63851–0489; tel. 573/359–1372, (Total facility includes 66 beds in nursing home–type unit) **A**9 10 **F**3 7 11 13 15 17 28 29 30 34 39 40 50 57 59 64 67 68 70 75 76 77 79 81 82 85 87 89 90 93 97 98 99 103 104 107 111 118 126 127 129 132 142 143 145 146 147 **P**6
Primary Contact: Kerry L. Noble, Administrator
COO: Larry Davis, Chief Operating Officer
CHR: Jackie Powell, Director Human Resources
Web address: www.pemiscot.org/
**Control:** County–Government, nonfederal **Service:** General Medical and Surgical

> **Staffed Beds:** 167 **Admissions:** 2197 **Census:** 67 **Outpatient Visits:** 32737
> **Births:** 53 **Total Expense ($000):** 29819 **Payroll Expense ($000):** 13457
> **Personnel:** 533

## HERMANN—Gasconade County

★ **HERMANN AREA DISTRICT HOSPITAL (261314)**, 509 West 18th Street, Zip 65041–0470, Mailing Address: P.O. Box 470, Zip 65041–0470; tel. 573/486–2191 **A**9 10 18 **F**3 11 15 18 28 29 30 34 35 40 41 44 45 53 56 57 59 62 63 64 67 68 69 71 75 77 78 81 85 86 87 89 90 93 96 97 104 107 111 113 118 126 127 128 129 131 132 134 142 145 **P**6
Primary Contact: Dan McKinney, Administrator
COO: Matt Siebert, Assistant Administrator of Ancillary Services
CFO: Denise Witthaus, Assistant Administrator Finance
CMO: Jeremy Tallery, D.O., Chief of Staff
CIO: Chris Gooch, Information Technology Director
CHR: Carol Schaefer, Human Resources
CNO: Sue Daller, R.N., Assistant Administrator of Nursing
Web address: www.hadh.org
**Control:** Hospital district or authority, Government, nonfederal **Service:** General Medical and Surgical

> **Staffed Beds:** 24 **Admissions:** 462 **Census:** 9 **Outpatient Visits:** 58839
> **Births:** 0 **Total Expense ($000):** 16907 **Payroll Expense ($000):** 7455
> **Personnel:** 170

## HOUSTON—Texas County

**TEXAS COUNTY MEMORIAL HOSPITAL (260024)**, 1333 South Sam Houston Boulevard, Zip 65483–2046; tel. 417/967–3311 **A**9 10 20 **F**3 7 13 15 28 29 34 40 45 53 57 59 62 63 64 70 76 81 85 86 87 89 93 97 107 111 113 118 126 128 129 132 142 147 **P**6
Primary Contact: Wesley E. Murray, Chief Executive Officer
CFO: Linda Pamperien, Chief Financial Officer
CMO: Charles Mueller, M.D., Chief of Staff
CHR: Anita Kuhn, Controller
Web address: www.tcmh.org
**Control:** County–Government, nonfederal **Service:** General Medical and Surgical

> **Staffed Beds:** 47 **Admissions:** 1873 **Census:** 18 **Outpatient Visits:** 121841
> **Births:** 269 **Total Expense ($000):** 27523 **Payroll Expense ($000):** 14962
> **Personnel:** 376

## INDEPENDENCE—Jackson County

✠ **CENTERPOINT MEDICAL CENTER (260095)**, 19600 East 39th Street, Zip 64057; tel. 816/698–7000 **A**1 2 9 10 **F**3 8 13 15 17 18 20 22 24 26 28 29 30 31 34 35 38 40 43 49 54 55 56 57 59 60 64 70 71 72 73 74 75 76 77 78 79 80 81 82 85 86 87 92 93 107 108 110 111 113 114 116 118 125 128 129 130 131 134 144 145 146 147 **S** HCA, Nashville, TN
Primary Contact: Carolyn W. Caldwell, President and Chief Executive Officer
COO: Phil Buttell, Chief Operating Officer
CFO: James H. Brown, Chief Financial Officer
CMO: Christopher Sullivan, M.D., Chief Medical Officer
CIO: Carl Sifers, Director Information Technology and System Services
CHR: Kyla Stoltz, Vice President Human Resources
Web address: www.centerpointmedical.com
**Control:** Corporation, Investor–owned, for–profit **Service:** General Medical and Surgical

> **Staffed Beds:** 221 **Admissions:** 13698 **Census:** 154 **Outpatient Visits:** 128213 **Births:** 1410 **Total Expense ($000):** 196348 **Payroll Expense ($000):** 63703 **Personnel:** 876

*Many Facility Codes have changed. Please refer to the AHA Guide Code Chart.* © 2012 AHA Guide

**MO**

## JEFFERSON CITY—Cole County

☒ **CAPITAL REGION MEDICAL CENTER (260047)**, 1125 Madison Street,
Zip 65101–5200, Mailing Address: P.O. Box 1128, Zip 65102–1128;
tel. 573/632–5000 **A**1 3 5 9 10 12 13 **F**3 5 11 13 15 18 20 22 24 28 29 30
31 32 34 35 36 38 40 45 46 47 48 49 51 53 54 56 57 58 59 61 62 64 65
66 70 73 74 75 76 77 78 79 80 81 85 87 89 90 92 93 94 97 99 100 102
104 107 108 110 111 113 117 119 120 128 129 130 131 134 143 145
146 **P**2 6 **S** University of Missouri Health Care, Columbia, MO
Primary Contact: Edward F. Farnsworth, FACHE, President
COO: Janet Weckenborg, FACHE, VP Operations
CFO: James McMillan, Vice President Finance
CMO: Lorenzo McKnelly, D.O., Chief of Staff
CIO: Jason Cecil, Chief Information Officer
CHR: Robert Mazur, Vice President Human Resources
CNO: Tawny Sandifer, R.N., Vice President Patient Care
Web address: www.crmc.org
**Control:** Other not–for–profit (including NFP Corporation) **Service:** General
Medical and Surgical

**Staffed Beds:** 114 **Admissions:** 7614 **Census:** 75 **Outpatient Visits:** 414830
**Births:** 784 **Total Expense ($000):** 155189 **Payroll Expense ($000):** 68020
**Personnel:** 1198

☒ **ST. MARYS HEALTH CENTER (260011)**, 100 St. Marys Medical Plaza,
Zip 65101–1602; tel. 573/761–7000 **A**1 9 10 19 **F**3 11 13 15 17 18 20 22
24 28 29 30 31 32 34 35 38 39 40 44 45 49 50 57 59 64 70 73 74 75 76
77 78 79 80 81 82 84 85 86 87 89 93 96 98 100 101 102 103 104 107 108
110 111 113 114 117 118 128 129 130 131 134 140 141 143 145 146 147
**P**6 **S** SSM Health Care, Saint Louis, MO
Primary Contact: R. Brent VanConia, President
COO: Anthony Houston, Executive Vice President
CMO: John Lucio, D.O., Vice President Medical Affairs
CHR: Susan Mankoski, Vice President Human Resources
CNO: Grace McBride, Vice President Acute Care Services
Web address: www.lethealingbegin.com
**Control:** Church–operated, Nongovernment, not–for profit **Service:** General
Medical and Surgical

**Staffed Beds:** 139 **Admissions:** 8666 **Census:** 93 **Outpatient Visits:** 228326
**Births:** 642 **Total Expense ($000):** 145844 **Payroll Expense ($000):** 48286
**Personnel:** 890

## JOPLIN—Newton County

★ ○ **FREEMAN HOSPITAL WEST (260137)**, 1102 West 32nd Street,
Zip 64804–3503; tel. 417/347–1111, (Includes FREEMAN HOSPITAL EAST, 932
East 34th Street, Zip 64804–3999; tel. 417/623–4640), (Total facility includes
32 beds in nursing home–type unit) **A**2 9 10 11 13 **F**3 11 13 15 17 18 20 22
24 26 28 29 30 31 34 35 36 37 38 39 40 42 43 44 45 46 47 48 49 50 54
56 57 58 59 60 61 62 64 65 68 70 71 72 74 75 76 77 78 79 81 82 84 85
86 87 89 90 93 96 97 98 100 102 103 107 108 110 111 113 114 118 123
127 128 129 130 131 134 143 144 145 146 147 **P**1 6 **S** Freeman Health
System, Joplin, MO
Primary Contact: Paula F. Baker, President and Chief Executive Officer
COO: Joe L. Kirk, Executive Vice President
CFO: Steve W. Graddy, Chief Financial Officer
CMO: Richard D. Schooler, M.D., Chief Medical Officer
CIO: Sue Annesser, Director Information Technology
CHR: Deborah Chiodo, Director Human Resources
Web address: www.freemanhealth.com
**Control:** Other not–for–profit (including NFP Corporation) **Service:** General
Medical and Surgical

**Staffed Beds:** 340 **Admissions:** 17643 **Census:** 249 **Outpatient Visits:**
695686 **Births:** 2381 **Total Expense ($000):** 376996 **Payroll Expense
($000):** 178106 **Personnel:** 2831

☐ **LANDMARK HOSPITAL OF JOPLIN (262016)**, 2040 West 32nd Street,
Zip 64804; tel. 417/627–1300 **A**1 9 10 **F**1 29 75 118 129 147 **S** Landmark
Hospitals, Cape Girardeau, MO
Primary Contact: Keith D'Amico, Chief Executive Officer
COO: Trish Shuler, Chief Clinical Officer
CFO: Richard H. Hogan, CPA, Chief Financial Officer
CMO: Ronald Williams, M.D., Medical Director
CHR: Teresa Woodward, Director Human Resources
Web address: www.landmarkhospitals.com
**Control:** Partnership, Investor–owned, for–profit **Service:** Long–Term Acute Care
hospital

**Staffed Beds:** 30 **Admissions:** 383 **Census:** 26 **Outpatient Visits:** 0 **Births:**
0 **Total Expense ($000):** 14413 **Payroll Expense ($000):** 5544 **Personnel:**
111

☒ △ **MERCY HOSPITAL JOPLIN (260001)**, 2817 South St. John's Boulevard,
Zip 64804–1626; tel. 417/781–2727, (Includes ST. JOHN'S REHABILITATION
CENTER, 2727 McClelland Boulevard, Zip 64804; tel. 417/659–6716), (Data for
304 days) **A**1 2 7 9 10 **F**3 4 5 7 11 12 13 15 17 18 20 22 24 26 28 29 30
31 34 35 37 38 39 40 43 44 45 49 50 51 54 57 58 59 60 61 62 63 64 65
66 68 70 74 75 76 77 78 79 81 82 83 84 85 86 87 90 93 94 97 98 99 100
101 102 103 104 105 106 107 108 111 113 114 115 118 119 120 122 125
126 128 129 130 131 133 134 143 145 146 147 **P**1 6 **S** Mercy Health,
Chesterfield, MO
Primary Contact: Gary W. Pulsipher, President and Chief Executive Officer
COO: Dottie Bringle, R.N., Chief Operating Officer and Chief Nursing Officer
CFO: Shelly Hunter, Chief Financial Officer
CIO: Robert Honeywell, Site Administrator
CHR: Scott Watson, JD, Vice President Human Resources and Support Services
Web address: www.stj.com
**Control:** Church–operated, Nongovernment, not–for profit **Service:** General
Medical and Surgical

**Staffed Beds:** 341 **Admissions:** 12200 **Census:** 203 **Outpatient Visits:**
130812 **Births:** 595 **Total Expense ($000):** 147309 **Payroll Expense
($000):** 59470 **Personnel:** 1437

## KANSAS CITY—Jackson County

☐ **CENTER FOR BEHAVIORAL MEDICINE (264008)**, 1000 East 24th Street,
Zip 64108–2776; tel. 816/512–7000 **A**1 3 5 10 **F**4 35 36 38 50 53 98
Primary Contact: Dick Gregory, Ph.D., Chief Executive Officer
COO: Scott Carter, Chief Operating Officer
CFO: Randy Riley, Chief Financial Officer
CMO: Stuart J. Munro, M.D., Clinical Director
CIO: Rob Curren, Director Information Technology
CHR: Silva Ward, Director Human Resources
Web address: www.dmhonline.dmh.state.mo.us
**Control:** State–Government, nonfederal **Service:** Psychiatric

**Staffed Beds:** 65 **Admissions:** 83 **Census:** 55 **Outpatient Visits:** 0 **Births:** 0
**Total Expense ($000):** 23012 **Payroll Expense ($000):** 12904 **Personnel:**
370

☒ **CHILDREN'S MERCY HOSPITALS AND CLINICS (263302)**, 2401 Gillham
Road, Zip 64108–4619; tel. 816/234–3000 **A**1 2 3 5 8 9 10 **F**3 7 8 9 11 12
16 19 20 21 22 23 24 25 26 27 29 30 31 32 34 35 36 39 40 41 43 44 48
49 50 54 55 57 58 59 60 61 62 64 65 68 72 73 74 75 77 78 79 81 82 84
85 86 87 88 89 90 91 92 93 94 96 97 100 101 104 107 108 111 113 116
117 118 129 130 131 133 135 137 138 140 141 143 144 145 147 **P**6 8
Primary Contact: Randall L. O'Donnell, Ph.D., President and Chief Executive Officer
COO: Jo W. Stueve, Co–Chief Operating Officer
CFO: Sandra A J Lawrence, Executive Vice President and Chief Financial Officer
CMO: V. Fred Burry, M.D., Executive Medical Director
CIO: Jean Ann Breedlove, Chief Information Officer
CHR: Dan Wright, Vice President Human Resources
Web address: www.childrensmercy.org
**Control:** Other not–for–profit (including NFP Corporation) **Service:** Children's
general

**Staffed Beds:** 265 **Admissions:** 12339 **Census:** 203 **Outpatient Visits:**
334044 **Births:** 19 **Total Expense ($000):** 693058 **Payroll Expense ($000):**
340267 **Personnel:** 4505

☐ **CRITTENTON CHILDREN'S CENTER (264018)**, 10918 Elm Avenue,
Zip 64134–4108; tel. 816/765–6600 **A**1 9 10 **F**5 29 30 32 34 35 68 75 77
86 87 98 99 100 101 102 104 106 129 131 145 **P**6 **S** Saint Luke's Health
System, Kansas City, MO
Primary Contact: Janine Hron, Chief Executive Officer
COO: JoAnn McDonough, Director Operations and Chief Nursing Officer
CFO: Willard Staron, Chief Financial Officer
CMO: Eileen Duggan, M.D., Medical Director
CIO: Deborah Gash, Vice President and Chief Information Officer
CHR: Shawna Roath, Director Human Resources
Web address: www.crittentonkc.org
**Control:** Other not–for–profit (including NFP Corporation) **Service:** Children's
hospital psychiatric

**Staffed Beds:** 54 **Admissions:** 2169 **Census:** 41 **Outpatient Visits:** 13819
**Births:** 0 **Total Expense ($000):** 22563 **Payroll Expense ($000):** 13317
**Personnel:** 211

**MO**

---

**Hospital, Medicare Provider Number, Address, Telephone, Approval, Facility, and Physician Codes, Health Care System**

★ American Hospital Association (AHA) membership
☐ The Joint Commission accreditation
◇ DNV Healthcare Inc. accreditation
○ American Osteopathic Association (AOA) accreditation
△ Commission on Accreditation of Rehabilitation Facilities (CARF) accreditation

☒ **KINDRED HOSPITAL KANSAS CITY (262011)**, 8701 Troost Avenue, Zip 64131–2767; tel. 816/995–2000 **A**1 9 10 **F**1 3 18 29 30 60 70 75 80 85 100 107 129 147 **S** Kindred Healthcare, Louisville, KY
Primary Contact: Aaron Anothayanontha, Chief Executive Officer
COO: Stephenie Hashmi, Chief Clinical Officer
CFO: Maureen Roach, Chief Financial Officer
Web address: www.kindredhospitalkc.com
**Control:** Corporation, Investor–owned, for–profit **Service:** Long–Term Acute Care hospital

**Staffed Beds:** 130 **Admissions:** 622 **Census:** 58 **Outpatient Visits:** 0 **Births:** 0 **Total Expense ($000):** 32234 **Payroll Expense ($000):** 10131 **Personnel:** 181

☒ **KINDRED HOSPITAL NORTHLAND (262018)**, 500 Northwest 68th Street, Zip 64118; tel. 816/420–6300 **A**1 9 10 **F**1 18 28 29 30 60 77 82 84 85 100 129 147 **S** Kindred Healthcare, Louisville, KY
Primary Contact: Alexander Gill, Interim Chief Executive Officer
CFO: Austin Walker, Accounting Manager
CMO: Sean R. Muldoon, M.D., Senior Vice President & Chief Medical Officer–Kindred Healthcare, Hospital Division
CHR: Jeffrey Sopko, West Region Director of HR
CNO: Julie Duben, Chief Clinical Officer
Web address: www.khnorthland.com
**Control:** Corporation, Investor–owned, for–profit **Service:** Long–Term Acute Care hospital

**Staffed Beds:** 35 **Admissions:** 416 **Census:** 31 **Outpatient Visits:** 0 **Births:** 0 **Total Expense ($000):** 16288 **Payroll Expense ($000):** 5385 **Personnel:** 118

**NORTHLAND LTAC HOSPITAL** See Kindred Hospital Northland

☒ **RESEARCH MEDICAL CENTER (260027)**, 2316 East Meyer Boulevard, Zip 64132–1136; tel. 816/276–4000 **A**1 2 3 5 9 10 **F**3 4 8 11 13 15 17 18 20 22 24 26 28 29 30 31 34 35 38 39 40 42 43 45 46 47 49 50 51 52 53 55 57 58 59 60 61 64 65 66 70 72 73 74 75 76 77 78 79 80 81 82 84 85 86 87 90 93 94 96 97 98 105 107 108 110 111 113 114 115 117 118 119 120 121 123 128 129 130 131 133 134 137 142 145 146 147 **S** HCA, Nashville, TN
Primary Contact: Kevin J. Hicks, President and Chief Executive Officer
COO: Jacqueline DeSouza, Chief Operating Officer
CFO: Susan Shreeve, Chief Financial Officer
CMO: George Liesmann, M.D., Chief Medical Officer
CIO: Tressy McKinney, Director Information Services
CHR: Dennis K. Johnson, Vice President Human Resources
Web address: www.researchmedicalcenter.com
**Control:** Corporation, Investor–owned, for–profit **Service:** General Medical and Surgical

**Staffed Beds:** 374 **Admissions:** 13904 **Census:** 200 **Outpatient Visits:** 149169 **Births:** 1529 **Total Expense ($000):** 311899 **Payroll Expense ($000):** 91455 **Personnel:** 1548

☒ **RESEARCH PSYCHIATRIC CENTER (264016)**, 2323 East 63rd Street, Zip 64130–3462; tel. 816/444–8161 **A**1 9 10 **F**4 5 29 35 87 98 99 100 101 102 103 104 105 129 **S** HCA, Nashville, TN
Primary Contact: Richard Failla, Chief Executive Officer
COO: Kevin Walker, Vice President Operations
CFO: Susan Shreeve, Chief Financial Officer
CMO: Steven Segraves, M.D., Medical Director
CIO: Matt Untch, Controller
CHR: Peggy Tyson, Director Human Resources
CNO: Carmen Kynard, R.N., Chief Nursing Officer
Web address: www.researchpsychiatriccenter.com
**Control:** Corporation, Investor–owned, for–profit **Service:** Psychiatric

**Staffed Beds:** 100 **Admissions:** 3850 **Census:** 72 **Outpatient Visits:** 8023 **Births:** 0 **Total Expense ($000):** 23111 **Payroll Expense ($000):** 10157 **Personnel:** 197

**SAINT LUKE'S CANCER INSTITUTE (260211)**, 4321 Washington, Medical Plaza III, Suite 5100, Zip 64111–3214; tel. 816/932–2823 **A**9 10 **F**3 15 34 35 57 59 64 71 78 85 86 94 107 111 113 116 118 119 120 122 123 129 131 135 142 145 **P**6 **S** Saint Luke's Health System, Kansas City, MO
Primary Contact: Julie L. Quirin, FACHE, Chief Executive Officer
Web address: www.saint–lukes.org
**Control:** Other not–for–profit (including NFP Corporation) **Service:** Cancer

**Staffed Beds:** 9 **Admissions:** 177 **Census:** 2 **Outpatient Visits:** 43936 **Births:** 0 **Payroll Expense ($000):** 12597 **Personnel:** 116

☒ **SAINT LUKE'S HOSPITAL OF KANSAS CITY (260138)**, 4401 Wornall Road, Zip 64111–3220; tel. 816/932–9886 **A**1 2 3 5 8 9 10 **F**3 9 11 12 13 14 15 17 18 20 22 24 26 28 29 30 31 32 34 35 36 37 40 43 44 45 46 47 48 49 50 53 55 56 57 58 59 60 61 62 64 65 66 68 70 71 72 73 74 75 76 77 78 79 81 82 84 85 86 87 90 91 92 93 94 95 96 97 100 101 102 104 107 108 110 111 113 114 115 116 117 118 122 123 125 128 129 130 131 134 136 137 138 140 145 146 147 **S** Saint Luke's Health System, Kansas City, MO
Primary Contact: Julie L. Quirin, FACHE, Chief Executive Officer
COO: Brad Simmons, Chief Operating Officer
CFO: Amy Nachtigal, Chief Financial Officer
CMO: John Yeast, M.D., Director Medical Affairs
CIO: Deborah Gash, Chief Information Officer
CHR: Doris Rogers, Vice President Human Resources
CNO: Debra White, Chief Nursing Officer
Web address: www.saint–lukes.org
**Control:** Church–operated, Nongovernment, not–for profit **Service:** General Medical and Surgical

**Staffed Beds:** 435 **Admissions:** 18211 **Census:** 265 **Outpatient Visits:** 352990 **Births:** 2357 **Total Expense ($000):** 483796 **Payroll Expense ($000):** 181175 **Personnel:** 3175

☒ **SAINT LUKE'S NORTH HOSPITAL – BARRY ROAD (260062)**, 5830 N.W. Barry Road, Zip 64154–2778; tel. 816/891–6000, (Includes SAINT LUKE'S NORTH HOSPITAL–SMITHVILLE CAMPUS, 601 South 169 Highway, Smithville, Zip 64089–9317; tel. 816/532–3700; Don Sipes, Chief Executive Officer) **A**1 9 10 **F**3 11 13 15 17 18 20 22 26 28 29 30 31 32 34 35 36 38 40 44 45 49 50 53 56 57 59 60 64 68 69 70 71 73 74 75 76 77 79 81 82 84 85 86 87 90 92 93 96 97 98 99 100 101 102 103 104 105 107 108 110 111 113 114 116 117 118 128 129 130 131 133 134 140 142 145 146 147 **S** Saint Luke's Health System, Kansas City, MO
Primary Contact: Kevin T. Trimble, FACHE, President and Chief Executive Officer
CFO: Julie Murphy, Chief Financial Officer
CIO: Carolyn Masoner, Director Information Services
CHR: Alan L. Abramovitz, Director Human Resources
Web address: www.saint–lukes.org
**Control:** Church–operated, Nongovernment, not–for profit **Service:** General Medical and Surgical

**Staffed Beds:** 137 **Admissions:** 6502 **Census:** 75 **Outpatient Visits:** 106168 **Births:** 823 **Total Expense ($000):** 98985 **Payroll Expense ($000):** 41264 **Personnel:** 749

☒ **SELECT SPECIALTY HOSPITAL–WESTERN MISSOURI (262014)**, 2316 East Meyer Boulevard, 3 West, Zip 64132; tel. 816/276–3300 **A**1 9 10 **F**1 3 29 77 84 85 86 147 **S** Select Medical Corporation, Mechanicsburg, PA
Primary Contact: Matthew Paul Pearson, Chief Executive Officer
Web address: www.selectmedicalcorp.com
**Control:** Corporation, Investor–owned, for–profit **Service:** Long–Term Acute Care hospital

**Staffed Beds:** 34 **Admissions:** 375 **Census:** 25 **Outpatient Visits:** 0 **Births:** 0 **Total Expense ($000):** 13976 **Payroll Expense ($000):** 5431 **Personnel:** 78

☒ **ST. JOSEPH MEDICAL CENTER (260085)**, 1000 Carondelet Drive, Zip 64114–4673; tel. 816/942–4400 **A**1 2 9 10 **F**3 11 13 15 17 18 20 22 24 26 28 29 30 31 34 35 36 40 45 46 47 49 50 51 56 57 59 60 64 68 70 71 72 74 75 76 77 78 79 80 81 82 84 85 86 87 90 96 107 108 109 110 111 113 114 115 117 118 128 129 131 134 145 146 147 **S** Ascension Health, Saint Louis, MO
Primary Contact: Michael A. Dorsey, FACHE, Chief Executive Officer
CFO: Steven R. Cleary, Vice President Finance
CMO: Stephens Stoops, M.D., Chief Medical Officer
CIO: Maggie Ratliff, Chief Information Officer
CHR: Dawn Bryant, Vice President Organizational Development
CHR: Dawn L. Bryant, Vice President Organizational Development
CNO: Debra Ohnoutka, Chief Nursing Officer
Web address: www.carondelethealth.org
**Control:** Other not–for–profit (including NFP Corporation) **Service:** General Medical and Surgical

**Staffed Beds:** 239 **Admissions:** 11251 **Census:** 149 **Outpatient Visits:** 120724 **Births:** 1256 **Total Expense ($000):** 173895 **Payroll Expense ($000):** 56098 **Personnel:** 976

MO

*Many Facility Codes have changed. Please refer to the AHA Guide Code Chart.* © 2012 AHA Guide

⊠ **TRUMAN MEDICAL CENTER–HOSPITAL HILL (260048)**, 2301 Holmes Street, Zip 64108–2640; tel. 816/404–1000 **A**1 2 3 5 8 9 10 **F**3 4 5 11 12 13 15 17 18 20 22 26 28 29 30 31 34 35 36 38 39 40 41 43 44 45 46 48 49 50 52 53 55 57 58 59 61 64 65 66 68 70 71 72 74 75 76 77 78 79 81 82 84 85 86 87 90 93 94 97 98 99 100 101 102 103 104 107 108 110 111 113 114 118 128 129 130 131 133 134 142 145 146 147 **P**5 6 **S** Truman Medical Centers, Kansas City, MO
Primary Contact: John W. Bluford, President and Chief Executive Officer
COO: Catherine D. Disch, Executive Vice President and Chief Operating Officer
CFO: Allen Johnson, Chief Financial Officer
CMO: Mark Steele, M.D., Chief Medical Officer
CIO: Mitzi Cardenas, Chief Information Officer
CHR: CiCi Rojas, Vice President Community Engagement
Web address: www.trumed.org
**Control:** Other not–for–profit (including NFP Corporation) **Service:** General Medical and Surgical

| Staffed Beds: 272 Admissions: 15353 Census: 200 Outpatient Visits: 588679 Births: 2076 Total Expense ($000): 315522 Payroll Expense ($000): 142524 Personnel: 2702 |
|---|

⊠ **TRUMAN MEDICAL CENTER–LAKEWOOD (260102)**, 7900 Lee's Summit Road, Zip 64139–1236; tel. 816/404–7000, (Total facility includes 212 beds in nursing home–type unit) **A**1 3 5 9 10 **F**3 4 5 6 11 13 15 29 30 32 34 35 36 38 39 40 41 44 45 50 53 54 56 57 58 59 64 65 66 67 68 70 71 74 75 76 77 79 81 82 85 86 87 89 90 93 94 96 97 98 99 100 101 102 103 104 107 113 118 128 129 130 131 133 134 142 145 146 **P**5 6 **S** Truman Medical Centers, Kansas City, MO
Primary Contact: John W. Bluford, President and Chief Executive Officer
COO: Charlie Shields, Chief Operating Officer
CFO: Allen Johnson, Chief Financial Officer
CFO: Daniel J. Williams, Senior Director Finance
CMO: Mark Steele, M.D., Chief Medical Officer
CIO: Mitzi Cardenas, Chief Information Officer
CHR: CiCi Rojas, Vice President Community Engagement
CNO: Lynette Wheeler, MSN, Chief Nursing Officer
Web address: www.trumanmed.org
**Control:** Other not–for–profit (including NFP Corporation) **Service:** General Medical and Surgical

| Staffed Beds: 310 Admissions: 5011 Census: 216 Outpatient Visits: 374655 Births: 804 Total Expense ($000): 116510 Payroll Expense ($000): 53151 Personnel: 845 |
|---|

⊠ **TWO RIVERS BEHAVIORAL HEALTH SYSTEM (264017)**, 5121 Raytown Road, Zip 64133–2141; tel. 816/382–6300 **A**1 9 10 **F**4 5 29 30 34 35 38 75 86 87 98 99 101 102 103 104 105 129 131 133 142 **S** Universal Health Services, Inc., King of Prussia, PA
Primary Contact: Scott Hullinger, Chief Executive Officer
CFO: Michael Delaney, Chief Financial Officer
CMO: Shahbaz Khan, M.D., Medical Director
CIO: Michael Witt, Director of Information Technology
CHR: Troy Angell, Director Human Resources
CNO: Rebecca Clark, Chief Nursing Officer
Web address: www.tworivershospital.com
**Control:** Corporation, Investor–owned, for–profit **Service:** Psychiatric

| Staffed Beds: 105 Admissions: 2804 Census: 48 Outpatient Visits: 6367 Births: 0 Total Expense ($000): 16444 Payroll Expense ($000): 7596 Personnel: 119 |
|---|

⊠ △ **VETERANS AFFAIRS MEDICAL CENTER**, 4801 East Linwood Boulevard, Zip 64128–2226; tel. 816/861–4700, (Nonreporting) **A**1 2 3 5 7 **S** Department of Veterans Affairs, Washington, DC
Primary Contact: Kent D. Hill, Director
CFO: Charles Henning, Program Director Business
Web address: www.va.gov/sta/guide/home.asp
**Control:** Veterans Affairs, Government, federal **Service:** General Medical and Surgical

| Staffed Beds: 157 |
|---|

**KENNETT—Dunklin County**

☐ **TWIN RIVERS REGIONAL MEDICAL CENTER (260015)**, 1301 First Street, Zip 63857–2508, Mailing Address: P.O. Box 728, Zip 63857–0728; tel. 573/888–4522 **A**1 9 10 **F**3 13 15 18 29 30 33 34 35 40 50 56 57 59 60 64 68 70 76 77 78 79 81 82 85 89 90 98 99 101 102 103 107 111 113 116 118 126 128 129 134 145 146 147 **S** Health Management Associates, Naples, FL
Primary Contact: Kenneth James, Chief Executive Officer
CFO: Tiffany Berry, Chief Financial Officer
CHR: Sherry Malone, Director Human Resources
Web address: www.twinriversmedctr.com
**Control:** Corporation, Investor–owned, for–profit **Service:** General Medical and Surgical

| Staffed Beds: 116 Admissions: 4644 Census: 45 Outpatient Visits: 75264 Births: 483 Total Expense ($000): 41842 Payroll Expense ($000): 15273 Personnel: 347 |
|---|

**KIRKSVILLE—Adair County**

★ ○ **NORTHEAST REGIONAL MEDICAL CENTER (260022)**, 315 South Osteopathy, Zip 63501–8599, Mailing Address: P.O. Box C8502, Zip 63501–8599; tel. 660/785–1000 **A**3 5 9 10 11 12 13 **F**3 12 13 15 20 28 29 30 34 35 40 43 45 46 49 50 51 53 57 59 60 62 64 68 70 74 75 76 77 79 81 82 85 86 87 89 90 93 107 108 111 118 126 128 129 130 131 132 134 145 146 147 **S** Community Health Systems, Inc., Franklin, TN
Primary Contact: Eric A. Barber, Chief Executive Officer
COO: Ranee C. Brayton, R.N., Associate Chief Executive Officer
CFO: Tom Luebbering, Chief Financial Officer
CMO: John Bailey, D.O., Chief of Staff
CIO: Chad Tatro, Supervisor Information Systems
CHR: Jim Bergman, Director Human Resources
CNO: Cindy Carter, Chief Nursing Officer
Web address: www.nermc.com
**Control:** Corporation, Investor–owned, for–profit **Service:** General Medical and Surgical

| Staffed Beds: 115 Admissions: 3368 Census: 36 Outpatient Visits: 76986 Births: 494 Total Expense ($000): 52406 Payroll Expense ($000): 17573 Personnel: 484 |
|---|

**LAKE SAINT LOUIS—St. Charles County**

⊠ **SSM ST. JOSEPH HOSPITAL WEST (260200)**, 100 Medical Plaza, Zip 63367–1366; tel. 636/625–5200 **A**1 2 9 10 **F**3 11 13 15 17 20 22 28 29 30 31 34 35 36 38 40 41 43 44 49 50 51 53 54 55 56 57 59 60 61 64 68 70 73 74 75 76 78 79 81 82 85 86 87 89 102 107 108 110 111 113 117 118 119 120 128 129 131 134 145 146 147 **P**6 8 **S** SSM Health Care, Saint Louis, MO
Primary Contact: Lisle Wescott, President
CFO: Hal Holder, Director Finance
CMO: Michael Handler, M.D., Vice President Medical Administration
CIO: Sharon Gardner, Manager Information Systems
CHR: Annie Kessler, Human Resources Consultant
Web address: www.ssmstjoseph.com
**Control:** Church–operated, Nongovernment, not–for profit **Service:** General Medical and Surgical

| Staffed Beds: 126 Admissions: 9102 Census: 87 Outpatient Visits: 122005 Births: 1072 Total Expense ($000): 123049 Payroll Expense ($000): 46807 Personnel: 713 |
|---|

**LAMAR—Barton County**

**BARTON COUNTY MEMORIAL HOSPITAL (261325)**, 29 N.W. First Lane, Zip 64759–8105; tel. 417/681–5100 **A**9 10 18 **F**3 11 15 18 28 30 31 34 35 36 39 40 44 45 57 59 64 68 75 77 79 81 85 86 87 89 90 93 97 107 108 110 111 113 118 126 127 128 129 130 131 132 134 142 147
Primary Contact: Rudy C. Snedigar, Administrator and Chief Executive Officer
COO: Virginia Rutledge, Assistant Administrator
CFO: Wendy Duvall, Chief Financial Officer
CIO: Brad Butler, Network Administrator
CHR: Sheila Boice, Director Human Resources
Web address: www.bcmh.net
**Control:** County–Government, nonfederal **Service:** General Medical and Surgical

| Staffed Beds: 25 Admissions: 1486 Census: 18 Outpatient Visits: 79465 Births: 0 Total Expense ($000): 21788 Payroll Expense ($000): 7356 Personnel: 210 |
|---|

MO

---

**Hospital, Medicare Provider Number, Address, Telephone, Approval, Facility, and Physician Codes, Health Care System**

★ American Hospital Association (AHA) membership
☐ The Joint Commission accreditation   ◇ DNV Healthcare Inc. accreditation
○ American Osteopathic Association (AOA) accreditation
△ Commission on Accreditation of Rehabilitation Facilities (CARF) accreditation

## LEBANON—Laclede County

☒ **MERCY HOSPITAL LEBANON (260059)**, 100 Hospital Drive, Zip 65536–9210; tel. 417/533–6100 **A**1 9 10 **F**3 11 13 15 28 29 30 31 32 35 36 37 40 50 53 57 59 64 65 68 70 71 75 76 77 78 79 81 82 83 85 86 87 89 90 93 107 108 111 113 118 128 129 130 131 132 134 143 145 146 147 **P**6 **S** Mercy Health, Chesterfield, MO
Primary Contact: Michael J. Gillen, FACHE, President
CFO: Douglas M. Hoban, Vice President and Chief Financial Officer
Web address: www.stjohnslebanon.com
**Control:** Church–operated, Nongovernment, not–for profit **Service:** General Medical and Surgical

**Staffed Beds:** 62 **Admissions:** 2403 **Census:** 21 **Outpatient Visits:** 104329 **Births:** 420 **Total Expense ($000):** 64800 **Payroll Expense ($000):** 28234 **Personnel:** 532

## LEE'S SUMMIT—Jackson County

☒ **LEE'S SUMMIT MEDICAL CENTER (260190)**, 2100 S.E. Blue Parkway, Zip 64063; tel. 816/282–5000 **A**1 9 10 **F**3 15 18 20 22 28 29 30 31 34 40 49 57 59 60 64 65 68 69 70 74 75 77 78 79 81 82 84 85 87 93 107 108 111 113 118 128 129 130 131 144 145 147 **S** HCA, Nashville, TN
Primary Contact: Jacqueline DeSouza, Chief Executive Officer
CFO: Matthew Leary, Chief Financial Officer
CIO: Evan Kenney, Manager Information Technology Systems
CHR: DeeDee Hawman, Director Human Resources
Web address: www.leessummitmedicalcenter.com
**Control:** Corporation, Investor–owned, for–profit **Service:** General Medical and Surgical

**Staffed Beds:** 64 **Admissions:** 3450 **Census:** 35 **Outpatient Visits:** 84346 **Births:** 0 **Total Expense ($000):** 60267 **Payroll Expense ($000):** 25993 **Personnel:** 298

☐ **SAINT LUKE'S EAST HOSPITAL (260216)**, 100 Ne Saint Lukes Boulevard, Zip 64086–6000; tel. 816/347–5000 **A**1 9 10 **F**3 13 15 17 18 20 22 26 28 29 30 31 34 35 38 40 45 49 50 56 57 59 60 64 68 70 73 74 75 76 78 79 80 81 82 84 85 86 87 92 93 94 96 107 108 110 111 113 116 117 118 125 128 129 131 144 145 146 147 **S** Saint Luke's Health System, Kansas City, MO
Primary Contact: Ronald L. Baker, Chief Executive Officer
COO: Gloria Solis, R.N., Chief Operating Officer and Chief Nursing Officer
Web address: www.saint–lukes.org
**Control:** Church–operated, Nongovernment, not–for profit **Service:** General Medical and Surgical

**Staffed Beds:** 125 **Admissions:** 7784 **Census:** 75 **Outpatient Visits:** 97557 **Births:** 1363 **Total Expense ($000):** 112555 **Payroll Expense ($000):** 41238 **Personnel:** 778

## LEXINGTON—Lafayette County

☒ **LAFAYETTE REGIONAL HEALTH CENTER (261320)**, 1500 State Street, Zip 64067–1107; tel. 660/259–2203 **A**1 9 10 18 **F**11 15 29 31 40 49 59 64 68 70 75 78 79 81 85 93 107 110 111 113 115 118 126 128 129 132 146 **P**6 **S** HCA, Nashville, TN
Primary Contact: Bret Kolman, CPA, Chief Executive Officer
COO: Darrel Box, VP of Operations
CFO: Teri James, Chief Financial Officer
CHR: Lee Tagai, Director Human Resources
CNO: Kim Leakey, R.N., Chief Nursing Officer
Web address: www.lafayetteregionalhealthcenter.com
**Control:** Corporation, Investor–owned, for–profit **Service:** General Medical and Surgical

**Staffed Beds:** 25 **Admissions:** 1170 **Census:** 11 **Outpatient Visits:** 79651 **Births:** 0 **Total Expense ($000):** 24838 **Payroll Expense ($000):** 9480 **Personnel:** 194

## LIBERTY—Clay County

☒ **LIBERTY HOSPITAL (260177)**, 2525 Glenn Hendren Drive, Zip 64068–9600, Mailing Address: P.O. Box 1002, Zip 64069–1002; tel. 816/781–7200, (Total facility includes 12 beds in nursing home–type unit) **A**1 2 9 10 **F**3 9 11 13 15 18 20 22 24 28 29 30 31 34 35 40 44 45 47 49 56 59 62 63 64 66 68 69 70 72 73 74 75 76 77 78 79 80 81 82 84 85 86 87 89 92 93 96 97 102 107 108 110 111 113 114 117 118 125 127 128 129 131 142 145 147
Primary Contact: David Feess, President and Chief Executive Officer
CFO: Erin Parde, Vice President, Finance and Operations
CHR: Patti L. Downey, Vice President, Human Resources
CNO: Lisa M. Vail, R.N., Vice President, Patient Care
Web address: www.Libertyhospital.org
**Control:** Hospital district or authority, Government, nonfederal **Service:** General Medical and Surgical

**Staffed Beds:** 250 **Admissions:** 13535 **Census:** 163 **Outpatient Visits:** 215078 **Births:** 1130 **Total Expense ($000):** 199415 **Payroll Expense ($000):** 88010 **Personnel:** 1361

## LOUISIANA—Pike County

☒ **PIKE COUNTY MEMORIAL HOSPITAL (261333)**, 2305 Georgia Street, Zip 63353–2559; tel. 573/754–5531 **A**1 9 10 18 **F**3 7 11 15 18 28 29 30 34 35 40 50 54 56 57 59 64 65 68 74 75 77 79 81 85 86 87 89 93 97 107 113 126 129 130 131 132 146 147
Primary Contact: Lorraine L. Harness, Administrator
CFO: Ann Perry, Chief Financial Officer
CIO: Jeremy Gruen, Director Information Systems
CHR: Dan Jones, Director Human Resources
Web address: www.pcmh–mo.org
**Control:** County–Government, nonfederal **Service:** General Medical and Surgical

**Staffed Beds:** 25 **Admissions:** 568 **Census:** 6 **Outpatient Visits:** 36991 **Births:** 0 **Total Expense ($000):** 13905 **Payroll Expense ($000):** 6532 **Personnel:** 159

## MACON—Macon County

★ **SAMARITAN MEMORIAL HOSPITAL (261313)**, 1205 North Missouri Street, Zip 63552–2095; tel. 660/385–8700 **A**9 10 18 **F**3 7 8 15 29 30 31 34 35 45 53 56 57 58 59 60 61 62 63 64 65 68 71 75 77 78 79 81 82 83 84 85 86 87 93 94 107 111 114 118 126 127 128 129 130 131 132 134 142 145 **P**5
Primary Contact: Bernard A. Orman, Jr., Administrator
CFO: Susan Spencer, Chief Financial Officer
CHR: Suzanne Britt, Director Human Resources
Web address: www.samaritanhospital.net
**Control:** County–Government, nonfederal **Service:** General Medical and Surgical

**Staffed Beds:** 25 **Admissions:** 567 **Census:** 10 **Outpatient Visits:** 57901 **Births:** 0 **Total Expense ($000):** 17215 **Payroll Expense ($000):** 7483 **Personnel:** 167

## MARSHALL—Saline County

★ **FITZGIBBON HOSPITAL (260142)**, 2305 South 65 Highway, Zip 65340–0250, Mailing Address: P.O. Box 250, Zip 65340–0250; tel. 660/886–7431 **A**3 5 9 10 **F**3 11 13 15 35 40 45 53 57 59 62 63 64 68 70 74 75 76 77 78 79 81 82 84 85 87 90 93 98 103 107 110 111 114 117 118 119 120 121 126 127 128 129 130 131 132 142 145 146
Primary Contact: Ronald A. Ott, Chief Executive Officer
COO: Dennis Sousley, Vice President of Clinical Services
CFO: Roberta Nienhueser, Chief Financial Officer
CMO: Shari Thompson, M.D., President Medical Staff
CIO: Tom Jones, Manager Information Technology
CHR: Myron Lite, Director Human Resources
CNO: Kathryn Lynne Ott, MSN, Vice President Patient Care Services/Chief Nursing Officer
Web address: www.fitzgibbon.org
**Control:** Other not–for–profit (including NFP Corporation) **Service:** General Medical and Surgical

**Staffed Beds:** 52 **Admissions:** 2332 **Census:** 23 **Outpatient Visits:** 104188 **Births:** 315 **Total Expense ($000):** 42871 **Payroll Expense ($000):** 18458 **Personnel:** 474

## MARYLAND HEIGHTS—St. Louis County

★ **RANKEN JORDAN – A PEDIATRIC SPECIALTY HOSPITAL (263303)**, (Specialty Hospital), 11365 Dorsett Road, Zip 63043–3411; tel. 314/872–6400 **A**9 10 **F**12 16 29 30 32 35 44 50 64 80 82 86 87 89 90 91 92 93 94 99 104 129 131 142 145 147 **P**6
Primary Contact: Laureen K. Tanner, R.N., MSN, FACHE, President and Chief Executive Officer
COO: Brett Moorehouse, FACHE, Vice President and Chief Operating Officer
CFO: Jean Bardwell, Vice President and Chief Financial Officer
CMO: Nicholas Holekamp, M.D., Medical Director
CIO: Jean Bardwell, Vice President and Chief Financial Officer
CHR: Thomas M. Irvin, Administrator Human Resources
Web address: www.rankenjordan.org
**Control:** Other not–for–profit (including NFP Corporation) **Service:** Children's rehabilitation

**Staffed Beds:** 34 **Admissions:** 221 **Census:** 29 **Outpatient Visits:** 6171 **Births:** 0 **Total Expense ($000):** 23485 **Payroll Expense ($000):** 12758 **Personnel:** 151

MO

*Many Facility Codes have changed. Please refer to the AHA Guide Code Chart.* © 2012 AHA Guide

## MARYVILLE—Nodaway County

☒ **ST. FRANCIS HOSPITAL AND HEALTH SERVICES (260050)**, 2016 South Main Street, Zip 64468–2655; tel. 660/562–2600 **A**1 5 9 10 20 **F**3 8 11 13 15 28 29 30 34 35 38 40 57 59 64 65 70 75 76 77 79 81 82 85 89 93 96 97 98 99 100 101 102 103 104 105 107 111 113 118 126 127 129 130 132 134 140 141 145 **P**6 **S** SSM Health Care, Saint Louis, MO
Primary Contact: Gray Cox, President
COO: Cathy New, Vice President Clinical Services
CFO: Jocelyn Skidmore, Director Finance
CMO: Shellie Faris, M.D., President Medical Staff
CIO: Dave Lewis, Director Information Services
CHR: Martha Archer, Director Human Resources
Web address: www.stfrancismaryville.com
**Control:** Church–operated, Nongovernment, not–for profit **Service:** General Medical and Surgical

**Staffed Beds:** 57 **Admissions:** 1546 **Census:** 20 **Outpatient Visits:** 93428 **Births:** 260 **Total Expense ($000):** 61494 **Payroll Expense ($000):** 26650 **Personnel:** 420

## MEMPHIS—Scotland County

★ **SCOTLAND COUNTY HOSPITAL (261310)**, 450 Sigler Avenue, Zip 63555–1726; tel. 660/465–8511, (Nonreporting) **A**9 10 18
Primary Contact: Marcia R. Dial, Administrator and Chief Executive Officer
CFO: Sheryl Templeton, Chief Financial Officer
CMO: Randy Tobler, M.D., Chief Medical Officer
CIO: Angela Schmitter, Director Health Information Management
CHR: Tammy Newland, Coordinator Human Resources
Web address: www.scotlandcountyhospital.com
**Control:** Hospital district or authority, Government, nonfederal **Service:** General Medical and Surgical

**Staffed Beds:** 25

**SCOTLAND COUNTY MEMORIAL HOSPITAL** See Scotland County Hospital

## MEXICO—Audrain County

☐ △ **AUDRAIN MEDICAL CENTER (260064)**, 620 East Monroe Street, Zip 65265–2919; tel. 573/582–5000 **A**1 2 7 9 10 **F**3 11 13 15 18 20 22 26 28 29 30 31 34 40 45 53 54 57 59 64 65 70 73 74 75 76 77 78 79 81 85 86 87 89 90 93 107 108 111 113 117 118 120 126 128 129 130 131 145 146 **P**6
Primary Contact: David A. Neuendorf, FACHE, President and Chief Executive Officer
COO: David A. Neuendorf, FACHE, President and Chief Executive Officer
CFO: Greg Shaw, Vice President and Chief Financial Officer
CMO: Michael Quinlan, M.D., Chief of Staff
CIO: Dawn Evans, Manager Information Technology
CHR: Christy Smiley, Director Human Resources
Web address: www.audrainmedicalcenter.com
**Control:** Other not–for–profit (including NFP Corporation) **Service:** General Medical and Surgical

**Staffed Beds:** 49 **Admissions:** 2579 **Census:** 24 **Outpatient Visits:** 160835 **Births:** 163 **Total Expense ($000):** 59055 **Payroll Expense ($000):** 22770 **Personnel:** 451

## MILAN—Sullivan County

★ **SULLIVAN COUNTY MEMORIAL HOSPITAL (261306)**, 630 West Third Street, Zip 63556–1076; tel. 660/265–4212, (Total facility includes 14 beds in nursing home–type unit) **A**9 10 18 **F**28 29 32 34 35 40 53 57 59 65 67 68 75 77 81 87 97 107 111 113 118 126 127 129 132 145 147 **P**5 6
Primary Contact: Martha Gragg, R.N., MSN, Chief Executive Officer
COO: Amy J. Michael, Chief Operating Officer
CFO: Amy J. Michael, Chief Operating Officer
CMO: Dale Essmyer, M.D., Chief of Staff
CMO: Thomas Williams, D.O., Chief of Staff
CIO: Jody Biston, Director Risk Management and Physician Clinic
CHR: Valerie Johnson, Director Human Resources
CHR: Billie Ryals, Human Resources Director
CNO: Carol Fordyce, Director of Patient Care Services
Web address: www.scmhospital.org
**Control:** City–County, Government, nonfederal **Service:** General Medical and Surgical

**Staffed Beds:** 39 **Admissions:** 355 **Census:** 20 **Outpatient Visits:** 18757 **Births:** 0 **Total Expense ($000):** 6449 **Payroll Expense ($000):** 2980 **Personnel:** 84

## MOBERLY—Randolph County

☒ **MOBERLY REGIONAL MEDICAL CENTER (260074)**, 1515 Union Avenue, Zip 65270–9449; tel. 660/263–8400 **A**1 9 10 20 **F**3 13 15 18 20 22 26 28 29 34 35 38 39 40 44 45 46 49 50 51 53 56 57 59 64 65 70 74 75 76 77 79 80 81 85 86 87 89 93 97 98 100 103 107 108 110 111 113 116 117 118 126 128 129 130 131 132 134 145 146 147 **S** Community Health Systems, Inc., Franklin, TN
Primary Contact: Christian Jones, Chief Executive Officer
CFO: Tracey Matheis, Chief Financial Officer
CMO: Philip Stitzer, D.O., Chief Medical Officer
CIO: Doris Whelan, Chief Information Officer
CHR: Tim Clark, Director Human Resources
Web address: www.moberlyhospital.com
**Control:** Corporation, Investor–owned, for–profit **Service:** General Medical and Surgical

**Staffed Beds:** 94 **Admissions:** 2933 **Census:** 42 **Outpatient Visits:** 49690 **Births:** 207 **Total Expense ($000):** 51682 **Payroll Expense ($000):** 15727 **Personnel:** 337

## MONETT—Barry County

☐ **COX MONETT (261329)**, 801 North Lincoln Avenue, Zip 65708–1641; tel. 417/235–3144 **A**1 9 10 18 **F**3 11 13 15 28 29 31 32 34 35 40 45 50 53 56 57 59 64 68 76 77 81 85 89 90 93 107 111 113 118 126 127 128 129 130 132 134 145 146 **P**6 **S** CoxHealth, Springfield, MO
Primary Contact: Genice Maroc, FACHE, Administrator and Chief Executive Officer
CFO: R. Martin Williams, Director Financial Services
CHR: Pamela Foland, Director Human Resources
Web address: www.coxhealth.com
**Control:** Other not–for–profit (including NFP Corporation) **Service:** General Medical and Surgical

**Staffed Beds:** 25 **Admissions:** 813 **Census:** 7 **Outpatient Visits:** 56394 **Births:** 282 **Total Expense ($000):** 28469 **Payroll Expense ($000):** 13509 **Personnel:** 239

## MOUNT VERNON—Lawrence County

☒ △ **MISSOURI REHABILITATION CENTER (262001)**, 600 North Main Street, Zip 65712–1004; tel. 417/466–3711 **A**1 7 9 10 **F**1 3 11 28 29 30 44 50 53 57 59 64 68 70 75 77 87 90 91 93 96 118 128 129 134 142 145 147 **P**6 **S** University of Missouri Health Care, Columbia, MO
Primary Contact: Steve Patterson, R.N., Executive Director
CFO: Amy Baker, Associate Director Finance Services
CMO: Jennie Gorham, D.O., Co–Medical Director
CIO: Tom Collier, Manager Information Systems
CHR: David Thiessen, Associate Director Support Services
CNO: Gail Getzendaner, Interim Director of Nursing
Web address: www.muhealth.org/~MOrehab
**Control:** State–Government, nonfederal **Service:** Long–Term Acute Care hospital

**Staffed Beds:** 79 **Admissions:** 313 **Census:** 40 **Outpatient Visits:** 58887 **Births:** 0 **Total Expense ($000):** 33036 **Payroll Expense ($000):** 17739 **Personnel:** 361

## MOUNTAIN VIEW—Howell County

☒ **MERCY ST. FRANCIS HOSPITAL (261335)**, 100 West Highway 60, Zip 65548–7125; tel. 417/934–7000 **A**1 9 10 18 **F**11 15 28 29 30 40 57 64 75 81 89 90 93 107 111 118 128 131 132 **P**6 **S** Mercy Health, Chesterfield, MO
Primary Contact: Jonathan O. Wade, President and Chief Executive Officer
CFO: Sherry Clouse Day, CPA, Chief Financial Officer
CMO: Barry Spoon, M.D., Chief of Staff
CIO: Jana Murray, Manager Medical Records
CHR: Tracy Smith, Director Human Resources
Web address: www.stjohns.com/aboutus/stfrancis.aspx
**Control:** Church–operated, Nongovernment, not–for profit **Service:** General Medical and Surgical

**Staffed Beds:** 20 **Admissions:** 499 **Census:** 7 **Outpatient Visits:** 18805 **Births:** 0 **Total Expense ($000):** 13818 **Payroll Expense ($000):** 6517 **Personnel:** 141

**MO**

---

**Hospital, Medicare Provider Number, Address, Telephone, Approval, Facility, and Physician Codes, Health Care System**

★ American Hospital Association (AHA) membership
☐ The Joint Commission accreditation      ◇ DNV Healthcare Inc. accreditation
○ American Osteopathic Association (AOA) accreditation
△ Commission on Accreditation of Rehabilitation Facilities (CARF) accreditation

### NEOSHO—Newton County

★ **FREEMAN NEOSHO HOSPITAL (261331)**, 113 West Hickory Street, Zip 64850–1705; tel. 417/455–4352 **A**9 10 18 **F**3 7 11 15 28 29 30 34 35 40 43 44 45 47 56 57 59 64 68 70 75 77 79 81 85 86 87 89 90 93 97 107 111 113 118 127 129 130 131 132 145 147 **S** Freeman Health System, Joplin, MO
Primary Contact: Daxton Holcomb, Chief Executive Officer
CFO: Steve W. Graddy, Chief Financial Officer
CMO: Rodney McFarland, M.D., Medical Director
CIO: Sue Annesser, Director Information Systems
CHR: Deborah Chiodo, Director Human Resources
Web address: www.freemanhealth.com
**Control:** Other not–for–profit (including NFP Corporation) **Service:** General Medical and Surgical

**Staffed Beds:** 25 **Admissions:** 1641 **Census:** 18 **Outpatient Visits:** 48065 **Births:** 0 **Total Expense ($000):** 22800 **Payroll Expense ($000):** 9577 **Personnel:** 192

### NEVADA—Vernon County

☐ **HEARTLAND BEHAVIORAL HEALTH SERVICES**, 1500 West Ashland Street, Zip 64772–1710; tel. 417/667–2666 **A**1 9 **F**98 99 101 102 **S** Universal Health Services, Inc., King of Prussia, PA
Primary Contact: Alyson Wysong–Harder, Chief Executive Officer
CFO: Terri Graves, Chief Financial Officer
CMO: Ahmad Tarar, M.D., Medical Director
CHR: Carri Compton–Ogle, Administrative Officer
Web address: www.heartlandbehavioral.com
**Control:** State–Government, nonfederal **Service:** Psychiatric

**Staffed Beds:** 37 **Admissions:** 1119 **Census:** 30 **Outpatient Visits:** 0 **Births:** 0 **Total Expense ($000):** 16421 **Payroll Expense ($000):** 7100 **Personnel:** 78

⊞ **NEVADA REGIONAL MEDICAL CENTER (260061)**, 800 South Ash Street, Zip 64772–3223; tel. 417/667–3355 **A**1 9 10 **F**3 11 13 15 18 26 27 28 29 30 31 32 34 35 39 40 41 45 50 54 57 59 62 63 64 65 69 70 74 75 76 77 78 79 81 82 84 85 86 87 89 90 91 93 94 96 98 101 102 103 104 107 110 111 113 118 126 128 129 130 131 132 134 142 143 145 147 **S** QHR, Brentwood, TN
Primary Contact: Judith K. Feuquay, Chief Executive Officer
CMO: Scott Beard, M.D., Chief of Staff
CIO: Jeffrey Price, Director Information Technology
CHR: Patty Gaughan, Human Resource Administrative Officer
Web address: www.nrmchealth.com
**Control:** City–Government, nonfederal **Service:** General Medical and Surgical

**Staffed Beds:** 71 **Admissions:** 2410 **Census:** 28 **Outpatient Visits:** 72169 **Births:** 330 **Total Expense ($000):** 33356 **Payroll Expense ($000):** 13387 **Personnel:** 324

### NORTH KANSAS CITY—Clay County

⊞ **NORTH KANSAS CITY HOSPITAL (260096)**, 2800 Clay Edwards Drive, Zip 64116–3220; tel. 816/691–2000 **A**1 2 9 10 **F**3 11 12 13 15 17 18 20 22 24 26 28 29 30 31 34 35 37 38 39 40 43 44 45 46 47 48 49 50 53 57 58 59 62 63 64 70 72 74 75 76 77 78 79 80 81 82 83 84 85 86 87 89 90 93 96 107 108 110 111 113 114 117 118 119 120 122 125 128 129 131 134 145 146
Primary Contact: Peggy Schmitt, President and Chief Executive Officer
COO: Jody Abbott, Senior Vice President and Chief Operating Officer
CFO: Jim McNey, Vice President Finance and Chief Financial Officer
CMO: Gary L. Carter, M.D., Medical Director of Quality
CIO: Art Fisk, Chief Information Officer
CHR: Beverly Johnson, Vice President Human Resources
CNO: Sarah G. Fields, R.N., Vice President Nursing
Web address: www.nkch.org
**Control:** City–Government, nonfederal **Service:** General Medical and Surgical

**Staffed Beds:** 409 **Admissions:** 21547 **Census:** 261 **Outpatient Visits:** 212844 **Births:** 1721 **Total Expense ($000):** 376260 **Payroll Expense ($000):** 141683 **Personnel:** 2474

### OSAGE BEACH—Camden County

⊞ **LAKE REGIONAL HEALTH SYSTEM (260186)**, 54 Hospital Drive, Zip 65065–3050; tel. 573/348–8000, (Total facility includes 16 beds in nursing home–type unit) **A**1 5 9 10 **F**3 11 12 13 15 17 18 20 22 24 28 29 30 31 32 34 35 38 39 40 43 44 45 48 49 50 51 53 57 59 60 62 64 65 68 70 74 75 76 77 78 79 81 82 84 85 86 87 89 93 96 107 108 110 111 113 114 117 118 120 126 127 128 129 130 131 134 143 144 145 147 **P**6
Primary Contact: Michael E. Henze, Chief Executive Officer
COO: Vicki L. Franklin, Senior Vice President and Chief Operating Officer
CFO: Dan Probstfield, Senior Vice President and Chief Financial Officer
CMO: Robert Hyatt, M.D., Senior Vice President Medical Affairs
CIO: Scott Poest, Chief Information Officer
CHR: Tom Williams, Director Human Resources
CNO: Janice L. Dungan, Sr Vice President Clinical Services
Web address: www.lakeregional.com
**Control:** Other not–for–profit (including NFP Corporation) **Service:** General Medical and Surgical

**Staffed Beds:** 116 **Admissions:** 6069 **Census:** 72 **Outpatient Visits:** 289502 **Births:** 725 **Total Expense ($000):** 171037 **Payroll Expense ($000):** 66820 **Personnel:** 1172

### OSCEOLA—St. Clair County

★ **SAC–OSAGE HOSPITAL (260147)**, Junction Highways 13 & Business 13, Zip 64776–0426, Mailing Address: P.O. Box 426, Zip 64776–0426; tel. 417/646–8181 **A**9 10 20 **F**3 7 8 11 15 29 30 34 35 40 49 57 69 75 77 79 81 83 89 90 93 107 111 118 126 127 132 145 **P**6
Primary Contact: Bryan D. Coffey, Chief Executive Officer
CMO: Niko van Zanten, M.D., Chief of Staff
CNO: Patricia Turner, R.N., Director of Nursing
Web address: www.sac–osagehospital.com
**Control:** Hospital district or authority, Government, nonfederal **Service:** General Medical and Surgical

**Staffed Beds:** 47 **Admissions:** 402 **Census:** 5 **Outpatient Visits:** 14311 **Births:** 0 **Total Expense ($000):** 7806 **Payroll Expense ($000):** 3637 **Personnel:** 81

### PERRYVILLE—Perry County

⊞ **PERRY COUNTY MEMORIAL HOSPITAL (261311)**, 434 North West Street, Zip 63775–1398; tel. 573/547–2536 **A**1 9 10 18 **F**3 7 8 11 13 15 29 30 31 34 35 40 44 48 51 53 54 56 57 59 62 64 66 68 75 76 77 78 79 81 85 87 89 90 92 93 97 99 100 101 102 103 104 107 111 113 116 118 128 129 130 131 132 134 142 143 144 146 147
Primary Contact: Patrick E. Carron, FACHE, President and Chief Executive Officer
COO: Lee Clinton, FACHE, Vice President Operations
CFO: Randall Wolf, Vice President Finance
CMO: Michael Steele, M.D., Chief of Staff
CIO: Ron Heuring, Director Information Systems
CHR: Christopher Wibbenmeyer, Director Human Resources
Web address: www.pchmo.org
**Control:** Other not–for–profit (including NFP Corporation) **Service:** General Medical and Surgical

**Staffed Beds:** 25 **Admissions:** 881 **Census:** 12 **Outpatient Visits:** 47111 **Births:** 142 **Total Expense ($000):** 26684 **Payroll Expense ($000):** 10408 **Personnel:** 293

### PILOT KNOB—Iron County

**IRON COUNTY HOSPITAL (261336)**, 301 North Highway 21, Zip 63663–0548, Mailing Address: P.O. Box 548, Zip 63663–0548; tel. 573/546–1260 **A**9 10 18 **F**11 15 40 57 90 93 107 111 118 126 127 129 132
Primary Contact: Cyndi Basler, Interim Chief Executive Officer
Web address: www.ironhospital.com
**Control:** Hospital district or authority, Government, nonfederal **Service:** General Medical and Surgical

**Staffed Beds:** 15 **Admissions:** 341 **Census:** 4 **Outpatient Visits:** 16618 **Births:** 0 **Total Expense ($000):** 8389 **Payroll Expense ($000):** 2040 **Personnel:** 63

### POPLAR BLUFF—Butler County

**BLACK RIVER MEDICAL CENTER**, 219 Physicians Park Drive, Zip 63901–3956; tel. 573/727–9080, (Nonreporting)
Primary Contact: Michael G. Burcham, Sr., President and CEO
**Control:** Other not–for–profit (including NFP Corporation) **Service:** General Medical and Surgical

**Staffed Beds:** 3

**MO**

*Many Facility Codes have changed. Please refer to the AHA Guide Code Chart.* © 2012 AHA Guide

⊞ **JOHN J. PERSHING VETERANS AFFAIRS MEDICAL CENTER**, 1500 North Westwood Boulevard, Zip 63901–3318; tel. 573/686–4151, (Total facility includes 40 beds in nursing home–type unit) **A**1 **F**3 5 11 15 29 30 33 34 36 38 39 40 41 45 53 54 56 59 62 63 64 65 75 77 79 81 83 84 86 87 90 93 94 97 100 104 107 111 113 118 126 127 129 134 142 143 145 146 147 **S** Department of Veterans Affairs, Washington, DC
Primary Contact: Marjorie Hedstrom, Director
COO: Stan Skorniak, MS, Associate Medical Center Director
CFO: Kristy Siebert, Manager Finance
CMO: Vijayachandran Nair, M.D., Chief of Staff
CIO: Janice Vernon, Supervisory Information Technology Specialist
CHR: Genise Denton, Manager Human Resources
Web address: www.poplarbluff.va.gov
**Control:** Veterans Affairs, Government, federal **Service:** General Medical and Surgical

**Staffed Beds:** 58 **Admissions:** 1673 **Census:** 40 **Outpatient Visits:** 101709 **Births:** 0 **Total Expense ($000):** 113959 **Payroll Expense ($000):** 35189 **Personnel:** 568

⊞ △ **POPLAR BLUFF REGIONAL MEDICAL CENTER (260119)**, 2620 North Westwood Boulevard, Zip 63901–3396, Mailing Address: P.O. Box 88, Zip 63902–0088; tel. 573/686–5311, (Includes POPLAR BLUFF REGIONAL MEDICAL CENTER–NORTH CAMPUS, 2620 North Westwood Boulevard, Zip 63901–2341; tel. 573/636–4111; POPLAR BLUFF REGIONAL MEDICAL CENTER–SOUTH CAMPUS, 621 Pine Boulevard, Zip 63901; tel. 573/785–7721) **A**1 2 7 9 10 19 **F**3 4 11 13 15 17 18 20 22 24 28 29 31 35 39 40 45 46 49 50 51 53 54 57 59 60 64 65 68 70 74 75 76 77 78 79 81 82 85 87 89 90 93 98 102 107 108 111 113 116 117 118 120 125 126 129 130 131 145 147 **P**6 **S** Health Management Associates, Naples, FL
Primary Contact: Charles L. Stewart, Chief Executive Officer
COO: Greg Carda, Chief Operating Officer
CFO: Mark Johnson, Chief Financial Officer
CMO: Austin Tinsley, M.D., Chief Medical Officer
CIO: Gary Dollins, Director Management Information Systems
CHR: Denise Rushin, Director Human Resources
Web address: www.poplarbluffregional.com
**Control:** Individual, Investor–owned, for–profit **Service:** General Medical and Surgical

**Staffed Beds:** 287 **Admissions:** 12028 **Census:** 137 **Outpatient Visits:** 154047 **Births:** 1199 **Total Expense ($000):** 132862 **Payroll Expense ($000):** 38093 **Personnel:** 905

### POTOSI—Washington County

★ **WASHINGTON COUNTY MEMORIAL HOSPITAL (261308)**, 300 Health Way, Zip 63664–1420; tel. 573/438–5451 **A**9 10 18 **F**3 11 15 28 29 34 35 40 45 57 59 64 65 68 74 75 77 79 81 87 90 93 97 98 104 106 107 108 111 113 118 126 128 129 132 143 144 145 146 147
Primary Contact: Leah Osbahr, Administrator
COO: Leah Osbahr, CEO
CFO: Debbie Pratt, Chief Financial Officer
CMO: James Hawk, M.D., Chief of Staff
CMO: James Weber, D.O., Chief of Staff
CIO: Andrew Schrum, Director Information Systems
CHR: Hopie Jenkins, Director Personnel
CNO: Beverly Williams, R.N., Chief Nursing Officer
Web address: www.wcmhosp.org
**Control:** County–Government, nonfederal **Service:** General Medical and Surgical

**Staffed Beds:** 25 **Admissions:** 682 **Census:** 10 **Outpatient Visits:** 49377 **Births:** 0 **Total Expense ($000):** 19563 **Payroll Expense ($000):** 10407 **Personnel:** 271

### RICHMOND—Ray County

**RAY COUNTY MEMORIAL HOSPITAL (261327)**, 904 Wollard Boulevard, Zip 64085–2229; tel. 816/470–5432 **A**9 10 18 **F**3 11 15 29 40 62 64 68 74 75 78 79 81 82 85 87 93 107 108 110 111 114 115 118 129 132 145
Primary Contact: Robert Littleton, Administrator
CFO: Donald Harr, Controller
CHR: Donna Strain, Director Human Resources
Web address: www.raycountyhospital.com
**Control:** County–Government, nonfederal **Service:** General Medical and Surgical

**Staffed Beds:** 25 **Admissions:** 969 **Census:** 11 **Outpatient Visits:** 18087 **Births:** 0 **Total Expense ($000):** 19641 **Payroll Expense ($000):** 8543 **Personnel:** 198

### ROLLA—Phelps County

⊞ △ **PHELPS COUNTY REGIONAL MEDICAL CENTER (260017)**, 1000 West Tenth Street, Zip 65401–2905; tel. 573/458–8899, (Total facility includes 18 beds in nursing home–type unit) **A**1 2 7 9 10 **F**3 7 8 11 13 15 17 18 20 26 28 29 30 31 34 35 39 40 45 47 48 49 51 57 59 60 63 68 70 73 74 75 76 77 78 79 81 85 86 89 90 93 96 98 100 101 102 103 104 107 110 111 113 115 117 118 119 120 122 126 127 128 130 131 134 142 143 145 147
Primary Contact: John Denbo, Chief Executive Officer
COO: Ellis Hawkins, Senior Vice President and Chief Operating Officer
CFO: Edward Clayton, Chief Financial Officer
CMO: Donald James, D.O., Chief Medical Officer
CIO: David Dawdy, Director Information Technology
CHR: Frank A. Lazzaro, III, Chief Human Resources Officer
CNO: Regenia Stull, R.N., Chief Nurse Executive
Web address: www.pcrmc.com
**Control:** County–Government, nonfederal **Service:** General Medical and Surgical

**Staffed Beds:** 217 **Admissions:** 7586 **Census:** 103 **Outpatient Visits:** 224609 **Births:** 859 **Total Expense ($000):** 151770 **Payroll Expense ($000):** 55586 **Personnel:** 1766

### SAINT CHARLES—St. Charles County

⊞ **CENTERPOINTE HOSPITAL (264012)**, 4801 Weldon Spring Parkway, Zip 63304–5611; tel. 636/441–7300 **A**1 9 10 **F**4 5 34 35 38 54 58 87 98 99 100 101 102 103 104 105 129 131 142
Primary Contact: Azfar Malik, M.D., Chief Executive Officer and Chief Medical Officer
COO: Susan Mathis, Chief Operating Officer
CFO: Tariq F. Malik, CPA, Acting Chief Financial Officer
CMO: Azfar Malik, M.D., Chief Executive Officer and Chief Medical Officer
CIO: Jennifer Bourn, Coordinator Health Information Systems
CHR: Kelli White, Manager Human Resources
Web address: www.centerpointehospital.com
**Control:** Corporation, Investor–owned, for–profit **Service:** Psychiatric

**Staffed Beds:** 104 **Admissions:** 2982 **Census:** 70 **Outpatient Visits:** 49626 **Births:** 0 **Total Expense ($000):** 28816 **Payroll Expense ($000):** 14930 **Personnel:** 232

⊞ **PROGRESS WEST HEALTHCARE CENTER (260219)**, Two Progress Point, Zip 63368–2208; tel. 636/344–2273 **A**1 10 **F**3 13 15 18 19 20 22 29 30 40 41 45 49 51 57 59 60 70 76 79 81 85 87 89 107 111 114 117 118 129 134 145 **S** BJC HealthCare, Saint Louis, MO
Primary Contact: John Antes, President
CFO: Glen Schweagel, Chief Financial Officer
CMO: Kenneth Hacker, M.D., Chief of Staff
CIO: Michael Kelly, Information Systems Account Executive
CHR: Janet Nystrom, Manager Human Resources
Web address: www.progresswesthealthcare.org
**Control:** Other not–for–profit (including NFP Corporation) **Service:** General Medical and Surgical

**Staffed Beds:** 42 **Admissions:** 3070 **Census:** 27 **Outpatient Visits:** 42299 **Births:** 527 **Total Expense ($000):** 62454 **Payroll Expense ($000):** 18421 **Personnel:** 299

★ **SELECT SPECIALTY HOSPITAL–ST. LOUIS (262013)**, 300 First Capitol Drive, Unit 1, Zip 63301–2844; tel. 636/947–5010 **A**9 10 **F**1 29 74 75 77 87 107 147 **S** Select Medical Corporation, Mechanicsburg, PA
Primary Contact: Jordan Tenenbaum, Chief Executive Officer
Web address: www.selectmedicalcorp.com
**Control:** Corporation, Investor–owned, for–profit **Service:** Long–Term Acute Care hospital

**Staffed Beds:** 33 **Admissions:** 346 **Census:** 29 **Outpatient Visits:** 0 **Births:** 0 **Total Expense ($000):** 16050 **Payroll Expense ($000):** 6141 **Personnel:** 119

**MO**

---

**Hospital, Medicare Provider Number, Address, Telephone, Approval, Facility, and Physician Codes, Health Care System**

★ American Hospital Association (AHA) membership
☐ The Joint Commission accreditation
◇ DNV Healthcare Inc. accreditation
○ American Osteopathic Association (AOA) accreditation
△ Commission on Accreditation of Rehabilitation Facilities (CARF) accreditation

✠ **SSM ST. JOSEPH HEALTH CENTER (260005)**, 300 First Capitol Drive, Zip 63301–2844; tel. 636/947–5000, (Includes SSM ST. JOSEPH HEALTH CENTER – WENTZVILLE, 500 Medical Drive, Wentzville, Zip 63385–3421; tel. 636/327–1000) **A**1 2 9 10 **F**3 4 5 11 13 15 17 18 20 22 24 26 28 29 30 31 34 35 36 38 39 40 43 44 45 46 49 50 51 53 55 56 57 58 59 60 61 64 68 70 73 74 75 76 78 79 81 82 85 86 87 90 96 97 98 99 100 101 102 103 104 105 107 108 110 111 113 116 117 118 119 120 128 129 131 133 134 142 145 146 147 **P**6 8 **S** SSM Health Care, Saint Louis, MO
Primary Contact: Gaspare Calvaruso, President
COO: Lee Bernstein, Executive Vice President and Chief Operating Officer
CFO: Hal Holder, Vice President Finance
CIO: Margaret Feilner, Director Information Services
CHR: Michael R. Garcia, Vice President Human Resources
Web address: www.ssmstjoseph.com
**Control:** Church–operated, Nongovernment, not–for profit **Service:** General Medical and Surgical

> **Staffed Beds: 331 Admissions: 15493 Census: 212 Outpatient Visits:** 144469 **Births:** 673 **Total Expense ($000):** 193179 **Payroll Expense ($000):** 71412 **Personnel:** 1247

### SAINT JOSEPH—Buchanan County

★ **HEARTLAND LONG TERM ACUTE CARE HOSPITAL (262019)**, 5325 Faraon Street, Zip 64506–3488; tel. 816/271–6000 **A**10 **F**1 3 29 86 129
Primary Contact: James Mikes, Administrator
Web address: www.heartland–health.com
**Control:** Other not–for–profit (including NFP Corporation) **Service:** Long–Term Acute Care hospital

> **Staffed Beds: 41 Admissions: 241 Census: 17 Outpatient Visits: 0 Births:** 0 **Total Expense ($000):** 11600 **Payroll Expense ($000):** 3448 **Personnel:** 58

✠ **HEARTLAND REGIONAL MEDICAL CENTER (260006)**, 5325 Faraon Street, Zip 64506–3488; tel. 816/271–6000 **A**1 2 5 9 10 20 **F**3 8 9 11 14 15 17 18 20 22 24 26 28 29 30 31 33 34 35 36 37 39 40 43 45 47 49 50 53 54 57 58 59 62 63 64 65 66 70 71 74 75 76 77 78 79 80 81 82 84 85 86 87 89 92 93 94 96 97 98 100 102 103 107 108 110 111 113 114 117 118 119 120 122 123 128 129 130 134 143 145 146 147 **P**6
Primary Contact: Samuel Mark Laney, M.D., President and Chief Executive Officer
COO: Curt Kretzinger, Chief Operating Officer
CFO: John P. Wilson, Chief Financial Officer
CIO: Joe Boyce, M.D., Chief Information Officer
CHR: Michael Pulido, Process Leader Human Resources
Web address: www.heartland–health.com
**Control:** Other not–for–profit (including NFP Corporation) **Service:** General Medical and Surgical

> **Staffed Beds: 352 Admissions: 19183 Census: 224 Outpatient Visits:** 959823 **Births:** 1712 **Total Expense ($000):** 442339 **Payroll Expense ($000):** 201271 **Personnel:** 2854

☐ **NORTHWEST MISSOURI PSYCHIATRIC REHABILITATION CENTER (264007)**, 3505 Frederick Avenue, Zip 64506–2914; tel. 816/387–2300 **A**1 10 **F**4 29 34 50 58 59 65 75 77 98 99 101 102 103 129 134 145 **P**6
Primary Contact: Dick Gregory, Ph.D., Chief Executive Officer
COO: Mary Attebury, Chief Operating Officer
CFO: Randy Riley, Fiscal and Administrative Manager
CMO: James B. Reynolds, M.D., Medical Director
CIO: Eduardo Abaricia, Director Information Technology
CHR: Mary Blakey Gorman, Director Human Resources
Web address: www.dmh.missouri.gov/hr/faclist.htm
**Control:** State–Government, nonfederal **Service:** Psychiatric

> **Staffed Beds: 108 Admissions: 71 Census: 107 Outpatient Visits:** 36 **Births:** 0 **Total Expense ($000):** 22426 **Payroll Expense ($000):** 10616 **Personnel:** 282

### SAINT LOUIS—St. Louis City County

✠ **BARNES–JEWISH HOSPITAL (260032)**, 1 Barnes–Jewish Hospital Plaza, Zip 63110–1003; tel. 314/747–3000, (Total facility includes 120 beds in nursing home–type unit) **A**1 2 3 5 8 9 10 **F**3 4 8 9 11 12 13 14 15 16 17 18 19 20 21 22 23 24 25 26 28 29 30 31 34 35 36 37 38 39 40 43 44 45 46 47 48 49 50 51 52 53 54 55 56 57 58 59 60 61 64 65 66 68 70 71 73 74 75 76 77 78 79 80 81 82 84 85 86 87 89 90 91 92 93 94 95 96 97 98 100 101 102 103 104 105 107 108 109 110 111 112 113 114 115 116 117 118 119 120 122 123 125 127 128 129 130 131 133 134 135 136 137 138 139 140 141 142 143 144 145 146 147 **P**6 **S** BJC HealthCare, Saint Louis, MO
Primary Contact: Richard J. Liekweg, President
CFO: Mark Krieger, Vice President and Chief Financial Officer
CMO: John Lynch, M.D., Vice President and Chief Medical Officer
CIO: Jerry Vuchak, Vice President Information Systems
CHR: John Beatty, Vice President Human Resources
CNO: Coreen Vlodarchyk, R.N., Vice President, Patient Care Services and Chief Nursing Officer
Web address: www.barnesjewish.org
**Control:** Other not–for–profit (including NFP Corporation) **Service:** General Medical and Surgical

> **Staffed Beds: 1305 Admissions: 55304 Census: 913 Outpatient Visits:** 689089 **Births:** 3421 **Total Expense ($000):** 1493801 **Payroll Expense ($000):** 460751 **Personnel:** 9571

✠ **BARNES–JEWISH WEST COUNTY HOSPITAL (260162)**, 12634 Olive Boulevard, Zip 63141–6337; tel. 314/996–8000 **A**1 3 5 9 10 **F**3 12 15 18 29 30 33 35 40 46 47 49 50 51 53 57 59 64 65 68 70 74 75 77 78 79 81 82 85 91 93 103 111 113 114 116 118 119 120 125 128 129 130 145 147 **S** BJC HealthCare, Saint Louis, MO
Primary Contact: Larry Tracy, FACHE, Chief Operating Officer
COO: Larry Tracy, FACHE, Chief Operating Officer
CFO: Diane M. Glen, Assistant Administrator
CMO: Sam B. Bhayani, Chief Medical Officer
CIO: Jerry Vuchak, Vice President Information Systems
CHR: Shelley Loring, Manager Human Resources
CNO: Marianne Fournie, R.N., Chief Nursing Officer
Web address: www.barnesjewishwestcounty.org
**Control:** Other not–for–profit (including NFP Corporation) **Service:** General Medical and Surgical

> **Staffed Beds: 77 Admissions: 2985 Census: 29 Outpatient Visits:** 89641 **Births:** 0 **Total Expense ($000):** 91382 **Payroll Expense ($000):** 27002 **Personnel:** 458

✠ **CHRISTIAN HOSPITAL (260180)**, 11133 Dunn Road, Zip 63136–6119; tel. 314/653–5000 **A**1 2 9 10 **F**3 5 7 8 11 15 17 18 20 22 24 26 28 29 30 31 34 35 40 42 45 46 47 49 50 51 53 54 56 57 58 59 60 63 65 68 69 70 71 74 75 77 78 79 80 81 82 84 85 86 87 90 92 93 94 96 98 100 101 102 103 104 105 107 110 111 113 114 116 117 119 120 122 125 128 129 131 134 145 146 147 **P**6 **S** BJC HealthCare, Saint Louis, MO
Primary Contact: Ronald B. McMullen, President
CFO: John Katsianis, Chief Financial Officer
CMO: Sebastian Rueckert, M.D., Chief Medical Officer
CIO: Michael Kelly, Vice President
CHR: Bryan Hartwick, Vice President Human Resources
CNO: Jennifer Cordia, Vice President and Chief Nursing Executive
Web address: www.bjc.org
**Control:** Other not–for–profit (including NFP Corporation) **Service:** General Medical and Surgical

> **Staffed Beds: 262 Admissions: 16025 Census: 236 Outpatient Visits:** 196355 **Births:** 0 **Total Expense ($000):** 280202 **Payroll Expense ($000):** 93202 **Personnel:** 1791

★ ○ **DES PERES HOSPITAL (260176)**, 2345 Dougherty Ferry Road, Zip 63122–3313; tel. 314/966–9100 **A**3 5 9 10 11 12 13 **F**3 12 15 17 18 20 22 24 26 29 30 31 34 35 36 40 44 49 50 54 56 57 58 59 60 64 68 69 70 74 75 77 79 81 85 86 87 93 103 107 111 113 118 129 130 131 134 142 145 147 **P**6 **S** TENET Healthcare Corporation, Dallas, TX
Primary Contact: John A. Grah, JD, FACHE, Chief Executive Officer
COO: Michael Kendrick, Chief Operating Officer
CFO: David Byrd, Chief Financial Officer
CMO: Karen Webb, M.D., Chief Medical Officer
CIO: Kay Hannon, Director Information Systems
CHR: Ron Birlew, Director Human Resources
Web address: www.despereshospital.com
**Control:** Corporation, Investor–owned, for–profit **Service:** General Medical and Surgical

> **Staffed Beds: 143 Admissions: 6535 Census: 78 Outpatient Visits:** 31257 **Births:** 0 **Total Expense ($000):** 122845 **Payroll Expense ($000):** 36925 **Personnel:** 593

☐ **HAWTHORN CHILDREN PSYCHIATRIC HOSPITAL**, 1901 Pennsylvania, Zip 63133; tel. 314/512–7800 **A**1 3 5 **F**98 99 106 **P**6
Primary Contact: Laurent D. Javois, Regional Executive Officer
COO: Marcia F. Perry, Chief Operating Officer
CFO: James D. Martin, Chief Financial Officer
CMO: Joshua Calhoun, M.D., Medical Director
CIO: Richard Moore, Director Information Technology
CHR: Donna Harris, Director Human Resources
Web address: www.dmh.missouri.gov/hcph/
**Control:** State–Government, nonfederal **Service:** Children's hospital psychiatric

> **Staffed Beds: 52 Admissions: 159 Census: 44 Outpatient Visits: 0 Births:** 0 **Total Expense ($000):** 14536 **Payroll Expense ($000):** 7543 **Personnel:** 228

✠ **KINDRED HOSPITAL–ST. LOUIS (262010)**, 4930 Lindell Boulevard, Zip 63108–1510; tel. 314/361–8700, (Includes KINDRED HOSPITAL ST. LOUIS–ST. ANTHONY'S, 10018 Kennerly Road, 3rd Floor, Zip 63128; tel. 314/525–8100; Robert S. Adcock, Chief Executive Officer) **A**1 9 10 **F**1 3 29 77 85 129 147 **S** Kindred Healthcare, Louisville, KY
Primary Contact: Stacy M. Howard, R.N., Chief Executive Officer
COO: Dakota Redd, R.N., Chief Clinical Officer
CFO: Maureen Roach, Senior Chief Financial Officer
CMO: Michael Holtzman, M.D., Medical Director
CIO: Thomas C. Christman, Director Plant Operations
CHR: Cindy Sander, Coordinator Human Resources
Web address: www.kindredstlouis.com/
**Control:** Corporation, Investor–owned, for–profit **Service:** Long–Term Acute Care hospital

> **Staffed Beds: 98 Admissions: 660 Census: 54 Outpatient Visits: 0 Births:** 0 **Total Expense ($000):** 32106 **Payroll Expense ($000):** 11832 **Personnel:** 204

**MO**

*Many Facility Codes have changed. Please refer to the AHA Guide Code Chart.* © 2012 AHA Guide

⌖ **MERCY HOSPITAL ST. LOUIS (260020)**, 615 South New Ballas Road, Zip 63141–8277; tel. 314/569–6000, (Includes MERCY CHILDREN'S HOSPITAL ST. LOUIS, 615 South New Ballas Road, Zip 63141–8221; tel. 314/251–6000), (Total facility includes 120 beds in nursing home–type unit) **A**1 2 3 5 8 9 10 **F**1 3 4 5 8 11 12 13 14 15 16 17 18 19 20 22 24 25 26 28 29 30 31 32 33 34 35 36 38 39 40 41 43 45 46 47 48 49 50 51 52 53 54 55 56 57 58 59 60 61 64 66 67 68 69 70 71 72 73 74 75 76 77 78 79 80 81 82 84 85 86 87 88 89 90 92 93 94 96 97 98 99 100 101 102 103 104 105 106 107 108 110 111 113 114 115 116 117 118 119 120 122 123 125 127 128 129 130 131 133 134 142 143 145 146 147 **P**6 8 **S** Mercy Health, Chesterfield, MO
Primary Contact: Jeffrey A. Johnston, President
COO: Eric J. Eoloff, Chief Operating Officer
CFO: Cheryl Matejka, Chief Financial Officer
CMO: Paul Hintze, M.D., Vice President Medical Affairs
CIO: Eugene Roth, Vice President Information Services
CHR: Rocky Ruello, Vice President Human Resources
Web address: www.mercy.net/stlouismo
**Control:** Other not–for–profit (including NFP Corporation) **Service:** General Medical and Surgical

**Staffed Beds:** 979 **Admissions:** 42132 **Census:** 652 **Outpatient Visits:** 837517 **Births:** 7830 **Total Expense ($000):** 725906 **Payroll Expense ($000):** 289155 **Personnel:** 4885

☐ **METROPOLITAN ST. LOUIS PSYCHIATRIC CENTER (264025)**, 5351 Delmar, Zip 63112–3198; tel. 314/877–0500 **A**1 3 5 10 **F**11 30 98 129 145
Primary Contact: Laurent D. Javois, Regional Executive Officer
COO: Anthony J. Cuneo, Chief Operating Officer
CFO: James D. Martin, Chief Financial Officer
CMO: Nicholas Nguyen, M.D., Interim Medical Director
CIO: Richard Moore, Director Information Technology
CHR: Donna Harris, Director Human Resources
Web address: www.dmh.missouri.gov/mpc
**Control:** State–Government, nonfederal **Service:** Psychiatric

**Staffed Beds:** 50 **Admissions:** 252 **Census:** 37 **Outpatient Visits:** 5 **Births:** 0 **Total Expense ($000):** 15665 **Payroll Expense ($000):** 7778 **Personnel:** 208

⌖ **MISSOURI BAPTIST MEDICAL CENTER (260108)**, 3015 North Ballas Road, Zip 63131–2329; tel. 314/996–5000 **A**1 2 3 5 9 10 **F**3 11 13 14 15 17 18 19 20 22 24 26 29 30 31 34 35 40 41 45 46 48 49 50 51 52 54 55 57 58 59 60 61 64 65 68 70 71 73 74 75 76 77 78 79 81 83 84 85 86 87 89 90 93 107 108 110 111 113 114 115 118 119 120 122 123 125 129 130 131 144 145 146 147 **P**6 **S** BJC HealthCare, Saint Louis, MO
Primary Contact: Joan Magruder, President
COO: Doug Black, Vice President Operations
CFO: Augusto A. Noronha, Vice President Finance and Chief Financial Officer
CMO: Timothy Ranney, M.D., Vice President Medical Affairs and Chief Medical Officer
CIO: Derrick Marcum, Director Information Systems
CHR: Sandra G. Young, Vice President Human Resources
CNO: Tim Mislan, MS, Vice President Patient Care Services
Web address: www.missouribaptistmedicalcenter.org
**Control:** Other not–for–profit (including NFP Corporation) **Service:** General Medical and Surgical

**Staffed Beds:** 448 **Admissions:** 22832 **Census:** 258 **Outpatient Visits:** 284289 **Total Expense ($000):** 426778 **Payroll Expense ($000):** 132249 **Personnel:** 2413

⌖ **SAINT LOUIS UNIVERSITY HOSPITAL (260105)**, 3635 Vista at Grand Boulevard, Zip 63110–0250, Mailing Address: P.O. Box 15250, Zip 63110–0250; tel. 314/577–8000 **A**1 2 3 5 8 9 10 **F**3 6 7 8 9 11 14 15 17 18 20 22 24 26 28 29 30 31 34 35 36 37 38 39 40 43 44 45 46 47 48 49 50 51 55 56 57 58 59 60 61 63 64 65 68 70 74 75 77 78 79 81 82 84 85 86 87 90 91 92 94 96 97 98 100 101 102 103 104 107 108 110 111 112 113 114 115 116 117 118 119 120 122 123 125 128 129 130 131 134 135 137 138 140 141 145 147 **P**1 **S** TENET Healthcare Corporation, Dallas, TX
Primary Contact: Phillip E. Sowa, Chief Executive Officer
COO: Dawn Anuszkiewicz, Chief Operating Officer
CFO: Raymond Alvey, Chief Financial Officer
CMO: Karen Webb, M.D., Chief Medical Officer
CIO: Patrick Brennan, Director Information System Technology
CHR: Vera W. Daniel, Chief Human Resources Officer
Web address: www.sluhospital.com
**Control:** Corporation, Investor–owned, for–profit **Service:** General Medical and Surgical

**Staffed Beds:** 332 **Admissions:** 15254 **Census:** 240 **Outpatient Visits:** 120489 **Births:** 0 **Total Expense ($000):** 387725 **Payroll Expense ($000):** 86508 **Personnel:** 1375

☐ **SHRINERS HOSPITALS FOR CHILDREN, ST. LOUIS (263304)**, 2001 South Lindbergh Boulevard, Zip 63131–3597; tel. 314/432–3600 **A**1 3 5 10 **F**3 29 34 57 59 64 65 68 74 75 79 80 85 86 87 89 93 94 97 129 130 131 145 147 **S** Shriners Hospitals for Children, Tampa, FL
Primary Contact: John Gloss, FACHE, Administrator
CFO: Sandra K. Lawson, Interim Director Fiscal Services
CMO: Perry L. Schoenecker, M.D., Chief of Staff
CIO: Jeanne Hall, Director Information Systems
CHR: Mark Venable, Interim Director Human Resources
Web address: www.shrinershq.org
**Control:** Other not–for–profit (including NFP Corporation) **Service:** Children's orthopedic

**Staffed Beds:** 42 **Admissions:** 701 **Census:** 9 **Outpatient Visits:** 11011 **Births:** 0 **Total Expense ($000):** 31056 **Payroll Expense ($000):** 11388 **Personnel:** 213

★ **SSM CARDINAL GLENNON CHILDREN'S MEDICAL CENTER**, 1465 South Grand Boulevard, Zip 63104–1095; tel. 314/577–5600 **A**3 5 9 **F**3 8 11 19 21 23 25 27 29 30 31 32 34 35 36 38 39 40 41 43 44 45 46 47 48 49 50 51 54 55 57 59 60 61 64 65 66 68 72 73 74 75 77 78 79 80 82 84 85 86 87 88 89 90 93 94 97 99 100 101 102 104 107 111 113 118 119 120 123 126 128 129 130 131 133 135 136 137 138 140 141 145 147 **P**6 8 **S** SSM Health Care, Saint Louis, MO
Primary Contact: Sherlyn Hailstone, MSN, R.N., FACHE, President
CFO: Karen Rewerts, Vice President Finance
CMO: Susan Heaney, M.D., Vice President Medical Affairs
CIO: Michael Paasch, Regional Vice President and Chief Information Officer
CHR: Mary Jane Brecklin, Network Vice President, South Operating Group
Web address: www.cardinalglennon.com
**Control:** Church–operated, Nongovernment, not–for profit **Service:** Children's general

**Staffed Beds:** 176 **Admissions:** 7314 **Census:** 131 **Outpatient Visits:** 220423 **Births:** 6 **Total Expense ($000):** 270249 **Payroll Expense ($000):** 95397 **Personnel:** 1514

⌖ **SSM ST. MARY'S HEALTH CENTER (260091)**, 6420 Clayton Road, Zip 63117–1811; tel. 314/768–8000 **A**1 2 5 8 9 10 **F**3 4 11 13 15 17 18 20 22 24 26 28 29 30 31 34 35 37 38 40 44 45 46 49 51 52 55 56 57 58 59 60 61 64 66 70 72 73 74 75 76 78 79 81 82 84 85 86 87 97 98 100 101 102 103 104 105 107 108 110 111 113 114 118 119 120 128 129 131 134 142 145 146 147 **P**6 8 **S** SSM Health Care, Saint Louis, MO
Primary Contact: Kathleen R. Becker, M.P.H., JD, President
CFO: Jo Bertram, Vice President Finance
CMO: Darren E. Wethers, M.D., President Medical Staff
CIO: Robert Curran, Director Health Information Management
Web address: www.stmarys–stlouis.com
**Control:** Church–operated, Nongovernment, not–for profit **Service:** General Medical and Surgical

**Staffed Beds:** 374 **Admissions:** 20083 **Census:** 265 **Outpatient Visits:** 178036 **Births:** 3061 **Total Expense ($000):** 281574 **Payroll Expense ($000):** 104846 **Personnel:** 1763

☐ **ST. ALEXIUS HOSPITAL – BROADWAY CAMPUS (260210)**, 3933 South Broadway, Zip 63118–4601; tel. 314/865–3333, (Includes SOUTHPOINTE HOSPITAL, 2639 Miami Street, Zip 63118–3929; tel. 314/772–1456) **A**1 6 9 10 **F**3 12 15 20 29 30 35 38 39 40 56 57 59 60 68 70 74 77 78 79 81 86 87 98 101 102 103 104 107 108 111 117 118 129 142 145 147 **P**6 **S** Success Healthcare, Boca Raton, FL
Primary Contact: Michael J. Motte, Chief Executive Officer
CFO: Matthew Brandt, Chief Financial Officer
CIO: Jennifer Schempp, Manager Information Systems
Web address: www.stalexiushospital.com
**Control:** Corporation, Investor–owned, for–profit **Service:** General Medical and Surgical

**Staffed Beds:** 189 **Admissions:** 5774 **Census:** 106 **Outpatient Visits:** 33346 **Births:** 0 **Total Expense ($000):** 68796 **Payroll Expense ($000):** 32831 **Personnel:** 676

☐ △ **ST. ALEXIUS HOSPITAL – FOREST PARK CAMPUS (260021)**, 6150 Oakland Avenue, Zip 63139–3215; tel. 314/768–3000, (Nonreporting) **A**1 3 5 7 9 10 **S** Success Healthcare, Boca Raton, FL
Primary Contact: Michael J. Motte, Chief Executive Officer
CHR: Kathaleen Clutts, Director Human Resources
Web address: www.stalexiushospital.com
**Control:** Corporation, Investor–owned, for–profit **Service:** Psychiatric

**Staffed Beds:** 178

**MO**

---

**Hospital, Medicare Provider Number, Address, Telephone, Approval, Facility, and Physician Codes, Health Care System**

★ American Hospital Association (AHA) membership
☐ The Joint Commission accreditation        ◇ DNV Healthcare Inc. accreditation
○ American Osteopathic Association (AOA) accreditation
△ Commission on Accreditation of Rehabilitation Facilities (CARF) accreditation

⊞ △ **ST. ANTHONY'S MEDICAL CENTER (260077)**, 10010 Kennerly Road, Zip 63128–2106; tel. 314/525–1000 **A**1 2 7 9 10 **F**3 4 5 8 11 12 13 15 17 18 20 22 24 26 28 29 30 31 32 34 35 37 38 40 41 42 43 47 49 50 51 53 54 56 57 59 60 61 62 63 64 65 68 69 70 73 74 75 76 77 78 79 80 81 82 84 85 86 87 89 90 91 92 93 94 95 96 97 98 99 100 101 102 103 104 105 107 108 110 111 113 117 118 119 120 121 122 123 128 129 130 131 134 142 143 145 146 147 **P**6
Primary Contact: James E. Gardner, Jr., Chief Executive Officer
CFO: John Skeans, Chief Financial Officer
CMO: David Morton, M.D., Chief Medical Officer
CIO: Jim Weldon, Chief Information Officer
CHR: Ann M. Bollone, Vice President Human Resources
CNO: Cathi Blise, Interim Chief Nursing Officer
Web address: www.stanthonysmedcenter.com
**Control:** Other not–for–profit (including NFP Corporation) **Service:** General Medical and Surgical

**Staffed Beds:** 599 **Admissions:** 27953 **Census:** 367 **Outpatient Visits:** 641039 **Births:** 1516 **Total Expense ($000):** 440351 **Payroll Expense ($000):** 199787 **Personnel:** 3461

**ST. JOHN'S MERCY CHILDREN'S HOSPITAL** See Mercy Children's Hospital St. Louis

**ST. JOHN'S MERCY MEDICAL CENTER** See Mercy Hospital St. Louis

⊞ △ **ST. LOUIS CHILDREN'S HOSPITAL (263301)**, One Children's Place, Zip 63110–1002; tel. 314/454–6000 **A**1 3 5 7 8 9 10 **F**3 5 7 11 16 17 19 20 21 22 23 25 26 27 29 30 31 32 34 35 38 39 40 41 42 43 44 45 46 47 48 49 50 54 57 58 59 60 61 62 63 64 65 68 71 72 74 75 77 78 79 81 82 83 84 85 86 87 88 89 90 92 93 99 100 101 102 104 107 108 109 111 112 113 114 118 128 130 131 133 134 135 136 137 138 139 140 141 142 143 144 145 147 **S** BJC HealthCare, Saint Louis, MO
Primary Contact: Lee F. Fetter, President and Senior Executive Officer
CFO: Doug Vanderslice, Vice President and Chief Financial Officer
CMO: F. Sessions Cole, M.D., Chief Medical Officer
CHR: David Cook, Vice President Human Resources
Web address: www.stlouischildrens.org
**Control:** Other not–for–profit (including NFP Corporation) **Service:** Children's general

**Staffed Beds:** 250 **Admissions:** 11588 **Census:** 196 **Outpatient Visits:** 157374 **Births:** 0 **Total Expense ($000):** 452145 **Payroll Expense ($000):** 135341 **Personnel:** 2638

☐ **ST. LOUIS PSYCHIATRIC REHABILITATION CENTER (264010)**, 5300 Arsenal Street, Zip 63139–1494; tel. 314/877–6500 **A**1 9 10 **F**11 30 39 50 53 65 68 75 86 87 98 100 101 106 129 142 145
Primary Contact: Laurent D. Javois, Regional Executive Officer
COO: H. Andrew Mannich, Chief Operating Officer
CFO: James D. Martin, Chief Financial Officer
CMO: Roy Wilson, M.D., Medical Director
CIO: Richard Moore, Director Information Technology
CHR: Donna Harris, Director Human Resources
Web address: www.dmh.missouri.gov
**Control:** State–Government, nonfederal **Service:** Psychiatric

**Staffed Beds:** 196 **Admissions:** 82 **Census:** 196 **Outpatient Visits:** 0 **Births:** 0 **Total Expense ($000):** 29914 **Payroll Expense ($000):** 16951 **Personnel:** 481

⊞ **THE REHABILITATION INSTITUTE OF ST. LOUIS (263028)**, 4455 Duncan Avenue, Zip 63110–1111; tel. 314/658–3800 **A**1 9 10 **F**29 44 56 58 64 68 74 75 79 82 87 90 91 93 94 100 129 131 142 145 147 **S** HEALTHSOUTH Corporation, Birmingham, AL
Primary Contact: Barbara Jacobsmeyer, Chief Executive Officer
COO: Jon McDowell, FACHE, Chief Operating Officer
CFO: Tara Diebling, Chief Financial Officer
CMO: David Carr, M.D., Physician Medical Director
CIO: Sherrie Marshall, Health Information Management Services Director
CHR: Christina Devine, Director Human Resources
CNO: Dakota Redd, R.N., Chief Nursing Officer
Web address: www.rehabinstitutestl.com
**Control:** Partnership, Investor–owned, for–profit **Service:** Rehabilitation

**Staffed Beds:** 96 **Admissions:** 1912 **Census:** 79 **Outpatient Visits:** 40143 **Births:** 0 **Total Expense ($000):** 31012 **Payroll Expense ($000):** 16430 **Personnel:** 316

⊞ △ **VETERANS AFFAIRS MEDICAL CENTER**, (Healthcare for our Veterans), 915 North Grand, Zip 63106–1621; tel. 314/652–4100, (Total facility includes 71 beds in nursing home–type unit) **A**1 3 5 7 **F**1 3 4 5 8 12 15 17 18 20 22 26 28 29 30 31 33 34 35 38 39 40 45 49 50 54 56 57 58 59 60 61 62 63 64 65 66 70 74 75 77 78 79 81 82 83 84 85 86 87 90 91 92 93 94 97 98 100 101 102 103 104 105 106 107 108 109 110 111 113 114 115 117 118 119 120 122 125 126 127 128 129 130 131 134 142 143 144 145 146 147
**S** Department of Veterans Affairs, Washington, DC
Primary Contact: RimaAnn O. Nelson, Director
CFO: Karen Westerheide, Chief Financial Officer
CMO: Nathan Ravi, M.D., Chief of Staff
CIO: Steve Warmbold, Director Information Management Service Line
CHR: Marie Lewis, Human Resources Liaison
Web address: www.va.gov/sta/guide/home.asp
**Control:** Veterans Affairs, Government, federal **Service:** General Medical and Surgical

**Staffed Beds:** 356 **Admissions:** 10699 **Census:** 268 **Outpatient Visits:** 687923 **Births:** 0 **Total Expense ($000):** 387833 **Payroll Expense ($000):** 232483 **Personnel:** 3603

### SAINT PETERS—St. Charles County

⊞ **BARNES–JEWISH ST. PETERS HOSPITAL (260191)**, 10 Hospital Drive, Zip 63376–1659; tel. 636/916–9000 **A**1 5 9 10 **F**3 8 11 13 15 18 20 22 28 29 30 31 34 35 40 41 49 57 59 64 70 75 76 77 78 79 81 85 86 87 90 93 107 108 110 111 113 114 117 118 119 120 122 123 128 129 131 134 145 146 147 **S** BJC HealthCare, Saint Louis, MO
Primary Contact: John Antes, President
COO: Ann Abad, Vice President Operations
CFO: Glen Schweagel, Vice President Finance
CMO: Dan Bergmann, M.D., Chief Medical Officer
CNO: Jill Skyles, R.N., Chief Nursing Officer
Web address: www.bjsph.org/
**Control:** Other not–for–profit (including NFP Corporation) **Service:** General Medical and Surgical

**Staffed Beds:** 113 **Admissions:** 6917 **Census:** 75 **Outpatient Visits:** 119261 **Births:** 488 **Total Expense ($000):** 123609 **Payroll Expense ($000):** 35630 **Personnel:** 776

### SALEM—Dent County

★ **SALEM MEMORIAL DISTRICT HOSPITAL (261318)**, Highway 72 North, Zip 65560–0774, Mailing Address: P.O. Box 774, Zip 65560–0774; tel. 573/729–6626, (Total facility includes 18 beds in nursing home–type unit) **A**9 10 18 **F**3 7 11 29 30 34 40 59 60 62 67 75 81 85 87 89 107 114 118 126 127 129 132 134 145
Primary Contact: Dennis P. Pryor, Administrator
CFO: Stephanie Wofford, Controller
CMO: Ryan Pharr, M.D., Chief Medical Staff
CHR: Gina Bobbitt, Director Human Resources
Web address: www.smdh.net
**Control:** Hospital district or authority, Government, nonfederal **Service:** General Medical and Surgical

**Staffed Beds:** 43 **Admissions:** 801 **Census:** 30 **Outpatient Visits:** 37547 **Births:** 0 **Total Expense ($000):** 18116 **Payroll Expense ($000):** 7481 **Personnel:** 171

### SEDALIA—Pettis County

⊞ **BOTHWELL REGIONAL HEALTH CENTER (260009)**, 601 East 14th Street, Zip 65301–1706, Mailing Address: P.O. Box 1706, Zip 65302–1706; tel. 660/826–8833, (Total facility includes 10 beds in nursing home–type unit) **A**1 9 10 **F**3 11 13 14 15 18 20 22 28 29 30 31 34 35 39 40 51 54 56 57 59 60 62 63 64 65 68 70 73 74 75 76 77 78 79 80 81 82 84 85 86 87 89 92 93 107 108 110 111 113 114 115 116 117 118 119 120 122 123 126 127 128 129 130 131 134 143 145 146 147
Primary Contact: John M. Dawes, FACHE, Chief Executive Officer
COO: Mark I. Hirshberg, Chief Operating Officer
CFO: David Halsell, Chief Financial Officer
CIO: Tom Fairfax, Director Information Systems
CHR: Deb Clemmer, Vice President Human Resources
Web address: www.brhc.org
**Control:** City–Government, nonfederal **Service:** General Medical and Surgical

**Staffed Beds:** 132 **Admissions:** 5669 **Census:** 66 **Outpatient Visits:** 183359 **Births:** 576 **Total Expense ($000):** 90723 **Payroll Expense ($000):** 38174 **Personnel:** 723

**MO**

## SIKESTON—Scott County

☐ △ **MISSOURI DELTA MEDICAL CENTER (260113)**, 1008 North Main Street, Zip 63801–5044; tel. 573/471–1600 **A**1 5 7 9 10 **F**3 11 13 15 18 28 29 30 31 32 34 35 39 40 44 50 51 53 54 56 57 59 62 64 68 70 74 75 76 77 78 79 81 82 84 85 86 87 89 90 93 97 98 103 107 108 109 110 111 114 115 116 117 118 126 128 129 130 131 143 145 146 147 **P**6
Primary Contact: Jason Schrumpf, President
CFO: Jon Branstetter, Vice President Finance
Web address: www.missouridelta.com
**Control:** Other not–for–profit (including NFP Corporation) **Service:** General Medical and Surgical

**Staffed Beds:** 160 **Admissions:** 4862 **Census:** 62 **Outpatient Visits:** 195875 **Births:** 515 **Total Expense ($000):** 83767 **Payroll Expense ($000):** 38940 **Personnel:** 782

## SPRINGFIELD—Greene County

☐ **LAKELAND BEHAVIORAL HEALTH SYSTEM (264024)**, 440 South Market Street, Zip 65806–2026; tel. 417/865–5581 **A**1 9 10 **F**98 99 129 **S** Acadia Healthcare Company, Inc., Franklin, TN
Primary Contact: Keith A. Furman, Chief Executive Officer
CFO: Rick Crump, Chief Financial Officer
CMO: Richard Aiken, M.D., Vice President and Medical Director
CHR: Dave England, Director Human Resources
Web address: www.lakeland–hospital.com
**Control:** Corporation, Investor–owned, for–profit **Service:** Children's hospital psychiatric

**Staffed Beds:** 66 **Admissions:** 1431 **Census:** 54 **Outpatient Visits:** 0 **Births:** 0 **Total Expense ($000):** 15043 **Payroll Expense ($000):** 8548 **Personnel:** 232

☒ △ **LESTER E. COX MEDICAL CENTERS (260040)**, 1423 North Jefferson Street, Zip 65802–1988; tel. 417/269–3000, (Includes LESTER E. COX MEDICAL CENTER NORTH, 1423 North Jefferson Avenue, Zip 65802; tel. 417/269–3000; LESTER E. COX MEDICAL CENTER SOUTH, 3801 South National Avenue, Zip 65807; tel. 417/269–6000) **A**1 2 7 9 10 **F**3 4 5 7 11 12 13 15 17 18 19 20 22 24 26 28 29 30 31 32 34 35 38 39 40 42 43 44 45 46 47 49 50 51 52 53 54 55 56 57 59 60 61 62 64 65 68 69 70 71 72 74 75 76 77 78 79 80 81 82 84 85 86 87 88 89 90 92 93 95 96 97 98 99 100 101 102 103 104 107 108 110 111 113 114 116 117 118 119 120 125 126 127 128 129 130 131 134 142 143 145 146 147 **P**3 6 **S** CoxHealth, Springfield, MO
Primary Contact: Steven D. Edwards, President and Chief Executive Officer
CFO: Jacob McWay, Senior Vice President and Chief Financial Officer
CMO: Dan Sontheimer, M.D., Vice President Medical Affairs
CIO: Bruce Robison, Vice President and Chief Information Officer
CHR: John Hursh, Vice President Human Resources
Web address: www.coxhealth.com
**Control:** Other not–for–profit (including NFP Corporation) **Service:** General Medical and Surgical

**Staffed Beds:** 646 **Admissions:** 31460 **Census:** 426 **Outpatient Visits:** 1315421 **Births:** 3324 **Total Expense ($000):** 845145 **Payroll Expense ($000):** 313064 **Personnel:** 6467

☒ △ **MERCY HOSPITAL SPRINGFIELD (260065)**, 1235 East Cherokee Street, Zip 65804–2263; tel. 417/820–2000, (Includes ST. JOHN'S CHILDREN'S HOSPITAL, 1235 East Cherokee Street, Zip 65804–2203; tel. 417/820–2000), (Total facility includes 25 beds in nursing home–type unit) **A**1 2 3 5 7 9 10 **F**3 5 6 7 8 9 11 12 13 15 16 17 18 20 22 24 26 28 30 31 34 36 38 39 40 43 44 48 49 50 51 53 54 55 56 57 59 60 61 62 63 64 65 68 70 71 72 73 74 75 76 77 78 79 81 82 84 85 86 87 88 89 90 91 93 94 97 98 100 101 102 103 104 107 108 111 113 115 116 117 118 119 120 122 123 125 127 128 129 130 131 133 134 142 143 145 146 147 **P**6 8 **S** Mercy Health, Chesterfield, MO
Primary Contact: Jon D. Swope, President and Chief Executive Officer
COO: Jay Guffey, Senior Vice President and Chief Operating Officer
CMO: Allan Allphin, M.D., Chief of Staff
CHR: Trisha Holbert, Vice President Human Resources
Web address: www.stjohns.com
**Control:** Church–operated, Nongovernment, not–for profit **Service:** General Medical and Surgical

**Staffed Beds:** 613 **Admissions:** 32334 **Census:** 444 **Outpatient Visits:** 616860 **Births:** 3026 **Total Expense ($000):** 772683 **Payroll Expense ($000):** 243815 **Personnel:** 5265

○ **OZARKS COMMUNITY HOSPITAL (260207)**, 2828 North National, Zip 65803–4306; tel. 417/837–4000 **A**9 10 11 **F**3 29 39 40 42 45 54 56 59 65 68 74 75 77 79 81 82 85 86 87 90 93 97 98 100 103 104 107 108 111 113 118 126 128 129 134 142 143 146 147 **P**6
Primary Contact: Paul Taylor, Administrator
CFO: Janet Taylor, CPA, Chief Financial Officer
Web address: www.ochonline.com
**Control:** Corporation, Investor–owned, for–profit **Service:** General Medical and Surgical

**Staffed Beds:** 35 **Admissions:** 1085 **Census:** 18 **Outpatient Visits:** 214497 **Births:** 0 **Total Expense ($000):** 51335 **Payroll Expense ($000):** 15271 **Personnel:** 523

☒ **SELECT SPECIALTY HOSPITAL–SPRINGFIELD (262017)**, 1630 East Primrose Street, Zip 65804; tel. 417/885–4700 **A**1 9 10 **F**1 3 29 45 70 85 90 107 147 **S** Select Medical Corporation, Mechanicsburg, PA
Primary Contact: Cynthia Whitten, R.N., Chief Executive Officer
CHR: Tonya Eddington, Coordinator Human Resources
Web address: www.selectspecialtyhospitals.com
**Control:** Corporation, Investor–owned, for–profit **Service:** Long–Term Acute Care hospital

**Staffed Beds:** 44 **Admissions:** 513 **Census:** 41 **Outpatient Visits:** 0 **Births:** 0 **Total Expense ($000):** 19850 **Payroll Expense ($000):** 6768 **Personnel:** 153

## STE. GENEVIEVE—Ste. Genevieve County

★ **STE. GENEVIEVE COUNTY MEMORIAL HOSPITAL (261330)**, 800 Suite Genevieve Drive, Zip 63670–0468; tel. 573/883–2751 **A**9 10 18 **F**3 11 13 15 18 28 29 31 34 35 38 39 40 50 53 56 57 59 62 64 65 68 75 76 77 78 79 81 82 85 86 87 89 92 93 107 111 114 118 126 128 129 130 131 132 134 145 146 147 **P**6
Primary Contact: Thomas Keim, Chief Executive Officer
CFO: Susan Eckenfels, Chief Financial Officer
CMO: Bhargav Kanani, M.D., Chief of Staff
CIO: Marsha Norris, Director Information Systems
CHR: Sarah Jo Kelley, Director Human Resources
Web address: www.stegenevievehospital.org
**Control:** County–Government, nonfederal **Service:** General Medical and Surgical

**Staffed Beds:** 25 **Admissions:** 1159 **Census:** 12 **Outpatient Visits:** 81884 **Births:** 108 **Total Expense ($000):** 29723 **Payroll Expense ($000):** 12975 **Personnel:** 266

## SULLIVAN—Crawford County

★ **MISSOURI BAPTIST SULLIVAN HOSPITAL (260115)**, 751 Sappington Bridge Road, Zip 63080–2354; tel. 573/468–4186 **A**9 10 **F**3 4 7 11 13 15 28 29 30 31 35 40 53 56 57 59 63 64 65 68 70 75 76 77 78 79 81 82 83 84 85 86 87 89 90 93 97 98 102 103 104 107 111 118 126 128 129 130 132 145 **S** BJC HealthCare, Saint Louis, MO
Primary Contact: Tony Schwarm, President
CFO: Christinia Lashmett, Director Financial Services
CMO: Roger Rembecki, M.D., Chief of Staff
CHR: Kathleen Reed, Manager Human Resources
Web address: www.missouribaptistsullivan.org
**Control:** Other not–for–profit (including NFP Corporation) **Service:** General Medical and Surgical

**Staffed Beds:** 56 **Admissions:** 2442 **Census:** 26 **Outpatient Visits:** 75578 **Births:** 283 **Total Expense ($000):** 43668 **Payroll Expense ($000):** 15133 **Personnel:** 349

## SWEET SPRINGS—Saline County

**I-70 COMMUNITY HOSPITAL (261334)**, 105 Hospital Drive, Zip 65351–2229; tel. 660/335–4700 **A**9 10 18 **F**3 11 29 34 35 40 45 57 59 64 65 68 75 83 85 87 89 90 93 107 111 118 126 127 128 129 132 142 **S** HMC/CAH Consolidated, Inc., Kansas City, MO
Primary Contact: Julie Davenport, Chief Executive Officer
CFO: Gary Clifton, Chief Financial Officer
CMO: Deborah Herrmann, M.D., Chief of Staff
CIO: Debra Harris, Director Medical Records
CHR: Diane Steinkuhler, Administrative Assistant Human Resources
Web address: www.i70medcenter.com
**Control:** Corporation, Investor–owned, for–profit **Service:** General Medical and Surgical

**Staffed Beds:** 15 **Admissions:** 252 **Census:** 3 **Outpatient Visits:** 11559 **Births:** 0 **Total Expense ($000):** 7100 **Payroll Expense ($000):** 3104 **Personnel:** 61

**MO**

---

**Hospital, Medicare Provider Number, Address, Telephone, Approval, Facility, and Physician Codes, Health Care System**

★ American Hospital Association (AHA) membership
☐ The Joint Commission accreditation
◇ DNV Healthcare Inc. accreditation
○ American Osteopathic Association (AOA) accreditation
△ Commission on Accreditation of Rehabilitation Facilities (CARF) accreditation

### TRENTON—Grundy County

**WRIGHT MEMORIAL HOSPITAL (261309)**, 191 Iowa Boulevard,
Zip 64683–8343, Mailing Address: P.O. Box 628, Zip 64683–0628;
tel. 660/358–5700 **A**9 10 18 **F**3 11 13 15 28 30 31 34 35 40 57 59 62 63
64 68 74 75 76 77 78 79 81 82 84 85 89 90 93 97 104 107 108 111 113
118 126 128 129 132 134 142 145 147 **P**1 **S** Saint Luke's Health System,
Kansas City, MO
Primary Contact: Gary W. Jordan, FACHE, Chief Executive Officer
CFO: Leslie Reed, Chief Financial Officer
CMO: Gerald C. Zabielski, M.D., Chief Medical Staff
CHR: Jenny Donovan, Director Human Resources
Web address: www.saintlukeshealthsystem.org
**Control:** Other not–for–profit (including NFP Corporation) **Service:** General
Medical and Surgical

**Staffed Beds:** 25 **Admissions:** 913 **Census:** 10 **Outpatient Visits:** 65055
**Births:** 155 **Total Expense ($000):** 23715 **Payroll Expense ($000):** 10119
**Personnel:** 198

### TROY—Lincoln County

☐ **LINCOLN COUNTY MEDICAL CENTER (261319)**, 1000 East Cherry Street,
Zip 63379–1513; tel. 636/528–8551 **A**1 9 10 18 **F**3 11 15 17 18 28 29 30
34 35 40 44 45 50 51 57 59 62 64 65 68 70 75 77 79 81 85 86 87 89 90
93 104 107 110 111 113 118 126 128 129 130 131 132 134 145 147 **P**6
Primary Contact: Patrick G. Bira, JD, FACHE, Chief Executive Officer
CIO: Travis Boyd, Manager Information Technology
CHR: Toni Price, Director Human Resources
Web address: www.lcmctroy.com
**Control:** County–Government, nonfederal **Service:** General Medical and Surgical

**Staffed Beds:** 25 **Admissions:** 1150 **Census:** 14 **Outpatient Visits:** 76256
**Births:** 0 **Total Expense ($000):** 30621 **Payroll Expense ($000):** 15704
**Personnel:** 291

### UNIONVILLE—Putnam County

★ **PUTNAM COUNTY MEMORIAL HOSPITAL (261305)**, 1926 Oak Street,
Zip 63565–1100, Mailing Address: P.O. Box 389, Zip 63565–0389;
tel. 660/947–2411 **A**9 10 18 **F**3 15 28 29 34 35 40 45 50 57 59 64 65 75
77 81 85 87 89 90 93 97 107 111 113 118 126 127 128 129 132 **P**6
Primary Contact: Cindy Cummings, Chief Executive Officer
CMO: W. Stephen Casady, M.D., Chief of Staff
CHR: Judy Green, Director Human Resources
Web address: www.pcmhosp.com
**Control:** County–Government, nonfederal **Service:** General Medical and Surgical

**Staffed Beds:** 15 **Admissions:** 229 **Census:** 3 **Outpatient Visits:** 15422
**Births:** 0 **Total Expense ($000):** 7940 **Payroll Expense ($000):** 3118
**Personnel:** 68

### WARRENSBURG—Johnson County

⊠ **WESTERN MISSOURI MEDICAL CENTER (260097)**, 403 Burkarth Road,
Zip 64093–3101; tel. 660/747–2500 **A**1 9 10 20 **F**3 8 11 12 13 15 17 18 28
29 30 31 32 34 35 40 45 47 57 59 61 64 65 68 70 75 76 77 78 79 81 82
85 89 90 93 102 107 108 110 111 114 117 118 126 128 129 130 131 132
134 145 146 147 **P**6
Primary Contact: John F. Smolen, FACHE, President and Chief Executive Officer
COO: Michael L. Gasparini, Vice President Clinical Services and Chief Operating
Officer
CFO: Terri Bradley, CPA, Vice President Financial Services and Chief Financial
Officer
CMO: Michael Misko, M.D., Vice President Medical Staff Services and Chief
Medical Officer
CIO: Carol McKinney, Director Information Services
CHR: Dennis Long, Director Human Resources
Web address: www.wmmc.com
**Control:** County–Government, nonfederal **Service:** General Medical and Surgical

**Staffed Beds:** 71 **Admissions:** 3118 **Census:** 30 **Outpatient Visits:** 122236
**Births:** 787 **Total Expense ($000):** 71750 **Payroll Expense ($000):** 28246
**Personnel:** 515

### WASHINGTON—Franklin County

⊠ **MERCY HOSPITAL WASHINGTON (260052)**, 901 East Fifth Street,
Zip 63090–3127; tel. 636/239–8000 **A**1 9 10 **F**3 4 8 11 12 13 14 15 17 18
20 22 28 29 30 31 32 34 35 40 43 46 48 49 50 52 57 59 61 64 66 68 69
70 73 75 76 77 78 79 81 82 84 85 87 89 90 93 94 96 97 99 100 101 104
107 108 110 111 113 115 117 118 120 123 126 128 129 130 131 133 134
143 145 146 147 **P**6 8 **S** Mercy Health, Chesterfield, MO
Primary Contact: Terri L. McLain, FACHE, President
COO: Joan Frost, R.N., Chief Operating Officer/Chief Nursing Officer
CFO: Cheryl Matejka, Chief Financial Officer
CMO: Thomas Riechers, M.D., Chief Medical Staff
CIO: Michael McCreary, Chief of Services
CHR: Frank Lenoir, Executive Director Human Resources
CNO: Joan Frost, R.N., Chief Operating Officer/Chief Nursing Officer
Web address: www.mercy.net
**Control:** Church–operated, Nongovernment, not–for profit **Service:** General
Medical and Surgical

**Staffed Beds:** 180 **Admissions:** 5582 **Census:** 49 **Outpatient Visits:** 149266
**Births:** 872 **Total Expense ($000):** 84926 **Payroll Expense ($000):** 37779
**Personnel:** 576

### WENTZVILLE—St. Charles County

**SSM ST. JOSEPH HEALTH CENTER – WENTZVILLE** See SSM St. Joseph
Health Center, Saint Charles

### WEST PLAINS—Howell County

⊠ **OZARKS MEDICAL CENTER (260078)**, 1100 Kentucky Avenue,
Zip 65775–2029, Mailing Address: P.O. Box 1100, Zip 65775–1100;
tel. 417/256–9111 **A**1 5 9 10 **F**2 3 5 7 11 13 15 17 18 20 22 24 28 29 30
31 34 38 40 44 45 49 57 59 61 62 63 64 68 70 74 75 76 77 78 79 81 82
84 85 86 87 89 90 93 94 98 99 100 101 102 103 104 107 108 110 111
114 117 118 119 120 126 128 129 130 131 134 143 144 145 146 147 **P**8
Primary Contact: David M. Zechman, FACHE, President and Chief Executive Officer
COO: Jeanne M. Looper, Chief Operating Officer
CFO: Michael Gross, Senior Vice President, Finance/Business Development
CMO: Edward R. Henegar, D.O., Vice President, Medical Affairs
CIO: Edward Boys, Chief Information Officer
CHR: Greg Shannon, Director Human Resources
CNO: Marcia Robson, R.N., Chief Nursing Officer
Web address: www.ozarksmedicalcenter.com
**Control:** Other not–for–profit (including NFP Corporation) **Service:** General
Medical and Surgical

**Staffed Beds:** 114 **Admissions:** 6198 **Census:** 62 **Outpatient Visits:** 522831
**Births:** 658 **Total Expense ($000):** 117081 **Payroll Expense ($000):** 56325
**Personnel:** 1093

### WINDSOR—Henry County

☐ **ROYAL OAKS HOSPITAL (264020)**, 307 North Main, Zip 65360–1449;
tel. 660/647–2182 **A**1 3 5 9 10 **F**30 98 99 100 101 102 103 104 105
Primary Contact: Alan W. Greiman, Administrator
Web address: www.royal–oaks–hospital.org
**Control:** Other not–for–profit (including NFP Corporation) **Service:** Psychiatric

**Staffed Beds:** 41 **Admissions:** 1382 **Census:** 29 **Outpatient Visits:** 0 **Births:**
0 **Total Expense ($000):** 10741 **Payroll Expense ($000):** 5929 **Personnel:**
155

**MO**

# MONTANA

## ANACONDA—Deer Lodge County

★ **COMMUNITY HOSPITAL OF ANACONDA (271335)**, 401 West Pennsylvania Street, Zip 59711–1931; tel. 406/563–8500, (Total facility includes 62 beds in nursing home–type unit) **A**9 10 18 **F**1 3 6 8 11 13 15 29 30 31 34 40 43 45 50 57 59 62 63 64 75 76 77 79 81 82 87 93 107 110 111 113 118 127 129 132 134 142 143 145 **P**6 **S** Providence Health & Services, Renton, WA
Primary Contact: Steve McNeece, Chief Executive Officer
COO: Laura Austin, Chief Financial Officer and Chief Operating Officer
CFO: Laura Austin, Chief Financial Officer and Chief Operating Officer
CMO: Shawna Baker, M.D., Chief of Staff
CIO: Laura Austin, Chief Financial Officer and Chief Operating Officer
CHR: Meg Hickey–Boynton, Director Human Resources and Marketing
CNO: Jamie Johnson, R.N., VP of Nursing
Web address: www.communityhospitalofanaconda.org
**Control:** Other not–for–profit (including NFP Corporation) **Service:** General Medical and Surgical

**Staffed Beds:** 87 **Admissions:** 1047 **Census:** 67 **Outpatient Visits:** 44878 **Births:** 36 **Total Expense ($000):** 29964 **Payroll Expense ($000):** 12463 **Personnel:** 227

## BAKER—Fallon County

**FALLON MEDICAL COMPLEX (271301)**, 202 South 4th Street West, Zip 59313–0820, Mailing Address: P.O. Box 820, Zip 59313–0820; tel. 406/778–3331, (Total facility includes 15 beds in nursing home–type unit) **A**9 10 18 **F**11 15 28 32 34 36 40 56 57 59 62 64 65 69 75 81 93 97 107 110 113 118 126 127 129 132 145 147 **P**6
Primary Contact: David Espeland, Chief Executive Officer
CFO: Selena Nelson, Chief Financial Officer
CMO: Darryl Espeland, D.O., Chief Medical Staff
Web address: www.fallonmedical.org
**Control:** Other not–for–profit (including NFP Corporation) **Service:** General Medical and Surgical

**Staffed Beds:** 40 **Admissions:** 276 **Census:** 31 **Outpatient Visits:** 19849 **Births:** 0 **Total Expense ($000):** 7504 **Payroll Expense ($000):** 3645 **Personnel:** 97

## BIG SANDY—Chouteau County

★ **BIG SANDY MEDICAL CENTER (271311)**, 166 Montana Avenue East, Zip 59520–8474, Mailing Address: P.O. Box 530, Zip 59520–0530; tel. 406/378–2188, (Total facility includes 22 beds in nursing home–type unit) **A**9 10 18 **F**40 64 93 126 127 132
Primary Contact: Harry Bold, Administrator
CFO: Nora Grubb, Chief Financial Officer
Web address: www.bsmc.org
**Control:** Other not–for–profit (including NFP Corporation) **Service:** General Medical and Surgical

**Staffed Beds:** 30 **Admissions:** 127 **Census:** 20 **Outpatient Visits:** 4825 **Births:** 0 **Total Expense ($000):** 3205 **Payroll Expense ($000):** 1800 **Personnel:** 38

## BIG TIMBER—Sweet Grass County

★ **PIONEER MEDICAL CENTER (271313)**, 301 West Seventh Avenue, Zip 59011–1228, Mailing Address: P.O. Box 1228, Zip 59011–1228; tel. 406/932–4603, (Total facility includes 35 beds in nursing home–type unit) **A**9 10 18 **F**2 7 10 34 35 40 41 45 57 59 63 64 65 69 75 77 93 97 126 127 129 130 131 132 **P**3 6
Primary Contact: Bren Lowe, Chief Executive Officer
CFO: Kyle Gee, Chief Financial Officer
CMO: Benjamin P. Bullington, M.D., Chief of Staff
CHR: Miki Gregorich, Director Human Resources
CNO: Randi Pike, Director of Nursing
Web address: www.pmcmt.org/
**Control:** County–Government, nonfederal **Service:** General Medical and Surgical

**Staffed Beds:** 60 **Admissions:** 175 **Census:** 39 **Outpatient Visits:** 7300 **Births:** 0 **Total Expense ($000):** 6016 **Payroll Expense ($000):** 2696 **Personnel:** 97

## BILLINGS—Yellowstone County

☐ **ADVANCED CARE HOSPITAL OF MONTANA (272001)**, 3528 Gabel Road, Zip 59102–7307; tel. 406/373–8000, (Nonreporting) **A**1 9 10 **S** Ernest Health, Inc., Albuquerque, NM
Primary Contact: Joseph McClure, Chief Executive Officer
Web address: www.achm.ernesthealth.com
**Control:** Corporation, Investor–owned, for–profit **Service:** Long–Term Acute Care hospital

**Staffed Beds:** 40

⊠ **BILLINGS CLINIC (270004)**, 2800 10th Avenue North, Zip 59101, Mailing Address: P.O. Box 37000, Zip 59107–7000; tel. 406/657–4000, (Total facility includes 125 beds in nursing home–type unit) **A**1 2 3 5 9 10 **F**3 7 8 9 10 11 13 15 17 18 20 22 24 26 28 29 30 31 32 34 35 36 38 40 43 44 45 46 48 49 50 51 52 54 55 56 57 58 59 60 61 63 64 65 66 68 70 71 72 74 75 76 77 78 79 81 82 84 85 86 87 91 92 93 97 98 99 100 101 102 103 104 105 107 108 110 111 113 114 115 116 117 118 119 120 123 125 127 128 129 130 131 133 134 142 143 145 146 147 **P**6
Primary Contact: Nicholas Wolter, M.D., President and Chief Executive Officer
CFO: Connie F. Prewitt, Chief Financial Officer
CMO: Mark C. Rumans, M.D., Physician in Chief
CIO: Chris E. Stevens, Chief Information Officer
CHR: Kellee J. Fisk, Vice President People Resources
Web address: www.billingsclinic.com
**Control:** Other not–for–profit (including NFP Corporation) **Service:** General Medical and Surgical

**Staffed Beds:** 388 **Admissions:** 14900 **Census:** 283 **Outpatient Visits:** 985846 **Births:** 1395 **Total Expense ($000):** 459992 **Payroll Expense ($000):** 225499 **Personnel:** 3059

⊠ △ **ST. VINCENT HEALTHCARE (270049)**, 1233 North 30th Street, Zip 59101–0165, Mailing Address: P.O. Box 35200, Zip 59107–5200; tel. 406/237–7000 **A**1 2 3 5 7 9 10 **F**3 8 11 12 13 15 17 18 19 20 22 24 28 29 30 32 34 35 36 37 38 39 40 43 44 45 47 49 50 51 56 57 59 60 61 64 68 70 71 72 74 75 76 77 78 79 81 82 85 86 87 88 89 90 92 93 97 99 100 101 103 104 107 108 111 113 117 118 125 128 129 130 131 133 134 142 143 144 145 146 147 **P**6 **S** Sisters of Charity of Leavenworth Health System, Denver, CO
Primary Contact: Jason Barker, Chief Executive Officer
CFO: Steve Ballock, Chief Financial Officer
CMO: Michael Schweitzer, M.D., Chief Medical Officer
CIO: Al Rooney, Director Information Systems
Web address: www.svh–mt.org
**Control:** Church–operated, Nongovernment, not–for profit **Service:** General Medical and Surgical

**Staffed Beds:** 206 **Admissions:** 11250 **Census:** 134 **Outpatient Visits:** 428683 **Births:** 1280 **Total Expense ($000):** 283314 **Payroll Expense ($000):** 112797 **Personnel:** 1691

## BOZEMAN—Gallatin County

⊠ **BOZEMAN DEACONESS HOSPITAL (270057)**, 915 Highland Boulevard, Zip 59715–6902; tel. 406/585–5000, (Nonreporting) **A**1 2 9 10 20
Primary Contact: Stan Moser, President and Chief Executive Officer
Web address: www.bozemandeaconess.org
**Control:** Other not–for–profit (including NFP Corporation) **Service:** General Medical and Surgical

**Staffed Beds:** 70

**MT**

---

**Hospital, Medicare Provider Number, Address, Telephone, Approval, Facility, and Physician Codes, Health Care System**

★ American Hospital Association (AHA) membership
☐ The Joint Commission accreditation   ◇ DNV Healthcare Inc. accreditation

○ American Osteopathic Association (AOA) accreditation
△ Commission on Accreditation of Rehabilitation Facilities (CARF) accreditation

**BUTTE—Silver Bow County**

✠ **ST. JAMES HEALTHCARE (270017)**, 400 South Clark Street,
Zip 59702–3300; tel. 406/723–2500 **A**1 9 10 **F**3 11 13 15 18 20 22 26 28
29 30 34 35 40 43 46 47 48 49 50 51 57 59 64 70 72 75 76 77 78 79 81
82 85 87 89 93 97 102 107 108 111 114 115 116 117 118 119 120 121
122 126 129 130 131 134 144 145 146 147 **P**6 **S** Sisters of Charity of
Leavenworth Health System, Denver, CO
Primary Contact: Charles T. Wright, President and Chief Executive Officer
CFO: Jay Doyle, Chief Financial Officer
CMO: Dennis Salisbury, M.D., Vice President for Medical Affairs
CHR: Trisha Palmer, Director
CNO: Shannon S. Holland, R.N., Vice President of Patient Care Service
Web address: www.stjameshealthcare.org
**Control:** Other not–for–profit (including NFP Corporation) **Service:** General
Medical and Surgical

**Staffed Beds:** 58 **Admissions:** 4319 **Census:** 38 **Outpatient Visits:** 74031
**Births:** 514 **Total Expense ($000):** 84095 **Payroll Expense ($000):** 29538
**Personnel:** 408

**CHESTER—Liberty County**

**LIBERTY MEDICAL CENTER (271334)**, 315 West Madison Avenue, Zip 59522,
Mailing Address: P.O. Box 705, Zip 59522–0705; tel. 406/759–5181 **A**9 10 18
**F**2 3 10 11 15 29 34 35 40 43 45 56 57 59 64 67 75 77 81 86 87 89 93 97
107 110 113 118 126 127 132 **P**6
Primary Contact: Ronald M. Gleason, Chief Executive Officer
CFO: Shari Meissner, Chief Financial Officer
CMO: Anna Earl, M.D., Chief of Staff
CIO: Marilyn Snyder, Chief Information Officer
CHR: Jane Allen, Director Human Resources and Payroll
Web address: www.lchnh.org
**Control:** Other not–for–profit (including NFP Corporation) **Service:** General
Medical and Surgical

**Staffed Beds:** 25 **Admissions:** 106 **Census:** 22 **Outpatient Visits:** 7279
**Births:** 0 **Total Expense ($000):** 6334 **Payroll Expense ($000):** 3324
**Personnel:** 85

**CHOTEAU—Teton County**

★ **TETON MEDICAL CENTER (271307)**, 915 4th Street North West,
Zip 59422–9123; tel. 406/466–5763, (Total facility includes 36 beds in nursing
home–type unit) **A**9 10 18 **F**2 3 15 34 35 40 41 53 54 56 57 59 63 64 68 87
93 107 126 127 129 130 132 142 145 **P**6
Primary Contact: Louie King, Interim Administrator
Web address: www.tetonmedicalcenter.net
**Control:** Hospital district or authority, Government, nonfederal **Service:** General
Medical and Surgical

**Staffed Beds:** 46 **Admissions:** 259 **Census:** 31 **Outpatient Visits:** 6979
**Births:** 0 **Total Expense ($000):** 6514 **Payroll Expense ($000):** 3496
**Personnel:** 94

**CIRCLE—McCone County**

★ **MCCONE COUNTY HEALTH CENTER (271305)**, 605 Sullivan Avenue,
Zip 59215, Mailing Address: P.O. Box 48, Zip 59215–0048; tel. 406/485–3381
**A**9 10 18 **F**2 3 11 40 41 65 132 134 142 145
Primary Contact: Nancy Rosaaen, Chief Executive Officer
CFO: Nancy Rosaaen, Chief Executive Officer
CHR: Jacque Gardner, Administrative Assistant, Clinic Manager, Co–Chief Financial
Officer and Chief Human Resources
**Control:** County–Government, nonfederal **Service:** General Medical and Surgical

**Staffed Beds:** 25 **Admissions:** 162 **Census:** 21 **Outpatient Visits:** 7765
**Births:** 0 **Total Expense ($000):** 3143 **Payroll Expense ($000):** 1327
**Personnel:** 40

**COLUMBUS—Stillwater County**

★ **STILLWATER COMMUNITY HOSPITAL (271330)**, 44 West Fourth Avenue
North, Zip 59019–0959, Mailing Address: P.O. Box 959, Zip 59019–0959;
tel. 406/322–5316 **A**9 10 18 **F**10 15 28 29 32 35 40 45 46 56 57 59 62 65
69 75 93 107 127 129 132 144 **P**1 3
Primary Contact: Tim Russell, Administrator
Web address: www.billingsclinic.com
**Control:** Other not–for–profit (including NFP Corporation) **Service:** General
Medical and Surgical

**Staffed Beds:** 23 **Admissions:** 234 **Census:** 4 **Outpatient Visits:** 9468
**Births:** 0 **Total Expense ($000):** 4500 **Payroll Expense ($000):** 1755
**Personnel:** 34

**CONRAD—Pondera County**

**PONDERA MEDICAL CENTER (271324)**, 805 Sunset Boulevard,
Zip 59425–1717, Mailing Address: P.O. Box 758, Zip 59425–0758;
tel. 406/271–3211, (Nonreporting) **A**9 10 18
Primary Contact: Mark L. Jones, Chief Executive Officer
CFO: Dave Doran, Chief Financial Officer
CMO: Peter Barran, M.D., Chief of Staff
CIO: Sean Kavawaha, Supervisor Information Technology and Information Systems
CHR: J. D. Duncan, Director Human Resources
Web address: www.ponderamedical.com
**Control:** Other not–for–profit (including NFP Corporation) **Service:** General
Medical and Surgical

**Staffed Beds:** 20

**CROW AGENCY—Big Horn County**

**CROW/NORTHERN CHEYENNE HOSPITAL (271339)**, P.O. Box 9,
Zip 59022–0009; tel. 406/638–2626, (Nonreporting) **A**10 18 **S** U. S. Indian
Health Service, Rockville, MD
Primary Contact: Yvonne Misiaszek, Service Unit Director
CMO: Jim Upchurch, M.D., Chief Medical Officer
CIO: Melanie Falls Down, Site Manager
Web address: www.ihs.gov/facilitiesservices/areaoffices/billings/crow/index.asp
**Control:** Public Health Service, Government, federal **Service:** General Medical
and Surgical

**Staffed Beds:** 24

**CULBERTSON—Roosevelt County**

★ **ROOSEVELT MEDICAL CENTER (271308)**, 818 Second Avenue East,
Zip 59218, Mailing Address: P.O. Box 419, Zip 59218–0419; tel. 406/787–6401
**A**9 10 18 **F**2 3 7 11 15 34 35 40 43 50 56 57 59 65 69 93 97 126 127 129
132 142 145 **P**6
Primary Contact: Audrey Stromberg, Administrator
CFO: Carolyn Casterline, Financial Director
Web address: www.roosmem.org
**Control:** Other not–for–profit (including NFP Corporation) **Service:** General
Medical and Surgical

**Staffed Beds:** 25 **Admissions:** 71 **Census:** 23 **Outpatient Visits:** 8078
**Births:** 0 **Total Expense ($000):** 4018 **Payroll Expense ($000):** 2348
**Personnel:** 69

**CUT BANK—Glacier County**

**NORTHERN ROCKIES MEDICAL CENTER (271337)**, 802 Second Street S.E.,
Zip 59427–3329; tel. 406/873–2251 **A**9 10 18 **F**8 11 29 34 40 50 57 59 64
65 66 81 89 91 93 97 107 108 118 126 128 129 132 **P**4 6
Primary Contact: Cherie Taylor, Chief Executive Officer
CFO: Treasure Berkram, Chief Financial Officer
CMO: Adron Medley, M.D., Chief Medical Staff
CHR: Kandie Lemieux, Administrative Assistant and Director Human Resources
Web address: www.nmrcinc.org
**Control:** Other not–for–profit (including NFP Corporation) **Service:** General
Medical and Surgical

**Staffed Beds:** 13 **Admissions:** 185 **Census:** 1 **Outpatient Visits:** 12924
**Births:** 0 **Total Expense ($000):** 6263 **Payroll Expense ($000):** 3719
**Personnel:** 73

**DEER LODGE—Powell County**

**POWELL COUNTY MEDICAL CENTER (271314)**, 1101 Texas Avenue,
Zip 59722–1828; tel. 406/846–2212 **A**9 10 18 **F**3 11 34 40 43 45 48 57 59
64 67 76 79 81 82 91 93 107 113 118 126 127 132 135 136 137 138 139
140 141 142 143 144 145 146 147 **P**6 **S** Cypress Health Systems, Benton, LA
Primary Contact: Alan Bird, Chief Executive Officer
CFO: Jaena Richards, Chief Financial Officer
CMO: Michelle Corbin, M.D., Chief of Staff
CIO: Chris Foster, Director Health Information Management
Web address: www.pcmh.org
**Control:** Other not–for–profit (including NFP Corporation) **Service:** General
Medical and Surgical

**Staffed Beds:** 16 **Admissions:** 267 **Census:** 4 **Outpatient Visits:** 8886
**Births:** 0 **Total Expense ($000):** 6088 **Payroll Expense ($000):** 2761
**Personnel:** 53

MT

## DILLON—Beaverhead County

★ **BARRETT HOSPITAL & HEALTHCARE (271318)**, 90 Highway 91 South, Zip 59725–3597; tel. 406/683–3000 **A**9 10 18 **F**3 13 15 24 28 29 32 34 35 37 38 40 43 44 45 50 57 59 62 63 64 65 68 70 75 77 79 81 82 83 84 85 86 87 89 93 94 97 107 108 110 111 114 117 118 119 127 129 130 131 132 145 147 **P**5 6 **S** HealthTech Management Services, Franklin, TN
Primary Contact: Ken Westman, Chief Executive Officer
CFO: Dick Achter, Chief Financial Officer
CMO: Cindy Christenson, Chief Clinical Officer
CIO: Dick Achter, Chief Financial Officer
Web address: www.barretthospital.org
**Control:** Hospital district or authority, Government, nonfederal **Service:** General Medical and Surgical

**Staffed Beds:** 20 **Admissions:** 752 **Census:** 5 **Outpatient Visits:** 30244 **Births:** 81 **Total Expense ($000):** 21278 **Payroll Expense ($000):** 11025 **Personnel:** 198

## EKALAKA—Carter County

**DAHL MEMORIAL HEALTHCARE ASSOCIATION (271302)**, 215 Sandy Street, Zip 59324, Mailing Address: P.O. Box 46, Zip 59324–0046; tel. 406/775–8730, (Total facility includes 23 beds in nursing home–type unit) **A**9 10 18 **F**2 7 40 41 57 59 65 69 126 127 129 130 132 134 142 145 147 **P**6
Primary Contact: Nadine Elmore, Chief Executive Officer
CFO: Nadine Elmore, Chief Executive Officer
CMO: Dale Diede, M.D., Medical Provider
CIO: Rhonda Knapp, Director Human Resources
CHR: Rhonda Knapp, Director Human Resources
Web address: www.dahlmemorial.com
**Control:** Other not–for–profit (including NFP Corporation) **Service:** General Medical and Surgical

**Staffed Beds:** 31 **Admissions:** 31 **Census:** 12 **Outpatient Visits:** 2576 **Births:** 0 **Total Expense ($000):** 1920 **Payroll Expense ($000):** 1084 **Personnel:** 34

## ENNIS—Madison County

**MADISON VALLEY MEDICAL CENTER (271329)**, 305 North Main Street, Zip 59729–0397, Mailing Address: P.O. Box 397, Zip 59729–0397; tel. 406/682–4222 **A**9 10 18 **F**3 11 40 57 67 104 107 118 127 132 134
Primary Contact: John Bishop, Chief Financial Officer
CFO: John Bishop, Chief Financial Officer
CMO: Cindy Sharp, M.D., Chief Medical Officer
CIO: Bo Nix, Chief Information Officer
Web address: www.mvhospital–clinic.com
**Control:** Hospital district or authority, Government, nonfederal **Service:** General Medical and Surgical

**Staffed Beds:** 10 **Admissions:** 100 **Census:** 1

## FORSYTH—Rosebud County

★ **ROSEBUD HEALTH CARE CENTER (271327)**, 383 North 17th Avenue, Zip 59327–0268, Mailing Address: P.O. Box 268, Zip 59327–0268; tel. 406/346–2161, (Total facility includes 31 beds in nursing home–type unit) **A**9 10 18 **F**2 30 32 34 40 41 43 45 50 57 59 75 93 97 107 126 127 130 131 132 142 143 144 145 147 **P**3 4 5
Primary Contact: Ryan Tooke, Interim Chief Executive Officer
CFO: Ryan Tooke, Chief Financial Officer
CMO: William Anderson, M.D., Medical Director
CHR: Karla Allies, Director Human Resources
Web address: www.rosebudhealthcare.com/
**Control:** Other not–for–profit (including NFP Corporation) **Service:** General Medical and Surgical

**Staffed Beds:** 55 **Admissions:** 411 **Census:** 37 **Outpatient Visits:** 11356 **Births:** 0 **Total Expense ($000):** 5758 **Payroll Expense ($000):** 3723

## FORT BENTON—Chouteau County

★ **MISSOURI RIVER MEDICAL CENTER (271304)**, 1501 St. Charles Street, Zip 59442–0249, Mailing Address: P.O. Box 249, Zip 59442–0249; tel. 406/622–3331, (Total facility includes 41 beds in nursing home–type unit) **A**9 10 18 **F**2 3 10 40 57 59 62 63 64 67 84 90 93 107 113 126 127 129 130 132 134 142 145 **P**5 **S** Benefis Health System, Great Falls, MT
Primary Contact: Jay Pottenger, Administrator
CFO: Lynn Asbeck, Manager Business Office
CHR: Carolyn Johnsrud, Manager Human Resources
Web address: www.mrmcfb.org
**Control:** Hospital district or authority, Government, nonfederal **Service:** General Medical and Surgical

**Staffed Beds:** 52 **Admissions:** 108 **Census:** 32 **Outpatient Visits:** 5514 **Births:** 0 **Total Expense ($000):** 5003 **Payroll Expense ($000):** 2750 **Personnel:** 82

## FORT HARRISON—Lewis and Clark County

⊞ **VETERANS AFFAIRS MONTANA HEALTH CARE SYSTEM**, 1892 Williams Street, Zip 59636, Mailing Address: P.O. Box 1500, Zip 59636–1500; tel. 406/442–6410, (Total facility includes 20 beds in nursing home–type unit) **A**1 **F**3 4 5 12 18 28 29 30 31 33 34 35 38 39 40 44 45 46 47 50 51 53 54 56 59 61 63 64 65 66 68 70 74 75 77 78 79 81 82 84 85 86 87 91 92 93 94 97 100 101 102 103 104 106 107 108 111 113 114 115 118 126 127 128 129 131 134 142 143 145 146 147 **S** Department of Veterans Affairs, Washington, DC
Primary Contact: Robin Korogi, Director
CFO: Brian Gustafson, Chief Financial Officer
CMO: Kurt Werner, M.D., Chief of Staff
CIO: Paul Gauthier, Chief Information Resources Management
CHR: Aggie Hamilton, Chief Human Resources
Web address: www.va.gov/sta/guide/home.asp
**Control:** Veterans Affairs, Government, federal **Service:** General Medical and Surgical

**Staffed Beds:** 65 **Admissions:** 2105 **Census:** 56 **Births:** 0

## GLASGOW—Valley County

⊞ **FRANCES MAHON DEACONESS HOSPITAL (271316)**, 621 Third Street South, Zip 59230–2699; tel. 406/228–3500 **A**1 9 10 18 **F**3 7 11 13 15 28 29 30 31 34 35 40 43 53 56 57 59 61 64 70 75 76 78 79 81 82 86 87 89 93 100 102 105 107 108 111 113 117 118 126 127 129 132 134 144 145 **P**6 7
Primary Contact: Randall G. Holom, Chief Executive Officer
COO: Ellen Guttenberg, Chief Operating Officer
CFO: Del Gienger, Director Financial Services
CMO: Gordon Bell, M.D., Chief of Staff
CIO: David L. Nixdorf, Director Support Services
CHR: Shelly Van Buren, Director Human Resources
CNO: Brenda Koessl, R.N., Director of Nursing Services
Web address: www.fmdh.org
**Control:** Other not–for–profit (including NFP Corporation) **Service:** General Medical and Surgical

**Staffed Beds:** 25 **Admissions:** 661 **Census:** 6 **Outpatient Visits:** 33395 **Births:** 126 **Total Expense ($000):** 18745 **Payroll Expense ($000):** 8766 **Personnel:** 163

## GLENDIVE—Dawson County

★ **GLENDIVE MEDICAL CENTER (271332)**, 202 Prospect Drive, Zip 59330–1999; tel. 406/345–3306, (Total facility includes 71 beds in nursing home–type unit) **A**9 10 18 **F**3 10 11 13 15 28 29 30 31 35 38 40 41 43 50 56 57 59 61 62 63 64 67 69 70 75 76 77 78 79 81 82 87 89 93 94 98 102 103 104 107 108 111 113 118 126 127 129 130 131 132 142 143 145 146 147 **P**6 7 8
Primary Contact: Scott A. Duke, Chief Executive Officer
CFO: Barbara Markham, Chief Financial Officer
CMO: Kevin Maxwell, M.D., Chief of Staff
CIO: Matthew Shahan, Director Information Systems
CHR: Joetta J. Pearcy, Human Resources Director
Web address: www.gmc.org
**Control:** Other not–for–profit (including NFP Corporation) **Service:** General Medical and Surgical

**Staffed Beds:** 96 **Admissions:** 1120 **Census:** 57 **Outpatient Visits:** 29891 **Births:** 141 **Total Expense ($000):** 28498 **Payroll Expense ($000):** 12155 **Personnel:** 247

**MT**

---

**Hospital, Medicare Provider Number, Address, Telephone, Approval, Facility, and Physician Codes, Health Care System**

★ American Hospital Association (AHA) membership
□ The Joint Commission accreditation ◇ DNV Healthcare Inc. accreditation

○ American Osteopathic Association (AOA) accreditation
△ Commission on Accreditation of Rehabilitation Facilities (CARF) accreditation

## GREAT FALLS—Cascade County

☒ △ **BENEFIS HOSPITALS (270012)**, 1101 26th Street South,
Zip 59405–5104; tel. 406/455–5000, (Includes BENEFIS HEALTH CARE–EAST
CAMPUS, 1101 26th Street, Zip 59405; tel. 406/761–1200; BENEFIS HEALTH
CARE–WEST CAMPUS, 500 15th Avenue South, Zip 59405, Mailing Address: P.O.
Box 5013, Zip 59403–5013; tel. 406/727–3333), (Total facility includes 146
beds in nursing home–type unit) **A**1 2 7 9 10 20 **F**3 4 5 6 8 11 12 13 15 17 18
20 22 24 28 29 30 31 34 35 37 38 40 43 45 48 49 50 54 55 56 57 58 59
60 61 62 63 64 65 70 71 72 73 74 75 76 77 78 79 80 81 82 83 84 85 86
87 88 89 90 92 93 96 97 98 100 101 102 103 104 105 107 108 110 111
113 114 118 119 120 122 123 125 126 127 128 129 130 131 132 133 134
135 140 142 143 144 145 146 **S** Benefis Health System, Great Falls, MT
Primary Contact: John H. Goodnow, Chief Executive Officer
COO: Julie Hickethier, R.N., Senior Vice President
CFO: Douglas Davenport, System Chief Financial Officer
CMO: Paul Dolan, M.D., Chief Medical Affairs Officer
CIO: Lee Roath, System Chief Information Officer
CHR: Terry Olinger, System Chief Human Resources Officer
Web address: www.benefis.org
**Control:** Other not–for–profit (including NFP Corporation) **Service:** General
Medical and Surgical

**Staffed Beds:** 438 **Admissions:** 12637 **Census:** 294 **Outpatient Visits:**
335652 **Births:** 1489 **Total Expense ($000):** 309960 **Payroll Expense**
**($000):** 126177 **Personnel:** 2099

**GREAT FALLS CLINIC MEDICAL CENTER (270086)**, 1411 9th Street South,
Zip 59405; tel. 406/216–8000 **A**9 10 **F**18 29 44 50 51 74 79 81 82 85 86
89 134
Primary Contact: Patrick M. Hermanson, Administrator
COO: Vicki Newmiller, Chief Operating Officer
CFO: Cheryl Cornwell, Chief Financial Officer
CMO: Nicholas Bonfilio, M.D., Chief of Staff
Web address: www.greatfallsclinicmedicalcenter.com
**Control:** Corporation, Investor–owned, for–profit **Service:** General Medical and
Surgical

**Staffed Beds:** 20 **Admissions:** 376 **Census:** 4 **Outpatient Visits:** 1210
**Births:** 0 **Total Expense ($000):** 10740 **Payroll Expense ($000):** 3019
**Personnel:** 88

## HAMILTON—Ravalli County

★ **MARCUS DALY MEMORIAL HOSPITAL (271340)**, 1200 Westwood Drive,
Zip 59840–2345; tel. 406/363–2211 **A**9 10 18 **F**1 3 7 8 11 13 15 17 28 30
34 35 40 45 50 57 59 62 63 64 65 70 74 75 76 77 79 81 83 84 89 93 97
102 105 107 110 111 114 118 126 127 128 129 130 131 132 143 144
145 147
Primary Contact: John M. Bartos, Chief Executive Officer
CFO: Donja Erdman, Chief Financial Officer
CMO: John Moreland, M.D., Chief Medical Officer
CIO: Brian Moreau, Director Data Processing
CHR: Debbie M. Morris, Director Human Resources
Web address: www.mdmh.org
**Control:** Other not–for–profit (including NFP Corporation) **Service:** General
Medical and Surgical

**Staffed Beds:** 37 **Admissions:** 1634 **Census:** 15 **Outpatient Visits:** 35308
**Births:** 149 **Total Expense ($000):** 35743 **Payroll Expense ($000):** 20123
**Personnel:** 397

## HARDIN—Big Horn County

★ **BIG HORN COUNTY MEMORIAL HOSPITAL (271338)**, 17 North Miles Avenue,
Zip 59034–2323; tel. 406/665–2310, (Total facility includes 36 beds in nursing
home–type unit) **A**9 10 18 **F**10 11 13 15 28 40 50 57 59 64 65 68 75 76 77
81 85 86 87 90 93 107 110 111 113 118 124 127 129 131 132 142 145
Primary Contact: George Minder, Chief Executive Officer
CFO: Roxie Cain, Chief Financial Officer
Web address: www.bighornhospital.org
**Control:** Other not–for–profit (including NFP Corporation) **Service:** General
Medical and Surgical

**Staffed Beds:** 61 **Admissions:** 310 **Census:** 49 **Outpatient Visits:** 7550
**Births:** 23 **Total Expense ($000):** 10955 **Payroll Expense ($000):** 6139
**Personnel:** 156

## HARLEM—Blaine County

**FORT BELKNAP U. S. PUBLIC HEALTH SERVICE INDIAN HOSPITAL**
**(271315)**, (Critical Access Hospital), 669 Agency Main Street, Zip 59526;
tel. 406/353–3100 **A**10 18 **F**7 40 75 107 110 **S** U. S. Indian Health Service,
Rockville, MD
Primary Contact: Steve Fox, Chief Executive Officer
CIO: Mikki Grant, Chief Information Officer
CHR: Mary H. Mount, Administrative Officer
Web address: www.ihs.gov
**Control:** PHS, Indian Service, Government, federal **Service:** General Medical and
Surgical

**Staffed Beds:** 6 **Admissions:** 32 **Census:** 1 **Outpatient Visits:** 9918 **Births:**
0

## HARLOWTON—Wheatland County

★ **WHEATLAND MEMORIAL HEALTHCARE (271321)**, 530 Third Street North
West, Zip 59036, Mailing Address: P.O. Box 287, Zip 59036–0287;
tel. 406/632–4351 **A**9 10 18 **F**15 30 32 34 35 40 43 50 56 57 59 61 64 65
75 77 85 87 93 97 107 110 117 118 126 129 131 132 134 142 145 146 **P**6
Primary Contact: Terri Donovan, Chief Executive Officer
CFO: Kathie Newland, Controller
CMO: Kris Cunningham, M.D., Chief of Staff
CIO: Russ Young, Network Administrator
CHR: Peggy Hiner, Executive Secretary and Manager Human Resources
CNO: Lauri Ann Cooney, Director Nursing
Web address: www.wheatlandmemorial.org
**Control:** Other not–for–profit (including NFP Corporation) **Service:** General
Medical and Surgical

**Staffed Beds:** 25 **Admissions:** 102 **Census:** 20 **Outpatient Visits:** 3867
**Births:** 0 **Total Expense ($000):** 5328 **Payroll Expense ($000):** 3049
**Personnel:** 71

## HAVRE—Hill County

★ **NORTHERN MONTANA HOSPITAL (270032)**, 30 13th Street,
Zip 59501–5222, Mailing Address: P.O. Box 1231, Zip 59501–1231;
tel. 406/265–2211, (Total facility includes 102 beds in nursing home–type unit)
**A**9 10 20 **F**10 11 13 15 28 29 34 35 36 38 40 50 53 56 57 59 60 63 64 68
70 75 76 77 79 81 82 84 85 89 93 97 99 101 102 103 104 105 107 108
110 111 113 117 118 126 127 128 129 131 132 134 145 147 **P**6
Primary Contact: David Henry, President and Chief Executive Officer
CFO: Kim Lucke, Vice President Finance
CHR: Bonnie O'Neill, Vice President Employee Services
CNO: Karen Pollington, VP Patient Care
Web address: www.nmhcare.org
**Control:** Other not–for–profit (including NFP Corporation) **Service:** General
Medical and Surgical

**Staffed Beds:** 129 **Admissions:** 1865 **Census:** 123 **Outpatient Visits:** 86026
**Births:** 372 **Total Expense ($000):** 48080 **Payroll Expense ($000):** 26546
**Personnel:** 490

## HELENA—Lewis And Clark County

☒ **SHODAIR CHILDREN'S HOSPITAL (274004)**, 2755 Colonial Drive,
Zip 59601–4926, Mailing Address: P.O. Box 5539, Zip 59604–5539;
tel. 406/444–7500 **A**1 9 10 **F**55 98 99 101 102 104 106 129 **P**6
Primary Contact: John P. Casey, Administrator
COO: John P. Casey, Administrator
CFO: Ron Wiens, Chief Financial Officer
CMO: Heather Zaluski, M.D., President Medical Staff
CIO: Judy Jackson, Director Health Information Management and Privacy Officer
Web address: www.shodairhospital.org
**Control:** Other not–for–profit (including NFP Corporation) **Service:** Children's
hospital psychiatric

**Staffed Beds:** 88 **Admissions:** 765 **Census:** 60 **Outpatient Visits:** 3814
**Births:** 0 **Total Expense ($000):** 19847 **Payroll Expense ($000):** 10924
**Personnel:** 159

☒ **ST. PETER'S HOSPITAL (270003)**, 2475 Broadway, Zip 59601;
tel. 406/442–2480 **A**1 2 9 10 20 **F**3 7 8 13 15 18 20 22 26 28 29 30 31 34
35 40 43 50 51 56 57 59 60 62 63 64 65 70 74 75 76 77 78 79 81 82 84
85 86 87 89 93 97 98 100 102 107 108 110 111 113 114 115 116 117 118
120 123 128 129 130 131 132 134 142 143 145 146 147 **P**6
Primary Contact: Thomas Gregg, Interim President and Chief Executive Officer
CFO: John Green, Vice President Finance
CIO: Tammy K. Buyok, Vice President Support Services
CHR: Thomas Gregg, Vice President Human Resources
Web address: www.stpetes.org
**Control:** Other not–for–profit (including NFP Corporation) **Service:** General
Medical and Surgical

**Staffed Beds:** 123 **Admissions:** 5377 **Census:** 58 **Outpatient Visits:** 173421
**Births:** 817 **Total Expense ($000):** 132925 **Payroll Expense ($000):** 52484
**Personnel:** 897

## JORDAN—Garfield County

**GARFIELD COUNTY HEALTH CENTER (271310)**, 332 Leavitt Avenue,
Zip 59337, Mailing Address: P.O. Box 389, Zip 59337–0389;
tel. 406/557–2500, (Nonreporting) **A**9 10 18
Primary Contact: Ronald W. Barnes, Chief Executive Officer
CFO: Sandi Williams, Manager Business Officer
CMO: Daniel Muniak, M.D., Chief Medical Officer
CIO: Sandi Williams, Manager Business Officer
**Control:** County–Government, nonfederal **Service:** General Medical and Surgical

**Staffed Beds:** 4

## KALISPELL—Flathead County

**HEALTHCENTER NORTHWEST** See The HealthCenter

**MT**

*Many Facility Codes have changed. Please refer to the AHA Guide Code Chart.* © 2012 AHA Guide

★ △ **KALISPELL REGIONAL MEDICAL CENTER (270051)**, 310 Sunnyview Lane, Zip 59901–3129; tel. 406/752–5111, (Includes PATHWAYS TREATMENT CENTER, 200 Heritage Way, Zip 59901; tel. 406/756–3950) **A**7 9 10 **F**3 4 5 8 12 13 15 18 20 22 24 26 28 29 30 31 34 35 36 40 43 45 46 48 49 50 56 57 58 59 62 63 64 70 72 74 75 76 77 78 79 81 85 86 87 90 93 96 98 99 100 101 102 103 104 105 107 108 113 114 117 118 119 120 122 125 128 129 130 131 142 143 144 145 146 147 **P**6
Primary Contact: Velinda Stevens, President
COO: Ted W. Hirsch, Senior Executive Director
CFO: Charles T. Pearce, Chief Financial and Information Officer
CHR: Deb Wilson, Director Human Resources
Web address: www.krmc.org
**Control:** Other not–for–profit (including NFP Corporation) **Service:** General Medical and Surgical

**Staffed Beds:** 163 **Admissions:** 7435 **Census:** 86 **Outpatient Visits:** 168711 **Births:** 642 **Total Expense ($000):** 168251 **Payroll Expense ($000):** 74293 **Personnel:** 1231

★ **THE HEALTHCENTER (270087)**, 320 Sunnyview Lane, Zip 59901–3129; tel. 406/751–7550 **A**9 10 **F**3 8 15 31 36 39 64 68 70 74 78 79 81 82 85 87 100 107 110 111 113 114 116 118 125 146 **P**2
Primary Contact: Tate J. Kreitinger, Chief Executive Officer
CMO: Craig Eddy, M.D., Chief Medical Officer
CIO: Charles T. Pearce, CFIO
CHR: Susan Stevens, Director Human Resources
CNO: Victoria Johnson, R.N., Nursing Director of Surgical and Medical Services
Web address: www.krmc.org
**Control:** Corporation, Investor–owned, for–profit **Service:** General Medical and Surgical

**Staffed Beds:** 30 **Admissions:** 787 **Census:** 5 **Outpatient Visits:** 38028 **Births:** 0 **Total Expense ($000):** 30502 **Payroll Expense ($000):** 6309 **Personnel:** 134

**LEWISTOWN—Fergus County**

★ **CENTRAL MONTANA MEDICAL CENTER (271345)**, 408 Wendell Avenue, Zip 59457–2261; tel. 406/535–7711, (Total facility includes 65 beds in nursing home–type unit) **A**9 10 18 **F**3 7 11 13 15 28 29 30 31 34 35 40 43 45 46 50 53 56 57 59 62 63 64 65 75 76 77 78 79 81 82 85 86 87 89 93 100 102 105 107 108 111 114 118 127 128 129 130 131 132 134 142 145 147 **P**6 **S** QHR, Brentwood, TN
Primary Contact: Lee Rhodes, Chief Executive Officer
COO: Dianne Scotten, Chief Clinical Officer
CFO: Alan Aldrich, Chief Financial Officer
CHR: Torie A. Lynch, Manager Human Resources
Web address: www.cmmccares.com
**Control:** Other not–for–profit (including NFP Corporation) **Service:** General Medical and Surgical

**Staffed Beds:** 90 **Admissions:** 1117 **Census:** 67 **Outpatient Visits:** 47675 **Births:** 100 **Total Expense ($000):** 24705 **Payroll Expense ($000):** 12549 **Personnel:** 312

**LIBBY—Lincoln County**

★ **ST. JOHN'S LUTHERAN HOSPITAL (271320)**, 350 Louisiana Avenue, Zip 59923–2130; tel. 406/293–0100 **A**9 10 18 **F**3 11 13 15 17 28 29 30 31 34 35 40 45 56 57 59 62 64 68 70 75 76 77 79 81 82 84 85 86 87 89 91 93 97 102 107 110 111 113 118 128 129 130 131 132 134 143 145 146 147 **P**6
Primary Contact: William Patten, Administrator and Chief Executive Officer
CFO: Steve Chavez, Chief Financial Officer
CMO: Jay Maloney, M.D., Chief of Staff
Web address: www.sjlh.com
**Control:** Other not–for–profit (including NFP Corporation) **Service:** General Medical and Surgical

**Staffed Beds:** 25 **Admissions:** 852 **Census:** 7 **Outpatient Visits:** 33380 **Births:** 107 **Total Expense ($000):** 23920 **Payroll Expense ($000):** 12414 **Personnel:** 207

**LIVINGSTON—Park County**

★ **LIVINGSTON MEMORIAL HOSPITAL (271317)**, 504 South 13th Street, Zip 59047–3727; tel. 406/222–3541 **A**9 10 18 **F**8 13 15 17 28 29 31 35 36 40 50 62 63 64 66 67 68 70 76 77 78 79 81 82 85 86 87 89 93 102 107 108 110 111 113 118 123 127 128 130 132 **P**3
Primary Contact: Samuel G. Pleshar, Chief Executive Officer
CFO: Melanie Emter, Director Finance
CMO: Michelle Donaldson, M.D., President Medical Staff
CHR: Connie Dunn, Director Human Resources
Web address: www.livingstonhealthcare.org
**Control:** Other not–for–profit (including NFP Corporation) **Service:** General Medical and Surgical

**Staffed Beds:** 25 **Admissions:** 889 **Census:** 9 **Outpatient Visits:** 22247 **Births:** 97 **Total Expense ($000):** 25751 **Payroll Expense ($000):** 14476 **Personnel:** 276

**MALTA—Phillips County**

★ **PHILLIPS COUNTY HOSPITAL (271312)**, 417 South Fourth East, Zip 59538, Mailing Address: P.O. Box 640, Zip 59538–0640; tel. 406/654–1100 **A**9 10 18 **F**15 28 29 30 31 32 34 35 40 43 45 56 58 59 62 64 65 67 78 93 97 107 113 126 127 129 132 147 **P**4
Primary Contact: Ward C. VanWichen, Chief Executive Officer
CFO: Stephanie Denham, Chief Financial Officer and Human Resources Officer
CMO: Ed Medina, M.D., Medical Director
CHR: Stephanie Denham, Chief Financial Officer and Human Resources Officer
CNO: Lonna Crowder, Director of Nursing
Web address: www.phillipscountyhospital.com
**Control:** Other not–for–profit (including NFP Corporation) **Service:** General Medical and Surgical

**Staffed Beds:** 6 **Admissions:** 174 **Census:** 1 **Outpatient Visits:** 6848 **Births:** 0 **Personnel:** 57

**MILES CITY—Custer County**

★ **HOLY ROSARY HEALTHCARE (271347)**, 2600 Wilson Street, Zip 59301–5094; tel. 406/233–2600, (Total facility includes 65 beds in nursing home–type unit) **A**9 10 **F**3 13 15 26 28 29 30 31 34 35 40 41 57 59 63 64 70 75 76 77 78 79 81 84 85 86 87 89 93 97 102 107 108 111 114 118 126 128 129 130 132 134 142 143 145 146 147 **P**6 **S** Sisters of Charity of Leavenworth Health System, Denver, CO
Primary Contact: Paul Lewis, Chief Executive Officer
CFO: Calvin Carey, VP Finance and Support Services
CHR: Cathy Rodenbaugh, Director Human Resources
CNO: Lisa Sanford, VP Patient Care/CNO
Web address: www.holyrosaryhealthcare.org
**Control:** Church–operated, Nongovernment, not–for profit **Service:** General Medical and Surgical

**Staffed Beds:** 90 **Admissions:** 1719 **Census:** 72 **Outpatient Visits:** 60665 **Births:** 239 **Total Expense ($000):** 37327 **Payroll Expense ($000):** 16529 **Personnel:** 284

**MISSOULA—Missoula County**

⊠ △ **COMMUNITY MEDICAL CENTER (270023)**, 2827 Fort Missoula Road, Zip 59804–7408; tel. 406/728–4100 **A**1 7 9 10 19 **F**2 3 11 13 17 18 20 22 26 28 29 30 31 34 35 37 40 43 45 46 47 48 49 51 54 57 59 64 65 68 70 72 73 74 75 76 77 78 79 81 82 83 84 85 87 88 89 90 91 92 93 94 96 97 107 108 110 114 115 116 117 118 125 129 131 133 134 142 143 144 145 146 147 **P**6 7
Primary Contact: Stephen G. Carlson, President and Chief Executive Officer
COO: Devin Huntley, Vice President Operations
CFO: David Richhart, Vice President Fiscal Services
CMO: Jonathan Weisul, M.D., Chief Medical Officer and Vice President Innovation
CIO: Leigh Thurston, Vice President Information Systems
CHR: Joe Schmier, Director Human Resources, Payroll & Employee Health
CNO: Jan Perry, R.N., Vice President Patient Care Services
Web address: www.communitymed.org
**Control:** Other not–for–profit (including NFP Corporation) **Service:** General Medical and Surgical

**Staffed Beds:** 137 **Admissions:** 5463 **Census:** 65 **Outpatient Visits:** 129888 **Births:** 1513 **Total Expense ($000):** 134909 **Payroll Expense ($000):** 56766 **Personnel:** 957

**MT**

**Hospital, Medicare Provider Number, Address, Telephone, Approval, Facility, and Physician Codes, Health Care System**

★ American Hospital Association (AHA) membership
□ The Joint Commission accreditation  ◇ DNV Healthcare Inc. accreditation
○ American Osteopathic Association (AOA) accreditation
△ Commission on Accreditation of Rehabilitation Facilities (CARF) accreditation

✠ △ **ST. PATRICK HOSPITAL (270014)**, 500 West Broadway,
Zip 59802–4096, Mailing Address: P.O. Box 4587, Zip 59806–4587;
tel. 406/543–7271 **A**1 2 5 7 9 10 19 **F**3 5 8 11 12 15 18 19 20 21 22 23 24
25 26 27 28 29 30 31 34 35 36 38 40 43 45 49 50 53 57 58 59 61 64 65
68 70 74 75 77 78 79 81 82 84 85 86 88 89 90 92 93 96 97 98 99 100
101 102 103 104 105 107 108 110 111 113 114 115 116 117 118 120 122
123 125 126 128 129 130 131 134 140 145 146 147 **P**6 **S** Providence
Health & Services, Renton, WA
Primary Contact: Jeff Fee, Chief Executive Officer
COO: Craig E. Aasved, Chief Operating Officer
CFO: Bruce Whitfield, Vice President and Chief Financial Officer
CHR: Karyn Trainor, Director Human Resources
Web address: www.saintpatrick.org
**Control:** Church–operated, Nongovernment, not–for profit **Service:** General
Medical and Surgical

**Staffed Beds:** 134 **Admissions:** 7908 **Census:** 104 **Outpatient Visits:**
154272 **Births:** 0 **Total Expense ($000):** 213882 **Payroll Expense ($000):**
61040 **Personnel:** 1336

**PHILIPSBURG—Granite County**

**GRANITE COUNTY MEDICAL CENTER (271303)**, 310 Sansome Street,
Zip 59858–0729, Mailing Address: P.O. Box 729, Zip 59858–0729;
tel. 406/859–3271, (Nonreporting) **A**9 10 18
Primary Contact: Jeff Prater, Chief Executive Officer
CFO: Susan Ossello, Chief Financial Officer
CMO: John Moore, M.D., Medical Director
Web address: www.gcmedcenter.org/
**Control:** County–Government, nonfederal **Service:** General Medical and Surgical

**Staffed Beds:** 9

**PLAINS—Sanders County**

★ **CLARK FORK VALLEY HOSPITAL (271323)**, 10 Kruger Road,
Zip 59859–0768, Mailing Address: P.O. Box 768, Zip 59859–0768;
tel. 406/826–4800, (Total facility includes 28 beds in nursing home–type unit) **A**9
10 18 **F**3 11 13 15 18 29 30 32 34 35 36 40 43 44 45 50 57 58 59 62 63
64 65 68 70 74 75 76 77 81 82 83 84 85 89 93 97 107 110 113 117 118
126 127 129 131 132 142 145 146 147 **P**6
Primary Contact: Gregory S. Hanson, M.D., Chief Executive Officer
CFO: Carla Neiman, Chief Financial Officer
CMO: Sharon Nichols, D.O., Chief of Staff
CIO: Carla Neiman, Chief Financial Officer
CHR: Barry Fowler, Director Human and System Resources
CNO: Dawn Lynch, R.N., Director of Patient Care Services
Web address: www.cfvh.org
**Control:** Other not–for–profit (including NFP Corporation) **Service:** General
Medical and Surgical

**Staffed Beds:** 44 **Admissions:** 362 **Census:** 25 **Outpatient Visits:** 37845
**Births:** 32 **Total Expense ($000):** 15068 **Payroll Expense ($000):** 7169
**Personnel:** 118

**PLENTYWOOD—Sheridan County**

**SHERIDAN MEMORIAL HOSPITAL (271322)**, 440 West Laurel Avenue,
Zip 59254–1596; tel. 406/765–1420, (Total facility includes 78 beds in nursing
home–type unit) **A**9 10 18 **F**3 7 11 13 15 17 35 40 57 59 62 63 75 77 81 93
107 110 113 118 126 127 129 131 132 144 145 146
Primary Contact: Sandra Christensen, Chief Executive Officer
Web address: www.sheridanhospital.org
**Control:** Other not–for–profit (including NFP Corporation) **Service:** General
Medical and Surgical

**Staffed Beds:** 110 **Admissions:** 340 **Census:** 56 **Outpatient Visits:** 10868
**Births:** 0 **Total Expense ($000):** 9910 **Payroll Expense ($000):** 5363

**POLSON—Lake County**

✠ **ST. JOSEPH HOSPITAL (271343)**, 6 Thirteenth Avenue East, Zip 59860–5316,
Mailing Address: P.O. Box 1010, Zip 59860–1010; tel. 406/883–5377 **A**1 9 10
18 **F**3 10 13 15 28 29 30 34 35 40 43 46 50 57 59 64 68 75 76 77 79 81
82 84 85 87 89 93 97 100 102 107 111 113 118 124 126 129 130 132 145
146 147 **P**6 **S** Providence Health & Services, Renton, WA
Primary Contact: James R. Kiser, II, Chief Executive Officer
COO: Colleen Nielsen, Director Operations
CFO: Kirk Bodlovic, Vice President and Chief Financial Officer
CMO: Kelly Bagnell, M.D., Chief of Staff
Web address: www.saintjoes.org
**Control:** Church–operated, Nongovernment, not–for profit **Service:** General
Medical and Surgical

**Staffed Beds:** 22 **Admissions:** 584 **Census:** 5 **Outpatient Visits:** 64447
**Births:** 118 **Total Expense ($000):** 24523 **Payroll Expense ($000):** 11514
**Personnel:** 198

**POPLAR—Roosevelt County**

★ **POPLAR COMMUNITY HOSPITAL (271300)**, H and Court Avenue, Zip 59255,
Mailing Address: P.O. Box 38, Zip 59255; tel. 406/768–3452 **A**9 10 18 **F**3 7 40
43 50 57 59 69 75 113 129 132 142 **P**3 6
Primary Contact: Margaret B. Norgaard, Chief Executive Officer
CHR: Annie Block, Director Human Resources
Web address: www.nemhs.net
**Control:** Other not–for–profit (including NFP Corporation) **Service:** General
Medical and Surgical

**Staffed Beds:** 20 **Admissions:** 150 **Census:** 8 **Outpatient Visits:** 9162
**Births:** 0 **Total Expense ($000):** 6376 **Payroll Expense ($000):** 2505
**Personnel:** 71

**RED LODGE—Carbon County**

★ **BEARTOOTH BILLINGS CLINIC (271326)**, 2525 North Broadway, Zip 59068,
Mailing Address: P.O. Box 590, Zip 59068–0590; tel. 406/446–2345 **A**9 10 18
**F**3 11 15 18 28 29 34 35 40 43 44 45 50 56 57 59 62 63 64 65 68 75 77
81 85 86 87 93 94 96 97 107 110 113 118 129 130 132 134 145 147 **P**6
Primary Contact: Kelley Evans, Chief Executive Officer
CFO: Kyle Gee, Chief Financial Officer
CMO: William George, M.D., Chief of Staff
CIO: Susan Scott, Director Medical Records
CHR: Katie Nordstrom, Director Human Resources
Web address: www.beartoothbillingsclinic.org
**Control:** Other not–for–profit (including NFP Corporation) **Service:** General
Medical and Surgical

**Staffed Beds:** 10 **Admissions:** 211 **Census:** 3 **Outpatient Visits:** 43473
**Births:** 0 **Total Expense ($000):** 9613 **Payroll Expense ($000):** 3032
**Personnel:** 74

**RONAN—Lake County**

★ **ST. LUKE COMMUNITY HOSPITAL (271325)**, 107 Sixth Avenue S.W.,
Zip 59864–2634; tel. 406/676–4441, (Total facility includes 75 beds in nursing
home–type unit) **A**9 10 18 **F**2 13 15 28 29 34 40 43 45 53 54 57 59 61 64 65
75 76 77 79 81 85 93 97 107 108 110 111 114 118 126 127 128 130 132
134 143 144 **P**6
Primary Contact: Shane H. Roberts, Chief Executive Officer
COO: Steve J. Todd, Chief Operating Officer
CFO: Paul Soukup, Chief Financial Officer
CMO: Paul D. Gochis, M.D., Chief of Staff
CHR: Theresa Jones, Manager Human Resources
Web address: www.stlukehealthnet.org
**Control:** Other not–for–profit (including NFP Corporation) **Service:** General
Medical and Surgical

**Staffed Beds:** 105 **Admissions:** 1260 **Census:** 65 **Outpatient Visits:** 77353
**Births:** 173 **Total Expense ($000):** 33192 **Payroll Expense ($000):** 16628
**Personnel:** 312

**ROUNDUP—Musselshell County**

★ **ROUNDUP MEMORIAL HEALTHCARE (271346)**, 1202 Third Street West,
Zip 59072–1816, Mailing Address: P.O. Box 40, Zip 59072–0040;
tel. 406/323–2301 **A**9 10 18 **F**11 29 34 40 45 57 59 65 85 87 97 107 118
126 129 131 132 145 **P**6
Primary Contact: Bradley Howell, Chief Executive Officer
CMO: Michael Flannery, M.D., Interim Chief of Staff
CHR: Rochelle Hatter, Chief Human Resources Officer
Web address: www.rmhmt.org/
**Control:** Other not–for–profit (including NFP Corporation) **Service:** General
Medical and Surgical

**Staffed Beds:** 25 **Admissions:** 92 **Census:** 19 **Outpatient Visits:** 6703
**Births:** 0 **Total Expense ($000):** 4913 **Payroll Expense ($000):** 2597
**Personnel:** 65

**SAINT MARY—Glacier County**

**U. S. PUBLIC HEALTH SERVICE BLACKFEET COMMUNITY HOSPITAL
(270074)**, Zip 59417–0760; Mailing Address: Browning, tel. 406/338–6100,
(Nonreporting) **A**5 10 **S** U. S. Indian Health Service, Rockville, MD
Primary Contact: Timothy Davis, Interim Chief Executive Officer
Web address: www.phs.ihs.gov
**Control:** PHS, Indian Service, Government, federal **Service:** General Medical and
Surgical

**Staffed Beds:** 25

**MT**

## SCOBEY—Daniels County

**DANIELS MEMORIAL HEALTHCARE CENTER (271342)**, 105 Fifth Avenue East, Zip 59263, Mailing Address: P.O. Box 400, Zip 59263–0400; tel. 406/487–2296, (Total facility includes 30 beds in nursing home–type unit) **A**9 10 18 **F**2 11 29 31 34 35 40 43 50 56 57 59 64 65 69 75 77 85 86 87 91 93 97 102 103 107 113 126 127 129 130 131 132 142 145 147 **P**6
Primary Contact: David Hubbard, Chief Executive Officer
CMO: Don Sawdey, M.D., Medical Director
CHR: Edith Huda, Director Human Resources
Web address: www.danielsmemorialhealthcare.org
**Control:** Hospital district or authority, Government, nonfederal **Service:** General Medical and Surgical

**Staffed Beds:** 54 **Admissions:** 213 **Census:** 30 **Outpatient Visits:** 5200 **Births:** 0 **Total Expense ($000):** 5972 **Payroll Expense ($000):** 3058 **Personnel:** 73

## SHELBY—Toole County

★ **MARIAS MEDICAL CENTER (271328)**, 640 Park Drive, Zip 59474–1663, Mailing Address: P.O. Box 915, Zip 59474–0915; tel. 406/434–3200, (Total facility includes 63 beds in nursing home–type unit) **A**9 10 18 **F**7 10 11 13 15 17 40 45 56 57 59 64 70 75 76 77 78 79 81 82 93 107 110 111 114 118 124 127 128 129 132
Primary Contact: Mark A. Cross, Chief Executive Officer
CFO: Melissa Ostberg, Chief Financial Officer
CMO: Charles G. Marlge, M.D., Chief of Staff
CIO: Jayce Yarn, Director Information Technology
CHR: Cindy Lamb, Director Human Resources
Web address: www.mmcmt.org
**Control:** County–Government, nonfederal **Service:** General Medical and Surgical

**Staffed Beds:** 88 **Admissions:** 526 **Census:** 46 **Outpatient Visits:** 11340 **Births:** 44 **Total Expense ($000):** 14223 **Payroll Expense ($000):** 6803 **Personnel:** 104

## SHERIDAN—Madison County

★ **RUBY VALLEY HOSPITAL (271319)**, 220 East Crofoot Street, Zip 59749, Mailing Address: P.O. Box 336, Zip 59749–0336; tel. 406/842–5453 **A**9 10 18 **F**2 11 28 29 34 35 38 40 50 56 57 59 64 65 66 71 75 77 82 86 90 91 93 97 118 126 127 129 132 134 146 147 **P**6
Primary Contact: John H. Semingson, Chief Executive Officer
CFO: Dennis Holschbach, Chief Financial Officer and Director Human Resources
CMO: Roman Hendrickson, M.D., Medical Director
CHR: Dennis Holschbach, Chief Financial Officer and Director Human Resources
CNO: Ted Woirhaye, R.N., Director of Nursing
Web address: www.rubyvalleyhospital.com/
**Control:** Hospital district or authority, Government, nonfederal **Service:** General Medical and Surgical

**Staffed Beds:** 8 **Admissions:** 228 **Census:** 3 **Outpatient Visits:** 5040 **Births:** 0 **Total Expense ($000):** 4143 **Payroll Expense ($000):** 2440 **Personnel:** 46

## SIDNEY—Richland County

★ **SIDNEY HEALTH CENTER (271344)**, 216 14th Avenue S.W., Zip 59270–3586; tel. 406/488–2100, (Total facility includes 93 beds in nursing home–type unit) **A**9 10 18 **F**2 3 13 15 17 28 30 31 34 35 40 45 50 56 57 59 62 63 64 70 75 76 78 79 81 82 84 85 86 87 89 93 96 107 108 110 114 118 119 120 121 122 124 127 128 129 132 143 144 145 146 147 **P**6 7
Primary Contact: Richard Haraldson, Chief Executive Officer
CFO: Tina Montgomery, Chief Financial Officer
CMO: Rajohn Karanjai, M.D., Chief Medical Officer
CIO: Brian Fay, Director Information Systems
CHR: Lisa Aisenbrey, Administrator Human Resources and Support Services
Web address: www.sidneyhealth.org
**Control:** Other not–for–profit (including NFP Corporation) **Service:** General Medical and Surgical

**Staffed Beds:** 118 **Admissions:** 1068 **Census:** 97 **Outpatient Visits:** 33614 **Births:** 116 **Total Expense ($000):** 42354 **Payroll Expense ($000):** 17324 **Personnel:** 420

## SUPERIOR—Mineral County

★ **MINERAL COMMUNITY HOSPITAL (271331)**, 1208 6th Avenue East, Zip 59872–9603, Mailing Address: P.O. Box 66, Zip 59872–0066; tel. 406/822–4841, (Nonreporting) **A**9 10 18
Primary Contact: Steven D. Carty, Chief Executive Officer
CFO: Cliff Case, Chief Financial Officer
CMO: Patrick Tufts, M.D., Medical Director
CHR: Stacy Conrow–Ververis, Director Human Resources
Web address: www.mineralcommunityhospital.com/
**Control:** Other not–for–profit (including NFP Corporation) **Service:** General Medical and Surgical

**Staffed Beds:** 25

## TERRY—Prairie County

**PRAIRIE COMMUNITY HEALTH CENTER** See Prairie Community Hospital

★ **PRAIRIE COMMUNITY HOSPITAL (271309)**, 312 South Adams Avenue, Zip 59349–0156, Mailing Address: P.O. Box 156, Zip 59349–0156; tel. 406/635–5511 **A**9 10 18 **F**3 11 32 34 40 57 59 65 67 69 75 87 90 126 127 132 134 145 146 147 **P**6
Primary Contact: Parker Powell, Administrator
CFO: Laurie Chandler, Financial Officer
CMO: Joseph M. Leal, Jr., M.D., Medical Director
CIO: Laurie Chandler, Chairman
CNO: Kay Schaaf, Chief Nursing Officer
Web address: www.prairiecommunityhospital.org/
**Control:** Hospital district or authority, Government, nonfederal **Service:** General Medical and Surgical

**Staffed Beds:** 21 **Admissions:** 21 **Census:** 20 **Outpatient Visits:** 3098 **Births:** 0 **Personnel:** 41

## TOWNSEND—Broadwater County

**BROADWATER HEALTH CENTER (271333)**, 110 North Oak Street, Zip 59644–2306; tel. 406/266–3186 **A**9 10 18 **F**3 11 67
Primary Contact: Joan Davis, R.N., Administrator
CFO: Lorrie Vennes, Chief Financial Officer
Web address: www.broadwaterhealthcenter.com
**Control:** County–Government, nonfederal **Service:** General Medical and Surgical

**Staffed Beds:** 44 **Admissions:** 78 **Census:** 1 **Births:** 0

## WARM SPRINGS—Deer Lodge County

**MONTANA STATE HOSPITAL (274086)**, 300 Garnet Way, Zip 59756–0300, Mailing Address: P.O. Box 300, Zip 59756–0300; tel. 406/693–7000 **A**10 **F**29 38 39 50 59 66 68 74 75 77 86 97 98 100 103 106 118 129 131 134 **P**6
Primary Contact: John W. Glueckert, Administrator
CFO: Tracey Sweeney, Director Business and Support Services
CMO: Thomas Gray, M.D., Medical Director
CIO: Billie Holmlund, Director Information Services
CHR: Todd Thun, Director Human Resources
Web address: www.msh.mt.gov
**Control:** State–Government, nonfederal **Service:** Psychiatric

**Staffed Beds:** 201 **Admissions:** 715 **Census:** 183 **Outpatient Visits:** 0 **Births:** 0 **Total Expense ($000):** 30438 **Payroll Expense ($000):** 16760 **Personnel:** 402

## WHITE SULPHUR SPRINGS—Meagher County

**MOUNTAINVIEW MEDICAL CENTER (271306)**, 16 West Main Street, Zip 59645, Mailing Address: P.O. Box Q, Zip 59645; tel. 406/547–3321, (Nonreporting) **A**9 10 18
Primary Contact: Aaron Rogers, Chief Executive Officer
Web address: www.mvmc.org
**Control:** Other not–for–profit (including NFP Corporation) **Service:** General Medical and Surgical

**Staffed Beds:** 25

**MT**

---

**Hospital, Medicare Provider Number, Address, Telephone, Approval, Facility, and Physician Codes, Health Care System**

★ American Hospital Association (AHA) membership
☐ The Joint Commission accreditation ◇ DNV Healthcare Inc. accreditation
○ American Osteopathic Association (AOA) accreditation
△ Commission on Accreditation of Rehabilitation Facilities (CARF) accreditation

## WHITEFISH—Flathead County

★ **NORTH VALLEY HOSPITAL (271336)**, 1600 Hospital Way, Zip 59937–7849;
tel. 406/863–3500 **A**9 10 18 **F**3 11 13 15 28 29 30 31 34 35 37 40 43 45
50 54 56 57 59 64 68 70 75 76 79 81 82 85 86 87 89 97 100 102 103 107
110 111 114 118 125 127 128 129 130 131 132 134 143 145 147 **P**5
**S** QHR, Brentwood, TN
Primary Contact: Jason A. Spring, FACHE, Chief Executive Officer
COO: Maura G. Fields, R.N., Chief Clinical Officer
CFO: Marilyn Hays, Chief Financial Officer
CFO: Randy Nightengale, Chief Financial Officer
CIO: Michael Barnes, Chief Information Officer
CHR: Susan Catt, Director Human Resources
Web address: www.nvhosp.org
**Control:** Other not–for–profit (including NFP Corporation) **Service:** General
Medical and Surgical

**Staffed Beds:** 25 **Admissions:** 1531 **Census:** 14 **Outpatient Visits:** 46805
**Births:** 464 **Total Expense ($000):** 37211 **Payroll Expense ($000):** 13093
**Personnel:** 222

## WOLF POINT—Roosevelt County

★ **TRINITY HOSPITAL (271341)**, 315 Knapp Street, Zip 59201–1826;
tel. 406/653–6500, (Total facility includes 60 beds in nursing home–type unit)
**A**10 18 **F**2 3 6 7 8 13 15 29 31 32 34 40 41 43 45 50 56 57 59 64 67 69
70 75 76 78 81 89 92 110 118 119 124 126 127 129 132 142 144
Primary Contact: Margaret B. Norgaard, Chief Executive Officer
Web address: www.nemhs.net
**Control:** Other not–for–profit (including NFP Corporation) **Service:** General
Medical and Surgical

**Staffed Beds:** 82 **Admissions:** 383 **Census:** 61 **Outpatient Visits:** 15158
**Births:** 134 **Total Expense ($000):** 12503 **Payroll Expense ($000):** 5638
**Personnel:** 168

MT

# NEBRASKA

## AINSWORTH—Brown County

**BROWN COUNTY HOSPITAL (281325)**, 945 East Zero Street,
Zip 69210–1547; tel. 402/387–2800 **A**9 10 18 **F**15 28 31 40 57 59 62 64 75
77 79 81 93 94 107 110 111 113 118 129 132
Primary Contact: Shannon Sorenson, Chief Executive Officer
CFO: Matt Sells, CPA, Chief Financial Officer
CMO: Annette Miller, M.D., Medical Staff Chairman
CIO: Mike Depko, Director Information Technology
CHR: Lisa Fischer, Director Human Resources
Web address: www.browncountyhospital.org
**Control:** County–Government, nonfederal **Service:** General Medical and Surgical

**Staffed Beds:** 18 **Admissions:** 202 **Census:** 2 **Outpatient Visits:** 9154
**Births:** 0 **Total Expense ($000):** 6149 **Payroll Expense ($000):** 2450
**Personnel:** 67

## ALBION—Boone County

★ **BOONE COUNTY HEALTH CENTER (281334)**, 723 West Fairview Street,
Zip 68620–1725, Mailing Address: P.O. Box 151, Zip 68620–0151;
tel. 402/395–2191 **A**9 10 18 **F**3 11 13 15 28 29 31 32 34 35 38 40 45 52
53 57 59 62 64 65 74 75 76 77 78 79 81 82 85 86 87 93 104 107 108 110
111 114 115 118 126 127 128 129 130 131 132 133 134 144 145 146 147
**P**5 6
Primary Contact: Victor N. Lee, FACHE, President and Chief Executive Officer
CFO: Mandy Kumm, Vice President Fiscal Services
CIO: Larry Zoucha, Chief Information Officer
CHR: Jennifer Beierman, Director Human Resources
Web address: www.boonecohealth.org
**Control:** County–Government, nonfederal **Service:** General Medical and Surgical

**Staffed Beds:** 25 **Admissions:** 778 **Census:** 8 **Outpatient Visits:** 83850
**Births:** 98 **Total Expense ($000):** 21379 **Payroll Expense ($000):** 10267
**Personnel:** 189

## ALLIANCE—Box Butte County

⊠ **BOX BUTTE GENERAL HOSPITAL (281360)**, 2101 Box Butte Avenue,
Zip 69301–0810, Mailing Address: P.O. Box 810, Zip 69301–0810;
tel. 308/762–6660 **A**1 9 10 18 **F**3 5 11 13 15 28 29 31 32 34 35 36 38 40
43 50 53 57 59 60 64 68 69 75 77 78 79 81 82 85 86 87 92 93 97 100
101 104 107 108 111 113 115 117 118 126 128 129 130 131 132 133 134
145 147
Primary Contact: Dan Griess, Chief Executive Officer
COO: Jim Parks, Chief Operating Officer
CFO: Tracy E. Jatczak, CPA, Chief Financial Officer
CMO: John J. Ruffing, Jr., M.D., Chief of Staff
CIO: Jim Parks, Chief Operating Officer
CHR: Rebecca Sisler, Director Human Resources
Web address: www.bbgh.org
**Control:** County–Government, nonfederal **Service:** General Medical and Surgical

**Staffed Beds:** 25 **Admissions:** 926 **Census:** 10 **Outpatient Visits:** 34501
**Births:** 84 **Total Expense ($000):** 23938 **Payroll Expense ($000):** 11087
**Personnel:** 241

## ALMA—Harlan County

★ **HARLAN COUNTY HEALTH SYSTEM (281300)**, 717 North Brown Street,
Zip 68920–0836, Mailing Address: P.O. Box 836, Zip 68920–0836;
tel. 308/928–2151 **A**9 10 18 **F**3 11 15 29 30 31 40 46 50 64 75 81 85 86
93 107 110 113 118 126 127 129 131 132 134 **P**6 **S** Great Plains Health
Alliance, Inc., Phillipsburg, KS
Primary Contact: Jeffrey D. Shelton, Chief Executive Officer
CFO: Sue Lans, Comptroller
CMO: Anton Smolik, M.D., Chief of Medical Staff
CIO: Bob Kentner, Coordinator Information Systems
CHR: Peg Howart, Coordinator Human Resources and Benefits
Web address: www.harlancountyhealth.com
**Control:** County–Government, nonfederal **Service:** General Medical and Surgical

**Staffed Beds:** 19 **Admissions:** 243 **Census:** 4 **Outpatient Visits:** 17224
**Births:** 0 **Total Expense ($000):** 7143 **Payroll Expense ($000):** 2951
**Personnel:** 58

## ATKINSON—Holt County

**WEST HOLT MEMORIAL HOSPITAL (281343)**, 406 West Neely Street,
Zip 68713–0200; tel. 402/925–2811, (Nonreporting) **A**9 10 18 **S** Faith Regional
Health Services, Norfolk, NE
Primary Contact: Michael F. Coyle, Chief Executive Officer
CFO: Karen Nollette, Chief Financial Officer
CMO: John Tubbs, M.D., Chief of Staff
CIO: Mark Johnson, Chief Information Officer
CHR: Margaret Linse, Administrative Secretary and Director Human Resources
Web address: www.westholtmed.org
**Control:** Other not–for–profit (including NFP Corporation) **Service:** General
Medical and Surgical

**Staffed Beds:** 18

## AUBURN—Nemaha County

★ **NEMAHA COUNTY HOSPITAL (281324)**, 2022 13th Street, Zip 68305–1799;
tel. 402/274–4366 **A**9 10 18 21 **F**1 3 4 7 11 12 13 15 16 17 28 29 30 31 35
40 43 62 64 67 68 70 72 73 74 75 76 77 78 79 80 81 82 85 87 88 89 90
93 94 98 107 110 111 113 116 118 127 128 132 134 140 146 147
Primary Contact: Marty Fattig, Administrator and Chief Executive Officer
COO: Kermit Moore, R.N., Chief Operating Officer and Chief Nursing Officer
CFO: Stacy Taylor, Chief Financial Officer
CHR: Susie Shupp, Director Human Resources
Web address: www.nchnet.org
**Control:** County–Government, nonfederal **Service:** General Medical and Surgical

**Staffed Beds:** 20 **Admissions:** 238 **Census:** 3 **Outpatient Visits:** 18980
**Births:** 0 **Total Expense ($000):** 9738 **Payroll Expense ($000):** 4008
**Personnel:** 71

## AURORA—Hamilton County

★ **MEMORIAL COMMUNITY HEALTH (281320)**, 1423 Seventh Street,
Zip 68818–1197; tel. 402/694–3171, (Total facility includes 48 beds in nursing
home–type unit) **A**9 10 18 **F**10 11 13 15 28 29 31 34 35 40 41 43 45 50 51
57 59 64 65 67 75 76 77 78 79 81 82 85 86 87 93 94 97 107 108 110 113
129 130 131 132 145 **P**6
Primary Contact: Diane R. Keller, Chief Executive Officer
CFO: Phil Fendt, Chief Financial Officer
CMO: Timothy Widhelm, M.D., Chief of Staff
CHR: Laurie Andrews, Chief Human Resources Officer
Web address: www.memorialcommunityhealth.org
**Control:** Other not–for–profit (including NFP Corporation) **Service:** General
Medical and Surgical

**Staffed Beds:** 64 **Admissions:** 363 **Census:** 44 **Outpatient Visits:** 21626
**Births:** 50 **Total Expense ($000):** 15260 **Payroll Expense ($000):** 7117
**Personnel:** 183

**MEMORIAL HOSPITAL** See Memorial Community Health

## BASSETT—Rock County

**ROCK COUNTY HOSPITAL (281333)**, 102 East South Street,
Zip 68714–5511; tel. 402/684–3366, (Total facility includes 30 beds in nursing
home–type unit) **A**9 10 18 **F**7 11 28 40 53 57 81 84 107 126 127 132
Primary Contact: Stacey A. Knox, Administrator
CMO: John I. Cherry, M.D., Chief of Staff
CHR: Jackie Carpenter, Office Manager
Web address: www.rockcountyhospital.com
**Control:** County–Government, nonfederal **Service:** General Medical and Surgical

**Staffed Beds:** 54 **Admissions:** 272 **Census:** 32 **Outpatient Visits:** 5216
**Births:** 0 **Total Expense ($000):** 5319 **Payroll Expense ($000):** 2741
**Personnel:** 79

NE

---

**Hospital, Medicare Provider Number, Address, Telephone, Approval, Facility, and Physician Codes, Health Care System**

★ American Hospital Association (AHA) membership
☐ The Joint Commission accreditation     ◇ DNV Healthcare Inc. accreditation

○ American Osteopathic Association (AOA) accreditation
△ Commission on Accreditation of Rehabilitation Facilities (CARF) accreditation

## BEATRICE—Gage County

☒ **BEATRICE COMMUNITY HOSPITAL AND HEALTH CENTER (281364)**, 4800 Hospital Parkway, Zip 68310–6906, Mailing Address: P.O. Box 278, Zip 68310–0278; tel. 402/228–3344 **A**1 9 10 18 **F**3 13 15 28 29 31 34 35 40 45 57 62 63 64 65 68 69 70 75 76 78 79 81 85 87 93 107 108 110 111 113 117 118 126 128 129 131 132 134 145 146
Primary Contact: Thomas W. Sommers, FACHE, President and Chief Executive Officer
CFO: Jon R. McMillan, Chief Financial Officer
CMO: Brett Studley, M.D., Chief of Staff
CHR: Charlotte Campbell, Chief Human Resources Officer
CNO: Julie L. Jones, R.N., Chief Nursing Officer
Web address: www.beatricecommunityhospital.com
**Control:** Other not-for-profit (including NFP Corporation) **Service:** General Medical and Surgical

**Staffed Beds:** 25 **Admissions:** 894 **Census:** 9 **Outpatient Visits:** 86884 **Births:** 138 **Total Expense ($000):** 36627 **Payroll Expense ($000):** 18066 **Personnel:** 316

## BELLEVUE—Sarpy County

☐ **BELLEVUE MEDICAL CENTER (280132)**, 2500 Bellevue Medical Center Drive, Zip 68123–1591; tel. 402/763–3000, (Nonreporting) **A**1 5 9 10
Primary Contact: Paulette Davidson, Chief Executive Officer
Web address: www.bellevuemed.com
**Control:** Partnership, Investor–owned, for–profit **Service:** General Medical and Surgical

**Staffed Beds:** 55

## BENKELMAN—Dundy County

★ **DUNDY COUNTY HOSPITAL (281340)**, 1313 North Cheyenne Street, Zip 69021, Mailing Address: P.O. Box 626, Zip 69021–0626; tel. 308/423–2204, (Nonreporting) **A**9 10 18
Primary Contact: Rita A. Jones, Chief Executive Officer
COO: Wendy Elkins, Director Operations
CFO: Dwana Roschewski, Director Fiscal Services
CMO: Lori Stonehocker, D.O., Chief Medical Staff
CIO: Anna Elliot, Head Information Technology
CHR: Sandy Noffsinger, Executive Assistant, Risk Manager and Director Marketing
Web address: www.bwtelcom.net/dch
**Control:** County–Government, nonfederal **Service:** General Medical and Surgical

**Staffed Beds:** 14

## BLAIR—Washington County

**MEMORIAL COMMUNITY HOSPITAL AND HEALTH SYSTEM (281359)**, 810 North 22nd Street, Zip 68008–1199, Mailing Address: P.O. Box 250, Zip 68008–0250; tel. 402/426–2182, (Nonreporting) **A**9 10 18 **S** Alegent Health, Omaha, NE
Primary Contact: Sally Harvey, R.N., Regional Administrator
CFO: Nicole Kreitel, Chief Financial Officer
CMO: John F. Simonson, M.D., President Medical Staff
CIO: DeeAnn Rosenau, Operations Director Information Technology and Revenue Cycle
CHR: Cathy Jenson, Human Resources Generalist
Web address: www.mchhs.org
**Control:** Other not-for-profit (including NFP Corporation) **Service:** General Medical and Surgical

**Staffed Beds:** 25

## BRIDGEPORT—Morrill County

**MORRILL COUNTY COMMUNITY HOSPITAL (281318)**, 1313 S Street, Zip 69336–0579, Mailing Address: P.O. Box 579, Zip 69336–0579; tel. 308/262–1616, (Nonreporting) **A**9 10 18
Primary Contact: Robin Stuart, Interim Administrator
Web address: www.morrillcountyhospital.org
**Control:** County–Government, nonfederal **Service:** General Medical and Surgical

**Staffed Beds:** 20

## BROKEN BOW—Custer County

**JENNIE M. MELHAM MEMORIAL MEDICAL CENTER (281365)**, 145 Memorial Drive, Zip 68822–1378, Mailing Address: P.O. Box 250, Zip 68822–0250; tel. 308/872–4100, (Nonreporting) **A**9 10 18
Primary Contact: Michael J. Steckler, President and Chief Executive Officer
CFO: Tim Schuckman, Chief Financial Officer
CIO: Tim Schuckman, Chief Financial Officer
Web address: www.brokenbow-ne.com/community/healthcare/melham.htm
**Control:** Other not-for-profit (including NFP Corporation) **Service:** General Medical and Surgical

**Staffed Beds:** 25

## CALLAWAY—Custer County

★ **CALLAWAY DISTRICT HOSPITAL (281335)**, 211 East Kimball, Zip 68825–0100, Mailing Address: P.O. Box 100, Zip 68825–0100; tel. 308/836–2228, (Nonreporting) **A**9 10 18
Primary Contact: Marvin Neth, Administrator
Web address: www.callaway-ne.com/hospital/
**Control:** Hospital district or authority, Government, nonfederal **Service:** General Medical and Surgical

**Staffed Beds:** 12

## CAMBRIDGE—Furnas County

★ **TRI VALLEY HEALTH SYSTEM (281348)**, 1305 West Highway 6 and 34, Zip 69022–0488, Mailing Address: P.O. Box 488, Zip 69022–0488; tel. 308/697–3329, (Nonreporting) **A**9 10 18 **S** HealthTech Management Services, Franklin, TN
Primary Contact: Roger W. Steinkruger, Chief Executive Officer
CFO: Diana Rippe, Financial Services Executive
CMO: Shelly Kasper-Cope, M.D., Chief of Staff
CIO: Doug Hall, Director Information Systems
CHR: Tammy Claussen, Human Resources Executive
Web address: www.trivalleyhealth.com
**Control:** Other not-for-profit (including NFP Corporation) **Service:** General Medical and Surgical

**Staffed Beds:** 51

## CENTRAL CITY—Merrick County

★ **LITZENBERG MEMORIAL COUNTY HOSPITAL (281328)**, 1715 26th Street, Zip 68826–9620; tel. 308/946–3015, (Nonreporting) **A**9 10 18
Primary Contact: Tad M. Hunt, MS, Chief Executive Officer
Web address: www.lmchealth.com
**Control:** County–Government, nonfederal **Service:** General Medical and Surgical

**Staffed Beds:** 20

## CHADRON—Dawes County

★ **CHADRON COMMUNITY HOSPITAL AND HEALTH SERVICES (281341)**, 825 Centennial Drive, Zip 69337–9400; tel. 308/432–5586 **A**5 9 10 18 **F**3 10 13 15 29 31 34 35 38 40 43 57 59 60 61 62 63 65 70 75 77 78 81 82 87 93 107 108 110 111 114 118 124 126 129 130 131 132 134 145 **P**5 8
Primary Contact: Harold L. Krueger, Jr., Chief Executive Officer
COO: Allen Van Driel, FACHE, Chief Operating Officer
CFO: Russ Bohnenkamp, Director Finance
CMO: Jerry McLain, M.D., Chief of Staff
CIO: Anna Turman, Chief Information Officer
CHR: Ellen Krueger, Director Human Resources
CNO: Cheryl Cassiday, R.N., Director of Nursing
Web address: www.chadronhospital.com
**Control:** Other not-for-profit (including NFP Corporation) **Service:** General Medical and Surgical

**Staffed Beds:** 25 **Admissions:** 632 **Census:** 5 **Outpatient Visits:** 3312 **Births:** 119 **Total Expense ($000):** 18590 **Payroll Expense ($000):** 6525 **Personnel:** 172

## COLUMBUS—Platte County

☒ **COLUMBUS COMMUNITY HOSPITAL (280111)**, 4600 38th Street, Zip 68601, Mailing Address: P.O. Box 1800, Zip 68602–1800; tel. 402/564–7118, (Total facility includes 4 beds in nursing home–type unit) **A**1 9 10 20 **F**3 8 11 13 15 17 28 29 34 35 37 38 39 40 43 45 57 59 62 63 64 65 68 69 70 75 76 77 79 81 82 84 85 86 87 93 107 108 110 111 114 117 118 126 127 128 129 130 131 132 134 145 147 **P**8
Primary Contact: Michael T. Hansen, FACHE, President and Chief Executive Officer
COO: James P. Goulet, Vice President Operations
CFO: J. Joseph Barbaglia, Vice President Financial Services
CMO: Mark Howerter, M.D., President Medical Staff
CIO: Cheryl Tira, Director Information Systems
CHR: Scott E. Messersmith, Director Human Resources
Web address: www.columbushosp.org
**Control:** Other not-for-profit (including NFP Corporation) **Service:** General Medical and Surgical

**Staffed Beds:** 51 **Admissions:** 2417 **Census:** 20 **Total Expense ($000):** 53522 **Payroll Expense ($000):** 24291

## COZAD—Dawson County

★ **COZAD COMMUNITY HOSPITAL (281327)**, 300 East 12th Street, Zip 69130–1505, Mailing Address: P.O. Box 108, Zip 69130–0108; tel. 308/784–2261 **A**9 10 18 **F**3 10 13 15 28 30 31 34 35 40 43 50 53 56 57 59 62 63 70 75 76 77 81 82 84 86 93 94 97 107 113 118 126 127 128 129 130 131 132 134 145 147 **P**6
Primary Contact: Lyle E. Davis, Administrator
Web address: www.cozadhealthcare.com
**Control:** Hospital district or authority, Government, nonfederal **Service:** General Medical and Surgical

**Staffed Beds:** 21 **Admissions:** 366 **Census:** 4 **Outpatient Visits:** 8725 **Births:** 39 **Total Expense ($000):** 10300 **Payroll Expense ($000):** 5367 **Personnel:** 116

*Many Facility Codes have changed. Please refer to the AHA Guide Code Chart.* © 2012 AHA Guide

**NE**

## CREIGHTON—Knox County

★ **AVERA CREIGHTON HOSPITAL (281331)**, 1503 Main Street,
Zip 68729–0186, Mailing Address: P.O. Box 186, Zip 68729–0186;
tel. 402/358–5700, (Total facility includes 47 beds in nursing home–type unit)
(Data for 150 days) **A**9 10 18 **F**8 11 15 28 29 31 34 35 40 45 46 50 53 56
57 59 62 64 65 75 77 78 81 84 90 93 107 110 126 127 129 130 132 145
146 147 **P**6 **S** Avera Health, Sioux Falls, SD
Primary Contact: Mark Schulte, Chief Executive Officer
CFO: Kim Hixson, Chief Financial Officer
CHR: Candace Timmerman, Director Human Resources
CNO: Jean M. Henes, R.N., Director of Nursing
Web address: www.avera.org/creighton/
**Control:** Other not–for–profit (including NFP Corporation) **Service:** General
Medical and Surgical

**Staffed Beds:** 54 **Admissions:** 167 **Census:** 46 **Outpatient Visits:** 5090
**Births:** 0 **Total Expense ($000):** 3881 **Payroll Expense ($000):** 1683
**Personnel:** 70

## CRETE—Saline County

★ **CRETE AREA MEDICAL CENTER (281354)**, 2910 Betten Drive,
Zip 68333–0220, Mailing Address: P.O. Box 220, Zip 68333–0220;
tel. 402/826–2102 **A**9 10 18 **F**13 15 28 29 31 34 40 43 57 59 64 65 68 78
79 81 93 97 107 111 113 116 118 126 128 129 130 132 142 145 146 **P**6
**S** BryanLGH Health System, Lincoln, NE
Primary Contact: Carol Friesen, Chief Executive Officer
CFO: Bryce Betke, Chief Financial Officer
CIO: Sheri Thompson, Director Information Technology
CHR: Bobbie Wilson, Director Human Resources
Web address: www.creteareamedicalcenter.com
**Control:** Other not–for–profit (including NFP Corporation) **Service:** General
Medical and Surgical

**Staffed Beds:** 24 **Admissions:** 386 **Census:** 4 **Outpatient Visits:** 50720
**Births:** 99 **Total Expense ($000):** 17073 **Payroll Expense ($000):** 7035
**Personnel:** 136

## DAVID CITY—Butler County

★ **BUTLER COUNTY HEALTH CARE CENTER (281332)**, 372 South Ninth Street,
Zip 68632–2116; tel. 402/367–1200, (Nonreporting) **A**9 10 18
Primary Contact: Donald T. Naiberk, Administrator
CFO: Ron Jones, Chief Financial Officer
CMO: Victor Thoendel, M.D., Chief Medical Officer
CIO: Cindy Neesen, Director of Information Technology
CHR: Andra Vandenberg, Director Human Resources
CNO: Sue M. Birkel, R.N., Director of Nursing
Web address: www.bchccnet.org
**Control:** County–Government, nonfederal **Service:** General Medical and Surgical

**Staffed Beds:** 25

## ELKHORN—Douglas County

**METHODIST WOMEN'S HOSPITAL** See Nebraska Methodist Hospital, Omaha

## FAIRBURY—Jefferson County

★ **JEFFERSON COMMUNITY HEALTH CENTER (281319)**, 2200 H Street,
Zip 68352–1119, Mailing Address: P.O. Box 277, Zip 68352–0277;
tel. 402/729–3351, (Total facility includes 39 beds in nursing home–type unit) **A**9
10 18 **F**2 3 13 15 28 29 30 31 34 35 40 42 44 50 53 57 59 62 75 76 77 78
79 81 85 86 87 93 107 110 113 118 127 129 130 131 132 134 145 **P**5
Primary Contact: William L. Welch, FACHE, Chief Executive Officer
CFO: Chad Jurgens, Chief Financial Officer
CIO: Dennis Ahl, Director Information Technology
CHR: Sandra A. Bauer, Director Human Resources
Web address: www.jchc.us
**Control:** Other not–for–profit (including NFP Corporation) **Service:** General
Medical and Surgical

**Staffed Beds:** 64 **Admissions:** 365 **Census:** 42 **Outpatient Visits:** 17820
**Births:** 37 **Total Expense ($000):** 15117 **Payroll Expense ($000):** 6018
**Personnel:** 158

## FALLS CITY—Richardson County

★ **COMMUNITY MEDICAL CENTER (281352)**, 3307 Barada Street,
Zip 68355–1599, Mailing Address: P.O. Box 399, Zip 68355–0399;
tel. 402/245–2428 **A**9 10 18 **F**3 13 15 28 31 34 35 40 43 45 57 59 75 76
78 81 85 93 97 107 111 118 126 129 132 134 **P**6
Primary Contact: Ryan C. Larsen, FACHE, Chief Executive Officer
CFO: Scott Sawyer, Chief Financial Officer
CIO: Karen Brown, Director Health Information
CHR: Shannon Weinmann, Director Human Resources
Web address: www.cmcfc.org
**Control:** Other not–for–profit (including NFP Corporation) **Service:** General
Medical and Surgical

**Staffed Beds:** 24 **Admissions:** 914 **Census:** 12 **Outpatient Visits:** 42245
**Births:** 57 **Total Expense ($000):** 17113 **Payroll Expense ($000):** 6495
**Personnel:** 155

## FRANKLIN—Franklin County

★ **FRANKLIN COUNTY MEMORIAL HOSPITAL (281311)**, 1406 Q Street,
Zip 68939–0315, Mailing Address: P.O. Box 315, Zip 68939–0315;
tel. 308/425–6221 **A**9 10 18 **F**3 11 17 28 30 31 34 35 40 43 45 50 57 59
64 65 72 75 77 79 81 93 97 107 118 126 128 129 131 132 **P**6
Primary Contact: Linda Bush, Chief Executive Officer
CFO: Amy Richards, Accounting
CMO: Linda Mazour, M.D., President
CIO: Cathy Webber, Chief Information Officer
Web address: www.fcmh.com
**Control:** County–Government, nonfederal **Service:** General Medical and Surgical

**Staffed Beds:** 14 **Admissions:** 173 **Census:** 2 **Births:** 0

## FREMONT—Dodge County

☐ **FREMONT AREA MEDICAL CENTER (280077)**, 450 East 23rd Street,
Zip 68025–2387; tel. 402/721–1610, (Nonreporting) **A**1 2 9 10
Primary Contact: Patrick M. Booth, Chief Executive Officer
CFO: David G. Hanen, Vice President and Chief Financial Officer
Web address: www.famc.org
**Control:** County–Government, nonfederal **Service:** General Medical and Surgical

**Staffed Beds:** 202

## FRIEND—Saline County

**WARREN MEMORIAL HOSPITAL (281330)**, 905 Second Street,
Zip 68359–1133; tel. 402/947–2541, (Total facility includes 46 beds in nursing
home–type unit) **A**9 10 18 **F**2 6 7 8 11 29 34 35 40 41 44 45 50 56 57 59 64
69 79 81 87 97 104 107 127 129 131 132 142 145
Primary Contact: John W. Wilson, Chief Executive Officer
CFO: Daniel R. Bartz, CPA, Chief Financial Officer
CMO: Roger Meyer, M.D., Chief of Staff
CIO: Mary Kay Carrithers, Manager Health Information
CHR: Jamie Tuttle, Coordinator Human Resources
Web address: www.warrenmemorialhospital.org
**Control:** City–Government, nonfederal **Service:** General Medical and Surgical

**Staffed Beds:** 60 **Admissions:** 29 **Census:** 41 **Outpatient Visits:** 16017
**Births:** 0 **Total Expense ($000):** 4758 **Payroll Expense ($000):** 2589

## GENEVA—Fillmore County

**FILLMORE COUNTY HOSPITAL (281301)**, 1900 F Street, Zip 68361–1325,
Mailing Address: P.O. Box 193, Zip 68361–0193; tel. 402/759–3167 **A**5 9 10
18 **F**7 13 14 15 28 29 31 34 35 37 40 41 45 46 47 48 50 56 57 59 64 65
74 75 77 78 79 81 91 92 93 103 107 110 113 114 115 116 117 118 128
129 131 132 142 147
Primary Contact: Paul Utemark, Chief Executive Officer
CFO: Jeanne Ackland, Manager Accounting and Acting Chief Financial Officer
CMO: John Jacobsen, M.D., Chief of Staff
CIO: Tyler Gewecke, Information Technology Technician
CHR: Ranee Hoarty, Business Manager Human Resources
Web address: www.fhsofgeneva.org
**Control:** County–Government, nonfederal **Service:** General Medical and Surgical

**Staffed Beds:** 25 **Admissions:** 468 **Census:** 6 **Outpatient Visits:** 25410
**Births:** 34 **Total Expense ($000):** 9594 **Payroll Expense ($000):** 3142
**Personnel:** 95

**NE**

---

**Hospital, Medicare Provider Number, Address, Telephone, Approval, Facility, and Physician Codes, Health Care System**

★ American Hospital Association (AHA) membership
☐ The Joint Commission accreditation ◇ DNV Healthcare Inc. accreditation

○ American Osteopathic Association (AOA) accreditation
△ Commission on Accreditation of Rehabilitation Facilities (CARF) accreditation

## GENOA—Nance County

**GENOA COMMUNITY HOSPITAL (281312)**, 706 Ewing Avenue, Zip 68640,
Mailing Address: P.O. Box 310, Zip 68640–0310; tel. 402/993–2283,
(Nonreporting) **A**9 10 18
Primary Contact: Mike Harris, Interim Administrator
CFO: Jennifer Wieck, Business Manager
CMO: Brian Buhlke, M.D., Medical Director
CHR: Kari Reeg, Manager Human Resources
**Control:** City–County, Government, nonfederal **Service:** General Medical and
Surgical

**Staffed Beds: 65**

## GORDON—Sheridan County

★ **GORDON MEMORIAL HOSPITAL (281358)**, 300 East Eighth Street,
Zip 69343–1123; tel. 308/282–0401, (Nonreporting) **A**9 10 18
Primary Contact: James LeBrun, Chief Executive Officer
CFO: Heidi Cushing, Director Finance
CMO: Christopher P. Costa, M.D., Chief of Staff
CIO: Ray Waldron, Director Information Technology
CHR: Shelley Beguin, Director Human Resources
Web address: www.gordonmemorial.org
**Control:** Hospital district or authority, Government, nonfederal **Service:** General
Medical and Surgical

**Staffed Beds: 25**

## GOTHENBURG—Dawson County

★ **GOTHENBURG MEMORIAL HOSPITAL (281313)**, 910 20th Street,
Zip 69138–1237, Mailing Address: P.O. Box 469, Zip 69138–0469;
tel. 308/537–3661, (Nonreporting) **A**9 10 18
Primary Contact: Kayleen Dudley, Interim Chief Executive Officer
CFO: Taci Bartlett, Chief Financial Officer
CMO: Craig Bartruff, M.D., Medical Director
CHR: Lisa Gieken, Director Human Resources
Web address: www.ghospital.org
**Control:** Hospital district or authority, Government, nonfederal **Service:** General
Medical and Surgical

**Staffed Beds: 12**

## GRAND ISLAND—Hall County

✠ **SAINT FRANCIS MEDICAL CENTER (280023)**, 2620 West Faidley Avenue,
Zip 68803–4297, Mailing Address: P.O. Box 9804, Zip 68802–9804;
tel. 308/384–4600, (Includes SAINT FRANCIS MEMORIAL HEALTH CENTER, 2116
West Faidley Avenue, Zip 68803, Mailing Address: P.O. Box 9804, Zip 68802;
tel. 308/384–4600), (Total facility includes 34 beds in nursing home–type unit)
**A**1 2 3 5 9 10 19 **F**3 4 5 7 8 10 11 12 13 15 17 18 20 22 28 30 31 34 35 40 43 45
46 47 51 53 59 60 63 64 65 68 70 72 74 75 76 77 78 79 81 82 84 85 89
90 91 97 104 105 110 119 120 122 127 128 129 131 134 144 145 147
**S** Catholic Health Initiatives, Englewood, CO
Primary Contact: Daniel P. McElligott, FACHE, President and Chief Executive
Officer
CFO: Lisa Webb, Vice President Finance and Chief Financial Officer
CMO: Mike Horn, M.D., Vice President Medical Affairs
CIO: Michael Foley, Director Information Systems
CHR: Lee Elliott, Vice President Human Resources and Fund Development
Web address: www.saintfrancisgi.org
**Control:** Church–operated, Nongovernment, not–for profit **Service:** General
Medical and Surgical

**Staffed Beds: 200 Admissions:** 6791 **Census:** 91 **Outpatient Visits:** 181738
**Births:** 956 **Total Expense ($000):** 132846 **Payroll Expense ($000):** 50735
**Personnel:** 951

## GRANT—Perkins County

★ **PERKINS COUNTY HEALTH SERVICES (281356)**, 900 Lincoln Avenue,
Zip 69140–9799; tel. 308/352–7200, (Includes GOLDEN OURS CONVALESCENT
HOME ), (Total facility includes 50 beds in nursing home–type unit) **A**9 10 18 **F**10
13 15 17 18 31 34 40 41 43 45 57 62 70 75 76 77 81 89 93 97 107 110
126 127 128 132 144 147 **P**6
Primary Contact: Pamela Holm, R.N., Administrator
COO: Tim Rowley, Chief Operating Officer
CFO: Tiffany Weber, Chief Financial Officer
CMO: Kristi Kohl, M.D., Chief Medical Officer
CIO: Jennifer Baumgartner, Chief Information Officer
CHR: Alicia Fraley, Chief Human Resources
CNO: Dana McArtor, R.N., Director of Nursing
Web address: www.pchsgrant.com
**Control:** Hospital district or authority, Government, nonfederal **Service:** General
Medical and Surgical

**Staffed Beds: 70 Admissions:** 367 **Census:** 49 **Outpatient Visits:** 12519
**Births:** 36 **Total Expense ($000):** 10545 **Payroll Expense ($000):** 4051
**Personnel:** 95

## HASTINGS—Adams County

**HASTINGS REGIONAL CENTER**, 4200 West Second Street, Zip 68901–9700,
Mailing Address: P.O. Box 579, Zip 68902–0579; tel. 402/462–1971,
(Nonreporting) **A**9
Primary Contact: William R. Gibson, Chief Executive Officer
COO: Marj A. Colburn, Facility Operating Officer, Risk Manager and Performance
Improvement Coordinator
CMO: Gene Wyse, D.O., Medical Director
CIO: Nancy Kinyoun, Director Health Information Management
CHR: LaDene Madson, Director Human Resources
Web address: www.dhhs.ne.gov
**Control:** State–Government, nonfederal **Service:** Other specialty

**Staffed Beds: 156**

✠ **MARY LANNING HEALTHCARE (280032)**, 715 North St. Joseph Avenue,
Zip 68901–4497; tel. 402/463–4521, (Nonreporting) **A**1 2 9 10
Primary Contact: Bradley D. Neet, FACHE, President and Chief Executive Officer
CMO: Joe Davis, M.D., Vice President Medical Affairs
CIO: George Sullivan, Director Management Information Systems
CHR: Bruce E. Cutright, MS, Vice President Human Resources
Web address: www.marylanning.org
**Control:** Other not–for–profit (including NFP Corporation) **Service:** General
Medical and Surgical

**Staffed Beds: 161**

## HEBRON—Thayer County

★ **THAYER COUNTY HEALTH SERVICES (281304)**, 120 Park Avenue,
Zip 68370–2019, Mailing Address: P.O. Box 49, Zip 68370–0049;
tel. 402/768–6041, (Nonreporting) **A**9 10 18
Primary Contact: Joyce Beck, Administrator
COO: Susan L. Moore, R.N., Director Nursing
CFO: Michael Pracheil, Chief Financial Officer
CMO: Michelle Kuhlmann, M.D., Director Medical Staff
CIO: Dan Engle, Chief Information Officer
Web address: www.thayercountyhealth.com
**Control:** County–Government, nonfederal **Service:** General Medical and Surgical

**Staffed Beds: 19**

## HENDERSON—York County

**HENDERSON HEALTH CARE SERVICES (281308)**, 1621 Front Street,
Zip 68371; tel. 402/723–4512, (Nonreporting) **A**9 10 18
Primary Contact: Cheryl Brown, Administrator
CMO: James M. Ohrt, M.D., Director Medical Staff
CHR: Lynette Friesen, Manager Human Resources
Web address: www.telcoweb.net/health
**Control:** Other not–for–profit (including NFP Corporation) **Service:** General
Medical and Surgical

**Staffed Beds: 56**

## HOLDREGE—Phelps County

✠ **PHELPS MEMORIAL HEALTH CENTER (281362)**, 1215 Tibbals Street,
Zip 68949–1255; tel. 308/995–2211 **A**1 9 10 18 **F**3 7 13 15 28 29 30 34 40
43 57 59 62 63 70 75 76 77 79 81 82 87 93 107 108 110 111 113 118 128
129 132 134 146 **S** QHR, Brentwood, TN
Primary Contact: Mark Harrel, Chief Executive Officer
CFO: Loren D. Schroder, Chief Financial Officer
CMO: Stuart Embury, M.D., Chief Medical Officer
CIO: Leora Smith, Information System and Health Information Management Team
Leader
CHR: Cindy Jackson, Director Human Resources
Web address: www.phelpsmemorial.com
**Control:** Other not–for–profit (including NFP Corporation) **Service:** General
Medical and Surgical

**Staffed Beds: 25 Admissions:** 1070 **Census:** 12 **Outpatient Visits:** 20197
**Births:** 110 **Total Expense ($000):** 22300 **Payroll Expense ($000):** 10100
**Personnel:** 189

## IMPERIAL—Chase County

**CHASE COUNTY COMMUNITY HOSPITAL (281351)**, 600 West 12th Street,
Zip 69033–0819, Mailing Address: P.O. Box 819, Zip 69033–0819;
tel. 308/882–7111, (Nonreporting) **A**9 10 18
Primary Contact: Lola Jones, R.N., Administrator
CFO: Renee Fink, CPA, Chief Financial Officer
CMO: Jonathan Richman, M.D., Chief of Staff
CIO: Jen Harris, Director Health Information Management
CHR: Julie Sharp, Supervisor Human Resources
Web address: www.chasecountyhospital.com
**Control:** County–Government, nonfederal **Service:** General Medical and Surgical

**Staffed Beds: 25**

**NE**

## KEARNEY—Buffalo County

**GOOD SAMARITAN HEALTH SYSTEMS** See Good Samaritan Hospital

✠ **GOOD SAMARITAN HOSPITAL (280009)**, 10 East 31st Street,
Zip 68847–2926, Mailing Address: P.O. Box 1990, Zip 68848–1990;
tel. 308/865–7100, (Includes RICHARD H. YOUNG HOSPITAL, 1755 Prairie View
Place, Zip 68848, Mailing Address: P.O. Box 1750, Zip 68848–1705;
tel. 308/865–2000), (Total facility includes 21 beds in nursing home–type unit)
**A**1 2 3 5 9 10 **F**3 7 9 12 13 15 18 20 22 24 28 29 30 31 34 35 40 43 44 45
46 48 49 50 51 53 57 58 59 60 65 69 70 71 72 74 75 76 77 78 79 80 81
82 83 84 85 86 87 89 90 92 93 98 99 101 102 103 104 107 108 110 111
113 114 115 116 117 118 119 120 122 123 125 127 128 129 131 133 134
145 147 **P**6 8 **S** Catholic Health Initiatives, Englewood, CO
Primary Contact: Michael H. Schnieders, President and Chief Executive Officer
CFO: George Harms, Chief Financial Officer
CIO: Tanya Arthur, Chief Information Officer
CHR: Robert Cunningham, Vice President Human Resources
Web address: www.gshs.org
**Control:** Church–operated, Nongovernment, not–for profit **Service:** General
Medical and Surgical

**Staffed Beds:** 229 **Admissions:** 10068 **Census:** 146 **Outpatient Visits:**
59735 **Births:** 949 **Total Expense ($000):** 180792 **Payroll Expense ($000):**
60847 **Personnel:** 1194

## KIMBALL—Kimball County

★ **KIMBALL HEALTH SERVICES (281305)**, 505 South Burg Street,
Zip 69145–1398; tel. 308/235–1952 **A**9 10 18 **F**3 34 40 42 43 45 57 59 64
65 81 85 93 97 107 113 126 129 132 145 147 **P**6
Primary Contact: Ken Hunter, R.N., Chief Executive Officer
CFO: David Usher, Chief Financial Officer
CMO: Richard Jay, M.D., Chief of Staff
CIO: Nicole Nielan, Director Information Technology
CHR: James R. Imler, Director Human Resources
CNO: Chad Jay, Chief Nursing Officer
Web address: www.kimballhealth.org
**Control:** County–Government, nonfederal **Service:** General Medical and Surgical

**Staffed Beds:** 12 **Admissions:** 220 **Census:** 2 **Outpatient Visits:** 13688
**Births:** 0 **Total Expense ($000):** 5945 **Payroll Expense ($000):** 3219
**Personnel:** 76

## LEXINGTON—Dawson County

★ **LEXINGTON REGIONAL HEALTH CENTER (281361)**, 1201 North Erie Street,
Zip 68850–0980, Mailing Address: P.O. Box 980, Zip 68850–0980;
tel. 308/324–5651, (Nonreporting) **A**9 10 18
Primary Contact: Leslie Marsh, Chief Executive Officer
CFO: Wade Eschenbrenner, Chief Financial Officer
CMO: Francisca Acosta–Carlson, M.D., Chief of Staff
CIO: Robb Hanna, Executive Director Information Technology
CHR: Jill Denker, Executive Director Human Resources
CNO: Dana Steiner, R.N., Executive Director of Nursing Services
Web address: www.lexingtonregional.org
**Control:** Hospital district or authority, Government, nonfederal **Service:** General
Medical and Surgical

**Staffed Beds:** 25

## LINCOLN—Lancaster County

✠ △ **BRYANLGH MEDICAL CENTER (280003)**, 1600 South 48th Street,
Zip 68506–1283; tel. 402/489–0200, (Includes BRYANLGH MEDICAL
CENTER–EAST, 1600 South 48th Street, Zip 68506–1299; tel. 402/489–0200;
BRYANLGH MEDICAL CENTER–WEST, 2300 South 16th Street, Zip 68502–3781;
tel. 402/475–1011) **A**1 2 7 9 10 **F**3 4 5 8 13 15 17 18 19 20 22 24 26 28 29
30 31 34 35 37 38 39 40 43 45 46 47 48–49 50 54 56 57 58 59 61 64 68
70 71 72 74 75 76 78 79 81 82 84 85 86 87 89 90 92 93 96 99 100
101 102 103 104 105 106 107 108 109 110 111 112 113 114 115 116 117
118 119 122 123 125 128 129 130 131 144 145 146 147 **S** BryanLGH Health
System, Lincoln, NE
Primary Contact: John T. Woodrich, President and Chief Operating Officer
CFO: Jennifer Lesoing–Lucs, Vice President and Chief Financial Officer
CMO: Carolyn Cody, M.D., Vice President Medical Affairs
CIO: Richard Marreel, Chief Information Officer
CHR: George A. Snider, Vice President Human Resources
Web address: www.bryanlgh.org
**Control:** Other not–for–profit (including NFP Corporation) **Service:** General
Medical and Surgical

**Staffed Beds:** 346 **Admissions:** 22107 **Census:** 262 **Outpatient Visits:**
217276 **Births:** 2588 **Total Expense ($000):** 420542 **Payroll Expense
($000):** 148262 **Personnel:** 2668

**LINCOLN DIVISION** See Veterans Affairs Nebraska–Western Iowa Health Care
System

**LINCOLN REGIONAL CENTER (284003)**, West Prospector Place and South
Folsom, Zip 68522–2299, Mailing Address: P.O. Box 94949, Zip 68509–4949;
tel. 402/479–5207, (Nonreporting) **A**9 10
Primary Contact: William R. Gibson, Chief Executive Officer
COO: Stacey Werth–Sweeney, Facility Operating Officer
CFO: Randy Willey, Business Manager
CMO: Vijay Dewan, M.D., Clinical Director
CHR: Scott Rasmussen, Director Human Resources
Web address: www.hhs.state.ne.us/beh/rc
**Control:** State–Government, nonfederal **Service:** Psychiatric

**Staffed Beds:** 253

**LINCOLN SURGICAL HOSPITAL (280127)**, 1710 South 70th Street, Suite 200,
Zip 68506; tel. 402/484–9090, (Nonreporting) **A**9 10
Primary Contact: Robb Linafelter, Chief Executive Officer
Web address: www.lincolnsurgery.com
**Control:** Corporation, Investor–owned, for–profit **Service:** Other specialty

**Staffed Beds:** 7

★ △ **MADONNA REHABILITATION HOSPITAL (282000)**, 5401 South Street,
Zip 68506–2150; tel. 402/489–7102, (Total facility includes 125 beds in nursing
home–type unit) **A**7 9 10 **F**1 6 10 27 28 29 32 34 35 36 50 53 54 56 57 58
59 63 64 67 74 75 77 79 84 86 87 90 91 92 93 94 95 96 127 129 130 131
142 145 147 **P**4 6
Primary Contact: Marsha Lommel, FACHE, President and Chief Executive Officer
COO: Paul Dongilli, Jr., Ph.D., Executive Vice President and Chief Operating Officer
CFO: Victor J. Witkowicz, Senior Vice President and Chief Financial Officer
CMO: Thomas Stadler, M.D., Vice President Medical Affairs and Chief Medical
Officer
CIO: David Rolfe, Chief Information Officer
CHR: Lou Ann Manske, Director Human Resources
Web address: www.madonna.org
**Control:** Other not–for–profit (including NFP Corporation) **Service:** Rehabilitation

**Staffed Beds:** 300 **Admissions:** 1747 **Census:** 219 **Outpatient Visits:** 54239
**Births:** 0 **Total Expense ($000):** 86887 **Payroll Expense ($000):** 55347
**Personnel:** 1156

★ **NEBRASKA HEART INSTITUTE AND HEART HOSPITAL (280128)**, 7500
South 91st Street, Zip 68526; tel. 402/327–2700, (Nonreporting) **A**9 10
**S** Catholic Health Initiatives, Englewood, CO
Primary Contact: Thomas Burnell, Chief Executive Officer
CFO: Dan Schonlau, Chief Financial Officer
CHR: Jamie N. Carlson, Chief Human Resources Officer
Web address: www.neheart.com
**Control:** Other not–for–profit (including NFP Corporation) **Service:** Heart

**Staffed Beds:** 52

**NEBRASKA PENAL AND CORRECTIONAL HOSPITAL**, 14th And Pioneer
Streets, Zip 68501; tel. 402/471–3161, (Nonreporting)
Primary Contact: George E. Lewis, M.D., Medical Officer
Web address: www.corrections.nebraska.gov
**Control:** State–Government, nonfederal **Service:** Hospital unit of an institution
(prison hospital, college infirmary, etc.)

**Staffed Beds:** 12

✠ **SAINT ELIZABETH REGIONAL MEDICAL CENTER (280020)**, 555 South 70th
Street, Zip 68510–2462; tel. 402/219–8000 **A**1 2 3 5 9 10 **F**3 8 11 12 13 15
16 18 20 22 24 26 28 29 30 31 34 35 37 39 40 44 45 46 47 48 49 50 51
55 58 59 60 61 64 65 68 70 72 74 75 76 78 79 80 81 84 85 86 87 89 92
107 108 110 111 113 114 115 116 117 118 119 120 122 123 125 128 129
131 134 143 144 145 146 147 **S** Catholic Health Initiatives, Englewood, CO
Primary Contact: Kim S. Moore, President and Chief Executive Officer
CFO: Jeanette Wojtalewicz, Vice President Finance
CMO: Cary Ward, M.D., Chief Medical Officer
CIO: Richard Bohaty, Director Information Technology
CHR: Cody Koch, Director Human Resources
Web address: www.saintelizabethonline.com
**Control:** Other not–for–profit (including NFP Corporation) **Service:** General
Medical and Surgical

**Staffed Beds:** 260 **Admissions:** 13465 **Census:** 152 **Outpatient Visits:**
103734 **Births:** 2338 **Total Expense ($000):** 209890 **Payroll Expense
($000):** 68813 **Personnel:** 1312

NE

---

**Hospital, Medicare Provider Number, Address, Telephone, Approval, Facility, and Physician Codes, Health Care System**

★ American Hospital Association (AHA) membership
□ The Joint Commission accreditation     ◇ DNV Healthcare Inc. accreditation
○ American Osteopathic Association (AOA) accreditation
△ Commission on Accreditation of Rehabilitation Facilities (CARF) accreditation

★ **VETERANS AFFAIRS NEBRASKA–WESTERN IOWA HEALTH CARE SYSTEM**, 600 South 70th Street, Zip 68510–2493; tel. 402/489–3802, (Includes LINCOLN DIVISION, 600 South 70th Street, tel. 402/489–3802), (Nonreporting) **A**9
**S** Department of Veterans Affairs, Washington, DC
Primary Contact: Nancy A. Gregory, Acting Director
CIO: David Daiker, Chief Information Resource Management
CHR: Dave Peters, Chief Human Resources Officer
Web address: www.nebraska.va.gov/visitors/lincoln.asp
**Control:** Veterans Affairs, Government, federal **Service:** General Medical and Surgical

| Staffed Beds: 186 |
| --- |

**LYNCH—Boyd County**

**NIOBRARA VALLEY HOSPITAL (281303)**, 401 South Fifth Street, Zip 68746–0118, Mailing Address: P.O. Box 118, Zip 68746–0118; tel. 402/569–2451 **A**9 10 18 **F**11 40 57 59 64 107 113 127 132 **P**5 **S** Faith Regional Health Services, Norfolk, NE
Primary Contact: Kelly Kalkowski, Chief Executive Officer
CFO: Martha Nelson, Chief Financial Officer
Web address: www.ci.lynch.ne.us/health.htm
**Control:** Other not–for–profit (including NFP Corporation) **Service:** General Medical and Surgical

| Staffed Beds: 20 Admissions: 43 Census: 1 Outpatient Visits: 1834 Births: 0 Total Expense ($000): 1856 Payroll Expense ($000): 802 |
| --- |

**MCCOOK—Red Willow County**

✠ **COMMUNITY HOSPITAL (281363)**, 1301 East H Street, Zip 69001–1328, Mailing Address: P.O. Box 1328, Zip 69001–1328; tel. 308/344–2650 **A**1 9 10 18 **F**3 11 13 15 28 31 34 35 37 40 43 57 59 62 63 64 68 74 75 77 78 79 81 82 85 86 87 94 107 110 111 113 118 123 126 128 129 131 132 145 146 147 **P**6
Primary Contact: James P. Ulrich, Jr., President and Chief Executive Officer
CFO: Troy Bruntz, Vice President Finance and Chief Financial Officer
CMO: Walter Eskildsen, M.D., Chief of Staff
CIO: Lori Beeby, Director Information Systems
CHR: Leanne R. Miller, Director Human Resources
CNO: Marta Hudson, R.N., VP Patient Care Services
Web address: www.chmccook.org
**Control:** Other not–for–profit (including NFP Corporation) **Service:** General Medical and Surgical

| Staffed Beds: 25 Admissions: 1069 Census: 9 Outpatient Visits: 30012 Births: 144 Total Expense ($000): 31053 Payroll Expense ($000): 11013 Personnel: 206 |
| --- |

**MINDEN—Kearney County**

★ **KEARNEY COUNTY HEALTH SERVICES (281306)**, 727 East First Street, Zip 68959–1705; tel. 308/832–3400, (Total facility includes 34 beds in nursing home–type unit) **A**9 10 18 **F**10 15 18 28 34 40 43 45 56 59 64 65 77 81 86 97 107 110 111 113 118 126 127 129 132 142 145 147
Primary Contact: Fred J. Meis, Chief Executive Officer
CFO: Rebekah Mussman, Chief Financial Officer
CMO: Eddie Pierce, M.D., Chief Medical Staff
CHR: Donna Dyke, Human Resources Officer
Web address: www.kchs.org
**Control:** County–Government, nonfederal **Service:** General Medical and Surgical

| Staffed Beds: 49 Admissions: 202 Census: 28 Births: 0 |
| --- |

**NEBRASKA CITY—Otoe County**

★ **ST. MARY'S COMMUNITY HOSPITAL (281342)**, 1314 Third Avenue, Zip 68410–1930; tel. 402/873–3321 **A**9 10 18 **F**3 13 15 17 28 31 35 40 45 64 67 68 69 70 75 76 78 79 81 82 85 87 89 107 110 111 113 117 118 127 128 131 132 134 147 **S** Catholic Health Initiatives, Englewood, CO
Primary Contact: Daniel J. Kelly, President and Chief Executive Officer
CFO: Shawn Closner, Vice President Finance
CMO: Jonathan Stelling, M.D., Chief Medical Officer
CNO: Brenda Jean Sebek, R.N., Chief Nursing Officer
Web address: www.stmaryshospitalnecity.org
**Control:** Church–operated, Nongovernment, not–for profit **Service:** General Medical and Surgical

| Staffed Beds: 18 Admissions: 503 Census: 5 Outpatient Visits: 30123 Births: 114 Total Expense ($000): 15011 Payroll Expense ($000): 5479 Personnel: 121 |
| --- |

**NELIGH—Antelope County**

★ **ANTELOPE MEMORIAL HOSPITAL (281326)**, 102 West Ninth Street, Zip 68756–0229, Mailing Address: P.O. Box 229, Zip 68756–0229; tel. 402/887–4151 **A**9 10 18 **F**7 13 28 35 36 40 53 56 59 62 63 64 68 76 77 79 81 89 93 107 118 126 127 129 130 132 146 **P**6
Primary Contact: Jack W. Green, Administrator
CFO: Martha Nelson, Chief Financial Officer
CMO: Troy Dawson, M.D., President Medical Staff
CIO: Kevin Trease, Chief Information Officer
CHR: Mary A. Schwager, Director Human Resources
CNO: Merry Sprout, R.N., Chief Nursing Officer
Web address: www.amhne.org/
**Control:** Other not–for–profit (including NFP Corporation) **Service:** General Medical and Surgical

| Staffed Beds: 25 Admissions: 396 Census: 6 Outpatient Visits: 33502 Births: 23 Total Expense ($000): 11766 Payroll Expense ($000): 5316 |
| --- |

**NORFOLK—Madison County**

✠ **FAITH REGIONAL HEALTH SERVICES (280125)**, 2700 West Norfolk Avenue, Zip 68701, Mailing Address: P.O. Box 869, Zip 68702–0869; tel. 402/644–7201, (Includes EAST CAMPUS, 1500 Koenigstein Avenue, tel. 402/371–3402; WEST CAMPUS, 2700 Norfolk Avenue, Mailing Address: P.O. Box 869, Zip 68702–0869; tel. 402/371–4880), (Total facility includes 93 beds in nursing home–type unit) **A**1 2 3 5 9 10 20 **F**3 5 8 13 15 18 20 22 24 26 28 29 30 31 32 34 35 39 40 43 44 45 46 48 49 50 51 53 54 56 57 59 61 62 63 64 68 70 72 73 74 75 76 77 78 79 81 82 83 84 85 86 87 89 90 93 96 97 98 100 101 102 103 104 105 107 108 110 111 113 114 116 117 118 119 120 122 126 128 129 130 131 134 142 145 146 147 **P**6 7 **S** Faith Regional Health Services, Norfolk, NE
Primary Contact: James J. Sinek, President and Chief Executive Officer
CFO: William C. Luke, Interim Chief Financial Officer
CMO: Dean O. French, M.D., Chief of Staff
CHR: Janet Pinkelman, Director Human Resources
Web address: www.frhs.org
**Control:** Other not–for–profit (including NFP Corporation) **Service:** General Medical and Surgical

| Staffed Beds: 146 Admissions: 4966 Census: 144 Outpatient Visits: 78437 Births: 931 Total Expense ($000): 128724 Payroll Expense ($000): 49186 Personnel: 969 |
| --- |

**NORFOLK REGIONAL CENTER (284004)**, 1700 North Victory Road, Zip 68701–6859, Mailing Address: P.O. Box 1209, Zip 68702–1209; tel. 402/370–3400, (Nonreporting) **A**9 10
Primary Contact: William R. Gibson, Chief Executive Officer
COO: Stephen O'Neill, Clinical Director
CFO: Randy Willey, Business Manager
CMO: Daniel Sturgis, Ph.D., Director Psychology
CIO: Marilyn Blunck, Director Health Information Management
CHR: Jim McElfresh, Manager Human Resources
Web address: www.hhss.ne.gov/beh/rc/nrcserv.htm
**Control:** State–Government, nonfederal **Service:** Psychiatric

| Staffed Beds: 179 |
| --- |

**NORTH PLATTE—Lincoln County**

✠ **GREAT PLAINS REGIONAL MEDICAL CENTER (280065)**, 601 West Leota Street, Zip 69101–6598, Mailing Address: P.O. Box 1167, Zip 69103–1167; tel. 308/696–8000, (Nonreporting) **A**1 2 3 5 9 10
Primary Contact: Gregory A. Nielsen, President
COO: Melvin McNea, Chief Operating Officer
CFO: Krystal Claymore, Chief Financial Officer
CIO: Jim Anderson, Chief Information Officer
CIO: Brandon Kelliher, IT Operations Officer
CHR: Kelly Hurt, VP Human Resources
Web address: www.gprmc.com
**Control:** Other not–for–profit (including NFP Corporation) **Service:** General Medical and Surgical

| Staffed Beds: 96 |
| --- |

**O'NEILL—Holt County**

★ **AVERA ST. ANTHONY'S HOSPITAL (281329)**, 302 North Second Street, Zip 68763–1514, Mailing Address: P.O. Box 270, Oneill, Zip 68763–0270; tel. 402/336–2611 **A**9 10 18 **F**3 8 13 15 28 29 30 31 32 34 35 38 40 45 46 48 52 56 57 59 60 61 62 64 65 68 74 75 76 77 78 79 81 82 86 87 91 93 94 96 107 108 111 112 113 118 119 123 126 128 129 130 132 134 142 145 147 **P**6 **S** Avera Health, Sioux Falls, SD
Primary Contact: Ronald J. Cork, President and Chief Executive Officer
CFO: Michael Garman, Chief Financial Officer
CMO: Preston Renshaw, M.D., Chief Medical Officer
CIO: Michael Garman, Chief Financial Officer
CHR: Crystal Kahle, Director Human Resources and Marketing
Web address: www.avera.org/st-anthonys
**Control:** Church–operated, Nongovernment, not–for profit **Service:** General Medical and Surgical

| Staffed Beds: 25 Admissions: 919 Census: 8 Outpatient Visits: 32749 Births: 165 Total Expense ($000): 25180 Payroll Expense ($000): 10461 Personnel: 233 |
| --- |

**NE**

## OAKLAND—Burt County

★ **OAKLAND MERCY HOSPITAL (281321)**, 601 East Second Street,
Zip 68045–1400; tel. 402/685–5601 **A**9 10 18 **F**11 15 28 29 30 31 34 35 40
44 50 57 59 75 81 93 97 107 118 126 127 129 131 132 134 147 **P**6
**S** Trinity Health, Novi, MI
Primary Contact: Roger W. Lenz, Interim Chief Executive Officer
CFO: David M A Jensen, Chief Financial Officer
CHR: Karolyn McEnroy, Business Office Manager
Web address: www.oaklandhospital.org
**Control:** Church–operated, Nongovernment, not–for profit **Service:** General
Medical and Surgical

**Staffed Beds:** 18 **Admissions:** 180 **Census:** 2 **Outpatient Visits:** 6928
**Births:** 0 **Total Expense ($000):** 5566 **Payroll Expense ($000):** 2871
**Personnel:** 56

## OGALLALA—Keith County

★ **OGALLALA COMMUNITY HOSPITAL (281355)**, 2601 North Spruce Street,
Zip 69153–2465; tel. 308/284–4011 **A**9 10 18 **F**3 13 15 18 19 29 30 31 35
40 43 46 57 59 76 77 78 79 81 85 87 89 93 97 107 110 113 118 128 132
147 **P**6 **S** Banner Health, Phoenix, AZ
Primary Contact: Sharon Lind, MSN, Chief Executive Officer
CFO: Dena Klockman, Chief Financial Officer
CMO: Kurt Johnson, M.D., Chief of Staff
CHR: Bethany Childers, Manager People Resources
Web address: www.bannerhealth.com
**Control:** Other not–for–profit (including NFP Corporation) **Service:** General
Medical and Surgical

**Staffed Beds:** 18 **Admissions:** 582 **Census:** 6 **Outpatient Visits:** 55132
**Births:** 79 **Total Expense ($000):** 15865 **Payroll Expense ($000):** 6827
**Personnel:** 113

## OMAHA—Douglas County

⊞ **ALEGENT HEALTH–BERGAN MERCY MEDICAL CENTER (280060)**, 7500
Mercy Road, Zip 68124–2319; tel. 402/398–6060, (Includes LASTING HOPE
RECOVERY CENTER, 415 South 25th Avenue, Zip 68131; tel. 402/717–5300;
Robin Conyers, Administrator) **A**1 2 3 5 9 10 **F**3 8 11 13 16 17 18 20 22 24
26 28 29 30 31 32 34 35 38 39 40 42 43 44 45 46 47 49 50 51 53 54 55
56 57 59 60 61 62 63 64 65 68 70 72 74 75 76 77 78 79 80 81 82 83 84
85 86 87 89 93 97 100 102 105 107 108 109 110 111 113 114 115 116
117 118 119 120 122 123 125 126 129 130 131 133 142 144 145 146 147
**P**6 8 **S** Alegent Health, Omaha, NE
Primary Contact: Marie E. Knedler, R.N., Vice President and Chief Operating
Officer
COO: Marie E. Knedler, R.N., Vice President and Chief Operating Officer
CFO: Amy Knott, Chief Financial Officer
CIO: Kenneth Lawonn, Senior Vice President Strategy & Technology
CHR: Nancy Wallace, Vice President Human Resources
CNO: Jane Carmody, R.N., Chief Nursing Officer
Web address: www.alegent.com/bergan
**Control:** Church–operated, Nongovernment, not–for profit **Service:** General
Medical and Surgical

**Staffed Beds:** 320 **Admissions:** 16464 **Census:** 228 **Outpatient Visits:**
223759 **Births:** 3464 **Total Expense ($000):** 298844 **Payroll Expense
($000):** 91821 **Personnel:** 1535

⊞ △ **ALEGENT HEALTH–IMMANUEL MEDICAL CENTER (280081)**, 6901
North 72nd Street, Zip 68122–1799; tel. 402/572–2121, (Total facility includes
165 beds in nursing home–type unit) **A**1 2 3 5 7 9 10 **F**3 4 5 6 11 12 13 15 17
18 20 22 26 28 29 30 31 32 34 35 36 37 38 39 40 42 43 44 45 49 50 53
56 57 58 59 62 63 68 70 72 73 74 75 76 77 78 79 80 81 82 83 84 85 86
87 88 89 90 92 93 96 97 98 99 100 101 102 103 104 105 106 107 108
109 110 111 113 114 116 117 118 119 120 122 123 125 127 128 129 130
131 133 135 141 144 145 146 147 **P**6 8 **S** Alegent Health, Omaha, NE
Primary Contact: Ann Schumacher, MSN, R.N., Vice President and Chief Operating
Officer
CFO: Tim H. Schnack, Chief Financial Officer
CIO: Kenneth Lawonn, Senior Vice President Strategy and Technology
CHR: Nancy Wallace, Vice President Human Resources
Web address: www.alegent.com/immanuel
**Control:** Church–operated, Nongovernment, not–for profit **Service:** General
Medical and Surgical

**Staffed Beds:** 285 **Admissions:** 9450 **Census:** 150 **Outpatient Visits:** 73157
**Births:** 572 **Total Expense ($000):** 164848 **Payroll Expense ($000):** 61998
**Personnel:** 1201

⊞ **ALEGENT HEALTH–LAKESIDE HOSPITAL (280130)**, 16901 Lakeside Hills
Court, Zip 68130–2318; tel. 402/717–8000 **A**1 2 9 10 **F**3 8 12 13 15 17 18
20 22 26 28 29 30 31 32 34 35 36 38 39 40 44 45 46 49 53 54 55 56 59
60 63 64 68 70 73 74 75 76 77 78 79 80 81 82 83 84 85 86 89 93 94 97
99 100 102 103 104 107 108 110 111 113 114 117 118 119 120 121 122
123 125 128 129 130 131 133 142 145 146 147 **P**8 **S** Alegent Health,
Omaha, NE
Primary Contact: Cindy Alloway, Vice President and Chief Operating Officer
COO: Cindy Alloway, Vice President and Chief Operating Officer
CFO: Timothy Meier, Chief Financial Officer
CMO: Patricia Murdock–Langan, Medical Director
CIO: Kenneth Lawonn, Senior Vice President and Chief Information Officer
CHR: Nancy Wallace, Vice President Human Resources
CNO: Jane Carmody, R.N., VP/Chief Nursing Executive
Web address: www.alegent.org
**Control:** Church–operated, Nongovernment, not–for profit **Service:** General
Medical and Surgical

**Staffed Beds:** 160 **Admissions:** 7037 **Census:** 67 **Outpatient Visits:** 165148
**Births:** 1155 **Total Expense ($000):** 104213 **Payroll Expense ($000):**
32105 **Personnel:** 773

☐ **BOYS TOWN NATIONAL RESEARCH HOSPITAL (283300)**, 555 North 30th
Street, Zip 68131–2136; tel. 402/498–6511 **A**1 3 5 9 10 **F**3 34 35 58 65 68
79 81 86 87 97 99 104 106 107 108 111 118 128 129 130 **P**6
Primary Contact: John K. Arch, FACHE, Administrator
CFO: Leigh Jean Koinzan, Director Finance
CMO: Patrick E. Brookhouser, M.D., Director and Chief Medical Officer
CIO: Ann Ducey, Chief Information Officer
CHR: Michael Gell, Director Human Resources
Web address: www.boystownhospital.org
**Control:** Other not–for–profit (including NFP Corporation) **Service:** Children's
general

**Staffed Beds:** 149 **Admissions:** 113 **Census:** 1 **Outpatient Visits:** 204339
**Births:** 0 **Total Expense ($000):** 80285 **Payroll Expense ($000):** 35899
**Personnel:** 800

⊞ **CHILDREN'S HOSPITAL AND MEDICAL CENTER (283301)**, 8200 Dodge
Street, Zip 68114–4113; tel. 402/955–5400 **A**1 3 5 9 10 **F**3 7 11 12 19 21 23
25 27 30 31 32 34 35 41 45 46 48 49 50 54 57 62 64 68 72 74 75 77
78 79 81 82 84 85 88 89 92 93 99 104 107 108 111 113 114 118 128 129
131 143 144 145 147 **P**6
Primary Contact: Gary A. Perkins, FACHE, President and Chief Executive Officer
COO: Kathy L. English, R.N., Executive Vice President and Chief Operating Officer
CFO: Michael Brown, Senior Vice President Finance and Chief Financial Officer
CMO: Carl H. Gumbiner, M.D., Senior Vice President Medical Affairs and Chief
Medical Officer
CIO: George Reynolds, M.D., Vice President, Chief Information Officer and Chief
Medical Information Officer
CHR: Corliss Lovstad, Vice President Human Resources
CNO: Debbie Arnow, VP Patient Care & Chief Nursing Officer
Web address: www.childrensomaha.org
**Control:** Other not–for–profit (including NFP Corporation) **Service:** Children's
general

**Staffed Beds:** 126 **Admissions:** 4417 **Census:** 86 **Outpatient Visits:** 287187
**Births:** 0 **Total Expense ($000):** 235504 **Payroll Expense ($000):** 100934
**Personnel:** 1522

⊞ **CREIGHTON UNIVERSITY MEDICAL CENTER (280030)**, 601 North 30th
Street, Zip 68131–2197; tel. 402/449–4000 **A**1 3 5 8 9 10 **F**3 11 12 13 15 17
18 19 20 21 22 23 24 25 26 27 28 29 30 31 32 34 35 37 38 40 41 43 45
46 47 48 49 50 51 52 54 56 57 58 59 60 61 64 68 70 72 73 74 76 77 78
79 81 85 86 87 88 89 91 92 93 94 96 97 100 102 107 110 111 113 114
117 118 119 120 122 123 125 129 131 135 140 145 146 147 **S** TENET
Healthcare Corporation, Dallas, TX
Primary Contact: Gary Honts, Chief Executive Officer
COO: Parveen Chand, Chief Operating Officer
CFO: Kerry Tolleson, Chief Financial Officer
CMO: Robert Dunlay, M.D., Chief Medical Officer
CIO: Rick Sweeney, Director Information Services
CHR: Kristine Nielsen, Interim Chief Human Resources Officer
CNO: Mary Anne McCrea, Chief Nursing Officer
Web address: www.saintjosephhospital.com
**Control:** Corporation, Investor–owned, for–profit **Service:** General Medical and
Surgical

**Staffed Beds:** 223 **Admissions:** 7859 **Census:** 107 **Outpatient Visits:** 85440
**Births:** 1149 **Total Expense ($000):** 176391 **Payroll Expense ($000):**
44545 **Personnel:** 832

---

**Hospital, Medicare Provider Number, Address, Telephone, Approval, Facility, and Physician Codes, Health Care System**

★ American Hospital Association (AHA) membership
☐ The Joint Commission accreditation ◇ DNV Healthcare Inc. accreditation
○ American Osteopathic Association (AOA) accreditation
△ Commission on Accreditation of Rehabilitation Facilities (CARF) accreditation

**NE**

★ ○ **DOUGLAS COUNTY COMMUNITY MENTAL HEALTH CENTER (284009),** 4102 Woolworth Avenue, Zip 68105–1899; tel. 402/444–7000 **A**9 10 11 **F**29 35 64 66 68 98 104 105 129 131 **P**6
Primary Contact: John Sheehan, Chief Executive Officer
CFO: DeDe Will, Director Finance
CMO: Sidney A. Kauzlarich, M.D., Medical Director
CIO: Dianne Wallace, County Information Manager
CHR: Lee A. Lazure, Director Civil Service Commission
CNO: Marti Christensen, Director of Psychiatric Nursing
Web address: www.co.douglas.ne.us
**Control:** County–Government, nonfederal **Service:** Psychiatric

**Staffed Beds:** 18 **Admissions:** 763 **Census:** 14 **Outpatient Visits:** 18717 **Births:** 0 **Total Expense ($000):** 6611 **Payroll Expense ($000):** 4844 **Personnel:** 77

**MIDWEST SURGICAL HOSPITAL (280131),** 7915 Farnam Drive, Zip 68114–4504; tel. 402/399–1900, (Nonreporting) **A**9 10
Primary Contact: Charles Livingston, Chief Executive Officer
Web address: www.mwsurgicalhospital.com
**Control:** Corporation, Investor–owned, for–profit **Service:** Surgical

**Staffed Beds:** 19

⊞ **NEBRASKA MEDICAL CENTER (280013),** 987400 Nebraska Medical Center, Zip 68198–7400; tel. 402/552–2000 **A**1 2 3 5 8 9 10 **F**3 11 12 13 15 16 17 18 20 22 24 26 28 29 30 31 34 35 37 38 40 41 43 45 46 47 48 49 50 53 54 57 58 59 60 61 64 68 70 72 74 75 76 77 78 79 80 81 82 84 85 86 87 88 89 92 93 94 96 97 98 101 107 108 110 111 113 114 115 116 117 118 119 120 122 123 125 128 129 130 131 134 135 136 137 138 140 141 145 146 147 **P**5 8
Primary Contact: Glenn A. Fosdick, FACHE, President and Chief Executive Officer
COO: Joe B. Graham, Chief Operating Officer
CFO: William S. Dinsmoor, Chief Financial Officer
CMO: Stephen B. Smith, M.D., Chief Medical Officer
CIO: Lianne Stevens, Vice President Information Technology
CHR: Nat Ponticello, Vice President Human Resources
CNO: Rosanna D. Morris, R.N., CNO & Senior VP Patient Care Services
Web address: www.nebraskamed.com
**Control:** Other not–for–profit (including NFP Corporation) **Service:** General Medical and Surgical

**Staffed Beds:** 511 **Admissions:** 25075 **Census:** 368 **Outpatient Visits:** 432245 **Births:** 2078 **Total Expense ($000):** 676414 **Payroll Expense ($000):** 254293 **Personnel:** 5545

⊞ △ **NEBRASKA METHODIST HOSPITAL (280040),** 8303 Dodge Street, Zip 68114–4108; tel. 402/354–4000, (Includes METHODIST WOMEN'S HOSPITAL, 707 North 190th Plaza, Elkhorn, Zip 68022–3974; tel. 402/815–4000; Susan Korth, M.P.H., Ph.D., Vice President and Chief Operating Officer) **A**1 2 3 5 7 9 10 **F**3 8 11 12 13 15 17 18 20 22 24 26 28 29 30 31 34 35 40 45 46 47 48 49 50 51 52 53 54 55 56 57 58 59 60 64 65 66 68 70 72 74 75 76 77 78 79 81 82 83 84 85 86 87 90 91 92 93 96 100 101 104 107 108 110 111 113 114 115 116 117 118 119 120 122 123 125 128 129 131 134 142 145 146 147 **P**8 **S** Nebraska Methodist Health System, Inc., Omaha, NE
Primary Contact: Stephen L. Goeser, FACHE, President and Chief Executive Officer
CFO: Linda K. Burt, Corporate Vice President Finance
CMO: William Shiffermiller, M.D., Vice President Medical Affairs
CIO: Roger Hertz, Vice President Information Technology
CHR: Holly Huerter, Vice President Human Resources
Web address: www.bestcare.org
**Control:** Other not–for–profit (including NFP Corporation) **Service:** General Medical and Surgical

**Staffed Beds:** 460 **Admissions:** 17188 **Census:** 237 **Outpatient Visits:** 317317 **Births:** 3505 **Total Expense ($000):** 386159 **Payroll Expense ($000):** 141942 **Personnel:** 2109

□ **NEBRASKA ORTHOPAEDIC HOSPITAL (280129),** 2808 South 143rd Plaza, Zip 68144–5611; tel. 402/637–0600 **A**1 3 5 9 10 **F**3 29 34 37 39 40 57 59 64 77 79 81 82 85 86 87 93 94 96 111 130 **P**6
Primary Contact: Tom Macy, FACHE, Chief Executive Officer
COO: Mark E. Longacre, FACHE, Chief Operating Officer
CFO: Anna McCaslin, Chief Financial Officer
CMO: Ian Crabb, M.D., Medical Director
CIO: Tim Pugsley, Manager Information Technology
CHR: Kathleen Kelley–Robinson, Manager Human Resources
Web address: www.neorthohospital.com
**Control:** Partnership, Investor–owned, for–profit **Service:** Orthopedic

**Staffed Beds:** 24 **Admissions:** 1410 **Census:** 11 **Outpatient Visits:** 58251 **Births:** 0 **Total Expense ($000):** 53659 **Payroll Expense ($000):** 16282 **Personnel:** 318

⊞ **SELECT SPECIALTY HOSPITAL–OMAHA (282001),** 1870 South 75th Street, Zip 68124–1700; tel. 402/361–5700, (Nonreporting) **A**1 9 10 **S** Select Medical Corporation, Mechanicsburg, PA
Primary Contact: Thomas N. Theroult, Chief Executive Officer
CMO: Guillermo Huerta, M.D., Chief Medical Officer
CMO: Antonio Saquaton, M.D., Chief Medical Officer
CIO: Cynde McCall, R.N., Chief Nursing Officer
CHR: Nicole Nelson, Human Resources Coordinator
CNO: Cynde McCall, R.N., Chief Nursing Officer
Web address: www.selectmedicalcorp.com
**Control:** Corporation, Investor–owned, for–profit **Service:** Long–Term Acute Care hospital

**Staffed Beds:** 52

⊞ **VETERANS AFFAIRS MEDICAL CENTER,** 4101 Woolworth Avenue, Zip 68105–1873; tel. 402/346–8800, (Total facility includes 76 beds in nursing home–type unit) **A**1 3 5 8 9 **F**3 5 7 12 18 20 22 26 29 30 31 34 35 38 39 40 45 46 47 48 49 50 51 53 54 56 57 58 59 60 61 62 63 64 65 66 67 68 70 74 75 77 78 79 81 82 84 85 86 87 92 93 94 97 98 101 102 103 104 105 106 107 108 109 111 113 114 115 116 118 126 127 128 129 131 134 142 143 144 145 146 147 **S** Department of Veterans Affairs, Washington, DC
Primary Contact: Nancy A. Gregory, Acting Director
COO: Katie Landwehr, Acting Associate Director
CFO: Kirk Kay, Chief Financial Officer
CMO: Thomas Lynch, M.D., Chief of Staff
CIO: John Horner, Manager Business Office
CHR: Cheryl M. DeWispelare, Chief Human Resources Officer
Web address: www.va.gov/sta/guide/home.asp
**Control:** Veterans Affairs, Government, federal **Service:** General Medical and Surgical

**Staffed Beds:** 100 **Admissions:** 2371 **Census:** 70 **Outpatient Visits:** 277432 **Births:** 0 **Personnel:** 2462

**ORD—Valley County**

★ **VALLEY COUNTY HEALTH SYSTEM (281353),** 2707 L. Street, Zip 68862–1675; tel. 308/728–4200, (Nonreporting) **A**9 10 18
Primary Contact: Ashley Woodward, Interim Chief Executive Officer
CFO: Ashley Woodward, Director Financial Services
CMO: Jennifer Bengston, M.D., Chief Medical Officer
CIO: Shane Molacek, Chief Information Officer
CHR: Tricia Richards, Director Human Resources
Web address: www.valleycountyhospital.org
**Control:** County–Government, nonfederal **Service:** General Medical and Surgical

**Staffed Beds:** 85

**OSCEOLA—Polk County**

**ANNIE JEFFREY MEMORIAL COUNTY HEALTH CENTER (281314),** 531 Beebe Street, Zip 68651, Mailing Address: P.O. Box 428, Zip 68651–0428; tel. 402/747–2031 **A**9 10 18 **F**67 70 76 80 89 90 127
Primary Contact: Joseph W. Lohrman, Chief Executive Officer
CFO: Joseph W. Lohrman, Chief Executive Officer
CMO: David Jameson, M.D., Chief of Staff
CIO: Frank Vrba, Chief Information Officer
CHR: Sue Leif, R.N., Director Human Resources
Web address: www.ajhc.org
**Control:** County–Government, nonfederal **Service:** General Medical and Surgical

**Staffed Beds:** 21 **Admissions:** 258 **Census:** 3

**OSHKOSH—Garden County**

**GARDEN COUNTY HEALTH SERVICES (281310),** 1100 West Second Street, Zip 69154; tel. 308/772–3283, (Nonreporting) **A**9 10 18
Primary Contact: Jimmie W. Hansel, Chief Executive Officer
CFO: Jennifer Moffat, Staff Accountant
CMO: Harold Keenan, M.D., Chief Medical Officer
CIO: DeeDee Waltman, Information Officer
CHR: Dodi Moffat, Supervisor Human Resources
Web address: www.gchealth.org
**Control:** County–Government, nonfederal **Service:** General Medical and Surgical

**Staffed Beds:** 10

**OSMOND—Pierce County**

★ **OSMOND GENERAL HOSPITAL (281347),** 402 North Maple Street, Zip 68765–0429, Mailing Address: P.O. Box 429, Zip 68765–0429; tel. 402/748–3393, (Nonreporting) **A**9 10 18
Primary Contact: Celine M. Mlady, Chief Executive Officer
CFO: Jodi Aschoff, Chief Financial Officer
CMO: David Mwebe, M.D., Chief of Staff
Web address: www.osmondhospital.com
**Control:** Other not–for–profit (including NFP Corporation) **Service:** General Medical and Surgical

**Staffed Beds:** 25

*Many Facility Codes have changed. Please refer to the AHA Guide Code Chart.* © 2012 AHA Guide

## PAPILLION—Sarpy County

⊠ **ALEGENT HEALTH–MIDLANDS HOSPITAL (280105)**, 11111 South 84th Street, Zip 68046–4122; tel. 402/593–3000 **A**1 2 9 10 **F**3 11 13 15 17 18 20 22 26 28 29 30 34 35 36 38 40 44 45 46 49 50 51 53 56 57 59 60 61 62 63 64 65 68 70 76 77 79 81 84 85 86 87 93 97 107 110 111 113 114 116 117 118 128 129 130 131 134 142 145 146 **P**6 8 **S** Alegent Health, Omaha, NE
Primary Contact: Kevin J. Nokels, FACHE, Vice President and Chief Operating Officer
COO: Kevin J. Nokels, FACHE, Vice President and Chief Operating Officer
CFO: Timothy Meier, Chief Financial Officer
CMO: Jeffrey Strohmyer, M.D., Chief Medical Officer
CIO: Kenneth Lawonn, Senior Vice President and Chief Information Officer
CHR: Nancy Wallace, Interim Senior Vice President Human Resources
Web address: www.alegent.org/midlands
**Control:** Church–operated, Nongovernment, not–for profit **Service:** General Medical and Surgical

**Staffed Beds:** 54 **Admissions:** 2192 **Census:** 19 **Outpatient Visits:** 70717 **Births:** 309 **Total Expense ($000):** 55528 **Payroll Expense ($000):** 16711 **Personnel:** 367

## PAWNEE CITY—Pawnee County

★ **PAWNEE COUNTY MEMORIAL HOSPITAL (281302)**, (Critical Access Hospital), 600 I Street, Zip 68420–3001, Mailing Address: P.O. Box 433, Zip 68420–0313; tel. 402/852–2231 **A**9 10 18 **F**15 18 28 30 31 34 40 43 45 57 59 65 75 77 79 82 93 97 102 107 110 113 118 126 129 131 132 134 146 **P**1
Primary Contact: James A. Kubik, Administrator
CHR: Jennifer Bartels, HR Director
CNO: Kris Meyer, R.N., Director of Nursing
**Control:** County–Government, nonfederal **Service:** General Medical and Surgical

**Staffed Beds:** 11 **Admissions:** 83 **Census:** 1 **Outpatient Visits:** 3758 **Births:** 0 **Total Expense ($000):** 6307 **Payroll Expense ($000):** 2462 **Personnel:** 63

## PENDER—Thurston County

★ **PENDER COMMUNITY HOSPITAL (281349)**, 100 Hospital Drive, Zip 68047–0100, Mailing Address: P.O. Box 100, Zip 68047–0100; tel. 402/385–3083, (Nonreporting) **A**9 10 18 **S** Trinity Health, Novi, MI
Primary Contact: Richard Thomason, FACHE, Chief Executive Officer
COO: Melissa Kelly, Chief Operating Officer
CFO: Melissa Kelly, Chief Financial Officer
CMO: Matt Timm, M.D., Medical Director
CIO: Teresa Heise, Coordinator Management Information Systems
CHR: Nancy Suhr, Manager Human Resources
CNO: Katie Peterson, R.N., Director of Nursing
Web address: www.pendercommunityhospital.com
**Control:** Hospital district or authority, Government, nonfederal **Service:** General Medical and Surgical

**Staffed Beds:** 67

## PLAINVIEW—Pierce County

**ALEGENT HEALTH PLAINVIEW HOSPITAL (281346)**, 704 North Third Street, Zip 68769, Mailing Address: P.O. Box 489, Zip 68769–0489; tel. 402/582–4245, (Nonreporting) **A**9 10 18 **S** Alegent Health, Omaha, NE
Primary Contact: Richard B. Gamel, Administrator
CFO: Rebecca Lambrecht, Manager Business Office and Chief Financial Officer
CMO: W. Brad Lockee, M.D., Chief of Staff
CHR: Diane Blair, Director Human Resources and Admissions
Web address: www.plainviewhealth.org
**Control:** Church–operated, Nongovernment, not–for profit **Service:** General Medical and Surgical

**Staffed Beds:** 16

## RED CLOUD—Webster County

**WEBSTER COUNTY COMMUNITY HOSPITAL (281316)**, Sixth Avenue and Franklin Street, Zip 68970–0465, Mailing Address: P.O. Box 465, Zip 68970–0465; tel. 402/746–5600, (Nonreporting) **A**9 10 18
Primary Contact: Marianna Harris, Administrator
CFO: Marcia Olson, Business Office Manager
CMO: Michele Durr, M.D., Medical Director
CIO: Eilleen Berry, Manager Information Technology
CHR: Marcia Olson, Business Office Manager
Web address: www.websterhospital.org
**Control:** County–Government, nonfederal **Service:** General Medical and Surgical

**Staffed Beds:** 16

## SAINT PAUL—Howard County

**HOWARD COUNTY COMMUNITY HOSPITAL** See Howard County Medical Center

★ **HOWARD COUNTY MEDICAL CENTER (281338)**, 1113 Sherman Street, Zip 68873–1536, Mailing Address: P.O. Box 406, Zip 68873–0406; tel. 308/754–4421 **A**9 10 18 **F**3 11 13 28 29 34 40 43 45 57 59 68 81 85 93 107 113 118 126 127 129 132 134 145
Primary Contact: Arlan D. Johnson, Chief Executive Officer
CFO: Thomas Parish, Chief Financial Officer
CMO: Jared Kramer, M.D., Chief of Staff
CIO: Kari Pierson, Manager
CHR: Shauna Graham, Director Human Resources
Web address: www.hcchmc.org
**Control:** County–Government, nonfederal **Service:** General Medical and Surgical

**Staffed Beds:** 25 **Admissions:** 348 **Census:** 7 **Outpatient Visits:** 22489 **Births:** 48 **Total Expense ($000):** 12897 **Payroll Expense ($000):** 6700

## SCHUYLER—Colfax County

★ **ALEGENT HEALTH–MEMORIAL HOSPITAL (281323)**, 104 West 17th Street, Zip 68661–1396; tel. 402/352–2441, (Nonreporting) **A**9 10 18 **S** Alegent Health, Omaha, NE
Primary Contact: Connie Peters, R.N., Operations Leader and Regional Health Administrator
CFO: Tim H. Schnack, Chief Financial Officer
CHR: Nancy Wallace, Vice President Human Resources
Web address: www.alegent.org
**Control:** Church–operated, Nongovernment, not–for profit **Service:** General Medical and Surgical

**Staffed Beds:** 25

## SCOTTSBLUFF—Scotts Bluff County

⊠ △ **REGIONAL WEST MEDICAL CENTER (280061)**, 4021 Avenue B, Zip 69361–4695; tel. 308/635–3711, (Total facility includes 18 beds in nursing home–type unit) **A**1 2 3 5 7 9 10 **F**8 11 12 14 15 17 28 29 30 40 43 45 47 62 64 65 68 69 70 72 74 76 77 78 81 85 89 90 92 93 98 107 108 110 111 113 114 118 119 120 127 128 129 145 146 147
Primary Contact: Todd Sorensen, M.D., Chief Executive Officer
CFO: David Griffiths, Vice President and Chief Financial Officer
CIO: Lisa Bewley, Vice President and Chief Information Officer
CHR: Steve Hodges, Vice President Human Resources
Web address: www.rwhs.org
**Control:** Other not–for–profit (including NFP Corporation) **Service:** General Medical and Surgical

**Staffed Beds:** 145 **Admissions:** 7271 **Census:** 85 **Outpatient Visits:** 351313 **Births:** 815 **Total Expense ($000):** 169978 **Payroll Expense ($000):** 60519 **Personnel:** 1146

## SEWARD—Seward County

★ **MEMORIAL HEALTH CARE SYSTEMS (281339)**, 300 North Columbia Avenue, Zip 68434–9907; tel. 402/643–2971 **A**9 10 18 **F**8 10 11 13 15 28 29 34 35 40 45 50 53 56 57 59 64 75 77 81 86 91 93 107 110 115 116 118 126 127 128 129 131 132 145 147 **P**6
Primary Contact: Roger J. Reamer, Chief Executive Officer
CFO: Greg Jerger, Chief Financial Officer
CMO: Tricia Sams, M.D., Medical Director
CIO: Carol Carlson, Director Marketing
Web address: www.mhcs.us
**Control:** Other not–for–profit (including NFP Corporation) **Service:** General Medical and Surgical

**Staffed Beds:** 36 **Admissions:** 790 **Census:** 15 **Outpatient Visits:** 29085 **Births:** 105 **Total Expense ($000):** 23061 **Payroll Expense ($000):** 11473 **Personnel:** 213

## SIDNEY—Cheyenne County

★ **SIDNEY REGIONAL MEDICAL CENTER (281357)**, 645 Osage Street, Zip 69162–1714; tel. 308/254–5825, (Nonreporting) **A**9 10 18
Primary Contact: Jason Petik, Chief Executive Officer
CFO: Kelly Utley, Chief Financial Officer
CMO: Mandy Shaw, M.D., Chief of Staff
Web address: www.sidneyrmc.com
**Control:** Other not–for–profit (including NFP Corporation) **Service:** General Medical and Surgical

**Staffed Beds:** 88

**NE**

## SUPERIOR—Nuckolls County

★ **BRODSTONE MEMORIAL HOSPITAL (281315)**, 520 East Tenth Street, Zip 68978–1225, Mailing Address: P.O. Box 187, Zip 68978–0187; tel. 402/879–3281, (Nonreporting) **A**9 10 18
Primary Contact: John E. Keelan, Administrator and Chief Executive Officer
COO: Dena C. Alvarez, R.N., COO & Chief Compliance Officer
CFO: Sandy Borden, Chief Financial Officer
CMO: Timothy Blecha, M.D., Medical Director
CIO: Tim Hiatt, Chief Information Officer
CHR: Jeremy Littrell, Director Human Resources
CNO: Kori Field, Director of Nursing
Web address: www.brodstonehospital.org
**Control:** Other not–for–profit (including NFP Corporation) **Service:** General Medical and Surgical

**Staffed Beds:** 25

## SYRACUSE—Otoe County

★ **COMMUNITY MEMORIAL HOSPITAL (281309)**, 1579 Midland Street, Zip 68446–9732, Mailing Address: P.O. Box N., Zip 68446–0518; tel. 402/269–2011 **A**9 10 18 **F**3 8 11 15 18 28 29 32 34 35 40 43 45 53 56 57 59 62 64 65 75 77 79 81 82 85 93 97 110 126 127 132 145 **P**6
Primary Contact: Michael Harvey, Chief Executive Officer
COO: Julie Werner, Chief Operating Officer
CFO: Michael Harvey, Chief Executive Officer
CFO: Jenn Seckinger, Chief Financial Officer
CMO: Zak Tempelmeyer, M.D., Chief Medical Staff
CIO: Matthew Steinblock, Systems Administrator
CHR: Karrie Beach, Director Human Resources
CNO: Pat Howell, Chief Nursing Officer
Web address: www.syracusecmh.org
**Control:** Hospital district or authority, Government, nonfederal **Service:** General Medical and Surgical

**Staffed Beds:** 10 **Admissions:** 120 **Census:** 1 **Outpatient Visits:** 13717 **Births:** 0 **Total Expense ($000):** 9558 **Payroll Expense ($000):** 4887 **Personnel:** 95

## TECUMSEH—Johnson County

★ **JOHNSON COUNTY HOSPITAL (281350)**, 202 High Street, Zip 68450–0599, Mailing Address: P.O. Box 599, Zip 68450–0599; tel. 402/335–3361, (Nonreporting) **A**9 10 18
Primary Contact: Diane Newman, Administrator
COO: Diane Newman, Administrator
CFO: Janice Oehm, Manager Business Office
CMO: Keith Shuey, M.D., Chief Medical Staff
CIO: Fred Pooch, Supervisor Information Technology
CHR: Susan Hessheimer, Director Human Resources
Web address: www.jchosp.com
**Control:** County–Government, nonfederal **Service:** General Medical and Surgical

**Staffed Beds:** 25

## TILDEN—Madison County

**TILDEN COMMUNITY HOSPITAL (281317)**, 308 West Second Street, Zip 68781–0340, Mailing Address: P.O. Box 340, Zip 68781–0340; tel. 402/368–5343, (Nonreporting) **A**9 10 18 **S** Faith Regional Health Services, Norfolk, NE
Primary Contact: Lon Knievel, Chief Executive Officer
CFO: Sarah Mitchell, Chief Financial Officer
CMO: Kelly Ellis, D.O., Chief Medical Officer
CIO: Sarah Mitchell, Chief Financial Officer
CHR: Lon Knievel, Chief Executive Officer
Web address: www.tildenhospital.org
**Control:** City–Government, nonfederal **Service:** General Medical and Surgical

**Staffed Beds:** 21

## VALENTINE—Cherry County

★ **CHERRY COUNTY HOSPITAL (281344)**, 510 North Green Street, Zip 69201–0410, Mailing Address: P.O. Box 410, Zip 69201–0410; tel. 402/376–2525, (Nonreporting) **A**5 9 10 18
Primary Contact: Brent A. Peterson, Administrator
CFO: Peggy Snell, Chief Finance Officer
**Control:** County–Government, nonfederal **Service:** General Medical and Surgical

**Staffed Beds:** 25

## WAHOO—Saunders County

★ **SAUNDERS MEDICAL CENTER (281307)**, 1760 County Road J., Zip 68066–4152; tel. 402/443–4191, (Nonreporting) **A**9 10 18
Primary Contact: Kenneth W. Archer, Chief Executive Officer
CMO: Leo L. Meduna, M.D., Chief Medical Officer
CIO: Carrie Stephens, Coordinator Information Systems
CHR: Karen Leise, Coordinator Human Resources
Web address: www.saundersmedicalcenter.com
**Control:** County–Government, nonfederal **Service:** General Medical and Surgical

**Staffed Beds:** 87

## WAYNE—Wayne County

★ **PROVIDENCE MEDICAL CENTER (281345)**, 1200 Providence Road, Zip 68787–1299; tel. 402/375–3800, (Nonreporting) **A**9 10 18
Primary Contact: H. Michael Hammond, Administrator
CFO: Dustin Peterson, Chief Financial Officer
CHR: Sonja Hunke, Director Human Resources
Web address: www.providencemedical.com
**Control:** Other not–for–profit (including NFP Corporation) **Service:** General Medical and Surgical

**Staffed Beds:** 25

## WEST POINT—Cuming County

★ **ST. FRANCIS MEMORIAL HOSPITAL (281322)**, 430 North Monitor Street, Zip 68788–1555; tel. 402/372–2404, (Total facility includes 63 beds in nursing home–type unit) **A**9 10 18 **F**3 6 11 13 15 28 29 30 31 34 35 40 43 45 53 57 59 62 63 64 68 75 76 77 78 79 81 82 85 86 90 92 93 94 98 99 100 103 107 111 113 118 126 127 129 130 131 132 134 145 146 147 **P**6
**S** Franciscan Sisters of Christian Charity Sponsored Ministries, Inc., Manitowoc, WI
Primary Contact: Ronald O. Briggs, FACHE, President and Chief Executive Officer
CFO: Dennis Dinslage, Vice President Finance and Chief Financial Officer
CMO: Scott Green, M.D., Chief of Staff
CIO: Jean Meiergerd, Chief Information Officer
CHR: Terri Ridder, Director Human Resources
Web address: www.fcswp.org
**Control:** Church–operated, Nongovernment, not–for profit **Service:** General Medical and Surgical

**Staffed Beds:** 92 **Admissions:** 574 **Census:** 67 **Outpatient Visits:** 67310 **Births:** 59 **Total Expense ($000):** 22386 **Payroll Expense ($000):** 11538 **Personnel:** 208

## WINNEBAGO—Thurston County

☐ **U. S. PUBLIC HEALTH SERVICE INDIAN HOSPITAL (280119)**, Highway 7577, Zip 68071; tel. 402/878–2231, (Nonreporting) **A**1 9 10 **S** U. S. Indian Health Service, Rockville, MD
Primary Contact: Sheriann Moore, Service Unit Director
CFO: Audrey Parker, Budget Analyst
Web address: www.ihs.gov
**Control:** PHS, Indian Service, Government, federal **Service:** General Medical and Surgical

**Staffed Beds:** 30

## YORK—York County

★ **YORK GENERAL HOSPITAL (281336)**, 2222 North Lincoln Avenue, Zip 68467–1095; tel. 402/362–6671, (Total facility includes 129 beds in nursing home–type unit) **A**9 10 18 **F**3 10 11 12 13 15 28 29 31 34 35 40 45 53 56 57 59 60 62 64 68 70 75 76 77 78 79 81 82 85 86 87 89 93 96 107 108 110 111 114 116 117 118 124 127 128 129 130 131 132 144 145 147
Primary Contact: Charles K. Schulz, Chief Executive Officer
COO: Jane Thompson, Administrator and Chief Operating Officer
CFO: Bob McQuistan, Vice President Finance
CMO: Daniel Growney, M.D., Chief of Staff
CIO: John Temple, Director Information Systems
CHR: Cathy Norquest, Director Human Resources
CNO: Jenny Obermier, VP, Director of Nursing
Web address: www.yorkgeneral.org
**Control:** Other not–for–profit (including NFP Corporation) **Service:** General Medical and Surgical

**Staffed Beds:** 154 **Admissions:** 1078 **Census:** 118 **Outpatient Visits:** 42916 **Births:** 123 **Total Expense ($000):** 35239 **Payroll Expense ($000):** 16528 **Personnel:** 389

NE

*Many Facility Codes have changed. Please refer to the AHA Guide Code Chart.*   © 2012 AHA Guide

# NEVADA

## BATTLE MOUNTAIN—Lander County

**BATTLE MOUNTAIN GENERAL HOSPITAL (291303)**, 535 South Humboldt Street, Zip 89820–1988; tel. 775/635–2550, (Nonreporting) **A**9 10 18
Primary Contact: Philip S. Hanna, Administrator
CFO: Cindy Fagg, Fiscal Officer
CMO: George Mardini, M.D., Chief of Staff
CIO: Terry Dunn, Director Information Technology
CHR: Lori Sherbondy, Director Human Resources
Web address: www.bmgh.org
**Control:** Hospital district or authority, Government, nonfederal **Service:** General Medical and Surgical

| Staffed Beds: 7 |
| --- |

## BOULDER CITY—Clark County

**BOULDER CITY HOSPITAL (291309)**, 901 Adams Boulevard, Zip 89005–2213; tel. 702/293–4111, (Total facility includes 39 beds in nursing home–type unit) **A**9 10 18 **F**1 29 34 40 57 62 70 93 105 107 111 118 129 132 145
Primary Contact: Tom Maher, Chief Executive Officer and Administrator
COO: Craig Bailey, MS, Chief Operating Officer
CFO: Frey Belete, Controller
CMO: Jim Chiang, M.D., Chief of Staff
CIO: Scott Brooks, Manager Information Technology
CHR: Dianna Todd, Director Human Resources
Web address: www.bouldercityhospital.org
**Control:** Other not–for–profit (including NFP Corporation) **Service:** General Medical and Surgical

| Staffed Beds: 63 Admissions: 443 Census: 38 Outpatient Visits: 16442 Births: 0 Total Expense ($000): 15332 Payroll Expense ($000): 8208 Personnel: 169 |
| --- |

## CALIENTE—Lincoln County

**GROVER C. DILS MEDICAL CENTER (291311)**, 700 North Spring Street, Zip 89008, Mailing Address: P.O. Box 1010, Zip 89008–1010; tel. 775/726–3171, (Nonreporting) **A**9 10 18
Primary Contact: Jason Bleak, Administrator and Chief Executive Officer
COO: Jason Bleak, Administrator and Chief Executive Officer
CFO: Sherlyn Fackrell, Finance Controller
CMO: R. William Katschke, Jr., M.D., Medical Director
CHR: Rozanne Mangum, Administrative Assistant and Director Human Resources
Web address: www.dilsmedicalcenter.org
**Control:** Other not–for–profit (including NFP Corporation) **Service:** Other specialty

| Staffed Beds: 20 |
| --- |

## CARSON CITY—Carson City County

**CARSON TAHOE CONTINUING CARE HOSPITAL (292008)**, 775 Fleischmann Way, 2nd Floor, Zip 89703; tel. 775/445–7795, (Nonreporting) **A**9 10
Primary Contact: Neal Duncan, Chief Executive Officer
Web address: www.carsontahoe.com
**Control:** Other not–for–profit (including NFP Corporation) **Service:** Long–Term Acute Care hospital

| Staffed Beds: 29 |
| --- |

☒ **CARSON TAHOE REGIONAL HEALTHCARE (290019)**, 1600 Medical Parkway, Zip 89703, Mailing Address: P.O. Box 2168, Zip 89702–2168; tel. 775/445–8672 **A**1 2 9 10 **F**3 4 5 8 11 13 15 17 18 20 22 24 28 29 30 31 34 35 38 40 42 48 49 57 59 64 65 68 70 74 75 76 77 78 79 81 85 86 87 89 90 91 93 98 99 100 101 102 103 104 105 107 108 111 113 118 119 120 122 123 129 131 134 143 145 146 147
Primary Contact: Edward L. Epperson, Chief Executive Officer
COO: Douglas Self, Chief Operating Officer
CFO: Ann Beck, Vice President Finance
CMO: Jeffrey Sanders, M.D., Chief of Staff
CIO: Cheri Glockner, Director Development
CHR: Carie Wilkens, Director of Human Resources
CNO: Cathy Dinauer, MSN, VP of Patient Care
Web address: www.carsontahoe.com
**Control:** Other not–for–profit (including NFP Corporation) **Service:** General Medical and Surgical

| Staffed Beds: 184 Admissions: 10157 Census: 123 Outpatient Visits: 193376 Births: 832 Total Expense ($000): 180367 Payroll Expense ($000): 70176 Personnel: 1073 |
| --- |

☐ **SIERRA SURGERY HOSPITAL (290051)**, 1400 Medical Parkway, Zip 89703; tel. 775/883–1700 **A**1 9 10 **F**3 15 29 34 39 51 64 65 68 79 81 82 85 107 110 111 118 144
Primary Contact: James R. Sergeant, Chief Executive Officer
CFO: Sheryl Hayden, Chief Financial Officer
Web address: www.sierrasurgery.com
**Control:** Partnership, Investor–owned, for–profit **Service:** Surgical

| Staffed Beds: 15 Admissions: 768 Census: 6 Outpatient Visits: 20077 Births: 0 Total Expense ($000): 30973 Payroll Expense ($000): 10047 Personnel: 144 |
| --- |

## ELKO—Elko County

☒ **NORTHEASTERN NEVADA REGIONAL HOSPITAL (290008)**, 2001 Errecart Boulevard, Zip 89801–3499; tel. 775/738–5151 **A**1 9 10 20 **F**3 8 11 13 15 18 20 29 30 31 34 35 40 44 45 50 57 59 64 65 68 75 76 77 78 79 81 82 85 86 87 89 93 103 107 108 110 111 114 118 128 131 134 147 **P**2 **S** LifePoint Hospitals, Inc., Brentwood, TN
Primary Contact: Gene Miller, Chief Executive Officer
COO: Ann Cariker, Chief Operating Officer
CFO: Grant Trollope, Chief Financial Officer
CIO: Jeff Morgan, Director Information Systems
CHR: Angela Chaffin, Director Human Resources
CNO: Dona E. Townsend, Chief Nursing Officer
Web address: www.nnrhospital.com
**Control:** Corporation, Investor–owned, for–profit **Service:** General Medical and Surgical

| Staffed Beds: 50 Admissions: 2450 Census: 18 Outpatient Visits: 51574 Births: 593 Total Expense ($000): 29124 Payroll Expense ($000): 16139 Personnel: 266 |
| --- |

## ELY—White Pine County

☒ **WILLIAM BEE RIRIE HOSPITAL (291302)**, 1500 Avenue H, Zip 89301–2699; tel. 775/289–3001 **A**1 9 10 18 **F**8 13 15 29 31 32 35 40 44 45 50 57 64 65 66 68 75 76 77 79 81 82 85 86 87 89 93 107 108 111 113 118 126 128 132 134 **P**6
Primary Contact: Jan Jensen, R.N., Chief Executive Officer and Administrator
CMO: G. N. Christensen, M.D., Chief Medical Officer
CIO: Destin Brandis, Chief Information Officer
CHR: Vicki Pereace, Manager Human Resources
Web address: www.elynevadahospital.org
**Control:** Hospital district or authority, Government, nonfederal **Service:** General Medical and Surgical

| Staffed Beds: 12 Admissions: 603 Census: 5 Outpatient Visits: 33718 Births: 88 Total Expense ($000): 25219 Payroll Expense ($000): 12582 Personnel: 92 |
| --- |

## FALLON—Churchill County

☒ **BANNER CHURCHILL COMMUNITY HOSPITAL (290006)**, 801 East Williams Avenue, Zip 89406–3052; tel. 775/867–7000 **A**1 9 10 20 **F**3 7 11 13 15 26 27 29 30 31 34 35 40 45 47 50 57 59 65 68 70 75 76 77 78 79 81 85 86 87 93 97 107 108 110 111 113 117 118 129 145 147 **P**6 **S** Banner Health, Phoenix, AZ
Primary Contact: John D'Angelo, Chief Executive Officer
CFO: Steven Fraker, Chief Financial Officer
CMO: Sukhbir Pannce, M.D., Chief Medical Officer
Web address: www.bannerhealth.com
**Control:** Other not–for–profit (including NFP Corporation) **Service:** General Medical and Surgical

| Staffed Beds: 40 Admissions: 2084 Census: 19 Outpatient Visits: 105828 Births: 391 Total Expense ($000): 41748 Payroll Expense ($000): 18445 Personnel: 287 |
| --- |

**NV**

---

**Hospital, Medicare Provider Number, Address, Telephone, Approval, Facility, and Physician Codes, Health Care System**

★ American Hospital Association (AHA) membership
☐ The Joint Commission accreditation          ◇ DNV Healthcare Inc. accreditation

○ American Osteopathic Association (AOA) accreditation
△ Commission on Accreditation of Rehabilitation Facilities (CARF) accreditation

---

### GARDNERVILLE—Douglas County

★ **CARSON VALLEY MEDICAL CENTER (291306)**, 1107 Highway 395,
Zip 89410; tel. 775/782–1600 **A**9 10 18 **F**11 15 29 31 34 35 40 45 47 48 50
53 54 56 57 59 60 64 68 70 75 77 79 81 93 103 107 108 110 111 114 117
118 126 128 129 131 132 134 143 145 147
Primary Contact: William R. Hale, Administrator
CFO: Marcus Armstrong, Chief Financial Officer
CNO: Linda Rowe, R.N., Chief Nursing Officer
Web address: www.carsonvalleymedicalcenter.com
**Control:** Other not–for–profit (including NFP Corporation) **Service:** General
Medical and Surgical

**Staffed Beds:** 23 **Admissions:** 813 **Census:** 8 **Outpatient Visits:** 114419
**Births:** 0 **Total Expense ($000):** 37029 **Payroll Expense ($000):** 13751
**Personnel:** 239

### HAWTHORNE—Mineral County

**MOUNT GRANT GENERAL HOSPITAL (291300)**, First and A Street,
Zip 89415, Mailing Address: P.O. Box 1510, Zip 89415–1510;
tel. 775/945–2461, (Nonreporting) **A**9 10 18
Primary Contact: Richard Munger, Administrator
Web address: www.mtgrantgenhospital.org/
**Control:** Other not–for–profit (including NFP Corporation) **Service:** General
Medical and Surgical

**Staffed Beds:** 11

### HENDERSON—Clark County

☒ **HEALTHSOUTH REHABILITATION HOSPITAL – HENDERSON (293032)**,
10301 Jeffreys Street, Zip 89052; tel. 702/939–9400, (Nonreporting) **A**1 10
**S** HEALTHSOUTH Corporation, Birmingham, AL
Primary Contact: Robert Bollard, Interim Chief Executive Officer
CFO: Robert Bollard, Chief Financial Officer
Web address: www.hendersonrehabhospital.com
**Control:** Corporation, Investor–owned, for–profit **Service:** Rehabilitation

**Staffed Beds:** 70

**SEVEN HILLS BEHAVIORAL INSTITUTE (294012)**, 3021 West Horizon Ridge
Parkway, Zip 89052–3990; tel. 702/646–5000, (Nonreporting) **S** Acadia
Healthcare Company, Inc., Franklin, TN
Primary Contact: John Hull, Chief Executive Officer
CMO: Keith Breiland, M.D., Medical Director
**Control:** Corporation, Investor–owned, for–profit **Service:** Psychiatric

**Staffed Beds:** 58

☒ **ST. ROSE DOMINICAN HOSPITALS – ROSE DE LIMA CAMPUS (290012)**,
102 East Lake Mead Parkway, Zip 89015–5524; tel. 702/616–5000 **A**1 9 10 **F**3
8 12 15 18 20 28 29 30 31 32 34 35 38 40 44 45 49 50 54 57 59 62 63 64
65 68 70 74 75 77 78 79 81 82 84 85 86 87 90 93 102 107 108 111 113
118 129 130 131 134 145 146 147 **S** Dignity Health, San Francisco, CA
Primary Contact: Allan M. Spooner, Interim President and Chief Executive Officer
COO: Teressa Conley, Vice President and Chief Operating Officer
CFO: Kevin Walters, Chief Financial Officer
CMO: Stephen K. Jones, M.D., Vice President Medical Staff Affairs
CIO: Sharon Hester, Site Manager Information Technology
Web address: www.strosecares.com
**Control:** Church–operated, Nongovernment, not–for profit **Service:** General
Medical and Surgical

**Staffed Beds:** 129 **Admissions:** 7161 **Census:** 90 **Outpatient Visits:** 42337
**Births:** 0 **Total Expense ($000):** 126157 **Payroll Expense ($000):** 57988
**Personnel:** 725

☒ **ST. ROSE DOMINICAN HOSPITALS – SIENA CAMPUS (290045)**, 3001 St.
Rose Parkway, Zip 89052; tel. 702/616–5000 **A**1 5 9 10 **F**3 7 13 15 18 20 21
22 23 24 26 28 29 30 31 32 34 35 38 40 41 43 44 45 50 54 57 59 60 64
68 70 72 74 75 76 77 78 79 81 82 83 84 85 86 87 88 89 93 102 107 108
110 111 113 114 118 125 129 130 131 133 134 145 146 147 **S** Dignity
Health, San Francisco, CA
Primary Contact: Rod A. Davis, FACHE, President and Chief Executive Officer
COO: Teressa Conley, Chief Operating Officer
CFO: Kevin Walters, Chief Financial Officer
CMO: Stephen K. Jones, M.D., Vice President Medical Staff Affairs
CIO: Sharon Hester, Site Manager Information Technology
CHR: LeRoy Walker, Vice President Human Resources
Web address: www.strosehospitals.com
**Control:** Church–operated, Nongovernment, not–for profit **Service:** General
Medical and Surgical

**Staffed Beds:** 219 **Admissions:** 17952 **Census:** 202 **Outpatient Visits:**
68991 **Births:** 3541 **Total Expense ($000):** 275013 **Payroll Expense**
**($000):** 119131 **Personnel:** 1515

### INCLINE VILLAGE—Washoe County

○ **INCLINE VILLAGE COMMUNITY HOSPITAL (291301)**, 880 Alder Avenue,
Zip 89450; tel. 775/833–4100, (Nonreporting) **A**5 9 10 11 18 **S** Tahoe Forest
Health System, Truckee, CA
Primary Contact: Judy Newland, R.N., Director
COO: Virginia Razo, Chief Operating Officer
CFO: Crystal Betts, Chief Financial Officer
CIO: Mark Griffiths, Director Management Information Systems
CHR: Jayne O'Flanagan, Director Human Resources
Web address: www.tfhd.com
**Control:** State–Government, nonfederal **Service:** General Medical and Surgical

**Staffed Beds:** 6

### LAS VEGAS—Clark County

☐ **CENTENNIAL HILLS HOSPITAL MEDICAL CENTER (290054)**, 6900 North
Durango Drive, Zip 89148; tel. 702/835–9700 **A**1 9 10 **F**3 11 13 15 20 22 26
29 30 34 35 38 40 45 46 49 50 57 59 60 64 65 68 70 73 75 76 77 79 81
85 107 108 110 111 112 113 114 118 123 129 145 146 **S** Universal Health
Services, Inc., King of Prussia, PA
Primary Contact: Sajit Pullarkat, Chief Executive Officer and Managing Director
Web address: www.centennialhillshospital.com
**Control:** Corporation, Investor–owned, for–profit **Service:** General Medical and
Surgical

**Staffed Beds:** 171 **Admissions:** 9192 **Census:** 97 **Outpatient Visits:** 50908
**Births:** 1453

☒ **COMPLEX CARE HOSPITAL AT TENAYA (292006)**, 2500 North Tenaya,
Zip 89128; tel. 702/562–2021, (Data for 153 days) **A**1 10 **F**1 29 60 82 84 91
118 147 **P**5 **S** LifeCare Management Services, Plano, TX
Primary Contact: Timothy C. Deaton, Administrator
CFO: Deborah Gerke, Chief Financial Officer
CMO: C. Dean Milne, D.O., Medical Director
CIO: Lynn Tunson, Manager Medical Records
CHR: Debra Tafoya, Director Human Resources
Web address: www.lifecare–hospitals.com
**Control:** Corporation, Investor–owned, for–profit **Service:** Long–Term Acute Care
hospital

**Staffed Beds:** 70 **Admissions:** 303 **Census:** 54 **Outpatient Visits:** 0 **Births:**
0 **Total Expense ($000):** 11154 **Payroll Expense ($000):** 4834 **Personnel:**
193

☐ **DESERT SPRINGS HOSPITAL MEDICAL CENTER (290022)**, 2075 East
Flamingo Road, Zip 89119–5121; tel. 702/733–8800, (Nonreporting) **A**1 9 10
**S** Universal Health Services, Inc., King of Prussia, PA
Primary Contact: Samuel Kaufman, Chief Executive Officer and Managing Director
CFO: Lynn Kennington, Chief Financial Officer
CMO: Adel R. Shehata, M.D., Medical Director
CIO: Tom Schoenig, System Director Information Services
CHR: Shirley A. Shadwick, Administrator Human Resources
Web address: www.desertspringshospital.net
**Control:** Corporation, Investor–owned, for–profit **Service:** General Medical and
Surgical

**Staffed Beds:** 346

**DESERT WILLOW TREATMENT CENTER**, 6171 West Charleston Boulevard,
Zip 89146; tel. 702/486–8900, (Nonreporting) **A**3 5
Primary Contact: Linda Santangelo, Ph.D., Director
**Control:** State–Government, nonfederal **Service:** Psychiatric

**Staffed Beds:** 58

**HARMON MEDICAL AND REHABILITATION HOSPITAL (290042)**, 2170 East
Harmon Avenue, Zip 89119; tel. 702/794–0100, (Nonreporting) **A**10
**S** Fundamental Long Term Care Holdings, LLC, Sparks Glencoe, MD
Primary Contact: Bonnie Essex Hillegass, Chief Executive Officer
**Control:** Corporation, Investor–owned, for–profit **Service:** Rehabilitation

**Staffed Beds:** 118

★ **HEALTHSOUTH DESERT CANYON REHABILITATION HOSPITAL (293033)**,
9175 West Oquendo Road, Zip 89148–1234; tel. 702/252–7342 **A**10 **F**3 29 77
79 90 91 93 **S** HEALTHSOUTH Corporation, Birmingham, AL
Primary Contact: Deanna Martin, MSN, Chief Executive Officer
Web address: www.healthsouthdesertcanyon.com
**Control:** Corporation, Investor–owned, for–profit **Service:** Rehabilitation

**Staffed Beds:** 50 **Admissions:** 997 **Census:** 36 **Outpatient Visits:** 2242
**Births:** 0 **Total Expense ($000):** 14437 **Payroll Expense ($000):** 6823
**Personnel:** 107

**NV**

✠ **HEALTHSOUTH REHABILITATION HOSPITAL–LAS VEGAS (293026)**, 1250 South Valley View Boulevard, Zip 89102–1861; tel. 702/877–8898 **A**1 10 **F**3 28 29 57 68 74 75 77 79 90 93 95 96 129 147 **S** HEALTHSOUTH Corporation, Birmingham, AL
Primary Contact: Josh D. Luke, Ph.D., FACHE, Chief Executive Officer
CFO: Sherilene DeLeon, Controller
CMO: Farzin Farhang, M.D., Medical Director
CHR: Gina Lewis, Director Human Resources
CNO: Elizabeth Solomon, R.N., Regional Quality/Risk Director and Interim Chief Nursing Officer
Web address: www.healthsouthlasvegas.com
**Control:** Corporation, Investor–owned, for–profit **Service:** Rehabilitation

**Staffed Beds: 79 Admissions: 1870 Census: 60 Outpatient Visits: 0 Births: 0 Total Expense ($000): 18071 Payroll Expense ($000): 10440 Personnel: 244**

☐ **HORIZON SPECIALTY HOSPITAL (292003)**, 640 Desert Lane, Zip 89106; tel. 702/382–3155 **A**1 9 10 **F**1 12 28 29 60 118 129 147 **S** Fundamental Long Term Care Holdings, LLC, Sparks Glencoe, MD
Primary Contact: Dave Tupper, Chief Executive Officer and Administrator
CFO: Darnell Bennett, Director Finance
CMO: Syed Rahman, M.D., Chief of Staff
CIO: Azena Ansi, Manager Health Information Management
CHR: Melvin Layugan, Director Human Resources
**Control:** Corporation, Investor–owned, for–profit **Service:** Long–Term Acute Care hospital

**Staffed Beds: 53 Admissions: 503 Census: 38 Outpatient Visits: 0 Births: 0 Total Expense ($000): 13178 Payroll Expense ($000): 4818 Personnel: 89**

**KINDRED HOSPITAL LAS VEGAS, DESERT SPRINGS CAMPUS** See Kindred Hospital Las Vegas–Sahara

✠ **KINDRED HOSPITAL LAS VEGAS–SAHARA (292002)**, 5110 West Sahara Avenue, Zip 89146–3406; tel. 702/871–1418, (Includes KINDRED HOSPITAL LAS VEGAS, DESERT SPRINGS CAMPUS, 2075 East Flamingo Road, Suite 114, Zip 89119; tel. 702/894–5728; KINDRED HOSPITAL–FLAMINGO, 2250 East Flamingo Road, Zip 89119; tel. 702/871–1418), (Nonreporting) **A**1 9 10 **S** Kindred Healthcare, Louisville, KY
Primary Contact: Christie Bond–Carafelli, Chief Executive Officer
CFO: William Lysaght, Chief Financial Officer
CMO: Paul Stewart, M.D., Medical Director
CHR: Jim Sturgeon, Area Director Human Resources
Web address: www.kindredhospitallvs.com/
**Control:** Corporation, Investor–owned, for–profit **Service:** Long–Term Acute Care hospital

**Staffed Beds: 238**

☐ **MONTEVISTA HOSPITAL (294009)**, 5900 West Rochelle Avenue, Zip 89103–3327; tel. 702/364–1111 **A**1 9 10 **F**5 98 99 102 103 104 105 129 **S** Strategic Behavioral Health, LLC, Memphis, TN
Primary Contact: Robert E. Marshall, Chief Executive Officer
CFO: Ben Winbery, Chief Financial Officer
CMO: William Bauer, M.D., Medical Director
CHR: Carol Nelson, Director Human Resources
Web address: www.montevistahospital.com
**Control:** Corporation, Investor–owned, for–profit **Service:** Psychiatric

**Staffed Beds: 80 Admissions: 3099 Census: 70 Outpatient Visits: 13118 Total Expense ($000): 15504 Payroll Expense ($000): 9188 Personnel: 205**

✠ **MOUNTAINVIEW HOSPITAL (290039)**, 3100 North Tenaya Way, Zip 89128–0436; tel. 702/255–5000 **A**1 5 9 10 **F**3 11 12 13 15 18 20 22 24 26 28 29 31 34 35 40 45 46 47 48 49 50 57 59 70 73 75 76 77 78 79 81 85 86 90 93 107 108 111 112 113 114 118 125 128 129 145 146 **P**1 **S** HCA, Nashville, TN
Primary Contact: William Wagnon, Chief Executive Officer
COO: J. D. Melchiode, Chief Operating Officer
CFO: Lana Arad, Chief Financial Officer
CMO: Jack Collier, M.D., Chief of Staff
CHR: Robert Nettles, Director Human Resources
Web address: www.mountainview–hospital.com
**Control:** Corporation, Investor–owned, for–profit **Service:** General Medical and Surgical

**Staffed Beds: 235 Admissions: 16300 Census: 199**

☐ **PROGRESSIVE HOSPITAL (292007)**, 4015 South McLeod Drive, Zip 89121; tel. 702/433–2200 **A**9 10 **F**1 29 30 85 91 129 147 **P**5
Primary Contact: Rosemary Thiele, Chief Executive Officer
Web address: www.progressivehospital.com/
**Control:** Partnership, Investor–owned, for–profit **Service:** Long–Term Acute Care hospital

**Staffed Beds: 24 Admissions: 190 Census: 13 Outpatient Visits: 0 Births: 0 Total Expense ($000): 6521 Payroll Expense ($000): 2889**

☐ **RED ROCK BEHAVIORAL HOSPITAL (294008)**, 5975 West Twain Avenue, Zip 89103–1237; tel. 702/214–8099 **A**1 9 10 **F**98 **S** Strategic Behavioral Health, LLC, Memphis, TN
Primary Contact: Bob Mash, Chief Executive Officer
Web address: www.redrockhospital.com
**Control:** Other not–for–profit (including NFP Corporation) **Service:** Psychiatric

**Staffed Beds: 21 Admissions: 520 Census: 17 Total Expense ($000): 3413 Payroll Expense ($000): 1946 Personnel: 51**

**REHABILITATION INSTITUTES OF NEVADA**, 1316 Eagle Meadow Court, Zip 89123; tel. 702/434–4444, (Nonreporting)
Primary Contact: Christopher A. Vito, President and Chief Executive Officer
**Control:** Corporation, Investor–owned, for–profit **Service:** Rehabilitation

**Staffed Beds: 25**

✠ **SOUTHERN HILLS HOSPITAL AND MEDICAL CENTER (290047)**, 9300 West Sunset Road, Zip 89148; tel. 702/880–2100 **A**1 9 10 **F**3 13 15 17 18 20 22 26 29 40 45 57 59 68 70 72 74 75 76 77 78 79 81 85 87 98 107 108 109 110 111 113 118 129 134 145 146 **P**5 **S** HCA, Nashville, TN
Primary Contact: Kimball Anderson, FACHE, Chief Executive Officer
COO: Andrea Davis, Assistant Administrator
CFO: Michael Herron, Chief Financial Officer
CIO: Joe Grandiosi, Director Information Technology
CHR: Tim Black, Director Human Resources
CNO: Natalie Ransom, Chief Nursing Officer
Web address: www.southernhillshospital.com
**Control:** Corporation, Investor–owned, for–profit **Service:** General Medical and Surgical

**Staffed Beds: 134 Admissions: 6368 Census: 68 Outpatient Visits: 22282 Births: 1387 Total Expense ($000): 84691 Payroll Expense ($000): 33554**

☐ **SOUTHERN NEVADA ADULT MENTAL HEALTH SERVICES (294002)**, 6161 West Charleston Boulevard, Zip 89146; tel. 702/486–6000 **A**1 3 5 10 **F**56 98 101 102 103 104 106
Primary Contact: James Northrop, Director
Web address: www.mhds.state.nv.us
**Control:** State–Government, nonfederal **Service:** Psychiatric

**Staffed Beds: 190 Admissions: 2959 Census: 157 Outpatient Visits: 50751 Births: 0 Total Expense ($000): 84985 Payroll Expense ($000): 38142 Personnel: 609**

☐ **SPRING MOUNTAIN SAHARA (294010)**, 5460 West Sahara, Zip 89146; tel. 702/216–8900 **A**1 9 10 **F**29 56 64 98 103 104 129 **S** Universal Health Services, Inc., King of Prussia, PA
Primary Contact: Darryl S. Dubroca, Chief Executive Officer and Managing Director
Web address: www.springmountainsahara.com
**Control:** Corporation, Investor–owned, for–profit **Service:** Psychiatric

**Staffed Beds: 30 Admissions: 782 Census: 23 Outpatient Visits: 1889 Births: 0 Total Expense ($000): 4412 Payroll Expense ($000): 2690 Personnel: 47**

☐ **SPRING MOUNTAIN TREATMENT CENTER (294011)**, 7000 West Spring Mountain Road, Zip 89117; tel. 702/873–2400 **A**1 9 10 **F**29 98 99 105 129 **S** Universal Health Services, Inc., King of Prussia, PA
Primary Contact: Darryl S. Dubroca, Chief Executive Officer and Managing Director
Web address: www.healthsouth.com
**Control:** Corporation, Investor–owned, for–profit **Service:** Psychiatric

**Staffed Beds: 82 Admissions: 2449 Census: 68 Outpatient Visits: 2189 Births: 0 Total Expense ($000): 11999 Payroll Expense ($000): 6710 Personnel: 162**

NV

---

**Hospital, Medicare Provider Number, Address, Telephone, Approval, Facility, and Physician Codes, Health Care System**

★ American Hospital Association (AHA) membership
☐ The Joint Commission accreditation
◇ DNV Healthcare Inc. accreditation
○ American Osteopathic Association (AOA) accreditation
△ Commission on Accreditation of Rehabilitation Facilities (CARF) accreditation

☐ **SPRING VALLEY HOSPITAL MEDICAL CENTER (290046)**, 5400 South Rainbow Boulevard, Zip 89118; tel. 702/853–3000, (Nonreporting) **A**1 9 10 **S** Universal Health Services, Inc., King of Prussia, PA
Primary Contact: Leonard Freehof, Chief Executive Officer and Managing Director
COO: Mason VanHouweling, Chief Operating Officer
CFO: Leanne Shields, Chief Financial Officer
CMO: Dan McBride, M.D., Chief of Staff
CHR: Angelique Davison, Administrator Human Resources
Web address: www.springvalleyhospital.com
**Control:** Corporation, Investor–owned, for–profit **Service:** General Medical and Surgical

**Staffed Beds:** 169

☒ **ST. ROSE DOMINICAN HOSPITALS – SAN MARTIN CAMPUS (290053)**, 8280 West Warm Springs Road, Zip 89113; tel. 702/492–8000 **A**1 9 10 **F**3 7 8 13 15 18 20 22 24 26 28 29 30 31 32 34 35 38 40 44 45 47 49 50 57 59 60 64 68 70 73 74 75 76 77 78 79 80 81 82 84 85 86 87 93 102 107 108 110 111 114 118 129 130 131 134 145 146 147 **S** Dignity Health, San Francisco, CA
Primary Contact: Victoria J. VanMeetren, President
COO: Teressa Conley, Chief Operating Officer
CFO: Kevin Walters, Chief Financial Officer
CMO: Stephen K. Jones, M.D., Chief Medical Officer
CIO: Sharon Hester, Site Manager Information Technology
CHR: LeRoy Walker, Vice President Human Resources
Web address: www.strosehospitals.org
**Control:** Church–operated, Nongovernment, not–for profit **Service:** General Medical and Surgical

**Staffed Beds:** 147 **Admissions:** 9129 **Census:** 97 **Outpatient Visits:** 31567 **Births:** 971 **Total Expense ($000):** 161092 **Payroll Expense ($000):** 59295 **Personnel:** 681

☐ **SUMMERLIN HOSPITAL MEDICAL CENTER (290041)**, 657 Town Center Drive, Zip 89144; tel. 702/233–7000, (Nonreporting) **A**1 9 10 **S** Universal Health Services, Inc., King of Prussia, PA
Primary Contact: Robert S. Freymuller, Chief Executive Officer
CFO: Vanessa Kochevar, Chief Financial Officer
Web address: www.summerlinhospital.org
**Control:** Corporation, Investor–owned, for–profit **Service:** General Medical and Surgical

**Staffed Beds:** 148

☒ △ **SUNRISE HOSPITAL AND MEDICAL CENTER (290003)**, 3186 Maryland Parkway, Zip 89109–2306, Mailing Address: P.O. Box 98530, Zip 89193–8530; tel. 702/731–8000, (Includes SUNRISE CHILDREN'S HOSPITAL ) **A**1 2 3 5 7 9 10 **F**3 12 13 15 17 18 19 20 21 22 23 24 25 26 27 29 30 31 34 35 39 40 41 43 45 46 49 57 58 59 60 61 64 65 68 70 72 74 75 76 77 78 79 81 82 83 85 88 89 90 92 107 108 110 111 113 114 115 116 117 118 123 125 128 129 131 134 145 146 147 **S** HCA, Nashville, TN
Primary Contact: Todd Sklamberg, President
CFO: Daniel Perritt, Chief Financial Officer
CMO: Katherine Keeley, M.D., Chief of Staff
CIO: Alan Burt, Director Information Services
Web address: www.sunrisehospital.com
**Control:** Corporation, Investor–owned, for–profit **Service:** General Medical and Surgical

**Staffed Beds:** 592 **Admissions:** 28676 **Census:** 431 **Outpatient Visits:** 160885 **Births:** 4121 **Total Expense ($000):** 442098 **Payroll Expense ($000):** 181789 **Personnel:** 2403

☒ **UNIVERSITY MEDICAL CENTER (290007)**, 1800 West Charleston Boulevard, Zip 89102–2386; tel. 702/383–2000 **A**1 2 3 5 8 9 10 **F**3 12 13 15 16 17 18 19 20 21 22 23 24 26 27 28 29 30 31 32 34 35 40 41 43 44 45 46 47 48 49 50 54 55 57 58 59 60 61 64 65 66 67 68 70 72 73 74 75 76 77 78 79 81 82 83 85 87 88 89 92 93 107 111 112 113 114 117 118 129 131 137 140 143 145 146 147 **P**1 8
Primary Contact: Brian G. Brannman, Chief Executive Officer
CFO: George Stevens, Chief Financial Officer
CMO: Dale Carrison, M.D., Chief of Staff
CIO: Ernie McKinley, Chief Information Officer
CHR: John Espinoza, Chief Human Resources Officer
Web address: www.umcsn.com
**Control:** County–Government, nonfederal **Service:** General Medical and Surgical

**Staffed Beds:** 541 **Admissions:** 25520 **Census:** 371 **Outpatient Visits:** 699741 **Births:** 3824 **Total Expense ($000):** 568181 **Payroll Expense ($000):** 223068 **Personnel:** 3457

☐ **VALLEY HOSPITAL MEDICAL CENTER (290021)**, 620 Shadow Lane, Zip 89106–4119; tel. 702/388–4000, (Nonreporting) **A**1 9 10 12 13 **S** Universal Health Services, Inc., King of Prussia, PA
Primary Contact: Jay Finnegan, Chief Executive Officer
CFO: Betsy A. Sponsler, Chief Financial Officer
CMO: Dost Wattoo, M.D., Chief of Staff
CIO: Tom Schoenig, Regional Director Information Services
CHR: Dana Thorne, Administrator Human Resources
Web address: www.valleyhospital.net
**Control:** Corporation, Investor–owned, for–profit **Service:** General Medical and Surgical

**Staffed Beds:** 365

**VEGAS VALLEY REHABILITATION HOSPITAL**, 2945 Casa Vegas, Zip 89109; tel. 702/735–7179, (Nonreporting) **S** Fundamental Long Term Care Holdings, LLC, Sparks Glencoe, MD
Primary Contact: Maureen Davis, Administrator
Web address: www.fundltc.com
**Control:** Corporation, Investor–owned, for–profit **Service:** Rehabilitation

**Staffed Beds:** 100

### LOVELOCK—Pershing County

**PERSHING GENERAL HOSPITAL (291304)**, 855 Sixth Street, Zip 89419, Mailing Address: P.O. Box 661, Zip 89419–0661; tel. 775/273–2621, (Total facility includes 25 beds in nursing home–type unit) **A**9 10 18 **F**40 57 97 103 107 113 126 127 129 132
Primary Contact: Patty Goldsworthy, Interim Chief Executive Officer and Administrator
CFO: Marjorie Skinner, Director Finance
CMO: Yousri Gadallah, M.D., Chief Medical Officer
CIO: Jim Weeldreyer, Manager Information Technology
CHR: Cynthia Hixenbaugh, Director Human Resources
Web address: www.pershinggenhospital.org
**Control:** Hospital district or authority, Government, nonfederal **Service:** Long–Term Acute Care hospital

**Staffed Beds:** 38 **Admissions:** 85 **Census:** 17 **Outpatient Visits:** 17251 **Births:** 0 **Total Expense ($000):** 9373 **Payroll Expense ($000):** 3596 **Personnel:** 77

### MESQUITE—Clark County

☒ **MESA VIEW REGIONAL HOSPITAL (291307)**, 1299 Bertha Howe Avenue, Zip 89027; tel. 702/346–8040 **A**1 9 10 18 **F**3 11 13 15 29 30 34 35 40 45 46 51 56 57 59 64 70 75 76 77 79 81 82 85 87 107 108 110 111 113 118 129 131 132 134 145 146 147 **P**7 **S** Community Health Systems, Inc., Franklin, TN
Primary Contact: Kapua Conley, Chief Executive Officer
CFO: Eric S. Hardy, Chief Financial Officer
CHR: Matthew Anderson, Director Human Resources
Web address: www.mesaviewhospital.com
**Control:** Corporation, Investor–owned, for–profit **Service:** General Medical and Surgical

**Staffed Beds:** 25 **Admissions:** 1108 **Census:** 8 **Outpatient Visits:** 20251 **Births:** 125 **Total Expense ($000):** 22855 **Payroll Expense ($000):** 10495 **Personnel:** 191

### NELLIS AFB—Clark County

☒ **MIKE O'CALLAGHAN FEDERAL HOSPITAL**, 4700 Las Vegas Boulevard North, Suite 2419, Zip 89191–6601; tel. 702/653–2000, (Nonreporting) **A**1 3 5 **S** Department of the Air Force, Washington, DC
Primary Contact: Colonel Christian Benjamin, USAF, MC, Commander
COO: Colonel Linnes L. Chester, USAF, Administrator
CFO: Major Kari Turkal–Barrett, Flight Commander Resource Management Officer
CMO: Lieutenant Colonel Markham Brown, M.D., Chief Medical Staff
CIO: Major Kevin Seeley, Chief Information Officer
Web address: www.lasvegas.va.gov/
**Control:** Air Force, Government, federal **Service:** General Medical and Surgical

**Staffed Beds:** 46

### NORTH LAS VEGAS—Clark County

**NORTH VISTA HOSPITAL (290005)**, 1409 East Lake Mead Boulevard, Zip 89030–7197; tel. 702/649–7711, (Nonreporting) **A**9 10 21 **S** IASIS Healthcare, Franklin, TN
Primary Contact: Richard L. Kilburn, Chief Executive Officer
COO: Michael Heindel, Chief Operating Officer
CFO: Kim Forbes–Daniels, Chief Financial Officer
Web address: www.northvistahospital.com
**Control:** Corporation, Investor–owned, for–profit **Service:** General Medical and Surgical

**Staffed Beds:** 198

★ **VETERANS AFFAIRS SOUTHERN NEVADA HEALTHCARE SYSTEM**, Zip 89036; tel. 702/636–3000, (Nonreporting) **A**5 **S** Department of Veterans Affairs, Washington, DC
Primary Contact: John Bright, Director
CFO: Richard O. Hays, Chief Fiscal Service
CMO: Ramanujam Komanduri, M.D., Chief of Staff
Web address: www.va.gov/sta/guide/home.asp
**Control:** Veterans Affairs, Government, federal **Service:** General Medical and Surgical

**Staffed Beds:** 57

NV

## PAHRUMP—Nye County

★ **DESERT VIEW HOSPITAL (291311)**, 360 South Lola Lane, Zip 89048; tel. 775/751–7500 **A**9 10 18 **F**15 18 29 34 40 57 79 81 86 87 107 111 118 129 132 147 **P**6 **S** Rural Health Group, Nephi, UT
Primary Contact: Susan Davila, Administrator and Chief Executive Officer
CMO: Fredric Siegel, M.D., Chief of Staff
CHR: Alecia Riddle, Manager Human Resources
CNO: Ellen Maborang, Chief Nursing Officer
Web address: www.desertviewhospital.com
**Control:** Corporation, Investor–owned, for–profit **Service:** General Medical and Surgical

**Staffed Beds:** 25 **Admissions:** 1734 **Census:** 14 **Outpatient Visits:** 23201 **Births:** 0 **Total Expense ($000):** 19332 **Payroll Expense ($000):** 6959 **Personnel:** 161

**DESERT VIEW REGIONAL MEDICAL CENTER** See Desert View Hospital

## RENO—Washoe County

☒ **RENOWN REGIONAL MEDICAL CENTER (290001)**, 1155 Mill Street, Zip 89502–1474; tel. 775/982–4100 **A**1 2 3 5 9 10 **F**3 5 11 13 15 17 18 19 20 21 22 23 24 25 26 27 28 29 30 31 32 34 35 37 40 41 43 45 49 54 56 57 58 59 60 61 62 64 65 66 68 70 72 73 74 75 76 77 78 79 81 82 84 85 86 87 88 89 93 99 100 101 102 103 104 105 107 108 109 110 111 113 114 117 118 119 120 122 123 125 129 130 131 134 143 144 145 146 147 **S** Renown Health, Reno, NV
Primary Contact: Gregory E. Boyer, Chief Executive Officer
COO: Kris Gaw, Chief Operating Officer
CFO: Sam King, Chief Financial Officer
CMO: Charles Johnson, M.D., Chief of Staff
CIO: Charles Scully, Chief Information Officer
CHR: Michelle Sanchez–Bickley, Vice President Human Resources
Web address: www.renown.org
**Control:** Other not–for–profit (including NFP Corporation) **Service:** General Medical and Surgical

**Staffed Beds:** 654 **Admissions:** 27333 **Census:** 394 **Outpatient Visits:** 260006 **Births:** 3422 **Total Expense ($000):** 455500 **Payroll Expense ($000):** 143242 **Personnel:** 2344

★ **RENOWN REHABILITATION HOSPITAL**, 1495 Mill Street, Zip 89502–1449; tel. 775/982–3500 **F**29 54 77 82 90 93 96 142 147 **P**5 6 **S** Renown Health, Reno, NV
Primary Contact: Blain Claypool, Chief Executive Officer
COO: Kris Gaw, Chief Operating Officer
CFO: Dawn Ahner, Chief Financial Officer
CIO: Charles Scully, Chief Information Officer
CHR: Michelle Sanchez–Bickley, Vice President Human Resources
CNO: Gail P. Green, R.N., Chief Nursing Officer
Web address: www.renown.org
**Control:** Other not–for–profit (including NFP Corporation) **Service:** Rehabilitation

**Staffed Beds:** 62 **Admissions:** 1005 **Census:** 40 **Outpatient Visits:** 21988 **Births:** 0 **Total Expense ($000):** 19516 **Payroll Expense ($000):** 10197 **Personnel:** 159

☒ **RENOWN SOUTH MEADOWS MEDICAL CENTER (290049)**, 10101 Double R Boulevard, Zip 89521; tel. 775/982–7000 **A**1 9 10 **F**8 10 12 29 30 35 39 40 46 49 68 70 74 75 79 81 85 87 93 97 107 108 111 118 124 129 130 145 **S** Renown Health, Reno, NV
Primary Contact: Blain Claypool, Chief Executive Officer
COO: Kris Gaw, Chief Operating Officer
CFO: Cora Case, Chief Financial Officer
CMO: Max Jackson, M.D., Chief Medical Officer
CIO: Charles Scully, Chief Information Officer
CHR: Michelle Sanchez–Bickley, Vice President Human Resources
CNO: Gail P. Green, R.N., Chief Nursing Officer
Web address: www.renown.org
**Control:** Other not–for–profit (including NFP Corporation) **Service:** General Medical and Surgical

**Staffed Beds:** 76 **Admissions:** 3022 **Census:** 27 **Outpatient Visits:** 53418 **Births:** 0 **Total Expense ($000):** 57274 **Payroll Expense ($000):** 19109 **Personnel:** 320

☒ **SAINT MARY'S REGIONAL MEDICAL CENTER (290009)**, 235 West Sixth Street, Zip 89503; tel. 775/770–3000 **A**1 2 3 5 9 10 **F**3 11 12 13 15 17 18 20 22 24 26 28 29 30 31 34 35 39 40 45 46 47 48 49 53 56 58 62 63 64 66 70 71 72 74 75 76 77 78 79 81 82 84 85 87 89 93 95 102 107 108 110 111 113 114 117 118 119 120 123 125 129 131 145 146 147 **S** Prime Healthcare Services, Ontario, CA
Primary Contact: Helen Lidholm, Chief Executive Officer
CFO: John R. Deakyne, Chief Financial Officer
CIO: Cindy Mullins, Director Information Technology
CHR: David Milovich, Vice President Human Resources
Web address: www.saintmarysreno.com
**Control:** Other not–for–profit (including NFP Corporation) **Service:** General Medical and Surgical

**Staffed Beds:** 272 **Admissions:** 12011 **Census:** 145 **Outpatient Visits:** 171109 **Births:** 2254 **Total Expense ($000):** 307151 **Payroll Expense ($000):** 115160 **Personnel:** 1354

☒ **TAHOE PACIFIC HOSPITALS (292004)**, 201 West Liberty Street, Suite 310, Zip 89501; tel. 775/355–5970, (Includes TAHOE PACIFIC HOSPITALS – WEST, 235 West Sixth Street, 5th Floor, Zip 89503–4548), (Nonreporting) **A**1 9 10 **S** LifeCare Management Services, Plano, TX
Primary Contact: Colin O'Sullivan, Administrator
COO: Theresa Fegan, Chief Clinical Officer
CFO: Nena Swenson, Financial Manager
CMO: T. Brian Callister, M.D., Chief Medical Officer
CIO: Kaylene Reeves, Director
CHR: Nelson Coy, Director Human Resources
Web address: www.lifecare–hospitals.com
**Control:** Corporation, Investor–owned, for–profit **Service:** General Medical and Surgical

**Staffed Beds:** 60

☒ **VETERANS AFFAIRS SIERRA NEVADA HEALTH CARE SYSTEM**, 1000 Locust Street, Zip 89502–2597; tel. 775/786–7200, (Nonreporting) **A**1 3 5 **S** Department of Veterans Affairs, Washington, DC
Primary Contact: Kurt W. Schlegelmilch, M.D., FACHE, Director
COO: Michael C. Tadych, Associate Director
CFO: Kathy Munday, Chief Financial Officer
CMO: Steven Brilliant, M.D., Chief of Staff
CIO: Jack Smith, Acting Chief Information Resources Management Service
CHR: Debbie Jenkins, Chief Human Resources Management Service
Web address: www.reno.va.gov
**Control:** Veterans Affairs, Government, federal **Service:** General Medical and Surgical

**Staffed Beds:** 64

☐ **WEST HILLS HOSPITAL (294003)**, 1240 East Ninth Street, Zip 89512–2997, Mailing Address: P.O. Box 30012, Zip 89520–3012; tel. 775/323–0478, (Nonreporting) **A**1 9 10 **S** Universal Health Services, Inc., King of Prussia, PA
Primary Contact: Steve Shell, Chief Executive Officer
CFO: Erich Koch, Chief Financial Officer
CMO: Philip Rich, M.D., Chief Medical Officer
CHR: Don Gay, Director Human Resources
Web address: www.westhillshospital.net
**Control:** Corporation, Investor–owned, for–profit **Service:** Psychiatric

**Staffed Beds:** 95

**WILLOW SPRINGS CENTER**, 690 Edison Way, Zip 89502–4135; tel. 775/858–3303 **A**3 5 **F**98 99 104 106
Primary Contact: Jim Serratt, Chief Executive Officer
CFO: Diahann Barrera, Chief Financial Officer
CMO: Jason Walenta, M.D., Medical Director
Web address: www.willowspringscenter.com
**Control:** Corporation, Investor–owned, for–profit **Service:** Children's hospital psychiatric

**Staffed Beds:** 116 **Admissions:** 411 **Census:** 94 **Outpatient Visits:** 9813 **Births:** 0

## SPARKS—Washoe County

☐ **NORTHERN NEVADA ADULT MENTAL HEALTH SERVICES (294000)**, 480 Galletti Way, Zip 89431–5574; tel. 775/688–2001 **A**1 3 5 9 10 **F**29 40 54 75 98 99 102 104 106 129 131
Primary Contact: Rosalyne Reynolds, Administrator
CFO: Elizabeth O'Brien, Chief Financial Officer
CIO: Lois Repass, Quality Assurance Specialist and Coordinator Performance Improvement
Web address: www.mhds.state.nv.us/
**Control:** State–Government, nonfederal **Service:** Psychiatric

**Staffed Beds:** 50 **Admissions:** 334 **Census:** 15 **Outpatient Visits:** 62293 **Births:** 0 **Total Expense ($000):** 29137 **Payroll Expense ($000):** 15822 **Personnel:** 237

NV

---

**Hospital, Medicare Provider Number, Address, Telephone, Approval, Facility, and Physician Codes, Health Care System**

★ American Hospital Association (AHA) membership
☐ The Joint Commission accreditation ◇ DNV Healthcare Inc. accreditation

○ American Osteopathic Association (AOA) accreditation
△ Commission on Accreditation of Rehabilitation Facilities (CARF) accreditation

☐ **NORTHERN NEVADA MEDICAL CENTER (290032)**, 2375 East Prater Way, Zip 89434–9900; tel. 775/331–7000, (Nonreporting) **A**1 9 10 **S** Universal Health Services, Inc., King of Prussia, PA
Primary Contact: Mark W. Crawford, Chief Executive Officer
COO: Tiffany Meert, Chief Operating Officer
CFO: Matthew Cova, Chief Financial Officer
CHR: Patricia Downs, Director Human Resources
Web address: www.nnmc.com
**Control:** Corporation, Investor–owned, for–profit **Service:** General Medical and Surgical

**Staffed Beds:** 80

### TONOPAH—Nye County

**NYE REGIONAL MEDICAL CENTER (290020)**, 825 South Main Street, Zip 89049, Mailing Address: P.O. Box 391, Zip 89049–0391; tel. 775/482–6233, (Nonreporting) **A**9 10 20
Primary Contact: Mercy Peterson, Interim Chief Executive Officer
CMO: Vincent Scoccia, D.O., Chief Medical Staff
CIO: Mercy Peterson, Assistant Administrator
CHR: Leilani Gordon, Director Human Resources and Payroll
Web address: www.nyeregional.org
**Control:** Corporation, Investor–owned, for–profit **Service:** General Medical and Surgical

**Staffed Beds:** 44

### WINNEMUCCA—Humboldt County

★ **HUMBOLDT GENERAL HOSPITAL (291308)**, 118 East Haskell Street, Zip 89445–3299; tel. 775/623–5222, (Nonreporting) **A**9 10 18
Primary Contact: James G. Parrish, FACHE, Chief Executive Officer
COO: Craig Prest, Director Operation Services
CFO: Larry Hutcheson, Chief Financial Officer and Director Administrative Services
CMO: Richard M. Ingle, M.D., Chief of Staff
CIO: Larry Hutcheson, Chief Financial Officer and Director Administrative Services
CHR: Rose Marie Green, Director Human Resources
Web address: www.hghospital.ws
**Control:** Hospital district or authority, Government, nonfederal **Service:** General Medical and Surgical

**Staffed Beds:** 52

### YERINGTON—Lyon County

**SOUTH LYON MEDICAL CENTER (290002)**, 213 South Whitacre, Zip 89447, Mailing Address: P.O. Box 940, Zip 89447–0940; tel. 775/463–2301, (Nonreporting) **A**9 10 20
Primary Contact: Kim O. Crandell, Administrator
Web address: www.southlyonmedicalcenter.org
**Control:** Other not–for–profit (including NFP Corporation) **Service:** General Medical and Surgical

**Staffed Beds:** 63

NV

# NEW HAMPSHIRE

## BERLIN—Coos County

**ANDROSCOGGIN VALLEY HOSPITAL (301310)**, 59 Page Hill Road,
Zip 03570–3531; tel. 603/752–2200 **A**9 10 18 **F**3 8 11 12 13 15 17 28 29
30 34 40 41 43 45 57 59 61 62 63 64 67 70 74 75 76 77 79 81 82 85 89
92 93 102 107 108 113 118 127 128 129 130 131 132 145 146 **P**6
Primary Contact: Russell G. Keene, Chief Executive Officer
CFO: Jeremy Roberge, Director Reimbursement
CMO: Keith M. Shute, M.D., Senior Vice President Medical Affairs and Clinical
Services
CIO: Linda M. Laperle, Vice President Administrative Services
CHR: James A. Wheeler, Vice President Human Relations and Community
Development
Web address: www.avhnh.org
**Control:** Other not–for–profit (including NFP Corporation) **Service:** General
Medical and Surgical

**Staffed Beds:** 25 **Admissions:** 1345 **Census:** 16 **Outpatient Visits:** 68244
**Births:** 137 **Total Expense ($000):** 51605 **Payroll Expense ($000):** 23886
**Personnel:** 330

## CLAREMONT—Sullivan County

**VALLEY REGIONAL HOSPITAL (301308)**, 243 Elm Street, Zip 03743–2099;
tel. 603/542–7771 **A**1 9 10 18 **F**2 3 11 13 14 15 28 29 34 35 38 40 45 49
50 51 54 57 59 62 63 64 68 70 74 75 76 77 79 81 84 85 87 93 97 104
107 108 110 113 117 118 129 131 132 134 145 146 **P**6
Primary Contact: Claire L. Bowen, Chief Executive Officer
CFO: Steven Monette, Chief Financial Officer
CMO: Carol F. Boerner, M.D., President Medical Staff
CIO: Patricia Witthaus, Director Information Services
CHR: Gregg Burdett, Vice President Administration and Physician Services
Web address: www.vrh.org
**Control:** Other not–for–profit (including NFP Corporation) **Service:** General
Medical and Surgical

**Staffed Beds:** 25 **Admissions:** 1131 **Census:** 13 **Outpatient Visits:** 83912
**Births:** 152 **Total Expense ($000):** 43458 **Payroll Expense ($000):** 18365
**Personnel:** 377

## COLEBROOK—Coos County

★ **UPPER CONNECTICUT VALLEY HOSPITAL (301300)**, 181 Corliss Lane,
Zip 03576–9533; tel. 603/237–4971 **A**9 10 18 **F**3 7 15 29 30 31 34 35 40
45 50 56 57 59 64 67 68 75 78 79 81 85 93 102 107 110 113 118 127 129
132 133 134 145 146 147 **P**6
Primary Contact: Charles White, Chief Administrative Officer
CMO: Gerald Westover, M.D., Medical Director
Web address: www.dartmouth–hitchcock.org/ucvh/
**Control:** Other not–for–profit (including NFP Corporation) **Service:** General
Medical and Surgical

**Staffed Beds:** 16 **Admissions:** 411 **Census:** 5 **Outpatient Visits:** 18041
**Births:** 0 **Total Expense ($000):** 13124 **Payroll Expense ($000):** 6060
**Personnel:** 90

## CONCORD—Merrimack County

**CONCORD HOSPITAL (300001)**, 250 Pleasant Street, Zip 03301–2598;
tel. 603/225–2711 **A**1 2 3 5 9 10 **F**3 8 12 13 14 15 17 18 20 22 24 26 28
29 30 31 33 34 35 36 37 38 39 40 42 43 44 46 49 50 51 53 54 55 56 57
58 59 61 64 65 66 68 69 70 71 74 75 76 77 78 79 80 81 82 83 84 85 86
87 89 93 97 98 99 100 101 102 103 104 105 107 108 110 111 113 114
117 118 119 120 125 128 129 130 131 133 134 143 144 145 146 147 **P**6
Primary Contact: Michael B. Green, President and Chief Executive Officer
COO: Joseph M. Conley, Chief Operating Officer
CFO: Bruce R. Burns, Chief Financial Officer
CMO: David F. Green, M.D., Chief Medical Officer
CIO: Deane Morrison, Chief Information Officer
CHR: Robin A. Moore, Vice President Human Resources
Web address: www.concordhospital.org
**Control:** Other not–for–profit (including NFP Corporation) **Service:** General
Medical and Surgical

**Staffed Beds:** 211 **Admissions:** 13004 **Census:** 149 **Outpatient Visits:**
630825 **Births:** 1349 **Total Expense ($000):** 365140 **Payroll Expense
($000):** 163439 **Personnel:** 2697

**HEALTHSOUTH REHABILITATION HOSPITAL (303027)**, 254 Pleasant Street,
Zip 03301–2508; tel. 603/226–9800, (Nonreporting) **A**1 10 **S** HEALTHSOUTH
Corporation, Birmingham, AL
Primary Contact: Catherine Devaney, Chief Executive Officer
CFO: Jeanine Chesley, Controller
CMO: Safwan Kazmouz, M.D., Chief Medical Director
CHR: Myra Nixon, Director Human Resources
CNO: Joseph Adamski, Chief Nursing Officer
Web address: www.healthsouthrehabconcordnh.com
**Control:** Corporation, Investor–owned, for–profit **Service:** Rehabilitation

**Staffed Beds:** 50

☐ **NEW HAMPSHIRE HOSPITAL (304000)**, 36 Clinton Street, Zip 03301–3861;
tel. 603/271–5300 **A**1 9 10 **F**3 29 30 39 56 57 61 68 74 75 77 86 87 98 99
101 103 129 134 145 **P**4 6
Primary Contact: Robert J. MacLeod, Chief Executive Officer
CFO: Jamie Dall, Director Finance and Support Operations
CMO: David G. Folks, M.D., Chief Medical Officer
CHR: Mark Bussiere, Administrator Human Resources
Web address: www.dhhs.state.nh.us./dhhs/default.htm
**Control:** State–Government, nonfederal **Service:** Psychiatric

**Staffed Beds:** 152 **Admissions:** 2305 **Census:** 152 **Outpatient Visits:** 0
**Births:** 0 **Total Expense ($000):** 64809 **Payroll Expense ($000):** 34675
**Personnel:** 675

## DERRY—Rockingham County

**PARKLAND MEDICAL CENTER (300017)**, One Parkland Drive,
Zip 03038–2750; tel. 603/432–1500, (Nonreporting) **A**1 2 9 10 **S** HCA,
Nashville, TN
Primary Contact: Tina Marie Legere, Chief Executive Officer
COO: Jeff Scionti, Chief Operating Officer
CIO: Brad George, Director Information Systems
CHR: Molly Lahti, Director Human Resources
Web address: www.parklandmedicalcenter.com
**Control:** Corporation, Investor–owned, for–profit **Service:** General Medical and
Surgical

**Staffed Beds:** 82

## DOVER—Strafford County

**WENTWORTH–DOUGLASS HOSPITAL (300018)**, 789 Central Avenue,
Zip 03820–2589; tel. 603/742–5252 **A**1 2 9 10 **F**3 11 13 17 18 20 22 28 29
30 31 32 34 35 36 39 40 42 43 44 45 46 47 49 50 51 53 54 55 57 58 59
61 64 65 68 70 73 74 75 76 77 78 79 81 82 84 85 86 87 89 92 93 94 97
107 108 111 113 114 117 118 119 120 122 123 125 128 129 130 131 134
142 143 144 145 146 147 **P**6 8
Primary Contact: Gregory J. Walker, Chief Executive Officer
COO: Daniel N. Dunn, Vice President Operations
CFO: Peter Walcek, Vice President Finance
CMO: Paul Cass, D.O., Chief Medical & Clinical Integration Officer
CIO: Jeffrey Pollock, Chief Information Officer
CHR: Erin Flanigan, Vice President Human Resources
CNO: Sheila Woolley, R.N., Vice President, Patient Care Services
Web address: www.wdhospital.com
**Control:** Other not–for–profit (including NFP Corporation) **Service:** General
Medical and Surgical

**Staffed Beds:** 128 **Admissions:** 6958 **Census:** 77 **Outpatient Visits:** 224840
**Births:** 929 **Total Expense ($000):** 209705 **Payroll Expense ($000):** 88700
**Personnel:** 1351

**NH**

---

**Hospital, Medicare Provider Number, Address, Telephone, Approval, Facility, and Physician Codes, Health Care System**

★ American Hospital Association (AHA) membership
☐ The Joint Commission accreditation     ◇ DNV Healthcare Inc. accreditation

○ American Osteopathic Association (AOA) accreditation
△ Commission on Accreditation of Rehabilitation Facilities (CARF) accreditation

---

## EXETER—Rockingham County

☒ **EXETER HOSPITAL (300023)**, 5 Alumni Drive, Zip 3833; tel. 603/778–7311 **A**1 2 9 10 19 21 **F**3 8 13 14 15 18 20 22 26 28 29 30 31 32 34 35 36 37 38 40 44 45 46 47 48 49 50 51 52 54 55 57 58 59 64 70 74 75 76 77 78 79 80 81 84 85 86 87 89 93 107 108 110 111 113 117 118 119 120 122 128 129 130 131 134 142 143 145 146 147
Primary Contact: Kevin J. Callahan, President and Chief Executive Officer
COO: Susan Burns–Tisdale, Senior Vice President Clinical Operations
CFO: Kevin J. O'Leary, Senior Vice President and Chief Financial Officer
CMO: Nancy Braese, D.O., President Medical Staff
CIO: David Briden, Chief Information Officer
CHR: Christopher Callahan, Vice President Human Resources
CNO: Susan Burns–Tisdale, Senior Vice President Clinical Operations, Interim CNO
Web address: www.ehr.org
**Control:** Other not–for–profit (including NFP Corporation) **Service:** General Medical and Surgical

**Staffed Beds:** 99 **Admissions:** 5781 **Census:** 62 **Outpatient Visits:** 175210 **Births:** 708 **Total Expense ($000):** 178201 **Payroll Expense ($000):** 66140 **Personnel:** 1087

## FRANKLIN—Merrimack County

★ **FRANKLIN REGIONAL HOSPITAL (301306)**, 15 Aiken Avenue, Zip 03235–1299; tel. 603/934–2060 **A**10 18 **F**11 15 18 29 30 31 34 35 36 40 44 46 47 48 49 50 57 58 59 61 64 66 68 70 74 75 77 78 79 81 82 83 84 85 86 87 93 97 99 100 101 102 103 107 115 118 126 127 128 129 130 131 132 134 143 145 146 147 **P**4 6 **S** LRGHealthcare, Laconia, NH
Primary Contact: Thomas Clairmont, President
CFO: Henry D. Lipman, Executive Vice President and Chief Financial Officer
CMO: Peter Walkley, M.D., Chief of Staff
CIO: Red Hutchinson, Chief Information Officer
Web address: www.lrgh.org
**Control:** Other not–for–profit (including NFP Corporation) **Service:** General Medical and Surgical

**Staffed Beds:** 25 **Admissions:** 998 **Census:** 13 **Outpatient Visits:** 72206 **Births:** 0 **Total Expense ($000):** 37950 **Payroll Expense ($000):** 13284 **Personnel:** 189

## GREENFIELD—Hillsborough County

**CROTCHED MOUNTAIN REHABILITATION CENTER**, 1 Verney Drive, Zip 03047–5000; tel. 603/547–3311, (Total facility includes 62 beds in nursing home–type unit) **F**2 3 10 29 30 35 36 38 39 50 53 54 57 75 77 86 87 90 91 93 99 100 104 106 129 130 131 134 142 145 147 **P**6
Primary Contact: Donald L. Shumway, Chief Executive Officer
COO: Michael Redmond, Senior Vice President and Chief Operating Officer
CFO: Joseph Fermano, Vice President Finance and Chief Financial Officer
CMO: W. Carl Cooley, M.D., Chief Medical Officer
CHR: Lorrie Rudis, Director Human Resources
Web address: www.cmf.org
**Control:** Other not–for–profit (including NFP Corporation) **Service:** Rehabilitation

**Staffed Beds:** 181 **Admissions:** 161 **Census:** 148 **Outpatient Visits:** 6446 **Births:** 0 **Total Expense ($000):** 41093 **Payroll Expense ($000):** 23296 **Personnel:** 654

## HAMPSTEAD—Rockingham County

☐ **HAMPSTEAD HOSPITAL (304001)**, 218 East Road, Zip 03841–2228; tel. 603/329–5311, (Nonreporting) **A**1 9 10
Primary Contact: Phillip J. Kubiak, President
COO: Cynthia A. Gove, Chief Operating Officer
CFO: John J. Whittier, Vice President Finance
CMO: Bienvenido Manzanero, M.D., Medical Director
CIO: Sandra J. Lucia, Director Health Information and Corporate Compliance Officer
CHR: Lisa M. Ryan, Coordinator Human Resources
Web address: www.hampsteadhospital.com
**Control:** Corporation, Investor–owned, for–profit **Service:** Psychiatric

**Staffed Beds:** 60

## KEENE—Cheshire County

☒ **CHESHIRE MEDICAL CENTER (300019)**, 580 Court Street, Zip 03431–1718; tel. 603/354–5400 **A**1 2 9 10 **F**3 12 13 15 17 18 28 29 30 31 34 35 38 40 43 44 45 46 49 51 53 56 57 59 61 64 65 68 70 74 75 76 77 78 79 81 82 84 85 86 87 89 90 91 92 93 94 96 97 98 99 100 101 102 103 104 105 107 108 110 111 113 114 117 118 120 128 129 130 131 132 134 145 146 147
Primary Contact: Arthur W. Nichols, President and Chief Executive Officer
CFO: Jill I. Batty, Chief Financial Officer
CMO: Don Caruso, M.D., Chief Medical Officer
CIO: Peter Malloy, Chief Information Officer
CHR: Julie Green, Vice President Human Resources
CNO: Cynthia Coughlin, MS, Chief Nursing Officer
Web address: www.cheshire–med.com
**Control:** Other not–for–profit (including NFP Corporation) **Service:** General Medical and Surgical

**Staffed Beds:** 140 **Admissions:** 4352 **Census:** 56 **Outpatient Visits:** 157746 **Births:** 437 **Total Expense ($000):** 143441 **Payroll Expense ($000):** 52988 **Personnel:** 1233

## LACONIA—Belknap County

★ **LAKES REGION GENERAL HOSPITAL (300005)**, 80 Highland Street, Zip 03246–3298; tel. 603/524–3211 **A**9 10 **F**3 5 7 8 11 13 15 18 28 29 30 31 32 34 35 36 39 40 43 44 45 46 47 48 49 50 53 56 57 58 59 60 61 64 66 68 70 74 75 76 77 78 79 81 82 83 84 85 86 87 89 93 97 98 99 100 101 102 103 107 113 117 118 128 129 130 131 132 134 143 145 146 147 **P**4 6 **S** LRGHealthcare, Laconia, NH
Primary Contact: Thomas Clairmont, President
CFO: Henry D. Lipman, Sr. VP/Financial Strategy and External Relations
CMO: Peter Walkley, M.D., Chief Medical Officer
CIO: Kevin Irish, Chief Information Officer
CHR: Suzanne Stiles, Chief Human Resources Officer & Sr. Vice President/Administrative and Support Services
CNO: Ellen Wolff, R.N., Chief Nursing Officer/Senior VP/Patient Care Services
Web address: www.lrgh.org
**Control:** Other not–for–profit (including NFP Corporation) **Service:** General Medical and Surgical

**Staffed Beds:** 104 **Admissions:** 4359 **Census:** 65 **Outpatient Visits:** 159050 **Births:** 406 **Total Expense ($000):** 159223 **Payroll Expense ($000):** 56307 **Personnel:** 868

## LANCASTER—Coos County

★ **WEEKS MEDICAL CENTER (301303)**, 173 Middle Street, Zip 03584–3561; tel. 603/788–4911 **A**9 10 18 **F**3 11 15 18 28 29 30 31 32 34 35 36 40 45 50 51 56 57 59 61 62 63 64 65 66 68 70 71 75 77 78 79 81 85 87 89 91 92 93 94 97 100 104 107 108 110 111 113 115 116 117 118 126 129 130 131 132 133 134 145 146 147 **P**6
Primary Contact: Scott W. Howe, Chief Executive Officer
CFO: Celeste Pitts, Chief Financial Officer
CMO: Lars Nielson, M.D., Chief Medical Officer
CIO: Darrell Bodnar, Director Information
CHR: Linda Rexford, Director Human Resources
CNO: Donna Walker, Chief Nurse Executive
Web address: www.weeksmedical.org
**Control:** Other not–for–profit (including NFP Corporation) **Service:** General Medical and Surgical

**Staffed Beds:** 25 **Admissions:** 858 **Census:** 10 **Outpatient Visits:** 77074 **Births:** 0 **Total Expense ($000):** 37854 **Payroll Expense ($000):** 19840 **Personnel:** 308

## LEBANON—Grafton County

★ **ALICE PECK DAY MEMORIAL HOSPITAL (301305)**, 10 Alice Peck Day Drive, Zip 03766–2650; tel. 603/448–3121 **A**9 10 18 **F**3 11 13 15 29 34 35 36 37 39 40 41 42 45 47 50 51 54 56 57 59 63 64 65 66 67 75 76 77 79 81 82 83 84 85 93 97 100 107 110 113 114 118 127 128 129 130 132 134 144 145 146 147 **P**5 6
Primary Contact: Harry G. Dorman, III, FACHE, President and Chief Executive Officer
COO: J. Todd Miller, Vice President and Chief Operating Officer
CFO: Evalie M. Crosby, CPA, Vice President Finance and Chief Financial Officer
CMO: Susan E. Mooney, M.D., Vice President and Chief Medical Officer
CIO: Lorraine Nichols, Director Information Services
CHR: Brenda Blair, Association Vice President Human Resources and Organizational Learning
CNO: Beverley A. Rankin, R.N., Vice President & Chief Nursing Officer
Web address: www.alicepeckday.org
**Control:** Other not–for–profit (including NFP Corporation) **Service:** General Medical and Surgical

**Staffed Beds:** 25 **Admissions:** 990 **Census:** 14 **Outpatient Visits:** 92585 **Births:** 276 **Total Expense ($000):** 46736 **Payroll Expense ($000):** 25598 **Personnel:** 358

☒ **DARTMOUTH–HITCHCOCK MEDICAL CENTER (300003)**, One Medical Center Drive, Zip 03756–0001; tel. 603/650–5000, (Includes CHILDREN'S HOSPITAL AT DARTMOUTH, One Medical Center Drive, Zip 03756; tel. 603/650–5000) **A**1 3 5 8 9 10 **F**3 5 6 7 8 9 11 12 13 14 15 17 18 19 20 21 22 23 24 25 26 27 28 29 30 31 32 34 35 36 37 38 39 40 41 43 44 45 46 47 48 49 50 51 52 53 54 55 56 57 58 59 60 61 63 64 65 66 68 70 71 72 74 75 76 77 78 79 80 81 82 84 85 86 87 88 89 91 92 93 94 96 97 98 99 100 101 102 103 104 105 107 108 110 111 113 114 115 116 117 118 119 120 122 123 125 128 129 130 131 133 134 135 137 140 141 142 144 145 146 147 **P**6
Primary Contact: James Weinstein, M.D., President and Chief Executive Officer
COO: Stephen J. LeBlanc, Chief Operating Officer
CFO: Daniel Jantzen, Chief Financial Officer
CMO: John R. Butterly, M.D., Medical Director
CIO: Peter A. Johnson, Vice President Information Services
CHR: Richard B. Davis, Chief Human Resources Officer
Web address: www.hitchcock.org
**Control:** Other not–for–profit (including NFP Corporation) **Service:** General Medical and Surgical

**Staffed Beds:** 381 **Admissions:** 19708 **Census:** 310 **Outpatient Visits:** 794632 **Births:** 1068 **Total Expense ($000):** 1010348 **Payroll Expense ($000):** 460808 **Personnel:** 5753

**NH**

**LITTLETON—Grafton County**

★ **LITTLETON REGIONAL HOSPITAL (301302)**, 600 Saint Johnsbury Road, Zip 03561–3436; tel. 603/444–9000 **A**9 10 18 **F**1 3 11 13 15 16 18 26 28 29 31 32 34 35 36 38 40 43 44 45 49 50 51 56 57 59 64 65 67 70 73 74 75 76 77 78 79 80 81 84 85 86 87 89 90 92 93 97 107 108 110 114 117 118 127 129 130 131 132 142 145 146 147 **P**6
Primary Contact: Warren K. West, FACHE, Chief Executive Officer
COO: Peter J. Wright, Chief Operating Officer
CFO: Robert L. Fotter, Chief Financial Officer
CIO: Scott Vachon, Director Information Technology
CHR: Georgene Novak, Director Human Resources
CNO: Linda Gilmore, Chief Nursing Officer/Chief Administrative Officer
Web address: www.littletonhospital.org
**Control:** Other not–for–profit (including NFP Corporation) **Service:** General Medical and Surgical

**Staffed Beds:** 25 **Admissions:** 1584 **Census:** 15 **Outpatient Visits:** 58319 **Births:** 308 **Total Expense ($000):** 61020 **Payroll Expense ($000):** 27741 **Personnel:** 383

**MANCHESTER—Hillsborough County**

⊞ **CATHOLIC MEDICAL CENTER (300034)**, 100 McGregor Street, Zip 03102–3770; tel. 603/668–3545 **A**1 2 9 10 **F**3 9 11 12 13 15 18 20 22 24 26 28 29 30 31 32 34 35 36 37 38 39 40 41 43 44 46 47 48 49 50 53 57 58 59 60 61 63 64 65 66 70 71 73 74 75 76 77 78 79 80 81 82 84 85 86 87 90 93 96 100 102 104 105 107 108 110 111 113 114 117 118 123 125 128 129 130 131 133 134 142 143 145 146 147 **P**6
Primary Contact: Joseph Pepe, M.D., Interim President and Chief Executive Officer
COO: Allen Ericson, Senior Vice President and Chief Operating Officer
CFO: Edward L. Dudley, III, Senior Vice President and Chief Financial Officer
CFO: Scott Watkins, Director, Employment/Employee Relations
CMO: Matthew Greenston, M.D., Interim Chief Medical Officer
CIO: Brian Tew, Vice President and Chief Information Officer
CNO: Robert A. Duhaime, R.N., Vice President–Operations/Chief Nurse Executive
Web address: www.catholicmedicalcenter.org
**Control:** Other not–for–profit (including NFP Corporation) **Service:** General Medical and Surgical

**Staffed Beds:** 233 **Admissions:** 9841 **Census:** 130 **Outpatient Visits:** 275425 **Births:** 1172 **Total Expense ($000):** 241599 **Payroll Expense ($000):** 112131 **Personnel:** 1460

⊞ △ **ELLIOT HOSPITAL (300012)**, One Elliot Way, Zip 03103–3599; tel. 603/669–5300 **A**1 2 7 9 10 **F**2 3 8 11 12 13 15 18 20 22 26 28 29 30 31 32 34 35 36 37 38 39 40 42 43 44 45 46 47 48 49 50 51 53 54 55 56 57 59 64 65 68 70 72 74 75 76 77 78 79 81 82 83 84 85 86 87 88 89 93 97 98 100 101 102 103 105 107 108 110 111 113 114 117 118 119 120 122 123 125 128 129 130 131 133 134 142 143 145 146 147 **P**6
Primary Contact: Douglas F. Dean, Jr., President and Chief Executive Officer
CFO: Richard Elwell, Senior Vice President and Chief Financial Officer
CMO: Greg Baxter, M.D., Vice President Medical Affairs
CIO: Denise Purington, Vice President and Chief Information Officer
CHR: Sabrina M. Granville, Vice President Human Resources
Web address: www.elliothospital.org
**Control:** Other not–for–profit (including NFP Corporation) **Service:** General Medical and Surgical

**Staffed Beds:** 279 **Admissions:** 12405 **Census:** 163 **Outpatient Visits:** 494556 **Births:** 1866 **Total Expense ($000):** 302271 **Payroll Expense ($000):** 117310 **Personnel:** 2704

★ **VETERANS AFFAIRS MEDICAL CENTER**, 718 Smyth Road, Zip 03104–4098; tel. 603/624–4366, (Nonreporting) **A**5 **S** Department of Veterans Affairs, Washington, DC
Primary Contact: Marc Levenson, M.D., Director
COO: Richard T. Rose, Associate Director
CFO: Frank Ryan, Chief Financial Officer
CMO: Andrew Breuder, M.D., Chief of Staff
CIO: John Foote, Chief Information Officer
CHR: Mary Ellen Kenney, Chief Human Services
Web address: www.va.gov/sta/guide/home.asp
**Control:** Veterans Affairs, Government, federal **Service:** Rehabilitation

**Staffed Beds:** 90

**NASHUA—Hillsborough County**

⊞ **SOUTHERN NEW HAMPSHIRE MEDICAL CENTER (300020)**, 8 Prospect Street, Zip 03060–3925, Mailing Address: P.O. Box 2014, Zip 03061–2014; tel. 603/577–2000 **A**1 2 3 5 9 10 **F**3 11 13 15 18 20 22 26 28 29 30 31 34 35 38 40 42 43 49 50 51 52 57 59 61 65 68 70 72 74 75 76 77 78 79 81 85 86 87 89 93 96 98 100 102 104 105 107 110 111 114 116 117 118 128 129 130 131 134 142 145 146 147 **P**6 8
Primary Contact: Thomas E. Wilhelmsen, Jr., President and Chief Executive Officer
CFO: Michael S. Rose, Senior Vice President Finance and Chief Financial Officer
CMO: Stephanie Wolf–Rosenblum, M.D., Chief Medical Officer
CIO: Andrew Watt, M.D., Vice President, Chief Information Officer and Chief Medical Information Officer
CHR: Merryll Rosenfeld, Vice President Human Resources
Web address: www.snhmc.org
**Control:** Other not–for–profit (including NFP Corporation) **Service:** General Medical and Surgical

**Staffed Beds:** 166 **Admissions:** 8540 **Census:** 100 **Outpatient Visits:** 232195 **Births:** 1460 **Total Expense ($000):** 167372 **Payroll Expense ($000):** 81700 **Personnel:** 1406

⊞ △ **ST. JOSEPH HOSPITAL (300011)**, 172 Kinsley Street, Zip 03061–2013; tel. 603/882–3000 **A**1 2 7 9 10 **F**2 3 7 11 13 15 18 20 28 29 30 31 32 34 35 36 40 42 43 44 49 50 51 54 56 57 59 61 62 63 64 65 68 70 74 75 76 77 78 79 81 82 83 84 85 86 87 89 90 93 97 98 103 104 107 108 110 111 114 115 116 118 125 128 129 131 134 145 146 147 **P**6 8 **S** Covenant Health Systems, Inc., Tewksbury, MA
Primary Contact: David Ross, President and Chief Executive Officer
COO: Pam Duchene, R.N., Vice President Patient Care Services
CFO: Richard Plamondon, Vice President Finance and Chief Financial Officer
CIO: Keith A. Choinka, Vice President Information Systems and Chief Information Officer
CHR: Jacqueline Woolley, Vice President Human Resources
Web address: www.stjosephhospital.com
**Control:** Church–operated, Nongovernment, not–for profit **Service:** General Medical and Surgical

**Staffed Beds:** 144 **Admissions:** 6490 **Census:** 94 **Outpatient Visits:** 201276 **Births:** 470 **Total Expense ($000):** 160456 **Payroll Expense ($000):** 66537 **Personnel:** 1042

**NEW LONDON—Merrimack County**

★ **NEW LONDON HOSPITAL (301304)**, 273 County Road, Zip 03257–4570; tel. 603/526–2911, (Total facility includes 58 beds in nursing home–type unit) **A**9 10 18 **F**3 7 11 15 18 29 30 31 32 34 40 41 45 50 51 54 56 57 59 64 67 70 74 75 77 78 79 81 82 84 85 87 93 94 97 100 102 107 110 111 113 118 126 127 128 129 130 132 133 145 146 147 **P**6
Primary Contact: Bruce King, President and Chief Executive Officer
COO: Terry Leblanc, Chief Operating Officer
CFO: Donald Griffin, CPA, Chief Financial Officer
CMO: Steven Powell, M.D., Chief Medical Officer
CIO: David Foss, Senior Director Information Systems
CHR: Catherine Bardier, Senior Director Human Resources
CNO: Trish Sweezey, R.N., Chief Nursing Officer
Web address: www.newlondonhospital.org
**Control:** Other not–for–profit (including NFP Corporation) **Service:** General Medical and Surgical

**Staffed Beds:** 83 **Admissions:** 1113 **Census:** 64 **Outpatient Visits:** 179036 **Births:** 0 **Total Expense ($000):** 54752 **Payroll Expense ($000):** 26770 **Personnel:** 438

**NORTH CONWAY—Carroll County**

**MEMORIAL HOSPITAL (301307)**, 3073 White Mountain Highway, Zip 03860–7101, Mailing Address: P.O. Box 5001, Zip 03860–5001; tel. 603/356–5461, (Total facility includes 45 beds in nursing home–type unit) **A**9 10 18 **F**3 11 13 15 28 29 30 31 34 35 36 40 43 45 50 51 57 59 64 67 68 70 75 76 77 78 79 81 82 85 86 87 90 94 96 97 105 107 110 114 118 127 129 130 131 132 143 145 146 **P**6
Primary Contact: Scott McKinnon, President and Chief Executive Officer
COO: Steven J. Wyrsch, R.N., Senior Vice President, Operations and Chief Operating Officer
CFO: John Newton, Vice President Financial and Support Services and Chief Financial Officer
CMO: Ray Rabideau, M.D., Medical Director
CIO: Curtis Kerbs, Vice President Information Services
CHR: Margaret Phillips, Director Human Resources
CNO: Ethnee Garner, Vice President Nursing Services
Web address: www.memorialhospitalnh.org
**Control:** Other not–for–profit (including NFP Corporation) **Service:** General Medical and Surgical

**Staffed Beds:** 70 **Admissions:** 1640 **Census:** 57 **Outpatient Visits:** 59935 **Births:** 244 **Total Expense ($000):** 58394 **Payroll Expense ($000):** 17468 **Personnel:** 381

**NH**

---

**Hospital, Medicare Provider Number, Address, Telephone, Approval, Facility, and Physician Codes, Health Care System**

★ American Hospital Association (AHA) membership
□ The Joint Commission accreditation  ◇ DNV Healthcare Inc. accreditation
○ American Osteopathic Association (AOA) accreditation
△ Commission on Accreditation of Rehabilitation Facilities (CARF) accreditation

## PETERBOROUGH—Hillsborough County

★ **MONADNOCK COMMUNITY HOSPITAL (301309)**, 452 Old Street Road, Zip 03458–1295; tel. 603/924–7191 **A**5 9 10 18 **F**3 13 15 28 29 30 31 34 35 36 38 39 40 41 44 45 50 53 56 57 59 64 65 70 74 75 76 77 78 79 81 82 85 86 87 89 93 97 99 100 101 102 103 104 107 108 110 114 117 118 129 130 131 132 133 134 145 146 147 **P**6
Primary Contact: Peter L. Gosline, Chief Executive Officer
CFO: Richard Scheinblum, Chief Financial Officer
CMO: Philip Vuocolo, M.D., Chief Medical Officer
CIO: Carol Roosa, Chief Information Officer
CHR: Michael Blood, VP Human Resources
CNO: Vicki Loughery, R.N., Chief Nursing Officer
Web address: www.monadnockhospital.org
**Control:** Other not–for–profit (including NFP Corporation) **Service:** General Medical and Surgical

**Staffed Beds:** 25 **Admissions:** 1415 **Census:** 13 **Outpatient Visits:** 77702 **Births:** 317 **Total Expense ($000):** 69760 **Payroll Expense ($000):** 30110 **Personnel:** 628

## PLYMOUTH—Grafton County

★ **SPEARE MEMORIAL HOSPITAL (301311)**, 16 Hospital Road, Zip 03264–1199; tel. 603/536–1120 **A**9 10 18 **F**3 13 15 26 28 29 30 31 32 34 35 39 40 45 53 54 55 57 59 64 70 75 76 77 78 79 81 84 85 93 94 97 107 110 113 118 126 128 129 130 131 132 143 145 146 **P**8
Primary Contact: Michelle McEwen, President and Chief Executive Officer
CFO: Richard F. Werkowski, Chief Financial Officer
CMO: Joseph Ebner, M.D., Chief Medical Officer
CIO: Alexis Jeannotte, Director Information Technology
CHR: Laurie Bolognani, Human Resources Officer
CNO: Kristine Hering, R.N., Chief Nursing Officer
Web address: www.spearehospital.com
**Control:** Other not–for–profit (including NFP Corporation) **Service:** General Medical and Surgical

**Staffed Beds:** 25 **Admissions:** 1277 **Census:** 12 **Outpatient Visits:** 75225 **Births:** 171 **Total Expense ($000):** 45313 **Payroll Expense ($000):** 20920 **Personnel:** 301

## PORTSMOUTH—Rockingham County

⊞ **PORTSMOUTH REGIONAL HOSPITAL (300029)**, 333 Borthwick Avenue, Zip 03801–7004; tel. 603/436–5110, (Nonreporting) **A**1 2 9 10 **S** HCA, Nashville, TN
Primary Contact: Anne Jamieson, FACHE, Chief Executive Officer
COO: Stuart Hemming, Chief Operating Officer
CFO: Richard Senger, Chief Financial Officer
CMO: Tim Pike, M.D., Chief Medical Officer
CIO: Ed Sovetskhy, Director Information Services
CHR: Jackie Brayton, Vice President Human Resources
Web address: www.portsmouthhospital.com
**Control:** Corporation, Investor–owned, for–profit **Service:** General Medical and Surgical

**Staffed Beds:** 165

## ROCHESTER—Strafford County

★ **FRISBIE MEMORIAL HOSPITAL (300014)**, 11 Whitehall Road, Zip 03867–3297; tel. 603/332–5211 **A**9 10 **F**3 7 11 13 17 18 20 21 28 29 31 32 34 35 40 42 45 46 49 50 56 57 59 64 68 70 75 76 77 78 79 81 82 83 86 87 89 93 97 98 103 104 105 107 111 114 116 117 118 128 129 131 134 145 146 **P**5 8
Primary Contact: Alvin D. Felgar, President and Chief Executive Officer
CFO: John A. Marzinzik, Vice President Finance
CMO: Susan Gaire, M.D., President Medical Staff
CHR: Carol Themelis, Vice President Human Resources
Web address: www.frisbiehospital.com
**Control:** Other not–for–profit (including NFP Corporation) **Service:** General Medical and Surgical

**Staffed Beds:** 82 **Admissions:** 3586 **Census:** 41 **Outpatient Visits:** 137864 **Births:** 397 **Total Expense ($000):** 108468 **Payroll Expense ($000):** 52256 **Personnel:** 802

## SALEM—Rockingham County

☐ △ **NORTHEAST REHABILITATION HOSPITAL (303026)**, 70 Butler Street, Zip 03079–3925; tel. 603/893–2900 **A**1 7 10 **F**29 30 34 35 54 57 62 64 68 74 75 77 79 82 85 86 87 90 93 95 96 129 130 131 134 145
Primary Contact: John F. Prochilo, Chief Executive Officer and Administrator
COO: Robert Kotsonis, Chief Operating Officer
CFO: Charles Champagne, Chief Financial Officer
CMO: James A. Whitlock, Jr., M.D., Medical Director
CIO: Larry Frank, Director Information Systems
CHR: Thomas A. Prince, Vice President Operations and Human Resources
CNO: Marie Sullivan, R.N., Chief Nursing Officer and Administrator
Web address: www.northeastrehab.com
**Control:** Corporation, Investor–owned, for–profit **Service:** Rehabilitation

**Staffed Beds:** 135 **Admissions:** 1778 **Census:** 68 **Outpatient Visits:** 172289 **Births:** 0 **Total Expense ($000):** 48498 **Payroll Expense ($000):** 27326 **Personnel:** 548

## WOLFEBORO—Carroll County

★ **HUGGINS HOSPITAL (301312)**, 240 South Main Street, Zip 03894–4455, Mailing Address: P.O. Box 912, Zip 03894–0912; tel. 603/569–7500, (Total facility includes 27 beds in nursing home–type unit) **A**9 10 18 **F**2 3 10 11 15 28 34 40 45 50 56 57 59 64 65 70 74 75 77 79 81 85 86 87 93 96 97 107 110 111 113 118 124 127 129 132 134 145 146 **P**6
Primary Contact: Michael Connelly, President
CFO: Jeremy Roberge, Chief Financial Officer
CMO: John Boornazian, M.D., Chief Medical Officer
CIO: Pam McGovern, Director Technology
CHR: Laura Stauss, Director of Human Resources
Web address: www.hugginshospital.org
**Control:** Other not–for–profit (including NFP Corporation) **Service:** General Medical and Surgical

**Staffed Beds:** 52 **Admissions:** 1279 **Census:** 29 **Outpatient Visits:** 143823 **Births:** 0 **Total Expense ($000):** 46922 **Payroll Expense ($000):** 19131 **Personnel:** 395

## WOODSVILLE—Grafton County

★ **COTTAGE HOSPITAL (301301)**, 90 Swiftwater Road, Zip 03785–2001, Mailing Address: P.O. Box 2001, Zip 03785–2001; tel. 603/747–9000 **A**9 10 18 **F**3 11 13 15 18 28 29 30 31 34 35 40 43 46 49 50 59 64 65 67 68 70 74 75 76 77 78 79 81 82 84 85 87 89 93 97 107 111 113 118 126 127 129 131 132 134 145 146 147
Primary Contact: Maria Ryan, Ph.D., Chief Executive Officer
COO: Lori Hughes, R.N., Chief Nursing Officer, Vice President Operations and Patient Care Services
CFO: Steven L. Plant, Chief Financial Officer
CIO: Rick Fredrick, Director Information Technology
CHR: Gerry J. Graham, Director Human Resources
CNO: Lori Hughes, R.N., Chief Nursing Officer, Vice President Operations & Patient Care Services
Web address: www.cottagehospital.org
**Control:** Other not–for–profit (including NFP Corporation) **Service:** General Medical and Surgical

**Staffed Beds:** 25 **Admissions:** 736 **Census:** 7 **Outpatient Visits:** 48200 **Births:** 90 **Total Expense ($000):** 27603 **Payroll Expense ($000):** 11696 **Personnel:** 211

**NH**

# NEW JERSEY

## ANCORA—Camden County

☐ **ANCORA PSYCHIATRIC HOSPITAL (314005)**, 301 Spring Garden Road, Zip 08037-9699; tel. 609/561-1700 **A**1 10 **F**30 39 56 68 75 87 97 98 129 134 142 145 **P**6 **S** Division of Mental Health and Addiction Services, Department of Human Services, State of New Jersey, Trenton, NJ
Primary Contact: Allan Boyer, Chief Executive Officer
COO: John Lubitsky, Deputy Chief Executive Officer Support Services
CFO: John Holmes, Business Manager
CMO: David Roat, D.O., Acting Medical Director
CIO: Charlene Ruberti, Director Information Technology Development
CHR: Alfred Filipini, Manager Human Resources
CNO: Catherine Jones, Chief Nursing Officer
Web address: www.peoplefirstnurses.nj.gov/ancora.htm
**Control:** State–Government, nonfederal **Service:** Psychiatric

**Staffed Beds:** 500 **Admissions:** 701 **Census:** 463 **Outpatient Visits:** 0 **Births:** 0 **Total Expense ($000):** 141205 **Payroll Expense ($000):** 85341 **Personnel:** 1616

## ATLANTIC CITY—Atlantic County

**ACUITY SPECIALTY HOSPITAL OF NEW JERSEY (312023)**, 1925 Pacific Avenue, Zip 08401-6713; tel. 609/441-8160, (Nonreporting) **A**10 21 **S** AcuityHealthcare, LP, Charlotte, NC
Primary Contact: Mary Beth Tubbs, Chief Executive Officer
Web address: www.acuityhealthcare.net
**Control:** Corporation, Investor–owned, for–profit **Service:** Long–Term Acute Care hospital

**Staffed Beds:** 30

⊠ **ATLANTICARE REGIONAL MEDICAL CENTER (310064)**, 1925 Pacific Avenue, Zip 08401-6713; tel. 609/441-8994, (Includes ATLANTICARE REGIONAL MEDICAL CENTER–MAINLAND DIVISION, Jimmie Leeds Road, Pomona, Zip 08240; tel. 609/652-1000) **A**1 2 9 10 **F**3 7 11 12 13 15 16 17 18 20 22 24 26 29 30 31 34 35 36 37 38 40 41 42 43 45 46 47 48 49 50 54 57 58 59 60 61 64 66 67 68 70 71 72 73 74 75 76 78 79 80 81 82 84 85 86 87 88 89 90 93 97 98 99 100 102 103 104 105 106 107 108 110 111 113 114 115 116 117 118 119 120 122 123 125 129 134 142 145 146 147 **P**6 **S** AtlantiCare, Egg Harbor Township, NJ
Primary Contact: Lori Herndon, President and Chief Executive Officer
COO: Lori Herndon, President and Chief Executive Officer
CFO: Walter Greiner, Chief Financial Officer
CMO: Marilouise Vendetti, M.D., Chief Medical Officer
CHR: Richard Lovering, Corporate Vice President Human Resources and Organizational Development
Web address: www.atlanticare.org
**Control:** Other not–for–profit (including NFP Corporation) **Service:** General Medical and Surgical

**Staffed Beds:** 538 **Admissions:** 29029 **Census:** 382 **Outpatient Visits:** 344506 **Births:** 2622 **Total Expense ($000):** 593206 **Payroll Expense ($000):** 259350 **Personnel:** 3510

## BAYONNE—Hudson County

☐ **BAYONNE MEDICAL CENTER (310025)**, 29 East 29th Street, Zip 07002-4699; tel. 201/858-5000, (Nonreporting) **A**1 2 6 10
Primary Contact: Mark Spektor, M.D., President and Chief Executive Officer
CFO: David Paulosky, Chief Financial Officer
CIO: Don Lutz, Chief Information Officer
CHR: Jennifer Dobin, Vice President Human Resources
Web address: www.bayonnemedicalcenter.org
**Control:** Corporation, Investor–owned, for–profit **Service:** General Medical and Surgical

**Staffed Beds:** 170

## BELLE MEAD—Somerset County

⊠ **CARRIER CLINIC (314012)**, 252 County Route 601, Zip 08502-0147, Mailing Address: P.O. Box 147, Zip 08502-0147; tel. 908/281-1000 **A**1 5 10 **F**4 5 98 99 100 101 102 103 **P**6
Primary Contact: C. Richard Sarle, CPA, FACHE, President and Chief Executive Officer
COO: Mary Pawlikowski, Chief Operating Officer
CFO: Randolph Jacobson, Chief Financial Officer
CMO: Marie Hasson, M.D., Medical Director
CIO: Peter Schwartz, Manager Information Services
CHR: Trish Toole, Vice President Administrative Services
CNO: Carol Kosztyo, R.N., Vice President, Patient Care Services
Web address: www.carrier.org
**Control:** Other not–for–profit (including NFP Corporation) **Service:** Psychiatric

**Staffed Beds:** 270 **Admissions:** 4979 **Census:** 207 **Outpatient Visits:** 379 **Births:** 0 **Total Expense ($000):** 54602 **Payroll Expense ($000):** 33741 **Personnel:** 608

**EAST MOUNTAIN HOSPITAL (314026)**, 40 East Mountain Road, Zip 8502; tel. 908/281-1500 **A**10 **F**38 87 98 102 106 129 142
Primary Contact: Michael Voorhees, MS, Executive Director
CFO: Randolph Jacobson, Chief Financial Officer
CMO: Bohdan Cehelyk, M.D., Chief Medical Officer
CIO: Peter Schwartz, Director Information Systems
CHR: Patricia Toole, Vice President Human Resources
CNO: Deborah Charette, Director of Nursing
**Control:** Other not–for–profit (including NFP Corporation) **Service:** Psychiatric

**Staffed Beds:** 16 **Admissions:** 406 **Census:** 15 **Outpatient Visits:** 0 **Births:** 0 **Total Expense ($000):** 4296 **Payroll Expense ($000):** 1916 **Personnel:** 26

## BELLEVILLE—Essex County

⊠ **CLARA MAASS MEDICAL CENTER (310009)**, One Clara Maass Drive, Zip 07109-3557; tel. 973/450-2000 **A**1 2 3 5 9 10 **F**1 3 4 8 11 12 13 15 16 17 18 19 20 22 28 29 30 31 34 35 38 40 42 43 44 47 49 50 51 55 56 57 58 59 60 61 62 63 64 66 67 68 70 72 73 74 75 76 78 79 80 81 82 85 86 87 88 89 90 91 92 93 94 98 100 101 102 103 107 108 110 111 113 114 115 116 117 118 119 120 122 127 128 129 131 142 145 146 147 **S** Barnabas Health, West Orange, NJ
Primary Contact: Mary Ellen Clyne, Ph.D., President and Chief Executive Officer
CIO: Michael McTigue, Chief Information Officer
Web address: www.sbhcs.com
**Control:** Other not–for–profit (including NFP Corporation) **Service:** General Medical and Surgical

**Staffed Beds:** 429 **Admissions:** 18726 **Census:** 232 **Outpatient Visits:** 354689 **Births:** 1610 **Total Expense ($000):** 208531 **Payroll Expense ($000):** 97794 **Personnel:** 1567

## BERKELEY HEIGHTS—Union County

★ **RUNNELLS SPECIALIZED HOSPITAL OF UNION COUNTY (314027)**, 40 Watchung Way, Zip 07922-2618; tel. 908/771-5700, (Nonreporting) **A**9 10
Primary Contact: Joan Wheeler, MSN, R.N., Administrator
CFO: Michael Drummond, Chief Financial Officer
CMO: Raymond Lanza, D.O., Medical Director
CIO: Margaret A. Salisbury, Director Marketing
CHR: Greg Hardoby, Director Personnel
CNO: Susan Palma, MS, Associate Administrator and Administrative Director Nursing
Web address: www.ucnj.org/runnells
**Control:** County–Government, nonfederal **Service:** General Medical and Surgical

**Staffed Beds:** 344

NJ

---

**Hospital, Medicare Provider Number, Address, Telephone, Approval, Facility, and Physician Codes, Health Care System**

★ American Hospital Association (AHA) membership
☐ The Joint Commission accreditation          ◇ DNV Healthcare Inc. accreditation

○ American Osteopathic Association (AOA) accreditation
△ Commission on Accreditation of Rehabilitation Facilities (CARF) accreditation

## BERLIN—Camden County

★ **VIRTUA BERLIN (310022)**, 100 Townsend Avenue, Zip 08009–9035;
tel. 856/322–3000 **A**9 10 **F**3 8 11 29 30 34 35 38 40 45 46 47 48 49 50 55
56 57 63 64 65 68 70 74 75 81 82 84 85 87 90 92 93 100 107 108 111
114 118 129 145 147 **S** Virtua Health, Marlton, NJ
Primary Contact: Gary L. Long, Chief Operating Officer
CFO: Robert Segin, Chief Financial Officer
CMO: John Matsinger, M.D., Medical Director
CIO: Alfred Campanella, Vice President and Chief Information Officer
CHR: Michael Pepe, Ph.D., Chief Human Resources Officer
Web address: www.virtua.org
**Control:** Other not–for–profit (including NFP Corporation) **Service:** General
Medical and Surgical

**Staffed Beds:** 82 **Admissions:** 4279 **Census:** 56 **Outpatient Visits:** 34136
**Births:** 0 **Total Expense ($000):** 74303 **Payroll Expense ($000):** 27918
**Personnel:** 324

## BLACKWOOD—Camden County

⊞ **CAMDEN COUNTY HEALTH SERVICES CENTER (314018)**, 425 Woodbury
Turnersville Road, Zip 08012–2960; tel. 856/374–6600, (Total facility includes
300 beds in nursing home–type unit) **A**1 9 10 **F**4 56 65 84 87 98 100 103 127
129 134 145 147 **P**6
Primary Contact: Kevin G. Halpern, Chief Executive Officer
COO: Gene Lynam, Chief Operating Officer and Treasurer
CFO: Gene Lynam, Chief Operating Officer and Treasurer
CMO: Michael S. DeShields, M.D., Director Medical Affairs
CIO: Richard Behm, Director Information Technology
CHR: Brian Eisen, Director Human Resources
Web address: www.cchsc.com
**Control:** County–Government, nonfederal **Service:** Psychiatric

**Staffed Beds:** 450 **Admissions:** 1265 **Census:** 421 **Outpatient Visits:** 31
**Births:** 0 **Total Expense ($000):** 75149 **Payroll Expense ($000):** 33966
**Personnel:** 494

## BOONTON TOWNSHIP—Morris County

**SAINT CLARE'S HOSPITAL/BOONTON TOWNSHIP** See Saint Clare's Health
System, Denville

## BRICK—Ocean County

☐ **SHORE REHABILITATION HOSPITAL (313033)**, 425 Jack Martin Boulevard,
Zip 08724–7732; tel. 732/836–4500, (Nonreporting) **A**1 10
Primary Contact: Amite Mohan, Executive Director
Web address: www.oceanmedicalcenter.com
**Control:** Other not–for–profit (including NFP Corporation) **Service:** Rehabilitation

**Staffed Beds:** 40

## BRICK TOWNSHIP—Ocean County

⊞ **OCEAN MEDICAL CENTER (310052)**, 425 Jack Martin Boulevard, Zip 8724;
tel. 732/840–2200 **A**1 2 9 10 **F**3 5 6 11 13 15 17 18 20 22 28 29 30 31 32
40 41 42 44 45 46 47 49 53 55 56 59 60 64 65 66 68 70 73 74 75 76 78
79 80 81 82 84 85 86 87 89 92 93 97 100 101 103 107 108 110 111 113
114 116 118 119 120 122 128 129 131 134 143 145 146 147 **P**7 **S** Meridian
Health, Neptune, NJ
Primary Contact: Dean Q. Lin, FACHE, President
COO: Regina Foley, R.N., Vice President Nursing and Operations
CFO: John Gantner, Executive Vice President Finance
CMO: James Clarke, M.D., Vice President Medical Affairs and Clinical
Effectiveness
CIO: Rebecca Weber, Senior Vice President and Chief Information Officer
Web address: www.meridianhealth.com
**Control:** Other not–for–profit (including NFP Corporation) **Service:** General
Medical and Surgical

**Staffed Beds:** 265 **Admissions:** 14097 **Census:** 188 **Outpatient Visits:**
151806 **Births:** 1008 **Total Expense ($000):** 206961 **Payroll Expense
($000):** 88942 **Personnel:** 1038

## BRIDGETON—Cumberland County

**BRIDGETON HEALTH CENTER** See South Jersey Healthcare – Regional Medical
Center, Vineland

## BROWNS MILLS—Burlington County

**DEBORAH HEART AND LUNG CENTER (310031)**, 200 Trenton Road,
Zip 08015–1799; tel. 609/893–6611, (Nonreporting) **A**3 5 9 10 13
Primary Contact: Joseph P. Chirichella, President and Chief Executive Officer
CFO: R. Grant Leidy, Vice President Finance
CMO: Lynn McGrath, M.D., Vice President Medical Affairs
CHR: James Carlino, Vice President Human Resources
Web address: www.deborah.org
**Control:** Other not–for–profit (including NFP Corporation) **Service:** Other specialty

**Staffed Beds:** 89

## CAMDEN—Camden County

⊞ **COOPER HEALTH SYSTEM (310014)**, One Cooper Plaza, Zip 08103–1489;
tel. 856/342–2000, (Includes CHILDEN'S REGIONAL HOSPITAL AT COOPER, One
Cooper Plaza, Zip 08103; tel. 800/826–6737) **A**1 2 3 5 8 9 10 13 **F**3 5 8 9 11
12 13 15 17 18 19 20 22 24 26 29 30 31 32 34 35 36 37 38 39 40 41 43
44 45 46 47 48 49 50 51 52 54 55 56 57 58 59 60 61 63 64 65 66 68 70
72 73 74 75 76 78 79 80 81 82 83 84 85 86 87 88 89 91 92 93 94 96 97
98 99 100 101 102 103 104 107 108 110 111 113 114 118 119 120 122
123 125 128 129 130 131 133 134 142 145 146 147 **P**6
Primary Contact: John P. Sheridan, Jr., President and Chief Executive Officer
COO: Adrienne Kirby, Ph.D., Chief Operating Officer
CFO: Douglas E. Shirley, Senior Executive Vice President and Chief Financial
Officer
CMO: Carolyn Bekes, M.D., Chief Medical Officer
CHR: Douglas Allen, Vice President Human Resources
Web address: www.cooperhealth.org
**Control:** Other not–for–profit (including NFP Corporation) **Service:** General
Medical and Surgical

**Staffed Beds:** 493 **Admissions:** 23157 **Census:** 340 **Outpatient Visits:**
249563 **Births:** 2188 **Total Expense ($000):** 578631 **Payroll Expense
($000):** 217326 **Personnel:** 4855

⊞ △ **OUR LADY OF LOURDES MEDICAL CENTER (310029)**, 1600 Haddon
Avenue, Zip 08103–3117; tel. 856/757–3500 **A**1 2 6 7 9 10 **F**3 11 12 13 15
17 18 20 22 24 26 28 29 30 31 32 34 35 36 37 38 40 44 47 49 50 55 56
57 58 59 60 61 64 65 66 68 70 71 72 73 74 75 76 78 79 81 82 84 85 86
87 90 95 96 97 100 107 108 110 111 113 114 117 118 125 129 131 133
134 137 138 141 145 146 147 **P**7 **S** Catholic Health East, Newtown Square, PA
Primary Contact: Alexander J. Hatala, President and Chief Executive Officer
COO: Mark Nessel, Chief Operating Officer
CFO: Michael Hammond, Chief Financial Officer
CMO: Alan R. Pope, M.D., Vice President Medical Affairs
CIO: Maureen Hetu, Chief Information Officer
CHR: Richard P. Kropp, Vice President Human Resources
CNO: Audrey Jadczak, R.N., Chief Nursing Officer
Web address: www.lourdesnet.org
**Control:** Other not–for–profit (including NFP Corporation) **Service:** General
Medical and Surgical

**Staffed Beds:** 391 **Admissions:** 13410 **Census:** 215 **Outpatient Visits:**
157505 **Births:** 1148 **Total Expense ($000):** 260013 **Payroll Expense
($000):** 97230 **Personnel:** 1587

## CAPE MAY COURT HOUSE—Cape May County

⊞ **CAPE REGIONAL MEDICAL CENTER (310011)**, Two Stone Harbor Boulevard,
Zip 08210–9990; tel. 609/463–2000 **A**1 2 9 10 **F**3 8 11 13 15 18 20 28 29
30 31 34 35 40 44 45 46 49 50 53 57 59 64 70 74 75 76 77 78 79 81 82
84 85 86 87 89 91 93 97 107 111 113 117 118 119 120 122 129 131 134
142 145 147
Primary Contact: Joanne Carrocino, FACHE, President and Chief Executive Officer
CFO: Mark Gill, Vice President Finance and Chief Financial Officer
CMO: Richard Falivena, D.O., Vice President Medical Affairs
CIO: Richard Wheatley, Chief Information Officer
CHR: Byron Hunter, Vice President Human Resources
Web address: www.caperegional.com
**Control:** Other not–for–profit (including NFP Corporation) **Service:** General
Medical and Surgical

**Staffed Beds:** 180 **Admissions:** 9705 **Census:** 98 **Outpatient Visits:** 150865
**Births:** 537 **Total Expense ($000):** 108095 **Payroll Expense ($000):** 47918
**Personnel:** 871

## CEDAR GROVE—Essex County

☐ **ESSEX COUNTY HOSPITAL CENTER (314020)**, 204 Grove Avenue,
Zip 07009–1436; tel. 973/571–2800, (Nonreporting) **A**1 10
Primary Contact: Lucia A. Guarini, Administrator
CFO: Lonnie Hughes, Comptroller
CMO: N. Elangovan, M.D., Medical Director
CIO: John Rosas, Compliance Officer
CHR: BettyAnn Jannuzzi, Supervisor Personnel
Web address: www.essexcountynj.org
**Control:** County–Government, nonfederal **Service:** Psychiatric

**Staffed Beds:** 180

**NJ**

## CHERRY HILL—Camden County

☒ ○ **KENNEDY MEMORIAL HOSPITALS–UNIVERSITY MEDICAL CENTER (310086)**, 2201 Chapel Avenue West, Zip 08002–2048, Mailing Address: P.O. Box 1916, Voorhees, Zip 08043–1916; tel. 856/488–6500, (Includes KENNEDY MEMORIAL HOSPITAL, 18 East Laurel Road, Stratford, Zip 08084; tel. 609/346–6000; KENNEDY MEMORIAL HOSPITAL, 435 Hurffville–Cross Keys Road, Turnersville, Zip 08012; tel. 609/582–2500) **A**1 9 10 11 12 **F**3 4 5 7 8 11 12 13 15 18 20 22 26 29 30 31 32 34 35 38 39 40 44 46 49 50 54 55 56 57 59 60 61 62 64 65 66 68 70 72 73 74 75 76 78 79 81 82 84 85 86 87 89 93 97 98 99 100 101 102 103 104 105 107 108 110 111 113 114 116 117 118 120 122 125 128 129 130 131 133 142 145 146 147
Primary Contact: Martin A. Bieber, President and Chief Executive Officer
COO: Paul A. Walker, Senior Vice President and Chief Operating Officer
CFO: Gary G. Terrinoni, Chief Financial Officer and Senior Vice President
CMO: Richard Boehler, M.D., Senior Vice President Medical Affairs and Chief Medical Officer
CIO: Thomas Balcavage, Vice President Information Systems and Chief Information Officer
CHR: Anneliese McMenamin, Vice President Human Resources
Web address: www.kennedyhealth.org
**Control:** Other not–for–profit (including NFP Corporation) **Service:** General Medical and Surgical

**Staffed Beds:** 495 **Admissions:** 31015 **Census:** 358 **Outpatient Visits:** 381268 **Births:** 1259 **Total Expense ($000):** 349165 **Payroll Expense ($000):** 178102 **Personnel:** 2867

## CHESTER—Morris County

**KESSLER INSTITUTE FOR REHABILITATION** See Kessler Institute for Rehabilitation, West Orange

## DENVILLE—Morris County

☒ **SAINT CLARE'S HEALTH SYSTEM (310050)**, 25 Pocono Road, Zip 07834–2954; tel. 973/625–6000, (Includes SAINT CLARE'S HOSPITAL/BOONTON TOWNSHIP, 130 Powerville Road, Boonton Township, Zip 07005; tel. 973/316–1800; SAINT CLARE'S HOSPITAL/DENVILLE, 25 Pocono Road, Zip 07834; tel. 973/625–6000; SAINT CLARE'S HOSPITAL/SUSSEX, 20 Walnut Street, Sussex, Zip 07461; tel. 973/702–2200; ST. CLARE'S HOSPITAL/DOVER, 400 West Blackwell Street, Dover, Zip 07801–3311; tel. 973/989–3000), (Total facility includes 118 beds in nursing home–type unit) **A**1 2 9 10 **F**1 3 4 5 7 10 11 12 13 14 15 18 20 22 26 28 29 30 31 32 34 35 36 38 40 41 44 45 46 47 48 49 50 51 54 56 57 58 59 61 62 64 65 66 67 68 70 71 73 74 75 76 77 78 79 81 82 83 84 85 86 87 89 90 92 93 97 98 99 100 101 102 103 104 105 106 107 108 109 110 111 112 113 115 116 117 118 119 120 122 124 125 126 127 128 129 130 131 133 134 142 144 145 146 **P**5 **S** Catholic Health Initiatives, Englewood, CO
Primary Contact: Leslie D. Hirsch, FACHE, President and Chief Executive Officer
COO: Suellyn Ellerbe, R.N., Executive Vice President, Chief Nursing Officer and Chief Operating Officer
CFO: Gordon A. King, Interim Chief Financial Officer
CMO: Alma Ratcliffe, M.D., Executive Vice President Medical Staff and Business Development
CIO: Tero Caamano, Director Information Technology
CHR: Gail C. Cohen, Vice President Human Resources
Web address: www.saintclares.org
**Control:** Church–operated, Nongovernment, not–for profit **Service:** General Medical and Surgical

**Staffed Beds:** 426 **Admissions:** 18932 **Census:** 246 **Outpatient Visits:** 255704 **Births:** 1435 **Total Expense ($000):** 305191 **Payroll Expense ($000):** 135937 **Personnel:** 2138

**SAINT CLARE'S HOSPITAL/DENVILLE** See Saint Clare's Health System

## DOVER—Morris County

☒ **KINDRED HOSPITAL–NEW JERSEY MORRIS COUNTY (312020)**, 400 West Blackwell Street, Zip 7801; tel. 973/537–3818, (Includes KINDRED HOSPITAL NEW JERSEY – RAHWAY, 865 Stone Street, Rahway, Zip 07065; tel. 732/453–2950; Sharon Rosetti, R.N., Chief Executive Officer; KINDRED HOSPITAL NEW JERSEY – WAYNE, 224 Hamburg Turnpike, Wayne, Zip 07470; tel. 973/636–7200; Alice M. O'Connor, R.N., Administrator), (Nonreporting) **A**1 10 **S** Kindred Healthcare, Louisville, KY
Primary Contact: Wayne D. Blanchard, Chief Executive Officer
CFO: Rishab Punjabi, Chief Financial Officer
CHR: Neil Rosner, Area Director Human Resources
Web address: www.khmorriscounty.com/
**Control:** Corporation, Investor–owned, for–profit **Service:** Long–Term Acute Care hospital

**Staffed Beds:** 117

## EAST ORANGE—Essex County

☒ **EAST ORANGE GENERAL HOSPITAL (310083)**, 300 Central Avenue, Zip 07019–2897; tel. 973/672–8400 **A**1 9 10 **F**4 5 7 10 11 15 18 28 29 31 34 35 38 40 45 46 53 57 59 60 61 68 70 71 77 81 84 90 93 97 98 99 102 104 105 106 107 108 110 111 113 118 129 142 147 **P**6
Primary Contact: Kevin J. Slavin, FACHE, President and Chief Executive Officer
CFO: Al Aboud, Chief Financial Officer
CMO: Valentine Burroughs, M.D., Chief Medical Officer
CIO: Thomas Ciccarelli, Chief Information Officer
CHR: Chester Banks, Director Human Resources
CNO: Mary Anne Marra, R.N., Vice President/Chief Nursing Officer
Web address: www.evh.org
**Control:** Other not–for–profit (including NFP Corporation) **Service:** General Medical and Surgical

**Staffed Beds:** 196 **Admissions:** 8043 **Census:** 150 **Outpatient Visits:** 96525 **Births:** 0 **Total Expense ($000):** 107605 **Payroll Expense ($000):** 58042

☒ △ **VETERANS AFFAIRS NEW JERSEY HEALTH CARE SYSTEM**, 385 Tremont Avenue, Zip 07018–1095; tel. 973/676–1000, (Includes EAST ORANGE DIVISION, 385 Tremont Avenue, tel. 973/676–1000; LYONS DIVISION, 151 Knollcroft Road, Lyons, Zip 07939–9998; tel. 908/647–0180), (Nonreporting) **A**1 2 3 5 7 8 **S** Department of Veterans Affairs, Washington, DC
Primary Contact: Kenneth H. Mizrach, Director
COO: Kenneth H. Mizrach, Director
CFO: Tyrone Taylor, Chief Financial Officer
CMO: Steven L. Lieberman, M.D., Chief of Staff
CIO: Marsha Evens, Acting Chief Information Resource Management
CHR: Joseph Capodiferro, Chief Human and Learning Resources
Web address: www.va.gov/sta/guide/home.asp
**Control:** Veterans Affairs, Government, federal **Service:** Other specialty

**Staffed Beds:** 414

## EDISON—Middlesex County

★ △ **JFK JOHNSON REHABILITATION INSTITUTE**, 65 James Street, Zip 08818–3059; tel. 732/321–7050, (Nonreporting) **A**7 **S** JFK Health System, Edison, NJ
Primary Contact: Anthony Cuzzola, Vice President Rehabilitation Services
CIO: Louis H. Hermans, Vice President Information Systems
Web address: www.solarishs.org
**Control:** Other not–for–profit (including NFP Corporation) **Service:** Rehabilitation

**Staffed Beds:** 92

☒ **JFK MEDICAL CENTER (310108)**, 65 James Street, Zip 08818–3059; tel. 732/321–7000, (Nonreporting) **A**1 2 3 5 9 10 **S** JFK Health System, Edison, NJ
Primary Contact: Raymond F. Fredericks, President and CEO
COO: Scott Gebhard, Executive Vice President and Chief Operating Officer
CFO: Richard C. Smith, Senior Vice President and Chief Financial Officer
CMO: William F. Oser, M.D., Senior Vice President and Chief Medical Officer
CIO: Louis H. Hermans, Vice President Information Systems
CHR: Shirley Higgins–Bowers, Vice President Human Resources
CNO: Patricia G. Rackovan, Senior Vice President & Chief Nurse Executive
Web address: www.jfkmc.org
**Control:** Other not–for–profit (including NFP Corporation) **Service:** General Medical and Surgical

**Staffed Beds:** 441

## ELIZABETH—Union County

☒ **TRINITAS REGIONAL MEDICAL CENTER (310027)**, 225 Williamson Street, Zip 7202; tel. 908/994–5000, (Includes TRINITAS HOSPITAL, 925 East Jersey Street, Zip 07201; tel. 908/994–5000; TRINITAS HOSPITAL – NEW POINT CAMPUS, 655 East Jersey Street, Zip 07206; tel. 201/351–9000), (Total facility includes 120 beds in nursing home–type unit) **A**1 2 6 9 10 13 **F**3 5 7 11 12 13 15 17 18 20 22 28 29 30 31 32 34 35 36 38 40 44 45 48 49 53 54 56 57 58 59 60 61 64 65 66 68 70 73 74 75 76 77 78 79 81 82 83 84 85 86 87 93 97 98 99 100 101 102 103 104 105 106 107 108 110 111 113 117 118 119 120 122 123 125 127 128 129 131 133 134 142 145 146 **P**6
Primary Contact: Gary S. Horan, FACHE, President and Chief Executive Officer
CFO: Karen Lumpp, Senior Vice President and Chief Financial Officer
CMO: William McHugh, M.D., Chief Medical Officer
CIO: Judy Comitto, Vice President Information Services and Chief Information Officer
CHR: Glenn Nacion, Vice President Human Resources
Web address: www.trinitashospital.com
**Control:** Other not–for–profit (including NFP Corporation) **Service:** General Medical and Surgical

**Staffed Beds:** 454 **Admissions:** 15860 **Census:** 380 **Outpatient Visits:** 431178 **Births:** 2331 **Total Expense ($000):** 284383 **Payroll Expense ($000):** 120959 **Personnel:** 2171

**NJ**

---

**Hospital, Medicare Provider Number, Address, Telephone, Approval, Facility, and Physician Codes, Health Care System**

★ American Hospital Association (AHA) membership
□ The Joint Commission accreditation          ◇ DNV Healthcare Inc. accreditation
○ American Osteopathic Association (AOA) accreditation
△ Commission on Accreditation of Rehabilitation Facilities (CARF) accreditation

## ELMER—Salem County

★ **SOUTH JERSEY HEALTHCARE – ELMER HOSPITAL (310069)**, 501 West Front Street, Zip 08318–1090; tel. 856/363–1000 **A**9 10 21 **F**3 11 12 13 15 28 29 30 34 38 40 44 50 57 59 64 68 70 74 75 76 77 78 79 81 82 85 86 87 89 93 107 108 110 111 118 129 130 131 133 145 146 147 **S** South Jersey Healthcare, Vineland, NJ
Primary Contact: Chester B. Kaletkowski, President and Chief Executive Officer
COO: John Bickings, Chief Operating Officer and Vice President Support Services
CFO: John A. DiAngelo, Senior Vice President Finance and Chief Financial Officer
CMO: Steven C. Linn, M.D., Chief Medical Officer
CIO: Thomas Pacek, Vice President Information Systems and Chief Information Officer
CHR: Erich Florentine, Chief People Officer
Web address: www.sjhealthcare.net
**Control:** Other not–for–profit (including NFP Corporation) **Service:** General Medical and Surgical

**Staffed Beds:** 88 **Admissions:** 3838 **Census:** 43 **Outpatient Visits:** 64478 **Births:** 328 **Total Expense ($000):** 58504 **Payroll Expense ($000):** 25854 **Personnel:** 323

## ENGLEWOOD—Bergen County

☒ **ENGLEWOOD HOSPITAL AND MEDICAL CENTER (310045)**, 350 Engle Street, Zip 07631–1898; tel. 201/894–3000 **A**1 2 3 5 9 10 **F**7 8 12 13 15 17 18 19 20 22 24 26 28 29 30 31 34 35 36 38 40 45 46 49 50 54 55 56 57 59 60 64 70 72 73 74 75 76 77 78 79 81 82 83 84 89 91 92 93 94 98 99 100 101 102 103 104 105 106 107 108 109 110 111 112 113 114 115 116 117 118 119 120 125 128 129 144 147 **P**6 7
Primary Contact: Douglas A. Duchak, President and Chief Executive Officer
COO: Warren Geller, Executive Vice President and Chief Operating Officer
CFO: Anthony T. Orlando, Senior Vice President Finance
CMO: Stephen Brunnquell, M.D., President Medical Staff
CIO: Ronald Fuschillo, Chief Information Officer
CHR: Patricia Wilson, Vice President Human Resources
CNO: Madelyn Pearson, R.N., Sr. Vice President Patient Care Services
Web address: www.englewoodhospital.com
**Control:** Other not–for–profit (including NFP Corporation) **Service:** General Medical and Surgical

**Staffed Beds:** 247 **Admissions:** 16500 **Census:** 233 **Outpatient Visits:** 419884 **Births:** 2300 **Total Expense ($000):** 339241 **Payroll Expense ($000):** 156390 **Personnel:** 2216

## FLEMINGTON—Hunterdon County

☒ **HUNTERDON MEDICAL CENTER (310005)**, 2100 Wescott Drive, Zip 08822–4604; tel. 908/788–6100 **A**1 2 3 5 9 10 **F**3 4 5 11 12 13 14 15 18 20 22 27 28 29 30 31 32 34 35 38 40 45 46 47 48 49 53 54 56 57 58 59 60 61 62 64 65 68 70 71 74 75 76 77 78 79 81 82 83 84 85 86 87 89 91 92 93 94 97 98 99 100 101 102 103 104 105 106 107 108 110 113 117 118 120 122 126 128 129 130 131 133 134 145 146 147 **P**1 5
Primary Contact: Robert P. Wise, FACHE, President and Chief Executive Officer
COO: Lawrence N. Grand, Executive Vice President and Chief Operating Officer
CFO: Daniel J. Deets, Chief Financial Officer
CIO: Glenn Mamary, Chief Information Officer
CHR: Violet Kocsis, Vice President Human Resources and Development
CNO: Patricia Steingall, R.N., Vice President, Patient Care Services
Web address: www.hunterdonhealthcare.org
**Control:** Other not–for–profit (including NFP Corporation) **Service:** General Medical and Surgical

**Staffed Beds:** 178 **Admissions:** 8279 **Census:** 99 **Outpatient Visits:** 560974 **Births:** 1056 **Total Expense ($000):** 222656 **Payroll Expense ($000):** 114235 **Personnel:** 1764

## FREEHOLD—Monmouth County

☒ **CENTRASTATE HEALTHCARE SYSTEM (310111)**, 901 West Main Street, Zip 07728–2549; tel. 732/431–2000 **A**1 2 3 5 9 10 **F**3 11 12 13 15 16 18 19 20 28 29 30 31 32 34 35 36 37 38 40 41 45 46 49 56 57 58 59 61 64 65 66 70 73 74 75 76 77 78 79 81 82 84 86 87 89 92 93 97 98 100 101 102 107 108 110 113 117 118 119 120 123 125 128 129 130 131 133 134 143 145 146 147
Primary Contact: John T. Gribbin, FACHE, President and Chief Executive Officer
COO: Daniel J. Messina, Ph.D., Senior Vice President and Chief Operating Officer
CFO: John Dellocono, Senior Vice President and Chief Financial Officer
CMO: Jack H. Dworkin, M.D., Vice President Medical Affairs and Chief Medical Officer
CIO: Indranil Ganguly, Vice President and Chief Information Officer
CHR: Fran Keane, Vice President Human Resources
Web address: www.centrastate.com
**Control:** Other not–for–profit (including NFP Corporation) **Service:** General Medical and Surgical

**Staffed Beds:** 273 **Admissions:** 14716 **Census:** 171 **Outpatient Visits:** 253140 **Births:** 1584 **Total Expense ($000):** 214587 **Payroll Expense ($000):** 89937 **Personnel:** 1411

## HACKENSACK—Bergen County

☒ **HACKENSACK UNIVERSITY MEDICAL CENTER (310001)**, 30 Prospect Avenue, Zip 07601–1912; tel. 201/996–2000, (Includes THE JOSEPH M. SANZARI CHILDREN'S HOSPITAL, 30 Prospect Avenue, Zip 07601–1914; tel. 201/996–2000) **A**1 2 3 5 8 9 10 **F**2 3 4 5 6 7 8 9 10 11 12 13 14 15 16 17 18 19 20 22 24 26 27 28 29 30 31 32 34 35 36 38 39 40 41 42 43 44 45 46 47 48 49 50 51 52 53 54 55 56 57 58 59 60 61 63 64 65 66 68 69 70 71 72 73 74 75 76 77 78 79 81 82 84 85 86 87 88 89 90 91 92 93 94 96 97 98 99 100 101 102 103 104 107 108 109 110 111 113 114 115 116 117 118 119 120 122 123 125 128 129 130 131 133 134 135 137 140 141 142 144 145 146 147 **P**1 5 6
Primary Contact: Robert C. Garrett, President and Chief Executive Officer
COO: Ketul J. Patel, Executive Vice President and Chief Operations and Strategy Officer
CFO: Robert Glenning, Executive Vice President Finance and Chief Financial Officer
CMO: Peter A. Gross, M.D., Senior Vice President and Chief Medical Officer
CHR: Nancy R. Corcoran, Senior Vice President Human Resources and Quality Service
Web address: www.humed.com
**Control:** Other not–for–profit (including NFP Corporation) **Service:** General Medical and Surgical

**Staffed Beds:** 694 **Admissions:** 71395 **Census:** 652 **Outpatient Visits:** 2990051 **Births:** 6212 **Total Expense ($000):** 1214565 **Payroll Expense ($000):** 543519 **Personnel:** 7292

## HACKETTSTOWN—Warren County

★ **HACKETTSTOWN REGIONAL MEDICAL CENTER (310115)**, 651 Willow Grove Street, Zip 07840–1792; tel. 908/852–5100, (Nonreporting) **A**9 10 **S** Adventist HealthCare, Rockville, MD
Primary Contact: Jason C. Coe, President and Chief Executive Officer
COO: Stella Visaggio, Chief Operating Officer
CFO: Robert Peterson, Chief Financial Officer
CMO: Kenneth Janowski, M.D., Chief Medical Officer
CIO: Dorothy Cox, Manager Information Systems
CHR: Jeanne Jepson, Director Human Resources
CNO: Linda Ambacher, Interim Chief Nursing Officer
Web address: www.hrmcnj.org
**Control:** Church–operated, Nongovernment, not–for profit **Service:** General Medical and Surgical

**Staffed Beds:** 111

## HAMILTON—Mercer County

☒ **ROBERT WOOD JOHNSON UNIVERSITY HOSPITAL AT HAMILTON (310110)**, One Hamilton Health Place, Zip 08690–3599; tel. 609/586–7900 **A**1 2 5 9 10 **F**3 8 9 11 12 13 15 17 18 20 22 26 28 29 30 31 32 34 35 36 39 40 41 44 46 47 48 49 50 51 53 54 55 56 57 58 59 60 61 63 64 65 66 68 69 70 71 73 74 75 76 77 78 79 81 82 84 85 86 87 92 93 96 97 100 102 103 107 108 110 111 113 114 115 116 117 118 119 120 122 123 128 129 130 131 133 134 142 143 144 145 146 147 **P**6 **S** Robert Wood Johnson Health System & Network, New Brunswick, NJ
Primary Contact: Anthony J. Cimino, President and Chief Executive Officer
COO: Barbara H. Smith, Senior Vice President & Chief Operating Officer
CFO: James M. Maher, Senior Vice President and Chief Financial Officer
CMO: Ronald Ryder, D.O., President of the Medical Staff
CNO: Lisa Breza, R.N., Vice President and Chief Nursing Officer
Web address: www.rwjhamilton.org
**Control:** Other not–for–profit (including NFP Corporation) **Service:** General Medical and Surgical

**Staffed Beds:** 242 **Admissions:** 13294 **Census:** 160 **Outpatient Visits:** 232639 **Births:** 1278 **Total Expense ($000):** 196709 **Payroll Expense ($000):** 83915 **Personnel:** 1165

**NJ**

*Many Facility Codes have changed. Please refer to the AHA Guide Code Chart.* © 2012 AHA Guide

## HOBOKEN—Hudson County

☐ **HOBOKEN UNIVERSITY MEDICAL CENTER (310040)**, 308 Willow Avenue, Zip 07030–3889; tel. 201/418–1000 **A**1 3 5 9 10 **F**2 5 7 11 12 13 14 15 18 19 28 29 30 31 32 34 35 38 40 41 45 46 47 48 49 50 54 55 56 57 59 60 61 64 66 68 70 73 74 75 76 77 78 79 81 82 84 85 87 89 90 92 93 94 96 97 98 99 100 101 102 103 104 105 107 108 110 111 114 117 118 129 130 131 133 145 146 147
Primary Contact: Phillip S. Schaengold, JD, President and Chief Executive Officer
CFO: Vincent Riccitelli, Vice President and Chief Financial Officer
CMO: Joseph Kozel, M.D., President Medical Staff
CIO: Lior Blik, Chief Information Officer
CHR: Yleana Contrera, Executive Director Human Resources
Web address: www.hobokenumc.com
**Control:** Corporation, Investor–owned, for–profit **Service:** General Medical and Surgical

**Staffed Beds:** 204 **Admissions:** 8828 **Census:** 108 **Outpatient Visits:** 122665 **Births:** 1466 **Total Expense ($000):** 145932 **Payroll Expense ($000):** 63737 **Personnel:** 911

## HOLMDEL—Monmouth County

☒ **BAYSHORE COMMUNITY HOSPITAL (310112)**, 727 North Beers Street, Zip 07733–1598; tel. 732/739–5900, (Total facility includes 13 beds in nursing home–type unit) **A**1 2 9 10 **F**3 8 11 12 15 18 20 28 29 30 31 40 41 45 49 50 51 53 56 60 64 65 66 68 70 74 75 78 79 81 82 84 85 87 89 92 93 97 107 108 110 111 113 115 116 117 118 127 128 129 131 134 144 145 146 147 **P**6 7 **S** Meridian Health, Neptune, NJ
Primary Contact: Anthony V. Cava, Executive Director
CMO: L. Scott Larsen, M.D., Vice President Medical Affairs
CIO: Dale Ragone, Interim Chief Information Officer
Web address: www.bchs.com
**Control:** Other not–for–profit (including NFP Corporation) **Service:** General Medical and Surgical

**Staffed Beds:** 142 **Admissions:** 7969 **Census:** 107 **Outpatient Visits:** 90664 **Births:** 0 **Total Expense ($000):** 101761 **Payroll Expense ($000):** 42943 **Personnel:** 618

## JERSEY CITY—Hudson County

☐ **CHRIST HOSPITAL (310016)**, 176 Palisade Avenue, Zip 07306–1196, Mailing Address: P.O. Box J–1, Zip 07306–1196; tel. 201/795–8200, (Nonreporting) **A**1 6 9 10 12 13
Primary Contact: Peter A. Kelly, President and Chief Executive Officer
CFO: George A. Popko, Senior Vice President and Chief Financial Officer
CMO: Bhavani P. Mekala, M.D., President Medical Staff
CIO: Marty Grossman, Director Information Technology
CHR: Eileen Clyne, Director Human Resources
Web address: www.christhospital.org
**Control:** Other not–for–profit (including NFP Corporation) **Service:** General Medical and Surgical

**Staffed Beds:** 381

☐ **LIBERTYHEALTH–JERSEY CITY MEDICAL CENTER (310074)**, 355 Grand Street, Zip 7302; tel. 201/915–2000, (Nonreporting) **A**1 3 5 9 10
Primary Contact: Joseph F. Scott, FACHE, President and Chief Executive Officer
CFO: Paul R. Goldberg, Chief Financial Officer
CMO: Kenneth Garay, M.D., Chief Medical Officer
CIO: Stephen Li, Vice President Management Information Systems
CHR: Mary Cataudella, Corporate Director Human Resources
Web address: www.libertyhcs.org
**Control:** Other not–for–profit (including NFP Corporation) **Service:** General Medical and Surgical

**Staffed Beds:** 269

## LAKEWOOD—Ocean County

☒ **KIMBALL MEDICAL CENTER (310084)**, 600 River Avenue, Zip 08701–4281; tel. 732/363–1900 **A**1 2 9 10 **F**3 11 13 18 20 28 29 30 31 32 34 35 36 38 39 40 43 44 50 56 57 58 59 60 61 64 68 70 73 74 75 76 77 78 79 81 82 84 86 87 89 93 96 97 98 100 101 102 103 104 105 107 108 111 113 116 118 129 130 131 132 133 134 145 146 147 **S** Barnabas Health, West Orange, NJ
Primary Contact: Michael Mimoso, FACHE, President and Chief Executive Officer
CFO: Thomas Percello, Chief Financial Officer
CMO: Todd Phillips, M.D., Interim Vice President, Medical Affairs
CIO: Chris Butler, Deputy CIO/System Vice President
CHR: Michele Schweers, Vice President Human Resources
CNO: Judy Colorado, R.N., Vice President, Patient Care Services
Web address: www.barnabashealth.org
**Control:** Other not–for–profit (including NFP Corporation) **Service:** General Medical and Surgical

**Staffed Beds:** 240 **Admissions:** 10791 **Census:** 164 **Outpatient Visits:** 113674 **Births:** 988 **Total Expense ($000):** 153138 **Payroll Expense ($000):** 64197 **Personnel:** 926

**SPECIALTY HOSPITAL AT KIMBALL**, 600 River Avenue, 4 West, Zip 8701; tel. 732/942–3588, (Nonreporting) **S** AcuteCare Health System, Lakewood, NJ
Primary Contact: Hilary Michaels, Executive Director
CFO: Richard L. Cassady, Chief Financial Officer
CMO: Howard Lebowitz, M.D., Chief Medical Officer
CHR: Mary Pat Napolitano, Director Human Resources
Web address: www.acutecarehs.com
**Control:** Corporation, Investor–owned, for–profit **Service:** Long–Term Acute Care hospital

**Staffed Beds:** 25

## LAWRENCEVILLE—Mercer County

☒ **ST. LAWRENCE REHABILITATION CENTER (313027)**, 2381 Lawrenceville Road, Zip 08648–2024; tel. 609/896–9500, (Total facility includes 57 beds in nursing home–type unit) **A**1 10 **F**29 30 34 57 64 68 90 93 96 108 127 129 131 142 145 147
Primary Contact: Darlene S. Hanley, R.N., President and Chief Executive Officer
COO: Shirley Pukala, R.N., Assistant Administrator of Operations
CFO: Thomas W. Boyle, Chief Financial Officer
CMO: Kevin McGuigan, M.D., Medical Director
CIO: Jane Millner, Director Community Relations and Development
CHR: John Levi, Director of Human Resources
CNO: Magdalena Sokolowski, R.N., Director of Nursing
Web address: www.slrc.org
**Control:** Church–operated, Nongovernment, not–for profit **Service:** Rehabilitation

**Staffed Beds:** 109 **Admissions:** 2449 **Census:** 97 **Outpatient Visits:** 21056 **Births:** 0 **Total Expense ($000):** 30796 **Payroll Expense ($000):** 17336 **Personnel:** 361

## LIVINGSTON—Essex County

☒ **SAINT BARNABAS MEDICAL CENTER (310076)**, 94 Old Short Hills Road, Zip 07039–5672; tel. 973/322–5000, (Nonreporting) **A**1 2 3 5 8 9 10 12 13 **S** Barnabas Health, West Orange, NJ
Primary Contact: John F. Bonamo, M.D., MS, Executive Director
CFO: Patrick Ahearn, Senior Vice President Finance and Administrative Services
CMO: Gregory Rokosz, D.O., Senior Vice President Medical and Academic Affairs
CIO: Michael McTigue, Chief Information Officer
CHR: Arnie Manzo, Vice President Human Resources
Web address: www.sbhcs.com
**Control:** Other not–for–profit (including NFP Corporation) **Service:** General Medical and Surgical

**Staffed Beds:** 597

**NJ**

---

**Hospital, Medicare Provider Number, Address, Telephone, Approval, Facility, and Physician Codes, Health Care System**

★ American Hospital Association (AHA) membership
☐ The Joint Commission accreditation
◇ DNV Healthcare Inc. accreditation
○ American Osteopathic Association (AOA) accreditation
△ Commission on Accreditation of Rehabilitation Facilities (CARF) accreditation

## LONG BRANCH—Monmouth County

⊠ **MONMOUTH MEDICAL CENTER (310075)**, 300 Second Avenue,
Zip 07740–6303; tel. 732/222–5200, (Includes CHILDREN'S HOSPITAL AT
MONMOUTH MEDICAL CENTER, 300 Second Avenue, tel. 732/222–5200) **A**1 2 3
5 8 9 10 **F**1 3 5 8 9 11 12 13 14 15 18 19 20 22 28 29 30 31 32 34 35 36
38 40 41 45 46 47 48 49 50 51 52 53 54 55 56 57 58 59 60 61 63 64 65
66 68 70 72 73 74 75 76 77 78 79 81 82 83 84 85 86 87 88 89 97 98 99
100 101 102 103 104 105 106 107 108 109 110 111 112 113 114 118 119
120 122 123 125 128 129 130 131 132 133 134 142 143 144 145 146 147
**P**5 6 7 8 **S** Barnabas Health, West Orange, NJ
Primary Contact: Frank J. Vozos, M.D., FACS, Executive Director
COO: Bill Arnold, Chief Operating Officer
CFO: Gerald Tofani, Chief Financial Officer
CMO: Eric Burkett, M.D., Vice President Medical Affairs
CIO: Paul Garrin, Chief Information Officer
CHR: Glenn Oppito, Vice President Human Resources
Web address: www.sbhcs.com
**Control:** Other not–for–profit (including NFP Corporation) **Service:** General
Medical and Surgical

**Staffed Beds:** 337 **Admissions:** 18609 **Census:** 230 **Outpatient Visits:**
184168 **Births:** 4422 **Total Expense ($000):** 300316 **Payroll Expense
($000):** 116161 **Personnel:** 1707

☐ **SPECIALTY HOSPITAL AT MONMOUTH (312017)**, 300 Second Avenue,
Zip 7740; tel. 732/923–5037, (Nonreporting) **A**1 10 **S** AcuteCare Health System,
Lakewood, NJ
Primary Contact: Violeta Peters, R.N., Chief Executive Officer
CFO: Kristin Prentiss, Chief Financial Officer
CMO: Eddie Santiago, M.D., Medical Director
CHR: Mary Pat Napolitano, Director Human Resources
Web address: www.acutecarehs.com
**Control:** Corporation, Investor–owned, for–profit **Service:** Long–Term Acute Care
hospital

**Staffed Beds:** 25

## LYONS—Somerset County

**LYONS DIVISION** See Veterans Affairs New Jersey Health Care System, East
Orange

## MANAHAWKIN—Ocean County

⊠ **SOUTHERN OCEAN MEDICAL CENTER (310113)**, 1140 Route 72 West,
Zip 08050–2499; tel. 609/978–8900, (Total facility includes 20 beds in nursing
home–type unit) **A**1 2 9 10 **F**3 11 12 13 15 18 20 28 29 30 31 32 40 44 45
46 51 54 56 59 64 65 66 68 70 72 73 74 76 77 78 79 81 82 84 85 86 87
88 90 92 93 97 98 107 108 110 111 113 117 118 127 128 129 131 134
143 145 146 147 **P**7 8 **S** Meridian Health, Neptune, NJ
Primary Contact: Joseph P. Coyle, President and Chief Executive Officer
COO: E. Joseph Hummel, Chief Strategy Officer
CFO: John Gantner, Executive Vice President Finance and Partner Company
Operations
CIO: Rebecca Weber, Senior Vice President and Chief Information Officer
Web address: www.soch.com
**Control:** Other not–for–profit (including NFP Corporation) **Service:** General
Medical and Surgical

**Staffed Beds:** 176 **Admissions:** 6582 **Census:** 90 **Outpatient Visits:** 148393
**Births:** 349 **Total Expense ($000):** 102478 **Payroll Expense ($000):** 48354
**Personnel:** 655

## MARLTON—Burlington County

☐ △ **MARLTON REHABILITATION HOSPITAL (313032)**, 92 Brick Road,
Zip 08053–2177; tel. 856/988–8778, (Nonreporting) **A**1 7 10 **S** Vibra
Healthcare, Mechanicsburg, PA
Primary Contact: Michael Long, MS, Chief Executive Officer
CFO: Stuart Moss, Chief Financial Officer
CMO: Kenneth Wu, M.D., Medical Director
CHR: Joanne Cornava, Director Human Resources
Web address: www.marltonrehab.com
**Control:** Corporation, Investor–owned, for–profit **Service:** Rehabilitation

**Staffed Beds:** 46

⊠ **VIRTUA MARLTON (313032)**, 90 Brick Road, Zip 08053–9697;
tel. 856/355–6000 **A**1 2 9 10 **F**20 22 26 29 31 40 45 49 56 60 64 68 70 75
78 79 81 82 84 85 87 93 107 111 118 128 129 145 **S** Virtua Health,
Marlton, NJ
Primary Contact: Gary L. Long, Chief Operating Officer
COO: Gary L. Long, Chief Operating Officer
CFO: Robert Segin, Executive Vice President & Chief Financial Officer
CMO: James P. Dwyer, D.O., Chief Medical Officer
CIO: Alfred Campanella, Chief Information Officer
CHR: Michael Pepe, Ph.D., Chief Human Resources
CNO: Ann Campbell, Chief Nursing Officer
Web address: www.virtua.org
**Control:** Other not–for–profit (including NFP Corporation) **Service:** General
Medical and Surgical

**Staffed Beds:** 192 **Admissions:** 10923 **Census:** 143 **Outpatient Visits:**
43554 **Births:** 0 **Total Expense ($000):** 201864 **Payroll Expense ($000):**
58890 **Personnel:** 796

☐ **WEISMAN CHILDREN'S REHABILITATION HOSPITAL (313302)**, 92 Brick
Road, 3rd Floor, Zip 8053; tel. 856/489–4520, (Nonreporting) **A**1 10
Primary Contact: Thomas J. Lonergan, Chief Executive Officer
CMO: Connie Domingo, M.D., Medical Director
CIO: Darren Pedersen, Coordinator Information Technology
CHR: Eileen Dumsha, Manager Employee Relations
Web address: www.weismanchildrens.com
**Control:** Corporation, Investor–owned, for–profit **Service:** Children's rehabilitation

**Staffed Beds:** 24

## MONTCLAIR—Essex County

☐ **HACKENSACK UNIVERSITY MEDICAL CENTER MOUNTAINSIDE (310054)**, 1
Bay Avenue, Zip 07042–4898; tel. 973/429–6000, (Nonreporting) **A**1 2 3 5 6
9 10
Primary Contact: John A. Fromhold, Chief Executive Officer
COO: Ed Devaney, Vice President and Chief Operating Officer
CHR: Fran Corridon, Vice President Human Resources and Shared Services
Web address: www.mountainsidenow.com
**Control:** Other not–for–profit (including NFP Corporation) **Service:** General
Medical and Surgical

**Staffed Beds:** 245

## MORRIS PLAINS—Morris County

☐ **GREYSTONE PARK PSYCHIATRIC HOSPITAL (314016)**, 59 Koch Avenue,
Zip 07950–1005; tel. 973/538–1800, (Nonreporting) **A**1 10 **S** Division of Mental
Health and Addiction Services, Department of Human Services, State of New
Jersey, Trenton, NJ
Primary Contact: Janet J. Monroe, R.N., Chief Executive Officer
COO: John Whitenack, Chief Operating Officer
CFO: Jack Frey, Business Manager
CMO: Milton Luria, M.D., Chief of Medicine
CHR: Jerri Casazza, Manager Human Resources
Web address: www.state.nj.us/humanservices/pfnurse/greystone.htm
**Control:** State–Government, nonfederal **Service:** Psychiatric

**Staffed Beds:** 557

## MORRISTOWN—Morris County

⊠ **MORRISTOWN MEDICAL CENTER (310015)**, 100 Madison Avenue,
Zip 07962–1956; tel. 973/971–5000, (Includes REHABILITATION INSTITUTE AT
THE MOUNT KEMBLE DIVISION ; GORYEB CHILDREN'S HOSPITAL, 100 Madison
Avenue, Zip 07960–6136; tel. 800/247–9580), (Total facility includes 40 beds in
nursing home–type unit) **A**1 2 3 5 8 9 10 **F**3 5 6 7 8 9 11 12 13 14 15 17 18
19 20 22 24 26 28 29 30 31 32 33 34 35 36 37 38 39 40 41 43 44 45 46
47 48 49 50 51 53 54 55 56 57 58 59 60 61 62 63 64 65 66 68 69 70 71
72 73 74 75 76 77 78 79 81 82 83 84 85 86 87 88 89 90 91 92 93 94 95
96 97 98 99 100 101 102 103 104 105 107 108 109 110 111 113 114 115
116 117 118 119 120 122 125 127 128 129 130 131 133 134 140 142 143
144 145 146 147 **P**3 5 6 **S** Atlantic Health, Morristown, NJ
Primary Contact: David J. Shulkin, M.D., President and Chief Executive Officer
COO: Joanne M. Conroy, M.D., Executive Vice President and Chief Operating
Officer
CFO: Kevin Shanley, Vice President Finance and Chief Financial Officer
CMO: Joanne M. Conroy, M.D., Executive Vice President and Chief Operating
Officer
CIO: Linda Reed, Vice President and Chief Information Officer
CHR: Andrew L. Kovach, Vice President Human Resources and Chief
Administrative Officer
Web address: www.atlantichealth.org/Morristown/
**Control:** Other not–for–profit (including NFP Corporation) **Service:** General
Medical and Surgical

**Staffed Beds:** 649 **Admissions:** 34440 **Census:** 527 **Outpatient Visits:**
306329 **Births:** 4034 **Total Expense ($000):** 727693 **Payroll Expense
($000):** 331732 **Personnel:** 5291

**NJ**

## MOUNT HOLLY—Burlington County

☒ **VIRTUA MEMORIAL (310057)**, 175 Madison Avenue, Zip 08060–2099; tel. 609/267–0700 **A**1 3 5 9 10 **F**5 11 13 15 17 18 23 28 29 30 31 40 41 45 48 49 56 57 59 60 70 73 74 75 76 77 78 81 85 86 87 89 93 98 102 105 107 108 110 111 113 114 117 118 119 123 125 128 129 142 145 146 147 **S** Virtua Health, Marlton, NJ
Primary Contact: Stephen Kolesk, M.D., Vice President and Chief Operating Officer
CFO: Robert Segin, Chief Financial Officer
CMO: James P. Dwyer, D.O., Executive Vice President and Chief Medical Officer
CHR: E. D. Dunn, Vice President Human Resources
Web address: www.virtua.org
**Control:** Other not–for–profit (including NFP Corporation) **Service:** General Medical and Surgical

**Staffed Beds:** 312 **Admissions:** 19252 **Census:** 248 **Outpatient Visits:** 174468 **Births:** 2598 **Total Expense ($000):** 262639 **Payroll Expense ($000):** 87006 **Personnel:** 1344

**VIRTUA MEMORIAL HOSPITAL BURLINGTON COUNTY** See Virtua Memorial

## NEPTUNE—Monmouth County

☒ **JERSEY SHORE UNIVERSITY MEDICAL CENTER (310073)**, 1945 Route 33, Zip 07754–0397; tel. 732/775–5500, (Includes K. HOVNANIAN CHILDREN'S HOSPITAL, 1945 State Route 33, Zip 07753–4859; tel. 800/560–9990) **A**1 2 3 5 8 9 10 13 **F**3 5 8 11 12 13 17 18 19 20 22 24 26 28 29 30 31 32 38 39 40 41 43 45 46 47 49 50 54 55 59 60 61 63 64 66 68 70 72 73 74 75 76 78 79 80 81 82 84 85 86 87 88 89 92 93 94 96 97 98 99 100 101 102 103 104 105 107 108 111 113 114 116 117 118 119 120 122 125 128 129 130 131 134 143 145 146 147 **P**7 **S** Meridian Health, Neptune, NJ
Primary Contact: Steven G. Littleson, FACHE, President
COO: Robert H. Adams, Vice President Operations
CFO: John Gantner, Executive Vice President Finance and Partner Company Operations
CMO: David Kountz, M.D., Senior Vice President Medical Affairs
CIO: Rebecca Weber, Senior Vice President and Chief Information Officer
Web address: www.meridianhealth.com
**Control:** Other not–for–profit (including NFP Corporation) **Service:** General Medical and Surgical

**Staffed Beds:** 540 **Admissions:** 27406 **Census:** 392 **Outpatient Visits:** 204807 **Births:** 2007 **Total Expense ($000):** 534961 **Payroll Expense ($000):** 203243 **Personnel:** 2563

## NEW BRUNSWICK—Middlesex County

☐ △ **CHILDREN'S SPECIALIZED HOSPITAL (313300)**, 200 Somerset Street, Zip 8901; tel. 732/258–7000, (Includes CHILDREN'S SPECIALIZED HOSPITAL, 150 New Providence Road, Mountainside, Zip 07092–2590; tel. 908/233–3720), (Nonreporting) **A**1 3 5 7 9 10 **S** Robert Wood Johnson Health System & Network, New Brunswick, NJ
Primary Contact: Amy B. Mansue, President and Chief Executive Officer
COO: Warren E. Moore, Executive Vice President and Chief Operating Officer
CFO: Joseph J. Dobosh, Jr., Vice President and Chief Financial Officer
CMO: Frank V. Castello, M.D., Medical Director
CIO: Pat DeMartino, Chief Information Officer
CHR: William Dwyer, Vice President Human Resources
Web address: www.childrens–specialized.org
**Control:** Other not–for–profit (including NFP Corporation) **Service:** Children's rehabilitation

**Staffed Beds:** 126

☒ **ROBERT WOOD JOHNSON UNIVERSITY HOSPITAL (310038)**, 1 Robert Wood Johnson Place, Zip 08903–2601; tel. 732/828–3000, (Includes BRISTOL–MYERS SQUIBB CHILDREN'S HOSPITAL, One Robert Wood Johnson Place, Zip 08901, Mailing Address: P.O. Box 2601, Zip 08903–2601; tel. 732/828–3000) **A**1 2 3 5 8 9 10 **F**3 6 7 8 9 11 12 13 14 15 17 18 19 20 22 24 26 28 29 30 31 32 34 35 37 38 39 40 41 43 44 45 46 47 48 49 50 51 52 53 54 55 56 57 58 59 60 61 62 63 64 65 66 68 70 71 72 73 74 75 76 77 78 79 81 82 84 85 86 87 88 89 91 92 93 94 96 97 99 100 102 104 107 108 109 110 111 112 113 114 115 116 117 118 119 120 122 123 125 128 129 130 131 133 134 135 136 137 140 141 142 143 145 146 147 **P**6 **S** Robert Wood Johnson Health System & Network, New Brunswick, NJ
Primary Contact: Stephen K. Jones, President and Chief Executive Officer
COO: Vincent D. Joseph, Executive Vice President and Chief Operating Officer
CFO: Paul D. Storiale, Senior Vice President Finance and Chief Financial Officer
CMO: Joshua M. Bershad, M.D., Senior Vice President Medical Affairs and Chief Medical Officer
CIO: Robert G. Irwin, Vice President Information Systems
CHR: Martin S. Everhart, Senior Vice President Human Resources
Web address: www.rwjuh.edu
**Control:** Other not–for–profit (including NFP Corporation) **Service:** General Medical and Surgical

**Staffed Beds:** 610 **Admissions:** 31452 **Census:** 497 **Outpatient Visits:** 245883 **Births:** 2267 **Total Expense ($000):** 725495 **Payroll Expense ($000):** 276089 **Personnel:** 3894

☒ **SAINT PETER'S UNIVERSITY HOSPITAL (310070)**, 254 Easton Avenue, Zip 08901–1780, Mailing Address: P.O. Box 591, Zip 08903–0591; tel. 732/745–8600 **A**1 2 3 5 8 9 10 **F**2 3 11 12 13 15 17 18 20 29 30 31 32 34 35 38 40 41 44 45 46 49 50 51 54 55 56 57 58 59 60 61 64 65 66 68 70 71 72 73 74 75 76 77 78 79 81 82 83 84 85 86 87 88 89 91 97 100 102 105 107 108 110 111 113 114 118 119 120 122 125 128 129 130 131 142 145 146 147 **P**3 6
Primary Contact: Ronald C. Rak, JD, Chief Executive Officer
COO: Patricia Carroll, Senior Vice President and Chief Operating Officer
CFO: Garrick J. Stoldt, Vice President and Chief Financial Officer
CMO: Anthony Passannante, Jr., M.D., Vice President, Chief Medical Officer and Co–Chief Quality Officer
CIO: Frank DiSanzo, Vice President and Chief Information Officer
CHR: Susan Ballestero, Vice President Human Resources
Web address: www.saintpetersuh.com
**Control:** Church–operated, Nongovernment, not–for profit **Service:** General Medical and Surgical

**Staffed Beds:** 384 **Admissions:** 21857 **Census:** 276 **Outpatient Visits:** 355668 **Births:** 5831 **Total Expense ($000):** 377453 **Payroll Expense ($000):** 186897 **Personnel:** 2674

## NEWARK—Essex County

☒ **NEWARK BETH ISRAEL MEDICAL CENTER (310002)**, 201 Lyons Avenue, Zip 07112–2027; tel. 973/926–7000, (Includes CHILDREN'S HOSPITAL OF NEW JERSEY, 201 Lyons Avenue, tel. 973/926–7000) **A**1 2 3 5 8 9 10 12 13 **F**2 3 12 15 17 18 19 20 21 22 23 24 25 26 28 29 30 31 32 34 38 39 40 41 42 46 48 49 50 55 56 57 58 59 60 61 64 68 70 72 73 74 75 76 77 78 79 80 81 86 87 88 89 92 93 97 98 99 100 101 102 104 105 107 108 110 111 113 114 116 118 119 130 131 134 136 137 139 140 141 142 145 146 147 **P**8 **S** Barnabas Health, West Orange, NJ
Primary Contact: John A. Brennan, M.D., M.P.H., President and Chief Executive Officer
COO: Darrell K. Terry, Sr., Senior Vice President Operations
CFO: Veronica Zeichner, Chief Financial Officer
CHR: Zach Lipner, Vice President Human Resources
Web address: www.sbhcs.com
**Control:** Other not–for–profit (including NFP Corporation) **Service:** General Medical and Surgical

**Staffed Beds:** 402 **Admissions:** 23633 **Census:** 411 **Outpatient Visits:** 301451 **Births:** 3442 **Total Expense ($000):** 495163 **Payroll Expense ($000):** 249919 **Personnel:** 3213

☒ **SAINT MICHAEL'S MEDICAL CENTER (310096)**, 111 Central Avenue, Zip 07102–2094; tel. 973/877–5549 **A**1 2 3 5 10 **F**3 5 12 15 17 18 20 22 24 26 29 30 31 34 35 37 38 40 45 47 48 49 50 51 57 58 59 60 61 64 66 68 70 74 75 77 78 79 81 82 85 86 87 91 92 93 97 98 100 102 104 107 108 110 111 113 118 120 125 128 129 131 142 143 145 146 147 **S** Catholic Health East, Newtown Square, PA
Primary Contact: David A. Ricci, President and Chief Executive Officer
CFO: John S. Grywalski, Jr., CPA, Chief Financial Officer
CMO: Sebastian Dovi, M.D., Interim Chief Medical Officer
CIO: Angelo Schittone, Chief Information Officer
CHR: Mary Beth Rose, Vice President Human Resources
Web address: www.smmcnj.org
**Control:** Church–operated, Nongovernment, not–for profit **Service:** General Medical and Surgical

**Staffed Beds:** 207 **Admissions:** 11090 **Census:** 163 **Outpatient Visits:** 86673 **Births:** 0 **Total Expense ($000):** 247049 **Payroll Expense ($000):** 85975 **Personnel:** 1231

☒ **UNIVERSITY OF MEDICINE AND DENTISTRY OF NEW JERSEY–UNIVERSITY HOSPITAL (310119)**, 150 Bergen Street, Zip 07103–2496; tel. 973/972–4300 **A**1 2 3 5 8 9 10 **F**1 3 4 7 11 15 16 17 18 20 22 24 26 28 29 30 31 32 34 35 36 37 38 39 40 41 43 44 45 46 47 49 50 52 55 56 57 58 59 60 61 64 65 66 67 68 70 71 72 73 74 75 76 77 78 79 80 81 82 84 85 86 87 88 89 90 92 93 94 97 98 100 102 103 107 108 110 111 112 113 116 118 120 122 123 125 127 129 130 131 132 133 134 138 142 143 144 145 146 147
Primary Contact: James R. Gonzalez, Acting President and Chief Executive Officer
CFO: Thomas M. Daly, Chief Financial Officer
CMO: Suzanne Atkin, M.D., Chief of Staff and Associate Dean Clinical Affairs
CIO: Richard Tunnell, Director Information Systems Technology and Health Management Information Systems
CHR: Gerard Garcia, Acting Vice President Human Resources
Web address: www.umdnj.edu
**Control:** State–Government, nonfederal **Service:** General Medical and Surgical

**Staffed Beds:** 357 **Admissions:** 18307 **Census:** 265 **Outpatient Visits:** 272630 **Births:** 1455 **Total Expense ($000):** 427711 **Payroll Expense ($000):** 261336 **Personnel:** 3020

**NJ**

---

**Hospital, Medicare Provider Number, Address, Telephone, Approval, Facility, and Physician Codes, Health Care System**

★ American Hospital Association (AHA) membership
☐ The Joint Commission accreditation ◇ DNV Healthcare Inc. accreditation
○ American Osteopathic Association (AOA) accreditation
△ Commission on Accreditation of Rehabilitation Facilities (CARF) accreditation

## NEWTON—Sussex County

☒ **NEWTON MEDICAL CENTER (310028)**, 175 High Street, Zip 07860–1004; tel. 973/383–2121, (Data for 275 days) **A**1 2 9 10 **F**3 4 5 6 8 9 11 12 13 14 15 17 18 19 20 22 24 26 28 29 30 31 32 33 34 35 37 38 39 40 41 44 45 46 47 48 49 50 51 53 54 55 56 57 58 59 60 61 62 64 65 66 68 69 70 71 72 73 74 75 76 77 78 79 81 82 83 85 86 87 88 89 91 92 93 94 95 96 97 98 99 100 101 102 103 104 105 106 107 108 110 111 113 117 118 125 128 129 130 131 133 134 142 144 145 146 147 **P**6 **S** Atlantic Health, Morristown, NJ
Primary Contact: Thomas J. Senker, FACHE, President and Chief Executive Officer
COO: Thomas J. Senker, FACHE, President and Chief Executive Officer
CFO: Kevin Lenahan, Director Corporate Accounting, Budgets, Grants and Reimbursements
CMO: David Lazarus, M.D., Medical Director Clinical Affairs
CIO: Linda Reed, Vice President Information Systems and Chief Information Officer
CHR: Andrew L. Kovach, Vice President Human Resources and Chief Administrative Officer
Web address: www.atlantichealth.org
**Control:** Other not–for–profit (including NFP Corporation) **Service:** General Medical and Surgical

**Staffed Beds: 140 Admissions: 8148 Census: 135 Outpatient Visits:** 183094 **Births: 558 Total Expense ($000): 125611 Payroll Expense ($000): 61600 Personnel: 774**

## NORTH BERGEN—Hudson County

☒ **PALISADES MEDICAL CENTER (310003)**, 7600 River Road, Zip 07047–6217; tel. 201/854–5000 **A**1 10 **F**3 7 8 11 12 13 15 18 20 28 29 30 31 34 35 38 40 45 56 57 59 68 70 73 74 75 76 77 78 79 81 84 85 86 87 89 91 92 93 102 104 107 111 114 118 128 129 131 142 145 146 147 **P**6
Primary Contact: Bruce J. Markowitz, President and Chief Executive Officer
COO: David J. Berkowitz, Vice President and Chief Operating Officer
CFO: John Calandriello, Vice President and Chief Financial Officer
CMO: Suresh Raina, M.D., Vice President Medical Staff and Chief Medical Officer
CIO: Glenn Hunsberger, Director Management Information Systems
CHR: Donna Cahill, Vice President Human Resources
Web address: www.palisadesmedical.org
**Control:** Other not–for–profit (including NFP Corporation) **Service:** General Medical and Surgical

**Staffed Beds: 176 Admissions: 9455 Census: 118 Outpatient Visits: 81298 Births: 1385 Total Expense ($000): 124331 Payroll Expense ($000): 59263 Personnel: 732**

## OLD BRIDGE—Middlesex County

**OLD BRIDGE DIVISION** See Raritan Bay Medical Center, Perth Amboy

## PARAMUS—Bergen County

☐ **BERGEN REGIONAL MEDICAL CENTER (310058)**, 230 East Ridgewood Avenue, Zip 07652–4131; tel. 201/967–4000, (Nonreporting) **A**1 10
Primary Contact: Joseph S. Orlando, President
COO: Susan Mendelowitz, Executive Vice President and Chief Operating Officer
CFO: Connie Magdangal, Executive Vice President and Chief Financial Officer
CMO: Robert M. Harris, M.D., President Medical and Dental Staff
CIO: Ronald Li, Vice President Management Information Systems
CHR: Guy Mennonna, Senior Vice President Human Resources
Web address: www.bergenregional.com
**Control:** County–Government, nonfederal **Service:** Psychiatric

**Staffed Beds: 432**

## PASSAIC—Passaic County

☒ **ST. MARY'S HOSPITAL (310006)**, 350 Boulevard, Zip 7055; tel. 973/365–4300 **A**1 9 10 **F**3 11 13 15 17 18 20 22 24 26 28 29 30 31 34 35 40 42 45 46 47 48 49 50 55 57 59 61 68 70 73 74 75 76 78 79 81 82 85 87 89 91 92 93 99 100 104 105 106 107 108 110 111 113 114 118 120 122 128 129 131 142 145
Primary Contact: Michael J. Sniffen, FACHE, President and Chief Executive Officer
COO: Edward Condit, Executive Vice President and Chief Operating Officer
CFO: Nicholas Lanza, Controller
CMO: Ronald Poblete, M.D., President Medical and Dental Staff
CHR: Cathy Lynch–Kilic, Vice President Human Resources
Web address: www.smh–passaic.org
**Control:** Other not–for–profit (including NFP Corporation) **Service:** General Medical and Surgical

**Staffed Beds: 269 Admissions: 8847 Census: 128 Outpatient Visits:** 142400 **Births: 1066 Total Expense ($000): 155078 Payroll Expense ($000): 66659 Personnel: 1144**

## PATERSON—Passaic County

★ **ST. JOSEPH'S REGIONAL MEDICAL CENTER (310019)**, 703 Main Street, Zip 07503–2691; tel. 973/754–2000, (Includes ST. JOSEPH'S CHILDREN'S HOSPITAL, 703 Main Street, Zip 07503–2621; tel. 973/754–2500; ST. JOSEPH'S WAYNE HOSPITAL, 224 Hamburg Turnpike, Wayne, Zip 07470–2100; tel. 973/942–6900; Daniel B. Kline, Administrator), (Total facility includes 151 beds in nursing home–type unit) **A**2 3 5 9 10 12 13 21 **F**3 5 7 8 11 12 13 14 15 17 18 19 20 21 22 23 24 25 26 27 28 29 30 31 32 34 35 37 38 39 40 41 43 44 45 46 47 48 49 50 54 55 56 57 58 59 60 61 62 63 64 65 66 68 70 71 72 73 74 75 76 77 78 79 81 82 83 84 85 86 87 88 89 90 92 93 96 97 98 99 100 101 102 103 104 105 107 108 109 110 111 112 113 114 115 116 117 118 119 120 122 125 128 129 130 131 132 133 134 142 143 144 145 146 147 **P**3 5 6
Primary Contact: William A. McDonald, President and Chief Executive Officer
COO: Gloria A. Kunze, R.N., Vice President Operations
CFO: Jack Robinson, Chief Financial Officer
CMO: James Labagnara, M.D., Vice President Medical Affairs
CIO: James Cavanagh, Chief Information Officer
CHR: John Bruno, Vice President Human Resources
Web address: www.stjosephshealth.org
**Control:** Church–operated, Nongovernment, not–for profit **Service:** General Medical and Surgical

**Staffed Beds: 700 Admissions: 33865 Census: 518 Outpatient Visits:** 291548 **Births: 3530 Total Expense ($000): 633968 Payroll Expense ($000): 310882 Personnel: 4415**

## PEAPACK—Somerset County

☐ **MATHENY MEDICAL AND EDUCATIONAL CENTER (312014)**, 65 Highland Avenue, Zip 7977, Mailing Address: P.O. Box 339, Zip 07977–0339; tel. 908/234–0011, (Nonreporting) **A**1 5 10
Primary Contact: Steven M. Proctor, President
COO: Christopher King, Director Operations and Administrative Services
CFO: Wayne Guberman, Director Finance
CMO: Gary E. Eddey, M.D., Medical Director
CIO: Ron Daniel, Manager Information Systems
CHR: Nancy Petrillo, Director Human Resources
Web address: www.matheny.org
**Control:** Other not–for–profit (including NFP Corporation) **Service:** Long–Term Acute Care hospital

**Staffed Beds: 101**

## PENNINGTON—Mercer County

☒ **CAPITAL HEALTH MEDICAL CENTER–HOPEWELL (310044)**, 1 Capital Way, Zip 8534; tel. 609/303–4000 **A**1 2 3 5 6 9 10 **F**3 7 11 13 15 18 19 20 28 29 30 31 34 35 40 41 45 46 47 49 50 51 55 57 58 59 60 64 66 68 69 70 73 74 75 76 77 78 79 81 82 84 85 86 87 89 90 97 102 107 108 109 110 111 113 115 116 118 120 122 123 125 129 131 144 145 146 147 **S** Capital Health, Trenton, NJ
Primary Contact: Al Maghazehe, Ph.D., FACHE, Chief Executive Officer
COO: Larry DiSanto, Executive Vice President and Chief Operating Officer
CFO: Ronald J. Guy, Chief Financial Officer
CMO: Robert Remstein, D.O., Vice President Medical Affairs
CIO: Eugene Grochala, Vice President Information Systems
CHR: J. Scott Clemmensen, Vice President Human Resources and Leadership Enhancement
Web address: www.capitalhealth.org
**Control:** Other not–for–profit (including NFP Corporation) **Service:** General Medical and Surgical

**Staffed Beds: 223 Admissions: 11080 Census: 128 Outpatient Visits:** 175000 **Births: 2107 Personnel: 1390**

## PERTH AMBOY—Middlesex County

☐ **CARE ONE AT RARITAN BAY MEDICAL CENTER (312018)**, 530 New Brunswick Avenue, Zip 08861–3654; tel. 732/324–6090, (Nonreporting) **A**1 10
Primary Contact: Sharon Bready, R.N., Chief Executive Officer
CFO: Richard Burguillos, Chief Financial Officer
Web address: www.care-one.com
**Control:** Corporation, Investor–owned, for–profit **Service:** Long–Term Acute Care hospital

**Staffed Beds: 30**

*Many Facility Codes have changed. Please refer to the AHA Guide Code Chart.*

© 2012 AHA Guide

**NJ**

✠ **RARITAN BAY MEDICAL CENTER (310039)**, 530 New Brunswick Avenue, Zip 8861; tel. 732/442–3700, (Includes OLD BRIDGE DIVISION, One Hospital Plaza, Old Bridge, Zip 08857; tel. 732/360–1000; PERTH AMBOY DIVISION, 530 New Brunswick Avenue, Zip 08861–3685; tel. 732/442–3700) **A**1 3 5 9 10 **F**5 7 9 11 12 13 15 18 20 22 26 29 30 31 34 35 36 38 39 40 45 46 49 50 51 54 56 57 59 60 61 64 65 66 68 70 74 75 76 77 78 79 81 82 87 89 92 93 94 97 98 100 101 102 103 104 107 108 110 111 116 118 128 129 131 142 145 146 147 **P**6
Primary Contact: Michael R. D'Agnes, President and Chief Executive Officer
COO: Vincent Costantino, Vice President Operations and Human Resources
CFO: Thomas Shanahan, Chief Financial Officer and Senior Vice President
CMO: Michael Ciencewicki, M.D., Vice President Medical Affairs
CHR: Vincent Costantino, Vice President Operations and Human Resources
Web address: www.rbmc.org
**Control:** Other not–for–profit (including NFP Corporation) **Service:** General Medical and Surgical

> **Staffed Beds:** 277 **Admissions:** 13990 **Census:** 192 **Outpatient Visits:** 152743 **Births:** 1216 **Total Expense ($000):** 197633 **Payroll Expense ($000):** 103911 **Personnel:** 1837

## PHILLIPSBURG—Warren County

✠ **ST. LUKE'S HOSPITAL – WARREN CAMPUS (310060)**, 185 Roseberry Street, Zip 08865–9955; tel. 908/859–6700 **A**1 2 3 5 9 10 13 **F**2 3 8 11 15 18 20 28 29 30 31 34 35 39 40 49 53 56 59 61 64 65 66 68 70 75 77 78 81 82 86 87 91 92 93 97 98 100 102 103 104 106 107 108 110 111 113 117 118 128 129 130 131 133 145 146 147 **P**7 **S** St. Luke's University Health Network, Bethlehem, PA
Primary Contact: Thomas H. Litz, FACHE, President an Chief Executive Officer
COO: Alice Wilson, FACHE, Vice President Administration
CFO: Carl M. Alberto, Vice President Finance and Chief Financial Officer
CMO: Edward Gilkey, M.D., Vice President Medical Affairs
CIO: Debbie Bowlby, Director Information Systems
CHR: Morgan G. Mahl, Director Human Resources
CNO: Gail Newton, R.N., Vice President Patient Care Services
Web address: www.warrenhospital.org
**Control:** Other not–for–profit (including NFP Corporation) **Service:** General Medical and Surgical

> **Staffed Beds:** 140 **Admissions:** 6490 **Census:** 79 **Outpatient Visits:** 128549 **Births:** 0 **Total Expense ($000):** 110180 **Payroll Expense ($000):** 44910 **Personnel:** 975

## PISCATAWAY—Middlesex County

**UNIVERSITY OF MEDICINE AND DENTISTRY OF NEW JERSEY, UNIVERSITY BEHAVIORAL HEALTHCARE (314011)**, 671 Hoes Lane, Zip 8855, Mailing Address: P.O. Box 1392, Zip 08855–1392; tel. 732/235–5900 **A**3 5 9 10 **F**2 5 6 29 35 40 41 75 87 98 99 101 102 103 104 105 106 129
Primary Contact: Christopher O. Kosseff, President and Chief Executive Officer
COO: Susan Furrer, PsyD, Acting Chief Operating Officer and Executive Director Behavioral Research and Training Institute
CFO: Alan Weinkrantz, Chief Financial Officer
CMO: Theresa Miskimen, M.D., Vice President Medical Services
CIO: Leon Garfinkel, Director Information Services
Web address: www.umdnj.edu
**Control:** State–Government, nonfederal **Service:** Psychiatric

> **Staffed Beds:** 48 **Admissions:** 1290 **Census:** 38 **Outpatient Visits:** 82507 **Births:** 0 **Personnel:** 70

## PLAINSBORO— County

**UNIVERSITY MEDICAL CENTER AT PRINCETON** See University Medical Center of Princeton at Plainsboro

✠ **UNIVERSITY MEDICAL CENTER OF PRINCETON AT PLAINSBORO (310010)**, One Plainsboro Road, Zip 8536; tel. 609/853–7100, (Includes ACUTE GENERAL HOSPITAL, MERWICK UNIT–EXTENDED CARE AND REHABILITATION, PRINCETON HOUSE UNIT–COMMUNITY MENTAL HEALTH AND SUBSTANCE ABUSE ) **A**1 2 3 5 9 10 **F**3 4 5 8 11 12 13 14 15 17 18 19 20 22 26 28 29 30 31 32 34 35 36 38 39 40 45 46 49 50 51 53 54 55 56 57 58 59 60 62 63 64 65 66 68 70 73 74 75 76 77 78 79 81 82 85 86 87 89 90 91 92 93 94 96 97 98 99 100 101 102 103 104 105 107 108 110 111 113 114 117 118 119 120 123 125 128 129 131 133 134 142 145 146 147 **P**6
Primary Contact: Mark T. Jones, President
CFO: Bruce Traub, Chief Financial Officer
CMO: Linda Sieglen, M.D., Vice President Medical Affairs
CIO: Anne Searle, Chief Information Officer
CHR: Marcia M. Telthorster, Vice President Human Resources
CNO: Susan G. Lorenz, R.N., Vice President, Patient Care Services & Chief Nursing Officer
Web address: www.princetonhcs.org
**Control:** Other not–for–profit (including NFP Corporation) **Service:** General Medical and Surgical

> **Staffed Beds:** 338 **Admissions:** 16693 **Census:** 254 **Outpatient Visits:** 768270 **Births:** 1920 **Total Expense ($000):** 311239 **Payroll Expense ($000):** 131950 **Personnel:** 2336

## POMONA—Atlantic County

**ATLANTICARE REGIONAL MEDICAL CENTER–MAINLAND DIVISION** See AtlantiCare Regional Medical Center, Atlantic City

✠ △ **BACHARACH INSTITUTE FOR REHABILITATION (313030)**, 61 West Jimmie Leeds Road, Zip 08240–0723, Mailing Address: P.O. Box 723, Zip 08240–0723; tel. 609/652–7000, (Nonreporting) **A**1 7 10
Primary Contact: Richard J. Kathrins, President and Chief Executive Officer
CFO: Jeanne Vuksta, Chief Financial Officer
CMO: Craig Anmuth, M.D., Medical Director
CIO: Jeff Rees, Director Information Systems
CHR: Diane Croshaw, Vice President Human Resources
Web address: www.bacharach.org
**Control:** Other not–for–profit (including NFP Corporation) **Service:** Rehabilitation

> **Staffed Beds:** 80

## POMPTON PLAINS—Morris County

✠ **CHILTON HOSPITAL (310017)**, 97 West Parkway, Zip 07444–1696; tel. 973/831–5000 **A**1 2 9 10 **F**3 7 11 12 13 15 17 18 19 20 22 28 29 30 31 32 34 35 38 40 41 44 45 47 49 50 54 57 59 64 65 66 70 73 74 75 76 77 78 79 81 82 84 85 86 87 89 93 97 102 107 108 109 110 111 113 114 117 118 120 122 125 128 129 130 131 134 145 146 147
Primary Contact: Deborah Zastocki, R.N., FACHE, President and Chief Executive Officer
COO: Thomas Scott, Chief Operating Officer
CFO: Michael Richetti, Chief Financial Officer
CMO: Charles Ross, M.D., Vice President Medical Affairs
CIO: Karen S. Smith, Director Information Services
CHR: Julia McGovern, Vice President Human Resources
Web address: www.chiltonmemorial.org
**Control:** Other not–for–profit (including NFP Corporation) **Service:** General Medical and Surgical

> **Staffed Beds:** 260 **Admissions:** 9353 **Census:** 129 **Outpatient Visits:** 167952 **Births:** 912 **Total Expense ($000):** 154568 **Payroll Expense ($000):** 75022 **Personnel:** 1109

## RAHWAY—Union County

**KINDRED HOSPITAL NEW JERSEY – RAHWAY** See Kindred Hospital–New Jersey Morris County, Dover

✠ **ROBERT WOOD JOHNSON UNIVERSITY HOSPITAL RAHWAY (310024)**, 865 Stone Street, Zip 07065–2797; tel. 732/381–4200, (Total facility includes 24 beds in nursing home–type unit) **A**1 10 **F**3 11 15 17 20 29 30 31 34 35 38 40 46 47 49 50 53 56 57 59 63 64 65 68 70 74 75 77 78 79 81 82 86 87 93 97 100 101 102 107 108 111 116 117 118 127 128 129 131 133 142 143 145 146 147 **S** Robert Wood Johnson Health System & Network, New Brunswick, NJ
Primary Contact: Kirk C. Tice, President and Chief Executive Officer
CFO: Peter Bihuniak, Vice President Finance
CMO: Radha Vinnakota, M.D., President Medical Staff
CIO: Denine Izzi, Site Manager Information Systems
CHR: Kathryn Tarantino, Vice President Administration
CNO: Lynn Kearney, VP Patient Services & Chief Nursing Officer
Web address: www.rwjuhr.com
**Control:** Other not–for–profit (including NFP Corporation) **Service:** General Medical and Surgical

> **Staffed Beds:** 163 **Admissions:** 6558 **Census:** 106 **Outpatient Visits:** 54621 **Births:** 0 **Total Expense ($000):** 98786 **Payroll Expense ($000):** 41338 **Personnel:** 736

NJ

---

**Hospital, Medicare Provider Number, Address, Telephone, Approval, Facility, and Physician Codes, Health Care System**

★ American Hospital Association (AHA) membership
☐ The Joint Commission accreditation
◇ DNV Healthcare Inc. accreditation
○ American Osteopathic Association (AOA) accreditation
△ Commission on Accreditation of Rehabilitation Facilities (CARF) accreditation

### RED BANK—Monmouth County

☒ △ **RIVERVIEW MEDICAL CENTER (310034)**, 1 Riverview Plaza,
Zip 07701–9982; tel. 732/741–2700 **A**1 2 7 9 10 **F**3 5 11 13 15 17 18 20 22
28 29 30 31 38 40 41 44 45 46 47 51 55 56 59 60 61 63 64 65 66 68 70
73 74 75 76 77 78 79 80 81 82 83 84 85 86 87 90 92 93 96 97 98 99 100
101 102 103 104 105 107 108 110 111 113 114 116 118 119 120 122 123
128 129 131 134 143 145 146 147 **P**7 **S** Meridian Health, Neptune, NJ
Primary Contact: Timothy J. Hogan, FACHE, President
COO: Kelly O'Brien, Vice President Operations
CFO: John Gantner, Executive Vice President Finance
CMO: Joseph Reichman, M.D., Vice President Medical Affairs and Clinical
Effectiveness
CIO: Rebecca Weber, Senior Vice President Information Technology
Web address: www.riverviewmedicalcenter.com
**Control:** Other not–for–profit (including NFP Corporation) **Service:** General
Medical and Surgical

**Staffed Beds:** 270 **Admissions:** 13867 **Census:** 193 **Outpatient Visits:**
139742 **Births:** 1448 **Total Expense ($000):** 211471 **Payroll Expense
($000):** 91226 **Personnel:** 1048

### RIDGEWOOD—Bergen County

☒ **VALLEY HOSPITAL (310012)**, 223 North Van Dien Avenue, Zip 07450–9982;
tel. 201/447–8000 **A**1 2 5 9 10 **F**3 8 11 12 13 15 17 18 19 20 22 24 26 28
29 30 31 32 34 35 36 37 38 40 41 45 46 47 48 49 50 51 52 53 54 55 56
57 58 59 60 61 64 65 66 68 69 70 72 73 74 75 76 77 78 79 80 81 82 84
85 86 87 88 89 92 93 94 96 97 100 101 102 103 107 108 109 110 111
112 113 114 115 117 118 119 120 122 123 125 128 129 130 131 133 134
142 144 145 146 147 **P**6
Primary Contact: Audrey Meyers, President and Chief Executive Officer
COO: Peter Diestel, Senior Vice President and Chief Operating Officer
CFO: Richard Keenan, Senior Vice President Finance and Chief Financial Officer
CMO: Mitchell Rubinstein, M.D., Vice President Medical Affairs
CIO: Eric R. Carey, Vice President Information Systems and Chief Information
Officer
CHR: Russell H. Showers, Vice President Human Resources
CNO: Ann Marie Leichman, R.N., Vice President Patient Care Services and Chief
Nursing Officer
Web address: www.valleyhealth.com
**Control:** Other not–for–profit (including NFP Corporation) **Service:** General
Medical and Surgical

**Staffed Beds:** 446 **Admissions:** 30971 **Census:** 366 **Outpatient Visits:**
327313 **Births:** 3085 **Total Expense ($000):** 526547 **Payroll Expense
($000):** 242797 **Personnel:** 3951

### ROCHELLE PARK—Bergen County

☒ **SELECT SPECIALTY HOSPITAL–NORTHEAST NEW JERSEY (312019)**, 96
Parkway, Zip 7662; tel. 201/221–2358, (Nonreporting) **A**1 10 **S** Select Medical
Corporation, Mechanicsburg, PA
Primary Contact: Barbara E. Hannan, Chief Executive Officer
Web address: www.selectmedicalcorp.com
**Control:** Corporation, Investor–owned, for–profit **Service:** Long–Term Acute Care
hospital

**Staffed Beds:** 59

### SADDLE BROOK—Bergen County

**KESSLER INSTITUTE FOR REHABILITATION** See Kessler Institute for
Rehabilitation, West Orange

### SALEM—Salem County

☒ **MEMORIAL HOSPITAL OF SALEM COUNTY (310091)**, 310 Woodstown Road,
Zip 08079–2080; tel. 856/935–1000, (Nonreporting) **A**1 9 10 **S** Community
Health Systems, Inc., Franklin, TN
Primary Contact: Richard Grogan, Chief Executive Officer
CFO: Donald Bevers, Chief Financial Officer
CIO: Brian McCarthy, Director Information Systems
Web address: www.salemhospitalnj.org
**Control:** Corporation, Investor–owned, for–profit **Service:** General Medical and
Surgical

**Staffed Beds:** 110

### SECAUCUS—Hudson County

**LIBERTYHEALTH–MEADOWLANDS HOSPITAL MEDICAL CENTER** See
Meadowlands Hospital Medical Center

---

☐ **MEADOWLANDS HOSPITAL MEDICAL CENTER (310118)**, 55 Meadowlands
Parkway, Zip 07094–1580; tel. 201/392–3100 **A**1 9 10 21 **F**3 8 13 15 29 30
35 40 44 45 46 54 70 73 74 76 81 87 89 90 107 111 114 118 128 129 142
144 145 146 147 **P**3
Primary Contact: Lynn McVey, President and Chief Executive Officer
COO: Martin W. Baicker, Senior Vice President and Administrator
CFO: Donald Parseghian, Chief Financial Officer
CMO: Kenneth Garay, M.D., Chief Medical Officer
CIO: James Yost, Director Management Information Systems
CHR: Mary Cataudella, Corporate Director Human Resources
Web address: www.meadowlandshospital.org
**Control:** Partnership, Investor–owned, for–profit **Service:** General Medical and
Surgical

**Staffed Beds:** 134 **Admissions:** 4514 **Census:** 67 **Outpatient Visits:** 41877
**Births:** 587 **Total Expense ($000):** 78866 **Payroll Expense ($000):** 36767

### SOMERS POINT—Atlantic County

☒ **SHORE MEDICAL CENTER (310047)**, 1 East New York Avenue,
Zip 08244–2387; tel. 609/653–3500 **A**1 2 9 10 **F**3 11 13 15 17 18 20 22 28
29 30 31 34 35 36 37 40 44 45 49 50 54 57 59 60 61 64 66 68 70 73 74
75 76 77 78 79 81 82 84 85 86 87 89 92 93 107 108 110 111 113 117 118
119 120 122 128 129 131 134 142 145 146 147
Primary Contact: Ronald W. Johnson, FACHE, President and Chief Executive
Officer
CFO: James T. Foley, CPA, Vice President and Chief Financial Officer
CMO: Peter R. Jungblut, M.D., Vice President Medical Affairs and Chief Medical
Officer
CMO: Jeanne M. Rowe, M.D., Chief Medical Officer
CIO: Fred Banner, Chief Information Officer
CHR: Alan Beatty, Vice President Human Resources
CNO: Joan Gavin, R.N., Chief Nursing Officer/Vice President, Patient Services
Web address: www.shoremedicalcenter.org
**Control:** Other not–for–profit (including NFP Corporation) **Service:** General
Medical and Surgical

**Staffed Beds:** 206 **Admissions:** 10730 **Census:** 120 **Outpatient Visits:**
102643 **Births:** 1129 **Total Expense ($000):** 190003 **Payroll Expense
($000):** 76800 **Personnel:** 1254

### SOMERVILLE—Somerset County

☒ **SOMERSET MEDICAL CENTER (310048)**, 110 Rehill Avenue,
Zip 08876–2598; tel. 908/685–2200 **A**1 2 3 5 9 10 **F**3 7 12 13 14 15 18 20
22 24 26 28 29 30 31 34 35 37 40 45 46 53 56 57 58 59 60 61 64 65 68
70 74 75 76 77 78 79 81 82 87 89 98 99 100 101 102 103 104 105 107
108 110 111 113 114 115 116 117 118 119 120 121 122 123 125 128 129
130 131 132 134 145 146 **P**3
Primary Contact: Kenneth Bateman, CPA, President and Chief Executive Officer
COO: Maureen Schneider, MSN, Senior Vice President Clinical Program
Development and Chief Operating Officer
CFO: James De Rosa, Vice President Finance
CMO: Richard Paris, M.D., Chief Medical Officer
CIO: Dave Dyer, Vice President and Chief Information Officer
CHR: Mary Ann Bross, Vice President Human Resources
Web address: www.smchealthwise.com
**Control:** State–Government, nonfederal **Service:** General Medical and Surgical

**Staffed Beds:** 250 **Admissions:** 14837 **Census:** 197 **Births:** 1091

### STRATFORD—Camden County

**KENNEDY MEMORIAL HOSPITAL** See Kennedy Memorial Hospitals–University
Medical Center, Cherry Hill

### SUMMIT—Union County

☒ **OVERLOOK MEDICAL CENTER (310051)**, 99 Beauvoir Avenue,
Zip 07902–0220; tel. 908/522–2000 **A**1 2 3 5 9 10 13 **F**3 5 6 7 8 9 11 12 13
14 15 17 18 19 20 22 28 29 30 31 32 34 35 36 37 38 39 40 41 42 44 45
46 47 48 49 50 51 53 54 55 56 57 58 59 60 61 62 63 64 65 66 68 69 70
71 72 73 74 75 76 77 78 79 81 82 83 84 85 86 87 89 92 93 94 96 97 98
99 100 101 102 103 104 105 107 108 109 110 111 113 114 115 116 117
118 119 120 122 123 125 128 129 130 131 133 134 142 143 144 145 146
147 **P**3 5 6 **S** Atlantic Health, Morristown, NJ
Primary Contact: Alan R. Lieber, President
COO: Mark Holtz, Chief Operating Officer
CFO: Kevin Lenahan, Vice President Finance and Chief Financial Officer
CMO: Norman Luka, M.D., Medical Director Clinical Affairs
CIO: Linda Reed, Vice President and Chief Information Officer
CHR: Andrew L. Kovach, Vice President Human Resources and Chief
Administrative Officer
CNO: Mary Patricia Sullivan, R.N., Chief Nursing Officer
Web address: www.atlantichealth.org/Overlook
**Control:** Other not–for–profit (including NFP Corporation) **Service:** General
Medical and Surgical

**Staffed Beds:** 299 **Admissions:** 22892 **Census:** 307 **Outpatient Visits:**
358712 **Births:** 2328 **Total Expense ($000):** 435934 **Payroll Expense
($000):** 215508 **Personnel:** 2830

**NJ**

☐ **SUMMIT OAKS HOSPITAL (314001)**, 19 Prospect Street, Zip 07902–0100; tel. 908/522–7000, (Nonreporting) **A**1 9 10 **S** Universal Health Services, Inc., King of Prussia, PA
Primary Contact: James P. Gallagher, Chief Executive Officer
Web address: www.summitoakshospital.com/
**Control:** Corporation, Investor–owned, for–profit **Service:** Psychiatric

| Staffed Beds: 90 |
|---|

### SUSSEX—Sussex County

**SAINT CLARE'S HOSPITAL/SUSSEX** See Saint Clare's Health System, Denville

### TEANECK—Bergen County

**HOLY NAME HOSPITAL** See Holy Name Medical Center

⊞ **HOLY NAME MEDICAL CENTER (310008)**, 718 Teaneck Road, Zip 07666–4281; tel. 201/833–3000 **A**1 2 6 9 10 **F**2 3 7 11 12 13 15 18 19 20 22 28 29 30 31 32 34 35 36 37 39 40 44 45 46 47 49 50 51 53 54 55 56 57 58 59 60 62 63 64 65 66 68 70 73 74 75 76 77 78 79 81 82 83 84 85 86 87 89 91 93 94 97 98 100 102 103 107 108 110 111 113 114 115 116 117 118 119 120 122 123 125 128 129 130 131 132 134 142 143 145 146 147 **P**4 5 7
Primary Contact: Michael Maron, President and Chief Executive Officer
CFO: Joseph M. Lemaire, Executive Vice President and Chief Financial Officer
CMO: Adam D. Jarrett, M.D., Executive Vice President and Chief Medical Officer
CIO: Michael Skvarenina, Assistant Vice President Information Systems
CHR: April Rodgers, Vice President, Human Resources
CNO: Sheryl A. Slonim, Executive Vice President and Chief Nursing Officer
Web address: www.holyname.org
**Control:** Other not–for–profit (including NFP Corporation) **Service:** General Medical and Surgical

| Staffed Beds: 318 Admissions: 20060 Census: 214 Outpatient Visits: 353111 Births: 1420 Total Expense ($000): 268057 Payroll Expense ($000): 119372 Personnel: 1987 |
|---|

### TINTON FALLS—Monmouth County

⊞ **REHABILITATION HOSPITAL OF TINTON FALLS (313035)**, 2 Centre Plaza, Zip 7724; tel. 732/460–5320 **A**1 10 **F**29 64 68 74 75 82 90 93 94 95 96 100 118 147 **S** HEALTHSOUTH Corporation, Birmingham, AL
Primary Contact: Linda A. Savino, MS, Chief Executive Officer
CFO: Lynne Traister, Controller
CMO: Todd Cooperman, M.D., Medical Director
CHR: Anita Saum, Director Human Resources
Web address: www.rehabnj.com
**Control:** Corporation, Investor–owned, for–profit **Service:** Rehabilitation

| Staffed Beds: 60 Admissions: 1382 Census: 47 Outpatient Visits: 10422 Births: 0 Total Expense ($000): 15801 Payroll Expense ($000): 9889 Personnel: 203 |
|---|

### TOMS RIVER—Ocean County

⊞ **COMMUNITY MEDICAL CENTER (310041)**, 99 Route 37 West, Zip 08755–6423; tel. 732/557–8051 **A**1 2 9 10 **F**3 11 12 13 15 17 18 20 22 28 29 30 31 32 34 35 36 38 40 43 44 47 48 49 50 53 54 55 56 57 58 59 60 61 62 63 64 68 69 70 73 74 75 76 77 78 79 80 81 83 84 85 86 87 89 92 93 96 100 102 107 108 109 110 111 113 114 117 118 119 120 122 123 125 127 128 129 131 132 133 134 142 145 146 147 **P**6 **S** Barnabas Health, West Orange, NJ
Primary Contact: Stephanie L. Bloom, FACHE, President and Chief Executive Officer
COO: Frank Gelormini, Chief Operating Officer
CFO: Mark Ostrander, Vice President Financial Services
CMO: John Crisanti, M.D., Vice President Medical Affairs
CIO: Shawn Fitzsimmons, Director Information Technology Services
CHR: Mary Deno, Vice President Human Resources
CNO: Fern Papalia, Vice President, Patient Care Services
Web address: www.barnabashealth.org
**Control:** Other not–for–profit (including NFP Corporation) **Service:** General Medical and Surgical

| Staffed Beds: 489 Admissions: 28741 Census: 395 Outpatient Visits: 350143 Births: 1591 Total Expense ($000): 318337 Payroll Expense ($000): 144234 Personnel: 3545 |
|---|

⊞ **HEALTHSOUTH REHABILITATION HOSPITAL OF TOMS RIVER (313029)**, 14 Hospital Drive, Zip 08755–6470; tel. 732/244–3100, (Nonreporting) **A**1 10 **S** HEALTHSOUTH Corporation, Birmingham, AL
Primary Contact: Patricia Ostaszewski, MS, Chief Executive Officer
COO: Patricia Ostaszewski, MS, Chief Executive Officer
CFO: Janet Turso, Controller
CMO: Joseph Stillo, M.D., Medical Director
CIO: Coleen Rossi, Director Quality Services
CHR: Lori Munyan, Director, Human Resources
CNO: Susan Castor, Chief Nursing Officer
Web address: www.rehabnj.com/tomsriver
**Control:** Corporation, Investor–owned, for–profit **Service:** Rehabilitation

| Staffed Beds: 129 |
|---|

⊞ **SAINT BARNABAS BEHAVIORAL HEALTH CENTER (314022)**, 1691 Highway 9, Zip 08755–1245; tel. 732/914–1688, (Nonreporting) **A**1 9 **S** Barnabas Health, West Orange, NJ
Primary Contact: Joe Hicks, Executive Director
Web address: www.barnabashealth.org/
**Control:** Corporation, Investor–owned, for–profit **Service:** Psychiatric

| Staffed Beds: 40 |
|---|

### TRENTON—Mercer County

⊞ **CAPITAL HEALTH REGIONAL MEDICAL CENTER (310092)**, 750 Brunswick Avenue, Zip 08638–4174; tel. 609/394–6000 **A**1 3 5 6 10 **F**3 7 11 13 15 18 19 28 29 30 32 34 35 39 40 42 43 45 47 48 49 51 57 58 59 60 66 68 70 72 73 74 75 76 77 79 81 82 84 85 87 89 90 96 97 98 99 100 101 102 105 107 108 110 111 112 113 114 115 118 129 145 146 147 **S** Capital Health, Trenton, NJ
Primary Contact: Al Maghazehe, Ph.D., FACHE, Chief Executive Officer
COO: Larry DiSanto, Executive Vice President and Chief Operating Officer
CFO: Shane Fleming, Chief Financial Officer
CMO: Robert Remstein, D.O., Vice President Medical Affairs
CIO: Eugene Grochala, Vice President Information Systems
CHR: J. Scott Clemmensen, Vice President Human Resources and Leadership Enhancement
CHR: Scott Clemmensen, Vice President Human Resources and Leadership Enhancement
CNO: Eileen M. Horton, Vice President, Patient Services/Chief Nursing Officer
Web address: www.capitalhealth.org
**Control:** Other not–for–profit (including NFP Corporation) **Service:** General Medical and Surgical

| Staffed Beds: 226 Admissions: 10548 Census: 153 Outpatient Visits: 176432 Births: 80 Personnel: 1769 |
|---|

⊞ **ST. FRANCIS MEDICAL CENTER (310021)**, 601 Hamilton Avenue, Zip 08629–1986; tel. 609/599–5000 **A**1 2 6 9 10 **F**2 3 11 12 15 17 18 20 22 24 26 29 30 31 34 35 40 45 46 48 49 50 56 57 58 59 60 61 62 64 65 66 68 69 70 71 74 75 78 79 81 82 84 85 86 87 92 93 97 98 99 100 101 102 103 104 105 107 108 110 111 113 114 117 118 120 122 123 128 129 131 134 142 143 145 146 147 **P**5 6 **S** Catholic Health East, Newtown Square, PA
Primary Contact: Gerard J. Jablonowski, President and Chief Executive Officer
CFO: Mark Kelly, Vice President Finance
CMO: C. James Romano, M.D., President Medical Staff
CIO: Richard Dowgun, Chief Information Officer
CHR: Laura James, Director Human Resources
Web address: www.stfrancismedical.com
**Control:** Church–operated, Nongovernment, not–for profit **Service:** General Medical and Surgical

| Staffed Beds: 163 Admissions: 6104 Census: 95 Outpatient Visits: 88706 Births: 0 Total Expense ($000): 123625 Payroll Expense ($000): 44913 Personnel: 881 |
|---|

☐ **TRENTON PSYCHIATRIC HOSPITAL (314013)**, Route 29 and Sullivan Way, Zip 08628–3425, Mailing Address: P.O. Box 7500, West Trenton, Zip 08628–7500; tel. 609/633–1500, (Nonreporting) **A**1 10 **S** Division of Mental Health and Addiction Services, Department of Human Services, State of New Jersey, Trenton, NJ
Primary Contact: Teresa A. McQuaide, Chief Executive Officer
COO: Christopher Morrison, Deputy Chief Executive Officer
CFO: Joseph Canale, Business Manager
CMO: Lawrence Rossi, M.D., Clinical Director
CIO: Scott Eustace, Director Health Information Technology
CHR: Marybeth Longo, Manager Human Resources
CNO: Colleen Birkhofer, Chief Nursing Officer
Web address: www.nj.gov/
**Control:** State–Government, nonfederal **Service:** Psychiatric

| Staffed Beds: 392 |
|---|

**NJ**

---

**Hospital, Medicare Provider Number, Address, Telephone, Approval, Facility, and Physician Codes, Health Care System**

★ American Hospital Association (AHA) membership
☐ The Joint Commission accreditation
◇ DNV Healthcare Inc. accreditation
○ American Osteopathic Association (AOA) accreditation
△ Commission on Accreditation of Rehabilitation Facilities (CARF) accreditation

**TURNERSVILLE—Camden County**

**KENNEDY MEMORIAL HOSPITAL** See Kennedy Memorial Hospitals–University Medical Center, Cherry Hill

**VINELAND—Cumberland County**

☒ **HEALTHSOUTH REHABILITATION HOSPITAL OF VINELAND (313036)**, 1237 West Sherman Avenue, Zip 8360; tel. 856/696–7100 **A**1 10 **F**29 34 59 68 74 75 79 82 86 90 93 96 129 131 147 **S** HEALTHSOUTH Corporation, Birmingham, AL
Primary Contact: Tammy Feuer, Chief Executive Officer
CMO: Eugenio Rocksmith, M.D., Medical Director
CHR: Dawn Pearson, Director Human Resources
Web address: www.rhsj.org
**Control:** Corporation, Investor–owned, for–profit **Service:** Rehabilitation

> **Staffed Beds:** 40 **Admissions:** 988 **Census:** 35 **Outpatient Visits:** 2833
> **Births:** 0 **Total Expense ($000):** 11536 **Payroll Expense ($000):** 6380
> **Personnel:** 117

★ **SOUTH JERSEY HEALTHCARE – REGIONAL MEDICAL CENTER (310032)**, 1505 West Sherman Avenue, Zip 8360; tel. 856/641–8000, (Includes BRIDGETON HEALTH CENTER, 333 Irving Avenue, Bridgeton, Zip 08302–2100; tel. 856/575–4500) **A**2 9 10 21 **F**3 8 11 12 13 15 17 18 20 28 29 30 34 35 37 38 40 42 44 49 50 54 57 59 60 64 68 70 72 73 74 75 76 77 78 79 81 82 85 86 87 89 93 98 99 100 101 102 103 104 105 107 108 110 111 113 114 117 118 119 120 122 125 129 130 131 133 145 146 147 **P**6 **S** South Jersey Healthcare, Vineland, NJ
Primary Contact: Chester B. Kaletkowski, President and Chief Executive Officer
COO: Elizabeth Sheridan, Chief Operating Officer
CFO: John A. DiAngelo, Senior Vice President Finance and Chief Financial Officer
CMO: Steven C. Linn, M.D., Chief Medical Officer
CIO: Thomas Pacek, Vice President Information Systems and Chief Information Officer
CHR: Erich Florentine, Chief People Officer
Web address: www.sjhealthcare.net
**Control:** Other not–for–profit (including NFP Corporation) **Service:** General Medical and Surgical

> **Staffed Beds:** 325 **Admissions:** 17535 **Census:** 230 **Outpatient Visits:** 302527 **Births:** 2046 **Total Expense ($000):** 296051 **Payroll Expense ($000):** 127267 **Personnel:** 1483

**VOORHEES—Camden County**

★ **VIRTUA VOORHEES (310022)**, 100 Bowman Drive, Zip 08043–9612; tel. 856/325–3000, (Includes VOORHEES PEDIATRIC FACILITY, 1304 Laurel Oak Road, Zip 08043–4310; tel. 888/873–5437) **A**3 5 10 **F**3 11 13 29 30 31 34 35 40 41 45 46 47 48 49 50 54 55 58 59 66 68 70 72 73 74 75 76 78 79 81 82 86 87 88 89 90 92 93 107 108 111 114 115 116 118 128 129 142 145 146 147 **S** Virtua Health, Marlton, NJ
Primary Contact: Michael S. Kotzen, Vice President and Chief Operating Officer
COO: Michael S. Kotzen, Vice President and Chief Operating Officer
CFO: Robert Rosvold, Director Finance
CMO: James P. Dwyer, D.O., Executive Vice President and Chief Medical Officer
CIO: Alfred Campanella, Chief Information Officer
Web address: www.virtua.org
**Control:** Other not–for–profit (including NFP Corporation) **Service:** General Medical and Surgical

> **Staffed Beds:** 398 **Admissions:** 19090 **Census:** 233 **Outpatient Visits:** 208088 **Births:** 4620 **Total Expense ($000):** 307436 **Payroll Expense ($000):** 110553 **Personnel:** 1477

**WAYNE—Passaic County**

**KINDRED HOSPITAL NEW JERSEY – WAYNE** See Kindred Hospital–New Jersey Morris County, Dover

**WEST ORANGE—Essex County**

☒ △ **KESSLER INSTITUTE FOR REHABILITATION (313025)**, 1199 Pleasant Valley Way, Zip 07052–1419; tel. 973/731–3600, (Includes KESSLER INSTITUTE FOR REHABILITATION, 201 Pleasant Hill Road, Chester, Zip 07930–2141; tel. 973/252–6300, Sue Kida, Chief Executive Officer; KESSLER INSTITUTE FOR REHABILITATION, 300 Market Street, Saddle Brook, Zip 07663–5309; tel. 201/368–6000; Philip J. Driscoll, Jr., Chief Executive Officer; KESSLER INSTITUTE FOR REHABILITATION, 1199 Pleasant Valley Way, Zip 07052–1424; tel. 973/731–3600; Bonnie Evans, Chief Executive Officer), (Nonreporting) **A**1 3 5 7 10 **S** Select Medical Corporation, Mechanicsburg, PA
Primary Contact: Robert Brehm, Division President
CMO: Bruce M. Gans, M.D., Executive Vice President and Chief Medical Officer
CHR: Ken Caldera, Director Human Resources
Web address: www.kessler-rehab.com
**Control:** Corporation, Investor–owned, for–profit **Service:** Rehabilitation

> **Staffed Beds:** 332

**KESSLER INSTITUTE FOR REHABILITATION** See Kessler Institute for Rehabilitation

**WESTAMPTON TOWNSHIP—Burlington County**

☐ **HAMPTON BEHAVIORAL HEALTH CENTER (314021)**, 650 Rancocas Road, Zip 08060–5613; Mailing Address: Mount Holly, tel. 609/267–7000 **A**1 9 10 **F**35 98 99 102 103 104 105 129 131 **P**6 **S** Universal Health Services, Inc., King of Prussia, PA
Primary Contact: Craig Hilton, Chief Executive Officer
COO: Joanne Aiello, Chief Operating Officer
CFO: Guy DiStefano, Chief Financial Officer
CMO: Charles Trigiani, D.O., Medical Director
CHR: Polly Costantini, Director Human Resources
Web address: www.hamptonhospital.com
**Control:** Corporation, Investor–owned, for–profit **Service:** Psychiatric

> **Staffed Beds:** 110 **Admissions:** 2650 **Census:** 100 **Outpatient Visits:** 15089
> **Births:** 0 **Total Expense ($000):** 19944 **Payroll Expense ($000):** 13047
> **Personnel:** 234

**WILLINGBORO—Burlington County**

☒ **LOURDES MEDICAL CENTER OF BURLINGTON COUNTY (310061)**, 218–A Sunset Road, Zip 08046–1162; tel. 609/835–2900 **A**1 2 9 10 13 **F**3 5 11 12 15 17 18 29 30 31 34 35 36 38 40 44 45 47 48 49 50 55 56 57 59 60 61 64 66 68 70 74 75 78 79 81 82 85 86 87 93 97 98 100 104 105 107 108 109 110 111 113 117 118 128 129 131 134 145 146 147 **S** Catholic Health East, Newtown Square, PA
Primary Contact: Mark Nessel, Executive Vice President and Chief Operating Officer
COO: Robert Ruggero, Senior Vice President Operations
CFO: Michael Hammond, Chief Financial Officer
CMO: Alan R. Pope, M.D., Vice President, Medical Affairs
CIO: Mike Elfert, Director Information Services
CHR: Richard P. Kropp, Vice President Human Resources
CHR: Janet Moran, Vice President Human Resources
CNO: Audrey Jadczak, R.N., Vice President/Chief Nursing Officer
Web address: www.lourdesnet.org
**Control:** Other not–for–profit (including NFP Corporation) **Service:** General Medical and Surgical

> **Staffed Beds:** 221 **Admissions:** 8101 **Census:** 121 **Outpatient Visits:** 111776 **Births:** 0 **Total Expense ($000):** 106460 **Payroll Expense ($000):** 42244 **Personnel:** 672

☐ **LOURDES SPECIALTY HOSPITAL OF SOUTHERN NEW JERSEY (312022)**, 218 Sunset Road, Zip 08046–1110; tel. 609/835–3650, (Nonreporting) **A**1 10
Primary Contact: Cheri Cowperthwait, Interim Chief Executive Officer
Web address: www.lourdesnet.org
**Control:** Corporation, Investor–owned, for–profit **Service:** Long–Term Acute Care hospital

> **Staffed Beds:** 30

**WOODBRIDGE—Middlesex County**

**WOODBRIDGE DEVELOPMENT CENTER**, Rahway Avenue, Zip 07095–3697, Mailing Address: P.O. Box 189, Zip 07095–0189; tel. 732/499–5951, (Nonreporting)
Primary Contact: Amy R. Bailon, M.D., Medical Director
Web address: www.state.nj.us/
**Control:** State–Government, nonfederal **Service:** Hospital unit within an institution for the mentally retarded

> **Staffed Beds:** 125

**WOODBURY—Gloucester County**

☒ **UNDERWOOD–MEMORIAL HOSPITAL (310081)**, 509 North Broad Street, Zip 08096–1697, Mailing Address: P.O. Box 359, Zip 08096–7359; tel. 856/845–0100 **A**1 3 5 9 10 **F**3 11 13 15 17 18 20 22 28 29 30 34 35 38 39 40 49 50 56 57 58 59 60 61 62 64 66 67 70 73 74 75 76 77 79 80 81 85 86 89 91 93 96 97 98 99 100 102 104 105 107 110 113 114 117 118 128 129 131 134 142 145 146 147 **P**6
Primary Contact: Eileen K. Cardile, R.N., MS, President and Chief Executive Officer
COO: John W. Graham, Executive Vice President and Chief Operating Officer
CFO: James R. Brant, Senior Vice President Finance and Chief Financial Officer
CIO: Robert Mizia, Director Information Systems and Chief Information Officer
CHR: Robert Manestrina, Vice President Human Resources
Web address: www.umhospital.org
**Control:** Other not–for–profit (including NFP Corporation) **Service:** General Medical and Surgical

> **Staffed Beds:** 240 **Admissions:** 12841 **Census:** 161 **Outpatient Visits:** 102405 **Births:** 941 **Total Expense ($000):** 169579 **Payroll Expense ($000):** 79227 **Personnel:** 1161

**NJ**

**WYCKOFF—Bergen County**

☒ **CHRISTIAN HEALTH CARE CENTER (314019)**, 301 Sicomac Avenue,
Zip 07481–2194; tel. 201/848–5200, (Total facility includes 292 beds in nursing
home–type unit) **A**1 9 10 **F**2 10 11 29 34 35 56 59 63 66 69 77 98 99 100
101 103 104 105 124 127 129 142 145 147
Primary Contact: Douglas A. Struyk, President and Chief Executive Officer
COO: Denise Ratcliffe, Executive Vice President and Chief Operating Officer
CFO: Kevin Stagg, Executive Vice President Finance and Chief Financial Officer
CMO: Howard Gilman, M.D., Medical Executive
CIO: Jennifer D'Angelo, Assistant Vice President Information Services
CHR: Bob Zierold, Senior Vice President Human Resources
CNO: Marianne Guerriero, Nurse Executive
Web address: www.chccnj.org
**Control:** Other not–for–profit (including NFP Corporation) **Service:** Psychiatric

**Staffed Beds:** 524 **Admissions:** 1871 **Census:** 498 **Outpatient Visits:** 42184
**Births:** 0 **Total Expense ($000):** 68740 **Payroll Expense ($000):** 40196
**Personnel:** 746

NJ

---

**Hospital, Medicare Provider Number, Address, Telephone, Approval, Facility, and Physician Codes, Health Care System**

★ American Hospital Association (AHA) membership
☐ The Joint Commission accreditation          ◇ DNV Healthcare Inc. accreditation

○ American Osteopathic Association (AOA) accreditation
△ Commission on Accreditation of Rehabilitation Facilities (CARF) accreditation

# NEW MEXICO

## ACOMA— County

☐ **ACOMA–CANONCITO–LAGUNA HOSPITAL (320070)**, 80B Veterans Boulevard, Zip 87034, Mailing Address: P.O. Box 130, San Fidel, Zip 87049–0130; tel. 505/552–5300, (Nonreporting) **A**1 10 **S** U. S. Indian Health Service, Rockville, MD
Primary Contact: William Thorne, Jr., Chief Executive Officer
Web address: www.ihs.gov/albuquerque/index.cfm?module=dsp_abq_acoma_canoncito_laguna
**Control:** PHS, Indian Service, Government, federal **Service:** General Medical and Surgical

**Staffed Beds:** 25

## ALAMOGORDO—Otero County

⊞ **GERALD CHAMPION REGIONAL MEDICAL CENTER (320004)**, 2669 North Scenic Drive, Zip 88310–8799; tel. 575/439–6100 **A**1 9 10 20 **F**3 8 9 11 13 18 29 30 31 34 35 40 43 45 50 51 56 57 58 59 64 70 74 75 76 77 78 79 81 85 86 87 97 98 101 103 104 105 107 108 111 113 115 116 118 128 129 131 132 141 145 146 **P**6 QHR, Brentwood, TN
Primary Contact: Robert J. Heckert, Jr., Chief Executive Officer
CFO: Morgan Hay, Chief Financial Officer
CMO: Arthur Austin, M.D., Vice President Medical Affairs
CIO: Ana Castro, Director Information Services and Clinical Information Services
CHR: Karen O'Brien, Director Human Resources
CNO: Martha C. Gorman, R.N., Vice President of Patient Care Services and Chief Nursing Officer
Web address: www.gcrmc.org
**Control:** Other not–for–profit (including NFP Corporation) **Service:** General Medical and Surgical

**Staffed Beds:** 86 **Admissions:** 4379 **Census:** 42 **Outpatient Visits:** 71053 **Births:** 593 **Total Expense ($000):** 95477 **Payroll Expense ($000):** 36992

## ALBUQUERQUE—Bernalillo County

⊞ **HEALTHSOUTH REHABILITATION HOSPITAL (323027)**, 7000 Jefferson Street N.E., Zip 87109–4313; tel. 505/344–9478 **A**1 9 10 **F**29 34 35 56 57 59 60 62 64 74 75 77 79 90 91 93 94 95 96 129 131 142 147 **S** HEALTHSOUTH Corporation, Birmingham, AL
Primary Contact: Sylvia K. Kelly, Chief Executive Officer
CFO: Byron Aten, Controller
CMO: Angela Walker, M.D., Medical Director
CHR: Victoria Otero, Director Human Resources
CNO: Veronica Gadomski, R.N., Chief Nursing Officer
Web address: www.healthsouthnewmexico.com
**Control:** Corporation, Investor–owned, for–profit **Service:** Rehabilitation

**Staffed Beds:** 87 **Admissions:** 1615 **Census:** 66 **Outpatient Visits:** 8745 **Births:** 0 **Total Expense ($000):** 19056 **Payroll Expense ($000):** 11985 **Personnel:** 226

⊞ **KINDRED HOSPITAL–ALBUQUERQUE (322002)**, 700 High Street N.E., Zip 87102–2565; tel. 505/242–4444, (Nonreporting) **A**1 9 10 **S** Kindred Healthcare, Louisville, KY
Primary Contact: Michael R. Shaw, Chief Executive Officer
CFO: Margaret Wantland, Chief Financial Officer
CMO: Jeffrey Dorf, M.D., Medical Director
CHR: Donald Whitney, Director Human Resources
CNO: Rhonda Lovato, R.N., Chief Clinical Officer
Web address: www.kindredalbuquerque.com/
**Control:** Corporation, Investor–owned, for–profit **Service:** Long–Term Acute Care hospital

**Staffed Beds:** 61

★ **LOVELACE MEDICAL CENTER (320009)**, 601 Martin Luther King Avenue N.E., Zip 87102–3670; tel. 505/727–8000, (Includes HEART HOSPITAL OF NEW MEXICO, 504 Elm Street, Zip 87102; tel. 505/724–2000; Ronald C. Winger, President), (Nonreporting) **A**9 10 **S** Ardent Health Services, Nashville, TN
Primary Contact: David S. Nevill, Chief Executive Officer
COO: Susan K. Rodgers, MSN, Chief Operating Officer
CFO: Gina Anderson, Chief Financial Officer
CFO: Brian Vaughan, Chief Financial Officer
CMO: Jean D. Remillard, M.D., Chief Medical Officer/Chief Quality Officer
CHR: Philip Espinosa, Human Resource Director
CHR: Randy Royster, Vice President Human Resources
CNO: Laurie S. Bigham, R.N., Chief Nursing Officer
Web address: www.lovelace.com
**Control:** Corporation, Investor–owned, for–profit **Service:** General Medical and Surgical

**Staffed Beds:** 263

★ △ **LOVELACE REHABILITATION HOSPITAL (323028)**, 505 Elm Street N.E., Zip 87102–2500; tel. 505/727–4700, (Nonreporting) **A**7 9 10 **S** Ardent Health Services, Nashville, TN
Primary Contact: Traci Willis, Chief Executive Officer
CFO: Andrea Solin, Chief Financial Officer
CHR: Becky Falance, Director Human Resources
Web address: www.lovelace.com
**Control:** Corporation, Investor–owned, for–profit **Service:** Rehabilitation

**Staffed Beds:** 80

⊞ **LOVELACE WESTSIDE HOSPITAL (320074)**, 10501 Golf Course Road N.W., Zip 87114–5000, Mailing Address: P.O. Box 25555, Zip 87125–0555; tel. 505/727–2000 **A**1 9 10 **F**3 12 13 15 29 39 40 42 57 68 70 75 79 81 85 86 87 107 110 111 113 114 118 134 145 **S** Ardent Health Services, Nashville, TN
Primary Contact: Troy Greer, Chief Executive Officer
COO: Karrie Brazaski, Chief Operating Officer and Chief Nursing Officer
CMO: William J. Mitchell, M.D., Chief Medical Officer
Web address: www.lovelacesandia.com
**Control:** Corporation, Investor–owned, for–profit **Service:** General Medical and Surgical

**Staffed Beds:** 80 **Admissions:** 2555 **Census:** 21 **Outpatient Visits:** 47986 **Births:** 217 **Total Expense ($000):** 50603 **Payroll Expense ($000):** 17272 **Personnel:** 324

⊞ **LOVELACE WOMEN'S HOSPITAL (320017)**, 4701 Montgomery Boulevard N.E., Zip 87109–1251, Mailing Address: P.O. Box 25555, Zip 87125–0555; tel. 505/727–7800, (Nonreporting) **A**1 9 10 **S** Ardent Health Services, Nashville, TN
Primary Contact: Sheri Milone, Chief Executive Officer and Administrator
COO: Janelle Raborn, Chief Operating Officer
CFO: Joseph Sereno, Chief Financial Officer
CHR: Carol Shelton, Director Human Resources
Web address: www.lovelace.com
**Control:** Corporation, Investor–owned, for–profit **Service:** General Medical and Surgical

**Staffed Beds:** 120

⊞ **PRESBYTERIAN HOSPITAL (320021)**, 1100 Central Avenue S.E., Zip 87106–4934, Mailing Address: P.O. Box 26666, Zip 87125–6666; tel. 505/841–1234 **A**1 2 3 5 9 10 **F**3 7 8 11 13 14 17 18 19 20 21 22 23 24 25 26 27 29 30 31 35 38 40 42 44 45 46 47 48 49 51 53 57 59 60 68 70 72 73 74 75 76 77 78 79 81 84 85 86 87 88 89 92 93 96 100 101 107 108 111 113 116 118 123 125 129 130 131 137 141 143 144 145 146 147 **P**6 **S** Presbyterian Healthcare Services, Albuquerque, NM
Primary Contact: Clay Holderman, Interim Administrator
COO: Clay Holderman, Chief Operating Officer–Central Delivery System
CFO: Paul Briggs, Executive Vice President and Chief Financial Officer
CFO: Donna Garcia, Vice President, Finance
CMO: Jayne McCormick, Chief Medical Officer CDS
CIO: Lee Marley, VP/Information Services Chief Application Officer
CHR: Lee Patchell, Lead Human Resources Business Partner
CNO: Ann L. Wright, R.N., Assistant Central Delivery System CNO
Web address: www.phs.org
**Control:** Other not–for–profit (including NFP Corporation) **Service:** General Medical and Surgical

**Staffed Beds:** 552 **Admissions:** 33538 **Census:** 408 **Outpatient Visits:** 1351145 **Births:** 4642 **Total Expense ($000):** 711323 **Payroll Expense ($000):** 330692 **Personnel:** 2963

★ **PRESBYTERIAN KASEMAN HOSPITAL**, 8300 Constitution Avenue N.E., Zip 87110–7624, Mailing Address: P.O. Box 26666, Zip 87125–6666; tel. 505/291–2000 **A**9 **F**3 5 15 29 30 31 40 50 53 56 63 64 65 68 75 78 81 82 84 85 86 87 93 97 98 99 100 101 102 103 104 105 107 108 111 113 114 115 116 118 119 120 122 127 128 129 131 133 145 147 **S** Presbyterian Healthcare Services, Albuquerque, NM
Primary Contact: Doyle Boykin, R.N., MSN, Administrator
COO: Paul Briggs, Executive VP/Chief Operating Officer
COO: David R. Scrase, M.D., Executive Senior Vice President and Chief Operating Officer
CFO: Dale Maxwell, Senior VP Chief Financial Officer
CMO: Eddie Benge, M.D., Vice President Medical Staff Affairs
CMO: Jayne McCormick, Chief Medical Officer CDS
CIO: Lee Marley, VP/Information Services Chief Application Officer
CHR: Cindy McGill, Senior Vice President Human Resources
Web address: www.phs.org
**Control:** Other not–for–profit (including NFP Corporation) **Service:** Surgical

**Staffed Beds:** 118 **Admissions:** 2282 **Census:** 68 **Outpatient Visits:** 100438 **Births:** 0 **Personnel:** 498

**NM**

**SPECIALTY HOSPITAL OF ALBUQUERQUE (322003)**, 235 Elm Street N.E., Zip 87102; tel. 505/842–5550 **A**9 10 **F**1 29 34 142 147 **S** Fundamental Long Term Care Holdings, LLC, Sparks Glencoe, MD
Primary Contact: William R. Fox, Chief Executive Officer
COO: Elizabeth Rees, Chief Clinical Officer
CFO: Julie Lenzo, Director Business Office
CMO: Jeffrey Ross, M.D., Medical Director
CHR: Robin Stendel–Freels, Coordinator Human Resources
**Control:** Partnership, Investor–owned, for–profit **Service:** Long–Term Acute Care hospital

**Staffed Beds: 24 Admissions: 226 Census: 19 Outpatient Visits: 0 Births:** 0

△ **TURQUOISE LODGE HOSPITAL**, 5901 Zuni Road S.E., Zip 87108–3073; tel. 505/841–8978, (Nonreporting) **A**7
Primary Contact: Michael Gutierrez, Executive Director
Web address: www.health.state.nm.us
**Control:** State–Government, nonfederal **Service:** Alcoholism and other chemical dependency

**Staffed Beds: 34**

⊠ **UNIVERSITY OF NEW MEXICO HOSPITALS (320001)**, 2211 Lomas Boulevard N.E., Zip 87106–2745; tel. 505/272–2111, (Includes CARRIE TINGLEY HOSPITAL, 1127 University Boulevard N.E., Zip 87102–1715; tel. 505/272–5200; Crystal Frantz, Executive Director; MENTAL HEALTH CENTER, 2600 Marble N.E., Zip 87131–2600; tel. 505/272–2800; UNIVERSITY OF NEW MEXICO CHILDREN'S PSYCHIATRIC HOSPITAL, 1001 Yale Boulevard N.E., Zip 87131–3830; tel. 505/272–2890; UNM CHILDREN'S HOSPITAL, 2211 Lomas Boulevard, N.E., tel. 505/272–2111) **A**1 2 3 5 8 9 10 **F**3 8 9 11 13 15 16 17 18 19 20 21 22 23 24 25 26 27 28 29 30 31 32 34 35 38 40 41 43 44 45 46 47 48 49 50 51 54 56 57 59 60 61 63 64 65 68 70 72 73 74 75 76 77 78 79 81 82 83 84 85 86 87 88 89 90 92 93 94 95 96 97 107 108 109 110 111 113 114 115 116 117 118 120 122 125 128 129 130 131 134 135 137 143 145 146 147
Primary Contact: Stephen W. McKernan, Chief Executive Officer
CFO: Ella Watt, Chief Financial Officer
CMO: Robert Katz, M.D., Vice President Clinical Affairs
CIO: Ron Margolis, Chief Information Officer
CHR: Jim Pendergast, Administrator Human Resources
Web address: www.unm.edu
**Control:** State–Government, nonfederal **Service:** General Medical and Surgical

**Staffed Beds: 537 Admissions: 25442 Census: 412 Outpatient Visits:** 581980 **Births: 3361 Total Expense ($000): 747986 Payroll Expense ($000): 291960 Personnel: 4892**

⊠ △ **VETERANS AFFAIRS MEDICAL CENTER**, 1501 San Pedro S.E., Zip 87108–5138; tel. 505/265–1711, (Nonreporting) **A**1 2 3 5 7 8 **S** Department of Veterans Affairs, Washington, DC
Primary Contact: George Marnell, Director
CFO: Michael McNeill, Chief Financial Management
CMO: Meghan Gerety, M.D., Chief of Staff
CIO: Ronald Ferrell, Chief Information Officer
CHR: Melvin Hooker, Chief Human Resources
Web address: www.southwest.va.gov/albuquerque/
**Control:** Veterans Affairs, Government, federal **Service:** General Medical and Surgical

**Staffed Beds: 281**

★ **ARTESIA GENERAL HOSPITAL (320030)**, 702 North 13th Street, Zip 88210–1199; tel. 575/748–3333, (Nonreporting) **A**9 10 20 **S** Community Hospital Corporation, Plano, TX
Primary Contact: Kenneth W. Randall, Chief Executive Officer
CFO: William Zemanek, Assistant Chief Financial Officer
CMO: Joe Salgado, M.D., Chief of Staff
CHR: Dawn Wright, Director Human Resources
Web address: www.artesiageneral.com
**Control:** Other not–for–profit (including NFP Corporation) **Service:** General Medical and Surgical

**Staffed Beds: 43**

⊠ **CARLSBAD MEDICAL CENTER (320063)**, 2430 West Pierce Street, Zip 88220–3597; tel. 575/887–4105, (Nonreporting) **A**1 9 10 **S** Community Health Systems, Inc., Franklin, TN
Primary Contact: Chad Campbell, Chief Executive Officer
CIO: Kenneth Kemp, Director Information Systems
CHR: Christina Beasley, Director Human Resources
Web address: www.carlsbadmedicalcenter.com
**Control:** Corporation, Investor–owned, for–profit **Service:** General Medical and Surgical

**Staffed Beds: 127**

★ **UNION COUNTY GENERAL HOSPITAL (321304)**, 300 Wilson Street, Zip 88415–3321, Mailing Address: P.O. Box 489, Zip 88415–0489; tel. 575/374–2585 **A**9 10 18 **F**3 11 13 29 31 35 40 45 50 57 59 62 64 65 68 70 76 81 82 85 87 89 93 97 102 107 113 118 128 129 132 143 144 147 **S** HealthTech Management Services, Franklin, TN
Primary Contact: Donald Weidemann, Administrator
CFO: Julie Price, Chief Financial Officer
CMO: Daniel Radunsky, M.D., Medical Staff President
CIO: Tim Justice, Chief Information Officer
CHR: Jill Swagerty, Director Human Resources
CNO: Stacye Bradley, R.N., Chief Nursing Officer
Web address: www.unioncountygeneral.com
**Control:** Other not–for–profit (including NFP Corporation) **Service:** General Medical and Surgical

**Staffed Beds: 21 Admissions: 288 Census: 3 Outpatient Visits: 11950 Births: 16 Total Expense ($000): 10967 Payroll Expense ($000): 4028 Personnel: 85**

⊠ **PLAINS REGIONAL MEDICAL CENTER (320022)**, 2100 Martin Luther King Boulevard, Zip 88101–9412, Mailing Address: P.O. Box 1688, Zip 88102–1688; tel. 575/769–2141 **A**1 9 10 **F**3 8 11 13 15 20 28 29 30 31 35 40 45 47 48 50 51 53 54 62 63 64 68 69 70 75 76 77 78 79 81 82 83 84 85 87 89 93 97 99 100 101 102 103 104 107 111 112 113 114 117 118 122 128 129 134 145 146 147 **P**6 **S** Presbyterian Healthcare Services, Albuquerque, NM
Primary Contact: Hoyt Skabelund, Administrator
CMO: Brian Willmon, M.D., Medical Director
CIO: Hoyt Skabelund, Administrator
CNO: Terri A. Marney, R.N., Director of Nursing
Web address: www.phs.org
**Control:** Other not–for–profit (including NFP Corporation) **Service:** General Medical and Surgical

**Staffed Beds: 106 Admissions: 5058 Census: 44 Outpatient Visits: 93159 Births: 1215 Total Expense ($000): 82237 Payroll Expense ($000): 29994 Personnel: 529**

**U. S. PUBLIC HEALTH SERVICE INDIAN HOSPITAL (320062)**, Zip 87313; tel. 505/786–5291, (Nonreporting) **A**10 **S** U. S. Indian Health Service, Rockville, MD
Primary Contact: Virgil Davis, Acting Chief Executive Officer
CFO: Darlene Kirk, Manager Finance
CIO: Jimmy Burbank, Chief Information Officer
CHR: Victoria Pablo, Human Resource Specialist
Web address: www.ihs.gov
**Control:** PHS, Indian Service, Government, federal **Service:** General Medical and Surgical

**Staffed Beds: 12**

⊠ **MIMBRES MEMORIAL HOSPITAL (320014)**, 900 West Ash Street, Zip 88030–4098, Mailing Address: P.O. Box 710, Zip 88031–0710; tel. 575/546–2761, (Nonreporting) **A**1 9 10 20 **S** Community Health Systems, Inc., Franklin, TN
Primary Contact: Steve Westenhofer, Chief Executive Officer
CFO: Suzanne Herbert, Chief Financial Officer
CHR: Johanna Gramer, Director Human Resources
CNO: Colonel Gwenda McClure, USAF, Chief Nursing Officer
Web address: www.mimbresmemorial.com
**Control:** Corporation, Investor–owned, for–profit **Service:** General Medical and Surgical

**Staffed Beds: 99**

**NM**

## ESPANOLA—Rio Arriba County

⊞ **ESPANOLA HOSPITAL (320011)**, 1010 Spruce Street, Zip 87532–2746; tel. 505/753–7111 **A**1 9 10 20 **F**3 7 8 11 13 15 29 30 32 34 35 40 45 50 53 57 59 62 64 65 68 70 75 76 79 81 85 89 93 107 108 110 113 114 117 118 128 145 **P**8 **S** Presbyterian Healthcare Services, Albuquerque, NM
Primary Contact: Brenda Romero, Administrator
Web address: www.phs.org
**Control:** Other not–for–profit (including NFP Corporation) **Service:** General Medical and Surgical

**Staffed Beds:** 80 **Admissions:** 2210 **Census:** 21 **Births:** 427 **Total Expense ($000):** 44624 **Payroll Expense ($000):** 22309 **Personnel:** 291

## FARMINGTON—San Juan County

⊞ **SAN JUAN REGIONAL MEDICAL CENTER (320005)**, 801 West Maple Street, Zip 87401–5630; tel. 505/609–2000, (Includes SAN JUAN REGIONAL MEDICAL CENTER REHABILITATION HOSPITAL, 525 South Schwartz, Zip 87401; tel. 505/609–2625) **A**1 2 5 9 10 21 **F**3 7 8 11 13 15 18 20 22 26 28 29 30 31 32 34 35 40 42 43 45 47 48 49 50 53 54 57 59 60 64 65 68 70 74 75 76 78 79 81 85 87 89 90 93 96 97 98 99 100 102 107 108 111 112 113 114 117 118 120 129 131 134 142 143 145 147 **P**5 6
Primary Contact: Rick D. Wallace, FACHE, President and Chief Executive Officer
COO: John Buffington, Chief Operating Officer
CFO: J. Michael Philips, Chief Strategy Officer
CMO: Robert Fabrey, M.D., Chief Medical Officer
CHR: Elizabeth Volkerding, Director Workforce Excellence
Web address: www.sanjuanregional.com
**Control:** Other not–for–profit (including NFP Corporation) **Service:** General Medical and Surgical

**Staffed Beds:** 198 **Admissions:** 10566 **Census:** 124 **Outpatient Visits:** 208713 **Births:** 1268 **Total Expense ($000):** 233945 **Payroll Expense ($000):** 111843 **Personnel:** 1641

## GALLUP—Mckinley County

⊞ **GALLUP INDIAN MEDICAL CENTER (320061)**, 516 East Nizhoni Boulevard, Zip 87301–5748, Mailing Address: P.O. Box 1337, Zip 87305–1337; tel. 505/722–1000, (Nonreporting) **A**1 5 9 10 **S** U. S. Indian Health Service, Rockville, MD
Primary Contact: Bennie C. Yazzie, Interim Chief Executive Officer
CFO: Agnes Kee, Financial Manager
CMO: Douglas G. Peter, M.D., Chief Medical Officer
CIO: Adrian C. Haven, Site Manager
CHR: Karen Lee, Director Human Resources
Web address:
www.ihs.gov/facilitiesservices/areaoffices/navajo/naihs-hcc-gallup.asp
**Control:** Public Health Service, Government, federal **Service:** General Medical and Surgical

**Staffed Beds:** 71

⊞ **REHOBOTH MCKINLEY CHRISTIAN HEALTH CARE SERVICES (320038)**, 1901 Red Rock Drive, Zip 87301–5683; tel. 505/863–7000 **A**1 5 9 10 20 **F**3 4 5 11 13 15 28 29 30 34 35 40 43 50 57 59 62 63 64 65 68 70 75 76 77 79 81 84 85 87 89 99 100 102 104 107 108 111 114 118 119 123 128 129 131 134 145 146
Primary Contact: Roger Gleisner, Interim Chief Executive Officer
CFO: Mark Hall, Chief Financial Officer
CMO: Mary L. Poel, M.D., Chief Medical Officer
CIO: Brett Mello, Chief Information Officer
CHR: George Laurin, Interim Chief Human Resources Officer
Web address: www.rmch.org
**Control:** Other not–for–profit (including NFP Corporation) **Service:** General Medical and Surgical

**Staffed Beds:** 80 **Admissions:** 3308 **Census:** 37 **Outpatient Visits:** 134587 **Births:** 495 **Total Expense ($000):** 60770 **Payroll Expense ($000):** 30182 **Personnel:** 504

## GRANTS—Cibola County

⊞ **CIBOLA GENERAL HOSPITAL (321308)**, 1016 East Roosevelt Avenue, Zip 87020–2118; tel. 505/287–4446, (Nonreporting) **A**1 9 10 18 20 **S** QHR, Brentwood, TN
Primary Contact: Michael Makosky, Chief Executive Officer
CFO: Jeff Rimel, Chief Financial Officer
CIO: Robert Volentine, Director Information Services
CHR: Sheila Cox, Director Human Resources
Web address: www.cibolahospital.com
**Control:** County–Government, nonfederal **Service:** General Medical and Surgical

**Staffed Beds:** 25

## HOBBS—Lea County

⊞ **LEA REGIONAL MEDICAL CENTER (320065)**, 5419 North Lovington Highway, Zip 88240–9125, Mailing Address: P.O. Box 3000, Zip 88241–9501; tel. 575/492–5000, (Nonreporting) **A**1 9 10 20 **S** Community Health Systems, Inc., Franklin, TN
Primary Contact: Timothy Thornell, FACHE, Chief Executive Officer
CFO: Steven Smith, Chief Financial Officer
CMO: Jesus Fonseca, M.D., Chief of Staff
CIO: Terry Purcell, Director Information Services
CIO: Terry Purcell, Director Information Services
CHR: Susan Hayes, Director Human Resources
CNO: Patrick A. Dunn, R.N., Chief Nursing Officer
Web address: www.learegionalmedical.com
**Control:** Corporation, Investor–owned, for–profit **Service:** General Medical and Surgical

**Staffed Beds:** 214

## LAS CRUCES—Dona Ana County

☐ **ADVANCED CARE HOSPITAL OF SOUTHERN NEW MEXICO (322004)**, 4451 East Lohman Avenue, Zip 88011; tel. 575/521–6600, (Nonreporting) **A**1 10 **S** Ernest Health, Inc., Albuquerque, NM
Primary Contact: Suzanne Quillen, R.N., Chief Executive Officer
Web address: www.achsnm.ernesthealth.com
**Control:** Corporation, Investor–owned, for–profit **Service:** Long–Term Acute Care hospital

**Staffed Beds:** 40

⊞ **MEMORIAL MEDICAL CENTER (320018)**, 2450 South Telshor Boulevard, Zip 88011–5076; tel. 575/522–8641 **A**1 9 10 **F**3 8 11 13 15 17 18 20 22 24 26 28 29 30 31 35 39 40 44 45 49 50 51 54 57 59 60 61 62 64 65 68 70 72 74 75 76 78 79 81 85 89 93 97 98 102 103 107 108 111 113 114 117 118 120 121 122 123 129 131 134 146 147 **S** LifePoint Hospitals, Inc., Brentwood, TN
Primary Contact: Paul F. Herzog, Chief Executive Officer
COO: Philip Rivera, Chief Operating Officer
CFO: James McGonnell, Chief Financial Officer
CMO: Bruce San Filippo, M.D., Chief Medical Officer
CIO: Berton Stevens, Director Information Systems
CHR: Laura Pierce, Chief Administrative Officer Human Resources
Web address: www.mmclc.org
**Control:** Corporation, Investor–owned, for–profit **Service:** General Medical and Surgical

**Staffed Beds:** 224 **Admissions:** 10872 **Census:** 142 **Outpatient Visits:** 172040 **Births:** 1690 **Total Expense ($000):** 161916 **Payroll Expense ($000):** 59990 **Personnel:** 1001

⊞ **MESILLA VALLEY HOSPITAL (324010)**, 3751 Del Rey Boulevard, Zip 88012–8526; tel. 575/382–3500 **A**1 9 10 **F**4 87 98 99 100 101 102 103 104 106 **S** Universal Health Services, Inc., King of Prussia, PA
Primary Contact: Brian Hemmert, Chief Executive Officer
CFO: Douglas Smith, Chief Financial Officer
CMO: Georgina Herrera, M.D., Medical Director
CHR: Linda Moya, Director Human Resources
Web address: www.mesillavalleyhospital.com
**Control:** Corporation, Investor–owned, for–profit **Service:** Psychiatric

**Staffed Beds:** 126 **Admissions:** 1965 **Census:** 75 **Outpatient Visits:** 16749 **Births:** 0 **Total Expense ($000):** 15817 **Payroll Expense ($000):** 8056 **Personnel:** 214

⊞ **MOUNTAINVIEW REGIONAL MEDICAL CENTER (320085)**, 4311 East Lohman Avenue, Zip 88011–8255; tel. 575/556–7600, (Nonreporting) **A**1 9 10 **S** Community Health Systems, Inc., Franklin, TN
Primary Contact: Denten Park, Chief Executive Officer
COO: Kathleen Cahill, Chief Operating Officer
CFO: Gene Alexander, Chief Financial Officer
CIO: Donald Harlow, Director of Information Services
CHR: Timothy C. Egan, Director, Human Resources
CNO: Gayle Nash, R.N., Chief Nursing Officer
Web address: www.mountainviewregional.com
**Control:** Corporation, Investor–owned, for–profit **Service:** General Medical and Surgical

**Staffed Beds:** 142

⊞ **REHABILITATION HOSPITAL OF SOUTHERN NEW MEXICO (323032)**, 4441 East Lohman Avenue, Zip 88011–8267; tel. 575/521–6400, (Nonreporting) **A**1 9 10 **S** Ernest Health, Inc., Albuquerque, NM
Primary Contact: Beverly Munoz, Chief Executive Officer
CFO: Jared Udall, Chief Financial Officer
CMO: Kimberly Encapera, M.D., Medical Director
CHR: Yolanda Mendoza, Director Human Resources
CNO: Yvonne Sandoval, Director of Nursing Operations
Web address: www.rhsnm.ernesthealth.com
**Control:** Corporation, Investor–owned, for–profit **Service:** Rehabilitation

**Staffed Beds:** 40

**NM**

*Many Facility Codes have changed. Please refer to the AHA Guide Code Chart.*
© 2012 AHA Guide

## LAS VEGAS—San Miguel County

✠ **ALTA VISTA REGIONAL HOSPITAL (320003)**, 104 Legion Drive, Zip 87701;
tel. 505/426–3500, (Nonreporting) **A**1 9 10 20 **S** Community Health Systems,
Inc., Franklin, TN
Primary Contact: Maridel Acosta, Chief Executive Officer
COO: Maridel Acosta, Chief Executive Officer
CFO: Leonard Tapia, Chief Financial Officer
CMO: Joseph Brown, M.D., Chief Medical Staff
CIO: Norman Wilder, Director Information Systems
CHR: Barbara Lujan, Director Human Resources
Web address: www.altavistaregionalhospital.com
**Control:** Corporation, Investor–owned, for–profit **Service:** General Medical and
Surgical

**Staffed Beds:** 52

☐ **NEW MEXICO BEHAVIORAL HEALTH INSTITUTE AT LAS VEGAS**, 3695 Hot
Springs Boulevard, Zip 87701–9575; tel. 505/454–2100, (Nonreporting) **A**1 9
Primary Contact: Steve Martinez, Executive Director and Administrator
CFO: Albino Martinez, Director Finance and Budget
Web address: www.health.state.nm.us
**Control:** State–Government, nonfederal **Service:** Psychiatric

**Staffed Beds:** 257

## LOS ALAMOS—Los Alamos County

✠ **LOS ALAMOS MEDICAL CENTER (320033)**, 3917 West Road,
Zip 87544–2293; tel. 505/661–9500, (Data for 360 days) **A**1 9 10 20 **F**3 11
13 15 28 29 30 31 34 35 40 45 50 57 59 68 70 75 76 78 79 81 82 85 86
87 89 91 93 97 107 110 111 113 118 123 129 145 **P**8 **S** LifePoint Hospitals,
Inc., Brentwood, TN
Primary Contact: Feliciano Jiron, Chief Executive Officer
CFO: Heather Teter, Chief Financial Officer
CMO: Sara Pasqualoni, M.D., Chief of Staff
CIO: Kevin Vigil, Director Information Systems
CHR: Jacqueline Carroll, Director Human Resources
Web address: www.losalamosmedicalcenter.com
**Control:** Corporation, Investor–owned, for–profit **Service:** General Medical and
Surgical

**Staffed Beds:** 38 **Admissions:** 1146 **Census:** 9 **Outpatient Visits:** 50028
**Births:** 215 **Total Expense ($000):** 38535 **Payroll Expense ($000):** 16415
**Personnel:** 217

## LOVINGTON—Lea County

★ **NOR–LEA GENERAL HOSPITAL (321305)**, 1600 North Main Avenue,
Zip 88260–2871; tel. 575/396–6611 **A**9 10 18 **F**3 9 11 15 18 26 28 29 30
31 32 34 35 39 40 45 46 49 50 54 57 59 64 66 68 74 75 77 78 81 89 93
97 99 103 107 108 110 111 113 118 126 128 129 131 132 134 146
147 **P**6
Primary Contact: David B. Shaw, Chief Executive Officer and Administrator
COO: Dan Hamilton, Director Inpatient Services
CFO: Allyson Roberts, CPA, Chief Financial Officer
CMO: Jeffrey Nelson, M.D., Chief of Staff
CIO: Brent Kelley, Director Information Technology
CHR: Carol DeArment, Director Human Resources
CNO: Cyndie Cribbs, Director of Nursing
Web address: www.nlgh.org
**Control:** Hospital district or authority, Government, nonfederal **Service:** General
Medical and Surgical

**Staffed Beds:** 18 **Admissions:** 816 **Census:** 6 **Outpatient Visits:** 144051
**Births:** 0 **Total Expense ($000):** 37681 **Payroll Expense ($000):** 16899
**Personnel:** 285

## MESCALERO—Otero County

☐ **MESCALERO PUBLIC HEALTH SERVICE INDIAN HOSPITAL (320058)**,
Zip 88340; tel. 505/671–4441, (Nonreporting) **A**1 9 10 **S** U. S. Indian Health
Service, Rockville, MD
Primary Contact: Dorlynn Simmons, Chief Executive Officer
CFO: Rainey Enjady, Administrative Officer
CIO: Kathy Murphy, Site Manager
Web address: www.ihs.gov
**Control:** Public Health Service, Government, federal **Service:** General Medical
and Surgical

**Staffed Beds:** 13

## PORTALES—Roosevelt County

**ROOSEVELT GENERAL HOSPITAL (320084)**, 42121 U.S. Highway 70,
Zip 88130, Mailing Address: P.O. Box 868, Zip 88130–0868;
tel. 575/359–1800, (Nonreporting) **A**9 10
Primary Contact: Larry E. Leaming, Ph.D., Chief Executive Officer
CFO: Eva Steven, Chief Financial Officer
CMO: Les Donaldson, M.D., Chief of Staff
CHR: Cindy Duncan, Director Human Resources
Web address: www.myrgh.org
**Control:** Hospital district or authority, Government, nonfederal **Service:** General
Medical and Surgical

**Staffed Beds:** 22

## RATON—Colfax County

★ **MINERS' COLFAX MEDICAL CENTER (321307)**, 200 Hospital Drive,
Zip 87740–2099; tel. 575/445–7700, (Includes MINERS' HOSPITAL OF NEW
MEXICO, Hospital Drive, Zip 87740, Mailing Address: Box 1067, Zip 87740;
tel. 505/445–2741), (Nonreporting) **A**9 10 18
Primary Contact: Charles Secora, M.D., Interim Chief Executive Officer
CFO: Albino Martinez, Director Budget and Finance
CIO: Richard Laner, Jr., Manager Information Systems
CHR: Jamie Johnson, Director Human Resources
Web address: www.minershosp.com
**Control:** County–Government, nonfederal **Service:** General Medical and Surgical

**Staffed Beds:** 33

## ROSWELL—Chaves County

✠ **EASTERN NEW MEXICO MEDICAL CENTER (320006)**, 405 West Country
Club Road, Zip 88201–5209; tel. 505/622–8170, (Nonreporting) **A**1 3 5 9 10
19 **S** Community Health Systems, Inc., Franklin, TN
CFO: Leanne Hacker, Chief Financial Officer
CMO: Jan Hobbs, M.D., Chief Medical Officer
CIO: Deepak Surl, Chief Information Officer
Web address: www.enmmc.com
**Control:** Corporation, Investor–owned, for–profit **Service:** General Medical and
Surgical

**Staffed Beds:** 149

☐ **NEW MEXICO REHABILITATION CENTER (323026)**, 31 Gail Harris Street,
Zip 88203–8190; tel. 575/347–3400, (Includes PECOS VALLEY LODGE, 31 Gail
Harris Avenue, Zip 88201; tel. 505/347–5491), (Nonreporting) **A**1 10
Primary Contact: Genia Devenport, Administrator
COO: Genia Devenport, Administrator
CFO: Janie Davies, Chief Financial Officer
CMO: Evan Nelson, M.D., Medical Director
CHR: Dorie Isler, Director Human Resources
**Control:** State–Government, nonfederal **Service:** Rehabilitation

**Staffed Beds:** 41

**ROSWELL REGIONAL HOSPITAL (320086)**, 117 East 19th Street, Zip 88201;
tel. 575/627–7000, (Nonreporting) **A**9 10 **S** Ardent Health Services, Nashville, TN
Primary Contact: Rod Schumacher, Chief Executive Officer
Web address: www.roswellregional.com
**Control:** Corporation, Investor–owned, for–profit **Service:** General Medical and
Surgical

**Staffed Beds:** 26

## RUIDOSO—Lincoln County

✠ **LINCOLN COUNTY MEDICAL CENTER (321306)**, 211 Sudderth Drive,
Zip 88345–6043, Mailing Address: P.O. Box 8000, Zip 88355–8000;
tel. 575/257–8200 **A**1 9 10 18 **F**7 11 13 15 29 30 35 39 40 45 46 53 56 57
59 64 68 70 76 77 78 81 85 87 91 93 103 107 110 111 114 118 131 134
145 147 **P**6 **S** Presbyterian Healthcare Services, Albuquerque, NM
Primary Contact: Alfred Santos, Administrator
CFO: Dudley McCauley, Controller
CMO: Chris Robinson, M.D., Chief of Staff
CHR: Deana Moses, Manager Human Resources
Web address: www.phs.org
**Control:** Other not–for–profit (including NFP Corporation) **Service:** General
Medical and Surgical

**Staffed Beds:** 25 **Admissions:** 1294 **Census:** 10 **Outpatient Visits:** 40321
**Births:** 359 **Total Expense ($000):** 30557 **Payroll Expense ($000):** 16793
**Personnel:** 220

**NM**

---

**Hospital, Medicare Provider Number, Address, Telephone, Approval, Facility, and Physician Codes, Health Care System**

★ American Hospital Association (AHA) membership
☐ The Joint Commission accreditation ◇ DNV Healthcare Inc. accreditation
○ American Osteopathic Association (AOA) accreditation
△ Commission on Accreditation of Rehabilitation Facilities (CARF) accreditation

## SANTA FE—Santa Fe County

✠ **CHRISTUS ST. VINCENT REGIONAL MEDICAL CENTER (320002)**, 455 St. Michael's Drive, Zip 87505–7663, Mailing Address: P.O. Box 2107, Zip 87504–2107; tel. 505/983–3361, (Nonreporting) **A**1 2 3 5 9 10 20 **S** CHRISTUS Health, Irving, TX
Primary Contact: Alex Valdez, JD, Chief Executive Officer
COO: Rick Crabtree, Chief Operating Officer
CFO: Rick Doxtator, Chief Financial Officer
CMO: Kevin C. Garrett, M.D., Chief Medical Officer
CHR: Barbara Roe, Vice President and Director Human Resources
Web address: www.stvin.org
**Control:** Other not–for–profit (including NFP Corporation) **Service:** General Medical and Surgical

| **Staffed Beds:** 195 |

☐ **PHS SANTA FE INDIAN HOSPITAL (320057)**, 1700 Cerrillos Road, Zip 87505–3554; tel. 505/988–9821, (Nonreporting) **A**1 5 9 10 **S** U. S. Indian Health Service, Rockville, MD
Primary Contact: Robert J. Lyon, Chief Executive Officer
CMO: Bret Smoker, M.D., Clinical Director
CIO: Vernita Jones, Site Manager
**Control:** Public Health Service, Government, federal **Service:** General Medical and Surgical

| **Staffed Beds:** 39 |

**PHYSICIANS MEDICAL CENTER OF SANTA FE HOSPITAL (320087)**, 2990 Rodeo Park Drive East, Zip 87505; tel. 505/428–5400, (Nonreporting) **A**9 10 **S** National Surgical Hospitals, Chicago, IL
Primary Contact: Lloyd Scarrow, Chief Executive Officer
Web address: www.pmchospital.com
**Control:** Individual, Investor–owned, for–profit **Service:** General Medical and Surgical

| **Staffed Beds:** 12 |

## SANTA ROSA—Guadalupe County

**GUADALUPE COUNTY HOSPITAL (320067)**, 720 Lake Drive, Zip 88435–2542, Mailing Address: P.O. Box 500, Zip 88435–0500; tel. 575/472–3417 **A**9 10 20 **F**3 29 34 35 40 57 59 65 68 87 107 113 118 129 131 **P**5
Primary Contact: Christina Campos, Administrator
COO: Christina Campos, Administrator
CFO: Bret Goebel, Finance Officer
CMO: Randal Brown, M.D., Chief of Staff
CIO: Kenneth Matthews, Manager Information Technology
CHR: Colleen Gallegos, Director Human Resources
**Control:** County–Government, nonfederal **Service:** General Medical and Surgical

| **Staffed Beds:** 10 **Admissions:** 252 **Census:** 2 **Births:** 0 **Total Expense ($000):** 7704 **Payroll Expense ($000):** 1484 |

## SANTA TERESA—Dona Ana County

✠ **PEAK BEHAVIORAL HEALTH SERVICES (324012)**, 5065 McNutt Road, Zip 88008–9442; tel. 575/589–3000 **A**1 9 10 **F**1 4 5 29 59 67 86 98 99 100 102 103 104 105 106 127 **S** Universal Health Services, Inc., King of Prussia, PA
Primary Contact: Jacob Cuellar, M.D., Chief Executive Officer
CFO: Espie Herrara, Chief Financial Officer
CHR: Mayra Lira, Human Resources Specialist
Web address: www.peakbehavioral.com/
**Control:** Corporation, Investor–owned, for–profit **Service:** Psychiatric

| **Staffed Beds:** 120 **Admissions:** 1122 **Census:** 75 **Outpatient Visits:** 0 **Births:** 0 |

## SHIPROCK—San Juan County

✠ **NORTHERN NAVAJO MEDICAL CENTER (320059)**, Zip 87420–0160; tel. 505/368–6001 **A**1 5 10 **F**3 5 8 13 15 29 30 32 34 35 46 54 57 59 65 70 73 74 75 76 77 79 81 82 83 84 85 86 87 89 93 97 99 100 104 110 118 133 143 146 147 **S** U. S. Indian Health Service, Rockville, MD
Primary Contact: Fannessa Comer, Chief Executive Officer
CFO: Paulette Chatto, Finance Officer
CMO: Stephen Bowers, M.D., Clinical Director
CIO: Roland Chapman, Chief Information Officer
CHR: Gloria Redhorse–Charley, Director Human Resources
Web address: www.home.nnmc.ihs.gov/
**Control:** PHS, Indian Service, Government, federal **Service:** General Medical and Surgical

| **Staffed Beds:** 62 **Admissions:** 3439 **Census:** 30 **Outpatient Visits:** 267450 **Births:** 584 **Total Expense ($000):** 98357 **Payroll Expense ($000):** 60430 **Personnel:** 978 |

## SILVER CITY—Grant County

✠ **GILA REGIONAL MEDICAL CENTER (320016)**, 1313 East 32nd Street, Zip 88061; tel. 575/538–4000 **A**1 9 10 20 **F**3 7 11 13 15 30 31 35 37 40 41 45 50 51 53 57 59 62 63 64 70 73 75 76 78 79 81 85 87 89 93 98 102 103 107 108 111 113 114 116 118 119 120 122 128 129 131 147 **P**5
Primary Contact: Brian S. Bentley, Chief Executive Officer
CFO: Craig Stewart, Chief Financial Officer
CIO: David Furnas, Chief Information Officer
CHR: Barbara Barela, Director Human Resources
CNO: Pam Fulks, R.N., Chief Nursing Officer
Web address: www.grmc.org
**Control:** County–Government, nonfederal **Service:** General Medical and Surgical

| **Staffed Beds:** 68 **Admissions:** 3088 **Census:** 29 **Outpatient Visits:** 77006 **Births:** 407 **Total Expense ($000):** 62386 **Payroll Expense ($000):** 27761 **Personnel:** 593 |

## SOCORRO—Socorro County

✠ **SOCORRO GENERAL HOSPITAL (321301)**, 1202 Highway 60 West, Zip 87801, Mailing Address: P.O. Box 1009, Zip 87801–1009; tel. 505/835–1140 **A**1 9 10 18 **F**3 8 11 13 15 29 30 34 35 40 45 57 59 62 63 64 68 75 77 81 83 85 91 93 100 103 107 113 129 131 132 133 134 146 **S** Presbyterian Healthcare Services, Albuquerque, NM
Primary Contact: Bo Beames, Administrator
CHR: Pam Miller–Balfour, Director Human Resources
Web address: www.phs.org
**Control:** Other not–for–profit (including NFP Corporation) **Service:** General Medical and Surgical

| **Staffed Beds:** 24 **Admissions:** 562 **Census:** 4 **Outpatient Visits:** 35437 **Births:** 149 **Total Expense ($000):** 22661 **Payroll Expense ($000):** 11568 **Personnel:** 167 |

## TAOS—Taos County

★ **HOLY CROSS HOSPITAL (320013)**, 1397 Weimer Road, Zip 87571–6284; tel. 575/758–8883 **A**9 10 20 21 **F**11 13 15 18 29 30 34 35 36 40 43 45 46 50 51 57 59 64 70 75 76 81 86 89 107 110 113 117 118 126 129 131 134 146 147 **P**8 **S** QHR, Brentwood, TN
Primary Contact: Peter A. Hofstetter, Chief Executive Officer
CFO: Richard Eisenring, Chief Financial Officer
CMO: Loretta Ortiz y Pino, M.D., Chief Medical Officer
CIO: Spencer Hamons, Chief Information Officer
CHR: Lisa Clark, Human Resources Officer
CNO: Mary Anna Abeyta, R.N., Chief Nursing/Clinical Services Officer
Web address: www.taoshospital.org
**Control:** Other not–for–profit (including NFP Corporation) **Service:** General Medical and Surgical

| **Staffed Beds:** 47 **Admissions:** 2473 **Census:** 22 **Outpatient Visits:** 66603 **Births:** 243 **Total Expense ($000):** 53873 **Payroll Expense ($000):** 23666 **Personnel:** 415 |

## TRUTH OR CONSEQUENCES—Sierra County

★ **SIERRA VISTA HOSPITAL (321300)**, 800 East Ninth Avenue, Zip 87901–1961; tel. 575/894–2111 **A**9 10 18 **F**7 11 15 30 34 40 54 57 59 65 67 93 99 102 104 107 110 118 126 127 129 132 **P**6
Primary Contact: Domenica Rush, Chief Executive Officer
CFO: Bret Gobel, Chief Financial Officer
CMO: James F. Malcolmson, M.D., Chief of Staff
CIO: Dan Morrell, Manager Information Systems
CHR: Mindee Holguin, Manager Human Resources
Web address: www.svhnm.org
**Control:** City–County, Government, nonfederal **Service:** General Medical and Surgical

| **Staffed Beds:** 25 **Admissions:** 394 **Census:** 4 **Outpatient Visits:** 21292 **Births:** 0 **Total Expense ($000):** 12197 **Payroll Expense ($000):** 6304 **Personnel:** 136 |

## TUCUMCARI—Quay County

★ **DR. DAN C. TRIGG MEMORIAL HOSPITAL (321302)**, 301 East Miel De Luna Avenue, Zip 88401–3810, Mailing Address: P.O. Box 608, Zip 88401–0608; tel. 575/461–7000 **A**9 10 18 **F**3 11 15 29 35 38 40 45 59 62 63 64 65 67 68 81 85 87 90 93 97 99 101 103 104 107 110 113 118 127 129 132 134 145 147 **P**6 **S** Presbyterian Healthcare Services, Albuquerque, NM
Primary Contact: Lance C. Labine, Administrator
Web address: www.phs.org
**Control:** Other not–for–profit (including NFP Corporation) **Service:** General Medical and Surgical

| **Staffed Beds:** 17 **Admissions:** 343 **Census:** 3 **Outpatient Visits:** 14525 **Births:** 7 **Total Expense ($000):** 14368 **Payroll Expense ($000):** 6729 **Personnel:** 97 |

**NM**

*Many Facility Codes have changed. Please refer to the AHA Guide Code Chart.* © 2012 AHA Guide

**ZUNI—McKinley County**

☐ **U. S. PUBLIC HEALTH SERVICE INDIAN HOSPITAL (320060)**, Route 301 North B. Street, Zip 87327, Mailing Address: P.O. Box 467, Zip 87327–0467; tel. 505/782–4431, (Nonreporting) **A**1 9 10 **S** U. S. Indian Health Service, Rockville, MD
Primary Contact: Jean Othole, Chief Executive Officer
CFO: Clyde Yatsattie, Administrative Officer
CMO: David Kessler, M.D., Clinical Director
CHR: Cynthia Tsalate, Human Resource Specialist
Web address: www.ihs.gov
**Control:** PHS, Indian Service, Government, federal **Service:** General Medical and Surgical

**Staffed Beds:** 32

NM

# NEW YORK

## ALBANY—Albany County

☒ **ALBANY MEDICAL CENTER (330013)**, 43 New Scotland Avenue, Zip 12208–3478; tel. 518/262–3125, (Includes ALBANY MEDICAL CENTER SOUTH–CLINICAL CAMPUS, 25 Hackett Boulevard, Zip 12208–3499; tel. 518/242–1200; Timothy W. Duffy, General Director) **A**1 2 3 5 8 9 10 **F**3 6 7 8 11 12 13 15 17 18 19 20 21 22 23 24 25 26 27 28 29 30 31 32 33 34 35 36 38 39 40 41 42 43 44 45 46 47 49 50 51 52 53 54 55 56 57 58 59 60 61 64 68 70 72 73 74 75 76 77 78 79 81 82 84 85 86 87 88 89 90 92 93 96 98 100 102 103 104 105 107 108 109 110 111 113 114 115 116 117 118 119 120 122 123 125 129 130 131 134 135 137 141 144 145 147 Primary Contact: James J. Barba, President and Chief Executive Officer COO: Bernadette R. Pedlow, Senior Vice President Business and Chief Operating Officer CFO: William C. Hasselbarth, Chief Financial Officer CMO: Dennis McKenna, M.D., Interim Vice President Medical Affairs CIO: George Hickman, Executive Vice President and Chief Information Officer CHR: Catherine Halakan, Senior Vice President Web address: www.amc.edu **Control:** Other not–for–profit (including NFP Corporation) **Service:** General Medical and Surgical

**Staffed Beds:** 644 **Admissions:** 32169 **Census:** 522 **Outpatient Visits:** 333967 **Births:** 2171 **Total Expense ($000):** 659129 **Payroll Expense ($000):** 229802 **Personnel:** 4423

★ **ALBANY MEMORIAL HOSPITAL (330003)**, 600 Northern Boulevard, Zip 12204–1083; tel. 518/471–3221, (Nonreporting) **A**5 9 10 **S** Catholic Health East, Newtown Square, PA Primary Contact: Steven P. Boyle, Executive Vice President COO: Karen Tassey, MS, Chief Operating Officer CFO: Lori Santos, Vice President Finance CMO: Daniel C. Silverman, M.D., Senior Vice President Medical Affairs CIO: Robert J. Duthe, Vice President Corporate Management Information Systems CHR: Barbara McCandless, Vice President Human Resources, Organization Development Web address: www.nehealth.com **Control:** Other not–for–profit (including NFP Corporation) **Service:** General Medical and Surgical

**Staffed Beds:** 165

☒ △ **ALBANY STRATTON VETERANS AFFAIRS MEDICAL CENTER**, 113 Holland Avenue, Zip 12208–3473; tel. 518/626–5000, (Total facility includes 41 beds in nursing home–type unit) **A**1 2 3 5 7 8 9 **F**2 3 4 5 12 15 17 18 20 28 29 30 31 34 35 39 40 45 46 47 50 54 56 57 58 59 60 61 62 63 64 65 68 70 74 75 77 78 79 81 82 83 84 86 87 91 92 93 94 97 98 100 102 103 104 105 106 107 108 109 111 114 117 127 128 129 131 134 142 145 146 147 **S** Department of Veterans Affairs, Washington, DC Primary Contact: Linda W. Weiss, MS, FACHE, Director COO: Donald W. Stuart, Associate Director CFO: Gerard Scorzelli, Chief Financial Officer CMO: Lourdes Irizarry, M.D., Chief of Staff CIO: Mike Mullahey, Operations Manager CHR: Kenneth Kio, Manager Human Resources CNO: Deborah Spath, R.N., Associate Director Patient and Nurses Services Web address: www.va.gov/sta/guide/home.asp **Control:** Veterans Affairs, Government, federal **Service:** General Medical and Surgical

**Staffed Beds:** 148 **Admissions:** 2779 **Census:** 45 **Outpatient Visits:** 311721 **Births:** 0 **Total Expense ($000):** 218339 **Payroll Expense ($000):** 120768 **Personnel:** 1243

☐ **CAPITAL DISTRICT PSYCHIATRIC CENTER (334046)**, 75 New Scotland Avenue, Zip 12208–3474; tel. 518/447–9611, (Nonreporting) **A**1 3 5 10 **S** New York State Office of Mental Health, Albany, NY Primary Contact: Lewis Campbell, Executive Director CMO: Beatrice Kovasznay, M.D., Clinical Director Web address: www.omh.ny.gov/omhweb/facilities/cdpc/facility.htm **Control:** State–Government, nonfederal **Service:** Psychiatric

**Staffed Beds:** 200

☒ **ST. PETER'S HOSPITAL (330057)**, 315 South Manning Boulevard, Zip 12208–1789; tel. 518/525–1550 **A**1 2 3 5 9 10 **F**4 5 8 11 12 13 15 17 18 19 20 21 22 23 24 25 26 27 28 29 30 31 34 35 36 37 38 39 40 45 46 47 48 49 50 51 53 54 56 57 59 60 61 62 63 64 65 66 68 69 70 71 72 73 74 75 76 77 78 79 81 82 84 85 86 87 89 90 91 92 93 97 107 108 109 110 111 113 114 115 116 117 118 119 120 122 123 125 128 129 131 132 134 142 144 145 146 147 **S** Catholic Health East, Newtown Square, PA Primary Contact: Steven P. Boyle, Executive Vice President CFO: James M. Gavin, Chief Financial Officer CMO: Robert Cella, M.D., Vice President Medical Affairs CIO: Jonathan Goldberg, Chief Information Officer CHR: Judy Gray, Vice President Human Resources Web address: www.sphcs.org **Control:** Church–operated, Nongovernment, not–for profit **Service:** General Medical and Surgical

**Staffed Beds:** 487 **Admissions:** 22765 **Census:** 332 **Outpatient Visits:** 496315 **Births:** 2645 **Total Expense ($000):** 426395 **Payroll Expense ($000):** 171360 **Personnel:** 3291

## ALEXANDRIA BAY—Jefferson County

★ **RIVER HOSPITAL (331309)**, 4 Fuller Street, Zip 13607–1316; tel. 315/482–2511, (Nonreporting) **A**9 10 18 Primary Contact: Ben Moore, III, President and Chief Executive Officer COO: William Connor, Assistant Administrator and Director Human Resources CFO: Traci Mintonye, Chief Financial Officer CMO: Prasad Yitta, M.D., Medical Director CIO: John Smithers, Network Specialist CHR: William Connor, Assistant Administrator and Director Human Resources CNO: Ann Narrow, Director of Nursing Web address: www.riverhospital.org **Control:** Other not–for–profit (including NFP Corporation) **Service:** General Medical and Surgical

**Staffed Beds:** 51

## AMITYVILLE—Suffolk County

☐ **SOUTH OAKS HOSPITAL (334027)**, 400 Sunrise Highway, Zip 11701–2508; tel. 631/264–4000 **A**1 9 10 **F**4 5 53 98 99 103 104 105 Primary Contact: Robert E. Detor, Chief Executive Officer CFO: Patricia Porter, Chief Financial Officer CMO: Yogendra Upadhyay, M.D., Senior Vice President Medical Affairs CHR: Pam Quiroga, Vice President Human Resources Web address: www.longislandhome.org **Control:** Other not–for–profit (including NFP Corporation) **Service:** Psychiatric

**Staffed Beds:** 233 **Admissions:** 4030 **Census:** 128 **Outpatient Visits:** 94788 **Births:** 0 **Total Expense ($000):** 45862 **Payroll Expense ($000):** 25657 **Personnel:** 498

## AMSTERDAM—Montgomery County

**ST. MARY'S AMSTERDAM CAMPUS** See St. Mary's Healthcare

☒ **ST. MARY'S HEALTHCARE (330047)**, 427 Guy Park Avenue, Zip 12010–1095; tel. 518/842–1900, (Includes ST. MARY'S AMSTERDAM CAMPUS, 4988 State Highway 30, Zip 12010–1699; tel. 518/842–3100), (Total facility includes 160 beds in nursing home–type unit) **A**1 9 10 **F**2 3 4 5 11 13 14 15 17 28 29 30 31 34 35 36 38 40 45 49 50 51 54 56 57 59 60 61 65 68 70 71 74 75 76 77 78 79 81 82 84 85 87 90 91 93 94 96 97 98 99 100 101 102 103 104 105 106 107 108 110 111 114 126 127 129 130 131 134 143 144 145 146 **S** Ascension Health, Saint Louis, MO Primary Contact: Victor Giulianelli, FACHE, President and Chief Executive Officer COO: Scott Bruce, Vice President Operations CFO: John Sagan, Vice President Finance CMO: Timothy Shoen, M.D., Vice President Medical Staff Services CIO: James DeGroff, Director Technology and Network Services CHR: Beth Case, Vice President Human Resources Web address: www.smha.org **Control:** Other not–for–profit (including NFP Corporation) **Service:** General Medical and Surgical

**Staffed Beds:** 310 **Admissions:** 6556 **Census:** 247 **Outpatient Visits:** 362956 **Births:** 501 **Total Expense ($000):** 128514 **Payroll Expense ($000):** 68402 **Personnel:** 1331

NY

*Many Facility Codes have changed. Please refer to the AHA Guide Code Chart.* © 2012 AHA Guide

## AUBURN—Cayuga County

✠ **AUBURN COMMUNITY HOSPITAL (330235)**, 17 Lansing Street,
Zip 13021–1943; tel. 315/255–7011, (Total facility includes 80 beds in nursing
home–type unit) **A**1 9 10 **F**1 12 13 15 26 28 29 30 31 34 35 40 49 54 55 57
59 64 70 76 78 79 81 82 89 98 103 107 108 110 111 113 118 128 129
131 143 145 146 147
Primary Contact: Scott A. Berlucchi, FACHE, President and Chief Executive Officer
COO: Thomas Filiak, Chief Operating Officer
CFO: John Baran, Chief Financial Officer
CMO: John A. Riccio, M.D., Chief Medical Officer
CIO: Chris Ryan, Chief Information Officer
CHR: Colleen McLaughlin, Director Employee Relations
Web address: www.auburnhospital.org
**Control:** Other not–for–profit (including NFP Corporation) **Service:** General
Medical and Surgical

> **Staffed Beds:** 179 **Admissions:** 5139 **Census:** 156 **Outpatient Visits:**
> 158806 **Births:** 398 **Total Expense ($000):** 84364 **Payroll Expense ($000):**
> 38523 **Personnel:** 674

## BATAVIA—Genesee County

✠ **UNITED MEMORIAL MEDICAL CENTER (330073)**, 127 North Street,
Zip 14020–2260; tel. 585/343–6030, (Includes UNITED MEMORIAL MEDICAL
CENTER–BANK STREET, 127 North Street, tel. 716/343–3131; UNITED
MEMORIAL MEDICAL CENTER–NORTH STREET, 16 Banks Street,
Zip 14020–1697; tel. 585/343–6030) **A**1 9 10 **F**3 4 8 13 14 15 17 18 19 28
29 30 31 32 34 35 39 40 43 49 50 54 57 59 64 65 70 75 76 77 79 81 82
85 86 89 93 97 107 111 113 114 116 118 128 129 130 134 143 145
146 147
Primary Contact: Mark C. Schoell, Chief Executive Officer
CFO: Robert Chiavetta, Vice President Finance
CMO: Michael Merrill, M.D., Interim Vice President Medical Affairs
CIO: Daniel O'Connor, Chief Information Officer
CHR: Sonja Gonyea, Director Human Resources
Web address: www.ummc.org
**Control:** Other not–for–profit (including NFP Corporation) **Service:** General
Medical and Surgical

> **Staffed Beds:** 131 **Admissions:** 4569 **Census:** 77 **Outpatient Visits:** 209739
> **Births:** 544 **Total Expense ($000):** 73883 **Payroll Expense ($000):** 31027
> **Personnel:** 631

★ **VETERANS AFFAIRS WESTERN NEW YORK HEALTHCARE
SYSTEM–BATAVIA DIVISION**, 222 Richmond Avenue, Zip 14020–1288;
tel. 585/297–1000, (Nonreporting) **A**5 9 **S** Department of Veterans Affairs,
Washington, DC
Primary Contact: Royce Calhoun, Assistant Director
Web address: www.buffalo.va.gov/batavia.asp
**Control:** Veterans Affairs, Government, federal **Service:** General Medical and
Surgical

> **Staffed Beds:** 128

## BATH—Steuben County

✠ **IRA DAVENPORT MEMORIAL HOSPITAL (330144)**, 7571 State Route 54,
Zip 14810–9590; tel. 607/776–8500, (Nonreporting) **A**1 9 10 21 **S** Arnot
Health, Elmira, NY
Primary Contact: James B. Watson, Chief Executive Officer
CMO: Dennis O'Connor, M.D., Medical Director
CIO: Hendrik Van der Horst, Chief Information Officer
CHR: Marybess Hazlett, Director Human Resources
Web address: www.davenportandtaylor.org
**Control:** Other not–for–profit (including NFP Corporation) **Service:** General
Medical and Surgical

> **Staffed Beds:** 156

✠ △ **VETERANS AFFAIRS MEDICAL CENTER**, 76 Veterans Avenue,
Zip 14810–0842; tel. 607/664–4000, (Total facility includes 124 beds in nursing
home–type unit) **A**1 7 9 **F**1 3 5 6 7 8 12 16 17 18 20 22 24 26 28 29 30 31
33 34 35 36 38 39 40 50 53 56 57 58 59 61 62 63 64 65 68 70 71 74 75
77 78 79 81 82 83 84 86 87 90 91 92 93 94 97 98 100 101 102 103 104
106 107 111 112 113 114 115 116 118 126 127 128 129 131 134 142 143
145 146 147 **P**6 **S** Department of Veterans Affairs, Washington, DC
Primary Contact: Michael J. Swartz, Medical Center Director
COO: David Krueger, Associate Director
CFO: Jill Haynes, Financial Coach
CMO: Felipe Diaz, M.D., Chief of Staff
CIO: Karen Clancy, Manager Information Systems Operations
CHR: Susan DeSalvo, Manager Human Resources
Web address: www.bath.va.gov
**Control:** Veterans Affairs, Government, federal **Service:** General Medical and
Surgical

> **Staffed Beds:** 359 **Admissions:** 1602 **Census:** 293 **Outpatient Visits:**
> 161184 **Births:** 0 **Total Expense ($000):** 95598 **Payroll Expense ($000):**
> 60459 **Personnel:** 744

## BAY SHORE—Suffolk County

✠ **SOUTHSIDE HOSPITAL (330043)**, 301 East Main Street, Zip 11706–8458;
tel. 631/968–3000 **A**1 2 3 5 9 10 **F**3 7 8 9 11 13 15 17 18 20 22 24 26 29
30 31 32 34 35 36 38 40 43 44 45 49 50 53 54 55 56 57 58 59 60 61 63
64 65 66 68 70 73 74 75 76 77 78 79 81 82 85 86 87 89 90 93 96 97 98
100 101 102 103 107 108 110 111 113 117 118 119 120 122 128 129 130
131 133 134 145 146 147 **P**6 **S** North Shore–Long Island Jewish Health
System, Great Neck, NY
CFO: Robert Power, Associate Executive Director Finance
CMO: Jay Enden, M.D., Medical Director
CIO: Lowney Mincy, Director Information Services
CHR: Anne J. Barrett, Associate Executive Director Human Resources
Web address: www.southsidehospital.org
**Control:** Other not–for–profit (including NFP Corporation) **Service:** General
Medical and Surgical

> **Staffed Beds:** 300 **Admissions:** 17204 **Census:** 231 **Outpatient Visits:**
> 149187 **Births:** 2434 **Total Expense ($000):** 343719 **Payroll Expense
> ($000):** 165015 **Personnel:** 2272

## BELLEROSE—Queens County, See New York City

## BETHPAGE—Nassau County

☐ **ST. JOSEPH HOSPITAL (330332)**, 4295 Hempstead Turnpike,
Zip 11714–5769; tel. 516/579–6000 **A**1 9 10 **F**3 8 15 17 18 29 30 34 35 40
45 46 49 50 51 56 57 59 60 64 65 68 69 70 74 75 79 81 85 86 87 89 93
107 108 111 113 118 128 129 130 131 145 147
Primary Contact: Drew Pallas, Executive Vice President and Chief Administrative
Officer
CMO: Lawrence A. Reduto, M.D., President and Chief Medical Officer
CIO: Blake Benz, Director Management Information Systems
CHR: Peter Chiacchiaro, Vice President Human Resources
Web address: www.newislandhospital.org
**Control:** Other not–for–profit (including NFP Corporation) **Service:** General
Medical and Surgical

> **Staffed Beds:** 140 **Admissions:** 7131 **Census:** 100 **Outpatient Visits:** 51613
> **Births:** 0 **Total Expense ($000):** 99743 **Payroll Expense ($000):** 45068
> **Personnel:** 705

## BINGHAMTON—Broome County

**BINGHAMTON GENERAL HOSPITAL** See United Health Services
Hospitals–Binghamton

☐ **GREATER BINGHAMTON HEALTH CENTER (334012)**, 425 Robinson Street,
Zip 13904–1735; tel. 607/724–1391 **A**1 10 **F**29 30 54 56 65 71 75 77 86 98
99 100 101 103 104 105 106 129 131 134 142 145 **P**1 **S** New York State
Office of Mental Health, Albany, NY
Primary Contact: Margaret R. Dugan, Executive Director
CFO: Cherry Randall, Business Officer
CIO: Timothy Lauve, Coordinator Mental Health Local Information Systems
CHR: Renee O'Brien, Director Human Resources
Web address: www.omh.ny.gov/omhweb/facilities/bipc/facility.htm
**Control:** State–Government, nonfederal **Service:** Psychiatric

> **Staffed Beds:** 115 **Admissions:** 346 **Census:** 116 **Outpatient Visits:** 37620
> **Births:** 0 **Personnel:** 372

**NY**

✠ **OUR LADY OF LOURDES MEMORIAL HOSPITAL (330011)**, 169 Riverside Drive, Zip 13905–4246; tel. 607/798–5111 **A**1 2 9 10 **F**3 11 12 13 15 18 19 28 29 30 32 34 35 36 39 40 44 45 46 47 49 50 51 53 54 56 57 59 60 62 63 64 65 66 68 70 71 74 75 76 77 78 79 81 84 85 86 87 89 93 97 99 100 101 103 104 107 108 110 111 113 114 117 118 119 120 122 123 125 126 128 129 130 131 133 134 142 143 144 145 146 147 **P**6 **S** Ascension Health, Saint Louis, MO
Primary Contact: David Patak, President and Chief Executive Officer
COO: Linda Miller, R.N., Senior Vice President Operations and Chief Nursing Officer
CFO: Gregg Hayton, Vice President Finance and Chief Financial Officer
CMO: Robert Taylor, III, M.D., Vice President Medical Affairs
CIO: John Laliberte, Assistant Vice President
CHR: Jim Silkworth, Chief Human Resources Officer
Web address: www.lourdes.com
**Control:** Church–operated, Nongovernment, not–for profit **Service:** General Medical and Surgical

Staffed Beds: 154 **Admissions:** 10192 **Census:** 115 **Outpatient Visits:** 1425023 **Births:** 1171 **Total Expense ($000):** 244422 **Payroll Expense ($000):** 109004 **Personnel:** 1747

**UNITED HEALTH SERVICES HOSPITALS–BINGHAMTON (330394)**, 10–42 Mitchell Avenue, Zip 13903–1678; tel. 607/763–6000, (Includes BINGHAMTON GENERAL HOSPITAL, 10–42 Mitchell Avenue, Zip 13903; tel. 607/762–2200; MEDICENTER, 600 High Avenue, Endicott, Zip 13760; tel. 607/754–7171; WILSON MEMORIAL REGIONAL MEDICAL CENTER, 33–57 Harrison Street, Johnson City, Zip 13790; tel. 607/763–6000) **A**8 9 10 12 13 **F**1 3 4 5 8 11 12 13 15 17 18 20 22 24 26 28 29 30 31 32 33 34 35 37 38 39 40 43 45 46 49 50 51 52 54 57 58 59 60 61 64 65 68 70 72 74 75 76 77 78 79 81 84 85 86 87 89 90 92 93 96 97 98 100 101 102 103 104 107 108 110 113 114 117 118 123 125 126 129 130 131 134 145 146 147 **P**3 **S** United Health Services, Binghamton, NY
Primary Contact: Matthew J. Salanger, President and Chief Executive Officer
Web address: www.uhs.net
**Control:** Other not–for–profit (including NFP Corporation) **Service:** General Medical and Surgical

Staffed Beds: 460 **Admissions:** 16672 **Census:** 279 **Outpatient Visits:** 381547 **Births:** 1601 **Total Expense ($000):** 411178 **Payroll Expense ($000):** 162890 **Personnel:** 3222

**BRENTWOOD—Suffolk County**

☐ **PILGRIM PSYCHIATRIC CENTER (334013)**, 998 Crooked Hill Road, Zip 11717–1087; tel. 631/761–3500, (Nonreporting) **A**1 10 **S** New York State Office of Mental Health, Albany, NY
Primary Contact: Dean R. Weinstock, R.N., Executive Director
COO: Kathy O'Keefe, Director Operations
CFO: Florence Corwin, Director for Administration
CMO: Inderjit Singh, M.D., Clinical Director
CIO: Douglas Cargonara, Ph.D., Chief Information Officer
CHR: Florence Corwin, Director Administration
Web address: www.omh.ny.gov/omhweb/facilities/pgpc/facility.htm
**Control:** State–Government, nonfederal **Service:** Psychiatric

Staffed Beds: 569

**BROCKPORT—Monroe County**

✠ **LAKESIDE MEMORIAL HOSPITAL (330037)**, 156 West Avenue, Zip 14420–1286; tel. 585/395–6095, (Nonreporting) **A**1 9 10
Primary Contact: Hugh Collins, Interim Chief Executive Officer
CMO: James E. Szalados, M.D., Vice President Medical Affairs
CIO: Dennis Gambill, Director Information Technology
CHR: James Cummings, Vice President Human Resources
CNO: Shawn Fisher, R.N., Director Clinical Services
Web address: www.lakesidehealth.com
**Control:** Other not–for–profit (including NFP Corporation) **Service:** General Medical and Surgical

Staffed Beds: 61

**BRONX—Bronx County, See New York City**

**BRONXVILLE—Westchester County**

✠ **LAWRENCE HOSPITAL CENTER (330061)**, 55 Palmer Avenue, Zip 10708–3403; tel. 914/787–1000 **A**1 2 5 9 10 **F**3 11 12 13 15 18 28 29 30 31 34 35 36 40 45 47 50 51 55 57 59 60 62 63 64 65 68 69 70 72 73 74 75 76 77 78 79 81 82 84 85 87 89 91 92 93 94 107 108 110 111 114 118 128 129 130 131 134 144 145 147
Primary Contact: Edward M. Dinan, President and Chief Executive Officer
COO: James Y. Lee, Executive Vice President and Chief Operating Officer
CFO: Murray Askinazi, Senior Vice President and Chief Financial Officer
CMO: Werner Roeder, M.D., Vice President Medical Affairs
CHR: Tom Mastroianni, Vice President Human Resources
CNO: Rose Ann O'Hare, R.N., Vice President Patient Services
Web address: www.lawrencehealth.org
**Control:** Other not–for–profit (including NFP Corporation) **Service:** General Medical and Surgical

Staffed Beds: 195 **Admissions:** 11328 **Census:** 151 **Outpatient Visits:** 166042 **Births:** 1632 **Total Expense ($000):** 173672 **Payroll Expense ($000):** 77585 **Personnel:** 931

**BROOKLYN—Kings County, See New York City**

**BUFFALO—Erie County**

**BRYLIN HOSPITALS (334022)**, 1263 Delaware Avenue, Zip 14209–2402; tel. 716/886–8200, (Nonreporting) **A**9 10
Primary Contact: Eric D. Pleskow, President and Chief Executive Officer
CFO: E. Paul Hettich, Chief Financial Officer
CMO: Balvinder Kang, M.D., Medical Director
CIO: Pawel Wieczorek, Director Information Technology
CHR: Jacquelyn Bixler, Vice President Human Resources
Web address: www.brylin.com
**Control:** Individual, Investor–owned, for–profit **Service:** Psychiatric

Staffed Beds: 88

☐ **BUFFALO PSYCHIATRIC CENTER (334052)**, 400 Forest Avenue, Zip 14213–1298; tel. 716/885–2261, (Nonreporting) **A**1 3 5 10 **S** New York State Office of Mental Health, Albany, NY
Primary Contact: Thomas Dodson, Executive Director
COO: Celia Spacone, M.D., Director Operations
CFO: Pamela Esposito, Director Quality Management and Acting Director Facility Administration
CMO: Jeffery Grace, M.D., Clinical Director
CIO: Anne Buchheit, Coordinator Mental Health Local Information Systems
CHR: Charles Siewert, Director Human Resources
Web address: www.omh.ny.gov
**Control:** State–Government, nonfederal **Service:** Psychiatric

Staffed Beds: 240

☐ **ERIE COUNTY MEDICAL CENTER (330219)**, 462 Grider Street, Zip 14215–3098; tel. 716/898–3000, (Nonreporting) **A**1 3 5 9 10
Primary Contact: Jody Lomeo, Chief Executive Officer
COO: Mark C. Barabas, President and Chief Operating Officer
CFO: Michael Sammarco, M.D., Chief Financial Officer
CMO: Brian Murray, M.D., Medical Director
CIO: Leslie Feidt, Chief Information Officer
CHR: Kathleen O'Hara, Vice President Human Resources
Web address: www.ecmc.edu
**Control:** County–Government, nonfederal **Service:** General Medical and Surgical

Staffed Beds: 1200

△ **KALEIDA HEALTH (330005)**, 100 High Street, Zip 14203–1154; tel. 716/859–5600, (Includes DE GRAFF MEMORIAL HOSPITAL, 445 Tremont Street, North Tonawanda, Zip 14120–0750, Mailing Address: P.O. Box 0750, Zip 14120–0750; tel. 716/694–4500; Tamara Owen, President; MILLARD FILLMORE SUBURBAN HOSPITAL, 1540 Maple Road, Williamsville, Zip 14221; tel. 716/688–3100; WOMEN AND CHILDREN'S HOSPITAL, 219 Bryant Street, Zip 14222–2099; tel. 716/878–7000; Cheryl Klass, President), (Total facility includes 380 beds in nursing home–type unit) **A**3 5 7 8 10 21 **F**2 3 5 8 9 11 12 13 15 17 18 19 20 21 22 23 24 25 26 29 30 31 32 34 35 36 37 39 40 41 43 44 45 46 49 50 51 54 55 56 57 58 59 60 61 62 63 64 65 66 68 70 71 72 73 74 75 76 77 78 79 81 82 83 84 85 86 87 88 89 90 92 93 94 96 97 98 99 100 101 102 103 104 105 107 108 109 110 111 112 113 114 115 116 117 118 125 127 129 130 131 134 137 141 142 144 145 146 147 **P**6
Primary Contact: James R. Kaskie, President and Chief Executive Officer
CFO: Joseph Kessler, Executive Vice President and Chief Financial Officer
CMO: Margaret Paroski, M.D., Executive Vice President and Chief Medical Officer
CIO: Francis Meyer, Vice President Information Systems Technology
Web address: www.kaleidahealth.org
**Control:** Other not–for–profit (including NFP Corporation) **Service:** General Medical and Surgical

Staffed Beds: 1541 **Admissions:** 63536 **Census:** 1317 **Outpatient Visits:** 617000 **Births:** 5614 **Total Expense ($000):** 1203832 **Payroll Expense ($000):** 521826 **Personnel:** 7923

✠ **MERCY HOSPITAL (330279)**, 565 Abbott Road, Zip 14220–2095;
tel. 716/826–7000, (Total facility includes 84 beds in nursing home–type unit) **A**1
3 5 9 10 **F**3 8 13 15 17 18 20 22 24 26 29 30 32 34 35 39 40 42 45 48 49
54 57 59 60 64 65 66 70 72 74 75 76 78 79 81 83 84 85 86 87 89 90 92
93 94 96 97 107 108 110 111 113 114 117 118 125 127 128 129 130 131
145 146 147 **P**5 6 **S** Catholic Health System, Buffalo, NY
Primary Contact: Charles J. Urlaub, President and Chief Executive Officer
COO: John J. Herman, Chief Operating Officer
CFO: James H. Dunlop, Jr., CPA, Senior Vice President Finance and Chief Financial
Officer
CMO: Timothy Gabryel, M.D., Vice President Medical Affairs and Medical Director
CIO: Michael Galang, M.D., Chief Information Officer
CHR: Joseph A. Scrivo, Jr., Director Human Resources
CNO: Kathleen Guarino, R.N., Vice President Patient Care Services
Web address: www.chsbuffalo.org
**Control:** Church–operated, Nongovernment, not–for profit **Service:** General
Medical and Surgical

**Staffed Beds:** 436 **Admissions:** 18769 **Census:** 345 **Outpatient Visits:**
406057 **Births:** 2392 **Total Expense ($000):** 305415 **Payroll Expense
($000):** 129049 **Personnel:** 1996

☐ **ROSWELL PARK CANCER INSTITUTE (330354)**, Elm and Carlton Streets,
Zip 14263–0001; tel. 716/845–2300 **A**1 2 3 5 8 9 10 **F**3 8 11 14 15 18 20
29 30 31 32 34 35 36 38 39 44 45 46 47 49 50 54 55 56 57 58 59 61 63
64 65 66 68 70 74 75 77 78 79 81 82 84 85 86 87 88 89 90 93 94 96 97
98 100 104 107 108 110 111 112 113 114 115 116 117 118 119 120 122
123 125 129 131 134 135 140 143 144 145 146 147 **P**6
Primary Contact: Donald L. Trump, M.D., President and Chief Executive Officer
COO: Joyce M. Yasko, Ph.D., Chief Operating Officer
CFO: Gregory McDonald, Vice President Finance and Chief Financial Officer
CMO: Judy Smith, M.D., Medical Director
CIO: Kevin Kimball, Vice President Information Technology
CHR: Vicki Garcia, Vice President Human Resources
CNO: Maureen Kelly, R.N., Chief Nursing Officer
Web address: www.roswellpark.org
**Control:** Hospital district or authority, Government, nonfederal **Service:** Cancer

**Staffed Beds:** 122 **Admissions:** 5156 **Census:** 100 **Outpatient Visits:**
202576 **Births:** 0 **Total Expense ($000):** 553680 **Payroll Expense ($000):**
216136 **Personnel:** 3343

✠ **SISTERS OF CHARITY HOSPITAL OF BUFFALO (330078)**, 2157 Main Street,
Zip 14214–2692; tel. 716/862–1000, (Total facility includes 80 beds in nursing
home–type unit) **A**1 2 3 5 9 10 12 13 **F**2 3 5 8 12 13 15 17 18 28 29 30 31
32 34 35 39 40 45 47 49 52 54 57 59 60 62 64 65 66 68 70 71 72 73 74
75 76 77 78 79 81 82 84 85 86 87 90 92 93 94 96 97 107 108 110 111
113 114 117 118 127 128 129 130 131 145 146 147 **P**5 6 **S** Catholic Health
System, Buffalo, NY
Primary Contact: Peter U. Bergmann, President and Chief Executive Officer
COO: Matthew Hamp, Chief Operating Officer
CFO: James H. Dunlop, Jr., CPA, Chief Financial Officer
CMO: Nady Shehata, M.D., Vice President Medical Affairs
CIO: Michael Galang, M.D., Chief Information Officer
CHR: David DeLorenzo, Senior Director Human Resources
CNO: Mary E. Dillon, MS, Vice President Patient Care Services
Web address: www.chsbuffalo.org
**Control:** Church–operated, Nongovernment, not–for profit **Service:** General
Medical and Surgical

**Staffed Beds:** 467 **Admissions:** 18031 **Census:** 322 **Outpatient Visits:**
624634 **Births:** 2961 **Total Expense ($000):** 290973 **Payroll Expense
($000):** 131606 **Personnel:** 2287

✠ △ **VETERANS AFFAIRS WESTERN NEW YORK HEALTHCARE
SYSTEM–BUFFALO DIVISION**, 3495 Bailey Avenue, Zip 14215–1129;
tel. 716/834–9200, (Nonreporting) **A**1 2 7 8 9 **S** Department of Veterans Affairs,
Washington, DC
Primary Contact: Craig Howard, Interim Director
CFO: Royce Calhoun, Business Manager
CMO: Miguel Rainstein, M.D., Acting Chief of Staff
CIO: Margaret Owczarzak, Facility Chief Information Officer
Web address: www.va.gov/visns/visn02
**Control:** Veterans Affairs, Government, federal **Service:** General Medical and
Surgical

**Staffed Beds:** 113

**WOMEN AND CHILDREN'S HOSPITAL** See KALEIDA Health

☐ **CATSKILL REGIONAL MEDICAL CENTER (331303)**, 8881 Route 97,
Zip 12723; tel. 845/887–5530, (Nonreporting) **A**1 9 10 18
Primary Contact: Chris L. White, Administrator
Web address: www.crmcny.org
**Control:** Other not–for–profit (including NFP Corporation) **Service:** General
Medical and Surgical

**Staffed Beds:** 25

✠ **F. F. THOMPSON HOSPITAL (330074)**, 350 Parrish Street, Zip 14424–1731;
tel. 585/396–6000, (Nonreporting) **A**1 9 10 **S** University of Rochester Medical
Center, Rochester, NY
Primary Contact: Michael Stapleton, R.N., MS, President and Chief Executive
Officer
CFO: Mark Prunoske, Chief Financial Officer and Senior Vice President Finance
CMO: Carlos Ortiz, M.D., Senior Vice President Medical Services
CIO: Mark Halladay, Director Information Services
CHR: Jennifer DeVault, Vice President Associate Services
Web address: www.thompsonhealth.com
**Control:** Other not–for–profit (including NFP Corporation) **Service:** General
Medical and Surgical

**Staffed Beds:** 267

**THOMPSON HEALTH** See F. F. Thompson Hospital

★ **VETERANS AFFAIRS MEDICAL CENTER**, 400 Fort Hill Avenue,
Zip 14424–1159; tel. 585/394–2000, (Total facility includes 116 beds in nursing
home–type unit) **A**3 5 **F**2 4 5 12 29 30 33 34 35 36 38 39 50 53 54 56 57 59
61 62 63 64 65 68 74 75 77 82 83 84 86 87 91 93 94 95 96 97 100 101
103 104 105 106 107 118 126 127 129 131 134 142 145 146 147
**S** Department of Veterans Affairs, Washington, DC
Primary Contact: Craig Howard, Director
CMO: Robert Babcock, M.D., Chief of Staff
CIO: Patricia Simon, Manager Information Systems
Web address: www.va.gov/sta/guide/home.asp
**Control:** Veterans Affairs, Government, federal **Service:** General Medical and
Surgical

**Staffed Beds:** 196 **Admissions:** 752 **Census:** 170 **Outpatient Visits:** 218581
**Births:** 0 **Total Expense ($000):** 120845 **Payroll Expense ($000):** 89157
**Personnel:** 897

**ARMS ACRES**, 75 Seminary Hill Road, Zip 10512–1921; tel. 845/225–3400,
(Nonreporting) **A**9
Primary Contact: Patrice Wallace–Moore, Chief Executive Officer and Executive
Director
CFO: Sultan Niazi, Chief Financial Officer
CMO: Fred Hesse, M.D., Medical Director
CIO: Dolores Watson, Director Health Information Management
CHR: Kim Halpin, Director Human Resources
CNO: Barbara Klein, R.N., Director of Nursing
Web address: www.armsacres.com
**Control:** Corporation, Investor–owned, for–profit **Service:** Alcoholism and other
chemical dependency

**Staffed Beds:** 146

✠ **PUTNAM HOSPITAL CENTER (330273)**, 670 Stoneleigh Avenue,
Zip 10512–3997; tel. 845/279–5711 **A**1 2 9 10 **F**3 11 12 13 15 28 29 30 31
32 33 34 35 38 40 49 51 54 57 59 60 63 64 68 70 74 75 76 78 79 81 82
85 86 87 89 93 98 99 100 101 102 103 104 105 107 108 111 113 115 116
118 119 120 128 129 130 131 134 145 146 147 **S** Health Quest Systems,
Inc., Lagrangeville, NY
Primary Contact: Maureen Zipparo, President and Chief Operating Officer
CFO: Anthony Mirdita, Chief Financial Officer
CMO: Ronald Tatelbaum, M.D., Interim Vice President Medical Affairs
CIO: Robert Diamond, Vice President and Chief Information Officer
CHR: Joan L. Calabrese, Director Human Resources
Web address: www.putnamhospital.org
**Control:** Other not–for–profit (including NFP Corporation) **Service:** General
Medical and Surgical

**Staffed Beds:** 164 **Admissions:** 7016 **Census:** 99 **Outpatient Visits:** 207159
**Births:** 434 **Total Expense ($000):** 148897 **Payroll Expense ($000):** 53895
**Personnel:** 782

**NY**

---

**Hospital, Medicare Provider Number, Address, Telephone, Approval, Facility, and Physician Codes, Health Care System**

★ American Hospital Association (AHA) membership
☐ The Joint Commission accreditation    ◇ DNV Healthcare Inc. accreditation

○ American Osteopathic Association (AOA) accreditation
△ Commission on Accreditation of Rehabilitation Facilities (CARF) accreditation

## CARTHAGE—Jefferson County

☐ **CARTHAGE AREA HOSPITAL (330263)**, 1001 West Street, Zip 13619–9703; tel. 315/493–1000, (Nonreporting) **A**1 9 10 20 21
Primary Contact: Adel Amir, Interim Chief Executive Officer
COO: Richard Duvall, Director Support Services and Chief Operating Officer
CMO: Mirza Ashraf, M.D., Medical Director
CIO: Skip Edie, Chief Information Officer
CHR: Richard Duvall, Director Support Services and Chief Operating Officer
Web address: www.carthagehospital.com
**Control:** Other not–for–profit (including NFP Corporation) **Service:** General Medical and Surgical

Staffed Beds: 78

## CASTLE POINT—Dutchess County

**VETERAN AFFAIRS HUDSON VALLEY HEALTH CARE SYSTEM–CASTLE POINT DIVISION** See Veterans Affairs Hudson Valley Health Care System–F.D. Roosevelt Hospital, Montrose

## CATSKILL—Greene County

**KAATERSKILL CARE** See Columbia Memorial Hospital, Hudson

## CLIFTON SPRINGS—Ontario County

★ **CLIFTON SPRINGS HOSPITAL AND CLINIC (330265)**, 2 Coulter Road, Zip 14432–1189; tel. 315/462–9561, (Nonreporting) **A**9 10 21
Primary Contact: John P. Galati, President and Chief Executive Officer
CFO: Arthur Dehey, Senior Vice President and Chief Financial Officer
CMO: Lewis Zulick, M.D., Vice President Medical Staff Affairs
CIO: David Markant, Director Information Systems
CHR: Kathy Babb, Manager Human Resources
CNO: Donna P. Smith, R.N., Vice President Patient Care Services and Chief Nursing Officer
Web address: www.cliftonspringshospital.org
**Control:** Other not–for–profit (including NFP Corporation) **Service:** General Medical and Surgical

Staffed Beds: 212

## COBLESKILL—Schoharie County

⊠ **COBLESKILL REGIONAL HOSPITAL (330268)**, 178 Grandview Drive, Zip 12043–5144; tel. 518/254–3456, (Nonreporting) **A**1 9 10 **S** Bassett Healthcare Network, Cooperstown, NY
Primary Contact: Eric H. Stein, FACHE, President and Chief Executive Officer
CFO: Leanna Jensen, Vice President Finance and Chief Financial Officer
CMO: Roy Korn, M.D., Medical Director
CIO: William Mackey, Director Information Systems
CHR: Randy Stark, Vice President Human Resources and Support Services
Web address: www.cobleskillhospital.org
**Control:** Other not–for–profit (including NFP Corporation) **Service:** General Medical and Surgical

Staffed Beds: 40

## COHOES—Albany County

**EDDY COHOES REHABILITATION CENTER (330407)**, 421 West Columbia Street, Zip 12047; tel. 518/237–5630, (Nonreporting) **A**10
Primary Contact: Laurie Mante, Administrator and Vice President
Web address: www.nehealth.com/Medical_Care/Eddy_Cohoes_Rehabilitation_Center/
**Control:** Other not–for–profit (including NFP Corporation) **Service:** Rehabilitation

Staffed Beds: 37

## COOPERSTOWN—Otsego County

⊠ **BASSETT MEDICAL CENTER (330136)**, One Atwell Road, Zip 13326–1394; tel. 607/547–3100 **A**1 2 3 5 8 9 10 **F**3 8 11 12 13 15 18 20 22 24 26 28 29 30 31 32 34 35 38 39 40 43 44 45 48 49 50 51 54 56 57 58 59 60 61 64 65 68 70 71 74 75 76 77 78 79 81 82 84 85 86 87 89 92 93 94 97 98 99 100 101 102 103 104 107 108 109 110 111 113 114 115 116 117 118 119 120 122 123 125 128 129 130 131 133 134 140 141 142 143 145 146 147 **P**6 **S** Bassett Healthcare Network, Cooperstown, NY
Primary Contact: William F. Streck, M.D., President and Chief Executive Officer
COO: Bertine C. McKenna, Ph.D., Executive Vice President and Chief Operating Officer
CFO: Nicholas Nicoletta, Corporate Vice President and Chief Financial Officer
CMO: Gerald D. Groff, M.D., Vice President Medical Affairs
CIO: Joseph Diver, Vice President Information Services and Chief Information Officer
CHR: Bruce W. Wilhelm, Vice President Human Resources
Web address: www.bassett.org
**Control:** Other not–for–profit (including NFP Corporation) **Service:** General Medical and Surgical

Staffed Beds: 164 Admissions: 9129 Census: 136 Outpatient Visits: 657579 Births: 826 Total Expense ($000): 380329 Payroll Expense ($000): 208897 Personnel: 2955

## CORNING—Steuben County

⊠ **CORNING HOSPITAL (330277)**, 176 Denison Parkway East, Zip 14830–2899; tel. 607/937–7200 **A**1 9 10 **F**3 8 11 13 15 28 29 31 32 34 35 37 38 40 44 45 49 50 53 57 59 64 70 75 76 77 78 79 81 82 87 89 92 93 100 107 108 110 111 114 118 119 120 123 128 129 130 131 134 144 145 146 147
**S** Guthrie Healthcare System, Sayre, PA
Primary Contact: Shirley P. Magana, President and Chief Operating Officer
COO: Shirley P. Magana, President and Chief Operating Officer
CFO: Francis M. Macafee, Vice President Finance and Chief Financial Officer
CMO: Chris Wentzel, M.D., Interim Medical Director
CIO: Carolyn Handrick, Manager Public Relations
CHR: Laura Manning, Administrative Director
CNO: Debra Raupers, MSN, Chief Nursing Officer
Web address: www.corninghospital.com
**Control:** Other not–for–profit (including NFP Corporation) **Service:** General Medical and Surgical

Staffed Beds: 82 Admissions: 4336 Census: 41 Outpatient Visits: 126084 Births: 375 Total Expense ($000): 67179 Payroll Expense ($000): 23485 Personnel: 506

## CORNWALL—Orange County

**ST. LUKE'S CORNWALL HOSPITAL – CORNWALL CAMPUS** See St. Luke's Cornwall Hospital, Newburgh

## CORTLAND—Cortland County

⊠ **CORTLAND REGIONAL MEDICAL CENTER (330175)**, 134 Homer Avenue, Zip 13045–1206; tel. 607/756–3500, (Total facility includes 82 beds in nursing home–type unit) **A**1 9 10 20 **F**2 3 11 13 15 28 29 30 35 40 45 49 50 54 56 57 59 62 64 68 70 76 77 79 81 82 85 86 87 89 91 93 96 98 100 102 107 108 110 111 113 114 117 118 127 129 130 131 132 134 143 145 146 147 **P**6
Primary Contact: Brian R. Mitteer, Chief Executive Officer
CFO: Denise Wrinn, Vice President Financial Services and Chief Financial Officer
CMO: Robert Karpman, M.D., Vice President Medical Affairs
CIO: Thomas Hallisey, Vice President Information Management
CHR: Jussi Maijala, Vice President Human Resources
CNO: Denise Mironti, Senior Vice President Patient Care Services
Web address: www.cortlandregional.org
**Control:** Other not–for–profit (including NFP Corporation) **Service:** General Medical and Surgical

Staffed Beds: 219 Admissions: 5408 Census: 171 Outpatient Visits: 134977 Births: 504 Total Expense ($000): 82789 Payroll Expense ($000): 37638 Personnel: 803

## CORTLANDT MANOR—Westchester County

☐ **HUDSON VALLEY HOSPITAL CENTER (330267)**, 1980 Crompond Road, Zip 10567–4182; tel. 914/737–9000 **A**1 9 10 **F**3 9 11 13 15 18 28 29 30 31 34 35 40 53 57 59 67 70 72 75 76 77 78 79 81 82 85 86 87 89 93 107 108 110 111 114 118 128 129 131 134 144 145 147 **P**2
Primary Contact: John C. Federspiel, President and Chief Executive Officer
COO: Deborah Neuendorf, Vice President Administration
CFO: Mark Webster, Vice President Finance
CMO: William Higgins, M.D., Vice President Medical Affairs
CIO: Bud Sorbello, Director Management Information Systems
CHR: Jeane L. Costella, Vice President
CNO: Kathleen Webster, R.N., Vice President Patient Services
Web address: www.hvhc.org
**Control:** Other not–for–profit (including NFP Corporation) **Service:** General Medical and Surgical

Staffed Beds: 128 Admissions: 6977 Census: 96 Outpatient Visits: 194508 Births: 892 Total Expense ($000): 135965 Payroll Expense ($000): 60822 Personnel: 1015

## CUBA—Allegany County

**CUBA MEMORIAL HOSPITAL (331301)**, 140 West Main Street, Zip 14727–1398; tel. 585/968–2000, (Nonreporting) **A**9 10 18
Primary Contact: Andrew Boser, Chief Executive Officer
CFO: Jack Ormond, Chief Financial Officer
Web address: www.cubamemorialhospital.com
**Control:** Other not–for–profit (including NFP Corporation) **Service:** General Medical and Surgical

Staffed Beds: 81

**NY**

## DANSVILLE—Livingston County

☒ **NICHOLAS H. NOYES MEMORIAL HOSPITAL (330238)**, 111 Clara Barton Street, Zip 14437–9503; tel. 585/335–6001, (Nonreporting) **A**1 9 10
Primary Contact: Amy Pollard, R.N., President and Chief Executive Officer
CFO: Jay T. Maslyn, Chief Financial Officer
CMO: Douglas Mayhle, M.D., Medical Director
CIO: John Dorak, Chief Information Officer
CHR: Jeanine Wilder, Director Human Resources
CNO: Tamara West, R.N., Vice President Patient Care
Web address: www.noyes-health.org
**Control:** Other not–for–profit (including NFP Corporation) **Service:** General Medical and Surgical

**Staffed Beds: 54**

## DELHI—Delaware County

☒ **O'CONNOR HOSPITAL (331305)**, 460 Andes Road, State Route 28, Zip 13753; tel. 607/746–0300 **A**1 9 10 18 **F**15 29 34 35 40 45 46 50 56 57 59 64 75 77 79 81 85 86 87 92 93 96 107 110 111 118 129 131 132 134 146 **S** Bassett Healthcare Network, Cooperstown, NY
Primary Contact: Daniel M. Ayres, Chief Executive Officer
CFO: Nicholas Nicoletta, Vice President and Chief Financial Officer
CMO: Alberto Gaitan, M.D., Medical Director
CHR: Barbara Green, Director Human Resources
CNO: Debra Neale, R.N., Chief Nursing Officer
Web address: www.oconnorhosp.org
**Control:** Other not–for–profit (including NFP Corporation) **Service:** General Medical and Surgical

**Staffed Beds: 16 Admissions: 434 Census: 7 Outpatient Visits: 34858 Births: 0 Total Expense ($000): 18261 Payroll Expense ($000): 6293 Personnel: 145**

## DIX HILLS—Suffolk County

☐ **SAGAMORE CHILDREN'S PSYCHIATRIC CENTER**, 197 Half Hollow Road, Zip 11746–5861; tel. 631/370–1700, (Nonreporting) **A**1 9 **S** New York State Office of Mental Health, Albany, NY
Primary Contact: Tom McOlvin, Executive Director
Web address: www.omh.ny.gov
**Control:** State–Government, nonfederal **Service:** Children's hospital psychiatric

**Staffed Beds: 69**

## DOBBS FERRY—Westchester County

**COMMUNITY HOSPITAL AT DOBBS FERRY (330036)**, 128 Ashford Avenue, Zip 10522–1896; tel. 914/693–0700, (Nonreporting) **A**10
Primary Contact: Ronald Corti, President and Chief Executive Officer
CFO: Dennis M. Keane, Vice President Finance and Chief Financial Officer
CMO: Francis C. Golier, M.D., Chief of Staff
CIO: Peter Weidner, Director Management Information Systems
CHR: Pam La France, Vice President Human Resources
Web address: www.riversidehealth.org
**Control:** Other not–for–profit (including NFP Corporation) **Service:** General Medical and Surgical

**Staffed Beds: 50**

## DUNKIRK—Chautauqua County

☒ **BROOKS MEMORIAL HOSPITAL (330229)**, 529 Central Avenue, Zip 14048–2599; tel. 716/366–1111 **A**1 9 10 **F**17 70 76
Primary Contact: Jonathan I. Lawrence, President and Chief Executive Officer
CFO: Ralph Webdale, Vice President Finance
CIO: Kathy Kucharski, Director Management Information Systems
CHR: Joan VanDette, Vice President Human Resources
Web address: www.brookshospital.org
**Control:** Other not–for–profit (including NFP Corporation) **Service:** General Medical and Surgical

**Staffed Beds: 65 Admissions: 2682 Census: 31 Outpatient Visits: 117026 Births: 643 Total Expense ($000): 41562 Payroll Expense ($000): 18741 Personnel: 411**

## EAST MEADOW—Nassau County

☒ **NASSAU UNIVERSITY MEDICAL CENTER (330027)**, 2201 Hempstead Turnpike, Zip 11554–1859; tel. 516/572–0123, (Total facility includes 589 beds in nursing home–type unit) **A**1 3 5 9 10 12 13 **F**3 4 5 7 8 9 11 12 13 14 15 16 17 18 19 20 26 29 30 31 34 35 38 39 40 43 44 45 46 47 48 49 50 52 56 57 58 59 60 61 63 64 65 66 68 70 71 72 73 74 75 76 77 78 79 81 82 83 84 85 87 88 89 90 92 93 94 96 97 98 99 100 101 102 103 104 106 107 108 110 111 113 114 117 118 120 127 129 130 131 134 142 143 144 145 146 147 **P**6
Primary Contact: Arthur A. Gianelli, President and Chief Executive Officer
CMO: Steven Walerstein, M.D., Executive Vice President and Medical Director
CIO: Ronald A. Tomo, Vice President and Chief Information Officer
CHR: Maureen Roarty, Vice President Human Resources
Web address: www.nuhealth.net
**Control:** Hospital district or authority, Government, nonfederal **Service:** General Medical and Surgical

**Staffed Beds: 1119 Admissions: 23531 Census: 946 Births: 1476**

## ELIZABETHTOWN—Essex County

☒ **ELIZABETHTOWN COMMUNITY HOSPITAL (331302)**, Park Street, Zip 12932–0277, Mailing Address: P.O. Box 277, Zip 12932–0277; tel. 518/873–6377 **A**1 9 10 18 **F**3 7 11 12 14 15 28 29 30 31 32 34 35 40 45 46 53 54 57 59 60 64 65 68 75 77 78 81 85 87 91 93 97 107 110 111 113 118 126 131 132 134 141 145 146 **P**6
Primary Contact: Rodney C. Boula, Administrator and Chief Executive Officer
COO: Matthew Nolan, Director Facilities and Operations
CFO: Alan Chardavoyne, Controller
CMO: Rob DeMuro, M.D., President Medical Staff
CHR: Michelle Meachem, Director Human Resources
Web address: www.ech.org
**Control:** Other not–for–profit (including NFP Corporation) **Service:** General Medical and Surgical

**Staffed Beds: 25 Admissions: 511 Census: 12 Outpatient Visits: 36853 Births: 0 Total Expense ($000): 17146 Payroll Expense ($000): 9240 Personnel: 134**

## ELLENVILLE—Ulster County

★ **ELLENVILLE REGIONAL HOSPITAL (331310)**, 10 Healthy Way, Zip 12428–5612; tel. 845/647–6400, (Nonreporting) **A**9 10 18
Primary Contact: Steven L. Kelley, President and Chief Executive Officer
CFO: Patricia Gavis, Chief Financial Officer
CMO: Helen Robinson, Chief Clinical Officer
CIO: Robert Rue, Controller
CHR: Deborah Briggs, Director Human Resources
Web address: www.ellenvilleregional.org
**Control:** Other not–for–profit (including NFP Corporation) **Service:** General Medical and Surgical

**Staffed Beds: 25**

## ELMHURST—Queens County, See New York City

## ELMIRA—Chemung County

★ **ARNOT OGDEN MEDICAL CENTER (330090)**, 600 Roe Avenue, Zip 14905–1629; tel. 607/737–4100, (Total facility includes 40 beds in nursing home–type unit) **A**2 6 9 10 21 **F**3 11 12 13 14 15 17 18 19 20 22 24 26 28 29 30 31 32 34 35 36 40 44 45 46 49 50 53 54 55 56 57 59 60 61 64 65 68 70 71 72 73 74 75 76 77 78 79 81 82 85 86 87 89 93 97 100 107 108 109 110 111 113 114 116 117 118 119 120 122 123 127 128 129 130 131 133 134 142 143 144 145 146 147 **P**6 **S** Arnot Health, Elmira, NY
Primary Contact: H. Fred Farley, R.N., Ph.D., FACHE, President and Chief Operating Officer
CFO: Ronald J. Kintz, Vice President and Treasurer
CMO: William Huffner, M.D., Vice President Medical Affairs
CIO: Gregg Martin, Manager Management Information Systems
CHR: Brian Forrest, Director Human Resources
CNO: Mary M. Vosburgh, R.N., Vice President Nursing and Chief Nursing Officer
Web address: www.aomc.org
**Control:** Other not–for–profit (including NFP Corporation) **Service:** General Medical and Surgical

**Staffed Beds: 244 Admissions: 11143 Census: 163 Outpatient Visits: 365319 Births: 1518 Total Expense ($000): 243928 Payroll Expense ($000): 128211 Personnel: 2055**

**NY**

---

**Hospital, Medicare Provider Number, Address, Telephone, Approval, Facility, and Physician Codes, Health Care System**

★ American Hospital Association (AHA) membership
☐ The Joint Commission accreditation ◇ DNV Healthcare Inc. accreditation

○ American Osteopathic Association (AOA) accreditation
△ Commission on Accreditation of Rehabilitation Facilities (CARF) accreditation

☐ **ELMIRA PSYCHIATRIC CENTER (334045)**, 100 Washington Street,
Zip 14901–2898; tel. 607/737–4739 **A**1 10 **F**39 54 64 98 99 101 103 104
106 131 **P**6 **S** New York State Office of Mental Health, Albany, NY
Primary Contact: Mark Stephany, Executive Director
COO: Shawn Rosno, Deputy Director Operations
CFO: J. Paul Bedzyk, Deputy Director Administration
CMO: Alec Whyte, M.D., Clinical Director
CIO: Edward Lorell, Facility Director Information
CHR: Patricia Santulli, Director Human Resources
Web address: www.omh.ny.gov/omhweb/facilities/elpc/facility.htm
**Control:** State–Government, nonfederal **Service:** Psychiatric

**Staffed Beds:** 100 **Admissions:** 288 **Census:** 86 **Outpatient Visits:** 106000
**Births:** 0 **Total Expense ($000):** 28832 **Payroll Expense ($000):** 20712
**Personnel:** 359

✠ **ST. JOSEPH'S HOSPITAL (330108)**, 555 St. Joseph's Boulevard,
Zip 14901–3223; tel. 607/733–6541, (Includes TWIN TIERS REHABILITATION
CENTER ), (Total facility includes 71 beds in nursing home–type unit) **A**1 9 10 **F**3
4 5 11 15 18 29 30 31 40 43 45 48 49 51 59 60 64 68 70 74 75 78 79 81
82 85 87 90 91 93 97 98 100 101 102 103 107 108 111 118 127 129 131
134 145 146 **S** Arnot Health, Elmira, NY
Primary Contact: H. Fred Farley, R.N., Ph.D., FACHE, President and Chief
Operating Officer
COO: H. Fred Farley, R.N., President and Chief Operating Officer
CFO: Ronald J. Kintz, Senior Vice President Finance and Chief Financial Officer
CMO: William Huffner, M.D., Chief Medical Officer and Senior Vice President
Medical Affairs
CIO: Gregg Martin, Chief Information Officer
CHR: Brian Forrest, Vice President Human Resources
CNO: Mary M. Vosburgh, R.N., Vice President Nursing and Chief Nursing Officer
Web address: www.stjosephs.org
**Control:** Other not–for–profit (including NFP Corporation) **Service:** General
Medical and Surgical

**Staffed Beds:** 212 **Admissions:** 4936 **Census:** 160 **Outpatient Visits:**
120797 **Total Expense ($000):** 62893 **Payroll Expense ($000):** 27441
**Personnel:** 551

### ENDICOTT—Broome County

**MEDICENTER** See United Health Services Hospitals–Binghamton, Binghamton

### FAR ROCKAWAY—Queens County, See New York City

### FLUSHING—Queens County, See New York City

### FOREST HILLS—Queens County, See New York City

### FRESH MEADOWS—Queens County

**CORNERSTONE OF MEDICAL ARTS CENTER HOSPITAL**, 159–05 Union
Turnpike, Zip 11366–1950; tel. 212/755–0200, (Nonreporting)
Primary Contact: Norman J. Sokolow, Chairman and Chief Executive Officer
COO: Thomas C. Puzo, President and Chief Operating Officer
CFO: Jeff OniFather, Chief Financial Officer
CMO: Sami Kaddouri, M.D., Medical Director
CHR: Gloria Burtch, Director Human Resources
Web address: www.cornerstoneny.com
**Control:** Corporation, Investor–owned, for–profit **Service:** Alcoholism and other
chemical dependency

**Staffed Beds:** 162

### GENEVA—Ontario County

✠ △ **GENEVA GENERAL HOSPITAL (330058)**, 196 North Street,
Zip 14456–1694; tel. 315/787–4000 **A**1 7 9 10 **F**3 8 11 13 15 17 18 28 29
30 31 32 34 35 40 45 49 50 54 57 59 60 61 64 66 69 70 74 75 76 77 78
79 81 85 86 87 90 92 93 96 97 107 108 110 111 114 117 118 128 129
131 134 145 146 **P**6 **S** Finger Lakes Health, Geneva, NY
Primary Contact: Jose Acevedo, M.D., President and Chief Executive Officer
COO: James Hiserodt, Senior Vice President Operations
CFO: Patricia Thompson, Treasurer and Chief Financial Officer
CMO: Jason Feinberg, M.D., Vice President Medical Affairs and Chief Medical
Officer
CIO: John Oates, Director Information Systems
CHR: Patrick R. Boyle, Vice President Human Resources
CNO: Eileen Gage, R.N., Vice President Nursing
Web address: www.flhealth.org
**Control:** Other not–for–profit (including NFP Corporation) **Service:** General
Medical and Surgical

**Staffed Beds:** 132 **Admissions:** 4084 **Census:** 49 **Outpatient Visits:** 472426
**Births:** 595 **Total Expense ($000):** 76702 **Payroll Expense ($000):** 43138
**Personnel:** 827

### GLEN COVE—Nassau County

✠ **GLEN COVE HOSPITAL (330181)**, 101 St. Andrews Lane, Zip 11542–2254;
tel. 516/674–7300 **A**1 2 3 5 9 10 **F**3 5 9 11 12 14 15 17 18 26 28 29 30 31
32 33 34 35 36 38 39 40 43 44 45 46 47 48 49 50 53 54 55 56 57 58 59
60 61 63 64 65 66 68 69 70 74 75 77 78 79 81 82 84 85 86 87 90 92 93
94 96 97 98 100 101 102 103 104 107 108 111 113 116 117 118 120 122
129 130 131 133 134 142 144 145 146 147 **P**6 **S** North Shore–Long Island
Jewish Health System, Great Neck, NY
Primary Contact: Dennis Connors, Executive Director
COO: Joshua Strugatz, Associate Executive Director Operations
CFO: Michele Frankel, Associate Executive Director Finance
CMO: George Dunn, M.D., Senior Vice President Medical Affairs
CHR: Thomas Salvo, Associate Executive Director Human Resources
CNO: Susan Kwiatek, Associate Executive Director Patient Care Services
Web address: www.northshorelij.com
**Control:** Other not–for–profit (including NFP Corporation) **Service:** General
Medical and Surgical

**Staffed Beds:** 265 **Admissions:** 9490 **Census:** 173 **Outpatient Visits:** 75636
**Births:** 0 **Total Expense ($000):** 188715 **Payroll Expense ($000):** 94576
**Personnel:** 1137

### GLEN OAKS—Queens County, See New York City

### GLENS FALLS—Warren County

✠ **GLENS FALLS HOSPITAL (330191)**, 100 Park Street, Zip 12801;
tel. 518/926–1000, (Nonreporting) **A**1 2 5 9 10
Primary Contact: David G. Kruczlnicki, President and Chief Executive Officer
COO: Dianne Shugrue, MSN, Senior Vice President Operations and Chief
Operating Officer
CFO: Jeffrey S. Treasure, Senior Vice President Finance and Chief Financial Officer
CMO: Robert M. Pickoff, M.D., Vice President Medical Affairs
CIO: Joan McFaul, Vice President Information Technology and Chief Information
Officer
CHR: Kathleen Smith, Interim Vice President Human Resources
CNO: Donna Kirker, R.N., Vice President Patient Services and Chief Nursing
Officer
Web address: www.glensfallshospital.org
**Control:** Other not–for–profit (including NFP Corporation) **Service:** General
Medical and Surgical

**Staffed Beds:** 335

### GLENVILLE—Schenectady County

**CONIFER PARK**, 79 Glenridge Road, Zip 12302–4523; tel. 518/399–6446 **A**9
**F**4 5 29
Primary Contact: Jeanne Gluchowski, Executive Director
COO: Jeanne Gluchowski, Executive Director
CFO: Jason Burczeuski, Controller
CMO: John Melbourne, M.D., Medical Director
CIO: Amy Kentera, Chief Information Officer
CHR: Maureen Fowler, Director Human Resources
Web address: www.libertymgt.com
**Control:** Corporation, Investor–owned, for–profit **Service:** Alcoholism and other
chemical dependency

**Staffed Beds:** 225 **Admissions:** 3760 **Census:** 198 **Outpatient Visits:**
105356 **Births:** 0 **Total Expense ($000):** 22031 **Payroll Expense ($000):**
14604 **Personnel:** 331

### GLOVERSVILLE—Fulton County

✠ **NATHAN LITTAUER HOSPITAL AND NURSING HOME (330276)**, 99 East
State Street, Zip 12078–1203; tel. 518/725–8621, (Total facility includes 84
beds in nursing home–type unit) **A**1 5 9 10 **F**3 8 11 13 15 18 28 29 30 31 32
34 35 36 37 40 45 46 50 53 54 57 59 61 64 65 70 74 75 76 77 78 79 81
82 85 86 87 89 93 97 107 108 110 114 117 118 123 127 129 130 131 134
144 145 146 **P**6
Primary Contact: Laurence E. Kelly, President and Chief Executive Officer
CFO: Henry Legendziewicz, Senior Vice President and Chief Financial Officer
CMO: Frederick Goldberg, M.D., Vice President Medical Affairs and Chief Medical
Officer
CIO: Martin Brown, Vice President Information Services and Chief Information
Officer
CHR: Lana Wydra, Vice President Human Resources
CNO: Regina Mulligan, Vice President Nursing
Web address: www.nlh.org
**Control:** Other not–for–profit (including NFP Corporation) **Service:** General
Medical and Surgical

**Staffed Beds:** 158 **Admissions:** 3611 **Census:** 134 **Outpatient Visits:**
231751 **Births:** 406 **Total Expense ($000):** 86212 **Payroll Expense ($000):**
45010 **Personnel:** 787

## GOUVERNEUR—St. Lawrence County

☒ **EDWARD JOHN NOBLE HOSPITAL OF GOUVERNEUR (330177)**, 77 West Barney Street, Zip 13642–1040; tel. 315/287–1000, (Total facility includes 40 beds in nursing home–type unit) **A**1 9 10 20 **F**3 8 11 13 15 29 30 32 34 35 36 38 39 40 43 45 50 54 55 56 57 59 61 64 65 70 71 75 76 77 79 81 85 86 87 89 93 97 107 108 110 111 113 118 126 127 129 130 131 132 134 142 145 146 147 **P**6
Primary Contact: Charles P. Conole, FACHE, Chief Executive Officer
COO: Charles P. Conole, FACHE, Chief Executive Officer
CFO: Joseph B. Vaganek, Chief Financial Officer
CMO: Donald Schuessler, M.D., Medical Director
CIO: Linda Fishel, Manager Information Services
CHR: Cathy Chirico, Director Human Resources
Web address: www.ejnoble.com
**Control:** Other not–for–profit (including NFP Corporation) **Service:** General Medical and Surgical

**Staffed Beds:** 87 **Admissions:** 1258 **Census:** 57 **Outpatient Visits:** 64852 **Births:** 121 **Total Expense ($000):** 22405 **Payroll Expense ($000):** 11256 **Personnel:** 226

## GREENPORT—Suffolk County

★ **EASTERN LONG ISLAND HOSPITAL (330088)**, 201 Manor Place, Zip 11944–1298; tel. 631/477–1000 **A**9 10 **F**3 4 17 18 28 29 31 34 35 40 45 47 49 53 56 59 64 68 70 74 78 79 81 82 85 93 97 98 100 102 103 106 107 110 111 118 129 131 134 145 **P**8
Primary Contact: Paul J. Connor, III, President and Chief Executive Officer
CFO: Robert A. Ragona, Vice President Finance
CMO: Lloyd Simon, M.D., Medical Director
CIO: Dan Scotto, Director Data Processing
CHR: August F. Menchini, Director Human Resources
CNO: D. Patricia Pispisa, Vice President Patient Care Services
Web address: www.elih.org
**Control:** Other not–for–profit (including NFP Corporation) **Service:** General Medical and Surgical

**Staffed Beds:** 90 **Admissions:** 3024 **Census:** 54 **Outpatient Visits:** 42009 **Births:** 0 **Total Expense ($000):** 43315 **Payroll Expense ($000):** 18446 **Personnel:** 286

## HAMILTON—Madison County

☒ **COMMUNITY MEMORIAL HOSPITAL (330249)**, 150 Broad Street, Zip 13346–9518; tel. 315/824–1100, (Nonreporting) **A**1 9 10
Primary Contact: David Felton, President and Chief Executive Officer
CFO: Richard S. Kirby, Executive Vice President and Chief Financial Officer
CMO: Michael S. Jastremski, M.D., Vice President Medical Affairs and Director Emergency Services
Web address: www.communitymemorial.org
**Control:** Other not–for–profit (including NFP Corporation) **Service:** General Medical and Surgical

**Staffed Beds:** 84

## HARRIS—Sullivan County

☒ **CATSKILL REGIONAL MEDICAL CENTER (330386)**, 68 Harris Bushville Road, Zip 12742–5030, Mailing Address: P.O. Box 800, Zip 12742–0800; tel. 845/794–3300, (Total facility includes 64 beds in nursing home–type unit) **A**1 2 9 10 **F**2 3 4 8 11 13 15 17 18 28 29 30 31 34 35 38 40 42 45 51 54 56 57 59 65 68 70 76 78 79 81 85 86 87 89 93 96 97 98 102 103 107 111 114 118 126 127 129 131 132 145 146 147
Primary Contact: Frederick H. Kuriger, FACHE, Chief Executive Officer
CFO: Mitchell Amado, Chief Financial Officer
CMO: Peter J. Panzarino, M.D., Chief Medical Officer
CIO: John Lynch, Vice President Chief Information Officer
CHR: Zigmund Nowicki, Director Human Resources
CNO: Barbara Gentile, Vice President Chief Nursing Officer
Web address: www.crmcny.org
**Control:** Other not–for–profit (including NFP Corporation) **Service:** General Medical and Surgical

**Staffed Beds:** 211 **Admissions:** 5825 **Census:** 131 **Outpatient Visits:** 107275 **Births:** 624 **Total Expense ($000):** 95263 **Payroll Expense ($000):** 43415 **Personnel:** 776

## HOLLISWOOD—Queens County, See New York City

## HORNELL—Steuben County

☒ **ST. JAMES MERCY HEALTH SYSTEM (330151)**, 411 Canisteo Street, Zip 14843–2197; tel. 607/324–8000, (Total facility includes 120 beds in nursing home–type unit) **A**1 9 10 20 **F**1 2 3 4 5 8 11 13 15 17 28 29 30 34 35 39 40 43 45 50 54 57 60 65 70 74 75 76 77 78 79 81 85 87 89 91 93 98 99 102 104 107 108 113 117 118 126 127 128 129 131 145 146 **P**1 **S** Catholic Health East, Newtown Square, PA
Primary Contact: Mary E. LaRowe, FACHE, President and Chief Executive Officer
CFO: Jennifer Sullivan, Senior Vice President Finance and Chief Financial Officer
CMO: Bradley Truax, M.D., Senior Vice President Medical Affairs and Chief Medical Officer
CIO: Bonnie Welch, Chief Information Officer
CNO: Patricia Uldrich, R.N., Chief Nursing Officer
Web address: www.stjamesmercy.org
**Control:** Other not–for–profit (including NFP Corporation) **Service:** General Medical and Surgical

**Staffed Beds:** 222 **Admissions:** 4805 **Census:** 163 **Outpatient Visits:** 184773 **Births:** 308 **Total Expense ($000):** 59197 **Payroll Expense ($000):** 28012

## HUDSON—Columbia County

**COLUMBIA MEMORIAL HOSPITAL (330094)**, 71 Prospect Avenue, Zip 12534–2907; tel. 518/828–7601, (Includes KAATERSKILL CARE, 161 Jefferson Heights, Catskill, Zip 12414; tel. 518/943–6363), (Total facility includes 120 beds in nursing home–type unit) **A**9 10 19 **F**8 11 13 15 18 29 30 34 35 36 37 39 40 45 46 48 49 50 51 54 56 57 59 60 61 63 64 68 70 71 74 75 76 77 78 79 81 82 85 86 87 92 93 97 98 99 100 102 107 108 110 111 113 114 115 116 118 124 126 127 128 129 130 134 143 145 146 147 **P**6
Primary Contact: Jane Ehrlich, President and Chief Executive Officer
COO: Jay P. Cahalan, Chief Operating Officer
CFO: Vincent Dingman, III, Chief Financial Officer
CMO: Norman Chapin, M.D., Medical Director
CIO: Cathleen Crowley, Chief Information Officer
CHR: Ray Jones, Vice President
Web address: www.columbiamemorial.com
**Control:** Other not–for–profit (including NFP Corporation) **Service:** General Medical and Surgical

**Staffed Beds:** 218 **Admissions:** 6497 **Census:** 200 **Outpatient Visits:** 352880 **Births:** 467 **Total Expense ($000):** 130380 **Payroll Expense ($000):** 68422 **Personnel:** 1245

## HUNTINGTON—Suffolk County

☒ **HUNTINGTON HOSPITAL (330045)**, 270 Park Avenue, Zip 11743–2799; tel. 631/351–2200 **A**1 2 9 10 **F**3 11 12 13 15 17 18 20 26 29 30 31 34 35 36 38 40 43 44 45 50 53 54 55 56 57 58 59 60 63 64 65 66 68 69 70 73 74 75 76 78 79 81 82 84 85 86 87 89 93 97 98 100 101 102 103 104 107 108 110 111 113 114 117 118 129 130 131 134 145 146 **P**6 **S** North Shore–Long Island Jewish Health System, Great Neck, NY
Primary Contact: Kevin F. Lawlor, President and Chief Executive Officer
COO: Thomas M. Hoeft, Executive Vice President and Chief Operating Officer
CFO: Michael Fagan, Chief Financial Officer
CMO: Michael Grosso, M.D., Senior Vice President Medical Affairs
CIO: Linda Fischer, Director Information Services
CHR: Michael J. Quartier, Vice President Administration and Human Resources
Web address: www.hunthosp.org
**Control:** Other not–for–profit (including NFP Corporation) **Service:** General Medical and Surgical

**Staffed Beds:** 299 **Admissions:** 16520 **Census:** 221 **Outpatient Visits:** 121249 **Births:** 1456 **Total Expense ($000):** 277188 **Payroll Expense ($000):** 133143 **Personnel:** 1849

## IRVING—Chautauqua County

○ **LAKE SHORE HEALTH CARE CENTER**, 845 Route 5 and 20, Zip 14081–9716; tel. 716/951–7000, (Total facility includes 120 beds in nursing home–type unit) **A**9 11 21 **F**2 3 4 5 11 15 40 42 62 70 80 98 127
Primary Contact: Louis J. Frascella, President and Chief Executive Officer
CMO: James Wild, M.D., Medical Director
CIO: Louis Di Rienzo, Chief Information Officer
CHR: Tracie Luther, Vice President Human Resources
Web address: www.tlchealth.org
**Control:** Other not–for–profit (including NFP Corporation) **Service:** General Medical and Surgical

**Staffed Beds:** 220 **Admissions:** 21455 **Census:** 156 **Outpatient Visits:** 61495 **Births:** 0 **Total Expense ($000):** 45628 **Payroll Expense ($000):** 20386 **Personnel:** 529

NY

---

**Hospital, Medicare Provider Number, Address, Telephone, Approval, Facility, and Physician Codes, Health Care System**

★ American Hospital Association (AHA) membership
☐ The Joint Commission accreditation        ◇ DNV Healthcare Inc. accreditation
○ American Osteopathic Association (AOA) accreditation
△ Commission on Accreditation of Rehabilitation Facilities (CARF) accreditation

## ITHACA—Tompkins County

✠ **CAYUGA MEDICAL CENTER AT ITHACA (330307)**, 101 Dates Drive,
Zip 14850–1342; tel. 607/274–4011 **A**1 2 5 9 10 **F**3 8 11 12 13 15 18 20 22
28 29 30 31 34 38 40 45 49 51 53 54 57 59 61 64 68 70 72 74 75 76 77
78 79 81 82 84 85 86 87 90 93 98 99 100 101 102 103 107 108 110 111
113 114 115 117 118 120 128 129 130 131 132 134 143 144 145 146
147 **P**6
Primary Contact: D. Rob Mackenzie, M.D., President and Chief Executive Officer
COO: D. Rob Mackenzie, M.D., President and Chief Executive Officer
CFO: John Rudd, Chief Financial Officer
CMO: David M. Evelyn, M.D., Vice President Medical Affairs
CIO: Anthony Votaw, Chief Information Officer
CHR: Alan Pedersen, Vice President Human Resources
Web address: www.cayugamed.org
**Control:** Other not–for–profit (including NFP Corporation) **Service:** General
Medical and Surgical

**Staffed Beds:** 190 **Admissions:** 6325 **Census:** 81 **Outpatient Visits:** 253390
**Births:** 836 **Total Expense ($000):** 171195 **Payroll Expense ($000):** 55120
**Personnel:** 1070

## JACKSON HEIGHTS—Queens County, See New York City

## JAMAICA—Queens County, See New York City

## JAMESTOWN—Chautauqua County

✠ **WOMAN'S CHRISTIAN ASSOCIATION HOSPITAL (330239)**, 207 Foote
Avenue, Zip 14702–9975, Mailing Address: P.O. Box 840, Zip 14702–0840;
tel. 716/487–0141 **A**1 2 9 10 **F**4 5 8 11 13 15 18 19 20 28 29 31 34 35 36
40 45 46 54 57 59 60 61 64 68 70 74 75 76 77 78 79 81 82 83 84 85 86
87 89 90 92 93 96 97 98 99 100 101 102 103 104 107 108 111 113 116
118 120 128 129 130 131 133 134 140 142 145 146 147
Primary Contact: Betsy T. Wright, President and Chief Executive Officer
CMO: Marlene Garone, M.D., Vice President Medical Affairs and Medical Director
CIO: Keith Robison, Chief Information Officer
CHR: Karen Bohall, Director Human Resources
Web address: www.wcahospital.org
**Control:** Other not–for–profit (including NFP Corporation) **Service:** General
Medical and Surgical

**Staffed Beds:** 222 **Admissions:** 7400 **Census:** 117 **Outpatient Visits:**
248000 **Births:** 631 **Total Expense ($000):** 101292 **Payroll Expense**
**($000):** 41605 **Personnel:** 1063

## JOHNSON CITY—Broome County

**WILSON MEMORIAL REGIONAL MEDICAL CENTER** See United Health Services
Hospitals–Binghamton, Binghamton

## KATONAH—Westchester County

☐ **FOUR WINDS HOSPITAL (334002)**, 800 Cross River Road, Zip 10536–3549;
tel. 914/763–8151, (Nonreporting) **A**1 9 10
Primary Contact: Martin A. Buccolo, Ph.D., Chief Executive Officer
COO: Moira Morrissey, Chief Operating Officer and General Counsel
CFO: Barry S. Weinstein, Chief Financial Officer
CMO: Jonathan Bauman, M.D., Chief Medical Officer
CIO: Barry S. Weinstein, Chief Financial Officer
CHR: Susan Cusano, Director Human Resources
Web address: www.fourwindshospital.com
**Control:** Partnership, Investor–owned, for–profit **Service:** Psychiatric

**Staffed Beds:** 175

## KENMORE—Erie County

✠ **KENMORE MERCY HOSPITAL (330102)**, 2950 Elmwood Avenue,
Zip 14217–1390; tel. 716/447–6100, (Total facility includes 160 beds in nursing
home–type unit) **A**1 9 10 **F**3 15 17 18 29 30 31 32 34 35 39 40 45 49 54 57
59 60 64 65 66 68 70 74 75 78 79 81 84 85 86 87 90 92 93 94 96 97 107
108 110 111 113 114 117 118 125 127 128 129 130 131 145 147 **P**5 6
**S** Catholic Health System, Buffalo, NY
Primary Contact: James M. Millard, President and Chief Executive Officer
COO: Walter Ludwig, Chief Operating Officer
CFO: James H. Dunlop, Jr., CPA, Senior Vice President and Chief Financial Officer
CMO: James Fitzpatrick, M.D., Vice President Medical Affairs
CHR: Pam Nicastro, Director Human Resources
Web address: www.chsbuffalo.org
**Control:** Church–operated, Nongovernment, not–for profit **Service:** General
Medical and Surgical

**Staffed Beds:** 315 **Admissions:** 8418 **Census:** 253 **Outpatient Visits:**
152090 **Births:** 0 **Total Expense ($000):** 135974 **Payroll Expense ($000):**
60112 **Personnel:** 999

## KINGSTON—Ulster County

☐ **BENEDICTINE HOSPITAL (330224)**, 105 Marys Avenue, Zip 12401–5894;
tel. 845/338–2500 **A**1 2 9 10 19 **F**3 4 8 11 15 18 20 29 30 31 34 35 36 45
49 50 54 56 57 59 63 64 66 68 70 74 75 78 79 81 83 84 85 86 87 90 98
105 107 108 110 113 118 119 120 122 128 129 130 131 145 146 147 **P**7
**S** HealthAlliance of the Hudson Valley, Kingston, NY
Primary Contact: David W. Lundquist, President and Chief Executive Officer
CFO: David Scarpino, Senior Vice President and Chief Financial Officer
CMO: Rafael Olazagasti, M.D., Vice President Medical Affairs and Network
Development
CIO: John Finch, Vice President Corporate Development
CHR: Heidi Rosborough, Manager Human Resources
Web address: www.benedictine.org
**Control:** Church–operated, Nongovernment, not–for profit **Service:** General
Medical and Surgical

**Staffed Beds:** 120 **Admissions:** 4323 **Census:** 85 **Outpatient Visits:** 77116
**Births:** 0 **Total Expense ($000):** 74159 **Payroll Expense ($000):** 25951
**Personnel:** 606

✠ **KINGSTON HOSPITAL (330004)**, 396 Broadway, Zip 12401–4692;
tel. 845/331–3131 **A**1 9 10 13 19 **F**3 8 11 13 15 18 20 28 29 30 34 35 36
40 45 49 50 54 56 57 59 60 63 64 68 70 74 75 76 77 79 81 82 83 84 85
86 87 89 92 93 102 107 108 110 111 113 114 118 129 130 131 134 145
146 147 **S** HealthAlliance of the Hudson Valley, Kingston, NY
Primary Contact: David W. Lundquist, President and Chief Executive Officer
COO: Charles Flinn, Chief Operating Officer
CFO: David Scarpino, Senior Vice President Finance and Chief Financial Officer
CMO: Frank Ehrlich, M.D., Chief Medical Officer
CIO: John Finch, Vice President Information Services
CHR: Greg M. Howard, Director Human Resource
CNO: Kathleen Lunney, R.N., Chief Nursing Officer
Web address: www.kingstonregionalhealth.org
**Control:** Other not–for–profit (including NFP Corporation) **Service:** General
Medical and Surgical

**Staffed Beds:** 150 **Admissions:** 9751 **Census:** 122 **Outpatient Visits:**
219520 **Births:** 521 **Total Expense ($000):** 105246 **Payroll Expense**
**($000):** 44949 **Personnel:** 900

## LEWISTON—Niagara County

✠ **MOUNT ST. MARY'S HOSPITAL AND HEALTH CENTER (330188)**, 5300
Military Road, Zip 14092–1903; tel. 716/297–4800, (Total facility includes 250
beds in nursing home–type unit) **A**1 9 10 **F**3 4 13 15 17 18 28 29 30 40 45 49
50 60 64 65 75 77 79 81 82 84 93 97 107 108 111 114 118 127 129 134
145 146 147 **P**5 **S** Ascension Health, Saint Louis, MO
Primary Contact: Judith A. Maness, FACHE, President and Chief Executive Officer
COO: Gary Tucker, Senior Vice President Operations and Chief Operating Officer
CFO: Michael F. Ickowski, Vice President Finance and Chief Financial Officer
CMO: Domonic F. Falsetti, M.D., Chief of Staff and Medical Director
CIO: Richard J. Witkowski, Director Management Information Systems
CHR: Deborah J. Serafin, Vice President Human Resources
Web address: www.msmh.org
**Control:** Other not–for–profit (including NFP Corporation) **Service:** General
Medical and Surgical

**Staffed Beds:** 425 **Admissions:** 6493 **Census:** 335 **Outpatient Visits:**
129494 **Births:** 254 **Total Expense ($000):** 109100 **Payroll Expense**
**($000):** 53129 **Personnel:** 720

## LITTLE FALLS—Herkimer County

★ **LITTLE FALLS HOSPITAL (331311)**, 140 Burwell Street, Zip 13365–1725;
tel. 315/823–1000, (Nonreporting) **A**9 10 18 **S** Bassett Healthcare Network,
Cooperstown, NY
Primary Contact: Michael L. Ogden, President and Chief Executive Officer
CFO: James Vielkind, Chief Financial Officer
CMO: Andrew Rauscher, M.D., Medical Director
CIO: Duane Merry, Chief Information Officer
CHR: Jack Fredericks, Vice President Human Resources
Web address: www.lfhny.org
**Control:** Other not–for–profit (including NFP Corporation) **Service:** General
Medical and Surgical

**Staffed Beds:** 59

## LITTLE NECK—Queens County, See New York City

*Many Facility Codes have changed. Please refer to the AHA Guide Code Chart.* © 2012 AHA Guide

## LOCKPORT—Niagara County

★ **EASTERN NIAGARA HEALTH SYSTEM (330163)**, 521 East Avenue, Zip 14094–3299; tel. 716/514–5700, (Includes EASTERN NIAGARA HOSPITAL INTER–COMMUNITY, 2600 William Street, Newfane, Zip 14108–1093; tel. 716/778–5111; EASTERN NIAGARA HOSPITAL LOCKPORT, 521 East Avenue, tel. 716/514–5700), (Nonreporting) **A**10
Primary Contact: Clare A. Haar, Chief Executive Officer
COO: David J. Di Bacco, Chief Operating Officer
CFO: Donald L. Kepner, Chief Financial Officer
CMO: Bruce J. Cusenz, M.D., Medical Director
CHR: Joseph J. DeFazio, Director Human Resources
Web address: www.enhs.org
**Control:** Other not–for–profit (including NFP Corporation) **Service:** General Medical and Surgical

| Staffed Beds: 171 |
|---|

## LONG BEACH—Nassau County

☐ **LONG BEACH MEDICAL CENTER (330225)**, 455 East Bay Drive, Zip 11561–2300, Mailing Address: P.O. Box 300, Zip 11561–2300; tel. 516/897–1000, (Total facility includes 200 beds in nursing home–type unit) **A**1 9 10 12 13 **F**3 4 5 8 9 11 13 15 29 30 31 34 35 36 38 39 40 45 46 49 50 53 56 57 58 59 60 61 62 64 65 66 68 70 74 75 78 79 81 82 85 86 87 89 90 91 92 93 94 97 98 99 100 101 102 103 104 106 107 108 111 113 117 118 127 129 130 131 133 134 142 144 145 147
Primary Contact: Douglas L. Melzer, Chief Executive Officer
CFO: Barry Stern, Chief Financial Officer
CMO: Harish Sood, M.D., Medical Director
CIO: Peter Genova, Chief Information Officer
CHR: Michelle Levine, Director Human Resources
CNO: Faye Duda, R.N., Chief Nursing Officer
Web address: www.lbmc.org
**Control:** Other not–for–profit (including NFP Corporation) **Service:** General Medical and Surgical

| Staffed Beds: 342 Admissions: 5300 Census: 263 Outpatient Visits: 92503 Births: 0 Total Expense ($000): 85613 Payroll Expense ($000): 46962 Personnel: 546 |
|---|

## LONG ISLAND CITY—Queens County, See New York City

## LOWVILLE—Lewis County

✠ **LEWIS COUNTY GENERAL HOSPITAL (330213)**, 7785 North State Street, Zip 13367–1297; tel. 315/376–5200, (Total facility includes 160 beds in nursing home–type unit) **A**1 9 10 20 **F**2 3 5 6 7 8 11 15 29 30 34 40 50 54 56 57 59 70 75 76 77 78 79 81 82 85 86 87 91 93 96 97 107 108 110 111 113 118 123 126 128 129 130 131 132 142 145 146 147 **P**6 8
Primary Contact: Eric Burch, Chief Executive Officer
CFO: Richard T. Lang, Chief Financial Officer
CMO: Catherine Williams, M.D., Medical Director
CIO: Rob Uttendorfsky, Director Information Management
CHR: Timothy J. Ryan, Jr., Director Human Resources
CNO: David Wood, Director Acute Care Services
Web address: www.lcgh.net
**Control:** County–Government, nonfederal **Service:** General Medical and Surgical

| Staffed Beds: 214 Admissions: 1690 Census: 171 Outpatient Visits: 123110 Births: 336 Total Expense ($000): 63851 Payroll Expense ($000): 24256 Personnel: 505 |
|---|

## MALONE—Franklin County

✠ **ALICE HYDE MEDICAL CENTER (330084)**, 133 Park Street, Zip 12953–0729, Mailing Address: P.O. Box 729, Zip 12953–0729; tel. 518/483–3000, (Total facility includes 75 beds in nursing home–type unit) **A**1 9 10 20 **F**3 11 13 15 17 18 28 29 31 34 35 36 39 40 45 50 57 59 60 64 68 70 75 76 77 78 79 81 82 84 85 86 87 90 93 97 107 108 110 111 114 116 118 120 123 126 127 128 129 130 131 134 142 145 147
Primary Contact: Douglas F. DiVello, President and Chief Executive Officer
CFO: Chris Frauenhofer, Vice President Finance
CFO: Michael Towle, Vice President Finance
CMO: Leonardo Dishman, M.D., Chief Medical Officer
CIO: Joel Benware, Chief Information Officer
CHR: Emily Campbell, Director Human Resources
CNO: John E. Aufdengarten, R.N., Vice President, Administration
CNO: Linda McClarigan, R.N., Vice President, Patient Care Services
Web address: www.alicehyde.com
**Control:** Other not–for–profit (including NFP Corporation) **Service:** General Medical and Surgical

| Staffed Beds: 135 Admissions: 3073 Census: 104 Outpatient Visits: 167641 Births: 314 Total Expense ($000): 69191 Payroll Expense ($000): 34670 Personnel: 591 |
|---|

## MANHASSET—Nassau County

**MANHASSET AMBULATORY CARE PAVILION** See Long Island Jewish Medical Center, New Hyde Park

✠ **NORTH SHORE UNIVERSITY HOSPITAL (330106)**, 300 Community Drive, Zip 11030–3816; tel. 516/562–0100 **A**1 2 3 5 8 9 10 **F**3 6 7 8 9 11 12 13 14 15 17 18 19 20 21 22 23 24 26 29 30 31 32 34 35 36 37 38 39 40 41 43 44 45 46 48 49 50 51 52 53 54 55 56 57 58 59 60 61 62 63 64 65 66 68 69 70 71 72 73 74 75 76 77 78 79 80 81 82 83 84 85 86 87 88 89 91 92 93 94 97 98 99 100 101 102 103 104 107 108 109 110 111 112 113 114 115 116 117 118 119 120 122 123 125 128 129 130 131 133 134 135 137 140 141 142 143 144 145 146 147 **P**6 **S** North Shore–Long Island Jewish Health System, Great Neck, NY
Primary Contact: Susan Somerville, R.N., Executive Director
CMO: Vicki LoPachin, M.D., Medical Director
CIO: Nympha Meindel, R.N., Chief Information Officer
CHR: Deirdre J. Duke, Associate Executive Director Human Resources
Web address: www.northshorelij.com
**Control:** Other not–for–profit (including NFP Corporation) **Service:** General Medical and Surgical

| Staffed Beds: 804 Admissions: 48787 Census: 758 Outpatient Visits: 716072 Births: 6163 Total Expense ($000): 1508981 Payroll Expense ($000): 729351 Personnel: 14386 |
|---|

## MANHATTAN—New York County, See New York City

## MARCY—Oneida County

☐ **CENTRAL NEW YORK PSYCHIATRIC CENTER**, Zip 13403; tel. 315/765–3600, (Nonreporting) **A**1 **S** New York State Office of Mental Health, Albany, NY
Primary Contact: Maureen Bosco, Interim Executive Director
Web address: www.omh.ny.gov
**Control:** State–Government, nonfederal **Service:** Psychiatric

| Staffed Beds: 226 |
|---|

## MARGARETVILLE—Delaware County

☐ **MARGARETVILLE HOSPITAL (331304)**, 42084 State Highway 28, Zip 12455–2820; tel. 845/586–2631 **A**1 9 10 18 **F**3 7 8 11 15 18 29 31 34 40 45 57 59 75 81 84 87 107 110 118 129 132 134 146 147 **S** HealthAlliance of the Hudson Valley, Kingston, NY
Primary Contact: Sandra A. Horan, Executive Director
CFO: David Scarpino, Chief Financial Officer
CHR: Linda Mead, Director Human Resources
Web address: www.margaretvillehospital.org
**Control:** Other not–for–profit (including NFP Corporation) **Service:** General Medical and Surgical

| Staffed Beds: 15 Admissions: 427 Census: 7 Outpatient Visits: 13859 Births: 0 Total Expense ($000): 10339 Payroll Expense ($000): 4324 Personnel: 104 |
|---|

## MASSENA—St. Lawrence County

✠ **MASSENA MEMORIAL HOSPITAL (330223)**, One Hospital Drive, Zip 13662–1097; tel. 315/764–1711 **A**1 9 10 20 **F**3 8 11 13 15 16 17 18 20 29 31 34 35 40 50 51 55 56 57 59 60 64 70 72 73 76 78 80 81 82 85 86 87 88 89 93 97 107 108 109 110 111 113 115 116 117 118 129 131 134 145 146 **P**3
Primary Contact: Charles F. Fahd, II, Chief Executive Officer
CFO: Sean Curtin, Interim Chief Financial Officer
CMO: Nimesh Desai, M.D., Medical Director
CIO: Jana Grose, Director Management Information Systems
CHR: Jonnie Dorothy, Senior Director Human Resources
CNO: Sue Beaulieu, Chief Nurse Executive
Web address: www.massenahospital.org
**Control:** City–Government, nonfederal **Service:** General Medical and Surgical

| Staffed Beds: 50 Admissions: 2677 Census: 28 Outpatient Visits: 122582 Births: 256 Total Expense ($000): 48300 Payroll Expense ($000): 21209 Personnel: 327 |
|---|

## MEDINA—Orleans County

✠ △ **MEDINA MEMORIAL HOSPITAL (330053)**, 200 Ohio Street, Zip 14103–1095; tel. 585/798–2000, (Nonreporting) **A**1 7 9 10
Primary Contact: James E. Sinner, President and Chief Executive Officer
CFO: Raj Mehta, Chief Financial Officer
CMO: Thomas J. Madejski, M.D., President Medical Staff
CHR: Mary Williams, Director Human Resources
Web address: www.medinamemorial.org
**Control:** Other not–for–profit (including NFP Corporation) **Service:** General Medical and Surgical

| Staffed Beds: 101 |
|---|

**NY**

---

### Hospital, Medicare Provider Number, Address, Telephone, Approval, Facility, and Physician Codes, Health Care System

★ American Hospital Association (AHA) membership
☐ The Joint Commission accreditation
◇ DNV Healthcare Inc. accreditation
○ American Osteopathic Association (AOA) accreditation
△ Commission on Accreditation of Rehabilitation Facilities (CARF) accreditation

## MIDDLETOWN—Orange County

☒ △ **ORANGE REGIONAL MEDICAL CENTER (330126)**, 707 East Main Street,
Zip 10940–2650; tel. 845/333–1000 **A**1 2 7 10 **F**3 5 8 11 12 13 15 17 18 19
20 22 26 28 29 30 31 34 35 40 49 51 54 55 57 59 60 64 68 70 74 75 76
77 78 79 80 81 82 83 84 85 86 87 89 90 93 96 98 99 100 101 102 103
104 105 107 108 110 111 113 114 116 117 118 119 120 122 123 128 129
131 134 143 145 146
Primary Contact: Scott Batulis, Chief Executive Officer
COO: Timothy P. Selz, Vice President
CFO: Mitch Amodo, Vice President and Chief Financial Officer
CMO: James Oxley, D.O., Vice President Medical Affairs
CIO: Shafiq Rab, Chief Information Officer
CHR: Deborah Carr, Vice President Human Resources
Web address: www.ormc.org
**Control:** Other not–for–profit (including NFP Corporation) **Service:** General
Medical and Surgical

**Staffed Beds:** 301 **Admissions:** 20412 **Census:** 293 **Outpatient Visits:**
162201 **Births:** 1607 **Total Expense ($000):** 332117 **Payroll Expense
($000):** 135425

## MINEOLA—Nassau County

☒ **WINTHROP–UNIVERSITY HOSPITAL (330167)**, 259 First Street,
Zip 11501–3957; tel. 516/663–0333, (Includes CHILDREN'S MEDICAL CENTER,
259 First Street, tel. 516/663–0333) **A**1 2 3 5 8 9 10 **F**3 5 8 9 11 12 13 14
15 17 18 19 20 22 24 26 28 29 30 31 32 34 35 38 39 40 41 43 44 45 46
47 48 49 50 51 53 54 55 56 57 58 59 60 61 62 63 64 65 66 68 69 70 71
72 73 74 75 76 77 78 79 81 82 84 85 86 87 88 89 92 93 94 97 100 107
108 110 111 113 114 115 116 117 118 119 120 122 123 125 128 129 130
131 133 134 141 144 145 146 147 **P**5
Primary Contact: John F. Collins, President and Chief Executive Officer
COO: Garry Schwall, Chief Operating Officer
CFO: Palmira Cataliotti, Vice President, Chief Financial Officer and Treasurer
CMO: Steven Fishbane, M.D., Chief Medical Officer
CIO: Nicholas Casabona, Chief Information Officer
CHR: George P. Rainer, Senior Vice President Human Resources
Web address: www.winthrop.org
**Control:** Other not–for–profit (including NFP Corporation) **Service:** General
Medical and Surgical

**Staffed Beds:** 509 **Admissions:** 33213 **Census:** 467 **Outpatient Visits:**
344618 **Births:** 4646 **Total Expense ($000):** 897746 **Payroll Expense
($000):** 325330 **Personnel:** 5865

## MONTOUR FALLS—Schuyler County

☒ **SCHUYLER HOSPITAL (331313)**, 220 Steuben Street, Zip 14865–9709;
tel. 607/535–7121, (Total facility includes 120 beds in nursing home–type unit)
**A**1 9 10 18 **F**11 12 15 18 29 30 34 35 40 45 57 59 64 68 70 75 76 77 79
81 82 85 93 94 97 107 110 111 113 118 127 128 129 130 132 134 145
146 147 **P**6
Primary Contact: Andrew R. Manzer, President and Chief Executive Officer
CMO: Michael Eisman, M.D., Medical Director
CHR: Troy Preston, Director Human Resources
Web address: www.schuylerhospital.org
**Control:** Other not–for–profit (including NFP Corporation) **Service:** General
Medical and Surgical

**Staffed Beds:** 145 **Admissions:** 1196 **Census:** 132 **Outpatient Visits:** 65535
**Births:** 102 **Total Expense ($000):** 32342 **Payroll Expense ($000):** 17248
**Personnel:** 352

## MONTROSE—Westchester County

☒ △ **VETERANS AFFAIRS HUDSON VALLEY HEALTH CARE SYSTEM–F.D.
ROOSEVELT HOSPITAL**, Zip 10548; tel. 914/737–4400, (Includes VETERAN
AFFAIRS HUDSON VALLEY HEALTH CARE SYSTEM–CASTLE POINT DIVISION,
Castle Point, Zip 12511–9999; tel. 914/831–2000; VETERANS AFFAIRS HUDSON
VALLEY HEALTH CARE SYSTEM–MONTROSE DIVISION, tel. 914/737–4400),
(Nonreporting) **A**1 3 5 7 **S** Department of Veterans Affairs, Washington, DC
Primary Contact: Gerald F. Culliton, Director
COO: John M. Grady, Associate Director
CFO: John Walsh, Chief Fiscal Services
CMO: Joanne J. Malina, M.D., Chief of Staff
CIO: Thomas Rooney, Chief Information Resource Management
CHR: Dardanella Russell, Chief Human Resources Management Service
Web address: www.va.gov/sta/guide/home.asp
**Control:** Veterans Affairs, Government, federal **Service:** Psychiatric

**Staffed Beds:** 356

## MOUNT KISCO—Westchester County

☒ **NORTHERN WESTCHESTER HOSPITAL (330162)**, 400 East Main Street,
Zip 10549–3477; tel. 914/666–1200 **A**1 2 5 9 10 **F**3 8 12 13 15 17 18 19 28
29 30 31 32 34 35 36 40 43 46 47 48 49 50 54 55 56 57 59 60 61 64 65
68 70 72 73 74 75 76 78 79 81 82 84 85 86 87 89 91 92 93 97 98 99 100
101 102 103 107 108 109 110 111 113 114 117 118 119 120 122 123 125
128 129 130 131 134 145 146 147
Primary Contact: Joel Seligman, President and Chief Executive Officer
CFO: John Partenza, Vice President and Treasurer
CMO: Marla Koroly, M.D., Chief Medical Officer and Senior Vice President Medical
Affairs
CIO: Sue Prince, Director Information Systems
CHR: Kerry Flynn Barrett, Vice President Human Resources
CNO: Lauraine Szekely, R.N., Senior Vice President, Patient Care
Web address: www.nwhc.net
**Control:** Other not–for–profit (including NFP Corporation) **Service:** General
Medical and Surgical

**Staffed Beds:** 189 **Admissions:** 10120 **Census:** 129 **Outpatient Visits:**
130936 **Births:** 1586

## MOUNT VERNON—Westchester County

☐ **MOUNT VERNON HOSPITAL (330086)**, 12 North Seventh Avenue,
Zip 10550–2098; tel. 914/664–8000, (Nonreporting) **A**1 3 5 9 10 **S** Sound
Shore Health System, New Rochelle, NY
Primary Contact: John R. Spicer, President and Chief Executive Officer
CFO: Albert M. Farina, Chief Financial Officer
CMO: Gary Ishkanian, M.D., Vice President Medical Affairs
CIO: Barbara Cooke, Director Health Information Systems
CHR: Dennis H. Ashley, Vice President Human Resources
Web address: www.sshsw.org
**Control:** Other not–for–profit (including NFP Corporation) **Service:** General
Medical and Surgical

**Staffed Beds:** 132

## NEW HAMPTON—Orange County

☐ **MID–HUDSON FORENSIC PSYCHIATRIC CENTER (334061)**, Route 17M,
Zip 10958, Mailing Address: P.O. Box 158, Zip 10958–0158;
tel. 845/374–8700, (Nonreporting) **A**1 10 **S** New York State Office of Mental
Health, Albany, NY
Primary Contact: Peggi Healy, Executive Director
Web address: www.omh.ny.gov
**Control:** State–Government, nonfederal **Service:** Psychiatric

**Staffed Beds:** 268

## NEW HYDE PARK—Queens County, See New York City

**NEW ROCHELLE—Westchester County**

✠ **SOUND SHORE MEDICAL CENTER OF WESTCHESTER (330184)**, 16 Guion Place, Zip 10801–5502; tel. 914/632–5000, (Nonreporting) **A**1 2 3 5 8 9 10 **S** Sound Shore Health System, New Rochelle, NY
Primary Contact: John R. Spicer, President and Chief Executive Officer
COO: John P. Mamangakis, Senior Vice President
CFO: Albert M. Farina, Senior Vice President and Chief Financial Officer
CMO: Richard Barone, M.D., Medical Director
CIO: Barbara Cooke, Director Health Information Systems
CHR: Dennis H. Ashley, Vice President Human Resources
CNO: Pamela M. Dupuis, R.N., Senior Vice President and Patient Care Services
Web address: www.sshsw.org
**Control:** Other not–for–profit (including NFP Corporation) **Service:** General Medical and Surgical

Staffed Beds: 356

**NEW YORK (Includes all hospitals located within the five boroughs)**
**BRONX** - Bronx County (Mailing Address - Bronx)
**BROOKLYN** - Kings County (Mailing Address - Brooklyn)
**MANHATTAN** - New York County (Mailing Address - New York)
**QUEENS** - Queens County (Mailing Addresses - Bellerose, Elmhurst, Far Rockaway, Flushing, Forest Hills, Glen Oaks, Holliswood, Jackson Heights, Jamaica, Little Neck, Long Island City, New Hyde Park, and Queens Village)
**RICHMOND VALLEY** - Richmond County (Mailing Address - Staten Island)

✠ **BELLEVUE HOSPITAL CENTER (330204)**, 462 First Avenue, Zip 10016–9198; tel. 212/562–4141 **A**1 3 5 8 9 10 **F**3 4 5 8 11 12 13 15 17 18 20 22 24 26 28 29 30 31 34 35 36 38 39 40 41 43 44 45 46 48 49 50 52 55 56 57 58 59 60 61 63 64 65 66 68 70 71 72 74 75 76 77 78 79 81 82 83 84 85 86 87 88 89 90 91 93 94 96 97 98 99 100 101 102 103 104 105 107 108 110 111 113 114 117 118 129 130 131 133 134 142 143 145 146 147 **S** New York City Health and Hospitals Corporation, New York, NY
Primary Contact: Lynda D. Curtis, Senior Vice President and Executive Director
COO: Steven Alexander, Chief Operating Officer
CFO: Aaron Cohen, Chief Financial Officer
CMO: Nate Link, M.D., Medical Director
CIO: Eli Tarlow, Chief Information Officer
CHR: Howard Kritz, Director Human Resources
CNO: Moftia Aujero, Chief Nurse Executive
Web address: www.nyc.gov/bellevue
**Control:** City–Government, nonfederal **Service:** General Medical and Surgical

Staffed Beds: 828 Admissions: 29575 Census: 689 Outpatient Visits: 637143 Births: 1827 Total Expense ($000): 730157 Payroll Expense ($000): 304610 Personnel: 4745

✠ **BETH ISRAEL MEDICAL CENTER (330169)**, First Avenue and 16th Street, Zip 10003–3803; tel. 212/420–2000, (Includes BETH ISRAEL MEDICAL CENTER–KINGS HIGHWAY DIVISION, 3201 Kings Highway, Brooklyn, Zip 11234; tel. 718/252–3000), (Total facility includes 28 beds in nursing home–type unit) **A**1 2 3 5 8 9 10 **F**3 4 5 7 8 9 11 13 14 15 17 18 19 20 22 24 26 28 29 30 31 32 33 34 35 36 38 39 40 41 43 44 45 46 47 48 49 50 51 52 54 55 57 58 59 60 61 64 65 66 68 70 72 74 75 76 77 78 79 80 81 82 83 84 85 86 87 88 89 90 92 93 94 96 97 98 99 100 101 102 103 104 107 108 110 111 113 114 117 118 119 120 122 125 128 129 130 131 134 140 143 144 145 146 147 **P**6 **S** Continuum Health Partners, New York, NY
Primary Contact: Harris M. Nagler, M.D., President
COO: Kevin Molloy, Senior Vice President and Chief Operating Officer
CFO: John Collura, Executive Vice President Financial Services and Chief Financial Officer
CMO: David Bernard, M.D., Chief Medical Officer
CIO: Bonnie Sessa, Vice President and Chief Information Officer
CHR: Marvin Russell, Corporate Senior Vice President Human Resources
Web address: www.bethisraelny.org
**Control:** Other not–for–profit (including NFP Corporation) **Service:** General Medical and Surgical

Staffed Beds: 840 Admissions: 55519 Census: 841 Outpatient Visits: 554269 Births: 3871 Total Expense ($000): 1433830 Payroll Expense ($000): 704125 Personnel: 8548

☐ **BRONX CHILDREN'S PSYCHIATRIC CENTER**, 1000 Waters Place, Bronx, Zip 10461–2799; tel. 718/239–3600, (Nonreporting) **A**1 **S** New York State Office of Mental Health, Albany, NY
Primary Contact: June Dacosta, Acting Executive Director
Web address: www.omh.ny.gov
**Control:** State–Government, nonfederal **Service:** Children's hospital psychiatric

Staffed Beds: 75

☐ **BRONX PSYCHIATRIC CENTER (334053)**, 1500 Waters Place, Bronx, Zip 10461–2796; tel. 718/931–0600, (Nonreporting) **A**1 3 5 10 **S** New York State Office of Mental Health, Albany, NY
Primary Contact: Pamela Turner, Executive Director
CFO: Robert Erway, Director for Administration
Web address: www.omh.ny.gov
**Control:** State–Government, nonfederal **Service:** Psychiatric

Staffed Beds: 450

✠ **BRONX–LEBANON HOSPITAL CENTER HEALTH CARE SYSTEM (330009)**, 1276 Fulton Avenue, Bronx, Zip 10456–3499; tel. 718/590–1800, (Includes BRONX–LEBANON SPECIAL CARE CENTER, 1265 Fulton Avenue, Zip 10465; tel. 718/579–7000; CONCOURSE DIVISION, 1650 Grand Concourse, Zip 10457; tel. 718/590–1800; FULTON DIVISION, 1276 Fulton Avenue, Zip 10456; tel. 718/590–1800; HIGHBRIDGE WOODYCREST CENTER, 936 Woodycrest Avenue, Zip 10452; tel. 718/293–3200), (Nonreporting) **A**1 3 5 8 9 10
Primary Contact: Miguel A. Fuentes, Jr., President and Chief Executive Officer
COO: Steven Anderman, Chief Operating Officer
CFO: Victor DeMarco, Chief Financial Officer
CMO: Milton A. Gumbs, M.D., Vice President and Medical Director
CIO: Ivan Durbak, Chief Information Officer
CHR: Selena Griffin–Mahon, Assistant Vice President Human Resources
Web address: www.bronxcare.org
**Control:** Other not–for–profit (including NFP Corporation) **Service:** General Medical and Surgical

Staffed Beds: 784

☐ **BROOKDALE HOSPITAL MEDICAL CENTER (330233)**, One Brookdale Plaza, Brooklyn, Zip 11212–3139; tel. 718/240–5000, (Total facility includes 448 beds in nursing home–type unit) **A**1 3 5 9 10 **F**2 5 8 10 12 13 14 15 17 18 19 20 21 22 28 29 30 31 32 34 35 38 39 40 41 43 46 50 51 52 54 55 56 57 58 59 60 61 62 63 64 65 66 69 70 71 72 73 74 75 76 77 78 79 80 81 82 84 85 86 87 88 89 93 96 97 98 99 100 101 102 103 104 105 106 107 108 110 111 118 125 127 128 129 130 131 133 134 144 145 146 147 **P**7
Primary Contact: Mark Toney, President and Chief Executive Officer
CFO: Mounir F. Doss, Executive Vice President and Chief Financial Officer
CMO: Richard Fogler, M.D., Chairman Surgery and Chief Medical Officer
CIO: Douglas Thompson, Director Information Systems
CHR: Max Sclair, Vice President Human Resources
Web address: www.brookdalehospital.org
**Control:** Other not–for–profit (including NFP Corporation) **Service:** General Medical and Surgical

Staffed Beds: 734 Admissions: 19251 Census: 737 Outpatient Visits: 242955 Births: 1547 Total Expense ($000): 522494 Payroll Expense ($000): 208058 Personnel: 1638

☐ **BROOKLYN CHILDREN'S PSYCHIATRIC CENTER**, 1819 Bergen Street, Brooklyn, Zip 11233–4513; tel. 718/221–4500, (Nonreporting) **A**1 3 5 **S** New York State Office of Mental Health, Albany, NY
Primary Contact: Diane Aman, Acting Executive Director
Web address: www.omh.ny.gov
**Control:** State–Government, nonfederal **Service:** Children's Psychiatric

Staffed Beds: 36

☐ **BROOKLYN HOSPITAL CENTER (330056)**, 121 DeKalb Avenue, Brooklyn, Zip 11201–5425; tel. 718/250–8000, (Nonreporting) **A**1 2 3 5 8 9 10 **S** New York Presbyterian Healthcare System, New York, NY
Primary Contact: Richard B. Becker, M.D., President, Chief Executive Officer and Interim Chief Medical Officer
COO: W. Trent Crable, Executive Vice President and Chief Operating Officer
CFO: Joseph Guarracino, Senior Vice President and Chief Financial Officer
CIO: Irene Farrelly, Vice President and Chief Information Officer
CHR: Ira Warm, Senior Vice President Human Resources
Web address: www.tbh.org
**Control:** Other not–for–profit (including NFP Corporation) **Service:** General Medical and Surgical

Staffed Beds: 374

---

**Hospital, Medicare Provider Number, Address, Telephone, Approval, Facility, and Physician Codes, Health Care System**

★ American Hospital Association (AHA) membership
☐ The Joint Commission accreditation
◇ DNV Healthcare Inc. accreditation
○ American Osteopathic Association (AOA) accreditation
△ Commission on Accreditation of Rehabilitation Facilities (CARF) accreditation

**NY**

✠ **CALVARY HOSPITAL (332006)**, 1740 Eastchester Road, Bronx, Zip 10461–2392; tel. 718/863–6900 **A**1 9 10 **F**1 29 30 35 39 62 63 64 68 74 78 82 84 87 118 120 129 131 133 145 147 **P**6
Primary Contact: Frank A. Calamari, President and Chief Executive Officer
COO: Richard J. Kutilek, Chief Operating Officer
CFO: Andrew Greco, Chief Financial Officer
CMO: Michael J. Brescia, M.D., Executive Medical Director
CIO: Patrick Martin, Director Information Systems
CHR: Michael T. Troncone, Chief Human Resources Officer
Web address: www.calvaryhospital.org
**Control:** Church–operated, Nongovernment, not–for profit **Service:** Long–Term Acute Care hospital

**Staffed Beds:** 225 **Admissions:** 3023 **Census:** 210 **Outpatient Visits:** 118973 **Births:** 0 **Total Expense ($000):** 108820 **Payroll Expense ($000):** 56149 **Personnel:** 764

✠ △ **COLER–GOLDWATER SPECIALTY HOSPITAL AND NURSING FACILITY (332008)**, One Main Street, Zip 10044; tel. 212/318–8000, (Includes COLER MEMORIAL HOSPITAL, Roosevelt Island, tel. 212/848–6000; GOLDWATER MEMORIAL HOSPITAL, Franklin D. Roosevelt Island, tel. 212/318–8000), (Total facility includes 1389 beds in nursing home–type unit) **A**1 3 5 7 10 **F**1 3 11 28 29 30 39 58 61 68 74 75 77 85 87 90 100 103 107 113 118 127 129 131 134 145 147 **P**4 **S** New York City Health and Hospitals Corporation, New York, NY
Primary Contact: Robert Hughes, Executive Director
CFO: Gloria Ranghelli, Deputy Chief Financial Officer
CMO: Yolanda Bruno, M.D., Medical Director
CHR: Howard Kritz, Director
Web address: www.coler–goldwater.org
**Control:** City–Government, nonfederal **Service:** General Medical and Surgical

**Staffed Beds:** 2016 **Admissions:** 2371 **Census:** 1802 **Outpatient Visits:** 0 **Births:** 0

**CONCOURSE DIVISION** See Bronx–Lebanon Hospital Center Health Care System, Bronx

✠ **CONEY ISLAND HOSPITAL (330196)**, 2601 Ocean Parkway, Brooklyn, Zip 11235–7795; tel. 718/616–3000 **A**1 3 5 8 9 10 12 13 **F**3 4 5 8 9 11 13 15 17 18 19 20 28 29 30 31 32 34 35 38 39 40 41 45 46 49 50 51 54 55 56 57 58 59 60 61 64 65 66 68 70 71 73 74 75 76 77 78 79 81 82 83 84 85 87 89 90 91 93 94 96 97 98 99 100 102 103 104 106 107 108 110 111 113 114 117 118 129 131 134 142 145 146 147 **S** New York City Health and Hospitals Corporation, New York, NY
Primary Contact: Arthur Wagner, Senior Vice President and Executive Director
COO: Mary Mong, R.N., Chief Operating Officer
CFO: Paul Pandolfini, Chief Financial Officer
CMO: John Maese, M.D., Chief Medical Officer
CIO: Silvana DeSimone, Chief Information Officer
CHR: Rodney Parker, Senior Associate Executive Director
Web address: www.ci.nyc.ny.us/html/hhc/html/coneyisland.html
**Control:** City–Government, nonfederal **Service:** General Medical and Surgical

**Staffed Beds:** 371 **Admissions:** 17917 **Census:** 332 **Outpatient Visits:** 363216 **Births:** 1267 **Total Expense ($000):** 369219 **Payroll Expense ($000):** 163483 **Personnel:** 2915

☐ **CREEDMOOR PSYCHIATRIC CENTER (334004)**, 79–25 Winchester Boulevard, Jamaica, Zip 11427–2199; tel. 718/264–3600 **A**1 10 **F**29 30 54 98 104 129 **S** New York State Office of Mental Health, Albany, NY
Primary Contact: William A. Fisher, M.D., Executive Director
CFO: Viodelda Ho–Shing, Deputy Director Administration
CIO: Connie Mitchell, Ph.D., Chief Information Officer
CHR: Rhonda Cicha, Director Human Resources
Web address: www.omh.ny.gov
**Control:** State–Government, nonfederal **Service:** Psychiatric

**Staffed Beds:** 380 **Admissions:** 280 **Census:** 392 **Births:** 0 **Total Expense ($000):** 131940 **Personnel:** 1054

✠ **ELMHURST HOSPITAL CENTER (330128)**, 79–01 Broadway, Elmhurst, Zip 11373–1329; tel. 718/334–4000 **A**1 2 3 5 8 9 10 **F**5 8 9 13 15 17 18 20 22 29 30 31 32 34 35 38 40 41 43 50 51 53 55 56 57 59 60 61 64 68 70 72 73 74 75 76 77 78 79 81 86 87 88 89 90 93 97 99 100 101 102 103 104 105 107 108 110 111 114 118 120 125 129 130 131 133 134 142 145 146 **P**6 **S** New York City Health and Hospitals Corporation, New York, NY
Primary Contact: Chris D. Constantino, Executive Director
COO: Wayne Zimmermann, Chief Operating Officer
CFO: Brian Stacey, Chief Financial Officer
CMO: Jasmin Moshirpur, M.D., Dean and Medical Director
CIO: Vincent Smith, Chief Information Officer
CHR: Jeannith Gangemi–Sosa, Associate Executive Director
CNO: Joann Gull, Chief Nursing Officer
Web address: www.elmhursthospitalcenter.org
**Control:** City–Government, nonfederal **Service:** General Medical and Surgical

**Staffed Beds:** 551 **Admissions:** 25563 **Census:** 462 **Outpatient Visits:** 703644 **Births:** 3748 **Total Expense ($000):** 574377 **Payroll Expense ($000):** 228413 **Personnel:** 3220

☐ **FLUSHING HOSPITAL MEDICAL CENTER (330193)**, 4500 Parsons Boulevard, Flushing, Zip 11355–2205; tel. 718/670–5000 **A**1 3 5 9 10 **F**3 4 5 7 8 11 13 15 17 18 29 30 31 32 34 35 36 39 40 41 45 56 57 59 60 61 64 65 68 70 71 72 74 75 76 77 78 79 81 82 84 85 87 89 91 92 93 97 98 100 101 102 103 104 107 110 111 113 118 129 131 134 145 146 147 **P**5 7
Primary Contact: Bruce J. Flanz, President and Chief Executive Officer
COO: Robert V. Levine, Executive Vice President and Chief Operating Officer
CFO: Mounir F. Doss, Executive Vice President and Chief Financial Officer
CMO: Peter Barra, M.D., Chief Medical Officer
CIO: Tony Gatto, Director Management Information Systems
CHR: Max Sclair, Vice President Human Resources
Web address: www.flushinghospital.org
**Control:** Other not–for–profit (including NFP Corporation) **Service:** General Medical and Surgical

**Staffed Beds:** 293 **Admissions:** 16604 **Census:** 261 **Outpatient Visits:** 166437 **Births:** 2874 **Total Expense ($000):** 267029 **Payroll Expense ($000):** 115414 **Personnel:** 1566

✠ **FOREST HILLS HOSPITAL (330353)**, 102–01 66th Road, Forest Hills, Zip 11375–2029; tel. 718/830–4000 **A**1 2 9 10 **F**3 8 12 13 15 18 29 30 31 34 35 37 38 40 43 45 46 49 50 51 52 55 57 58 59 60 64 65 66 68 70 73 74 75 76 77 78 79 81 82 84 85 86 87 97 100 102 107 111 113 118 123 129 131 134 142 145 146 147 **P**6 **S** North Shore–Long Island Jewish Health System, Great Neck, NY
Primary Contact: Rita Mercieca, R.N., Executive Director
COO: Mark J. Solazzo, Senior Vice President and Chief Operating Officer
CFO: Robert S. Shapiro, Senior Vice President and Chief Financial Officer
CMO: Lawrence Smith, M.D., Senior Vice President and Chief Medical Officer
CIO: John Bosco, Vice President and Chief Information Officer
CHR: Joseph Cabral, Vice President and Chief Human Resources Officer
Web address: www.northshorelij.com
**Control:** Other not–for–profit (including NFP Corporation) **Service:** General Medical and Surgical

**Staffed Beds:** 242 **Admissions:** 16738 **Census:** 219 **Outpatient Visits:** 72746 **Births:** 2333 **Total Expense ($000):** 204860 **Payroll Expense ($000):** 98199 **Personnel:** 1315

**FULTON DIVISION** See Bronx–Lebanon Hospital Center Health Care System, Bronx

**GOLDWATER MEMORIAL HOSPITAL** See Coler–Goldwater Specialty Hospital and Nursing Facility

☐ **GRACIE SQUARE HOSPITAL (334048)**, 420 East 76th Street, Zip 10021–3104; tel. 212/988–4400, (Nonreporting) **A**1 9 10 **S** New York Presbyterian Healthcare System, New York, NY
Primary Contact: Frank Bruno, Chief Executive Officer
Web address: www.nygsh.org
**Control:** Other not–for–profit (including NFP Corporation) **Service:** Psychiatric

**Staffed Beds:** 157

✠ △ **HARLEM HOSPITAL CENTER (330240)**, 506 Lenox Avenue, Zip 10037–1894; tel. 212/939–1000, (Includes HARLEM GENERAL CARE UNIT AND HARLEM PSYCHIATRIC UNIT ) **A**1 3 5 7 8 9 10 **F**2 3 4 5 8 11 12 13 15 16 17 18 19 22 29 30 31 32 34 35 38 39 40 41 43 44 45 49 50 52 53 55 57 58 59 60 61 62 64 65 68 70 71 72 73 74 75 76 77 78 79 80 81 82 84 85 86 87 88 89 90 93 94 95 96 97 98 99 100 101 102 104 107 108 110 111 113 117 118 129 131 133 134 140 141 143 145 146 147 **S** New York City Health and Hospitals Corporation, New York, NY
Primary Contact: Denise C. Soares, R.N., Executive Director
Web address: www.nyc.gov/html/hhc/harlem
**Control:** City–Government, nonfederal **Service:** General Medical and Surgical

**Staffed Beds:** 272 **Admissions:** 11986 **Census:** 201 **Outpatient Visits:** 329656 **Births:** 1066 **Total Expense ($000):** 345516 **Payroll Expense ($000):** 151270 **Personnel:** 2208

☐ **HOLLISWOOD HOSPITAL (334055)**, 87–37 Palermo Street, Jamaica, Zip 11423–1209; tel. 718/776–8181, (Nonreporting) **A**1 10 **S** Liberty Management Group, Inc.
Primary Contact: Alan Eskenazi, Chief Executive Officer
CMO: Jeffrey Borenstein, M.D., Medical Director
CHR: Dorothy A. Muller, Director Human Resources
Web address: www.holliswoodhospital.com
**Control:** Corporation, Investor–owned, for–profit **Service:** Psychiatric

**Staffed Beds:** 125

**NY**

*Many Facility Codes have changed. Please refer to the AHA Guide Code Chart.* © 2012 AHA Guide

★ **HOSPITAL FOR SPECIAL SURGERY (330270)**, 535 East 70th Street, Zip 10021–4898; tel. 212/606–1000 **A**3 5 8 9 10 **F**3 8 9 29 30 32 33 34 35 36 37 38 43 44 50 53 54 56 57 58 59 64 66 68 74 75 77 79 80 81 82 84 85 86 87 89 92 93 94 97 100 107 109 111 113 114 115 116 117 118 120 122 125 129 130 131 133 140 141 145 146 **P**8 **S** New York Presbyterian Healthcare System, New York, NY
Primary Contact: Louis A. Shapiro, President and Chief Executive Officer
COO: Lisa Goldstein, Executive Vice President and Chief Operating Officer
CFO: Stacey Malakoff, Executive Vice President and Chief Financial Officer
CMO: Thomas P. Sculco, M.D., Surgeon–in–Chief and Medical Director
CIO: Jamie Mooney, Vice President and Chief Information Officer
CHR: Bruce Slawitsky, Vice President Human Resources
CNO: Stephanie J. Goldberg, MSN, Senior Vice President and Chief Nursing Officer
Web address: www.hss.edu
**Control:** Other not–for–profit (including NFP Corporation) **Service:** Orthopedic

**Staffed Beds:** 188 **Admissions:** 13457 **Census:** 146 **Outpatient Visits:** 320727 **Births:** 0 **Total Expense ($000):** 614823 **Payroll Expense ($000):** 252823 **Personnel:** 3391

☐ **INTERFAITH MEDICAL CENTER (330397)**, 1545 Atlantic Avenue, Brooklyn, Zip 11213; tel. 718/613–4000, (Nonreporting) **A**1 3 5 9 10
Primary Contact: Laura Gaffney, President and Chief Executive Officer
CFO: Gregg Dixon, CPA, Chief Financial Officer
CMO: Jochanan Weisenfreund, M.D., Senior Vice President Academic and Medical Affairs
CIO: Mark Lederman, Chief Information Officer
CHR: Venra Mathurin, Vice President Human Resources
Web address: www.interfaithmedical.com
**Control:** Other not–for–profit (including NFP Corporation) **Service:** General Medical and Surgical

**Staffed Beds:** 277

**JACK D WEILER HOSPITAL OF ALBERT EINSTEIN COLLEGE OF MEDICINE**
See Montefiore Medical Center, Bronx

⊠ **JACOBI MEDICAL CENTER (330127)**, 1400 Pelham Parkway South, Bronx, Zip 10461–1197; tel. 718/918–5000 **A**1 3 8 9 10 **F**3 4 5 8 11 12 13 15 16 17 18 26 29 30 31 32 34 35 38 39 40 41 43 44 45 46 47 50 51 55 56 57 58 59 60 61 62 64 65 66 68 70 72 73 74 75 76 77 78 79 80 81 82 84 85 87 88 89 90 92 93 94 96 97 98 99 100 101 102 103 104 107 108 110 111 113 116 118 129 130 131 133 134 143 145 146 147 **P**6 **S** New York City Health and Hospitals Corporation, New York, NY
Primary Contact: William P. Walsh, Senior Vice President and Executive Director
COO: Christopher Fugazy, Chief Operating Officer
CFO: Kathy Garramone, Chief Financial Officer
CMO: Joseph Skarzynski, M.D., Medical Director
CIO: Diane Carr, Chief Information Officer
CHR: Dolores Leite, Chief Human Resource Executive
CNO: Ellen O'Connor, Chief Nursing Officer
Web address: www.nyc.gov/html/hhc/jacobi/home.html
**Control:** City–Government, nonfederal **Service:** General Medical and Surgical

**Staffed Beds:** 457 **Admissions:** 20083 **Census:** 374 **Outpatient Visits:** 464025 **Births:** 2072 **Total Expense ($000):** 607426 **Payroll Expense ($000):** 253022 **Personnel:** 3867

⊠ **JAMAICA HOSPITAL MEDICAL CENTER (330014)**, 8900 Van Wyck Expressway, Jamaica, Zip 11418–2832; tel. 718/206–6000 **A**1 3 5 9 10 13 **F**1 3 7 11 13 15 17 18 19 20 22 26 29 30 31 34 35 36 39 40 43 44 45 49 50 52 53 54 55 56 57 58 59 60 61 62 64 65 66 68 70 71 72 73 74 75 76 77 78 79 80 81 82 83 84 85 86 87 89 90 92 93 94 96 97 98 100 101 102 103 104 107 108 110 111 113 114 117 118 129 130 131 133 134 142 143 145 146 **P**5 7 8
Primary Contact: Bruce J. Flanz, President and Chief Executive Officer
CFO: Mounir F. Doss, Executive Vice President and Chief Financial Officer
CMO: Anthony Di Maria, M.D., Medical Director
CIO: Richard Hlavenka, Director Management Information Systems
CHR: Max Sclair, Vice President Human Resources
Web address: www.Jamaicahospital.org
**Control:** Other not–for–profit (including NFP Corporation) **Service:** General Medical and Surgical

**Staffed Beds:** 424 **Admissions:** 22674 **Census:** 345 **Outpatient Visits:** 361176 **Births:** 2713 **Total Expense ($000):** 538493 **Payroll Expense ($000):** 221145 **Personnel:** 2974

⊠ **KINGS COUNTY HOSPITAL CENTER (330202)**, 451 Clarkson Avenue, Brooklyn, Zip 11203–2097; tel. 718/245–3131 **A**1 2 3 5 8 9 10 **F**3 4 5 8 9 11 12 13 15 17 18 19 20 24 26 28 29 30 31 32 34 35 38 39 40 41 43 46 47 49 50 51 52 53 56 57 58 59 60 61 64 65 68 70 71 72 73 74 75 76 77 78 79 80 81 82 83 84 85 86 87 88 89 90 91 92 93 94 97 98 99 100 101 102 103 104 106 107 108 110 111 113 114 115 118 119 120 122 128 129 130 131 133 134 142 143 144 145 146 147 **P**6 **S** New York City Health and Hospitals Corporation, New York, NY
Primary Contact: Antonio D. Martin, Senior Vice President and Executive Director
COO: Roslyn Weinstein, Chief Operating Officer
CFO: Julian John, Chief Financial Officer
CMO: Abha Agrawal, M.D., Medical Director
CIO: Dino Civan, Chief Information Officer
CHR: Raquel Ayala, Deputy Executive Director Network and Human Resources
Web address: www.ci.nyc.ny.us/html/hhc/html/kings.html
**Control:** City–Government, nonfederal **Service:** General Medical and Surgical

**Staffed Beds:** 601 **Admissions:** 25101 **Census:** 515 **Outpatient Visits:** 760749 **Births:** 2602 **Total Expense ($000):** 729808 **Payroll Expense ($000):** 381283 **Personnel:** 5253

☐ **KINGSBORO PSYCHIATRIC CENTER (334058)**, 681 Clarkson Avenue, Brooklyn, Zip 11203–2125; tel. 718/221–7395, (Nonreporting) **A**1 3 5 10 **S** New York State Office of Mental Health, Albany, NY
Primary Contact: James McCummings, Executive Director
COO: James McCummings, Executive Director
CFO: Yinusa Awolowo, Business Officer
CMO: Jeffery Lucey, M.D., Clinical Director
CIO: George Gavora, Director Program Evaluation
CHR: Geraldine Cody, Director Human Resources
Web address: www.omh.ny.gov/omhweb/facilities/kbpc/facility/htm
**Control:** State–Government, nonfederal **Service:** Psychiatric

**Staffed Beds:** 290

⊠ △ **KINGSBROOK JEWISH MEDICAL CENTER (330201)**, 585 Schenectady Avenue, Brooklyn, Zip 11203–1891; tel. 718/604–5000, (Total facility includes 492 beds in nursing home–type unit) **A**1 3 5 7 9 10 **F**3 8 15 17 18 28 29 30 34 35 39 40 45 46 48 49 50 54 56 57 59 60 61 64 65 68 70 74 75 77 78 79 80 81 82 84 85 87 89 90 91 92 93 94 96 97 98 100 101 103 104 107 108 110 111 113 114 118 127 129 130 134 142 145 146 147
Primary Contact: Linda Brady, M.D., President and Chief Executive Officer
COO: Robert Dubicki, Executive Vice President and Chief Operating Officer
CFO: John Schmitt, Senior Vice President and Chief Financial Officer
CMO: Sibte Burney, M.D., Senior Vice President Medical Affairs and Chief Medical Officer
CIO: Daniel Morreale, Vice President and Chief Information Officer
CHR: John McKeon, Vice President Human Resources
CNO: Jane Lederer, R.N., Vice President and Chief Nursing Officer
Web address: www.kingsbrook.org
**Control:** Other not–for–profit (including NFP Corporation) **Service:** General Medical and Surgical

**Staffed Beds:** 775 **Admissions:** 11824 **Census:** 683 **Outpatient Visits:** 123366 **Births:** 0 **Total Expense ($000):** 261172 **Payroll Expense ($000):** 136823 **Personnel:** 1900

★ **LENOX HILL HOSPITAL (330119)**, 100 East 77th Street, Zip 10075–1850; tel. 212/434–2000, (Includes MANHATTAN EYE, EAR AND THROAT HOSPITAL, 210 East 64th Street, Zip 10021–9885; tel. 212/838–9200; Philip P. Rosenthal, Executive Director) **A**3 5 8 9 10 **F**7 8 9 11 12 13 14 15 17 18 20 22 24 26 29 30 31 32 34 35 37 38 39 40 43 44 47 48 49 50 51 54 55 58 59 60 61 62 63 64 65 66 68 70 72 74 75 76 77 78 79 81 82 84 85 86 87 89 91 92 93 94 97 98 99 100 101 102 103 104 105 107 108 111 114 116 117 118 125 129 130 131 134 142 145 146 147 **P**6 **S** North Shore–Long Island Jewish Health System, Great Neck, NY
Primary Contact: Frank J. Danza, Executive Director
COO: Philip P. Rosenthal, Executive Director
CFO: Michael P. Breslin, Executive Vice President and Chief Financial Officer
CMO: Marc L. Napp, M.D., Vice President Medical Affairs
CIO: Beth Dituro, Divisional Chief Information Officer
CHR: Glenn Courounis, Vice President Human Resources
Web address: www.lenoxhillhospital.org
**Control:** Other not–for–profit (including NFP Corporation) **Service:** General Medical and Surgical

**Staffed Beds:** 539 **Admissions:** 29222 **Census:** 383 **Outpatient Visits:** 186627 **Births:** 4186 **Total Expense ($000):** 643761 **Payroll Expense ($000):** 298786 **Personnel:** 4023

**NY**

---

**Hospital, Medicare Provider Number, Address, Telephone, Approval, Facility, and Physician Codes, Health Care System**

★ American Hospital Association (AHA) membership
☐ The Joint Commission accreditation          ◇ DNV Healthcare Inc. accreditation

◯ American Osteopathic Association (AOA) accreditation
△ Commission on Accreditation of Rehabilitation Facilities (CARF) accreditation

✠ **LINCOLN MEDICAL AND MENTAL HEALTH CENTER (330080)**, 234 East 149th Street, Bronx, Zip 10451–5504; tel. 718/579–5700 **A**1 2 3 5 8 9 10 **F**3 5 8 11 13 15 18 19 29 30 31 32 34 35 38 39 40 41 43 45 50 55 56 57 58 59 60 61 64 65 66 68 70 71 72 73 74 75 76 77 78 79 81 82 84 86 87 88 89 93 97 98 99 100 101 102 103 104 107 108 110 111 113 114 118 129 131 133 134 142 143 145 146 147 **P**4 **S** New York City Health and Hospitals Corporation, New York, NY
Primary Contact: Iris Jimenez–Hernandez, Senior Vice President and Executive Director
COO: Lauren Johnston, Deputy Executive Director
CFO: Victor Bekker, Chief Financial Officer
CMO: Melissa Schori, M.D., Medical Director
CIO: Maricar Barrameda, Chief Information Officer
CHR: Jeannith Gangemi–Sosa, Senior Associate Executive Director
Web address: www.nyc.gov/html/hhc/lincoln/
**Control:** City–Government, nonfederal **Service:** General Medical and Surgical

**Staffed Beds:** 335 **Admissions:** 23456 **Census:** 257 **Outpatient Visits:** 603973 **Births:** 2461 **Total Expense ($000):** 395357 **Payroll Expense ($000):** 196536 **Personnel:** 3218

✠ **LONG ISLAND JEWISH MEDICAL CENTER (330195)**, 270–05 76th Avenue, New Hyde Park, Zip 11040–1496; tel. 718/470–7000, (Includes MANHASSET AMBULATORY CARE PAVILION, 1554 Northern Boulevard, Manhasset, Zip 11030; tel. 516/365–2070; STEVEN AND ALEXANDRA COHEN CHILDREN'S MEDICAL CENTER OF NEW YORK, 270–05 76th Avenue, Zip 11040; tel. 718/470–3000; ZUCKER HILLSIDE HOSPITAL, 75–59 263rd Street, Glen Oaks, Zip 11004; tel. 718/470–8000) **A**1 2 3 5 8 9 10 13 **F**2 3 5 6 7 8 9 10 11 12 13 14 15 17 18 19 20 21 22 23 24 25 26 27 29 30 31 32 34 35 38 39 40 41 43 44 45 46 47 48 49 50 51 52 53 54 55 56 57 58 59 60 61 62 63 64 65 66 68 70 72 73 74 75 76 77 78 79 81 82 83 84 85 86 87 88 89 92 93 97 98 99 100 101 102 103 104 105 106 107 108 109 110 111 113 114 115 116 117 118 119 120 122 123 125 128 129 130 131 133 134 135 140 141 142 143 145 146 147 **P**6 **S** North Shore–Long Island Jewish Health System, Great Neck, NY
Primary Contact: Chantal Weinhold, Executive Director
CMO: Jeremy Boal, M.D., Medical Director
CIO: Jim Bosco, Chief Information Officer
CHR: Ronald W. Stone, Regional Chief Human Resource Officer
Web address: www.lij.edu
**Control:** Other not–for–profit (including NFP Corporation) **Service:** General Medical and Surgical

**Staffed Beds:** 840 **Admissions:** 46094 **Census:** 780 **Outpatient Visits:** 694297 **Births:** 4969 **Total Expense ($000):** 1399943 **Payroll Expense ($000):** 675450 **Personnel:** 14501

✠ **LUTHERAN MEDICAL CENTER (330306)**, 150 55th Street, Brooklyn, Zip 11220–2559; tel. 718/630–7000 **A**1 3 5 9 10 13 **F**3 4 5 7 8 11 12 13 14 15 17 18 20 22 29 30 31 32 34 35 36 38 39 40 43 49 50 51 55 58 59 60 61 62 63 64 65 66 68 70 71 72 73 74 75 76 77 78 79 81 82 83 84 85 86 87 89 90 91 92 93 94 97 98 100 101 102 103 104 107 108 111 113 118 120 124 128 129 130 131 142 145 146 147 **P**6
Primary Contact: Wendy Z. Goldstein, President and Chief Executive Officer
COO: Claudia Caine, Executive Vice President and Chief Operating Officer
CFO: Richard Langfelder, Executive Vice President and Chief Financial Officer
CMO: Beth Raucher, M.D., Senior Vice President and Chief Medical Officer
CIO: Steve Art, Senior Vice President and Chief Information Officer
CHR: Frank Scheets, Senior Vice President
Web address: www.lmcmc.com
**Control:** Church–operated, Nongovernment, not–for profit **Service:** General Medical and Surgical

**Staffed Beds:** 393 **Admissions:** 24111 **Census:** 345 **Outpatient Visits:** 705140 **Births:** 4298 **Total Expense ($000):** 517339 **Payroll Expense ($000):** 247119 **Personnel:** 3768

✠ **MAIMONIDES MEDICAL CENTER (330194)**, 4802 Tenth Avenue, Brooklyn, Zip 11219–2916; tel. 718/283–6000, (Includes MAIMONIDES INFANTS AND CHILDREN'S HOSPITAL OF BROOKLYN, 4802 Tenth Avenue, tel. 718/283–6000) **A**1 2 3 5 8 9 10 12 13 **F**2 3 7 8 9 11 12 13 14 15 17 18 19 20 22 24 26 28 29 30 31 32 34 35 38 39 40 41 44 45 46 47 48 49 50 51 52 54 55 56 57 58 59 60 61 64 65 66 68 70 72 73 74 75 76 77 78 79 81 82 84 85 86 87 88 89 91 92 93 96 97 99 100 101 102 103 104 107 108 110 111 113 114 115 116 117 118 119 120 122 123 125 128 129 130 131 133 134 144 145 146 147 **P**5 6
Primary Contact: Pamela S. Brier, President and Chief Executive Officer
COO: Mark McDougle, Executive Vice President and Chief Operating Officer
CFO: Robert Naldi, Chief Financial Officer
CMO: Samuel Kopel, M.D., Medical Director
CIO: Walter Fahey, Chief Information Officer
CHR: Marc Leff, Vice President Human Resources
Web address: www.maimonidesmed.org/
**Control:** Other not–for–profit (including NFP Corporation) **Service:** General Medical and Surgical

**Staffed Beds:** 641 **Admissions:** 38565 **Census:** 586 **Outpatient Visits:** 430973 **Births:** 8005 **Total Expense ($000):** 971563 **Payroll Expense ($000):** 476048 **Personnel:** 5641

☐ **MANHATTAN PSYCHIATRIC CENTER–WARD'S ISLAND (334054)**, 600 East 125th Street, Zip 10035–9998; tel. 646/672–6767, (Nonreporting) **A**1 3 5 10 **S** New York State Office of Mental Health, Albany, NY
Primary Contact: Stephen Rabinowitz, Executive Director
Web address: www.omh.ny.gov
**Control:** State–Government, nonfederal **Service:** Psychiatric

**Staffed Beds:** 745

✠ **MEMORIAL SLOAN–KETTERING CANCER CENTER (330154)**, 1275 York Avenue, Zip 10065; tel. 212/639–2000 **A**1 2 3 5 8 9 10 **F**3 11 14 15 29 31 32 34 35 36 37 39 44 45 46 47 49 50 54 55 56 57 58 59 60 61 64 66 68 70 74 75 77 78 79 81 82 84 85 86 87 89 92 93 94 96 99 100 103 104 107 108 110 111 112 113 114 115 116 117 118 119 120 122 123 125 129 131 134 135 141 142 143 144 145 146 147
Primary Contact: Craig B. Thompson, M.D., President and Chief Executive Officer
COO: John R. Gunn, Executive Vice President and Chief Operating Officer
CFO: Michael Gutnick, Senior Vice President Finance
CMO: Robert E. Wittes, M.D., Physician in Chief
CIO: Patricia Skarulis, Vice President Information Systems
CHR: Dennis Dowdell, Vice President Human Resources
Web address: www.mskcc.org
**Control:** Other not–for–profit (including NFP Corporation) **Service:** Cancer

**Staffed Beds:** 470 **Admissions:** 24487 **Census:** 386 **Outpatient Visits:** 1279969 **Births:** 0 **Total Expense ($000):** 2048968 **Payroll Expense ($000):** 808239 **Personnel:** 10284

✠ **METROPOLITAN HOSPITAL CENTER (330199)**, 1901 First Avenue, Zip 10029–7404; tel. 212/423–6262, (Includes METROPOLITAN GENERAL CARE UNIT, METROPOLITAN DRUG DETOXIFICATION AND METROPOLITAN PSYCHIATRIC UNIT ) **A**1 3 5 8 9 10 **F**3 4 5 8 9 11 12 13 15 17 18 19 28 29 30 31 32 34 35 38 39 40 41 43 44 45 46 49 50 51 53 54 55 56 57 58 59 60 61 64 65 66 68 70 72 73 74 75 76 77 78 79 81 82 83 84 85 87 88 89 90 92 93 96 97 98 99 100 101 102 103 104 105 107 108 110 111 114 118 129 131 132 133 134 143 144 145 146 147 **S** New York City Health and Hospitals Corporation, New York, NY
Primary Contact: Meryl Weinberg, Executive Director
COO: Gregory Atwater, Chief Operating Officer
CFO: Elizabeth Guzman, Chief Financial Officer
CMO: Richard Stone, M.D., Medical Director
CIO: Don Lee, Chief Information Officer
CHR: April Alexander, Director Human Resources
Web address: www.nyc.gov/html/hhc/metropolitan.html
**Control:** City–Government, nonfederal **Service:** General Medical and Surgical

**Staffed Beds:** 349 **Admissions:** 13542 **Census:** 237 **Outpatient Visits:** 449289 **Births:** 1347 **Total Expense ($000):** 309212 **Payroll Expense ($000):** 140269 **Personnel:** 2448

✠ **MONTEFIORE MEDICAL CENTER (330059)**, 111 East 210th Street, Bronx, Zip 10467–2401; tel. 718/920–4321, (Includes CHILDREN'S HOSPITAL OF MONTEFIORE, 3415 Bainbridge Avenue, Zip 10467–2403; tel. 718/741–2426; JACK D WEILER HOSPITAL OF ALBERT EINSTEIN COLLEGE OF MEDICINE, 1825 Eastchester Road, Zip 10461–2373; tel. 718/904–2000; MONTEFIORE MEDICAL CENTER – NORTH DIVISION, 600 East 233rd Street, Zip 10466–2697; tel. 718/920–9000) **A**1 3 5 8 9 10 **F**3 4 5 6 7 8 9 12 13 14 15 17 18 19 20 21 22 23 24 25 26 27 28 29 30 31 32 34 35 36 37 38 39 40 41 42 43 45 46 47 48 49 50 51 52 53 54 55 56 57 58 59 60 61 62 63 64 65 66 68 70 71 72 73 74 75 76 77 78 79 80 81 82 83 84 85 86 87 88 89 90 92 93 94 95 96 97 98 99 100 101 102 103 104 107 108 110 111 113 114 115 116 117 118 119 120 122 123 125 128 129 130 131 133 134 135 136 137 138 140 141 142 143 144 145 146 147 **P**5 6
Primary Contact: Steven M. Safyer, M.D., President and Chief Executive Officer
COO: Robert B. Conaty, Executive Vice President Operations
CFO: Joel A. Perlman, Executive Vice President Finance
CMO: Gary Kalkut, M.D., Senior Vice President and Chief Medical Officer
CIO: Jack Wolf, Vice President Information Systems
Web address: www.montefiore.org
**Control:** Other not–for–profit (including NFP Corporation) **Service:** General Medical and Surgical

**Staffed Beds:** 1418 **Admissions:** 83480 **Census:** 1328 **Outpatient Visits:** 1853618 **Births:** 6670 **Total Expense ($000):** 2878966 **Payroll Expense ($000):** 1336865 **Personnel:** 16414

**MORGAN STANLEY CHILDREN'S HOSPITAL OF NEW YORK–PRESBYTERIAN**
See New York–Presbyterian Hospital

✠ △ **MOUNT SINAI HOSPITAL (330024)**, One Gustave L. Levy Place, Zip 10029–6574; tel. 212/241–6500, (Includes KRAVIS CHILDREN'S HOSPITAL, One Gustave L. Levy Pl, Zip 10029, Mailing Address: PO Box 1153, Zip 10002–0916; tel. 800/637–4624) **A**1 3 5 7 8 9 10 **F**3 4 6 7 8 9 11 12 13 14 15 17 18 19 20 21 22 23 24 25 26 27 28 29 30 31 32 34 35 36 37 38 39 40 41 42 43 44 45 46 47 48 49 50 51 52 54 55 56 57 58 59 60 61 62 63 64 65 66 68 70 71 72 73 74 75 76 77 78 79 80 81 82 83 84 85 86 87 88 89 90 91 92 93 94 95 96 97 98 99 100 101 102 103 104 105 107 108 110 111 113 114 115 116 117 118 119 120 122 123 125 128 129 130 131 133 134 135 136 137 138 140 141 142 143 144 145 146 147 **P**5 6
Primary Contact: Wayne Keathley, M.P.H., President and Chief Operating Officer
COO: Wayne Keathley, M.P.H., President and Chief Operating Officer
CFO: Donald Scanlon, Chief Financial Officer
CMO: Ira Nash, M.D., Chief Medical Officer
CIO: Jack Nelson, Senior Vice President and Chief Information Officer
CHR: Jane Maksoud, Senior Vice President Human Resources and Labor Relations
Web address: www.mountsinai.org
**Control:** Other not–for–profit (including NFP Corporation) **Service:** General Medical and Surgical

**Staffed Beds:** 1031 **Admissions:** 52910 **Census:** 867 **Outpatient Visits:** 641892 **Births:** 5963 **Total Expense ($000):** 1461149 **Payroll Expense ($000):** 575154 **Personnel:** 7611

☐ **NEW YORK COMMUNITY HOSPITAL (330019)**, 2525 Kings Highway, Brooklyn, Zip 11229–1798, Mailing Address: 2513 Avenue O, Zip 11210–5230; tel. 718/692–5300, (Nonreporting) **A**1 9 10 **S** New York Presbyterian Healthcare System, New York, NY
Primary Contact: Lin H. Mo, President and Chief Executive Officer
COO: Una E. Morrissey, R.N., Senior Vice President, Chief Nursing Officer and Chief Operating Officer
CFO: Leonardo Tamburello, Divisional Chief Financial Officer
CMO: Herbert Rader, M.D., Vice President and Medical Director
CIO: Edward B. Stolyar, D.O., Director Management Information Systems
CHR: Steve Meyers, Director Human Resources
Web address: www.nych.com
**Control:** Other not–for–profit (including NFP Corporation) **Service:** General Medical and Surgical

**Staffed Beds:** 125

✠ **NEW YORK DOWNTOWN HOSPITAL (330064)**, 170 William Street, Zip 10038–2649; tel. 212/312–5000 **A**1 3 5 9 10 **F**7 8 13 15 29 30 34 35 40 45 46 49 54 56 57 58 59 60 61 64 65 66 68 70 73 74 75 76 77 78 79 81 83 85 87 93 97 107 108 110 111 113 114 118 119 129 142 144 145 146 147 **P**6
Primary Contact: Jeffrey Menkes, President and Chief Executive Officer
COO: Anthony Alfano, Senior Vice President and Chief Operating Officer
CMO: Steven G. Friedman, M.D., Interim Chief Medical Officer and Chair, Department of Surgery
CIO: Frank Negro, Interim Chief Information Officer
CHR: Anthony Alfano, Senior Vice President Operations and Chief Human Resources Officer
CNO: Kit Yuen, R.N., Interim Chief Nursing Officer
Web address: www.downtownhospital.org
**Control:** Other not–for–profit (including NFP Corporation) **Service:** General Medical and Surgical

**Staffed Beds:** 128 **Admissions:** 5181 **Census:** 114 **Outpatient Visits:** 94054 **Births:** 2763 **Total Expense ($000):** 204393 **Payroll Expense ($000):** 85343

✠ **NEW YORK EYE AND EAR INFIRMARY (330100)**, 310 East 14th Street, Zip 10003–4201; tel. 212/979–4000 **A**1 3 5 9 10 **F**11 29 30 34 35 43 44 50 54 57 58 59 64 65 66 68 74 81 82 85 86 91 92 93 94 107 113 118 128 129 131 141 145 **P**8 **S** Continuum Health Partners, New York, NY
Primary Contact: D. McWilliams Kessler, President and Chief Executive Officer
COO: Allan Fine, Senior Vice President and Chief Strategy and Operations Officer
CFO: Charles Figliozzi, CPA, Vice President and Chief Financial Officer
CMO: J. Robert Rosenthal, M.D., Senior Vice President Medical Affairs
CIO: Don Ushak, Director Information Systems
CHR: Susan Singer, Director Human Resources
Web address: www.nyee.edu
**Control:** Other not–for–profit (including NFP Corporation) **Service:** Eye, ear, nose, and throat

**Staffed Beds:** 32 **Admissions:** 823 **Census:** 5 **Outpatient Visits:** 224101 **Births:** 0 **Total Expense ($000):** 128358 **Payroll Expense ($000):** 55626 **Personnel:** 850

☐ **NEW YORK HOSPITAL QUEENS (330055)**, 56–45 Main Street, Flushing, Zip 11355–5000; tel. 718/670–1231 **A**1 2 3 5 9 10 **F**3 7 8 11 12 13 14 15 17 18 19 20 22 24 26 28 29 30 31 32 34 35 36 37 39 40 41 43 44 45 46 47 48 49 50 51 52 53 54 55 56 57 58 59 60 61 64 65 68 70 71 72 73 74 75 76 77 78 79 80 81 82 84 85 86 87 88 89 92 93 97 100 107 108 110 111 113 114 115 116 117 118 119 120 121 122 125 129 130 131 134 141 142 143 145 146 147 **S** New York Presbyterian Healthcare System, New York, NY
Primary Contact: Stephen S. Mills, President and Chief Executive Officer
COO: John E. Sciortino, Senior Vice President and Chief Operating Officer
CFO: Kevin J. Ward, Vice President and Chief Financial Officer
CMO: Stephen Rimar, M.D., Senior Vice President Medical Affairs
CIO: Thomas Kemp, Chief Information Officer
CHR: Lorraine Orlando, Vice President Human Resources
Web address: www.nyhq.org
**Control:** Other not–for–profit (including NFP Corporation) **Service:** General Medical and Surgical

**Staffed Beds:** 519 **Admissions:** 36086 **Census:** 497 **Outpatient Visits:** 278024 **Births:** 4139 **Total Expense ($000):** 625794 **Payroll Expense ($000):** 289351 **Personnel:** 3373

✠ **NEW YORK METHODIST HOSPITAL (330236)**, 506 Sixth Street, Brooklyn, Zip 11215–3609; tel. 718/780–3000, (Nonreporting) **A**1 2 3 5 8 9 10 **S** New York Presbyterian Healthcare System, New York, NY
Primary Contact: Mark J. Mundy, President and Chief Executive Officer
COO: Lauren Yedvab, Senior Vice President
CFO: Edward A. Zaidberg, Senior Vice President Finance
CMO: Stanley Sherbell, M.D., Executive Vice President Medical Affairs
CIO: Joseph Saverese, Director Information Systems
CHR: Dennis Buchanan, Vice President Human Resources
CNO: Rebecca L. Flood, R.N., Senior Vice President Nursing
Web address: www.nym.org
**Control:** Other not–for–profit (including NFP Corporation) **Service:** General Medical and Surgical

**Staffed Beds:** 591

☐ **NEW YORK STATE PSYCHIATRIC INSTITUTE (334009)**, 1051 Riverside Drive, Zip 10032–1007; tel. 212/543–5000, (Nonreporting) **A**1 3 5 10 **S** New York State Office of Mental Health, Albany, NY
Primary Contact: Jeffrey A. Lieberman, M.D., Executive Director
COO: Janelle Dierkens, Chief Administration Officer
CFO: Jonathan Segal, Chief Financial Officer
CMO: David Lowenthal, M.D., Clinical Director
CIO: Joseph Grun, Chief Information Officer
CHR: Rebecca Dechabert, Acting Director Personnel
Web address: www.nyspi.org
**Control:** State–Government, nonfederal **Service:** Psychiatric

**Staffed Beds:** 58

☐ **NEW YORK WESTCHESTER SQUARE MEDICAL CENTER (330316)**, 2475 Saint Raymonds Avenue, Bronx, Zip 10461–3124; tel. 718/430–7300 **A**1 5 9 10 **F**3 7 8 15 17 18 29 30 31 34 35 39 40 42 45 49 56 57 59 60 68 74 75 78 79 81 87 93 102 107 111 118 129 145 147 **S** New York Presbyterian Healthcare System, New York, NY
Primary Contact: Alan Kopman, FACHE, President and Chief Executive Officer
CFO: Elliott Gamberg, Vice President Finance
CMO: Louis C. Rose, M.D., Chief Medical Officer
CIO: Mary O'Brien, Director Information Systems and Telecommunications
CHR: Barbara DeAngelo, Director Human Resources
Web address: www.nywsmc.org
**Control:** Other not–for–profit (including NFP Corporation) **Service:** General Medical and Surgical

**Staffed Beds:** 140 **Admissions:** 5789 **Census:** 105 **Outpatient Visits:** 37045 **Total Expense ($000):** 79216 **Payroll Expense ($000):** 34498 **Personnel:** 553

NY

**Hospital, Medicare Provider Number, Address, Telephone, Approval, Facility, and Physician Codes, Health Care System**

★ American Hospital Association (AHA) membership
☐ The Joint Commission accreditation
◇ DNV Healthcare Inc. accreditation
○ American Osteopathic Association (AOA) accreditation
△ Commission on Accreditation of Rehabilitation Facilities (CARF) accreditation

☒ △ **NEW YORK–PRESBYTERIAN HOSPITAL (330101)**, 525 East 68th Street, Zip 10065–4870; tel. 212/746–5454, (Includes MORGAN STANLEY CHILDREN'S HOSPITAL OF NEW YORK–PRESBYTERIAN, 3959 Broadway, Zip 10032–3784; tel. 212/305–2500; NEW YORK–PRESBYTERIAN HOSPITAL, WESTCHESTER DIVISION, 21 Bloomingdale Road, White Plains, Zip 10605; tel. 914/682–9100; NEW YORK–PRESBYTERIAN HOSPITAL/WEILL CORNELL MEDICAL CENTER, 525 East 68th Street, Zip 10021–4885; tel. 212/746–5454; NEW YORK–PRESBYTERIAN/COLUMBIA UNIVERSITY MEDICAL CENTER, 161 Fort Washington Avenue, Zip 10032; tel. 212/305–2500; PAYNE WHITNEY PSYCHIATRIC CLINIC, 525 East 68th Street, Zip 10021; tel. 212/746–3800; THE ALLEN PAVILION, 5141 Broadway, Zip 10032; tel. 212/932–5000) **A**1 2 3 5 7 8 9 10 **F**3 4 5 6 7 8 9 11 12 13 14 15 16 17 18 19 20 21 22 23 24 25 26 27 28 29 30 31 32 34 35 36 37 38 39 40 41 43 44 45 46 47 48 49 50 51 52 53 54 55 56 57 58 59 60 61 64 66 68 70 72 73 74 75 76 77 78 79 80 81 82 84 85 86 87 88 89 90 92 93 94 96 97 98 99 100 101 102 103 104 105 107 108 109 110 111 112 113 114 115 116 117 118 119 120 122 123 125 128 129 130 131 133 134 135 136 137 138 140 141 142 143 144 145 146 147 **S** New York Presbyterian Healthcare System, New York, NY
Primary Contact: Steven J. Corwin, M.D., Chief Executive Officer
CFO: Phyllis R. Lantos, Executive Vice President, Chief Financial Officer and Treasurer
CMO: Laura Forese, M.D., Senior Vice President and Chief Medical Officer
CIO: Aurelia Boyer, Senior Vice President and Chief Information Officer
CHR: G. Thomas Ferguson, Senior Vice President and Chief Human Resources Officer
Web address: www.nyp.org
**Control:** Other not–for–profit (including NFP Corporation) **Service:** General Medical and Surgical

**Staffed Beds:** 2264 **Admissions:** 105339 **Census:** 1892 **Outpatient Visits:** 1830183 **Births:** 12514 **Total Expense ($000):** 3457135 **Payroll Expense ($000):** 1668635 **Personnel:** 19024

☒ **NORTH CENTRAL BRONX HOSPITAL (330385)**, 3424 Kossuth Avenue, Bronx, Zip 10467–2489; tel. 718/519–3500 **A**1 8 9 10 **F**3 5 8 11 12 13 15 18 28 29 30 32 34 35 38 39 40 41 43 44 45 46 48 50 51 55 56 57 58 59 60 61 64 65 66 68 70 72 73 74 75 76 77 78 79 80 81 82 84 85 87 92 93 94 96 97 98 99 100 101 102 103 104 105 107 108 110 111 114 118 129 130 131 134 143 145 146 147 **P**6 **S** New York City Health and Hospitals Corporation, New York, NY
Primary Contact: William P. Walsh, Executive Director
COO: Sheldon McLeod, Chief Operating Officer
CFO: Kathy Garramone, Chief Financial Officer
CMO: Joseph Skarzynski, M.D., Medical Director
CIO: Diane Carr, Chief Information Officer
CHR: Dolores Leite, Chief Human Resource Executive
CNO: Elizabeth Gerdts, Chief Nursing Officer
Web address: www.ci.nyc.ny.us/html/hhc/html/northcentralbronx.html
**Control:** City–Government, nonfederal **Service:** General Medical and Surgical

**Staffed Beds:** 213 **Admissions:** 7442 **Census:** 126 **Outpatient Visits:** 252045 **Births:** 1647 **Total Expense ($000):** 169737 **Payroll Expense ($000):** 78335 **Personnel:** 1290

**NYU HOSPITAL FOR JOINT DISEASES** See NYU Langone Medical Center's Hospital for Joint Diseases

☒ **NYU LANGONE MEDICAL CENTER (330214)**, 550 First Avenue, Zip 10016–6402; tel. 212/263–7300, (Includes NYU CHILDREN'S HOSPITAL, 545 First Avenue, Zip 10016–6401; tel. 212/263–7300; NYU LANGONE MEDICAL CENTER'S HOSPITAL FOR JOINT DISEASES, 301 East 17th Street, Zip 10003–3890; tel. 212/598–6000; David A. Dibner, FACHE, Senior Vice President Hospital Operations and Musculoskeletal Strategic Area; RUSK INSTITUTE, 400 East 34th Street, Zip 10016) **A**1 5 8 9 10 **F**3 5 6 8 9 11 12 13 14 15 17 18 19 20 21 22 23 24 25 26 27 28 29 30 31 32 34 35 36 37 38 39 40 41 43 44 45 46 47 48 49 50 52 53 54 55 56 57 58 59 60 61 63 64 65 66 68 70 72 73 74 75 76 77 78 79 80 81 82 84 85 86 87 88 89 90 91 92 93 95 96 97 98 99 100 101 102 103 104 107 108 110 111 113 114 115 116 117 118 119 120 122 123 125 128 129 130 131 133 134 135 137 138 140 144 145 146 147 **P**5 6
Primary Contact: Robert I. Grossman, M.D., Chief Executive Officer
COO: Bernard Birnbaum, M.D., Senior Vice President, Vice Dean and Chief Hospital Operations
CFO: Michael Burke, Senior Vice President and Corporate Chief Financial Officer
CMO: Robert Press, M.D., Chief Medical Officer
CHR: Nancy Sanchez, Senior Vice President and Vice Dean Human Resources
Web address: www.nyumedicalcenter.org
**Control:** Other not–for–profit (including NFP Corporation) **Service:** General Medical and Surgical

**Staffed Beds:** 806 **Admissions:** 37929 **Census:** 596 **Outpatient Visits:** 666877 **Births:** 4789 **Total Expense ($000):** 1560456 **Payroll Expense ($000):** 588975 **Personnel:** 7882

**PAYNE WHITNEY PSYCHIATRIC CLINIC** See New York–Presbyterian Hospital

☐ **QUEENS CHILDREN'S PSYCHIATRIC CENTER**, 74–03 Commonwealth Boulevard, Jamaica, Zip 11426–1890; tel. 718/264–4506, (Nonreporting) **A**1 **S** New York State Office of Mental Health, Albany, NY
Primary Contact: June Dacosta, Acting Executive Director
CMO: David M. Rube, M.D., Clinical Director
CIO: Ed Yunusov, Coordinator Facility Information Center
Web address: www.omh.ny.gov
**Control:** State–Government, nonfederal **Service:** Children's hospital psychiatric

**Staffed Beds:** 84

☒ **QUEENS HOSPITAL CENTER (330231)**, 82–68 164th Street, Jamaica, Zip 11432–1104; tel. 718/883–3000 **A**1 2 3 5 8 9 10 **F**4 5 8 11 13 15 30 31 32 34 35 38 39 40 43 50 53 54 56 57 59 61 64 68 70 72 73 76 77 78 81 87 90 93 97 98 99 100 102 103 104 105 107 111 115 118 128 129 133 134 145 146 **P**6 **S** New York City Health and Hospitals Corporation, New York, NY
Primary Contact: Julius Wool, Executive Director
COO: Robert Rossdale, Deputy Executive Director
CFO: Brian Stacey, Chief Financial Officer
CMO: Jasmin Moshirpur, M.D., Chief Medical Officer
CIO: Vincent Smith, Chief Information Officer
CHR: Jeannith Gangemi–Sosa, Senior Associate Executive Director
CNO: Joan Gabriele, Deputy Executive Director
Web address: www.nyc.gov/html/hhc/qhc/html/home/home.shtml
**Control:** City–Government, nonfederal **Service:** General Medical and Surgical

**Staffed Beds:** 303 **Admissions:** 15669 **Census:** 257 **Outpatient Visits:** 427435 **Births:** 2042 **Total Expense ($000):** 333878 **Payroll Expense ($000):** 136551 **Personnel:** 1877

☒ **RICHMOND UNIVERSITY MEDICAL CENTER (330028)**, 355 Bard Avenue, Staten Island, Zip 10310–1664; tel. 718/818–1234 **A**1 2 3 5 9 10 **F**3 4 5 7 11 13 14 15 17 18 19 20 26 29 30 31 32 34 35 38 40 43 45 47 49 50 51 55 56 57 58 59 61 64 65 66 68 70 71 72 73 74 75 76 77 78 79 81 82 84 88 89 92 93 94 98 99 100 101 102 103 104 107 108 109 110 111 113 114 118 129 130 131 133 134 142 143 145 146 147 **P**4
Primary Contact: Richard J. Murphy, President and Chief Executive Officer
CMO: Edward Arsura, M.D., Chief Medical Officer
CHR: Patricia Caldari, Vice President
Web address: www.rumcsi.org
**Control:** Other not–for–profit (including NFP Corporation) **Service:** General Medical and Surgical

**Staffed Beds:** 384 **Admissions:** 18527 **Census:** 285 **Outpatient Visits:** 127163 **Births:** 2967 **Total Expense ($000):** 285418 **Payroll Expense ($000):** 137618 **Personnel:** 1914

☐ **ROCKEFELLER UNIVERSITY HOSPITAL (330387)**, 1230 York Avenue, Zip 10021–6399; tel. 212/327–8000, (Nonreporting) **A**1 10
Primary Contact: James G. Krueger, M.D., Ph.D., Chief Executive Officer
CMO: Barbara O'Sullivan, M.D., Medical Director
Web address: www.rucares.org
**Control:** Other not–for–profit (including NFP Corporation) **Service:** Other specialty

**Staffed Beds:** 40

**ROOSEVELT HOSPITAL** See St. Luke's–Roosevelt Hospital Center

☐ **SOUTH BEACH PSYCHIATRIC CENTER (334043)**, 777 Seaview Avenue, Staten Island, Zip 10305–3409; tel. 718/667–2300, (Nonreporting) **A**1 3 5 10 **S** New York State Office of Mental Health, Albany, NY
Primary Contact: Thomas Uttaro, Executive Director
COO: Eileen Klein, Ph.D., Deputy Director Operations
CFO: Jeffrey Einbond, Director Facility Administration
CHR: George Bouquio, Director Human Resources
Web address: www.omh.ny.gov
**Control:** State–Government, nonfederal **Service:** Psychiatric

**Staffed Beds:** 340

☒ **ST. BARNABAS HOSPITAL (330399)**, 183rd Street & Third Avenue, Bronx, Zip 10457–9998; tel. 718/960–9000, (Total facility includes 199 beds in nursing home–type unit) **A**1 3 5 6 9 10 12 13 **F**2 3 4 5 7 8 11 13 15 18 20 26 28 29 30 31 32 34 35 36 38 39 40 43 44 45 46 47 48 49 50 51 54 55 56 57 58 59 60 61 64 65 66 68 70 71 72 74 75 76 77 78 79 81 82 85 86 87 89 93 97 98 99 100 102 103 104 107 108 109 111 113 114 116 117 118 119 120 121 122 123 129 130 131 133 134 144 145 146 147 **P**6
Primary Contact: Scott Cooper, M.D., Chief Executive Officer
COO: Len Walsh, Executive Vice President and Chief Operating Officer
CFO: Todd Gorlewski, Senior Vice President and Chief Financial Officer
CMO: Jerry Balentine, D.O., Executive Vice President and Chief Medical Director
CIO: Noah Caldwell, Senior Vice President and Chief Information Officer
CHR: Marc Wolf, Director Human Resources
CNO: Denise Richardson, R.N., Senior Vice President and Chief Nursing Officer
Web address: www.stbarnabashospital.org
**Control:** Other not–for–profit (including NFP Corporation) **Service:** General Medical and Surgical

**Staffed Beds:** 660 **Admissions:** 21138 **Census:** 247

☐ **ST. JOHN'S EPISCOPAL HOSPITAL–SOUTH SHORE (330395)**, 327 Beach 19th Street, Far Rockaway, Zip 11691–4423; tel. 718/869–7000, (Data for 364 days) **A**1 3 5 9 10 12 13 **F**3 4 8 11 15 17 29 30 31 34 35 40 49 50 51 56 57 58 59 60 61 64 65 66 68 70 73 74 75 76 78 79 81 82 84 85 86 87 89 92 93 97 98 100 102 103 104 105 107 108 110 111 114 118 129 131 145 147
Primary Contact: Nelson Toebbe, Chief Executive Officer
COO: Patrick L. Sullivan, Chief Operating Officer
CFO: Kathleen Garcia, Controller
CMO: Raymond Pastore, M.D., Chief Medical Officer
CIO: Michael J. Piro, Chief Information Officer
CHR: Roger Franco, Director Human Resources
Web address: www.ehs.org
**Control:** Church–operated, Nongovernment, not–for profit **Service:** General Medical and Surgical

**Staffed Beds:** 241 **Admissions:** 10104 **Census:** 203 **Outpatient Visits:** 145289 **Births:** 876 **Total Expense ($000):** 181139 **Payroll Expense ($000):** 88379 **Personnel:** 1180

☒ **ST. LUKE'S–ROOSEVELT HOSPITAL CENTER (330046)**, 1111 Amsterdam Avenue, Zip 10025–1716; tel. 212/523–4000, (Includes ROOSEVELT HOSPITAL, 1000 Tenth Avenue, Zip 10019; tel. 212/523–5700; ST. LUKE'S HOSPITAL CENTER, 1111 Amsterdam Avenue, Zip 10025; tel. 212/523–4000) **A**1 2 3 5 8 9 10 **F**3 4 5 7 8 9 11 12 13 14 15 17 18 20 22 24 26 29 30 31 32 34 35 38 39 40 41 43 44 46 49 50 52 55 56 57 58 59 60 61 64 65 66 68 70 72 74 75 76 77 78 79 81 82 84 85 86 87 89 90 92 93 94 96 97 98 99 100 101 102 103 104 105 107 108 110 111 112 113 117 118 119 120 123 125 129 130 131 133 134 137 143 144 145 146 147 **P**6 **S** Continuum Health Partners, New York, NY
Primary Contact: Frank J. Cracolici, President
COO: Timothy Day, Chief Administrative Officer
CFO: John Collura, Executive Vice President and Chief Financial Officer
CMO: Robert A. Catalano, M.D., Chief Medical Officer
CIO: Mark Moroses, Vice President and Chief Information Officer
CHR: Marvin Russell, Senior Vice President Human Resources
Web address: www.slrhc.org
**Control:** Other not–for–profit (including NFP Corporation) **Service:** General Medical and Surgical

**Staffed Beds:** 711 **Admissions:** 44109 **Census:** 698 **Outpatient Visits:** 638372 **Births:** 6696 **Total Expense ($000):** 1203447 **Payroll Expense ($000):** 578571 **Personnel:** 6019

☒ △ **STATEN ISLAND UNIVERSITY HOSPITAL (330160)**, 475 Seaview Avenue, Staten Island, Zip 10305–3436; tel. 718/226–9000 **A**1 2 3 5 7 8 9 10 **F**3 4 5 7 8 11 12 13 14 15 16 17 18 19 20 22 24 26 28 29 30 31 32 34 35 36 38 39 40 41 43 44 49 50 51 52 54 55 56 57 58 59 60 61 63 64 65 66 68 70 72 73 74 75 76 77 78 79 81 82 84 85 86 87 88 89 90 91 92 93 94 95 96 97 98 100 101 102 103 104 105 107 108 110 111 113 114 115 116 117 118 119 120 122 123 125 128 129 131 133 134 145 146 147 **P**6 **S** North Shore–Long Island Jewish Health System, Great Neck, NY
Primary Contact: Anthony C. Ferreri, President and Chief Executive Officer
COO: Donna Proske, MS, Executive Vice President, Chief Operating Officer and Chief Nursing Executive
CFO: Thomas Reca, Sr., Senior Vice President Finance and Chief Financial Officer
CMO: Mark Jarrett, M.D., Chief Medical Officer
CIO: Kathy Kania, Chief Information Officer
CHR: Margaret Dialto, Vice President Human Resources
Web address: www.siuh.edu
**Control:** Other not–for–profit (including NFP Corporation) **Service:** General Medical and Surgical

**Staffed Beds:** 663 **Admissions:** 42476 **Census:** 585 **Outpatient Visits:** 393124 **Births:** 3069 **Total Expense ($000):** 757108 **Payroll Expense ($000):** 385547 **Personnel:** 5024

**STEVEN AND ALEXANDRA COHEN CHILDREN'S MEDICAL CENTER OF NEW YORK** See Long Island Jewish Medical Center, New Hyde Park

☒ **SUNY DOWNSTATE MEDICAL CENTER UNIVERSITY HOSPITAL OF BROOKLYN (330350)**, 445 Lenox Road, Brooklyn, Zip 11203–2017; tel. 718/270–1000, (Nonreporting) **A**1 2 3 5 8 10
Primary Contact: Debra D. Carey, Chief Executive Officer
COO: David Conley, Chief Administrative Officer
CFO: Gerry Dantis, Assistant Vice President Finance
CMO: Michael Lucchesi, M.D., Interim Chief Medical Officer
CIO: Ernest P. Weber, Jr., Interim Chief Information Officer
CHR: Hendrina Goeloe–Alston, Assistant Vice President Personnel
Web address: www.downstate.edu
**Control:** State–Government, nonfederal **Service:** General Medical and Surgical

**Staffed Beds:** 360

**TERENCE CARDINAL COOKE HEALTH CARE CENTER (332022)**, 1249 Fifth Avenue, Zip 10029–4413; tel. 212/360–1000, (Nonreporting) **A**10
Primary Contact: James Karkenny, Chief Executive Officer
Web address: www.tcchcc.org/
**Control:** Church–operated, Nongovernment, not–for profit **Service:** Long–Term Acute Care hospital

**Staffed Beds:** 28

**THE ALLEN PAVILION** See New York–Presbyterian Hospital

**THE MOUNT SINAI HOSPITAL OF QUEENS (330258)**, 25–10 30th Avenue, Long Island City, Zip 11102–2448; tel. 718/932–1000 **A**10 **F**3 8 15 18 29 30 31 32 34 35 40 43 45 49 50 54 56 57 59 60 62 63 64 65 66 68 70 74 75 77 79 80 81 82 83 84 85 86 87 93 100 107 111 118 129 134 145 146 147 **P**6
Primary Contact: Caryn A. Schwab, Executive Director
COO: Judy Trilivas, Vice President and Chief Operating Officer
CFO: Salvatore Morello, Vice President Finance
CMO: David M. Nierman, M.D., Vice President and Chief Medical Officer
CIO: Jack Abuin, Director Management Information Systems
CHR: Norma Calame, Director Human Resources
Web address: www.mshq.org
**Control:** Other not–for–profit (including NFP Corporation) **Service:** General Medical and Surgical

**Staffed Beds:** 192 **Admissions:** 10238 **Census:** 158 **Outpatient Visits:** 114213 **Births:** 0 **Total Expense ($000):** 142650 **Payroll Expense ($000):** 74838 **Personnel:** 1072

☒ **UNIVERSITY HOSPITAL OF BROOKLYN AT LONG ISLAND COLLEGE HOSPITAL (330152)**, 339 Hicks Street, Brooklyn, Zip 11201–5509; tel. 718/780–1000, (Nonreporting) **A**1 2 3 5 8 9 10
Primary Contact: Debra D. Carey, Interim Chief Executive Officer
COO: John Byrne, Executive Vice President and Chief Operating Officer
CFO: Tomas Del Rio, Vice President Finance
CIO: Hal Wachter, Director Information Systems
Web address: www.downstate.edu/lich/
**Control:** State–Government, nonfederal **Service:** General Medical and Surgical

**Staffed Beds:** 337

☒ △ **VETERANS ADMINISTRATION NEW YORK HARBOR HEALTHCARE SYSTEM**, 800 Poly Place, Brooklyn, Zip 11209–7104; tel. 718/630–3500, (Includes VETERANS AFFAIRS MEDICAL CENTER, 423 East 23rd Street, New York, Zip 10010–5050; tel. 212/686–7500), (Total facility includes 179 beds in nursing home–type unit) **A**1 2 3 5 7 8 **F**2 3 4 5 7 8 9 15 17 18 20 22 24 26 28 29 30 31 34 35 38 39 40 45 46 48 49 53 54 56 57 58 59 60 61 62 63 64 65 68 70 74 75 77 78 79 80 81 82 83 84 85 86 87 90 91 92 93 94 96 97 98 100 101 102 103 104 105 107 109 111 113 114 117 118 119 120 127 129 130 131 134 142 145 146 147 **P**6 **S** Department of Veterans Affairs, Washington, DC
Primary Contact: Martina A. Parauda, Director
CFO: Daniel Downey, Chief Fiscal Service
CIO: Maria Schay, Chief Information Officer
Web address: www.nyharbor.va.gov
**Control:** Veterans Affairs, Government, federal **Service:** General Medical and Surgical

**Staffed Beds:** 517 **Admissions:** 10603 **Census:** 392 **Outpatient Visits:** 736146 **Births:** 0 **Total Expense ($000):** 700727 **Payroll Expense ($000):** 316603 **Personnel:** 3731

☒ △ **VETERANS AFFAIRS MEDICAL CENTER**, 130 West Kingsbridge Road, Bronx, Zip 10468–3992; tel. 718/584–9000, (Total facility includes 84 beds in nursing home–type unit) **A**1 2 3 5 7 8 **F**3 5 8 9 11 12 17 18 29 30 31 33 34 35 36 37 38 39 40 43 44 45 46 48 49 50 51 53 54 56 57 58 59 60 61 62 63 64 65 68 70 74 75 77 78 79 80 81 82 83 84 85 86 87 90 91 92 93 94 95 96 97 98 100 101 102 103 104 107 109 111 113 114 117 118 119 122 129 131 134 142 145 146 147 **S** Department of Veterans Affairs, Washington, DC
Primary Contact: Maryann Musumeci, Director
CFO: Gregory Angelo, Chief Fiscal Program
CMO: Clive Rosendorff, M.D., Chief Medical Program
CIO: Linda Bund, Chief Information Officer and Director Education
CHR: Peter Tinker, Chief Human Resources Officer
Web address: www.va.gov/sta/guide/home.asp
**Control:** Veterans Affairs, Government, federal **Service:** General Medical and Surgical

**Staffed Beds:** 325 **Admissions:** 4312 **Census:** 177 **Outpatient Visits:** 328617 **Births:** 0 **Total Expense ($000):** 269374 **Payroll Expense ($000):** 138638 **Personnel:** 1903

⊞ **WOODHULL MEDICAL AND MENTAL HEALTH CENTER (330396)**, 760 Broadway, Brooklyn, Zip 11206–5383; tel. 718/963–8000 **A**1 3 5 8 9 10 **F**3 4 5 8 11 15 29 30 31 34 35 38 39 40 41 43 45 46 48 49 53 54 55 56 57 58 59 60 61 64 65 66 68 70 71 72 73 74 75 76 77 78 79 81 82 83 84 85 86 87 89 93 94 97 98 99 100 101 102 103 104 107 111 118 129 131 134 142 145 146 **P**6 **S** New York City Health and Hospitals Corporation, New York, NY
Primary Contact: George M. Proctor, Senior Vice President and Executive Director
COO: Eve Borzon, R.N., Chief Operating Officer
CFO: Milton Nunez, Chief Financial Officer
CMO: Edward Fishkin, M.D., Medical Director
CIO: Cynthia Bianchi, Chief Information Officer
CHR: Yvette Villanueva, Senior Associate Executive Director
Web address: www.nyc.gov/html/hhc
**Control:** City–County, Government, nonfederal **Service:** General Medical and Surgical

**Staffed Beds:** 346 **Admissions:** 15809 **Census:** 296 **Outpatient Visits:** 536983 **Births:** 2185 **Total Expense ($000):** 411428 **Payroll Expense ($000):** 174953 **Personnel:** 2786

☐ **WYCKOFF HEIGHTS MEDICAL CENTER (330221)**, 374 Stockholm Street, Brooklyn, Zip 11237–4099; tel. 718/963–7272, (Nonreporting) **A**1 3 5 9 10 12 13
Primary Contact: Ramon J. Rodriguez, President and Chief Executive Officer
COO: Frances Heaney, R.N., Executive Vice President and Chief Operating Officer
CFO: Leon Kozlowski, Vice President Finance and Chief Financial Officer
CMO: Mounzer Tchelebi, M.D., Medical Director
CIO: Cletis Earle, Vice President and Chief Information Officer
CHR: Margaret E. Cornelius, Vice President Human Resources
Web address: www.wyckoffhospital.org
**Control:** Other not–for–profit (including NFP Corporation) **Service:** General Medical and Surgical

**Staffed Beds:** 279

**ZUCKER HILLSIDE HOSPITAL** See Long Island Jewish Medical Center, New Hyde Park

### NEWARK—Wayne County

⊞ **NEWARK–WAYNE COMMUNITY HOSPITAL (330030)**, 1200 Driving Park Avenue, Zip 14513, Mailing Address: P.O. Box 111, Zip 14513–0111; tel. 315/332–2022, (Total facility includes 180 beds in nursing home–type unit) **A**1 9 10 **F**2 3 8 11 13 15 28 29 30 34 35 38 40 43 44 50 54 55 56 57 59 61 64 68 70 74 75 76 77 79 80 81 85 86 87 90 93 97 98 100 102 103 107 110 111 113 117 118 127 129 130 131 134 145 146 147 **P**5 7 **S** Rochester General Health System, Rochester, NY
Primary Contact: Mark F. Klyczek, President and Chief Executive Officer
CFO: Paula Tinch, Interim Chief Financial Officer
CMO: Richard Gangemi, M.D., Senior Vice President Academic, Medical Affairs and Chief Medical Officer
CIO: Chris Teumer, Vice President and Chief Information Officer
CHR: Janine Schue, Senior Vice President People Resources
CNO: Cheryl Sheridan, R.N., Senior Vice President and Chief Nursing Officer
Web address: www.rochestergeneral.org
**Control:** Other not–for–profit (including NFP Corporation) **Service:** General Medical and Surgical

**Staffed Beds:** 270 **Admissions:** 4194 **Census:** 229 **Outpatient Visits:** 155347 **Births:** 427 **Total Expense ($000):** 74117 **Payroll Expense ($000):** 36781 **Personnel:** 642

### NEWBURGH—Orange County

⊞ **ST. LUKE'S CORNWALL HOSPITAL (330264)**, 70 Dubois Street, Zip 12550–4851; tel. 845/561–4400, (Includes ST. LUKE'S CORNWALL HOSPITAL – CORNWALL CAMPUS, 19 Laurel Avenue, Cornwall, Zip 12518–1499; tel. 845/534–7711; ST. LUKE'S CORNWALL HOSPITAL – NEWBURGH CAMPUS, 70 Dubois Street, Zip 12550–4898; tel. 845/561–4400) **A**1 2 9 10 **F**3 11 13 15 18 20 22 28 29 31 34 35 36 37 40 44 46 49 50 51 54 55 57 59 64 68 70 72 74 75 76 77 78 79 81 82 84 85 86 87 89 93 96 100 102 107 108 110 113 114 117 118 125 128 129 131 134 145 147 **P**4
Primary Contact: Allan E. Atzrott, FACHE, President and Chief Executive Officer
COO: Robert Ross, Executive Vice President and Chief Operating Officer
CFO: Mary Elizabeth Duffy, Senior Vice President and Chief Financial Officer
CMO: Christine Jelalian, M.D., Medical Director
CIO: Jane Lake, Director Materials Management
CHR: Deborah Turner, Vice President Human Resources
Web address: www.stlukescornwallhospital.org
**Control:** Other not–for–profit (including NFP Corporation) **Service:** General Medical and Surgical

**Staffed Beds:** 202 **Admissions:** 11411 **Census:** 148 **Outpatient Visits:** 163958 **Births:** 978 **Total Expense ($000):** 178141 **Payroll Expense ($000):** 72323 **Personnel:** 1005

### NIAGARA FALLS—Niagara County

**NIAGARA FALLS MEMORIAL MEDICAL CENTER (330065)**, 621 Tenth Street, Zip 14302–0708, Mailing Address: P.O. Box 708, Zip 14302–0708; tel. 716/278–4000, (Nonreporting) **A**3 5 9 10 13
Primary Contact: Joseph A. Ruffolo, President and Chief Executive Officer
CMO: Fatma Patel, M.D., Vice President Medical Affairs
CIO: Diane Martin–Pratt, Director Information Systems
Web address: www.nfmmc.org
**Control:** Other not–for–profit (including NFP Corporation) **Service:** General Medical and Surgical

**Staffed Beds:** 288

### NORTH TONAWANDA—Niagara County

**DE GRAFF MEMORIAL HOSPITAL** See KALEIDA Health, Buffalo

### NORTHPORT—Suffolk County

⊞ △ **VETERANS AFFAIRS MEDICAL CENTER**, 79 Middleville Road, Zip 11768–2293; tel. 631/261–4400, (Total facility includes 170 beds in nursing home–type unit) **A**1 2 3 5 7 8 **F**3 5 8 12 18 20 29 30 31 33 34 35 36 38 39 40 44 45 46 47 49 50 51 53 56 57 58 59 60 61 62 64 65 68 70 71 74 75 77 78 79 81 82 83 84 85 86 87 90 91 92 93 94 95 96 97 98 100 101 102 103 104 105 106 107 108 111 115 117 118 120 121 126 127 128 129 131 132 134 143 145 146 147 **S** Department of Veterans Affairs, Washington, DC
Primary Contact: Philip C. Moschitta, Director
COO: Maria Favale, FACHE, Associate Director
CFO: Mary Pat Hessman, Chief Fiscal
CMO: Edward Mack, M.D., Chief of Staff
CIO: Robert Ziskin, Chief Information Officer
CHR: Edward Yankowski, Chief Human Resources Management Service
CNO: Rosie Chatman, R.N., Associate Director Patient and Nursing Services
Web address: www.va.gov/sta/guide/home.asp
**Control:** Veterans Affairs, Government, federal **Service:** General Medical and Surgical

**Staffed Beds:** 502 **Admissions:** 3651 **Census:** 248 **Outpatient Visits:** 541622 **Births:** 0 **Total Expense ($000):** 278117 **Payroll Expense ($000):** 182797 **Personnel:** 1789

### NORWICH—Chenango County

○ **CHENANGO MEMORIAL HOSPITAL (330033)**, 179 North Broad Street, Zip 13815–1097; tel. 607/337–4111, (Nonreporting) **A**9 10 11 **S** United Health Services, Binghamton, NY
Primary Contact: Drake M. Lamen, M.D., President and Chief Executive Officer
COO: Drake M. Lamen, M.D., President and Chief Executive Officer
CFO: Robert R. McCarthy, Vice President Finance and Chief Financial Officer
CMO: Michael F. Trevisani, M.D., Vice President Medical Affairs and Chief Medical Officer
CIO: Tracy McCumber, Manager Information Systems
CHR: Anne L. English, Director Human Resources
CNO: Dru Cavanagh, R.N., Vice President Patient Care Services and Chief Nursing Officer
Web address: www.uhs.net/cmh
**Control:** Other not–for–profit (including NFP Corporation) **Service:** General Medical and Surgical

**Staffed Beds:** 138

### NYACK—Rockland County

☐ **NYACK HOSPITAL (330104)**, 160 North Midland Avenue, Zip 10960–1998; tel. 845/348–2000 **A**1 2 5 9 10 **F**4 5 8 11 13 14 15 17 29 30 31 40 43 46 59 65 69 70 72 75 77 78 79 81 82 93 107 108 111 115 117 118 128 129 134 145 147 **P**6 **S** New York Presbyterian Healthcare System, New York, NY
Primary Contact: David H. Freed, President and Chief Executive Officer
CFO: John Burke, Chief Financial Officer
CMO: Michael E. Rader, M.D., Vice President and Medical Director
CIO: John Volanto, Vice President and Chief Information Officer
CHR: Mary K. Shinick, Vice President Human Resources
CNO: Mary Ann Anderson, R.N., Chief Nursing Officer
Web address: www.nyackhospital.org
**Control:** Other not–for–profit (including NFP Corporation) **Service:** General Medical and Surgical

**Staffed Beds:** 375 **Admissions:** 14708 **Census:** 183 **Outpatient Visits:** 174964 **Births:** 1784 **Total Expense ($000):** 202462 **Payroll Expense ($000):** 95326 **Personnel:** 1455

**NY**

## OCEANSIDE—Nassau County

⊠ **SOUTH NASSAU COMMUNITIES HOSPITAL (330198)**, One Healthy Way, Zip 11572–1551; tel. 516/632–3000 **A**1 2 3 5 9 10 13 **F**3 5 11 12 13 15 17 18 20 22 26 28 29 30 31 34 35 37 38 40 41 43 44 45 46 47 49 50 54 55 56 57 58 59 60 62 64 66 68 69 70 73 74 75 76 77 78 79 81 82 83 84 85 87 89 91 92 93 97 98 99 100 102 103 104 105 107 108 109 110 111 113 114 117 118 119 120 122 123 125 128 129 130 131 134 144 145 147
Primary Contact: Joseph A. Quagliata, President and Chief Executive Officer
COO: Joseph Lamantia, Executive Vice President and Chief Operating Officer
CFO: Mark A. Bogen, Senior Vice President and Chief Financial Officer
CMO: Linda Efferen, M.D., Senior Vice President and Chief Medical Officer
CIO: John Mertz, Chief Information Officer
CHR: Paul Giordano, Vice President Human Resources
CNO: Sue Penque, R.N., Senior Vice President and Chief Nursing Officer
Web address: www.southnassau.org
**Control:** Other not–for–profit (including NFP Corporation) **Service:** General Medical and Surgical

**Staffed Beds:** 385 **Admissions:** 20788 **Census:** 316 **Outpatient Visits:** 378368 **Births:** 1712 **Total Expense ($000):** 367623 **Payroll Expense ($000):** 176650 **Personnel:** 2352

## OGDENSBURG—St. Lawrence County

★ **CLAXTON–HEPBURN MEDICAL CENTER (330211)**, 214 King Street, Zip 13669–1142; tel. 315/393–3600 **A**2 9 10 20 21 **F**3 11 13 15 28 29 30 31 34 35 36 38 40 44 45 50 51 53 54 56 57 59 60 61 64 70 74 75 76 77 78 79 81 82 85 86 87 90 91 92 93 94 96 97 98 100 101 102 103 104 107 108 110 111 113 117 118 120 122 128 129 130 131 132 133 134 144 145 146 147 **P**6 7
Primary Contact: Mark Webster, President and Chief Executive Officer
COO: Vicki Perrine, Chief Operating Officer and Vice President Clinical Services
CFO: Kelley Tiernan, Chief Financial Officer
CMO: Gary Hart, M.D., Chief Medical Officer
CIO: James Flood, Director Information Systems
CHR: Lou–Ann McNally, Director Human Resources
CNO: David Ferris, Chief Nursing Officer and Vice President Patient Care Services
Web address: www.claxtonhepburn.org
**Control:** Other not–for–profit (including NFP Corporation) **Service:** General Medical and Surgical

**Staffed Beds:** 130 **Admissions:** 3693 **Census:** 60 **Outpatient Visits:** 176723 **Births:** 338 **Total Expense ($000):** 89667 **Payroll Expense ($000):** 39121 **Personnel:** 628

☐ **ST. LAWRENCE PSYCHIATRIC CENTER (334003)**, 1 Chimney Point Drive, Zip 13669–2291; tel. 315/541–2001, (Nonreporting) **A**1 5 10 **S** New York State Office of Mental Health, Albany, NY
Primary Contact: Samua A. Bastien, IV, Ph.D., Executive Director
CFO: Timothy J. Lamitie, Deputy Director Administration
CMO: Harishankar Sanghi, M.D., Clinical Director
CIO: Christopher Ashwood, Coordinator Information Systems
CHR: Geri Koutner–Rausch, Director Human Resources
Web address: www.omh.ny.gov/omhweb/facilities/slpc/facility.htm
**Control:** State–Government, nonfederal **Service:** Psychiatric

**Staffed Beds:** 146

## OLEAN—Cattaraugus County

⊠ **OLEAN GENERAL HOSPITAL (330103)**, 515 Main Street, Zip 14760–1513; tel. 716/373–2600 **A**1 3 5 9 10 **F**3 8 11 13 15 17 18 22 28 29 30 31 34 35 38 39 40 45 46 47 48 49 50 51 53 54 57 58 59 60 61 62 64 65 70 74 75 76 77 78 79 81 82 84 85 86 87 89 92 93 94 97 98 100 101 102 103 107 108 109 110 111 114 115 116 117 118 120 128 129 130 131 132 133 134 142 143 144 145 146 147 **S** Upper Allegheny Health System, Olean, NY
Primary Contact: Timothy J. Finan, FACHE, President and Chief Executive Officer
COO: Ronald Mornelli, Senior Vice President Operations and Chief Operating Officer
CFO: Richard G. Braun, Jr., CPA, Senior Vice President and Chief Financial Officer
CMO: William Mills, M.D., Senior Vice President Quality and Professional Affairs
CIO: Jason Yaworsky, Senior Vice President Information Systems and Chief Information Officer
CHR: Timothy M. McNamara, Senior Vice President Human Resources
CNO: Jeff S. Zewe, R.N., Vice President Patient Care Services and Chief Nursing Officer
Web address: www.ogh.org
**Control:** Other not–for–profit (including NFP Corporation) **Service:** General Medical and Surgical

**Staffed Beds:** 186 **Admissions:** 6923 **Census:** 97 **Outpatient Visits:** 166720 **Births:** 790 **Total Expense ($000):** 96648 **Payroll Expense ($000):** 39299 **Personnel:** 763

## ONEIDA—Madison County

⊠ **ONEIDA HEALTHCARE (330115)**, 321 Genesee Street, Zip 13421–2611; tel. 315/363–6000, (Total facility includes 160 beds in nursing home–type unit) **A**1 9 10 **F**3 11 13 15 18 29 34 40 45 49 50 54 57 59 64 65 70 74 75 76 77 79 81 87 89 91 92 93 97 107 108 111 114 116 117 118 125 127 128 129 134 145 **P**6
Primary Contact: Gene Morreale, President and Chief Executive Officer
COO: Paul A. Scopac, Vice President of Operations and Chief Operating Officer
CFO: Vincent S. Maneen, Chief Financial Officer
CFO: Dewey R. Rowlands, Vice President Finance and Chief Financial Officer
CMO: Dan J. Vick, M.D., Vice President of Medical Affairs and Chief Medical Officer
CIO: Mary McGuirl, Director Information Systems
CHR: John G. Margo, Vice President Human Resources
CNO: Janis Kohlbrenner, R.N., Vice President Clinical Services and Chief Nursing Officer
Web address: www.oneidahealthcare.org
**Control:** Other not–for–profit (including NFP Corporation) **Service:** General Medical and Surgical

**Staffed Beds:** 231 **Admissions:** 3411 **Census:** 187 **Outpatient Visits:** 152913 **Births:** 549 **Total Expense ($000):** 82251 **Payroll Expense ($000):** 37178 **Personnel:** 537

## ONEONTA—Otsego County

⊠ **AURELIA OSBORN FOX MEMORIAL HOSPITAL (330085)**, 1 Norton Avenue, Zip 13820–2629; tel. 607/432–2000, (Total facility includes 131 beds in nursing home–type unit) **A**1 9 10 21 **F**2 3 11 13 15 17 26 28 29 30 34 35 39 40 45 46 47 48 50 51 53 54 56 57 59 64 65 68 70 74 75 76 77 81 85 86 87 89 93 96 97 104 107 108 110 111 114 117 118 119 120 122 127 128 129 143 145 146 **P**6 **S** Bassett Healthcare Network, Cooperstown, NY
Primary Contact: John R. Remillard, President
CFO: Mark J. Wright, Vice President Finance
CMO: Benjamin Friedell, Vice President Medical Affairs
CIO: Joseph Phillips, Director Information Systems
CHR: Keith Valk, Vice President Human Resources
CNO: Robbin Scobie, Vice President Nursing
Web address: www.aofoxhospital.com
**Control:** Other not–for–profit (including NFP Corporation) **Service:** General Medical and Surgical

**Staffed Beds:** 220 **Admissions:** 3729 **Census:** 169 **Outpatient Visits:** 238695 **Births:** 330 **Total Expense ($000):** 83024 **Payroll Expense ($000):** 38156 **Personnel:** 735

## ORANGEBURG—Rockland County

☐ **ROCKLAND CHILDREN'S PSYCHIATRIC CENTER**, 599 Convent Road, Zip 10962; tel. 845/359–7400, (Nonreporting) **A**1 3 5 **S** New York State Office of Mental Health, Albany, NY
Primary Contact: Raul Silva, M.D., Executive Director
COO: Kenneth Perrotte, Director Operations
CFO: Peter Gorey, Administrative Coordinator
CMO: Sadhana Sardana, M.D., Clinical Director
CIO: Mary Pivonka, Director Quality Management
Web address: www.omh.ny.gov/
**Control:** State–Government, nonfederal **Service:** Children's hospital psychiatric

**Staffed Beds:** 54

☐ **ROCKLAND PSYCHIATRIC CENTER (334015)**, 140 Old Orangeburg Road, Zip 10962–0071; tel. 845/359–1000, (Nonreporting) **A**1 3 5 10 **S** New York State Office of Mental Health, Albany, NY
Primary Contact: James H. Bopp, Executive Director
Web address: www.omh.ny.gov/
**Control:** State–Government, nonfederal **Service:** Psychiatric

**Staffed Beds:** 525

## OSSINING—Westchester County

**OSSINING CORRECTIONAL FACILITIES HOSPITAL**, 354 Hunter Street, Zip 10562–5498; tel. 914/941–0108, (Nonreporting)
Primary Contact: John Perilli, M.D., Health Services Director
**Control:** State–Government, nonfederal **Service:** Hospital unit of an institution (prison hospital, college infirmary, etc.)

**Staffed Beds:** 25

NY

---

**Hospital, Medicare Provider Number, Address, Telephone, Approval, Facility, and Physician Codes, Health Care System**

★ American Hospital Association (AHA) membership
☐ The Joint Commission accreditation    ◇ DNV Healthcare Inc. accreditation
○ American Osteopathic Association (AOA) accreditation
△ Commission on Accreditation of Rehabilitation Facilities (CARF) accreditation

---

**STONY LODGE HOSPITAL (334059)**, 40 Croton Dam Road, Zip 10562–2644,
Mailing Address: P.O. Box 1250, Briarcliff Manor, Zip 10510–0327;
tel. 914/941–7400, (Nonreporting) **A**9 10
Primary Contact: Kevin F. Czipo, Executive Director and Chief Executive Officer
CMO: Emil R. Pincus, M.D., Medical Director
CHR: Anne Alley, Director Human Resources
Web address: www.stonylodge.com
**Control:** Corporation, Investor–owned, for–profit **Service:** Psychiatric

| Staffed Beds: 50 |
|---|

### OSWEGO—Oswego County

✠ **OSWEGO HOSPITAL (330218)**, 110 West Sixth Street, Zip 13126–9985;
tel. 315/349–5511 **A**1 9 10 20 **F**3 8 11 13 15 17 28 29 34 38 40 45 46 49
50 54 57 59 64 70 74 75 76 77 79 80 81 84 85 86 87 89 93 97 98 99 100
101 102 103 104 107 108 110 111 114 117 118 129 130 131 134 143 145
147 **P**6
Primary Contact: Ann C. Gilpin, President and Chief Executive Officer
COO: Nancy Deavers, R.N., Vice President and Chief Operating Officer
CFO: Eric Campbell, Chief Financial Officer
CMO: Renato Mandanas, M.D., Vice President Medical Affairs
CIO: Major Barry Ryle, Chief Information Officer
CNO: Valerie Favata, R.N., Chief Nursing Officer
Web address: www.oswegohealth.org
**Control:** Other not–for–profit (including NFP Corporation) **Service:** General
Medical and Surgical

| Staffed Beds: 132 Admissions: 5656 Census: 75 Outpatient Visits: 361685 |
|---|
| Births: 667 Total Expense ($000): 95755 Payroll Expense ($000): 46783 |
| Personnel: 851 |

### PATCHOGUE—Suffolk County

★ **BROOKHAVEN MEMORIAL HOSPITAL MEDICAL CENTER (330141)**, 101
Hospital Road, Zip 11772–4897; tel. 631/654–7100, (Nonreporting) **A**9 10 12
13 21
Primary Contact: Thomas Ockers, President and Chief Executive Officer
COO: Richard T. Margulis, Executive Vice President and Chief Operating Officer
CFO: Brenda Farrell, Vice President Finance
CMO: Ronald Klein, M.D., Vice President and Chief Medical Officer
CIO: Marc Gibbs, Interim Chief Information Officer
CHR: Susan C. Hever, Director Human Resources
CNO: Kim K. Mendez, Ed.D., Vice President and Chief Nursing Officer
Web address: www.bmhmc.org
**Control:** Other not–for–profit (including NFP Corporation) **Service:** General
Medical and Surgical

| Staffed Beds: 306 |
|---|

### PENN YAN—Yates County

★ **SOLDIERS AND SAILORS MEMORIAL HOSPITAL OF YATES COUNTY
(331314)**, 418 North Main Street, Zip 14527–1085; tel. 315/531–2000 **A**9 10
18 **F**2 3 11 15 18 28 29 34 35 38 40 45 46 54 56 57 59 62 64 65 66 68 70
75 81 87 93 97 98 100 101 102 103 104 105 106 107 110 113 118 127
129 131 132 134 142 145 146 **P**6 **S** Finger Lakes Health, Geneva, NY
Primary Contact: Jose Acevedo, M.D., President and Chief Executive Officer
COO: Frank Korich, Vice President and Site Administrator
CFO: Patricia Thompson, Treasurer and Chief Financial Officer
CMO: Jason Feinberg, M.D., Vice President Medical Affairs and Chief Medical
Officer
CIO: John Oates, Director Information Systems
CHR: Patrick R. Boyle, Vice President Human Resources
CNO: Eileen Gage, R.N., Vice President Nursing
Web address: www.flhealth.org
**Control:** Other not–for–profit (including NFP Corporation) **Service:** General
Medical and Surgical

| Staffed Beds: 186 Admissions: 1094 Census: 153 Outpatient Visits: |
|---|
| 184030 Births: 0 Total Expense ($000): 31440 Payroll Expense ($000): |
| 15022 Personnel: 364 |

### PLAINVIEW—Nassau County

✠ **PLAINVIEW HOSPITAL (330331)**, 888 Old Country Road, Zip 11803–4978;
tel. 516/719–3000 **A**1 2 10 12 13 **F**3 9 13 15 17 18 29 30 31 34 35 36 38
40 43 44 45 46 49 50 57 58 60 64 65 68 69 70 71 74 75 76 78 79 81
84 85 86 87 97 101 102 107 108 110 111 116 118 129 131 134 145 147
**P**6 **S** North Shore–Long Island Jewish Health System, Great Neck, NY
Primary Contact: Michael Fener, Executive Director
CMO: Alan Mensch, M.D., Senior Vice President Medical Affairs
CIO: Nicholas O'Connor, Vice President and Chief Information Officer
Web address: www.northshorelij.com
**Control:** Other not–for–profit (including NFP Corporation) **Service:** General
Medical and Surgical

| Staffed Beds: 204 Admissions: 12042 Census: 174 Outpatient Visits: |
|---|
| 58795 Births: 1329 Total Expense ($000): 194806 Payroll Expense |
| ($000): 90974 Personnel: 1215 |

### PLATTSBURGH—Clinton County

✠ **CHAMPLAIN VALLEY PHYSICIANS HOSPITAL MEDICAL CENTER (330250)**,
75 Beekman Street, Zip 12901–1438; tel. 518/561–2000, (Total facility includes
90 beds in nursing home–type unit) **A**1 2 9 10 **F**3 7 8 11 13 14 15 17 18 20
22 24 26 28 29 30 31 32 34 35 37 38 39 40 43 44 45 46 49 51 53 54 57
59 60 61 64 65 66 70 74 75 76 77 78 79 81 82 83 84 85 86 87 89 93 94
97 98 99 100 101 102 104 106 107 108 110 111 113 116 117 118 119
120 122 125 127 128 129 130 131 134 143 145 146 147 **P**1 5 7
Primary Contact: Stephens M. Mundy, President and Chief Executive Officer
COO: Debra Donahue, Senior Vice President and Chief Operating Officer
CFO: Joyce Rafferty, Vice President Finance
CMO: Richard Dal Col, Vice President and Chief Medical Officer
CIO: Wouter Rietsema, M.D., Chief Quality and Information Officer
CHR: Michelle Lebeau, Vice President Human Resources
CNO: Debra Donahue, Senior Vice President and Chief Operating Officer
Web address: www.cvph.org
**Control:** Other not–for–profit (including NFP Corporation) **Service:** General
Medical and Surgical

| Staffed Beds: 341 Admissions: 10509 Census: 267 Outpatient Visits: |
|---|
| 341131 Births: 913 Total Expense ($000): 276043 Payroll Expense |
| ($000): 129366 Personnel: 1851 |

### POMONA—Rockland County

☐ **SUMMIT PARK HOSPITAL AND NURSING CARE CENTER (332014)**, 50
Sanatorium Road, Building A., Zip 10970; tel. 845/364–2700, (Nonreporting) **A**1
9 10
Primary Contact: Richard J. Maloney, M.P.H., Commissioner
COO: Richard J. Maloney, M.P.H., Commissioner
CFO: Chris Kopf, Chief Fiscal Officer
CMO: Paul Mercurio, M.D., Medical Director
CHR: Mary Hagan, Director Human Resources
Web address: www.co.rockland.ny.us
**Control:** County–Government, nonfederal **Service:** Long–Term Acute Care
hospital

| Staffed Beds: 408 |
|---|

### PORT JEFFERSON—Suffolk County

✠ **JOHN T. MATHER MEMORIAL HOSPITAL (330185)**, 75 North Country Road,
Zip 11777–2190; tel. 631/473–1320 **A**1 2 9 10 **F**5 8 12 14 15 17 29 34 35
36 37 38 40 44 49 51 55 56 57 59 60 64 69 70 75 77 78 79 81 82 85
87 93 98 99 100 102 103 104 105 107 108 110 111 113 114 117 118 119
125 128 129 131 145 146 147
Primary Contact: Kenneth D. Roberts, President
COO: Kevin J. Murray, Senior Vice President
CFO: Joseph Wisnoski, Vice President Finance and Chief Financial Officer
CMO: Joan Faro, M.D., Chief Medical Officer
CIO: Thomas Heiman, Assistant Vice President Information Services
CHR: Diane Marotta, Vice President Human Resources
CNO: Marie Mulligan, R.N., Vice President Nursing
Web address: www.matherhospital.com
**Control:** Other not–for–profit (including NFP Corporation) **Service:** General
Medical and Surgical

| Staffed Beds: 248 Admissions: 12451 Census: 200 Outpatient Visits: |
|---|
| 123041 Births: 0 Total Expense ($000): 243161 Payroll Expense ($000): |
| 125641 Personnel: 1943 |

☐ △ **ST. CHARLES HOSPITAL (330246)**, 200 Belle Terre Road,
Zip 11777–1928; tel. 631/474–6000, (Nonreporting) **A**1 2 7 9 10 **S** Catholic
Health Services of Long Island, Rockville Centre, NY
Primary Contact: James O'Connor, Executive Vice President
COO: Ronald Weingartner, Chief Operating Officer
CFO: Frank Fox, Vice President Finance and Chief Financial Officer
CFO: Frank Fox, Vice President Finance and Chief Financial Officer
CIO: Felix Pabon–Ramirez, Chief Information Officer
CHR: Mark Boehrer, Director Human Resources
Web address: www.stcharleshospital.chsli.org
**Control:** Church–operated, Nongovernment, not–for profit **Service:** General
Medical and Surgical

| Staffed Beds: 289 |
|---|

### PORT JERVIS—Orange County

✠ **BON SECOURS COMMUNITY HOSPITAL (330135)**, 160 East Main Street,
Zip 12771–2245, Mailing Address: P.O. Box 1014, Zip 12771–1014;
tel. 845/858–7000, (Nonreporting) **A**1 2 9 10 **S** Bon Secours Health System,
Inc., Marriottsville, MD
Primary Contact: Jeff Reilly, Senior Vice President Operations
COO: Gaynor Rosenstein, Vice President Operations
CFO: Stephen D. Majetich, CPA, Senior Vice President and Chief Financial Officer
CMO: Jeffrey Auerbach, D.O., Medical Director
CHR: Kim Hirkaler, Director Human Resources
Web address: www.bonsecourscommunityhosp.org
**Control:** Church–operated, Nongovernment, not–for profit **Service:** General
Medical and Surgical

| Staffed Beds: 187 |
|---|

*Many Facility Codes have changed. Please refer to the AHA Guide Code Chart.* © 2012 AHA Guide

## POTSDAM—St. Lawrence County

★ **CANTON–POTSDAM HOSPITAL (330197)**, 50 Leroy Street, Zip 13676–1799; tel. 315/265–3300 **A**9 10 20 21 **F**3 4 5 8 11 13 14 15 18 26 28 29 30 31 34 35 38 39 40 43 46 54 57 59 64 65 68 71 74 75 76 77 78 79 81 82 86 87 92 93 96 97 98 100 102 104 105 107 108 110 111 114 116 117 118 120 122 126 127 128 129 130 131 132 134 142 144 145 146 147 **P**6
Primary Contact: David B. Acker, FACHE, President and Chief Executive Officer
CFO: Richard Jacobs, Vice President Finance and Chief Financial Officer
CMO: Robert T. Rogers, II, M.D., Medical Director
CIO: Jorge C. Grillo, Chief Information Officer
CHR: A. Jack Davis, Vice President Human Resources
CNO: Cathy Ann Schantz, MSN, Vice President Patient Care Services and Chief Nursing Officer
Web address: www.cphospital.org
**Control:** Other not–for–profit (including NFP Corporation) **Service:** General Medical and Surgical

**Staffed Beds:** 94 **Admissions:** 4416 **Census:** 53 **Outpatient Visits:** 206714 **Births:** 371 **Total Expense ($000):** 87563 **Payroll Expense ($000):** 41563 **Personnel:** 758

## POUGHKEEPSIE—Dutchess County

△ **SAINT FRANCIS HOSPITAL AND HEALTH CENTERS (330067)**, 241 North Road, Zip 12601–1154; tel. 845/483–5000 **A**2 7 9 10 21 **F**1 3 4 8 11 12 15 17 18 20 22 29 30 31 32 34 35 36 37 40 43 45 46 49 50 55 56 57 60 61 62 63 64 65 66 68 70 74 75 77 78 79 80 81 82 85 86 87 89 90 91 93 98 99 100 101 102 103 104 107 108 111 114 117 118 128 129 130 131 132 133 134 143 145 147
Primary Contact: Robert L. Savage, President and Chief Executive Officer
CFO: Will de la Pena, Chief Financial Officer
CMO: J. Keith Festa, M.D., Vice President Medical Affairs
CIO: Joseph McCann, Chief Information Officer
CHR: Helen Rinaudo, Vice President Human Resources
CNO: Patricia Nocket, Assistant Vice President Clinical Nursing Services
Web address: www.sfhhc.org
**Control:** Church–operated, Nongovernment, not–for profit **Service:** General Medical and Surgical

**Staffed Beds:** 322 **Admissions:** 8655 **Census:** 163 **Outpatient Visits:** 206999 **Births:** 0 **Total Expense ($000):** 146079 **Payroll Expense ($000):** 69307 **Personnel:** 1183

⊠ **VASSAR BROTHERS MEDICAL CENTER (330023)**, 45 Reade Place, Zip 12601–3947; tel. 845/454–8500 **A**1 2 9 10 **F**3 8 11 13 14 15 17 18 20 22 24 26 29 30 31 32 34 35 36 39 40 46 49 50 51 54 55 56 57 58 59 60 63 64 66 68 70 72 74 75 76 77 78 79 81 82 84 85 86 87 89 93 97 107 108 110 111 113 114 118 119 120 123 125 128 129 131 134 145 146 147 **S** Health Quest Systems, Inc., Lagrangeville, NY
Primary Contact: Janet L. Ready, President and Chief Operating Officer
CFO: Maryann Kepple, Chief Financial Officer
CMO: Stephen A. Katz, M.D., Chief Medical Officer and Senior Vice President Medical Affairs
CIO: Robert Diamond, Chief Information Officer
CHR: Jeffrey McDonough, Assistant Vice President Human Resources
CNO: Margaret M. Cusumano, R.N., Chief Nursing Officer and Vice President Care Services
Web address: www.health–quest.org
**Control:** Other not–for–profit (including NFP Corporation) **Service:** General Medical and Surgical

**Staffed Beds:** 365 **Admissions:** 19238 **Census:** 263 **Outpatient Visits:** 245751 **Births:** 2248 **Total Expense ($000):** 367980 **Payroll Expense ($000):** 118516 **Personnel:** 1740

## QUEENS—Queens County, See New York City

## QUEENS VILLAGE—Queens County, See New York City

## RHINEBECK—Dutchess County

⊠ △ **NORTHERN DUTCHESS HOSPITAL (330049)**, 6511 Springbrook Avenue, Zip 12572–5002, Mailing Address: P.O. Box 5002, Zip 12572–5002; tel. 845/876–3001 **A**1 7 9 10 **F**3 9 11 13 15 18 28 29 30 34 35 36 37 40 50 53 54 56 57 59 64 68 70 74 75 76 77 79 81 82 85 90 93 107 108 111 113 118 128 129 130 131 134 145 146 **S** Health Quest Systems, Inc., Lagrangeville, NY
Primary Contact: Denise George, R.N., President and Chief Executive Officer
CFO: Alan Mossoff, Chief Financial Officer
CMO: John Sabia, M.D., Medical Director
CIO: Catherine Schuster, Chief Information Officer
CHR: Eileen Miller, Director Human Resources
Web address: www.health–quest.org/home_nd.cfm?id=9
**Control:** Other not–for–profit (including NFP Corporation) **Service:** General Medical and Surgical

**Staffed Beds:** 68 **Admissions:** 3325 **Census:** 42 **Outpatient Visits:** 63518 **Births:** 880 **Total Expense ($000):** 61099 **Payroll Expense ($000):** 21463 **Personnel:** 439

## RICHMOND VALLEY—Richmond County, See New York City

## RIVERHEAD—Suffolk County

☐ **PECONIC BAY MEDICAL CENTER (330107)**, 1300 Roanoke Avenue, Zip 11901–2031; tel. 631/548–6000, (Total facility includes 60 beds in nursing home–type unit) **A**1 9 10 12 13 **F**7 11 12 13 15 29 30 31 34 40 45 46 47 49 50 57 59 60 61 64 68 70 74 75 76 77 78 79 80 81 84 85 86 87 90 93 96 107 108 110 111 114 117 118 125 127 129 130 131 142 145 146 147 **P**7
Primary Contact: Andrew J. Mitchell, President and Chief Executive Officer
COO: Ronald McManus, Senior Vice President Clinical Services and Business Entities
CFO: Michael O'Donnell, Chief Financial Officer
CMO: Richard Kubiak, M.D., Vice President Medical Affairs
CIO: Arthur Crowe, Director Information Systems
CHR: Monica Chestnut–Rauls, Vice President Human Resources
CNO: Gerard Zunno, R.N., Vice President Patient Care Services
Web address: www.pbmchealth.org
**Control:** Other not–for–profit (including NFP Corporation) **Service:** General Medical and Surgical

**Staffed Beds:** 176 **Admissions:** 8228 **Census:** 141 **Outpatient Visits:** 94919 **Births:** 410 **Total Expense ($000):** 129342 **Payroll Expense ($000):** 52807 **Personnel:** 848

## ROCHESTER—Monroe County

⊠ **HIGHLAND HOSPITAL OF ROCHESTER (330164)**, 1000 South Avenue, Zip 14620–2733; tel. 585/473–2200 **A**1 3 5 9 10 **F**5 8 12 13 15 18 29 30 31 34 35 37 38 39 40 43 45 46 49 50 54 55 56 57 59 61 63 64 65 68 70 74 75 76 77 78 79 81 82 83 84 85 86 87 97 100 107 108 109 110 111 112 113 114 118 119 120 121 122 125 129 133 144 145 146 **P**6 **S** University of Rochester Medical Center, Rochester, NY
Primary Contact: Steven I. Goldstein, President and Chief Executive Officer
COO: Cindy Becker, Vice President and Chief Operating Officer
CFO: Leonard J. Shute, Chief Financial Officer
CMO: Raymond Mayewski, M.D., Chief Medical Officer
CIO: D. Jerome Powell, M.D., Chief Information Officer
CHR: Kathleen Gallucci, Chief Human Resources
Web address: www.stronghealth.com
**Control:** Hospital district or authority, Government, nonfederal **Service:** General Medical and Surgical

**Staffed Beds:** 261 **Admissions:** 16109 **Census:** 194 **Outpatient Visits:** 252491 **Births:** 2968 **Total Expense ($000):** 260249 **Payroll Expense ($000):** 122184 **Personnel:** 2004

⊠ **ROCHESTER GENERAL HOSPITAL (330125)**, 1425 Portland Avenue, Zip 14621–3099; tel. 585/922–4000 **A**1 2 9 10 **F**3 5 8 9 11 12 13 14 15 17 18 20 22 24 26 28 29 30 31 32 34 35 36 38 39 40 41 43 44 47 49 50 51 54 55 56 57 58 59 60 61 64 66 68 70 73 74 75 76 77 78 79 80 81 82 84 85 86 87 89 90 92 93 96 97 98 99 100 101 102 103 104 107 108 110 111 113 114 117 118 119 120 122 123 125 129 130 131 133 134 144 145 146 147 **P**5 7 **S** Rochester General Health System, Rochester, NY
Primary Contact: Robert Nesselbush, President
CMO: Richard Gangemi, M.D., Senior Vice President Academic and Medical Affairs
CIO: David Kamowski, Senior Vice President and Chief Information Officer
CHR: Janine Schue, Senior Vice President Human Resources
CNO: Cheryl Sheridan, R.N., Senior Vice President Patient Care Services
Web address: www.rochestergeneral.org
**Control:** Other not–for–profit (including NFP Corporation) **Service:** General Medical and Surgical

**Staffed Beds:** 520 **Admissions:** 31138 **Census:** 470 **Outpatient Visits:** 1448410 **Births:** 2422 **Total Expense ($000):** 672934 **Payroll Expense ($000):** 326822 **Personnel:** 5204

NY

**Hospital, Medicare Provider Number, Address, Telephone, Approval, Facility, and Physician Codes, Health Care System**

★ American Hospital Association (AHA) membership
☐ The Joint Commission accreditation
◇ DNV Healthcare Inc. accreditation
○ American Osteopathic Association (AOA) accreditation
△ Commission on Accreditation of Rehabilitation Facilities (CARF) accreditation

☐ **ROCHESTER PSYCHIATRIC CENTER (334020)**, 1111 Elmwood Avenue,
Zip 14620–3005; tel. 585/241–1200, (Nonreporting) **A**1 3 5 10 **S** New York
State Office of Mental Health, Albany, NY
Primary Contact: Michael P. Zuber, Ph.D., Executive Director
COO: Joseph Coffey, Director Facility Administration
CFO: Rosanne Minnis, Business Officer
CMO: Laurence Guttmacher, M.D., Clinical Director
CIO: Stephen Font, Coordinator Information Systems
CHR: Christine Hally, Director Human Resources
Web address: www.omh.ny.gov/omhweb/facilities/ropc/facility.htm
**Control:** State–Government, nonfederal **Service:** Psychiatric

**Staffed Beds:** 180

☒ △ **STRONG MEMORIAL HOSPITAL OF THE UNIVERSITY OF ROCHESTER
(330285)**, 601 Elmwood Avenue, Zip 14642–0002; tel. 585/275–2100,
(Includes GOLISANO CHILDREN'S HOSPITAL, 601 Elmwood Avenue, Zip 14610;
tel. 585/275–2182) **A**1 2 3 5 7 8 9 10 **F**3 5 6 8 9 11 12 13 14 15 16 17 18
19 20 21 22 23 24 25 26 27 28 29 30 31 32 33 34 35 38 39 40 41 43 44
45 46 47 48 49 50 51 52 53 54 55 56 57 58 59 61 63 64 65 66 68 70 71
72 73 74 75 76 77 78 79 81 82 83 84 85 86 87 88 89 90 91 92 93 94 96
97 98 99 100 101 102 103 104 105 107 108 110 111 113 114 115 116
117 118 119 120 122 123 125 128 129 130 131 133 134 135 136 137 138
140 141 142 143 145 146 147 **P**5 6 **S** University of Rochester Medical Center,
Rochester, NY
Primary Contact: Steven I. Goldstein, President and Chief Executive Officer
COO: Kathleen M. Parrinello, Ph.D., Chief Operating Officer
CFO: Leonard J. Shute, Chief Financial Officer
CMO: Raymond Mayewski, M.D., Chief Medical Officer
CIO: D. Jerome Powell, M.D., Chief Information Officer
CHR: Charles J. Murphy, Associate Vice President Human Resources
Web address: www.urmc.rochester.edu
**Control:** Other not–for–profit (including NFP Corporation) **Service:** General
Medical and Surgical

**Staffed Beds:** 750 **Admissions:** 38029 **Census:** 686 **Outpatient Visits:**
1316944 **Births:** 2979 **Total Expense ($000):** 1036438 **Payroll Expense
($000):** 416721 **Personnel:** 8181

☒ **UNITY HOSPITAL (330226)**, 1555 Long Pond Road, Zip 14626–4182;
tel. 585/723–7000, (Nonreporting) **A**1 2 3 5 9 10
Primary Contact: Warren Hern, President and Chief Executive Officer
COO: Stewart C. Putnam, Executive Vice President and Chief Operating Officer
CFO: Tom Crilly, Executive Vice President and Chief Financial Officer
CMO: James Haley, M.D., Senior Vice President and Chief Medical Officer
CIO: John Glynn, Senior Vice President and Chief Information Officer
CHR: Maryalice Keller, Vice President Brand and Talent Management
CNO: Jane McCormack, R.N., Vice President, Chief Nursing Officer and Nursing
and Patient Care Services
Web address: www.unityhealth.org
**Control:** Other not–for–profit (including NFP Corporation) **Service:** General
Medical and Surgical

**Staffed Beds:** 441

### ROCKVILLE CENTRE—Nassau County

☐ **MERCY MEDICAL CENTER (330259)**, 1000 North Village Avenue,
Zip 11570–1000; tel. 516/705–2525 **A**1 2 9 10 **F**5 11 12 13 14 15 18 20 26
28 29 30 31 34 35 36 37 38 39 40 43 44 45 50 54 56 57 59 60 63 64 65
66 68 72 73 74 75 77 78 79 80 81 82 84 85 87 90 92 93 94 97 98 100
101 102 103 104 105 107 108 109 110 111 113 114 115 116 117 118 119
120 123 125 127 128 129 130 131 134 143 144 145 146 147 **S** Catholic
Health Services of Long Island, Rockville Centre, NY
Primary Contact: Alan D. Guerci, M.D., Chief Executive Officer
COO: Ronald Steimel, Vice President Administration and Chief Operating Officer
CFO: William C. Armstrong, Senior Vice President and Chief Financial Officer
CMO: John Reilly, M.D., Vice President Medical Affairs and Chief Medical Officer
CIO: Marcy Dunn, Vice President Information Services and Chief Information
Officer
CHR: Allison Cianciotto Croyle, Vice President of Human Resources
CNO: Renee Mauriello, R.N., Vice President, Patient Care Services
Web address: www.mercymedicalcenter.chsli.org
**Control:** Church–operated, Nongovernment, not–for profit **Service:** General
Medical and Surgical

**Staffed Beds:** 196 **Admissions:** 10919 **Census:** 199 **Outpatient Visits:**
111629 **Births:** 1249

### ROME—Oneida County

★ ○ **ROME MEMORIAL HOSPITAL (330215)**, 1500 North James Street,
Zip 13440–2844; tel. 315/338–7000, (Total facility includes 82 beds in nursing
home–type unit) **A**9 10 11 **F**3 5 8 13 15 18 26 27 29 30 31 34 35 37 40 46
49 56 57 59 61 64 65 66 70 74 75 76 77 78 79 80 81 84 85 86 87 89 93
97 99 101 102 103 106 107 108 110 111 114 117 118 119 120 122 127
128 129 130 131 134 145 146 147 **P**6
Primary Contact: Basil Ariglio, President and Chief Executive Officer
COO: Raymond Carnevale, Senior Vice President and Chief Operating Officer
CFO: Nicholas Mayhew, Vice President and Chief Financial Officer
CMO: Waleed Albert, M.D., Chief Medical Officer
CIO: Bruce Peterson, Chief Information Officer
CHR: Regina Chambers, Assistant Vice President Human Resource
CNO: Durinda Durr, Vice President and Chief Nursing Officer
Web address: www.romehospital.org
**Control:** Other not–for–profit (including NFP Corporation) **Service:** General
Medical and Surgical

**Staffed Beds:** 203 **Admissions:** 5309 **Census:** 129 **Outpatient Visits:**
150557 **Births:** 640 **Total Expense ($000):** 82921 **Payroll Expense ($000):**
39491 **Personnel:** 872

### ROSLYN—Nassau County

☒ **ST. FRANCIS HOSPITAL (330182)**, 100 Port Washington Boulevard,
Zip 11576–1353; tel. 516/562–6000 **A**1 9 10 **F**3 7 11 15 17 18 19 20 21 22
23 24 26 27 28 29 30 31 34 35 36 37 38 39 40 43 44 45 46 47 49 50 53
54 56 57 58 59 60 61 62 63 64 65 66 68 70 71 74 75 77 78 79 80 81 82
84 85 86 87 89 93 94 97 100 102 107 108 109 110 111 113 114 115 116
117 118 123 125 129 130 131 134 140 144 145 146 147 **P**6 **S** Catholic
Health Services of Long Island, Rockville Centre, NY
Primary Contact: Alan D. Guerci, M.D., Chief Executive Officer
COO: Ruth Hennessey, Executive Vice President and Chief Administrative Officer
CFO: William C. Armstrong, Vice President and Chief Financial Officer
CMO: Jack Soterakis, M.D., Executive Vice President Medical Affairs
CIO: Marcy Dunn, Vice President Information Services and Chief Information
Officer
CHR: Barbara Fierro, Director, Human Resources
CNO: Ann S. Cella, R.N., Senior Vice President, Patient Care Services
Web address: www.stfrancisheartcenter.chsli.org
**Control:** Church–operated, Nongovernment, not–for profit **Service:** General
Medical and Surgical

**Staffed Beds:** 312 **Admissions:** 18003 **Census:** 298 **Outpatient Visits:**
175225 **Births:** 0 **Total Expense ($000):** 470762 **Payroll Expense ($000):**
214297 **Personnel:** 2674

### RYE—Westchester County

☒ **RYE HOSPITAL CENTER (334033)**, 754 Boston Post Road, Zip 10580–2724;
tel. 914/967–4567 **A**1 9 10 **F**98 99 103 129 145
Primary Contact: Jack C. Schoenholtz, M.D., President, Chief Executive Officer,
Administrator and Medical Director
CFO: John Marcogliese, Vice President Financial Operations
Web address: www.ryehospitalcenter.org
**Control:** Corporation, Investor–owned, for–profit **Service:** Psychiatric

**Staffed Beds:** 34 **Admissions:** 265 **Census:** 26 **Outpatient Visits:** 0 **Births:**
0 **Total Expense ($000):** 6388 **Payroll Expense ($000):** 3331 **Personnel:**
68

### SARANAC LAKE—Franklin County

☒ ○ **ADIRONDACK MEDICAL CENTER (330079)**, 2233 State Route 86,
Zip 12983, Mailing Address: P.O. Box 471, Zip 12983–0471;
tel. 518/891–4141, (Total facility includes 194 beds in nursing home–type unit)
**A**1 9 10 11 **F**3 8 9 12 13 15 18 28 29 30 31 34 35 37 38 39 40 41 42 43
45 46 49 54 56 57 59 60 64 70 71 74 75 76 77 78 79 81 82 84 85 86 89
90 92 93 94 97 98 102 103 104 107 108 110 111 113 115 118 126 127
128 129 130 131 134 145 146 147 **P**1 5 **S** HealthTech Management Services,
Franklin, TN
Primary Contact: Chandler M. Ralph, President and Chief Executive Officer
COO: Cynthia McGuire, Chief Operating Officer
CFO: Patrick M. Facteau, Chief Financial Officer
CMO: William Viscardo, M.D., Chief Medical Officer
CHR: MaDena DuChemin, Chief Human Resources Officer
Web address: www.amccares.org
**Control:** Other not–for–profit (including NFP Corporation) **Service:** General
Medical and Surgical

**Staffed Beds:** 271 **Admissions:** 2820 **Census:** 210 **Outpatient Visits:**
121830 **Births:** 177 **Total Expense ($000):** 97760 **Payroll Expense ($000):**
43048 **Personnel:** 690

### SARATOGA SPRINGS—Saratoga County

☐ **FOUR WINDS HOSPITAL (334049)**, 30 Crescent Avenue, Zip 12866;
tel. 518/584–3600, (Nonreporting) **A**1 9 10
Primary Contact: David J. Woodlock, Administrator
Web address: www.fourwindshospital.com
**Control:** Corporation, Investor–owned, for–profit **Service:** Children's hospital
psychiatric

**Staffed Beds:** 83

NY

*Many Facility Codes have changed. Please refer to the AHA Guide Code Chart.* © 2012 AHA Guide

✠ **SARATOGA HOSPITAL (330222)**, 211 Church Street, Zip 12866–1003; tel. 518/587–3222, (Total facility includes 36 beds in nursing home–type unit) **A**1 5 9 10 **F**3 8 12 13 15 17 18 20 29 30 31 34 35 37 38 40 45 47 49 50 54 56 57 59 64 68 70 74 75 76 77 78 79 81 82 85 92 93 94 96 97 98 100 101 102 103 106 107 108 110 111 113 114 115 116 118 119 120 125 127 129 130 131 134 143 144 145 146 **P**6
Primary Contact: Angelo G. Calbone, President and Chief Executive Officer
CFO: Gary Foster, Vice President and Chief Financial Officer
CMO: Joyce L. Peabody, M.D., Vice President and Chief Medical Officer
CIO: John Mangona, Chief Information Officer and Compliance Officer
CHR: Jeffrey M. Methven, Vice President Ambulatory Services and Chief Human Resources Officer
Web address: www.saratogacare.org
**Control:** Other not–for–profit (including NFP Corporation) **Service:** General Medical and Surgical

**Staffed Beds: 199 Admissions: 9554 Census: 165 Outpatient Visits: 236946 Births: 757 Total Expense ($000): 191219 Payroll Expense ($000): 84706 Personnel: 1563**

### SCHENECTADY—Schenectady County

✠ **ELLIS HOSPITAL (330153)**, 1101 Nott Street, Zip 12308–2425; tel. 518/243–4000, (Includes BELLEVUE WOMAN'S CARE CENTER, 2210 Troy Road, Zip 12309–4797; tel. 518/346–9400; ELLIS HOSPITAL HEALTH CENTER, 600 McClellan Street, Zip 12304–1090; tel. 518/382–2000), (Total facility includes 82 beds in nursing home–type unit) **A**1 3 5 9 10 **F**8 10 12 13 15 18 20 22 24 26 28 29 30 31 38 39 40 64 65 68 70 72 74 75 76 77 78 79 81 82 83 84 89 93 98 99 100 101 102 103 104 107 108 110 111 113 114 116 118 120 125 127 128 129 145 146 147 **P**6
Primary Contact: James W. Connolly, President and Chief Executive Officer
COO: Paul A. Milton, Executive Vice President and Chief Operating Officer
CFO: Daniel Rinaldi, Chief Financial Officer
CMO: David Liebers, M.D., Chief Medical Officer and Vice President Medical Affairs
CIO: David Snyder, Chief Information Officer and Vice President Information Technology
CHR: Joseph Giansante, Vice President Human Resources
Web address: www.ellismedicine.org
**Control:** Other not–for–profit (including NFP Corporation) **Service:** General Medical and Surgical

**Staffed Beds: 431 Admissions: 21465 Census: 357 Outpatient Visits: 494430 Births: 2441 Total Expense ($000): 318656 Payroll Expense ($000): 174369**

**ELLIS HOSPITAL HEALTH CENTER** See Ellis Hospital

**ELLIS HOSPITAL MCCLELLAN CAMPUS** See Ellis Hospital Health Center

✠ △ **SUNNYVIEW REHABILITATION HOSPITAL (330406)**, 1270 Belmont Avenue, Zip 12308–2104; tel. 518/382–4500 **A**1 3 5 7 9 10 **F**3 28 29 53 56 57 59 64 74 79 90 93 94 118 129 131 134 145 **P**5 **S** Catholic Health East, Newtown Square, PA
Primary Contact: Edward Eisenman, Chief Executive Officer
CFO: Kristin Signor, Director Finance
CMO: Lynne T. Nicolson, M.D., Medical Director
CIO: Patrick Clark, Manager Information Technology
CHR: Meghan Glowa, Director Human Resources
Web address: www.sunnyview.org
**Control:** Other not–for–profit (including NFP Corporation) **Service:** Rehabilitation

**Staffed Beds: 115 Admissions: 2472 Census: 90 Outpatient Visits: 54406 Births: 0 Total Expense ($000): 43619 Payroll Expense ($000): 25180 Personnel: 543**

### SLEEPY HOLLOW—Westchester County

✠ **PHELPS MEMORIAL HOSPITAL CENTER (330261)**, 701 North Broadway, Zip 10591–1020; tel. 914/366–3000, (Nonreporting) **A**1 5 9 10
Primary Contact: Keith F. Safian, President and Chief Executive Officer
COO: Bruce B. Davidow, Senior Vice President and Chief Operating Officer
CFO: Vincent DeSantis, Vice President Finance
CMO: Lawrence L. Faltz, M.D., Senior Vice President Medical Affairs and Medical Director
CHR: Joanne Sturans, Vice President Human Resources
Web address: www.phelpshospital.org
**Control:** Other not–for–profit (including NFP Corporation) **Service:** General Medical and Surgical

**Staffed Beds: 228**

### SMITHTOWN—Suffolk County

☐ **ST. CATHERINE OF SIENA MEDICAL CENTER (330401)**, 50 Route 25–A, Zip 11787–1348; tel. 631/862–3000, (Nonreporting) **A**1 9 10 **S** Catholic Health Services of Long Island, Rockville Centre, NY
Primary Contact: Dennis Verzi, Executive Director
CFO: Dan Macksood, Regional Vice President and Chief Financial Officer
CHR: Danielle A. Robbins, Vice President Human Resources
Web address: www.stcatherinemedicalcenter.org
**Control:** Church–operated, Nongovernment, not–for profit **Service:** General Medical and Surgical

**Staffed Beds: 503**

### SOUTHAMPTON—Suffolk County

✠ **SOUTHAMPTON HOSPITAL (330340)**, 240 Meeting House Lane, Zip 11968–5090; tel. 631/726–8200 **A**1 9 10 12 13 **F**3 8 12 13 15 18 28 29 30 31 34 35 36 37 40 44 45 46 50 60 61 65 68 70 74 75 76 77 78 79 81 82 84 85 86 87 89 93 107 108 110 111 114 117 118 129 130 131 134 144 145 147 **P**4 6 8
Primary Contact: Robert S. Chaloner, President and Chief Executive Officer
COO: Frederic Weinbaum, M.D., Executive Vice President Operations and Chief Medical Officer
CFO: Chris Schulteis, Vice President/Chief Financial Officer
CMO: Frederic Weinbaum, M.D., Executive Vice President Operations and Chief Medical Officer
CIO: William Bifulco, Vice President/Chief Information Officer
CHR: Paul Robert Davin, Vice President, Human Resources
CNO: Patricia Darcey, R.N., Vice President/Chief Nursing Officer
Web address: www.southamptonhospital.org
**Control:** Other not–for–profit (including NFP Corporation) **Service:** General Medical and Surgical

**Staffed Beds: 80 Admissions: 5505 Census: 52 Outpatient Visits: 630385 Births: 687 Total Expense ($000): 98809 Payroll Expense ($000): 49420 Personnel: 785**

### SPRINGVILLE—Erie County

**BERTRAND CHAFFEE HOSPITAL (330111)**, 224 East Main Street, Zip 14141–1497; tel. 716/592–2871, (Nonreporting) **A**9 10
Primary Contact: Nils Gunnersen, Administrator
CMO: J. Matthew Baker, M.D., President Medical Staff
CHR: Mary Beth Brown, Director Human Resources
Web address: www.chaffeehospitalandhome.com
**Control:** Other not–for–profit (including NFP Corporation) **Service:** General Medical and Surgical

**Staffed Beds: 24**

### STAR LAKE—St. Lawrence County

★ **CLIFTON–FINE HOSPITAL (331307)**, Oswegatchie Trail, Zip 13690, Mailing Address: 1014 Oswegatchie Trail, Zip 13690–0010; tel. 315/848–3351, (Nonreporting) **A**9 10 18
Primary Contact: Robert P. Kimmes, Chief Executive Officer
CFO: Nancy Russell, Chief Financial Officer
CMO: David Welch, M.D., Medical Director
CIO: Steve Potter, Manager Business and Information Systems
CNO: Michelle Bristol, Director of Nursing
Web address: www.cliftonfinehospital.org
**Control:** Other not–for–profit (including NFP Corporation) **Service:** General Medical and Surgical

**Staffed Beds: 20**

### STATEN ISLAND—Richmond County, See New York City

---

**Hospital, Medicare Provider Number, Address, Telephone, Approval, Facility, and Physician Codes, Health Care System**

★ American Hospital Association (AHA) membership
☐ The Joint Commission accreditation   ◇ DNV Healthcare Inc. accreditation
○ American Osteopathic Association (AOA) accreditation
△ Commission on Accreditation of Rehabilitation Facilities (CARF) accreditation

**NY**

## STONY BROOK—Suffolk County

⊞ **STONY BROOK UNIVERSITY MEDICAL CENTER (330393)**, State University of New York, Zip 11794–8410; tel. 631/444–1077 **A**1 2 3 5 8 9 10 **F**3 6 7 8 9 11 12 13 14 15 16 17 18 19 20 22 24 26 28 29 30 31 32 34 35 38 39 40 41 43 44 45 46 47 48 49 50 51 52 54 55 56 57 58 59 60 61 64 65 66 67 68 70 72 74 75 76 77 78 79 81 82 84 85 86 87 88 89 93 96 97 98 99 100 101 102 103 104 105 107 108 110 111 113 114 115 116 117 118 119 120 121 122 123 125 128 129 130 131 133 134 135 137 140 142 144 145 146 147 **P**1 6
Primary Contact: Fred S. Sganga, Interim Chief Executive Officer
COO: Carol Gomes, Director Operations
CFO: Gary E. Bie, Chief Financial Officer
CMO: Todd Griffin, M.D., Chief Medical Officer
CIO: Jane Tsui–Wu, Interim Chief Information Officer
CHR: Elizabeth McCoy, Chief Human Resources Management
CNO: Lee Anne Xippolitos, R.N., Chief Nursing Officer
Web address: www.stonybrookmedicalcenter.org
**Control:** State–Government, nonfederal **Service:** General Medical and Surgical

**Staffed Beds:** 652 **Admissions:** 31257 **Census:** 512 **Outpatient Visits:** 445853 **Births:** 3812 **Total Expense ($000):** 858880 **Payroll Expense ($000):** 397532 **Personnel:** 5724

## SUFFERN—Rockland County

⊞ **GOOD SAMARITAN HOSPITAL (330158)**, 255 Lafayette Avenue, Zip 10901–4869; tel. 845/368–5000, (Nonreporting) **A**1 2 9 10 **S** Bon Secours Health System, Inc., Marriottsville, MD
Primary Contact: Philip A. Patterson, Chief Executive Officer
COO: Gerry Durney, Chief Operating Officer
CFO: Melinda Hancock, Interim Chief Financial Officer
CMO: Rodney W. Williams, M.D., Vice President Medical Affairs
CIO: Deborah K. Marshall, Vice President Public Relations
CHR: Pamela Tarulli, Senior Vice President Human Resources
Web address: www.goodsamhosp.org
**Control:** Church–operated, Nongovernment, not–for profit **Service:** General Medical and Surgical

**Staffed Beds:** 308

## SYOSSET—Nassau County

★ **SYOSSET HOSPITAL**, 221 Jericho Turnpike, Zip 11791–4567; tel. 516/496–6400 **A**9 **F**3 12 15 18 29 30 34 35 36 38 40 43 44 45 50 57 58 59 64 65 68 70 74 79 81 82 84 85 87 97 98 100 101 102 107 108 118 129 131 134 145 147 **P**6 **S** North Shore–Long Island Jewish Health System, Great Neck, NY
Primary Contact: Michael Fener, Executive Director
COO: Mark J. Solazzo, Regional Chief Operating Officer
CFO: Richard Reilly, Deputy Executive Director
CMO: Randolph DiLorenzo, M.D., Medical Director
CHR: Andrew S. Goldberg, Associate Executive Director
Web address: www.northshorelij.com
**Control:** Other not–for–profit (including NFP Corporation) **Service:** General Medical and Surgical

**Staffed Beds:** 75 **Admissions:** 4285 **Census:** 58 **Outpatient Visits:** 37107 **Births:** 0 **Total Expense ($000):** 114912 **Payroll Expense ($000):** 53631 **Personnel:** 622

## SYRACUSE—Onondaga County

**COMMUNITY–GENERAL HOSPITAL OF GREATER SYRACUSE** See Upstate University Hospital at Community General

★ **CROUSE HOSPITAL (330203)**, 736 Irving Avenue, Zip 13210–1690; tel. 315/470–7111 **A**3 5 9 10 21 **F**3 4 5 8 11 12 13 15 18 19 20 21 22 23 26 27 29 31 34 35 36 37 40 49 50 56 59 60 70 72 74 75 76 77 78 79 81 84 86 87 89 93 96 107 108 110 113 114 115 116 117 118 125 128 129 131 134 143 144 145 146 147
Primary Contact: Paul J. Kronenberg, M.D., President and Chief Executive Officer
CFO: Kimberly Boynton, Chief Financial Officer
CMO: Ronald Stahl, M.D., Chief Medical Officer
CHR: John Bergemann, Director Human Resources
Web address: www.crouse.org
**Control:** Other not–for–profit (including NFP Corporation) **Service:** General Medical and Surgical

**Staffed Beds:** 487 **Admissions:** 20806 **Census:** 326 **Outpatient Visits:** 311895 **Births:** 4171 **Total Expense ($000):** 346104 **Payroll Expense ($000):** 153650 **Personnel:** 2308

☐ **RICHARD H. HUTCHINGS PSYCHIATRIC CENTER (334001)**, 620 Madison Street, Zip 13210–2319; tel. 315/426–3632, (Nonreporting) **A**1 3 5 10 **S** New York State Office of Mental Health, Albany, NY
Primary Contact: Colleen A. Sawyer, R.N., MSN, Executive Director
COO: David Peppel, Director Operations
CFO: Robert Stapleton, Director Administration
CMO: Mark Cattalani, M.D., Clinical Director
CIO: Neil Nemi, Administrator Facility Information Center
CHR: Katherine Herron, Director Human Resources
Web address: www.omh.ny.gov
**Control:** State–Government, nonfederal **Service:** Psychiatric

**Staffed Beds:** 131

★ **ST. JOSEPH'S HOSPITAL HEALTH CENTER (330140)**, 301 Prospect Avenue, Zip 13203–1807; tel. 315/448–5111 **A**3 5 9 10 21 **F**8 12 13 14 15 18 20 22 24 26 28 29 30 31 34 35 38 39 40 45 46 48 49 50 53 54 57 58 59 60 62 64 66 68 70 72 73 74 75 76 77 78 79 81 82 83 84 87 92 93 94 97 98 99 100 101 102 104 107 108 110 113 114 117 118 128 129 130 131 134 143 144 145 146 147 **S** Sisters of Saint Francis, Syracuse, NY
Primary Contact: Kathryn H. Ruscitto, President
COO: Mary W. Brown, Senior Vice President Operations
CFO: Michael Shaffer, Vice President Fiscal Services
CMO: Sandra Sulik, M.D., Vice President Medical Affairs
CIO: Charles Fennell, Vice President Information Management
CHR: Frank Panzetta, Director Human Resources
CNO: AnneMarie Czyz, R.N., Vice President for Clinical and Educational Services
Web address: www.sjhsyr.org
**Control:** Other not–for–profit (including NFP Corporation) **Service:** General Medical and Surgical

**Staffed Beds:** 431 **Admissions:** 24171 **Census:** 359 **Outpatient Visits:** 593934 **Births:** 1994 **Total Expense ($000):** 458898 **Payroll Expense ($000):** 205285 **Personnel:** 3511

★ **UPSTATE UNIVERSITY HOSPITAL (330241)**, 750 East Adams Street, Zip 13210–2342; tel. 315/464–5540, (Includes UPSTATE UNIVERSITY HOSPITAL AT COMMUNITY GENERAL, 4900 Broad Road, Zip 13215–2293; tel. 315/492–5011; Thomas P. Quinn, President and Chief Executive Officer) **A**2 8 9 10 21 **F**3 9 11 12 15 16 17 18 19 20 22 23 24 25 26 28 29 30 31 32 34 35 38 39 40 41 43 44 45 46 47 48 49 50 51 52 54 55 56 57 58 59 60 61 64 66 68 70 74 75 76 77 78 79 81 82 84 85 86 87 88 89 90 92 93 95 97 98 99 100 101 102 103 104 105 107 108 110 111 113 114 117 118 119 120 121 122 123 125 128 129 130 131 133 134 135 137 144 145 146 147
Primary Contact: John B. McCabe, M.D., Chief Executive Officer
COO: Paul E. Seale, FACHE, Chief Operating Officer
CFO: Stuart M. Wright, CPA, Chief Financial Officer
CMO: David Duggan, M.D., Medical Director
CMO: David Duggan, M.D., Medical Director
CIO: Terry Wagner, Chief Information Officer
CHR: Eric Frost, Associate Vice President Human Resources
CNO: Katharine Mooney, R.N., Chief Nursing Officer
Web address: www.upstate.edu/hospital
**Control:** State–Government, nonfederal **Service:** General Medical and Surgical

**Staffed Beds:** 617 **Admissions:** 24347 **Census:** 423 **Outpatient Visits:** 508230 **Births:** 505 **Total Expense ($000):** 695759 **Payroll Expense ($000):** 269736 **Personnel:** 3927

⊞ △ **VETERANS AFFAIRS MEDICAL CENTER**, 800 Irving Avenue, Zip 13210–2716; tel. 315/425–4400, (Total facility includes 48 beds in nursing home–type unit) **A**1 3 5 7 8 **F**2 3 5 17 18 20 22 26 28 29 30 31 33 34 35 36 38 39 40 44 45 46 49 51 54 56 57 58 59 60 61 62 63 64 65 70 71 74 75 77 78 79 80 81 82 83 84 85 86 87 90 91 92 93 94 96 97 98 100 101 102 103 104 106 107 108 111 114 118 126 128 129 130 131 134 142 145 146 147 **P**6 **S** Department of Veterans Affairs, Washington, DC
Primary Contact: James Cody, Director
CFO: Elisabeth Kittell, Chief Financial Officer
CMO: William Marx, M.D., Chief of Staff
CIO: James Nichols, Chief Information Officer
CHR: Mark Antinelli, Manager Human Resources
Web address: www.syracuse.va.gov
**Control:** Veterans Affairs, Government, federal **Service:** General Medical and Surgical

**Staffed Beds:** 154 **Admissions:** 4905 **Census:** 89 **Outpatient Visits:** 454946 **Births:** 0 **Total Expense ($000):** 208005 **Payroll Expense ($000):** 97305

## TICONDEROGA—Essex County

★ **MOSES LUDINGTON HOSPITAL (331306)**, 1019 Wicker Street, Zip 12883–1097; tel. 518/585–2831 **A**9 10 18 **F**11 15 28 35 39 40 42 57 63 64 74 78 79 81 93 107 110 118 129 130 131 132 142 145
Primary Contact: William E. Holmes, Chief Executive Officer
CMO: Cornelia Sue Freyhofer, M.D., Medical Director
CIO: Lisa Busby, Manager Information Systems
CHR: Tamara Evens, Director Human Resources
Web address: www.mosesludington.com
**Control:** Other not–for–profit (including NFP Corporation) **Service:** General Medical and Surgical

**Staffed Beds:** 15 **Admissions:** 230 **Census:** 2 **Outpatient Visits:** 24754 **Births:** 0 **Total Expense ($000):** 11902 **Payroll Expense ($000):** 5618 **Personnel:** 132

**NY**

## TROY—Rensselaer County

★ **SAMARITAN HOSPITAL (330180)**, 2215 Burdett Avenue, Zip 12180–2475; tel. 518/271–3300 **A**5 9 10 **F**3 4 8 11 15 17 18 20 22 29 30 31 38 40 49 50 60 63 68 70 74 75 77 78 81 83 84 85 87 93 94 98 102 103 104 107 108 110 111 113 114 118 119 120 125 129 145 146 **S** Catholic Health East, Newtown Square, PA
Primary Contact: Norman E. Dascher, Jr., Chief Executive Officer
CFO: Daniel A. Kochie, CPA, Chief Financial Officer
CMO: Daniel C. Silverman, M.D., Chief Medical Officer, Acute Care Troy
CIO: Karen LeBlanc, Director, Applications
CHR: Barbara McCandless, Corporate Vice President Human Resources
CNO: Jacqueline Priore, Chief Nursing Officer
Web address: www.nehealth.com
**Control:** Other not–for–profit (including NFP Corporation) **Service:** General Medical and Surgical

**Staffed Beds:** 134 **Admissions:** 7257 **Census:** 127 **Outpatient Visits:** 301604 **Births:** 389 **Total Expense ($000):** 115998 **Payroll Expense ($000):** 56260 **Personnel:** 1054

☒ **ST. MARY'S HOSPITAL (330232)**, 1300 Massachusetts Avenue, Zip 12180–1695; tel. 518/268–5000, (Includes SETON HEALTH SYSTEM–ST. MARY'S HOSPITAL, 1300 Massachusetts Avenue, Zip 12180; tel. 518/272–5000), (Total facility includes 120 beds in nursing home–type unit) **A**1 9 10 **F**3 4 8 12 15 17 18 28 29 30 31 34 35 40 45 46 47 48 49 50 51 54 55 56 57 58 59 60 61 62 63 64 65 66 68 74 75 77 78 79 81 82 83 84 85 86 87 88 93 97 107 108 110 111 113 114 118 127 128 129 131 132 134 143 144 145 146 147 **S** Catholic Health East, Newtown Square, PA
Primary Contact: Norman E. Dascher, Jr., Executive Vice President
CFO: Scott St George, Senior Vice President and Chief Financial Officer
CMO: Richard Rubin, M.D., Chief Medical Officer
CHR: Kathleen Occhiogrosso, Vice President Human Resources
Web address: www.setonhealth.org
**Control:** Church–operated, Nongovernment, not–for profit **Service:** General Medical and Surgical

**Staffed Beds:** 293 **Admissions:** 6794 **Census:** 212 **Outpatient Visits:** 450932 **Births:** 554 **Total Expense ($000):** 139084 **Payroll Expense ($000):** 71282 **Personnel:** 1261

## UTICA—Oneida County

★ △ **FAXTON–ST. LUKE'S HEALTHCARE (330044)**, 1656 Champlin Avenue, Zip 13502–4830, Mailing Address: P.O. Box 479, Zip 13503–0479; tel. 315/624–6000, (Includes FAXTON CAMPUS, 1676 Sunset Avenue, Zip 13502–5475; tel. 315/624–6200; ST. LUKE'S CAMPUS, Zip 13413; tel. 315/624–6000) **A**2 7 9 10 21 **F**3 12 13 15 17 18 20 22 28 29 30 31 32 34 35 39 40 44 45 49 50 53 57 59 60 64 65 67 68 70 73 75 76 77 78 79 81 82 84 89 90 91 92 93 96 97 98 102 107 108 110 111 113 115 116 117 118 119 120 122 123 129 131 134 143 145 146
Primary Contact: Scott H. Perra, President and Chief Executive Officer
COO: Steven J. Brown, Senior Vice President and Chief Operating Officer
CFO: Michael Haile, Senior Vice President and Chief Financial Officer
CMO: Daniel Kopp, M.D., Senior Vice President and Chief Medical Officer
CIO: Kevin Mahoney, Vice President and Chief Information Officer
CHR: Tony Scibelli, Vice President Human Resources and Operations
Web address: www.mvnhealth.com
**Control:** Other not–for–profit (including NFP Corporation) **Service:** General Medical and Surgical

**Staffed Beds:** 319 **Admissions:** 15541 **Census:** 215 **Outpatient Visits:** 488446 **Births:** 2110

☐ **MOHAWK VALLEY PSYCHIATRIC CENTER (334021)**, 1400 Noyes Street, Zip 13502–3803; tel. 315/738–3800, (Nonreporting) **A**1 10 **S** New York State Office of Mental Health, Albany, NY
Primary Contact: Colleen A. Sawyer, R.N., MSN, Executive Director
Web address: www.omh.ny.gov/omhweb/facilities/mvpc/facility.htm
**Control:** State–Government, nonfederal **Service:** Psychiatric

**Staffed Beds:** 614

★ **ST. ELIZABETH MEDICAL CENTER (330245)**, 2209 Genesee Street, Zip 13501–5999; tel. 315/798–8100 **A**9 10 12 13 21 **F**3 8 11 15 16 17 18 20 22 24 26 29 30 32 34 36 37 38 40 43 45 47 49 50 54 57 58 59 61 62 64 65 66 68 70 74 75 77 79 80 81 85 86 87 89 90 92 93 97 98 100 102 103 107 108 110 113 114 117 118 126 128 129 130 131 145 146 147 **P**6 **S** Sisters of Saint Francis, Syracuse, NY
Primary Contact: Richard H. Ketcham, FACHE, President and Chief Executive Officer
COO: Robert Scholefield, Chief Operating Officer
CFO: Louis Aiello, Chief Financial Officer
CMO: Albert D'Accurzio, M.D., Medical Director
CIO: Robert Gillette, Chief Information Officer
CHR: Patrick Buckley, Vice President Human Resources
CNO: Varinya Sheppard, R.N., Chief Nursing Officer
Web address: www.stemc.org
**Control:** Church–operated, Nongovernment, not–for profit **Service:** General Medical and Surgical

**Staffed Beds:** 181 **Admissions:** 11973 **Census:** 159 **Outpatient Visits:** 448509 **Births:** 0 **Total Expense ($000):** 196483 **Payroll Expense ($000):** 92094 **Personnel:** 1762

**ST. LUKE'S CAMPUS** See Faxton–St. Luke's Healthcare

## VALHALLA—Westchester County

☒ **BLYTHEDALE CHILDREN'S HOSPITAL (333301)**, 95 Bradhurst Avenue, Zip 10595–1697; tel. 914/592–7555, (Nonreporting) **A**1 10
Primary Contact: Larry L. Levine, President and Chief Executive Officer
COO: Maureen Desimone, Chief Operating Officer
CFO: John Canning, Chief Financial Officer
CMO: Joelle Mast, Ph.D., Chief Medical Officer
CHR: Ronald Gallo, Director Human Resources
Web address: www.blythedale.org
**Control:** Other not–for–profit (including NFP Corporation) **Service:** Children's rehabilitation

**Staffed Beds:** 92

☐ **WESTCHESTER MEDICAL CENTER (330234)**, 100 Woods Road, Zip 10595–1530; tel. 914/493–7000, (Includes MARIA FARERI CHILDREN'S HOSPITAL, 95 Grasslands Road, Zip 10595–1652; tel. 866/962–7337) **A**1 3 5 8 9 10 **F**3 8 12 13 14 15 16 17 18 19 20 21 22 23 24 25 26 27 28 29 30 31 32 34 35 36 37 38 39 40 41 43 44 45 46 47 48 49 50 52 54 55 56 57 58 59 60 61 64 65 66 68 70 71 72 73 74 75 76 77 78 79 81 82 84 85 86 87 88 89 90 91 92 94 97 98 99 100 101 102 103 104 107 108 110 111 113 114 117 118 119 120 122 123 125 128 129 130 131 133 134 135 136 137 138 140 141 144 145 146 147 **P**6
Primary Contact: Michael D. Israel, President and Chief Executive Officer
COO: Gary F. Brudnicki, Senior Executive Vice President, Chief Operating Officer and Chief Financial Officer
CFO: Gary F. Brudnicki, Senior Executive Vice President, Chief Operating Officer and Chief Financial Officer
CMO: Renee Garrick, M.D., Chief Medical Officer
CIO: John Moustakakis, Senior Vice President Information Systems and Chief Information Officer
CHR: Paul S. Hochenberg, Senior Vice President Human Resources
Web address: www.worldclassmedicine.com
**Control:** Hospital district or authority, Government, nonfederal **Service:** General Medical and Surgical

**Staffed Beds:** 643 **Admissions:** 22728 **Census:** 535 **Outpatient Visits:** 153753 **Births:** 923 **Total Expense ($000):** 805535 **Payroll Expense ($000):** 357672 **Personnel:** 3451

## VALLEY STREAM—Nassau County

☒ **FRANKLIN HOSPITAL (330372)**, 900 Franklin Avenue, Zip 11580–2190; tel. 516/256–6000, (Total facility includes 120 beds in nursing home–type unit) **A**1 2 9 10 **F**2 3 11 12 17 18 26 29 30 31 34 35 40 42 43 45 49 50 56 57 58 59 60 62 63 64 65 68 70 74 75 77 78 79 81 82 83 84 85 86 87 92 94 97 98 100 102 103 107 108 111 113 117 118 127 129 131 134 142 145 147 **P**6 **S** North Shore–Long Island Jewish Health System, Great Neck, NY
Primary Contact: Catherine Hottendorf, R.N., MS, Executive Director
COO: Mark J. Solazzo, Executive Vice President and Chief Operating Officer
CFO: Elizabeth Zubko, Associate Executive Director Finance
CMO: Anthony J. Shallash, M.D., Interim Medical Director
CIO: John Bosco, Chief Information Officer
CHR: Karina Norr–McPhillips, Associate Executive Director Human Resources
CNO: Barbara Popkin, R.N., Associate Executive Director Patient Care Services
Web address: www.northshorelij.com
**Control:** Other not–for–profit (including NFP Corporation) **Service:** General Medical and Surgical

**Staffed Beds:** 356 **Admissions:** 12695 **Census:** 291 **Outpatient Visits:** 71717 **Births:** 0 **Total Expense ($000):** 181084 **Payroll Expense ($000):** 88153 **Personnel:** 1388

**NY**

---

**Hospital, Medicare Provider Number, Address, Telephone, Approval, Facility, and Physician Codes, Health Care System**

★ American Hospital Association (AHA) membership
☐ The Joint Commission accreditation   ◇ DNV Healthcare Inc. accreditation

○ American Osteopathic Association (AOA) accreditation
△ Commission on Accreditation of Rehabilitation Facilities (CARF) accreditation

---

## WALTON—Delaware County

**DELAWARE VALLEY HOSPITAL (331312)**, 1 Titus Place, Zip 13856–1498; tel. 607/865–2100 **A**9 10 18 **F**3 4 5 8 11 15 18 19 28 34 35 36 40 45 57 58 59 64 65 75 77 83 85 93 97 107 110 113 118 129 131 132 145 **S** United Health Services, Binghamton, NY
Primary Contact: Dru Cavanagh, R.N., Interim Chief Executive Officer
CFO: Paul Summers, Chief Financial Officer
CMO: Michael F. Trevisani, M.D., Executive Vice President and Chief Medical Officer
CIO: James Armstrong, Manager Information Technology
CHR: Dru Cavanagh, R.N., Interim Chief Executive Officer
CNO: Victoria Conkling, Vice President Chief Nursing Officer
Web address: www.uhs.net
**Control:** Other not–for–profit (including NFP Corporation) **Service:** General Medical and Surgical

**Staffed Beds:** 25 **Admissions:** 816 **Census:** 12 **Outpatient Visits:** 87419 **Births:** 0 **Total Expense ($000):** 14637 **Payroll Expense ($000):** 8122 **Personnel:** 168

## WARSAW—Wyoming County

**WYOMING COUNTY COMMUNITY HOSPITAL (330008)**, 400 North Main Street, Zip 14569–1025; tel. 585/786–8940, (Nonreporting) **A**1 9 10 20
Primary Contact: Donald T. Eichenauer, Chief Executive Officer
COO: Lori Roche, Chief Operating Officer
CFO: Paula Parker, Chief Financial Officer
CMO: Scott Treutlein, M.D., Medical Director
CIO: Jane Beechler, Director Healthcare Information Systems
CHR: Denise M. Morley, Director Human Resources
CNO: Dawn James, Director of Nursing
Web address: www.wcchs.net
**Control:** County–Government, nonfederal **Service:** General Medical and Surgical

**Staffed Beds:** 75

## WARWICK—Orange County

**ST. ANTHONY COMMUNITY HOSPITAL (330205)**, 15 Maple Avenue, Zip 10990–1028; tel. 845/986–2276, (Nonreporting) **A**1 9 10 **S** Bon Secours Health System, Inc., Marriottsville, MD
Primary Contact: Jeff Reilly, Senior Vice President Operations
CFO: Stephen D. Majetich, CPA, Chief Financial Officer
Web address: www.stanthonycommunityhosp.org
**Control:** Church–operated, Nongovernment, not–for profit **Service:** General Medical and Surgical

**Staffed Beds:** 73

## WATERTOWN—Jefferson County

**SAMARITAN MEDICAL CENTER (330157)**, 830 Washington Street, Zip 13601–4034; tel. 315/785–4000 **A**1 9 10 12 13 20 **F**3 5 8 13 15 18 20 29 30 31 35 40 49 51 57 60 64 68 70 73 74 75 76 77 78 79 81 82 87 89 90 93 97 98 99 100 102 103 104 107 108 111 113 115 118 119 120 126 128 129 134 145 146 147 **P**6
Primary Contact: Thomas H. Carman, President and Chief Executive Officer
CFO: Paul Kraeger, Vice President Finance and Chief Financial Officer
CMO: Spencer P. Falcon, M.D., Vice President Medical Affairs
CIO: M. Andrew Short, Vice President Information Services
CHR: Thomas Shatraw, Director Human Resources
Web address: www.samaritanhealth.com
**Control:** Other not–for–profit (including NFP Corporation) **Service:** General Medical and Surgical

**Staffed Beds:** 212 **Admissions:** 8619 **Census:** 147 **Outpatient Visits:** 234489 **Births:** 1629 **Total Expense ($000):** 167921 **Payroll Expense ($000):** 77176 **Personnel:** 1308

## WELLSVILLE—Allegany County

**JONES MEMORIAL HOSPITAL (330096)**, 191 North Main Street, Zip 14895–1197, Mailing Address: P.O. Box 72, Zip 14895–0072; tel. 585/593–1100 **A**1 9 10 20 **F**3 8 11 13 15 17 28 29 30 31 34 35 36 40 43 57 59 61 64 68 70 75 76 77 78 79 81 82 85 89 93 97 107 110 113 118 128 130 131 132 145 146
Primary Contact: Eva Benedict, President and Chief Executive Officer
CFO: Tracy Gates, Chief Financial Officer
CMO: Frank Edwards, M.D., Medical Director
CIO: Tracy Gates, Chief Financial Officer
CHR: Brenda Sobeck, Director of Human Resources
CNO: Donna Bliven, Vice President Patient Management Services
Web address: www.jmhny.org
**Control:** Other not–for–profit (including NFP Corporation) **Service:** General Medical and Surgical

**Staffed Beds:** 55 **Admissions:** 2101 **Census:** 18 **Outpatient Visits:** 144345 **Births:** 295 **Total Expense ($000):** 32115 **Payroll Expense ($000):** 15658 **Personnel:** 309

## WEST HAVERSTRAW—Rockland County

△ **HELEN HAYES HOSPITAL (330405)**, Route 9W, Zip 10993–1127; tel. 845/786–4000, (Total facility includes 25 beds in nursing home–type unit) **A**1 5 7 10 **F**9 28 29 30 34 35 39 44 53 57 58 59 64 65 74 77 79 81 82 86 87 90 91 92 93 94 100 118 127 129 130 131 134 142 145 146 147 **P**6
Primary Contact: Val S. Gray, Chief Executive Officer
COO: Edmund Zybert, Chief Operating Officer
CFO: Richard Buhowski, Chief Financial Officer
CMO: John T. Pellicone, M.D., Medical Director
CIO: Virgil Ennis, Chief Information Officer
CHR: Kathleen Martucci, Director Human Resources
Web address: www.helenhayeshospital.org
**Control:** State–Government, nonfederal **Service:** Rehabilitation

**Staffed Beds:** 155 **Admissions:** 2549 **Census:** 104 **Outpatient Visits:** 67688 **Births:** 0 **Total Expense ($000):** 76471 **Payroll Expense ($000):** 34248 **Personnel:** 584

## WEST ISLIP—Suffolk County

**GOOD SAMARITAN HOSPITAL MEDICAL CENTER (330286)**, 1000 Montauk Highway, Zip 11795–4927; tel. 631/376–3000, (Nonreporting) **A**1 2 9 10 12 13 **S** Catholic Health Services of Long Island, Rockville Centre, NY
Primary Contact: Nancy B. Simmons, Executive Vice President and Chief Administrative Officer
CFO: Dan Macksood, Regional Senior Vice President and Chief Financial Officer
CMO: Jerome Weiner, M.D., Senior Vice President Medical Affairs
CIO: Marcy Dunn, Vice President Information Services and Chief Information Officer
CHR: Lori Spina, Vice President Human Resources
Web address: www.good–samaritan–hospital.org
**Control:** Church–operated, Nongovernment, not–for profit **Service:** General Medical and Surgical

**Staffed Beds:** 531

## WEST POINT—Orange County

**KELLER ARMY COMMUNITY HOSPITAL**, 900 Washington Road, Zip 10996–1197, Mailing Address: U.S. Military Academy, Building 900, Zip 10996–1197; tel. 845/938–5169, (Nonreporting) **A**1 3 5 **S** Department of the Army, Office of the Surgeon General, Falls Church, VA
Primary Contact: Colonel Beverly Land, Commanding Officer
COO: Lieutenant Colonel Thomas Bell, Deputy Commander Administration
CFO: Russell DeVries, Chief Business Operations
CMO: Lieutenant Colonel Michael Doyle, M.D., Deputy Commander Clinical Services
CIO: Patrick McGuinness, Chief Information Management
CHR: Margaret Greco, Chief Human Resources
Web address: www.kach.amedd.army.mil/
**Control:** Army, Government, federal **Service:** General Medical and Surgical

**Staffed Beds:** 31

## WEST SENECA—Erie County

**WESTERN NEW YORK CHILDREN'S PSYCHIATRIC CENTER**, 1010 East and West Road, Zip 14224–3602; tel. 716/677–7000, (Nonreporting) **A**1 3 5 **S** New York State Office of Mental Health, Albany, NY
Primary Contact: Kathe Hayes, Executive Director
COO: David Privett, Deputy Director
CMO: Patrick Stein, M.D., Clinical Director
CIO: Dan Hrubiak, Associate Computer Program Analyst
CHR: Charles Siewert, Director Human Resources
Web address: www.omh.ny.gov
**Control:** State–Government, nonfederal **Service:** Children's hospital psychiatric

**Staffed Beds:** 46

## WESTFIELD—Chautauqua County

★ **WESTFIELD MEMORIAL HOSPITAL (330166)**, 189 East Main Street, Zip 14787–1195; tel. 716/326–4921, (Nonreporting) **A**9 10 **S** Saint Vincent Health System, Erie, PA
Primary Contact: Scott Whalen, Ph.D., FACHE, President and Chief Executive Officer
COO: Karen Surkala, Vice President
CFO: Henry J. Ward, Vice President and Chief Financial Officer
CMO: Russell Elwell, M.D., Medical Director
CIO: Cindy Harper, Director Information Systems
Web address: www.wmhinc.org
**Control:** Other not–for–profit (including NFP Corporation) **Service:** General Medical and Surgical

**Staffed Beds:** 4

*Many Facility Codes have changed. Please refer to the AHA Guide Code Chart.* © 2012 AHA Guide

**WHITE PLAINS—Westchester County**

☒ △ **BURKE REHABILITATION HOSPITAL (330404)**, 785 Mamaroneck Avenue,
Zip 10605–2523; tel. 914/597–2500, (Nonreporting) **A**1 3 5 7 10
Primary Contact: Mary Beth Walsh, M.D., Chief Executive Officer
COO: Brian M. Swift, Senior Administrator Plant Operations
CFO: John Stewart, Director Finance
CMO: Mary Beth Walsh, M.D., Chief Executive Officer
CIO: Cathy Dwyer, Senior Administrator Information Systems
CHR: Annette Bucci, Senior Administrator Human Resources
CNO: Marie Spencer, Chief Nursing Officer and Senior Administrator
Web address: www.burke.org
**Control:** Other not–for–profit (including NFP Corporation) **Service:** Rehabilitation

| Staffed Beds: 150 |
|---|

**NEW YORK–PRESBYTERIAN HOSPITAL, WESTCHESTER DIVISION** See New
York–Presbyterian Hospital, New York

☒ **WHITE PLAINS HOSPITAL CENTER (330304)**, 41 East Post Road,
Zip 10601–4699; tel. 914/681–0600, (Nonreporting) **A**1 2 9 10
Primary Contact: Jon B. Schandler, President and Chief Executive Officer
COO: Edward F. Leonard, Executive Vice President and Chief Operating Officer
CFO: John Sciurba, Vice President and Chief Financial Officer
CMO: Michael Palumbo, M.D., Executive Vice President and Medical Director
CHR: John Sanchez, Vice President Human Resources
Web address: www.wphospital.org
**Control:** Other not–for–profit (including NFP Corporation) **Service:** General
Medical and Surgical

| Staffed Beds: 292 |
|---|

**WILLIAMSVILLE—Erie County**

**MILLARD FILLMORE SUBURBAN HOSPITAL** See KALEIDA Health, Buffalo

**YONKERS—Westchester County**

**ANDRUS PAVILION** See St. John's Riverside Hospital

☐ **ST. JOHN'S RIVERSIDE HOSPITAL (330208)**, 967 North Broadway,
Zip 10701–1399; tel. 914/964–4444, (Includes ANDRUS PAVILION, 967 North
Broadway, tel. 914/964–4444; PARKCARE PAVILION, Two Park Avenue,
Zip 10703–3497; tel. 914/964–7300), (Total facility includes 120 beds in
nursing home–type unit) **A**1 9 10 **F**3 4 5 8 11 12 13 15 18 29 30 31 34 35 36
37 39 40 45 46 49 50 51 54 55 57 59 60 61 64 65 68 70 73 74 75 76 77
78 79 81 82 83 84 85 87 91 92 93 107 108 110 111 113 114 117 118 119
127 128 129 131 134 142 145 146 147
Primary Contact: James Foy, President and Chief Executive Officer
COO: Lynn M. Nelson, R.N., Chief Operating Officer
CFO: Dennis M. Keane, Vice President Finance and Chief Financial Officer
CMO: Paul Antonecchia, M.D., Vice President Medical Affairs
CIO: Peter Weidner, Director Management Information Systems
CHR: Pam La France, Vice President Human Resources
Web address: www.riversidehealth.org
**Control:** Other not–for–profit (including NFP Corporation) **Service:** General
Medical and Surgical

| Staffed Beds: 480 Admissions: 19778 Census: 301 Outpatient Visits: 219439 Births: 1585 Total Expense ($000): 222960 Payroll Expense ($000): 105334 Personnel: 2033 |
|---|

☒ **ST. JOSEPH'S MEDICAL CENTER (330006)**, 127 South Broadway,
Zip 10701–4006; tel. 914/378–7000, (Nonreporting) **A**1 3 5 9 10
Primary Contact: Michael J. Spicer, President and Chief Executive Officer
CFO: James J. Curcuruto, Senior Vice President Finance
CMO: Nicholas De Robertis, M.D., Medical Director
CIO: Deborah Di Bernardo, Chief Information Officer
CHR: Dean Civitello, Vice President Human Resources, Public Relations and
Development
CNO: Jeffry E. Foltz, R.N., Vice President for Nursing
Web address: www.saintjosephs.org
**Control:** Other not–for–profit (including NFP Corporation) **Service:** General
Medical and Surgical

| Staffed Beds: 394 |
|---|

**NY**

| **Hospital, Medicare Provider Number, Address, Telephone, Approval, Facility, and Physician Codes, Health Care System** |
|---|
| ★ American Hospital Association (AHA) membership      ○ American Osteopathic Association (AOA) accreditation |
| ☐ The Joint Commission accreditation      ◇ DNV Healthcare Inc. accreditation      △ Commission on Accreditation of Rehabilitation Facilities (CARF) accreditation |

# NORTH CAROLINA

### AHOSKIE—Hertford County

✠ **VIDANT ROANOKE–CHOWAN HOSPITAL (340099)**, 500 South Academy Street, Zip 27910–3261, Mailing Address: P.O. Box 1385, Zip 27910–1385; tel. 252/209–3000 **A**1 9 10 **F**3 8 11 13 15 28 29 30 34 35 40 45 46 53 56 57 59 64 68 70 75 76 77 79 81 82 85 86 87 92 93 98 100 102 103 107 108 110 111 113 118 128 129 131 145 147 **S** Vidant Health, Greenville, NC
Primary Contact: Susan S. Lassiter, President
CFO: Jon Graham, Chief Financial Officer
CMO: Luis Rodriguez, M.D., Chief of Staff
CHR: Debbie Sisler, Director Human Resources
CNO: Nettie Evans, Vice President Patient Care Services
Web address: www.vidanthealth.com
**Control:** Other not–for–profit (including NFP Corporation) **Service:** General Medical and Surgical

**Staffed Beds:** 103 **Admissions:** 5233 **Census:** 63 **Outpatient Visits:** 66043 **Births:** 402 **Total Expense ($000):** 61929 **Payroll Expense ($000):** 25057 **Personnel:** 579

### ALBEMARLE—Stanly County

✠ **STANLY REGIONAL MEDICAL CENTER (340119)**, 301 Yadkin Street, Zip 28001–3448, Mailing Address: P.O. Box 1489, Zip 28002–1489; tel. 704/984–4000 **A**1 9 10 **F**3 11 12 13 15 17 20 28 29 30 31 34 35 39 40 45 49 57 59 60 61 62 63 64 68 70 74 75 76 77 78 79 81 82 85 86 89 90 91 93 98 100 101 102 103 107 108 111 118 122 128 129 130 131 145 147 **S** Carolinas HealthCare System, Charlotte, NC
Primary Contact: Alfred P. Taylor, Chief Executive Officer
COO: Brian Freeman, Vice President of Operations
CFO: Nick Samilo, Vice President Fiscal Services and Chief Financial Officer
CMO: Michael Bohnsack, M.D., Chief of Staff
CIO: Brian Freeman, Vice President of Operations
CHR: Paul Morlock, Vice President Human Resources
CNO: Judy Doran, R.N., Vice President of Hospital Services and Chief Nurse Executive
Web address: www.stanly.org
**Control:** Other not–for–profit (including NFP Corporation) **Service:** General Medical and Surgical

**Staffed Beds:** 102 **Admissions:** 4991 **Census:** 54 **Outpatient Visits:** 84613 **Births:** 685 **Total Expense ($000):** 84986 **Payroll Expense ($000):** 32862 **Personnel:** 635

### ASHEBORO—Randolph County

✠ **RANDOLPH HOSPITAL (340123)**, 364 White Oak Street, Zip 27203–5400, Mailing Address: P.O. Box 1048, Zip 27204–1048; tel. 336/625–5151 **A**1 2 9 10 **F**3 13 15 20 28 29 30 31 34 35 39 40 44 45 48 49 50 57 58 59 61 62 64 65 68 70 71 74 75 76 77 78 79 80 81 84 85 86 87 89 91 92 93 94 95 97 107 109 110 111 113 114 117 118 119 120 122 128 129 130 131 134 145 147 **P**6
Primary Contact: Steve E. Eblin, Chief Executive Officer
CFO: Lynwood R. White, Vice President Finance
CMO: Robert Dough, M.D., Chief of Staff
CIO: Angela Burgess, Chief Information Officer
Web address: www.randolphhospital.org
**Control:** Other not–for–profit (including NFP Corporation) **Service:** General Medical and Surgical

**Staffed Beds:** 122 **Admissions:** 6308 **Census:** 70 **Outpatient Visits:** 145942 **Births:** 820 **Total Expense ($000):** 92726 **Payroll Expense ($000):** 40571 **Personnel:** 969

### ASHEVILLE—Buncombe County

★ **ASHEVILLE SPECIALTY HOSPITAL (342017)**, 428 Biltmore Avenue, 4th Floor, Zip 28801; tel. 828/213–5400 **A**10 **F**1 3 29 30 36 77 82 85 147 **S** Mission Health System, Asheville, NC
Primary Contact: Robert C. Desotelle, President and Chief Executive Officer
COO: Michelle Stillman, Director of Care Management
CFO: Gregg Dixon, CPA, Chief Financial Officer
CMO: Joseph Aiello, M.D., Chief of Staff
CIO: Dorothy L. Porter, Director of Compliance/Risk/Quality
CHR: Jennifer Calloway, Human Resources Coordinator
CNO: Wanda Miller, R.N., Director of Clinical Services
Web address: www.ashevillespecialtyhospital.org
**Control:** Partnership, Investor–owned, for–profit **Service:** Long–Term Acute Care hospital

**Staffed Beds:** 31 **Admissions:** 356 **Census:** 24 **Outpatient Visits:** 0 **Births:** 0 **Total Expense ($000):** 12453 **Payroll Expense ($000):** 6129 **Personnel:** 93

✠ △ **CAREPARTNERS HEALTH SERVICES (343025)**, 68 Sweeten Creek Road, Zip 28803–1599, Mailing Address: P.O. Box 5779, Zip 28813–5779; tel. 828/277–4800 **A**1 7 10 21 **F**2 29 30 34 36 44 50 56 57 59 62 63 64 68 77 79 82 84 87 90 93 94 119 129 130 131 142 145 147 **P**5
Primary Contact: Tracy Buchanan, Chief Executive Officer
COO: Gary Bowers, Chief Operating Officer
CFO: Diann Bolick, Chief Financial Officer
CIO: Drake Thomas, Chief Information Officer
CHR: Karen Vernon–Young, Vice President Human Resources and Communications
Web address: www.carepartners.org
**Control:** Other not–for–profit (including NFP Corporation) **Service:** Rehabilitation

**Staffed Beds:** 80 **Admissions:** 1215 **Census:** 47 **Outpatient Visits:** 42042 **Births:** 0 **Total Expense ($000):** 19243 **Payroll Expense ($000):** 12402 **Personnel:** 157

✠ **CHARLES GEORGE VETERANS AFFAIRS MEDICAL CENTER**, 1100 Tunnel Road, Zip 28805–2087; tel. 828/298–7911, (Nonreporting) **A**1 3 5 **S** Department of Veterans Affairs, Washington, DC
Primary Contact: Cynthia Breyfogle, Director
CMO: MaryAnn Curl, M.D., Interim Chief of Staff
CIO: Carla McLendon, Director Information Resource Management Services
CHR: Melissa Bragg, Chief Human Resources Management
Web address: www.asheville.va.gov/
**Control:** Veterans Affairs, Government, federal **Service:** General Medical and Surgical

**Staffed Beds:** 116

✠ **MISSION HOSPITAL (340002)**, 509 Biltmore Avenue, Zip 28801–4690; tel. 828/213–1111, (Includes MEMORIAL MISSION HOSPITAL, 509 Biltmore Avenue, tel. 828/255–4000; MISSION CHILDREN'S HOSPITAL, 509 Biltmore Avenue, Zip 28801–4601; tel. 828/213–1740; ST. JOSEPH'S HOSPITAL, 428 Biltmore Avenue, Zip 28801–9839; tel. 828/255–3100) **A**1 2 9 10 **F**3 7 8 11 12 13 15 17 18 19 20 22 24 26 28 29 30 31 32 34 35 36 37 39 40 43 44 45 46 47 48 49 50 51 53 54 55 56 57 58 59 60 61 64 65 68 70 71 72 73 74 75 76 77 78 79 80 81 82 84 85 86 87 88 89 91 92 93 95 96 97 98 99 100 101 102 103 104 105 107 108 110 111 113 114 115 116 117 118 119 120 122 123 125 128 129 130 131 133 134 141 142 145 146 147 **P**6 **S** Mission Health System, Asheville, NC
Primary Contact: Ronald A. Paulus, M.D., President and Chief Executive Officer
COO: Brian W. Aston, Chief Operating Officer
CFO: Charles F. Ayscue, Senior Vice President Finance and Chief Financial Officer
CMO: Alan Baumgarten, M.D., Chief of Staff
CIO: D. Arlo Jennings, Ph.D., Chief Information Officer
CHR: Maria Roloff, Vice President Human Resources
Web address: www.missionhospitals.org
**Control:** Other not–for–profit (including NFP Corporation) **Service:** General Medical and Surgical

**Staffed Beds:** 744 **Admissions:** 38104 **Census:** 550 **Outpatient Visits:** 356996 **Births:** 4016 **Total Expense ($000):** 732077 **Payroll Expense ($000):** 298001 **Personnel:** 5705

### BELHAVEN—Beaufort County

★ **VIDANT PUNGO HOSPITAL (341310)**, 202 East Water Street, Zip 27810–9998; tel. 252/943–2111, (Total facility includes 10 beds in nursing home–type unit) **A**9 10 18 **F**3 7 15 29 35 40 56 85 87 93 104 107 110 114 118 127 128 129 132 145 **S** Vidant Health, Greenville, NC
Primary Contact: Harvey Case, President
CFO: Gerald Hardison, Director Finance
CMO: Gregory Jones, M.D., Chief of Staff
CIO: Jenny Brown, Director Human Resources and Public Relations
CHR: Jenny Brown, Director Human Resources and Public Relations
Web address: www.pungodistricthospital.org
**Control:** Other not–for–profit (including NFP Corporation) **Service:** General Medical and Surgical

**Staffed Beds:** 35 **Admissions:** 731 **Census:** 16 **Outpatient Visits:** 10555 **Births:** 0 **Total Expense ($000):** 10984 **Payroll Expense ($000):** 5588

### BLACK MOUNTAIN—Buncombe County

**JULIAN F. KEITH ALCOHOL AND DRUG ABUSE TREATMENT CENTER (344023)**, 201 Tabernacle Road, Zip 28711–2599; tel. 828/669–3400, (Nonreporting) **A**10
Primary Contact: W. Douglas Baker, Director
CFO: Jackie Maurer, Fiscal Officer
CMO: Anthony Burnett, M.D., Medical Director
CHR: Faye Hamlin, Manager Human Resources
Web address: www.jfkadatc.net
**Control:** State–Government, nonfederal **Service:** Alcoholism and other chemical dependency

**Staffed Beds:** 110

*Many Facility Codes have changed. Please refer to the AHA Guide Code Chart.*   © 2012 AHA Guide

## BLOWING ROCK—Watauga County

⊠ **BLOWING ROCK HOSPITAL (341321)**, 418 Chestnut Street, Zip 28605–0148, Mailing Address: P.O. Box 148, Zip 28605–0148; tel. 828/295–3136, (Includes DAVANT REHABILITATION AND EXTENDED CARE CENTER ), (Total facility includes 72 beds in nursing home–type unit) **A**1 9 10 18 **F**39 40 64 75 87 91 93 127 129 132 142 145 147 **S** Appalachian Regional Healthcare System, Boone, NC
Primary Contact: Timothy R. Ford, Chief Executive Officer
CFO: Kevin B. May, Chief Financial Officer
CMO: Charles Davant, III, M.D., Chief Medical Officer
CIO: Mike Quinto, Chief Information Officer
CHR: Roxane Greer, Coordinator Human Resources
CNO: Elizabeth Hayes, R.N., Director of Patient Services
Web address: www.apprhs.org
**Control:** Other not–for–profit (including NFP Corporation) **Service:** General Medical and Surgical

**Staffed Beds:** 97 **Admissions:** 276 **Census:** 68 **Outpatient Visits:** 2158 **Births:** 0 **Total Expense ($000):** 9309 **Payroll Expense ($000):** 4090 **Personnel:** 110

## BOILING SPRINGS—Cleveland County

**CRAWLEY MEMORIAL HOSPITAL (342019)**, 315 West College Avenue, Zip 28017, Mailing Address: P.O. Box 996, Zip 28017–0996; tel. 704/434–9466, (Total facility includes 10 beds in nursing home–type unit) **A**9 10 **F**1 29 85 87 127 **S** Carolinas HealthCare System, Charlotte, NC
Primary Contact: Brian Gwyn, President and Chief Executive Officer
COO: Brian Gwyn, President and Chief Executive Officer
CFO: Christine M. Martin, Chief Financial Officer
CMO: Charles M. Tomlinson, M.D., Vice President and Chief Medical Officer
CIO: Theresa Bridges, Chief Information Officer
CHR: Debra Kale, Vice President Human Resources
CNO: Veronica Poole–Adams, R.N., Vice President and Chief Nursing Officer
Web address: www.carolinas.org
**Control:** Other not–for–profit (including NFP Corporation) **Service:** Long–Term Acute Care hospital

**Staffed Beds:** 51 **Admissions:** 206 **Census:** 14 **Outpatient Visits:** 10 **Births:** 0 **Total Expense ($000):** 7290 **Payroll Expense ($000):** 2674 **Personnel:** 60

## BOLIVIA—Brunswick County

⊠ **BRUNSWICK NOVANT MEDICAL CENTER (340158)**, 240 Hospital Drive N.E., Zip 28462; tel. 910/721–1000 **A**1 9 10 **F**3 11 13 15 18 26 28 29 30 34 35 40 45 46 57 59 64 70 75 76 79 80 81 85 87 93 96 102 107 108 110 111 113 117 118 129 134 145 **S** Novant Health, Winston–Salem, NC
Primary Contact: Shelbourn Stevens, President
CFO: Joan Thomas, Chief Financial Officer
CMO: Robert Hassler, M.D., Director Medical Affairs
CIO: Pamela Parrish, Director Information Systems
Web address: www.brunswicknovant.org
**Control:** Other not–for–profit (including NFP Corporation) **Service:** General Medical and Surgical

**Staffed Beds:** 60 **Admissions:** 3284 **Census:** 32 **Outpatient Visits:** 108581 **Births:** 409 **Total Expense ($000):** 59163 **Payroll Expense ($000):** 18714 **Personnel:** 383

## BOONE—Watauga County

⊠ **WATAUGA MEDICAL CENTER (340051)**, 336 Deerfield Road, Zip 28607–5008, Mailing Address: P.O. Box 2600, Zip 28607–2600; tel. 828/262–4100 **A**1 2 9 10 **F**3 5 13 15 17 18 20 22 26 28 29 30 31 32 34 35 38 40 44 45 46 47 48 49 50 53 54 57 59 62 64 70 73 75 77 78 81 82 84 85 86 87 89 90 91 92 93 96 107 108 110 111 113 114 117 118 119 120 121 122 123 128 129 130 131 134 143 144 145 146 147 **P**6 8 **S** Appalachian Regional Healthcare System, Boone, NC
Primary Contact: Chuck Mantooth, President
CFO: Kevin B. May, Chief Financial Officer
CMO: Herman A. Godwin, Jr., M.D., Senior Vice President and Medical Director
CIO: Mike Quinto, Chief Information Officer
CHR: Amy Crabbe, Senior Vice President Human Resources
CNO: Claire P. Cline, M.P.H., Senior Vice President Patient Care Services/CNO
Web address: www.apprhs.org
**Control:** Other not–for–profit (including NFP Corporation) **Service:** General Medical and Surgical

**Staffed Beds:** 99 **Admissions:** 4670 **Census:** 48 **Outpatient Visits:** 118341 **Births:** 569 **Total Expense ($000):** 98125 **Payroll Expense ($000):** 34705 **Personnel:** 638

## BREVARD—Transylvania County

⊠ **TRANSYLVANIA REGIONAL HOSPITAL (341319)**, 260 Hospital Drive, Zip 28712–1116; tel. 828/884–9111, (Total facility includes 10 beds in nursing home–type unit) **A**1 9 10 18 **F**2 3 11 13 15 28 29 30 31 34 35 36 40 45 49 53 56 57 59 62 63 64 70 76 78 79 80 81 85 97 107 110 111 113 118 127 129 131 132 145 **P**6 **S** Mission Health System, Asheville, NC
Primary Contact: Robert J. Bednarek, President and Chief Executive Officer
COO: Rebecca W. Carter, MSN, Vice President Patient Care and Chief Operating Officer
CFO: Linda Coye, Chief Financial Officer
CFO: Marc Nakagawa, Vice President and Chief Financial Officer
CMO: Jim Kelling, M.D., Chief of Staff
CIO: Ed Coye, Director Information Technology
CHR: Mark L. Emory, System Director Human Resources
CNO: Rebecca W. Carter, MSN, Vice President Patient Care and Chief Operating Officer
Web address: www.trhospital.org
**Control:** Other not–for–profit (including NFP Corporation) **Service:** General Medical and Surgical

**Staffed Beds:** 52 **Admissions:** 1966 **Census:** 18 **Outpatient Visits:** 53771 **Births:** 124 **Total Expense ($000):** 59441 **Payroll Expense ($000):** 19660 **Personnel:** 507

## BRYSON CITY—Swain County

★ **MEDWEST – SWAIN (341305)**, 45 Plateau Street, Zip 28713–6784; tel. 828/488–2155 **A**9 10 18 **F**8 11 15 29 30 35 40 44 45 57 59 62 63 68 75 77 81 82 84 85 91 93 107 118 129 132 145 147 **S** MedWest Health System, Sylva, NC
Primary Contact: J. Michael Poore, Chief Executive Officer
CFO: Steve Heatherly, Executive Vice President Finance and Operations
CMO: David Zimmerman, M.D., Chief of Staff
CIO: Dale Chernich, Chief Information Officer
Web address: www.westcare.org
**Control:** Other not–for–profit (including NFP Corporation) **Service:** General Medical and Surgical

**Staffed Beds:** 25 **Admissions:** 475 **Census:** 4 **Outpatient Visits:** 21826 **Births:** 0 **Total Expense ($000):** 8425 **Payroll Expense ($000):** 4368 **Personnel:** 87

## BURGAW—Pender County

⊠ **PENDER MEMORIAL HOSPITAL (341307)**, 507 East Freemont Street, Zip 28425–5131; tel. 910/259–5451, (Total facility includes 43 beds in nursing home–type unit) **A**1 9 10 18 **F**3 11 15 29 34 40 42 45 57 59 62 64 68 81 85 86 87 93 96 107 113 118 127 129 132 134 142 145 147 **S** New Hanover Regional Medical Center, Wilmington, NC
Primary Contact: Ruth Glaser, President
CFO: Chris Riggs, Chief Financial Officer
CMO: Joseph Cooper, M.D., Chief of Staff
CHR: Lori McKoy, Business Partner
CNO: Katherine Haddix–Hill, R.N., Chief Nursing Officer/Chief Operating Officer
Web address: www.pendermemorial.org
**Control:** County–Government, nonfederal **Service:** General Medical and Surgical

**Staffed Beds:** 68 **Admissions:** 891 **Census:** 48 **Outpatient Visits:** 26004 **Births:** 0 **Total Expense ($000):** 23318 **Payroll Expense ($000):** 10667 **Personnel:** 282

## BURLINGTON—Alamance County

⊠ **ALAMANCE REGIONAL MEDICAL CENTER (340070)**, 1240 Huffman Mill Road, Zip 27216–0202, Mailing Address: P.O. Box 202, Zip 27216–0202; tel. 336/538–7000 **A**1 2 9 10 **F**3 8 9 12 13 15 18 20 22 24 28 29 30 31 32 34 35 36 38 39 40 44 45 46 47 49 50 53 55 56 57 58 59 60 64 68 70 73 74 76 77 78 79 81 82 84 85 86 87 89 91 93 94 96 97 98 100 101 102 103 107 108 110 111 113 116 117 118 119 120 122 129 130 131 134 143 144 145 146 147
Primary Contact: John G. Currin, Jr., President
COO: John G. Currin, Jr., President
CFO: Rex Street, Senior Vice President and Chief Financial Officer
CMO: Andrew Lamb, M.D., Chief of Staff
CIO: Jesse Long, Director Information Technology
CHR: Dick Donahey, Senior Vice President Human Resources
Web address: www.armc.com
**Control:** Other not–for–profit (including NFP Corporation) **Service:** General Medical and Surgical

**Staffed Beds:** 218 **Admissions:** 12247 **Census:** 139 **Outpatient Visits:** 122091 **Births:** 1227 **Total Expense ($000):** 205533 **Payroll Expense ($000):** 81656 **Personnel:** 1857

---

**Hospital, Medicare Provider Number, Address, Telephone, Approval, Facility, and Physician Codes, Health Care System**

★ American Hospital Association (AHA) membership
□ The Joint Commission accreditation    ◇ DNV Healthcare Inc. accreditation

○ American Osteopathic Association (AOA) accreditation
△ Commission on Accreditation of Rehabilitation Facilities (CARF) accreditation

**NC**

## BURNSVILLE—Yancey County

**YANCEY COMMUNITY MEDICAL CENTER (341301)**, 800 Medical Campus Drive, Zip 28714–9010; tel. 828/682–6136, (Nonreporting) **A**9 10
Primary Contact: Dena Hensley, Administrator
**Control:** Other not–for–profit (including NFP Corporation) **Service:** General Medical and Surgical

Staffed Beds: 6

## BUTNER—Granville County

☐ **CENTRAL REGIONAL HOSPITAL (344001)**, 300 Veazey Road, Zip 27509–1668; tel. 919/764–2000 **A**1 9 10 **F**3 30 39 74 75 98 99 103 106 118 129 142 145 **P**6
Primary Contact: Michael Hennike, Chief Executive Officer
**Control:** State–Government, nonfederal **Service:** Psychiatric

Staffed Beds: 382 Admissions: 2313 Census: 375 Outpatient Visits: 0 Births: 0 Total Expense ($000): 172891 Payroll Expense ($000): 95969 Personnel: 2032

☐ **JOHN UMSTEAD HOSPITAL (344004)**, 1003 12th Street, Zip 27509–1626; tel. 919/575–7211, (Includes ALCOHOL AND DRUG ABUSE TREATMENT CENTER, 205 West E Street, Zip 27509; tel. 919/575–7928; Cliff Hood, Director), (Nonreporting) **A**1 3 5 9 10
Primary Contact: Patricia L. Christian, Ph.D., R.N., Chief Executive Officer
Web address: www.juh.dhhs.state.nc.us
**Control:** State–Government, nonfederal **Service:** Psychiatric

Staffed Beds: 514

## CAMP LEJEUNE—Onslow County

☒ **NAVAL HOSPITAL**, Zip 28547–0100; tel. 910/450–4300, (Nonreporting) **A**1
**S** Bureau of Medicine and Surgery, Department of the Navy, Washington, DC
Primary Contact: Captain Daniel J. Zinder, Commanding Officer
Web address: www.med.navy.mil/sites/nhcl
**Control:** Navy, Government, federal **Service:** General Medical and Surgical

Staffed Beds: 117

## CARY—Wake County

☒ △ **WAKEMED CARY HOSPITAL (340173)**, 1900 Kildaire Farm Road, Zip 27518; tel. 919/350–2300, (Total facility includes 36 beds in nursing home–type unit) **A**1 7 9 10 **F**3 7 11 12 13 15 18 20 22 24 26 28 29 30 31 34 35 40 42 43 44 45 48 49 50 54 57 59 61 64 68 70 72 73 74 75 76 77 79 81 82 85 86 92 93 107 108 111 113 114 117 118 125 127 129 131 145 146 **P**6 **S** WakeMed Health & Hospitals, Raleigh, NC
Primary Contact: David C. Coulter, Senior Vice President and Chief Executive Officer
CFO: Michael D. DeVaughn, Senior Vice President and Chief Financial Officer
CMO: West Lawson, M.D., Chief Medical Officer
CIO: Denton Arledge, Vice President and Chief Information Officer
CHR: Jeanene R. Martin, M.P.H., Senior Vice President Human Resources
Web address: www.wakemed.org
**Control:** Other not–for–profit (including NFP Corporation) **Service:** General Medical and Surgical

Staffed Beds: 192 Admissions: 10614 Census: 152 Outpatient Visits: 257959 Births: 2458 Total Expense ($000): 165732 Payroll Expense ($000): 63621 Personnel: 1095

## CHAPEL HILL—Orange County

☒ △ **UNIVERSITY OF NORTH CAROLINA HOSPITALS (340061)**, 101 Manning Drive, Zip 27514–4220; tel. 919/966–4131, (Includes NORTH CAROLINA CHILDREN'S AND WOMEN'S HOSPITAL ; NORTH CAROLINA CHILDREN'S HOSPITAL, 101 Manning Drive, tel. 919/966–4131; NORTH CAROLINA NEUROSCIENCES HOSPITAL, University Campus, Zip 27514; tel. 919/966–1141) **A**1 2 3 5 7 8 9 10 **F**3 4 5 7 8 9 10 11 12 13 14 15 16 17 18 19 20 21 22 23 24 25 26 27 28 29 30 31 32 34 35 36 38 39 40 41 43 44 45 46 47 48 49 50 52 53 54 55 56 57 58 59 60 61 62 63 64 65 66 68 70 72 73 74 75 76 77 78 79 80 81 82 84 85 86 87 88 89 90 91 92 93 96 97 98 99 100 101 102 103 104 105 107 108 110 111 113 114 115 116 117 118 119 120 122 123 125 128 129 130 131 133 134 135 136 137 138 139 140 141 142 144 145 146 147
Primary Contact: Gary L. Park, President
COO: Brian Goldstein, M.D., Executive Vice President and Chief Operating Officer
CFO: Christopher Ellington, Executive Vice President and Chief Financial Officer
CIO: J. P. Kichak, Vice President Information Services
CHR: William Rotella, Vice President Human Resources
Web address: www.unchealthcare.org
**Control:** State–Government, nonfederal **Service:** General Medical and Surgical

Staffed Beds: 799 Admissions: 37826 Census: 636 Outpatient Visits: 834445 Births: 3509 Total Expense ($000): 959751 Payroll Expense ($000): 435426 Personnel: 7562

## CHARLOTTE—Mecklenburg County

☒ **CAROLINAS MEDICAL CENTER (340113)**, 1000 Blythe Boulevard, Zip 28203–5871, Mailing Address: P.O. Box 32861, Zip 28232–2861; tel. 704/355–2000, (Includes LEVINE CHILDREN'S HOSPITAL, 1000 Blythe Boulevard, Zip 28203; tel. 704/381–2000) **A**1 2 3 5 6 8 9 10 **F**3 7 8 12 13 15 17 18 19 20 21 22 23 24 25 26 27 28 29 30 31 32 34 35 36 37 38 39 40 41 43 44 45 46 47 48 49 50 52 54 55 56 57 58 59 60 61 62 64 65 66 68 70 71 72 73 74 75 76 77 78 79 80 81 82 83 84 85 86 87 88 89 90 93 96 97 98 99 100 101 102 103 104 105 107 108 111 113 114 115 116 117 118 119 120 122 123 125 128 129 130 131 133 134 135 136 137 138 140 141 142 144 145 146 147 **P**6 **S** Carolinas HealthCare System, Charlotte, NC
Primary Contact: Spencer Lilly, Interim President
CFO: Greg A. Gombar, Chief Financial Officer
CMO: Roger A. Ray, M.D., Executive Vice President and Chief Medical Officer
CIO: Craig Richardville, Senior Vice President and Chief Information Officer
CHR: Debra Plousha–Moore, Senior Vice President Human Resources
Web address: www.carolinasmedicalcenter.org
**Control:** Hospital district or authority, Government, nonfederal **Service:** General Medical and Surgical

Staffed Beds: 874 Admissions: 49194 Census: 777 Outpatient Visits: 798460 Births: 5858 Total Expense ($000): 1780017 Payroll Expense ($000): 625912 Personnel: 10050

☒ △ **CAROLINAS MEDICAL CENTER–MERCY (340098)**, 2001 Vail Avenue, Zip 28207–1289; tel. 704/304–5000, (Includes CAROLINAS MEDICAL CENTER–PINEVILLE, 10628 Park Road, Zip 28210; tel. 704/543–2000; Christopher R. Hummer, President) **A**1 2 7 9 10 **F**4 12 13 18 20 22 24 26 29 30 31 34 40 42 44 45 49 50 57 59 60 64 65 68 70 72 74 75 76 78 79 81 82 84 85 86 87 93 107 108 111 113 114 117 118 125 128 129 144 145 147 **S** Carolinas HealthCare System, Charlotte, NC
Primary Contact: D. Channing Roush, President
COO: Joseph G. Piemont, Executive Vice President and Chief Operating Officer
CFO: Greg A. Gombar, Chief Financial Officer
CMO: Michael Ruhlen, M.D., Chief Medical Officer
CIO: Craig Richardville, Senior Vice President
CHR: Pia Walker, Director Human Resources
Web address: www.carolinashealthcare.org
**Control:** Hospital district or authority, Government, nonfederal **Service:** General Medical and Surgical

Staffed Beds: 303 Admissions: 17654 Census: 204 Outpatient Visits: 197374 Births: 2596 Total Expense ($000): 329907 Payroll Expense ($000): 114881 Personnel: 1848

☒ **CAROLINAS MEDICAL CENTER–UNIVERSITY (340166)**, 8800 North Tryon Street, Zip 28262–8415, Mailing Address: P.O. Box 560727, Zip 28256–0727; tel. 704/863–6000 **A**1 2 9 10 **F**8 13 18 20 26 29 30 31 34 40 44 45 49 50 57 59 60 64 65 68 70 72 74 75 76 78 79 81 82 84 85 86 87 93 107 111 113 114 117 118 125 128 129 144 145 147 **S** Carolinas HealthCare System, Charlotte, NC
Primary Contact: William H. Leonard, President
CFO: Greg A. Gombar, Chief Financial Officer
CIO: John J. Knox, III, Senior Vice President and Chief Information Officer
Web address: www.carolinashealthcare.org
**Control:** Hospital district or authority, Government, nonfederal **Service:** General Medical and Surgical

Staffed Beds: 130 Admissions: 5990 Census: 56 Outpatient Visits: 125057 Births: 1477 Total Expense ($000): 119721 Payroll Expense ($000): 44496 Personnel: 720

☒ △ **CAROLINAS REHABILITATION (343026)**, 1100 Blythe Boulevard, Zip 28203–5864; tel. 704/355–4300 **A**1 7 9 10 **F**30 64 74 77 79 82 90 91 93 95 128 129 130 131 145 **P**1 **S** Carolinas HealthCare System, Charlotte, NC
Primary Contact: Robert G. Larrison, Jr., President
COO: Todd Bennett, Vice President
CFO: William Hopkins, Director Finance
CMO: William Bockenek, M.D., Medical Director
CIO: Craig Richardville, Chief Information Officer
CHR: Jami J. Herzberg, Assistant Vice President
CNO: Susan Chase, Vice President
Web address: www.carolinasrehabilitation.org
**Control:** Other not–for–profit (including NFP Corporation) **Service:** Rehabilitation

Staffed Beds: 169 Admissions: 2742 Census: 117 Outpatient Visits: 63109 Births: 0 Total Expense ($000): 68178 Payroll Expense ($000): 32967 Personnel: 652

☐ **CAROLINAS SPECIALTY HOSPITAL (342015)**, 2001 Vail Avenue, 7th Floor, Zip 28207; tel. 704/379–6450, (Nonreporting) **A**1 10 **S** AcuityHealthcare, LP, Charlotte, NC
Primary Contact: Susan R. Davis, Chief Executive Officer
Web address: www.cshnc.org
**Control:** Corporation, Investor–owned, for–profit **Service:** Long–Term Acute Care hospital

Staffed Beds: 38

✠ **PRESBYTERIAN HOSPITAL (340053)**, 200 Hawthorne Lane, Zip 28204–2528, Mailing Address: P.O. Box 33549, Zip 28233–3549; tel. 704/384–4000, (Includes PRESBYTERIAN HEMBY CHILDREN'S HOSPITAL, 200 Hawthorne Lane, Zip 28204–2515; tel. 704/384–5134) **A**1 2 9 10 **F**3 5 7 8 11 12 13 15 17 18 19 20 22 24 26 28 29 30 31 32 34 35 36 38 40 45 46 47 48 49 53 54 55 56 57 58 59 60 61 63 64 65 68 70 71 72 73 74 75 76 77 78 79 81 82 84 85 86 87 88 89 91 92 93 98 99 100 101 102 103 104 105 107 108 110 111 113 114 115 116 117 118 119 120 123 125 128 129 131 134 141 142 143 144 145 146 147 **P**6 **S** Novant Health, Winston–Salem, NC
Primary Contact: Derrick Mark Billings, President
COO: Amy Vance, Executive Vice President and Chief Operating Officer
CFO: Mark Moyer, Vice President and Chief Financial Officer
CMO: Stephen Wallenhaupt, M.D., Executive Vice President Medical Affairs
CIO: David B. Garrett, Senior Vice President Information Technology
CHR: Janet Smith–Hill, Senior Vice President Human Resources
Web address: www.presbyterian.org
**Control:** Other not–for–profit (including NFP Corporation) **Service:** General Medical and Surgical

**Staffed Beds: 582 Admissions: 29082 Census: 444 Outpatient Visits: 385718 Births: 4946 Total Expense ($000): 505825 Payroll Expense ($000): 185689 Personnel: 3228**

✠ **PRESBYTERIAN–ORTHOPAEDIC HOSPITAL (340153)**, 1901 Randolph Road, Zip 28207–1195; tel. 704/316–2000, (Total facility includes 16 beds in nursing home–type unit) **A**1 9 10 **F**3 11 29 30 37 44 50 51 64 68 75 79 81 82 86 87 97 107 111 113 118 127 129 130 131 145 **S** Novant Health, Winston–Salem, NC
Primary Contact: Mike Riley, Senior Vice President and Chief Operating Officer
CFO: Tammy Geist, Chief Financial Officer
CIO: Shelia Cook, Director Information Systems
Web address: www.novanthealth.org
**Control:** Other not–for–profit (including NFP Corporation) **Service:** Orthopedic

**Staffed Beds: 80 Admissions: 3506 Census: 38 Outpatient Visits: 25538 Births: 0 Total Expense ($000): 80567 Payroll Expense ($000): 20400 Personnel: 352**

### CHEROKEE—Swain County

✠ **CHEROKEE INDIAN HOSPITAL (340156)**, 1 Hospital Road, Zip 28719, Mailing Address: 1 Hospital Drive, Zip 28719; tel. 828/497–9163, (Nonreporting) **A**1 10
Primary Contact: Casey Cooper, Chief Executive Officer
COO: Beth Greene, Chief Operating Officer
CFO: Chrissy Arch, Chief Financial Officer
CMO: Michael E. Toedt, M.D., Director Clinical Services
CIO: Anthony Taylor, Manager Information Technology
**Control:** Other not–for–profit (including NFP Corporation) **Service:** General Medical and Surgical

**Staffed Beds: 28**

### CLINTON—Sampson County

✠ **SAMPSON REGIONAL MEDICAL CENTER (340024)**, 607 Beaman Street, Zip 28328–2697, Mailing Address: P.O. Box 260, Zip 28329–0260; tel. 910/592–8511, (Total facility includes 30 beds in nursing home–type unit) **A**1 9 10 **F**3 7 8 13 14 15 28 29 30 34 35 38 40 44 45 46 48 50 53 57 59 62 64 65 68 70 76 77 78 79 81 82 85 86 87 89 93 97 107 108 111 113 114 118 120 122 127 128 129 130 131 134 142 143 145 146 147
Primary Contact: David J. Masterson, Chief Executive Officer
COO: Geraldine H. Shipp, Director of Risk Management
CFO: Jerry Heinzman, Senior Vice President and Chief Financial Officer
CMO: Shawn Howerton, M.D., President Medical Staff
CIO: Kelly Lucas, Chief Information Officer
CHR: Michael W. Gilpin, Vice President Human Resources
CNO: Rebecca Willis, Chief Nursing Officer
Web address: www.sampsonrmc.org
**Control:** County–Government, nonfederal **Service:** General Medical and Surgical

**Staffed Beds: 105 Admissions: 3696 Census: 63 Outpatient Visits: 76792 Births: 447 Total Expense ($000): 49093 Payroll Expense ($000): 29725 Personnel: 578**

### CLYDE—Haywood County

✠ **MEDWEST – HAYWOOD (340184)**, 262 Leroy George Drive, Zip 28721–9434; tel. 828/456–7311 **A**1 9 10 **F**3 11 15 18 20 28 29 30 31 34 35 38 40 44 45 46 50 51 53 54 57 59 62 63 64 65 68 70 71 74 75 76 77 78 79 81 82 84 85 86 87 93 98 100 101 102 107 108 111 113 117 118 128 129 130 131 143 145 146 147 **P**8 **S** MedWest Health System, Sylva, NC
Primary Contact: John Young, Interim CEO
COO: Teresa Reynolds, Chief Operating Officer
CFO: Rose Coyne, Interim CFO
CMO: Tyson Smith, M.D., Chief Medical Officer
CIO: Greg Copen, Chief Information Officer
CHR: Janet Millsaps, Vice President Human Resources
CNO: Dwayne Hooks, Jr., R.N., Chief Nursing Officer
Web address: www.haymed.org
**Control:** Hospital district or authority, Government, nonfederal **Service:** General Medical and Surgical

**Staffed Beds: 146 Admissions: 6315 Census: 61 Outpatient Visits: 246973 Births: 360 Total Expense ($000): 85639 Payroll Expense ($000): 43215 Personnel: 814**

### COLUMBUS—Polk County

✠ **ST. LUKE'S HOSPITAL (341322)**, 101 Hospital Drive, Zip 28722–9473; tel. 828/894–3311 **A**1 9 10 18 **F**3 11 15 29 30 34 35 40 45 56 57 59 62 64 70 75 77 79 81 85 93 98 103 106 107 108 113 118 129 132 134 145 147 **S** Carolinas HealthCare System, Charlotte, NC
Primary Contact: Kenneth A. Shull, FACHE, Chief Executive Officer
CFO: Christine M. Martin, Chief Financial Officer
CMO: James Holleman, M.D., Chief of Staff
CIO: David Pearson, Chief Information Officer
CHR: Amy Arledge, Vice President Support Services
Web address: www.saintlukeshospital.com
**Control:** Other not–for–profit (including NFP Corporation) **Service:** General Medical and Surgical

**Staffed Beds: 35 Admissions: 1568 Census: 24 Outpatient Visits: 23523 Births: 0 Total Expense ($000): 24707 Payroll Expense ($000): 10374 Personnel: 313**

### CONCORD—Cabarrus County

✠ **CAROLINAS MEDICAL CENTER–NORTHEAST (340001)**, 920 Church Street North, Zip 28025–2983; tel. 704/403–3000 **A**1 2 9 10 **F**3 5 7 8 9 11 12 13 14 15 17 18 20 22 24 26 28 29 30 31 32 34 35 36 37 38 40 43 44 45 47 48 49 50 51 53 54 55 56 57 58 59 60 61 63 64 65 66 68 70 71 72 73 74 75 76 77 78 79 80 81 82 84 85 86 87 88 89 93 97 98 99 100 102 103 104 105 107 108 110 111 112 113 114 115 116 117 118 120 122 123 125 128 129 130 131 134 142 144 145 146 147 **P**6 **S** Carolinas HealthCare System, Charlotte, NC
Primary Contact: Phyllis A. Wingate, Division President
COO: Bill Hubbard, Vice President, Operations
CFO: James Ramsey, Vice President Finance
CMO: Jean Wright, M.D., Chief Medical Officer
CIO: Keith McNeice, Vice President and Chief Information Officer
CHR: Lesley Chambless, Assistant Vice President Workforce Relations
CNO: Kate Grew, MSN, Vice President/Chief Nurse Executive
Web address: www.carolinashealthcare.org
**Control:** Hospital district or authority, Government, nonfederal **Service:** General Medical and Surgical

**Staffed Beds: 450 Admissions: 22260 Census: 279 Outpatient Visits: 506342 Births: 2627 Total Expense ($000): 371410 Payroll Expense ($000): 155270 Personnel: 2847**

### DANBURY—Stokes County

✠ **PIONEER COMMUNITY HOSPITAL OF STOKES (341317)**, 1570 Highway 8 and 89 North, Zip 27016, Mailing Address: P.O. Box 10, Zip 27016–0010; tel. 336/593–2831, (Nonreporting) **A**1 9 10 18 21 **S** Pioneer Health Services, Magee, MS
Primary Contact: James R. White, Jr., Chief Executive Officer
CMO: Samuel C. Newsome, M.D., President Medical Staff
CHR: Lashaunda Lash, Manager Human Resources
Web address: www.pchstokes.com
**Control:** Corporation, Investor–owned, for–profit **Service:** General Medical and Surgical

**Staffed Beds: 25**

**Hospital, Medicare Provider Number, Address, Telephone, Approval, Facility, and Physician Codes, Health Care System**

★ American Hospital Association (AHA) membership
□ The Joint Commission accreditation          ◇ DNV Healthcare Inc. accreditation
○ American Osteopathic Association (AOA) accreditation
△ Commission on Accreditation of Rehabilitation Facilities (CARF) accreditation

NC

© 2012 AHA Guide          *Many Facility Codes have changed. Please refer to the AHA Guide Code Chart.*          Hospitals **A451**

## DUNN—Harnett County

**BETSY JOHNSON REGIONAL HOSPITAL (340071)**, 800 Tilghman Drive, Zip 28334–5599, Mailing Address: Drawer 1706, Zip 28335–1706; tel. 910/892–7161 **A**1 9 10 **F**3 11 13 15 18 28 29 30 35 39 40 45 50 56 57 59 68 70 73 75 76 77 79 81 82 85 86 87 89 92 93 96 107 108 110 111 113 117 118 128 129 134 145 147 **S** WakeMed Health & Hospitals, Raleigh, NC
Primary Contact: Kenneth E. Bryan, President and Chief Executive Officer
COO: Kenneth E. Bryan, President and Chief Executive Officer
CFO: Robin Nichols, Chief Financial Officer
CMO: Wallace J. Horne, M.D., Vice President Medical Affairs
CIO: Tim Krieger, Director Information Systems
CHR: Sondra Davis, Vice President Human Resources & System Development
CNO: Vicki Allen, R.N., Chief Nursing Officer & Vice President Patient Care Services
Web address: www.bjrh.org
**Control:** Other not–for–profit (including NFP Corporation) **Service:** General Medical and Surgical

**Staffed Beds:** 89 **Admissions:** 6468 **Census:** 68 **Outpatient Visits:** 94060 **Births:** 737 **Total Expense ($000):** 77148 **Payroll Expense ($000):** 35720 **Personnel:** 599

## DURHAM—Durham County

**DUKE UNIVERSITY HOSPITAL (340030)**, 2301 Erwin Road, Zip 27710–0001, Mailing Address: P.O. Box 3708, Zip 27710–3708; tel. 919/684–8111, (Includes DUKE CHILDREN'S HOSPITAL & HEALTH CENTER, 2301 Erwin Road, Mailing Address: PO Box 3708, Zip 27702; tel. 919/684–8111) **A**1 2 3 5 8 9 10 **F**3 5 6 7 8 9 11 13 15 16 17 18 19 20 21 22 23 24 25 26 27 28 29 30 31 32 34 35 36 37 38 39 40 41 43 44 45 46 47 48 49 50 51 52 53 54 55 56 57 58 59 60 61 64 65 66 68 70 72 73 74 75 76 77 78 79 80 81 82 84 85 86 87 88 89 91 92 93 94 95 96 97 98 99 100 101 102 103 104 107 108 110 111 113 114 115 116 117 118 119 120 122 123 125 126 128 129 130 131 133 134 135 136 137 138 139 140 141 143 144 145 146 147 **P**1 **S** Duke University Health System, Durham, NC
Primary Contact: Kevin W. Sowers, R.N., MSN, Chief Executive Officer
CFO: Sabrina Olsen, Chief Financial Officer
CMO: Thomas Owens, M.D., Chief Medical Officer
CIO: Asif Ahmad, Chief Information Officer
CHR: Deborah Page, Chief Human Resources Officer
Web address: www.dukehealth.org
**Control:** Other not–for–profit (including NFP Corporation) **Service:** General Medical and Surgical

**Staffed Beds:** 813 **Admissions:** 38098 **Census:** 682 **Outpatient Visits:** 1170589 **Births:** 2894 **Total Expense ($000):** 1561484 **Payroll Expense ($000):** 554803 **Personnel:** 9114

**DURHAM REGIONAL HOSPITAL (340155)**, 3643 North Roxboro Road, Zip 27704–2763; tel. 919/470–4000 **A**1 3 5 6 9 10 **F**3 8 11 12 13 15 17 18 20 22 24 26 28 29 30 31 34 35 40 44 45 47 50 51 57 59 60 64 66 68 70 73 74 75 76 77 78 79 80 81 82 84 85 87 90 96 98 100 102 105 107 108 110 111 114 117 118 119 120 122 123 125 129 130 131 145 146 147 **P**6 **S** Duke University Health System, Durham, NC
Primary Contact: Kerry Watson, President
CFO: Jonathan B. Hoy, Chief Financial Officer
CMO: Lisa C. Pickett, M.D., Chief Medical Officer
CIO: Terry Mears, Director Information Systems
CHR: Richard J. Walsh, Ph.D., Chief Human Resources Officer
Web address: www.durhamregional.org
**Control:** Other not–for–profit (including NFP Corporation) **Service:** General Medical and Surgical

**Staffed Beds:** 202 **Admissions:** 15369 **Census:** 202 **Outpatient Visits:** 125763 **Births:** 2239 **Total Expense ($000):** 257291 **Payroll Expense ($000):** 107421 **Personnel:** 1974

**DURHAM VETERANS AFFAIRS MEDICAL CENTER**, 508 Fulton Street, Zip 27705–3897; tel. 919/286–0411, (Total facility includes 120 beds in nursing home–type unit) **A**1 3 5 8 **F**3 5 11 12 15 17 20 24 26 28 29 30 31 33 34 35 38 39 40 44 50 51 54 56 57 58 59 60 61 63 64 65 66 70 74 75 77 78 79 81 82 84 86 87 93 94 97 98 100 101 102 103 104 107 108 109 110 111 112 113 114 115 116 117 118 119 120 123 125 126 127 128 129 131 134 144 145 146 147 **S** Department of Veterans Affairs, Washington, DC
Primary Contact: DeAnne Seekins, Director
COO: Rudy Klopfer, Associate Director
CFO: David Kuboushek, Chief, Fiscal Service
CMO: John D. Shelburne, M.D., Chief of Staff
CIO: Toby Dickerson, Chief Information Resources Management Services
CIO: Conrad Raber, Chief Information Resources Management Service
CHR: Jerry Freeman, Chief, Human Resources Management Services
CNO: Kathryn M. Ward–Presson, R.N., Associate Director for Patient Care Services
Web address: www.va.gov
**Control:** Veterans Affairs, Government, federal **Service:** General Medical and Surgical

**Staffed Beds:** 265 **Admissions:** 7124 **Census:** 112 **Outpatient Visits:** 532781 **Births:** 0 **Total Expense ($000):** 419295 **Payroll Expense ($000):** 205947 **Personnel:** 1998

**NORTH CAROLINA SPECIALTY HOSPITAL (340049)**, 3916 Ben Franklin Boulevard, Zip 27704; tel. 919/956–9300 **A**1 9 10 **F**3 64 79 81 82 85 86 87 118 125 129 134 **S** National Surgical Hospitals, Chicago, IL
Primary Contact: Randi L. Shults, Chief Executive Officer
CFO: Bill Wilson, Chief Financial Officer
CMO: Thomas Dimmig, M.D., Medical Director
CHR: Deborah Wheeler, Director Human Resources
CNO: John Medlin, Chief Nursing Officer
Web address: www.ncspecialty.com
**Control:** Partnership, Investor–owned, for–profit **Service:** General Medical and Surgical

**Staffed Beds:** 18 **Admissions:** 1654 **Census:** 11 **Outpatient Visits:** 11677 **Births:** 0 **Total Expense ($000):** 31052 **Payroll Expense ($000):** 9722 **Personnel:** 143

**SELECT SPECIALTY HOSPITAL–DURHAM (342018)**, 3643 North Roxboro Road, 6th Floor, Zip 27704; tel. 919/470–9137, (Nonreporting) **A**1 10 **S** Select Medical Corporation, Mechanicsburg, PA
Primary Contact: Robert F. Jernigan, Jr., Chief Executive Officer
Web address: www.selectmedicalcorp.com
**Control:** Corporation, Investor–owned, for–profit **Service:** Long–Term Acute Care hospital

**Staffed Beds:** 30

## EDEN—Rockingham County

**MOREHEAD MEMORIAL HOSPITAL (340060)**, 117 East King's Highway, Zip 27288–5299; tel. 336/623–9711, (Total facility includes 121 beds in nursing home–type unit) **A**1 2 9 10 **F**3 11 13 15 18 26 28 29 30 31 34 35 36 40 45 47 48 49 50 57 59 64 68 70 73 74 75 76 77 78 79 81 85 87 89 90 93 97 107 108 110 111 113 117 118 121 122 127 128 129 131 134 142 145 146 147 **S** QHR, Brentwood, TN
Primary Contact: Carl Martin, President and Chief Executive Officer
CFO: Dan Elmer, Vice President Finance
CHR: Tom Stevens, Director Personnel
Web address: www.morehead.us
**Control:** Other not–for–profit (including NFP Corporation) **Service:** General Medical and Surgical

**Staffed Beds:** 214 **Admissions:** 6104 **Census:** 176 **Outpatient Visits:** 168331 **Births:** 552 **Total Expense ($000):** 87888 **Payroll Expense ($000):** 41229 **Personnel:** 835

## EDENTON—Chowan County

**VIDANT CHOWAN HOSPITAL (341318)**, 211 Virginia Road, Zip 27932–0629, Mailing Address: P.O. Box 629, Zip 27932–0629; tel. 252/482–8451, (Total facility includes 32 beds in nursing home–type unit) **A**1 9 10 18 **F**3 11 13 15 18 19 28 29 30 31 34 35 40 45 46 56 57 59 64 70 74 75 76 77 78 79 81 82 85 89 93 107 108 110 111 113 118 127 129 131 132 134 145 146 **S** Vidant Health, Greenville, NC
Primary Contact: Jeffrey N. Sackrison, FACHE, President
COO: Jeffery Dial, Chief Operating Officer
CFO: Brian Harvill, Vice President Financial Services
CMO: William Hope, IV, M.D., Chief of Medical Staff
CIO: Megan Booth–Mills, Director Planning and Marketing
CHR: Debbie Swicegood, Director Human Resources
CNO: Cindy Coker, M.P.H., Vice President, Patient Care Services
Web address: www.vidanthealth.com
**Control:** Other not–for–profit (including NFP Corporation) **Service:** General Medical and Surgical

**Staffed Beds:** 67 **Admissions:** 1847 **Census:** 46 **Outpatient Visits:** 40984 **Births:** 325 **Total Expense ($000):** 43416 **Payroll Expense ($000):** 18721 **Personnel:** 397

## ELIZABETH CITY—Pasquotank County

**ALBEMARLE HEALTH (340109)**, 1144 North Road Street, Zip 27909, Mailing Address: P.O. Box 1587, Zip 27906–1587; tel. 252/335–0531 **A**1 9 10 **F**3 13 15 17 18 20 28 29 30 31 34 35 39 40 45 53 57 59 64 68 70 74 75 76 77 78 79 81 84 86 87 92 93 94 107 108 111 114 117 118 120 128 129 131 145 146 147 **S** Vidant Health, Greenville, NC
Primary Contact: Sharon M. Tanner, President
COO: Jan King Robinson, VP, Operations
CFO: Raymond Owings, Vice President Finance
CMO: Daniel S. Terryberry, M.D., Chief Medical Officer
CIO: Steve Clark, Chief Information Officer
CHR: Brenda Rosecrans, Director, Human Resources
CNO: Dan Drake, VP, Patient Care Services
Web address: www.albemarlehealth.org
**Control:** Hospital district or authority, Government, nonfederal **Service:** General Medical and Surgical

**Staffed Beds:** 140 **Admissions:** 5022 **Census:** 60 **Outpatient Visits:** 134852 **Births:** 697 **Total Expense ($000):** 84942 **Payroll Expense ($000):** 38937 **Personnel:** 842

## ELIZABETHTOWN—Bladen County

**BLADEN COUNTY HOSPITAL** See Cape Fear Valley – Bladen County Hospital

*Many Facility Codes have changed. Please refer to the AHA Guide Code Chart.*     © 2012 AHA Guide

✠ **CAPE FEAR VALLEY – BLADEN COUNTY HOSPITAL (341315)**, 501 South Poplar Street, Zip 28337–0398, Mailing Address: P.O. Box 398, Zip 28337–0398; tel. 910/862–5100, (Nonreporting) **A**1 9·10 18 **S** Cape Fear Valley Health System, Fayetteville, NC
Primary Contact: Cameron Highsmith, Chief Executive Officer
COO: Cameron Highsmith, Chief Executive Officer
CFO: Sandra Williams, Chief Financial Officer
CMO: Pearly Graham Hoskins, M.D., President Medical Staff
CIO: Craig Kellum, Director Management Information Systems
CHR: Ginger Parks, Director Human Resources
Web address: www.bchn.org
**Control:** County–Government, nonfederal **Service:** General Medical and Surgical

| Staffed Beds: 26 |

### ELKIN—Surry County

✠ **HUGH CHATHAM MEMORIAL HOSPITAL (340097)**, 180 Parkwood Drive, Zip 28621–0560, Mailing Address: P.O. Box 560, Zip 28621–0560; tel. 336/527–7000, (Total facility includes 127 beds in nursing home–type unit) **A**1 9 10 **F**3 6 10 11 13 15 28 29 30 34 40 45 57 59 62 63 64 68 70 75 76 81 85 87 91 93 96 97 107 108 110 111 113 117 118 119 120 124 126 127 128 129 131 132 133 134 145 146 147 **S** Alliant Management Services, Louisville, KY
Primary Contact: David Loving, Chief Executive Officer
CMO: Stephen Isaacs, M.D., Chief of Staff
CIO: Lee Powe, Director Management Information Systems
CHR: Jeff Seaford, Director Human Resources
Web address: www.hughchatham.org
**Control:** Other not–for–profit (including NFP Corporation) **Service:** General Medical and Surgical

| Staffed Beds: 208 Admissions: 4812 Census: 156 Outpatient Visits: 67479 Births: 519 Total Expense ($000): 68086 Payroll Expense ($000): 24610 Personnel: 683 |

### FAYETTEVILLE—Cumberland County

✠ △ **CAPE FEAR VALLEY MEDICAL CENTER (340028)**, 1638 Owen Drive, Zip 28304–3431, Mailing Address: P.O. Box 2000, Zip 28302–2000; tel. 910/615–4000, (Includes SOUTHEASTERN REGIONAL REHABILITATION CENTER ; BEHAVIORAL HEALTH CARE OF CAPE FEAR VALLEY HEALTH SYSTEM, 3425 Melrose Road, Zip 28304–1695; tel. 910/609–3000; SOUTHEASTERN REGIONAL REHABILITATION CENTER, 1638 Owen Drive, Zip 28304; tel. 910/609–4000) **A**1 2 3 5 7 9 10 13 **F**1 7 8 12 14 15 17 18 20 22 24 26 28 29 30 31 34 40 43 51 53 54 56 57 59 60 62 63 64 65 68 70 71 72 73 74 75 76 77 78 79 80 81 82 83 84 85 86 87 88 89 90 91 92 93 96 97 98 99 100 102 103 104 107 108 110 111 113 114 115 116 118 119 120 122 123 125 126 128 129 130 131 134 142 143 144 145 146 147 **P**6 **S** Cape Fear Valley Health System, Fayetteville, NC
Primary Contact: Michael Nagowski, President and Chief Executive Officer
CFO: Sandra Williams, Chief Financial Officer
CMO: Richard S. Taylor, M.D., Chief Medical Officer
CHR: William B. Pryor, Senior Vice President Human Resources
Web address: www.capefearvalley.com
**Control:** Other not–for–profit (including NFP Corporation) **Service:** General Medical and Surgical

| Staffed Beds: 666 Admissions: 33968 Census: 587 Outpatient Visits: 543201 Births: 4741 Total Expense ($000): 540795 Payroll Expense ($000): 287887 Personnel: 4603 |

**HIGHSMITH–RAINEY SPECIALTY HOSPITAL (342014)**, 150 Robeson Street, Zip 28301–5570; tel. 910/615–1000, (Nonreporting) **A**10 **S** Cape Fear Valley Health System, Fayetteville, NC
Primary Contact: Michael Nagowski, President and Chief Executive Officer
Web address: www.capefearvalley.com
**Control:** Other not–for–profit (including NFP Corporation) **Service:** Long–Term Acute Care hospital

| Staffed Beds: 133 |

✠ **VETERANS AFFAIRS MEDICAL CENTER**, 2300 Ramsey Street, Zip 28301–3899; tel. 910/488–2120, (Nonreporting) **A**1 **S** Department of Veterans Affairs, Washington, DC
Primary Contact: Elizabeth Goolsby, Director
COO: James Galkowski, Associate Director for Operations
CFO: Patrick Bullard, Chief Financial Officer
CMO: Anna B. Teague, M.D., Chief of Staff
CIO: Kenneth Williams, Chief Information Officer
CHR: Joseph Whaley, Chief, Human Resources Management Service
CNO: Joyce Alexander–Hines, R.N., Associate Director, Patient Care Services
Web address: www.fayettevillenc.va.gov
**Control:** Veterans Affairs, Government, federal **Service:** General Medical and Surgical

| Staffed Beds: 56 |

### FORT BRAGG—Cumberland County

✠ **WOMACK ARMY MEDICAL CENTER**, Normandy Drive, Zip 28307–5000; tel. 910/907–6000, (Nonreporting) **A**1 3 5 **S** Department of the Army, Office of the Surgeon General, Falls Church, VA
Primary Contact: Colonel Brian Canfield, Commander
Web address: www.wamc.amedd.army.mil/
**Control:** Army, Government, federal **Service:** General Medical and Surgical

| Staffed Beds: 156 |

### FRANKLIN—Macon County

✠ **ANGEL MEDICAL CENTER (341326)**, 120 Riverview Street, Zip 28734, Mailing Address: P.O. Box 1209, Zip 28744; tel. 828/524–8411 **A**1 9 10 18 **F**3 8 11 13 15 18 28 29 30 31 34 35 36 40 45 49 57 59 62 63 64 70 75 76 77 78 79 81 82 83 84 85 86 87 91 92 93 107 108 110 111 113 117 118 123 128 131 132 134 143 145 146 147 **P**6 **S** Mission Health System, Asheville, NC
Primary Contact: Martin Wadewitz, Interim Chief Executive Officer
COO: Martin Wadewitz, Chief Operations Officer/ Vice President, Operations
CFO: Jeff W. Rush, Interim Vice President Finance
CIO: Gary Hanold, Director Management Information Systems
CHR: Mark Garber, Vice President, Human Resources
CNO: Sheila C. Price, R.N., Chief Nursing Officer/Vice President of Nursing
Web address: www.angelmed.org
**Control:** Hospital district or authority, Government, nonfederal **Service:** General Medical and Surgical

| Staffed Beds: 25 Admissions: 1622 Census: 16 Outpatient Visits: 85655 Births: 163 Total Expense ($000): 39542 Payroll Expense ($000): 20669 Personnel: 383 |

### GASTONIA—Gaston County

✠ **GASTON MEMORIAL HOSPITAL (340032)**, 2525 Court Drive, Zip 28054–2142, Mailing Address: P.O. Box 1747, Zip 28053–1747; tel. 704/834–2000 **A**1 2 9 10 **F**3 13 15 17 18 20 22 24 26 28 29 30 31 34 35 40 44 45 49 50 53 57 58 59 60 64 70 72 73 74 75 76 78 79 81 82 87 89 91 92 93 94 96 98 99 100 101 102 107 108 110 111 113 114 115 116 117 118 119 120 122 125 129 131 134 145 146 147
Primary Contact: Randall L. Kelley, President and Chief Executive Officer
COO: Douglas R. Luckett, Executive Vice President and Chief Operating Officer
CFO: David O'Connor, Executive Vice President and Chief Financial Officer
CIO: Mike Johnson, Assistant Vice President, Chief Information Officer
CHR: Elizabeth McCraw, Vice President, Human Resources
Web address: www.caromont.org
**Control:** Other not–for–profit (including NFP Corporation) **Service:** General Medical and Surgical

| Staffed Beds: 394 Admissions: 23035 Census: 246 Outpatient Visits: 330469 Births: 2584 Total Expense ($000): 296037 Payroll Expense ($000): 132036 Personnel: 2256 |

### GOLDSBORO—Wayne County

☐ **CHERRY HOSPITAL (344026)**, 201 Stevens Mill Road, Zip 27530–1057; tel. 919/731–3200 **A**1 9 10 **F**30 39 98 99 103 108 145
Primary Contact: Luckey Welsh, Interim Director
COO: Richard Courliss, Chief Support Services
CFO: Susie Sherrod Sanders, Budget Officer
CMO: Kimberly Johnson, M.D., Clinical Director
CIO: Lisa Pettus, Manager Information Systems
CHR: Angela Crawford, Director Human Resources
Web address: www.cherryhospital.org
**Control:** State–Government, nonfederal **Service:** Psychiatric

| Staffed Beds: 251 Admissions: 1311 Census: 166 Outpatient Visits: 506 Births: 0 Total Expense ($000): 68007 Payroll Expense ($000): 41407 Personnel: 1035 |

✠ **WAYNE MEMORIAL HOSPITAL (340010)**, 2700 Wayne Memorial Drive, Zip 27534, Mailing Address: P.O. Box 8001, Zip 27533; tel. 919/736–1110 **A**1 9 10 **F**3 8 13 15 20 28 29 30 31 32 34 35 39 40 49 50 57 58 59 60 64 65 68 70 71 73 74 76 77 78 79 81 82 85 86 89 93 96 98 101 102 103 104 107 108 110 111 113 117 118 125 128 129 131 133 134 142 145 146 147 **P**6
Primary Contact: J. William Paugh, President and Chief Executive Officer
COO: Thomas A. Bradshaw, Vice President Operations
CFO: Rebecca W. Craig, Vice President and Chief Financial Officer
CIO: Lori Cole, Director Information Management
CHR: Richard K. Rogers, FACHE, Vice President Human Resources
CNO: Shirley S. Harkey, R.N., Vice President, Patient Services
Web address: www.waynehealth.org
**Control:** Other not–for–profit (including NFP Corporation) **Service:** General Medical and Surgical

| Staffed Beds: 274 Admissions: 11674 Census: 146 Outpatient Visits: 149578 Births: 1506 Total Expense ($000): 171051 Payroll Expense ($000): 73915 Personnel: 1515 |

---

**Hospital, Medicare Provider Number, Address, Telephone, Approval, Facility, and Physician Codes, Health Care System**

★ American Hospital Association (AHA) membership
☐ The Joint Commission accreditation ◇ DNV Healthcare Inc. accreditation
○ American Osteopathic Association (AOA) accreditation
△ Commission on Accreditation of Rehabilitation Facilities (CARF) accreditation

**NC**

## GREENSBORO—Guilford County

✠ △ **CONE HEALTH (340091)**, 1200 North Elm Street, Zip 27401–1020; tel. 336/832–7000, (Includes ANNIE PENN HOSPITAL, 618 South Main Street, Reidsville, Zip 27320–5094; tel. 336/951–4000; Mickey Foster, Chief Executive Officer; BEHAVIORAL HEALTH CENTER, 700 Walter Reed Drive, Zip 27403–1129; tel. 336/832–9600; Troy Chisolm, Vice President and Administrator; MOSES H. CONE MEMORIAL HOSPITAL, 1200 North Elm Street, Zip 27401; tel. 336/832–7000; Judith A. Schanel, R.N., MSN, FACHE, President; WESLEY LONG COMMUNITY HOSPITAL, 501 North Elam Avenue, Zip 27403; tel. 336/832–1000; Paul A. Jeffrey, Vice President and Administrator; WOMEN'S HOSPITAL OF GREENSBORO, 801 Green Valley Road, Zip 27408; tel. 336/832–6500), (Total facility includes 92 beds in nursing home–type unit) **A**1 2 3 5 7 9 10 **F**3 5 7 8 11 12 13 15 17 18 20 22 24 26 28 29 30 31 32 34 35 37 39 40 41 42 43 44 45 46 47 49 50 54 56 57 58 59 60 61 63 64 66 68 70 72 74 75 76 77 78 79 80 81 82 83 84 85 86 87 88 89 90 92 93 95 96 97 98 99 100 101 102 103 104 107 108 110 111 113 114 116 117 118 119 120 122 123 125 127 128 129 130 131 133 134 143 144 145 146 147 **P**6 8
Primary Contact: R. Timothy Rice, President and Chief Executive Officer
CMO: William Bowman, M.D., Vice President Medical Affairs
CIO: John Jenkins, Vice President and Chief Information Officer
CHR: Noel F. Burt, Ph.D., Chief Human Resources Officer
Web address: www.conehealth.com
**Control:** Other not–for–profit (including NFP Corporation) **Service:** General Medical and Surgical

**Staffed Beds:** 1044 **Admissions:** 49082 **Census:** 726 **Outpatient Visits:** 648640 **Births:** 5960 **Total Expense ($000):** 834375 **Payroll Expense ($000):** 355636 **Personnel:** 7264

✠ **KINDRED HOSPITAL–GREENSBORO (342012)**, 2401 Southside Boulevard, Zip 27406–3311; tel. 336/271–2800, (Nonreporting) **A**1 9 10 **S** Kindred Healthcare, Louisville, KY
Primary Contact: Derek Murzyn, Chief Executive Officer
CFO: Michael Nelson, Chief Financial Officer
CMO: Percy E. Jones, M.D., Chief of Staff
CIO: Little Shuford, Manager Medical Information
CHR: Michele Roberts, Hospital Recruiter
Web address: www.khgreensboro.com
**Control:** Corporation, Investor–owned, for–profit **Service:** General Medical and Surgical

**Staffed Beds:** 124

✠ **SELECT SPECIALTY HOSPITAL–GREENSBORO (342020)**, 1200 North Elm Street, 5th Floor, Zip 27401; tel. 336/832–8571 **A**1 10 **F**1 147 **S** Select Medical Corporation, Mechanicsburg, PA
Primary Contact: Deana Knight, Chief Executive Officer
CHR: Karen Tracey, Chief Human Resources
CNO: Robin Clark, Chief Nursing Officer
Web address: www.selectmedicalcorp.com
**Control:** Corporation, Investor–owned, for–profit **Service:** Long–Term Acute Care hospital

**Staffed Beds:** 30 **Admissions:** 270 **Census:** 19 **Births:** 0

## GREENVILLE—Pitt County

**PITT COUNTY MEMORIAL HOSPITAL** See Vidant Medical Center

✠ △ **VIDANT MEDICAL CENTER (340040)**, 2100 Stantonsburg Road, Zip 27834, Mailing Address: P.O. Box 6028, Zip 27835–6028; tel. 252/847–4100, (Includes UNIVERSITY HEALTH SYSTEMS CHILDREN'S HOSPITAL, 2100 Stantonsburg Road, Zip 27834–2818, Mailing Address: PO Box 6028, Zip 27835–6028; tel. 252/847–4100) **A**1 2 3 5 7 8 9 10 **F**3 7 12 13 14 15 17 18 19 20 21 22 23 24 25 26 27 28 29 30 31 32 34 35 38 40 41 42 43 44 45 46 47 48 49 50 51 52 54 55 56 59 60 61 64 65 67 68 70 72 73 74 75 76 77 78 79 80 81 82 83 84 85 86 87 88 89 90 92 93 94 95 96 97 98 100 101 102 103 104 107 108 111 113 114 115 116 117 118 123 125 128 129 130 131 133 134 135 137 142 143 144 145 146 147 **P**6 **S** Vidant Health, Greenville, NC
Primary Contact: Steven Lawler, President
CFO: Jack W. Holsten, Chief Financial Officer
CMO: Ernest Larkin, M.D., Chief Medical Officer
CIO: Stuart James, Chief Information Officer
CHR: Tyree Walker, Chief Human Resources Officer
Web address: www.uhseast.com
**Control:** Other not–for–profit (including NFP Corporation) **Service:** General Medical and Surgical

**Staffed Beds:** 847 **Admissions:** 44352 **Census:** 690 **Outpatient Visits:** 373359 **Births:** 3592 **Total Expense ($000):** 887515 **Payroll Expense ($000):** 322520 **Personnel:** 7388

**WALTER B. JONES ALCOHOL AND DRUG ABUSE TREATMENT CENTER (344024)**, 2577 West Fifth Street, Zip 27834–7813; tel. 252/830–3426 **A**10 **F**4 29 34 35 38 59 66 75 82 86 87 96 100 129 134 142 **P**6
Primary Contact: Theresa Edmondson, Director
CFO: Tom Basnight, Chief Financial Officer
CMO: Gary Leonhardt, M.D., Clinical Director
Web address: www.ncdhhs.gov
**Control:** State–Government, nonfederal **Service:** Alcoholism and other chemical dependency

**Staffed Beds:** 80 **Admissions:** 1631 **Census:** 65 **Outpatient Visits:** 0 **Births:** 0 **Total Expense ($000):** 11189 **Payroll Expense ($000):** 7887 **Personnel:** 152

## HAMLET—Richmond County

☐ **SANDHILLS REGIONAL MEDICAL CENTER (340106)**, 1000 West Hamlet Avenue, Zip 28345–4522, Mailing Address: P.O. Box 1109, Zip 28345–1109; tel. 910/205–8000 **A**1 9 10 **F**3 7 8 18 29 34 35 40 49 57 59 64 70 75 79 81 82 87 98 102 103 104 105 106 107 108 111 113 117 118 129 134 145 **P**6 **S** Health Management Associates, Naples, FL
Primary Contact: Michael H. McNair, Chief Executive Officer
COO: Thomas Roddy, Assistant Administrator
CHR: Jenny La Fave, Director
Web address: www.hma–corp.com
**Control:** Corporation, Investor–owned, for–profit **Service:** General Medical and Surgical

**Staffed Beds:** 64 **Admissions:** 3280 **Census:** 37 **Outpatient Visits:** 13812 **Births:** 0 **Total Expense ($000):** 28315 **Payroll Expense ($000):** 11259 **Personnel:** 187

## HENDERSON—Vance County

✠ △ **MARIA PARHAM MEDICAL CENTER (340132)**, 566 Ruin Creek Road, Zip 27536–2957; tel. 252/438–4143, (Nonreporting) **A**1 7 9 10 **S** Duke LifePoint Healthcare, Brentwood, TN
Primary Contact: Robert G. Singletary, President and Chief Executive Officer
COO: Jay Kennedy, Chief Operating Officer
CFO: Jim Chatman, Chief Financial Officer
CIO: Randy Williams, Director Management Information Systems
CHR: Tonya Jones, Vice President Human Resources
CNO: Cindy Faulkner, Chief Nursing Officer
Web address: www.mariaparham.com
**Control:** Other not–for–profit (including NFP Corporation) **Service:** General Medical and Surgical

**Staffed Beds:** 102

## HENDERSONVILLE—Henderson County

✠ **MARGARET R. PARDEE MEMORIAL HOSPITAL (340017)**, 800 North Justice Street, Zip 28791; tel. 828/696–1000 **A**1 2 9 10 21 **F**2 3 4 11 13 15 18 22 28 29 30 31 34 35 36 38 39 40 44 45 46 47 48 49 50 56 57 58 59 62 63 65 68 69 70 74 75 76 77 78 79 81 82 85 86 87 89 93 94 97 98 100 101 102 103 104 107 108 110 111 113 114 117 118 120 122 128 129 130 131 134 142 143 145 146 147 **P**6
Primary Contact: James M. Kirby, II, Chief Executive Officer
CFO: Alan House, Chief Financial Officer
CMO: Robert Kiskaddon, M.D., Chief Medical Officer
CHR: Hope Reynolds, Executive Director Human Resources and Support Services
Web address: www.pardeehospital.org
**Control:** County–Government, nonfederal **Service:** General Medical and Surgical

**Staffed Beds:** 161 **Admissions:** 7466 **Census:** 79 **Outpatient Visits:** 237476 **Births:** 355 **Total Expense ($000):** 134654 **Payroll Expense ($000):** 54493 **Personnel:** 1037

★ ○ **PARK RIDGE HEALTH (340023)**, 100 Hospital Drive, Zip 28792–5272; tel. 828/684–8501 **A**2 9 10 11 19 **F**3 11 13 15 18 28 29 30 31 32 34 35 40 43 45 46 47 48 49 50 56 57 59 62 65 68 70 71 75 76 77 78 79 80 81 82 83 85 87 93 94 98 101 102 103 104 105 107 108 110 111 113 114 117 118 128 129 130 131 134 141 145 146 147 **P**6 **S** Adventist Health System Sunbelt Health Care Corporation, Altamonte Springs, FL
Primary Contact: Jimm Bunch, President and Chief Executive Officer
CFO: Karsten Randolph, Vice President Finance/Chief Financial Officer
CIO: Lee Strickland, Regional Director Information Technology
CHR: Brandon M. Nudd, Director, Organizational Development
CNO: Craig Lindsey, R.N., Vice President Clinical Services/Chief Nursing Officer
Web address: www.parkridgehealth.org
**Control:** Other not–for–profit (including NFP Corporation) **Service:** General Medical and Surgical

**Staffed Beds:** 98 **Admissions:** 4014 **Census:** 60 **Outpatient Visits:** 351834 **Births:** 587 **Total Expense ($000):** 117777 **Payroll Expense ($000):** 49386 **Personnel:** 847

*Many Facility Codes have changed. Please refer to the AHA Guide Code Chart.* © 2012 AHA Guide

## HICKORY—Catawba County

☒ △ **CATAWBA VALLEY MEDICAL CENTER (340143)**, 810 Fairgrove Church Road S.E., Zip 28602–9643; tel. 828/326–3000 **A**1 2 5 7 9 10 **F**3 5 11 12 13 15 18 20 22 26 28 29 30 31 34 35 36 37 39 40 44 45 46 47 48 49 50 51 53 54 56 57 59 61 64 65 66 68 70 71 73 74 75 76 77 78 79 81 82 84 85 86 87 89 90 91 92 93 96 97 98 100 101 102 103 104 107 108 109 110 111 113 114 116 117 118 119 120 121 122 123 125 128 129 130 131 134 142 143 144 145 146 147
Primary Contact: J. Anthony Rose, President and Chief Executive Officer
COO: Scott Echelberger, Vice President, Operations
CFO: David J. Boone, Senior Vice President, Finance
CIO: Jerry Reardon, Director Information Systems
CHR: Phyllis Johnston, Director
CNO: Edward L. Beard, MSN, Senior Vice President, Patient Care Services & CNO
Web address: www.catawbavalleymc.org
**Control:** County–Government, nonfederal **Service:** General Medical and Surgical

**Staffed Beds:** 213 **Admissions:** 10083 **Census:** 129 **Outpatient Visits:** 189605 **Births:** 1685 **Total Expense ($000):** 151499 **Payroll Expense ($000):** 78724 **Personnel:** 1275

☒ **FRYE REGIONAL MEDICAL CENTER (340116)**, 420 North Center Street, Zip 28601–5049; tel. 828/322–6070, (Includes FRYE REGIONAL MEDICAL CENTER–SOUTH CAMPUS, One Third Avenue N.W., Zip 28601, Mailing Address: P.O. Box 369, Zip 28603; tel. 704/315–5777) **A**1 2 9 10 **F**11 12 13 15 17 18 20 22 24 26 28 29 30 31 34 35 37 40 45 46 49 54 57 59 64 68 70 72 74 75 76 77 78 79 81 82 85 86 87 89 90 93 96 98 101 103 107 108 110 111 113 114 117 118 125 127 128 129 130 131 143 145 146 147 **P**6 **S** TENET Healthcare Corporation, Dallas, TX
Primary Contact: Michael R. Blackburn, Chief Executive Officer
COO: Rich Ellis, Chief Operating Officer
CFO: Sherry Henderson, Vice President Financial Services and Chief Financial Officer
CMO: Frank C. Smeeks, M.D., Chief Medical Officer
CHR: Liz Elich, Vice President Human Resources
Web address: www.fryemedctr.com
**Control:** Corporation, Investor–owned, for–profit **Service:** General Medical and Surgical

**Staffed Beds:** 306 **Admissions:** 12081 **Census:** 173 **Outpatient Visits:** 131525 **Births:** 527 **Personnel:** 1236

## HIGH POINT—Guilford County

☒ △ **HIGH POINT REGIONAL HEALTH SYSTEM (340004)**, 601 North Elm Street, Zip 27262–4398, Mailing Address: P.O. Box HP–5, Zip 27261; tel. 336/878–6000 **A**1 2 7 9 10 **F**3 4 5 7 8 11 12 13 15 17 18 20 22 24 26 28 29 30 31 34 35 40 43 44 45 49 50 51 52 53 54 57 58 59 60 62 64 66 68 70 71 73 74 75 76 77 78 79 80 81 82 84 85 86 87 90 93 94 96 98 100 101 102 103 104 107 108 109 110 111 113 114 115 116 117 118 119 120 125 129 130 131 134 143 144 145 146 147 **P**6
Primary Contact: Jeffrey S. Miller, President and Chief Executive Officer
COO: Martha Barham, Vice President and Chief Operating Officer
COO: Gregory W. Taylor, M.D., Vice President and Chief Operating Officer
CFO: Kimberly Crews, Vice President Finance and Chief Financial Officer
CMO: L. Dale Williams, M.D., Vice President and Chief Medical Director
CHR: Katherine Burns, Vice President Human Resources
CNO: Tammi Erving–Mengel, Vice President, Chief Nursing Officer
Web address: www.highpointregional.com
**Control:** Other not–for–profit (including NFP Corporation) **Service:** General Medical and Surgical

**Staffed Beds:** 335 **Admissions:** 14647 **Census:** 206 **Outpatient Visits:** 249611 **Births:** 1468 **Total Expense ($000):** 234526 **Payroll Expense ($000):** 91701 **Personnel:** 2027

## HIGHLANDS—Macon County

☒ **HIGHLANDS–CASHIERS HOSPITAL (341316)**, 190 Hospital Drive, Zip 28741–7600, Mailing Address: P.O. Drawer 190, Zip 28741–0190; tel. 828/526–1200, (Total facility includes 84 beds in nursing home–type unit) **A**1 9 10 18 **F**1 3 8 11 15 29 30 34 35 40 45 46 49 53 54 56 57 59 75 79 81 82 93 111 112 114 115 117 118 128 129 132 134 145 146 147 **P**6
Primary Contact: Craig B. James, Chief Executive Officer
COO: Frank Leslie, Vice President Operations
CFO: Michael E. Daiken, Chief Financial Officer
CIO: Mike Brown, IT Manager
CHR: Amanda Talley, Human Resources Director
CNO: Eileen Lipham, Chief Nursing Officer
Web address: www.hchospital.org
**Control:** Other not–for–profit (including NFP Corporation) **Service:** General Medical and Surgical

**Staffed Beds:** 108 **Admissions:** 398 **Census:** 76 **Outpatient Visits:** 11721 **Births:** 0 **Total Expense ($000):** 23087 **Payroll Expense ($000):** 11160 **Personnel:** 234

## HUNTERSVILLE—Mecklenburg County

☒ **PRESBYTERIAN HOSPITAL HUNTERSVILLE (340183)**, 10030 Gilead Road, Zip 28078, Mailing Address: P.O. Box 3508, Zip 28070–3508; tel. 704/316–4000 **A**1 9 10 **F**3 8 11 12 13 18 20 26 29 30 31 34 35 40 45 50 57 59 64 68 70 73 75 76 77 78 79 81 82 85 86 87 89 93 96 100 102 107 108 110 111 113 117 118 125 128 129 131 134 145 146 **S** Novant Health, Winston–Salem, NC
Primary Contact: Tanya S. Blackmon, President
CFO: Jason Yanni, Senior Financial Analyst
CMO: David Cook, M.D., Chief Medical Officer
CIO: Richard B. McKnight, Senior Vice President and Chief Information Officer
CHR: Tracy Craig, Director Human Resources
Web address: www.novanthealth.org
**Control:** Other not–for–profit (including NFP Corporation) **Service:** General Medical and Surgical

**Staffed Beds:** 60 **Admissions:** 5598 **Census:** 56 **Outpatient Visits:** 144619 **Births:** 1092 **Total Expense ($000):** 95885 **Payroll Expense ($000):** 32164 **Personnel:** 536

## JACKSONVILLE—Onslow County

☐ **BRYNN MARR HOSPITAL (344016)**, 192 Village Drive, Zip 28546–7299; tel. 910/577–1400, (Nonreporting) **A**1 9 10 **S** Universal Health Services, Inc., King of Prussia, PA
Primary Contact: Jay Kortemeyer, Chief Executive Officer
COO: Cynthia Waun, Chief Operating Officer and Risk Manager
CFO: David Warmerdam, Chief Financial Officer
CMO: Ashraf Mikhail, M.D., Medical Director
CIO: Cynthia Waun, Chief Operating Officer and Risk Manager
CHR: Jeff Nardo, Director Human Resources
Web address: www.brynnmarr.org
**Control:** Corporation, Investor–owned, for–profit **Service:** Psychiatric

**Staffed Beds:** 87

☒ **ONSLOW MEMORIAL HOSPITAL (340042)**, 317 Western Boulevard, Zip 28540–6379, Mailing Address: P.O. Box 1358, Zip 28541–1358; tel. 910/577–2345 **A**1 9 10 **F**3 8 11 13 15 20 28 29 34 40 45 46 47 48 49 54 57 59 60 64 68 70 72 73 75 76 77 79 81 82 84 85 86 87 89 93 107 108 110 111 116 117 118 125 128 129 130 131 134 145 146 147 **P**8
Primary Contact: Ed Piper, Chief Executive Officer
CFO: Roy Smith, Chief Financial Officer
CMO: Elizabeth D'Angelo, M.D., Chief of Staff
CIO: Christina Feak, Chief Information Officer
CHR: Sue Kegley, Director Human Resources
CNO: Crystal Hayden, R.N., Chief Nursing Officer
Web address: www.onslow.org
**Control:** Hospital district or authority, Government, nonfederal **Service:** General Medical and Surgical

**Staffed Beds:** 144 **Admissions:** 9603 **Census:** 98 **Outpatient Visits:** 130981 **Births:** 2128 **Total Expense ($000):** 91430 **Payroll Expense ($000):** 51973 **Personnel:** 1117

## JEFFERSON—Ashe County

☒ **ASHE MEMORIAL HOSPITAL (341325)**, 200 Hospital Avenue, Zip 28640–9244; tel. 336/846–7101, (Total facility includes 60 beds in nursing home–type unit) **A**1 9 10 18 **F**3 8 11 13 15 28 30 34 35 40 45 46 48 53 57 59 64 75 76 80 81 85 86 89 93 107 108 111 113 117 118 126 127 129 131 132 134 140 141 145 **S** QHR, Brentwood, TN
Primary Contact: R. D. Williams, Administrator and Chief Executive Officer
COO: Joe Thore, Chief Operating Officer
CFO: Joy McClure, Chief Financial Officer
CMO: Christopher Campbell, M.D., Chief of Staff
CIO: William Baldwin, Chief Information Officer
CHR: Sherry Cox, Chief Human Resources Officer
Web address: www.ashememorial.org
**Control:** Other not–for–profit (including NFP Corporation) **Service:** General Medical and Surgical

**Staffed Beds:** 85 **Admissions:** 1582 **Census:** 66 **Outpatient Visits:** 50293 **Births:** 94 **Total Expense ($000):** 29624 **Payroll Expense ($000):** 13777 **Personnel:** 302

---

**Hospital, Medicare Provider Number, Address, Telephone, Approval, Facility, and Physician Codes, Health Care System**

★ American Hospital Association (AHA) membership
☐ The Joint Commission accreditation       ◇ DNV Healthcare Inc. accreditation
○ American Osteopathic Association (AOA) accreditation
△ Commission on Accreditation of Rehabilitation Facilities (CARF) accreditation

NC

## KENANSVILLE—Duplin County

⊞ **VIDANT DUPLIN HOSPITAL (340120)**, 401 North Main Street,
Zip 28349–9989, Mailing Address: P.O. Box 278, Zip 28349–0278;
tel. 910/296–0941 **A**1 9 10 **F**3 11 13 15 18 19 29 30 34 35 39 40 45 56 57
59 68 70 75 76 77 79 81 91 93 97 98 101 102 103 107 108 110 111 114
118 128 129 130 134 145 146 **S** Vidant Health, Greenville, NC
Primary Contact: Jay Briley, Chief Executive Officer
CFO: Lucinda Crawford, Vice President Financial Services
CMO: Danny Pate, M.D., Chief Medical Staff
CIO: Lucinda Crawford, Vice President Financial Services
CHR: Pansy Chase, Director Human Resources
Web address: www.vidanthealth.com
**Control:** Other not–for–profit (including NFP Corporation) **Service:** General
Medical and Surgical

| | |
|---|---|
| **Staffed Beds:** 74 **Admissions:** 3320 **Census:** 43 **Outpatient Visits:** 50408 **Births:** 547 **Total Expense ($000):** 21061 **Payroll Expense ($000):** 14895 **Personnel:** 364 | |

## KINGS MOUNTAIN—Cleveland County

⊞ **KINGS MOUNTAIN HOSPITAL (340037)**, 706 West King Street,
Zip 28086–2708; tel. 980/487–5000, (Total facility includes 10 beds in nursing
home–type unit) **A**1 9 10 **F**3 4 15 17 29 30 40 45 46 49 67 70 79 81 82 85
89 93 98 107 111 113 118 127 129 132 145 147 **S** Carolinas HealthCare
System, Charlotte, NC
Primary Contact: Brian Gwyn, President
COO: Sheri Deshazo, Chief Operating Officer
CFO: Terry Edwards, Controller
CHR: Debra Kale, Director Human Resources
Web address: www.carolinas.org
**Control:** County–Government, nonfederal **Service:** General Medical and Surgical

| | |
|---|---|
| **Staffed Beds:** 72 **Admissions:** 2786 **Census:** 39 **Outpatient Visits:** 48236 **Births:** 0 **Total Expense ($000):** 33168 **Payroll Expense ($000):** 14320 **Personnel:** 273 | |

## KINSTON—Lenoir County

**CASWELL CENTER**, 2415 West Vernon Avenue, Zip 28504–3321;
tel. 252/208–4000, (Nonreporting)
Primary Contact: Leon Owens, Director
CFO: Jim Hall, Budget Officer
CMO: Tony Bright, M.D., Administrator Medical Services
CHR: Ken Lafone, Director Human Resources
Web address: www.caswellcenter.org
**Control:** State–Government, nonfederal **Service:** Institution for mental retardation

| | |
|---|---|
| **Staffed Beds:** 829 | |

☐ **LENOIR MEMORIAL HOSPITAL (340027)**, 100 Airport Road, Zip 28501–1634,
Mailing Address: P.O. Box 1678, Zip 28503–1678; tel. 252/522–7000, (Total
facility includes 26 beds in nursing home–type unit) **A**1 2 9 10 **F**3 8 11 13 18 20
28 29 30 31 34 35 38 40 43 45 47 48 49 50 53 56 57 59 60 61 64 65 68
70 74 75 76 77 78 79 80 81 82 85 86 87 89 90 93 102 107 108 111 113
114 117 118 119 120 122 127 128 129 131 133 134 142 144 145 147
Primary Contact: Gary E. Black, President and Chief Executive Officer
CFO: Sarah Mayo, Vice President Financial and Information Services
CMO: Wayne Jarman, M.D., President Medical Staff
CIO: Karl Vanderstouw, Director Management Information Systems
CHR: Jim Dobbins, Vice President Human Resources
CNO: Rosalind S. McDonald, MSN, Vice President Nursing Services
Web address: www.lenoirmemorial.org
**Control:** Other not–for–profit (including NFP Corporation) **Service:** General
Medical and Surgical

| | |
|---|---|
| **Staffed Beds:** 218 **Admissions:** 7829 **Census:** 118 **Outpatient Visits:** 82788 **Births:** 469 **Total Expense ($000):** 99925 **Payroll Expense ($000):** 44373 **Personnel:** 852 | |

## LAURINBURG—Scotland County

⊞ **SCOTLAND HEALTH CARE SYSTEM (340008)**, 500 Lauchwood Drive,
Zip 28352–5599; tel. 910/291–7000, (Total facility includes 50 beds in nursing
home–type unit) **A**1 2 9 10 **F**3 11 13 15 18 28 29 31 34 37 40 45 54 57 59
64 66 70 71 73 74 75 76 77 78 79 81 82 85 86 87 89 90 93 96 97 107
110 111 113 114 118 119 120 122 126 127 129 131 134 142 143 144 145
146 147 **P**8 **S** Carolinas HealthCare System, Charlotte, NC
Primary Contact: Gregory C. Wood, Chief Executive Officer
CFO: Matthew Pracht, Vice President Finance
CMO: Brian Parkes, M.D., Chief Medical Officer
CIO: Bryan Kincaid, Director Information Systems
CHR: Ann Locklear, Vice President, Human Resources
CNO: Lane Harrington, R.N., Vice President Patient Care Services
Web address: www.scotlandhealth.org
**Control:** Other not–for–profit (including NFP Corporation) **Service:** General
Medical and Surgical

| | |
|---|---|
| **Staffed Beds:** 152 **Admissions:** 6232 **Census:** 104 **Outpatient Visits:** 184063 **Births:** 683 **Total Expense ($000):** 102267 **Payroll Expense ($000):** 40198 **Personnel:** 954 | |

## LENOIR—Caldwell County

⊞ **CALDWELL MEMORIAL HOSPITAL (340041)**, 321 Mulberry Street S.W.,
Zip 28645–5720, Mailing Address: P.O. Box 1890, Zip 28645–1890;
tel. 828/757–5100 **A**1 2 9 10 **F**3 8 11 13 15 18 20 28 29 34 35 37 40 46 49
51 53 55 57 59 64 65 70 74 75 76 77 79 81 85 87 89 93 97 107 108 110
111 114 117 118 128 130 134 143 145 146 147 **P**6
Primary Contact: Laura J. Easton, R.N., President and Chief Executive Officer
CFO: Donald F. Gardner, Vice President Finance/Chief Financial Officer
CMO: Edward Pearce, M.D., Chief of Staff
CIO: Nathan White, Director Information Systems
CHR: Rebecca Smith, Vice President and Chief Operating Officer
CNO: Sharon M. Kimball, R.N., Vice President and Chief Nursing Officer
Web address: www.caldwell–mem.org
**Control:** Other not–for–profit (including NFP Corporation) **Service:** General
Medical and Surgical

| | |
|---|---|
| **Staffed Beds:** 74 **Admissions:** 3614 **Census:** 48 **Outpatient Visits:** 33311 **Births:** 511 **Total Expense ($000):** 87272 **Payroll Expense ($000):** 38186 **Personnel:** 765 | |

## LEXINGTON—Davidson County

**LEXINGTON MEMORIAL HOSPITAL** See Wake Forest Baptist Health–Lexington
Medical Center

⊞ **WAKE FOREST BAPTIST HEALTH–LEXINGTON MEDICAL CENTER
(340096)**, 250 Hospital Drive, Zip 27292–6728, Mailing Address: P.O. Box
1817, Zip 27293–1817; tel. 336/248–5161 **A**1 9 10 **F**3 11 12 13 15 17 18 28
29 30 32 34 35 40 45 47 49 50 51 57 59 64 68 70 74 75 76 77 79 80 81
82 85 86 87 89 90 93 107 110 111 118 123 128 129 130 131 134
143 145 146 147 **P**6 **S** Wake Forest Baptist Health, Winston–Salem, NC
Primary Contact: Steven C. Snelgrove, Chief Executive Officer
CFO: Danny Squires, Vice President and Chief Financial Officer
CMO: Gordon Kammire, M.D., Chief of Staff
CIO: Kevin Buchanan, Chief Information Officer
Web address: www.lexingtonmemorial.com
**Control:** Other not–for–profit (including NFP Corporation) **Service:** General
Medical and Surgical

| | |
|---|---|
| **Staffed Beds:** 69 **Admissions:** 3509 **Census:** 28 **Outpatient Visits:** 87447 **Births:** 676 **Total Expense ($000):** 56822 **Payroll Expense ($000):** 27291 **Personnel:** 702 | |

## LINCOLNTON—Lincoln County

⊞ **CAROLINAS MEDICAL CENTER–LINCOLN (340145)**, 433 McAlister Road,
Zip 28092; tel. 980/212–2000 **A**1 9 10 **F**3 8 11 13 15 18 26 27 28 29 30 31
34 35 40 44 45 50 51 54 57 59 64 68 70 73 74 75 76 77 78 79 81 82 85
87 91 93 94 96 107 108 110 111 113 114 117 118 128 129 130 131 134
145 147 **P**6 **S** Carolinas HealthCare System, Charlotte, NC
Primary Contact: Peter W. Acker, President
COO: Teresa C. Watson, Vice President Administration
CFO: Jarrett Morris, Vice President Finance
CIO: Jarrett Morris, Vice President Finance
CHR: Lesley Chambless, Vice President Human Resources
Web address: www.cmc–lincoln.org
**Control:** Hospital district or authority, Government, nonfederal **Service:** General
Medical and Surgical

| | |
|---|---|
| **Staffed Beds:** 90 **Admissions:** 3726 **Census:** 45 **Outpatient Visits:** 96612 **Births:** 379 **Total Expense ($000):** 69949 **Payroll Expense ($000):** 31503 **Personnel:** 592 | |

## LINVILLE—Avery County

⊞ **CHARLES A. CANNON MEMORIAL HOSPITAL (341323)**, 434 Hospital Drive,
Zip 28646, Mailing Address: P.O. Box 767, Zip 28646; tel. 828/737–7000 **A**1 9
10 18 **F**3 8 11 13 15 18 28 29 30 31 40 45 64 68 70 76 77 81 85 89 91 93
98 102 104 106 107 113 118 128 129 132 134 145 146 **P**8 **S** Appalachian
Regional Healthcare System, Boone, NC
Primary Contact: Carmen Lacey, MSN, R.N., President
CFO: Kevin B. May, System Director Finance
CMO: Thomas M. Haizlip, Jr., M.D., Chief of Staff
CIO: Mike Quinto, Chief Information Officer
CHR: Amy Crabbe, Vice President Human Resources
Web address: www.apprhs.org
**Control:** Other not–for–profit (including NFP Corporation) **Service:** General
Medical and Surgical

| | |
|---|---|
| **Staffed Beds:** 35 **Admissions:** 2160 **Census:** 26 **Outpatient Visits:** 27566 **Births:** 113 **Total Expense ($000):** 17326 **Payroll Expense ($000):** 8866 **Personnel:** 178 | |

**NC**

## LOUISBURG—Franklin County

✠ **FRANKLIN REGIONAL MEDICAL CENTER (340036)**, 100 Hospital Drive, Zip 27549–2256, Mailing Address: P.O. Box 609, Zip 27549–0609; tel. 919/497–8401 **A**1 9 10 **F**3 11 12 15 18 29 34 40 44 45 49 50 57 59 67 70 74 75 79 81 82 85 86 90 107 108 110 111 113 117 118 127 128 129 145 **S** Novant Health, Winston–Salem, NC
Primary Contact: Jody Morris, President and Chief Executive Officer
CIO: Kim Webster, Manager Information Systems
CHR: Joanna Holder, Director Human Resources
Web address: www.franklinregional.org
**Control:** Other not–for–profit (including NFP Corporation) **Service:** General Medical and Surgical

**Staffed Beds:** 70 **Admissions:** 1198 **Census:** 12 **Outpatient Visits:** 36214
**Births:** 0 **Total Expense ($000):** 28374 **Payroll Expense ($000):** 10876
**Personnel:** 183

## LUMBERTON—Robeson County

✠ **SOUTHEASTERN REGIONAL MEDICAL CENTER (340050)**, 300 West 27th Street, Zip 28358–3017, Mailing Address: P.O. Box 1408, Zip 28359–1408; tel. 910/671–5000, (Total facility includes 115 beds in nursing home–type unit) **A**1 2 9 10 **F**3 5 7 9 12 13 17 18 20 22 24 28 29 30 31 34 35 40 45 48 49 50 53 54 57 59 60 61 62 63 64 67 68 70 71 72 73 76 77 78 79 80 81 82 83 85 87 89 92 93 98 102 103 107 108 111 113 114 117 118 119 120 126 127 128 129 130 131 143 145 147
Primary Contact: Joann Anderson, President and Chief Executive Officer
CFO: C. Thomas Johnson, III, Vice President Organizational Development and Chief Financial Officer
CMO: Jim Parker, M.D., President Medical Staff
CIO: Eric Harper, Chief Information Officer
CHR: Joseph W. Glezen, Director Human Resources
Web address: www.srmc.org
**Control:** Other not–for–profit (including NFP Corporation) **Service:** General Medical and Surgical

**Staffed Beds:** 373 **Admissions:** 14416 **Census:** 297 **Outpatient Visits:** 426413 **Births:** 1480 **Total Expense ($000):** 169250 **Payroll Expense ($000):** 87831 **Personnel:** 2085

## MARION—Mcdowell County

✠ **MCDOWELL HOSPITAL (340087)**, 430 Rankin Drive, Zip 28752–6568, Mailing Address: P.O. Box 730, Zip 28752–0730; tel. 828/659–5000 **A**1 9 10 **F**3 11 13 15 28 29 30 31 34 35 39 40 45 48 50 54 57 59 64 65 68 70 75 76 77 78 79 81 82 85 87 90 93 107 108 110 113 118 126 129 130 131 132 145 **P**6 **S** Mission Health System, Asheville, NC
Primary Contact: Lynn Ingram Boggs, President and Chief Executive Officer
COO: Jason Clapsaddle, Vice President Operations
CFO: Clint Stewart, Vice President Finance/Business Operations
CMO: Robert Morrow, M.D., Chief of Staff
CIO: Andrew Cooper, Manager, Information Services
CHR: Teresa McCarthy, Interim Director Human Resources
CNO: Kathy Hefner, Vice President Clinical Operations
Web address: www.mcdhospital.org
**Control:** Other not–for–profit (including NFP Corporation) **Service:** General Medical and Surgical

**Staffed Beds:** 49 **Admissions:** 1831 **Census:** 18 **Outpatient Visits:** 113458
**Births:** 112 **Total Expense ($000):** 36607 **Payroll Expense ($000):** 18747
**Personnel:** 387

## MATTHEWS—Mecklenburg County

✠ **PRESBYTERIAN HOSPITAL MATTHEWS (340171)**, 1500 Matthews Township Parkway, Zip 28105–4656, Mailing Address: P.O. Box 3310, Zip 28106–3310; tel. 704/384–6500 **A**1 9 10 **F**3 11 12 13 15 18 20 22 26 29 30 31 34 35 36 40 45 49 56 57 59 64 68 70 73 75 76 77 78 79 81 82 84 85 86 87 92 93 107 108 110 111 113 115 116 118 125 128 129 131 143 144 145 146 147 **S** Novant Health, Winston–Salem, NC
Primary Contact: Roland R. Bibeau, President
COO: Amy Vance, Executive Vice President and Chief Operating Officer
CFO: Greg Klein, Senior Director Finance
CMO: Thomas Zweng, M.D., Senior Vice President Medical Affairs
CIO: David B. Garrett, Chief Information Officer
CHR: Susan Kennedy, Manager Human Resources
Web address: www.presbyterian.org
**Control:** Other not–for–profit (including NFP Corporation) **Service:** General Medical and Surgical

**Staffed Beds:** 117 **Admissions:** 7957 **Census:** 87 **Outpatient Visits:** 201328
**Births:** 1346 **Total Expense ($000):** 115974 **Payroll Expense ($000):** 40942 **Personnel:** 744

## MOCKSVILLE—Davie County

✠ **WAKE FOREST BAPTIST HEALTH–DAVIE HOSPITAL (341313)**, 223 Hospital Street, Zip 27028–2038, Mailing Address: P.O. Box 1209, Zip 27028–1209; tel. 336/751–8100 **A**1 9 10 18 **F**3 15 30 34 35 40 59 64 79 81 85 107 113 118 129 132 **S** Wake Forest Baptist Health, Winston–Salem, NC
Primary Contact: Kevin Walsh, Administrator
CFO: Terry R. Bowman, Chief Financial Officer
CMO: Mark Keller, M.D., President Medical Staff
CHR: Linda Pate, Director Human Resources
Web address: www.daviehospital.org
**Control:** Other not–for–profit (including NFP Corporation) **Service:** General Medical and Surgical

**Staffed Beds:** 25 **Admissions:** 285 **Census:** 6 **Outpatient Visits:** 15596
**Births:** 0 **Total Expense ($000):** 10504 **Payroll Expense ($000):** 3977
**Personnel:** 146

## MONROE—Union County

✠ **CAROLINAS MEDICAL CENTER–UNION (340130)**, 600 Hospital Drive, Zip 28112–6000, Mailing Address: P.O. Box 5003, Zip 28111–5003; tel. 704/283–3100, (Total facility includes 70 beds in nursing home–type unit) **A**1 2 9 10 **F**3 4 5 8 11 13 18 20 26 28 29 30 31 34 35 39 40 42 45 49 56 57 59 62 64 66 67 70 73 74 75 76 77 78 79 81 82 85 86 87 89 93 107 108 111 113 114 117 118 119 120 122 127 128 129 131 134 143 145 146 147 **S** Carolinas HealthCare System, Charlotte, NC
Primary Contact: Michael Lutes, President
CFO: John G. Moore, Vice President and Chief Financial Officer
CMO: Dan Hagler, M.D., Vice President and Chief Medical Officer
CIO: Lisa Sykes, Director Information Services
CHR: Rhonda McFarland, Director Human Resources
Web address: www.cmc–union.org
**Control:** Hospital district or authority, Government, nonfederal **Service:** General Medical and Surgical

**Staffed Beds:** 239 **Admissions:** 9405 **Census:** 163 **Outpatient Visits:** 179433 **Births:** 1236 **Total Expense ($000):** 149920 **Payroll Expense ($000):** 60751 **Personnel:** 1176

## MOORESVILLE—Iredell County

☐ **LAKE NORMAN REGIONAL MEDICAL CENTER (340129)**, 171 Fairview Road, Zip 28117–9500, Mailing Address: P.O. Box 3250, Zip 28117–3250; tel. 704/660–4000, (Nonreporting) **A**1 2 9 10 19 **S** Health Management Associates, Naples, FL
Primary Contact: Greg Lowe, Chief Executive Officer
CFO: James Stoner, Chief Financial Officer
CHR: Christine McKenzie, Director Human Resources
Web address: www.lnrmc.com
**Control:** Corporation, Investor–owned, for–profit **Service:** General Medical and Surgical

**Staffed Beds:** 103

## MOREHEAD CITY—Carteret County

✠ **CARTERET GENERAL HOSPITAL (340142)**, 3500 Arendell Street, Zip 28557–1619, Mailing Address: P.O. Box 1619, Zip 28557–1619; tel. 252/808–6000, (Total facility includes 104 beds in nursing home–type unit) **A**1 9 10 **F**3 7 11 12 13 15 18 28 29 30 31 34 35 40 45 46 54 57 59 62 63 64 65 68 70 75 76 77 78 79 81 82 84 85 86 87 89 91 92 93 97 107 108 110 111 113 114 117 118 119 120 122 127 128 129 131 134 142 143 144 145 147
Primary Contact: Richard A. Brvenik, FACHE, President
CFO: Joanie King, Chief Financial Officer
CMO: Leon M. Morrison, M.D., Vice President Medical Staff Services
CIO: Kyle Marek, Manager Information Services
CHR: Elizabeth Beswick, Vice President Human Resources and Public Relations
Web address: www.ccgh.org
**Control:** County–Government, nonfederal **Service:** General Medical and Surgical

**Staffed Beds:** 208 **Admissions:** 6480 **Census:** 120 **Outpatient Visits:** 164784 **Births:** 826 **Total Expense ($000):** 96051 **Payroll Expense ($000):** 46999 **Personnel:** 898

## MORGANTON—Burke County

☐ **BROUGHTON HOSPITAL (344025)**, 1000 South Sterling Street, Zip 28655–3999; tel. 828/433–2111, (Nonreporting) **A**1 5 9 10
Primary Contact: Thomas J. Mahle, Chief Executive Officer
CFO: Jonathan Berry, Chief Support Services and Chief Financial Officer
CMO: George Krebs, M.D., Chief Medical Officer
CIO: Phil Shirley, Director Information Resource Management
CHR: Mary Ragsdale, Director Human Resources
Web address: www.broughtonhospital.org
**Control:** State–Government, nonfederal **Service:** Psychiatric

**Staffed Beds:** 370

---

**Hospital, Medicare Provider Number, Address, Telephone, Approval, Facility, and Physician Codes, Health Care System**

★ American Hospital Association (AHA) membership
☐ The Joint Commission accreditation        ◇ DNV Healthcare Inc. accreditation

○ American Osteopathic Association (AOA) accreditation
△ Commission on Accreditation of Rehabilitation Facilities (CARF) accreditation

**NC**

⊞ **GRACE HOSPITAL (340075)**, 2201 South Sterling Street, Zip 28655–4058; tel. 828/580–5000, (Nonreporting) **A**1 2 9 10 **S** Carolinas HealthCare System, Charlotte, NC
Primary Contact: Kenneth W. Wood, President and Chief Executive Officer
COO: Kathy C. Bailey, Ph.D., Sr. Vice President, Chief Operating Officer
CFO: Robert Fritts, Chief Financial Officer
CMO: Joe Mazzola, D.O., Sr. Vice President Medical Affairs/Chief Quality Officer
CHR: David Shirlen, Vice President Human Resources
CNO: Susan Brown, R.N., Sr. Vice President, Chief Nursing Officer
Web address: www.gracehcs.org
**Control:** Other not–for–profit (including NFP Corporation) **Service:** General Medical and Surgical

| Staffed Beds: 117 |
|---|

### MOUNT AIRY—Surry County

⊞ **NORTHERN HOSPITAL OF SURRY COUNTY (340003)**, 830 Rockford Street, Zip 27030–5365, Mailing Address: P.O. Box 1101, Zip 27030–1101; tel. 336/719–7000, (Total facility includes 33 beds in nursing home–type unit) **A**1 9 10 **F**3 11 13 15 18 20 29 30 31 34 35 39 40 45 50 51 56 57 59 64 65 70 74 75 76 77 79 80 81 82 85 86 87 93 102 107 108 110 111 113 114 116 117 118 127 128 129 130 131 132 144 145 146 147 **P**6 **S** QHR, Brentwood, TN
Primary Contact: William B. James, Chief Executive Officer
CFO: Robert G. Hetrick, Chief Financial Officer
CMO: Scott Corbin, M.D., Chief of Staff
CIO: Robert Hall, Chief Information Officer
CHR: Jeannie Moore, Director Human Resources
CNO: Robin Hodgin, R.N., Chief Administrator of Patient Care Services
Web address: www.northernhospital.com
**Control:** Hospital district or authority, Government, nonfederal **Service:** General Medical and Surgical

| Staffed Beds: 108 Admissions: 4944 Census: 82 Outpatient Visits: 173159 Births: 454 Total Expense ($000): 75756 Payroll Expense ($000): 31282 Personnel: 639 |
|---|

### MURPHY—Cherokee County

⊞ **MURPHY MEDICAL CENTER (340160)**, 3990 U.S. Highway 64 East Alt, Zip 28906–7917; tel. 828/837–8161, (Nonreporting) **A**1 9 10 **S** Carolinas HealthCare System, Charlotte, NC
Primary Contact: Michael Stevenson, Administrator
COO: Toni Lovingood, Chief Operating Officer
CFO: Steve Gilgen, Chief Financial Officer
CMO: Jeffrey H. Martin, M.D., Chief of Staff
CIO: Connie Stalcup, Manager Information Systems
CHR: Russ Paine, Human Resources Officer
CNO: Teresa Bowleg, R.N., Chief Nursing Officer
Web address: www.murphymedical.org
**Control:** Other not–for–profit (including NFP Corporation) **Service:** General Medical and Surgical

| Staffed Beds: 191 |
|---|

### NAGS HEAD—Dare County

⊞ **THE OUTER BANKS HOSPITAL (341324)**, 4800 South Croatan Highway, Zip 27959–9704; tel. 252/449–4511, (Nonreporting) **A**1 9 10 18 **S** Vidant Health, Greenville, NC
Primary Contact: Ronald A. Sloan, FACHE, President
CFO: Todd Warlitner, Vice President Business Operations
CMO: Roger Lever, M.D., President Medical Staff
CHR: Mary Kelley, Director Human Resources
CNO: Judy Bruno, R.N., Vice President, Clinical Operations
Web address: www.theouterbankshospital.com
**Control:** Other not–for–profit (including NFP Corporation) **Service:** General Medical and Surgical

| Staffed Beds: 61 |
|---|

### NEW BERN—Craven County

⊞ △ **CAROLINAEAST MEDICAL CENTER (340131)**, 2000 Neuse Boulevard, Zip 28560–3499, Mailing Address: P.O. Box 12157, Zip 28561–2157; tel. 252/633–8111 **A**1 2 7 9 10 **F**3 7 11 13 15 17 18 20 22 24 26 28 29 30 31 34 35 40 45 47 48 49 54 57 59 60 61 62 64 67 68 70 74 75 76 77 78 79 81 85 87 89 90 92 93 94 96 98 100 101 102 103 104 105 107 108 110 111 113 114 115 116 117 118 119 120 122 125 128 129 131 134 142 145 146 147 **P**6
Primary Contact: G. Raymond Leggett, Chief Executive Officer
COO: Rosanne Leahy, Vice President Nursing Services
CMO: Ronald B. May, M.D., Vice President Medical Affairs
CIO: Tim Ludwig, Vice President Ancillary Services
CHR: Bruce A. Martin, Vice President Human Resources
Web address: www.carolinaeasthealth.com
**Control:** Hospital district or authority, Government, nonfederal **Service:** General Medical and Surgical

| Staffed Beds: 350 Admissions: 14509 Census: 179 Outpatient Visits: 168984 Births: 1363 Total Expense ($000): 219605 Payroll Expense ($000): 87851 Personnel: 1512 |
|---|

### NORTH WILKESBORO—Wilkes County

⊞ **WILKES REGIONAL MEDICAL CENTER (340064)**, 1370 West D Street, Zip 28659–3506, Mailing Address: P.O. Box 609, Zip 28659–0609; tel. 336/651–8100, (Nonreporting) **A**1 9 10 **S** Carolinas HealthCare System, Charlotte, NC
Primary Contact: J. Gene Faile, Chief Executive Officer
CFO: Marlin Markham, Chief Financial Officer
CMO: Ashton Molai, M.D., Chief Medical Officer
CIO: Carl Espenship, Director Facility Services
CHR: Vanya Baker, Director
Web address: www.wilkesregional.org
**Control:** Hospital district or authority, Government, nonfederal **Service:** General Medical and Surgical

| Staffed Beds: 98 |
|---|

### OXFORD—Granville County

⊞ **GRANVILLE HEALTH SYSTEM (340127)**, 1010 College Street, Zip 27565–2507, Mailing Address: P.O. Box 947, Zip 27565–0947; tel. 919/690–3000, (Total facility includes 80 beds in nursing home–type unit) **A**1 9 10 **F**2 3 7 11 13 15 18 19 29 30 31 34 35 38 39 40 45 50 54 55 56 57 59 64 66 70 75 76 77 78 79 81 82 85 86 93 99 100 101 103 104 107 108 110 111 117 118 123 126 127 128 129 131 132 142 143 145 146 147 **P**3 6 8
Primary Contact: L. Lee Isley, Chief Executive Officer
COO: Cristina Rigsbee, Chief Operating Officer
CFO: Jeffrey Armstrong, CPA, Chief Financial Officer
CMO: James Williams, M.D., Chief Medical Staff
CIO: Geoff Tanthorey, Director Information Systems
CHR: Scott C. Thomas, Administrative Director Human Resources/Communication
CNO: Maria Calloway, R.N., Chief Nursing Officer
Web address: www.granvillemedical.com
**Control:** County–Government, nonfederal **Service:** General Medical and Surgical

| Staffed Beds: 142 Admissions: 2838 Census: 95 Outpatient Visits: 59814 Births: 361 Total Expense ($000): 54600 Payroll Expense ($000): 26343 Personnel: 521 |
|---|

### PINEHURST—Moore County

⊞ △ **FIRSTHEALTH MOORE REGIONAL HOSPITAL (340115)**, 155 Memorial Drive, Zip 28374–8710, Mailing Address: P.O. Box 3000, Zip 28374–3000; tel. 910/715–1000 **A**1 2 7 9 10 19 **F**3 4 5 11 12 13 15 17 18 20 22 24 26 28 29 30 31 34 35 40 44 45 46 48 49 50 51 53 54 56 57 58 59 60 64 65 68 70 72 74 75 76 77 78 79 81 82 86 87 89 90 93 96 98 99 100 101 102 103 104 105 107 108 111 113 114 117 118 119 120 125 128 129 131 133 134 142 143 145 146 147 **S** FirstHealth of the Carolinas, Pinehurst, NC
Primary Contact: David J. Kilarski, Chief Executive Officer
CFO: Lynn S. DeJaco, Chief Financial Officer
CMO: John F. Krahnert, M.D., Chief Medical Officer
CIO: David B. Dillehunt, Chief Information Officer
CHR: Dan Biediger, Vice President Human Resources
Web address: www.firsthealth.org
**Control:** Other not–for–profit (including NFP Corporation) **Service:** General Medical and Surgical

| Staffed Beds: 379 Admissions: 20652 Census: 270 Outpatient Visits: 184331 Births: 1589 Total Expense ($000): 327608 Payroll Expense ($000): 125736 Personnel: 2793 |
|---|

### PLYMOUTH—Washington County

⊞ **WASHINGTON COUNTY HOSPITAL (341314)**, 958 U.S. Highway 64 East, Zip 27962–9591; tel. 252/793–4135, (Nonreporting) **A**1 9 10 18 **S** HMC/CAH Consolidated, Inc., Kansas City, MO
Primary Contact: Harley Smith, President
CFO: Al Arrowood, Chief Financial Officer
CMO: Robert Venable, M.D., Chief Medical Staff
CIO: Christina Craft, Director Information Systems
CHR: Harley Smith, Director Human Resources
CNO: Kimberly Manning, Chief Nursing Officer
Web address: www.wchonline.com
**Control:** County–Government, nonfederal **Service:** General Medical and Surgical

| Staffed Beds: 25 |
|---|

### RALEIGH—Wake County

**CENTRAL PRISON HOSPITAL**, 1300 Western Boulevard, Zip 27606–2148; tel. 919/733–0800, (Nonreporting)
Primary Contact: Thomas J. Hawkins, Administrator
CFO: Annette Goforth, Manager Administrative Services
CMO: Olushola Metiko, M.D., Medical Director
Web address: www.doc.state.nc.us/dop/prisons/central.htm
**Control:** State–Government, nonfederal **Service:** Hospital unit of an institution (prison hospital, college infirmary, etc.)

| Staffed Beds: 230 |
|---|

**NC**

*Many Facility Codes have changed. Please refer to the AHA Guide Code Chart.*
© 2012 AHA Guide

**DOROTHEA DIX HOSPITAL**, 3601 Mail Service Center, Zip 27699–3601; tel. 919/733–5540, (Nonreporting) **A**9
Primary Contact: James Osberg, III, Ph.D., Director
CFO: Jean Yardley, Budget Officer
CMO: Scott Mann, M.D., Medical Director
CHR: Mosella Jamerson, Director Human Resources
**Control:** State–Government, nonfederal **Service:** Psychiatric

**Staffed Beds: 443**

✠ **DUKE RALEIGH HOSPITAL (340073)**, 3400 Wake Forest Road, Zip 27609–7373, Mailing Address: P.O. Box 28280, Zip 27611–8280; tel. 919/954–3000 **A**1 2 9 10 **F**3 11 12 15 18 20 22 26 28 29 30 31 34 35 36 39 40 44 45 46 47 49 50 51 53 55 57 58 59 60 64 68 70 74 75 77 78 79 80 81 82 84 85 87 92 93 96 100 101 102 107 108 110 111 114 116 117 118 119 120 122 125 128 129 130 131 134 145 147 **P**6 **S** Duke University Health System, Durham, NC
Primary Contact: Douglas B. Vinsel, FACHE, Chief Executive Officer
COO: Richard Gannotta, Chief Operating Officer
CMO: Ted Kunstling, M.D., Chief Medical Officer
CIO: Janis Curtis, Interim Director Information Technology
CHR: Don Barnes, Chief Human Resources Officer
Web address: www.dukehealthraleigh.org
**Control:** Other not–for–profit (including NFP Corporation) **Service:** General Medical and Surgical

**Staffed Beds: 148 Admissions: 7385 Census: 86 Outpatient Visits: 134893 Births: 1 Total Expense ($000): 225554 Payroll Expense ($000): 73040 Personnel: 1270**

☐ **HOLLY HILL HOSPITAL (344014)**, 3019 Falstaff Road, Zip 27610–1812; tel. 919/250–7000, (Nonreporting) **A**1 9 10 **S** Universal Health Services, Inc., King of Prussia, PA
Primary Contact: Robert L. Turner, Ph.D., Chief Executive Officer
CFO: Ron Howard, Chief Financial Officer
CMO: Thomas Cornwall, M.D., Medical Director
CHR: Maria Teresa Sulit, Director Human Resources
Web address: www.hollyhillhospital.com
**Control:** Corporation, Investor–owned, for–profit **Service:** Psychiatric

**Staffed Beds: 152**

**LARRY B. ZIEVERINK, SR. ALCOHOLISM TREATMENT CENTER**, 3000 Falstaff Road, Zip 27610–1897; tel. 919/250–1500 **F**3 4 29 34 35 36 38 44 50 57 59 61 75 77 86 100 101 129 131 134 **P**6
Primary Contact: Martin D. Woodward, Director Acute Care Services
COO: Martin D. Woodward, Director Acute Care Services
CFO: Paul Gross, Human Services and Finance Officer
CMO: Enrique Lopez, M.D., Medical Director
CIO: Wil A. Glenn, Director Communications
Web address: www.wakegov.com/county/family/atc
**Control:** County–Government, nonfederal **Service:** Alcoholism and other chemical dependency

**Staffed Beds: 16 Admissions: 687 Census: 17 Outpatient Visits: 0 Births: 0 Total Expense ($000): 2858 Payroll Expense ($000): 2038 Personnel: 16**

✠ △ **REX HEALTHCARE (340114)**, 4420 Lake Boone Trail, Zip 27607–6599; tel. 919/784–3100, (Total facility includes 227 beds in nursing home–type unit) **A**1 2 7 9 10 **F**3 7 8 11 12 13 14 15 17 18 20 22 24 26 28 29 30 31 32 34 35 36 40 44 45 46 47 48 49 50 53 54 56 57 58 59 60 62 64 65 66 68 70 73 74 75 76 77 78 79 81 82 84 85 86 87 89 92 93 96 97 100 102 107 108 110 111 113 114 115 116 117 118 119 120 122 125 127 128 129 130 131 134 141 142 143 144 145 146 147 **P**6
Primary Contact: David W. Strong, President
COO: Steve W. Burriss, Chief Operating Officer
CFO: Bernadette Spong, Chief Financial Officer
CMO: Linda H. Butler, M.D., Chief Medical Officer
CHR: Sylvia D. Hackett, Vice President Human Resources
CNO: Mary Lou Powell, MSN, Chief Nursing Officer
Web address: www.rexhealth.com
**Control:** Other not–for–profit (including NFP Corporation) **Service:** General Medical and Surgical

**Staffed Beds: 660 Admissions: 28405 Census: 490 Outpatient Visits: 609923 Births: 5849 Total Expense ($000): 582472 Payroll Expense ($000): 254769 Personnel: 4120**

✠ △ **WAKEMED RALEIGH CAMPUS (340069)**, 3000 New Bern Avenue, Zip 27610–1295; tel. 919/350–8000, (Total facility includes 19 beds in nursing home–type unit) **A**1 3 5 7 9 10 **F**3 7 8 9 11 12 13 15 17 18 20 22 24 26 28 29 30 31 32 34 35 37 38 40 41 42 43 44 45 48 49 50 53 54 56 57 58 59 60 61 62 63 64 65 66 68 70 71 72 73 74 75 76 77 78 79 81 82 85 86 87 88 89 90 92 93 96 97 107 108 110 111 113 114 117 118 125 127 129 130 131 133 134 142 143 145 146 147 **P**6 **S** WakeMed Health & Hospitals, Raleigh, NC
Primary Contact: William K. Atkinson, II, Ph.D., President and Chief Executive Officer
COO: Thomas Gettinger, Executive Vice President and Chief Operating Officer
CFO: Michael D. DeVaughn, Senior Vice President Finance and Chief Financial Officer
CMO: West Lawson, M.D., Chief Medical Officer
CIO: Denton Arledge, Vice President and Chief Information Officer
CHR: Jeanene R. Martin, M.P.H., Senior Vice President Human Resources
Web address: www.wakemed.org
**Control:** Other not–for–profit (including NFP Corporation) **Service:** General Medical and Surgical

**Staffed Beds: 647 Admissions: 36357 Census: 554 Outpatient Visits: 929001 Births: 4782 Total Expense ($000): 768729 Payroll Expense ($000): 384115 Personnel: 5935**

**REIDSVILLE—Rockingham County**

**ANNIE PENN HOSPITAL** See Cone Health, Greensboro

**ROANOKE RAPIDS—Halifax County**

✠ **HALIFAX REGIONAL MEDICAL CENTER (340151)**, 250 Smith Church Road, Zip 27870, Mailing Address: P.O. Box 1089, Zip 27870; tel. 252/535–8011 **A**1 9 10 **F**3 11 13 15 18 20 23 29 31 34 35 38 39 40 45 48 49 50 54 57 58 59 60 61 64 65 66 68 69 70 75 76 77 78 79 81 84 85 86 91 93 94 97 98 101 102 103 104 106 107 108 109 110 111 113 118 123 126 128 129 131 134 145 147 **P**6
Primary Contact: William Mahone, V, President and Chief Executive Officer
CFO: Sherry Jensen, Chief Financial Officer
CIO: Robert Gordon, Manager Information Systems
CHR: James B. Wood, Chief Human Resources Officer
CNO: Karen Daniels, MSN, Chief Nursing Officer
Web address: www.halifaxmedicalcenter.org
**Control:** Other not–for–profit (including NFP Corporation) **Service:** General Medical and Surgical

**Staffed Beds: 142 Admissions: 6853 Census: 93 Outpatient Visits: 82086 Births: 624 Total Expense ($000): 80528 Payroll Expense ($000): 34447 Personnel: 815**

**ROCKINGHAM—Richmond County**

★ **FIRSTHEALTH RICHMOND MEMORIAL HOSPITAL (340035)**, 925 Long Drive, Zip 28379–4815; tel. 910/417–3000 **A**9 10 **F**3 13 15 18 20 28 29 30 34 35 40 45 46 47 48 49 50 53 57 59 64 70 75 76 77 81 82 85 87 89 92 93 96 107 108 110 111 113 118 119 128 130 131 133 134 144 145 146 147 **S** FirstHealth of the Carolinas, Pinehurst, NC
Primary Contact: John J. Jackson, President
COO: Allison Duckworth, Chief Operating Officer and Chief Nursing Officer
CFO: John D. Price, Chief Financial Officer
CMO: George Bussey, M.D., Chief Medical Officer
Web address: www.firsthealth.org
**Control:** Other not–for–profit (including NFP Corporation) **Service:** General Medical and Surgical

**Staffed Beds: 91 Admissions: 2929 Census: 25 Outpatient Visits: 59819 Births: 397 Total Expense ($000): 36609 Payroll Expense ($000): 18090 Personnel: 324**

**ROCKY MOUNT—Nash County**

✠ **LIFECARE HOSPITALS OF NORTH CAROLINA (342013)**, 1051 Noell Lane, Zip 27804–1761; tel. 252/451–2300 **A**1 10 **F**1 3 18 29 74 75 77 79 82 85 147 **S** LifeCare Management Services, Plano, TX
Primary Contact: Kevin S. Cooper, R.N., Administrator
COO: Robyn Perkerson, Chief Clinical Officer
CMO: Daniel Crocker, M.D., Chief Medical Officer
CHR: Vicky Goode, Director Human Resources
CNO: Brandee Chappell, Director of Nursing
Web address: www.lifecare–hospitals.com
**Control:** Corporation, Investor–owned, for–profit **Service:** Long–Term Acute Care hospital

**Staffed Beds: 40 Admissions: 470 Census: 38 Outpatient Visits: 0 Births: 0 Total Expense ($000): 17864 Payroll Expense ($000): 7811 Personnel: 146**

---

**Hospital, Medicare Provider Number, Address, Telephone, Approval, Facility, and Physician Codes, Health Care System**

★ American Hospital Association (AHA) membership
☐ The Joint Commission accreditation
◇ DNV Healthcare Inc. accreditation
○ American Osteopathic Association (AOA) accreditation
△ Commission on Accreditation of Rehabilitation Facilities (CARF) accreditation

NC

☐ **NASH HEALTH CARE SYSTEMS (340147)**, 2460 Curtis Ellis Drive, Zip 27804–2297; tel. 252/443–8000 **A**1 2 9 10 F3 4 5 11 12 13 15 18 20 22 28 29 30 31 34 35 38 40 45 47 48 49 50 53 57 59 60 63 64 70 73 74 75 76 77 78 79 80 81 82 84 85 86 87 89 90 93 94 96 98 100 101 102 103 104 107 108 110 111 113 116 117 118 120 122 125 128 129 130 131 134 145 146 147 **P**6
Primary Contact: Larry H. Chewning, III, President and Chief Executive Officer
COO: Brad Weisner, Executive Vice President and Chief Operating Officer
CFO: Al Hooks, Senior Vice President and Chief Financial Officer
CMO: David Gorby, M.D., Interim Senior Vice President & Chief Medical Officer/VP Patient Safety & Quality
CIO: David Hinkle, Senior Vice President and Chief Information Officer
CHR: Cam Blalock, Senior Vice President Corporate Services
CNO: Leslie Hall, R.N., Senior Vice President–Chief Nursing Officer
Web address: www.nhcs.org
**Control:** Hospital district or authority, Government, nonfederal **Service:** General Medical and Surgical

**Staffed Beds:** 290 **Admissions:** 12479 **Census:** 173 **Outpatient Visits:** 176545 **Births:** 1223 **Total Expense ($000):** 203091 **Payroll Expense ($000):** 89813 **Personnel:** 1640

### ROXBORO—Person County

⊞ **PERSON MEMORIAL HOSPITAL (340159)**, 615 Ridge Road, Zip 27573–4630; tel. 336/599–2121, (Total facility includes 60 beds in nursing home–type unit) **A**1 9 10 F3 11 15 28 29 31 34 40 45 57 59 64 70 75 77 78 79 81 82 85 87 93 96 103 104 107 108 111 113 117 118 127 128 129 131 145 **S** Duke LifePoint Healthcare, Brentwood, TN
Primary Contact: Chad Brown, M.P.H., Chief Executive Officer
CFO: Neal Bolton, Chief Financial Officer
CMO: Kenneth Flowe, M.D., Chief Medical Officer
CIO: Cameron Bellamy, CIS Manager
CHR: Mary Drumwright, Director Human Resources
CNO: Jan Ramey, MSN, Chief Nursing Officer
Web address: www.personhospital.com
**Control:** Other not–for–profit (including NFP Corporation) **Service:** General Medical and Surgical

**Staffed Beds:** 110 **Admissions:** 2019 **Census:** 79 **Outpatient Visits:** 45697 **Births:** 0

### RUTHERFORDTON—Rutherford County

⊞ **RUTHERFORD REGIONAL MEDICAL CENTER (340013)**, 288 South Ridgecrest Avenue, Zip 28139–3097; tel. 828/286–5000 **A**1 2 9 10 19 F3 11 13 15 18 20 28 29 30 31 34 35 40 45 48 49 50 53 57 59 62 64 70 74 75 76 77 78 79 81 82 85 86 87 89 93 97 98 100 101 102 104 106 107 108 110 111 113 114 115 116 117 118 123 129 130 131 134 145 146 147 **S** QHR, Brentwood, TN
Primary Contact: Cindy D. Buck, Interim Chief Executive Officer
CFO: Cindy D. Buck, Chief Financial Officer
CMO: Dean Backstrom, M.D., Vice President Medical Affairs
CIO: Tommy Finley, Chief Information Officer
CHR: Jim H. Rowell, Vice President Human Resources
Web address: www.rutherfordhosp.org
**Control:** Other not–for–profit (including NFP Corporation) **Service:** General Medical and Surgical

**Staffed Beds:** 116 **Admissions:** 5508 **Census:** 54 **Outpatient Visits:** 173585 **Births:** 547 **Total Expense ($000):** 83180 **Payroll Expense ($000):** 39392 **Personnel:** 773

### SALISBURY—Rowan County

⊞ **ROWAN REGIONAL MEDICAL CENTER (340015)**, 612 Mocksville Avenue, Zip 28144–2799; tel. 704/210–5000 **A**1 9 10 F3 6 8 11 13 15 17 18 20 22 26 28 29 30 31 32 34 35 40 44 45 46 48 49 50 51 56 57 59 60 61 63 64 68 70 71 73 74 75 76 77 78 79 81 84 85 86 87 90 91 92 93 94 96 98 100 102 107 108 110 111 113 115 116 117 118 119 120 122 129 130 131 134 145 146 147 **P**2 **S** Novant Health, Winston–Salem, NC
Primary Contact: Dari Caldwell, President
COO: Sean M. Sanz, Chief Operating Officer
CMO: David N. Smith, M.D., Vice President Medical Affairs
CHR: Jerry Clevenger, Vice President Human Resources
Web address: www.rowan.org
**Control:** Other not–for–profit (including NFP Corporation) **Service:** General Medical and Surgical

**Staffed Beds:** 196 **Admissions:** 9137 **Census:** 113 **Outpatient Visits:** 307568 **Births:** 758 **Total Expense ($000):** 152776 **Payroll Expense ($000):** 57878 **Personnel:** 1064

⊞ △ **VETERANS AFFAIRS MEDICAL CENTER**, 1601 Brenner Avenue, Zip 28144–2559; tel. 704/638–9000, (Nonreporting) **A**1 3 5 7 **S** Department of Veterans Affairs, Washington, DC
Primary Contact: Anthony L. Dawson, FACHE, Interim Director
COO: Anthony L. Dawson, FACHE, Associate Director
CFO: Steve Patil, Chief Financial Officer
CIO: Deborah Gunn, Chief Information Officer
CHR: Sandra Fischer, Director Human Resources
Web address: www.salisbury.va.gov
**Control:** Veterans Affairs, Government, federal **Service:** Psychiatric

**Staffed Beds:** 171

### SANFORD—Lee County

⊞ **CENTRAL CAROLINA HOSPITAL (340020)**, 1135 Carthage Street, Zip 27330–4111; tel. 919/774–2100, (Nonreporting) **A**1 9 10 **S** TENET Healthcare Corporation, Dallas, TX
Primary Contact: Doug Doris, Chief Executive Officer
COO: David Clay, Chief Operating Officer
CFO: Lyra Howalt, Chief Financial Officer
CMO: David Katzin, M.D., Chief Medical Officer
CIO: Jimmy Whitaker, Director Information Systems
CHR: Joseph F. Eastman, Director Human Resources
CNO: Ursula Lawrence, MSN, Chief Nursing Officer
Web address: www.centralcarolinahosp.com
**Control:** Corporation, Investor–owned, for–profit **Service:** General Medical and Surgical

**Staffed Beds:** 116

### SCOTLAND NECK—Halifax County

★ **OUR COMMUNITY HOSPITAL (341302)**, 921 Junior High Road, Zip 27874–0405, Mailing Address: Box 405, Zip 27874–0405; tel. 252/826–4144, (Nonreporting) **A**9 10 18
Primary Contact: Thomas K. Majure, Administrator
CFO: Angela Hicks, Controller
CMO: Cornelius Artis, M.D., Chief Medical Officer
CIO: Dana Mobley, Chief Information Officer
CNO: Claudia Giddings, R.N., Chief Nursing Officer
Web address: www.och–bltc.org
**Control:** Other not–for–profit (including NFP Corporation) **Service:** General Medical and Surgical

**Staffed Beds:** 100

### SHELBY—Cleveland County

⊞ **CLEVELAND REGIONAL MEDICAL CENTER (340021)**, 201 East Grover Street, Zip 28150; tel. 704/487–3000, (Total facility includes 120 beds in nursing home–type unit) **A**1 2 9 10 19 F1 3 8 11 13 15 18 20 28 29 30 31 32 34 35 38 39 40 43 44 47 48 49 50 51 56 57 59 61 64 65 67 70 74 75 76 77 78 79 80 81 82 85 86 87 89 93 102 106 107 108 110 111 113 114 117 118 120 122 127 129 130 131 134 142 144 145 146 147 **S** Carolinas HealthCare System, Charlotte, NC
Primary Contact: Brian Gwyn, President and Chief Executive Officer
COO: Veronica Poole–Adams, R.N., Vice President, Chief Operating Officer and Chief Nursing Executive
CFO: Rose Coyne, Vice President and Chief Financial Officer
CIO: Craig Richardville, Chief Information Officer
CHR: Debra Kale, Vice President Human Resources
Web address: www.clevelandregional.org
**Control:** Hospital district or authority, Government, nonfederal **Service:** General Medical and Surgical

**Staffed Beds:** 364 **Admissions:** 9078 **Census:** 204 **Outpatient Visits:** 136750 **Births:** 1017 **Total Expense ($000):** 144684 **Payroll Expense ($000):** 59509 **Personnel:** 1201

### SILER CITY—Chatham County

⊞ **CHATHAM HOSPITAL (341311)**, 475 Progress Boulevard, Zip 27344, Mailing Address: P.O. Box 649, Zip 27344; tel. 919/799–4000 **A**1 9 10 18 F3 15 18 28 29 30 34 35 40 45 57 59 68 70 75 77 81 85 92 93 107 110 111 113 118 128 129 132 134 145
Primary Contact: Robert A. Enders, Jr., President
CFO: Brock Simonds, Interim Chief Financial Officer
CMO: James Davis, M.D., Chief Medical Staff
CIO: Louis Manz, Director Information and Communication Services
CHR: Jodie Solow, Director Human Resources
CNO: Linda B. Ellington, R.N., Interim Vice President and Chief Nursing Officer
Web address: www.chathamhospital.org
**Control:** Other not–for–profit (including NFP Corporation) **Service:** General Medical and Surgical

**Staffed Beds:** 25 **Admissions:** 683 **Census:** 8 **Outpatient Visits:** 36818 **Births:** 1 **Total Expense ($000):** 15243 **Payroll Expense ($000):** 8618 **Personnel:** 214

**NC**

## SMITHFIELD—Johnston County

✠ **JOHNSTON HEALTH (340090)**, 509 North Bright Leaf Boulevard, Zip 27577–1376, Mailing Address: P.O. Box 1376, Zip 27577–1376; tel. 919/934–8171 **A**1 9 10 **F**3 8 11 13 15 17 18 20 26 28 29 30 31 34 35 40 42 45 50 53 54 56 57 59 60 61 62 63 64 68 70 73 74 75 76 79 81 82 85 86 87 89 92 93 97 98 100 107 108 110 111 113 114 118 119 120 121 125 128 129 131 143 145 146 147 **P**6 **S** QHR, Brentwood, TN
Primary Contact: Charles W. Elliott, Jr., Chief Executive Officer
COO: Ruth Marler, Chief Operating Officer/Chief Nursing Officer
CFO: Edward A. Klein, Chief Financial Officer
CIO: Teresa Chappell, Chief Information Officer
CHR: Timothy A. Hays, Vice President Human Resources
CNO: Ruth Marler, Chief Operating Officer/Chief Nursing Officer
Web address: www.johnstonhealth.org
**Control:** Hospital district or authority, Government, nonfederal **Service:** General Medical and Surgical

**Staffed Beds:** 147 **Admissions:** 8660 **Census:** 106 **Outpatient Visits:** 157409 **Births:** 1362 **Total Expense ($000):** 153444 **Payroll Expense ($000):** 60130 **Personnel:** 1091

## SOUTHPORT—Brunswick County

✠ **J. ARTHUR DOSHER MEMORIAL HOSPITAL (341327)**, 924 North Howe Street, Zip 28461–3099; tel. 910/457–3800, (Total facility includes 57 beds in nursing home–type unit) **A**1 9 10 18 **F**3 15 28 30 34 35 40 45 46 47 53 54 57 59 65 68 75 77 79 81 84 85 92 93 94 107 110 113 118 127 128 129 131 132 142 145
Primary Contact: Edgar Haywood, III, Chief Executive Officer
COO: Lynda Stanley, Senior Vice President and Chief Operating Officer
CFO: Dennis J. Coffey, CPA, Senior Vice President and Chief Financial Officer
CMO: Brad L. Hilaman, M.D., Chief of Staff
CIO: Susan Shomaker, Director Information Management Systems
CHR: Pat Aderhold, Director Human Resources
Web address: www.dosher.org
**Control:** Other not–for–profit (including NFP Corporation) **Service:** General Medical and Surgical

**Staffed Beds:** 82 **Admissions:** 1250 **Census:** 62 **Outpatient Visits:** 59974 **Births:** 0 **Total Expense ($000):** 32523 **Payroll Expense ($000):** 13240 **Personnel:** 300

## SPARTA—Alleghany County

✠ **ALLEGHANY MEMORIAL HOSPITAL (341320)**, 233 Doctors Street, Zip 28675–0009, Mailing Address: P.O. Box 9, Zip 28675–0009; tel. 336/372–5511 **A**1 9 10 18 **F**3 15 29 30 34 35 40 43 45 57 59 64 67 77 79 81 82 87 90 93 97 107 111 118 128 129 130 132 134 145 **P**5 **S** QHR, Brentwood, TN
Primary Contact: James F. Heitzenrater, FACHE, Chief Executive Officer
CFO: Katie Myers, Chief Financial Officer
CMO: Jack Cahn, M.D., Chief Medical Staff
CIO: Darlene Keith, Chief Information Systems
CHR: John Spencer, Director Human Resources
Web address: www.amhsparta.org
**Control:** Other not–for–profit (including NFP Corporation) **Service:** General Medical and Surgical

**Staffed Beds:** 25 **Admissions:** 708 **Census:** 7 **Outpatient Visits:** 27678 **Births:** 0 **Total Expense ($000):** 11270 **Payroll Expense ($000):** 4526 **Personnel:** 139

## SPRUCE PINE—Mitchell County

✠ **BLUE RIDGE REGIONAL HOSPITAL (340011)**, 125 Hospital Drive, Zip 28777, Mailing Address: P.O. Box 9, Zip 28777; tel. 828/765–4201 **A**1 9 10 **F**3 13 15 17 28 29 30 31 32 34 35 39 40 43 45 46 50 53 54 57 59 64 66 70 75 76 77 78 79 81 82 85 87 90 93 96 97 107 108 111 113 117 118 126 127 128 129 130 131 132 134 143 144 145 146 147 **P**6 **S** Mission Health System, Asheville, NC
Primary Contact: Oscar K. Weinmeister, III, Chief Executive Officer
CFO: Jonathan Smith, Chief Financial Officer
CMO: David Hoeppner, M.D., Chief of Staff
CIO: Pam Blevins, R.N., Director, Clinical Informatics
CHR: Thomas White, Director Human Resources
CNO: A. Jane Edwards, MSN, Vice President, Patient Care Services
Web address: www.spchospital.org
**Control:** Other not–for–profit (including NFP Corporation) **Service:** General Medical and Surgical

**Staffed Beds:** 42 **Admissions:** 2056 **Census:** 17 **Outpatient Visits:** 109246 **Births:** 127 **Total Expense ($000):** 34777 **Payroll Expense ($000):** 17594 **Personnel:** 374

## STATESVILLE—Iredell County

☐ **DAVIS REGIONAL MEDICAL CENTER (340144)**, 218 Old Mocksville Road, Zip 28625–1930, Mailing Address: P.O. Box 1823, Zip 28687–1823; tel. 704/873–0281, (Nonreporting) **A**1 9 10 19 **S** Health Management Associates, Naples, FL
Primary Contact: Vincent T. Cherry, Jr., Chief Executive Officer
CFO: Kyle Johnson, Chief Financial Officer
CMO: Seema Garcha, M.D., Chief of Staff
CIO: Janie Stikeleather, Director Marketing and Community Relations
CHR: Lana Smith, Director Human Resources
Web address: www.davisregional.com
**Control:** Corporation, Investor–owned, for–profit **Service:** General Medical and Surgical

**Staffed Beds:** 131

✠ **IREDELL MEMORIAL HOSPITAL (340039)**, 557 Brookdale Drive, Zip 28677–1828, Mailing Address: P.O. Box 1828, Zip 28687–1828; tel. 704/873–5661, (Total facility includes 48 beds in nursing home–type unit) **A**1 2 9 10 **F**3 11 13 15 17 18 20 22 28 29 30 31 32 34 35 40 41 45 47 49 50 56 57 58 59 60 62 64 68 70 74 75 76 77 78 79 81 82 85 86 87 89 93 97 107 108 111 113 114 116 117 118 119 120 122 127 128 129 131 134 145 146 147 **P**6
Primary Contact: Ed Rush, President and Chief Executive Officer
CFO: Fred W. Karnap, Vice President Finance
CMO: James Bradford, M.D., President Medical Staff
CIO: Myers M. David, Chief Information Officer
CHR: John Green, Vice President Human Resources
Web address: www.iredellmemorial.org
**Control:** Other not–for–profit (including NFP Corporation) **Service:** General Medical and Surgical

**Staffed Beds:** 211 **Admissions:** 9632 **Census:** 154 **Outpatient Visits:** 153830 **Births:** 825 **Total Expense ($000):** 137632 **Payroll Expense ($000):** 63123 **Personnel:** 1001

## SYLVA—Jackson County

✠ **MEDWEST – HARRIS (340016)**, 68 Hospital Road, Zip 28779–2795; tel. 828/586–7000 **A**1 9 10 **F**3 7 8 11 13 15 28 30 34 35 40 46 50 54 62 63 64 68 70 72 75 76 77 78 79 81 82 84 85 86 87 89 93 107 108 110 111 113 118 119 120 128 129 130 134 142 143 145 146 147 **S** MedWest Health System, Sylva, NC
Primary Contact: J. Michael Poore, Chief Executive Officer
CMO: Dwayne Hooks, Jr., R.N., Chief Clinical Officer
CIO: Dale Chernich, Chief Information Officer
CHR: Janet Millsaps, Chief Human Resources Officer
Web address: www.westcare.org
**Control:** Other not–for–profit (including NFP Corporation) **Service:** General Medical and Surgical

**Staffed Beds:** 86 **Admissions:** 3802 **Census:** 36 **Outpatient Visits:** 176707 **Births:** 661 **Total Expense ($000):** 88103 **Payroll Expense ($000):** 45550 **Personnel:** 771

## TARBORO—Edgecombe County

✠ △ **VIDANT EDGECOMBE HOSPITAL (340107)**, 111 Hospital Drive, Zip 27886–2011; tel. 252/641–7700 **A**1 2 7 9 10 **F**3 11 12 13 15 29 30 31 39 40 50 57 59 70 73 75 76 78 79 81 82 85 87 89 90 92 93 96 107 110 111 118 126 129 130 131 134 144 145 **S** Vidant Health, Greenville, NC
Primary Contact: Wendell H. Baker, Jr., President
CFO: Charles Alford, Vice President Financial Services
CMO: Barry Bunn, M.D., Chief of Staff
CHR: Kadie Moore, Director Human Resources
CNO: Patrick Heins, Vice President Patient Care Services
Web address: www.VidantHealth.com
**Control:** Other not–for–profit (including NFP Corporation) **Service:** General Medical and Surgical

**Staffed Beds:** 117 **Admissions:** 4354 **Census:** 46 **Outpatient Visits:** 53824 **Births:** 433 **Total Expense ($000):** 61087 **Payroll Expense ($000):** 24027 **Personnel:** 556

## THOMASVILLE—Davidson County

✚ **THOMASVILLE MEDICAL CENTER (340085)**, 207 Old Lexington Road,
Zip 27360–3428, Mailing Address: P.O. Box 789, Zip 27361–0789;
tel. 336/472–2000 **A**1 9 10 **F**13 15 20 28 29 30 34 35 40 45 47 48 56 57
59 64 70 74 75 76 77 79 81 85 86 87 89 93 98 103 104 107 108 111 113
117 118 128 131 134 145 146 **P**6 **S** Novant Health, Winston–Salem, NC
Primary Contact: Kathie A. Johnson, R.N., MS, Ph.D., President and Chief
Executive Officer
CNO: Christina Grabus, R.N., Chief Nursing Officer
Web address: www.thomasvillemedicalcenter.org
**Control:** Other not–for–profit (including NFP Corporation) **Service:** General
Medical and Surgical

**Staffed Beds:** 101 **Admissions:** 4137 **Census:** 56 **Outpatient Visits:** 138091
**Births:** 612 **Total Expense ($000):** 62467 **Payroll Expense ($000):** 24183
**Personnel:** 507

## TROY—Montgomery County

✚ **FIRSTHEALTH MONTGOMERY MEMORIAL HOSPITAL (341303)**, 520 Allen
Street, Zip 27371–2802, Mailing Address: P.O. Box 486, Zip 27371–0486;
tel. 910/572–1301, (Nonreporting) **A**1 9 10 18 **S** FirstHealth of the Carolinas,
Pinehurst, NC
Primary Contact: Beth Walker, R.N., President
CFO: Bryan Hawkins, Controller
CHR: Tina H. Thompson, Coordinator Human Resources
Web address: www.firsthealth.org
**Control:** Other not–for–profit (including NFP Corporation) **Service:** General
Medical and Surgical

**Staffed Beds:** 25

## VALDESE—Burke County

✚ **VALDESE GENERAL HOSPITAL (340055)**, 720 Malcolm Boulevard, Zip 28690,
Mailing Address: P.O. Box 700, Zip 28690–0700; tel. 828/874–2251, (Total
facility includes 104 beds in nursing home–type unit) **A**1 2 9 10 **F**3 8 15 18 28
29 30 31 35 40 41 45 46 57 59 64 70 74 75 77 78 79 81 82 84 85 87 93
107 108 109 110 111 114 115 116 117 118 120 127 128 129 134 142 145
146 147 **S** Carolinas HealthCare System, Charlotte, NC
Primary Contact: Kenneth W. Wood, President and Chief Executive Officer
COO: Kathy C. Bailey, Ph.D., Sr. Vice President, Chief Operating Officer
CFO: Robert Fritts, Sr. Vice President, Chief Financial Officer
CFO: Robert Fritts, Chief Financial Officer
CMO: Dorwyn Croon, M.D., President Medical Staff
CMO: Joe Mazzola, D.O., Sr. Vice President Medical Affairs/Chief Quality Officer
CHR: Phil Satey, Vice President Human Resources
CHR: David Shirlen, Vice President Human Resources
CNO: Susan Brown, R.N., Sr. Vice President, Chief Nursing Officer
Web address: www.blueridgehealth.org
**Control:** Other not–for–profit (including NFP Corporation) **Service:** General
Medical and Surgical

**Staffed Beds:** 155 **Admissions:** 2187 **Census:** 119 **Outpatient Visits:** 71506
**Births:** 0 **Total Expense ($000):** 65846 **Payroll Expense ($000):** 19852
**Personnel:** 351

## WADESBORO—Anson County

✚ **ANSON COMMUNITY HOSPITAL (340084)**, 500 Morven Road,
Zip 28170–2745; tel. 704/694–5131, (Total facility includes 95 beds in nursing
home–type unit) **A**1 9 10 **F**11 15 28 29 30 34 35 40 57 59 62 64 65 71 77 81
86 87 93 97 107 110 113 118 127 129 131 132 134 144 145 **S** Carolinas
HealthCare System, Charlotte, NC
Primary Contact: Frederick G. Thompson, Ph.D., President
CFO: John G. Moore, Chief Financial Officer
CMO: A. Niazi, M.D., Chief of Staff
CIO: Lisa Sykes, IS/Communications Director
CHR: Sherri McRorie, Director Human Resources
CNO: Paula Stegall, R.N., Chief Nurse Executive
Web address: www.carolinasmedicalcenter.org
**Control:** Hospital district or authority, Government, nonfederal **Service:** General
Medical and Surgical

**Staffed Beds:** 125 **Admissions:** 888 **Census:** 86 **Outpatient Visits:** 26245
**Births:** 0 **Total Expense ($000):** 22819 **Payroll Expense ($000):** 10267
**Personnel:** 242

## WASHINGTON—Beaufort County

**BEAUFORT COUNTY HOSPITAL** See Vidant Beaufort Hospital

★ **VIDANT BEAUFORT HOSPITAL (340186)**, 628 East 12th Street,
Zip 27889–3409; tel. 252/975–4100 **A**9 10 **F**3 5 7 9 13 15 26 27 28 29 30
31 34 35 36 38 40 49 53 57 59 62 64 65 69 70 75 76 78 79 81 82 85 86
87 93 97 98 99 100 101 102 104 107 108 109 111 114 117 118 128 129
131 134 142 143 144 145 **S** Vidant Health, Greenville, NC
Primary Contact: Harvey Case, President
CMO: Jay Manning, M.D., Chief of Staff
CIO: Amy Boyd, Information Systems Manager
CHR: Penny Coltrain, Director Human Resources
CNO: Lynne Fisher, R.N., Vice President of Patient Care Services
Web address: www.beaufortregionalhealthsystem.org
**Control:** Hospital district or authority, Government, nonfederal **Service:** General
Medical and Surgical

**Staffed Beds:** 95 **Admissions:** 3415 **Census:** 37 **Outpatient Visits:** 86038
**Births:** 355 **Total Expense ($000):** 74175 **Payroll Expense ($000):** 26210
**Personnel:** 571

## WHITEVILLE—Columbus County

✚ **COLUMBUS REGIONAL HEALTHCARE SYSTEM (340068)**, 500 Jefferson
Street, Zip 28472–9987; tel. 910/642–8011 **A**1 9 10 19 **F**3 11 13 15 18 28
29 30 31 34 35 40 45 54 57 59 64 70 74 75 76 79 81 85 86 87 89 91 97
107 108 111 113 118 125 128 129 131 145 147 **S** Carolinas HealthCare
System, Charlotte, NC
Primary Contact: Henry Hawthorne, III, President and Chief Executive Officer
COO: A. Todd Howell, Chief Operating Officer
CFO: Carl Biber, Chief Financial Officer
CMO: Craig M. Slater, M.D., Chief Medical Officer
CIO: Lisa Ward, Director Management Information Systems
CHR: Ginger Scott, Vice President Human Resources
Web address: www.crhealthcare.org
**Control:** Hospital district or authority, Government, nonfederal **Service:** General
Medical and Surgical

**Staffed Beds:** 107 **Admissions:** 5293 **Census:** 63 **Outpatient Visits:** 115240
**Births:** 282 **Total Expense ($000):** 57437 **Payroll Expense ($000):** 27840
**Personnel:** 616

## WILLIAMSTON—Martin County

✚ **MARTIN GENERAL HOSPITAL (340133)**, 310 South McCaskey Road,
Zip 27892–2150, Mailing Address: P.O. Box 1128, Zip 27892–1128;
tel. 252/809–6179 **A**1 9 10 **F**3 11 13 15 29 34 35 40 45 50 56 57 59 61 64
65 70 76 77 79 81 82 87 92 93 97 107 111 118 128 132 146 **S** Community
Health Systems, Inc., Franklin, TN
Primary Contact: Jodi Beauregard, Chief Executive Officer
CFO: Craig R. Fichter, Chief Financial Officer
CIO: James Griffin, Manager Information Systems
CNO: Molly Well, Chief Nursing Officer
Web address: www.martingeneral.com
**Control:** Corporation, Investor–owned, for–profit **Service:** General Medical and
Surgical

**Staffed Beds:** 49 **Admissions:** 2222 **Census:** 20 **Outpatient Visits:** 41405
**Births:** 184 **Total Expense ($000):** 23228 **Payroll Expense ($000):** 11573
**Personnel:** 233

## WILMINGTON—New Hanover County

✚ △ **NEW HANOVER REGIONAL MEDICAL CENTER (340141)**, 2131 South
17th Street, Zip 28401–7483, Mailing Address: P.O. Box 1990,
Zip 28402–9000; tel. 910/343–7000, (Includes CAPE FEAR HOSPITAL, 5301
Wrightsville Avenue, Zip 28403–6599; tel. 910/452–8100) **A**1 2 7 9 10 12 13
**F**3 7 8 11 12 13 15 17 18 20 22 24 26 28 29 30 31 34 35 36 37 39 40 43
44 45 46 48 49 50 53 54 56 57 58 59 60 61 64 65 66 68 70 72 73 74 75
76 77 78 79 80 81 82 84 85 86 87 88 89 90 92 93 94 96 97 98 100 101
102 103 107 108 110 111 113 114 116 117 118 119 120 122 125 129 130
131 134 143 145 146 147 **S** New Hanover Regional Medical Center,
Wilmington, NC
Primary Contact: John K. Barto, Jr., President and Chief Executive Officer
COO: Matthew Heywood, Chief Operating Officer
CFO: Edwin J. Ollie, Executive Vice President and Chief Financial Officer
CMO: Sam Spicer, M.D., Vice President Medical Affairs
CIO: Avery Cloud, Vice President and Chief Information Officer
CHR: Keith A. Strawn, Vice President Human Resources
Web address: www.nhhn.org
**Control:** County–Government, nonfederal **Service:** General Medical and Surgical

**Staffed Beds:** 709 **Admissions:** 36026 **Census:** 484 **Outpatient Visits:**
314055 **Births:** 3958 **Total Expense ($000):** 601211 **Payroll Expense
($000):** 224987 **Personnel:** 3910

**WILMINGTON TREATMENT CENTER (340168)**, 2520 Troy Drive,
Zip 28401–7643; tel. 910/762–2727, (Nonreporting) **A**9 10
Primary Contact: Charles S. Sharp, Chief Executive Officer
COO: Paige Bottom, Director Operations
CFO: Virginia Powell, Director Finance
CMO: Patrick Martin, M.D., Medical Director
Web address: www.wilmtreatment.com
**Control:** Corporation, Investor–owned, for–profit **Service:** Alcoholism and other
chemical dependency

**Staffed Beds:** 94

**NC**

*Many Facility Codes have changed. Please refer to the AHA Guide Code Chart.* © 2012 AHA Guide

## WILSON—Wilson County

**TRIANGLE EAST NURSING CARE CENTER** See WilMed Nursing Care Center

✠ **WILSON MEDICAL CENTER (340126)**, 1705 Tarboro Street, S.W.,
Zip 27893–3428; tel. 252/399–8040 **A**1 2 9 10 19 **F**3 11 13 15 18 19 20 26
28 29 30 31 34 39 40 45 47 48 49 57 60 64 70 73 74 75 76 77 78 79 81
82 83 84 85 86 87 89 90 92 93 94 97 98 101 102 103 107 108 110 111
113 114 117 118 119 120 122 126 128 129 131 134 145 147 **P**6
Primary Contact: Richard E. Hudson, FACHE, President and Chief Executive Officer
CFO: Lynn Lambert, Chief Financial Officer
CMO: Rick Guarino, M.D., Vice President Medical Affairs
CIO: Brian Dietrick, Director Information Systems
CHR: Denise O'Hara, Vice President Human Resources
CNO: Melinda Laird, MS, Vice President Clinical Services
Web address: www.wilmed.org
**Control:** Other not–for–profit (including NFP Corporation) **Service:** General
Medical and Surgical

> **Staffed Beds:** 220 **Admissions:** 8153 **Census:** 91 **Outpatient Visits:** 149398
> **Births:** 998 **Total Expense ($000):** 124359 **Payroll Expense ($000):** 53096
> **Personnel:** 1094

## WINDSOR—Bertie County

✠ **VIDANT BERTIE HOSPITAL (341304)**, 1403 South King Street,
Zip 27983–1726, Mailing Address: P.O. Box 40, Zip 27983–1726;
tel. 252/794–6600 **A**1 9 10 18 **F**3 15 29 30 34 35 40 45 57 59 64 77 78 79
81 82 93 94 97 107 132 134 145 **S** Vidant Health, Greenville, NC
Primary Contact: Jeffrey N. Sackrison, FACHE, President
COO: Jeffery Dial, Chief Operating Officer
CFO: Mike Dacus, Vice President Financial Services
CFO: Brian Harvill, Vice President Financial Services
CMO: William Ballance, M.D., Chief of Medical Staff
CIO: Megan Booth–Mills, Director Planning and Marketing
CHR: Mary Beth Hill, Coordinator Human Resources
CNO: Patricia Taylor, Director, Patient Care Services
Web address: www.vidanthealth.com
**Control:** Other not–for–profit (including NFP Corporation) **Service:** General
Medical and Surgical

> **Staffed Beds:** 6 **Admissions:** 452 **Census:** 4 **Outpatient Visits:** 18533
> **Births:** 0 **Total Expense ($000):** 14955 **Payroll Expense ($000):** 7066
> **Personnel:** 126

## WINSTON SALEM—Forsyth County

**BRENNER CHILDREN'S HOSPITAL & HEALTH SERVICES** See Wake Forest
Baptist Medical Center, Winston–Salem

## WINSTON–SALEM—Forsyth County

✠ **FORSYTH MEDICAL CENTER (340014)**, 3333 Silas Creek Parkway,
Zip 27103–3090; tel. 336/718–5000, (Includes KERNERSVILLE MEDICAL
CENTER, 2911750 Kernersville Medical Parkway, Kernersville, Zip 27284–2932,
Mailing Address: 1750 Kernersville Medical Parkway, Zip 27284–2932;
tel. 336/564–4000; Joanne Allen, R.N., President) **A**1 2 3 5 9 10 **F**3 4 5 7 8 9
10 13 14 17 18 20 22 24 26 28 29 30 31 32 34 35 37 38 40 42 43 44 45
46 49 50 53 54 56 57 58 59 60 61 64 65 66 67 68 70 71 72 74 75 76 77
78 79 80 81 82 83 84 85 88 89 90 93 96 98 100 101 102 103 104 105
107 108 109 111 112 113 114 115 116 117 118 119 120 122 123 125 127
129 130 131 134 142 145 146 147 **P**6 **S** Novant Health, Winston–Salem, NC
Primary Contact: Jeffery T. Lindsay, Chief Executive Officer
COO: Paul Hammes, Senior Vice President and Chief Operating Officer
CMO: Elms Allen, M.D., Senior Vice President Medical Affairs
CIO: David B. Garrett, Chief Information Officer
CHR: Janet Smith–Hill, Senior Vice President Human Resources
Web address: www.novanthealth.org
**Control:** Other not–for–profit (including NFP Corporation) **Service:** General
Medical and Surgical

> **Staffed Beds:** 681 **Admissions:** 40938 **Census:** 637 **Outpatient Visits:**
> 367770 **Births:** 6283 **Total Expense ($000):** 617401 **Payroll Expense**
> **($000):** 229740 **Personnel:** 4474

✠ **MEDICAL PARK HOSPITAL (340148)**, 1950 South Hawthorne Road,
Zip 27103–3993; tel. 336/718–0600 **A**1 2 9 10 **F**3 29 35 64 68 74 78 79 80
81 82 85 89 125 129 130 145 **S** Novant Health, Winston–Salem, NC
Primary Contact: Teresa Carter, Vice President and Chief Operating Officer
COO: Jeffery T. Lindsay, Executive Vice President and Chief Operating Officer
CMO: Elms Allen, M.D., Senior Vice President Medical Affairs
CHR: Vasilia Perimenis, Vice President Human Resources
Web address: www.novanthealth.org
**Control:** Other not–for–profit (including NFP Corporation) **Service:** General
Medical and Surgical

> **Staffed Beds:** 22 **Admissions:** 773 **Census:** 8 **Outpatient Visits:** 39836
> **Births:** 0 **Total Expense ($000):** 43310 **Payroll Expense ($000):** 12384
> **Personnel:** 212

☐ **OLD VINEYARD BEHAVIORAL HEALTH SERVICES (344007)**, 3637 Old
Vineyard Road, Zip 27104–4842; tel. 336/794–3550 **A**1 9 10 **F**29 75 87 98 99
101 102 103 104 105 129 **P**5 **S** Universal Health Services, Inc., King of
Prussia, PA
Primary Contact: Kevin Patton, Chief Executive Officer
CFO: Ernest C. Priddy, III, Chief Financial Officer
CMO: Raj Thotakura, M.D., Medical Director
CHR: Jackie Pennino, Director Human Resources
CNO: Carol Fisher, Director of Nursing
Web address: www.oldvineyard.net
**Control:** Corporation, Investor–owned, for–profit **Service:** Psychiatric

> **Staffed Beds:** 102 **Admissions:** 2570 **Census:** 59 **Outpatient Visits:** 3621
> **Births:** 0 **Total Expense ($000):** 14124 **Payroll Expense ($000):** 7025
> **Personnel:** 224

✠ **SELECT SPECIALTY HOSPITAL–WINSTON–SALEM (342016)**, 3333 Silas
Creek Parkway, 6th Floor, Zip 27103; tel. 336/718–6300, (Nonreporting) **A**1 10
**S** Select Medical Corporation, Mechanicsburg, PA
Primary Contact: Marion Reef, Chief Executive Officer
CHR: Sherry Meacham, Coordinator Human Resources
Web address: www.selectmedicalcorp.com
**Control:** Corporation, Investor–owned, for–profit **Service:** Long–Term Acute Care
hospital

> **Staffed Beds:** 42

✠ **WAKE FOREST BAPTIST MEDICAL CENTER (340047)**, Medical Center
Boulevard, Zip 27157–0001; tel. 336/716–2011, (Includes BRENNER
CHILDREN'S HOSPITAL & HEALTH SERVICES, Medical Center Boulevard, Winston
Salem, Zip 27157, Mailing Address: One Medical Center Boulevard, Zip 27157;
tel. 336/716–2255) **A**1 3 5 8 9 10 **F**3 5 6 7 8 9 11 12 15 16 17 18 19 20 21
22 23 24 25 26 27 28 29 30 31 32 33 34 35 36 37 38 39 40 41 43 44 45
46 47 48 49 50 52 53 54 55 56 57 58 59 60 61 64 65 66 67 68 70 71 72
73 74 75 77 78 79 80 81 82 83 84 85 86 87 88 89 90 92 93 95 96 97 98
99 100 101 102 103 104 107 108 110 111 113 114 115 116 117 118 119
120 122 123 125 128 129 130 131 132 133 134 135 136 137 140 141 142
143 144 145 146 147 **P**1 6 **S** Wake Forest Baptist Health, Winston–Salem, NC
Primary Contact: Sanjay K. Saha, Executive Vice President, Operations
CFO: Gina B. Ramsey, Vice President Financial Services and Chief Financial Officer
CMO: Patricia L. Adams, M.D., Chief Professional Services
CIO: Paul M. LoRusso, Vice President Information Services and Chief Information
Officer
Web address: www.wfubmc.edu
**Control:** Other not–for–profit (including NFP Corporation) **Service:** General
Medical and Surgical

> **Staffed Beds:** 853 **Admissions:** 38511 **Census:** 651 **Outpatient Visits:**
> 382557 **Births:** 0 **Total Expense ($000):** 974424 **Payroll Expense ($000):**
> 393379 **Personnel:** 7383

**WAKE FOREST UNIVERSITY HEALTH SERVICE (349803)**, Medical Center
Boulevard, Zip 27109, Mailing Address: P.O. Box 7386, Zip 27109–7386;
tel. 336/758–5937, (Nonreporting) **A**2
Primary Contact: Cecil Price, M.D., Director
Web address: www.wfu.edu
**Control:** Other not–for–profit (including NFP Corporation) **Service:** Hospital unit of
an institution (prison hospital, college infamary, etc.)

> **Staffed Beds:** 6

## YADKINVILLE—Yadkin County

**HOOTS MEMORIAL HOSPITAL** See Yadkin Valley Community Hospital

✠ **YADKIN VALLEY COMMUNITY HOSPITAL (341308)**, 624 West Main Street,
Zip 27055–7804, Mailing Address: P.O. Box 68, Zip 27055–0068;
tel. 336/679–2041, (Nonreporting) **A**1 9 10 18 **S** HMC/CAH Consolidated, Inc.,
Kansas City, MO
Primary Contact: Frederick L. Soule, Interim Chief Executive Officer
CFO: Julie Norman, Chief Financial Officer
CHR: Bruce Niemeyer, Director Human Resources
Web address: www.hmccah.com
**Control:** Other not–for–profit (including NFP Corporation) **Service:** General
Medical and Surgical

> **Staffed Beds:** 22

---

**Hospital, Medicare Provider Number, Address, Telephone, Approval, Facility, and Physician Codes, Health Care System**

★ American Hospital Association (AHA) membership
☐ The Joint Commission accreditation
◇ DNV Healthcare Inc. accreditation
○ American Osteopathic Association (AOA) accreditation
△ Commission on Accreditation of Rehabilitation Facilities (CARF) accreditation

**NC**

# NORTH DAKOTA

### ASHLEY—Mcintosh County

★ **ASHLEY MEDICAL CENTER (351322)**, 612 North Center Avenue, Zip 58413–0556, Mailing Address: P.O. Box 450, Zip 58413–0450; tel. 701/288–3433, (Nonreporting) **A**9 10 18
Primary Contact: Jerry Lepp, Acting Chief Executive Officer
COO: Craig Lambrecht, M.D., Chief Operating Officer
CFO: Jerry Lepp, Chief Financial Officer
CMO: Udom Tinsa, M.D., Medical Director
Web address: www.amctoday.org
**Control:** Other not–for–profit (including NFP Corporation) **Service:** General Medical and Surgical

| Staffed Beds: 64 |
| --- |

### BELCOURT—Rolette County

☐ **PUBLIC HEALTH SERVICE INDIAN HOSPITAL – QUENTIN N. BURDICK MEMORIAL HEALTH FACILITY (350063)**, 2 Blocks North of Highway 5, Zip 58316, Mailing Address: P.O. Box 160, Zip 58316–0160; tel. 701/477–6111, (Nonreporting) **A**1 5 9 10 **S** U. S. Indian Health Service, Rockville, MD
Primary Contact: RoxAnne LaVallie–Unabia, Chief Executive Officer
CFO: Peggy Poitra, Financial Management Specialist
CMO: Monica Mayer, M.D., Clinical Director
CIO: Duane Marcellais, Information Technology Specialist
CHR: Donna Belgarde, Human Resources Specialist
Web address: www.ihs.gov
**Control:** Public Health Service, Government, federal **Service:** General Medical and Surgical

| Staffed Beds: 27 |
| --- |

### BISMARCK—Burleigh County

★ △ **MEDCENTER ONE (350015)**, 300 North Seventh Street, Zip 58501–4439, Mailing Address: P.O. Box 5525, Zip 58506–5525; tel. 701/323–6000, (Total facility includes 18 beds in nursing home–type unit) **A**2 3 5 7 9 10 **F**3 9 11 12 13 15 17 18 20 22 24 26 28 29 30 31 32 33 34 35 36 37 40 43 44 45 46 47 48 49 51 52 53 56 57 58 59 60 61 62 63 64 65 69 70 72 73 74 75 76 77 78 79 81 82 84 85 86 87 88 89 90 91 92 93 95 96 97 98 99 100 101 102 103 104 105 107 108 109 110 111 113 114 117 118 125 127 128 129 130 131 137 143 144 145 146 147 **P**6 **S** Sanford Health, Sioux Falls, SD
Primary Contact: Craig Lambrecht, M.D., President and Chief Executive Officer
CFO: Paul Morth, Vice President Finance
CMO: Anthoney M. Tello, M.D., Medical Director
CIO: John Miller, Vice President Information Services
CHR: Scott D. Boehm, Vice President Human Resources
Web address: www.medcenterone.com
**Control:** Other not–for–profit (including NFP Corporation) **Service:** General Medical and Surgical

| Staffed Beds: 218 Admissions: 9991 Census: 132 Outpatient Visits: 464219 Births: 765 Total Expense ($000): 298226 Payroll Expense ($000): 157880 Personnel: 2438 |
| --- |

⊠ △ **ST. ALEXIUS MEDICAL CENTER (350002)**, 900 East Broadway, Zip 58501–4586, Mailing Address: P.O. Box 5510, Zip 58506–5510; tel. 701/530–7000, (Total facility includes 19 beds in nursing home–type unit) **A**1 2 3 5 7 9 10 **F**3 8 9 11 12 13 15 17 18 19 20 21 22 23 24 25 26 28 29 30 32 34 35 38 40 43 49 53 56 57 58 59 60 62 63 64 68 70 72 73 74 75 76 77 78 79 81 82 85 86 88 89 90 91 92 93 94 98 99 100 101 102 103 104 105 107 110 111 113 116 118 126 127 128 131 133 134 144 145 146 147 **P**8 **S** Benedictine Sisters of the Annunciation, Bismarck, ND
Primary Contact: Gary P. Miller, President and Chief Executive Officer
CFO: Gary P. Miller, President and Chief Executive Officer
CMO: Shiraz Hyder, M.D., Director Medical Affairs
CIO: Todd Bortke, Director Information Systems
CHR: Wanda Pfaff, Vice President Human Resources
Web address: www.st.alexius.org
**Control:** Church–operated, Nongovernment, not–for profit **Service:** General Medical and Surgical

| Staffed Beds: 281 Admissions: 10578 Census: 130 Outpatient Visits: 231601 Births: 1394 Total Expense ($000): 229664 Payroll Expense ($000): 109867 Personnel: 1883 |
| --- |

### BOTTINEAU—Bottineau County

☐ **ST. ANDREW'S HEALTH CENTER (351307)**, 316 Ohmer Street, Zip 58318–1018; tel. 701/228–9300 **A**5 9 10 18 **F**15 28 29 30 34 35 40 45 47 50 56 57 64 75 81 83 87 97 107 110 124 126 127 129 130 131 132 134 142 143 145 147 **P**5 **S** Sisters of Mary of the Presentation Health System, Fargo, ND
Primary Contact: Jodi Atkinson, President and Chief Executive Officer
CHR: Brenda Arneson, Administrative Assistant
Web address: www.standrewshealth.com
**Control:** Church–operated, Nongovernment, not–for profit **Service:** General Medical and Surgical

| Staffed Beds: 25 Admissions: 145 Census: 1 Outpatient Visits: 7288 Births: 0 Total Expense ($000): 6121 Payroll Expense ($000): 2383 Personnel: 88 |
| --- |

### BOWMAN—Bowman County

**SOUTHWEST HEALTHCARE SERVICES (351313)**, 802 2nd Street Northwest, Zip 58623–4483, Mailing Address: P.O. Drawer C, Zip 58623; tel. 701/523–5265, (Nonreporting) **A**9 10 18
Primary Contact: Dennis Goebel, Chief Executive Officer
CFO: Becky Hansen, Chief Financial Officer
Web address: www.swhealthcare.net
**Control:** Other not–for–profit (including NFP Corporation) **Service:** General Medical and Surgical

| Staffed Beds: 89 |
| --- |

### CANDO—Towner County

★ **TOWNER COUNTY MEDICAL CENTER (351331)**, State Highway 281 North, Zip 58324, Mailing Address: P.O. Box 688, Zip 58324–0688; tel. 701/968–4411, (Nonreporting) **A**5 9 10 18
Primary Contact: Tammy Larson, Interim Chief Executive Officer
CFO: Tammy Larson, Chief Financial Officer
CMO: Russ Petty, M.D., Chief of Staff
CHR: Pat Klingenberg, Director Human Resources
Web address: www.tcmedcenter.org
**Control:** Other not–for–profit (including NFP Corporation) **Service:** General Medical and Surgical

| Staffed Beds: 20 |
| --- |

### CARRINGTON—Foster County

★ **CARRINGTON HEALTH CENTER (351318)**, 800 North Fourth Street, Zip 58421–1217, Mailing Address: P.O. Box 461, Zip 58421–0461; tel. 701/652–3141, (Total facility includes 19 beds in nursing home–type unit) **A**5 9 10 18 **F**1 3 4 7 11 12 15 16 17 28 29 30 31 34 35 40 41 43 45 56 57 59 64 66 67 68 70 72 73 75 76 80 81 85 88 89 90 93 98 107 110 113 118 126 127 129 131 132 142 145 147 **P**6 **S** Catholic Health Initiatives, Englewood, CO
Primary Contact: Mariann Doeling, R.N., Administrator
COO: Brenda Rask, Vice President Operations
CFO: Jennifer Hoornaert, Chief Financial Officer
CMO: Michael J. Page, M.D., Chief Medical Officer
CIO: Keith Stauffer, Regional Chief Information Officer
CHR: Allison Lindgren, Chief Human Resources
CNO: Christine Schroeder, R.N., Chief Nursing Officer
Web address: www.carringtonhealthcenter.org
**Control:** Church–operated, Nongovernment, not–for profit **Service:** General Medical and Surgical

| Staffed Beds: 49 Admissions: 382 Census: 20 Outpatient Visits: 22534 Births: 0 Total Expense ($000): 13674 Payroll Expense ($000): 7178 Personnel: 142 |
| --- |

### CAVALIER—Pembina County

★ **PEMBINA COUNTY MEMORIAL HOSPITAL AND WEDGEWOOD MANOR (351319)**, 301 Mountain Street East, Zip 58220–4015, Mailing Address: P.O. Box 380, Zip 58220–0380; tel. 701/265–8461, (Total facility includes 50 beds in nursing home–type unit) **A**5 9 10 18 **F**1 2 3 4 16 17 28 29 31 40 42 43 45 56 59 65 67 68 70 72 73 76 78 80 81 82 84 85 86 87 88 89 90 93 97 98 107 113 118 126 127 129 130 131 132 134 145 **P**5
Primary Contact: Everett A. Butler, Chief Executive Officer
CMO: K. S. Sumra, M.D., Chief of Staff
CIO: Robert Heidt, Director Information Systems
Web address: www.cavalierhospital.com
**Control:** Other not–for–profit (including NFP Corporation) **Service:** General Medical and Surgical

| Staffed Beds: 75 Admissions: 329 Census: 51 Outpatient Visits: 15788 Births: 0 Total Expense ($000): 10198 Payroll Expense ($000): 4035 Personnel: 130 |
| --- |

*Many Facility Codes have changed. Please refer to the AHA Guide Code Chart.*    © 2012 AHA Guide

## COOPERSTOWN—Griggs County

**COOPERSTOWN MEDICAL CENTER (351306)**, 1200 Roberts Avenue, Zip 58425; tel. 701/797–2221, (Nonreporting) **A**9 10 18
Primary Contact: Gregory Stomp, Chief Executive Officer
CFO: Ken Smith, Chief Financial Officer
CMO: Jeffrey Peterson, M.D., Medical Director
CHR: Pamela VenHuizen, Chief Human Resources Officer
Web address: www.coopermc.com
**Control:** Other not–for–profit (including NFP Corporation) **Service:** General Medical and Surgical

**Staffed Beds:** 10

## CROSBY—Divide County

**ST. LUKE'S HOSPITAL (351325)**, 702 First Street Southwest, Zip 58730–0010, Mailing Address: P.O. Box 10, Zip 58730–0010; tel. 701/965–6384, (Nonreporting) **A**5 9 10 18
Primary Contact: Leslie O. Urvand, Administrator
Web address: www.dcstlukes.org/
**Control:** Other not–for–profit (including NFP Corporation) **Service:** General Medical and Surgical

**Staffed Beds:** 12

## DEVILS LAKE—Ramsey County

✠ **MERCY HOSPITAL (351333)**, 1031 Seventh Street N.E., Zip 58301–2798; tel. 701/662–2131 **A**1 5 9 10 18 **F**3 11 13 17 28 29 30 34 35 40 42 43 45 50 53 57 70 75 76 81 87 89 93 107 108 111 113 117 118 129 130 131 132 145 147 **S** Catholic Health Initiatives, Englewood, CO
Primary Contact: James L. Marshall, Chief Executive Officer
CHR: Tanya Knutson, Director Human Resources
Web address: www.mercyhospitaldl.com
**Control:** Other not–for–profit (including NFP Corporation) **Service:** General Medical and Surgical

**Staffed Beds:** 25 **Admissions:** 1133 **Census:** 15 **Outpatient Visits:** 24297 **Births:** 360 **Total Expense ($000):** 18378 **Payroll Expense ($000):** 8414 **Personnel:** 149

## DICKINSON—Stark County

✠ **ST. JOSEPH'S HOSPITAL AND HEALTH CENTER (351336)**, 30 Seventh Street West, Zip 58601–4399; tel. 701/456–4000 **A**1 5 9 10 18 **F**3 8 11 13 15 28 29 30 34 35 40 43 53 57 59 62 63 64 70 75 76 79 81 84 85 86 87 89 97 107 108 111 113 118 126 128 129 131 132 145 **S** Catholic Health Initiatives, Englewood, CO
Primary Contact: Reed Reyman, President and Chief Executive Officer
CFO: William Schneider, Chief Financial Officer
CMO: Thomas Arnold, M.D., Chief Medical Officer
CHR: Denise Lutz, Chief Human Resources Officer
CNO: Michelle Hinrichs, Chief Nursing Officer
Web address: www.stjoeshospital.org
**Control:** Church–operated, Nongovernment, not–for profit **Service:** General Medical and Surgical

**Staffed Beds:** 25 **Admissions:** 1736 **Census:** 16 **Outpatient Visits:** 37215 **Births:** 362 **Total Expense ($000):** 39290 **Payroll Expense ($000):** 16121 **Personnel:** 339

## ELGIN—Grant County

**JACOBSON MEMORIAL HOSPITAL CARE CENTER (351314)**, 601 East Street North, Zip 58533–0376, Mailing Address: P.O. Box 367, Zip 58533–0367; tel. 701/584–2792, (Nonreporting) **A**9 10 18
Primary Contact: Jim Opdahl, Administrator
CFO: Brandon Vaughan, Chief Financial Officer
CMO: Kent Diehl, M.D., Chief of Staff
CHR: Theo Stoller, Director Human Resources
Web address: www.jacobsonhospital.org
**Control:** Other not–for–profit (including NFP Corporation) **Service:** General Medical and Surgical

**Staffed Beds:** 46

## FARGO—Cass County

✠ **ESSENTIA HEALTH FARGO (350070)**, 3000 32nd Avenue South, Zip 58103; tel. 701/364–8000 **A**1 2 5 9 10 **F**3 8 11 12 13 15 18 20 22 24 26 28 29 30 31 32 33 34 35 38 39 40 43 45 46 47 48 49 50 51 52 54 55 56 57 58 59 60 61 64 65 68 70 71 72 74 75 76 77 78 79 81 82 83 84 85 86 87 89 91 92 93 94 95 96 97 107 108 110 111 113 114 117 118 119 120 121 123 129 130 131 134 142 143 145 146 147 **P**6 **S** Essentia Health, Duluth, MN
Primary Contact: Greg Glasner, M.D., Chief Executive Officer
COO: Kevin M. Pitzer, Chief Administrative Officer
CFO: Dennis Fuhrman, Vice President Finance
CMO: Michael Briggs, M.D., Chief Medical Officer
CIO: Ken Gilles, Chief Information Officer
CHR: Keith Wahlund, Vice President Human Resources
Web address: www.essentiahealth.com
**Control:** Other not–for–profit (including NFP Corporation) **Service:** General Medical and Surgical

**Staffed Beds:** 117 **Admissions:** 7652 **Census:** 80 **Outpatient Visits:** 35762 **Births:** 1304 **Total Expense ($000):** 243145 **Payroll Expense ($000):** 118320 **Personnel:** 1908

**INNOVIS HEALTH** See Essentia Health Fargo

✠ **KINDRED HOSPITAL FARGO (352004)**, 1720 University Drive South, Zip 58103; tel. 701/241–9099, (Nonreporting) **A**1 9 10 **S** Kindred Healthcare, Louisville, KY
Primary Contact: Custer Huseby, Chief Executive Officer
Web address: www.khfargo.com
**Control:** Corporation, Investor–owned, for–profit **Service:** Long–Term Acute Care hospital

**Staffed Beds:** 31

**MERITCARE MEDICAL CENTER** See Sanford Medical Center Fargo

✠ **PRAIRIE ST. JOHN'S (354004)**, 510 4th Street South, Zip 58103–1914; tel. 701/476–7200, (Nonreporting) **A**1 9 10 **S** Universal Health Services, Inc., King of Prussia, PA
Primary Contact: Gregory LaFrancois, Chief Executive Officer
COO: Jennifer Faul, Chief Operating Officer
CFO: Tom Eide, Chief Financial Officer
CMO: Eduardo Meza, M.D., Medical Director
CHR: Michelle A. Parkinson, Director Human Resources
Web address: www.prairie–stjohns.com
**Control:** Corporation, Investor–owned, for–profit **Service:** Psychiatric

**Staffed Beds:** 89

✠ △ **SANFORD MEDICAL CENTER FARGO (350011)**, 801 Broadway North, Zip 58122; tel. 701/234–2000, (Includes MERITCARE SOUTH UNIVERSITY, 1720 South University Drive, Zip 58103–4994; tel. 701/280–4100) **A**1 2 3 5 7 8 9 10 **F**3 7 8 9 11 12 13 15 17 18 19 20 21 22 23 24 25 26 27 28 29 30 31 35 39 40 43 44 45 46 48 49 50 51 52 53 54 55 56 58 60 61 62 63 64 65 68 70 72 73 74 75 76 78 79 80 81 82 83 84 85 87 88 89 90 91 92 93 96 97 98 99 101 102 104 105 107 111 112 113 114 115 116 117 118 119 120 122 123 125 128 129 130 134 137 141 142 145 147 **P**6 **S** Sanford Health, Sioux Falls, SD
Primary Contact: Dennis C. Millirons, FACHE, President
COO: Bruce Pitts, M.D., Executive Vice President Clinical Services
CFO: Lisa Carlson, Chief Financial Officer
CMO: Rhonda L. Ketterling, M.D., Chief Medical Officer
CIO: Craig Hewit, Executive Partner Information Technology and Chief Information Officer
Web address: www.sanfordhealth.org
**Control:** Other not–for–profit (including NFP Corporation) **Service:** General Medical and Surgical

**Staffed Beds:** 456 **Admissions:** 24431 **Census:** 313 **Outpatient Visits:** 367527 **Births:** 2307 **Total Expense ($000):** 389365 **Payroll Expense ($000):** 129220 **Personnel:** 2587

**TRIUMPH HOSPITAL – FARGO** See Kindred Hospital Fargo

---

**Hospital, Medicare Provider Number, Address, Telephone, Approval, Facility, and Physician Codes, Health Care System**

★ American Hospital Association (AHA) membership
☐ The Joint Commission accreditation     ◇ DNV Healthcare Inc. accreditation
○ American Osteopathic Association (AOA) accreditation
△ Commission on Accreditation of Rehabilitation Facilities (CARF) accreditation

⊠ **VETERANS AFFAIRS HEALTH CARE SYSTEM**, 2101 Elm Street North,
Zip 58102–2498; tel. 701/232–3241 **A**1 2 3 5 **F**3 4 5 11 12 18 28 29 30 31
35 38 39 40 44 45 48 53 56 57 58 59 60 61 62 65 70 74 75 77 78 79 81
84 85 86 87 91 92 93 94 97 98 100 102 103 104 107 108 111 114 117
118 127 129 131 134 143 145 146 147 **P**6 **S** Department of Veterans Affairs,
Washington, DC
Primary Contact: Michael J. Murphy, Director
COO: Dale DeKrey, MS, Associate Director Operations and Resources
CFO: Roger Sayler, Finance Officer
CMO: J. Brian Hancock, M.D., Chief of Staff
CIO: Michael Hayes, Chief Information Resource Management
CIO: Raymond Nelson, Acting Chief Information Resource Management
CHR: Jason Wells, Chief Human Resources Management Service
CNO: Julie Bruhn, R.N., Associate Director Patient Care and Nurse Executive
Web address: www.va.gov/sta/guide/home.asp
**Control:** Veterans Affairs, Government, federal **Service:** General Medical and
Surgical

**Staffed Beds:** 77 **Admissions:** 2025 **Census:** 29 **Outpatient Visits:** 242484
**Births:** 0 **Total Expense ($000):** 183746 **Payroll Expense ($000):** 54785
**Personnel:** 901

**FORT YATES—Sioux County**

☐ **U. S. PUBLIC HEALTH SERVICE INDIAN HOSPITAL (350064)**, N 10 North
River Road, Zip 58538, Mailing Address: P.O. Box J, Zip 58538;
tel. 701/854–3831, (Nonreporting) **A**1 5 9 10 **S** U. S. Indian Health Service,
Rockville, MD
Primary Contact: Lisa Guardipee, Director
CFO: William Condon, Deputy Administrative Officer
Web address: www.ihs.gov
**Control:** PHS, Indian Service, Government, federal **Service:** General Medical and
Surgical

**Staffed Beds:** 14

**GARRISON—Mclean County**

★ **GARRISON MEMORIAL HOSPITAL (351303)**, 407 Third Avenue S.E.,
Zip 58540–7235; tel. 701/463–2275, (Nonreporting) **A**5 9 10 18 **S** Benedictine
Sisters of the Annunciation, Bismarck, ND
Primary Contact: Dean Mattern, President and Chief Executive Officer
CFO: Tod Graeber, Controller
CMO: Vern Harchenko, M.D., Chief of Staff
CNO: Beth Hetletved, Director of Nurses
Web address: www.garrisonmh.com
**Control:** Other not–for–profit (including NFP Corporation) **Service:** General
Medical and Surgical

**Staffed Beds:** 22

**GRAFTON—Walsh County**

★ **UNITY MEDICAL CENTER (351320)**, 164 West 13th Street, Zip 58237–1896;
tel. 701/352–1620 **A**5 9 10 18 **F**3 11 28 31 34 35 40 45 57 59 71 78 81 86
87 107 113 126 127 128 129 131 132 134 142 **P**5
Primary Contact: Everett A. Butler, Chief Executive Officer
CFO: Rachel Ray, Chief Financial Officer
Web address: www.unitymedcenter.com
**Control:** Other not–for–profit (including NFP Corporation) **Service:** General
Medical and Surgical

**Staffed Beds:** 17 **Admissions:** 287 **Census:** 2 **Outpatient Visits:** 40745
**Births:** 0 **Total Expense ($000):** 7554 **Payroll Expense ($000):** 3823
**Personnel:** 79

**GRAND FORKS—Grand Forks County**

⊠ △ **ALTRU HEALTH SYSTEM (350019)**, 1200 South Columbia Road,
Zip 58201–4032, Mailing Address: P.O. Box 6002, Zip 58206–6002;
tel. 701/780–5000, (Includes ALTRU HOSPITAL, 1200 South Columbia Road,
Zip 58201; tel. 701/780–5000; ALTRU REHABILITATION CENTER, 1300 South
Columbia Road, Zip 58201; tel. 701/780–2311) **A**1 2 3 5 7 9 10 20 **F**3 5 7 8
10 11 12 13 14 15 18 20 22 24 28 29 30 31 32 34 35 36 37 38 40 43 44
45 48 49 50 52 53 56 57 58 59 60 61 62 63 64 65 66 69 70 71 72 74
75 76 77 78 79 81 82 83 84 85 86 87 90 91 92 93 94 96 97 98 99 100
101 102 103 104 105 107 108 111 113 115 116 118 119 120 123 124 128
129 130 131 134 142 143 144 145 146 147 **P**6
Primary Contact: David R. Molmen, Chief Executive Officer
CFO: Dwight Thompson, Chief Financial Officer
CMO: James Van Looy, M.D., Chief Medical Executive
CIO: Mark Waind, Administrative Director Information Services
CHR: Lee Lindquist, Administrative Director Human Services
Web address: www.altru.org
**Control:** Other not–for–profit (including NFP Corporation) **Service:** General
Medical and Surgical

**Staffed Beds:** 264 **Admissions:** 13987 **Census:** 169 **Outpatient Visits:**
607615 **Births:** 1518 **Total Expense ($000):** 366049 **Payroll Expense
($000):** 209417 **Personnel:** 2927

**RICHARD P. STADTER PSYCHIATRIC CENTER (354005)**, 1451 44th Avenue
South, Zip 58201; tel. 701/772–2500, (Nonreporting) **A**9 10 21
Primary Contact: Thomas Peterson, M.D., Chief Executive Officer
COO: Bonnie Peterson, Chief Operating Officer and Vice President Clinical
Services
CFO: Darin Ohe, Chief Financial Officer
CMO: Thomas Peterson, M.D., Chief Executive Officer
CHR: Dan Bjerknes, Director Human Resources
Web address: www.stadtercenter.com
**Control:** Corporation, Investor–owned, for–profit **Service:** Psychiatric

**Staffed Beds:** 34

**HARVEY—Wells County**

★ **ST. ALOISIUS MEDICAL CENTER (351327)**, 325 East Brewster Street,
Zip 58341–1653; tel. 701/324–4651, (Total facility includes 95 beds in nursing
home–type unit) **A**5 9 10 18 **F**13 15 28 30 40 45 53 56 57 59 70 76 77 81 85
93 107 110 113 124 127 129 130 131 132 145 146 **S** Sisters of Mary of the
Presentation Health System, Fargo, ND
Primary Contact: Rockford Zastoupil, President and Chief Executive Officer
CFO: Sandra Teubner, Chief Financial Officer
Web address: www.staloisius.com
**Control:** Church–operated, Nongovernment, not–for profit **Service:** General
Medical and Surgical

**Staffed Beds:** 120 **Admissions:** 541 **Census:** 98 **Outpatient Visits:** 8084
**Births:** 18 **Total Expense ($000):** 13105 **Payroll Expense ($000):** 6145
**Personnel:** 244

**HAZEN—Mercer County**

★ **SAKAKAWEA MEDICAL CENTER (351310)**, 510 Eighth Avenue N.E.,
Zip 58545–4637; tel. 701/748–2225, (Nonreporting) **A**5 9 10 18
Primary Contact: Darrold Bertsch, Chief Executive Officer
CFO: Renae Snyder, Chief Financial Officer
CHR: Cheryl Axtman, Administrative Assistant
CNO: Marcie Schulz, Director Patient Care
Web address: www.sakmedcenter.com
**Control:** Other not–for–profit (including NFP Corporation) **Service:** General
Medical and Surgical

**Staffed Beds:** 18

**HETTINGER—Adams County**

**WEST RIVER REGIONAL MEDICAL CENTER (351330)**, 1000 Highway 12,
Zip 58639–7530; tel. 701/567–4561, (Nonreporting) **A**5 9 10 18
Primary Contact: James K. Long, CPA, Administrator and Chief Executive Officer
CFO: Karan Ehlers, Chief Financial Officer
CMO: John Joyce, M.D., Chief of Staff
CIO: Julia Gochenour, Manager Information Systems
CHR: Christi Miller, Manager Human Resources
Web address: www.wrhs.com
**Control:** Other not–for–profit (including NFP Corporation) **Service:** General
Medical and Surgical

**Staffed Beds:** 25

**HILLSBORO—Traill County**

★ **HILLSBORO MEDICAL CENTER (351329)**, 12 Third Street S.E., Zip 58045,
Mailing Address: P.O. Box 609, Zip 58045–0609; tel. 701/636–3200,
(Nonreporting) **A**5 9 10 18 **S** Sanford Health, Sioux Falls, SD
Primary Contact: Jac McTaggart, Chief Executive Officer
CFO: Darlene Swanson, Business Manager
CMO: Charles J. Breen, M.D., Medical Director
CIO: Darlene Swanson, Business Manager
CHR: Jenny Jacobson, Manager Human Resources
Web address: www.hillsboromedicalcenter.com
**Control:** Other not–for–profit (including NFP Corporation) **Service:** General
Medical and Surgical

**Staffed Beds:** 52

**JAMESTOWN—Stutsman County**

⊠ **JAMESTOWN REGIONAL MEDICAL CENTER (351335)**, 2422 20th Street
S.W., Zip 58401–6201; tel. 701/252–1050 **A**1 5 9 10 18 **F**3 11 13 15 31 34
35 40 43 44 50 53 57 59 62 63 64 70 75 76 77 81 82 84 85 86 87 89 93
107 108 110 111 113 114 117 118 129 131 132 134 145
Primary Contact: Todd R. Hudspeth, President and Chief Executive Officer
CMO: Debra Geier, M.D., President Medical Staff
CIO: Jeremey Schiele, Chief Information Officer
CHR: Ricki Ramlo, Vice President Human Resources
CNO: Cindy Gohner, Vice President Clinical Services
Web address: www.jamestownhospital.com
**Control:** Other not–for–profit (including NFP Corporation) **Service:** General
Medical and Surgical

**Staffed Beds:** 25 **Admissions:** 1258 **Census:** 10 **Outpatient Visits:** 26108
**Births:** 305 **Total Expense ($000):** 25520 **Payroll Expense ($000):** 12760
**Personnel:** 249

*Many Facility Codes have changed. Please refer to the AHA Guide Code Chart.* © 2012 AHA Guide

☐ **NORTH DAKOTA STATE HOSPITAL (354003)**, 2605 Circle Drive S.E.,
Zip 58401–6905; tel. 701/253–3964, (Nonreporting) **A**1 5 9 10
Primary Contact: Alex Schweitzer, Superintendent and Chief Executive Officer
CFO: Gene O. Wahl, Chief Financial Officer
Web address: www.nd.gov/
**Control:** State–Government, nonfederal **Service:** Psychiatric

| Staffed Beds: 140 |
| --- |

### KENMARE—Ward County

★ **KENMARE COMMUNITY HOSPITAL (351305)**, 317 First Avenue N.W.,
Zip 58746–7104, Mailing Address: P.O. Box 697, Zip 58746–0697;
tel. 701/385–4296, (Nonreporting) **A**9 10 18
Primary Contact: Margaret Shawn Smothers, Administrator
COO: Bev Heninger, Director Nursing
CFO: Kevin Seehafer, Chief Financial Officer
CMO: Jesse Sabitti, M.D., Chief Medical Officer
CIO: Alan Okerson, Director Information Technology
CHR: Ranae Ehlke, Administrative Secretary and Coordinator Risk Management
and Human Resources
Web address: www.kenmarend.net/hospital.htm
**Control:** Other not–for–profit (including NFP Corporation) **Service:** General
Medical and Surgical

| Staffed Beds: 37 |
| --- |

### LANGDON—Cavalier County

★ **CAVALIER COUNTY MEMORIAL HOSPITAL (351323)**, 909 Second Street,
Zip 58249–2407; tel. 701/256–6100, (Nonreporting) **A**5 9 10 18
Primary Contact: Lawrence Blue, Administrator and Chief Executive Officer
COO: Lawrence Blue, Administrator and Chief Executive Officer
CFO: Julie Feil, Accountant
CMO: Suresh Patel, M.D., Chief Medical Officer
CIO: Mary Jane Domres, Director Materials Management and Administrator
Information Technology
CHR: Andrea Jacobson, Human Resource Officer
Web address: www.cavaliercountyhospital.com
**Control:** Other not–for–profit (including NFP Corporation) **Service:** General
Medical and Surgical

| Staffed Beds: 25 |
| --- |

### LINTON—Emmons County

**LINTON HOSPITAL (351328)**, 518 North Broadway, Zip 58552–7308, Mailing
Address: P.O. Box 850, Zip 58552–0850; tel. 701/254–4511, (Nonreporting) **A**5
9 10 18
Primary Contact: Lowell D. Herfindahl, Interim Chief Executive Officer
CFO: Beverly Vilhauer, Chief Operating Officer and Chief Financial Officer
CMO: Edgar Oliveira, M.D., Chief Medical Staff
CHR: Sue Meidinger, Manager Business Office
Web address: www.lintonhospital.com
**Control:** Other not–for–profit (including NFP Corporation) **Service:** General
Medical and Surgical

| Staffed Beds: 14 |
| --- |

### LISBON—Ransom County

★ **LISBON AREA HEALTH SERVICES (351311)**, 905 Main Street,
Zip 58054–0353, Mailing Address: P.O. Box 353, Zip 58054–0353;
tel. 701/683–5241, (Nonreporting) **A**5 9 10 18 **S** Catholic Health Initiatives,
Englewood, CO
Primary Contact: Peggy Larson, Administrator
COO: Sheri Heinisch, Compliance Officer
CFO: Amber Stowman, Controller
CHR: Janet Froemke, Human Resources Officer
Web address: www.lisbonhospital.com
**Control:** Church–operated, Nongovernment, not–for profit **Service:** General
Medical and Surgical

| Staffed Beds: 25 |
| --- |

### MANDAN—Morton County

⊠ **KINDRED HOSPITAL–CENTRAL DAKOTAS (352005)**, 1000 18th Street N.W.,
Zip 58554; tel. 701/667–2000, (Nonreporting) **A**1 9 10 **S** Kindred Healthcare,
Louisville, KY
Primary Contact: April Bishop, Chief Executive Officer
Web address: www.khcentraldakotas.com
**Control:** Corporation, Investor–owned, for–profit **Service:** Long–Term Acute Care
hospital

| Staffed Beds: 41 |
| --- |

**TRIUMPH HOSPITAL – CENTRAL DAKOTAS** See Kindred Hospital–Central
Dakotas

### MAYVILLE—Traill County

**MERITCARE MAYVILLE UNION HOSPITAL** See Sanford Medical Center Mayville

★ **SANFORD MEDICAL CENTER MAYVILLE (351309)**, 42 Sixth Avenue S.E.,
Zip 58257–1598; tel. 701/786–3800, (Nonreporting) **A**5 9 10 18 **S** Sanford
Health, Sioux Falls, SD
Primary Contact: Roger Baier, Chief Executive Officer
CMO: James Mehus, M.D., Chief of Staff
Web address: www.unionhospital.com
**Control:** Other not–for–profit (including NFP Corporation) **Service:** General
Medical and Surgical

| Staffed Beds: 18 |
| --- |

### MCVILLE—Nelson County

**NELSON COUNTY HEALTH SYSTEM (351308)**, 200 Main Street,
Zip 58254–4002, Mailing Address: P.O. Box 367, Zip 58254–0367;
tel. 701/322–4328, (Nonreporting) **A**9 10 18
Primary Contact: Cathy Swenson, Chief Executive Officer
CFO: Steve Forde, Chief Financial Officer
CMO: Erling Martinson, M.D., Medical Director
Web address: www.nelsoncountyhealthsystem.org
**Control:** Other not–for–profit (including NFP Corporation) **Service:** General
Medical and Surgical

| Staffed Beds: 58 |
| --- |

### MINOT—Ward County

⊠ △ **TRINITY HEALTH (350006)**, One Burdick Expressway West, Zip 58701,
Mailing Address: P.O. Box 5020, Zip 58702–5020; tel. 701/857–5000, (Includes
TRINITY HOSPITAL–ST. JOSEPH'S, 407 3rd Street S.E., Zip 58702–5001;
tel. 701/857–2000), (Nonreporting) **A**1 2 3 5 7 9 10
Primary Contact: John M. Kutch, President
CFO: Kevin Seehafer, Chief Financial Officer
CHR: Paul Simonson, Vice President
Web address: www.trinityhealth.org
**Control:** Other not–for–profit (including NFP Corporation) **Service:** General
Medical and Surgical

| Staffed Beds: 584 |
| --- |

### NORTHWOOD—Grand Forks County

**SANFORD NORTHWOOD DEACONESS HEALTH CENTER (351312)**, 4 North
Park Street, Zip 58267–0190, Mailing Address: P.O. Box 190, Zip 58267–0190;
tel. 701/587–6060, (Nonreporting) **A**5 9 10 18 **S** Sanford Health, Sioux Falls, SD
Primary Contact: Pete Antonson, Chief Executive Officer
CMO: Jon Berg, M.D., Chief of Staff
CIO: Chad Peterson, Chief Information Officer
Web address: www.ndhc.net
**Control:** Church–operated, Nongovernment, not–for profit **Service:** General
Medical and Surgical

| Staffed Beds: 73 |
| --- |

### OAKES—Dickey County

★ **OAKES COMMUNITY HOSPITAL (351315)**, 1200 North Seventh Street,
Zip 58474–2502; tel. 701/742–3291, (Nonreporting) **A**5 9 10 18 **S** Catholic
Health Initiatives, Englewood, CO
Primary Contact: Lee Boyles, Chief Executive Officer
CFO: Becki Thompson, Controller
CMO: Vani Nagala, M.D., Chief Medical Officer
CIO: Terry Engel, Manager Information Technology
CHR: Julie Entzminger, Manager Human Resources
Web address: www.oakeshospital.com
**Control:** Other not–for–profit (including NFP Corporation) **Service:** General
Medical and Surgical

| Staffed Beds: 20 |
| --- |

---

**Hospital, Medicare Provider Number, Address, Telephone, Approval, Facility, and Physician Codes, Health Care System**

★ American Hospital Association (AHA) membership
☐ The Joint Commission accreditation
◇ DNV Healthcare Inc. accreditation
○ American Osteopathic Association (AOA) accreditation
△ Commission on Accreditation of Rehabilitation Facilities (CARF) accreditation

## PARK RIVER—Walsh County

★ **FIRST CARE HEALTH CENTER (351326)**, 115 Vivian Street, Zip 58270–0708, Mailing Address: PO Box I., Zip 58270; tel. 701/284–7500 **A**5 9 10 18 **F**11 15 28 29 30 31 34 35 40 45 50 59 64 65 68 77 81 93 104 107 110 111 113 118 126 129 132 **P**6
Primary Contact: Louise Dryburgh, Chief Executive Officer
CFO: Layne Ensrude, Chief Financial Officer
CMO: Olukayode S. Omotunde, M.D., Chief Medical Staff
CNO: Amy Burianek, Director Nurses
Web address: www.firstcarehc.com
**Control:** Other not–for–profit (including NFP Corporation) **Service:** General Medical and Surgical

**Staffed Beds:** 14 **Admissions:** 314 **Census:** 6 **Outpatient Visits:** 29158 **Births:** 0 **Total Expense ($000):** 8676 **Payroll Expense ($000):** 3073 **Personnel:** 74

## ROLLA—Rolette County

**PRESENTATION MEDICAL CENTER (351316)**, 213 Second Avenue N.E., Zip 58367–7153, Mailing Address: P.O. Box 759, Zip 58367–0759; tel. 701/477–3161 **A**5 9 10 18 **F**1 3 8 11 15 28 29 30 31 34 35 40 41 42 45 50 57 59 64 66 78 79 81 85 87 89 91 92 93 97 107 110 111 113 118 127 129 130 132 134 146 147 **P**6 **S** Sisters of Mary of the Presentation Health System, Fargo, ND
Primary Contact: Michael Pfeifer, Chief Executive Officer
CFO: Paula Wilkie, Chief Financial Officer
CMO: Norman Gardner, M.D., President Medical Staff
CHR: Holly Cahill, Director Human Resources
Web address: www.pmc–rolla.com
**Control:** Church–operated, Nongovernment, not–for profit **Service:** General Medical and Surgical

**Staffed Beds:** 25 **Admissions:** 196 **Census:** 6 **Outpatient Visits:** 10150 **Births:** 0 **Total Expense ($000):** 7548 **Payroll Expense ($000):** 3243 **Personnel:** 83

## RUGBY—Pierce County

★ **HEART OF AMERICA MEDICAL CENTER (351332)**, 800 Main Avenue South, Zip 58368–2198; tel. 701/776–5261, (Nonreporting) **A**5 9 10 18
Primary Contact: Jeff Lingerfelt, Chief Executive Officer
CFO: Bonnie Kuehnemund, Comptroller
CIO: Jeremy Schonebery, Director Information Technology
Web address: www.hamc.com
**Control:** Other not–for–profit (including NFP Corporation) **Service:** General Medical and Surgical

**Staffed Beds:** 20

## STANLEY—Mountrail County

★ **MOUNTRAIL COUNTY MEDICAL CENTER (351301)**, 615 6th Street S.E., Zip 58784–4323, Mailing Address: P.O. Box 399, Zip 58784–0399; tel. 701/628–2424, (Nonreporting) **A**9 10 18
Primary Contact: Ryan Mickelson, Chief Executive Officer
CFO: Ramona Edwards, Chief Financial Officer
CMO: Tyrone Langager, M.D., Chief Medical Officer
CIO: Krystle Clark, Director Medical Records
CHR: Linda Halvorson, Director Human Resources
Web address: www.stanleyhealth.org
**Control:** Other not–for–profit (including NFP Corporation) **Service:** General Medical and Surgical

**Staffed Beds:** 11

## TIOGA—Williams County

★ **TIOGA MEDICAL CENTER (351300)**, 810 North Welo Street, Zip 58852–0159, Mailing Address: P.O. Box 159, Zip 58852–0159; tel. 701/664–3305, (Nonreporting) **A**3 5 9 10 18
Primary Contact: Randall K. Pederson, Chief Executive Officer
CMO: Swami P. Gade, M.D., Medical Director
CHR: Mary Ann Holm, Office Clerk
Web address: www.tiogahealth.org
**Control:** Other not–for–profit (including NFP Corporation) **Service:** General Medical and Surgical

**Staffed Beds:** 55

## TURTLE LAKE—McLean County

**COMMUNITY MEMORIAL HOSPITAL (351304)**, 220 Fifth Avenue, Zip 58575–4005, Mailing Address: P.O. Box 280, Zip 58575–0280; tel. 701/448–2331 **A**9 10 18 **F**2 3 11 12 28 34 40 53 59 64 67 93 107 126 127 132 **P**6
Primary Contact: Dean Mattern, President and Chief Executive Officer
CFO: Karen Aafedt, Assistant Administrator and Controller
Web address: www.wrtc.com/cullum/hospital
**Control:** Church–operated, Nongovernment, not–for profit **Service:** General Medical and Surgical

**Staffed Beds:** 25 **Admissions:** 100 **Census:** 15 **Outpatient Visits:** 6186 **Births:** 0 **Total Expense ($000):** 3094 **Payroll Expense ($000):** 1775 **Personnel:** 52

## VALLEY CITY—Barnes County

★ **MERCY HOSPITAL (351324)**, 570 Chautauqua Boulevard, Zip 58072–3199; tel. 701/845–6400 **A**5 9 10 18 **F**3 11 28 29 30 32 34 40 43 45 50 64 75 77 81 84 85 86 87 92 93 107 110 113 129 130 131 132 145 147 **S** Catholic Health Initiatives, Englewood, CO
Primary Contact: Keith E. Heuser, Administrator
COO: Camille Settelmeyer, Assistant Administrator Clinical Services
CFO: Beth Smith, Controller
CHR: Lesley Erlandson, Human Resources Generalist
Web address: www.mercyhospitalvalleycity.org
**Control:** Church–operated, Nongovernment, not–for profit **Service:** General Medical and Surgical

**Staffed Beds:** 19 **Admissions:** 538 **Census:** 10 **Outpatient Visits:** 15914 **Births:** 0 **Total Expense ($000):** 11317 **Payroll Expense ($000):** 5345 **Personnel:** 112

## WATFORD CITY—Mckenzie County

★ **MCKENZIE COUNTY HEALTHCARE SYSTEM (351302)**, 516 North Main Street, Zip 58854–0548; tel. 701/842–3000 **A**9 10 18 **F**3 11 28 29 34 40 43 50 57 59 62 64 81 93 94 97 107 113 118 126 128 130 132 145
Primary Contact: Daniel R. Kelly, Chief Executive Officer
CFO: Colette Anderson, Manager Finance
CMO: Gary Ramage, M.D., Chief Medical Officer
CIO: Karn Pederson, Manager Health Information Management
CHR: Becky Smith, Manager Human Resources
Web address: www.mckenziehealth.com
**Control:** Other not–for–profit (including NFP Corporation) **Service:** General Medical and Surgical

**Staffed Beds:** 24 **Admissions:** 170 **Census:** 2 **Outpatient Visits:** 9990 **Total Expense ($000):** 5703 **Payroll Expense ($000):** 4648 **Personnel:** 171

## WILLISTON—Williams County

⊞ **MERCY MEDICAL CENTER (351334)**, 1301 15th Avenue West, Zip 58801–3896; tel. 701/774–7400 **A**1 5 9 10 18 **F**3 28 29 30 31 34 40 57 59 60 62 63 65 70 75 76 77 78 79 81 82 91 92 93 97 104 107 108 110 111 113 118 128 129 132 **S** Catholic Health Initiatives, Englewood, CO
Primary Contact: Matthew Grimshaw, Chief Executive Officer
CFO: Kerry Monson, Vice President Finance and Chief Financial Officer
CMO: William Brunsman, M.D., Chief of Staff
CIO: Sean Key, Director Information Technology
CHR: Mary Banta, Director Human Resources
Web address: www.mercy–williston.org
**Control:** Church–operated, Nongovernment, not–for profit **Service:** General Medical and Surgical

**Staffed Beds:** 25 **Admissions:** 1538 **Census:** 13

## WISHEK—Mcintosh County

★ **WISHEK COMMUNITY HOSPITAL AND CLINICS (351321)**, 1007 Fourth Avenue South, Zip 58495–7527, Mailing Address: P.O. Box 647, Zip 58495–0647; tel. 701/452–2326 **A**5 9 10 18 **F**3 7 11 15 17 18 28 29 30 32 34 35 36 40 44 45 50 53 56 57 59 60 62 63 64 65 67 68 75 81 83 87 90 91 92 93 97 107 111 113 126 127 129 130 132 142 145 146 **P**3 6
Primary Contact: Jim Opdahl, Interim Chief Executive Officer
CFO: Sahlenia Braun, Chief Financial Officer
CMO: Edgar Oliveira, M.D., Chief of Staff
CIO: Kari Buchholz, Director Health Information Management
CHR: Shar Bauer, Executive Secretary
Web address: www.wishekhospital.com
**Control:** Other not–for–profit (including NFP Corporation) **Service:** General Medical and Surgical

**Staffed Beds:** 17 **Admissions:** 283 **Census:** 3 **Outpatient Visits:** 15194 **Births:** 0 **Total Expense ($000):** 6051 **Payroll Expense ($000):** 2895 **Personnel:** 81

# OHIO

## AKRON—Summit County

✠ **AKRON CHILDREN'S HOSPITAL (363303)**, One Perkins Square,
Zip 44308–1062; tel. 330/543–1000 **A**1 2 3 5 8 9 10 13 **F**3 7 11 16 18 19
21 23 25 27 29 30 31 32 33 34 35 36 38 39 40 41 42 43 44 50 54 55 57
58 59 60 61 62 63 64 65 66 68 72 73 74 75 77 78 79 80 81 82 84 85 86
87 88 89 91 92 93 94 96 97 98 99 100 101 102 104 105 107 108 111 112
113 115 116 117 118 128 129 130 131 133 134 135 140 142 143 145
147 **P**6
Primary Contact: William H. Considine, President
COO: Grace Wakulchik, R.N., Chief Operating Officer
CFO: Michael Trainer, Chief Financial Officer
CMO: Michael Bird, M.D., Vice President Medical Services
CIO: Tom Ogg, Vice President Information Services and Chief Information Officer
CHR: Walter Schwoeble, Vice President Human Resources
CNO: Lisa Aurilio, R.N., Vice President Patient Services and Chief Nursing Officer
Web address: www.akronchildrens.org
**Control:** Other not–for–profit (including NFP Corporation) **Service:** Children's
general

| Staffed Beds: 372 **Admissions:** 9656 **Census:** 192 **Outpatient Visits:**
660187 **Births:** 0 **Total Expense ($000):** 473533 **Payroll Expense ($000):**
237266 **Personnel:** 3581 |

✠ **AKRON GENERAL MEDICAL CENTER (360027)**, 400 Wabash Avenue,
Zip 44307–2433; tel. 330/344–6000 **A**1 2 3 5 8 9 10 **F**3 5 11 12 13 14 15
17 18 20 22 24 26 28 29 30 31 34 35 36 38 39 40 42 43 44 45 46 48 49
50 51 52 53 54 55 56 57 58 59 60 61 64 65 66 68 70 71 73 74 75 76 77
78 79 81 82 84 85 86 87 91 92 93 94 96 97 98 100 101 102 103 104 105
107 108 109 110 111 113 114 115 116 117 118 119 120 122 123 125 128
129 130 131 133 134 142 144 145 146 147 **P**6 8 **S** Akron General Health
System, Akron, OH
Primary Contact: Alan Papa, President
CFO: Stephen M. Gary, Senior Vice President and Chief Financial officer
CMO: David Peter, M.D., Senior Vice President Medical Affairs and Chief Medical
Director
CIO: David Fiser, Vice President and Chief Information Officer
CHR: Don Corpora, Senior Vice President Human Resources
CNO: Beverly Bokovitz, R.N., Senior Vice President and Chief Nursing Officer
Web address: www.akrongeneral.org
**Control:** Other not–for–profit (including NFP Corporation) **Service:** General
Medical and Surgical

| Staffed Beds: 474 **Admissions:** 23291 **Census:** 297 **Outpatient Visits:**
542248 **Births:** 3269 **Total Expense ($000):** 426480 **Payroll Expense
($000):** 184359 **Personnel:** 2992 |

✠ **SELECT SPECIALTY HOSPITAL–AKRON (362027)**, 200 East Market Street,
Zip 44308; tel. 330/761–7500, (Nonreporting) **A**1 10 **S** Select Medical
Corporation, Mechanicsburg, PA
Primary Contact: Kimberly A. Thomas, JD, MSN, R.N., Chief Executive Officer
Web address: www.selectmedicalcorp.com
**Control:** Corporation, Investor–owned, for–profit **Service:** Long–Term Acute Care
hospital

| Staffed Beds: 60 |

**SUMMA AKRON CITY HOSPITAL** See Summa Health System

✠ **SUMMA HEALTH SYSTEM (360020)**, 525 East Market Street,
Zip 44309–2090; tel. 330/375–3000, (Includes SUMMA AKRON CITY HOSPITAL,
525 East Market Street, Mailing Address: P.O. Box 2090, Zip 44309–2090;
tel. 330/375–3000; SUMMA SAINT THOMAS HOSPITAL, 444 North Main Street,
Zip 44310; tel. 330/375–3000) **A**1 2 3 8 9 10 **F**1 2 3 4 5 6 7 8 9 11 12 13
15 17 18 20 22 24 26 28 29 30 31 33 34 35 36 37 38 39 40 41 42 43 44
45 46 47 48 49 50 51 52 53 54 55 56 57 58 59 60 61 62 63 64 65 66 68
70 71 72 74 75 76 77 78 79 80 81 82 83 84 85 86 87 90 92 93 96 97 98
99 100 101 102 103 104 105 107 108 109 110 111 113 114 115 116 117
118 119 120 122 123 125 128 129 130 131 132 134 142 143 144 145 146
147 **P**6 8 **S** Summa Health System, Akron, OH
Primary Contact: Thomas J. Strauss, President and Chief Executive Officer
COO: Robert Harrigan, Vice President and Chief Operating Officer
CMO: Dale Murphy, M.D., Vice President Medical Affairs
CIO: Greg Kall, Chief Information Officer
CHR: Kyle Klawitter, Vice President Human Resources
Web address: www.summahealth.org
**Control:** Other not–for–profit (including NFP Corporation) **Service:** General
Medical and Surgical

| Staffed Beds: 461 **Admissions:** 32431 **Census:** 432 **Outpatient Visits:**
432623 **Births:** 2992 **Total Expense ($000):** 606820 **Payroll Expense
($000):** 234793 **Personnel:** 5023 |

**SUMMA SAINT THOMAS HOSPITAL** See Summa Health System

## ALLIANCE—Stark County

☐ **ALLIANCE COMMUNITY HOSPITAL (360131)**, 200 East State Street,
Zip 44601–4399; tel. 330/596–6000, (Total facility includes 68 beds in nursing
home–type unit) **A**1 2 5 9 10 **F**3 8 11 13 15 28 29 30 31 34 35 36 40 45 49
50 51 56 57 59 60 62 63 64 68 69 70 74 75 76 77 79 81 82 85 86 87 90
93 96 98 103 107 108 110 111 114 117 118 127 128 129 131 134 142
145 146 147 **P**5 7 8
Primary Contact: Stanley W. Jonas, Chief Executive Officer
COO: Amy Antonacci, Vice President Nursing Services
CFO: Dale Wells, Senior Vice President Finance and Operations
CMO: Ashraf Ahmed, M.D., Senior Vice President Physician and Hospital Services
CIO: David W. Shroades, Vice President Technology Services
CHR: Connie Poulton, Vice President Colleague Relations
Web address: www.achosp.org
**Control:** Other not–for–profit (including NFP Corporation) **Service:** General
Medical and Surgical

| Staffed Beds: 196 **Admissions:** 4344 **Census:** 113 **Outpatient Visits:**
163138 **Births:** 402 **Total Expense ($000):** 88224 **Payroll Expense ($000):**
39751 **Personnel:** 825 |

## AMHERST—Lorain County

☐ **SPECIALTY HOSPITAL OF LORAIN (362025)**, 254 Cleveland Avenue,
Zip 44001; tel. 440/988–6260, (Nonreporting) **A**1 10
Primary Contact: Julia M. Meeks, Chief Operating Officer
**Control:** Other not–for–profit (including NFP Corporation) **Service:** Long–Term
Acute Care hospital

| Staffed Beds: 30 |

## ARCHBOLD—Fulton County

**ARCHBOLD HOSPITAL** See Community Hospitals and Wellness Centers, Bryan

## ASHLAND—Ashland County

✠ **SAMARITAN REGIONAL HEALTH SYSTEM (360002)**, 1025 Center Street,
Zip 44805–4011; tel. 419/289–0491 **A**1 5 9 10 **F**11 13 15 29 30 31 34 35
40 50 51 54 57 59 62 64 68 70 75 76 77 78 79 81 86 87 93 107 108 111
113 118 128 129 130 131 145 146
Primary Contact: Danny L. Boggs, President and Chief Executive Officer
CFO: Mary Griest, Vice President Finance and Chief Financial Officer
CMO: Philip Myers, M.D., Vice President Medical Affairs
CIO: Alec Williams, Chief Information Officer
CHR: Alyce Legg, Vice President Human Resources
Web address: www.samaritanhospital.org
**Control:** Other not–for–profit (including NFP Corporation) **Service:** General
Medical and Surgical

| Staffed Beds: 49 **Admissions:** 2358 **Census:** 17 **Outpatient Visits:** 145114
**Births:** 375 **Total Expense ($000):** 73446 **Payroll Expense ($000):** 24919
**Personnel:** 524 |

## ASHTABULA—Ashtabula County

☐ **ASHTABULA COUNTY MEDICAL CENTER (360125)**, 2420 Lake Avenue,
Zip 44004–4954; tel. 440/997–2262, (Total facility includes 16 beds in nursing
home–type unit) **A**1 2 5 9 10 20 **F**3 11 13 15 18 20 28 29 30 31 34 35 38 40
45 49 50 51 53 57 59 61 62 63 64 68 70 74 75 76 77 78 79 80 81 82 83
84 85 86 87 89 93 97 98 100 102 103 104 105 107 108 111 113 115 116
117 118 127 128 129 130 131 134 145 147 **P**4 5 8
Primary Contact: Michael J. Habowski, President and Chief Executive Officer
CFO: Phil Pawlowski, Vice President Finance and Chief Financial Officer
CMO: Timothy O'Brien, M.D., Chief of Staff
CIO: David Jacobs, Director Information Systems
CHR: Robert Sincich, Vice President Human Resources
Web address: www.acmchealth.org
**Control:** Other not–for–profit (including NFP Corporation) **Service:** General
Medical and Surgical

| Staffed Beds: 156 **Admissions:** 5450 **Census:** 58 **Outpatient Visits:** 201059
**Births:** 444 **Total Expense ($000):** 91937 **Payroll Expense ($000):** 41160
**Personnel:** 679 |

---

**OH**

## ATHENS—Athens County

☐ **APPALACHIAN BEHAVIORAL HEALTHCARE (364027)**, 100 Hospital Drive, Zip 45701–2301; tel. 740/594–5000, (Nonreporting) **A**1 9 10 **S** Ohio Department of Mental Health, Columbus, OH
Primary Contact: Jane E. Krason, R.N., Chief Executive Officer
CMO: Mark F. McGee, M.D., Chief Clinical Officer
CHR: Amy Grover, Director
Web address: www.mh.state.oh.us
**Control:** State–Government, nonfederal **Service:** Psychiatric

| Staffed Beds: 224 |
| --- |

⊠ **O'BLENESS MEMORIAL HOSPITAL (360014)**, 55 Hospital Drive, Zip 45701–2302; tel. 740/593–5551 **A**1 9 10 12 13 **F**3 13 15 18 20 28 31 34 37 40 51 57 59 65 66 68 70 75 76 78 79 80 81 85 93 94 107 108 110 111 114 118 125 129 145 147 **P**4 **S** OhioHealth, Columbus, OH
Primary Contact: Greg Long, Chief Executive Officer
CFO: Robert Melaragno, Vice President Finance
CIO: Kristine Barr, Vice President Communication Services
CHR: Sandie Leasure, Senior Vice President Human Resources
Web address: www.obleness.org
**Control:** Other not–for–profit (including NFP Corporation) **Service:** General Medical and Surgical

| Staffed Beds: 132 Admissions: 2845 Census: 10 Outpatient Visits: 112106 Births: 598 Total Expense ($000): 59241 Payroll Expense ($000): 18833 Personnel: 427 |
| --- |

## BARBERTON—Summit County

⊠ **SUMMA BARBERTON CITIZENS HOSPITAL (360019)**, 155 Fifth Street N.E., Zip 44203–3332; tel. 330/615–3000, (Total facility includes 20 beds in nursing home–type unit) **A**1 2 3 5 9 10 **F**3 8 13 14 15 17 18 20 22 24 26 28 29 30 31 34 35 39 40 44 46 47 48 49 50 51 53 54 56 57 58 59 60 61 63 64 68 70 74 75 76 77 78 79 81 82 85 86 87 90 91 92 93 97 98 100 102 103 107 108 110 111 113 115 116 117 118 127 128 130 131 134 145 146 147 **P**6 8 **S** Summa Health System, Akron, OH
Primary Contact: Thomas DeBord, President
CFO: Charles Alderson, Chief Financial Officer
CMO: Jeffrey Morris, M.D., Medical Director
CIO: David Lynch, Regional Director Information Systems
CHR: Don Argiro, Regional Director Human Resources
CNO: Kathy Jobe, R.N., Chief Nursing Officer and Vice President Patient Care Services
Web address: www.barbhosp.com
**Control:** Other not–for–profit (including NFP Corporation) **Service:** General Medical and Surgical

| Staffed Beds: 212 Admissions: 9718 Census: 136 Outpatient Visits: 477655 Births: 655 Total Expense ($000): 140741 Payroll Expense ($000): 55283 Personnel: 1096 |
| --- |

## BARNESVILLE—Belmont County

⊠ **BARNESVILLE HOSPITAL (361321)**, 639 West Main Street, Zip 43713–0309, Mailing Address: P.O. Box 309, Zip 43713–0309; tel. 740/425–3941 **A**1 9 10 18 **F**3 11 15 17 28 29 30 31 34 35 39 40 41 45 50 57 59 64 65 69 70 74 75 77 78 79 81 85 86 87 89 91 93 107 108 113 118 127 128 129 132 134 144 145 **P**6
Primary Contact: Richard L. Doan, FACHE, Chief Executive Officer
COO: David Phillips, Chief Operating Officer
CFO: Willie Cooper–Lohr, Chief Financial Officer
CMO: David J. Hilliard, D.O., Chief of Staff
CIO: Tiffany Gramby, Director Health Information Management and Privacy Officer
CHR: Beth K. Brill, Director Human Resources
CNO: Cynthia Touvelle, R.N., Senior Director Care Management and Chief Nursing Officer
Web address: www.barnesvillehospital.com
**Control:** Other not–for–profit (including NFP Corporation) **Service:** General Medical and Surgical

| Staffed Beds: 25 Admissions: 1313 Census: 12 Outpatient Visits: 36131 Births: 0 Total Expense ($000): 18508 Payroll Expense ($000): 8522 Personnel: 209 |
| --- |

## BATAVIA—Clermont County

⊠ **MERCY HOSPITAL CLERMONT (360236)**, 3000 Hospital Drive, Zip 45103–1921; tel. 513/732–8200, (Nonreporting) **A**1 2 9 10 **S** Catholic Health Partners, Cincinnati, OH
Primary Contact: Gayle M. Heintzelman, President and Chief Executive Officer
CFO: Will Woodward, Director Finance
CMO: Howard Bell, M.D., Chief of Staff
CHR: Shelly Sherman, Director Human Resources
Web address: www.e–mercy.com
**Control:** Church–operated, Nongovernment, not–for profit **Service:** General Medical and Surgical

| Staffed Beds: 119 |
| --- |

## BEACHWOOD—Cuyahoga County

★ **UNIVERSITY HOSPITALS AHUJA MEDICAL CENTER (360359)**, 3999 Richmond Road, Zip 44122–6805; tel. 216/593–5500, (Data for 306 days) **A**9 10 **F**3 15 18 20 22 24 26 29 30 34 35 36 40 41 42 45 46 47 48 49 50 51 56 57 59 60 61 65 68 70 74 75 77 79 81 82 85 87 107 108 109 110 111 114 118 125 129 143 144 145 147 **S** University Hospitals, Cleveland, OH
Primary Contact: Susan V. Juris, President
Web address: www.uhhospitals.org/ahuja/tabid/7051/uhahujamedicalcenter.aspx
**Control:** Other not–for–profit (including NFP Corporation) **Service:** General Medical and Surgical

| Staffed Beds: 92 Admissions: 4009 Census: 49 Outpatient Visits: 54547 Births: 0 Total Expense ($000): 84205 Payroll Expense ($000): 32446 Personnel: 671 |
| --- |

## BEAVERCREEK—Rock County County

★ **SOIN MEDICAL CENTER**, 3535 Pentagon Boulevard, Zip 45431; tel. 937/702–4000, (Nonreporting) **S** Kettering Health Network, Dayton, OH
Primary Contact: Terry M. Burns, President
Web address: www.khnetwork.org/soin
**Control:** Other not–for–profit (including NFP Corporation) **Service:** General Medical and Surgical

| Staffed Beds: 63 |
| --- |

## BELLAIRE—Belmont County

☐ **BELMONT COMMUNITY HOSPITAL (360153)**, 4697 Harrison Street, Zip 43906–1338, Mailing Address: P.O. Box 653, Zip 43906–0653; tel. 740/671–1200, (Nonreporting) **A**1 9 10
Primary Contact: John DeBlasis, Senior Administrator
CFO: James B. Murdy, Chief Financial Officer
CMO: Charles L. Geiger, D.O., Chief of Staff
CHR: Donna Moore, Director Human Resources
Web address: www.wheelinghospital.org/facilities/bch/
**Control:** Other not–for–profit (including NFP Corporation) **Service:** General Medical and Surgical

| Staffed Beds: 66 |
| --- |

## BELLEFONTAINE—Logan County

⊠ **MARY RUTAN HOSPITAL (360197)**, 205 Palmer Avenue, Zip 43311–2281; tel. 937/592–4015 **A**1 3 5 9 10 20 21 **F**3 11 13 14 15 18 20 28 29 30 31 32 34 40 50 54 57 59 64 66 68 70 75 76 77 78 79 81 82 85 86 87 89 107 108 110 111 113 118 128 129 131 134 145 146
Primary Contact: Mandy C. Goble, President and Chief Executive Officer
CFO: Ron Carmin, Vice President Fiscal Affairs
CMO: Grant Varian, M.D., Medical Director
CIO: Robert Reynolds, Director Information Systems
CHR: Tim Froebe, Vice President Human Resources
Web address: www.maryrutan.org
**Control:** Other not–for–profit (including NFP Corporation) **Service:** General Medical and Surgical

| Staffed Beds: 100 Admissions: 1839 Census: 15 Outpatient Visits: 117024 Births: 349 Total Expense ($000): 73249 Payroll Expense ($000): 28633 Personnel: 548 |
| --- |

## BELLEVUE—Sandusky County

⊠ **BELLEVUE HOSPITAL (360107)**, 1400 West Main Street, Zip 44811–1028, Mailing Address: P.O. Box 8004, Zip 44811–8004; tel. 419/483–4040 **A**1 2 5 9 10 **F**3 11 13 15 28 31 34 35 40 41 46 50 56 57 59 61 62 68 70 74 75 76 77 79 81 82 85 89 93 107 108 110 111 113 117 118 126 128 129 130 131 132 134 142 145 **P**8
Primary Contact: Michael Winthrop, President
CFO: Timothy Buit, Vice President of Finance and Chief Financial Officer
CMO: J. Andrew Huddleston, D.O., President Medical Staff
CIO: Kim Stults, Director Education
CHR: Deborah Ganci, Vice President Human Resources
Web address: www.bellevuehospital.com
**Control:** Other not–for–profit (including NFP Corporation) **Service:** General Medical and Surgical

| Staffed Beds: 50 Admissions: 2079 Census: 19 Outpatient Visits: 79018 Births: 345 Total Expense ($000): 42414 Payroll Expense ($000): 16138 Personnel: 339 |
| --- |

## BLUFFTON—Allen County

⊠ **BLUFFTON HOSPITAL (361322)**, 139 Garau Street, Zip 45817–0048;
tel. 419/358–9010 **A**1 9 **F**13 15 18 34 40 45 70 76 81 82 93 107 110 118
129 145 146 **S** Blanchard Valley Health System, Findlay, OH
Primary Contact: William D. Watkins, Chief Administrative Officer
CFO: David Cytlak, Vice President Finance
CMO: William H. Kose, M.D., Vice President Quality and Medical Affairs
CIO: David Cytlak, Vice President Finance
CHR: Ryan Fisher, Director Human Resources
CNO: Barbara J. Pasztor, R.N., Vice President Nursing and Patient Care Services
Web address: www.bvhealthsystem.org
**Control:** Other not–for–profit (including NFP Corporation) **Service:** General
Medical and Surgical

**Staffed Beds: 25 Admissions:** 389 **Census:** 3 **Outpatient Visits:** 40046
**Births:** 246 **Total Expense ($000):** 14165 **Payroll Expense ($000):** 7733
**Personnel:** 119

## BOARDMAN—Mahoning County

☐ **GREENBRIAR REHABILITATION HOSPITAL (363032)**, 8064 South Avenue,
Suite One, Zip 44512; tel. 330/726–3700, (Nonreporting) **A**1 9 10
Primary Contact: Daphne Bonner, Administrator
**Control:** Corporation, Investor–owned, for–profit **Service:** Rehabilitation

**Staffed Beds: 29**

**MAHONING VALLEY HOSPITAL** See Vibra Hospital of Mahoning Valley

⊠ **ST. ELIZABETH BOARDMAN HEALTH CENTER (360276)**, 8401 Market
Street, Zip 44512–6777; tel. 330/729–2929 **A**1 9 10 **F**3 8 11 15 18 29 30 34
35 40 45 46 59 60 67 68 70 74 75 77 78 79 81 82 84 85 87 93 107 108
110 111 113 118 119 120 128 129 130 145 147 **P**3 **S** Catholic Health
Partners, Cincinnati, OH
Primary Contact: Eugenia Aubel, President
CFO: Donald E. Kline, Senior Vice President Finance
CMO: Nicholas Kreatsoulas, M.D., Vice President Medical Affairs
CIO: Charles Folkwein, Vice President Ancillary Services
CHR: Molly Seals, Senior Vice President Human Resources and Learning
Web address:
www.ehealthconnection.com/regions/youngstown/content/show_facility.asp?facility_id=
190
**Control:** Church–operated, Nongovernment, not–for profit **Service:** General
Medical and Surgical

**Staffed Beds: 128 Admissions:** 8444 **Census:** 97 **Outpatient Visits:** 80470
**Births:** 0 **Total Expense ($000):** 83390 **Payroll Expense ($000):** 28750
**Personnel:** 561

☐ **VIBRA HOSPITAL OF MAHONING VALLEY (362023)**, 8049 South Avenue,
Zip 44512; tel. 330/726–5000, (Nonreporting) **A**1 10 **S** Vibra Healthcare,
Mechanicsburg, PA
Primary Contact: Mary Lou Sankovich, R.N., MSN, Chief Executive Officer and
Chief Nursing Officer
Web address: www.mahoningvalleyhospital.com
**Control:** Corporation, Investor–owned, for–profit **Service:** Long–Term Acute Care
hospital

**Staffed Beds: 45**

## BORDMAN—Mahoning County

**SELECT SPECIALTY HOSPITAL–YOUNGSTOWN, BOARDMAN CAMPUS** See
Select Specialty Hospital–Youngstown, Youngstown

## BOWLING GREEN—Wood County

⊠ **WOOD COUNTY HOSPITAL (360029)**, 950 West Wooster Street,
Zip 43402–2603; tel. 419/354–8900 **A**1 3 5 9 10 **F**3 11 12 13 15 17 28 29
30 32 34 35 40 44 45 46 50 57 59 64 65 68 69 70 75 76 77 79 81 82 85
87 89 93 107 108 110 111 113 114 117 118 128 129 130 131 134 143
145 146 147 **P**8
Primary Contact: Stanley R. Korducki, President
COO: Carole Matthews, Vice President Patient Care
CFO: Karol Bortel, Vice President Financial Services
CIO: Joanne White, Chief Information Officer
CHR: Frank Day, Vice President Patient Services
Web address: www.woodcountyhospital.org
**Control:** Other not–for–profit (including NFP Corporation) **Service:** General
Medical and Surgical

**Staffed Beds: 102 Admissions:** 3656 **Census:** 32 **Outpatient Visits:** 114331
**Births:** 315 **Total Expense ($000):** 66422 **Payroll Expense ($000):** 28559
**Personnel:** 689

## BRYAN—Williams County

☐ **COMMUNITY HOSPITALS AND WELLNESS CENTERS (360121)**, 433 West
High Street, Zip 43506–1679; tel. 419/636–1131, (Includes ARCHBOLD
HOSPITAL, 121 Westfield Drive, Archbold, Zip 43502; tel. 419/445–4415;
BRYAN HOSPITAL, 433 West High Street, Zip 43506; tel. 419/636–1131;
MONTPELIER HOSPITAL, 909 East Snyder Avenue, Montpelier, Zip 43543;
tel. 419/485–3154), (Nonreporting) **A**1 2 5 9 10
Primary Contact: Philip L. Ennen, Vice President and Chief Executive Officer
CFO: Leroy P. Feather, Vice President Finance
CIO: Greg Slattery, Vice President Information
CHR: Mary Ann Potts, Director Personnel
Web address: www.chwchospital.com
**Control:** Other not–for–profit (including NFP Corporation) **Service:** General
Medical and Surgical

**Staffed Beds: 113**

## BUCYRUS—Crawford County

⊠ **BUCYRUS COMMUNITY HOSPITAL (361316)**, 629 North Sandusky Avenue,
Zip 44820–1821; tel. 419/562–4677, (Nonreporting) **A**1 5 9 10 18 21 **S** Avita
Health System, Galion, OH
Primary Contact: Jerome Morasko, Chief Executive Officer
COO: Andy Daniels, Chief Operating Officer
CMO: Michael A. Johnson, M.D., Chief of Staff
CIO: Joann Riedlinger, Vice President Nursing and Manager Information Systems
CHR: Jeanne Perkins, Vice President Nursing and Interim Manager Human
Resources
Web address: www.bchonline.org
**Control:** Other not–for–profit (including NFP Corporation) **Service:** General
Medical and Surgical

**Staffed Beds: 25**

## CADIZ—Harrison County

⊠ **HARRISON COMMUNITY HOSPITAL (361311)**, 951 East Market Street,
Zip 43907–9799; tel. 740/942–4631 **A**1 9 10 18 **F**7 11 15 18 28 29 30 31
34 40 45 47 50 51 53 57 58 59 62 64 65 68 74 75 78 79 81 82 85 86 87
93 97 107 108 110 111 113 118 129 131 132 134 142 145 146 147
Primary Contact: Terry M. Carson, Chief Executive Officer
CFO: Sally Huff, Controller
CMO: Isam Tabbah, M.D., Chief of Staff
CHR: Marcella Evans, Director Human Resources
CNO: Elizabeth Kovacs, R.N., Director of Nursing
Web address: www.harrisoncommunity.com
**Control:** Other not–for–profit (including NFP Corporation) **Service:** General
Medical and Surgical

**Staffed Beds: 25 Admissions:** 462 **Census:** 7 **Outpatient Visits:** 40408
**Births:** 0 **Total Expense ($000):** 15267 **Payroll Expense ($000):** 6583
**Personnel:** 173

## CAMBRIDGE—Guernsey County

⊠ **SOUTHEASTERN OHIO REGIONAL MEDICAL CENTER (360203)**, 1341 North
Clark Street, Zip 43725–9614, Mailing Address: P.O. Box 610, Zip 43725–0610;
tel. 740/439–8000 **A**1 2 9 10 20 **F**3 7 11 13 15 18 20 28 29 30 31 32 34 35
40 43 46 48 49 51 57 59 60 62 63 64 65 66 70 75 76 77 78 79 81 82 83
84 85 86 87 91 93 96 97 107 108 110 111 113 115 117 118 128 129 130
131 134 143 145 146 147 **P**6 8
Primary Contact: Raymond M. Chorey, President and Chief Executive Officer
CFO: Donald P. Huelskamp, Vice President Finance and Chief Financial Officer
CMO: E. Edwin Conaway, M.D., Vice President Medical Affairs and Chief Medical
Officer
CIO: Kevin Ludwigsen, Interim Chief Information Officer
CHR: Ann Rollman, Vice President Human Resources
CNO: Angela S. Long, Vice President Clinical Services and Chief Nursing Officer
Web address: www.seormc.org
**Control:** Other not–for–profit (including NFP Corporation) **Service:** General
Medical and Surgical

**Staffed Beds: 95 Admissions:** 4469 **Census:** 39 **Outpatient Visits:** 127981
**Births:** 474 **Total Expense ($000):** 69561 **Payroll Expense ($000):** 27786
**Personnel:** 633

**OH**

## CANAL WINCHESTER—Fairfield County

☐ **DILEY RIDGE MEDICAL CENTER (360358)**, 7911 Diley Road, Zip 43110–9653; tel. 614/838–7911 **A**1 9 10 **F**3 15 29 30 35 40 50 54 64 68 85 87 107 110 111 113 118 129 146
Primary Contact: Jodi Wilson, Site Administrator
Web address: www.dileyridgemedicalcenter.com
**Control:** Other not–for–profit (including NFP Corporation) **Service:** General Medical and Surgical

**Staffed Beds: 10 Admissions: 58 Census: 1 Outpatient Visits: 35243 Births: 0 Total Expense ($000): 10210 Payroll Expense ($000): 3364 Personnel: 89**

## CANTON—Stark County

☐ **ACUTE CARE SPECIALTY HOSPITAL OF AULTMAN (362032)**, 2600 Sixth Street, S.W., Zip 44710; tel. 330/363–4000 **A**1 10 **F**1 29 30 39
Primary Contact: Jackie Toth, Administrator
Web address: www.aultman.org
**Control:** Other not–for–profit (including NFP Corporation) **Service:** Long–Term Acute Care hospital

**Staffed Beds: 30 Admissions: 218 Census: 15 Outpatient Visits: 0 Births: 0 Total Expense ($000): 7855 Payroll Expense ($000): 3654 Personnel: 52**

☒ △ **AULTMAN HOSPITAL (360084)**, 2600 Sixth Street S.W., Zip 44710–1702; tel. 330/452–9911, (Includes AULTMAN HOSPITAL PEDIATRIC SERVICES, 2600 Sixth Street, S.W., tel. 330/363–5455), (Total facility includes 60 beds in nursing home–type unit) **A**1 2 3 5 7 9 10 13 **F**3 7 8 11 12 13 14 15 17 18 20 22 24 26 28 29 30 31 34 35 39 40 43 44 45 48 49 50 51 53 54 55 56 57 58 59 60 61 62 63 64 68 70 71 72 74 75 76 77 78 79 81 82 83 84 85 86 87 89 90 93 96 97 98 102 103 104 105 106 107 108 109 110 111 113 116 117 118 119 120 122 125 127 128 129 130 131 132 133 134 142 143 144 145 146 147 **P**6 **S** Aultman Health Foundation, Canton, OH
Primary Contact: Edward J. Roth, III, President and Chief Executive Officer
COO: Christopher Remark, Chief Operating Officer
CFO: Mark Wright, Vice President
CHR: Sue Olivera, Vice President
Web address: www.aultman.com
**Control:** Other not–for–profit (including NFP Corporation) **Service:** General Medical and Surgical

**Staffed Beds: 612 Admissions: 25539 Census: 395 Outpatient Visits: 494356 Births: 2458 Total Expense ($000): 399144 Payroll Expense ($000): 178191 Personnel: 4318**

☒ △ **MERCY MEDICAL CENTER (360070)**, 1320 Mercy Drive N.W., Zip 44708–2641; tel. 330/489–1000 **A**1 2 3 5 7 9 10 **F**3 11 13 15 17 18 20 22 24 26 28 29 30 31 34 35 39 40 43 44 46 49 50 51 53 54 56 57 59 60 62 63 64 66 68 70 72 73 74 75 76 77 78 79 80 81 82 84 85 86 87 89 90 91 92 93 96 97 98 100 102 107 108 111 114 115 116 117 118 119 120 121 122 125 128 129 130 131 134 142 143 145 146 147 **P**6 7 **S** Sisters of Charity Health System, Cleveland, OH
Primary Contact: Thomas E. Cecconi, President and Chief Executive Officer
COO: Jeffrey Smith, Senior Vice President and Chief Operating Officer
CFO: Michael S. Rieger, Vice President and Chief Financial Officer
CMO: David Gormsen, D.O., Chief Medical Officer
CNO: Barbara Yingling, R.N., Vice President and Chief Nursing Officer
Web address: www.cantonmercy.org
**Control:** Other not–for–profit (including NFP Corporation) **Service:** General Medical and Surgical

**Staffed Beds: 337 Admissions: 15158 Census: 209 Outpatient Visits: 616903 Births: 1590 Total Expense ($000): 275352 Payroll Expense ($000): 109399 Personnel: 2112**

☒ **SELECT SPECIALTY HOSPITAL–CANTON (362016)**, 1320 Mercy Drive N.W., Zip 44708; tel. 330/489–8189, (Nonreporting) **A**1 10 **S** Select Medical Corporation, Mechanicsburg, PA
Primary Contact: Dawne Wheeler, Chief Executive Officer
Web address: www.selectmedicalcorp.com
**Control:** Corporation, Investor–owned, for–profit **Service:** Long–Term Acute Care hospital

**Staffed Beds: 30**

## CHARDON—Geauga County

☐ **HEATHERHILL CARE COMMUNITIES (362014)**, 12340 Bass Lake Road, Zip 44024–8327; tel. 440/285–4040, (Nonreporting) **A**1 9 10
Primary Contact: Jim Homa, Chief Executive Officer
COO: Linton Sharpnack, R.N., Director Nursing
CFO: Rebecca Ivcic, Chief Financial Officer
CMO: Donald Goddard, M.D., Chief Medical Officer
CHR: Danialle Lynce, Manager Human Resources
Web address: www.heatherhill.com
**Control:** Other not–for–profit (including NFP Corporation) **Service:** General Medical and Surgical

**Staffed Beds: 214**

☒ **UNIVERSITY HOSPITALS GEAUGA MEDICAL CENTER (360192)**, 13207 Ravenna Road, Zip 44024–7032; tel. 440/269–6000 **A**1 2 9 10 **F**3 8 11 12 13 14 15 18 20 22 26 28 29 30 31 34 35 37 39 40 44 49 50 51 54 56 57 59 60 64 65 68 70 74 75 76 77 78 79 81 82 85 86 87 93 98 102 107 108 110 111 113 114 115 116 117 118 123 129 131 134 145 147 **S** University Hospitals, Cleveland, OH
Primary Contact: M. Steven Jones, President
COO: M. Steven Jones, President
CFO: Paul Amantea, Director Finance
CMO: David Kosnosky, M.D., Chief Medical Officer
CIO: Lou Ciraldo, Information Services Representative
CHR: Danialle Lynce, Manager Human Resources
CNO: Peggy A. Kuhar, R.N., Chief Nursing Officer
Web address: www.uhhospitals.org/geauga/
**Control:** Other not–for–profit (including NFP Corporation) **Service:** General Medical and Surgical

**Staffed Beds: 126 Admissions: 7536 Census: 80 Outpatient Visits: 101597 Births: 1093 Total Expense ($000): 96609 Payroll Expense ($000): 36310 Personnel: 694**

## CHILLICOTHE—Ross County

☒ **ADENA HEALTH SYSTEM (360159)**, 272 Hospital Road, Zip 45601–9031; tel. 740/779–7500 **A**1 2 5 9 10 19 21 **F**3 5 8 11 13 15 17 18 20 22 24 26 28 29 30 31 32 34 35 38 40 41 45 46 49 56 57 60 61 62 63 64 68 70 73 74 75 76 77 78 79 80 81 82 84 85 87 89 93 96 97 98 99 100 102 104 107 108 110 111 113 114 116 117 118 119 120 122 127 128 129 130 131 132 134 143 144 145 146 147 **P**6
Primary Contact: Mark H. Shuter, President and Chief Executive Officer
CFO: Keith T. Coleman, Chief Financial Officer
CMO: John Fortney, M.D., Chief Medical Officer
CIO: Mark Moffitt, Chief Information Officer
CHR: Eric Perdue, Chief Human Resource Officer
CNO: Judith Henson, Chief Nursing Officer
Web address: www.adena.org
**Control:** Other not–for–profit (including NFP Corporation) **Service:** General Medical and Surgical

**Staffed Beds: 254 Admissions: 13942 Census: 127 Outpatient Visits: 462216 Births: 1148 Total Expense ($000): 358792 Payroll Expense ($000): 159969 Personnel: 2028**

☒ **VETERANS AFFAIRS MEDICAL CENTER**, 17273 State Route 104, Zip 45601–8608; tel. 740/773–1141, (Total facility includes 162 beds in nursing home–type unit) **A**1 5 9 **F**3 5 18 28 29 30 33 34 35 36 38 39 44 45 47 50 53 54 56 57 59 61 62 63 64 65 67 74 75 77 79 80 81 82 84 86 87 93 94 96 97 98 100 101 102 103 104 105 106 107 108 111 114 118 126 127 128 129 131 134 142 143 145 146 147 **P**6 **S** Department of Veterans Affairs, Washington, DC
Primary Contact: Jeffrey T. Gering, Medical Center Director
COO: Keith Sullivan, Associate Director
CFO: Rick Deckard, Chief Fiscal Service
CMO: Deborah Meesig, M.D., Chief of Staff
CIO: William Gawler, Chief Information Officer
CHR: Angela Young, Human Resources Officer
Web address: www.va.gov/sta/guide/home.asp
**Control:** Veterans Affairs, Government, federal **Service:** Psychiatric

**Staffed Beds: 297 Admissions: 4310 Census: 250 Outpatient Visits: 319739 Births: 0 Total Expense ($000): 189361 Payroll Expense ($000): 89853 Personnel: 1196**

## CINCINNATI—Hamilton County

☐ **BETHESDA NORTH HOSPITAL (360179)**, 10500 Montgomery Road, Zip 45242–4402; tel. 513/865–1111 **A**1 2 3 5 9 10 **F**3 5 9 11 13 15 17 18 20 22 24 26 28 29 30 31 34 35 36 37 38 39 40 41 42 43 44 45 46 47 48 49 50 53 54 55 56 57 58 59 60 61 63 64 65 66 68 70 71 73 74 75 76 77 78 79 81 82 84 85 86 87 90 91 92 93 94 96 97 100 101 102 104 107 108 110 111 113 114 115 116 117 118 119 120 122 123 125 128 129 130 131 133 134 140 142 143 144 145 146 147 **P**6
Primary Contact: Sher McClanahan, Chief Operating Officer
CFO: Craig Rucker, Senior Vice President and Chief Financial Officer
CMO: Georges Feghali, M.D., Senior Vice President Quality and Chief Medical Officer
CIO: Rick Moore, Chief Information Officer
Web address: www.trihealth.com
**Control:** Other not–for–profit (including NFP Corporation) **Service:** General Medical and Surgical

**Staffed Beds: 375 Admissions: 24123 Census: 263 Outpatient Visits: 263657 Births: 4116 Total Expense ($000): 399284 Payroll Expense ($000): 138252 Personnel: 3182**

*Many Facility Codes have changed. Please refer to the AHA Guide Code Chart.* © 2012 AHA Guide

⊠ △ **CHRIST HOSPITAL (360163)**, 2139 Auburn Avenue, Zip 45219–2906; tel. 513/585–2000 **A**1 2 3 5 7 9 10 **F**3 6 8 9 11 12 13 15 17 18 20 22 24 26 28 29 30 31 34 35 36 37 38 39 40 44 45 46 47 48 49 50 51 52 53 54 55 56 57 58 59 60 61 64 65 66 68 70 73 74 75 76 77 78 79 80 81 82 83 84 85 86 87 90 92 93 94 96 97 98 99 100 101 102 103 104 105 107 108 110 111 113 114 115 116 117 118 119 120 122 123 125 129 130 131 134 137 140 142 143 144 145 146 147 **P**6
Primary Contact: Susan Croushore, President and Chief Executive Officer
COO: Victor DiPilla, Vice President and Chief Business Development Officer
CFO: Chris Bergman, Chief Financial Officer
CMO: Bernard B. Gawne, M.D., Vice President and Chief Medical Officer
CIO: Alex Vaillancourt, Chief Information Officer
CHR: Rick Tolson, Chief Administrative Officer and Chief Human Resources Officer
CNO: Deborah Marie Hayes, R.N., Chief Hospital Officer and Chief Nursing Officer
Web address: www.thechristhospital.com
**Control:** Other not–for–profit (including NFP Corporation) **Service:** General Medical and Surgical

**Staffed Beds:** 526 **Admissions:** 25343 **Census:** 305 **Outpatient Visits:** 273454 **Births:** 2987 **Total Expense ($000):** 532722 **Payroll Expense ($000):** 186188 **Personnel:** 2878

⊠ △ **CINCINNATI CHILDREN'S HOSPITAL MEDICAL CENTER (363300)**, 3333 Burnet Avenue, Zip 45229–3039; tel. 513/636–4200, (Includes DIVISION OF ADOLESCENT MEDICINE, CINCINNATI CENTER FOR DEVELOPMENTAL DISORDERS, AND CONVALESCENT HOSPITAL FOR CHILDREN ; CHILDREN'S HOSPITAL, Elland and Bethesda Avenues, Zip 45229) **A**1 2 3 5 7 8 9 10 **F**3 7 9 11 12 17 18 19 20 21 22 23 24 25 26 27 28 29 30 31 32 34 35 36 37 38 39 40 41 42 43 44 48 49 50 51 54 55 57 58 59 60 61 62 63 64 65 66 68 72 74 75 77 78 79 81 82 84 85 86 87 88 89 90 91 92 93 94 95 96 97 98 99 100 101 102 104 105 106 107 108 111 112 113 114 115 116 117 118 125 128 129 130 131 133 134 135 136 137 138 140 141 143 145 147 **P**1
Primary Contact: Michael Fisher, President and Chief Executive Officer
CFO: Scott J. Hamlin, Chief Financial Officer
CIO: Marianne Speight, Vice President Information System and Chief Information Officer
Web address: www.cincinnatichildrens.org
**Control:** Other not–for–profit (including NFP Corporation) **Service:** Children's general

**Staffed Beds:** 512 **Admissions:** 17844 **Census:** 339 **Outpatient Visits:** 1069416 **Births:** 11 **Total Expense ($000):** 1590503 **Payroll Expense ($000):** 797449 **Personnel:** 12996

⊠ △ **DRAKE CENTER (362004)**, 151 West Galbraith Road, Zip 45216–1015; tel. 513/418–2500, (Total facility includes 83 beds in nursing home–type unit) **A**1 3 5 7 10 **F**1 3 6 10 11 29 30 34 35 36 44 50 53 57 58 59 60 64 68 74 75 77 82 85 86 87 91 92 93 94 95 96 100 107 111 113 118 124 127 129 131 145 147 **P**5 **S** UC Health, Cincinnati, OH
Primary Contact: Debra C. Hampton, Ph.D., Vice President, Administration and Chief Nursing Officer
CFO: Duane Pifko, Interim Director Financial Services
CHR: Sharon Hancock, Director Human Resources
Web address: www.drakecenter.uchealth.com
**Control:** Other not–for–profit (including NFP Corporation) **Service:** Long–Term Acute Care hospital

**Staffed Beds:** 269 **Admissions:** 1948 **Census:** 156 **Outpatient Visits:** 41583 **Births:** 0 **Total Expense ($000):** 76546 **Payroll Expense ($000):** 37458 **Personnel:** 696

☐ **EVENDALE MEDICAL CENTER (360350)**, 3155 Glendale Milford Road, Zip 45241–3134; tel. 513/454–2222, (Nonreporting) **A**1 9
Primary Contact: Kelvin Hanger, Chief Executive Officer
Web address: www.evendalemedical.com
**Control:** Other not–for–profit (including NFP Corporation) **Service:** Other specialty

**Staffed Beds:** 29

⊠ △ **GOOD SAMARITAN HOSPITAL (360134)**, 375 Dixmyth Avenue, Zip 45220–2489; tel. 513/862–1400 **A**1 2 3 5 7 8 9 10 **F**2 3 5 6 9 11 12 13 15 17 18 20 22 24 26 28 29 30 31 34 35 36 37 38 39 40 41 42 44 45 46 47 48 49 50 53 54 55 56 57 58 59 60 61 63 64 65 66 68 70 71 72 74 75 76 77 78 79 81 82 84 85 86 87 90 91 92 93 94 96 97 98 99 100 101 102 103 104 105 106 107 108 110 111 113 114 115 116 117 118 120 122 125 128 129 130 131 133 134 140 142 143 144 145 146 147 **P**6 **S** Catholic Health Initiatives, Englewood, CO
Primary Contact: David Dornheggen, Chief Operating Officer
COO: Gerald P. Oliphant, Executive Vice President and Chief Operating Officer
CFO: Craig Rucker, Senior Vice President and Chief Financial Officer
CMO: Georges Feghali, M.D., Senior Vice President Quality and Chief Medical Officer
CIO: Rick Moore, Chief Information Officer
CHR: Walter L. McLarty, Chief Human Resources Officer
Web address: www.trihealth.com
**Control:** Church–operated, Nongovernment, not–for profit **Service:** General Medical and Surgical

**Staffed Beds:** 520 **Admissions:** 26833 **Census:** 352 **Outpatient Visits:** 206099 **Births:** 6596 **Total Expense ($000):** 440599 **Payroll Expense ($000):** 159160 **Personnel:** 2946

★ **HEALTHSOUTH REHABILITATION HOSPITAL AT DRAKE (363034)**, 151 West Galbraith Road, Zip 45216–1015; tel. 513/418–5600, (Nonreporting) **S** HEALTHSOUTH Corporation, Birmingham, AL
Primary Contact: Mark S. Brodeur, FACHE, Chief Executive Officer
CFO: Scott Corder, Controller
CMO: Mark Goddard, M.D., Medical Director
CHR: Jason Sparks, Director, Human Resources
CNO: Kathy McNally, Chief Nursing Officer
Web address: www.healthsouthatdrake.com
**Control:** Corporation, Investor–owned, for–profit **Service:** Rehabilitation

**Staffed Beds:** 40

⊠ **MERCY HOSPITAL ANDERSON (360001)**, 7500 State Road, Zip 45255–2492; tel. 513/624–4500, (Nonreporting) **A**1 2 9 10 **S** Catholic Health Partners, Cincinnati, OH
Primary Contact: Patricia A. Schroer, President and Chief Executive Officer
COO: Gyasi Chisley, Site Administrator and Chief Operating Officer
CFO: Deborah Bloomfield, Chief Financial Officer
CMO: Leonard M. Randolph, Jr., M.D., Senior Vice President and Chief Medical Officer
CIO: Matt Eversole, Regional Vice President Information Services
CHR: Maggie Lund, Divisional Senior Vice President Human Resources
Web address: www.e–mercy.com
**Control:** Church–operated, Nongovernment, not–for profit **Service:** General Medical and Surgical

**Staffed Beds:** 188

⊠ **MERCY HOSPITAL MOUNT AIRY (360234)**, 2446 Kipling Avenue, Zip 45239–6650; tel. 513/853–5000 **A**1 2 9 10 **F**3 11 12 15 18 20 28 29 30 31 34 37 40 45 46 49 50 51 56 57 58 59 60 64 68 70 74 75 77 78 79 81 82 84 85 87 90 91 92 98 99 106 107 108 110 111 113 114 115 117 118 129 145 146 147 **S** Catholic Health Partners, Cincinnati, OH
Primary Contact: Michael R. Stephens, President and Market Leader
CMO: Leonard M. Randolph, Jr., M.D., Senior Vice President and Divisional Chief Medical Officer
CIO: Yousuf Ahmad, Divisional Senior Vice President
CHR: Maggie Lund, Regional Vice President Human Resources
Web address: www.e–mercy.com
**Control:** Other not–for–profit (including NFP Corporation) **Service:** General Medical and Surgical

**Staffed Beds:** 170 **Admissions:** 6781 **Census:** 79 **Outpatient Visits:** 41274 **Births:** 0 **Total Expense ($000):** 74491 **Payroll Expense ($000):** 28864 **Personnel:** 592

⊠ **MERCY HOSPITAL WESTERN HILLS (360113)**, 3131 Queen City Avenue, Zip 45238–2396; tel. 513/389–5000 **A**1 2 9 10 **F**3 11 15 18 20 28 29 30 31 34 35 40 42 45 46 47 49 50 53 56 57 58 59 60 62 64 68 70 74 75 77 78 79 81 82 84 85 87 90 92 93 94 98 103 106 107 108 110 111 113 114 117 118 129 145 146 **S** Catholic Health Partners, Cincinnati, OH
Primary Contact: Michael R. Stephens, President and Market Leader
Web address: www.e–mercy.com
**Control:** Other not–for–profit (including NFP Corporation) **Service:** General Medical and Surgical

**Staffed Beds:** 156 **Admissions:** 6753 **Census:** 84 **Outpatient Visits:** 59836 **Total Expense ($000):** 74039 **Payroll Expense ($000):** 32750 **Personnel:** 602

---

**Hospital, Medicare Provider Number, Address, Telephone, Approval, Facility, and Physician Codes, Health Care System**

★ American Hospital Association (AHA) membership
☐ The Joint Commission accreditation   ◇ DNV Healthcare Inc. accreditation
◯ American Osteopathic Association (AOA) accreditation
△ Commission on Accreditation of Rehabilitation Facilities (CARF) accreditation

OH

✠ **REGENCY HOSPITAL OF CINCINNATI (362034)**, 311 Straight Street, Zip 45219; tel. 513/559–5900, (Nonreporting) **A**1 10 **S** Select Medical Corporation, Mechanicsburg, PA
Primary Contact: Angie Holden, Chief Executive Officer
CMO: Sunil Dama, M.D., Medical Director
CHR: Elizabeth M. Wilson, Coordinator Human Resources
Web address: www.regencyhospital.com
**Control:** Corporation, Investor–owned, for–profit **Service:** Long–Term Acute Care hospital

| Staffed Beds: 31 |
|---|

✠ **SELECT SPECIALTY HOSPITAL–CINCINNATI (362019)**, 375 Dixmyth Avenue, Zip 45220; tel. 513/872–4444, (Nonreporting) **A**1 9 10 **S** Select Medical Corporation, Mechanicsburg, PA
Primary Contact: Salvatore Iweimrin, R.N., Chief Executive Officer
Web address: www.selectmedicalcorp.com
**Control:** Corporation, Investor–owned, for–profit **Service:** Long–Term Acute Care hospital

| Staffed Beds: 35 |
|---|

☐ **SHRINERS HOSPITALS FOR CHILDREN, SHRINERS BURNS HOSPITAL, CINCINNATI (363308)**, 3229 Burnet Avenue, Zip 45229–3095; tel. 513/872–6000, (Nonreporting) **A**1 10 **S** Shriners Hospitals for Children, Tampa, FL
Primary Contact: Ronald R. Hitzler, Administrator
CFO: James Lester, Director Fiscal Services
CMO: Richard J. Kagan, M.D., Chief of Staff
CIO: Mark Washam, Chief Information Officer
CHR: Sally Skillman, Director Human Resources
Web address: www.shrinershq.org
**Control:** Other not–for–profit (including NFP Corporation) **Service:** Children's other specialty

| Staffed Beds: 30 |
|---|

✠ **SUMMIT BEHAVIORAL HEALTHCARE (364035)**, 1101 Summit Road, Zip 45237–2652; tel. 513/948–3600, (Nonreporting) **A**1 9 10 **S** Ohio Department of Mental Health, Columbus, OH
Primary Contact: Elizabeth Banks, Chief Executive Officer
COO: Jeff Amend, Chief Operating Officer
CFO: Steven Burns, Director Fiscal Services
CMO: Lawrence Ostrowski, M.D., Chief Clinical Officer
CIO: Eric Bradley, Director Computer Information Services
CHR: Rhonda Milton, Director Human Resources
Web address: www.mh.state.oh.us/
**Control:** State–Government, nonfederal **Service:** Psychiatric

| Staffed Beds: 284 |
|---|

✠ **THE JEWISH HOSPITAL (360016)**, 4777 East Galbraith Road, Zip 45236–2725; tel. 513/686–3000 **A**1 2 3 5 9 10 **F**3 11 12 15 18 20 22 24 26 28 29 30 31 33 34 35 37 39 40 45 46 47 49 50 60 64 66 68 70 74 75 78 79 81 82 84 85 87 91 92 93 97 100 107 108 110 111 114 117 118 119 122 123 125 129 130 131 134 135 145 **P**6 **S** Catholic Health Partners, Cincinnati, OH
Primary Contact: Steve Holman, President
COO: Pam VanSant, Vice President and Chief Operating Officer
Web address: www.jewishhospitalcincinnati.com/
**Control:** Other not–for–profit (including NFP Corporation) **Service:** General Medical and Surgical

| Staffed Beds: 209 Admissions: 11403 Census: 136 Outpatient Visits: 90312 Total Expense ($000): 185281 Payroll Expense ($000): 68659 Personnel: 1162 |
|---|

✠ **UNIVERSITY HOSPITAL (360003)**, 234 Goodman Street, Zip 45219–2316; tel. 513/584–1000 **A**1 2 3 5 8 10 **F**3 6 7 9 11 12 13 15 16 17 18 20 22 24 26 28 29 30 31 34 35 36 37 38 39 40 43 44 45 46 47 48 49 50 52 53 54 55 56 57 58 59 60 61 63 64 66 68 70 71 72 74 75 76 77 78 79 80 81 82 84 85 86 87 92 93 94 97 98 100 101 102 103 104 107 108 110 111 112 113 114 115 116 117 118 119 120 122 123 125 129 130 131 133 137 138 140 141 142 145 146 147 **S** UC Health, Cincinnati, OH
Primary Contact: W. Brian Gibler, M.D., President and Chief Executive Officer
COO: Nancy Barone, Vice President and Executive Director Operations and Strategic Planning
CFO: Doug Arvin, Vice President Financial Services
CMO: Robert Wones, M.D., Vice President and Associate Chief of Staff
CIO: Jay Brown, Vice President and Chief Information Officer
CHR: Clarence Pauley, Vice President Human Resources
Web address: www.universityhospital.uchealth.com
**Control:** Other not–for–profit (including NFP Corporation) **Service:** General Medical and Surgical

| Staffed Beds: 466 Admissions: 30079 Census: 390 Outpatient Visits: 314416 Births: 2484 Total Expense ($000): 629246 Payroll Expense ($000): 219057 Personnel: 4097 |
|---|

✠ △ **VETERANS AFFAIRS MEDICAL CENTER**, 3200 Vine Street, Zip 45220–2288; tel. 513/475–6300, (Total facility includes 64 beds in nursing home–type unit) **A**1 2 3 5 7 8 **F**1 3 4 5 8 12 15 18 20 22 24 26 28 29 30 31 33 34 35 36 37 38 39 40 42 44 45 46 47 48 50 51 53 54 55 56 57 58 59 60 61 62 63 64 65 68 70 71 74 75 77 78 79 81 82 83 84 85 86 87 91 92 93 94 97 98 100 101 102 103 104 105 106 107 108 111 113 114 115 116 118 125 126 128 129 131 134 142 143 144 145 146 147 **S** Department of Veterans Affairs, Washington, DC
Primary Contact: Linda D. Smith, Director
COO: David Ninneman, Associate Director
CFO: Sandra Selvidge, Chief Fiscal Service
CMO: Robert E. Falcone, M.D., Chief of Staff
CIO: Vique Caro, Chief Information Officer
CHR: Sandra Stenger, Acting Chief Human Resources
CNO: Katheryn Cook, R.N., Nurse Executive
Web address: www.cincinnati.va.gov/
**Control:** Veterans Affairs, Government, federal **Service:** General Medical and Surgical

| Staffed Beds: 269 Admissions: 6182 Census: 224 Outpatient Visits: 520717 Births: 0 Total Expense ($000): 180682 Payroll Expense ($000): 141065 Personnel: 1984 |
|---|

**CIRCLEVILLE—Pickaway County**

✠ **BERGER HEALTH SYSTEM (360170)**, 600 North Pickaway Street, Zip 43113–1447; tel. 740/474–2126 **A**1 5 9 10 **F**3 13 15 18 22 28 29 30 31 32 34 35 36 40 45 49 50 51 54 56 57 59 60 63 64 65 68 70 74 75 76 77 78 79 80 81 82 85 86 87 90 92 93 107 108 110 111 113 114 115 116 118 123 128 129 130 131 134 142 144 145 146 147
Primary Contact: Tim Colburn, President and Chief Executive Officer
CFO: Tom Scherer, Interim Vice President Finance
CMO: Brett Call, D.O., Chief of Staff
CIO: Andy Chileski, Chief Information Officer and Vice President Facilities
CHR: Suzanne Welker, Chief Human Resources Officer and Vice President Marketing Strategy
CNO: Brenda M. Strittmatter, Patient Services Officer
Web address: www.bergerhealth.com
**Control:** City–County, Government, nonfederal **Service:** General Medical and Surgical

| Staffed Beds: 79 Admissions: 2709 Census: 27 Outpatient Visits: 105688 Births: 367 Total Expense ($000): 66125 Payroll Expense ($000): 22111 Personnel: 498 |
|---|

**CLEVELAND—Cuyahoga County**

**CLEVELAND CAMPUS** See Northcoast Behavioral Healthcare System, Northfield

✠ △ **CLEVELAND CLINIC CHILDREN'S HOSPITAL FOR REHABILITATION (363304)**, 2801 Martin Luther King Jr. Drive, Zip 44104–3865; tel. 216/448–6400 **A**1 7 9 10 **F**16 28 29 30 32 34 35 36 50 57 60 68 69 74 75 80 82 86 89 90 93 94 96 100 129 131 142 145 147 **S** Cleveland Clinic Health System, Cleveland, OH
Primary Contact: Michael J. McHugh, M.D., Medical Director
COO: Alec G. Kulik, Administrator
CFO: Debra Nyikes, Director Finance and Chief Financial Officer
CMO: Roberta Bauer, M.D., Acting Chair Medical Staff
CIO: C. Martin Harris, M.D., Chief Information Officer
CHR: Jan Hlahol, Manager Human Resources
Web address: www.clevelandclinic.org/childrenshospital
**Control:** Other not–for–profit (including NFP Corporation) **Service:** Children's rehabilitation

| Staffed Beds: 25 Admissions: 227 Census: 14 Outpatient Visits: 51924 Births: 0 Total Expense ($000): 29942 Payroll Expense ($000): 17238 Personnel: 312 |
|---|

✠ △ **CLEVELAND CLINIC FOUNDATION (360180)**, 9500 Euclid Avenue, Zip 44195–5108; tel. 216/444–2200, (Includes CLEVELAND CLINIC CHILDREN'S HOSPITAL, 9500 Euclid Avenue, Zip 44103; tel. 800/223–2273) **A**1 3 5 7 8 9 10 **F**3 4 5 7 8 9 12 14 15 17 18 19 20 21 22 23 24 25 26 27 28 29 30 31 32 33 34 35 36 37 38 39 40 44 45 46 47 48 49 50 51 52 53 54 55 56 57 58 59 60 61 62 63 64 65 66 68 70 71 72 73 74 75 76 77 78 79 80 81 82 83 84 85 86 87 88 89 90 91 92 93 94 96 97 100 101 102 103 104 105 107 108 109 110 111 112 113 114 115 116 117 118 119 120 122 123 125 126 128 129 130 131 133 134 135 136 137 138 139 140 141 142 143 144 145 146 147 **P**6 **S** Cleveland Clinic Health System, Cleveland, OH
Primary Contact: Delos Cosgrove, M.D., President and Chief Executive Officer
CFO: Steven Glass, Chief Financial Officer
CMO: Joseph Hahn, M.D., Chief of Staff
CIO: C. Martin Harris, M.D., Chief Information Officer
CHR: Joseph Patrnchak, Chief Human Resources Officer
Web address: www.clevelandclinic.org
**Control:** Other not–for–profit (including NFP Corporation) **Service:** General Medical and Surgical

| Staffed Beds: 1267 Admissions: 52885 Census: 941 Outpatient Visits: 4311183 Births: 17 Total Expense ($000): 3534147 Payroll Expense ($000): 1884718 Personnel: 26731 |
|---|

*Many Facility Codes have changed. Please refer to the AHA Guide Code Chart.* © 2012 AHA Guide

✠ **FAIRVIEW HOSPITAL (360077)**, 18101 Lorain Avenue, Zip 44111–5656;
tel. 216/476–7000, (Total facility includes 11 beds in nursing home–type unit) **A**1
2 3 5 9 10 13 **F**2 8 13 15 17 18 19 20 22 24 26 28 29 30 31 32 34 35 40
41 43 45 46 49 50 51 53 56 57 58 59 60 64 65 66 68 70 71 72 74 75 76
78 79 81 82 85 86 87 89 92 93 97 98 99 102 107 108 110 111 113 114
115 116 117 118 119 120 125 127 129 130 131 134 142 145 146
**S** Cleveland Clinic Health System, Cleveland, OH
Primary Contact: Janice Murphy, President
COO: John C. Mills, Senior Vice President Operations
CFO: Ankit Chhabra, Director Finance
CMO: Neil Smith, M.D., Chief Medical Officer
CIO: C. Martin Harris, M.D., Chief Information Officer
CHR: Ann Beatty, Director Human Resources
CNO: Deborah C. Small, R.N., Chief Nursing Officer
Web address: www.fairviewhospital.org
**Control:** Other not–for–profit (including NFP Corporation) **Service:** General
Medical and Surgical

**Staffed Beds: 375 Admissions: 21755 Census: 275 Outpatient Visits:**
273828 **Births:** 4156 **Total Expense ($000):** 310523 **Payroll Expense
($000):** 135938 **Personnel:** 1978

**GRACE HOSPITAL (362015)**, 2307 West 14th Street, Zip 44113–3698;
tel. 216/687–1500, (Nonreporting) **A**10
Primary Contact: Rajive Khanna, Chief Executive Officer
COO: Rajive Khanna, Chief Executive Officer
CMO: John Nickels, M.D., President Medical Staff
CIO: Mary Zimpfer, Vice President Quality Management
Web address: www.gracehospital.org
**Control:** Other not–for–profit (including NFP Corporation) **Service:** Long–Term
Acute Care hospital

**Staffed Beds: 87**

**HANNA HOUSE SKILLED NURSING FACILITY** See University Hospitals Case
Medical Center

✠ **HILLCREST HOSPITAL (360230)**, 6780 Mayfield Road, Zip 44124–2202;
tel. 440/312–4500 **A**1 2 9 10 **F**3 11 13 15 17 18 20 22 24 26 28 29 30 31
34 35 38 40 41 43 46 49 50 51 55 57 59 60 64 65 68 69 70 72 74 75 76
77 78 79 81 82 84 85 86 89 93 97 100 107 108 110 111 113 114 115 116
118 119 120 125 128 129 130 131 134 142 144 145 146 147 **S** Cleveland
Clinic Health System, Cleveland, OH
Primary Contact: Jeffrey A. Leimgruber, President
Web address: www.hillcresthospital.org
**Control:** Other not–for–profit (including NFP Corporation) **Service:** General
Medical and Surgical

**Staffed Beds: 406 Admissions: 20983 Census: 273 Outpatient Visits:**
233058 **Births:** 3544 **Total Expense ($000):** 307256 **Payroll Expense
($000):** 119983 **Personnel:** 1926

✠ **KINDRED HOSPITAL CLEVELAND–GATEWAY (362026)**, 2351 East 22nd
Street, 7th Floor, Zip 44115; tel. 216/363–2671, (Includes KINDRED HOSPITAL
OF CLEVELAND, 11900 Fairhill Road, Zip 44120–1062; tel. 216/983–8030;
Steve Jakubcanin, Executive Director), (Nonreporting) **A**1 10 **S** Kindred
Healthcare, Louisville, KY
Primary Contact: Ian Cooper, Chief Executive Officer
Web address: www.kindredgateway.com
**Control:** Corporation, Investor–owned, for–profit **Service:** Long–Term Acute Care
hospital

**Staffed Beds: 153**

**KINDRED HOSPITAL OF CLEVELAND** See Kindred Hospital Cleveland–Gateway

✠ **LUTHERAN HOSPITAL (360087)**, 1730 West 25th Street, Zip 44113–3170;
tel. 216/696–4300 **A**1 9 10 **F**3 9 15 29 30 34 37 40 50 56 57 58 59 60 65
70 74 75 77 79 81 82 85 86 87 93 98 103 104 107 111 113 118 128 129
130 131 134 142 145 147 **S** Cleveland Clinic Health System, Cleveland, OH
Primary Contact: Brian Donley, M.D., President
COO: Kris Bennett, Chief Operating Officer
CFO: Don Urbancsik, Director Finance
CMO: Ronald Golovan, M.D., Vice President Medical Operations
CIO: C. Martin Harris, M.D., Chief Information Officer
CHR: Sheree Laborie, Director Human Resources
CNO: Denise Minor, R.N., Chief Nursing Officer
Web address: www.lutheranhospital.org
**Control:** Other not–for–profit (including NFP Corporation) **Service:** General
Medical and Surgical

**Staffed Beds: 182 Admissions: 6856 Census: 99 Outpatient Visits: 57567
Births:** 0 **Total Expense ($000):** 83409 **Payroll Expense ($000):** 38306
**Personnel:** 612

✠ △ **METROHEALTH MEDICAL CENTER (360059)**, 2500 MetroHealth Drive,
Zip 44109–1998; tel. 216/778–7800, (Total facility includes 294 beds in nursing
home–type unit) **A**1 2 3 5 7 8 9 10 13 **F**3 5 6 7 8 9 11 12 13 15 16 17 18 19
20 22 24 26 27 28 29 30 31 32 34 35 36 38 39 40 43 44 45 46 47 49 50
51 52 53 54 55 56 57 58 59 60 61 63 64 65 66 68 70 71 72 74 75 76 77
78 79 80 81 82 83 84 85 86 87 88 89 90 91 92 93 94 95 96 97 98 99 100
101 102 103 104 105 107 108 110 111 113 114 115 116 117 118 120 122
127 128 129 130 131 133 134 142 143 145 146 147 **P**6
Primary Contact: Mark J. Moran, President and Chief Executive Officer
COO: Edward Hills, D.D.S., Interim Chief Operating Officer
CFO: Jeffrey Rooney, Chief Financial Officer
CMO: Alfred Connors, Senior Vice President Medical Affairs and Chief Medical
Officer
CIO: James Schlesinger, Interim Chief Information Officer
CHR: Debbie Warman, Vice President Human Resources
CNO: Mavis Bechtle, MSN, Vice President and Chief Nursing Officer
Web address: www.metrohealth.org
**Control:** County–Government, nonfederal **Service:** General Medical and Surgical

**Staffed Beds: 861 Admissions: 25577 Census: 602 Outpatient Visits:**
965800 **Births:** 2879 **Total Expense ($000):** 658260 **Payroll Expense
($000):** 410710 **Personnel:** 5226

**RAINBOW BABIES AND CHILDREN'S HOSPITAL** See University Hospitals Case
Medical Center

✠ **REGENCY HOSPITAL CLEVELAND EAST (362029)**, 4200 Interchange
Corporate Center Road, Zip 44128–5631; tel. 216/910–3800, (Includes
REGENCY HOSPITAL OF AKRON, 155 Fifth Street N.E., Barberton, Zip 44203;
tel. 330/615–3792; Timothy Rolsen, Chief Executive Officer; REGENCY HOSPITAL
OF CLEVELAND – WEST, 6990 Engle Road, Middleburg Heights,
Zip 44130–3420; tel. 440/202–4200; Barbara Wojtala, Chief Executive Officer;
REGENCY HOSPITAL OF RAVENNA, 6847 North Chestnut Street, Ravenna,
Zip 44266; tel. 330/296–2350; Timothy Rolsen, Chief Executive Officer),
(Nonreporting) **A**1 10 **S** Select Medical Corporation, Mechanicsburg, PA
Primary Contact: Barbara Wojtala, Chief Executive Officer
Web address: www.regencyhospital.com/
**Control:** Corporation, Investor–owned, for–profit **Service:** Long–Term Acute Care
hospital

**Staffed Beds: 44**

**SAINT LUKE'S MEDICAL CENTER** See St. Vincent Charity Medical Center

☐ **ST. VINCENT CHARITY MEDICAL CENTER (360037)**, 2351 East 22nd Street,
Zip 44115–3111; tel. 216/861–6200, (Includes SAINT LUKE'S MEDICAL CENTER,
11311 Shaker Boulevard, Zip 44104–3805; tel. 216/368–7000) **A**1 2 5 9 10 **F**3
4 5 12 15 17 18 20 22 24 28 29 30 31 33 34 35 37 39 40 42 45 50 54 56
57 59 60 61 62 64 65 66 68 70 71 74 75 77 78 79 81 82 84 85 86 87 93
97 98 100 102 103 107 108 110 113 117 118 129 145 147 **P**4 **S** Sisters of
Charity Health System, Cleveland, OH
Primary Contact: David Perse, M.D., President
COO: Beverly Lozar, Vice President Professional and Support Services
CFO: Matthew Rish, Vice President Finance
CIO: Robin Stursa, Chief Information Officer
CHR: Gary Lazroff, Vice President Human Resources
Web address: www.svch.net
**Control:** Other not–for–profit (including NFP Corporation) **Service:** General
Medical and Surgical

**Staffed Beds: 203 Admissions: 7446 Census: 101 Outpatient Visits:**
154154 **Births:** 0 **Total Expense ($000):** 141270 **Payroll Expense ($000):**
56503 **Personnel:** 1057

✠ **UNIVERSITY HOSPITALS BEDFORD MEDICAL CENTER (360115)**, 44 Blaine
Avenue, Zip 44146–2709; tel. 440/735–3900 **A**1 2 10 **F**8 14 15 20 29 34 35
40 43 44 49 50 57 59 60 65 66 68 69 70 75 77 79 81 82 86 87 89 93 96
97 107 108 109 110 111 113 115 116 117 118 128 129 131 132 134 142
145 146 147 **S** University Hospitals, Cleveland, OH
Primary Contact: Laurie Delgado, President
COO: Michelle Giltner, Director Professional and Support Staff Services
CFO: Gigi Umbel, Director Finance
CMO: Marwan Hilal, M.D., Chief Medical Officer
CNO: James Williams, Chief Nursing Officer
Web address: www.uhbedford.org
**Control:** Other not–for–profit (including NFP Corporation) **Service:** General
Medical and Surgical

**Staffed Beds: 77 Admissions: 3489 Census: 43 Outpatient Visits: 80378
Births:** 0 **Total Expense ($000):** 46816 **Payroll Expense ($000):** 20900
**Personnel:** 335

⊠ **UNIVERSITY HOSPITALS CASE MEDICAL CENTER (360137)**, 11100 Euclid Avenue, Zip 44106–2602; tel. 216/844–1000, (Includes ALFRED AND NORMA LERNER TOWER, BOLWELL HEALTH CENTER, HANNA PAVILION, LAKESIDE HOSPITAL, SAMUEL MATHER PAVILION ; HANNA HOUSE SKILLED NURSING FACILITY, 11100 Euclid Avenue, Zip 44106; RAINBOW BABIES AND CHILDREN'S HOSPITAL, 2074 Abington Road, Zip 44106; tel. 216/844–3911; UNIVERSITY MACDONALD WOMEN'S HOSPITAL, Abington Road, Zip 44106), (Total facility includes 38 beds in nursing home–type unit) **A**1 2 3 5 8 9 10 **F**2 3 5 6 8 9 10 11 12 13 14 15 17 18 19 20 21 22 23 24 25 26 27 28 29 30 31 32 34 35 36 37 38 39 40 41 42 43 44 45 46 47 48 49 50 51 52 53 54 55 56 57 58 59 60 61 62 64 65 66 68 70 71 72 73 74 75 76 77 78 79 81 82 83 84 85 86 87 89 90 91 92 93 94 96 97 98 99 100 101 102 103 104 105 107 108 109 110 111 112 113 114 115 116 117 118 119 120 122 123 125 127 128 129 130 131 133 134 135 136 137 138 139 140 141 142 143 144 145 146 147 **S** University Hospitals, Cleveland, OH
Primary Contact: Fred C. Rothstein, M.D., President
COO: Ron Dziedzicki, R.N., Chief Support Services Officer
CFO: Sonia Salvino, Vice President Finance
CMO: Michael Anderson, M.D., Chief Medical Officer
CHR: Julie Chester, Director Human Resources
Web address: www.UHhospitals.org
**Control:** Other not–for–profit (including NFP Corporation) **Service:** General Medical and Surgical

**Staffed Beds:** 777 **Admissions:** 39056 **Census:** 630 **Outpatient Visits:** 1113710 **Births:** 3692 **Total Expense ($000):** 1074186 **Payroll Expense ($000):** 411052 **Personnel:** 7296

⊠ ○ **UNIVERSITY HOSPITALS RICHMOND MEDICAL CENTER (360075)**, 27100 Chardon Road, Zip 44143–1116; tel. 440/585–6500 **A**1 9 10 11 12 13 **F**3 8 15 18 20 26 29 34 35 40 47 48 49 50 51 59 60 64 67 68 70 74 75 77 79 81 82 85 87 90 91 92 93 100 102 105 107 111 115 117 118 128 129 145 147 **P**5 **S** University Hospitals, Cleveland, OH
Primary Contact: Laurie Delgado, President
CFO: Scott Platz, Director Finance
CMO: Rosemary Lienung, M.D., Chief Medical Officer
CHR: Stephanie W. Neonakis, Manager
Web address: www.uhrichmond.org
**Control:** Other not–for–profit (including NFP Corporation) **Service:** General Medical and Surgical

**Staffed Beds:** 60 **Admissions:** 3224 **Census:** 36 **Outpatient Visits:** 57454 **Births:** 0 **Total Expense ($000):** 55493 **Payroll Expense ($000):** 23521 **Personnel:** 407

⊠ △ **VETERANS AFFAIRS MEDICAL CENTER**, 10701 East Boulevard, Zip 44106–1702; tel. 216/791–3800, (Total facility includes 160 beds in nursing home–type unit) **A**1 2 3 5 7 8 **F**1 2 3 4 5 6 7 8 9 10 11 12 15 17 18 20 22 24 26 28 29 30 31 34 35 36 37 38 39 40 42 44 45 46 47 48 49 50 51 54 56 57 58 59 60 61 62 63 64 65 66 67 68 70 71 74 75 77 78 79 80 81 82 83 84 85 86 87 90 91 92 93 94 95 96 97 98 100 101 102 103 104 105 106 107 108 110 111 112 113 114 115 116 117 118 119 120 122 127 128 129 131 134 142 143 145 146 147 **S** Department of Veterans Affairs, Washington, DC
Primary Contact: Susan Fuehrer, Director
COO: Sean Nelson, Deputy Director
CFO: Gene DeAngelis, Chief Fiscal Service
CMO: Murray Altose, M.D., Chief of Staff
CIO: Steve Gaj, Facility Chief Information Officer
CHR: Charles Franks, Chief Human Resources
Web address: www.va.gov/sta/guide/home.asp
**Control:** Veterans Affairs, Government, federal **Service:** General Medical and Surgical

**Staffed Beds:** 592 **Admissions:** 11308 **Census:** 524 **Outpatient Visits:** 1412760 **Births:** 0 **Total Expense ($000):** 809785 **Payroll Expense ($000):** 325648 **Personnel:** 4510

**COLDWATER—Mercer County**

⊠ **MERCER COUNTY JOINT TOWNSHIP COMMUNITY HOSPITAL (360058)**, 800 West Main Street, Zip 45828–1698; tel. 419/678–2341 **A**1 9 10 **F**3 7 11 12 13 15 18 28 29 30 31 34 35 40 42 44 45 47 50 51 54 55 57 59 61 62 64 65 68 70 75 76 77 78 79 81 82 85 87 92 93 94 97 107 108 110 111 113 117 118 129 130 131 132 133 134 142 143 144 145 146 147 **P**3
Primary Contact: Paula J. Detterman, FACHE, Chief Executive Officer
CFO: George Boyles, Vice President Finance and Chief Financial Officer
CMO: Craig Dues, D.O., Chief Medical Officer
CIO: Kyle Rindler, Director Information Systems
CHR: Ed Sweetnich, Director Human Resources
CNO: Lisa R. Klenke, R.N., Vice President Patient Care Services
Web address: www.mercer–health.com
**Control:** Hospital district or authority, Government, nonfederal **Service:** General Medical and Surgical

**Staffed Beds:** 60 **Admissions:** 1932 **Census:** 13 **Outpatient Visits:** 65453 **Births:** 336 **Total Expense ($000):** 41532 **Payroll Expense ($000):** 16391 **Personnel:** 384

**COLUMBUS—Franklin County**

⊠ ○ **DOCTORS HOSPITAL (360152)**, 5100 West Broad Street, Zip 43228–1607; tel. 614/544–1000 **A**1 2 9 10 11 12 13 **F**3 15 17 18 20 22 24 26 28 29 30 31 40 42 45 46 47 48 49 50 64 65 66 68 70 73 74 75 76 77 78 79 81 82 85 87 92 93 97 100 101 102 107 108 110 111 113 114 118 119 120 125 129 130 134 144 145 146 **P**1 3 5 7 **S** OhioHealth, Columbus, OH
Primary Contact: Michael L. Reichfield, President
CFO: Troy Hammett, Vice President and Chief Financial Officer
CMO: Dean Colwell, D.O., Vice President Medical Affairs
CIO: Michael Krouse, Chief Information Officer
CHR: David Sullivan, Director Human Resources
Web address: www.ohiohealth.com
**Control:** Church–operated, Nongovernment, not–for profit **Service:** General Medical and Surgical

**Staffed Beds:** 213 **Admissions:** 9480 **Census:** 106 **Outpatient Visits:** 281025 **Births:** 875 **Total Expense ($000):** 200376 **Payroll Expense ($000):** 99934 **Personnel:** 1260

⊠ **GRANT MEDICAL CENTER (360017)**, 111 South Grant Avenue, Zip 43215–1898; tel. 614/566–9000 **A**1 2 8 9 10 **F**3 7 8 9 11 13 15 17 18 20 22 24 26 28 29 30 31 34 35 36 37 40 42 43 45 46 47 48 49 50 53 54 56 57 58 59 60 61 64 66 67 68 70 72 74 75 76 78 79 81 82 83 84 85 86 87 97 100 102 107 108 109 110 111 113 114 115 116 118 119 120 122 123 125 128 129 130 131 134 142 143 145 146 147 **P**1 3 5 7 **S** OhioHealth, Columbus, OH
Primary Contact: Vinson Yates, President
COO: Michael Lawson, Senior Vice President Operations
CMO: Greg Morrison, M.D., Vice President Medical Affairs
CIO: Michael Krouse, Chief Information Officer
CHR: Linda Simpson, Vice President Human Resources
CNO: Donna Hanly, R.N., Senior Vice President and Chief Nursing Officer
Web address: www.ohiohealth.com
**Control:** Church–operated, Nongovernment, not–for profit **Service:** General Medical and Surgical

**Staffed Beds:** 392 **Admissions:** 22199 **Census:** 243 **Outpatient Visits:** 614590 **Births:** 2532 **Total Expense ($000):** 467542 **Payroll Expense ($000):** 218615 **Personnel:** 2518

⊠ **JAMES CANCER HOSPITAL AND SOLOVE RESEARCH INSTITUTE (360242)**, 300 West Tenth Avenue, Zip 43210–1240; tel. 614/293–3300 **A**1 2 3 5 8 9 10 **F**3 7 15 29 30 31 32 34 35 36 37 38 39 44 46 47 48 49 50 52 54 55 57 58 59 61 62 64 66 68 70 71 74 75 77 78 79 81 82 84 85 86 87 93 97 100 107 108 110 111 112 113 114 115 116 117 118 119 120 122 123 125 129 131 133 134 135 140 142 143 144 145 146 147 **P**6 **S** Ohio State University Health System, Columbus, OH
Primary Contact: Michael Caligiuri, Chief Executive Officer
COO: Dennis J. Smith, Chief Operating Officer
CFO: Bell Julian, Associate Executive Director and Chief Financial Officer
CIO: Twyla Pohar, Manager Computer Systems
CHR: Jill Hannah, Director Human Resources
Web address: www.jamesline.com
**Control:** State–Government, nonfederal **Service:** Cancer

**Staffed Beds:** 209 **Admissions:** 10368 **Census:** 178 **Outpatient Visits:** 239155 **Births:** 0 **Total Expense ($000):** 470459 **Payroll Expense ($000):** 113504 **Personnel:** 2432

⊠ △ **MOUNT CARMEL (360035)**, 793 West State Street, Zip 43222–1551; tel. 614/234–5000, (Includes MOUNT CARMEL EAST HOSPITAL, 6001 East Broad Street, Zip 43213; tel. 614/234–6000; Claus von Zychlin, President; MOUNT CARMEL WEST HOSPITAL, 793 West State Street, Zip 43222; tel. 614/234–5000; Sean McKibben, President and CEO) **A**1 2 3 5 7 9 10 **F**3 11 12 13 15 17 18 20 22 24 26 29 30 31 34 35 37 40 43 44 45 46 47 48 49 50 54 55 57 58 59 61 63 64 65 66 68 70 72 74 75 76 78 79 81 83 84 85 86 87 90 92 94 96 97 98 100 101 102 103 104 107 108 109 110 111 113 114 115 116 117 118 119 120 122 125 129 130 131 144 145 146 147 **P**6 8 **S** Trinity Health, Novi, MI
Primary Contact: Claus von Zychlin, President and Chief Executive Officer
COO: Mary R. Trimmer, Interim Chief Operating Officer
CFO: Russell W. Gardner, Chief Financial Officer
CIO: Cindy Sheets, Chief Information Officer
Web address: www.mountcarmelhealth.com
**Control:** Church–operated, Nongovernment, not–for profit **Service:** General Medical and Surgical

**Staffed Beds:** 729 **Admissions:** 38355 **Census:** 458 **Outpatient Visits:** 432586 **Births:** 3453 **Total Expense ($000):** 619242 **Payroll Expense ($000):** 205826 **Personnel:** 4899

**OH**

☒ △ **NATIONWIDE CHILDREN'S HOSPITAL (363305)**, 700 Children's Drive, Zip 43205–2696; tel. 614/722–2000 **A**1 3 5 7 8 9 10 **F**3 7 8 12 16 17 18 19 20 21 22 23 24 25 26 27 28 29 30 31 32 34 35 38 39 40 41 43 44 45 48 50 53 54 55 57 58 59 60 61 62 63 64 65 66 68 71 72 74 75 77 78 79 81 82 83 84 85 86 87 88 89 90 92 93 97 99 100 101 102 104 107 108 111 112 113 114 117 118 128 129 130 131 132 133 134 135 136 137 139 140 142 143 145 147 **P**6 8
Primary Contact: Steve Allen, M.D., Chief Executive Officer
COO: Rick Miller, President and Chief Operating Officer
CFO: Tim Robinson, Executive Vice President, Chief Financial and Administrative Officer and Treasurer
CMO: Richard Brilli, M.D., Chief Medical Officer
CIO: Denise Zabawski, Vice President Information Services and Chief Information Officer
CHR: Jose Balderrama, Vice President Human Resources
Web address: www.nationwidechildrens.org
**Control:** Other not–for–profit (including NFP Corporation) **Service:** Children's general

**Staffed Beds:** 451 **Admissions:** 20434 **Census:** 331 **Outpatient Visits:** 952937 **Births:** 0 **Total Expense ($000):** 538190 **Payroll Expense ($000):** 324939 **Personnel:** 5965

☐ **OHIO HOSPITAL FOR CHILD AND ADOLESCENT PSYCHIATRY (364041)**, 880 Greenlawn Avenue, Zip 43223–2616; tel. 614/449–9664 **A**1 9 10 **F**98 99 103 105 **S** Behavioral Centers of America, Nashville, TN
Primary Contact: Roxanne Jividen, Chief Executive Officer
Web address: www.bca–corp.com
**Control:** Corporation, Investor–owned, for–profit **Service:** Psychiatric

**Staffed Beds:** 68 **Admissions:** 2702 **Census:** 62 **Outpatient Visits:** 3567 **Births:** 0 **Total Expense ($000):** 12317 **Payroll Expense ($000):** 5514 **Personnel:** 178

☒ △ **OHIO STATE UNIVERSITY MEDICAL CENTER (360085)**, 370 West 9th Avenue, Zip 43210–1240; tel. 614/293–8000, (Includes OHIO STATE UNIVERSITY HOSPITALS EAST, 1492 East Broad Street, Zip 43205–1546; tel. 614/257–3000) **A**1 3 5 7 8 9 10 **F**3 4 5 6 7 8 9 11 12 13 15 16 17 18 20 22 24 26 28 29 30 31 33 34 35 36 37 38 39 40 43 44 45 46 47 48 49 50 51 52 53 54 55 56 57 58 59 60 61 62 64 65 66 68 70 72 73 74 75 76 77 78 79 80 81 82 84 85 86 87 90 91 92 93 94 95 96 97 98 99 100 101 102 103 104 105 107 108 110 111 112 113 114 117 118 125 128 129 130 131 133 134 136 137 138 140 141 142 143 144 145 146 147 **P**6 **S** Ohio State University Health System, Columbus, OH
Primary Contact: Peter E. Geier, Chief Executive Officer
COO: Jay D. Kasey, Chief Operating Officer
CFO: Michael Rutherford, Chief Financial Officer
CMO: Hagop Mekhjian, M.D., Medical Director
CIO: Herb Smaltz, Chief Information Officer
CHR: Les Ridout, Human Resources Officer
Web address: www.osumedcenter.edu
**Control:** State–Government, nonfederal **Service:** General Medical and Surgical

**Staffed Beds:** 976 **Admissions:** 46501 **Census:** 723 **Outpatient Visits:** 857837 **Births:** 4122 **Total Expense ($000):** 1193248 **Payroll Expense ($000):** 375322 **Personnel:** 9718

☒ **REGENCY HOSPITAL OF COLUMBUS (362037)**, 1430 South High Street, Zip 43207–1045; tel. 614/456–0300, (Nonreporting) **A**1 10 **S** Select Medical Corporation, Mechanicsburg, PA
Primary Contact: Sara Poling, Chief Executive Officer
Web address: www.regencyhospital.com/
**Control:** Corporation, Investor–owned, for–profit **Service:** Long–Term Acute Care hospital

**Staffed Beds:** 43

☒ △ **RIVERSIDE METHODIST HOSPITAL (360006)**, 3535 Olentangy River Road, Zip 43214–3998; tel. 614/566–5000 **A**1 2 3 5 7 8 9 10 **F**3 7 8 11 12 13 14 15 17 18 20 22 24 26 28 29 30 31 33 34 35 36 37 38 39 40 42 43 44 45 46 47 48 49 50 51 53 54 55 56 57 58 59 60 61 62 63 64 65 66 68 69 70 71 72 74 75 76 77 78 79 80 81 82 83 84 85 86 87 90 91 92 93 94 96 97 98 100 102 103 104 107 108 110 111 113 114 115 116 118 119 120 122 123 125 129 131 134 142 143 144 145 146 **P**1 3 5 7 **S** OhioHealth, Columbus, OH
Primary Contact: Stephen Markovich, M.D., President
COO: Brian Jepson, Chief Operating Officer
CFO: Peter Bury, Vice President Finance
CMO: Leonard J. Lozada, M.D., Vice President Medical Affairs
CIO: Michael Krouse, Chief Information Officer
CHR: Shereen Solaiman, Vice President Human Resources
CNO: Karen Robeano, MS, Chief Nursing Officer
Web address: www.ohiohealth.com
**Control:** Church–operated, Nongovernment, not–for profit **Service:** General Medical and Surgical

**Staffed Beds:** 796 **Admissions:** 44644 **Census:** 507 **Outpatient Visits:** 792812 **Births:** 6103 **Total Expense ($000):** 778082 **Payroll Expense ($000):** 323823 **Personnel:** 4547

☒ **SELECT SPECIALTY HOSPITAL–COLUMBUS (362022)**, 1087 Dennison Avenue, Zip 43201; tel. 614/458–9000, (Includes SELECT SPECIALTY HOSPITAL–COLUMBUS, MOUNT CARMEL CAMPUS, 793 West State Street, Zip 43222–1551; tel. 614/234–0950), (Nonreporting) **A**1 10 **S** Select Medical Corporation, Mechanicsburg, PA
Primary Contact: Gene Cashman, Chief Executive Officer
CMO: Victoria Ruff, M.D., Medical Director
CHR: Charles Pankowski, Manager Human Resources
Web address: www.selectmedicalcorp.com
**Control:** Corporation, Investor–owned, for–profit **Service:** Long–Term Acute Care hospital

**Staffed Beds:** 176

**SELECT SPECIALTY HOSPITAL–COLUMBUS, MOUNT CARMEL CAMPUS** See Select Specialty Hospital–Columbus

☒ **TWIN VALLEY BEHAVIORAL HEALTHCARE (364007)**, 2200 West Broad Street, Zip 43223–1295; tel. 614/752–0333 **A**1 9 10 **F**29 30 39 65 68 87 98 100 101 104 105 129 131 134 145 **S** Ohio Department of Mental Health, Columbus, OH
Primary Contact: Karen Woods–Nyce, Chief Executive Officer
COO: David Blahnik, Chief Operating Officer
CFO: John Eardley, Chief Financial Officer
CMO: R. Alan Freeland, M.D., Chief Clinical Officer
CIO: Missy McGarvey, Director Computer Information Systems
CHR: Marcia McKeen, Director Human Resources
CNO: Michael Breakwell, R.N., Nurse Executive
Web address: www.mh.state.oh.us/ibhs/bhos/tvbh.html
**Control:** State–Government, nonfederal **Service:** Psychiatric

**Staffed Beds:** 248 **Admissions:** 1461 **Census:** 175 **Outpatient Visits:** 0 **Births:** 0 **Total Expense ($000):** 48370 **Payroll Expense ($000):** 26432 **Personnel:** 428

**CONCORD TOWNSHIP—Lake County**

☒ △ **LAKE HEALTH (360098)**, 7590 Auburn Road, Zip 44077–3472; tel. 440/375–8100 **A**1 2 7 9 10 **F**3 8 11 13 15 18 20 22 24 26 28 29 30 34 35 40 42 44 45 49 50 51 53 54 56 57 58 59 60 62 63 64 65 68 69 70 73 74 75 76 77 79 81 82 85 86 87 90 93 97 98 100 101 102 103 107 108 110 111 113 115 116 117 118 128 129 130 131 132 134 142 143 145 146 147 **P**1
Primary Contact: Cynthia Moore–Hardy, President and Chief Executive Officer
CMO: Theodore Nichols, M.D., Senior Vice President Medical Affairs
CIO: Gerald Peters, Vice President Information Technologies and Chief Information Officer
Web address: www.lhs.net
**Control:** Other not–for–profit (including NFP Corporation) **Service:** General Medical and Surgical

**Staffed Beds:** 357 **Admissions:** 18794 **Census:** 226 **Outpatient Visits:** 418432 **Births:** 1949 **Total Expense ($000):** 303333 **Payroll Expense ($000):** 112479 **Personnel:** 2413

---

**Hospital, Medicare Provider Number, Address, Telephone, Approval, Facility, and Physician Codes, Health Care System**

★ American Hospital Association (AHA) membership
☐ The Joint Commission accreditation
◇ DNV Healthcare Inc. accreditation
○ American Osteopathic Association (AOA) accreditation
△ Commission on Accreditation of Rehabilitation Facilities (CARF) accreditation

## CONNEAUT—Ashtabula County

⊠ **UNIVERSITY HOSPITALS CONNEAUT MEDICAL CENTER (361308)**, 158 West Main Road, Zip 44030–2039; tel. 440/593–1131 **A**1 9 10 18 **F**3 7 11 15 18 28 29 34 35 37 40 51 59 64 70 75 77 78 79 81 82 86 87 93 107 110 111 113 118 129 131 132 134 142 145 146 147 **S** University Hospitals, Cleveland, OH
Primary Contact: Robert David, President and Chief Executive Officer
COO: Richard Trice, Director Operations
CFO: Wendy Snyder, Director Finance
CMO: Gary Huston, D.O., Chief Medical Officer
CIO: Stephanie Cleversy, Manager Health Information Services
CHR: Barbara Gurto, Manager Human Resources
CNO: Karen McNeil, Chief Nursing Officer
Web address: www.uhhospitals.org
**Control:** Other not–for–profit (including NFP Corporation) **Service:** General Medical and Surgical

**Staffed Beds:** 25 **Admissions:** 722 **Census:** 7 **Outpatient Visits:** 129920 **Births:** 0 **Total Expense ($000):** 24846 **Payroll Expense ($000):** 10267 **Personnel:** 162

## COSHOCTON—Coshocton County

☐ **COSHOCTON COUNTY MEMORIAL HOSPITAL (360109)**, 1460 Orange Street, Zip 43812–6330, Mailing Address: P.O. Box 1330, Zip 43812–6330; tel. 740/622–6411, (Nonreporting) **A**1 5 9 10 20
Primary Contact: Robert Miller, Chief Executive Officer
CFO: Robin Nichols, Chief Financial Officer
CMO: Tammy S. Alverson, M.D., Chief of Staff
CIO: Seth Peterson, Director Information Services
CHR: Rick Davis, Chief Operating Officer and Support Services
Web address: www.ccmh.net
**Control:** Other not–for–profit (including NFP Corporation) **Service:** General Medical and Surgical

**Staffed Beds:** 109

## CUYAHOGA FALLS—Summit County

**CUYAHOGA FALLS GENERAL HOSPITAL** See Summa Western Reserve Hospital

★ △ **EDWIN SHAW REHAB (360241)**, 330 Broadway Street East, Zip 44221–3342; tel. 330/436–0910, (Nonreporting) **A**5 7 9 10 **S** Akron General Health System, Akron, OH
Primary Contact: Kim Strubel, Vice President
CFO: Debbie Gorbach, Vice President and Treasurer
CMO: Michael J. Delahanty, D.O., Medical Director
CHR: Heather Sans, Human Resource Generalist
Web address: www.edwinshaw.com
**Control:** County–Government, nonfederal **Service:** Rehabilitation

**Staffed Beds:** 38

○ **SUMMA WESTERN RESERVE HOSPITAL (360150)**, 1900 23rd Street, Zip 44223–1499; tel. 330/971–7000 **A**9 10 11 12 13 **F**3 18 20 29 30 31 35 40 45 54 57 58 59 60 63 64 65 66 68 70 74 75 77 78 79 81 82 85 93 96 97 107 108 111 113 118 128 129 142 143 145 147 **P**6 **S** Summa Health System, Akron, OH
Primary Contact: Robert Kent, D.O., President and Chief Executive Officer
CFO: Jill Hiner, Vice President and Chief Financial Officer
CMO: Charles Feunning, M.D., President Medical Staff
CHR: Heather Milicevic, Director Human Resources
Web address: www.westernreservehospital.org
**Control:** Partnership, Investor–owned, for–profit **Service:** General Medical and Surgical

**Staffed Beds:** 105 **Admissions:** 3695 **Census:** 42 **Outpatient Visits:** 113090 **Births:** 0 **Total Expense ($000):** 92768 **Payroll Expense ($000):** 34728 **Personnel:** 652

## DAYTON—Montgomery County

☐ **CHILDREN'S MEDICAL CENTER (363306)**, One Children's Plaza, Zip 45404–1815; tel. 937/641–3000 **A**1 2 3 5 8 9 10 **F**3 7 11 19 21 29 30 31 32 34 35 39 40 41 43 44 45 50 54 55 57 58 59 60 61 62 63 64 65 66 72 74 75 77 78 79 81 82 84 85 86 87 88 89 93 97 107 111 114 118 128 129 131 133 134 143 145 **P**6
Primary Contact: David Kinsaul, President and Chief Executive Officer
COO: Matthew P. Graybill, Chief Operating Officer
CFO: David T. Miller, Vice President and Chief Financial Officer
CMO: Thomas Murphy, M.D., Vice President Medical Affairs
CIO: Beth Fredette, Chief Information Officer
Web address: www.childrensdayton.org
**Control:** Other not–for–profit (including NFP Corporation) **Service:** Children's general

**Staffed Beds:** 133 **Admissions:** 6744 **Census:** 81 **Outpatient Visits:** 267291 **Births:** 0 **Total Expense ($000):** 174506 **Payroll Expense ($000):** 76334 **Personnel:** 1584

☐ △ **DAYTON REHABILITATION INSTITUTE (363033)**, One Elizabeth Place, Zip 45417–3445; tel. 937/424–8200, (Nonreporting) **A**1 7
Primary Contact: Randy J. Kitchen, Chief Executive Officer
Web address: www.reliantdayton.com
**Control:** Other not–for–profit (including NFP Corporation) **Service:** Rehabilitation

**Staffed Beds:** 50

⊠ **GOOD SAMARITAN HOSPITAL (360052)**, 2222 Philadelphia Drive, Zip 45406–1813; tel. 937/734–2612 **A**1 2 3 5 9 10 **F**3 11 13 15 17 18 20 22 24 26 28 29 30 31 36 37 40 44 45 46 49 50 54 55 56 58 60 61 64 66 70 73 74 75 76 77 78 79 80 81 82 83 85 86 87 92 93 96 97 98 100 101 102 103 104 107 108 109 110 111 113 114 117 118 125 128 129 130 131 143 144 145 146 147 **P**6 **S** Catholic Health Initiatives, Englewood, CO
Primary Contact: Eloise Broner, President and Chief Executive Officer
CFO: Thomas F. Curtin, Vice President and Chief Financial Officer
CMO: Daniel L. Schoulties, M.D., Vice President Medical Affairs
CIO: Mikki Clancy, Vice President and Chief Information Officer
CHR: William Linesch, Vice President Human Resources
CNO: Mary E. Garman, R.N., Chief Nursing Officer and Vice President Operations
Web address: www.goodsamdayton.com
**Control:** Church–operated, Nongovernment, not–for profit **Service:** General Medical and Surgical

**Staffed Beds:** 400 **Admissions:** 18829 **Census:** 240 **Outpatient Visits:** 295573 **Births:** 1094 **Total Expense ($000):** 315623 **Payroll Expense ($000):** 124460 **Personnel:** 2677

★ ○ △ **GRANDVIEW MEDICAL CENTER (360133)**, 405 Grand Avenue, Zip 45405–4796; tel. 937/226–3200, (Includes SOUTHVIEW HOSPITAL AND FAMILY HEALTH CENTER, 1997 Miamisburg–Centerville Road, Zip 45459–3800; tel. 937/439–6000) **A**2 7 9 10 11 12 13 **F**3 4 5 8 11 12 13 18 20 22 24 28 29 30 31 32 34 35 36 37 38 39 40 42 44 45 47 48 49 50 53 54 57 58 59 60 61 62 63 64 65 66 68 70 72 73 74 75 76 77 78 79 80 81 82 85 86 87 90 93 96 97 98 100 101 102 103 104 105 107 108 110 111 113 114 115 116 117 118 119 120 122 123 125 128 129 130 131 134 140 143 144 145 146 147 **P**7 8 **S** Kettering Health Network, Dayton, OH
Primary Contact: Richard Haas, FACHE, President
CFO: Todd Anderson, Chief Financial Officer
CMO: Tom Hardy, D.O., Vice President Medical Affairs
CHR: Karen Borgert, Vice President Human Resources
Web address: www.khnetwork.org
**Control:** Church–operated, Nongovernment, not–for profit **Service:** General Medical and Surgical

**Staffed Beds:** 317 **Admissions:** 14240 **Census:** 169 **Outpatient Visits:** 308288 **Births:** 1849 **Total Expense ($000):** 230324 **Payroll Expense ($000):** 92932 **Personnel:** 1913

⊠ **KINDRED HOSPITAL–DAYTON (362033)**, One Elizabeth Place, 5th Floor, Zip 45408; tel. 937/222–5963, (Nonreporting) **A**1 9 10 **S** Kindred Healthcare, Louisville, KY
Primary Contact: Lynn Schoen, Chief Executive Officer
CMO: Felipe Rubio, M.D., Medical Director
Web address: www.khdayton.com
**Control:** Corporation, Investor–owned, for–profit **Service:** Long–Term Acute Care hospital

**Staffed Beds:** 67

⊠ △ **MIAMI VALLEY HOSPITAL (360051)**, One Wyoming Street, Zip 45409–2793; tel. 937/208–8000 **A**1 2 3 5 7 8 9 10 **F**1 2 3 4 5 12 13 15 16 17 18 20 22 24 26 28 29 30 31 34 35 37 39 40 42 43 44 46 47 48 49 50 53 54 55 56 57 58 59 60 61 64 67 68 70 72 73 74 75 76 78 79 80 81 82 84 85 86 87 88 89 90 91 92 93 96 98 100 101 102 103 104 105 107 108 110 111 112 113 114 115 116 117 118 123 125 127 128 129 130 131 132 133 134 135 137 140 142 145 146 147
Primary Contact: Bobbie Gerhart, President and Chief Executive Officer
COO: Joann Ringer, Chief Operating Officer
CFO: Scott Shelton, Executive Vice President and Chief Financial Officer
CMO: Gary Collier, M.D., Vice President Medical Affairs and Chief Medical Officer
CIO: Mikki Clancy, Vice President and Chief Information Officer
CHR: William Linesch, Vice President Human Resources
Web address: www.miamivalleyhospital.com
**Control:** Other not–for–profit (including NFP Corporation) **Service:** General Medical and Surgical

**Staffed Beds:** 840 **Admissions:** 34489 **Census:** 543 **Outpatient Visits:** 310672 **Births:** 4834 **Total Expense ($000):** 755612 **Payroll Expense ($000):** 310138 **Personnel:** 5716

**SOUTHVIEW HOSPITAL AND FAMILY HEALTH CENTER** See Grandview Medical Center

☐ **THE MEDICAL CENTER AT ELIZABETH PLACE (360274)**, One Elizabeth Place, Zip 45408; tel. 937/660–3100, (Nonreporting) **A**1 10
Primary Contact: Alexander M. Rintoul, Chief Executive Officer
Web address: www.mcep.us
**Control:** Partnership, Investor–owned, for–profit **Service:** General Medical and Surgical

**Staffed Beds:** 26

*Many Facility Codes have changed. Please refer to the AHA Guide Code Chart.*
© 2012 AHA Guide

☒ △ **VETERANS AFFAIRS MEDICAL CENTER**, 4100 West Third Street, Zip 45428–1002; tel. 937/268–6511, (Total facility includes 225 beds in nursing home–type unit) **A**1 2 3 5 7 8 **F**2 3 5 20 22 29 30 31 33 34 35 36 38 39 40 45 46 47 48 49 53 56 57 58 59 60 61 62 63 64 65 68 70 71 74 75 77 78 79 81 82 83 84 85 86 87 91 92 93 94 95 96 97 98 100 101 102 103 104 106 107 108 109 111 112 113 114 115 116 117 118 119 120 121 122 123 126 127 128 129 131 134 143 145 146 147 **S** Department of Veterans Affairs, Washington, DC
Primary Contact: Glenn A. Costie, FACHE, Director
COO: Terry Taylor, Associate Director
CFO: Lawrence Andrews, Chief Fiscal Services
CMO: William Germann, M.D., Acting Chief of Staff
CIO: Susan Sherer, Chief Information Resource Management
CHR: Jerry A. Erwin, Chief Human Resources Management Service
Web address: www.va.gov/sta/guide/home.asp
**Control:** Veterans Affairs, Government, federal **Service:** General Medical and Surgical

**Staffed Beds:** 370 **Admissions:** 6619 **Census:** 295 **Outpatient Visits:** 425140 **Births:** 0 **Total Expense ($000):** 329431 **Payroll Expense ($000):** 145248 **Personnel:** 1984

### DEFIANCE—Defiance County

☒ **MERCY HOSPITAL OF DEFIANCE (360270)**, 1404 East Second Street, Zip 43512; tel. 419/782–8444 **A**1 9 10 **F**3 8 29 30 34 40 45 46 57 64 65 68 74 75 79 81 82 85 87 97 128 134 145 **P**8 **S** Catholic Health Partners, Cincinnati, OH
Primary Contact: Sonya Selhorst, Administrator
CFO: Samantha M. Platzke, Senior Vice President Finance and Chief Financial Officer
CMO: William C. Reeves, D.O., Chief of Staff
CHR: Marilyn Reineke, Director Human Resources
Web address: www.ehealthconnection.com/regions/toledo/
**Control:** Partnership, Investor–owned, for–profit **Service:** General Medical and Surgical

**Staffed Beds:** 23 **Admissions:** 2202 **Census:** 13 **Outpatient Visits:** 12396 **Births:** 0 **Personnel:** 123

☒ **PROMEDICA DEFIANCE REGIONAL HOSPITAL (361328)**, 1200 Ralston Avenue, Zip 43512–1396; tel. 419/783–6955 **A**1 5 9 10 18 **F**3 11 13 15 18 20 28 31 32 34 40 43 57 59 64 66 68 70 75 76 77 78 79 81 85 86 87 93 98 100 101 102 103 104 105 107 108 110 111 113 117 118 128 129 131 134 143 145 146 **S** ProMedica Health System, Toledo, OH
Primary Contact: Gary Cates, President and Chief Executive Officer
CMO: Kermit Erwin, M.D., Medical Director
CIO: Stephanie Sonnenberg, Director Information Management Systems
CHR: Linda Shaffer, Director Human Resources
Web address: www.promedica.org
**Control:** Other not–for–profit (including NFP Corporation) **Service:** General Medical and Surgical

**Staffed Beds:** 35 **Admissions:** 2241 **Census:** 17 **Outpatient Visits:** 73393 **Births:** 634 **Total Expense ($000):** 45271 **Payroll Expense ($000):** 13081 **Personnel:** 216

### DELAWARE—Delaware County

☒ △ **GRADY MEMORIAL HOSPITAL (360210)**, 561 West Central Avenue, Zip 43015–1485; tel. 740/615–1000 **A**1 2 7 9 10 **F**3 13 15 18 20 26 28 29 30 31 34 35 39 40 44 45 46 48 50 54 57 58 59 64 65 66 68 70 74 75 76 77 78 79 81 82 83 84 85 86 87 92 93 96 97 102 107 108 109 110 111 113 118 123 129 130 131 134 145 146 147 **P**1 3 5 7 **S** OhioHealth, Columbus, OH
Primary Contact: Bruce P. Hagen, President
COO: Bob Walsh, R.N., Chief Operating Officer
CFO: David Hensel, Director Financial Operations
CMO: Barbara Evert, M.D., Vice President Medical Affairs
CIO: Michael Krouse, Chief Information Officer Information Services
CHR: Beth Crow, Associate Relations Representative
CNO: Elizabeth A. Biegler, R.N., Chief Nursing Officer
Web address: www.ohiohealth.com
**Control:** Church–operated, Nongovernment, not–for profit **Service:** General Medical and Surgical

**Staffed Beds:** 61 **Admissions:** 2624 **Census:** 24 **Outpatient Visits:** 169810 **Births:** 386 **Total Expense ($000):** 69505 **Payroll Expense ($000):** 28599 **Personnel:** 400

### DENNISON—Tuscarawas County

**TEN LAKES CENTER (364042)**, 819 North First Street, 3rd Floor, Zip 44621; tel. 740/922–7499, (Nonreporting) **A**9 10 **S** Behavioral Centers of America, Nashville, TN
Primary Contact: Laura Blackburn, Administrator
Web address: www.tenlakescenter.com/
**Control:** Corporation, Investor–owned, for–profit **Service:** Psychiatric

**Staffed Beds:** 16

☒ **TRINITY HOSPITAL TWIN CITY (361302)**, 819 North First Street, Zip 44621–1098; tel. 740/922–2800 **A**1 9 10 18 **F**11 15 18 28 30 34 35 40 50 59 64 70 75 77 81 85 86 87 89 97 107 113 118 127 128 129 132 145 146 **P**4 **S** Sylvania Franciscan Health, Toledo, OH
Primary Contact: Joseph J. Mitchell, President
CFO: Angela Trammell, Controller
CMO: Jose Martinez, M.D., Chief of Staff
CHR: Lauren Castello, Director Human Resources
Web address: www.twincityhospital.org
**Control:** Church–operated, Nongovernment, not–for profit **Service:** General Medical and Surgical

**Staffed Beds:** 25 **Admissions:** 329 **Census:** 3 **Outpatient Visits:** 15489 **Births:** 0 **Total Expense ($000):** 10391 **Payroll Expense ($000):** 4402 **Personnel:** 194

### DOVER—Tuscarawas County

★ **UNION HOSPITAL (360010)**, 659 Boulevard, Zip 44622–2077; tel. 330/343–3311 **A**5 9 10 19 21 **F**3 8 11 13 14 15 28 29 34 35 40 50 53 57 59 62 64 70 75 76 77 78 79 80 81 82 85 86 89 90 93 107 108 110 111 117 118 119 128 129 130 131 145 147 **P**6 8
Primary Contact: Bruce James, Chief Executive Officer
CFO: Eugene A. Thorn, III, Vice President Finance and Chief Financial Officer
CMO: Thomas J. Kelly, M.P.H., Vice President Medical Affairs
CIO: David Baumgardner, Director Information Management
CHR: Darwin K. Smith, Vice President Human Resources
CNO: Diana Boyd, Vice President Nursing
Web address: www.unionhospital.org
**Control:** Other not–for–profit (including NFP Corporation) **Service:** General Medical and Surgical

**Staffed Beds:** 154 **Admissions:** 5920 **Census:** 65 **Outpatient Visits:** 302075 **Births:** 706 **Total Expense ($000):** 104351 **Payroll Expense ($000):** 42734 **Personnel:** 923

### DUBLIN—Franklin County

☒ **DUBLIN METHODIST HOSPITAL (360348)**, 7500 Hospital Drive, Zip 43016; tel. 614/544–8000 **A**1 9 10 **F**3 13 15 18 29 30 34 35 40 45 46 57 59 62 68 70 75 76 77 79 81 82 85 87 90 97 107 110 111 114 118 129 131 134 145 146 **P**1 3 5 7 **S** OhioHealth, Columbus, OH
Primary Contact: Bruce P. Hagen, President
COO: Steve Bunyard, Chief Operating Officer
CFO: Michael Bichimer, Director Financial Operations
CMO: Barbara Evert, M.D., Vice President Medical Affairs
CIO: Michael Krouse, Senior Vice President Chief Information Officer
CHR: Diane Shaub, Director Human Resources
CNO: Elizabeth A. Biegler, R.N., Chief Nursing Officer
Web address: www.ohiohealth.com
**Control:** Church–operated, Nongovernment, not–for profit **Service:** General Medical and Surgical

**Staffed Beds:** 92 **Admissions:** 4720 **Census:** 37 **Outpatient Visits:** 69038 **Births:** 1375 **Total Expense ($000):** 97172 **Payroll Expense ($000):** 33896 **Personnel:** 486

### EAST LIVERPOOL—Columbiana County

☒ **EAST LIVERPOOL CITY HOSPITAL (360096)**, 425 West Fifth Street, Zip 43920–2498; tel. 330/385–7200, (Total facility includes 20 beds in nursing home–type unit) **A**1 9 10 **F**3 11 13 15 18 28 29 30 31 32 34 35 39 40 44 45 49 50 51 57 59 60 64 70 74 75 76 77 78 79 81 85 86 87 89 93 97 107 108 109 111 114 118 127 129 131 134 145 147 **P**5
Primary Contact: Kenneth Cochran, R.N., FACHE, President and Chief Executive Officer
CFO: Kyle Johnson, Vice President Finance
CMO: Mark Swift, D.O., President Medical Staff
CIO: Frank Mader, Director Information Services
CHR: Pam Smith, Director Human Resources
CNO: Patrick Beaver, R.N., Vice President Patient Care and Chief Nursing Officer
Web address: www.elch.org
**Control:** Other not–for–profit (including NFP Corporation) **Service:** General Medical and Surgical

**Staffed Beds:** 109 **Admissions:** 4968 **Census:** 52 **Outpatient Visits:** 103832 **Births:** 252 **Total Expense ($000):** 60499 **Payroll Expense ($000):** 23643 **Personnel:** 504

**Hospital, Medicare Provider Number, Address, Telephone, Approval, Facility, and Physician Codes, Health Care System**

★ American Hospital Association (AHA) membership
☐ The Joint Commission accreditation ◇ DNV Healthcare Inc. accreditation
○ American Osteopathic Association (AOA) accreditation
△ Commission on Accreditation of Rehabilitation Facilities (CARF) accreditation

**OH**

## ELYRIA—Lorain County

☒ **EMH ELYRIA MEDICAL CENTER (360145)**, 630 East River Street, Zip 44035–5902; tel. 440/329–7500 **A**1 2 9 10 **F**3 8 11 12 13 15 17 18 20 22 24 26 28 29 30 31 34 37 40 42 50 53 54 57 59 62 64 68 70 73 74 75 76 77 78 79 81 82 85 86 87 89 92 93 94 98 107 108 110 111 113 114 117 118 125 128 129 130 134 145 147 **P**6 7 8
Primary Contact: Donald S. Sheldon, M.D., President and Chief Executive Officer
CFO: James M. Simone, Vice President and Chief Financial Officer
CIO: Char Wray, Vice President Chief Clinical Operations and Chief Information Officer
CHR: Daniel Miller, Vice President Human Resources
CNO: Jill Cooksey, Vice President Chief Nursing Officer
Web address: www.emh–healthcare.org
**Control:** Other not–for–profit (including NFP Corporation) **Service:** General Medical and Surgical

**Staffed Beds:** 266 **Admissions:** 14807 **Census:** 168 **Outpatient Visits:** 251120 **Births:** 877 **Total Expense ($000):** 185571 **Payroll Expense ($000):** 74092 **Personnel:** 1607

## EUCLID—Cuyahoga County

☒ △ **EUCLID HOSPITAL (360082)**, 18901 Lake Shore Boulevard, Zip 44119–1090; tel. 216/531–9000, (Total facility includes 40 beds in nursing home–type unit) **A**1 2 7 9 10 **F**3 15 17 18 20 26 28 29 30 31 34 35 39 40 45 49 50 56 57 59 60 62 64 70 74 75 77 78 79 81 82 85 87 90 91 93 94 96 98 100 102 103 104 107 108 111 113 117 118 127 129 130 145 147
**S** Cleveland Clinic Health System, Cleveland, OH
Primary Contact: Mark Froimson, President
COO: Rich Lea, Vice President Operations
CFO: Don Urbancsik, Director Finance
CMO: Marita Volk, M.D., Director Medical Services and Chief of Staff
CHR: Gloria Donnelly, Director Human Resources
Web address: www.euclidhospital.org
**Control:** Other not–for–profit (including NFP Corporation) **Service:** General Medical and Surgical

**Staffed Beds:** 231 **Admissions:** 8491 **Census:** 152 **Outpatient Visits:** 86547 **Births:** 0 **Total Expense ($000):** 102112 **Payroll Expense ($000):** 48152 **Personnel:** 723

## FAIRFIELD—Butler County

☒ **MERCY HEALTH – FAIRFIELD HOSPITAL (360056)**, 3000 Mack Road, Zip 45014; tel. 513/870–7000 **A**1 2 9 10 **F**3 8 11 13 15 17 18 20 22 24 28 29 30 31 34 35 40 44 49 50 54 57 59 64 65 68 70 73 74 75 76 77 78 79 81 82 84 85 87 90 93 107 108 110 111 113 114 117 118 125 129 131 134 145 146 147 **S** Catholic Health Partners, Cincinnati, OH
Primary Contact: Thomas S. Urban, Market Leader and President
COO: Patricia Davis–Hagens, R.N., Vice President Operations and Nursing, Chief Operating Officer and Chief Nursing Officer
CFO: Robin Yon, Site Finance Director
CMO: John Kennedy, M.D., Vice President Medical Affairs
CIO: Yousuf Ahmad, Divisional Senior Vice President and Chief Network Transformation Officer
CHR: Maggie Lund, Divisional Senior Vice President Human Resources
CNO: Patricia Davis–Hagens, R.N., Vice President Operations and Nursing, Chief Operating Officer and Chief Nursing Officer
Web address: www.e–mercy.com
**Control:** Church–operated, Nongovernment, not–for profit **Service:** General Medical and Surgical

**Staffed Beds:** 228 **Admissions:** 15370 **Census:** 149 **Outpatient Visits:** 202689 **Births:** 2044 **Total Expense ($000):** 175141 **Payroll Expense ($000):** 63287 **Personnel:** 1147

## FINDLAY—Hancock County

☒ **BLANCHARD VALLEY HOSPITAL (360095)**, 1900 South Main Street, Zip 45840; tel. 419/423–4500, (Includes BLANCHARD VALLEY HOSPITAL, 1900 South Main Street, tel. 419/423–4500) **A**1 2 3 5 9 10 19 **F**3 11 13 15 17 18 20 22 24 28 29 30 31 34 35 40 41 42 43 46 48 49 50 59 60 64 70 72 74 76 77 78 79 81 82 83 84 85 86 87 93 94 96 97 98 103 107 108 111 113 115 116 117 118 119 125 128 129 130 131 133 134 145 146 147 **P**5
**S** Blanchard Valley Health System, Findlay, OH
Primary Contact: Scott C. Malaney, President and Chief Executive Officer
COO: Christopher E. Press, FACHE, President, Blanchard Valley Regional Health Center
CFO: David Cytlak, Chief Financial Officer
CMO: William H. Kose, M.D., Senior Vice President Medical Affairs
CHR: Douglas DeFrain, Director Human Resources
Web address: www.bvhealthsystem.org
**Control:** Other not–for–profit (including NFP Corporation) **Service:** General Medical and Surgical

**Staffed Beds:** 181 **Admissions:** 7657 **Census:** 74 **Outpatient Visits:** 244046 **Births:** 1106 **Total Expense ($000):** 158773 **Payroll Expense ($000):** 69936 **Personnel:** 1082

## FOSTORIA—Hancock County

☒ **PROMEDICA FOSTORIA COMMUNITY HOSPITAL (361318)**, 501 Van Buren Street, Zip 44830–0907, Mailing Address: P.O. Box 907, Zip 44830–0907; tel. 419/435–7734 **A**1 5 9 10 18 **F**3 11 13 15 28 31 32 34 35 40 45 46 57 59 60 62 64 66 68 70 75 76 78 79 81 85 86 89 93 94 96 97 107 108 110 111 114 116 117 118 127 128 129 130 131 132 134 143 145 **P**7
**S** ProMedica Health System, Toledo, OH
Primary Contact: Daniel Schwanke, President
COO: Tom Borer, Vice President Operations
CFO: Ken Swint, Vice President Finance and Chief Financial Officer
CMO: Terrence Fondessy, M.D., Vice President Medical Affairs
CIO: David G. Selman, Corporate Vice President Information Resources
CHR: Charles McDowell, Corporate Vice President Human Resources
Web address: www.promedica.org
**Control:** Other not–for–profit (including NFP Corporation) **Service:** General Medical and Surgical

**Staffed Beds:** 25 **Admissions:** 1337 **Census:** 12 **Outpatient Visits:** 79916 **Births:** 176 **Total Expense ($000):** 36395 **Payroll Expense ($000):** 11025 **Personnel:** 204

## FREMONT—Sandusky County

☒ **MEMORIAL HOSPITAL (360156)**, 715 South Taft Avenue, Zip 43420–3200; tel. 419/332–7321 **A**1 2 5 9 10 **F**8 11 13 14 19 29 30 32 34 35 38 40 51 53 56 57 59 62 63 69 75 76 80 81 82 89 92 93 100 101 103 104 107 110 111 114 117 118 128 129 130 131 145 146 147 **P**1 **S** QHR, Brentwood, TN
Primary Contact: Wesley W. Oswald, Interim Chief Executive Officer
CFO: Rick Ruppel, Chief Financial Officer
CIO: Dustin Hufford, Chief Information Officer
CHR: Warrenette Parthemore, Director Human Resources
CNO: Jill A. Trosin, R.N., Chief Nursing Officer
Web address: www.memorialhcs.org
**Control:** Other not–for–profit (including NFP Corporation) **Service:** General Medical and Surgical

**Staffed Beds:** 71 **Admissions:** 2134 **Census:** 17 **Outpatient Visits:** 80448 **Births:** 373 **Total Expense ($000):** 60984 **Payroll Expense ($000):** 25539

○ **PHYSICIAN'S CHOICE HOSPITAL – FREMONT (360356)**, 2390 Enterprise Street, Zip 43420–8507; tel. 567/201–2911, (Nonreporting) **A**11
Primary Contact: Jerome McTague, M.D., JD, Administrator and Chief Executive Officer
Web address: www.physicianschoicehospital.com
**Control:** Partnership, Investor–owned, for–profit **Service:** Other specialty

**Staffed Beds:** 8

## GALION—Crawford County

★ **GALION COMMUNITY HOSPITAL (361325)**, 269 Portland Way South, Zip 44833–2399; tel. 419/468–4841, (Nonreporting) **A**9 10 18 21 **S** Avita Health System, Galion, OH
Primary Contact: Jerome Morasko, President and Chief Executive Officer
CFO: D. Eric Draime, Vice President and Chief Financial Officer
CIO: Andy Daniels, Vice President Non–Clinical Operations and Information Systems
CHR: Traci L. Oswald, Vice President Human Resources
Web address: www.galionhospital.org
**Control:** Other not–for–profit (including NFP Corporation) **Service:** General Medical and Surgical

**Staffed Beds:** 35

## GALLIPOLIS—Gallia County

☐ △ **HOLZER MEDICAL CENTER (360054)**, 100 Jackson Pike, Zip 45631–1563; tel. 740/446–5000 **A**1 2 5 7 9 10 19 **F**3 8 12 13 17 18 20 22 24 26 29 30 31 34 35 40 45 49 53 57 59 62 63 64 70 76 77 78 79 81 85 87 89 90 93 96 107 108 113 114 117 118 129 131 145 147 **P**6
Primary Contact: James R. Phillipe, President
CFO: Kenneth G. Payne, Chief Financial Officer
CMO: John Viall, M.D., Vice President Medical Affairs
CIO: John Allen, Chief Information Officer
CHR: Lisa Halley, Vice President Human Resources
Web address: www.holzer.org
**Control:** Other not–for–profit (including NFP Corporation) **Service:** General Medical and Surgical

**Staffed Beds:** 181 **Admissions:** 6828 **Census:** 72 **Outpatient Visits:** 70734 **Births:** 622 **Total Expense ($000):** 104483 **Payroll Expense ($000):** 33130 **Personnel:** 932

*Many Facility Codes have changed. Please refer to the AHA Guide Code Chart.* © 2012 AHA Guide

### GARFIELD HEIGHTS—Cuyahoga County

✠ △ **MARYMOUNT HOSPITAL (360143)**, 12300 McCracken Road, Zip 44125–2975; tel. 216/581–0500 **A**1 2 7 10 **F**3 8 11 15 28 29 30 31 34 35 38 39 40 42 44 47 48 49 50 51 53 54 55 56 57 58 59 60 61 63 64 65 68 69 70 74 75 77 78 79 81 82 85 86 87 93 96 97 98 99 100 101 102 103 104 105 107 108 111 113 115 116 117 118 123 129 130 131 134 142 145 147 **S** Cleveland Clinic Health System, Cleveland, OH
Primary Contact: Joanne Zeroske, President and Chief Executive Officer
COO: William D. Keckan, Chief Operating Officer
CFO: Mike Benich, Controller
CMO: George V. Topalsky, M.D., Vice President Medical Operations
CIO: Ralph A. Cagna, Director Information Technology Operations, Cleveland Clinic Health System South Market
CHR: Doris A. Zajec, Human Resources Business Partner
CNO: Barbara Zinner, Interim Chief Nursing Officer
Web address: www.marymount.org
**Control:** Other not–for–profit (including NFP Corporation) **Service:** General Medical and Surgical

**Staffed Beds:** 232 **Admissions:** 11572 **Census:** 155 **Outpatient Visits:** 122944 **Births:** 253 **Total Expense ($000):** 143928 **Payroll Expense ($000):** 61576 **Personnel:** 966

### GENEVA—Ashtabula County

✠ **UNIVERSITY HOSPITALS GENEVA MEDICAL CENTER (361307)**, 870 West Main Street, Zip 44041–1295; tel. 440/466–1141 **A**1 9 10 18 **F**3 7 11 15 18 29 34 35 40 46 51 59 64 68 70 75 77 78 79 81 82 86 87 93 107 110 111 113 118 128 129 131 132 134 142 145 146 **S** University Hospitals, Cleveland, OH
Primary Contact: Robert David, President and Chief Executive Officer
CFO: Wendy Snyder, Director Finance
CMO: Amitabh Goel, M.D., Chief Medical Officer
CIO: Stephanie Cleversy, Manager Health Information Systems
CHR: Kate Van Stratton, Manager Human Resources
CNO: Karen McNeil, Chief Nursing Officer
CNO: Richard Trice, Director Operations
Web address: www.uhhs.com
**Control:** Other not–for–profit (including NFP Corporation) **Service:** General Medical and Surgical

**Staffed Beds:** 25 **Admissions:** 1449 **Census:** 15 **Outpatient Visits:** 186239 **Births:** 0 **Total Expense ($000):** 32433 **Payroll Expense ($000):** 13410 **Personnel:** 205

### GEORGETOWN—Brown County

☐ **SOUTHWEST REGIONAL MEDICAL CENTER (360116)**, 425 Home Street, Zip 45121–1407; tel. 937/378–7500 **A**1 9 10 **F**3 11 12 13 15 29 34 37 40 45 47 50 57 59 62 64 70 73 75 76 77 79 81 85 86 87 89 90 93 97 107 108 110 111 113 117 118 126 128 129 143 145 146 147 **P**6
Primary Contact: Michael C. Patterson, Chief Executive Officer
Web address: www.swrmed.org
**Control:** Corporation, Investor–owned, for–profit **Service:** General Medical and Surgical

**Staffed Beds:** 59 **Admissions:** 528 **Census:** 8 **Outpatient Visits:** 53536 **Births:** 207 **Total Expense ($000):** 31541 **Payroll Expense ($000):** 13832 **Personnel:** 306

### GREEN SPRINGS—Sandusky County

☐ **ST. FRANCIS HEALTH CARE CENTRE (362007)**, 401 North Broadway, Zip 44836–9653; tel. 419/639–2626, (Nonreporting) **A**1 9 10
Primary Contact: Kim D. Eicher, Chief Executive Officer
CFO: Douglas Morris, Chief Financial Officer
CMO: John Yuhas, D.O., Medical Director
CHR: Joan E. Schmidt, Director Human Resources
Web address: www.sfhcc.org
**Control:** Church–operated, Nongovernment, not–for profit **Service:** General Medical and Surgical

**Staffed Beds:** 186

### GREENFIELD—Highland County

☐ △ **ADENA GREENFIELD MEDICAL CENTER (361304)**, 550 Mirabeau Street, Zip 45123–1617; tel. 937/981–9400, (Nonreporting) **A**1 7 9 10 18 21
Primary Contact: Sandra L. Smith, Administrator
COO: Jeff Graham, Chief Operating Officer
CFO: Ralph W. Sorrell, Sr., Chief Financial Officer
CIO: Marcus Bost, Director Information Services and Chief Information Officer
CHR: Brandt Lippert, Vice President Human Resources
Web address: www.adena.org
**Control:** Other not–for–profit (including NFP Corporation) **Service:** General Medical and Surgical

**Staffed Beds:** 25

### GREENVILLE—Darke County

★ ○ **WAYNE HOSPITAL (360044)**, 835 Sweitzer Street, Zip 45331–1077; tel. 937/548–1141 **A**2 9 10 11 **F**3 8 11 13 15 29 30 31 34 35 39 40 41 45 57 58 59 64 70 75 76 77 78 79 81 83 84 85 86 89 93 107 108 110 111 113 117 118 128 129 130 131 132 134 145 146 147 **P**1
Primary Contact: Wayne G. Deschambeau, President and Chief Executive Officer
CFO: Dennis Lockard, Vice President Fiscal Services and Chief Financial Officer
CMO: Guillermo Trevino, M.D., President Medical Staff
CIO: Shelton Monger, Director Information Technology
CHR: Peggy Schwartz, Vice President Human Resources
CNO: Kimberlee Freeman, R.N., Vice President Patient Care Services and Chief Nursing Officer
Web address: www.waynehealthcare.org
**Control:** Other not–for–profit (including NFP Corporation) **Service:** General Medical and Surgical

**Staffed Beds:** 73 **Admissions:** 2264 **Census:** 18 **Outpatient Visits:** 83804 **Births:** 319 **Total Expense ($000):** 48707 **Payroll Expense ($000):** 19239 **Personnel:** 454

### GROVEPORT—Franklin County

☐ **BARIX CLINICS OF OHIO (360258)**, 3964 Hamilton Square Boulevard, Zip 43125–9119; tel. 614/834–6800, (Nonreporting) **A**1 10
Primary Contact: Goran Dragolovic, Chief Executive Officer
Web address: www.barixclinics.com/contact_us/ohio.jsp
**Control:** Individual, Investor–owned, for–profit **Service:** Surgical

**Staffed Beds:** 24

### HAMILTON—Butler County

☐ **BUTLER COUNTY MEDICAL CENTER (360269)**, 3125 Hamilton Mason Road, Zip 45011–5307; tel. 513/894–8888, (Nonreporting) **A**1 9 10
Primary Contact: Ajay Mangal, M.D., Chief Executive Officer
COO: Mary Ann Gellenbeck, Chief Operating Officer
CFO: Michael L. Griffin, Chief Financial Officer
CHR: Amy Turner, Director Human Resources
Web address: www.bcsurg.com
**Control:** Corporation, Investor–owned, for–profit **Service:** Surgical

**Staffed Beds:** 8

✠ **FORT HAMILTON HOSPITAL (360132)**, 630 Eaton Avenue, Zip 45013–2770; tel. 513/867–2000 **A**1 2 9 10 **F**1 3 4 8 11 13 15 16 17 18 20 22 28 29 30 31 34 35 40 44 45 46 47 49 50 57 59 61 62 67 68 70 72 73 74 75 76 78 79 80 81 84 85 87 88 89 90 93 98 101 102 103 104 105 107 108 110 111 114 115 116 117 118 119 120 121 122 123 127 128 129 131 142 143 145 146 147 **S** Kettering Health Network, Dayton, OH
Primary Contact: Jennifer Swenson, President
CHR: Joseph Geigle, Director Human Resources
Web address: www.khnetwork.org/fort_hamilton
**Control:** Other not–for–profit (including NFP Corporation) **Service:** General Medical and Surgical

**Staffed Beds:** 187 **Admissions:** 8212 **Census:** 101 **Outpatient Visits:** 85989 **Births:** 608 **Personnel:** 800

### HICKSVILLE—Defiance County

✠ **COMMUNITY MEMORIAL HOSPITAL (361301)**, 208 North Columbus Street, Zip 43526–1299; tel. 419/542–6692, (Nonreporting) **A**1 9 10 18
Primary Contact: Melvin H. Fahs, Chief Executive Officer
CFO: Susan Hobeck, Chief Financial Officer
CIO: Chuck Bohlmann, Chief Information Officer
CHR: Michelle Waggoner, Vice President Human Resources and Physician Services
CNO: Jane Zachrich, Chief Nursing Officer
Web address: www.cmhosp.com
**Control:** Hospital district or authority, Government, nonfederal **Service:** General Medical and Surgical

**Staffed Beds:** 25

---

**Hospital, Medicare Provider Number, Address, Telephone, Approval, Facility, and Physician Codes, Health Care System**

★ American Hospital Association (AHA) membership
☐ The Joint Commission accreditation
◇ DNV Healthcare Inc. accreditation
○ American Osteopathic Association (AOA) accreditation
△ Commission on Accreditation of Rehabilitation Facilities (CARF) accreditation

## HILLSBORO—Highland County

**HIGHLAND DISTRICT HOSPITAL (361332)**, 1275 North High Street, Zip 45133–8571; tel. 937/393–6100 **A**1 9 10 18 **F**3 11 13 15 29 30 31 34 35 40 45 47 49 57 59 62 64 74 76 77 78 79 81 85 86 87 92 93 94 96 98 103 107 111 117 118 126 129 130 131 134 145 147 **P**3
Primary Contact: James E. Baer, FACHE, President and Chief Executive Officer
CFO: Randal Lennartz, Vice President Finance
CMO: Linda R. Welder, M.D., Chief of Staff
CHR: Julie Pence, Associate Director Human Resources
CNO: Timothy Parry, R.N., Vice President Nursing
Web address: www.hdh.org
**Control:** Hospital district or authority, Government, nonfederal **Service:** General Medical and Surgical

> **Staffed Beds:** 25 **Admissions:** 2114 **Census:** 20 **Outpatient Visits:** 84660
> **Births:** 396 **Total Expense ($000):** 31604 **Payroll Expense ($000):** 13619
> **Personnel:** 303

## JACKSON—Jackson County

**HOLZER MEDICAL CENTER – JACKSON (361320)**, 500 Burlington Road, Zip 45640–9360; tel. 740/288–4625 **A**1 9 10 18 **F**3 29 30 32 35 37 39 40 54 57 59 64 70 75 79 81 82 85 86 87 93 97 107 113 118 129 132 145 **P**3
Primary Contact: James R. Phillippe, II, President
CFO: Kevin Yeager, Vice President Fiscal Services
CMO: Nimal Dutla, M.D., Chief Medical Staff
CHR: Sandy Carlisle, Manager Human Resources
Web address: www.holzer.org
**Control:** Other not–for–profit (including NFP Corporation) **Service:** General Medical and Surgical

> **Staffed Beds:** 24 **Admissions:** 1358 **Census:** 13 **Outpatient Visits:** 47716
> **Births:** 0 **Total Expense ($000):** 33482 **Payroll Expense ($000):** 13325
> **Personnel:** 236

## KENTON—Hardin County

**HARDIN MEMORIAL HOSPITAL (361315)**, 921 East Franklin Street, Zip 43326–2099; tel. 419/673–0761 **A**1 9 10 18 **F**11 15 29 30 34 40 45 57 59 61 75 77 78 79 81 86 87 93 97 102 107 108 110 111 113 115 118 128 129 130 131 132 145 146 **S** OhioHealth, Columbus, OH
Primary Contact: Mark R. Seckinger, Administrator and Chief Executive Officer
CFO: Ron Snyder, Chief Financial Officer
Web address: www.hardinmemorial.org
**Control:** Other not–for–profit (including NFP Corporation) **Service:** General Medical and Surgical

> **Staffed Beds:** 25 **Admissions:** 1008 **Census:** 12 **Outpatient Visits:** 59390
> **Births:** 0 **Total Expense ($000):** 19570 **Payroll Expense ($000):** 8844
> **Personnel:** 190

## KETTERING—Montgomery County

△ **KETTERING MEDICAL CENTER (360079)**, 3535 Southern Boulevard,. Zip 45429; tel. 937/298–4331, (Total facility includes 100 beds in nursing home–type unit) **A**1 2 3 5 7 8 9 10 **F**3 4 5 6 8 10 11 12 13 15 17 18 20 22 24 26 28 29 30 31 32 34 35 36 37 38 39 40 42 43 44 45 46 47 48 49 50 51 52 53 54 56 57 58 59 60 61 62 63 64 65 66 67 68 70 71 72 73 74 75 76 77 78 79 80 81 82 84 85 86 87 90 91 92 93 96 97 98 99 100 101 102 103 104 107 110 111 113 114 115 116 117 118 119 120 122 123 124 125 127 128 129 130 131 134 140 142 144 145 146 147 **P**7 8 **S** Kettering Health Network, Dayton, OH
Primary Contact: Roy G. Chew, Ph.D., President
COO: Brett Spenst, Vice President Finance and Operations
CFO: Brett Spenst, Vice President Finance and Operations
CMO: Gregory Wise, M.D., Vice President Medical Affairs
CIO: Jon Russell, Vice President Information Systems
CHR: Beverly Morris, Vice President Human Resources
CNO: Brenda Kuhn, Ph.D., Vice President Patient Care Services
Web address: www.kmcnetwork.org
**Control:** Church–operated, Nongovernment, not–for profit **Service:** General Medical and Surgical

> **Staffed Beds:** 515 **Admissions:** 19517 **Census:** 277 **Outpatient Visits:** 293011 **Births:** 2467 **Total Expense ($000):** 476318 **Payroll Expense ($000):** 197894 **Personnel:** 2761

## LAKEWOOD—Cuyahoga County

△ **LAKEWOOD HOSPITAL (360212)**, 14519 Detroit Avenue, Zip 44107–4383; tel. 216/521–4200, (Total facility includes 25 beds in nursing home–type unit) **A**1 2 7 9 10 **F**13 15 20 22 26 28 29 30 34 35 40 45 46 49 50 56 57 59 60 64 65 68 69 70 74 75 76 77 79 81 82 85 86 87 90 93 97 98 100 101 102 103 107 108 111 117 118 127 129 131 133 142 145 146 147 **S** Cleveland Clinic Health System, Cleveland, OH
Primary Contact: Robert Weil, M.D., President
COO: Shannan Ritchie, Chief Operating Officer
CFO: Ankit Chhabra, Director Finance
CMO: Charles Garven, M.D., Vice President Medical Operations
CIO: C. Martin Harris, M.D., Chief Information Officer
CHR: Sheree Laborie, Director Human Resources
CNO: Mary R. Sauer, R.N., Chief Nursing Officer
Web address: www.lakewoodhospital.org
**Control:** Other not–for–profit (including NFP Corporation) **Service:** General Medical and Surgical

> **Staffed Beds:** 250 **Admissions:** 8908 **Census:** 140 **Outpatient Visits:** 148600 **Births:** 702 **Total Expense ($000):** 123469 **Payroll Expense ($000):** 55736 **Personnel:** 795

## LANCASTER—Fairfield County

△ **FAIRFIELD MEDICAL CENTER (360072)**, 401 North Ewing Street, Zip 43130–3371; tel. 740/687–8000 **A**1 2 5 7 9 10 13 **F**3 8 9 11 13 15 18 20 22 24 26 28 29 30 34 35 38 40 41 44 45 47 48 49 50 53 54 57 59 64 70 74 75 76 77 78 79 81 82 83 84 85 87 89 93 96 97 98 102 104 107 108 110 111 113 114 115 116 117 118 128 129 130 131 134 144 145 146 147
Primary Contact: Mina H. Ubbing, President and Chief Executive Officer
COO: Howard Sniderman, Chief Operating Officer
CFO: Sky Gettys, Chief Financial Officer
CMO: Steve Cox, M.D., Chief Medical Officer
CIO: Jean Robertson, M.D., Chief Information Officer
CNO: Cynthia Pearsall, Chief Nursing Officer
Web address: www.fmchealth.org
**Control:** Other not–for–profit (including NFP Corporation) **Service:** General Medical and Surgical

> **Staffed Beds:** 222 **Admissions:** 10429 **Census:** 109 **Outpatient Visits:** 247151 **Births:** 1056 **Total Expense ($000):** 188829 **Payroll Expense ($000):** 78481 **Personnel:** 1564

## LIMA—Allen County

**INSTITUTE FOR ORTHOPAEDIC SURGERY (360263)**, 801 Medical Drive, Suite B., Zip 45804; tel. 419/224–7586, (Nonreporting) **A**1 9 10 **S** Catholic Health Partners, Cincinnati, OH
Primary Contact: Sally Rhodes, R.N., MSN, Administrative Director
CFO: Sally Rhodes, R.N., Administrative Director
CMO: Mark McDonald, M.D., President
CHR: Pat Farmer, Coordinator Human Resources and Safety Officer
Web address: www.ioshospital.com
**Control:** Partnership, Investor–owned, for–profit **Service:** Orthopedic

> **Staffed Beds:** 8

**KINDRED HOSPITAL LIMA (362020)**, 730 West Market Street, 6th Floor, Zip 45801; tel. 419/224–1888, (Nonreporting) **A**1 9 10 **S** Kindred Healthcare, Louisville, KY
Primary Contact: Kris Karns, FACHE, Ph.D., Chief Executive Officer
Web address: www.khlima.com
**Control:** Corporation, Investor–owned, for–profit **Service:** Long–Term Acute Care hospital

> **Staffed Beds:** 26

△ **LIMA MEMORIAL HEALTH SYSTEM (360009)**, 1001 Bellefontaine Avenue, Zip 45804–2899; tel. 419/228–3335, (Total facility includes 17 beds in nursing home–type unit) **A**1 2 7 9 10 **F**3 11 13 15 17 18 20 22 24 28 29 30 31 34 35 36 40 43 45 46 47 48 49 50 54 57 58 59 60 62 63 64 65 68 69 70 73 74 75 76 77 78 79 81 82 84 85 86 89 90 93 96 107 108 110 111 113 116 118 119 120 128 129 130 131 145 146 147 **P**6 8
Primary Contact: Michael D. Swick, President and Chief Executive Officer
COO: Robert Armstrong, Senior Vice President and Chief Operating Officer
CFO: Eric Pohjala, Vice President and Chief Financial Officer
CMO: C. Lynn Thompson, M.D., Vice President Medical Affairs
CIO: Cheryl Homan, Administrative Director
CHR: Tillie Schiffler, Director Human Resources
CNO: Ann–Marie J. Pohl, R.N., Vice President and Chief Nursing Officer
Web address: www.limamemorial.org
**Control:** Other not–for–profit (including NFP Corporation) **Service:** General Medical and Surgical

> **Staffed Beds:** 242 **Admissions:** 7828 **Census:** 99 **Outpatient Visits:** 261731 **Births:** 591 **Total Expense ($000):** 142296 **Payroll Expense ($000):** 52282 **Personnel:** 1042

☐ **OAKWOOD CORRECTIONAL FACILITY**, 3200 North West Street,
Zip 45801–2000; tel. 419/225–8052, (Nonreporting) **A**1
Primary Contact: Christopher Yanai, Warden and Chief Executive Officer
CFO: Thomas Ferry, Business Administrator
CHR: Glenda Turner, Director Personnel
Web address: www.drc.state.oh.us/public/ocf.htm
**Control:** State–Government, nonfederal **Service:** Psychiatric

**Staffed Beds:** 61

☒ △ **ST. RITA'S MEDICAL CENTER (360066)**, 730 West Market Street,
Zip 45801–4670; tel. 419/227–3361 **A**1 2 7 9 10 **F**3 4 5 9 11 13 15 17 18
20 22 24 26 28 29 30 31 32 34 35 36 39 40 42 43 45 46 47 49 50 53 54
56 57 58 59 60 61 62 63 64 66 68 70 72 73 74 75 76 77 78 79 81 82 84
85 86 87 89 90 92 93 96 98 100 101 102 103 107 108 110 111 113 114
115 116 117 118 119 120 125 127 128 129 130 131 134 143 145 146 147
**P**6 8 **S** Catholic Health Partners, Cincinnati, OH
Primary Contact: Robert O. Baxter, President
COO: Brian Smith, Executive Vice President and Chief Operating Officer
CMO: Herbert Schumm, M.D., Vice President Medical Affairs
CHR: Will Cason, Vice President Human Resources
Web address: www.stritas.org
**Control:** Church–operated, Nongovernment, not–for profit **Service:** General
Medical and Surgical

**Staffed Beds:** 415 **Admissions:** 20160 **Census:** 231 **Outpatient Visits:**
420788 **Births:** 1553 **Total Expense ($000):** 328361 **Payroll Expense
($000):** 117167 **Personnel:** 2425

**TRIUMPH HOSPITAL LIMA** See Kindred Hospital Lima

## LODI—Medina County

☒ **LODI COMMUNITY HOSPITAL (361303)**, 225 Elyria Street, Zip 44254–1096;
tel. 330/948–1222 **A**1 9 10 18 **F**3 11 15 26 29 30 34 35 40 45 46 57 59 64
65 69 75 77 79 81 82 93 96 97 107 113 118 127 128 129 131 132 145 **P**1
6 **S** Akron General Health System, Akron, OH
Primary Contact: Thomas Whelan, President
COO: Dana Kocsis, R.N., Vice President Nursing and Operations
CFO: Alan A. Ganci, Director Finance and Controller
CMO: David Peter, M.D., Senior Vice President Medical Affairs and Chief Medical
Officer
CIO: Robb Baldauf, Coordinator Information Systems
CHR: Lynn Moraca, Director Human Resources
CNO: Beverly Bokovitz, R.N., Senior Vice President and Chief Nursing Officer
Web address: www.lodihospital.org
**Control:** Other not–for–profit (including NFP Corporation) **Service:** General
Medical and Surgical

**Staffed Beds:** 25 **Admissions:** 412 **Census:** 7 **Outpatient Visits:** 27818
**Births:** 0 **Total Expense ($000):** 14009 **Payroll Expense ($000):** 6882
**Personnel:** 116

## LOGAN—Hocking County

☒ **HOCKING VALLEY COMMUNITY HOSPITAL (361330)**, 601 State Route 664
North, Zip 43138–0966, Mailing Address: P.O. Box 966, Zip 43138–0966;
tel. 740/380–8000, (Total facility includes 18 beds in nursing home–type unit) **A**1
9 10 18 **F**3 8 11 15 28 29 31 34 40 56 57 59 64 70 75 77 78 79 81 85 86
93 98 103 107 111 114 117 118 127 128 129 132 134 143 145 146 147
**P**1 3
Primary Contact: LeeAnn Lucas–Helber, President
CFO: Steve Berkhouse, Chief Financial Officer
CMO: Duane Mast, M.D., Medical Director
CIO: John Burgess, Director Information Services
CHR: Robert Schmidt, Director Human Resources
CNO: Julie Stuck, R.N., Vice President Patient Services
Web address: www.hvch.org
**Control:** County–Government, nonfederal **Service:** General Medical and Surgical

**Staffed Beds:** 53 **Admissions:** 1412 **Census:** 31 **Outpatient Visits:** 70147
**Births:** 0 **Total Expense ($000):** 33081 **Payroll Expense ($000):** 13821
**Personnel:** 316

## LONDON—Madison County

☒ **MADISON COUNTY HOSPITAL (360189)**, 210 North Main Street,
Zip 43140–1115; tel. 740/845–7000 **A**1 9 10 **F**11 13 15 18 29 31 34 35 38
40 45 53 57 59 64 70 75 76 77 78 79 81 82 85 86 87 89 93 94 96 107
108 110 111 113 117 118 128 129 130 131 134 145 146
Primary Contact: Fred L. Kolb, Chief Executive Officer
CFO: Michael Browning, Chief Financial Officer
CMO: Robert Mueller, M.D., Chief of Staff
CIO: Dennis Vogt, Director Information Technology
CHR: Becky Rozell, Chief Human Resources Officer
CNO: Jennifer Piccione, Chief Nursing and Clinical Services Officer
Web address: www.madisoncountyhospital.org
**Control:** Other not–for–profit (including NFP Corporation) **Service:** General
Medical and Surgical

**Staffed Beds:** 55 **Admissions:** 1373 **Census:** 12 **Outpatient Visits:** 37826
**Births:** 280 **Total Expense ($000):** 26101 **Payroll Expense ($000):** 11273
**Personnel:** 236

## LORAIN—Lorain County

☒ △ **MERCY REGIONAL MEDICAL CENTER (360172)**, 3700 Kolbe Road,
Zip 44053–1697; tel. 440/960–4000, (Nonreporting) **A**1 2 7 9 10 **S** Catholic
Health Partners, Cincinnati, OH
Primary Contact: Edwin M. Oley, President and Chief Executive Officer
CFO: Gary Wengerd, Vice President Finance and Chief Financial Officer
CMO: Donald Blanford, M.D., Chief Medical Officer
CHR: Sarah Nickell, Vice President Human Resources
Web address: www.community–health–partners.com
**Control:** Church–operated, Nongovernment, not–for profit **Service:** General
Medical and Surgical

**Staffed Beds:** 259

## MANSFIELD—Richland County

☒ **KINDRED HOSPITAL OF CENTRAL OHIO (362021)**, 335 Glessner Avenue, 5th
Floor, Zip 44903; tel. 419/526–0777, (Nonreporting) **A**1 10 **S** Kindred
Healthcare, Louisville, KY
Primary Contact: Kris Karns, FACHE, Ph.D., Chief Executive Officer
Web address: www.khcentralohio.com/
**Control:** Corporation, Investor–owned, for–profit **Service:** Long–Term Acute Care
hospital

**Staffed Beds:** 33

☐ **MEDCENTRAL – MANSFIELD HOSPITAL (360118)**, 335 Glessner Avenue,
Zip 44903–2265; tel. 419/526–8000, (Includes MANSFIELD HOSPITAL, 335
Glessner Avenue, tel. 419/526–8000) **A**1 2 5 9 10 **F**3 5 8 11 13 15 17 18 20
22 24 26 28 29 30 31 32 34 35 38 39 40 43 44 45 46 47 48 49 50 51 53
54 55 56 57 58 59 61 62 63 64 65 70 73 74 75 76 77 78 79 81 82 85 86
87 89 90 92 93 96 98 99 100 101 102 103 104 105 107 108 110 111 113
115 116 117 118 119 120 121 122 123 128 129 130 131 132 134 143 145
146 147 **P**3 **S** MedCentral Health System, Mansfield, OH
Primary Contact: James E. Meyer, President and Chief Executive Officer
CMO: Terry Weston, M.D., Vice President Physician Services
CIO: Mike Mistretta, Vice President Information Systems and Chief Information
Officer
CHR: Beth Hildreth, Vice President Human Resources
Web address: www.medcentral.org
**Control:** Other not–for–profit (including NFP Corporation) **Service:** General
Medical and Surgical

**Staffed Beds:** 268 **Admissions:** 12765 **Census:** 168 **Outpatient Visits:**
270402 **Births:** 1017 **Personnel:** 1719

## MARIETTA—Washington County

★ ○ △ **MARIETTA MEMORIAL HOSPITAL (360147)**, 401 Matthew Street,
Zip 45750–1699; tel. 740/374–1400, (Nonreporting) **A**2 5 7 9 10 11
Primary Contact: J. Scott Cantley, President and Chief Executive Officer
CFO: Eric L. Young, Vice President Finance and Chief Financial Officer
CMO: Michael Nill, M.D., President Medical Staff
CIO: Andy Altenburger, Chief Information Officer
CHR: Dee Ann Gehlauf, Senior Vice President Business and Organization
Development
Web address: www.mmhospital.org
**Control:** Other not–for–profit (including NFP Corporation) **Service:** General
Medical and Surgical

**Staffed Beds:** 152

---

**Hospital, Medicare Provider Number, Address, Telephone, Approval, Facility, and Physician Codes, Health Care System**

★ American Hospital Association (AHA) membership      ○ American Osteopathic Association (AOA) accreditation
☐ The Joint Commission accreditation    ◇ DNV Healthcare Inc. accreditation      △ Commission on Accreditation of Rehabilitation Facilities (CARF) accreditation

★ ○ **SELBY GENERAL HOSPITAL (361319)**, 1106 Colegate Drive, Zip 45750–1323; tel. 740/568–2000 **A**9 10 11 18 **F**3 29 30 34 35 40 45 56 57 59 64 68 69 70 75 77 79 81 82 85 86 87 104 107 108 111 116 118 129 132 134 145 **P**5
Primary Contact: Stephen Smith, Administrator
CFO: Eric L. Young, Chief Financial Officer
CMO: David Spears, D.O., Chief of Staff
CHR: Cindy Hall, Coordinator Human Resources
CNO: Misti Spencer, Director Inpatient Services
Web address: www.selbygeneral.org
**Control:** Other not–for–profit (including NFP Corporation) **Service:** General Medical and Surgical

**Staffed Beds:** 25 **Admissions:** 1257 **Census:** 13 **Outpatient Visits:** 28719 **Births:** 0 **Total Expense ($000):** 25396 **Payroll Expense ($000):** 10065 **Personnel:** 198

### MARION—Marion County

⊠ △ **OHIOHEALTH MARION GENERAL HOSPITAL (360011)**, 1000 McKinley Park Drive, Zip 43302–6397; tel. 740/383–8400 **A**1 2 7 9 10 19 **F**3 15 18 20 22 24 26 28 29 30 31 35 40 53 57 59 60 62 63 68 70 72 73 74 75 76 78 79 81 87 89 98 104 105 107 111 113 118 129 131 134 145 147 **S** OhioHealth, Columbus, OH
Primary Contact: John W. Sanders, President
COO: Joseph Hooper, Vice President Operations
CFO: Steven Brown, Vice President Finance
CMO: Richard Flaksman, M.D., Vice President Medical Affairs
CIO: Chris King, Director Information Services
CHR: Linda Alesi, Director Human Resources
CNO: Eric Wallis, R.N., Vice President Patient Care and Chief Nursing Officer
Web address: www.ohiohealth.com/mariongeneral
**Control:** Other not–for–profit (including NFP Corporation) **Service:** General Medical and Surgical

**Staffed Beds:** 170 **Admissions:** 8172 **Census:** 83 **Outpatient Visits:** 86248 **Births:** 1075 **Total Expense ($000):** 115584 **Payroll Expense ($000):** 49319 **Personnel:** 875

### MARTINS FERRY—Belmont County

□ **EAST OHIO REGIONAL HOSPITAL (360080)**, 90 North Fourth Street, Zip 43935–1648; tel. 740/633–1100, (Total facility includes 61 beds in nursing home–type unit) **A**1 9 10 **F**3 11 13 15 20 28 29 30 31 34 35 37 40 43 44 45 49 53 57 59 64 68 70 74 75 76 77 79 81 82 85 87 107 108 110 111 113 114 117 118 127 128 129 130 131 132 134 145 147 **P**5 6 **S** Ohio Valley Health Services and Education Corporation, Wheeling, WV
Primary Contact: George G. Couch, FACHE, President and Chief Executive Officer
COO: Kelly Bettem, Assistant Chief Operating Officer
CFO: Tom Feldman, Chief Financial Officer
CIO: Karen Wayrauch, Interim Director Information Systems
CHR: James R. Stultz, Senior Vice President Human Resources
Web address: www.eorh–online.com
**Control:** Other not–for–profit (including NFP Corporation) **Service:** General Medical and Surgical

**Staffed Beds:** 172 **Admissions:** 3701 **Census:** 84 **Outpatient Visits:** 147978 **Births:** 291 **Total Expense ($000):** 57079 **Payroll Expense ($000):** 24684 **Personnel:** 604

### MARYSVILLE—Union County

★ **MEMORIAL HOSPITAL OF UNION COUNTY (360092)**, 500 London Avenue, Zip 43040–1594; tel. 937/644–6115, (Nonreporting) **A**5 9 10 21
Primary Contact: Olas A. Hubbs, III, FACHE, President and Chief Executive Officer
COO: Laurie A. Whittington, Chief Operating Officer
CFO: Jeffrey Ehlers, Chief Financial Officer
CMO: Matthew Hazelbaker, M.D., President Medical Staff
CIO: Carl Zani, Director Information Systems
CHR: Carman Wirtz, Vice President Human Resources
CNO: Robin Slattman, Chief Nursing Officer
Web address: www.memorialhosp.org
**Control:** County–Government, nonfederal **Service:** General Medical and Surgical

**Staffed Beds:** 56

### MASON—Warren County

⊠ **LINDNER CENTER OF HOPE (364044)**, 4075 Old Western Row Road, Zip 45040–3104; tel. 513/536–0311 **A**1 9 10 **F**4 29 30 35 53 98 99 101 103 104 105 106 111 129 133 **P**6
Primary Contact: Paul Keck, M.D., President and Chief Executive Officer
COO: Brian Owens, Chief Operating Officer
CFO: David McAdams, Chief Financial Officer
CIO: Cliff McClintick, Chief Information Officer
CHR: Debbie A. Strawser, Director Human Resources
Web address: www.lindnercenterofhope.org
**Control:** Other not–for–profit (including NFP Corporation) **Service:** Psychiatric

**Staffed Beds:** 64 **Admissions:** 1816 **Census:** 38 **Outpatient Visits:** 17653 **Births:** 0 **Total Expense ($000):** 29317 **Payroll Expense ($000):** 14930 **Personnel:** 229

### MASSILLON—Stark County

★ ○ △ **AFFINITY MEDICAL CENTER (360151)**, 875 Eighth Street N.E., Zip 44646–8503, Mailing Address: P.O. Box 805, Zip 44648–8503; tel. 330/832–8761, (Nonreporting) **A**7 9 10 11 12 13 **S** Community Health Systems, Inc., Franklin, TN
Primary Contact: Ronald L. Bierman, Chief Executive Officer
CFO: James Hutchinson, CPA, Chief Financial Officer
Web address: www.affinitymedicalcenter.com
**Control:** Corporation, Investor–owned, for–profit **Service:** General Medical and Surgical

**Staffed Beds:** 112

□ **HEARTLAND BEHAVIORAL HEALTHCARE (364031)**, 3000 Erie Street, Zip 44646–7993, Mailing Address: P.O. Box 540, Zip 44648–0540; tel. 330/833–3135 **A**1 5 9 10 **F**86 87 98 103 129 145 **P**6 **S** Ohio Department of Mental Health, Columbus, OH
Primary Contact: James Ignelzi, Interim Chief Executive Officer
CFO: Patricia Eddleman, Fiscal Officer
CMO: Steven Thomson, M.D., Medical Director
CIO: Robert Hobart, Director Management Information Systems
CHR: Jerald Wilhite, Administrator Human Resources
Web address: www.mh.state.oh.us/ibhs/bhos/hoh.html
**Control:** State–Government, nonfederal **Service:** Psychiatric

**Staffed Beds:** 130 **Admissions:** 905 **Census:** 112 **Outpatient Visits:** 0 **Births:** 0 **Total Expense ($000):** 24889 **Payroll Expense ($000):** 14396 **Personnel:** 224

### MAUMEE—Lucas County

□ **ARROWHEAD BEHAVIORAL HEALTH HOSPITAL (364036)**, 1725 Timber Line Road, Zip 43537–4015; tel. 419/891–9333, (Nonreporting) **A**1 9 10 **S** Universal Health Services, Inc., King of Prussia, PA
Primary Contact: Elyssia Lowe–Narayan, Chief Executive Officer
CFO: Kim Blackwell, Chief Financial Officer
CMO: Siva Yechoor, M.D., Medical Director
CIO: Lynette Box, Director Medical Records
CHR: Eunice Russell, Manager Human Resources
Web address: www.arrowheadbehavioral.com
**Control:** Corporation, Investor–owned, for–profit **Service:** Other specialty

**Staffed Beds:** 42

⊠ **PROMEDICA ST. LUKE'S HOSPITAL (360090)**, 5901 Monclova Road, Zip 43537–1899; tel. 419/893–5911 **A**1 2 3 5 9 10 **F**1 3 4 11 13 15 16 17 18 20 22 24 26 28 29 30 31 34 35 40 45 46 48 49 56 57 59 64 67 68 70 72 73 74 76 77 78 79 80 81 82 85 86 87 88 89 92 93 98 100 107 108 111 113 117 118 125 127 128 129 130 131 133 134 142 145 146 147 **P**6 8 **S** ProMedica Health System, Toledo, OH
Primary Contact: Daniel L. Wakeman, President
COO: Lori Johnston, Chief Financial Officer and Chief Operating Officer
CFO: Lori Johnston, Chief Financial Officer and Chief Operating Officer
CMO: Stephen Bazeley, M.D., Vice President Medical Affairs
CIO: Patricia Swint, Director Information Technology
CHR: Connie Sessler, Director Human Resources
CNO: Theresa Konwinski, R.N., Vice President Patient Care
Web address: www.stlukeshospital.com
**Control:** Other not–for–profit (including NFP Corporation) **Service:** General Medical and Surgical

**Staffed Beds:** 209 **Admissions:** 11680 **Census:** 122 **Outpatient Visits:** 260380 **Births:** 852 **Total Expense ($000):** 163336 **Payroll Expense ($000):** 64320 **Personnel:** 1364

### MEDINA—Medina County

⊠ **MEDINA HOSPITAL (360091)**, 1000 East Washington Street, Zip 44256–2170; tel. 330/725–1000 **A**1 2 5 9 10 **F**3 7 13 15 18 20 28 29 30 31 34 35 40 50 57 59 60 62 64 66 70 74 75 76 77 78 81 82 85 86 93 96 107 111 113 115 118 128 129 130 131 132 134 143 145 146 147 **S** Cleveland Clinic Health System, Cleveland, OH
Primary Contact: Thomas Tulisiak, M.D., President
COO: Vicky Snyder, Chief Operating Officer and Chief Financial Officer
CFO: Vicky Snyder, Chief Operating Officer and Chief Financial Officer
CMO: Rick Shewbridge, M.D., Vice President Medical Operations
CIO: David Ingram, Director Management Information Systems
CHR: Amy Clark, Vice President Human Resources
CNO: Mary Kennedy, Chief Nursing Officer
Web address: www.medinahospital.org
**Control:** Other not–for–profit (including NFP Corporation) **Service:** General Medical and Surgical

**Staffed Beds:** 110 **Admissions:** 6248 **Census:** 67 **Outpatient Visits:** 102312 **Births:** 983 **Total Expense ($000):** 85777 **Payroll Expense ($000):** 40586 **Personnel:** 697

## MIAMISBURG—Montgomery County

☒ **LIFECARE HOSPITAL OF DAYTON (362028)**, 4000 Miamisburg–Centerville Road, Zip 45342; tel. 937/384–8300, (Nonreporting) **A**1 9 10 **S** LifeCare Management Services, Plano, TX
Primary Contact: Russell Dean, Chief Executive Officer
CMO: Richard Gregg, M.D., Medical Director
CHR: Pam Fannin, Coordinator Human Resources
Web address: www.lifecare–hospitals.com
**Control:** Corporation, Investor–owned, for–profit **Service:** Long–Term Acute Care hospital

**Staffed Beds: 44**

☒ **SYCAMORE MEDICAL CENTER (360239)**, 4000 Miamisburg–Centerville Road, Zip 45342; tel. 937/866–0551 **A**1 9 10 **F**3 5 8 11 12 15 18 20 28 29 30 31 32 34 35 36 38 39 40 42 44 45 47 48 49 50 53 54 56 57 58 59 60 61 62 63 64 65 66 68 70 74 75 77 78 79 81 82 83 85 86 87 93 97 98 99 100 101 102 104 105 107 108 110 111 113 114 117 118 124 128 129 130 131 133 134 140 145 146 147 **P**7 8 **S** Kettering Health Network, Dayton, OH
Primary Contact: Mark T. Smith, JD, CPA, President
CMO: Gregory Wise, M.D., Vice President Medical Affairs
CIO: Jon Russell, Chief Information Officer
CHR: Beverly Morris, Vice President Human Resources
Web address: www.khnetwork.org
**Control:** Church–operated, Nongovernment, not–for profit **Service:** General Medical and Surgical

**Staffed Beds: 163 Admissions: 7671 Census: 90 Outpatient Visits: 117920 Births: 0 Total Expense ($000): 72958 Payroll Expense ($000): 32410 Personnel: 771**

## MIDDLEBURG HEIGHTS—Cuyahoga County

☐ **SOUTHWEST GENERAL HEALTH CENTER (360155)**, 18697 Bagley Road, Zip 44130–3497; tel. 440/816–8000 **A**1 2 9 10 **F**3 5 7 11 13 15 17 18 20 22 24 26 28 29 30 31 32 34 35 36 37 38 39 40 42 43 44 45 49 50 51 53 54 56 57 59 60 62 63 64 65 66 68 70 74 75 76 77 78 79 81 82 85 86 87 90 91 92 93 94 98 99 100 101 102 103 104 105 107 108 110 111 113 114 117 118 119 120 122 125 127 128 129 130 131 133 134 142 143 145 146 147 **P**6
Primary Contact: Thomas A. Selden, FACHE, President and Chief Executive Officer
CFO: Mary Ann Freas, Vice President and Chief Financial Officer
CMO: Marilyn McNamara, M.D., Vice President Medical Affairs
CIO: Teresa Rini Barber, Vice President Support Services
CHR: Judy Murphy, Director Human Resources
Web address: www.swgeneral.com
**Control:** Other not–for–profit (including NFP Corporation) **Service:** General Medical and Surgical

**Staffed Beds: 316 Admissions: 15633 Census: 207 Outpatient Visits: 399164 Births: 1128 Total Expense ($000): 251162 Payroll Expense ($000): 100780 Personnel: 1991**

## MIDDLETOWN—Warren County

☐ △ **ATRIUM MEDICAL CENTER (360076)**, One Medical Center Drive, Zip 45005–1066; tel. 513/424–2111 **A**1 2 7 9 10 21 **F**3 8 11 13 15 17 18 20 22 24 26 28 29 30 31 34 37 40 43 45 46 47 49 50 51 54 56 57 59 60 70 72 73 74 75 76 77 78 79 81 82 85 86 87 90 92 93 96 98 99 100 101 102 103 104 105 107 108 111 113 114 115 116 117 118 123 125 129 130 143 145 146 **P**8
Primary Contact: Carol Turner, President and Chief Executive Officer
CFO: Tom Maloney, Chief Financial Officer
CMO: Mark Williams, M.D., Chief Medical Officer
CHR: Ted Ripperger, Administrative Director Human Resources
Web address: www.atriummedcenter.org
**Control:** Other not–for–profit (including NFP Corporation) **Service:** General Medical and Surgical

**Staffed Beds: 314 Admissions: 11875 Census: 152 Outpatient Visits: 205169 Births: 973 Total Expense ($000): 220540 Payroll Expense ($000): 76570 Personnel: 1565**

## MILLERSBURG—Holmes County

☐ **POMERENE HOSPITAL (360148)**, 981 Wooster Road, Zip 44654–1094; tel. 330/674–1015 **A**1 9 10 **F**3 11 13 15 29 30 34 35 40 53 55 57 59 68 70 75 76 77 79 81 85 89 93 107 108 110 113 117 118 128 129 130 134 143 145 147 **P**7
Primary Contact: Tony Snyder, Administrator and Chief Executive Officer
CFO: Jason Justus, Vice President Finance and Chief Financial Officer
CMO: Yasser Omran, M.D., President Medical Staff
CIO: Mark Jacobs, Director Information Services
CHR: Rebecca Ragon, Coordinator Public Relations and Marketing
Web address: www.pomerenehospital.org
**Control:** County–Government, nonfederal **Service:** General Medical and Surgical

**Staffed Beds: 40 Admissions: 1693 Census: 17 Outpatient Visits: 38175 Births: 512 Total Expense ($000): 24473 Payroll Expense ($000): 11190 Personnel: 245**

## MONTPELIER—Williams County

△ **COMMUNITY HOSPITALS AND WELLNESS CENTERS–MONTPELIER (361327)**, 909 East Snyder Avenue, Zip 43543; tel. 419/385–3154, (Nonreporting) **A**7 9 10 18
Primary Contact: Philip L. Ennen, President and Chief Executive Officer
Web address: www.chwchospital.com
**Control:** Corporation, Investor–owned, for–profit **Service:** General Medical and Surgical

**Staffed Beds: 35**

**MONTPELIER HOSPITAL** See Community Hospitals and Wellness Centers, Bryan

## MOUNT GILEAD—Morrow County

☐ **MORROW COUNTY HOSPITAL (361313)**, 651 West Marion Road, Zip 43338–1027; tel. 419/946–5015, (Nonreporting) **A**1 5 9 10 18 **S** OhioHealth, Columbus, OH
Primary Contact: Christopher Truax, Chief Executive Officer
CFO: Joe Schueler, Chief Financial Officer
Web address: www.morrowcountyhospital.com
**Control:** County–Government, nonfederal **Service:** General Medical and Surgical

**Staffed Beds: 53**

## MOUNT VERNON—Knox County

☒ **KNOX COMMUNITY HOSPITAL (360040)**, 1330 Coshocton Road, Zip 43050–1495; tel. 740/393–9000 **A**1 2 9 10 20 **F**3 11 13 15 18 20 22 26 28 29 30 31 34 35 40 44 45 50 51 53 57 59 64 68 69 70 75 76 77 78 79 81 82 83 84 85 86 87 89 93 96 97 107 108 110 111 113 116 117 118 119 120 128 129 131 133 143 145 146 **P**6 **S** QHR, Brentwood, TN
Primary Contact: Bruce D. White, Chief Executive Officer
COO: Bruce M. Behner, Chief Operating Officer
CFO: Michael Ambrosiani, Chief Financial Officer
CMO: Judy Schwartz, M.D., Chief Medical Officer
CIO: Kwi Holland, Vice President Information Services
CHR: Lisa Bragg, Vice President Human Resources
CNO: Sandra Beidelschies, MSN, Chief Nursing Officer
Web address: www.knoxcommhosp.org
**Control:** Other not–for–profit (including NFP Corporation) **Service:** General Medical and Surgical

**Staffed Beds: 87 Admissions: 3390 Census: 34 Outpatient Visits: 99520 Births: 359 Total Expense ($000): 105636 Payroll Expense ($000): 47302 Personnel: 815**

## NAPOLEON—Henry County

☒ **HENRY COUNTY HOSPITAL (361309)**, 1600 East Riverview Avenue, Zip 43545–9399; tel. 419/592–4015 **A**1 5 9 10 18 **F**3 5 11 13 15 28 29 31 34 35 36 40 53 57 59 64 65 68 70 75 76 78 79 81 82 85 86 87 93 99 100 101 104 107 108 113 118 129 131 132 134 145
Primary Contact: Kimberly Bordenkircher, Chief Executive Officer
COO: Michelle Rychener, Chief Operating Officer
CFO: Mary Clapp, Controller
CHR: Jennifer A. Fisher, Manager Human Resources
CNO: Patricia Frank, Chief Nursing Officer
Web address: www.henrycountyhospital.org
**Control:** Other not–for–profit (including NFP Corporation) **Service:** General Medical and Surgical

**Staffed Beds: 25 Admissions: 857 Census: 10 Outpatient Visits: 67195 Births: 139 Total Expense ($000): 23728 Payroll Expense ($000): 9357 Personnel: 181**

---

**Hospital, Medicare Provider Number, Address, Telephone, Approval, Facility, and Physician Codes, Health Care System**

★ American Hospital Association (AHA) membership
☐ The Joint Commission accreditation ◇ DNV Healthcare Inc. accreditation
○ American Osteopathic Association (AOA) accreditation
△ Commission on Accreditation of Rehabilitation Facilities (CARF) accreditation

**OH**

## NELSONVILLE—Athens County

★ ○ **DOCTORS HOSPITAL NELSONVILLE (361305)**, 1950 Mount Saint Mary Drive, Zip 45764–1193; tel. 740/753–1931 **A**9 10 11 18 **F**3 15 29 40 45 50 57 59 64 75 79 81 84 87 96 97 107 108 110 113 117 129 132 147 **P**6 **S** OhioHealth, Columbus, OH
Primary Contact: LaMar L. Wyse, Chief Operating Officer
COO: LaMar L. Wyse, Chief Operating Officer
CFO: Shannon M. Atha, Director Finance
CMO: Marjorie Devol, M.D., Chief of Staff
CIO: Danny Canter, Manager Information Systems
CHR: Terry Wilson, Director Human Resources and Compliance
CNO: Sandy Wood, Director Patient Care Services
Web address: www.ohiohealth.com
**Control:** Other not–for–profit (including NFP Corporation) **Service:** General Medical and Surgical

**Staffed Beds:** 25 **Admissions:** 551 **Census:** 9 **Outpatient Visits:** 36517 **Births:** 0 **Total Expense ($000):** 16501 **Payroll Expense ($000):** 7585 **Personnel:** 153

## NEW ALBANY—Franklin County

⊞ **MOUNT CARMEL NEW ALBANY SURGICAL HOSPITAL (360266)**, 7333 Smith's Mill Road, Zip 43054; tel. 614/775–6600 **A**1 9 10 **F**29 34 35 44 57 58 59 64 65 68 74 75 79 81 85 86 87 94 107 111 113 145 **P**6 8 **S** Trinity Health, Novi, MI
Primary Contact: Richard D'Enbeau, Chief Operating Officer
Web address: www.newalbanysurgicalhospital.com
**Control:** Church–operated, Nongovernment, not–for profit **Service:** General Medical and Surgical

**Staffed Beds:** 60 **Admissions:** 4851 **Census:** 27 **Outpatient Visits:** 13812 **Births:** 0 **Total Expense ($000):** 83063 **Payroll Expense ($000):** 11437 **Personnel:** 212

## NEWARK—Licking County

☐ **LICKING MEMORIAL HOSPITAL (360218)**, 1320 West Main Street, Zip 43055–3699; tel. 740/348–4000 **A**1 2 9 10 **F**1 3 4 5 13 15 16 17 18 20 22 26 28 29 30 31 32 34 35 40 41 45 49 50 53 57 59 62 64 65 67 68 70 72 73 74 75 76 77 78 79 80 81 82 84 85 86 87 88 89 90 92 93 97 98 100 101 102 104 105 106 107 108 110 111 113 114 117 118 127 129 131 134 143 145 146 147 **P**6
Primary Contact: Robert A. Montagnese, President and Chief Executive Officer
CFO: Cindy Webster, Vice President Financial Services
CMO: Craig Cairns, M.D., Vice President Medical Affairs
CIO: Sallie Arnett, Vice President Information Systems
CHR: Anne Peterson, Vice President Human Resources and Support Services
Web address: www.lmhealth.org
**Control:** Other not–for–profit (including NFP Corporation) **Service:** General Medical and Surgical

**Staffed Beds:** 199 **Admissions:** 6867 **Census:** 58 **Outpatient Visits:** 286809 **Births:** 974 **Total Expense ($000):** 128493 **Payroll Expense ($000):** 51838 **Personnel:** 1168

**MEDICAL CENTER OF NEWARK (360347)**, 2000 Tamarack Road, Zip 43055; tel. 740/522–7800 **A**9 10 **F**3 18 29 31 34 35 45 48 51 57 58 59 63 65 68 74 78 79 81 82 91 107 111 113 118 147
Primary Contact: Michael Greene, Chief Executive Officer
Web address: www.mcnohio.com
**Control:** Partnership, Investor–owned, for–profit **Service:** General Medical and Surgical

**Staffed Beds:** 20 **Admissions:** 561 **Census:** 5 **Outpatient Visits:** 30695 **Births:** 0 **Total Expense ($000):** 19288 **Payroll Expense ($000):** 5487 **Personnel:** 131

## NORTHFIELD—Summit County

☐ **NORTHCOAST BEHAVIORAL HEALTHCARE SYSTEM (364011)**, 1756 Sagamore Road, Zip 44067–1086; tel. 330/467–7131, (Includes CLEVELAND CAMPUS, 1708 Southpoint Drive, Cleveland, Zip 44109–1999; tel. 216/787–0500; NORTHFIELD CAMPUS, 1756 Sagamore Road, Zip 44067, Mailing Address: P.O. Box 305, Zip 44067–0305; tel. 330/467–7131; TOLEDO CAMPUS, 930 South Detroit Avenue, Toledo, Zip 43614–2701; tel. 419/381–1881) **A**1 3 10 **F**30 53 65 75 77 82 98 106 129 134 145 **S** Ohio Department of Mental Health, Columbus, OH
Primary Contact: David Celletti, Chief Executive Officer
CFO: Jeff Comfort, Vice President Administration
CIO: Karl Donenwirth, Vice President Information Services
Web address: www.mh.state.oh.us
**Control:** State–Government, nonfederal **Service:** Psychiatric

**Staffed Beds:** 260 **Admissions:** 1698 **Census:** 260 **Outpatient Visits:** 0 **Births:** 0 **Total Expense ($000):** 52963 **Payroll Expense ($000):** 27478 **Personnel:** 484

## NORWALK—Huron County

⊞ ○ **FISHER–TITUS MEDICAL CENTER (360065)**, 272 Benedict Avenue, Zip 44857–2374; tel. 419/668–8101, (Total facility includes 69 beds in nursing home–type unit) **A**1 2 5 9 10 11 19 **F**3 10 11 13 15 18 20 28 29 31 34 35 36 39 40 43 45 49 50 51 56 57 58 59 62 64 68 70 74 75 76 77 78 79 81 82 85 86 87 92 93 94 96 97 107 108 110 111 114 117 118 127 129 130 131 134 145 146 147 **P**2 6 7
Primary Contact: Patrick J. Martin, President and Chief Executive Officer
COO: Lorna Strayer, Senior Vice President Administration and Business Development
CFO: Duane L. Woods, Jr., Chief Financial Officer
CMO: Gary L. Moorman, D.O., Vice President Medical Affairs
CIO: John Britton, Director Information Services
CHR: Phillip Annarino, Vice President Human Resources
CNO: Cherie Spragg, R.N., Senior Vice President Nursing Services
Web address: www.fisher–titus.com
**Control:** Other not–for–profit (including NFP Corporation) **Service:** General Medical and Surgical

**Staffed Beds:** 147 **Admissions:** 4485 **Census:** 106 **Outpatient Visits:** 159056 **Births:** 615 **Total Expense ($000):** 100167 **Payroll Expense ($000):** 40376 **Personnel:** 753

## OBERLIN—Lorain County

⊞ **MERCY ALLEN HOSPITAL (361306)**, 200 West Lorain Street, Zip 44074–1077; tel. 440/775–1211, (Nonreporting) **A**1 9 10 18 **S** Catholic Health Partners, Cincinnati, OH
Primary Contact: Susan Bowers, R.N., President and Chief Nursing Officer
CFO: Donald E. Kline, Chief Financial Officer and Vice President Operations
CMO: Eric Jenkins, M.D., Chief of Staff
CIO: Sami Othman, Regional Site Director Information Process Services
CHR: Amie Richason, Chief Human Resources Officer
CNO: Susan Bowers, R.N., President and Chief Nursing Officer
Web address: www.mercyonline.org/mercy_allen_hospital.aspx
**Control:** Other not–for–profit (including NFP Corporation) **Service:** General Medical and Surgical

**Staffed Beds:** 25

## OREGON—Lucas County

⊞ △ **MERCY ST. CHARLES HOSPITAL (360081)**, 2600 Navarre Avenue, Zip 43616–3297; tel. 419/696–7200 **A**1 2 7 9 10 **F**3 11 13 15 17 18 28 29 30 31 34 35 40 43 44 46 47 48 49 51 53 56 57 59 60 64 66 68 70 71 73 74 75 76 77 78 79 81 82 84 85 86 87 90 92 93 94 97 98 100 101 102 103 107 109 110 111 113 114 115 116 118 122 124 128 129 131 132 145 146 147 **P**8 **S** Catholic Health Partners, Cincinnati, OH
Primary Contact: Robert E. Gospodarek, President and Chief Executive Officer
COO: Jeffrey Dempsey, Vice President Operations
CFO: Robert Moon, Senior Vice President Northern Region and Chief Financial Officer
CMO: Krishna Ragothaman, M.D., Chief of Staff
CIO: Michael Shork, M.D., Director Information Systems Services
CHR: Gary George, Regional Vice President Human Resources
CNO: Judy Zbierajewski, Chief Nursing Officer and Vice President Patient Care
Web address: www.mercyweb.org
**Control:** Church–operated, Nongovernment, not–for profit **Service:** General Medical and Surgical

**Staffed Beds:** 271 **Admissions:** 9639 **Census:** 147 **Outpatient Visits:** 225571 **Births:** 449 **Personnel:** 895

⊞ **PROMEDICA BAY PARK HOSPITAL (360259)**, 2801 Bay Park Drive, Zip 43616; tel. 419/690–7900 **A**1 9 10 **F**3 11 13 15 18 20 29 30 31 34 35 40 44 45 49 50 51 57 58 59 64 68 70 74 75 76 77 78 79 81 82 85 86 87 92 93 107 108 110 111 113 116 117 118 123 128 129 130 131 134 145 146 147 **S** ProMedica Health System, Toledo, OH
Primary Contact: Holly L. Bristoll, President
CFO: David Brewer, Director Finance
CMO: David Lindstrom, M.D., Vice President Medical Affairs
CIO: David G. Selman, Corporate Vice President Information Resources
CHR: Kara Zimmerly, Manager Human Resources
CNO: Maurine Weis, Vice President Patient Care Service and Chief Nursing Officer
Web address: www.promedica.org
**Control:** Other not–for–profit (including NFP Corporation) **Service:** General Medical and Surgical

**Staffed Beds:** 72 **Admissions:** 3560 **Census:** 39 **Outpatient Visits:** 101128 **Births:** 616 **Total Expense ($000):** 73367 **Payroll Expense ($000):** 22054 **Personnel:** 395

**ST. CHARLES MERCY HOSPITAL** See Mercy St. Charles Hospital

*Many Facility Codes have changed. Please refer to the AHA Guide Code Chart.* © 2012 AHA Guide

## ORRVILLE—Wayne County

⊠ **AULTMAN ORRVILLE HOSPITAL (361323)**, 832 South Main Street, Zip 44667–2208; tel. 330/682–3010 **A**1 9 10 18 **F**3 8 11 13 15 24 29 30 34 35 40 45 47 50 51 53 57 59 68 70 75 76 77 79 81 82 85 86 87 89 93 107 108 110 111 113 117 118 127 128 129 130 131 132 134 142 145 146 **P**1 5 **S** Aultman Health Foundation, Canton, OH
Primary Contact: Marchelle Suppan, DPM, President and Chief Executive Officer
COO: Judy Erb, Vice President Patient Care Services and Chief Nursing Officer
CFO: Adam M. Luntz, Vice President Finance and Chief Financial Officer
CIO: Roger Mutchler, Manager Information Technology
CHR: Lori Kotewicz, Supervisor Human Resources
CNO: Judy Erb, Vice President Patient Services and Chief Nursing Officer
Web address: www.aultmanorrville.org
**Control:** Other not–for–profit (including NFP Corporation) **Service:** General Medical and Surgical

**Staffed Beds:** 25 **Admissions:** 715 **Census:** 6 **Outpatient Visits:** 46614 **Births:** 290 **Total Expense ($000):** 13087 **Payroll Expense ($000):** 8867 **Personnel:** 187

## OXFORD—Butler County

★ ○ **MCCULLOUGH–HYDE MEMORIAL HOSPITAL (360046)**, 110 North Poplar Street, Zip 45056–1292; tel. 513/523–2111 **A**9 10 11 **F**3 11 13 15 28 29 30 31 32 34 35 36 40 45 47 49 54 57 59 64 65 69 70 74 75 76 77 78 79 81 82 85 89 93 94 107 108 110 111 113 117 118 128 129 130 131 134 142 143 145 146 147
Primary Contact: Bryan D. Hehemann, President and Chief Executive Officer
CFO: John R. Clements, Vice President and Chief Financial Officer
CIO: Kathy Dickman, Director Information Technology
CHR: Dennis Johnson, Director Human Resources
CNO: Pamela Collins, Vice President Chief Patient Services Officer
Web address: www.mhmh.org
**Control:** Other not–for–profit (including NFP Corporation) **Service:** General Medical and Surgical

**Staffed Beds:** 45 **Admissions:** 2608 **Census:** 25 **Outpatient Visits:** 86909 **Births:** 408 **Total Expense ($000):** 56366 **Payroll Expense ($000):** 22394 **Personnel:** 394

## PARMA—Cuyahoga County

⊠ △ **PARMA COMMUNITY GENERAL HOSPITAL (360041)**, 7007 Powers Boulevard, Zip 44129–5495; tel. 440/743–3000, (Total facility includes 11 beds in nursing home–type unit) **A**1 2 7 9 10 **F**2 3 8 10 11 12 13 15 17 18 20 22 24 26 28 29 30 31 32 34 35 36 40 44 45 49 50 51 53 56 57 58 59 62 63 64 65 68 69 70 71 74 75 76 77 78 79 81 82 85 86 87 90 93 96 98 100 101 103 107 108 111 113 114 117 118 119 120 125 127 129 130 131 134 142 143 145 146 147 **P**6
Primary Contact: Terrence G. Deis, President and Chief Executive Officer
CFO: Barry L. Franklin, Executive Vice President and Chief Financial Officer
CMO: Dale Cowan, M.D., Vice President Medical Affairs
CIO: Barry L. Franklin, Executive Vice President and Chief Financial Officer
CHR: Ralph Knull, Vice President Human Resources
CNO: Pam Falasco, Vice President, Chief Nursing Officer
Web address: www.parmahospital.org
**Control:** Other not–for–profit (including NFP Corporation) **Service:** General Medical and Surgical

**Staffed Beds:** 279 **Admissions:** 14557 **Census:** 182 **Outpatient Visits:** 229443 **Births:** 430 **Total Expense ($000):** 175552 **Payroll Expense ($000):** 73076 **Personnel:** 1586

## PAULDING—Paulding County

☐ **PAULDING COUNTY HOSPITAL (361300)**, 1035 West Wayne Street, Zip 45879–9220; tel. 419/399–4080 **A**1 9 10 18 **F**3 11 15 28 29 31 40 51 53 57 59 62 64 69 77 78 79 81 85 93 107 110 111 113 118 127 128 129 132 142 143 145 147
Primary Contact: Gary W. Adkins, Chief Executive Officer
COO: Randy Ruge, Chief Operating Officer
CFO: Rob Goshia, Chief Financial Officer
CMO: Wendell J. Spangler, M.D., Chief of Staff
CIO: Dan Kaufman, Director Information Services
CHR: Melanie Rittenour, Director Human Resources
Web address: www.pauldingcountyhospital.com
**Control:** County–Government, nonfederal **Service:** General Medical and Surgical

**Staffed Beds:** 25 **Admissions:** 524 **Census:** 7 **Outpatient Visits:** 28447 **Births:** 0 **Total Expense ($000):** 18574 **Payroll Expense ($000):** 8756 **Personnel:** 188

## PORT CLINTON—Ottawa County

⊠ **H. B. MAGRUDER MEMORIAL HOSPITAL (361314)**, 615 Fulton Street, Zip 43452–2034; tel. 419/734–3131, (Nonreporting) **A**1 5 9 10 18
Primary Contact: Michael E. Long, Chief Executive Officer
CFO: J. Todd Almendinger, Vice President Finance and Chief Financial Officer
CMO: Panju Prithviraj, M.D., President Medical Staff
CHR: Jennifer Capizzi, Director Human Resources
Web address: www.magruderhospital.com
**Control:** Other not–for–profit (including NFP Corporation) **Service:** General Medical and Surgical

**Staffed Beds:** 25

## PORTSMOUTH—Scioto County

⊠ △ **SOUTHERN OHIO MEDICAL CENTER (360008)**, 1805 27th Street, Zip 45662–2400; tel. 740/356–5000 **A**1 2 5 7 9 10 13 **F**3 11 13 15 17 18 20 22 24 26 28 29 30 31 34 35 37 38 40 41 44 45 46 49 50 53 54 57 59 62 63 64 65 68 70 74 75 76 77 78 79 81 83 84 85 86 87 89 90 92 97 100 102 104 107 108 109 110 111 113 114 115 116 117 118 119 120 121 122 123 124 128 129 130 131 134 143 144 145 **P**3
Primary Contact: Randal M. Arnett, President and Chief Executive Officer
COO: Claudia L. Burchett, R.N., Vice President Patient Services
CFO: Dean Wray, Vice President Finance
CMO: Kendall Stewart, M.D., Medical Director
CIO: Brent Richard, Administrative Director Information Systems
CHR: Vicki Noel, Vice President Human Resources
Web address: www.somc.org
**Control:** Other not–for–profit (including NFP Corporation) **Service:** General Medical and Surgical

**Staffed Beds:** 230 **Admissions:** 11816 **Census:** 139 **Outpatient Visits:** 257906 **Births:** 1145 **Total Expense ($000):** 229739 **Payroll Expense ($000):** 85341 **Personnel:** 1913

## PROCTORVILLE—Lawrence County

☐ **THREE GABLES SURGERY CENTER (360261)**, 5897 County Road 107, Zip 45669–8852; tel. 740/886–9911 **A**1 9 10 **F**3 8 34 45 48 57 59 64 65 81 82 93 107 111 113 128 **P**8
Primary Contact: Tony Alouise, Chief Executive Officer
Web address: www.threegablessurgery.com
**Control:** Partnership, Investor–owned, for–profit **Service:** General Medical and Surgical

**Staffed Beds:** 8 **Admissions:** 250 **Census:** 1 **Outpatient Visits:** 4705 **Births:** 0 **Total Expense ($000):** 10548 **Payroll Expense ($000):** 3440 **Personnel:** 62

## RAVENNA—Portage County

☐ **ROBINSON MEMORIAL HOSPITAL (360078)**, 6847 North Chestnut Street, Zip 44266–1204, Mailing Address: P.O. Box 1204, Zip 44266–1204; tel. 330/297–0811, (Nonreporting) **A**1 2 3 5 9 10 **S** Summa Health System, Akron, OH
Primary Contact: Stephen Colecchi, President and Chief Executive Officer
COO: Richard Clough, Chief Operating Officer
CFO: Carl Ebner, Vice President Finance
CMO: Stephen Francis, M.D., Vice President Medical Affairs
CIO: David Baldwin, Chief Information Officer
CHR: Pamela Mackintosh, Vice President Human Resources
Web address: www.robinsonmemorial.org
**Control:** County–Government, nonfederal **Service:** General Medical and Surgical

**Staffed Beds:** 141

## ROCK CREEK—Ashtabula County

**GLENBEIGH HOSPITAL AND OUTPATIENT CENTERS (360245)**, 2863 Route 45, Zip 44084, Mailing Address: P.O. Box 298, Zip 44084–0298; tel. 440/563–3400 **A**9 10 **F**4 5 29 30 34 36 53 54 57 75 86 87 100 129 131 134 **P**5
Primary Contact: Patricia Weston–Hall, Chief Executive Officer
CFO: Phil Pawlowski, Chief Financial Officer
CIO: Linda Advey, Manager Information Systems
CHR: Shirley Deary, Director Human Resources
Web address: www.glenbeigh.com
**Control:** Other not–for–profit (including NFP Corporation) **Service:** Alcoholism and other chemical dependency

**Staffed Beds:** 113 **Admissions:** 2563 **Census:** 66 **Outpatient Visits:** 65174 **Births:** 0 **Total Expense ($000):** 14586 **Payroll Expense ($000):** 7851 **Personnel:** 205

---

**Hospital, Medicare Provider Number, Address, Telephone, Approval, Facility, and Physician Codes, Health Care System**

★ American Hospital Association (AHA) membership
☐ The Joint Commission accreditation    ◇ DNV Healthcare Inc. accreditation
○ American Osteopathic Association (AOA) accreditation
△ Commission on Accreditation of Rehabilitation Facilities (CARF) accreditation

**OH**

### SAINT MARYS—Auglaize County

**JOINT TOWNSHIP DISTRICT MEMORIAL HOSPITAL (360032)**, 200 St. Clair Street, Zip 45885–2400; tel. 419/394–3335, (Total facility includes 15 beds in nursing home–type unit) **A**9 10 21 **F**3 7 8 11 12 13 15 28 29 30 31 32 34 35 36 40 41 42 43 51 53 57 59 62 63 64 70 75 77 78 79 81 82 83 84 85 87 90 93 97 107 108 110 114 118 127 128 129 130 131 134 142 143 145 146 147
Primary Contact: Kevin W. Harlan, President
CFO: Jeffrey W. Vossler, Vice President Financial Services
CIO: DeWayne Marsee, Director Information Systems
CHR: Art Swain, Vice President Support Services
Web address: www.grandlakehealth.org
**Control:** Other not–for–profit (including NFP Corporation) **Service:** General Medical and Surgical

**Staffed Beds:** 57 **Admissions:** 2055 **Census:** 17 **Outpatient Visits:** 108785 **Births:** 299 **Total Expense ($000):** 58699 **Payroll Expense ($000):** 20891 **Personnel:** 477

### SALEM—Columbiana County

⊠ **SALEM COMMUNITY HOSPITAL (360185)**, 1995 East State Street, Zip 44460–0121; tel. 330/332–1551, (Total facility includes 15 beds in nursing home–type unit) **A**1 5 9 10 **F**3 11 13 15 18 28 29 30 31 40 45 49 51 57 59 64 70 74 75 76 77 78 79 81 82 85 89 92 93 107 108 111 113 114 116 117 118 127 128 129 131 134 144 145 147
Primary Contact: Steven T. Ruwoldt, Chief Executive Officer
CFO: Mike Giangardella, Vice President Finance and Administration
CMO: Anita Hackstedde, M.D., Vice President Medical Affairs
CIO: Mark L'Italien, Director Information Services
CHR: Barb Hirst, Vice President Human Resources and Chief Nursing Officer
CNO: Barb Hirst, Vice President Human Resources and Chief Nursing Officer
Web address: www.salemhosp.com
**Control:** Other not–for–profit (including NFP Corporation) **Service:** General Medical and Surgical

**Staffed Beds:** 140 **Admissions:** 5012 **Census:** 65 **Outpatient Visits:** 128719 **Births:** 601 **Total Expense ($000):** 96856 **Payroll Expense ($000):** 41963 **Personnel:** 758

### SANDUSKY—Erie County

○ **FIRELANDS REGIONAL HEALTH SYSTEM (360025)**, 1111 Hayes Avenue, Zip 44870; tel. 419/557–7400, (Includes FIRELANDS REGIONAL MEDICAL CENTER – MAIN CAMPUS, 1111 Hayes Avenue, tel. 419/557–7400; FIRELANDS REGIONAL MEDICAL CENTER SOUTH CAMPUS, 1912 Hayes Avenue, Zip 44870–4736; tel. 419/557–7000) **A**2 6 9 10 11 12 13 19 **F**3 5 8 11 13 15 18 20 22 24 28 29 31 34 35 38 40 43 45 47 48 49 50 56 57 58 59 60 61 62 64 65 68 70 73 74 75 76 77 78 79 81 82 85 86 87 89 90 92 93 96 98 99 100 101 102 103 104 105 107 108 110 111 113 114 117 118 119 120 122 123 128 129 130 131 134 142 145 146 147 **P**8
Primary Contact: Martin Tursky, President and Chief Executive Officer
COO: Tamara Jackson, R.N., Senior Vice President and Chief Nursing Officer
CFO: Daniel J. Moncher, Vice President and Chief Financial Officer
CMO: Brenda Violette, M.D., Director Medical Staff
CIO: Robert Ayres, Director Information Systems
CHR: James Sennish, Vice President Human Resources
Web address: www.firelands.com
**Control:** Other not–for–profit (including NFP Corporation) **Service:** General Medical and Surgical

**Staffed Beds:** 236 **Admissions:** 8318 **Census:** 112 **Outpatient Visits:** 276788 **Births:** 704 **Total Expense ($000):** 194318 **Payroll Expense ($000):** 77160 **Personnel:** 1552

### SEAMAN—Adams County

⊠ **ADAMS COUNTY REGIONAL MEDICAL CENTER (361326)**, 230 Medical Center Drive, Zip 45679–8002; tel. 937/386–3400 **A**1 9 10 18 **F**11 15 28 29 30 31 34 35 40 53 54 57 59 62 64 65 75 77 78 79 81 82 92 93 104 107 111 114 115 118 128 130 131 132 134 145 147
Primary Contact: Saundra J. Stevens, Chief Executive Officer
CFO: Scott D. Smith, Chief Financial Officer
CHR: Joyce Porter, Chief Human Resources Officer
CNO: Sharon Ashley, MSN, Chief Nursing Officer
Web address: www.acrmc.com
**Control:** County–Government, nonfederal **Service:** General Medical and Surgical

**Staffed Beds:** 25 **Admissions:** 956 **Census:** 9 **Outpatient Visits:** 61478 **Births:** 0 **Total Expense ($000):** 26186 **Payroll Expense ($000):** 9119 **Personnel:** 256

### SHELBY—Richland County

☐ **MEDCENTRAL – SHELBY HOSPITAL (361324)**, 199 West Main Street, Zip 44875–1490; tel. 419/342–5015 **A**1 9 10 18 **F**3 11 13 15 18 29 31 34 35 40 57 59 64 68 69 70 75 76 78 79 81 93 107 113 118 129 132 145 **S** MedCentral Health System, Mansfield, OH
Primary Contact: Ron Distl, Chief Executive Officer
Web address: www.medcentral.org/body.cfm?id=153
**Control:** Other not–for–profit (including NFP Corporation) **Service:** General Medical and Surgical

**Staffed Beds:** 25 **Admissions:** 1271 **Census:** 12 **Outpatient Visits:** 35364 **Births:** 174 **Personnel:** 148

### SIDNEY—Shelby County

★ ○ **WILSON MEMORIAL HOSPITAL (360013)**, 915 West Michigan Street, Zip 45365–2491; tel. 937/498–2311 **A**9 10 11 **F**3 11 13 15 28 29 30 31 40 45 46 49 56 57 59 62 63 64 68 70 75 76 77 78 79 81 85 86 87 89 93 98 103 107 108 111 117 118 123 128 129 130 131 134 143 145 146 **P**6
Primary Contact: Thomas J. Boecker, President and Chief Executive Officer
COO: Craig Lannoye, Vice President Operations
CFO: Douglas Bomba, Vice President Finance
CMO: Paul Thorpe, M.D., Chief of Staff
CIO: Larry Meyers, Chief Information Officer
CHR: John R. Eve, Human Resources Officer
Web address: www.wilsonhospital.com
**Control:** Other not–for–profit (including NFP Corporation) **Service:** General Medical and Surgical

**Staffed Beds:** 71 **Admissions:** 2675 **Census:** 29 **Outpatient Visits:** 141047 **Births:** 767 **Total Expense ($000):** 61457 **Payroll Expense ($000):** 23997 **Personnel:** 624

### SPRINGFIELD—Clark County

☐ **OHIO VALLEY MEDICAL CENTER (360355)**, 100 West Main Street, Zip 45502–1312; tel. 937/521–3900, (Nonreporting) **A**1 9 10
Primary Contact: Steve Eisentrager, Administrator
Web address: www.myovmc.com/
**Control:** Partnership, Investor–owned, for–profit **Service:** General Medical and Surgical

**Staffed Beds:** 24

⊠ **SPRINGFIELD REGIONAL MEDICAL CENTER (360086)**, 100 Medical Center Drive, Zip 45504–2687; tel. 937/325–0531, (Includes SPRINGFIELD REGIONAL MEDICAL CENTER – FOUNTAIN CAMPUS, 1343 North Fountain Boulevard, Zip 45501–1380; tel. 937/390–5000; Mark S. Wiener, President) **A**1 2 6 9 10 **F**3 5 8 11 12 13 15 17 18 20 22 24 26 28 29 30 31 34 35 37 40 45 49 51 59 61 63 64 68 70 74 75 76 77 78 79 81 82 83 84 85 86 87 89 90 93 107 108 110 111 113 114 117 118 119 120 125 126 128 129 130 131 134 145 146 147 **P**6 **S** Catholic Health Partners, Cincinnati, OH
Primary Contact: Mark S. Wiener, President
CFO: John F. Dempsey, Vice President and Chief Financial Officer
CIO: Yousuf Ahmad, Chief Information Officer
CHR: Cherie Lamborn, Interim Vice President Human Resources
Web address: www.communityhospital.com
**Control:** Church–operated, Nongovernment, not–for profit **Service:** General Medical and Surgical

**Staffed Beds:** 254 **Admissions:** 14465 **Census:** 170 **Outpatient Visits:** 319041 **Births:** 1340 **Total Expense ($000):** 205046 **Payroll Expense ($000):** 71716 **Personnel:** 1267

### STEUBENVILLE—Jefferson County

☐ **ACUITY SPECIALTY HOSPITAL – OHIO VALLEY (362035)**, 380 Summit Avenue, 3rd Floor, Zip 43952; tel. 740/283–7600, (Nonreporting) **A**1 9 10 **S** AcuityHealthcare, LP, Charlotte, NC
Primary Contact: Judy Weaver, MS, Chief Executive Officer
Web address: www.acuityhealthcare.net
**Control:** Corporation, Investor–owned, for–profit **Service:** Long–Term Acute Care hospital

**Staffed Beds:** 40

☐ **LIFE LINE HOSPITAL (362039)**, 200 School Street, Zip 43953–9610; tel. 740/346–2600 **A**1 10 **F**1 3 29 45 64 75 81 85 87 93 96 100 107 111 115 118 128 129 147
Primary Contact: Susan T. Colpo, Chief Executive Officer
Web address: www.llhospital.com
**Control:** Partnership, Investor–owned, for–profit **Service:** Long–Term Acute Care hospital

**Staffed Beds:** 36 **Admissions:** 425 **Census:** 28 **Outpatient Visits:** 119370 **Births:** 0 **Total Expense ($000):** 20729 **Payroll Expense ($000):** 8956 **Personnel:** 221

✠ △ **TRINITY HEALTH SYSTEM (360211)**, 380 Summit Avenue, Zip 43952–2699; tel. 740/283–7000, (Includes TRINITY MEDICAL CENTER EAST, 380 Summit Avenue, tel. 740/283–7000; TRINITY MEDICAL CENTER WEST, 4000 Johnson Road, Zip 43952–2393; tel. 740/264–8000) **A**1 2 6 7 9 10 **F**3 4 5 11 12 13 15 17 18 20 22 24 26 28 29 30 31 32 34 35 38 40 45 46 47 49 51 54 56 57 59 62 64 65 70 74 75 76 77 78 79 81 85 86 87 89 90 92 93 94 96 97 98 99 100 101 102 103 104 105 107 108 110 111 113 114 116 117 118 119 120 122 127 128 129 130 131 134 143 145 146 147 **P**6 **S** Sylvania Franciscan Health, Toledo, OH
Primary Contact: Fred B. Brower, President and Chief Executive Officer
CFO: Elizabeth Allen, Vice President Finance
CMO: Ivan Wright, M.D., Vice President Medical Affairs
CIO: Tom Kiger, Director Information Systems
CHR: Lewis C. Musso, Vice President Human Resources
Web address: www.trinityhealth.com
**Control:** Other not–for–profit (including NFP Corporation) **Service:** General Medical and Surgical

**Staffed Beds:** 319 **Admissions:** 10837 **Census:** 180 **Outpatient Visits:** 248217 **Births:** 552 **Total Expense ($000):** 180385 **Payroll Expense ($000):** 74150 **Personnel:** 1606

### SYLVANIA—Lucas County

✠ △ **PROMEDICA FLOWER HOSPITAL (360074)**, 5200 Harroun Road, Zip 43560–2196; tel. 419/824–1444 **A**1 2 3 5 7 9 10 **F**2 3 11 12 13 15 18 20 24 28 29 30 31 34 35 36 38 40 43 47 48 49 50 57 58 59 60 64 65 67 68 70 75 76 77 78 79 81 82 84 85 86 87 90 91 92 93 94 96 97 98 100 101 102 103 107 108 109 110 111 113 115 116 117 118 119 120 122 123 128 129 130 131 142 145 146 **S** ProMedica Health System, Toledo, OH
Primary Contact: Alan Sattler, President
CFO: Kathleen S. Hanley, Chief Financial Officer
CIO: David G. Selman, Vice President Information
CHR: Charles McDowell, Chief Human Resources Officer
Web address: www.promedica.org
**Control:** Other not–for–profit (including NFP Corporation) **Service:** General Medical and Surgical

**Staffed Beds:** 218 **Admissions:** 10088 **Census:** 142 **Outpatient Visits:** 188741 **Births:** 1109 **Total Expense ($000):** 180101 **Payroll Expense ($000):** 61461 **Personnel:** 1242

✠ **REGENCY HOSPITAL OF TOLEDO (362036)**, 5220 Alexis Road, Zip 43560–2504; tel. 419/318–5700, (Nonreporting) **A**1 3 5 10 **S** Select Medical Corporation, Mechanicsburg, PA
Primary Contact: Patrick J. Murtha, Chief Executive Officer
Web address: www.regencyhospital.com
**Control:** Corporation, Investor–owned, for–profit **Service:** Long–Term Acute Care hospital

**Staffed Beds:** 35

### TIFFIN—Seneca County

✠ **MERCY TIFFIN HOSPITAL (360089)**, 45 St. Lawrence Drive, Zip 44883–0727; tel. 419/455–7000 **A**1 2 5 9 10 **F**3 11 12 13 15 18 19 28 29 30 31 34 35 36 40 46 49 50 51 56 57 59 62 64 66 68 70 74 75 76 78 79 81 82 83 84 85 86 87 89 97 107 108 110 111 114 117 118 120 122 123 128 129 131 132 133 134 144 145 146 147 **S** Catholic Health Partners, Cincinnati, OH
Primary Contact: Dale E. Thornton, M.P.H., President and Chief Executive Officer
CMO: Wesley Hedges, M.D., President Medical Staff
CHR: Diana Olson, Chief Human Resources Officer
Web address: www.mercyweb.org
**Control:** Church–operated, Nongovernment, not–for profit **Service:** General Medical and Surgical

**Staffed Beds:** 51 **Admissions:** 2097 **Census:** 25 **Outpatient Visits:** 96666 **Births:** 360 **Total Expense ($000):** 52107 **Payroll Expense ($000):** 17355 **Personnel:** 359

### TOLEDO—Lucas County

☐ **ADVANCED SPECIALTY HOSPITAL OF TOLEDO (362038)**, 1015 Garden Lake Parkway, Zip 43614–2779; tel. 419/381–0037, (Nonreporting) **A**1 10
Primary Contact: Alan Fisher, Chief Executive Officer
Web address: www.advancedspecialtyhospitals.com
**Control:** Corporation, Investor–owned, for–profit **Service:** Long–Term Acute Care hospital

**Staffed Beds:** 40

✠ **MERCY ST. ANNE HOSPITAL (360262)**, 3404 West Sylvania Avenue, Zip 43623; tel. 419/407–2663 **A**1 2 9 10 **F**3 15 18 29 30 31 34 35 36 38 40 46 56 57 59 64 65 68 70 74 75 78 79 81 84 85 86 92 97 107 108 110 111 113 115 116 117 118 128 129 130 131 145 146 **P**8 **S** Catholic Health Partners, Cincinnati, OH
Primary Contact: Bradley J. Bertke, President and Chief Executive Officer
CFO: Samantha Platzke, Chief Financial Officer
CMO: Erich Pontasch, M.D., Chief of Staff
CHR: Gary George, Regional Vice President Human Resources
Web address: www.mercyweb.org
**Control:** Church–operated, Nongovernment, not–for profit **Service:** General Medical and Surgical

**Staffed Beds:** 96 **Admissions:** 4853 **Census:** 53 **Outpatient Visits:** 234050 **Births:** 0 **Personnel:** 554

✠ ○ **MERCY ST. VINCENT MEDICAL CENTER (360112)**, 2213 Cherry Street, Zip 43608–2691; tel. 419/251–3232, (Includes MERCY CHILDREN'S HOSPITAL, 2213 Cherry Street, tel. 419/251–8000) **A**1 2 3 5 9 10 11 12 13 **F**3 7 8 11 12 13 15 16 17 18 19 20 21 22 23 24 25 26 28 29 30 32 34 35 38 39 40 41 43 44 45 46 48 49 50 51 54 56 57 58 59 60 61 64 65 66 68 70 72 74 75 76 77 78 79 81 82 83 84 85 86 87 88 89 92 93 97 98 100 101 102 103 104 105 107 108 110 111 113 114 115 117 118 125 128 129 130 131 133 134 140 145 146 147 **P**8 **S** Catholic Health Partners, Cincinnati, OH
Primary Contact: Kevin S. Cook, President and Chief Executive Officer
CFO: Samantha M. Platzke, Senior Vice President Finance and Chief Financial Officer
CMO: David R. Franzblau, M.D., Chief Medical Officer
CHR: Gary George, Regional Vice President Human Resources
Web address: www.mercyweb.org
**Control:** Church–operated, Nongovernment, not–for profit **Service:** General Medical and Surgical

**Staffed Beds:** 431 **Admissions:** 19254 **Census:** 236 **Outpatient Visits:** 407078 **Births:** 1003 **Personnel:** 2728

☐ **NORTHWEST OHIO PSYCHIATRIC HOSPITAL (364014)**, 930 Detroit Avenue, Zip 43614–2701; tel. 419/381–1881, (Nonreporting) **A**1 10 **S** Ohio Department of Mental Health, Columbus, OH
Primary Contact: Mychail Scheramic, M.D., Chief Executive Officer
Web address: www.mh.state.oh.us/
**Control:** State–Government, nonfederal **Service:** Psychiatric

**Staffed Beds:** 24

✠ **PROMEDICA TOLEDO HOSPITAL (360068)**, 2142 North Cove Boulevard, Zip 43606–3896; tel. 419/291–4000, (Includes PROMEDICA WILDWOOD ORTHOPAEDIC AND SPINE HOSPITAL, 2901 North Reynolds Road, Zip 43615; tel. 419/578–7700; Holly L. Bristoll, President; TOLEDO CHILDREN'S HOSPITAL, 2142 North Cove Boulevard, Zip 43606), (Total facility includes 25 beds in nursing home–type unit) **A**1 3 5 9 10 13 **F**3 7 8 9 11 12 13 15 17 18 19 20 21 22 23 24 25 26 27 29 30 31 32 34 35 36 38 39 40 43 48 49 50 51 52 53 54 55 57 58 59 60 64 65 67 68 70 71 72 74 75 76 77 78 79 81 82 84 85 86 87 88 89 91 92 93 94 96 97 98 99 100 101 102 104 105 107 108 109 110 111 113 114 117 118 122 125 127 128 129 130 131 133 134 142 143 145 146 147 **S** ProMedica Health System, Toledo, OH
Primary Contact: Kevin C. Webb, Ph.D., President
CFO: Gary Akenberger, Senior Vice President Finance
CMO: Neeraj Kanwal, M.D., Vice President Medical Affairs
CIO: David G. Selman, Chief Information Officer
CHR: Randy Schimmoeller, Vice President Human Resources
Web address: www.promedica.org
**Control:** Other not–for–profit (including NFP Corporation) **Service:** General Medical and Surgical

**Staffed Beds:** 616 **Admissions:** 29889 **Census:** 428 **Outpatient Visits:** 684016 **Births:** 3712 **Total Expense ($000):** 639641 **Payroll Expense ($000):** 214403 **Personnel:** 4498

✠ △ **THE UNIVERSITY OF TOLEDO MEDICAL CENTER (360048)**, 3000 Arlington Avenue, Zip 43614–5805; tel. 419/383–4000 **A**1 2 3 5 7 8 9 10 **F**3 8 11 15 17 18 20 22 24 26 28 29 30 31 32 34 35 36 37 38 39 40 43 44 45 46 47 49 54 56 57 58 59 60 61 64 65 70 74 75 77 78 79 81 82 84 85 87 89 90 91 92 93 96 97 98 99 100 101 102 103 104 105 107 108 110 111 113 114 117 118 120 123 125 128 129 130 131 133 134 137 145 146 147
Primary Contact: Scott Scarborough, Ph.D., CPA, Interim Executive Director
CFO: Daniel Morissette, Senior Vice President Finance and Administration
CMO: Ronald McGinnis, M.D., Medical Director
CIO: Lawrence Burns, Vice President Institutional Advancement
CHR: William Logie, Vice President Human Resources
Web address: www.utoledo.edu
**Control:** State–Government, nonfederal **Service:** General Medical and Surgical

**Staffed Beds:** 227 **Admissions:** 11559 **Census:** 160 **Outpatient Visits:** 255293 **Births:** 0 **Total Expense ($000):** 235328 **Payroll Expense ($000):** 99047 **Personnel:** 2050

**TOLEDO CAMPUS** See Northcoast Behavioral Healthcare System, Northfield

---

**Hospital, Medicare Provider Number, Address, Telephone, Approval, Facility, and Physician Codes, Health Care System**

★ American Hospital Association (AHA) membership
☐ The Joint Commission accreditation
◇ DNV Healthcare Inc. accreditation
○ American Osteopathic Association (AOA) accreditation
△ Commission on Accreditation of Rehabilitation Facilities (CARF) accreditation

---

**OH**

### TROY—Miami County

☐ △ **UPPER VALLEY MEDICAL CENTER (360174)**, 3130 North County Road 25A, Zip 45373–1309; tel. 937/440–4000, (Includes DETTMER HOSPITAL, 3130 North Dixie Highway, Zip 45373–1039; tel. 937/440–7500), (Nonreporting) **A**1 2 5 7 9 10
Primary Contact: Thomas Parker, Chief Executive Officer
CFO: Tim Snider, Senior Vice President and Chief Financial Officer
CMO: Dan Bailey, M.D., Vice President Medical Affairs and Chief Medical Officer
CIO: William Watercutter, Director Management Information System
CHR: Tracy Moser, Director Human Resources
Web address: www.uvmc.com
**Control:** Other not–for–profit (including NFP Corporation) **Service:** General Medical and Surgical

**Staffed Beds:** 168

### UPPER SANDUSKY—Wyandot County

★ **WYANDOT MEMORIAL HOSPITAL (361329)**, 885 North Sandusky Avenue, Zip 43351–1098; tel. 419/294–4991 **A**9 10 18 **F**3 11 13 15 17 18 28 29 31 34 35 40 45 53 57 59 64 65 74 75 76 77 78 79 81 82 85 86 87 89 92 93 97 107 108 110 111 114 116 117 118 123 128 129 131 132 134 145 147 **P**6
Primary Contact: Joseph A. D'Ettorre, Chief Executive Officer
COO: Ty Shaull, Chief Operating Officer
CFO: Alan H. Yeates, Vice President Fiscal Services
CMO: Keri Harris, M.D., Chief of Staff
CHR: Vickie Underwood, Director Human Resources
Web address: www.wyandotmemorial.org
**Control:** Hospital district or authority, Government, nonfederal **Service:** General Medical and Surgical

**Staffed Beds:** 25 **Admissions:** 721 **Census:** 8 **Outpatient Visits:** 50141
**Births:** 94 **Total Expense ($000):** 24669 **Payroll Expense ($000):** 9396
**Personnel:** 182

### URBANA—Champaign County

★ **MERCY MEMORIAL HOSPITAL (361312)**, 904 Scioto Street, Zip 43078–2200; tel. 937/653–5231, (Nonreporting) **A**9 10 18 **S** Catholic Health Partners, Cincinnati, OH
Primary Contact: Karen S. Gorby, R.N., MSN, FACHE, Administrator
Web address: www.health–partners.org
**Control:** Church–operated, Nongovernment, not–for profit **Service:** General Medical and Surgical

**Staffed Beds:** 25

### VAN WERT—Van Wert County

☒ **VAN WERT COUNTY HOSPITAL (360071)**, 1250 South Washington Street, Zip 45891–2599; tel. 419/238–2390 **A**1 5 9 10 **F**8 13 15 28 31 34 35 39 40 53 54 57 59 70 72 76 79 81 85 89 93 107 108 118 126 128 129 145 **P**7 8
Primary Contact: Mark J. Minick, President and Chief Executive Officer
CFO: Michael T. Holliday, Vice President Fiscal and Administrative Services
CMO: Scott Jarvis, M.D., President Medical Staff
CIO: Jerry Borton, Manager Information
CHR: Joyce Pothast, Vice President Human and Environmental Services
Web address: www.vanwerthospital.org
**Control:** Other not–for–profit (including NFP Corporation) **Service:** General Medical and Surgical

**Staffed Beds:** 79 **Admissions:** 1379 **Census:** 12 **Outpatient Visits:** 61081
**Births:** 160 **Total Expense ($000):** 38418 **Payroll Expense ($000):** 12228
**Personnel:** 304

### WADSWORTH—Medina County

☐ **SUMMA WADSWORTH–RITTMAN HOSPITAL (360195)**, 195 Wadsworth Road, Zip 44281–9505; tel. 330/331–1000 **A**1 5 9 10 **F**3 8 11 15 18 29 30 31 34 35 38 40 44 45 46 47 48 49 57 59 60 62 64 68 70 74 75 77 78 79 81 82 85 86 87 90 91 93 96 97 107 108 109 110 111 114 118 128 129 130 131 134 142 145 146 147 **P**6 8 **S** Summa Health System, Akron, OH
Primary Contact: Thomas DeBord, President
CFO: Charles Alderson, Chief Financial Officer
CMO: Jeffrey Morris, M.D., Vice President Medical Affairs
CIO: David Lynch, Regional Director Information Services
CHR: Don Argiro, Regional Director Human Resources
Web address: www.wrhhs.org
**Control:** Other not–for–profit (including NFP Corporation) **Service:** General Medical and Surgical

**Staffed Beds:** 62 **Admissions:** 2725 **Census:** 32 **Outpatient Visits:** 87932
**Births:** 0 **Total Expense ($000):** 50126 **Payroll Expense ($000):** 19045
**Personnel:** 373

**WADSWORTH–RITTMAN HOSPITAL** See Summa Wadsworth–Rittman Hospital

### WARREN—Trumbull County

☒ △ **HILLSIDE REHABILITATION HOSPITAL (363026)**, 8747 Squires Lane N.E., Zip 44484–1649; tel. 330/841–3700, (Nonreporting) **A**1 5 7 9 10 **S** Community Health Systems, Inc., Franklin, TN
Primary Contact: Marilyn Titus, Vice President and Chief Operating Officer
COO: Marilyn Titus, Vice President and Chief Operating Officer
CFO: Lisa Medovich, Senior Vice President and Chief Financial Officer
CMO: Cynthia DiMauro, M.D., Medical Director
CIO: Timothy Roe, Chief Information Officer
CHR: Lisa Johnson, Vice President Human Resources
Web address: www.valleycarehealth.net
**Control:** Corporation, Investor–owned, for–profit **Service:** Rehabilitation

**Staffed Beds:** 65

☒ ○ **ST. JOSEPH HEALTH CENTER (360161)**, 667 Eastland Avenue S.E., Zip 44484–4531; tel. 330/841–4000 **A**1 2 9 10 11 12 13 **F**3 5 8 11 12 13 15 28 29 30 31 35 40 42 43 44 45 46 50 51 53 54 56 57 59 60 61 64 66 68 69 70 75 76 77 78 79 81 82 85 86 87 89 93 97 107 108 109 111 113 115 116 117 118 119 120 122 128 129 131 134 142 143 145 146 147 **P**3 **S** Catholic Health Partners, Cincinnati, OH
Primary Contact: John Finizio, President
COO: Robert W. Shroder, President and Chief Executive Officer
CFO: Donald E. Kline, Senior Vice President Finance
CMO: Nicholas Kreatsoulas, M.D., Vice President Medical Affairs
CIO: Charles Folkwein, Vice President Ancillary Services
CHR: Molly Seals, Senior Vice President Human Resources and Learning
Web address: www.hmpartners.org
**Control:** Church–operated, Nongovernment, not–for profit **Service:** General Medical and Surgical

**Staffed Beds:** 138 **Admissions:** 7962 **Census:** 98 **Outpatient Visits:** 170156
**Births:** 711 **Total Expense ($000):** 113140 **Payroll Expense ($000):** 39765
**Personnel:** 771

☒ **TRUMBULL MEMORIAL HOSPITAL (360055)**, 1350 East Market Street, Zip 44482–6628; tel. 330/841–9011, (Nonreporting) **A**1 2 5 9 10 **S** Community Health Systems, Inc., Franklin, TN
Primary Contact: Robert G. Wolleben, Chief Executive Officer
CFO: Lisa Medovich, Senior Vice President and Chief Financial Officer
CMO: Thomas L. James, M.D., Senior Vice President and Chief Medical Officer
CIO: Barry Fitts, Chief Information Officer
CHR: Laurie Barber, Director Human Resources
Web address: www.valleycarehealth.net
**Control:** Corporation, Investor–owned, for–profit **Service:** General Medical and Surgical

**Staffed Beds:** 292

### WARRENSVILLE HEIGHTS—Cuyahoga County

☒ ○ **SOUTH POINTE HOSPITAL (360144)**, 20000 Harvard Road, Zip 44122–7099; tel. 216/491–6000 **A**1 2 9 10 11 12 13 **F**11 15 18 20 26 28 29 30 31 34 35 36 38 39 40 42 44 50 51 54 57 58 59 60 61 64 65 66 68 69 70 75 77 78 79 81 82 84 85 86 87 92 93 97 100 102 107 108 110 111 114 116 118 129 130 131 134 142 143 145 147 **S** Cleveland Clinic Health System, Cleveland, OH
Primary Contact: Brian J. Harte, M.D., President
COO: Andrea Jacobs, Chief Operating Officer
CFO: Lindsay Bird, Director Finance
CMO: Arun Gupta, M.D., Vice President Medical Affairs
CIO: Ralph A. Cagna, Director Information Technology
CHR: Doris A. Zajec, Director Human Resources
Web address: www.southpointehospital.org
**Control:** Other not–for–profit (including NFP Corporation) **Service:** General Medical and Surgical

**Staffed Beds:** 172 **Admissions:** 8615 **Census:** 134 **Outpatient Visits:** 136138 **Births:** 0 **Total Expense ($000):** 125309 **Payroll Expense ($000):** 55830 **Personnel:** 939

### WASHINGTON COURT HOUSE—Fayette County

☒ **FAYETTE COUNTY MEMORIAL HOSPITAL (361331)**, 1430 Columbus Avenue, Zip 43160–1791; tel. 740/335–1210 **A**1 9 10 18 **F**3 7 11 15 18 29 30 34 35 36 40 45 57 59 64 68 70 74 75 77 78 79 81 85 86 87 89 93 94 96 97 102 107 110 113 118 126 128 129 130 131 132 134 145 147 **P**4 **S** Trinity Health, Novi, MI
Primary Contact: Lyndon J. Christman, President and Chief Executive Officer
CFO: Thomas McDermott, Vice President Finance
CMO: William Stevenson, M.D., Chief of Staff
CIO: Bruce Denen, Manager Data Processing
CHR: Earlene Christensen, Director Human Resources
Web address: www.fcmh.org
**Control:** County–Government, nonfederal **Service:** General Medical and Surgical

**Staffed Beds:** 25 **Admissions:** 1007 **Census:** 11 **Outpatient Visits:** 81727
**Births:** 0 **Total Expense ($000):** 36932 **Payroll Expense ($000):** 14871
**Personnel:** 340

## WAUSEON—Fulton County

✠ **FULTON COUNTY HEALTH CENTER (361333)**, 725 South Shoop Avenue, Zip 43567–1701; tel. 419/335–2015, (Total facility includes 71 beds in nursing home–type unit) **A**1 2 5 9 10 18 **F**3 8 11 13 15 18 20 26 28 29 31 34 40 53 57 59 67 69 70 75 76 77 78 79 81 87 89 93 98 101 102 103 104 105 107 108 111 114 117 118 124 127 128 129 130 131 134 145 147
Primary Contact: E. Dean Beck, Administrator
COO: Patti Finn, Assistant Administrator
CFO: Darrell Topmiller, Director Finance
CIO: Larry Hefflinger, Director Information Systems
CHR: Kristy Snyder, Director Human Resources
Web address: www.fultoncountyhealthcenter.org
**Control:** Other not–for–profit (including NFP Corporation) **Service:** General Medical and Surgical

**Staffed Beds:** 106 **Admissions:** 2036 **Census:** 82 **Outpatient Visits:** 160213 **Births:** 270 **Total Expense ($000):** 57507 **Payroll Expense ($000):** 23002 **Personnel:** 655

## WAVERLY—Pike County

○ **PIKE COMMUNITY HOSPITAL (361334)**, 100 Dawn Lane, Zip 45690–9138; tel. 740/947–2186 **A**9 10 11 18 **F**11 15 34 35 54 81 93 107 111 113 118 129 132 145 **P**6
Primary Contact: Craig E. Solle, President and Chief Executive Officer
COO: Tina Perko, Vice President Operations
CFO: Sharon Novak, CPA, Vice President Finance
CHR: Berna Brock, Vice President Human Resources
Web address: www.pikecommunityhospital.org
**Control:** Other not–for–profit (including NFP Corporation) **Service:** General Medical and Surgical

**Staffed Beds:** 25 **Admissions:** 716 **Census:** 6 **Outpatient Visits:** 16830 **Births:** 0 **Total Expense ($000):** 17727 **Payroll Expense ($000):** 7742 **Personnel:** 234

## WEST CHESTER—Butler County

★ **UC HEALTH SURGICAL HOSPITAL (360271)**, 7750 University Court, Zip 45069; tel. 513/475–8300 **A**9 10 **F**3 15 64 79 81 82 85 86 107 110 111 114 118 128 146 **S** UC Health, Cincinnati, OH
Primary Contact: Lesley Gilbertson, M.D., Executive and Medical Director
COO: Sara Deem, Director Operations
CFO: Tom Ducro, Chief Financial Officer
CMO: Lesley Gilbertson, M.D., Executive and Medical Director
CIO: Steve Knost, Manager Facilities
CHR: Penny Elder, Manager Human Resources
Web address: www.surgicalhospital.uchealth.com
**Control:** Other not–for–profit (including NFP Corporation) **Service:** General Medical and Surgical

**Staffed Beds:** 8 **Admissions:** 158 **Census:** 1 **Outpatient Visits:** 23522 **Births:** 0 **Total Expense ($000):** 9313 **Payroll Expense ($000):** 3307 **Personnel:** 66

✠ **WEST CHESTER HOSPITAL (360354)**, 7700 University Drive, Zip 45069–2505; tel. 513/298–3000 **A**1 10 **F**3 12 15 18 20 22 24 26 29 30 31 34 35 40 44 45 47 48 49 50 57 58 59 60 64 68 70 74 75 78 79 81 82 85 86 87 92 107 108 110 111 114 116 118 123 125 129 130 131 144 145 146 147 **S** UC Health, Cincinnati, OH
Primary Contact: Kevin Joseph, M.D., Chief Executive Officer
COO: Tom G. Daskalakis, Chief Operating Officer
Web address: www.westchesterhospital.uchealth.com
**Control:** Other not–for–profit (including NFP Corporation) **Service:** General Medical and Surgical

**Staffed Beds:** 126 **Admissions:** 6280 **Census:** 63 **Outpatient Visits:** 53688 **Births:** 0 **Total Expense ($000):** 123891 **Payroll Expense ($000):** 31932 **Personnel:** 564

## WESTERVILLE—Franklin County

✠ **MOUNT CARMEL ST. ANN'S (360012)**, 500 South Cleveland Avenue, Zip 43081–8998; tel. 614/898–4000 **A**1 2 3 5 9 10 **F**3 11 13 15 18 20 22 26 29 30 31 34 35 37 40 44 45 46 47 48 49 50 54 55 57 58 59 61 63 64 65 66 68 70 74 75 76 78 79 81 83 84 85 86 87 93 94 97 100 101 102 107 108 109 110 111 113 114 115 117 118 119 122 123 125 129 130 131 144 145 146 147 **P**6 8 **S** Trinity Health, Novi, MI
Primary Contact: Claus von Zychlin, Executive Vice President and Chief Operating Officer
Web address: www.mountcarmelhealth.com
**Control:** Church–operated, Nongovernment, not–for profit **Service:** General Medical and Surgical

**Staffed Beds:** 250 **Admissions:** 19516 **Census:** 176 **Outpatient Visits:** 207788 **Births:** 4458 **Total Expense ($000):** 225760 **Payroll Expense ($000):** 80599 **Personnel:** 1461

## WESTLAKE—Cuyahoga County

□ **ST. JOHN MEDICAL CENTER (360123)**, 29000 Center Ridge Road, Zip 44145–5293; tel. 440/835–8000 **A**1 2 10 12 13 **F**3 8 13 15 17 18 20 22 24 26 28 29 30 31 34 35 39 40 43 44 45 47 49 50 51 56 57 59 64 65 68 70 71 74 75 76 78 79 80 81 82 84 85 86 87 89 92 93 100 107 108 110 111 113 114 118 129 131 142 143 145 146 147 **P**4 **S** Sisters of Charity Health System, Cleveland, OH
Primary Contact: William A. Young, Jr., President and Chief Executive Officer
CFO: Allen R. Tracy, Senior Vice President and Chief Financial Officer
CMO: Michael Dobrovich, M.D., Chief Medical Officer
CIO: James H. Carroll, Chief Information Officer
CHR: Gary Lazroff, Vice President Human Resources
Web address: www.sjws.net
**Control:** Other not–for–profit (including NFP Corporation) **Service:** General Medical and Surgical

**Staffed Beds:** 182 **Admissions:** 11727 **Census:** 115 **Outpatient Visits:** 178482 **Births:** 677 **Total Expense ($000):** 133883 **Payroll Expense ($000):** 53590 **Personnel:** 1178

**ST. JOHN WEST SHORE HOSPITAL** See St. John Medical Center

## WILLARD—Huron County

✠ **MERCY WILLARD HOSPITAL (361310)**, 1100 Neal Zick Road, Zip 44890–9287; tel. 419/964–5000 **A**1 5 9 10 18 **F**3 5 15 18 28 30 34 35 40 46 57 59 70 74 75 77 79 81 84 85 87 89 93 107 111 113 116 118 128 129 130 131 132 134 142 144 145 146 **S** Catholic Health Partners, Cincinnati, OH
Primary Contact: B. Lynn Detterman, Chief Executive Officer
CFO: Cindy Dennison, Senior Director Rural Division
CMO: Bill Back, M.D., Chief of Staff
CHR: Diana Olson, Chief Human Resources Officer
Web address: www.mercyweb.org
**Control:** Church–operated, Nongovernment, not–for profit **Service:** General Medical and Surgical

**Staffed Beds:** 25 **Admissions:** 535 **Census:** 9 **Outpatient Visits:** 36811 **Births:** 2 **Total Expense ($000):** 20194 **Payroll Expense ($000):** 8086 **Personnel:** 165

## WILLOUGHBY—Lake County

□ **WINDSOR–LAURELWOOD CENTER FOR BEHAVIORAL MEDICINE (364029)**, 35900 Euclid Avenue, Zip 44094–4648; tel. 440/953–3000, (Nonreporting) **A**1 9 10 **S** Universal Health Services, Inc., King of Prussia, PA
Primary Contact: Daniel Aranda, Chief Executive Officer
CFO: Robin Stough, Chief Financial Officer
CMO: Leonard Barley, M.D., Chief Medical Officer
CIO: Andrew Johnson, Information Technology and Purchasing Officer
CHR: Greg Kennedy, Manager Human Resources
Web address: www.windsorlaurelwood.com
**Control:** Individual, Investor–owned, for–profit **Service:** Psychiatric

**Staffed Beds:** 152

## WILMINGTON—Clinton County

□ △ **CLINTON MEMORIAL HOSPITAL (360175)**, 610 West Main Street, Zip 45177–0600; tel. 937/382–6611 **A**1 2 3 5 7 9 10 **F**3 11 13 15 18 29 30 31 34 35 36 40 45 50 51 56 59 62 64 68 70 74 75 76 78 79 81 82 85 86 87 90 93 96 97 107 108 111 114 118 120 123 128 129 130 131 145 147 **P**5 **S** RegionalCare Hospital Partners, Brentwood, TN
Primary Contact: Michael C. Choo, M.D., Chief Executive Officer
CMO: Michael C. Choo, M.D., Chief Executive Officer
CHR: Mary Ann Foland, Manager Human Resources
Web address: www.cmhregional.com
**Control:** Corporation, Investor–owned, for–profit **Service:** General Medical and Surgical

**Staffed Beds:** 85 **Admissions:** 4490 **Census:** 39 **Outpatient Visits:** 125681 **Births:** 640 **Total Expense ($000):** 91943 **Payroll Expense ($000):** 29736 **Personnel:** 613

## WOOSTER—Wayne County

□ **WOOSTER COMMUNITY HOSPITAL (360036)**, 1761 Beall Avenue, Zip 44691–2342; tel. 330/263–8100 **A**1 2 5 9 10 19 **F**3 11 13 14 15 20 26 28 29 30 31 32 34 35 40 45 49 51 53 57 59 61 62 64 70 74 75 76 77 78 79 81 85 86 87 89 90 92 93 107 108 110 111 113 114 117 118 128 129 131 134 142 145 146 147 **P**3 7 **S** QHR, Brentwood, TN
Primary Contact: William E. Sheron, Chief Executive Officer
Web address: www.woosterhospital.org
**Control:** City–Government, nonfederal **Service:** General Medical and Surgical

**Staffed Beds:** 150 **Admissions:** 5802 **Census:** 50

---

**Hospital, Medicare Provider Number, Address, Telephone, Approval, Facility, and Physician Codes, Health Care System**

★ American Hospital Association (AHA) membership
□ The Joint Commission accreditation          ◇ DNV Healthcare Inc. accreditation
○ American Osteopathic Association (AOA) accreditation
△ Commission on Accreditation of Rehabilitation Facilities (CARF) accreditation

### WRIGHT–PATTERSON AFB—Greene County

✖ **WRIGHT PATTERSON MEDICAL CENTER**, 4881 Sugar Maple Drive, Zip 45433–5529; tel. 937/257–9144 **A**1 2 3 5 **F**3 5 7 11 12 13 18 19 20 29 30 31 32 33 34 35 36 38 39 40 43 44 45 46 47 48 49 50 57 58 59 60 61 64 65 70 74 75 76 77 78 79 81 82 86 87 93 94 97 99 100 101 102 103 104 107 108 109 110 111 114 116 118 119 121 122 128 129 130 131 134 140 141 145 146 **S** Department of the Air Force, Washington, DC
Primary Contact: Brent Erickson, Administrator
COO: Brent Erickson, Administrator
CFO: Major Vigil Scott, Resource Management Flight Commander
CMO: Colonel William Venanzi, M.D., Chief Medical Officer
CIO: Matt Osborne, Flight Chief Medical Information Systems
CHR: Rhonda Buie, Chief Civilian Personnel
Web address: www.wpafb.af.mil/units/wpmc/
**Control:** Air Force, Government, federal **Service:** General Medical and Surgical

| |
|---|
| **Staffed Beds:** 52 **Admissions:** 4077 **Census:** 25 |

### XENIA—Greene County

✖ △ **GREENE MEMORIAL HOSPITAL (360026)**, 1141 North Monroe Drive, Zip 45385–1600; tel. 937/352–2000 **A**1 2 3 5 7 9 10 **F**3 5 8 11 12 15 18 20 28 29 30 31 34 35 40 42 43 44 45 46 50 54 56 57 59 63 64 65 68 69 70 71 74 75 77 78 79 81 82 85 86 87 90 92 93 94 97 98 100 101 102 103 107 108 111 117 118 120 128 129 130 131 134 140 142 143 145 146 147 **P**7 **S** Kettering Health Network, Dayton, OH
Primary Contact: Terry M. Burns, President
CIO: Pam Holiday, Director Management Information Systems
CHR: Amanda Koch, Director Human Resources
Web address: www.greenehealth.org
**Control:** Church–operated, Nongovernment, not–for profit **Service:** General Medical and Surgical

| |
|---|
| **Staffed Beds:** 89 **Admissions:** 4212 **Census:** 51 **Outpatient Visits:** 129818 **Births:** 0 **Total Expense ($000):** 71867 **Payroll Expense ($000):** 30893 **Personnel:** 622 |

### YOUNGSTOWN—Trumbull County

☐ **BELMONT PINES HOSPITAL (364038)**, 615 Churchill–Hubbard Road, Zip 44505–1379; tel. 330/759–2700, (Nonreporting) **A**1 9 10 **S** Universal Health Services, Inc., King of Prussia, PA
Primary Contact: George H. Perry, Ph.D., Chief Executive Officer
CFO: Robin Stough, Chief Financial Officer
CMO: Phillip Maiden, M.D., Medical Director
Web address: www.belmontpines.com
**Control:** Corporation, Investor–owned, for–profit **Service:** Psychiatric

| |
|---|
| **Staffed Beds:** 46 |

✖ **NORTHSIDE MEDICAL CENTER (360141)**, 500 Gypsy Lane, Zip 44501–0240; tel. 330/884–1000, (Includes NORTHSIDE MEDICAL CENTER, 500 Gypsy Lane, tel. 330/747–1444), (Nonreporting) **A**1 2 3 5 8 9 10 **S** Community Health Systems, Inc., Franklin, TN
Primary Contact: David J. Fikse, Chief Executive Officer
COO: Michael Seelman, Chief Operating Officer
CFO: Lisa Medovich, Senior Vice President and Chief Financial Officer
CMO: Jay Osborne, M.D., Senior Vice President Medical Affairs
CIO: Timothy Roe, Chief Information Officer
CHR: Lavern H. Carrera, Senior Vice President Human Resources
Web address: www.valleycarehealth.net
**Control:** Corporation, Investor–owned, for–profit **Service:** General Medical and Surgical

| |
|---|
| **Staffed Beds:** 373 |

**NORTHSIDE MEDICAL CENTER** See Northside Medical Center

✖ **SELECT SPECIALTY HOSPITAL–YOUNGSTOWN (362024)**, 1044 Belmont Avenue, Zip 44501; tel. 330/480–2349, (Includes SELECT SPECIALTY HOSPITAL–YOUNGSTOWN, BOARDMAN CAMPUS, 8401 Market Street, 7th Floor, Bordman, Zip 44512–6725; Mailing Address: Youngstown, tel. 330/729–1700), (Nonreporting) **A**1 10 **S** Select Medical Corporation, Mechanicsburg, PA
Primary Contact: Sharon Noro, Chief Executive Officer
Web address: www.selectmedicalcorp.com
**Control:** Corporation, Investor–owned, for–profit **Service:** Long–Term Acute Care hospital

| |
|---|
| **Staffed Beds:** 51 |

✖ △ **ST. ELIZABETH HEALTH CENTER (360064)**, 1044 Belmont Avenue, Zip 44504–1096, Mailing Address: P.O. Box 1790, Zip 44501–1790; tel. 330/746–7211 **A**1 2 3 5 7 9 10 **F**3 7 8 11 12 13 14 15 17 18 20 22 24 26 28 29 30 31 32 34 35 39 40 42 43 44 45 46 49 50 51 53 54 56 57 58 59 60 61 64 66 67 68 69 70 71 74 75 76 77 78 79 81 82 83 84 85 86 87 89 90 93 96 97 98 100 101 102 103 104 106 107 108 109 110 111 113 114 115 116 117 118 119 120 122 123 125 128 129 130 131 134 142 145 146 147 **P**3 **S** Catholic Health Partners, Cincinnati, OH
Primary Contact: Robert W. Shroder, President and Chief Executive Officer
COO: Donald E. Koenig, Jr., Executive Vice President and Chief Operating Officer
CFO: Donald E. Kline, Senior Vice President Finance
CMO: Nicholas Kreatsoulas, M.D., Senior Vice President and Chief Medical Officer
CIO: Charles Folkwein, Senior Vice President Ancillary Services and Information Technology
CHR: Molly Seals, Senior Vice President Human Resources and Learning
Web address: www.hmpartners.org
**Control:** Church–operated, Nongovernment, not–for profit **Service:** General Medical and Surgical

| |
|---|
| **Staffed Beds:** 429 **Admissions:** 18789 **Census:** 250 **Outpatient Visits:** 284934 **Births:** 1736 **Total Expense ($000):** 268271 **Payroll Expense ($000):** 90570 **Personnel:** 2239 |

☐ **SURGICAL HOSPITAL AT SOUTHWOODS (360352)**, 7630 Southern Boulevard, Zip 44512–5633; tel. 330/729–8000, (Nonreporting) **A**1 9
Primary Contact: Ed Muransky, Owner
Web address: www.surgeryatsouthwoods.com/
**Control:** Other not–for–profit (including NFP Corporation) **Service:** Surgical

| |
|---|
| **Staffed Beds:** 12 |

### ZANESVILLE—Muskingum County

★ ○ △ **GENESIS HEALTHCARE SYSTEM (360039)**, 2951 Maple Avenue, Zip 43701–2881; tel. 740/454–5000, (Includes BETHESDA HOSPITAL, 2951 Maple Avenue, Zip 43701–1465; tel. 614/454–4000; GOOD SAMARITAN MEDICAL AND REHABILITATION CENTER, 800 Forest Avenue, tel. 614/454–5000), (Total facility includes 17 beds in nursing home–type unit) **A**2 5 7 9 10 11 19 **F**3 5 8 11 13 15 17 18 20 22 24 26 28 29 30 31 32 34 35 36 40 44 45 46 47 48 50 51 54 58 59 60 63 64 65 68 70 73 74 75 76 77 78 79 80 81 82 83 84 85 86 87 89 90 91 92 93 94 96 98 99 100 101 102 103 104 105 107 108 110 111 113 114 115 116 117 118 119 120 122 123 125 127 128 129 130 131 134 143 145 146 147 **P**6 8 **S** Franciscan Sisters of Christian Charity Sponsored Ministries, Inc., Manitowoc, WI
Primary Contact: Matthew J. Perry, President and Chief Executive Officer
CFO: Paul Masterson, Chief Financial Officer
CIO: Ed Romito, Director Information Systems
Web address: www.genesishcs.com
**Control:** Other not–for–profit (including NFP Corporation) **Service:** General Medical and Surgical

| |
|---|
| **Staffed Beds:** 358 **Admissions:** 16991 **Census:** 191 **Outpatient Visits:** 304181 **Births:** 1370 **Total Expense ($000):** 260455 **Payroll Expense ($000):** 109186 **Personnel:** 2544 |

✖ **SELECT SPECIALTY HOSPITAL–ZANESVILLE (362031)**, 800 Forest Avenue, 6th Floor, Zip 43701; tel. 740/588–7888, (Nonreporting) **A**1 10 **S** Select Medical Corporation, Mechanicsburg, PA
Primary Contact: Linda Supplee, Chief Executive Officer
Web address: www.selectmedicalcorp.com
**Control:** Corporation, Investor–owned, for–profit **Service:** Long–Term Acute Care hospital

| |
|---|
| **Staffed Beds:** 35 |

*Many Facility Codes have changed. Please refer to the AHA Guide Code Chart.* © 2012 AHA Guide

# OKLAHOMA

## ADA—Pontotoc County

⊠ **CHICKASAW NATION MEDICAL CENTER (370180)**, 1921 Stonecipher Drive, Zip 74820–3439; tel. 580/436–3980, (Nonreporting) **A**1 10
Primary Contact: Judy Goforth Parker, Ph.D., Administrator
CFO: Marty Wafford, Chief Financial Officer
CMO: Richard McClain, M.D., Chief Medical Officer
CIO: Carol McCurdy, Chief Information Officer
CHR: Jalinda Kelley, Director
CNO: Heather Summers, Director
Web address: www.chickasaw.net
**Control:** Other not–for–profit (including NFP Corporation) **Service:** General Medical and Surgical

**Staffed Beds:** 51

☐ **ROLLING HILLS HOSPITAL (374016)**, 1000 Rolling Hills Lane, Zip 74820–9415; tel. 580/436–3600, (Nonreporting) **A**1 9 10 **S** Acadia Healthcare Company, Inc., Franklin, TN
Primary Contact: John Baker, Chief Executive Officer
CMO: Robert Morton, M.D., Medical Director
CIO: Sherry Barnes, Director Health Information and Quality Management
CHR: Timothy Blackwell, Manager Human Resources
Web address: www.rollinghillshospital.com
**Control:** Corporation, Investor–owned, for–profit **Service:** Psychiatric

**Staffed Beds:** 44

⊠ △ **VALLEY VIEW REGIONAL HOSPITAL (370020)**, 430 North Monta Vista, Zip 74820–4610; tel. 580/332–2323 **A**1 2 7 9 10 **F**3 7 11 15 17 18 29 30 31 34 35 40 41 43 45 69 70 72 75 76 77 78 79 81 87 89 90 93 98 102 103 107 110 111 113 115 118 119 120 126 128 129 130 132 144 145 146 147 **P**3 6 **S** Mercy Health, Chesterfield, MO
Primary Contact: W. Kent Rogers, Chief Executive Officer
CFO: Mary Krause, Vice President Finance
CMO: Donald Davies, M.D., Chief of Staff
CIO: Chad Henderson, Interim Director Management Information Systems
CHR: Katrina Simpson, Director Human Resources
Web address: www.valleyviewregional.com
**Control:** Other not–for–profit (including NFP Corporation) **Service:** General Medical and Surgical

**Staffed Beds:** 131 **Admissions:** 4709 **Census:** 59 **Outpatient Visits:** 39776 **Births:** 566 **Total Expense ($000):** 63311 **Payroll Expense ($000):** 28034 **Personnel:** 615

## ALTUS—Jackson County

⊠ **JACKSON COUNTY MEMORIAL HOSPITAL (370022)**, 1200 East Pecan Street, Zip 73521–6192, Mailing Address: P.O. Box 8190, Zip 73522–8190; tel. 580/379–5000, (Total facility includes 16 beds in nursing home–type unit) **A**1 3 5 9 10 **F**3 10 11 13 15 29 30 34 35 40 43 45 49 56 57 59 62 63 64 65 68 70 75 76 77 78 79 81 85 86 87 90 93 100 101 103 104 107 110 111 113 118 127 128 129 131 132 134 144 145 146 147 **P**6
Primary Contact: William G. Wilson, President and Chief Executive Officer
COO: Jim King, Executive Vice President and Chief Operating Officer
CFO: Nancy Davidson, Senior Vice President and Chief Financial Officer
CMO: Melinda Powers, D.O., Chief of Staff
CIO: Dena Daniel, Director Information Systems
CHR: Richard Pope, Vice President Human Resources
CNO: Kay Bolding, R.N., Vice President Patient Care Services and Chief Nursing Officer
Web address: www.jcmh.com
**Control:** Hospital district or authority, Government, nonfederal **Service:** General Medical and Surgical

**Staffed Beds:** 85 **Admissions:** 4214 **Census:** 43 **Outpatient Visits:** 156820 **Births:** 466 **Total Expense ($000):** 59588 **Payroll Expense ($000):** 34533 **Personnel:** 686

## ALVA—Woods County

**SHARE MEDICAL CENTER (370080)**, 800 Share Drive, Zip 73717–3699, Mailing Address: P.O. Box 727, Zip 73717–0727; tel. 580/327–2800, (Total facility includes 65 beds in nursing home–type unit) **A**9 10 20 **F**3 15 29 34 35 40 45 57 59 62 63 64 67 69 81 85 87 93 97 100 104 107 110 118 128 129 132 145 147 **S** QHR, Brentwood, TN
Primary Contact: Kandice K. Allen, R.N., Interim Chief Executive Officer
CFO: Albert Wiss, Chief Financial Officer
CMO: Kirt Bierig, D.O., Chief of Staff
CHR: Kristi Moorman, Supervisor Human Resources
Web address: www.smcok.com
**Control:** Hospital district or authority, Government, nonfederal **Service:** General Medical and Surgical

**Staffed Beds:** 90 **Admissions:** 418 **Census:** 53 **Outpatient Visits:** 16852 **Births:** 0 **Total Expense ($000):** 11258 **Payroll Expense ($000):** 5124 **Personnel:** 143

## ANADARKO—Caddo County

**PHYSICIANS' HOSPITAL IN ANADARKO (371314)**, 1002 Central Boulevard East, Zip 73005–4496; tel. 405/247–2551, (Nonreporting) **A**9 10 18 **S** Southern Plains Medical Group, Oklahoma City, OK
Primary Contact: Richard Carter, M.D., Chief Executive Officer
**Control:** Partnership, Investor–owned, for–profit **Service:** General Medical and Surgical

**Staffed Beds:** 25

## ANTLERS—Pushmataha County

**PUSHMATAHA HOSPITAL & HOME HEALTH (370083)**, 510 East Main Street, Zip 74523–3262, Mailing Address: P.O. Box 518, Zip 74523–3262; tel. 580/298–3341 **A**9 10 **F**3 11 29 39 40 45 46 50 57 62 81 85 89 107 118 134 144
Primary Contact: Mark E. Rogers, Chief Executive Officer and Administrator
CFO: Stephen Poe, Chief Financial Officer
CMO: G. Wayne Flatt, D.O., Chief Medical Director
CHR: Pat McCarty, Director Human Resources
Web address: www.pushhospital.com
**Control:** State–Government, nonfederal **Service:** General Medical and Surgical

**Staffed Beds:** 25 **Admissions:** 665 **Census:** 6 **Outpatient Visits:** 5804 **Births:** 1 **Total Expense ($000):** 7013 **Payroll Expense ($000):** 3668 **Personnel:** 52

## ARDMORE—Carter County

⊠ **MERCY HOSPITAL ARDMORE (370047)**, 1011 14th Avenue N.W., Zip 73401–1828; tel. 580/223–5400 **A**1 9 10 **F**3 8 11 13 15 18 20 22 28 29 30 31 34 40 41 43 45 57 59 62 70 74 76 78 79 81 82 83 84 85 87 89 90 93 107 108 110 111 113 116 117 118 119 120 122 128 129 145 147 **P**6 **S** Mercy Health, Chesterfield, MO
Primary Contact: Mindy Burdick, FACHE, President
COO: Ryan Barnard, Chief Operating Officer
CFO: Karen Hendren, Vice President of Finance
CMO: Pam Kimbrough, M.D., Vice President Medical Affairs
CHR: Melinda Sharum, Director of Human Resources
CNO: Rhonda Jean Hanan, Vice President of Patient Care
Web address: www.mercyok.net
**Control:** Church–operated, Nongovernment, not–for profit **Service:** General Medical and Surgical

**Staffed Beds:** 190 **Admissions:** 8164 **Census:** 102 **Outpatient Visits:** 127502 **Births:** 909 **Total Expense ($000):** 110242 **Payroll Expense ($000):** 39446 **Personnel:** 788

## ATOKA—Atoka County

★ **ATOKA COUNTY MEDICAL CENTER (371300)**, 1501 South Virginia Avenue, Zip 74525–3298; tel. 580/889–3333, (Nonreporting) **A**9 10 18
Primary Contact: Paul Reano, Chief Executive Officer
CFO: Jamie McGaugh, Controller
CMO: Bruce Rumbaugh, M.D., Director Patient Care
CHR: Naomi Farris, Director Human Resources
Web address: www.atoka–hosp.otnnet.net
**Control:** Hospital district or authority, Government, nonfederal **Service:** General Medical and Surgical

**Staffed Beds:** 25

---

**Hospital, Medicare Provider Number, Address, Telephone, Approval, Facility, and Physician Codes, Health Care System**

★ American Hospital Association (AHA) membership
☐ The Joint Commission accreditation
◇ DNV Healthcare Inc. accreditation
○ American Osteopathic Association (AOA) accreditation
△ Commission on Accreditation of Rehabilitation Facilities (CARF) accreditation

**OK**

## BARTLESVILLE—Washington County

★ **JANE PHILLIPS MEDICAL CENTER (370018)**, 3500 East Frank Phillips Boulevard, Zip 74006–2411; tel. 918/333–7200 **A**3 5 9 10 19 21 **F**3 11 13 15 17 18 20 22 24 28 29 30 31 34 35 40 43 46 49 50 51 53 57 58 59 60 61 62 64 68 74 75 76 77 78 79 81 82 84 85 86 87 90 92 93 96 98 102 103 107 111 113 114 115 116 117 118 120 122 126 128 129 130 134 142 144 145 146 147 **P**4 **S** Marian Health System, Tulsa, OK
Primary Contact: David R. Stire, President and Chief Executive Officer
CFO: Mike Moore, Chief Financial Officer
CIO: Rob Poole, Director
CHR: Jennifer Workman, Director Human Resources
Web address: www.jpmc.org
**Control:** Church–operated, Nongovernment, not–for profit **Service:** General Medical and Surgical

| | |
|---|---|
| **Staffed Beds:** 140 **Admissions:** 5930 **Census:** 66 **Outpatient Visits:** 78238 **Births:** 670 **Total Expense ($000):** 98585 **Payroll Expense ($000):** 37986 **Personnel:** 806 | |

## BEAVER—Beaver County

**BEAVER COUNTY MEMORIAL HOSPITAL (371322)**, 212 East Eighth Street, Zip 73932, Mailing Address: P.O. Box 640, Zip 73932–0640; tel. 580/625–4551, (Nonreporting) **A**9 10 18
Primary Contact: Brent Meyers, Administrator
Web address: www.beavercountyhospitalauthority.org
**Control:** Hospital district or authority, Government, nonfederal **Service:** General Medical and Surgical

| | |
|---|---|
| **Staffed Beds:** 24 | |

## BETHANY—Oklahoma County

△ **THE CHILDREN'S CENTER (373302)**, 6800 N.W. 39th Expressway, Zip 73008–2513; tel. 405/789–6711 **A**7 10 **F**1 29 39 59 75 79 90 91 93 107 129 145 147 **P**6
Primary Contact: Albert Gray, Chief Executive Officer
Web address: www.thechildrens–center.org
**Control:** Other not–for–profit (including NFP Corporation) **Service:** Children's general

| | |
|---|---|
| **Staffed Beds:** 120 **Admissions:** 254 **Census:** 106 **Outpatient Visits:** 9200 **Births:** 0 **Total Expense ($000):** 23191 **Payroll Expense ($000):** 14466 **Personnel:** 392 | |

## BLACKWELL—Kay County

⊠ **INTEGRIS BLACKWELL REGIONAL HOSPITAL (370030)**, 710 South 13th Street, Zip 74631–3700; tel. 580/363–2311 **A**1 9 10 **F**11 13 15 29 30 34 40 57 59 62 76 79 81 107 127 132 145 **P**5 6 **S** Health Management Associates, Naples, FL
Primary Contact: Julie M. McCormack, R.N., Administrator
CFO: Sheryl Schmidtberger, Chief Financial Officer
CMO: Samuel Hague, M.D., Chief of Staff
CHR: Karen Ware, Director Human Resources
Web address: www.integris–health.com
**Control:** Other not–for–profit (including NFP Corporation) **Service:** General Medical and Surgical

| | |
|---|---|
| **Staffed Beds:** 31 **Admissions:** 946 **Census:** 10 **Personnel:** 97 | |

## BOISE CITY—Cimarron County

**CIMARRON MEMORIAL HOSPITAL (371307)**, 100 South Ellis Street, Zip 73933; tel. 580/544–2501 **A**9 10 18 **F**15 29 32 34 40 50 57 59 65 66 68 75 85 89 90 93 97 107 113 126 128 129 132 147 **P**6
Primary Contact: David M. Peyok, Chief Executive Officer
Web address: www.cimarronmemorialhospital.org
**Control:** County–Government, nonfederal **Service:** General Medical and Surgical

| | |
|---|---|
| **Staffed Beds:** 25 **Admissions:** 205 **Census:** 2 **Outpatient Visits:** 9878 **Births:** 0 **Total Expense ($000):** 3624 **Payroll Expense ($000):** 1925 **Personnel:** 46 | |

## BRISTOW—Creek County

**BRISTOW MEDICAL CENTER (370041)**, 700 West 7th Avenue, Suite 6, Zip 74010–2302; tel. 918/367–2215, (Nonreporting) **A**9 10
Primary Contact: Jan Winter, Chief Executive Officer
CFO: Robin Van Vickle, Chief Financial Officer
Web address: www.bristowmedcenter.com
**Control:** Corporation, Investor–owned, for–profit **Service:** General Medical and Surgical

| | |
|---|---|
| **Staffed Beds:** 17 | |

## BROKEN ARROW—Tulsa County

★ **ST. JOHN BROKEN ARROW (370235)**, 1000 West Boise Circle, Zip 74012–4900; tel. 918/994–8100 **A**9 10 21 **F**3 8 11 14 15 18 29 30 34 35 37 40 45 50 57 59 64 68 74 79 81 84 85 87 89 93 94 107 108 110 111 114 118 129 131 134 145 **P**1 5 **S** Marian Health System, Tulsa, OK
Primary Contact: David L. Phillips, Chief Executive Officer
CFO: Lex S. Anderson, Chief Financial Officer
CMO: Todd Hoffman, M.D., Medical Director
CNO: Martha Mars, R.N., Director of Nursing
Web address: www.stjohnbrokenarrow.com
**Control:** Corporation, Investor–owned, for–profit **Service:** General Medical and Surgical

| | |
|---|---|
| **Staffed Beds:** 44 **Admissions:** 2303 **Census:** 13 **Outpatient Visits:** 45950 **Births:** 0 **Total Expense ($000):** 49552 **Payroll Expense ($000):** 11241 **Personnel:** 234 | |

## BUFFALO—Harper County

★ **HARPER COUNTY COMMUNITY HOSPITAL (371324)**, Highway 64 North, Zip 73834, Mailing Address: P.O. Box 60, Zip 73834–0060; tel. 580/735–2555 **A**9 10 18 **F**40 69 75 76 81 87 89 93 107 127 132 134 147 **P**5 6
Primary Contact: Karen Ives, Administrator
CFO: Georganna Buss, Chief Financial Officer
Web address: www.hcchospital.com/
**Control:** County–Government, nonfederal **Service:** General Medical and Surgical

| | |
|---|---|
| **Staffed Beds:** 16 **Admissions:** 253 **Census:** 2 **Births:** 4 | |

## CARNEGIE—Caddo County

★ **CARNEGIE TRI–COUNTY MUNICIPAL HOSPITAL (371334)**, 102 North Broadway, Zip 73015, Mailing Address: P.O. Box 97, Zip 73015–0097; tel. 580/654–1050, (Nonreporting) **A**9 10 18
Primary Contact: Shane Dunning, Administrator
**Control:** City–Government, nonfederal **Service:** General Medical and Surgical

| | |
|---|---|
| **Staffed Beds:** 19 | |

## CHEYENNE—Roger Mills County

★ **ROGER MILLS MEMORIAL HOSPITAL (371303)**, Fifth and L. L Males Avenue, Zip 73628; tel. 580/497–3336 **A**9 10 18 **F**3 7 34 40 57 59 65 93 107 126 132
Primary Contact: Marilyn Bryan, Administrator
CFO: Lois Wilson, Controller
Web address: www.rogermillsmemorialhospital.com/
**Control:** Hospital district or authority, Government, nonfederal **Service:** General Medical and Surgical

| | |
|---|---|
| **Staffed Beds:** 15 **Admissions:** 52 **Census:** 1 **Outpatient Visits:** 3477 **Births:** 0 **Total Expense ($000):** 3889 **Payroll Expense ($000):** 1869 **Personnel:** 48 | |

## CHICKASHA—Grady County

★ **GRADY MEMORIAL HOSPITAL (370054)**, 2220 West Iowa Avenue, Zip 73018–2738; tel. 405/224–2300 **A**5 9 10 19 **F**3 8 11 13 15 17 29 30 34 35 40 43 45 57 59 69 70 73 76 79 81 82 85 89 93 107 110 111 113 114 118 126 127 128 129 131 132 143 145 146 **P**6
Primary Contact: Michael Nunamaker, FACHE, Chief Executive Officer
CFO: Linda Hart, Vice President Finance
CMO: Bruce Storms, M.D., Chief of Staff
CIO: Sylvia Ho, Director Information Services
CHR: Steve Hutchens, Vice President General Services
Web address: www.gradymem.org
**Control:** Hospital district or authority, Government, nonfederal **Service:** General Medical and Surgical

| | |
|---|---|
| **Staffed Beds:** 52 **Admissions:** 1899 **Census:** 17 **Outpatient Visits:** 114048 **Births:** 313 **Total Expense ($000):** 39399 **Payroll Expense ($000):** 18492 **Personnel:** 353 | |

## CLAREMORE—Rogers County

☐ **CLAREMORE INDIAN HOSPITAL (370173)**, 101 South Moore Avenue, Zip 74017–5091; tel. 918/342–6200 **A**1 5 10 **F**3 13 15 30 34 39 40 45 50 59 64 68 70 75 76 77 81 86 89 93 97 107 114 118 129 134 146 **S** U. S. Indian Health Service, Rockville, MD
Primary Contact: George Valliere, Chief Executive Officer
CFO: LaLana Spears, Supervisor Accounting
CMO: Paul Mobley, D.O., Clinical Director
CIO: David Ponder, Information Technology Officer
CHR: Jamelle King, Director Human Resources
Web address: www.ihs.gov
**Control:** PHS, Indian Service, Government, federal **Service:** General Medical and Surgical

| | |
|---|---|
| **Staffed Beds:** 46 **Admissions:** 956 **Census:** 8 **Outpatient Visits:** 206604 **Births:** 232 | |

*Many Facility Codes have changed. Please refer to the AHA Guide Code Chart.*

© 2012 AHA Guide

OK

⊞ **HILLCREST HOSPITAL CLAREMORE (370039)**, 1202 North Muskogee Place, Zip 74017–3036; tel. 918/341–2556 **A**1 9 10 **F**3 11 13 15 20 22 26 28 29 30 34 35 37 40 45 49 51 57 59 64 70 74 76 77 79 81 82 85 86 87 93 98 103 107 108 110 111 118 125 127 128 129 130 132 134 144 145 146 147 **S** Ardent Health Services, Nashville, TN
Primary Contact: David Chaussard, Chief Executive Officer
CIO: Celeste Rodden, Chief Information Officer
CHR: Pat Goad, Director Human Resources
CNO: Dava Baldridge, Chief Nursing Officer
Web address: www.hillcrestclaremore.com
**Control:** Corporation, Investor–owned, for–profit **Service:** General Medical and Surgical

> **Staffed Beds:** 89 **Admissions:** 2813 **Census:** 29 **Outpatient Visits:** 46965 **Births:** 549 **Total Expense ($000):** 33516 **Payroll Expense ($000):** 13520 **Personnel:** 379

### CLEVELAND—Pawnee County

**CLEVELAND AREA HOSPITAL (371320)**, 1401 West Pawnee Street, Zip 74020–3019; tel. 918/358–2501 **A**9 10 18 **F**11 29 34 40 53 57 59 64 77 81 87 89 93 107 113 118 129 132
Primary Contact: James Clough, Chief Executive Officer
CFO: Jon Davis, Chief Financial Officer
CMO: Jason Sims, M.D., Chief Medical Officer
CHR: Sherry Brown, Director Human Resources
Web address: www.clevelandareahospital.com
**Control:** Hospital district or authority, Government, nonfederal **Service:** General Medical and Surgical

> **Staffed Beds:** 14 **Admissions:** 486 **Census:** 4 **Outpatient Visits:** 13405 **Births:** 0 **Total Expense ($000):** 5808 **Payroll Expense ($000):** 5466 **Personnel:** 74

### CLINTON—Custer County

⊞ **INTEGRIS CLINTON REGIONAL HOSPITAL (370029)**, 100 North 30th Street, Zip 73601–3117, Mailing Address: P.O. Box 1569, Zip 73601–1569; tel. 580/323–2363 **A**1 9 10 **F**3 11 13 15 29 30 31 34 40 45 59 62 63 70 75 76 77 78 81 86 90 93 96 107 108 111 113 118 120 122 128 129 130 131 132 145 146 147 **P**6 **S** Health Management Associates, Naples, FL
Primary Contact: Darcey O'Brien, Chief Executive Officer
CFO: Richard Foster, Chief Financial Officer
Web address: www.integris–health.com
**Control:** Other not–for–profit (including NFP Corporation) **Service:** General Medical and Surgical

> **Staffed Beds:** 49 **Admissions:** 1629 **Census:** 15 **Outpatient Visits:** 21171 **Births:** 217 **Total Expense ($000):** 24519 **Payroll Expense ($000):** 10265 **Personnel:** 178

### COALGATE—Coal County

★ **COAL COUNTY GENERAL HOSPITAL (371319)**, 6 North Covington Street, Zip 74538–2002, Mailing Address: P.O. Box 326, Zip 74538; tel. 580/927–2327 **A**9 10 18 **F**40 57 59 107 113 118 132
Primary Contact: Billy Johnson, Chief Executive Officer
CFO: Jamie Massie, Chief Financial Officer
Web address: www.hillcrest.com
**Control:** Other not–for–profit (including NFP Corporation) **Service:** General Medical and Surgical

> **Staffed Beds:** 20 **Admissions:** 774 **Census:** 8 **Outpatient Visits:** 4662 **Births:** 0 **Total Expense ($000):** 3935 **Payroll Expense ($000):** 1844 **Personnel:** 49

### CORDELL—Washita County

★ **CORDELL MEMORIAL HOSPITAL (371325)**, 1220 North Glenn English Street, Zip 73632–2010; tel. 580/832–3339 **A**9 10 18 **F**7 40 57 59 65 89 107 127 132
Primary Contact: Charles H. Greene, Jr., Administrator
CFO: Sue Kelley, Chief Financial Officer
**Control:** City–Government, nonfederal **Service:** General Medical and Surgical

> **Staffed Beds:** 25 **Admissions:** 257 **Census:** 2 **Outpatient Visits:** 4679 **Births:** 0 **Total Expense ($000):** 3839 **Payroll Expense ($000):** 1716 **Personnel:** 41

### CUSHING—Payne County

⊞ **CUSHING REGIONAL HOSPITAL (370099)**, 1027 East Cherry Street, Zip 74023–4101, Mailing Address: P.O. Box 1409, Zip 74023–1409; tel. 918/225–2915, (Nonreporting) **A**1 9 10 **S** Ardent Health Services, Nashville, TN
Primary Contact: Randy DuBois, Chief Executive Officer
COO: Abigail Kendall, Chief Nursing Officer and Chief Operating Officer
CFO: Brandon Bullard, Chief Financial Officer
Web address: www.hillcrest.com
**Control:** Corporation, Investor–owned, for–profit **Service:** General Medical and Surgical

> **Staffed Beds:** 95

### DRUMRIGHT—Creek County

**DRUMRIGHT REGIONAL HOSPITAL (371331)**, 610 West Bypass, Zip 74030–5957; tel. 918/382–2300 **A**9 10 18 **F**3 15 18 29 34 35 40 45 57 59 64 77 79 81 93 107 108 111 115 116 118 126 128 129 132 **P**3 6 **S** HMC/CAH Consolidated, Inc., Kansas City, MO
Primary Contact: Darrel Morris, Chief Executive Officer
CFO: Mark Conrath, Chief Financial Officer
Web address: www.drumrighthospital.com
**Control:** Corporation, Investor–owned, for–profit **Service:** General Medical and Surgical

> **Staffed Beds:** 15 **Admissions:** 625 **Census:** 7 **Outpatient Visits:** 4493 **Births:** 0 **Total Expense ($000):** 8219 **Payroll Expense ($000):** 3683 **Personnel:** 71

### DUNCAN—Stephens County

⊞ △ **DUNCAN REGIONAL HOSPITAL (370023)**, 1407 North Whisenant Drive, Zip 73533–1650, Mailing Address: P.O. Box 2000, Zip 73534–2000; tel. 580/252–5300, (Total facility includes 16 beds in nursing home–type unit) **A**1 5 7 9 10 20 **F**3 8 11 13 28 29 30 34 35 40 43 45 46 47 51 53 62 63 64 68 70 75 76 77 79 81 85 87 89 90 93 96 98 103 104 107 108 111 113 117 118 127 128 129 130 131 145 147 **P**6
Primary Contact: Jay R. Johnson, FACHE, President and Chief Executive Officer
CFO: Douglas R. Volinski, Vice President and Chief Financial Officer
CIO: Roger Neal, Vice President and Chief Information Officer
CHR: Mark Rhoades, Vice President and Chief Human Resources Officer
CNO: Cindy Rauh, R.N., Vice President and Chief Nursing Officer
Web address: www.duncanregional.com
**Control:** Other not–for–profit (including NFP Corporation) **Service:** General Medical and Surgical

> **Staffed Beds:** 124 **Admissions:** 4729 **Census:** 59 **Outpatient Visits:** 95076 **Births:** 500 **Total Expense ($000):** 72200 **Payroll Expense ($000):** 28140 **Personnel:** 714

### DURANT—Bryan County

⊞ **MEDICAL CENTER OF SOUTHEASTERN OKLAHOMA (370014)**, 1800 University Boulevard, Zip 74701–3006, Mailing Address: P.O. Box 1207, Zip 74702–1207; tel. 580/924–3080 **A**1 9 10 13 19 **F**3 8 11 13 15 17 20 28 29 39 40 45 51 56 59 62 70 74 75 76 79 80 81 85 86 87 89 93 107 108 110 111 114 117 118 128 129 134 144 145 146 147 **P**8 **S** Health Management Associates, Naples, FL
Primary Contact: Patricia Dorris, Executive Director
CFO: Cindy Rios, Chief Financial Officer
CMO: Kevin Gordon, M.D., Chief of Staff
CIO: Katy Stinson, Director Information Services
Web address: www.mymcso.com
**Control:** Corporation, Investor–owned, for–profit **Service:** General Medical and Surgical

> **Staffed Beds:** 148 **Admissions:** 7160 **Census:** 71 **Outpatient Visits:** 59086 **Births:** 1146 **Personnel:** 426

### EDMOND—Oklahoma County

**EDMOND MEDICAL CENTER** See OU Medical Center Edmond

★ **INTEGRIS HEALTH EDMOND (370236)**, 4801 Integris Parkway, Zip 73034–8864; tel. 405/657–3000, (Nonreporting) **S** INTEGRIS Health, Oklahoma City, OK
Primary Contact: Avilla Williams, MS, President
Web address: www.integrisok.com/edmond
**Control:** Other not–for–profit (including NFP Corporation) **Service:** General Medical and Surgical

> **Staffed Beds:** 40

---

**Hospital, Medicare Provider Number, Address, Telephone, Approval, Facility, and Physician Codes, Health Care System**

★ American Hospital Association (AHA) membership
□ The Joint Commission accreditation     ◇ DNV Healthcare Inc. accreditation
○ American Osteopathic Association (AOA) accreditation
△ Commission on Accreditation of Rehabilitation Facilities (CARF) accreditation

**OK**

☐ **LTAC OF EDMOND (372005)**, 1100 East Ninth Street, Zip 73034–5755; tel. 405/341–8150, (Data for 354 days) **A**1 9 10 **F**1 3 29 34 56 60 118 129 134 142 147 **P**8 **S** AMG Integrated Healthcare Management, Lafayette, LA
Primary Contact: Ginger Creech, Chief Executive Officer
CFO: Rowena Davidson, Manager Business Office
CMO: Brian Levy, M.D., Medical Director
CHR: Pam Grimes, Director Human Resources
Web address: www.amgihm.com
**Control:** Corporation, Investor–owned, for–profit **Service:** Long–Term Acute Care hospital

**Staffed Beds:** 37 **Admissions:** 305 **Census:** 20 **Outpatient Visits:** 0 **Births:** 0 **Total Expense ($000):** 9324 **Payroll Expense ($000):** 3961

**OU MEDICAL CENTER EDMOND** See OU Medical Center, Oklahoma City

**SUMMIT MEDICAL CENTER (370225)**, 1800 South Renaissance Boulevard, Zip 73013–3023; tel. 405/359–2400, (Nonreporting) **A**10
Primary Contact: Curtis Summers, Chief Executive Officer
Web address: www.summitmedcenter.com/
**Control:** Corporation, Investor–owned, for–profit **Service:** Other specialty

**Staffed Beds:** 15

### EL RENO—Canadian County

★ **MERCY HOSPITAL EL RENO (370011)**, 2115 Parkview Drive, Zip 73036–2199, Mailing Address: P.O. Box 129, Zip 73036–0129; tel. 405/262–2640 **A**9 10 **F**3 7 8 30 35 40 45 46 50 62 64 65 77 79 81 82 85 93 107 131 134 145 **P**6 **S** Mercy Health, Chesterfield, MO
Primary Contact: Doug Danker, Administrator
CMO: Michael Dean Sullivan, M.D., Chief of Staff
CIO: Karen Heldreth, Director Data Processing
CHR: Wendy Ward, Director Human Resources
Web address: www.mercyok.net
**Control:** Church–operated, Nongovernment, not–for profit **Service:** General Medical and Surgical

**Staffed Beds:** 48 **Admissions:** 728 **Census:** 6 **Outpatient Visits:** 37337 **Births:** 78 **Total Expense ($000):** 13135 **Payroll Expense ($000):** 7421 **Personnel:** 128

**PARKVIEW HOSPITAL** See Mercy Hospital El Reno

### ELK CITY—Beckham County

☒ **GREAT PLAINS REGIONAL MEDICAL CENTER (370019)**, 1801 West Third Street, Zip 73644–5145, Mailing Address: P.O. Box 2339, Zip 73648–2339; tel. 580/225–2511 **A**1 9 10 **F**3 11 13 15 18 20 26 29 30 31 34 35 40 43 44 45 47 50 51 56 57 59 62 64 68 70 75 76 77 78 79 81 82 85 86 87 89 91 93 96 98 100 101 102 103 107 108 110 111 114 117 118 119 120 122 128 129 130 131 134 142 145 146 147
Primary Contact: Don Ikner, Chief Executive Officer
CMO: Craig Phelps, M.D., Chief of Staff
CIO: Terry Davis, Chief Information Officer
CHR: Misty Carter, Director Human Resources
Web address: www.gprmc–ok.com
**Control:** Other not–for–profit (including NFP Corporation) **Service:** General Medical and Surgical

**Staffed Beds:** 50 **Admissions:** 2393 **Census:** 25 **Outpatient Visits:** 58435 **Births:** 453 **Total Expense ($000):** 43120 **Payroll Expense ($000):** 16765 **Personnel:** 356

### ENID—Garfield County

**INTEGRIS BASS BEHAVIORAL HEALTH SYSTEM** See Integris Bass Meadowlake

☒ **INTEGRIS BASS BAPTIST HEALTH CENTER (370016)**, 600 South Monroe Street, Zip 73701–7211, Mailing Address: P.O. Box 3168, Zip 73702–3168; tel. 580/233–2300 **A**1 5 9 10 13 19 **F**3 11 13 15 17 18 20 22 24 28 29 30 31 35 40 43 45 49 57 62 68 70 74 75 76 77 78 79 81 85 98 99 103 107 108 111 113 116 117 118 119 120 126 127 128 131 143 145 146 147 **S** INTEGRIS Health, Oklahoma City, OK
Primary Contact: Jeffrey S. Tarrant, FACHE, President
CFO: Rebecca Tucker, Chief Financial Officer
Web address: www.integris–health.com
**Control:** Other not–for–profit (including NFP Corporation) **Service:** General Medical and Surgical

**Staffed Beds:** 167 **Admissions:** 4915 **Census:** 99 **Outpatient Visits:** 55375 **Births:** 936 **Total Expense ($000):** 97183 **Payroll Expense ($000):** 43264 **Personnel:** 705

☐ **INTEGRIS BASS PAVILION (372016)**, 401 South Third Street, Zip 73701–5737; tel. 580/249–4260 **A**1 9 10 **F**1 11 29 30 40 43 68 75 77 82 85 93 130 145 147 **S** INTEGRIS Health, Oklahoma City, OK
Primary Contact: Jeffrey S. Tarrant, FACHE, President
CFO: Rebecca Tucker, Chief Financial Officer
CMO: Edward Herrman, M.D., Assistant Administrator Patient Care Services
CHR: Tera L. Latta, Director Human Resources
Web address: www.integris–health.com/integris/en–us/locations/bass–enid
**Control:** Other not–for–profit (including NFP Corporation) **Service:** General Medical and Surgical

**Staffed Beds:** 24 **Admissions:** 251 **Census:** 18 **Outpatient Visits:** 1916 **Births:** 0 **Total Expense ($000):** 9496 **Payroll Expense ($000):** 3828 **Personnel:** 65

☐ △ **ST. MARY'S REGIONAL MEDICAL CENTER (370026)**, 305 South Fifth Street, Zip 73701–5899, Mailing Address: P.O. Box 232, Zip 73702–0232; tel. 580/233–6100 **A**1 5 7 9 10 **F**3 11 13 15 17 18 20 22 28 29 30 31 34 35 39 40 42 43 45 49 51 54 57 59 60 61 68 69 70 72 74 75 76 78 79 81 82 85 86 90 93 107 108 110 111 113 114 117 118 127 128 129 130 131 145 146 **S** Universal Health Services, Inc., King of Prussia, PA
Primary Contact: Stanley D. Tatum, FACHE, Chief Executive Officer
COO: Nicholas Crafts, Chief Operating Officer
CFO: Vanessa Kochevar, Chief Financial Officer
CMO: Seth Switzen, M.D., Chief of Staff
CIO: Conrad Ramirez, Director Information Services
CHR: Linda Hoag, Director Human Resources
Web address: www.stmarysregional.com
**Control:** Corporation, Investor–owned, for–profit **Service:** General Medical and Surgical

**Staffed Beds:** 163 **Admissions:** 5683 **Census:** 84 **Outpatient Visits:** 67293 **Births:** 322 **Total Expense ($000):** 72611 **Payroll Expense ($000):** 30338 **Personnel:** 608

### EUFAULA—McIntosh County

**EPIC MEDICAL CENTER (370169)**, 1 Hospital Drive, Zip 74432–4010, Mailing Address: P.O. Box 629, Zip 74432–0629; tel. 918/689–2535 **A**9 10 **F**3 34 40 45 81
Primary Contact: Vicki Schaff, Chief Operating Officer
COO: Vicki Schaff, Chief Operating Officer
CFO: Phyllis Eakle, Chief Financial Officer
CMO: Ed Farrow, M.D., Chief Medical Staff
Web address: www.epichealthcare.net
**Control:** Corporation, Investor–owned, for–profit **Service:** General Medical and Surgical

**Staffed Beds:** 33 **Admissions:** 90 **Census:** 1 **Outpatient Visits:** 10779 **Births:** 0 **Total Expense ($000):** 2905 **Payroll Expense ($000):** 1774 **Personnel:** 40

### FAIRFAX—Osage County

★ **FAIRFAX COMMUNITY HOSPITAL (371318)**, Taft Avenue and Highway 18, Zip 74637–4028, Mailing Address: P.O. Box 219, Zip 74637–0219; tel. 918/642–3291 **A**9 10 18 **F**3 11 29 40 45 57 81 93 107 116 128 132 145 **S** HMC/CAH Consolidated, Inc., Kansas City, MO
Primary Contact: Tina Steele, Chief Executive Officer and Chief Financial Officer
COO: Linda Thompson, Chief Operating Officer
CFO: Tina Steele, Chief Executive Officer and Chief Financial Officer
CMO: Arman Janloo, M.D., Chief Medical Staff
CIO: Lisa Drymon, Manager
CHR: Sharon Binkley, Director Human Resources
Web address: www.fairfaxmemorialhospital.com
**Control:** Corporation, Investor–owned, for–profit **Service:** General Medical and Surgical

**Staffed Beds:** 15 **Admissions:** 207 **Census:** 3 **Outpatient Visits:** 5649 **Total Expense ($000):** 4333 **Payroll Expense ($000):** 1907 **Personnel:** 39

**FAIRFAX MEMORIAL HOSPITAL** See Fairfax Community Hospital

### FAIRVIEW—Major County

**FAIRVIEW REGIONAL MEDICAL CENTER (371329)**, 523 East State Road, Zip 73737–1498, Mailing Address: P.O. Box 548, Zip 73737–0548; tel. 580/227–3721 **A**9 10 18 **F**3 28 34 40 43 45 57 59 64 65 69 75 77 81 82 84 85 91 93 107 113 126 127 130 132 134 145 **P**6
Primary Contact: Roger Knak, Administrator
CFO: Jamie Eitzen, Chief Financial Officer
CMO: Solomon Ali, M.D., Chief of Staff
CHR: Macky Martin, Director Human Resources
Web address: www.fairviewregional.net
**Control:** Hospital district or authority, Government, nonfederal **Service:** General Medical and Surgical

**Staffed Beds:** 25 **Admissions:** 236 **Census:** 4 **Outpatient Visits:** 10146 **Births:** 0 **Total Expense ($000):** 5732 **Payroll Expense ($000):** 3104 **Personnel:** 96

*Many Facility Codes have changed. Please refer to the AHA Guide Code Chart.*

## FORT SILL—Comanche County

✉ **REYNOLDS ARMY COMMUNITY HOSPITAL**, 4301 Mow Way Road,
Zip 73503–6300; tel. 580/458–3000, (Nonreporting) **A**1 3 5 **S** Department of
the Army, Office of the Surgeon General, Falls Church, VA
Primary Contact: Colonel Jennifer L. Bedick, Commander
COO: Lieutenant Colonel Paul Roberts, Chief of Staff and Deputy Commander for
Administration
CFO: Captain Shelley Mizelle, Chief Resource Management Division
CMO: Colonel Donald Mondragon, M.D., Deputy Commander Clinical Services
CIO: Major Eric McClung, Chief Information Management Division
CHR: Homer Williams, Chief Civilian Personnel Branch
Web address: www.rach.sill.amedd.army.mil
**Control:** Army, Government, federal **Service:** General Medical and Surgical

**Staffed Beds:** 43

## FORT SUPPLY— County

**NORTHWEST CENTER FOR BEHAVIORAL HEALTH (374001)**, 1222 Tenth
Street, Zip 73841–0001; tel. 580/766–2311 **A**9 10 **F**5 98 102 104 106 **P**6
**S** Oklahoma Department of Mental Health and Substance Abuse Services,
Oklahoma City, OK
Primary Contact: Trudy Hoffman, Executive Director
Web address: www.ncbhok.org/
**Control:** State–Government, nonfederal **Service:** Psychiatric

**Staffed Beds:** 28 **Admissions:** 610 **Census:** 24 **Outpatient Visits:** 35996
**Births:** 0 **Total Expense ($000):** 13406 **Payroll Expense ($000):** 6925
**Personnel:** 187

## FREDERICK—Tillman County

★ **MEMORIAL HOSPITAL AND PHYSICIAN GROUP (370051)**, 319 East
Josephine Avenue, Zip 73542–2220; tel. 580/335–7565, (Total facility includes
30 beds in nursing home–type unit) **A**9 10 20 **F**11 29 40 59 62 64 67 81 89 93
107 113 118 132 **P**6
Primary Contact: Michael J. Carter, Chief Executive Officer
COO: Cindy Duncan, Chief Operating Officer
Web address: www.frederickhospital.com
**Control:** Hospital district or authority, Government, nonfederal **Service:** General
Medical and Surgical

**Staffed Beds:** 55 **Admissions:** 638 **Census:** 33 **Outpatient Visits:** 33173
**Births:** 2 **Total Expense ($000):** 8008 **Payroll Expense ($000):** 3990
**Personnel:** 116

## GROVE—Delaware County

✉ **INTEGRIS GROVE GENERAL HOSPITAL (370113)**, 1001 East 18th Street,
Zip 74344–2907; tel. 918/786–2243 **A**1 9 10 20 **F**3 7 11 13 29 30 40 54 57
62 64 70 77 79 81 85 107 110 111 113 118 124 128 145 146 **S** INTEGRIS
Health, Oklahoma City, OK
Primary Contact: Greg Martin, President
CFO: Kevin Cox, Chief Financial Officer
CMO: James Rutter, M.D., Chief of Staff
CHR: Vicki Cossairt, Director Human Resources
CNO: Angela Bidleman, R.N., Chief Nursing Officer
Web address: www.integris-health.com
**Control:** Other not–for–profit (including NFP Corporation) **Service:** General
Medical and Surgical

**Staffed Beds:** 58 **Admissions:** 3222 **Census:** 28 **Outpatient Visits:** 55729
**Births:** 323 **Total Expense ($000):** 49749 **Payroll Expense ($000):** 17584
**Personnel:** 306

## GUTHRIE—Logan County

★ **MERCY HOSPITAL LOGAN COUNTY (371317)**, Highway 33 West at Academy
Road, Zip 73044–3700, Mailing Address: P.O. Box 1017, Zip 73044–1017;
tel. 405/282–6700 **A**9 10 18 **F**3 8 11 15 29 30 34 40 49 50 59 62 64 65 79
81 85 93 97 107 110 111 113 118 126 128 129 130 132 147 **P**6 **S** Mercy
Health, Chesterfield, MO
Primary Contact: Joshua Tucker, Chief Executive Officer
CMO: Stephen Travis, M.D., Chief of Staff
CHR: Mary Jo Messelt, Director Human Resources
Web address: www.loganmedicalcenter.com
**Control:** County–Government, nonfederal **Service:** General Medical and Surgical

**Staffed Beds:** 25 **Admissions:** 985 **Census:** 15 **Outpatient Visits:** 95390
**Births:** 0 **Total Expense ($000):** 24027 **Payroll Expense ($000):** 11796
**Personnel:** 220

## GUYMON—Texas County

★ **MEMORIAL HOSPITAL OF TEXAS COUNTY (370138)**, 520 Medical Drive,
Zip 73942–4438; tel. 580/338–6515 **A**9 10 20 **F**3 11 13 15 29 34 40 43 45
57 59 62 63 64 65 68 70 75 76 79 81 82 85 89 93 102 107 108 110 111
113 118 130 132 146 147 **P**6
Primary Contact: Lee Hughes, Chief Executive Officer
CFO: Jamie R. Jacoby, Chief Financial Officer
Web address: www.mhtcguymon.org
**Control:** County–Government, nonfederal **Service:** General Medical and Surgical

**Staffed Beds:** 14 **Admissions:** 1203 **Census:** 9 **Outpatient Visits:** 46494
**Births:** 341 **Total Expense ($000):** 20086 **Payroll Expense ($000):** 8621
**Personnel:** 161

## HEALDTON—Carter County

★ **MERCY HOSPITAL HEALDTON (371310)**, 3462 Hospital Road, Zip 73438,
Mailing Address: P.O. Box 928, Zip 73438; tel. 580/229–0701 **A**9 10 18 **F**3 29
34 40 64 93 107 113 132 **P**6 **S** Mercy Health, Chesterfield, MO
Primary Contact: Jeremy A. Jones, Administrator
CMO: Mark Newey, D.O., Chief of Staff
CHR: Melinda Sharum, Director Human Resources
Web address: www.mercyok.com
**Control:** Church–operated, Nongovernment, not–for profit **Service:** General
Medical and Surgical

**Staffed Beds:** 22 **Admissions:** 173 **Census:** 5 **Outpatient Visits:** 11346
**Births:** 0 **Total Expense ($000):** 4170 **Payroll Expense ($000):** 2574
**Personnel:** 38

## HENRYETTA—Okmulgee County

★ **HENRYETTA MEDICAL CENTER (370183)**, Dewey Bartlett & Main Streets,
Zip 74437–6820, Mailing Address: P.O. Box 1269, Zip 74437–1269;
tel. 918/650–1100 **A**9 10 **F**3 15 29 40 45 54 56 62 64 65 68 79 81 85 87
93 98 102 103 107 111 113 118 127 128 129 132 142 147 **P**6 **S** Ardent
Health Services, Nashville, TN
Primary Contact: Dee Renshaw, Chief Executive Officer
CFO: Brandon Bullard, Chief Financial Officer
Web address: www.henryettamedicalcenter.com
**Control:** Corporation, Investor–owned, for–profit **Service:** General Medical and
Surgical

**Staffed Beds:** 41 **Admissions:** 1171 **Census:** 19 **Outpatient Visits:** 29082
**Births:** 2 **Total Expense ($000):** 15454 **Payroll Expense ($000):** 7434
**Personnel:** 163

## HOBART—Kiowa County

★ **ELKVIEW GENERAL HOSPITAL (370153)**, 429 West Elm Street,
Zip 73651–1615; tel. 580/726–3324 **A**9 10 20 **F**3 15 28 29 31 34 35 40 45
56 59 62 79 81 85 89 93 107 108 110 111 114 117 118 128 132 145
147 **P**6
Primary Contact: Corey Lively, Chief Executive Officer
COO: Harold Moad, Chief Operating Officer
CFO: Lisa Hart, Chief Financial Officer
CMO: Samatha Jackson, M.D., Chief of Staff
CIO: Chris Clark, Chief Technology Officer
CHR: Sharon Moad, Director Personnel
**Control:** Hospital district or authority, Government, nonfederal **Service:** General
Medical and Surgical

**Staffed Beds:** 38 **Admissions:** 1339 **Census:** 14 **Outpatient Visits:** 11522
**Births:** 2 **Total Expense ($000):** 11100 **Payroll Expense ($000):** 6939
**Personnel:** 161

## HOLDENVILLE—Hughes County

★ **HOLDENVILLE GENERAL HOSPITAL (371321)**, 100 McDougal Drive,
Zip 74848–2822; tel. 405/379–4200 **A**9 10 18 **F**3 11 29 30 40 45 48 51 57
59 64 81 82 93 97 107 111 119 126 128 132 134 142 145 147 **P**6
Primary Contact: Roberta Jeffrey, Chief Executive Officer
CMO: Tom Osborn, D.O., Chief Medical Staff
CIO: Mike Combs, Manager Information Technology
CHR: Heather Heard, Director Human Resources
CNO: Shirley Orr, R.N., Chief Nursing Officer
Web address: www.holdenvillegeneral.org
**Control:** City–Government, nonfederal **Service:** General Medical and Surgical

**Staffed Beds:** 25 **Admissions:** 589 **Census:** 6 **Outpatient Visits:** 29639
**Births:** 0 **Total Expense ($000):** 9021 **Payroll Expense ($000):** 4237
**Personnel:** 114

---

**Hospital, Medicare Provider Number, Address, Telephone, Approval, Facility, and Physician Codes, Health Care System**

★ American Hospital Association (AHA) membership
☐ The Joint Commission accreditation     ◇ DNV Healthcare Inc. accreditation

○ American Osteopathic Association (AOA) accreditation
△ Commission on Accreditation of Rehabilitation Facilities (CARF) accreditation

## HOLLIS—Harmon County

★ **HARMON MEMORIAL HOSPITAL (370036)**, 400 East Chestnut Street, Zip 73550–2030, Mailing Address: P.O. Box 791, Zip 73550–0791; tel. 580/688–3363, (Nonreporting) **A**9 10 20
Primary Contact: Sheila Lewis, Administrator
CFO: Willie Mae Copeland, Chief Financial Officer
CMO: Akram Abraham, M.D., Chief of Staff
CHR: Abbey Welch, Director Human Resources
**Control:** Hospital district or authority, Government, nonfederal **Service:** General Medical and Surgical

**Staffed Beds:** 72

## HUGO—Choctaw County

**CHOCTAW MEMORIAL HOSPITAL (370100)**, 1405 East Kirk Street, Zip 74743–3603; tel. 580/317–9500, (Nonreporting) **A**9 10
Primary Contact: Marcia O'Connor, Chief Executive Officer
CIO: Andy Richmond, Director Information Technology
CHR: Darlene Galyon, Director Human Resources
Web address: www.choctawmemorial.com
**Control:** Hospital district or authority, Government, nonfederal **Service:** General Medical and Surgical

**Staffed Beds:** 34

**LANE FROST HEALTH AND REHABILITATION CENTER (372017)**, 2815 East Jackson Street, Zip 74743; tel. 580/326–9200, (Nonreporting) **A**10
Primary Contact: Robert F. Berry, Chief Executive Officer
Web address: www.lanefrosthealth.com/
**Control:** Other not–for–profit (including NFP Corporation) **Service:** Long–Term Acute Care hospital

**Staffed Beds:** 25

## IDABEL—Mccurtain County

★ **MCCURTAIN MEMORIAL HOSPITAL (370048)**, 1301 Lincoln Road, Zip 74745–7341; tel. 580/286–7623 **A**9 10 20 **F**3 11 13 15 28 29 30 40 49 53 62 64 70 75 76 81 87 93 98 103 107 110 111 113 118 127 129 132 **P**6 8
Primary Contact: Bristol Messer, Chief Executive Officer
CFO: Ray B. Whitmore, Chief Financial Officer
CMO: Michael C. West, M.D., Chief of Staff
CIO: Dana A. Stowell, Chief Information Officer
CHR: Frank Drobil, Director Human Resources
Web address: www.mmhok.com
**Control:** Other not–for–profit (including NFP Corporation) **Service:** General Medical and Surgical

**Staffed Beds:** 77 **Admissions:** 2098 **Census:** 19 **Outpatient Visits:** 38232 **Births:** 301 **Total Expense ($000):** 19107 **Payroll Expense ($000):** 9663 **Personnel:** 243

## KINGFISHER—Kingfisher County

★ **KINGFISHER REGIONAL HOSPITAL (371313)**, 1000 Kingfisher Regional Hospital Drive, Zip 73750–3528, Mailing Address: P.O. Box 59, Zip 73750–0059; tel. 405/375–3141 **A**9 10 18 **F**3 29 35 40 59 71 81 91 93 107 111 113 118 128 132 145 **S** Mercy Health, Chesterfield, MO
Primary Contact: Nancy Schmid, Chief Executive Officer
CFO: Amy Harmon, Chief Financial Officer
CMO: Brett Krablin, M.D., Chief of Staff
CIO: Rose Sherwood, Information Technology Specialist
CHR: Carolyn Bjerke, Director Human Resources
Web address: www.kingfisherhospital.com
**Control:** Other not–for–profit (including NFP Corporation) **Service:** General Medical and Surgical

**Staffed Beds:** 25 **Admissions:** 702 **Census:** 12 **Outpatient Visits:** 9181 **Births:** 70 **Total Expense ($000):** 16276 **Payroll Expense ($000):** 5141 **Personnel:** 92

## LAWTON—Comanche County

⊠ △ **COMANCHE COUNTY MEMORIAL HOSPITAL (370056)**, 3401 West Gore Boulevard, Zip 73505–0129, Mailing Address: P.O. Box 129, Zip 73502–0129; tel. 580/355–8620, (Total facility includes 135 beds in nursing home–type unit) **A**1 2 3 5 7 9 10 **F**3 7 8 11 12 13 15 17 18 20 22 24 26 28 29 30 31 32 34 35 40 43 45 47 49 50 51 54 56 57 58 59 62 64 65 66 68 70 74 75 76 77 78 79 80 81 82 84 85 86 90 91 92 93 98 103 104 107 108 110 111 113 114 115 116 117 118 119 120 122 123 126 127 128 129 130 131 133 134 142 143 145 146 147 **P**6
Primary Contact: Randall K. Segler, FACHE, Chief Executive Officer
CFO: David Blackmon, Chief Financial Officer
CMO: Richard Campbell, M.D., President Medical Staff
CIO: Ron Noreen, Director Information Services
CHR: Donna Wade, Senior Director Human Resources
Web address: www.ccmhonline.com
**Control:** Hospital district or authority, Government, nonfederal **Service:** General Medical and Surgical

**Staffed Beds:** 380 **Admissions:** 11094 **Census:** 265 **Outpatient Visits:** 154437 **Births:** 1226 **Total Expense ($000):** 205712 **Payroll Expense ($000):** 84918 **Personnel:** 1275

**JIM TALIAFERRO COMMUNITY MENTAL HEALTH (374008)**, 602 S.W. 37th Street, Zip 73505; tel. 580/248–5780, (Nonreporting) **A**9 10
Primary Contact: Randy May, Interim Executive Director
**Control:** State–Government, nonfederal **Service:** Psychiatric

**Staffed Beds:** 26

☐ **LAWTON INDIAN HOSPITAL (370170)**, 1515 Lawrie Tatum Road, Zip 73507–3099; tel. 580/353–0350, (Nonreporting) **A**1 10 **S** U. S. Indian Health Service, Rockville, MD
Primary Contact: Greg Ketcher, Administrator
CFO: Sarabeth Sahmaunt, Supervisory Accountant
CMO: Bryce Poolaw, M.D., Clinical Director
CIO: Steve Barse, Chief Information Officer
CHR: Twylla Jimboy, Supervisor Human Resources
Web address: www.ihs.gov
**Control:** PHS, Indian Service, Government, federal **Service:** General Medical and Surgical

**Staffed Beds:** 26

☐ △ **SOUTHWESTERN MEDICAL CENTER (370097)**, 5602 S.W. Lee Boulevard, Zip 73505–9635; tel. 580/531–4700 **A**1 2 3 5 7 9 10 **F**3 11 13 14 18 29 30 31 34 35 40 43 51 56 57 59 60 64 68 70 74 76 77 78 79 80 81 82 85 87 89 90 91 92 93 97 98 99 101 102 103 104 106 107 108 111 113 114 117 118 122 123 128 129 130 132 145 146 147 **P**6 8 **S** Capella Healthcare, Franklin, TN
Primary Contact: Stephen O. Hyde, FACHE, Chief Executive Officer
CFO: Lisa Clarke, Interim Chief Financial Officer
CMO: Steve Snell, M.D., Chief of Staff
CIO: Kent Lewis, Director Information Services
CHR: Helen Hooper, Director Human Resources
Web address: www.swmconline.com
**Control:** Corporation, Investor–owned, for–profit **Service:** General Medical and Surgical

**Staffed Beds:** 178 **Admissions:** 4576 **Census:** 87 **Outpatient Visits:** 42243 **Births:** 514 **Total Expense ($000):** 69335 **Payroll Expense ($000):** 26830 **Personnel:** 436

## LINDSAY—Garvin County

**LINDSAY MUNICIPAL HOSPITAL (370214)**, Highway 19 West, Zip 73052, Mailing Address: P.O. Box 888, Zip 73052–0888; tel. 405/756–1404, (Nonreporting) **A**9 10
Primary Contact: Norma N. Howard, Chief Executive Officer
**Control:** City–Government, nonfederal **Service:** General Medical and Surgical

**Staffed Beds:** 26

## MADILL—Marshall County

⊞ **INTEGRIS MARSHALL COUNTY MEDICAL CENTER (371326)**, 1 Hospital Drive, Zip 73446, Mailing Address: P.O. Box 827, Zip 73446–0827; tel. 580/795–3384 **A**1 9 10 18 **F**3 11 29 30 34 35 40 41 45 50 57 59 64 81 82 87 93 107 111 113 118 126 129 131 132 134 145 **P**6 **S** Health Management Associates, Naples, FL
Primary Contact: Matthew M. Lyden, Chief Executive Officer
CFO: Thomas Briggs, Chief Financial Officer
CMO: Joe Potter, M.D., Chief of Staff
CHR: Lori Friend, Director Human Resources
CNO: Holly Bain, Chief Nursing Officer
Web address: www.integrismarshallcounty.com
**Control:** Other not–for–profit (including NFP Corporation) **Service:** General Medical and Surgical

**Staffed Beds:** 21 **Admissions:** 676 **Census:** 6 **Outpatient Visits:** 16057 **Births:** 0 **Total Expense ($000):** 9780 **Payroll Expense ($000):** 4898 **Personnel:** 93

## MANGUM—Greer County

**QUARTZ MOUNTAIN MEDICAL CENTER (371330)**, One Wickersham Drive, Zip 73554–9116, Mailing Address: P.O. Box 280, Zip 73554–0280; tel. 580/782–3353 **A**9 10 18 **F**29 40 41 45 54 57 68 81 107 111 118 126 127 128 132 147 **P**6
Primary Contact: Lindsay Crabb, Chief Executive Officer
COO: Danny Avery, Chief Financial Officer and Chief Operating Officer
CIO: Gregg Burnam, Chief Information Officer and Manager Business Office
Web address: www.mangumhealth.com
**Control:** Individual, Investor–owned, for–profit **Service:** General Medical and Surgical

**Staffed Beds:** 25 **Admissions:** 271 **Census:** 4 **Outpatient Visits:** 13508 **Births:** 0 **Total Expense ($000):** 6739 **Payroll Expense ($000):** 3406 **Personnel:** 59

*Many Facility Codes have changed. Please refer to the AHA Guide Code Chart.*

## MARIETTA—Love County

★ **MERCY HEALTH LOVE COUNTY (371306)**, 300 Wanda Street, Zip 73448–1200; tel. 580/276–3347 **A**9 10 18 **F**3 29 34 40 50 57 59 84 107 118 126 127 132 134 142 145 147 **S** Mercy Health, Chesterfield, MO
Primary Contact: Richard Barker, Administrator
CMO: J. T. O'Connor, M.D., Medical Director
CIO: Connie Graham, Public Information Officer
Web address: www.mercyhealthlovecounty.com
**Control:** Church–operated, Nongovernment, not–for profit **Service:** General Medical and Surgical

| | |
|---|---|
| **Staffed Beds:** 25 **Admissions:** 435 **Census:** 8 **Outpatient Visits:** 24613 **Births:** 0 **Total Expense ($000):** 11707 **Payroll Expense ($000):** 6863 **Personnel:** 130 | |

## MCALESTER—Pittsburg County

**CARL ALBERT COMMUNITY MENTAL HEALTH CENTER (374006)**, 1101 East Monroe Avenue, Zip 74501–4826; tel. 918/426–7800, (Nonreporting) **A**10
Primary Contact: Debbie Moran, Executive Director
CFO: Konnie Taylor, Chief Financial Officer
CMO: William Mings, M.D., Medical Director
CHR: Judy Allen, Human Resource Specialist
Web address: www.odmhsas.org
**Control:** State–Government, nonfederal **Service:** Psychiatric

| | |
|---|---|
| **Staffed Beds:** 15 | |

★ △ **MCALESTER REGIONAL HEALTH CENTER (370034)**, One Clark Bass Boulevard, Zip 74501–4267, Mailing Address: P.O. Box 1228, Zip 74502–1228; tel. 918/426–1800 **A**7 9 10 21 **F**2 3 10 11 13 15 18 20 29 30 34 35 40 43 45 49 51 53 54 56 57 59 61 62 64 68 69 70 75 76 77 79 81 82 85 86 90 92 103 104 105 107 109 110 111 112 113 114 116 117 118 124 126 127 128 129 131 134 143 145 146 147
Primary Contact: David N. Keith, FACHE, President and Chief Executive Officer
CFO: Melissa Walker, Senior Vice President and Chief Financial Officer
CIO: Frank Hilbert, Senior Vice President and Chief Information Officer
CHR: Steven Brooks, Vice President Human Resources
CNO: Danny Hardman, Senior Vice President and Chief Nursing Officer
Web address: www.mrhcok.com
**Control:** City–Government, nonfederal **Service:** General Medical and Surgical

| | |
|---|---|
| **Staffed Beds:** 143 **Admissions:** 4930 **Census:** 62 **Outpatient Visits:** 82368 **Births:** 591 **Total Expense ($000):** 67394 **Payroll Expense ($000):** 31750 **Personnel:** 691 | |

## MIAMI—Ottawa County

⊞ **INTEGRIS BAPTIST REGIONAL HEALTH CENTER (370004)**, 200 Second Street S.W., Zip 74354–6830, Mailing Address: P.O. Box 1207, Zip 74355–1207; tel. 918/542–6611 **A**1 9 10 20 **F**3 5 7 11 13 15 26 29 30 31 34 35 40 43 50 51 56 57 59 62 63 64 66 70 75 76 77 79 81 85 86 89 90 93 98 100 101 102 103 104 105 107 108 111 114 118 124 128 129 130 131 132 143 145 146 147 **P**5 7 **S** INTEGRIS Health, Oklahoma City, OK
Primary Contact: Joel A. Hart, FACHE, President
COO: Randy Jobe, Chief Operating Officer
CFO: Amy Marsh, Chief Financial Officer
CMO: Matt Osborn, M.D., Chief of Staff
CHR: Jamil Haynes, Regional Director Human Resources
Web address: www.integris–health.com
**Control:** Other not–for–profit (including NFP Corporation) **Service:** General Medical and Surgical

| | |
|---|---|
| **Staffed Beds:** 84 **Admissions:** 3354 **Census:** 33 **Outpatient Visits:** 73128 **Births:** 359 **Total Expense ($000):** 48401 **Payroll Expense ($000):** 22988 **Personnel:** 371 | |

★ **WILLOW CREST HOSPITAL (374017)**, 130 A Street S.W., Zip 74354–6800; tel. 918/542–1836 **A**9 10 **F**29 75 98 99 101 102 106 129 132 **P**6
Primary Contact: Anne G. Anthony, FACHE, President and Chief Executive Officer
COO: Steven Goodman, Chief Operating Officer
CFO: Cindy Bell, Director Finance
CMO: Mark Elkington, M.D., Chief Medical Officer
CIO: Steven Goodman, Chief Operating Officer
CHR: Kathy Henderson, Director Human Resources, Media and Public Relations
Web address: www.willowcresthospital.com
**Control:** Corporation, Investor–owned, for–profit **Service:** Children's hospital psychiatric

| | |
|---|---|
| **Staffed Beds:** 75 **Admissions:** 560 **Census:** 50 **Outpatient Visits:** 0 **Births:** 0 **Total Expense ($000):** 6633 **Payroll Expense ($000):** 4248 **Personnel:** 120 | |

## MIDWEST CITY—Oklahoma County

☐ **MIDWEST REGIONAL MEDICAL CENTER (370094)**, 2825 Parklawn Drive, Zip 73110–4258; tel. 405/610–4411 **A**1 3 5 9 10 **F**3 7 8 11 13 14 15 17 18 20 22 24 28 29 30 31 34 40 43 46 49 50 57 59 70 74 76 77 78 79 81 85 86 87 91 92 93 98 100 101 102 107 108 110 111 113 114 117 118 125 129 131 142 145 146 **P**6 **S** Health Management Associates, Naples, FL
Primary Contact: Stan V. Holm, FACHE, Chief Executive Officer
CFO: Shea Sutherland, Chief Financial Officer
CMO: Dan Donnell, M.D., Chief of Staff
CHR: Angela C. Giese, Director Human Resources
Web address: www.midwestregional.com
**Control:** Corporation, Investor–owned, for–profit **Service:** General Medical and Surgical

| | |
|---|---|
| **Staffed Beds:** 255 **Admissions:** 13224 **Census:** 151 **Outpatient Visits:** 122194 **Births:** 696 **Total Expense ($000):** 140399 **Payroll Expense ($000):** 52473 **Personnel:** 931 | |

☐ **SPECIALTY HOSPITAL OF MIDWEST CITY (372012)**, 8210 National Avenue, Zip 73110; tel. 405/739–0800 **A**1 9 10 **F**1 18 29 65 75 77 79 85 86 87 147 **P**5 **S** Encore Healthcare, Columbia, MD
Primary Contact: Chad Lovett, Chief Executive Officer
CFO: Lisa Griffis, Chief Financial Officer and Business Office Manager
Web address: www.specialtyhospitalmidwestcity.com/specialty_midwest/index.aspx
**Control:** Corporation, Investor–owned, for–profit **Service:** Long–Term Acute Care hospital

| | |
|---|---|
| **Staffed Beds:** 31 **Admissions:** 297 **Census:** 19 **Outpatient Visits:** 0 **Births:** 0 **Total Expense ($000):** 10168 **Payroll Expense ($000):** 3203 **Personnel:** 81 | |

## MOORE—Cleveland County

**MOORE MEDICAL CENTER** See Norman Regional Health System, Norman

## MUSKOGEE—Muskogee County

⊠ **JACK C. MONTGOMERY VETERANS AFFAIRS MEDICAL CENTER**, 1011 Honor Heights Drive, Zip 74401–1318; tel. 918/683–3261 **A**1 2 5 **F**3 5 8 18 29 30 31 34 35 36 38 39 40 44 48 50 53 54 56 57 58 59 60 61 63 64 65 70 74 75 77 78 79 81 82 83 84 85 86 87 90 92 93 94 96 97 98 100 101 102 103 104 107 108 118 126 129 131 132 134 142 145 146 147 **S** Department of Veterans Affairs, Washington, DC
Primary Contact: Bryan C. Matthews, Acting Director
CFO: Robert Wood, Chief Fiscal Services
CMO: Karen Gribbin, M.D., Chief of Staff
CIO: Gary Duvall, Chief Information Resource Management
CHR: Kay DeCamp, Chief Human Resources Officer
Web address: www.muskogee.va.gov
**Control:** Veterans Affairs, Government, federal **Service:** General Medical and Surgical

| | |
|---|---|
| **Staffed Beds:** 111 **Admissions:** 5084 **Census:** 78 **Outpatient Visits:** 392946 **Births:** 0 **Total Expense ($000):** 240363 **Payroll Expense ($000):** 109419 **Personnel:** 1338 | |

☐ **MUSKOGEE COMMUNITY HOSPITAL (370232)**, 2900 North Main Street, Zip 74401–4078; tel. 918/687–7777 **A**1 9 10 **F**3 11 12 15 29 30 31 32 34 35 40 45 46 47 48 49 57 59 64 65 68 74 75 77 78 79 81 82 85 86 87 107 108 110 111 113 114 118 119 120 123 128 129 131 143 145 146 147 **P**5 **S** Capella Healthcare, Franklin, TN
Primary Contact: Mark Roberts, President
Web address: www.mch–ok.com
**Control:** Partnership, Investor–owned, for–profit **Service:** General Medical and Surgical

| | |
|---|---|
| **Staffed Beds:** 45 **Admissions:** 1531 **Census:** 16 **Outpatient Visits:** 21893 **Births:** 93 **Personnel:** 261 | |

☐ **MUSKOGEE REGIONAL MEDICAL CENTER (370025)**, 300 Rockefeller Drive, Zip 74401–5081; tel. 918/682–5501 **A**1 2 9 10 **F**3 8 11 13 15 18 20 22 29 30 31 35 40 43 45 46 47 48 49 51 57 59 60 62 64 68 70 74 75 76 77 78 79 81 85 86 87 89 90 96 98 100 102 105 107 108 111 113 114 118 119 120 122 128 129 130 132 143 145 146 147 **S** Capella Healthcare, Franklin, TN
Primary Contact: Kevin N. Fowler, Chief Executive Officer
COO: Holly Clark, Chief Operating Officer
CFO: Patty Doles, Chief Financial Officer
CHR: Linda Mathis, Director Human Resources
Web address: www.muskogeehealth.com
**Control:** Corporation, Investor–owned, for–profit **Service:** General Medical and Surgical

| | |
|---|---|
| **Staffed Beds:** 194 **Admissions:** 8172 **Census:** 104 **Births:** 680 **Total Expense ($000):** 90400 **Payroll Expense ($000):** 33288 **Personnel:** 678 | |

---

**Hospital, Medicare Provider Number, Address, Telephone, Approval, Facility, and Physician Codes, Health Care System**

★ American Hospital Association (AHA) membership
☐ The Joint Commission accreditation
◇ DNV Healthcare Inc. accreditation
○ American Osteopathic Association (AOA) accreditation
△ Commission on Accreditation of Rehabilitation Facilities (CARF) accreditation

OK

**SOLARA HOSPITAL OF MUSKOGEE (372022)**, 351 South 40th Street, Zip 74401–4916; tel. 918/682–6161 **A**9 10 **F**1 3 29 40 77 85 96 129 147 **S** Solara Healthcare, Dallas, TX
Primary Contact: Craig Koele, Chief Executive Officer
CMO: David Kyger, M.D., Chief Medical Officer
Web address: www.solarahc.com
**Control:** Corporation, Investor–owned, for–profit **Service:** Long–Term Acute Care hospital

**Staffed Beds:** 41 **Admissions:** 512 **Census:** 40 **Outpatient Visits:** 5 **Births:** 0 **Total Expense ($000):** 12316 **Payroll Expense ($000):** 5475 **Personnel:** 110

### NORMAN—Cleveland County

**CENTRAL OKLAHOMA COMMUNITY MENTAL HEALTH CENTER**, 909 East Alameda Street, Zip 73071–5229, Mailing Address: P.O. Box 400, Zip 73070–0400; tel. 405/360–5100, (Nonreporting) **A**9
Primary Contact: Lawrence Gross, Executive Director
Web address: www.cocmhc.org
**Control:** State–Government, nonfederal **Service:** Psychiatric

**Staffed Beds:** 28

☐ **GRIFFIN MEMORIAL HOSPITAL (374000)**, 900 East Main Street, Zip 73071–5305, Mailing Address: P.O. Box 151, Zip 73070–0151; tel. 405/321–4880 **A**1 10 **F**40 98 102 103 129 **P**6 **S** Oklahoma Department of Mental Health and Substance Abuse Services, Oklahoma City, OK
Primary Contact: Randy May, Executive Director
CFO: Bob Mathew, Director Finance
CMO: Stan Ardoin, M.D., Medical Director
Web address: www.odmhsas.org
**Control:** State–Government, nonfederal **Service:** Psychiatric

**Staffed Beds:** 120 **Admissions:** 1874 **Census:** 106 **Outpatient Visits:** 228 **Births:** 0 **Total Expense ($000):** 26593 **Payroll Expense ($000):** 14136 **Personnel:** 353

**J. D. MCCARTY CENTER FOR CHILDREN WITH DEVELOPMENTAL DISABILITIES (373300)**, 2002 East Robinson, Zip 73071–5264; tel. 405/307–2800 **A**10 **F**3 35 64 65 75 77 87 90 91 93 129 134 145
Primary Contact: Vicki Kuerstersteffen, Chief Executive Officer
CFO: Ken Younkin, Comptroller
CMO: Thomas Thurston, M.D., Medical Director
CIO: Joel Mann, Administrator Information Systems
CHR: Debbie Barrett, Director Human Resources
Web address: www.jdmc.org
**Control:** State–Government, nonfederal **Service:** Children's rehabilitation

**Staffed Beds:** 36 **Admissions:** 208 **Census:** 32 **Outpatient Visits:** 6661 **Births:** 0 **Total Expense ($000):** 16980 **Payroll Expense ($000):** 8069 **Personnel:** 225

✠ △ **NORMAN REGIONAL HEALTH SYSTEM (370008)**, 901 North Porter Street, Zip 73071–6482, Mailing Address: P.O. Box 1308, Zip 73070–1308; tel. 405/307–1000, (Includes MOORE MEDICAL CENTER, 700 South Telephone Road, Moore, Zip 73160; tel. 405/793–9355; Ryan Gehris, Chief Administrative Officer; NORMAN REGIONAL HOSPITAL, 901 North Porter Street, Mailing Address: P.O. Box 1308, Zip 73070–1308; tel. 405/307–1000) **A**1 2 7 9 10 **F**3 7 11 12 13 15 17 18 20 22 24 28 29 30 31 32 34 35 36 37 39 40 42 43 44 45 47 48 49 50 53 54 55 56 57 58 59 62 63 64 65 69 70 72 74 75 76 77 78 79 80 81 82 83 84 85 86 87 89 90 93 94 96 97 98 100 101 102 103 107 110 111 113 114 116 117 118 119 122 125 126 128 129 130 131 134 142 144 145 146 147 **P**5 6 8
Primary Contact: David D. Whitaker, FACHE, President and Chief Executive Officer
COO: Greg Terrell, Senior Vice President and Chief Operating Officer
CFO: Ken Hopkins, Vice President Finance and Chief Financial Officer
CMO: William McMillan, M.D., Vice President Medical Affairs
CIO: John Meharg, Director Health Information Technology
CHR: Jim Beyer, Director Human Resources
Web address: www.normanregional.com
**Control:** Hospital district or authority, Government, nonfederal **Service:** General Medical and Surgical

**Staffed Beds:** 388 **Admissions:** 17185 **Census:** 209 **Outpatient Visits:** 384166 **Births:** 2990 **Total Expense ($000):** 286848 **Payroll Expense ($000):** 126452 **Personnel:** 2314

✠ **NORMAN SPECIALTY HOSPITAL (372021)**, 1210 West Robinson Street, Zip 73069–7401; tel. 405/321–8824 **A**1 9 10 **F**1 90 129 147 **P**8
Primary Contact: Talitha Glosemeyer, M.P.H., Administrator
CFO: Stephanie Wortham, Director Financial Services
CMO: Mehan Shahsavari, M.D., Chief of Staff
CHR: Sandy Carroll, Coordinator Human Resources
Web address: www.normanspecialtyhospital.com
**Control:** Individual, Investor–owned, for–profit **Service:** Long–Term Acute Care hospital

**Staffed Beds:** 50 **Admissions:** 544 **Census:** 39 **Outpatient Visits:** 2 **Births:** 0 **Personnel:** 162

### NOWATA—Nowata County

**JANE PHILLIPS NOWATA HEALTH CENTER (371305)**, 237 South Locust Street, Zip 74048–0426, Mailing Address: P.O. Box 426, Zip 74048–0426; tel. 918/273–3102 **A**9 10 18 **F**3 40 43 118 127 132 **P**5
Primary Contact: Scott Upton, Administrator
CMO: David Caughell, M.D., Chief of Staff
Web address: www.jpmc.org
**Control:** Church–operated, Nongovernment, not–for profit **Service:** General Medical and Surgical

**Staffed Beds:** 13 **Admissions:** 184 **Census:** 5 **Outpatient Visits:** 3010 **Births:** 0 **Total Expense ($000):** 2615 **Payroll Expense ($000):** 1654 **Personnel:** 35

### OKEENE—Blaine County

★ **OKEENE MUNICIPAL HOSPITAL (371327)**, 207 East F Street, Zip 73763, Mailing Address: P.O. Box 489, Zip 73763–0489; tel. 580/822–4417 **A**9 10 18 **F**3 29 34 40 45 50 59 64 68 81 85 93 97 107 111 118 129 131 132 145 **P**6
Primary Contact: Shelly Dunham, R.N., Chief Executive Officer
COO: Pat Lorenz, Chief Operating Officer
CFO: Sandra Lamle, Chief Financial Officer
CHR: Barbara Creps, Director Human Resources and Accounting
CNO: Tamara Fischer, Chief Nursing Officer
Web address: www.okeenehospital.com
**Control:** Hospital district or authority, Government, nonfederal **Service:** General Medical and Surgical

**Staffed Beds:** 17 **Admissions:** 393 **Census:** 7 **Outpatient Visits:** 22922 **Births:** 0 **Total Expense ($000):** 6064 **Payroll Expense ($000):** 2616 **Personnel:** 60

### OKEMAH—Okfuskee County

★ **CREEK NATION COMMUNITY HOSPITAL (371333)**, 309 North 14th Street, Zip 74859–2028; tel. 918/623–1424, (Nonreporting) **A**9 10 18
Primary Contact: Cynthia Tainpeah, Administrator
COO: Seneca Smith, Chief Operating Officer
CFO: Tyler McIntosh, Chief Financial Officer
CMO: Lawrence Vark, M.D., Chief Medical Officer
CHR: Mickey Romine, Manager
**Control:** Other not–for–profit (including NFP Corporation) **Service:** General Medical and Surgical

**Staffed Beds:** 18

### OKLAHOMA CITY—Oklahoma County

☐ **CEDAR RIDGE HOSPITAL (374023)**, 6501 N.E. 50th Street, Zip 73141; tel. 405/605–6111 **A**1 9 10 **F**34 57 59 71 75 98 99 100 101 102 103 104 106 **S** Universal Health Services, Inc., King of Prussia, PA
Primary Contact: Kevan Finley, Chief Executive Officer
Web address: www.cedarridgebhs.com
**Control:** Corporation, Investor–owned, for–profit **Service:** Psychiatric

**Staffed Beds:** 116 **Admissions:** 2191 **Census:** 79 **Outpatient Visits:** 0 **Births:** 0

**CHILDREN'S HOSPITAL OF OKLAHOMA** See OU Medical Center

☐ **COMMUNITY HOSPITAL (370203)**, 3100 S.W. 89th Street, Zip 73159–7900; tel. 405/378–3755, (Nonreporting) **A**1 9 10 21
Primary Contact: Brian L. Clemens, President and Chief Executive Officer
Web address: www.communityhospitalokc.com
**Control:** Corporation, Investor–owned, for–profit **Service:** General Medical and Surgical

**Staffed Beds:** 40

✠ △ **DEACONESS HOSPITAL (370032)**, 5501 North Portland Avenue, Zip 73112–2099; tel. 405/604–6000 **A**1 2 7 9 10 **F**3 8 11 12 13 15 17 18 20 22 24 28 29 30 31 34 35 40 41 43 45 46 47 49 50 52 56 57 59 60 70 72 73 74 75 76 78 79 80 81 83 84 85 86 87 89 90 93 97 98 101 102 103 107 108 109 110 111 113 118 119 125 127 128 129 131 134 145 146 147 **P**8 **S** Community Health Systems, Inc., Franklin, TN
Primary Contact: Cathryn A. Hibbs, FACHE, Chief Executive Officer
CIO: Don Bandy, Director Information Technology
CHR: Ellen Gifford, Director Human Resources
Web address: www.deaconessokc.com
**Control:** Partnership, Investor–owned, for–profit **Service:** General Medical and Surgical

**Staffed Beds:** 273 **Admissions:** 9950 **Census:** 144 **Outpatient Visits:** 71721 **Births:** 1132 **Total Expense ($000):** 119982 **Payroll Expense ($000):** 48474 **Personnel:** 1059

**EVERETT TOWER** See OU Medical Center

⊠ △ **INTEGRIS BAPTIST MEDICAL CENTER (370028)**, 3300 N.W.
Expressway, Zip 73112–4418; tel. 405/949–3011, (Includes INTEGRIS MENTAL
HEALTH SYSTEM–SPENCER, 2601 North Spencer Road, Spencer,
Zip 73084–3699, Mailing Address: P.O. Box 11137, Oklahoma City,
Zip 73136–0137; tel. 405/717–9800) **A**1 2 3 5 7 9 10 **F**3 8 11 12 13 15 16
17 18 20 22 24 26 28 29 30 31 32 34 35 36 38 39 40 43 44 45 46 49 50
52 54 55 56 57 58 59 60 62 63 64 68 70 71 72 74 75 76 77 78 79 80 81
82 83 84 85 86 87 88 89 92 93 96 97 98 99 100 101 102 104 106 107 108
110 111 113 114 115 117 118 119 120 122 123 128 129 130 131 132 133
134 136 137 138 139 140 141 142 145 146 147 **P**5 7 **S** INTEGRIS Health,
Oklahoma City, OK
Primary Contact: Chris Hammes, FACHE, President
CFO: Wentz J. Miller, Jr., Managing Director and Chief Financial Officer
CMO: James P. White, M.D., Chief Medical Officer
CIO: John Delano, Vice President Chief Information Officer
CHR: Robert Quiring, Vice President Human Resources
Web address: www.integrisok.com
**Control:** Other not–for–profit (including NFP Corporation) **Service:** General
Medical and Surgical

**Staffed Beds:** 569 **Admissions:** 23231 **Census:** 404 **Outpatient Visits:**
174682 **Births:** 2394 **Total Expense ($000):** 534168 **Payroll Expense
($000):** 187949 **Personnel:** 3395

⊠ △ **INTEGRIS SOUTHWEST MEDICAL CENTER (370106)**, 4401 South
Western, Zip 73109–3441; tel. 405/636–7000 **A**1 2 7 9 10 13 **F**3 11 13 15 18
20 22 24 28 29 30 31 32 34 35 38 39 40 43 46 47 49 50 57 58 59 60 62
64 68 69 70 74 75 76 77 78 79 80 81 82 85 86 87 90 93 96 100 102 107
108 110 111 113 118 119 120 122 123 128 129 130 131 132 133 134 142
143 145 146 147 **S** INTEGRIS Health, Oklahoma City, OK
Primary Contact: James D. Moore, FACHE, Chief Executive Officer
CFO: Errol Mitchell, Vice President
CIO: John Delano, Vice President and Chief Information Officer
CHR: Lynn Ketch, Director
Web address: www.integris–health.com
**Control:** Other not–for–profit (including NFP Corporation) **Service:** General
Medical and Surgical

**Staffed Beds:** 305 **Admissions:** 12625 **Census:** 191 **Outpatient Visits:**
166468 **Births:** 1073 **Total Expense ($000):** 215217 **Payroll Expense
($000):** 82894 **Personnel:** 1161

⊠ **KINDRED HOSPITAL– OKLAHOMA CITY (372004)**, 1407 North Robinson
Avenue, Zip 73103–4823; tel. 405/232–8000, (Includes KINDRED
HOSPITAL–OKLAHOMA CITY SOUTH, 2129 S.W. 59th Street, Zip 73119;
tel. 405/713–5955) **A**1 3 5 9 10 **F**29 40 46 60 68 70 85 87 118 129 144
147 **S** Kindred Healthcare, Louisville, KY
Primary Contact: Gayla Campbell, Chief Executive Officer
Web address: www.kindredoklahoma.com
**Control:** Corporation, Investor–owned, for–profit **Service:** General Medical and
Surgical

**Staffed Beds:** 93 **Admissions:** 799 **Census:** 43 **Outpatient Visits:** 0 **Births:**
0 **Total Expense ($000):** 26211 **Payroll Expense ($000):** 10640
**Personnel:** 198

⊠ **LAKESIDE WOMEN'S HOSPITAL (370199)**, 11200 North Portland Avenue,
Zip 73120–5045; tel. 405/936–1500 **A**1 9 10 **F**3 12 13 15 30 35 40 45 59
64 76 81 85 87 110 118 125 128 131 146 **P**6
Primary Contact: Kelley Brewer, R.N., MSN, Chief Executive Officer
CFO: Darla McCallister, Chief Financial Officer
CMO: Lisa Wasemiller–Smith, M.D., Chief Medical Officer
CHR: Renee Beene, Manager Human Resources
Web address: www.lakeside-wh.net
**Control:** Corporation, Investor–owned, for–profit **Service:** Obstetrics and
gynecology

**Staffed Beds:** 23 **Admissions:** 1567 **Census:** 9 **Outpatient Visits:** 2803
**Births:** 1386 **Total Expense ($000):** 19779 **Payroll Expense ($000):** 7258
**Personnel:** 137

**MCBRIDE CLINIC ORTHOPEDIC HOSPITAL (370222)**, 9600 Broadway
Extension, Zip 73114–7408; tel. 405/486–2100 **A**10 **F**3 29 40 64 68 77 79 81
82 85 86 87 90 91 107 111 113 128 129 130
Primary Contact: Mark Galliart, Chief Executive Officer
COO: Christine H. Weigel, R.N., Clinical Operating Officer
CFO: Annie Bassett, Director Finance
CMO: Thomas Janssen, M.D., Chief of Staff
CIO: Ronnie Green, Director Information Systems
CHR: Cathy Witham, Director Human Resources
Web address: www.mcbrideclinicorthopedichospital.com
**Control:** Corporation, Investor–owned, for–profit **Service:** Orthopedic

**Staffed Beds:** 78 **Admissions:** 3129 **Census:** 28 **Outpatient Visits:** 145321
**Births:** 0 **Total Expense ($000):** 80424 **Payroll Expense ($000):** 29172
**Personnel:** 644

⊠ △ **MERCY HOSPITAL OKLAHOMA CITY (370013)**, 4300 West Memorial
Road, Zip 73120–8362; tel. 405/755–1515 **A**1 2 7 9 10 **F**3 11 13 15 28 29
30 31 32 34 35 39 40 41 43 45 49 50 53 55 57 58 59 60 61 62 63 64 65
68 70 72 74 75 76 77 78 79 81 82 83 84 85 86 87 89 90 91 92 93 94 96
100 101 107 108 110 111 114 116 117 118 119 120 123 125 128 129 130
131 133 134 142 145 146 147 **P**6 **S** Mercy Health, Chesterfield, MO
Primary Contact: Jim Gebhart, Jr., FACHE, President
COO: Aaron Steffens, Chief Operating Officer
CFO: Jon Vitiello, Chief Financial Officer
CMO: Mark Johnson, M.D., Chief Medical Officer
CIO: Ellen Stephens, Vice President Information Services
CHR: Becky J. Payton, Vice President Human Resources
CNO: Linda T. Fanning, R.N., Chief Nursing Officer
Web address: www.mercyok.net
**Control:** Church–operated, Nongovernment, not–for profit **Service:** General
Medical and Surgical

**Staffed Beds:** 369 **Admissions:** 17406 **Census:** 259 **Outpatient Visits:**
258296 **Births:** 3026 **Total Expense ($000):** 290924 **Payroll Expense
($000):** 108595 **Personnel:** 1993

☐ **NORTHWEST SURGICAL HOSPITAL (370192)**, 9204 North May Avenue,
Zip 73120–4419; tel. 405/848–1918, (Nonreporting) **A**1 9 10 21
Primary Contact: Brian L. Clemens, Chief Executive Officer
CFO: Cindy Thompson, Chief Financial Officer
CMO: Jimmy Conway, M.D., President Medical Staff
Web address: www.nwsurgicalokc.com/
**Control:** Corporation, Investor–owned, for–profit **Service:** Orthopedic

**Staffed Beds:** 9

☐ **OKLAHOMA CENTER FOR ORTHOPEDIC AND MULTI–SPECIALTY SURGERY
(370212)**, 8100 South Walker, Suite C., Zip 73139, Mailing Address: P.O. Box
890609, Zip 73189; tel. 405/602–6500, (Nonreporting) **A**1 9 10 **S** United
Surgical Partners International, Addison, TX
Primary Contact: Teri Philbrick, Chief Executive Officer
CFO: Donna Avant, Chief Financial Officer
CHR: Sherry Wagner, Director Human Resources
Web address: www.okla-sc.com/
**Control:** Corporation, Investor–owned, for–profit **Service:** Orthopedic

**Staffed Beds:** 10

☐ **OKLAHOMA HEART HOSPITAL (370215)**, 4050 West Memorial Road,
Zip 73120; tel. 405/608–3200 **A**1 9 10 21 **F**17 18 20 22 24 26 28 29 30 34
35 40 64 68 74 75 81 86 87 100 102 107 108 115 116 145 **P**2
Primary Contact: John Harvey, M.D., President and Chief Executive Officer
COO: Peggy Tipton, Chief Operating Officer and Chief Nursing Officer
CFO: Carol Walker, Chief Financial Officer
CMO: John Harvey, M.D., President and Chief Executive Officer
CIO: Steve Miller, Chief Information Officer
CHR: Katherine Wynn, Director Human Resource
Web address: www.okheart.com
**Control:** Corporation, Investor–owned, for–profit **Service:** Heart

**Staffed Beds:** 99 **Admissions:** 8990 **Census:** 87 **Outpatient Visits:** 19598
**Births:** 0 **Total Expense ($000):** 153715 **Payroll Expense ($000):** 52335
**Personnel:** 1416

☐ **OKLAHOMA HEART HOSPITAL SOUTH CAMPUS (370234)**, 5200 East I–240
Service Road, Zip 73135; tel. 405/628–6000 **A**1 10 21 **F**17 18 20 22 24 26
28 29 30 34 35 40 64 68 74 75 81 82 100 107 115 116 145 **P**6
Primary Contact: John Harvey, M.D., President and Chief Executive Officer
Web address: www.okheart.com
**Control:** Corporation, Investor–owned, for–profit **Service:** Heart

**Staffed Beds:** 46 **Admissions:** 4986 **Census:** 39 **Outpatient Visits:** 13571
**Births:** 0 **Total Expense ($000):** 67853 **Payroll Expense ($000):** 26148
**Personnel:** 353

☐ **OKLAHOMA SPINE HOSPITAL (370206)**, 14101 Parkway Commons Drive,
Zip 73134; tel. 405/749–2700, (Nonreporting) **A**1 10 21
Primary Contact: Kevin Blaylock, Chief Executive Officer
Web address: www.oklahomaspine.com
**Control:** Corporation, Investor–owned, for–profit **Service:** Other specialty

**Staffed Beds:** 12

**Hospital, Medicare Provider Number, Address, Telephone, Approval, Facility, and Physician Codes, Health Care System**

★ American Hospital Association (AHA) membership
☐ The Joint Commission accreditation          ◇ DNV Healthcare Inc. accreditation

○ American Osteopathic Association (AOA) accreditation
△ Commission on Accreditation of Rehabilitation Facilities (CARF) accreditation

**OK**

⊠ **ORTHOPEDIC HOSPITAL (370220)**, 1044 S.W. 44th Street, Suite 620, Zip 73109–3609; tel. 405/631–3085 **A**10 **F**3 40 79 81 82 87 **P**8
Primary Contact: Denny Oreb, Interim Chief Executive Officer
CFO: Patti Bode, Chief Financial Officer
CMO: Joel L. Frazier, M.D., Medical Director
CIO: Reza Tavasoli, Information Officer
Web address: www.ortho–ok.com
**Control:** Corporation, Investor–owned, for–profit **Service:** Orthopedic

**Staffed Beds:** 8 **Admissions:** 162 **Census:** 1 **Outpatient Visits:** 895 **Births:** 0 **Total Expense ($000):** 5719 **Payroll Expense ($000):** 1885 **Personnel:** 28

⊠ **OU MEDICAL CENTER (370093)**, 1200 Everett Drive, Zip 73104–5047, Mailing Address: P.O. Box 26307, Zip 73126–0307; tel. 405/271–3636, (Includes CHILDREN'S HOSPITAL OF OKLAHOMA, 940 N.E. 13th Street, Zip 73104, Mailing Address: P.O. Box 26307, Zip 73126; tel. 405/271–6165; EVERETT TOWER, 1200 Everett Drive, Zip 73104; tel. 405/271–4700; OU MEDICAL CENTER EDMOND, 1 South Bryant Avenue, Edmond, Zip 73034–6309; tel. 405/341–6100; Jordan Herget, Chief Executive Officer; PRESBYTERIAN TOWER, 700 N.E. 13th Street, Zip 73104–5070; tel. 405/271–5100) **A**1 2 3 5 8 9 10 **F**3 8 11 12 13 15 17 19 20 21 22 23 24 25 26 27 28 29 30 31 32 34 35 37 38 39 40 41 43 45 46 47 48 49 50 51 52 55 56 57 58 59 60 61 63 64 65 66 68 70 72 74 75 76 77 78 79 81 82 83 84 85 86 87 88 89 91 92 93 94 96 97 98 100 102 103 105 107 108 110 111 113 114 115 116 117 118 119 120 122 123 125 128 129 130 131 134 135 137 138 141 143 144 145 146 147 **S** HCA, Nashville, TN
Primary Contact: Cole C. Eslyn, FACHE, President and Chief Executive Officer
COO: Rebecca Benoit, Chief Operating Officer
CFO: Jim Watson, Chief Financial Officer
CMO: Curt Steinhart, M.D., Chief Medical Officer
CIO: Larry Forsyth, Director Information Services
CHR: Laura Land, Chief Human Resources Officer
Web address: www.oumedcenter.com
**Control:** Corporation, Investor–owned, for–profit **Service:** General Medical and Surgical

**Staffed Beds:** 750 **Admissions:** 28602 **Census:** 484 **Outpatient Visits:** 306552 **Births:** 4085 **Total Expense ($000):** 652062 **Payroll Expense ($000):** 187768 **Personnel:** 3569

**PRESBYTERIAN TOWER** See OU Medical Center

⊠ **SELECT SPECIALTY HOSPITAL–OKLAHOMA CITY (372009)**, 3524 N.W. 56th Street, Zip 73112–4510; tel. 405/606–6700 **A**1 9 10 **F**1 3 12 29 40 74 75 79 85 87 107 118 129 147 **S** Select Medical Corporation, Mechanicsburg, PA
Primary Contact: Connie Strickland, Chief Executive Officer
Web address: www.selectmedicalcorp.com
**Control:** Corporation, Investor–owned, for–profit **Service:** Long–Term Acute Care hospital

**Staffed Beds:** 72 **Admissions:** 741 **Census:** 54 **Outpatient Visits:** 0 **Total Expense ($000):** 23839 **Payroll Expense ($000):** 9144 **Personnel:** 198

⊠ △ **ST. ANTHONY HOSPITAL (370037)**, 1000 North Lee Street, Zip 73102–1080, Mailing Address: P.O. Box 205, Zip 73101–0205; tel. 405/272–7000, (Includes BONE AND JOINT HOSPITAL, 1111 North Dewey Avenue, Zip 73103–2609; tel. 405/272–9671; Chad S. Aduddell, President) **A**1 2 3 5 7 9 10 12 13 **F**3 4 8 12 13 15 17 18 20 22 24 26 28 29 30 31 34 35 40 43 44 45 47 49 50 51 56 57 58 59 64 65 67 68 70 74 75 76 77 78 79 81 82 84 85 86 87 90 93 96 97 98 99 100 101 102 103 104 105 107 108 110 111 113 114 118 119 120 122 123 125 128 129 130 131 134 137 145 **S** SSM Health Care, Saint Louis, MO
Primary Contact: Joe Hodges, President
COO: Marti Jourden, FACHE, Chief Quality Officer
CFO: Shasta Manuel, Executive Director Finance
CMO: Kersey Winfree, M.D., Chief Medical Officer
CIO: Kevin Olson, Director Information Systems
CHR: Cynthia Brundise, Vice President Human Resources
Web address: www.saintsok.com
**Control:** Church–operated, Nongovernment, not–for profit **Service:** General Medical and Surgical

**Staffed Beds:** 499 **Admissions:** 17049 **Census:** 308 **Outpatient Visits:** 173230 **Births:** 1420 **Total Expense ($000):** 311826 **Payroll Expense ($000):** 117897 **Personnel:** 1904

☐ **SURGICAL HOSPITAL OF OKLAHOMA (370201)**, 100 S.E. 59th Street, Zip 73129; tel. 405/634–9300 **A**1 10 **F**3 40 81 128
Primary Contact: Phil Ross, Chief Executive Officer
Web address: www.sh–ok.com/
**Control:** Partnership, Investor–owned, for–profit **Service:** General Medical and Surgical

**Staffed Beds:** 12 **Admissions:** 205 **Census:** 1 **Outpatient Visits:** 4125 **Births:** 0 **Total Expense ($000):** 11190 **Payroll Expense ($000):** 3613 **Personnel:** 66

⊠ **VALIR REHABILITATION HOSPITAL (373025)**, 700 N.W. Seventh Street, Zip 73102–1212; tel. 405/236–3131 **A**1 10 **F**28 29 30 35 40 54 68 75 86 87 90 91 93 96 100 118 142
Primary Contact: Scott Brown, Interim Chief Executive Officer
COO: Ginger Castleberry, Chief Operating Officer
CFO: Scott Brown, Chief Financial Officer
CMO: Tonya Washburn, M.D., Medical Director
CIO: Mark Dickey, Director Business Development
CHR: Bill Turner, Vice President Human Resources
Web address: www.valir.com
**Control:** Corporation, Investor–owned, for–profit **Service:** Rehabilitation

**Staffed Beds:** 45 **Admissions:** 871 **Census:** 27 **Outpatient Visits:** 4800 **Births:** 0 **Total Expense ($000):** 12282 **Payroll Expense ($000):** 6952 **Personnel:** 165

⊠ △ **VETERANS AFFAIRS MEDICAL CENTER**, 921 N.E. 13th Street, Zip 73104–5028; tel. 405/456–1000 **A**1 2 3 5 7 8 9 **F**2 3 5 6 8 9 10 12 17 18 20 22 24 26 28 29 30 31 34 35 38 39 40 44 45 47 48 49 50 53 54 56 57 58 59 60 61 62 63 64 65 67 68 70 71 74 75 77 78 79 80 81 82 83 84 85 86 87 90 91 93 94 96 97 98 100 101 102 103 104 105 106 107 111 113 114 115 116 118 129 131 134 142 143 145 146 147 **S** Department of Veterans Affairs, Washington, DC
Primary Contact: David P. Wood, FACHE, Medical Center Director
CFO: James Hurst, Chief Fiscal Service
CMO: Mark Huycke, M.D., Chief of Staff
CIO: Lindsay Buell, Chief Information Management Services
CHR: Kyle Inhofe, Chief Human Resources Officer
Web address: www.oklahoma.va.gov
**Control:** Veterans Affairs, Government, federal **Service:** General Medical and Surgical

**Staffed Beds:** 192 **Admissions:** 6867 **Census:** 148 **Outpatient Visits:** 494288 **Births:** 0 **Total Expense ($000):** 274973 **Payroll Expense ($000):** 191029 **Personnel:** 2038

**OKMULGEE—Okmulgee County**

**GEORGE NIGH REHABILITATION CENTER** See George Nigh Rehabilitation Institute

○ **GEORGE NIGH REHABILITATION INSTITUTE (373026)**, 900 East Airport Road, Zip 74447–9762, Mailing Address: P.O. Box 1118, Zip 74447–1118; tel. 918/756–9211, (Total facility includes 8 beds in nursing home–type unit) **A**10 11 **F**1 28 29 34 56 57 82 90 93 94 96 127 129 134 142 145 147 **P**5
Primary Contact: Gala McBee, Administrator
CFO: Djogan Djogan, Chief Financial Officer
CHR: Denaye Atwell, Manager Human Resources
Web address: www.gnrc.ouhsc.edu
**Control:** State–Government, nonfederal **Service:** Rehabilitation

**Staffed Beds:** 38 **Admissions:** 362 **Census:** 16 **Outpatient Visits:** 6590 **Births:** 0 **Total Expense ($000):** 6178 **Payroll Expense ($000):** 3597 **Personnel:** 93

★ **OKMULGEE MEMORIAL HOSPITAL (370057)**, 1401 Morris Drive, Zip 74447–6419, Mailing Address: P.O. Box 1038, Zip 74447–1038; tel. 918/756–4233 **A**9 10 **F**3 11 15 29 30 34 40 43 45 50 56 57 59 62 68 79 81 83 85 87 89 92 93 98 103 106 107 108 114 118 127 129 132 145 **P**6 **S** QHR, Brentwood, TN
Primary Contact: George N. Miller, Jr., Chief Executive Officer
CFO: John W. Crawford, Chief Financial Officer
CMO: Michael Sandlin, M.D., Chief of Staff
CIO: Sharon Riker, Manager Data Processing
CHR: Stacey R. Burton, Director Human Resources
Web address: www.okmulgeehospital.com
**Control:** Other not–for–profit (including NFP Corporation) **Service:** General Medical and Surgical

**Staffed Beds:** 36 **Admissions:** 1270 **Census:** 20 **Outpatient Visits:** 30751 **Births:** 0 **Total Expense ($000):** 17109 **Payroll Expense ($000):** 8732 **Personnel:** 201

**OWASSO—Tulsa County**

★ **BAILEY MEDICAL CENTER (370228)**, 10502 North 110th East Avenue, Zip 74055; tel. 918/376–8000 **A**9 10 **F**3 12 13 15 18 29 34 40 45 51 57 70 76 79 81 94 107 108 110 111 114 118 128 131 145 146 **S** Ardent Health Services, Nashville, TN
Primary Contact: Keith Mason, Chief Executive Officer
CFO: Becky Speight, Chief Financial Officer
CHR: Rachel Steward, Manager Human Resources
Web address: www.baileymedicalcenter.com
**Control:** Corporation, Investor–owned, for–profit **Service:** General Medical and Surgical

**Staffed Beds:** 37 **Admissions:** 1285 **Census:** 10 **Outpatient Visits:** 26902 **Births:** 312 **Total Expense ($000):** 27161 **Payroll Expense ($000):** 9571 **Personnel:** 172

★ **ST. JOHN OWASSO (370227)**, 12451 East 100th Street North,
Zip 74055–4600; tel. 918/274–5000 **A**9 10 **F**3 11 13 15 18 29 30 34 35 40
45 57 59 64 68 76 79 81 85 87 93 107 108 110 111 113 114 118 129 130
131 145 **P**5 6 **S** Marian Health System, Tulsa, OK
Primary Contact: David L. Phillips, President and Chief Executive Officer
CFO: Lex S. Anderson, Chief Financial Officer
CMO: Tim Hepner, M.D., Medical Director
CIO: Mike Reeves, Chief Information Officer
CNO: Dan Hall, R.N., Director of Nursing
Web address: www.stjohnowasso.com
**Control:** Church–operated, Nongovernment, not–for profit **Service:** General
Medical and Surgical

**Staffed Beds:** 36 **Admissions:** 1789 **Census:** 11 **Outpatient Visits:** 52346
**Births:** 390 **Total Expense ($000):** 25664 **Payroll Expense ($000):** 10312
**Personnel:** 210

### PAULS VALLEY—Garvin County

★ **PAULS VALLEY GENERAL HOSPITAL (370156)**, 100 Valley Drive,
Zip 73075–6613, Mailing Address: P.O. Box 368, Zip 73075–0368;
tel. 405/238–5501, (Nonreporting) **A**9 10 20
Primary Contact: Bridget Cosby, Chief Executive Officer
CIO: Craig Bowie, Information Technology Manager
CHR: Kari Kuykendall, Human Resources Specialist
CNO: Karla Brown, Interim Chief Nursing Officer
Web address: www.pvgh.net
**Control:** City–Government, nonfederal **Service:** General Medical and Surgical

**Staffed Beds:** 50

### PAWHUSKA—Osage County

**PAWHUSKA HOSPITAL (371309)**, 1101 East 15th Street, Zip 74056–1920;
tel. 918/287–3232 **A**9 10 18 **F**11 29 34 40 50 57 64 68 90 93 107 127 132
134 147
Primary Contact: Karen Arrowsmith, Administrator
CMO: Mike Priest, M.D., Chief of Staff
**Control:** Church–operated, Nongovernment, not–for profit **Service:** General
Medical and Surgical

**Staffed Beds:** 27 **Admissions:** 117 **Census:** 2 **Outpatient Visits:** 7893
**Births:** 0 **Personnel:** 45

### PERRY—Noble County

★ **PERRY MEMORIAL HOSPITAL (370139)**, 501 North 14th Street,
Zip 73077–5099; tel. 580/336–3541 **A**9 10 20 **F**3 11 15 30 34 40 45 57 59
62 64 79 81 85 93 107 111 113 118 132 145 147 **S** QHR, Brentwood, TN
Primary Contact: Terry W. Shambles, Interim Chief Executive Officer
CFO: Terry W. Shambles, Chief Financial Officer
CMO: Michael Hartwig, M.D., Chief of Staff
CHR: Robin Webb, Director Human Resources
Web address: www.pmh–ok.org
**Control:** Hospital district or authority, Government, nonfederal **Service:** General
Medical and Surgical

**Staffed Beds:** 26 **Admissions:** 554 **Census:** 9 **Outpatient Visits:** 16476
**Births:** 0 **Total Expense ($000):** 6448 **Payroll Expense ($000):** 3348
**Personnel:** 100

### PONCA CITY—Kay County

⊞ **PONCA CITY MEDICAL CENTER (370006)**, 1900 North 14th Street,
Zip 74601–2099; tel. 580/765–3321 **A**1 9 10 19 **F**3 13 15 20 28 29 30 31
34 35 40 43 46 49 51 53 56 57 59 64 65 66 68 69 70 74 75 76 77 78 79
81 82 85 89 90 93 97 107 110 111 113 116 117 118 128 129 130 131 132
134 144 145 146 147 **S** Community Health Systems, Inc., Franklin, TN
Primary Contact: R. Andrew Wachtel, FACHE, Chief Executive Officer
COO: Nikia Beene, Assistant Chief Executive Officer
CFO: Geoff Blomeley, Interim Chief Financial Officer
CIO: Rob Dreussi, Interim Director Information Systems
CHR: Lisa Zaloudek, Chief Human Resources Officer
CNO: Jeanne Stara, R.N., Chief Nursing Officer
Web address: www.poncamedcenter.com
**Control:** Corporation, Investor–owned, for–profit **Service:** General Medical and
Surgical

**Staffed Beds:** 72 **Admissions:** 3546 **Census:** 30 **Outpatient Visits:** 63543
**Births:** 637 **Total Expense ($000):** 50281 **Payroll Expense ($000):** 17666
**Personnel:** 341

### POTEAU—Le Flore County

★ **EASTERN OKLAHOMA MEDICAL CENTER (370040)**, 105 Wall Street,
Zip 74953–4428, Mailing Address: P.O. Box 1148, Zip 74953–1148;
tel. 918/647–8161 **A**9 10 **F**3 11 13 15 29 34 40 45 50 57 59 62 68 70 76
81 85 86 87 89 93 107 110 111 113 114 118 145 **P**4
Primary Contact: Terry Buckner, Chief Executive Officer
CFO: Nancy Frier, Chief Financial Officer
CMO: Dennis Carter, M.D., Chief of Staff
CIO: Michael C. Huggins, Administrator Network System
CHR: Michele Oglesby, Manager Human Resources
**Control:** County–Government, nonfederal **Service:** General Medical and Surgical

**Staffed Beds:** 84 **Admissions:** 2616 **Census:** 29 **Outpatient Visits:** 28800
**Personnel:** 222

### PRAGUE—Lincoln County

★ **PRAGUE COMMUNITY HOSPITAL (371301)**, 1322 Klabzuba Avenue,
Zip 74864–9005, Mailing Address: P.O. Box S., Zip 74864–1090;
tel. 405/567–4922 **A**9 10 18 **F**18 29 34 40 43 45 57 59 64 68 70 81 89 93
107 111 118 126 127 128 129 131 132 **P**6 **S** HMC/CAH Consolidated, Inc.,
Kansas City, MO
Primary Contact: Joan Walters, R.N., MSN, Administrator
CFO: Doug Erickson, Chief Financial Officer
CMO: Darryl Jackson, D.O., Chief of Staff
CIO: Rhonda Whitnum, Director Health Improvement Management
CHR: Angie Brezny, Director Human Resources
Web address: www.praguehospital.com
**Control:** Corporation, Investor–owned, for–profit **Service:** General Medical and
Surgical

**Staffed Beds:** 19 **Admissions:** 343 **Census:** 4 **Outpatient Visits:** 2931
**Births:** 0 **Total Expense ($000):** 5400 **Payroll Expense ($000):** 2905
**Personnel:** 57

### PRYOR—Mayes County

⊞ **INTEGRIS MAYES COUNTY MEDICAL CENTER (370015)**, 111 North Bailey
Street, Zip 74361–4211, Mailing Address: P.O. Box 278, Zip 74362–0278;
tel. 918/825–1600, (Nonreporting) **A**1 9 10 **S** Health Management Associates,
Naples, FL
Primary Contact: Douglas K. Weaver, FACHE, President
CFO: Kristy McCollough, Assistant Administrator and Chief Financial Officer
CMO: Lora Collier, M.D., Chief Medical Staff
CHR: Jamil Haynes, Director Human Resources
Web address: www.integris–health.com
**Control:** Partnership, Investor–owned, for–profit **Service:** General Medical and
Surgical

**Staffed Beds:** 39

### PURCELL—Mcclain County

★ **PURCELL MUNICIPAL HOSPITAL (370158)**, 1500 North Green Avenue,
Zip 73080–1699, Mailing Address: P.O. Box 511, Zip 73080–0511;
tel. 405/527–6524 **A**9 10 **F**3 11 13 15 18 29 30 35 40 45 48 57 59 64 65
76 77 79 81 82 86 87 89 93 110 113 118 126 129 131 132 **P**8
Primary Contact: James T. Berry, Chief Executive Officer
COO: Lisa Roberts, Chief Operating Officer
CFO: Jennifer Warren, Chief Financial Officer
CMO: Heather Lynch, M.D., Chief of Staff
CIO: Jennifer Coates, Coordinator Information Technology
CHR: Tara Selfridge, Manager Human Resources
Web address: www.purcellhospital.com
**Control:** City–Government, nonfederal **Service:** General Medical and Surgical

**Staffed Beds:** 30 **Admissions:** 1281 **Census:** 12 **Outpatient Visits:** 43519
**Births:** 39 **Total Expense ($000):** 12289 **Payroll Expense ($000):** 5520
**Personnel:** 134

---

**Hospital, Medicare Provider Number, Address, Telephone, Approval, Facility, and Physician Codes, Health Care System**

★ American Hospital Association (AHA) membership
☐ The Joint Commission accreditation          ◇ DNV Healthcare Inc. accreditation
○ American Osteopathic Association (AOA) accreditation
△ Commission on Accreditation of Rehabilitation Facilities (CARF) accreditation

OK

## SALLISAW—Sequoyah County

**SEQUOYAH MEMORIAL HOSPITAL (370112)**, 213 East Redwood Street, Zip 74955–2811, Mailing Address: P.O. Box 505, Zip 74955–0505; tel. 918/774–1100 **A**9 10 **F**29 30 40 43 57 62 63 64 65 81 93 107 111 112 118 128 131 134 145
Primary Contact: Debra R. Knoke, Chief Executive Officer
COO: Debra R. Knoke, Chief Executive Officer
CFO: Glenn Click, Chief Financial Officer
CMO: William E. Wood, M.D., Chief of Staff
CIO: Gary McClanahan, Chief Information Officer
CHR: David Martin, Supervisor Human Resources
Web address: www.sequoyahmemorial.com/home.php
**Control:** Hospital district or authority, Government, nonfederal **Service:** General Medical and Surgical

**Staffed Beds:** 26 **Admissions:** 1012 **Census:** 8 **Outpatient Visits:** 21026
**Births:** 1 **Total Expense ($000):** 14769 **Payroll Expense ($000):** 7239
**Personnel:** 182

## SAPULPA—Creek County

★ **ST. JOHN SAPULPA (371312)**, 519 South Division Street, Zip 74066–4501, Mailing Address: P.O. Box 1368, Zip 74067–1368; tel. 918/224–4280 **A**9 10 18 **F**3 8 11 15 29 30 34 35 39 40 45 49 57 64 75 77 79 81 85 86 93 107 110 111 118 129 132 134 145 **S** Marian Health System, Tulsa, OK
Primary Contact: Valerie Round, Chief Executive Officer
CMO: Roger D. Wilson, M.D., Medical Director
Web address: www.sjmc.org
**Control:** Church–operated, Nongovernment, not–for profit **Service:** General Medical and Surgical

**Staffed Beds:** 25 **Admissions:** 1918 **Census:** 17 **Outpatient Visits:** 30366
**Births:** 0 **Total Expense ($000):** 16616 **Payroll Expense ($000):** 7129
**Personnel:** 170

## SAYRE—Beckham County

★ **SAYRE MEMORIAL HOSPITAL (370103)**, 911 Hospital Drive, Zip 73662–1206; tel. 580/928–5541, (Nonreporting) **A**9 10
Primary Contact: Wallace N. Boyd, Chief Executive Officer
CFO: Brenda K. Doyel, Chief Financial Officer
Web address: www.sayrehospital.org
**Control:** Other not–for–profit (including NFP Corporation) **Service:** General Medical and Surgical

**Staffed Beds:** 46

## SEILING—Dewey County

★ **SEILING COMMUNITY HOSPITAL (371332)**, Highway 60 N.E., Zip 73663, Mailing Address: P.O. Box 720, Zip 73663–0720; tel. 580/922–7361 **A**9 10 18 **F**40 41 65 107 111 118 128 132 **P**5 **S** HMC/CAH Consolidated, Inc., Kansas City, MO
Primary Contact: Larry Troxell, Chief Executive Officer
CFO: Nancy Freed, Chief Financial Officer
CMO: Kenneth Duffy, M.D., Medical Director
CHR: Sandy Landreth, Director Human Resources
**Control:** Corporation, Investor–owned, for–profit **Service:** General Medical and Surgical

**Staffed Beds:** 18 **Admissions:** 229 **Census:** 2 **Outpatient Visits:** 6249
**Births:** 0 **Total Expense ($000):** 3472 **Payroll Expense ($000):** 1742
**Personnel:** 34

## SEMINOLE—Seminole County

⊞ **INTEGRIS SEMINOLE MEDICAL CENTER (370229)**, 2401 Wrangler Boulevard, Zip 74868–1917; tel. 405/303–4000 **A**1 9 10 **F**3 11 15 18 29 30 34 35 40 41 51 57 59 65 68 79 81 82 93 102 107 108 110 111 113 118 129 134 145 147 **P**6 **S** Health Management Associates, Naples, FL
Primary Contact: C. David Hill, President
CMO: Nikki Chawla, M.D., Medical Director
CHR: Lori Friend, Human Resources Director
CNO: Barbara Lewis, Chief Nursing Officer
Web address: www.hma.com
**Control:** Other not–for–profit (including NFP Corporation) **Service:** General Medical and Surgical

**Staffed Beds:** 32 **Admissions:** 658 **Census:** 6 **Outpatient Visits:** 20472
**Births:** 6 **Total Expense ($000):** 13413 **Payroll Expense ($000):** 4950
**Personnel:** 93

## SHATTUCK—Ellis County

★ **NEWMAN MEMORIAL HOSPITAL (370007)**, 905 South Main Street, Zip 73858–9205; tel. 580/938–2551 **A**9 10 20 **F**3 11 13 15 29 30 35 39 40 53 57 59 62 64 65 69 76 81 87 93 104 107 111 114 118 128 129 132 145 **P**6
Primary Contact: Gary W. Mitchell, DPH, FACHE, Chief Executive Officer
COO: Kevin O'Brien, Chief Operating Officer
CMO: Barbara H. Miller, M.D., Chief Medical Officer
CNO: Denise Ketterman, R.N., Chief Nursing Officer
Web address: www.newmanmemorialhospital.org
**Control:** Other not–for–profit (including NFP Corporation) **Service:** General Medical and Surgical

**Staffed Beds:** 27 **Admissions:** 603 **Census:** 4 **Outpatient Visits:** 45386
**Births:** 191 **Total Expense ($000):** 9645 **Payroll Expense ($000):** 3938
**Personnel:** 86

## SHAWNEE—Pottawatomie County

**SOLARA HOSPITAL OF SHAWNEE (372019)**, 1900 Gordon Cooper Drive, 2nd Floor, Zip 74801; tel. 405/395–5800, (Nonreporting) **A**9 10 **S** Solara Healthcare, Dallas, TX
Primary Contact: Michael E. Gerten, Chief Executive Officer
COO: Michael E. Gerten, Chief Executive Officer
CMO: Phillip A. Haddad, M.D., Chief Medical Officer
Web address: www.solarahc.com
**Control:** Corporation, Investor–owned, for–profit **Service:** Long–Term Acute Care hospital

**Staffed Beds:** 34

★ **ST. ANTHONY SHAWNEE HOSPITAL (370149)**, 1102 West MacArthur Street, Zip 74804–1744; tel. 405/273–2270 **A**2 9 10 19 21 **F**3 11 13 15 18 20 29 30 34 35 40 43 45 50 57 59 60 64 65 68 69 70 75 76 77 79 81 82 87 90 93 94 107 110 111 113 118 120 122 128 129 130 131 134 143 145 146 147 **P**5 6 **S** SSM Health Care, Saint Louis, MO
Primary Contact: Charles E. Skillings, President and Chief Executive Officer
COO: Thomas Keller, Executive Vice President and Chief Operating Officer
CFO: Jennifer Pierce, Administrative Director of Finance
CMO: Gaynell Anderson, M.D., Medical Director
CIO: Linda E. Brown, Vice President of Support Services
CHR: Michael Spears, Vice President of Human Resources
CNO: Angela Mohr, R.N., Vice President of Nursing
Web address: www.stanthonyshawnee.com
**Control:** Other not–for–profit (including NFP Corporation) **Service:** General Medical and Surgical

**Staffed Beds:** 131 **Admissions:** 5063 **Census:** 47 **Outpatient Visits:** 101154
**Births:** 984 **Total Expense ($000):** 56184 **Payroll Expense ($000):** 23187
**Personnel:** 490

**UNITY HEALTH CENTER** See St. Anthony Shawnee Hospital

## SPENCER—Oklahoma County

**INTEGRIS MENTAL HEALTH SYSTEM–SPENCER** See Integris Baptist Medical Center, Oklahoma City

## STIGLER—Haskell County

**HASKELL COUNTY COMMUNITY HOSPITAL (371335)**, 401 Northwest H Street, Zip 74462–1625, Mailing Address: P.O. Box 728, Zip 74462–0728; tel. 918/967–4682, (Nonreporting) **A**9 10 18 **S** HMC/CAH Consolidated, Inc., Kansas City, MO
Primary Contact: Scott McIntyre, FACHE, Chief Executive Officer
CMO: Mark McCurry, M.D., Chief of Staff
CIO: Steve Hurst, Information Technology Specialist
Web address: www.hchs.otnnet.net
**Control:** Corporation, Investor–owned, for–profit **Service:** General Medical and Surgical

**Staffed Beds:** 32

**HASKELL COUNTY HEALTHCARE SYSTEM** See Haskell County Community Hospital

**OK**

## STILLWATER—Payne County

★ △ **STILLWATER MEDICAL CENTER (370049)**, 1323 West Sixth Avenue, Zip 74074–4399, Mailing Address: P.O. Box 2408, Zip 74076–2408; tel. 405/372–1480 **A**7 9 10 21 **F**3 8 11 13 15 18 20 22 28 29 31 34 35 39 40 43 45 46 47 48 49 50 51 53 56 62 65 68 69 70 74 75 76 79 81 82 85 87 90 91 93 94 107 108 110 111 114 116 118 128 129 134 145 147 **P**6 7
Primary Contact: Jerry G. Moeller, FACHE, President and Chief Executive Officer
CFO: Alan Lovelace, Vice President and Chief Financial Officer
CMO: Woody Jenkins, M.D., Chief of Medical Staff
CIO: Chris Roark, Chief Information Officer
CHR: Keith Hufnagel, Director Human Resources
CNO: Liz Michael, Vice President Patient Care Services and Chief Nursing Officer
Web address: www.stillwater-medical.org
**Control:** Hospital district or authority, Government, nonfederal **Service:** General Medical and Surgical

**Staffed Beds:** 87 **Admissions:** 4402 **Census:** 48 **Outpatient Visits:** 120431 **Births:** 974 **Total Expense ($000):** 90957 **Payroll Expense ($000):** 38582 **Personnel:** 806

## STILWELL—Adair County

**MEMORIAL HOSPITAL (370178)**, 1401 West Locust, Zip 74960, Mailing Address: P.O. Box 272, Zip 74960; tel. 918/696–3101, (Nonreporting) **A**9 10
Primary Contact: Alan L. Adams, President
Web address: www.stilwellmemorialhospital.com
**Control:** Corporation, Investor–owned, for–profit **Service:** General Medical and Surgical

**Staffed Beds:** 30

## STROUD—Lincoln County

**STROUD REGIONAL MEDICAL CENTER (371316)**, Highway 66 West, Zip 74079, Mailing Address: P.O. Box 530, Zip 74079–0530; tel. 918/968–3571 **A**9 10 18 **F**3 8 11 29 30 34 35 40 41 43 45 57 59 64 81 89 107 113 127 129 132 **P**5 **S** Southern Plains Medical Group, Oklahoma City, OK
Primary Contact: Regina Peters, Chief Executive Officer
COO: Regina Peters, Chief Executive Officer
CFO: Richard E. Rentsch, President
CMO: Ken Darvin, M.D., Chief of Staff
CIO: Donna Buchanan, Director Nursing
CHR: Leannette Raffety, Administrative Generalist
**Control:** Other not–for–profit (including NFP Corporation) **Service:** General Medical and Surgical

**Staffed Beds:** 25 **Admissions:** 3468 **Census:** 14 **Outpatient Visits:** 14603 **Births:** 0 **Personnel:** 55

## SULPHUR—Murray County

★ **ARBUCKLE MEMORIAL HOSPITAL (371328)**, 2011 West Broadway Street, Zip 73086–4221; tel. 580/622–2161 **A**9 10 18 **F**29 32 40 45 56 57 81 87 93 107 118 128 132 134 147 **P**6 **S** Mercy Health, Chesterfield, MO
Primary Contact: Darin Farrell, Chief Executive Officer
CFO: Denise Hancock, Chief Financial Officer
CMO: Teresa Lynn, D.O., Chief of Staff
CIO: Tiffany Sands, Manager Health Information
CHR: Sallie Tomlinson, Manager Human Resources
Web address: www.arbucklehospital.com/
**Control:** County–Government, nonfederal **Service:** General Medical and Surgical

**Staffed Beds:** 10 **Admissions:** 508 **Census:** 5 **Outpatient Visits:** 30989 **Births:** 0 **Total Expense ($000):** 13472 **Payroll Expense ($000):** 5423 **Personnel:** 112

## TAHLEQUAH—Cherokee County

★ **TAHLEQUAH CITY HOSPITAL (370089)**, 1400 East Downing Street, Zip 74464–3324, Mailing Address: P.O. Box 1008, Zip 74465–1008; tel. 918/456–0641 **A**9 10 13 20 **F**3 7 11 13 15 17 18 20 22 24 28 29 30 31 35 39 40 43 45 46 47 49 51 57 59 60 70 75 76 77 78 79 80 81 82 85 87 89 90 93 97 98 103 107 108 110 111 113 114 118 119 120 122 128 129 145 146 147 **P**6
Primary Contact: Brian K. Woodliff, President and Chief Executive Officer
COO: David McClain, Executive Vice President Operations
CFO: Julie Newman, Vice President Finance
CIO: Julie Newman, Vice President Finance
CHR: Phyllis Smith, Vice President Human Resources
Web address: www.tch-ok.org
**Control:** City–Government, nonfederal **Service:** General Medical and Surgical

**Staffed Beds:** 90 **Admissions:** 4667 **Census:** 50 **Outpatient Visits:** 83408 **Births:** 343 **Total Expense ($000):** 64583 **Payroll Expense ($000):** 21973 **Personnel:** 650

⊞ **WILLIAM W. HASTINGS INDIAN HOSPITAL (370171)**, 100 South Bliss Avenue, Zip 74464–3399; tel. 918/458–3100 **A**1 10 21 **F**3 5 11 12 15 29 30 32 34 35 38 39 40 41 44 45 46 47 48 50 55 57 59 61 64 65 68 70 75 76 77 79 81 82 85 86 87 93 97 100 101 102 104 107 110 113 118 128 129 130 131 134 140 142 143 145 146 147 **P**6 **S** U. S. Indian Health Service, Rockville, MD
Primary Contact: Charles Grim, D.D.S., Chief Executive Officer
CNO: Valerie J. Rogers, Director of Nursing
**Control:** PHS, Indian Service, Government, federal **Service:** General Medical and Surgical

**Staffed Beds:** 58 **Admissions:** 2122 **Census:** 18 **Outpatient Visits:** 306085 **Births:** 773 **Total Expense ($000):** 83974 **Payroll Expense ($000):** 40425 **Personnel:** 637

## TALIHINA—Latimer County

⊞ **CHOCTAW NATION HEALTH CARE CENTER (370172)**, One Choctaw Way, Zip 74571–2022; tel. 918/567–7000, (Nonreporting) **A**1 10
Primary Contact: Teresa Jackson, Chief Executive Officer
COO: Todd Hallmark, Chief Operating Officer
CMO: Jason Hill, M.D., Chief Medical Officer
CIO: Skip Leader, Chief Information Officer
CHR: Evelyn Jones, Director Human Resources
Web address: www.choctawnationhealth.com
**Control:** Other not–for–profit (including NFP Corporation) **Service:** General Medical and Surgical

**Staffed Beds:** 37

## TISHOMINGO—Johnston County

**JOHNSTON MEMORIAL HOSPITAL** See Mercy Hospital Tishomingo

★ **MERCY HOSPITAL TISHOMINGO (371304)**, 1000 South Byrd Street, Zip 73460–3299; tel. 580/371–2327, (Data for 181 days) **A**9 10 18 **F**3 29 40 132 **S** Mercy Health, Chesterfield, MO
Primary Contact: Richard Barker, Interim Chief Executive Officer
CFO: Lisa Dowling, Manager Finance
CHR: Arlita Hummelke, Manager Human Resources
Web address: www.mercy.net/
**Control:** Church–operated, Nongovernment, not–for profit **Service:** General Medical and Surgical

**Staffed Beds:** 25 **Admissions:** 209 **Census:** 4 **Outpatient Visits:** 2428 **Births:** 0 **Total Expense ($000):** 1834 **Payroll Expense ($000):** 1064 **Personnel:** 41

## TULSA—Tulsa County

**BROOKHAVEN HOSPITAL (374012)**, 201 South Garnett Road, Zip 74128–1805; tel. 918/438–4257 **A**10 **F**4 5 29 30 77 98 104 106 129 131
Primary Contact: Rolf B. Gainer, Chief Executive Officer and Administrator
CFO: Kenneth Pierce, Chief Financial Officer
CMO: Mark Gage, D.O., Medical Director
CHR: Mike Atkinson, Director Administrative Services
Web address: www.brookhavenhospital.com
**Control:** Corporation, Investor–owned, for–profit **Service:** Psychiatric

**Staffed Beds:** 64 **Admissions:** 1008 **Census:** 45 **Outpatient Visits:** 2908 **Births:** 0 **Total Expense ($000):** 9600 **Payroll Expense ($000):** 5276 **Personnel:** 154

★ **CONTINUOUS CARE CENTERS OF TULSA (372011)**, 1923 South Utica Avenue, 4 South, Zip 74104–6510; tel. 918/744–3047, (Includes CONTINUOUS CARE CENTERS OF OKLAHOMA, 744 West Ninth Street, 9th Floor, Zip 74127; tel. 918/599–4604) **A**9 10 **F**1 3 29 40 50 65 75 79 82 84 85 87 96 129 147 **P**8
Primary Contact: Raymond L. Replogle, President and Chief Executive Officer
COO: Mike Harris, Chief Operating Officer
CFO: Basil Wyatt, Chief Financial Officer
CMO: Mark Myers, M.D., Chief Medical Officer
CIO: Dana Jetton, Chief Information Officer
CHR: Donna Nagel, Director Human Resources
Web address: www.cccok.com
**Control:** Other not–for–profit (including NFP Corporation) **Service:** General Medical and Surgical

**Staffed Beds:** 46 **Admissions:** 442 **Census:** 31 **Outpatient Visits:** 0 **Births:** 0 **Total Expense ($000):** 16105 **Payroll Expense ($000):** 5620 **Personnel:** 91

---

**Hospital, Medicare Provider Number, Address, Telephone, Approval, Facility, and Physician Codes, Health Care System**

★ American Hospital Association (AHA) membership
☐ The Joint Commission accreditation
◇ DNV Healthcare Inc. accreditation
○ American Osteopathic Association (AOA) accreditation
△ Commission on Accreditation of Rehabilitation Facilities (CARF) accreditation

✠ **HILLCREST MEDICAL CENTER (370001)**, 1120 South Utica, Zip 74104–4090; tel. 918/579–1000 **A**1 3 5 9 10 **F**3 7 8 11 13 15 16 17 18 20 22 24 26 28 29 30 31 32 34 35 37 39 40 43 45 49 50 51 53 56 57 58 59 60 61 62 64 68 70 72 74 75 76 77 78 79 80 81 83 84 85 86 87 89 90 93 95 96 98 99 100 101 102 105 106 107 108 110 111 112 113 114 115 116 117 118 119 120 122 123 128 129 130 131 134 142 144 145 146 147 **S** Ardent Health Services, Nashville, TN
Primary Contact: Jason Fahrlander, FACHE, Chief Executive Officer
CMO: Steven Landgarten, M.D., Chief Medical Officer
Web address: www.hillcrest.com
**Control:** Corporation, Investor–owned, for–profit **Service:** General Medical and Surgical

**Staffed Beds:** 537 **Admissions:** 24117 **Census:** 339 **Outpatient Visits:** 118307 **Births:** 3266 **Total Expense ($000):** 320066 **Payroll Expense ($000):** 121585 **Personnel:** 1827

✠ **KINDRED HOSPITAL TULSA (372018)**, 3219 South 79th East Avenue, Zip 74145–1343; tel. 918/663–8183 **A**1 9 10 **F**1 3 29 40 60 68 75 87 94 100 107 108 113 129 142 147 **P**5 **S** Kindred Healthcare, Louisville, KY
Primary Contact: Lee A. Simpson, Jr., Chief Executive Officer
CFO: Lee A. Simpson, Jr., Chief Executive Officer
Web address: www.khtulsa.com
**Control:** Corporation, Investor–owned, for–profit **Service:** Long–Term Acute Care hospital

**Staffed Beds:** 60 **Admissions:** 501 **Census:** 36 **Outpatient Visits:** 3 **Births:** 0 **Total Expense ($000):** 16223 **Payroll Expense ($000):** 7539 **Personnel:** 129

✠ **LAUREATE PSYCHIATRIC CLINIC AND HOSPITAL (374020)**, 6655 South Yale Avenue, Zip 74136–3329; tel. 918/481–4000, (Nonreporting) **A**1 3 5 9 10 **S** Saint Francis Health System, Tulsa, OK
Primary Contact: William Schloss, Senior Vice President
COO: William Schloss, Senior Vice President
CFO: Barry L. Steichen, Executive Vice President, Chief Administrative Officer and Chief Financial Officer
CMO: Peter Aran, M.D., Senior Vice President and Chief Medical Officer
CIO: Mark Stastny, Vice President Information Technology
CHR: Amy B. Adams, Executive Director Human Resources
CNO: Lynn A. Sund, R.N., Senior Vice President, Administrator and Chief Nursing Executive
Web address: www.laureate.com
**Control:** Other not–for–profit (including NFP Corporation) **Service:** Psychiatric

**Staffed Beds:** 75

**MEADOWBROOK SPECIALTY HOSPITAL OF TULSA** See Kindred Hospital Tulsa

**OKLAHOMA NEUROSPECIALTY CENTER**, 2408 E. 81st Street, Suite 2600, Zip 74137; tel. 918/477–5111, (Nonreporting) **A**9
Primary Contact: Frank Lewis, Ph.D., Chief Executive Officer
Web address: www.ok.neurospecialty.com
**Control:** Corporation, Investor–owned, for–profit **Service:** General Medical and Surgical

**Staffed Beds:** 18

✠ ○ **OKLAHOMA STATE UNIVERSITY MEDICAL CENTER (370078)**, 744 West Ninth Street, Zip 74127–9990; tel. 918/599–1000 **A**1 9 10 11 12 13 **F**3 8 13 15 18 20 22 24 26 28 29 30 31 34 35 40 45 47 49 50 56 57 59 64 65 68 70 71 72 74 75 76 77 78 79 81 82 84 85 87 89 92 93 96 97 107 108 110 111 114 118 128 129 134 145 147 **P**6
Primary Contact: Jan Slater, Chief Executive Officer
CFO: Wayne Walthall, Interim Chief Financial Officer
CMO: Damon Baker, D.O., Chief Medical Officer
CHR: Sunny J. Benjamin, Director Human Resources
Web address: www.osu–medcenter.com
**Control:** City–Government, nonfederal **Service:** General Medical and Surgical

**Staffed Beds:** 180 **Admissions:** 7007 **Census:** 87 **Outpatient Visits:** 71457 **Births:** 613 **Total Expense ($000):** 115479 **Payroll Expense ($000):** 51124 **Personnel:** 1053

**OKLAHOMA SURGICAL HOSPITAL (370210)**, 2408 East 81st Street, Suite 300, Zip 74137–4215; tel. 918/477–5000 **A**10 **F**3 12 29 30 34 35 40 41 45 50 51 64 68 74 75 79 81 82 85 86 87 93 94 107 108 111 113 118 125 129 130 **P**2
Primary Contact: Rick Ferguson, Chief Executive Officer
COO: Beverly Pickett, R.N., Chief Nursing Officer
CFO: Dub Cleland, Chief Financial Officer
Web address: www.oklahomasurgicalhospital.com
**Control:** Partnership, Investor–owned, for–profit **Service:** General Medical and Surgical

**Staffed Beds:** 49 **Admissions:** 3311 **Census:** 20 **Outpatient Visits:** 22472 **Births:** 0 **Total Expense ($000):** 66297 **Payroll Expense ($000):** 14968 **Personnel:** 324

**PARKSIDE HOSPITAL (374021)**, 1620 East 12th Street, Zip 74120–5407; tel. 918/582–2131 **A**5 9 10 **F**3 5 29 30 98 99 102 104 105 106 **P**6
Primary Contact: Debra Moore, Chief Executive Officer
CFO: Jim White, Chief Financial Officer
CMO: John White, M.D., Medical Director
CIO: Nita Gould, Director Information Services
CHR: David Patterson, Director Human Resources
Web address: www.parksideinc.org
**Control:** Other not–for–profit (including NFP Corporation) **Service:** Psychiatric

**Staffed Beds:** 70 **Admissions:** 1513 **Census:** 61 **Outpatient Visits:** 22836 **Births:** 0 **Total Expense ($000):** 11452 **Payroll Expense ($000):** 7322 **Personnel:** 185

**PINNACLE SPECIALTY HOSPITAL (370233)**, 2408 East 81st Street, Suite 600, Zip 74137–4200; tel. 918/392–2780, (Nonreporting)
Primary Contact: Mark Starns, Administrator
Web address: www.pinnaclespecialtyhospital.com/
**Control:** Partnership, Investor–owned, for–profit **Service:** General Medical and Surgical

**Staffed Beds:** 4

**SAINT FRANCIS HEART HOSPITAL** See Saint Francis Hospital

✠ **SAINT FRANCIS HOSPITAL (370091)**, 6161 South Yale Avenue, Zip 74136–1902; tel. 918/494–2200, (Includes CHILDREN'S HOSPITAL AT SAINT FRANCIS, 6161 South Yale Avenue, tel. 918/502–6714; SAINT FRANCIS HEART HOSPITAL, 6161 South Yale Avenue, tel. 918/502–2022) **A**1 2 3 5 9 10 **F**3 7 8 11 12 13 15 17 18 19 20 21 22 23 24 25 26 27 28 29 30 31 32 35 37 39 40 41 43 44 45 46 47 49 50 51 54 55 56 57 58 60 61 64 66 68 69 70 72 73 74 75 76 77 78 79 80 81 82 83 84 85 86 87 88 89 90 93 107 108 110 111 112 113 114 115 117 118 119 120 122 123 125 128 129 130 131 134 135 137 140 145 147 **P**6 **S** Saint Francis Health System, Tulsa, OK
Primary Contact: Lynn A. Sund, R.N., MS, Senior Vice President, Administrator and Chief Nursing Executive
COO: Lynn A. Sund, R.N., Senior Vice President, Administrator and Chief Nursing Executive
CFO: Barry L. Steichen, Executive Vice President and Chief Financial Officer
CMO: Peter Aran, M.D., Senior Vice President and Chief Medical Officer
CIO: Mark Stastny, Vice President Information Technology
CHR: Amy B. Adams, Executive Director Human Resources
Web address: www.saintfrancis.com
**Control:** Other not–for–profit (including NFP Corporation) **Service:** General Medical and Surgical

**Staffed Beds:** 774 **Admissions:** 41820 **Census:** 578 **Outpatient Visits:** 254790 **Births:** 3800 **Total Expense ($000):** 561124 **Payroll Expense ($000):** 220794 **Personnel:** 4759

✠ **SAINT FRANCIS HOSPITAL SOUTH (370218)**, 10501 East 91St. Streeet, Zip 74133–5790; tel. 918/455–3535 **A**1 10 **F**13 15 18 20 22 29 34 40 49 57 64 70 79 81 82 92 107 108 110 111 113 114 118 129 145 **P**6 **S** Saint Francis Health System, Tulsa, OK
Primary Contact: David S. Weil, Senior Vice President and Administrator
Web address: www.sfh–ba.com
**Control:** Other not–for–profit (including NFP Corporation) **Service:** General Medical and Surgical

**Staffed Beds:** 60 **Admissions:** 2881 **Census:** 26 **Outpatient Visits:** 31867 **Births:** 809 **Total Expense ($000):** 43456 **Payroll Expense ($000):** 16971 **Personnel:** 253

✠ **SELECT SPECIALTY HOSPITAL–TULSA MIDTOWN (372007)**, 1125 South Trenton Avenue, Zip 74104; tel. 918/579–7300 **A**1 9 10 **F**1 3 29 34 35 75 129 147 **P**8 **S** Select Medical Corporation, Mechanicsburg, PA
Primary Contact: Linda Tiemens, Chief Executive Officer
CFO: Bryon Briggs, Assistant Chief Financial Officer
Web address: www.selectmedicalcorp.com
**Control:** Corporation, Investor–owned, for–profit **Service:** Long–Term Acute Care hospital

**Staffed Beds:** 56 **Admissions:** 429 **Census:** 30 **Outpatient Visits:** 0 **Births:** 0 **Total Expense ($000):** 15129 **Payroll Expense ($000):** 5879 **Personnel:** 108

**SHADOW MOUNTAIN BEHAVIORAL HEALTH SYSTEM**, 6262 South Sheridan Road, Zip 74133–4055; tel. 918/492–8200 **A**9 **F**40 41 42 54 59 98 99 101 102 104 106 **P**6 **S** Universal Health Services, Inc., King of Prussia, PA
Primary Contact: Mike Kistler, Chief Executive Officer
COO: Selena Stockley, Chief Operating Officer
CFO: Kirt Penrod, Chief Financial Officer
CMO: Dean Martin, M.D., Medical Director
CHR: Duane Harris, Director Human Resources
Web address: www.shadowmountainbhs.com
**Control:** Corporation, Investor–owned, for–profit **Service:** Children's hospital psychiatric

**Staffed Beds:** 202 **Admissions:** 1741 **Census:** 188 **Outpatient Visits:** 16904 **Births:** 0 **Total Expense ($000):** 31227 **Payroll Expense ($000):** 12368 **Personnel:** 356

*Many Facility Codes have changed. Please refer to the AHA Guide Code Chart.*

✠ **SOUTHCREST HOSPITAL (370202)**, 8801 South 101st East Avenue, Zip 74133–5716; tel. 918/294–4000 **A**1 9 10 **F**3 13 15 18 20 22 24 28 29 30 34 40 43 49 51 54 57 59 70 75 76 79 81 85 86 87 93 97 107 108 110 111 113 114 117 118 123 128 129 130 145 146 147 **S** Ardent Health Services, Nashville, TN
Primary Contact: Joseph H. Neely, FACHE, Chief Executive Officer
COO: Kyle McCann, Chief Operating Officer
CFO: Matt Romero, Vice President Finance and Chief Financial Officer
CMO: Gregory R. Pittman, M.D., Chief of Staff
CIO: Frank Evans, Director Information Services
CHR: Rebecca Hert, Director Human Resources
Web address: www.southcresthospital.com
**Control:** Corporation, Investor–owned, for–profit **Service:** General Medical and Surgical

**Staffed Beds:** 160 **Admissions:** 7694 **Census:** 86 **Outpatient Visits:** 83740 **Births:** 1667 **Total Expense ($000):** 97318 **Payroll Expense ($000):** 34694 **Personnel:** 663

☐ **SOUTHWESTERN REGIONAL MEDICAL CENTER (370190)**, 10109 East 79th Street, Zip 74133–4564; tel. 918/286–5000 **A**1 2 10 **F**3 15 29 30 31 33 34 35 36 40 44 45 46 47 48 49 50 57 58 59 63 64 68 70 74 75 77 78 81 82 84 85 86 87 93 97 100 104 107 108 110 111 112 113 116 117 118 119 120 122 123 128 129 131 134 144 145 147 **S** Cancer Treatment Centers of America, Schaumburg, IL
Primary Contact: Steve Mackin, President and Chief Executive Officer
CFO: David Hedges, Chief Financial Officer
CMO: James P. Flynn, M.D., President Medical Staff
CHR: Wendy Whelan, Director Talent
Web address: www.cancercenter.com
**Control:** Corporation, Investor–owned, for–profit **Service:** Cancer

**Staffed Beds:** 43 **Admissions:** 845 **Census:** 14 **Outpatient Visits:** 62710 **Births:** 0 **Personnel:** 760

✠ **ST. JOHN MEDICAL CENTER (370114)**, 1923 South Utica Avenue, Zip 74104–6502; tel. 918/744–2345 **A**1 2 3 5 9 10 **F**3 8 9 11 12 13 14 15 17 18 19 20 22 24 26 28 29 30 31 34 35 37 40 43 45 46 47 48 49 50 51 53 54 56 57 58 59 60 61 65 66 68 70 71 72 73 74 75 76 77 78 79 80 81 82 84 85 86 87 88 89 90 93 94 96 97 100 104 107 108 110 111 113 114 115 116 117 118 119 120 122 123 125 128 129 130 131 134 137 140 142 144 145 146 147 **P**6 7 8 **S** Marian Health System, Tulsa, OK
Primary Contact: S. Charles Anderson, President and Chief Executive Officer
CFO: Lex S. Anderson, Chief Financial Officer
CMO: William Allred, M.D., Vice President Medical Affairs
CIO: Mike Reeves, Vice President
CHR: Page Bachman, Corporate Vice President
Web address: www.sjmc.org
**Control:** Church–operated, Nongovernment, not–for profit **Service:** General Medical and Surgical

**Staffed Beds:** 547 **Admissions:** 27564 **Census:** 398 **Outpatient Visits:** 395031 **Births:** 1907 **Total Expense ($000):** 432630 **Payroll Expense ($000):** 149307 **Personnel:** 3136

✠ **TULSA SPINE AND SPECIALTY HOSPITAL (370216)**, 6901 South Olympia Avenue, Zip 74132–1843; tel. 918/388–5701, (Nonreporting) **A**1 10
Primary Contact: Terry L. Woodbeck, Administrator
CFO: Thom Biby, Chief Financial Officer
CMO: David Fell, M.D., Chief Medical Officer
Web address: www.tulsaspinehospital.com
**Control:** Corporation, Investor–owned, for–profit **Service:** General Medical and Surgical

**Staffed Beds:** 21

### VINITA—Craig County

★ **CRAIG GENERAL HOSPITAL (370065)**, 735 North Foreman Street, Zip 74301–1418, Mailing Address: P.O. Box 326, Zip 74301–0326; tel. 918/256–7551 **A**9 10 20 **F**3 11 13 15 29 30 31 34 35 40 53 56 57 59 64 65 69 76 81 85 87 89 98 103 104 107 110 111 114 118 126 127 129 130 131 132 134 143 145 147
Primary Contact: B. Joe Gunn, Ed.D., FACHE, Interim Chief Executive Officer
CFO: James Brasel, Chief Financial Officer
CMO: Ed Allensworth, M.D., Medical Director
CIO: Steven Chase, Chief Information Officer
CHR: Marsha Emerson, Chief Support Officer
Web address: www.craiggeneralhospital.com
**Control:** Hospital district or authority, Government, nonfederal **Service:** General Medical and Surgical

**Staffed Beds:** 56 **Admissions:** 1898 **Census:** 25 **Outpatient Visits:** 34189 **Births:** 76 **Total Expense ($000):** 23478 **Payroll Expense ($000):** 10929 **Personnel:** 241

**OKLAHOMA FORENSIC CENTER**, 24800 South 4420 Road, Zip 74301, Mailing Address: P.O. Box 69, Zip 74301–0069; tel. 918/256–7841 **F**30 87 98 129 **P**1 **S** Oklahoma Department of Mental Health and Substance Abuse Services, Oklahoma City, OK
Primary Contact: William T. Burkett, Chief Executive Officer
CFO: Miriam Harris, Director Finance
CHR: Julie Jacobs, Director Human Resources
**Control:** State–Government, nonfederal **Service:** Psychiatric

**Staffed Beds:** 200 **Admissions:** 217 **Census:** 155 **Outpatient Visits:** 0 **Births:** 0 **Total Expense ($000):** 20362 **Payroll Expense ($000):** 9395 **Personnel:** 275

### WAGONER—Wagoner County

**WAGONER COMMUNITY HOSPITAL (370166)**, 1200 West Cherokee Street, Zip 74467–4624, Mailing Address: P.O. Box 407, Zip 74477–0407; tel. 918/485–5514 **A**9 10 **F**3 11 15 29 30 34 40 41 45 49 50 56 57 59 64 65 68 70 74 75 79 81 82 85 87 89 98 102 103 104 107 108 113 118 129 134 145 147
Primary Contact: Jimmy Leopard, FACHE, Chief Executive Officer
CFO: Rod Shook, Chief Financial Officer
CMO: John Perry, M.D., Chief of Staff
CHR: Barnetta Pofahl, Director Human Resources
Web address: www.wagonerhospital.com
**Control:** Hospital district or authority, Government, nonfederal **Service:** General Medical and Surgical

**Staffed Beds:** 100 **Admissions:** 2999 **Census:** 34 **Outpatient Visits:** 20329 **Births:** 0 **Total Expense ($000):** 13907 **Payroll Expense ($000):** 6827 **Personnel:** 155

### WATONGA—Blaine County

★ **WATONGA MUNICIPAL HOSPITAL (371302)**, 500 North Nash Boulevard, Zip 73772–0370, Mailing Address: Box 370, Zip 73772–0370; tel. 580/623–7211 **A**9 10 18 **F**7 11 29 30 40 56 93 107 118 132
Primary Contact: Cindy Carmichael, Interim Chief Executive Officer
CFO: Gene Kaberline, Chief Financial Officer
CIO: Alisha Glazier, Compliance Officer and Director Health Information Management
CHR: Tim Prepieri, Director Human Resources
Web address: www.watongahospital.com
**Control:** City–Government, nonfederal **Service:** General Medical and Surgical

**Staffed Beds:** 17 **Admissions:** 509 **Census:** 4 **Outpatient Visits:** 7728 **Births:** 0 **Total Expense ($000):** 3679 **Payroll Expense ($000):** 2443 **Personnel:** 46

### WAURIKA—Jefferson County

★ **JEFFERSON COUNTY HOSPITAL (371311)**, Highway 70 and 81, Zip 73573–3075, Mailing Address: P.O. Box 90, Zip 73573–0090; tel. 580/228–2344 **A**9 10 18 **F**11 35 40 107 118 126 132 **P**6
Primary Contact: Jane McDowell, FACHE, Administrator
CFO: Richard Tallon, Chief Financial Officer
CMO: Rob Linzman, D.O., Chief of Staff
CIO: Nikki McGahey, Information Officer
Web address: www.jeffersoncountyhospital.net
**Control:** Hospital district or authority, Government, nonfederal **Service:** General Medical and Surgical

**Staffed Beds:** 25 **Admissions:** 282 **Census:** 3 **Outpatient Visits:** 12273 **Births:** 0 **Total Expense ($000):** 3173 **Payroll Expense ($000):** 1779 **Personnel:** 40

### WEATHERFORD—Custer County

★ **WEATHERFORD REGIONAL HOSPITAL (371323)**, 3701 East Main Street, Zip 73096; tel. 580/772–5551 **A**9 10 18 **F**3 11 13 15 29 34 40 45 64 68 75 76 77 81 86 87 93 107 111 114 118 129 132 134 143 145 146 147 **P**6
Primary Contact: Debbie Howe, Chief Executive Officer
CFO: Stephanie Helton, Chief Financial Officer
CMO: Michael Aaron, M.D., Chief of Staff
CIO: Claudia Wright, Director Health Information Management
CHR: Tawnya Paden, Director Human Resources
Web address: www.weatherfordhospital.com
**Control:** Hospital district or authority, Government, nonfederal **Service:** General Medical and Surgical

**Staffed Beds:** 25 **Admissions:** 947 **Census:** 9 **Outpatient Visits:** 24174 **Births:** 234 **Total Expense ($000):** 17096 **Payroll Expense ($000):** 6749 **Personnel:** 152

---

**Hospital, Medicare Provider Number, Address, Telephone, Approval, Facility, and Physician Codes, Health Care System**

★ American Hospital Association (AHA) membership
☐ The Joint Commission accreditation      ◇ DNV Healthcare Inc. accreditation
○ American Osteopathic Association (AOA) accreditation
△ Commission on Accreditation of Rehabilitation Facilities (CARF) accreditation

**OK**

### WILBURTON—Latimer County

**LATIMER COUNTY GENERAL HOSPITAL (370072)**, 806 Highway 2 North,
Zip 74578–3698; tel. 918/465–2391 **A**9 10 **F**3 30 40 43 62 107 108 118
145 **P**5
Primary Contact: Dody Goad, Administrator
CMO: Richard Valbuena, M.D., Medical Director
**Control:** County–Government, nonfederal **Service:** General Medical and Surgical

**Staffed Beds:** 33 **Admissions:** 581 **Census:** 5 **Outpatient Visits:** 11597
**Births:** 0 **Total Expense ($000):** 7241 **Payroll Expense ($000):** 3816
**Personnel:** 77

### WOODWARD—Woodward County

☒ **WOODWARD REGIONAL HOSPITAL (370002)**, 900 17th Street,
Zip 73801–2448; tel. 580/256–5511 **A**1 9 10 20 **F**13 15 29 30 31 32 34 35
40 43 45 50 57 59 64 68 69 70 75 76 77 79 81 85 93 107 108 110 111
113 118 123 128 129 130 132 134 145 **P**6 **S** Community Health Systems,
Inc., Franklin, TN
Primary Contact: David T. Wallace, Chief Executive Officer
CFO: Tom Early, Chief Financial Officer
Web address: www.woodwardhospital.com
**Control:** Corporation, Investor–owned, for–profit **Service:** General Medical and
Surgical

**Staffed Beds:** 44 **Admissions:** 1417 **Census:** 13 **Outpatient Visits:** 34839
**Births:** 161 **Total Expense ($000):** 24429 **Payroll Expense ($000):** 9077
**Personnel:** 202

### YUKON—Canadian County

☒ **INTEGRIS CANADIAN VALLEY HOSPITAL (370211)**, 1201 Health Center
Parkway, Zip 73099–6381; tel. 405/717–6800 **A**1 9 10 **F**3 13 15 29 30 40 45
46 49 59 60 64 68 70 76 79 81 87 93 97 107 108 110 111 117 118 129
134 145 147 **S** INTEGRIS Health, Oklahoma City, OK
Primary Contact: Rex Van Meter, President
CFO: Cindy White, CPA, Assistant Vice President and Chief Financial Officer
CMO: Glen Hyde, M.D., Chief of Staff
CHR: Kimberly Brown, Human Resources Recruiter Generalist
Web address: www.integris–health.com
**Control:** Other not–for–profit (including NFP Corporation) **Service:** General
Medical and Surgical

**Staffed Beds:** 75 **Admissions:** 3146 **Census:** 28 **Outpatient Visits:** 56153
**Births:** 902 **Total Expense ($000):** 56186 **Payroll Expense ($000):** 23036
**Personnel:** 286

*Many Facility Codes have changed. Please refer to the AHA Guide Code Chart.*
© 2012 AHA Guide

# OREGON

## ALBANY—Linn County

★ **SAMARITAN ALBANY GENERAL HOSPITAL (380022)**, 1046 West Sixth Avenue, Zip 97321–1999; tel. 541/812–4000 **A**9 10 21 **F**3 11 12 13 15 18 28 29 30 31 34 35 36 40 43 45 47 49 53 57 59 63 64 70 75 76 78 79 81 84 85 86 87 89 93 97 107 111 113 116 118 128 129 131 134 144 145 146 147 **P**6 **S** Samaritan Health Services, Corvallis, OR
Primary Contact: David G. Triebes, Chief Executive Officer
CFO: Daniel B. Smith, Vice President Finance
Web address: www.samhealth.org
**Control:** Other not–for–profit (including NFP Corporation) **Service:** General Medical and Surgical

**Staffed Beds:** 70 **Admissions:** 3446 **Census:** 28 **Outpatient Visits:** 97334 **Births:** 623 **Total Expense ($000):** 105886 **Payroll Expense ($000):** 43573 **Personnel:** 770

## ASHLAND—Jackson County

★ **ASHLAND COMMUNITY HOSPITAL (380005)**, 280 Maple Street, Zip 97520–1593; tel. 541/201–4000 **A**9 10 21 **F**3 8 11 13 15 29 30 34 35 36 40 43 48 49 50 54 62 63 64 65 68 70 75 76 79 81 82 84 85 86 87 93 97 107 110 113 118 129 131 144 145 146 147 **P**6
Primary Contact: Mark E. Marchetti, President and Chief Executive Officer
CFO: Arebi Garsa, Chief Financial Officer
CMO: Miriam Soriano, M.D., Chief Medical Staff
CHR: Karen Herwig, Vice President Human Resources
Web address: www.ashlandhospital.org
**Control:** Other not–for–profit (including NFP Corporation) **Service:** General Medical and Surgical

**Staffed Beds:** 36 **Admissions:** 1544 **Census:** 14 **Outpatient Visits:** 58697 **Births:** 340 **Total Expense ($000):** 49069 **Payroll Expense ($000):** 20493 **Personnel:** 259

## ASTORIA—Clatsop County

☒ **COLUMBIA MEMORIAL HOSPITAL (381320)**, 2111 Exchange Street, Zip 97103–3329; tel. 503/325–4321 **A**1 9 10 18 **F**3 8 11 13 15 18 19 28 29 30 31 34 35 36 40 41 42 43 44 46 50 51 53 57 58 59 62 63 64 68 70 75 76 77 78 79 81 85 86 87 89 93 97 107 108 110 111 113 114 118 129 130 131 133 134 142 143 145 146 147 **P**6
Primary Contact: Erik Thorsen, Chief Executive Officer
CFO: Guy Rivers, Chief Financial Officer
CMO: Robert Holland, M.D., President Professional Staff
CHR: Cheryl Martin, Manager Human Resources
Web address: www.columbiamemorial.org
**Control:** Other not–for–profit (including NFP Corporation) **Service:** General Medical and Surgical

**Staffed Beds:** 25 **Admissions:** 1651 **Census:** 12 **Outpatient Visits:** 114000 **Births:** 343 **Total Expense ($000):** 59222 **Payroll Expense ($000):** 26140 **Personnel:** 430

## BAKER CITY—Baker County

☒ **SAINT ALPHONSUS MEDICAL CENTER – BAKER CITY (381315)**, 3325 Pocahontas Road, Zip 97814–1464; tel. 541/523–6461, (Total facility includes 40 beds in nursing home–type unit) **A**1 9 10 18 **F**3 11 13 15 29 34 35 37 40 43 44 45 57 59 64 67 70 76 77 79 81 82 85 91 93 107 110 113 118 127 128 130 132 142 145 146 147 **S** Trinity Health, Novi, MI
Primary Contact: H. Ray Gibbons, FACHE, Chief Executive Officer
CFO: Robert D. Wehling, Interim Chief Financial Officer
CHR: Jerry Nickell, Vice President Human Resource and Mission
Web address: www.stelizabethhealth.com
**Control:** Other not–for–profit (including NFP Corporation) **Service:** General Medical and Surgical

**Staffed Beds:** 65 **Admissions:** 1149 **Census:** 40 **Outpatient Visits:** 32105 **Births:** 125 **Total Expense ($000):** 25872 **Payroll Expense ($000):** 11814 **Personnel:** 229

**ST. ELIZABETH HEALTH SERVICES** See Saint Alphonsus Medical Center – Baker City

## BANDON—Coos County

★ **SOUTHERN COOS HOSPITAL AND HEALTH CENTER (381304)**, 900 11th Street S.E., Zip 97411–9114; tel. 541/347–2426 **A**9 10 18 **F**1 3 15 35 40 45 50 57 65 67 68 75 81 82 85 87 107 110 113 118 127 129 131 132 134 147
Primary Contact: James A. Wathen, Chief Executive Officer
CFO: Alan Dow, Interim Chief Financial Officer
Web address: www.southerncoos.org
**Control:** Hospital district or authority, Government, nonfederal **Service:** General Medical and Surgical

**Staffed Beds:** 19 **Admissions:** 414 **Census:** 3 **Outpatient Visits:** 12424 **Births:** 0 **Total Expense ($000):** 15709 **Payroll Expense ($000):** 7772 **Personnel:** 148

## BEND—Deschutes County

☒ **ST. CHARLES MEDICAL CENTER – BEND (380047)**, 2500 N.E. Neff Road, Zip 97701–6015; tel. 541/382–4321 **A**1 2 5 9 10 19 **F**3 8 11 12 13 18 20 22 24 26 28 29 30 31 34 35 36 37 38 40 43 45 49 50 51 57 59 60 62 63 64 65 67 68 70 72 74 75 76 77 78 79 81 82 84 85 86 89 90 93 98 100 101 102 104 106 107 108 111 113 114 115 116 117 118 120 122 123 128 129 131 134 144 145 147 **S** St. Charles Health System, Inc., Bend, OR
Primary Contact: Jay Henry, Chief Executive Officer
COO: Rick Martin, Vice President of Ancillary and Support Services
CFO: Karen Shepard, Senior Vice President Finance and Chief Financial Officer
CMO: Michel Boileau, M.D., Chief Clinical Officer
CIO: William Winnenberg, Chief Information Officer
CHR: Rebecca Morgan, Senior Director Human Resources
CNO: Timothy D. Eixenberger, R.N., Chief Nursing Officer
Web address: www.scmc.org
**Control:** Other not–for–profit (including NFP Corporation) **Service:** General Medical and Surgical

**Staffed Beds:** 261 **Admissions:** 14711 **Census:** 162 **Outpatient Visits:** 174896 **Births:** 1663 **Total Expense ($000):** 400574 **Payroll Expense ($000):** 151213 **Personnel:** 2002

## BURNS—Harney County

★ **HARNEY DISTRICT HOSPITAL (381307)**, 557 West Washington Street, Zip 97720–1497; tel. 541/573–7281 **A**9 10 18 **F**3 7 13 15 29 31 34 35 40 43 45 57 59 64 65 70 71 75 76 78 81 82 85 102 107 111 113 118 128 131 132 145 **P**5
Primary Contact: Jim Bishop, Chief Executive Officer
CMO: Kevin Johnston, M.D., Chief Medical Staff
CHR: Sammie Masterson, Chief Human Resources Officer
Web address: www.harneydh.com
**Control:** Hospital district or authority, Government, nonfederal **Service:** General Medical and Surgical

**Staffed Beds:** 20 **Admissions:** 444 **Census:** 5 **Outpatient Visits:** 18544 **Births:** 57 **Total Expense ($000):** 14276 **Payroll Expense ($000):** 5800 **Personnel:** 114

## CLACKAMAS—Clackamas County

☒ **SUNNYSIDE MEDICAL CENTER (380091)**, 10180 S.E. Sunnyside Road, Zip 97015–9303; tel. 503/652–2880 **A**1 2 10 **F**3 11 12 13 17 18 20 22 24 26 30 31 34 37 40 45 46 47 49 51 60 61 64 68 70 74 75 76 77 78 79 81 84 85 86 87 93 94 97 102 107 108 111 113 114 118 129 140 145 146 147 **P**6 **S** Kaiser Foundation Hospitals, Oakland, CA
Primary Contact: Susan Mullaney, Administrator
COO: Gary Petersen, Chief Operating Officer
CFO: Rolf Norman, Chief Financial Officer
CMO: Rick Olson, M.D., Chief of Staff
CIO: Mark A. Burmester, Vice President Strategy and Communications
CHR: Rich Smith, Vice President Human Resources
Web address: www.kaiserpermanente.org
**Control:** Other not–for–profit (including NFP Corporation) **Service:** General Medical and Surgical

**Staffed Beds:** 283 **Admissions:** 19096 **Census:** 190 **Outpatient Visits:** 64592 **Births:** 1868 **Total Expense ($000):** 388486 **Payroll Expense ($000):** 139491 **Personnel:** 2145

**OR**

## COOS BAY—Coos County

✠ **BAY AREA HOSPITAL (380090)**, 1775 Thompson Road, Zip 97420–2198; tel. 541/269–8111 **A**1 2 9 10 **F**3 11 12 13 15 18 28 31 34 35 37 40 43 45 46 50 51 54 57 59 62 68 70 72 73 74 75 76 77 78 79 81 83 84 85 89 91 92 93 98 99 100 101 102 104 107 108 110 111 116 117 118 119 120 122 128 129 131 134 141 145 147
Primary Contact: Paul Janke, FACHE, President and Chief Executive Officer
CMO: Bill Moriarty, M.D., Chief Medical Officer
CIO: Bob Adams, Director Information Services
CHR: Suzie Q. McDaniel, Director Human Resources
Web address: www.bayareahospital.org
**Control:** Hospital district or authority, Government, nonfederal **Service:** General Medical and Surgical

| | |
|---|---|
| **Staffed Beds:** 127 **Admissions:** 6195 **Census:** 63 **Outpatient Visits:** 88148 **Births:** 624 **Total Expense ($000):** 110175 **Payroll Expense ($000):** 54824 **Personnel:** 819 | |

## COQUILLE—Coos County

★ **COQUILLE VALLEY HOSPITAL (381312)**, 940 East Fifth Street, Zip 97423–1699; tel. 541/396–3101 **A**9 10 18 **F**3 11 13 15 29 34 35 40 43 45 46 50 57 59 62 70 75 76 79 81 85 86 87 107 113 117 118 131 132 134 147 **P**6
Primary Contact: Dennis G. Zielinski, Chief Executive Officer and Administrator
CFO: Gail Ludington, Chief Financial Officer
CMO: James Sinnott, M.D., Chief Medical Staff
CIO: Curt Carpenter, Manager Information Technology
CHR: Monte Johnston, Manager Human Resources
Web address: www.cvhospital.org
**Control:** Hospital district or authority, Government, nonfederal **Service:** General Medical and Surgical

| | |
|---|---|
| **Staffed Beds:** 25 **Admissions:** 516 **Census:** 4 **Outpatient Visits:** 21558 **Births:** 21 **Total Expense ($000):** 12111 **Payroll Expense ($000):** 6024 **Personnel:** 110 | |

## CORVALLIS—Benton County

★ **GOOD SAMARITAN REGIONAL MEDICAL CENTER (380014)**, 3600 N.W. Samaritan Drive, Zip 97330–3737, Mailing Address: P.O. Box 1068, Zip 97339–1068; tel. 541/768–5111 **A**2 9 10 12 13 19 21 **F**3 5 8 11 12 13 15 18 20 22 24 26 28 29 30 31 34 36 37 40 43 46 47 49 50 53 54 57 59 60 62 64 68 70 73 74 75 76 77 78 79 81 82 84 85 86 87 89 93 97 98 100 101 102 104 107 108 110 111 113 114 117 118 119 120 122 123 125 128 129 130 131 134 143 144 145 146 147 **P**6 **S** Samaritan Health Services, Corvallis, OR
Primary Contact: Steven W. Jasperson, Chief Executive Officer
CFO: Daniel B. Smith, Vice President Finance
CIO: Bob Power, Vice President Information Services
CHR: Sheryl Helms, Vice President Human Resources
Web address: www.samhealth.org
**Control:** Other not–for–profit (including NFP Corporation) **Service:** General Medical and Surgical

| | |
|---|---|
| **Staffed Beds:** 165 **Admissions:** 9626 **Census:** 116 **Outpatient Visits:** 181258 **Births:** 1063 **Total Expense ($000):** 314986 **Payroll Expense ($000):** 130113 **Personnel:** 1511 | |

## COTTAGE GROVE—Lane County

★ **COTTAGE GROVE COMMUNITY HOSPITAL (381301)**, 1515 Village Drive, Zip 97424–9700; tel. 541/942–0511 **A**9 10 18 **F**3 11 15 29 30 32 34 35 40 50 56 57 58 59 64 65 66 68 75 82 84 93 97 107 110 114 118 129 131 145 146 **P**6 **S** PeaceHealth, Bellevue, WA
Primary Contact: MaryAnne McMurren, R.N., Administrator and Chief Executive Officer
Web address: www.peacehealth.org
**Control:** Church–operated, Nongovernment, not–for profit **Service:** General Medical and Surgical

| | |
|---|---|
| **Staffed Beds:** 14 **Admissions:** 413 **Census:** 3 **Outpatient Visits:** 37997 **Births:** 0 **Total Expense ($000):** 26484 **Payroll Expense ($000):** 9169 **Personnel:** 138 | |

## DALLAS—Polk County

**WEST VALLEY HOSPITAL (381308)**, 525 S.E. Washington Street, Zip 97338–2899, Mailing Address: P.O. Box 378, Zip 97338–0378; tel. 503/623–8301 **A**9 10 18 **F**3 11 15 35 40 42 43 50 59 64 75 79 81 85 93 107 108 110 111 113 118 130 131 132 142 145 147 **P**6 **S** Salem Health, Salem, OR
Primary Contact: Robert C. Brannigan, Administrator
COO: Robert C. Brannigan, Administrator
CFO: Aaron Crane, Chief Financial Officer
CMO: David Holloway, M.D., Chief Medical Officer
CIO: Ken Kudla, Chief Information Officer
CHR: Beverly Bow, Vice President Human Resources
Web address: www.westvalleyhospital.org
**Control:** Other not–for–profit (including NFP Corporation) **Service:** General Medical and Surgical

| | |
|---|---|
| **Staffed Beds:** 6 **Admissions:** 113 **Census:** 1 **Outpatient Visits:** 73158 **Total Expense ($000):** 19501 **Payroll Expense ($000):** 9255 **Personnel:** 108 | |

## ENTERPRISE—Wallowa County

★ **WALLOWA MEMORIAL HOSPITAL (381306)**, 601 Medical Parkway, Zip 97828–1167; tel. 541/426–3111, (Total facility includes 32 beds in nursing home–type unit) **A**3 5 9 10 18 **F**3 7 11 13 15 29 30 31 34 35 40 43 45 46 56 57 59 62 64 67 68 75 76 78 79 81 82 85 93 102 107 110 113 118 127 128 130 131 132 134 142 147
Primary Contact: David L. Harman, Chief Executive Officer
CFO: Lexi M. Fields, Chief Financial Officer
CMO: Kirsten Caine, M.D., Chief Medical Staff
CIO: John Straughan, Director Information Technology
CHR: Linda Childers, Director Human Resources
Web address: www.wchcd.org
**Control:** Hospital district or authority, Government, nonfederal **Service:** General Medical and Surgical

| | |
|---|---|
| **Staffed Beds:** 57 **Admissions:** 675 **Census:** 25 **Outpatient Visits:** 18866 **Births:** 50 **Total Expense ($000):** 16564 **Payroll Expense ($000):** 7438 **Personnel:** 130 | |

## EUGENE—Lane County

✠ △ **SACRED HEART MEDICAL CENTER (380033)**, 1255 Hilyard Street, Zip 97401–3700, Mailing Address: P.O. Box 10905, Zip 97440–0905; tel. 541/686–7300 **A**1 7 9 10 **F**3 11 29 30 31 34 35 40 44 50 62 63 64 68 70 75 82 84 85 90 91 92 93 98 99 100 101 102 103 104 107 113 118 122 129 131 145 147 **P**6 **S** PeaceHealth, Bellevue, WA
Primary Contact: Thomas A. Reitinger, Interim Chief Executive Officer
CFO: Wendy Apland, Interim Chief Financial Officer
CMO: Bill Moshofsky, M.D., Chief of Staff
CIO: Don McMillan, Chief Information Officer
CHR: Craig J. Mills, Vice President Human Resources
Web address: www.peacehealth.org
**Control:** Church–operated, Nongovernment, not–for profit **Service:** General Medical and Surgical

| | |
|---|---|
| **Staffed Beds:** 93 **Admissions:** 2661 **Census:** 53 **Outpatient Visits:** 107436 **Births:** 0 **Total Expense ($000):** 91953 **Payroll Expense ($000):** 39971 **Personnel:** 1124 | |

**SERENITY LANE**, 616 East 16th, Zip 97401–4357; tel. 541/687–1110, (Nonreporting)
Primary Contact: Peter J. Asmuth, Executive Director and Administrator
CMO: Ron Schwerzler, M.D., Director Medical Services
CIO: Josh Bolton, Chief Information Officer
Web address: www.serenitylane.org
**Control:** Other not–for–profit (including NFP Corporation) **Service:** Alcoholism and other chemical dependency

| | |
|---|---|
| **Staffed Beds:** 55 | |

## FLORENCE—Lane County

★ **PEACE HARBOR HOSPITAL (381316)**, 400 Ninth Street, Zip 97439–7398; tel. 541/997–8412 **A**9 10 18 **F**11 13 15 28 29 30 34 35 40 43 45 50 57 59 62 63 64 68 70 76 77 79 81 85 93 97 107 108 110 111 113 117 118 131 132 134 145 146 147 **P**6 **S** PeaceHealth, Bellevue, WA
Primary Contact: Rick Yecny, Chief Executive Officer
CMO: Ron Shearer, M.D., Regional Medical Director
CIO: Ginni Boughal, Director Health Information and Information Technology
CHR: Don Bourland, Vice President Human Resources
Web address: www.peacehealth.org
**Control:** Church–operated, Nongovernment, not–for profit **Service:** General Medical and Surgical

| | |
|---|---|
| **Staffed Beds:** 21 **Admissions:** 1029 **Census:** 9 **Outpatient Visits:** 87932 **Births:** 58 **Total Expense ($000):** 55425 **Payroll Expense ($000):** 30146 **Personnel:** 438 | |

## FOREST GROVE—Washington County

**TUALITY FOREST GROVE HOSPITAL** See Tuality Healthcare, Hillsboro

## GOLD BEACH—Curry County

★ **CURRY GENERAL HOSPITAL (381322)**, 94220 Fourth Street, Zip 97444–9990; tel. 541/247–6621 **A**9 10 18 **F**3 10 11 13 15 28 29 34 35 40 43 56 57 59 64 65 70 75 76 79 81 82 98 105 107 113 118 126 132 134 143 145 146 147
Primary Contact: William I. McMillan, FACHE, Chief Executive Officer
COO: A. Alexander Gorman, Director Operations
CFO: Mark Sayler, Chief Financial Officer
CIO: Kwang Veloso, Director Information Systems
CHR: Terri Tomberlin, Manager Human Resources
Web address: www.curryhealthnetwork.com
**Control:** Hospital district or authority, Government, nonfederal **Service:** General Medical and Surgical

| | |
|---|---|
| **Staffed Beds:** 22 **Admissions:** 750 **Census:** 8 **Outpatient Visits:** 49455 **Births:** 65 **Total Expense ($000):** 23686 **Payroll Expense ($000):** 11914 **Personnel:** 189 | |

*Many Facility Codes have changed. Please refer to the AHA Guide Code Chart.* © 2012 AHA Guide

## GRANTS PASS—Josephine County

★ **THREE RIVERS MEDICAL CENTER (380002)**, 500 S.W. Ramsey Avenue, Zip 97527; tel. 541/472–7000 **A**9 10 21 **F**11 13 15 20 21 22 23 28 29 30 31 34 35 40 43 45 46 50 57 59 64 65 70 75 76 78 81 87 93 102 107 108 110 111 117 118 121 129 131 142 145 146 147 **P**6 **S** Asante Health System, Medford, OR
Primary Contact: Win Howard, Chief Executive Officer
COO: David Kinyon, Vice President of Operations and Outpatient Services
CFO: Marvin Haas, Chief Administration and Finance Officer
CMO: Kenneth Lindsey, M.D., Vice President of Medical Affairs
CIO: Mark Hetz, Chief Information Officer
CHR: Gregg Edwards, Chief People Officer
CNO: Kristin Gillen, R.N., Vice President of Patient Care Services
Web address: www.asante.org
**Control:** Other not–for–profit (including NFP Corporation) **Service:** General Medical and Surgical

**Staffed Beds:** 107 **Admissions:** 6759 **Census:** 60 **Outpatient Visits:** 206922 **Births:** 705 **Total Expense ($000):** 121959 **Payroll Expense ($000):** 44101 **Personnel:** 622

## GRESHAM—Multnomah County

⊞ **LEGACY MOUNT HOOD MEDICAL CENTER (380025)**, 24800 S.E. Stark, Zip 97030–0154; tel. 503/667–1122 **A**1 2 9 10 **F**3 11 13 15 18 20 22 26 28 29 30 31 32 35 38 40 44 45 46 49 50 56 57 59 60 64 68 70 74 75 76 77 78 79 81 85 86 87 93 100 101 102 107 108 110 111 113 117 118 119 120 128 129 131 145 146 147 **P**8 **S** Legacy Health, Portland, OR
Primary Contact: Gretchen Nichols, R.N., Chief Administrative Officer
COO: Mike Newcomb, D.O., Senior Vice President and Chief Operating Officer
CMO: Jack Cioffi, M.D., Senior Vice President and Chief Medical Officer
CIO: Glen Lutz, Senior Vice President and Chief Information Officer
CHR: Sonja Steves, Senior Vice President Human Resources
Web address: www.legacyhealth.org
**Control:** Other not–for–profit (including NFP Corporation) **Service:** General Medical and Surgical

**Staffed Beds:** 90 **Admissions:** 4990 **Census:** 47 **Outpatient Visits:** 76769 **Births:** 992 **Total Expense ($000):** 88795 **Payroll Expense ($000):** 34008 **Personnel:** 478

## HEPPNER—Morrow County

**PIONEER MEMORIAL HOSPITAL (381310)**, 564 East Pioneer Drive, Zip 97836, Mailing Address: P.O. Box 9, Zip 97836; tel. 541/676–9133 **A**9 10 18 **F**3 7 17 34 35 40 45 50 57 59 62 63 64 66 68 69 75 97 107 118 126 132 142 147 **P**6
Primary Contact: Michael Blauer, Administrator
CFO: Nicole Mahoney, Chief Financial Officer
CIO: Shawn Cutsforth, Information Systems Officer
CHR: Patti Allstott, Administrative Coordinator Human Resources and Grant Writer
Web address: www.morrowcountyhealthdistrict.org
**Control:** Hospital district or authority, Government, nonfederal **Service:** General Medical and Surgical

**Staffed Beds:** 21 **Admissions:** 104 **Census:** 7 **Outpatient Visits:** 5565 **Births:** 0 **Total Expense ($000):** 7125 **Payroll Expense ($000):** 4010 **Personnel:** 57

## HERMISTON—Umatilla County

★ **GOOD SHEPHERD HEALTH CARE SYSTEM (381325)**, 610 N.W. 11th Street, Zip 97838–9696; tel. 541/667–3400 **A**9 10 18 21 **F**3 8 11 13 15 28 29 30 31 34 35 37 40 43 45 50 53 57 59 62 63 64 65 68 70 75 76 77 78 79 81 84 85 86 89 93 97 107 108 110 111 113 118 126 128 129 130 131 132 134 140 142 145 146 147 **P**3 4 7
Primary Contact: Dennis E. Burke, President and Chief Executive Officer
COO: David T. Hughes, FACHE, Senior Vice President Operations and Chief Operating Officer
CFO: Jan D. Peter, Vice President Fiscal Services and Chief Financial Officer
CMO: Richard Flaiz, M.D., President Medical Staff
CIO: Rob Rizk, Information Technology Director
CHR: Kelly Sanders, Vice President Human Resources
CNO: Theresa Brock, Vice President Nursing
Web address: www.gshealth.org
**Control:** Other not–for–profit (including NFP Corporation) **Service:** General Medical and Surgical

**Staffed Beds:** 25 **Admissions:** 2242 **Census:** 16 **Outpatient Visits:** 65019 **Births:** 558 **Total Expense ($000):** 54520 **Payroll Expense ($000):** 23512 **Personnel:** 377

## HILLSBORO—Washington County

⊞ **TUALITY HEALTHCARE (380021)**, 335 S.E. Eighth Avenue, Zip 97123–4246; tel. 503/681–1111, (Includes TUALITY COMMUNITY HOSPITAL, 335 S.E. Eighth Avenue, Zip 97123, Mailing Address: P.O. Box 309, Zip 97123; tel. 503/681–1111; TUALITY FOREST GROVE HOSPITAL, 1809 Maple Street, Forest Grove, Zip 97116–1995; tel. 503/357–2173) **A**1 5 9 10 **F**3 11 13 15 17 18 20 22 24 26 28 29 30 31 32 34 35 36 37 40 44 45 47 49 50 53 54 56 57 59 62 64 68 70 71 74 75 76 77 78 79 80 81 82 85 86 87 93 97 98 100 103 104 107 108 111 113 117 118 128 129 130 131 134 142 143 144 145 146 147 **P**1 6
Primary Contact: Richard Stenson, President and Chief Executive Officer
COO: Manuel S. Berman, Administrator and Chief Operating Officer
CFO: Tim Fleischmann, Chief Financial Officer
CMO: Darell Lumaco, M.D., Chief of Staff
CIO: John Stoneburg, Chief Information Officer
CHR: Kathy Ratliffe, Director Human Resources
Web address: www.tuality.com
**Control:** Other not–for–profit (including NFP Corporation) **Service:** General Medical and Surgical

**Staffed Beds:** 148 **Admissions:** 5162 **Census:** 62 **Outpatient Visits:** 252554 **Births:** 1096 **Total Expense ($000):** 160671 **Payroll Expense ($000):** 75032 **Personnel:** 1130

## HOOD RIVER—Hood River County

⊞ **PROVIDENCE HOOD RIVER MEMORIAL HOSPITAL (381318)**, 811 13th Street, Zip 97031–1204, Mailing Address: P.O. Box 149, Zip 97031–0149; tel. 541/386–3911 **A**1 9 10 18 **F**2 3 5 8 9 10 11 12 13 15 28 29 30 31 34 35 36 40 43 45 47 48 53 54 56 57 59 60 64 65 68 70 71 75 76 77 79 81 85 86 92 97 99 100 101 102 104 107 108 110 111 113 117 118 124 128 131 132 133 134 142 145 146 147 **P**6 **S** Providence Health & Services, Renton, WA
Primary Contact: Edward E. Freysinger, Chief Executive Officer
CFO: Ron Guth, Chief Financial Officer
CHR: Catherine Bourgault, Director Human Resources
Web address: www.providence.org/hoodriver
**Control:** Church–operated, Nongovernment, not–for profit **Service:** General Medical and Surgical

**Staffed Beds:** 25 **Admissions:** 1604 **Census:** 12 **Outpatient Visits:** 145033 **Births:** 404 **Total Expense ($000):** 63222 **Payroll Expense ($000):** 23106 **Personnel:** 380

## JOHN DAY—Grant County

★ **BLUE MOUNTAIN HOSPITAL (381305)**, 170 Ford Road, Zip 97845–2009; tel. 541/575–1311, (Total facility includes 48 beds in nursing home–type unit) **A**3 5 9 10 18 **F**3 7 8 11 13 15 17 29 30 31 34 35 36 40 41 43 45 56 57 59 62 63 64 67 68 70 75 76 81 82 86 87 93 107 110 111 113 118 126 127 129 130 131 132 134 142 144 147 **P**6 **S** HealthTech Management Services, Franklin, TN
Primary Contact: Robert Houser, FACHE, Chief Executive Officer
CMO: Keith Thomas, M.D., Chief of Staff
CIO: Marci Brown, Director Information Technology
CHR: Verlene Davis, Director Human Resources
Web address: www.bluemountainhospital.org
**Control:** Hospital district or authority, Government, nonfederal **Service:** General Medical and Surgical

**Staffed Beds:** 64 **Admissions:** 368 **Census:** 33 **Outpatient Visits:** 22509 **Births:** 46 **Total Expense ($000):** 16825 **Payroll Expense ($000):** 9142 **Personnel:** 163

## KLAMATH FALLS—Klamath County

★ **SKY LAKES MEDICAL CENTER (380050)**, 2865 Daggett Avenue, Zip 97601–1180; tel. 541/882–6311 **A**2 3 5 9 10 21 **F**3 8 11 12 13 15 18 20 22 29 30 31 34 35 37 40 43 44 45 46 47 48 50 51 53 54 56 57 59 61 62 64 68 70 71 74 75 76 77 78 79 81 83 84 85 86 87 93 94 96 97 100 102 107 108 110 111 112 113 114 115 116 117 118 119 120 122 129 130 131 133 134 140 141 144 145 146 147 **P**6
Primary Contact: Paul R. Stewart, President and Chief Executive Officer
CFO: Richard Rico, Vice President and Chief Financial Officer
CMO: Rick Zwartverwer, M.D., Vice President Medical Affairs
CIO: David Chabner, Director Information Services
CHR: Don York, Vice President Human Resources
CNO: Annette E. Cole, R.N., Vice President and Chief Nursing Officer
Web address: www.skylakes.org
**Control:** Other not–for–profit (including NFP Corporation) **Service:** General Medical and Surgical

**Staffed Beds:** 100 **Admissions:** 5596 **Census:** 54 **Outpatient Visits:** 217825 **Births:** 850 **Total Expense ($000):** 148618 **Payroll Expense ($000):** 59398 **Personnel:** 939

---

**Hospital, Medicare Provider Number, Address, Telephone, Approval, Facility, and Physician Codes, Health Care System**

★ American Hospital Association (AHA) membership
☐ The Joint Commission accreditation ◇ DNV Healthcare Inc. accreditation
○ American Osteopathic Association (AOA) accreditation
△ Commission on Accreditation of Rehabilitation Facilities (CARF) accreditation

**OR**

## LA GRANDE—Union County

✠ **GRANDE RONDE HOSPITAL (381321)**, 900 Sunset Drive, Zip 97850–1362, Mailing Address: P.O. Box 3290, Zip 97850–3290; tel. 541/963–8421 **A**1 9 10 18 **F**3 8 11 13 15 17 29 30 31 34 37 39 40 41 43 44 45 50 53 54 57 59 62 63 64 66 70 74 75 76 77 78 79 81 82 85 86 87 89 93 96 97 107 108 110 111 113 117 118 127 129 130 131 132 134 145 146 147 **P**6
Primary Contact: James A. Mattes, President and Chief Executive Officer
CFO: Wade Weis, Senior Director Finance
CIO: Parhez Sattar, Senior Director Information Technology
CHR: Kristi Puckett, Director Human Resources
Web address: www.grh.org
**Control:** Other not–for–profit (including NFP Corporation) **Service:** General Medical and Surgical

**Staffed Beds:** 25 **Admissions:** 1567 **Census:** 15 **Outpatient Visits:** 83695 **Births:** 270 **Total Expense ($000):** 54313 **Payroll Expense ($000):** 28140 **Personnel:** 397

## LAKEVIEW—Lake County

★ **LAKE DISTRICT HOSPITAL (381309)**, 700 South J Street, Zip 97630–1679; tel. 541/947–2114, (Total facility includes 47 beds in nursing home–type unit) **A**5 9 10 18 **F**11 13 15 30 35 40 43 46 57 59 62 63 64 67 68 76 81 93 107 111 118 127 129 131 132 134 143 145 147 **P**4
Primary Contact: Gordon Ensley, Chief Executive Officer
COO: Charles Tveit, Chief Operating Officer
CFO: Ken Landau, Chief Financial Officer
CMO: C. Scott Graham, D.O., Chief of Staff
CHR: Linda Michaelson, Director Human Resources
Web address: www.lakehealthdistrict.org
**Control:** Hospital district or authority, Government, nonfederal **Service:** General Medical and Surgical

**Staffed Beds:** 71 **Admissions:** 553 **Census:** 25 **Outpatient Visits:** 25369 **Births:** 61 **Total Expense ($000):** 15531 **Payroll Expense ($000):** 7212 **Personnel:** 126

## LEBANON—Linn County

★ **SAMARITAN LEBANON COMMUNITY HOSPITAL (381323)**, 525 North Santiam Highway, Zip 97355–4363, Mailing Address: P.O. Box 739, Zip 97355–0739; tel. 541/258–2101 **A**9 10 18 21 **F**3 11 13 15 18 28 29 30 31 34 35 40 43 44 45 46 47 50 53 59 60 64 68 70 75 76 78 79 81 82 83 85 86 87 89 92 93 97 107 108 110 111 113 117 118 129 130 131 134 143 145 146 147 **P**6 **S** Samaritan Health Services, Corvallis, OR
Primary Contact: Becky A. Pape, R.N., Chief Executive Officer
CFO: Daniel B. Smith, Vice President Finance
CMO: Rick Salisbury, M.D., President Medical Staff
CIO: Bob Power, Vice President Information Services
CHR: Connie Erwin, Manager
Web address: www.samhealth.org
**Control:** Other not–for–profit (including NFP Corporation) **Service:** General Medical and Surgical

**Staffed Beds:** 25 **Admissions:** 1915 **Census:** 16 **Outpatient Visits:** 148849 **Births:** 329 **Total Expense ($000):** 70139 **Payroll Expense ($000):** 36247 **Personnel:** 440

## LINCOLN CITY—Lincoln County

★ **SAMARITAN NORTH LINCOLN HOSPITAL (381302)**, 3043 N.E. 28th Street, Zip 97367–4523, Mailing Address: P.O. Box 767, Zip 97367–0767; tel. 541/994–3661 **A**9 10 18 21 **F**3 8 11 13 15 29 30 34 35 40 43 50 51 57 59 62 63 64 67 68 70 75 76 79 81 84 85 86 87 90 93 97 107 108 110 111 113 117 118 126 127 129 131 132 134 143 145 147 **P**6 **S** Samaritan Health Services, Corvallis, OR
Primary Contact: Marty Cahill, Chief Executive Officer
CFO: Kathryn Doksum, Director Finance
CMO: Michael Halferty, M.D., President Medical Staff
CHR: Lauri Bolton, Director Human Resources
Web address: www.samhealth.org
**Control:** Other not–for–profit (including NFP Corporation) **Service:** General Medical and Surgical

**Staffed Beds:** 25 **Admissions:** 1043 **Census:** 7 **Outpatient Visits:** 74995 **Births:** 144 **Total Expense ($000):** 39398 **Payroll Expense ($000):** 21834 **Personnel:** 297

## MADRAS—Jefferson County

★ **MOUNTAIN VIEW HOSPITAL DISTRICT (381324)**, 470 N.E. A Street, Zip 97741–1844; tel. 541/475–3882 **A**9 10 18 **F**3 13 15 29 30 34 35 37 40 43 45 50 57 59 62 63 64 67 68 70 75 76 77 79 80 81 84 85 87 89 90 98 107 110 113 118 127 129 131 132 134 145 **P**7 **S** St. Charles Health System, Inc., Bend, OR
Primary Contact: Jeanine Gentry, Chief Executive Officer
CFO: Martha Bewley, Chief Financial Officer
CMO: Thomas Manning, M.D., Medical Director
CIO: Burt Ridge, Director of Information Technology
CHR: JoDee Tittle, Human Resources Director
CNO: Christine Gish, R.N., Acute Care Director
Web address: www.mvhd.org
**Control:** Hospital district or authority, Government, nonfederal **Service:** General Medical and Surgical

**Staffed Beds:** 25 **Admissions:** 1028 **Census:** 10 **Outpatient Visits:** 26490 **Births:** 196 **Total Expense ($000):** 21996 **Payroll Expense ($000):** 13256 **Personnel:** 218

## MCMINNVILLE—Yamhill County

☐ **WILLAMETTE VALLEY MEDICAL CENTER (380071)**, 2700 S.E. Stratus Avenue, Zip 97128–6498; tel. 503/472–6131 **A**1 2 9 10 **F**3 11 12 13 15 18 20 26 27 28 29 30 31 34 35 40 43 46 50 56 57 58 59 60 64 65 70 74 75 76 77 78 79 81 82 84 85 87 92 93 107 108 110 111 113 114 117 118 119 122 123 128 129 131 134 145 146 147 **P**5 6 **S** Capella Healthcare, Franklin, TN
Primary Contact: Daniel Ordyna, Chief Executive Officer
CFO: Cory Rhoades, Chief Financial Officer
CIO: Diane Farrow, Manager Information Technology and Systems
CHR: Drew Burke, Director Human Resources
Web address: www.wvmcweb.com
**Control:** Corporation, Investor–owned, for–profit **Service:** General Medical and Surgical

**Staffed Beds:** 88 **Admissions:** 4057 **Census:** 37 **Outpatient Visits:** 112413 **Births:** 550 **Total Expense ($000):** 71675 **Payroll Expense ($000):** 25924 **Personnel:** 448

## MEDFORD—Jackson County

✠ △ **PROVIDENCE MEDFORD MEDICAL CENTER (380075)**, 1111 Crater Lake Avenue, Zip 97504–6241; tel. 541/732–5000 **A**1 2 7 9 10 **F**3 11 13 15 17 18 20 22 29 30 31 32 34 35 40 43 45 49 50 55 56 57 59 61 62 63 64 68 70 74 75 76 77 78 79 81 82 84 85 86 87 90 92 93 96 97 102 107 110 113 114 117 118 119 120 122 123 125 129 131 142 145 146 147 **P**6 **S** Providence Health & Services, Renton, WA
Primary Contact: Thomas S. Hanenburg, Chief Executive
COO: Brian J. Herwig, Chief Operating Officer
CFO: Chris Pizzi, Assistant Administrator Fiscal Services
CHR: Julie Levison, Director Human Resources
CNO: Jane E. Hanson, R.N., Chief Nursing Officer
Web address: www.providence.org
**Control:** Church–operated, Nongovernment, not–for profit **Service:** General Medical and Surgical

**Staffed Beds:** 113 **Admissions:** 6420 **Census:** 66 **Outpatient Visits:** 293241 **Births:** 520 **Total Expense ($000):** 152496 **Payroll Expense ($000):** 58824 **Personnel:** 893

★ **ROGUE VALLEY MEDICAL CENTER (380018)**, 2825 East Barnett Road, Zip 97504–8332; tel. 541/789–7000 **A**2 9 10 21 **F**11 12 13 15 17 18 19 20 21 22 23 24 25 26 27 28 29 30 31 32 34 35 37 40 43 45 46 50 51 57 58 59 63 64 65 70 72 74 75 76 78 79 81 82 84 85 86 87 89 90 93 94 98 100 102 107 108 110 111 112 114 118 119 120 121 125 129 131 142 145 146 147 **P**6 **S** Asante Health System, Medford, OR
Primary Contact: Scott A. Kelly, Chief Executive Officer
COO: Jose Romo, Vice President of Operations
CFO: Mark Collins, Interim Chief Finance Officer
CMO: Jamie Grebosky, M.D., Vice President of Medical Affairs
CIO: Mark Hetz, Chief Information Officer
CHR: Gregg Edwards, Chief People Officer
CNO: Jo Lynn Wallace, Vice President of Nursing
Web address: www.asante.org
**Control:** Other not–for–profit (including NFP Corporation) **Service:** General Medical and Surgical

**Staffed Beds:** 307 **Admissions:** 14414 **Census:** 180 **Outpatient Visits:** 357003 **Births:** 1556 **Total Expense ($000):** 331619 **Payroll Expense ($000):** 109372 **Personnel:** 1595

*Many Facility Codes have changed. Please refer to the AHA Guide Code Chart.* © 2012 AHA Guide

## MILWAUKIE—Clackamas County

☒ **PROVIDENCE MILWAUKIE HOSPITAL (380082)**, 10150 S.E. 32nd Avenue,
Zip 97222–6516; tel. 503/513–8300 **A**1 2 3 5 9 10 **F**3 13 15 29 30 34 35 36
40 44 45 46 50 53 54 57 59 63 64 68 70 71 74 75 76 77 79 81 82 84 85
87 89 91 92 93 97 100 105 107 108 111 113 114 118 128 129 130 131
132 134 145 146 147 **P**6 **S** Providence Health & Services, Renton, WA
Primary Contact: Keith Hyde, Chief Executive Officer
CFO: Elizabeth Sublette, Chief Financial Officer
CHR: Joann M. Pfister, Director Human Resources
CNO: Lauren M. Bridge, R.N., Chief Nurse Executive
Web address: www.providence.org
**Control:** Church–operated, Nongovernment, not–for profit **Service:** General
Medical and Surgical

**Staffed Beds:** 64 **Admissions:** 3274 **Census:** 27 **Outpatient Visits:** 211392
**Births:** 520 **Total Expense ($000):** 83066 **Payroll Expense ($000):** 31047
**Personnel:** 405

## NEWBERG—Yamhill County

☒ **PROVIDENCE NEWBERG MEDICAL CENTER (380037)**, 1001 Providence
Drive, Zip 97132–7485; tel. 503/537–1555 **A**1 9 10 **F**3 11 13 15 18 20 29 30
34 35 40 45 49 50 57 59 60 64 68 70 75 76 77 79 81 85 87 93 100 107
108 110 111 113 117 118 128 129 131 134 145 146 147 **P**6 **S** Providence
Health & Services, Renton, WA
Primary Contact: Alan C. Olive, Chief Executive Officer
CFO: Jack R. Sumner, Assistant Administrator Finance
CMO: George Weghorst, M.D., Chief Medical Officer
CIO: Laureen O'Brien, Chief Information Officer
CHR: Cheryl Gebhart, Director Human Resources Providence Health Plan and
Providence Medical Group
Web address: www.phsor.org
**Control:** Church–operated, Nongovernment, not–for profit **Service:** General
Medical and Surgical

**Staffed Beds:** 40 **Admissions:** 2399 **Census:** 20 **Outpatient Visits:** 192878
**Births:** 571 **Total Expense ($000):** 84149 **Payroll Expense ($000):** 28115
**Personnel:** 404

## NEWPORT—Lincoln County

★ **SAMARITAN PACIFIC COMMUNITIES HOSPITAL (381314)**, 930 S.W. Abbey
Street, Zip 97365–4820, Mailing Address: P.O. Box 945, Zip 97365–4820;
tel. 541/265–2244 **A**9 10 18 21 **F**3 8 11 13 15 17 28 29 30 31 34 35 40 43
45 47 50 54 60 62 63 64 70 75 76 77 78 79 81 84 85 87 89 92 93 97 107
110 111 113 118 128 129 131 132 134 143 145 146 147 **P**6 **S** Samaritan
Health Services, Corvallis, OR
Primary Contact: David C. Bigelow, PharmD, Chief Executive Officer
CHR: Penny Dunne, R.N., Director Human Resources
Web address: www.samhealth.org
**Control:** Other not–for–profit (including NFP Corporation) **Service:** General
Medical and Surgical

**Staffed Beds:** 25 **Admissions:** 1418 **Census:** 11 **Outpatient Visits:** 87514
**Births:** 190 **Total Expense ($000):** 60100 **Payroll Expense ($000):** 28623
**Personnel:** 402

## ONTARIO—Malheur County

**HOLY ROSARY MEDICAL CENTER** See Saint Alphonsus Medical Center –
Ontario

☒ **SAINT ALPHONSUS MEDICAL CENTER – ONTARIO (380052)**, 351 S.W.
Ninth Street, Zip 97914–2693; tel. 541/881–7000 **A**1 5 9 10 **F**3 11 12 13 15
18 29 30 32 34 35 40 43 44 45 46 50 51 54 56 57 59 62 63 64 65 66 68
70 75 76 77 79 81 82 87 93 97 107 108 110 113 117 118 128 129 130
131 134 143 145 146 147 **P**6 **S** Trinity Health, Novi, MI
Primary Contact: Richard L. Palagi, Chief Executive Officer
CFO: Paul Vachek, Vice President of Finance/Operations
CHR: Brenda Munsey, Senior Human Resources Business Partner
CNO: Nancy Greer, R.N., Chief Nursing Officer
Web address: www.holyrosary–ontario.org
**Control:** Church–operated, Nongovernment, not–for profit **Service:** General
Medical and Surgical

**Staffed Beds:** 49 **Admissions:** 3002 **Census:** 24 **Outpatient Visits:** 70431
**Births:** 589 **Total Expense ($000):** 53925 **Payroll Expense ($000):** 22117
**Personnel:** 389

## OREGON CITY—Clackamas County

☒ **PROVIDENCE WILLAMETTE FALLS MEDICAL CENTER (380038)**, 1500
Division Street, Zip 97045–1597; tel. 503/656–1631 **A**1 9 10 **F**13 15 29 30 34
35 36 40 44 45 46 50 53 54 57 59 63 64 68 70 74 75 76 77 78 79 81 82
84 85 87 91 92 93 97 100 107 108 111 113 118 129 130 131 132 134 145
146 **P**5 6 **S** Providence Health & Services, Renton, WA
Primary Contact: Russ Reinhard, Chief Executive
CFO: Elizabeth Sublette, Chief Finance Officer
CMO: Kevin Jamison, M.D., Chief Medical Officer
CHR: Joann M. Pfister, Director Human Resources
Web address: www.providence.org/pwfmc
**Control:** Church–operated, Nongovernment, not–for profit **Service:** General
Medical and Surgical

**Staffed Beds:** 89 **Admissions:** 4275 **Census:** 33 **Outpatient Visits:** 158266
**Births:** 983 **Total Expense ($000):** 94966 **Payroll Expense ($000):** 37473
**Personnel:** 508

## PENDLETON—Umatilla County

**BLUE MOUNTAIN RECOVERY CENTER (384011)**, 2600 Westgate,
Zip 97801–9613; tel. 541/276–0810, (Nonreporting) **A**10
Primary Contact: Kerry Kelly, Superintendent
COO: Kerry Kelly, Superintendent
CFO: Dan Grant, Manager Business Office
CMO: Peter Davidson, M.D., Chief Medical Officer
CHR: Billy Martin, Human Resource Analyst
**Control:** State–Government, nonfederal **Service:** Psychiatric

**Staffed Beds:** 60

☒ **ST. ANTHONY HOSPITAL (381319)**, 1601 S.E. Court Avenue,
Zip 97801–3297; tel. 541/276–5121 **A**1 5 9 10 18 **F**3 13 15 29 30 31 35 39
40 43 45 51 53 54 57 59 62 63 64 65 68 75 76 77 78 79 81 85 86 87 93
97 107 108 110 111 114 117 118 126 128 129 130 131 132 133 134 143
145 **P**6 **S** Catholic Health Initiatives, Englewood, CO
Primary Contact: Jim Schlenker, Interim President and Chief Executive Officer
CFO: Jim Schlenker, Vice President and Chief Financial Officer
CMO: Malcolm Townsley, M.D., Chief of Staff
CHR: Janeen K. Reding, Director Human Resources
Web address: www.sahpendleton.org
**Control:** Church–operated, Nongovernment, not–for profit **Service:** General
Medical and Surgical

**Staffed Beds:** 25 **Admissions:** 1694 **Census:** 15 **Outpatient Visits:** 47102
**Births:** 315 **Total Expense ($000):** 43440 **Payroll Expense ($000):** 19104
**Personnel:** 307

## PORTLAND—Multnomah County

☒ **ADVENTIST MEDICAL CENTER (380060)**, 10123 S.E. Market Street,
Zip 97216–2599; tel. 503/257–2500 **A**1 2 9 10 **F**3 11 13 15 17 18 20 22 24
26 28 29 30 31 34 35 36 40 44 45 49 53 54 57 58 59 62 63 64 70 71 74
75 76 77 78 79 81 84 85 86 87 93 94 97 98 100 102 107 108 110 111 113
114 117 118 120 122 125 128 129 130 131 134 143 145 146 147 **P**6 7
**S** Adventist Health, Roseville, CA
Primary Contact: Thomas Russell, Chief Executive Officer
COO: Ronald K. Benfield, Chief Operating Officer
CFO: V. Mark Perry, Chief Financial Officer
CMO: Wesley E. Rippey, M.D., Chief Medical Officer
CHR: Herbert Hill, Director Human Resources
Web address: www.adventisthealthnw.com
**Control:** Church–operated, Nongovernment, not–for profit **Service:** General
Medical and Surgical

**Staffed Beds:** 252 **Admissions:** 11531 **Census:** 119 **Outpatient Visits:**
424668 **Births:** 1175 **Total Expense ($000):** 267640 **Payroll Expense
($000):** 118005 **Personnel:** 1627

☐ **CEDAR HILLS HOSPITAL (384012)**, 10300 S.W. Eastridge Street,
Zip 97225–5004; tel. 503/944–5000, (Nonreporting) **A**1 9 10 **S** Ascend Health
Corporation, New York, NY
Primary Contact: Michael Sherbun, Ph.D., Chief Executive Officer
Web address: www.cedarhillshospital.com
**Control:** Corporation, Investor–owned, for–profit **Service:** Psychiatric

**Staffed Beds:** 78

**DOERNBECHER CHILDREN'S HOSPITAL** See OHSU Hospital

**GOOD SAMARITAN HOSPITAL AND MEDICAL CENTER** See Legacy Good
Samaritan Hospital and Medical Center

---

**Hospital, Medicare Provider Number, Address, Telephone, Approval, Facility, and Physician Codes, Health Care System**

★ American Hospital Association (AHA) membership
☐ The Joint Commission accreditation          ◇ DNV Healthcare Inc. accreditation

○ American Osteopathic Association (AOA) accreditation
△ Commission on Accreditation of Rehabilitation Facilities (CARF) accreditation

☒ △ **LEGACY EMANUEL HOSPITAL AND HEALTH CENTER (380007)**, 2801 North Gantenbein Avenue, Zip 97227–1674; tel. 503/413–2200, (Includes RANDALL CHILDREN'S HOSPITAL, 2801 North Gantenbein Avenue, Zip 97227–1623; tel. 503/413–2200) **A**1 2 3 5 7 9 10 **F**3 11 13 15 16 18 19 20 21 22 23 24 25 26 27 29 30 31 32 34 35 38 40 41 43 44 45 46 47 49 50 51 53 54 56 57 59 60 61 64 65 66 68 70 72 73 74 75 76 77 78 79 80 81 83 84 85 86 87 88 89 93 97 98 99 100 101 102 105 107 108 110 111 112 113 117 118 125 126 129 131 143 145 146 147 **P**8 **S** Legacy Health, Portland, OR
Primary Contact: Lori Morgan, M.D., Chief Administrative Officer
CFO: Pamela S. Vukovich, Senior Vice President, Chief Financial Officer and Treasurer
CIO: Dick Gibson, Senior Vice President and Chief Information Officer
CHR: Sonja Steves, Senior Vice President Human Resources and Marketing
Web address: www.legacyhealth.org
**Control:** Other not–for–profit (including NFP Corporation) **Service:** General Medical and Surgical

Staffed Beds: 406 Admissions: 18437 Census: 275 Births: 1801 Total Expense ($000): 536961 Payroll Expense ($000): 240137 Personnel: 3214

☒ **LEGACY GOOD SAMARITAN HOSPITAL AND MEDICAL CENTER (380017)**, 1015 N.W. 22nd Avenue, Zip 97210–3099; tel. 503/413–7711, (Includes GOOD SAMARITAN HOSPITAL AND MEDICAL CENTER, 1015 N.W. 22nd Avenue, Zip 97210; tel. 503/229–7711; REHABILITATION INSTITUTE OF OREGON, 2010 N.W. Kearney Street, Zip 97209; tel. 503/226–3774) **A**1 2 3 5 9 10 **F**3 8 11 12 13 15 18 20 22 24 26 28 29 30 31 34 35 38 40 44 45 46 47 48 49 50 51 53 55 56 57 58 59 60 61 64 65 66 68 70 74 75 76 77 78 79 80 81 82 83 84 85 86 87 90 91 93 96 97 98 100 101 102 103 107 108 110 111 113 115 116 117 118 119 120 122 123 125 128 129 131 134 137 141 144 145 146 147 **P**8 **S** Legacy Health, Portland, OR
Primary Contact: Tony Melaragno, M.D., Chief Administrative Officer
CFO: Pamela S. Vukovich, Senior Vice President, Chief Financial Officer and Treasurer
CIO: C. Matthew Calais, Senior Vice President and Chief Information Officer
CHR: Sonja Steves, Vice President Marketing
Web address: www.legacyhealth.org
**Control:** Other not–for–profit (including NFP Corporation) **Service:** General Medical and Surgical

Staffed Beds: 249 Admissions: 11315 Census: 147 Outpatient Visits: 166467 Births: 1114 Total Expense ($000): 270508 Payroll Expense ($000): 97741 Personnel: 1385

☒ **OHSU HOSPITAL (380009)**, 3181 S.W. Sam Jackson Park Road, Zip 97201–3098; tel. 503/494–8311, (Includes DOERNBECHER CHILDREN'S HOSPITAL, 3181 S.W. Sam Jackson Park Road, Zip 97201) **A**1 2 3 5 8 9 10 **F**3 5 6 8 9 11 12 13 15 17 18 19 21 23 24 25 26 27 28 29 30 31 32 33 34 35 36 37 38 39 40 41 43 44 45 46 47 48 49 50 51 52 53 54 55 56 57 58 59 60 61 64 65 66 68 70 71 72 74 75 76 77 78 79 81 82 83 84 85 86 87 88 89 91 92 93 94 95 97 98 99 100 101 102 103 104 105 106 107 108 109 110 111 112 113 114 115 116 117 118 119 120 122 123 125 128 129 130 131 133 134 135 136 137 138 140 141 143 144 145 146 147 **P**1
Primary Contact: Peter F. Rapp, Vice President and Executive Director
COO: Cynthia M. Grueber, Chief Operating Officer
CFO: Diana Gernhart, Chief Financial Officer
CMO: Charles M. Kilo, M.D., Chief Medical Officer
CIO: Bridget Haggerty, Chief Information Officer
CHR: Priscilla B. Andres, Director Human Resources
Web address: www.ohsu.edu
**Control:** Hospital district or authority, Government, nonfederal **Service:** General Medical and Surgical

Staffed Beds: 537 Admissions: 28686 Census: 444 Outpatient Visits: 698621 Births: 2291 Total Expense ($000): 1012447 Payroll Expense ($000): 375932 Personnel: 5664

☒ **PROVIDENCE PORTLAND MEDICAL CENTER (380061)**, 4805 N.E. Glisan Street, Zip 97213–2967; tel. 503/215–5526 **A**1 2 3 5 9 10 **F**3 4 5 9 13 15 17 18 20 22 24 26 29 30 31 34 35 36 37 38 40 44 45 46 49 50 51 53 54 56 57 58 59 60 61 62 63 64 65 66 68 70 73 74 75 76 77 78 79 81 82 84 85 86 87 90 93 97 98 99 100 102 103 104 105 107 108 109 110 111 113 115 116 117 118 120 122 123 125 128 131 132 134 135 136 144 145 146 147 **P**6 **S** Providence Health & Services, Renton, WA
Primary Contact: Theron Park, Chief Executive Officer
COO: James Arp, Chief Operating Officer
CFO: Eric Olson, Chief Financial Officer
CIO: Laureen O'Brien, Chief Information Officer
CHR: Jeannie Mikulic, Director Human Resources
Web address: www.providence.org
**Control:** Church–operated, Nongovernment, not–for profit **Service:** General Medical and Surgical

Staffed Beds: 412 Admissions: 21699 Census: 284 Outpatient Visits: 1245107 Births: 2411 Total Expense ($000): 608691 Payroll Expense ($000): 209810 Personnel: 2834

☒ **PROVIDENCE ST. VINCENT MEDICAL CENTER (380004)**, 9205 S.W. Barnes Road, Zip 97225–6661; tel. 503/216–1234, (Includes CHILDREN AT PROVIDENCE ST. VINCENT, 9205 S.W. Barnes Road, Zip 97225–6603; tel. 503/216–4400) **A**1 2 3 5 9 10 **F**3 5 13 15 17 18 20 22 24 26 28 29 30 31 34 35 36 37 38 40 44 45 46 47 48 49 50 51 53 54 56 57 58 59 60 61 64 65 68 70 72 74 75 76 77 78 79 81 82 83 84 85 86 87 89 91 92 93 97 98 100 102 103 104 105 107 108 109 110 111 112 113 114 115 116 117 118 119 120 122 125 128 129 130 131 132 134 145 146 147 **P**6
**S** Providence Health & Services, Renton, WA
Primary Contact: Janice Burger, Administrator
CFO: William Olson, Director Finance
CIO: Kate Chester, Senior Coordinator Public Relations
Web address: www.providence.org/portland/hospitals
**Control:** Church–operated, Nongovernment, not–for profit **Service:** General Medical and Surgical

Staffed Beds: 552 Admissions: 28617 Census: 354 Outpatient Visits: 777196 Births: 4922 Total Expense ($000): 682041 Payroll Expense ($000): 221613 Personnel: 3001

**REHABILITATION INSTITUTE OF OREGON** See Legacy Good Samaritan Hospital and Medical Center

☐ **SHRINERS HOSPITALS FOR CHILDREN, PORTLAND (383300)**, 3101 S.W. Sam Jackson Park Road, Zip 97239; tel. 503/241–5090 **A**1 3 5 10 **F**3 34 35 37 50 58 64 68 75 77 79 81 85 86 87 89 91 93 94 129 131 133 145 147 **P**6 **S** Shriners Hospitals for Children, Tampa, FL
Primary Contact: J. Craig Patchin, Administrator
CFO: Mark Knudsen, Director Fiscal Services
CMO: Michael Aiona, M.D., Chief of Staff
CIO: Carl Montante, Director Information Systems and Information Technology
CHR: Rhonda Smith, Director Human Resources
CNO: Suzanne Diers, R.N., Director Patient Care Services
Web address: www.shcc.org
**Control:** Other not–for–profit (including NFP Corporation) **Service:** Children's general

Staffed Beds: 8 Admissions: 674 Census: 6 Outpatient Visits: 13033 Births: 0 Personnel: 226

☒ **VETERANS AFFAIRS MEDICAL CENTER**, 3710 S.W. U.S. Veterans Hospital Road, Zip 97239, Mailing Address: P.O. Box 1034, Zip 97207–1034; tel. 503/220–8262, (Nonreporting) **A**1 2 3 5 8 **S** Department of Veterans Affairs, Washington, DC
Primary Contact: John E. Patrick, Director
CFO: Annette Barkema, Chief Financial Officer
CMO: Thomas Anderson, M.D., Chief of Staff
CIO: James Horner, Chief Information Officer
CHR: Melody Mikutowski, Chief Human Resources Management
Web address: www.va.gov/sta/guide/home.asp
**Control:** Veterans Affairs, Government, federal **Service:** General Medical and Surgical

Staffed Beds: 149

☐ **VIBRA SPECIALTY HOSPITAL OF PORTLAND (382004)**, 10300 N.E. Hancock Street, Zip 97220; tel. 503/257–5500, (Nonreporting) **A**1 9 10 **S** Vibra Healthcare, Mechanicsburg, PA
Primary Contact: Tina Key, Chief Executive Officer
Web address: www.vibrahealthcare.com
**Control:** Corporation, Investor–owned, for–profit **Service:** Long–Term Acute Care hospital

Staffed Beds: 60

**PRINEVILLE—Crook County**

★ **PIONEER MEMORIAL HOSPITAL (381313)**, 1201 N.E. Elm Street, Zip 97754–1206; tel. 541/447–6254 **A**9 10 18 **F**3 11 15 29 34 35 40 43 45 50 59 63 64 65 70 75 79 81 82 84 86 87 97 107 113 118 128 131 132 134 145 **S** St. Charles Health System, Inc., Bend, OR
Primary Contact: Robert Gomes, Chief Executive Officer
COO: Jim Kirkbride, Director of Support Services
CFO: Karen Shepard, Senior Vice President and Chief Financial Officer
CMO: Michel Boileau, M.D., Chief Clinical Officer
CIO: William Winnenberg, Chief Information Officer
CHR: Rebecca Morgan, Senior Director Human Resources
CNO: Karen Reed, Chief Nursing Officer
Web address: www.stcharleshealthcare.org
**Control:** Other not–for–profit (including NFP Corporation) **Service:** General Medical and Surgical

Staffed Beds: 25 Admissions: 786 Census: 8 Outpatient Visits: 34947 Births: 0 Total Expense ($000): 18535 Payroll Expense ($000): 10748 Personnel: 175

*Many Facility Codes have changed. Please refer to the AHA Guide Code Chart.* © 2012 AHA Guide

**OR**

## REDMOND—Deschutes County

✠ **ST. CHARLES MEDICAL CENTER – REDMOND (380040)**, 1253 N.W. Canal Boulevard, Zip 97756–1395; tel. 541/548–8131 **A**1 9 10 20 **F**3 11 13 29 30 34 40 43 45 47 51 57 59 62 64 70 75 76 81 82 84 85 92 93 102 107 108 113 118 129 134 145 147 **P**4 7 **S** St. Charles Health System, Inc., Bend, OR
Primary Contact: Robert Gomes, Chief Executive Officer
COO: Jim Kirkbride, Director of Support Services
CFO: Karen Shepard, Senior Vice President Finance and Chief Financial Officer
CMO: Michel Boileau, M.D., Chief Clinical Officer
CIO: William Winnenberg, Chief Information Officer
CHR: Rebecca Morgan, Senior Director Human Resources
CNO: Karen Reed, Interim Chief Nursing Officer
Web address: www.stcharleshealthcare.org
**Control:** Other not–for–profit (including NFP Corporation) **Service:** General Medical and Surgical

**Staffed Beds:** 48 **Admissions:** 2256 **Census:** 17 **Outpatient Visits:** 62806 **Births:** 327 **Total Expense ($000):** 59067 **Payroll Expense ($000):** 26100 **Personnel:** 375

## REEDSPORT—Douglas County

**LOWER UMPQUA HOSPITAL DISTRICT (381311)**, 600 Ranch Road, Zip 97467–1795; tel. 541/271–2171 **A**9 10 18 **F**3 7 11 15 29 34 35 37 40 43 45 46 70 75 77 81 85 87 93 107 108 113 117 118 126 129 131 132 134 142 145 **P**6
Primary Contact: Sandra Reese, Administrator
CFO: John Chivers, Chief Financial Officer
CMO: Ronald Vail, M.D., Chief of Staff
CIO: Timothy Picou, Manager Information Technology
Web address: www.lowerumpquahospital.com
**Control:** Hospital district or authority, Government, nonfederal **Service:** General Medical and Surgical

**Staffed Beds:** 16 **Admissions:** 642 **Census:** 6 **Outpatient Visits:** 22643 **Births:** 0 **Total Expense ($000):** 17024 **Payroll Expense ($000):** 7085 **Personnel:** 122

## ROSEBURG—Douglas County

✠ **MERCY MEDICAL CENTER (380027)**, 2700 Stewart Parkway, Zip 97471–1297; tel. 541/673–0611 **A**1 2 9 10 **F**3 8 11 13 15 17 18 19 20 21 22 23 24 25 26 27 28 29 30 31 32 34 35 37 38 40 43 44 45 46 47 48 49 50 51 54 56 57 59 60 61 62 63 64 65 68 70 74 75 76 77 78 79 81 82 84 85 86 87 89 93 96 102 107 108 110 111 113 114 117 118 128 129 131 134 142 145 146 147 **P**6 **S** Catholic Health Initiatives, Englewood, CO
Primary Contact: Kelly C. Morgan, President and Chief Executive Officer
COO: Debbie Boswell, Chief Operating Officer and Chief Nursing Officer
CFO: John Kasberger, Vice President and Chief Financial Officer
CMO: Jason Gray, M.D., Chief Medical Officer
CIO: Kathleen Nickel, Director Communications
CHR: Deb Lightcap, Director Human Resources
CNO: Debbie Boswell, Chief Operating Officer and Chief Nursing Officer
Web address: www.mercyrose.org
**Control:** Church–operated, Nongovernment, not–for profit **Service:** General Medical and Surgical

**Staffed Beds:** 141 **Admissions:** 7514 **Census:** 81 **Outpatient Visits:** 284126 **Births:** 911 **Total Expense ($000):** 133467 **Payroll Expense ($000):** 51185 **Personnel:** 817

✠ △ **VETERANS AFFAIRS ROSEBURG HEALTHCARE SYSTEM**, 913 N.W. Garden Valley Boulevard, Zip 97470–6513; tel. 541/440–1000, (Nonreporting) **A**1 7 **S** Department of Veterans Affairs, Washington, DC
Primary Contact: Carol Bogedain, FACHE, Director
Web address: www.va.gov/sta/guide/home.asp
**Control:** Veterans Affairs, Government, federal **Service:** General Medical and Surgical

**Staffed Beds:** 88

## SALEM—Marion County

☐ **OREGON STATE HOSPITAL (384008)**, 2600 Center Street N.E., Zip 97301–2682; tel. 503/945–2870, (Nonreporting) **A**1 3 5 10
Primary Contact: Greg Roberts, Superintendent
Web address: www.oregon.gov/dhs/mentalhealth/osh/main.shtml
**Control:** State–Government, nonfederal **Service:** Psychiatric

**Staffed Beds:** 638

✠ **SALEM HOSPITAL (380051)**, 665 Winter Street S.E., Zip 97301–3959, Mailing Address: P.O. Box 14001, Zip 97309–5014; tel. 503/561–5200, (Includes PSYCHIATRIC MEDICINE CENTER, 1127 Oak Street S.E., Zip 97301, Mailing Address: P.O. Box 14001, Zip 97309–5014; REGIONAL REHABILITATION CENTER, 2561 Center Street N.E., Zip 97301, Mailing Address: P.O. Box 14001, Zip 97309–5014; tel. 503/370–5986) **A**1 2 9 10 **F**3 11 12 13 15 17 18 19 20 22 24 26 28 29 30 31 34 35 36 37 38 40 43 45 46 47 48 49 50 53 54 55 56 57 58 59 64 66 67 68 70 72 74 75 76 77 78 79 81 82 84 85 88 87 89 90 91 92 93 94 95 96 97 98 99 100 102 103 104 105 106 107 108 109 110 111 112 113 114 115 116 117 118 119 120 121 122 123 125 128 129 130 131 134 143 144 145 146 147 **P**6 **S** Salem Health, Salem, OR
Primary Contact: Norman F. Gruber, President and Chief Executive Officer
COO: Cheryl R. Nester Wolfe, R.N., Senior Vice President Operations and Chief Nursing Officer
CFO: Aaron Crane, Chief Financial Officer
CMO: W. David Holloway, M.D., Chief Medical Officer
CIO: Ken Kudla, Chief Information Officer
CHR: Beverly Bow, Vice President Human Resources
Web address: www.salemhospital.org
**Control:** Other not–for–profit (including NFP Corporation) **Service:** General Medical and Surgical

**Staffed Beds:** 459 **Admissions:** 23189 **Census:** 277 **Outpatient Visits:** 520167 **Births:** 3199 **Total Expense ($000):** 522579 **Payroll Expense ($000):** 220389 **Personnel:** 3129

## SEASIDE—Clatsop County

✠ **PROVIDENCE SEASIDE HOSPITAL (381303)**, 725 South Wahanna Road, Zip 97138–7735; tel. 503/717–7000, (Total facility includes 20 beds in nursing home–type unit) **A**1 9 10 18 **F**3 12 13 15 30 31 32 34 35 40 45 46 57 59 61 64 65 66 67 68 70 75 76 78 79 81 82 84 85 86 87 92 93 97 104 107 108 110 111 113 118 126 127 131 132 134 142 145 146 147 **P**6 **S** Providence Health & Services, Renton, WA
Primary Contact: Krista Farnham, Chief Executive
COO: Kenneth Boucher, Associate Administrator
CFO: Pamela Hayes, Director Finance
CMO: Timothy Opie, M.D., President Professional Staff
CHR: Marti Hanen, Director Human Resources
Web address: www.providence.org
**Control:** Church–operated, Nongovernment, not–for profit **Service:** General Medical and Surgical

**Staffed Beds:** 47 **Admissions:** 937 **Census:** 26 **Outpatient Visits:** 115282 **Births:** 149 **Total Expense ($000):** 44998 **Payroll Expense ($000):** 22348 **Personnel:** 324

## SILVERTON—Marion County

✠ **SILVERTON HOSPITAL (380029)**, 342 Fairview Street, Zip 97381–1993; tel. 503/873–1500 **A**1 9 10 **F**3 11 13 15 20 26 28 29 30 34 35 40 43 47 50 53 54 57 59 64 65 66 68 70 75 76 77 79 81 85 86 87 89 107 108 110 111 113 114 118 123 126 128 129 130 131 134 142 143 145 146 147
Primary Contact: Richard M. Cagen, Administrator
COO: Jeffrey D. Lorenz, Vice President Corporate Services
CFO: Jeff Fritsche, Chief Financial Officer
CMO: James Nealon, M.D., President Medical Staff
CIO: Lentz Farrell, Information Services Specialist
CHR: Jim M. Washam, Director Human Resources
Web address: www.silvertonhospital.org
**Control:** Other not–for–profit (including NFP Corporation) **Service:** General Medical and Surgical

**Staffed Beds:** 48 **Admissions:** 3429 **Census:** 25 **Outpatient Visits:** 142071 **Births:** 1677 **Total Expense ($000):** 94133 **Payroll Expense ($000):** 49830 **Personnel:** 767

## SPRINGFIELD—Lane County

✠ **MCKENZIE–WILLAMETTE MEDICAL CENTER (380020)**, 1460 G Street, Zip 97477–4197; tel. 541/726–4400 **A**1 9 10 **F**3 11 13 17 18 20 22 24 28 29 30 31 34 35 39 40 41 43 45 47 48 49 50 57 59 70 73 76 78 79 81 82 85 87 93 107 108 111 114 117 118 125 128 129 131 145 146 147 **P**6 **S** Community Health Systems, Inc., Franklin, TN
Primary Contact: Maurine Cate, Chief Executive Officer
COO: Randy Burrows, Director Administrative Services
CFO: Jason McLaughlin, Chief Financial Officer
CIO: Mike Allen, Director Information Technology
CHR: Megan A. O'Leary, Vice President Human Resources and Rehabilitation Services
Web address: www.mckweb.com
**Control:** Corporation, Investor–owned, for–profit **Service:** General Medical and Surgical

**Staffed Beds:** 113 **Admissions:** 6161 **Census:** 57 **Outpatient Visits:** 55410 **Births:** 591 **Total Expense ($000):** 103019 **Payroll Expense ($000):** 41935 **Personnel:** 530

---

**Hospital, Medicare Provider Number, Address, Telephone, Approval, Facility, and Physician Codes, Health Care System**

★ American Hospital Association (AHA) membership
☐ The Joint Commission accreditation  ◇ DNV Healthcare Inc. accreditation
○ American Osteopathic Association (AOA) accreditation
△ Commission on Accreditation of Rehabilitation Facilities (CARF) accreditation

---

OR

✠ **SACRED HEART MEDICAL CENTER AT RIVERBEND (380102)**, 3333 Riverbend Drive, Zip 97477–8800; tel. 541/222–7300 **A**1 9 10 **F**3 11 12 13 15 18 20 22 24 26 28 29 30 31 34 35 37 40 43 45 46 47 49 50 51 53 54 56 57 58 59 60 61 62 63 64 68 70 72 74 75 76 77 78 79 81 82 83 84 85 87 89 91 92 93 99 100 101 102 103 104 107 108 111 113 114 117 118 119 123 125 128 129 130 131 134 145 146 147 **P**6 **S** PeaceHealth, Bellevue, WA
Primary Contact: John Hill, Chief Executive Officer
COO: Roger Saydack, Interim Chief Operating Officer
CFO: Wendy Apland, Regional Vice President of Finance/Chief Financial Officer
CIO: Tom Fricks, Interim Senior Vice President of Information Technology
CHR: Craig J. Mills, Regional Vice President of Culture and People
Web address: www.peacehealth.org
**Control:** Church–operated, Nongovernment, not–for profit **Service:** General Medical and Surgical

**Staffed Beds:** 388 **Admissions:** 26661 **Census:** 277 **Outpatient Visits:** 92466 **Births:** 2889 **Total Expense ($000):** 475354 **Payroll Expense ($000):** 143370 **Personnel:** 2092

### STAYTON—Marion County

✠ **SANTIAM MEMORIAL HOSPITAL (380056)**, 1401 North 10th Avenue, Zip 97383–1399; tel. 503/769–2175 **A**1 9 10 **F**3 7 11 13 15 29 30 40 41 43 50 65 76 81 85 87 89 107 111 114 118 127 129 132 134 142 **P**8
Primary Contact: Terry L. Fletchall, Administrator
COO: Maggie Hudson, Director Operations and Financial Services
CFO: Rachael Seeder, Controller
CMO: Thomas VanVeen, M.D., Chief Medical Officer
Web address: www.santiamhospital.com
**Control:** Other not–for–profit (including NFP Corporation) **Service:** General Medical and Surgical

**Staffed Beds:** 40 **Admissions:** 1049 **Census:** 8 **Outpatient Visits:** 34854 **Births:** 152 **Personnel:** 218

### THE DALLES—Wasco County

✠ △ **MID–COLUMBIA MEDICAL CENTER (380001)**, 1700 East 19th Street, Zip 97058–3316; tel. 541/296–1111 **A**1 2 7 9 10 **F**11 12 13 15 17 18 19 28 29 30 31 32 34 35 36 40 43 45 46 47 50 51 57 59 62 64 65 66 68 70 75 76 77 78 79 81 82 83 84 86 87 89 90 91 92 93 97 99 100 101 104 107 108 109 110 111 113 114 117 118 119 120 122 126 128 129 130 131 132 134 143 144 145 146 147 **P**4
Primary Contact: Duane Francis, President and Chief Executive Officer
COO: Randy Skov, Vice President
CFO: Don Arbon, Vice President Finance
CMO: Judy Richardson, M.D., President Medical Staff
CIO: Erick Larson, Vice President and Chief Information Officer
CHR: Christine Espy, Director Human Resources
Web address: www.mcmc.net
**Control:** Other not–for–profit (including NFP Corporation) **Service:** General Medical and Surgical

**Staffed Beds:** 49 **Admissions:** 2043 **Census:** 18 **Outpatient Visits:** 123746 **Births:** 277 **Total Expense ($000):** 76711 **Payroll Expense ($000):** 37906 **Personnel:** 482

### TILLAMOOK—Tillamook County

✠ **TILLAMOOK COUNTY GENERAL HOSPITAL (381317)**, 1000 Third Street, Zip 97141–3430; tel. 503/842–4444 **A**1 9 10 18 **F**2 3 7 13 15 17 18 29 30 31 33 34 35 40 43 45 50 57 59 64 68 75 76 77 78 79 81 85 87 93 94 102 107 108 110 111 114 118 126 129 131 132 134 144 145 147 **S** Adventist Health, Roseville, CA
Primary Contact: Larry Davy, President and Chief Executive Officer
CFO: Walt Larson, Vice President Finance
Web address: www.tcgh.com
**Control:** Church–operated, Nongovernment, not–for profit **Service:** General Medical and Surgical

**Staffed Beds:** 25 **Admissions:** 1329 **Census:** 11 **Outpatient Visits:** 65097 **Births:** 157 **Total Expense ($000):** 51494 **Payroll Expense ($000):** 23087 **Personnel:** 332

### TUALATIN—Clackamas County

✠ **LEGACY MERIDIAN PARK HOSPITAL (380089)**, 19300 S.W. 65th Avenue, Zip 97062–9741; tel. 503/692–1212 **A**1 2 9 10 **F**3 11 13 15 18 20 22 28 29 30 31 32 34 35 38 40 44 45 46 49 50 51 56 57 59 60 64 68 70 74 75 76 77 78 79 80 81 85 86 87 93 107 108 110 111 113 114 115 116 117 118 119 120 125 128 129 131 144 145 146 147 **P**8 **S** Legacy Health, Portland, OR
Primary Contact: Allyson Anderson, Chief Administrative Officer
COO: Mike Newcomb, D.O., Senior Vice President and Chief Operating Officer
CFO: David Eager, Senior Vice President, Chief Financial Officer
CMO: Lewis Low, M.D., Senior Vice President and Chief Medical Officer
CIO: John Jay Kenagy, Ph.D., Senior Vice President and Chief Information Officer
CHR: Sonja Steves, Vice President Human Resources and Marketing
CNO: Carol Bradley, MSN, Senior Vice President and Chief Nursing Officer
Web address: www.legacyhealth.org
**Control:** Other not–for–profit (including NFP Corporation) **Service:** General Medical and Surgical

**Staffed Beds:** 130 **Admissions:** 7377 **Census:** 71 **Outpatient Visits:** 98908 **Births:** 874 **Total Expense ($000):** 137412 **Payroll Expense ($000):** 46181 **Personnel:** 667

*Many Facility Codes have changed. Please refer to the AHA Guide Code Chart.* © 2012 AHA Guide

# PENNSYLVANIA

## ABINGTON—Montgomery County

⊠ **ABINGTON MEMORIAL HOSPITAL (390231)**, 1200 Old York Road,
Zip 19001–3720; tel. 215/481–2000 **A**1 2 3 5 6 9 10 12 13 **F**3 6 8 9 11 12
13 15 17 18 19 20 22 24 26 28 29 30 31 32 34 35 36 37 38 39 40 43 44
45 46 49 50 52 53 54 55 56 57 58 59 60 61 62 63 64 65 66 68 70 72 74
75 76 77 78 79 80 81 82 83 84 85 86 87 89 90 91 92 93 94 96 97 98 99
100 101 102 103 104 107 108 110 111 113 114 117 118 119 120 122 123
125 128 129 130 131 134 145 146 147 **P**6
Primary Contact: Laurence M. Merlis, President and Chief Executive Officer
COO: Margaret M. McGoldrick, Executive Vice President and Administrator
CFO: Michael Walsh, Senior Vice President Finance and Chief Financial Officer
CMO: John J. Kelly, M.D., Chief of Staff
CIO: Alison Ferren, Vice President Information Technology and Chief Information
Officer
CHR: Meghan Patton, Vice President Human Resources
Web address: www.amh.org
**Control:** Other not–for–profit (including NFP Corporation) **Service:** General
Medical and Surgical

**Staffed Beds:** 632 **Admissions:** 36250 **Census:** 447 **Outpatient Visits:**
605990 **Births:** 5130 **Total Expense ($000):** 664161 **Payroll Expense
($000):** 309767 **Personnel:** 4049

## ALLENTOWN—Lehigh County

☐ △ **GOOD SHEPHERD REHABILITATION HOSPITAL (393035)**, 850 South 5th
Street, Zip 18103–3308; tel. 610/776–3299 **A**1 3 5 7 9 10 **F**28 29 30 32 34
35 36 53 54 56 57 58 59 64 65 66 68 74 75 77 82 86 87 90 91 92 93 94
95 96 107 111 118 129 130 131 142 145 147 **P**1 **S** Good Shepherd
Rehabilitation Network, Allentown, PA
Primary Contact: Sally T. Gammon, FACHE, President and Chief Executive Officer
CFO: Daniel Confalone, Chief Financial Officer
Web address: www.goodshepherdrehab.org
**Control:** Other not–for–profit (including NFP Corporation) **Service:** Rehabilitation

**Staffed Beds:** 102 **Admissions:** 1908 **Census:** 75 **Outpatient Visits:** 203549
**Births:** 0 **Total Expense ($000):** 73962 **Payroll Expense ($000):** 26486
**Personnel:** 956

⊠ **LEHIGH VALLEY HOSPITAL (390133)**, 1200 South Cedar Crest Boulevard,
Zip 18105–6248, Mailing Address: P.O. Box 689, Zip 18105–1556;
tel. 610/402–8000, (Includes LEHIGH VALLEY HEALTH NETWORK PEDIATRICS,
17th and Chew Streets, Zip 18102, Mailing Address: PO Box 7017,
Zip 18105–7017; tel. 610/402–2273) **A**1 2 3 5 8 9 10 **F**3 6 8 9 11 12 13 15
16 17 18 19 20 22 24 26 28 29 30 31 32 34 35 36 37 38 39 40 41 43 44
45 46 47 48 49 50 51 53 54 55 56 57 58 59 60 61 62 63 64 65 66 68 70
71 72 74 76 77 78 79 80 81 82 84 85 86 87 88 89 90 92 93 96 97 98 99
100 102 105 106 107 108 110 113 114 117 118 119 120 122 123 125 127
128 129 130 131 133 134 137 140 141 142 145 146 147 **P**5 6 8 **S** Lehigh
Valley Health Network, Allentown, PA
Primary Contact: Ronald W. Swinfard, M.D., President and Chief Executive Officer
COO: Terry Ann Capuano, R.N., Chief Operating Officer
CIO: Harry Lukens, Senior Vice President and Chief Information Officer
CHR: Mary Kay Grim, Senior Vice President Human Resources
Web address: www.lvhhn.org
**Control:** Other not–for–profit (including NFP Corporation) **Service:** General
Medical and Surgical

**Staffed Beds:** 783 **Admissions:** 44435 **Census:** 656 **Outpatient Visits:**
324417 **Births:** 3740 **Total Expense ($000):** 909342 **Payroll Expense
($000):** 296060 **Personnel:** 5947

☐ △ **SACRED HEART HOSPITAL (390197)**, 421 West Chew Street,
Zip 18102–3490; tel. 610/776–4500, (Total facility includes 16 beds in nursing
home–type unit) **A**1 2 3 5 7 9 10 13 **F**3 11 12 13 15 18 20 22 24 28 29 30
31 32 34 35 38 39 40 43 45 46 47 49 50 56 57 63 64 66 68 74
75 76 77 78 79 80 81 82 84 85 87 91 92 93 97 98 100 101 102 103 107
108 111 113 118 120 127 128 129 131 134 142 145 146 147 **P**8
Primary Contact: John L. Nespoli, Chief Executive Officer
CMO: Farrokh Sadr, M.D., Chief Medical Officer
CIO: Tracy Burkhart, Vice President Information Services
CHR: Joseph Mikitka, Vice President Human Resources
Web address: www.shh.org
**Control:** Other not–for–profit (including NFP Corporation) **Service:** General
Medical and Surgical

**Staffed Beds:** 141 **Admissions:** 6252 **Census:** 105 **Outpatient Visits:**
160619 **Births:** 265 **Total Expense ($000):** 98164 **Payroll Expense ($000):**
38965 **Personnel:** 857

**ST LUKE'S HOSPITAL – ALLENTOWN CAMPUS** See St. Luke's University
Hospital – Bethlehem Campus, Bethlehem

**SURGICAL SPECIALTY CENTER AT COORDINATED HEALTH (390321)**, 1503
North Cedar Crest Boulevard, Zip 18104–2302; tel. 610/861–8080,
(Nonreporting) **A**9 10
Primary Contact: Emil Dilorio, M.D., Chief Executive Officer
Web address: www.coordinatedhealth.com
**Control:** Other not–for–profit (including NFP Corporation) **Service:** Surgical

**Staffed Beds:** 20

☐ **WESTFIELD HOSPITAL (390318)**, 4815 West Tilghman Street,
Zip 18104–9374; tel. 610/973–8400, (Nonreporting) **A**1 9 10
Primary Contact: Yasin N. Khan, M.D., Chief Executive Officer
Web address: www.westfieldhospital.com
**Control:** Corporation, Investor–owned, for–profit **Service:** General Medical and
Surgical

**Staffed Beds:** 26

## ALTOONA—Blair County

⊠ ○ **ALTOONA REGIONAL HEALTH SYSTEM (390073)**, 620 Howard Avenue,
Zip 16601–4804; tel. 814/889–2011 **A**1 2 9 10 11 12 13 **F**3 5 8 11 12 13 15
18 20 22 24 26 28 29 30 31 32 34 35 37 38 40 43 45 47 48 49 50 51 54
55 56 57 59 60 64 65 66 68 70 73 74 75 76 77 78 79 81 83 84 85 86 87
89 90 93 98 100 101 102 103 107 108 111 113 114 115 116 117 118 119
120 122 123 128 129 130 131 134 145 146 147
Primary Contact: Gerald Murray, President and Chief Executive Officer
COO: Ron McConnell, Chief Operating Officer
CFO: Charles Zorger, Senior Vice President Finance
CMO: David Cowger, M.D., Senior Vice President Quality and Medical Affairs and
Chief Medical Officer
CIO: Dale Fuller, Vice President and Chief Information Officer
CHR: Gary Naugle, Senior Vice President Human Resources
Web address: www.altoonaregional.org
**Control:** Other not–for–profit (including NFP Corporation) **Service:** General
Medical and Surgical

**Staffed Beds:** 433 **Admissions:** 18964 **Census:** 249 **Outpatient Visits:**
364263 **Births:** 1132 **Total Expense ($000):** 318177 **Payroll Expense
($000):** 124751 **Personnel:** 2149

⊠ **HEALTHSOUTH REHABILITATION HOSPITAL OF ALTOONA (393040)**, 2005
Valley View Boulevard, Zip 16602–4598; tel. 814/944–3535, (Nonreporting) **A**1
10 **S** HEALTHSOUTH Corporation, Birmingham, AL
Primary Contact: Scott Filler, Chief Executive Officer
CFO: George Berger, Controller
CMO: Rakesh Patel, D.O., Medical Director
CIO: Kathleen Edwards, Manager Information Systems Operation
CHR: Christine Filer, Director Human Resources
Web address: www.healthsouthaltoona.com
**Control:** Corporation, Investor–owned, for–profit **Service:** Rehabilitation

**Staffed Beds:** 70

⊠ **JAMES E. VAN ZANDT VETERANS AFFAIRS MEDICAL CENTER**, 2907
Pleasant Valley Boulevard, Zip 16602–4305; tel. 814/943–8164, (Nonreporting)
**A**1 9 **S** Department of Veterans Affairs, Washington, DC
Primary Contact: Charles T. Becker, Acting Director
COO: Charles T. Becker, Acting Director
CFO: Teresa Waksmonski, Chief Fiscal Service
CMO: Santha Kurian, M.D., Chief of Staff
CIO: Shawn Nocita, Chief Information Resource Management
CHR: Nicole Albus, Chief Human Resources
Web address: www.altoona.va.gov
**Control:** Veterans Affairs, Government, federal **Service:** General Medical and
Surgical

**Staffed Beds:** 68

---

**Hospital, Medicare Provider Number, Address, Telephone, Approval, Facility, and Physician Codes, Health Care System**

★ American Hospital Association (AHA) membership
☐ The Joint Commission accreditation ◇ DNV Healthcare Inc. accreditation

○ American Osteopathic Association (AOA) accreditation
△ Commission on Accreditation of Rehabilitation Facilities (CARF) accreditation

**PA**

### AMBLER—Montgomery County

☐ **HORSHAM CLINIC (394034)**, 722 East Butler Pike, Zip 19002–2310;
tel. 215/643–7800, (Nonreporting) **A**1 9 10 **S** Universal Health Services, Inc.,
King of Prussia, PA
Primary Contact: Phyllis Weisfield, Chief Executive Officer and Managing Director
CFO: Robert Chavez, Chief Financial Officer
CMO: James B. Congdon, M.D., Medical Director
CIO: Suzanne Scholz, Director Medical Records
CHR: Kathleen Nichelson, Director Human Resources
CNO: Linda Starr, Director of Nursing
Web address: www.horshamclinic.com
**Control:** Individual, Investor–owned, for–profit **Service:** Psychiatric

| Staffed Beds: 138 |
| --- |

### ASHLAND—Schuylkill County

**SAINT CATHERINE MEDICAL CENTER FOUNTAIN SPRINGS (390313)**, 101
Broad Street, Zip 17921–2147; tel. 570/875–2000, (Nonreporting) **A**9 10
**S** Saint Catherine Healthcare, LLC, Ashland, PA
Primary Contact: Daniel A. Colon, President and Chief Executive Officer
CFO: Merlyn E. Knapp, Chief Financial Officer
CMO: John W. Stefovic, M.D., President Medical Staff
Web address: www.stchc.com/scmcfs
**Control:** Corporation, Investor–owned, for–profit **Service:** General Medical and
Surgical

| Staffed Beds: 79 |
| --- |

### BEAVER—Beaver County

☐ **HERITAGE VALLEY BEAVER (390036)**, 1000 Dutch Ridge Road,
Zip 15009–9727; tel. 724/728–7000, (Nonreporting) **A**1 9 10 12 13 **S** Heritage
Valley Health System, Beaver, PA
Primary Contact: Norman F. Mitry, President and Chief Executive Officer
COO: Rosemary Nolan, R.N., Chief Operating Officer and Chief Nursing Officer
CFO: Bryan J. Randall, Vice President Finance and Chief Financial Officer
CMO: John Cinicola, M.D., Chief Medical Officer
CIO: David Carleton, Chief Information Officer
CHR: Bruce Edwards, Vice President Human Resources
CNO: Marcia L. Ferrero, MS, Chief Nursing Officer
Web address: www.heritagevalley.org
**Control:** Other not–for–profit (including NFP Corporation) **Service:** General
Medical and Surgical

| Staffed Beds: 312 |
| --- |

✠ **KINDRED HOSPITAL–HERITAGE VALLEY (392043)**, 1000 Dutch Ridge Road,
Zip 15009; tel. 724/773–8480, (Nonreporting) **A**1 9 10 **S** Kindred Healthcare,
Louisville, KY
Primary Contact: Rodney B. Jones, Administrator
CFO: Kevin Varley, Chief Financial Officer
CMO: Jeffrey Erukhimou, M.D., Medical Director
Web address: www.kindredhospitalhv.com/
**Control:** Corporation, Investor–owned, for–profit **Service:** Long–Term Acute Care
hospital

| Staffed Beds: 35 |
| --- |

### BENSALEM—Bucks County

**LIVENGRIN FOUNDATION**, 4833 Hulmeville Road, Zip 19020–3099;
tel. 215/638–5200, (Nonreporting) **A**9
Primary Contact: Richard M. Pine, President and Chief Executive Officer
CFO: James D. Flis, Chief Financial Officer
CMO: William J. Lorman, Ph.D., Clinical Director
CIO: William Miller, Coordinator Management Information Systems
Web address: www.livengrin.org
**Control:** Other not–for–profit (including NFP Corporation) **Service:** Alcoholism and
other chemical dependency

| Staffed Beds: 76 |
| --- |

**ROTHMAN SPECIALTY HOSPITAL (390322)**, 3300 Tillman Drive,
Zip 19020–2071; tel. 215/244–7400, (Nonreporting)
Primary Contact: Michael A. West, Chief Executive Officer
Web address: www.rothmanspecialtyhospital.com/
**Control:** Partnership, Investor–owned, for–profit **Service:** Surgical

| Staffed Beds: 24 |
| --- |

### BERWICK—Columbia County

✠ **BERWICK HOSPITAL CENTER (390072)**, 701 East 16th Street,
Zip 18603–2397; tel. 570/759–5000, (Total facility includes 240 beds in nursing
home–type unit) **A**1 9 10 **F**3 13 15 20 28 29 31 34 39 40 46 56 57 59 62 63
64 70 74 75 76 77 78 79 81 82 85 93 98 102 103 107 110 111 113 116
118 127 128 129 131 132 145 146 147 **P**6 **S** Community Health Systems,
Inc., Franklin, TN
Primary Contact: Ronald R. Beer, Chief Executive Officer
CFO: Jay Graham, Interim Chief Financial Officer
CMO: Frank Giugliano, M.D., Chief of Staff
CHR: Jackie Ridall, Director Human Resources
Web address: www.berwick–hospital.com
**Control:** Corporation, Investor–owned, for–profit **Service:** General Medical and
Surgical

| Staffed Beds: 341 Admissions: 3505 Census: 217 Outpatient Visits: 88646 |
| --- |
| Births: 80 Personnel: 455 |

### BETHLEHEM—Lehigh County

☐ **GOOD SHEPHERD SPECIALTY HOSPITAL (392033)**, 2545 Schoenersville
Road, 3rd Floor, Zip 18017; tel. 484/884–5051 **A**1 9 10 **F**1 3 **P**5 **S** Good
Shepherd Rehabilitation Network, Allentown, PA
Primary Contact: Lisa Marsilio, Vice President and Administrator
Web address: www.goodshepherdrehab.org
**Control:** Other not–for–profit (including NFP Corporation) **Service:** Long–Term
Acute Care hospital

| Staffed Beds: 32 Admissions: 400 Census: 29 Outpatient Visits: 0 Births: |
| --- |
| 0 Total Expense ($000): 15568 Payroll Expense ($000): 5315 Personnel: |
| 81 |

✠ **LEHIGH VALLEY HOSPITAL–MUHLENBERG (390263)**, 2545 Schoenersville
Road, Zip 18017–7300; tel. 484/884–2201 **A**1 2 9 10 12 13 **F**3 11 12 15 17
18 20 22 24 26 28 29 30 31 34 35 36 37 38 39 40 44 45 49 50 51 53 54
57 58 59 60 62 63 64 65 68 70 74 77 78 79 80 81 82 84 85 86 87 90 92
93 96 97 102 106 107 108 110 111 113 114 117 118 119 120 122 123
128 129 130 131 133 134 142 145 147 **P**5 6 8 **S** Lehigh Valley Health
Network, Allentown, PA
Primary Contact: Ronald W. Swinfard, M.D., President and Chief Executive Officer
COO: Terry Ann Capuano, R.N., Chief Operating Officer
CMO: Thomas Whalen, M.D., Chief Medical Officer
CIO: Harry Lukens, Senior Vice President and Chief Information Officer
CHR: Mary Kay Grim, Senior Vice President Human Resources
Web address: www.lvhn.org
**Control:** Other not–for–profit (including NFP Corporation) **Service:** General
Medical and Surgical

| Staffed Beds: 168 Admissions: 10534 Census: 143 Outpatient Visits: |
| --- |
| 167799 Births: 0 Total Expense ($000): 188942 Payroll Expense ($000): |
| 68036 Personnel: 1261 |

☐ △ **ST. LUKE'S UNIVERSITY HOSPITAL – BETHLEHEM CAMPUS (390049)**,
801 Ostrum Street, Zip 18015–1065; tel. 610/954–4000, (Includes ST LUKE'S
HOSPITAL – ALLENTOWN CAMPUS, 1736 Hamilton Street, Allentown,
Zip 18104–5656; tel. 610/770–8300) **A**1 2 3 5 6 7 8 9 10 12 13 **F**3 9 11 12
13 15 17 18 19 20 22 24 26 27 28 29 30 31 32 34 35 36 37 38 39 40 42
43 44 45 46 47 48 49 50 51 52 53 54 55 56 57 58 59 60 61 63 64 65 66
68 70 71 72 73 74 75 76 77 78 79 81 82 84 85 86 87 89 90 93 96 97 98
99 100 101 102 103 104 105 107 108 109 110 111 114 116 117 118 119
120 122 123 125 128 129 130 131 133 134 143 144 145 146 147 **P**6 8
**S** St. Luke's University Health Network, Bethlehem, PA
Primary Contact: Richard A. Anderson, President and Chief Executive Officer
COO: Carol Kuplen, R.N., Chief Operating Officer and Chief Nursing Officer
CFO: Tom Lichtenwalner, Vice President Finance
CMO: Jeffrey Jahre, M.D., Vice President Medical and Academic Affairs
CIO: Chad Brisendine, Chief Information Officer
CHR: Robert Zimmel, Senior Vice President Human Resources
Web address: www.slhn–lehighvalley.org
**Control:** Other not–for–profit (including NFP Corporation) **Service:** General
Medical and Surgical

| Staffed Beds: 581 Admissions: 34166 Census: 391 Outpatient Visits: |
| --- |
| 789728 Births: 4151 Total Expense ($000): 465177 Payroll Expense |
| ($000): 233083 Personnel: 4218 |

*Many Facility Codes have changed. Please refer to the AHA Guide Code Chart.* © 2012 AHA Guide

## BLOOMSBURG—Columbia County

★ **GEISINGER–BLOOMSBURG HOSPITAL (390003)**, 549 Fair Street, Zip 17815–1419; tel. 570/387–2100 **A**9 10 **F**3 11 13 15 18 26 28 29 30 31 34 35 36 40 44 45 50 51 56 57 59 64 65 68 70 75 76 77 78 79 81 82 85 87 93 98 99 101 102 103 107 108 110 111 114 117 118 123 128 129 131 134 **S** Geisinger Health System, Danville, PA
Primary Contact: Lissa Bryan–Smith, Chief Administrative Officer
COO: Joseph M. DeVito, Vice President Finance and Chief Operating Officer
CFO: Joseph M. DeVito, Vice President Finance and Chief Operating Officer
CMO: James Joseph, M.D., President Medical Staff
CIO: Thomas Wray, Director Information
CHR: Mary Lenzini Howe, Vice President Human Resources
Web address: www.bloomhealth.net
**Control:** Other not–for–profit (including NFP Corporation) **Service:** General Medical and Surgical

**Staffed Beds:** 72 **Admissions:** 2807 **Census:** 32 **Outpatient Visits:** 85484
**Births:** 303 **Total Expense ($000):** 38463 **Payroll Expense ($000):** 16284
**Personnel:** 364

## BRADFORD—Mckean County

★ **BRADFORD REGIONAL MEDICAL CENTER (390118)**, 116 Interstate Parkway, Zip 16701–1036; tel. 814/368–4143, (Total facility includes 95 beds in nursing home–type unit) **A**9 10 **F**3 5 8 11 13 15 18 20 28 29 31 34 35 39 40 45 47 49 50 53 56 57 59 62 63 64 65 70 75 76 77 78 79 81 82 84 85 86 87 93 97 98 100 101 102 103 104 105 107 108 110 111 113 116 117 118 127 128 129 130 131 134 145 146 147 **P**6 **S** Upper Allegheny Health System, Olean, NY
Primary Contact: Timothy J. Finan, FACHE, President and Chief Executive Officer
COO: David A. Kobis, Senior Vice President and Chief Operating Officer
CFO: Richard G. Braun, Jr., CPA, Senior Vice President and Chief Financial Officer
CMO: William Mills, M.D., Senior Vice President Quality and Professional Affairs
CIO: Jason Yaworsky, Chief Information Officer
CHR: Timothy M. McNamara, Senior Vice President Human Resources
Web address: www.brmc.com
**Control:** Other not–for–profit (including NFP Corporation) **Service:** General Medical and Surgical

**Staffed Beds:** 182 **Admissions:** 3367 **Census:** 131 **Outpatient Visits:** 126026 **Births:** 282 **Total Expense ($000):** 63489 **Payroll Expense ($000):** 27099 **Personnel:** 541

## BRISTOL—Bucks County

☐ **LOWER BUCKS HOSPITAL (390070)**, 501 Bath Road, Zip 19007–3190; tel. 215/785–9200 **A**1 9 10 **F**3 8 11 13 15 18 20 22 24 26 28 29 30 40 41 50 62 65 70 72 74 76 77 79 81 85 87 89 92 93 98 102 107 108 109 110 111 113 118 128 129 131 134 145 147
Primary Contact: Albert Mezzaroba, Chief Executive Officer
CFO: Michael Olivieri, Chief Financial Officer
CMO: Omid Rowshan, M.D., President Medical Staff
CIO: John McHale, Vice President Management Information Systems
CHR: Kellie Pearson, Director Human Resources
Web address: www.lowerbuckshospital.org
**Control:** Other not–for–profit (including NFP Corporation) **Service:** General Medical and Surgical

**Staffed Beds:** 150 **Admissions:** 7541 **Census:** 85 **Outpatient Visits:** 74888
**Births:** 987 **Total Expense ($000):** 91502 **Payroll Expense ($000):** 39674
**Personnel:** 671

## BROOKVILLE—Jefferson County

**BROOKVILLE HOSPITAL (391312)**, 100 Hospital Road, Zip 15825–1367; tel. 814/849–2312 **A**9 10 18 **F**3 11 15 18 28 29 30 34 35 39 40 45 46 57 59 62 64 65 75 77 79 81 82 85 86 93 98 102 103 104 107 108 110 113 117 118 126 128 129 130 131 132 144 145.
Primary Contact: Rose Campbell, R.N., President
CFO: Julie Peer, Vice President Finance
CMO: Timothy Pendleton, M.D., President Medical Staff
CIO: Benjamin Reynolds, Director Information Systems
CHR: Warren Thrush, Coordinator Human Resources
Web address: www.brookvillehospital.org
**Control:** Other not–for–profit (including NFP Corporation) **Service:** General Medical and Surgical

**Staffed Beds:** 35 **Admissions:** 1292 **Census:** 17 **Outpatient Visits:** 82644
**Births:** 0 **Total Expense ($000):** 26350 **Payroll Expense ($000):** 9591
**Personnel:** 245

## BRYN MAWR—Montgomery County

⊠ **BRYN MAWR HOSPITAL (390139)**, 130 South Bryn Mawr Avenue, Zip 19010–3160; tel. 484/337–3000, (Nonreporting) **A**1 2 3 5 9 10 13 **S** Main Line Health, Bryn Mawr, PA
Primary Contact: Andrea F. Gilbert, FACHE, President
COO: Andrea F. Gilbert, FACHE, President
CFO: Michael J. Buongiorno, Executive Vice President Finance and Chief Financial Officer
CMO: Donald C. Arthur, M.D., Chief Medical Officer
CIO: Karen A. Thomas, R.N., Vice President and Chief Information Officer
CHR: Terry Dougherty, Director Human Resources
Web address: www.brynmawrhospital.org
**Control:** Other not–for–profit (including NFP Corporation) **Service:** General Medical and Surgical

**Staffed Beds:** 319

## BUTLER—Butler County

★ **BUTLER HEALTH SYSTEM (390168)**, 1 Hospital Way, Zip 16001–4697; tel. 724/283–6666, (Total facility includes 25 beds in nursing–type unit) **A**2 9 10 **F**3 4 5 11 15 18 20 22 24 26 28 29 31 32 35 40 45 57 59 70 74 76 79 81 82 85 87 93 98 100 103 107 108 111 113 117 118 127 128 129 131 134 145 146 147 **P**6
Primary Contact: Ken DeFurio, President and Chief Executive Officer
CFO: Anne Krebs, Chief Financial Officer
CMO: John C. Reefer, M.D., Director
CIO: Chuck Oleson, Chief Information Officer
CHR: Thomas A. Genevro, Vice President Human Resources
Web address: www.butlerhealthsystem.org
**Control:** Other not–for–profit (including NFP Corporation) **Service:** General Medical and Surgical

**Staffed Beds:** 322 **Admissions:** 13136 **Census:** 178 **Outpatient Visits:** 484577 **Births:** 645 **Total Expense ($000):** 203305 **Payroll Expense ($000):** 77300 **Personnel:** 1387

★ △ **VA BUTLER HEALTHCARE**, 325 New Castle Road, Zip 16001–2480; tel. 724/287–4781, (Nonreporting) **A**7 9 **S** Department of Veterans Affairs, Washington, DC
Primary Contact: Patricia Nealon, Director
COO: Richard W. Cotter, Associate Director Operations
CFO: Doug George, Chief Financial Officer
CMO: Timothy R. Burke, M.D., Chief of Staff
CIO: Kirk Hastings, Chief Information Technology
CHR: Michelle Dominski, Human Resources Officer
Web address: www.butler.va.gov
**Control:** Veterans Affairs, Government, federal **Service:** Other specialty

**Staffed Beds:** 66

**VETERANS AFFAIRS MEDICAL CENTER** See VA Butler Healthcare

## CAMP HILL—Cumberland County

⊠ **HOLY SPIRIT HOSPITAL (390004)**, 503 North 21st Street, Zip 17011–2204; tel. 717/763–2100 **A**1 9 10 **F**3 8 11 13 14 15 17 18 20 22 24 26 28 29 30 31 34 35 37 38 40 44 46 49 50 54 57 58 59 61 62 63 64 65 70 72 73 74 75 76 77 78 79 80 81 82 84 85 86 87 93 94 96 98 99 100 101 102 103 104 105 107 108 110 111 113 114 118 125 128 129 131 133 134 143 144 145 146 147 **P**6
Primary Contact: Sister Romaine Niemeyer, President and Chief Executive Officer
COO: Richard Schaffner, Senior Vice President and Chief Operating Officer
CFO: Manuel J. Evans, Senior Vice President Finance and Chief Financial Officer
CMO: Joseph Torchia, M.D., Senior Vice President Medical Affairs and Chief Medical Officer
CIO: Edith Dees, Vice President Information Services and Chief Information Officer
CHR: William Shartle, Senior Vice President Human Resources
Web address: www.hsh.org
**Control:** Other not–for–profit (including NFP Corporation) **Service:** General Medical and Surgical

**Staffed Beds:** 290 **Admissions:** 15015 **Census:** 196 **Outpatient Visits:** 262212 **Births:** 1203 **Total Expense ($000):** 242920 **Payroll Expense ($000):** 105429 **Personnel:** 1895

---

**Hospital, Medicare Provider Number, Address, Telephone, Approval, Facility, and Physician Codes, Health Care System**

★ American Hospital Association (AHA) membership
☐ The Joint Commission accreditation     ◇ DNV Healthcare Inc. accreditation
○ American Osteopathic Association (AOA) accreditation
△ Commission on Accreditation of Rehabilitation Facilities (CARF) accreditation

✠ **SELECT SPECIALTY HOSPITAL–CENTRAL PENNSYLVANIA (392039)**, 503 North 21st Street, 5th Floor, Zip 17011; tel. 717/972–4575, (Includes SELECT SPECIALTY HOSPITAL–HARRISBURG, 2501 NorthThird Street, Landis Building, Harrisburg, Zip 17110–1904; tel. 717/724–6605; SELECT SPECIALTY HOSPITAL–YORK, 1001 South George Street, York, Zip 17403–3676; tel. 717/851–2661; Marcia Medlin, Chief Executive Officer), (Nonreporting) **A**1 9 10 **S** Select Medical Corporation, Mechanicsburg, PA
Primary Contact: Claudia Ann Eisenmann, Chief Executive Officer
Web address: www.selectmedicalcorp.com
**Control:** Corporation, Investor–owned, for–profit **Service:** Long–Term Acute Care hospital

| Staffed Beds: 92 |
| --- |

**STATE CORRECTIONAL INSTITUTION AT CAMP HILL**, 2500 Lisburn Road, Zip 17011–8005, Mailing Address: P.O. Box 200, Zip 17001–0200; tel. 717/737–4531, (Nonreporting)
Primary Contact: Kathy Montag, Administrator Health Care
Web address: www.cor.state.pa.us/
**Control:** State–Government, nonfederal **Service:** Other specialty

| Staffed Beds: 34 |
| --- |

### CANONSBURG—Washington County

✠ **CANONSBURG GENERAL HOSPITAL (390160)**, 100 Medical Boulevard, Zip 15317–9762; tel. 724/745–6100, (Nonreporting) **A**1 9 10 **S** West Penn Allegheny Health System, Pittsburgh, PA
Primary Contact: Terry Wiltrout, Chief Executive Officer
CFO: Gene Trout, Chief Financial Officer
CMO: Thomas B. Corkery, D.O., Chief Medical Officer
CIO: David Vincent, Director Information Systems
CHR: Martha L. Clister, Director Human Resources
Web address: www.wpahs.org
**Control:** Other not–for–profit (including NFP Corporation) **Service:** General Medical and Surgical

| Staffed Beds: 60 |
| --- |

### CARLISLE—Cumberland County

☐ **CARLISLE REGIONAL MEDICAL CENTER (390058)**, 361 Alexander Spring Road, Zip 17015–6940; tel. 717/249–1212, (Nonreporting) **A**1 9 10 **S** Health Management Associates, Naples, FL
Primary Contact: John Kristel, Chief Executive Officer
CFO: Jeffrey Morgan, Associate Executive Director and Chief Financial Officer
CMO: Howard Alster, M.D., President Medical Staff
CIO: Kemp Beatty, Director Information Management
Web address: www.carlislermc.com/default.aspx
**Control:** Corporation, Investor–owned, for–profit **Service:** General Medical and Surgical

| Staffed Beds: 165 |
| --- |

### CENTRE HALL—Centre County

✠ **MEADOWS PSYCHIATRIC CENTER (394040)**, 132 The Meadows Drive, Zip 16828–9231; tel. 814/364–2161, (Nonreporting) **A**1 9 10 **S** Universal Health Services, Inc., King of Prussia, PA
Primary Contact: Thomas Kenny, Chief Executive Officer
CMO: Nalin Patel, M.D., Medical Director
CHR: Kimberly J. Tate, Director Human Resources
Web address: www.themeadows.net
**Control:** Corporation, Investor–owned, for–profit **Service:** Psychiatric

| Staffed Beds: 101 |
| --- |

### CHAMBERSBURG—Franklin County

✠ **CHAMBERSBURG HOSPITAL (390151)**, 112 North Seventh Street, Zip 17201–1720; tel. 717/267–3000 **A**1 2 9 10 19 **F**3 11 12 13 15 17 18 20 22 28 29 30 31 34 35 36 37 38 39 40 45 49 50 53 54 56 57 59 61 64 65 68 70 74 75 76 77 78 79 81 82 83 84 85 86 87 89 90 91 93 94 95 97 98 99 100 101 102 103 104 107 108 110 111 113 116 117 118 119 120 122 125 128 129 130 131 134 143 145 146 147 **P**6 8 **S** Summit Health, Chambersburg, PA
Primary Contact: Norman B. Epstein, FACHE, President
COO: John P. Massimilla, FACHE, Vice President Administration
CFO: Patrick W. O'Donnell, CPA, Senior Vice President and Chief Operating Officer
CMO: Thomas Anderson, M.D., Vice President Medical Affairs
CIO: Michele Zeigler, Vice President and Chief Information Officer
CHR: Louis J. Gregorio, FACHE, Vice President Human Resources
Web address: www.summithealth.org
**Control:** Other not–for–profit (including NFP Corporation) **Service:** General Medical and Surgical

| Staffed Beds: 240 Admissions: 12447 Census: 141 Outpatient Visits: 333811 Births: 1407 Total Expense ($000): 218042 Payroll Expense ($000): 93238 Personnel: 1490 |
| --- |

### CLARION—Clarion County

★ ○ **CLARION HOSPITAL (390093)**, One Hospital Drive, Zip 16214–8501; tel. 814/226–9500 **A**9 10 11 12 13 **F**3 7 11 13 15 29 30 31 35 40 48 49 51 57 59 64 70 76 77 78 79 81 82 84 85 90 107 108 111 114 118 128 129 131 132 134 144 145 147 **S** QHR, Brentwood, TN
Primary Contact: Byron Quinton, Chief Executive Officer
CFO: Vincent M. Lamorella, Chief Financial Officer
CHR: Michael Wienand, Manager Human Resources
Web address: www.clarionhospital.org
**Control:** Other not–for–profit (including NFP Corporation) **Service:** General Medical and Surgical

| Staffed Beds: 77 Admissions: 2740 Census: 30 Outpatient Visits: 127403 Births: 249 Total Expense ($000): 48206 Payroll Expense ($000): 17436 Personnel: 482 |
| --- |

☐ **CLARION PSYCHIATRIC CENTER (394043)**, 2 Hospital Drive, Zip 16214–8502; tel. 814/226–9545, (Nonreporting) **A**1 9 10 **S** Universal Health Services, Inc., King of Prussia, PA
Primary Contact: Robert Scheffler, Chief Executive Officer
CFO: Shelly Rhoades, Chief Financial Officer
CMO: Maher Ayyash, M.D., Chief Medical Officer
CHR: Dianne C. Bilunka, Director Human Resources
Web address: www.clarioncenter.com
**Control:** Corporation, Investor–owned, for–profit **Service:** Psychiatric

| Staffed Beds: 74 |
| --- |

### CLARKS SUMMIT—Lackawanna County

☐ **CLARKS SUMMIT STATE HOSPITAL (394012)**, 1451 Hillside Drive, Zip 18411–9504; tel. 570/586–2011, (Nonreporting) **A**1 10
Primary Contact: Thomas P. Comerford, Jr., Superintendent
COO: Gordon Weber, Chief Operating Officer
CMO: David Waibel, M.D., Medical Director
CHR: William Abda, Chief Human Resources Officer
Web address: www.dpw.state.pa.us/
**Control:** State–Government, nonfederal **Service:** Psychiatric

| Staffed Beds: 242 |
| --- |

### CLEARFIELD—Clearfield County

**CLEARFIELD HOSPITAL (390052)**, 809 Turnpike Avenue, Zip 16830–1232, Mailing Address: P.O. Box 992, Zip 16830–0992; tel. 814/765–5341, (Nonreporting) **A**9 10
Primary Contact: Gary Macioce, President and Chief Executive Officer
CFO: Pat Cressley, Vice President and Chief Financial Officer
CMO: Gregory Sheffo, M.D., Chief Medical Officer
CIO: Terry Trinidad, Director Management Information Systems
CHR: Robert J. McKee, Vice President and Chief Human Resources Officer
CNO: Kathy Bedger, Chief Nursing Officer
Web address: www.clearfieldhosp.org
**Control:** Other not–for–profit (including NFP Corporation) **Service:** General Medical and Surgical

| Staffed Beds: 96 |
| --- |

### COALDALE—Schuylkill County

☐ **ST. LUKE'S HOSPITAL – MINERS CAMPUS (390183)**, 360 West Ruddle Street, Zip 18218–1027; tel. 570/645–2131, (Total facility includes 48 beds in nursing home–type unit) **A**1 9 10 **F**3 15 18 28 29 31 34 40 45 49 51 53 54 56 57 59 60 62 64 65 68 70 75 77 78 79 81 85 86 93 107 108 110 111 114 117 118 126 127 128 129 130 131 144 145 147 **P**6 8 **S** St. Luke's University Health Network, Bethlehem, PA
Primary Contact: William E. Moyer, President
COO: Joel Fagerstrom, Executive Vice President and Chief Operating Officer
CFO: Michele Levitz, Director Finance
CMO: Glenn Freed, D.O., Medical Director
CIO: Chad Brisendine, Vice President and Chief Information Officer
CHR: Susan Van Why, Director Human Resources
CNO: Kimberly Sargent, Vice President Patient Services
Web address: www.slhn.org
**Control:** Other not–for–profit (including NFP Corporation) **Service:** General Medical and Surgical

| Staffed Beds: 92 Admissions: 1808 Census: 65 Outpatient Visits: 104035 Births: 0 Total Expense ($000): 38748 Payroll Expense ($000): 16126 Personnel: 335 |
| --- |

### COATESVILLE—Chester County

✠ **BRANDYWINE HOSPITAL (390076)**, 201 Reeceville Road, Zip 19320–1536; tel. 610/383–8000, (Nonreporting) **A**1 2 6 9 10 **S** Community Health Systems, Inc., Franklin, TN
Primary Contact: Bryan Burklow, Chief Executive Officer
COO: Jill Tillman, Assistant Chief Executive Officer
CFO: Jay Graham, Interim Chief Financial Officer
Web address: www.brandywinehospital.com
**Control:** Corporation, Investor–owned, for–profit **Service:** General Medical and Surgical

| Staffed Beds: 164 |
| --- |

*Many Facility Codes have changed. Please refer to the AHA Guide Code Chart.* © 2012 AHA Guide

☒ △ **VETERANS AFFAIRS MEDICAL CENTER**, 1400 Black Horse Hill Road, Zip 19320–2040; tel. 610/384–7711, (Nonreporting) **A**1 7 9 **S** Department of Veterans Affairs, Washington, DC
Primary Contact: Gary W. Devansky, Director
CFO: Tony Wolfgang, Chief Financial Officer
CMO: James F. Tischler, M.D., Chief of Staff
CIO: Eugene Doria, Chief Information Officer
CHR: George Pearson, Director Human Resources Management Service
Web address: www.va.gov/sta/guide/home.asp
**Control:** Veterans Affairs, Government, federal **Service:** Alcoholism and other chemical dependency

**Staffed Beds: 306**

### CONNELLSVILLE—Fayette County

**HIGHLANDS HOSPITAL (390184)**, 401 East Murphy Avenue, Zip 15425–2700; tel. 724/628–1500 **A**9 10 **F**3 11 12 15 29 30 34 35 36 39 40 44 45 46 49 50 51 53 56 57 59 61 64 65 70 75 77 79 81 85 87 89 93 98 99 100 101 102 103 107 108 113 118 128 129 131 132 142 145
Primary Contact: Michelle P. Cunningham, Chief Executive Officer
CFO: John Andursky, Chief Financial Officer
CMO: Richard Grimaldi, President Medical Staff
CIO: John Andursky, Chief Financial Officer
CHR: Mary June Krosoff, Chief Human Resources Officer
CNO: Tammy Donaldson, Director of Nursing
Web address: www.highlandshospital.org
**Control:** Other not–for–profit (including NFP Corporation) **Service:** General Medical and Surgical

**Staffed Beds: 71 Admissions: 2543 Census: 33 Outpatient Visits: 58311 Births: 0 Total Expense ($000): 23160 Payroll Expense ($000): 10036 Personnel: 269**

### CORRY—Erie County

**CORRY MEMORIAL HOSPITAL (391308)**, 612 West Smith Street, Zip 16407–1196; tel. 814/664–4641, (Nonreporting) **A**9 10 18
Primary Contact: Barbara Nichols, R.N., President and Chief Executive Officer
CFO: Michael Heller, Chief Financial Officer
CIO: Ken O'Day, Supervisor Information Systems
CHR: Gary Webb, Director Human Resources
Web address: www.corryhospital.com
**Control:** Other not–for–profit (including NFP Corporation) **Service:** General Medical and Surgical

**Staffed Beds: 25**

### COUDERSPORT—Potter County

☒ **CHARLES COLE MEMORIAL HOSPITAL (391313)**, 1001 East Second Street, Zip 16915–8161; tel. 814/274–9300, (Total facility includes 49 beds in nursing home–type unit) **A**1 9 10 18 **F**3 10 11 13 15 28 29 30 31 35 40 45 48 49 53 57 59 62 63 64 70 76 77 78 79 81 82 87 92 93 98 103 107 108 111 113 118 120 126 127 128 129 130 131 132 144 145 146 147 **P**6
Primary Contact: Edward C. Pitchford, President and Chief Executive Officer
COO: Cynthia Hardesty, Vice President and Chief Nursing Executive
CFO: Ron Rapp, Controller
CMO: Michael E. Callahan, M.D., President Medical Staff
CIO: Geoff Mazur, Director Information Technology
CHR: J. Thomas Noe, Director Human Resources
Web address: www.charlescolehospital.com
**Control:** Other not–for–profit (including NFP Corporation) **Service:** General Medical and Surgical

**Staffed Beds: 84 Admissions: 1907 Census: 67 Outpatient Visits: 229147 Births: 240 Total Expense ($000): 66530 Payroll Expense ($000): 23831 Personnel: 494**

### CRANBERRY—Butler County

**UPMC PASSAVANT CRANBERRY** See UPMC Passavant, Pittsburgh

### DANVILLE—Montour County

☐ **DANVILLE STATE HOSPITAL (394004)**, 200 State Hospital Drive, Zip 17821–9198; tel. 570/271–4500, (Nonreporting) **A**1 10
Primary Contact: Theresa Long, Chief Executive Officer
COO: Thomas J. Burk, Chief Operating Officer
CFO: Patricia Riegert, Director Fiscal Services
CMO: Anthony Montecalvo, M.D., Chief Medical Executive
CHR: Thomas J. Burk, Chief Operating Officer
CNO: Brenda Lahout, Chief Nurse Executive
Web address: www.dpw.state.pa.us/foradults/statehospitals/danvillestatehospital/index.htm
**Control:** State–Government, nonfederal **Service:** Psychiatric

**Staffed Beds: 170**

☒ **GEISINGER HEALTHSOUTH REHABILITATION HOSPITAL (393047)**, 2 Rehab Lane, Zip 17821; tel. 570/271–6733, (Nonreporting) **A**1 9 10 **S** HEALTHSOUTH Corporation, Birmingham, AL
Primary Contact: Lorie Dillon, Chief Executive Officer
CFO: Sally Shipierski, Controller
CMO: Greg Burke, M.D., Medical Director
CHR: Christian Shirley, Director Human Resources
Web address: www.geisingerhealthsouth.com
**Control:** Corporation, Investor–owned, for–profit **Service:** Rehabilitation

**Staffed Beds: 42**

☒ **GEISINGER MEDICAL CENTER (390006)**, 100 North Academy Avenue, Zip 17822–2201; tel. 570/271–6211, (Includes GEISINGER–SHAMOKIN AREA COMMUNITY HOSPITAL, 4200 Hospital Road, Coal Township, Zip 17866–9697; tel. 570/644–4200; Thomas R. Harlow, FACHE, President and Chief Executive Officer) **A**1 2 3 5 8 9 10 13 19 **F**3 7 8 9 11 12 13 15 17 18 19 20 21 22 23 24 25 26 27 28 29 30 31 32 34 35 36 38 39 40 43 44 45 46 47 48 49 50 51 52 53 54 55 57 58 59 60 61 64 65 70 71 72 73 74 75 76 77 78 79 80 81 82 84 85 86 87 88 89 93 94 97 98 99 100 101 102 103 104 105 107 108 110 111 113 114 115 116 117 118 119 120 122 123 125 126 128 129 130 131 133 134 135 137 138 140 141 144 145 146 147 **P**6 **S** Geisinger Health System, Danville, PA
Primary Contact: Thomas P. Sokola, Chief Administrative Officer
COO: Frank J. Trembulak, Executive Vice President and Chief Operating Officer
CFO: Kevin F. Brennan, CPA, Executive Vice President and Chief Financial Officer
CIO: Frank Richards, Chief Information Officer
CHR: Richard E. Merkle, Chief Human Resources Officer
Web address: www.geisinger.org
**Control:** Other not–for–profit (including NFP Corporation) **Service:** General Medical and Surgical

**Staffed Beds: 475 Admissions: 26028 Census: 359 Outpatient Visits: 822583 Births: 1749 Total Expense ($000): 773052 Payroll Expense ($000): 213869 Personnel: 5182**

☒ **SELECT SPECIALTY HOSPITAL–DANVILLE (392047)**, 100 North Academy Avenue, 3rd Floor, Zip 17822–3050; tel. 570/214–9653, (Nonreporting) **A**1 9 10 **S** Select Medical Corporation, Mechanicsburg, PA
Primary Contact: Brian Mann, Chief Executive Officer
Web address: www.selectmedicalcorp.com
**Control:** Corporation, Investor–owned, for–profit **Service:** Long–Term Acute Care hospital

**Staffed Beds: 30**

### DARBY—Delaware County

☒ **KINDRED HOSPITAL–DELAWARE COUNTY (392032)**, 1500 Lansdowne Avenue, 6th Floor, Zip 19023; tel. 610/237–5780, (Nonreporting) **A**1 9 10 **S** Kindred Healthcare, Louisville, KY
Primary Contact: Deborah Karn, Chief Executive Officer
COO: Susan Ferguson, Chief Operating Officer
CFO: Thomas A. McMullen, Chief Financial Officer
CMO: Joanne Connaughton, M.D., Chief Medical Officer
CHR: Neil Rosner, Area Director Human Resources
Web address: www.kindreddelco.com/
**Control:** Corporation, Investor–owned, for–profit **Service:** Long–Term Acute Care hospital

**Staffed Beds: 39**

☒ △ **MERCY FITZGERALD HOSPITAL (390156)**, 1500 South Lansdowe Avenue, Zip 19023; tel. 610/237–4000, (Includes MERCY FITZGERALD HOSPITAL, 1500 South Lansdowe Avenue, tel. 610/237–4000; MERCY PHILADELPHIA HOSPITAL, 501 South 54th Street, Philadelphia, Zip 19143; tel. 215/748–9000) **A**1 2 3 7 9 10 12 13 **F**3 4 5 11 12 15 18 20 22 24 26 28 29 30 31 34 35 38 40 45 49 50 51 53 54 55 57 58 59 61 64 65 66 69 70 75 77 78 79 81 82 85 86 87 90 91 92 93 96 97 98 100 101 102 103 104 107 108 110 111 113 114 117 118 119 120 122 123 129 131 134 144 145 146 147 **S** Catholic Health East, Newtown Square, PA
Primary Contact: Kathryn Conallen, Executive Director
COO: Ruth Thomas, Chief Operating Officer
CFO: Don Snenk, Chief Financial Officer
CMO: Jeff Komins, M.D., Chief Medical Officer
CIO: Jeff Byda, Vice President Information Technology
Web address: www.mercyhealth.org
**Control:** Church–operated, Nongovernment, not–for profit **Service:** General Medical and Surgical

**Staffed Beds: 391 Admissions: 20010 Census: 257 Outpatient Visits: 226382 Births: 0 Total Expense ($000): 315533 Payroll Expense ($000): 121593 Personnel: 2111**

---

**Hospital, Medicare Provider Number, Address, Telephone, Approval, Facility, and Physician Codes, Health Care System**

★ American Hospital Association (AHA) membership
☐ The Joint Commission accreditation  ◇ DNV Healthcare Inc. accreditation
○ American Osteopathic Association (AOA) accreditation
△ Commission on Accreditation of Rehabilitation Facilities (CARF) accreditation

**PA**

### DOWNINGTOWN—Chester County

**ST. JOHN VIANNEY HOSPITAL**, 151 Woodbine Road, Zip 19335–3057; tel. 610/269–2600, (Nonreporting) **A**9
Primary Contact: Edward Maguire, Administrator
Web address: www.sjvcenter.org
**Control:** Church–operated, Nongovernment, not–for profit **Service:** Psychiatric

**Staffed Beds:** 42

### DOYLESTOWN—Bucks County

⊞ **DOYLESTOWN HOSPITAL (390203)**, 595 West State Street, Zip 18901–2597; tel. 215/345–2200, (Total facility includes 127 beds in nursing home–type unit) **A**1 2 9 10 **F**3 8 10 13 15 17 18 20 22 24 26 28 29 30 31 34 35 40 45 49 50 54 56 57 58 59 62 63 64 70 73 74 75 76 77 78 79 81 82 84 85 86 92 93 94 96 107 108 110 111 113 114 116 117 118 123 124 125 127 129 130 131 140 145 146 147 **P**5 6 8
Primary Contact: Richard A. Reif, President and Chief Executive Officer
COO: Eleanor Wilson, R.N., Vice President and Chief Operating Officer
CFO: Daniel Upton, Vice President and Chief Financial Officer
CMO: Scott S. Levy, M.D., Vice President and Chief Medical Officer
CIO: Richard Lang, Ed.D., Vice President and Chief Information Officer
CHR: Barbara Hebel, Vice President Human Resources
Web address: www.dh.org
**Control:** Other not–for–profit (including NFP Corporation) **Service:** General Medical and Surgical

**Staffed Beds:** 374 **Admissions:** 12860 **Census:** 201 **Outpatient Visits:** 302731 **Births:** 1256 **Total Expense ($000):** 229478 **Payroll Expense ($000):** 91495 **Personnel:** 1668

☐ **FOUNDATIONS BEHAVIORAL HEALTH (394038)**, 833 East Butler Avenue, Zip 18901–2280; tel. 215/345–0444, (Nonreporting) **A**1 9 10 **S** Universal Health Services, Inc., King of Prussia, PA
Primary Contact: Robert Weinhold, Chief Executive Officer
Web address: www.fbh.com
**Control:** Other not–for–profit (including NFP Corporation) **Service:** Children's hospital psychiatric

**Staffed Beds:** 102

### DREXEL HILL—Delaware County

⊞ ○ **DELAWARE COUNTY MEMORIAL HOSPITAL (390081)**, 501 North Lansdowne Avenue, Zip 19026–1114; tel. 610/284–8100 **A**1 2 3 5 9 10 11 12 **F**3 7 9 11 13 15 17 18 28 29 30 31 34 35 36 40 44 45 46 49 50 51 55 56 57 58 59 60 61 62 63 64 68 72 74 75 76 77 78 79 81 84 85 86 87 90 92 93 94 96 97 100 107 108 109 110 111 113 114 115 116 117 118 119 120 122 128 129 130 131 133 134 142 145 146 147 **P**6 **S** Crozer–Keystone Health System, Springfield, PA
Primary Contact: William McCune, President
CFO: Richard I. Bennett, Senior Vice President and Chief Financial Officer
CMO: Seth Malin, M.D., President Medical and Dental Staff
CIO: Robert E. Wilson, Vice President and Chief Information Officer
Web address: www.crozer.org
**Control:** Other not–for–profit (including NFP Corporation) **Service:** General Medical and Surgical

**Staffed Beds:** 213 **Admissions:** 9752 **Census:** 137 **Outpatient Visits:** 167679 **Births:** 1529 **Total Expense ($000):** 183982 **Payroll Expense ($000):** 70222 **Personnel:** 900

### DU BOIS—Clearfield County

⊞ **DUBOIS REGIONAL MEDICAL CENTER (390086)**, 100 Hospital Avenue, Zip 15801–1440, Mailing Address: P.O. Box 447, Zip 15801–0447; tel. 814/371–2200, (Nonreporting) **A**1 2 9 10 19
Primary Contact: John Sutika, President
CMO: Gary Dugan, M.D., Vice President Medical Affairs
CIO: Thomas Johnson, Manager Management Information Systems
CHR: Robert J. McKee, Vice President Human Resources
Web address: www.drmc.org
**Control:** Other not–for–profit (including NFP Corporation) **Service:** General Medical and Surgical

**Staffed Beds:** 203

### EAGLEVILLE—Montgomery County

★ **EAGLEVILLE HOSPITAL (390278)**, 100 Eagleville Road, Zip 19408–0045, Mailing Address: P.O. Box 45, Zip 19408–0045; tel. 610/539–6000 **A**5 9 10 **F**4 29 34 35 50 61 68 75 86 98 100 101 103 129 131 133 142 145 146 **P**6
Primary Contact: Maureen King Pollock, Chief Executive Officer
COO: Lois Chepak, R.N., Chief Clinical Officer
CFO: Alfred Salvitti, Chief Financial Officer
CMO: Robert Wilson, D.O., Director Medical Services
CIO: Richard R. Mitchell, Director Information Technology
CHR: Zoe Yousaitis, Director Human Resources
Web address: www.eaglevillehospital.org
**Control:** Other not–for–profit (including NFP Corporation) **Service:** Alcoholism and other chemical dependency

**Staffed Beds:** 84 **Admissions:** 1536 **Census:** 43 **Outpatient Visits:** 0 **Births:** 0 **Total Expense ($000):** 28338 **Payroll Expense ($000):** 16883 **Personnel:** 373

### EAST STROUDSBURG—Monroe County

⊞ △ **POCONO MEDICAL CENTER (390201)**, 206 East Brown Street, Zip 18301–3006; tel. 570/421–4000 **A**1 2 7 9 10 **F**3 11 12 13 14 15 17 18 20 22 24 26 28 29 30 31 32 34 35 36 38 39 40 43 45 46 48 49 50 54 55 56 57 59 61 64 65 66 70 72 74 75 76 77 78 79 81 82 83 84 85 86 87 89 92 93 97 98 100 101 102 103 107 108 110 111 113 114 117 118 119 120 122 123 125 129 131 134 143 145 147
Primary Contact: Kathleen E. Kuck, R.N., President and Chief Executive Officer
COO: Susan Labus, Chief Operating Officer
CFO: Michael Wilk, Vice President Financial Services and Chief Financial Officer
CIO: Joseph Fisne, Chief Information Officer
CHR: Lynn M. Lansdowne, Vice President Human Resources
Web address: www.pmchealthsystem.org
**Control:** Other not–for–profit (including NFP Corporation) **Service:** General Medical and Surgical

**Staffed Beds:** 231 **Admissions:** 11982 **Census:** 142 **Outpatient Visits:** 264027 **Births:** 888 **Total Expense ($000):** 211255 **Payroll Expense ($000):** 85058 **Personnel:** 1582

### EASTON—Northampton County

⊞ **EASTON HOSPITAL (390162)**, 250 South 21st Street, Zip 18042–3892; tel. 610/250–4000, (Nonreporting) **A**1 2 3 5 9 10 **S** Community Health Systems, Inc., Franklin, TN
Primary Contact: Brian Finestein, Chief Executive Officer
CFO: James Washecka, Chief Financial Officer
CMO: David Lyon, M.D., Chief Medical Officer
CIO: Kenneth Castle, Chief Information Officer
CHR: Lori Ofner, Vice President Human Resources
Web address: www.easton–hospital.com
**Control:** Other not–for–profit (including NFP Corporation) **Service:** General Medical and Surgical

**Staffed Beds:** 231

⊞ **KINDRED HOSPITAL EASTON (392034)**, 250 South 21st Street, 3rd Floor, Zip 18042; tel. 610/250–4724, (Nonreporting) **A**1 9 10 **S** Kindred Healthcare, Louisville, KY
Primary Contact: Louise Cassidy, Chief Executive Officer
Web address: www.kheaston.com/
**Control:** Corporation, Investor–owned, for–profit **Service:** Long–Term Acute Care hospital

**Staffed Beds:** 31

**ST. LUKE'S HOSPITAL – ANDERSON CAMPUS (390326)**, 1872 Riverside Circle, Zip 18045–5669; tel. 484/503–3000, (Nonreporting) **S** St. Luke's University Health Network, Bethlehem, PA
Primary Contact: Edward Nawrocki, President
CMO: Justin P. Psaila, M.D., Vice President Medical Affairs
CNO: Darla Frack, R.N., Chief Nursing Officer
Web address: www.mystlukesonline.org
**Control:** Other not–for–profit (including NFP Corporation) **Service:** General Medical and Surgical

**Staffed Beds:** 108

**TRIUMPH HOSPITAL EASTON** See Kindred Hospital Easton

### ELLWOOD CITY—Lawrence County

**ELLWOOD CITY HOSPITAL (390008)**, 724 Pershing Street, Zip 16117–1474; tel. 724/752–0081, (Nonreporting) **A**9 10
Primary Contact: Raymond J. Beck, President and Chief Executive Officer
COO: Carolyn Izzo, Senior Vice President and Chief Operating Officer
CFO: Christopher M. Little, Vice President and Chief Financial Officer
CIO: Bryan O'Shaughnessy, Chief Information Officer
CHR: Paul Landman, Director Human Resources
Web address: www.TheEllwoodCityHospital.org
**Control:** Other not–for–profit (including NFP Corporation) **Service:** General Medical and Surgical

**Staffed Beds:** 95

*Many Facility Codes have changed. Please refer to the AHA Guide Code Chart.* © 2012 AHA Guide

**EPHRATA—Lancaster County**

☐ **EPHRATA COMMUNITY HOSPITAL (390225)**, 169 Martin Avenue,
Zip 17522–1002, Mailing Address: P.O. Box 1002, Zip 17522–1002;
tel. 717/733–0311 **A**1 2 9 10 **F**11 12 13 15 18 20 28 29 30 31 34 35 36 40
42 49 50 51 54 57 59 60 61 62 64 69 70 72 74 75 76 77 78 79 80 81 82
85 86 87 89 90 97 98 99 100 101 102 103 107 108 111 113 114 117 118
120 128 129 131 134 143 145 146 147 **P**6 8
Primary Contact: John M. Porter, Jr., President and Chief Executive Officer
COO: Robert Graupensperger, Executive Vice President
CFO: John A. Holmes, Chief Financial Officer
CMO: Vincent D. Glielmi, D.O., Senior Vice President Medical Affairs
CIO: John Jabour, Chief Information Officer
CHR: Barbara Mumma, Vice President Human Resources
CNO: Marcia A. Hansen, R.N., Vice President Patient Services and Chief Nursing
Officer
Web address: www.ephratahospital.org
**Control:** Other not–for–profit (including NFP Corporation) **Service:** General
Medical and Surgical

**Staffed Beds: 134 Admissions: 6918 Census: 75 Outpatient Visits: 405040
Births: 764 Total Expense ($000): 191338 Payroll Expense ($000): 85554
Personnel: 1774**

**ERIE—Erie County**

**HAMOT MEDICAL CENTER** See UPMC Hamot

☒ **HEALTHSOUTH REHABILITATION HOSPITAL OF ERIE (393046)**, 143 East
Second Street, Zip 16507–1501; tel. 814/878–1200 **A**1 10 **F**90 91 129
**S** HEALTHSOUTH Corporation, Birmingham, AL
Primary Contact: Lucretia Atti, Interim Chief Executive Officer
CFO: Lori Gibbens, Controller
CMO: Douglas Grisier, D.O., Medical Director
CIO: Sharon Zielinski, Manager Health Information
CHR: William Robinson, Director Human Resources
Web address: www.healthsoutherie.com
**Control:** Corporation, Investor–owned, for–profit **Service:** Rehabilitation

**Staffed Beds: 100 Admissions: 1808 Census: 71 Outpatient Visits: 0
Births: 0 Personnel: 239**

○ **MILLCREEK COMMUNITY HOSPITAL (390198)**, 5515 Peach Street,
Zip 16509–2695; tel. 814/864–4031, (Nonreporting) **A**9 10 11 12 13
Primary Contact: Mary L. Eckert, President and Chief Executive Officer
CFO: Richard P. Olinger, Chief Financial Officer
CMO: John J. Kalata, D.O., Chief of Staff
CIO: Cheryl Girardier, Director Information Technology
CHR: Polly Momeyer, Manager Human Resources
CNO: Katie Agresti, R.N., Director Patient Care Services
Web address: www.millcreekcommunityhospital.com
**Control:** Other not–for–profit (including NFP Corporation) **Service:** General
Medical and Surgical

**Staffed Beds: 145**

★ **SAINT VINCENT HEALTH CENTER (390009)**, 232 West 25th Street,
Zip 16544–0002; tel. 814/452–5000, (Total facility includes 14 beds in nursing
home–type unit) **A**2 9 10 12 13 **F**3 5 8 9 11 12 13 15 17 18 20 22 24 26 28
29 30 31 32 33 34 35 36 38 39 40 42 44 45 46 48 49 50 51 53 54 56 57
58 59 60 61 62 63 64 65 66 68 70 72 74 75 76 77 78 79 80 81 82 83 84
85 86 87 90 93 96 97 98 100 101 102 103 104 107 108 110 111 113
114 116 117 118 119 120 122 123 125 127 128 129 130 131 132 134 141
143 145 146 147 **P**3 6 7 **S** Saint Vincent Health System, Erie, PA
Primary Contact: Scott Whalen, Ph.D., FACHE, President and Chief Executive
Officer
COO: Thomas Fucci, Chief Operating Officer
CFO: Al Mansfield, Chief Financial Officer
CMO: Richard Cogley, M.D., Senior Vice President Medical Affairs and Chief
Medical Officer
CIO: Richard B. Ong, Chief Information Officer
Web address: www.svhs.org
**Control:** Other not–for–profit (including NFP Corporation) **Service:** General
Medical and Surgical

**Staffed Beds: 486 Admissions: 17839 Census: 251 Outpatient Visits:
181648 Births: 1869 Total Expense ($000): 264999 Payroll Expense
($000): 86033 Personnel: 1971**

☒ **SELECT SPECIALTY HOSPITAL–ERIE (392037)**, 252 West 11th Street,
Zip 16501; tel. 814/874–5300, (Nonreporting) **A**1 9 10 **S** Select Medical
Corporation, Mechanicsburg, PA
Primary Contact: Anne Frew, Chief Executive Officer
Web address: www.selectmedicalcorp.com
**Control:** Corporation, Investor–owned, for–profit **Service:** Long–Term Acute Care
hospital

**Staffed Beds: 50**

☐ **SHRINERS HOSPITALS FOR CHILDREN, ERIE**, 1645 West 8th Street,
Zip 16505–5007; tel. 814/875–8700, (Nonreporting) **A**1 **S** Shriners Hospitals for
Children, Tampa, FL
Primary Contact: Charles Walczak, FACHE, Administrator
CFO: Karen L. Wagner, CPA, Director Fiscal Services
CMO: John Lubahn, M.D., Chief of Staff
CIO: Maureen Hubert, Manager Management Information Services
CHR: Chris DeSantis, Manager Human Resources
Web address: www.shrinershq.org
**Control:** Other not–for–profit (including NFP Corporation) **Service:** Children's
orthopedic

**Staffed Beds: 30**

☐ **UPMC HAMOT (390063)**, 201 State Street, Zip 16550–0002;
tel. 814/877–6000 **A**1 2 3 5 8 9 10 13 **F**3 9 11 12 13 15 17 18 20 22 24 26
28 29 30 31 34 35 36 37 38 39 40 43 44 45 46 47 48 49 50 51 56 57 58
59 60 61 62 63 64 65 66 68 70 72 74 75 76 77 78 79 80 81 82 84 85 86
87 89 91 92 93 96 100 107 108 110 111 113 114 117 118 123 125 128
129 130 131 134 140 145 146 147 **P**6 8 **S** UPMC, Pittsburgh, PA
Primary Contact: John T. Malone, President and Chief Executive Officer
COO: V. James Fiorenzo, Executive Vice President and Chief Operating Officer
CFO: Stephen M. Danch, Chief Financial Officer
CMO: Richard Long, M.D., Chief Medical Officer
CIO: Joseph Butler, Vice President and Chief Information Officer
CHR: Joseph Butler, Vice President and Chief Information Officer
Web address: www.hamot.org
**Control:** Other not–for–profit (including NFP Corporation) **Service:** General
Medical and Surgical

**Staffed Beds: 387 Admissions: 16777 Census: 225 Outpatient Visits:
351195 Births: 1456 Total Expense ($000): 303906 Payroll Expense
($000): 107597 Personnel: 2403**

☒ **VETERANS AFFAIRS MEDICAL CENTER**, 135 East 38th Street,
Zip 16504–1559; tel. 814/860–2576, (Nonreporting) **A**1 9 **S** Department of
Veterans Affairs, Washington, DC
Primary Contact: Michael Adelman, M.D., Director
CFO: Joann Pritchard, Chief Financial Officer
CMO: Anthony Behm, D.O., Chief of Staff
CIO: Sean Rowand, Chief Information Officer
CHR: Lynn Nies, Human Resources Officer
Web address: www.va.gov/sta/guide/home.asp
**Control:** Veterans Affairs, Government, federal **Service:** General Medical and
Surgical

**Staffed Beds: 26**

**EVERETT—Bedford County**

☐ **UPMC BEDFORD MEMORIAL (390117)**, 10455 Lincoln Highway,
Zip 15537–7046; tel. 814/623–6161 **A**1 9 10 20 **F**3 8 11 13 15 18 28 29 30
34 35 39 40 41 45 48 50 51 56 57 59 61 64 65 68 70 71 74 75 76 77 78
79 81 85 86 87 89 93 97 102 104 107 108 111 113 118 128 129 130 131
132 134 145 146 **S** UPMC, Pittsburgh, PA
Primary Contact: Roger P. Winn, President
CFO: Mario Wilfong, Vice President Finance and Administration
CIO: Mark Wiley, Manager Information Systems Development
CHR: Michelle A. Speck, Vice President Human Resources
CNO: Paula Thomas, R.N., Vice President Patient Services
Web address: www.upmcbedfordmemorial.com
**Control:** Other not–for–profit (including NFP Corporation) **Service:** General
Medical and Surgical

**Staffed Beds: 27 Admissions: 2099 Census: 16 Outpatient Visits: 99659
Births: 272 Total Expense ($000): 38407 Payroll Expense ($000): 15555
Personnel: 302**

**FARRELL—Mercer County**

**SHENANGO VALLEY CAMPUS** See UPMC Horizon, Greenville

**FORT WASHINGTON—Montgomery County**

☐ **BROOKE GLEN BEHAVIORAL HOSPITAL (394049)**, 7170 Lafayette Avenue,
Zip 19034–0209; tel. 215/641–5300, (Nonreporting) **A**1 3 5 9 10 **S** Universal
Health Services, Inc., King of Prussia, PA
Primary Contact: Neil Callahan, Chief Executive Officer
COO: William R. Mason, Chief Operating Officer
CFO: Robert Zagerman, Chief Financial Officer
CMO: Chand Nair, M.D., Medical Director
CHR: Dawn Kownacki, Director Human Resources
Web address: www.brookeglenbehavioral.com
**Control:** Corporation, Investor–owned, for–profit **Service:** Psychiatric

**Staffed Beds: 146**

**PA**

---

**Hospital, Medicare Provider Number, Address, Telephone, Approval, Facility, and Physician Codes, Health Care System**

★ American Hospital Association (AHA) membership
☐ The Joint Commission accreditation   ◇ DNV Healthcare Inc. accreditation
○ American Osteopathic Association (AOA) accreditation
△ Commission on Accreditation of Rehabilitation Facilities (CARF) accreditation

**PA**

### GETTYSBURG—Adams County

☒ **GETTYSBURG HOSPITAL (390065)**, 147 Gettys Street, Zip 17325–2534;
tel. 717/334–2121 **A**1 9 10 **F**3 8 11 13 15 18 20 27 28 29 30 31 34 35 40
45 48 50 51 54 59 60 64 65 68 70 75 76 77 78 79 81 82 85 87 93 102
107 108 110 111 113 114 117 118 128 129 130 131 133 134 145 146 **P**8
**S** WellSpan Health, York, PA
Primary Contact: Jane E. Hyde, President
COO: Joseph H. Edgar, Senior Vice President Operations
CMO: Charles Marley, D.O., Vice President Medical Affairs
CIO: Robin Kimple, Director Information Services
CHR: Kim Brister, Director Human Resources
Web address: www.wellspan.org
**Control:** Other not–for–profit (including NFP Corporation) **Service:** General
Medical and Surgical

**Staffed Beds:** 76 **Admissions:** 4174 **Census:** 46 **Outpatient Visits:** 204645
**Births:** 507 **Total Expense ($000):** 116575 **Payroll Expense ($000):** 44442
**Personnel:** 739

### GREENSBURG—Westmoreland County

☐ **EXCELA HEALTH WESTMORELAND HOSPITAL (390145)**, 532 West
Pittsburgh Street, Zip 15601–2282; tel. 724/832–4000 **A**1 9 10 **F**3 5 8 9 11
12 13 15 17 18 20 22 24 26 28 29 30 32 34 35 36 38 40 44 45 47 48 49
50 51 56 57 59 61 64 65 68 70 73 74 75 76 77 78 79 81 82 84 85 86 87
89 90 92 93 96 97 98 100 101 102 103 104 105 107 108 110 111 113 114
117 118 128 129 130 131 133 134 142 145 146 147 **S** Excela Health,
Greensburg, PA
Primary Contact: Ronald H. Ott, President
COO: Samuel Raneri, Senior Vice President Operations and Business Development
CFO: Jeffrey T. Curry, Executive Vice President and Chief Financial Officer
CMO: Jerome Granato, M.D., Chief Medical Officer
CIO: Otto Salguero, Chief Information Officer
CHR: John Caverno, Chief Human Resources Officer
Web address: www.excelahealth.org
**Control:** Other not–for–profit (including NFP Corporation) **Service:** General
Medical and Surgical

**Staffed Beds:** 359 **Admissions:** 19054 **Census:** 258 **Outpatient Visits:**
384283 **Births:** 1773 **Total Expense ($000):** 224789 **Payroll Expense
($000):** 94286 **Personnel:** 2050

### GREENVILLE—Mercer County

☐ ○ **UPMC HORIZON (390178)**, 110 North Main Street, Zip 16125–1726;
tel. 724/588–2100, (Includes GREENVILLE CAMPUS, 110 North Main Street,
Zip 16125–1795; tel. 724/588–2100; SHENANGO VALLEY CAMPUS, 2200
Memorial Drive, Farrell, Zip 16121–1398; tel. 724/981–3500), (Total facility
includes 25 beds in nursing home–type unit) **A**1 2 9 10 11 13 **F**3 11 12 13 15
18 20 28 29 30 31 32 34 35 39 40 44 47 49 50 53 54 56 57 59 64 68 70
74 75 76 77 78 79 81 82 85 86 87 90 92 93 97 107 108 110 111 113 114
115 116 117 118 120 122 127 128 129 130 131 134 145 146 147 **S** UPMC,
Pittsburgh, PA
Primary Contact: Donald R. Owrey, President
CFO: David Shulik, Vice President and Chief Financial Officer
CMO: Samuel Daisley, D.O., Vice President Medical Affairs
CHR: Connie Mayle, Vice President Administrative Services
Web address: www.horizon.upmc.com
**Control:** Other not–for–profit (including NFP Corporation) **Service:** General
Medical and Surgical

**Staffed Beds:** 187 **Admissions:** 7749 **Census:** 107 **Outpatient Visits:**
189231 **Births:** 783 **Total Expense ($000):** 118603 **Payroll Expense
($000):** 38986 **Personnel:** 772

### GROVE CITY—Mercer County

**GROVE CITY MEDICAL CENTER (390266)**, 631 North Broad Street Extension,
Zip 16127–4603; tel. 724/450–7000, (Total facility includes 20 beds in nursing
home–type unit) **A**9 10 **F**3 8 12 15 18 20 28 29 31 34 35 40 45 46 50 51 54
57 59 60 62 64 70 75 76 78 79 81 82 87 93 107 108 110 111 114 116 117
118 123 126 127 128 129 131 134 145 146 147 **P**6
Primary Contact: Robert Jackson, Jr., Chief Executive Officer
CFO: David Poland, Vice President Finance
CMO: Armando Sciullo, D.O., Chief of Staff
CIO: Philip Swartwood, Director Information Systems
CHR: Donald Henley, Vice President Human Resources and Social Services
Web address: www.gcmcpa.org
**Control:** Other not–for–profit (including NFP Corporation) **Service:** General
Medical and Surgical

**Staffed Beds:** 109 **Admissions:** 2163 **Census:** 31 **Outpatient Visits:** 116527
**Births:** 264 **Total Expense ($000):** 44236 **Payroll Expense ($000):** 17850
**Personnel:** 409

### HANOVER—York County

☒ **HANOVER HOSPITAL (390233)**, 300 Highland Avenue, Zip 17331–2297;
tel. 717/637–3711 **A**1 9 10 **F**3 7 11 13 15 18 20 28 29 30 31 32 34 35 40
44 45 47 49 50 51 53 54 56 57 59 61 64 65 68 70 74 75 76 77 78 79 81
84 85 86 87 89 90 93 96 107 108 110 111 113 114 117 118 128 129 130
131 133 134 142 143 145 146 147
Primary Contact: James Wissler, President and Chief Executive Officer
COO: Michael A. Hockenberry, Vice President Operations
CFO: Michael W. Gaskins, Executive Vice President and Chief Financial Officer
CMO: Michael H. Ader, M.D., Vice President Medical Affairs
CIO: Pamela Owens, Director Health Information Management
CHR: Christine Miller, Vice President Human Resources
CNO: M. Patricia Saunders, R.N., Vice President Nursing
Web address: www.hanoverhospital.org
**Control:** Other not–for–profit (including NFP Corporation) **Service:** General
Medical and Surgical

**Staffed Beds:** 106 **Admissions:** 5512 **Census:** 69 **Outpatient Visits:** 198825
**Births:** 545 **Total Expense ($000):** 126582 **Payroll Expense ($000):** 50485
**Personnel:** 963

### HARRISBURG—Dauphin County

**COMMUNITY HOSPITAL** See Pinnacle Health System

☐ **PENNSYLVANIA PSYCHIATRIC HOSPITAL (394051)**, 2501 North Third
Street, Zip 17110–1904; tel. 717/782–6420, (Nonreporting) **A**1 3 5 10
Primary Contact: William Daly, Interim Chief Executive Officer
Web address: www.ppimhs.org/
**Control:** Partnership, Investor–owned, for–profit **Service:** Psychiatric

**Staffed Beds:** 73

☐ **PINNACLE HEALTH SYSTEM (390067)**, 111 South Front Street,
Zip 17101–2010, Mailing Address: P.O. Box 8700, Zip 17105–8700;
tel. 717/782–3131, (Includes COMMUNITY HOSPITAL, 4300 Londonderry Road,
Zip 17109–5397, Mailing Address: P.O. Box 3000, Zip 17105–3000;
tel. 717/652–3000; HARRISBURG HOSPITAL, 111 South Front Street,
Zip 17101–2099; tel. 717/782–3131; POLYCLINIC HOSPITAL, 2501 North Third
Street, Zip 17110–1904; tel. 717/782–4141; Roger Longenderfer, M.D.,
President and Chief Executive Officer) **A**1 2 3 5 8 9 10 12 13 **F**3 7 11 12 13 14
15 17 18 20 22 24 26 28 29 30 31 32 35 36 37 40 44 45 48 49 50 54 56
57 58 59 60 61 64 65 66 68 70 72 74 75 76 77 78 79 81 82 84 85 86 87
89 90 93 96 97 107 108 110 111 113 114 116 118 120 122 125 129 131
133 134 137 141 142 145 146 **P**6
Primary Contact: Michael A. Young, FACHE, President and Chief Executive Officer
COO: Philip Guarneschelli, Senior Vice President and Chief Operating Officer
CFO: William H. Pugh, Senior Vice President Corporate Finance and Chief Financial
Officer
CMO: Dana Kellis, M.D., Senior Vice President Medical Affairs and Chief Medical
Officer
CIO: Steven Roth, Vice President Informatics and Chief Information Officer
CHR: Thomas Kess, Vice President Human Resources
Web address: www.pinnaclehealth.org
**Control:** Other not–for–profit (including NFP Corporation) **Service:** General
Medical and Surgical

**Staffed Beds:** 571 **Admissions:** 29474 **Census:** 384 **Outpatient Visits:**
545398 **Births:** 4001 **Personnel:** 4218

**POLYCLINIC HOSPITAL** See Pinnacle Health System

**SELECT SPECIALTY HOSPITAL–HARRISBURG** See Select Specialty
Hospital–Central Pennsylvania, Camp Hill

### HASTINGS—Cambria County

**MINERS MEDICAL CENTER (390130)**, 290 Haida Avenue, Zip 16646, Mailing
Address: P.O. Box 689, Zip 16646–0689; tel. 814/247–3100 **A**9 10 20 **F**3 15
18 29 30 35 36 40 45 48 56 57 59 64 70 75 78 79 81 86 92 93 96 97 102
107 108 110 113 118 128 129 130 132 143 145 **P**8 **S** Conemaugh Health
System, Johnstown, PA
Primary Contact: William R. Crowe, President
CFO: Kimberly Semelsberger, Vice President Financial Operations
CIO: James Homerski, Director Information Services
CHR: John Fresh, Vice President Human Resources
Web address: www.minersmedicalcenter.org
**Control:** Other not–for–profit (including NFP Corporation) **Service:** General
Medical and Surgical

**Staffed Beds:** 30 **Admissions:** 876 **Census:** 10 **Outpatient Visits:** 50699
**Births:** 2 **Total Expense ($000):** 17347 **Payroll Expense ($000):** 5353
**Personnel:** 140

*Many Facility Codes have changed. Please refer to the AHA Guide Code Chart.* © 2012 AHA Guide

**PA**

## HAZLETON—Luzerne County

★ ○ **HAZLETON GENERAL HOSPITAL (390185)**, 700 East Broad Street, Zip 18201–6897; tel. 570/501–4000 **A**9 10 11 **F**3 8 11 12 13 15 28 29 30 31 34 35 40 50 53 54 57 58 59 60 62 64 68 69 70 75 76 77 78 79 81 82 85 86 87 89 90 93 107 108 110 111 113 117 118 123 128 129 130 131 134 142 145 146 147
Primary Contact: James Edwards, President
COO: John R. Fletcher, Vice President and Chief Operating Officer
CFO: William Bauer, Vice President Finance and Chief Financial Officer
CMO: Anthony Valente, M.D., Vice President Medical Affairs
CIO: Carl Shoener, Chief Information Officer
CHR: Elizabeth Perrong, Vice President Human Resources
Web address: www.ghha.org
**Control:** Other not–for–profit (including NFP Corporation) **Service:** General Medical and Surgical

**Staffed Beds:** 141 **Admissions:** 6456 **Census:** 88 **Outpatient Visits:** 156633 **Births:** 650 **Total Expense ($000):** 88136 **Payroll Expense ($000):** 37784 **Personnel:** 586

## HERSHEY—Dauphin County

✠ **PENN STATE MILTON S. HERSHEY MEDICAL CENTER (390256)**, 500 University Drive, Zip 17033–0850, Mailing Address: P.O. Box 850, Zip 17033–0850; tel. 717/531–8521, (Includes PENN STATE CHILDREN'S HOSPITAL, 500 University Drive, Zip 17033–2360; tel. 717/531–8521) **A**1 2 3 5 8 9 10 **F**3 4 5 6 7 8 9 11 12 13 14 15 17 18 19 20 21 22 23 24 25 26 27 28 29 30 31 32 34 35 36 37 38 40 41 43 44 45 46 47 48 49 50 51 52 53 54 55 56 57 58 59 60 61 64 65 66 68 70 72 73 74 75 76 77 78 79 80 81 82 84 85 86 87 88 89 90 91 92 93 96 97 98 99 100 101 102 103 104 105 106 107 108 109 110 111 113 114 115 116 117 118 119 120 122 123 125 128 129 130 131 133 134 135 136 137 138 140 141 142 143 144 145 146 147 **P**6
Primary Contact: Harold L. Paz, M.D., Chief Executive Officer
COO: Alan L. Brechbill, Executive Director
CFO: Kevin Haley, Chief Financial Officer
CMO: Carol V. Freer, M.D., Chief Medical Officer
CIO: Thomas Abendroth, M.D., Chief Information Officer
CHR: Charles Wilson, Chief Human Resources Officer
Web address: www.pennstatehershey.org/web/guest/home
**Control:** Other not–for–profit (including NFP Corporation) **Service:** General Medical and Surgical

**Staffed Beds:** 469 **Admissions:** 25119 **Census:** 385 **Outpatient Visits:** 499143 **Births:** 1775 **Total Expense ($000):** 801842 **Payroll Expense ($000):** 329159 **Personnel:** 7328

## HONESDALE—Wayne County

★ **WAYNE MEMORIAL HOSPITAL (390125)**, 601 Park Street, Zip 18431–1498; tel. 570/253–8100 **A**2 9 10 **F**3 11 13 15 18 28 30 31 34 35 36 37 39 40 45 46 48 49 50 51 53 54 56 57 59 61 62 63 64 65 75 76 77 78 79 81 86 89 90 92 93 99 100 101 102 103 104 107 108 110 111 114 115 116 118 123 128 129 130 131 132 133 134 145 146 147 **P**6
Primary Contact: David L. Hoff, Chief Executive Officer
COO: John D. Conte, Director Facility Services
CFO: Michael J. Clifford, Director Finance
CMO: George Tietjen, M.D., Chief of Staff
CIO: Tom Hoffman, Manager Information Systems
CHR: Elizabeth McDonald, Director Human Resources
Web address: www.wmh.org
**Control:** Other not–for–profit (including NFP Corporation) **Service:** General Medical and Surgical

**Staffed Beds:** 104 **Admissions:** 3375 **Census:** 43 **Outpatient Visits:** 115678 **Births:** 381 **Total Expense ($000):** 65273 **Payroll Expense ($000):** 26713 **Personnel:** 534

## HUMMELSTOWN—Dauphin County

✠ **PENN STATE HERSHEY REHABILITATION HOSPITAL (393053)**, 1135 Old West Chocolate Avenue, Zip 17036; tel. 717/832–2600, (Nonreporting) **A**1 9 10 **S** Select Medical Corporation, Mechanicsburg, PA
Primary Contact: Mary A. Zweifel, Chief Executive Officer
Web address: www.psh–rehab.com
**Control:** Corporation, Investor–owned, for–profit **Service:** Rehabilitation

**Staffed Beds:** 32

## HUNTINGDON—Huntingdon County

✠ **J. C. BLAIR MEMORIAL HOSPITAL (390056)**, 1225 Warm Springs Avenue, Zip 16652–2398; tel. 814/643–2290 **A**1 9 10 20 **F**3 11 13 15 18 29 34 35 40 49 57 59 64 68 70 75 76 81 85 86 87 89 96 98 99 100 102 103 104 105 107 108 110 111 113 117 118 128 129 131 132 134 145 147 **P**7 **S** QHR, Brentwood, TN
Primary Contact: Lisa Mallon, Interim President and Chief Executive Officer
CFO: Michael Widener, Chief Financial Officer
CMO: Christopher Patitsas, M.D., Chief of Staff
CHR: Michael Hubert, Vice President Human Resources
Web address: www.jcblair.org
**Control:** Other not–for–profit (including NFP Corporation) **Service:** General Medical and Surgical

**Staffed Beds:** 72 **Admissions:** 2224 **Census:** 27 **Outpatient Visits:** 118711 **Births:** 219 **Total Expense ($000):** 39489 **Payroll Expense ($000):** 17293 **Personnel:** 328

## INDIANA—Indiana County

★ **INDIANA REGIONAL MEDICAL CENTER (390173)**, 835 Hospital Road, Zip 15701–0788, Mailing Address: P.O. Box 788, Zip 15701–0788; tel. 724/357–7000 **A**9 10 20 **F**3 11 15 18 28 29 30 31 32 34 35 40 44 46 47 49 53 56 57 59 64 65 70 71 74 75 76 77 78 79 81 82 83 84 85 87 89 90 91 98 102 103 107 108 111 113 114 117 118 119 120 122 123 128 129 131 143 145 147 **P**4 6
Primary Contact: Stephen A. Wolfe, President and Chief Executive Officer
COO: Dominic Paccapaniccia, Chief Operating Officer
CFO: Robert Gongaware, Senior Vice President Finance
CMO: Bruce A. Bush, M.D., Senior Vice President Medical Affairs
CIO: Wade Patrick, Senior Vice President Information Services
CHR: Matt Reading, Director Human Resources
Web address: www.indianarmc.org
**Control:** Other not–for–profit (including NFP Corporation) **Service:** General Medical and Surgical

**Staffed Beds:** 164 **Admissions:** 7671 **Census:** 94 **Outpatient Visits:** 249976 **Births:** 631 **Total Expense ($000):** 127572 **Payroll Expense ($000):** 56435 **Personnel:** 869

## JEFFERSON HILLS—Allegheny County

☐ **JEFFERSON REGIONAL MEDICAL CENTER (390265)**, 565 Coal Valley Road, Zip 15025–3703, Mailing Address: Box 18119, Pittsburgh, Zip 15236–0119; tel. 412/469–5000, (Nonreporting) **A**1 9 10
Primary Contact: John Dempster, President and Chief Executive Officer
COO: James C. Cooper, Chief Operating Officer
CFO: Joanne A. Hahey, Senior Vice President and Chief Financial Officer
CMO: Richard F. Collins, M.D., Executive Vice President and Chief Medical Officer
CIO: James Witenske, Chief Information Officer
CHR: Rosanne C. Saunders, Senior Vice President and Chief Human Resources Officer
CNO: Louise Urban, R.N., Senior Vice President Patient Care Services and Chief Nursing Officer
Web address: www.jeffersonregional.com
**Control:** Other not–for–profit (including NFP Corporation) **Service:** General Medical and Surgical

**Staffed Beds:** 373

## JERSEY SHORE—Lycoming County

✠ **JERSEY SHORE HOSPITAL (391300)**, 1020 Thompson Street, Zip 17740–1794; tel. 570/398–0100 **A**1 9 10 18 **F**3 15 18 28 29 30 35 40 45 59 75 77 79 81 82 85 93 107 108 110 111 114 118 128 129 130 132 134 143 144 145 **P**7 **S** QHR, Brentwood, TN
Primary Contact: Carey W. Plummer, President and Chief Executive Officer
CFO: Mark Rice, CPA, Controller
CMO: Steven E. Katz, M.D., Chief Medical Officer
CIO: Christine Haas, Manager Information Technology
CHR: Trudi Alexander, Director Human Resources
Web address: www.jsh.org
**Control:** Other not–for–profit (including NFP Corporation) **Service:** General Medical and Surgical

**Staffed Beds:** 25 **Admissions:** 1014 **Census:** 11 **Outpatient Visits:** 85521 **Births:** 0 **Total Expense ($000):** 27943 **Payroll Expense ($000):** 10554 **Personnel:** 257

---

**Hospital, Medicare Provider Number, Address, Telephone, Approval, Facility, and Physician Codes, Health Care System**

★ American Hospital Association (AHA) membership
☐ The Joint Commission accreditation
◇ DNV Healthcare Inc. accreditation
○ American Osteopathic Association (AOA) accreditation
△ Commission on Accreditation of Rehabilitation Facilities (CARF) accreditation

**PA**

## JOHNSTOWN—Cambria County

☐ **MEMORIAL MEDICAL CENTER (390110)**, 1086 Franklin Street, Zip 15905–4398; tel. 814/534–9000, (Includes GOOD SAMARITAN MEDICAL CENTER, 1020 Franklin Street, Zip 15905–4186; tel. 814/533–1000; MEMORIAL MEDICAL CENTER – LEE CAMPUS, 320 Main Street, Zip 15901–1601; tel. 814/533–0123) **A**1 2 5 6 9 10 12 13 **F**3 5 8 11 12 13 14 15 17 18 20 22 24 28 29 30 31 32 34 35 40 42 43 44 45 46 49 50 51 53 54 55 56 57 59 61 62 63 64 68 70 72 74 75 76 77 78 79 81 82 83 84 85 86 87 89 90 91 92 93 97 98 99 100 101 102 103 104 107 108 110 111 113 114 117 118 126 128 129 130 131 133 134 143 144 145 146 147 **S** Conemaugh Health System, Johnstown, PA
Primary Contact: Steven E. Tucker, President and Chief Operating Officer
COO: Steven E. Tucker, President and Chief Operating Officer
CFO: Edward De Pasquale, Chief Financial Officer
CMO: David J. Carlson, D.O., Chief Medical Officer
CIO: Joseph Dado, Chief Information Officer
CHR: Mary York, Vice President Human Resources
Web address: www.conemaugh.org
**Control:** Other not–for–profit (including NFP Corporation) **Service:** General Medical and Surgical

**Staffed Beds:** 525 **Admissions:** 24432 **Census:** 388 **Outpatient Visits:** 480729 **Births:** 1291 **Total Expense ($000):** 360712 **Payroll Expense ($000):** 143527 **Personnel:** 3357

**MEMORIAL MEDICAL CENTER – LEE CAMPUS** See Memorial Medical Center

☒ **SELECT SPECIALTY HOSPITAL–JOHNSTOWN (392031)**, 320 Main Street, Zip 15901; tel. 814/534–7300, (Nonreporting) **A**1 9 10 **S** Select Medical Corporation, Mechanicsburg, PA
Primary Contact: Kelly Blake, Chief Executive Officer
CMO: Gary Davidson, M.D., Medical Director
Web address: www.selectmedicalcorp.com
**Control:** Corporation, Investor–owned, for–profit **Service:** Long–Term Acute Care hospital

**Staffed Beds:** 39

## KANE—Mckean County

**KANE COMMUNITY HOSPITAL (390104)**, 4372 Route 6, Zip 16735–3060; tel. 814/837–8585 **A**9 10 20 **F**3 11 12 15 17 28 29 30 31 34 35 40 41 45 46 50 53 57 59 62 64 65 70 75 77 79 81 82 85 89 91 93 107 108 110 111 113 116 117 118 127 128 129 130 131 132 134 144 145 146 **P**4 6
Primary Contact: J. Gary Rhodes, FACHE, Chief Executive Officer
CFO: Angela Hadzega, Chief Financial Officer
CMO: Linda Rettger, M.D., President Medical Staff
CIO: Margaret Twidale, Manager Information Systems
CHR: Marsha Keller, Director Human Resources
CNO: Pam Bray, Director of Nursing and Director Inpatient Services
Web address: www.kanehosp.com
**Control:** Other not–for–profit (including NFP Corporation) **Service:** General Medical and Surgical

**Staffed Beds:** 31 **Admissions:** 1016 **Census:** 12 **Outpatient Visits:** 31892 **Births:** 0 **Total Expense ($000):** 17364 **Payroll Expense ($000):** 8175 **Personnel:** 181

## KITTANNING—Armstrong County

**ACMH HOSPITAL (390163)**, One Nolte Drive, Zip 16201–7111; tel. 724/543–8500, (Nonreporting) **A**2 9 10 19
Primary Contact: John I. Lewis, President and Chief Executive Officer
CFO: Patrick Burns, Vice President Finance
CMO: Harold Altman, M.D., Chief Medical Officer
CIO: Dianne Emminger, Vice President Information Services
CHR: Anne Remaley, Vice President Human Resources
Web address: www.acmh.org
**Control:** Other not–for–profit (including NFP Corporation) **Service:** General Medical and Surgical

**Staffed Beds:** 170

## LANCASTER—Lancaster County

☒ **LANCASTER GENERAL HEALTH (390100)**, 555 North Duke Street, Zip 17604–3555, Mailing Address: P.O. Box 3555, Zip 17604–3555; tel. 717/544–5511 **A**1 2 3 5 9 10 **F**3 11 12 13 14 15 18 20 22 24 26 28 29 30 31 34 35 36 37 39 40 43 44 45 46 47 49 50 51 54 55 56 57 58 59 60 61 64 65 66 68 70 72 73 74 75 76 77 78 79 80 81 82 85 86 87 89 91 92 93 96 97 98 100 102 107 108 110 112 113 114 116 117 118 119 120 122 123 125 128 129 131 134 140 141 144 145 146 147 **P**6
Primary Contact: Thomas E. Beeman, Ph.D., FACHE, President and Chief Executive Officer
COO: Marion A. McGowan, Executive Vice President and Chief Operating Officer
CFO: F. Joseph Byorick, Senior Vice President Finance and Chief Financial Officer
CMO: Lee M. Duke, II, M.D., Senior Vice President and Chief Physician Executive
CIO: Gary Davidson, Senior Vice President and Chief Information Officer
CHR: Regina Mingle, Senior Vice President and Chief Leadership Officer
Web address: www.lancastergeneral.org
**Control:** Other not–for–profit (including NFP Corporation) **Service:** General Medical and Surgical

**Staffed Beds:** 623 **Admissions:** 33277 **Census:** 440 **Outpatient Visits:** 1311740 **Births:** 4329 **Total Expense ($000):** 752054 **Payroll Expense ($000):** 300060 **Personnel:** 4805

☐ **LANCASTER REGIONAL MEDICAL CENTER (390061)**, 250 College Avenue, Zip 17603, Mailing Address: P.O. Box 3434, Zip 17604–3434; tel. 717/291–8211 **A**1 9 10 **F**2 3 15 18 20 22 24 26 28 29 30 31 34 35 37 40 45 47 48 49 50 51 56 57 59 64 68 70 74 75 77 78 79 81 82 84 85 87 90 91 92 93 96 98 100 101 102 103 107 108 110 111 113 118 120 125 128 129 130 134 145 **S** Health Management Associates, Naples, FL
Primary Contact: Bob Moore, FACHE, Chief Executive Officer
COO: Deborah J. Willwerth, R.N., Chief Operating Officer
CFO: Mike Johnson, Chief Financial Officer
CMO: N. A. Mastropietro, M.D., Medical Director
CHR: Brian Hoffman, Director Human Resources
CNO: Tami Lee, MSN, Chief Nursing Officer
Web address: www.lancasterregional.com
**Control:** Corporation, Investor–owned, for–profit **Service:** General Medical and Surgical

**Staffed Beds:** 150 **Admissions:** 4882 **Census:** 79 **Outpatient Visits:** 89857 **Births:** 0 **Total Expense ($000):** 82702 **Payroll Expense ($000):** 29491 **Personnel:** 588

☐ **LANCASTER REHABILITATION HOSPITAL (393054)**, 675 Good Drive, Zip 17601–2426; tel. 717/406–3000, (Nonreporting) **A**1 10 **S** Centerre Healthcare, Brentwood, TN
Primary Contact: Tammy L. Ober, Chief Executive Officer
CFO: David Stark, Chief Financial Officer
CHR: Lisa Andrews, Director Human Resources
Web address: www.lancastergeneral.org
**Control:** Corporation, Investor–owned, for–profit **Service:** Rehabilitation

**Staffed Beds:** 10

## LANGHORNE—Bucks County

**BUCKS COUNTY CAMPUS** See Aria Health, Philadelphia

☒ **ST. MARY MEDICAL CENTER (390258)**, 1201 Langhorne–Newtown Road, Zip 19047–1234; tel. 215/710–2000 **A**1 2 9 10 **F**15 17 18 20 22 24 26 28 29 30 31 32 34 35 40 41 43 53 55 56 57 59 64 70 72 74 75 76 77 78 79 81 82 84 86 87 89 90 91 92 93 94 107 108 110 111 113 114 115 116 117 118 120 122 123 128 129 131 134 145 146 147 **S** Catholic Health East, Newtown Square, PA
Primary Contact: Gregory T. Wozniak, President and Chief Executive Officer
CFO: Gail Kosyla, Chief Financial Officer and Vice President Finance
CMO: Joseph Conroy, M.D., Vice President Medical Affairs
CIO: Marian Moran, Chief Information Officer
CHR: Mary Sweeney, Vice President Colleague Services and Development
Web address: www.stmaryhealthcare.org
**Control:** Church–operated, Nongovernment, not–for profit **Service:** General Medical and Surgical

**Staffed Beds:** 315 **Admissions:** 23824 **Census:** 286 **Outpatient Visits:** 280473 **Births:** 2016 **Total Expense ($000):** 355915 **Payroll Expense ($000):** 143953 **Personnel:** 2553

*Many Facility Codes have changed. Please refer to the AHA Guide Code Chart.* © 2012 AHA Guide

**PA**

## LANSDALE—Montgomery County

**ABINGTON HEALTH LANSDALE HOSPITAL (390012)**, 100 Medical Campus Drive, Zip 19446–1200; tel. 215/368–2100 **A**1 2 9 10 **F**3 8 11 15 18 28 29 30 31 34 35 39 40 45 49 50 57 59 64 65 69 70 74 78 79 81 82 85 90 93 107 111 113 118 128 129 131 145 146 147 **P**6
Primary Contact: Gary R. Candia, Ph.D., FACHE, Chief Executive Officer
COO: Katie Farrell, Chief Operating Officer
CFO: Raymond Leichner, Director Finance
CMO: Joseph Kraynak, M.D., Chief Medical Officer
CIO: Joan Lauman, Manager Clinical Systems
CHR: John Coker, Director Human Resource
Web address: www.amh.org/lansdale/index.aspx
**Control:** Other not–for–profit (including NFP Corporation) **Service:** General Medical and Surgical

**Staffed Beds:** 127 **Admissions:** 5881 **Census:** 61 **Outpatient Visits:** 87840 **Births:** 2 **Total Expense ($000):** 72160 **Payroll Expense ($000):** 31981 **Personnel:** 486

## LATROBE—Westmoreland County

**EXCELA LATROBE AREA HOSPITAL (390219)**, One Mellon Way, Zip 15650–1096; tel. 724/537–1000 **A**1 2 3 5 9 10 13 **F**3 8 11 12 15 29 30 34 35 38 40 44 45 48 49 50 51 53 56 57 59 60 64 65 68 70 74 75 77 78 79 81 82 85 86 87 92 93 97 98 99 100 101 104 107 108 110 111 113 114 117 118 125 128 129 131 133 134 142 145 146 147 **P**6 **S** Excela Health, Greensburg, PA
Primary Contact: Michael D. Busch, Executive Vice President and Chief Operating Officer
COO: Samuel Raneri, Senior Vice President Operations and Business Development
CFO: Jeffrey T. Curry, Executive Vice President and Chief Financial Officer
CMO: Jerome Granato, M.D., Chief Medical Officer
CIO: Otto Salguero, Chief Information Officer
CHR: Jill Clements, Vice President Human Resources
Web address: www.excelahealth.org
**Control:** Other not–for–profit (including NFP Corporation) **Service:** General Medical and Surgical

**Staffed Beds:** 153 **Admissions:** 7920 **Census:** 88 **Outpatient Visits:** 254025 **Births:** 0 **Total Expense ($000):** 116712 **Payroll Expense ($000):** 40417 **Personnel:** 955

**SELECT SPECIALTY HOSPITAL–LAUREL HIGHLANDS (392036)**, 121 West Second Street, Zip 15650; tel. 724/539–3230, (Nonreporting) **A**1 9 10 **S** Select Medical Corporation, Mechanicsburg, PA
Primary Contact: Anthony Martino, Chief Executive Officer
Web address: www.selectmedicalcorp.com
**Control:** Corporation, Investor–owned, for–profit **Service:** Long–Term Acute Care hospital

**Staffed Beds:** 40

## LEBANON—Lebanon County

**THE GOOD SAMARITAN HOSPITAL (390066)**, Fourth and Walnut Streets, Zip 17042–1281, Mailing Address: P.O. Box 1281, Zip 17042–1281; tel. 717/270–7500, (Total facility includes 19 beds in nursing home–type unit) **A**1 3 5 9 10 **F**3 8 11 13 14 15 17 18 20 22 24 26 28 29 30 31 34 35 39 40 50 51 53 54 57 59 60 62 63 64 68 70 75 76 77 78 79 80 81 82 85 87 89 90 92 93 94 96 97 107 108 110 111 113 117 118 127 128 129 131 134 143 145 147 **P**8
Primary Contact: Robert J. Longo, FACHE, President and Chief Executive Officer
COO: William Hendrick, Senior Vice President and Chief Operating Officer
CFO: Robert J. Richards, Vice President Finance and Chief Financial Officer
CMO: Robert D. Shaver, M.D., Vice President Medical Affairs
CIO: Louis Eaglehouse, Site Director and Chief Information Officer
CHR: Kimberly Feeman, Vice President Human Resources
Web address: www.gshleb.org
**Control:** Other not–for–profit (including NFP Corporation) **Service:** General Medical and Surgical

**Staffed Beds:** 158 **Admissions:** 8983 **Census:** 116 **Outpatient Visits:** 268138 **Births:** 884 **Total Expense ($000):** 157562 **Payroll Expense ($000):** 54538 **Personnel:** 1208

**△ VETERANS AFFAIRS MEDICAL CENTER**, 1700 South Lincoln Avenue, Zip 17042–7529; tel. 717/272–6621, (Nonreporting) **A**1 2 3 5 7 9
**S** Department of Veterans Affairs, Washington, DC
Primary Contact: Robert W. Callahan, Jr., Director
COO: William H. Mills, Associate Director
CFO: John Beistline, Assistant Chief Fiscal
CMO: Kanan Chatterjee, M.D., Chief of Staff
CIO: Debra Stickler, Chief Information Officer
CHR: Raymer Kent, Manager Human Resources
Web address: www.lebanon.va.gov
**Control:** Veterans Affairs, Government, federal **Service:** General Medical and Surgical

**Staffed Beds:** 213

## LEHIGHTON—Carbon County

**△ GNADEN HUETTEN MEMORIAL HOSPITAL (390194)**, 211 North 12th Street, Zip 18235–1138; tel. 610/377–1300, (Total facility includes 91 beds in nursing home–type unit) **A**1 7 9 10 **F**3 11 15 28 29 30 34 35 40 50 57 59 62 64 65 68 70 74 75 77 79 81 82 85 87 89 90 93 94 97 98 102 107 111 113 115 116 118 123 127 129 131 132 134 145 146 147 **S** Blue Mountain Health System, Lehighton, PA
Primary Contact: Andrew E. Harris, Chief Executive Officer
CMO: Clement McGinley, M.D., Vice President Medical Affairs
CIO: Maria Nunnes, Director Information Systems
CHR: Terry Purcell, Vice President Support Services and Ambulatory Care
Web address: www.bluemountainhealthsystem.org
**Control:** Other not–for–profit (including NFP Corporation) **Service:** General Medical and Surgical

**Staffed Beds:** 186 **Admissions:** 3202 **Census:** 131 **Outpatient Visits:** 53548 **Births:** 0 **Total Expense ($000):** 55844 **Payroll Expense ($000):** 23156 **Personnel:** 652

## LEWISBURG—Union County

**EVANGELICAL COMMUNITY HOSPITAL (390013)**, One Hospital Drive, Zip 17837–9350; tel. 570/522–2000 **A**9 10 19 **F**3 11 12 13 15 18 19 20 22 28 29 30 31 34 35 40 45 49 50 51 53 54 57 59 63 64 65 68 74 75 76 77 78 79 81 82 85 86 87 89 90 93 94 96 97 107 108 110 111 113 114 117 118 128 129 130 131 134 143 145 147 **P**7
Primary Contact: Michael N. O'Keefe, President and Chief Executive Officer
COO: Kendra A. Aucker, Vice President Operations
CFO: Jim Stopper, Interim Chief Financial Officer
CMO: J. Lawrence Ginsburg, M.D., Vice President Medical Affairs
CIO: Dale Moyer, Vice President Information Systems
CHR: Glenn Eisenhauer, Vice President
Web address: www.evanhospital.com
**Control:** Other not–for–profit (including NFP Corporation) **Service:** General Medical and Surgical

**Staffed Beds:** 127 **Admissions:** 5923 **Census:** 53 **Outpatient Visits:** 221883 **Births:** 1002 **Total Expense ($000):** 111350 **Payroll Expense ($000):** 45768 **Personnel:** 1051

**U. S. PENITENTIARY INFIRMARY**, Route 7, Zip 17837–9303; tel. 570/523–1251, (Nonreporting)
Primary Contact: Arnold Reyes, Administrator
**Control:** Department of Justice, Government, federal **Service:** Hospital unit of an institution (prison hospital, college infirmary, etc.)

**Staffed Beds:** 17

## LEWISTOWN—Mifflin County

**LEWISTOWN HOSPITAL (390048)**, 400 Highland Avenue, Zip 17044–1198; tel. 717/248–5411 **A**1 2 5 6 9 10 **F**3 11 12 13 15 17 18 19 28 29 30 31 34 35 40 50 51 57 59 64 68 70 71 74 75 76 78 79 81 82 85 86 89 97 98 99 100 101 102 103 107 108 110 111 113 115 116 117 118 120 123 128 129 131 134 145 146 147 **P**6
Primary Contact: Kay A. Hamilton, R.N., MS, President and Chief Executive Officer
COO: Kirk E. Thomas, Vice President Operations
CFO: Randy E. Tewksbury, Vice President Finance
CMO: Daniel Reifsnyder, M.D., President Medical and Dental Staff
CIO: Ronald M. Cowan, Vice President Information Systems
CHR: N. Sue Reinke, Vice President Human Resources
Web address: www.lewistownhospital.org
**Control:** Other not–for–profit (including NFP Corporation) **Service:** General Medical and Surgical

**Staffed Beds:** 123 **Admissions:** 5192 **Census:** 55 **Outpatient Visits:** 240885 **Births:** 497 **Total Expense ($000):** 85300 **Payroll Expense ($000):** 34640 **Personnel:** 723

---

**Hospital, Medicare Provider Number, Address, Telephone, Approval, Facility, and Physician Codes, Health Care System**

★ American Hospital Association (AHA) membership
□ The Joint Commission accreditation  ◇ DNV Healthcare Inc. accreditation
○ American Osteopathic Association (AOA) accreditation
△ Commission on Accreditation of Rehabilitation Facilities (CARF) accreditation

**LITITZ—Lancaster County**

☐ **HEART OF LANCASTER REGIONAL MEDICAL CENTER (390068)**, 1500 Highlands Drive, Zip 17543; tel. 717/625–5000, (Nonreporting) **A**1 9 10 12 13 **S** Health Management Associates, Naples, FL
Primary Contact: James Machado, Administrator
CIO: David Fisher, Director Information Systems
Web address: www.heartoflancaster.com
**Control:** Corporation, Investor–owned, for–profit **Service:** General Medical and Surgical

Staffed Beds: 139

**LOCK HAVEN—Clinton County**

☒ **LOCK HAVEN HOSPITAL (390071)**, 24 Cree Drive, Zip 17745–2699; tel. 570/893–5000, (Nonreporting) **A**1 9 10 **S** Community Health Systems, Inc., Franklin, TN
Primary Contact: John A. Zidansek, Chief Executive Officer
CFO: Paige Adkins, Chief Financial Officer
CMO: Rajesh Patel, M.D., Chief of Staff
CIO: Judy Chapman, Interim Director Information Systems
CHR: Lynn Moon, Director Human Resources
Web address: www.lockhavenhospital.com
**Control:** Corporation, Investor–owned, for–profit **Service:** General Medical and Surgical

Staffed Beds: 59

**MALVERN—Chester County**

☒ △ **BRYN MAWR REHABILITATION HOSPITAL (393025)**, 414 Paoli Pike, Zip 19355–3300, Mailing Address: P.O. Box 3007, Zip 19355–0707; tel. 484/596–5400 **A**1 7 9 10 **F**3 28 29 30 34 68 75 82 87 90 91 92 93 94 95 96 100 118 129 131 142 145 147 **P**5 **S** Main Line Health, Bryn Mawr, PA
Primary Contact: Donna Phillips, President
CFO: Michael J. Buongiorno, Vice President Finance and Treasurer
CMO: John Kraus, M.D., Chief Medical Officer
CIO: Karen A. Thomas, R.N., Chief Information Officer
Web address: www.brynmawrrehab.org
**Control:** Other not–for–profit (including NFP Corporation) **Service:** Rehabilitation

Staffed Beds: 148 Admissions: 2841 Census: 119 Outpatient Visits: 57828 Births: 0 Total Expense ($000): 59959 Payroll Expense ($000): 31863 Personnel: 515

**DEVEREUX CHILDREN'S BEHAVIORAL HEALTH CENTER**, 655 Sugartown Road, Zip 19355–0275, Mailing Address: P.O. Box 275, Zip 19355–0275; tel. 610/296–6820 **A**9 **F**29 98 99 106 **P**6 **S** Devereux, Villanova, PA
Primary Contact: David E. Woodward, Executive Director
COO: Howard Jarden, Ph.D., Assistant Executive Director
CFO: David Schultheis, Chief Financial Officer
CMO: Jacquelyn Zavodnick, M.D., Medical Director
CIO: MaryLou Hettinger, Director Quality Management
CHR: Sean Maher, Director Human Resources
Web address: www.devereux.org
**Control:** Other not–for–profit (including NFP Corporation) **Service:** Children's hospital psychiatric

Staffed Beds: 33 Admissions: 496 Census: 24 Outpatient Visits: 0 Births: 0 Total Expense ($000): 5168 Payroll Expense ($000): 2833 Personnel: 55

☐ **MALVERN INSTITUTE**, 940 King Road, Zip 19355–3167; tel. 610/647–0330, (Nonreporting) **A**1 9
Primary Contact: Richard Mangano, Administrator and Chief Executive Officer
CFO: Janet Corley, Accountant
Web address: www.malverninstitute.com
**Control:** Corporation, Investor–owned, for–profit **Service:** Alcoholism and other chemical dependency

Staffed Beds: 40

**MC CONNELLSBURG—Fulton County**

★ **FULTON COUNTY MEDICAL CENTER (391303)**, 214 Peach Orchard Road, Zip 17233–8559; tel. 717/485–3155, (Nonreporting) **A**9 10 18
Primary Contact: Jason F. Hawkins, President and Chief Executive Officer
COO: William Buterbaugh, Director Support Services
CFO: Deborah A. Shughart, Vice President and Chief Financial Officer
CMO: Sharon E. Martin, M.D., President Medical Staff
CIO: Harold M. Gress, Jr., Manager Management Information Systems
CHR: Cheryl Rose, Manager Human Resources
Web address: www.fcmcpa.org
**Control:** Other not–for–profit (including NFP Corporation) **Service:** General Medical and Surgical

Staffed Beds: 88

**MCKEES ROCKS—Allegheny County**

☒ **OHIO VALLEY GENERAL HOSPITAL (390157)**, 25 Heckel Road, Zip 15136–1694; tel. 412/777–6161 **A**1 6 9 10 **F**3 10 15 18 20 29 30 40 45 49 51 59 65 70 75 77 79 81 82 85 87 90 92 93 98 103 107 108 111 117 118 128 129 142 145 147 **P**6
Primary Contact: David W. Scott, President and Chief Executive Officer
CFO: Tad Tefera, Vice President Finance
CIO: Lynn Aumer, Director Information Management
CHR: Vicki Mell, Vice President Human Resources
Web address: www.ohiovalleyhospital.org
**Control:** Other not–for–profit (including NFP Corporation) **Service:** General Medical and Surgical

Staffed Beds: 138 Admissions: 3709 Census: 56 Outpatient Visits: 122853 Births: 0 Total Expense ($000): 66471 Payroll Expense ($000): 23348 Personnel: 454

**MCKEESPORT—Allegheny County**

☒ **SELECT SPECIALTY HOSPITAL–MCKEESPORT (392045)**, 1500 Fifth Avenue, Zip 15132; tel. 412/664–2900, (Nonreporting) **A**1 9 10 **S** Select Medical Corporation, Mechanicsburg, PA
Primary Contact: John St. Leger, Chief Executive Officer
Web address: www.selectmedicalcorp.com
**Control:** Corporation, Investor–owned, for–profit **Service:** Long–Term Acute Care hospital

Staffed Beds: 30

☐ **UPMC MCKEESPORT (390002)**, 1500 Fifth Avenue, Zip 15132–2422; tel. 412/664–2000, (Total facility includes 19 beds in nursing home–type unit) **A**1 3 5 9 10 12 13 **F**3 8 11 15 17 18 20 28 29 30 31 32 34 35 37 40 49 50 54 56 57 59 60 61 62 64 65 66 68 70 74 75 77 78 79 81 84 85 86 87 90 93 96 97 98 100 101 102 103 107 111 113 114 117 118 120 127 128 129 130 131 133 134 142 145 146 147 **S** UPMC, Pittsburgh, PA
Primary Contact: Cynthia M. Dorundo, President
COO: Merle Taylor, Vice President Operations
CFO: Christopher Stockhausen, Chief Financial Officer
CMO: R. Curtis Waligura, D.O., Vice President Medical Affairs, Chief Medical Officer
CIO: Joyce Krut, Vice President Information Systems
CHR: Mark P. Frick, Vice President Human Resources
CNO: Cheryl A. Como, R.N., Vice President Patient Services and Chief Nursing Officer
Web address: www.mckeesport.upmc.com
**Control:** Other not–for–profit (including NFP Corporation) **Service:** General Medical and Surgical

Staffed Beds: 231 Admissions: 10758 Census: 180 Outpatient Visits: 127330 Births: 0 Total Expense ($000): 123635 Payroll Expense ($000): 62173 Personnel: 908

**MEADOWBROOK—Montgomery County**

☐ **HOLY REDEEMER HOSPITAL AND MEDICAL CENTER (390097)**, 1648 Huntingdon Pike, Zip 19046–8001; tel. 215/947–3000, (Total facility includes 21 beds in nursing home–type unit) **A**1 2 5 10 21 **F**3 10 11 13 15 17 18 20 22 29 30 31 34 35 39 40 41 44 45 46 49 50 53 57 58 59 61 62 63 64 69 70 72 74 75 76 77 78 79 81 82 84 85 86 87 89 92 93 97 98 100 103 107 108 109 110 113 114 116 117 118 119 120 122 127 128 129 130 131 133 134 140 142 145 146 147
Primary Contact: Michael B. Laign, President and Chief Executive Officer
COO: Michele L. Urofsky, Executive Vice President and Chief Administrative Officer
CFO: Russell R. Wagner, Senior Vice President and Chief Financial Officer
CMO: Anthony V. Coletta, M.D., Executive Vice President and Chief Medical Officer
CIO: Donald F. Friel, Executive Vice President
CHR: Joseph J. Cassidy, Vice President
Web address: www.holyredeemer.com
**Control:** Other not–for–profit (including NFP Corporation) **Service:** General Medical and Surgical

Staffed Beds: 263 Admissions: 13668 Census: 181 Outpatient Visits: 328375 Births: 2837 Total Expense ($000): 184789 Payroll Expense ($000): 77619 Personnel: 1396

**MEADVILLE—Crawford County**

★ **MEADVILLE MEDICAL CENTER (390113)**, 751 Liberty Street, Zip 16335–2559; tel. 814/333–5000, (Total facility includes 32 beds in nursing home–type unit) **A**2 9 10 12 13 21 **F**3 4 5 11 13 15 16 18 20 22 28 29 30 31 35 36 38 40 45 46 49 53 57 59 63 64 70 75 76 77 78 79 81 82 85 86 87 89 90 91 93 98 99 103 107 110 111 113 114 117 118 119 127 128 129 130 131 143 145 146 147 **P**6 7
Primary Contact: Philip Pandolph, Chief Executive Officer
CMO: Denise Johnson, M.D., Medical Director
CIO: Mark Mahoney, Manager Information Systems
CHR: Greg Maras, Vice President Human Resources
Web address: www.mmchs.org
**Control:** Other not–for–profit (including NFP Corporation) **Service:** General Medical and Surgical

Staffed Beds: 208 Admissions: 7481 Census: 111 Outpatient Visits: 227630 Births: 519 Total Expense ($000): 137485 Payroll Expense ($000): 51731 Personnel: 1074

PA

**MECHANICSBURG—Cumberland County**

**HEALTHSOUTH REGIONAL SPECIALTY HOSPITAL** See LifeCare Hospitals of Mechanicsburg

✠ **HEALTHSOUTH REHABILITATION HOSPITAL OF MECHANICSBURG (393031)**, 175 Lancaster Boulevard, Zip 17055–0736, Mailing Address: P.O. Box 2016, Zip 17055–2016; tel. 717/691–3700, (Nonreporting) **A**1 9 10 **S** HEALTHSOUTH Corporation, Birmingham, AL
Primary Contact: Mark Freeburn, Chief Executive Officer
CMO: Michael Lupinacci, M.D., Medical Director
CHR: David Staskin, Director Human Resources
Web address: www.healthsouthpa.com
**Control:** Corporation, Investor–owned, for–profit **Service:** Rehabilitation

| **Staffed Beds:** 75 |

✠ **LIFECARE HOSPITALS OF MECHANICSBURG (392038)**, 4950 Wilson Lane, Zip 17055; tel. 717/697–7706, (Data for 153 days) **A**1 9 10 **F**1 3 7 12 18 29 60 68 75 77 91 **P**5 **S** LifeCare Management Services, Plano, TX
Primary Contact: Nicholas Mezza, Chief Executive Officer
CFO: Jay Shoen, Controller
CHR: David Staskin, Director Human Resources
Web address: www.lifecare–hospitals.com/hospital.php?id=20
**Control:** Corporation, Investor–owned, for–profit **Service:** Long–Term Acute Care hospital

| **Staffed Beds:** 68 **Admissions:** 171 **Census:** 28 **Outpatient Visits:** 0 **Births:** 0 **Total Expense ($000):** 5546 **Payroll Expense ($000):** 2533 **Personnel:** 126 |

**MEDIA—Delaware County**

✠ **RIDDLE HOSPITAL (390222)**, 1068 West Baltimore Pike, Zip 19063–5177; tel. 484/227–9400, (Total facility includes 23 beds in nursing home–type unit) **A**1 2 9 10 **F**3 7 11 13 15 20 22 28 29 31 34 35 39 40 44 45 46 49 50 53 54 56 57 59 61 64 65 68 70 72 74 75 76 77 78 79 80 81 82 85 86 87 92 93 96 97 100 107 108 111 113 114 117 118 127 128 129 130 131 133 134 142 145 146 147 **P**6 **S** Main Line Health, Bryn Mawr, PA
Primary Contact: Gary L. Perecko, President
COO: James Paradis, Vice President Administration
CMO: Joseph D. Hope, D.O., President Medical Staff
CHR: Mary Louise Ciciretti, Director Human Resources
Web address: www.riddlehospital.org
**Control:** Other not–for–profit (including NFP Corporation) **Service:** General Medical and Surgical

| **Staffed Beds:** 209 **Admissions:** 10935 **Census:** 136 **Outpatient Visits:** 60126 **Births:** 976 **Total Expense ($000):** 166552 **Payroll Expense ($000):** 64132 **Personnel:** 884 |

**RIDDLE MEMORIAL HOSPITAL** See Riddle Hospital

**MEYERSDALE—Somerset County**

**MEYERSDALE MEDICAL CENTER (391302)**, 200 Hospital Drive, Zip 15552–1249; tel. 814/634–5911 **A**9 10 18 **F**15 18 29 34 40 46 50 57 59 64 75 81 107 113 118 126 129 131 132 145 147 **S** Conemaugh Health System, Johnstown, PA
Primary Contact: Mary L. Libengood, President
CFO: Heather Smith, Director Finance
CMO: Nathan Thomas, M.D., President Medical Staff
Web address: www.conemaugh.org
**Control:** Other not–for–profit (including NFP Corporation) **Service:** General Medical and Surgical

| **Staffed Beds:** 20 **Admissions:** 383 **Census:** 5 **Outpatient Visits:** 43740 **Births:** 0 **Total Expense ($000):** 11255 **Payroll Expense ($000):** 4206 **Personnel:** 90 |

**MONONGAHELA—Washington County**

✠ **MONONGAHELA VALLEY HOSPITAL (390147)**, 1163 Country Club Road, Route 88, Zip 15063–1095; tel. 724/258–1000 **A**1 2 9 10 **F**3 8 9 11 12 15 17 18 20 22 28 29 30 31 32 34 35 39 40 45 48 49 50 51 54 56 57 59 61 64 68 70 74 75 77 78 79 80 81 82 85 86 87 89 90 92 93 96 98 100 101 102 103 107 108 110 113 114 117 118 119 120 122 128 129 130 131 133 134 145 146 147 **P**8
Primary Contact: Louis J. Panza, Jr., President and Chief Executive Officer
COO: Patrick J. Alberts, Senior Vice President and Chief Operating Officer
CFO: Daniel F. Simmons, Senior Vice President and Treasurer
CIO: Sandra Osborne, Director Information Systems
CHR: David Clark, Vice President Human Resources
Web address: www.monvalleyhospital.com
**Control:** Other not–for–profit (including NFP Corporation) **Service:** General Medical and Surgical

| **Staffed Beds:** 210 **Admissions:** 8587 **Census:** 125 **Outpatient Visits:** 273495 **Births:** 0 **Total Expense ($000):** 111162 **Payroll Expense ($000):** 48236 **Personnel:** 1055 |

**MONROEVILLE—Allegheny County**

✠ **FORBES REGIONAL HOSPITAL (390267)**, 2570 Haymaker Road, Zip 15146–3513; tel. 412/858–2000 **A**1 3 5 9 10 **F**3 7 8 11 13 15 17 18 20 22 24 26 29 30 31 34 35 36 37 40 45 46 49 50 51 57 59 63 64 65 68 69 70 73 74 75 76 78 79 81 82 84 85 86 87 89 90 91 92 93 98 100 101 102 103 107 108 110 111 113 114 118 122 123 125 129 131 132 145 147 **S** West Penn Allegheny Health System, Pittsburgh, PA
Primary Contact: Reese Jackson, President and Chief Executive Officer
COO: Thomas B. Moser, Chief Operating Officer
CFO: James A. Kanuch, Vice President Finance
CIO: Sharon Lewis, Director Information Systems
CHR: Tanya Ulrich, Director Human Resources
Web address: www.wpahs.org
**Control:** Other not–for–profit (including NFP Corporation) **Service:** General Medical and Surgical

| **Staffed Beds:** 310 **Admissions:** 15447 **Census:** 219 **Outpatient Visits:** 179635 **Births:** 811 **Total Expense ($000):** 155582 **Payroll Expense ($000):** 58861 **Personnel:** 1155 |

**HEALTHSOUTH HOSPITAL OF PITTSBURGH** See LifeCare Hospitals of Pittsburgh – Monroeville

✠ **LIFECARE HOSPITALS OF PITTSBURGH – MONROEVILLE (392041)**, 2380 McGinley Road, Zip 15146–4400; tel. 412/856–2400, (Data for 153 days) **A**1 9 10 **F**29 93 107 **P**5 **S** LifeCare Management Services, Plano, TX
Primary Contact: Richard Pletz, Administrator
CMO: Robert Crossey, D.O., Chief Medical Officer
CIO: Justin Armstrong, Chief Information Officer
CHR: Chelsea Webber, Director Human Resources
Web address: www.lifecare–hospitals.com/hospital.php?id=8
**Control:** Corporation, Investor–owned, for–profit **Service:** Long–Term Acute Care hospital

| **Staffed Beds:** 87 **Admissions:** 193 **Census:** 33 **Outpatient Visits:** 2272 **Births:** 0 **Total Expense ($000):** 7308 **Payroll Expense ($000):** 3086 **Personnel:** 164 |

**WESTERN PENNSYLVANIA HOSPITAL – FORBES REGIONAL CAMPUS** See Forbes Regional Hospital

**MONTROSE—Susquehanna County**

**ENDLESS MOUNTAIN HEALTH SYSTEMS (391306)**, 25 Grow Avenue, Zip 18801–1106; tel. 570/278–3801, (Nonreporting) **A**9 10 18
Primary Contact: Rexford Catlin, Chief Executive Officer
CIO: Gary Passmore, Chief Information Officer
CHR: Paula Anderson, Administrative Director Human Resources
Web address: www.endlesscare.org
**Control:** Other not–for–profit (including NFP Corporation) **Service:** General Medical and Surgical

| **Staffed Beds:** 21 |

**MOUNT GRETNA—Lebanon County**

☐ **PHILHAVEN (394020)**, 283 South Butler Road, Zip 17064–0550, Mailing Address: P.O. Box 550, Zip 17064–0550; tel. 717/273–8871 **A**1 9 10 **F**30 98 99 100 101 102 103 104 105 106 129 145 **P**6
Primary Contact: Phil Hess, Chief Executive Officer
COO: Phil Hess, Chief Executive Officer
CFO: Matt Rogers, Chief Financial Officer
CMO: Francis D. Sparrow, M.D., Medical Director
CIO: Lori Nolt, Director Information Technology
CHR: Denis Orthaus, Director Human Resources
Web address: www.philhaven.org
**Control:** Church–operated, Nongovernment, not–for profit **Service:** Psychiatric

| **Staffed Beds:** 97 **Admissions:** 2042 **Census:** 77 **Outpatient Visits:** 82249 **Births:** 0 **Total Expense ($000):** 54068 **Payroll Expense ($000):** 34363 **Personnel:** 865 |

**PA**

---

**Hospital, Medicare Provider Number, Address, Telephone, Approval, Facility, and Physician Codes, Health Care System**

★ American Hospital Association (AHA) membership
☐ The Joint Commission accreditation ◇ DNV Healthcare Inc. accreditation

○ American Osteopathic Association (AOA) accreditation
△ Commission on Accreditation of Rehabilitation Facilities (CARF) accreditation

**PA**

## MOUNT PLEASANT—Westmoreland County

☐ **EXCELA FRICK HOSPITAL (390217)**, 508 South Church Street,
Zip 15666–1790; tel. 724/547–1500 **A**1 9 10 **F**3 8 12 15 29 30 34 35 40 45
49 57 59 64 65 68 70 74 75 77 78 79 81 85 86 87 92 93 96 102 107 108
110 111 113 117 118 128 129 131 134 142 145 147 **S** Excela Health,
Greensburg, PA
Primary Contact: Ronald H. Ott, President
COO: Samuel Raneri, Senior Vice President Operations and Business Development
CFO: Jeffrey T. Curry, Executive Vice President and Chief Financial Officer
CMO: Jerome Granato, M.D., Chief Medical Officer
CIO: Otto Salguero, Chief Information Officer
CHR: John Caverno, Chief Human Resources Officer
Web address: www.frickhospital.org
**Control:** Other not–for–profit (including NFP Corporation) **Service:** General
Medical and Surgical

| | |
|---|---|
| **Staffed Beds:** 65 **Admissions:** 3562 **Census:** 44 **Outpatient Visits:** 121179 **Births:** 0 **Total Expense ($000):** 45819 **Payroll Expense ($000):** 17207 **Personnel:** 366 | |

## MUNCY—Lycoming County

★ **MUNCY VALLEY HOSPITAL (391301)**, 215 East Water Street,
Zip 17756–8700; tel. 570/546–8282, (Total facility includes 136 beds in nursing
home–type unit) **A**9 10 18 **F**6 11 34 40 44 50 56 57 59 64 68 81 86 87 93
107 108 118 127 129 132 143 145 **P**7 **S** Susquehanna Health System,
Williamsport, PA
Primary Contact: Ronald J. Reynolds, President
CFO: Charles J. Santangelo, CPA, Executive Vice President and Chief Financial
Officer
CMO: George A. Manchester, M.D., Executive Vice President and Chief Medical
Officer
CIO: Karen M. Armstrong, FACHE, Senior Vice President and Chief Information
Officer
CHR: Glenn C. Mechling, FACHE, Senior Vice President Human Resources
Web address: www.susquehannahealth.org
**Control:** Other not–for–profit (including NFP Corporation) **Service:** General
Medical and Surgical

| | |
|---|---|
| **Staffed Beds:** 156 **Admissions:** 1144 **Census:** 141 **Outpatient Visits:** 32026 **Births:** 0 **Total Expense ($000):** 34525 **Payroll Expense ($000):** 12596 **Personnel:** 264 | |

## NANTICOKE—Luzerne County

★ **SPECIAL CARE HOSPITAL (392025)**, 128 West Washington Street,
Zip 18634–3113; tel. 570/735–5000, (Nonreporting) **A**9 10 **S** Community Health
Systems, Inc., Franklin, TN
Primary Contact: Robert D. Williams, Chief Executive Officer
CFO: Stephen Franko, Chief Financial Officer
Web address: www.specialcarehospital.net
**Control:** Corporation, Investor–owned, for–profit **Service:** Long–Term Acute Care
hospital

| | |
|---|---|
| **Staffed Beds:** 64 | |

## NATRONA HEIGHTS—Allegheny County

☒ **ALLEGHENY VALLEY HOSPITAL (390032)**, 1301 Carlisle Street,
Zip 15065–1152; tel. 724/224–5100 **A**1 2 6 9 10 **F**3 11 14 15 17 18 24 28
29 30 31 34 35 38 39 40 44 45 47 49 50 51 54 56 57 58 59 64 65 68 70
74 75 77 78 79 80 81 85 86 87 92 93 96 98 100 101 102 103 107 108 111
113 116 117 118 119 120 122 128 129 131 132 134 142 143 145 146 147
**S** West Penn Allegheny Health System, Pittsburgh, PA
Primary Contact: Ned Laubacher, President and Chief Executive Officer
COO: Michael Harlovic, R.N., Senior Vice President and Chief Operating Officer
CFO: George Sandora, Vice President Finance
CMO: Radha Kambhampati, M.D., Vice President Medical Affairs
CIO: Linda Fergus, Manager Information Technology
CHR: A. Jack Davis, Director Human Resources
Web address: www.wpahs.org
**Control:** Other not–for–profit (including NFP Corporation) **Service:** General
Medical and Surgical

| | |
|---|---|
| **Staffed Beds:** 228 **Admissions:** 9086 **Census:** 130 **Outpatient Visits:** 213248 **Births:** 1 **Total Expense ($000):** 99698 **Payroll Expense ($000):** 41530 **Personnel:** 937 | |

## NEW CASTLE—Lawrence County

☒ **JAMESON HOSPITAL (390016)**, 1211 Wilmington Avenue, Zip 16105–2516;
tel. 724/658–9001, (Total facility includes 20 beds in nursing home–type unit) **A**1
6 9 10 19 **F**3 8 11 12 13 15 18 20 22 28 29 30 31 32 34 35 38 40 44 45
49 50 51 54 56 57 59 63 64 65 68 70 75 76 77 79 81 82 85 86 87 90 91
93 94 96 98 99 101 102 103 105 107 108 110 111 113 114 117 118 127
128 129 131 134 145 146
Primary Contact: Douglas Danko, President and Chief Executive Officer
CFO: James Aubel, Chief Financial Officer
CMO: Mohammad Ali, M.D., President Medical Staff
CIO: Frank Divito, Manager Information Systems
CHR: Neil A. Chessin, Vice President
Web address: www.jamesonhealth.org
**Control:** Other not–for–profit (including NFP Corporation) **Service:** General
Medical and Surgical

| | |
|---|---|
| **Staffed Beds:** 238 **Admissions:** 9604 **Census:** 127 **Outpatient Visits:** 295662 **Births:** 460 **Total Expense ($000):** 103010 **Payroll Expense ($000):** 44997 **Personnel:** 1023 | |

## NORRISTOWN—Montgomery County

☒ ○ **MERCY SUBURBAN HOSPITAL (390116)**, 2701 DeKalb Pike,
Zip 19401–1820; tel. 610/278–2000 **A**1 2 9 10 11 12 13 **F**3 11 15 18 28 29
30 31 34 40 46 50 54 56 57 59 64 70 74 75 77 78 79 81 82 84 85 87 93
98 103 107 108 110 111 113 114 117 118 127 128 129 131 134 145 146
147 **S** Catholic Health East, Newtown Square, PA
Primary Contact: Jeffrey Snyder, Chief Executive Officer
COO: Carol Fluegge, Chief Operating Officer
CFO: Peter B. Kenniff, CPA, Chief Financial Officer
CMO: Wayne Miller, D.O., Associate Chief Medical Officer
CIO: Michael Yulich, Director Information Services
CHR: Gretchen Pendleton, Chief Human Resources Officer
Web address: www.mercyhealth.org
**Control:** Church–operated, Nongovernment, not–for profit **Service:** General
Medical and Surgical

| | |
|---|---|
| **Staffed Beds:** 126 **Admissions:** 5899 **Census:** 78 **Outpatient Visits:** 30103 **Births:** 0 **Total Expense ($000):** 107972 **Payroll Expense ($000):** 39898 **Personnel:** 781 | |

☐ **MONTGOMERY COUNTY EMERGENCY SERVICE (394033)**, 50 Beech Drive,
Zip 19403–5421; tel. 610/279–6100 **A**1 9 10 **F**4 5 7 29 35 38 50 64 98 99
100 101 102 103 104 129 **P**6
Primary Contact: Rocio Nell, M.D., Chief Executive Officer
COO: William Myers, Chief Operating Officer
CFO: William Myers, Chief Operating Officer
CHR: Karen Mossop, Director Human Resources
Web address: www.mces.org
**Control:** Other not–for–profit (including NFP Corporation) **Service:** Psychiatric

| | |
|---|---|
| **Staffed Beds:** 81 **Admissions:** 2372 **Census:** 67 **Outpatient Visits:** 3046 **Births:** 0 **Total Expense ($000):** 15973 **Payroll Expense ($000):** 10493 **Personnel:** 203 | |

☒ **MONTGOMERY HOSPITAL MEDICAL CENTER (390108)**, 1301 Powell Street,
Zip 19401–3377, Mailing Address: P.O. Box 992, Zip 19404–0992;
tel. 610/270–2000 **A**1 2 3 5 9 10 **F**3 11 13 15 17 18 20 22 28 29 30 31 34
35 37 40 41 45 50 57 59 60 62 63 65 66 70 72 74 75 76 77 78 79 81 82
83 84 85 86 87 91 92 93 94 98 100 101 103 107 108 110 111 114 118
119 120 121 123 128 129 131 134 142 145 146 **P**6 **S** Albert Einstein
Healthcare Network, Philadelphia, PA
Primary Contact: Timothy M. Casey, President and Chief Executive Officer
CFO: Edward Ladely, Senior Vice President and Chief Financial Officer
CIO: Ed Hemschoot, Director Information Systems
CHR: Murray Swim, Chief Human Resources Officer
Web address: www.montgomeryhospital.org
**Control:** Other not–for–profit (including NFP Corporation) **Service:** General
Medical and Surgical

| | |
|---|---|
| **Staffed Beds:** 177 **Admissions:** 6295 **Census:** 72 **Outpatient Visits:** 158992 **Births:** 1058 **Total Expense ($000):** 93673 **Payroll Expense ($000):** 40273 **Personnel:** 856 | |

☐ **NORRISTOWN STATE HOSPITAL (394001)**, 1001 Sterigere Street,
Zip 19401–5300; tel. 610/270–1000, (Nonreporting) **A**1 3 5 9 10
Primary Contact: Gerald P. Kent, Chief Executive Officer
COO: Gary Raisner, Chief Operating Officer
CMO: Mia Marcovici, M.D., Chief Medical Officer
CHR: Richard Szczurowski, Director Human Resources
**Control:** State–Government, nonfederal **Service:** Psychiatric

| | |
|---|---|
| **Staffed Beds:** 394 | |

*Many Facility Codes have changed. Please refer to the AHA Guide Code Chart.* © 2012 AHA Guide

**PA**

⊠ **VALLEY FORGE MEDICAL CENTER AND HOSPITAL (390272)**, 1033 West Germantown Pike, Zip 19403–3905; tel. 610/539–8500 **A**1 10 **F**3 4 29 61 68 75 82 100 129 131 147 **P**6
Primary Contact: Marian W. Colcher, President and Chief Executive Officer
CFO: Gregg Y. Slocum, Chief Financial Officer
CMO: Robert E. Colcher, M.D., Medical Director
CHR: Frederick D. Jackes, Assistant Administrator and Director Human Resources
Web address: www.vfmc.net
**Control:** Corporation, Investor–owned, for–profit **Service:** Alcoholism and other chemical dependency

**Staffed Beds:** 86 **Admissions:** 2187 **Census:** 76 **Outpatient Visits:** 0 **Births:** 0 **Total Expense ($000):** 11420 **Payroll Expense ($000):** 7359 **Personnel:** 152

### OAKDALE—Allegheny County

⊠ **KINDRED HOSPITAL–PITTSBURGH (392028)**, 7777 Steubenville Pike, Zip 15071–3409; tel. 412/494–5500, (Nonreporting) **A**1 9 10 **S** Kindred Healthcare, Louisville, KY
Primary Contact: John T. Burton, Administrator
CFO: Kevin Varley, Chief Financial Officer
CMO: Ravi Alagar, M.D., Medical Director
CIO: Kurt Segeleon, Director Health Information Management
CHR: Nancy Smocynski, Director Payroll, Personnel and Human Resources
Web address: www.kindredhospitalpittsburgh.com/
**Control:** Corporation, Investor–owned, for–profit **Service:** Long–Term Acute Care hospital

**Staffed Beds:** 63

### OREFIELD—Lehigh County

**KIDSPEACE CHILDREN'S HOSPITAL (394047)**, 5300 Kids Peace Drive, Zip 18069–2044; tel. 610/799–8800 **A**9 10 **F**29 38 98 99 100 101 102 104 105 106 **P**6
Primary Contact: William R. Isemann, President and Chief Executive Officer
CFO: Tim Richards, Executive Vice President and Chief Financial Officer
Web address: www.kidspeace.org
**Control:** Other not–for–profit (including NFP Corporation) **Service:** Children's hospital psychiatric

**Staffed Beds:** 80 **Admissions:** 1881 **Census:** 69 **Outpatient Visits:** 7000 **Births:** 0 **Total Expense ($000):** 17469 **Payroll Expense ($000):** 7731 **Personnel:** 176

### PALMERTON—Carbon County

☐ **PALMERTON HOSPITAL (390019)**, 135 Lafayette Avenue, Zip 18071–1596; tel. 610/826–3141 **A**1 9 10 **F**2 3 11 12 15 28 29 34 35 40 44 46 47 49 50 56 57 59 64 65 68 70 74 75 77 79 81 85 86 87 92 93 97 98 102 103 107 108 110 118 128 129 131 134 145 **S** Blue Mountain Health System, Lehighton, PA
Primary Contact: Andrew E. Harris, Chief Executive Officer
CFO: Andrea Andrae, Chief Financial Officer
CMO: Patrick Hanley, D.O., Interim Vice President Medical Affairs
CIO: Steve Kinkaid, Director Information Systems
CHR: Terry Purcell, Vice President Ambulatory Care and Support Services
Web address: www.bmhs.com
**Control:** Other not–for–profit (including NFP Corporation) **Service:** General Medical and Surgical

**Staffed Beds:** 60 **Admissions:** 2078 **Census:** 30 **Outpatient Visits:** 48063 **Births:** 0 **Total Expense ($000):** 26635 **Payroll Expense ($000):** 11610 **Personnel:** 317

### PAOLI—Chester County

⊠ **PAOLI HOSPITAL (390153)**, 255 West Lancaster Avenue, Zip 19301–1763; tel. 484/565–1000 **A**1 2 9 10 **F**3 8 13 15 18 20 22 24 26 28 29 30 31 34 35 38 40 43 46 47 48 49 50 51 54 57 59 60 61 62 63 64 65 68 70 72 74 75 76 77 78 79 80 81 82 84 85 86 87 93 94 102 107 108 109 110 111 112 113 114 115 116 117 118 119 120 121 122 123 125 128 129 134 135 142 143 145 146 147 **P**5 **S** Main Line Health, Bryn Mawr, PA
Primary Contact: Barbara J. Tachovsky, President
CFO: John Doyle, Vice President Finance
CMO: Donald C. Arthur, M.D., Chief Medical Officer
CIO: Karen A. Thomas, R.N., Vice President and Chief Information Officer
CHR: Deborah Fedora, Director Human Resources
Web address: www.mainlinehealth.org
**Control:** Other not–for–profit (including NFP Corporation) **Service:** General Medical and Surgical

**Staffed Beds:** 222 **Admissions:** 14656 **Census:** 148 **Outpatient Visits:** 289632 **Births:** 2343 **Total Expense ($000):** 214042 **Payroll Expense ($000):** 73345 **Personnel:** 1028

### PECKVILLE—Lackawanna County

★ **MID–VALLEY HOSPITAL (391311)**, 1400 Main Street, Zip 18452–2009; tel. 570/383–5500, (Nonreporting) **A**9 10 18 **S** Community Health Systems, Inc., Franklin, TN
Primary Contact: Ann Marie Stevens, Chief Executive Officer
CFO: James G. Brittain, Chief Financial Officer
CMO: Rajan Mulloth, M.D., President Medical Staff
CIO: Edward Roman, Chief Information Officer and Chief Privacy Officer
CHR: Michele Dean, Human Resources Specialist
Web address: www.mth.org
**Control:** Corporation, Investor–owned, for–profit **Service:** General Medical and Surgical

**Staffed Beds:** 25

### PHILADELPHIA—Philadelphia County

**ALBERT EINSTEIN MEDICAL CENTER** See Einstein Medical Center Philadelphia

⊠ △ **ARIA HEALTH (390115)**, 10800 Knights Road, Zip 19114–4200; tel. 215/612–4000, (Includes BUCKS COUNTY CAMPUS, 380 North Oxford Valley Road, Langhorne, Zip 19047–8399; tel. 215/949–5000; FRANKFORD CAMPUS, Frankford Avenue and Wakeling Street, Zip 19124; tel. 215/831–2000) **A**1 6 7 10 12 13 **F**3 5 11 12 14 15 17 18 20 22 24 26 28 29 30 31 32 34 35 36 39 40 43 44 45 46 48 49 53 54 57 59 61 62 64 65 66 68 69 70 74 75 77 78 79 80 81 82 85 86 87 92 93 94 96 97 98 100 101 102 103 104 107 108 110 113 114 115 116 117 118 119 120 122 123 125 126 128 129 130 131 134 142 143 144 145 146 147 **P**6
Primary Contact: Kathleen Kinslow, Ed.D., President and Chief Executive Officer
CFO: Robert J. Crossin, Vice President Finance
CMO: Domenick Bucci, M.D., Medical Director
CIO: Joseph Olszewski, Director Information Services
Web address: www.ariahealth.org
**Control:** Other not–for–profit (including NFP Corporation) **Service:** General Medical and Surgical

**Staffed Beds:** 485 **Admissions:** 25806 **Census:** 353 **Outpatient Visits:** 312863 **Births:** 0 **Total Expense ($000):** 393010 **Payroll Expense ($000):** 167133 **Personnel:** 2807

☐ **BELMONT CENTER FOR COMPREHENSIVE TREATMENT (394023)**, 4200 Monument Road, Zip 19131–1625; tel. 215/877–2000 **A**1 3 5 9 10 **F**5 29 34 58 98 99 103 104 105 129 145 **P**6 **S** Albert Einstein Healthcare Network, Philadelphia, PA
Primary Contact: Sharon A. Bergen, Chief Operating Officer
COO: Sharon A. Bergen, Chief Operating Officer
CFO: Guy Romaniello, Director Fiscal Services
CMO: Lawrence A. Real, M.D., Medical Director
CHR: Kymm Steliga, Human Resources Specialist
Web address: www.einstein.edu
**Control:** Other not–for–profit (including NFP Corporation) **Service:** Psychiatric

**Staffed Beds:** 147 **Admissions:** 3754 **Census:** 133 **Outpatient Visits:** 60332 **Births:** 0 **Total Expense ($000):** 37996 **Payroll Expense ($000):** 23355 **Personnel:** 378

⊠ **CHESTNUT HILL HOSPITAL (390026)**, 8835 Germantown Avenue, Zip 19118–2718; tel. 215/248–8200 **A**1 2 3 5 9 10 **F**3 12 15 17 18 26 29 30 31 34 35 37 38 40 45 47 48 49 50 54 56 57 58 59 60 64 70 74 75 77 78 79 81 82 84 85 86 87 90 91 92 93 96 97 107 108 109 110 111 113 114 118 119 120 125 128 129 130 131 145 146 147 **P**6 **S** Community Health Systems, Inc., Franklin, TN
Primary Contact: John D. Cacciamani, Chief Executive Officer
COO: Andrew Goldfrach, Assistant Chief Executive Officer
CFO: Debbie Konarski, Chief Financial Officer
CMO: John Scanlon, DPM, Chief Medical Officer
CIO: Beth Crossley, Director Information Systems
CHR: James Como, Director Human Resources
Web address: www.chhealthsystem.com
**Control:** Corporation, Investor–owned, for–profit **Service:** General Medical and Surgical

**Staffed Beds:** 135 **Admissions:** 6694 **Census:** 72 **Births:** 0

---

**Hospital, Medicare Provider Number, Address, Telephone, Approval, Facility, and Physician Codes, Health Care System**

★ American Hospital Association (AHA) membership
☐ The Joint Commission accreditation
◇ DNV Healthcare Inc. accreditation
○ American Osteopathic Association (AOA) accreditation
△ Commission on Accreditation of Rehabilitation Facilities (CARF) accreditation

**PA**

☐ **CHILDREN'S HOSPITAL OF PHILADELPHIA (393303)**, 3401 Civic Center Boulevard, Zip 19104–4399; tel. 215/590–1000 **A**1 3 5 8 9 10 **F**3 7 8 11 13 17 18 19 20 21 22 23 24 25 26 27 28 29 30 31 32 34 35 37 38 39 40 41 43 44 45 46 48 50 54 55 57 58 59 60 61 62 64 65 66 68 71 72 74 75 76 77 78 79 81 82 83 84 85 86 87 88 89 90 91 92 93 96 97 99 100 101 102 104 107 108 111 112 113 114 115 116 117 118 125 128 129 130 131 133 135 136 137 138 139 143 145 147 **P**6
Primary Contact: Steven M. Altschuler, M.D., President and Chief Executive Officer
COO: Madeline Bell, Executive Vice President and Chief Operating Officer
CFO: Thomas Todorow, Chief Financial Officer
CMO: Michael Apkon, M.D., Senior Vice President and Chief Medical Officer
CIO: Bryan Wolf, M.D., Senior Vice President and Chief Information Officer
CHR: Robert Croner, Executive Vice President and Chief Human Resources Officer
Web address: www.chop.edu
**Control:** Other not–for–profit (including NFP Corporation) **Service:** Children's general

**Staffed Beds:** 469 **Admissions:** 28401 **Census:** 400 **Outpatient Visits:** 1142200 **Births:** 322 **Total Expense ($000):** 1398924 **Payroll Expense ($000):** 654844 **Personnel:** 9093

☐ **EASTERN REGIONAL MEDICAL CENTER (390312)**, 1331 East Wyoming Avenue, Zip 19124; tel. 800/294–8333, (Nonreporting) **A**1 10 **S** Cancer Treatment Centers of America, Schaumburg, IL
Primary Contact: John McNeil, President and Chief Executive Officer
Web address: www.cancercenter.com
**Control:** Corporation, Investor–owned, for–profit **Service:** Long–Term Acute Care hospital

**Staffed Beds:** 22

☐ **EINSTEIN MEDICAL CENTER PHILADELPHIA (390142)**, 5501 Old York Road, Zip 19141–3098; tel. 215/456–7890, (Includes EINSTEIN MEDICAL CENTER ELKINS PARK, 60 East Township Line Road, Elkins Park, Zip 19027–2220; tel. 215/663–6000; Ruth Lefton, Chief Operating Officer), (Total facility includes 78 beds in nursing home–type unit) **A**1 2 3 5 8 9 10 12 13 **F**3 8 11 12 13 15 17 18 20 22 24 26 29 30 31 32 34 35 36 39 40 41 43 45 46 47 48 49 50 55 56 57 59 60 61 64 65 66 68 70 72 74 75 76 78 79 81 82 84 85 86 87 90 92 93 95 96 97 98 100 103 107 108 111 113 114 118 119 120 122 123 125 127 128 129 130 131 133 134 135 137 138 141 144 145 146 147 **P**6 **S** Albert Einstein Healthcare Network, Philadelphia, PA
Primary Contact: Barry R. Freedman, President and Chief Executive Officer
COO: A. Susan Bernini, Chief Operating Officer
CFO: Brian Derrick, Chief Financial Officer
CIO: Kenneth Levitan, Vice President Information Systems
CHR: Lynne R. Kornblatt, Vice President Human Resources
Web address: www.einstein.edu
**Control:** Other not–for–profit (including NFP Corporation) **Service:** General Medical and Surgical

**Staffed Beds:** 652 **Admissions:** 28898 **Census:** 539 **Outpatient Visits:** 503920 **Births:** 3077 **Total Expense ($000):** 667928 **Payroll Expense ($000):** 290759 **Personnel:** 5675

☐ **FAIRMOUNT BEHAVIORAL HEALTH SYSTEM (394027)**, 561 Fairthorne Avenue, Zip 19128–2499; tel. 215/487–4000 **A**1 9 10 **F**4 98 99 102 105 129 **P**6 **S** Universal Health Services, Inc., King of Prussia, PA
Primary Contact: Charles McLister, Chief Executive Officer
COO: Jennifer Riedel, Chief Operating Officer
CFO: Anthony Tortella, Chief Financial Officer
CMO: Silvia Gratz, D.O., Chief Medical Officer
CIO: Anthony Tortella, Chief Financial Officer
CHR: Theresa Mahoney, Director Human Resources
Web address: www.fairmountbhs.com
**Control:** Corporation, Investor–owned, for–profit **Service:** Psychiatric

**Staffed Beds:** 239 **Admissions:** 6232 **Census:** 211 **Outpatient Visits:** 7408 **Births:** 0 **Total Expense ($000):** 37129 **Payroll Expense ($000):** 22578 **Personnel:** 413

✠ **FOX CHASE CANCER CENTER–AMERICAN ONCOLOGIC HOSPITAL (390196)**, 333 Cottman Avenue, Zip 19111; tel. 215/728–6900 **A**1 2 3 5 8 9 10 **F**3 8 11 15 29 30 31 34 35 36 45 46 47 49 50 55 57 58 59 60 61 64 68 70 71 74 75 77 78 79 81 82 84 85 86 87 93 100 104 107 108 109 110 111 113 114 115 116 117 118 119 120 122 123 125 129 131 134 143 144 145 146 147 **P**6 **S** Temple University Health System, Philadelphia, PA
Primary Contact: Michael V. Seiden, President and Chief Executive Officer
COO: Gary J. Weyhmuller, Chief Operating Officer
CFO: Joseph Hediger, Chief Financial Officer
CMO: J. Robert Beck, M.D., Chief Medical Officer
CIO: Michael Sweeney, Chief Information Officer
Web address: www.fccc.edu
**Control:** Other not–for–profit (including NFP Corporation) **Service:** General Medical and Surgical

**Staffed Beds:** 65 **Admissions:** 4827 **Census:** 61 **Outpatient Visits:** 88497 **Births:** 0 **Total Expense ($000):** 207188 **Payroll Expense ($000):** 52441 **Personnel:** 1043

✠ **FRIENDS HOSPITAL (394008)**, 4641 Roosevelt Boulevard, Zip 19124–2343; tel. 215/831–4600, (Nonreporting) **A**1 3 5 9 10 **S** Universal Health Services, Inc., King of Prussia, PA
Primary Contact: Geoff Botak, Chief Executive Officer
COO: Diane Carugati, Chief Operating Officer
CFO: Alfred P. Salvitti, Chief Financial Officer
CMO: Marc Rothman, M.D., Medical Director
CIO: John Healy, Manager Information Technology
CHR: Paul Cavanaugh, Director Human Resources
Web address: www.friendshospital.com
**Control:** Corporation, Investor–owned, for–profit **Service:** Psychiatric

**Staffed Beds:** 219

☐ **GIRARD MEDICAL CENTER (392026)**, Girard Avenue at Eighth Street, Zip 19122; tel. 215/787–2000, (Nonreporting) **A**1 9 10
Primary Contact: Marlene Walsh, Vice President and Administrator
Web address: www.nphs.com
**Control:** Other not–for–profit (including NFP Corporation) **Service:** Long–Term Acute Care hospital

**Staffed Beds:** 163

☐ **GOOD SHEPHERD PENN PARTNERS SPECIALTY HOSPITAL AT RITTENHOUSE (392050)**, 1800 Lombard Street, Zip 19146–1414; tel. 877/969–7342 **A**1 9 10 **F**1 3 28 29 30 34 57 59 64 77 85 86 87 95 96 129 130 131 134 147 **P**5 **S** Good Shepherd Rehabilitation Network, Allentown, PA
Primary Contact: Linda Dean, Chief Executive Officer
Web address: www.phillyrehab.com/longterm
**Control:** Partnership, Investor–owned, for–profit **Service:** Long–Term Acute Care hospital

**Staffed Beds:** 38 **Admissions:** 311 **Census:** 26 **Outpatient Visits:** 89104 **Births:** 0 **Total Expense ($000):** 54360 **Personnel:** 124

✠ **HAHNEMANN UNIVERSITY HOSPITAL (390290)**, Broad and Vine Streets, Zip 19102–1192; tel. 215/762–7000 **A**1 2 3 5 8 9 10 **F**3 8 12 13 14 15 17 18 20 22 24 26 28 29 31 34 35 40 43 44 48 49 50 51 57 58 59 60 64 65 70 72 74 75 76 77 78 79 80 81 82 85 87 91 92 97 98 100 102 103 105 107 108 110 111 113 114 118 119 120 122 123 125 128 129 130 131 135 136 137 138 141 143 146 147 **P**6 **S** TENET Healthcare Corporation, Dallas, TX
Primary Contact: Michael P. Halter, Chief Executive Officer
COO: James B. Burke, Chief Operating Officer
CFO: Brian Reilly, Chief Financial Officer
CMO: George Amrom, M.D., Vice President Medical Affairs
CIO: Tom Nataloni, Senior Director Information Technology
CHR: Steven Simmons, Chief Human Resources Officer
Web address: www.hahnemannhospital.com
**Control:** Corporation, Investor–owned, for–profit **Service:** General Medical and Surgical

**Staffed Beds:** 496 **Admissions:** 19738 **Census:** 313 **Outpatient Visits:** 108570 **Births:** 2213 **Personnel:** 2566

✠ △ **HOSPITAL OF THE UNIVERSITY OF PENNSYLVANIA (390111)**, 3400 Spruce Street, Zip 19104–4206; tel. 215/662–4000 **A**1 5 7 8 9 10 **F**3 7 8 9 11 12 13 14 15 17 18 20 21 22 23 24 25 26 29 30 31 34 35 36 37 38 39 40 43 44 45 46 47 48 49 50 51 52 54 55 56 57 58 59 60 61 62 63 64 65 66 68 70 72 73 74 75 76 77 78 79 80 81 82 84 85 86 87 90 91 92 96 97 100 101 102 104 107 108 109 110 111 113 114 115 116 117 118 119 120 121 122 123 125 128 129 130 131 133 134 135 136 137 138 139 140 141 142 144 145 146 147 **P**6 **S** University of Pennsylvania Health System, Philadelphia, PA
Primary Contact: Garry L. Scheib, Executive Director
COO: Albert P. Black, Jr., Chief Operating Officer
CFO: Keith Kasper, Chief Financial Officer
CMO: Patrick J. Brennan, M.D., Senior Vice President and Chief Medical Officer
CIO: Michael Restuccia, Chief Information Officer
CHR: Patricia J. Wren, Chief Human Resources Officer
Web address: www.pennhealth.com
**Control:** Other not–for–profit (including NFP Corporation) **Service:** General Medical and Surgical

**Staffed Beds:** 782 **Admissions:** 37849 **Census:** 686 **Outpatient Visits:** 1038837 **Births:** 4395 **Total Expense ($000):** 1824005 **Payroll Expense ($000):** 730379 **Personnel:** 11794

✠ **JEANES HOSPITAL (390080)**, 7600 Central Avenue, Zip 19111–2499; tel. 215/728–2000 **A**1 5 9 10 **F**3 11 12 15 18 20 22 24 26 28 29 30 31 34 35 40 44 45 56 57 59 60 62 65 68 70 74 75 77 78 79 81 82 85 90 91 92 93 107 108 110 111 113 114 115 116 118 119 123 128 129 131 144 145 147 **P**6 **S** Temple University Health System, Philadelphia, PA
Primary Contact: Linda J. Grass, Executive Director and Chief Executive Officer
CFO: Gerald P. Oetzel, Chief Financial Officer
CMO: Andrea C. McCoy, M.D., Chief Medical Officer
CIO: Arthur C. Papacostas, M.D., Vice President and Chief Information Officer
CHR: Elisabeth Donahue, Associate Director Human Resources
Web address: www.jeanes.com
**Control:** Other not–for–profit (including NFP Corporation) **Service:** General Medical and Surgical

**Staffed Beds:** 176 **Admissions:** 9065 **Census:** 118 **Outpatient Visits:** 113215 **Births:** 0 **Total Expense ($000):** 162401 **Payroll Expense ($000):** 59831 **Personnel:** 983

☐ **KENSINGTON HOSPITAL (390025)**, 136 West Diamond Street, Zip 19122–1721; tel. 215/426–8100, (Nonreporting) **A**1 9 10
Primary Contact: Eileen Hause, Chief Executive Officer
CFO: Kenneth Biddle, Controller
CMO: Luis F. Vera, M.D., Medical Director
CHR: Maria Dimichele, Administrative Assistant
CNO: Aleyamma John, R.N., Director of Nursing
**Control:** State–Government, nonfederal **Service:** General Medical and Surgical

**Staffed Beds:** 33

⊠ **KINDRED HOSPITAL SOUTH PHILADELPHIA (392046)**, 1930 South Broad Street, Zip 19145–2304; tel. 267/570–5200, (Nonreporting) **A**1 9 10 **S** Kindred Healthcare, Louisville, KY
Primary Contact: Garrett Arneson, Chief Executive Officer
CFO: Teresa A. Gresko, Chief Financial Officer
CIO: Charles Schechterly, Director Information Systems
CHR: Maryann Kenkelen, Vice President Human Resources and Tenant Services
Web address: www.khsouthphilly.com
**Control:** Corporation, Investor–owned, for–profit **Service:** General Medical and Surgical

**Staffed Beds:** 58

⊠ **KINDRED HOSPITAL–PHILADELPHIA (392027)**, 6129 Palmetto Street, Zip 19111–5729; tel. 215/722–8555, (Nonreporting) **A**1 9 10 **S** Kindred Healthcare, Louisville, KY
Primary Contact: Garrett Arneson, Interim Chief Executive Officer
COO: Sandra Collins, Chief Clinical Officer
CFO: Thomas A. McMullen, Chief Financial Officer
Web address: www.kindredphila.com/
**Control:** Corporation, Investor–owned, for–profit **Service:** Long–Term Acute Care hospital

**Staffed Beds:** 109

⊠ △ **MAGEE REHABILITATION HOSPITAL (393038)**, 1513 Race Street, Zip 19102–1177; tel. 215/587–3000 **A**1 3 5 7 9 10 **F**2 11 29 30 35 60 64 68 74 75 77 79 82 86 90 91 92 93 96 129 131 145 147 **P**6 **S** Jefferson Health System, Radnor, PA
Primary Contact: Jack A. Carroll, Ph.D., President and Chief Executive Officer
CFO: Patricia A. Underwood, Chief Financial Officer
CMO: Guy Fried, M.D., Chief Medical Officer
CHR: Scott Agostini, Director
Web address: www.mageerehab.org
**Control:** Other not–for–profit (including NFP Corporation) **Service:** Rehabilitation

**Staffed Beds:** 96 **Admissions:** 1143 **Census:** 78 **Outpatient Visits:** 58291 **Births:** 0 **Total Expense ($000):** 54336 **Payroll Expense ($000):** 30874 **Personnel:** 478

**MERCY PHILADELPHIA HOSPITAL** See Mercy Fitzgerald Hospital, Darby

**METHODIST HOSPITAL** See Thomas Jefferson University Hospital

⊠ △ **NAZARETH HOSPITAL (390204)**, 2601 Holme Avenue, Zip 19152–2096; tel. 215/335–6000, (Total facility includes 28 beds in nursing home–type unit) **A**1 7 9 10 **F**3 15 18 20 22 29 30 31 34 35 37 39 40 45 49 50 53 56 57 58 59 64 65 70 74 75 77 78 79 80 81 82 84 85 86 87 90 93 97 100 107 108 110 111 113 114 117 118 119 120 127 129 130 131 134 145 147 **P**7 **S** Catholic Health East, Newtown Square, PA
Primary Contact: Nancy Cherone, Interim Chief Executive Officer
CFO: David Wajda, Chief Financial Officer
CMO: James Blute, III, M.D., Chief Medical Officer
CIO: Christine Brutschea, Chief Information Technology
CHR: Mary Ellen Cockerham, Vice President Human Resources
Web address: www.nazarethhospital.org
**Control:** Other not–for–profit (including NFP Corporation) **Service:** General Medical and Surgical

**Staffed Beds:** 233 **Admissions:** 10420 **Census:** 153 **Outpatient Visits:** 153053 **Births:** 0 **Total Expense ($000):** 145267 **Payroll Expense ($000):** 60360 **Personnel:** 1055

**NORTH PHILADELPHIA HEALTH SYSTEM (390132)**, 1524 West Girard Avenue, Zip 19130–1615; tel. 215/787–9000, (Includes ST. JOSEPH'S HOSPITAL, Girard Avenue at Sixteenth Street, Zip 19130; tel. 215/787–9000; Catherine Kutzler, R.N., Vice President and Administrator), (Nonreporting) **A**9 10
Primary Contact: George J. Walmsley, III, CPA, President and Chief Executive Officer
CFO: Ronald Kaplan, Chief Financial Officer
CIO: Tony Iero, Director Management Information Systems
CHR: James Gloner, Senior Vice President
Web address: www.nphs.com
**Control:** Other not–for–profit (including NFP Corporation) **Service:** General Medical and Surgical

**Staffed Beds:** 315

⊠ **PENN PRESBYTERIAN MEDICAL CENTER (390223)**, 51 North 39th Street, Zip 19104–2699; tel. 215/662–8000, (Total facility includes 26 beds in nursing home–type unit) **A**1 3 5 9 10 **F**3 4 5 7 9 11 12 15 17 18 20 22 24 26 29 30 31 32 34 35 36 37 39 40 44 45 46 49 50 54 56 57 58 59 60 61 62 63 64 65 66 68 70 74 75 77 78 79 81 82 84 85 86 87 92 93 94 97 98 100 104 105 107 108 109 110 111 113 114 117 118 125 127 129 130 131 133 134 140 141 142 145 146 147 **P**6 **S** University of Pennsylvania Health System, Philadelphia, PA
Primary Contact: Michele M. Volpe, Executive Director and Chief Executive Officer
COO: Robert J. Russell, Associate Executive Director Operations
CFO: Anthony Zumpano, Chief Financial Officer
CMO: Ana Pujols–McKee, M.D., Chief Medical Officer and Associate Executive Director
CIO: Theresa Hiltunen, Entity Information Officer
CHR: Gail Kimble, Chief Human Resource Officer
Web address: www.pennmedicine.org/pmc/
**Control:** Other not–for–profit (including NFP Corporation) **Service:** General Medical and Surgical

**Staffed Beds:** 331 **Admissions:** 16810 **Census:** 225 **Outpatient Visits:** 138346 **Births:** 0 **Total Expense ($000):** 425152 **Payroll Expense ($000):** 150510 **Personnel:** 1721

⊠ **PENNSYLVANIA HOSPITAL (390226)**, 800 Spruce Street, Zip 19107–6192; tel. 215/829–3000, (Total facility includes 21 beds in nursing home–type unit) **A**1 3 5 9 10 13 **F**3 6 8 9 11 12 14 15 17 18 20 22 24 26 29 30 31 34 35 36 37 38 40 44 45 46 50 52 53 54 55 56 57 58 59 60 61 63 64 65 68 70 72 74 75 76 77 78 79 80 81 82 84 85 86 87 97 98 100 101 102 103 104 107 108 110 111 113 114 115 116 117 118 119 120 122 123 125 127 128 129 130 131 133 134 135 140 141 145 146 147 **P**6 **S** University of Pennsylvania Health System, Philadelphia, PA
Primary Contact: R. Michael Buckley, M.D., Executive Director
COO: Deborah L. Staples, Chief Operating Officer
CFO: Frank Anastasi, Chief Financial Officer
CMO: Daniel Feinberg, M.D., Chief Medical Officer
CIO: Linda Sinisi, Entity Information Officer
CHR: Denise Mariotti, Chief Human Resources Officer
Web address: www.pahosp.com
**Control:** Other not–for–profit (including NFP Corporation) **Service:** General Medical and Surgical

**Staffed Beds:** 474 **Admissions:** 23520 **Census:** 341 **Outpatient Visits:** 183253 **Births:** 4842 **Total Expense ($000):** 466276 **Payroll Expense ($000):** 167037 **Personnel:** 2448

☐ **ROXBOROUGH MEMORIAL HOSPITAL (390304)**, 5800 Ridge Avenue, Zip 19128–1737; tel. 215/483–9900, (Nonreporting) **A**1 6 9 10 **S** Prime Healthcare Services, Ontario, CA
Primary Contact: Peter J. Adamo, Chief Executive Officer
CFO: Timothy Richards, Chief Financial Officer
Web address: www.roxboroughmemorial.com
**Control:** Corporation, Investor–owned, for–profit **Service:** General Medical and Surgical

**Staffed Beds:** 137

⊠ **SHRINERS HOSPITALS FOR CHILDREN, PHILADELPHIA (393309)**, 3551 North Broad Street, Zip 19140–4105; tel. 215/430–4000 **A**1 3 5 10 **F**29 35 57 58 64 65 68 74 75 77 79 81 82 85 88 89 91 92 93 94 96 118 129 131 132 142 145 **S** Shriners Hospitals for Children, Tampa, FL
Primary Contact: Ernest N. Perilli, Administrator
CFO: Mario Salvati, Director Fiscal Services
CMO: Randal Betz, M.D., Chief of Staff
CIO: Mark Morrison, Director Support Services
CHR: Wanda Amaro, Director Human Resources
Web address: www.shrinershq.org
**Control:** Other not–for–profit (including NFP Corporation) **Service:** Children's orthopedic

**Staffed Beds:** 39 **Admissions:** 910 **Census:** 12 **Outpatient Visits:** 11392 **Births:** 0 **Personnel:** 288

⊠ **ST. CHRISTOPHER'S HOSPITAL FOR CHILDREN (393307)**, 3601 A. Street, Zip 19134–1043; tel. 215/427–5000 **A**1 3 5 8 9 10 **F**3 7 16 17 19 21 23 25 27 29 30 31 32 34 35 39 41 43 44 50 55 58 59 60 61 68 72 73 74 75 77 78 79 80 81 84 88 89 93 97 99 102 107 111 112 114 118 128 129 130 131 135 137 145 **S** TENET Healthcare Corporation, Dallas, TX
Primary Contact: Carolyn Jackson, Chief Executive Officer
COO: Maria Scenna, Chief Operating Officer
CFO: Gil Cottle, Chief Financial Officer
CMO: Barbara Hoffman, M.D., Chief Medical Officer
CIO: Steve Landis, Director Information Services
CHR: Lisa Coulter, Director Human Resources
Web address: www.stchristophershospital.com
**Control:** Corporation, Investor–owned, for–profit **Service:** Children's general

**Staffed Beds:** 181 **Admissions:** 11429 **Census:** 128 **Births:** 0

**PA**

---

**Hospital, Medicare Provider Number, Address, Telephone, Approval, Facility, and Physician Codes, Health Care System**

★ American Hospital Association (AHA) membership
☐ The Joint Commission accreditation
◇ DNV Healthcare Inc. accreditation
○ American Osteopathic Association (AOA) accreditation
△ Commission on Accreditation of Rehabilitation Facilities (CARF) accreditation

**TEMPLE UNIVERSITY HOSPITAL (390027)**, 3401 North Broad Street, Zip 19140–5192; tel. 215/707–2000, (Includes TEMPLE UNIVERSITY HOSPITAL – EPISCOPAL DIVISION, 100 East Lehigh Avenue, Zip 19125–1098; tel. 215/427–7000) **A**1 2 3 5 6 8 9 10 **F**3 11 12 13 15 16 17 18 20 22 24 26 28 29 30 31 34 35 37 38 40 41 42 43 44 45 46 47 48 49 50 55 56 57 58 59 60 61 64 68 70 72 73 74 75 76 77 78 79 81 82 83 84 85 86 87 90 92 93 94 97 98 100 101 102 104 107 108 110 111 113 114 117 118 119 120 122 123 125 128 129 130 131 134 135 136 137 138 139 140 141 144 145 146 147 **P**4 **S** Temple University Health System, Philadelphia, PA
Primary Contact: John N. Kastanis, FACHE, Interim Chief Executive Officer
CFO: Edward Chabalowski, Chief Financial Officer
CIO: Arthur C. Papacostas, M.D., Vice President and Chief Information Officer
Web address: www.tuh.templehealth.org/content/default.htm
**Control:** Other not–for–profit (including NFP Corporation) **Service:** General Medical and Surgical

**Staffed Beds:** 730 **Admissions:** 35247 **Census:** 541 **Outpatient Visits:** 324377 **Births:** 3512 **Total Expense ($000):** 775283 **Payroll Expense ($000):** 282663 **Personnel:** 4255

△ **THOMAS JEFFERSON UNIVERSITY HOSPITAL (390174)**, 211 S. 9th Street, Suite 300, Zip 19107–5096; tel. 215/955–6000, (Includes METHODIST HOSPITAL, 2301 South Broad Street, Zip 19148; tel. 215/952–9000) **A**1 2 3 5 7 8 9 10 **F**3 5 6 7 8 9 11 12 13 14 15 17 18 20 22 24 26 28 29 30 31 32 34 35 36 37 38 39 40 43 44 45 46 47 48 49 50 51 52 53 54 55 56 57 58 59 61 64 66 68 70 72 73 74 75 76 77 78 79 80 81 82 84 85 86 87 89 90 92 93 94 96 97 98 100 101 102 103 104 107 108 109 110 111 113 114 115 116 117 118 119 120 122 123 125 128 129 130 131 134 135 136 137 138 140 141 142 144 145 146 147 **P**6 8.**S** Jefferson Health System, Radnor, PA
Primary Contact: David P. McQuaid, FACHE, President and Chief Operating Officer
COO: David P. McQuaid, FACHE, President and Chief Operating Officer
CFO: Neil Lubarsky, Senior Vice President Finance
CMO: Geno Merli, M.D., Chief Medical Officer
CIO: Stephen Tranquillo, Chief Information Officer
CHR: Mary Ellen Keeney, Vice President Human Resources
Web address: www.jeffersonhospital.org
**Control:** Other not–for–profit (including NFP Corporation) **Service:** General Medical and Surgical

**Staffed Beds:** 930 **Admissions:** 46321 **Census:** 713 **Outpatient Visits:** 472851 **Births:** 1986 **Total Expense ($000):** 1334649 **Payroll Expense ($000):** 456629 **Personnel:** 7255

**TRIUMPH HOSPITAL PHILADELPHIA** See Kindred Hospital South Philadelphia

△ **VETERANS AFFAIRS MEDICAL CENTER**, 3900 Woodland Avenue, Zip 19104–4594; tel. 215/823–5800, (Nonreporting) **A**1 2 3 5 7 8 9 **S** Department of Veterans Affairs, Washington, DC
Primary Contact: Joseph M. Dalpiaz, Director
COO: Jeffrey Beiler, Associate Director
CFO: Graciela McDaniel, Chief Financial Officer
CMO: Dave Oslin, M.D., Chief of Staff
CIO: Adrienne Ficchi, Vice President Information Management
CHR: Gerald Morelli, Director Human Resources
**Control:** Veterans Affairs, Government, federal **Service:** General Medical and Surgical

**Staffed Beds:** 134

**PHOENIXVILLE HOSPITAL (390127)**, 140 Nutt Road, Zip 19460–3900, Mailing Address: P.O. Box 3001, Zip 19460–0916; tel. 610/983–1000 **A**1 2 9 10 **F**3 8 11 12 13 15 17 18 20 22 24 26 28 29 31 32 35 36 38 39 40 45 49 51 56 57 59 61 64 69 70 72 74 75 76 77 78 79 81 82 85 86 87 93 100 102 107 108 111 117 118 129 131 133 134 145 146 147 **S** Community Health Systems, Inc., Franklin, TN
Primary Contact: Stephen M. Tullman, Chief Executive Officer
COO: Cheryl Kreider, Chief Operating Officer
CFO: Jacqueline Nalls, Chief Financial Officer
CMO: David Stepansky, M.D., Chief Medical Officer
CIO: Terry Murphy, Director Information Services
CHR: Denise Chiolo, Chief Human Resources Officer
Web address: www.phoenixvillehospital.com
**Control:** Corporation, Investor–owned, for–profit **Service:** General Medical and Surgical

**Staffed Beds:** 118 **Admissions:** 7721 **Census:** 83 **Outpatient Visits:** 118432 **Births:** 887 **Total Expense ($000):** 144272 **Payroll Expense ($000):** 43744 **Personnel:** 669

**ALLEGHENY GENERAL HOSPITAL (390050)**, 320 East North Avenue, Zip 15212–4756; tel. 412/359–3131 **A**1 2 3 5 8 9 10 **F**3 7 8 9 11 12 15 17 18 19 20 22 24 26 28 29 30 31 32 34 35 36 38 39 40 41 43 44 45 46 47 48 49 50 51 53 54 55 57 58 59 61 62 63 64 65 66 68 70 74 75 77 78 79 80 81 82 84 85 86 87 88 89 92 93 94 95 96 97 99 100 101 102 103 104 105 107 108 109 110 111 113 114 115 116 117 118 119 120 122 123 125 128 129 130 131 133 134 136 137 138 139 141 142 144 145 146 147 **P**6 **S** West Penn Allegheny Health System, Pittsburgh, PA
Primary Contact: Judith F. Zedreck, R.N., Interim Chief Executive Officer
COO: Judith F. Zedreck, R.N., Interim Chief Executive Officer
CFO: James A. Kanuch, Vice President
CMO: Tony Farah, M.D., President Medical Staff
CIO: John Foley, Chief Information Officer
CHR: John Lasky, Vice President Human Resources
Web address: www.wpahs.org
**Control:** Other not–for–profit (including NFP Corporation) **Service:** General Medical and Surgical

**Staffed Beds:** 366 **Admissions:** 23975 **Census:** 362 **Outpatient Visits:** 444321 **Births:** 0 **Total Expense ($000):** 577872 **Payroll Expense ($000):** 195318 **Personnel:** 3503

☐ **CHILDREN'S HOSPITAL OF PITTSBURGH OF UPMC (393302)**, 4401 Penn Avenue, Zip 15224–1334; tel. 412/692–5325 **A**1 3 5 9 10 **F**3 8 12 17 19 22 23 24 25 27 28 29 30 31 32 34 35 39 40 41 43 45 46 48 49 50 53 54 55 57 59 60 64 66 68 71 72 74 75 77 78 79 81 82 84 86 87 88 89 93 97 100 107 108 109 111 114 115 116 117 118 119 120 122 123 125 128 129 130 131 133 134 135 136 137 138 139 140 141 142 143 145 **S** UPMC, Pittsburgh, PA
Primary Contact: Christopher Gessner, President
COO: Christopher Gessner, President
Web address: www.chp.edu
**Control:** Other not–for–profit (including NFP Corporation) **Service:** Children's general

**Staffed Beds:** 296 **Admissions:** 13687 **Census:** 210 **Outpatient Visits:** 631499 **Births:** 0 **Total Expense ($000):** 433780 **Payroll Expense ($000):** 133220

**EYE AND EAR HOSPITAL OF PITTSBURGH** See UPMC Presbyterian Shadyside

**HEALTHSOUTH HARMARVILLE REHABILITATION HOSPITAL (393027)**, Guys Run Road, Zip 15238–0460, Mailing Address: P.O. Box 11460, Zip 15238–0460; tel. 412/828–1300, (Total facility includes 40 beds in nursing home–type unit) **A**1 10 **F**29 30 60 62 64 77 90 93 94 95 96 100 127 131 145 147 **S** HEALTHSOUTH Corporation, Birmingham, AL
Primary Contact: Kenneth J. Anthony, Chief Executive Officer
CFO: Beth Miller, Controller
CMO: Thomas Franz, M.D., Medical Director
CHR: Ethel Black, Director Human Resources
Web address: www.healthsouthharmarville.com
**Control:** Corporation, Investor–owned, for–profit **Service:** Rehabilitation

**Staffed Beds:** 202 **Admissions:** 2313 **Census:** 112 **Outpatient Visits:** 18807 **Births:** 0 **Total Expense ($000):** 31140 **Payroll Expense ($000):** 17350 **Personnel:** 386

**KINDRED HOSPITAL PITTSBURGH–NORTH SHORE (392049)**, 1004 Arch Street, Zip 15212–5235; tel. 412/323–5800, (Nonreporting) **A**1 9 10 **S** Kindred Healthcare, Louisville, KY
Primary Contact: Rodney B. Jones, Interim Administrator
Web address: www.kindrednorthshore.com/
**Control:** Corporation, Investor–owned, for–profit **Service:** Long–Term Acute Care hospital

**Staffed Beds:** 111

**LIFECARE HOSPITALS OF PITTSBURGH (392024)**, 225 Penn Avenue, Zip 15221–2148; tel. 412/247–2424, (Includes LIFECARE HOSPITALS OF PITTSBURGH – SUBURBAN CAMPUS, 100 South Jackson Avenue, 4th Floor, Zip 15202–3428; Richard Pletz, Administrator), (Total facility includes 40 beds in nursing home unit) **A**1 9 10 **F**1 3 29 30 85 87 103 107 113 127 129 145 147 **P**5 **S** LifeCare Management Services, Plano, TX
Primary Contact: Richard Pletz, Administrator
CFO: Nikki Aykul, Manager Business Office
CMO: Steven Sotos, M.D., President Medical Staff
CIO: George Fitzgerald, Regional Director Information Systems
CHR: Robin Arslanpay, Director Human Resources
Web address: www.lifecare–hospitals.com
**Control:** Corporation, Investor–owned, for–profit **Service:** Long–Term Acute Care hospital

**Staffed Beds:** 236 **Admissions:** 1596 **Census:** 121 **Outpatient Visits:** 0 **Births:** 0 **Total Expense ($000):** 51364 **Payroll Expense ($000):** 23792 **Personnel:** 525

*Many Facility Codes have changed. Please refer to the AHA Guide Code Chart.*   © 2012 AHA Guide

PA

✉ **MAGEE–WOMENS HOSPITAL OF UPMC (390114)**, 300 Halket Street, Zip 15213–3108; tel. 412/641–1000, (Total facility includes 20 beds in nursing home–type unit) **A**1 2 3 5 8 9 10 **F**3 11 12 13 15 29 30 31 34 35 40 44 45 46 49 52 54 55 56 57 58 59 64 65 66 68 70 72 74 75 76 78 79 80 81 82 84 85 86 87 97 107 108 110 111 114 116 118 119 120 122 125 129 130 131 133 134 145 146 147 **S** UPMC, Pittsburgh, PA
Primary Contact: Leslie C. Davis, President
CFO: Eileen Simmons, Chief Financial Officer
CMO: Dennis English, M.D., Vice President Medical Affairs
CIO: Lou Baverso, Chief Information Officer
CHR: Kelli Reale, Vice President Human Resources
CNO: Maribeth McLaughlin, R.N., Vice President Patient Care Services
Web address: www.magee.edu
**Control:** Other not–for–profit (including NFP Corporation) **Service:** Obstetrics and gynecology

**Staffed Beds:** 318 **Admissions:** 20513 **Census:** 229 **Outpatient Visits:** 334951 **Births:** 10160 **Total Expense ($000):** 374331 **Payroll Expense ($000):** 101770 **Personnel:** 2191

✉ **SELECT SPECIALTY HOSPITAL–PITTSBURGH/UPMC (392044)**, 200 Lothrop Street, E824, Zip 15213; tel. 412/586–9800, (Nonreporting) **A**1 9 10 **S** Select Medical Corporation, Mechanicsburg, PA
Primary Contact: Anthony Martino, Interim Chief Executive Officer
Web address: www.selectmedicalcorp.com
**Control:** Corporation, Investor–owned, for–profit **Service:** Long–Term Acute Care hospital

**Staffed Beds:** 32

☐ **SOUTHWOOD PSYCHIATRIC HOSPITAL**, 2575 Boyce Plaza Road, Zip 15241–3925; tel. 412/257–2290 **A**1 9 **F**98 99 106 **P**6 **S** Acadia Healthcare Company, Inc., Franklin, TN
Primary Contact: Stephen J. Quigley, Chief Executive Officer
CFO: Frank Urban, Chief Financial Officer
CMO: Allan W. Clark, M.D., Medical Director
CHR: Erin J. Frohnhofer, Director Human Resources
Web address: www.southwoodhospital.com
**Control:** Corporation, Investor–owned, for–profit **Service:** Children's hospital psychiatric

**Staffed Beds:** 112 **Admissions:** 1337 **Census:** 101 **Outpatient Visits:** 33120 **Births:** 0 **Total Expense ($000):** 13582 **Payroll Expense ($000):** 8538 **Personnel:** 219

✉ **ST. CLAIR MEMORIAL HOSPITAL (390228)**, 1000 Bower Hill Road, Zip 15243–1873; tel. 412/942–4000 **A**1 2 9 10 **F**3 8 11 12 13 15 17 18 20 22 24 26 28 29 30 31 32 34 35 38 40 44 45 49 50 51 53 54 56 57 59 60 61 64 65 67 70 73 74 75 76 77 78 79 81 82 84 85 86 87 89 90 92 93 96 98 100 101 102 103 105 107 108 110 111 113 114 118 125 128 129 131 133 134 142 145 146 147
Primary Contact: James M. Collins, President and Chief Executive Officer
COO: Michael J. Flanagan, Senior Vice President and Chief Operating Officer
CFO: Richard C. Chesnos, Senior Vice President Finance and Chief Financial Officer
CMO: G. Alan Yeasted, M.D., Senior Vice President and Chief Medical Officer
CIO: Richard Schaeffer, Vice President Information Systems and Chief Information Officer
CHR: Andrea Kalina, Vice President Human Resources and Organizational Advancement
Web address: www.stclair.org
**Control:** Other not–for–profit (including NFP Corporation) **Service:** General Medical and Surgical

**Staffed Beds:** 315 **Admissions:** 16679 **Census:** 217 **Outpatient Visits:** 339826 **Births:** 1266 **Total Expense ($000):** 216380 **Payroll Expense ($000):** 86569 **Personnel:** 1664

★ **THE CHILDREN'S HOME OF PITTSBURGH (393304)**, 5324 Penn Avenue, Zip 15224; tel. 412/441–4884, (Nonreporting) **A**9 10
Primary Contact: Pamela R. Schanwald, Chief Executive Officer
COO: Kimberly Reblock, M.D., Chief Operating Officer
CFO: Kimberly A. Phillips, Chief Financial Officer
CMO: Frederick C. Sherman, M.D., Chief Medical Officer
Web address: www.childrenshomepgh.org
**Control:** Other not–for–profit (including NFP Corporation) **Service:** Children's general

**Staffed Beds:** 15

★ △ **THE CHILDREN'S INSTITUTE OF PITTSBURGH (393308)**, 1405 Shady Avenue, Zip 15217–1350; tel. 412/420–2400, (Nonreporting) **A**7 10
Primary Contact: David K. Miles, President and Chief Executive Officer
COO: Jane T. Keim, Vice President Operations
CFO: Jody Mulvihill, Vice President Finance
CMO: Maryanne Henderson, D.O., Medical Director
CIO: Sharon Dorogy, Director Health Information Management
CHR: Bob Brown, Director Human Resources
Web address: www.amazingkids.org
**Control:** Other not–for–profit (including NFP Corporation) **Service:** Children's rehabilitation

**Staffed Beds:** 69

☐ △ **UPMC MERCY (390028)**, 1400 Locust Street, Zip 15219–5166; tel. 412/232–8111 **A**1 3 5 6 7 8 9 10 12 13 **F**3 4 8 13 15 16 17 18 19 20 22 24 26 28 29 30 31 32 34 35 36 39 40 43 44 45 49 50 51 54 57 58 59 60 61 62 64 65 66 68 70 72 74 75 76 77 78 79 81 82 84 85 86 87 90 91 92 93 94 95 96 97 98 101 102 107 108 111 113 114 115 117 118 125 128 129 140 141 145 146 147 **P**6 **S** UPMC, Pittsburgh, PA
Primary Contact: Will L. Cook, President
CFO: Jack Gaenzle, Senior Vice President Finance and Administration
CIO: Stephen D. Adams, Executive Vice President and Chief Information Officer
CHR: Kristen Bell, Director Human Resources
Web address: www.upmc.com/HospitalsFacilities/HFHome/Hospitals/Mercy/
**Control:** Other not–for–profit (including NFP Corporation) **Service:** General Medical and Surgical

**Staffed Beds:** 488 **Admissions:** 21486 **Census:** 360 **Outpatient Visits:** 203473 **Births:** 1470 **Total Expense ($000):** 364468 **Payroll Expense ($000):** 115318 **Personnel:** 2370

**UPMC MONTEFIORE** See UPMC Presbyterian Shadyside

☐ **UPMC PASSAVANT (390107)**, 9100 Babcock Boulevard, Zip 15237–5815; tel. 412/367–6700, (Includes UPMC PASSAVANT CRANBERRY, One St. Francis Way, Cranberry, Zip 16066; tel. 724/772–5300; Teresa G. Petrick, President) **A**1 2 9 10 **F**3 11 15 17 18 20 22 24 26 28 29 30 31 34 35 40 42 43 46 47 48 49 51 56 57 59 62 63 64 65 68 70 74 75 77 78 79 81 82 83 84 85 86 87 90 92 107 109 111 113 116 117 118 120 125 127 128 129 131 132 134 142 143 144 145 146 147 **S** UPMC, Pittsburgh, PA
Primary Contact: David T. Martin, President
COO: Marcie S. Caplan, Vice President
CFO: Dennis Tomassetti, Chief Financial Officer
CMO: James W. Boyle, M.D., Chief Medical Officer
CIO: Karen Borosky, Vice President and Chief Information Officer
CHR: Gary Mignosna, Vice President Human Resources
Web address: www.upmc.edu/passavant
**Control:** Other not–for–profit (including NFP Corporation) **Service:** General Medical and Surgical

**Staffed Beds:** 412 **Admissions:** 17883 **Census:** 260 **Outpatient Visits:** 289220 **Births:** 0 **Total Expense ($000):** 321428 **Personnel:** 1753

☐ **UPMC PRESBYTERIAN SHADYSIDE (390164)**, 200 Lothrop Street, Zip 15213–2585; tel. 412/647–2345, (Includes EYE AND EAR HOSPITAL OF PITTSBURGH, 200 Lothrop Street, Zip 15213–2592; tel. 412/647–2345; UPMC MONTEFIORE, 3459 Fifth Avenue, Zip 15213; tel. 412/647–2345; John Innocenti, Sr., President and Chief Executive Officer; UPMC PRESBYTERIAN HOSPITAL, 200 Lothrop Street, Zip 15213; tel. 412/647–2345; UPMC SHADYSIDE, 5230 Centre Avenue, Zip 15232–1381; tel. 412/623–2121; WESTERN PSYCHIATRIC INSTITUTE AND CLINIC, 3811 O'Hara Street, Zip 15213–2593; tel. 412/624–2100), (Total facility includes 23 beds in nursing home–type unit) **A**1 2 5 6 8 9 10 12 13 **F**2 3 5 6 7 8 9 10 11 12 14 15 17 18 19 20 22 24 25 26 28 29 30 31 32 33 34 35 36 37 38 39 40 42 43 44 45 46 47 48 49 50 51 52 53 54 55 56 57 58 59 60 61 62 63 64 65 66 68 69 70 71 74 75 77 78 79 80 81 82 83 84 85 86 87 89 90 91 92 93 94 97 98 99 100 101 102 103 104 105 106 107 108 109 110 111 112 113 114 115 116 117 118 119 120 122 123 125 127 128 129 130 131 133 134 135 136 137 138 139 140 141 142 143 144 145 146 147 **P**6 **S** UPMC, Pittsburgh, PA
Primary Contact: John Innocenti, Sr., President and Chief Executive Officer
COO: James Terwilliger, Vice President Operations
CMO: Margaret Reidy, M.D., Vice President Medical Affairs
CIO: James Venturella, Chief Information Officer
CHR: Louis Goodman, Vice President Human Resources
Web address: www.upmc.edu
**Control:** Other not–for–profit (including NFP Corporation) **Service:** General Medical and Surgical

**Staffed Beds:** 1763 **Admissions:** 63930 **Census:** 1268 **Outpatient Visits:** 1189471 **Births:** 0 **Total Expense ($000):** 1929869 **Payroll Expense ($000):** 494334 **Personnel:** 15151

---

**Hospital, Medicare Provider Number, Address, Telephone, Approval, Facility, and Physician Codes, Health Care System**

★ American Hospital Association (AHA) membership
☐ The Joint Commission accreditation
◇ DNV Healthcare Inc. accreditation
◯ American Osteopathic Association (AOA) accreditation
△ Commission on Accreditation of Rehabilitation Facilities (CARF) accreditation

**PA**

☐ **UPMC ST. MARGARET (390102)**, 815 Freeport Road, Zip 15215–3301; tel. 412/784–4000 **A**1 2 3 5 6 9 10 13 **F**3 6 8 9 11 12 15 18 20 29 30 31 34 35 37 40 44 49 50 51 54 56 57 58 59 60 61 63 64 65 68 70 74 75 77 78 79 81 82 84 85 86 87 90 94 97 102 103 104 107 108 111 113 114 117 118 120 128 129 130 131 133 134 145 **S** UPMC, Pittsburgh, PA
Primary Contact: Teresa G. Petrick, President
COO: Douglass Harrison, Vice President Operations
CFO: Thomas M. Newman, Vice President Finance
CMO: John Lagnese, M.D., Vice President Medical Affairs
CIO: Charles M. Rudek, Chief Information Officer
CHR: Tracey Stange Kolo, Vice President Human Resources
CNO: Mary C. Barkhymer, R.N., Vice President Patient Care Services and Chief Nursing Officer
Web address: www.stmargaret.upmc.com
**Control:** Other not–for–profit (including NFP Corporation) **Service:** General Medical and Surgical

**Staffed Beds:** 249 **Admissions:** 15108 **Census:** 203 **Outpatient Visits:** 209754 **Births:** 0 **Total Expense ($000):** 221501 **Payroll Expense ($000):** 74476 **Personnel:** 1444

✠ △ **VETERANS AFFAIRS PITTSBURGH HEALTHCARE SYSTEM**, University Drive, Zip 15240–1001; tel. 412/688–6000, (Includes VETERANS AFFAIRS MEDICAL CENTER, 7180 Highland Drive, Zip 15206–1297; tel. 412/365–4900; VETERANS AFFAIRS MEDICAL CENTER, University Drive C, tel. 412/688–6000), (Nonreporting) **A**1 2 7 8 9 **S** Department of Veterans Affairs, Washington, DC
Primary Contact: Terry Gerigk Wolf, Director
CFO: James Baker, Vice President Business Support Services
CMO: Rajiv Jain, M.D., Chief of Staff
CIO: Dewaine Beard, Chief Information Officer
CHR: Marie Colosimo, Human Resources Officer
Web address: www.pittsburgh.va.gov/
**Control:** Veterans Affairs, Government, federal **Service:** Psychiatric

**Staffed Beds:** 447

✠ **WESTERN PENNSYLVANIA HOSPITAL (390090)**, 4800 Friendship Avenue, Zip 15224–1722; tel. 412/578–5000, (Nonreporting) **A**1 2 3 5 6 8 9 10 12 13 **S** West Penn Allegheny Health System, Pittsburgh, PA
Primary Contact: Duke Rupert, President and Chief Executive Officer
CFO: James A. Kanuch, Vice President Finance
CMO: Marian R. Block, M.D., Chief Quality Officer
CIO: Joyce Polovich, Manager Information Systems
CHR: Sally Carozza, Director Human Resources
Web address: www.wpahs.org
**Control:** Other not–for–profit (including NFP Corporation) **Service:** General Medical and Surgical

**Staffed Beds:** 439

**WESTERN PSYCHIATRIC INSTITUTE AND CLINIC** See UPMC Presbyterian Shadyside

### PLEASANT GAP—Centre County

✠ **HEALTHSOUTH NITTANY VALLEY REHABILITATION HOSPITAL (393039)**, 550 West College Avenue, Zip 16823–7401; tel. 814/359–3421 **A**1 9 10 **F**29 34 44 59 75 86 87 90 91 93 94 95 96 129 131 134 **S** HEALTHSOUTH Corporation, Birmingham, AL
Primary Contact: Susan Hartman, Chief Executive Officer
CMO: Richard Allatt, M.D., Medical Director
CHR: Jody Hay, Director Human Resources
Web address: www.nittanyvalleyrehab.com
**Control:** Corporation, Investor–owned, for–profit **Service:** Rehabilitation

**Staffed Beds:** 73 **Admissions:** 901 **Census:** 32 **Outpatient Visits:** 21219 **Births:** 0 **Total Expense ($000):** 12825 **Payroll Expense ($000):** 7220 **Personnel:** 141

### POTTSTOWN—Montgomery County

✠ **POTTSTOWN MEMORIAL MEDICAL CENTER (390123)**, 1600 East High Street, Zip 19464–5093; tel. 610/327–7000 **A**1 2 9 10 **F**3 9 13 15 18 29 30 31 34 35 38 40 44 45 49 50 51 54 55 56 57 59 60 64 68 70 74 75 76 77 78 79 81 82 85 89 91 92 93 97 98 100 107 111 115 116 118 123 124 127 130 131 134 145 146 147 **P**6 **S** Community Health Systems, Inc., Franklin, TN
Primary Contact: Sharif Omar, Chief Executive Officer
COO: Sharif Omar, Chief Operating Officer
CFO: Michael Zwetschkenbaum, Chief Financial Officer
CMO: Richard F. Saylor, M.D., Chief Medical Officer
CIO: Ron Peterson, Chief Information Officer
CHR: Ruta Ore, Director Human Resources
Web address: www.pottstownmemorial.com
**Control:** Corporation, Investor–owned, for–profit **Service:** General Medical and Surgical

**Staffed Beds:** 234 **Admissions:** 9934 **Census:** 126 **Outpatient Visits:** 129469 **Births:** 621 **Total Expense ($000):** 107118 **Payroll Expense ($000):** 50277 **Personnel:** 768

### POTTSVILLE—Schuylkill County

✠ △ **SCHUYLKILL MEDICAL CENTER – EAST NORWEGIAN STREET (390031)**, 700 East Norwegian Street, Zip 17901–2710; tel. 570/621–4000 **A**1 2 7 9 10 **F**3 5 11 15 18 29 30 31 34 39 40 49 56 57 59 64 70 74 75 77 78 79 81 85 86 90 93 98 100 103 107 108 109 110 111 114 117 118 129 131 134 145 146 147 **P**6 **S** Schuylkill Health System, Pottsville, PA
Primary Contact: John E. Simodejka, President and Chief Executive Officer
CFO: Diane Boris, Vice President and Chief Financial Officer
CIO: Karen Rarick, Director Information Technology
CHR: Martin Treasure, Director Human Resources
Web address: www.schuylkillhealth.com
**Control:** Other not–for–profit (including NFP Corporation) **Service:** General Medical and Surgical

**Staffed Beds:** 126 **Admissions:** 5314 **Census:** 86 **Outpatient Visits:** 120233 **Births:** 0 **Total Expense ($000):** 60009 **Payroll Expense ($000):** 27567 **Personnel:** 527

✠ **SCHUYLKILL MEDICAL CENTER – SOUTH JACKSON STREET (390030)**, 420 South Jackson Street, Zip 17901–3625; tel. 570/621–5000, (Total facility includes 11 beds in nursing home–type unit) **A**1 2 6 9 10 19 **F**3 11 13 15 18 19 28 29 30 32 34 35 38 40 45 46 49 51 54 56 57 59 64 70 74 75 76 77 78 79 81 82 85 86 89 92 93 96 98 99 100 101 102 103 104 105 107 108 110 111 114 117 118 127 128 129 130 131 145 146 **P**6 **S** Schuylkill Health System, Pottsville, PA
Primary Contact: John E. Simodejka, President and Chief Executive Officer
CFO: Diane Boris, Chief Financial Officer
CIO: Karen Rarick, Director Information Systems
CHR: Martin Treasure, Director Human Resources
Web address: www.schuylkillhealth.com
**Control:** Other not–for–profit (including NFP Corporation) **Service:** General Medical and Surgical

**Staffed Beds:** 191 **Admissions:** 7697 **Census:** 106 **Outpatient Visits:** 118277 **Births:** 1033 **Total Expense ($000):** 86369 **Payroll Expense ($000):** 39290 **Personnel:** 741

### PUNXSUTAWNEY—Jefferson County

**PUNXSUTAWNEY AREA HOSPITAL (390199)**, 81 Hillcrest Drive, Zip 15767–2616; tel. 814/938–1800 **A**9 10 **F**3 13 15 18 29 30 34 35 40 45 50 51 57 59 60 61 62 68 70 74 75 76 77 79 81 82 85 86 93 107 108 110 111 113 115 116 117 118 129 131 132 147 **P**6
Primary Contact: Daniel D. Blough, Jr., Chief Executive Officer
CFO: Jack Sisk, Chief Financial Officer
CMO: Dajani Zuhd, M.D., President Medical Staff
CIO: Chuck States, Director Information Systems
CHR: Barbara Kostok, Manager Human Resources
Web address: www.pah.org
**Control:** Other not–for–profit (including NFP Corporation) **Service:** General Medical and Surgical

**Staffed Beds:** 44 **Admissions:** 1942 **Census:** 20 **Outpatient Visits:** 97306 **Total Expense ($000):** 32155 **Payroll Expense ($000):** 17081 **Personnel:** 343

### QUAKERTOWN—Bucks County

☐ **ST. LUKE'S HOSPITAL – QUAKERTOWN CAMPUS (390035)**, 1021 Park Avenue, Zip 18951–1573; tel. 215/538–4500 **A**1 2 9 10 **F**3 11 15 18 28 29 30 31 34 38 40 44 45 49 50 51 53 54 56 57 59 60 64 65 66 68 69 70 74 75 77 78 79 81 82 85 86 87 93 98 99 100 102 103 107 108 110 111 114 117 118 128 129 131 134 142 144 145 147 **P**6 8 **S** St. Luke's University Health Network, Bethlehem, PA
Primary Contact: Edward Nawrocki, President
CFO: Theresa Corrado, Director Finance
CMO: Thomas Filipowicz, M.D., Medical Director
CIO: Chad Brisendine, Chief Information Officer
CHR: Shelley Maley, Director Human Resources
Web address: www.slhhn.org
**Control:** Other not–for–profit (including NFP Corporation) **Service:** General Medical and Surgical

**Staffed Beds:** 57 **Admissions:** 3464 **Census:** 41 **Outpatient Visits:** 109072 **Births:** 0 **Total Expense ($000):** 48595 **Payroll Expense ($000):** 18248 **Personnel:** 299

### READING—Berks County

**HAVEN BEHAVIORAL HEALTH OF EASTERN PENNSYLVANIA (394052)**, 145 North 6th Street, 3rd Floor, Zip 19601–3096; tel. 610/406–4340, (Nonreporting) **S** Haven Behavioral Healthcare, Nashville, TN
Primary Contact: John Baker, Interim Chief Executive Officer
CMO: Mark Putnam, M.D., Medical Director
CHR: Kathy Copenhaver, Director Human Resources
Web address: www.havenbehavioralhospital.com
**Control:** Corporation, Investor–owned, for–profit **Service:** Psychiatric

**Staffed Beds:** 48

**PA**

⊞ **HEALTHSOUTH READING REHABILITATION HOSPITAL (393026)**, 1623 Morgantown Road, Zip 19607–9455; tel. 610/796–6000, (Nonreporting) **A**1 9 10 **S** HEALTHSOUTH Corporation, Birmingham, AL
Primary Contact: Richard Kruczek, Chief Executive Officer
CFO: Jason Pulaski, Controller
CMO: Patti Brown, M.D., Medical Director
CHR: Edward Werner, Director Human Resources
Web address: www.healthsouthreading.com
**Control:** Corporation, Investor–owned, for–profit **Service:** Rehabilitation

**Staffed Beds:** 60

⊞ **ST. JOSEPH MEDICAL CENTER (390096)**, 2500 Bernville Road, Zip 19605, Mailing Address: P.O. Box 316, Zip 19603–0316; tel. 610/378–2000, (Includes ST. JOSEPH MEDICAL CENTER–DOWNTOWN READING, 145 North Sixth Street, Zip 19601, Mailing Address: P.O. Box 316, Zip 19603–0316; tel. 610/376–2100) **A**1 2 9 10 12 13 **F**3 13 15 18 20 22 24 26 28 29 30 31 32 34 35 39 40 44 45 49 50 51 53 54 57 58 59 64 66 68 70 72 74 75 76 77 78 79 81 85 87 89 93 97 107 108 111 113 114 115 116 117 118 119 120 129 130 131 134 143 145 146 147 **P**6 **S** Catholic Health Initiatives, Englewood, CO
Primary Contact: John R. Morahan, FACHE, President and Chief Executive Officer
CFO: Lim David, Vice President Finance and Chief Financial Officer
CMO: Samuel Alfano, D.O., Vice President Medical Affairs
CIO: Bart Rowe, Director Information Technology
CHR: Scott Mengle, Vice President Human Resources
Web address: www.thefutureofhealthcare.org
**Control:** Church–operated, Nongovernment, not–for profit **Service:** General Medical and Surgical

**Staffed Beds:** 180 **Admissions:** 8450 **Census:** 105 **Outpatient Visits:** 322276 **Births:** 800 **Total Expense ($000):** 173288 **Payroll Expense ($000):** 63196 **Personnel:** 1326

**RENOVO—Clinton County**

**BUCKTAIL MEDICAL CENTER (391304)**, 1001 Pine Street, Zip 17764–1620; tel. 570/923–1000, (Total facility includes 43 beds in nursing home–type unit) **A**9 10 18 **F**3 7 11 34 40 42 54 56 59 65 66 69 97 126 127 129 132 142 145
Primary Contact: Thomas Foster, Chief Executive Officer
CFO: Wendy Janerella, Controller
CMO: Alvin Berlot, M.D., Medical Director
Web address: www.bucktailmed.org
**Control:** Other not–for–profit (including NFP Corporation) **Service:** General Medical and Surgical

**Staffed Beds:** 64 **Admissions:** 153 **Census:** 34 **Outpatient Visits:** 10197 **Births:** 0 **Total Expense ($000):** 5871 **Payroll Expense ($000):** 2570 **Personnel:** 80

**RIDLEY PARK—Delaware County**

**TAYLOR HOSPITAL** See Crozer–Chester Medical Center, Upland

**ROARING SPRING—Blair County**

⊞ **NASON HOSPITAL (390062)**, 105 Nason Drive, Zip 16673–1202; tel. 814/224–2141 **A**1 9 10 **F**3 11 13 15 29 30 34 35 40 45 51 57 59 62 63 64 68 70 74 75 76 77 79 81 82 85 92 107 108 111 113 118 129 131 132 134 145 146 147 **P**3
Primary Contact: Garrett W. Hoover, FACHE, President and Chief Executive Officer
CFO: Raymond C. Askey, CPA, Vice President Fiscal Services
CIO: Brian Lilly, Director Information Systems
CHR: Lorie Smith, Director Human Resources
Web address: www.nasonhospital.org
**Control:** Other not–for–profit (including NFP Corporation) **Service:** General Medical and Surgical

**Staffed Beds:** 45 **Admissions:** 2059 **Census:** 19 **Outpatient Visits:** 105794 **Births:** 538 **Total Expense ($000):** 29264 **Payroll Expense ($000):** 11475 **Personnel:** 259

**ROYERSFORD—Montgomery County**

**PHYSICIANS CARE SURGICAL HOSPITAL (390324)**, 454 Enterprise Drive, Zip 19468–1200; tel. 610/495–3330, (Nonreporting)
Primary Contact: David Orskey, Administrator
Web address: www.phycarehospital.com
**Control:** Partnership, Investor–owned, for–profit **Service:** Surgical

**Staffed Beds:** 12

**SAINT MARYS—Elk County**

★ **ELK REGIONAL HEALTH CENTER (390154)**, 763 Johnsonburg Road, Zip 15857–3498; tel. 814/788–8000, (Total facility includes 138 beds in nursing home–type unit) **A**9 10 20 **F**3 6 11 13 15 20 28 29 30 34 35 40 44 45 56 57 59 70 76 77 79 81 82 85 86 87 89 93 98 100 103 107 108 110 111 117 118 127 128 129 130 132 134 143 145 146 147
Primary Contact: Gregory P. Bauer, President and Chief Executive Officer
CFO: Laurie MacDonald, Vice President Finance
CMO: David Johe, M.D., President Medical Staff
CIO: Mary Ann Schwabenbauer, Director Information Technology
CHR: Seanna D'Amore, Director Human Resources
Web address: www.elkregional.org
**Control:** Other not–for–profit (including NFP Corporation) **Service:** General Medical and Surgical

**Staffed Beds:** 218 **Admissions:** 3410 **Census:** 162 **Outpatient Visits:** 158612 **Births:** 188 **Total Expense ($000):** 70116 **Payroll Expense ($000):** 33774 **Personnel:** 747

**SAYRE—Bradford County**

⊞ **ROBERT PACKER HOSPITAL (390079)**, 1 Guthrie Square, Zip 18840–1698; tel. 570/888–6666 **A**1 2 3 5 9 10 12 13 19 **F**3 11 12 13 15 17 18 20 22 24 26 28 29 30 31 34 37 38 40 43 45 47 49 50 51 57 58 59 60 61 64 68 70 73 74 75 76 78 79 81 82 85 86 87 89 92 93 98 99 100 101 102 103 105 107 108 110 111 113 114 115 116 117 118 119 120 122 125 128 129 131 140 141 144 145 147 **S** Guthrie Healthcare System, Sayre, PA
Primary Contact: Marie T. Droege, President
CFO: Minh Dang, Vice President Finance
CIO: Dale Swingle, Vice President Information Services
CHR: Frank Pinkosky, Senior Vice President
Web address: www.guthrie.org
**Control:** Other not–for–profit (including NFP Corporation) **Service:** General Medical and Surgical

**Staffed Beds:** 238 **Admissions:** 13695 **Census:** 173 **Outpatient Visits:** 155408 **Births:** 724 **Total Expense ($000):** 215068 **Payroll Expense ($000):** 63702 **Personnel:** 1177

**SCRANTON—Lackawanna County**

⊞ △ **ALLIED SERVICES REHABILITATION HOSPITAL (393030)**, 475 Morgan Highway, Zip 18501–1103, Mailing Address: P.O. Box 1103, Zip 18501–1103; tel. 570/348–1300 **A**1 7 10 **F**11 29 34 53 56 59 64 74 75 77 78 79 86 87 90 91 93 94 96 129 142 145
Primary Contact: Jackie Fletcher–Brozena, Senior Vice President and Chief Operating Officer
CFO: Michael Avvisato, Senior Vice President and Chief Financial Officer
CMO: Gregory Basting, M.D., Vice President Medical Affairs
CIO: John Regula, Chief Information Officer
CHR: Susan D. Montross, Vice President Human Resources
Web address: www.allied–services.org
**Control:** Other not–for–profit (including NFP Corporation) **Service:** Rehabilitation

**Staffed Beds:** 117 **Admissions:** 2097 **Census:** 59 **Outpatient Visits:** 93774 **Births:** 0 **Total Expense ($000):** 33626 **Payroll Expense ($000):** 15960 **Personnel:** 360

**COMMUNITY MEDICAL CENTER HEALTHCARE SYSTEM** See Geisinger–Community Medical Center

⊞ **GEISINGER–COMMUNITY MEDICAL CENTER (390001)**, 1800 Mulberry Street, Zip 18510–2369; tel. 570/969–8000 **A**1 3 5 9 10 **F**3 11 15 17 18 20 22 24 26 28 29 30 31 34 35 38 40 42 43 44 45 46 49 50 56 57 58 59 64 68 70 74 75 77 78 79 81 82 85 86 87 89 92 93 97 98 102 103 107 108 109 110 111 113 114 117 118 123 129 131 134 145 146 147 **S** Geisinger Health System, Danville, PA
Primary Contact: Robert P. Steigmeyer, President and Chief Executive Officer
COO: Barbara Bossi, Senior Vice President Operations and Patient Care Services
CFO: Thomas Kelly, Interim Chief Financial Officer
CHR: Lois Wolfe, Director Human Resources
Web address: www.cmchealthsys.org
**Control:** Other not–for–profit (including NFP Corporation) **Service:** General Medical and Surgical

**Staffed Beds:** 232 **Admissions:** 11898 **Census:** 150 **Outpatient Visits:** 89977 **Births:** 0 **Total Expense ($000):** 156594 **Payroll Expense ($000):** 64619 **Personnel:** 1019

**MERCY HOSPITAL OF SCRANTON** See Regional Hospital of Scranton

---

**Hospital, Medicare Provider Number, Address, Telephone, Approval, Facility, and Physician Codes, Health Care System**

★ American Hospital Association (AHA) membership
□ The Joint Commission accreditation      ◇ DNV Healthcare Inc. accreditation
○ American Osteopathic Association (AOA) accreditation
△ Commission on Accreditation of Rehabilitation Facilities (CARF) accreditation

**PA**

☒ △ **MOSES TAYLOR HOSPITAL (390119)**, 700 Quincy Avenue, Zip 18510–1724; tel. 570/340–2100 **A**1 3 5 7 9 10 **F**3 11 13 15 18 28 29 30 31 34 40 49 51 56 57 59 61 62 64 65 66 68 70 72 74 75 76 77 78 79 81 82 85 86 87 89 93 98 103 107 108 110 111 113 114 118 128 129 131 134 145 146 147 **P**6 **S** Community Health Systems, Inc., Franklin, TN
Primary Contact: Justin Davis, Chief Executive Officer
CFO: Thomas Kelly, Jr., Chief Financial Officer
CIO: Edward Roman, Chief Information Officer and Chief Privacy Officer
CHR: Paul Gionfriddo, MS, Vice President Human Resources
Web address: www.mth.org
**Control:** Other not–for–profit (including NFP Corporation) **Service:** General Medical and Surgical

**Staffed Beds:** 217 **Admissions:** 10554 **Census:** 136 **Outpatient Visits:** 172317 **Births:** 2728 **Total Expense ($000):** 124896 **Payroll Expense ($000):** 47403 **Personnel:** 1084

☒ **REGIONAL HOSPITAL OF SCRANTON (390237)**, 746 Jefferson Avenue, Zip 18510–1624; tel. 570/348–7100, (Nonreporting) **A**1 2 3 5 9 10 12 **S** Community Health Systems, Inc., Franklin, TN
Primary Contact: Brooks Turkel, Chief Executive Officer
CFO: Stephen Franko, Vice President Finance and Chief Financial Officer
CMO: Anthony Yanni, M.D., Vice President Medical Affairs
CIO: Jorge Coronel, Chief Information Officer
CHR: Elizabeth Leo, Vice President Human Resources
Web address: www.regionalhospitalofscranton.net
**Control:** Corporation, Investor–owned, for–profit **Service:** General Medical and Surgical

**Staffed Beds:** 224

**SELLERSVILLE—Bucks County**

☒ **GRAND VIEW HOSPITAL (390057)**, 700 Lawn Avenue, Zip 18960–1576, Mailing Address: P.O. Box 902, Zip 18960–0902; tel. 215/453–4000 **A**1 2 9 10 **F**3 7 11 13 15 18 19 28 29 31 32 34 35 37 40 44 45 49 50 54 56 57 59 61 62 63 64 65 68 70 71 73 74 76 77 78 79 81 82 84 85 86 87 89 90 93 96 107 108 110 111 113 114 116 117 118 120 122 129 130 131 134 144 145 146 147 **P**6
Primary Contact: Stuart H. Fine, Chief Executive Officer
CFO: Michael Keen, Senior Vice President and Chief Financial Officer
CMO: Jane Ferry, M.D., Vice President Medical Affairs
CIO: Jane Doll Loveless, Vice President Information Services
Web address: www.gvh.org
**Control:** Other not–for–profit (including NFP Corporation) **Service:** General Medical and Surgical

**Staffed Beds:** 202 **Admissions:** 9679 **Census:** 106 **Outpatient Visits:** 310814 **Births:** 1688 **Total Expense ($000):** 171439 **Payroll Expense ($000):** 84121 **Personnel:** 1369

**SENECA—Venango County**

☐ **UPMC NORTHWEST (390091)**, 100 Fairfield Drive, Zip 16346; tel. 814/676–7600, (Total facility includes 16 beds in nursing home–type unit) **A**1 2 9 10 19 **F**3 6 8 10 11 13 15 18 28 29 30 31 34 35 40 43 45 47 50 56 57 59 62 63 64 65 68 70 74 75 76 78 79 81 82 83 84 85 86 87 89 90 93 96 97 98 100 101 102 103 107 108 110 111 113 117 118 120 127 129 130 131 134 143 144 145 146 147 **S** UPMC, Pittsburgh, PA
Primary Contact: David Gibbons, President
COO: David J. Patton, Vice President Operations
CFO: W. Roger McCauley, Senior Vice President Administration and Chief Financial Officer
CMO: John Shonnard, M.D., Medical Director
CHR: Courtney Cox, Vice President Human Resources
Web address: www.northwest.upmc.com
**Control:** Other not–for–profit (including NFP Corporation) **Service:** General Medical and Surgical

**Staffed Beds:** 180 **Admissions:** 7226 **Census:** 103 **Outpatient Visits:** 175227 **Births:** 486 **Total Expense ($000):** 84379 **Payroll Expense ($000):** 29488 **Personnel:** 636

**SEWICKLEY—Allegheny County**

☒ **HEALTHSOUTH REHABILITATION HOSPITAL (393045)**, 303 Camp Meeting Road, Zip 15143–8322; tel. 412/741–9500 **A**1 10 **F**29 34 56 57 59 60 64 65 74 75 87 90 91 92 93 95 96 100 131 145 147 **S** HEALTHSOUTH Corporation, Birmingham, AL
Primary Contact: Leah Laffey, MSN, R.N., Chief Executive Officer
CFO: Jim Steinkirchner, Regional Controller
CMO: Shelana Gibbs–McElvy, M.D., Medical Director
CIO: Annette Gratzmiller, Director Information Services
CHR: Kathy Mischler, Director Human Resources
Web address: www.healthsouthsewickley.com
**Control:** Corporation, Investor–owned, for–profit **Service:** Rehabilitation

**Staffed Beds:** 44 **Admissions:** 726 **Census:** 30 **Outpatient Visits:** 3778 **Births:** 0 **Total Expense ($000):** 8859 **Payroll Expense ($000):** 4791 **Personnel:** 72

☐ **SEWICKLEY VALLEY HOSPITAL, (A DIVISION OF VALLEY MEDICAL FACILITIES) (390037)**, 720 Blackburn Road, Zip 15143–1459; tel. 412/741–6600, (Nonreporting) **A**1 6 9 10 **S** Heritage Valley Health System, Beaver, PA
Primary Contact: Norman F. Mitry, President and Chief Executive Officer
COO: Rosemary Nolan, R.N., Chief Operating Officer and Chief Nursing Officer
CFO: Bryan J. Randall, Vice President Finance and Chief Financial Officer
CMO: Oliver Hayes, D.O., Chief Medical Officer
CIO: David Carleton, Chief Information Officer
CHR: Bruce Edwards, Vice President Human Resources
CNO: Linda Homyk, Chief Nursing Officer
Web address: www.heritagevalley.org
**Control:** Other not–for–profit (including NFP Corporation) **Service:** General Medical and Surgical

**Staffed Beds:** 171

**SHARON—Mercer County**

☒ **SHARON REGIONAL HEALTH SYSTEM (390211)**, 740 East State Street, Zip 16146–3395; tel. 724/983–3911, (Total facility includes 38 beds in nursing home–type unit) **A**1 2 6 9 10 **F**3 5 11 12 13 15 17 18 19 20 22 24 26 28 29 30 31 34 35 38 39 40 44 45 47 48 49 50 51 54 56 57 58 59 60 62 63 64 65 70 73 74 75 76 77 78 79 80 81 82 84 85 86 87 89 90 92 93 96 98 99 100 101 102 103 104 105 107 108 110 111 113 114 117 118 119 120 122 126 127 128 129 130 131 133 134 145 146 147 **P**6 8
Primary Contact: Linde Finsrud Wilson, Chief Executive Officer
COO: John R. Janoso, President and Chief Operating Officer
CFO: Jeffrey Chrobak, Vice President Finance and Chief Financial Officer
CHR: John Davidson, Vice President Human Resources
Web address: www.sharonregional.com
**Control:** Other not–for–profit (including NFP Corporation) **Service:** General Medical and Surgical

**Staffed Beds:** 239 **Admissions:** 10391 **Census:** 149 **Outpatient Visits:** 345498 **Births:** 266 **Total Expense ($000):** 178047 **Payroll Expense ($000):** 62568 **Personnel:** 1419

**SHICKSHINNY—Luzerne County**

**CLEAR BROOK LODGE**, 890 Bethel Road, Zip 18655; tel. 570/864–3116, (Nonreporting)
Primary Contact: Nicholas Colangelo, Chief Executive Officer
Web address: www.clearbrookinc.com
**Control:** Other not–for–profit (including NFP Corporation) **Service:** Alcoholism and other chemical dependency

**Staffed Beds:** 65

**SHIPPENSBURG—Franklin County**

**ROXBURY TREATMENT CENTER (394050)**, 601 Roxbury Road, Zip 17257–9302; tel. 800/648–4673, (Nonreporting) **A**10 **S** Universal Health Services, Inc., King of Prussia, PA
Primary Contact: Geoff Botak, Chief Executive Officer
Web address: www.roxburyhospital.com
**Control:** Corporation, Investor–owned, for–profit **Service:** Psychiatric

**Staffed Beds:** 94

**SOMERSET—Somerset County**

★ **SOMERSET HOSPITAL (390039)**, 225 South Center Avenue, Zip 15501–2088; tel. 814/443–5000 **A**9 10 20 **F**8 11 13 15 17 18 20 22 26 28 29 30 32 34 35 40 45 49 50 53 57 59 62 63 64 68 74 76 77 79 80 81 82 85 86 87 89 93 97 98 99 100 103 104 107 108 111 114 118 128 129 130 131 132 134 140 145 146 147 **P**3 8
Primary Contact: Michael J. Farrell, FACHE, Chief Executive Officer
COO: Craig M. Saylor, Vice President and Chief Operating Officer
CFO: Ron Park, Chief Financial Officer
CIO: Jonathan Bauer, Director Information Services
CHR: Sharon Glover, Director Human Resources
Web address: www.somersethospital.com
**Control:** Other not–for–profit (including NFP Corporation) **Service:** General Medical and Surgical

**Staffed Beds:** 111 **Admissions:** 4115 **Census:** 53 **Outpatient Visits:** 147432 **Births:** 354 **Total Expense ($000):** 63387 **Payroll Expense ($000):** 25574 **Personnel:** 593

**SPRINGFIELD—Delaware County**

**SPRINGFIELD HOSPITAL** See Crozer-Chester Medical Center, Upland

**STATE COLLEGE—Centre County**

☒ **MOUNT NITTANY MEDICAL CENTER (390268)**, 1800 Park Avenue,
Zip 16803–6797; tel. 814/231–7000 **A**1 2 3 5 9 10 **F**3 7 13 15 17 20 22 28
29 30 31 35 40 51 57 59 64 68 70 73 74 75 76 77 78 79 80 81 82 85 87
89 93 98 100 101 102 107 108 111 113 114 117 118 120 128 129 131
134 142 143 145 147
Primary Contact: Steven E. Brown, FACHE, President and Chief Executive Officer
CFO: Richard Wisniewski, Senior Vice President Finance and Chief Financial Officer
CMO: Jeffrey Ratner, M.D., Senior Vice President Medical Affairs
CIO: Kenneth Bixel, Vice President and Chief Information Officer
CHR: Jerry Dittmann, Vice President Human Resources
Web address: www.mountnittany.org
**Control:** Other not–for–profit (including NFP Corporation) **Service:** General
Medical and Surgical

> **Staffed Beds:** 205 **Admissions:** 12029 **Census:** 137 **Outpatient Visits:**
> 219844 **Births:** 1291 **Total Expense ($000):** 239826 **Payroll Expense**
> **($000):** 96053 **Personnel:** 1263

**SUNBURY—Northumberland County**

☒ **SUNBURY COMMUNITY HOSPITAL (390084)**, 350 North Eleventh Street,
Zip 17801–1611; tel. 570/286–3333, (Nonreporting) **A**1 9 10 **S** Community
Health Systems, Inc., Franklin, TN
Primary Contact: Jeff Hunt, Chief Executive Officer
CIO: Scott Yucha, Director Information Technology
CHR: Talia Beatty, Director Human Resources
Web address: www.sunburyhospital.com
**Control:** Other not–for–profit (including NFP Corporation) **Service:** General
Medical and Surgical

> **Staffed Beds:** 76

**SUSQUEHANNA—Susquehanna County**

**BARNES–KASSON COUNTY HOSPITAL (391309)**, 2872 Turnpike Street,
Zip 18847–2771; tel. 570/853–3135, (Nonreporting) **A**9 10 18
Primary Contact: Sara F. Adornato, Executive Director
CFO: Sara F. Adornato, Executive Director
CMO: Warren DeWitt, M.D., Chief Medical Officer
CIO: John Sepcoski, Director Information Technology
CHR: William D. Iveson, Jr., Clinical Operations Officer and Director Human
Resources
Web address: www.barnes–kasson.org
**Control:** Other not–for–profit (including NFP Corporation) **Service:** General
Medical and Surgical

> **Staffed Beds:** 83

**TITUSVILLE—Crawford County**

★ **TITUSVILLE AREA HOSPITAL (390122)**, 406 West Oak Street,
Zip 16354–1404; tel. 814/827–1851, (Nonreporting) **A**9 10 20
Primary Contact: Anthony J. Nasralla, FACHE, President and Chief Executive
Officer
CFO: Paul Mattis, Vice President Finance
CMO: William Sonnenberg, M.D., President Medical Staff
CIO: Deanna Callahan, Director Information Systems
CHR: Jeffrey Saintz, Vice President Human Resources
Web address: www.titusvillehospital.org
**Control:** Other not–for–profit (including NFP Corporation) **Service:** General
Medical and Surgical

> **Staffed Beds:** 50

**TORRANCE—Westmoreland County**

☐ **TORRANCE STATE HOSPITAL (394026)**, Torrance Road, Zip 15779–0111,
Mailing Address: P.O. Box 111, Zip 15779–0111; tel. 724/459–8000 **A**1 10 **F**39
98 106 129 134 142 145 146 147
Primary Contact: Edna I. McCutcheon, Chief Executive Officer
COO: R. Brad Snyder, Chief Operating Officer
CFO: Michael Yahner, Chief Financial Officer
CMO: Herbert G. Chissell, M.D., Chief Medical Officer
Web address: www.dpw.state.pa.us
**Control:** State–Government, nonfederal **Service:** Psychiatric

> **Staffed Beds:** 358 **Admissions:** 354 **Census:** 304 **Outpatient Visits:** 0
> **Births:** 0 **Total Expense ($000):** 69575 **Payroll Expense ($000):** 33424
> **Personnel:** 649

**TOWANDA—Bradford County**

**MEMORIAL HOSPITAL (390236)**, One Hospital Drive, Zip 18848–9702;
tel. 570/265–2191, (Nonreporting) **A**9 10 **S** QHR, Brentwood, TN
Primary Contact: Gary A. Baker, President
CFO: William K. Rohrbach, Vice President Fiscal Affairs
CMO: Constance Sweet, M.D., President Medical Staff
CHR: Linda Berry, Vice President Human Resources
Web address: www.memorialhospital.org
**Control:** Other not–for–profit (including NFP Corporation) **Service:** General
Medical and Surgical

> **Staffed Beds:** 183

**TRANSFER—Mercer County**

**EDGEWOOD SURGICAL HOSPITAL (390307)**, 239 Edgewood Drive Extension,
Zip 16154; tel. 724/646–0400, (Nonreporting) **A**9 10
Primary Contact: Michael Torn, Chief Executive Officer
Web address: www.edgewoodsurgical.com
**Control:** Corporation, Investor–owned, for–profit **Service:** Surgical

> **Staffed Beds:** 10

**TROY—Bradford County**

★ ○ **TROY COMMUNITY HOSPITAL (391305)**, 101 Elmira Street,
Zip 16947–1271; tel. 570/297–2121 **A**9 10 11 18 **F**3 11 15 28 30 34 40 45
50 57 64 75 81 85 87 93 96 107 110 111 118 128 129 132 134 145 147
**S** Guthrie Healthcare System, Sayre, PA
Primary Contact: Staci Covey, R.N., MS, President
CFO: Bernie Smith, Chief Financial Officer
CMO: Vance A. Good, M.D., Chief Medical Staff
Web address: www.guthrie.org
**Control:** Other not–for–profit (including NFP Corporation) **Service:** General
Medical and Surgical

> **Staffed Beds:** 25 **Admissions:** 739 **Census:** 21 **Outpatient Visits:** 30717
> **Births:** 0 **Total Expense ($000):** 12142 **Payroll Expense ($000):** 4497
> **Personnel:** 88

**TUNKHANNOCK—Wyoming County**

☒ **TYLER MEMORIAL HOSPITAL (390192)**, 880 State Road 6 West,
Zip 18657–6149; tel. 570/836–2161, (Nonreporting) **A**1 9 10 **S** Community
Health Systems, Inc., Franklin, TN
Primary Contact: Denise S. Gieski, MS, Chief Executive Officer
CFO: Stephen Franko, Chief Financial Officer
CMO: Brenda Goodrich, D.O., Chief of Staff
Web address: www.tylermemorialhospital.net
**Control:** Corporation, Investor–owned, for–profit **Service:** General Medical and
Surgical

> **Staffed Beds:** 58

**TYRONE—Blair County**

**TYRONE HOSPITAL (391307)**, 187 Hospital Drive, Zip 16686–1808;
tel. 814/684–1255 **A**9 10 18 **F**3 15 40 75 77 79 81 82 93 107 118 129
132 145
Primary Contact: Stephen Gildea, Chief Executive Officer
CFO: Michael Zenone, Chief Financial Officer
CMO: Jerome DeJulia, M.D., Chief Medical Officer
Web address: www.tyronehospital.org
**Control:** Other not–for–profit (including NFP Corporation) **Service:** General
Medical and Surgical

> **Staffed Beds:** 25 **Admissions:** 630 **Census:** 7 **Outpatient Visits:** 43098
> **Births:** 0 **Total Expense ($000):** 18194 **Payroll Expense ($000):** 9788
> **Personnel:** 156

**PA**

---

**Hospital, Medicare Provider Number, Address, Telephone, Approval, Facility, and Physician Codes, Health Care System**

★ American Hospital Association (AHA) membership
☐ The Joint Commission accreditation ◇ DNV Healthcare Inc. accreditation
○ American Osteopathic Association (AOA) accreditation
△ Commission on Accreditation of Rehabilitation Facilities (CARF) accreditation

## UNIONTOWN—Fayette County

✠ **UNIONTOWN HOSPITAL (390041)**, 500 West Berkeley Street, Zip 15401–5596; tel. 724/430–5000, (Total facility includes 38 beds in nursing home–type unit) **A**1 9 10 **F**11 13 15 18 20 22 26 28 29 35 40 45 49 51 54 59 64 70 73 74 75 76 78 79 81 84 89 90 92 93 95 96 98 102 103 104 107 108 110 111 113 114 117 118 127 129 131 134 145 147
Primary Contact: Paul Bacharach, President and Chief Executive Officer
CFO: Steven P. Handy, CPA, Senior Vice President, Chief Financial Officer and Chief Information Officer
CIO: Steven P. Handy, CPA, Senior Vice President, Chief Financial Officer and Chief Information Officer
CHR: James Proud, Vice President Human Resources and Marketing
Web address: www.uniontownhospital.com
**Control:** Other not–for–profit (including NFP Corporation) **Service:** General Medical and Surgical

**Staffed Beds:** 231 **Admissions:** 11092 **Census:** 143 **Outpatient Visits:** 255111 **Births:** 989 **Total Expense ($000):** 129419 **Payroll Expense ($000):** 48622 **Personnel:** 1140

## UPLAND—Delaware County

✠ ○ **CROZER–CHESTER MEDICAL CENTER (390180)**, One Medical Center Boulevard, Zip 19013–3995; tel. 610/447–2000, (Includes SPRINGFIELD HOSPITAL, 190 West Sproul Road, Springfield, Zip 19064–2097; tel. 610/328–8700; TAYLOR HOSPITAL, 175 East Chester Pike, Ridley Park, Zip 19078–2212; tel. 610/595–6000) **A**1 2 3 5 8 9 10 11 12 13 **F**2 3 5 6 7 8 11 12 13 14 15 16 17 18 20 22 24 26 28 29 30 31 32 34 35 37 38 40 41 43 44 45 46 49 50 51 52 54 55 56 57 58 59 61 62 63 64 65 66 68 70 72 74 75 76 77 78 79 81 82 83 84 85 86 87 89 90 92 93 94 96 97 98 99 100 101 102 103 104 105 107 108 109 110 111 113 114 115 116 117 118 119 120 122 123 125 128 129 130 131 133 134 142 145 146 147 **P**6 **S** Crozer–Keystone Health System, Springfield, PA
Primary Contact: Patrick Gavin, President
CMO: Sat Arora, M.D., President Medical and Dental Staff
CIO: Robert E. Wilson, Vice President and Chief Information Officer
Web address: www.crozer.org
**Control:** Other not–for–profit (including NFP Corporation) **Service:** General Medical and Surgical

**Staffed Beds:** 507 **Admissions:** 27921 **Census:** 378 **Outpatient Visits:** 400177 **Births:** 1871 **Total Expense ($000):** 541656 **Payroll Expense ($000):** 210705 **Personnel:** 2910

## WARREN—Warren County

**WARREN GENERAL HOSPITAL (390146)**, Two Crescent Park West, Zip 16365–0068, Mailing Address: P.O. Box 68, Zip 16365–0068; tel. 814/723–4973, (Nonreporting) **A**9 10
Primary Contact: John P. Papalia, FACHE, Chief Executive Officer
COO: Randy California, Chief Operating Officer
CFO: Murray S. Marsh, Jr., Chief Financial Officer
CMO: Dale McNett, M.D., Medical Director
CIO: Rick Setili, Manager Information Systems
CHR: Stacy Ryan, Corporate Director Human Resources
CNO: Trudy Bloomquist, Director of Nursing
Web address: www.wgh.org
**Control:** Other not–for–profit (including NFP Corporation) **Service:** General Medical and Surgical

**Staffed Beds:** 105

☐ **WARREN STATE HOSPITAL (394016)**, 33 Main Drive, Zip 16365–5001; tel. 814/723–5500 **A**1 10 **F**4 30 39 50 56 75 77 82 86 98 100 101 103 127 129 131 134 142 145 **P**1
Primary Contact: Charlotte M. Uber, Chief Executive Officer
COO: Tim Taylor, Chief Operating Officer
CFO: Terry Crambes, Manager Finance
CMO: Asha Prabhu, M.D., Chief Medical Officer
CIO: Karen Byler, Information Technician
CHR: Nancy Saullo, Director Human Resources
Web address: www.dpw.pa.gov
**Control:** State–Government, nonfederal **Service:** Psychiatric

**Staffed Beds:** 190 **Admissions:** 124 **Census:** 172 **Outpatient Visits:** 0 **Births:** 0 **Total Expense ($000):** 41612 **Payroll Expense ($000):** 21200 **Personnel:** 394

## WASHINGTON—Washington County

✠ **WASHINGTON HOSPITAL (390042)**, 155 Wilson Avenue, Zip 15301–3398; tel. 724/225–7000 **A**1 3 5 6 9 10 13 **F**3 5 11 13 15 18 20 22 24 26 28 29 30 31 32 34 35 36 38 39 40 45 46 49 50 53 54 56 57 59 60 61 63 64 65 70 74 75 76 77 78 79 81 82 83 84 85 86 89 90 91 92 93 94 96 97 98 99 100 101 102 103 107 108 110 111 113 114 118 129 130 131 133 134 145 146 147 **P**1 7
Primary Contact: Gary B. Weinstein, President and Chief Executive Officer
COO: Brook Ward, Executive Vice President
CFO: Michael J. Roney, Vice President Finance and Chief Financial Officer
CMO: Paul T. Cullen, M.D., Vice President Medical Affairs
CIO: Rodney Louk, Vice President Information Systems
CHR: Barbara A. McCullough, Vice President Human Resources
Web address: www.washingtonhospital.org
**Control:** Other not–for–profit (including NFP Corporation) **Service:** General Medical and Surgical

**Staffed Beds:** 260 **Admissions:** 14679 **Census:** 175 **Outpatient Visits:** 677477 **Births:** 1008 **Total Expense ($000):** 221382 **Payroll Expense ($000):** 96601 **Personnel:** 1626

## WAYNESBORO—Franklin County

✠ **WAYNESBORO HOSPITAL (390138)**, 501 East Main Street, Zip 17268–2394; tel. 717/765–4000 **A**1 9 10 **F**3 11 13 15 29 30 34 40 45 49 50 54 57 59 64 65 68 74 75 76 77 79 81 85 86 87 91 92 93 94 107 108 110 111 114 117 118 129 130 131 132 134 145 146 147 **P**8 **S** Summit Health, Chambersburg, PA
Primary Contact: Melissa Dubrow, Interim Administrative Officer
CFO: Patrick W. O'Donnell, CPA, Vice President Finance
CMO: Thomas Anderson, M.D., Vice President Medical Affairs
CIO: Michele Zeigler, Vice President Information Services
CHR: Jennifer Knight, Manager Human Resources
Web address: www.summithealth.org
**Control:** Other not–for–profit (including NFP Corporation) **Service:** General Medical and Surgical

**Staffed Beds:** 64 **Admissions:** 2715 **Census:** 26 **Outpatient Visits:** 108221 **Births:** 443 **Total Expense ($000):** 51853 **Payroll Expense ($000):** 26997 **Personnel:** 438

## WAYNESBURG—Greene County

☐ **SOUTHWEST REGIONAL MEDICAL CENTER (390150)**, 350 Bonar Avenue, Zip 15370–1608; tel. 724/627–3101, (Nonreporting) **A**1 9 10 **S** RegionalCare Hospital Partners, Brentwood, TN
Primary Contact: Cynthia Cowie, Chief Executive Officer
COO: Janel Mudry, Chief Operating Officer
CFO: James C. Rutkowski, Chief Financial Officer
CMO: Jamie Boris, M.D., President Medical Staff
CIO: Chris Zaglama, Director Information Services
CHR: Lisa Petro, Director Human Resources
Web address: www.sw–rmc.com
**Control:** Corporation, Investor–owned, for–profit **Service:** General Medical and Surgical

**Staffed Beds:** 77

## WELLSBORO—Tioga County

✠ **SOLDIERS AND SAILORS MEMORIAL HOSPITAL (390043)**, 32–36 Central Avenue, Zip 16901–1899; tel. 570/724–1631 **A**1 9 10 20 **F**3 11 13 15 17 28 40 48 49 64 65 70 75 76 79 81 85 93 98 102 103 104 107 108 110 111 114 117 118 128 129 145 **P**7
Primary Contact: Jan E. Fisher, President and Chief Executive Officer
CFO: Ronald Gilbert, Jr., Chief Financial Officer
CMO: Walter Laibinis, M.D., Chief Medical Officer
CIO: Joe Bubacz, Chief Information Officer
CHR: Gene Yajko, Director Human Resources
Web address: www.laurelhs.org
**Control:** Other not–for–profit (including NFP Corporation) **Service:** General Medical and Surgical

**Staffed Beds:** 83 **Admissions:** 2471 **Census:** 29 **Outpatient Visits:** 106396 **Births:** 285 **Total Expense ($000):** 42737 **Payroll Expense ($000):** 17926 **Personnel:** 456

## WERNERSVILLE—Berks County

☐ **WERNERSVILLE STATE HOSPITAL (394014)**, Route 422, Zip 19565–0300, Mailing Address: P.O. Box 300, Zip 19565–0300; tel. 610/678–3411 **A**1 10 **F**30 39 75 77 98 103 129 134 145
Primary Contact: Andrea Kepler, Chief Executive Officer
COO: Cheryl Benson, Chief Operating Officer
CMO: Dale K. Adair, M.D., Chief Medical Officer
CIO: William Edwards, Information Technology Generalist
CHR: Melvin McMinn, Director Human Resources
Web address: www.dpw.state.pa.us/
**Control:** State–Government, nonfederal **Service:** Psychiatric

**Staffed Beds:** 275 **Admissions:** 74 **Census:** 260 **Outpatient Visits:** 0 **Births:** 0 **Total Expense ($000):** 53388 **Payroll Expense ($000):** 28858 **Personnel:** 572

**PA**

## WEST CHESTER—Chester County

☒ **CHESTER COUNTY HOSPITAL (390179)**, 701 East Marshall Street, Zip 19380–4412; tel. 610/431–5000 **A**1 2 3 5 9 10 **F**3 11 13 15 17 18 20 22 24 26 28 29 31 32 34 35 40 41 45 49 50 55 56 57 59 62 63 64 65 68 69 70 72 75 76 77 78 79 81 82 84 85 86 87 89 92 93 97 107 108 110 111 113 114 117 118 120 122 129 130 131 133 134 145 146 147 **P**6
Primary Contact: Michael J. Duncan, System Chief Executive Officer
COO: Michael Barber, System Chief Operating Officer
CFO: Kenneth E. Flickinger, System Chief Financial Officer
CMO: Richard D. Donze, D.O., Senior Vice President Medical Affairs
CHR: Jacqueline Felicetti, Director Human Resources
Web address: www.cchosp.com
**Control:** Other not–for–profit (including NFP Corporation) **Service:** General Medical and Surgical

| |
|---|
| **Staffed Beds:** 220 **Admissions:** 14204 **Census:** 164 **Outpatient Visits:** 444383 **Births:** 2459 **Total Expense ($000):** 227537 **Payroll Expense ($000):** 95090 **Personnel:** 1583 |

☒ **LIFECARE HOSPITALS OF CHESTER COUNTY (392048)**, 400 East Marshall Street, Zip 19380; tel. 484/826–0400, (Nonreporting) **A**1 9 10 **S** LifeCare Management Services, Plano, TX
Primary Contact: Rosalie Cox, Administrator
Web address: www.lifecare–hospitals.com
**Control:** Corporation, Investor–owned, for–profit **Service:** Long–Term Acute Care hospital

| |
|---|
| **Staffed Beds:** 39 |

## WEST GROVE—Chester County

☒ **JENNERSVILLE REGIONAL HOSPITAL (390220)**, 1015 West Baltimore Pike, Zip 19390–9459; tel. 610/869–1000 **A**1 2 9 10 **F**3 11 13 15 29 35 40 49 50 51 57 59 70 74 75 76 79 81 82 85 87 92 93 107 108 110 111 114 118 128 129 130 131 132 144 145 146 **P**6 **S** Community Health Systems, Inc., Franklin, TN
Primary Contact: Charles A. Davis, Chief Executive Officer
COO: Matthew Gooch, Chief Operating Officer
CFO: Brent Smith, Chief Financial Officer
CMO: Michael Barkasy, M.D., Chief of Staff
CIO: Joanne Sciotti, Director Information Technology
CHR: Nancy Newcomb, Director Human Resources
Web address: www.jennersville.com
**Control:** Corporation, Investor–owned, for–profit **Service:** General Medical and Surgical

| |
|---|
| **Staffed Beds:** 59 **Admissions:** 2868 **Census:** 34 **Outpatient Visits:** 15039 **Births:** 425 **Total Expense ($000):** 47440 **Payroll Expense ($000):** 18401 **Personnel:** 263 |

## WEST READING—Berks County

☒ △ **READING HOSPITAL AND MEDICAL CENTER (390044)**, Sixth Avenue and Spruce Street, Zip 19611–1428, Mailing Address: P.O. Box 16052, Zip 19612–6052; tel. 610/988–8000 **A**1 2 3 5 6 7 8 9 10 12 13 **F**3 5 8 11 12 13 15 18 20 22 24 26 28 29 30 31 34 35 37 40 41 42 43 44 45 46 48 49 50 54 56 57 58 59 60 61 62 64 66 68 70 72 73 74 75 76 77 78 79 81 82 84 85 86 87 89 90 92 93 94 96 97 98 99 100 101 102 103 104 105 106 107 108 110 111 113 114 115 116 117 118 119 120 122 123 124 125 127 128 129 130 131 134 143 145 146 147 **P**6 8
Primary Contact: Clinton Matthews, President and Chief Executive Officer
CFO: Richard W. Jones, Chief Financial Officer
CMO: M. Joseph Grennan, Jr., M.D., Senior Vice President and Chief Medical Officer
CIO: Jayashree Raman, Vice President and Chief Information Officer
Web address: www.readinghospital.org
**Control:** Other not–for–profit (including NFP Corporation) **Service:** General Medical and Surgical

| |
|---|
| **Staffed Beds:** 711 **Admissions:** 30285 **Census:** 455 **Outpatient Visits:** 1024996 **Births:** 3495 **Total Expense ($000):** 654820 **Payroll Expense ($000):** 271613 **Personnel:** 4973 |

## WILKES BARRE—Luzerne County

☒ **GEISINGER WYOMING VALLEY MEDICAL CENTER (390270)**, 1000 East Mountain Boulevard, Zip 18711–0027; tel. 570/808–7300 **A**1 2 3 5 9 10 13 **F**3 7 8 11 12 13 15 17 18 19 20 22 24 25 28 29 30 31 32 34 37 39 40 42 43 44 45 46 49 50 54 57 59 64 65 68 70 74 75 76 77 78 79 80 81 82 83 84 85 86 87 89 90 92 93 96 100 107 108 111 113 115 116 118 119 120 122 125 128 129 130 131 134 137 141 143 145 146 147 **P**6 **S** Geisinger Health System, Danville, PA
Primary Contact: John J. Buckley, Chief Administrative Officer
CFO: Thomas A. Bielecki, Chief Financial Officer
CMO: Steven Pierdon, M.D., Executive Vice President and Chief Medical Officer
CIO: Frank Richards, Chief Information Officer
CHR: Margaret Heffers, Assistant Vice President Human Resources
Web address: www.geisinger.org
**Control:** Other not–for–profit (including NFP Corporation) **Service:** General Medical and Surgical

| |
|---|
| **Staffed Beds:** 242 **Admissions:** 12868 **Census:** 165 **Outpatient Visits:** 588889 **Births:** 1382 **Total Expense ($000):** 334004 **Payroll Expense ($000):** 76706 **Personnel:** 1796 |

☒ **KINDRED HOSPITAL–WYOMING VALLEY (392042)**, 575 North River Street, 7th Floor, Zip 18764–0999; tel. 570/552–7620, (Nonreporting) **A**1 9 10 **S** Kindred Healthcare, Louisville, KY
Primary Contact: Sharon Yurkiewicz, Chief Executive Officer
Web address: www.kindredhospitalwv.com/
**Control:** Corporation, Investor–owned, for–profit **Service:** Long–Term Acute Care hospital

| |
|---|
| **Staffed Beds:** 36 |

## WILKES–BARRE—Luzerne County

**CLEAR BROOK MANOR**, 1100 East Northampton Street, Zip 18702–9803; tel. 570/823–1171, (Nonreporting)
Primary Contact: Robert Piccone, President
Web address: www.clearbrookinc.com
**Control:** Other not–for–profit (including NFP Corporation) **Service:** Alcoholism and other chemical dependency

| |
|---|
| **Staffed Beds:** 50 |

☒ **FIRST HOSPITAL WYOMING VALLEY (394039)**, 562 Wyoming Avenue, Zip 18704–3721; tel. 570/552–3900 **A**1 10 **F**42 98 99 103 104 105 **P**6 **S** Community Health Systems, Inc., Franklin, TN
Primary Contact: Mark Schor, Chief Executive Officer
COO: Richard Sapolis, Director Clinical Operations
CMO: Steven R. Kafrissen, M.D., Medical Director
Web address: www.firsthospital.net/Pages/home.aspx
**Control:** Corporation, Investor–owned, for–profit **Service:** Psychiatric

| |
|---|
| **Staffed Beds:** 107 **Admissions:** 3609 **Census:** 91 **Outpatient Visits:** 0 **Births:** 0 **Personnel:** 112 |

☒ **JOHN HEINZ INSTITUTE OF REHABILITATION MEDICINE (393036)**, 150 Mundy Street, Zip 18702–6830; tel. 570/826–3800, (Total facility includes 21 beds in nursing home–type unit) **A**1 10 **F**3 11 29 30 32 35 54 57 59 62 64 68 75 77 82 86 90 91 92 93 129 130 131 142 145 147
Primary Contact: Jackie Fletcher–Brozena, Senior Vice President and Chief Operating Officer
CFO: Mike Avvisato, Vice President and Chief Financial Officer
CMO: Gregory Basting, M.D., Vice President Medical Affairs
CIO: John Regula, Chief Information Officer
CHR: Susan D. Montross, Vice President Human Resources
Web address: www.allied–services.org
**Control:** Other not–for–profit (including NFP Corporation) **Service:** Rehabilitation

| |
|---|
| **Staffed Beds:** 71 **Admissions:** 1813 **Census:** 58 **Outpatient Visits:** 98685 **Births:** 0 **Total Expense ($000):** 32659 **Payroll Expense ($000):** 17161 **Personnel:** 378 |

---

**PA**

⊞ △ **VETERANS AFFAIRS MEDICAL CENTER**, 1111 East End Boulevard,
Zip 18711–0030; tel. 570/824–3521, (Total facility includes 105 beds in nursing
home–type unit) **A**1 2 3 5 7 9 **F**2 3 5 8 10 11 12 28 29 30 34 35 38 39 40 44
50 53 54 56 57 58 59 60 61 62 63 64 65 68 70 74 75 77 78 79 81 82 83
84 86 87 92 93 94 97 98 100 101 102 103 104 107 111 113 114 117 118
127 128 129 131 134 145 146 **P**6 **S** Department of Veterans Affairs,
Washington, DC
Primary Contact: Margaret B. Kaplan, Director
COO: C. Gene Molino, Associate Director
CFO: Donald E. Foote, Fiscal Officer
CMO: Mirza Z. Ali, M.D., Chief of Staff
CIO: David Longmore, Chief Information Officer
CHR: Dawn P. DeMorrow, Chief Human Resources Service
Web address: www.va.gov/vamcwb
**Control:** Veterans Affairs, Government, federal **Service:** General Medical and
Surgical

**Staffed Beds:** 173 **Admissions:** 3622 **Census:** 136 **Outpatient Visits:**
378967 **Total Expense ($000):** 226962 **Payroll Expense ($000):** 78658
**Personnel:** 905

★ **WILKES–BARRE GENERAL HOSPITAL (390137)**, 575 North River Street,
Zip 18764–0001; tel. 570/829–8111, (Includes WILKES–BARRE GENERAL
HOSPITAL, 575 North River Street, Zip 18764; tel. 570/829–8111) **A**2 3 5 9 10
13 **F**3 4 8 12 13 15 17 18 20 22 24 28 29 30 31 34 37 40 44 45 46 48 49
50 53 54 56 57 59 61 64 66 70 73 74 75 76 78 79 81 85 86 87 89 90 93
107 108 110 111 112 113 114 115 117 118 119 120 122 123 125 128 129
131 144 145 146 147 **S** Community Health Systems, Inc., Franklin, TN
Primary Contact: Cornelio R. Catena, President and Chief Executive Officer
COO: Robert P. Hoffman, Vice President and Director Patient Care Services
CFO: Maggie Koehler, Senior Vice President and Chief Financial Officer
CMO: Ragupathy Veluswamy, M.D., Vice President Medical Affairs
CIO: Chris Galanda, Chief Information Officer
CHR: James Carmody, Vice President Human Resources
Web address: www.wvhc.org
**Control:** Corporation, Investor–owned, for–profit **Service:** General Medical and
Surgical

**Staffed Beds:** 372 **Admissions:** 17016 **Census:** 230 **Outpatient Visits:**
516634 **Births:** 1187 **Total Expense ($000):** 248256 **Payroll Expense
($000):** 84675 **Personnel:** 1946

**WYOMING VALLEY HEALTH CARE SYSTEM** See Wilkes–Barre General Hospital

**WILLIAMSPORT—Lycoming County**

★ **DIVINE PROVIDENCE HOSPITAL (394048)**, 1100 Grampian Boulevard,
Zip 17701–1995; tel. 570/326–8000 **A**2 9 10 **F**10 11 15 31 35 38 44 50 51
53 54 56 59 62 63 64 66 68 75 77 78 79 81 82 83 84 86 87 93 98 99 100
103 107 108 110 111 114 118 119 120 128 129 130 131 133 145 146 147
**P**7 **S** Susquehanna Health System, Williamsport, PA
Primary Contact: Robert E. Kane, Administrator and Chief Executive Officer
COO: Neil G. Armstrong, FACHE, Vice President and Chief Operating Officer
Web address: www.susquehannahealth.org
**Control:** Other not–for–profit (including NFP Corporation) **Service:** Psychiatric

**Staffed Beds:** 31 **Admissions:** 810 **Census:** 17 **Outpatient Visits:** 287766
**Births:** 0 **Total Expense ($000):** 75077 **Payroll Expense ($000):** 20130
**Personnel:** 285

**WILLIAMSPORT HOSPITAL AND MEDICAL CENTER** See Williamsport Regional
Medical Center

⊞ △ **WILLIAMSPORT REGIONAL MEDICAL CENTER (390045)**, 700 High
Street, Zip 17701–3109; tel. 570/321–1000 **A**1 2 7 9 10 13 **F**7 9 11 12 13 15
17 18 20 22 24 26 28 29 30 32 34 35 37 38 40 44 45 46 49 50 52 53 56
57 58 59 60 61 65 68 70 73 74 75 76 77 79 81 85 86 87 89 90 91 92 93
94 96 97 107 108 110 113 114 115 116 117 118 119 120 122 123 125
129 131 133 134 142 143 145 146 **P**7 **S** Susquehanna Health System,
Williamsport, PA
Primary Contact: Neil G. Armstrong, FACHE, President
COO: Neil G. Armstrong, FACHE, President
CFO: Charles J. Santangelo, CPA, Executive Vice President and Chief Financial
Officer
CMO: George A. Manchester, M.D., Executive Vice President Medical Affairs
CIO: Karen M. Armstrong, FACHE, Senior Vice President and Chief Information
Officer
CHR: Glenn C. Mechling, FACHE, Senior Vice President Human Resources
**Control:** Other not–for–profit (including NFP Corporation) **Service:** General
Medical and Surgical

**Staffed Beds:** 224 **Admissions:** 11391 **Census:** 133 **Outpatient Visits:**
167008 **Births:** 1092 **Total Expense ($000):** 195115 **Payroll Expense
($000):** 74821 **Personnel:** 1256

**WINDBER—Somerset County**

★ **WINDBER MEDICAL CENTER (390112)**, 600 Somerset Avenue,
Zip 15963–1331; tel. 814/467–3000 **A**9 10 **F**3 8 12 13 15 18 26 28 29 30
32 34 35 36 40 45 53 55 56 57 58 59 62 63 64 70 75 76 77 79 81 83 84
85 86 91 92 93 107 110 111 114 116 117 118 126 128 129 130 131 134
145 146
Primary Contact: Barbara J. Cliff, Ph.D., FACHE, President and Chief Executive
Officer
COO: Holly Rigby, Senior Vice President and Chief Operating Officer
CFO: Linda Fanale, Chief Financial Officer
CMO: Kim Marley, M.D., Chief Medical Officer
CIO: Renee Adams, Director Information Technology
CHR: Jamie Brock, Director Human Resources
Web address: www.windbercare.org
**Control:** Other not–for–profit (including NFP Corporation) **Service:** General
Medical and Surgical

**Staffed Beds:** 53 **Admissions:** 1764 **Census:** 16 **Outpatient Visits:** 109090
**Births:** 232 **Total Expense ($000):** 48053 **Payroll Expense ($000):** 21268
**Personnel:** 440

**WYNNEWOOD—Montgomery County**

**LANKENAU HOSPITAL** See Lankenau Medical Center

⊞ **LANKENAU MEDICAL CENTER (390195)**, 100 Lancaster Avenue West,
Zip 19096–3411; tel. 484/476–2000, (Total facility includes 22 beds in nursing
home–type unit) **A**1 2 3 5 8 10 12 13 **F**3 11 13 15 17 18 20 22 24 26 28 29
30 31 34 35 39 40 43 45 48 49 50 54 55 56 57 58 59 64 66 68 70 72 73
74 75 76 77 78 79 81 82 84 85 86 87 91 92 93 97 107 108 110 111 113
114 117 118 119 120 122 123 125 127 128 129 131 134 137 144 145 147
**P**7 **S** Main Line Health, Bryn Mawr, PA
Primary Contact: Phillip D. Robinson, Chief Executive Officer
CFO: Michael J. Buongiorno, Vice President Finance
CMO: Thomas G. McCarter, Jr., M.D., Chief Medical Officer
CIO: Karen A. Thomas, R.N., Acting Vice President and Chief Information Officer
CHR: Eileen McAnally, Senior Vice President Human Resources
Web address: www.mainlinehealth.org
**Control:** Other not–for–profit (including NFP Corporation) **Service:** General
Medical and Surgical

**Staffed Beds:** 353 **Admissions:** 20195 **Census:** 253 **Outpatient Visits:**
288057 **Births:** 2811 **Total Expense ($000):** 346409 **Payroll Expense
($000):** 117708 **Personnel:** 2104

**WYOMISSING—Berks County**

☐ **SURGICAL INSTITUTE OF READING (390316)**, 2752 Century Boulevard,
Zip 19610–3345; tel. 610/378–8800 **A**1 9 10 **F**3 8 29 45 79 81 82 85 86
107 113
Primary Contact: Debbie Beissel, Administrator
CFO: Cheryl Peterson, Business Office Manager
CHR: Megan Schaffer, Administrative Assistant
Web address: www.sireading.com
**Control:** Partnership, Investor–owned, for–profit **Service:** Surgical

**Staffed Beds:** 15 **Admissions:** 557 **Census:** 4 **Births:** 0

**YORK—York County**

⊞ **HEALTHSOUTH REHABILITATION HOSPITAL OF YORK (393037)**, 1850
Normandie Drive, Zip 17408–1534; tel. 717/767–6941, (Nonreporting) **A**1 9 10
**S** HEALTHSOUTH Corporation, Birmingham, AL
Primary Contact: Steven Alwine, Chief Executive Officer
CFO: Tracey Claxton, Controller
CMO: Bruce Sicilia, M.D., Medical Director
CIO: Courtney E. Stoner, Director Marketing Operations
CHR: Sarah Arthur, Director Human Resources
Web address: www.healthsouthyork.com
**Control:** Corporation, Investor–owned, for–profit **Service:** Rehabilitation

**Staffed Beds:** 90

★ ○ **MEMORIAL HOSPITAL (390101)**, 325 South Belmont Street,
Zip 17403–2609, Mailing Address: P.O. Box 15118, Zip 17405–7118;
tel. 717/843–8623 **A**9 10 11 12 13 **F**3 7 11 13 15 18 20 22 26 29 30 35 38
40 45 48 54 56 57 58 59 62 63 66 68 70 75 76 77 78 79 81 85 86
89 92 93 96 108 110 117 118 123 125 128 129 130 131 134 145 **P**6
**S** Community Health Systems, Inc., Franklin, TN
Primary Contact: Sally J. Dixon, President and Chief Executive Officer
CIO: James Mahoney, Chief Information Officer
CHR: Corey Hudak, Director Human Resources
Web address: www.mhyork.org
**Control:** Other not–for–profit (including NFP Corporation) **Service:** General
Medical and Surgical

**Staffed Beds:** 100 **Admissions:** 4802 **Census:** 56 **Outpatient Visits:** 166338
**Total Expense ($000):** 97852 **Payroll Expense ($000):** 44356 **Personnel:**
832

*Many Facility Codes have changed. Please refer to the AHA Guide Code Chart.* © 2012 AHA Guide

**OSS ORTHOPAEDIC SPECIALTY HOSPITAL (390325)**, 1861 Powder Mill Road, Zip 17402–4723; tel. 717/718–2000 **F**29 64 79 81 87 93 129 134 **P**8
Primary Contact: Todd M. Lord, Chief Executive Officer
Web address: www.osshospital.com
**Control:** Partnership, Investor–owned, for–profit **Service:** Orthopedic

**Staffed Beds:** 30 **Admissions:** 1268 **Census:** 8 **Outpatient Visits:** 3405 **Births:** 0 **Total Expense ($000):** 24460 **Payroll Expense ($000):** 5310 **Personnel:** 128

**SELECT SPECIALTY HOSPITAL–YORK** See Select Specialty Hospital–Central Pennsylvania, Camp Hill

⊞ **YORK HOSPITAL (390046)**, 1001 South George Street, Zip 17405–3645; tel. 717/851–2345, (Includes WELLSPAN SURGERY AND REHABILLITATION HOSPITAL, 55 Monument Road, Zip 17403–5023; tel. 717/812–6100; Barbara Yarrish, R.N., Vice President, Operations) **A**1 2 3 5 8 9 10 12 13 **F**3 5 7 11 12 13 14 15 17 18 20 22 24 26 28 29 30 31 34 35 39 40 43 44 45 46 48 49 50 54 55 56 57 58 59 60 61 64 65 66 68 70 72 74 75 76 77 78 79 81 82 84 85 86 87 89 92 93 97 98 99 100 101 102 103 104 107 108 110 111 113 114 116 117 118 119 120 122 123 125 128 129 130 131 134 145 147 **S** WellSpan Health, York, PA
Primary Contact: Keith Noll, President
COO: Raymond Rosen, FACHE, Vice President Operations
CFO: Michael F. O'Connor, Senior Vice President Finance
CMO: Peter M. Hartmann, M.D., Vice President Medical Affairs
CIO: R. Hai Baker, M.D., Vice President and Chief Information Officer
CHR: Robert J. Batory, Vice President Human Resources
Web address: www.wellspan.org
**Control:** Other not–for–profit (including NFP Corporation) **Service:** General Medical and Surgical

**Staffed Beds:** 549 **Admissions:** 28428 **Census:** 388 **Outpatient Visits:** 865000 **Births:** 3181 **Total Expense ($000):** 710006 **Payroll Expense ($000):** 245161 **Personnel:** 4021

# RHODE ISLAND

## CRANSTON—Providence County

☐ **ELEANOR SLATER HOSPITAL (412001)**, John O. Pastore Center, 111 Howard Avenue, Zip 02920–0269, Mailing Address: P.O. Box 8269, Zip 02920–8269; tel. 401/462–3085, (Nonreporting) **A**1 9 10
Primary Contact: Paul J. Despres, Chief Executive Officer
CMO: Charlene Tate, M.D., Chief Medical Staff and Clinical Services
Web address: www.bhddh.ri.gov/esh/
**Control:** State-Government, nonfederal **Service:** General Medical and Surgical

| Staffed Beds: 495 |
| --- |

## EAST PROVIDENCE—Providence County

☐ **EMMA PENDLETON BRADLEY HOSPITAL (414003)**, 1011 Veterans Memorial Parkway, Zip 02915–5099; tel. 401/432–1000, (Nonreporting) **A**1 3 5 9 10 **S** Lifespan Corporation, Providence, RI
Primary Contact: Daniel J. Wall, President and Chief Executive Officer
CFO: Mamie Wakefield, Vice President Finance and Chief Financial Officer
CMO: Henry T. Sachs, III, M.D., Medical Director
CIO: Carole Cotter, Senior Vice President and Chief Information Officer
CHR: Rob Duval, Chief Human Resources Officer
Web address: www.lifespan.org
**Control:** Other not-for-profit (including NFP Corporation) **Service:** Children's hospital psychiatric

| Staffed Beds: 51 |
| --- |

## NEWPORT—Newport County

☐ △ **NEWPORT HOSPITAL (410006)**, 11 Friendship Street, Zip 02840–2299; tel. 401/846–6400 **A**1 2 7 9 10 21 **F**3 8 11 13 15 28 29 30 31 34 35 40 45 49 51 53 54 56 57 59 60 64 68 70 74 75 76 77 78 79 81 82 85 86 89 90 91 92 93 96 97 98 100 102 103 104 105 107 108 110 111 113 117 118 128 129 131 134 145 146 147 **S** Lifespan Corporation, Providence, RI
Primary Contact: August B. Cordeiro, FACHE, President and Chief Executive Officer
CFO: Frank J. Byrne, Director Finance and Treasurer
CMO: Terrence R. McWilliams, M.D., Vice President Medical Affairs
CHR: Barbara J. Arcangeli, Vice President Human Resources
CNO: Paula Gillette, MSN, Vice President Patient Care Services and Chief Nursing Officer
Web address: www.newporthospital.org
**Control:** Other not-for-profit (including NFP Corporation) **Service:** General Medical and Surgical

| Staffed Beds: 119 Admissions: 4903 Census: 69 Outpatient Visits: 87520 Births: 583 Total Expense ($000): 107306 Payroll Expense ($000): 47309 Personnel: 614 |
| --- |

## NORTH PROVIDENCE—Providence County

☐ △ **ST. JOSEPH HEALTH SERVICES OF RHODE ISLAND (410005)**, 200 High Service Avenue, Zip 02904–5199; tel. 401/456–3000, (Includes OUR LADY OF FATIMA HOSPITAL, 200 High Service Avenue, Zip 02904; tel. 401/456–3000; ST. JOSEPH HOSPITAL FOR SPECIALTY CARE, 21 Peace Street, Providence, Zip 02907; tel. 401/456–3000) **A**1 2 6 7 9 10 **F**3 8 10 15 18 26 28 29 30 31 34 35 39 40 44 45 47 49 50 51 54 59 60 63 64 65 66 68 70 74 75 77 78 79 81 82 85 86 87 90 93 96 97 98 101 102 103 104 105 107 108 110 111 113 114 118 123 129 131 140 143 145 146 147
Primary Contact: Kenneth H. Belcher, President and Chief Executive Officer
CHR: Darlene Souza, Vice President
Web address: www.saintjosephri.com
**Control:** Other not-for-profit (including NFP Corporation) **Service:** General Medical and Surgical

| Staffed Beds: 231 Admissions: 8226 Census: 151 Outpatient Visits: 235108 Births: 0 Total Expense ($000): 159748 Payroll Expense ($000): 73967 Personnel: 1053 |
| --- |

## NORTH SMITHFIELD—Providence County

**LANDMARK MEDICAL CENTER–FOGARTY UNIT** See Landmark Medical Center, Woonsocket

☐ **REHABILITATION HOSPITAL OF RHODE ISLAND (413025)**, 116 Eddie Dowling Highway, Zip 2896; tel. 401/766–0800, (Nonreporting) **A**1 9 10
Primary Contact: Richard Charest, Chief Executive Officer
COO: Demetra Ouellette, Chief Operating Officer
CFO: Matthew Cotti, Chief Financial Officer
CMO: Jorge Mayoral, M.D., Medical Director
CIO: Colleen Ryan, Chief Information Officer and Vice President Professional Services
CHR: Mona M. Willis, Director Human Resources
Web address: www.rhri.net
**Control:** Partnership, Investor–owned, for-profit **Service:** Rehabilitation

| Staffed Beds: 70 |
| --- |

## PAWTUCKET—Providence County

⊠ △ **MEMORIAL HOSPITAL OF RHODE ISLAND (410001)**, 111 Brewster Street, Zip 02860–4499; tel. 401/729–2000, (Nonreporting) **A**1 2 3 5 7 8 9 10
Primary Contact: Arthur J. DeBlois, Interim President and Chief Executive Officer
COO: Shelley A. MacDonald Gallagher, R.N., Senior Vice President Operations
CFO: Michael Ryan, Senior Vice President Finance
CMO: Andrew Artenstein, M.D., Chief Medical Officer
CIO: Lisa Mahar, Director Information Systems
CHR: Lisa Pratt, Vice President Human Resources
Web address: www.mhri.org
**Control:** Other not-for-profit (including NFP Corporation) **Service:** General Medical and Surgical

| Staffed Beds: 159 |
| --- |

## PROVIDENCE—Providence County

⊠ **BUTLER HOSPITAL (414000)**, 345 Blackstone Boulevard, Zip 02906–4829; tel. 401/455–6200 **A**1 3 5 9 10 **F**4 5 29 30 34 35 38 40 44 50 56 57 59 68 74 75 81 86 98 99 101 102 103 104 105 129 131 134 145 **P**6 **S** Care New England Health System, Providence, RI
Primary Contact: Patricia R. Recupero, M.D., JD, President and Chief Executive Officer
COO: Walter Dias, Vice President and Chief Operating Officer
CFO: Bonnie Baker, Vice President Finance and Chief Financial Officer
CMO: Steven Rasmussen, M.D., Medical Director
CIO: Cedric T. Priebe, M.D., Vice President and Chief Information Officer
CHR: Timothy Bigelow, Director Human Resources
Web address: www.butler.org
**Control:** Other not-for-profit (including NFP Corporation) **Service:** Psychiatric

| Staffed Beds: 117 Admissions: 5782 Census: 122 Outpatient Visits: 41239 Births: 0 Total Expense ($000): 93432 Payroll Expense ($000): 53607 Personnel: 735 |
| --- |

☐ **MIRIAM HOSPITAL (410012)**, 164 Summit Avenue, Zip 02906–2895; tel. 401/793–2500 **A**1 2 3 5 8 9 10 **F**8 11 12 15 17 18 20 22 26 28 29 30 31 34 35 40 45 46 49 50 53 54 56 57 58 59 60 61 64 65 66 67 68 70 74 75 77 78 79 81 82 84 85 87 92 93 97 100 104 107 108 110 111 113 114 117 118 125 129 131 134 145 146 147 **P**3 5 6 **S** Lifespan Corporation, Providence, RI
Primary Contact: Arthur J. Sampson, FACHE, Executive Director
COO: Maria Ducharme, R.N., Interim Chief Nursing Officer
CFO: Mamie Wakefield, Chief Financial Officer
CMO: R. William Corwin, M.D., Vice President and Chief Medical Officer
CIO: Carole Cotter, Vice President and Chief Information Officer
CHR: Nancy McMahon, Vice President Human Resources
Web address: www.lifespan.org
**Control:** Other not-for-profit (including NFP Corporation) **Service:** General Medical and Surgical

| Staffed Beds: 247 Admissions: 14614 Census: 183 Outpatient Visits: 111344 Births: 0 Total Expense ($000): 382158 Payroll Expense ($000): 155483 Personnel: 1857 |
| --- |

☐ **RHODE ISLAND HOSPITAL (410007)**, 593 Eddy Street, Zip 02903–4900; tel. 401/444–4000, (Includes HASBRO CHILDREN'S HOSPITAL, 593 Eddy Street, Zip 02903–4923; tel. 401/444–4000) **A**1 2 3 5 8 9 10 **F**3 6 7 8 11 12 15 16 17 18 19 20 21 22 23 24 26 29 30 31 32 34 35 38 39 40 41 43 45 46 47 48 49 50 51 53 54 55 56 57 58 59 60 61 64 65 66 68 70 74 75 77 78 79 81 82 84 85 86 87 88 89 92 93 94 97 98 99 100 101 102 103 104 105 107 108 110 111 113 114 115 116 117 118 119 120 122 123 128 129 130 131 133 134 137 141 144 145 147 **P**3 5 6 **S** Lifespan Corporation, Providence, RI
Primary Contact: Timothy J. Babineau, M.D., President and Chief Executive Officer
COO: Fredrick Macri, Executive Vice President
CFO: Mamie Wakefield, Senior Vice President and Chief Financial Officer
CMO: John B. Murphy, M.D., Vice President Medical Affairs and Chief Medical Officer
CIO: Carole Cotter, Senior Vice President and Chief Information Officer
CHR: Louis Sperling, Vice President Human Resources
Web address: www.lifespan.org
**Control:** Other not-for-profit (including NFP Corporation) **Service:** General Medical and Surgical

| Staffed Beds: 672 Admissions: 35140 Census: 521 Outpatient Visits: 351603 Total Expense ($000): 1020640 Payroll Expense ($000): 464300 Personnel: 5522 |
| --- |

*Many Facility Codes have changed. Please refer to the AHA Guide Code Chart.* © 2012 AHA Guide

✠ **ROGER WILLIAMS MEDICAL CENTER (410004)**, 825 Chalkstone Avenue, Zip 02908–4735; tel. 401/456–2000 **A**1 2 3 5 8 9 10 **F**3 4 5 8 12 15 18 26 29 30 31 34 35 37 40 45 46 47 48 49 50 51 56 57 58 59 60 61 62 64 65 68 70 74 75 78 79 81 82 84 85 86 87 92 97 98 100 101 102 103 104 105 107 108 110 111 113 114 117 118 128 129 130 131 134 135 145 146 147 **P**5 8
Primary Contact: Kenneth H. Belcher, President and Chief Executive Officer
CFO: Addy Kane, Chief Financial Officer
CMO: Elaine Jones, M.D., President Medical Staff
CIO: Susan Cerrone Abely, Vice President and Chief Information Officer
Web address: www.rwmc.com
**Control:** Other not–for–profit (including NFP Corporation) **Service:** General Medical and Surgical

**Staffed Beds:** 177 **Admissions:** 7608 **Census:** 95 **Outpatient Visits:** 170614 **Births:** 0 **Total Expense ($000):** 147266 **Payroll Expense ($000):** 65410 **Personnel:** 1032

**ST. JOSEPH HOSPITAL FOR SPECIALTY CARE** See St. Joseph Health Services of Rhode Island, North Providence

✠ **VETERANS AFFAIRS MEDICAL CENTER**, 830 Chalkstone Avenue, Zip 02908–4799; tel. 401/273–7100 **A**1 2 3 5 9 **F**5 8 18 28 29 30 31 34 35 39 40 45 46 49 50 51 54 55 56 58 60 61 62 64 65 66 68 70 74 75 77 78 79 81 82 83 84 86 87 92 93 94 97 98 101 102 103 104 105 107 108 111 113 114 117 118 126 128 129 131 134 135 136 137 138 139 140 141 143 145 146 147 **S** Department of Veterans Affairs, Washington, DC
Primary Contact: Vincent Ng, Director
Web address: www.providence.va.gov/
**Control:** Veterans Affairs, Government, federal **Service:** General Medical and Surgical

**Staffed Beds:** 73 **Admissions:** 3384 **Census:** 56 **Outpatient Visits:** 368975 **Births:** 0 **Personnel:** 1225

✠ **WOMEN & INFANTS HOSPITAL OF RHODE ISLAND (410010)**, 101 Dudley Street, Zip 02905–2499; tel. 401/274–1100 **A**1 2 3 5 8 9 10 **F**3 5 11 13 15 29 30 31 34 35 36 38 40 44 45 46 50 52 54 55 57 58 59 63 64 65 66 68 71 72 73 75 76 77 78 81 82 84 85 86 87 97 98 100 101 104 105 107 110 111 113 118 125 129 131 133 134 142 145 146 **P**5 6 8 **S** Care New England Health System, Providence, RI
Primary Contact: Constance A. Howes, President and Chief Executive Officer
COO: Mark Marcantano, Executive Vice President and Chief Operating Officer
CMO: Raymond Powrie, M.D., Senior Vice President Quality and Clinical Effectiveness
CIO: Cedric T. Priebe, M.D., Senior Vice President and Chief Information Officer
CHR: Paul F. Heffernan, Vice President Human Resources
Web address: www.womenandinfants.org
**Control:** Other not–for–profit (including NFP Corporation) **Service:** Obstetrics and gynecology

**Staffed Beds:** 247 **Admissions:** 13289 **Census:** 167 **Outpatient Visits:** 171943 **Births:** 8502 **Total Expense ($000):** 412770 **Payroll Expense ($000):** 186773 **Personnel:** 2127

**WAKEFIELD—Washington County**

☐ **SOUTH COUNTY HOSPITAL (410008)**, 100 Kenyon Avenue, Zip 02879–4299; tel. 401/782–8000 **A**1 2 9 10 **F**3 11 13 15 20 28 29 31 34 35 36 37 38 40 45 49 51 53 54 56 57 59 64 65 70 74 75 76 77 78 79 81 85 86 87 89 93 102 103 104 107 108 110 111 113 118 125 128 129 130 131 132 134 142 143 145 146 147 **P**4 6
Primary Contact: Louis R. Giancola, President and Chief Executive Officer
CFO: Thomas Breen, Vice President and Chief Financial Officer
CMO: Joseph J. O'Neill, M.D., Vice President Medical Affairs
CIO: Gary Croteau, Assistant Vice President and Chief Information Officer
CHR: Maggie Thomas, Vice President Human Resources and Practice Management
Web address: www.schospital.com
**Control:** Other not–for–profit (including NFP Corporation) **Service:** General Medical and Surgical

**Staffed Beds:** 77 **Admissions:** 4844 **Census:** 50 **Outpatient Visits:** 179483 **Births:** 416 **Total Expense ($000):** 106712 **Payroll Expense ($000):** 42522 **Personnel:** 600

**WARWICK—Kent County**

✠ △ **KENT COUNTY MEMORIAL HOSPITAL (410009)**, 455 Tollgate Road, Zip 02886–2770; tel. 401/737–7000 **A**1 2 7 9 10 13 **F**3 11 12 13 15 17 18 20 22 28 29 30 31 32 34 35 36 39 40 41 45 46 47 48 49 50 51 56 57 58 59 60 61 64 65 68 70 73 74 75 76 77 78 79 81 82 85 86 87 89 90 93 96 97 98 100 102 103 107 108 110 111 113 117 118 128 129 130 131 142 145 146 147 **P**6 8 **S** Care New England Health System, Providence, RI
Primary Contact: Sandra L. Coletta, President and Chief Executive Officer
CFO: Paul Beaudoin, Senior Vice President Finance and Chief Financial Officer
CIO: Cedric T. Priebe, M.D., Senior Vice President and Chief Information Officer
CHR: Marilyn J. Walsh, Vice President Human Resources
Web address: www.kentri.org
**Control:** Other not–for–profit (including NFP Corporation) **Service:** General Medical and Surgical

**Staffed Beds:** 306 **Admissions:** 14598 **Census:** 218 **Outpatient Visits:** 212729 **Births:** 1087 **Total Expense ($000):** 288794 **Payroll Expense ($000):** 124245 **Personnel:** 1457

**WESTERLY—Washington County**

★ **WESTERLY HOSPITAL (410013)**, 25 Wells Street, Zip 02891–2934; tel. 401/596–6000, (Nonreporting) **A**2 9 10 21
Primary Contact: Charles S. Kinney, President and Chief Executive Officer
COO: Jeanne LaChance, Executive Vice President
CIO: Nancy Barisano, Chief Information Officer
CHR: Jodie Tate, Director Human Resources
Web address: www.westerlyhospital.org
**Control:** Other not–for–profit (including NFP Corporation) **Service:** General Medical and Surgical

**Staffed Beds:** 100

**WOONSOCKET—Providence County**

☐ **LANDMARK MEDICAL CENTER (410011)**, 115 Cass Avenue, Zip 02895–4731; tel. 401/769–4100, (Includes LANDMARK MEDICAL CENTER–FOGARTY UNIT, Eddie Dowling Highway, North Smithfield, Zip 02896; Mailing Address: Woonsocket, tel. 401/766–0800; LANDMARK MEDICAL CENTER–WOONSOCKET UNIT, 115 Cass Avenue, Zip 02895; tel. 401/769–4100), (Nonreporting) **A**1 2 9 10
Primary Contact: Richard Charest, President
CFO: Dana Diggins, Chief Financial Officer
CMO: Stanley Balon, M.D., President Medical Staff
CIO: Colleen Ryan, Director Management Information Systems
CHR: Mona M. Willis, Director Human Resources
Web address: www.landmarkmedical.org
**Control:** Other not–for–profit (including NFP Corporation) **Service:** General Medical and Surgical

**Staffed Beds:** 133

**RI**

---

**Hospital, Medicare Provider Number, Address, Telephone, Approval, Facility, and Physician Codes, Health Care System**

★ American Hospital Association (AHA) membership
☐ The Joint Commission accreditation   ◇ DNV Healthcare Inc. accreditation
○ American Osteopathic Association (AOA) accreditation
△ Commission on Accreditation of Rehabilitation Facilities (CARF) accreditation

# SOUTH CAROLINA

## ABBEVILLE—Abbeville County

☒ **ABBEVILLE AREA MEDICAL CENTER (421301)**, 420 Thomson Circle,
Zip 29620–5656, Mailing Address: P.O. Box 887, Zip 29620–0887;
tel. 864/366–5011 **A**1 9 10 18 **F**3 15 17 28 29 30 35 40 51 53 56 57 59 62
64 67 70 74 75 77 79 81 85 87 89 90 107 108 110 113 118 126 127 128
129 131 132 134 145 146 147 **P**4 5 **S** QHR, Brentwood, TN
Primary Contact: Richard D. Osmus, Chief Executive Officer
CFO: Timothy Wren, Chief Financial Officer
CMO: Michael Turner, M.D., Chief of Staff
CIO: Tim Stewart, Chief Information Officer
CHR: Alice Rigney, Chief Human Resources Officer
Web address: www.abbevilleareamc.com
**Control:** County–Government, nonfederal **Service:** General Medical and Surgical

> **Staffed Beds:** 25 **Admissions:** 733 **Census:** 7 **Outpatient Visits:** 12770
> **Births:** 0 **Total Expense ($000):** 29817 **Payroll Expense ($000):** 12469
> **Personnel:** 311

## AIKEN—Aiken County

☐ **AIKEN REGIONAL MEDICAL CENTERS (420082)**, 302 University Parkway,
Zip 29801–2757; tel. 803/641–5000, (Includes AURORA PAVILION, 655 Medical
Park Drive, Zip 29801; tel. 803/641–5900) **A**1 5 9 10 **F**3 4 5 11 12 15 18 20
22 24 29 30 31 34 35 40 46 49 56 57 58 64 70 73 74 76 77 78 79 80
81 85 86 87 89 98 99 100 101 102 103 104 105 107 108 110 111 113 114
118 120 122 128 129 130 131 134 145 146 147 **S** Universal Health Services,
Inc., King of Prussia, PA
Primary Contact: Carlos Milanes, Chief Executive Officer and Managing Director
COO: Scott Ansede, Chief Operating Officer
Web address: www.aikenregional.com
**Control:** Corporation, Investor–owned, for–profit **Service:** General Medical and
Surgical

> **Staffed Beds:** 256 **Admissions:** 12448 **Census:** 169 **Outpatient Visits:**
> 141934 **Births:** 1122 **Total Expense ($000):** 141567 **Payroll Expense**
> **($000):** 50353 **Personnel:** 869

## ANDERSON—Anderson County

☒ **ANMED HEALTH MEDICAL CENTER (420027)**, 800 North Fant Street,
Zip 29621–5793; tel. 864/512–1000, (Includes ANMED HEALTH WOMEN'S AND
CHILDREN'S HOSPITAL, 2000 East Greenville Street, Zip 29621;
tel. 864/512–1000) **A**1 2 3 5 9 10 **F**3 4 5 11 12 13 14 15 17 18 20 22 24 26
28 29 30 31 34 35 37 39 40 43 45 46 48 49 50 51 53 54 56 57 58 59 60
61 62 64 65 68 70 71 73 74 75 76 77 78 79 81 84 85 86 87 89 90 91 97
98 100 101 102 103 104 105 107 108 110 111 113 114 116 117 118 120
122 125 126 128 129 130 131 134 143 145 146 147 **S** AnMed Health,
Anderson, SC
Primary Contact: John A. Miller, Jr., FACHE, Chief Executive Officer
COO: William T. Manson, III, President
CFO: Jerry A. Parrish, Vice President
CMO: Mike Tillirson, D.O., Executive Vice President and Chief Medical Officer
CIO: Kathy Hammond, Director Information Services
CHR: Doug Douglas, Vice President Human Resources
Web address: www.anmedhealth.org
**Control:** Other not–for–profit (including NFP Corporation) **Service:** General
Medical and Surgical

> **Staffed Beds:** 382 **Admissions:** 19262 **Census:** 248 **Outpatient Visits:**
> 676466 **Births:** 1985 **Total Expense ($000):** 414027 **Payroll Expense**
> **($000):** 153872 **Personnel:** 3273

☒ **ANMED HEALTH REHABILITATION HOSPITAL (423029)**, 1 Spring Back Way,
Zip 29621; tel. 864/716–2600 **A**1 10 **F**3 29 30 56 74 75 79 90 91 95 96
**S** HEALTHSOUTH Corporation, Birmingham, AL
Primary Contact: Michele M. Skripps, R.N., Administrator
CFO: Julie Saylors, Controller
CMO: William Vogentiz, M.D., Medical Director
CHR: Tara Myers, Director Human Resources
Web address: www.anmedrehab.com
**Control:** Corporation, Investor–owned, for–profit **Service:** Rehabilitation

> **Staffed Beds:** 45 **Admissions:** 1186 **Census:** 42 **Births:** 0 **Total Expense**
> **($000):** 11242 **Payroll Expense ($000):** 6273 **Personnel:** 173

☐ **PATRICK B. HARRIS PSYCHIATRIC HOSPITAL (424011)**, 130 Highway 252,
Zip 29622; tel. 864/231–2600 **A**1 10 **F**35 57 86 87 98 100 101 102 103 129
142 145
Primary Contact: John Fletcher, Chief Executive Officer
Web address: www.patrickbharrispsychiatrichospital.com/index.htm
**Control:** State–Government, nonfederal **Service:** Psychiatric

> **Staffed Beds:** 114 **Admissions:** 878 **Census:** 113 **Personnel:** 305

## BARNWELL—Barnwell County

☐ **BARNWELL COUNTY HOSPITAL (420016)**, 811 Reynolds Road,
Zip 29812–1555; tel. 803/259–1000 **A**1 9 10 20 **F**3 15 29 34 35 40 45 49
57 59 64 65 70 77 81 86 87 89 90 93 107 108 111 118 126 128 145
Primary Contact: Mary T. Valliant, R.N., MS, Chief Executive Officer
CFO: Troy Pickens, Chief Financial Officer
CMO: Dean Koukos, M.D., Chief Medical Staff
CIO: Randal Padgett, Manager Information Systems
CHR: Sherry Donaldson, Director Human Resources
CNO: Marsha Gantt, Interim Chief Nursing Officer
Web address: www.bchospital.org
**Control:** County–Government, nonfederal **Service:** General Medical and Surgical

> **Staffed Beds:** 33 **Admissions:** 872 **Census:** 7 **Births:** 0 **Personnel:** 138

## BEAUFORT—Beaufort County

☒ **BEAUFORT MEMORIAL HOSPITAL (420067)**, 955 Ribaut Road,
Zip 29902–5441; tel. 843/522–5200, (Nonreporting) **A**1 2 9 10
Primary Contact: Richard Kirk Toomey, FACHE, President and Chief Executive
Officer
CFO: Jeffrey L. White, Senior Vice President and Chief Financial Officer
CMO: Paul Mazzeo, M.D., Chief of Staff
CIO: Edward Ricks, Vice President and Chief Information Officer
CHR: David Homyk, Vice President Human Resources
Web address: www.bmhsc.org
**Control:** County–Government, nonfederal **Service:** General Medical and Surgical

> **Staffed Beds:** 203

☒ **NAVAL HOSPITAL BEAUFORT**, 1 Pinckney Boulevard, Zip 29902–6148;
tel. 843/228–5301, (Nonreporting) **A**1 5 **S** Bureau of Medicine and Surgery,
Department of the Navy, Washington, DC
Primary Contact: Captain J. R. Queen, MSC, USN, Commanding Officer
Web address: www.beaufortnavalhospital.com/
**Control:** Navy, Government, federal **Service:** General Medical and Surgical

> **Staffed Beds:** 20

## BENNETTSVILLE—Marlboro County

☒ **MARLBORO PARK HOSPITAL (420054)**, 1138 Cheraw Highway,
Zip 29512–0738; tel. 843/479–2881 **A**1 9 10 **F**3 13 15 17 18 29 34 35 40
45 57 59 64 65 70 75 76 77 79 81 85 86 87 89 98 103 107 108 118 126
127 129 131 132 134 145 146 **S** Community Health Systems, Inc., Franklin, TN
Primary Contact: Ronnie Daves, Chief Executive Officer
CMO: Cindy Crittendon, M.D., Chief of Staff
CIO: Rod McLaurin, Director Information Systems
CHR: Christi Meggs, Director Human Resources
Web address: www.marlboroparkhospital.com
**Control:** Corporation, Investor–owned, for–profit **Service:** General Medical and
Surgical

> **Staffed Beds:** 102 **Admissions:** 1529 **Census:** 14 **Outpatient Visits:** 13950
> **Total Expense ($000):** 23691 **Payroll Expense ($000):** 9968 **Personnel:**
> 184

## CAMDEN—Kershaw County

☒ **KERSHAWHEALTH (420048)**, 1315 Roberts Street, Zip 29020–3737, Mailing
Address: P.O. Box 7003, Zip 29021–7003; tel. 803/432–4311, (Total facility
includes 96 beds in nursing home–type unit) **A**1 9 10 **F**3 7 11 13 15 20 24 28
29 30 31 32 34 35 40 44 45 46 47 49 50 51 54 57 59 61 62 63 64 67 68
70 75 76 77 78 79 81 85 86 87 89 90 93 97 108 110 111 113 114 118 126
127 128 129 131 142 143 145 146 147
Primary Contact: Donnie J. Weeks, FACHE, President and Chief Executive Officer
COO: Mike Bunch, Executive Vice President, Chief Operating Officer and Chief
Financial Officer
CHR: Angela F. Nettles, Director Human Resources
Web address: www.kershawhealth.com
**Control:** County–Government, nonfederal **Service:** General Medical and Surgical

> **Staffed Beds:** 215 **Admissions:** 5968 **Census:** 160 **Births:** 407 **Total**
> **Expense ($000):** 110725 **Payroll Expense ($000):** 46529 **Personnel:** 1050

*Many Facility Codes have changed. Please refer to the AHA Guide Code Chart.*
© 2012 AHA Guide

**SC**

**CHARLESTON—Charleston County**

✠ **BON SECOURS ST. FRANCIS HOSPITAL (420065)**, 2095 Henry Tecklenburg Drive, Zip 29414–0001; tel. 843/402–1000 **A**1 9 10 **F**3 7 12 13 14 15 20 28 29 30 31 34 35 40 43 45 46 47 48 49 50 51 56 57 59 60 64 68 70 73 74 75 76 77 78 79 80 81 82 84 85 86 87 89 100 107 108 110 111 113 117 118 129 130 131 144 145 146 147 **S** Carolinas HealthCare System, Charlotte, NC
Primary Contact: Allen P. Carroll, Senior Vice President and Chief Executive Officer
CFO: Bret Johnson, Chief Financial Officer
CMO: Steven D. Shapiro, M.D., Chief Medical Officer
CIO: Michael Taylor, Chief Information Officer
CHR: Douglas Harrison, Vice President Human Resources
Web address: www.ropersaintfrancis.com
**Control:** Other not–for–profit (including NFP Corporation) **Service:** General Medical and Surgical

**Staffed Beds:** 179 **Admissions:** 8798 **Census:** 92 **Outpatient Visits:** 144075 **Births:** 1845 **Total Expense ($000):** 138074 **Payroll Expense ($000):** 51285 **Personnel:** 987

★ **HEALTHSOUTH REHABILITATION HOSPITAL OF CHARLESTON (423027)**, 9181 Medcom Street, Zip 29406–9168; tel. 843/820–7777 **A**10 **F**9 29 35 54 56 57 64 65 77 82 86 90 95 96 131 142 145 147 **S** HEALTHSOUTH Corporation, Birmingham, AL
Primary Contact: Troy Powell, Chief Executive Officer
CFO: Beckye Lariviere, Controller
CMO: William Livesay, Jr., D.O., Medical Director
CHR: Donna White, Director Human Resources
Web address: www.healthsouthcharleston.com
**Control:** Corporation, Investor–owned, for–profit **Service:** Rehabilitation

**Staffed Beds:** 46 **Admissions:** 978 **Census:** 34 **Total Expense ($000):** 11421 **Payroll Expense ($000):** 6123 **Personnel:** 130

★ **KINDRED HOSPITAL–CHARLESTON (422005)**, 326 Calhoun Street, 3rd Floor, Zip 29401; tel. 843/876–8670 **A**10 **F**1 3 17 29 35 60 70 90 147 **S** Kindred Healthcare, Louisville, KY
Primary Contact: Jennifer Sheets, R.N., Chief Executive Officer
CFO: Julia Smith, Chief Financial Officer
CMO: Athena Beldecos, M.D., Medical Director
CHR: Julia Taylor, Area Director Human Resources
Web address: www.khcharleston.com
**Control:** Corporation, Investor–owned, for–profit **Service:** Long–Term Acute Care hospital

**Staffed Beds:** 55 **Admissions:** 228 **Census:** 27 **Outpatient Visits:** 0 **Births:** 0 **Total Expense ($000):** 12807 **Payroll Expense ($000):** 6523 **Personnel:** 109

✠ **MUSC MEDICAL CENTER OF MEDICAL UNIVERSITY OF SOUTH CAROLINA (420004)**, 169 Ashley Avenue, Zip 29425; tel. 843/792–2300, (Includes MUSC CHILDREN'S HOSPITAL, 171 Ashley Avenue, Zip 29425–8908; tel. 843/792–1414) **A**1 2 3 4 5 6 7 9 10 **F**1 3 4 5 6 7 9 10 11 12 13 15 16 17 18 19 20 21 22 23 24 25 26 27 28 29 30 31 32 34 35 37 38 39 40 41 43 44 45 46 47 48 49 50 51 52 53 54 55 56 57 59 60 61 64 66 68 70 71 72 73 74 75 76 77 78 79 80 81 82 84 85 86 87 88 89 92 97 98 99 100 101 102 103 104 105 107 108 109 110 111 113 114 115 116 117 118 119 120 122 123 125 127 128 129 130 131 133 134 135 136 137 138 139 140 141 143 144 145 146 147
Primary Contact: W. Stuart Smith, Executive Director and Vice President Clinical Operations
CFO: Lisa P. Montgomery, Administrator Finance and Support Services
CMO: Patrick J. Cawley, M.D., Medical Director
CIO: Frank Clark, Chief Information Officer
CHR: Betts Ellis, Administrator Institutional Relations
Web address: www.muschealth.com
**Control:** State–Government, nonfederal **Service:** General Medical and Surgical

**Staffed Beds:** 712 **Admissions:** 32783 **Census:** 581 **Outpatient Visits:** 957399 **Births:** 2218 **Total Expense ($000):** 1027686 **Payroll Expense ($000):** 377623 **Personnel:** 6353

☐ **PALMETTO LOWCOUNTRY BEHAVIORAL HEALTH (424006)**, 2777 Speissegger Drive, Zip 29405–8299; tel. 843/747–5830, (Total facility includes 32 beds in nursing home–type unit) **A**1 10 **F**4 5 29 64 98 99 101 102 103 104 105 129 131 **S** Universal Health Services, Inc., King of Prussia, PA
Primary Contact: Cherie Tolley, Chief Executive Officer
COO: Marc Turner, Chief Operating Officer
CFO: Stan Markowski, Chief Financial Officer
CMO: Steven Lopez, M.D., Chief Medical Officer
CHR: Josh Smith, Vice President Human Resources
Web address: www.plbhs.com
**Control:** Corporation, Investor–owned, for–profit **Service:** Psychiatric

**Staffed Beds:** 112 **Admissions:** 2573 **Census:** 77 **Outpatient Visits:** 4946 **Births:** 0 **Total Expense ($000):** 13033 **Payroll Expense ($000):** 8045

✠ **RALPH H. JOHNSON VETERANS AFFAIRS MEDICAL CENTER**, 109 Bee Street, Zip 29401–5799; tel. 843/577–5011, (Nonreporting) **A**1 2 3 5 8 **S** Department of Veterans Affairs, Washington, DC
Primary Contact: Carolyn L. Adams, Director
CFO: Cassandra Helfer, Chief Financial Officer
CMO: Florence N. Hutchison, M.D., Chief of Staff
CIO: Michael Cortright, Chief Information Officer
Web address: www.va.gov/sta/guide/home.asp
**Control:** Veterans Affairs, Government, federal **Service:** General Medical and Surgical

**Staffed Beds:** 98

✠ △ **ROPER HOSPITAL (420087)**, 316 Calhoun Street, Zip 29401–1125; tel. 843/724–2000 **A**1 2 7 9 10 **F**3 7 8 11 13 14 15 17 18 20 22 24 26 28 29 30 31 34 35 40 42 43 45 49 50 51 54 55 56 57 59 60 61 62 64 65 68 69 70 73 74 75 76 77 78 79 80 81 82 84 85 86 87 90 92 96 100 107 108 110 111 113 114 116 117 118 119 120 122 123 125 128 129 130 131 134 135 140 142 143 145 146 147 **S** Carolinas HealthCare System, Charlotte, NC
Primary Contact: Matthew J. Severance, FACHE, Chief Executive Officer
CFO: Bret Johnson, Chief Financial Officer
CMO: Steven D. Shapiro, M.D., Vice President Medical Affairs
CIO: Michael Taylor, Chief Information Officer
CHR: Douglas Harrison, Vice President Human Resources
CHR: Douglas Harrison, Vice President Human Resources
Web address: www.ropersaintfrancis.com
**Control:** Other not–for–profit (including NFP Corporation) **Service:** General Medical and Surgical

**Staffed Beds:** 342 **Admissions:** 15471 **Census:** 230 **Outpatient Visits:** 259103 **Births:** 677 **Total Expense ($000):** 341331 **Payroll Expense ($000):** 118117 **Personnel:** 2245

✠ **TRIDENT MEDICAL CENTER (420079)**, 9330 Medical Plaza Drive, Zip 29406–9195; tel. 843/797–7000, (Includes MONCKS CORNER MEDICAL CENTER, 401 North Live Oak Drive, Highway 17A, Moncks Corner, Zip 29461–5603; tel. 843/761–8721; SUMMERVILLE MEDICAL CENTER, 295 Midland Parkway, Summerville, Zip 29485–8104; tel. 843/832–5000; Louis Caputo, Chief Executive Officer) **A**1 2 3 5 9 10 **F**3 12 13 15 16 18 20 22 24 26 28 29 30 31 34 35 39 40 42 43 45 46 47 48 49 50 54 55 56 57 59 60 61 64 70 72 73 74 75 76 77 78 79 80 81 85 86 87 89 90 107 108 110 111 113 114 116 117 118 119 120 122 125 128 129 130 131 134 144 145 146 147 **S** HCA, Nashville, TN
Primary Contact: Todd Gallati, FACHE, President and Chief Executive Officer
CFO: Teresa Finch, Chief Financial Officer
CIO: Susan Murray, Director Information Services
CHR: Joe B. Hill, Jr., Vice President Human Resources
Web address: www.tridenthealthsystem.com
**Control:** Corporation, Investor–owned, for–profit **Service:** General Medical and Surgical

**Staffed Beds:** 403 **Admissions:** 21260 **Census:** 252 **Births:** 3043 **Total Expense ($000):** 307363 **Payroll Expense ($000):** 97939 **Personnel:** 1663

**CHERAW—Chesterfield County**

✠ **CHESTERFIELD GENERAL HOSPITAL (420062)**, 711 Chesterfield Highway, Zip 29520; tel. 843/537–7881 **A**1 9 10 **F**3 11 13 15 18 19 28 29 30 34 35 40 45 56 57 59 64 65 70 75 76 77 79 81 85 86 87 89 90 97 102 107 108 113 117 118 127 129 131 132 134 145 146 147 **S** Community Health Systems, Inc., Franklin, TN
Primary Contact: Jeff Reece, Chief Executive Officer
CFO: Nathan Crabdree, Chief Financial Officer
CMO: David Bersinger, M.D., Chief of Staff
Web address: www.chesterfieldgeneral.com
**Control:** Corporation, Investor–owned, for–profit **Service:** General Medical and Surgical

**Staffed Beds:** 59 **Admissions:** 2348 **Census:** 23 **Outpatient Visits:** 31005 **Births:** 160 **Total Expense ($000):** 27711 **Payroll Expense ($000):** 10969 **Personnel:** 221

**CHESTER—Chester County**

☐ **CHESTER REGIONAL MEDICAL CENTER (420019)**, 1 Medical Park Drive, Zip 29706–9799; tel. 803/581–3151, (Total facility includes 100 beds in nursing home–type unit) **A**1 9 10 **F**1 15 18 20 22 24 28 29 34 35 40 53 56 57 59 64 65 70 75 77 79 81 85 86 87 89 90 107 108 113 118 127 128 129 130 131 134 145 **S** Health Management Associates, Naples, FL
Primary Contact: Page H. Vaughan, Chief Executive Officer
CIO: Rick Lewis, Chief Information Officer
Web address: www.chospital.org
**Control:** Corporation, Investor–owned, for–profit **Service:** General Medical and Surgical

**Staffed Beds:** 136 **Admissions:** 1811 **Census:** 95 **Outpatient Visits:** 17886 **Births:** 0 **Personnel:** 224

SC

---

**Hospital, Medicare Provider Number, Address, Telephone, Approval, Facility, and Physician Codes, Health Care System**

★ American Hospital Association (AHA) membership
☐ The Joint Commission accreditation　　◇ DNV Healthcare Inc. accreditation

○ American Osteopathic Association (AOA) accreditation
△ Commission on Accreditation of Rehabilitation Facilities (CARF) accreditation

**CLINTON—Laurens County**

✠ **LAURENS COUNTY HEALTH CARE SYSTEM (420038)**, Highway 76 East, Zip 29325–2331, Mailing Address: P.O. Box 976, Zip 29325–0976; tel. 864/833–9100, (Includes LAURENS COUNTY HOSPITAL, Zip 29325; tel. 803/833–9100), (Total facility includes 14 beds in nursing home–type unit) **A**1 9 10 **F**3 11 13 15 17 18 28 29 30 34 35 40 46 48 57 59 61 64 70 75 76 77 79 80 81 85 87 89 90 107 108 110 118 127 128 129 131 134 140 145 146 147
Primary Contact: Richard E. D'Alberto, FACHE, Chief Executive Officer
COO: Kay Swisher, Vice President and Chief Operating Officer
CFO: William Grant, Vice President Fiscal and Support Services
CMO: Mike Wiggins, M.D., Chief of Staff
CIO: Joel Bradley, Director Information Systems
CHR: Robin Callas, Director Human Resources
Web address: www.lchcs.org
**Control:** Hospital district or authority, Government, nonfederal **Service:** General Medical and Surgical

**Staffed Beds:** 90 **Admissions:** 2973 **Census:** 41 **Births:** 306 **Total Expense ($000):** 59702 **Payroll Expense ($000):** 23366 **Personnel:** 203

**WHITTEN CENTER**, Highway 76 East, Zip 29325, Mailing Address: P.O. Box 239, Zip 29325; tel. 864/833–2733, (Nonreporting)
Primary Contact: William Killion, Chief Executive Officer
**Control:** State–Government, nonfederal **Service:** Institution for mental retardation

**Staffed Beds:** 22

**COLUMBIA—Richland County**

**EARLE E. MORRIS ALCOHOL AND DRUG TREATMENT CENTER**, 610 Faison Drive, Zip 29203–3298; tel. 803/935–7100 **F**4 29 39 53 61 67 74 75 87 98 129 131 145
Primary Contact: George McConnell, Director
Web address: www.state.sc.us/dmh/morris_village/
**Control:** State–Government, nonfederal **Service:** Alcoholism and other chemical dependency

**Staffed Beds:** 131 **Admissions:** 1512 **Census:** 112 **Births:** 0 **Personnel:** 160

☐ **G. WERBER BRYAN PSYCHIATRIC HOSPITAL (424005)**, 220 Faison Drive, Zip 29203–3295; tel. 803/935–7146 **A**1 10 **F**4 30 50 74 75 97 98 101 103 129 131 134 145
Primary Contact: Harvey Miller, Director
COO: Jaclyn Upfield, Chief Operating Officer
CIO: Sam Livingston, Information Resource Consultant
CHR: Kim Church, Manager Human Resources
Web address: www.scdmh.org
**Control:** State–Government, nonfederal **Service:** Psychiatric

**Staffed Beds:** 198 **Admissions:** 758 **Census:** 184 **Personnel:** 435

✠ **HEALTHSOUTH REHABILITATION HOSPITAL (423025)**, 2935 Colonial Drive, Zip 29203–6811; tel. 803/254–7777 **A**1 10 **F**2 29 34 35 54 56 57 59 64 74 75 77 79 86 87 90 91 92 95 96 129 130 131 147 **S** HEALTHSOUTH Corporation, Birmingham, AL
Primary Contact: James H. Rogers, FACHE, Regional Vice President
CFO: Jessica Burriss, Chief Financial Officer
CMO: Devin Troyer, M.D., Medical Director
CHR: Luanne Burton, Director Human Resources
Web address: www.healthsouthcolumbia.com
**Control:** Corporation, Investor–owned, for–profit **Service:** Rehabilitation

**Staffed Beds:** 96 **Admissions:** 1546 **Census:** 55 **Births:** 0 **Total Expense ($000):** 17003 **Payroll Expense ($000):** 9350 **Personnel:** 225

**INTERMEDICAL HOSPITAL OF SOUTH CAROLINA (422006)**, Taylor at Marion Street, Zip 29220, Mailing Address: PO BOX 11069, Zip 29211–1069; tel. 803/296–3757 **A**9 10 **F**1 3 29 34 57 58 85 129 147
Primary Contact: Armando Colombo, Chief Executive Officer
Web address: www.intermedicalhospital.com
**Control:** Other not–for–profit (including NFP Corporation) **Service:** Long–Term Acute Care hospital

**Staffed Beds:** 35 **Admissions:** 278 **Census:** 21 **Total Expense ($000):** 10492 **Payroll Expense ($000):** 3442

✠ **PALMETTO HEALTH BAPTIST (420086)**, Taylor at Marion Street, Zip 29220–0001; tel. 803/296–5010, (Total facility includes 22 beds in nursing home–type unit) **A**1 2 3 5 9 10 **F**1 3 5 11 12 13 15 18 20 29 30 31 34 35 40 45 47 48 49 51 54 57 59 61 62 63 64 68 70 71 72 73 74 75 76 77 78 79 80 81 82 84 85 86 87 89 90 98 99 100 101 102 103 104 105 107 108 110 111 112 113 114 115 116 117 118 123 127 129 131 144 145 146 147 **S** Palmetto Health, Columbia, SC
Primary Contact: James M. Bridges, Executive Vice President and Chief Operating Officer
COO: James M. Bridges, Executive Vice President and Chief Operating Officer
CFO: Paul K. Duane, Executive Vice President and Chief Financial Officer
CMO: Mark J. Mayson, M.D., Medical Director
CIO: Michelle Edwards, Executive Vice President Information Technology
CHR: Trip Gregory, Senior Vice President Human Resources
Web address: www.palmettohealth.org
**Control:** Other not–for–profit (including NFP Corporation) **Service:** General Medical and Surgical

**Staffed Beds:** 451 **Admissions:** 17907 **Census:** 274 **Outpatient Visits:** 52118 **Births:** 3494 **Total Expense ($000):** 333691 **Payroll Expense ($000):** 127600 **Personnel:** 2166

✠ **PALMETTO HEALTH RICHLAND (420018)**, Five Richland Medical Park Drive, Zip 29203–6897; tel. 803/434–7000, (Includes PALMETTO HEALTH CHILDREN'S HOSPITAL, Five Richland Medical Park Drive, Zip 29203–6863; tel. 803/434–6882) **A**1 2 3 5 8 9 10 **F**2 3 4 5 6 11 13 15 17 18 20 22 24 28 29 30 31 32 34 35 39 40 43 45 46 54 55 56 57 59 60 61 64 68 70 72 73 74 75 76 77 78 79 81 86 87 88 89 90 97 98 99 100 101 102 103 104 105 107 108 110 111 113 117 118 120 125 128 129 130 131 133 134 142 145 146 147 **S** Palmetto Health, Columbia, SC
Primary Contact: Stan Hickson, FACHE, Executive Vice President and Chief Operating Officer
CFO: Paul K. Duane, Executive Vice President and Chief Financial Officer
CMO: Jennifer Risinger, M.D., Chief of Staff
CHR: Trip Gregory, Senior Vice President Human Resources
Web address: www.palmettohealth.org
**Control:** Other not–for–profit (including NFP Corporation) **Service:** General Medical and Surgical

**Staffed Beds:** 669 **Admissions:** 31023 **Census:** 537 **Outpatient Visits:** 452635 **Births:** 2202 **Total Expense ($000):** 667438 **Payroll Expense ($000):** 244100 **Personnel:** 4415

✠ **PROVIDENCE HOSPITAL (420026)**, 2435 Forest Drive, Zip 29204–2098; tel. 803/865–4500, (Includes PROVIDENCE HOSPITAL NORTHEAST, 120 Gateway Corporate Boulevard, Zip 29203–9611; tel. 803/865–4500; Ryan Hall, Vice President) **A**1 9 10 21 **F**3 8 11 13 15 17 20 22 24 26 28 29 30 34 35 38 40 44 45 49 50 54 57 58 59 61 64 68 70 74 75 76 79 80 81 85 86 87 89 90 92 93 94 100 107 108 111 113 117 118 128 129 130 131 140 145 146 147 P5 **S** Sisters of Charity Health System, Cleveland, OH
Primary Contact: George A. Zara, President and Chief Executive Officer
CFO: David K. Stewart, Senior Vice President and Chief Financial Officer
CMO: Wayne Sribnick, M.D., Senior Vice President and Chief Medical Officer
CIO: Lib Cumbee, Director Information Systems
CHR: Richard W. Grooms, Jr., Vice President Human Resources
Web address: www.provhosp.com
**Control:** Church–operated, Nongovernment, not–for profit **Service:** General Medical and Surgical

**Staffed Beds:** 314 **Admissions:** 12053 **Census:** 157 **Births:** 602 **Total Expense ($000):** 281439 **Payroll Expense ($000):** 76386 **Personnel:** 1345

**SOUTH CAROLINA DEPARTMENT OF CORRECTIONS HOSPITAL**, 4344 Broad River Road, Zip 29210–4098; tel. 803/896–8567, (Nonreporting)
Primary Contact: John Solomon, M.D., Director
Web address: www.doc.sc.gov/
**Control:** State–Government, nonfederal **Service:** Hospital unit of an institution (prison hospital, college infirmary, etc.)

**Staffed Beds:** 70

☐ **WILLIAM S. HALL PSYCHIATRIC INSTITUTE (424003)**, 1800 Colonial Drive, Zip 29203–6827; tel. 803/898–1693 **A**1 5 10 **F**4 30 74 75 98 99 104 129 145
Primary Contact: Angela Forand, Director
COO: Doug Glover, Controller
CFO: Doug Glover, Controller
CMO: Phyllis Bryant–Mobley, M.D., Director Medical Services
CIO: Mesa Foard, Director Information technology
CHR: Kim Church, Manager Human Resources
Web address: www.scdmh.org
**Control:** State–Government, nonfederal **Service:** Psychiatric

**Staffed Beds:** 38 **Admissions:** 438 **Census:** 31 **Personnel:** 200

*Many Facility Codes have changed. Please refer to the AHA Guide Code Chart.*

© 2012 AHA Guide

✠ △ **WM. JENNINGS BRYAN DORN VETERANS AFFAIRS MEDICAL CENTER**, 6439 Garners Ferry Road, Zip 29209–1639; tel. 803/776–4000, (Nonreporting) **A**1 2 3 5 7 9 **S** Department of Veterans Affairs, Washington, DC
Primary Contact: Rebecca J. Wiley, R.N., Director
COO: Rebecca J. Stackhouse, Associate Director
CFO: James Cavanaugh, Chief Finance Officer
CMO: Alfred Boykin, M.D., Chief of Staff
CIO: David C. Owings, Director Information Management Service Line
CHR: Phyllis Jones, Chief Human Resources
Web address: www.columbiasc.va.gov/
**Control:** Veterans Affairs, Government, federal **Service:** General Medical and Surgical

> **Staffed Beds:** 109

### CONWAY—Horry County

★ **CONWAY MEDICAL CENTER (420049)**, 300 Singleton Ridge Road, Zip 29526–9175, Mailing Address: P.O. Box 829, Zip 29528–0829; tel. 843/347–7111, (Total facility includes 113 beds in nursing home–type unit) **A**9 10 21 **F**1 3 8 11 12 13 15 18 20 26 28 29 30 34 35 40 45 46 49 50 51 53 57 59 60 61 68 70 71 73 75 76 77 79 81 84 85 86 87 89 90 107 110 111 113 114 117 118 127 128 129 131 134 144 145 146
Primary Contact: Philip A. Clayton, President and Chief Executive Officer
CFO: Bret Barr, Vice President Fiscal Services
CMO: Preston Strosnider, M.D., Vice President Medical Affairs
CIO: Mickey Waters, Director Information Technology
CHR: Craig Hyman, Vice President Human Resources
Web address: www.conwaymedicalcenter.com
**Control:** Other not–for–profit (including NFP Corporation) **Service:** General Medical and Surgical

> **Staffed Beds:** 287 **Admissions:** 8200 **Census:** 205 **Outpatient Visits:** 56906 **Births:** 1246 **Total Expense ($000):** 126781 **Payroll Expense ($000):** 46420 **Personnel:** 940

☐ **LIGHTHOUSE CARE CENTER OF CONWAY (424002)**, 152 Waccamaw Medical Park Drive, Zip 29526–8901; tel. 843/347–8871 **A**1 9 10 **F**4 98 99 101 102 103 106 127 **S** Universal Health Services, Inc., King of Prussia, PA
Primary Contact: Thomas L. Ryba, Chief Executive Officer
CFO: Chris Frater, Chief Financial Officer
CMO: William Van Horn, M.D., Medical Director
CIO: Chris Frater, Chief Financial Officer
CHR: Lois Woodall, Director Human Resources
CNO: Penny Muckenfuss, Chief Nursing Officer
Web address: www.lighthousecarecenterofconway.com/
**Control:** Corporation, Investor–owned, for–profit **Service:** Psychiatric

> **Staffed Beds:** 52 **Admissions:** 2084 **Census:** 47 **Outpatient Visits:** 0 **Births:** 0

### DARLINGTON—Darlington County

**MCLEOD MEDICAL CENTER–DARLINGTON** See McLeod Regional Medical Center, Florence

### DILLON—Dillon County

✠ **MCLEOD MEDICAL CENTER DILLON (420005)**, 301 East Jackson Street, Zip 29536–2509, Mailing Address: P.O. Box 1327, Zip 29536–1327; tel. 843/774–4111 **A**1 9 10 **F**3 11 15 28 29 30 32 34 35 40 50 57 59 64 68 70 75 76 79 81 82 85 87 89 90 107 111 113 118 129 131 133 134 145 146 147 **P**6
Primary Contact: Deborah Locklair, FACHE, Administrator
CFO: Fulton Ervin, Senior Vice President and Chief Financial Officer
CMO: Walter B. Blum, M.D., Chief of Staff
CIO: Jenean Blackmon, Assistant Vice President and Chief Information Officer
CHR: Cynthia Causey, Associate Administrator Human and Mission Services
Web address: www.mcleodhealth.org
**Control:** Other not–for–profit (including NFP Corporation) **Service:** General Medical and Surgical

> **Staffed Beds:** 63 **Admissions:** 2792 **Census:** 27 **Births:** 285 **Total Expense ($000):** 35128 **Payroll Expense ($000):** 14215 **Personnel:** 293

### EASLEY—Pickens County

✠ **BAPTIST EASLEY HOSPITAL (420015)**, 200 Fleetwood Drive, Zip 29640–2076, Mailing Address: P.O. Box 2129, Zip 29641–2129; tel. 864/442–7200 **A**1 9 10 **F**3 11 13 15 20 28 29 30 35 39 40 56 57 58 59 64 70 75 76 79 81 85 86 87 89 107 108 113 118 129 131 133 145 146 **P**1 **S** Palmetto Health, Columbia, SC
Primary Contact: Roddey E. Gettys, III, Chief Executive Officer
COO: Roddey E. Gettys, III, Chief Executive Officer
CFO: J. Larry Pope, Vice President Finance
CMO: Scott Parker, M.D., Medical Director
CHR: Elizabeth Parsons, Human Resources Business Partner
Web address: www.palmettohealth.org
**Control:** Other not–for–profit (including NFP Corporation) **Service:** General Medical and Surgical

> **Staffed Beds:** 89 **Admissions:** 4771 **Census:** 56 **Outpatient Visits:** 46627 **Total Expense ($000):** 81814 **Payroll Expense ($000):** 29983 **Personnel:** 800

### EDGEFIELD—Edgefield County

★ **EDGEFIELD COUNTY HOSPITAL (421304)**, 300 Ridge Medical Plaza, Zip 29824; tel. 803/637–3174 **A**9 10 18 **F**3 11 34 35 40 45 57 59 65 66 68 75 77 79 81 90 97 107 113 118 126 127 129 131 132 145
Primary Contact: Patricia C. Robinson, Chief Executive Officer
CFO: William Garry, Chief Financial Officer
CMO: W. Hugh Morgan, M.D., Chief Medical Staff
CIO: Faye Burton, Director Health Information Management
CHR: Leslie G. Seigler, Executive Assistant and Coordinator Human Resources
Web address: www.myech.org
**Control:** County–Government, nonfederal **Service:** General Medical and Surgical

> **Staffed Beds:** 25 **Admissions:** 450 **Census:** 7 **Births:** 0 **Total Expense ($000):** 11850 **Payroll Expense ($000):** 5897 **Personnel:** 177

### FAIRFAX—Allendale County

★ **ALLENDALE COUNTY HOSPITAL (421300)**, 1787 Allendale Fairfax Highway, Zip 29827–0278, Mailing Address: P.O. Box 218, Zip 29827–0218; tel. 803/632–3311, (Total facility includes 44 beds in nursing home–type unit) **A**9 10 18 **F**3 15 34 35 40 45 48 57 59 61 64 67 68 75 86 87 90 97 107 113 118 126 127 129 132 146 **P**6
Primary Contact: M. K. Hiatt, Administrator
Web address: www.allendalecountyhospital.com/
**Control:** County–Government, nonfederal **Service:** General Medical and Surgical

> **Staffed Beds:** 69 **Admissions:** 351 **Census:** 44 **Outpatient Visits:** 36654 **Births:** 0 **Total Expense ($000):** 11163 **Payroll Expense ($000):** 5980 **Personnel:** 161

### FLORENCE—Florence County

✠ △ **CAROLINAS HOSPITAL SYSTEM (420091)**, 805 Pamplico Highway, Zip 29505–6050, Mailing Address: P.O. Box 100550, Zip 29502–0550; tel. 843/674–5000, (Total facility includes 42 beds in nursing home–type unit) **A**1 7 9 10 **F**4 5 6 8 11 13 15 17 20 22 24 28 29 30 31 32 34 35 38 39 40 43 45 53 55 56 57 59 60 61 62 63 64 68 70 71 72 73 74 75 76 77 78 79 81 82 86 87 88 89 90 97 98 103 104 107 108 110 111 113 114 115 116 117 118 120 122 127 128 129 130 131 134 142 143 145 146 147 **S** Community Health Systems, Inc., Franklin, TN
Primary Contact: Darcy Craven, Interim President
CFO: Steve Embree, Chief Financial Officer
CMO: James Brennan, M.D., Chief of Staff
CIO: Marty Parker, Chief Information Officer
CHR: Tammy Dickerson, Director Human Resources
Web address: www.carolinashospital.com
**Control:** Corporation, Investor–owned, for–profit **Service:** General Medical and Surgical

> **Staffed Beds:** 436 **Admissions:** 12829 **Census:** 269 **Births:** 855 **Total Expense ($000):** 185181 **Payroll Expense ($000):** 67482 **Personnel:** 1207

✠ **HEALTHSOUTH REHABILITATION HOSPITAL (423026)**, 900 East Cheves Street, Zip 29506–2704; tel. 843/679–9000 **A**1 10 **F**9 29 34 35 56 57 59 64 75 77 82 86 87 90 91 92 95 96 129 130 131 147 **S** HEALTHSOUTH Corporation, Birmingham, AL
Primary Contact: Thom King, Chief Executive Officer
CFO: Robert Wheeler, Controller
CMO: Adora Matthews, M.D., Medical Director
CHR: Susan Trantham, Director Human Resources
Web address: www.healthsouthflorence.com
**Control:** Corporation, Investor–owned, for–profit **Service:** Rehabilitation

> **Staffed Beds:** 88 **Admissions:** 1122 **Census:** 44 **Outpatient Visits:** 2376 **Total Expense ($000):** 13061 **Payroll Expense ($000):** 7049 **Personnel:** 161

---

**Hospital, Medicare Provider Number, Address, Telephone, Approval, Facility, and Physician Codes, Health Care System**

★ American Hospital Association (AHA) membership
☐ The Joint Commission accreditation   ◇ DNV Healthcare Inc. accreditation
○ American Osteopathic Association (AOA) accreditation
△ Commission on Accreditation of Rehabilitation Facilities (CARF) accreditation

SC

✠ **MCLEOD REGIONAL MEDICAL CENTER (420051)**, 555 East Cheves Street, Zip 29502–2617, Mailing Address: P.O. Box 100551, Zip 29502–0551; tel. 843/777–2000, (Includes MCLEOD MEDICAL CENTER–DARLINGTON, 701 Cashua Ferry Road, Darlington, Zip 29532–8488, Mailing Address: P.O. Box 1859, Zip 29540; tel. 843/395–1100; Pat Godbold, Administrator) **A**1 2 3 5 9 10 **F**1 3 7 8 11 13 15 17 18 20 22 24 26 28 29 30 31 32 34 35 38 39 40 43 45 46 47 48 49 50 53 54 56 57 58 59 60 61 62 63 64 66 67 68 70 71 72 73 74 75 76 77 78 79 81 82 84 85 86 87 88 89 90 92 93 94 96 97 98 100 101 102 103 104 107 108 110 111 113 114 115 118 120 126 127 128 129 130 131 132 134 142 144 145 146 147 **P**6
Primary Contact: Robert L. Colones, President and Chief Executive Officer
COO: Ronald L. Boring, Senior Vice President and Chief Operating Officer
CFO: Fulton Ervin, Chief Financial Officer
CMO: Alva W. Whitehead, M.D., Vice President Medical Services
CIO: Jenean Blackmon, Associate Vice President and Chief Information Officer
CHR: Jeannette Glenn, Vice President Human Resources, Education and Training
Web address: www.mcleodhealth.org
**Control:** Other not–for–profit (including NFP Corporation) **Service:** General Medical and Surgical

**Staffed Beds: 565 Admissions: 24181 Census: 370 Births: 2068 Total Expense ($000): 505829 Payroll Expense ($000): 157273 Personnel: 3109**

✠ **REGENCY HOSPITAL OF FLORENCE (422007)**, 121 East Cedar Street, Zip 29506; tel. 843/661–3499 **A**1 9 10 **F**1 3 29 34 35 57 58 70 77 80 82 84 85 90 100 118 127 129 147 **P**5 **S** Select Medical Corporation, Mechanicsburg, PA
Primary Contact: Darrell Jones, Chief Executive Officer
COO: Alisa Jett, Director Clinical Services
CMO: Vinod Tona, M.D., President Medical Staff
CHR: Tina Stokes, Manager Human Resources
Web address: www.regencyhospital.com
**Control:** Corporation, Investor–owned, for–profit **Service:** Long–Term Acute Care hospital

**Staffed Beds: 40 Admissions: 441 Census: 32 Outpatient Visits: 0 Births: 0 Personnel: 125**

**FORT JACKSON—Richland County**

✠ **MONCRIEF ARMY COMMUNITY HOSPITAL**, 4500 Stuart Street, Zip 29207–5720; tel. 803/751–2160, (Nonreporting) **A**1 3 5 **S** Department of the Army, Office of the Surgeon General, Falls Church, VA
Primary Contact: Colonel Ramona Fiorey, MSN, M.P.H., Commander
CMO: Lieutenant Colonel Larry Andrew, M.D., Deputy Commander Clinical Services
Web address: www.moncrief.amedd.army.mil
**Control:** Army, Government, federal **Service:** General Medical and Surgical

**Staffed Beds: 60**

**GAFFNEY—Cherokee County**

✠ **UPSTATE CAROLINA MEDICAL CENTER (420043)**, 1530 North Limestone Street, Zip 29340–4738; tel. 864/487–4271 **A**1 9 10 **F**3 7 8 11 15 29 30 35 40 45 46 51 57 59 64 67 70 75 76 79 81 82 85 86 87 89 107 108 110 111 113 118 128 129 134 145 146 147 **S** Novant Health, Winston–Salem, NC
Primary Contact: Kimberly Taylor, Chief Operating Officer
CMO: Steven Lewis, M.D., Chief of Staff
CIO: Richard Bledsoe, Director Information Systems
CHR: Connie Gibson, R.N., Director Human Resources
Web address: www.upstatecarolina.org
**Control:** Corporation, Investor–owned, for–profit **Service:** General Medical and Surgical

**Staffed Beds: 125 Admissions: 3338 Census: 35 Outpatient Visits: 38512 Births: 383 Total Expense ($000): 44458 Payroll Expense ($000): 17145 Personnel: 371**

**GEORGETOWN—Georgetown County**

✠ **GEORGETOWN MEMORIAL HOSPITAL (420020)**, 606 Black River Road, Zip 29440–3368, Mailing Address: Drawer 421718, Zip 29442–1718; tel. 843/527–7000 **A**1 2 3 5 9 10 19 **F**3 11 12 13 15 17 18 20 22 26 28 29 30 31 32 34 35 39 40 45 50 52 54 56 57 59 60 61 64 65 68 70 73 74 75 76 77 78 79 81 82 84 85 86 87 89 90 97 100 102 107 108 109 110 111 114 117 118 129 130 131 134 145 146 147 **S** Georgetown Hospital System, Georgetown, SC
Primary Contact: Bruce P. Bailey, Chief Executive Officer
COO: Gayle L. Resetar, Vice President and Chief Operating Officer
CFO: Terry L. Kiser, Vice President and Chief Financial Officer
CMO: Roy E. Gilbreath, M.D., Vice President Medical Affairs
CIO: Frank Scafidi, Vice President and Chief Information Officer
CHR: James F. Harper, Vice President and Chief Human Resources Officer
Web address: www.georgetownhospitalsystem.org
**Control:** Other not–for–profit (including NFP Corporation) **Service:** General Medical and Surgical

**Staffed Beds: 136 Admissions: 5725 Census: 64 Outpatient Visits: 139062 Births: 372 Total Expense ($000): 101057 Payroll Expense ($000): 43423 Personnel: 783**

**GREENVILLE—Greenville County**

✠ △ **BON SECOURS ST. FRANCIS HEALTH SYSTEM (420023)**, One St. Francis Drive, Zip 29601–3207; tel. 864/255–1000, (Includes BON SECOURS ST. FRANCIS EASTSIDE, 125 Commonwealth Drive, Zip 29615–4812; tel. 864/675–4000) **A**1 2 7 9 10 **F**1 3 12 13 15 17 18 20 22 24 26 28 29 30 31 34 35 36 40 44 45 49 50 57 59 60 64 68 70 73 74 75 76 77 78 79 80 81 82 84 85 86 87 89 90 93 96 107 108 110 111 113 114 118 125 127 129 130 131 134 135 144 145 146 147 **P**6 **S** Bon Secours Health System, Inc., Marriottsville, MD
Primary Contact: Mark S. Nantz, FACHE, Chief Executive Officer
CFO: Ronnie Hyatt, Senior Vice President Finance and Chief Financial Officer
CMO: Mary Jo Cagle, M.D., Chief Medical Officer
CIO: Rita Hooker, Administrative Director Information Services
CHR: Lisa C. Slayton, Senior Vice President Human Resources
Web address: www.stfrancishealth.org
**Control:** Other not–for–profit (including NFP Corporation) **Service:** General Medical and Surgical

**Staffed Beds: 331 Admissions: 18405 Census: 215 Outpatient Visits: 92006 Births: 2293 Total Expense ($000): 325491 Payroll Expense ($000): 123642 Personnel: 1401**

✠ △ **GREENVILLE MEMORIAL HOSPITAL (420078)**, 701 Grove Road, Zip 29605–4295; tel. 864/455–7000, (Includes CHILDREN'S HOSPITAL, 701 Grove Road, Zip 29605–5611; tel. 864/455–7000; MARSHALL I. PICKENS HOSPITAL, 701 Grove Road, Zip 29605–5601; tel. 864/455–8988; ROGER C. PEACE REHABILITATION HOSPITAL, 701 Grove Road, tel. 864/455–7000), (Total facility includes 44 beds in nursing home–type unit) **A**1 2 3 5 7 8 9 10 **F**1 3 4 5 11 13 15 17 18 19 20 22 24 26 28 29 30 31 34 35 36 38 39 40 41 43 44 45 46 47 48 49 50 52 53 54 56 57 58 59 61 62 64 65 66 68 70 72 73 74 75 76 77 78 79 81 83 84 85 86 87 88 89 90 92 96 97 98 99 100 101 102 103 104 105 106 107 110 111 113 114 117 118 125 127 128 129 131 133 134 135 140 141 144 145 146 147 **P**6 **S** Greenville Hospital System, Greenville, SC
Primary Contact: Paul F. Johnson, President
CNO: Michelle T. Smith, R.N., Chief Nursing Officer
Web address: www.ghs.org
**Control:** Other not–for–profit (including NFP Corporation) **Service:** General Medical and Surgical

**Staffed Beds: 786 Admissions: 34780 Census: 688 Outpatient Visits: 451051 Births: 4851 Total Expense ($000): 682107 Payroll Expense ($000): 202382 Personnel: 5260**

✠ **PATEWOOD MEMORIAL HOSPITAL (420102)**, 175 Patewood Drive, Zip 29605; tel. 864/797–1000 **A**1 9 10 **F**3 11 29 30 37 50 54 64 77 81 85 107 113 118 127 129 145 **P**6 **S** Greenville Hospital System, Greenville, SC
Primary Contact: Beverly J. Haines, R.N., Interim President
Web address: www.ghs.org/patewood
**Control:** Other not–for–profit (including NFP Corporation) **Service:** General Medical and Surgical

**Staffed Beds: 36 Admissions: 1067 Census: 7 Outpatient Visits: 2388 Births: 0 Total Expense ($000): 38724 Payroll Expense ($000): 9053 Personnel: 161**

✠ **REGENCY HOSPITAL OF GREENVILLE (422009)**, One St. Francis Drive, 4th Floor, Zip 29601; tel. 864/255–1438 **A**1 9 10 **F**1 3 29 34 56 57 60 75 77 82 85 86 87 90 127 129 147 **S** Select Medical Corporation, Mechanicsburg, PA
Primary Contact: Stephanie James, Chief Executive Officer
Web address: www.regencyhospital.com
**Control:** Corporation, Investor–owned, for–profit **Service:** Long–Term Acute Care hospital

**Staffed Beds: 32 Admissions: 334 Census: 25 Outpatient Visits: 0 Births: 0**

☐ **SHRINERS HOSPITALS FOR CHILDREN, GREENVILLE**, 950 West Faris Road, Zip 29605–4277; tel. 864/271–3444 **A**1 3 5 **F**59 64 68 75 77 79 81 85 87 89 90 127 129 130 145 147 **P**6 **S** Shriners Hospitals for Children, Tampa, FL
Primary Contact: Randall R. Romberger, Administrator
CFO: John Conti, Director Finance
CMO: Peter J. Stasikelis, M.D., Chief of Staff
CHR: Willis E. Tisdale, Director Human Resources
CNO: Ranae M. Thompson, MSN, Director Patient Care Services
Web address: www.shrinershospitalsforchildren.org
**Control:** Other not–for–profit (including NFP Corporation) **Service:** Children's orthopedic

**Staffed Beds: 24 Admissions: 458 Census: 3 Outpatient Visits: 30753 Births: 0 Personnel: 157**

*Many Facility Codes have changed. Please refer to the AHA Guide Code Chart.* © 2012 AHA Guide

## GREENWOOD—Greenwood County

☐ **GREENWOOD REGIONAL REHABILITATION HOSPITAL (423030)**, 1530 Parkway, Zip 29646; tel. 864/330–9070, (Total facility includes 12 beds in nursing home–type unit) **A**1 10 **F**1 3 29 75 90 127 129 131 142 147 **S** Ernest Health, Inc., Albuquerque, NM
Primary Contact: Timothy Kagle, Chief Executive Officer
Web address: www.grrh.ernesthealth.com
**Control:** Corporation, Investor–owned, for–profit **Service:** Rehabilitation

**Staffed Beds:** 46 **Admissions:** 1005 **Census:** 36 **Outpatient Visits:** 0 **Births:** 0 **Total Expense ($000):** 12465 **Payroll Expense ($000):** 5667 **Personnel:** 124

✠ **SELF REGIONAL HEALTHCARE (420071)**, 1325 Spring Street, Zip 29646–3860; tel. 864/725–4111 **A**1 2 3 5 9 10 **F**3 8 11 12 13 15 17 18 20 22 24 26 28 29 30 31 32 34 35 39 40 43 49 50 53 54 57 59 60 62 64 68 70 72 73 74 75 76 77 78 79 80 81 82 84 86 87 89 90 97 98 102 107 108 110 111 113 114 118 119 120 122 123 125 128 129 130 131 133 134 143 145 146 147 **P**5 8
Primary Contact: James A. Pfeiffer, FACHE, President and Chief Executive Officer
COO: Fred L. Latham, Executive Vice President and Chief Operating Officer
CFO: Camie Patterson, Senior Vice President Operations and Chief Financial Officer
CMO: F Gregory Mappin, M.D., Vice President Medical Affairs
CIO: Chuck McDevitt, Chief Information Officer
CHR: Michael Dixon, Director Human Resources
Web address: www.selfregional.org
**Control:** City–County, Government, nonfederal **Service:** General Medical and Surgical

**Staffed Beds:** 326 **Admissions:** 13374 **Census:** 159 **Outpatient Visits:** 54729 **Births:** 1543 **Total Expense ($000):** 297315 **Payroll Expense ($000):** 105524 **Personnel:** 2041

## GREER—Greenville County

☐ **CAROLINA CENTER FOR BEHAVIORAL HEALTH (424010)**, 2700 East Phillips Road, Zip 29650–4816; tel. 864/235–2335 **A**1 9 10 **F**4 5 56 98 99 100 101 102 103 104 105 129 **P**6 **S** Universal Health Services, Inc., King of Prussia, PA
Primary Contact: John Willingham, Chief Executive Officer and Managing Director
CFO: Jeff Skelton, Chief Financial Officer
CMO: Ralph Castriotta, M.D., Medical Director
CHR: George Hammett, Director Human Resources
Web address: www.thecarolinacenter.com
**Control:** Corporation, Investor–owned, for–profit **Service:** Psychiatric

**Staffed Beds:** 112 **Admissions:** 3155 **Census:** 94 **Births:** 0 **Total Expense ($000):** 17948 **Payroll Expense ($000):** 9949 **Personnel:** 233

✠ **GREER MEMORIAL HOSPITAL (420033)**, 830 South Bumcombe Road, Zip 29650–2400; tel. 864/848–8200, (Includes ROGER HUNTINGTON NURSING CENTER ) **A**1 9 10 **F**1 3 11 13 15 18 28 29 30 34 35 40 43 44 47 49 50 57 59 61 64 65 68 70 76 77 79 81 82 85 86 87 89 107 110 111 113 118 127 128 129 145 146 **P**6 **S** Greenville Hospital System, Greenville, SC
Primary Contact: John F. Mansure, FACHE, President
Web address: www.ghs.org
**Control:** Other not–for–profit (including NFP Corporation) **Service:** General Medical and Surgical

**Staffed Beds:** 70 **Admissions:** 3603 **Census:** 33 **Outpatient Visits:** 102948 **Births:** 600 **Total Expense ($000):** 68871 **Payroll Expense ($000):** 21929 **Personnel:** 374

✠ **VILLAGE HOSPITAL (420103)**, 250 Westmoreland Road, Zip 29651; tel. 864/530–6000 **A**1 9 10 **F**1 3 11 15 18 29 30 34 35 37 40 45 49 50 54 57 59 64 68 70 74 75 77 79 81 82 84 85 86 87 90 107 108 110 111 113 114 118 127 129 145 **S** Spartanburg Regional Healthcare System, Spartanburg, SC
Primary Contact: J. Philip Feisal, Chief Executive Officer
Web address: www.villageatpelham.com
**Control:** Hospital district or authority, Government, nonfederal **Service:** General Medical and Surgical

**Staffed Beds:** 34 **Admissions:** 1441 **Census:** 14 **Outpatient Visits:** 32573 **Births:** 0 **Total Expense ($000):** 37329 **Payroll Expense ($000):** 12535 **Personnel:** 339

## HARDEEVILLE—Jasper County

✠ **COASTAL CAROLINA HOSPITAL (420101)**, 1000 Medical Center Drive, Zip 29927; tel. 843/784–8000 **A**1 9 10 **F**1 3 11 15 28 29 30 34 35 40 46 47 49 51 57 59 64 70 74 75 77 79 81 85 89 90 107 108 111 113 118 126 127 129 130 132 145 146 147 **S** TENET Healthcare Corporation, Dallas, TX
Primary Contact: William J. Masterton, Chief Executive Officer
COO: Shelly L. Weilenman, R.N., Chief Nursing Officer
CFO: Drew Shea, Assistant Chief Financial Officer
CIO: Carnel Aiken, Director Information Systems
CHR: Darlene Nester, Market Chief Human Resources Officer
Web address: www.coastalhospital.com
**Control:** Corporation, Investor–owned, for–profit **Service:** General Medical and Surgical

**Staffed Beds:** 41 **Admissions:** 1483 **Census:** 14 **Outpatient Visits:** 47814 **Births:** 0 **Total Expense ($000):** 28730 **Payroll Expense ($000):** 10055 **Personnel:** 209

## HARTSVILLE—Darlington County

☐ **CAROLINA PINES REGIONAL MEDICAL CENTER (420010)**, 1304 West Bobo Newsom Highway, Zip 29550–4710; tel. 843/339–2100 **A**1 9 10 **F**3 11 13 15 20 28 29 30 34 35 40 43 46 49 57 59 60 64 70 73 74 75 76 79 81 82 85 86 87 89 90 107 108 111 114 117 118 128 129 130 131 145 146 147 **S** Health Management Associates, Naples, FL
Primary Contact: J. Timothy Browne, FACHE, Chief Executive Officer
CFO: Michael Cherry, Chief Financial Officer
CIO: Denise Barefoot, Director Health Information Systems
CHR: Charlotte Adams, Director Associate Resources
Web address: www.cprmc.com
**Control:** Corporation, Investor–owned, for–profit **Service:** General Medical and Surgical

**Staffed Beds:** 99 **Admissions:** 5323 **Census:** 50 **Outpatient Visits:** 37043 **Births:** 563 **Total Expense ($000):** 62093 **Payroll Expense ($000):** 22651 **Personnel:** 443

## HILTON HEAD ISLAND—Beaufort County

✠ **HILTON HEAD HOSPITAL (420080)**, 25 Hospital Center Boulevard, Zip 29926–2738; tel. 843/681–6122 **A**1 9 10 20 **F**3 11 13 15 17 18 20 22 24 26 28 29 30 32 34 35 40 46 47 48 49 50 51 53 54 57 59 60 61 64 65 68 70 74 76 77 78 79 81 84 85 86 87 89 96 107 110 111 113 114 117 118 127 129 130 131 134 145 146 147 **S** TENET Healthcare Corporation, Dallas, TX
Primary Contact: Mark T. O'Neil, Jr., President and Chief Executive Officer
CFO: Cassie Ball, Chief Financial Officer
CMO: Glenn Neil Love, M.D., Medical Director
CIO: Stephen Brendler, Director Information Systems
CHR: Darlene Nester, Chief Human Resources Officer
Web address: www.hiltonheadregional.com
**Control:** Partnership, Investor–owned, for–profit **Service:** General Medical and Surgical

**Staffed Beds:** 93 **Admissions:** 5019 **Census:** 49 **Births:** 667 **Total Expense ($000):** 86165 **Payroll Expense ($000):** 22159 **Personnel:** 513

## KINGSTREE—Williamsburg County

✠ **WILLIAMSBURG REGIONAL HOSPITAL (421303)**, 500 Nelson Boulevard, Zip 29556–4027; tel. 843/355–8888 **A**1 9 10 18 **F**1 3 11 15 29 30 31 34 35 40 44 50 56 57 59 64 68 77 78 81 86 87 89 90 93 94 97 103 104 107 113 118 126 127 128 129 132 134 145 147
Primary Contact: Mitchell D. Monsour, Interim Chief Executive Officer
COO: Dan Harrington, Chief Operating Officer and Director Human Resources
CFO: Judy Gamble, Chief Financial Officer
CMO: Frank Trefney, M.D., Chief Medical Staff
CIO: Jamie Newsom, Director Information Systems
Web address: www.wmbgrh.com/
**Control:** Other not–for–profit (including NFP Corporation) **Service:** General Medical and Surgical

**Staffed Beds:** 25 **Admissions:** 962 **Census:** 17 **Outpatient Visits:** 19352 **Births:** 0 **Total Expense ($000):** 15079 **Payroll Expense ($000):** 6026 **Personnel:** 168

SC

---

**Hospital, Medicare Provider Number, Address, Telephone, Approval, Facility, and Physician Codes, Health Care System**

★ American Hospital Association (AHA) membership
☐ The Joint Commission accreditation    ◇ DNV Healthcare Inc. accreditation

○ American Osteopathic Association (AOA) accreditation
△ Commission on Accreditation of Rehabilitation Facilities (CARF) accreditation

## LAKE CITY—Florence County

★ **LAKE CITY COMMUNITY HOSPITAL (420066)**, 258 North Ron McNair Boulevard, Zip 29560–1029, Mailing Address: P.O. Box 1479, Zip 29560–1479; tel. 843/374–2036 **A**9 10 **F**11 15 28 29 30 34 35 40 50 56 57 59 61 64 69 75 77 79 81 86 90 107 108 111 113 118 126 129 145
Primary Contact: Henry McCutcheon, Chief Executive Officer
CFO: Henry McCutcheon, Chief Executive Officer
CMO: Daniel DeCamps, M.D., Chief of Staff
CIO: Kimberly Glover, Director Information Systems
CHR: Anne Poston, Human Resources Officer
Web address: www.lcchospital.org
**Control:** Hospital district or authority, Government, nonfederal **Service:** General Medical and Surgical

**Staffed Beds:** 30 **Admissions:** 950 **Census:** 9 **Outpatient Visits:** 17010
**Total Expense ($000):** 15696 **Payroll Expense ($000):** 6609 **Personnel:** 168

## LANCASTER—Lancaster County

✠ **SPRINGS MEMORIAL HOSPITAL (420036)**, 800 West Meeting Street, Zip 29720–2298; tel. 803/286–1214, (Total facility includes 14 beds in nursing home–type unit) **A**1 5 9 10 **F**1 3 8 11 13 15 17 18 20 29 31 34 35 40 43 47 48 49 51 57 59 60 62 63 64 68 70 73 74 75 76 78 79 81 85 89 90 102 107 108 110 111 113 114 117 118 127 128 131 134 145 146 **S** Community Health Systems, Inc., Franklin, TN
Primary Contact: Douglas T. Arbour, Chief Executive Officer
CFO: Nathan Crabtree, Chief Financial Officer
CMO: Keith Shealy, M.D., Chief of Staff
CIO: Chrys Steele, Director Information Systems
CHR: Trent Elmore, Director Human Resources
Web address: www.springsmemorial.com
**Control:** Corporation, Investor–owned, for–profit **Service:** General Medical and Surgical

**Staffed Beds:** 186 **Admissions:** 7892 **Census:** 99 **Outpatient Visits:** 39082
**Births:** 701 **Total Expense ($000):** 89149 **Payroll Expense ($000):** 28744
**Personnel:** 653

## LORIS—Horry County

✠ **MCLEOD LORIS HEALTHCARE (420064)**, 3655 Mitchell Street, Box 690001, Zip 29569–9601; tel. 843/716–7000, (Total facility includes 88 beds in nursing home–type unit) **A**1 9 10 **F**1 3 11 15 17 18 20 28 29 30 32 34 40 44 50 53 57 59 60 64 65 68 70 74 75 76 77 79 80 81 82 84 85 86 87 89 90 96 107 108 110 111 114 117 118 126 127 128 129 130 131 133 134 145 147 **P**6
Primary Contact: Edward D. Tinsley, III, Chief Executive Officer
COO: Arnold Green, Senior Vice President and Chief Operating Officer
CFO: Fred O. Todd, Senior Vice President Finance
CMO: James N. Craigie, M.D., Vice President Medical Affairs
CHR: Teresa Pougnaud, Vice President Human Resources
Web address: www.lorishealth.org
**Control:** Hospital district or authority, Government, nonfederal **Service:** General Medical and Surgical

**Staffed Beds:** 193 **Admissions:** 3528 **Census:** 117 **Outpatient Visits:** 109237 **Births:** 427 **Total Expense ($000):** 99865 **Payroll Expense ($000):** 40032 **Personnel:** 676

## MANNING—Clarendon County

✠ **CLARENDON MEMORIAL HOSPITAL (420069)**, 10 Hospital Street, Zip 29102–3153, Mailing Address: P.O. Box 550, Zip 29102–0550; tel. 803/435–8463 **A**1 9 10 **F**1 3 7 11 13 15 28 29 30 35 39 40 45 50 53 54 56 57 59 62 64 65 67 70 75 76 77 79 81 82 85 89 90 91 96 107 108 110 111 113 117 118 126 127 128 129 131 134 142 145 146 147
Primary Contact: Edward R. Frye, Jr., Chief Executive Officer
COO: Eleyce Winn, Assistant Administrator
CFO: Richard Stokes, CPA, Chief Financial Officer
CMO: Beryl Bachus Keith, M.D., Chief of Staff
CIO: Pat Kolb, Manager Information Technology
CHR: Gail R. Duke, Director Human Resources
Web address: www.clarendonhealth.com
**Control:** Hospital district or authority, Government, nonfederal **Service:** General Medical and Surgical

**Staffed Beds:** 56 **Admissions:** 2570 **Census:** 31 **Outpatient Visits:** 138747
**Births:** 615 **Personnel:** 519

## MOUNT PLEASANT—Charleston County

✠ **EAST COOPER MEDICAL CENTER (420089)**, 2000 Hospital Drive, Zip 29464–3294; tel. 843/881–0100 **A**1 5 9 10 **F**3 13 15 18 29 31 34 35 40 43 46 57 58 59 64 70 73 74 75 76 77 78 79 80 81 82 84 85 86 90 107 108 110 111 113 114 118 128 129 130 131 134 145 146 147 **S** TENET Healthcare Corporation, Dallas, TX
Primary Contact: Jason P. Alexander, FACHE, Chief Executive Officer
CFO: Steve Woodford, Chief Financial Officer
CMO: W. John Langley, M.D., Chairman
CIO: Jack Goynes, Director Information Resources
CHR: Mike Gilpen, Director Human Resources
Web address: www.eastcoopermedctr.com
**Control:** Corporation, Investor–owned, for–profit **Service:** General Medical and Surgical

**Staffed Beds:** 140 **Admissions:** 4559 **Census:** 42 **Outpatient Visits:** 58031
**Births:** 1428 **Total Expense ($000):** 100754 **Payroll Expense ($000):** 26137 **Personnel:** 434

**EAST COOPER REGIONAL MEDICAL CENTER** See East Cooper Medical Center

✠ **MOUNT PLEASANT HOSPITAL (420104)**, 3500 North Highway 17, Zip 29466–9123; tel. 843/606–7000 **A**1 9 10 **F**3 7 13 15 29 30 34 40 45 57 68 70 75 76 79 81 84 85 86 87 89 107 108 110 111 114 117 118 128 142 146 147 **S** Carolinas HealthCare System, Charlotte, NC
Primary Contact: John Sullivan, Chief Executive Officer
Web address: www.mymountpleasanthospital.com
**Control:** Other not–for–profit (including NFP Corporation) **Service:** General Medical and Surgical

**Staffed Beds:** 50 **Admissions:** 1340 **Census:** 10 **Outpatient Visits:** 29651
**Births:** 369 **Total Expense ($000):** 44535 **Payroll Expense ($000):** 13974 **Personnel:** 268

## MULLINS—Marion County

**MARION COUNTY MEDICAL CENTER** See Marion Regional Hospital

✠ **MARION REGIONAL HOSPITAL (420055)**, 2829 East Highway 76, Zip 29574–6035, Mailing Address: P.O. Drawer 1150, Marion, Zip 29571–1150; tel. 843/431–2000 **A**1 9 10 **F**1 3 13 15 18 28 29 30 34 40 45 46 51 70 76 77 79 81 82 85 86 89 90 107 118 127 128 129 134 145 147 **P**6 **S** Community Health Systems, Inc., Franklin, TN
Primary Contact: David Cope, Chief Executive Officer
CFO: Alta DuBose, Chief Financial Officer
CMO: Alvin Abinsay, M.D., Chief Medical Staff
CIO: Charlie Grantham, Manager Information Systems
CHR: Kay White, Director Human Resources and Diversity
Web address: www.carolinashospitalmarion.com/Pages/Home.aspx
**Control:** Corporation, Investor–owned, for–profit **Service:** General Medical and Surgical

**Staffed Beds:** 124 **Admissions:** 3425 **Census:** 33 **Outpatient Visits:** 24490
**Total Expense ($000):** 61399 **Payroll Expense ($000):** 18902 **Personnel:** 333

## MURRELLS INLET—Georgetown County

✠ △ **WACCAMAW COMMUNITY HOSPITAL (420098)**, 4070 Highway 17 Bypass, Zip 29576, Mailing Address: P.O. Drawer 3350, Zip 29576; tel. 843/652–1000 **A**1 2 9 10 **F**3 11 13 15 17 18 29 30 31 32 35 37 39 40 45 50 51 56 60 61 65 68 70 73 74 75 76 77 78 79 81 82 84 85 86 87 89 90 96 97 100 102 107 108 109 110 111 114 117 118 129 145 146 147 **S** Georgetown Hospital System, Georgetown, SC
Primary Contact: Gayle L. Resetar, Chief Operating Officer
CFO: Terry L. Kiser, Chief Financial Officer
CIO: Gary Praznik, Chief Information Officer
Web address: www.gmhsc.com
**Control:** Other not–for–profit (including NFP Corporation) **Service:** General Medical and Surgical

**Staffed Beds:** 169 **Admissions:** 8413 **Census:** 116 **Outpatient Visits:** 87361
**Births:** 584 **Total Expense ($000):** 119697 **Payroll Expense ($000):** 33056 **Personnel:** 614

## MYRTLE BEACH—Horry County

✠ **GRAND STRAND REGIONAL MEDICAL CENTER (420085)**, 809 82nd Parkway, Zip 29572–1413; tel. 843/692–1000 **A**1 2 9 10 19 **F**3 11 13 15 17 18 20 22 24 26 28 29 30 31 34 35 37 39 40 42 43 46 47 49 50 54 56 57 59 60 64 70 73 74 75 76 77 78 79 81 82 85 86 87 89 90 107 108 110 111 113 114 117 118 125 129 131 134 145 146 **S** HCA, Nashville, TN
Primary Contact: Doug White, Chief Executive Officer
CFO: Turner Wortham, Chief Financial Officer
Web address: www.grandstrandmed.com
**Control:** Corporation, Investor–owned, for–profit **Service:** General Medical and Surgical

**Staffed Beds:** 221 **Admissions:** 15235 **Census:** 177 **Births:** 1005 **Total Expense ($000):** 177072 **Personnel:** 1050

*Many Facility Codes have changed. Please refer to the AHA Guide Code Chart.* © 2012 AHA Guide

## NEWBERRY—Newberry County

☒ **NEWBERRY COUNTY MEMORIAL HOSPITAL (420053)**, 2669 Kinard Street, Zip 29108–0497, Mailing Address: P.O. Box 497, Zip 29108–0497; tel. 803/276–7570 **A**1 9 10 20 **F**1 3 7 11 13 15 17 28 29 30 31 32 34 35 40 45 47 53 56 57 59 64 68 70 75 76 77 78 79 81 82 85 86 87 89 90 103 104 107 108 109 110 111 113 118 127 128 129 132 134 142 145 146 147 **P**6 **S** QHR, Brentwood, TN
Primary Contact: Ronald J. Vigus, Chief Executive Officer
CFO: Steve Anderson, Interim Chief Financial Officer
CMO: Oscar Lovelace, M.D., Chief of Staff
CIO: David Wolff, Director Information Technology
CHR: Dyan Bowman, Director Human Resources
Web address: www.newberryhospital.org
**Control:** County–Government, nonfederal **Service:** General Medical and Surgical

**Staffed Beds:** 32 **Admissions:** 2292 **Census:** 25 **Outpatient Visits:** 65912 **Births:** 334 **Total Expense ($000):** 43177 **Payroll Expense ($000):** 17139 **Personnel:** 369

## ORANGEBURG—Orangeburg County

☒ **REGIONAL MEDICAL CENTER (420068)**, 3000 St. Matthews Road, Zip 29118–1470; tel. 803/395–2200 **A**1 2 9 10 19 **F**3 11 13 14 15 17 18 20 28 29 30 31 32 34 35 39 40 43 44 45 46 47 48 50 53 57 59 60 61 62 65 68 70 73 74 75 76 77 78 79 81 82 84 85 86 87 89 90 97 98 100 101 102 103 107 108 110 111 113 114 118 120 126 128 129 130 131 133 134 143 145 146 147 **S** QHR, Brentwood, TN
Primary Contact: Thomas C. Dandridge, FACHE, President and Chief Executive Officer
CFO: Cheryl S. Mason, Chief Financial Officer
CIO: Marilyn Tremblay, Director Information
CHR: Howard Harris, Vice President Human Resources
Web address: www.trmchealth.org
**Control:** City–County, Government, nonfederal **Service:** General Medical and Surgical

**Staffed Beds:** 286 **Admissions:** 10848 **Census:** 156 **Outpatient Visits:** 68432 **Births:** 1210 **Total Expense ($000):** 183563 **Payroll Expense ($000):** 81105 **Personnel:** 1275

☐ **WILLIAM J. MCCORD ADOLESCENT AND TREATMENT CENTER (424013)**, 910 Cook Road, Zip 29116, Mailing Address: P.O. Box 1166, Zip 29116–1166; tel. 803/534–2328 **A**1 10 **F**4 5 34 35 38 57 61 98 99 131 133 134
Primary Contact: Michael Dennis, Director
Web address: www.mccordcenter.com
**Control:** Other not–for–profit (including NFP Corporation) **Service:** Psychiatric

**Staffed Beds:** 15 **Admissions:** 118 **Census:** 14 **Outpatient Visits:** 0 **Births:** 0 **Personnel:** 45

## PICKENS—Pickens County

★ **CANNON MEMORIAL HOSPITAL (420011)**, 123 West G. Acker Drive, Zip 29671–2739, Mailing Address: P.O. Box 188, Zip 29671–0188; tel. 864/878–4791, (Nonreporting) **A**9 10 21 **S** Carolinas HealthCare System, Charlotte, NC
Primary Contact: Norman G. Rentz, President and Chief Executive Officer
CFO: Mary F. Arnette, Chief Financial Officer
CMO: Daniel J. Dahlhausen, M.D., Chief of Staff
CHR: Lisa G. Bryant, Director Human Resources
Web address: www.cannonhospital.org
**Control:** Other not–for–profit (including NFP Corporation) **Service:** General Medical and Surgical

**Staffed Beds:** 42

## ROCK HILL—York County

☒ **HEALTHSOUTH REHABILITATION HOSPITAL (423028)**, 1795 Dr. Frank Gaston Boulevard, Zip 29732; tel. 803/326–3500 **A**1 10 **F**29 56 64 75 90 95 129 **S** HEALTHSOUTH Corporation, Birmingham, AL
Primary Contact: Anthony W. Jackson, Chief Executive Officer
Web address: www.healthsouthrockhill.com
**Control:** Corporation, Investor–owned, for–profit **Service:** Rehabilitation

**Staffed Beds:** 46 **Admissions:** 1005 **Census:** 37 **Total Expense ($000):** 10555 **Payroll Expense ($000):** 5875 **Personnel:** 91

☒ **PIEDMONT MEDICAL CENTER (420002)**, 222 Herlong Avenue, Zip 29732–1952; tel. 803/329–1234 **A**1 2 9 10 **F**3 7 11 12 13 15 17 18 20 22 24 28 29 30 31 34 35 40 43 45 49 50 57 59 60 64 70 73 74 75 76 77 78 79 81 82 85 86 89 90 98 100 102 107 108 110 111 113 114 117 118 129 131 134 145 146 147 **S** TENET Healthcare Corporation, Dallas, TX
Primary Contact: Charles F. Miller, President and Chief Executive Officer
COO: Claudia Douglass, Chief Operating Officer
CFO: Jay M. Pennisson, Chief Financial Officer
CMO: Richard Patteson, M.D., Chief Medical Officer
CIO: Joel Dean, Director Information Services
CHR: Donald L. Currier, Vice President Human Resources
Web address: www.piedmontmedicalcenter.com
**Control:** Corporation, Investor–owned, for–profit **Service:** General Medical and Surgical

**Staffed Beds:** 281 **Admissions:** 14901 **Census:** 186 **Outpatient Visits:** 61017 **Total Expense ($000):** 197698 **Payroll Expense ($000):** 70444 **Personnel:** 966

## SENECA—Oconee County

☒ **OCONEE MEDICAL CENTER (420009)**, 298 Memorial Drive, Zip 29672–9499; tel. 864/882–3351, (Includes LILA DOYLE NURSING CARE FACILITY ), (Total facility includes 120 beds in nursing home–type unit) **A**1 9 10 **F**3 7 11 13 15 20 28 29 30 31 34 35 40 54 56 57 59 61 62 63 64 67 70 71 74 75 76 77 78 79 81 82 85 86 87 89 90 97 100 107 108 113 118 127 129 131 134 142 145 147 **P**8
Primary Contact: Jeanne L. Ward, Ed.D., R.N., President and Chief Executive Officer
COO: Hunter Kome, Vice President Operations
CFO: Kevin Herbert, Chief Financial Officer
CMO: Conrad K. Shuler, M.D., Chief Medical Officer
CIO: Jay Hansen, Director Information Services
CHR: Thomas C. Conley, Senior Director Human Resources
Web address: www.oconeemed.org
**Control:** Other not–for–profit (including NFP Corporation) **Service:** General Medical and Surgical

**Staffed Beds:** 248 **Admissions:** 7750 **Census:** 193 **Outpatient Visits:** 48333 **Births:** 574 **Personnel:** 1162

## SIMPSONVILLE—Greenville County

☒ **HILLCREST MEMORIAL HOSPITAL (420037)**, 729 S.E. Main Street, Zip 29681–3280; tel. 864/454–6100 **A**1 9 10 **F**1 3 11 12 15 18 29 30 35 40 44 45 50 57 58 59 61 64 68 70 79 81 85 86 90 107 110 111 113 118 128 129 131 134 145 **P**6 **S** Greenville Hospital System, Greenville, SC
Primary Contact: Eric Bour, M.D., President
CFO: Pam DeVore, Financial Manager
Web address: www.ghs.org
**Control:** Other not–for–profit (including NFP Corporation) **Service:** General Medical and Surgical

**Staffed Beds:** 43 **Admissions:** 2002 **Census:** 18 **Outpatient Visits:** 66027 **Births:** 0 **Total Expense ($000):** 46029 **Payroll Expense ($000):** 13908 **Personnel:** 225

## SPARTANBURG—Spartanburg County

☒ △ **MARY BLACK MEMORIAL HOSPITAL (420083)**, 1700 Skylyn Drive, Zip 29307–1061, Mailing Address: P.O. Box 3217, Zip 29304–3217; tel. 864/573–3000 **A**1 7 9 10 **F**3 11 13 15 18 19 20 29 31 34 35 37 40 45 46 47 49 50 54 57 59 64 70 73 75 76 77 78 79 81 85 86 87 89 90 98 103 107 108 109 110 111 113 114 117 118 123 125 127 129 130 140 141 145 146 147 **P**8 **S** Community Health Systems, Inc., Franklin, TN
Primary Contact: Douglas J. Moyer, Chief Executive Officer
COO: David Cope, Chief Operating Officer
CFO: Richard A. Meyer, Chief Financial Officer
CIO: Jeff Nash, Director Information Technology and Services
CHR: Amy Martin, Director Human Resources
Web address: www.maryblack.org
**Control:** Corporation, Investor–owned, for–profit **Service:** General Medical and Surgical

**Staffed Beds:** 181 **Admissions:** 7041 **Census:** 94 **Outpatient Visits:** 45868 **Births:** 964 **Personnel:** 764

☒ **SPARTANBURG HOSPITAL FOR RESTORATIVE CARE (422004)**, 389 Serpentine Drive, Zip 29303–3026; tel. 864/560–3280 **A**1 9 10 **F**1 29 30 31 35 57 59 60 68 70 75 77 79 82 84 85 87 90 118 127 129 147 **S** Spartanburg Regional Healthcare System, Spartanburg, SC
Primary Contact: Anita M. Butler, Chief Executive Officer
Web address: www.srhs.com
**Control:** Hospital district or authority, Government, nonfederal **Service:** Long–Term Acute Care hospital

**Staffed Beds:** 91 **Admissions:** 383 **Census:** 33 **Total Expense ($000):** 22368 **Payroll Expense ($000):** 11400 **Personnel:** 200

---

**Hospital, Medicare Provider Number, Address, Telephone, Approval, Facility, and Physician Codes, Health Care System**

★ American Hospital Association (AHA) membership
☐ The Joint Commission accreditation
◇ DNV Healthcare Inc. accreditation
○ American Osteopathic Association (AOA) accreditation
△ Commission on Accreditation of Rehabilitation Facilities (CARF) accreditation

**SC**

★ **SPARTANBURG REGIONAL MEDICAL CENTER (420007)**, 101 East Wood Street, Zip 29303–3016; tel. 864/560–6000, (Total facility includes 25 beds in nursing home–type unit) **A**2 3 5 9 10 13 **F**3 7 11 12 13 15 17 18 20 22 24 26 28 29 30 31 34 35 36 37 38 39 40 43 45 46 47 48 49 50 53 54 56 57 58 59 60 61 62 63 64 65 66 68 70 71 72 73 74 75 76 77 78 79 81 82 83 84 85 86 87 88 89 90 97 98 99 100 101 102 103 104 105 107 108 110 111 113 114 116 117 118 119 120 122 123 125 128 129 130 131 134 142 143 144 145 146 147 **P**1 2 **S** Spartanburg Regional Healthcare System, Spartanburg, SC
Primary Contact: J. Philip Feisal, Senior Vice President Acute Care Hospitals
CMO: Robert Flandry, M.D., Vice President and Chief Medical Officer
CHR: Kathy Sinclair, Vice President Human Resources
Web address: www.spartanburgregional.com
**Control:** Hospital district or authority, Government, nonfederal **Service:** General Medical and Surgical

**Staffed Beds:** 539 **Admissions:** 27324 **Census:** 412 **Outpatient Visits:** 122694 **Births:** 2763 **Total Expense ($000):** 561273 **Payroll Expense ($000):** 208590 **Personnel:** 3524

### SUMTER—Sumter County

✦ **TUOMEY HEALTHCARE SYSTEM (420070)**, 129 North Washington Street, Zip 29150–4983; tel. 803/774–9000, (Total facility includes 18 beds in nursing home–type unit) **A**1 9 10 **F**3 13 15 20 28 29 30 31 32 34 35 40 48 49 50 51 54 56 59 60 62 63 64 68 70 73 75 76 77 78 79 80 81 85 86 87 89 90 93 102 107 108 110 111 113 116 118 120 127 128 129 130 131 134 145 146 147 **P**6
Primary Contact: Jay Cox, FACHE, President and Chief Executive Officer
COO: Gregg Martin, Senior Vice President and Chief Operating Officer
CFO: Michael H. Winiarski, FACHE, Vice President and Chief Financial Officer
CMO: Gene Dickerson, M.D., Vice President Medical Affairs
CIO: Cheryl Martin, Chief Information Officer
CHR: Letitia Pringle–Miller, Administrative Director
Web address: www.tuomey.com
**Control:** Other not–for–profit (including NFP Corporation) **Service:** General Medical and Surgical

**Staffed Beds:** 260 **Admissions:** 8848 **Census:** 197 **Outpatient Visits:** 131855 **Births:** 1284

### TRAVELERS REST—Greenville County

✦ **NORTH GREENVILLE HOSPITAL (422008)**, 807 North Main Street, Zip 29690–0628; tel. 864/834–5132 **A**1 9 10 **F**1 3 15 29 30 34 35 40 44 50 58 64 68 75 79 85 86 87 107 110 111 113 127 129 145 147 **P**6
Primary Contact: Michael Batchelor, President
Web address: www.ghs.org
**Control:** Other not–for–profit (including NFP Corporation) **Service:** Long–Term Acute Care hospital

**Staffed Beds:** 29 **Admissions:** 281 **Census:** 23 **Outpatient Visits:** 38989 **Births:** 0 **Total Expense ($000):** 24914 **Payroll Expense ($000):** 8511 **Personnel:** 152

☐ **SPRINGBROOK BEHAVIORAL HEALTH SYSTEM (424007)**, One Havenwood Lane, Zip 29690, Mailing Address: P.O. Box 1005, Zip 29690–1005; tel. 864/834–8013, (Total facility includes 68 beds in nursing home–type unit) **A**1 9 10 **F**98 99 104 106 129
Primary Contact: C. Keith Jackson, Chief Executive Officer
CFO: Bart Bennett, Chief Financial Officer
CMO: April Richardson, M.D., Medical Director
CIO: Lateka Benson, Manager Health Information
CHR: Steve Ivester, Director Human Resources
CNO: Francine Lopomo, R.N., Director of Nursing
Web address: www.springbrookbehavioral.com
**Control:** Corporation, Investor–owned, for–profit **Service:** Psychiatric

**Staffed Beds:** 88 **Admissions:** 555 **Census:** 69 **Outpatient Visits:** 1452 **Births:** 0 **Personnel:** 178

### UNION—Union County

✦ **WALLACE THOMSON HOSPITAL (420039)**, 322 West South Street, Zip 29379–2857, Mailing Address: P.O. Box 789, Zip 29379–0789; tel. 864/427–0351, (Total facility includes 112 beds in nursing home–type unit) **A**1 9 10 **F**1 3 7 13 15 29 34 35 40 57 59 64 69 70 75 76 79 81 82 86 87 89 107 111 118 128 129 134 145 146
Primary Contact: Hamilton Hudson, Interim Chief Executive Officer
CFO: Jeff W. Rush, Chief Financial Officer
CIO: Billy Helmandollar, Director Information Services
CHR: Michelle Helton, Director Human Resources
Web address: www.wallacethomson.com
**Control:** Hospital district or authority, Government, nonfederal **Service:** General Medical and Surgical

**Staffed Beds:** 171 **Admissions:** 2701 **Census:** 135 **Outpatient Visits:** 35343 **Births:** 65 **Total Expense ($000):** 31829 **Payroll Expense ($000):** 11469 **Personnel:** 389

### VARNVILLE—Hampton County

★ **HAMPTON REGIONAL MEDICAL CENTER (420072)**, 503 Carolina Avenue West, Zip 29944, Mailing Address: P.O. Box 338, Zip 29944–0338; tel. 803/943–2771 **A**9 10 20 **F**15 17 18 24 28 29 34 35 40 57 59 64 67 70 77 79 81 90 107 108 110 111 113 118 126 128 129 145
Primary Contact: Dave H. Hamill, President and Chief Executive Officer
Web address: www.hamptonregional.com
**Control:** Other not–for–profit (including NFP Corporation) **Service:** General Medical and Surgical

**Staffed Beds:** 32 **Admissions:** 972 **Census:** 10 **Outpatient Visits:** 12630 **Personnel:** 168

### WALTERBORO—Colleton County

✦ **COLLETON MEDICAL CENTER (420030)**, 501 Robertson Boulevard, Zip 29488–5714; tel. 843/782–2000 **A**1 9 10 20 **F**3 11 13 15 18 26 29 30 32 34 35 36 40 45 47 49 56 57 59 60 64 65 68 70 75 76 77 79 81 82 85 86 87 89 90 96 98 102 107 108 110 111 113 118 128 129 130 131 145 146 147 **P**5 **S** HCA, Nashville, TN
Primary Contact: Mitchell P. Mongell, FACHE, Chief Executive Officer
COO: Tony Taylor, Vice President Operations
CFO: Ronnie Midgett, Chief Financial Officer
CMO: Kim Rakes–Stephens, M.D., Chief Medical Staff
CHR: Alysia Price, Director Human Resources
Web address: www.colletonmedical.com
**Control:** Corporation, Investor–owned, for–profit **Service:** General Medical and Surgical

**Staffed Beds:** 131 **Admissions:** 4495 **Census:** 59 **Outpatient Visits:** 28786 **Births:** 339 **Total Expense ($000):** 57686 **Payroll Expense ($000):** 19600 **Personnel:** 320

### WEST COLUMBIA—Lexington County

★ **LEXINGTON MEDICAL CENTER (420073)**, 2720 Sunset Boulevard, Zip 29169–4816; tel. 803/791–2000 **A**2 9 10 21 **F**3 11 12 13 15 18 20 22 28 29 30 31 32 34 35 38 39 40 43 44 45 48 49 50 53 54 57 58 59 60 61 64 68 70 73 74 75 76 77 78 79 80 81 82 85 86 87 89 90 92 107 108 110 111 113 114 117 118 119 120 122 126 128 129 130 131 134 140 141 143 144 145 146 147 **P**6
Primary Contact: Michael J. Biediger, FACHE, President and Chief Executive Officer
COO: Tod Augsburger, Senior Vice President and Chief Operating Officer
CFO: Melinda Kruzner, Chief Financial Officer
CMO: Aubrey Miller, M.D., Chief of Staff
CHR: Kathy A. Howell, Vice President Human Resources
Web address: www.lexmed.com
**Control:** Hospital district or authority, Government, nonfederal **Service:** General Medical and Surgical

**Staffed Beds:** 377 **Admissions:** 18511 **Census:** 247 **Outpatient Visits:** 113126 **Births:** 2946 **Total Expense ($000):** 374734 **Payroll Expense ($000):** 151730 **Personnel:** 2996

☐ **THREE RIVERS BEHAVIORAL HEALTH (424008)**, 2900 Sunset Boulevard, Zip 29169–3422; tel. 803/796–9911, (Total facility includes 20 beds in nursing home–type unit) **A**1 9 10 **F**4 5 35 98 99 100 101 103 104 105 106 **S** Universal Health Services, Inc., King of Prussia, PA
Primary Contact: Jeffrey Barnett, Chief Executive Officer
CFO: Christopher Jensen, Chief Financial Officer
CMO: Cheryl Dodds, M.D., Medical Director
CHR: Nita Sundberg, Director Human Resources
CNO: Regena Sellers, Chief Nursing Officer
Web address: www.threeriversbehavioral.org
**Control:** Corporation, Investor–owned, for–profit **Service:** Psychiatric

**Staffed Beds:** 98 **Admissions:** 2485 **Census:** 91 **Outpatient Visits:** 0 **Births:** 0 **Personnel:** 152

### WINNSBORO—Fairfield County

☐ **FAIRFIELD MEMORIAL HOSPITAL (421302)**, 102 U.S. Highway 321 By–Pass N., Zip 29180–9251, Mailing Address: P.O. Box 620, Zip 29180–0620; tel. 803/635–5548, (Nonreporting) **A**1 5 9 10 18
Primary Contact: Michael Williams, FACHE, Administrator
CFO: Anne Bass, Chief Financial Officer
CMO: Larry D. Cantey, M.D., Chief Medical Officer
CIO: Reynolds Searle, Director Information Systems
CHR: Shawna Martin Lyde, Director Human Resources
Web address: www.fairfieldmemorial.com
**Control:** County–Government, nonfederal **Service:** General Medical and Surgical

**Staffed Beds:** 25

**SC**

# SOUTH DAKOTA

## ABERDEEN—Brown County

★ △ **AVERA ST. LUKE'S HOSPITAL (430014)**, 305 South State Street, Zip 57402–4450; tel. 605/622–5000, (Total facility includes 137 beds in nursing home–type unit) **A**2 7 9 10 20 **F**2 3 5 7 10 11 13 15 17 18 20 22 28 29 30 31 32 34 35 36 39 40 45 46 48 56 57 59 60 61 62 63 64 70 71 74 75 76 77 78 79 81 82 84 85 86 87 89 90 92 93 96 97 98 99 100 101 102 103 104 107 108 110 111 113 114 117 118 119 120 122 124 126 127 128 129 130 131 132 134 145 146 147 **P**6 **S** Avera Health, Sioux Falls, SD
Primary Contact: Todd Forkel, President and Chief Executive Officer
COO: K. C. DeBoer, Vice President
CFO: Geoff Durst, Vice President Finance
CMO: John Fritz, D.O., Vice President Medical Affairs
CIO: Julie Kusler, Manager Information Services
CHR: Mary Davis, Vice President
Web address: www.averastlukes.org
**Control:** Church–operated, Nongovernment, not–for profit **Service:** General Medical and Surgical

**Staffed Beds:** 270 **Admissions:** 6100 **Census:** 201 **Outpatient Visits:** 257853 **Births:** 744 **Total Expense ($000):** 147134 **Payroll Expense ($000):** 72780 **Personnel:** 1110

**DAKOTA PLAINS SURGICAL CENTER (430092)**, 701 8th Avenue N.W., Suite C., Zip 57401; tel. 605/225–3300, (Nonreporting) **A**9 10
Primary Contact: Charles Livingston, Administrator
**Control:** Corporation, Investor–owned, for–profit **Service:** Surgical

**Staffed Beds:** 15

## ARMOUR—Douglas County

**DOUGLAS COUNTY MEMORIAL HOSPITAL (431305)**, 708 Eighth Street, Zip 57313–2102; tel. 605/724–2159 **A**9 10 18 **F**3 7 10 13 15 28 31 34 35 40 45 53 57 59 62 64 65 69 76 77 81 93 107 111 118 126 132 **P**6
Primary Contact: Heath Brouwer, Administrator
CFO: Dorothy Spease, Manager Business Office
Web address: www.dcmhsd.org
**Control:** Other not–for–profit (including NFP Corporation) **Service:** General Medical and Surgical

**Staffed Beds:** 11 **Admissions:** 251 **Census:** 2 **Outpatient Visits:** 10836 **Births:** 28 **Total Expense ($000):** 7875 **Payroll Expense ($000):** 3247 **Personnel:** 73

## BOWDLE—Edmunds County

★ **BOWDLE HOSPITAL (431318)**, 8001 West Fifth Street, Zip 57428–0566, Mailing Address: P.O. Box 556, Zip 57428–0556; tel. 605/285–6146, (Total facility includes 36 beds in nursing home–type unit) **A**9 10 18 **F**2 7 10 28 40 45 53 59 65 126 127 132
Primary Contact: Sandy Schlechter, Chief Executive Officer
CMO: Janice Lumnitz, M.D., Chief of Staff
CIO: Kim Miller, Chief Information Officer
Web address: www.bowdlehc.com
**Control:** City–Government, nonfederal **Service:** General Medical and Surgical

**Staffed Beds:** 48 **Admissions:** 283 **Census:** 36 **Outpatient Visits:** 3532 **Births:** 0 **Total Expense ($000):** 3177 **Payroll Expense ($000):** 2054 **Personnel:** 76

## BRITTON—Marshall County

★ **MARSHALL COUNTY HEALTHCARE CENTER AVERA (431312)**, 413 Ninth Street, Zip 57430; tel. 605/448–2253 **A**9 10 18 **F**10 11 28 29 34 35 40 41 53 57 59 62 64 65 77 86 87 132 145 **P**5 **S** Avera Health, Sioux Falls, SD
Primary Contact: Nick Fosness, Chief Executive Officer
Web address: www.avera.org
**Control:** Other not–for–profit (including NFP Corporation) **Service:** General Medical and Surgical

**Staffed Beds:** 18 **Admissions:** 230 **Census:** 3 **Outpatient Visits:** 5453 **Births:** 0 **Total Expense ($000):** 4986 **Payroll Expense ($000):** 2278 **Personnel:** 79

## BROOKINGS—Brookings County

★ **BROOKINGS HEALTH SYSTEM (430008)**, 300 22nd Avenue, Zip 57006–2496; tel. 605/696–9000, (Total facility includes 79 beds in nursing home–type unit) **A**9 10 20 **F**3 7 11 13 28 29 30 31 32 34 35 40 43 45 57 59 62 63 64 69 70 75 76 77 81 84 85 87 89 93 96 107 111 113 117 118 124 126 127 128 129 131 132 145 146 147
Primary Contact: Jason R. Merkley, Chief Executive Officer
CFO: Kevin Coffey, Chief Financial Officer
CMO: Merritt Warren, M.D., Medical Director and Chief of Staff
CHR: September Bessler, Manager Human Resources
Web address: www.brookingshealth.org
**Control:** City–Government, nonfederal **Service:** General Medical and Surgical

**Staffed Beds:** 128 **Admissions:** 1076 **Census:** 81 **Outpatient Visits:** 9860 **Births:** 248 **Total Expense ($000):** 29885 **Payroll Expense ($000):** 15020 **Personnel:** 331

## BURKE—Gregory County

★ **COMMUNITY MEMORIAL HOSPITAL (431309)**, 809 Jackson Street, Zip 57523, Mailing Address: P.O. Box 319, Zip 57523–0319; tel. 605/775–2621 **A**9 10 18 **F**3 11 28 31 34 40 57 59 65 67 87 97 107 113 126 127 132 **P**5 **S** Sanford Health, Sioux Falls, SD
Primary Contact: Jim Frank, Chief Executive Officer
CMO: Teresa Marts, M.D., Chief Medical Staff
CHR: Tami Lyon, Director Human Resources
Web address: www.sanfordhealth.org
**Control:** Other not–for–profit (including NFP Corporation) **Service:** General Medical and Surgical

**Staffed Beds:** 16 **Admissions:** 208 **Census:** 5 **Outpatient Visits:** 1736 **Births:** 0 **Total Expense ($000):** 3674 **Payroll Expense ($000):** 1822 **Personnel:** 51

## CANTON—Lincoln County

★ **SANFORD CANTON–INWOOD MEDICAL CENTER (431333)**, 440 North Hiawatha Drive, Zip 57013–9404; tel. 605/987–2621 **A**9 10 18 **F**10 28 40 45 59 64 71 77 81 93 107 129 132 **S** Sanford Health, Sioux Falls, SD
Primary Contact: Eric C. Hilmoe, Chief Executive Officer
CFO: Paul Gerhart, Chief Financial Officer
Web address: www.sanfordcantoninwood.org
**Control:** Other not–for–profit (including NFP Corporation) **Service:** General Medical and Surgical

**Staffed Beds:** 18 **Admissions:** 268 **Census:** 3 **Outpatient Visits:** 19293 **Births:** 0 **Total Expense ($000):** 5861 **Payroll Expense ($000):** 2655 **Personnel:** 75

## CHAMBERLAIN—Brule County

★ **SANFORD MEDICAL CENTER CHAMBERLAIN (431329)**, 300 South Byron Boulevard, Zip 57325–9741; tel. 605/234–5511, (Total facility includes 44 beds in nursing home–type unit) **A**9 10 18 **F**3 8 13 15 18 19 28 29 31 34 35 40 43 50 57 59 68 70 75 76 77 78 81 85 86 89 93 100 101 102 103 107 113 118 129 130 132 145 147 **P**6 **S** Sanford Health, Sioux Falls, SD
Primary Contact: Maureen K. Cadwell, Chief Executive Officer
CFO: Erica Peterson, Chief Financial Officer
CMO: John Jones, M.D., Chief Medical Staff
CHR: Dorothy Hieb, Director Human Resources
Web address: www.sanfordmiddakota.org
**Control:** Other not–for–profit (including NFP Corporation) **Service:** General Medical and Surgical

**Staffed Beds:** 69 **Admissions:** 487 **Census:** 47 **Outpatient Visits:** 29675 **Births:** 61 **Total Expense ($000):** 18558 **Payroll Expense ($000):** 7598 **Personnel:** 157

**SANFORD MID DAKOTA MEDICAL CENTER** See Sanford Medical Center Chamberlain

SD

**Hospital, Medicare Provider Number, Address, Telephone, Approval, Facility, and Physician Codes, Health Care System**

★ American Hospital Association (AHA) membership
□ The Joint Commission accreditation ◇ DNV Healthcare Inc. accreditation
○ American Osteopathic Association (AOA) accreditation
△ Commission on Accreditation of Rehabilitation Facilities (CARF) accreditation

## CLEAR LAKE—Deuel County

★ **SANFORD DEUEL COUNTY MEDICAL CENTER (431307)**, 701 Third Avenue
South, Zip 57226–2016; tel. 605/874–2141 **A**9 10 18 **F**3 11 28 29 32 34 35
40 45 50 53 57 59 62 64 65 67 68 81 86 87 89 90 92 97 98 107 118 126
127 132 134 143 146 147 **P**6 **S** Sanford Health, Sioux Falls, SD
Primary Contact: Robert J. Salmon, Chief Executive Officer
CFO: Allison Nelson, Chief Financial Officer
CMO: Terrance Smith, M.D., Chairman Medical Staff
Web address: www.sanforddeuelcounty.org
**Control:** Other not–for–profit (including NFP Corporation) **Service:** General
Medical and Surgical

**Staffed Beds: 10 Admissions: 203 Census: 3 Outpatient Visits:** 15196
**Births:** 0 **Total Expense ($000):** 5052 **Payroll Expense ($000):** 2474
**Personnel:** 45

## CUSTER—Custer County

★ **CUSTER REGIONAL HOSPITAL (431323)**, 1039 Montgomery Street,
Zip 57730–1397; tel. 605/673–2229 **A**9 10 18 **F**6 10 15 29 34 35 40 41 56
57 59 64 65 67 68 71 77 79 87 89 90 92 93 94 97 107 110 111 113 118
126 127 129 132 134 142 143 145 147 **S** Regional Health, Rapid City, SD
Primary Contact: Veronica Schmidt, Chief Executive Officer
Web address: www.regionalhealth.com
**Control:** Other not–for–profit (including NFP Corporation) **Service:** General
Medical and Surgical

**Staffed Beds: 87 Admissions: 232 Census: 2 Outpatient Visits:** 21194
**Births:** 0 **Personnel:** 90

## DAKOTA DUNES—Union County

**SIOUXLAND SURGERY CENTER (430089)**, 600 North Sioux Point Road,
Zip 57049–5000; tel. 605/232–3332, (Nonreporting) **A**9 10
Primary Contact: Greg Miner, Administrator
Web address: www.siouxlandsurg.com/
**Control:** Corporation, Investor–owned, for–profit **Service:** Other specialty

**Staffed Beds: 40**

## DE SMET—Kingsbury County

★ **AVERA DE SMET MEMORIAL HOSPITAL (431332)**, 306 Prairie Avenue S.W.,
Zip 57231, Mailing Address: P.O. Box 160, Zip 57231; tel. 605/854–3329 **A**9
10 18 **F**3 15 28 34 35 40 59 68 77 93 132 **P**6 **S** Avera Health, Sioux Falls, SD
Primary Contact: Janice Schardin, R.N., MS, Administrator and Chief Executive
Officer
Web address: www.desmetmemorial.org
**Control:** Other not–for–profit (including NFP Corporation) **Service:** General
Medical and Surgical

**Staffed Beds: 14 Admissions: 96 Census: 1 Outpatient Visits:** 10447
**Births:** 0 **Total Expense ($000):** 3167 **Payroll Expense ($000):** 1381
**Personnel:** 22

## DEADWOOD—Lawrence County

★ **LEAD–DEADWOOD REGIONAL HOSPITAL (431320)**, 61 Charles Street,
Zip 57732–1303; tel. 605/722–6101 **A**9 10 18 **F**3 7 10 15 28 29 30 31 34
35 40 43 59 64 65 68 69 71 77 78 81 85 87 93 94 97 107 113 114 116
118 119 120 124 132 147 **S** Regional Health, Rapid City, SD
Primary Contact: Sherry Bea Smith, R.N., Chief Executive Officer and Chief
Financial Officer
CFO: Sherry Bea Smith, R.N., Chief Executive Officer and Chief Financial Officer
CMO: Elizabeth Sayler, M.D., Chief of Staff
CHR: Kathryn L. Shockey, Director Human Resources
Web address: www.regionalhealth.com
**Control:** State–Government, nonfederal **Service:** General Medical and Surgical

**Staffed Beds: 18 Admissions: 330 Census: 4 Outpatient Visits:** 11347
**Births:** 0 **Total Expense ($000):** 8517 **Payroll Expense ($000):** 4216
**Personnel:** 79

## DELL RAPIDS—Minnehaha County

**AVERA DELLS AREA HEALTH CENTER** See Avera Dells Area Hospital

★ **AVERA DELLS AREA HOSPITAL (431331)**, 909 North Iowa Avenue,
Zip 57022–1231; tel. 605/428–5431 **A**9 10 18 **F**3 11 15 28 34 35 40 45 53
57 59 64 65 75 81 86 92 93 97 107 110 127 131 132 145 147 **P**6 **S** Avera
Health, Sioux Falls, SD
Primary Contact: Lindsay Leischner, R.N., Administrator and Chief Executive
Officer
CFO: Kory Holt, Division Controller Network Operations
CMO: Matt Herber, M.D., Chief of Staff
CIO: Thelma Haak, Manager Health Information
CHR: Dawn Ingalls, Regional Manager Human Resources
Web address: www.avera.org
**Control:** Other not–for–profit (including NFP Corporation) **Service:** General
Medical and Surgical

**Staffed Beds: 23 Admissions: 294 Census: 4 Outpatient Visits:** 15974
**Births:** 0 **Total Expense ($000):** 4929 **Payroll Expense ($000):** 1956
**Personnel:** 46

## EAGLE BUTTE—Dewey County

**U. S. PUBLIC HEALTH SERVICE INDIAN HOSPITAL (430083)**, 317 Main
Street, Zip 57625–1012, Mailing Address: P.O. Box 1012, Zip 57625–1012;
tel. 605/964–7724, (Nonreporting) **A**10 **S** U. S. Indian Health Service,
Rockville, MD
Primary Contact: Charlene Red Thunder, Chief Executive Officer
CFO: Lisa Deal, Budget Analyst
Web address: www.ihs.gov
**Control:** Public Health Service, Government, federal **Service:** General Medical
and Surgical

**Staffed Beds: 11**

## EUREKA—Mcpherson County

★ **EUREKA COMMUNITY HEALTH SERVICES AVERA (431308)**, 410 Ninth
Street, Zip 57437–0517, Mailing Address: P.O. Box 517, Zip 57437–0517;
tel. 605/284–2661 **A**9 10 18 **F**10 28 35 40 45 59 62 65 77 81 93 132
**S** Avera Health, Sioux Falls, SD
Primary Contact: Robert A. Dockter, Administrator
CFO: Joyce Schwingler, Chief Financial Officer
Web address: www.avera.org
**Control:** Other not–for–profit (including NFP Corporation) **Service:** General
Medical and Surgical

**Staffed Beds: 6 Admissions: 115 Census: 1 Outpatient Visits:** 6387 **Births:**
0 **Total Expense ($000):** 2231 **Payroll Expense ($000):** 876 **Personnel:** 32

## FAULKTON—Faulk County

**FAULKTON AREA MEDICAL CENTER (431301)**, 1300 Oak Street, Zip 57438,
Mailing Address: P.O. Box 100, Zip 57438–0100; tel. 605/598–6263 **A**9 10 18
**F**3 17 28 29 40 45 57 59 77 93 97 107 126 132 **P**5
Primary Contact: Jay A. Jahnig, Chief Executive Officer
COO: Jay A. Jahnig, Chief Executive Officer
CFO: Susan Miller, Financial Administrator
CMO: K. A. Bartholomew, M.D., Medical Director
CIO: Cheryl Arthurs, Health Information Transcriptionist
CHR: Susan Miller, Financial Administrator
Web address: www.faulktonmedical.org
**Control:** Other not–for–profit (including NFP Corporation) **Service:** General
Medical and Surgical

**Staffed Beds: 12 Admissions: 340 Census: 5 Outpatient Visits:** 11467
**Births:** 0 **Total Expense ($000):** 6731 **Payroll Expense ($000):** 2874
**Personnel:** 63

## FLANDREAU—Moody County

★ **AVERA FLANDREAU HOSPITAL (431310)**, 214 North Prairie Street,
Zip 57028–1243; tel. 605/997–2433 **A**9 10 18 **F**3 28 31 34 35 40 45 57 59
64 65 75 81 86 92 93 97 107 118 126 127 131 132 145 147 **P**6 **S** Avera
Health, Sioux Falls, SD
Primary Contact: Lindsay Leischner, R.N., Administrator and Chief Executive
Officer
CFO: Kory Holt, Division Controller Network Operations
CMO: Gary Bruning, M.D., President Medical Staff
CIO: Brittney Luze, Director Health Information
CHR: Mona Schafer, Regional Manager Human Resources
Web address: www.flandreaumedical.org
**Control:** Other not–for–profit (including NFP Corporation) **Service:** General
Medical and Surgical

**Staffed Beds: 18 Admissions: 216 Census: 1 Outpatient Visits:** 13109
**Births:** 0 **Total Expense ($000):** 4192 **Payroll Expense ($000):** 1803
**Personnel:** 44

**AVERA FLANDREAU MEDICAL CENTER** See Avera Flandreau Hospital

## FORT MEADE—Meade County

⊠ △ **VETERANS AFFAIRS BLACK HILLS HEALTH CARE SYSTEM**, 113
Comanche Road, Zip 57741–1099; tel. 605/720–7170, (Includes VETERANS
AFFAIRS MEDICAL CENTER, 500 North Fifth Street, Hot Springs, Zip 57747;
tel. 605/745–2052), (Nonreporting) **A**1 5 7 9 **S** Department of Veterans Affairs,
Washington, DC
Primary Contact: Stephen R. DiStasio, Acting Director
COO: Stephen R. DiStasio, Associate Director Operations
CFO: Bill Gambill, Chief Financial Officer
CHR: Marg McCaleb, Chief Human Resources Management
Web address: www.va.gov/sta/guide/home.asp
**Control:** Veterans Affairs, Government, federal **Service:** General Medical and
Surgical

**Staffed Beds: 308**

**SD**

*Many Facility Codes have changed. Please refer to the AHA Guide Code Chart.* © 2012 AHA Guide

**FREEMAN—Hutchinson County**

★ **FREEMAN REGIONAL HEALTH SERVICES (431313)**, 510 East Eighth Street, Zip 57029–0370, Mailing Address: P.O. Box 370, Zip 57029–0370; tel. 605/925–4000, (Total facility includes 53 beds in nursing home–type unit) **A**9 10 18 **F**2 3 6 11 15 28 30 31 34 35 40 45 49 56 57 58 64 65 68 69 70 75 77 78 79 81 82 86 89 90 93 107 113 118 124 126 127 129 132 142 145
Primary Contact: Daniel Gran, Chief Executive Officer
CFO: Neil Frizzell, Chief Financial Officer
Web address: www.freemanregional.com
**Control:** Other not–for–profit (including NFP Corporation) **Service:** General Medical and Surgical

**Staffed Beds:** 78 **Admissions:** 240 **Census:** 56 **Outpatient Visits:** 8508 **Births:** 0 **Total Expense ($000):** 7930 **Payroll Expense ($000):** 3686 **Personnel:** 128

**GETTYSBURG—Potter County**

★ **GETTYSBURG MEMORIAL HOSPITAL (431302)**, 606 East Garfield Avenue, Zip 57442–1398; tel. 605/765–2480, (Total facility includes 50 beds in nursing home–type unit) **A**9 10 18 **F**3 6 11 28 29 30 34 35 36 40 50 59 64 67 75 77 79 81 82 86 87 93 107 124 127 129 131 132 145 **S** Catholic Health Initiatives, Englewood, CO
Primary Contact: Mark Schmidt, President and Chief Executive Officer
Web address: www.st–marys.com
**Control:** Church–operated, Nongovernment, not–for profit **Service:** General Medical and Surgical

**Staffed Beds:** 60 **Admissions:** 135 **Census:** 52 **Outpatient Visits:** 6002 **Births:** 0 **Total Expense ($000):** 5469 **Payroll Expense ($000):** 2500 **Personnel:** 71

**GREGORY—Gregory County**

★ **AVERA GREGORY HOSPITAL (431338)**, 400 Park Avenue, Zip 57533–0400, Mailing Address: P.O. Box 408, Zip 57533–0408; tel. 605/835–8394, (Total facility includes 38 beds in nursing home–type unit) **A**9 10 18 **F**3 13 15 17 28 29 30 31 34 35 40 43 45 56 57 59 60 70 75 76 77 78 79 81 82 86 87 89 107 110 127 128 129 130 131 132 142 146 **S** Avera Health, Sioux Falls, SD
Primary Contact: Anthony Timanus, Chief Executive Officer
CFO: Trish Keiser, Comptroller
CMO: Rich Kafka, M.D., Chief Medical Officer
CIO: Justin Keegan, Director Support Services
CHR: Carol Postulka, Administrative Coordinator
Web address: www.gregoryhealthcare.org
**Control:** Church–operated, Nongovernment, not–for profit **Service:** General Medical and Surgical

**Staffed Beds:** 63 **Admissions:** 659 **Census:** 44 **Outpatient Visits:** 15707 **Births:** 1 **Total Expense ($000):** 12401 **Payroll Expense ($000):** 5713 **Personnel:** 132

**HOT SPRINGS—Fall River County**

★ **FALL RIVER HOSPITAL (431322)**, 1201 Highway 71 South, Zip 57747–8800; tel. 605/745–3159, (Includes CASTLE MANOR ) **A**9 10 18 **F**3 28 34 40 43 45 56 57 59 64 65 74 79 81 93 102 107 113 118 126 127 128 130 131 132 145 147 **P**6
Primary Contact: Tricia Uhlir, Chief Executive Officer
CFO: Jesse Naze, Chief Financial Officer
CMO: Heather Preuss, M.D., Medical Director
CHR: Cindy Trent, Manager Personnel
Web address: www.fallriverhealthservices.com
**Control:** Other not–for–profit (including NFP Corporation) **Service:** General Medical and Surgical

**Staffed Beds:** 25 **Admissions:** 271 **Census:** 10 **Outpatient Visits:** 18842 **Births:** 0 **Total Expense ($000):** 12035 **Payroll Expense ($000):** 4735 **Personnel:** 97

**VETERANS AFFAIRS MEDICAL CENTER** See Veterans Affairs Black Hills Health Care System, Fort Meade

**HURON—Beadle County**

★ **HURON REGIONAL MEDICAL CENTER (431335)**, 172 Fourth Street S.E., Zip 57350–2590; tel. 605/353–6200 **A**9 10 18 **F**3 11 13 14 15 28 29 30 31 34 35 40 43 45 57 59 60 62 63 64 68 70 75 76 77 78 79 81 85 86 89 93 102 107 108 110 111 114 117 118 129 131 132 145 147 **P**6 **S** QHR, Brentwood, TN
Primary Contact: John L. Single, Chief Executive Officer
CFO: Marcia Zwanziger, Vice President Finance
CMO: Cy Haatvedt, M.D., Chief of Staff
CHR: Rhonda Hanson, Director Human Resources
Web address: www.huronregional.org
**Control:** Other not–for–profit (including NFP Corporation) **Service:** General Medical and Surgical

**Staffed Beds:** 25 **Admissions:** 1359 **Census:** 13 **Outpatient Visits:** 55559 **Births:** 343 **Total Expense ($000):** 28185 **Payroll Expense ($000):** 12460 **Personnel:** 246

**MADISON—Lake County**

★ **MADISON COMMUNITY HOSPITAL (431300)**, 917 North Washington Avenue, Zip 57042–1696; tel. 605/256–6551 **A**9 10 18 **F**7 11 13 15 28 31 34 35 40 41 43 57 59 62 64 70 75 76 77 81 82 85 89 93 107 108 110 113 118 128 131 132 134 142 144 145 147 **P**5
Primary Contact: Tamara Miller, Administrator
CFO: Teresa Mallett, Director Accounting and Health Information Management
Web address: www.madisonhospital.com
**Control:** Other not–for–profit (including NFP Corporation) **Service:** General Medical and Surgical

**Staffed Beds:** 25 **Admissions:** 500 **Census:** 7 **Outpatient Visits:** 23837 **Births:** 42 **Total Expense ($000):** 11697 **Payroll Expense ($000):** 5603 **Personnel:** 134

**MARTIN—Bennett County**

**BENNETT COUNTY HOSPITAL AND NURSING HOME (431314)**, (Critical Access Hospital), 102 Major Allen Street, Zip 57551, Mailing Address: P.O. Box 70, Zip 57551; tel. 605/685–6622, (Total facility includes 43 beds in nursing home–type unit) **A**9 10 18 **F**2 7 10 29 30 34 35 40 41 50 53 57 59 62 65 66 67 68 84 90 92 93 127 129 130 132 142
Primary Contact: Debbie Klesack, Interim Chief Executive Officer
CFO: Jean Kirk, Chief Financial Officer
CMO: Peter Knowles–Smith, M.D., Medical Director
CIO: Jean Kirk, Chief Financial Officer
CHR: T. J. Porter, Director Human Resources
Web address: www.bennettcountyhospital.com/
**Control:** Other not–for–profit (including NFP Corporation) **Service:** General Medical and Surgical

**Staffed Beds:** 54 **Admissions:** 172 **Census:** 38 **Outpatient Visits:** 2327 **Births:** 2 **Total Expense ($000):** 6023 **Payroll Expense ($000):** 4241

**MILBANK—Grant County**

★ **MILBANK AREA HOSPITAL AVERA (431326)**, 901 East Virgil Avenue, Zip 57252; tel. 605/432–4538, (Includes ST. WILLIAM HOME FOR THE AGED ), (Nonreporting) **A**9 10 18 **S** Avera Health, Sioux Falls, SD
Primary Contact: Natalie Gauer, Administrator
CFO: Jamie Schaefer, Vice President Finance
CMO: Kevin Bjordahl, M.D., Chief Medical Officer
CHR: Mona Schafer, Regional Manager Human Resources
Web address: www.averamilbank.org
**Control:** Other not–for–profit (including NFP Corporation) **Service:** General Medical and Surgical

**Staffed Beds:** 25

**MILLER—Hand County**

★ **AVERA HAND COUNTY MEMORIAL HOSPITAL & CLINIC (431337)**, 300 West Fifth Street, Zip 57362–1238; tel. 605/853–2421 **A**9 10 18 **F**8 11 15 17 28 29 34 35 40 42 43 45 46 50 53 56 57 59 64 74 77 79 81 86 87 93 107 113 118 127 128 131 132 145 147 **P**5 **S** Avera Health, Sioux Falls, SD
Primary Contact: Bryan Breitling, Administrator
CFO: Debbie Pullman, Director Finance
CMO: Joel Huber, M.D., Chief of Staff
CIO: Janice Purrington, Coordinator Medical Records
Web address: www.avera.org
**Control:** Other not–for–profit (including NFP Corporation) **Service:** General Medical and Surgical

**Staffed Beds:** 19 **Admissions:** 381 **Census:** 4 **Outpatient Visits:** 12390 **Births:** 0 **Total Expense ($000):** 5182 **Payroll Expense ($000):** 2650 **Personnel:** 44

**SD**

## MITCHELL—Davison County

☒ **AVERA QUEEN OF PEACE HOSPITAL (430013)**, 525 North Foster,
Zip 57301–2999; tel. 605/995–2000, (Total facility includes 111 beds in nursing
home–type unit) **A**1 2 9 10 **F**3 10 12 13 15 28 29 30 31 34 35 39 40 43 48
50 53 56 57 59 62 63 64 65 69 70 71 75 76 77 78 79 81 82 85 86 89 93
94 96 102 107 110 111 113 117 118 120 122 124 126 127 128 129 130
131 132 134 143 145 146 147 **P**6 **S** Avera Health, Sioux Falls, SD
Primary Contact: Thomas A. Clark, President and Chief Executive Officer
CFO: Patrick Clark, Senior Vice President Finance and Support Services
CMO: Mark Reynen, D.O., President Medical Staff
CIO: Patti Brooks, Director Information Systems
CHR: Rita Lemon, Director Human Resources
Web address: www.averaqueenofpeace.org
**Control:** Church–operated, Nongovernment, not–for profit **Service:** General
Medical and Surgical

**Staffed Beds: 196 Admissions: 2687 Census: 136 Outpatient Visits:**
112859 **Births:** 473 **Total Expense ($000):** 77197 **Payroll Expense ($000):**
37333 **Personnel:** 600

## MOBRIDGE—Walworth County

★ **MOBRIDGE REGIONAL HOSPITAL (431325)**, 1401 Tenth Avenue West,
Zip 57601–1199, Mailing Address: P.O. Box 580, Zip 57601–0580;
tel. 605/845–3692 **A**9 10 18 **F**3 7 8 10 11 13 15 17 28 31 34 35 40 43 45
54 56 57 59 62 64 65 67 70 75 76 81 89 93 97 107 110 113 118 124 126
127 128 129 132 **P**6
Primary Contact: Angelia K. Svihovec, Chief Executive Officer
CFO: Renae Tisdall, Chief Financial Officer
CMO: Travis Henderson, M.D., Chief of Staff
CIO: Brian Schaefbauer, Director Information Technology
CHR: Keri Wientjes, Director Human Resources
Web address: www.mobridgehospital.org
**Control:** Other not–for–profit (including NFP Corporation) **Service:** General
Medical and Surgical

**Staffed Beds: 25 Admissions: 744 Census: 7 Outpatient Visits:** 29453
**Births:** 60 **Total Expense ($000):** 12625 **Payroll Expense ($000):** 6934
**Personnel:** 140

## PARKSTON—Hutchinson County

★ **AVERA ST. BENEDICT HOSPITAL (431330)**, 401 West Glynn Drive,
Zip 57366–2031; tel. 605/928–3311, (Total facility includes 75 beds in nursing
home–type unit) **A**9 10 18 **F**2 3 8 10 13 15 28 29 30 31 32 34 35 38 40 45
53 56 57 59 64 65 69 81 82 83 85 86 87 89 107 110 111 113 115 118 127
128 129 130 131 132 134 145 147 **P**6 **S** Avera Health, Sioux Falls, SD
Primary Contact: Gale N. Walker, President and Chief Executive Officer
CFO: Rita Blasius, Assistant Administrator and Chief Financial Officer
CMO: Richard Honke, M.D., Chief of Staff
CIO: Adam Popp, Director Information Systems
CHR: Phyllis Ehler, Director Human Resources
Web address: www.averastbenedict.org
**Control:** Church–operated, Nongovernment, not–for profit **Service:** General
Medical and Surgical

**Staffed Beds: 100 Admissions: 499 Census: 79 Outpatient Visits:** 20747
**Births:** 35 **Total Expense ($000):** 15245 **Payroll Expense ($000):** 7919
**Personnel:** 162

## PHILIP—Haakon County

**HANS P. PETERSON MEMORIAL HOSPITAL** See Philip Health Services

★ **PHILIP HEALTH SERVICES (431319)**, 503 West Pine Street, Zip 57567,
Mailing Address: P.O. Box 790, Zip 57567–0790; tel. 605/859–2511, (Total
facility includes 30 beds in nursing home–type unit) **A**9 10 18 **F**10 11 40 57 59
62 85 93 107 113 118 126 127 129 130 132 147 **P**6 **S** Regional Health, Rapid
City, SD
Primary Contact: Kent Olson, Administrator and Chief Executive Officer
Web address: www.rcrh.org/Facilities/Hospitals/HPPMemorial.asp
**Control:** Other not–for–profit (including NFP Corporation) **Service:** General
Medical and Surgical

**Staffed Beds: 48 Admissions: 259 Census: 42 Outpatient Visits:** 9208
**Births:** 0 **Total Expense ($000):** 7644 **Payroll Expense ($000):** 4169
**Personnel:** 101

## PIERRE—Hughes County

☒ **ST. MARY'S HEALTHCARE CENTER (430015)**, 800 East Dakota Avenue,
Zip 57501–3313; tel. 605/224–3100, (Total facility includes 105 beds in nursing
home–type unit) **A**1 9 10 20 **F**2 3 8 13 15 28 29 30 31 34 38 40 41 43 45 48
49 50 59 60 64 68 70 71 76 77 78 79 81 82 83 84 85 87 93 96 97 107
110 111 113 118 124 127 128 129 131 132 134 145 147 **P**5 **S** Catholic
Health Initiatives, Englewood, CO
Primary Contact: Joseph Messmer, Interim Chief Executive Officer
CFO: Adam Paul, Vice President Finance
CMO: Denise Hanisch, M.D., Chief of Staff
CIO: Jamie Raske, Information Technology Lead
CHR: Paul Marso, Vice President Human Resources
Web address: www.st–marys.com
**Control:** Other not–for–profit (including NFP Corporation) **Service:** General
Medical and Surgical

**Staffed Beds: 164 Admissions: 1769 Census: 96 Outpatient Visits:** 47609
**Births:** 408 **Total Expense ($000):** 39242 **Payroll Expense ($000):** 15999
**Personnel:** 336

## PINE RIDGE—Shannon County

**U. S. PUBLIC HEALTH SERVICE INDIAN HOSPITAL (430081)**, East Highway
18, Zip 57770, Mailing Address: P.O. Box 1201, Zip 57770–1201;
tel. 605/867–5131, (Nonreporting) **A**10 **S** U. S. Indian Health Service,
Rockville, MD
Primary Contact: William Pourier, Service Unit Director
CFO: Sophia Conny, Deputy Administrative Officer
CMO: Jan Colton, M.D., Acting Clinical Director
CHR: Annabelle Blackbear, Human Resources Specialist
Web address: www.ihs.gov
**Control:** Public Health Service, Government, federal **Service:** General Medical
and Surgical

**Staffed Beds: 45**

## PLATTE—Charles Mix County

★ **PLATTE HEALTH CENTER AVERA (431306)**, 601 East Seventh,
Zip 57369–2123, Mailing Address: P.O. Box 200, Zip 57369–0200;
tel. 605/337–3364, (Total facility includes 48 beds in nursing home–type unit) **A**9
10 18 **F**1 3 11 13 15 28 31 34 40 41 45 57 59 62 64 65 68 78 81 107 110
113 118 126 127 128 129 130 132 147 **P**6 **S** Avera Health, Sioux Falls, SD
Primary Contact: Mark Burket, Chief Executive Officer
CFO: Jerry Hoffman, Chief Financial Officer
Web address: www.phcavera.org
**Control:** Other not–for–profit (including NFP Corporation) **Service:** General
Medical and Surgical

**Staffed Beds: 65 Admissions: 295 Census: 50 Outpatient Visits:** 22440
**Births:** 25 **Total Expense ($000):** 10917 **Payroll Expense ($000):** 5565
**Personnel:** 92

## RAPID CITY—Pennington County

**BLACK HILLS SURGERY CENTER (430091)**, 216 Anamaria Drive, Zip 57701,
Mailing Address: 1868 Lombardy Drive, Zip 57701; tel. 605/721–4900,
(Nonreporting) **A**9 10
Primary Contact: Franklin Shobe, Administrator and Chief Executive Officer
Web address: www.bhsc.com
**Control:** Partnership, Investor–owned, for–profit **Service:** General Medical and
Surgical

**Staffed Beds: 26**

**INDIAN HEALTH SERVICE HOSPITAL (430082)**, 3200 Canyon Lake Drive,
Zip 57702–8197; tel. 605/355–2280, (Nonreporting) **A**10 **S** U. S. Indian Health
Service, Rockville, MD
Primary Contact: Helen Thompson, Interim Director
CFO: Helen Thompson, Administrative Officer
Web address: www.ihs.gov
**Control:** PHS, Indian Service, Government, federal **Service:** General Medical and
Surgical

**Staffed Beds: 5**

**SD**

⊠ △ **RAPID CITY REGIONAL HOSPITAL (430077)**, 353 Fairmont Boulevard, Zip 57701–7393, Mailing Address: P.O. Box 6000, Zip 57709–6000; tel. 605/719–1000 **A**1 3 5 7 9 10 **F**3 5 11 12 13 15 17 18 20 22 24 26 28 29 30 31 34 35 36 38 40 43 44 45 46 47 48 49 51 56 57 58 59 60 62 63 64 65 66 68 70 72 73 74 75 76 77 78 79 80 81 82 84 85 86 87 88 89 90 92 93 98 99 100 101 102 104 107 108 110 111 114 118 119 120 121 122 123 128 129 130 131 134 140 142 145 147 **P**1 5 6 **S** Regional Health, Rapid City, SD
Primary Contact: Timothy H. Sughrue, Chief Executive Officer
COO: Robert Baxter, Chief Operating Officer
CFO: Mark Thompson, Vice President Financial Services
CMO: Robert Allen, M.D., Vice President Medical Affairs
CIO: Richard Latuchie, Vice President Business Development
CHR: Robert McGlone, Vice President Human Resources
Web address: www.rcrh.org
**Control:** Other not–for–profit (including NFP Corporation) **Service:** General Medical and Surgical

**Staffed Beds:** 374 **Admissions:** 16837 **Census:** 263 **Outpatient Visits:** 171189 **Births:** 2231 **Total Expense ($000):** 321433 **Payroll Expense ($000):** 139749 **Personnel:** 2493

**SAME DAY SURGERY CENTER (430093)**, 651 Cathedral Drive, Zip 57701; tel. 605/719–5000, (Nonreporting) **A**9 10
Primary Contact: Doris Fritts, R.N., Executive Director
Web address: www.samedaysurgerycenter.org
**Control:** Corporation, Investor–owned, for–profit **Service:** Surgical

**Staffed Beds:** 8

### REDFIELD—Spink County

**COMMUNITY MEMORIAL HOSPITAL (431316)**, 110 West Tenth Avenue, Zip 57469–0420, Mailing Address: P.O. Box 420, Zip 57469–0420; tel. 605/472–1110 **A**9 10 18 **F**7 8 11 17 28 34 35 40 45 53 56 57 59 62 64 65 67 75 77 81 84 85 89 93 97 107 113 118 126 127 129 130 131 132 145 **P**6
Primary Contact: Nicholas R. Brandner, Chief Executive Officer
CFO: Lynn Moller, Chief Financial Officer
Web address: www.redfield–sd.com/hospital.html
**Control:** City–Government, nonfederal **Service:** General Medical and Surgical

**Staffed Beds:** 23 **Admissions:** 409 **Census:** 6 **Outpatient Visits:** 18190 **Births:** 0 **Total Expense ($000):** 10601 **Payroll Expense ($000):** 5231 **Personnel:** 106

### ROSEBUD—Todd County

**U. S. PUBLIC HEALTH SERVICE INDIAN HOSPITAL (430084)**, Highway 18, Soldier Creek Road, Zip 57570; tel. 605/747–2231, (Nonreporting) **A**10 **S** U. S. Indian Health Service, Rockville, MD
Primary Contact: Shelly Harris, Chief Executive Officer
COO: Romeo Vivit, Chief Surgeon
CMO: Valerie Parker, M.D., Clinical Director
CHR: Michelle Zephier, Human Resource Specialist
Web address: www.ihs.gov
**Control:** PHS, Indian Service, Government, federal **Service:** General Medical and Surgical

**Staffed Beds:** 35

### SCOTLAND—Bon Homme County

★ **LANDMANN–JUNGMAN MEMORIAL HOSPITAL AVERA (431317)**, 600 Billars Street, Zip 57059–2026; tel. 605/583–2226 **A**9 10 18 **F**11 34 35 40 45 53 59 65 77 93 97 107 113 118 124 126 129 131 132 **P**7 **S** Avera Health, Sioux Falls, SD
Primary Contact: Lee Baldwin, Administrator and Chief Executive Officer
CFO: Darcy Kepplinger, Manager Business Office
Web address: www.ljmh.org
**Control:** Other not–for–profit (including NFP Corporation) **Service:** General Medical and Surgical

**Staffed Beds:** 19 **Admissions:** 80 **Census:** 1 **Outpatient Visits:** 6000 **Births:** 0

### SIOUX FALLS—Lincoln County

☐ **AVERA HEART HOSPITAL OF SOUTH DAKOTA (430095)**, 4500 West 69th Street, Zip 57108–8148; tel. 605/977–7000, (Nonreporting) **A**1 9 10
Primary Contact: Jon Soderholm, President
CFO: Jean White, Vice President Finance
Web address: www.southdakotaheart.com
**Control:** Partnership, Investor–owned, for–profit **Service:** General Medical and Surgical

**Staffed Beds:** 55

⊠ △ **AVERA MCKENNAN HOSPITAL AND UNIVERSITY HEALTH CENTER (430016)**, 800 East 21st Street, Zip 57105–1096, Mailing Address: P.O. Box 5045, Zip 57117–5045; tel. 605/322–8000, (Includes AVERA CHILDREN'S HOSPITAL, 800 East 21st Street, Zip 57105–1016, Mailing Address: PO Box 5045, Zip 57117–5045; tel. 605/322–5437), (Total facility includes 90 beds in nursing home–type unit) **A**1 2 3 5 7 8 9 10 **F**3 5 7 8 10 11 12 13 15 18 19 20 21 22 23 24 29 30 31 32 34 35 36 38 39 40 41 43 44 46 49 50 53 54 55 56 57 58 59 60 61 63 64 65 66 67 68 70 71 72 74 75 76 77 78 79 81 82 84 85 86 87 88 89 90 92 93 94 96 97 98 99 100 101 102 103 104 105 107 108 110 111 113 114 115 116 117 118 119 120 122 123 124 125 127 128 129 131 133 134 135 137 140 141 142 143 144 145 146 147 **P**6 8 **S** Avera Health, Sioux Falls, SD
Primary Contact: David Kapaska, D.O., Regional President
COO: Judy Blauwet, M.P.H., Senior Vice President Operations and Chief Nursing Officer
CFO: Julie Norton, Chief Financial Officer
CIO: Kristin Gross, Director Information Technology Center
CHR: Bill McLean, Senior Vice President Human Resources
Web address: www.averamckennan.org
**Control:** Church–operated, Nongovernment, not–for profit **Service:** General Medical and Surgical

**Staffed Beds:** 400 **Admissions:** 20642 **Census:** 295 **Outpatient Visits:** 229643 **Births:** 1910 **Total Expense ($000):** 579275 **Payroll Expense ($000):** 275148 **Personnel:** 3562

**CHILDRENS CARE HOSPITAL AND SCHOOL (433300)**, (Pediatric Speciality Hospital), 2501 West 26th Street, Zip 57105–2498; tel. 605/782–2300 **A**9 10 **F**3 64 75 80 90 91 93 94 129 145
Primary Contact: Dianna Rajski, President and Chief Executive Officer
CFO: John Clark, Chief Financial Officer
CMO: Christiane Maroun, M.D., Chief of Staff
CHR: Tiffany Reilly, Director Human Resources
Web address: www.cchs.org
**Control:** Other not–for–profit (including NFP Corporation) **Service:** Children's other specialty

**Staffed Beds:** 114 **Admissions:** 26 **Census:** 67 **Outpatient Visits:** 15064 **Total Expense ($000):** 26366 **Payroll Expense ($000):** 15150 **Personnel:** 32

⊠ △ **SANFORD UNIVERSITY OF SOUTH DAKOTA MEDICAL CENTER (430027)**, 1305 West 18th Street, Zip 57105–0496, Mailing Address: P.O. Box 5039, Zip 57117–5039; tel. 605/333–1000, (Includes SANFORD CHILDREN'S HOSPITAL, 1600 West 22nd Street, Zip 57105, Mailing Address: PO Box 5039, Zip 57117–5039; tel. 605/333–1000) **A**1 2 3 5 7 8 9 10 **F**3 7 8 9 11 10 14 17 18 19 20 21 22 23 24 25 26 27 28 29 30 31 32 34 35 37 38 40 43 44 45 46 48 49 50 51 52 53 55 56 57 58 59 60 61 63 64 65 70 71 72 73 74 75 76 77 78 79 80 81 82 84 85 86 87 88 89 90 91 92 93 94 96 107 108 110 111 113 114 115 116 117 118 119 120 122 123 125 128 129 130 131 133 134 137 140 142 145 146 147 **S** Sanford Health, Sioux Falls, SD
Primary Contact: Charles O'Brien, M.D., President
COO: Randy Bury, Chief Operating Officer
CFO: Jeff Sandene, Chief Finance
CMO: Ken Aspaas, M.D., Chief Medical Officer
CIO: Arlyn Broekhuis, Vice President and Chief Information Officer
CHR: Evan Burkett, Chief Human Resource Officer
Web address: www.sanfordhealth.org
**Control:** Other not–for–profit (including NFP Corporation) **Service:** General Medical and Surgical

**Staffed Beds:** 478 **Admissions:** 23886 **Census:** 295 **Outpatient Visits:** 368518 **Births:** 3158 **Total Expense ($000):** 479302 **Payroll Expense ($000):** 197739 **Personnel:** 4407

⊠ **SELECT SPECIALTY HOSPITAL–SIOUX FALLS (432002)**, 1325 South Cliff Avenue, Suite 3300, Zip 57105; tel. 605/322–3500, (Nonreporting) **A**1 9 10 **S** Select Medical Corporation, Mechanicsburg, PA
Primary Contact: Carol Ulmer, Chief Executive Officer
Web address: www.selectmedicalcorp.com
**Control:** Corporation, Investor–owned, for–profit **Service:** Long–Term Acute Care hospital

**Staffed Beds:** 21

**SIOUX FALLS SURGICAL CENTER (430090)**, 910 East 20th Street, Zip 57105; tel. 605/334–6730, (Nonreporting) **A**9 10
Primary Contact: Donald A. Schellpfeffer, M.D., Chief Executive Officer
CFO: Kyle Goldammer, Chief Financial Officer
CMO: Donald A. Schellpfeffer, M.D., Medical Director
Web address: www.sfsurgical.com
**Control:** Partnership, Investor–owned, for–profit **Service:** General Medical and Surgical

**Staffed Beds:** 35

**SD**

---

**Hospital, Medicare Provider Number, Address, Telephone, Approval, Facility, and Physician Codes, Health Care System**

★ American Hospital Association (AHA) membership
☐ The Joint Commission accreditation          ◇ DNV Healthcare Inc. accreditation
○ American Osteopathic Association (AOA) accreditation
△ Commission on Accreditation of Rehabilitation Facilities (CARF) accreditation

✠ **SIOUX FALLS VA HEALTH CARE SYSTEM**, 2501 West 22nd Street, Zip 57105–9920, Mailing Address: P.O. Box 5046, Zip 57117–5046; tel. 605/336–3230, (Total facility includes 58 beds in nursing home–type unit) **A**1 3 5 9 **F**1 5 8 12 18 29 30 31 33 35 39 40 45 50 56 58 59 60 61 62 64 65 70 74 75 77 78 79 81 82 84 85 86 87 93 94 97 98 100 102 103 104 105 107 108 111 118 126 128 129 134 142 145 146 **P**6 **S** Department of Veterans Affairs, Washington, DC
Primary Contact: Patrick Kelly, Director
COO: Sara Ackert, Associate Director
CFO: Daniel Hubbard, Chief Financial Officer
CMO: Victor Waters, M.D., Chief of Staff
CIO: Eric Heiser, Chief Information Resource Management
CHR: Betsy Geiver, Chief Human Resources Officer
Web address: www.siouxfalls.va.gov
**Control:** Veterans Affairs, Government, federal **Service:** General Medical and Surgical

**Staffed Beds:** 98 **Admissions:** 2750 **Census:** 81 **Outpatient Visits:** 271237
**Births:** 0

### SISSETON—Roberts County

★ **COTEAU DES PRAIRIES HOSPITAL (431339)**, 205 Orchard Drive, Zip 57262–2398; tel. 605/698–7647 **A**9 10 18 **F**13 28 31 34 35 40 53 57 59 62 64 70 75 76 77 81 86 89 90 93 107 118 126 132 **P**6
Primary Contact: Dan C. Ellis, Chief Executive Officer
Web address: www.cdphospital.com
**Control:** Other not–for–profit (including NFP Corporation) **Service:** General Medical and Surgical

**Staffed Beds:** 25 **Admissions:** 494 **Census:** 4 **Outpatient Visits:** 39939
**Births:** 170 **Total Expense ($000):** 11409 **Payroll Expense ($000):** 5372
**Personnel:** 108

### SPEARFISH—Lawrence County

★ **SPEARFISH REGIONAL HOSPITAL (430048)**, 1440 North Main Street, Zip 57783–1504; tel. 605/644–4000 **A**9 10 20 **F**3 11 13 15 28 29 31 34 40 45 57 59 62 63 70 75 76 79 81 84 85 89 93 97 107 108 110 111 113 118 127 128 129 131 132 134 145 146 147 **P**6 **S** Regional Health, Rapid City, SD
Primary Contact: Larry W. Veitz, Chief Executive Officer
Web address: www.regionalhealth.com
**Control:** Other not–for–profit (including NFP Corporation) **Service:** General Medical and Surgical

**Staffed Beds:** 34 **Admissions:** 1525 **Census:** 12 **Outpatient Visits:** 28991
**Births:** 459 **Total Expense ($000):** 25684 **Payroll Expense ($000):** 10842
**Personnel:** 195

★ **SPEARFISH REGIONAL SURGERY CENTER (430094)**, 1316 North 10th Street, Zip 57783; tel. 605/642–3113 **A**9 10 **F**8 39 45 51 57 74 79 81 82
Primary Contact: Michael DeLano, Administrator
COO: Matthew Long, Chief Operating Officer
CFO: Jeff Roehrich, Chief Financial Officer
CMO: Richard Keim, M.D., Chief Medical Officer
CIO: Bill Stoeckman, Chief Information Officer
CHR: Pat Akin, Chief Human Resource Officer
Web address: www.rcrh.org
**Control:** Other not–for–profit (including NFP Corporation) **Service:** General Medical and Surgical

**Staffed Beds:** 4 **Admissions:** 65 **Census:** 1 **Outpatient Visits:** 1985 **Births:** 0 **Total Expense ($000):** 4575 **Payroll Expense ($000):** 2007 **Personnel:** 42

### STURGIS—Meade County

★ **STURGIS REGIONAL HOSPITAL (431321)**, 949 Harmon Street, Zip 57785–2452; tel. 605/720–2400, (Total facility includes 84 beds in nursing home–type unit) **A**9 10 18 **F**11 15 28 29 40 46 77 81 82 93 107 110 111 113 118 127 131 132 147 **S** Regional Health, Rapid City, SD
Primary Contact: Van D. Hyde, MS, Chief Executive Officer
CFO: Jodie Mitchell, Facility Financial Director
CMO: Constance Stock, M.D., Chief of Staff
CHR: Ginger Chord, Coordinator Human Resources
Web address: www.rcrh.org/Facilities/Hospitals/SCHCC/Default.asp
**Control:** Other not–for–profit (including NFP Corporation) **Service:** General Medical and Surgical

**Staffed Beds:** 109 **Admissions:** 767 **Census:** 93 **Outpatient Visits:** 9739
**Births:** 0 **Total Expense ($000):** 14472 **Payroll Expense ($000):** 7354
**Personnel:** 187

### TYNDALL—Bon Homme County

★ **ST. MICHAEL'S HOSPITAL AVERA (431327)**, 410 West 16th Avenue, Zip 57066, Mailing Address: P.O. Box 27, Zip 57066–0027; tel. 605/589–3341 **A**9 10 18 **F**3 15 28 31 34 40 45 53 57 59 64 65 67 70 77 81 86 89 92 93 94 107 110 118 126 127 128 130 132 147 **P**6 **S** Avera Health, Sioux Falls, SD
Primary Contact: Carol Deurmier, Chief Executive Officer
CFO: Lisa Ronke, Director Finance
CMO: Herbert A. Saloum, M.D., Medical Director
Web address: www.avera.org/
**Control:** Church–operated, Nongovernment, not–for profit **Service:** General Medical and Surgical

**Staffed Beds:** 25 **Admissions:** 219 **Census:** 10 **Outpatient Visits:** 10054
**Births:** 0 **Total Expense ($000):** 7808 **Payroll Expense ($000):** 3023
**Personnel:** 63

### VERMILLION—Clay County

★ **SANFORD VERMILLION MEDICAL CENTER (431336)**, 20 South Plum Street, Zip 57069–3346; tel. 605/624–2611, (Total facility includes 66 beds in nursing home–type unit) **A**9 10 18 **F**15 29 35 40 43 59 67 81 91 92 93 97 107 115 118 128 129 130 131 132 134 **P**8 **S** Sanford Health, Sioux Falls, SD
Primary Contact: Timothy J. Tracy, Chief Executive Officer
CFO: Valerie Osterberg, Chief Financial Officer
CMO: Roy Mortinsen, M.D., Chief of Staff
CIO: Mary C. Merrigan, Manager Public Relations
CHR: Cindy Benzel, Manager Human Resources
CNO: Jeff Berens, MS, Chief Nursing Officer
Web address: www.sanfordvermillion.org
**Control:** Other not–for–profit (including NFP Corporation) **Service:** General Medical and Surgical

**Staffed Beds:** 114 **Admissions:** 620 **Census:** 71 **Outpatient Visits:** 38291
**Births:** 103 **Total Expense ($000):** 16513 **Payroll Expense ($000):** 7402
**Personnel:** 144

### VIBORG—Turner County

★ **PIONEER MEMORIAL HOSPITAL AND HEALTH SERVICES (431328)**, 315 North Washington Street, Zip 57070–2002, Mailing Address: P.O. Box 368, Zip 57070–0368; tel. 605/326–5161, (Total facility includes 52 beds in nursing home–type unit) **A**9 10 18 **F**6 10 15 28 30 34 40 43 45 53 56 57 59 63 65 69 75 79 81 87 97 107 111 118 124 126 127 129 131 132 **P**6 **S** Sanford Health, Sioux Falls, SD
Primary Contact: Georgia C. Pokorney, Chief Executive Officer
CFO: Anne Christiansen, Chief Financial Officer
CMO: Curtis Mark, M.D., Chief Medical Officer
Web address: www.pioneermemorial.org
**Control:** Other not–for–profit (including NFP Corporation) **Service:** General Medical and Surgical

**Staffed Beds:** 64 **Admissions:** 168 **Census:** 52 **Outpatient Visits:** 30013
**Births:** 0 **Total Expense ($000):** 12125 **Payroll Expense ($000):** 6333
**Personnel:** 148

### WAGNER—Charles Mix County

★ **WAGNER COMMUNITY MEMORIAL HOSPITAL AVERA (431315)**, 513 Third Street S.W., Zip 57380, Mailing Address: P.O. Box 280, Zip 57380–0280; tel. 605/384–3611 **A**9 10 18 **F**3 11 15 17 18 28 31 34 40 43 45 57 59 64 67 70 75 77 81 93 97 107 110 113 118 124 127 129 132 147 **P**6 **S** Avera Health, Sioux Falls, SD
Primary Contact: Bryan Slaba, Chief Executive Officer
CFO: Lisa Weisser, Supervisor Finance
CIO: Bernadette Koupal, Supervisor Business Office, Coordinator Information Systems and Administrative Assistant
CHR: Marcia Podzimek, Chief Human Resources Officer
Web address: www.avera.org
**Control:** Other not–for–profit (including NFP Corporation) **Service:** General Medical and Surgical

**Staffed Beds:** 20 **Admissions:** 351 **Census:** 3 **Outpatient Visits:** 10455
**Births:** 0 **Total Expense ($000):** 7249 **Payroll Expense ($000):** 3048
**Personnel:** 67

### WATERTOWN—Codington County

★ **PRAIRIE LAKES HEALTHCARE SYSTEM (430005)**, 401 9th Avenue N.W., Zip 57201–6210, Mailing Address: P.O. Box 1210, Zip 57201–1210; tel. 605/882–7000 **A**9 10 20 **F**3 7 12 13 18 20 22 28 29 30 31 34 35 38 40 43 50 57 58 59 60 62 63 76 77 78 79 80 81 82 83 84 85 86 87 89 93 107 108 111 113 118 119 120 122 123 129 131 132 145 146 147
Primary Contact: Jill Fuller, R.N., Ph.D., President and Chief Executive Officer
CFO: David Hinderaker, Chief Financial Officer
CMO: Daniel Reiffenberger, M.D., Chief Medical Staff
CIO: Grant Tillett, Director Information Technologies
CHR: Nathan Lake, Vice President Human Resources
Web address: www.prairielakes.com
**Control:** Other not–for–profit (including NFP Corporation) **Service:** General Medical and Surgical

**Staffed Beds:** 81 **Admissions:** 3443 **Census:** 32 **Outpatient Visits:** 82088
**Births:** 614 **Total Expense ($000):** 68488 **Payroll Expense ($000):** 28196
**Personnel:** 578

SD

*Many Facility Codes have changed. Please refer to the AHA Guide Code Chart.*

## WEBSTER—Day County

★ **SANFORD MEDICAL CENTER WEBSTER (431311)**, 1401 West 1st Street,
Zip 57274–1816, Mailing Address: P.O. Box 489, Zip 57274–0489;
tel. 605/345–3336 **A**9 10 18 **F**15 28 29 34 35 40 43 57 59 63 64 70 71 77
81 86 87 91 93 97 107 108 111 113 118 126 127 129 130 132 147 **P**6
**S** Sanford Health, Sioux Falls, SD
Primary Contact: David Rogers, Chief Executive Officer
CFO: Sheryl L. Pappas, Chief Financial Officer
Web address: www.sanfordhealth.org
**Control:** Other not–for–profit (including NFP Corporation) **Service:** General
Medical and Surgical

**Staffed Beds:** 20 **Admissions:** 186 **Census:** 1 **Outpatient Visits:** 16119
**Births:** 0 **Total Expense ($000):** 6756 **Payroll Expense ($000):** 3203
**Personnel:** 68

**SANFORD WEBSTER MEDICAL CENTER** See Sanford Medical Center Webster

## WESSINGTON SPRINGS—Jerauld County

★ **AVERA WESKOTA MEMORIAL HOSPITAL (431324)**, 604 First Street N.E.,
Zip 57382; tel. 605/539–1201 **A**9 10 18 **F**3 15 28 31 35 40 53 57 59 64 75
77 81 85 93 107 113 118 127 129 130 131 132 **P**5 **S** Avera Health, Sioux
Falls, SD
Primary Contact: Gaea Blue, Administrator and Chief Executive Officer
CFO: Linda Jager, Director Finance
CMO: Thomas Dean, M.D., Chief of Staff
Web address: www.averaweskota.org
**Control:** Other not–for–profit (including NFP Corporation) **Service:** General
Medical and Surgical

**Staffed Beds:** 23 **Admissions:** 153 **Census:** 2 **Outpatient Visits:** 5869
**Births:** 0 **Total Expense ($000):** 3654 **Payroll Expense ($000):** 1603
**Personnel:** 34

## WINNER—Tripp County

★ **WINNER REGIONAL HEALTHCARE CENTER (431334)**, 745 East Eighth
Street, Zip 57580–2677; tel. 605/842–7100, (Total facility includes 79 beds in
nursing home–type unit) **A**9 10 18 **F**13 15 17 28 31 34 35 40 47 56 57 59 62
64 65 75 76 78 79 81 85 87 107 108 113 118 126 127 130 131 132 147
**P**3 5 **S** Sanford Health, Sioux Falls, SD
Primary Contact: John M. Osse, Interim Chief Executive Officer
CFO: Phil Husher, Chief Financial Officer
CMO: Thomas Kosina, M.D., Chief of Staff
CHR: Karleen Flakus, Director Human Resources
Web address: www.winnerregional.org
**Control:** Other not–for–profit (including NFP Corporation) **Service:** General
Medical and Surgical

**Staffed Beds:** 104 **Admissions:** 858 **Census:** 84 **Outpatient Visits:** 5635
**Births:** 198 **Total Expense ($000):** 16259 **Payroll Expense ($000):** 7148
**Personnel:** 209

## YANKTON—Yankton County

☒ **AVERA SACRED HEART HOSPITAL (430012)**, 501 Summit Avenue,
Zip 57078–3899; tel. 605/668–8000, (Total facility includes 187 beds in nursing
home–type unit) **A**1 2 5 9 10 **F**2 3 8 10 13 15 20 22 28 29 30 31 34 35 40
45 51 53 54 56 57 59 60 62 63 64 65 68 70 75 76 77 78 79 80 81 82 84
85 87 89 90 93 96 97 107 108 110 111 114 115 116 117 118 120 122 124
126 127 128 129 130 131 132 134 145 147 **S** Avera Health, Sioux Falls, SD
Primary Contact: Pamela J. Rezac, Regional President
COO: Douglas R. Ekeren, Vice President Planning and Development
CFO: Jamie Schaefer, Vice President Finance
CMO: Barry A. Graham, M.D., Vice President Medical Affairs
CIO: Kathy Quinlivan, Director Management Information Systems
CHR: Kimberly Jensen, Vice President Human Resources
Web address: www.averasacredheart.com
**Control:** Church–operated, Nongovernment, not–for profit **Service:** General
Medical and Surgical

**Staffed Beds:** 293 **Admissions:** 4394 **Census:** 225 **Outpatient Visits:** 98992
**Births:** 548 **Total Expense ($000):** 94079 **Payroll Expense ($000):** 43652
**Personnel:** 768

**LEWIS AND CLARK SPECIALTY HOSPITAL (430096)**, 2601 Fox Run Parkway,
Zip 57078; tel. 605/665–5100, (Nonreporting) **A**9 10
Primary Contact: Michelle J. Jordan, Administrator
CFO: Terry Steichen, Business Officer
CHR: Elizabeth Steichen, Human Resources
Web address: www.lewisandclarkspecialty.com
**Control:** Corporation, Investor–owned, for–profit **Service:** Other specialty

**Staffed Beds:** 6

**SD**

# TENNESSEE

## ASHLAND CITY—Cheatham County

☒ **TRISTAR ASHLAND CITY MEDICAL CENTER (441311)**, 313 North Main Street, Zip 37015–1347; tel. 615/792–3030 **A**1 9 10 18 **F**3 15 29 30 40 45 81 93 107 111 118 122 129 132 **S** HCA, Nashville, TN
Primary Contact: Darrell White, R.N., Administrator
COO: Micki J. Slingerland, Chief Operating Officer
CFO: David A. Summers, Chief Financial Officer
CMO: Ravi Chari, M.D., Chief Medical Officer
CIO: David Archer, Director Information Systems
Web address: www.tristarcentennial.com
**Control:** Corporation, Investor–owned, for–profit **Service:** General Medical and Surgical

**Staffed Beds:** 12 **Admissions:** 182 **Census:** 4 **Outpatient Visits:** 20348 **Births:** 0 **Total Expense ($000):** 3500 **Payroll Expense ($000):** 3382 **Personnel:** 48

## ATHENS—Mcminn County

☒ **ATHENS REGIONAL MEDICAL CENTER (440068)**, 1114 West Madison Avenue, Zip 37303–4150, Mailing Address: P.O. Box 250, Zip 37371–0250; tel. 423/745–1411 **A**1 9 10 **F**3 11 13 15 28 29 30 31 34 35 37 40 41 43 44 45 46 48 50 51 54 57 59 61 64 65 68 70 73 74 75 76 77 78 79 81 84 85 86 89 90 93 102 107 108 110 111 113 114 115 116 117 118 125 128 129 131 132 134 145 146 147 **P**7 **S** LifePoint Hospitals, Inc., Brentwood, TN
Primary Contact: John R. Workman, Chief Executive Officer
CFO: David Alley, Chief Financial Officer
Web address: www.athensrmc.com
**Control:** Corporation, Investor–owned, for–profit **Service:** General Medical and Surgical

**Staffed Beds:** 63 **Admissions:** 2299 **Census:** 23 **Outpatient Visits:** 80716 **Births:** 409 **Total Expense ($000):** 31380 **Payroll Expense ($000):** 13342 **Personnel:** 289

## BARTLETT—Shelby County

☒ **SAINT FRANCIS HOSPITAL–BARTLETT (440228)**, 2986 Kate Bond Road, Zip 38133–4003; tel. 901/820–7000 **A**1 9 10 **F**3 11 13 15 18 20 29 30 31 34 35 38 40 44 45 49 50 57 59 60 64 68 70 72 74 75 76 77 78 79 81 85 86 87 93 107 108 110 111 113 118 129 130 145 146 147 **S** TENET Healthcare Corporation, Dallas, TX
Primary Contact: Jeremy Clark, Chief Executive Officer
COO: Gwen Bonner, Chief Operating Officer
CMO: Thomas W. Ratliff, M.D., President Medical Staff
CIO: Mike Hadley, Director Information Systems
CHR: Deb Lollar, Director Human Resources
Web address: www.saintfrancisbartlett.com
**Control:** Corporation, Investor–owned, for–profit **Service:** General Medical and Surgical

**Staffed Beds:** 100 **Admissions:** 5998 **Census:** 85 **Outpatient Visits:** 61304 **Births:** 790

## BOLIVAR—Hardeman County

☒ **BOLIVAR GENERAL HOSPITAL (440181)**, 650 Nuckolls Road, Zip 38008–1532, Mailing Address: P.O. Box 509, Zip 38008–0509; tel. 731/658–3100 **A**1 9 10 **F**3 15 29 30 35 40 45 57 59 64 75 81 87 93 107 118 129 131 132 145 **S** West Tennessee Healthcare, Jackson, TN
Primary Contact: Ruby Kirby, Administrator
CFO: Terry Swindell, Controller
CMO: Suara Rahaman, M.D., Chief Medical Staff
Web address: www.wth.net
**Control:** Hospital district or authority, Government, nonfederal **Service:** General Medical and Surgical

**Staffed Beds:** 21 **Admissions:** 342 **Census:** 3 **Outpatient Visits:** 16362 **Births:** 1 **Total Expense ($000):** 4519 **Payroll Expense ($000):** 2963 **Personnel:** 72

☐ **WESTERN MENTAL HEALTH INSTITUTE (444008)**, 11100 Old Highway 64, West, Zip 38008–1554; tel. 731/228–2000, (Nonreporting) **A**1 10
Primary Contact: Roger Pursley, Chief Executive Officer
CFO: Richard Taylor, Chief Financial Officer
CMO: Doug King, M.D., Director Clinical Services
CIO: Earl Bates, Director Information Technology
CHR: Barry Young, Director Human Resources
**Control:** State–Government, nonfederal **Service:** Psychiatric

**Staffed Beds:** 247

## BRISTOL—Sullivan County

☒ **SELECT SPECIALTY HOSPITAL–TRICITIES (442016)**, One Medical Park Boulevard, 5th Floor, Zip 37620–8964; tel. 423/844–5900, (Nonreporting) **A**1 9 10 **S** Select Medical Corporation, Mechanicsburg, PA
Primary Contact: Megan Schmidt, Chief Executive Officer
Web address: www.selectmedicalcorp.com
**Control:** Corporation, Investor–owned, for–profit **Service:** General Medical and Surgical

**Staffed Beds:** 33

☒ **WELLMONT BRISTOL REGIONAL MEDICAL CENTER (440012)**, 1 Medical Park Boulevard, Zip 37620–7430; tel. 423/844–1121 **A**1 2 3 5 9 10 **F**3 11 12 13 15 17 18 20 22 24 28 29 30 31 34 35 37 38 39 40 43 45 46 47 48 49 50 51 54 56 57 58 59 60 61 62 63 64 67 70 73 74 75 76 77 78 79 80 81 82 83 84 85 86 87 89 90 91 92 93 94 96 97 98 99 100 101 102 103 107 108 109 110 111 114 115 116 117 118 119 120 122 123 125 128 129 130 131 134 143 144 145 146 147 **P**5 **S** Wellmont Health System, Kingsport, TN
Primary Contact: Barton A. Hove, President
COO: Greg Neal, Chief Operating Officer
CFO: Troy Clark, Vice President Finance and Operations
CMO: Jack Butterworth, M.D., Vice President Medical Affairs
CIO: Dallas Rinehart, Director Operations and Information Services
CHR: Hamlin J. Wilson, Senior Vice President Human Resources
Web address: www.wellmont.org
**Control:** Other not–for–profit (including NFP Corporation) **Service:** General Medical and Surgical

**Staffed Beds:** 348 **Admissions:** 15970 **Census:** 200 **Outpatient Visits:** 149653 **Births:** 844 **Total Expense ($000):** 213380 **Payroll Expense ($000):** 67318 **Personnel:** 1604

## BROWNSVILLE—Haywood County

☒ **HAYWOOD PARK COMMUNITY HOSPITAL (440174)**, 2545 North Washington Avenue, Zip 38012–1610; tel. 731/772–4110 **A**1 9 10 **F**15 29 40 45 64 81 87 93 107 111 113 118 128 132 144 145 **S** Community Health Systems, Inc., Franklin, TN
Primary Contact: Jeremy Gray, Chief Executive Officer
CFO: Richard Read, Chief Financial Officer
CMO: Daniel Cofie, M.D., Chief of Staff
CHR: Phyllis Cozart, Director Human Resources
Web address: www.haywoodparkcommunity.com
**Control:** Corporation, Investor–owned, for–profit **Service:** General Medical and Surgical

**Staffed Beds:** 36 **Admissions:** 816 **Census:** 6 **Outpatient Visits:** 10025 **Births:** 0 **Total Expense ($000):** 8471 **Payroll Expense ($000):** 3836 **Personnel:** 79

## CAMDEN—Benton County

☒ **CAMDEN GENERAL HOSPITAL (441316)**, 175 Hospital Drive, Zip 38320–1617; tel. 731/584–6135 **A**1 9 10 18 **F**3 15 29 30 35 40 57 59 64 75 79 81 85 87 93 107 111 118 129 131 132 145 **S** West Tennessee Healthcare, Jackson, TN
Primary Contact: Denny R. Smith, Administrator
COO: James E. Ross, Chief Operating Officer
CFO: Terry Swindell, Chief Financial Officer
CMO: Jon R. Winter, D.O., Chief of Staff
CIO: Jeff Frieling, Vice President Information Systems
CHR: Barry Phillips, Executive Director Human Resources
Web address: www.wth.net
**Control:** Hospital district or authority, Government, nonfederal **Service:** General Medical and Surgical

**Staffed Beds:** 12 **Admissions:** 354 **Census:** 6 **Outpatient Visits:** 14774 **Births:** 0 **Total Expense ($000):** 4883 **Payroll Expense ($000):** 2828 **Personnel:** 69

## CARTHAGE—Smith County

☒ **RIVERVIEW REGIONAL MEDICAL CENTER NORTH (440186)**, 158 Hospital Drive, Zip 37030–1096; tel. 615/735–1560, (Nonreporting) **A**1 9 10 **S** LifePoint Hospitals, Inc., Brentwood, TN
Primary Contact: Jimmy D. Stuart, Administrator
CHR: Gina Anderson, Human Resources Officer
Web address: www.myriverviewmedical.com/
**Control:** Corporation, Investor–owned, for–profit **Service:** General Medical and Surgical

**Staffed Beds:** 63

**TN**

*Many Facility Codes have changed. Please refer to the AHA Guide Code Chart.*  © 2012 AHA Guide

✠ **RIVERVIEW REGIONAL MEDICAL CENTER SOUTH (441307)**, 130 Lebanon Highway, Zip 37030–2955; tel. 615/735–9815, (Nonreporting) **A**1 9 10 18 **S** LifePoint Hospitals, Inc., Brentwood, TN
Primary Contact: Jimmy D. Stuart, Administrator
Web address: www.myriverviewmedical.com
**Control:** Corporation, Investor–owned, for–profit **Service:** General Medical and Surgical

**Staffed Beds:** 25

### CELINA—Clay County

☐ **CUMBERLAND RIVER HOSPITAL (440141)**, 100 Old Jefferson Street, Zip 38551–4040, Mailing Address: P. O. Box 427, Zip 38551–0427; tel. 931/243–3581, (Nonreporting) **A**1 9 10
Primary Contact: Andrea Rich–McLerran, Chief Executive Officer
CFO: Tricia Strong, Chief Financial Officer
CMO: Roberto Mauricio, M.D., Chief of Staff
CIO: Margie Boone, Registered Health Information Technician
CHR: Susan Renodin Deaton, Chief Human Resources Officer
Web address: www.cumberlandriverhospital.com
**Control:** Corporation, Investor–owned, for–profit **Service:** General Medical and Surgical

**Staffed Beds:** 34

### CENTERVILLE—Hickman County

✠ **HICKMAN COMMUNITY HOSPITAL (441300)**, 135 East Swan Street, Zip 37033–1446; tel. 931/729–4271, (Total facility includes 40 beds in nursing home–type unit) **A**1 9 10 18 **F**29 30 34 35 40 41 45 56 57 59 62 64 65 67 77 81 86 87 89 90 93 104 107 118 126 127 129 132 134 147 **P**6 **S** Ascension Health, Saint Louis, MO
Primary Contact: Jack M. Keller, Administrator
COO: Jack M. Keller, Administrator
CFO: Craig Sullivan, Chief Financial Officer
CMO: Marek Durakiewicz, M.D., Chief of Staff
CIO: Kevin Campbell, Administrator Compliance and Mission
CHR: Dorothy Yokley, Assistant Administrator
Web address: www.hickmanhospital.com
**Control:** Other not–for–profit (including NFP Corporation) **Service:** General Medical and Surgical

**Staffed Beds:** 65 **Admissions:** 483 **Census:** 35 **Outpatient Visits:** 10600 **Births:** 0 **Total Expense ($000):** 15128 **Payroll Expense ($000):** 7295 **Personnel:** 116

### CHATTANOOGA—Hamilton County

✠ **ERLANGER MEDICAL CENTER (440104)**, 632 Morrison Springs Road, Zip 37415; tel. 423/778–7000, (Includes ERLANGER EAST HOSPITAL, 1755 Gunbarrel Road, Zip 37421; tel. 423/778–8700; Teresa Radeker, Administrator; ERLANGER NORTH HOSPITAL, 632 Morrison Springs Road, tel. 615/778–3300; T. C. THOMPSON CHILDREN'S HOSPITAL, 910 Blackford Street, Zip 37403; tel. 615/778–6011; Cynthia Rhodes, Administrator; WILLIE D. MILLER EYE CENTER, 975 East Third Street, Zip 37403; tel. 615/778–6011) **A**1 2 3 5 8 9 10 **F**3 8 11 12 13 14 15 17 18 19 20 21 22 23 24 25 26 27 28 29 30 31 32 34 35 37 38 39 40 41 43 44 45 47 49 50 54 55 57 59 60 61 64 68 70 72 74 75 76 77 78 79 80 81 82 85 86 87 88 89 93 96 97 98 103 107 108 110 111 113 114 117 118 119 120 122 123 125 128 129 130 131 137 143 144 145 146 147 **S** Erlanger Health System, Chattanooga, TN
Primary Contact: Charlesetta Woodard–Thompson, President and Chief Executive Officer
CFO: Britt Tabor, Senior Vice President and Chief Financial Officer
CMO: Cy Huffman, M.D., Chief Medical Officer
CIO: Laurene Vamprine, Senior Vice President Information Systems
CHR: Gregg Gentry, Senior Vice President Human Resources
Web address: www.erlanger.org
**Control:** Hospital district or authority, Government, nonfederal **Service:** General Medical and Surgical

**Staffed Beds:** 538 **Admissions:** 27705 **Census:** 378 **Outpatient Visits:** 258688 **Births:** 5288 **Total Expense ($000):** 517347 **Payroll Expense ($000):** 229160 **Personnel:** 4293

**ERLANGER WOMEN'S EAST HOSPITAL** See Erlanger East Hospital

✠ **HEALTHSOUTH CHATTANOOGA REHABILITATION HOSPITAL (440162)**, 2412 McCallie Avenue, Zip 37404–3398; tel. 423/698–0221 **A**1 10 **F**29 34 59 60 75 90 92 95 96 131 145 147 **S** HEALTHSOUTH Corporation, Birmingham, AL
Primary Contact: Scott Rowe, Chief Executive Officer
COO: Scott Rowe, Chief Executive Officer
CFO: Karen Klassen, Controller
CMO: Amjad Munir, M.D., Medical Director
CIO: Denise Smith, Director Health Information
CHR: Deborah Hersom, Director Human Resources
Web address: www.healthsouthchattanooga.com
**Control:** Corporation, Investor–owned, for–profit **Service:** Rehabilitation

**Staffed Beds:** 46 **Admissions:** 1027 **Census:** 36 **Outpatient Visits:** 0 **Births:** 0 **Total Expense ($000):** 10342 **Payroll Expense ($000):** 5972 **Personnel:** 124

✠ **KINDRED HOSPITAL–CHATTANOOGA (442007)**, 709 Walnut Street, Zip 37402–1916; tel. 423/266–7721, (Nonreporting) **A**1 9 10 **S** Kindred Healthcare, Louisville, KY
Primary Contact: William J. Bryant, Chief Executive Officer
COO: Rick Rheinheimer, Chief Clinical Officer
CFO: Julia Smith, Chief Financial Officer
CMO: Randy Heisser, M.D., Medical Director
CHR: Kellie McCampbell, Coordinator Human Resources
Web address: www.kindredchattanooga.com/
**Control:** Corporation, Investor–owned, for–profit **Service:** Long–Term Acute Care hospital

**Staffed Beds:** 44

✠ **MEMORIAL HEALTH CARE SYSTEM (440091)**, 2525 De Sales Avenue, Zip 37404–1161; tel. 423/495–2525, (Includes MEMORIAL HOSPITAL HIXSON, 2051 Hamill Road, Hixson, Zip 37343–4026; tel. 423/495–7100), (Nonreporting) **A**1 2 9 10 **S** Catholic Health Initiatives, Englewood, CO
Primary Contact: James M. Hobson, President and Chief Executive Officer
COO: Debra L. Moore, Senior Vice President
CFO: David Winchester, Interim Vice President and Chief Financial Officer
CMO: S. Gale Fellowes, M.D., Chief Medical Officer
CIO: David Peterson, Regional Chief Information Officer
CHR: Brad Pope, Vice President Human Resources
Web address: www.memorial.org
**Control:** Church–operated, Nongovernment, not–for profit **Service:** General Medical and Surgical

**Staffed Beds:** 336

☐ **MOCCASIN BEND MENTAL HEALTH INSTITUTE (444002)**, 100 Moccasin Bend Road, Zip 37405–4415; tel. 423/265–2271 **A**1 10 **F**30 34 50 56 59 65 75 77 86 87 98 100 101 102 103 129 131 134 142 145
Primary Contact: William L. Ventress, Chief Executive Officer
COO: Rob Cotterman, Assistant Superintendent Program Services
CMO: Terry R. Holmes, M.D., Clinical Director
CIO: Mickey Williams, Manager Information Technology
CHR: Cynthia Honeycutt, Director Human Resources
Web address: www.state.tn.us/mental/mhs/mbhmhi/moc.htm
**Control:** State–Government, nonfederal **Service:** Psychiatric

**Staffed Beds:** 150 **Admissions:** 2137 **Census:** 102 **Outpatient Visits:** 0 **Births:** 0 **Total Expense ($000):** 23597 **Payroll Expense ($000):** 13077 **Personnel:** 357

✠ **PARKRIDGE MEDICAL CENTER (440156)**, 2333 McCallie Avenue, Zip 37404–3258; tel. 423/698–6061, (Includes EAST RIDGE HOSPITAL, 941 Spring Creek Road, East Ridge, Zip 37412, Mailing Address: P.O. Box 91229, Zip 37412–6229; tel. 423/855–3500; Jarrett B. Millsaps, Jr., Chief Executive Officer; PARKRIDGE VALLEY HOSPTIAL, 2200 Morris Hill Road, Zip 37421; tel. 423/894–4220) **A**1 2 9 10 **F**3 5 13 15 18 20 22 24 26 28 29 30 31 39 40 45 46 49 51 56 57 58 59 60 70 72 75 76 77 78 79 81 85 90 93 98 99 103 104 105 106 107 108 110 111 113 114 118 120 125 128 129 130 145 147 **S** HCA, Nashville, TN
Primary Contact: Darrell W. Moore, Chief Executive Officer
COO: Jim L. Coleman, Jr., Chief Operating Officer
CIO: Paul Marsh, Director Information Systems
CHR: Carole Hoffman, Vice President
Web address: www.parkridgemedicalcenter.com
**Control:** Corporation, Investor–owned, for–profit **Service:** General Medical and Surgical

**Staffed Beds:** 433 **Admissions:** 14481 **Census:** 255 **Outpatient Visits:** 126529 **Births:** 1448 **Total Expense ($000):** 182875 **Payroll Expense ($000):** 71821 **Personnel:** 1249

**TN**

---

**Hospital, Medicare Provider Number, Address, Telephone, Approval, Facility, and Physician Codes, Health Care System**

★ American Hospital Association (AHA) membership
☐ The Joint Commission accreditation   ◇ DNV Healthcare Inc. accreditation
○ American Osteopathic Association (AOA) accreditation
△ Commission on Accreditation of Rehabilitation Facilities (CARF) accreditation

⊞ △ **SISKIN HOSPITAL FOR PHYSICAL REHABILITATION (443025)**, One Siskin Plaza, Zip 37403–1306; tel. 423/634–1200, (Total facility includes 29 beds in nursing home–type unit) **A**1 7 10 **F**29 35 53 54 59 64 75 82 90 93 127 129 131 145 147 **P**4
Primary Contact: Robert P. Main, President and Chief Executive Officer
COO: Linda Knudson Lind, Senior Vice President and Chief Operating Officer
CFO: Carol Arnhart, Controller and Chief Financial Officer
CMO: David N. Bowers, M.D., Medical Director
CHR: M. Debby Barker, Director Human Resources
Web address: www.siskinrehab.org
**Control:** Other not–for–profit (including NFP Corporation) **Service:** Rehabilitation

> **Staffed Beds:** 109 **Admissions:** 2146 **Census:** 74 **Outpatient Visits:** 32806 **Births:** 0 **Total Expense ($000):** 26942 **Payroll Expense ($000):** 15225 **Personnel:** 275

**T. C. THOMPSON CHILDREN'S HOSPITAL** See Erlanger Medical Center

**WILLIE D. MILLER EYE CENTER** See Erlanger Medical Center

## CLARKSVILLE—Montgomery County

⊞ **GATEWAY MEDICAL CENTER (440035)**, 651 Dunlop Lane, Zip 37040–5015, Mailing Address: P.O. Box 31629, Zip 37040–0028; tel. 931/502–1000, (Nonreporting) **A**1 2 9 10 **S** Community Health Systems, Inc., Franklin, TN
Primary Contact: Timothy Puthoff, Chief Executive Officer
COO: Corey Ewing, Chief Operating Officer
CFO: Scott Pfister, Chief Financial Officer
CMO: Thomas L. Ely, D.O., Chief Medical Officer
CIO: Frank Ruotolo, Chief Information Officer
CHR: Richard H. Johnson, Director Human Resources
Web address: www.ghsystem.com
**Control:** Partnership, Investor–owned, for–profit **Service:** General Medical and Surgical

> **Staffed Beds:** 247

## CLEVELAND—Bradley County

⊞ **SKYRIDGE MEDICAL CENTER (440185)**, 2305 Chambliss Avenue N.W., Zip 37311–3847, Mailing Address: P.O. Box 3060, Zip 37320–3060; tel. 423/559–6000, (Includes SKYRIDGE MEDICAL CENTER – WESTSIDE CAMPUS, 2800 Westside Drive N.W., Zip 37312–3599; tel. 423/339–4100; R. Coleman Foss, Chief Executive Officer) **A**1 9 10 **F**3 5 13 15 18 20 22 28 29 30 31 34 35 39 40 45 49 50 57 59 60 64 68 70 76 77 78 79 81 82 85 87 89 93 98 104 105 107 108 110 111 113 114 117 118 123 128 134 145 147 **S** Community Health Systems, Inc., Franklin, TN
Primary Contact: R. Coleman Foss, Chief Executive Officer
COO: Bernadette De Prez, Chief Operating Officer
CFO: Bill Ziesmer, Chief Financial Officer
CMO: Stephen Jackson, M.D., Chief of Staff
CHR: Kristine Godfrey, Director Human Resources
Web address: www.skyridgemedicalcenter.net
**Control:** Corporation, Investor–owned, for–profit **Service:** General Medical and Surgical

> **Staffed Beds:** 208 **Admissions:** 9483 **Census:** 108 **Outpatient Visits:** 113469 **Births:** 1030 **Personnel:** 823

## COLLIERVILLE—Shelby County

★ **BAPTIST MEMORIAL HOSPITAL–COLLIERVILLE (440217)**, 1500 West Poplar Avenue, Zip 38017–0601; tel. 901/861–9400 **A**9 10 **F**3 15 29 30 31 35 40 45 53 57 59 60 70 75 77 79 81 85 91 92 93 96 107 108 110 111 113 117 118 128 134 144 145 146 147 **S** Baptist Memorial Health Care Corporation, Memphis, TN
Primary Contact: Kyle Armstrong, Administrator
CFO: Terri Seago, Chief Financial Officer
CIO: Doug Reiselt, Vice President and Chief Information Officer
CHR: Brenda Johnson, Director Human Resources
Web address: www.bmhcc.org
**Control:** Other not–for–profit (including NFP Corporation) **Service:** General Medical and Surgical

> **Staffed Beds:** 81 **Admissions:** 2451 **Census:** 28 **Outpatient Visits:** 28540 **Births:** 0 **Total Expense ($000):** 44098 **Payroll Expense ($000):** 18053 **Personnel:** 300

## COLUMBIA—Maury County

⊞ **MAURY REGIONAL HOSPITAL (440073)**, 1224 Trotwood Avenue, Zip 38401–4802; tel. 931/381–1111, (Total facility includes 19 beds in nursing home–type unit) **A**1 2 9 10 19 **F**7 8 11 13 15 17 18 20 22 24 28 29 30 31 34 35 40 44 45 46 48 50 51 54 57 59 60 62 64 68 70 73 74 75 76 77 78 79 80 81 85 86 87 89 93 97 107 108 111 113 115 116 117 118 120 122 127 128 129 130 131 134 143 145 146 147
Primary Contact: Robert Otwell, Chief Executive Officer
CFO: Nick Swift, Chief Financial Officer
CMO: Charles A. Ball, M.D., Chief Medical Officer
CIO: Terry Phillips, Director Information Technology
CHR: Kaye Brewer, Director Human Resources
Web address: www.mauryregional.com
**Control:** County–Government, nonfederal **Service:** General Medical and Surgical

> **Staffed Beds:** 225 **Admissions:** 13819 **Census:** 149 **Outpatient Visits:** 214892 **Births:** 1483 **Total Expense ($000):** 216405 **Payroll Expense ($000):** 91347 **Personnel:** 1784

## COOKEVILLE—Putnam County

⊞ **COOKEVILLE REGIONAL MEDICAL CENTER (440059)**, 1 Medical Center Boulevard, Zip 38501–1795, Mailing Address: P.O. Box 340, Zip 38503–0340; tel. 931/528–2541, (Nonreporting) **A**1 2 9 10 19
Primary Contact: Menachem Langer, M.D., Chief Executive Officer
CFO: Paul Korth, Chief Financial Officer
CIO: Les Bernstein, Director Information Systems
CHR: Angel Lewis, Executive Director Human Resources
Web address: www.crmchealth.org
**Control:** City–Government, nonfederal **Service:** General Medical and Surgical

> **Staffed Beds:** 217

## COPPERHILL—Polk County

☐ **COPPER BASIN MEDICAL CENTER (441315)**, 144 Medical Center Drive, Zip 37317, Mailing Address: P.O. Box 990, Zip 37317–0990; tel. 423/496–5511, (Nonreporting) **A**1 9 10 18
Primary Contact: Alexander B. Altman, III, Chief Executive Officer and Chief Financial Officer
CFO: Alexander B. Altman, III, Chief Executive Officer and Chief Financial Officer
CMO: Allen Uhlik, M.D., Chief of Staff
CIO: Matt Deal, Director Maintenance
CHR: Kathy Pack, Manager Human Resources
Web address: www.copperbasin.org
**Control:** Other not–for–profit (including NFP Corporation) **Service:** General Medical and Surgical

> **Staffed Beds:** 25

## COVINGTON—Tipton County

⊞ **BAPTIST MEMORIAL HOSPITAL–TIPTON (440131)**, 1995 Highway 51 South, Zip 38019–3635; tel. 901/476–2621 **A**1 9 10 **F**3 8 11 15 29 30 31 34 35 40 45 57 59 65 70 74 75 76 77 78 79 81 85 87 89 93 100 107 108 110 111 113 116 118 119 120 128 129 131 134 145 147 **P**6 **S** Baptist Memorial Health Care Corporation, Memphis, TN
Primary Contact: William A. Tuttle, Interim Chief Executive Officer
CFO: Monique Hart, Chief Financial Officer
CMO: James W. Martin, D.D.S., Chief of Staff
CHR: Myra Cousar, Director Human Resources
Web address: www.bmhcc.org
**Control:** Other not–for–profit (including NFP Corporation) **Service:** General Medical and Surgical

> **Staffed Beds:** 50 **Admissions:** 1515 **Census:** 14 **Outpatient Visits:** 40486 **Births:** 387 **Total Expense ($000):** 23717 **Payroll Expense ($000):** 9943 **Personnel:** 214

## CROSSVILLE—Cumberland County

⊞ **CUMBERLAND MEDICAL CENTER (440009)**, 421 South Main Street, Zip 38555–5031; tel. 931/484–9511 **A**1 2 9 10 20 **F**3 8 11 13 15 18 20 28 29 30 31 34 35 40 41 48 49 51 53 54 57 59 62 64 66 68 70 74 75 76 77 78 79 80 81 85 86 87 89 90 93 96 97 107 111 113 118 119 120 128 129 131 134 145 146 147
Primary Contact: Barry Wagner, D.O., President and Chief Executive Officer
CFO: Larry E. Moore, Chief Financial Officer
CIO: Joe Lowe, Director Management Information Systems
CHR: Pat Whittenburg, Director Human Resources and Corporate Compliance Officer
Web address: www.cmchealthcare.org
**Control:** Other not–for–profit (including NFP Corporation) **Service:** General Medical and Surgical

> **Staffed Beds:** 165 **Admissions:** 6045 **Census:** 71 **Outpatient Visits:** 94690 **Births:** 706 **Total Expense ($000):** 83016 **Payroll Expense ($000):** 40415 **Personnel:** 881

*Many Facility Codes have changed. Please refer to the AHA Guide Code Chart.* © 2012 AHA Guide

## DAYTON—Rhea County

✠ **RHEA MEDICAL CENTER (441310)**, 9400 Rhea County Highway,
Zip 37321–7922; tel. 423/775–1121, (Nonreporting) **A**1 9 10 18 **S** QHR,
Brentwood, TN
Primary Contact: Kennedy L. Croom, Jr., Administrator and Chief Executive Officer
CFO: Harv Sanders, Chief Financial Officer
CMO: Chetan Shah, M.D., Chief of Staff
CHR: Peri Meadows, Director Human Resources
Web address: www.rheamedical.org
**Control:** County–Government, nonfederal **Service:** General Medical and Surgical

**Staffed Beds:** 25

## DICKSON—Dickson County

✠ **HORIZON MEDICAL CENTER (440046)**, 111 Highway 70 East,
Zip 37055–2080; tel. 615/446–0446, (Nonreporting) **A**1 2 9 10 **S** HCA,
Nashville, TN
Primary Contact: John A. Marshall, Chief Executive Officer
CFO: Clarence Gray, Chief Financial Officer
CIO: Rick Stoker, Director Management Information Systems
CHR: Sheila Kight, Director Human Resources
Web address: www.horizonmedicalcenter.com
**Control:** Corporation, Investor–owned, for–profit **Service:** General Medical and Surgical

**Staffed Beds:** 130

## DYERSBURG—Dyer County

✠ **DYERSBURG REGIONAL MEDICAL CENTER (440072)**, 400 East Tickle
Street, Zip 38024–3120; tel. 731/285–2410 **A**1 9 10 20 **F**7 8 13 15 18 20 29
34 39 40 45 46 47 48 49 50 51 57 59 60 70 75 76 77 79 81 82 87 89 91
92 93 97 107 108 109 110 111 113 114 118 119 120 126 128 129 130
132 142 143 144 145 146 147 **P**4 5 6 **S** Community Health Systems, Inc.,
Franklin, TN
Primary Contact: Ben Youree, Interim Chief Executive Officer
COO: Ben Youree, Assistant Chief Executive Officer
CFO: Terri Warren, Chief Financial Officer
CMO: Doreen Feldhouse, M.D., Chief of Staff
CIO: Russ Shephard, Senior Systems Analyst
CHR: Beverly Ray, Director Human Resources
Web address: www.dyersburgregionalmc.com
**Control:** Corporation, Investor–owned, for–profit **Service:** General Medical and Surgical

**Staffed Beds:** 110 **Admissions:** 5298 **Census:** 44 **Outpatient Visits:** 88000
**Births:** 499 **Total Expense ($000):** 52719 **Payroll Expense ($000):** 20789
**Personnel:** 599

## EAST RIDGE—Hamilton County

**EAST RIDGE HOSPITAL** See Parkridge Medical Center, Chattanooga

## ELIZABETHTON—Carter County

☐ **SYCAMORE SHOALS HOSPITAL (440018)**, 1501 West Elk Avenue,
Zip 37643–2874; tel. 423/542–1300 **A**1 9 10 **F**3 11 13 15 29 30 35 40 44
50 53 56 57 59 62 64 68 70 74 76 77 78 79 81 86 87 93 98 103 107 108
111 113 118 128 129 131 134 145 146 **S** Mountain States Health Alliance,
Johnson City, TN
Primary Contact: Dwayne Taylor, Chief Executive Officer
COO: Melanie Stanton, R.N., Chief Nursing Officer
CFO: Brad Logan, Chief Financial Officer
CMO: Morris H. Seligman, M.D., Chief Medical Officer and Chief Medical
Information Officer
CIO: Paul Merrywell, Chief Information Officer
CHR: Sharon Sheppard, Manager Human Resources
Web address: www.msha.com
**Control:** Other not–for–profit (including NFP Corporation) **Service:** General
Medical and Surgical

**Staffed Beds:** 79 **Admissions:** 3641 **Census:** 42 **Outpatient Visits:** 70995
**Births:** 479 **Total Expense ($000):** 33215 **Payroll Expense ($000):** 17310
**Personnel:** 320

## ERIN—Houston County

✠ **PATIENTS' CHOICE MEDICAL CENTER OF ERIN (441312)**, 5001 East Main
Street, Zip 37061–0489, Mailing Address: P.O. Box 489, Zip 37061–0489;
tel. 931/289–4211, (Nonreporting) **A**1 9 10 18 **S** Alliant Management Services,
Louisville, KY
Primary Contact: Gladys Anderson, Interim CEO
CFO: Shannon Allison, Chief Financial Officer
CMO: Erin Chambers, M.D., Chief Medical Officer
CHR: Reta Brady, Administrative Assistant and Manager Human Resources
Web address: www.pcmc–erintn.com/
**Control:** Corporation, Investor–owned, for–profit **Service:** General Medical and
Surgical

**Staffed Beds:** 25

## ERWIN—Unicoi County

✠ **UNICOI COUNTY MEMORIAL HOSPITAL (440001)**, 100 Greenway Circle,
Zip 37650–2196, Mailing Address: P.O. Box 802, Zip 37650–0802;
tel. 423/743–3141, (Nonreporting) **A**1 9 10
Primary Contact: Jim S. Pate, President and Chief Executive Officer
CFO: Toni Buchanan, Chief Financial Officer
CMO: Charles Miller, D.O., Chief of Staff
CIO: Spencer Levleit, Director Information Technology
CHR: Susan Broyles, Director Human Resources and Safety
Web address: www.ucmhnet.org
**Control:** Other not–for–profit (including NFP Corporation) **Service:** General
Medical and Surgical

**Staffed Beds:** 83

## ETOWAH—Mcminn County

✠ **WOODS MEMORIAL HOSPITAL (440054)**, 886 Highway 411 North,
Zip 37331–1912; tel. 423/263–3600, (Nonreporting) **A**1 9 10 **S** LifePoint
Hospitals, Inc., Brentwood, TN
Primary Contact: John R. Workman, Chief Executive Officer
CMO: Charles B. Cox, M.D., Chief of Staff
Web address: www.woodshospital.org
**Control:** Partnership, Investor–owned, for–profit **Service:** General Medical and
Surgical

**Staffed Beds:** 30

## FAYETTEVILLE—Lincoln County

★ **LINCOLN COUNTY HEALTH SYSTEM (440102)**, 106 Medical Center
Boulevard, Zip 37334–2684; tel. 931/438–1100, (Total facility includes 294
beds in nursing home–type unit) **A**9 10 **F**2 3 7 10 11 13 15 18 29 30 34 35 40
45 50 53 56 57 59 62 63 64 67 70 74 75 76 77 79 81 85 93 98 103 104
107 108 110 111 113 117 118 127 128 131 142 145 147 **S** QHR,
Brentwood, TN
Primary Contact: Jamie W. Guin, Jr., Chief Executive Officer
CFO: David Groce, Associate Administrator and Chief Financial Officer
CMO: Linda Jackson, M.D., Chief of Staff
CHR: Wendy Nogler, Director Human Resources
Web address: www.lchealthsystem.com
**Control:** County–Government, nonfederal **Service:** General Medical and Surgical

**Staffed Beds:** 353 **Admissions:** 2283 **Census:** 256 **Outpatient Visits:** 58705
**Births:** 273 **Total Expense ($000):** 35263 **Payroll Expense ($000):** 18334
**Personnel:** 557

## FRANKLIN—Williamson County

☐ **ROLLING HILLS HOSPITAL (444007)**, 2014 Quail Hollow Circle,
Zip 37067–5967; tel. 615/628–5700, (Nonreporting) **A**1 10 **S** Universal Health
Services, Inc., King of Prussia, PA
Primary Contact: Richard A. Bangert, Chief Executive Officer
Web address: www.rollinghillshospital.org/
**Control:** Corporation, Investor–owned, for–profit **Service:** Psychiatric

**Staffed Beds:** 80

☐ **WILLIAMSON MEDICAL CENTER (440029)**, 4321 Carothers Parkway,
Zip 37067–8542; tel. 615/435–5000, (Nonreporting) **A**1 2 9 10
Primary Contact: Dennis E. Miller, FACHE, Chief Executive Officer
COO: Julie Miller, Chief Operating Officer
CFO: Donald Webb, Chief Financial Officer
CMO: Starling C. Evins, M.D., Chief of Staff
CIO: Steve Dycus, Director Marketing and Public Relations
CHR: Phyllis Molyneux, Associate Administrator Human Resources and Education
Web address: www.williamsonmedicalcenter.org
**Control:** County–Government, nonfederal **Service:** General Medical and Surgical

**Staffed Beds:** 184

**TN**

---

**Hospital, Medicare Provider Number, Address, Telephone, Approval, Facility, and Physician Codes, Health Care System**

★ American Hospital Association (AHA) membership
☐ The Joint Commission accreditation ◇ DNV Healthcare Inc. accreditation
○ American Osteopathic Association (AOA) accreditation
△ Commission on Accreditation of Rehabilitation Facilities (CARF) accreditation

## GALLATIN—Sumner County

⊠ **SUMNER REGIONAL MEDICAL CENTER (440003)**, 555 Hartsville Pike, Zip 37066–2449, Mailing Address: P.O. Box 1558, Zip 37066–1558; tel. 615/452–4210, (Nonreporting) **A**1 2 9 10 **S** LifePoint Hospitals, Inc., Brentwood, TN
Primary Contact: Mary Jo Lewis, FACHE, President and Chief Executive Officer
CFO: David Wilhoite, CPA, Senior Vice President Finance and Chief Financial Officer
CIO: David Young, Vice President External Operations
Web address: www.sumner.org
**Control:** Corporation, Investor–owned, for–profit **Service:** General Medical and Surgical

**Staffed Beds:** 145

## GERMANTOWN—Shelby County

⊠ △ **BAPTIST REHABILITATION–GERMANTOWN (440147)**, 2100 Exeter Road, Zip 38138–3978; tel. 901/757–1350, (Total facility includes 18 beds in nursing home–type unit) **A**1 7 9 10 **F**3 29 30 34 35 54 57 59 64 68 75 77 79 86 87 90 91 92 93 96 107 111 113 118 127 129 130 131 142 145 147 **S** Baptist Memorial Health Care Corporation, Memphis, TN
Primary Contact: Brian Hogan, Interim Chief Executive Officer
CMO: Sunita Jain, M.D., Chief Medical Officer
CNO: Brian Hogan, Chief Nursing Officer
Web address: www.bmhcc.org
**Control:** Other not–for–profit (including NFP Corporation) **Service:** Rehabilitation

**Staffed Beds:** 58 **Admissions:** 967 **Census:** 35 **Outpatient Visits:** 11527 **Births:** 0 **Total Expense ($000):** 23539 **Payroll Expense ($000):** 11813 **Personnel:** 219

**METHODIST LE BONHEUR GERMANTOWN HOSPITAL** See Methodist Healthcare Memphis Hospitals, Memphis

## GREENEVILLE—Greene County

⊠ **LAUGHLIN MEMORIAL HOSPITAL (440025)**, 1420 Tusculum Boulevard, Zip 37745–5825; tel. 423/787–5000, (Total facility includes 90 beds in nursing home–type unit) **A**1 2 9 10 19 **F**3 11 12 28 31 34 35 37 40 45 46 48 49 50 56 57 59 62 64 68 70 73 74 75 76 77 78 79 81 85 86 87 89 93 107 108 110 111 113 114 117 118 120 122 127 128 129 130 131 133 134 145 146
Primary Contact: Charles H. Whitfield, Jr., President and Chief Executive Officer
CFO: Mark Compton, Chief Financial Officer
CHR: Robert Roark, Director Human Resources
Web address: www.laughlinmemorial.org
**Control:** Other not–for–profit (including NFP Corporation) **Service:** General Medical and Surgical

**Staffed Beds:** 224 **Admissions:** 3588 **Census:** 124 **Outpatient Visits:** 118393 **Births:** 228 **Total Expense ($000):** 70133 **Payroll Expense ($000):** 29014 **Personnel:** 602

⊠ **TAKOMA REGIONAL HOSPITAL (440050)**, 401 Takoma Avenue, Zip 37743–4647; tel. 423/639–3151 **A**1 9 10 **F**3 11 13 15 29 30 40 45 57 70 75 76 81 87 89 90 93 98 103 107 108 110 111 118 130 143 147 **S** Adventist Health System Sunbelt Health Care Corporation, Altamonte Springs, FL
Primary Contact: Daniel Wolcott, President
CFO: Tom VandenHoven, Chief Financial Officer
CMO: Frederick Myers, M.D., Chief Medical Officer
CHR: Jack Lister, Director Human Resources
Web address: www.takoma.org
**Control:** Church–operated, Nongovernment, not–for profit **Service:** General Medical and Surgical

**Staffed Beds:** 100 **Admissions:** 2275 **Census:** 29 **Outpatient Visits:** 175395 **Births:** 242 **Personnel:** 435

## HARRIMAN—Roane County

⊠ **ROANE MEDICAL CENTER (440031)**, 412 Devonia Street, Zip 37748–0489, Mailing Address: P.O. Box 489, Zip 37748–0489; tel. 865/882–1323 **A**1 9 10 **F**15 70 81 **S** Covenant Health, Knoxville, TN
Primary Contact: Gaye Jolly, Chief Executive Officer
CFO: Janice Bardill, Chief Financial Officer
CIO: Janice Bardill, Chief Financial Officer
CHR: Joyce Marsalis, Manager Human Resources
Web address: www.roanemedical.com
**Control:** Other not–for–profit (including NFP Corporation) **Service:** General Medical and Surgical

**Staffed Beds:** 36 **Admissions:** 1973 **Census:** 20 **Outpatient Visits:** 52821 **Births:** 0 **Total Expense ($000):** 26277 **Payroll Expense ($000):** 12381 **Personnel:** 268

## HARTSVILLE—Trousdale County

⊠ **TROUSDALE MEDICAL CENTER (441301)**, 500 Church Street, Zip 37074–1744; tel. 615/374–2221, (Nonreporting) **A**1 9 10 18 **S** LifePoint Hospitals, Inc., Brentwood, TN
Primary Contact: William D. Mize, Interim Chief Executive Officer
COO: William D. Mize, Chief Operating Officer
CFO: David Wilhoite, CPA, Senior Vice President Finance and Chief Financial Officer
CIO: David Young, Senior Vice President Planning and Technology
CHR: Amy Overstreet, Director Human Resources
Web address: www.trousdale.org
**Control:** Corporation, Investor–owned, for–profit **Service:** General Medical and Surgical

**Staffed Beds:** 25

## HENDERSONVILLE—Sumner County

⊠ **HENDERSONVILLE MEDICAL CENTER (440194)**, 355 New Shackle Island Road, Zip 37075–2479; tel. 615/338–1000 **A**1 9 10 **F**3 13 15 18 20 22 26 29 30 40 45 46 48 49 50 54 64 70 74 75 76 79 81 82 85 87 93 107 110 111 113 114 118 129 145 146 **S** HCA, Nashville, TN
Primary Contact: Regina Bartlett, Chief Executive Officer
COO: Kenneth C. Donahey, Chief Operating Officer
CFO: Michael Morrison, Chief Financial Officer
CMO: Randy Howard, M.D., Chief of Staff
CIO: Hal Schultheis, Director Information Systems
CHR: Jennifer Burden, Vice President Human Resources
Web address: www.hendersonvillemedicalcenter.com
**Control:** Corporation, Investor–owned, for–profit **Service:** General Medical and Surgical

**Staffed Beds:** 81 **Admissions:** 4718 **Census:** 51 **Outpatient Visits:** 50797 **Births:** 598 **Total Expense ($000):** 63452 **Payroll Expense ($000):** 25723 **Personnel:** 365

## HERMITAGE—Davidson County

⊠ **SUMMIT MEDICAL CENTER (440150)**, 5655 Frist Boulevard, Zip 37076–2053; tel. 615/316–3000 **A**1 2 9 10 **F**3 11 13 15 18 20 22 26 28 29 30 31 34 35 37 38 39 40 43 45 46 47 48 49 50 53 56 57 59 61 64 70 72 74 75 76 77 78 79 80 81 82 85 87 89 93 98 100 102 107 108 110 111 113 114 117 118 120 122 123 125 128 129 130 134 144 145 146 147 **P**6 **S** HCA, Nashville, TN
Primary Contact: Jeffrey T. Whitehorn, Chief Executive Officer
COO: Greg Caples, Chief Operating Officer
CFO: Timothy Stanfill, Chief Financial Officer
Web address: www.summitmedctr.com
**Control:** Corporation, Investor–owned, for–profit **Service:** General Medical and Surgical

**Staffed Beds:** 188 **Admissions:** 9916 **Census:** 109 **Outpatient Visits:** 108314 **Births:** 1197 **Total Expense ($000):** 115775 **Payroll Expense ($000):** 42614 **Personnel:** 708

## HUMBOLDT—Gibson County

⊠ **HUMBOLDT GENERAL HOSPITAL (440115)**, 3525 Chere Carol Road, Zip 38343–3699; tel. 731/784–2321 **A**1 9 10 **F**3 15 29 30 35 40 57 59 64 68 75 81 85 87 93 107 118 129 131 132 145 **S** West Tennessee Healthcare, Jackson, TN
Primary Contact: Sherry Scruggs, Administrator
CFO: Terry Swindell, Chief Financial Officer
CMO: Ernesto Chioco, M.D., Chief of Staff
Web address: www.wth.net
**Control:** Hospital district or authority, Government, nonfederal **Service:** General Medical and Surgical

**Staffed Beds:** 30 **Admissions:** 668 **Census:** 7 **Outpatient Visits:** 15386 **Births:** 0 **Total Expense ($000):** 3658 **Payroll Expense ($000):** 3653 **Personnel:** 84

## HUNTINGDON—Carroll County

⊠ **BAPTIST MEMORIAL HOSPITAL–HUNTINGDON (440016)**, 631 R.B. Wilson Drive, Zip 38344–1727; tel. 731/986–4461 **A**1 9 10 **F**3 7 15 28 29 30 34 35 40 50 57 59 61 62 63 64 65 68 70 75 77 79 81 82 83 85 86 87 93 102 107 111 113 117 118 129 130 131 132 134 144 145 147 **S** Baptist Memorial Health Care Corporation, Memphis, TN
Primary Contact: Susan M. Breeden, Administrator and Chief Executive Officer
CFO: Sharron Holland, Chief Financial Officer
CHR: Kim King, Director Human Resources and Public Relations
Web address: www.bmhcc.org
**Control:** Other not–for–profit (including NFP Corporation) **Service:** General Medical and Surgical

**Staffed Beds:** 33 **Admissions:** 845 **Census:** 10 **Outpatient Visits:** 19204 **Births:** 0 **Total Expense ($000):** 12971 **Payroll Expense ($000):** 6229 **Personnel:** 186

**TN**

*Many Facility Codes have changed. Please refer to the AHA Guide Code Chart.* © 2012 AHA Guide

## JACKSON—Madison County

⊠ △ **JACKSON–MADISON COUNTY GENERAL HOSPITAL (440002)**, 620 Skyline Drive, Zip 38301; tel. 731/541–5000 **A**1 2 3 5 7 9 10 19 **F**3 7 8 11 13 15 17 18 20 22 24 26 28 29 30 31 34 35 40 45 46 47 48 49 51 56 57 58 59 60 63 64 65 66 68 70 72 74 75 76 77 78 79 80 81 82 83 84 85 86 87 88 89 90 92 93 94 96 97 107 108 110 111 112 114 115 116 117 118 119 120 123 125 128 129 130 131 134 144 145 146 147 **P**5 8 **S** West Tennessee Healthcare, Jackson, TN
Primary Contact: Bobby Arnold, President and Chief Executive Officer
COO: James E. Ross, Vice President and Chief Operating Officer
CFO: Jeff Blankenship, CPA, Vice President and Chief Financial Officer
CMO: Lucius Wright, M.D., Chief of Staff
CIO: Jeff Frieling, Vice President and Chief Information Officer
Web address: www.wth.org
**Control:** Hospital district or authority, Government, nonfederal **Service:** General Medical and Surgical

**Staffed Beds:** 619 **Admissions:** 27132 **Census:** 420 **Outpatient Visits:** 177278 **Births:** 2778 **Total Expense ($000):** 436439 **Payroll Expense ($000):** 187698 **Personnel:** 3832

★ **PATHWAYS OF TENNESSEE (444010)**, 238 Summar Drive, Zip 38301–3906; tel. 731/541–8200 **A**10 **F**4 5 29 35 38 57 59 98 99 100 101 102 103 104 131 133 **S** West Tennessee Healthcare, Jackson, TN
Primary Contact: Pam Henson, Executive Director
CMO: Doug King, M.D., Medical Director
CIO: Jeff Frieling, Chief Information Officer
CHR: Barry Phillips, Director Human Resources
Web address: www.wth.net
**Control:** Hospital district or authority, Government, nonfederal **Service:** Psychiatric

**Staffed Beds:** 25 **Admissions:** 691 **Census:** 8 **Outpatient Visits:** 141428 **Births:** 0 **Total Expense ($000):** 16280 **Payroll Expense ($000):** 9225 **Personnel:** 242

⊠ **REGIONAL HOSPITAL OF JACKSON (440189)**, 367 Hospital Boulevard, Zip 38305–2080; tel. 731/661–2000 **A**1 9 10 **F**13 15 18 20 22 29 34 39 40 45 49 56 57 59 60 62 64 70 74 75 76 77 78 79 81 82 89 92 93 97 107 108 110 111 112 113 114 118 128 129 131 146 **S** Community Health Systems, Inc., Franklin, TN
Primary Contact: Stephen Grubbs, Chief Executive Officer
CFO: Richard Read, Chief Financial Officer
CHR: Joel R. Windham, Director Human Resources
Web address: www.regionalhospitaljackson.com/Pages/Home.aspx
**Control:** Corporation, Investor–owned, for–profit **Service:** General Medical and Surgical

**Staffed Beds:** 120 **Admissions:** 6383 **Census:** 64 **Personnel:** 650

## JAMESTOWN—Fentress County

☐ **JAMESTOWN REGIONAL MEDICAL CENTER (440083)**, 436 Central Avenue West, Zip 38556–3031, Mailing Address: P.O. Box 1500, Zip 38556–1500; tel. 931/879–8171, (Nonreporting) **A**1 9 10 20 **S** Health Management Associates, Naples, FL
Primary Contact: Kimberly L. Anthony, Chief Executive Officer
CMO: Mark Hendrixson, M.D., Chief Medical Officer
CIO: Rick Smith, Director Information Systems
CHR: Shelia Russell, Director Human Resources
Web address: www.jamestownregional.org
**Control:** Corporation, Investor–owned, for–profit **Service:** General Medical and Surgical

**Staffed Beds:** 85

## JASPER—Marion County

☐ **GRANDVIEW MEDICAL CENTER (440064)**, 1000 Highway 28, Zip 37347–3638; tel. 423/837–9500, (Nonreporting) **A**1 9 10 **S** Capella Healthcare, Franklin, TN
Primary Contact: Bruce A. Baldwin, Chief Executive Officer
CFO: Debbie Hennessee, Chief Financial Officer
Web address: www.grandviewhospital.com
**Control:** Corporation, Investor–owned, for–profit **Service:** General Medical and Surgical

**Staffed Beds:** 68

## JEFFERSON CITY—Jefferson County

⊠ **JEFFERSON MEMORIAL HOSPITAL (440056)**, 110 Hospital Drive, Zip 37760–5281; tel. 865/471–2500, (Nonreporting) **A**1 9 10 **S** Health Management Associates, Naples, FL
Primary Contact: David V. Bunch, President
COO: Carol C. Wolfenbarger, R.N., Chief Operating Officer and Chief Nursing Executive
CFO: Roseann M. Devault, Chief Financial Officer
Web address: www.hma.com/content/jefferson–memorial–hospital
**Control:** Corporation, Investor–owned, for–profit **Service:** General Medical and Surgical

**Staffed Beds:** 54

**ST. MARY'S JEFFERSON MEMORIAL HOSPITAL** See Jefferson Memorial Hospital

## JELLICO—Campbell County

⊠ **JELLICO COMMUNITY HOSPITAL (440180)**, 188 Hospital Lane, Zip 37762–4400; tel. 423/784–7252 **A**1 9 10 **F**3 7 11 13 15 29 30 34 35 40 43 44 48 50 53 54 57 59 62 64 65 68 70 75 76 77 81 85 86 87 93 97 107 108 110 111 113 118 129 130 131 132 133 134 142 145 147 **P**6 **S** Adventist Health System Sunbelt Health Care Corporation, Altamonte Springs, FL
Primary Contact: Erik Wangsness, Chief Executive Officer
COO: Pamela Hodge, R.N., Chief Nursing Officer and Coordinator Performance Improvement
CFO: William Villegas, Chief Financial Officer
CMO: Geogy Thomas, M.D., Chief of Staff
CIO: Derek Brown, Chief Information Officer
CHR: Vince Vannett, Director Human Resources
Web address: www.jellicohospital.com
**Control:** Other not–for–profit (including NFP Corporation) **Service:** General Medical and Surgical

**Staffed Beds:** 31 **Admissions:** 1765 **Census:** 18 **Outpatient Visits:** 51794 **Births:** 161 **Total Expense ($000):** 26794 **Payroll Expense ($000):** 10770 **Personnel:** 322

## JOHNSON CITY—Washington County

⊠ **FRANKLIN WOODS COMMUNITY HOSPITAL (440184)**, 300 MedTech Parkway, Zip 37604–2277; tel. 423/302–1000, (Total facility includes 34 beds in nursing home–type unit) (Data for 354 days) **A**1 9 10 **F**3 13 29 30 35 40 44 50 56 59 68 70 74 76 77 79 81 86 87 93 97 107 108 111 113 117 118 127 129 142 145 **S** Mountain States Health Alliance, Johnson City, TN
Primary Contact: Tony Benton, Chief Executive Officer
Web address: www.msha.com
**Control:** Other not–for–profit (including NFP Corporation) **Service:** General Medical and Surgical

**Staffed Beds:** 114 **Admissions:** 4476 **Census:** 70 **Outpatient Visits:** 38555 **Births:** 862 **Total Expense ($000):** 48102 **Payroll Expense ($000):** 21490 **Personnel:** 375

⊠ **JOHNSON CITY MEDICAL CENTER (440063)**, 400 North State of Franklin Road, Zip 37604–6094; tel. 423/431–6111, (Includes NISWONGER CHILDREN'S HOSPITAL, 400 North State Of Franklin Road, Zip 37604–6035; tel. 423/431–6111), (Total facility includes 13 beds in nursing home–type unit) **A**1 2 3 5 8 9 10 **F**3 7 8 11 12 13 15 17 18 19 20 21 22 23 24 25 26 28 29 30 31 32 34 35 39 40 43 44 46 47 48 49 50 51 53 54 55 56 57 58 59 60 61 62 63 64 68 70 72 74 75 76 77 78 79 81 82 84 85 86 87 88 89 93 97 100 102 107 108 111 113 114 116 117 118 120 122 123 127 128 129 130 131 133 134 137 140 141 142 145 146 147 **P**6 **S** Mountain States Health Alliance, Johnson City, TN
Primary Contact: David E. Nicely, Chief Executive Officer
CFO: Shane Hilton, Vice President and Chief Financial Officer
CHR: Jamie Parsons, Vice President Human Resources
Web address: www.msha.com
**Control:** Other not–for–profit (including NFP Corporation) **Service:** General Medical and Surgical

**Staffed Beds:** 514 **Admissions:** 26079 **Census:** 365 **Outpatient Visits:** 255178 **Births:** 1343 **Total Expense ($000):** 330378 **Payroll Expense ($000):** 126109 **Personnel:** 2405

**NORTH SIDE HOSPITAL** See Franklin Woods Community Hospital

△ **QUILLEN REHABILITATION HOSPITAL**, 2511 Wesley Street, Zip 37601–1723; tel. 423/283–0700 **A**7 **F**3 29 30 68 74 79 86 90 93 129 131 **S** Mountain States Health Alliance, Johnson City, TN
Primary Contact: Ann Fleming, Senior Vice President
Web address: www.msha.com
**Control:** Other not–for–profit (including NFP Corporation) **Service:** Rehabilitation

**Staffed Beds:** 47 **Admissions:** 648 **Census:** 23 **Outpatient Visits:** 13271 **Births:** 0 **Total Expense ($000):** 4776 **Payroll Expense ($000):** 4392 **Personnel:** 87

**TN**

---

**Hospital, Medicare Provider Number, Address, Telephone, Approval, Facility, and Physician Codes, Health Care System**

★ American Hospital Association (AHA) membership
☐ The Joint Commission accreditation
◇ DNV Healthcare Inc. accreditation
○ American Osteopathic Association (AOA) accreditation
△ Commission on Accreditation of Rehabilitation Facilities (CARF) accreditation

**WOODRIDGE HOSPITAL**, 403 State of Franklin Road, Zip 37604–6034; tel. 423/431–7060 **A**3 5 **F**29 30 68 86 98 100 101 103 104 105 129 131 **S** Mountain States Health Alliance, Johnson City, TN
Primary Contact: Grace Pereira, Interim Chief Executive Officer
COO: Kim Moore, Director Operations
CFO: John Doyle, Assistant Vice President and Chief Financial Officer
CMO: Terry Borel, M.D., Medical Director
CIO: Ed Herbert, Vice President Marketing and Communications
Web address: www.msha.com
**Control:** Other not–for–profit (including NFP Corporation) **Service:** Psychiatric

Staffed Beds: 84 Admissions: 3430 Census: 54 Outpatient Visits: 2216
Births: 0 Total Expense ($000): 13813 Payroll Expense ($000): 7706
Personnel: 140

### KINGSPORT—Sullivan County

☒ **HEALTHSOUTH REHABILITATION HOSPITAL (443027)**, 113 Cassel Drive, Zip 37660–3775; tel. 423/246–7240, (Nonreporting) **A**1 10 **S** HEALTHSOUTH Corporation, Birmingham, AL
Primary Contact: Susan Glenn, Chief Executive Officer
CFO: Natalie Tilson, Controller
CMO: James P. Little, M.D., Medical Director
CIO: Natalie Tilson, Controller
CHR: Joyce Jones, Director Human Resources
Web address: www.healthsouthkingsport.com
**Control:** Corporation, Investor–owned, for–profit **Service:** Rehabilitation

Staffed Beds: 50

☐ **INDIAN PATH MEDICAL CENTER (440176)**, 2000 Brookside Drive, Zip 37660–4627; tel. 423/857–7000, (Total facility includes 20 beds in nursing home–type unit) **A**1 9 10 **F**3 5 8 11 13 15 18 20 29 30 35 38 40 49 50 51 56 57 59 60 64 68 70 73 74 75 76 77 78 79 81 86 87 93 97 100 101 102 103 104 105 107 108 111 113 117 118 122 127 128 129 130 131 145 146 147 **S** Mountain States Health Alliance, Johnson City, TN
Primary Contact: Monty E. McLaurin, President and Chief Executive Officer
CFO: Pat Hale, Chief Financial Officer
CMO: Frank Lauro, M.D., Chief Medical Officer
CIO: Matthew Grissinger, Site Manager Information Systems
CHR: Kevin M. Smith, Director Human Resources
CNO: Susan Fannon, Chief Nursing Officer
Web address: www.msha.com
**Control:** Other not–for–profit (including NFP Corporation) **Service:** General Medical and Surgical

Staffed Beds: 189 Admissions: 6823 Census: 81 Outpatient Visits: 147883
Births: 878 Total Expense ($000): 81435 Payroll Expense ($000): 33063
Personnel: 621

☒ **WELLMONT HOLSTON VALLEY MEDICAL CENTER (440017)**, 130 West Ravine Street, Zip 37660, Mailing Address: P.O. Box 238, Zip 37662–0238; tel. 423/224–4000 **A**1 2 3 5 9 10 **F**3 11 12 13 15 17 18 19 20 22 24 26 28 29 30 31 32 34 35 40 43 48 49 50 51 54 55 57 58 59 60 61 64 65 68 70 72 74 75 76 77 78 79 81 82 83 84 85 87 88 89 92 93 107 108 110 111 113 114 115 116 117 118 119 120 121 122 125 128 129 130 131 134 145 146 147 **S** Wellmont Health System, Kingsport, TN
Primary Contact: Virginia Frank, President and Chief Executive Officer
COO: Martha O'Regan Chill, Executive Vice President Operations
CFO: Brad H. Price, Vice President Finance and Operations
CMO: J. Dale Sargent, M.D., Chief Medical Officer
CIO: Kent Petty, Chief Information Officer
CHR: Hamlin J. Wilson, Senior Vice President Human Resources
Web address: www.wellmont.org
**Control:** Other not–for–profit (including NFP Corporation) **Service:** General Medical and Surgical

Staffed Beds: 345 Admissions: 19313 Census: 248 Outpatient Visits: 190293 Births: 993 Total Expense ($000): 284797 Payroll Expense ($000): 79396 Personnel: 1663

### KNOXVILLE—Knox County

☐ **EAST TENNESSEE CHILDREN'S HOSPITAL (443303)**, 2018 Clinch Avenue, Zip 37916–2393, Mailing Address: P.O. Box 15010, Zip 37901–5010; tel. 865/541–8000 **A**1 9 10 **F**3 11 29 30 31 32 35 39 40 41 43 44 54 57 58 59 62 64 68 72 74 75 77 78 79 81 82 85 86 87 88 89 93 94 97 107 111 118 128 129 131 145 **P**8
Primary Contact: Keith D. Goodwin, President and Chief Executive Officer
COO: Rudolph McKinley, Jr., Vice President Operations and Chief Operating Officer
CFO: Zane Goodrich, Vice President Finance
CMO: Joe Childs, M.D., Vice President Medical Services
CIO: John Hanks, Director Information Systems
CHR: Sue Wilburn, Vice President Human Resources and Organizational Development
CNO: Laura P. Barnes, MSN, Vice President Patient Care Services and Chief Nursing Officer
Web address: www.etch.com
**Control:** Other not–for–profit (including NFP Corporation) **Service:** Children's general

Staffed Beds: 152 Admissions: 5832 Census: 98 Outpatient Visits: 170757
Births: 0 Total Expense ($000): 140608 Payroll Expense ($000): 67657
Personnel: 1283

☒ △ **FORT SANDERS REGIONAL MEDICAL CENTER (440125)**, 1901 West Clinch Avenue, Zip 37916–2307; tel. 865/541–1111, (Total facility includes 24 beds in nursing home–type unit) **A**1 2 7 9 10 **F**3 11 13 15 17 18 20 22 24 26 28 29 30 31 34 35 40 45 46 47 48 49 50 51 54 55 56 57 58 59 60 61 64 68 74 75 76 77 78 79 80 81 84 85 86 87 90 91 92 93 94 96 100 102 107 108 110 111 113 114 117 118 125 127 128 129 130 131 135 140 141 145 146 147 **P**6 7 **S** Covenant Health, Knoxville, TN
Primary Contact: Keith Altshuler, President and Chief Administrative Officer
Web address: www.covenanthealth.com
**Control:** Other not–for–profit (including NFP Corporation) **Service:** General Medical and Surgical

Staffed Beds: 402 Admissions: 16621 Census: 259 Outpatient Visits: 212282 Births: 2752 Total Expense ($000): 248267 Payroll Expense ($000): 84427 Personnel: 1701

**MERCY MEDICAL CENTER WEST** See Turkey Creek Medical Center

☒ **PARKWEST MEDICAL CENTER (440173)**, 9352 Park West Boulevard, Zip 37923–4325, Mailing Address: P.O. Box 22993, Zip 37933–0993; tel. 865/373–1000 **A**1 2 9 10 **F**3 8 11 12 13 15 17 18 20 22 24 28 29 30 31 40 45 46 47 49 50 51 56 60 64 68 70 74 76 77 78 79 81 82 84 85 87 98 103 107 110 111 114 118 125 128 129 130 134 145 146 147 **P**6 7 **S** Covenant Health, Knoxville, TN
Primary Contact: Rick Lassiter, President and Chief Administrative Officer
COO: Emlyn Cobble, Vice President and Chief Support Officer
CFO: Scott Hamilton, Vice President and Chief Financial Officer
CHR: Randall Carr, Director Human Resources
Web address: www.yesparkwest.com
**Control:** Other not–for–profit (including NFP Corporation) **Service:** General Medical and Surgical

Staffed Beds: 297 Admissions: 17058 Census: 212 Outpatient Visits: 151271 Births: 1648 Total Expense ($000): 223209 Payroll Expense ($000): 73415 Personnel: 1559

☒ △ **PHYSICIANS REGIONAL MEDICAL CENTER (440120)**, 900 East Oak Hill Avenue, Zip 37917–4556; tel. 865/545–8000, (Includes NORTH KNOXVILLE MEDICAL CENTER, 7565 Dannaher Way, Powell, Zip 37849–4029; tel. 865/859–7000; Rob Followell, Chief Executive Officer), (Data for 92 days) **A**1 2 7 9 10 **F**8 13 15 17 18 20 22 24 26 28 29 30 31 34 35 40 49 51 53 54 56 57 59 60 61 62 63 64 70 73 74 75 76 77 78 79 80 81 82 83 84 85 86 87 90 92 93 96 98 100 103 105 107 108 110 111 113 114 116 117 118 119 120 122 125 127 128 129 130 131 145 146 147 **S** Health Management Associates, Naples, FL
Primary Contact: Karen Metz, Chief Executive Officer
CFO: Rhonda Maynard, Chief Financial Officer
CIO: Tom Lakins, Director Information Systems
CHR: Marty Margetts, Senior Vice President Human Resources
Web address: www.hma.com/content/physicians–regional–medical–center
**Control:** Corporation, Investor–owned, for–profit **Service:** General Medical and Surgical

Staffed Beds: 243 Admissions: 4097 Census: 203 Outpatient Visits: 51402
Births: 324 Total Expense ($000): 47185 Payroll Expense ($000): 15587
Personnel: 1364

☒ **SELECT SPECIALTY HOSPITAL–KNOXVILLE (442012)**, 1901 Clinch Avenue, Suite 404, Zip 37916–2307; tel. 865/541–2615, (Nonreporting) **A**1 9 10 **S** Select Medical Corporation, Mechanicsburg, PA
Primary Contact: Vanda Scott, Chief Executive Officer
COO: Steve Plumlee, Chief Operating Officer
CFO: Lynne Rudisill, Controller
CMO: Brantly Burns, M.D., Medical Director
CIO: Vanda Scott, Chief Executive Officer
CHR: Shara Johnson, Coordinator Human Resources
Web address: www.selectmedicalcorp.com
**Control:** Corporation, Investor–owned, for–profit **Service:** Long–Term Acute Care hospital

Staffed Beds: 35

☒ **SELECT SPECIALTY HOSPITAL–NORTH KNOXVILLE (442015)**, 900 East Oak Hill Avenue, Zip 37917; tel. 865/541–2615, (Nonreporting) **A**1 9 10 **S** Select Medical Corporation, Mechanicsburg, PA
Primary Contact: Vanda Scott, Chief Executive Officer
COO: Steve Plumlee, Chief Operating Officer
CFO: Lynne Rudisill, Controller
CMO: Jeff Summers, M.D., Medical Director
CHR: Hope Franklin, Coordinator Human Resources
Web address: www.selectmedicalcorp.com
**Control:** Corporation, Investor–owned, for–profit **Service:** Long–Term Acute Care hospital

Staffed Beds: 33

TN

*Many Facility Codes have changed. Please refer to the AHA Guide Code Chart.* © 2012 AHA Guide

✠ **THE UNIVERSITY OF TENNESSEE MEDICAL CENTER (440015)**, 1924 Alcoa Highway, Box 81, Zip 37920–6900; tel. 865/305–9000 **A**1 2 3 5 8 9 10 13 **F**3 8 11 12 13 14 15 17 18 19 20 21 22 23 24 25 26 27 28 29 30 31 34 35 36 39 40 43 45 46 47 48 49 50 51 53 54 55 56 57 58 59 60 61 62 63 64 68 70 71 72 74 75 76 77 78 79 81 82 84 85 87 88 91 92 93 94 96 97 107 108 109 110 111 113 114 115 116 117 118 119 120 121 122 123 125 128 129 130 131 134 137 140 141 143 144 145 146 147 **P**6
Primary Contact: Joseph Landsman, President and Chief Executive Officer
COO: David Hall, Senior Vice President and Chief Operating Officer
CFO: Thomas Fisher, Senior Vice President and Chief Financial Officer
CMO: John W. Lacey, III, M.D., Senior Vice President and Chief Medical Officer
CIO: Douglas Fain, Director Computer Services
CHR: Betty Gissel, Vice President Human Resources
Web address: www.utmedicalcenter.org
**Control:** Other not–for–profit (including NFP Corporation) **Service:** General Medical and Surgical

**Staffed Beds:** 515 **Admissions:** 23629 **Census:** 376 **Outpatient Visits:** 193408 **Births:** 2822 **Total Expense ($000):** 480640 **Payroll Expense ($000):** 193429 **Personnel:** 3075

✠ **TURKEY CREEK MEDICAL CENTER (440226)**, 10820 Parkside Drive, Zip 37922–1956; tel. 865/218–7011, (Nonreporting) **A**1 9 10 **S** Health Management Associates, Naples, FL
Primary Contact: Lance W. Jones, Chief Executive Officer
Web address: www.hma.com/content/turkey–creek–medical–center
**Control:** Corporation, Investor–owned, for–profit **Service:** General Medical and Surgical

**Staffed Beds:** 101

## LA FOLLETTE—Campbell County

✠ **LAFOLLETTE MEDICAL CENTER (440033)**, 923 East Central Avenue, Zip 37766–3106, Mailing Address: P.O. Box 1301, Zip 37766–1301; tel. 423/907–1200, (Nonreporting) **A**1 9 10 **S** Health Management Associates, Naples, FL
Primary Contact: Mark Cain, Chief Executive Officer
COO: Sara Heatherly–Lloyd, Chief Operating Officer
CFO: Glenn McGuire, Chief Financial Officer
CMO: Michael Hill, M.D., Chief of Staff
CIO: Doug Kibler, Management Information Systems Specialist
CHR: Bess Stout, Director Human Resources
Web address: www.hma.com/content/lafollette–medical–center
**Control:** Corporation, Investor–owned, for–profit **Service:** General Medical and Surgical

**Staffed Beds:** 164

## LAFAYETTE—Macon County

✠ **MACON COUNTY GENERAL HOSPITAL (441305)**, 204 Medical Drive, Zip 37083–1799, Mailing Address: P.O. Box 378, Zip 37083–0378; tel. 615/666–2147 **A**1 9 10 18 21 **F**3 15 18 29 30 34 40 57 59 65 75 77 81 86 93 107 113 118 127 129 131 132 145 **S** QHR, Brentwood, TN
Primary Contact: Dennis A. Wolford, FACHE, Chief Executive Officer
CFO: Thomas J. Kidd, Assistant Administrator and Chief Financial Officer
Web address: www.mcgh.net
**Control:** Other not–for–profit (including NFP Corporation) **Service:** General Medical and Surgical

**Staffed Beds:** 25 **Admissions:** 823 **Census:** 9 **Outpatient Visits:** 23581 **Births:** 0

## LAWRENCEBURG—Lawrence County

✠ **CROCKETT HOSPITAL (440175)**, 1607 South Locust Avenue, Zip 38464–4011, Mailing Address: P.O. Box 847, Zip 38464–0847; tel. 931/762–6571, (Nonreporting) **A**1 9 10 **S** LifePoint Hospitals, Inc., Brentwood, TN
Primary Contact: Jeff Noblin, FACHE, Chief Executive Officer
CFO: John W. Copeland, Chief Financial Officer
CIO: Jason Weaver, Director Information Systems
CHR: Robert Augustin, Director Human Resources
Web address: www.crocketthospital.com
**Control:** Corporation, Investor–owned, for–profit **Service:** General Medical and Surgical

**Staffed Beds:** 90

## LEBANON—Wilson County

✠ **UNIVERSITY MEDICAL CENTER (440193)**, 1411 Baddour Parkway, Zip 37087–2595; tel. 615/444–8262, (Includes MCFARLAND SPECIALTY HOSPITAL, 500 Park Avenue, Zip 37087–3720; tel. 615/449–0500) **A**1 5 9 10 **F**3 8 9 13 14 15 18 20 28 29 30 31 34 39 40 41 44 45 47 49 50 51 54 56 57 59 60 61 64 65 68 70 74 75 76 77 79 81 82 85 86 87 90 93 96 98 102 103 106 107 108 110 111 113 114 117 118 125 128 129 130 134 140 145 146 **S** Health Management Associates, Naples, FL
Primary Contact: Saad Ehtisham, R.N., FACHE, Chief Executive Officer
COO: Michael G. Morrical, Chief Operating Officer
CMO: Andrew Jordan, M.D., Chief of Staff
CIO: Adrian Fung, Director Information Systems
Web address: www.universitymedicalcenter.com
**Control:** Corporation, Investor–owned, for–profit **Service:** General Medical and Surgical

**Staffed Beds:** 245 **Admissions:** 6938 **Census:** 103 **Outpatient Visits:** 100426 **Births:** 842 **Personnel:** 661

## LENOIR CITY—Loudon County

✠ **FORT LOUDOUN MEDICAL CENTER (440110)**, 550 Fort Loudoun Medical Center Drive, Zip 37772–5673; tel. 865/271–6000 **A**1 9 10 **F**3 11 15 28 29 30 34 35 40 45 46 47 55 57 59 68 70 77 79 81 85 102 107 110 111 118 131 134 145 **S** Covenant Health, Knoxville, TN
Primary Contact: Jeffrey Feike, President and Chief Administrative Officer
Web address: www.covenanthealth.com
**Control:** Other not–for–profit (including NFP Corporation) **Service:** General Medical and Surgical

**Staffed Beds:** 40 **Admissions:** 1817 **Census:** 18 **Outpatient Visits:** 72595 **Births:** 0 **Total Expense ($000):** 22893 **Payroll Expense ($000):** 10587 **Personnel:** 235

## LEWISBURG—Marshall County

☐ **MARSHALL MEDICAL CENTER (441309)**, 1080 North Ellington Parkway, Zip 37091–2227, Mailing Address: P.O. Box 1609, Zip 37091–1609; tel. 931/359–6241 **A**1 9 10 18 **F**3 11 15 29 30 34 40 50 56 57 59 68 75 77 81 92 93 108 110 111 113 118 128 130 132 134 145
Primary Contact: Phyllis Brown, Chief Executive Officer
CFO: Kyle Jones, Controller
CMO: Tim Nash, M.D., Chief of Staff
CHR: Joyce Gentile, Human Resource Benefits Specialist
Web address: www.mauryregional.com
**Control:** County–Government, nonfederal **Service:** General Medical and Surgical

**Staffed Beds:** 12 **Admissions:** 290 **Census:** 3 **Outpatient Visits:** 41612 **Births:** 0 **Total Expense ($000):** 12753 **Payroll Expense ($000):** 6025 **Personnel:** 134

## LEXINGTON—Henderson County

✠ **HENDERSON COUNTY COMMUNITY HOSPITAL (440008)**, 200 West Church Street, Zip 38351–2014; tel. 731/968–3646 **A**1 9 10 **F**3 7 15 29 34 40 45 81 107 111 113 118 126 132 134 145 **S** Community Health Systems, Inc., Franklin, TN
Primary Contact: Jack S. Buck, Chief Executive Officer
CFO: Leonard Binkley, Jr., Interim Chief Financial Officer
CHR: John Degi, Director Human Resources
Web address: www.hendersoncchospital.com
**Control:** Corporation, Investor–owned, for–profit **Service:** General Medical and Surgical

**Staffed Beds:** 36 **Admissions:** 934 **Census:** 8 **Outpatient Visits:** 18935 **Births:** 0 **Total Expense ($000):** 12067 **Payroll Expense ($000):** 5221 **Personnel:** 112

## LINDEN—Perry County

**PERRY COMMUNITY HOSPITAL (440040)**, 2718 Squirrel Hollow Drive, Zip 37096–9100; tel. 931/589–2121, (Nonreporting) **A**9 10
Primary Contact: John B. Avery, III, Administrator
**Control:** Other not–for–profit (including NFP Corporation) **Service:** General Medical and Surgical

**Staffed Beds:** 53

**TN**

---

**Hospital, Medicare Provider Number, Address, Telephone, Approval, Facility, and Physician Codes, Health Care System**

★ American Hospital Association (AHA) membership
☐ The Joint Commission accreditation   ◇ DNV Healthcare Inc. accreditation
○ American Osteopathic Association (AOA) accreditation
△ Commission on Accreditation of Rehabilitation Facilities (CARF) accreditation

## LIVINGSTON—Overton County

★ **LIVINGSTON REGIONAL HOSPITAL (440187)**, 315 Oak Street, Zip 38570,
Mailing Address: P.O. Box 550, Zip 38570–0550; tel. 931/823–5611 **A**9 10 **F**3
13 15 17 29 30 34 35 39 40 46 55 56 57 70 75 76 77 78 79 81 87 90 93
98 103 107 110 111 117 118 128 129 130 132 144 145 146 **S** LifePoint
Hospitals, Inc., Brentwood, TN
Primary Contact: Michael J. Meadows, Chief Executive Officer
COO: Michelle Watson, Chief Operating Officer and Chief Nursing Officer
CFO: Joseph Ross, Chief Financial Officer
CMO: Trueman Smith, M.D., Chief Medical Officer
CIO: Joseph Ross, Chief Financial Officer
CHR: Valerie Guimaraes, Director Human Resources
Web address: www.livingstonhospital.com
**Control:** Corporation, Investor–owned, for–profit **Service:** General Medical and
Surgical

**Staffed Beds: 82 Admissions: 3285 Census: 45 Outpatient Visits:** 39008
**Births:** 331 **Total Expense ($000):** 24799 **Payroll Expense ($000):** 12321
**Personnel:** 245

## LOUISVILLE—Blount County

**PENINSULA HOSPITAL**, 2347 Jones Bend Road, Zip 37777–5213, Mailing
Address: P.O. Box 2000, Zip 37777–2000; tel. 865/970–9800 **F**4 5 29 30 35
38 50 64 68 71 86 87 98 99 101 104 129 **P**6
Primary Contact: Teresa Gomez, Chief Nursing Officer
CFO: Sonja Jones, Chief Financial Officer
CMO: Kris Houser, M.D., Medical Director
CIO: Roger Ricker, Director Marketing and Public Relations
CHR: Angie Montgomery, Director Human Resources
Web address: www.peninsula–hospital.org
**Control:** Other not–for–profit (including NFP Corporation) **Service:** Psychiatric

**Staffed Beds: 141 Admissions: 4305 Census: 67 Outpatient Visits:** 87170
**Births:** 0 **Total Expense ($000):** 30556 **Payroll Expense ($000):** 16353
**Personnel:** 363

## MADISON—Davidson County

★ **SKYLINE MADISON CAMPUS (440135)**, 500 Hospital Drive, Zip 37115–5032;
tel. 615/769–5000, (Nonreporting) **A**9 10 **S** HCA, Nashville, TN
Primary Contact: Steve Otto, Chief Executive Officer
COO: Jill Howard, R.N., Chief Operating Officer
CFO: Bradley Schultz, Chief Financial Officer
CMO: L. Brett Babat, M.D., Chief Medical Officer
CHR: Andy Hooper, Director Human Resources
Web address: www.skylinemadison.com
**Control:** Corporation, Investor–owned, for–profit **Service:** General Medical and
Surgical

**Staffed Beds:** 284

## MANCHESTER—Coffee County

○ **MEDICAL CENTER OF MANCHESTER (441308)**, 481 Interstate Drive,
Zip 37355–3108, Mailing Address: P.O. Box 1409, Zip 37349–4409;
tel. 931/728–6354, (Nonreporting) **A**9 10 11 18
Primary Contact: Robert J. Couch, Chief Executive Officer
CMO: W. D. Daniel, D.O., Chief of Staff
CHR: Shelly Turner, Chief Clinical Services Officer
**Control:** Corporation, Investor–owned, for–profit **Service:** General Medical and
Surgical

**Staffed Beds:** 25

**UNITED REGIONAL MEDICAL CENTER (440007)**, 1001 McArthur Drive,
Zip 37355–2455, Mailing Address: P.O. Box 1079, Zip 37349–1079;
tel. 931/728–3586 **A**9 10 **F**3 11 15 18 29 30 34 39 40 45 46 50 54 57 59
65 77 81 82 85 87 89 107 108 111 113 116 118 128 129 132 147
Primary Contact: Martha Logan, Chief Executive Officer
CFO: Pam Jernigan, Chief Financial Officer
CMO: Gary Bryant, M.D., Chief of Staff
CIO: Matt Burks, Director Information Technology
CHR: Nolan Hayes, Director Human Resources
Web address: www.urmchealthcare.com
**Control:** Corporation, Investor–owned, for–profit **Service:** General Medical and
Surgical

**Staffed Beds: 36 Admissions: 1328 Census: 12 Outpatient Visits:** 23962
**Births:** 0 **Total Expense ($000):** 14441 **Payroll Expense ($000):** 6183
**Personnel:** 146

## MARTIN—Weakley County

⊞ **HEALTHSOUTH CANE CREEK REHABILITATION HOSPITAL (443030)**, 180
Mt Pelia Road, Zip 38237–3812; tel. 731/587–4231 **A**1 10 **F**34 56 74 75 79
90 91 94 95 96 142 147 **S** HEALTHSOUTH Corporation, Birmingham, AL
Primary Contact: Eric Garrard, Chief Executive Officer
CFO: Bethany Smith, Controller
CMO: William Eason, M.D., Medical Director
CIO: Jan Gill, Director Health Information Management Systems
CHR: Sharon Shihady, Director Human Resources
Web address: www.healthsouthcanecreek.com
**Control:** Corporation, Investor–owned, for–profit **Service:** Rehabilitation

**Staffed Beds: 40 Admissions: 719 Census: 27 Outpatient Visits: 0 Births:**
0 **Total Expense ($000):** 6593 **Payroll Expense ($000):** 3735 **Personnel:**
101

⊞ **VOLUNTEER COMMUNITY HOSPITAL (440061)**, 161 Mount Pelia Road,
Zip 38237–3811; tel. 731/587–4261, (Nonreporting) **A**1 9 10 **S** Community
Health Systems, Inc., Franklin, TN
Primary Contact: Clyde Wood, Chief Executive Officer
CMO: Suresh Thota, M.D., Chief of Staff
CHR: Tammie Bell, Director Human Resources
Web address: www.volunteercommunityhospital.com
**Control:** Corporation, Investor–owned, for–profit **Service:** General Medical and
Surgical

**Staffed Beds:** 65

## MARYVILLE—Blount County

⊞ **BLOUNT MEMORIAL HOSPITAL (440011)**, 907 East Lamar Alexander
Parkway, Zip 37804–5016, (Total facility includes 76 beds in
nursing home–type unit) **A**1 2 9 10 **F**3 4 10 11 12 13 15 17 18 20 22 26 28
29 30 31 32 35 38 40 43 45 46 49 53 54 56 57 59 62 63 64 67 68 70 74
75 76 77 78 79 80 81 82 84 85 86 87 90 93 96 97 98 99 100 101 102 103
104 105 107 108 110 111 113 114 115 116 117 118 119 120 121 122 124
125 127 128 129 130 131 133 134 145 146 147 **P**6 7
Primary Contact: Don Heinemann, Administrator and Chief Executive Officer
CFO: David E. Avriett, Assistant Administrator
CMO: G. Harold Naramore, M.D., Chief Medical Officer and In house Legal
Counsel
CHR: Chris Wilkes, MS, Director Human Resources
Web address: www.blountmemorial.org
**Control:** County–Government, nonfederal **Service:** General Medical and Surgical

**Staffed Beds: 314 Admissions: 13293 Census: 222 Outpatient Visits:**
183759 **Births:** 775 **Total Expense ($000):** 181852 **Payroll Expense
($000):** 84075 **Personnel:** 1765

## MC MINNVILLE—Warren County

□ **RIVER PARK HOSPITAL (440151)**, 1559 Sparta Street, Zip 37110–1316;
tel. 931/815–4000, (Nonreporting) **A**1 9 10 **S** Capella Healthcare, Franklin, TN
Primary Contact: Timothy W. McGill, Chief Executive Officer
CFO: Christina Patterson, Chief Financial Officer
CMO: Randal D. Rampp, M.D., Chief Medical Officer
CIO: Jeff Johnson, Director Information Systems
CHR: Deeann Johnson, Director Human Resources
Web address: www.riverparkhospital.com
**Control:** Corporation, Investor–owned, for–profit **Service:** General Medical and
Surgical

**Staffed Beds:** 125

## MCKENZIE—Carroll County

⊞ **MCKENZIE REGIONAL HOSPITAL (440182)**, 161 Hospital Drive,
Zip 38201–1636; tel. 731/352–5344 **A**1 9 10 **F**3 29 40 53 76 81 85 89 93
107 118 130 132 145 **S** Community Health Systems, Inc., Franklin, TN
Primary Contact: Darrell Blaylock, Chief Executive Officer
CFO: Kevin Harvey, Chief Financial Officer
CHR: Joyce Hamilton, Director Human Resources
Web address: www.mckenzieregionalhospital.com
**Control:** Corporation, Investor–owned, for–profit **Service:** General Medical and
Surgical

**Staffed Beds: 34 Admissions: 1726 Census: 13 Outpatient Visits:** 14407
**Births:** 389 **Total Expense ($000):** 11960 **Payroll Expense ($000):** 5653
**Personnel:** 122

**TN**

*Many Facility Codes have changed. Please refer to the AHA Guide Code Chart.*  © 2012 AHA Guide

## MEMPHIS—Shelby County

✠ **BAPTIST MEMORIAL HOSPITAL – MEMPHIS (440048)**, 6019 Walnut Grove Road, Zip 38120–2173; tel. 901/226–5000, (Total facility includes 35 beds in nursing home–type unit) **A**1 2 3 5 9 10 **F**3 8 18 20 22 24 26 28 29 30 31 40 46 47 60 63 68 70 74 75 78 79 81 83 84 85 89 92 93 96 107 111 113 114 115 116 117 118 119 120 122 123 125 127 136 140 145 147 **S** Baptist Memorial Health Care Corporation, Memphis, TN
Primary Contact: Derick Ziegler, Administrator and Chief Executive Officer
CFO: Cyndi Pittman, Chief Financial Officer
CMO: Christian C. Patrick, M.D., Chief Medical Officer
CIO: Doug Reiselt, Vice President and Chief Information Officer
CHR: Jerry Barbaree, Director Human Resources
Web address: www.baptistonline.org
**Control:** Other not–for–profit (including NFP Corporation) **Service:** General Medical and Surgical

**Staffed Beds:** 642 **Admissions:** 26972 **Census:** 511 **Outpatient Visits:** 62373 **Births:** 0 **Total Expense ($000):** 402666 **Payroll Expense ($000):** 155347 **Personnel:** 3084

★ **BAPTIST MEMORIAL HOSPITAL FOR WOMEN (440222)**, 6225 Humphreys Boulevard, Zip 38120–2373; tel. 901/227–9000 **A**9 10 **F**3 12 13 15 29 30 34 35 46 55 57 59 64 68 70 71 72 73 76 81 82 86 87 107 108 110 118 123 129 131 134 145 146 **S** Baptist Memorial Health Care Corporation, Memphis, TN
Primary Contact: Anita Vaughn, Administrator and Chief Executive Officer
CFO: Margaret Williams, Chief Financial Officer
CMO: Christine Mestemacher, M.D., President Medical Staff
CHR: Karen Ingram, Director Human Resources
Web address: www.bmhcc.org
**Control:** Other not–for–profit (including NFP Corporation) **Service:** Obstetrics and gynecology

**Staffed Beds:** 140 **Admissions:** 6764 **Census:** 74 **Outpatient Visits:** 39881 **Births:** 4945 **Total Expense ($000):** 66292 **Payroll Expense ($000):** 30122 **Personnel:** 575

✠ **BAPTIST MEMORIAL RESTORATIVE CARE HOSPITAL (442010)**, 6019 Walnut Grove Road, Zip 38120–2113; tel. 901/226–1400 **A**1 9 10 **F**1 3 29 68 75 129 147 **S** Baptist Memorial Health Care Corporation, Memphis, TN
Primary Contact: Janice Hill, R.N., Administrator
Web address: www.baptistonline.org/facilities/restorativecare
**Control:** Other not–for–profit (including NFP Corporation) **Service:** General Medical and Surgical

**Staffed Beds:** 30 **Admissions:** 204 **Census:** 23 **Outpatient Visits:** 0 **Births:** 0 **Total Expense ($000):** 13786 **Payroll Expense ($000):** 4616 **Personnel:** 86

☐ **DELTA MEDICAL CENTER (440159)**, 3000 Getwell Road, Zip 38118–2299; tel. 901/369–8100, (Nonreporting) **A**1 9 10
Primary Contact: Mary Hammons, Chief Executive Officer
CFO: Glen Roberts, Chief Financial Officer
CMO: David Richardson, M.D., Chief of Staff
CIO: Patrick Duffee, Director Medical Information Systems
CHR: Karyn Erickson, Director Human Resources
Web address: www.deltamedcenter.com
**Control:** Corporation, Investor–owned, for–profit **Service:** General Medical and Surgical

**Staffed Beds:** 170

✠ **HEALTHSOUTH REHABILITATION HOSPITAL (443031)**, 4100 Austin Peay Highway, Zip 38128–2502; tel. 901/213–5400 **A**1 10 **F**28 29 30 90 **S** HEALTHSOUTH Corporation, Birmingham, AL
Primary Contact: Brad Kennedy, Chief Executive Officer
CFO: Valerie Jones, Chief Financial Officer
CMO: Donald Sullivan, M.D., Medical Director
CHR: Matthew Richardson, Director Human Resources
Web address: www.healthsouthnorthmemphis.com
**Control:** Corporation, Investor–owned, for–profit **Service:** Rehabilitation

**Staffed Beds:** 40 **Admissions:** 1075 **Census:** 37 **Outpatient Visits:** 0 **Births:** 0 **Total Expense ($000):** 9597 **Payroll Expense ($000):** 5575 **Personnel:** 117

✠ **HEALTHSOUTH REHABILITATION HOSPITAL OF MEMPHIS (443029)**, 1282 Union Avenue, Zip 38104–3414; tel. 901/722–2000 **A**1 10 **F**3 28 29 30 34 60 75 87 90 93 95 96 **S** HEALTHSOUTH Corporation, Birmingham, AL
Primary Contact: Michael L. Pierce, Chief Executive Officer
CFO: Valerie Jones, Chief Financial Officer
CMO: Dale Cunningham, M.D., Medical Director
CHR: Sandra Milburn, Director Human Resources
Web address: www.healthsouthmemphis.com
**Control:** Partnership, Investor–owned, for–profit **Service:** Rehabilitation

**Staffed Beds:** 72 **Admissions:** 1582 **Census:** 53 **Outpatient Visits:** 7303 **Births:** 0 **Total Expense ($000):** 16773 **Payroll Expense ($000):** 8645 **Personnel:** 185

**LAKESIDE BEHAVIORAL HEALTH SYSTEM (444004)**, 2911 Brunswick Road, Zip 38133–4199; tel. 901/377–4700 **A**10 **F**4 5 38 98 99 100 101 102 103 104 105 106 **S** Universal Health Services, Inc., King of Prussia, PA
Primary Contact: Shelley A. Nowak, Chief Executive Officer
COO: Joy Golden, Chief Operating Officer
CFO: Felicia Swauncy, Chief Financial Officer
CMO: C. Hal Brunt, M.D., Medical Director
CIO: Kevin Pendleton, Chief Information Technology
CHR: James Miller, Director Human Resources
Web address: www.lakesidebhs.com
**Control:** Corporation, Investor–owned, for–profit **Service:** Psychiatric

**Staffed Beds:** 311 **Admissions:** 6820 **Census:** 173 **Outpatient Visits:** 22618 **Births:** 0 **Total Expense ($000):** 33755 **Payroll Expense ($000):** 15151 **Personnel:** 369

**LE BONHEUR CHILDREN'S HOSPITAL** See Methodist Healthcare Memphis Hospitals

☐ **MEMPHIS MENTAL HEALTH INSTITUTE (444001)**, 865 Poplar Avenue, Zip 38105–4626, Mailing Address: P.O. Box 40966, Zip 38174–0966; tel. 901/577–1800 **A**1 5 10 **F**3 50 86 87 98 101 103 129 145 **P**6
Primary Contact: Lisa Daniel, Interim Chief Executive Officer
COO: Clyde Slate, Assistant Superintendent Administrative Services
CFO: Linda White, Director Fiscal Services
CMO: Kayla Fisher, M.D., Medical Director
CHR: Randy Durham, Director Personnel
Web address: www.tn.gov/mental/mhs/mhs2.html
**Control:** State–Government, nonfederal **Service:** Psychiatric

**Staffed Beds:** 75 **Admissions:** 1853 **Census:** 56 **Outpatient Visits:** 0 **Births:** 0 **Total Expense ($000):** 19032 **Payroll Expense ($000):** 10331 **Personnel:** 233

☐ **METHODIST EXTENDED CARE HOSPITAL (442013)**, 225 South Claybrook Street, Zip 38104–3537; tel. 901/516–2152 **A**1 10 **F**1 3 29 30 75 131 147 **S** Methodist Le Bonheur Healthcare, Memphis, TN
Primary Contact: Sandra Bailey–DeLeeuw, Administrator
COO: Sandra Hugueley, Assistant Administrator and Chief Nursing Officer
CFO: Kris Sanders, Chief Financial Officer
CMO: Hany Mounir Habashy, M.D., Chief Medical Director
CHR: Tina Sims, Director Human Resources
CNO: Sandra Hugueley, Assistant Administrator and Chief Nursing Officer
Web address: www.methodisthealth.org
**Control:** Other not–for–profit (including NFP Corporation) **Service:** Long–Term Acute Care hospital

**Staffed Beds:** 36 **Admissions:** 467 **Census:** 31 **Outpatient Visits:** 0 **Total Expense ($000):** 14310 **Payroll Expense ($000):** 6583 **Personnel:** 132

**TN**

---

**Hospital, Medicare Provider Number, Address, Telephone, Approval, Facility, and Physician Codes, Health Care System**

★ American Hospital Association (AHA) membership
☐ The Joint Commission accreditation      ◇ DNV Healthcare Inc. accreditation
○ American Osteopathic Association (AOA) accreditation
△ Commission on Accreditation of Rehabilitation Facilities (CARF) accreditation

☐ **METHODIST HEALTHCARE MEMPHIS HOSPITALS (440049)**, 1265 Union Avenue, Zip 38104; tel. 901/516–7000, (Includes LE BONHEUR CHILDREN'S HOSPITAL, 50 North Dunlap Street, Zip 38103; tel. 901/287–5437; Meri Armour, Chief Executive Officer; METHODIST HEALTHCARE–NORTH HOSPITAL, 3960 New Covington Pike, Zip 38128; tel. 901/384–5389; William A. Kenley, Chief Executive Officer and Administrator; METHODIST HEALTHCARE–SOUTH HOSPITAL, 1300 Wesley Drive, Zip 38116; tel. 901/516–3081; Michael O. Ugwueke, Administrator; METHODIST LE BONHEUR GERMANTOWN HOSPITAL, 7691 Poplar Avenue, Germantown, Zip 38138; tel. 901/516–6000), (Total facility includes 20 beds in nursing home–type unit) **A**1 2 3 5 8 9 10 **F**3 7 8 11 12 13 15 17 18 19 20 21 22 23 24 25 26 27 28 29 30 31 32 34 35 37 38 39 40 41 43 44 45 46 47 48 49 50 54 55 56 57 58 59 60 61 64 65 66 68 70 71 72 73 74 75 76 77 78 79 80 81 82 84 85 86 87 88 89 92 93 96 97 98 99 100 101 102 103 104 105 107 108 110 111 112 113 114 115 116 117 118 119 120 122 123 125 127 128 129 130 134 135 137 138 140 141 142 143 144 145 146 147 **P**5 6 8 **S** Methodist Le Bonheur Healthcare, Memphis, TN
Primary Contact: Kevin M. Spiegel, FACHE, Chief Executive Officer
CFO: Chris J. McLean, Chief Financial Officer
CMO: Robin Womeodu, M.D., Chief Medical Officer
CIO: Andy Fowler, Senior Vice President Information Systems
CHR: Carol Ross–Spang, Senior Vice President
Web address: www.methodisthealth.org
**Control:** Other not–for–profit (including NFP Corporation) **Service:** General Medical and Surgical

**Staffed Beds:** 1321 **Admissions:** 62229 **Census:** 970 **Outpatient Visits:** 571064 **Births:** 5039 **Total Expense ($000):** 1102261 **Payroll Expense ($000):** 409297 **Personnel:** 7483

☒ **REGIONAL MEDICAL CENTER AT MEMPHIS (440152)**, 877 Jefferson Avenue, Zip 38103–2897; tel. 901/545–7100 **A**1 3 5 8 9 10 **F**3 11 13 15 16 18 20 22 29 30 34 35 39 40 43 44 45 49 50 57 58 59 61 64 68 70 71 72 73 74 75 76 77 79 80 81 85 86 87 90 92 93 97 107 108 110 111 113 118 129 133 140 145 146 147
Primary Contact: Reginald W. Coopwood, M.D., President and Chief Executive Officer
COO: Rob Sumter, Executive Vice President and Chief Operating Officer
CFO: Rick Wagers, Senior Executive Vice President and Chief Financial Officer
CMO: Jack D. McCue, M.D., Senior Vice President and Interim Chief Medical Officer
CHR: Fred Boyd, Interim Vice President Human Resources
Web address: www.the–med.org
**Control:** Other not–for–profit (including NFP Corporation) **Service:** General Medical and Surgical

**Staffed Beds:** 325 **Admissions:** 13258 **Census:** 249 **Outpatient Visits:** 125497 **Births:** 3596 **Total Expense ($000):** 204773 **Payroll Expense ($000):** 113257 **Personnel:** 1979

☒ **SAINT FRANCIS HOSPITAL (440183)**, 5959 Park Avenue, Zip 38119–5198, Mailing Address: P.O. Box 171808, Zip 38187–1808; tel. 901/765–1000 **A**1 2 3 5 9 10 **F**3 8 11 12 13 15 17 18 20 22 24 26 28 29 30 31 34 35 38 39 40 44 45 46 47 48 49 50 51 54 56 57 58 59 60 64 68 70 72 74 75 76 77 78 79 81 82 84 85 86 87 90 93 97 98 99 100 101 102 103 104 107 108 110 111 113 114 115 116 117 118 120 122 125 128 129 130 131 140 142 145 146 147 **P**5 6 8 **S** TENET Healthcare Corporation, Dallas, TX
Primary Contact: David L. Archer, Chief Executive Officer
COO: Audrey Gregory, R.N., Chief Operating Officer
CFO: Bradley Robertson, Chief Financial Officer
CMO: Michael Lachina, M.D., Chief Medical Officer
CIO: Mike Hadley, Chief Information Officer
CHR: Everett Liddell, Vice President Human Resources
Web address: www.saintfrancishosp.com
**Control:** Corporation, Investor–owned, for–profit **Service:** General Medical and Surgical

**Staffed Beds:** 511 **Admissions:** 15703 **Census:** 256 **Outpatient Visits:** 119528 **Births:** 1769 **Total Expense ($000):** 212892 **Payroll Expense ($000):** 75013 **Personnel:** 1367

☒ **SELECT SPECIALTY HOSPITAL–MEMPHIS (442014)**, 5959 Park Avenue, 12th Floor, Zip 38119–5200; tel. 901/765–1245, (Nonreporting) **A**1 9 10 **S** Select Medical Corporation, Mechanicsburg, PA
Primary Contact: Mark A. Kelly, Chief Executive Officer
Web address: www.selectmedicalcorp.com
**Control:** Corporation, Investor–owned, for–profit **Service:** Long–Term Acute Care hospital

**Staffed Beds:** 38

☒ **ST. JUDE CHILDREN'S RESEARCH HOSPITAL (443302)**, 262 Danny Thomas Place, Zip 38105–3678; tel. 901/595–3300, (Nonreporting) **A**1 3 5 9 10
Primary Contact: William E. Evans, PharmD, Director
CFO: Mike Canarios, Vice President and Chief Financial Officer
CMO: Joseph Laver, M.D., Executive Vice President and Chief Medical Officer
CIO: Clayton Naeve, Vice President and Chief Information Officer
CHR: Mary Anna Quinn, Vice President
Web address: www.stjude.org
**Control:** Other not–for–profit (including NFP Corporation) **Service:** Children's other specialty

**Staffed Beds:** 56

☒ △ **VETERANS AFFAIRS MEDICAL CENTER**, 1030 Jefferson Avenue, Zip 38104–2193; tel. 901/523–8990 **A**1 3 5 7 8 **F**3 4 5 17 18 20 22 24 28 29 30 31 34 35 38 39 40 45 47 49 51 56 57 58 59 60 61 62 64 65 70 74 75 77 78 79 80 81 82 83 84 85 86 87 92 93 94 97 98 100 101 102 103 104 105 106 107 111 113 114 115 116 117 118 121 128 129 134 145 146 147 **P**6 **S** Department of Veterans Affairs, Washington, DC
Primary Contact: James L. Robinson, III, PsyD, Director
COO: Marlin Angell, Associate Director
CMO: Margarethe Hagemann, M.D., Chief of Staff
CIO: Jenny Pangle, Chief Officer Information and Technology
CHR: Brenda Cabunoc, Chief Human Resource Management Services
Web address: www.memphis.va.gov
**Control:** Veterans Affairs, Government, federal **Service:** General Medical and Surgical

**Staffed Beds:** 280 **Admissions:** 6986 **Census:** 169 **Outpatient Visits:** 535699 **Births:** 0 **Personnel:** 3826

## MILAN—Gibson County

☒ **MILAN GENERAL HOSPITAL (440060)**, 4039 Highland Street, Zip 38358–3483; tel. 731/686–1591 **A**1 9 10 **F**3 15 29 30 35 40 45 57 59 64 68 70 81 85 87 93 96 107 118 129 131 132 145 **S** West Tennessee Healthcare, Jackson, TN
Primary Contact: Sherry Scruggs, Administrator
CMO: Kenneth Tozier, M.D., Chief of Surgery
Web address: www.wth.org
**Control:** Hospital district or authority, Government, nonfederal **Service:** General Medical and Surgical

**Staffed Beds:** 28 **Admissions:** 315 **Census:** 4 **Outpatient Visits:** 13338 **Births:** 0 **Total Expense ($000):** 6165 **Payroll Expense ($000):** 3371 **Personnel:** 72

## MORRISTOWN—Hamblen County

☒ **LAKEWAY REGIONAL HOSPITAL (440067)**, 726 McFarland Street, Zip 37814–3990; tel. 423/586–2302, (Nonreporting) **A**1 9 10 19 **S** Community Health Systems, Inc., Franklin, TN
Primary Contact: Priscilla Millis, Chief Executive Officer
CMO: Paul Cardali, M.D., Chief of Staff
CHR: Deirdre Helton, Director Human Resources
Web address: www.lakewayregionalhospital.com
**Control:** Corporation, Investor–owned, for–profit **Service:** General Medical and Surgical

**Staffed Beds:** 135

☒ **MORRISTOWN–HAMBLEN HEALTHCARE SYSTEM (440030)**, 908 West Fourth North Street, Zip 37814–3894, Mailing Address: P.O. Box 1178, Zip 37816–1178; tel. 423/586–4231, (Nonreporting) **A**1 9 10 **S** Covenant Health, Knoxville, TN
Primary Contact: Gordon Lintz, Chief Administrative Officer
CFO: James Alwell, Interim Vice President and Chief Financial Officer
CIO: Tim Krieger, Director Information Systems
CHR: Derek Winkle, Director Human Resources
Web address: www.mhhs1.org
**Control:** Other not–for–profit (including NFP Corporation) **Service:** General Medical and Surgical

**Staffed Beds:** 143

## MOUNTAIN CITY—Johnson County

★ **JOHNSON COUNTY COMMUNITY HOSPITAL (441304)**, 1901 South Shady Street, Zip 37683–2271; tel. 423/727–1100 **A**9 10 18 **F**3 15 28 30 35 40 44 50 68 86 93 97 107 **P**6 **S** Mountain States Health Alliance, Johnson City, TN
Primary Contact: Lisa Heaton, Administrator and Chief Nursing Officer
Web address: www.msha.com
**Control:** Other not–for–profit (including NFP Corporation) **Service:** General Medical and Surgical

**Staffed Beds:** 2 **Admissions:** 20 **Census:** 1 **Outpatient Visits:** 36870 **Births:** 0 **Total Expense ($000):** 6144 **Payroll Expense ($000):** 3740 **Personnel:** 58

## MOUNTAIN HOME—Washington County

☒ **JAMES H. QUILLEN VETERANS AFFAIRS MEDICAL CENTER**, Zip 37684–5002; tel. 423/926–1171, (Nonreporting) **A**1 2 3 5 8 **S** Department of Veterans Affairs, Washington, DC
Primary Contact: Charlene S. Ehret, FACHE, Director
CFO: Brian P. Fuchs, Chief Fiscal Service
CMO: David Reagan, M.D., Chief of Staff
CIO: Karen Perry, Chief Information Resource Management Services
CHR: Patsy Fish, Chief Human Resources Management
Web address: www.va.gov
**Control:** Veterans Affairs, Government, federal **Service:** General Medical and Surgical

**Staffed Beds:** 483

*Many Facility Codes have changed. Please refer to the AHA Guide Code Chart.*       © 2012 AHA Guide

TN

## MURFREESBORO—Rutherford County

**ALVIN C. YORK CAMPUS** See Veterans Affairs Tennessee Valley Healthcare System, Nashville

✠ **MIDDLE TENNESSEE MEDICAL CENTER (440053)**, 1700 Medical Center Parkway, Zip 37129–2245; tel. 615/396–4100, (Nonreporting) **A**1 2 3 5 9 10 **S** Ascension Health, Saint Louis, MO
Primary Contact: Gordon B. Ferguson, President and Chief Executive Officer
COO: Elizabeth Lemons, Chief Operating Officer
CFO: Martha Tolbert Rowland, Vice President Finance
CMO: Andy Brown, M.D., Vice President Medical Affairs
CIO: Dan West, Director Information Technology Systems
CHR: Carol Bragdon, Director Human Resources
Web address: www.mtmc.org
**Control:** Church–operated, Nongovernment, not–for profit **Service:** General Medical and Surgical

**Staffed Beds:** 286

## NASHVILLE—Davidson County

✠ **BAPTIST HOSPITAL (440133)**, 2000 Church Street, Zip 37236–0002; tel. 615/284–5555, (Nonreporting) **A**1 2 3 5 9 10 **S** Ascension Health, Saint Louis, MO
Primary Contact: Bernard Sherry, President and Chief Executive Officer
COO: Renee A. Kessler, Chief Operating Officer
CFO: Carrie Teaford, Vice President Finance
CMO: William Thompson, M.D., Chief Medical Officer
CIO: Jim Drew, Chief Information Officer
CHR: Martha Underwood, Chief Human Resources Officer
Web address: www.baptisthospital.com
**Control:** Other not–for–profit (including NFP Corporation) **Service:** General Medical and Surgical

**Staffed Beds:** 425

**CENTENNIAL MEDICAL CENTER** See Tristar Centennial Medical Center

✠ **KINDRED HOSPITAL–NASHVILLE (442006)**, 1412 County Hospital Road, Zip 37218; tel. 615/687–2600, (Nonreporting) **A**1 10 **S** Kindred Healthcare, Louisville, KY
Primary Contact: William P. Macri, Chief Executive Officer
COO: Lisa Manor, Chief Clinical Officer
CFO: Philip L. Jones, Chief Financial Officer
CMO: Clyde Heflin, M.D., Chief Medical Officer
CHR: Robyn Dunman, Coordinator Human Resources
Web address: www.khnashville.com/
**Control:** Corporation, Investor–owned, for–profit **Service:** Long–Term Acute Care hospital

**Staffed Beds:** 58

☐ **MIDDLE TENNESSEE MENTAL HEALTH INSTITUTE (444014)**, 221 Stewarts Ferry Pike, Zip 37214–3325; tel. 615/902–7535 **A**1 3 5 10 **F**30 75 77 98 101 102 103 106
Primary Contact: Candace L. Gilligan, Chief Executive Officer
CFO: Mark Stanley, Director Fiscal Services
CMO: Mohammad S. Jahan, M.D., Clinical Director
CHR: Margie Dunn, Director Human Resources
Web address: www.tn.gov/mental/mhs/mhs2.html
**Control:** State–Government, nonfederal **Service:** Psychiatric

**Staffed Beds:** 195 **Admissions:** 2745 **Census:** 163 **Outpatient Visits:** 0 **Births:** 0 **Total Expense ($000):** 43121 **Payroll Expense ($000):** 23961 **Personnel:** 569

**MONROE CARELL JR. CHILDREN'S HOSPITAL AT VANDERBILT** See Vanderbilt Hospital and Clinics

✠ **NASHVILLE GENERAL HOSPITAL (440111)**, 1818 Albion Street, Zip 37208–2918; tel. 615/341–4000, (Nonreporting) **A**1 2 3 5 9 10
Primary Contact: Jason E. Boyd, FACHE, Interim Chief Executive Officer
COO: Jason E. Boyd, FACHE, Chief Operating Officer
CHR: Diana Wohlfardt, Director Human Resources
Web address: www.nashvilleha.org
**Control:** City–County, Government, nonfederal **Service:** General Medical and Surgical

**Staffed Beds:** 98

**PSYCHIATRIC HOSPITAL AT VANDERBILT** See Vanderbilt Hospital and Clinics

✠ **SAINT THOMAS HOSPITAL (440082)**, 4220 Harding Road, Zip 37205–2095, Mailing Address: P.O. Box 380, Zip 37202–0380; tel. 615/222–2111, (Nonreporting) **A**1 2 3 5 9 10 **S** Ascension Health, Saint Louis, MO
Primary Contact: Dawn Rudolph, Chief Executive Officer
COO: Don King, Chief Operating Officer
CFO: Lisa Davis, Vice President Finance
CMO: Dale Batchelor, M.D., Chief Medical Officer
CIO: Chris Young, Vice President and Chief Information Officer
CHR: Stephanie C. Stewart, Executive Director, Human Resources
Web address: www.stthomas.org
**Control:** Church–operated, Nongovernment, not–for profit **Service:** General Medical and Surgical

**Staffed Beds:** 395

✠ **SELECT SPECIALTY HOSPITAL–NASHVILLE (442011)**, 2000 Hayes Street, Zip 37203–2318; tel. 615/284–4599, (Nonreporting) **A**1 9 10 **S** Select Medical Corporation, Mechanicsburg, PA
Primary Contact: Michael McAlister, Chief Executive Officer
Web address: www.selectmedicalcorp.com
**Control:** Corporation, Investor–owned, for–profit **Service:** Long–Term Acute Care hospital

**Staffed Beds:** 47

✠ △ **SKYLINE MEDICAL CENTER (440006)**, 3441 Dickerson Pike, Zip 37207–2539; tel. 615/769–2000, (Nonreporting) **A**1 2 7 9 10 **S** HCA, Nashville, TN
Primary Contact: Steve Otto, Chief Executive Officer
COO: Michael Ehrat, Chief Operating Officer
CFO: Bradley Schultz, Chief Financial Officer
CMO: L. Brett Babat, M.D., Chief Medical Officer
CHR: Andy Hooper, Director Human Resources
Web address: www.skylinemedicalcenter.com
**Control:** Corporation, Investor–owned, for–profit **Service:** General Medical and Surgical

**Staffed Beds:** 295

✠ **SOUTHERN HILLS MEDICAL CENTER (440197)**, 391 Wallace Road, Zip 37211–4859; tel. 615/781–4000 **A**1 2 9 10 **F**15 18 20 22 29 30 31 34 35 40 44 45 47 49 50 54 56 57 58 59 60 64 65 69 70 74 75 77 78 79 81 85 87 90 93 94 96 97 107 108 110 111 113 118 128 129 132 134 145 146 147 **S** HCA, Nashville, TN
Primary Contact: Thomas H. Ozburn, Chief Executive Officer
COO: Richard Tumlin, Chief Operating Officer
CFO: Chuck Bennett, Chief Financial Officer
CMO: Jonathan Rotker, M.D., Chief of Staff
CIO: Ronnie Gannon, Director Information Services
CHR: Gary Briggs, Director Human Resources
Web address: www.southernhills.com
**Control:** Corporation, Investor–owned, for–profit **Service:** General Medical and Surgical

**Staffed Beds:** 101 **Admissions:** 3553 **Census:** 43 **Outpatient Visits:** 77187 **Births:** 1 **Total Expense ($000):** 64151 **Payroll Expense ($000):** 25915 **Personnel:** 426

**THE CENTER FOR SPINAL SURGERY (440218)**, 2011 Murphy Avenue Suite 400, Zip 37203; tel. 615/341–7500, (Nonreporting) **A**9 10
Primary Contact: Kathy Watson, R.N., Administrator and Chief Nursing Officer
CFO: Angie Crow, Financial Director
CMO: Everette Howell, M.D., Chief Medical Officer
Web address: www.centerforspinalsurgery.com
**Control:** Partnership, Investor–owned, for–profit **Service:** General Medical and Surgical

**Staffed Beds:** 23

✠ **TRISTAR CENTENNIAL MEDICAL CENTER (440161)**, 2300 Patterson Street, Zip 37203–1528; tel. 615/342–1000 **A**1 2 3 5 9 10 **F**3 12 13 15 17 18 20 22 24 26 28 29 30 31 35 40 41 51 53 54 56 59 60 70 71 72 73 74 75 76 77 78 79 81 82 85 86 87 89 98 103 106 107 108 110 111 113 114 115 117 118 120 125 128 129 131 135 137 145 146 **S** HCA, Nashville, TN
Primary Contact: Thomas L. Herron, FACHE, Chief Executive Officer
COO: Micki J. Slingerland, Chief Operating Officer
CFO: David A. Summers, Chief Financial Officer
CMO: Ravi Chari, M.D., Chief Medical Officer
CHR: Patricia Knight, Vice President Human Resources
Web address: www.tristarcentennial.com
**Control:** Corporation, Investor–owned, for–profit **Service:** General Medical and Surgical

**Staffed Beds:** 584 **Admissions:** 23139 **Census:** 382 **Outpatient Visits:** 171150 **Births:** 2613 **Total Expense ($000):** 361601 **Payroll Expense ($000):** 131590

TN

---

**Hospital, Medicare Provider Number, Address, Telephone, Approval, Facility, and Physician Codes, Health Care System**

★ American Hospital Association (AHA) membership
☐ The Joint Commission accreditation
◇ DNV Healthcare Inc. accreditation
○ American Osteopathic Association (AOA) accreditation
△ Commission on Accreditation of Rehabilitation Facilities (CARF) accreditation

✠ **VANDERBILT HOSPITAL AND CLINICS (440039)**, 1211 22nd Avenue North, Zip 37232–2102; tel. 615/322–5000, (Includes MONROE CARELL JR. CHILDREN'S HOSPITAL AT VANDERBILT, 2200 Children's Way, Zip 37232; tel. 615/936–1000; Luke Gregory, Chief Executive Officer; PSYCHIATRIC HOSPITAL AT VANDERBILT, 1601 23rd Avenue South, Zip 37212–3198; tel. 615/320–7770) **A**1 2 3 5 8 9 10 **F**2 3 4 5 6 7 8 9 11 12 13 15 16 17 18 19 20 21 22 23 24 25 26 27 28 29 30 31 32 34 35 36 37 38 39 40 41 42 43 44 45 46 47 48 49 50 51 52 53 54 55 56 57 58 59 60 61 62 63 64 65 66 68 70 72 74 75 76 77 78 79 80 81 82 84 85 86 87 88 89 90 91 92 93 94 95 96 97 98 99 100 101 102 103 104 105 106 107 108 109 110 111 113 114 115 116 117 118 119 120 122 123 125 128 129 130 131 133 134 135 136 137 138 139 140 141 142 143 145 146 147 **P**1 5 6 7 **S** Vanderbilt Healthcare, Nashville, TN
Primary Contact: David R. Posch, Chief Executive Officer
CFO: Warren E. Beck, Associate Vice Chancellor Health Affairs and Senior Vice President Finance
CMO: Paul Sternberg, M.D., Professor and Chairman
CIO: William Stead, Associate Vice Chancellor for Health Affairs, Director Informatics Center and Chief Strategy and Information Officer
CHR: Lenon J. Coleman, Interim Chief Human Resources Officer
Web address: www.mc.vanderbilt.edu
**Control:** Other not–for–profit (including NFP Corporation) **Service:** General Medical and Surgical

**Staffed Beds:** 909 **Admissions:** 49174 **Census:** 754 **Outpatient Visits:** 1696382 **Births:** 3279 **Total Expense ($000):** 1657594 **Payroll Expense ($000):** 572873 **Personnel:** 11990

✠ **VANDERBILT STALLWORTH REHABILITATION HOSPITAL (443028)**, 2201 Childrens Way, Zip 37212–3165; tel. 615/320–7600, (Nonreporting) **A**1 5 9 10 **S** HEALTHSOUTH Corporation, Birmingham, AL
Primary Contact: Susan Heath, Chief Executive Officer
CFO: Peggy Belyeu, Controller
CMO: Bob Coxe, M.D., Medical Director
CHR: Ruth Beasley, Director Human Resources
Web address: www.vanderbiltstallworthrehab.com
**Control:** Corporation, Investor–owned, for–profit **Service:** Rehabilitation

**Staffed Beds:** 80

✠ **VETERANS AFFAIRS TENNESSEE VALLEY HEALTHCARE SYSTEM**, 1310 24th Avenue South, Zip 37212–2637; tel. 615/327–4751, (Includes ALVIN C. YORK CAMPUS, 3400 Lebanon Pike, Murfreesboro, Zip 37129–1236; tel. 615/867–6000; NASHVILLE CAMPUS, 1310 24th Avenue South, tel. 615/327–4751), (Nonreporting) **A**1 2 3 5 8 **S** Department of Veterans Affairs, Washington, DC
Primary Contact: Juan A. Morales, R.N., MSN, Health System Director
COO: Gary D. Trende, FACHE, Chief Operating Officer
CFO: Jim A. Hayes, Chief Fiscal Service
CMO: Michael Doukas, Chief of Staff
CHR: Shirley F. Pettite, Chief, Human Resources
Web address: www.tennesseevalley.va.gov
**Control:** Veterans Affairs, Government, federal **Service:** General Medical and Surgical

**Staffed Beds:** 260

### NEWPORT—Cocke County

**BAPTIST HOSPITAL OF COCKE COUNTY** See Newport Medical Center

✠ **NEWPORT MEDICAL CENTER (440153)**, 435 Second Street, Zip 37821–3799; tel. 423/625–2200, (Nonreporting) **A**1 9 10 **S** Health Management Associates, Naples, FL
Primary Contact: Spencer Thomas, Chief Executive Officer
CFO: Jon Richards, Chief Financial Officer
CMO: Constantino Diaz, M.D., Chief of Staff
CHR: Gina Kinkaid, Vice President Human Resources
Web address: www.hma.com/content/newport–medical–center
**Control:** Corporation, Investor–owned, for–profit **Service:** General Medical and Surgical

**Staffed Beds:** 47

### OAK RIDGE—Anderson County

✠ **METHODIST MEDICAL CENTER OF OAK RIDGE (440034)**, 990 Oak Ridge Turnpike, Zip 37830–6976, Mailing Address: P.O. Box 2529, Zip 37831–2529; tel. 865/835–1000 **A**1 2 9 10 **F**3 11 13 15 17 18 20 22 24 26 28 29 30 31 34 35 40 45 49 51 57 59 60 61 64 65 68 70 74 75 76 77 78 79 81 82 84 85 86 87 89 92 93 100 107 108 110 111 113 114 115 116 117 118 119 120 122 125 128 129 130 131 134 140 141 145 146 147 **P**6 7 **S** Covenant Health, Knoxville, TN
Primary Contact: Michael Belbeck, President and Chief Administrative Officer
COO: Suzanne Koehler, Vice President and Chief Support Officer
CFO: Julie Utterback, Vice President and Chief Financial Officer
CHR: Rick Akens, Director Human Resources
Web address: www.mmcoakridge.com
**Control:** Other not–for–profit (including NFP Corporation) **Service:** General Medical and Surgical

**Staffed Beds:** 255 **Admissions:** 11108 **Census:** 141 **Outpatient Visits:** 158687 **Births:** 625 **Total Expense ($000):** 146920 **Payroll Expense ($000):** 54567 **Personnel:** 1006

✠ **RIDGEVIEW PSYCHIATRIC HOSPITAL AND CENTER (444003)**, 240 West Tyrone Road, Zip 37830–6571; tel. 865/482–1076, (Nonreporting) **A**10
Primary Contact: Robert J. Benning, Chief Executive Officer
COO: Brian Buuck, Chief Operating Officer
CFO: Mary Claire Duff, CPA, Chief Financial Officer
CMO: Renu Bhateja, M.D., President Medical Staff
CHR: Julie M. Wright, Director Human Resources
Web address: www.ridgeviewresources.com
**Control:** Other not–for–profit (including NFP Corporation) **Service:** Psychiatric

**Staffed Beds:** 20

### PARIS—Henry County

✠ **HENRY COUNTY MEDICAL CENTER (440132)**, 301 Tyson Avenue, Zip 38242–4544, Mailing Address: P.O. Box 1030, Zip 38242–1030; tel. 731/642–1220, (Total facility includes 150 beds in nursing home–type unit) **A**1 9 10 **F**3 7 11 13 15 17 18 20 28 29 30 31 32 34 35 39 40 51 53 57 59 62 63 64 67 68 70 76 77 78 79 81 82 85 86 87 89 93 98 102 103 107 108 111 113 117 118 120 127 128 129 130 131 132 134 145 147
Primary Contact: Thomas H. Gee, Administrator
CFO: Lisa Casteel, Chief Financial Officer
CIO: Pam Ridley, Director Information Systems
CHR: Edwin L. Ledden, Assistant Administrator
Web address: www.hcmc–tn.org
**Control:** Hospital district or authority, Government, nonfederal **Service:** General Medical and Surgical

**Staffed Beds:** 251 **Admissions:** 4392 **Census:** 176 **Outpatient Visits:** 77547 **Births:** 374 **Total Expense ($000):** 67626 **Payroll Expense ($000):** 29343 **Personnel:** 656

### PARSONS—Decatur County

☐ **DECATUR COUNTY GENERAL HOSPITAL (440070)**, 969 Tennessee Avenue South, Zip 38363–1649, Mailing Address: P.O. Box 250, Zip 38363–0250; tel. 731/847–3031, (Nonreporting) **A**1 9 10
Primary Contact: John M. Carruth, Chief Executive Officer
CFO: Donna Hayes, Controller
CMO: Tom Hamilton, M.D., Chief of Staff
CHR: Shelley Bartholomew, Director Human Resources
Web address: www.dcgh.org
**Control:** County–Government, nonfederal **Service:** General Medical and Surgical

**Staffed Beds:** 40

### PIKEVILLE—Bledsoe County

☐ **ERLANGER BLEDSOE HOSPITAL (441306)**, 71 Wheeler Avenue, Zip 37367, Mailing Address: P.O. Box 699, Zip 37367–0699; tel. 423/447–2112 **A**1 9 10 18 **F**3 15 29 34 40 50 54 56 57 59 64 65 86 93 107 110 118 129 132 **S** Erlanger Health System, Chattanooga, TN
Primary Contact: Stephanie Boynton, Administrator
CMO: Arturo L. Quito, M.D., Chief of Staff
CIO: Debbie Rains, Coordinator Health Information Management
CHR: Patsy Brown, Site Coordinator Human Resources
Web address: www.erlanger.org
**Control:** Hospital district or authority, Government, nonfederal **Service:** General Medical and Surgical

**Staffed Beds:** 25 **Admissions:** 226 **Census:** 7 **Outpatient Visits:** 12684 **Births:** 0 **Total Expense ($000):** 8483 **Payroll Expense ($000):** 3285 **Personnel:** 67

### POWELL—Knox County

**MERCY MEDICAL CENTER NORTH** See North Knoxville Medical Center

### PULASKI—Giles County

✠ **HILLSIDE HOSPITAL (440020)**, 1265 East College Street, Zip 38478–4500; tel. 931/363–7531 **A**1 9 10 **F**3 11 13 15 17 28 29 30 34 40 56 57 59 68 70 75 76 77 79 81 85 93 98 103 107 108 110 111 113 118 128 129 130 131 132 134 142 145 146 147 **S** LifePoint Hospitals, Inc., Brentwood, TN
Primary Contact: Roxana J. Pool, R.N., M.P.H., Chief Executive Officer
CFO: Donald Gavin, Chief Financial Officer
CHR: Jane Petty, Director Human Resources
Web address: www.hillsidehospital.com
**Control:** Corporation, Investor–owned, for–profit **Service:** General Medical and Surgical

**Staffed Beds:** 50 **Admissions:** 1473 **Census:** 19 **Outpatient Visits:** 31238 **Births:** 127 **Total Expense ($000):** 23731 **Payroll Expense ($000):** 9056 **Personnel:** 252

TN

## RIPLEY—Lauderdale County

☒ **LAUDERDALE COMMUNITY HOSPITAL (441314)**, 326 Asbury Avenue, Zip 38063–9701; tel. 731/221–2200 **A**1 9 10 18 **F**1 3 11 15 29 30 34 35 40 45 57 59 64 74 75 77 79 81 85 87 89 93 107 113 118 129 131 132 133 134 145 147 **S** HMC/CAH Consolidated, Inc., Kansas City, MO
Primary Contact: Scott Tongate, Chief Executive Officer
CFO: Jim Sneed, Chief Financial Officer
CMO: Syed A. Zaidi, M.D., Chief of Staff
CIO: Jim Vaden, Director Information Systems
CHR: Gail Henderson, Manager Human Resources
Web address: www.lauderdalehospital.com/
**Control:** Corporation, Investor–owned, for–profit **Service:** General Medical and Surgical

**Staffed Beds:** 25 **Admissions:** 590 **Census:** 9 **Outpatient Visits:** 18543 **Births:** 0 **Total Expense ($000):** 13070 **Payroll Expense ($000):** 5787 **Personnel:** 146

## ROGERSVILLE—Hawkins County

☒ **WELLMONT HAWKINS COUNTY MEMORIAL HOSPITAL (440032)**, 851 Locust Street, Zip 37857–2407, Mailing Address: P.O. Box 130, Zip 37857–0130; tel. 423/921–7000 **A**1 5 9 10 **F**3 11 15 29 30 34 40 45 47 70 75 77 79 81 91 93 107 108 118 128 129 132 145 147 **S** Wellmont Health System, Kingsport, TN
Primary Contact: Greg Neal, President and Chief Executive Officer
CFO: Dale Poe, Chief Financial Officer
CHR: Robin Poteete, Manager Human Resources
Web address: www.wellmont.org
**Control:** Other not–for–profit (including NFP Corporation) **Service:** General Medical and Surgical

**Staffed Beds:** 50 **Admissions:** 1603 **Census:** 14 **Outpatient Visits:** 19857 **Total Expense ($000):** 20408 **Payroll Expense ($000):** 6552 **Personnel:** 176

## SAVANNAH—Hardin County

☒ **HARDIN MEDICAL CENTER (440109)**, 935 Wayne Road, Zip 38372–1937; tel. 731/926–8000, (Nonreporting) **A**1 9 10
Primary Contact: Charlotte Burns, Administrator and Chief Executive Officer
CFO: Mike Harbor, Chief Financial Officer
CMO: Gilbert M. Thayer, M.D., Chief Medical Staff
CIO: Jacob Bomar, Director Information Technology
CHR: Jimmy Davis, Director Human Resources
Web address: www.hardinmedicalcenter.org
**Control:** County–Government, nonfederal **Service:** General Medical and Surgical

**Staffed Beds:** 119

## SELMER—Mcnairy County

☒ **MCNAIRY REGIONAL HOSPITAL (440051)**, 705 East Poplar Avenue, Zip 38375–1828; tel. 731/645–3221, (Nonreporting) **A**1 9 10 **S** Community Health Systems, Inc., Franklin, TN
Primary Contact: Pamela W. Roberts, Chief Executive Officer
CFO: Meredith Jones, Chief Financial Officer
CMO: Ryan Bartz, D.O., Chief of Staff
CHR: Linda Durham, Director Human Resources
Web address: www.mcnairyregionalhospital.com
**Control:** Other not–for–profit (including NFP Corporation) **Service:** General Medical and Surgical

**Staffed Beds:** 45

## SEVIERVILLE—Sevier County

☒ **LECONTE MEDICAL CENTER (440081)**, 742 Middle Creek Road, Zip 37862–5019, Mailing Address: P.O. Box 8005, Zip 37864–8005; tel. 865/446–7000, (Total facility includes 54 beds in nursing home–type unit) **A**1 9 10 **F**3 11 13 15 18 20 28 29 30 31 34 35 40 45 47 50 51 53 57 59 61 64 67 68 70 75 76 78 79 81 85 87 93 97 107 110 111 113 118 127 128 129 130 134 145 146 147 **P**6 7 **S** Covenant Health, Knoxville, TN
Primary Contact: Ellen Wilhoit, President and Chief Administrative Officer
COO: Rick Carringer, Vice President Finance and Support Services
CFO: Rick Carringer, Vice President Finance and Support Services
CMO: Curtis Burke, M.D., Chief of Staff
CIO: Amanda Brabson, Director Marketing and Public Relations
CHR: Steve Bramble, Director Human Resources
Web address: www.lecontemedicalcenter.com
**Control:** Other not–for–profit (including NFP Corporation) **Service:** General Medical and Surgical

**Staffed Beds:** 123 **Admissions:** 3856 **Census:** 76 **Outpatient Visits:** 119664 **Births:** 948 **Total Expense ($000):** 46937 **Payroll Expense ($000):** 22120 **Personnel:** 460

## SEWANEE—Franklin County

**EMERALD–HODGSON HOSPITAL** See Southern Tennessee Medical Center, Winchester

## SHELBYVILLE—Bedford County

☒ **HERITAGE MEDICAL CENTER (440137)**, 2835 Highway 231 North, Zip 37160–7327; tel. 931/685–5433, (Nonreporting) **A**1 9 10 **S** Community Health Systems, Inc., Franklin, TN
Primary Contact: Daniel Buckner, Interim Chief Executive Officer
CIO: Debbie Sudduth, Director Information Services
Web address: www.heritagemedicalcenter.com
**Control:** County–Government, nonfederal **Service:** General Medical and Surgical

**Staffed Beds:** 70

## SMITHVILLE—Dekalb County

☐ **DEKALB COMMUNITY HOSPITAL (440148)**, 520 West Main Street, Zip 37166–0640, Mailing Address: P.O. Box 640, Zip 37166–0640; tel. 615/215–5000, (Nonreporting) **A**1 9 10 **S** Capella Healthcare, Franklin, TN
Primary Contact: Robert M. Luther, Interim Chief Executive Officer
CMO: Hugh Don Cripps, M.D., Chief of Staff
CHR: Gingie Braswell, Director Human Resources
Web address: www.dekalbcommunityhospital.com
**Control:** Corporation, Investor–owned, for–profit **Service:** General Medical and Surgical

**Staffed Beds:** 52

## SMYRNA—Rutherford County

☒ **STONECREST MEDICAL CENTER (440227)**, 200 StoneCrest Boulevard, Zip 37167–6810; tel. 615/768–2000, (Nonreporting) **A**1 2 9 10 **S** HCA, Nashville, TN
Primary Contact: Mark E. Sims, Chief Executive Officer
COO: Zachary McCluskey, Chief Operating Officer
CFO: Joseph E. Bowman, Chief Financial Officer
CMO: Corbi Milligan, M.D., Chief of Staff
CHR: Cynthia Adams, Vice President Human Resources
Web address: www.stonecrestmedical.com
**Control:** Corporation, Investor–owned, for–profit **Service:** General Medical and Surgical

**Staffed Beds:** 101

## SNEEDVILLE—Hancock County

★ **WELLMONT HANCOCK COUNTY HOSPITAL (441313)**, 1519 Main Street, Zip 37869–3657; tel. 423/733–5000, (Nonreporting) **A**9 10 18 **S** Wellmont Health System, Kingsport, TN
Primary Contact: Fred L. Pelle, FACHE, President and Chief Executive Officer
COO: Tracey Moffatt, Chief Operating Officer
CFO: Dale Poe, Chief Financial Officer
CMO: J. Dale Sargent, M.D., Chief Medical Officer
CIO: Kent Petty, Chief Information Officer
CHR: Robin Poteete, Manager Human Resources
Web address: www.wellmont.org/Hospitals/Hancock–County–Hospital.aspx
**Control:** Other not–for–profit (including NFP Corporation) **Service:** General Medical and Surgical

**Staffed Beds:** 10

## SOMERVILLE—Fayette County

☐ **METHODIST HEALTHCARE–FAYETTE HOSPITAL (440168)**, 214 Lakeview Drive, Zip 38068–9737; tel. 901/516–4000 **A**1 9 10 **F**3 8 15 29 34 35 40 45 57 59 64 68 75 81 85 87 93 107 113 118 132 145 147 **S** Methodist Le Bonheur Healthcare, Memphis, TN
Primary Contact: David Crislip, Administrator
CFO: Jane George, Controller
CMO: Barton Thrasher, M.D., Chief of Staff
CHR: Joanell West, Human Resources Generalist
Web address: www.methodisthealth.org
**Control:** Other not–for–profit (including NFP Corporation) **Service:** General Medical and Surgical

**Staffed Beds:** 10 **Admissions:** 308 **Census:** 3 **Outpatient Visits:** 13556 **Births:** 0 **Total Expense ($000):** 9165 **Payroll Expense ($000):** 4087 **Personnel:** 60

**TN**

---

**Hospital, Medicare Provider Number, Address, Telephone, Approval, Facility, and Physician Codes, Health Care System**

★ American Hospital Association (AHA) membership
☐ The Joint Commission accreditation ◇ DNV Healthcare Inc. accreditation
○ American Osteopathic Association (AOA) accreditation
△ Commission on Accreditation of Rehabilitation Facilities (CARF) accreditation

---

## SPARTA—White County

☐ **HIGHLANDS MEDICAL CENTER (440192)**, 401 Sewell Road,
Zip 38583–1299; tel. 931/738–9211, (Nonreporting) **A**1 9 10 **S** Capella
Healthcare, Franklin, TN
Primary Contact: William Little, Chief Executive Officer
CFO: Tim Lynch, Interim Chief Financial Officer
CMO: Ronald Cunliffe, D.O., Chief of Staff
CIO: Glenn Wade, Director Information Systems
CHR: Kent Frisbee, Director Human Resources
Web address: www.whitecountyhospital.com
**Control:** Corporation, Investor–owned, for–profit **Service:** General Medical and
Surgical

**Staffed Beds:** 44

## SPRINGFIELD—Robertson County

✠ **NORTHCREST MEDICAL CENTER (440065)**, 100 North Crest Drive,
Zip 37172–3961; tel. 615/384–2411, (Nonreporting) **A**1 9 10
Primary Contact: Scott Raynes, President and Chief Executive Officer
COO: Randy Mills, Vice President Operations and Business Development
CFO: James A. Schmidt, Chief Financial Officer
CMO: Jonathan Kroser, M.D., Chief of Staff
CIO: Randy Davis, Chief Information Officer
CHR: Amber King, Director Human Resources
Web address: www.northcrest.com
**Control:** Other not–for–profit (including NFP Corporation) **Service:** General
Medical and Surgical

**Staffed Beds:** 81

## SWEETWATER—Monroe County

✠ **SWEETWATER HOSPITAL (440084)**, 304 Wright Street, Zip 37874–2897;
tel. 865/213–8200, (Nonreporting) **A**1 9 10
Primary Contact: Scott Bowman, Administrator
Web address: www.sweetwaterhospital.org
**Control:** Other not–for–profit (including NFP Corporation) **Service:** General
Medical and Surgical

**Staffed Beds:** 59

## TAZEWELL—Claiborne County

✠ **CLAIBORNE COUNTY HOSPITAL (440057)**, 1850 Old Knoxville Road,
Zip 37879–3625; tel. 423/626–4211, (Nonreporting) **A**1 9 10 20
Primary Contact: Tim S. Brown, Chief Executive Officer
CFO: Tracee McFarland, Chief Financial Officer
CHR: Susan Stone, Director Human Resources
Web address: www.claibornehospital.org
**Control:** County–Government, nonfederal **Service:** General Medical and Surgical

**Staffed Beds:** 62

## TRENTON—Gibson County

✠ **GIBSON GENERAL HOSPITAL (440047)**, 200 Hospital Drive, Zip 38382–3313;
tel. 731/855–7900 **A**1 9 10 **F**3 15 29 30 35 40 57 59 64 68 75 81 87 93
107 118 129 131 132 145 **S** West Tennessee Healthcare, Jackson, TN
Primary Contact: Sherry Scruggs, Administrator
CFO: Terry Swindell, Controller
CMO: Thomas Nelson, M.D., Director Emergency Room
CHR: Judy Hime, Director Human Resources
Web address: www.wth.net
**Control:** Hospital district or authority, Government, nonfederal **Service:** General
Medical and Surgical

**Staffed Beds:** 32 **Admissions:** 384 **Census:** 4 **Outpatient Visits:** 11863
**Births:** 1 **Total Expense ($000):** 5397 **Payroll Expense ($000):** 3176
**Personnel:** 78

## TULLAHOMA—Coffee County

☐ **HARTON REGIONAL MEDICAL CENTER (440144)**, 1801 North Jackson
Street, Zip 37388–2201; tel. 931/393–3000, (Nonreporting) **A**1 9 10 19
**S** Health Management Associates, Naples, FL
Primary Contact: William R. Spray, Chief Executive Officer
COO: Tracy Byers, Chief Operating Officer
CFO: Shaun Adams, Chief Financial Officer
CMO: Michael Tepedino, M.D., Chief of Staff
CIO: Donald Cooper, Director Information Systems
CHR: Lenore Blackwell, Director Human Resources
Web address: www.hartonmedicalcenter.com
**Control:** Corporation, Investor–owned, for–profit **Service:** Rehabilitation

**Staffed Beds:** 104

## UNION CITY—Obion County

✠ **BAPTIST MEMORIAL HOSPITAL–UNION CITY (440130)**, 1201 Bishop Street,
Zip 38261–5403, Mailing Address: P.O. Box 310, Zip 38281–0310;
tel. 731/885–2410 **A**1 9 10 **F**4 5 7 11 13 15 18 20 26 29 30 35 40 45 48 50
51 53 63 70 75 76 79 80 81 82 84 85 87 89 91 93 98 99 100 101 102 104
105 107 108 110 111 113 117 118 123 129 134 145 **P**3 **S** Baptist Memorial
Health Care Corporation, Memphis, TN
Primary Contact: Barry Bondurant, Administrator and Chief Executive Officer
CFO: Mike Perryman, Chief Financial Officer
CMO: James Batey, M.D., President Medical Staff
CIO: David Mercer, Coordinator Information Systems
CHR: Nicky Thomas, Director Human Resources
Web address: www.bmhcc.org
**Control:** Other not–for–profit (including NFP Corporation) **Service:** General
Medical and Surgical

**Staffed Beds:** 88 **Admissions:** 2898 **Census:** 26 **Outpatient Visits:** 41530
**Births:** 265 **Total Expense ($000):** 37873 **Payroll Expense ($000):** 15269
**Personnel:** 376

## WAVERLY—Humphreys County

**THREE RIVERS HOSPITAL (441303)**, 451 Highway 13 South,
Zip 37185–2149, Mailing Address: P.O. Box 437, Zip 37185–2149;
tel. 931/296–4203 **A**9 10 18 **F**3 15 29 34 40 45 57 59 64 81 91 103 107
113 118 129 132 134 147
Primary Contact: Freda Russell, Interim Chief Executive Officer
CFO: Sandra Patrick, Chief Financial Officer
CMO: Patrick J. Murphy, M.D., Chief of Staff
CHR: Linda Rawlings, Director Human Resources and Personnel
Web address: www.threerivershospital.org
**Control:** Other not–for–profit (including NFP Corporation) **Service:** General
Medical and Surgical

**Staffed Beds:** 25 **Admissions:** 587 **Census:** 9 **Outpatient Visits:** 22131
**Births:** 0 **Total Expense ($000):** 8256 **Payroll Expense ($000):** 3643
**Personnel:** 87

## WAYNESBORO—Wayne County

☐ **WAYNE MEDICAL CENTER (440010)**, 103 J. V. Mangubat Drive, Zip 38485,
Mailing Address: P.O. Box 580, Zip 38485–0580; tel. 931/722–5411,
(Nonreporting) **A**1 9 10 20
Primary Contact: Gerald Faircloth, Chief Executive Officer
CFO: Michael A. Sears, Chief Financial Officer
CMO: Esmeraldo Herrera, M.D., Chief of Staff
CHR: Vicki Petty, Manager Human Resources
Web address: www.mauryregional.com
**Control:** Other not–for–profit (including NFP Corporation) **Service:** General
Medical and Surgical

**Staffed Beds:** 78

## WINCHESTER—Franklin County

✠ **SOUTHERN TENNESSEE MEDICAL CENTER (440058)**, 185 Hospital Road,
Zip 37398–2404; tel. 931/967–8200, (Includes EMERALD–HODGSON HOSPITAL,
1260 University Avenue, Sewanee, Zip 37375–2303; tel. 931/598–5691; Ralph
Underwood, Administrator), (Total facility includes 46 beds in nursing home–type
unit) **A**1 9 10 **F**3 13 15 20 29 34 38 40 45 46 48 56 57 59 70 74 75 76 77
79 81 85 86 87 90 93 98 103 107 108 110 111 113 118 127 128 129 134
145 146 147 **S** LifePoint Hospitals, Inc., Brentwood, TN
Primary Contact: J. Phillip Young, FACHE, Chief Executive Officer
COO: Heather L. Harper, Chief Operating Officer
CFO: Steve Moore, Chief Financial Officer
CIO: James Payne, Director Information Systems
CHR: Linda Tipps, Director Human Resources
Web address: www.southerntennessee.com
**Control:** Corporation, Investor–owned, for–profit **Service:** General Medical and
Surgical

**Staffed Beds:** 153 **Admissions:** 6101 **Census:** 86 **Outpatient Visits:** 63483
**Births:** 355 **Total Expense ($000):** 52447 **Payroll Expense ($000):** 22703
**Personnel:** 408

## WOODBURY—Cannon County

☐ **STONES RIVER HOSPITAL (440200)**, 324 Doolittle Road, Zip 37190–1140;
tel. 615/563–4001, (Nonreporting) **A**1 9 10 **S** Capella Healthcare, Franklin, TN
Primary Contact: Robert M. Luther, Interim Chief Executive Officer
CMO: J. C. Wall, M.D., Chief of Staff
CHR: Brian Woods, Director Human Resources
Web address: www.stonesriverhospital.com
**Control:** Corporation, Investor–owned, for–profit **Service:** General Medical and
Surgical

**Staffed Beds:** 60

**TN**

# TEXAS

## ABILENE—Taylor County

✠ **ABILENE REGIONAL MEDICAL CENTER (450558)**, 6250 U.S. Highway 83, Zip 79606–5299; tel. 325/428–1000, (Total facility includes 25 beds in nursing home–type unit) **A**1 9 10 **F**8 11 13 15 17 18 20 22 24 26 28 29 30 31 34 35 40 41 43 46 49 50 51 53 56 57 59 64 68 70 72 75 76 77 78 79 81 85 86 87 89 93 107 108 110 111 113 114 117 118 127 129 131 134 145 146 147 **P**3 **S** Community Health Systems, Inc., Franklin, TN
Primary Contact: Michael D. Murphy, Chief Executive Officer
CFO: Ron Bennett, Chief Financial Officer
CIO: Dennis Newquist, Director Information Systems
CHR: Edwin Winkelmeyer, Director Human Resources
Web address: www.abileneregional.com
**Control:** Corporation, Investor–owned, for–profit **Service:** General Medical and Surgical

**Staffed Beds:** 205 **Admissions:** 7060 **Census:** 89 **Outpatient Visits:** 68705 **Births:** 1286 **Total Expense ($000):** 90022 **Payroll Expense ($000):** 35101 **Personnel:** 666

✠ **ACADIA ABILENE HOSPITAL (454098)**, 4225 Woods Place, Zip 79602–7991, Mailing Address: P.O. Box 5559, Zip 79608; tel. 325/698–6600 **A**1 9 10 **F**4 5 29 34 54 56 57 64 86 87 98 99 101 103 104 105 129 **P**4 **S** Acadia Healthcare Company, Inc., Franklin, TN
Primary Contact: Shana Hisaw, Chief Operating Officer
Web address: www.acadiaabilene.com
**Control:** Corporation, Investor–owned, for–profit **Service:** Psychiatric

**Staffed Beds:** 58 **Admissions:** 1683 **Census:** 49 **Outpatient Visits:** 5655 **Births:** 0 **Total Expense ($000):** 9235 **Payroll Expense ($000):** 4078 **Personnel:** 106

**HENDRICK CENTER FOR EXTENDED CARE (452029)**, 1900 Pine Street, Zip 79601; tel. 325/670–2384 **A**10 **F**1 29 31 68 85 129
Primary Contact: Tim Riley, Vice President
**Control:** Church–operated, Nongovernment, not–for profit **Service:** Long–Term Acute Care hospital

**Staffed Beds:** 19 **Admissions:** 217 **Census:** 17 **Outpatient Visits:** 0 **Births:** 0 **Total Expense ($000):** 5385 **Payroll Expense ($000):** 1644 **Personnel:** 33

✠ **HENDRICK HEALTH SYSTEM (450229)**, 1900 Pine Street, Zip 79601–2432; tel. 325/670–2000, (Total facility includes 20 beds in nursing home–type unit) **A**1 9 10 **F**3 11 12 13 14 15 17 18 20 22 24 26 28 29 30 31 32 34 35 36 39 40 43 44 45 48 49 50 51 53 56 57 59 60 61 62 64 68 70 73 74 75 76 77 78 79 80 81 85 86 87 88 89 90 92 93 96 97 102 107 108 110 111 113 114 117 118 122 127 128 129 131 134 142 145 146 147
Primary Contact: Tim Lancaster, FACHE, President and Chief Executive Officer
CFO: Stephen Kimmel, Senior Vice President and Chief Financial Officer
CMO: Steve Faehnle, M.D., Vice President Medical Affairs
CHR: Mike McBroom, FACHE, Vice President Human Resources
Web address: www.ehendrick.org
**Control:** Church–operated, Nongovernment, not–for profit **Service:** General Medical and Surgical

**Staffed Beds:** 364 **Admissions:** 15374 **Census:** 233 **Outpatient Visits:** 274621 **Births:** 1433 **Total Expense ($000):** 214919 **Payroll Expense ($000):** 96310 **Personnel:** 1891

☐ **RELIANT REHABILITATION HOSPITAL ABILENE (673039)**, 6401 Directors Parkway, Zip 79606–5869; tel. 325/691–1600 **A**1 9 10 **F**3 74 79 82 87 90 91 129 134 **S** Reliant Healthcare Partners, Addison, TX
Primary Contact: Lisa M. Nelson, R.N., MS, Chief Executive Officer
Web address: www.reliantabilene.com
**Control:** Partnership, Investor–owned, for–profit **Service:** Rehabilitation

**Staffed Beds:** 30 **Admissions:** 443 **Census:** 14 **Outpatient Visits:** 545 **Births:** 0 **Total Expense ($000):** 6314 **Payroll Expense ($000):** 2600 **Personnel:** 46

## ADDISON—Dallas County

**METHODIST HOSPITAL FOR SURGERY (670073)**, 17101 North Dallas Parkway, Zip 75001–7103; tel. 469/248–3900 **A**21 **F**3 29 30 35 40 70 81 93 107 111 112 118 129 145 **P**2 **S** Methodist Health System, Dallas, TX
Primary Contact: Chris Shoup, President
CFO: Jade Andrews, Chief Financial Officer
CMO: Rajiv Pandit, M.D., Medical Director
CIO: Ronda Kirk Johnson, Manager Health Information Management
CNO: Patti Griffith, R.N., Chief Nursing Officer
Web address: www.methodisthospitalforsurgery.com/
**Control:** Corporation, Investor–owned, for–profit **Service:** Surgical

**Staffed Beds:** 32 **Admissions:** 1270 **Census:** 10 **Outpatient Visits:** 5802 **Births:** 0 **Total Expense ($000):** 47628 **Payroll Expense ($000):** 8728 **Personnel:** 142

## ALICE—Jim Wells County

✠ **CHRISTUS SPOHN HOSPITAL ALICE (450828)**, 2500 East Main Street, Zip 78332–4169; tel. 361/661–8000 **A**1 9 10 20 **F**3 11 13 15 18 20 22 28 29 30 35 39 40 43 45 46 49 50 57 59 68 70 75 76 77 79 81 84 85 86 87 89 93 97 98 100 101 102 103 107 108 111 113 118 126 129 145 147 **P**7 8 **S** CHRISTUS Health, Irving, TX
Primary Contact: Mark Casanova, Vice President and Chief Operating Officer
COO: Mark Casanova, Vice President and Chief Operating Officer
CFO: Michael Guajardo, Director Finance
CMO: Alejandro Lopez, Jr., M.D., Chief of Staff
CIO: Jean Deanoglis, Director Management Information Systems
CHR: Emily Diaz–Lopez, Director Human Resources
Web address: www.christusspohn.org/locations_alice.htm
**Control:** Church–operated, Nongovernment, not–for profit **Service:** General Medical and Surgical

**Staffed Beds:** 114 **Admissions:** 3632 **Census:** 41 **Outpatient Visits:** 51780 **Births:** 452 **Total Expense ($000):** 49013 **Payroll Expense ($000):** 20137 **Personnel:** 278

## ALLEN—Collin County

✠ **TEXAS HEALTH PRESBYTERIAN HOSPITAL ALLEN (450840)**, 1105 Central Expressway North, Zip 75013; tel. 972/747–1000 **A**1 9 10 **F**3 13 15 28 29 30 34 35 38 40 47 51 54 55 57 59 64 65 70 73 74 75 76 79 81 93 107 110 111 114 117 118 125 128 129 131 134 145 146 147 **S** Texas Health Resources, Arlington, TX
Primary Contact: Sheila A. McKinney, President
CFO: Dan Rich, Director Finance
CMO: Kimberly Barksdale, M.D., President Medical Staff
CHR: Sharon Chisholm, Director Human Resources
Web address: www.texashealth.org
**Control:** Other not–for–profit (including NFP Corporation) **Service:** General Medical and Surgical

**Staffed Beds:** 73 **Admissions:** 4270 **Census:** 38 **Outpatient Visits:** 50996 **Births:** 1264 **Total Expense ($000):** 59436 **Payroll Expense ($000):** 25244 **Personnel:** 340

☐ **TWIN CREEKS REHABILITATION HOSPITAL (673025)**, 1001 Raintree Circle, Zip 75013; tel. 972/908–2015 **A**1 9 10 **F**3 28 29 30 34 40 56 59 60 74 75 79 87 90 91 94 96 100 129 131 145 147
Primary Contact: Bill Kaupas, Interim Chief Executive Officer
Web address: www.twincreekshosp.com/
**Control:** Partnership, Investor–owned, for–profit **Service:** Rehabilitation

**Staffed Beds:** 39 **Admissions:** 529 **Census:** 18 **Outpatient Visits:** 2 **Births:** 0 **Total Expense ($000):** 7715 **Payroll Expense ($000):** 3597 **Personnel:** 116

## ALPINE—Brewster County

✠ **BIG BEND REGIONAL MEDICAL CENTER (451378)**, 2600 Highway 118 North, Zip 79830–2002; tel. 432/837–3447 **A**1 9 10 18 **F**3 29 30 34 35 40 43 45 49 57 59 64 75 76 81 85 93 107 113 118 131 132 145 146 147 **P**6 **S** Community Health Systems, Inc., Franklin, TN
Primary Contact: Michael J. Ellis, Chief Executive Officer
Web address: www.bigbendhealthcare.com
**Control:** Corporation, Investor–owned, for–profit **Service:** General Medical and Surgical

**Staffed Beds:** 25 **Admissions:** 985 **Census:** 8 **Outpatient Visits:** 13103 **Births:** 171 **Total Expense ($000):** 18429 **Payroll Expense ($000):** 5701 **Personnel:** 97

TX

---

**Hospital, Medicare Provider Number, Address, Telephone, Approval, Facility, and Physician Codes, Health Care System**

★ American Hospital Association (AHA) membership
☐ The Joint Commission accreditation ◇ DNV Healthcare Inc. accreditation
○ American Osteopathic Association (AOA) accreditation
△ Commission on Accreditation of Rehabilitation Facilities (CARF) accreditation

---

## ALVIN—Brazoria County

**ALVIN DIAGNOSTIC AND URGENT CARE CENTER** See Clear Lake Regional Medical Center, Webster

## AMARILLO—Potter County

✠ **AMARILLO VETERANS AFFAIRS HEALTH CARE SYSTEM**, 6010 West Amarillo Boulevard, Zip 79106–1992; tel. 806/355–9703, (Nonreporting) **A**1 2 3 5 9 **S** Department of Veterans Affairs, Washington, DC
Primary Contact: Andrew Welch, Director
COO: Lance Robinson, Associate Director
CMO: James Gray, M.D., Chief Medical Service
CIO: Modesto Baca, Chief Information Officer
CHR: Ken Creamer, Chief Human Resource
Web address: www.va.gov/sta/guide/home.asp
**Control:** Veterans Affairs, Government, federal **Service:** General Medical and Surgical

> **Staffed Beds:** 69

✠ **BAPTIST ST. ANTHONY HEALTH SYSTEM (450231)**, 1600 Wallace Boulevard, Zip 79106–1799; tel. 806/212–2000 **A**1 2 3 5 9 10 21 **F**3 7 8 11 12 13 15 17 18 19 20 22 24 26 28 29 30 31 34 35 40 45 46 48 49 51 53 54 57 59 62 63 64 70 72 74 75 76 77 78 79 81 82 85 86 87 88 89 90 91 93 96 107 108 110 111 113 114 116 118 125 128 129 130 144 145 146 147
Primary Contact: Bob Williams, President and Chief Executive Officer
COO: Michael Cruz, Vice President Operations
CFO: Brian Walton, Vice President and Chief Financial Officer
CMO: Bill Neilson, M.D., Vice President Medical Affairs
CHR: Cheryl L. Jones, Director Human Resources and Education
Web address: www.bsahs.org
**Control:** Church–operated, Nongovernment, not–for profit **Service:** General Medical and Surgical

> **Staffed Beds:** 448 **Admissions:** 21253 **Census:** 257 **Outpatient Visits:** 156715 **Births:** 2517 **Total Expense ($000):** 250124 **Payroll Expense ($000):** 92441 **Personnel:** 2459

✠ **KINDRED HOSPITAL–AMARILLO (452060)**, 7501 Wallace Boulevard, Zip 79124–2150; tel. 806/467–7000 **A**1 9 10 **F**1 3 26 29 34 35 45 46 50 56 57 59 60 61 70 74 75 77 79 82 84 85 86 87 96 107 108 113 129 147 **P**8 **S** Kindred Healthcare, Louisville, KY
Primary Contact: Kay E. Peck, Ph.D., Chief Executive Officer
CFO: Michael Smesny, Region Chief Financial Officer
CMO: Pablo Rodrigues, M.D., Medical Director
CHR: Brandon Ammons, Director Human Resources
Web address: www.khamarillo.com/
**Control:** Corporation, Investor–owned, for–profit **Service:** General Medical and Surgical

> **Staffed Beds:** 72 **Admissions:** 626 **Census:** 55 **Outpatient Visits:** 0 **Births:** 0 **Total Expense ($000):** 23117 **Payroll Expense ($000):** 9130 **Personnel:** 244

★ **KINDRED REHABILITATION HOSPITAL (453096)**, 7200 West 9th Avenue, Zip 79106; tel. 806/468–2900 **A**9 10 **F**3 29 56 60 75 77 82 87 90 91 96 129 142 147 **S** Kindred Healthcare, Louisville, KY
Primary Contact: Kay E. Peck, Ph.D., Chief Executive Officer
Web address: www.khrehabamarillo.com/
**Control:** Partnership, Investor–owned, for–profit **Service:** Rehabilitation

> **Staffed Beds:** 42 **Admissions:** 590 **Census:** 18 **Outpatient Visits:** 0 **Births:** 0 **Total Expense ($000):** 6392 **Payroll Expense ($000):** 3662 **Personnel:** 114

✠ **NORTHWEST TEXAS HEALTHCARE SYSTEM (450209)**, 1501 South Coulter Avenue, Zip 79106–1790, Mailing Address: P.O. Box 1110, Zip 79105–1110; tel. 806/354–1000, (Includes CHILDREN'S HOSPITAL, 1501 South Coulter Street, Zip 79106–1770; tel. 806/354–1000; PSYCHIATRIC PAVILION, 7201 Evans, Zip 79106) **A**1 2 3 5 9 10 **F**3 4 5 11 13 15 17 18 20 22 24 25 26 28 29 30 31 32 34 35 37 38 39 40 43 44 45 46 48 49 50 54 56 57 59 60 61 64 66 67 68 70 72 74 75 76 77 78 79 81 84 86 88 89 92 93 94 97 98 99 100 101 102 103 104 105 107 108 110 111 113 114 117 118 128 129 131 134 145 146 147 **P**6 **S** Universal Health Services, Inc., King of Prussia, PA
Primary Contact: Sharon Oxendale, Interim Chief Executive Officer and Managing Director
COO: Sharon Oxendale, Chief Operating Officer
CFO: Raymond Grenier, Chief Financial Officer
CMO: Nathan Goldstein, III, M.D., Chief Medical Officer
CIO: Sam Mason, Director Management Information Systems
CHR: Charlyn Snow, Director Human Resources
Web address: www.nwtexashealthcare.com
**Control:** Corporation, Investor–owned, for–profit **Service:** General Medical and Surgical

> **Staffed Beds:** 426 **Admissions:** 18932 **Census:** 250 **Outpatient Visits:** 243227 **Births:** 2242 **Total Expense ($000):** 253831 **Payroll Expense ($000):** 86109 **Personnel:** 1702

**NORTHWEST TEXAS SURGERY CENTER (450796)**, 3501 South Soncy Road Suite 118, Zip 79119–6405; tel. 806/359–7999 **A**9 10 **F**39 40 68 79 81 82 85 93 125 130
Primary Contact: Clay Weiss, Administrator
**Control:** Corporation, Investor–owned, for–profit **Service:** General Medical and Surgical

> **Staffed Beds:** 4 **Admissions:** 99 **Census:** 1 **Outpatient Visits:** 4272 **Births:** 0 **Total Expense ($000):** 8961 **Payroll Expense ($000):** 2779 **Personnel:** 50

**PHYSICIANS SURGICAL HOSPITAL – PANHANDLE CAMPUS**, 7100 West 9th Avenue, Zip 79106–1704; tel. 806/212–0247, (Nonreporting)
Primary Contact: Brad McCall, President and Chief Executive Officer
CFO: Whitt Holder, Chief Financial Officer
CNO: Debbie Inman, Chief Nursing Officer
Web address: www.physurg.com/
**Control:** Partnership, Investor–owned, for–profit **Service:** General Medical and Surgical

> **Staffed Beds:** 11

**PHYSICIANS SURGICAL HOSPITAL – QUAIL CREEK (450875)**, 6819 Plum Creek, Zip 79124; tel. 806/354–6100 **A**9 10 **F**29 30 40 44 50 68 75 79 81 85 89 129 134
Primary Contact: Brad McCall, President and Chief Executive Officer
CFO: Whitt Holder, Chief Financial Officer
CNO: Debbie Inman, Chief Nursing Officer
Web address: www.physurg.com
**Control:** Corporation, Investor–owned, for–profit **Service:** Surgical

> **Staffed Beds:** 39 **Admissions:** 1536 **Census:** 9 **Outpatient Visits:** 12823 **Births:** 0 **Total Expense ($000):** 34661 **Payroll Expense ($000):** 8865 **Personnel:** 154

☐ **PLUM CREEK SPECIALTY HOSPITAL (452066)**, 5601 Plum Creek Drive, Zip 79124–1801; tel. 806/351–1000 **A**1 9 10 **F**1 29 75 77 85 86 129 147 **S** Encore Healthcare, Columbia, MD
Primary Contact: Billy Blasingame, Chief Executive Officer
Web address: www.specialtyhospital–plumcreek.net
**Control:** Corporation, Investor–owned, for–profit **Service:** Long–Term Acute Care hospital

> **Staffed Beds:** 47 **Admissions:** 254 **Census:** 21 **Outpatient Visits:** 0 **Births:** 0 **Total Expense ($000):** 9856 **Payroll Expense ($000):** 2829 **Personnel:** 97

**SPECIALTY HOSPITAL AT PLUM CREEK** See Plum Creek Specialty Hospital

## ANAHUAC—Chambers County

★ **CHAMBERS COUNTY PUBLIC HOSPITAL DISTRICT 1 (451320)**, 200 Hospital Drive, Zip 77514, Mailing Address: P.O. Box 398, Zip 77514; tel. 409/267–3143 **A**9 10 18 **F**3 8 11 29 34 35 40 43 45 47 50 53 54 56 57 59 70 80 81 86 87 88 89 107 111 113 118 127 129 132 145 146 **P**3 7
Primary Contact: Theresa Cheaney, Interim Chief Executive Officer
CFO: Theresa Cheaney, Controller
CMO: Leonidas Andres, M.D., Chief of Staff
Web address: www.chambershealth.org
**Control:** Hospital district or authority, Government, nonfederal **Service:** General Medical and Surgical

> **Staffed Beds:** 14 **Admissions:** 226 **Census:** 3 **Outpatient Visits:** 35302 **Births:** 0 **Total Expense ($000):** 6647 **Payroll Expense ($000):** 4236 **Personnel:** 100

## ANDREWS—Andrews County

✠ **PERMIAN REGIONAL MEDICAL CENTER (450144)**, Northeast By–Pass, Zip 79714, Mailing Address: P.O. Box 2108, Zip 79714–2108; tel. 432/523–2200 **A**1 9 10 20 21 **F**3 11 13 15 29 34 35 36 38 40 43 44 50 53 56 57 59 62 64 68 70 73 75 76 77 81 82 84 85 86 87 89 93 97 107 108 110 111 114 118 126 128 129 130 131 132 134 143 144 145 147 **P**6 7
Primary Contact: Russell Tippin, Chief Executive Officer
CFO: Sandra Cox, Controller
CIO: Dan Smart, Chief Information Management Officer
CHR: Pam McCormick, Director Human Resources
Web address: www.permianregional.com
**Control:** Hospital district or authority, Government, nonfederal **Service:** General Medical and Surgical

> **Staffed Beds:** 44 **Admissions:** 942 **Census:** 8 **Outpatient Visits:** 26097 **Births:** 269 **Total Expense ($000):** 30969 **Payroll Expense ($000):** 15129 **Personnel:** 247

## ANGLETON—Brazoria County

**ANGLETON DANBURY MEDICAL CENTER (450591)**, 132 East Hospital Drive, Zip 77515–4197; tel. 979/849–7721 **A**1 9 10 **F**3 11 13 15 18 28 29 30 34 35 36 40 43 45 46 49 53 57 59 64 65 68 70 74 75 76 77 79 81 82 85 86 87 91 93 107 108 111 113 114 118 129 131 134 145 **P**1
Primary Contact: David A. Bleakney, Administrator
CFO: William D. Garwood, III, Associate Administrator and Chief Financial Officer
CHR: Paula Tobon-Stevens, Associate Administrator
Web address: www.admc.org
**Control:** Hospital district or authority, Government, nonfederal **Service:** General Medical and Surgical

**Staffed Beds:** 51 **Admissions:** 3473 **Census:** 22 **Outpatient Visits:** 44435 **Births:** 340 **Total Expense ($000):** 18015 **Payroll Expense ($000):** 11867 **Personnel:** 233

## ANSON—Jones County

★ **ANSON GENERAL HOSPITAL (450078)**, 101 Avenue J, Zip 79501–2198; tel. 325/823–3231 **A**9 10 **F**7 11 29 40 45 62 75 77 81 89 107 126 132 **P**8
Primary Contact: Pamela Gonzales, Chief Operating Officer
CFO: Rick McDonald, Chief Financial Officer
CIO: Lynna B. Cox, Director Health Information Services
**Control:** City–Government, nonfederal **Service:** General Medical and Surgical

**Staffed Beds:** 35 **Admissions:** 397 **Census:** 7 **Outpatient Visits:** 16233 **Births:** 0 **Total Expense ($000):** 6149 **Payroll Expense ($000):** 3454 **Personnel:** 113

## ARANSAS PASS—San Patricio County

**CARE REGIONAL MEDICAL CENTER (450605)**, 1711 West Wheeler Avenue, Zip 78336–4536; tel. 361/758–8585 **A**9 10 **F**3 4 11 15 18 29 34 35 40 43 44 45 50 56 57 59 64 65 68 70 75 77 78 79 81 85 86 87 90 93 97 98 101 102 103 107 108 113 118 129 131 132 142 145 147
Primary Contact: Jacob Quintana, Administrator
CHR: Sherry Gwynn, Administrative Director Human Resources
Web address: www.crmctx.com
**Control:** Corporation, Investor–owned, for–profit **Service:** General Medical and Surgical

**Staffed Beds:** 52 **Admissions:** 1416 **Census:** 17 **Outpatient Visits:** 22704 **Births:** 0 **Total Expense ($000):** 11906 **Payroll Expense ($000):** 5963 **Personnel:** 166

**NORTH BAY HOSPITAL** See Care Regional Medical Center

## ARLINGTON—Tarrant County

**ARLINGTON REHABILITATION HOSPITAL** See Kindred Rehabilitation Hospital Arlington

☐ **BAYLOR ORTHOPEDIC AND SPINE HOSPITAL AT ARLINGTON (670067)**, 707 Highlander Boulevard, Zip 76015–4319; tel. 817/583–7100 **A**1 9 10 **F**3 29 40 75 79 81 82 85 86 87 107 111 **S** Baylor Health Care System, Dallas, TX
Primary Contact: Allan Beck, Chief Executive Officer
Web address: www.baylorarlington.com
**Control:** Partnership, Investor–owned, for–profit **Service:** General Medical and Surgical

**Staffed Beds:** 24 **Admissions:** 898 **Census:** 4 **Outpatient Visits:** 4677 **Births:** 0 **Total Expense ($000):** 23230 **Payroll Expense ($000):** 5158 **Personnel:** 80

⊞ **HEALTHSOUTH REHABILITATION HOSPITAL OF ARLINGTON (453040)**, 3200 Matlock Road, Zip 76015–2911; tel. 817/468–4000 **A**1 9 10 **F**3 29 64 74 75 77 79 82 90 91 93 94 95 96 128 129 130 131 **S** HEALTHSOUTH Corporation, Birmingham, AL
Primary Contact: Mark S. Deno, Chief Executive Officer
CFO: Kathy Dickerson, Chief Financial Officer
CMO: Rizwan Shah, M.D., Medical Director
CHR: Nancy Rosiles, Coordinator Human Resources
Web address: www.healthsoutharlington.com
**Control:** Corporation, Investor–owned, for–profit **Service:** Rehabilitation

**Staffed Beds:** 65 **Admissions:** 1454 **Census:** 51 **Outpatient Visits:** 9194 **Births:** 0 **Total Expense ($000):** 18918 **Payroll Expense ($000):** 10033 **Personnel:** 218

⊞ **KINDRED HOSPITAL TARRANT COUNTY–ARLINGTON (452028)**, 1000 North Cooper Street, Zip 76011–5540; tel. 817/548–3400 **A**1 9 10 **F**1 3 29 30 40 56 57 77 80 82 93 129 147 **S** Kindred Healthcare, Louisville, KY
Primary Contact: Christina Richard, Administrator
CFO: Jennifer Penland, Controller
CMO: Bernard A. McGowen, M.D., Medical Director
Web address: www.kindredhospitalarl.com/
**Control:** Corporation, Investor–owned, for–profit **Service:** Long–Term Acute Care hospital

**Staffed Beds:** 78 **Admissions:** 668 **Census:** 54 **Outpatient Visits:** 388 **Births:** 0 **Total Expense ($000):** 19018 **Payroll Expense ($000):** 9434 **Personnel:** 205

⊞ **KINDRED REHABILITATION HOSPITAL ARLINGTON (453094)**, 2601 West Randol Mill Road, Zip 76012; tel. 817/804–4400 **A**1 9 10 **F**3 29 34 57 59 74 75 86 87 90 94 96 129 131 145 147 **S** Kindred Healthcare, Louisville, KY
Primary Contact: Chetan Bhasin, Chief Executive Officer
Web address: www.khrehabarlington.com
**Control:** Corporation, Investor–owned, for–profit **Service:** Rehabilitation

**Staffed Beds:** 24 **Admissions:** 614 **Census:** 19 **Outpatient Visits:** 0 **Births:** 0 **Total Expense ($000):** 6260 **Payroll Expense ($000):** 4013 **Personnel:** 78

⊞ **MEDICAL CENTER OF ARLINGTON (450675)**, 3301 Matlock Road, Zip 76015–2998; tel. 817/465–3241 **A**1 2 9 10 **F**3 11 12 13 15 17 18 20 22 24 26 28 29 31 34 35 39 40 43 45 46 47 48 49 50 56 57 59 64 68 70 72 74 75 76 78 79 81 82 85 86 87 92 93 107 108 110 111 113 114 117 118 125 129 130 131 134 143 144 145 146 147 **S** HCA, Nashville, TN
Primary Contact: Winston Borland, President and Chief Executive Officer
CFO: Jeff Ardemagni, Chief Financial Officer
CMO: Randy Davidson, M.D., Chief of Staff
CIO: Tammy Phillips, Director Information Services
CHR: Jerry L. McMorrough, Vice President Human Resources
Web address: www.medicalcenterarlington.com
**Control:** Corporation, Investor–owned, for–profit **Service:** General Medical and Surgical

**Staffed Beds:** 297 **Admissions:** 13487 **Census:** 184 **Outpatient Visits:** 88409 **Births:** 3956 **Total Expense ($000):** 171724 **Payroll Expense ($000):** 65875 **Personnel:** 1001

☐ **MILLWOOD HOSPITAL (454012)**, 1011 North Cooper Street, Zip 76011–5517; tel. 817/261–3121 **A**1 9 10 **F**4 5 29 30 35 54 56 71 87 98 99 100 101 102 103 104 105 129 131 **S** Universal Health Services, Inc., King of Prussia, PA
Primary Contact: Jon C. O'Shaughnessy, Chief Executive Officer
CFO: Jeff Epperson, Chief Financial Officer
CMO: Ernest Brownlee, M.D., Medical Director
CIO: Linda Jones, Director Medical Records
CHR: Shirley Spurlock, Director Human Resources
Web address: www.millwoodhospital.com
**Control:** Partnership, Investor–owned, for–profit **Service:** Psychiatric

**Staffed Beds:** 122 **Admissions:** 4428 **Census:** 93 **Outpatient Visits:** 25204 **Births:** 0 **Total Expense ($000):** 22873 **Payroll Expense ($000):** 10149 **Personnel:** 241

**SUNDANCE HOSPITAL (454113)**, 7000 U.S. Highway 287 South, Zip 76001; tel. 817/583–8080, (Nonreporting) **A**10
Primary Contact: Puskoor Kumar, M.D., Administrator
Web address: www.sundancehealthcare.com
**Control:** Corporation, Investor–owned, for–profit **Service:** Psychiatric

**Staffed Beds:** 30

⊞ **TEXAS HEALTH ARLINGTON MEMORIAL HOSPITAL (450064)**, 800 West Randol Mill Road, Zip 76012–2503; tel. 817/548–6100 **A**1 9 10 **F**3 11 12 13 15 17 18 20 22 24 26 28 29 30 31 34 35 37 40 45 46 47 48 49 51 53 54 57 59 60 63 64 65 68 70 72 74 75 76 77 78 79 81 82 85 86 87 93 100 107 108 110 111 113 114 117 118 123 129 131 134 135 145 146 147 **S** Texas Health Resources, Arlington, TX
Primary Contact: Kirk King, FACHE, President
COO: Sandra L. Harris, R.N., Senior Vice President and Chief Operating Officer
CMO: Robert N. Cluck, M.D., Vice President and Medical Director
CHR: Yvonne Kyler, Director Human Resources
Web address: www.arlingtonmemorial.org
**Control:** Other not–for–profit (including NFP Corporation) **Service:** General Medical and Surgical

**Staffed Beds:** 289 **Admissions:** 12968 **Census:** 178 **Outpatient Visits:** 100345 **Births:** 1834 **Total Expense ($000):** 232139 **Payroll Expense ($000):** 96912 **Personnel:** 1462

TX

**Hospital, Medicare Provider Number, Address, Telephone, Approval, Facility, and Physician Codes, Health Care System**

★ American Hospital Association (AHA) membership
☐ The Joint Commission accreditation ◇ DNV Healthcare Inc. accreditation
○ American Osteopathic Association (AOA) accreditation
△ Commission on Accreditation of Rehabilitation Facilities (CARF) accreditation

© 2012 AHA Guide *Many Facility Codes have changed. Please refer to the AHA Guide Code Chart.* Hospitals **A579**

**TX**

**TEXAS HEALTH HEART & VASCULAR HOSPITAL ARLINGTON (670071)**, 811 Wright Street, Zip 76012–4708; tel. 817/960–3500 **F**3 17 18 20 22 24 26 28 29 30 60 64 65 68 81 85 117 118 134
Primary Contact: Sherri Emerson, Chief Executive Officer
**Control:** Partnership, Investor–owned, for–profit **Service:** Heart

> **Staffed Beds:** 26 **Admissions:** 1096 **Census:** 14 **Outpatient Visits:** 2523
> **Births:** 0 **Total Expense ($000):** 42739 **Payroll Expense ($000):** 7973
> **Personnel:** 122

☒ **USMD HOSPITAL AT ARLINGTON (450872)**, 801 West Interstate 20, Zip 76017–5851; tel. 817/472–3400 **A**1 9 10 **F**3 12 29 34 35 39 40 45 49 50 51 57 58 59 64 70 74 75 78 79 81 82 85 87 92 107 108 111 113 118 123 125 131 **S** USMD Inc., Irving, TX
Primary Contact: Marcia Crim, R.N., MSN, Chief Executive Officer
COO: Marcia Crim, R.N., Chief Nursing Officer and Chief Operating Officer
CFO: Gordon Davis, Vice President Finance
CMO: James Ward, M.D., President Medical Staff
CIO: Bob Rick, Vice President Information Technology
CHR: Alex Stefanowicz, Vice President Human Resources
Web address: www.usmdhospital.com
**Control:** Partnership, Investor–owned, for–profit **Service:** General Medical and Surgical

> **Staffed Beds:** 34 **Admissions:** 1988 **Census:** 11 **Outpatient Visits:** 34601
> **Births:** 0 **Total Expense ($000):** 67976 **Payroll Expense ($000):** 13296
> **Personnel:** 305

### ASPERMONT—Stonewall County

**STONEWALL MEMORIAL HOSPITAL (451318)**, 821 North Broadway, Zip 79502–2913, Mailing Address: P.O. Box C, Zip 79502–0902; tel. 940/989–3551 **A**9 10 18 **F**3 29 34 40 41 57 59 64 97 104 118 126 127 132 **P**6
Primary Contact: James E. Ferguson, Chief Executive Officer
CFO: Debra Meador, Assistant Administrator
CMO: Daniel Hadzie, M.D., Chief of Staff
Web address: www.smhdhealth.org/
**Control:** Hospital district or authority, Government, nonfederal **Service:** General Medical and Surgical

> **Staffed Beds:** 12 **Admissions:** 102 **Census:** 2 **Outpatient Visits:** 10988
> **Births:** 0 **Total Expense ($000):** 5459 **Payroll Expense ($000):** 1876
> **Personnel:** 56

### ATHENS—Henderson County

☒ **EAST TEXAS MEDICAL CENTER ATHENS (450389)**, 2000 South Palestine Street, Zip 75751–5610; tel. 903/676–1000 **A**1 9 10 **F**3 11 15 18 20 26 29 40 42 43 45 49 50 51 57 64 65 66 70 74 75 76 77 78 79 81 85 86 89 107 108 110 111 113 114 118 126 129 131 144 **P**7 **S** East Texas Medical Center Regional Healthcare System, Tyler, TX
Primary Contact: Patrick L. Wallace, Administrator
CFO: David A. Travis, Chief Financial Officer
CHR: Jennifer Rummel, Director Human Resources
Web address: www.etmc.org
**Control:** Other not–for–profit (including NFP Corporation) **Service:** General Medical and Surgical

> **Staffed Beds:** 117 **Admissions:** 6793 **Census:** 67 **Outpatient Visits:** 101332
> **Births:** 809 **Total Expense ($000):** 46738 **Payroll Expense ($000):** 24317
> **Personnel:** 470

### ATLANTA—Cass County

★ **ATLANTA MEMORIAL HOSPITAL (450615)**, 1007 South William Street, Zip 75551–3245; tel. 903/799–3000 **A**9 10 **F**3 11 15 29 30 32 34 35 40 43 45 53 57 59 62 64 68 70 75 77 81 87 91 93 98 100 103 107 110 111 113 118 128 129 131 132 145 147 **P**8
Primary Contact: Deborah Robison, R.N., Interim Chief Executive Officer
CFO: Jackie Rainey, Assistant Administrator and Controller
CIO: Rick Mauldin, Director Information Services
CHR: Debra Embry, Associate Administrator Employee Services
Web address: www.atlantamemorial.com
**Control:** Hospital district or authority, Government, nonfederal **Service:** General Medical and Surgical

> **Staffed Beds:** 37 **Admissions:** 1065 **Census:** 15 **Outpatient Visits:** 34991
> **Births:** 0 **Total Expense ($000):** 14145 **Payroll Expense ($000):** 7871
> **Personnel:** 174

### AUSTIN—Travis County

**AUSTIN LAKES HOSPITAL (454069)**, 1025 East 32nd Street, Zip 78705–2714; tel. 512/544–5253 **A**9 10 **F**98 103 105 129 **S** Universal Health Services, Inc., King of Prussia, PA
Primary Contact: Ramona Key, Chief Executive Officer
Web address: www.austinlakeshospital.com
**Control:** Corporation, Investor–owned, for–profit **Service:** Psychiatric

> **Staffed Beds:** 54 **Admissions:** 2942 **Census:** 51 **Outpatient Visits:** 6609
> **Births:** 0 **Total Expense ($000):** 10928 **Payroll Expense ($000):** 6045
> **Personnel:** 135

☐ **AUSTIN STATE HOSPITAL (454084)**, 4110 Guadalupe Street, Zip 78751–4296; tel. 512/452–0381 **A**1 3 5 10 **F**29 30 39 40 50 56 59 65 68 75 82 86 98 99 101 102 103 129 131 142 145 **P**1 **S** Texas Department of State Health Services, Austin, TX
Primary Contact: Carl Schock, Superintendent
CMO: Ross Taylor, M.D., Clinical Director
CIO: Cindy Reed, Director Community Relations
Web address: www.mhmr.state.tx.us
**Control:** State–Government, nonfederal **Service:** Psychiatric

> **Staffed Beds:** 314 **Admissions:** 3014 **Census:** 183 **Outpatient Visits:** 0
> **Births:** 0 **Total Expense ($000):** 66894 **Payroll Expense ($000):** 34506
> **Personnel:** 858

☐ **AUSTIN SURGICAL HOSPITAL (450871)**, 3003 Bee Caves Road, Zip 78746–5542; tel. 512/314–3800 **A**1 9 10 **F**3 29 37 40 51 59 64 65 68 70 77 79 81 82 85 107 111 118 147 **P**2
Primary Contact: Gregg Magers, Chief Executive Officer
CFO: Lawrence Oldham, Chief Financial Officer
CMO: Brannon Smoot, M.D., Medical Director
CHR: Marilyn Jennings, Director Human Resources
Web address: www.austinsurgicalhospital.com
**Control:** Partnership, Investor–owned, for–profit **Service:** Orthopedic

> **Staffed Beds:** 23 **Admissions:** 896 **Census:** 6 **Outpatient Visits:** 4766
> **Births:** 0 **Total Expense ($000):** 20969 **Payroll Expense ($000):** 6285
> **Personnel:** 105

☒ **CENTRAL TEXAS REHABILITATION HOSPITAL (673027)**, 1201 West 38th Street, 8th Floor, Zip 78705–1006; tel. 512/406–6300 **A**1 9 10 **F**3 29 74 79 82 90 91 96 129 131 147 **S** Kindred Healthcare, Louisville, KY
Primary Contact: Peggy Barrett, R.N., Chief Executive Officer
COO: Lisa Kunz, R.N., Chief Nursing Officer
CMO: Mary Ann Gonzales, M.D., Medical Director
CIO: Peggy Barrett, R.N., Chief Executive Officer
CHR: Liza Cuero, Coordinator Human Resources
CNO: Lisa Kunz, R.N., Chief Nursing Officer
Web address: www.khrehabcentraltexas.com/
**Control:** Partnership, Investor–owned, for–profit **Service:** Rehabilitation

> **Staffed Beds:** 20 **Admissions:** 513 **Census:** 18 **Outpatient Visits:** 0 **Births:**
> 0 **Total Expense ($000):** 8696 **Payroll Expense ($000):** 3583 **Personnel:**
> 57

☐ **CORNERSTONE HOSPITAL OF AUSTIN (452034)**, 4207 Burnet Road, Zip 78756–3396; tel. 512/706–1900, (Includes CORNERSTONE HOSPITAL OF AUSTIN, 1005 East 32nd Street, Zip 78705; tel. 512/867–5822; Edward J. Sherwood, M.D., Chief Executive Officer) **A**1 9 10 **F**1 3 29 30 75 77 87 91 129 147 **S** Cornerstone Healthcare Group, Dallas, TX
Primary Contact: Michael Hutka, Interim Chief Executive Officer
CFO: Gregory Taylor, Chief Financial Officer
CMO: David Pohl, M.D., Chief of Staff
Web address: www.chghospitals.com/cha.html
**Control:** Corporation, Investor–owned, for–profit **Service:** Long–Term Acute Care hospital

> **Staffed Beds:** 128 **Admissions:** 623 **Census:** 46 **Outpatient Visits:** 0 **Births:**
> 0 **Total Expense ($000):** 17464 **Payroll Expense ($000):** 7151 **Personnel:**
> 139

☒ **DELL CHILDREN'S MEDICAL CENTER OF CENTRAL TEXAS (453310)**, 4900 Mueller Boulevard, Zip 78723–3079; tel. 512/324–0000 **A**1 2 3 5 9 10 **F**3 11 19 21 23 25 27 29 30 31 32 34 35 37 39 40 41 43 44 49 50 54 58 59 60 61 64 65 68 71 72 74 75 77 78 79 80 81 82 84 85 86 87 88 89 93 100 104 107 111 112 113 114 117 118 128 129 130 131 134 142 145 147 **P**3 8 **S** Ascension Health, Saint Louis, MO
Primary Contact: Robert I. Bonar, Jr., President and Chief Executive Officer
COO: Sister Teresa George, Vice President and Chief Operating Officer
Web address: www.dellchildrens.net
**Control:** Church–operated, Nongovernment, not–for profit **Service:** Children's general

> **Staffed Beds:** 176 **Admissions:** 8424 **Census:** 110 **Outpatient Visits:**
> 333607 **Births:** 0 **Total Expense ($000):** 286436 **Payroll Expense ($000):**
> 141951 **Personnel:** 2290

☒ **HEALTHSOUTH REHABILITATION HOSPITAL OF AUSTIN (453044)**, 1215 Red River Street, Zip 78701–1921; tel. 512/474–5700 **A**1 9 10 **F**29 56 62 74 75 77 79 86 87 90 91 147 **S** HEALTHSOUTH Corporation, Birmingham, AL
Primary Contact: Duke Saldivar, Chief Executive Officer
CFO: Pamela McLaughlin, Chief Financial Officer
CMO: Elena Arizmendez, M.D., Executive Medical Director
CHR: Debbie Belcher, Director Human Resources
CNO: Mary Ann Lee, Chief Nursing Officer
Web address: www.healthsouthaustin.com
**Control:** Corporation, Investor–owned, for–profit **Service:** Rehabilitation

> **Staffed Beds:** 55 **Admissions:** 1103 **Census:** 41 **Outpatient Visits:** 21014
> **Births:** 0 **Total Expense ($000):** 17134 **Payroll Expense ($000):** 8965
> **Personnel:** 170

*Many Facility Codes have changed. Please refer to the AHA Guide Code Chart.* © 2012 AHA Guide

☐ **NORTHWEST HILLS SURGICAL HOSPITAL (450808)**, 6818 Austin Center Boulevard, Zip 78731–3158; tel. 512/346–1994 **A**1 9 10 **F**40 45 64 79 81
CFO: Jenny Salome, Chief Financial Officer and Assistant Administrator
Web address: www.northwesthillssurgical.com
**Control:** Partnership, Investor–owned, for–profit **Service:** General Medical and Surgical

**Staffed Beds:** 8 **Admissions:** 577 **Census:** 2 **Outpatient Visits:** 8995 **Births:** 0 **Total Expense ($000):** 21889 **Payroll Expense ($000):** 4277 **Personnel:** 77

☒ **SETON MEDICAL CENTER AUSTIN (450056)**, 1201 West 38th Street, Zip 78705–1006; tel. 512/324–1000 **A**1 2 3 5 9 10 **F**3 11 12 13 15 18 20 22 24 26 28 29 30 31 34 35 37 40 43 44 45 46 49 50 53 54 57 58 59 60 61 64 68 70 72 74 75 76 77 78 79 81 82 84 85 86 87 93 107 108 111 113 114 118 129 130 131 134 136 145 147 **P**3 8 **S** Ascension Health, Saint Louis, MO
Primary Contact: Gregory Hartman, President and Chief Executive Officer
COO: Charlotte Thrasher, Vice President and Chief Operating Officer
CFO: Douglas D. Waite, Chief Financial Officer
CMO: Samson Jesudass, M.D., Vice President Medical Affairs
CIO: Gerry Lewis, Chief Information Officer
CHR: Trennis Jones, Vice President Human Resources
Web address: www.seton.net
**Control:** Church–operated, Nongovernment, not–for profit **Service:** General Medical and Surgical

**Staffed Beds:** 425 **Admissions:** 20656 **Census:** 271 **Births:** 3129 **Total Expense ($000):** 315621 **Payroll Expense ($000):** 134442 **Personnel:** 2629

☒ **SETON NORTHWEST HOSPITAL (450867)**, 11113 Research Boulevard, Zip 78759–5236; tel. 512/324–6000 **A**1 2 9 10 **F**3 11 12 13 15 18 29 30 31 34 35 36 37 40 43 44 45 47 49 50 51 57 59 64 68 70 73 74 75 76 77 78 79 81 85 86 87 93 107 111 113 118 128 129 130 131 134 145 147 **P**3 8 **S** Ascension Health, Saint Louis, MO
Primary Contact: Michelle Robertson, R.N., President and Chief Executive Officer
CFO: Douglas D. Waite, Chief Financial Officer
CMO: Ed LeBlanc, M.D., Vice President Medical Affairs
CIO: Gerry Lewis, Chief Information Officer
CHR: Trennis Jones, Senior Vice President and Chief Administrative Officer
Web address: www.seton.net
**Control:** Church–operated, Nongovernment, not–for profit **Service:** General Medical and Surgical

**Staffed Beds:** 121 **Admissions:** 5186 **Census:** 49 **Outpatient Visits:** 92427 **Births:** 885 **Total Expense ($000):** 75564 **Payroll Expense ($000):** 36204 **Personnel:** 672

☒ **SETON SHOAL CREEK HOSPITAL (454029)**, 3501 Mills Avenue, Zip 78731–6391; tel. 512/324–2000 **A**1 9 10 **F**4 5 29 30 34 68 86 87 98 99 100 101 103 104 129 131 134 **P**3 8 **S** Ascension Health, Saint Louis, MO
Primary Contact: Alan Isaacson, Vice President and Chief Operating Officer
COO: Alan Isaacson, Vice President and Chief Operating Officer
CFO: Douglas D. Waite, Chief Financial Officer
CMO: Kari Wolfe, M.D., Medical Director
CIO: Gerry Lewis, Chief Information Officer
CHR: Thomas Wilken, Vice President Human Resources
Web address: www.seton.net
**Control:** Church–operated, Nongovernment, not–for profit **Service:** Psychiatric

**Staffed Beds:** 84 **Admissions:** 4424 **Census:** 65 **Outpatient Visits:** 21315 **Births:** 0 **Total Expense ($000):** 23891 **Payroll Expense ($000):** 13907 **Personnel:** 286

☒ **SETON SOUTHWEST HEALTHCARE CENTER (450865)**, 7900 F. M. 1826, Zip 78737; tel. 512/324–9000 **A**1 9 10 **F**3 11 13 15 29 30 34 35 36 40 43 44 45 50 57 59 64 68 71 75 76 79 81 82 85 87 93 107 111 114 118 128 129 130 131 134 145 **P**3 8 **S** Ascension Health, Saint Louis, MO
Primary Contact: Mary Faria, FACHE, Administrator
Web address: www.seton.net
**Control:** Church–operated, Nongovernment, not–for profit **Service:** General Medical and Surgical

**Staffed Beds:** 17 **Admissions:** 1371 **Census:** 10 **Outpatient Visits:** 31590 **Births:** 667 **Total Expense ($000):** 32541 **Payroll Expense ($000):** 13350 **Personnel:** 242

☒ **ST. DAVID'S MEDICAL CENTER (450431)**, 919 East 32nd Street, Zip 78705–2709, Mailing Address: P.O. Box 4039, Zip 78765–4039; tel. 512/476–7111, (Includes HEART HOSPITAL OF AUSTIN, 3801 North Lamar Boulevard, Zip 78756–4080; tel. 512/407–7000; David Laird, Chief Executive Officer; ST. DAVID'S GEORGETOWN HOSPITAL, 2000 Scenic Drive, Georgetown, Zip 78626–7726; tel. 512/943–3000; Hugh Brown, Chief Executive Officer) **A**1 2 3 5 9 10 **F**3 8 11 12 13 15 17 18 20 22 24 26 28 29 30 31 34 35 37 39 40 45 46 47 48 49 53 56 57 58 59 61 64 68 70 72 73 74 75 76 77 78 79 81 85 86 87 90 93 107 108 109 110 111 113 114 115 118 125 129 130 131 134 145 146 147 **S** HCA, Nashville, TN
Primary Contact: Donald H. Wilkerson, Chief Executive Officer
COO: Richard A. Hammett, Chief Operating Officer
CFO: Cindy Brouillette, Chief Financial Officer
CMO: John Marietta, M.D., Chief Medical Officer
CIO: Debi Castleberry, Director Information System
CHR: De De Juel, Director Human Resources
Web address: www.stdavids.com
**Control:** Other not–for–profit (including NFP Corporation) **Service:** General Medical and Surgical

**Staffed Beds:** 458 **Admissions:** 22852 **Census:** 297 **Outpatient Visits:** 151257 **Births:** 4999 **Total Expense ($000):** 360102 **Payroll Expense ($000):** 128054 **Personnel:** 2234

☒ **ST. DAVID'S NORTH AUSTIN MEDICAL CENTER (450809)**, 12221 North MoPac Expressway, Zip 78758–2496; tel. 512/901–1000 **A**1 9 10 **F**3 11 12 13 15 18 20 22 24 26 28 29 30 31 34 35 40 42 43 47 49 53 54 56 57 59 64 70 72 73 74 75 76 77 78 79 81 82 84 85 86 87 90 93 107 108 111 113 114 117 118 125 129 130 131 137 143 144 145 146 147 **S** HCA, Nashville, TN
Primary Contact: Allen Harrison, Chief Executive Officer
COO: Sheri Dube, Chief Operating Officer
CFO: Cindy Sexton, Chief Financial Officer
CMO: Kenneth W. Mitchell, M.D., Medical Director
CIO: Marshall Pearson, Director Management Information Systems
CHR: Julie Hajek, Director Human Resources
Web address: www.northaustin.com
**Control:** Other not–for–profit (including NFP Corporation) **Service:** General Medical and Surgical

**Staffed Beds:** 332 **Admissions:** 16476 **Census:** 229 **Outpatient Visits:** 125504 **Births:** 5496 **Total Expense ($000):** 211124 **Payroll Expense ($000):** 73046 **Personnel:** 1239

☒ **ST. DAVID'S REHABILITATION CENTER (453038)**, 1005 East 32nd Street, Zip 78705–2705, Mailing Address: P.O. Box 4270, Zip 78765–4270; tel. 512/544–5100 **A**1 9 10 **F**29 30 35 36 64 77 90 93 96 130 131 147 **S** HCA, Nashville, TN
Primary Contact: Diane Owens, Administrator
COO: Richard A. Hammett, Chief Operating Officer
CFO: Cindy Brouillette, Chief Financial Officer
CMO: John Marietta, M.D., Chief Medical Officer
CIO: Debi Castleberry, Director Information System
CHR: De De Juel, Director Human Resources
Web address: www.stdavids.com
**Control:** Other not–for–profit (including NFP Corporation) **Service:** Rehabilitation

**Staffed Beds:** 64 **Admissions:** 1470 **Census:** 57 **Outpatient Visits:** 41146 **Births:** 0 **Total Expense ($000):** 25561 **Payroll Expense ($000):** 12990 **Personnel:** 210

☒ **ST. DAVID'S SOUTH AUSTIN MEDICAL CENTER (450713)**, 901 West Ben White Boulevard, Zip 78704–6903; tel. 512/447–2211 **A**1 2 9 10 **F**3 11 12 13 15 17 18 20 22 24 26 28 29 30 31 34 35 40 42 43 45 46 47 48 49 54 56 57 59 64 70 73 74 75 76 77 78 79 81 82 85 87 93 107 108 110 111 113 114 117 118 125 128 129 131 143 145 146 147 **P**7 8 **S** HCA, Nashville, TN
Primary Contact: Todd E. Steward, Chief Executive Officer
COO: Brett Matens, Chief Operating Officer
CFO: Wesley D. Fountain, Chief Financial Officer
CMO: Albert Gros, M.D., Chief Medical Officer
CIO: Richard Lear, Director Information Systems
CHR: Lisa Talbot, Director Human Resources
Web address: www.southaustinmc.com
**Control:** Other not–for–profit (including NFP Corporation) **Service:** General Medical and Surgical

**Staffed Beds:** 222 **Admissions:** 13619 **Census:** 169 **Outpatient Visits:** 119420 **Births:** 1650 **Total Expense ($000):** 152844 **Payroll Expense ($000):** 59613 **Personnel:** 1073

**TX**

**Hospital, Medicare Provider Number, Address, Telephone, Approval, Facility, and Physician Codes, Health Care System**

★ American Hospital Association (AHA) membership
☐ The Joint Commission accreditation          ◇ DNV Healthcare Inc. accreditation
○ American Osteopathic Association (AOA) accreditation
△ Commission on Accreditation of Rehabilitation Facilities (CARF) accreditation

© 2012 AHA Guide          *Many Facility Codes have changed. Please refer to the AHA Guide Code Chart.*          Hospitals **A581**

□ △ **TEXAS NEUROREHAB CENTER (452038)**, 1106 West Dittmar, Zip 78745–6388, Mailing Address: P.O. Box 150459, Zip 78715–0459; tel. 512/444–4835 **A**1 7 9 10 **F**1 10 29 43 54 74 75 79 93 108 129 147 **P**5 **S** Universal Health Services, Inc., King of Prussia, PA
Primary Contact: Edgar E. Prettyman, PsyD, Chief Executive Officer
COO: Omar Correa, Chief Operating Officer
CFO: Omar Correa, Chief Financial Officer
CMO: James Boysen, M.D., Executive Medical Director
CHR: Colleen Lewis, Director Human Resources
Web address: www.texasneurorehab.com
**Control:** Partnership, Investor–owned, for–profit **Service:** General Medical and Surgical

**Staffed Beds:** 47 **Admissions:** 519 **Census:** 42 **Outpatient Visits:** 4408 **Births:** 0 **Total Expense ($000):** 12264 **Payroll Expense ($000):** 7319 **Personnel:** 303

**THE HOSPITAL AT WESTLAKE MEDICAL CENTER (670006)**, 5656 Bee Caves Road, Zip 78746; tel. 512/327–0000 **A**9 10 **F**3 18 20 22 24 26 28 29 37 39 40 45 51 53 58 64 68 70 75 77 79 81 82 85 92 93 107 111 113 118 125 128 129 130 147
Primary Contact: Rip Miller, Chief Executive Officer
CFO: Julie Churchill, Director Financial Services
CMO: Tom Burns, M.D., Chief of Staff
CHR: Kellie Bryson, Director Human Resources
Web address: www.westlakemedical.com
**Control:** Partnership, Investor–owned, for–profit **Service:** General Medical and Surgical

**Staffed Beds:** 23 **Admissions:** 959 **Census:** 8 **Outpatient Visits:** 12212 **Births:** 0 **Total Expense ($000):** 32851 **Payroll Expense ($000):** 10601 **Personnel:** 175

⊠ **UNIVERSITY MEDICAL CENTER AT BRACKENRIDGE (450124)**, 601 East 15th Street, Zip 78701–1996; tel. 512/324–7000 **A**1 2 3 5 9 10 **F**3 11 13 15 18 20 22 24 26 29 30 31 34 35 37 39 40 43 44 45 47 49 50 55 57 58 59 60 61 64 65 66 68 70 71 72 74 75 76 77 78 79 81 82 84 85 87 93 97 100 104 107 108 110 111 113 114 117 118 123 129 131 134 142 145 147 **P**3 8 **S** Ascension Health, Saint Louis, MO
Primary Contact: Gregory Hartman, President and Chief Executive Officer
COO: Kate Henderson, Vice President and Chief Operating Officer
CFO: Douglas D. Waite, Chief Financial Officer
CMO: Jim Lindsey, M.D., Senior Vice President Medical Affairs
CIO: Gerry Lewis, Chief Information Officer
Web address: www.seton.net
**Control:** Church–operated, Nongovernment, not–for profit **Service:** General Medical and Surgical

**Staffed Beds:** 241 **Admissions:** 13638 **Census:** 176 **Outpatient Visits:** 572618 **Births:** 1516 **Total Expense ($000):** 441452 **Payroll Expense ($000):** 214372 **Personnel:** 2447

### AZLE—Tarrant County

⊠ **TEXAS HEALTH HARRIS METHODIST HOSPITAL AZLE (450419)**, 108 Denver Trail, Zip 76020–3614; tel. 817/444–8600 **A**1 9 10 **F**3 11 15 29 30 34 35 40 43 45 57 59 63 64 65 70 75 77 79 81 82 85 93 107 110 113 118 129 130 134 145 146 147 **S** Texas Health Resources, Arlington, TX
Primary Contact: Bob S. Ellzey, FACHE, President
CFO: Brian Blessing, Chief Financial Officer
CMO: Kristi Kuenstler, M.D., Chief of Staff
CIO: Edward Marx, Vice President and Chief Information Officer
CHR: Jan Flavin, Director Human Resources
Web address: www.harrismethodisthospitals.org
**Control:** Other not–for–profit (including NFP Corporation) **Service:** General Medical and Surgical

**Staffed Beds:** 31 **Admissions:** 1754 **Census:** 15 **Outpatient Visits:** 34355 **Births:** 1 **Total Expense ($000):** 29758 **Payroll Expense ($000):** 13854 **Personnel:** 222

### BALLINGER—Runnels County

**BALLINGER MEMORIAL HOSPITAL (451310)**, 608 Avenue B, Zip 76821–2499, Mailing Address: P.O. Box 617, Zip 76821–0617; tel. 325/365–2531 **A**9 10 18 **F**3 7 11 28 34 40 43 50 53 54 56 57 59 64 65 68 75 77 87 93 101 103 104 107 113 126 129 132 142 147 **P**5
Primary Contact: Lance W. Keilers, Administrator
CFO: Josilyn Peterson, Chief Financial Officer
CHR: Roselyn Hudgens, Director Human Resources
Web address: www.ballingerhospital.org
**Control:** Hospital district or authority, Government, nonfederal **Service:** General Medical and Surgical

**Staffed Beds:** 16 **Admissions:** 179 **Census:** 3 **Outpatient Visits:** 26100 **Births:** 0 **Total Expense ($000):** 5352 **Payroll Expense ($000):** 2702 **Personnel:** 75

### BAY CITY—Matagorda County

⊠ **MATAGORDA REGIONAL MEDICAL CENTER (450465)**, 104 7th Street, Zip 77414–4853; tel. 979/245–6383 **A**1 9 10 20 **F**3 11 13 15 18 20 22 28 29 30 32 34 38 39 40 43 46 47 50 51 53 56 57 59 64 65 66 68 70 75 76 77 79 81 82 85 86 89 93 98 103 107 108 110 111 113 118 129 131 134 145 146 147 **S** QHR, Brentwood, TN
Primary Contact: Steven L. Smith, Chief Executive Officer
CFO: Bryan Prochnow, Chief Financial Officer
CIO: Mary Ann Cervantes, District Director Management Information Systems
CHR: Cindy Krebs, District Director Human Resources
Web address: www.matagordaregional.org
**Control:** Hospital district or authority, Government, nonfederal **Service:** General Medical and Surgical

**Staffed Beds:** 58 **Admissions:** 2828 **Census:** 32 **Outpatient Visits:** 34241 **Births:** 375 **Total Expense ($000):** 43652 **Payroll Expense ($000):** 16590 **Personnel:** 276

### BAYTOWN—Harris County

★ **SAN JACINTO METHODIST HOSPITAL (450424)**, 4401 Garth Road, Zip 77521–2122; tel. 281/420–8600, (Includes SAN JACINTO METHODIST HOSPITAL – ALEXANDER, 1700 James Bowie Drive, Zip 77520–3386; tel. 281/420–6100), (Total facility includes 30 beds in nursing home–type unit) **A**2 9 10 13 21 **F**3 8 11 12 13 15 18 20 22 24 26 28 29 30 31 34 35 38 40 44 48 49 50 53 57 59 61 64 65 70 73 74 75 76 77 78 79 80 81 82 85 86 87 89 90 91 93 97 98 102 103 107 108 110 111 113 114 115 116 117 118 119 120 122 123 127 128 129 131 144 145 146 147 **P**3 **S** The Methodist Hospital System, Houston, TX
Primary Contact: Donna Gares, R.N., President and Chief Executive Officer
CFO: Jonathan Sturgis, Chief Financial Officer
CMO: Bruce Kennedy, M.D., Chief Medical Officer
CHR: Sherri Davis–Sampson, Director Human Resources
Web address: www.methodisthealth.com
**Control:** Other not–for–profit (including NFP Corporation) **Service:** General Medical and Surgical

**Staffed Beds:** 275 **Admissions:** 12843 **Census:** 167 **Outpatient Visits:** 141627 **Births:** 1579 **Total Expense ($000):** 178830 **Payroll Expense ($000):** 82630 **Personnel:** 1341

### BEAUMONT—Jefferson County

★ **BAPTIST HOSPITALS OF SOUTHEAST TEXAS (450346)**, 3080 College Street, Zip 77701–4689, Mailing Address: P.O. Box 1591, Zip 77704–1591; tel. 409/212–5000, (Includes BAPTIST HOSPITALS OF SOUTHEAST TEXAS FANNIN BEHAVIORAL HEALTH CENTER, 3250 Fannin Street, Zip 77701; tel. 409/212–7000) **A**9 10 21 **F**3 4 5 11 13 15 17 18 20 22 24 26 28 29 30 31 34 35 37 40 45 48 49 51 55 59 60 64 70 72 73 74 75 76 77 78 79 81 85 86 87 88 89 90 93 94 96 98 99 100 101 102 103 104 105 107 108 110 111 114 116 117 118 119 120 122 129 131 134 143 145 146 147 **P**6 **S** Community Hospital Corporation, Plano, TX
Primary Contact: David N. Parmer, President and Chief Executive Officer
COO: Guy Giesecke, Chief Operations Officer
CFO: Gary Troutman, CPA, Chief Financial Officer
CIO: Troy Napier, Chief Information Officer
CHR: Jennifer Barroeta, Chief Human Resources Officer
Web address: www.mhbh.org
**Control:** Other not–for–profit (including NFP Corporation) **Service:** General Medical and Surgical

**Staffed Beds:** 394 **Admissions:** 17235 **Census:** 225 **Outpatient Visits:** 130690 **Births:** 1715 **Total Expense ($000):** 186468 **Payroll Expense ($000):** 75296 **Personnel:** 1325

**BEAUMONT BONE AND JOINT INSTITUTE (670007)**, 3650 Laurel Street, Zip 77707; tel. 409/838–0346 **A**9 10 **F**3 40 79 81 129 130 140
Primary Contact: Duane N. Hill, Chief Executive Officer
Web address: www.orthodoc.aaos.org/bbji/
**Control:** Partnership, Investor–owned, for–profit **Service:** General Medical and Surgical

**Staffed Beds:** 6 **Admissions:** 1 **Census:** 1 **Outpatient Visits:** 5542 **Births:** 0 **Total Expense ($000):** 7196 **Payroll Expense ($000):** 1816 **Personnel:** 46

**TX**

*Many Facility Codes have changed. Please refer to the AHA Guide Code Chart.* © 2012 AHA Guide

✠ **CHRISTUS HOSPITAL–ST. ELIZABETH (450034)**, 2830 Calder Avenue, Zip 77702–1809, Mailing Address: P.O. Box 5405, Zip 77726–5405; tel. 409/892–7171, (Includes CHRISTUS HOSPITAL–ST. MARY, 3600 Gates Boulevard, Port Arthur, Zip 77642–3601, Mailing Address: P.O. Box 3696, Zip 77643–3696; tel. 409/985–7431; Wayne Moore, Administrator) **A**1 2 9 10 **F**3 11 13 15 17 18 20 22 24 26 28 29 30 31 34 35 36 38 40 43 44 49 50 51 53 54 57 59 60 64 70 72 74 75 76 77 78 79 81 82 83 85 86 87 88 89 93 94 107 108 111 113 117 118 123 128 129 131 143 145 146 147 **P**8 **S** CHRISTUS Health, Irving, TX
Primary Contact: Paul Trevino, Administrator
CFO: Shawn Adams, Assistant Administrator Finance
CMO: Rick Tyler, M.D., Vice President Medical Affairs
CIO: Robert Jacobs, Regional Director Information Management
CHR: Charles Foster, Regional Director Human Resources
Web address: www.christushospital.org
**Control:** Church–operated, Nongovernment, not–for profit **Service:** General Medical and Surgical

**Staffed Beds:** 456 **Admissions:** 20658 **Census:** 263 **Outpatient Visits:** 347134 **Births:** 1775 **Total Expense ($000):** 351232 **Payroll Expense ($000):** 110308 **Personnel:** 1777

✠ **DUBUIS HOSPITAL OF BEAUMONT (452042)**, 2830 Calder Avenue, 4th Floor, Zip 77702; tel. 409/899–8154 **A**1 9 10 **F**1 3 18 29 30 31 129 147 **P**5 **S** Dubuis Health System, Houston, TX
Primary Contact: Tim Freeman, Administrator
Web address: www.dubuis.org
**Control:** Church–operated, Nongovernment, not–for profit **Service:** Long–Term Acute Care hospital

**Staffed Beds:** 51 **Admissions:** 589 **Census:** 42 **Outpatient Visits:** 0 **Births:** 0 **Total Expense ($000):** 17142 **Payroll Expense ($000):** 6514 **Personnel:** 116

**HARBOR HOSPITAL OF SOUTHEAST TEXAS (452093)**, 860 South 8th Street, Zip 77701; tel. 409/840–3200 **A**9 10 **F**1 3 29 30 35 45 85 129 147
Primary Contact: Thomas M. Harlan, Chief Executive Officer
Web address: www.communityhospitalcorp.com
**Control:** Partnership, Investor–owned, for–profit **Service:** General Medical and Surgical

**Staffed Beds:** 30 **Admissions:** 357 **Census:** 24 **Outpatient Visits:** 0 **Births:** 0 **Total Expense ($000):** 11829 **Payroll Expense ($000):** 5373 **Personnel:** 81

✠ **HEALTHSOUTH REHABILITATION HOSPITAL OF BEAUMONT (453048)**, 3340 Plaza 10 Boulevard, Zip 77707–2551; tel. 409/835–0835 **A**1 9 10 **F**3 28 29 30 62 64 74 75 77 79 87 90 91 93 95 96 129 130 131 147 **S** HEALTHSOUTH Corporation, Birmingham, AL
Primary Contact: H. J. Gaspard, Chief Executive Officer
CFO: Tracey Allen, Chief Financial Officer
CMO: Linda C. Smith, M.D., Medical Director
Web address: www.healthsouthbeaumont.com
**Control:** Corporation, Investor–owned, for–profit **Service:** Rehabilitation

**Staffed Beds:** 61 **Admissions:** 847 **Census:** 30 **Births:** 0 **Total Expense ($000):** 12506 **Payroll Expense ($000):** 6235 **Personnel:** 119

**MEMORIAL HERMANN BAPTIST FANNIN BEHAVIORAL HEALTH CENTER**
See Baptist Hospitals of Southeast Texas Fannin Behavioral Health Center

### BEDFORD—Fort Worth–Arlington County

**RELIANT REHABILITATION HOSPITAL MID–CITIES (673044)**, 2304 State Highway 121, Zip 76021; tel. 817/684–2000 **F**3 29 40 64 90 131
Primary Contact: Robert M. Smart, Chief Executive Officer
CFO: Mary Mwaniki, Chief Financial Officer
CMO: Toni Willis, M.D., Medical Director
CHR: Christie Moore, Director Human Resources
Web address: www.relianthcp.com
**Control:** Partnership, Investor–owned, for–profit **Service:** Rehabilitation

**Staffed Beds:** 60 **Admissions:** 1050 **Census:** 33 **Outpatient Visits:** 2243 **Births:** 0 **Total Expense ($000):** 10313 **Payroll Expense ($000):** 6695 **Personnel:** 88

✠ **TEXAS HEALTH HARRIS METHODIST HOSPITAL HURST–EULESS–BEDFORD (450639)**, 1600 Hospital Parkway, Zip 76022–6913, Mailing Address: P.O. Box 669, Zip 76095–0669; tel. 817/685–4000, (Includes HARRIS METHODIST–SPRINGWOOD, 1608 Hospital Parkway, Zip 76022; tel. 817/355–7700) **A**1 2 9 10 **F**4 5 9 11 12 13 15 18 20 22 24 26 28 29 30 31 34 35 40 47 49 53 60 64 70 72 74 75 76 78 79 80 81 82 86 87 93 98 99 100 101 102 103 104 105 106 107 108 111 113 117 118 125 128 129 130 131 133 134 145 146 147 **S** Texas Health Resources, Arlington, TX
Primary Contact: Deborah Paganelli, President
COO: Alice Landers, Administrative Director Operations
CFO: Shelly Miland, Vice President Finance and Chief Financial Officer
CMO: Bob Nowland, M.D., Chief of Staff
CHR: Dale Smith, Director Human Resources
Web address: www.texashealth.org
**Control:** Other not–for–profit (including NFP Corporation) **Service:** General Medical and Surgical

**Staffed Beds:** 259 **Admissions:** 14236 **Census:** 172 **Outpatient Visits:** 85071 **Births:** 1913 **Total Expense ($000):** 214171 **Payroll Expense ($000):** 90222 **Personnel:** 1348

### BEEVILLE—Bee County

✠ **CHRISTUS SPOHN HOSPITAL BEEVILLE (450082)**, 1500 East Houston Street, Zip 78102–5312; tel. 361/354–2000 **A**1 9 10 20 **F**3 11 13 15 29 30 32 34 35 40 43 45 50 57 59 64 70 75 76 77 79 81 85 86 87 93 97 107 108 111 113 118 129 131 145 146 147 **S** CHRISTUS Health, Irving, TX
Primary Contact: Raymond Ramos, Vice President and Chief Operating Officer
Web address: www.christusspohn.org
**Control:** Church–operated, Nongovernment, not–for profit **Service:** General Medical and Surgical

**Staffed Beds:** 49 **Admissions:** 1906 **Census:** 20 **Outpatient Visits:** 37929 **Births:** 367 **Total Expense ($000):** 28422 **Payroll Expense ($000):** 12671 **Personnel:** 179

### BELLAIRE—Harris County

**FIRST STREET HOSPITAL (670029)**, 4801 Bissonnet, Zip 77401–4028; tel. 713/275–1111 **A**10 21 **F**3 12 29 37 40 42 45 64 68 79 81 85 87 107 111 113 118 125 129
Primary Contact: Sharon McDonough, Chief Executive Officer
Web address: www.firststreethospital.com
**Control:** Partnership, Investor–owned, for–profit **Service:** General Medical and Surgical

**Staffed Beds:** 19 **Admissions:** 1082 **Census:** 4 **Outpatient Visits:** 38376 **Births:** 0 **Total Expense ($000):** 17440 **Payroll Expense ($000):** 6210 **Personnel:** 231

☐ **HOUSTON ORTHOPEDIC AND SPINE HOSPITAL (670012)**, 5410 West Loop South, Zip 77401; tel. 713/314–4500, (Nonreporting) **A**1 10
Primary Contact: Andrew Knizley, Chief Executive Officer
CMO: L. V. Ansell, M.D., Medical Director
Web address: www.foundationsurgicalhospital.com
**Control:** Partnership, Investor–owned, for–profit **Service:** General Medical and Surgical

**Staffed Beds:** 64

### BELLVILLE—Austin County

✠ **BELLVILLE GENERAL HOSPITAL (450253)**, 44 North Cummings Street, Zip 77418–1347; tel. 979/865–3141 **A**1 9 10 **F**3 11 15 29 40 43 45 50 57 59 64 65 68 75 80 81 107 111 113 118 126 132 145
Primary Contact: Michael Morris, Administrator
CMO: Christophe Gay, M.D., Chief of Staff
CHR: Jacqueline McEuen, Coordinator Human Resources
Web address: www.bellvillehospital.com
**Control:** Other not–for–profit (including NFP Corporation) **Service:** General Medical and Surgical

**Staffed Beds:** 25 **Admissions:** 532 **Census:** 5 **Outpatient Visits:** 65765 **Births:** 0 **Total Expense ($000):** 9576 **Payroll Expense ($000):** 3629 **Personnel:** 88

**TX**

---

**Hospital, Medicare Provider Number, Address, Telephone, Approval, Facility, and Physician Codes, Health Care System**

★ American Hospital Association (AHA) membership
☐ The Joint Commission accreditation   ◇ DNV Healthcare Inc. accreditation
○ American Osteopathic Association (AOA) accreditation
△ Commission on Accreditation of Rehabilitation Facilities (CARF) accreditation

## BELTON—Bell County

**CEDAR CREST HOSPITAL (454114)**, 3500 I–35 South, Zip 76513; tel. 254/939–2100 **A**9 10 **F**29 30 34 35 59 68 86 87 98 99 100 101 103 104 105 106 129 142 **P**4 **S** Behavioral Centers of America, Nashville, TN
Primary Contact: Ingrid Whittle, Chief Executive Officer
CFO: Barry Combs, Chief Financial Officer
CMO: Karen Brooks, M.D., Medical Director
CIO: Melanie Orsag, Director Health Information Services
CHR: Jackie Burk, Director Human Resources
Web address: www.cedarcresthospital.com
**Control:** Corporation, Investor–owned, for–profit **Service:** Psychiatric

**Staffed Beds:** 50 **Admissions:** 987 **Census:** 23 **Outpatient Visits:** 1503 **Births:** 0 **Total Expense ($000):** 2755 **Payroll Expense ($000):** 1603 **Personnel:** 91

## BIG LAKE—Reagan County

★ **REAGAN MEMORIAL HOSPITAL (451301)**, 805 North Main Street, Zip 76932–3999; tel. 325/884–2561 **A**9 10 18 **F**3 40 43 53 57 93 107 129 132 **P**5
Primary Contact: Bobby Ewell, Chief Executive Officer
CMO: Joseph Sudolcan, M.D., Medical Director
**Control:** Hospital district or authority, Government, nonfederal **Service:** General Medical and Surgical

**Staffed Beds:** 8 **Admissions:** 47 **Census:** 1 **Outpatient Visits:** 3788 **Births:** 0 **Total Expense ($000):** 6642 **Payroll Expense ($000):** 2595 **Personnel:** 40

## BIG SPRING—Howard County

☐ **BIG SPRING STATE HOSPITAL (454000)**, 1901 North Highway 87, Zip 79720–0283; tel. 432/267–8216 **A**1 3 5 9 10 **F**30 56 59 68 75 77 86 87 98 101 102 103 106 129 131 134 145 **P**6 **S** Texas Department of State Health Services, Austin, TX
Primary Contact: Edward Moughon, Superintendent
CFO: Adrienne Bides, Assistant Chief Financial Officer and Budget Analyst
CMO: Ba Han, M.D., Clinical Director
CIO: Elizabeth Correa, Director Information Management
CHR: Lorie Couch, Assistant Superintendent
CNO: Stormy Ward, Chief Nurse Executive
Web address: www.dshs.state.tx.us/mhhospitals/BigSpringSH/default.shtm
**Control:** State–Government, nonfederal **Service:** Psychiatric

**Staffed Beds:** 200 **Admissions:** 890 **Census:** 186 **Outpatient Visits:** 0 **Births:** 0 **Total Expense ($000):** 37983 **Payroll Expense ($000):** 19570 **Personnel:** 551

⊠ **SCENIC MOUNTAIN MEDICAL CENTER (450653)**, 1601 West 11th Place, Zip 79720–4198; tel. 432/263–1211 **A**1 9 10 20 **F**3 11 13 15 20 29 30 34 39 40 43 45 51 57 59 64 65 68 69 70 75 76 77 79 81 85 87 89 93 94 97 107 110 111 113 118 128 129 132 145 146 147 **P**6 **S** Community Health Systems, Inc., Franklin, TN
Primary Contact: Larry Rodgers, Chief Executive Officer
CFO: Michael Ruff, Chief Financial Officer
CMO: Steve Saeed Ahmed, M.D., Chief of Staff
CHR: Dwight Linton, Director Human Resources
Web address: www.smmccares.com
**Control:** Corporation, Investor–owned, for–profit **Service:** General Medical and Surgical

**Staffed Beds:** 75 **Admissions:** 3049 **Census:** 30 **Outpatient Visits:** 28816 **Births:** 233 **Total Expense ($000):** 31464 **Payroll Expense ($000):** 14006 **Personnel:** 221

⊠ **WEST TEXAS VA HEALTH CARE SYSTEM**, 300 Veterans Boulevard, Zip 79720–5500; Mailing Address: Big Springs, tel. 432/263–7361, (Nonreporting) **A**1 3 5 9 **S** Department of Veterans Affairs, Washington, DC
Primary Contact: Daniel L. Marsh, Director
CFO: Ray Olivas, Chief Fiscal Service
CMO: Martin Schnier, D.O., Chief of Staff
CIO: Mike McKinley, Information Security Officer
CHR: Anna Osborne, Chief Human Resources Management Service
Web address: www.bigspring.va.gov/about/
**Control:** Veterans Affairs, Government, federal **Service:** General Medical and Surgical

**Staffed Beds:** 149

## BONHAM—Fannin County

☐ **RED RIVER REGIONAL HOSPITAL (451370)**, 504 Lipscomb Boulevard, Zip 75418–4096, Mailing Address: P.O. Box C., Zip 75418–0180; tel. 903/583–8585 **A**1 9 10 18 21 **F**3 11 15 28 29 30 34 35 40 46 50 57 59 64 65 70 75 81 87 93 107 108 110 111 117 118 129 132 134 145
Primary Contact: David Conejo, Chief Executive Officer
CFO: Jay Hodges, Chief Financial Officer
CMO: Michael Brown, D.O., Chief of Staff
CIO: Jack Farguson, Director Information Technology
CHR: Brenda Bagley, Director Human Resources
CNO: William Kiefer, Chief Nursing Officer
Web address: www.redriverregional.com/
**Control:** Partnership, Investor–owned, for–profit **Service:** General Medical and Surgical

**Staffed Beds:** 25 **Admissions:** 944 **Census:** 10 **Outpatient Visits:** 12328 **Births:** 0 **Total Expense ($000):** 13961 **Payroll Expense ($000):** 5656 **Personnel:** 103

**SAM RAYBURN MEMORIAL VETERANS CENTER** See Veterans Affairs North Texas Health Care System, Dallas

## BORGER—Hutchinson County

**GOLDEN PLAINS COMMUNITY HOSPITAL (451369)**, 200 South McGee Street, Zip 79007–4022; tel. 806/273–1100 **A**9 10 18 **F**11 13 15 29 30 34 35 40 43 45 50 54 57 59 62 64 65 66 68 70 75 76 77 79 81 85 86 87 93 107 108 111 126 129 130 131 132 145 146 147 **P**6
Primary Contact: Dennis D. Jack, President and Chief Executive Officer
COO: Melody Henderson, R.N., Chief Operating Officer and Chief Nursing Officer
CFO: Dennis P. Kilday, Chief Financial Officer
CMO: Bard Rogers, M.D., Chief of Staff
CHR: Sally Mason, Director Human Resources
Web address: www.goldenplains.org
**Control:** Corporation, Investor–owned, for–profit **Service:** General Medical and Surgical

**Staffed Beds:** 25 **Admissions:** 899 **Census:** 7 **Outpatient Visits:** 44914 **Births:** 237 **Total Expense ($000):** 20417 **Payroll Expense ($000):** 7419 **Personnel:** 186

## BOWIE—Montague County

★ **BOWIE MEMORIAL HOSPITAL (450497)**, 705 East Greenwood Avenue, Zip 76230–3199; tel. 940/872–1126 **A**9 10 **F**3 10 11 15 28 29 40 43 45 53 57 62 63 64 70 75 81 82 84 93 103 107 114 118 128 129 130 131 132 147 **P**4
Primary Contact: T. Kim Lee, CPA, Chief Executive Officer
CMO: Gary Evans, M.D., Chief of Staff
CIO: Randell Cox, Director Data Processing
CHR: Mary Bates, Director Human Resources
Web address: www.bowiememorial.com
**Control:** Hospital district or authority, Government, nonfederal **Service:** General Medical and Surgical

**Staffed Beds:** 44 **Admissions:** 958 **Census:** 13 **Outpatient Visits:** 30804 **Births:** 0 **Total Expense ($000):** 7460 **Payroll Expense ($000):** 5801 **Personnel:** 170

## BRADY—Mcculloch County

**HEART OF TEXAS MEMORIAL HOSPITAL (451348)**, 2008 Nine Road, Zip 76825–1150, Mailing Address: P.O. Box 1150, Zip 76825–1150; tel. 325/597–2901 **A**9 10 18 **F**11 15 28 40 43 45 53 57 64 81 93 103 107 111 113 118 126 128 132 **P**4
Primary Contact: Tim Jones, Interim Chief Executive Officer
CFO: Brad Burnett, Chief Financial Officer
CMO: Pete Castro, D.O., Chief of Staff
**Control:** Hospital district or authority, Government, nonfederal **Service:** General Medical and Surgical

**Staffed Beds:** 25 **Admissions:** 348 **Census:** 3 **Outpatient Visits:** 32219 **Births:** 0 **Total Expense ($000):** 8843 **Payroll Expense ($000):** 3489 **Personnel:** 86

## BRECKENRIDGE—Stephens County

**STEPHENS MEMORIAL HOSPITAL (450498)**, 200 South Geneva Street, Zip 76424–4799; tel. 254/559–2242 **A**9 10 20 **F**3 7 8 11 15 28 30 34 35 40 43 45 50 53 56 57 59 63 64 68 69 81 85 87 89 93 97 103 107 113 129 132 145
Primary Contact: Shane Kernell, Administrator
CMO: Dwight J. Nichols, M.D., Chief of Staff
CIO: Bobby Thompson, Director Information Technology
CHR: Michelle Funderburg, Director Human Resources
Web address: www.smhtx.com
**Control:** County–Government, nonfederal **Service:** General Medical and Surgical

**Staffed Beds:** 21 **Admissions:** 658 **Census:** 8 **Outpatient Visits:** 19351 **Births:** 0 **Total Expense ($000):** 10000 **Payroll Expense ($000):** 4402 **Personnel:** 143

**TX**

*Many Facility Codes have changed. Please refer to the AHA Guide Code Chart.* © 2012 AHA Guide

**BRENHAM—Washington County**

✠ **SCOTT & WHITE HOSPITAL – BRENHAM (450187)**, 700 Medical Parkway, Zip 77833–5498; tel. 979/836–6173 **A**1 9 10 **F**3 11 13 29 30 32 34 35 40 43 44 50 51 53 56 57 59 64 65 70 75 76 77 78 79 80 81 85 86 87 93 107 108 110 113 118 126 128 129 131 132 134 145 **P**6 **S** Scott & White Healthcare, Temple, TX
Primary Contact: John L. Simms, President and Chief Executive Officer
COO: John L. Simms, President and Chief Executive Officer
CFO: Jane Wellmann, Chief Financial Officer
CMO: Donald Draehn, M.D., Chief of Staff
CIO: Sharon Schwartz, Director Medical Records
CHR: Bob Schubert, Director Human Resources
Web address: www.swbrenham.org
**Control:** Other not–for–profit (including NFP Corporation) **Service:** General Medical and Surgical

> **Staffed Beds:** 60 **Admissions:** 1781 **Census:** 16 **Outpatient Visits:** 33175 **Births:** 372 **Total Expense ($000):** 29384 **Payroll Expense ($000):** 13202 **Personnel:** 255

**BRIDGEPORT—Wise County**

**NORTH TEXAS COMMUNITY HOSPITAL (670052)**, 1904 Doctors Hospital Drive, Zip 76426; tel. 940/683–0300 **A**9 10 21 **F**3 11 13 18 19 29 30 34 40 45 51 57 59 64 68 70 75 76 79 81 85 93 107 108 110 111 114 118 120 128 129 134 145 146
Primary Contact: Max L. Ludeke, FACHE, Chief Executive Officer
Web address: www.ntchospital.org
**Control:** Other not–for–profit (including NFP Corporation) **Service:** General Medical and Surgical

> **Staffed Beds:** 21 **Admissions:** 1179 **Census:** 9 **Outpatient Visits:** 18552 **Births:** 211 **Total Expense ($000):** 15795 **Payroll Expense ($000):** 7439 **Personnel:** 167

**BROWNFIELD—Terry County**

★ **BROWNFIELD REGIONAL MEDICAL CENTER (450399)**, 705 East Felt Street, Zip 79316–3439; tel. 806/637–3551 **A**9 10 20 **F**3 7 13 28 29 30 34 40 43 45 50 53 57 59 62 64 65 68 75 76 80 81 85 86 87 89 90 93 97 102 107 118 126 129 134 147 **P**4
Primary Contact: Mike Click, Administrator
CFO: Josh Savage, Chief Financial Officer
CIO: Sheryl Holcombe, Administrative Assistant
CHR: Avis DePoyster, Director Human Resources
Web address: www.brownfield–rmc.org
**Control:** Hospital district or authority, Government, nonfederal **Service:** General Medical and Surgical

> **Staffed Beds:** 26 **Admissions:** 956 **Census:** 8 **Outpatient Visits:** 53380 **Births:** 133 **Total Expense ($000):** 12770 **Payroll Expense ($000):** 6097 **Personnel:** 208

**BROWNSVILLE—Cameron County**

☐ **BROWNSVILLE DOCTORS HOSPITAL (450841)**, 4750 North Expressway, Zip 78526; tel. 956/554–2000, (Nonreporting) **A**1 9 10
Primary Contact: C. Lynn Anderson, M.D., Interim Chief Executive Officer
COO: C. Lynn Anderson, M.D., Interim Operating Officer and Chairman of the Board
CFO: Rusty Young, Chief Financial Officer
CMO: Manuel G. Guajardo, M.D., Medical Director
CIO: Rusty Young, Chief Financial Officer
CHR: Eddie Melendez, Director Human Resources
Web address: www.brownsvilledoctorshospital.com
**Control:** Partnership, Investor–owned, for–profit **Service:** General Medical and Surgical

> **Staffed Beds:** 56

**SOLARA HOSPITAL HARLINGEN–BROWNSVILLE CAMPUS**, 333 Lorenaly Drive, Zip 78526; tel. 956/546–0808, (Nonreporting) **A**9 **S** Cornerstone Healthcare Group, Dallas, TX
Primary Contact: Paul E. Qualls, Jr., Chief Executive Officer
COO: Ken W. McGee, Vice President Hospital Development
CFO: A. Shane Wells, Chief Financial Officer
CMO: Ann B. McCracken, M.D., Chief Medical Director
CIO: Adam Davis, Chief Information Officer
CHR: Dan Perkins, Director Human Resources
Web address: www.solarahc.com/shcbr.html
**Control:** Corporation, Investor–owned, for–profit **Service:** Long–Term Acute Care hospital

> **Staffed Beds:** 41

☐ **SOUTH TEXAS REHABILITATION HOSPITAL (453092)**, 425 East Alton Gloor Boulevard, Zip 78526; tel. 956/554–6000 **A**1 9 10 **F**3 28 29 34 35 59 64 75 77 86 87 90 93 94 96 129 131 147 **P**6 **S** Ernest Health, Inc., Albuquerque, NM
Primary Contact: Jessie Eason Smedley, Chief Executive Officer
COO: Mary Valdez, Chief Operating Officer
CFO: Sue Thomsen, Chief Financial Officer
CMO: Christopher Wilson, M.D., Inpatient Medical Director
CIO: Deborah Alcocer, Chief Information Officer
CHR: Tony Rodriguez, Director Human Resources
CNO: Cheryl Sexton, Director Nursing Operations
Web address: www.strh.ernesthealth.com
**Control:** Partnership, Investor–owned, for–profit **Service:** Rehabilitation

> **Staffed Beds:** 40 **Admissions:** 851 **Census:** 34 **Outpatient Visits:** 3022 **Births:** 0 **Total Expense ($000):** 13505 **Payroll Expense ($000):** 6356 **Personnel:** 118

✠ **VALLEY BAPTIST MEDICAL CENTER–BROWNSVILLE (450028)**, 1040 West Jefferson Street, Zip 78520–5829, Mailing Address: P.O. Box 3590, Zip 78523–3590; tel. 956/698–5400, (Total facility includes 11 beds in nursing home–type unit) **A**1 9 10 **F**3 11 13 15 18 20 22 24 26 28 29 30 34 35 39 40 43 44 45 49 50 54 56 57 59 60 63 64 65 70 72 73 74 75 76 77 79 81 82 84 85 86 87 89 93 98 100 101 102 103 104 105 106 107 109 110 111 112 113 114 117 128 129 131 145 146 147 **P**8 **S** Valley Baptist Health System, Harlingen, TX
Primary Contact: Leslie Bingham, Senior Vice President and Chief Executive Officer
CFO: Glen Boles, Chief Financial Officer
CIO: Carlos Morales, Manager Data Processing
Web address: www.valleybaptist.net/brownsville/
**Control:** Other not–for–profit (including NFP Corporation) **Service:** General Medical and Surgical

> **Staffed Beds:** 240 **Admissions:** 11774 **Census:** 138 **Outpatient Visits:** 52825 **Births:** 1636 **Total Expense ($000):** 129818 **Payroll Expense ($000):** 36996 **Personnel:** 687

✠ **VALLEY REGIONAL MEDICAL CENTER (450662)**, 100A Alton Gloor Boulevard, Zip 78526–3346, Mailing Address: P.O. Box 3710, Zip 78523–3710; tel. 956/350–7101 **A**1 9 10 **F**3 11 13 15 18 20 22 24 26 29 30 31 32 34 35 39 40 43 44 45 47 49 50 53 57 59 60 61 64 65 68 70 72 73 74 75 76 77 78 79 81 82 84 85 86 87 89 93 107 108 110 111 114 117 118 129 131 134 142 145 146 147 **P**7 **S** HCA, Nashville, TN
Primary Contact: Susan Andrews, Chief Executive Officer
COO: Steven C. Hoelscher, Chief Operating Officer
CFO: Marcia Patterson, Chief Financial Officer
CHR: Margie Salazar, Director Human Resources
CNO: Holley Tyler, R.N., Chief Nursing Officer
Web address: www.valleyregionalmedicalcenter.com
**Control:** Partnership, Investor–owned, for–profit **Service:** General Medical and Surgical

> **Staffed Beds:** 214 **Admissions:** 9915 **Census:** 121 **Outpatient Visits:** 60596 **Births:** 2557 **Total Expense ($000):** 127866 **Payroll Expense ($000):** 44937 **Personnel:** 688

**BROWNWOOD—Brown County**

✠ **BROWNWOOD REGIONAL MEDICAL CENTER (450587)**, 1501 Burnet Drive, Zip 76801–5933, Mailing Address: P.O. Box 760, Zip 76804–0760; tel. 325/646–8541, (Total facility includes 20 beds in nursing home–type unit) **A**1 9 10 20 **F**3 11 13 15 18 20 26 28 29 30 31 35 39 40 45 48 49 50 51 53 54 56 57 59 64 68 70 74 75 76 77 78 79 81 82 85 86 87 93 97 107 108 111 113 118 120 122 127 128 129 131 145 146 147 **P**3 8 **S** Community Health Systems, Inc., Franklin, TN
Primary Contact: Claude E. Camp, III, Chief Executive Officer
CMO: Tim Moore, M.D., Chief of Staff
CIO: Paul Ferguson, Director Information Systems
CHR: Mikeana Bailey, Director Human Resources
Web address: www.brmc–cares.com
**Control:** Partnership, Investor–owned, for–profit **Service:** General Medical and Surgical

> **Staffed Beds:** 168 **Admissions:** 5692 **Census:** 71 **Outpatient Visits:** 64928 **Births:** 663 **Total Expense ($000):** 55734 **Payroll Expense ($000):** 23797 **Personnel:** 503

**TX**

---

**Hospital, Medicare Provider Number, Address, Telephone, Approval, Facility, and Physician Codes, Health Care System**

★ American Hospital Association (AHA) membership
☐ The Joint Commission accreditation
◇ DNV Healthcare Inc. accreditation
○ American Osteopathic Association (AOA) accreditation
△ Commission on Accreditation of Rehabilitation Facilities (CARF) accreditation

## BRYAN—Brazos County

✠ **CHRISTUS DUBUIS HOSPITAL OF BRYAN (452113)**, 1600 Joseph Drive, 2nd Floor, Zip 77802; tel. 979/821–5000 **A**1 9 10 **F**1 3 29 30 34 42 75 82 86 87 91 129 **P**8 **S** Dubuis Health System, Houston, TX
Primary Contact: Randy E. Johnson, Administrator
Web address: www.dubuis.org
**Control:** Church–operated, Nongovernment, not–for profit **Service:** Long–Term Acute Care hospital

| | |
|---|---|
| **Staffed Beds:** 30 **Admissions:** 211 **Census:** 14 **Outpatient Visits:** 0 **Births:** 0 **Total Expense ($000):** 6930 **Payroll Expense ($000):** 2678 **Personnel:** 52 | |

✠ **ST. JOSEPH REGIONAL HEALTH CENTER (450011)**, 2801 Franciscan Drive, Zip 77802–2599; tel. 979/776–3777 **A**1 2 3 5 9 10 **F**3 7 11 12 13 15 17 18 20 22 24 28 29 30 31 32 34 35 37 40 42 43 44 45 46 48 49 50 53 54 57 59 64 65 68 70 74 75 76 77 78 79 80 81 85 86 87 89 90 93 96 107 110 111 113 117 118 120 122 123 125 126 128 129 130 131 134 142 143 145 147 **S** Sylvania Franciscan Health, Toledo, OH
Primary Contact: Kathleen R. Krusie, Chief Executive Officer
CFO: Lisa McNair, CPA, Senior Vice President and Chief Financial Officer
CMO: Mark Montgomery, M.D., Vice President Quality and Medical Affairs
CIO: John Phillips, Vice President Information Services
CHR: Michael Costa, Vice President Human Resources
Web address: www.st–joseph.org
**Control:** Church–operated, Nongovernment, not–for profit **Service:** General Medical and Surgical

| | |
|---|---|
| **Staffed Beds:** 238 **Admissions:** 17579 **Census:** 186 **Outpatient Visits:** 364030 **Births:** 2214 **Total Expense ($000):** 247143 **Payroll Expense ($000):** 89833 **Personnel:** 1700 | |

☐ **THE PHYSICIANS CENTRE HOSPITAL (450834)**, 3131 University Drive East, Zip 77802–3473; tel. 979/731–3100 **A**1 9 10 **F**3 12 15 34 35 40 44 45 50 51 59 64 68 74 75 79 81 82 85 86 87 89 107 111 113 118 129 130 131 134
Primary Contact: Kori Rich, Chief Executive Officer
CIO: Shawn Clark, Director Information Systems
CHR: LeeAnn Ford, Director Human Resources and Imaging
Web address: www.thephysicianscentre.com
**Control:** Corporation, Investor–owned, for–profit **Service:** General Medical and Surgical

| | |
|---|---|
| **Staffed Beds:** 16 **Admissions:** 500 **Census:** 3 **Outpatient Visits:** 11246 **Births:** 0 **Total Expense ($000):** 14916 **Payroll Expense ($000):** 4294 **Personnel:** 79 | |

## BURNET—Burnet County

✠ **SETON HIGHLAND LAKES (451365)**, 3201 South Water Street, Zip 78611–7219, Mailing Address: P.O. Box 1219, Zip 78611–7219; tel. 512/715–3000 **A**1 9 10 18 **F**3 11 15 18 28 29 30 34 35 44 50 57 59 62 63 64 65 66 68 70 71 74 75 77 78 79 81 82 84 85 86 87 91 92 93 97 107 110 111 114 118 126 129 131 132 134 145 147 **P**3 8 **S** Ascension Health, Saint Louis, MO
Primary Contact: Michelle Robertson, R.N., President and Chief Executive Officer
CFO: Douglas D. Waite, Senior Vice President and Chief Financial Officer
CIO: Gerry Lewis, Chief Information Officer
Web address: www.seton.net
**Control:** Church–operated, Nongovernment, not–for profit **Service:** General Medical and Surgical

| | |
|---|---|
| **Staffed Beds:** 25 **Admissions:** 1598 **Census:** 14 **Outpatient Visits:** 94899 **Births:** 0 **Total Expense ($000):** 45424 **Payroll Expense ($000):** 19909 **Personnel:** 409 | |

## CALDWELL—Burleson County

✠ **BURLESON ST. JOSEPH HEALTH CENTER (451305)**, 1101 Woodson Drive, Zip 77836–1052, Mailing Address: P.O. Box 360, Zip 77836–0360; tel. 979/567–3245 **A**1 9 10 18 **F**3 7 11 14 29 30 34 35 40 43 57 59 64 68 93 107 113 129 132 142 **P**5 6 **S** Sylvania Franciscan Health, Toledo, OH
Primary Contact: John Hughson, Chief Executive Officer
CFO: Lisa McNair, CPA, Senior Vice President and Chief Financial Officer
CMO: Barker Stigler, M.D., Chief of Staff
CIO: John Phillips, Vice President Information Systems
CHR: Doni Roper, Director Human Resources
Web address: www.st–joseph.org/
**Control:** Church–operated, Nongovernment, not–for profit **Service:** General Medical and Surgical

| | |
|---|---|
| **Staffed Beds:** 25 **Admissions:** 308 **Census:** 5 **Outpatient Visits:** 17031 **Births:** 0 **Total Expense ($000):** 8409 **Payroll Expense ($000):** 4051 **Personnel:** 76 | |

## CAMERON—Milam County

**CENTRAL TEXAS HOSPITAL (450770)**, 806 North Crockett Avenue, Zip 76520–2599; tel. 254/697–6591 **A**9 10 **F**3 11 29 40 54 59 64 65 89 107 108 113 118 126 127 132 143 145 **P**8
Primary Contact: Tariq Mahmood, Chief Executive Officer
CFO: Joe White, Chief Financial Officer
Web address: www.centexhospital.com
**Control:** Corporation, Investor–owned, for–profit **Service:** General Medical and Surgical

| | |
|---|---|
| **Staffed Beds:** 34 **Admissions:** 913 **Census:** 9 **Outpatient Visits:** 5433 **Births:** 0 **Total Expense ($000):** 4482 **Payroll Expense ($000):** 2291 **Personnel:** 79 | |

## CANADIAN—Hemphill County

**HEMPHILL COUNTY HOSPITAL (450578)**, 1020 South Fourth Street, Zip 79014–3315; tel. 806/323–6422 **A**9 10 20 **F**2 7 29 35 40 45 56 57 62 63 64 68 69 87 89 93 97 102 107 108 129 132 145 147
Primary Contact: Christy Francis, Administrator
Web address: www.hchdst.org
**Control:** Hospital district or authority, Government, nonfederal **Service:** General Medical and Surgical

| | |
|---|---|
| **Staffed Beds:** 19 **Admissions:** 308 **Census:** 3 **Outpatient Visits:** 13391 **Births:** 0 **Total Expense ($000):** 6543 **Payroll Expense ($000):** 2911 **Personnel:** 84 | |

## CARRIZO SPRINGS—Dimmit County

**DIMMIT COUNTY MEMORIAL HOSPITAL (450620)**, 704 Hospital Drive, Zip 78834–3836; tel. 830/876–2424 **A**9 10 20 **F**11 13 40 43 45 57 62 64 70 76 81 87 89 93 107 114 118
Primary Contact: Ernest Flores, Jr., Administrator
CFO: Alma Melendez, Controller
Web address: www.dcmhospital.org
**Control:** Other not–for–profit (including NFP Corporation) **Service:** General Medical and Surgical

| | |
|---|---|
| **Staffed Beds:** 35 **Admissions:** 1137 **Census:** 7 **Outpatient Visits:** 19877 **Births:** 230 **Total Expense ($000):** 10582 **Payroll Expense ($000):** 4437 **Personnel:** 141 | |

## CARROLLTON—Denton County

✠ **BAYLOR MEDICAL CENTER AT CARROLLTON (450730)**, 4343 North Josey Lane, Zip 75010–4691; tel. 972/492–1010 **A**1 9 10 **F**3 11 12 13 15 18 20 29 30 31 35 40 48 49 50 52 54 55 56 57 59 64 70 72 73 74 75 76 77 78 79 81 82 85 86 87 93 107 108 111 113 114 117 118 128 129 130 131 134 145 146 147
Primary Contact: Michael Sanborn, MS, FACHE, President
CFO: Norma Ramos, Chief Financial Officer
CIO: Paul Ratcliff, Director Information Services
CHR: Sheila K. Richards, Director Human Resources
Web address: www.baylorhealth.com
**Control:** Corporation, Investor–owned, for–profit **Service:** General Medical and Surgical

| | |
|---|---|
| **Staffed Beds:** 115 **Admissions:** 6423 **Census:** 72 **Outpatient Visits:** 74249 **Births:** 1598 **Total Expense ($000):** 100990 **Payroll Expense ($000):** 41462 **Personnel:** 602 | |

✠ **SELECT SPECIALTY HOSPITAL–DALLAS (452022)**, 2329 West Parker Road, Zip 75010; tel. 469/892–1400 **A**1 9 10 **F**1 3 29 40 56 74 75 77 85 91 107 113 129 147 **S** Select Medical Corporation, Mechanicsburg, PA
Primary Contact: Curt L. Roberts, Chief Executive Officer
Web address: www.selectmedical.com
**Control:** Corporation, Investor–owned, for–profit **Service:** Long–Term Acute Care hospital

| | |
|---|---|
| **Staffed Beds:** 60 **Admissions:** 542 **Census:** 39 **Outpatient Visits:** 0 **Births:** 0 **Total Expense ($000):** 22148 **Payroll Expense ($000):** 9173 **Personnel:** 154 | |

## CARTHAGE—Panola County

✠ **EAST TEXAS MEDICAL CENTER CARTHAGE (450210)**, 409 Cottage Road, Zip 75633–1466, Mailing Address: P.O. Box 549, Zip 75633–0549; tel. 903/693–3841 **A**1 9 10 20 **F**3 8 11 13 15 28 29 30 34 35 40 43 45 50 57 59 64 65 70 75 76 81 85 89 107 108 110 111 114 118 126 128 144 145 146 **S** East Texas Medical Center Regional Healthcare System, Tyler, TX
Primary Contact: Gary Mikeal Hudson, Administrator
COO: Gary Mikeal Hudson, Administrator
CMO: A. R. Barrett, D.O., Chief of Staff
CIO: Renee Lawhorn, Director Medical Records
CHR: Mitzi Shuttlesworth, Director Human Resources
Web address: www.etmc.org
**Control:** Other not–for–profit (including NFP Corporation) **Service:** General Medical and Surgical

| | |
|---|---|
| **Staffed Beds:** 37 **Admissions:** 1331 **Census:** 8 **Outpatient Visits:** 72275 **Births:** 148 **Total Expense ($000):** 17205 **Payroll Expense ($000):** 8116 **Personnel:** 157 | |

**TX**

*Many Facility Codes have changed. Please refer to the AHA Guide Code Chart.*
© 2012 AHA Guide

## CEDAR PARK—Williamson County

⊞ **CEDAR PARK REGIONAL MEDICAL CENTER (670043)**, 1401 Medical Parkway, Zip 78613–7763; tel. 512/528–7000 **A**1 9 10 **F**3 12 13 15 20 29 34 35 40 45 47 49 50 57 59 68 70 75 76 77 78 79 81 82 85 87 93 107 108 110 111 114 118 125 131 134 145 146 147 **S** Community Health Systems, Inc., Franklin, TN
Primary Contact: Tim P. Adams, FACHE, Chief Executive Officer
COO: Jeremy Barclay, Chief Operating Officer
CFO: Erich Wallschlaeger, Chief Financial Officer
CIO: Brad Hoar, Director Information and Technology
CHR: Amy D. Reeves, Director Human Resources
Web address: www.cedarparkregional.com
**Control:** Corporation, Investor–owned, for–profit **Service:** General Medical and Surgical

**Staffed Beds:** 77 **Admissions:** 3650 **Census:** 31 **Outpatient Visits:** 33513 **Total Expense ($000):** 58103 **Payroll Expense ($000):** 20495 **Personnel:** 344

## CENTER—Shelby County

**SHELBY REGIONAL MEDICAL CENTER (450839)**, 602 Hurst Street, Zip 75935–3414, Mailing Address: P.O. Box 1749, Zip 75935–1749; tel. 936/598–2781, (Nonreporting) **A**9 10
Primary Contact: Tariq Mahmood, Chief Executive Officer
Web address: www.shelbyregional.com
**Control:** Partnership, Investor–owned, for–profit **Service:** General Medical and Surgical

**Staffed Beds:** 44

## CHANNELVIEW—Harris County

⊞ **KINDRED HOSPITAL EAST HOUSTON (452075)**, 15101 East Freeway, Zip 77530; tel. 832/200–5500, (Includes KINDRED HOSPITAL BAYTOWN, 1700 James Bowie Drive, 3rd Floor, Baytown, Zip 77520; tel. 281/420–7800; Robert Notarini, Chief Executive Officer) **A**1 9 10 **F**1 3 29 45 57 64 75 77 81 85 93 107 118 147 **S** Kindred Healthcare, Louisville, KY
Primary Contact: Angel Gradney, Chief Executive Officer
Web address: www.kheasthouston.com
**Control:** Corporation, Investor–owned, for–profit **Service:** Long–Term Acute Care hospital

**Staffed Beds:** 230 **Admissions:** 2135 **Census:** 150 **Outpatient Visits:** 2924 **Births:** 0 **Total Expense ($000):** 75434 **Payroll Expense ($000):** 27683 **Personnel:** 456

## CHILDRESS—Childress County

★ **CHILDRESS REGIONAL MEDICAL CENTER (450369)**, Highway 83 North, Zip 79201–5800, Mailing Address: P.O. Box 1030, Zip 79201–1030; tel. 940/937–6371 **A**9 10 20 **F**7 8 13 15 29 32 34 35 40 43 45 50 56 57 59 60 61 62 63 64 65 66 76 79 81 85 86 87 89 93 107 111 118 126 128 129 132
Primary Contact: John Henderson, Administrator
COO: Holly Holcomb, Chief Operating Officer
CFO: Kathy McLain, Chief Financial Officer
CMO: R. D. Caldwell, M.D., Chief of Staff
CHR: Gayle Cannon, Director Human Resources
Web address: www.childresshospital.com
**Control:** Hospital district or authority, Government, nonfederal **Service:** General Medical and Surgical

**Staffed Beds:** 39 **Admissions:** 1254 **Census:** 9 **Outpatient Visits:** 89749 **Births:** 261 **Total Expense ($000):** 23152 **Payroll Expense ($000):** 9644 **Personnel:** 258

## CHILLICOTHE—Hardeman County

★ **CHILLICOTHE HOSPITAL DISTRICT (451326)**, 303 Avenue I, Zip 79225, Mailing Address: P.O. Box 370, Zip 79225–0370; tel. 940/852–5131 **A**9 10 18 **F**29 34 40 43 45 57 59 69 89 131 132 **P**5
Primary Contact: Linda Hall, Administrator
CFO: Linda Hall, Administrator
CMO: Weldon Glidden, M.D., Chief of Staff
CIO: Kathy Busby, Medical Record Technician
CHR: Linda Hall, Administrator
Web address: www.chillicothehospital.org
**Control:** Hospital district or authority, Government, nonfederal **Service:** General Medical and Surgical

**Staffed Beds:** 13 **Admissions:** 75 **Census:** 1 **Outpatient Visits:** 6803 **Births:** 0 **Total Expense ($000):** 2000 **Payroll Expense ($000):** 971 **Personnel:** 24

## CLARKSVILLE—Red River County

★ **EAST TEXAS MEDICAL CENTER CLARKSVILLE (450188)**, 3000 West Main Street, Zip 75426, Mailing Address: P.O. Box 1270, Zip 75426–1270; tel. 903/427–6400 **A**9 10 **F**11 17 26 29 34 39 40 43 44 45 54 56 57 59 64 68 75 81 85 86 87 107 108 114 117 118 126 128 129 134 144 145 **P**8 **S** East Texas Medical Center Regional Healthcare System, Tyler, TX
Primary Contact: John S. Hart, Administrator
CFO: James Hines, Chief Financial Officer
CMO: Ravi K. Sreerama, M.D., Chief of Staff
CIO: James Hines, Chief Financial Officer
CHR: Susan Hill, Director Human Resources
Web address: www.etmc.org
**Control:** Other not–for–profit (including NFP Corporation) **Service:** General Medical and Surgical

**Staffed Beds:** 36 **Admissions:** 1484 **Census:** 14 **Outpatient Visits:** 17218 **Births:** 0 **Total Expense ($000):** 8193 **Payroll Expense ($000):** 4988 **Personnel:** 113

## CLEBURNE—Johnson County

⊞ **TEXAS HEALTH HARRIS METHODIST HOSPITAL CLEBURNE (450148)**, 201 Walls Drive, Zip 76033–4007; tel. 817/641–2551 **A**1 9 10 **F**3 11 13 15 29 32 34 35 40 43 44 45 46 49 50 51 56 57 59 64 65 68 70 75 76 77 79 81 85 89 93 107 108 110 113 118 123 128 129 145 147 **S** Texas Health Resources, Arlington, TX
Primary Contact: Blake Kretz, President
CFO: James E. Frosch, Director Finance
CHR: Dianne Mayfield, Director
Web address: www.texashealth.org
**Control:** Other not–for–profit (including NFP Corporation) **Service:** General Medical and Surgical

**Staffed Beds:** 85 **Admissions:** 3784 **Census:** 38 **Outpatient Visits:** 43621 **Births:** 602 **Total Expense ($000):** 56569 **Payroll Expense ($000):** 23219 **Personnel:** 288

## CLEVELAND—Liberty County

⊞ **CLEVELAND REGIONAL MEDICAL CENTER (450296)**, 300 East Crockett Street, Zip 77327–4062, Mailing Address: P.O. Box 1688, Zip 77328–1688; tel. 281/593–1811 **A**1 9 10 **F**3 11 13 15 18 29 30 34 35 40 41 43 50 57 59 62 64 68 70 74 75 76 77 79 81 85 87 92 107 108 113 118 129 131 132 145 **P**6
Primary Contact: G. Wayne Schuler, Chief Executive Officer
Web address: www.clevelandregionalmedicalcenter.com
**Control:** Partnership, Investor–owned, for–profit **Service:** General Medical and Surgical

**Staffed Beds:** 98 **Admissions:** 3085 **Census:** 23 **Outpatient Visits:** 23711 **Births:** 379 **Total Expense ($000):** 25873 **Payroll Expense ($000):** 12345 **Personnel:** 232

**DOCTORS DIAGNOSTIC HOSPITAL (670018)**, 1017 South Travis Street, Zip 77327–5152; tel. 281/622–2900, (Nonreporting) **A**9 10
Primary Contact: S. Jeffrey Ackerman, M.D., Chief Executive Officer
Web address: www.doctorsdiagnostichospital.com
**Control:** Partnership, Investor–owned, for–profit **Service:** General Medical and Surgical

**Staffed Beds:** 6

## CLIFTON—Bosque County

★ **GOODALL–WITCHER HEALTHCARE (450052)**, 101 South Avenue T, Zip 76634–1897, Mailing Address: P.O. Box 549, Zip 76634–0549; tel. 254/675–8322 **A**9 10 20 **F**3 11 13 15 29 30 34 35 36 40 43 45 53 57 59 62 64 65 68 76 77 81 93 107 108 113 118 126 129 132 145 146 147 **P**3
Primary Contact: Clarence Fields, Jr., FACHE, President and Chief Executive Officer
CFO: Vickie Gloff, Accountant
Web address: www.gwhf.org
**Control:** Other not–for–profit (including NFP Corporation) **Service:** General Medical and Surgical

**Staffed Beds:** 33 **Admissions:** 903 **Census:** 11 **Outpatient Visits:** 39889 **Births:** 100 **Total Expense ($000):** 16903 **Payroll Expense ($000):** 6396 **Personnel:** 175

TX

**Hospital, Medicare Provider Number, Address, Telephone, Approval, Facility, and Physician Codes, Health Care System**

★ American Hospital Association (AHA) membership
☐ The Joint Commission accreditation  ◇ DNV Healthcare Inc. accreditation
○ American Osteopathic Association (AOA) accreditation
△ Commission on Accreditation of Rehabilitation Facilities (CARF) accreditation

## COLEMAN—Coleman County

★ **COLEMAN COUNTY MEDICAL CENTER (451347)**, 310 South Pecos Street, Zip 76834–4159; tel. 325/625–2135 **A**9 10 18 **F**7 8 11 13 29 40 68 77 81 107 113 127 132 **P**5
Primary Contact: Michael W. Pruitt, Interim Administrator
CIO: Raul Hurtado, Chief Information Officer
CHR: Sue Titsworth, Director Human Resources
Web address: www.colemantexas.org/hospital.html
**Control:** Hospital district or authority, Government, nonfederal **Service:** General Medical and Surgical

> **Staffed Beds:** 25 **Admissions:** 519 **Census:** 6 **Outpatient Visits:** 4783
> **Births:** 29 **Total Expense ($000):** 7676 **Payroll Expense ($000):** 3875
> **Personnel:** 102

## COLLEGE STATION—Brazos County

☒ **COLLEGE STATION MEDICAL CENTER (450299)**, 1604 Rock Prairie Road, Zip 77845–8345, Mailing Address: P.O. Box 10000, Zip 77842–3500; tel. 979/764–5100 **A**1 2 5 9 10 **F**3 11 13 15 18 20 22 24 26 28 29 30 31 34 40 43 45 46 49 53 57 61 70 72 74 76 77 78 79 81 82 84 85 87 89 90 93 107 108 111 113 114 117 118 125 126 128 129 130 131 134 145 146 147 **P**7 **S** Community Health Systems, Inc., Franklin, TN
Primary Contact: Thomas W. Jackson, Chief Executive Officer
CFO: Wayne Colson, Chief Financial Officer
CHR: Sharon Bond, Director Human Resources
Web address: www.csmedcenter.com
**Control:** Corporation, Investor–owned, for–profit **Service:** General Medical and Surgical

> **Staffed Beds:** 166 **Admissions:** 5877 **Census:** 56 **Outpatient Visits:** 52831
> **Births:** 1491 **Total Expense ($000):** 106828 **Payroll Expense ($000):** 43215 **Personnel:** 736

## COLORADO CITY—Mitchell County

★ **MITCHELL COUNTY HOSPITAL (451342)**, 997 West Interstate 20, Zip 79512–2685; tel. 325/728–3431 **A**9 10 18 **F**3 7 11 28 29 40 43 45 50 59 64 68 81 93 107 118 132 145 **P**6
Primary Contact: Robbie Dewberry, Chief Executive Officer
CFO: Joe Wright, Chief Financial Officer
CMO: Dee A. Roach, M.D., Chief of Staff
CIO: Bo Everett, Director Human Resources and Information Technology
CHR: Bo Everett, Director Human Resources and Information Technology
Web address: www.mitchellcountyhospital.com
**Control:** Hospital district or authority, Government, nonfederal **Service:** General Medical and Surgical

> **Staffed Beds:** 25 **Admissions:** 703 **Census:** 9 **Outpatient Visits:** 30407
> **Births:** 1 **Total Expense ($000):** 13937 **Payroll Expense ($000):** 8289
> **Personnel:** 164

## COLUMBUS—Colorado County

★ **COLUMBUS COMMUNITY HOSPITAL (450370)**, 110 Shult Drive, Zip 78934–3010; tel. 979/732–2371 **A**5 9 10 **F**3 11 13 15 29 31 40 43 56 57 62 68 76 79 81 89 107 108 113 118 126 129 132 134
Primary Contact: Robert Thomas, Administrator
CFO: Regina Wicke, Chief Financial Officer
CMO: David Wilkinson, M.D., Chief of Staff
CIO: Regina Wicke, Chief Financial Officer
CHR: Janie Hammonds, Human Resources Officer
Web address: www.columbusch.com
**Control:** Other not–for–profit (including NFP Corporation) **Service:** General Medical and Surgical

> **Staffed Beds:** 40 **Admissions:** 1146 **Census:** 11 **Outpatient Visits:** 70648
> **Births:** 215 **Total Expense ($000):** 20844 **Payroll Expense ($000):** 7218
> **Personnel:** 149

## COMANCHE—Comanche County

★ **COMANCHE COUNTY MEDICAL CENTER (450234)**, 10201 Highway 16, Zip 76442–4462; tel. 254/879–4900 **A**9 10 20 **F**8 11 15 28 29 30 40 43 45 49 50 57 59 64 65 68 70 75 77 79 81 82 84 85 87 93 107 111 114 118 126 128 129 131 132 134 142 144 145 147 **P**4
Primary Contact: Kevin Storey, Chief Executive Officer
CFO: Cleo Cagle, Chief Financial Officer
CMO: Todd Davis, D.O., Chief of Staff
CIO: Ismelda Garza, Director Information Systems
CHR: Peggy Jordan, Director Human Resources
Web address: www.comanchecmc.org
**Control:** Other not–for–profit (including NFP Corporation) **Service:** General Medical and Surgical

> **Staffed Beds:** 25 **Admissions:** 1115 **Census:** 10 **Outpatient Visits:** 22915
> **Total Expense ($000):** 20124 **Payroll Expense ($000):** 6994 **Personnel:** 172

## COMMERCE—Hunt County

☒ **HUNT REGIONAL COMMUNITY HOSPITAL (451321)**, 2900 Sterling Hart Drive, Zip 75428; tel. 903/886–3161 **A**1 9 10 18 **F**3 11 29 30 40 41 43 57 75 85 87 93 104 105 107 113 118 129 132 145 **P**6
Primary Contact: Michael R. Klepin, Administrator
COO: John Heatherly, Assistant Administrator Support Services
CFO: Jeri Rich, Assistant Administrator and Chief Financial Officer
CMO: Richard Selvaggi, M.D., Chief of Staff
CIO: Joe Hartley, Director Information Systems
CHR: Stacey Lane, Director Human Resources
Web address: www.huntregional.org
**Control:** Hospital district or authority, Government, nonfederal **Service:** General Medical and Surgical

> **Staffed Beds:** 24 **Admissions:** 355 **Census:** 4 **Outpatient Visits:** 7690
> **Births:** 0 **Total Expense ($000):** 6668 **Payroll Expense ($000):** 2630
> **Personnel:** 42

## CONROE—Montgomery County

☐ **ASPIRE BEHAVIORAL HEALTH OF CONROE (454112)**, 2006 South Loop 336 West, Suite 500, Zip 77304–3315; tel. 936/647–3500 **A**1 9 10 **F**5 29 40 56 98 102 103 104 105 129
Primary Contact: Linda Corcoran, Chief Executive Officer
**Control:** Partnership, Investor–owned, for–profit **Service:** Psychiatric

> **Staffed Beds:** 30 **Admissions:** 381 **Census:** 10 **Outpatient Visits:** 648
> **Births:** 0 **Total Expense ($000):** 2593 **Payroll Expense ($000):** 2204
> **Personnel:** 49

☒ **CONROE REGIONAL MEDICAL CENTER (450222)**, 504 Medical Boulevard, Zip 77304, Mailing Address: P.O. Box 1538, Zip 77305–1538; tel. 936/539–1111 **A**1 9 10 13 **F**3 11 12 13 15 17 18 20 22 24 26 28 29 31 34 35 40 41 43 45 46 53 54 57 59 64 68 70 72 73 74 75 76 78 79 81 82 85 86 89 91 93 107 108 111 113 114 117 118 120 123 128 129 131 134 145 146 147 **P**7 **S** HCA, Nashville, TN
Primary Contact: Jerry A. Nash, Chief Executive Officer
COO: Eric Becker, Chief Operating Officer
CFO: Thomas A. Holt, Chief Financial Officer
CIO: Daniel Andresen, Director Information Services
CHR: Diana Howell, Director Human Resources
Web address: www.conroeregional.com
**Control:** Partnership, Investor–owned, for–profit **Service:** General Medical and Surgical

> **Staffed Beds:** 292 **Admissions:** 14757 **Census:** 202 **Outpatient Visits:** 106680 **Births:** 1095 **Total Expense ($000):** 199069 **Payroll Expense ($000):** 69295 **Personnel:** 1025

☒ **HEALTHSOUTH REHABILITATION HOSPITAL OF NORTH HOUSTON (453059)**, 18550 I 45 South, Zip 77384; tel. 281/364–2000 **A**1 10 **F**3 29 35 44 57 59 62 64 68 75 77 79 82 86 87 90 91 93 129 131 147 **S** HEALTHSOUTH Corporation, Birmingham, AL
Primary Contact: Krista Uselman, Chief Executive Officer
CMO: Ben Agana, M.D., Medical Director
CHR: Valerie Wells, Manager Human Resources
Web address: www.healthsouth.com
**Control:** Corporation, Investor–owned, for–profit **Service:** Rehabilitation

> **Staffed Beds:** 84 **Admissions:** 1067 **Census:** 40 **Outpatient Visits:** 14548
> **Births:** 0 **Total Expense ($000):** 14105 **Payroll Expense ($000):** 8338
> **Personnel:** 126

☐ **SOLARA HOSPITAL CONROE (452107)**, 1500 Grand Lake Drive, Zip 77304; tel. 936/523–1800 **A**1 9 10 **F**1 3 34 39 40 74 75 79 85 86 87 91 129 147 **S** Solara Healthcare, Dallas, TX
Primary Contact: Steve Hockert, Chief Executive Officer
Web address: www.solarahc.com/shcco.html
**Control:** Partnership, Investor–owned, for–profit **Service:** Long–Term Acute Care hospital

> **Staffed Beds:** 41 **Admissions:** 517 **Census:** 36 **Outpatient Visits:** 7 **Births:** 0 **Total Expense ($000):** 15209 **Payroll Expense ($000):** 6076 **Personnel:** 126

## CORINTH—Denton County

**ATRIUM MEDICAL CENTER OF CORINTH (452111)**, 3305 Corinth Parkway, Zip 76208–5380; tel. 940/270–4100 **A**10 21 **F**1 3 28 29 40 45 47 60 64 68 70 75 77 86 87 96 107 111 113 118 147 **P**2
Primary Contact: Dorothy J. Elford, Chief Executive Officer
COO: Kathy Mason, Chief Operating Officer
CFO: Melissa Dovel, Manager Human Resources
CFO: Anbu Nachimuthu, Chief Financial Officer
CMO: Jalil Kahn, M.D., Chief of Staff
CIO: Wendy Keller, Director Health Information Management
CNO: Michelle Gray, Nurse Executive
Web address: www.atriumhealthcare.net
**Control:** Corporation, Investor–owned, for–profit **Service:** Long–Term Acute Care hospital

> **Staffed Beds:** 57 **Admissions:** 630 **Census:** 46 **Outpatient Visits:** 2528
> **Births:** 0 **Total Expense ($000):** 24937 **Payroll Expense ($000):** 9355
> **Personnel:** 169

**TX**

## CORPUS CHRISTI—Nueces County

☒ △ **CHRISTUS SPOHN HOSPITAL CORPUS CHRISTI MEMORIAL (450046)**, 2606 Hospital Boulevard, Zip 78405–1818, Mailing Address: P.O. Box 5280, Zip 78465–5280; tel. 361/902–4000, (Includes CHRISTUS SPOHN HOSPITAL CORPUS CHRISTI SHORELINE, 600 Elizabeth Street, Zip 78404–2235; tel. 361/881–3000; Paul Gaden, Chief Executive Officer; CHRISTUS SPOHN HOSPITAL CORPUS CHRISTUS SOUTH, 5950 Saratoga, Zip 78414–4100; tel. 361/985–5000), (Total facility includes 24 beds in nursing home–type unit) **A**1 2 3 5 7 9 10 **F**3 8 11 13 15 17 18 20 22 24 26 28 29 30 35 36 37 38 39 40 43 45 46 47 48 49 50 51 53 54 56 60 64 66 68 70 72 73 74 75 76 77 79 81 85 87 90 93 97 98 99 100 101 102 103 107 108 111 113 117 118 126 127 129 145 146 147 **S** CHRISTUS Health, Irving, TX
Primary Contact: Paul Gaden, Vice President and Chief Operating Officer
CFO: Scott Merryman, Chief Financial Officer
CMO: Richard Davis, M.D., Regional Chief Medical Officer
CHR: Mary LaFrancois, Vice President Human Resources
Web address: www.christusspohn.org
**Control:** Church–operated, Nongovernment, not–for profit **Service:** General Medical and Surgical

> **Staffed Beds:** 800 **Admissions:** 34386 **Census:** 524 **Outpatient Visits:** 317037 **Births:** 2923 **Total Expense ($000):** 514961 **Payroll Expense ($000):** 198448 **Personnel:** 3214

☒ **CORPUS CHRISTI MEDICAL CENTER (450788)**, 3315 South Alameda Street, Zip 78411–1883, Mailing Address: P.O. Box 8991, Zip 78468–8991; tel. 361/761–1400, (Includes BAYVIEW BEHAVIORAL HOSPITAL, 6629 Wooldridge Road, Zip 78414; tel. 361/986–9444; Jamie Molbert, Associate Administrator; CORPUS CHRISTI MEDICAL CENTER BAY AREA, 7101 South Padre Island Drive, Zip 78412–4999; tel. 361/985–1200) **A**1 9 10 12 13 **F**3 11 12 13 15 17 18 20 22 24 26 28 29 30 31 34 35 37 38 40 44 49 50 53 57 58 59 64 68 70 72 73 74 75 76 77 78 79 81 85 86 87 93 97 98 99 100 101 102 103 104 107 108 110 111 113 114 117 118 119 120 125 129 130 131 145 146 **P**3 8 **S** HCA, Nashville, TN
Primary Contact: Jay Woodall, Chief Executive Officer
CFO: Chris Nicosia, Chief Financial Officer
CMO: Scott McKinstry, M.D., Chief of Staff
CIO: Sharon Orton, Director Information Services and Technology
CHR: Michael Conwill, Director Human Resources
Web address: www.ccmedicalcenter.com
**Control:** Partnership, Investor–owned, for–profit **Service:** General Medical and Surgical

> **Staffed Beds:** 453 **Admissions:** 16397 **Census:** 205 **Outpatient Visits:** 93732 **Births:** 3721 **Total Expense ($000):** 209971 **Payroll Expense ($000):** 73231 **Personnel:** 1497

☐ **CORPUS CHRISTI SPECIALTY HOSPITAL (452036)**, 1310 Third Street, Zip 78404–2208; tel. 361/888–4323 **A**1 9 10 **F**1 3 29 129 147 **P**5 **S** Encore Healthcare, Columbia, MD
Primary Contact: Judy Wolfe, Chief Executive Officer
CFO: Cynthia Barron, Manager Business Office
CMO: Raymond Acebo, M.D., Director Medical Staff
CHR: Carmen Newton, Manager Human Resources
Web address: www.encore–healthcare.com
**Control:** Corporation, Investor–owned, for–profit **Service:** Long–Term Acute Care hospital

> **Staffed Beds:** 31 **Admissions:** 219 **Census:** 17 **Outpatient Visits:** 0 **Births:** 0 **Total Expense ($000):** 7603 **Payroll Expense ($000):** 3121 **Personnel:** 39

☒ **DRISCOLL CHILDREN'S HOSPITAL (453301)**, 3533 South Alameda Street, Zip 78411–1785, Mailing Address: P.O. Box 6530, Zip 78466–6530; tel. 361/694–5000 **A**1 3 5 9 10 13 **F**3 7 11 12 19 21 23 25 27 29 30 31 32 34 35 38 39 40 41 49 50 54 55 57 58 59 60 61 64 65 68 72 74 75 77 78 79 81 82 85 86 87 88 89 92 93 97 99 104 107 108 111 113 117 118 126 129 130 131 133 137 142 143 145 147
Primary Contact: Steve Woerner, Chief Executive Officer
COO: Donna Quinn, Vice President Operations and Quality
CFO: Eric Hamon, Chief Financial Officer
CIO: Miguel Perez, Director Information Systems
CHR: Bill Larsen, Vice President Human Resources
Web address: www.driscollchildrens.org
**Control:** Other not–for–profit (including NFP Corporation) **Service:** Children's general

> **Staffed Beds:** 162 **Admissions:** 4973 **Census:** 71 **Outpatient Visits:** 120747 **Births:** 0 **Total Expense ($000):** 183526 **Payroll Expense ($000):** 78033 **Personnel:** 1687

☒ **DUBUIS HOSPITAL OF CORPUS CHRISTI (452086)**, 600 Elizabeth Street, 3rd Floor, Zip 78404; tel. 361/881–3223 **A**1 9 10 **F**1 3 29 30 31 75 82 84 87 96 103 147 **P**5 **S** Dubuis Health System, Houston, TX
Primary Contact: Diane Kaiser, Administrator
Web address: www.dubuis.org
**Control:** Church–operated, Nongovernment, not–for profit **Service:** Long–Term Acute Care hospital

> **Staffed Beds:** 22 **Admissions:** 244 **Census:** 18 **Outpatient Visits:** 0 **Births:** 0 **Total Expense ($000):** 9135 **Payroll Expense ($000):** 3467 **Personnel:** 64

☒ **KINDRED HOSPITAL–CORPUS CHRISTI (452092)**, 6226 Saratoga Boulevard, Zip 78414–3421; tel. 361/986–1600 **A**1 9 10 **F**1 3 29 30 34 35 45 57 59 60 61 64 70 74 75 77 79 82 85 86 87 93 97 100 107 129 145 147 **S** Kindred Healthcare, Louisville, KY
Primary Contact: Diana Schultz, Chief Executive Officer
CFO: Eva De La Paz, Chief Financial Officer
CMO: Salim Surani, M.D., Medical Director
CHR: Kasey Parkey, Coordinator Payroll and Benefits
Web address: www.khcorpuschristi.com/
**Control:** Corporation, Investor–owned, for–profit **Service:** Long–Term Acute Care hospital

> **Staffed Beds:** 68 **Admissions:** 593 **Census:** 40 **Outpatient Visits:** 663 **Births:** 0 **Total Expense ($000):** 18100 **Payroll Expense ($000):** 7287 **Personnel:** 131

**SOUTH TEXAS SURGICAL HOSPITAL (670061)**, 6130 Parkway Drive, Zip 78414–2455; tel. 361/993–2000 **A**9 10 **F**3 29 40 45 54 64 67 68 75 79 81 82 85 118 129 **S** National Surgical Hospitals, Chicago, IL
Primary Contact: James Murphy, Chief Executive Officer
Web address: www.nshinc.com
**Control:** Partnership, Investor–owned, for–profit **Service:** General Medical and Surgical

> **Staffed Beds:** 20 **Admissions:** 759 **Census:** 7 **Outpatient Visits:** 3613 **Births:** 0 **Personnel:** 186

## CORSICANA—Navarro County

☒ **NAVARRO REGIONAL HOSPITAL (450447)**, 3201 West State Highway 22, Zip 75110–2469; tel. 903/654–6800 **A**1 9 10 19 **F**3 11 13 14 15 18 29 30 34 35 39 40 43 45 47 49 50 51 57 59 60 64 68 70 75 76 79 81 82 85 93 107 108 110 111 113 118 128 131 134 145 147 **P**7 **S** Community Health Systems, Inc., Franklin, TN
Primary Contact: Xavier Villarreal, Chief Executive Officer
CFO: Marco Rodriguez, Chief Financial Officer
CIO: Marco Rodriguez, Chief Financial Officer
CHR: Linda Gould, Director Human Resources
Web address: www.navarrohospital.com
**Control:** Partnership, Investor–owned, for–profit **Service:** General Medical and Surgical

> **Staffed Beds:** 148 **Admissions:** 3856 **Census:** 34 **Outpatient Visits:** 40784 **Births:** 470 **Total Expense ($000):** 40658 **Payroll Expense ($000):** 14722 **Personnel:** 275

## CRANE—Crane County

★ ○ **CRANE MEMORIAL HOSPITAL (451353)**, 1310 South Alford Street, Zip 79731–3899; tel. 432/558–3555 **A**9 10 11 18 **F**3 29 32 34 40 57 59 64 65 68 75 81 86 97 107 118 126 132 144 146 147 **P**6
Primary Contact: Dianne Yeager, Chief Executive Officer
CMO: Jay Sigel, M.D., Chief Medical Staff
Web address: www.cranememorial.org
**Control:** Hospital district or authority, Government, nonfederal **Service:** General Medical and Surgical

> **Staffed Beds:** 25 **Admissions:** 205 **Census:** 2 **Outpatient Visits:** 8072 **Births:** 0 **Total Expense ($000):** 3640 **Payroll Expense ($000):** 2072 **Personnel:** 43

## CROCKETT—Houston County

☒ **EAST TEXAS MEDICAL CENTER CROCKETT (450580)**, 1100 Loop 304 East, Zip 75835–1810; tel. 936/546–3862 **A**1 9 10 20 **F**3 11 13 15 28 29 32 35 40 43 46 50 54 57 58 59 61 64 70 75 76 81 87 97 107 108 111 113 117 118 128 132 145 **P**7 **S** East Texas Medical Center Regional Healthcare System, Tyler, TX
Primary Contact: Terry Cutler, Administrator and Chief Operating Officer
Web address: www.etmc.org
**Control:** Other not–for–profit (including NFP Corporation) **Service:** General Medical and Surgical

> **Staffed Beds:** 49 **Admissions:** 1972 **Census:** 20 **Outpatient Visits:** 67466 **Births:** 199 **Total Expense ($000):** 16726 **Payroll Expense ($000):** 7687 **Personnel:** 165

**TX**

---

**Hospital, Medicare Provider Number, Address, Telephone, Approval, Facility, and Physician Codes, Health Care System**

★ American Hospital Association (AHA) membership
☐ The Joint Commission accreditation ◇ DNV Healthcare Inc. accreditation
○ American Osteopathic Association (AOA) accreditation
△ Commission on Accreditation of Rehabilitation Facilities (CARF) accreditation

## CROSBYTON—Crosby County

**CROSBYTON CLINIC HOSPITAL (451345)**, 710 West Main Street, Zip 79322–2143; tel. 806/675–2382 **A**9 10 18 **F**7 29 34 40 50 57 59 63 64 68 87 93 111 118 124 126 129 132 147 **P**6
Primary Contact: Debra Miller, Administrator
CFO: Cherie Parkhill, Chief Financial Officer
CMO: Steve B. Alley, M.D., Chief of Staff
CHR: Jane Wheeless, Director Human Resources
CNO: Anna Bradford, R.N., Chief Nursing Officer
Web address: www.crosbytonclinichospital.com
**Control:** Other not–for–profit (including NFP Corporation) **Service:** General Medical and Surgical

**Staffed Beds:** 25 **Admissions:** 319 **Census:** 4 **Outpatient Visits:** 17287 **Births:** 0 **Total Expense ($000):** 5268 **Payroll Expense ($000):** 2525 **Personnel:** 69

## CUERO—Dewitt County

★ **CUERO COMMUNITY HOSPITAL (450597)**, 2550 North Esplanade Street, Zip 77954–4716; tel. 361/275–6191 **A**9 10 **F**3 7 11 13 15 29 34 40 43 45 57 59 62 64 68 70 75 76 77 79 81 85 86 93 103 107 108 111 114 117 118 128 129 130
Primary Contact: Darryl Stefka, Administrator
CFO: Greg Pritchett, Controller
CIO: Arthur Mueller, Director Management Information Systems
CHR: Wanda Kolodziejcyk, Director Human Resources
Web address: www.cuerohosp.org
**Control:** Hospital district or authority, Government, nonfederal **Service:** General Medical and Surgical

**Staffed Beds:** 35 **Admissions:** 1799 **Census:** 17 **Outpatient Visits:** 138238 **Births:** 153 **Total Expense ($000):** 22467 **Payroll Expense ($000):** 11316 **Personnel:** 330

## CYPRESS—Harris County

☐ **NORTH CYPRESS MEDICAL CENTER (670024)**, 21214 Northwest Freeway, Zip 77429–3373; tel. 832/912–3500 **A**1 10 **F**3 8 12 15 18 20 22 24 26 28 29 31 34 35 36 37 39 40 42 44 45 46 47 48 49 50 51 57 59 60 64 70 74 75 77 78 79 81 82 85 86 87 93 96 107 108 109 110 111 113 114 115 116 117 118 119 120 122 123 128 129 130 131 145 147
Primary Contact: Robert Behar, M.D., Chief Executive Officer
Web address: www.ncmc–hospital.com
**Control:** Partnership, Investor–owned, for–profit **Service:** General Medical and Surgical

**Staffed Beds:** 139 **Admissions:** 8417 **Census:** 104 **Outpatient Visits:** 191634 **Births:** 0 **Total Expense ($000):** 217669 **Payroll Expense ($000):** 72992 **Personnel:** 1365

## DALHART—Hartley County

★ **COON MEMORIAL HOSPITAL AND HOME (451331)**, 1411 Denver Avenue, Zip 79022–4809, Mailing Address: P.O. Box 2014, Zip 79022–6014; tel. 806/244–4571 **A**9 10 18 **F**3 7 10 11 13 30 34 35 40 43 45 50 53 57 59 62 63 64 65 68 69 71 76 77 79 81 82 83 85 87 89 90 93 97 103 107 113 118 124 126 130 132 142 143 145 147 **P**5
Primary Contact: Leroy Schaffner, Chief Executive Officer
CFO: Donny Pettit, Chief Financial Officer
CMO: Randy Herring, M.D., Chief of Staff
CIO: Joshua Gray, Director Information Technology
CHR: Dee Dawn McCormick, Director Personnel and Human Resources
Web address: www.coonmemorial.org
**Control:** Hospital district or authority, Government, nonfederal **Service:** General Medical and Surgical

**Staffed Beds:** 21 **Admissions:** 520 **Census:** 5 **Outpatient Visits:** 13625 **Births:** 95 **Total Expense ($000):** 21279 **Payroll Expense ($000):** 8254 **Personnel:** 168

## DALLAS—Dallas County

**A. WEBB ROBERTS HOSPITAL** See Baylor University Medical Center

✠ △ **BAYLOR INSTITUTE FOR REHABILITATION (453036)**, 909 North Washington Avenue, Zip 75246–1520; tel. 214/820–9300, (Data for 273 days) **A**1 7 9 10 **F**3 29 30 35 44 62 64 65 68 74 77 85 86 87 90 92 93 94 96 129 130 131 134 142 147 **S** Baylor Health Care System, Dallas, TX
Primary Contact: Jon C. Skinner, Chief Executive Officer
COO: David Smith, Vice President Rehabilitation Services
CFO: Ted Bolcavage, Vice President and Division Controller
CMO: Amy Wilson, M.D., Medical Director
CIO: James Talalai, Senior Vice President and Chief Information Officer
CHR: Karen Hill, Director Human Resources
Web address: www.bhcs.com
**Control:** Other not–for–profit (including NFP Corporation) **Service:** Rehabilitation

**Staffed Beds:** 87 **Admissions:** 1140 **Census:** 72 **Outpatient Visits:** 29521 **Births:** 0 **Total Expense ($000):** 37670 **Payroll Expense ($000):** 18492 **Personnel:** 430

☐ **BAYLOR JACK AND JANE HAMILTON HEART AND VASCULAR HOSPITAL (450851)**, 621 North Hall Street, Zip 75226–1339; tel. 214/820–0600 **A**1 9 10 **F**3 11 18 20 21 22 26 28 29 30 34 35 57 58 59 64 68 75 81 85 86 87 93 96 100 107 114 118 131 134
Primary Contact: Nancy Vish, Ph.D., President
CFO: Julius Wicke, III, Vice President Finance and Hospital Financial Officer
CMO: Kevin Wheelan, M.D., Medical Director
CHR: Kim Krause, Director Human Resources
Web address: www.baylorhearthospital.com
**Control:** Partnership, Investor–owned, for–profit **Service:** General Medical and Surgical

**Staffed Beds:** 64 **Admissions:** 2131 **Census:** 18 **Outpatient Visits:** 20679 **Births:** 0 **Total Expense ($000):** 79341 **Payroll Expense ($000):** 21132 **Personnel:** 313

✠ **BAYLOR MEDICAL CENTER AT UPTOWN (450422)**, 2727 East Lemmon Avenue, Zip 75204–2895; tel. 214/443–3000 **A**1 9 10 **F**40 68 79 81 82 85 107 111 **S** United Surgical Partners International, Addison, TX
Primary Contact: Matt Chance, Administrator
COO: Diane Boyne, Chief Nursing Officer
CFO: Andra Manning, Manager Business Office
CMO: Mark Armstrong, M.D., Medical Director
CIO: Chris Guitte, Director Information Technology
CHR: Robert Talbot, Director Human Resources
Web address: www.bmcuptown.com
**Control:** Partnership, Investor–owned, for–profit **Service:** General Medical and Surgical

**Staffed Beds:** 24 **Admissions:** 1075 **Census:** 6 **Outpatient Visits:** 4386 **Births:** 0 **Total Expense ($000):** 34539 **Payroll Expense ($000):** 6833 **Personnel:** 104

✠ **BAYLOR SPECIALTY HOSPITAL (452017)**, 3504 Swiss Avenue, Zip 75204–6224; tel. 214/820–9700 **A**1 9 10 **F**1 30 50 75 77 85 93 112 129 144 147 **S** Baylor Health Care System, Dallas, TX
Primary Contact: Elizabeth Youngblood, President
CFO: Robert Knowlton, Vice President
CMO: Michael Highbaugh, M.D., Medical Director
CHR: Karen Hill, Coordinator Human Resources
Web address: www.bhcs.com
**Control:** Other not–for–profit (including NFP Corporation) **Service:** General Medical and Surgical

**Staffed Beds:** 61 **Admissions:** 582 **Census:** 45 **Outpatient Visits:** 0 **Births:** 0 **Total Expense ($000):** 27896 **Payroll Expense ($000):** 10711 **Personnel:** 206

✠ **BAYLOR UNIVERSITY MEDICAL CENTER (450021)**, 3500 Gaston Avenue, Zip 75246–2088; tel. 214/820–0111, (Includes A. WEBB ROBERTS HOSPITAL, Zip 75246; ERIK AND MARGARET JONSSON HOSPITAL, Zip 75246; GEORGE W. TRUETT MEMORIAL HOSPITAL, 3500 Gaston Avenue, Zip 75246; KARL AND ESTHER HOBLITZELLE MEMORIAL HOSPITAL, 3500 Gaston Avenue, Zip 75246) **A**1 2 3 5 8 9 10 **F**3 6 11 12 13 14 15 17 18 20 22 24 26 28 29 30 31 34 35 36 37 38 39 40 43 44 45 46 47 48 49 50 51 54 55 56 57 58 59 60 61 63 64 65 66 68 70 72 74 75 76 78 79 80 81 82 84 85 86 87 90 91 92 94 95 96 97 102 107 108 110 111 112 113 114 115 116 117 118 119 120 122 123 125 128 129 130 131 134 135 136 137 138 139 140 141 142 143 144 145 146 147 **S** Baylor Health Care System, Dallas, TX
Primary Contact: John B. McWhorter, III, President
COO: James D. Thaxton, Chief Operating Officer
CFO: Jay Whitfield, Chief Financial Officer
CMO: Irving Prengler, M.D., Vice President Medical Staff Affairs
CHR: Queen Greene, Director Human Resources
Web address: www.baylorhealth.com
**Control:** Other not–for–profit (including NFP Corporation) **Service:** General Medical and Surgical

**Staffed Beds:** 933 **Admissions:** 37580 **Census:** 652 **Outpatient Visits:** 297988 **Births:** 4251 **Total Expense ($000):** 885541 **Payroll Expense ($000):** 303614 **Personnel:** 4162

✠ **CHILDREN'S MEDICAL CENTER OF DALLAS (453302)**, 1935 Medical District Drive, Zip 75235–7794; tel. 214/456–7000 **A**1 3 5 8 9 10 **F**3 7 8 11 12 17 19 21 23 25 27 29 30 31 32 34 35 38 39 40 41 43 44 45 46 47 48 49 50 51 54 55 57 58 59 60 61 64 65 66 68 72 74 75 77 78 79 81 82 84 85 86 87 88 89 91 92 93 94 97 98 99 100 101 102 104 105 106 107 108 111 113 115 116 117 118 125 126 128 129 130 131 133 135 136 137 138 139 140 141 142 143 144 145 147
Primary Contact: Christopher J. Durovich, President and Chief Executive Officer
COO: Douglas G. Hock, Senior Vice President Operations
CFO: Ray R. Dziesinski, Senior Vice President and Chief Financial Officer
CMO: Julio Perez–Foutan, M.D., Executive Vice President Medical Affairs
CIO: Pamela Arora, Vice President Information Systems
CHR: Jim Herring, Senior Vice President
Web address: www.childrens.com
**Control:** Other not–for–profit (including NFP Corporation) **Service:** Children's general

**Staffed Beds:** 442 **Admissions:** 26588 **Census:** 274 **Outpatient Visits:** 530817 **Births:** 0 **Total Expense ($000):** 796822 **Payroll Expense ($000):** 374853 **Personnel:** 5399

**TX**

*Many Facility Codes have changed. Please refer to the AHA Guide Code Chart.* © 2012 AHA Guide

☐ **DALLAS MEDICAL CENTER (450379)**, Seven Medical Parkway, Zip 75234, Mailing Address: P.O. Box 819094, Zip 75381–9094; tel. 972/247–1000 **A**1 10 **F**3 11 12 15 17 18 24 29 34 39 40 44 50 58 61 65 68 70 74 77 78 79 81 82 84 85 86 91 107 108 110 111 113 118 128 129 130 131 145 147 **P**5 **S** Physician Synergy Group, Irving, TX
Primary Contact: Raji Kumar, Chief Executive Officer
CFO: Karen Bomersbach, Chief Financial Officer
CIO: Mary Jo Tallant–Ball, Director Health Information Systems
CHR: Stephanie S. Talley, Associate Administrator and Director Human Resources
Web address: www.dallasmedcenter.com
**Control:** Corporation, Investor–owned, for–profit **Service:** General Medical and Surgical

> **Staffed Beds:** 89 **Admissions:** 3146 **Census:** 27 **Outpatient Visits:** 40369 **Births:** 0 **Total Expense ($000):** 27445 **Payroll Expense ($000):** 15845 **Personnel:** 294

★ **DOCTORS HOSPITAL AT WHITE ROCK LAKE (450678)**, 9440 Poppy Drive, Zip 75218–3694; tel. 214/324–6100 **A**1 9 10 **F**3 8 11 12 13 15 17 18 20 22 24 26 28 29 30 31 34 35 37 40 45 47 49 50 53 56 57 59 64 70 72 73 74 75 76 77 78 79 81 82 85 93 107 108 110 111 114 118 128 129 131 134 145 146 147 **S** TENET Healthcare Corporation, Dallas, TX
Primary Contact: G. Scott Manis, Chief Executive Officer
COO: Chakilla Robinson–White, Chief Operating Officer
CFO: Roger D. Hutchins, Chief Financial Officer
CMO: Dwight A. Lee, M.D., Chief Medical Officer
CIO: Dianne Yarborough, Director Information Systems
CHR: Marlene Urbach, Chief Human Resources Officer
Web address: www.doctorshospitaldallas.com
**Control:** Partnership, Investor–owned, for–profit **Service:** General Medical and Surgical

> **Staffed Beds:** 163 **Admissions:** 7213 **Census:** 79 **Outpatient Visits:** 68591 **Births:** 1237 **Total Expense ($000):** 93067 **Payroll Expense ($000):** 34859 **Personnel:** 522

○ **FOREST PARK MEDICAL CENTER (670057)**, 11990 North Central Expressway, Zip 75243–3714; tel. 972/234–1900 **A**10 11 **F**3 12 29 30 40 45 47 49 64 68 70 75 77 79 81 82 85 87 107 111 114 118 125 129 131 **P**8
Primary Contact: Susie Edler, Chief Executive Officer
Web address: www.forestparkmc.com/
**Control:** Partnership, Investor–owned, for–profit **Service:** General Medical and Surgical

> **Staffed Beds:** 84 **Admissions:** 3578 **Census:** 15 **Outpatient Visits:** 9202 **Births:** 0 **Total Expense ($000):** 118817 **Payroll Expense ($000):** 20559 **Personnel:** 461

○ **GLOBALREHAB HOSPITAL – DALLAS (673033)**, 1340 Empire Central Drive, Zip 75247–4022; tel. 214/879–7300 **A**11 **F**29 68 75 90 91 96 100 129 147 **S** GLOBALREHAB, Dallas, TX
Primary Contact: Ellen Shankles, Chief Executive Officer
Web address: www.globalrehabhospitals.com
**Control:** Individual, Investor–owned, for–profit **Service:** Rehabilitation

> **Staffed Beds:** 42 **Admissions:** 878 **Census:** 33 **Outpatient Visits:** 0 **Births:** 0 **Total Expense ($000):** 15150 **Payroll Expense ($000):** 7370 **Personnel:** 81

☒ **GREEN OAKS HOSPITAL (454094)**, 7808 Clodus Fields Drive, Zip 75251–2206; tel. 972/991–9504 **A**1 9 10 **F**4 5 29 54 87 98 99 102 103 104 105 129 131 **P**5 **S** HCA, Nashville, TN
Primary Contact: Thomas M. Collins, President, Chairman and Chief Executive Officer
COO: Pam Whitley, R.N., Chief Operating Officer and Chief Nursing Officer
CFO: Scott Cook, Chief Financial Officer
CMO: Joel Holiner, M.D., Executive Medical Director
CIO: Chebon Bravo, Director Information Systems
CHR: Kevin Adkins, Director Human Resources
Web address: www.greenoakspsych.com
**Control:** Corporation, Investor–owned, for–profit **Service:** Psychiatric

> **Staffed Beds:** 106 **Admissions:** 5655 **Census:** 105 **Outpatient Visits:** 30417 **Births:** 0 **Total Expense ($000):** 31153 **Payroll Expense ($000):** 17451 **Personnel:** 291

★ **KINDRED HOSPITAL DALLAS CENTRAL (452108)**, 8050 Meadows Road, Zip 75231; tel. 469/232–6500 **A**9 10 **F**1 3 29 40 45 75 77 85 87 96 107 113 129 147 **S** Kindred Healthcare, Louisville, KY
Primary Contact: Justin Smith, Interim Chief Executive Officer
Web address: www.khdallascentral.com/
**Control:** Corporation, Investor–owned, for–profit **Service:** Long–Term Acute Care hospital

> **Staffed Beds:** 60 **Admissions:** 518 **Census:** 33 **Outpatient Visits:** 10 **Births:** 0 **Total Expense ($000):** 19025 **Payroll Expense ($000):** 8904 **Personnel:** 152

**KINDRED HOSPITAL DALLAS–WALNUT HILL** See Kindred Hospital–Dallas

☒ **KINDRED HOSPITAL–DALLAS (452015)**, 9525 Greenville Avenue, Zip 75243–4116; tel. 214/355–2600, (Includes KINDRED HOSPITAL DALLAS–WALNUT HILL, 8200 Walnut Hill Lane, Zip 75231; tel. 214/345–6500) **A**1 9 10 **F**1 3 29 40 70 107 129 147 **P**5 **S** Kindred Healthcare, Louisville, KY
Primary Contact: Brenda Rowe, Chief Executive Officer
CFO: Jean McDowell, Chief Financial Officer
Web address: www.khdallas.com
**Control:** Partnership, Investor–owned, for–profit **Service:** Long–Term Acute Care hospital

> **Staffed Beds:** 100 **Admissions:** 417 **Census:** 31 **Outpatient Visits:** 0 **Births:** 0 **Total Expense ($000):** 18143 **Payroll Expense ($000):** 7660 **Personnel:** 147

☒ **KINDRED HOSPITAL–WHITE ROCK (452071)**, 9440 Poppy Drive, 5th Floor, Zip 75218; tel. 214/324–6562 **A**1 9 10 **F**1 29 85 86 87 129 147 **P**5 **S** Kindred Healthcare, Louisville, KY
Primary Contact: Justin Smith, Administrator
COO: Kim Chipman, Chief Clinical Officer
CFO: Jennifer Penland, Controller
CMO: Mark Ferris, M.D., Medical Director
Web address: www.khwhiterock.com
**Control:** Partnership, Investor–owned, for–profit **Service:** Long–Term Acute Care hospital

> **Staffed Beds:** 25 **Admissions:** 264 **Census:** 20 **Outpatient Visits:** 0 **Births:** 0 **Total Expense ($000):** 10046 **Payroll Expense ($000):** 4248 **Personnel:** 72

☒ **LIFECARE HOSPITALS OF DALLAS (452044)**, 6161 Harry Hines Boulevard, Suite 100, Zip 75235–5369; tel. 214/525–6300 **A**1 9 10 **F**1 3 26 29 30 45 64 147 **S** LifeCare Management Services, Plano, TX
Primary Contact: Jay Lindsey, Chief Executive Officer
CFO: Karin Bradford, Chief Financial Officer
CHR: Cathy Greenwood, Manager Human Resources
Web address: www.lifecare–hospitals.com
**Control:** Partnership, Investor–owned, for–profit **Service:** Long–Term Acute Care hospital

> **Staffed Beds:** 60 **Admissions:** 413 **Census:** 28 **Outpatient Visits:** 236 **Births:** 0 **Total Expense ($000):** 15234 **Payroll Expense ($000):** 7559 **Personnel:** 139

**LIFECARE HOSPITALS OF NORTH TEXAS** See LifeCare Hospitals of Dallas

**MARY SHIELS HOSPITAL** See Baylor Medical Center at Uptown

☒ **MEDICAL CITY DALLAS HOSPITAL (450647)**, 7777 Forest Lane, Zip 75230–2598; tel. 972/566–7000, (Includes MEDICAL CITY CHILDREN'S HOSPITAL, 7777 Forest Lane, Zip 75230–2505; tel. 972/566–7000) **A**1 2 3 5 9 10 **F**3 8 11 12 13 15 17 18 19 20 21 22 23 24 25 26 27 28 29 30 31 34 35 37 40 41 44 45 46 47 49 50 51 55 56 57 58 59 60 64 65 68 70 72 73 74 75 76 77 78 79 81 82 84 85 86 87 88 89 93 96 107 108 110 111 113 114 115 116 117 118 125 128 129 131 134 135 136 137 140 141 145 146 147 **P**6 7 **S** HCA, Nashville, TN
Primary Contact: Erol R. Akdamar, President and Chief Executive Officer
CFO: Mark Atchley, Vice President and Chief Financial Officer
CMO: Mark Hebert, M.D., President Medical Staff
CIO: Troy Sypien, Director Information Technology and Systems
CHR: Jenifer K. Tertel, Director Human Resources
Web address: www.medicalcityhospital.com
**Control:** Corporation, Investor–owned, for–profit **Service:** General Medical and Surgical

> **Staffed Beds:** 592 **Admissions:** 24902 **Census:** 374 **Outpatient Visits:** 158877 **Births:** 3194 **Total Expense ($000):** 405304 **Payroll Expense ($000):** 158777 **Personnel:** 2073

☒ **METHODIST CHARLTON MEDICAL CENTER (450723)**, 3500 West Wheatland Road, Zip 75237–3460, Mailing Address: P.O. Box 225357, Zip 75222–5357; tel. 214/947–7777 **A**1 9 10 13 **F**3 11 13 15 20 22 29 30 31 34 35 40 46 47 49 50 53 58 59 60 64 68 70 73 74 76 78 79 81 82 84 85 86 87 97 107 108 111 113 117 118 129 130 131 145 147 **P**1 6 7 **S** Methodist Health System, Dallas, TX
Primary Contact: Jonathan S. Davis, FACHE, President
CFO: Michael J. Schaefer, Executive Vice President and Chief Financial Officer
CMO: Allan Van Horn, M.D., President Medical Staff
CIO: Pamela McNutt, Vice President Information Systems
CHR: John S. Lacy, Senior Vice President Human Resources
Web address: www.mhs.com
**Control:** Other not–for–profit (including NFP Corporation) **Service:** General Medical and Surgical

> **Staffed Beds:** 258 **Admissions:** 12874 **Census:** 174 **Outpatient Visits:** 145610 **Births:** 1707 **Total Expense ($000):** 184946 **Payroll Expense ($000):** 87647 **Personnel:** 1380

---

**Hospital, Medicare Provider Number, Address, Telephone, Approval, Facility, and Physician Codes, Health Care System**

★ American Hospital Association (AHA) membership
☐ The Joint Commission accreditation
◇ DNV Healthcare Inc. accreditation
○ American Osteopathic Association (AOA) accreditation
△ Commission on Accreditation of Rehabilitation Facilities (CARF) accreditation

**TX**

✠ **METHODIST DALLAS MEDICAL CENTER (450051)**, 1441 North Beckley Avenue, Zip 75203–1201, Mailing Address: P.O. Box 655999, Zip 75265–5999; tel. 214/947–8181 **A**1 2 3 5 8 9 10 **F**3 11 12 13 15 17 18 20 22 24 26 28 29 30 31 34 35 37 40 43 45 46 47 48 49 50 53 54 58 59 60 64 66 68 70 72 74 76 78 79 81 82 84 85 87 92 93 97 107 108 110 111 117 118 125 129 131 137 138 141 145 147 **P**1 6 7 **S** Methodist Health System, Dallas, TX
Primary Contact: Laura Irvine, President
COO: Pamela Stoyanoff, Executive Vice President and Chief Operating Officer
CFO: Randy Walker, Vice President
CIO: Pamela McNutt, Senior Vice President and Chief Information Officer
CHR: Jackie Middleton, Vice President Human Resources
Web address: www.mhd.com
**Control:** Other not–for–profit (including NFP Corporation) **Service:** General Medical and Surgical

| | |
|---|---|
| **Staffed Beds:** 420 **Admissions:** 18015 **Census:** 258 **Outpatient Visits:** 155760 **Births:** 3400 **Total Expense ($000):** 343213 **Payroll Expense ($000):** 147914 **Personnel:** 2372 | |

☐ **METHODIST REHABILITATION HOSPITAL (673031)**, 3020 West Wheatland Road, Zip 75237–3537; tel. 972/708–8604 **A**1 9 10 **F**29 30 60 90 91 93 96 **S** Methodist Health System, Dallas, TX
Primary Contact: Barbara Mobley, Chief Executive Officer
Web address: www.methodist–rehab.com
**Control:** Partnership, Investor–owned, for–profit **Service:** Rehabilitation

| | |
|---|---|
| **Staffed Beds:** 40 **Admissions:** 901 **Census:** 30 **Outpatient Visits:** 11361 **Births:** 0 **Total Expense ($000):** 14541 **Payroll Expense ($000):** 7176 **Personnel:** 128 | |

☐ **NORTH CENTRAL SURGICAL CENTER (670049)**, 9301 North Central Expressway, Suite 100, Zip 75231; tel. 214/265–2810 **A**1 9 10 **F**3 40 45 79 81 82 85 107 111 113 114 118
Primary Contact: Suzanne Greever, Chief Executive Officer
COO: Keli Odom, Chief Operating Officer
CFO: Lisa Gildon, Chief Financial Officer
CMO: Stuart Simon, M.D., Medical Director
Web address: www.northcentral–sc.com/
**Control:** Partnership, Investor–owned, for–profit **Service:** Surgical

| | |
|---|---|
| **Staffed Beds:** 23 **Admissions:** 888 **Census:** 5 **Outpatient Visits:** 12046 **Births:** 0 **Total Expense ($000):** 48426 **Payroll Expense ($000):** 11383 **Personnel:** 221 | |

✠ **OUR CHILDREN'S HOUSE AT BAYLOR (453308)**, 3504 Swiss Avenue, Zip 75204–6224; tel. 214/820–9838 **A**1 9 10 **F**3 29 30 32 34 35 39 50 54 58 59 74 75 81 85 86 87 89 90 93 112 128 129 131 142 144 145 147 **S** Baylor Health Care System, Dallas, TX
Primary Contact: Elizabeth Youngblood, President
COO: Fabian Polo, Chief Operating Officer
CFO: Robert Knowlton, Vice President Finance
CMO: Andrew Gelfand, M.D., Medical Director
CHR: Karen Hill, Coordinator Human Resources
Web address: www.bhcs.com
**Control:** Other not–for–profit (including NFP Corporation) **Service:** Children's general

| | |
|---|---|
| **Staffed Beds:** 54 **Admissions:** 357 **Census:** 21 **Outpatient Visits:** 137278 **Births:** 0 **Total Expense ($000):** 35283 **Payroll Expense ($000):** 18394 **Personnel:** 296 | |

✠ **PARKLAND HEALTH & HOSPITAL SYSTEM (450015)**, 5201 Harry Hines Boulevard, Zip 75235–7731; tel. 214/590–8000 **A**1 2 3 5 8 9 10 **F**3 8 9 11 12 13 15 16 17 18 20 22 24 26 28 29 30 31 34 35 38 39 40 42 43 46 47 48 49 50 51 52 54 55 56 57 58 59 61 64 65 66 68 70 71 72 74 75 76 77 78 79 80 81 82 84 85 86 87 90 91 92 93 94 97 98 99 100 101 102 103 107 108 111 112 113 114 115 116 117 118 128 129 130 131 133 134 137 140 141 142 143 145 146 147 **P**1
Primary Contact: Thomas C. Royer, M.D., Interim Chief Executive Officer
CMO: John Jay Shannon, M.D., Chief Medical Officer
CIO: Jack Kowitt, Senior Vice President and Chief Information Officer
CNO: Mary K. Eagen, R.N., Executive Vice President, Chief Nursing Officer
Web address: www.parklandhospital.com
**Control:** Hospital district or authority, Government, nonfederal **Service:** General Medical and Surgical

| | |
|---|---|
| **Staffed Beds:** 784 **Admissions:** 37290 **Census:** 572 **Outpatient Visits:** 1245061 **Births:** 12391 **Total Expense ($000):** 1237477 **Payroll Expense ($000):** 553595 **Personnel:** 9054 | |

☐ **PINE CREEK MEDICAL CENTER (450894)**, 9032 Harry Hines Boulevard, Zip 75235; tel. 214/231–2273 **A**1 9 10 **F**3 12 29 30 34 40 42 45 49 51 64 79 81 82 85 93 107 111 113 **S** Physician Synergy Group, Irving, TX
Primary Contact: Corazon Ramirez, M.D., Chief Executive Officer
CFO: Michael Conroy, Chief Financial Officer
CIO: Kevin Carney, Senior Information Systems Analyst
Web address: www.pinecreekmedicalcenter.com
**Control:** Partnership, Investor–owned, for–profit **Service:** General Medical and Surgical

| | |
|---|---|
| **Staffed Beds:** 18 **Admissions:** 1216 **Census:** 7 **Outpatient Visits:** 4686 **Births:** 0 **Total Expense ($000):** 29419 **Payroll Expense ($000):** 8996 **Personnel:** 138 | |

**RELIANT REHABILITATION HOSPITAL DALLAS (673043)**, 7930 Northaven Road, Zip 75230–3331; tel. 214/706–8200 **F**3 29 40 64 68 74 75 77 86 87 90 91 93 96 118 129 147
Primary Contact: Randy Penny, Chief Executive Officer
CFO: Mary Mwaniki, Chief Financial Officer
CMO: Anna Freed–Sigurdsson, M.D., Medical Director
CIO: James E. King, Corporate Director Information Technology
CHR: Ieesha Cannida, Director Human Resources
CNO: Nancy Faas, R.N., Chief Nursing Officer
Web address: www.relianthcp.com
**Control:** Partnership, Investor–owned, for–profit **Service:** Rehabilitation

| | |
|---|---|
| **Staffed Beds:** 60 **Admissions:** 741 **Census:** 24 **Outpatient Visits:** 2516 **Births:** 0 **Total Expense ($000):** 12388 **Payroll Expense ($000):** 5190 **Personnel:** 73 | |

**SOUTH HAMPTON COMMUNITY HOSPITAL (670002)**, 2929 South Hampton Road, Zip 75224; tel. 214/623–4400 **A**9 10 **F**3 12 29 30 34 40 45 46 47 49 50 51 56 60 64 70 79 81 85 89 93 107 108 111 114 118 128 129 147 **S** Renaissance Healthcare Systems, Houston, TX
Primary Contact: Steven Walker, Chief Executive Officer
Web address: www.shchospital.com
**Control:** Partnership, Investor–owned, for–profit **Service:** General Medical and Surgical

| | |
|---|---|
| **Staffed Beds:** 90 **Admissions:** 1921 **Census:** 24 **Outpatient Visits:** 19959 **Births:** 0 **Total Expense ($000):** 29682 **Payroll Expense ($000):** 12154 **Personnel:** 205 | |

✠ △ **TEXAS HEALTH PRESBYTERIAN HOSPITAL DALLAS (450462)**, 8200 Walnut Hill Lane, Zip 75231–4402; tel. 214/345–6789 **A**1 2 3 5 7 9 10 **F**3 5 11 12 13 15 17 18 19 20 22 24 26 28 29 30 31 32 34 35 36 37 38 40 44 45 46 47 49 50 51 52 53 54 55 56 57 58 59 60 61 62 63 64 65 66 68 70 72 74 75 76 77 78 79 80 81 82 85 86 87 90 91 92 93 94 95 96 97 98 100 101 102 103 104 105 107 108 110 111 112 113 114 117 118 123 125 128 129 130 131 134 142 143 144 145 146 147 **P**6 **S** Texas Health Resources, Arlington, TX
Primary Contact: Britt Berrett, President and Chief Executive Officer
COO: James A. Berg, Senior Vice President and Chief Quality Officer
CFO: Mark Meyer, Vice President and Chief Financial Officer
CMO: Mark Lester, M.D., Vice President and Chief Quality Officer
CHR: Connie Wright, Director Human Resources
CNO: Cole Edmonson, R.N., Vice President and Chief Nursing Officer
Web address: www.texashealth.org
**Control:** Other not–for–profit (including NFP Corporation) **Service:** General Medical and Surgical

| | |
|---|---|
| **Staffed Beds:** 631 **Admissions:** 27353 **Census:** 424 **Outpatient Visits:** 386172 **Births:** 5556 **Total Expense ($000):** 541155 **Payroll Expense ($000):** 195050 **Personnel:** 2831 | |

**TEXAS HOSPITAL FOR ADVANCED MEDICINE** See Dallas Medical Center

☐ **TEXAS INSTITUTE FOR SURGERY AT TEXAS HEALTH PRESBYTERIAN DALLAS (450889)**, 7115 Greenville Avenue, Zip 75231–5101; tel. 214/647–5300 **A**1 9 10 **F**40 51 64 79 81 107 128 **P**2
Primary Contact: David Helfer, President
CFO: Andrew Summers, Vice President Business Operations
CMO: Presley Mock, M.D., Chief of Staff
CHR: Jack Martin, Director Human Resources
CNO: Joy Dier, R.N., Vice President Clinical Services and Chief Nursing Officer
Web address: www.texasinstituteforsurgery.com
**Control:** Partnership, Investor–owned, for–profit **Service:** General Medical and Surgical

| | |
|---|---|
| **Staffed Beds:** 9 **Admissions:** 71 **Census:** 1 **Outpatient Visits:** 12281 **Births:** 0 **Total Expense ($000):** 38131 **Payroll Expense ($000):** 8477 **Personnel:** 138 | |

✠ **TEXAS SCOTTISH RITE HOSPITAL FOR CHILDREN**, 2222 Welborn Street, Zip 75219–9982, Mailing Address: P.O. Box 190567, Zip 75219–0567; tel. 214/559–5000 **A**1 3 5 **F**3 9 11 29 30 34 35 39 44 50 53 58 64 68 74 75 77 79 81 85 86 87 89 92 94 107 111 114 118 129 131 142 145 147 **P**6
Primary Contact: Robert L. Walker, President and Chief Executive Officer
CFO: John T. Schoonmaker, Senior Vice President and Chief Financial Officer
CMO: Steve Richards, M.D., Chief Medical Officer
CIO: Hunt Gregg, Director Information Systems
CHR: James D. Sturgis, Director Human Resources
Web address: www.tsrhc.org
**Control:** Other not–for–profit (including NFP Corporation) **Service:** Children's orthopedic

| | |
|---|---|
| **Staffed Beds:** 52 **Admissions:** 1853 **Census:** 20 **Outpatient Visits:** 37878 **Births:** 0 **Total Expense ($000):** 97507 **Personnel:** 774 | |

**TX**

*Many Facility Codes have changed. Please refer to the AHA Guide Code Chart.* © 2012 AHA Guide

☐ **TEXAS SPECIALTY HOSPITAL AT DALLAS (452067)**, 7955 Harry Hines Boulevard, Zip 75235–3395; tel. 214/637–0000 **A**1 9 10 **F**1 29 30 64 75 85 87 147 **S** Fundamental Long Term Care Holdings, LLC, Sparks Glencoe, MD
Primary Contact: Glenna Carver, R.N., Chief Executive Officer
CFO: Diana B. Smith, Chief Financial Officer
CMO: Gary E. Goff, M.D., Medical Director
CHR: Ginger Davenport, Director Human Resources
Web address: www.thicare.com
**Control:** Corporation, Investor–owned, for–profit **Service:** Long–Term Acute Care hospital

**Staffed Beds:** 62 **Admissions:** 191 **Census:** 12 **Outpatient Visits:** 391
**Births:** 0 **Total Expense ($000):** 9307 **Payroll Expense ($000):** 2631
**Personnel:** 47

☐ **TIMBERLAWN MENTAL HEALTH SYSTEM (454081)**, 4600 Samuell Boulevard, Zip 75228–6800; tel. 214/381–7181 **A**1 9 10 **F**4 5 54 56 59 64 87 98 99 100 101 102 103 104 105 129 131 142 **S** Universal Health Services, Inc., King of Prussia, PA
Primary Contact: Craig Nuckles, Chief Executive Officer, Managing and Regional Vice President
CFO: Lori Verbeke, Chief Financial Officer
CMO: John Pascoe, M.D., Executive Medical Director
CIO: Angela L. Pruitt, Director Health Information Management and Quality Improvement
CHR: Winnie Boehnke, Director Human Resources
Web address: www.timberlawn.com
**Control:** Corporation, Investor–owned, for–profit **Service:** Psychiatric

**Staffed Beds:** 144 **Admissions:** 5793 **Census:** 120 **Outpatient Visits:** 18721
**Births:** 0 **Total Expense ($000):** 22253 **Payroll Expense ($000):** 10309
**Personnel:** 233

✖ △ **UNIVERSITY OF TEXAS SOUTHWESTERN MEDICAL CENTER (450766)**, 5323 Harry Hines Boulevard, Zip 75390–9265; tel. 214/645–5555, (Includes UNIVERSITY OF TEXAS SOUTHWESTERN MEDICAL CENTER – ST. PAUL, 5909 Harry Hines Boulevard, Zip 75390–9200; tel. 214/645–5555; UNIVERSITY OF TEXAS SOUTHWESTERN MEDICAL CENTER – ZALE LIPSHY, 5151 Harry Hines Boulevard, tel. 214/645–5555; Daniel Podolsky, M.D., President) **A**1 2 3 5 7 8 9 10 **F**3 6 7 8 9 11 12 13 15 17 18 20 22 24 26 28 29 30 31 34 35 36 38 39 40 44 45 46 47 48 49 50 52 53 54 55 56 57 58 59 60 61 62 64 65 66 68 70 71 72 74 75 76 77 78 79 80 81 82 84 85 86 87 90 91 92 93 94 95 96 97 98 99 100 101 102 103 104 107 108 109 110 111 113 114 115 116 117 118 119 120 122 123 125 128 129 130 131 134 135 136 137 138 139 140 141 142 144 145 146 147 **P**5 6
Primary Contact: John Warner, M.D., Chief Executive Officer
CMO: Steven Leach, M.D., Chief Medical Officer
CIO: Suresh Gunasekaran, Assistant Vice President Information Resources
CHR: William Behrendt, Ph.D., Vice President Human Resources
Web address: www.utsouthwestern.edu
**Control:** State–Government, nonfederal **Service:** General Medical and Surgical

**Staffed Beds:** 464 **Admissions:** 20003 **Census:** 332 **Outpatient Visits:** 229176 **Births:** 1452 **Total Expense ($000):** 481884 **Payroll Expense ($000):** 181756 **Personnel:** 2903

✖ △ **VETERANS AFFAIRS NORTH TEXAS HEALTH CARE SYSTEM**, 4500 South Lancaster Road, Zip 75216–7167; tel. 214/742–8387, (Includes SAM RAYBURN MEMORIAL VETERANS CENTER, 1201 East Ninth Street, Bonham, Zip 75418–4091; tel. 903/583–2111), (Nonreporting) **A**1 2 3 5 7 9 **S** Department of Veterans Affairs, Washington, DC
Primary Contact: Mark Doskocil, Acting Director
CFO: Garry Martin, Chief Fiscal
CIO: Lucy Rogers, Chief Information Resource Management Systems
Web address: www.va.gov/sta/guide/home.asp
**Control:** Veterans Affairs, Government, federal **Service:** General Medical and Surgical

**Staffed Beds:** 875

### DE SOTO—Dallas County

✖ **SELECT SPECIALTY HOSPITAL–SOUTH DALLAS (452078)**, 800 Kirnwood Drive, Zip 75115; tel. 972/780–6500 **A**1 9 10 **F**1 3 29 40 85 107 129 147 **S** Select Medical Corporation, Mechanicsburg, PA
Primary Contact: Jeff Jennings, Chief Executive Officer
Web address: www.selectmedicalcorp.com
**Control:** Corporation, Investor–owned, for–profit **Service:** Long–Term Acute Care hospital

**Staffed Beds:** 100 **Admissions:** 535 **Census:** 37 **Outpatient Visits:** 0 **Births:** 0 **Total Expense ($000):** 20325 **Payroll Expense ($000):** 7188 **Personnel:** 124

### DECATUR—Wise County

✖ **WISE REGIONAL HEALTH SYSTEM (450271)**, 2000 South FM 51, Zip 76234–3702; tel. 940/627–5921 **A**1 2 9 10 **F**3 11 12 13 15 17 18 20 22 24 26 28 29 30 31 32 34 40 43 45 47 49 51 53 54 56 57 59 60 64 70 74 75 76 77 78 79 81 85 87 89 90 93 96 97 98 103 104 107 108 110 111 113 114 115 117 118 128 129 130 131 134 146 147 **P**7
Primary Contact: Stephen M. Summers, CPA, FACHE, Chief Executive Officer
COO: Leon Fuqua, Assistant Administrator
CFO: Jim Eaton, Chief Financial Officer
CMO: Jon Walker, M.D., Chief of Staff
CIO: Joe Arispie, Director Information Systems
CHR: Mike McQuiston, Director Human Resources
Web address: www.wiseregional.com
**Control:** Hospital district or authority, Government, nonfederal **Service:** General Medical and Surgical

**Staffed Beds:** 133 **Admissions:** 4899 **Census:** 57 **Outpatient Visits:** 169595
**Births:** 480 **Total Expense ($000):** 117042 **Payroll Expense ($000):** 40373
**Personnel:** 896

### DEL RIO—Val Verde County

✖ **VAL VERDE REGIONAL MEDICAL CENTER (450154)**, 801 Bedell Avenue, Zip 78840–4112; tel. 830/775–8566 **A**1 9 10 20 **F**3 7 11 13 15 18 20 29 30 34 35 40 43 46 48 54 57 59 63 73 75 76 77 79 81 84 85 87 89 93 96 107 108 110 111 113 118 128 130 131 132 145 146
Primary Contact: Marc Strode, Chief Executive Officer
CHR: John Furman, Director Human Resources
Web address: www.vvrmc.org
**Control:** Hospital district or authority, Government, nonfederal **Service:** General Medical and Surgical

**Staffed Beds:** 80 **Admissions:** 3212 **Census:** 30 **Outpatient Visits:** 49519
**Births:** 902 **Total Expense ($000):** 42440 **Payroll Expense ($000):** 19392
**Personnel:** 411

### DENISON—Grayson County

☐ **TEXOMA MEDICAL CENTER (450324)**, 5016 U.S. Highway 75 S., Zip 75020–2035, Mailing Address: P.O. Box 890, Zip 75021–0890; tel. 903/416–4000 **A**1 9 10 **F**3 11 12 13 15 17 18 20 22 24 28 29 30 31 34 40 41 43 45 46 47 49 50 53 57 59 62 64 70 74 75 76 77 78 79 81 85 86 89 90 93 96 98 99 100 101 102 103 104 105 107 108 110 111 114 118 128 129 131 143 144 145 146 147 **P**6 7 **S** Universal Health Services, Inc., King of Prussia, PA
Primary Contact: Ronald T. Seal, Chief Executive Officer
COO: Justin Kendrick, Chief Operating Officer
CFO: Bobby Pruiett, Chief Financial Officer
CMO: Robert Sanders, M.D., Chief Medical Officer
CHR: Minnie Burkhardt, Associate Administrator
Web address: www.texomamedicalcenter.net
**Control:** Corporation, Investor–owned, for–profit **Service:** General Medical and Surgical

**Staffed Beds:** 251 **Admissions:** 9837 **Census:** 158 **Outpatient Visits:** 67879
**Births:** 697 **Total Expense ($000):** 129030 **Payroll Expense ($000):** 52741
**Personnel:** 1089

### DENTON—Denton County

✖ **DENTON REGIONAL MEDICAL CENTER (450634)**, 3535 South 1–35 East, Zip 76210; tel. 940/384–3535 **A**1 2 9 10 **F**3 12 13 18 20 22 24 26 28 29 30 34 35 40 43 45 46 47 49 50 57 59 64 66 68 69 70 74 75 76 77 79 81 82 84 85 86 87 93 95 96 107 108 111 113 117 118 125 129 131 134 145 146 147 **S** HCA, Nashville, TN
Primary Contact: Caleb F. O'Rear, Chief Executive Officer
COO: Jeffrey T. Lawrence, Chief Operating Officer
CMO: Filippo Masciarelli, M.D., Chief of Staff
CHR: Jenna Sutherland, Manager Human Resources
Web address: www.dentonregional.com
**Control:** Partnership, Investor–owned, for–profit **Service:** General Medical and Surgical

**Staffed Beds:** 208 **Admissions:** 10677 **Census:** 131 **Outpatient Visits:** 99928 **Births:** 975 **Total Expense ($000):** 126774 **Payroll Expense ($000):** 50928 **Personnel:** 688

☐ **INTEGRITY TRANSITIONAL HOSPITAL (452109)**, 2813 South Mayhill Road, Zip 76208; tel. 940/320–2300 **A**1 9 10 **F**1 3 29 40 42 77 84 86 87 91 129 147 **P**5
Primary Contact: Christy Carver, Administrator
Web address: www.ithdenton.com
**Control:** Partnership, Investor–owned, for–profit **Service:** General Medical and Surgical

**Staffed Beds:** 54 **Admissions:** 310 **Census:** 21 **Outpatient Visits:** 0 **Births:** 0 **Total Expense ($000):** 10115 **Payroll Expense ($000):** 3963 **Personnel:** 74

TX

---

**Hospital, Medicare Provider Number, Address, Telephone, Approval, Facility, and Physician Codes, Health Care System**

★ American Hospital Association (AHA) membership
☐ The Joint Commission accreditation    ◇ DNV Healthcare Inc. accreditation

○ American Osteopathic Association (AOA) accreditation
△ Commission on Accreditation of Rehabilitation Facilities (CARF) accreditation

**TX**

**MAYHILL HOSPITAL (670010)**, 2809 South Mayhill Road, Zip 76208–5910; tel. 940/239–3000 **A**9 10 **F**4 29 40 56 82 98 102 103 104 129 **S** Ascend Health Corporation, New York, NY
Primary Contact: Susan M. Young, Chief Executive Officer
CFO: Lori Davis, Chief Financial Officer
CMO: Gary Watts, M.D., Chief Medical Officer
CIO: Darla Powell, Administrative Assistant
CHR: Kashion Lewis, Director Human Resources
Web address: www.mayhillhospital.com
**Control:** Partnership, Investor–owned, for–profit **Service:** Psychiatric

**Staffed Beds:** 59 **Admissions:** 1019 **Census:** 26 **Outpatient Visits:** 2333 **Births:** 0 **Total Expense ($000):** 6968 **Payroll Expense ($000):** 2635 **Personnel:** 60

**NORTH TEXAS HOSPITAL (450893)**, 2801 South Mayhill Road, Zip 76208–5910; tel. 940/220–0600 **A**9 10 21 **F**3 12 29 40 45 47 49 51 74 79 81 82 85 107 111 113 117 118 125 147 **S** Cirrus Health, Dallas, TX
Primary Contact: Judith Schiros, Chief Executive Officer and Administrator
Web address: www.northtexashospital.com
**Control:** Partnership, Investor–owned, for–profit **Service:** General Medical and Surgical

**Staffed Beds:** 16 **Admissions:** 453 **Census:** 2 **Outpatient Visits:** 9474 **Births:** 0 **Total Expense ($000):** 25245 **Payroll Expense ($000):** 6673 **Personnel:** 77

☒ **SELECT REHABILITATION HOSPITAL OF DENTON (673036)**, 2620 Scripture Street, Zip 76201; tel. 940/297–6500 **A**1 9 10 **F**3 29 40 60 64 68 74 75 77 79 87 90 93 96 134 147 **P**6 **S** Select Medical Corporation, Mechanicsburg, PA
Primary Contact: Michele Powell, Chief Executive Officer
Web address: www.selectrehab–denton.com/
**Control:** Corporation, Investor–owned, for–profit **Service:** Rehabilitation

**Staffed Beds:** 44 **Admissions:** 767 **Census:** 26 **Outpatient Visits:** 1475 **Births:** 0 **Total Expense ($000):** 12018 **Payroll Expense ($000):** 7042 **Personnel:** 90

☒ **TEXAS HEALTH PRESBYTERIAN HOSPITAL DENTON (450743)**, 3000 I. 35 North, Zip 76201–3798; tel. 940/898–7000 **A**1 9 10 **F**3 11 12 13 15 18 20 22 24 26 28 29 30 31 34 35 40 45 46 48 49 57 59 70 72 74 75 76 78 79 81 82 85 86 89 93 107 108 110 111 113 114 117 118 128 129 130 131 134 144 145 146 147 **S** Texas Health Resources, Arlington, TX
Primary Contact: Stan C. Morton, FACHE, President
COO: Jeff Reecer, Chief Operating Officer
CFO: David B. Meltzer, Chief Financial Officer
CMO: Bob Schwab, M.D., Chief Quality Officer
CIO: Ellen Painter, Director Marketing
CHR: Donna Coleman, Director Human Resources
Web address: www.dentonhospital.com
**Control:** Other not–for–profit (including NFP Corporation) **Service:** General Medical and Surgical

**Staffed Beds:** 208 **Admissions:** 9627 **Census:** 119 **Outpatient Visits:** 69890 **Births:** 1932 **Total Expense ($000):** 149169 **Payroll Expense ($000):** 55382 **Personnel:** 832

☒ **UNIVERSITY BEHAVIORAL HEALTH OF DENTON (454104)**, 2026 West University Drive, Zip 76201–0644; tel. 940/320–8100 **A**1 9 10 **F**4 5 54 98 100 102 103 104 105 **S** Ascend Health Corporation, New York, NY
Primary Contact: Susan M. Young, Chief Executive Officer
CFO: Cathi Ledet, Comptroller
CMO: Atique Khan, M.D., Medical Director
CIO: Elizabeth Pratt, Director Health Information Management
CHR: Russell Allison, Human Resources Representative
CNO: Patricia Brewer, Chief Nursing Officer
Web address: www.ubhdenton.net
**Control:** Partnership, Investor–owned, for–profit **Service:** Psychiatric

**Staffed Beds:** 104 **Admissions:** 3230 **Census:** 90 **Outpatient Visits:** 11847 **Births:** 0 **Total Expense ($000):** 15605 **Payroll Expense ($000):** 9103 **Personnel:** 219

**DENVER CITY—Yoakum County**

★ **YOAKUM COUNTY HOSPITAL (451308)**, 412 Mustang Avenue, Zip 79323–2750, Mailing Address: P.O. Box 1130, Zip 79323–1130; tel. 806/592–2121 **A**9 10 18 **F**3 11 13 28 29 34 35 40 43 50 53 57 59 60 62 64 76 81 87 89 93 107 114 118 126 128 132 145 **P**6
Primary Contact: Chris Ekrem, Chief Executive Officer
CFO: Suann Parrish, Chief Financial Officer
CMO: Dan Khan, M.D., Chief Medical Officer
CIO: Todd Carrillo, Chief Information Officer
CHR: Teresa Howard, Manager Human Resources
Web address: www.ych.us
**Control:** County–Government, nonfederal **Service:** General Medical and Surgical

**Staffed Beds:** 22 **Admissions:** 627 **Census:** 7 **Outpatient Visits:** 59650 **Births:** 128 **Total Expense ($000):** 19791 **Payroll Expense ($000):** 7005 **Personnel:** 172

**DESOTO—Dallas County**

☐ **HICKORY TRAIL HOSPITAL (454065)**, 2000 Old Hickory Trail, Zip 75115–2242; tel. 972/298–7323 **A**1 9 10 **F**4 5 29 38 98 99 103 104 105 129 **S** Universal Health Services, Inc., King of Prussia, PA
Primary Contact: Mercy Estevez, Chief Executive Officer
CFO: Terri Logsdon, Chief Financial Officer
CMO: Manoochehr Khatami, M.D., Medical Director
CHR: Sarah Warren, Coordinator Human Resources
Web address: www.hickorytrail.com
**Control:** Corporation, Investor–owned, for–profit **Service:** Psychiatric

**Staffed Beds:** 86 **Admissions:** 2958 **Census:** 64 **Outpatient Visits:** 10555 **Births:** 0 **Total Expense ($000):** 11932 **Payroll Expense ($000):** 7796 **Personnel:** 226

☐ **VIBRA SPECIALTY HOSPITAL OF DALLAS (452097)**, 2700 Walker Way, Zip 75115–2088; tel. 214/638–1500 **A**1 9 10 **F**1 3 29 75 77 87 91 129 147 **S** Vibra Healthcare, Mechanicsburg, PA
Primary Contact: Paul P. Hall, Jr., Chief Executive Officer and Chief Clinical Officer
CFO: Donald Trimble, CPA, Chief Financial Officer
CMO: Lauren McDonald, M.D., Medical Director and Medical Staff President
CHR: Tim Lozier, Director Human Resources
Web address: www.vibrahealthcare.com
**Control:** Corporation, Investor–owned, for–profit **Service:** Long–Term Acute Care hospital

**Staffed Beds:** 60 **Admissions:** 469 **Census:** 37 **Outpatient Visits:** 2665 **Births:** 0 **Total Expense ($000):** 19386 **Payroll Expense ($000):** 7835 **Personnel:** 102

**DILLEY—Frio County**

☐ **COMMUNITY GENERAL HOSPITAL (450813)**, 230 West Miller, Zip 78017; tel. 830/965–2003 **A**1 9 10 **F**1 3 4 16 17 29 34 40 57 59 64 67 70 72 73 80 88 89 90 97 98 107 126 127 147 **P**5
Primary Contact: Syed Parvez, M.D., Administrator
**Control:** Corporation, Investor–owned, for–profit **Service:** General Medical and Surgical

**Staffed Beds:** 18 **Admissions:** 675 **Census:** 4 **Outpatient Visits:** 5439 **Births:** 0 **Total Expense ($000):** 2749 **Payroll Expense ($000):** 1385 **Personnel:** 46

**DIMMITT—Castro County**

★ **PLAINS MEMORIAL HOSPITAL (451350)**, 310 West Halsell Street, Zip 79027–1846, Mailing Address: P.O. Box 278, Zip 79027–0278; tel. 806/647–2191 **A**9 10 18 **F**7 32 34 35 40 43 53 57 59 64 65 69 75 77 81 82 85 86 87 93 97 107 113 118 126 129 132 134 147 **P**6
Primary Contact: Linda Rasor, R.N., Chief Executive Officer
COO: Peggy A. Bradley, Chief Operating Officer
CFO: Milton Wilhite, Chief Financial Officer
CMO: Daniel Griffis, M.D., Medical Director
CIO: Milton Wilhite, Chief Financial Officer
CHR: Debbie Underwood, Manager Human Resources
Web address: www.plainsmemorial.com
**Control:** Hospital district or authority, Government, nonfederal **Service:** General Medical and Surgical

**Staffed Beds:** 25 **Admissions:** 351 **Census:** 5 **Outpatient Visits:** 30834 **Births:** 0 **Personnel:** 93

**DUMAS—Moore County**

☐ **MOORE COUNTY HOSPITAL DISTRICT (450221)**, 224 East Second Street, Zip 79029–3808; tel. 806/935–7171 **A**1 9 10 20 **F**3 7 11 13 15 28 34 35 39 40 43 46 50 51 57 59 62 63 70 75 76 77 79 81 85 86 89 91 93 107 111 114 118 129 130 131 132 145 146 147
Primary Contact: Jeff Turner, FACHE, Chief Executive Officer
COO: Yvonne Blue, Chief Operations Officer
CFO: John E. Bailey, Chief Financial Officer
CHR: Ashleigh Wiswell, Director Human Resources
CNO: Stacey Cropley, M.D., Chief Nursing Officer
Web address: www.mchd.net
**Control:** Hospital district or authority, Government, nonfederal **Service:** General Medical and Surgical

**Staffed Beds:** 47 **Admissions:** 1087 **Census:** 9 **Outpatient Visits:** 30158 **Births:** 269 **Total Expense ($000):** 23459 **Payroll Expense ($000):** 11503 **Personnel:** 245

## EAGLE LAKE—Colorado County

★ **RICE MEDICAL CENTER (451312)**, 600 South Austin Road, Zip 77434-3298, Mailing Address: P.O. Box 277, Zip 77434-0277; tel. 979/234-5571 **A**9 10 18 **F**11 13 15 29 40 43 57 59 64 65 70 76 79 81 107 118 126 132 **P**6 **S** CHRISTUS Health, Irving, TX
Primary Contact: James D. Janek, Chief Executive Officer
CFO: Noble Anderson, Director Patient Financial Services
CMO: Ray Cantu, D.O., Chief of Staff
CHR: Darilyn Henderson, Human Resources Officer
Web address: www.ricemedicalcenter.org
**Control:** Corporation, Investor-owned, for-profit **Service:** General Medical and Surgical

**Staffed Beds:** 15 **Admissions:** 334 **Census:** 4 **Outpatient Visits:** 13787 **Births:** 36 **Total Expense ($000):** 10899 **Payroll Expense ($000):** 3073 **Personnel:** 88

## EAGLE PASS—Maverick County

☐ **FORT DUNCAN REGIONAL MEDICAL CENTER (450092)**, 3333 North Foster Maldonado Boulevard, Zip 78852-5893; tel. 830/773-5321 **A**1 9 10 **F**3 13 15 29 35 40 43 46 57 59 60 64 65 68 70 75 76 77 79 81 86 87 89 90 93 107 110 111 113 118 128 129 145 146 147 **S** Universal Health Services, Inc., King of Prussia, PA
Primary Contact: Rene Lopez, Chief Executive Officer
COO: Richard Prati, Chief Operating Officer
CFO: Joel Morales, Chief Financial Officer
CMO: David Land, D.O., Chief Medical Staff
CIO: Tony Hernandez, Director Information Technology
CHR: Daisy Rodriquez, Director Human Resources
CNO: Wilma Carbonel Mason, Chief Nursing Officer
Web address: www.fortduncanmedicalcenter.com
**Control:** Corporation, Investor-owned, for-profit **Service:** General Medical and Surgical

**Staffed Beds:** 101 **Admissions:** 5163 **Census:** 58 **Outpatient Visits:** 41987 **Births:** 1119 **Total Expense ($000):** 47866 **Payroll Expense ($000):** 19759 **Personnel:** 357

## EASTLAND—Eastland County

★ **EASTLAND MEMORIAL HOSPITAL (450411)**, 304 South Daugherty Street, Zip 76448-2609, Mailing Address: P.O. Box 897, Zip 76448-0897; tel. 254/629-2601 **A**9 10 20 **F**7 11 15 28 30 34 40 43 49 50 53 56 57 59 64 65 68 75 81 85 86 87 93 107 111 118 129 130 145 147
Primary Contact: Ted Matthews, Chief Executive Officer
Web address: www.eastlandmemorial.com
**Control:** Hospital district or authority, Government, nonfederal **Service:** General Medical and Surgical

**Staffed Beds:** 36 **Admissions:** 1112 **Census:** 12 **Outpatient Visits:** 23065 **Births:** 2 **Total Expense ($000):** 9698 **Payroll Expense ($000):** 5904 **Personnel:** 154

## EDEN—Concho County

**CONCHO COUNTY HOSPITAL (451325)**, 614 Eaker Street, Zip 76837-0359, Mailing Address: P.O. Box 987, Zip 76837-0987; tel. 325/869-5911 **A**9 10 18 **F**3 40 43 50 57 59 68 77 87 107 132 145
Primary Contact: Dudley R. White, Administrator and Chief Executive Officer
CFO: Melanie Lozano, Chief Financial Officer
Web address: www.conchocountyhospital.com
**Control:** Hospital district or authority, Government, nonfederal **Service:** General Medical and Surgical

**Staffed Beds:** 16 **Admissions:** 74 **Census:** 1 **Outpatient Visits:** 4487 **Births:** 0 **Total Expense ($000):** 3143 **Payroll Expense ($000):** 1351 **Personnel:** 28

## EDINBURG—Hidalgo County

⌧ **CORNERSTONE REGIONAL HOSPITAL (450825)**, 2302 Cornerstone Boulevard, Zip 78539-8471; tel. 956/618-4444 **A**1 9 10 **F**3 8 29 37 39 40 45 46 51 57 64 74 79 81 82 85 87 118 **P**8 **S** Universal Health Services, Inc., King of Prussia, PA
Primary Contact: Alma Medina, R.N., Chief Executive Officer
COO: Silvia Guerrero, Chief Accountant
CFO: Chris Garza, Director Patient Financial Services
CMO: John G. Orfanos, M.D., Chief of Staff
CHR: Erika Betancourt, Coordinator Human Resources
Web address: www.southtexashealthsystem.com/Facilities/Cornerstone-Regional-Hospital
**Control:** Partnership, Investor-owned, for-profit **Service:** General Medical and Surgical

**Staffed Beds:** 14 **Admissions:** 440 **Census:** 3 **Outpatient Visits:** 2481 **Births:** 0 **Total Expense ($000):** 10966 **Payroll Expense ($000):** 2769 **Personnel:** 74

☐ **DOCTOR'S HOSPITAL AT RENAISSANCE (450869)**, 5501 South McColl Road, Zip 78539-9152; tel. 956/362-7360 **A**1 9 10 **F**3 12 13 15 17 18 20 22 24 26 28 29 30 31 34 35 38 39 40 45 46 47 49 50 51 57 58 59 60 64 65 70 72 73 74 75 76 77 78 79 81 82 84 85 87 88 89 90 93 96 98 99 100 101 102 103 107 108 110 111 112 113 114 115 116 117 118 119 120 122 123 125 129 131 144 145 146 147 **P**3 8
Primary Contact: Lawrence Gelman, M.D., Chief Executive Officer
COO: Marissa Castaneda, Chief Operating Officer and Director Marketing
CFO: Susan S. Turley, Chief Financial Officer
Web address: www.dhr-rgv.com
**Control:** Partnership, Investor-owned, for-profit **Service:** General Medical and Surgical

**Staffed Beds:** 506 **Admissions:** 29924 **Census:** 378 **Outpatient Visits:** 199233 **Births:** 8713 **Total Expense ($000):** 318477 **Payroll Expense ($000):** 141264 **Personnel:** 2949

☐ **SOUTH TEXAS HEALTH SYSTEM (450119)**, 1102 West Trenton Road, Zip 78539-9105; tel. 956/388-6000, (Includes EDINBURG CHILDREN'S HOSPITAL, 1400 West Trenton Road, Zip 78539; tel. 956/388-8000; EDINBURG REGIONAL MEDICAL CENTER, 1102 West Trenton Road, Zip 78539-6199; tel. 956/388-6000; MCALLEN HEART HOSPITAL, 1900 South D. Street, McAllen, Zip 78503; tel. 956/994-2000; MCALLEN MEDICAL CENTER, 301 West Expressway 83, McAllen, Zip 78503-3045; tel. 956/632-4000; SOUTH TEXAS BEHAVIORAL HEALTH CENTER, 2101 West Trenton Road, Zip 78539; tel. 956/388-1300; Joe Rodriguez, Chief Executive Officer) **A**1 9 10 **F**3 4 11 12 13 15 17 18 20 22 24 26 29 30 31 34 35 37 38 39 40 41 43 45 46 47 48 49 50 53 57 59 60 68 70 72 74 75 76 77 78 79 81 85 86 87 88 89 90 96 98 99 100 101 102 103 104 107 108 110 111 113 114 118 128 129 134 137 145 147 **P**6 8 **S** Universal Health Services, Inc., King of Prussia, PA
Primary Contact: Linda Resendez, R.N., Chief Executive Officer
COO: Mike Adams, Chief Operating Officer
CMO: Humberto Hidalgo, M.D., Chief of Staff
CIO: Rosie L. Mendiola, Director Information Systems
CHR: Cindi Mistrot, Associate Administrator
Web address: www.southtexashealthsystem.com
**Control:** Partnership, Investor-owned, for-profit **Service:** General Medical and Surgical

**Staffed Beds:** 775 **Admissions:** 25545 **Census:** 336 **Outpatient Visits:** 92501 **Births:** 1354 **Total Expense ($000):** 292413 **Payroll Expense ($000):** 97553 **Personnel:** 1969

## EDNA—Jackson County

★ **JACKSON COUNTY HOSPITAL DISTRICT (451363)**, 1013 South Wells Street, Zip 77957-4098; tel. 361/782-7800 **A**9 10 18 **F**15 34 40 43 45 50 56 57 59 62 64 65 68 75 81 87 93 103 104 107 110 111 113 118 126 128 129 130 132 145 147 **P**8
Primary Contact: Bill Jones, Administrator
CFO: William Satrom, Chief Financial Officer
CMO: Deepinder Judge, M.D., Chief of Staff
CIO: Donna Coleman, Director Professional Services
CIO: Donna Coleman, Director Professional Services
CHR: Mindy Curlee, Coordinator Human Resources
Web address: www.jchd.org
**Control:** Hospital district or authority, Government, nonfederal **Service:** General Medical and Surgical

**Staffed Beds:** 25 **Admissions:** 453 **Census:** 4 **Outpatient Visits:** 15033 **Births:** 0 **Total Expense ($000):** 13181 **Payroll Expense ($000):** 4654 **Personnel:** 113

## EL CAMPO—Wharton County

**EL CAMPO MEMORIAL HOSPITAL (450694)**, 303 Sandy Corner Road, Zip 77437-9535; tel. 979/543-6251 **A**9 10 **F**3 11 15 29 34 35 40 45 56 57 59 60 62 64 68 70 75 77 79 81 85 86 93 97 107 108 110 111 113 118 126 128 129 130 131 132 147 **P**6
Primary Contact: Tisha Zalman, Chief Executive Officer
CFO: Gwynn Wigginton, Controller
CMO: Patrick Johnson, D.O., Chief of Staff
CHR: Pat Trigg, Coordinator Personnel and Credentialing
CNO: Desiree Vrazel, Director of Nurses
Web address: www.ecmh.org
**Control:** Hospital district or authority, Government, nonfederal **Service:** General Medical and Surgical

**Staffed Beds:** 30 **Admissions:** 678 **Census:** 7 **Outpatient Visits:** 54183 **Births:** 0 **Total Expense ($000):** 14982 **Payroll Expense ($000):** 5840 **Personnel:** 123

**TX**

**Hospital, Medicare Provider Number, Address, Telephone, Approval, Facility, and Physician Codes, Health Care System**

★ American Hospital Association (AHA) membership
☐ The Joint Commission accreditation
◇ DNV Healthcare Inc. accreditation
○ American Osteopathic Association (AOA) accreditation
△ Commission on Accreditation of Rehabilitation Facilities (CARF) accreditation

## EL PASO—El Paso County

☐ **EAST EL PASO PHYSICIANS MEDICAL CENTER (450877)**, 1416 George Dieter Drive, Zip 79936–7601; tel. 915/598–4240, (Nonreporting) **A**1 9 10
Primary Contact: Alfredo Ontiveros, Jr., Chief Executive Officer
CFO: Chris Barela, Controller
CIO: Louie Aguilera, Director Information Technology
CHR: Janice Harris, Director Human Resources
Web address: www.physiciansmedcenter.com
**Control:** Partnership, Investor–owned, for–profit **Service:** General Medical and Surgical

**Staffed Beds:** 40

**EL PASO CHILDREN'S HOSPITAL**, 4845 Alameda Avenue, Zip 79905; tel. 915/298–5444, (Nonreporting)
Primary Contact: Lawrence Duncan, Chief Executive Officer
COO: Elias Armendariz, Vice President Operations
CFO: David Mier, Chief Financial Officer
CMO: Bradley Fuhrman, M.D., Physician in Chief
CIO: Janina Prada, Director Information Technology
CHR: Natalia Chaparro, Manager Human Resources
CNO: Paul Ocon, R.N., Chief Nursing Officer
Web address: www.elpasochildrens.org
**Control:** Other not–for–profit (including NFP Corporation) **Service:** Children's general

**Staffed Beds:** 122

**EL PASO LTAC HOSPITAL (452103)**, 1221 North Cotton Street, 3rd Floor, Zip 79902–3015; tel. 915/496–9687 **A**9 10 **F**1 3 29 30 34 57 60 75 77 82 84 85 86 87 91 100 103 118 129 147
Primary Contact: Evelyn G. Stewart, Chief Executive Officer
**Control:** Partnership, Investor–owned, for–profit **Service:** Long–Term Acute Care hospital

**Staffed Beds:** 33 **Admissions:** 320 **Census:** 21 **Outpatient Visits:** 0 **Births:** 0 **Total Expense ($000):** 6531 **Payroll Expense ($000):** 2514 **Personnel:** 69

☐ **EL PASO PSYCHIATRIC CENTER (454100)**, 4615 Alameda Avenue, Zip 79905–2702; tel. 915/532–2202 **A**1 3 5 9 10 **F**29 98 99 103 129 **P**6 **S** Texas Department of State Health Services, Austin, TX
Primary Contact: Zulema Carrillo, Chief Executive Officer
CFO: David Osterhout, Assistant Superintendent and Chief Financial Officer
CMO: Nicolas Baida–Fragoso, M.D., Clinical Director
**Control:** State–Government, nonfederal **Service:** Psychiatric

**Staffed Beds:** 77 **Admissions:** 769 **Census:** 71 **Outpatient Visits:** 0 **Births:** 0 **Total Expense ($000):** 18870 **Payroll Expense ($000):** 9418 **Personnel:** 246

☐ **EL PASO SPECIALTY HOSPITAL (450845)**, 1755 Curie Drive, Zip 79902–2919; tel. 915/544–3636 **A**1 9 10 **F**3 29 34 35 40 57 59 64 68 75 79 81 82 85 87 129 130 147 **S** National Surgical Hospitals, Chicago, IL
Primary Contact: James Wilcox, Chief Executive Officer
CFO: Greg Watters, Chief Financial Officer
CMO: David Mansfield, M.D., Chief of Staff
CNO: Anne Harvey, MSN, Chief Nursing Officer
Web address: www.elpasospecialtyhospital.com
**Control:** Partnership, Investor–owned, for–profit **Service:** Orthopedic

**Staffed Beds:** 27 **Admissions:** 916 **Census:** 7 **Outpatient Visits:** 15305 **Births:** 0 **Total Expense ($000):** 26838 **Payroll Expense ($000):** 6482 **Personnel:** 134

☐ △ **HIGHLANDS REGIONAL REHABILITATION HOSPITAL (453086)**, 1395 George Dieter Drive, Zip 79936; tel. 915/298–7222 **A**1 7 9 10 **F**3 29 30 34 57 59 64 74 75 79 86 87 90 93 96 100 129 131 142 145 147
Primary Contact: Robert Ward, Chief Executive Officer
Web address: www.highlandsrehab.com
**Control:** Partnership, Investor–owned, for–profit **Service:** Rehabilitation

**Staffed Beds:** 41 **Admissions:** 767 **Census:** 23 **Outpatient Visits:** 5573 **Births:** 0 **Total Expense ($000):** 11539 **Payroll Expense ($000):** 5453 **Personnel:** 141

⊞ **KINDRED HOSPITAL EL PASO (452079)**, 1740 Curie Drive, Zip 79902; tel. 915/351–9044 **A**1 9 10 **F**3 29 30 34 70 75 77 87 129 147 **S** Kindred Healthcare, Louisville, KY
Primary Contact: Aleen D. Arabit, Chief Executive Officer
CFO: Michael Smesny, Chief Financial Officer
CMO: Mauricio Jimenez, M.D., Chief Medical Officer
CHR: Laura Anchondo, Administrator Human Resources
Web address: www.khelpaso.com
**Control:** Corporation, Investor–owned, for–profit **Service:** Long–Term Acute Care hospital

**Staffed Beds:** 62 **Admissions:** 733 **Census:** 50 **Outpatient Visits:** 389 **Births:** 0 **Total Expense ($000):** 18957 **Payroll Expense ($000):** 8495 **Personnel:** 118

⊞ **LAS PALMAS DEL SOL HEALTHCARE (450107)**, 1801 North Oregon Street, Zip 79902–3591; tel. 915/521–1200, (Includes DEL SOL MEDICAL CENTER, 10301 West Gateway Boulevard, Zip 79925–7798; tel. 915/595–9000; Jacob Cintron, FACHE, Chief Executive Officer; LAS PALMAS REHABILITATION HOSPITAL, 300 Waymore Drive, Zip 79902–1628; tel. 915/577–2600) **A**1 5 9 10 **F**1 4 11 12 13 15 16 17 18 20 22 24 28 29 30 31 34 35 36 40 43 46 50 51 53 54 56 57 59 61 64 65 67 68 70 72 73 74 75 76 77 78 79 80 81 86 87 88 89 90 93 98 107 108 111 114 117 118 120 129 130 131 137 141 145 146 147 **S** HCA, Nashville, TN
Primary Contact: Hank Hernandez, Chief Executive Officer
COO: Don Karl, Chief Operating Officer
Web address: www.laspalmashealth.com
**Control:** Partnership, Investor–owned, for–profit **Service:** General Medical and Surgical

**Staffed Beds:** 550 **Admissions:** 28220 **Census:** 378 **Outpatient Visits:** 243314 **Births:** 4818 **Total Expense ($000):** 347359 **Payroll Expense ($000):** 124643 **Personnel:** 2081

☐ **MESA HILLS SPECIALTY HOSPITAL (452035)**, 2311 North Oregon Street, Zip 79902–3216; tel. 915/545–1823 **A**1 9 10 **F**1 8 29 34 54 56 57 58 59 61 64 65 74 75 77 82 83 84 85 86 87 91 94 129 142 147 **S** Encore Healthcare, Columbia, MD
Primary Contact: William Balay, Jr., Chief Executive Officer
COO: Elena Pino, Chief Operating Officer and Chief Nursing Officer
CFO: Priscilla Carter, Chief Financial Officer
Web address: www.ihs–inc.com
**Control:** Corporation, Investor–owned, for–profit **Service:** Long–Term Acute Care hospital

**Staffed Beds:** 32 **Admissions:** 283 **Census:** 22 **Outpatient Visits:** 3977 **Births:** 0 **Total Expense ($000):** 11609 **Payroll Expense ($000):** 3668 **Personnel:** 54

⊞ **PROVIDENCE MEMORIAL HOSPITAL (450002)**, 2001 North Oregon Street, Zip 79902–3368; tel. 915/577–6011, (Includes CHILDREN'S HOSPITAL AT PROVIDENCE, 2001 North Oregon Street, Zip 79902–3320; tel. 915/577–7746) **A**1 2 9 10 **F**3 11 12 13 14 15 17 18 19 20 21 22 23 24 25 28 29 30 31 32 34 35 40 41 43 44 45 46 49 50 51 54 57 59 63 64 65 70 72 73 74 75 76 77 78 79 81 82 84 85 86 87 88 89 91 92 93 107 108 110 111 113 117 118 125 128 129 131 133 134 144 145 146 147 **P**1 **S** TENET Healthcare Corporation, Dallas, TX
Primary Contact: John Harris, Chief Executive Officer
CFO: Charles Hondley, Chief Financial Officer
CIO: Ray Davis, Administrative Director
CHR: Mark Thomasson, Vice President Human Resources
Web address: www.sphn.com
**Control:** Partnership, Investor–owned, for–profit **Service:** General Medical and Surgical

**Staffed Beds:** 359 **Admissions:** 18451 **Census:** 220 **Outpatient Visits:** 184517 **Births:** 3839 **Total Expense ($000):** 240726 **Payroll Expense ($000):** 80528 **Personnel:** 1402

⊞ **SIERRA MEDICAL CENTER (450668)**, 1625 Medical Center Drive, Zip 79902–5044; tel. 915/747–4000 **A**1 2 5 9 10 **F**3 11 13 15 17 18 20 22 24 26 28 29 30 31 34 35 40 43 44 45 46 47 48 49 50 54 57 59 61 64 68 69 70 72 74 75 76 77 78 79 81 85 86 89 107 108 110 111 113 114 117 118 123 129 131 133 143 144 145 146 147 **P**1 **S** TENET Healthcare Corporation, Dallas, TX
Primary Contact: Edmundo Castaneda, Chief Executive Officer
CFO: Enrique Bernal, Chief Financial Officer
CHR: Linda Wallace, Director Human Resources
Web address: www.sphn.com
**Control:** Partnership, Investor–owned, for–profit **Service:** General Medical and Surgical

**Staffed Beds:** 334 **Admissions:** 10931 **Census:** 138 **Outpatient Visits:** 97099 **Births:** 1951 **Total Expense ($000):** 142266 **Payroll Expense ($000):** 58638 **Personnel:** 854

⊞ **SIERRA PROVIDENCE EAST MEDICAL CENTER (670047)**, 2400 Trawood Drive, Zip 79936; tel. 915/577–8000 **A**1 2 5 9 10 **F**3 13 15 18 20 22 26 29 30 31 34 35 40 45 46 47 49 50 57 59 60 63 64 68 70 72 73 74 75 76 77 79 81 85 86 87 93 107 108 111 114 118 129 133 145 147 **P**1 **S** TENET Healthcare Corporation, Dallas, TX
Primary Contact: Sally Hurt–Steffen, MSN, R.N., Chief Executive Officer
Web address: www.sphn.com
**Control:** Individual, Investor–owned, for–profit **Service:** General Medical and Surgical

**Staffed Beds:** 110 **Admissions:** 6924 **Census:** 77 **Outpatient Visits:** 63109 **Births:** 1402 **Total Expense ($000):** 82159 **Payroll Expense ($000):** 30355 **Personnel:** 517

**TRIUMPH HOSPITAL EL PASO** See Kindred Hospital El Paso

*Many Facility Codes have changed. Please refer to the AHA Guide Code Chart.*
© 2012 AHA Guide

TX

☐ **UNIVERSITY BEHAVIORAL HEALTH OF EL PASO (454109)**, 1900 Denver Avenue, Zip 79902–3008; tel. 915/544–4000 **A**1 3 5 9 10 **F**4 98 99 103 104 105 **S** Ascend Health Corporation, New York, NY
Primary Contact: Selene Quintana–Hammon, Chief Executive Officer
Web address: www.ubhelpaso.com/
**Control:** Corporation, Investor–owned, for–profit **Service:** Psychiatric

**Staffed Beds:** 163 **Admissions:** 3792 **Census:** 120 **Outpatient Visits:** 14728 **Births:** 0 **Total Expense ($000):** 19778 **Payroll Expense ($000):** 10573 **Personnel:** 271

⊞ **UNIVERSITY MEDICAL CENTER OF EL PASO (450024)**, 4815 Alameda Avenue, Zip 79905–2794, Mailing Address: P.O. Box 20009, Zip 79998–0009; tel. 915/544–1200 **A**1 2 3 5 8 9 10 **F**3 8 11 13 15 17 18 20 22 24 26 28 29 30 31 34 35 37 39 40 43 45 46 47 48 49 50 51 53 54 57 59 60 61 64 65 68 70 72 73 74 75 76 77 79 81 85 86 87 88 89 92 93 94 97 100 102 107 110 111 113 117 118 125 126 129 133 142 143 144 145 146 147 **P**6
Primary Contact: James N. Valenti, FACHE, President and Chief Executive Officer
COO: James N. Valenti, FACHE, President and Chief Executive Officer
CMO: Carmela Morales, M.D., Chief of Staff
CIO: Janina Prada, Director Information Services
CHR: Gilbert Blancas, Director Human Resources
Web address: www.thomasoncares.org
**Control:** Hospital district or authority, Government, nonfederal **Service:** General Medical and Surgical

**Staffed Beds:** 296 **Admissions:** 16679 **Census:** 207 **Outpatient Visits:** 643777 **Births:** 3754 **Total Expense ($000):** 275656 **Payroll Expense ($000):** 111271 **Personnel:** 2158

⊞ **WILLIAM BEAUMONT ARMY MEDICAL CENTER**, 5005 North Piedras Street, Zip 79920–5001; tel. 915/742–2121, (Nonreporting) **A**1 2 3 5 9 **S** Department of the Army, Office of the Surgeon General, Falls Church, VA
Primary Contact: Colonel Dennis Doyle, Commanding Officer
COO: Colonel James J. Leech, Commander
CMO: Colonel Homer Lemar, M.D., Deputy Commander Clinical Services
CIO: Major Rion Koon, Chief Information Management Division
Web address: www.wbamc.amedd.army.mil
**Control:** Army, Government, federal **Service:** General Medical and Surgical

**Staffed Beds:** 209

### ELDORADO—Schleicher County

★ **SCHLEICHER COUNTY MEDICAL CENTER (451304)**, 400 West Murchison, Zip 76936, Mailing Address: P.O. Box V., Zip 76936–1246; tel. 325/853–2507 **A**9 10 18 **F**11 34 40 43 57 59 60 90 107 126 127 132 142 147 **S** Preferred Management Corporation, Shawnee, OK
Primary Contact: Paul Burke, Administrator
CFO: Larry Stephens, Chief Financial Officer
CMO: Gordy Day, M.D., Medical Director
CHR: Beverly Minor, Chief Human Resources
Web address: www.scmc.us
**Control:** Corporation, Investor–owned, for–profit **Service:** General Medical and Surgical

**Staffed Beds:** 14 **Admissions:** 106 **Census:** 1 **Outpatient Visits:** 8287 **Births:** 0 **Total Expense ($000):** 4430 **Payroll Expense ($000):** 1860 **Personnel:** 46

### ELECTRA—Wichita County

★ **ELECTRA MEMORIAL HOSPITAL (451343)**, 1207 South Bailey Street, Zip 76360–3221, Mailing Address: P.O. Box 1112, Zip 76360–1112; tel. 940/495–3981 **A**9 10 18 **F**3 7 11 32 40 43 45 50 53 56 57 59 62 64 65 66 75 77 81 93 97 107 113 118 128 129 130 132 146 147
Primary Contact: Jan A. Reed, CPA, Administrator and Chief Executive Officer
CFO: Rebecca McCain, Chief Financial Officer and Assistant Administrator
Web address: www.electrahospital.com
**Control:** Hospital district or authority, Government, nonfederal **Service:** General Medical and Surgical

**Staffed Beds:** 22 **Admissions:** 372 **Census:** 5 **Outpatient Visits:** 20989 **Births:** 0 **Total Expense ($000):** 7328 **Payroll Expense ($000):** 4522 **Personnel:** 106

### ENNIS—Ellis County

⊞ **ENNIS REGIONAL MEDICAL CENTER (450833)**, 2201 West Lampasas Street, Zip 75119–5644; tel. 972/875–0900 **A**1 9 10 **F**3 11 13 15 18 29 34 40 43 45 50 51 57 59 68 70 76 77 79 81 82 85 93 94 107 110 111 114 118 145 **S** LifePoint Hospitals, Inc., Brentwood, TN
Primary Contact: David Anderson, Chief Executive Officer
CFO: Jack Wilcox, Chief Financial Officer
CMO: Ralph W. Blair, Jr., M.D., Chief of Staff
CHR: James Dopson, Director Human Resources
Web address: www.ennisregional.com
**Control:** Partnership, Investor–owned, for–profit **Service:** General Medical and Surgical

**Staffed Beds:** 58 **Admissions:** 2270 **Census:** 17 **Outpatient Visits:** 32587 **Births:** 735 **Total Expense ($000):** 25046 **Payroll Expense ($000):** 10216 **Personnel:** 189

### FAIRFIELD—Freestone County

★ **EAST TEXAS MEDICAL CENTER FAIRFIELD (450658)**, 125 Newman Street, Zip 75840–1499; tel. 903/389–2121 **A**9 10 20 **F**15 28 40 57 59 75 81 82 107 114 118 126 129 131 132 **P**7 **S** East Texas Medical Center Regional Healthcare System, Tyler, TX
Primary Contact: Ruth Cook, Administrator
CFO: David A. Travis, Chief Financial Officer
CMO: J. Michael Orms, M.D., Chief of Staff
CHR: Jennifer Rummel, Director Human Resources
Web address: www.etmc.org
**Control:** Other not–for–profit (including NFP Corporation) **Service:** General Medical and Surgical

**Staffed Beds:** 20 **Admissions:** 628 **Census:** 6 **Outpatient Visits:** 38814 **Births:** 0 **Total Expense ($000):** 7780 **Payroll Expense ($000):** 4080 **Personnel:** 91

### FLORESVILLE—Wilson County

**CONNALLY MEDICAL CENTER (450108)**, 499 10th Street, Zip 78114–3175; tel. 830/393–1300 **A**9 10 **F**3 15 29 34 35 40 43 45 57 59 62 64 70 75 81 82 85 86 87 107 108 111 113 118 129 131 132 145
Primary Contact: Jerome M. Brooks, Chief Executive Officer
COO: Thomas Repino, Executive Director Ancillary Services
CIO: Kim Schultz, Manager Information
CHR: Dane Bonecutter, Director Human Resources
CNO: Celeste Brizzee, Chief Nursing Officer
Web address: www.connallymmc.org
**Control:** Hospital district or authority, Government, nonfederal **Service:** General Medical and Surgical

**Staffed Beds:** 17 **Admissions:** 1168 **Census:** 8 **Outpatient Visits:** 67579 **Births:** 2 **Total Expense ($000):** 17004 **Payroll Expense ($000):** 8422 **Personnel:** 195

### FLOWER MOUND—Denton County

**CONTINUUM REHABILITATION HOSPITAL OF NORTH TEXAS (673047)**, 3100 Peters Colony Road, Zip 75022–2949; tel. 214/513–0310, (Nonreporting) **A**21
Primary Contact: Patrick Lee, Chief Executive Officer
Web address: www.continuumhs.com
**Control:** Corporation, Investor–owned, for–profit **Service:** Rehabilitation

**Staffed Beds:** 41

**TEXAS HEALTH PRESBYTERIAN HOSPITAL FLOWER MOUND**, 4400 Long Prairie Road, Zip 75028–1892; tel. 469/322–7000 **A**9 21 **F**3 13 15 18 20 29 30 31 40 45 49 70 73 74 76 77 78 79 81 85 107 108 110 111 114 118 129 145 146
Primary Contact: Spencer Turner, Chief Executive Officer
COO: Shelley R. Tobey, R.N., Chief Operating Officer and Chief Nursing Officer
CFO: Tom Howard, Chief Financial Officer
CHR: Nicole Schweigert, Director Human Resources
CNO: Shelley R. Tobey, R.N., Chief Operating Officer and Chief Nursing Officer
Web address: www.phfmtexas.com/
**Control:** Partnership, Investor–owned, for–profit **Service:** General Medical and Surgical

**Staffed Beds:** 72 **Admissions:** 2793 **Census:** 28 **Outpatient Visits:** 21002 **Births:** 646 **Total Expense ($000):** 60443 **Payroll Expense ($000):** 19278 **Personnel:** 311

**TX**

---

**Hospital, Medicare Provider Number, Address, Telephone, Approval, Facility, and Physician Codes, Health Care System**

★ American Hospital Association (AHA) membership
☐ The Joint Commission accreditation    ◇ DNV Healthcare Inc. accreditation
○ American Osteopathic Association (AOA) accreditation
△ Commission on Accreditation of Rehabilitation Facilities (CARF) accreditation

## FORT HOOD—Bell County

✠ **CARL R. DARNALL ARMY MEDICAL CENTER**, 36000 Darnall Loop, Zip 76544–5095; tel. 254/288–8000, (Nonreporting) **A**1 2 3 5 9 **S** Department of the Army, Office of the Surgeon General, Falls Church, VA
Primary Contact: Colonel Patrick D. Sargent, Commander
COO: Colonel Cynthia O'Connell, M.D., Chief of Staff
CFO: Major David Rollins, Chief Resource Management
CMO: Colonel Kimberly Kesling, Deputy Commander Clinical Service
CIO: Christopher Henry, Chief Information Management
CHR: Charles Burton, Chief Human Resources
Web address: www.crdamc.amedd.army.mil
**Control:** Army, Government, federal **Service:** General Medical and Surgical

Staffed Beds: 109

## FORT SAM HOUSTON—Bexar County

**BROOKE ARMY MEDICAL CENTER** See San Antonio Military Medical Center

✠ **SAN ANTONIO MILITARY MEDICAL CENTER**, 3851 Roger Brookes Drive, Zip 78234–6200; tel. 210/916–4141, (Nonreporting) **A**1 2 3 5 9 **S** Department of the Army, Office of the Surgeon General, Falls Church, VA
Primary Contact: Colonel Noel J. Cardenas, FACHE, Commander
CFO: Lieutenant Colonel Talford Mindingal, Chief Resource Management Division
CMO: Colonel Carlos Angueira, Deputy Commander Clinical Services
CIO: Lieutenant Colonel Hailey Windham, Chief Information Management
CHR: Rose Juarez, Chief Civilian Personnel Branch
Web address: www.bamc.amedd.army.mil
**Control:** Army, Government, federal **Service:** General Medical and Surgical

Staffed Beds: 226

## FORT STOCKTON—Pecos County

★ **PECOS COUNTY MEMORIAL HOSPITAL (450178)**, 387 West I. H–10, Zip 79735–8912, Mailing Address: P.O. Box 1648, Zip 79735–1648; tel. 432/336–2004 **A**9 10 20 **F**3 11 13 29 35 40 43 53 57 59 62 65 75 76 81 93 107 118 126 128 129 **P**5 6
Primary Contact: Jim Horton, Chief Executive Officer
CFO: Leticia Fox, Chief Financial Officer
CMO: Subodh Mallik, M.D., Chief of Staff
CHR: Diana Mesa, Director Human Resources
Web address: www.pcmhfs.com
**Control:** County–Government, nonfederal **Service:** General Medical and Surgical

Staffed Beds: 27 Admissions: 1407 Census: 11 Outpatient Visits: 44841 Births: 146 Total Expense ($000): 20717 Payroll Expense ($000): 8905 Personnel: 224

## FORT WORTH—Tarrant County

✠ **BAYLOR ALL SAINTS MEDICAL CENTER AT FORT WORTH (450137)**, 1400 Eighth Avenue, Zip 76104–4192; tel. 817/926–2544 **A**1 2 9 10 **F**3 11 13 15 17 18 20 22 24 26 28 29 30 31 34 35 36 38 40 45 46 47 49 53 54 59 64 68 70 72 73 74 75 76 77 78 79 80 81 82 84 86 87 90 93 96 97 98 100 101 102 103 104 105 107 108 111 113 114 118 123 125 129 130 131 134 137 138 141 145 146 147 **S** Baylor Health Care System, Dallas, TX
Primary Contact: Steven R. Newton, President
COO: David G. Klein, M.D., Chief Operating Officer
CFO: Preshie Wilson, Vice President Finance
CIO: Sandy Vaughn, Director Information Services
CHR: Julie Strittmatter, Director Human Resources
Web address: www.baylorhealth.com
**Control:** Other not–for–profit (including NFP Corporation) **Service:** General Medical and Surgical

Staffed Beds: 606 Admissions: 21616 Census: 266 Outpatient Visits: 114108 Births: 5767 Total Expense ($000): 374610 Payroll Expense ($000): 132099 Personnel: 1661

☐ **BAYLOR SURGICAL HOSPITAL AT FORT WORTH (450880)**, 750 12th Avenue, Zip 76104; tel. 817/334–5050 **A**1 9 10 **F**3 29 40 45 51 64 65 75 77 79 81 82 85 86 87 107 111 113 118 140
Primary Contact: Roger Rhodes, Chief Executive Officer
Web address: www.mcsh–hospital.com
**Control:** Partnership, Investor–owned, for–profit **Service:** General Medical and Surgical

Staffed Beds: 22 Admissions: 918 Census: 6 Outpatient Visits: 11650 Births: 0 Total Expense ($000): 44446 Payroll Expense ($000): 8536 Personnel: 153

✠ **COOK CHILDREN'S MEDICAL CENTER (453300)**, 801 Seventh Avenue, Zip 76104–2796; tel. 682/885–4000 **A**1 3 5 9 10 **F**3 7 8 19 21 23 25 27 29 30 31 32 34 35 38 39 40 43 44 45 48 50 51 54 55 57 58 59 60 61 64 68 72 73 74 75 77 78 79 80 81 82 84 85 86 87 88 89 90 93 97 98 99 100 101 102 104 105 106 107 108 111 112 113 117 118 128 129 130 131 133 135 137 142 145 **P**6
Primary Contact: Rick W. Merrill, President and Chief Executive Officer
CFO: Richard P. Goode, Chief Financial Officer
CMO: James C. Cunningham, M.D., Chief Medical Officer
CIO: Tracy Waller, Interim Chief Information Officer
CHR: Frank J. Rossi, Senior Vice President Human Resources
Web address: www.cookchildrens.org
**Control:** Other not–for–profit (including NFP Corporation) **Service:** Children's general

Staffed Beds: 302 Admissions: 11939 Census: 200 Outpatient Visits: 278860 Births: 0 Total Expense ($000): 508102 Payroll Expense ($000): 186559 Personnel: 3108

○ **GLOBALREHAB HOSPITAL – FORT WORTH (673035)**, 6601 Harris Parkway, Zip 76132–6108; tel. 817/433–9600 **A**11 **F**3 28 29 75 90 129 **S** GLOBALREHAB, Dallas, TX
Primary Contact: Brigid Greenberg, Interim Chief Executive Officer
Web address: www.globalrehabhospitals.com
**Control:** Corporation, Investor–owned, for–profit **Service:** Rehabilitation

Staffed Beds: 42 Admissions: 1003 Census: 35 Outpatient Visits: 0 Births: 0 Total Expense ($000): 14759 Payroll Expense ($000): 7290 Personnel: 112

✠ **HEALTHSOUTH REHABILITATION HOSPITAL (453041)**, 1212 West Lancaster Avenue, Zip 76102–4510; tel. 817/870–2336 **A**1 9 10 **F**3 29 64 74 75 77 79 82 86 90 91 93 95 96 100 129 130 147 **S** HEALTHSOUTH Corporation, Birmingham, AL
Primary Contact: Trent Pierce, R.N., Chief Executive Officer
CFO: Sherry Hapney, Chief Financial Officer
CMO: Patrick Donovan, M.D., Director Medical Staff
CHR: Tara Kleas, Director Human Resources
Web address: www.healthsouthfortworth.com
**Control:** Corporation, Investor–owned, for–profit **Service:** Rehabilitation

Staffed Beds: 60 Admissions: 916 Census: 33 Outpatient Visits: 7310 Births: 0 Total Expense ($000): 11877 Payroll Expense ($000): 7051 Personnel: 125

✠ **HEALTHSOUTH REHABILITATION HOSPITAL–CITYVIEW (453042)**, 6701 Oakmont Boulevard, Zip 76132–2957; tel. 817/370–4700 **A**1 9 10 **F**3 29 30 54 62 68 77 82 90 91 93 94 95 96 117 129 130 147 **S** HEALTHSOUTH Corporation, Birmingham, AL
Primary Contact: Deborah Hopps, Chief Executive Officer
Web address: www.healthsouthcityview.com
**Control:** Corporation, Investor–owned, for–profit **Service:** Rehabilitation

Staffed Beds: 62 Admissions: 1029 Census: 37 Outpatient Visits: 8994 Births: 0 Total Expense ($000): 14580 Payroll Expense ($000): 8391 Personnel: 130

✠ **HUGULEY MEMORIAL MEDICAL CENTER (450677)**, 11801 South Freeway, Zip 76134, Mailing Address: P.O. Box 6337, Zip 76115–0337; tel. 817/293–9110 **A**1 9 10 **F**3 5 13 15 17 18 20 22 24 28 29 30 31 32 34 35 38 40 44 49 51 53 54 56 57 59 60 62 64 68 70 71 75 76 77 78 79 80 81 82 85 86 87 89 93 98 100 101 102 103 104 105 107 108 110 111 113 117 118 119 120 129 131 134 145 146 147 **S** Adventist Health System Sunbelt Health Care Corporation, Altamonte Springs, FL
Primary Contact: Kenneth A. Finch, President and Chief Executive Officer
CFO: Dan Enderson, Chief Financial Officer
CMO: Edward Laue, M.D., Chief Medical Officer
CIO: David Smith, Manager Data Center
CHR: Leah Foley, Director Human Resources
Web address: www.huguley.org
**Control:** Church–operated, Nongovernment, not–for profit **Service:** General Medical and Surgical

Staffed Beds: 188 Admissions: 9412 Census: 111 Outpatient Visits: 130902 Births: 883 Total Expense ($000): 132972 Payroll Expense ($000): 51856 Personnel: 970

**JOHN PETER SMITH HOSPITAL** See JPS Health Network

*Many Facility Codes have changed. Please refer to the AHA Guide Code Chart.* © 2012 AHA Guide

TX

★ **JPS HEALTH NETWORK (450039)**, 1500 South Main Street, Zip 76104–4917; tel. 817/921–3431, (Includes JOHN PETER SMITH HOSPITAL, 1500 South Main Street, Zip 76104; tel. 817/921–3431; TRINITY SPRINGS PAVILION, 1500 South Main Street, tel. 817/927–3636; Lilly Wong, Director Psychiatry), (Total facility includes 15 beds in nursing home–type unit) **A**3 5 8 10 **F**3 8 11 13 15 17 18 20 22 24 26 28 29 30 31 32 34 35 36 37 38 39 40 43 44 45 49 50 54 55 56 57 58 59 60 61 64 65 66 68 70 72 74 75 76 77 78 79 80 81 82 85 86 87 89 91 92 93 97 98 99 100 101 102 103 104 107 108 110 111 113 114 117 118 119 120 122 123 125 127 129 130 131 133 134 141 142 143 145 146 147 **P**3
Primary Contact: Robert Earley, President and Chief Executive Officer
COO: Bill Whitman, Chief Operating Officer
CFO: David Salsberry, Chief Financial Officer
CMO: Gary Floyd, M.D., Executive Vice President Medical Affairs and Chief Medical Officer
CIO: James Pennington, Chief Information Officer
CHR: Rose Thomason, Interim Vice President Human Resources
Web address: www.jpshealthnet.org
**Control:** Hospital district or authority, Government, nonfederal **Service:** General Medical and Surgical

**Staffed Beds:** 517 **Admissions:** 28042 **Census:** 403 **Outpatient Visits:** 1092520 **Births:** 5670 **Total Expense ($000):** 652798 **Payroll Expense ($000):** 244485 **Personnel:** 4106

⊞ **KINDRED HOSPITAL TARRANT COUNTY–FORT WORTH SOUTHWEST (452088)**, 7800 Oakmont Boulevard, Zip 76132–4299; tel. 817/346–0094 **A**1 9 10 **F**1 3 28 29 80 107 129 134 147 **S** Kindred Healthcare, Louisville, KY
Primary Contact: Anna Rojas, Chief Executive Officer
CFO: Tom Spencer, Chief Financial Officer
CMO: Henry Cunningham, M.D., President Medical Staff
CHR: Joy Raines, Coordinator Human Resources
Web address: www.kindredhospitalfwsw.com/
**Control:** Corporation, Investor–owned, for–profit **Service:** Long–Term Acute Care hospital

**Staffed Beds:** 74 **Admissions:** 801 **Census:** 60 **Outpatient Visits:** 82 **Births:** 0 **Total Expense ($000):** 21892 **Payroll Expense ($000):** 10283 **Personnel:** 192

⊞ **KINDRED HOSPITAL–FORT WORTH (452088)**, 815 Eighth Avenue, Zip 76104; tel. 817/332–4812, (Nonreporting) **A**1 9 10 **S** Kindred Healthcare, Louisville, KY
Primary Contact: Angela Harris, Chief Executive Officer
CFO: Susan Popp, Controller
CMO: Stuart McDonald, M.D., President Medical Staff
CIO: Norma Warner, Area Director Health Information Management
CHR: Nicole Newpower, Coordinator Human Resources
Web address: www.kindredfortworth.com/
**Control:** Corporation, Investor–owned, for–profit **Service:** Long–Term Acute Care hospital

**Staffed Beds:** 67

⊞ **PLAZA MEDICAL CENTER OF FORT WORTH (450672)**, 900 Eighth Avenue, Zip 76104–3986; tel. 817/336–2100 **A**1 2 9 10 12 13 **F**3 11 12 17 18 20 22 24 26 28 29 30 31 34 35 36 37 40 45 47 48 49 50 57 58 59 68 70 74 75 77 78 79 80 81 85 87 93 96 107 108 111 114 116 117 118 128 129 131 144 145 147 **P**8 **S** HCA, Nashville, TN
Primary Contact: Clay Franklin, Chief Executive Officer
COO: Greg Haralson, Chief Operating Officer
CFO: Elia Stokes, Chief Financial Officer
CMO: Amir Malik, M.D., Cardiologist
CIO: Kelley Fredrickson, Director Information Services
CHR: Cyndi Roberts, Director Human Resources
Web address: www.plazamedicalcenter.com
**Control:** Partnership, Investor–owned, for–profit **Service:** General Medical and Surgical

**Staffed Beds:** 219 **Admissions:** 11504 **Census:** 157 **Outpatient Visits:** 37881 **Births:** 0 **Total Expense ($000):** 173768 **Payroll Expense ($000):** 57666 **Personnel:** 823

⊞ **REGENCY HOSPITAL OF FORT WORTH (452099)**, 6801 Oakmont Boulevard, Zip 76132–3918; tel. 817/840–2500 **A**1 9 10 **F**1 3 29 45 75 77 85 86 87 129 147 **P**5 **S** Select Medical Corporation, Mechanicsburg, PA
Primary Contact: Brad Ervin, Chief Executive Officer
Web address: www.regencyhospital.com
**Control:** Corporation, Investor–owned, for–profit **Service:** Long–Term Acute Care hospital

**Staffed Beds:** 44 **Admissions:** 448 **Census:** 31 **Outpatient Visits:** 0 **Births:** 0 **Total Expense ($000):** 16716 **Payroll Expense ($000):** 6997 **Personnel:** 122

⊞ △ **TEXAS HEALTH HARRIS METHODIST HOSPITAL FORT WORTH (450135)**, 1301 Pennsylvania Avenue, Zip 76104–2122; tel. 817/250–2000 **A**1 2 7 9 10 **F**3 11 12 13 15 17 18 20 22 24 26 28 29 30 31 34 35 36 40 42 43 45 46 47 48 49 50 52 53 54 55 56 57 58 59 60 64 68 70 71 72 74 75 76 77 78 79 81 83 84 85 86 87 90 93 95 96 100 107 108 110 111 113 114 115 116 117 118 123 125 129 130 131 134 137 140 144 145 146 147 **P**8 **S** Texas Health Resources, Arlington, TX
Primary Contact: Lillie Biggins, R.N., President
CFO: Richard Humphrey, Vice President Finance
CMO: Harold Berenzweig, M.D., Vice President Medical and Information Management
CHR: Joseph Condon, Director Human Resources
Web address: www.texashealth.org
**Control:** Other not–for–profit (including NFP Corporation) **Service:** General Medical and Surgical

**Staffed Beds:** 620 **Admissions:** 33637 **Census:** 482 **Outpatient Visits:** 155981 **Births:** 3072 **Total Expense ($000):** 613309 **Payroll Expense ($000):** 223329 **Personnel:** 3919

⊞ **TEXAS HEALTH HARRIS METHODIST HOSPITAL SOUTHWEST FORT WORTH (450779)**, 6100 Harris Parkway, Zip 76132–4199; tel. 817/433–5000 **A**1 9 10 **F**3 11 13 15 18 20 29 30 34 35 38 40 45 49 50 59 64 68 70 72 75 76 77 78 79 81 82 84 85 86 87 93 102 107 108 110 111 113 117 118 125 128 129 144 145 146 **S** Texas Health Resources, Arlington, TX
Primary Contact: Brett McClung, President
COO: Allen Tseng, Administrative Director
CMO: Robert Lilli, M.D., Chief of Staff
CHR: Jody Thomas, Director Human Resources
Web address: www.texashealth.org
**Control:** Church–operated, Nongovernment, not–for profit **Service:** General Medical and Surgical

**Staffed Beds:** 143 **Admissions:** 10324 **Census:** 106 **Outpatient Visits:** 81393 **Births:** 2895 **Total Expense ($000):** 132670 **Payroll Expense ($000):** 51137 **Personnel:** 699

⊞ **TEXAS HEALTH SPECIALTY HOSPITAL (452018)**, 1301 Pennsylvania Avenue, 4th Floor, Zip 76104–2190; tel. 817/250–5500 **A**1 9 10 **F**1 3 44 87 129 147 **S** Texas Health Resources, Arlington, TX
Primary Contact: Susan Louise Baldwin, R.N., FACHE, President and Chief Nursing Officer
CFO: Vicki L. Galati, Chief Financial Officer
CMO: John Pender, M.D., Medical Director
CHR: Crystal Galloway, Human Resources Generalist
CNO: Susan Louise Baldwin, R.N., President and Chief Nursing Officer
Web address: www.texashealth.org
**Control:** Church–operated, Nongovernment, not–for profit **Service:** Long–Term Acute Care hospital

**Staffed Beds:** 10 **Admissions:** 99 **Census:** 8 **Outpatient Visits:** 0 **Births:** 0 **Total Expense ($000):** 6547 **Payroll Expense ($000):** 2903 **Personnel:** 39

**TEXAS REHABILITATION HOSPITAL OF FORT WORTH (673048)**, 425 Alabama Avenue, Zip 76104–1022; tel. 817/820–3400, (Data for 245 days) **A**10 **F**3 29 74 79 90 91 96 129 131 147
Primary Contact: Russell Bailey, Chief Executive Officer
Web address: www.texasrehabhospital.com/
**Control:** Corporation, Investor–owned, for–profit **Service:** Rehabilitation

**Staffed Beds:** 50 **Admissions:** 501 **Census:** 26 **Outpatient Visits:** 0 **Births:** 0 **Personnel:** 125

☐ **USMD HOSPITAL AT FORT WORTH (670046)**, 5900 Dirks Road, Zip 76132; tel. 817/433–9100 **A**1 9 10 **F**3 29 39 40 51 64 68 81 85 89 107 113 118 129 **S** USMD Inc., Irving, TX
Primary Contact: Stephanie Atkins–Guidry, Administrator
CHR: Alex Stefanowicz, Vice President Human Resources
CNO: Stephanie Atkins–Guidry, Administrator and Chief Nursing Officer
Web address: www.usmdfortworth.com/
**Control:** Partnership, Investor–owned, for–profit **Service:** Surgical

**Staffed Beds:** 8 **Admissions:** 579 **Census:** 4 **Outpatient Visits:** 5683 **Births:** 0 **Total Expense ($000):** 28831 **Payroll Expense ($000):** 4311 **Personnel:** 110

**TX**

---

**Hospital, Medicare Provider Number, Address, Telephone, Approval, Facility, and Physician Codes, Health Care System**

★ American Hospital Association (AHA) membership
☐ The Joint Commission accreditation
◇ DNV Healthcare Inc. accreditation
○ American Osteopathic Association (AOA) accreditation
△ Commission on Accreditation of Rehabilitation Facilities (CARF) accreditation

## FREDERICKSBURG—Gillespie County

✉ **HILL COUNTRY MEMORIAL HOSPITAL (450604)**, 1020 South State Highway 16, Zip 78624–4471, Mailing Address: P.O. Box 835, Zip 78624–0835; tel. 830/997–4353 **A**1 9 10 20 **F**3 11 13 15 20 28 29 30 31 32 34 35 37 40 43 45 46 48 49 50 51 53 57 59 62 63 64 68 70 74 75 76 77 78 79 81 82 84 85 86 87 90 93 96 107 108 110 111 113 117 118 123 128 129 130 131 132 134 144 145 147 **P**8
Primary Contact: Michael R. Williams, D.O., M.D., Chief Executive Officer
COO: Debbye Wallace, Chief Operating Officer
CFO: Mark Jones, Chief Financial Officer
CMO: Jose A. Lopez, M.D., Chief of Staff
CIO: Holly Schmidt, Chief Information Officer
CHR: Erin Cates, Director Human Resources
Web address: www.hcmhs.org
**Control:** Other not–for–profit (including NFP Corporation) **Service:** General Medical and Surgical

**Staffed Beds:** 54 **Admissions:** 2936 **Census:** 28 **Outpatient Visits:** 74761 **Births:** 497 **Total Expense ($000):** 59055 **Payroll Expense ($000):** 26014 **Personnel:** 498

## FRIONA—Parmer County

**PARMER COUNTY COMMUNITY HOSPITAL** See Parmer Medical Center

**PARMER MEDICAL CENTER (451300)**, 1307 Cleveland Avenue, Zip 79035–1121; tel. 806/250–2754 **A**9 10 18 **F**34 40 43 57 64 75 77 89 91 93 107 118 129 132 147 **S** Preferred Management Corporation, Shawnee, OK
Primary Contact: B. Lance Gatlin, FACHE, Administrator
Web address: www.pcchtx.com
**Control:** Other not–for–profit (including NFP Corporation) **Service:** General Medical and Surgical

**Staffed Beds:** 15 **Admissions:** 174 **Census:** 3 **Outpatient Visits:** 9556 **Births:** 0 **Personnel:** 64

## FRISCO—Collin County

☐ **BAYLOR INSTITUTE FOR REHABILITATION AT FRISCO (673046)**, 2990 Legacy Drive, Zip 75034–6066; tel. 469/888–5100 **A**1 10 **F**29 30 34 36 75 90 91 93 96 129 131 147
Primary Contact: Mark D. Boles, Chief Executive Officer
Web address: www.baylorhealth.com/bir
**Control:** Partnership, Investor–owned, for–profit **Service:** Rehabilitation

**Staffed Beds:** 44 **Admissions:** 403 **Census:** 15 **Outpatient Visits:** 1519 **Births:** 0 **Total Expense ($000):** 9149 **Payroll Expense ($000):** 4695 **Personnel:** 93

☐ **BAYLOR MEDICAL CENTER AT FRISCO (450853)**, 5601 Warren Parkway, Zip 75034; tel. 214/407–5000 **A**1 9 10 **F**3 13 29 34 40 51 54 57 64 68 72 74 75 76 79 81 85 87 107 111 113 118 143 **S** United Surgical Partners International, Addison, TX
Primary Contact: William A. Keaton, Chief Executive Officer
CFO: Kevin Coats, Chief Financial Officer
CMO: Jimmy Laferney, M.D., Vice President Medical Staff Affairs
CIO: Steve Young, Director Information Systems
CHR: Margaret Garcia, Manager Human Resources
CNO: Randi Elliott MSN, Chief Nursing Officer
Web address: www.bmcf.com
**Control:** Partnership, Investor–owned, for–profit **Service:** General Medical and Surgical

**Staffed Beds:** 68 **Admissions:** 4570 **Census:** 40 **Outpatient Visits:** 27922 **Births:** 2494 **Total Expense ($000):** 113320 **Payroll Expense ($000):** 33593 **Personnel:** 550

✉ **CENTENNIAL MEDICAL CENTER (450885)**, 12505 Lebanon Road, Zip 75035–8298; tel. 972/963–3333 **A**1 9 10 **F**3 13 15 18 20 22 24 29 31 34 35 40 45 46 47 48 49 50 51 57 59 70 72 74 76 78 79 81 85 86 89 93 97 107 108 110 111 113 114 118 123 129 130 145 146 147 **S** TENET Healthcare Corporation, Dallas, TX
Primary Contact: Joe D. Thomason, Chief Executive Officer
COO: Paul Abraham, Chief Operating Officer
CFO: Blaise Bondi, Chief Financial Officer
CMO: Robert Hendler, M.D., Regional Chief Medical Officer
CHR: Stephanie S. Talley, Director Human Resources
Web address: www.centennialmedcenter.com
**Control:** Corporation, Investor–owned, for–profit **Service:** General Medical and Surgical

**Staffed Beds:** 118 **Admissions:** 4967 **Census:** 62 **Outpatient Visits:** 38088 **Births:** 977 **Total Expense ($000):** 82777 **Payroll Expense ($000):** 27213 **Personnel:** 580

**FOREST PARK MEDICAL CENTER FRISCO**, 5500 Frisco Square Boulevard, Zip 75034–3305; tel. 214/618–0500, (Nonreporting)
Primary Contact: Julie A. Camp, R.N., Chief Executive Officer
**Control:** Corporation, Investor–owned, for–profit **Service:** Surgical

**Staffed Beds:** 30

## GAINESVILLE—Cooke County

★ **NORTH TEXAS MEDICAL CENTER (450090)**, 1900 Hospital Boulevard, Zip 76240–2002; tel. 940/665–1751 **A**9 10 20 **F**3 11 13 15 28 29 30 34 35 40 43 45 50 59 60 62 64 68 70 75 76 77 79 81 85 87 93 104 107 108 110 111 114 117 118 126 129 131 132 134 145 146 147
Primary Contact: Randy B. Bacus, FACHE, Chief Executive Officer
CFO: Kelly Hayes, Chief Financial Officer
CHR: Teresa Krebs, Director Human Resources
Web address: www.ntmconline.net
**Control:** Hospital district or authority, Government, nonfederal **Service:** General Medical and Surgical

**Staffed Beds:** 60 **Admissions:** 1864 **Census:** 16 **Outpatient Visits:** 39492 **Births:** 489 **Total Expense ($000):** 23062 **Payroll Expense ($000):** 11604 **Personnel:** 278

## GALVESTON—Galveston County

☐ **SHRINERS HOSPITALS FOR CHILDREN, GALVESTON BURNS HOSPITAL (453311)**, (Burn Care), 815 Market Street, Zip 77550–2725; tel. 409/770–6600 **A**1 3 5 10 **F**3 11 16 29 34 64 68 75 77 81 82 86 93 99 100 129 145 147 **S** Shriners Hospitals for Children, Tampa, FL
Primary Contact: David A. Ferrell, Chief Executive Officer
COO: Mary Jaco, R.N., Director Patient Care Services and Chief Operating Officer
CFO: Lona Pope, Director Financial Services
CMO: David N. Herndon, M.D., Chief of Staff
CHR: Lynn Clements, Director Human Resources
CNO: Mary Jaco, R.N., Director Patient Care Services and Chief Operating Officer
Web address: www.shrinershq.org
**Control:** Other not–for–profit (including NFP Corporation) **Service:** Children's other specialty

**Staffed Beds:** 30 **Admissions:** 1416 **Census:** 8 **Outpatient Visits:** 8663 **Births:** 0 **Total Expense ($000):** 16194 **Payroll Expense ($000):** 5324 **Personnel:** 194

✉ **UNIVERSITY OF TEXAS MEDICAL BRANCH HOSPITALS (450018)**, 301 University Boulevard, Zip 77555–0128; tel. 409/772–1011 **A**1 2 5 8 9 10 13 **F**3 11 12 13 14 15 16 17 18 19 20 21 22 23 24 25 26 28 29 30 31 32 34 35 36 38 40 41 43 44 45 46 49 50 51 52 53 54 55 56 57 58 59 60 61 64 65 66 68 70 71 72 73 74 75 76 77 78 79 81 82 84 85 86 87 88 89 90 93 94 97 99 100 101 102 103 104 107 108 110 111 113 114 116 117 118 119 120 122 123 125 128 129 130 131 133 134 136 137 138 139 140 141 142 143 144 145 146 147 **P**6 **S** University of Texas System, Austin, TX
Primary Contact: Donna K. Sollenberger, Executive Vice President and Chief Executive Officer
CFO: William Elger, Executive Vice President and Chief Business and Finance Officer
CMO: Steve Quach, M.D., Chief Medical Officer
CIO: Ralph Farr, Chief Information Officer
CHR: Ronald McKinley, Ph.D., Vice President Human Resources and Employee Services
Web address: www.utmb.edu
**Control:** State–Government, nonfederal **Service:** General Medical and Surgical

**Staffed Beds:** 428 **Admissions:** 25017 **Census:** 338 **Outpatient Visits:** 681624 **Births:** 7057 **Total Expense ($000):** 478527 **Payroll Expense ($000):** 223078 **Personnel:** 3473

## GARLAND—Dallas County

✉ **BAYLOR MEDICAL CENTER AT GARLAND (450280)**, 2300 Marie Curie Drive, Zip 75042–5706; tel. 972/487–5000 **A**1 9 10 **F**3 11 13 15 18 20 22 24 26 28 29 30 34 35 40 45 47 50 54 57 59 60 64 65 66 70 72 74 75 76 77 78 79 81 82 84 85 86 87 90 93 94 107 108 110 111 113 117 118 128 129 131 134 144 145 146 147 **S** Baylor Health Care System, Dallas, TX
Primary Contact: Thomas J. Trenary, President
COO: Barbara Vaughn, Interim Chief Nursing Officer and Chief Operating Officer
CFO: Mike Winter, Vice President and Chief Financial Officer
CMO: Jeffrey Kopita, M.D., Chief Medical Officer and Vice President Medical Affairs
CIO: Michael Larsen, Director Information Systems
CHR: Laura Settles, Director Human Resources
Web address: www.baylorhealth.com
**Control:** Other not–for–profit (including NFP Corporation) **Service:** General Medical and Surgical

**Staffed Beds:** 240 **Admissions:** 10432 **Census:** 134 **Outpatient Visits:** 120315 **Births:** 1337 **Total Expense ($000):** 184048 **Payroll Expense ($000):** 72695 **Personnel:** 1079

## GATESVILLE—Coryell County

☐ **CORYELL MEMORIAL HOSPITAL (451379)**, 1507 West Main Street, Zip 76528–1098; tel. 254/865–8251 **A**1 9 10 18 **F**3 7 10 11 15 18 20 28 40 43 50 53 57 62 65 70 81 82 87 93 97 107 111 114 118 124 126 128 129 132 **P**4 6
Primary Contact: David Byrom, Chief Executive Officer
COO: David Byrom, Chief Executive Officer
CFO: Carol Jones, Controller and Manager Business Office
CMO: J D Sheffield, D.O., President Medical Staff
CIO: Mike Huckabee, Network Administrator
CHR: Paula Smithhart, Director Human Resources
CNO: Jeanne Griffith, Chief Nursing Officer
Web address: www.cmhos.org
**Control:** Hospital district or authority, Government, nonfederal **Service:** General Medical and Surgical

**Staffed Beds:** 25 **Admissions:** 896 **Census:** 7 **Outpatient Visits:** 57951
**Births:** 0 **Total Expense ($000):** 21209 **Payroll Expense ($000):** 10048
**Personnel:** 306

## GILMER—Upshur County

★ **EAST TEXAS MEDICAL CENTER–GILMER (450884)**, 712 North Wood Street, Zip 75644–1751; tel. 903/841–7100 **A**9 10 **F**3 11 29 30 40 43 50 57 59 68 85 87 97 107 108 111 114 118 126 **S** East Texas Medical Center Regional Healthcare System, Tyler, TX
Primary Contact: Jorge E. Leal, Administrator
CFO: Thomas O'Gorman, Jr., Chief Financial Officer
CHR: William Henry, Director Human Resources
Web address: www.etmc.org
**Control:** Other not–for–profit (including NFP Corporation) **Service:** General Medical and Surgical

**Staffed Beds:** 35 **Admissions:** 696 **Census:** 6 **Outpatient Visits:** 30708
**Births:** 0 **Total Expense ($000):** 11170 **Payroll Expense ($000):** 3697
**Personnel:** 78

## GLEN ROSE—Somervell County

✠ **GLEN ROSE MEDICAL CENTER (450451)**, 1021 Holden Street, Zip 76043–4937, Mailing Address: P.O. Box 2099, Zip 76043–2099; tel. 254/897–2215, (Total facility includes 118 beds in nursing home–type unit) **A**1 9 10 **F**15 29 34 40 42 43 45 56 57 59 65 79 81 90 93 103 104 107 108 110 111 112 118 126 128 129 131 132 142 145 **P**7
Primary Contact: Ray Reynolds, Chief Executive Officer
COO: Mo S. Sheldon, Chief Operating Officer
CHR: Janice Nickell, Administrative Assistant
Web address: www.glenrosemedicalcenter.com
**Control:** County–Government, nonfederal **Service:** General Medical and Surgical

**Staffed Beds:** 134 **Admissions:** 822 **Census:** 99 **Outpatient Visits:** 100017
**Births:** 0 **Total Expense ($000):** 15473 **Payroll Expense ($000):** 8561
**Personnel:** 151

## GONZALES—Gonzales County

★ **MEMORIAL HOSPITAL (450235)**, 1110 Sarah Dewitt Drive, Zip 78629–2021, Mailing Address: P.O. Box 587, Zip 78629–0587; tel. 830/672–7581 **A**9 10 **F**3 11 13 15 29 30 34 35 38 40 43 53 57 59 62 64 65 68 70 75 76 77 81 85 87 93 97 107 111 114 118 126 128 129 131 132 147 **S** QHR, Brentwood, TN
Primary Contact: Charles Norris, Chief Executive Officer
CFO: Patty Stewart, Chief Financial Officer
CMO: Commie Hisey, D.O., Chief of Staff
CHR: Joni Leland, Director Human Resources
Web address: www.gonzaleshealthcare.com
**Control:** Hospital district or authority, Government, nonfederal **Service:** General Medical and Surgical

**Staffed Beds:** 32 **Admissions:** 1034 **Census:** 8 **Outpatient Visits:** 61839
**Births:** 167 **Total Expense ($000):** 22075 **Payroll Expense ($000):** 9409
**Personnel:** 228

## GRAHAM—Young County

★ **GRAHAM REGIONAL MEDICAL CENTER (450085)**, 1301 Montgomery Road, Zip 76450–4224, Mailing Address: P.O. Box 1390, Zip 76450–1390; tel. 940/549–3400 **A**9 10 20 **F**7 11 13 15 28 29 40 43 46 53 57 59 62 63 70 75 76 79 81 85 89 93 104 107 111 114 118 126 129 132 134 **P**5
Primary Contact: Steve L. Hartgraves, Administrator and Chief Executive Officer
CFO: Bonnie Blevins, Chief Financial Officer
CIO: Jeff Clark, Director Information Systems
CHR: Judy Guinn, Chief Human Resources Officer
Web address: www.grahamrmc.com
**Control:** City–Government, nonfederal **Service:** General Medical and Surgical

**Staffed Beds:** 37 **Admissions:** 1225 **Census:** 11 **Outpatient Visits:** 65240
**Births:** 261 **Total Expense ($000):** 18749 **Payroll Expense ($000):** 9207
**Personnel:** 197

## GRANBURY—Hood County

✠ **LAKE GRANBURY MEDICAL CENTER (450596)**, 1310 Paluxy Road, Zip 76048–5655; tel. 817/573–2273 **A**1 9 10 **F**3 8 11 12 13 15 18 20 22 26 28 29 30 34 37 40 43 45 49 53 57 59 64 70 74 75 76 77 79 81 82 85 86 93 107 108 110 111 113 117 118 125 128 132 145 146 **S** Community Health Systems, Inc., Franklin, TN
Primary Contact: David Orcutt, Chief Executive Officer
COO: Vicky Cha, Assistant Chief Executive Officer
CIO: Kevin Myers, Director Information Systems
CHR: Carol Langley, Director Human Resources
Web address: www.lakegranburymedicalcenter.com
**Control:** Corporation, Investor–owned, for–profit **Service:** General Medical and Surgical

**Staffed Beds:** 83 **Admissions:** 2443 **Census:** 20 **Outpatient Visits:** 43340
**Births:** 506 **Total Expense ($000):** 28812 **Payroll Expense ($000):** 15261
**Personnel:** 277

## GRAND SALINE—Van Zandt County

**COZBY–GERMANY HOSPITAL (450283)**, 707 North Waldrip Street, Zip 75140–1555; tel. 903/962–4242, (Nonreporting) **A**9 10 20
Primary Contact: Patty Vasquez, Administrator
CMO: Irfan Rana, M.D., Chief of Staff
CIO: Suzi Walker, Manager Business Office
CHR: Lee Anne Sanders, Director Human Resources
Web address: www.cozbygermanyhospital.com
**Control:** Other not–for–profit (including NFP Corporation) **Service:** General Medical and Surgical

**Staffed Beds:** 24

## GRAPEVINE—Tarrant County

✠ **BAYLOR REGIONAL MEDICAL CENTER AT GRAPEVINE (450563)**, 1650 West College Street, Zip 76051–1650; tel. 817/481–1588 **A**1 9 10 **F**3 11 12 13 15 18 20 22 24 26 28 29 30 31 34 35 40 45 46 47 48 49 56 57 59 61 64 65 70 72 74 75 76 77 78 79 80 81 82 86 87 107 108 110 111 113 114 118 125 128 129 130 131 134 144 145 146 **S** Baylor Health Care System, Dallas, TX
Primary Contact: Doug Lawson, President
COO: Chris York, FACHE, Chief Operating Officer
CFO: Preshie Wilson, Vice President Finance Services
CMO: Thomas Purgett, M.D., Chief Medical Staff
CIO: David Krzjci, Director Information Systems
CHR: Donna Stark, Director Human Resources
Web address: www.bhcs.com
**Control:** Other not–for–profit (including NFP Corporation) **Service:** General Medical and Surgical

**Staffed Beds:** 274 **Admissions:** 12809 **Census:** 162 **Outpatient Visits:** 90624 **Births:** 2986 **Total Expense ($000):** 213565 **Payroll Expense ($000):** 78350 **Personnel:** 1179

☐ **ETHICUS HOSPITAL – GRAPEVINE (452110)**, 4201 William D. Tate Avenue, Zip 76051; tel. 817/288–1300 **A**1 9 10 **F**1 3 29 30 40 60 64 68 74 75 77 84 85 87 93 96 107 118 129 147
Primary Contact: Robbye N. Dubois, Chief Executive Officer
Web address: www.ethicusgrapevine.com
**Control:** Partnership, Investor–owned, for–profit **Service:** Long–Term Acute Care hospital

**Staffed Beds:** 46 **Admissions:** 524 **Census:** 44 **Outpatient Visits:** 38 **Births:** 0 **Total Expense ($000):** 24984 **Payroll Expense ($000):** 11972
**Personnel:** 164

## GREENVILLE—Hunt County

☐ **GLEN OAKS HOSPITAL (454050)**, 301 Division Street, Zip 75401–4101; tel. 903/454–6000 **A**1 9 10 **F**4 5 29 34 40 68 98 99 100 101 102 103 104 105 **S** Universal Health Services, Inc., King of Prussia, PA
Primary Contact: Joel Klein, Chief Executive Officer and Managing Director
CFO: Lowell K. Hudson, Chief Financial Officer
CMO: David Lucas, R.N., Director of Nursing
CMO: Satish Narayan, M.D., Medical Director
CHR: Joe Carson, Director Human Resources
Web address: www.glenoakshospital.com
**Control:** Corporation, Investor–owned, for–profit **Service:** Psychiatric

**Staffed Beds:** 54 **Admissions:** 1700 **Census:** 42 **Outpatient Visits:** 5514
**Births:** 0 **Total Expense ($000):** 7334 **Payroll Expense ($000):** 3959
**Personnel:** 90

**TX**

---

**Hospital, Medicare Provider Number, Address, Telephone, Approval, Facility, and Physician Codes, Health Care System**

★ American Hospital Association (AHA) membership
☐ The Joint Commission accreditation ◇ DNV Healthcare Inc. accreditation
○ American Osteopathic Association (AOA) accreditation
△ Commission on Accreditation of Rehabilitation Facilities (CARF) accreditation

✠ **HUNT MEMORIAL HOSPITAL DISTRICT (450352)**, 4215 Joe Ramsey Boulevard, Zip 75401–7899, Mailing Address: P.O. Box 1059, Zip 75403–1059; tel. 903/408–5000, (Includes HUNT MEMORIAL HOSPITAL DISTRICT, 4215 Joe Ramsey Boulevard, Zip 75403–1059, Mailing Address: Drawer 1059, Zip 75403–1059; tel. 903/408–5000) **A**1 9 10 **F**3 8 11 13 15 28 29 30 31 34 35 40 41 43 45 46 49 50 53 57 59 62 68 70 73 75 76 77 78 79 81 82 84 85 86 87 90 93 98 103 104 107 108 110 111 113 114 116 117 118 120 122 128 129 131 132 145 147 **P**6
Primary Contact: Richard Carter, District Chief Executive Officer
COO: Michael R. Klepin, Administrator
CFO: Jeri Rich, Assistant Administrator and Chief Financial Officer
CMO: James H. Sandin, M.D., Assistant Administrator Medical Affairs
CIO: Joe Hartley, Director Information Systems
CHR: John Heatherly, Assistant Administrator Support Services
Web address: www.huntregional.org
**Control:** Hospital district or authority, Government, nonfederal **Service:** General Medical and Surgical

**Staffed Beds:** 206 **Admissions:** 6947 **Census:** 86 **Outpatient Visits:** 118640 **Births:** 1071 **Total Expense ($000):** 101324 **Payroll Expense ($000):** 41117 **Personnel:** 781

### GROESBECK—Limestone County

★ **LIMESTONE MEDICAL CENTER (451303)**, 701 Mcclintic Drive, Zip 76642–2128; tel. 254/729–3281 **A**9 10 18 **F**3 7 11 28 32 34 35 40 41 43 45 57 64 65 75 77 84 85 90 93 96 97 104 107 113 126 128 129 132 134 145 147
Primary Contact: Penny Gray, Administrator and Chief Executive Officer
COO: Larry Price, Assistant Administrator
CFO: Mike Williams, Accountant
CIO: Byong Lee, Manager Information Technology and PACS Administrator
CHR: Jean Koester, Manager Human Resources
CNO: Jean Wragge, Director of Nurses
Web address: www.lmchospital.com
**Control:** Hospital district or authority, Government, nonfederal **Service:** General Medical and Surgical

**Staffed Beds:** 20 **Admissions:** 319 **Census:** 8 **Outpatient Visits:** 19663 **Births:** 0 **Total Expense ($000):** 16609 **Payroll Expense ($000):** 7022 **Personnel:** 182

### GROVES—Jefferson County

○ **RENAISSANCE HOSPITAL (450123)**, 5500 39th Street, Zip 77619–9805; tel. 409/962–5733 **A**9 10 11 **F**3 17 18 20 22 24 29 40 45 46 47 57 60 64 70 79 81 82 85 87 107 108 111 113 117 118 **S** Renaissance Healthcare Systems, Houston, TX
Primary Contact: Eileen Nguyen, Administrator
CFO: John Murphy, Chief Financial Officer
Web address: www.renhealthcare.org
**Control:** Individual, Investor–owned, for–profit **Service:** General Medical and Surgical

**Staffed Beds:** 28 **Admissions:** 986 **Census:** 15 **Outpatient Visits:** 9776 **Births:** 0 **Personnel:** 166

### HALLETTSVILLE—Lavaca County

**LAVACA MEDICAL CENTER (451376)**, 1400 North Texana Street, Zip 77964–2099; tel. 361/798–3671 **A**9 10 18 **F**11 15 29 34 40 41 43 53 56 57 59 64 65 68 77 80 81 85 86 87 93 97 107 111 113 118 126 132 134 145 147
Primary Contact: James Vanek, Chief Executive Officer
**Control:** Hospital district or authority, Government, nonfederal **Service:** General Medical and Surgical

**Staffed Beds:** 25 **Admissions:** 556 **Census:** 6 **Outpatient Visits:** 22640 **Births:** 0 **Total Expense ($000):** 13948 **Payroll Expense ($000):** 5205 **Personnel:** 124

### HAMILTON—Hamilton County

★ **HAMILTON GENERAL HOSPITAL (450754)**, 400 North Brown Street, Zip 76531–1518; tel. 254/386–1600 **A**9 10 20 **F**3 7 11 28 34 40 43 44 45 50 53 56 57 59 64 68 79 80 81 82 85 86 93 97 103 104 107 113 126 129 131
Primary Contact: Michele Cathey, Administrator and Chief Executive Officer
CFO: Brenda Denison, Chief Financial Officer
CIO: Chad Reinert, Director Information Technology
CHR: Emily Dossey, Director Human Resources
CNO: Debra Martin, Director of Nursing
Web address: www.hamiltonhospital.org
**Control:** Hospital district or authority, Government, nonfederal **Service:** General Medical and Surgical

**Staffed Beds:** 34 **Admissions:** 1811 **Census:** 17 **Outpatient Visits:** 97725 **Births:** 0 **Total Expense ($000):** 19858 **Payroll Expense ($000):** 8497 **Personnel:** 192

### HAMLIN—Jones County

**HAMLIN MEMORIAL HOSPITAL (450243)**, 632 Northwest Second Street, Zip 79520–3831, Mailing Address: P.O. Box 400, Zip 79520–0400; tel. 325/576–3646 **A**9 10 **F**3 7 11 28 29 40 43 64 68 69 93 107 132 134 145 147 **P**5
Primary Contact: Patricia Barnett, Chief Executive Officer
CMO: Krishna Sunkavalle, M.D., Chief Medical Officer
Web address: www.hamlinedc.org
**Control:** Hospital district or authority, Government, nonfederal **Service:** General Medical and Surgical

**Staffed Beds:** 23 **Admissions:** 187 **Census:** 3 **Outpatient Visits:** 4275 **Births:** 0 **Total Expense ($000):** 3145 **Payroll Expense ($000):** 1846 **Personnel:** 70

### HARLINGEN—Cameron County

☐ **HARLINGEN MEDICAL CENTER (450855)**, 5501 South Expressway 77, Zip 78550; tel. 956/365–1000 **A**1 9 10 **F**3 12 13 15 17 18 20 22 24 29 30 40 43 49 50 51 57 59 64 68 70 74 75 76 79 81 85 86 89 107 108 110 111 113 114 117 118 128 129 145 146 147 **P**2 **S** Prime Healthcare Services, Ontario, CA
Primary Contact: Todd Mann, President and Chief Executive Officer
COO: Brenda Ivory, Vice President Clinical Services and Chief Operating Officer
CFO: Harvey Torres, Vice President Finance and Chief Financial Officer
CMO: Hugo Blake, M.D., Chief Medical Staff
CHR: Diane Elizondo, Director Human Resources
Web address: www.hmcrgv.com
**Control:** Partnership, Investor–owned, for–profit **Service:** General Medical and Surgical

**Staffed Beds:** 88 **Admissions:** 5619 **Census:** 51 **Outpatient Visits:** 71992 **Births:** 1145 **Total Expense ($000):** 68681 **Payroll Expense ($000):** 25913 **Personnel:** 441

☐ **RIO GRANDE STATE CENTER/SOUTH TEXAS HEALTH CARE SYSTEM (454088)**, 1401 South Rangerville Road, Zip 78552–7638; tel. 956/364–8000, (Includes RIO GRANDE STATE CENTER, 1401 South Rangerville Road, tel. 956/364–8000; SOUTH TEXAS HEALTH CARE SYSTEM, 1401 Rangerville Road, Zip 78552–7609; tel. 956/364–8000) **A**1 9 10 **F**15 30 53 54 57 65 66 68 75 87 97 98 101 107 118 129 131 134 142 145 146 **P**6 **S** Texas Department of State Health Services, Austin, TX
Primary Contact: Sonia Hernandez–Keeble, Superintendent
CFO: Tom Garza, Director Fiscal and Support
CMO: David Moron, M.D., Clinical Director
CIO: Blas Ortiz, Jr., Assistant Superintendent and Public Information Officer
CHR: Irma Garcia, Job Coordinator
Web address: www.dshs.state.tx.us/mhospital/riograndesc/default.shtm
**Control:** State–Government, nonfederal **Service:** Psychiatric

**Staffed Beds:** 128 **Admissions:** 1110 **Census:** 52 **Outpatient Visits:** 62971 **Births:** 0 **Total Expense ($000):** 15649 **Payroll Expense ($000):** 7848 **Personnel:** 483

**SOLARA HOSPITAL HARLINGEN (452101)**, 508 Victoria Lane, Zip 78550–3225; tel. 956/425–9600 **A**9 10 **F**1 3 29 30 34 35 75 85 86 129 147 **S** Solara Healthcare, Dallas, TX
Primary Contact: Paul E. Qualls, Jr., Chief Executive Officer
CFO: Laura Nowell, Vice President Accounting and Finance
CMO: Ann B. McCracken, M.D., President Medical Staff
CIO: Adam Davis, Chief Information Officer
CHR: Lydia Cantu–Lopez, Human Resources Representative
Web address: www.solarahc.com/shcha.html
**Control:** Partnership, Investor–owned, for–profit **Service:** Long–Term Acute Care hospital

**Staffed Beds:** 82 **Admissions:** 751 **Census:** 54 **Outpatient Visits:** 0 **Births:** 0 **Total Expense ($000):** 25635 **Payroll Expense ($000):** 9723 **Personnel:** 190

✠ **VALLEY BAPTIST MEDICAL CENTER–HARLINGEN (450033)**, 2101 Pease Street, Zip 78550–8307, Mailing Address: P.O. Drawer 2588, Zip 78551–2588; tel. 956/389–1100 **A**1 3 5 9 10 **F**3 11 12 13 14 15 17 18 20 22 24 26 28 29 30 31 34 35 39 40 43 44 45 46 47 48 49 50 51 54 56 57 59 60 63 64 65 68 70 71 72 73 74 75 76 77 78 79 81 82 84 85 86 87 88 89 90 91 92 93 94 100 103 104 107 108 110 111 112 113 114 118 125 128 129 131 143 145 146 147 **P**8 **S** Valley Baptist Health System, Harlingen, TX
Primary Contact: William D. Adams, Senior Vice President and Chief Executive Officer
CFO: Joe Beck, Chief Financial Officer
CMO: E. Chandler Deal, M.D., Vice President Medical Affairs and Chief Medical Officer
CIO: Jim Barbaglia, Chief Information Officer
CHR: Irma L. Pye, Senior Vice President and Chief Human Resource Officer
Web address: www.valleybaptist.net
**Control:** Other not–for–profit (including NFP Corporation) **Service:** General Medical and Surgical

**Staffed Beds:** 416 **Admissions:** 18583 **Census:** 262 **Outpatient Visits:** 93691 **Births:** 1945 **Total Expense ($000):** 244830 **Payroll Expense ($000):** 68075 **Personnel:** 1262

*Many Facility Codes have changed. Please refer to the AHA Guide Code Chart.* © 2012 AHA Guide

**TX**

## HASKELL—Haskell County

**HASKELL MEMORIAL HOSPITAL (451341)**, 1 North Avenue N,
Zip 79521–5499, Mailing Address: P.O. Box 1117, Zip 79521–1117;
tel. 940/864–2621 **A**9 10 18 **F**11 28 29 34 35 40 45 56 57 59 68 75 77 86
87 93 118 129 130 132 145 **P**1
Primary Contact: Fran McCown, Administrator
CHR: Emily Moore, Director Human Resources and Information Technology
CNO: Charolotte Welch, Chief Nursing Officer
**Control:** Hospital district or authority, Government, nonfederal **Service:** General
Medical and Surgical

**Staffed Beds:** 25 **Admissions:** 297 **Census:** 3 **Outpatient Visits:** 7160
**Births:** 0 **Total Expense ($000):** 3700 **Payroll Expense ($000):** 1843
**Personnel:** 59

## HEMPHILL—Sabine County

☒ **SABINE COUNTY HOSPITAL (451361)**, Highway 83 West, Zip 75948, Mailing
Address: P.O. Box 750, Zip 75948–0750; tel. 409/787–3300 **A**1 9 10 18 **F**34
40 43 50 57 59 64 68 75 83 84 91 92 93 94 107 113 118 126 132
**S** Preferred Management Corporation, Shawnee, OK
Primary Contact: Diana Taylor, Administrator
COO: Deanna Lathrop, Assistant Administrator
CFO: Cindy Erickson, Chief Financial Officer
CMO: Grover C. Winslow, M.D., Chief of Staff
CIO: Margaret Moore, Manager Business Office
Web address: www.sabinecountyhospital.com/
**Control:** Corporation, Investor–owned, for–profit **Service:** General Medical and
Surgical

**Staffed Beds:** 25 **Admissions:** 321 **Census:** 4 **Outpatient Visits:** 21041
**Births:** 0 **Total Expense ($000):** 5883 **Payroll Expense ($000):** 2774
**Personnel:** 80

## HENDERSON—Rusk County

☒ **EAST TEXAS MEDICAL CENTER HENDERSON (450475)**, 300 Wilson Street,
Zip 75652–5956; tel. 903/657–7541 **A**1 9 10 **F**3 8 11 13 15 28 29 30 34 35
37 40 43 45 50 57 59 64 65 70 75 76 79 81 85 107 108 110 111 114 118
126 128 132 144 145 146 147 **S** East Texas Medical Center Regional
Healthcare System, Tyler, TX
Primary Contact: Mark Leitner, Chief Executive Officer
COO: Carla Degges, R.N., Chief Clinical Officer
CFO: Phillip A. Caron, Chief Financial Officer
CHR: William Henry, Director Human Resources
Web address: www.etmc.org/etmchenderson
**Control:** Other not–for–profit (including NFP Corporation) **Service:** General
Medical and Surgical

**Staffed Beds:** 47 **Admissions:** 1509 **Census:** 15 **Outpatient Visits:** 45642
**Births:** 210 **Total Expense ($000):** 21592 **Payroll Expense ($000):** 9295
**Personnel:** 179

## HENRIETTA—Clay County

**CLAY COUNTY MEMORIAL HOSPITAL (451362)**, 310 West South Street,
Zip 76365–3346; tel. 940/538–5621 **A**9 10 18 **F**7 8 11 28 34 35 40 50 53
57 62 68 80 81 90 93 107 111 118 129 131 132 **P**5
Primary Contact: Jeff Huskey, Chief Executive Officer and Administrator
COO: Michael Clark, Director Operations
CFO: Debra Haehn, Chief Financial Officer
CMO: Mitchell Wolfe, M.D., Chief of Staff
CIO: Larry Evangelista, Supervisor Information Technology
CHR: Linda Burleson, Administrative Secretary
Web address: www.ccmhospital.com
**Control:** County–Government, nonfederal **Service:** General Medical and Surgical

**Staffed Beds:** 25 **Admissions:** 257 **Census:** 2 **Outpatient Visits:** 7701
**Births:** 0 **Total Expense ($000):** 4736 **Payroll Expense ($000):** 2890
**Personnel:** 82

## HEREFORD—Deaf Smith County

**HEREFORD REGIONAL MEDICAL CENTER (450155)**, 801 East Third Street,
Zip 79045–5727; tel. 806/364–2141 **A**9 10 **F**3 7 11 13 15 29 35 40 43 50
57 59 62 65 70 76 77 81 85 93 107 113 118 126 129 132 146 **P**5
Primary Contact: Nathan A. Flood, Chief Executive Officer
COO: Meri Killingsworth, Chief Operating Officer
CFO: Greg Reinart, Chief Financial Officer
Web address: www.herefordregional.com
**Control:** Hospital district or authority, Government, nonfederal **Service:** General
Medical and Surgical

**Staffed Beds:** 35 **Admissions:** 739 **Census:** 7 **Outpatient Visits:** 71400
**Births:** 314 **Total Expense ($000):** 16489 **Payroll Expense ($000):** 6854
**Personnel:** 179

## HILLSBORO—Hill County

☒ **HILL REGIONAL HOSPITAL (450192)**, 101 Circle Drive, Zip 76645–2670;
tel. 254/580–8500 **A**1 9 10 **F**3 13 15 17 18 19 29 34 35 40 43 45 50 57 59
64 65 68 70 75 76 77 79 81 86 87 88 89 93 107 117 118 132 145 146
**S** Community Health Systems, Inc., Franklin, TN
Primary Contact: Jan McClure, Chief Executive Officer
CFO: Judy Culp, Chief Financial Officer
CHR: Becky Hale, Director Human Resources
Web address: www.chs.net
**Control:** Corporation, Investor–owned, for–profit **Service:** General Medical and
Surgical

**Staffed Beds:** 66 **Admissions:** 1970 **Census:** 17 **Outpatient Visits:** 22066
**Births:** 294 **Total Expense ($000):** 30097 **Payroll Expense ($000):** 10139
**Personnel:** 167

## HONDO—Medina County

**MEDINA COMMUNITY HOSPITAL** See Medina Regional Hospital

**MEDINA REGIONAL HOSPITAL (451330)**, 3100 Avenue E., Zip 78861–3599;
tel. 830/426–7700 **A**9 10 18 **F**3 11 13 15 29 34 35 40 43 45 50 57 59 64
76 81 87 93 97 107 111 113 118 126 132 145 **P**4
Primary Contact: Janice Simons, FACHE, Chief Executive Officer
COO: Dale Semar, Controller
CFO: Kevin Frosch, Chief Financial Officer
CMO: John Meyer, M.D., Chief of Staff
CIO: Michael Smith, Director Support Services and Information Technology
CHR: Sharon Garcia, Human Resources Representative
Web address: www.medinahospital.net
**Control:** Hospital district or authority, Government, nonfederal **Service:** General
Medical and Surgical

**Staffed Beds:** 25 **Admissions:** 823 **Census:** 7 **Outpatient Visits:** 92620
**Births:** 191 **Total Expense ($000):** 19367 **Payroll Expense ($000):** 7178
**Personnel:** 181

## HOUSTON—Harris County

☐ **BEHAVIORAL HOSPITAL OF BELLAIRE (454107)**, 5314 Dashwood Drive,
Zip 77081–4603; tel. 713/600–9500 **A**1 9 10 **F**4 5 56 98 100 103 104 105
**S** Ascend Health Corporation, New York, NY
Primary Contact: Lawrence Story, Chief Executive Officer
Web address: www.bhbhospital.com
**Control:** Corporation, Investor–owned, for–profit **Service:** Psychiatric

**Staffed Beds:** 70 **Admissions:** 1875 **Census:** 59 **Outpatient Visits:** 14713
**Births:** 0 **Total Expense ($000):** 13967 **Payroll Expense ($000):** 8190
**Personnel:** 179

**BEN TAUB GENERAL HOSPITAL** See Harris County Hospital District

**CHILDREN'S MEMORIAL HERMANN HOSPITAL** See Memorial Hermann –
Texas Medical Center

**CORNERSTONE HOSPITAL OF HOUSTON – BELLAIRE (452032)**, 5314
Dashwood, Zip 77081; tel. 713/295–5300, (Includes CORNERSTONE HOSPITAL
OF HOUSTON AT CLEARLAKE, 709 Medical Center Boulevard, Webster,
Zip 77598; tel. 281/332–3322; Steve Flaherty, Chief Executive Officer) **A**9 10 **F**1
3 29 65 85 86 87 91 129 147 **S** Cornerstone Healthcare Group, Dallas, TX
Primary Contact: James Camp, R.N., Chief Executive Officer
COO: Ken W. McGee, Vice President Operations
CFO: A. Shane Wells, Chief Financial Officer
CMO: Mark Barlow, M.D., Chief Medical Officer and President Medical Staff
CIO: Kent Chambless, Chief Information Officer
CHR: Margaret Blunt, Director Human Resources
Web address: www.chghospitals.com
**Control:** Partnership, Investor–owned, for–profit **Service:** Long–Term Acute Care
hospital

**Staffed Beds:** 130 **Admissions:** 1282 **Census:** 90 **Outpatient Visits:** 0
**Births:** 0 **Total Expense ($000):** 39596 **Payroll Expense ($000):** 14220
**Personnel:** 272

☒ **CORNERSTONE HOSPITAL OF SOUTH HOUSTON (452055)**, 1919 Labranch
7GWS Street, Zip 77002; tel. 713/756–8660 **A**1 9 10 **F**1 3 29 65 68 77 85 86
87 147 **S** Cornerstone Healthcare Group, Dallas, TX
Primary Contact: Sharon Stuart, R.N., Chief Executive Officer
COO: Sam D. Barkman, Vice President Operations
Web address: www.chghospitals.com
**Control:** Church–operated, Nongovernment, not–for profit **Service:** Long–Term
Acute Care hospital

**Staffed Beds:** 30 **Admissions:** 167 **Census:** 11 **Outpatient Visits:** 0 **Births:**
0 **Total Expense ($000):** 5804 **Payroll Expense ($000):** 2540 **Personnel:**
37

**TX**

☐ **CYPRESS CREEK HOSPITAL (454108)**, 17750 Cali Drive, Zip 77090–2700; tel. 281/586–7600 **A**1 9 10 **F**4 5 29 30 64 71 87 98 99 100 102 104 105 129 131 **S** Universal Health Services, Inc., King of Prussia, PA
Primary Contact: Brian Brooker, Chief Executive Officer
CFO: Carol Neilson–Beale, Chief Financial Officer
CMO: Marshall Lucas, M.D., Medical Director
CHR: Brenda Dominguez, Director Human Resources
CNO: Shazetta Richardson, Director of Nursing
Web address: www.cypresscreekhospital.com
**Control:** Corporation, Investor–owned, for–profit **Service:** Psychiatric

**Staffed Beds:** 96 **Admissions:** 4089 **Census:** 87 **Outpatient Visits:** 7292 **Births:** 0 **Total Expense ($000):** 22374 **Payroll Expense ($000):** 10662 **Personnel:** 209

✉ **CYPRESS FAIRBANKS MEDICAL CENTER (450716)**, 10655 Steepletop Drive, Zip 77065–4297; tel. 281/890–4285 **A**1 9 10 **F**3 11 12 13 15 18 20 22 24 28 29 30 31 34 40 42 45 46 47 49 50 53 57 59 64 70 72 74 75 76 77 78 79 81 82 85 87 89 93 107 108 110 111 112 113 114 117 118 123 128 129 130 131 143 144 145 146 147 **P**8 **S** TENET Healthcare Corporation, Dallas, TX
Primary Contact: Terry J. Wheeler, Chief Executive Officer
COO: Jaikumar Krishnaswamy, Chief Operating Officer
CFO: James Wright, M.D., Chief Financial Officer
CMO: Marcus Barnett, M.D., Chief of Staff
CIO: Donna Cain, Director Information Systems Department
CHR: Lorinnsa Bridges Kee, Director Human Resource
Web address: www.cyfairhospital.com
**Control:** Corporation, Investor–owned, for–profit **Service:** General Medical and Surgical

**Staffed Beds:** 181 **Admissions:** 8712 **Census:** 95 **Outpatient Visits:** 94474 **Births:** 3021 **Total Expense ($000):** 108227 **Payroll Expense ($000):** 45287 **Personnel:** 697

☐ **DOCTOR'S HOSPITAL – TIDWELL (450803)**, 510 West Tidwell Road, Zip 77091–4399; tel. 713/691–1111, (Includes DOCTORS HOSPITAL PARKWAY, 233 West Parker Road, Zip 77076–2999; tel. 281/765–2600) **A**1 9 10 **F**11 13 15 18 20 22 26 29 34 39 40 44 45 46 47 49 50 57 59 60 68 70 74 75 77 79 81 85 93 96 107 111 113 118 142 147
Primary Contact: Michael R. Bullard, Chief Executive Officer
COO: Farida Moeen, M.D., Chief Operating Officer
CFO: Theresa Eatherly, Chief Financial Officer
CMO: Cesar Ortega, M.D., Chief of Staff
CIO: Dell Davis, Director Information Systems
CHR: Carolyn Washington, Director of Human Resources
Web address: www.dhthou.com/
**Control:** Partnership, Investor–owned, for–profit **Service:** General Medical and Surgical

**Staffed Beds:** 89 **Admissions:** 4190 **Census:** 39 **Outpatient Visits:** 23148 **Births:** 1232 **Total Expense ($000):** 40537 **Payroll Expense ($000):** 18318 **Personnel:** 350

**DUBUIS HOSPITAL OF HOUSTON** See Cornerstone Hospital of South Houston

★ △ **HARRIS COUNTY HOSPITAL DISTRICT (450289)**, 2525 Holly Hall Street, Zip 77054–4108, Mailing Address: P.O. Box 66769, Zip 77266–6769; tel. 713/566–6403, (Includes BEN TAUB GENERAL HOSPITAL, 1504 Taub Loop, Zip 77030; tel. 713/873–2300; LYNDON B JOHNSON GENERAL HOSPITAL, 5656 Kelley, Zip 77026; tel. 713/566–5000; Jesse Lee Tucker, Administrator; QUENTIN MEASE HOSPITAL, 3601 North MacGregor, Zip 77004; tel. 713/873–3700; Jeffrey Webster, Administrator), (Total facility includes 24 beds in nursing home–type unit) **A**2 3 5 7 8 9 10 **F**3 5 7 13 15 17 18 20 22 24 26 29 30 31 32 34 35 39 40 43 45 46 49 50 51 54 55 56 57 58 59 60 61 64 65 68 70 71 72 73 74 75 76 77 78 79 81 82 84 87 88 89 90 91 92 93 94 97 98 99 100 101 102 103 104 107 110 111 112 113 114 117 118 119 120 123 127 128 129 131 133 134 142 143 144 145 146 147 **P**6
Primary Contact: David S. Lopez, FACHE, President and Chief Executive Officer
COO: George V. Masi, Chief Operating Officer
CFO: Michael Norby, Interim Chief Financial Officer
CMO: Fred Sutton, M.D., Chief Medical Officer
CIO: Tim Tindle, Chief Information Officer
CHR: Lou Gould, Vice President Human Resources
Web address: www.hchdonline.com
**Control:** Hospital district or authority, Government, nonfederal **Service:** General Medical and Surgical

**Staffed Beds:** 825 **Admissions:** 36686 **Census:** 578 **Outpatient Visits:** 1636623 **Births:** 7662 **Total Expense ($000):** 708853 **Payroll Expense ($000):** 456702 **Personnel:** 6812

☐ **HEALTHBRIDGE CHILDREN'S HOSPITAL OF HOUSTON (453309)**, 2929 Woodland Park Drive, Zip 77082; tel. 281/293–7774 **A**1 9 10 21 **F**3 29 74 75 79 85 87 89 93 100 129 145 147 **S** Nexus Health Systems, Houston, TX
Primary Contact: Joseph Rafferty, Chief Executive Officer
CMO: Robert Yetman, M.D., Medical Director
CHR: Guy Murdock, Vice President Human Resources
Web address: www.healthbridgehouston.com/
**Control:** Partnership, Investor–owned, for–profit **Service:** Children's general

**Staffed Beds:** 40 **Admissions:** 337 **Census:** 26 **Outpatient Visits:** 305 **Births:** 0 **Total Expense ($000):** 13547 **Payroll Expense ($000):** 5646 **Personnel:** 108

★ **HEALTHSOUTH REHABILITATION HOSPITAL OF CYPRESS (673050)**, 13031 Wortham Center Drive, Zip 77065–5662; tel. 832/280–2512, (Nonreporting) **A**10 **S** HEALTHSOUTH Corporation, Birmingham, AL
Primary Contact: Sheila A. Kramer, Chief Executive Officer
Web address: www.healthsouthcypress.com
**Control:** Corporation, Investor–owned, for–profit **Service:** Rehabilitation

**Staffed Beds:** 40

☐ **HOUSTON HOSPITAL FOR SPECIALIZED SURGERY (450797)**, 5445 La Branch Street, Zip 77004–6836; tel. 713/528–6800 **A**1 3 5 9 10 **F**3 8 40 45 46 47 48 49 74 79 81 82
Primary Contact: Walter W. Topp, III, Administrator
CFO: Deborah Jones, Controller
Web address: www.scasurgery.com
**Control:** Partnership, Investor–owned, for–profit **Service:** General Medical and Surgical

**Staffed Beds:** 7 **Admissions:** 132 **Census:** 1 **Outpatient Visits:** 5277 **Births:** 0 **Total Expense ($000):** 12639 **Payroll Expense ($000):** 3667 **Personnel:** 86

✉ **HOUSTON NORTHWEST MEDICAL CENTER (450638)**, 710 FM 1960 Road West, Zip 77090–3402; tel. 281/440–1000 **A**1 2 3 5 9 10 **F**3 8 11 12 13 15 18 20 22 24 26 28 29 30 31 34 40 43 45 46 49 50 54 59 64 65 70 72 74 75 77 78 79 81 82 84 85 86 87 89 91 92 93 96 102 107 108 109 110 111 112 113 114 115 116 117 118 125 128 129 131 134 143 144 145 146 147 **S** TENET Healthcare Corporation, Dallas, TX
Primary Contact: Linda Mercier, R.N., MSN, Chief Executive Officer
COO: Juan Fresquez, Chief Operating Officer
CFO: Sean B. Gallagher, Chief Financial Officer
CIO: Terry Janis, Director Information Systems
CHR: Judy White House, Director Human Resources
Web address: www.hnmc.com
**Control:** Partnership, Investor–owned, for–profit **Service:** General Medical and Surgical

**Staffed Beds:** 339 **Admissions:** 16761 **Census:** 206 **Outpatient Visits:** 135914 **Births:** 2802 **Total Expense ($000):** 224345 **Payroll Expense ($000):** 83700 **Personnel:** 1305

☐ **INTRACARE NORTH HOSPITAL (454083)**, 1120 Cypress Station Drive, Zip 77090–3031; tel. 281/893–7200 **A**1 9 10 **F**5 98 99 100 101 103 104 105
Primary Contact: Rob Yates, Chief Executive Officer
CFO: Fred Chan, Chief Financial Officer
CMO: Javier Ruiz, M.D., Medical Director
Web address: www.intracare.org
**Control:** Other not–for–profit (including NFP Corporation) **Service:** Psychiatric

**Staffed Beds:** 68 **Admissions:** 2190 **Census:** 41 **Outpatient Visits:** 3975 **Births:** 0 **Total Expense ($000):** 9317 **Payroll Expense ($000):** 5141 **Personnel:** 201

✉ **KINDRED HOSPITAL MIDTOWN (452027)**, 105 Drew Avenue, Zip 77006; tel. 713/529–8922 **A**1 9 10 **F**1 3 29 75 77 85 87 96 129 147 **S** Kindred Healthcare, Louisville, KY
Primary Contact: James Poullard, Chief Executive Officer
Web address: www.khmidtown.com
**Control:** Corporation, Investor–owned, for–profit **Service:** Long–Term Acute Care hospital

**Staffed Beds:** 40 **Admissions:** 202 **Census:** 15 **Outpatient Visits:** 0 **Births:** 0 **Total Expense ($000):** 8605 **Payroll Expense ($000):** 4128 **Personnel:** 62

★ **KINDRED HOSPITAL NORTH HOUSTON (452074)**, 7407 North Freeway, Zip 77076–1314; tel. 832/200–6000, (Includes KINDRED HOSPITAL SPRING, 205 Hollow Tree Lane, Zip 77090; tel. 832/249–2700; Eric Cantrell, Chief Executive Officer; TRIUMPH HOSPITAL WEST HOUSTON, 8850 Long Point Road, 6th Floor, Zip 77055; tel. 713/365–7800) **A**9 10 **F**1 3 18 29 30 31 42 45 49 60 64 70 74 75 78 79 85 86 87 91 93 94 107 118 129 147 **S** Kindred Healthcare, Louisville, KY
Primary Contact: Michael B. Davis, Chief Executive Officer
COO: Erin O'Malley, M.D., Chief Clinical Officer
CFO: Terry Hohmann, Chief Financial Officer
CMO: Erin O'Malley, M.D., Chief Clinical Officer
CIO: William Elsesser, Director Professional Relations
CHR: Charles Lopez, Director Human Resources
Web address: www.khnorthhouston.com
**Control:** Partnership, Investor–owned, for–profit **Service:** Long–Term Acute Care hospital

**Staffed Beds:** 288 **Admissions:** 1479 **Census:** 101 **Outpatient Visits:** 499 **Births:** 0 **Total Expense ($000):** 57712 **Payroll Expense ($000):** 21822 **Personnel:** 510

*Many Facility Codes have changed. Please refer to the AHA Guide Code Chart.* © 2012 AHA Guide

TX

⊞ **KINDRED HOSPITAL–HOUSTON (452023)**, 6441 Main Street, Zip 77030–1596; tel. 713/790–0500 **A**1 5 9 10 **F**1 3 29 30 31 64 70 75 77 85 107 129 147 **S** Kindred Healthcare, Louisville, KY
Primary Contact: Robert Stein, Chief Executive Officer
CFO: Sara Langlitz, Controller
Web address: www.khhouston.com/
**Control:** Corporation, Investor–owned, for–profit **Service:** Long–Term Acute Care hospital

**Staffed Beds:** 105 **Admissions:** 882 **Census:** 67 **Outpatient Visits:** 1 **Births:** 0 **Total Expense ($000):** 31122 **Payroll Expense ($000):** 13182 **Personnel:** 225

⊞ **KINDRED HOSPITAL–HOUSTON NORTHWEST (452039)**, 11297 Fallbrook Drive, Zip 77065–4292; tel. 281/897–8114 **A**1 9 10 **F**1 3 29 57 64 70 77 87 93 107 113 129 147 **P**5 **S** Kindred Healthcare, Louisville, KY
Primary Contact: Mary Anne Craig, Chief Executive Officer
Web address: www.khhoustonnw.com/
**Control:** Corporation, Investor–owned, for–profit **Service:** Long–Term Acute Care hospital

**Staffed Beds:** 84 **Admissions:** 861 **Census:** 59 **Outpatient Visits:** 94 **Births:** 0 **Total Expense ($000):** 30345 **Payroll Expense ($000):** 11960 **Personnel:** 182

**LYNDON B JOHNSON GENERAL HOSPITAL** See Harris County Hospital District

⊞ **MEMORIAL HERMANN – TEXAS MEDICAL CENTER (450068)**, 6411 Fannin Street, Zip 77030–1501; tel. 713/704–4000, (Includes CHILDREN'S MEMORIAL HERMANN HOSPITAL, 6411 Fannin, Zip 77030; tel. 713/704–5437), (Total facility includes 8 beds in nursing home–type unit) **A**1 2 3 5 8 9 10 **F**3 7 12 13 15 16 17 18 19 20 21 22 23 24 25 26 27 28 29 30 31 32 34 35 36 37 39 40 43 44 45 46 47 48 49 50 51 55 56 57 58 59 60 61 62 64 68 70 72 73 74 75 76 77 78 79 81 82 84 85 86 87 88 89 90 91 92 93 96 97 99 100 102 103 107 108 109 110 111 113 114 115 116 117 118 123 125 127 128 129 130 131 133 134 137 138 140 141 142 143 145 146 147 **P**5 6 **S** Memorial Hermann Healthcare System, Houston, TX
Primary Contact: Craig Cordola, Chief Executive Officer
COO: Tom Flanagan, Chief Operating Officer
CFO: William Pack, Chief Financial Officer
CMO: Jeffrey Katz, M.D., Chief Medical Officer
CIO: David Bradshaw, Chief Information Officer
CHR: Vivian Kardow, Chief Human Resources Officer
Web address: www.mhhs.org
**Control:** Other not–for–profit (including NFP Corporation) **Service:** General Medical and Surgical

**Staffed Beds:** 868 **Admissions:** 33961 **Census:** 615 **Outpatient Visits:** 148277 **Births:** 4935 **Total Expense ($000):** 818546 **Payroll Expense ($000):** 280736 **Personnel:** 3723

⊞ **MEMORIAL HERMANN MEMORIAL CITY MEDICAL CENTER (450610)**, 921 Gessner Road, Zip 77024–2501; tel. 713/242–3000 **A**1 2 9 10 **F**3 12 13 15 18 20 22 24 26 28 29 30 31 34 35 37 40 41 43 45 46 49 51 56 57 59 60 65 70 72 74 75 76 77 78 79 80 81 82 84 85 87 89 107 108 110 111 113 114 116 117 118 119 120 122 123 125 128 129 130 131 134 143 145 146 **P**5 6 **S** Memorial Hermann Healthcare System, Houston, TX
Primary Contact: Keith N. Alexander, Chief Executive Officer
COO: James Witt, Chief Operations Officer
CFO: Lisa Kendler, Chief Financial Officer
CMO: Donald Gibson, M.D., Chief Medical Officer
CIO: David Bradshaw, Chief Information, Planning and Marketing Officer
CHR: Suzanne S. Meier, System Director, Compensation and Human Resources Technology
Web address: www.memorialhermann.org
**Control:** Other not–for–profit (including NFP Corporation) **Service:** General Medical and Surgical

**Staffed Beds:** 377 **Admissions:** 19733 **Census:** 223 **Outpatient Visits:** 227906 **Births:** 2968 **Total Expense ($000):** 328510 **Payroll Expense ($000):** 102542 **Personnel:** 1306

⊞ **MEMORIAL HERMANN NORTHWEST HOSPITAL (450184)**, 1635 North Loop West, Zip 77008; tel. 713/867–3380, (Includes MEMORIAL HERMANN SOUTHEAST HOSPITAL, 11800 Astoria Boulevard, Zip 77089–6041; tel. 281/929–6100; Erin Asprec, Chief Executive Officer; MEMORIAL HERMANN SOUTHWEST HOSPITAL, 7600 Beechnut, Zip 77074–1850; tel. 713/456–5000; George Gaston, Chief Executive Officer; MEMORIAL HERMANN THE WOODLANDS HOSPITAL, 9250 Pinecroft Drive, The Woodlands, Zip 77380–3225; tel. 281/364–2300) **A**1 2 3 5 9 10 **F**3 8 11 12 13 15 17 18 19 20 22 24 26 28 29 30 31 34 35 36 37 40 41 42 43 44 45 46 47 48 49 50 51 54 55 56 57 58 59 60 62 63 64 65 68 69 70 72 73 74 75 76 77 78 79 80 81 82 83 84 86 87 89 90 91 92 93 96 98 100 101 102 103 104 107 108 109 110 111 113 114 115 116 117 118 119 120 122 123 125 128 129 130 131 134 142 145 146 147 **P**5 6 **S** Memorial Hermann Healthcare System, Houston, TX
Primary Contact: Gary Kerr, Chief Executive Officer
CFO: Roger Faculak, Chief Financial Officer
CMO: Maurice Leibman, M.D., Chief Medical Officer
CIO: David Bradshaw, Chief Information Officer
CHR: Terry Henske, Director Human Resources
Web address: www.mhbh.org
**Control:** Other not–for–profit (including NFP Corporation) **Service:** General Medical and Surgical

**Staffed Beds:** 1172 **Admissions:** 53824 **Census:** 673 **Outpatient Visits:** 451411 **Births:** 11462 **Total Expense ($000):** 695977 **Payroll Expense ($000):** 320346 **Personnel:** 4422

**MEMORIAL HERMANN SOUTHEAST HOSPITAL** See Memorial Hermann Northwest Hospital

**MEMORIAL HERMANN SOUTHWEST HOSPITAL** See Memorial Hermann Northwest Hospital

☐ **MENNINGER CLINIC**, 2801 Gessner, Zip 77080–2503; tel. 713/275–5000 **A**1 3 5 **F**30 98 99 101 129
Primary Contact: Ian Aitken, President and Chief Executive Officer
COO: Shawna Morris, Senior Vice President Operations and Chief Operating Officer
CFO: Kenneth Klein, CPA, Senior Vice President Finance and Chief Financial Officer
CMO: John M. Oldham, M.D., Senior Vice President and Chief of Staff
CIO: Kenneth Klein, CPA, Senior Vice President Finance and Chief Financial Officer
CHR: Shawna Morris, Senior Vice President Operations and Chief Operating Officer
Web address: www.menningerclinic.com
**Control:** Other not–for–profit (including NFP Corporation) **Service:** Psychiatric

**Staffed Beds:** 102 **Admissions:** 806 **Census:** 78 **Outpatient Visits:** 0 **Births:** 0 **Total Expense ($000):** 37059 **Payroll Expense ($000):** 16016 **Personnel:** 271

★ **METHODIST WEST HOUSTON HOSPITAL (670077)**, 18500 Katy Freeway, Zip 77094–1110; tel. 832/522–1000 **A**10 21 **F**3 8 13 15 18 20 22 24 26 29 30 31 40 45 49 50 51 57 59 60 68 70 72 75 76 78 79 81 82 85 87 93 107 108 109 110 111 112 113 114 118 119 120 122 123 125 129 130 131 134 **P**1 **S** The Methodist Hospital System, Houston, TX
Primary Contact: Wayne M. Voss, Chief Executive Officer
Web address: www.methodisthealth.com
**Control:** Other not–for–profit (including NFP Corporation) **Service:** General Medical and Surgical

**Staffed Beds:** 75 **Admissions:** 2802 **Census:** 27 **Outpatient Visits:** 35188 **Births:** 551 **Total Expense ($000):** 83510 **Payroll Expense ($000):** 28882 **Personnel:** 518

⊞ **METHODIST WILLOWBROOK HOSPITAL (450844)**, 18220 Tomball Parkway, Zip 77070; tel. 281/477–1000 **A**1 9 10 **F**3 8 12 13 15 18 20 22 24 26 28 29 30 31 35 36 37 40 44 45 46 49 59 64 65 70 73 74 75 76 77 78 79 80 81 85 86 87 89 93 96 107 108 110 111 113 114 118 119 120 122 123 125 129 130 131 134 145 146 147 **S** The Methodist Hospital System, Houston, TX
Primary Contact: Beryl O. Ramsey, FACHE, Chief Executive Officer
CHR: Sherene Thompson, Director Human Resources
Web address: www.methodisthealth.com
**Control:** Other not–for–profit (including NFP Corporation) **Service:** General Medical and Surgical

**Staffed Beds:** 195 **Admissions:** 13597 **Census:** 150 **Outpatient Visits:** 113133 **Births:** 2814 **Total Expense ($000):** 189920 **Payroll Expense ($000):** 73288 **Personnel:** 1229

**TX**

---

☒ △ **MICHAEL E. DEBAKEY VETERANS AFFAIRS MEDICAL CENTER**, 2002 Holcombe Boulevard, Zip 77030–4298; tel. 713/791–1414, (Nonreporting) **A**1 2 3 5 7 8 9 **S** Department of Veterans Affairs, Washington, DC
Primary Contact: Adam C. Walmus, Director
COO: Francisco Vazquez, Associate Director
CFO: Alisa Cooper, Manager Financial Resources
CMO: Jagadeesh S. Kalavar, M.D., Chief of Staff
CIO: Kevin Lenamond, Information Management Service Line Executive
CHR: Kathy Salazar, Manager Human Resources
Web address: www.houston.va.gov
**Control:** Veterans Affairs, Government, federal **Service:** General Medical and Surgical

| | |
|---|---|
| **Staffed Beds:** 739 | |

☒ **PARK PLAZA HOSPITAL (450659)**, 1313 Hermann Drive, Zip 77004–7092; tel. 713/527–5000 **A**1 2 9 10 **F**3 12 13 15 18 20 22 29 31 34 35 40 45 49 50 56 57 59 60 70 73 74 76 78 79 81 85 92 107 108 110 111 113 114 117 118 119 120 122 128 129 131 145 146 147 **S** TENET Healthcare Corporation, Dallas, TX
Primary Contact: John Tressa, R.N., MSN, Chief Executive Officer
COO: Mary Jo Goodman, Chief Operating Officer
CFO: Kirk Pogue, Chief Financial Officer
CIO: Terry Janis, Assistant Vice President
CHR: Lori Knowles, Director Human Resources
Web address: www.parkplazahospital.com
**Control:** Partnership, Investor–owned, for–profit **Service:** General Medical and Surgical

**Staffed Beds:** 208 **Admissions:** 5794 **Census:** 75 **Outpatient Visits:** 46200 **Births:** 853 **Total Expense ($000):** 97706 **Payroll Expense ($000):** 34223 **Personnel:** 587

☒ **PLAZA SPECIALTY HOSPITAL (452046)**, 1300 Binz, Zip 77004; tel. 713/285–1000 **A**1 9 10 **F**1 3 29 31 56 63 68 70 75 77 78 82 84 85 87 129 147 **P**8 **S** TENET Healthcare Corporation, Dallas, TX
Primary Contact: Steven Barr, R.N., MSN, Chief Executive Officer
CFO: Charles R. Handley, Chief Financial Officer
CMO: Wasae S. Tabibi, M.D., President Medical Staff
CIO: Steve Peacock, Assistant Vice President
Web address: www.plazaspecialtyhospital.com
**Control:** Corporation, Investor–owned, for–profit **Service:** Long–Term Acute Care hospital

**Staffed Beds:** 56 **Admissions:** 345 **Census:** 26 **Outpatient Visits:** 0 **Births:** 0 **Total Expense ($000):** 20515 **Payroll Expense ($000):** 5522 **Personnel:** 89

**QUENTIN MEASE HOSPITAL** See Harris County Hospital District

**RENAISSANCE HOSPITAL – HOUSTON** See St. Anthony's Hospital

☐ **RIVERSIDE GENERAL HOSPITAL (450446)**, 3204 Ennis Street, Zip 77004–3299; tel. 713/526–2441 **A**1 9 10 **F**4 43 54 64 87 98 99 100 101 102 103 104 105 129 142 145 **P**5
Primary Contact: Earnest Gibson, III, Administrator
CFO: Manny Ignacio, Controller
Web address: www.riversidegeneral.org
**Control:** Other not–for–profit (including NFP Corporation) **Service:** Psychiatric

**Staffed Beds:** 89 **Admissions:** 1230 **Census:** 32 **Outpatient Visits:** 17600 **Births:** 0 **Total Expense ($000):** 32753 **Payroll Expense ($000):** 8968 **Personnel:** 226

☒ **SELECT SPECIALTY HOSPITAL–HOUSTON (452049)**, 1917 Ashland Street, Zip 77008–3994; tel. 713/861–6161, (Includes SELECT SPECIALTY HOSPITAL–HOUSTON MEDICAL CENTER, 2130 West Holcombe, Zip 77030–1502; tel. 713/218–2300; Vivian Bond, Administrator; SELECT SPECIALTY HOSPITAL–HOUSTON WEST, 9430 Old Katy Road, Zip 77055; tel. 713/984–2273; Sandra Stephens, R.N., Administrator) **A**1 9 10 **F**1 3 29 34 40 45 50 57 59 60 64 70 81 85 87 91 93 107 113 118 129 147 **S** Select Medical Corporation, Mechanicsburg, PA
Primary Contact: Jesse Ruiz, Chief Executive Officer
CFO: Traci Jameson, Manager Finance
CMO: Chi C. Mao, M.D., Medical Director
CHR: Pamela Simpson, Director Human Resources
Web address: www.selectmedicalcorp.com
**Control:** Partnership, Investor–owned, for–profit **Service:** Long–Term Acute Care hospital

**Staffed Beds:** 277 **Admissions:** 1908 **Census:** 136 **Outpatient Visits:** 1638 **Births:** 0 **Total Expense ($000):** 72490 **Payroll Expense ($000):** 30251 **Personnel:** 593

**SELECT SPECIALTY HOSPITAL–HOUSTON MEDICAL CENTER** See Select Specialty Hospital–Houston

**SELECT SPECIALTY HOSPITAL–HOUSTON WEST** See Select Specialty Hospital–Houston

☐ **SHRINERS HOSPITALS FOR CHILDREN, HOUSTON (453312)**, 6977 Main Street, Zip 77030–3701; tel. 713/797–1616 **A**1 3 5 10 **F**3 29 30 35 50 64 66 68 74 75 77 79 81 86 87 89 93 94 96 129 130 131 133 142 145 147 **P**6 **S** Shriners Hospitals for Children, Tampa, FL
Primary Contact: David A. Ferrell, Chief Executive Officer
COO: Cathy Moniaci, Chief Operating Officer
CFO: Lona Pope, Director Fiscal Services
CMO: Douglas A. Barnes, M.D., Chief of Staff
CHR: Lynn Clements, Director Human Resources
Web address: www.shrinershospitals.org
**Control:** Other not–for–profit (including NFP Corporation) **Service:** Children's orthopedic

**Staffed Beds:** 40 **Admissions:** 183 **Census:** 6 **Outpatient Visits:** 9961 **Births:** 0 **Total Expense ($000):** 13676 **Payroll Expense ($000):** 6269 **Personnel:** 175

☐ **SPRING BRANCH MEDICAL CENTER (450630)**, 8850 Long Point Road, Zip 77055–3082; tel. 713/467–6555, (Data for 334 days) **A**1 5 9 10 **F**3 13 15 18 26 29 40 41 43 50 70 72 76 78 79 81 82 85 107 108 111 116 120 123 129 145 146
Primary Contact: Marty McVey, Chief Executive Officer
Web address: www.springbranchmedical.com
**Control:** Individual, Investor–owned, for–profit **Service:** General Medical and Surgical

**Staffed Beds:** 36 **Admissions:** 510 **Census:** 4 **Outpatient Visits:** 9322 **Births:** 57 **Personnel:** 259

**ST. ANTHONY'S HOSPITAL (450795)**, 2807 Little York Road, Zip 77093–3495; tel. 713/697–7777 **A**9 10 **F**12 26 29 34 35 40 43 45 46 49 50 56 57 59 60 61 64 65 68 70 75 79 81 82 85 91 92 93 105 107 113 118 129 134 142 145 **S** Renaissance Healthcare Systems, Houston, TX
Primary Contact: Jason B. Fisher, Chief Executive Officer
COO: Nora Peralta, Chief Nursing Officer
CFO: John Lucia, Chief Financial Officer
CMO: Rafael Borges, M.D., Chief of Staff
CIO: Bill DuBrul, Director Information Technology
CHR: Cathy McCue, Director Human Resources
Web address: www.stanthonyshouston.com
**Control:** Partnership, Investor–owned, for–profit **Service:** General Medical and Surgical

**Staffed Beds:** 39 **Admissions:** 1485 **Census:** 13 **Outpatient Visits:** 11426 **Births:** 0 **Personnel:** 174

☐ **ST. JOSEPH MEDICAL CENTER (450035)**, 1401 St. Joseph Parkway, Zip 77002–8321; tel. 713/757–1000, (Total facility includes 18 beds in nursing home–type unit) **A**1 3 5 9 10 21 **F**3 11 12 13 14 15 17 18 20 22 24 26 28 29 30 31 34 35 36 37 39 40 42 44 45 46 47 48 49 50 51 56 57 58 59 60 61 63 64 65 66 68 70 74 75 76 77 78 79 81 82 84 85 86 87 90 93 94 97 98 101 102 103 107 108 111 113 114 115 116 117 118 120 123 127 128 129 130 131 134 142 143 145 146 147 **P**8 **S** IASIS Healthcare, Franklin, TN
Primary Contact: Patrick J. Mathews, Chief Executive Officer and Chief Financial Officer
COO: Laura Fortin, Chief Operating Officer
CFO: Patrick J. Mathews, Chief Executive Officer and Chief Financial Officer
CIO: Robin Brown, Chief Information Officer and Compliance Officer
CHR: Kris Clatanoff, Director Human Resources
Web address: www.sjmctx.com
**Control:** Partnership, Investor–owned, for–profit **Service:** General Medical and Surgical

**Staffed Beds:** 384 **Admissions:** 16940 **Census:** 235 **Outpatient Visits:** 102985 **Births:** 4898 **Total Expense ($000):** 229879 **Payroll Expense ($000):** 86025 **Personnel:** 1579

☒ **ST. LUKE'S EPISCOPAL HOSPITAL (450193)**, 6720 Bertner Avenue, Zip 77030–2697, Mailing Address: P.O. Box 20269, Zip 77225–0269; tel. 832/355–1000 **A**1 2 3 5 8 11 12 13 14 15 17 18 20 22 24 26 28 29 30 31 34 35 36 37 39 40 42 44 45 46 47 48 49 50 51 56 57 58 59 60 61 63 64 65 66 68 70 74 75 76 77 78 79 81 82 84 85 86 87 90 92 96 97 100 107 108 110 111 112 113 114 117 118 119 120 122 123 125 128 129 130 131 134 136 137 138 139 141 144 145 146 147 **P**5 8 **S** St. Luke's Episcopal Health System, Houston, TX
Primary Contact: Margaret M. Van Bree, Dr.PH, Chief Executive Officer
CFO: William Brosius, Vice President and Chief Financial Officer
CMO: Angela Shippy, M.D., Vice President Medical Affairs
CIO: James Albin, Interim Chief Information Officer
CHR: Deborah H. Mahannah, Vice President Human Resources
Web address: www.stlukestexas.com
**Control:** Church–operated, Nongovernment, not–for profit **Service:** General Medical and Surgical

**Staffed Beds:** 711 **Admissions:** 34333 **Census:** 545 **Outpatient Visits:** 274672 **Births:** 2861 **Total Expense ($000):** 780462 **Payroll Expense ($000):** 290028 **Personnel:** 3434

*Many Facility Codes have changed. Please refer to the AHA Guide Code Chart.* © 2012 AHA Guide

★ **ST. LUKE'S HOSPITAL AT THE VINTAGE (670075)**, 20171 Chasewood Park Drive, Zip 77070; tel. 832/534–5000 **A**9 10 21 **F**3 13 15 18 20 22 26 29 30 34 35 40 41 45 49 56 57 60 64 70 72 74 75 76 77 81 85 107 108 110 111 113 114 117 118 129 145 146 **P**5 **S** St. Luke's Episcopal Health System, Houston, TX
Primary Contact: Francis X. Speidel, M.D., Chief Executive Officer
Web address: www.stlukesvintage.com/
**Control:** Corporation, Investor–owned, for–profit **Service:** General Medical and Surgical

**Staffed Beds:** 78 **Admissions:** 2172 **Census:** 23 **Outpatient Visits:** 28030 **Births:** 262 **Total Expense ($000):** 57081 **Payroll Expense ($000):** 17968 **Personnel:** 283

⊠ **TEXAS CHILDREN'S HOSPITAL (453304)**, 6621 Fannin Street, Zip 77030–2399, Mailing Address: Box 300630, Zip 77230–0630; tel. 832/824–1000 **A**1 3 5 8 9 10 **F**3 7 11 12 17 19 21 23 25 27 29 30 31 32 34 38 39 40 41 43 48 50 57 58 59 60 61 64 65 68 71 72 73 74 75 77 78 79 80 81 84 85 86 87 88 89 92 93 95 96 97 99 100 101 104 107 108 111 113 114 117 118 128 129 130 131 133 135 136 137 138 139 140 142 143 145 147
Primary Contact: Mark A. Wallace, President and Chief Executive Officer
COO: Randall P. Wright, Executive Vice President and Chief Operating Officer
CFO: Benjamin B. Melson, CPA, Executive Vice President and Chief Financial Officer
CMO: Mark W. Kline, M.D., Physician in Chief
CHR: Linda W. Aldred, Senior Vice President
Web address: www.texaschildrenshospital.org
**Control:** Other not–for–profit (including NFP Corporation) **Service:** Children's general

**Staffed Beds:** 491 **Admissions:** 21661 **Census:** 380 **Outpatient Visits:** 1562284 **Births:** 0 **Total Expense ($000):** 1003247 **Payroll Expense ($000):** 410532 **Personnel:** 4962

⊠ **TEXAS ORTHOPEDIC HOSPITAL (450804)**, 7401 Main Street, Zip 77030–4509; tel. 713/799–8600 **A**1 3 5 9 10 **F**3 29 30 40 59 64 68 70 79 81 82 85 86 87 90 93 94 97 107 111 114 118 145 **S** HCA, Nashville, TN
Primary Contact: Trent Lind, Chief Executive Officer
CFO: Jill Birdsong, Chief Financial Officer
CMO: James B. Bennett, M.D., Chief of Staff
Web address: www.texasorthopedic.com
**Control:** Partnership, Investor–owned, for–profit **Service:** Orthopedic

**Staffed Beds:** 49 **Admissions:** 2817 **Census:** 22 **Outpatient Visits:** 35838 **Births:** 0 **Total Expense ($000):** 67194 **Payroll Expense ($000):** 21565 **Personnel:** 348

☐ **TEXAS SPECIALTY HOSPITAL AT HOUSTON (452043)**, 6160 South Loop East, Zip 77087–1010; tel. 713/640–2400 **A**1 9 10 **F**1 3 4 29 30 67 70 75 77 85 87 90 98 127 129 147 **S** Fundamental Long Term Care Holdings, LLC, Sparks Glencoe, MD
Primary Contact: Michael Higginbotham, Chief Executive Officer
CFO: Betty Priestley, Manager Business Office
CMO: Alfred Louis, M.D., Chief Medical Staff
CHR: Laura Garza, Director Human Resources
Web address: www.thicare.com
**Control:** Corporation, Investor–owned, for–profit **Service:** Long–Term Acute Care hospital

**Staffed Beds:** 25 **Admissions:** 242 **Census:** 18 **Outpatient Visits:** 0 **Births:** 0 **Total Expense ($000):** 10183 **Payroll Expense ($000):** 3187 **Personnel:** 56

⊠ **THE METHODIST HOSPITAL (450358)**, 6565 Fannin Street, Zip 77030–2707; tel. 713/790–3311, (Total facility includes 25 beds in nursing home–type unit) **A**1 2 3 5 8 9 10 21 **F**3 6 8 9 11 12 13 14 15 17 18 20 22 24 26 28 29 30 31 33 34 35 36 37 39 40 41 42 44 45 46 47 48 49 50 51 53 54 55 56 57 58 59 60 61 63 64 65 67 68 70 73 74 75 76 77 78 79 80 81 82 83 84 85 86 87 90 92 93 96 97 98 100 101 102 103 104 105 107 108 110 111 112 113 114 115 116 117 118 119 120 121 122 123 125 127 128 129 130 131 134 135 136 137 138 139 140 141 142 144 145 146 147 **P**8 **S** The Methodist Hospital System, Houston, TX
Primary Contact: Roberta Schwartz, Executive Vice President
CMO: Dirk Sostman, M.D., Executive Vice President, Chief Medical Officer and Chief Academic Officer
CIO: Timothy L. Thompson, Sr., Senior Vice President and Chief Information Officer
CHR: Lauren P. Rykert, Senior Vice President
Web address: www.methodisthealth.com
**Control:** Other not–for–profit (including NFP Corporation) **Service:** General Medical and Surgical

**Staffed Beds:** 884 **Admissions:** 36586 **Census:** 618 **Outpatient Visits:** 336689 **Births:** 1375 **Total Expense ($000):** 1129250 **Payroll Expense ($000):** 324907 **Personnel:** 6068

⊠ **THE WOMAN'S HOSPITAL OF TEXAS (450674)**, 7600 Fannin Street, Zip 77054–1906; tel. 713/790–1234 **A**1 5 9 10 **F**3 7 8 13 15 29 30 34 40 46 50 53 58 68 70 72 73 75 76 77 81 85 86 87 93 107 108 110 111 117 118 125 129 131 145 146 **S** HCA, Nashville, TN
Primary Contact: Linda B. Russell, Chief Executive Officer
COO: Jennifer Garza, Chief Operating Officer
CMO: Eberhard Lotze, M.D., Chief Medical Officer
CIO: Mark Schlicher, Director Information Technology and Services
CHR: Arnita Crawford, Director Human Resources
Web address: www.womanshospital.com
**Control:** Partnership, Investor–owned, for–profit **Service:** Obstetrics and gynecology

**Staffed Beds:** 367 **Admissions:** 13632 **Census:** 199 **Outpatient Visits:** 55485 **Births:** 9477 **Total Expense ($000):** 150306 **Payroll Expense ($000):** 75932 **Personnel:** 794

★ △ **TIRR MEMORIAL HERMANN (453025)**, 1333 Moursund Street, Zip 77030–3405; tel. 713/799–5000 **A**3 5 7 9 10 **F**11 29 30 34 35 44 50 52 54 58 59 60 64 68 74 75 77 79 82 86 87 90 91 93 95 96 97 100 104 107 118 129 130 131 145 147 **P**5 6 **S** Memorial Hermann Healthcare System, Houston, TX
Primary Contact: Carl E. Josehart, Chief Executive Officer
COO: Mary Ann Euliarte, R.N., Chief Operating Officer and Chief Nursing Officer
CFO: Barrie Strickland, Chief Financial Officer
CMO: Gerard E. Francisco, M.D., Medical Director
CIO: Andy Draper, Director Information Systems
CHR: Vivian Kardow, Chief Human Resources Officer
Web address: www.memorialhermann.org/locations/tirr.html
**Control:** Other not–for–profit (including NFP Corporation) **Service:** Rehabilitation

**Staffed Beds:** 119 **Admissions:** 1154 **Census:** 91 **Outpatient Visits:** 12740 **Births:** 0 **Total Expense ($000):** 69913 **Payroll Expense ($000):** 36540 **Personnel:** 501

**TOPS SURGICAL SPECIALTY HOSPITAL (450774)**, 17080 Red Oak Drive, Zip 77090; tel. 281/539–2900 **A**9 10 **F**3 15 29 39 40 45 46 64 68 78 79 81 85 89 107 108 110 111 113 118 141 **S** United Surgical Partners International, Addison, TX
Primary Contact: Samuel H. Rossmann, Chief Executive Officer
CFO: Daniel Smith, Chief Financial Officer
CMO: Thomas Barton, M.D., Medical Director
CIO: Maud Jones, Manager Medical Records
CHR: Ashley Monzingo, Human Resources, Accounts Payable and Payroll
CNO: Andrea Wappelhorst, Chief Nursing Officer
Web address: www.tops–hospital.com
**Control:** Partnership, Investor–owned, for–profit **Service:** General Medical and Surgical

**Staffed Beds:** 16 **Admissions:** 622 **Census:** 4 **Outpatient Visits:** 37465 **Births:** 0 **Total Expense ($000):** 25545 **Payroll Expense ($000):** 7692 **Personnel:** 155

**TRIUMPH HOSPITAL CENTRAL** See Kindred Hospital Midtown

**TRIUMPH HOSPITAL NORTH HOUSTON** See Kindred Hospital North Houston

**TRIUMPH HOSPITAL NORTHWEST** See Kindred Hospital Spring

☐ **UNIVERSITY GENERAL HOSPITAL (670019)**, 7501 Fannin Street, Zip 77054; tel. 713/375–7000 **A**1 9 10 **F**3 12 18 20 22 29 40 45 49 57 59 67 70 75 79 81 82 85 86 107 108 111 114 118 129 131 147
Primary Contact: Charles D. Schuetz, Chief Executive Officer
Web address: www.ughospital.com
**Control:** Partnership, Investor–owned, for–profit **Service:** General Medical and Surgical

**Staffed Beds:** 69 **Admissions:** 3267 **Census:** 32 **Outpatient Visits:** 11785 **Births:** 0 **Total Expense ($000):** 68500 **Payroll Expense ($000):** 20985 **Personnel:** 234

⊠ **UNIVERSITY OF TEXAS HARRIS COUNTY PSYCHIATRIC CENTER (454076)**, 2800 South MacGregor Way, Zip 77021–1000, Mailing Address: P.O. Box 20249, Zip 77225–0249; tel. 713/741–5000 **A**1 5 9 10 **F**29 30 34 35 57 58 68 75 86 87 98 99 100 101 103 106 129 145 **P**6 **S** University of Texas System, Austin, TX
Primary Contact: Jair C. Soares, M.D., Executive Director
COO: Lois Jean Moore, FACHE, Administrator
CFO: Vanessa McKeon, Interim Chief Financial Officer
CMO: R. Andrew Harper, M.D., Medical Director
CIO: Geri Konigsberg, Director Public Information
CHR: Sherri Orioli, Director Personnel Systems
Web address: www.uth.tmc.edu
**Control:** State–Government, nonfederal **Service:** Psychiatric

**Staffed Beds:** 211 **Admissions:** 7701 **Census:** 174 **Outpatient Visits:** 0 **Births:** 0 **Total Expense ($000):** 36513 **Payroll Expense ($000):** 22917 **Personnel:** 381

**TX**

⊠ **UNIVERSITY OF TEXAS M.D. ANDERSON CANCER CENTER (450076)**, 1515 Holcombe Boulevard, Box 91, Zip 77030–4095; tel. 713/792–2121 **A**1 2 3 5 8 9 10 **F**3 8 11 14 15 18 20 29 30 31 32 34 35 36 37 38 39 40 44 45 46 47 48 49 50 54 55 57 58 59 60 63 64 66 68 70 71 74 75 77 78 79 80 81 82 83 84 85 86 87 88 89 92 93 96 97 99 100 101 102 104 107 108 110 111 112 113 114 115 116 117 118 119 120 121 122 123 125 128 129 131 133 134 135 140 144 145 146 147 **P**6 **S** University of Texas System, Austin, TX
Primary Contact: Ronald A. DePinho, M.D., President
CFO: Dwain Morris, Vice President and Chief Financial Officer
CMO: Thomas Burke, M.D., Executive Vice President and Physician–in–Chief
CIO: Lynn H. Vogel, Vice President and Chief Information Officer
CHR: Shibu Varghese, Vice President Human Resources
Web address: www.mdanderson.org
**Control:** State–Government, nonfederal **Service:** Cancer

**Staffed Beds: 607 Admissions: 25230 Census: 494 Outpatient Visits:** 1200025 **Births:** 0 **Total Expense ($000):** 3087811 **Payroll Expense ($000):** 1418469 **Personnel:** 17942

⊠ **WEST HOUSTON MEDICAL CENTER (450644)**, 12141 Richmond Avenue, Zip 77082–2499; tel. 281/558–3444 **A**1 9 10 **F**3 11 12 13 15 18 20 22 24 26 28 29 30 31 39 40 42 45 46 47 48 49 50 51 56 57 59 60 64 70 73 74 75 76 77 78 79 80 81 82 85 90 93 96 98 102 103 107 110 111 114 115 116 117 118 120 123 128 129 131 144 145 146 147 **S** HCA, Nashville, TN
Primary Contact: Todd Caliva, Chief Executive Officer
CFO: Stanley K. Nord, Chief Financial Officer
CMO: Magdy Rizk, M.D., Chief of Staff
CIO: Sergio Almeida, Director Information Systems
CHR: Carol Melville, Director Human Resources
Web address: www.westhoustonmedical.com
**Control:** Partnership, Investor–owned, for–profit **Service:** General Medical and Surgical

**Staffed Beds: 227 Admissions: 10370 Census: 141 Outpatient Visits:** 103038 **Births:** 2253 **Total Expense ($000):** 124672 **Payroll Expense ($000):** 57047 **Personnel:** 748

☐ **WEST OAKS HOSPITAL (454026)**, 6500 Hornwood Drive, Zip 77074–5095; tel. 713/995–0909 **A**1 3 5 9 10 **F**5 29 54 56 64 68 98 99 100 101 103 104 105 131 **S** Universal Health Services, Inc., King of Prussia, PA
Primary Contact: Tim C. Simmons, Chief Executive Officer
CFO: Christy Amy, Chief Financial Officer
CMO: George Santos, M.D., Executive Medical Director
CHR: Janice Webster, Director Human Resources
Web address: www.westoakshospital.com
**Control:** Corporation, Investor–owned, for–profit **Service:** Psychiatric

**Staffed Beds: 144 Admissions: 5938 Census: 119 Outpatient Visits:** 27092 **Births:** 0 **Total Expense ($000):** 23598 **Payroll Expense ($000):** 14495 **Personnel:** 247

**WESTBURY COMMUNITY HOSPITAL (450674)**, 5556 Gasmer Drive, Zip 77035–4502; tel. 713/422–2625 **A**21 **F**3 5 29 35 38 64 68 98 99 100 101 102 103 104 105 129
Primary Contact: Jeff Jeffery Parsons, Administrator
Web address: www.westburyhospital.com
**Control:** Corporation, Investor–owned, for–profit **Service:** Psychiatric

**Staffed Beds: 137 Admissions: 1424 Census: 28 Outpatient Visits:** 69137 **Births:** 0 **Total Expense ($000):** 20787 **Payroll Expense ($000):** 12068 **Personnel:** 254

**HUMBLE—Harris County**

⊠ **HEALTHSOUTH REHABILITATION HOSPITAL (453029)**, 19002 McKay Drive, Zip 77338–5701; tel. 281/446–6148 **A**1 9 10 **F**29 56 64 75 77 82 86 87 90 91 92 93 95 96 129 131 142 147 **S** HEALTHSOUTH Corporation, Birmingham, AL
Primary Contact: Angela L. Simmons, Chief Executive Officer
CFO: Dave Renneker, Chief Financial Officer
CMO: Emile Mathurin, Jr., M.D., Medical Director
CHR: Valerie Wells, Manager Human Resources
Web address: www.healthsouthhumble.com
**Control:** Corporation, Investor–owned, for–profit **Service:** Rehabilitation

**Staffed Beds: 60 Admissions: 1178 Census: 45 Outpatient Visits:** 7123 **Births:** 0 **Total Expense ($000):** 13244 **Payroll Expense ($000):** 8054 **Personnel:** 149

☐ **ICON HOSPITAL (670048)**, 19211 Mckay Boulevard, Zip 77338–5502; tel. 281/883–5500 **A**1 9 10 **F**1 3 29 40 77 85 91 129 134 147 **S** AcuityHealthcare, LP, Charlotte, NC
Primary Contact: Kiley P. Cedotal, Chief Executive Officer
Web address: www.acuityhealthcare.net
**Control:** Partnership, Investor–owned, for–profit **Service:** General Medical and Surgical

**Staffed Beds: 42 Admissions: 533 Census: 38 Outpatient Visits:** 0 **Births:** 0 **Total Expense ($000):** 18349 **Payroll Expense ($000):** 8398 **Personnel:** 161

★ **KINDRED REHABILITATION HOSPITAL NORTHEAST HOUSTON**, 18839 McKay Road, Zip 77338; tel. 281/964–6600, (Nonreporting) **S** Kindred Healthcare, Louisville, KY
Primary Contact: Jeffrey Smith, Chief Executive Officer
Web address: www.khrehabnortheasthouston.com
**Control:** Corporation, Investor–owned, for–profit **Service:** Rehabilitation

**Staffed Beds: 46**

⊠ **MEMORIAL HERMANN NORTHEAST (450684)**, 18951 North Memorial Drive, Zip 77338–4297; tel. 281/540–7700 **A**1 2 9 10 **F**3 11 12 13 15 18 20 22 24 26 29 30 31 34 35 36 37 40 45 46 49 53 54 56 57 59 64 70 72 73 74 75 76 77 78 79 80 81 85 86 87 93 107 108 109 110 111 113 114 118 119 120 122 128 129 131 134 145 146 147 **P**5 6 **S** Memorial Hermann Healthcare System, Houston, TX
Primary Contact: Louis G. Smith, Jr., Chief Executive Officer
COO: Louis G. Smith, Jr., Chief Executive Officer
CMO: Susan Curling, M.D., Chief Medical Officer
CHR: Stephanie Foster, Director Human Resources
Web address: www.memorialhermann.org
**Control:** Other not–for–profit (including NFP Corporation) **Service:** General Medical and Surgical

**Staffed Beds: 227 Admissions: 9016 Census: 116 Outpatient Visits:** 88763 **Births:** 1204 **Total Expense ($000):** 96799 **Payroll Expense ($000):** 54830 **Personnel:** 758

**HUNTSVILLE—Walker County**

⊠ **HUNTSVILLE MEMORIAL HOSPITAL (450347)**, 110 Memorial Hospital Drive, Zip 77340–4362, Mailing Address: P.O. Box 4001, Zip 77342–4001; tel. 936/291–3411 **A**1 9 10 **F**3 5 8 11 13 15 26 28 29 31 32 34 35 39 40 45 46 50 53 54 56 57 59 62 64 65 66 68 70 75 76 77 78 79 81 82 85 86 87 89 90 91 92 93 97 100 101 103 107 108 110 111 113 114 117 118 126 129 130 131 140 141 145 146 147
Primary Contact: Sally I. Nelson, Chief Executive Officer
COO: Tripp Montalbo, Chief Operating Officer
CFO: Robert Gray, Assistant Administrator Financial Services
CIO: John Heeman, Director Information Systems
CHR: Diane L. Stevens, MS, Director Human Resources and Compliance Officer
Web address: www.huntsvillememorial.com
**Control:** Other not–for–profit (including NFP Corporation) **Service:** General Medical and Surgical

**Staffed Beds: 96 Admissions: 3525 Census: 39 Outpatient Visits:** 93643 **Births:** 517 **Total Expense ($000):** 62578 **Payroll Expense ($000):** 28489 **Personnel:** 424

**HURST—Tarrant County**

☐ **COOK CHILDREN'S NORTHEAST HOSPITAL (670045)**, 6316 Precinct Line Road, Zip 76054; tel. 817/605–2500 **A**1 9 10 **F**3 39 40 41 45 48 64 68 79 81 89 107 111 113 118 143
Primary Contact: Candace Grantham, Chief Executive Officer
Web address: www.cookchildrens.org
**Control:** Corporation, Investor–owned, for–profit **Service:** Children's general

**Staffed Beds: 3 Admissions: 30 Census: 1 Outpatient Visits:** 57894 **Births:** 0 **Total Expense ($000):** 20428 **Payroll Expense ($000):** 10836 **Personnel:** 157

☐ **SOUTHWEST SURGICAL HOSPITAL (450886)**, 1612 Hurst Town Center Drive, Zip 76054–6236; tel. 817/345–4100 **A**1 9 10 **F**3 12 29 33 34 40 41 45 47 51 57 59 65 68 75 77 79 81 82 85 86 87 107 113 118 128 129 130 145 147 **S** National Surgical Hospitals, Chicago, IL
Primary Contact: Harold Stigler, Chief Executive Officer
CFO: Michelle Brost, Financial Officer
CMO: Dale Brancel, D.O., Chief of Staff
CHR: Donna Irvin, Director Human Resources
Web address: www.swsurgery.com
**Control:** Partnership, Investor–owned, for–profit **Service:** Surgical

**Staffed Beds: 23 Admissions: 283 Census: 2 Outpatient Visits:** 5160 **Births:** 0 **Total Expense ($000):** 16647 **Payroll Expense ($000):** 4418 **Personnel:** 78

**IRAAN—Pecos County**

**IRAAN GENERAL HOSPITAL (451307)**, 600 349 North, Zip 79744, Mailing Address: P.O. Box 665, Zip 79744–2057; tel. 432/639–2871 **A**9 10 18 **F**28 40 43 56 57 59 64 65 75 86 93 104 107 118 126 129 132
Primary Contact: Teresa Callahan, R.N., MSN, Chief Executive Officer
CFO: Tami Burks, Chief Fiscal Services
CMO: Robert W. Garcia, M.D., Chief Medical Officer
CHR: Cathy Tucker, Director Human Resources
Web address: www.igh–hospital.com
**Control:** Hospital district or authority, Government, nonfederal **Service:** General Medical and Surgical

**Staffed Beds: 13 Admissions: 29 Census: 1 Outpatient Visits:** 12452 **Births:** 0 **Total Expense ($000):** 6554 **Payroll Expense ($000):** 2269 **Personnel:** 47

**TX**

## IRVING—Dallas County

☒ **BAYLOR MEDICAL CENTER AT IRVING (450079)**, 1901 North MacArthur Boulevard, Zip 75061; tel. 972/579–8100 **A**1 9 10 **F**3 11 12 13 15 17 18 20 22 24 26 28 29 30 31 34 35 40 45 46 47 49 54 55 57 58 59 64 65 70 73 74 75 76 77 78 79 80 81 82 84 85 86 87 90 93 94 100 107 108 110 111 113 114 115 116 117 118 119 120 121 125 128 129 140 142 145 146 147 **S** Baylor Health Care System, Dallas, TX
Primary Contact: Cindy K. Schamp, President
COO: Brenda K. Blain, MSN, Chief Nursing Officer and Chief Operating Officer
CFO: Lucy Catala, Vice President Finance
CMO: Jeffrey Embrey, M.D., Vice President Medical Affairs
CHR: Lisa Seay, Director Human Resources
CNO: Brenda K. Blain, MSN, Chief Nursing Officer and Chief Operating Officer
Web address: www.baylorhealth.com
**Control:** Other not–for–profit (including NFP Corporation) **Service:** General Medical and Surgical

**Staffed Beds:** 222 **Admissions:** 10319 **Census:** 130 **Outpatient Visits:** 106784 **Births:** 1880 **Total Expense ($000):** 187698 **Payroll Expense ($000):** 68815 **Personnel:** 969

☐ **IRVING COPPELL SURGICAL HOSPITAL (450874)**, 400 West Interstate 635, Zip 75063; tel. 972/868–4000 **A**1 9 10 **F**3 40 51 64 68 75 81 85 100 107 111 113 118 **P**2 **S** United Surgical Partners International, Addison, TX
Primary Contact: Deonna Unell, Chief Executive Officer
CFO: Gabrielle Holland, Chief Financial Officer
CMO: Scott McGraw, M.D., Medical Director
Web address: www.ic–sh.com
**Control:** Partnership, Investor–owned, for–profit **Service:** General Medical and Surgical

**Staffed Beds:** 12 **Admissions:** 350 **Census:** 2 **Outpatient Visits:** 6933 **Births:** 0 **Total Expense ($000):** 23875 **Payroll Expense ($000):** 4355 **Personnel:** 92

☒ **LAS COLINAS MEDICAL CENTER (450822)**, 6800 North MacArthur Boulevard, Zip 75039–2422; tel. 972/969–2000 **A**1 9 10 **F**3 8 13 15 18 20 22 24 28 29 30 31 34 35 40 43 45 46 47 48 49 50 57 59 60 64 68 70 72 73 74 75 76 78 79 81 87 93 100 102 107 108 110 111 113 117 118 125 128 129 131 145 146 **S** HCA, Nashville, TN
Primary Contact: Daniela Decell, Chief Executive Officer
COO: Chip Zahn, Chief Operating Officer
CFO: Nick Galt, Chief Financial Officer
Web address: www.lascolinasmedical.com
**Control:** Corporation, Investor–owned, for–profit **Service:** General Medical and Surgical

**Staffed Beds:** 90 **Admissions:** 4961 **Census:** 46 **Outpatient Visits:** 50294 **Births:** 1685 **Total Expense ($000):** 62669 **Payroll Expense ($000):** 24091 **Personnel:** 374

## JACKSBORO—Jack County

**FAITH COMMUNITY HOSPITAL (450241)**, 717 Magnolia Street, Zip 76458–1111; tel. 940/567–6633 **A**9 10 20 **F**7 11 28 40 43 57 77 93 107 118 126 129 132 **P**6
Primary Contact: Frank Beaman, Administrator
CFO: James Bartlett, Chief Financial Officer
CMO: S. Jamal, M.D., Medical Director
CIO: Bradlee Landis, Chief Information Officer
CHR: James Bartlett, Human Resources
CNO: Joy Henry, R.N., Director Nurses
Web address: www.faithcommunityhospital.com
**Control:** Hospital district or authority, Government, nonfederal **Service:** General Medical and Surgical

**Staffed Beds:** 17 **Admissions:** 433 **Census:** 4 **Outpatient Visits:** 17673 **Births:** 0 **Total Expense ($000):** 5323 **Payroll Expense ($000):** 2691 **Personnel:** 69

## JACKSONVILLE—Cherokee County

☒ **EAST TEXAS MEDICAL CENTER JACKSONVILLE (450194)**, 501 South Ragsdale Street, Zip 75766–2413; tel. 903/541–5000 **A**1 9 10 20 **F**3 8 11 13 15 18 20 26 29 31 34 35 37 39 40 42 43 45 50 57 59 64 65 70 75 76 79 81 82 85 107 108 110 111 114 118 126 128 144 145 146 147 **S** East Texas Medical Center Regional Healthcare System, Tyler, TX
Primary Contact: Jack R. Endres, Administrator
CFO: Phillip A. Caron, Chief Financial Officer
CHR: Elysia Epperson, Director Human Resources
Web address: www.etmc.org
**Control:** Other not–for–profit (including NFP Corporation) **Service:** General Medical and Surgical

**Staffed Beds:** 38 **Admissions:** 2167 **Census:** 20 **Outpatient Visits:** 60607 **Births:** 461 **Total Expense ($000):** 21415 **Payroll Expense ($000):** 11144 **Personnel:** 201

☒ **MOTHER FRANCES HOSPITAL – JACKSONVILLE (451319)**, 2026 South Jackson, Zip 75766; tel. 903/541–4500 **A**1 9 10 18 **F**3 8 15 18 28 29 30 32 34 35 39 40 43 45 50 53 56 57 59 64 65 68 77 79 81 82 85 93 97 107 108 110 111 113 118 128 129 144 146 **P**5 6 7 8 **S** Trinity Mother Frances Hospitals and Clinics, Tyler, TX
Primary Contact: Thomas N. Cammack, Jr., Chief Administrative Officer
COO: Michael Lewis, Chief Operating Officer
CFO: William L. Bellenfant, Chief Financial Officer
CMO: Matthew Vierkant, M.D., President Medical Staff
CIO: Lee Portwood, Chief Information Officer
CHR: Davlin King, Team Leader Human Resources
Web address: www.tmfhs.org
**Control:** Other not–for–profit (including NFP Corporation) **Service:** General Medical and Surgical

**Staffed Beds:** 21 **Admissions:** 1203 **Census:** 10 **Outpatient Visits:** 71991 **Births:** 0 **Total Expense ($000):** 28922 **Payroll Expense ($000):** 7741 **Personnel:** 141

## JASPER—Jasper County

☒ **CHRISTUS JASPER MEMORIAL HOSPITAL (450573)**, 1275 Marvin Hancock Drive, Zip 75951–4995; tel. 409/384–5461 **A**1 9 10 **F**3 11 13 15 29 30 34 40 43 50 51 57 59 64 70 76 77 79 81 83 89 90 107 111 118 126 129 134 145 **P**8 **S** CHRISTUS Health, Irving, TX
Primary Contact: Deborah Wiegand, R.N., Administrator
CFO: Libby Lewis, Chief Financial Officer
CHR: Kay Powell, Director Human Resources
Web address: www.christusjasper.org
**Control:** Church–operated, Nongovernment, not–for profit **Service:** General Medical and Surgical

**Staffed Beds:** 50 **Admissions:** 1827 **Census:** 17 **Outpatient Visits:** 79683 **Births:** 368 **Total Expense ($000):** 26311 **Payroll Expense ($000):** 11228 **Personnel:** 224

## JOURDANTON—Atascosa County

☒ **SOUTH TEXAS REGIONAL MEDICAL CENTER (450165)**, 1905 Highway 97 East, Zip 78026–1504; tel. 830/769–3515 **A**1 9 10 20 **F**3 11 13 15 18 20 28 29 30 34 35 39 40 43 45 57 59 64 68 70 75 76 77 79 81 85 93 107 108 110 111 113 118 126 128 129 131 132 145 146 147 **P**6 **S** Community Health Systems, Inc., Franklin, TN
Primary Contact: James R. Resendez, Chief Executive Officer
COO: Gerardo Flores, R.N., Chief Operating Officer and Chief Nursing Officer
CFO: Gary Redmon, Chief Financial Officer
CMO: Edward Blackmon, M.D., Chief of Staff
CHR: Carrie Steinle, Chief Human Resources
CNO: Gerardo Flores, R.N., Chief Operating Officer and Chief Nursing Officer
Web address: www.strmc.com
**Control:** Corporation, Investor–owned, for–profit **Service:** General Medical and Surgical

**Staffed Beds:** 67 **Admissions:** 2271 **Census:** 20 **Outpatient Visits:** 72280 **Births:** 267 **Total Expense ($000):** 36895 **Payroll Expense ($000):** 17727 **Personnel:** 289

## JUNCTION—Kimble County

★ **KIMBLE HOSPITAL (451306)**, 2101 Main Street, Zip 76849–2101; tel. 325/446–3321 **A**9 10 18 **F**3 29 34 40 41 43 57 59 93 107 126 132 **S** Preferred Management Corporation, Shawnee, OK
Primary Contact: Steve Bowen, Chief Executive Officer
COO: Teena Hagood, Chief Nursing Officer
CFO: Larry Stephens, Chief Financial Officer
CMO: Ben Udall, M.D., Chief of Staff
CIO: Anna Henry, Chief Information Officer
CHR: Hope Lamb, Manager Human Resources
Web address: www.kimblehospital.org/
**Control:** Corporation, Investor–owned, for–profit **Service:** General Medical and Surgical

**Staffed Beds:** 15 **Admissions:** 219 **Census:** 2 **Outpatient Visits:** 45935 **Births:** 1 **Total Expense ($000):** 4953 **Payroll Expense ($000):** 2601 **Personnel:** 65

**TX**

---

**Hospital, Medicare Provider Number, Address, Telephone, Approval, Facility, and Physician Codes, Health Care System**

★ American Hospital Association (AHA) membership
☐ The Joint Commission accreditation
◇ DNV Healthcare Inc. accreditation
◯ American Osteopathic Association (AOA) accreditation
△ Commission on Accreditation of Rehabilitation Facilities (CARF) accreditation

## KATY—Harris County

⊠ **CHRISTUS ST. CATHERINE HOSPITAL (450832)**, 701 Fry Road, Zip 77450; tel. 281/599–5700 **A**1 2 9 10 **F**3 11 12 13 15 17 18 29 30 34 35 40 54 57 59 61 64 69 70 75 76 77 78 79 81 82 84 86 87 89 90 93 107 108 110 111 113 114 116 118 123 128 129 130 131 134 145 146 147 **S** CHRISTUS Health, Irving, TX
Primary Contact: Jack H. McCabe, FACHE, Administrator
CFO: Nancy Brock, Chief Financial Officer
CHR: James A. Fitch, Director Human Resources
Web address: www.christusstcatherine.org
**Control:** Church–operated, Nongovernment, not–for profit **Service:** General Medical and Surgical

**Staffed Beds:** 102 **Admissions:** 6132 **Census:** 64 **Outpatient Visits:** 85151 **Births:** 1132 **Total Expense ($000):** 105502 **Payroll Expense ($000):** 36200 **Personnel:** 584

⊠ **MEMORIAL HERMANN KATY HOSPITAL (450847)**, 23900 Katy Freeway, Zip 77494; tel. 281/644–7000 **A**1 9 10 **F**3 8 11 13 15 29 30 35 39 40 43 45 46 49 57 59 61 64 65 66 68 69 70 73 75 76 77 79 81 89 93 102 107 108 111 113 117 118 129 131 145 146 **P**5 6 **S** Memorial Hermann Healthcare System, Houston, TX
Primary Contact: Brian S. Barbe, Chief Executive Officer
CFO: Lisa Kendler, Chief Financial Officer
Web address: www.memorialhermann.org
**Control:** Other not–for–profit (including NFP Corporation) **Service:** General Medical and Surgical

**Staffed Beds:** 142 **Admissions:** 9489 **Census:** 93 **Outpatient Visits:** 84873 **Births:** 2701 **Total Expense ($000):** 100607 **Payroll Expense ($000):** 50479 **Personnel:** 749

⊠ **MEMORIAL HERMANN REHABILITATION HOSPITAL – KATY (673038)**, 21720 Kingsland Boulevard, Zip 77450–2513; tel. 281/579–5555 **A**1 9 10 **F**3 29 64 79 90 92 93 107 111 113 118 129 130 147 **S** Memorial Hermann Healthcare System, Houston, TX
Primary Contact: Noelle Lopez, Executive Director
Web address: www.memorialhermann.com
**Control:** Partnership, Investor–owned, for–profit **Service:** Rehabilitation

**Staffed Beds:** 35 **Admissions:** 697 **Census:** 25 **Outpatient Visits:** 9684 **Births:** 0 **Total Expense ($000):** 18612 **Payroll Expense ($000):** 7841 **Personnel:** 116

## KAUFMAN—Kaufman County

⊠ **TEXAS HEALTH PRESBYTERIAN HOSPITAL KAUFMAN (450292)**, 850 Ed Hall Drive, Zip 75142, Mailing Address: P.O. Box 1108, Zip 75142–1108; tel. 972/932–7200 **A**1 9 10 **F**3 8 11 13 15 29 30 34 35 40 43 45 50 57 59 65 68 70 75 76 79 81 82 85 86 87 93 102 107 108 111 113 117 118 129 131 134 145 147 **P**5 **S** Texas Health Resources, Arlington, TX
Primary Contact: Patsy Youngs, President
CMO: Prabha Mohan, M.D., President Medical Staff
CHR: Carolyn Whitehurst, Director Human Resources
Web address: www.texashealth.org
**Control:** Other not–for–profit (including NFP Corporation) **Service:** General Medical and Surgical

**Staffed Beds:** 68 **Admissions:** 2326 **Census:** 22 **Outpatient Visits:** 39144 **Births:** 291 **Total Expense ($000):** 31806 **Payroll Expense ($000):** 12671 **Personnel:** 218

## KENEDY—Karnes County

★ **OTTO KAISER MEMORIAL HOSPITAL (451364)**, 3349 South Highway 181, Zip 78119–5240; tel. 830/583–3401 **A**9 10 **F**3 11 15 29 30 34 40 45 46 57 62 64 68 77 81 93 107 111 113 118 129 132 134 147 **P**8
Primary Contact: Nathan Tudor, Administrator and Chief Executive Officer
CFO: Beverly Montez, Manager Business Office
Web address: www.okmh.net
**Control:** Hospital district or authority, Government, nonfederal **Service:** General Medical and Surgical

**Staffed Beds:** 21 **Admissions:** 465 **Census:** 6 **Outpatient Visits:** 16048 **Births:** 0 **Total Expense ($000):** 9501 **Payroll Expense ($000):** 4890 **Personnel:** 118

## KERMIT—Winkler County

**WINKLER COUNTY MEMORIAL HOSPITAL (451314)**, 821 Jeffee Drive, Zip 79745–4696, Mailing Address: Drawer H, Zip 79745–6008; tel. 432/586–5864 **A**9 10 18 **F**3 32 34 36 40 57 59 64 65 69 93 97 107 113 118 126 132
Primary Contact: William E. Ernst, Administrator
CFO: Wannah Hartley, Controller
CMO: K. Pham, M.D., Chief of Staff
CIO: Keith Palmer, Assistant Administrator
**Control:** County–Government, nonfederal **Service:** General Medical and Surgical

**Staffed Beds:** 19 **Admissions:** 236 **Census:** 2 **Outpatient Visits:** 7452 **Births:** 0 **Total Expense ($000):** 7426 **Payroll Expense ($000):** 2960 **Personnel:** 77

## KERRVILLE—Kerr County

**KERRVILLE DIVISION** See South Texas Veterans Health Care System, San Antonio

☐ **KERRVILLE STATE HOSPITAL (454014)**, 721 Thompson Drive, Zip 78028–5154; tel. 830/896–2211 **A**1 3 5 9 10 **F**11 30 34 39 44 50 56 65 68 75 86 87 97 98 101 103 129 131 134 145 **S** Texas Department of State Health Services, Austin, TX
Primary Contact: Jay Norwood, Acting Superintendent
CMO: Janet E. TRUE, M.D., Clinical Director
Web address: www.dshs.state.tx.us/lmhhospitals/kerrvillesh
**Control:** State–Government, nonfederal **Service:** Psychiatric

**Staffed Beds:** 202 **Admissions:** 74 **Census:** 198 **Outpatient Visits:** 0 **Births:** 0 **Total Expense ($000):** 36625 **Payroll Expense ($000):** 20022 **Personnel:** 541

⊠ **PETERSON REGIONAL MEDICAL CENTER (450007)**, 551 Hill Country Drive, Zip 78028–5398; tel. 830/896–4200 **A**1 9 10 **F**3 8 11 13 15 18 20 26 29 30 31 34 35 39 40 44 45 49 54 57 59 62 63 64 65 68 70 74 75 76 77 78 79 80 81 82 84 85 86 87 90 93 96 100 107 108 110 111 113 114 118 129 130 131 134 145 146 147 **P**1 3
Primary Contact: James Patrick Murray, FACHE, Chief Executive Officer
COO: Stephen Pautler, FACHE, Chief Operating Officer
CFO: Robert H. Walther, Chief Financial Officer
CMO: Eileen Toloza, M.D., Chief of Staff
CIO: Richard Cruthirds, Director Information Systems
CHR: Buddy Volpe, Director Human Resources
Web address: www.petersonrmc.com
**Control:** Other not–for–profit (including NFP Corporation) **Service:** General Medical and Surgical

**Staffed Beds:** 124 **Admissions:** 4836 **Census:** 67 **Outpatient Visits:** 134731 **Births:** 357 **Total Expense ($000):** 94503 **Payroll Expense ($000):** 38365 **Personnel:** 824

## KILGORE—Gregg County

**ALLEGIANCE SPECIALTY HOSPITAL OF KILGORE (450488)**, 1612 South Henderson Boulevard, Zip 75662–3594; tel. 903/984–3505 **A**9 10 21 **F**3 29 34 35 56 57 59 98 101 103 104 129 **S** Allegiance Health Management, Shreveport, LA
Primary Contact: Sherry Bustin, Chief Executive Officer
CHR: Becky Wilson, Manager Human Resources
Web address: www.ahmgt.com
**Control:** Corporation, Investor–owned, for–profit **Service:** Psychiatric

**Staffed Beds:** 60 **Admissions:** 517 **Census:** 18 **Outpatient Visits:** 21740 **Births:** 0 **Total Expense ($000):** 7706 **Payroll Expense ($000):** 3123 **Personnel:** 98

## KILLEEN—Bell County

⊠ **METROPLEX ADVENTIST HOSPITAL (450152)**, 2201 South Clear Creek Road, Zip 76549–4110; tel. 254/526–7523 **A**1 9 10 **F**3 8 11 12 13 15 18 20 22 26 28 29 30 34 35 39 40 46 48 49 54 57 59 62 65 68 70 71 75 76 77 78 79 81 82 85 86 87 89 93 98 99 100 101 102 103 104 105 107 108 111 113 114 117 118 128 129 130 131 134 145 146 147 **P**8 **S** Adventist Health System Sunbelt Health Care Corporation, Altamonte Springs, FL
Primary Contact: Carlyle L. E. Walton, Chief Executive Officer
CFO: Penny Johnson, Chief Financial Officer
CMO: Frederick Barnett, M.D., Chief of Staff
CIO: Dale Koebnick, Director Management Information Systems and Patient Access
CHR: Brenda Coley, Executive Director
Web address: www.mplex.org
**Control:** Church–operated, Nongovernment, not–for profit **Service:** General Medical and Surgical

**Staffed Beds:** 177 **Admissions:** 9066 **Census:** 87 **Outpatient Visits:** 120373 **Births:** 1725 **Total Expense ($000):** 108078 **Payroll Expense ($000):** 46060 **Personnel:** 1038

## KINGSVILLE—Kleberg County

⊠ **CHRISTUS SPOHN HOSPITAL KLEBERG (450163)**, 1311 General Cavazos Boulevard, Zip 78363–1197; tel. 361/595–1661 **A**1 9 10 20 **F**3 11 13 15 29 30 34 35 40 41 43 53 54 57 59 64 65 66 70 74 75 76 77 81 85 86 87 93 102 106 107 108 110 118 129 145 **S** CHRISTUS Health, Irving, TX
Primary Contact: Norman L. McBride, FACHE, Vice President and Chief Operating Officer
CFO: Lauralinda Moore, Manager Finance
CHR: Candace Jefferson, Manager Human Resources
Web address: www.christusspohn.org
**Control:** Church–operated, Nongovernment, not–for profit **Service:** General Medical and Surgical

**Staffed Beds:** 77 **Admissions:** 3841 **Census:** 47 **Outpatient Visits:** 31832 **Births:** 356 **Total Expense ($000):** 30387 **Payroll Expense ($000):** 18425 **Personnel:** 258

TX

## KINGWOOD—Harris County

**KINGWOOD MEDICAL CENTER (450775)**, 22999 U.S. Highway 59 North, Zip 77339; tel. 281/348–8000 **A**1 9 10 **F**3 11 13 15 18 20 22 24 26 28 29 30 31 34 35 40 49 50 51 56 57 59 60 61 64 68 70 72 74 75 76 77 78 79 81 82 84 85 87 89 90 92 97 102 107 108 110 111 113 114 118 123 128 129 131 142 143 145 146 **P**7 **S** HCA, Nashville, TN
Primary Contact: Melinda Stephenson, Chief Executive Officer
COO: Megan Marietta, Chief Operating Officer
CFO: Bryan R. Lee, Chief Financial Officer
CMO: J. Mario Villafani, M.D., Chief of Staff
Web address: www.kingwoodmedical.com
**Control:** Corporation, Investor–owned, for–profit **Service:** General Medical and Surgical

**Staffed Beds:** 248 **Admissions:** 13275 **Census:** 174 **Outpatient Visits:** 81763 **Births:** 2253 **Total Expense ($000):** 140685 **Payroll Expense ($000):** 56949 **Personnel:** 742

**KINGWOOD PINES HOSPITAL (454103)**, 2001 Ladbrook Drive, Zip 77339; tel. 281/358–1495 **A**1 9 10 **F**4 5 29 38 56 59 75 86 87 98 99 100 101 102 103 104 105 129 131 **S** Universal Health Services, Inc., King of Prussia, PA
Primary Contact: James Burroughs, Chief Executive Officer
CFO: Richard Kurzenberger, Chief Financial Officer
CMO: Gary E. Miller, M.D., Medical Director
CHR: Adrienne Livingston, Director Human Resources
Web address: www.kingwoodpines.com
**Control:** Corporation, Investor–owned, for–profit **Service:** Psychiatric

**Staffed Beds:** 116 **Admissions:** 3584 **Census:** 78 **Outpatient Visits:** 3015 **Births:** 0 **Total Expense ($000):** 19853 **Payroll Expense ($000):** 8986 **Personnel:** 188

**KINGWOOD SPECIALTY HOSPITAL** See Memorial Hermann Surgical Hospital Kingwood

**MEMORIAL HERMANN SURGICAL HOSPITAL KINGWOOD (670005)**, 300 Kingwood Medical Drive, Zip 77339; tel. 281/312–4000 **A**1 9 10 **F**3 40 45 51 64 68 79 81 82 85 86 87
Primary Contact: Marc Celia, R.N., MS, FACHE, Chief Executive Officer
Web address: www.memorialhermannkingwood.com
**Control:** Corporation, Investor–owned, for–profit **Service:** General Medical and Surgical

**Staffed Beds:** 10 **Admissions:** 205 **Census:** 1 **Outpatient Visits:** 5366 **Births:** 0 **Total Expense ($000):** 24522 **Payroll Expense ($000):** 3487 **Personnel:** 60

## KNOX CITY—Knox County

**KNOX COUNTY HOSPITAL (450746)**, 701 South Fifth Street, Zip 79529; Mailing Address: P.O. Box 608, Zip 79529–0608; tel. 940/657–3535 **A**9 10 20 **F**7 11 28 32 40 43 57 59 62 126 132 **P**6
Primary Contact: Stephan A. Kuehler, Administrator
CFO: Dan Offutt, Manager Finance
CMO: Shirley Barretto, M.D., Chief of Staff
CIO: Sue Marion, Manager Business Office
Web address: www.knoxcountyhospital–texas.com
**Control:** Hospital district or authority, Government, nonfederal **Service:** General Medical and Surgical

**Staffed Beds:** 14 **Admissions:** 186 **Census:** 2 **Outpatient Visits:** 33789 **Births:** 0 **Total Expense ($000):** 5509 **Payroll Expense ($000):** 2612 **Personnel:** 72

## KYLE—Hays County

**SETON MEDICAL CENTER HAYS (670056)**, 6001 Kyle Parkway, Zip 78640–6112, Mailing Address: 6001 Kyle Prkway, Zip 78640–6112; tel. 512/504–5000 **A**1 9 10 **F**3 11 13 15 18 20 22 24 28 29 30 35 40 44 45 46 49 50 60 65 68 70 72 74 75 76 77 78 79 81 82 85 107 110 111 113 114 118 128 129 134 142 145 147 **P**3 8 **S** Ascension Health, Saint Louis, MO
Primary Contact: Herb Dyer, Chief Executive Officer and Chief Operating Officer
COO: Herb Dyer, Chief Executive Officer and Chief Operating Officer
Web address: www.seton.net
**Control:** Church–operated, Nongovernment, not–for profit **Service:** General Medical and Surgical

**Staffed Beds:** 84 **Admissions:** 4618 **Census:** 50 **Outpatient Visits:** 39287 **Births:** 600 **Total Expense ($000):** 86470 **Payroll Expense ($000):** 36653 **Personnel:** 686

## LA GRANGE—Fayette County

★ **ST. MARK'S MEDICAL CENTER (670004)**, One St. Mark's Place, Zip 78945; tel. 979/242–2200 **A**3 5 9 10 **F**3 8 11 12 13 15 29 30 34 40 43 45 50 56 57 59 68 70 74 75 76 79 81 82 84 85 87 89 93 107 110 111 113 118 127 128 129 132 144 145 146 **S** Community Hospital Corporation, Plano, TX
Primary Contact: Nathan Staggs, President and Chief Executive Officer
COO: Carol Drozd, Chief Operating Officer
CFO: Dennis Boyd, Chief Financial Officer
CMO: Russell Juno, M.D., Chief of Staff
CHR: Tammy Oehlke, Director Human Resources
Web address: www.smmctx.org
**Control:** Other not–for–profit (including NFP Corporation) **Service:** General Medical and Surgical

**Staffed Beds:** 48 **Admissions:** 2305 **Census:** 24 **Outpatient Visits:** 50164 **Births:** 317 **Total Expense ($000):** 25472 **Payroll Expense ($000):** 8859 **Personnel:** 175

## LAKE JACKSON—Brazoria County

**BRAZOSPORT REGIONAL HEALTH SYSTEM (450072)**, 100 Medical Drive, Zip 77566–9983; tel. 979/297–4411 **A**1 2 9 10 **F**3 11 12 13 15 18 20 22 24 28 29 30 31 34 37 40 41 43 45 47 49 50 51 57 59 60 62 64 65 68 70 74 75 76 77 78 79 81 82 85 86 89 90 91 93 94 107 108 110 111 113 116 117 118 119 120 122 128 129 131 145 146 147 **P**8 **S** QHR, Brentwood, TN
Primary Contact: Daniel L. Buche, Chief Executive Officer
COO: Al Guevara, Vice President Operations
CFO: Chuck Jeffress, Vice President Fiscal Services
CMO: Adam Corley, M.D., Chief of Staff
CIO: Todd Edwards, Director Information Management Systems
CHR: Christopher Calia, Director Human Resources
Web address: www.brhs.org
**Control:** Other not–for–profit (including NFP Corporation) **Service:** General Medical and Surgical

**Staffed Beds:** 103 **Admissions:** 5245 **Census:** 53 **Outpatient Visits:** 130278 **Births:** 627 **Total Expense ($000):** 71375 **Payroll Expense ($000):** 31644 **Personnel:** 544

## LAMESA—Dawson County

**MEDICAL ARTS HOSPITAL (450489)**, 2200 North Bryan Avenue, Zip 79331–3145; tel. 806/872–2183 **A**9 10 20 **F**11 13 28 29 30 35 40 43 45 50 57 59 62 64 75 76 81 87 93 97 107 111 113 118 126 129 132 144 145 147 **P**6
Primary Contact: Letha Hughes, Chief Executive Officer
CFO: Steve Brock, Chief Financial Officer
CMO: Fidel Ogeda, M.D., Chief of Staff
CHR: Jo Beth Smith, Director Human Resources
Web address: www.medicalartshospital.org
**Control:** Hospital district or authority, Government, nonfederal **Service:** General Medical and Surgical

**Staffed Beds:** 22 **Admissions:** 686 **Census:** 9 **Outpatient Visits:** 91295 **Births:** 90 **Total Expense ($000):** 22387 **Payroll Expense ($000):** 7549 **Personnel:** 223

## LAMPASAS—Lampasas County

**ROLLINS–BROOK COMMUNITY HOSPITAL (451323)**, 608 North Key Avenue, Zip 76550, Mailing Address: P.O. Box 589, Zip 76550; tel. 512/556–3682 **A**1 9 10 18 **F**3 15 29 30 35 40 57 59 61 75 77 81 87 93 107 111 113 118 129 131 132 145 147 **P**8 **S** Adventist Health System Sunbelt Health Care Corporation, Altamonte Springs, FL
Primary Contact: Jeffrey D. Villanueva, Vice President and Administrator
CFO: Janice Hagensicker, Chief Financial Officer
CHR: Brenda Coley, Executive Director
Web address: www.mplex.org
**Control:** Church–operated, Nongovernment, not–for profit **Service:** General Medical and Surgical

**Staffed Beds:** 35 **Admissions:** 759 **Census:** 10 **Outpatient Visits:** 17012 **Births:** 0 **Total Expense ($000):** 12855 **Payroll Expense ($000):** 4474 **Personnel:** 126

**TX**

---

**Hospital, Medicare Provider Number, Address, Telephone, Approval, Facility, and Physician Codes, Health Care System**

★ American Hospital Association (AHA) membership
☐ The Joint Commission accreditation
◇ DNV Healthcare Inc. accreditation
◯ American Osteopathic Association (AOA) accreditation
△ Commission on Accreditation of Rehabilitation Facilities (CARF) accreditation

## LAREDO—Webb County

☐ **DOCTORS HOSPITAL OF LAREDO (450643)**, 10700 McPherson Road, Zip 78045; tel. 956/523–2000 **A**1 2 9 10 **F**3 11 12 13 15 18 20 22 26 29 30 31 32 34 37 39 40 43 45 48 49 50 54 57 59 60 63 64 70 71 72 74 75 76 77 78 79 81 85 87 89 90 91 93 107 108 111 113 118 120 128 129 131 145 **P**5 **S** Universal Health Services, Inc., King of Prussia, PA
Primary Contact: Elmo Lopez, Jr., Chief Executive Officer
COO: Eladio Montalvo, Chief Operating Officer
CFO: Dinah Gonzalez, Chief Financial Officer
CMO: Juan F. Montalvo, M.D., Chief of Staff
CIO: Maribel Mata, Director Information Services
CHR: Roseann Figueroa, Director Human Resources
Web address: www.doctorshosplaredo.com
**Control:** Partnership, Investor–owned, for–profit **Service:** General Medical and Surgical

**Staffed Beds: 183 Admissions: 9279 Census: 104 Outpatient Visits: 89180 Births: 2638 Total Expense ($000): 85951 Payroll Expense ($000): 35666 Personnel: 695**

☒ **LAREDO MEDICAL CENTER (450029)**, 1700 East Saunders Avenue, Zip 78041–5401, Mailing Address: Drawer 2068, Zip 78044–2068; tel. 956/796–5000, (Total facility includes 18 beds in nursing home–type unit) **A**1 9 10 **F**3 8 11 12 13 15 18 20 22 24 26 28 29 30 31 34 35 37 40 43 45 46 49 50 51 53 54 56 57 59 60 64 68 70 72 74 75 76 77 78 79 81 85 86 87 89 90 91 92 93 96 107 108 110 111 113 118 119 120 122 127 128 131 134 145 146 147 **S** Community Health Systems, Inc., Franklin, TN
Primary Contact: Timothy E. Schmidt, Chief Executive Officer
COO: John E. Ulbricht, Chief Operating Officer
CFO: Ed Romero, Chief Financial Officer
CIO: Joe Rivera, Chief Information Technology Officer
CHR: Michael W. Hartley, Director Human Resources
Web address: www.laredomedical.com
**Control:** Corporation, Investor–owned, for–profit **Service:** General Medical and Surgical

**Staffed Beds: 326 Admissions: 16695 Census: 225 Outpatient Visits: 174197 Births: 3352 Total Expense ($000): 161337 Payroll Expense ($000): 53537 Personnel: 1315**

☐ **LAREDO SPECIALTY HOSPITAL (452096)**, 2005 Bustamente Street, Zip 78041–5470; tel. 956/753–5353 **A**1 10 **F**3 29 30 53 70 75 77 85 86 87 91 96 129 147 **S** Ernest Health, Inc., Albuquerque, NM
Primary Contact: Mario Rodriguez, Chief Executive Officer
COO: Bernadette Hernandez, R.N., Chief Operating Officer
CFO: Robert Voss, Chief Financial Officer
CMO: Marisa Guerrero, Director Human Resources
CMO: Benson Huang, M.D., Medical Director
CNO: Bernadette Hernandez, R.N., Chief Operating Officer and Chief Nursing Officer
Web address: www.lsh.ernesthealth.com
**Control:** Partnership, Investor–owned, for–profit **Service:** General Medical and Surgical

**Staffed Beds: 60 Admissions: 482 Census: 33 Outpatient Visits: 0 Births: 0 Total Expense ($000): 16706 Payroll Expense ($000): 5932 Personnel: 119**

## LEAGUE CITY—Galveston County

☐ **DEVEREUX TEXAS TREATMENT NETWORK (454085)**, 1150 Devereux Drive, Zip 77573–2043; tel. 281/335–1000 **A**1 9 10 **F**4 5 29 32 35 38 43 53 54 59 64 75 86 87 98 99 100 101 102 104 105 106 129 131 133 **S** Devereux, Villanova, PA
Primary Contact: Pamela E. Helm, Executive Director
Web address: www.devereux.org
**Control:** Other not–for–profit (including NFP Corporation) **Service:** Children's hospital psychiatric

**Staffed Beds: 57 Admissions: 489 Census: 62 Outpatient Visits: 4487 Births: 0 Total Expense ($000): 11441 Payroll Expense ($000): 3839 Personnel: 80**

## LEVELLAND—Hockley County

★ **COVENANT HOSPITAL–LEVELLAND (450755)**, 1900 South College Avenue, Zip 79336–6508; tel. 806/894–4963 **A**9 10 **F**11 13 15 29 30 34 40 43 45 50 54 57 59 64 65 68 75 76 77 81 82 85 86 87 89 90 91 93 97 107 111 118 126 129 132 145 **P**4 **S** Covenant Health System, Lubbock, TX
Primary Contact: Jerry Osburn, Administrator
CFO: John Dolan, Chief Financial Officer
CMO: Stephanie Kubacak, M.D., Chief of Staff
CIO: Kevin Elmore, Chief Information Officer
CHR: Kathy McDonald, Director Personnel
Web address: www.covenanthealth.org
**Control:** Church–operated, Nongovernment, not–for profit **Service:** General Medical and Surgical

**Staffed Beds: 22 Admissions: 981 Census: 9 Outpatient Visits: 37986 Births: 272 Total Expense ($000): 19148 Payroll Expense ($000): 7728 Personnel: 217**

## LEWISVILLE—Denton County

☒ **MEDICAL CENTER OF LEWISVILLE (450669)**, 500 West Main, Zip 75057–3699; tel. 972/420–1000 **A**1 9 10 **F**3 13 15 18 20 26 28 29 30 31 34 35 40 42 46 49 57 59 68 70 72 74 75 76 78 79 81 85 87 89 93 107 108 110 111 113 117 118 128 129 130 131 134 145 146 147 **P**5 **S** HCA, Nashville, TN
Primary Contact: Ashley McClellan, Chief Executive Officer
CFO: Lisa Brodbeck, Chief Financial Officer
CIO: Shirley Archambeault, Chief Information Officer
CHR: Dara Biegert, Assistant Vice President Human Resources
Web address: www.lewisvillemedical.com
**Control:** Corporation, Investor–owned, for–profit **Service:** General Medical and Surgical

**Staffed Beds: 182 Admissions: 8075 Census: 93 Outpatient Visits: 64271 Births: 1766 Total Expense ($000): 123348 Payroll Expense ($000): 44870 Personnel: 674**

## LIBERTY—Liberty County

☐ **LIBERTY DAYTON REGIONAL MEDICAL CENTER (451375)**, 1353 North Travis, Zip 77575–1353; tel. 936/336–7316 **A**1 9 10 18 **F**3 29 40 45 56 64 81 85 107 114 127 129 132
Primary Contact: Ray Mason, Interim Chief Executive Officer
CFO: Hal Mayo, Chief Financial Officer
CMO: Don Callens, M.D., Chief Medical Officer
CNO: Mark Nichols, R.N., Director of Nurses
Web address: www.libertydaytonrmc.com
**Control:** Hospital district or authority, Government, nonfederal **Service:** General Medical and Surgical

**Staffed Beds: 17 Admissions: 387 Census: 3 Outpatient Visits: 16325 Births: 0 Total Expense ($000): 3463 Payroll Expense ($000): 1443 Personnel: 59**

## LINDEN—Cass County

★ **GOOD SHEPHERD MEDICAL CENTER–LINDEN (451302)**, 404 North Kaufman Street, Zip 75563–5235; tel. 903/756–5561 **A**9 10 18 **F**3 11 13 28 29 30 34 40 43 45 49 50 57 64 68 75 76 77 81 85 87 93 94 97 102 107 108 110 113 118 126 129 130 131 132 134 142 145 147 **S** Good Shepherd Health System, Longview, TX
Primary Contact: Carla Roadcap, R.N., MSN, Chief Executive Officer
CMO: Donald Simmons, M.D., Chief Medical Staff
Web address: www.gsmclinden.org
**Control:** Other not–for–profit (including NFP Corporation) **Service:** General Medical and Surgical

**Staffed Beds: 25 Admissions: 494 Census: 6 Outpatient Visits: 32164 Births: 0 Total Expense ($000): 10694 Payroll Expense ($000): 4217 Personnel: 83**

## LITTLEFIELD—Lamb County

★ **LAMB HEALTHCARE CENTER (450698)**, 1500 South Sunset, Zip 79339–4899; tel. 806/385–6411 **A**9 10 20 **F**13 29 35 40 43 45 57 59 64 66 75 76 81 86 87 89 107 113 118 126 131 132 133 146 **P**6
Primary Contact: Jo Nell Wischkaemper, Administrator
CFO: Cindy Klein, Chief Financial Officer
CMO: Isabel Molina, M.D., Chief Medical Officer
CHR: Joan Williams, Administrative Assistant
Web address: www.littlefieldtexas.org/LL_LHC.html
**Control:** County–Government, nonfederal **Service:** General Medical and Surgical

**Staffed Beds: 41 Admissions: 652 Census: 8 Outpatient Visits: 23512 Births: 154 Total Expense ($000): 10278 Payroll Expense ($000): 4256 Personnel: 136**

## LIVINGSTON—Polk County

☐ **MEMORIAL MEDICAL CENTER – LIVINGSTON (450395)**, 1717 Highway 59 Bypass, Zip 77351–1257, Mailing Address: P.O. Box 1257, Zip 77351–1257; tel. 936/329–8700 **A**1 9 10 **F**3 11 13 15 29 34 35 40 43 45 46 50 57 59 62 64 68 70 74 75 76 79 81 85 87 89 107 108 110 111 113 118 128 129 131 145 **S** Memorial Health System of East Texas, Lufkin, TX
Primary Contact: David LeMonte, Chief Executive Officer
CFO: Kristi Gay, Chief Financial Officer
CMO: C. K. Mani, M.D., Chief of Staff
CHR: Ray G. Grossman, Vice President Human Resources
Web address: www.memorialhealth.org
**Control:** Other not–for–profit (including NFP Corporation) **Service:** General Medical and Surgical

**Staffed Beds: 66 Admissions: 2386 Census: 25 Outpatient Visits: 52332 Births: 318 Total Expense ($000): 40045 Payroll Expense ($000): 16020 Personnel: 271**

TX

*Many Facility Codes have changed. Please refer to the AHA Guide Code Chart.* © 2012 AHA Guide

## LLANO—Llano County

★ **SCOTT & WHITE HOSPITAL – LLANO (450219)**, 200 West Ollie Street, Zip 78643–2628; tel. 325/247–5040 **A**9 10 20 **F**3 7 11 12 13 15 32 34 35 40 43 45 57 59 62 75 76 77 81 85 87 93 107 113 118 126 128 129 134 145 **S** Scott & White Healthcare, Temple, TX
Primary Contact: Kevin Leeper, Chief Executive Officer
COO: Linda Meredith, MSN, Chief Operating Officer
CFO: Jason Cole, Director Finance
CMO: Kim Russell, M.D., Chief of Staff
CIO: Rodney Lott, Director Management Information Systems and Facility Operations
CHR: Pearl Oestreich, Director Human Resources
CNO: Reta Hunt, Director of Nursing
Web address: www.llanomemorial.org
**Control:** Other not–for–profit (including NFP Corporation) **Service:** General Medical and Surgical

**Staffed Beds:** 26 **Admissions:** 885 **Census:** 6 **Outpatient Visits:** 109353 **Births:** 265 **Total Expense ($000):** 23057 **Payroll Expense ($000):** 11750 **Personnel:** 301

## LOCKNEY—Floyd County

★ **W. J. MANGOLD MEMORIAL HOSPITAL (451337)**, 320 North Main Street, Zip 79241–0037, Mailing Address: Box 37, Zip 79241–0037; tel. 806/652–3373 **A**9 10 18 **F**3 13 35 40 43 45 53 57 59 62 64 65 76 81 85 93 97 107 111 118 126 129 132 147 **P**4
Primary Contact: Sharon Hunt, Administrator
CFO: Sharon Hunt, Administrator
CIO: Larry Mullins, Chief Information Officer
CHR: Marsha Allen, Director Human Resources
Web address: www.mangoldmemorial.org
**Control:** Hospital district or authority, Government, nonfederal **Service:** General Medical and Surgical

**Staffed Beds:** 25 **Admissions:** 620 **Census:** 7 **Outpatient Visits:** 34861 **Births:** 68 **Total Expense ($000):** 9317 **Payroll Expense ($000):** 4592 **Personnel:** 123

## LONGVIEW—Gregg County

**BEHAVIORAL HOSPITAL OF LONGVIEW (454105)**, 22 Bermuda Lane, Zip 75605; tel. 903/291–3456 **A**10 **F**29 98 100 101 103 129
Primary Contact: Denise Allen, Administrator
Web address: www.longviewhospital.com
**Control:** Corporation, Investor–owned, for–profit **Service:** Psychiatric

**Staffed Beds:** 41 **Admissions:** 725 **Census:** 34 **Outpatient Visits:** 76 **Births:** 0 **Total Expense ($000):** 7271 **Payroll Expense ($000):** 3529 **Personnel:** 102

✠ △ **GOOD SHEPHERD MEDICAL CENTER (450037)**, 700 East Marshall Avenue, Zip 75601–5571; tel. 903/315–2000 **A**1 7 9 10 **F**3 7 11 13 15 18 20 22 24 26 28 29 30 31 32 33 44 40 43 45 46 49 50 51 53 54 56 57 59 60 61 64 68 70 71 72 73 74 75 76 77 78 79 80 81 82 85 86 87 89 90 92 93 97 102 107 108 111 113 114 117 118 128 129 130 131 134 142 143 145 146 147 **P**8 **S** Good Shepherd Health System, Longview, TX
Primary Contact: Edward D. Banos, President and Chief Executive Officer
CFO: Patricia Keel, Chief Financial Officer
CIO: Ralph Holcomb, Chief Information Officer
CHR: Sandie Feriggno, Director Human Resources
Web address: www.gsmc.org
**Control:** Other not–for–profit (including NFP Corporation) **Service:** General Medical and Surgical

**Staffed Beds:** 399 **Admissions:** 19723 **Census:** 262 **Outpatient Visits:** 163351 **Births:** 2550 **Total Expense ($000):** 248745 **Payroll Expense ($000):** 93498 **Personnel:** 1783

✠ **LONGVIEW REGIONAL MEDICAL CENTER (450702)**, 2901 North Fourth Street, Zip 75605–5191, Mailing Address: P.O. Box 14000, Zip 75607–4000; tel. 903/758–1818, (Total facility includes 15 beds in nursing home–type unit) **A**1 9 10 **F**3 8 11 12 13 17 18 20 22 24 28 29 30 31 34 37 40 43 45 46 47 49 50 57 59 61 64 65 67 70 74 75 76 78 79 81 84 85 86 87 89 107 108 111 113 114 117 118 123 125 127 129 145 147 **P**8 **S** Community Health Systems, Inc., Franklin, TN
Primary Contact: Jim R. Kendrick, Chief Executive Officer
COO: Jill Bayless–Berney, MSN, Chief Operating Officer
CFO: Todd Johnson, Chief Financial Officer
CMO: Timothy Tobin, M.D., Chief of Staff
CIO: Keith Jarvis, Director Information Systems
CHR: Stella Barrow, Director Human Resources
Web address: www.longviewregional.com
**Control:** Corporation, Investor–owned, for–profit **Service:** General Medical and Surgical

**Staffed Beds:** 127 **Admissions:** 6069 **Census:** 70 **Outpatient Visits:** 53672 **Births:** 969 **Total Expense ($000):** 92411 **Payroll Expense ($000):** 35668 **Personnel:** 674

✠ **SELECT SPECIALTY HOSPITAL–LONGVIEW (452087)**, 700 East Marshall Avenue, 1st Floor, Zip 75601; tel. 903/315–1111 **A**1 9 10 **F**1 3 28 29 40 75 77 85 91 92 129 147 **S** Select Medical Corporation, Mechanicsburg, PA
Primary Contact: Robert A. Turner, Chief Executive Officer
Web address: www.selectmedicalcorp.com
**Control:** Corporation, Investor–owned, for–profit **Service:** Long–Term Acute Care hospital

**Staffed Beds:** 32 **Admissions:** 445 **Census:** 31 **Outpatient Visits:** 0 **Births:** 0 **Total Expense ($000):** 14996 **Payroll Expense ($000):** 6015 **Personnel:** 117

## LUBBOCK—Lubbock County

✠ **COVENANT CHILDREN'S HOSPITAL (453306)**, 4000 24th Street, Zip 79410–1218; tel. 806/725–1011 **A**1 3 5 9 10 **F**3 19 21 23 25 27 30 31 32 40 41 43 50 59 72 73 81 89 **S** Covenant Health System, Lubbock, TX
Primary Contact: Christopher J. Dougherty, Chief Executive Officer
CMO: Scott Robins, M.D., Chief Medical Officer
CIO: Jim Reid, Vice President and Chief Information Officer
CHR: Rodney Cates, Senior Vice President Human Resources
Web address: www.covenanthealth.org
**Control:** Other not–for–profit (including NFP Corporation) **Service:** Children's general

**Staffed Beds:** 73 **Admissions:** 2713 **Census:** 51 **Outpatient Visits:** 31462 **Births:** 0 **Total Expense ($000):** 54156 **Payroll Expense ($000):** 17633 **Personnel:** 206

✠ **COVENANT MEDICAL CENTER (450040)**, 3615 19th Street, Zip 79410–1201, Mailing Address: P.O. Box 1201, Zip 79408–1201; tel. 806/725–0000, (Includes COVENANT MEDICAL CENTER–LAKESIDE, 4000 24th Street, Zip 79410–1894; tel. 806/725–0000) **A**1 2 3 5 6 9 10 **F**5 7 12 13 15 17 18 20 22 24 26 28 29 30 31 34 35 39 40 43 46 47 48 49 50 51 53 54 55 57 58 59 60 61 63 64 65 68 70 71 74 75 76 77 78 79 80 81 82 83 84 85 86 87 90 91 93 94 96 98 102 105 107 108 109 111 113 114 115 116 118 119 120 122 128 129 130 131 134 142 143 145 146 147 **P**6 8 **S** Covenant Health System, Lubbock, TX
Primary Contact: Richard H. Parks, FACHE, President and Chief Executive Officer
CFO: John A. Grigson, Senior Vice President and Chief Financial Officer
CMO: Scott Robins, M.D., Chief Medical Officer
CIO: Jim Reid, Vice President and Chief Information Officer
CHR: Rodney Cates, Senior Vice President Human Resources
Web address: www.covenanthealth.org
**Control:** Other not–for–profit (including NFP Corporation) **Service:** General Medical and Surgical

**Staffed Beds:** 607 **Admissions:** 28393 **Census:** 375 **Outpatient Visits:** 345987 **Births:** 2685 **Total Expense ($000):** 460901 **Payroll Expense ($000):** 137937 **Personnel:** 3131

**COVENANT SPECIALTY HOSPITAL (452102)**, 3815 20th Street, Zip 79410; tel. 806/725–9200 **A**10 **F**1 3 29 30 31 60 63 68 75 77 78 79 87 118 129 142 147 **S** Covenant Health System, Lubbock, TX
Primary Contact: Walt Cathey, Administrator
Web address: www.covenanthealth.org/view/Facilities/Specialty_Hospital
**Control:** Partnership, Investor–owned, for–profit **Service:** Long–Term Acute Care hospital

**Staffed Beds:** 56 **Admissions:** 512 **Census:** 36 **Outpatient Visits:** 0 **Births:** 0 **Personnel:** 124

☐ **GRACE MEDICAL CENTER (450162)**, 2412 50th Street, Zip 79412–2494; tel. 806/788–4100, (Nonreporting) **A**1 3 5 9 10
Primary Contact: Charley O. Trimble, Chief Executive Officer
CMO: Howard Beck, M.D., Chief of Staff
CIO: Jason Derouen, Director Management Information Systems
CHR: Sally Charles, Coordinator Human Resources
Web address: www.gracehealthsystem.com
**Control:** Partnership, Investor–owned, for–profit **Service:** General Medical and Surgical

**Staffed Beds:** 77

☐ **LLANO SPECIALTY HOSPITAL OF LUBBOCK (452050)**, 1409 9th Street, Zip 79401–2601; tel. 806/767–9133 **A**1 9 10 **F**1 12 29 65 75 91 129 147 **S** Fundamental Long Term Care Holdings, LLC, Sparks Glencoe, MD
Primary Contact: Dennis Fleenor, R.N., Chief Executive Officer
CFO: Robert Stanley, Chief Financial Officer
CMO: Enrique Rodriguez, M.D., Medical Director
CHR: Jerrie Yoakum, Director Human Resources
CNO: Charalene Ruble, Chief Nursing Officer
Web address: www.fundltc.com/Healthcare%20Facility%20Locator/facility_page.aspx?locationID=190
**Control:** Corporation, Investor–owned, for–profit **Service:** Long–Term Acute Care hospital

**Staffed Beds:** 30 **Admissions:** 72 **Census:** 5 **Outpatient Visits:** 0 **Births:** 0 **Total Expense ($000):** 3525 **Payroll Expense ($000):** 1481 **Personnel:** 30

**LUBBOCK HEART HOSPITAL (450876)**, 4810 North Loop 289, Zip 79416; tel. 806/687–7777 **A**3 5 9 10 **F**3 17 18 20 22 24 26 29 34 40 45 57 58 59 81 83 107 108 114 118 128 134 145 147
Primary Contact: Roy C. Vinson, Chief Executive Officer
Web address: www.lubbockhearthospital.com
**Control:** Partnership, Investor–owned, for–profit **Service:** General Medical and Surgical

**Staffed Beds:** 62 **Admissions:** 3687 **Census:** 37 **Outpatient Visits:** 11660 **Births:** 0 **Total Expense ($000):** 50447 **Payroll Expense ($000):** 16744 **Personnel:** 303

☐ **SUNRISE CANYON HOSPITAL (454093)**, 1602 10th Street, Zip 79408–2828, Mailing Address: P.O. Box 2828, Zip 79408–2828; tel. 806/740–1407, (Data for 344 days) **A**1 10 **F**86 98 101 103 129 142
Primary Contact: Leonard Valderaz, Administrator
CFO: Beth Lawson, Chief Financial Officer and Director Governmental Affairs
CMO: Marsha Spalding, M.D., Medical Director
CIO: Tim Carroll, Chief Information Officer
CHR: Barbara McCann, Director Human Resources
Web address: www.lrl.mhmr.state.tx.us
**Control:** Other not–for–profit (including NFP Corporation) **Service:** Psychiatric

**Staffed Beds:** 30 **Admissions:** 502 **Census:** 19 **Outpatient Visits:** 0 **Births:** 0 **Total Expense ($000):** 6069 **Payroll Expense ($000):** 2049 **Personnel:** 44

**TEXAS SPECIALTY HOSPITAL AT LUBBOCK (452116)**, 4302 Princeton Street, Zip 79415–1304; tel. 806/723–8700 **A**9 10 **F**1 3 12 29 60 92 147 **S** Fundamental Long Term Care Holdings, LLC, Sparks Glencoe, MD
Primary Contact: Deanna Graves, Chief Executive Officer
CFO: Robert Stanley, Chief Financial Officer
CNO: Jennifer Reeves, Chief Nursing Officer
**Control:** Corporation, Investor–owned, for–profit **Service:** Long–Term Acute Care hospital

**Staffed Beds:** 37 **Admissions:** 343 **Census:** 23 **Outpatient Visits:** 0 **Births:** 0 **Total Expense ($000):** 8390 **Payroll Expense ($000):** 3293 **Personnel:** 81

**TRUSTPOINT HOSPITAL (670050)**, 4302 Princeton Street, Zip 79415–1304; tel. 806/749–2222 **A**3 5 9 10 **F**3 29 34 35 40 56 57 64 68 74 75 77 79 85 86 87 90 91 93 94 96 98 103 129 134 147
Primary Contact: Craig Bragg, Chief Executive Officer
Web address: www.trustpointhospital.com/
**Control:** Partnership, Investor–owned, for–profit **Service:** Rehabilitation

**Staffed Beds:** 71 **Admissions:** 1413 **Census:** 46 **Outpatient Visits:** 10 **Births:** 0 **Total Expense ($000):** 16299 **Payroll Expense ($000):** 6772 **Personnel:** 190

✠ **UNIVERSITY MEDICAL CENTER (450686)**, 602 Indiana Avenue, Zip 79415–3364, Mailing Address: P.O. Box 5980, Zip 79408–5980; tel. 806/775–8200 **A**1 2 3 5 8 9 10 **F**3 7 8 11 12 13 15 16 17 18 19 20 21 22 23 24 26 27 28 29 30 35 40 43 45 46 47 48 49 50 51 54 57 58 59 60 62 64 65 66 68 70 72 74 75 76 77 78 79 81 84 85 86 87 88 89 93 94 96 97 107 108 109 110 111 113 114 115 116 117 118 119 120 121 122 123 129 130 131 135 140 143 145 146 147
Primary Contact: David G. Allison, President and Chief Executive Officer
COO: Mark Funderburk, Executive Vice President and Administrator
CFO: Jeff Dane, Executive Vice President and Chief Financial Officer
CIO: Bill Eubanks, Senior Vice President and Chief Information Officer
CHR: Adrienne Cozart, Vice President Human Resources
Web address: www.umchealthsystem.com
**Control:** Hospital district or authority, Government, nonfederal **Service:** General Medical and Surgical

**Staffed Beds:** 401 **Admissions:** 24568 **Census:** 296 **Outpatient Visits:** 246854 **Births:** 2343 **Total Expense ($000):** 157426 **Payroll Expense ($000):** 143133 **Personnel:** 2524

**LUFKIN—Angelina County**

✠ **MEMORIAL MEDICAL CENTER – LUFKIN (450211)**, 1201 West Frank Avenue, Zip 75904–3357, Mailing Address: P.O. Box 1447, Zip 75902–1447; tel. 936/634–8111 **A**1 2 9 10 19 **F**3 11 12 13 14 15 17 18 20 21 22 23 24 26 28 29 30 31 34 35 37 38 40 44 45 47 48 49 50 51 56 57 59 60 61 62 63 64 68 70 71 73 74 75 76 77 78 79 81 82 83 84 85 86 87 90 91 92 93 97 100 101 102 107 108 110 111 112 113 114 115 116 118 120 125 128 129 131 134 142 143 145 146 147 **P**7 **S** Memorial Health System of East Texas, Lufkin, TX
Primary Contact: Gary N. Looper, President and Chief Executive Officer
CFO: Kristi Gay, Chief Financial Officer
CHR: Tanya Tyler, Vice President Human Resources
Web address: www.memorialhealth.org
**Control:** Other not–for–profit (including NFP Corporation) **Service:** General Medical and Surgical

**Staffed Beds:** 217 **Admissions:** 7848 **Census:** 103 **Outpatient Visits:** 140281 **Births:** 627 **Total Expense ($000):** 130607 **Payroll Expense ($000):** 37917 **Personnel:** 811

**MEMORIAL SPECIALTY HOSPITAL (452031)**, 1201 West Frank Avenue, Zip 75904; tel. 936/639–7975 **A**9 10 **F**1 3 29 31 50 61 68 74 75 85 86 129 144 **S** Memorial Health System of East Texas, Lufkin, TX
Primary Contact: Leslie Leach, Administrator
CFO: Kristi Gay, Chief Financial Officer
CMO: David Todd, M.D., President Medical Staff
CHR: Tanya Tyler, Vice President Human Resources
Web address: www.memorialhealth.org
**Control:** Other not–for–profit (including NFP Corporation) **Service:** Long–Term Acute Care hospital

**Staffed Beds:** 26 **Admissions:** 300 **Census:** 22 **Outpatient Visits:** 0 **Births:** 0 **Total Expense ($000):** 9021 **Payroll Expense ($000):** 4803 **Personnel:** 69

✠ **WOODLAND HEIGHTS MEDICAL CENTER (450484)**, 505 South John Redditt Drive, Zip 75904–3157, Mailing Address: P.O. Box 150610, Zip 75915–0610; tel. 936/634–8311, (Total facility includes 15 beds in nursing home–type unit) **A**1 9 10 19 **F**3 8 11 12 13 15 17 18 20 22 24 26 28 29 30 34 35 40 41 46 49 50 51 53 57 59 64 68 70 74 75 76 77 78 79 81 82 85 86 87 93 102 107 108 111 113 114 117 118 127 128 129 130 145 146 147 **S** Community Health Systems, Inc., Franklin, TN
Primary Contact: Casey Robertson, Chief Executive Officer
CFO: Sam Minkowitz, Chief Financial Officer
CMO: Jansen Todd, D.O., Chief of Staff
CIO: Virginia DeLardonis, Director Information Systems
CHR: Sally McKinney, Director Human Resources
Web address: www.woodlandheights.net
**Control:** Partnership, Investor–owned, for–profit **Service:** General Medical and Surgical

**Staffed Beds:** 115 **Admissions:** 4904 **Census:** 61 **Outpatient Visits:** 41881 **Births:** 740 **Total Expense ($000):** 62851 **Payroll Expense ($000):** 27640 **Personnel:** 514

**LULING—Caldwell County**

✠ **SETON EDGAR B. DAVIS HOSPITAL (451371)**, 130 Hays Street, Zip 78648–3207; tel. 830/875–7000 **A**1 9 10 18 **F**3 11 15 18 29 30 35 40 43 44 45 50 56 68 71 75 79 81 84 85 87 93 97 103 107 111 113 118 126 129 132 134 142 145 **P**3 8 **S** Ascension Health, Saint Louis, MO
Primary Contact: Neal Kelley, Administrator
COO: Neal Kelley, Administrator
CFO: Douglas D. Waite, Chief Financial Officer
CMO: Martin E. Weiner, M.D., Chief of Staff
CIO: Gerry Lewis, Chief Information Officer
CHR: Cheryl Williams, Director Human Resources
Web address: www.seton.net
**Control:** Church–operated, Nongovernment, not–for profit **Service:** General Medical and Surgical

**Staffed Beds:** 25 **Admissions:** 1243 **Census:** 14 **Outpatient Visits:** 67103 **Births:** 0 **Total Expense ($000):** 28090 **Payroll Expense ($000):** 13332 **Personnel:** 278

☐ **WARM SPRINGS SPECIALTY HOSPITAL (452062)**, 200 Memorial Drive, Zip 78648; tel. 830/875–8400 **A**1 9 10 **F**1 3 29 53 64 93 96 129 132 **S** Post Acute Medical, LLC, Camp Hill, PA
Primary Contact: Jason Carter, Chief Executive Officer
CFO: James Asberry, Chief Financial Officer
Web address: www.warmsprings.org
**Control:** Partnership, Investor–owned, for–profit **Service:** Long–Term Acute Care hospital

**Staffed Beds:** 34 **Admissions:** 420 **Census:** 29 **Outpatient Visits:** 9815 **Births:** 0 **Total Expense ($000):** 15006 **Payroll Expense ($000):** 5869 **Personnel:** 143

### MADISONVILLE—Madison County

⊠ **MADISON ST. JOSEPH HEALTH CENTER (451316)**, 100 West Cross Street, Zip 77864–0698, Mailing Address: Box 698, Zip 77864–0698; tel. 936/348–2631 **A**1 9 10 18 **F**3 11 15 30 40 43 57 59 64 68 75 82 93 107 108 110 118 129 132 134 145 147 **P**5 **S** Sylvania Franciscan Health, Toledo, OH
Primary Contact: Reed Edmundson, Administrator
COO: Reed Edmundson, Administrator
CFO: Bruce Thacker, Controller
CMO: Grover Hubley, M.D., President Medical Staff
CIO: Jana Ard, R.N., Director Clinical Resource Management
CHR: Doni Roper, Director Human Resources
Web address: www.st–joseph.org
**Control:** Church–operated, Nongovernment, not–for profit **Service:** General Medical and Surgical

**Staffed Beds:** 25 **Admissions:** 522 **Census:** 10 **Outpatient Visits:** 20252 **Births:** 0 **Total Expense ($000):** 9648 **Payroll Expense ($000):** 4967 **Personnel:** 92

### MANSFIELD—Tarrant County

⊠ **KINDRED HOSPITAL–MANSFIELD (452019)**, 1802 Highway 157 North, Zip 76063–9555; tel. 817/473–6101 **A**1 9 10 **F**3 12 29 30 40 45 46 60 70 75 79 81 82 85 107 108 129 131 147 **S** Kindred Healthcare, Louisville, KY
Primary Contact: Susan Schaetti, Administrator
CFO: Judy Baker, Chief Financial Officer
Web address: www.kindredmansfield.com
**Control:** Corporation, Investor–owned, for–profit **Service:** General Medical and Surgical

**Staffed Beds:** 55 **Admissions:** 346 **Census:** 25 **Outpatient Visits:** 529 **Births:** 0 **Total Expense ($000):** 12335 **Payroll Expense ($000):** 5907 **Personnel:** 108

⊠ **METHODIST MANSFIELD MEDICAL CENTER (670023)**, 2700 East Broad Street, Zip 76063–5899; tel. 682/622–2000 **A**1 9 10 **F**3 11 13 15 18 20 22 29 30 31 34 35 37 40 46 48 49 50 58 59 60 68 70 71 74 76 78 79 81 82 84 85 87 93 97 107 108 110 111 114 117 118 129 131 145 **P**1 6 7 **S** Methodist Health System, Dallas, TX
Primary Contact: John E. Phillips, FACHE, President and Chief Executive Officer
CFO: Michael J. Schaefer, Executive Vice President and Chief Financial Officer
CMO: Adam L. Myers, M.D., Chief Medical Officer
CIO: Pamela McNutt, Senior Vice President and Chief Information Officer
CHR: Judy K. Laister, Director, Human Resources
Web address: www.methodisthealthsystem.org
**Control:** Other not–for–profit (including NFP Corporation) **Service:** General Medical and Surgical

**Staffed Beds:** 130 **Admissions:** 6829 **Census:** 78 **Outpatient Visits:** 62683 **Births:** 1535 **Total Expense ($000):** 95121 **Payroll Expense ($000):** 42000 **Personnel:** 624

### MARLIN—Falls County

★ **FALLS COMMUNITY HOSPITAL AND CLINIC (450348)**, 322 Coleman Street, Zip 76661–2358, Mailing Address: P.O. Box 60, Zip 76661–0060; tel. 254/803–3561 **A**9 10 20 **F**3 11 32 33 34 35 36 40 43 45 53 56 57 59 64 65 66 68 75 82 87 91 93 97 99 103 104 107 113 126 128 130 132 134 145 147
Primary Contact: Willis L. Reese, Administrator
COO: Julie Sharp, Chief Operations Officer
CFO: Willis L. Reese, Administrator
CMO: James Scott Crockett, M.D., Chief of Staff
CIO: Julie Sharp, Chief Operations Officer
CHR: Peggy Polster, Manager Personnel and Administrative Assistant
Web address: www.fallshospital.com
**Control:** Other not–for–profit (including NFP Corporation) **Service:** General Medical and Surgical

**Staffed Beds:** 32 **Admissions:** 740 **Census:** 7 **Outpatient Visits:** 67046 **Births:** 0 **Total Expense ($000):** 12504 **Payroll Expense ($000):** 5798 **Personnel:** 142

### MARSHALL—Harrison County

☐ **GOOD SHEPHERD MEDICAL CENTER–MARSHALL (450032)**, 811 South Washington Avenue, Zip 75670–5336, Mailing Address: P.O. Box 1599, Zip 75671–1599; tel. 903/927–6000 **A**1 9 10 **F**3 11 13 15 18 28 29 30 34 35 40 43 49 50 53 54 57 59 60 64 65 68 70 75 77 79 80 81 86 87 89 90 93 97 102 103 107 108 110 111 114 118 126 128 129 130 131 144 145 146 147 **P**7 8 **S** Good Shepherd Health System, Longview, TX
Primary Contact: Russell J. Collier, FACHE, President and Chief Executive Officer
COO: Ray Delk, FACHE, Vice President Operations
CFO: Patricia Keel, Chief Financial Officer
CMO: John McDonald, D.O., President and Chief of Medical Staff
CIO: Walter Grimes, Director Information Technology
CHR: Ginger Garrett, Regional Director Human Resources
CNO: Paula Brandon, MSN, Vice President Patient Care Services
Web address: www.gsmcmarshall.org
**Control:** Other not–for–profit (including NFP Corporation) **Service:** General Medical and Surgical

**Staffed Beds:** 142 **Admissions:** 4024 **Census:** 41 **Outpatient Visits:** 86380 **Births:** 578 **Total Expense ($000):** 56188 **Payroll Expense ($000):** 18365 **Personnel:** 397

### MCALLEN—Hidalgo County

**LIFECARE HOSPITALS OF SOUTH TEXAS–MCALLEN** See Lifecare Hospitals of South Texas–North McAllen

⊠ **LIFECARE HOSPITALS OF SOUTH TEXAS–NORTH MCALLEN (452063)**, 5101 North Jackson, Zip 78504; tel. 956/926–7000, (Includes LIFECARE HOSPITALS OF SOUTH TEXAS–MCALLEN, 2001 South M Street, Zip 78503; tel. 956/688–4300; Michelle Lozano, Adminstrator) **A**1 9 10 **F**1 3 29 57 75 77 84 85 87 147 **S** LifeCare Management Services, Plano, TX
Primary Contact: Michelle Lozano, Administrator
Web address: www.lifecare–hospitals.com
**Control:** Corporation, Investor–owned, for–profit **Service:** Long–Term Acute Care hospital

**Staffed Beds:** 94 **Admissions:** 821 **Census:** 62 **Outpatient Visits:** 0 **Births:** 0 **Total Expense ($000):** 27043 **Payroll Expense ($000):** 11259 **Personnel:** 197

⊠ **RIO GRANDE REGIONAL HOSPITAL (450711)**, 101 East Ridge Road, Zip 78503–1299; tel. 956/632–6000 **A**1 9 10 **F**3 8 11 12 13 15 18 19 20 21 22 23 24 25 26 29 30 31 34 35 39 40 41 43 45 46 49 50 51 54 56 57 59 60 64 68 70 71 72 73 74 75 76 78 79 81 85 87 88 89 93 107 108 110 111 113 118 129 131 145 146 147 **P**7 **S** HCA, Nashville, TN
Primary Contact: Gregory A. Seiler, Chief Executive Officer
COO: David Elgarico, Chief Operating Officer
CFO: William Saller, Chief Financial Officer
CIO: Carlos Leal, Chief Information Officer
CHR: Marjorie Whittemore, Director Human Resources
Web address: www.riohealth.com
**Control:** Partnership, Investor–owned, for–profit **Service:** General Medical and Surgical

**Staffed Beds:** 320 **Admissions:** 15960 **Census:** 184 **Outpatient Visits:** 78123 **Births:** 2932 **Total Expense ($000):** 122167 **Payroll Expense ($000):** 59100 **Personnel:** 887

**SOLARA HOSPITAL MCALLEN (452095)**, 301 West Expressway 83, Zip 78503–3045; tel. 956/632–4880 **A**9 10 **F**1 3 29 56 74 75 82 87 91 147 **P**5 **S** Solara Healthcare, Dallas, TX
Primary Contact: Jack Boggess, Chief Executive Officer
Web address: www.solarahc.com/shcmc.html
**Control:** Corporation, Investor–owned, for–profit **Service:** Long–Term Acute Care hospital

**Staffed Beds:** 78 **Admissions:** 735 **Census:** 54 **Outpatient Visits:** 0 **Births:** 0 **Total Expense ($000):** 20690 **Payroll Expense ($000):** 8300 **Personnel:** 159

**TX**

**Hospital, Medicare Provider Number, Address, Telephone, Approval, Facility, and Physician Codes, Health Care System**

★ American Hospital Association (AHA) membership
☐ The Joint Commission accreditation
◇ DNV Healthcare Inc. accreditation
○ American Osteopathic Association (AOA) accreditation
△ Commission on Accreditation of Rehabilitation Facilities (CARF) accreditation

© 2012 AHA Guide *Many Facility Codes have changed. Please refer to the AHA Guide Code Chart.* Hospitals **A615**

## MCCAMEY—Upton County

★ **MCCAMEY COUNTY HOSPITAL DISTRICT (451309)**, Highway 305 South, Zip 79752, Mailing Address: P.O. Box 1200, Zip 79752–1200; tel. 432/652–8626, (Total facility includes 30 beds in nursing home–type unit) **A**9 10 18 **F**3 40 53 59 64 65 66 93 126 127 132
Primary Contact: Jaime Ramirez, Chief Executive Officer
COO: Tana Robertson, Chief Operating Officer
CFO: Judith Gulihur, Director Human Resources and Chief Financial Officer
CMO: Ramon Domingo, M.D., Chief of Staff
CIO: Larry Rollins, Supervisor Information Technology
CHR: Judith Gulihur, Director Human Resources and Chief Financial Officer
Web address: www.mccameyhospital.org
**Control:** Hospital district or authority, Government, nonfederal **Service:** General Medical and Surgical

**Staffed Beds:** 44 **Admissions:** 74 **Census:** 26 **Outpatient Visits:** 8126 **Births:** 0 **Total Expense ($000):** 6877 **Payroll Expense ($000):** 3846 **Personnel:** 64

## MCKINNEY—Collin County

⌧ **MEDICAL CENTER OF MCKINNEY (450403)**, 4500 Medical Center Drive, Zip 75069–3499; tel. 972/547–8000, (Includes WYSONG CAMPUS, 130 South Central Expressway, Zip 75070; tel. 972/548–5300) **A**1 9 10 **F**3 4 5 11 13 15 18 20 22 24 28 29 30 31 34 40 45 56 57 59 60 64 68 70 74 75 76 77 78 79 81 82 85 87 90 93 96 97 98 102 103 107 108 111 113 114 118 120 128 129 130 131 145 146 147 **S** HCA, Nashville, TN
Primary Contact: Ernest C. Lynch, III, Chief Executive Officer
COO: LaSharndra Barbarin, Chief Operating Officer
CFO: Dwayne Ray, Chief Financial Officer
CIO: Kevin Fletcher, Director Information Systems
CHR: Senta Miles, Director Human Resources
Web address: www.medicalcenterofmckinney.com
**Control:** Partnership, Investor–owned, for–profit **Service:** General Medical and Surgical

**Staffed Beds:** 224 **Admissions:** 11983 **Census:** 163 **Outpatient Visits:** 79524 **Births:** 1088 **Total Expense ($000):** 122904 **Payroll Expense ($000):** 51878 **Personnel:** 826

☐ **METHODIST MCKINNEY HOSPITAL (670069)**, 8000 West Eldorado Parkway, Zip 75070–5940; tel. 972/569–2700 **A**1 9 10 **F**3 15 29 34 40 45 51 70 75 79 81 82 85 107 111 118 129 **S** Methodist Health System, Dallas, TX
Primary Contact: Joseph Minissale, Interim President
CFO: Rebecca Chaisson, Interim Chief Financial Officer
CHR: Rory Money, Manager Human Resources
Web address: www.methodistmckinneyhospital.com
**Control:** Partnership, Investor–owned, for–profit **Service:** General Medical and Surgical

**Staffed Beds:** 23 **Admissions:** 489 **Census:** 3 **Outpatient Visits:** 7184 **Births:** 0 **Total Expense ($000):** 20135 **Payroll Expense ($000):** 5464 **Personnel:** 83

**THE HOSPITAL AT CRAIG RANCH (670063)**, 6045 Alma Road, Zip 75070–2188; tel. 469/854–8000 **A**9 10 21 **F**3 8 29 40 51 64 68 70 75 79 81 82 85 89 107 113 118
Primary Contact: Glenda Mendoza, Acting Chief Executive Officer
Web address: www.hospitalcraigranch.com
**Control:** Corporation, Investor–owned, for–profit **Service:** General Medical and Surgical

**Staffed Beds:** 24 **Admissions:** 302 **Census:** 2 **Outpatient Visits:** 3312 **Births:** 0 **Total Expense ($000):** 22671 **Payroll Expense ($000):** 5948 **Personnel:** 97

## MESQUITE—Dallas County

☐ **DALLAS REGIONAL MEDICAL CENTER (450688)**, 1011 North Galloway Avenue, Zip 75149–2433; tel. 214/320–7000 **A**1 9 10 **F**3 12 15 18 20 22 24 26 29 30 34 35 40 43 46 47 49 50 54 56 57 59 64 68 70 74 75 79 80 81 85 86 87 97 107 108 110 111 113 118 125 129 130 134 145 146 **S** Health Management Associates, Naples, FL
Primary Contact: Matthew T. Caldwell, Chief Executive Officer
CFO: Gene Winters, Chief Financial Officer
CMO: Srinivas Gunukula, M.D., Chief of Staff
CNO: Tina Pollock, R.N., Chief Nursing Officer
Web address: www.dallasregionalmedicalcenter.com
**Control:** Corporation, Investor–owned, for–profit **Service:** General Medical and Surgical

**Staffed Beds:** 85 **Admissions:** 5103 **Census:** 62 **Outpatient Visits:** 63640 **Births:** 6 **Total Expense ($000):** 64635 **Payroll Expense ($000):** 25872 **Personnel:** 417

**MESQUITE REHABILITATION HOSPITAL (673045)**, 1023 North Belt Line Road, Zip 75149–1788; tel. 972/216–2400 **F**3 28 29 30 34 35 57 59 64 82 90 91 93 96 147 **S** Ernest Health, Inc., Albuquerque, NM
Primary Contact: Brenda M. Antwine, Chief Executive Officer
Web address: www.mesquiterehab.ernesthealth.com
**Control:** Corporation, Investor–owned, for–profit **Service:** Rehabilitation

**Staffed Beds:** 20 **Admissions:** 408 **Census:** 16 **Outpatient Visits:** 470 **Births:** 0 **Total Expense ($000):** 5625 **Payroll Expense ($000):** 3175 **Personnel:** 51

☐ **MESQUITE SPECIALTY HOSPITAL (452100)**, 1024 North Galloway Avenue, Zip 75149–2434; tel. 972/216–2300 **A**1 9 10 **F**1 3 29 64 74 75 77 79 85 87 93 129 134 147 **S** Ernest Health, Inc., Albuquerque, NM
Primary Contact: Brenda M. Antwine, Chief Executive Officer
Web address: www.msh.ernesthealth.com
**Control:** Partnership, Investor–owned, for–profit **Service:** Long–Term Acute Care hospital

**Staffed Beds:** 40 **Admissions:** 441 **Census:** 31 **Outpatient Visits:** 1876 **Births:** 0 **Total Expense ($000):** 14547 **Payroll Expense ($000):** 6845 **Personnel:** 122

## MEXIA—Limestone County

⌧ **PARKVIEW REGIONAL HOSPITAL (450400)**, 600 South Bonham, Zip 76667–3608; tel. 254/562–0408 **A**1 9 10 20 **F**3 11 15 29 30 34 35 40 43 45 51 53 56 57 59 64 65 70 75 77 78 79 81 85 86 87 93 97 98 103 107 108 110 111 113 118 126 129 131 132 145 **P**5 6 **S** LifePoint Hospitals, Inc., Brentwood, TN
Primary Contact: Kevin Zachary, Chief Executive Officer
CFO: Michael Herr, Chief Financial Officer
CMO: Greg Newman, M.D., Chief of Staff
Web address: www.parkviewregional.com
**Control:** Partnership, Investor–owned, for–profit **Service:** General Medical and Surgical

**Staffed Beds:** 58 **Admissions:** 1179 **Census:** 14 **Outpatient Visits:** 21561 **Births:** 0 **Total Expense ($000):** 16880 **Payroll Expense ($000):** 8197 **Personnel:** 183

## MIDLAND—Midland County

**ALLEGIANCE SPECIALTY HOSPITAL PERMIAN BASIN**, 207 Tradewinds Boulevard, Zip 79706–2807; tel. 432/699–3215 **A**21 **F**34 40 56 57 64 68 98 101 103 104 129 131 134 **S** Allegiance Health Management, Shreveport, LA
Primary Contact: Cheryl Rayl, Chief Executive Officer
Web address: www.ahmgt.com
**Control:** Corporation, Investor–owned, for–profit **Service:** Psychiatric

**Staffed Beds:** 48 **Admissions:** 687 **Census:** 18 **Outpatient Visits:** 11134 **Births:** 0 **Total Expense ($000):** 7620 **Payroll Expense ($000):** 3592 **Personnel:** 90

☐ **BCA PERMIAN BASIN (454110)**, 3300 South FM 1788, Zip 79706–2601; tel. 432/561–5915 **A**1 9 10 **F**29 35 98 99 100 101 103 105 129 131 **P**6 **S** Behavioral Centers of America, Nashville, TN
Primary Contact: John Flanagan, Chief Executive Officer
Web address: www.bcapermianbasin.com/
**Control:** Corporation, Investor–owned, for–profit **Service:** Psychiatric

**Staffed Beds:** 64 **Admissions:** 1890 **Census:** 33 **Outpatient Visits:** 1460 **Births:** 0 **Total Expense ($000):** 8498 **Payroll Expense ($000):** 3744 **Personnel:** 86

⌧ **HEALTHSOUTH REHABILITATION HOSPITAL MIDLAND–ODESSA (453057)**, 1800 Heritage Boulevard, Zip 79707–9750; tel. 432/520–1600 **A**1 5 9 10 **F**3 29 57 59 62 64 74 75 90 93 129 142 147 **S** HEALTHSOUTH Corporation, Birmingham, AL
Primary Contact: Christopher Wortham, Chief Executive Officer
CFO: Nichole Dykes, Chief Financial Officer and Controller
CMO: Mark A. Fredrickson, M.D., Medical Director
CHR: Tina Parker, Director Human Resources
Web address: www.healthsouthmidland.com
**Control:** Corporation, Investor–owned, for–profit **Service:** Rehabilitation

**Staffed Beds:** 60 **Admissions:** 1159 **Census:** 41 **Outpatient Visits:** 6333 **Births:** 0 **Total Expense ($000):** 12520 **Payroll Expense ($000):** 8068 **Personnel:** 148

**TX**

★ **MIDLAND MEMORIAL HOSPITAL (450133)**, 2200 West Illinois Avenue, Zip 79701–6499; tel. 432/685–1111, (Includes MIDLAND MEMORIAL HOSPITAL–WEST CAMPUS, 4214 Andrews Highway, Zip 79703; tel. 432/522–3270) **A**2 3 5 9 10 21 **F**3 8 11 13 15 17 18 20 22 24 28 29 30 31 32 34 35 40 43 45 49 50 56 57 59 61 64 68 70 73 74 75 76 77 78 79 80 81 82 85 86 87 88 89 93 97 107 108 111 113 114 115 116 117 118 123 125 128 129 130 131 134 144 145 146 147 **P**8
Primary Contact: Russell Meyers, President and Chief Executive Officer
CFO: Stephen Bowerman, Chief Financial Officer
CIO: David Whiles, Director Health Information Systems
CHR: Cori Hyatt, Director Human Resources
Web address: www.midland–memorial.com
**Control:** Hospital district or authority, Government, nonfederal **Service:** General Medical and Surgical

**Staffed Beds:** 225 **Admissions:** 10977 **Census:** 128 **Outpatient Visits:** 151462 **Births:** 1938 **Total Expense ($000):** 191843 **Payroll Expense ($000):** 79325 **Personnel:** 1283

**MIDLAND MEMORIAL HOSPITAL (450133)**, 4214 Andrews Highway, Zip 79703–4861; tel. 432/685–1584, (Nonreporting) **A**9 10
Primary Contact: Russell Meyers, President and Chief Executive Officer
CFO: Lawrence A. Sanz, Senior Vice President Finance and Chief Financial Officer
CIO: David Whiles, Director Health Information Systems
CHR: Cori Hyatt, Director Human Resources
Web address: www.midland–memorial.com
**Control:** Corporation, Investor–owned, for–profit **Service:** General Medical and Surgical

**Staffed Beds:** 86

⊞ **SELECT SPECIALTY HOSPITAL–MIDLAND (452084)**, 4214 Andrews Highway, Suite 320, Zip 79703; tel. 432/522–3364 **A**1 9 10 **F**1 3 28 29 91 147 **S** Select Medical Corporation, Mechanicsburg, PA
Primary Contact: Connie K. Siffring, Chief Executive Officer
Web address: www.selectmedicalcorp.com
**Control:** Corporation, Investor–owned, for–profit **Service:** Long–Term Acute Care hospital

**Staffed Beds:** 29 **Admissions:** 275 **Census:** 21 **Outpatient Visits:** 0 **Births:** 0 **Total Expense ($000):** 8382 **Payroll Expense ($000):** 3758 **Personnel:** 69

**MINERAL WELLS—Palo Pinto County**

⊞ **PALO PINTO GENERAL HOSPITAL (450565)**, 400 S.W. 25th Avenue, Zip 76067–9685; tel. 940/328–6403 **A**1 9 10 **F**11 13 15 17 18 28 29 32 34 40 43 46 51 53 54 57 59 62 63 64 65 66 68 69 71 74 75 76 77 78 79 81 84 86 87 91 93 107 108 111 113 118 126 128 129 130 132 134 145 146 **P**1
Primary Contact: Harris W. Brooks, Administrator and Chief Executive Officer
CFO: Dee Waldow, Chief Financial Officer
CMO: Chuck Myers, M.D., Chief of Staff
CHR: Barbara Stagner, Director Human Resources
Web address: www.ppgh.com
**Control:** Hospital district or authority, Government, nonfederal **Service:** General Medical and Surgical

**Staffed Beds:** 42 **Admissions:** 2108 **Census:** 18 **Outpatient Visits:** 132262 **Births:** 355 **Total Expense ($000):** 34676 **Payroll Expense ($000):** 15152 **Personnel:** 300

**MISSION—Hidalgo County**

⊞ △ **MISSION REGIONAL MEDICAL CENTER (450176)**, 900 South Bryan Road, Zip 78572–6613; tel. 956/323–9000 **A**1 7 9 10 **F**3 11 12 13 15 18 20 22 29 30 31 34 35 40 43 45 46 49 50 51 57 59 60 64 65 66 68 70 72 74 75 76 77 79 81 85 87 89 90 93 96 107 108 110 111 114 118 129 131 145 146 147 **P**8
Primary Contact: Javier Iruegas, Chief Executive Officer
COO: Carlos Trevino, Chief Operating Officer
CFO: Timothy J. McVey, Chief Financial Officer
CMO: Philip J. Fracica, M.D., Chief Medical Officer
CIO: Sri Yarramsetti, Director Information Systems
CHR: Susan Willars, Vice President Human Resources
Web address: www.missionrmc.org
**Control:** Other not–for–profit (including NFP Corporation) **Service:** General Medical and Surgical

**Staffed Beds:** 245 **Admissions:** 11192 **Census:** 155 **Outpatient Visits:** 70368 **Births:** 2331 **Total Expense ($000):** 112782 **Payroll Expense ($000):** 55866 **Personnel:** 997

**MONAHANS—Ward County**

**WARD MEMORIAL HOSPITAL (451373)**, 406 South Gary Street, Zip 79756–4798, Mailing Address: P.O. Box 40, Zip 79756–0040; tel. 432/943–2511 **A**9 10 18 **F**3 11 40 42 43 45 64 65 66 81 82 89 93 107 113 118 126 130 132 147 **P**6
Primary Contact: Padraic White, Interim Administrator
CFO: Leticia Rodriguez, Controller
CHR: Donna Lemon, Director Human Resources
Web address: www.wardmemorial.org
**Control:** County–Government, nonfederal **Service:** General Medical and Surgical

**Staffed Beds:** 25 **Admissions:** 479 **Census:** 5 **Outpatient Visits:** 22759 **Births:** 0 **Total Expense ($000):** 6389 **Payroll Expense ($000):** 4493 **Personnel:** 97

**MORTON—Cochran County**

**COCHRAN MEMORIAL HOSPITAL (451366)**, 201 East Grant Street, Zip 79346–3444; tel. 806/266–5565 **A**9 10 18 **F**34 40 57 59 65 126 **P**5 6
Primary Contact: Larry Turney, Administrator
CHR: Niona Tunney, Director Human Resources
**Control:** Hospital district or authority, Government, nonfederal **Service:** General Medical and Surgical

**Staffed Beds:** 13 **Admissions:** 19 **Census:** 1 **Outpatient Visits:** 6074 **Births:** 0 **Total Expense ($000):** 3065 **Payroll Expense ($000):** 1556 **Personnel:** 45

**MOUNT PLEASANT—Titus County**

⊞ **TITUS REGIONAL MEDICAL CENTER (450080)**, 2001 North Jefferson Avenue, Zip 75455–2398; tel. 903/577–6000, (Total facility includes 7 beds in nursing home–type unit) **A**1 9 10 19 **F**3 7 11 12 13 15 18 19 20 24 26 28 29 30 34 35 39 40 43 45 47 50 51 53 54 56 57 58 59 64 68 70 73 74 75 76 78 79 81 82 85 89 90 93 97 98 103 108 110 111 113 114 116 117 118 120 122 126 127 128 129 131 134 146 147
Primary Contact: Ronald D. Davis, Chief Executive Officer
CFO: Duane Shafer, Chief Financial Officer
CMO: Milan Sekulic, M.D., Chief of Staff
CIO: David Stone, Director Information Systems
CHR: Tony Piazza, Director Human Resources
Web address: www.titusregional.com
**Control:** Hospital district or authority, Government, nonfederal **Service:** General Medical and Surgical

**Staffed Beds:** 92 **Admissions:** 4621 **Census:** 57 **Outpatient Visits:** 204072 **Births:** 1016 **Total Expense ($000):** 56011 **Payroll Expense ($000):** 27885 **Personnel:** 590

**MOUNT VERNON—Franklin County**

★ **EAST TEXAS MEDICAL CENTER–MOUNT VERNON (450373)**, 500 Highway 37 South, Zip 75457–3602, Mailing Address: P.O. Box 477, Zip 75457–0477; tel. 903/537–8000 **A**9 10 **F**3 29 34 35 40 43 45 47 50 57 63 64 65 68 75 79 81 82 84 85 86 87 97 102 107 108 113 118 126 **P**7 **S** East Texas Medical Center Regional Healthcare System, Tyler, TX
Primary Contact: David Bailey, Administrator
CFO: Margaret Haak–Muse, Chief Financial Officer and Assistant Administrator
CMO: Michael Walker, D.O., Chief of Staff
CHR: Kathy Shelton, Director Human Resources
Web address: www.etmc.org
**Control:** Other not–for–profit (including NFP Corporation) **Service:** General Medical and Surgical

**Staffed Beds:** 30 **Admissions:** 553 **Census:** 5 **Outpatient Visits:** 14481 **Births:** 0 **Total Expense ($000):** 5960 **Payroll Expense ($000):** 2368 **Personnel:** 54

**MUENSTER—Cooke County**

**MUENSTER MEMORIAL HOSPITAL (451335)**, 605 North Maple Street, Zip 76252–2424, Mailing Address: P.O. Box 370, Zip 76252–0370; tel. 940/759–2271 **A**9 10 18 **F**11 35 40 43 45 53 57 59 62 64 65 75 77 81 93 107 113 118 126 129 132 145 **P**8
Primary Contact: Michael Kent, Chief Executive Officer
CFO: Richard Teeter, Chief Financial Officer
CMO: J. Stephen Jones, M.D., Chief of Staff
CIO: Sheri Hutchins, Director Health Information Management
**Control:** Hospital district or authority, Government, nonfederal **Service:** General Medical and Surgical

**Staffed Beds:** 18 **Admissions:** 298 **Census:** 8 **Outpatient Visits:** 5228 **Births:** 0 **Total Expense ($000):** 7176 **Payroll Expense ($000):** 4892 **Personnel:** 107

**TX**

**Hospital, Medicare Provider Number, Address, Telephone, Approval, Facility, and Physician Codes, Health Care System**

★ American Hospital Association (AHA) membership
□ The Joint Commission accreditation          ◇ DNV Healthcare Inc. accreditation
○ American Osteopathic Association (AOA) accreditation
△ Commission on Accreditation of Rehabilitation Facilities (CARF) accreditation

## MULESHOE—Bailey County

★ **MULESHOE AREA MEDICAL CENTER (451372)**, 708 South First Street, Zip 79347; tel. 806/272–4524 **A**9 10 18 **F**3 8 11 29 34 35 40 43 45 50 59 64 65 68 69 75 77 81 93 107 113 118 126 129 132
Primary Contact: David Burke, Administrator and Chief Executive Officer
CMO: Bruce Purdy, M.D., Chief of Staff
CHR: Suzanne Nichols, Director Human Resources
Web address: www.mahdtx.org
**Control:** Hospital district or authority, Government, nonfederal **Service:** General Medical and Surgical

**Staffed Beds:** 25 **Admissions:** 718 **Census:** 5 **Outpatient Visits:** 31095 **Births:** 0 **Total Expense ($000):** 7501 **Payroll Expense ($000):** 3025 **Personnel:** 120

## NACOGDOCHES—Nacogdoches County

✠ **NACOGDOCHES MEDICAL CENTER (450656)**, 4920 N.E. Stallings, Zip 75965–1200, Mailing Address: P.O. Box 631604, Zip 75963–1604; tel. 936/569–9481 **A**1 9 10 19 **F**11 13 15 18 20 22 24 26 29 31 34 35 39 40 43 45 46 49 51 56 57 59 60 64 70 74 75 76 77 78 79 81 82 85 86 87 93 107 108 110 111 114 117 118 120 122 128 129 130 131 134 145 146 147 **S** TENET Healthcare Corporation, Dallas, TX
Primary Contact: Gary L. Stokes, Chief Executive Officer
COO: Collin LeMaistre, Chief Operating Officer
CFO: Rhonda Rogers, Chief Financial Officer
CMO: Dolamu Sokunbi, M.D., Chief of Staff
CIO: Teresa Simon, Director Information Systems
CHR: Teresa Farrell, Director Human Resources
Web address: www.nacmedicalcenter.com
**Control:** Partnership, Investor–owned, for–profit **Service:** General Medical and Surgical

**Staffed Beds:** 109 **Admissions:** 4330 **Census:** 45 **Outpatient Visits:** 47510 **Births:** 591 **Total Expense ($000):** 54317 **Payroll Expense ($000):** 19548 **Personnel:** 348

☐ **NACOGDOCHES MEMORIAL HOSPITAL (450508)**, 1204 North Mound Street, Zip 75961–4061; tel. 936/564–4611 **A**1 9 10 19 **F**3 7 11 13 15 18 20 22 24 26 28 29 30 31 34 35 40 43 46 47 49 50 57 59 61 64 68 70 74 76 77 78 79 80 81 85 86 89 90 93 96 107 108 110 111 113 117 118 125 128 129 131 145 146 147
Primary Contact: Tim Hayward, Administrator
CFO: Jane Ann Bridges, Chief Financial Officer
CNO: Beth Knight, Chief Nursing Officer
Web address: www.nacmem.org
**Control:** Hospital district or authority, Government, nonfederal **Service:** General Medical and Surgical

**Staffed Beds:** 136 **Admissions:** 6290 **Census:** 85 **Outpatient Visits:** 72930 **Births:** 848 **Total Expense ($000):** 92855 **Payroll Expense ($000):** 36886 **Personnel:** 810

## NASSAU BAY—Harris County

✠ **CHRISTUS ST. JOHN HOSPITAL (450709)**, 18300 St. John Drive, Zip 77058–6302; tel. 281/333–5503 **A**1 2 3 5 9 10 **F**3 11 13 15 18 20 22 24 26 28 29 30 34 35 40 44 45 49 51 53 54 57 59 60 62 63 64 65 66 68 69 70 71 73 74 75 76 77 78 79 81 82 83 84 85 86 87 93 107 108 110 111 113 114 118 129 130 131 145 146 147 **P**8 **S** CHRISTUS Health, Irving, TX
Primary Contact: Thomas Permetti, Regional Chief Operating Officer and Administrator
COO: Nancy Pittman, MS, Chief Operating Officer and Chief Nursing Executive
CFO: David Witt, Chief Financial Officer
CMO: Harold Gottlieb, M.D., Medical Director
CHR: Charles Foster, Region Vice President Human Resources
CNO: Nancy Pittman, MS, Chief Operating Officer and Chief Nursing Officer
Web address: www.christusstjohn.org
**Control:** Other not–for–profit (including NFP Corporation) **Service:** General Medical and Surgical

**Staffed Beds:** 121 **Admissions:** 6001 **Census:** 69 **Outpatient Visits:** 136409 **Births:** 611 **Total Expense ($000):** 94170 **Payroll Expense ($000):** 38359 **Personnel:** 614

## NAVASOTA—Grimes County

✠ **GRIMES ST. JOSEPH HEALTH CENTER (451322)**, 210 South Judson Street, Zip 77868–3704; tel. 936/825–6585 **A**1 9 10 18 **F**3 29 34 40 43 57 59 75 77 81 93 107 111 118 129 131 132 134 145 **S** Sylvania Franciscan Health, Toledo, OH
Primary Contact: Dia Copeland, Administrator
COO: Anthony D. Pfitzer, FACHE, Chief Executive Officer
CFO: Lisa McNair, CPA, Senior Vice President and Chief Financial Officer
CMO: Jamie Benton, M.D., Chief of Staff
CIO: John Phillips, Vice President Information System
CHR: Michael Costa, Director Human Resources
Web address: www.st–joseph.org
**Control:** Church–operated, Nongovernment, not–for profit **Service:** General Medical and Surgical

**Staffed Beds:** 18 **Admissions:** 537 **Census:** 9 **Outpatient Visits:** 18450 **Births:** 0 **Total Expense ($000):** 9000 **Payroll Expense ($000):** 4469 **Personnel:** 92

## NEDERLAND—Jefferson County

**PROMISE SPECIALTY HOSPITAL OF SOUTHEAST TEXAS (452083)**, 2600 Highway 365, Zip 77627–6237; tel. 409/726–8700, (Data for 335 days) **A**9 10 **F**1 3 29 30 35 40 70 75 129 147 **S** Promise Healthcare, Boca Raton, FL
Primary Contact: Gayla Quillin, Administrator
Web address: www.promise–southeasttexas.com
**Control:** Corporation, Investor–owned, for–profit **Service:** Long–Term Acute Care hospital

**Staffed Beds:** 36 **Admissions:** 254 **Census:** 22 **Outpatient Visits:** 0 **Births:** 0 **Total Expense ($000):** 11552 **Payroll Expense ($000):** 4683 **Personnel:** 87

## NEW BRAUNFELS—Comal County

✠ **CHRISTUS SANTA ROSA HOSPITAL – NEW BRAUNFELS (450059)**, 600 North Union Avenue, Zip 78130–4191; tel. 830/606–9111, (Nonreporting) **A**1 9 10 **S** CHRISTUS Health, Irving, TX
Primary Contact: Jim D. Wesson, Vice President and Administrator
CMO: James C. Martin, M.D., Vice President and Chief Medical Officer
CIO: Steve Martin, Chief Information Officer
Web address: www.christussantarosa.org
**Control:** Other not–for–profit (including NFP Corporation) **Service:** General Medical and Surgical

**Staffed Beds:** 112

**GULF STATES LONG TERM ACUTE CARE OF NEW BRAUNFELS** See Hill Country Specialty Hospital

☐ **HILL COUNTRY SPECIALTY HOSPITAL (452106)**, 1445 Hanz Drive, Zip 78130; tel. 830/627–7600 **A**1 9 10 **F**1 3 29 30 34 85 129 147
Primary Contact: Brenda Miles, Chief Executive Officer
Web address: www.hillcountryspecialty.com/
**Control:** Partnership, Investor–owned, for–profit **Service:** Long–Term Acute Care hospital

**Staffed Beds:** 40 **Admissions:** 313 **Census:** 20 **Outpatient Visits:** 0 **Births:** 0 **Total Expense ($000):** 11803 **Payroll Expense ($000):** 4412 **Personnel:** 71

**NEW BRAUNFELS REGIONAL REHABILITATION HOSPITAL (673049)**, 2041 Sundance Parkway, Zip 78130–2779; tel. 830/625–6700, (Nonreporting) **S** Ernest Health, Inc., Albuquerque, NM
Primary Contact: Jennifer Malatek, Chief Executive Officer
CFO: Robert Voss, Chief Financial Officer
CMO: Maria R. Lomba, Medical Director
CHR: Laura Granger, Director, Human Resources
CNO: Denise Benningfield–Crelia, Director, Nursing Operations
Web address: www.nbrrh.ernesthealth.com
**Control:** Corporation, Investor–owned, for–profit **Service:** Rehabilitation

**Staffed Beds:** 20

## NOCONA—Montague County

**NOCONA GENERAL HOSPITAL (450641)**, 100 Park Road, Zip 76255–3616; tel. 940/825–3235 **A**9 10 **F**7 11 15 28 29 30 34 35 40 43 50 53 57 59 62 64 75 81 82 86 87 93 97 107 108 113 118 129 132 145 147 **P**5
Primary Contact: Lance Meekins, Administrator
CFO: Lance Meekins, Administrator
CMO: Chance Dingler, M.D., Chief Medical Officer
CHR: Paula Monkres, Administrative Assistant and Director Human Resources
Web address: www.noconageneral.com/
**Control:** Hospital district or authority, Government, nonfederal **Service:** General Medical and Surgical

**Staffed Beds:** 25 **Admissions:** 727 **Census:** 8 **Outpatient Visits:** 15600 **Births:** 0 **Total Expense ($000):** 6198 **Payroll Expense ($000):** 3811 **Personnel:** 104

## NORTH RICHLAND HILLS—Tarrant County

✠ **NORTH HILLS HOSPITAL (450087)**, 4401 Booth Calloway Road, Zip 76180–7399; tel. 817/255–1000 **A**1 9 10 **F**3 8 12 13 15 17 18 20 22 24 28 29 30 31 34 37 40 42 45 49 53 56 57 59 64 70 74 75 76 77 78 79 81 85 86 87 93 107 108 110 111 114 117 118 129 131 134 145 146 147 **P**3 **S** HCA, Nashville, TN
Primary Contact: Randy Moresi, Chief Executive Officer
CFO: William Saller, Chief Financial Officer
CMO: Paul Kim, M.D., Chief of Staff
CIO: Ruben Castro, Associate Administrator and Facility Information Security Officer
CHR: Cynthia Dang, Vice President Human Resources
Web address: www.northhillshospital.com
**Control:** Partnership, Investor–owned, for–profit **Service:** General Medical and Surgical

**Staffed Beds:** 176 **Admissions:** 8303 **Census:** 92 **Outpatient Visits:** 79234 **Births:** 943 **Total Expense ($000):** 110384 **Payroll Expense ($000):** 42779 **Personnel:** 586

*Many Facility Codes have changed. Please refer to the AHA Guide Code Chart.* © 2012 AHA Guide

## ODESSA—Ector County

☐ **BASIN HEALTHCARE CENTER (670066)**, 900 East 4th Street, Zip 79761–5255; tel. 432/362–9900 **A**1 9 10 **F**3 8 29 39 40 45 81 82 98 107 111 113 118
Primary Contact: Keith Abbott, Chief Executive Officer
CFO: Carl Flanagan, CPA, Chief Financial Officer
CMO: Richard Bartlett, M.D., Chief Medical Officer
CIO: Carl Flanagan, CPA, Chief Financial Officer
CHR: Gail Knous, Chief Executive Officer and Chief Compliance Officer
**Control:** Corporation, Investor–owned, for–profit **Service:** General Medical and Surgical

**Staffed Beds:** 14 **Admissions:** 536 **Census:** 3 **Outpatient Visits:** 9823 **Births:** 0 **Total Expense ($000):** 9590 **Payroll Expense ($000):** 3418 **Personnel:** 87

⊠ **MEDICAL CENTER HEALTH SYSTEM (450132)**, 500 West Fourth Street, Zip 79761–5059, Mailing Address: P.O. Drawer 7239, Zip 79760–7239; tel. 432/640–4000 **A**1 2 3 5 8 9 10 **F**3 8 11 12 13 15 17 18 20 22 24 26 28 29 30 31 34 35 39 40 43 46 47 48 49 50 53 54 57 59 64 65 66 68 70 71 72 74 75 76 77 78 79 81 85 87 89 90 93 107 111 113 114 115 116 117 118 125 128 129 130 131 134 143 145 146 147 **P**6 8
Primary Contact: William W. Webster, FACHE, Chief Executive Officer
COO: Tony Ruiz, Chief Operating Officer
CFO: Robert Abernethy, Chief Financial Officer
CMO: Bruce Becker, M.D., Chief Medical Officer
CIO: Gary Barnes, Chief Information Officer
CHR: Harvey Hudspeth, Executive Director Human Resources
Web address: www.mchodessa.com
**Control:** Hospital district or authority, Government, nonfederal **Service:** General Medical and Surgical

**Staffed Beds:** 306 **Admissions:** 14194 **Census:** 194 **Outpatient Visits:** 276411 **Births:** 1091 **Total Expense ($000):** 140816 **Payroll Expense ($000):** 84354 **Personnel:** 1601

**MEDICAL CENTER HOSPITAL** See Medical Center Health System

**ODESSA REGIONAL MEDICAL CENTER (450661)**, 520 East Sixth Street, Zip 79761–4565, Mailing Address: P.O. Box 4859, Zip 79760–4859; tel. 432/582–8000 **A**5 9 10 21 **F**3 8 13 15 17 18 19 20 21 22 23 24 25 29 34 35 40 43 46 49 50 52 55 57 59 64 72 75 76 79 81 85 86 87 89 90 107 108 111 114 118 123 129 143 145 146 **P**8 **S** IASIS Healthcare, Franklin, TN
Primary Contact: Stacey L. Gerig, Chief Executive Officer
CFO: Michael Metts, Chief Financial Officer
CHR: Jill Sparkman, Director Human Resources
Web address: www.odessaregionalmedicalcenter.com
**Control:** Partnership, Investor–owned, for–profit **Service:** General Medical and Surgical

**Staffed Beds:** 194 **Admissions:** 6594 **Census:** 89 **Outpatient Visits:** 44353 **Births:** 2527 **Total Expense ($000):** 135259 **Payroll Expense ($000):** 33817 **Personnel:** 599

⊠ **REGENCY HOSPITAL OF ODESSA (452085)**, 318 North Alleghaney, Suite 202, Zip 79761; tel. 432/552–4000 **A**1 9 10 **F**1 29 30 85 129 147 **P**5 **S** Select Medical Corporation, Mechanicsburg, PA
Primary Contact: Don Cubb, Chief Executive Officer
Web address: www.regencyhospital.com
**Control:** Corporation, Investor–owned, for–profit **Service:** Long–Term Acute Care hospital

**Staffed Beds:** 36 **Admissions:** 348 **Census:** 23 **Outpatient Visits:** 0 **Births:** 0 **Total Expense ($000):** 11267 **Payroll Expense ($000):** 4790 **Personnel:** 58

## OLNEY—Young County

★ **HAMILTON HOSPITAL (451354)**, 903 West Hamilton Street, Zip 76374–1725, Mailing Address: P.O. Box 158, Zip 76374–0158; tel. 940/564–5521 **A**9 10 18 **F**7 11 13 28 29 30 40 43 53 57 76 77 81 86 89 93 107 113 118 126 129 132 145 147
Primary Contact: Michael H. Huff, Chief Executive Officer
CMO: Mark L. Mankins, M.D., Chief of Staff
Web address: www.olneyhamiltonhospital.com
**Control:** Hospital district or authority, Government, nonfederal **Service:** General Medical and Surgical

**Staffed Beds:** 25 **Admissions:** 741 **Census:** 10 **Outpatient Visits:** 12841 **Births:** 13 **Total Expense ($000):** 7866 **Payroll Expense ($000):** 4663 **Personnel:** 115

## ORANGE—Orange County

★ **BAPTIST ORANGE HOSPITAL (450005)**, 608 Strickland Drive, Zip 77630–4717; tel. 409/883–9361 **A**9 10 21 **F**3 13 15 18 29 30 34 35 39 40 45 57 59 64 70 75 76 79 81 85 89 93 107 108 111 114 117 118 129 145 146 147 **S** Community Hospital Corporation, Plano, TX
Primary Contact: Jarren Garrett, Chief Administrative Officer
CFO: Gary Troutman, CPA, Chief Financial Officer
CMO: Miguel Castellanos, M.D., Chief of Staff
CIO: Troy Napier, Director
CHR: Jennifer Barroeta, Manager Human Resources
Web address: www.baptistorangehospital.org
**Control:** Other not–for–profit (including NFP Corporation) **Service:** General Medical and Surgical

**Staffed Beds:** 40 **Admissions:** 2062 **Census:** 20 **Outpatient Visits:** 34064 **Births:** 213 **Total Expense ($000):** 30808 **Payroll Expense ($000):** 10823 **Personnel:** 197

**MEMORIAL HERMANN BAPTIST ORANGE HOSPITAL** See Baptist Orange Hospital

## PALACIOS—Matagorda County

**PALACIOS COMMUNITY MEDICAL CENTER (451332)**, 311 Green Street, Zip 77465–3214; tel. 361/972–2511 **A**9 10 18 **F**3 29 30 34 35 38 40 44 50 54 56 57 59 65 66 68 86 87 107 113 118 126 131 132 145
Primary Contact: Don Bates, Chief Executive Officer
CFO: Cherri Waites, Chief Financial Officer
CIO: Lisa Henderson, Administrative Assistant
CHR: Lisa Henderson, Administrative Assistant
Web address: www.palacioshospital.com
**Control:** Other not–for–profit (including NFP Corporation) **Service:** General Medical and Surgical

**Staffed Beds:** 11 **Admissions:** 380 **Census:** 3 **Outpatient Visits:** 8197 **Births:** 0 **Total Expense ($000):** 4450 **Payroll Expense ($000):** 2155 **Personnel:** 47

## PALESTINE—Anderson County

★ **PALESTINE REGIONAL MEDICAL CENTER–EAST (450747)**, 2900 South Loop 256, Zip 75801–6958; tel. 903/731–1000 **A**9 10 20 **F**3 7 11 13 15 18 20 22 26 28 29 30 34 40 43 44 47 48 49 50 51 56 57 59 63 70 76 79 81 82 85 86 87 89 90 93 96 97 98 100 101 102 103 104 107 108 110 111 113 117 118 128 129 130 132 142 145 146 147 **S** LifePoint Hospitals, Inc., Brentwood, TN
Primary Contact: Alan E. George, Chief Executive Officer
CFO: Louis D. Ferguson, Chief Financial Officer
CIO: Rebecca Chou, Director Information Systems
CHR: Rhonda Beard, Director Human Resources
Web address: www.palestineregional.com
**Control:** Partnership, Investor–owned, for–profit **Service:** General Medical and Surgical

**Staffed Beds:** 113 **Admissions:** 6069 **Census:** 61 **Outpatient Visits:** 67008 **Births:** 841 **Total Expense ($000):** 47657 **Payroll Expense ($000):** 24607 **Personnel:** 477

⊠ **PALESTINE REGIONAL REHABILITATION CENTER (453089)**, 4000 South Loop 256, Zip 75801–8467, Mailing Address: P.O. Box 4070, Zip 75802–4070; tel. 903/731–5100, (Nonreporting) **A**1 10 **S** LifePoint Hospitals, Inc., Brentwood, TN
Primary Contact: Ronald Safford, Administrator
CHR: Rhonda Beard, Director Human Resources
Web address: www.palestineregional.com
**Control:** Corporation, Investor–owned, for–profit **Service:** Rehabilitation

**Staffed Beds:** 12

**TX**

## PAMPA—Gray County

☐ **PAMPA REGIONAL MEDICAL CENTER (450099)**, One Medical Plaza, Zip 79065; tel. 806/665–3721 **A**1 9 10 20 **F**3 11 12 13 15 16 18 20 22 29 30 40 45 51 57 58 59 65 68 70 75 76 77 79 81 82 85 86 87 93 96 98 103 104 107 108 111 114 117 118 129 131 145 146 147 **P**6 **S** Prime Healthcare Services, Ontario, CA
Primary Contact: Richard L. McConahy, Interim Chief Executive Officer
CFO: Paul Christenson, Chief Financial Officer
CMO: David Hampton, M.D., Chief Medical Staff
CIO: Joy Patton, Chief Information Services
CHR: Debbie Dixon, Director Human Resources
CNO: Catherine Kenney, Chief Nursing Officer
Web address: www.prmctx.com
**Control:** Partnership, Investor–owned, for–profit **Service:** General Medical and Surgical

**Staffed Beds:** 32 **Admissions:** 2023 **Census:** 22 **Outpatient Visits:** 35229 **Births:** 203 **Total Expense ($000):** 29178 **Payroll Expense ($000):** 10941 **Personnel:** 255

## PARIS—Lamar County

⊠ **DUBUIS HOSPITAL OF PARIS (452082)**, 865 Deshong Drive, 5th Floor, Zip 75462; tel. 903/782–2960 **A**1 9 10 **F**1 3 29 30 85 145 147 **S** Dubuis Health System, Houston, TX
Primary Contact: Kathie Reese, Administrator
CMO: James E. Gulde, M.D., Medical Director
Web address: www.dubuis.org
**Control:** Church–operated, Nongovernment, not–for profit **Service:** Long–Term Acute Care hospital

**Staffed Beds:** 25 **Admissions:** 190 **Census:** 13 **Outpatient Visits:** 0 **Births:** 0 **Total Expense ($000):** 4881 **Payroll Expense ($000):** 1744 **Personnel:** 39

☐ **PARIS REGIONAL MEDICAL CENTER (450196)**, 820 Clarksville Street, Zip 75460–9070; tel. 903/785–4521, (Includes PARIS REGIONAL MEDICAL CENTER, 865 Deshong Drive, Zip 75462–2097; tel. 903/737–1111; PARIS REGIONAL MEDICAL CENTER–SOUTH CAMPUS, 820 Clarksville Street, Mailing Address: P.O. Box 9070, Zip 75461–9070; tel. 903/785–4521) **A**1 9 10 19 **F**3 8 11 13 15 17 18 20 22 24 26 28 29 30 31 34 35 36 39 40 45 49 51 55 57 59 60 65 66 68 70 72 74 76 77 78 79 81 82 85 86 87 89 90 91 93 97 98 102 103 107 108 111 114 118 126 129 131 134 143 144 145 146 147 **P**5 **S** RegionalCare Hospital Partners, Brentwood, TN
Primary Contact: Billy Porter, Chief Executive Officer
CFO: Ken Miller, Chief Financial Officer
CMO: Richard Bercher, M.D., Chief Medical Officer
CHR: Cheryl Perry, Director Human Resources
Web address: www.parisrmc.com
**Control:** Partnership, Investor–owned, for–profit **Service:** General Medical and Surgical

**Staffed Beds:** 226 **Admissions:** 8396 **Census:** 108 **Outpatient Visits:** 86837 **Births:** 667 **Total Expense ($000):** 99409 **Payroll Expense ($000):** 33511 **Personnel:** 796

## PASADENA—Harris County

⊠ **BAYSHORE MEDICAL CENTER (450097)**, 4000 Spencer Highway, Zip 77504–1294; tel. 713/359–2000, (Includes EAST HOUSTON REGIONAL MEDICAL CENTER, 13111 East Freeway, Houston, Zip 77015–5820; tel. 713/393–2000; Alice G. Adams, R.N., Chief Executive Officer) **A**1 2 3 5 9 10 **F**3 12 13 15 17 18 20 28 29 31 34 35 39 40 41 42 43 47 49 51 55 56 57 59 60 64 70 72 74 75 76 77 78 79 81 82 84 86 89 90 91 93 98 100 102 103 107 108 111 113 114 115 116 117 118 119 120 122 128 129 130 143 145 146 147 **S** HCA, Nashville, TN
Primary Contact: Jeffrey S. Holland, Chief Executive Officer
COO: Jeanna Barnard, Chief Operating Officer
CFO: John Armour, Chief Financial Officer
CMO: Harold Walton, M.D., Chief of Staff
CIO: Clifford Ferguson, Director Information Technology and Systems
Web address: www.bayshoremedical.com
**Control:** Partnership, Investor–owned, for–profit **Service:** General Medical and Surgical

**Staffed Beds:** 476 **Admissions:** 19306 **Census:** 252 **Outpatient Visits:** 171912 **Births:** 3862 **Total Expense ($000):** 219997 **Payroll Expense ($000):** 94792 **Personnel:** 1468

★ **KINDRED HOSPITAL–BAY AREA**, 4801 East Sam Houston Parkway South, Zip 77505–3955; tel. 281/991–5463 **A**9 **F**1 3 29 30 34 45 46 47 60 64 70 77 93 107 113 129 131 145 147 **P**5 **S** Kindred Healthcare, Louisville, KY
Primary Contact: Anne R. Leon, Administrator
CHR: Nellie Moen, Coordinator Human Resources
Web address: www.khbayareahouston.com/
**Control:** Corporation, Investor–owned, for–profit **Service:** Long–Term Acute Care hospital

**Staffed Beds:** 74 **Admissions:** 944 **Census:** 64 **Outpatient Visits:** 29 **Births:** 0 **Total Expense ($000):** 25442 **Payroll Expense ($000):** 11724 **Personnel:** 178

**PATIENTS MEDICAL CENTER** See St. Luke's Patients Medical Center

★ **ST. LUKE'S PATIENTS MEDICAL CENTER (670031)**, 4600 East Sam Houston Parkway South, Zip 77505; tel. 713/948–7000 **A**9 10 21 **F**12 15 18 20 22 24 29 30 31 35 40 45 46 54 64 70 74 77 81 82 91 93 94 107 111 113 114 115 116 118 128 129 145 146 147 **S** St. Luke's Episcopal Health System, Houston, TX
Primary Contact: William Simmons, President and Chief Executive Officer
Web address: www.stlukestexas.com
**Control:** Corporation, Investor–owned, for–profit **Service:** General Medical and Surgical

**Staffed Beds:** 61 **Admissions:** 3778 **Census:** 46 **Outpatient Visits:** 45471 **Births:** 0 **Total Expense ($000):** 53638 **Payroll Expense ($000):** 22624 **Personnel:** 362

○ **SURGERY SPECIALTY HOSPITALS OF AMERICA (450831)**, 4301B Vista, Zip 77504; tel. 713/378–3000 **A**10 11 **F**3 12 29 40 45 68 70 75 79 81 85 107 118 128 131 **P**8 **S** Dynacq Healthcare, Inc., Houston, TX
Primary Contact: Celia Barrera, Administrator
**Control:** Partnership, Investor–owned, for–profit **Service:** General Medical and Surgical

**Staffed Beds:** 37 **Admissions:** 143 **Census:** 1 **Outpatient Visits:** 1086 **Births:** 0 **Personnel:** 97

## PEARSALL—Frio County

★ **FRIO REGIONAL HOSPITAL (450293)**, 200 South I. H. 35, Zip 78061–3998; tel. 830/334–3617 **A**9 10 **F**3 8 15 29 35 40 43 45 53 59 62 64 68 76 77 81 87 93 107 113 118 129 147
Primary Contact: Michael S. Thompson, Chief Executive Officer
CHR: Cayce Morse, Administrative Assistant
Web address: www.frioregionalhospital.com
**Control:** Other not–for–profit (including NFP Corporation) **Service:** General Medical and Surgical

**Staffed Beds:** 22 **Admissions:** 404 **Census:** 3 **Outpatient Visits:** 20356 **Births:** 106 **Total Expense ($000):** 10168 **Payroll Expense ($000):** 3498 **Personnel:** 109

## PECOS—Reeves County

**REEVES COUNTY HOSPITAL (451377)**, 2323 Texas Street, Zip 79772–7338; tel. 432/447–3551 **A**9 10 18 **F**3 11 13 35 40 43 57 60 64 68 70 76 81 87 89 93 107 113 118 126 129 130 132 145 146 147
Primary Contact: Albert LaRochelle, Chief Executive Officer
CFO: Frank Seals, Chief Financial Officer
CMO: W. J. Bang, M.D., Chief of Staff
CHR: Nadine Smith, Director Human Resources
Web address: www.reevescountyhospital.com
**Control:** Hospital district or authority, Government, nonfederal **Service:** General Medical and Surgical

**Staffed Beds:** 25 **Admissions:** 854 **Census:** 8 **Outpatient Visits:** 37888 **Births:** 56 **Total Expense ($000):** 15073 **Payroll Expense ($000):** 7070 **Personnel:** 157

## PERRYTON—Ochiltree County

★ **OCHILTREE GENERAL HOSPITAL (451359)**, 3101 Garrett Drive, Zip 79070–5393; tel. 806/435–3606 **A**9 10 18 **F**10 11 13 15 35 40 43 57 59 62 63 64 69 76 81 85 89 93 107 108 113 118 126 129 132 142 145 146 **P**1
Primary Contact: Jeff Barnhart, Chief Executive Officer
CIO: Dyan Harrison, Manager Health Information
Web address: www.ochiltreehospital.com
**Control:** Hospital district or authority, Government, nonfederal **Service:** General Medical and Surgical

**Staffed Beds:** 25 **Admissions:** 710 **Census:** 9 **Outpatient Visits:** 40430 **Births:** 195 **Total Expense ($000):** 13241 **Payroll Expense ($000):** 5665 **Personnel:** 178

## PITTSBURG—Camp County

★ **EAST TEXAS MEDICAL CENTER PITTSBURG (451367)**, 2701 Highway 271 North, Zip 75686–1032; tel. 903/946–5000 **A**9 10 18 **F**3 11 12 28 29 35 40 43 45 50 57 59 64 68 70 81 85 89 92 93 97 107 108 111 114 118 126 128 129 132 **P**6 **S** East Texas Medical Center Regional Healthcare System, Tyler, TX
Primary Contact: W. Perry Henderson, Administrator
CFO: Thomas O'Gorman, Jr., Assistant Administrator and Chief Financial Officer
CMO: W. R. Christensen, M.D., Chief of Staff
CIO: Paula Anthony, Vice President Information Services
CHR: Kathy Shelton, Director Human Resources
Web address: www.etmc.org
**Control:** Other not–for–profit (including NFP Corporation) **Service:** General Medical and Surgical

**Staffed Beds:** 25 **Admissions:** 1266 **Census:** 14 **Outpatient Visits:** 74883 **Births:** 0 **Total Expense ($000):** 26753 **Payroll Expense ($000):** 9237 **Personnel:** 215

**TX**

*Many Facility Codes have changed. Please refer to the AHA Guide Code Chart.* © 2012 AHA Guide

## PLAINVIEW—Hale County

**ALLEGIANCE BEHAVIORAL HEALTH CENTER OF PLAINVIEW (454101)**, 2601 Dimmit Road, 4th Floor, Zip 79072; tel. 806/296-9191 **A**10 **F**29 35 56 64 98 101 103 104 **S** Allegiance Health Management, Shreveport, LA
Primary Contact: Glenn G. Hoffman, MS, Chief Executive Officer
COO: Don Cameron, Chief Operating Officer
CFO: Jim Turgeon, Vice President Finance
CMO: Victor A. Gutierrez, M.D., Medical Director
CIO: Richard Merk, Executive Vice President
CHR: Rob Lindsey, Jr., Vice President Human Resources
Web address: www.ahmgt.com
**Control:** Corporation, Investor-owned, for-profit **Service:** Psychiatric

> **Staffed Beds:** 20 **Admissions:** 252 **Census:** 11 **Outpatient Visits:** 37733
> **Births:** 0 **Total Expense ($000):** 4635 **Payroll Expense ($000):** 2070
> **Personnel:** 33

⊞ **COVENANT HOSPITAL PLAINVIEW (450539)**, 2601 Dimmitt Road, Zip 79072-1833; tel. 806/296-5531 **A**1 9 10 20 **F**3 11 13 15 29 30 32 34 35 40 43 44 50 51 54 56 57 59 61 64 65 68 70 75 76 77 79 81 85 86 87 93 97 107 108 113 117 118 126 128 129 130 131 132 133 145 147 **S** Covenant Health System, Lubbock, TX
Primary Contact: Alan N. King, FACHE, President and Chief Executive Officer
CFO: Clay Taylor, Chief Financial Officer
CMO: Sergio Lara, M.D., Chief Medical Officer
CIO: Tim Branch, Manager Information Technology
Web address: www.covenantplainview.org
**Control:** Church-operated, Nongovernment, not-for profit **Service:** General Medical and Surgical

> **Staffed Beds:** 68 **Admissions:** 2098 **Census:** 17 **Outpatient Visits:** 90558
> **Births:** 521 **Total Expense ($000):** 28891 **Payroll Expense ($000):** 9773
> **Personnel:** 276

## PLANO—Collin County

⊞ **BAYLOR REGIONAL MEDICAL CENTER AT PLANO (450890)**, 4700 Alliance Boulevard, Zip 75093; tel. 469/814-2000 **A**1 2 9 10 **F**3 12 15 29 30 34 35 40 45 46 47'49 54 57 58 59 64 70 74 75 77 78 79 80 81 82 84 85 86 87 107 108 110 111 113 117 118 125 128 129 130 131 144 145 146 147 **S** Baylor Health Care System, Dallas, TX
Primary Contact: Jerri Garison, R.N., President
COO: Ellen Pitcher, MSN, Chief Operating Officer and Chief Nursing Officer
CFO: Deanne Kindered, Vice President Finance
CMO: Bradley M. Leonard, M.D., Vice President Medical Affairs
CHR: Tamara DeFer, Director Human Resources
Web address: www.baylorhealth.com
**Control:** Other not-for-profit (including NFP Corporation) **Service:** General Medical and Surgical

> **Staffed Beds:** 112 **Admissions:** 5395 **Census:** 78 **Outpatient Visits:** 48975
> **Births:** 0 **Total Expense ($000):** 153009 **Payroll Expense ($000):** 47739
> **Personnel:** 683

⊞ **HEALTHSOUTH PLANO REHABILITATION HOSPITAL (453047)**, 2800 West 15th Street, Zip 75075-7526; tel. 972/612-9000 **A**1 9 10 **F**34 57 59 62 90 93 95 96 100 128 129 131 147 **S** HEALTHSOUTH Corporation, Birmingham, AL
Primary Contact: Jennifer Lynn Brewer, Chief Executive Officer
CFO: Catrina Madkins, Controller and Chief Financial Officer
CMO: Omar Colon, M.D., Medical Director
Web address: www.healthsouthplano.com
**Control:** Corporation, Investor-owned, for-profit **Service:** Rehabilitation

> **Staffed Beds:** 65 **Admissions:** 1343 **Census:** 47 **Outpatient Visits:** 17530
> **Births:** 0 **Total Expense ($000):** 18056 **Payroll Expense ($000):** 10041
> **Personnel:** 211

★ **MEDICAL CENTER OF PLANO (450651)**, 3901 West 15th Street, Zip 75075-7799; tel. 972/596-6800 **A**2 9 10 **F**3 11 12 13 15 18 20 22 24 26 28 29 30 31 34 35 40 43 45 46 48 49 51 53 54 55 57 58 59 60 64 70 72 74 75 76 78 79 81 82 84 85 86 87 89 93 107 108 110 111 112 113 114 116 117 118 123 125 128 129 131 134 144 145 146 147 **P**5 **S** HCA, Nashville, TN
Primary Contact: Troy Villarreal, Chief Executive Officer
COO: Glenn Wallace, Chief Operating Officer
CFO: W. Patrick Whitmore, Chief Financial Officer
CMO: Ann Arnold, M.D., Medical Director
CIO: Michael Gfeller, Director Information Systems
CHR: Shanna Warren, Director Human Resources
Web address: www.medicalcenterplano.com
**Control:** Partnership, Investor-owned, for-profit **Service:** General Medical and Surgical

> **Staffed Beds:** 306 **Admissions:** 16491 **Census:** 235 **Outpatient Visits:** 113637 **Births:** 2103 **Total Expense ($000):** 232916 **Payroll Expense ($000):** 87789 **Personnel:** 1374

☐ **PLANO SPECIALTY HOSPITAL (452054)**, 1621 Coit Road, Zip 75075; tel. 972/758-5200 **A**1 9 10 **F**1 3 29 45 75 82 84 85 86 87 96 129 134 147 **S** Encore Healthcare, Columbia, MD
Primary Contact: Jerry Amato, Chief Executive Officer
CFO: Deanna Lankford, Business Office Manager
CHR: Robbie McCranie, Director Human Resources
Web address: www.planospecialtyhospital.com
**Control:** Corporation, Investor-owned, for-profit **Service:** Long-Term Acute Care hospital

> **Staffed Beds:** 43 **Admissions:** 340 **Census:** 22 **Outpatient Visits:** 0 **Births:** 0 **Total Expense ($000):** 11793 **Payroll Expense ($000):** 3757 **Personnel:** 74

☐ **TEXAS HEALTH CENTER FOR DIAGNOSTIC & SURGERY (450891)**, 6020 West Parker Road, Zip 75093; tel. 972/403-2700 **A**1 2 9 10 **F**3 29 40 42 45 54 64 79 81 82 85 87 107 111 113 118 128
Primary Contact: Larry Robertson, Chief Executive Officer
CFO: Douglas Browning, Chief Financial Officer
CHR: Cookie Tedder, Human Resources Manager
CNO: Ellen Baldwin, R.N., Chief Nursing Officer
Web address: www.thcds.com
**Control:** Partnership, Investor-owned, for-profit **Service:** General Medical and Surgical

> **Staffed Beds:** 18 **Admissions:** 804 **Census:** 4 **Outpatient Visits:** 16349
> **Births:** 0 **Total Expense ($000):** 44830 **Payroll Expense ($000):** 9791
> **Personnel:** 143

⊞ **TEXAS HEALTH PRESBYTERIAN HOSPITAL PLANO (450771)**, 6200 West Parker Road, Zip 75093-7914; tel. 972/981-8000 **A**1 9 10 **F**3 12 13 15 18 20 22 24 26 29 30 31 32 34 35 37 38 40 43 44 45 48 49 50 52 54 55 57 58 59 60 64 68 70 72 74 75 76 77 78 79 81 85 86 87 89 93 96 107 108 110 111 113 114 117 118 129 131 134 144 145 146 147 **P**8 **S** Texas Health Resources, Arlington, TX
Primary Contact: Mike Evans, R.N., MS, President
CFO: Ray Cassens, Vice President and Chief Financial Officer
CMO: Alfred Rodriguez, M.D., President Medical Staff
CIO: Susan Anderson, Director Information Systems
CHR: Angie Noel, Administrative Director Human Resources
Web address: www.texashealth.org
**Control:** Other not-for-profit (including NFP Corporation) **Service:** General Medical and Surgical

> **Staffed Beds:** 338 **Admissions:** 15273 **Census:** 219 **Outpatient Visits:** 79234 **Births:** 3869 **Total Expense ($000):** 260569 **Payroll Expense ($000):** 93699 **Personnel:** 1189

**THE HEART HOSPITAL BAYLOR PLANO (670025)**, 1100 Allied Drive, Zip 75093; tel. 469/814-3278 **A**9 10 **F**3 18 20 22 24 26 28 29 30 34 40 57 64 75 78 79 81 82 84 85 86 87 91 92 93 94 95 96 97 107 108 110 111 112 113 114 115 116 117 118 119 120 122 123 125 129 136 145 146
Primary Contact: Mark Valentine, President and Chief Executive Officer
CFO: Bryan Nichols, Chief Financial Officer
CMO: Trent Pettijohn, M.D., Chief Medical Officer
CIO: Nayan Patel, Director Information Systems
CHR: Michael Ramey, Director Human Resources
CNO: Susan Moats, R.N., Vice President of Patient Care Services and Chief Nursing Officer
Web address: www.thehearthospital.com
**Control:** Partnership, Investor-owned, for-profit **Service:** General Medical and Surgical

> **Staffed Beds:** 116 **Admissions:** 3174 **Census:** 47 **Outpatient Visits:** 14260
> **Births:** 0 **Total Expense ($000):** 133624 **Payroll Expense ($000):** 40813
> **Personnel:** 571

## PORT ARTHUR—Jefferson County

★ **CHRISTUS DUBUIS HOSPITAL OF PORT ARTHUR**, 3600 Gates Boulevard, Zip 77642; tel. 409/989-5300, (Nonreporting) **A**9 **S** Dubuis Health System, Houston, TX
Primary Contact: Barbara Flournoy, Administrator
Web address: www.dubuis.org
**Control:** Church-operated, Nongovernment, not-for profit **Service:** Other specialty

> **Staffed Beds:** 15

**DUBUIS HOSPITAL OF PORT ARTHUR** See Christus Dubuis Hospital of Port Arthur

**TX**

---

**Hospital, Medicare Provider Number, Address, Telephone, Approval, Facility, and Physician Codes, Health Care System**

★ American Hospital Association (AHA) membership
☐ The Joint Commission accreditation  ◇ DNV Healthcare Inc. accreditation
○ American Osteopathic Association (AOA) accreditation
△ Commission on Accreditation of Rehabilitation Facilities (CARF) accreditation

---

**THE MEDICAL CENTER OF SOUTHEAST TEXAS (450518)**, 2555 Jimmy Johnson Boulevard, Zip 77640; tel. 409/724–7389 **A**9 10 21 **F**3 8 11 13 15 17 18 20 22 24 28 29 30 34 35 40 44 45 47 49 50 56 57 59 64 72 74 76 77 79 81 82 85 86 87 89 90 91 92 93 94 98 101 102 103 104 105 107 108 110 111 113 114 118 129 131 134 147 **P**2 **S** IASIS Healthcare, Franklin, TN
Primary Contact: Matthew S. Roberts, Chief Executive Officer
COO: Chris McMahon, Chief Operating Officer
CFO: William Whiddon, Chief Financial Officer
CMO: Nidal Buheis, M.D., Chief of Staff
CIO: Bryan Hebert, Director Information Systems
CHR: Carol Hebert, Director Human Resources
Web address: www.medicalcentersetexas.com
**Control:** Partnership, Investor–owned, for–profit **Service:** General Medical and Surgical

**Staffed Beds:** 185 **Admissions:** 7036 **Census:** 87 **Outpatient Visits:** 52803 **Births:** 1191 **Total Expense ($000):** 90604 **Payroll Expense ($000):** 32812 **Personnel:** 617

### PORT LAVACA—Calhoun County

★ **MEMORIAL MEDICAL CENTER (451356)**, 815 North Virginia Street, Zip 77979–3025, Mailing Address: P.O. Box 25, Zip 77979–0025; tel. 361/552–6713 **A**9 10 18 **F**3 11 13 15 18 29 30 32 34 35 40 43 44 45 46 49 50 57 59 64 65 68 70 75 76 77 78 79 81 84 85 86 87 93 107 108 111 114 117 118 128 129 131 132 133 134 145 146 147
Primary Contact: Jason Anglin, Chief Executive Officer
CFO: Rick Hart, Chief Financial Officer
CMO: Jeannine Griffin, M.D., Chief of Staff
Web address: www.mmcportlavaca.com
**Control:** County–Government, nonfederal **Service:** General Medical and Surgical

**Staffed Beds:** 25 **Admissions:** 1354 **Census:** 15 **Outpatient Visits:** 34038 **Births:** 109 **Total Expense ($000):** 20075 **Payroll Expense ($000):** 7892 **Personnel:** 171

### QUANAH—Hardeman County

★ **HARDEMAN COUNTY MEMORIAL HOSPITAL (451352)**, 402 Mercer Street, Zip 79252–4026, Mailing Address: P.O. Box 90, Zip 79252–0090; tel. 940/663–2795 **A**9 10 18 **F**3 11 28 29 30 34 40 43 45 50 56 57 59 62 63 64 75 77 87 93 100 101 103 104 107 126 129 132 **P**5
Primary Contact: Carol Lively, Chief Executive Officer
CFO: Butch Hall, Chief Financial Officer
CMO: Kevin Lane, D.O., Chief of Staff
Web address: www.quanahnet.com\hospital\navbarframe.htm
**Control:** Hospital district or authority, Government, nonfederal **Service:** General Medical and Surgical

**Staffed Beds:** 18 **Admissions:** 342 **Census:** 5 **Outpatient Visits:** 28962 **Births:** 0 **Total Expense ($000):** 9456 **Payroll Expense ($000):** 5274 **Personnel:** 123

### QUITMAN—Wood County

★ **EAST TEXAS MEDICAL CENTER–QUITMAN (451380)**, 117 Winnsboro Street, Zip 75783–2144, Mailing Address: P.O. Box 1000, Zip 75783–1000; tel. 903/763–6300 **A**9 10 18 **F**3 11 15 29 30 35 40 43 45 50 57 59 64 65 68 79 81 85 87 107 108 110 111 114 118 126 128 129 132 **S** East Texas Medical Center Regional Healthcare System, Tyler, TX
Primary Contact: Warren Robicheaux, Administrator
CFO: Tania LeMons, Controller
CMO: James D. Dopson, M.D., Chief Medical Staff
CHR: William Henry, Director Human Resources
Web address: www.etmc.org
**Control:** Other not–for–profit (including NFP Corporation) **Service:** General Medical and Surgical

**Staffed Beds:** 25 **Admissions:** 1134 **Census:** 12 **Outpatient Visits:** 39036 **Births:** 0 **Total Expense ($000):** 14396 **Payroll Expense ($000):** 5311 **Personnel:** 117

### RANKIN—Upton County

★ **RANKIN HOSPITAL DISTRICT (451329)**, 1105 Elizabeth Street, Zip 79778, Mailing Address: P.O. Box 327, Zip 79778–0327; tel. 432/693–2443 **A**9 10 18 **F**35 40 59 64 65 68 89 93 97
Primary Contact: Wayne Ogburn, FACHE, Administrator
CFO: Tami Burks, Comptroller
CMO: Thomas J. Curvin, M.D., Chief of Staff
**Control:** Hospital district or authority, Government, nonfederal **Service:** General Medical and Surgical

**Staffed Beds:** 10 **Admissions:** 13 **Census:** 1 **Outpatient Visits:** 1210 **Births:** 0 **Personnel:** 34

### REFUGIO—Refugio County

**REFUGIO COUNTY MEMORIAL HOSPITAL (451317)**, 107 Swift Street, Zip 78377–2425; tel. 361/526–2321 **A**9 10 18 **F**3 7 29 40 43 57 61 64 75 81 86 87 93 97 107 118 126 132 **P**6
Primary Contact: Louis R. Willeke, Administrator
Web address: www.refugiohospital.com/
**Control:** Hospital district or authority, Government, nonfederal **Service:** General Medical and Surgical

**Staffed Beds:** 20 **Admissions:** 126 **Census:** 2 **Outpatient Visits:** 25600 **Births:** 0 **Total Expense ($000):** 12073 **Payroll Expense ($000):** 4590 **Personnel:** 120

### RICHARDSON—Dallas County

⊞ **METHODIST RICHARDSON MEDICAL CENTER (450537)**, 401 West Campbell Road, Zip 75080–3416; tel. 972/498–4000 **A**1 2 9 10 **F**3 4 5 11 13 15 17 18 20 22 24 29 30 31 34 35 38 40 42 46 49 54 55 56 57 59 64 65 68 70 74 75 76 77 78 79 81 82 85 86 87 93 97 98 100 101 102 103 104 105 107 108 109 110 111 112 114 115 116 118 119 120 122 123 125 128 129 130 131 134 145 146 147 **P**1 **S** Methodist Health System, Dallas, TX
Primary Contact: E. Kenneth Hutchenrider, President
CFO: Bob Simpson, Vice President Finance
CIO: Terri Morris, Manager Information Systems
CHR: Shannan Gulbis, Director Human Resources
Web address: www.richardsonregional.com
**Control:** Other not–for–profit (including NFP Corporation) **Service:** General Medical and Surgical

**Staffed Beds:** 147 **Admissions:** 5948 **Census:** 75 **Outpatient Visits:** 60526 **Births:** 474 **Total Expense ($000):** 116588 **Payroll Expense ($000):** 42522 **Personnel:** 677

⊞ **RELIANT REHABILITATION HOSPITAL NORTH TEXAS (673029)**, 3351 Waterview Parkway, Zip 75080; tel. 972/398–5700 **A**1 9 10 **F**3 29 30 40 90 91 93 96 **S** Reliant Healthcare Partners, Addison, TX
Primary Contact: Jim Ransom, Chief Executive Officer
CFO: Mary Mwaniki, Chief Financial Officer
CMO: Richard Jones, M.D., Medical Director
Web address: www.relianthcp.com
**Control:** Partnership, Investor–owned, for–profit **Service:** Rehabilitation

**Staffed Beds:** 50 **Admissions:** 1161 **Census:** 42 **Outpatient Visits:** 11979 **Births:** 0 **Total Expense ($000):** 16285 **Payroll Expense ($000):** 8028 **Personnel:** 113

### RICHMOND—Fort Bend County

☐ △ **OAKBEND MEDICAL CENTER (450330)**, 1705 Jackson Street, Zip 77469–3289; tel. 281/341–3000, (Total facility includes 26 beds in nursing home–type unit) **A**1 2 7 9 10 **F**3 11 13 15 18 20 22 24 26 29 30 31 34 35 40 42 43 45 46 47 49 50 56 57 59 64 65 70 72 74 75 76 78 79 81 82 85 87 89 93 98 102 103 107 108 109 110 111 114 117 118 127 128 129 131 145 146 147 **P**6
Primary Contact: Joe Freudenberger, Chief Executive Officer
CFO: James R. Shallock, Chief Financial Officer
CMO: Douglas Thibodeaux, M.D., Chief Medical Officer
CHR: Nancy Retzlaff, Director Human Resources
Web address: www.oakbendmedcenter.org
**Control:** Hospital district or authority, Government, nonfederal **Service:** General Medical and Surgical

**Staffed Beds:** 195 **Admissions:** 5833 **Census:** 74 **Outpatient Visits:** 55061 **Births:** 1265 **Total Expense ($000):** 55470 **Payroll Expense ($000):** 26816 **Personnel:** 525

### RIO GRANDE CITY—Starr County

★ **STARR COUNTY MEMORIAL HOSPITAL (450654)**, 2753 Hospital Court, Zip 78582–9801, Mailing Address: P.O. Box 78, Zip 78582–0078; tel. 956/487–5561 **A**9 10 20 **F**7 11 13 15 29 30 34 40 43 45 46 50 57 59 64 65 66 68 75 76 79 80 81 89 107 111 113 118 126 129 134 144 147
Primary Contact: Thalia H. Munoz, Administrator
CFO: Rafael Olivares, Controller
Web address: www.starrcountyhospital.com
**Control:** Hospital district or authority, Government, nonfederal **Service:** General Medical and Surgical

**Staffed Beds:** 47 **Admissions:** 1846 **Census:** 17 **Outpatient Visits:** 55930 **Births:** 379 **Total Expense ($000):** 23656 **Payroll Expense ($000):** 9971 **Personnel:** 256

TX

## ROCKDALE—Milam County

**LITTLE RIVER MEDICAL CENTER (451357)**, 1700 Brazos Street, Zip 76567-2517, Mailing Address: Drawer 1010, Zip 76567-1010; tel. 512/446-4500 **A**9 10 18 **F**11 15 18 20 22 26 28 29 40 54 57 59 64 65 68 75 77 79 81 82 83 84 85 87 93 96 97 107 108 110 111 114 118 126 129 130 132 147
Primary Contact: Jeffrey Madison, Chief Executive Officer
CMO: John Weed, III, M.D., Medical Director
CHR: Crystal Foley, Director Human Resources
Web address: www.lrhealthcare.com
**Control:** Corporation, Investor-owned, for-profit **Service:** General Medical and Surgical

**Staffed Beds:** 21 **Admissions:** 480 **Census:** 9 **Outpatient Visits:** 50246 **Births:** 2 **Total Expense ($000):** 23627 **Payroll Expense ($000):** 8015 **Personnel:** 190

## ROCKWALL—Rockwall County

✠ **PRESBYTERIAN HOSPITAL OF ROCKWALL (670044)**, 3150 Horizon Road, Zip 75032; tel. 469/698-1000 **A**1 9 10 **F**3 12 13 15 29 30 40 45 46 47 49 50 67 68 70 75 76 77 79 81 85 93 107 108 110 111 114 118 129 145 146
Primary Contact: Kenneth R. Teel, President
Web address: www.phrtexas.com
**Control:** Corporation, Investor-owned, for-profit **Service:** General Medical and Surgical

**Staffed Beds:** 50 **Admissions:** 3684 **Census:** 33 **Outpatient Visits:** 34207 **Births:** 763 **Total Expense ($000):** 68898 **Personnel:** 403

## ROTAN—Fisher County

**FISHER COUNTY HOSPITAL DISTRICT (451313)**, 774 State Highway 70 North, Zip 79546-4019, Mailing Address: P.O. Drawer F, Zip 79546-4019; tel. 325/735-2256 **A**9 10 18 **F**7 28 32 34 35 40 43 50 53 56 57 59 64 66 75 93 97 107 118 126 132 **P**6
Primary Contact: Steve Lefevre, Administrator
CFO: Debbie Hull, Chief Financial Officer
CMO: C. M. Callan, M.D., Chief of Staff
Web address: www.fishercountyhospital.com
**Control:** Hospital district or authority, Government, nonfederal **Service:** General Medical and Surgical

**Staffed Beds:** 10 **Admissions:** 101 **Census:** 1 **Outpatient Visits:** 21442 **Births:** 0 **Total Expense ($000):** 6956 **Payroll Expense ($000):** 3238 **Personnel:** 72

## ROUND ROCK—Williamson County

☐ **RELIANT REHABILITATION HOSPITAL CENTRAL TEXAS (673032)**, 1400 Hester's Crossing, Zip 78681; tel. 512/244-4400, (Total facility includes 25 beds in nursing home-type unit) **A**1 9 10 **F**3 29 64 68 74 75 79 90 91 93 94 95 96 100 103 127 129 130 147 **S** Reliant Healthcare Partners, Addison, TX
Primary Contact: Abraham Sims, Interim Chief Executive Officer
Web address: www.reliantcentraltx.com/
**Control:** Partnership, Investor-owned, for-profit **Service:** Rehabilitation

**Staffed Beds:** 75 **Admissions:** 1637 **Census:** 56 **Outpatient Visits:** 9067 **Births:** 0 **Total Expense ($000):** 18385 **Payroll Expense ($000):** 9530 **Personnel:** 105

✠ **SCOTT & WHITE HOSPITAL AT ROUND ROCK (670034)**, 300 University Boulevard, Zip 78665-1032; tel. 512/509-0200 **A**1 5 9 10 **F**3 13 15 18 20 22 26 29 30 31 34 35 40 45 46 47 49 51 54 57 59 60 64 68 70 74 75 76 78 79 81 82 85 87 93 97 99 100 104 107 110 111 114 115 118 129 130 143 145 146 147 **P**6 **S** Scott & White Healthcare, Temple, TX
Primary Contact: Ernest L. Bovio, Jr., Chief Executive Officer
CFO: Jason Cole, Senior Director Finance
CMO: Bud Chumbley, M.D., Chief Medical Officer
CHR: Brenda Cox, Director Human Resources
Web address: www.scottandwhite.org
**Control:** Other not-for-profit (including NFP Corporation) **Service:** General Medical and Surgical

**Staffed Beds:** 74 **Admissions:** 4115 **Census:** 37 **Outpatient Visits:** 315237 **Births:** 612 **Total Expense ($000):** 118992 **Payroll Expense ($000):** 42293 **Personnel:** 841

✠ **SETON MEDICAL CENTER WILLIAMSON (670041)**, 201 Seton Parkway, Zip 78665; tel. 512/324-4000 **A**1 5 9 10 **F**3 11 12 13 15 18 20 22 24 26 28 29 30 31 34 35 37 40 43 44 45 46 49 50 51 53 54 57 58 59 60 64 68 70 72 74 75 76 77 78 79 81 82 84 85 86 87 93 96 107 108 110 111 113 114 118 123 125 128 129 130 131 134 145 146 147 **P**3 8 **S** Ascension Health, Saint Louis, MO
Primary Contact: Michelle Robertson, R.N., President and Chief Executive Officer
CFO: Douglas D. Waite, Senior Vice President and Chief Financial Officer
CMO: Hugh V. Gilmore, M.D., Vice President Medical Affairs
CIO: Gerry Lewis, Chief Information Officer
CHR: Thomas Wilken, Vice President Human Resources
Web address: www.seton.net/williamson
**Control:** Church-operated, Nongovernment, not-for profit **Service:** General Medical and Surgical

**Staffed Beds:** 135 **Admissions:** 7308 **Census:** 73 **Outpatient Visits:** 56397 **Births:** 940 **Total Expense ($000):** 136860 **Payroll Expense ($000):** 50863 **Personnel:** 972

✠ **ST. DAVID'S ROUND ROCK MEDICAL CENTER (450718)**, 2400 Round Rock Avenue, Zip 78681-4097; tel. 512/341-1000 **A**1 2 5 9 10 **F**3 11 13 15 18 22 24 26 28 29 30 31 34 35 40 43 47 49 57 59 64 70 73 74 75 76 77 78 79 80 81 84 85 86 87 90 93 107 108 110 111 113 114 118 128 129 131 143 145 146 147 **P**7 8 **S** HCA, Nashville, TN
Primary Contact: Deborah L. Ryle, Administrator and Chief Executive Officer
COO: Tad Hatton, Chief Operating Officer
CFO: Cindy Sexton, Chief Financial Officer
CMO: David Martin, M.D., Vice President Medical Staff Affairs
CHR: Amy Noak, Director Human Resources
Web address: www.stdavids.com
**Control:** Other not-for-profit (including NFP Corporation) **Service:** General Medical and Surgical

**Staffed Beds:** 156 **Admissions:** 7489 **Census:** 83 **Outpatient Visits:** 69261 **Births:** 1719 **Total Expense ($000):** 107660 **Payroll Expense ($000):** 37357 **Personnel:** 593

## ROWLETT—Rockwall County

✠ **LAKE POINTE MEDICAL CENTER (450742)**, 6800 Scenic Drive, Zip 75088-4552, Mailing Address: P.O. Box 1550, Zip 75030-1550; tel. 972/412-2273 **A**1 9 10 **F**3 12 13 15 18 22 29 30 32 34 40 43 45 49 50 53 54 57 59 60 70 72 73 74 75 76 77 78 79 81 85 86 93 107 108 110 111 113 114 116 117 118 119 120 128 129 130 143 145 146 147 **S** TENET Healthcare Corporation, Dallas, TX
Primary Contact: J. Eric Evans, Chief Executive Officer
COO: Jeffrey Patterson, Chief Operating Officer
CFO: Bryan Forry, Chief Financial Officer
CMO: Christopher Cottrell, M.D., Chief of Staff
CIO: Robert Williams, Director Information Systems
CHR: David Olmstead, Associate Administrator and Director Human Resources
Web address: www.lakepointemedical.com
**Control:** Corporation, Investor-owned, for-profit **Service:** General Medical and Surgical

**Staffed Beds:** 112 **Admissions:** 6434 **Census:** 61 **Outpatient Visits:** 76618 **Births:** 1237 **Total Expense ($000):** 74826 **Payroll Expense ($000):** 28305 **Personnel:** 500

## RUSK—Cherokee County

☐ **RUSK STATE HOSPITAL (454009)**, 805 North Dickinson, Zip 75785, Mailing Address: P.O. Box 318, Zip 75785-0318; tel. 903/683-3421 **A**1 9 10 **F**3 30 39 44 50 68 75 86 87 98 103 106 129 134 145 147 **P**6 **S** Texas Department of State Health Services, Austin, TX
Primary Contact: Ted Debbs, Administrator
COO: Lynda Roberson, Senior Program Director
CFO: Frances Long, Chief Financial Officer
CMO: Douglas Johnson, M.D., Clinical Director
CIO: Glenda Bruce, Director Community Relations
Web address: www.mhmr.state.tx.us
**Control:** State-Government, nonfederal **Service:** Psychiatric

**Staffed Beds:** 290 **Admissions:** 914 **Census:** 305 **Outpatient Visits:** 0 **Births:** 0 **Total Expense ($000):** 57778 **Payroll Expense ($000):** 30836 **Personnel:** 916

**TX**

---

**Hospital, Medicare Provider Number, Address, Telephone, Approval, Facility, and Physician Codes, Health Care System**

★ American Hospital Association (AHA) membership
☐ The Joint Commission accreditation      ◇ DNV Healthcare Inc. accreditation
○ American Osteopathic Association (AOA) accreditation
△ Commission on Accreditation of Rehabilitation Facilities (CARF) accreditation

## SAN ANGELO—Tom Green County

☐ **RIVER CREST HOSPITAL (454064)**, 1636 Hunters Glen Road,
Zip 76901–5016; tel. 325/949–5722 **A**1 9 10 **F**4 5 87 98 99 100 101 102
103 104 105 129 131 **S** Universal Health Services, Inc., King of Prussia, PA
Primary Contact: Shelah Adams, Chief Executive Officer
CFO: Frank Urban, Chief Financial Officer
CMO: John Crowley, M.D., Medical Director
CHR: Brenda Coats, Director Human Resources
Web address: www.rivercresthospital.com
**Control:** Corporation, Investor–owned, for–profit **Service:** Psychiatric

**Staffed Beds:** 80 **Admissions:** 1727 **Census:** 37 **Outpatient Visits:** 1548
**Births:** 0 **Total Expense ($000):** 7686 **Payroll Expense ($000):** 3838
**Personnel:** 89

⊠ △ **SAN ANGELO COMMUNITY MEDICAL CENTER (450340)**, 3501
Knickerbocker Road, Zip 76904–7698; tel. 325/949–9511 **A**1 2 7 9 10 **F**3 8 11
13 15 18 20 22 24 28 29 30 31 34 37 40 43 45 49 51 53 54 57 59 60 63
64 68 70 72 74 75 76 78 79 81 82 84 85 89 90 93 107 108 110 111 117
118 128 129 130 134 143 144 145 147 **P**8 **S** Community Health Systems,
Inc., Franklin, TN
Primary Contact: America S. Farrell, FACHE, Interim Chief Executive Officer
CFO: Richard Ervin, Chief Financial Officer
CHR: Lisa Bibb, Director Human Resources
Web address: www.sacmc.com
**Control:** Partnership, Investor–owned, for–profit **Service:** General Medical and
Surgical

**Staffed Beds:** 131 **Admissions:** 5770 **Census:** 69 **Outpatient Visits:** 83890
**Births:** 925 **Total Expense ($000):** 75174 **Payroll Expense ($000):** 31928
**Personnel:** 627

⊠ △ **SHANNON MEDICAL CENTER (450571)**, 120 East Harris Street,
Zip 76903–5976; tel. 325/653–6741, (Includes SHANNON MEDICAL CENTER–
ST. JOHN'S CAMPUS, 2018 Pulliam Street, Zip 76905–5197;
tel. 915/659–7100), (Total facility includes 24 beds in nursing home–type unit)
**A**1 2 3 5 7 9 10 **F**3 7 8 11 13 15 18 20 22 24 26 28 29 30 31 32 34 35 37
38 40 43 45 49 50 51 53 54 56 57 58 59 60 61 62 64 68 70 72 74 74 75
76 77 78 79 80 81 82 84 85 86 87 89 90 92 93 94 96 98 100 101 102 103
107 108 110 111 113 114 116 118 126 127 128 129 130 131 133 143 144
145 146 147 **P**6
Primary Contact: Bryan Horner, President and Chief Executive Officer
CFO: Shane Plymell, Chief Financial Officer
CMO: Irvin Zeitler, D.O., Vice President Medical Affairs
CIO: Tom Perkins, Chief Information Officer
CHR: Teresa Morgan, Assistant Vice President Human Resources
Web address: www.shannonhealth.com
**Control:** Other not–for–profit (including NFP Corporation) **Service:** General
Medical and Surgical

**Staffed Beds:** 278 **Admissions:** 11585 **Census:** 156 **Outpatient Visits:**
111193 **Births:** 1062 **Total Expense ($000):** 184091 **Payroll Expense
($000):** 72669 **Personnel:** 1516

## SAN ANTONIO—Bexar County

☐ **ACUITY HOSPITAL OF SOUTH TEXAS (452040)**, 718 Lexington Avenue,
Zip 78212–4768; tel. 210/572–4600 **A**1 9 10 **F**1 3 29 91 147 **P**8
**S** AcuityHealthcare, LP, Charlotte, NC
Primary Contact: Scott Galliardt, Chief Executive Officer
CFO: Wayne Hegwood, Chief Financial Officer
CFO: Lydia Washington, Controller
CMO: Lovelesh Manocha, M.D., Chief Medical Officer
CHR: Yolanda Ochoa, Director Human Resources
CNO: Emilie Kilpatrick, Chief Clinical Officer
Web address: www.acuityhealthcare.net
**Control:** Corporation, Investor–owned, for–profit **Service:** Long–Term Acute Care
hospital

**Staffed Beds:** 30 **Admissions:** 384 **Census:** 27 **Outpatient Visits:** 0 **Births:**
0 **Total Expense ($000):** 12415 **Payroll Expense ($000):** 6035 **Personnel:**
100

⊠ △ **BAPTIST HEALTH SYSTEM (450058)**, 111 Dallas Street,
Zip 78205–1230; tel. 210/297–7000, (Includes NORTH CENTRAL BAPTIST
HOSPITAL, 520 Madison Oak Drive, Zip 78258–3912; tel. 210/297–4000;
NORTHEAST BAPTIST HOSPITAL, 8811 Village Drive, Zip 78217–5440;
tel. 210/297–2000; Matthew Stone, Chief Executive Officer; SOUTHEAST
BAPTIST HOSPITAL, 4214 East Southcross Boulevard, Zip 78222–3740;
tel. 210/297–3000; Andrew M. Harris, Chief Executive Officer; ST. LUKE'S
BAPTIST HOSPITAL, 7930 Floyd Curl Drive, Zip 78229–0100;
tel. 210/297–5000; Graham D. Reeve, Chief Executive Officer) **A**1 2 3 5 7 9 10
**F**3 11 12 13 14 15 17 18 19 20 22 24 26 28 29 30 31 35 37 38 40 41 43
44 45 46 47 50 55 56 57 59 60 64 65 68 70 72 73 74 75 76 77 78 79 80
81 82 85 86 87 88 89 90 91 92 93 95 96 98 101 102 103 107 108 111 113
114 115 116 118 123 125 128 129 131 134 144 145 146 147 **P**8
**S** Vanguard Health System, Nashville, TN
Primary Contact: David S. Goldberg, President
COO: Philip J. Noel, III, Assistant Administrator and Chief Operating Officer
CFO: Linda Kirks, Chief Financial Officer
CMO: Carol Wratten, M.D., Interim Chief Medical Officer
CIO: Gary Davis, Vice President Information Systems
CHR: Sarah Spinharney, Senior Vice President
Web address: www.baptisthealthsystem.com
**Control:** Partnership, Investor–owned, for–profit **Service:** General Medical and
Surgical

**Staffed Beds:** 1342 **Admissions:** 63438 **Census:** 774 **Outpatient Visits:**
288607 **Births:** 10169 **Total Expense ($000):** 711581 **Payroll Expense
($000):** 292513 **Personnel:** 5668

⊠ **CHRISTUS SANTA ROSA HEALTH CARE (450237)**, 333 North Santa Rosa
Street, Zip 78207–3108; tel. 210/704–4184, (Includes CHRISTUS SANTA ROSA
CHILDREN'S HOSPITAL, 333 North Santa Rosa Street, Zip 78207;
tel. 210/704–2011; Marcy Doderer, Vice President and Administrator; CHRISTUS
SANTA ROSA REHABILITATION HOSPITAL, 2827 Babcock Road, Zip 78229–4813;
tel. 210/705–6300) **A**1 3 5 9 10 **F**3 8 11 12 13 15 18 19 20 21 22 23 24 25
26 27 28 29 30 32 34 35 37 39 40 41 43 45 46 48 49 54 55 56 57 58 59
60 63 64 65 67 70 71 72 73 74 75 76 77 78 79 80 81 82 83 84 85 86 87
88 89 90 93 96 97 104 107 108 110 111 113 114 116 117 118 125 128
129 131 133 136 137 138 139 141 145 146 **P**6 **S** CHRISTUS Health, Irving, TX
Primary Contact: Patrick Brian Carrier, President and Chief Executive Officer
COO: Val Baciarelli, Chief Operating Officer
CFO: Shawn Barnett, Vice President and Chief Financial Officer
CMO: James C. Martin, M.D., Vice President and Chief Medical Officer
CIO: Steve Martin, Chief Information Officer
CHR: Fernando Fleites, Vice President Human Resources
Web address: www.christussantarosa.org
**Control:** Church–operated, Nongovernment, not–for profit **Service:** General
Medical and Surgical

**Staffed Beds:** 778 **Admissions:** 32305 **Census:** 455 **Outpatient Visits:**
412728 **Births:** 3690 **Total Expense ($000):** 548526 **Payroll Expense
($000):** 202344 **Personnel:** 3355

**CLARITY CHILD GUIDANCE CENTER**, 8535 Tom Slick, Zip 78229–3363;
tel. 210/616–0300 **A**5 9 **F**29 41 98 99 101 102 104 105 106 129
Primary Contact: Frederick W. Hines, President
CFO: Michael Bernick, Vice President Finance
CMO: Graham Rogeness, M.D., Medical Director
CHR: Gina Massey, Vice President Human Resources
Web address: www.claritycgc.org
**Control:** Other not–for–profit (including NFP Corporation) **Service:** Children's
hospital psychiatric

**Staffed Beds:** 52 **Admissions:** 1632 **Census:** 38 **Outpatient Visits:** 12269
**Births:** 0 **Total Expense ($000):** 15067 **Payroll Expense ($000):** 9171
**Personnel:** 221

☐ **FOUNDATION SURGICAL HOSPITAL OF SAN ANTONIO (670054)**, 9522
Huebner Road, Zip 78240; tel. 210/478–5400, (Nonreporting) **A**1 10 21
Primary Contact: Robert Trussell, Administrator
Web address: www.fshsanantonio.com/bariatric–foundation–surgical.html
**Control:** Corporation, Investor–owned, for–profit **Service:** General Medical and
Surgical

**Staffed Beds:** 20

○ **GLOBALREHAB HOSPITAL – SAN ANTONIO (673040)**, 19126 Stonehue
Road, Zip 78258–3490; tel. 210/482–3400 **A**9 10 11 **F**3 29 75 90 96 129
**S** GLOBALREHAB, Dallas, TX
Primary Contact: Travis Rich, Chief Executive Officer
Web address: www.globalrehabhospitals.com
**Control:** Partnership, Investor–owned, for–profit **Service:** Rehabilitation

**Staffed Beds:** 42 **Admissions:** 891 **Census:** 32 **Outpatient Visits:** 0 **Births:**
0 **Total Expense ($000):** 14027 **Payroll Expense ($000):** 6778 **Personnel:**
109

*Many Facility Codes have changed. Please refer to the AHA Guide Code Chart.* © 2012 AHA Guide

☒ **HEALTHSOUTH REHABILITATION INSTITUTE OF SAN ANTONIO (453031)**, 9119 Cinnamon Hill, Zip 78240–5401; tel. 210/691–0737 **A**1 9 10 **F**29 62 64 75 90 91 93 94 96 129 131 147 **P**5 **S** HEALTHSOUTH Corporation, Birmingham, AL
Primary Contact: Scott Butcher, Chief Executive Officer
CFO: Larry Spriggs, Controller
CMO: Richard Senelick, M.D., Medical Director
CHR: Vanessa Tejada, Manager Human Resources
Web address: www.hsriosa.com
**Control:** Corporation, Investor–owned, for–profit **Service:** Rehabilitation

**Staffed Beds:** 96 **Admissions:** 1323 **Census:** 55 **Outpatient Visits:** 11933 **Births:** 0 **Total Expense ($000):** 19648 **Payroll Expense ($000):** 10135 **Personnel:** 191

☒ **KINDRED HOSPITAL–SAN ANTONIO (452016)**, 3636 Medical Drive, Zip 78229–3184; tel. 210/616–0616 **A**1 9 10 **F**1 3 29 30 70 85 87 129 147 **S** Kindred Healthcare, Louisville, KY
Primary Contact: Katherine Eskew, Chief Executive Officer
CFO: Erin Russell, Controller
CMO: Charles Duncan, M.D., Medical Director
CHR: Brian Mosley, Coordinator Human Resources and Payroll Benefits
Web address: www.khsanantonio.com/
**Control:** Corporation, Investor–owned, for–profit **Service:** Long–Term Acute Care hospital

**Staffed Beds:** 59 **Admissions:** 483 **Census:** 36 **Outpatient Visits:** 12 **Births:** 0 **Total Expense ($000):** 20305 **Payroll Expense ($000):** 7744 **Personnel:** 133

☐ **LAUREL RIDGE TREATMENT CENTER (454060)**, 17720 Corporate Woods Drive, Zip 78259–3500; tel. 210/491–9400 **A**1 3 5 9 10 **F**5 29 35 38 75 77 98 99 100 101 103 105 106 129 131 **S** Universal Health Services, Inc., King of Prussia, PA
Primary Contact: Dan Thomas, Chief Executive Officer
COO: Shawn Owens, Chief Operating Officer
CFO: Laura Brown, Chief Financial Officer
CMO: Benigno J. Fernandez, M.D., Executive Medical Director
CHR: Brenda Frederick, Director Human Resources
CNO: Kathy Rosetta, Chief Nursing Officer
Web address: www.laurelridgetc.com
**Control:** Partnership, Investor–owned, for–profit **Service:** Psychiatric

**Staffed Beds:** 190 **Admissions:** 6123 **Census:** 155 **Outpatient Visits:** 16932 **Births:** 0 **Total Expense ($000):** 40761 **Payroll Expense ($000):** 18185 **Personnel:** 339

☒ **LIFECARE HOSPITALS OF SAN ANTONIO (452059)**, 8026 Floyd Curl Drive, Zip 78229–3915; tel. 210/690–7000 **A**1 9 10 **F**1 3 29 45 75 77 85 86 87 96 97 107 113 129 147 **S** LifeCare Management Services, Plano, TX
Primary Contact: Randell G. Stokes, Administrator
Web address: www.lifecare–hospitals.com
**Control:** Corporation, Investor–owned, for–profit **Service:** Long–Term Acute Care hospital

**Staffed Beds:** 62 **Admissions:** 628 **Census:** 54 **Outpatient Visits:** 0 **Births:** 0 **Total Expense ($000):** 27164 **Payroll Expense ($000):** 11786 **Personnel:** 237

☒ **METHODIST AMBULATORY SURGERY HOSPITAL (450780)**, 9150 Huebner Road, Suite 100, Zip 78240–1545; tel. 210/575–5000 **A**1 9 10 **F**3 29 37 40 68 79 81 85 87 **P**8 **S** HCA, Nashville, TN
Primary Contact: Elaine F. Morris, Administrator
CFO: Tim Carr, Chief Financial Officer
Web address: www.mas.sahealth.com
**Control:** Partnership, Investor–owned, for–profit **Service:** General Medical and Surgical

**Staffed Beds:** 23 **Admissions:** 784 **Census:** 6 **Outpatient Visits:** 9491 **Births:** 0 **Total Expense ($000):** 24708 **Payroll Expense ($000):** 7013 **Personnel:** 115

☒ **METHODIST HOSPITAL (450388)**, 7700 Floyd Curl Drive, Zip 78229–3993; tel. 210/575–4000, (Includes METHODIST CHILDREN'S HOSPITAL OF SOUTH TEXAS, 7700 Floyd Curl Drive, Zip 78229–3383; tel. 210/575–7000; Mark McLoone, Chief Executive Officer; METHODIST SPECIALTY AND TRANSPLANT HOSPITAL, 8026 Floyd Curl Drive, Zip 78229–3915; tel. 210/575–4000; METROPOLITAN METHODIST HOSPITAL, 1310 McCullough Avenue, Zip 78212–2617; tel. 210/757–2200; Dominic J. Dominguez, Interim Chief Executive Officer; NORTHEAST METHODIST HOSPITAL, 12412 Judson Road, Live Oak, Zip 78233–3255; tel. 210/650–4949) **A**1 2 3 5 9 10 **F**3 4 5 8 11 12 13 15 17 18 19 20 21 22 23 24 25 26 27 28 29 30 31 34 35 38 40 41 42 43 44 45 46 47 48 49 51 53 54 56 57 58 59 60 64 65 68 70 72 74 75 76 77 78 79 80 81 82 84 85 86 87 88 89 90 93 95 96 98 100 101 102 103 104 105 107 108 111 113 114 118 120 123 125 126 128 129 131 134 135 136 137 138 141 142 144 145 146 147 **P**7 **S** HCA, Nashville, TN
Primary Contact: Gay Nord, Chief Executive Officer
COO: Michael E. Beaver, Chief Operating Officer
CFO: Nancy Meadows, Chief Financial Officer
CMO: Russell Woodward, M.D., Chief Medical Officer
CIO: Eddie Cuellar, Vice President Information Systems
CHR: Nancy Edgar, Vice President Human Resources
Web address: www.sahealth.com
**Control:** Partnership, Investor–owned, for–profit **Service:** General Medical and Surgical

**Staffed Beds:** 1484 **Admissions:** 74904 **Census:** 1016 **Outpatient Visits:** 431528 **Births:** 8807 **Total Expense ($000):** 1008735 **Payroll Expense ($000):** 343797 **Personnel:** 5755

☒ **METHODIST STONE OAK HOSPITAL (670055)**, 1139 East Sonterra Boulevard, Zip 78258; tel. 210/638–2100 **A**1 9 10 **F**3 13 15 18 20 22 24 29 30 31 34 38 40 44 45 46 47 49 57 59 60 64 65 68 70 72 74 75 76 77 78 79 80 81 82 85 86 87 107 108 111 114 117 118 125 129 144 145 146 **S** HCA, Nashville, TN
Primary Contact: Dean M. Alexander, Chief Executive Officer
Web address: www.stoneoakhealth.com
**Control:** Partnership, Investor–owned, for–profit **Service:** General Medical and Surgical

**Staffed Beds:** 134 **Admissions:** 7932 **Census:** 81 **Outpatient Visits:** 35881 **Births:** 1066 **Total Expense ($000):** 114196 **Payroll Expense ($000):** 31636 **Personnel:** 470

**METHODIST TEXSAN HOSPITAL (450878)**, 6700 IH–10 West, Zip 78201; tel. 210/736–6700, (Nonreporting) **A**9 10
Primary Contact: P. Craig Desmond, President
Web address: www.texsanhearthospital.com
**Control:** Corporation, Investor–owned, for–profit **Service:** General Medical and Surgical

**Staffed Beds:** 75

☐ **NIX HEALTH CARE SYSTEM (450130)**, 414 Navarro Street, Zip 78205–2522; tel. 210/271–1800 **A**1 3 5 9 10 **F**3 5 12 15 18 20 22 24 26 29 30 31 35 40 44 45 49 56 57 59 60 62 64 68 70 74 75 78 79 81 82 85 87 90 93 97 98 99 103 107 108 111 113 117 118 128 129 141 142 145 146 147 Primary Contact: John F. Strieby, Chief Executive Officer
COO: Thomas Klawiter, Senior Vice President and Chief Operating Officer
CFO: Lester Surrock, Chief Financial Officer
CMO: Lisa A. Davis, M.D., Chief of Staff
CIO: Steve Kinkaid, Vice President Technology
CHR: Richard Lance, Vice President Human Resources
Web address: www.nixhealth.com
**Control:** Partnership, Investor–owned, for–profit **Service:** General Medical and Surgical

**Staffed Beds:** 160 **Admissions:** 7423 **Census:** 113 **Outpatient Visits:** 132193 **Births:** 0 **Total Expense ($000):** 94734 **Payroll Expense ($000):** 33092 **Personnel:** 712

☐ **PROMISE HOSPITAL OF SAN ANTONIO (452090)**, 7400 Barlite Boulevard, 2nd Floor, Zip 78224; tel. 210/921–3550 **A**1 9 10 **F**1 3 29 30 87 129 147 **S** Promise Healthcare, Boca Raton, FL
Primary Contact: Karen Pitcher, Vice President and Chief Executive Officer
CHR: Margaret Silva, Executive Assistant and Coordinator Human Resources
CNO: Sharon Schirmer, R.N., Chief Clinical Officer
Web address: www.promise–sanantonio.com
**Control:** Corporation, Investor–owned, for–profit **Service:** Long–Term Acute Care hospital

**Staffed Beds:** 26 **Admissions:** 169 **Census:** 13 **Outpatient Visits:** 0 **Births:** 0 **Total Expense ($000):** 7138 **Payroll Expense ($000):** 3437 **Personnel:** 73

**TX**

---

**Hospital, Medicare Provider Number, Address, Telephone, Approval, Facility, and Physician Codes, Health Care System**

★ American Hospital Association (AHA) membership
☐ The Joint Commission accreditation  ◇ DNV Healthcare Inc. accreditation
◯ American Osteopathic Association (AOA) accreditation
△ Commission on Accreditation of Rehabilitation Facilities (CARF) accreditation

☐ **SAN ANTONIO STATE HOSPITAL (454011)**, 6711 South New Braunfels, Suite 100, Zip 78223–3006; tel. 210/531–7711 **A**1 5 9 10 **F**30 39 53 56 57 59 68 75 77 86 87 98 99 100 101 103 106 129 131 134 145 **P**1 **S** Texas Department of State Health Services, Austin, TX
Primary Contact: Robert C. Arizpe, Superintendent
CFO: Janie Rabago, Chief Accountant
CMO: Terresa Stallworth, M.D., Clinical Director
CIO: Chris Stanush, Director Information Management
CHR: Renee Bourland, Human Resources Specialist
CNO: Maria DC Ostrander, R.N., Chief Nurse Executive
Web address: www.dshs.state.tx.us
**Control:** State–Government, nonfederal **Service:** Psychiatric

**Staffed Beds:** 302 **Admissions:** 1839 **Census:** 276 **Outpatient Visits:** 0 **Births:** 0 **Total Expense ($000):** 60595 **Payroll Expense ($000):** 33287 **Personnel:** 839

☒ **SELECT SPECIALTY HOSPITAL–SAN ANTONIO (452073)**, 111 Dallas Street, 4th Floor, Zip 78205; tel. 210/297–7185 **A**1 9 10 **F**1 29 147 **P**8 **S** Select Medical Corporation, Mechanicsburg, PA
Primary Contact: Sean Stricker, Chief Executive Officer
Web address: www.selectmedicalcorp.com
**Control:** Corporation, Investor–owned, for–profit **Service:** Long–Term Acute Care hospital

**Staffed Beds:** 44 **Admissions:** 518 **Census:** 39 **Outpatient Visits:** 0 **Births:** 0 **Total Expense ($000):** 20055 **Payroll Expense ($000):** 6926 **Personnel:** 132

☐ **SOUTH TEXAS SPINE AND SURGICAL HOSPITAL (450856)**, 18600 Hardy Oak Boulevard, Zip 78258; tel. 210/507–4090 **A**1 5 9 10 **F**3 29 40 41 64 75 77 79 81 85 86 87 **S** National Surgical Hospitals, Chicago, IL
Primary Contact: Debbie Kelly, Chief Executive Officer
CFO: Sylvia Garcia, Chief Accounting Officer
CHR: Sally Hall, Manager Human Resources
Web address: www.shst.net
**Control:** Partnership, Investor–owned, for–profit **Service:** General Medical and Surgical

**Staffed Beds:** 30 **Admissions:** 1121 **Census:** 8 **Outpatient Visits:** 2644 **Births:** 0 **Total Expense ($000):** 26064 **Payroll Expense ($000):** 5361 **Personnel:** 97

☒ △ **SOUTH TEXAS VETERANS HEALTH CARE SYSTEM**, 7400 Merton Minter Boulevard, Zip 78284–5799; tel. 210/617–5140, (Includes KERRVILLE DIVISION, 3600 Memorial Boulevard, Kerrville, Zip 78028; tel. 210/896–2020; SAN ANTONIO DIVISION, 7400 Merton Minter Boulevard, tel. 210/617–5300), (Nonreporting) **A**1 3 5 7 8 9 **S** Department of Veterans Affairs, Washington, DC
Primary Contact: Marie L. Weldon, FACHE, Director
CFO: I. M. Rachal, Chief Fiscal Service
CMO: Richard Bauer, M.D., Chief of Staff
CIO: Simon Willett, Director Administrative Operations
CHR: Leslie Cruthirds, Chief Human Resource Management Service
Web address: www.vasthcs.med.va.gov
**Control:** Veterans Affairs, Government, federal **Service:** General Medical and Surgical

**Staffed Beds:** 838

**SOUTHWEST GENERAL HOSPITAL (450697)**, 7400 Barlite Boulevard, Zip 78224–1399; tel. 210/921–2000 **A**9 10 21 **F**3 12 13 15 18 20 22 24 26 29 30 35 37 40 43 44 45 46 49 50 51 54 56 57 59 60 64 65 70 72 74 75 76 77 78 79 80 81 85 87 90 93 98 100 102 103 105 107 108 110 111 113 114 118 125 128 129 131 134 145 146 147 **S** IASIS Healthcare, Franklin, TN
Primary Contact: Gregory Padilla, Chief Executive Officer
COO: Trey Klawiter, Chief Operating Officer
CFO: Joe Sereno, Interim Chief Financial Officer
CMO: Damaso Oliva, M.D., Chief Medical Officer
CIO: Sam Sowder, Director Information Systems
CHR: Christina Rivera, Director Human Resources
Web address: www.swgeneralhospital.com
**Control:** Corporation, Investor–owned, for–profit **Service:** General Medical and Surgical

**Staffed Beds:** 265 **Admissions:** 9985 **Census:** 134 **Outpatient Visits:** 84594 **Births:** 1861 **Total Expense ($000):** 108030 **Payroll Expense ($000):** 41273 **Personnel:** 612

**ST. LUKE'S BAPTIST HOSPITAL** See Baptist Health System

☐ **TEXAS CENTER FOR INFECTIOUS DISEASE (452033)**, 2303 S.E. Military Drive, Zip 78223–3597; tel. 210/534–8857 **A**1 10 **F**1 3 29 30 50 53 54 61 64 68 75 87 129 131 134 142 145 **P**4 6 **S** Texas Department of State Health Services, Austin, TX
Primary Contact: James N. Elkins, FACHE, Director
COO: Peggy Perry, Assistant Director
CFO: Glenda Armstrong–Huff, Assistant Superintendent
CMO: David Griffith, M.D., Medical Director
CIO: Andre Avant, Facility Automation Manager
CHR: Gerald Shackelford, Staff Support Specialist
CNO: Rebecca Sanchez, R.N., Director of Nursing
Web address: www.dshs.state.tx.us/tcid
**Control:** State–Government, nonfederal **Service:** Tuberculosis and other respiratory diseases

**Staffed Beds:** 75 **Admissions:** 78 **Census:** 39 **Outpatient Visits:** 874 **Births:** 0 **Total Expense ($000):** 12866 **Payroll Expense ($000):** 5766 **Personnel:** 165

☒ **UNIVERSITY HEALTH SYSTEM (450213)**, 4502 Medical Drive, Zip 78229–4493; tel. 210/358–4000, (Includes UNIVERSITY HEALTH CENTER – DOWNTOWN, 4502 Medical Drive, tel. 210/358–3400; UNIVERSITY HOSPITAL, 4502 Medical Drive, tel. 210/358–4000) **A**1 2 3 5 8 9 10 **F**3 4 7 11 13 14 15 16 17 18 20 22 24 26 28 29 30 31 32 34 35 38 40 41 43 44 45 46 47 48 49 50 51 52 53 54 55 56 57 58 59 61 64 65 66 68 70 72 73 74 75 76 77 78 79 80 81 82 83 84 85 86 87 88 89 90 92 93 96 98 100 101 102 107 109 110 111 113 114 117 118 123 125 128 129 131 134 137 138 139 140 141 142 143 144 145 146 147 **P**6
Primary Contact: George B. Hernandez, Jr., President and Chief Executive Officer
COO: Chris Vasquez, Executive Vice President and Chief Operating Officer
CFO: Peggy Deming, Executive Vice President and Chief Financial Officer
CIO: Bill Phillips, Vice President Information Services
CHR: Theresa Scepanski, Vice President People and Organizational Development
Web address: www.universityhealthsystem.com
**Control:** Hospital district or authority, Government, nonfederal **Service:** General Medical and Surgical

**Staffed Beds:** 379 **Admissions:** 19799 **Census:** 349 **Outpatient Visits:** 2075105 **Births:** 2864 **Total Expense ($000):** 847530 **Payroll Expense ($000):** 254780 **Personnel:** 5269

☐ **VICTORY MEDICAL CENTER – SAN ANTONIO (670021)**, 4243 East Southcross Boulevard, Zip 78222; tel. 210/368–7400 **A**1 10 **F**3 8 12 29 40 45 75 79 81 82 85 86 87 131
Primary Contact: Paul H. Ballard, Chief Executive Officer
Web address: www.innovahealth.net
**Control:** Partnership, Investor–owned, for–profit **Service:** Surgical

**Staffed Beds:** 9 **Admissions:** 488 **Census:** 3 **Outpatient Visits:** 926 **Births:** 0 **Total Expense ($000):** 33871 **Payroll Expense ($000):** 4120 **Personnel:** 73

☐ **WARM SPRINGS REHABILITATION HOSPITAL (453035)**, 5101 Medical Drive, Zip 78229–6098; tel. 210/616–0100, (Total facility includes 4 beds in nursing home–type unit) **A**1 5 9 10 **F**3 11 29 30 57 64 68 74 75 79 82 90 91 93 94 96 127 129 131 145 147 **S** Post Acute Medical, LLC, Camp Hill, PA
Primary Contact: Dennis Falck, Chief Executive Officer
CFO: James Asberry, Chief Financial Officer
CMO: Alex Willingham, M.D., Medical Director
CIO: Rick Marek, Vice President Medical Information Systems
CHR: Waynea Finley, System Director Human Resources
Web address: www.warmsprings.org
**Control:** Partnership, Investor–owned, for–profit **Service:** Rehabilitation

**Staffed Beds:** 64 **Admissions:** 1414 **Census:** 52 **Outpatient Visits:** 29350 **Births:** 0 **Total Expense ($000):** 23645 **Payroll Expense ($000):** 11773 **Personnel:** 232

**SAN AUGUSTINE—San Augustine County**

**MEMORIAL MEDICAL CENTER – SAN AUGUSTINE (451360)**, 511 East Hospital Street, Zip 75972–2121, Mailing Address: P.O. Box 658, Zip 75972–0658; tel. 936/275–3446 **A**9 10 18 **F**29 35 40 57 59 64 102 107 118 131 132 **S** Memorial Health System of East Texas, Lufkin, TX
Primary Contact: Darlene Williams, R.N., Administrator
CFO: Kristi Gay, Chief Financial Officer
Web address: www.memorialhealth.org
**Control:** Other not–for–profit (including NFP Corporation) **Service:** General Medical and Surgical

**Staffed Beds:** 18 **Admissions:** 371 **Census:** 3 **Outpatient Visits:** 16659 **Births:** 0 **Total Expense ($000):** 5948 **Payroll Expense ($000):** 2824 **Personnel:** 50

*Many Facility Codes have changed. Please refer to the AHA Guide Code Chart.* © 2012 AHA Guide

## SAN MARCOS—Hays County

☒ **CENTRAL TEXAS MEDICAL CENTER (450272)**, 1301 Wonder World Drive, Zip 78666–7544; tel. 512/353–8979 **A**1 9 10 **F**3 5 11 13 15 18 20 29 30 32 34 35 39 40 43 44 45 49 50 51 56 57 59 60 62 63 64 65 68 70 72 75 76 77 79 80 81 82 85 86 87 92 93 94 103 107 108 111 113 115 116 117 118 128 129 130 131 145 146 147 **P**6 8 **S** Adventist Health System Sunbelt Health Care Corporation, Altamonte Springs, FL
Primary Contact: Sam Huenergardt, President and Chief Executive Officer
CFO: Richard Boggess, Chief Financial Officer
CHR: Debbie D. Cox, Administrative Director Human Resources
Web address: www.ctmc.org
**Control:** Church–operated, Nongovernment, not–for profit **Service:** General Medical and Surgical

**Staffed Beds:** 178 **Admissions:** 4637 **Census:** 44 **Outpatient Visits:** 66164 **Births:** 1001 **Total Expense ($000):** 78578 **Payroll Expense ($000):** 29399 **Personnel:** 544

## SEGUIN—Guadalupe County

☒ **GUADALUPE REGIONAL MEDICAL CENTER (450104)**, 1215 East Court Street, Zip 78155–5189; tel. 830/379–2411 **A**1 9 10 **F**3 5 11 13 15 18 28 29 30 31 34 40 43 45 46 49 50 51 53 56 59 60 62 63 64 68 70 74 75 76 77 78 79 81 82 84 85 86 87 92 93 102 103 104 107 108 110 111 112 113 117 118 128 129 131 142 144 145 147 **P**1
Primary Contact: Robert Haynes, FACHE, Chief Executive Officer
COO: Lauren Carter, Associate Administrator
CFO: Penny Wallace, Chief Financial Officer
CMO: Steve White, M.D., Chief Medical Officer
CIO: Steve Ratliff, Director Information
CHR: Fay Bennett, Director Human Resources
Web address: www.grmedcenter.com
**Control:** City–County, Government, nonfederal **Service:** General Medical and Surgical

**Staffed Beds:** 110 **Admissions:** 4575 **Census:** 46 **Outpatient Visits:** 126920 **Births:** 711 **Total Expense ($000):** 77967 **Payroll Expense ($000):** 29748 **Personnel:** 622

## SEMINOLE—Gaines County

★ **MEMORIAL HOSPITAL (451358)**, 209 N.W. Eighth Street, Zip 79360–3447; tel. 432/758–5811 **A**9 10 18 **F**3 10 11 13 28 29 30 32 34 35 40 43 45 53 56 57 59 62 63 64 65 75 76 81 83 97 102 107 113 118 129 130 131 132 142 145 146 147
Primary Contact: Betsy Briscoe, Chief Executive Officer
CFO: Traci Anderson, Chief Financial Officer
CMO: Jean–Pierre Letellier, M.D., Chief of Staff
Web address: www.seminolehospitaldistrict.com
**Control:** Hospital district or authority, Government, nonfederal **Service:** General Medical and Surgical

**Staffed Beds:** 25 **Admissions:** 800 **Census:** 10 **Outpatient Visits:** 39539 **Births:** 202 **Total Expense ($000):** 20055 **Payroll Expense ($000):** 6055 **Personnel:** 170

## SEYMOUR—Baylor County

**SEYMOUR HOSPITAL (450586)**, 200 Stadium Drive, Zip 76380–2344; tel. 940/889–5572 **A**9 10 20 **F**2 3 7 11 13 14 28 29 34 36 40 43 45 50 53 56 57 59 62 64 65 66 68 70 75 76 81 85 86 87 93 94 100 102 103 104 107 118 126 129 132 134 145 146 147 **P**1
Primary Contact: Leslie Hardin, Chief Executive Officer and Chief Financial Officer
CFO: Leslie Hardin, Chief Executive Officer and Chief Financial Officer
CMO: Richard Niles, M.D., Chief of Staff
CHR: Linda Moore, Manager Human Resources
Web address: www.seymourhospital.com/
**Control:** Hospital district or authority, Government, nonfederal **Service:** General Medical and Surgical

**Staffed Beds:** 38 **Admissions:** 528 **Census:** 7 **Outpatient Visits:** 31171 **Births:** 48 **Total Expense ($000):** 8211 **Payroll Expense ($000):** 4495 **Personnel:** 117

## SHAMROCK—Wheeler County

**SHAMROCK GENERAL HOSPITAL (451340)**, 1000 South Main Street, Zip 79079–2896; tel. 806/256–2114 **A**9 10 18 **F**7 11 29 32 40 43 63 65 68 93 107 118 126 129 132 **P**4
Primary Contact: Wiley M. Fires, Administrator
CFO: Wiley M. Fires, Administrator
CHR: Cecille Williams, Assistant Administrator
**Control:** Hospital district or authority, Government, nonfederal **Service:** General Medical and Surgical

**Staffed Beds:** 13 **Admissions:** 115 **Census:** 1 **Outpatient Visits:** 18052 **Births:** 1 **Total Expense ($000):** 4495 **Payroll Expense ($000):** 2021 **Personnel:** 74

## SHENANDOAH—Montgomery County

☐ **NEXUS SPECIALTY HOSPITAL**, 123 Vision Park Boulevard, Zip 77384; tel. 281/364–0317 **A**1 9 21 **F**1 3 29 64 70 74 75 85 100 107 114 118 129 131 147 **S** Nexus Health Systems, Houston, TX
Primary Contact: Erin Cassidy, Chief Executive Officer
COO: Guido J. Cubellis, Chief Operating Officer
CFO: Julia Hatton, Chief Financial Officer
CMO: Ather Siddiqi, M.D., Medical Director
CIO: Deepak Chaudhry, Vice President Information Technology
CHR: Guy Murdock, Vice President Human Resources
CNO: Natalie Munoz, Director of Clinical Services
Web address: www.nexusspecialty.com
**Control:** Partnership, Investor–owned, for–profit **Service:** Long–Term Acute Care hospital

**Staffed Beds:** 75 **Admissions:** 662 **Census:** 53 **Outpatient Visits:** 12 **Births:** 0 **Total Expense ($000):** 26181 **Payroll Expense ($000):** 10944 **Personnel:** 217

☐ **RELIANT REHABILITATION HOSPITAL NORTH HOUSTON (673034)**, 117 Vision Park Boulevard, Zip 77384–3001; tel. 936/444–1700 **A**1 9 10 **F**29 60 64 68 75 77 90 91 93 94 95 96 129 147 **S** Reliant Healthcare Partners, Addison, TX
Primary Contact: Abraham Sims, Chief Executive Officer
CFO: Terri Weiss, Chief Financial Officer
Web address: www.reliantnorthhouston.com/
**Control:** Partnership, Investor–owned, for–profit **Service:** Rehabilitation

**Staffed Beds:** 60 **Admissions:** 1704 **Census:** 49 **Outpatient Visits:** 11806 **Births:** 0 **Total Expense ($000):** 25141 **Payroll Expense ($000):** 9516 **Personnel:** 163

## SHERMAN—Grayson County

**CARRUS REHABILITATION HOSPITAL (673041)**, 1810 West U.S. Highway 82, Suite 100, Zip 75092–7069; tel. 903/870–2600 **A**10 21 **F**3 29 40 41 44 65 74 75 77 79 85 86 87 90 91 96 129 **S** Carrus Hospitals, Sherman, TX
Primary Contact: Ronald E. Dorris, Chief Executive Officer
Web address: www.carrushospital.com
**Control:** Corporation, Investor–owned, for–profit **Service:** Rehabilitation

**Staffed Beds:** 24 **Admissions:** 441 **Census:** 16 **Outpatient Visits:** 0 **Births:** 0 **Total Expense ($000):** 5322 **Payroll Expense ($000):** 2299 **Personnel:** 31

**CARRUS SPECIALTY HOSPITAL (452041)**, 1810 West U.S. Highway 82, Zip 75092–7069; tel. 903/870–2600 **A**9 10 21 **F**1 3 29 40 41 44 56 65 74 75 77 78 79 83 85 86 87 91 128 129 147 **S** Carrus Hospitals, Sherman, TX
Primary Contact: Ronald E. Dorris, Chief Executive Officer
CFO: Michael Exline, Chief Financial Officer
CHR: Diane Swenson, Director of Staff Services and Chief Nursing Officer
CNO: Diane Swenson, Director of Staff Services and Chief Nursing Officer
Web address: www.carrushospital.com
**Control:** Corporation, Investor–owned, for–profit **Service:** Long–Term Acute Care hospital

**Staffed Beds:** 16 **Admissions:** 189 **Census:** 13 **Outpatient Visits:** 171 **Births:** 0 **Total Expense ($000):** 7275 **Payroll Expense ($000):** 2559 **Personnel:** 43

**HERITAGE PARK SURGICAL HOSPITAL (670076)**, 3601 North Calais Street, Zip 75090; tel. 903/870–0999 **A**21 **F**8 29 34 35 40 46 49 51 54 57 68 79 81 82 85 86 87 107 111 113 118 128 **P**8
Primary Contact: DeAnn Sutton, Chief Executive Officer
Web address: www.heritageparksurgicalhospital.com
**Control:** State–Government, nonfederal **Service:** General Medical and Surgical

**Staffed Beds:** 12 **Admissions:** 251 **Census:** 2 **Outpatient Visits:** 18892 **Births:** 0 **Total Expense ($000):** 23026 **Payroll Expense ($000):** 5398 **Personnel:** 135

**LIFE CENTER SPECIALTY HOSPITAL (673037)**, 1111 Gallagher Drive, Zip 75090–1713; tel. 903/870–7000, (Nonreporting) **A**9 10
Primary Contact: Louis Bradley, Chief Executive Officer
Web address: www.lifecenterhospital.org
**Control:** Other not–for–profit (including NFP Corporation) **Service:** Other specialty

**Staffed Beds:** 59

**TX**

---

**Hospital, Medicare Provider Number, Address, Telephone, Approval, Facility, and Physician Codes, Health Care System**

★ American Hospital Association (AHA) membership
☐ The Joint Commission accreditation ◇ DNV Healthcare Inc. accreditation

○ American Osteopathic Association (AOA) accreditation
△ Commission on Accreditation of Rehabilitation Facilities (CARF) accreditation

⊠ **TEXAS HEALTH PRESBYTERIAN HOSPITAL–WNJ (450469)**, 500 North Highland Avenue, Zip 75092–7354; tel. 903/870–4611 **A**1 9 10 **F**3 11 13 15 17 18 20 22 24 26 28 29 30 31 35 40 41 45 49 53 54 56 57 58 59 61 64 70 74 76 77 78 79 80 81 84 86 87 89 93 96 100 103 106 107 108 111 117 118 126 129 131 145 146 147 **S** LHP Hospital Group, Plano, TX
Primary Contact: Vance V. Reynolds, FACHE, CPA, Chief Executive Officer
CFO: Mitch Mulvehill, Senior Vice President and Chief Financial Officer
CMO: Gary Marlow, M.D., President Medical Staff
CIO: Tom Fitzgerald, Manager Information Technology Service Delivery
CHR: Linda Creswell, Director Human Resources
Web address: www.wnj.org
**Control:** Partnership, Investor–owned, for–profit **Service:** General Medical and Surgical

**Staffed Beds:** 215 **Admissions:** 7601 **Census:** 94 **Outpatient Visits:** 48416 **Births:** 631 **Total Expense ($000):** 97901 **Payroll Expense ($000):** 40268 **Personnel:** 650

**WILSON N. JONES MEDICAL CENTER** See Texas Health Presbyterian Hospital–WNJ

### SMITHVILLE—Bastrop County

★ **SETON SMITHVILLE REGIONAL HOSPITAL (450143)**, 800 East Highway 71, Zip 78957; tel. 512/237–3214 **A**9 10 **F**3 11 15 29 40 43 53 57 59 62 64 68 70 77 79 81 87 93 107 108 110 111 113 118 129 145 147 **P**4 6
**S** Ascension Health, Saint Louis, MO
Primary Contact: Grady Hooper, Chief Executive Officer
CFO: Noralene Corder, Chief Financial Officer
CHR: Debbie Adkins, Director Human Resources
Web address: www.srhnet.org
**Control:** Hospital district or authority, Government, nonfederal **Service:** General Medical and Surgical

**Staffed Beds:** 12 **Admissions:** 695 **Census:** 7 **Outpatient Visits:** 81984 **Births:** 0 **Total Expense ($000):** 18307 **Payroll Expense ($000):** 9527 **Personnel:** 237

### SNYDER—Scurry County

★ **COGDELL MEMORIAL HOSPITAL (450073)**, 1700 Cogdell Boulevard, Zip 79549–6198; tel. 325/573–6374 **A**9 10 20 **F**8 11 13 15 18 19 29 30 34 40 43 45 46 47 48 49 50 53 56 57 59 62 64 65 68 70 75 76 77 79 81 85 86 87 91 92 93 97 107 108 111 114 118 126 129 130 131 132 144 145 146 147 **P**6
Primary Contact: William W. Weldon, Ph.D., Interim Chief Executive Officer
CFO: John Everett, Chief Financial Officer
CMO: Robert Rakov, M.D., Chief Medical Officer
CHR: Linda Warren, Director Human Resources
Web address: www.cogdellhospital.com
**Control:** Hospital district or authority, Government, nonfederal **Service:** General Medical and Surgical

**Staffed Beds:** 49 **Admissions:** 883 **Census:** 8 **Outpatient Visits:** 54880 **Births:** 205 **Total Expense ($000):** 25615 **Payroll Expense ($000):** 8694 **Personnel:** 194

### SONORA—Sutton County

★ **LILLIAN M. HUDSPETH MEMORIAL HOSPITAL (451324)**, 308 Hudspeth Avenue, Zip 76950–3399, Mailing Address: P.O. Box 455, Zip 76950–0455; tel. 325/387–2521 **A**9 10 18 **F**3 7 11 12 15 18 28 29 30 32 34 35 40 43 44 45 50 53 57 59 64 65 66 68 74 75 79 86 87 89 90 93 96 97 107 110 111 114 118 126 130 131 132 133 134 146 147
Primary Contact: Keith L. Butler, Chief Executive Officer
CFO: Michelle Schaefer, Chief Financial Officer
CMO: Mark Edwards, M.D., Chief Medical Officer
Web address: www.sonora–hospital.org
**Control:** Hospital district or authority, Government, nonfederal **Service:** General Medical and Surgical

**Staffed Beds:** 12 **Admissions:** 314 **Census:** 3 **Outpatient Visits:** 6667 **Births:** 0 **Total Expense ($000):** 7912 **Payroll Expense ($000):** 3250 **Personnel:** 67

### SOUTHLAKE—Tarrant County

☐ **TEXAS HEALTH HARRIS METHODIST HOSPITAL SOUTHLAKE (450888)**, 1545 East Southlake Boulevard, Zip 76092–6422; tel. 817/748–8700 **A**1 9 10 **F**3 29 30 40 64 74 79 81 85 107 111 113 118 129 145 **P**2
Primary Contact: Traci Bernard, President
CFO: Gorman Warren, Chief Financial Officer
CMO: David Taunton, M.D., Chief of Staff
CIO: Joey Sudomir, Chief Information Officer
CHR: Kenneth Drinkwater, Director Human Resources
Web address: www.texashealthsouthlake.com
**Control:** Corporation, Investor–owned, for–profit **Service:** General Medical and Surgical

**Staffed Beds:** 18 **Admissions:** 852 **Census:** 6 **Outpatient Visits:** 12728 **Births:** 0 **Total Expense ($000):** 44678 **Payroll Expense ($000):** 9794 **Personnel:** 139

### SPEARMAN—Hansford County

★ **HANSFORD HOSPITAL (451344)**, 707 South Roland Street, Zip 79081–3441; tel. 806/659–2535 **A**9 10 18 **F**11 31 32 34 40 43 56 57 59 62 63 64 65 68 69 78 93 107 126 129 132 **P**6
Primary Contact: Jonathan D. Bailey, Chief Executive Officer
CFO: Scott Beedy, Chief Financial Officer
CMO: Mark Garnett, M.D., Chief of Staff
CHR: Jackie Nelson, Director Human Resources
Web address: www.hchd.net
**Control:** Hospital district or authority, Government, nonfederal **Service:** General Medical and Surgical

**Staffed Beds:** 20 **Admissions:** 231 **Census:** 3 **Outpatient Visits:** 23164 **Births:** 0 **Total Expense ($000):** 8008 **Payroll Expense ($000):** 3382 **Personnel:** 83

### SPRING—Montgomery County

**NEXUS SPECIALTY HOSPITAL THE WOODLANDS (452057)**, 9182 Six Pines Drive, Zip 77380–3670; tel. 281/364–0317, (Nonreporting)
Primary Contact: Erin Cassidy, Chief Executive Officer
COO: Guido J. Cubellis, Chief Operating Officer
CFO: Julia Hatton, Chief Financial Officer
CMO: Ather Siddiqi, M.D., Medical Director
CIO: Deepak Chaudhry, Vice President Information Technology
CHR: Guy Murdock, Vice President Human Resources
CNO: Natalie Munoz, Director of Clinical Services
Web address: www.nexusspecialty.com
**Control:** Partnership, Investor–owned, for–profit **Service:** General Medical and Surgical

**Staffed Beds:** 21

### STAFFORD—Fort Bend County

**ATRIUM MEDICAL CENTER (452114)**, 11929 West Airport Boulevard, Zip 77477–2451; tel. 281/207–8200 **A**21 **F**1 3 29 45 46 56 60 83 85 105 107 113 118 147
Primary Contact: Danny Cox, Chief Executive Officer
Web address: www.atriummedicalcenter.com
**Control:** Partnership, Investor–owned, for–profit **Service:** Long–Term Acute Care hospital

**Staffed Beds:** 68 **Admissions:** 644 **Census:** 42 **Outpatient Visits:** 19800 **Births:** 0 **Total Expense ($000):** 22039 **Payroll Expense ($000):** 9100 **Personnel:** 183

### STAMFORD—Jones County

**STAMFORD MEMORIAL HOSPITAL (450306)**, 1601 Columbia Street, Zip 79553, Mailing Address: P.O. Box 911, Zip 79553–0911; tel. 325/773–2725 **A**9 10 **F**11 28 30 34 35 40 41 43 50 53 57 59 62 64 65 68 81 89 93 126 132 145 147 **P**4
Primary Contact: Richard G. DeFoore, FACHE, Chief Executive Officer
CFO: Elizabeth Miller, CPA, Chief Financial Officer
CMO: Michael Hart, M.D., Medical Director
CIO: Birgitta Neal, Data Entry and Information Technologist
CHR: Cheryl Hertel, Coordinator Human Resources
Web address: www.stamfordmemorialhospital.com
**Control:** Hospital district or authority, Government, nonfederal **Service:** General Medical and Surgical

**Staffed Beds:** 25 **Admissions:** 340 **Census:** 4 **Outpatient Visits:** 25620 **Births:** 0 **Total Expense ($000):** 8434 **Payroll Expense ($000):** 4306 **Personnel:** 162

### STANTON—Martin County

**MARTIN COUNTY HOSPITAL DISTRICT (451333)**, 610 North St. Peter Street, Zip 79782, Mailing Address: P.O. Box 640, Zip 79782–0640; tel. 432/756–3345 **A**9 10 18 **F**7 40 43 57 62 76 81 89 107 118 126 132
Primary Contact: Paul McKinney, Administrator
CFO: Alison Israel, Controller
Web address: www.martinch.com/
**Control:** Hospital district or authority, Government, nonfederal **Service:** General Medical and Surgical

**Staffed Beds:** 20 **Admissions:** 125 **Census:** 1 **Outpatient Visits:** 10909 **Births:** 0 **Total Expense ($000):** 7188 **Payroll Expense ($000):** 3467 **Personnel:** 98

**TX**

**STEPHENVILLE—Erath County**

☒ **TEXAS HEALTH HARRIS METHODIST HOSPITAL STEPHENVILLE (450351)**, 411 North Belknap Street, Zip 76401–3415; tel. 254/965–1500 **A**1 9 10 20 **F**3 8 11 13 15 29 30 34 35 40 41 43 45 51 57 59 65 70 75 76 77 79 81 82 86 89 93 94 108 111 113 117 118 129 134 144 145 146 147 **S** Texas Health Resources, Arlington, TX
Primary Contact: Christopher Leu, Chief Executive Officer
CFO: Carol Cross, Chief Financial Officer
CMO: Jeffrey Edwards, M.D., Chief of Staff
CHR: Kimberly Leondar, Director Human Resources
Web address: www.texashealth.org
**Control:** Other not–for–profit (including NFP Corporation) **Service:** General Medical and Surgical

**Staffed Beds:** 54 **Admissions:** 2022 **Census:** 18 **Outpatient Visits:** 31950 **Births:** 458 **Total Expense ($000):** 36996 **Payroll Expense ($000):** 14058 **Personnel:** 191

**SUGAR LAND—Fort Bend County**

☒ **HEALTHSOUTH SUGAR LAND REHABILITATION HOSPITAL (673042)**, 1325 Highway 6, Zip 77478; tel. 281/276–7574 **A**1 9 10 **F**3 29 34 35 57 75 87 90 95 96 129 147 **S** HEALTHSOUTH Corporation, Birmingham, AL
Primary Contact: Nicholas Hardin, Chief Executive Officer
Web address: www.healthsouthsugarland.com
**Control:** Corporation, Investor–owned, for–profit **Service:** Rehabilitation

**Staffed Beds:** 50 **Admissions:** 948 **Census:** 35 **Outpatient Visits:** 0 **Births:** 0 **Total Expense ($000):** 13816 **Payroll Expense ($000):** 6453 **Personnel:** 136

☒ **KINDRED HOSPITAL SUGAR LAND (452080)**, 1550 First Colony Boulevard, Zip 77479; tel. 281/275–6000 **A**1 9 10 **F**1 3 29 31 35 40 45 57 65 75 77 85 87 91 94 107 129 147 **S** Kindred Healthcare, Louisville, KY
Primary Contact: Lorene Perona, Chief Executive Officer
COO: Roberta Consolver, Chief Clinical Officer
CFO: Steven Bryan, Chief Financial Officer
CMO: Subodh Bhuchar, M.D., Chief of Staff
CIO: Artie Dmello, Director Case Management
CHR: Craig King, Coordinator Human Resources
Web address: www.khsugarland.com
**Control:** Corporation, Investor–owned, for–profit **Service:** General Medical and Surgical

**Staffed Beds:** 171 **Admissions:** 1962 **Census:** 143 **Outpatient Visits:** 541 **Births:** 0 **Total Expense ($000):** 71754 **Payroll Expense ($000):** 26947 **Personnel:** 440

☒ **MEMORIAL HERMANN SUGAR LAND HOSPITAL (450848)**, 17500 West Grand Parkway South, Zip 77479; tel. 281/725–5000 **A**1 9 10 **F**3 8 11 13 14 15 20 22 29 30 34 35 36 37 39 40 41 43 44 45 46 47 48 49 50 51 53 54 55 56 57 59 60 62 63 64 68 70 72 74 75 76 77 78 79 81 82 85 86 87 89 91 92 93 97 107 108 109 110 111 112 113 115 116 118 123 128 129 130 145 146 147 **P**5 6 **S** Memorial Hermann Healthcare System, Houston, TX
Primary Contact: Jim Brown, Chief Executive Officer
CFO: Daniel Goggin, Chief Financial Officer
CMO: William Riley, Jr., M.D., Chief of Staff
CHR: Robert Blake, Chief Human Resources Officer Southwest Market
Web address: www.memorialhermann.org
**Control:** Other not–for–profit (including NFP Corporation) **Service:** General Medical and Surgical

**Staffed Beds:** 77 **Admissions:** 4108 **Census:** 37 **Outpatient Visits:** 51106 **Births:** 1133 **Total Expense ($000):** 66445 **Payroll Expense ($000):** 26025 **Personnel:** 315

☒ **METHODIST SUGAR LAND HOSPITAL (450820)**, 16655 S.W. Freeway, Zip 77479–2343; tel. 281/274–7000 **A**1 9 10 21 **F**3 13 15 18 20 22 24 26 29 30 31 34 35 37 40 49 50 51 53 57 59 60 64 68 70 73 74 75 76 77 78 79 81 82 85 87 93 96 107 108 110 111 113 114 118 119 120 122 125 129 130 131 145 146 **S** The Methodist Hospital System, Houston, TX
Primary Contact: Christopher Siebenaler, Administrator and Chief Executive Officer
CFO: Lowell Stanton, Chief Financial Officer
CMO: Jeffrey Jackson, M.D., Medical Director
CHR: Luis Mario Garcia, Jr., Director Human Resources
Web address: www.methodisthealth.com
**Control:** Other not–for–profit (including NFP Corporation) **Service:** General Medical and Surgical

**Staffed Beds:** 207 **Admissions:** 11597 **Census:** 131 **Outpatient Visits:** 143847 **Births:** 2218 **Total Expense ($000):** 205025 **Payroll Expense ($000):** 73374 **Personnel:** 1315

☒ **ST. LUKE'S SUGAR LAND HOSPITAL (670053)**, 1317 Lake Pointe Parkway, Zip 77478; tel. 281/637–7000 **A**1 9 10 21 **F**3 13 15 18 20 22 26 29 30 34 35 37 39 40 41 42 44 45 46 49 50 57 60 64 68 70 72 74 75 76 79 81 82 85 107 108 110 114 118 128 129 145 146 147 **P**5 **S** St. Luke's Episcopal Health System, Houston, TX
Primary Contact: Bryan J. Hargis, FACHE, Chief Executive Officer
Web address: www.stlukessugarland.com
**Control:** Partnership, Investor–owned, for–profit **Service:** General Medical and Surgical

**Staffed Beds:** 84 **Admissions:** 4118 **Census:** 44 **Outpatient Visits:** 25519 **Births:** 870 **Total Expense ($000):** 89512 **Payroll Expense ($000):** 23561 **Personnel:** 318

**SUGAR LAND REHABILITATION HOSPITAL** See HEALTHSOUTH Sugar Land Rehabilitation Hospital

☐ **SUGAR LAND SURGICAL HOSPITAL (450860)**, 1211 Highway 6, Suite 70, Zip 77478; tel. 281/243–1000 **A**1 9 10 **F**3 29 40 45 59 64 75 79 81 82 85 86 87 89 92 111 118 129 **P**2 **S** United Surgical Partners International, Addison, TX
Primary Contact: Daniel Smith, Interim Chief Executive Officer
CFO: Raquel Hebert, Business Manager
CMO: Ken Thomson, M.D., Medical Director
Web address: www.sugarlandhospital.com
**Control:** Partnership, Investor–owned, for–profit **Service:** General Medical and Surgical

**Staffed Beds:** 6 **Admissions:** 385 **Census:** 3 **Outpatient Visits:** 7595 **Births:** 0 **Total Expense ($000):** 21754 **Payroll Expense ($000):** 5624 **Personnel:** 150

**TRIUMPH HOSPITAL SOUTHWEST** See Kindred Hospital Sugar Land

**SULPHUR SPRINGS—Hopkins County**

★ **HOPKINS COUNTY MEMORIAL HOSPITAL (450236)**, 115 Airport Road, Zip 75482–0115; tel. 903/885–7671 **A**9 10 **F**1 7 11 13 15 28 29 34 35 40 43 56 59 63 70 73 74 76 80 81 84 87 93 96 107 108 111 117 118 129 145 **P**6
Primary Contact: Michael McAndrew, Chief Executive Officer
COO: Donna Geiken Wallace, Chief Operating Officer and Chief Financial Officer
CFO: Donna Geiken Wallace, Chief Operating Officer and Chief Financial Officer
CMO: Darren Arnecke, Chief Medical Staff
CIO: Brandon Gauntt, Director Information Systems
CHR: Donna Rudzik, Director Human Resources
Web address: www.hcmh.com
**Control:** Hospital district or authority, Government, nonfederal **Service:** General Medical and Surgical

**Staffed Beds:** 50 **Admissions:** 3364 **Census:** 32 **Outpatient Visits:** 63104 **Births:** 849 **Total Expense ($000):** 48825 **Payroll Expense ($000):** 17591 **Personnel:** 448

**SUNNYVALE—Dallas County**

☐ **TEXAS REGIONAL MEDICAL CENTER**, 231 South Collins Road, Zip 75182–4624; tel. 972/892–3000 **A**1 9 **F**3 13 15 18 20 22 24 29 34 35 40 45 49 57 59 64 70 74 75 76 79 80 81 82 85 87 107 108 110 111 113 114 118 129 134 145 146 147 **P**8
Primary Contact: Terry J. Fontenot, Chief Executive Officer
CFO: Ben Dunford, Chief Financial Officer
Web address: www.texasregionalmedicalcenter.com
**Control:** Partnership, Investor–owned, for–profit **Service:** General Medical and Surgical

**Staffed Beds:** 70 **Admissions:** 6121 **Census:** 50 **Outpatient Visits:** 29357 **Births:** 1242 **Total Expense ($000):** 72885 **Payroll Expense ($000):** 23084 **Personnel:** 426

**SWEENY—Brazoria County**

**SWEENY COMMUNITY HOSPITAL (451311)**, 305 North McKinney Street, Zip 77480–2895; tel. 979/548–1500 **A**9 10 18 **F**3 7 10 11 15 29 34 35 40 43 45 56 57 59 65 69 70 75 81 85 93 103 104 107 110 113 118 129 131 132 142 144 147
Primary Contact: William H. Barnes, Administrator
CFO: Hong Wade, Chief Financial Officer
CMO: Fabio Aglieco, D.O., Chief of Staff
CIO: Stuart Butler, Director Information Technology
CHR: Grace Baty, Director Human Resources
Web address: www.sweenyhospital.org
**Control:** Hospital district or authority, Government, nonfederal **Service:** General Medical and Surgical

**Staffed Beds:** 14 **Admissions:** 344 **Census:** 2 **Outpatient Visits:** 17859 **Births:** 0 **Total Expense ($000):** 7757 **Payroll Expense ($000):** 5942 **Personnel:** 157

TX

**Hospital, Medicare Provider Number, Address, Telephone, Approval, Facility, and Physician Codes, Health Care System**

★ American Hospital Association (AHA) membership
☐ The Joint Commission accreditation          ◇ DNV Healthcare Inc. accreditation
○ American Osteopathic Association (AOA) accreditation
△ Commission on Accreditation of Rehabilitation Facilities (CARF) accreditation

## SWEETWATER—Nolan County

✠ **ROLLING PLAINS MEMORIAL HOSPITAL (450055)**, 200 East Arizona Street, Zip 79556–7199, Mailing Address: P.O. Box 690, Zip 79556–0690; tel. 325/235–1701 **A**1 9 10 20 **F**3 11 13 15 28 29 34 35 40 43 59 62 70 76 81 85 89 93 97 107 108 110 113 118 129 131 132 134 145
Primary Contact: Donna Boatright, MSN, Administrator
CFO: Rhonda Guelker, Senior Director Finance
CMO: Frederick Kassis, M.D., Chief of Staff
CHR: Gay Nell Cherry, Director Human Resources
Web address: www.rpmh.net
**Control:** Hospital district or authority, Government, nonfederal **Service:** General Medical and Surgical

**Staffed Beds:** 52 **Admissions:** 1384 **Census:** 15 **Outpatient Visits:** 87014 **Births:** 137 **Total Expense ($000):** 22422 **Payroll Expense ($000):** 11232 **Personnel:** 251

## TAHOKA—Lynn County

★ **LYNN COUNTY HOSPITAL DISTRICT (451351)**, 2600 Lockwood, Zip 79373–1310, Mailing Address: Box 1310, Zip 79373–1310; tel. 806/998–4533 **A**9 10 18 **F**3 7 10 13 29 32 34 35 40 43 44 53 54 56 57 59 64 65 66 75 76 86 89 93 97 107 132 146 147 **P**5 8
Primary Contact: Jimmy L. Morris, Chief Executive Officer and Administrator
CFO: Donna Raindl, Manager Business Office
CMO: Donald Freitag, M.D., Chief Medical Officer
CIO: Tim Pledger, Director Information Technology
CHR: Amy Schuknecht, Manager Human Resources
Web address: www.lchdhealthcare.org
**Control:** Hospital district or authority, Government, nonfederal **Service:** General Medical and Surgical

**Staffed Beds:** 19 **Admissions:** 149 **Census:** 5 **Outpatient Visits:** 31432 **Births:** 0 **Total Expense ($000):** 5523 **Payroll Expense ($000):** 2773 **Personnel:** 73

## TAYLOR—Williamson County

**JOHNS COMMUNITY HOSPITAL** See Scott & White Hospital – Taylor

✠ **SCOTT & WHITE HOSPITAL – TAYLOR (451374)**, 305 Mallard Lane, Zip 76574–1208; tel. 512/352–7611 **A**1 9 10 18 **F**3 11 15 18 29 34 40 41 43 45 57 59 62 64 81 85 86 93 97 107 108 110 113 118 128 129 131 132 147 **P**6 **S** Scott & White Healthcare, Temple, TX
Primary Contact: Kevin E. Smith, Chief Operating Officer
CIO: Tim Tarbell, Assistant Administrator Support Services
Web address: www.swtaylor.org
**Control:** Other not-for-profit (including NFP Corporation) **Service:** General Medical and Surgical

**Staffed Beds:** 23 **Admissions:** 584 **Census:** 10 **Outpatient Visits:** 37342 **Births:** 0 **Total Expense ($000):** 13502 **Payroll Expense ($000):** 6513 **Personnel:** 120

## TEMPLE—Bell County

✠ △ **CENTRAL TEXAS VETERANS HEALTHCARE SYSTEM**, 1901 Veterans Memorial Drive, Zip 76504–7493; tel. 254/778–4811, (Includes OLIN E. TEAGUE VETERANS' CENTER, 1901 South First Street, Zip 76504; tel. 817/778–4811; WACO VETERANS AFFAIRS HOSPITAL, 4800 Memorial Drive, Waco, Zip 76711–1397; tel. 254/752–6581), (Nonreporting) **A**1 2 3 5 7 8 9 **S** Department of Veterans Affairs, Washington, DC
Primary Contact: Thomas C. Smith, III, FACHE, Director
COO: Russell E. Lloyd, Associate Director Resources
CFO: Amy Maynard, Acting Chief Finance Service
CMO: William F. Harper, M.D., Chief of Staff
CIO: Sandra Wright, Acting Chief Information Technology Services
CHR: James Basso, Chief Human Resources Officer
Web address: www.central-texas.med.va.gov
**Control:** Veterans Affairs, Government, federal **Service:** General Medical and Surgical

**Staffed Beds:** 1532

**CHILDREN'S HOSPITAL AT SCOTT & WHITE** See Scott and White Memorial Hospital

**OLIN E. TEAGUE VETERANS' CENTER** See Central Texas Veterans Healthcare System

★ **SCOTT AND WHITE CONTINUING CARE HOSPITAL (670030)**, 546 North Kegley Road, Zip 76502; tel. 254/215–0900 **A**9 10 **F**1 3 29 30 50 60 68 85 87 107 118 129 147 **P**6 **S** Scott & White Healthcare, Temple, TX
Primary Contact: Kimberly K. Langston, R.N., Executive Associate Director and Administrator
Web address: www.sw.org/location/temple–cch
**Control:** Other not-for-profit (including NFP Corporation) **Service:** Long–Term Acute Care hospital

**Staffed Beds:** 50 **Admissions:** 402 **Census:** 34 **Outpatient Visits:** 0 **Births:** 0 **Total Expense ($000):** 19426 **Payroll Expense ($000):** 7840 **Personnel:** 133

## SCOTT AND WHITE MEMORIAL HOSPITAL (450054)

✠ **SCOTT AND WHITE MEMORIAL HOSPITAL (450054)**, 2401 South 31st Street, Zip 76508–0002; tel. 254/724–2111, (Includes CHILDREN'S HOSPITAL AT SCOTT & WHITE, 2401 South 31st Street, Zip 76508–0001; tel. 877/724–5437; KING'S DAUGHTERS HOSPITAL, 1901 S.W. H. K. Dodgen Loop, Zip 76502–1896; tel. 254/771–8600; John Boyd, III, M.D., Chief Executive Officer), (Total facility includes 49 beds in nursing home–type unit) **A**1 2 3 5 8 9 10 **F**3 5 7 9 11 12 13 14 15 17 18 19 20 21 22 24 26 27 28 29 30 31 32 34 35 36 37 38 39 40 43 44 45 46 47 48 49 50 51 52 54 55 56 57 58 59 60 61 62 63 64 65 68 70 72 73 74 75 76 77 78 79 81 82 84 85 86 87 88 89 91 92 93 96 97 98 100 102 103 104 105 107 108 110 111 113 114 115 116 117 118 119 120 122 123 125 127 128 129 130 131 133 134 135 136 137 138 140 141 143 144 145 146 147 **P**6 **S** Scott & White Healthcare, Temple, TX
Primary Contact: Patricia M. Currie, FACHE, Chief Hospital Services
CIO: William McCombs, III, Ph.D., Chief Information Officer
Web address: www.sw.org
**Control:** Other not-for-profit (including NFP Corporation) **Service:** General Medical and Surgical

**Staffed Beds:** 603 **Admissions:** 30753 **Census:** 441 **Outpatient Visits:** 1324821 **Births:** 3157 **Total Expense ($000):** 687212 **Payroll Expense ($000):** 286603 **Personnel:** 6444

## TERRELL—Kaufman County

**RENAISSANCE HOSPITAL TERRELL (450683)**, 1551 Highway 34 South, Zip 75160–4833; tel. 972/563–7611 **A**9 10 **F**3 11 18 19 29 30 34 40 45 46 47 48 57 64 70 73 75 76 78 79 81 82 85 86 87 89 107 113 114 118 142 145 147 **P**5 **S** Renaissance Healthcare Systems, Houston, TX
Primary Contact: Sean Astolfo, Administrator
CMO: Reba Williams–White, M.D., Chief of Staff
CHR: Patsy Branscum, Director Human Resources
Web address: www.terrell–hospital.com
**Control:** Corporation, Investor–owned, for–profit **Service:** General Medical and Surgical

**Staffed Beds:** 102 **Admissions:** 1539 **Census:** 12 **Outpatient Visits:** 11194 **Births:** 55

☐ **TERRELL STATE HOSPITAL (454006)**, 1200 East Brin Street, Zip 75160–2938; tel. 972/524–6452 **A**1 5 9 10 **F**30 34 39 57 68 75 86 87 98 99 100 101 103 129 131 134 145 **P**6 **S** Texas Department of State Health Services, Austin, TX
Primary Contact: Joe Finch, PsyD, Superintendent
CFO: Mike Verseckes, Financial Officer
CMO: Anthony Claxton, M.D., Clinical Director
CIO: Lisa Knox, Manager Facility Automation
Web address: www.dshs.state.tx.us/mhhospitals/terrellsh
**Control:** State–Government, nonfederal **Service:** Psychiatric

**Staffed Beds:** 316 **Admissions:** 2713 **Census:** 305 **Outpatient Visits:** 0 **Births:** 0 **Total Expense ($000):** 71989 **Payroll Expense ($000):** 34785 **Personnel:** 886

## TEXARKANA—Bowie County

✠ **CHRISTUS ST. MICHAEL HEALTH SYSTEM (450801)**, 2600 St. Michael Drive, Zip 75503–2372; tel. 903/614–1000 **A**1 2 9 10 **F**3 11 13 15 17 18 20 22 24 29 30 31 34 35 40 41 43 45 49 51 53 56 57 59 60 64 65 68 70 71 72 74 75 76 77 78 79 80 81 82 84 85 86 87 89 92 96 97 107 108 109 110 111 113 114 117 118 119 120 121 122 123 125 128 129 130 131 134 142 145 146 147 **P**8 **S** CHRISTUS Health, Irving, TX
Primary Contact: Chris Karam, President and Chief Executive Officer
CFO: Shawn Barnett, Vice President and Chief Financial Officer
CMO: Mike Finley, M.D., Chief Medical Officer
CIO: Alana Higgins, Regional Information Management Executive
CHR: Pam Kennedy, Vice President Regional Human Resources and Organizational Department
Web address: www.christusstmichael.org
**Control:** Church–operated, Nongovernment, not–for profit **Service:** General Medical and Surgical

**Staffed Beds:** 312 **Admissions:** 15042 **Census:** 179 **Outpatient Visits:** 154602 **Births:** 1490 **Total Expense ($000):** 222989 **Payroll Expense ($000):** 69218 **Personnel:** 1648

✠ **CHRISTUS ST. MICHAEL REHABILITATION HOSPITAL (453065)**, 2400 St. Michael Drive, Zip 75503; tel. 903/614–4000 **A**1 9 10 **F**11 18 28 29 30 34 35 57 59 65 68 75 77 79 82 85 87 90 93 96 131 134 142 147 **S** CHRISTUS Health, Irving, TX
Primary Contact: Aloma Gender, R.N., MSN, Administrator and Chief Nursing Officer
CFO: Shawn Barnett, Vice President and Chief Financial Officer
CMO: Richard Sharp, M.D., Medical Director
CHR: Karen Williams, Director Human Resources
Web address: www.christusstmichael.org
**Control:** Church–operated, Nongovernment, not–for profit **Service:** Rehabilitation

**Staffed Beds:** 50 **Admissions:** 1110 **Census:** 37 **Outpatient Visits:** 43975 **Births:** 0 **Total Expense ($000):** 21230 **Payroll Expense ($000):** 9347 **Personnel:** 188

*Many Facility Codes have changed. Please refer to the AHA Guide Code Chart.*   © 2012 AHA Guide

✠ **DUBUIS HOSPITAL OF TEXARKANA (452061)**, 2400 St. Michael Drive, 2nd Floor, Zip 75503–2372; tel. 903/614–7600 **A**1 9 10 **F**1 3 29 77 82 84 86 87 129 147 **S** Dubuis Health System, Houston, TX
Primary Contact: Holly Powell, Administrator
Web address: www.dubuis.org
**Control:** Church–operated, Nongovernment, not–for profit **Service:** Long–Term Acute Care hospital

**Staffed Beds:** 49 **Admissions:** 481 **Census:** 37 **Outpatient Visits:** 0 **Births:** 0 **Total Expense ($000):** 14277 **Payroll Expense ($000):** 4817 **Personnel:** 102

✠ **HEALTHSOUTH REHABILITATION HOSPITAL OF TEXARKANA (453053)**, 515 West 12th Street, Zip 75501–4416; tel. 903/793–0088 **A**1 9 10 **F**3 28 29 62 64 74 77 79 87 90 91 93 94 95 96 100 129 130 142 147 **P**5 **S** HEALTHSOUTH Corporation, Birmingham, AL
Primary Contact: Jerry Jasper, Chief Executive Officer
CFO: Phylis Buck, Controller
CMO: Mark A. Wren, M.D., Medical Director
CHR: Ann R. Clapp, Director Human Resources
Web address: www.healthsouthtexarkana.com
**Control:** Corporation, Investor–owned, for–profit **Service:** Rehabilitation

**Staffed Beds:** 60 **Admissions:** 874 **Census:** 33 **Outpatient Visits:** 12082 **Births:** 0 **Total Expense ($000):** 10167 **Payroll Expense ($000):** 6024 **Personnel:** 135

☐ **WADLEY REGIONAL MEDICAL CENTER (450200)**, 1000 Pine Street, Zip 75501–5170; tel. 903/798–8000 **A**1 2 9 10 **F**3 11 12 13 15 18 20 22 24 28 29 30 31 34 35 40 44 45 49 50 51 55 56 57 59 60 61 64 65 68 70 71 73 74 75 76 77 79 81 82 85 86 89 98 103 107 108 110 111 113 114 118 125 129 131 145 146 147 **P**2 8 **S** IASIS Healthcare, Franklin, TN
Primary Contact: Thomas D. Gilbert, Chief Executive Officer
CFO: Steve Winegeart, Chief Financial Officer
CMO: G. Peter Dingeldein, M.D., Chief Medical Officer
CHR: Debby Butler, Director Human Resources
Web address: www.wadleyhealth.com
**Control:** Partnership, Investor–owned, for–profit **Service:** General Medical and Surgical

**Staffed Beds:** 157 **Admissions:** 7222 **Census:** 85 **Outpatient Visits:** 90315 **Births:** 1221 **Total Expense ($000):** 94808 **Payroll Expense ($000):** 31462 **Personnel:** 665

## THE WOODLANDS—Montgomery County

**MEMORIAL HERMANN THE WOODLANDS HOSPITAL** See Memorial Hermann Northwest Hospital, Houston

★ **ST. LUKE'S LAKESIDE HOSPITAL (670059)**, 17400 St. Luke's Way, Zip 77384; tel. 936/266–9000 **A**9 10 21 **F**3 18 20 22 26 29 30 34 35 40 50 57 59 64 68 75 79 81 87 94 107 111 114 118 129 130 134 **S** St. Luke's Episcopal Health System, Houston, TX
Primary Contact: Debra F. Sukin, Chief Executive Officer
Web address: www.stlukeslakeside.com/
**Control:** Corporation, Investor–owned, for–profit **Service:** General Medical and Surgical

**Staffed Beds:** 30 **Admissions:** 873 **Census:** 6 **Outpatient Visits:** 9441 **Births:** 0 **Total Expense ($000):** 40414 **Payroll Expense ($000):** 6758 **Personnel:** 102

✠ **ST. LUKE'S THE WOODLANDS HOSPITAL (450862)**, 17200 St. Luke's Way, Zip 77384; tel. 936/266–2000 **A**1 9 10 21 **F**3 11 12 13 15 18 20 22 24 26 29 30 34 35 38 40 41 45 49 50 57 58 59 64 68 70 72 74 75 76 78 79 81 82 85 86 87 89 93 107 108 109 110 111 113 117 118 123 125 128 129 130 134 144 145 146 **P**5 6 **S** St. Luke's Episcopal Health System, Houston, TX
Primary Contact: Debra F. Sukin, Chief Executive Officer
CFO: Mary Sue Lipham, Controller
CMO: Jefy Mathew, M.D., Chief of Staff
Web address: www.stlukeswoodlands.com
**Control:** Church–operated, Nongovernment, not–for profit **Service:** General Medical and Surgical

**Staffed Beds:** 154 **Admissions:** 8861 **Census:** 103 **Outpatient Visits:** 59237 **Births:** 1853 **Total Expense ($000):** 124449 **Payroll Expense ($000):** 43092 **Personnel:** 835

## THROCKMORTON—Throckmorton County

★ **THROCKMORTON COUNTY MEMORIAL HOSPITAL (451339)**, 802 North Minter Street, Zip 76483–5357, Mailing Address: P.O. Box 729, Zip 76483–0729; tel. 940/849–2151 **A**9 10 18 **F**7 40 41 43 64 65 68 75 87 126 127 132 **P**5 6
Primary Contact: Michael Curtis, Administrator and Chief Executive Officer
CFO: Silvia A. Tipton, Chief Financial Officer and Director Human Resources
CMO: Craig Beasley, M.D., Chief of Staff and Medical Officer
CIO: Amber Myer, Director Medical Records
CHR: Silvia A. Tipton, Chief Financial Officer and Director Human Resources
**Control:** County–Government, nonfederal **Service:** General Medical and Surgical

**Staffed Beds:** 14 **Admissions:** 135 **Census:** 2 **Outpatient Visits:** 4981 **Births:** 0 **Total Expense ($000):** 2532 **Payroll Expense ($000):** 1098 **Personnel:** 39

## TOMBALL—Harris County

★ **TOMBALL REGIONAL MEDICAL CENTER (450670)**, 605 Holderrieth Street, Zip 77375–0889, Mailing Address: P.O. Box 889, Zip 77377–0889; tel. 281/401–7500, (Total facility includes 17 beds in nursing home–type unit) **A**9 10 21 **F**2 3 8 10 11 13 15 17 18 20 22 24 28 29 30 34 40 44 45 46 47 48 49 50 51 52 53 57 59 60 62 64 70 72 74 75 76 78 79 80 81 82 85 86 87 89 90 91 94 96 98 102 103 107 108 110 111 113 114 118 119 120 122 123 124 127 128 129 130 131 134 145 147 **S** Community Health Systems, Inc., Franklin, TN
Primary Contact: Bud Wethington, Chief Executive Officer
COO: Keith Barber, CPA, Chief Operating Officer and Chief Financial Officer
CFO: Keith Barber, CPA, Chief Operating Officer and Chief Financial Officer
CMO: Rodney Light, M.D., Chief Medical Officer
CIO: Marlene Pezzia, Director
CHR: Marcia Moore, Vice President
Web address: www.tomballregionalmedicalcenter.com
**Control:** Hospital district or authority, Government, nonfederal **Service:** General Medical and Surgical

**Staffed Beds:** 289 **Admissions:** 9943 **Census:** 144 **Outpatient Visits:** 80270 **Births:** 721 **Total Expense ($000):** 156125 **Payroll Expense ($000):** 64658 **Personnel:** 1081

## TRINITY—Trinity County

★ **EAST TEXAS MEDICAL CENTER TRINITY (450749)**, 317 Prospect Drive, Zip 75862, Mailing Address: P.O. Box 3169, Zip 75862; tel. 936/744–1100 **A**9 10 **F**11 29 40 43 64 107 113 114 118 126 145 **P**7 **S** East Texas Medical Center Regional Healthcare System, Tyler, TX
Primary Contact: Brett Kirkham, Administrator
CFO: Jerry A. Dominguez, CPA, Chief Financial Officer
CMO: David Mandel, M.D., Chief of Staff
CHR: Kathy Turner, Director Human Resources
Web address: www.etmc.org
**Control:** Other not–for–profit (including NFP Corporation) **Service:** General Medical and Surgical

**Staffed Beds:** 22 **Admissions:** 610 **Census:** 7 **Outpatient Visits:** 32599 **Births:** 0 **Total Expense ($000):** 8412 **Payroll Expense ($000):** 3538 **Personnel:** 55

## TROPHY CLUB—Denton County

☐ **BAYLOR MEDICAL CENTER AT TROPHY CLUB (450883)**, 2850 East State Highway 114, Zip 76262; tel. 817/837–4600 **A**1 9 10 **F**3 12 29 40 64 70 75 79 81 85 87 107 108 111 113 117 120 122 131 140 **S** Cirrus Health, Dallas, TX
Primary Contact: Melanie Chick, Chief Executive Officer
CFO: Jonathan Saunders, Chief Financial Officer
CMO: Mike Stanton, D.O., Medical Director
CIO: Scot Bradford, Chief Information Officer
CNO: Tina Huddleston, Chief Nursing Officer
Web address: www.tc–mc.com
**Control:** Partnership, Investor–owned, for–profit **Service:** General Medical and Surgical

**Staffed Beds:** 20 **Admissions:** 539 **Census:** 3 **Outpatient Visits:** 6559 **Births:** 0 **Total Expense ($000):** 28098 **Payroll Expense ($000):** 6097 **Personnel:** 139

**TX**

---

**Hospital, Medicare Provider Number, Address, Telephone, Approval, Facility, and Physician Codes, Health Care System**

★ American Hospital Association (AHA) membership
☐ The Joint Commission accreditation ◇ DNV Healthcare Inc. accreditation
○ American Osteopathic Association (AOA) accreditation
△ Commission on Accreditation of Rehabilitation Facilities (CARF) accreditation

## TULIA—Swisher County

★ **SWISHER MEMORIAL HOSPITAL DISTRICT (451349)**, 539 Southeast Second, Zip 79088-2403, Mailing Address: P.O. Box 808, Zip 79088-0808; tel. 806/995-3581 **A**9 10 18 **F**3 7 10 11 29 34 35 40 43 50 53 57 59 62 64 68 93 107 114 126 129 132 **P**4
Primary Contact: Debbie King, Chief Executive Officer
CFO: Connie Wilhelm, Chief Financial Officer
CIO: Brad Roberts, Network Administrator
Web address: www.swisherhospital.com
**Control:** Hospital district or authority, Government, nonfederal **Service:** General Medical and Surgical

**Staffed Beds: 20 Admissions: 366 Census: 5 Outpatient Visits: 32137 Births: 0 Total Expense ($000): 9629 Payroll Expense ($000): 4296 Personnel: 98**

## TYLER—Smith County

✠ △ **EAST TEXAS MEDICAL CENTER REHABILITATION CENTER (453072)**, 701 Olympic Plaza Circle, Zip 75701-1996; tel. 903/596-3000 **A**1 7 9 10 **F**3 28 29 30 34 53 57 75 86 90 91 93 96 129 130 131 147 **S** East Texas Medical Center Regional Healthcare System, Tyler, TX
Primary Contact: Eddie L. Howard, Vice President and Chief Operating Officer
CFO: James Blanton, Chief Financial Officer
CMO: Jerry Schwarzbach, M.D., Medical Director
CIO: Paula Anthony, Vice President Information Services
CHR: Mike Gray, Corporate Vice President Human Resources
Web address: www.etmc.org
**Control:** Other not-for-profit (including NFP Corporation) **Service:** Rehabilitation

**Staffed Beds: 49 Admissions: 1030 Census: 38 Outpatient Visits: 64824 Births: 0 Total Expense ($000): 25786 Payroll Expense ($000): 12257 Personnel: 199**

✠ **EAST TEXAS MEDICAL CENTER SPECIALTY HOSPITAL (452051)**, 1000 South Beckham, 5th Floor, Zip 75701; tel. 903/596-3600 **A**1 9 10 **F**1 3 29 30 75 84 129 147 **S** East Texas Medical Center Regional Healthcare System, Tyler, TX
Primary Contact: Eddie L. Howard, Vice President, Chief Operating Officer and Administrator
CFO: James Blanton, Chief Financial Officer
CMO: J. David Johnson, M.D., Chief of Staff
CIO: Paula Anthony, Vice President Information Services
CHR: Mike Gray, Corporate Vice President Human Resources
Web address: www.etmc.org
**Control:** Other not-for-profit (including NFP Corporation) **Service:** Long-Term Acute Care hospital

**Staffed Beds: 36 Admissions: 392 Census: 29 Outpatient Visits: 0 Births: 0 Total Expense ($000): 14730 Payroll Expense ($000): 4790 Personnel: 83**

✠ **EAST TEXAS MEDICAL CENTER TYLER (450083)**, 1000 South Beckham Street, Zip 75701-1996, Mailing Address: Box 6400, Zip 75711-6400; tel. 903/597-0351, (Includes EAST TEXAS MEDICAL CENTER BEHAVIORAL HEALTH CENTER, 4101 University Boulevard, Zip 75701-6600; tel. 903/566-8668; Jerry W. Echols, Administrator and Chief Executive Officer) **A**1 2 3 5 9 10 **F**3 5 8 11 12 13 15 17 18 20 22 24 26 28 29 30 31 35 37 38 40 42 43 44 45 46 47 48 49 51 54 56 58 59 60 61 64 65 68 70 71 73 74 75 76 78 79 80 81 82 84 85 86 87 89 93 98 99 100 101 102 103 104 105 107 110 111 113 114 116 117 118 119 120 122 123 125 128 129 131 137 140 144 145 146 147 **S** East Texas Medical Center Regional Healthcare System, Tyler, TX
Primary Contact: Robert B. Evans, Administrator and Chief Executive Officer
CFO: Byron Hale, Chief Financial Officer
CMO: John Andrews, M.D., Chief of Staff
CIO: Paula Anthony, Vice President Information Services
CHR: Mike Gray, Corporate Vice President Human Resources
Web address: www.etmc.org
**Control:** Other not-for-profit (including NFP Corporation) **Service:** General Medical and Surgical

**Staffed Beds: 450 Admissions: 20496 Census: 322 Outpatient Visits: 144536 Births: 805 Total Expense ($000): 377755 Payroll Expense ($000): 126027 Personnel: 3129**

✠ **MOTHER FRANCES HOSPITAL – TYLER (450102)**, 800 East Dawson Street, Zip 75701-2036; tel. 903/593-8441 **A**1 2 9 10 **F**3 7 8 11 12 13 18 19 20 22 24 26 28 29 30 31 32 34 37 40 43 45 46 47 48 49 50 51 53 54 55 59 60 64 66 68 70 72 73 74 75 76 77 78 79 80 81 82 83 84 85 86 87 89 93 102 107 108 110 111 113 114 118 123 125 126 128 129 130 131 133 143 145 146 147 **P**5 6 7 8 **S** Trinity Mother Frances Hospitals and Clinics, Tyler, TX
Primary Contact: Laura Owen, Senior Vice President and Chief Executive Officer
COO: Laura Owen, Senior Vice President and Chief Operating Officer
CHR: Randy Perdue, Assistant Vice President
Web address: www.tmfhs.org
**Control:** Other not-for-profit (including NFP Corporation) **Service:** General Medical and Surgical

**Staffed Beds: 392 Admissions: 22986 Census: 304 Outpatient Visits: 527951 Births: 2568 Total Expense ($000): 436958 Payroll Expense ($000): 143598 Personnel: 3340**

**TEXAS SPINE & JOINT HOSPITAL (450864)**, 1814 Roseland Boulevard, Suite 100, Zip 75701; tel. 903/525-3300 **A**10 **F**8 29 39 40 77 79 81 82 85 107 111 113 118
Primary Contact: Tony Wahl, Chief Executive Officer
CFO: Greg Cummings, Chief Financial Officer
CMO: Duane Lee Griffith, M.D., Chief of Staff
CNO: Deborah Pelton, R.N., Chief Nursing Officer
Web address: www.tsjh.org
**Control:** Partnership, Investor-owned, for-profit **Service:** Orthopedic

**Staffed Beds: 20 Admissions: 1379 Census: 9 Outpatient Visits: 17162 Births: 0 Total Expense ($000): 50121 Payroll Expense ($000): 10973 Personnel: 255**

✠ **TRINITY MOTHER FRANCES REHABILITATION HOSPITAL (453056)**, 3131 Troup Highway, Zip 75701-8352; tel. 903/510-7000 **A**1 9 10 **F**3 9 28 29 56 62 64 74 75 77 79 82 87 90 91 93 95 96 129 130 131 142 146 147 **S** HEALTHSOUTH Corporation, Birmingham, AL
Primary Contact: Sharla Anderson, Chief Executive Officer
CFO: Michael G. Treadway, Controller
CMO: Bradley Merritt, M.D., Medical Director
Web address: www.tmfrehabhospital.com
**Control:** Partnership, Investor-owned, for-profit **Service:** Rehabilitation

**Staffed Beds: 74 Admissions: 1876 Census: 64 Outpatient Visits: 16356 Births: 0 Total Expense ($000): 18227 Payroll Expense ($000): 10423 Personnel: 191**

**TYLER CONTINUECARE HOSPITAL AT MOTHER FRANCES (452091)**, 800 East Dawson, 4th Floor, Zip 75701; tel. 903/531-4080 **A**9 10 **F**1 3 29 34 59 74 75 77 85 86 87 129 134 147 **P**4 **S** Trinity Mother Frances Hospitals and Clinics, Tyler, TX
Primary Contact: Stephanie Hyde, Chief Executive Officer
Web address: www.continuecare.org
**Control:** Other not-for-profit (including NFP Corporation) **Service:** General Medical and Surgical

**Staffed Beds: 51 Admissions: 672 Census: 49 Outpatient Visits: 0 Births: 0 Total Expense ($000): 22922 Payroll Expense ($000): 9602 Personnel: 154**

✠ **UNIVERSITY OF TEXAS HEALTH SCIENCE CENTER AT TYLER (450690)**, 11937 Highway 271, Zip 75708-3154; tel. 903/877-7777 **A**1 5 9 10 **F**3 8 11 15 18 20 22 24 26 28 29 30 31 32 34 35 40 42 43 45 46 49 50 53 56 57 58 59 64 65 68 70 74 75 77 78 79 81 85 86 87 93 97 107 108 110 111 113 114 117 118 128 129 134 145 146 147 **P**6 **S** University of Texas System, Austin, TX
Primary Contact: Kirk A. Calhoun, M.D., President
COO: Robert Marshall, Vice President and Chief Operating Officer
CFO: Vernon Moore, Chief Business and Finance
CMO: David Coultas, M.D., Vice President Clinical Affairs
CIO: Vernon Moore, Chief Business and Finance
CHR: Georgia Melton, Associate Vice President Human Resources
Web address: www.uthct.edu
**Control:** State-Government, nonfederal **Service:** General Medical and Surgical

**Staffed Beds: 116 Admissions: 2320 Census: 29 Outpatient Visits: 203972 Births: 0 Total Expense ($000): 118866 Payroll Expense ($000): 54550 Personnel: 791**

## UVALDE—Uvalde County

✠ **UVALDE COUNTY HOSPITAL AUTHORITY (450177)**, 1025 Garner Field Road, Zip 78801-1025; tel. 830/278-6251 **A**1 9 10 20 **F**3 11 13 15 17 18 29 30 39 40 43 45 50 56 57 59 63 64 68 70 76 81 85 86 87 89 90 93 104 107 108 111 114 117 118 126 129 131 132 145 146 147 **P**3
Primary Contact: James E. Buckner, Jr., FACHE, Administrator
CFO: Valerie Lopez, CPA, Controller
CIO: Carolina Velasquez, Chief Information Officer
CHR: Charla Carter, Director Human Resources
Web address: www.umhtx.org
**Control:** Hospital district or authority, Government, nonfederal **Service:** General Medical and Surgical

**Staffed Beds: 48 Admissions: 1986 Census: 20 Outpatient Visits: 65552 Births: 382 Total Expense ($000): 45470 Payroll Expense ($000): 18955 Personnel: 447**

## VAN HORN—Culberson County

★ **CULBERSON HOSPITAL (451338)**, Eisenhower-Farm Market Road 2185, Zip 79855, Mailing Address: P.O. Box 609, Zip 79855-0609; tel. 432/283-2760 **A**9 10 18 **F**3 7 34 40 43 56 57 59 65 66 68 93 107 113 118 126 132 **P**6 **S** Preferred Management Corporation, Shawnee, OK
Primary Contact: Jared Chanski, Administrator
CMO: John A. Thomas, M.D., Chief Medical Staff
Web address: www.culbersonhospital.org
**Control:** Corporation, Investor-owned, for-profit **Service:** General Medical and Surgical

**Staffed Beds: 14 Admissions: 107 Census: 2 Outpatient Visits: 10373 Births: 0 Total Expense ($000): 4809 Payroll Expense ($000): 2355 Personnel: 61**

*Many Facility Codes have changed. Please refer to the AHA Guide Code Chart.* © 2012 AHA Guide

## VERNON—Wilbarger County

☐ **NORTH TEXAS STATE HOSPITAL**, Highway 70 Northwest, Zip 76384, Mailing Address: P.O. Box 2231, Zip 76385–2231; tel. 940/552–9901 **A**1 **F**11 30 39 44 56 57 68 75 86 87 96 98 99 103 129 131 134 145 **P**6 **S** Texas Department of State Health Services, Austin, TX
Primary Contact: James E. Smith, Superintendent
CFO: William Lowery, Financial Officer
CIO: Crystal Dennstedt, Information Officer
Web address: www.mhmr.state.tx.us
**Control:** State–Government, nonfederal **Service:** Psychiatric

**Staffed Beds:** 603 **Admissions:** 2330 **Census:** 578 **Outpatient Visits:** 0 **Births:** 0 **Total Expense ($000):** 113237 **Payroll Expense ($000):** 65202 **Personnel:** 1933

**WILBARGER GENERAL HOSPITAL (450584)**, 920 Hillcrest Drive, Zip 76384–3196; tel. 940/552–9351 **A**9 10 20 **F**3 11 15 29 34 35 40 43 45 54 56 57 60 62 75 81 85 86 87 93 98 101 103 104 107 111 114 118 123 126 129 131 132 142 145 147 **P**5
Primary Contact: Jonathon Voelkel, Administrator
CFO: Richard Thieman, Chief Financial Officer
CIO: Ed Nary, Director Information Technology and Chief Compliance Officer
CHR: Cathie Bristo, Director Human Resources
Web address: www.wghospital.com
**Control:** Hospital district or authority, Government, nonfederal **Service:** General Medical and Surgical

**Staffed Beds:** 27 **Admissions:** 995 **Census:** 13 **Outpatient Visits:** 21697 **Births:** 0 **Total Expense ($000):** 17470 **Payroll Expense ($000):** 8454 **Personnel:** 215

## VICTORIA—Victoria County

★ **CITIZENS MEDICAL CENTER (450023)**, 2701 Hospital Drive, Zip 77901–5749; tel. 361/573–9181, (Total facility includes 20 beds in nursing home–type unit) **A**2 9 10 21 **F**1 3 4 8 11 12 13 15 16 17 18 20 22 24 28 29 30 31 34 35 38 40 41 43 49 54 56 57 59 60 64 65 66 67 70 72 73 74 75 76 77 78 79 80 81 84 85 86 87 88 89 90 93 94 97 98 100 101 102 103 105 107 108 109 111 113 114 115 116 117 118 119 120 126 127 129 130 131 134 143 145 146 147 **P**6
Primary Contact: David P. Brown, Administrator
CFO: Phillip Hacker, Chief Financial Officer
CHR: Jim Heger, Director Human Resources
Web address: www.citizensmedicalcenter.org
**Control:** County–Government, nonfederal **Service:** General Medical and Surgical

**Staffed Beds:** 296 **Admissions:** 9604 **Census:** 123 **Outpatient Visits:** 88763 **Births:** 875 **Total Expense ($000):** 130102 **Payroll Expense ($000):** 57264 **Personnel:** 1053

⊞ **DETAR HEALTHCARE SYSTEM (450147)**, 506 East San Antonio Street, Zip 77901–6060, Mailing Address: P.O. Box 2089, Zip 77902–2089; tel. 361/575–7441, (Includes DETAR HOSPITAL NORTH, 101 Medical Drive, Zip 77904–3198; tel. 361/573–6100; William R. Blanchard, Chief Executive Officer), (Total facility includes 16 beds in nursing home–type unit) **A**1 9 10 **F**3 12 13 15 18 20 22 24 28 29 30 31 39 40 41 43 47 49 51 53 56 64 70 72 74 75 76 77 78 79 81 82 85 86 87 89 90 91 93 98 100 101 103 107 108 110 111 113 117 118 125 127 129 131 145 146 147 **P**3 5 8 **S** Community Health Systems, Inc., Franklin, TN
Primary Contact: William R. Blanchard, Chief Executive Officer
CFO: Donald E. Hagan, Chief Financial Officer
CMO: James R. Brand, M.D., Chief of Staff
CIO: Kim Tompkins, Director Information Services
CHR: Kristina Elsik, Director Human Resources
Web address: www.detar.com
**Control:** Corporation, Investor–owned, for–profit **Service:** General Medical and Surgical

**Staffed Beds:** 222 **Admissions:** 8654 **Census:** 102 **Outpatient Visits:** 83339 **Births:** 1126 **Total Expense ($000):** 102110 **Payroll Expense ($000):** 43374 **Personnel:** 834

⊞ **KINDRED HOSPITAL VICTORIA (452056)**, 506 East San Antonio Street, 3rd Floor, Zip 77901–6060; tel. 361/575–1445 **A**1 9 10 **F**1 3 29 30 31 42 82 85 86 87 97 129 147 **P**2 **S** Kindred Healthcare, Louisville, KY
Primary Contact: Tammy Barben, Chief Executive Officer
CHR: Rachel Reeves, Manager Human Resources
Web address: www.khvictoria.com
**Control:** Corporation, Investor–owned, for–profit **Service:** General Medical and Surgical

**Staffed Beds:** 23 **Admissions:** 297 **Census:** 21 **Outpatient Visits:** 0 **Births:** 0 **Total Expense ($000):** 8974 **Payroll Expense ($000):** 3869 **Personnel:** 66

☐ **WARM SPRINGS SPECIALTY HOSPITAL OF VICTORIA (452094)**, 102 Medical Drive, Zip 77904; tel. 361/576–6200 **A**1 9 10 **F**1 3 29 75 77 85 93 94 96 147 **S** Post Acute Medical, LLC, Camp Hill, PA
Primary Contact: Brian Holt, Chief Executive Officer
CFO: James Asberry, Chief Financial Officer
CMO: Behram Khan, M.D., Medical Director
CHR: Waynea Finley, Corporate Director Human Resources
Web address: www.warmsprings.org
**Control:** Partnership, Investor–owned, for–profit **Service:** Long–Term Acute Care hospital

**Staffed Beds:** 26 **Admissions:** 363 **Census:** 25 **Outpatient Visits:** 10877 **Births:** 0 **Total Expense ($000):** 12541 **Payroll Expense ($000):** 4682 **Personnel:** 103

## WACO—Mclennan County

⊞ △ **HILLCREST BAPTIST MEDICAL CENTER (450101)**, 100 Hillcrest Medical Boulevard, Zip 76712–8897; tel. 254/202–2000, (Includes HILLCREST BAPTIST MEDICAL CENTER – HERRING AVENUE CAMPUS, 3000 HERRING AVENUE, ZIP 76708 ) **A**1 2 3 5 7 9 10 **F**3 9 11 12 13 15 18 20 22 24 26 28 29 30 31 34 40 43 44 45 49 50 51 53 54 56 57 59 60 61 64 68 70 72 74 75 76 78 79 81 82 84 85 86 87 89 90 93 96 97 102 107 108 110 111 113 114 115 116 117 118 127 128 129 130 131 144 145 146 147 **P**6 **S** Scott & White Healthcare, Temple, TX
Primary Contact: Glenn A. Robinson, Chief Executive Officer
COO: Jim Gebhart, FACHE, Chief Operating Officer
CFO: Richard Perkins, Chief Financial Officer
CIO: Richard Warren, Chief Information Officer
CHR: Bob Brace, Director Human Resources
Web address: www.hillcrest.net
**Control:** Other not–for–profit (including NFP Corporation) **Service:** General Medical and Surgical

**Staffed Beds:** 260 **Admissions:** 12588 **Census:** 166 **Outpatient Visits:** 142221 **Births:** 2696 **Total Expense ($000):** 183500 **Payroll Expense ($000):** 66645 **Personnel:** 1282

⊞ **PROVIDENCE HEALTH CENTER (450042)**, 6901 Medical Parkway, Zip 76712–7998, Mailing Address: P.O. Box 2589, Zip 76702–2589; tel. 254/751–4000, (Includes DEPAUL CENTER, 301 Londonderry Drive, Zip 76712; tel. 254/776–5970; Keith Hopkins, Vice President), (Total facility includes 341 beds in nursing home–type unit) **A**1 2 3 5 9 10 **F**2 3 4 5 6 8 9 10 11 12 13 15 18 20 22 24 26 28 29 30 31 34 35 38 40 41 44 45 46 48 49 50 53 54 56 57 58 59 61 62 64 67 68 70 74 75 76 77 78 79 81 85 86 87 89 93 97 98 99 100 101 102 103 104 105 107 108 110 113 114 118 124 127 129 131 134 143 145 146 147 **P**5 6 **S** Ascension Health, Saint Louis, MO
Primary Contact: Kent A. Keahey, FACHE, President and Chief Executive Officer
CFO: Karen K. Richardson, Senior Vice President and Chief Financial Officer
CMO: T. Marc Barrett, M.D., Senior Vice President Medical Affairs
CIO: Jay Scherler, Director Information Systems and Vice President Business Services
CHR: Chuck Sivess, Vice President Human Resources
Web address: www.providence.net
**Control:** Church–operated, Nongovernment, not–for profit **Service:** General Medical and Surgical

**Staffed Beds:** 647 **Admissions:** 18212 **Census:** 501 **Outpatient Visits:** 341385 **Births:** 1296 **Total Expense ($000):** 259363 **Payroll Expense ($000):** 106521 **Personnel:** 2002

**WACO VETERANS AFFAIRS HOSPITAL** See Central Texas Veterans Healthcare System, Temple

## WAXAHACHIE—Ellis County

⊞ **BAYLOR MEDICAL CENTER AT WAXAHACHIE (450372)**, 1405 West Jefferson Street, Zip 75165–2275; tel. 972/923–7000 **A**1 9 10 **F**3 11 12 15 28 29 30 34 35 40 41 53 57 59 64 65 68 70 71 74 75 77 78 79 81 82 84 85 93 107 108 110 111 113 118 123 128 129 134 146 147 **S** Baylor Health Care System, Dallas, TX
Primary Contact: Jay Fox, President
COO: Cindy Murray, R.N., Chief Nursing Officer and Chief Operating Officer
CFO: Steve Roussel, Vice President Finance
CMO: Valerie Goman, M.D., President Medical Staff
CIO: Gary Beazley, Coordinator Information Systems
CHR: Marcos Ramirez, Manager Human Resources
Web address: www.bhcs.com
**Control:** Other not–for–profit (including NFP Corporation) **Service:** General Medical and Surgical

**Staffed Beds:** 54 **Admissions:** 2986 **Census:** 32 **Outpatient Visits:** 68100 **Births:** 0 **Total Expense ($000):** 65682 **Payroll Expense ($000):** 24956 **Personnel:** 359

**TX**

---

**Hospital, Medicare Provider Number, Address, Telephone, Approval, Facility, and Physician Codes, Health Care System**

★ American Hospital Association (AHA) membership
☐ The Joint Commission accreditation
◇ DNV Healthcare Inc. accreditation
○ American Osteopathic Association (AOA) accreditation
△ Commission on Accreditation of Rehabilitation Facilities (CARF) accreditation

## WEATHERFORD—Parker County

☒ **WEATHERFORD REGIONAL MEDICAL CENTER (450203)**, 713 East Anderson Street, Zip 76086–9971; tel. 817/596–8751 **A**1 9 10 **F**3 13 29 31 34 35 40 43 45 57 59 70 75 76 77 78 79 81 82 85 93 107 111 113 114 118 129 131 132 134 143 145 147 **P**8 **S** Community Health Systems, Inc., Franklin, TN
Primary Contact: Cory Countryman, Interim Chief Executive Officer
CFO: Nancy Cooke, Chief Financial Officer
CMO: Jon–Paul Harmer, M.D., Chief Medical Staff
CIO: Merri Kober, Director Information Services
CHR: Richard Aguirre, Administrative Director Human Resources
Web address: www.weatherfordregional.com
**Control:** Corporation, Investor–owned, for–profit **Service:** General Medical and Surgical

**Staffed Beds:** 82 **Admissions:** 4745 **Census:** 44 **Outpatient Visits:** 57368 **Births:** 503 **Total Expense ($000):** 65398 **Payroll Expense ($000):** 20131 **Personnel:** 403

## WEBSTER—Harris County

☒ **CLEAR LAKE REGIONAL MEDICAL CENTER (450617)**, 500 Medical Center Boulevard, Zip 77598–4286; tel. 281/332–2511, (Includes ALVIN DIAGNOSTIC AND URGENT CARE CENTER, 301 Medic Lane, Alvin, Zip 77511–5597; tel. 281/331–6141; MAINLAND MEDICAL CENTER, 6801 E F Lowry Expressway, Texas City, Zip 77591; tel. 409/938–5000; Robert A. Heifner, Administrator) **A**1 3 5 9 10 **F**3 11 13 15 17 18 20 22 24 26 28 29 30 31 34 35 40 41 42 44 45 46 47 49 50 51 54 56 57 59 60 64 70 72 74 75 76 77 78 79 81 83 85 86 87 88 89 90 93 96 98 100 101 103 104 107 108 110 111 113 114 117 118 123 125 128 129 131 134 145 146 147 **S** HCA, Nashville, TN
Primary Contact: Stephen K. Jones, Jr., FACHE, Chief Executive Officer
CFO: Jeff Sliwinski, Chief Financial Officer
CMO: Richard Marietta, M.D., Medical Director
CIO: Ley Samson, Director Management Information Systems
CHR: Brad Horst, Director Human Resources
Web address: www.clearlakermc.com
**Control:** Partnership, Investor–owned, for–profit **Service:** General Medical and Surgical

**Staffed Beds:** 655 **Admissions:** 30282 **Census:** 398 **Outpatient Visits:** 220070 **Births:** 4327 **Total Expense ($000):** 336674 **Payroll Expense ($000):** 147456 **Personnel:** 2467

**CLEAR LAKE REHABILITATION HOSPITAL** See Kindred Rehabilitation Hospital Clear Lake

**HOUSTON PHYSICIANS HOSPITAL (670008)**, 333 North Texas Avenue, Zip 77598; tel. 281/557–5620 **A**5 9 10 **F**3 29 40 51 64 68 74 79 81 82 85 86 91 93 107 111 113 140
Primary Contact: Michele Dionne, Chief Executive Officer
Web address: www.houstonphysicianshospital.com
**Control:** Corporation, Investor–owned, for–profit **Service:** General Medical and Surgical

**Staffed Beds:** 21 **Admissions:** 730 **Census:** 4 **Outpatient Visits:** 11529 **Births:** 0 **Total Expense ($000):** 33213 **Payroll Expense ($000):** 8048 **Personnel:** 180

☒ **KINDRED REHABILITATION HOSPITAL CLEAR LAKE (453052)**, 655 East Medical Center Boulevard, Zip 77598–4328; tel. 281/286–1500 **A**1 9 10 **F**3 29 64 74 75 79 90 93 95 129 130 131 142 145 147 **S** Kindred Healthcare, Louisville, KY
Primary Contact: Dale R. Mulder, President and Chief Executive Officer
CFO: Barbara Franco, Chief Financial Officer
CMO: Michael Rosenblatt, M.D., Medical Director
CIO: Barbara Franco, Chief Financial Officer
CHR: Dalia Nandin, Manager Human Resources
Web address: www.khrehabclearlake.com/
**Control:** Corporation, Investor–owned, for–profit **Service:** Rehabilitation

**Staffed Beds:** 60 **Admissions:** 1059 **Census:** 39 **Outpatient Visits:** 7426 **Births:** 0 **Total Expense ($000):** 14534 **Payroll Expense ($000):** 7470 **Personnel:** 118

## WEIMAR—Colorado County

★ **COLORADO–FAYETTE MEDICAL CENTER (450438)**, 400 Youens Drive, Zip 78962–9561; tel. 979/725–9531 **A**3 5 9 10 **F**11 15 29 34 40 45 57 59 62 65 77 79 80 81 93 107 111 118 126 128 132
Primary Contact: Steven Gularte, Chief Executive Officer
CFO: Vicki Lewis, Chief Financial Officer
CMO: Juan Carlos Ortega, M.D., Chief of Staff
Web address: www.cfmc–online.com
**Control:** Other not–for–profit (including NFP Corporation) **Service:** General Medical and Surgical

**Staffed Beds:** 15 **Admissions:** 903 **Census:** 11 **Outpatient Visits:** 9295 **Births:** 0 **Total Expense ($000):** 10445 **Payroll Expense ($000):** 3958 **Personnel:** 111

## WELLINGTON—Collingsworth County

★ **COLLINGSWORTH GENERAL HOSPITAL (451355)**, 1013 15th Street, Zip 79095–3703, Mailing Address: P.O. Box 1112, Zip 79095–1112; tel. 806/447–2521 **A**9 10 18 **F**3 16 36 40 43 57 59 68 93 97 107 113 126 132 **S** Preferred Management Corporation, Shawnee, OK
Primary Contact: Candy Powell, Administrator
CFO: Larry Stephens, Chief Financial Officer
CMO: David E. Haacke, M.D., Chief of Staff
CIO: Thomas T. Ng, Chief Information Officer
CHR: Christie O'Rear, Human Resources Officer
Web address: www.collingsworthgeneral.net
**Control:** Corporation, Investor–owned, for–profit **Service:** General Medical and Surgical

**Staffed Beds:** 13 **Admissions:** 329 **Census:** 4 **Outpatient Visits:** 14757 **Births:** 0 **Total Expense ($000):** 5149 **Payroll Expense ($000):** 2348 **Personnel:** 58

## WESLACO—Hidalgo County

☒ **KNAPP MEDICAL CENTER (450128)**, 1401 East Eighth Street, Zip 78596–6640, Mailing Address: P.O. Box 1110, Zip 78599–1110; tel. 956/968–8567 **A**1 9 10 **F**3 8 11 12 13 15 18 19 20 29 30 31 34 35 39 40 43 44 46 49 50 51 56 57 59 60 63 64 70 73 74 75 76 77 78 79 81 82 84 85 86 87 89 93 107 108 110 111 113 114 117 118 129 130 131 133 134 142 145 146 147 **P**8
Primary Contact: James A. Summersett, III, FACHE, President and Chief Executive Officer
CIO: Gary Light, Chief Information Officer
CHR: Emmett Craig, Chief Human Resources Officer
Web address: www.knappmed.org
**Control:** Other not–for–profit (including NFP Corporation) **Service:** General Medical and Surgical

**Staffed Beds:** 202 **Admissions:** 10434 **Census:** 97 **Outpatient Visits:** 70218 **Births:** 1865 **Total Expense ($000):** 98281 **Payroll Expense ($000):** 42090 **Personnel:** 827

△ **WESLACO REHABILITATION HOSPITAL (453091)**, 906 South James Street, Zip 78596; tel. 956/969–2222 **A**7 9 10 **F**3 29 30 77 90 91 129
Primary Contact: Maggie E. Barreiro, Administrator
CFO: Leo Dan Perez, Controller
CMO: Pedro McDougal, M.D., Medical Director
CHR: Debbie Pendleton, Human Resources Specialist
CNO: Rita Mata–Guerrero, Nurse Director
Web address: www.weslacorehabhospital.com
**Control:** Partnership, Investor–owned, for–profit **Service:** Rehabilitation

**Staffed Beds:** 32 **Admissions:** 605 **Census:** 21 **Outpatient Visits:** 0 **Births:** 0 **Total Expense ($000):** 5964 **Payroll Expense ($000):** 4823 **Personnel:** 88

## WHARTON—Wharton County

☐ **GULF COAST MEDICAL CENTER (450214)**, 10141 Highway 59, Zip 77488–3004; tel. 979/282–6100 **A**1 9 10 **F**11 18 20 22 29 40 43 49 64 70 76 77 78 79 81 82 93 98 103 107 108 113 117 118 120 128 129 145 147 **S** Signature Hospital Corporation, Houston, TX
Primary Contact: Martin R. Slack, Chief Executive Officer
CFO: Gary Williams, Chief Financial Officer
CHR: Loretta Flynn, Director Human Resources
Web address: www.gulfcoastmedical.com
**Control:** Partnership, Investor–owned, for–profit **Service:** General Medical and Surgical

**Staffed Beds:** 59 **Admissions:** 1658 **Census:** 20 **Outpatient Visits:** 24014 **Births:** 227 **Total Expense ($000):** 26950 **Payroll Expense ($000):** 9874 **Personnel:** 200

## WHEELER—Wheeler County

★ **PARKVIEW HOSPITAL (451334)**, 1000 Sweetwater Street, Zip 79096, Mailing Address: P.O. Box 1030, Zip 79096–1030; tel. 806/826–5581 **A**9 10 18 **F**3 7 10 39 40 59 62 65 68 89 93 107 113 118 127 129 132 147
Primary Contact: Ann Fagan–Cook, Administrator and Chief Executive Officer
CIO: Ann Fagan Cook, Chief Information Officer
Web address: www.parkviewhosp.org
**Control:** Hospital district or authority, Government, nonfederal **Service:** General Medical and Surgical

**Staffed Beds:** 16 **Admissions:** 371 **Census:** 3 **Outpatient Visits:** 2246 **Births:** 0 **Total Expense ($000):** 6138 **Payroll Expense ($000):** 3098 **Personnel:** 101

**TX**

*Many Facility Codes have changed. Please refer to the AHA Guide Code Chart.* © 2012 AHA Guide

## WHITNEY—Hill County

**LAKE WHITNEY MEDICAL CENTER (450270)**, 200 North San Jacinto Street, Zip 76692-2388, Mailing Address: P.O. Box 458, Zip 76692-0458; tel. 254/694-3165 **A**9 10 **F**3 5 7 11 35 40 41 56 62 64 65 68 87 89 99 100 101 102 103 104 107 113 126 129 132 145 147 **P**5 6
Primary Contact: Ruth Ann Crow, Administrator
COO: Tariq Mahmood, Chief Executive Officer
CFO: Joe White, Chief Financial Officer
CMO: Aman Ali Shah, M.D., Chief Medical Staff
CIO: Patricia Daniel, Chief Information Officer
CHR: Darleen Towers, Director Human Resources
Web address: www.lakewhitneychamber.com
**Control:** Corporation, Investor-owned, for-profit **Service:** General Medical and Surgical

**Staffed Beds:** 25 **Admissions:** 1031 **Census:** 9 **Outpatient Visits:** 6753 **Births:** 0 **Total Expense ($000):** 7296 **Payroll Expense ($000):** 2956 **Personnel:** 100

## WICHITA FALLS—Wichita County

☒ **HEALTHSOUTH REHABILITATION HOSPITAL–WICHITA FALLS (453054)**, 3901 Armory Road, Zip 76302-2204; tel. 940/720-5700 **A**1 9 10 **F**3 28 29 44 50 53 62 64 68 74 75 77 79 82 86 87 90 91 92 93 95 96 131 142 145 147 **S** HEALTHSOUTH Corporation, Birmingham, AL
Primary Contact: Michael L. Bullitt, Chief Executive Officer
CFO: Tom Box, CPA, Chief Financial Officer
CMO: Virgil Frardo, M.D., Medical Director
CIO: Mary Walker, Manager Information Technology
CHR: Kathleen Pirtle, Director Human Resources
Web address: www.healthsouthwichitafalls.com
**Control:** Partnership, Investor-owned, for-profit **Service:** Rehabilitation

**Staffed Beds:** 63 **Admissions:** 1331 **Census:** 49 **Outpatient Visits:** 12298 **Births:** 0 **Total Expense ($000):** 14586 **Payroll Expense ($000):** 7875 **Personnel:** 180

☐ **KELL WEST REGIONAL HOSPITAL (450827)**, 5420 Kell West Boulevard, Zip 76310-1610; tel. 940/692-5888 **A**1 9 10 **F**3 31 39 40 49 50 51 74 75 78 79 81 82 85 87 91 93 107 108 113 118 129 **P**5
Primary Contact: Jerry Myers, M.D., Chief Executive Officer
CFO: Fran Lindemann, Director Finance
Web address: www.kellwest.com
**Control:** Partnership, Investor-owned, for-profit **Service:** General Medical and Surgical

**Staffed Beds:** 41 **Admissions:** 1186 **Census:** 11 **Outpatient Visits:** 30141 **Births:** 0 **Total Expense ($000):** 25721 **Payroll Expense ($000):** 8711 **Personnel:** 223

**NORTH TEXAS STATE HOSPITAL, WICHITA FALLS CAMPUS (454008)**, 6515 Lake Road, Zip 76308-5419, Mailing Address: Box 300, Zip 76307-0300; tel. 940/692-1220, (Nonreporting) **A**5 9 10
Primary Contact: James E. Smith, Superintendent
CFO: Bill Lowery, Chief Financial Officer
CMO: Lauren Parsons, M.D., Clinical Director
CIO: Crystal Dennstedt, Chief Information Officer
Web address: www.mhmr.state.tx.us
**Control:** State-Government, nonfederal **Service:** Psychiatric

**Staffed Beds:** 381

☐ **RED RIVER HOSPITAL (454018)**, 1505 Eighth Street, Zip 76301-3106; tel. 940/322-3171 **A**1 9 10 **F**4 5 29 75 86 87 98 99 101 103 104 105 129 131 **S** Acadia Healthcare Company, Inc., Franklin, TN
Primary Contact: Robert Mansfield, Chief Executive Officer
CFO: Lee Mitchell, Chief Financial Officer
CMO: Harvey C. Martin, M.D., Medical Director
CIO: Fay Helton, Director Medical Records
CHR: Tracy Fehr, Executive Assistant and Director Human Resources
CNO: Amy Frate, Director of Nursing
Web address: www.redriverhospital.com
**Control:** Corporation, Investor-owned, for-profit **Service:** Psychiatric

**Staffed Beds:** 66 **Admissions:** 1804 **Census:** 60 **Outpatient Visits:** 204 **Births:** 0 **Total Expense ($000):** 9129 **Payroll Expense ($000):** 5288 **Personnel:** 130

☐ **TEXAS SPECIALTY HOSPITAL AT WICHITA FALLS (452068)**, 1103 Grace Street, Zip 76301-4414; tel. 940/720-6633 **A**1 9 10 **F**1 3 29 30 31 56 75 77 82 85 86 87 91 100 129 142 147 **S** Fundamental Long Term Care Holdings, LLC, Sparks Glencoe, MD
Primary Contact: Delnita Bray, Administrator
CFO: Debbie Herder, Controller
CMO: Robert McBroom, M.D., Medical Director
CIO: Gail McIlroy, Director Medical Records
CNO: Deanna Dowling, R.N., Chief Nursing Officer
Web address: www.thicare.com
**Control:** Corporation, Investor-owned, for-profit **Service:** Long-Term Acute Care hospital

**Staffed Beds:** 31 **Admissions:** 255 **Census:** 18 **Outpatient Visits:** 0 **Births:** 0 **Total Expense ($000):** 6726 **Payroll Expense ($000):** 2347 **Personnel:** 70

☒ **UNITED REGIONAL HEALTH CARE SYSTEM (450010)**, 1600 11th Street, Zip 76301-4307; tel. 940/764-7000, (Includes UNITED REGIONAL HEALTH CARE SYSTEM–EIGHTH STREET CAMPUS, 1600 Eighth Street, Zip 76301-3164; UNITED REGIONAL HEALTH CARE SYSTEM–ELEVENTH STREET CAMPUS, 1600 11th Street, Zip 76301-9988; tel. 940/764-0055) **A**1 2 3 5 9 10 **F**3 11 12 13 15 17 18 20 21 22 24 26 28 29 30 31 32 34 35 37 39 40 43 44 45 46 47 48 49 50 51 53 57 59 60 61 64 65 68 70 73 74 75 76 77 78 79 80 81 82 84 85 86 87 89 92 93 102 107 110 111 113 114 115 116 117 118 125 129 130 131 133 145 146 147 **P**3
Primary Contact: Phyllis A. Cowling, CPA, President and Chief Executive Officer
COO: Nancy Townley, R.N., Senior Vice President Operations
CFO: Robert M. Pert, Vice President Finance and Chief Financial Officer
CMO: Scott Hoyer, M.D., Vice President Quality and Chief Medical Officer
CIO: Jerry Marshall, Director Information Systems
CHR: Kristi Faulkner, Director Human Resources
Web address: www.urhcs.org
**Control:** Other not-for-profit (including NFP Corporation) **Service:** General Medical and Surgical

**Staffed Beds:** 272 **Admissions:** 15253 **Census:** 165 **Outpatient Visits:** 133250 **Births:** 2180 **Total Expense ($000):** 249393 **Payroll Expense ($000):** 97952 **Personnel:** 1547

## WINNIE—Chambers County

**WINNIE COMMUNITY HOSPITAL (451328)**, 538 Broadway, Zip 77665-1249, Mailing Address: P.O. Box 1249, Zip 77665-1249; tel. 409/296-6000 **A**9 10 18 **F**3 29 34 40 59 65 107 132 145 **P**6
Primary Contact: Daniel Yancy, Administrator and Chief Executive Officer
CFO: Julie Harris, Chief Financial Officer
CMO: Leonidas Andres, M.D., Chief of Staff
CHR: Anha Simon, Director Human Resources
Web address: www.winniehospital.com
**Control:** Partnership, Investor-owned, for-profit **Service:** General Medical and Surgical

**Staffed Beds:** 25 **Admissions:** 501 **Census:** 5 **Outpatient Visits:** 22433 **Total Expense ($000):** 7203 **Payroll Expense ($000):** 2987 **Personnel:** 66

## WINNSBORO—Wood County

☒ **MOTHER FRANCES HOSPITAL – WINNSBORO (451380)**, 719 West Coke Road, Zip 75494-0628, Mailing Address: P.O. Box 628, Zip 75494-0628; tel. 903/342-5227 **A**1 9 10 18 **F**3 15 18 29 30 34 40 43 45 56 57 59 64 68 70 75 79 81 82 85 87 93 98 100 101 103 104 107 110 113 126 128 129 130 131 132 145 147 **P**5 6 7 8 **S** Trinity Mother Frances Hospitals and Clinics, Tyler, TX
Primary Contact: Janet Coates, President and Chief Executive Officer
CFO: Renae Thomas, Chief Financial Officer
CMO: Mark A. Clothier, M.D., President Medical Staff
Web address: www.tmfhs.org
**Control:** Other not-for-profit (including NFP Corporation) **Service:** General Medical and Surgical

**Staffed Beds:** 35 **Admissions:** 867 **Census:** 12 **Outpatient Visits:** 16627 **Births:** 0 **Total Expense ($000):** 17012 **Payroll Expense ($000):** 5492 **Personnel:** 115

**TEXAS HEALTH PRESBYTERIAN HOSPITAL WINNSBORO** See Mother Frances Hospital – Winnsboro

**TX**

---

**Hospital, Medicare Provider Number, Address, Telephone, Approval, Facility, and Physician Codes, Health Care System**

★ American Hospital Association (AHA) membership
☐ The Joint Commission accreditation
◇ DNV Healthcare Inc. accreditation
○ American Osteopathic Association (AOA) accreditation
△ Commission on Accreditation of Rehabilitation Facilities (CARF) accreditation

## WINTERS—Runnels County

**NORTH RUNNELS HOSPITAL (451315)**, 7821 East Highway 53, Zip 79567, Mailing Address: P.O. Box 185, Zip 79567–0185; tel. 325/754–5551 **A**9 10 18 **F**7 11 40 57 59 62 65 66 68 97 118 126 132 **P**5
Primary Contact: Sidney Tucker, Chief Executive Officer
CFO: Judy Espitia, Chief Financial Officer
CMO: Sarah Endicott, M.D., Chief of Staff
**Control:** Hospital district or authority, Government, nonfederal **Service:** General Medical and Surgical

**Staffed Beds:** 21 **Admissions:** 221 **Census:** 2 **Outpatient Visits:** 11347 **Births:** 0 **Total Expense ($000):** 3626 **Payroll Expense ($000):** 2094 **Personnel:** 48

## WOODVILLE—Tyler County

★ **TYLER COUNTY HOSPITAL (450460)**, 1100 West Bluff Street, Zip 75979–4799, Mailing Address: P.O. Box 549, Zip 75979–0549; tel. 409/283–8141 **A**9 10 20 **F**3 11 30 35 40 43 46 57 59 64 81 107 113 118 126 145 **P**5
Primary Contact: Sandra Gayle Wright, R.N., Ed.D., Chief Executive Officer
CFO: Richard Wallace, Assistant Administrator, Chief Financial Officer and Controller
CMO: James Brown, M.D., President
CIO: Rachel Haygood, Director Information Technology
CHR: Jan Thomsen, Director Human Resources
Web address: www.tchospital.us
**Control:** Hospital district or authority, Government, nonfederal **Service:** General Medical and Surgical

**Staffed Beds:** 25 **Admissions:** 774 **Census:** 7 **Outpatient Visits:** 18767 **Births:** 1 **Total Expense ($000):** 10426 **Payroll Expense ($000):** 4341 **Personnel:** 122

## YOAKUM—Lavaca County

★ **YOAKUM COMMUNITY HOSPITAL (451346)**, 1200 Carl Ramert Drive, Zip 77995–4198, Mailing Address: P.O. Box 753, Zip 77995–0753; tel. 361/293–2321 **A**9 10 18 **F**3 11 13 15 29 34 35 40 43 56 57 59 64 70 76 79 81 85 86 93 107 108 111 113 118 128 131 132 133 145 147 **S** Community Hospital Corporation, Plano, TX
Primary Contact: Karen Barber, Chief Executive Officer
CFO: Robert Foret, Chief Financial Officer
CMO: Timothy Wagner, M.D., Chief Medical Staff
CHR: Karen Roznovsky, Director Human Resources
Web address: www.yoakumhospital.org
**Control:** Other not–for–profit (including NFP Corporation) **Service:** General Medical and Surgical

**Staffed Beds:** 25 **Admissions:** 1067 **Census:** 13 **Outpatient Visits:** 20563 **Births:** 69 **Total Expense ($000):** 14133 **Payroll Expense ($000):** 5961 **Personnel:** 95

**TX**

*Many Facility Codes have changed. Please refer to the AHA Guide Code Chart.*

# UTAH

## AMERICAN FORK—Utah County

☒ **AMERICAN FORK HOSPITAL (460023)**, 170 North 1100 East,
Zip 84003–2096; tel. 801/855–3300 **A**1 9 10 **F**3 13 15 29 31 32 34 38 39
40 43 44 45 48 54 57 59 62 64 70 72 75 76 77 78 81 82 85 86 87 89 107
110 111 113 115 116 118 122 127 129 130 131 133 143 145 146 147
**S** Intermountain Healthcare, Inc, Salt Lake City, UT
Primary Contact: Michael R. Olson, Administrator
CFO: Rodney Lisonbee, Chief Financial Officer
CMO: Paul H. Robinson, M.D., Medical Director
CIO: Diane Rindlisbacher, Manager Information Systems
CHR: Nate Bigler, Director Human Resource
Web address: www.intermountainhealthcare.org
**Control:** Other not–for–profit (including NFP Corporation) **Service:** General
Medical and Surgical

> **Staffed Beds:** 88 **Admissions:** 6670 **Census:** 54 **Outpatient Visits:** 176199
> **Births:** 3044 **Total Expense ($000):** 93790 **Payroll Expense ($000):** 30877
> **Personnel:** 659

## BEAVER—Beaver County

**BEAVER VALLEY HOSPITAL (460035)**, 1109 North 100 West, Zip 84713,
Mailing Address: P.O. Box 1670, Zip 84713–1670; tel. 435/438–2531,
(Nonreporting) **A**9 10 20
Primary Contact: Craig Val Davidson, Chief Executive Officer and Administrator
Web address: www.beaverutah.net
**Control:** City–Government, nonfederal **Service:** General Medical and Surgical

> **Staffed Beds:** 49

## BLANDING—San Juan County

**BLUE MOUNTAIN HOSPITAL (461310)**, 802 South 200 West,
Zip 84511–3910; tel. 435/678–3993 **A**9 10 18 **F**30 40 41 45 47 48 49 50 57
60 76 78 81 105 109 110 111 118 132 145 **P**4 6 7
Primary Contact: Donna Singer, Chief Executive Officer
COO: Donna Jensen, Director Clinical Services
CFO: Jeremy Lyman, Chief Financial Director
CMO: L. Val Jones, M.D., Medical Director
CIO: Billy Xaochay, Manager Information Technology
CHR: Gail M. Northern, Director Human Resources
Web address: www.bmhutah.com
**Control:** Other not–for–profit (including NFP Corporation) **Service:** General
Medical and Surgical

> **Staffed Beds:** 11 **Admissions:** 312 **Census:** 3 **Outpatient Visits:** 4686
> **Births:** 125 **Total Expense ($000):** 9058 **Payroll Expense ($000):** 2670

## BOUNTIFUL—Davis County

☒ **LAKEVIEW HOSPITAL (460042)**, 630 East Medical Drive, Zip 84010–4996;
tel. 801/299–2200, (Nonreporting) **A**1 9 10 **S** HCA, Nashville, TN
Primary Contact: Rand Kerr, Chief Executive Officer
COO: Troy Wood, Chief Operating Officer
CFO: Wayne Dalton, Chief Financial Officer
CIO: Brent Barton, Director Information Technology
CHR: Julie Isom, Director Human Resources
Web address: www.lakeviewhospital.com
**Control:** Corporation, Investor–owned, for–profit **Service:** General Medical and
Surgical

> **Staffed Beds:** 116

**SOUTH DAVIS COMMUNITY HOSPITAL (462003)**, 401 South 400 East,
Zip 84010; tel. 801/295–2361, (Nonreporting) **A**9 10
Primary Contact: Richard G. Bennett, Administrator
CFO: Daniel J. Foster, Chief Financial Officer
CMO: Scott Southworth, M.D., Medical Director
CHR: Jamey Sulser, Director Human Resources
Web address: www.sdch.com
**Control:** Other not–for–profit (including NFP Corporation) **Service:** Long–Term
Acute Care hospital

> **Staffed Beds:** 176

## BRIGHAM CITY—Box Elder County

☒ **BRIGHAM CITY COMMUNITY HOSPITAL (460017)**, 950 South Medical Drive,
Zip 84302; tel. 435/734–9471, (Nonreporting) **A**1 9 10 **S** HCA, Nashville, TN
Primary Contact: Richard Spuhler, Chief Executive Officer
CMO: Carey Lloyd, M.D., Chief Medical Officer
CIO: Steve Reichard, Manager Information Systems
CHR: Kathy Worley, Director Human Resources
Web address: www.brighamcityhospital.com
**Control:** Corporation, Investor–owned, for–profit **Service:** General Medical and
Surgical

> **Staffed Beds:** 39

## CEDAR CITY—Iron County

☒ **VALLEY VIEW MEDICAL CENTER (460007)**, 1303 North Main Street,
Zip 84720–3462; tel. 435/868–5000 **A**1 9 10 20 **F**8 11 13 15 18 28 29 31
35 70 76 89 **S** Intermountain Healthcare, Inc, Salt Lake City, UT
Primary Contact: Jason Wilson, Administrator
CFO: Reed Sargent, Assistant Administrator Finance
Web address: www.ihc.com
**Control:** Other not–for–profit (including NFP Corporation) **Service:** General
Medical and Surgical

> **Staffed Beds:** 48 **Admissions:** 3745 **Census:** 18

## DELTA—Millard County

★ **DELTA COMMUNITY MEDICAL CENTER (461300)**, 126 South White Sage
Avenue, Zip 84624–8928; tel. 435/864–5591 **A**9 10 18 **F**3 8 11 13 15 31 34
40 41 42 45 54 57 59 68 75 76 81 82 86 87 89 107 110 132 144 145 146
147 **P**5 **S** Intermountain Healthcare, Inc, Salt Lake City, UT
Primary Contact: James E. Beckstrand, Administrator
CFO: Chris Thompson, Chief Financial Officer
Web address: www.ihc.com
**Control:** Other not–for–profit (including NFP Corporation) **Service:** General
Medical and Surgical

> **Staffed Beds:** 18 **Admissions:** 271 **Census:** 2 **Outpatient Visits:** 15656
> **Births:** 105 **Total Expense ($000):** 6566 **Payroll Expense ($000):** 2571
> **Personnel:** 45

## FILLMORE—Millard County

★ **FILLMORE COMMUNITY MEDICAL CENTER (461301)**, 674 South Highway
99, Zip 84631–9701; tel. 435/743–5591 **A**9 10 18 **F**3 8 11 13 15 29 31 34
38 40 41 50 56 57 59 62 63 64 67 68 75 76 81 82 86 87 89 93 107 110
118 127 132 144 145 146 147 **S** Intermountain Healthcare, Inc, Salt Lake
City, UT
Primary Contact: James E. Beckstrand, Administrator
CFO: Chris Thompson, Chief Financial Officer
Web address: www.ihc.com
**Control:** Other not–for–profit (including NFP Corporation) **Service:** General
Medical and Surgical

> **Staffed Beds:** 19 **Admissions:** 196 **Census:** 12 **Outpatient Visits:** 9683
> **Births:** 29 **Total Expense ($000):** 5868 **Payroll Expense ($000):** 2359
> **Personnel:** 50

## GUNNISON—Sanpete County

★ **GUNNISON VALLEY HOSPITAL (461306)**, 64 East 100 North, Zip 84634,
Mailing Address: P.O. Box 759, Zip 84634–0759; tel. 435/528–7246 **A**9 10 18
**F**7 18 34 35 40 56 57 59 62 63 64 65 76 78 79 81 97 107 113 128 129
132 **P**6
Primary Contact: Mark F. Dalley, Administrator
CFO: Brian Murray, Chief Financial Officer
CHR: David Peterson, Manager Human Resources
Web address: www.gvhospital.org
**Control:** County–Government, nonfederal **Service:** General Medical and Surgical

> **Staffed Beds:** 25 **Admissions:** 876 **Census:** 9 **Outpatient Visits:** 32543
> **Births:** 197 **Total Expense ($000):** 15675 **Payroll Expense ($000):** 6934
> **Personnel:** 170

**UT**

**HEBER CITY—Wasatch County**

★ **HEBER VALLEY MEDICAL CENTER (461307)**, 1485 South Highway 40,
Zip 84032–3522; tel. 435/654–2500, (Nonreporting) **A**9 10 18 **S** Intermountain
Healthcare, Inc, Salt Lake City, UT
Primary Contact: Steve Anderson, Administrator
Web address: www.ihc.com
**Control:** Other not–for–profit (including NFP Corporation) **Service:** General
Medical and Surgical

| Staffed Beds: 19 |
|---|

**KANAB—Kane County**

**KANE COUNTY HOSPITAL (461309)**, 355 North Main Street,
Zip 84741–3238; tel. 435/644–5811, (Nonreporting) **A**9 10 18
Primary Contact: Sherrie Pandya, Administrator
CFO: Stephen Howells, Chief Financial Officer
CMO: Darin Ott, D.O., Chief of Staff
CHR: Laurali Noteman, Director Human Resources
Web address: www.kanecountyhospital.net
**Control:** Hospital district or authority, Government, nonfederal **Service:** General
Medical and Surgical

| Staffed Beds: 25 |
|---|

**LAYTON—Davis County**

**DAVIS HOSPITAL AND MEDICAL CENTER (460041)**, 1600 West Antelope
Drive, Zip 84041–1142; tel. 801/807–1000 **A**9 10 21 **F**3 11 12 13 15 17 18
20 22 26 28 29 31 34 35 40 45 46 47 48 49 55 57 59 64 65 68 70 72 73
74 75 76 77 78 79 81 82 85 86 87 89 90 93 94 98 102 105 107 108 109
110 111 113 114 115 116 118 119 128 129 145 146 147 **S** IASIS
Healthcare, Franklin, TN
Primary Contact: Michael E. Jensen, President and Chief Executive Officer
CFO: Jared Spackman, Chief Financial Officer
CMO: Shay Holley, M.D., President Medical Staff
CIO: Shane Williams, Director Information Systems
CHR: Kevin Mansfield, Director Human Resources
Web address: www.davishospital.com
**Control:** Corporation, Investor–owned, for–profit **Service:** General Medical and
Surgical

| Staffed Beds: 200 Admissions: 6323 Census: 59 Outpatient Visits: 171302 |
|---|
| Births: 1936 Personnel: 567 |

**LOGAN—Cache County**

☒ **LOGAN REGIONAL HOSPITAL (460015)**, 1400 North 500 East,
Zip 84341–2499; tel. 435/716–1000, (Total facility includes 10 beds in nursing
home–type unit) **A**1 9 10 **F**3 8 11 13 14 15 18 20 22 28 29 31 32 34 35 36
37 40 43 45 46 49 50 51 57 59 60 64 66 68 70 72 74 75 76 77 78 79 81
82 85 86 87 89 91 93 97 98 99 100 101 102 103 104 105 107 108 109
110 111 113 114 118 119 120 122 127 128 129 130 131 134 145 146 147
**P**6 **S** Intermountain Healthcare, Inc, Salt Lake City, UT
Primary Contact: Michael A. Clark, Administrator and Chief Executive Officer
COO: Brandon McBride, Chief Operating Officer
CFO: Alan Robinson, Chief Financial Officer
CMO: Todd A. Brown, M.D., Medical Director
CIO: Dave Felts, Chief Information Systems
CHR: Jolene Clonts, Director Human Resources
Web address: www.loganregionalhospital.org
**Control:** Other not–for–profit (including NFP Corporation) **Service:** General
Medical and Surgical

| Staffed Beds: 135 Admissions: 7093 Census: 58 Outpatient Visits: 296796 |
|---|
| Births: 2578 Total Expense ($000): 115708 Payroll Expense ($000): |
| 39673 Personnel: 899 |

**MILFORD—Beaver County**

★ **MILFORD VALLEY MEMORIAL HOSPITAL (461305)**, 451 North Main Street,
Zip 84751–0640, Mailing Address: P.O. Box 640, Zip 84751;
tel. 435/387–2411, (Nonreporting) **A**9 10 18
Primary Contact: Craig Val Davidson, Chief Executive Officer
**Control:** Hospital district or authority, Government, nonfederal **Service:** General
Medical and Surgical

| Staffed Beds: 25 |
|---|

**MOAB—Grand County**

★ **MOAB REGIONAL HOSPITAL (461302)**, 450 West Williams Way,
Zip 84532–2297; tel. 435/719–3500 **A**9 10 18 **F**3 13 15 29 30 31 34 35 40
43 45 57 59 63 64 65 66 68 75 76 79 81 82 85 86 89 90 97 107 110 111
114 118 127 129 130 131 132 143 147 **P**6
Primary Contact: Roy E. Barraclough, Administrator and Chief Executive Officer
COO: Vicki Gigliotti, Chief Clinical Officer
CFO: Ken Knight, Chief Financial Officer
CMO: Jonas Munger, M.D., Chief Medical Staff
CIO: Mike Foster, Manager Information Systems
CHR: Becky Striblen, Director Human Resources
Web address: www.amhmoab.org
**Control:** Other not–for–profit (including NFP Corporation) **Service:** General
Medical and Surgical

| Staffed Beds: 17 Admissions: 708 Census: 7 Outpatient Visits: 19954 |
|---|
| Births: 92 Personnel: 143 |

**MONTICELLO—San Juan County**

**SAN JUAN HOSPITAL (461308)**, 380 West 100 North, Zip 84535, Mailing
Address: P.O. Box 308, Zip 84535–0308; tel. 435/587–2116, (Nonreporting) **A**9
10 18
Primary Contact: Phillip W. Lowe, Chief Executive Officer
CFO: Lyman Duncan, Chief Financial Officer
CMO: James Redd, M.D., Chief Medical Officer
Web address: www.sanjuanhealthservices.org/
**Control:** County–Government, nonfederal **Service:** General Medical and Surgical

| Staffed Beds: 25 |
|---|

**MOUNT PLEASANT—Sanpete County**

★ **SANPETE VALLEY HOSPITAL (461303)**, 1100 South Medical Drive,
Zip 84647–2222; tel. 435/462–2441 **A**9 10 18 **F**3 13 15 18 29 34 35 40 41
45 50 54 56 57 59 63 64 65 68 75 76 79 81 82 87 89 107 110 113 118
127 128 129 132 142 145 **S** Intermountain Healthcare, Inc, Salt Lake City, UT
Primary Contact: Mark L. Allen, FACHE, Administrator
CFO: Chris Thompson, Chief Financial Officer
CMO: Allen Day, M.D., President Medical Staff
CIO: Michael Ence, Computer Specialist
CHR: Heather Hafen, Manager Human Resources
Web address: www.intermountainhealthcare.com
**Control:** Other not–for–profit (including NFP Corporation) **Service:** General
Medical and Surgical

| Staffed Beds: 19 Admissions: 575 Census: 6 Outpatient Visits: 29562 |
|---|

**MURRAY—Salt Lake County**

☐ △ **INTERMOUNTAIN MEDICAL CENTER (460010)**, 5121 South Cottonwood
Street, Zip 84157; tel. 801/507–7000 **A**1 2 3 5 7 9 10 **F**3 7 8 12 13 15 17 18
20 22 24 26 28 29 30 31 34 35 37 39 40 43 44 45 46 47 48 49 50 51 52
53 54 55 56 57 58 59 60 61 63 64 70 72 74 75 76 77 78 79 81 82 84
85 86 87 90 91 92 93 94 96 97 100 102 107 108 109 110 111 112 113
114 116 117 118 119 120 121 122 123 125 128 129 130 131 136 137 138
140 141 145 146 147 **P**6 **S** Intermountain Healthcare, Inc, Salt Lake City, UT
Primary Contact: David Grauer, Administrator
COO: Kelly L. Duffin, Operations Manager
Web address: www.intermountainhealthcare.org
**Control:** Other not–for–profit (including NFP Corporation) **Service:** General
Medical and Surgical

| Staffed Beds: 452 Admissions: 27489 Census: 316 Outpatient Visits: |
|---|
| 648155 Births: 4432 Total Expense ($000): 605664 Payroll Expense |
| ($000): 217080 Personnel: 3679 |

☒ **THE ORTHOPEDIC SPECIALTY HOSPITAL (460049)**, 5848 South 300 East,
Zip 84107; tel. 801/314–4100 **A**1 9 10 **F**3 9 29 32 34 35 37 53 57 58 59 68
74 75 77 79 81 85 86 87 91 93 94 107 111 113 118 129 130 133 134 145
**P**6 **S** Intermountain Healthcare, Inc, Salt Lake City, UT
Primary Contact: Bryan Johnson, Administrator
CFO: Ronald Jensen, Manager Finance
CMO: Jon Sundin, M.D., Medical Director
CIO: David Baird, Chief Information Officer
CHR: Tina Tasso, Manager Human Resources
Web address: www.intermountainhealthcare.org
**Control:** Other not–for–profit (including NFP Corporation) **Service:** Orthopedic

| Staffed Beds: 36 Admissions: 1804 Census: 11 Outpatient Visits: 58842 |
|---|
| Births: 0 Total Expense ($000): 57549 Payroll Expense ($000): 14584 |
| Personnel: 334 |

*Many Facility Codes have changed. Please refer to the AHA Guide Code Chart.* © 2012 AHA Guide

UT

## NEPHI—Juab County

★ **CENTRAL VALLEY MEDICAL CENTER (461304)**, 48 West 1500 North,
Zip 84648; tel. 435/623–3000 **A**9 10 18 **F**3 13 15 34 35 40 41 43 45 50 57
62 63 64 65 75 76 77 79 81 82 85 86 89 93 94 97 107 110 113 118 127
128 129 130 132 146 147 **P**6 **S** Rural Health Group, Nephi, UT
Primary Contact: Mark R. Stoddard, President
COO: John E. Gledhill, Chief Operating Officer
CFO: Brent Davis, Chief Financial Officer
CMO: James Rosenbeck, D.O., Chief of Staff
CIO: Ken Richens, Chief Information Officer
CHR: Brian Allsop, Director Human Resources
Web address: www.cvmed.net
**Control:** Other not–for–profit (including NFP Corporation) **Service:** General
Medical and Surgical

**Staffed Beds:** 25 **Admissions:** 1099 **Census:** 11 **Outpatient Visits:** 31258
**Births:** 162 **Total Expense ($000):** 24901 **Payroll Expense ($000):** 7297
**Personnel:** 204

## NORTH LOGAN—Cache County

☐ **CACHE VALLEY SPECIALTY HOSPITAL (460054)**, 2380 North 400 East,
Zip 84341; tel. 435/713–9700, (Nonreporting) **A**1 9 10 **S** National Surgical
Hospitals, Chicago, IL
Primary Contact: John C. Worley, Jr., Chief Executive Officer
CFO: David S. Geary, Chief Financial Officer
CMO: Brian Nelson, M.D., Chief Medical Officer
Web address: www.cvsh.com
**Control:** Corporation, Investor–owned, for–profit **Service:** General Medical and
Surgical

**Staffed Beds:** 15

## OGDEN—Weber County

✠ **MCKAY-DEE HOSPITAL CENTER (460004)**, 4401 Harrison Boulevard,
Zip 84403; tel. 801/387–2800 **A**1 2 9 10 **F**3 8 11 12 13 15 17 18 20 22 24
26 28 29 30 31 34 35 38 39 40 43 44 45 46 49 50 51 53 54 55 57 58 59
60 61 64 65 66 67 68 70 72 74 75 76 77 78 79 81 82 84 85 86 87 89 90
91 93 97 98 99 100 101 102 103 104 105 106 107 108 110 111 113 114
115 116 118 119 120 122 125 128 129 130 131 133 134 143 145 146 147
**P**6 **S** Intermountain Healthcare, Inc, Salt Lake City, UT
Primary Contact: Timothy T. Pehrson, Chief Executive Officer
CFO: Doug Smith, Chief Financial Officer
CMO: Richard Arbogast, M.D., Chief Medical Officer
CIO: Mary Gathers, Director Information Systems
CHR: Karen Burnett, Regional Director Human Resources
Web address: www.mckay–dee.org
**Control:** Other not–for–profit (including NFP Corporation) **Service:** General
Medical and Surgical

**Staffed Beds:** 311 **Admissions:** 19091 **Census:** 191 **Outpatient Visits:**
249546 **Births:** 3922 **Total Expense ($000):** 302533 **Payroll Expense
($000):** 103467 **Personnel:** 2074

✠ **OGDEN REGIONAL MEDICAL CENTER (460005)**, 5475 South 500 East,
Zip 84405–6978; tel. 801/479–2111, (Nonreporting) **A**1 9 10 **S** HCA,
Nashville, TN
Primary Contact: Mark B. Adams, Chief Executive Officer
CFO: Judd Taylor, Chief Financial Officer
CMO: Michael Diehl, M.D., President
CIO: Sarah Dewitt, Director
CHR: Chris Bissenden, Director Human Resources
Web address: www.ogdenregional.com
**Control:** Corporation, Investor–owned, for–profit **Service:** General Medical and
Surgical

**Staffed Beds:** 167

## OREM—Utah County

✠ **OREM COMMUNITY HOSPITAL (460043)**, 331 North 400 West,
Zip 84057–1999; tel. 801/224–4080 **A**1 9 10 **F**3 11 13 15 29 32 35 38 39
40 43 44 54 59 64 68 75 76 81 82 86 87 93 97 107 111 118 131 134 145
**S** Intermountain Healthcare, Inc, Salt Lake City, UT
Primary Contact: Steven Badger, R.N., Administrator
CFO: Rodney Lisonbee, Chief Financial Officer
CMO: Neil Whitaker, M.D., Chief Medical Director
CIO: Diane Rindlisbacher, Manager Information Systems
CHR: Pam Niece, Director Human Resources
Web address: www.intermountainhealthcare.org
**Control:** Other not–for–profit (including NFP Corporation) **Service:** General
Medical and Surgical

**Staffed Beds:** 18 **Admissions:** 1363 **Census:** 8 **Outpatient Visits:** 49052
**Births:** 1309 **Total Expense ($000):** 23403 **Payroll Expense ($000):** 8707
**Personnel:** 187

✠ **TIMPANOGOS REGIONAL HOSPITAL (460052)**, 750 West 800 North,
Zip 84059–3660; tel. 801/714–6000 **A**1 9 10 **F**3 13 15 17 18 19 20 22 24
26 28 29 39 40 43 45 47 48 49 57 59 60 70 72 73 74 75 76 78 79 81 85
87 89 102 107 108 110 111 113 118 125 129 140 145 **P**6 **S** HCA,
Nashville, TN
Primary Contact: Keith D. Tintle, Chief Executive Officer
Web address: www.timpanogosregionalhospital.com
**Control:** Corporation, Investor–owned, for–profit **Service:** General Medical and
Surgical

**Staffed Beds:** 117 **Admissions:** 4371 **Census:** 41 **Outpatient Visits:** 27946
**Births:** 1681 **Total Expense ($000):** 58863 **Payroll Expense ($000):** 22733
**Personnel:** 392

## PANGUITCH—Garfield County

★ **GARFIELD MEMORIAL HOSPITAL AND CLINICS (460033)**, 200 North 400
East, Zip 84759, Mailing Address: P.O. Box 389, Zip 84759–0389;
tel. 435/676–8811, (Total facility includes 27 beds in nursing home–type unit) **A**9
10 20 **F**2 13 15 29 32 34 35 40 45 56 57 59 64 65 67 75 76 81 87 97 107
110 118 126 127 128 129 131 132 147 **P**6 **S** Intermountain Healthcare, Inc,
Salt Lake City, UT
Primary Contact: Alberto Vasquez, Administrator
CFO: Reed Sargent, Assistant Administrator Finance
Web address: www.ihc.com/xp/ihc/garfield
**Control:** Other not–for–profit (including NFP Corporation) **Service:** General
Medical and Surgical

**Staffed Beds:** 41 **Admissions:** 345 **Census:** 28 **Outpatient Visits:** 33954
**Births:** 22 **Total Expense ($000):** 9485 **Payroll Expense ($000):** 4625
**Personnel:** 96

## PARK CITY—Summit County

✠ **PARK CITY MEDICAL CENTER (460057)**, 900 Round Valley Drive,
Zip 84060–7552; tel. 435/658–7000 **A**1 9 10 **F**3 13 15 18 29 34 35 36 38
40 43 45 48 50 51 53 57 59 65 68 74 75 76 79 81 82 85 87 89 93 96 102
107 108 110 111 114 118 128 129 130 134 145 146 **P**6 **S** Intermountain
Healthcare, Inc, Salt Lake City, UT
Primary Contact: Robert W. Allen, Chief Executive Officer
COO: Steve Anderson, Chief Operating Officer
CFO: Craig Mills, Senior Financial Advisor
CHR: Bruce Dent, Director Human Resources
Web address: www.intermountainhealthcare.org
**Control:** Other not–for–profit (including NFP Corporation) **Service:** General
Medical and Surgical

**Staffed Beds:** 26 **Admissions:** 1353 **Census:** 7 **Outpatient Visits:** 75765
**Births:** 264 **Total Expense ($000):** 45608 **Payroll Expense ($000):** 14013
**Personnel:** 270

## PAYSON—Utah County

✠ **MOUNTAIN VIEW HOSPITAL (460013)**, 1000 East 100 North,
Zip 84651–1690; tel. 801/465–7000, (Nonreporting) **A**1 9 10 **S** HCA,
Nashville, TN
Primary Contact: Kevin Johnson, Chief Executive Officer
COO: Kimball Anderson, FACHE, Chief Operating Officer
CFO: Steven R. Schramm, Chief Financial Officer
CMO: Joseph Dinkins, M.D., Chief Medical Staff
CHR: Wally Trotter, Director Human Resources
Web address: www.mvhpayson.com
**Control:** Corporation, Investor–owned, for–profit **Service:** General Medical and
Surgical

**Staffed Beds:** 114

## PRICE—Carbon County

✠ **CASTLEVIEW HOSPITAL (460011)**, 300 North Hospital Drive,
Zip 84501–4200; tel. 435/637–4800, (Nonreporting) **A**1 9 10 20 **S** LifePoint
Hospitals, Inc., Brentwood, TN
Primary Contact: Mark Holyoak, Chief Executive Officer
CFO: Ryan Moynier, Chief Financial Officer
CMO: Sterling Potter, M.D., Chief of Staff
CIO: Keenan Johnson, Director Information Systems
CHR: David Donaldson, Director Human Resources
Web address: www.castleviewhospital.net
**Control:** Corporation, Investor–owned, for–profit **Service:** General Medical and
Surgical

**Staffed Beds:** 57

**UT**

---

**Hospital, Medicare Provider Number, Address, Telephone, Approval, Facility, and Physician Codes, Health Care System**

★ American Hospital Association (AHA) membership
☐ The Joint Commission accreditation ◇ DNV Healthcare Inc. accreditation
◯ American Osteopathic Association (AOA) accreditation
△ Commission on Accreditation of Rehabilitation Facilities (CARF) accreditation

## PROVO—Utah County

☐ **UTAH STATE HOSPITAL (464001)**, 1300 East Center Street, Zip 84606–3554, Mailing Address: P.O. Box 270, Zip 84603–0270; tel. 801/344–4400 **A**1 10 **F**30 34 56 75 77 86 87 91 98 99 100 101 103 129 134 142 145 **P**6
Primary Contact: Dallas Earnshaw, Chief Executive Officer
COO: Dallas Earnshaw, Chief Executive Officer
CFO: Robert Burton, Manager Finance
CMO: Richard Spencer, M.D., Clinical Director
CIO: Jill Hill, Director Information Technology
CHR: David Gardner, Manager Human Resources
Web address: www.ush.utah.gov
**Control:** State–Government, nonfederal **Service:** Psychiatric

**Staffed Beds:** 329 **Admissions:** 415 **Census:** 307 **Outpatient Visits:** 0
**Births:** 0 **Total Expense ($000):** 55210 **Payroll Expense ($000):** 28236
**Personnel:** 788

⊞ △ **UTAH VALLEY REGIONAL MEDICAL CENTER (460001)**, 1034 North 500 West, Zip 84604–3337; tel. 801/357–7850 **A**1 2 7 9 10 **F**3 11 13 15 17 18 20 21 22 23 24 25 28 29 30 31 32 34 35 38 39 40 43 44 45 48 49 50 51 53 54 56 57 58 59 60 61 62 63 64 68 69 70 72 74 75 76 77 78 81 82 84 85 86 87 88 89 90 91 92 93 94 97 98 99 100 101 102 103 104 105 107 108 110 111 113 114 115 116 117 118 120 122 128 129 130 131 132 133 143 145 146 147 **P**6 **S** Intermountain Healthcare, Inc, Salt Lake City, UT
Primary Contact: Steve Smoot, Administrator
CFO: Rodney Lisonbee, Chief Financial Officer
CMO: Neil Whitaker, M.D., Medical Director
CIO: Diane Rindlisbacher, Director Information Systems
Web address: www.utahvalleyregional.org
**Control:** Other not–for–profit (including NFP Corporation) **Service:** General Medical and Surgical

**Staffed Beds:** 367 **Admissions:** 19282 **Census:** 231 **Outpatient Visits:** 353860 **Births:** 4286 **Total Expense ($000):** 363290 **Payroll Expense ($000):** 131554 **Personnel:** 2841

☐ **UTAH VALLEY SPECIALTY HOSPITAL (462005)**, 306 West River Bend Lane, Zip 84604; tel. 801/226–8880, (Nonreporting) **A**1 9 10 **S** Ernest Health, Inc., Albuquerque, NM
Primary Contact: Marie Prothero, R.N., MSN, Chief Executive Officer
Web address: www.uvsh.ernesthealth.com
**Control:** Corporation, Investor–owned, for–profit **Service:** Long–Term Acute Care hospital

**Staffed Beds:** 40

## RICHFIELD—Sevier County

⊞ **SEVIER VALLEY MEDICAL CENTER (460026)**, 1000 North Main Street, Zip 84701–1843; tel. 435/896–8271 **A**1 9 10 20 **F**3 8 13 15 29 34 35 40 45 57 59 62 63 64 68 75 76 77 79 81 82 89 92 97 107 108 111 117 118 128 132 145 **P**5 6 **S** Intermountain Healthcare, Inc, Salt Lake City, UT
Primary Contact: Gary E. Beck, Administrator
CFO: Chris Thompson, Chief Financial Officer
CHR: Katey Nelson, Director Human Resources
Web address: www.intermountain.com
**Control:** Other not–for–profit (including NFP Corporation) **Service:** General Medical and Surgical

**Staffed Beds:** 27 **Admissions:** 871 **Census:** 6 **Outpatient Visits:** 51731
**Births:** 218 **Total Expense ($000):** 19376 **Payroll Expense ($000):** 6079
**Personnel:** 133

## RIVERTON—Salt Lake County

⊞ **RIVERTON HOSPITAL (460058)**, 3741 West 12600 South, Zip 84065–7215; tel. 801/285–4000 **A**1 9 10 **F**3 13 15 29 31 34 39 40 43 44 45 46 47 48 49 50 51 57 59 64 68 70 76 78 79 81 85 86 87 89 93 94 97 107 108 110 111 113 114 117 118 128 129 130 145 146 147 **S** Intermountain Healthcare, Inc, Salt Lake City, UT
Primary Contact: Blair Kent, Administrator
Web address: www.intermountainhealthcare.org/
**Control:** Other not–for–profit (including NFP Corporation) **Service:** General Medical and Surgical

**Staffed Beds:** 92 **Admissions:** 4270 **Census:** 29 **Outpatient Visits:** 111951
**Births:** 2244 **Total Expense ($000):** 61547 **Payroll Expense ($000):** 20794
**Personnel:** 403

## ROOSEVELT—Duchesne County

★ **UINTAH BASIN MEDICAL CENTER (460019)**, 250 West 300 North, 75–2, Zip 84066; tel. 435/722–6163, (Total facility includes 90 beds in nursing home–type unit) **A**9 10 20 **F**6 7 11 13 15 17 35 40 43 45 50 52 53 54 57 59 60 62 63 70 73 76 77 79 81 84 85 87 89 93 107 110 111 113 117 118 127 128 129 130 131 134 143 145 146 147 **P**7
Primary Contact: Bradley D. LeBaron, FACHE, President and Chief Executive Officer
CFO: Brent Hales, Chief Financial Officer
CMO: Gary B. White, M.D., Chief Medical Staff
CHR: Randall Bennett, Assistant Administrator
Web address: www.ubmc.org
**Control:** Other not–for–profit (including NFP Corporation) **Service:** General Medical and Surgical

**Staffed Beds:** 124 **Admissions:** 1814 **Census:** 85 **Outpatient Visits:** 62870
**Births:** 546 **Total Expense ($000):** 59377 **Payroll Expense ($000):** 19585
**Personnel:** 505

## SAINT GEORGE—Washington County

⊞ △ **DIXIE REGIONAL MEDICAL CENTER (460021)**, 1380 East Medical Center Drive, Zip 84790; tel. 435/251–1000, (Includes DIXIE REGIONAL MEDICAL CENTER, 544 South 400 East, St. George, Zip 84770) **A**1 2 7 9 10 **F**3 7 11 12 13 15 18 19 20 21 22 23 24 25 28 29 31 34 35 38 40 43 45 46 50 53 54 57 59 64 67 68 70 72 74 75 76 77 78 79 80 81 82 83 84 85 89 90 93 98 102 107 108 110 111 113 114 116 118 119 120 128 129 130 131 134 145 146 147 **P**5 **S** Intermountain Healthcare, Inc, Salt Lake City, UT
Primary Contact: Terri Kane, Administrator
CFO: Mary Hatch, Chief Financial Officer
CMO: Steven Van Norman, M.D., Medical Director
CIO: Lance Bedingfield, Director Information Services
CHR: Vicki Wilson, Chief Human Resources Officer
Web address: www.intermountainhealthcare.org
**Control:** Other not–for–profit (including NFP Corporation) **Service:** General Medical and Surgical

**Staffed Beds:** 261 **Admissions:** 14391 **Census:** 142 **Outpatient Visits:** 454888 **Births:** 2241 **Total Expense ($000):** 288625 **Payroll Expense ($000):** 91682 **Personnel:** 1816

## SALT LAKE CITY—Salt Lake County

⊞ **LDS HOSPITAL (460006)**, Eighth Avenue and C Street, Zip 84143–0001; tel. 801/408–1100 **A**1 2 3 5 9 10 **F**3 4 5 7 8 12 13 15 18 28 29 30 31 34 35 38 39 40 43 45 46 48 50 51 52 53 54 55 56 57 58 59 60 61 63 64 65 66 68 70 73 74 75 76 77 78 79 81 84 85 86 87 89 91 92 93 94 98 100 101 102 103 104 105 107 108 109 110 111 113 114 116 118 119 120 128 129 130 131 135 145 146 147 **P**6 **S** Intermountain Healthcare, Inc, Salt Lake City, UT
Primary Contact: Jim Sheets, Administrator
CFO: David M. Larsen, Chief Financial Officer
CMO: William L. Hamilton, M.D., Chief Medical Officer
CIO: David Baird, Chief Information Officer
CHR: Nancy Adams, Chief Human Resources Officer
Web address: www.intermountainhealthcare.org
**Control:** Other not–for–profit (including NFP Corporation) **Service:** General Medical and Surgical

**Staffed Beds:** 236 **Admissions:** 10201 **Census:** 113 **Outpatient Visits:** 247222 **Births:** 2675 **Total Expense ($000):** 196824 **Payroll Expense ($000):** 70370 **Personnel:** 1280

⊞ **PRIMARY CHILDREN'S MEDICAL CENTER (463301)**, 100 North Mario Capecchi Drive, Zip 84113–1100; tel. 801/662–1000 **A**1 3 5 9 10 **F**3 5 9 11 17 19 21 23 25 27 29 30 31 32 34 35 36 38 39 40 41 43 44 45 48 49 50 54 55 58 59 61 64 65 68 72 74 75 77 78 79 81 82 84 85 86 87 88 89 92 93 96 98 99 100 101 102 104 105 106 107 108 111 113 114 115 116 117 118 123 128 129 131 133 135 136 137 138 140 141 145 147 **S** Intermountain Healthcare, Inc, Salt Lake City, UT
Primary Contact: Katy Welkie, R.N., Administrator and Chief Executive Officer
CFO: Jeremiah Radandt, Chief Financial Officer
CMO: Ed Clark, M.D., Medical Director
CIO: Joe Hales, Director Information Systems
CHR: Albert Bennett Buckworth, Director Human Resources
Web address: www.intermountainhealthcare.org
**Control:** Other not–for–profit (including NFP Corporation) **Service:** Children's general

**Staffed Beds:** 289 **Admissions:** 13550 **Census:** 191 **Outpatient Visits:** 331931 **Births:** 0 **Total Expense ($000):** 363744 **Payroll Expense ($000):** 143123 **Personnel:** 2671

**PROMISE SPECIALTY HOSPITAL OF SALT LAKE (462004)**, 1050 East South Temple, 3rd Floor, Zip 84102; tel. 801/350–4110, (Nonreporting) **A**9 10 **S** Promise Healthcare, Boca Raton, FL
Primary Contact: Linda Hook, Chief Executive Officer
Web address: www.promise-saltlake.com
**Control:** Corporation, Investor–owned, for–profit **Service:** Long–Term Acute Care hospital

**Staffed Beds:** 32

*Many Facility Codes have changed. Please refer to the AHA Guide Code Chart.*
© 2012 AHA Guide

**UT**

**SALT LAKE BEHAVIORAL HEALTH (464013)**, 3802 South 700 East, Zip 84106–1182; tel. 801/264–6000, (Nonreporting) **A**9 10 **S** Ascend Health Corporation, New York, NY
Primary Contact: Michael Rowley, Chief Executive Officer
Web address: www.saltlakebehavioralhealth.com
**Control:** Corporation, Investor–owned, for–profit **Service:** Psychiatric

Staffed Beds: 118

**SALT LAKE REGIONAL MEDICAL CENTER (460003)**, 1050 East South Temple, Zip 84102–1599; tel. 801/350–4111, (Nonreporting) **A**1 3 5 9 10 21 **S** IASIS Healthcare, Franklin, TN
Primary Contact: Jeff Frandsen, Chief Executive Officer
CFO: Steven Payne, Chief Financial Officer
CMO: Wanda Updike, M.D., Chief of Staff
CIO: Mark Runyan, Director Information Services
CHR: Carolyn Livingston, Director Human Resources
Web address: www.saltlakeregional.com
**Control:** Corporation, Investor–owned, for–profit **Service:** General Medical and Surgical

Staffed Beds: 132

**SHRINERS HOSPITALS FOR CHILDREN–INTERMOUNTAIN (463302)**, Fairfax Road & Virginia Street, Zip 84103–4399; tel. 801/536–3500 **A**1 3 5 10 **F**3 11 29 34 35 50 57 58 59 64 68 74 75 77 79 80 81 82 85 86 87 89 90 93 94 118 129 130 131 142 145 **P**1 **S** Shriners Hospitals for Children, Tampa, FL
Primary Contact: Kevin Martin, R.N., M.P.H., Administrator
CFO: Randy Lindberg, Director Fiscal Services
CMO: Jacques D'Astous, M.D., Chief of Staff
CIO: Mike Allen, Director Information Technology
CHR: Russ Crockett, Director Human Resources
Web address: www.shriners.org
**Control:** Other not–for–profit (including NFP Corporation) **Service:** Children's orthopedic

Staffed Beds: 40 Admissions: 1241 Census: 7 Outpatient Visits: 18026
Births: 0

**ST. MARK'S HOSPITAL (460047)**, 1200 East 3900 South, Zip 84124–1390; tel. 801/268–7111 **A**1 2 9 10 **F**3 8 11 12 13 14 15 17 18 20 22 24 26 28 29 30 31 34 35 36 38 40 42 46 49 50 53 56 57 58 59 60 64 65 67 70 72 73 74 75 76 77 78 79 80 81 82 84 85 86 87 102 107 108 110 111 113 114 117 118 123 125 127 128 129 131 134 144 145 146 147 **S** HCA, Nashville, TN
Primary Contact: Steven B. Bateman, Chief Executive Officer
COO: Matt Dixon, Chief Operating Officer
CFO: Bryan McKinley, Chief Financial Officer
CMO: J. Eric Vanderhooft, M.D., President Medical Staff
CIO: Jesse Trujillo, Chief Information Officer
CHR: Robyn Opheikens, Assistant Administrator Human Resources
Web address: www.stmarkshospital.com
**Control:** Corporation, Investor–owned, for–profit **Service:** General Medical and Surgical

Staffed Beds: 317 Admissions: 15111 Census: 168 Outpatient Visits: 143949 Births: 3176 Personnel: 1246

△ **UNIVERSITY OF UTAH HEALTH CARE – HOSPITAL AND CLINICS (460009)**, 50 North Medical Drive, Zip 84132–0002; tel. 801/581–2121 **A**1 3 5 7 9 10 **F**3 6 7 9 12 13 15 16 17 18 20 22 24 26 28 29 30 34 35 36 37 38 39 40 42 43 44 45 46 47 48 49 50 52 53 54 55 56 57 58 59 60 61 62 64 65 68 70 71 72 73 74 75 76 77 78 79 80 81 82 83 84 85 86 87 89 90 91 92 93 94 96 97 98 100 101 102 103 104 107 108 110 111 112 113 114 115 116 117 118 119 120 122 123 125 128 129 130 131 133 134 135 136 137 138 139 140 141 142 143 144 145 146 147 **P**1
Primary Contact: David Entwistle, Chief Executive Officer
COO: Quinn McKenna, Chief Operating Officer
CFO: Gordon Crabtree, Chief Financial Officer
CMO: Thomas Miller, M.D., Medical Director
CIO: James Turnbull, Vice President and Chief Information Officer
CHR: Sherri Hollingsworth, Chief Human Resources Officer
Web address: www.uuhsc.utah.edu
**Control:** State–Government, nonfederal **Service:** General Medical and Surgical

Staffed Beds: 476 Admissions: 23860 Census: 370 Outpatient Visits: 1097335 Births: 3713 Total Expense ($000): 850112 Payroll Expense ($000): 310034 Personnel: 6152

**UNIVERSITY OF UTAH NEUROPSYCHIATRIC INSTITUTE (464009)**, 501 Chipeta Way, Zip 84108–1225; tel. 801/583–2500 **A**1 3 5 9 10 **F**4 5 30 34 35 54 57 64 75 98 99 100 101 103 104 105 129 **P**1 5 6
Primary Contact: Ross Van Vranken, Chief Executive Officer
CFO: Becky Schaefer, Chief Financial Officer
CMO: Michael Lowry, M.D., Medical Director
Web address: www.med.utah.edu/uni
**Control:** State–Government, nonfederal **Service:** Psychiatric

Staffed Beds: 90 Admissions: 3427 Census: 76 Outpatient Visits: 28161
Births: 0 Total Expense ($000): 40772 Payroll Expense ($000): 15103
Personnel: 508

△ **VETERANS AFFAIRS SALT LAKE CITY HEALTH CARE SYSTEM**, 500 Foothill Drive, Zip 84148–0002; tel. 801/582–1565 **A**1 3 5 7 **F**3 4 5 8 12 18 20 22 24 28 29 30 34 35 36 38 39 40 44 45 46 47 48 49 50 53 54 56 57 58 59 60 61 62 64 65 70 71 74 75 77 78 79 81 82 83 84 85 86 87 90 92 93 94 96 97 98 100 101 102 103 104 105 106 107 108 109 111 113 114 115 116 117 118 126 128 129 131 132 134 136 142 143 145 146 147 **P**6 **S** Department of Veterans Affairs, Washington, DC
Primary Contact: Steven W. Young, Director
COO: Roy Hawkins, Acting Associate Director
CFO: Val Martin, Director Financial Management Services Center
CMO: Ronald J. Gebhart, M.D., Chief of Staff
CIO: Lisa Leonelis, Chief Information Officer
CHR: Lisa Porter, Director Human Resources, Leadership and Education
Web address: www.saltlakecity.va.gov/
**Control:** Veterans Affairs, Government, federal **Service:** General Medical and Surgical

Staffed Beds: 121 Admissions: 6180 Census: 98 Outpatient Visits: 638866
Births: 0 Total Expense ($000): 390807 Payroll Expense ($000): 177507
Personnel: 1940

**SANDY—Salt Lake County**

**ALTA VIEW HOSPITAL (460044)**, 9660 South 1300 East, Zip 84094–3793; tel. 801/501–2600 **A**1 2 9 10 **F**3 8 12 13 15 29 34 35 38 39 40 43 44 45 46 47 48 49 50 53 54 56 57 59 64 68 70 75 76 78 79 81 85 86 87 92 93 102 107 108 110 111 114 118 128 129 131 134 140 142 145 146 **S** Intermountain Healthcare, Inc, Salt Lake City, UT
Primary Contact: Becky Kapp, Administrator
CFO: Todd Sanders, Manager Finance
CHR: Diane Holman, Manager Human Resources
Web address: www.intermountainhealthcare.org
**Control:** Other not–for–profit (including NFP Corporation) **Service:** General Medical and Surgical

Staffed Beds: 71 Admissions: 3898 Census: 29 Outpatient Visits: 139049
Births: 1350 Total Expense ($000): 75465 Payroll Expense ($000): 25180
Personnel: 463

**HEALTHSOUTH REHABILITATION HOSPITAL OF UTAH (463025)**, 8074 South 1300 East, Zip 84094–0743; tel. 801/561–3400, (Nonreporting) **A**1 10 **S** HEALTHSOUTH Corporation, Birmingham, AL
Primary Contact: Philip Eaton, Chief Executive Officer
CFO: Daren Woolstenhulme, Chief Financial Officer
CMO: Joseph VickRoy, M.D., Medical Director
CHR: Troy Jensen, Director Human Resources
Web address: www.healthsouthutah.com
**Control:** Corporation, Investor–owned, for–profit **Service:** Rehabilitation

Staffed Beds: 105

**TOOELE—Tooele County**

**MOUNTAIN WEST MEDICAL CENTER (460014)**, 2055 North Main, Zip 84074–2794; tel. 435/843–3600, (Nonreporting) **A**1 9 10 **S** Community Health Systems, Inc., Franklin, TN
Primary Contact: Tim Moran, Interim Chief Executive Officer
CFO: Scott Banks, Chief Financial Officer
CMO: James Antinori, M.D., Chief of Staff
CHR: James Glade, Director Human Resources
Web address: www.mountainwestmc.com
**Control:** Corporation, Investor–owned, for–profit **Service:** General Medical and Surgical

Staffed Beds: 31

UT

### TREMONTON—Box Elder County

★ **BEAR RIVER VALLEY HOSPITAL (460039)**, 905 North 1000 West,
Zip 84337–2497; tel. 435/207–4500, (Nonreporting) **A**9 10 **S** Intermountain
Healthcare, Inc, Salt Lake City, UT
Primary Contact: Eric Packer, Administrator
CHR: Joy Sadler, Director Human Resources
Web address: www.ihc.com
**Control:** Other not–for–profit (including NFP Corporation) **Service:** General
Medical and Surgical

**Staffed Beds:** 14

### VERNAL—Uintah County

⊞ **ASHLEY REGIONAL MEDICAL CENTER (460030)**, 150 West 100 North,
Zip 84078–2036; tel. 435/789–3342, (Nonreporting) **A**1 9 10 20 **S** LifePoint
Hospitals, Inc., Brentwood, TN
Primary Contact: Si Hutt, Chief Executive Officer
CFO: Chad Labrum, Chief Financial Officer
CMO: Nolan Brooksby, M.D., Chief of Staff
CIO: Mark Rich, Director Information Services
CHR: Deena Mansfield, Director Human Resources
Web address: www.ashleyregional.com
**Control:** Corporation, Investor–owned, for–profit **Service:** General Medical and
Surgical

**Staffed Beds:** 39

### WEST JORDAN—Salt Lake County

☐ **JORDAN VALLEY MEDICAL CENTER (460051)**, 3580 West 9000 South,
Zip 84088–8811; tel. 801/561–8888 **A**1 9 10 21 **F**3 12 15 17 18 20 22 28
29 30 31 34 35 37 39 40 41 45 46 48 49 50 51 53 57 59 60 64 70 72 73
74 75 76 77 79 85 87 89 90 91 93 98 107 108 110 111 114 118 125 128
130 134 145 146 147 **S** IASIS Healthcare, Franklin, TN
Primary Contact: Bryanie W. Swilley, Jr., Chief Executive Officer
COO: Jon Butterfield, Chief Operating Officer
CFO: Kurt Shipley, Chief Financial Officer
CMO: B. Dee Allred, M.D., President Medical Staff
Web address: www.jordanvalleymc.com
**Control:** Partnership, Investor–owned, for–profit **Service:** General Medical and
Surgical

**Staffed Beds:** 183 **Admissions:** 6536 **Census:** 61 **Outpatient Visits:** 91853
**Births:** 2382 **Total Expense ($000):** 74827 **Payroll Expense ($000):** 28740

### WEST VALLEY CITY—Salt Lake County

**PIONEER VALLEY HOSPITAL**, 3460 South Pioneer Parkway, Zip 84120–2648;
tel. 801/964–3100, (Nonreporting) **S** IASIS Healthcare, Franklin, TN
Primary Contact: Bryanie W. Swilley, Jr., Chief Executive Officer
COO: Jon Butterfield, Chief Operating Officer
CFO: Kurt Shipley, Chief Financial Officer
CMO: B. Dee Allred, M.D., President Medical Staff
CIO: Jodi DeJong, Director Marketing
CHR: Misty Birch, Director Human Resources
Web address: www.pioneervalleyhospital.com
**Control:** Corporation, Investor–owned, for–profit **Service:** General Medical and
Surgical

**Staffed Beds:** 101

UT

# VERMONT

## BENNINGTON—Bennington County

✠ **SOUTHWESTERN VERMONT MEDICAL CENTER (470012)**, 100 Hospital
Drive, Zip 05201–5004; tel. 802/442–6361, (Nonreporting) **A**1 2 9 10
Primary Contact: Thomas A. Dee, Chief Executive Officer
CMO: Mark Novotny, M.D., Chief Medical Officer
CIO: Richard Ogilvie, Chief Information Officer
CHR: Craig Ghidotti, Vice President Human Resources
Web address: www.svhealthcare.org
**Control:** Other not–for–profit (including NFP Corporation) **Service:** General
Medical and Surgical

**Staffed Beds:** 85

## BERLIN—Washington County

✠ **CENTRAL VERMONT MEDICAL CENTER (470001)**, 130 Fisher Road,
Zip 05602–9516, Mailing Address: P.O. Box 547, Barre, Zip 05641–0547;
tel. 802/371–4100, (Total facility includes 153 beds in nursing home–type unit)
**A**1 9 10 **F**3 8 11 13 15 28 29 30 31 34 35 36 40 43 44 45 46 49 50 51 52
53 57 58 59 64 65 70 74 75 76 77 78 81 82 84 85 87 93 94 96 97 98 99
100 102 104 107 108 110 111 113 114 115 116 117 118 127 129 130 131
134 142 145 146 147 **P**6 8
Primary Contact: Judith C. Tartaglia, President and Chief Executive Officer
COO: Nancy Lothian, Chief Operating Officer
CFO: Cheyenne Follard, Chief Financial Officer
CMO: Philip Brown, D.O., Vice President Medical Affairs
CHR: Patricia Rickard, Vice President Human Resources
Web address: www.cvmc.org/
**Control:** Other not–for–profit (including NFP Corporation) **Service:** General
Medical and Surgical

**Staffed Beds:** 240 **Admissions:** 3775 **Census:** 190 **Outpatient Visits:**
297793 **Births:** 384 **Total Expense ($000):** 111618 **Payroll Expense**
**($000):** 51961 **Personnel:** 749

## BRATTLEBORO—Windham County

★ **BRATTLEBORO MEMORIAL HOSPITAL (470011)**, 17 Belmont Avenue,
Zip 05301–3498; tel. 802/257–0341 **A**9 10 **F**3 8 11 13 14 15 17 18 28 29
30 31 34 35 39 40 45 49 52 53 57 59 64 68 70 74 75 76 77 78 79 81 85
87 93 107 108 110 113 117 118 129 130 131 134 145 146 147
Primary Contact: Steven R. Gordon, President and Chief Executive Officer
CFO: Michael Rogers, Vice President Fiscal Services
CMO: David Albright, M.D., Chief Medical Officer
CIO: Jonathan Farina, Chief Information Officer
CHR: Michael Kelliher, Vice President Human Resources
Web address: www.bmhvt.org
**Control:** Other not–for–profit (including NFP Corporation) **Service:** General
Medical and Surgical

**Staffed Beds:** 32 **Admissions:** 1675 **Census:** 18 **Outpatient Visits:** 90485
**Births:** 334 **Total Expense ($000):** 59723 **Payroll Expense ($000):** 24255
**Personnel:** 346

✠ **BRATTLEBORO RETREAT (474001)**, Anna Marsh Lane, Zip 5301, Mailing
Address: P.O. Box 803, Zip 05302–0803; tel. 802/257–7785, (Nonreporting) **A**1
5 9 10
Primary Contact: Robert E. Simpson, Jr., M.P.H., President and Chief Executive
Officer
CFO: John E. Blaha, Vice President Finance and Chief Financial Officer
CMO: Frederick Engstrom, M.D., Medical Director
CHR: Kathleen Brooks, Director Human Resources
Web address: www.brattlebororetreat.org
**Control:** Other not–for–profit (including NFP Corporation) **Service:** Psychiatric

**Staffed Beds:** 93

## BURLINGTON—Chittenden County

✠ **FLETCHER ALLEN HEALTH CARE (470003)**, 111 Colchester Avenue,
Zip 05401–1473; tel. 802/847–0000, (Includes FANNY ALLEN CAMPUS, 101
College Parkway, Colchester, Zip 05446–3035; tel. 802/655–1234; MEDICAL
CENTER HOSPITAL CAMPUS, Colchester Avenue, Zip 05401; tel. 802/847–2345;
VERMONT CHILDREN'S HOSPITAL, 111 Colchester Avenue, tel. 802/847–0000)
**A**1 2 3 5 8 9 10 **F**3 4 5 6 7 9 11 12 13 15 16 17 18 19 20 21 22 23 24 25
26 28 29 30 31 32 34 35 36 37 39 40 43 44 45 46 47 48 49 50 51 52 54
55 56 57 58 59 60 61 63 64 65 66 68 70 72 73 74 75 76 77 78 79 81 82
84 85 86 87 88 89 90 91 92 93 94 96 97 98 99 100 101 102 103 104 105
107 108 110 111 113 114 115 116 117 118 119 120 122 123 125 128 129
130 131 134 135 137 140 141 142 143 144 145 146 147 **P**6
Primary Contact: John R. Brumsted, M.D., President and Chief Executive Officer
COO: Sandra L. Dalton, R.N., Senior Vice President Patient Care Services and
Chief Nursing Officer
CFO: Roger Deshaies, Chief Financial Officer
CMO: Stephen Leffler, Chief Medical Officer
CIO: Charles H. Podesta, Vice President Information Services
CHR: Paul Macuga, Chief Human Resources Officer
Web address: www.fletcherallen.org
**Control:** Other not–for–profit (including NFP Corporation) **Service:** General
Medical and Surgical

**Staffed Beds:** 419 **Admissions:** 19800 **Census:** 307 **Outpatient Visits:**
1312936 **Births:** 2175 **Total Expense ($000):** 833826 **Payroll Expense**
**($000):** 426487 **Personnel:** 5859

## MIDDLEBURY—Addison County

✠ **PORTER MEDICAL CENTER (471307)**, 115 Porter Drive, Zip 05753–8423;
tel. 802/388–4701 **A**1 9 10 18 **F**3 8 11 13 15 18 26 29 40 43 45 50 59 64
68 70 75 76 79 81 85 86 93 97 107 108 111 113 114 118 129 132 145 **P**6
Primary Contact: James L. Daily, President
CFO: Marilyn A. Olejnik, Vice President Finance
CMO: Mike Kiernan, M.D., President Medical Staff
CIO: Ronald Hallman, Vice President Development and Public Relations
CHR: Dan Arseneau, Vice President Human Resources
Web address: www.portermedical.org
**Control:** Other not–for–profit (including NFP Corporation) **Service:** General
Medical and Surgical

**Staffed Beds:** 25 **Admissions:** 1554 **Census:** 13 **Total Expense ($000):**
60989 **Personnel:** 493

## MORRISVILLE—Lamoille County

★ **COPLEY HOSPITAL (471305)**, 528 Washington Highway, Zip 05661–8973;
tel. 802/888–8888 **A**9 10 18 **F**13 15 28 29 30 31 34 35 39 40 58 59 64 65
70 74 75 76 77 78 79 81 85 86 93 107 110 111 118 128 129 130 132 134
145 147
Primary Contact: Melvyn Patashnick, President and Chief Executive Officer
CFO: Rassoul Rangaviz, Chief Financial Officer
CMO: Joel Silverstein, M.D., Chief Medical Officer
CIO: Greg Ward, Senior Director Clinical Services
CHR: April E. Tuck, Senior Director Human Resources
Web address: www.copleyvt.org
**Control:** Other not–for–profit (including NFP Corporation) **Service:** General
Medical and Surgical

**Staffed Beds:** 25 **Admissions:** 1639 **Census:** 13 **Outpatient Visits:** 70246
**Births:** 218 **Total Expense ($000):** 47554 **Payroll Expense ($000):** 23852
**Personnel:** 315

**VT**

---

**Hospital, Medicare Provider Number, Address, Telephone, Approval, Facility, and Physician Codes, Health Care System**

★ American Hospital Association (AHA) membership
☐ The Joint Commission accreditation ◇ DNV Healthcare Inc. accreditation
○ American Osteopathic Association (AOA) accreditation
△ Commission on Accreditation of Rehabilitation Facilities (CARF) accreditation

## NEWPORT—Orleans County

★ **NORTH COUNTRY HOSPITAL AND HEALTH CENTER (471304)**, 189 Prouty Drive, Zip 05855–9326; tel. 802/334–7331 **A**9 10 18 **F**11 13 15 28 30 31 34 40 45 53 70 74 75 76 77 78 79 81 82 84 89 93 104 107 108 110 111 118 126 127 128 129 130 132 134 145 147
Primary Contact: Claudio D. Fort, President and Chief Executive Officer
CFO: Andre Bissonnette, Vice President Finance
CMO: Thomas Moseley, M.D., President Medical Staff
CIO: Ervin Goodwin, Manager Information Services
CHR: William Perket, Vice President Human Resources
Web address: www.nchsi.org
**Control:** Other not–for–profit (including NFP Corporation) **Service:** General Medical and Surgical

**Staffed Beds:** 25 **Admissions:** 1637 **Census:** 15 **Outpatient Visits:** 82479 **Total Expense ($000):** 69963 **Payroll Expense ($000):** 33813 **Personnel:** 505

## RANDOLPH—Orange County

★ **GIFFORD MEDICAL CENTER (471301)**, 44 South Main Street, Zip 05060–1381, Mailing Address: P.O. Box 2000, Zip 05060–2000; tel. 802/728–7000, (Total facility includes 30 beds in nursing home–type unit) **A**2 9 10 18 **F**2 3 8 11 13 28 29 30 31 32 33 34 35 38 40 45 49 50 51 54 56 57 59 64 65 66 67 68 70 74 75 76 77 78 79 81 82 83 84 85 86 87 89 93 96 97 107 108 111 113 118 126 127 129 130 131 132 134 145 146 147 **P**6
Primary Contact: Joseph L. Woodin, President and Chief Executive Officer
CFO: David Sanville, Vice President Finance
CMO: Joshua Plavin, M.D., Director Medical Staff
CIO: John Brugger, Director Information Systems
CHR: Christopher J. Lackney, Director Human Resources
Web address: www.giffordmed.org
**Control:** Other not–for–profit (including NFP Corporation) **Service:** General Medical and Surgical

**Staffed Beds:** 82 **Admissions:** 1595 **Census:** 47 **Outpatient Visits:** 69707 **Births:** 216 **Total Expense ($000):** 54302 **Payroll Expense ($000):** 28121 **Personnel:** 432

## RUTLAND—Rutland County

⊞ **RUTLAND REGIONAL MEDICAL CENTER (470005)**, 160 Allen Street, Zip 05701–4595; tel. 802/775–7111 **A**1 2 9 10 **F**13 15 18 20 22 23 24 28 29 31 34 40 45 47 48 49 51 55 57 59 61 64 70 76 77 78 79 81 82 83 84 85 87 90 91 93 94 98 100 101 104 107 108 111 114 115 116 117 118 128 129 145 146 147
Primary Contact: Thomas W. Huebner, President
CFO: Ed Ogorzalek, Chief Financial Officer
CIO: John Kijewski, Vice President and Chief Information Officer
Web address: www.rrmc.org
**Control:** Other not–for–profit (including NFP Corporation) **Service:** General Medical and Surgical

**Staffed Beds:** 134 **Admissions:** 6239 **Census:** 92 **Outpatient Visits:** 174679 **Births:** 6239 **Total Expense ($000):** 185872 **Personnel:** 1132

## SAINT ALBANS—Franklin County

⊞ **NORTHWESTERN MEDICAL CENTER (470024)**, 133 Fairfield Street, Zip 05478–1726; tel. 802/524–5911, (Nonreporting) **A**1 2 9 10 20 **S** QHR, Brentwood, TN
Primary Contact: Jill Berry Bowen, President and Chief Executive Officer
COO: Leo Gaudreau, Manager Plant and Property
CFO: Ted D. Sirotta, Chief Financial Officer
CIO: Stephen C. Stata, Interim Chief Technology Officer
CHR: Mary Lou Beaulieu, Director Human Resources and Compliance Officer
Web address: www.northwesternmedicalcenter.org
**Control:** Other not–for–profit (including NFP Corporation) **Service:** General Medical and Surgical

**Staffed Beds:** 20

## SAINT JOHNSBURY—Caledonia County

★ **NORTHEASTERN VERMONT REGIONAL HOSPITAL (471303)**, 1315 Hospital Drive, Zip 05819–9962, Mailing Address: PO Box 905, Zip 05819–0905; tel. 802/748–8141 **A**9 10 18 **F**3 11 13 15 18 26 28 29 30 34 35 40 41 44 45 50 51 59 63 64 65 68 70 74 75 76 77 79 81 84 86 87 89 93 107 108 110 111 114 117 118 126 129 130 131 132 134 145 146 **P**6
Primary Contact: Paul R. Bengtson, Chief Executive Officer
CFO: Robert Hersey, Chief Financial Officer
CIO: Andrea Lott, Vice President Information Services
CHR: Betty Ann Gwatkin, Vice President Human Resources
Web address: www.nvrh.org
**Control:** Other not–for–profit (including NFP Corporation) **Service:** General Medical and Surgical

**Staffed Beds:** 25 **Admissions:** 1505 **Census:** 13 **Outpatient Visits:** 153930 **Births:** 221 **Total Expense ($000):** 56524 **Payroll Expense ($000):** 25385 **Personnel:** 334

## SPRINGFIELD—Windsor County

**SPRINGFIELD HOSPITAL (471306)**, 25 Ridgewood Road, Zip 05156–2003, Mailing Address: P.O. Box 2003, Zip 05156–2003; tel. 802/885–2151, (Nonreporting) **A**9 10 18
Primary Contact: Glenn D. Cordner, Chief Executive Officer
CFO: Laverne Lindamood, Director Finance
CMO: Mark C. Hamilton, M.D., President Medical Staff
Web address: www.springfieldhospital.org
**Control:** Other not–for–profit (including NFP Corporation) **Service:** General Medical and Surgical

**Staffed Beds:** 35

## TOWNSHEND—Windham County

★ **GRACE COTTAGE HOSPITAL (471300)**, 185 Grafton Road, Zip 05353–0216, Mailing Address: P.O. Box 216, Zip 05353–0216; tel. 802/365–7357, (Nonreporting) **A**9 10 18
Primary Contact: Mick Brant, Chief Executive Officer
CFO: Stephen A. Brown, Chief Financial Officer
CMO: Timothy Shafer, M.D., Medical Director
CIO: Tony Marques, Director Information Systems
CHR: Tim McNulty, Vice President Human Resources
Web address: www.gracecottage.org
**Control:** Other not–for–profit (including NFP Corporation) **Service:** General Medical and Surgical

**Staffed Beds:** 19

## WHITE RIVER JUNCTION—Windsor County

⊞ **VETERANS AFFAIRS MEDICAL CENTER**, 215 North Main Street, Zip 05009–0001; tel. 802/291–6206 **A**1 3 5 8 **F**3 5 8 9 12 18 20 29 30 31 34 35 36 38 39 40 44 45 46 49 50 53 54 56 57 58 59 60 61 62 63 64 65 70 74 75 77 78 79 81 82 84 85 86 87 93 94 95 96 97 98 100 101 102 103 104 105 107 108 111 114 117 118 126 129 131 134 140 142 143 145 146 147 **P**1 6 **S** Department of Veterans Affairs, Washington, DC
Primary Contact: Robert M. Walton, Director
CFO: Joan Wilmot, Chief Fiscal Officer
CMO: Thomas Parrino, M.D., Chief of Staff
CIO: Matthew Rafus, Chief Information Officer
CHR: Barbara Nadeau, Chief Human Resources
Web address: www.va.gov/sta/guide/home.asp
**Control:** Veterans Affairs, Government, federal **Service:** General Medical and Surgical

**Staffed Beds:** 60 **Admissions:** 2408 **Census:** 40 **Outpatient Visits:** 228632 **Births:** 0 **Total Expense ($000):** 160688 **Payroll Expense ($000):** 66012 **Personnel:** 785

## WINDSOR—Windsor County

★ **MT. ASCUTNEY HOSPITAL AND HEALTH CENTER (471302)**, 289 County Road, Zip 05089–9702; tel. 802/674–6711, (Total facility includes 25 beds in nursing home–type unit) **A**9 10 18 **F**3 8 10 11 15 28 29 30 31 32 34 35 36 40 41 44 45 49 50 54 56 57 59 63 64 65 66 68 69 70 71 75 77 78 79 81 82 84 85 86 87 90 91 92 93 94 96 97 100 104 107 110 111 114 118 124 127 129 131 132 133 134 142 145 147 **P**6
Primary Contact: Kevin Donovan, Chief Executive Officer
COO: Bennett J. Beres, Chief Operating Officer
CMO: Catherine Schneider, M.D., Chief Medical Officer
CIO: Scott Schreier, Chief Information Officer
CHR: Jean Martaniuk, Director Personnel
Web address: www.mtascutneyhospital.org
**Control:** Other not–for–profit (including NFP Corporation) **Service:** General Medical and Surgical

**Staffed Beds:** 60 **Admissions:** 1156 **Census:** 51 **Outpatient Visits:** 90431 **Births:** 0 **Total Expense ($000):** 45717 **Payroll Expense ($000):** 21743 **Personnel:** 370

**VT**

*Many Facility Codes have changed. Please refer to the AHA Guide Code Chart.* © 2012 AHA Guide

# VIRGINIA

## ABINGDON—Washington County

✠ **JOHNSTON MEMORIAL HOSPITAL (490053)**, 16000 Johnston Memorial Drive, Zip 24211; tel. 276/676–7000 **A**1 2 9 10 **F**3 11 13 14 15 34 35 37 40 49 50 51 54 57 59 61 62 64 68 70 73 74 75 76 77 78 79 81 82 85 86 87 93 103 107 108 110 111 113 114 117 118 120 122 129 130 131 134 145 146 147 **S** Mountain States Health Alliance, Johnson City, TN
Primary Contact: Sean S. McMurray, FACHE, Vice President and Chief Executive Officer
COO: Stephen K. Givens, Chief Operating Officer
CFO: Timothy Evans, Chief Financial Officer
CMO: Kevin Armstrong, M.D., President Medical Staff
CHR: Jackie G. Phipps, Director Human Resources
Web address: www.jmh.org
**Control:** Other not–for–profit (including NFP Corporation) **Service:** General Medical and Surgical

**Staffed Beds:** 100 **Admissions:** 6222 **Census:** 60 **Outpatient Visits:** 136952 **Births:** 687 **Total Expense ($000):** 89057 **Payroll Expense ($000):** 33816 **Personnel:** 715

## ALDIE—Loudoun County

★ **HEALTHSOUTH REHABILITATION HOSPITAL OF NORTHERN VIRGINIA (493033)**, 24430 Millstream Drive, Zip 20105–3098; tel. 703/957–2000, (Nonreporting) **S** HEALTHSOUTH Corporation, Birmingham, AL
Primary Contact: Christina Stover, Chief Executive Officer
Web address: www.healthsouthnorthernvirginia.com
**Control:** Corporation, Investor–owned, for–profit **Service:** Rehabilitation

**Staffed Beds:** 40

## ALEXANDRIA—Alexandria City County

✠ **INOVA ALEXANDRIA HOSPITAL (490040)**, 4320 Seminary Road, Zip 22304–1594; tel. 703/504–3167 **A**1 2 9 10 **F**3 11 13 14 15 17 18 20 22 24 26 28 29 30 31 34 35 38 39 40 42 44 45 48 49 50 51 55 57 59 60 61 63 64 65 66 68 69 70 72 74 75 76 77 78 79 80 81 82 84 85 86 87 89 92 93 100 101 102 107 108 110 111 113 114 116 117 118 119 120 122 123 128 129 130 131 134 144 145 146 147 **P**6 **S** Inova Health System, Falls Church, VA
Primary Contact: Christine Candio, Chief Executive Officer
COO: Daniel W. Jackson, Chief Operating Officer
CFO: Todd Lockcuff, Chief Financial Officer
CMO: John R. Audett, M.D., Chief Medical Officer
CIO: Geoffrey Brown, Senior Vice President Information Services
CHR: Hugo Aguas, Vice President Human Resources
Web address: www.inova.org
**Control:** Other not–for–profit (including NFP Corporation) **Service:** General Medical and Surgical

**Staffed Beds:** 334 **Admissions:** 15680 **Census:** 197 **Outpatient Visits:** 277080 **Births:** 3985 **Total Expense ($000):** 283607 **Payroll Expense ($000):** 118240 **Personnel:** 1741

✠ △ **INOVA MOUNT VERNON HOSPITAL (490122)**, 2501 Parker's Lane, Zip 22306; tel. 703/664–7000 **A**1 2 3 5 7 9 10 **F**3 5 11 14 15 18 24 26 28 29 30 31 34 35 37 38 39 40 44 45 48 49 50 51 55 57 58 59 60 61 63 64 65 66 68 69 70 74 75 77 78 79 80 81 82 84 85 86 87 90 91 92 93 94 96 98 100 101 102 103 104 105 107 108 110 111 113 114 117 118 129 130 131 134 144 145 147 **S** Inova Health System, Falls Church, VA
Primary Contact: Barbara J. Doyle, R.N., MS, Senior Vice President and Chief Executive Officer
CFO: Tammy Razmic, Associate Administrator Finance and Chief Financial Officer
CHR: Bev Sugar, Associate Administrator and Director Human Resources
Web address: www.inova.org
**Control:** Other not–for–profit (including NFP Corporation) **Service:** General Medical and Surgical

**Staffed Beds:** 237 **Admissions:** 8256 **Census:** 144 **Outpatient Visits:** 84116 **Births:** 0 **Total Expense ($000):** 158321 **Payroll Expense ($000):** 64799 **Personnel:** 953

## ARLINGTON—Arlington County

**CAPITAL HOSPICE (490129)**, 4715 15th Street North, Zip 22205–2640; tel. 703/538–2065, (Nonreporting) **A**3
Primary Contact: Malene S. Davis, R.N., President and Chief Executive Officer
CFO: David Schwind, Chief Financial Officer
CIO: Diane Rigsby, Chief Information Officer
Web address: www.capitalhospice.org
**Control:** Other not–for–profit (including NFP Corporation) **Service:** Other specialty

**Staffed Beds:** 15

✠ **VIRGINIA HOSPITAL CENTER – ARLINGTON (490050)**, 1701 North George Mason Drive, Zip 22205–3698; tel. 703/558–5000 **A**1 2 3 5 9 10 **F**3 4 5 8 11 12 13 15 17 18 20 22 24 26 28 29 30 31 34 35 37 38 40 45 46 48 49 50 51 54 57 59 60 61 62 64 65 66 68 70 72 73 74 75 76 78 79 81 84 85 86 87 89 90 92 93 94 95 96 97 98 102 104 105 107 110 111 113 114 115 116 117 118 119 120 122 123 125 128 129 131 134 143 144 145 146 147 **P**6
Primary Contact: James B. Cole, Chief Executive Officer
COO: Carl Bahnlein, Executive Vice President and Chief Operating Officer
CFO: Robin Norman, Senior Vice President and Chief Financial Officer
CMO: Archie McPherson, M.D., Vice President and Chief Medical Officer
CIO: David Crutchfield, Vice President and Chief Information Officer
CHR: Michael Malone, Vice President and Chief Human Resources Officer
Web address: www.virginiahospitalcenter.com
**Control:** Other not–for–profit (including NFP Corporation) **Service:** General Medical and Surgical

**Staffed Beds:** 342 **Admissions:** 21029 **Census:** 240 **Outpatient Visits:** 310901 **Births:** 4247 **Total Expense ($000):** 323222 **Payroll Expense ($000):** 128002 **Personnel:** 1993

## BEDFORD—Bedford City County

✠ **BEDFORD MEMORIAL HOSPITAL (490088)**, 1613 Oakwood Street, Zip 24523–0688, Mailing Address: P.O. Box 688, Zip 24523–0688; tel. 540/586–2441, (Total facility includes 111 beds in nursing home–type unit) **A**1 9 10 **F**2 3 11 15 18 19 28 29 30 34 35 40 57 59 63 67 70 81 84 85 93 97 107 118 127 129 133 142 144 145 **S** Carilion Clinic, Roanoke, VA
Primary Contact: Patti Jurkus, President and Chief Executive Officer
CFO: Donald E. Lorton, Executive Vice President
CMO: E. Allen Joslyn, M.D., Chief Medical Officer
Web address: www.bmhva.com
**Control:** Other not–for–profit (including NFP Corporation) **Service:** General Medical and Surgical

**Staffed Beds:** 124 **Admissions:** 1807 **Census:** 114 **Outpatient Visits:** 25559 **Births:** 0 **Total Expense ($000):** 30732 **Payroll Expense ($000):** 13098 **Personnel:** 300

## BIG STONE GAP—Wise County

✠ **WELLMONT LONESOME PINE HOSPITAL (490114)**, 1990 Holton Avenue East, Zip 24219–3350; tel. 276/523–3111 **A**1 9 10 13 **F**3 11 13 15 18 29 30 31 34 35 40 49 50 57 59 63 68 70 76 77 78 79 81 85 87 89 93 97 107 111 115 116 117 118 119 120 122 129 145 **S** Wellmont Health System, Kingsport, TN
Primary Contact: David L. Brash, Interim President
CFO: Sheila Fleenor, Controller
CMO: Elizabeth Cooperstein, M.D., Chief Medical Officer
Web address: www.wellmont.org
**Control:** Other not–for–profit (including NFP Corporation) **Service:** General Medical and Surgical

**Staffed Beds:** 60 **Admissions:** 2392 **Census:** 20 **Outpatient Visits:** 34206 **Births:** 219 **Total Expense ($000):** 32838 **Payroll Expense ($000):** 9373 **Personnel:** 202

**VA**

---

**Hospital, Medicare Provider Number, Address, Telephone, Approval, Facility, and Physician Codes, Health Care System**

★ American Hospital Association (AHA) membership
☐ The Joint Commission accreditation          ◇ DNV Healthcare Inc. accreditation
○ American Osteopathic Association (AOA) accreditation
△ Commission on Accreditation of Rehabilitation Facilities (CARF) accreditation

## BLACKSBURG—Montgomery County

☒ **MONTGOMERY REGIONAL HOSPITAL (490110)**, 3700 South Main Street, Zip 24060–7081, Mailing Address: P.O. Box 90004, Zip 24062–9004; tel. 540/951–1111 **A**1 9 10 12 13 **F**3 13 15 17 18 20 22 28 29 30 31 34 35 36 37 40 43 45 48 49 54 55 57 59 64 70 74 75 76 78 79 81 82 85 86 89 93 107 108 110 111 113 114 117 118 129 130 131 145 146 147 **S** HCA, Nashville, TN
Primary Contact: Scott Hill, Chief Executive Officer
COO: David Cashwell, Chief Operating Officer
CFO: Timothy W. Haasken, Chief Financial Officer
CMO: C. Y. Davis, M.D., Chief Medical Officer
CHR: Kristie Walker, Director Human Resources
Web address: www.mrhospital.com
**Control:** Corporation, Investor–owned, for–profit **Service:** General Medical and Surgical

**Staffed Beds:** 103 **Admissions:** 4103 **Census:** 42 **Outpatient Visits:** 70604 **Births:** 455

## BRISTOL—Bristol City County

★ **REHABILITATION HOSPITAL OF SOUTHWEST VIRGINIA (493034)**, 103 North Street, Zip 24201–3201; tel. 276/642–7900, (Nonreporting) **A**10 **S** HEALTHSOUTH Corporation, Birmingham, AL
Primary Contact: Georgeanne Cole, Chief Executive Officer
Web address: www.rehabilitationhospitalswvirginia.com
**Control:** Partnership, Investor–owned, for–profit **Service:** Rehabilitation

**Staffed Beds:** 25

## BURKEVILLE—Nottoway County

☐ **PIEDMONT GERIATRIC HOSPITAL (490134)**, 5001 East Patrick Henry Highway, Zip 23922–0427, Mailing Address: P.O. Box 427, Zip 23922–0427; tel. 434/767–4401, (Nonreporting) **A**1 9 10 **S** Virginia Department of Mental Health, Richmond, VA
Primary Contact: Stephen M. Herrick, Ph.D., Director
CFO: James G. Ayers, Chief Financial Officer
CMO: Hugo Falcon, M.D., Director Medical Services
CHR: Michael Wimsatt, Director Human Resources
Web address: www.pgh.dmhmrsas.virginia.gov
**Control:** State–Government, nonfederal **Service:** Other specialty

**Staffed Beds:** 150

## CATAWBA—Roanoke County

☐ **CATAWBA HOSPITAL (490135)**, 5525 Catawba Hospital Drive, Zip 24070–2115, Mailing Address: P.O. Box 200, Zip 24070–0200; tel. 540/375–4200 **A**1 9 10 **F**29 30 35 38 39 44 50 68 75 77 98 103 129 145 **P**6 **S** Virginia Department of Mental Health, Richmond, VA
Primary Contact: Walton F. Mitchell, III, Director
COO: Charles Law, Chief Operating Officer
CFO: Cecil Hardin, CPA, Chief Financial Officer
CMO: Yad Jabbarpour, M.D., Chief of Staff
CIO: Charles Law, Chief Operating Officer
CHR: Patricia Ebbett, Chief Human Resources Officer
Web address: www.catawba.dmhmrsas.virginia.gov
**Control:** State–Government, nonfederal **Service:** Psychiatric

**Staffed Beds:** 110 **Admissions:** 322 **Census:** 100 **Outpatient Visits:** 0 **Births:** 0 **Total Expense ($000):** 20398 **Payroll Expense ($000):** 11612 **Personnel:** 264

## CHARLOTTESVILLE—Charlottesville City County

☒ **MARTHA JEFFERSON HOSPITAL (490077)**, 500 Martha Jefferson Drive, Zip 22911; tel. 434/654–7000 **A**1 2 3 5 9 10 **F**3 8 12 13 15 18 20 22 26 28 29 30 31 34 35 36 40 42 45 46 48 49 50 52 54 57 59 64 68 70 74 75 76 78 79 81 82 84 85 86 87 89 92 93 94 97 107 108 110 111 113 114 117 118 119 120 122 123 128 129 131 134 144 145 146 147 **P**1 **S** Sentara Healthcare, Norfolk, VA
Primary Contact: James E. Haden, President and Chief Executive Officer
COO: Elliot H. Kuida, Vice President and Chief Operating Officer
CFO: J. Michael Burris, Vice President Corporate Services and Chief Financial Officer
CMO: F. Michael Ashby, M.D., Vice President and Medical Director
CIO: Marijo Lecker, Vice President
CHR: Susan M. Cabell-Mains, Vice President Administration
Web address: www.marthajefferson.org
**Control:** Other not–for–profit (including NFP Corporation) **Service:** General Medical and Surgical

**Staffed Beds:** 139 **Admissions:** 10858 **Census:** 94 **Outpatient Visits:** 428210 **Births:** 1695 **Total Expense ($000):** 207697 **Payroll Expense ($000):** 89609 **Personnel:** 1427

**TRANSITIONAL CARE HOSPITAL (492011)**, 2965 Ivy Road (250 West), Zip 22903–9330; tel. 434/924–7897, (Data for 330 days) **F**1 3 29 85 94 113 129 145 147 **P**3 **S** UVA Health System, Charlottesville, VA
Primary Contact: Michelle Hereford, Administrator
Web address: www.uvahealth.com/services/transitional–care–hospital
**Control:** State–Government, nonfederal **Service:** Long–Term Acute Care hospital

**Staffed Beds:** 20 **Admissions:** 61 **Census:** 7 **Outpatient Visits:** 0 **Births:** 0 **Total Expense ($000):** 9234 **Payroll Expense ($000):** 2986 **Personnel:** 62

☒ **UNIVERSITY OF VIRGINIA MEDICAL CENTER (490009)**, 1215 Lee Street, Zip 22908–0001, Mailing Address: P.O. Box 800809, Zip 22908–0809; tel. 434/924–0211, (Includes UNIVERSITY OF VIRGINIA CHILDREN'S HOSPITAL, PO Box 800566, Zip 22901; tel. 434/982–4453) **A**1 2 3 5 8 9 10 **F**3 5 6 7 8 9 11 12 13 15 17 18 19 20 21 22 23 24 25 26 27 28 30 31 32 34 35 36 37 38 39 40 41 43 44 45 46 47 48 49 50 51 52 54 55 56 57 58 59 60 61 62 64 65 66 68 70 71 72 74 75 76 77 78 79 80 81 82 83 84 85 86 87 88 89 90 91 92 93 94 97 98 99 100 101 102 103 104 107 108 110 111 113 114 115 116 117 118 119 120 122 123 125 128 129 130 131 133 134 136 137 138 139 140 141 142 144 145 146 147 **P**3 4 **S** UVA Health System, Charlottesville, VA
Primary Contact: R. Edward Howell, Vice President and Chief Executive Officer
COO: Robert Cofield, Dr.PH, Chief Operating Officer and Associate Vice President
CFO: Larry Fitzgerald, Chief Financial Officer
CMO: Jonathon D. Truwit, M.D., Chief Medical Officer
CIO: Barbara Baldwin, Chief Information Officer
CHR: John Boswell, Associate Chief Human Resources
Web address: www.healthsystem.virginia.edu
**Control:** State–Government, nonfederal **Service:** General Medical and Surgical

**Staffed Beds:** 570 **Admissions:** 28041 **Census:** 454 **Outpatient Visits:** 1635284 **Births:** 1662 **Total Expense ($000):** 955266 **Payroll Expense ($000):** 348780 **Personnel:** 6114

☒ **UVA–HEALTHSOUTH REHABILITATION HOSPITAL (493029)**, 515 Ray C. Hunt Drive, Zip 22903; tel. 434/244–2000 **A**1 3 5 10 **F**90 91 93 94 95 96 147 **S** HEALTHSOUTH Corporation, Birmingham, AL
Primary Contact: Thomas J. Cook, Chief Executive Officer
Web address: www.uvahealthsouth.com
**Control:** Partnership, Investor–owned, for–profit **Service:** Rehabilitation

**Staffed Beds:** 50 **Admissions:** 1045 **Census:** 38 **Outpatient Visits:** 25403 **Births:** 0 **Total Expense ($000):** 17236 **Payroll Expense ($000):** 11006

## CHESAPEAKE—Chesapeake City County

☒ **CHESAPEAKE REGIONAL MEDICAL CENTER (490120)**, 736 Battlefield Boulevard North, Zip 23320–4941, Mailing Address: P.O. Box 2028, Zip 23327–2028; tel. 757/312–8121 **A**1 2 9 10 **F**3 6 8 10 11 12 13 15 18 20 22 26 28 29 30 31 34 35 36 40 44 45 46 49 50 53 54 56 57 59 61 62 63 64 65 68 69 70 71 73 74 75 76 77 78 79 81 84 85 86 87 89 91 93 98 100 101 102 103 107 108 110 111 113 114 117 118 119 120 122 128 129 131 134 140 141 142 145 146 147 **P**6
Primary Contact: Wynn L. Dixon, Jr., Chief Executive Officer
COO: Wynn L. Dixon, Jr., Chief Executive Officer
CFO: Michael Corcoran, Chief Financial Officer
CMO: Cynthia Romero, M.D., Chief Medical Officer
CIO: Ken Deans, Chief Information Officer
Web address: www.chesapeakeregional.com
**Control:** Hospital district or authority, Government, nonfederal **Service:** General Medical and Surgical

**Staffed Beds:** 310 **Admissions:** 16848 **Census:** 231 **Outpatient Visits:** 188653 **Births:** 2698 **Total Expense ($000):** 236730 **Payroll Expense ($000):** 100842 **Personnel:** 1983

## CHRISTIANSBURG—Montgomery County

☒ **CARILION NEW RIVER VALLEY MEDICAL CENTER (490042)**, 2900 Lamb Circle, Zip 24073–5041, Mailing Address: P.O. Box 5, Radford, Zip 24143–0005; tel. 540/731–2000 **A**1 9 10 19 **F**5 12 13 15 18 28 29 30 31 35 40 43 47 48 49 50 51 59 62 63 64 70 74 75 76 77 79 81 84 85 89 93 98 102 103 104 105 107 108 110 111 113 114 116 118 128 129 134 145 146 147 **S** Carilion Clinic, Roanoke, VA
Primary Contact: John S. Piatkowski, M.D., President and Chief Executive Officer
CFO: Rob Vaughan, Chief Financial Officer
CMO: Dennis Means, M.D., Vice President Medical Affairs
CIO: Daniel Borchi, Chief Information Officer
CHR: Patti Jurkus, Director Human Resources
Web address: www.carilionclinic.org
**Control:** Other not–for–profit (including NFP Corporation) **Service:** General Medical and Surgical

**Staffed Beds:** 146 **Admissions:** 7837 **Census:** 83 **Outpatient Visits:** 85208 **Births:** 1148 **Total Expense ($000):** 126365 **Payroll Expense ($000):** 40279 **Personnel:** 807

**VA**

*Many Facility Codes have changed. Please refer to the AHA Guide Code Chart.* © 2012 AHA Guide

## CLINTWOOD—Dickenson County

○ **DICKENSON COMMUNITY HOSPITAL (491303)**, 312 Hospital Drive,
Zip 24228, Mailing Address: P.O. Box 1440, Zip 24228–1440;
tel. 276/926–0300 **A**9 10 11 18 **F**3 11 29 30 40 43 50 57 64 68 75 85 86
97 107 118 129 132 145 **P**6 **S** Mountain States Health Alliance, Johnson
City, TN
Primary Contact: Mark T. Leonard, Chief Executive Officer
CFO: Stephen Sawyer, Chief Financial Officer
CMO: Erin Mullins, D.O., Chief Medical Staff
CHR: Valeri J. Colyer, Director Human Resources
Web address: www.dchosp.com
**Control:** Other not–for–profit (including NFP Corporation) **Service:** General
Medical and Surgical

**Staffed Beds:** 2 **Admissions:** 1 **Census:** 1 **Outpatient Visits:** 22606 **Births:**
0 **Total Expense ($000):** 4566 **Payroll Expense ($000):** 2565 **Personnel:**
40

## CULPEPER—Culpeper County

✠ **CULPEPER REGIONAL HOSPITAL (490019)**, 501 Sunset Lane,
Zip 22701–3917, Mailing Address: P.O. Box 592, Zip 22701–0592;
tel. 540/829–4100 **A**1 3 5 9 10 **F**3 7 8 11 13 15 18 28 29 30 34 35 36 37
38 40 45 50 54 57 59 64 68 70 74 75 76 77 78 79 81 82 83 84 85 87 93
97 102 107 108 110 111 113 118 119 120 122 129 131 132 134 142 145
147 **P**6 8
Primary Contact: H. Lee Kirk, Jr., President and Chief Executive Officer
COO: Thomas Saul, Interim Chief Operating Officer
CFO: Samuel Morgan, Senior Vice President Financial Operations
CMO: Sok Yi, M.D., President Medical Staff
CIO: Brian Rock, Director Information Systems
CHR: Susan Edwards, Vice President Human Resources
Web address: www.culpeperhospital.com
**Control:** Other not–for–profit (including NFP Corporation) **Service:** General
Medical and Surgical

**Staffed Beds:** 67 **Admissions:** 3278 **Census:** 35 **Outpatient Visits:** 60165
**Births:** 354 **Total Expense ($000):** 59435 **Payroll Expense ($000):** 26407
**Personnel:** 546

## DANVILLE—Danville City County

✠ **DANVILLE REGIONAL MEDICAL CENTER (490075)**, 142 South Main Street,
Zip 24541–2922; tel. 434/799–2100, (Nonreporting) **A**1 2 6 9 10 12 13
**S** LifePoint Hospitals, Inc., Brentwood, TN
Primary Contact: Eric Deaton, Chief Executive Officer
CFO: Mark T. Anderson, Chief Financial Officer
CMO: James F. Starling, M.D., Chief Medical Officer
CIO: David Cartwright, Director Management Information Systems
Web address: www.danvilleregional.org
**Control:** Other not–for–profit (including NFP Corporation) **Service:** General
Medical and Surgical

**Staffed Beds:** 151

☐ **SOUTHERN VIRGINIA MENTAL HEALTH INSTITUTE (494017)**, 382 Taylor
Drive, Zip 24541–4023; tel. 434/799–6220 **A**1 9 10 **F**34 50 57 68 75 77 86
87 98 101 129 131 145 **P**6 **S** Virginia Department of Mental Health,
Richmond, VA
Primary Contact: David M. Lyon, Director
CFO: Wade Hopkins, Administrator
CMO: B. R. Ashby, Jr., M.D., President and Chief Executive Officer
CIO: Bracken Jones, Director Information Technology
CHR: Pauline Wasiuk, Director Human Resources
Web address: www.svmhi.dmhmrsas.virginia.gov
**Control:** State–Government, nonfederal **Service:** Psychiatric

**Staffed Beds:** 72 **Admissions:** 325 **Census:** 55 **Outpatient Visits:** 0 **Births:**
0

## EMPORIA—Emporia City County

✠ **SOUTHERN VIRGINIA REGIONAL MEDICAL CENTER (490097)**, 727 North
Main Street, Zip 23847–1274; tel. 434/348–4400 **A**1 9 10 **F**3 11 15 26 28 29
30 31 39 40 45 49 57 59 62 64 70 77 78 79 81 82 85 89 93 98 103 107
114 118 123 128 129 132 145 147 **S** Community Health Systems, Inc.,
Franklin, TN
Primary Contact: Britton Phelps, Chief Executive Officer
CFO: Elmer Polite, Chief Financial Officer
CMO: Michael S. Anderson, M.D., Chief of Staff
CIO: Tracy Bullock, Director Management Information Systems
CHR: Becky Parrish, Director Human Resources
Web address: www.svrmc.com
**Control:** Corporation, Investor–owned, for–profit **Service:** General Medical and
Surgical

**Staffed Beds:** 80 **Admissions:** 2939 **Census:** 36 **Outpatient Visits:** 24005
**Births:** 0 **Total Expense ($000):** 34338 **Payroll Expense ($000):** 12496
**Personnel:** 292

## FAIRFAX—Fairfax County

✠ **INOVA FAIR OAKS HOSPITAL (490101)**, 3600 Joseph Siewick Drive,
Zip 22033–1798; tel. 703/391–3600 **A**1 2 3 5 9 10 **F**3 11 12 13 14 15 18 29
30 31 32 34 35 37 38 39 40 44 45 47 48 49 50 51 54 55 57 59 60 61 62
63 64 65 66 68 69 70 72 74 75 76 77 78 79 80 81 82 84 85 86 87 89 92
93 100 101 102 107 108 110 111 113 114 117 118 125 128 129 130 131
134 145 146 147 **S** Inova Health System, Falls Church, VA
Primary Contact: John L. Fitzgerald, Chief Executive Officer
CFO: Bill Bane, Assistant Vice President and Chief Financial Officer
CMO: G. Michael Lynch, M.D., Chief Medical Officer
CIO: Geoffrey Brown, Chief Information Officer
CHR: Jennifer Gertenbach, Director Human Resources
Web address: www.inova.org
**Control:** Other not–for–profit (including NFP Corporation) **Service:** General
Medical and Surgical

**Staffed Beds:** 196 **Admissions:** 12818 **Census:** 120 **Outpatient Visits:**
115815 **Births:** 3638 **Total Expense ($000):** 214899 **Payroll Expense
($000):** 78577 **Personnel:** 1105

## FALLS CHURCH—Fairfax County

✠ **DOMINION HOSPITAL (494023)**, 2960 Sleepy Hollow Road, Zip 22044–2030;
tel. 703/536–2000, (Nonreporting) **A**1 9 10 **S** HCA, Nashville, TN
Primary Contact: Suzanne B. Jackson, FACHE, Chief Executive Officer
CFO: Edward R. Stojakovich, Chief Financial Officer
CMO: Gary Litovitz, M.D., Medical Director
CIO: Leslie Gilliam, Director Health Information Management
CHR: Lesley Channell, Assistant Vice President Human Resources
Web address: www.dominionhospital.com
**Control:** Corporation, Investor–owned, for–profit **Service:** Psychiatric

**Staffed Beds:** 94

✠ **INOVA FAIRFAX HOSPITAL (490063)**, 3300 Gallows Road, Zip 22042–3300;
tel. 703/776–4001, (Includes INOVA FAIRFAX HOSPITAL FOR CHILDREN, 3300
Gallows Road, Zip 22042–3307; tel. 703/776–4002) **A**1 2 3 5 8 9 10 **F**3 4 5 8
11 12 13 14 15 17 18 19 20 21 22 23 24 25 26 27 28 29 30 31 32 34 35
36 37 38 39 40 41 42 43 44 45 46 47 48 49 50 51 54 55 56 57 58 59 60
61 63 64 65 66 68 69 71 72 73 74 75 76 77 78 79 80 81 82 83 84 85 86
87 88 89 92 93 94 96 97 98 99 100 101 102 103 104 105 107 108 109
110 111 113 114 116 117 118 119 120 122 123 125 128 129 130 131 133
134 135 136 137 139 140 141 144 145 146 147 **P**6 **S** Inova Health System,
Falls Church, VA
Primary Contact: L. Reuven Pasternak, M.D., M.P.H., Chief Executive Officer
COO: Rodney N. Huebbers, Campus Administrator
CFO: Ronald Ewald, Chief Financial Officer
CMO: Joseph Hallal, M.D., Chief Medical Officer
CIO: Geoffrey Brown, Vice President Information Systems
CHR: Ken Hull, Director Human Resources
Web address: www.inova.org
**Control:** Other not–for–profit (including NFP Corporation) **Service:** General
Medical and Surgical

**Staffed Beds:** 927 **Admissions:** 48092 **Census:** 678 **Outpatient Visits:**
355182 **Births:** 10244 **Total Expense ($000):** 1065807 **Payroll Expense
($000):** 414989 **Personnel:** 5595

**VA**

---

**Hospital, Medicare Provider Number, Address, Telephone, Approval, Facility, and Physician Codes, Health Care System**

★ American Hospital Association (AHA) membership
☐ The Joint Commission accreditation
◇ DNV Healthcare Inc. accreditation
○ American Osteopathic Association (AOA) accreditation
△ Commission on Accreditation of Rehabilitation Facilities (CARF) accreditation

☐ **NORTHERN VIRGINIA MENTAL HEALTH INSTITUTE (494010)**, 3302 Gallows Road, Zip 22042–3398; tel. 703/207–7110 **A**1 3 5 9 10 **F**11 29 30 35 44 50 59 68 75 77 87 98 101 129 131 145 **S** Virginia Department of Mental Health, Richmond, VA
Primary Contact: R. Maxilimien del Rio, M.D., Facility Director
CFO: Anne Baxter, Director Fiscal Services
CMO: R. Maxilimien del Rio, M.D., Medical Director
CHR: Betsy Thompson, Director Human Resources
Web address: www.nvmhi.dmhmrsas.virginia.gov
**Control:** State–Government, nonfederal **Service:** Psychiatric

**Staffed Beds: 123 Admissions: 873 Census: 118 Outpatient Visits: 0 Births: 0 Total Expense ($000): 24030 Payroll Expense ($000): 16288**

**FARMVILLE—Prince Edward County**

☒ **CENTRA SOUTHSIDE COMMUNITY HOSPITAL (490090)**, 800 Oak Street, Zip 23901–1199; tel. 434/392–8811 **A**1 5 9 10 20 **F**3 11 13 15 28 29 30 34 35 40 43 44 45 50 57 59 62 64 70 75 76 77 79 81 85 86 87 89 93 107 108 110 114 117 118 128 129 131 132 145 146 147 **P**6 **S** Centra Health, Inc., Lynchburg, VA
Primary Contact: E. W. Tibbs, President and Chief Executive Officer
CFO: William L. Bass, Jr., Vice President Finance and Chief Financial Officer
Web address: www.centrasouthside.com
**Control:** Other not–for–profit (including NFP Corporation) **Service:** General Medical and Surgical

**Staffed Beds: 86 Admissions: 4945 Census: 40 Outpatient Visits: 119115 Births: 410 Total Expense ($000): 63737 Payroll Expense ($000): 29146 Personnel: 469**

**SOUTHSIDE COMMUNITY HOSPITAL** See Centra Southside Community Hospital

**FISHERSVILLE—Augusta County**

☒ **AUGUSTA HEALTH (490018)**, 78 Medical Center Drive, Zip 22939–2332, Mailing Address: P.O. Box 1000, Zip 22939–1000; tel. 540/932–4000 **A**1 2 3 5 9 10 **F**3 5 7 11 13 15 17 18 20 22 28 29 30 31 34 35 36 39 40 45 46 48 49 50 51 53 54 56 57 58 59 61 62 63 64 68 70 74 75 76 77 78 79 81 82 85 86 87 89 90 91 92 93 96 97 98 100 101 102 103 104 105 107 108 110 111 113 114 117 118 119 120 122 127 128 129 130 131 134 143 144 145 146 147 **P**6
Primary Contact: Mary N. Mannix, FACHE, President and Chief Executive Officer
CFO: John R. Heider, Vice President Finance
CMO: Fred Castello, M.D., Chief Medical Officer
CIO: Velma Carroll, Chief Information Officer
CHR: Sue Krzastek, Vice President Human Resources
Web address: www.augustahealth.com
**Control:** Other not–for–profit (including NFP Corporation) **Service:** General Medical and Surgical

**Staffed Beds: 224 Admissions: 11757 Census: 140 Outpatient Visits: 542078 Births: 1233 Total Expense ($000): 245357 Payroll Expense ($000): 100605 Personnel: 1902**

**WOODROW WILSON REHABILITATION CENTER**, Zip 22939–1500; tel. 540/332–7000, (Nonreporting) **A**5
Primary Contact: Richard Luck, Ed.D., Facility Director
COO: Richard Luck, Ed.D., Facility Director
CFO: Ernie Steidle, Chief Operating Officer
CMO: Mammen Mathew, M.D., Chief Rehabilitation Medicine
CIO: Keith Burt, Director Marketing
CHR: Debbie Mitchell, Director Human Resources
Web address: www.wwrc.net
**Control:** State–Government, nonfederal **Service:** Rehabilitation

**Staffed Beds: 30**

**FORT BELVOIR—Fairfax County**

☒ **DEWITT ARMY COMMUNITY HOSPITAL**, 9501 Farrell Road, Zip 22060–5901, Mailing Address: 9501 Farrell Road, Suite GC11, Zip 22060–5901; tel. 703/805–0510, (Nonreporting) **A**1 3 5 **S** Department of the Army, Office of the Surgeon General, Falls Church, VA
Primary Contact: Colonel Susan Annicelli, Commander
CMO: Lieutenant Colonel Mark D. Harris, Deputy Commander Clinical Services
CIO: Terrance Branch, Chief Information Management
Web address: www.dewitt.wramc.amedd.army.mil
**Control:** Army, Government, federal **Service:** General Medical and Surgical

**Staffed Beds: 46**

**FRANKLIN—Franklin City County**

☒ **SOUTHAMPTON MEMORIAL HOSPITAL (490092)**, 100 Fairview Drive, Zip 23851–1206, Mailing Address: P.O. Box 817, Zip 23851–0817; tel. 757/569–6100, (Nonreporting) **A**1 9 10 20 **S** Community Health Systems, Inc., Franklin, TN
Primary Contact: Phil A. Wright, II, Chief Executive Officer
CFO: Steve Ramey, Chief Financial Officer
CMO: Daniel Peak, M.D., Chief Medical Staff
CHR: E. Al Parrish, Director Human Resources
Web address: www.smhfranklin.com
**Control:** Corporation, Investor–owned, for–profit **Service:** General Medical and Surgical

**Staffed Beds: 72**

**FREDERICKSBURG—Fredericksburg City County**

☒ **HEALTHSOUTH REHABILITATION HOSPITAL OF FREDERICKSBURG (493032)**, 300 Park Hill Drive, Zip 22401–3387; tel. 540/368–7300, (Nonreporting) **A**1 10 **S** HEALTHSOUTH Corporation, Birmingham, AL
Primary Contact: Donna Z. Phillips, M.D., Chief Executive Officer
Web address: www.fredericksburgrehabhospital.com
**Control:** Corporation, Investor–owned, for–profit **Service:** Rehabilitation

**Staffed Beds: 40**

☒ **MARY WASHINGTON HOSPITAL (490022)**, 1001 Sam Perry Boulevard, Zip 22401–3354; tel. 540/741–1100 **A**1 2 9 10 **F**3 5 13 15 17 18 20 22 24 26 28 29 30 31 34 35 36 40 42 43 44 45 46 48 49 50 54 57 58 59 62 64 68 70 71 72 74 75 76 77 78 79 81 84 85 86 87 89 91 93 96 97 98 99 100 101 102 104 105 107 108 109 110 111 112 113 114 117 118 119 120 122 123 125 128 129 130 131 134 145 146 147 **P**6 **S** Mary Washington Healthcare, Fredericksburg, VA
Primary Contact: Fred M. Rankin, III, President and Chief Executive Officer
COO: Walter J. Kiwall, Executive Vice President and Chief Operating Officer
CFO: Sean Barden, Executive Vice President and Chief Financial Officer
CMO: J. Thomas Ryan, M.D., Executive Vice President and Chief Medical Officer
CHR: Kathryn S. Wall, Executive Vice President Human Resources and Organizational Development
Web address: www.mwhc.org
**Control:** Other not–for–profit (including NFP Corporation) **Service:** General Medical and Surgical

**Staffed Beds: 437 Admissions: 23133 Census: 309 Outpatient Visits: 361074 Births: 3091 Total Expense ($000): 410223 Payroll Expense ($000): 138099 Personnel: 2326**

**SNOWDEN AT FREDERICKSBURG**, 1200 Sam Perry Boulevard, Zip 22401; tel. 540/741–3900, (Nonreporting) **A**9
Primary Contact: Charles Scercy, Chief Executive Officer
Web address: www.snowdenmentalhealth.com
**Control:** Other not–for–profit (including NFP Corporation) **Service:** Psychiatric

**Staffed Beds: 30**

☒ **SPOTSYLVANIA REGIONAL MEDICAL CENTER (490141)**, 4600 Spotsylvania Parkway, Zip 22408; tel. 540/834–1500, (Nonreporting) **A**1 9 10 **S** HCA, Nashville, TN
Primary Contact: Timothy C. Tobin, FACHE, President and Chief Executive Officer
COO: Terika Richardson, M.P.H., Associate Administrator
CFO: Sean Thomson, CPA, Chief Financial Officer
Web address: www.spotsrmc.com
**Control:** Corporation, Investor–owned, for–profit **Service:** General Medical and Surgical

**Staffed Beds: 100**

**FRONT ROYAL—Warren County**

☒ **WARREN MEMORIAL HOSPITAL (490033)**, 1000 North Shenandoah Avenue, Zip 22630–3598; tel. 540/636–0300, (Total facility includes 120 beds in nursing home–type unit) **A**1 9 10 13 **F**3 11 13 15 28 29 30 34 35 36 40 50 53 54 56 57 59 64 65 67 70 75 76 77 79 81 82 85 86 87 93 96 107 108 111 113 117 118 127 129 131 134 143 145 146 147 **P**6 **S** Valley Health System, Winchester, VA
Primary Contact: Patrick B. Nolan, President and Chief Executive Officer
CFO: Phillip Graybeal, Chief Financial Officer
CMO: Robert Meltvedt, Jr., M.D., Vice President Medical Affairs
Web address: www.valleyhealthlink.com
**Control:** Other not–for–profit (including NFP Corporation) **Service:** General Medical and Surgical

**Staffed Beds: 166 Admissions: 2964 Census: 137 Outpatient Visits: 90505 Births: 401 Total Expense ($000): 60196 Payroll Expense ($000): 24032 Personnel: 327**

**VA**

*Many Facility Codes have changed. Please refer to the AHA Guide Code Chart.* © 2012 AHA Guide

## GALAX—Galax City County

**☒ TWIN COUNTY REGIONAL HOSPITAL (490115)**, 200 Hospital Drive, Zip 24333–2283; tel. 276/236–8181 **A1** 9 10 20 **F3** 9 13 14 15 28 29 30 31 32 34 35 40 45 50 51 53 57 62 63 64 65 68 70 75 76 77 78 79 81 85 87 89 93 94 98 100 101 102 103 104 107 108 111 113 117 118 126 128 129 131 132 134 145 146 147 **P5** 8 **S** Duke LifePoint Healthcare, Brentwood, TN
Primary Contact: Jon D. Applebaum, President and Chief Executive Officer
COO: Sandy Moretz, R.N., Chief Operating Officer and Vice President Patient Care Services
CFO: Stephanie Bryant, Chief Financial Officer
CIO: Jack Roberts, Director Information Systems
CHR: Kay P. Cochran, Vice President Human Resources
Web address: www.tcrh.org
**Control:** Other not–for–profit (including NFP Corporation) **Service:** General Medical and Surgical

**Staffed Beds:** 86 **Admissions:** 3504 **Census:** 39 **Outpatient Visits:** 74320 **Births:** 316 **Total Expense ($000):** 46897 **Payroll Expense ($000):** 22177 **Personnel:** 593

## GLOUCESTER—Gloucester County

**☒ RIVERSIDE WALTER REED HOSPITAL (490130)**, 7519 Hospital Drive, Zip 23061–4178, Mailing Address: P.O. Box 1130, Zip 23061–1130; tel. 804/693–8800 **A1** 9 10 **F3** 11 15 28 29 35 40 43 44 45 49 50 51 57 59 63 64 70 75 77 79 81 85 86 87 92 93 107 108 110 111 113 117 118 119 120 122 129 131 145 **P6** **S** Riverside Health System, Newport News, VA
Primary Contact: Megan K. Moore, Vice President and Administrator
CHR: Kent Taylor, Director Human Resources
Web address: www.riversideonline.com
**Control:** Other not–for–profit (including NFP Corporation) **Service:** General Medical and Surgical

**Staffed Beds:** 30 **Admissions:** 2740 **Census:** 29 **Outpatient Visits:** 92869 **Births:** 0 **Total Expense ($000):** 41194 **Payroll Expense ($000):** 15311 **Personnel:** 272

## GRUNDY—Buchanan County

**☒ BUCHANAN GENERAL HOSPITAL (490127)**, 1535 Slate Creek Road, Zip 24614–6974; tel. 276/935–1000 **A1** 9 10 20 **F3** 15 18 40 41 45 57 59 62 70 81 93 107 108 114 118 128 129 131 134 145
Primary Contact: Robert D. Ruchti, R.N., Interim Chief Executive Officer
CFO: Kim Boyd, Chief Financial Officer
CMO: Diana Hursch, M.D., Chief of Staff
CIO: Rita Ramey, Director Information Systems
CHR: Wanda Stiltner, Director Human Resources
Web address: www.bgh.org
**Control:** Other not–for–profit (including NFP Corporation) **Service:** General Medical and Surgical

**Staffed Beds:** 134 **Admissions:** 1697 **Census:** 19 **Outpatient Visits:** 43842 **Births:** 0 **Total Expense ($000):** 21413 **Payroll Expense ($000):** 9698 **Personnel:** 217

## HAMPTON—Hampton City County

**☐ RIVERSIDE BEHAVIORAL HEALTH CENTER (494001)**, 2244 Executive Drive, Zip 23666–2430; tel. 757/827–1001, (Nonreporting) **A1** 5 9 10 **S** Riverside Health System, Newport News, VA
Primary Contact: Allan D. Erbe, Administrator
COO: William B. Downey, Chief Operating Officer
CMO: Phillip Schlobohm, M.D., Executive Medical Director
CHR: Amy Barrack, Director Human Resources
Web address: www.riversideonline.com
**Control:** Other not–for–profit (including NFP Corporation) **Service:** Psychiatric

**Staffed Beds:** 79

**☒ SENTARA CAREPLEX HOSPITAL (490093)**, 3000 Coliseum Drive, Zip 23666–5963; tel. 757/736–1000 **A1** 2 3 5 9 10 **F3** 8 11 12 15 18 20 22 26 28 29 30 31 34 35 36 37 39 40 41 42 43 44 45 47 49 50 53 54 57 58 59 60 61 63 64 65 68 70 71 74 75 77 78 79 80 81 82 83 84 85 86 87 92 93 94 96 100 107 108 110 111 113 115 116 117 118 119 120 122 128 129 130 131 143 145 146 147 **S** Sentara Healthcare, Norfolk, VA
Primary Contact: Debra A. Flores, R.N., MS, President and Administrator
COO: Chet Hart, Vice President Operations
CFO: Cheryl Larner, Chief Financial Officer
CMO: Arthur Greene, M.D., Vice President Medical Affairs
CIO: Thomas Ewing, Director Information Technology
CHR: David Kidd, Manager Human Resources
Web address: www.sentara.com
**Control:** Other not–for–profit (including NFP Corporation) **Service:** General Medical and Surgical

**Staffed Beds:** 182 **Admissions:** 9144 **Census:** 126 **Outpatient Visits:** 386223 **Births:** 0 **Total Expense ($000):** 196898 **Payroll Expense ($000):** 74751 **Personnel:** 1193

**☒ U. S. AIR FORCE HOSPITAL**, 77 Nealy Avenue, Zip 23665–2080; tel. 757/764–6969, (Nonreporting) **A1** **S** Department of the Air Force, Washington, DC
Primary Contact: Colonel Eric Stone, Commander
COO: Colonel Jerome Wizda, Commander
CFO: Major Travis Ingrodi, Flight Commander Resource Management
CMO: Colonel Paul Gourley, M.D., Chief Hospital Services
CIO: Lieutenant Elliot Blackman, Chief Information Management and Technology
CHR: Michael Dietz, Chief Hospital Administration
Web address: www.jble.af.mil
**Control:** Air Force, Government, federal **Service:** General Medical and Surgical

**Staffed Beds:** 65

**☒ △ VETERANS AFFAIRS MEDICAL CENTER**, 100 Emancipation Drive, Zip 23667–0001; tel. 757/722–9961, (Total facility includes 119 beds in nursing home–type unit) **A1** 3 5 7 **F3** 5 8 10 12 15 18 20 22 26 28 29 30 31 34 35 36 38 39 40 43 44 45 46 50 51 53 54 56 57 58 59 60 61 62 63 64 65 66 70 71 74 75 77 78 79 81 82 83 84 85 86 87 91 92 93 94 97 98 99 100 101 102 104 105 106 107 111 113 115 116 118 126 127 128 129 131 132 134 142 145 146 147 **P6** **S** Department of Veterans Affairs, Washington, DC
Primary Contact: DeAnne Seekins, Director
COO: Lorraine B. Price, Associate Director
CFO: Terry Grew, Chief Business Office
CMO: Val Gibberman, M.D., Acting Chief of Staff
CIO: Cary Parks, Chief Information Resource Management
Web address: www.va.gov/sta/guide/home.asp
**Control:** Veterans Affairs, Government, federal **Service:** General Medical and Surgical

**Staffed Beds:** 395 **Admissions:** 3790 **Census:** 331 **Outpatient Visits:** 437640 **Births:** 0 **Total Expense ($000):** 313647 **Payroll Expense ($000):** 145000

## HARRISONBURG—Harrisonburg City County

**☒ ROCKINGHAM MEMORIAL HOSPITAL (490004)**, 2010 Health Campus Drive, Zip 22801–3293; tel. 540/433–4100 **A1** 2 5 9 10 **F3** 5 8 11 12 13 15 17 18 20 22 24 26 28 29 30 31 32 34 35 36 40 44 45 49 50 53 54 55 56 57 59 62 63 64 68 70 71 73 74 76 77 78 79 81 82 84 85 86 87 89 93 97 98 99 102 104 105 107 110 111 113 114 117 118 119 120 128 129 130 131 134 144 145 146 **P6** 8 **S** Sentara Healthcare, Norfolk, VA
Primary Contact: James D. Krauss, President and Chief Executive Officer
COO: Richard L. Haushalter, Chief Operating Officer
CMO: Dale Carroll, M.D., Senior Vice President Medical Affairs and Performance Improvement
CIO: Mike Rozmus, Director Information Systems
CHR: Mark Zimmerman, Vice President Human Resources Development and Support Services
Web address: www.rmhonline.com
**Control:** Other not–for–profit (including NFP Corporation) **Service:** General Medical and Surgical

**Staffed Beds:** 238 **Admissions:** 14686 **Census:** 152 **Outpatient Visits:** 357412 **Births:** 1688 **Total Expense ($000):** 327145 **Payroll Expense ($000):** 131338 **Personnel:** 2272

## HOPEWELL—Hopewell City County

**☒ JOHN RANDOLPH MEDICAL CENTER (490020)**, 411 West Randolph Road, Zip 23860–2938; tel. 804/541–1600 **A1** 2 9 10 **F3** 5 11 15 17 18 20 28 29 30 31 34 38 40 44 45 49 50 51 54 57 59 61 64 70 74 75 77 78 79 81 85 86 87 92 93 96 98 100 101 102 103 105 106 107 108 113 114 117 118 129 130 131 134 143 145 147 **P6** **S** HCA, Nashville, TN
Primary Contact: Dia Nichols, Chief Executive Officer
CFO: Chigger Bynum, Chief Financial Officer
CHR: MaDena DuChemin, Assistant Administrator Human Resources
Web address: www.johnrandolphmed.com
**Control:** Corporation, Investor–owned, for–profit **Service:** General Medical and Surgical

**Staffed Beds:** 118 **Admissions:** 4842 **Census:** 73 **Outpatient Visits:** 64857 **Births:** 0 **Personnel:** 433

**VA**

## HOT SPRINGS—Bath County

✠ **BATH COMMUNITY HOSPITAL (491300)**, 83 Park Drive, Zip 24445, Mailing Address: P.O. Box Z., Zip 24445–0750; tel. 540/839–7000 **A**1 9 10 18 **F**3 7 15 28 30 35 40 45 49 50 53 57 59 64 75 77 79 81 92 93 94 102 107 111 118 126 127 128 129 130 132 134 142
Primary Contact: Deborah Lipes, R.N., Chief Executive Officer
CFO: Mark Hall, Chief Financial Officer
CMO: James Redington, M.D., Chief of Staff
CIO: Tracy Bartley, Manager Information Technology
CHR: Patricia Foutz, Director Human Resources
Web address: www.bcchospital.org
**Control:** Other not–for–profit (including NFP Corporation) **Service:** General Medical and Surgical

**Staffed Beds:** 25 **Admissions:** 473 **Census:** 6 **Outpatient Visits:** 11028 **Births:** 0 **Total Expense ($000):** 11406 **Payroll Expense ($000):** 5835 **Personnel:** 136

## KILMARNOCK—Lancaster County

✠ **RAPPAHANNOCK GENERAL HOSPITAL (490123)**, 101 Harris Drive, Zip 22482, Mailing Address: P.O. Box 1449, Zip 22482–1449; tel. 804/435–8000, (Nonreporting) **A**1 9 10 20
Primary Contact: James M. Holmes, Jr., President and Chief Executive Officer
Web address: www.rgh–hospital.com
**Control:** Other not–for–profit (including NFP Corporation) **Service:** General Medical and Surgical

**Staffed Beds:** 76

## LEBANON—Russell County

☐ **RUSSELL COUNTY MEDICAL CENTER (490002)**, 58 Carroll Street, Zip 24266, Mailing Address: P.O. Box 3600, Zip 24266–0200; tel. 276/883–8000 **A**1 9 10 **F**3 11 15 29 30 35 38 40 50 54 56 57 59 62 63 64 68 70 75 81 82 84 85 93 97 98 100 102 103 104 107 108 111 113 117 118 129 131 132 145 147 **S** Mountain States Health Alliance, Johnson City, TN
Primary Contact: Edward C. Greene, Jr., Assistant Vice President and Administrator
COO: Edward C. Greene, Jr., Assistant Vice President and Administrator
CMO: Louis Dizon, M.D., Chief of Staff
CHR: Phyllis Kiser, Director Human Resources
Web address: www.rcmc.net
**Control:** Other not–for–profit (including NFP Corporation) **Service:** General Medical and Surgical

**Staffed Beds:** 78 **Admissions:** 3066 **Census:** 36 **Outpatient Visits:** 31739 **Births:** 0 **Total Expense ($000):** 20875 **Payroll Expense ($000):** 10114 **Personnel:** 224

## LEESBURG—Loudoun County

✠ **INOVA LOUDOUN HOSPITAL (490043)**, 44045 Riverside Parkway, Zip 20176–2799, Mailing Address: P.O. Box 6000, Zip 20177–0600; tel. 703/858–6000, (Total facility includes 100 beds in nursing home–type unit) **A**1 2 5 9 10 **F**3 4 5 11 13 14 15 18 20 22 26 28 29 30 31 32 34 35 37 38 39 40 41 42 44 45 48 49 50 54 55 57 59 60 61 63 64 65 66 67 68 70 71 72 74 75 76 77 78 79 81 82 84 85 86 87 89 92 93 96 98 101 102 103 104 105 107 108 110 111 113 114 117 118 119 120 122 125 127 129 130 131 134 145 146 147 **P**6 **S** Inova Health System, Falls Church, VA
Primary Contact: Patrick Walters, Interim Chief Executive Officer
COO: Susan Carroll, Chief Operating Officer
CFO: Glenn Zirbser, Chief Financial Officer
CMO: Christopher Chiantella, M.D., Chief of Staff
CIO: Nancy Mengel, Director Information Technology
CHR: Sarah Pavik, Director Human Resources and Guest Services
Web address: www.inova.org
**Control:** Other not–for–profit (including NFP Corporation) **Service:** General Medical and Surgical

**Staffed Beds:** 290 **Admissions:** 12032 **Census:** 226 **Outpatient Visits:** 161678 **Births:** 2672 **Total Expense ($000):** 212861 **Payroll Expense ($000):** 88896 **Personnel:** 1380

## LEXINGTON—Lexington City County

✠ **CARILION STONEWALL JACKSON HOSPITAL (491304)**, 1 Health Circle, Zip 24450–2492; tel. 540/458–3300 **A**1 9 10 18 **F**7 8 11 15 28 29 34 35 40 45 48 49 50 53 56 57 59 62 70 75 77 79 81 85 87 93 107 108 110 111 114 118 128 129 132 145 **S** Carilion Clinic, Roanoke, VA
Primary Contact: Charles E. Carr, Chief Executive Officer
CMO: Lyle McClung, M.D., Chief of Staff
Web address: www.carilionclinic.com
**Control:** Other not–for–profit (including NFP Corporation) **Service:** General Medical and Surgical

**Staffed Beds:** 25 **Admissions:** 1321 **Census:** 14 **Outpatient Visits:** 30944 **Births:** 0 **Total Expense ($000):** 27891 **Payroll Expense ($000):** 9817 **Personnel:** 211

## LOW MOOR—Alleghany County

✠ **LEWISGALE HOSPITAL ALLEGHANY (490126)**, One ARH Lane, Zip 24457, Mailing Address: P.O. Box 7, Zip 24457–0007; tel. 540/862–6011, (Nonreporting) **A**1 9 10 20 **S** HCA, Nashville, TN
Primary Contact: Greg T. Madsen, Chief Executive Officer
CFO: Tim Prestridge, Chief Financial Officer
CMO: Hassan Honainy, M.D., President Medical Staff
CIO: Jeffrey Steelman, Director Information Systems
Web address: www.alleghanyregional.com
**Control:** Corporation, Investor–owned, for–profit **Service:** General Medical and Surgical

**Staffed Beds:** 146

## LURAY—Page County

✠ **PAGE MEMORIAL HOSPITAL (491307)**, 200 Memorial Drive, Zip 22835–1005; tel. 540/743–4561 **A**1 9 10 18 **F**3 7 8 11 15 29 30 34 35 40 43 53 56 57 59 60 64 66 68 74 75 77 79 81 85 90 93 107 108 110 111 113 118 126 127 128 132 142 145 **P**2 **S** Valley Health System, Winchester, VA
Primary Contact: N. Travis Clark, President
CFO: Phillip Graybeal, Chief Financial Officer
Web address: www.pagememorialhospital.org
**Control:** Other not–for–profit (including NFP Corporation) **Service:** General Medical and Surgical

**Staffed Beds:** 25 **Admissions:** 646 **Census:** 5 **Outpatient Visits:** 86274 **Births:** 0 **Total Expense ($000):** 20645 **Payroll Expense ($000):** 10087 **Personnel:** 174

## LYNCHBURG—Lynchburg City County

**CENTER FOR RESTORATIVE CARE AND REHABILITATION (492010)**, 3300 Rivermont Avenue, Zip 24503–2030; tel. 434/200–1799, (Nonreporting) **A**10
Primary Contact: Kay Bowling, Chief Executive Officer
**Control:** Partnership, Investor–owned, for–profit **Service:** Long–Term Acute Care hospital

**Staffed Beds:** 36

**CENTRA HEALTH** See Centra Lynchburg General Hospital

✠ **CENTRA LYNCHBURG GENERAL HOSPITAL (490021)**, 1920 Atherholt Road, Zip 24501–1104; tel. 434/200–4700, (Includes LYNCHBURG GENERAL HOSPITAL, 1901 Tate Springs Road, Zip 24501–1167; tel. 434/200–3000; VIRGINIA BAPTIST HOSPITAL, 3300 Rivermont Avenue, Zip 24503–2053; tel. 434/200–4000), (Total facility includes 447 beds in nursing home–type unit) **A**1 2 3 5 6 9 10 **F**1 2 3 5 6 7 8 10 11 13 15 17 18 19 20 22 24 26 28 29 30 31 34 35 37 38 40 43 44 45 46 48 49 50 53 56 57 59 60 61 62 63 64 67 68 69 70 71 72 74 75 76 77 78 79 80 81 82 84 85 86 87 89 90 93 94 98 99 100 102 103 104 105 106 107 108 109 110 111 113 114 116 117 118 119 120 122 123 124 125 126 127 128 129 134 142 143 145 146 147 **P**7 **S** Centra Health, Inc., Lynchburg, VA
Primary Contact: W. Michael Bryant, President and Chief Executive Officer
CFO: Lewis C. Addison, Senior Vice President and Chief Financial Officer
CMO: Chalmers Nunn, M.D., Chief Medical Officer and Senior Vice President
CIO: Ben Clark, Vice President and Chief Information Officer
CHR: Jan Walker, Director Human Resources
Web address: www.centrahealth.com
**Control:** Other not–for–profit (including NFP Corporation) **Service:** General Medical and Surgical

**Staffed Beds:** 1081 **Admissions:** 32078 **Census:** 802 **Outpatient Visits:** 482744 **Births:** 2611 **Total Expense ($000):** 554892 **Payroll Expense ($000):** 251984 **Personnel:** 4263

## MADISON HEIGHTS—Amherst County

**CENTRAL VIRGINIA TRAINING CENTER (490108)**, 210 East Colony Road, Zip 24572–2005, Mailing Address: P.O. Box 1098, Lynchburg, Zip 24505–1098; tel. 434/947–6326, (Nonreporting) **A**10 **S** Virginia Department of Mental Health, Richmond, VA
Primary Contact: Denise D. Micheletti, R.N., Director
COO: Denise D. Micheletti, R.N., Director
CFO: Charles Felmlee, Assistant Director Fiscal Services
CMO: Balraj Bawa, M.D., Assistant Director Medical Services
CHR: Burchkhard Blob, Manager Human Resources
Web address: www.cvtc.dmhmrsas.virginia.gov/
**Control:** State–Government, nonfederal **Service:** Institution for mental retardation

**Staffed Beds:** 1112

**VA**

*Many Facility Codes have changed. Please refer to the AHA Guide Code Chart.*  © 2012 AHA Guide

## MANASSAS—Manassas City County

☒ **PRINCE WILLIAM HOSPITAL (490045)**, 8700 Sudley Road, Zip 20110–4418,
Mailing Address: P.O. Box 2610, Zip 20108–0867; tel. 703/369–8000 **A**1 2 9
10 **F**3 5 8 10 11 15 18 19 20 22 26 28 29 30 31 32 34 35 36 38 39 40
42 44 45 49 50 51 53 54 57 59 62 64 65 68 70 72 74 75 76 77 78 79 81
82 85 86 87 89 93 97 98 99 100 102 103 104 107 110 111 113 114 118
128 129 131 133 134 145 146 147 **P**7 **S** Novant Health, Winston–Salem, NC
Primary Contact: Melissa Robson, President
COO: Melissa Robson, President
CFO: Robert Riley, Chief Financial Officer
CMO: S. Marc Krenytzky, M.D., Vice President Medical Affairs
CIO: Velma Carroll, Interim Chief Information Officer
CHR: Terry Lovell, Vice President Human Resources
Web address: www.pwhs.org
**Control:** Other not–for–profit (including NFP Corporation) **Service:** General
Medical and Surgical

**Staffed Beds:** 168 **Admissions:** 10247 **Census:** 107 **Outpatient Visits:**
217759 **Births:** 2247 **Total Expense ($000):** 171797 **Payroll Expense
($000):** 76634 **Personnel:** 1009

## MARION—Smyth County

☐ **SMYTH COUNTY COMMUNITY HOSPITAL (490038)**, 243 Medical Park Drive,
Zip 24354, Mailing Address: P.O. Box 880, Zip 24354–0880;
tel. 276/378–1000, (Total facility includes 109 beds in nursing home–type unit)
**A**1 9 10 **F**3 10 11 15 28 29 30 34 40 46 47 48 56 57 59 62 64 65 67 68 70
75 77 79 81 82 84 85 87 90 93 97 107 111 118 127 129 131 132 134 145
147 **S** Mountain States Health Alliance, Johnson City, TN
Primary Contact: Lindy P. White, President and Chief Executive Officer
CFO: John Jeter, Chief Financial Officer
Web address:
www.msha.com/hospitals/smyth_county_community_hospital_l_marion_va.aspx
**Control:** Other not–for–profit (including NFP Corporation) **Service:** General
Medical and Surgical

**Staffed Beds:** 151 **Admissions:** 2415 **Census:** 124 **Outpatient Visits:** 97393
**Births:** 78 **Total Expense ($000):** 38124 **Payroll Expense ($000):** 17390
**Personnel:** 266

☐ **SOUTHWESTERN VIRGINIA MENTAL HEALTH INSTITUTE (490105)**, 340
Bagley Circle, Zip 24354–3390; tel. 276/783–1200, (Nonreporting) **A**1 9 10
**S** Virginia Department of Mental Health, Richmond, VA
Primary Contact: Cynthia McClaskey, Ph.D., Director
CIO: Kim Ratliff, Director Health Information Management
Web address: www.swvmhi.dmhmrsas.virginia.gov/
**Control:** State–Government, nonfederal **Service:** Psychiatric

**Staffed Beds:** 266

## MARTINSVILLE—Martinsville City County

★ **MEMORIAL HOSPITAL (490079)**, 320 Hospital Drive, Zip 24112–1981, Mailing
Address: P.O. Box 4788, Zip 24115–4788; tel. 276/666–7200, (Nonreporting)
**A**2 9 10 19 **S** LifePoint Hospitals, Inc., Brentwood, TN
Primary Contact: Grady W. Philips, III, Chief Executive Officer
CFO: Brandy Hanners, Chief Financial Officer
CIO: Jeff Butker, Chief Information Officer
CHR: Sherry Schofield, Director Human Resources
Web address: www.martinsvillehospital.com
**Control:** Corporation, Investor–owned, for–profit **Service:** General Medical and
Surgical

**Staffed Beds:** 220

## MECHANICSVILLE—Hanover County

☒ **BON SECOURS MEMORIAL REGIONAL MEDICAL CENTER (490069)**, 8260
Atlee Road, Zip 23116–1844; tel. 804/764–6000, (Nonreporting) **A**1 2 5 9 10
**S** Bon Secours Health System, Inc., Marriottsville, MD
Primary Contact: Michael Robinson, Chief Executive Officer
CFO: Peter Gallagher, Vice President and Chief Financial Officer
CMO: Roger Cappello, M.D., Vice President Medical Affairs
CHR: Bonnie Shelor, Vice President Human Resources
Web address: www.bonsecours.com
**Control:** Church–operated, Nongovernment, not–for profit **Service:** General
Medical and Surgical

**Staffed Beds:** 225

☒ **SHELTERING ARMS REHABILITATION HOSPITAL (493025)**, 8254 Atlee
Road, Zip 23116–1844; tel. 804/764–7055 **A**1 10 **F**29 30 34 53 54 55 57 59
68 74 77 79 86 87 90 92 93 95 96 129 130 131 142 145 **P**6
Primary Contact: James E. Sok, FACHE, President and Chief Executive Officer
COO: Michael J. McDonnell, Vice President and Chief Operating Officer
CMO: Hillary Hawkins, M.D., Medical Director
CHR: Ellen B. Vance, Vice President and Chief Human Resource Officer
Web address: www.shelteringarms.com
**Control:** Other not–for–profit (including NFP Corporation) **Service:** Rehabilitation

**Staffed Beds:** 68 **Admissions:** 1751 **Census:** 60 **Outpatient Visits:** 81390
**Births:** 0 **Total Expense ($000):** 53711 **Payroll Expense ($000):** 31995
**Personnel:** 564

## MIDLOTHIAN—Chesterfield County

☒ **BON SECOURS ST. FRANCIS MEDICAL CENTER (490136)**, 13710 St.
Francis Boulevard, Zip 23114–3267; tel. 804/594–7300, (Nonreporting) **A**1 2 9
10 **S** Bon Secours Health System, Inc., Marriottsville, MD
Primary Contact: Mark M. Gordon, Executive Vice President
COO: Peter J. Bernard, Chief Executive Officer
CFO: Peter Gallagher, Chief Financial Officer
CIO: Mike Lokie, Project Director
CHR: Paul Catucci, Administrative Director Human Resources
Web address: www.bonsecours.com/sfmc/default.asp
**Control:** Other not–for–profit (including NFP Corporation) **Service:** General
Medical and Surgical

**Staffed Beds:** 130

☐ **SHELTERING ARMS HOSPITAL SOUTH (493030)**, 13700 St. Francis
Boulevard, Suite 400, Zip 23114–3222; tel. 804/764–1000, (Nonreporting)
**A**1 10
Primary Contact: James E. Sok, FACHE, President and Chief Executive Officer
COO: Michael J. McDonnell, Vice President and Chief Operations Officer
CFO: Mike Dacus, Vice President and Chief Financial Officer
CMO: Timothy Silver, M.D., Medical Director
CHR: Ellen B. Vance, Vice President Human Resources
CNO: Cheryl D. Lee, R.N., Vice President Patient Care Services, Chief Executive
Nurse and Compliance Officer
Web address: www.shelteringarms.com
**Control:** Other not–for–profit (including NFP Corporation) **Service:** Rehabilitation

**Staffed Beds:** 28

## NASSAWADOX—Northampton County

☐ **RIVERSIDE SHORE MEMORIAL HOSPITAL (490037)**, 9507 Hospital Avenue,
Zip 23413–1821, Mailing Address: P.O. Box 17, Zip 23413–0017;
tel. 757/414–8000, (Total facility includes 13 beds in nursing home–type unit) **A**1
2 9 10 20 **F**2 3 11 15 28 29 30 31 34 40 45 50 62 70 75 76 77 78 79 81
82 85 93 102 103 105 107 110 111 117 118 127 128 129 131 132 134
145 147 **P**6 **S** Riverside Health System, Newport News, VA
Primary Contact: Joseph P. Zager, Vice President and Administrator
CFO: Wade Broughman, Chief Financial Officer
CMO: Charles Goldstein, M.D., President Medical Staff
CIO: Rob Gayman, Director Information Systems
CHR: Nicole Miller, Director Human Resources
Web address: www.shorehealthservices.org
**Control:** Other not–for–profit (including NFP Corporation) **Service:** General
Medical and Surgical

**Staffed Beds:** 48 **Admissions:** 3551 **Census:** 42 **Outpatient Visits:** 80047
**Births:** 515 **Total Expense ($000):** 52096 **Payroll Expense ($000):** 22180
**Personnel:** 326

**SHORE MEMORIAL HOSPITAL** See Riverside Shore Memorial Hospital

## NEW KENT—New Kent County

☐ **CUMBERLAND HOSPITAL (493300)**, 9407 Cumberland Road,
Zip 23124–0150; tel. 804/966–2242, (Nonreporting) **A**1 10 **S** Universal Health
Services, Inc., King of Prussia, PA
Primary Contact: Patrice Gay Brooks, Chief Executive Officer
CFO: Joanne Rial, Chief Financial Officer
CMO: Daniel N. Davidow, M.D., Medical Director
CIO: Towanda Brown, Director Standards and Regulatory Compliance
CHR: Lauren Bonner, Director Human Resources
Web address: www.cumberlandhospital.com
**Control:** Corporation, Investor–owned, for–profit **Service:** Children's rehabilitation

**Staffed Beds:** 132

**VA**

---

**Hospital, Medicare Provider Number, Address, Telephone, Approval, Facility, and Physician Codes, Health Care System**

★ American Hospital Association (AHA) membership
☐ The Joint Commission accreditation ◇ DNV Healthcare Inc. accreditation
○ American Osteopathic Association (AOA) accreditation
△ Commission on Accreditation of Rehabilitation Facilities (CARF) accreditation

## NEWPORT NEWS—Newport News City County

**HAMPTON ROADS SPECIALTY HOSPITAL (492008)**, 245 Chesapeake Avenue, Zip 23607–6038; tel. 757/534–5000, (Nonreporting) **A**10 **S** Riverside Health System, Newport News, VA
Primary Contact: Courtney Detwiler, R.N., Administrator
Web address: www.hamptonroadsspecialtyhospital.com
**Control:** Other not–for–profit (including NFP Corporation) **Service:** Long–Term Acute Care hospital

**Staffed Beds: 25**

**KEYSTONE NEWPORT NEWS**, 17579 Warwick Boulevard, Zip 23603–1343; tel. 757/888–0400, (Nonreporting)
Primary Contact: Robert J. Lehmann, Chief Executive Officer
Web address: www.keystonenewportnews.com
**Control:** Corporation, Investor–owned, for–profit **Service:** Psychiatric

**Staffed Beds: 68**

✠ **MARY IMMACULATE HOSPITAL (490041)**, 2 Bernardine Drive, Zip 23602–4499; tel. 757/886–6000, (Includes ST. FRANCIS NURSING CENTER ), (Total facility includes 115 beds in nursing home–type unit) **A**1 9 10 **F**3 5 11 12 13 15 18 20 22 24 26 28 29 30 31 34 40 44 45 46 50 57 59 61 63 64 67 68 70 73 74 75 76 77 78 79 81 82 84 85 86 87 91 93 102 107 108 111 113 117 118 129 130 131 142 144 145 146 147 **P**6 **S** Bon Secours Health System, Inc., Marriottsville, MD
Primary Contact: Patricia L. Robertson, Executive Vice President
COO: Darlene Stephenson, Vice President Operations
CFO: Greg Simia, Chief Financial Officer
CIO: Terri Spence, Vice President Information Services
CHR: John Mashinski, Vice President Human Resources
Web address: www.bonsecourshamptonroads.com
**Control:** Other not–for–profit (including NFP Corporation) **Service:** General Medical and Surgical

**Staffed Beds: 232 Admissions: 9684 Census: 184 Outpatient Visits: 54973 Births: 1588 Total Expense ($000): 154872 Payroll Expense ($000): 43235 Personnel: 760**

☐ **RIVERSIDE REGIONAL MEDICAL CENTER (490052)**, 500 J. Clyde Morris Boulevard, Zip 23601–1929; tel. 757/594–2000, (Includes RIVERSIDE PSYCHIATRIC INSTITUTE ) **A**1 2 3 5 6 9 10 13 **F**3 11 12 13 15 17 18 20 22 24 26 28 29 30 31 32 35 38 39 40 43 44 45 49 50 51 54 55 56 57 58 59 60 61 62 63 64 70 72 74 75 76 77 78 79 81 82 85 86 87 89 92 93 97 107 108 110 111 113 114 115 116 117 118 119 120 122 123 125 128 129 131 140 141 143 145 146 147 **P**6 **S** Riverside Health System, Newport News, VA
Primary Contact: Patrick Parcells, Senior Vice President and Administrator
COO: William B. Downey, Chief Operating Officer
CFO: Wade Broughman, Executive Vice President and Chief Financial Officer
CMO: Barry L. Gross, M.D., Executive Vice President and Chief Medical Officer
CIO: John T. Stanley, Vice President Planning and Information Systems
CHR: Larry Boyles, Senior Vice President
Web address: www.riverside–online.com
**Control:** Other not–for–profit (including NFP Corporation) **Service:** General Medical and Surgical

**Staffed Beds: 188 Admissions: 15814 Census: 185 Outpatient Visits: 414021 Births: 2785 Total Expense ($000): 384466 Payroll Expense ($000): 143040 Personnel: 1215**

✠ △ **RIVERSIDE REHABILITATION INSTITUTE (493027)**, 245 Chesapeake Avenue, Zip 23607–6038; tel. 757/928–8000 **A**1 7 10 **F**3 29 30 43 57 64 77 82 87 90 91 93 94 96 129 131 145 **P**6 **S** Riverside Health System, Newport News, VA
Primary Contact: Edward Heckler, Administrator
COO: William B. Downey, President and Chief Executive Officer
CFO: Wade Broughman, Executive Vice President and Chief Financial Officer
CMO: C. Renee Moss, M.D., Chief Medical Officer
CIO: John T. Stanley, Vice President Planning and Information Systems
CHR: Ashleigh Andrews, Manager Human Resources
Web address: www.riverside–online.com
**Control:** Other not–for–profit (including NFP Corporation) **Service:** Rehabilitation

**Staffed Beds: 30 Admissions: 726 Census: 30 Outpatient Visits: 13277 Births: 0 Total Expense ($000): 13147 Payroll Expense ($000): 7599 Personnel: 130**

## NORFOLK—Norfolk City County

✠ **BON SECOURS–DEPAUL MEDICAL CENTER (490011)**, 150 Kingsley Lane, Zip 23505–4650; tel. 757/889–5000, (Total facility includes 24 beds in nursing home–type unit) **A**1 2 3 5 9 10 **F**3 11 13 15 18 20 22 29 30 31 34 35 40 44 45 46 50 51 54 56 57 59 61 64 68 70 74 75 76 78 79 81 82 84 85 86 87 93 97 102 107 108 110 111 113 114 116 117 118 119 120 127 128 129 130 131 142 144 145 146 147 **P**6 **S** Bon Secours Health System, Inc., Marriottsville, MD
Primary Contact: John E. Barrett, III, Chief Executive Officer
COO: David P. Setchel, Vice President Operations
CFO: Greg Simia, Interim Chief Financial Officer
CIO: Lynne Zultanky, Director Corporate Communications and Media Relations
CHR: John Mashinski, Senior Vice President Human Resources
Web address: www.bonsecourshamptonroads.com
**Control:** Other not–for–profit (including NFP Corporation) **Service:** General Medical and Surgical

**Staffed Beds: 238 Admissions: 7770 Census: 102 Outpatient Visits: 94485 Births: 1058 Total Expense ($000): 166400 Payroll Expense ($000): 49913 Personnel: 900**

☐ **CHILDREN'S HOSPITAL OF THE KING'S DAUGHTERS (493301)**, 601 Children's Lane, Zip 23507–1910; tel. 757/668–7000 **A**1 3 5 9 10 **F**3 7 8 9 12 16 17 19 21 23 25 27 29 30 31 32 34 35 39 40 41 44 45 48 50 54 55 57 58 59 60 61 64 68 72 73 74 75 77 78 79 80 81 82 84 85 86 87 88 89 90 91 92 93 94 97 99 100 102 104 107 108 111 114 118 128 129 130 131 133 135 137 140 144 145 147 **P**8
Primary Contact: James D. Dahling, President and Chief Executive Officer
CFO: Dennis Ryan, Senior Vice President and Chief Financial Officer
CMO: Arno Zaritsky, M.D., Senior Vice President Clinical Services
CIO: Deborah Barnes, Vice President and Chief Information Officer
CHR: David Bowers, Vice President Human Resources and Support Services
CNO: Jo-Ann Burke, R.N., Vice President Patient Care Services
Web address: www.chkd.org
**Control:** Other not–for–profit (including NFP Corporation) **Service:** Children's general

**Staffed Beds: 206 Admissions: 5482 Census: 141 Outpatient Visits: 202546 Births: 0 Total Expense ($000): 250200 Payroll Expense ($000): 112026 Personnel: 2194**

**HOSPITAL FOR EXTENDED RECOVERY (492007)**, 600 Gresham Drive, Suite 700, Zip 23507; tel. 757/388–1700, (Nonreporting) **A**9 10
Primary Contact: Linda B. O'Neil, R.N., Chief Executive Officer
**Control:** Other not–for–profit (including NFP Corporation) **Service:** Long–Term Acute Care hospital

**Staffed Beds: 35**

**LAKE TAYLOR TRANSITIONAL CARE HOSPITAL (492001)**, 1309 Kempsville Road, Zip 23502–2286; tel. 757/461–5001, (Total facility includes 192 beds in nursing home–type unit) **A**3 5 10 **F**1 3 11 29 30 39 61 67 79 82 84 85 96 127 129 145 147
Primary Contact: Thomas J. Orsini, President and Chief Executive Officer
CFO: Robert W. Fogg, Director Finance
CMO: Antoine A. Arrage, M.D., Director Medical Services
CIO: Mark Davis, Director Information Systems
CHR: LeeAnn Lowman, Director Human Resources
Web address: www.laketaylor.org
**Control:** Hospital district or authority, Government, nonfederal **Service:** Long–Term Acute Care hospital

**Staffed Beds: 293 Admissions: 1350 Census: 234 Outpatient Visits: 0 Births: 0 Total Expense ($000): 32330 Payroll Expense ($000): 14516 Personnel: 364**

**NORFOLK PSYCHIATRIC CENTER**, 860 Kempsville Road, Zip 23502–3980; tel. 757/461–4565, (Nonreporting)
Primary Contact: Arlene Manzella, Administrator
**Control:** Corporation, Investor–owned, for–profit **Service:** Psychiatric

**Staffed Beds: 77**

✠ **SENTARA LEIGH HOSPITAL (490046)**, 830 Kempsville Road, Zip 23502–3920; tel. 757/261–6000 **A**1 2 3 5 9 10 **F**3 8 9 11 12 13 15 18 20 22 26 28 29 30 31 34 35 36 37 38 39 40 41 44 45 46 47 48 49 50 51 54 57 58 59 60 61 63 64 68 70 71 74 75 76 77 78 79 81 82 84 85 86 87 92 93 94 96 97 100 102 107 108 110 111 113 115 116 117 118 125 129 130 131 140 143 144 145 146 147 **P**6 **S** Sentara Healthcare, Norfolk, VA
Primary Contact: Teresa L. Edwards, Vice President and Administrator
COO: Howard P. Kern, President and Chief Operating Officer
CFO: Robert Broermann, Senior Vice President and Chief Financial Officer
CMO: Gary R. Yates, M.D., Senior Vice President and Chief Medical Officer
CIO: Bert Reese, Chief Information Officer
CHR: Michael V. Taylor, Senior Vice President Human Resources
Web address: www.sentara.com
**Control:** Other not–for–profit (including NFP Corporation) **Service:** General Medical and Surgical

**Staffed Beds: 238 Admissions: 14828 Census: 178 Outpatient Visits: 387415 Births: 2219 Total Expense ($000): 204850 Payroll Expense ($000): 81235 Personnel: 1228**

**VA**

*Many Facility Codes have changed. Please refer to the AHA Guide Code Chart.*
© 2012 AHA Guide

☒ **SENTARA NORFOLK GENERAL HOSPITAL (490007)**, 600 Gresham Drive, Zip 23507; tel. 757/388–3000 **A1** 2 3 5 6 7 8 9 **F**3 7 11 12 13 15 16 17 18 20 22 24 26 28 29 30 31 34 35 36 38 39 40 41 43 44 45 46 47 48 49 50 51 54 56 57 58 59 60 61 63 64 65 66 68 70 71 74 75 76 77 78 79 81 82 84 85 86 87 90 93 94 98 99 100 101 102 103 104 105 106 107 108 110 111 113 114 115 116 117 118 119 120 122 123 125 128 129 130 131 134 135 136 137 140 141 145 146 147 **P**6 **S** Sentara Healthcare, Norfolk, VA
Primary Contact: Mary L. Blunt, Corporate Vice President and Administrator
CFO: Robert Broermann, Senior Vice President and Chief Financial Officer
CMO: Gary R. Yates, M.D., Chief Medical Officer
CIO: Bert Reese, Chief Information Officer
Web address: www.sentara.com
**Control:** Other not–for–profit (including NFP Corporation) **Service:** General Medical and Surgical

**Staffed Beds:** 491 **Admissions:** 24808 **Census:** 401 **Outpatient Visits:** 549726 **Births:** 2744 **Total Expense ($000):** 574886 **Payroll Expense ($000):** 203496 **Personnel:** 3286

### NORTON—Norton City County

☒ **MOUNTAIN VIEW REGIONAL MEDICAL CENTER (490027)**, 310 Third Street N.E., Zip 24273–1137; tel. 276/679–9100, (Total facility includes 44 beds in nursing home–type unit) **A**1 9 10 **F**3 11 15 18 28 29 30 34 35 40 48 49 50 57 59 63 68 70 77 79 81 85 87 92 93 97 107 111 114 116 117 118 128 129 130 145 **S** Wellmont Health System, Kingsport, TN
Primary Contact: David L. Brash, System Regional Vice President and President
COO: Donna Jennings, Vice President Quality and Ancillary Services
CFO: David R. Jones, Interim Chief Financial Officer
CMO: Kathleen Deponte, M.D., Chief of Staff
CIO: Wade Freeman, Regional Site Director
CHR: Bobby Collins, Director Human Resources
Web address: www.wellmont.org
**Control:** Other not–for–profit (including NFP Corporation) **Service:** General Medical and Surgical

**Staffed Beds:** 118 **Admissions:** 1876 **Census:** 51 **Outpatient Visits:** 38687 **Births:** 0 **Total Expense ($000):** 23959 **Payroll Expense ($000):** 6338 **Personnel:** 188

○ △ **NORTON COMMUNITY HOSPITAL (490001)**, 100 15th Street N.W., Zip 24273–1616; tel. 276/679–9600 **A**7 9 10 11 13 **F**3 11 12 13 15 28 29 30 32 34 35 36 38 40 50 51 53 54 56 57 59 62 64 65 68 70 75 76 77 79 81 82 85 86 87 90 93 97 107 111 113 117 118 128 129 130 131 132 133 134 145 146 147 **S** Mountain States Health Alliance, Johnson City, TN
Primary Contact: Mark T. Leonard, Chief Executive Officer
CFO: Stephen Sawyer, Chief Financial Officer
CMO: Allen Mullens, M.D., Chief Medical Staff
CIO: Judy Lawson, Director Information Services
CHR: Valeri J. Colyer, Director Human Resources
Web address: www.nchosp.org
**Control:** Other not–for–profit (including NFP Corporation) **Service:** General Medical and Surgical

**Staffed Beds:** 40 **Admissions:** 4386 **Census:** 38 **Outpatient Visits:** 96610 **Births:** 418 **Total Expense ($000):** 39130 **Payroll Expense ($000):** 20600 **Personnel:** 362

### PEARISBURG—Giles County

☒ **CARILION GILES COMMUNITY HOSPITAL (491302)**, 159 Hartley Way, Zip 24134–2471; tel. 540/921–6000 **A**1 9 10 18 **F**3 11 12 13 15 28 29 34 35 39 40 45 50 57 59 64 65 68 70 75 81 82 85 86 87 90 93 96 107 108 110 111 114 118 127 129 131 132 134 142 145 146 **S** Carilion Clinic, Roanoke, VA
Primary Contact: James E. Tyler, Vice President and Administrator
CMO: John Tamminen, M.D., President Medical Staff
CHR: Carrie Boggess, Human Resource Generalist
Web address: www.carilion.com
**Control:** Other not–for–profit (including NFP Corporation) **Service:** General Medical and Surgical

**Staffed Beds:** 25 **Admissions:** 1185 **Census:** 15 **Outpatient Visits:** 23769 **Births:** 0 **Total Expense ($000):** 23640 **Payroll Expense ($000):** 8391 **Personnel:** 175

### PENNINGTON GAP—Lee County

☒ **LEE REGIONAL MEDICAL CENTER (490012)**, 1800 Combs Road, Zip 24277–1808, Mailing Address: P.O. Box 589, Zip 24277–0589; tel. 276/546–1440, (Nonreporting) **A**1 9 10 **S** Wellmont Health System, Kingsport, TN
Primary Contact: Ron Prewitt, President
Web address: www.wellmont.org/Hospitals/Lee–Regional–Medical–Center.aspx
**Control:** Other not–for–profit (including NFP Corporation) **Service:** General Medical and Surgical

**Staffed Beds:** 58

### PETERSBURG—Petersburg City County

☐ **CENTRAL STATE HOSPITAL**, 26317 West Washington Street, Zip 23803, Mailing Address: P.O. Box 4030, Zip 23803–4030; tel. 804/524–7000 **A**1 5 9 **F**30 77 87 98 102 106 129 142 **P**6 **S** Virginia Department of Mental Health, Richmond, VA
Primary Contact: Charles M. Davis, M.D., Ph.D., Director
CMO: Ronald O. Forbes, M.D., Medical Director
CHR: Tracy Salisbury, Director Human Resources
Web address: www.csh.dmhmrsas.virginia.gov
**Control:** State–Government, nonfederal **Service:** Psychiatric

**Staffed Beds:** 277 **Admissions:** 484 **Census:** 242 **Outpatient Visits:** 0 **Births:** 0 **Total Expense ($000):** 48989 **Payroll Expense ($000):** 30683 **Personnel:** 706

☒ **HEALTHSOUTH REHABILITATION HOSPITAL OF PETERSBURG (493031)**, 95 Pinehill Boulevard, Zip 23805–9233; tel. 804/504–8100, (Nonreporting) **A**1 10 **S** HEALTHSOUTH Corporation, Birmingham, AL
Primary Contact: Scott Rotsted, Chief Executive Officer
Web address: www.healthsouthpetersburg.com
**Control:** Corporation, Investor–owned, for–profit **Service:** Rehabilitation

**Staffed Beds:** 40

**HIRAM W. DAVIS MEDICAL CENTER (490104)**, 26317 West Washington Street, Zip 23803–2727, Mailing Address: P.O. Box 4030, Zip 23803–0030; tel. 804/524–7344, (Nonreporting) **A**10 **S** Virginia Department of Mental Health, Richmond, VA
Primary Contact: Bill Hawkins, Director
COO: Brenda Buenvenida, Facility Administrator
CFO: Bob Kaufman, Fiscal Officer
CHR: Tracy Salisbury, Director Human Resources
**Control:** State–Government, nonfederal **Service:** Long–Term Acute Care hospital

**Staffed Beds:** 10

☒ **POPLAR SPRINGS HOSPITAL (494022)**, 350 Poplar Drive, Zip 23805–9367; tel. 804/733–6874, (Nonreporting) **A**1 9 10 **S** Universal Health Services, Inc., King of Prussia, PA
Primary Contact: Richard Clark, Chief Executive Officer
COO: Kate McBride, Chief Operating Officer
CFO: Bettie Hill, Chief Financial Officer
CMO: Thresa Simon, M.D., Medical Director
CHR: Morris Mitchell, Director Human Resources
Web address: www.poplarsprings.com
**Control:** Corporation, Investor–owned, for–profit **Service:** Psychiatric

**Staffed Beds:** 120

☒ **SOUTHSIDE REGIONAL MEDICAL CENTER (490067)**, 200 Medical Park Boulevard, Zip 23805; tel. 804/765–5000, (Total facility includes 20 beds in nursing home–type unit) **A**1 6 9 10 **F**3 11 12 13 15 18 20 22 26 28 29 30 31 34 40 43 45 46 47 48 49 50 54 56 57 59 60 64 70 72 74 75 76 77 78 79 81 82 85 86 87 89 93 97 98 101 102 104 105 107 108 110 111 113 114 117 118 120 123 129 130 131 134 143 145 146 147 **P**6 **S** Community Health Systems, Inc., Franklin, TN
Primary Contact: Michael Yungmann, Chief Executive Officer
CFO: Charles Coder, Chief Financial Officer
CMO: Boyd Wickizer, Jr., M.D., Chief Medical Officer
CHR: Irene Buskey, Director Human Resources
Web address: www.srmconline.com
**Control:** Corporation, Investor–owned, for–profit **Service:** General Medical and Surgical

**Staffed Beds:** 300 **Admissions:** 12753 **Census:** 175 **Outpatient Visits:** 111970 **Births:** 1369 **Total Expense ($000):** 129133 **Payroll Expense ($000):** 62894 **Personnel:** 1386

**VA**

---

**Hospital, Medicare Provider Number, Address, Telephone, Approval, Facility, and Physician Codes, Health Care System**

★ American Hospital Association (AHA) membership
☐ The Joint Commission accreditation
◇ DNV Healthcare Inc. accreditation
○ American Osteopathic Association (AOA) accreditation
△ Commission on Accreditation of Rehabilitation Facilities (CARF) accreditation

## PORTSMOUTH—Portsmouth City County

⊞ △ **BON SECOURS MARYVIEW MEDICAL CENTER (490017)**, 3636 High Street, Zip 23707–3270; tel. 757/398–2200, (Total facility includes 120 beds in nursing home–type unit) **A**1 2 3 5 7 9 10 **F**3 4 5 8 11 12 13 15 17 18 20 22 24 26 28 29 30 31 34 35 36 38 40 42 44 45 46 50 51 54 57 59 61 62 63 64 66 67 68 70 74 75 76 77 78 79 81 82 84 85 86 87 90 91 93 96 97 98 99 100 101 102 103 104 105 106 107 108 110 111 113 114 117 118 120 125 127 128 129 130 131 133 134 142 144 145 146 **P**6 **S** Bon Secours Health System, Inc., Marriottsville, MD
Primary Contact: Joseph M. Oddis, Chief Executive Officer
COO: Robert Guanci, Vice President Operations
CFO: Greg Simia, Chief Financial Officer
CMO: Warren Austin, M.D., Vice President Medical Affairs
CIO: Terri Spence, Chief Information Officer
CHR: Vickie Humphries, Director Human Resources
Web address: www.bonsecourshamptonroads.com
**Control:** Other not–for–profit (including NFP Corporation) **Service:** General Medical and Surgical

| **Staffed Beds:** 466 **Admissions:** 13233 **Census:** 291 **Outpatient Visits:** 145509 **Births:** 1060 **Total Expense ($000):** 289324 **Payroll Expense ($000):** 100014 **Personnel:** 1756 |

★ **NAVAL MEDICAL CENTER**, 620 John Paul Jones Circle, Zip 23708–2197; tel. 757/953–5000, (Nonreporting) **A**2 3 5 **S** Bureau of Medicine and Surgery, Department of the Navy, Washington, DC
Primary Contact: Rear Admiral Elaine Wagner, M.D., Commander
COO: Commander David Collins, Director for Administration
CFO: Commander Carlos J. Martinez, Director Resource Management
CMO: Commander Thomas Mooney, M.D., President Executive Committee Medical Staff
CIO: Lieutenant Colonel Karen Albany, Chief Information Officer
CHR: Jane Ackiss, Site Manager Human Resources
Web address: www.nmcp.med.navy.mil
**Control:** Navy, Government, federal **Service:** General Medical and Surgical

| **Staffed Beds:** 274 |

## PULASKI—Pulaski County

⊞ **LEWISGALE HOSPITAL AT PULASKI (490116)**, 2400 Lee Highway, Zip 24301–0759, Mailing Address: P.O. Box 759, Zip 24301–0759; tel. 540/994–8100, (Nonreporting) **A**1 2 9 10 **S** HCA, Nashville, TN
Primary Contact: Mark Nichols, FACHE, Chief Executive Officer
CMO: Stuart Goldstein, D.O., Chief of Staff
CIO: Dan Cheverton, Director Information Systems
CHR: Jana Beckner, Director Human Resources
Web address: www.pch–va.com/
**Control:** Corporation, Investor–owned, for–profit **Service:** General Medical and Surgical

| **Staffed Beds:** 54 |

## RESTON—Fairfax County

⊞ **RESTON HOSPITAL CENTER (490107)**, 1850 Town Center Parkway, Zip 20190–3219; tel. 703/689–9000 **A**1 2 9 10 **F**3 12 13 15 18 20 22 26 29 30 31 34 35 36 37 39 40 44 45 46 47 48 49 51 53 57 58 59 64 69 70 72 74 75 76 77 78 79 81 82 85 86 87 89 92 93 107 108 109 110 113 114 117 118 119 120 122 125 129 130 131 134 140 144 145 146 147 **P**6 **S** HCA, Nashville, TN
Primary Contact: Tim McManus, President and Chief Executive Officer
COO: Jane Raymond, Vice President and Chief Operating Officer
CFO: Edward R. Stojakovich, Chief Financial Officer
CMO: Walter R. Zolkiwsky, M.D., Vice President Medical Affairs
CIO: Paresh Shah, Director Information Systems
CHR: Lesley Channell, Assistant Vice President Human Resources
Web address: www.restonhospital.com
**Control:** Corporation, Investor–owned, for–profit **Service:** General Medical and Surgical

| **Staffed Beds:** 187 **Admissions:** 11992 **Census:** 128 **Outpatient Visits:** 112960 **Births:** 3303 **Total Expense ($000):** 212224 **Payroll Expense ($000):** 65918 **Personnel:** 963 |

## RICHLANDS—Tazewell County

⊞ **CLINCH VALLEY MEDICAL CENTER (490060)**, 6801 Governor G. C. Peery Highway, Zip 24641–2194; tel. 276/596–6000, (Total facility includes 14 beds in nursing home–type unit) **A**1 9 10 **F**3 13 14 15 17 18 19 20 28 29 30 31 34 35 39 40 41 45 49 56 57 59 64 70 74 75 76 77 78 79 81 85 86 87 89 93 94 97 107 108 110 111 113 114 117 118 119 120 127 128 129 131 133 134 142 145 146 147 **S** LifePoint Hospitals, Inc., Brentwood, TN
Primary Contact: David B. Darden, Chief Executive Officer
COO: Peter Mulkey, Chief Operating Officer
CFO: Bob Barrett, Chief Financial Officer
CMO: Larry Mitchell, M.D., Chief of Staff
CIO: Chris Perkins, Director Information Services
CHR: John Knowles, Director Human Resources
Web address: www.clinchvalleymedicalcenter.com
**Control:** Corporation, Investor–owned, for–profit **Service:** General Medical and Surgical

| **Staffed Beds:** 111 **Admissions:** 4795 **Census:** 51 **Outpatient Visits:** 63428 **Births:** 437 **Personnel:** 457 |

## RICHMOND—Henrico County

⊞ **BON SECOURS ST. MARY'S HOSPITAL (490059)**, 5801 Bremo Road, Zip 23226–1907; tel. 804/285–2011, (Includes BON SECOURS ST. MARY'S CHILDREN'S SERVICES, 5801 Bremo Road, tel. 804/285–2011) **A**1 2 3 5 9 10 **F**3 8 11 12 13 15 17 18 20 22 24 26 28 29 30 31 34 36 37 40 41 44 45 46 47 49 50 51 56 57 59 60 63 64 70 72 73 74 75 76 78 79 80 81 82 84 85 86 87 88 89 98 102 103 107 108 110 111 113 114 115 116 117 118 119 120 122 123 125 130 131 144 145 146 147 **P**6 8 **S** Bon Secours Health System, Inc., Marriottsville, MD
Primary Contact: Toni R. Ardabell, R.N., Chief Executive Officer
COO: Thomas L. Koenig, Vice President and Chief Operating Officer
CFO: Peter Gallagher, Chief Financial Officer
CMO: Mark Bladergroen, M.D., Vice President Medical Affairs
CIO: Jeff Burke, Chief Information Officer
CHR: Paul Catucci, Director Human Resources
Web address: www.bonsecours.com
**Control:** Church–operated, Nongovernment, not–for profit **Service:** General Medical and Surgical

| **Staffed Beds:** 391 **Admissions:** 22283 **Census:** 272 **Outpatient Visits:** 158359 **Births:** 2316 **Total Expense ($000):** 414388 **Payroll Expense ($000):** 129786 **Personnel:** 2006 |

⊞ **BON SECOURS–RICHMOND COMMUNITY HOSPITAL (490094)**, 1500 North 28th Street, Zip 23223–5396, Mailing Address: P.O. Box 27184, Zip 23261–7184; tel. 804/225–1700 **A**1 6 9 10 **F**4 5 15 18 28 29 30 31 34 35 38 40 49 57 61 70 71 74 77 81 84 85 98 100 102 104 107 108 110 111 113 114 118 129 142 145 **S** Bon Secours Health System, Inc., Marriottsville, MD
Primary Contact: Michael Robinson, Executive Vice President and Administrator
CFO: Peter Gallagher, Senior Vice President and Chief Financial Officer
CIO: Jeff Burke, Chief Information Officer
CHR: Shelia White, Director Human Resources
Web address: www.bonsecours.com
**Control:** Church–operated, Nongovernment, not–for profit **Service:** General Medical and Surgical

| **Staffed Beds:** 101 **Admissions:** 2854 **Census:** 41 **Outpatient Visits:** 48582 **Births:** 0 **Total Expense ($000):** 50066 **Payroll Expense ($000):** 16381 **Personnel:** 251 |

★ **CHILDREN'S HOSPITAL OF RICHMOND (493302)**, 2924 Brook Road, Zip 23220–1298; tel. 804/321–7474, (Nonreporting) **A**3 5 9 10
Primary Contact: Leslie G. Wyatt, Senior Vice President Children's Services and Executive Director
COO: Leslie G. Wyatt, Senior Vice President Children's Services and Executive Director
CFO: Samuel G. Weidman, Executive Vice President and Chief Financial Officer
CMO: Eugene A. Monasterio, M.D., Medical Director
CIO: Greg Friedman, Director Information Technology
CHR: Karen Bennett, Vice President Human Resources and Compliance
Web address: www.chrichmond.org
**Control:** Other not–for–profit (including NFP Corporation) **Service:** Children's rehabilitation

| **Staffed Beds:** 36 |

⊞ **CJW MEDICAL CENTER (490112)**, 7101 Jahnke Road, Zip 23225–4044; tel. 804/320–3911, (Includes CHIPPENHAM MEDICAL CENTER, 7101 Jahnke Road, Zip 23225; tel. 804/320–3911; JOHNSTON–WILLIS HOSPITAL, 1401 Johnston–Willis Drive, Zip 23235; tel. 804/330–2000), (Nonreporting) **A**1 2 5 9 10 **S** HCA, Nashville, TN
Primary Contact: Tim McManus, Interim Chief Executive Officer
COO: Betsy Blair, R.N., Chief Operating Officer
CFO: Lynn Strader, Chief Financial Officer
CMO: Georgean DeBlois, M.D., Chairman Medical Staff
CIO: Tracy Hechler, Healthcare Director Information Services
CHR: Kris Lukish, Human Resources Officer
Web address: www.cjwmedical.com
**Control:** Corporation, Investor–owned, for–profit **Service:** General Medical and Surgical

| **Staffed Beds:** 758 |

**VA**

**HALLMARK YOUTHCARE – RICHMOND**, 12800 West Creek Parkway, Zip 23238–1116; tel. 804/784–2200, (Nonreporting)
Primary Contact: A. Scott Cork, Chief Executive Officer
Web address: www.hallmarkyouthcare.org
**Control:** Corporation, Investor–owned, for–profit **Service:** Psychiatric

Staffed Beds: 84

☒ **HEALTHSOUTH REHABILITATION HOSPITAL OF VIRGINIA (493028)**, 5700 Fitzhugh Avenue, Zip 23226–1877; tel. 804/288–5700, (Nonreporting) **A**1 10 **S** HEALTHSOUTH Corporation, Birmingham, AL
Primary Contact: Jeff Ruskan, II, Chief Executive Officer
CFO: Alan M. Phillips, Controller
CMO: Roger Giordano, M.D., Medical Director
CIO: Faye Encke, Director Information Management
CHR: Tonya Ferguson, Director Human Resources
Web address: www.healthsouthrichmond.com
**Control:** Corporation, Investor–owned, for–profit **Service:** Rehabilitation

Staffed Beds: 40

☒ **HENRICO DOCTORS' HOSPITAL (490118)**, 1602 Skipwith Road, Zip 23229–5205; tel. 804/289–4500, (Includes HENRICO DOCTORS' HOSPITAL – FOREST, 1602 Skipwith Road, Zip 23229–5298; tel. 804/289–4500; HENRICO DOCTORS' HOSPITAL – PARHAM, 7700 East Parham Road, Zip 23294–4301; tel. 804/747–5600; HENRICO DOCTORS' HOSPITAL – RETREAT CAMPUS, 2621 Grove Avenue, Zip 23220–4308; tel. 804/254–5100) **A**1 2 9 10 **F**3 8 12 13 15 17 18 20 22 24 26 28 29 30 31 34 35 37 40 42 44 45 46 50 51 54 55 57 64 65 68 70 71 72 73 74 75 76 77 78 79 81 85 86 87 89 90 93 96 97 107 108 109 110 111 112 113 114 118 119 120 122 125 128 129 130 131 134 137 140 143 144 145 146 147 **S** HCA, Nashville, TN
Primary Contact: Patrick J. Farrell, Chief Executive Officer
COO: Lisa R. Valentine, Chief Operating Officer
CFO: Christopher Denton, Chief Financial Officer
CIO: Daniel Patton, Director Information Systems
CHR: Steven Burgess, Administrator Human Resources
Web address: www.henricodoctorshospital.com
**Control:** Corporation, Investor–owned, for–profit **Service:** General Medical and Surgical

Staffed Beds: 488 Admissions: 18689 Census: 291 Outpatient Visits: 138064 Births: 3381 Personnel: 1880

☒ △ **HUNTER HOLMES MCGUIRE VETERANS AFFAIRS MEDICAL CENTER**, 1201 Broad Rock Boulevard, Zip 23249–0002; tel. 804/675–5000, (Nonreporting) **A**1 2 3 5 7 8 **S** Department of Veterans Affairs, Washington, DC
Primary Contact: Charles E. Sepich, FACHE, Director
COO: David P. Budinger, Associate Director
CFO: Roger T. Vergne, Chief Fiscal Service
CMO: Judy Brannen, M.D., Interim Chief of Staff
CIO: David Dahlstrand, Associate Chief of Staff Information Technology
CHR: Heather Moody, Chief Human Resource Management
Web address: www.va.gov/sta/guide/home.asp
**Control:** Veterans Affairs, Government, federal **Service:** General Medical and Surgical

Staffed Beds: 317

**JOHNSTON–WILLIS HOSPITAL** See CJW Medical Center

☒ **KINDRED HOSPITAL RICHMOND (492009)**, 2220 Edward Holland Drive, Zip 23230–2519; tel. 804/678–7000, (Nonreporting) **A**1 9 10 **S** Kindred Healthcare, Louisville, KY
Primary Contact: Greg Floyd, Chief Executive Officer
Web address: www.kindredrichmond.com/
**Control:** Corporation, Investor–owned, for–profit **Service:** Long–Term Acute Care hospital

Staffed Beds: 60

☒ **VCU HEALTH SYSTEM (490032)**, 1250 East Marshall Street, Zip 23219, Mailing Address: P.O. Box 980510, Zip 23298–0510; tel. 804/828–9000, (Includes VCU HEALTH SYSTEM CHILDREN'S MEDICAL CENTER, 1001 East Marshall Street, Zip 23219–1918, Mailing Address: PO Box 980646, Zip 23298–0646; tel. 804/828–9602) **A**1 3 5 8 9 10 **F**2 3 4 6 7 8 9 11 12 13 15 16 17 18 19 20 21 22 23 24 25 26 27 28 29 30 31 32 34 35 36 37 38 39 40 41 43 44 45 46 47 48 49 50 51 52 54 55 56 57 58 59 60 61 62 64 66 68 70 71 72 73 74 75 76 78 79 80 81 82 83 84 85 86 87 88 89 90 92 93 96 97 98 99 100 101 102 103 104 105 107 108 109 110 111 113 114 115 116 117 118 119 120 122 123 125 128 129 130 131 133 134 135 136 137 138 140 141 142 143 144 145 146 147 **P**6
Primary Contact: John Duval, Chief Executive Officer
COO: Deborah W. Davis, Chief Operating Officer
CFO: Dominic J. Pulco, Executive Vice President Finance and Chief Financial Officer
CMO: Ron Clark, M.D., Vice President Clinical Activities and Chief Medical Officer
CIO: Richard Pollack, Vice President Information Services
CHR: Maria Curran, Vice President Human Resources
Web address: www.vcuhealth.org
**Control:** Hospital district or authority, Government, nonfederal **Service:** General Medical and Surgical

Staffed Beds: 747 Admissions: 31412 Census: 543 Outpatient Visits: 644974 Births: 2273 Total Expense ($000): 918151 Payroll Expense ($000): 341473 Personnel: 7058

**ROANOKE—Roanoke County**

☒ **CARILION MEDICAL CENTER (490024)**, Belleview at Jefferson Street, Zip 24014, Mailing Address: P.O. Box 13367, Zip 24033–3367; tel. 540/981–7000, (Includes CARILION CLINIC CHILDREN'S HOSPITAL, 1906 Belleview Avenue, S.E., Zip 24014–1838; tel. 540/981–7000; CARILION ROANOKE COMMUNITY HOSPITAL, 101 Elm Avenue S.E., Zip 24013–2230, Mailing Address: P.O. Box 12946, Zip 24029–2946; tel. 540/985–8000; ROANOKE MEMORIAL REHABILITATION CENTER, South Jefferson and McClanahan Streets, Mailing Address: P.O. Box 13367, Zip 24033; tel. 703/342–4541) **A**1 2 3 5 8 9 10 12 13 **F**3 5 7 8 9 11 12 13 17 18 20 22 24 26 28 29 30 31 32 33 34 35 36 37 38 39 40 41 42 43 44 45 46 47 48 49 50 51 52 53 54 55 56 57 58 59 60 61 62 63 64 65 66 68 70 71 72 73 74 75 76 77 78 79 81 82 83 84 85 86 87 88 90 92 93 96 97 98 99 100 101 102 103 104 106 107 108 110 111 113 114 115 116 117 118 119 120 122 123 125 128 129 130 131 133 134 142 143 145 146 147 **P**6 **S** Carilion Clinic, Roanoke, VA
Primary Contact: Nancy Howell Agee, President and Chief Executive Officer
CFO: Donald E. Lorton, Executive Vice President and Chief Financial Officer
CMO: Mark D. Werner, M.D., Executive Vice President and Chief Medical Officer
CIO: Daniel Barchi, Senior Vice President and Chief Information Officer
CHR: Jeanne S. Armentrout, Vice President Human Resources
Web address: www.carilionclinic.org
**Control:** Other not–for–profit (including NFP Corporation) **Service:** General Medical and Surgical

Staffed Beds: 624 Admissions: 34908 Census: 496 Outpatient Visits: 216228 Births: 3300 Total Expense ($000): 834599 Payroll Expense ($000): 355868 Personnel: 5400

**ROCKY MOUNT—Franklin County**

☒ **CARILION FRANKLIN MEMORIAL HOSPITAL (490089)**, 180 Floyd Avenue, Zip 24151–1389; tel. 540/483–5277 **A**1 9 10 **F**11 15 28 29 30 34 35 40 50 59 62 63 68 70 75 77 81 84 87 93 107 110 114 118 129 131 134 145 **S** Carilion Clinic, Roanoke, VA
Primary Contact: William D. Jacobsen, Chief Executive Officer
Web address: www.carilion.com
**Control:** Other not–for–profit (including NFP Corporation) **Service:** General Medical and Surgical

Staffed Beds: 32 Admissions: 1752 Census: 16 Outpatient Visits: 38340 Births: 146 Total Expense ($000): 34220 Payroll Expense ($000): 12463 Personnel: 237

**SALEM—Salem City County**

☒ **LEWIS–GALE MEDICAL CENTER (490048)**, 1900 Electric Road, Zip 24153–7494; tel. 540/776–4000, (Includes LEWIS–GALE PAVILION, 1902 Braeburn Drive, Zip 24153–7391; tel. 703/772–2800), (Nonreporting) **A**1 2 9 10 **S** HCA, Nashville, TN
Primary Contact: Victor Giovanetti, President and Chief Executive Officer
COO: Charlotte C. Tyson, Chief Operating Officer
CFO: Angela D. Reynolds, Chief Financial Officer
CMO: Joseph Nelson, M.D., President Medical Staff
CIO: Beth Cole, Director Information Services
CHR: Dale Beaudoin, Vice President Human Resources
Web address: www.lewis–gale.com
**Control:** Corporation, Investor–owned, for–profit **Service:** General Medical and Surgical

Staffed Beds: 521

**VA**

---

✠ **VETERANS AFFAIRS MEDICAL CENTER**, 1970 Roanoke Boulevard, Zip 24153–6478; tel. 540/982–2463, (Nonreporting) **A**1 2 3 5 8 **S** Department of Veterans Affairs, Washington, DC
Primary Contact: Miguel H. LaPuz, M.D., Director
CFO: Codie Walker, Chief Financial Officer
CMO: Maureen McCarthy, M.D., Chief of Staff
CIO: Sharon Collins, Chief Information Officer
CHR: Timothy McGuigan, Chief Human Resources
Web address: www.salem.va.gov
**Control:** Veterans Affairs, Government, federal **Service:** General Medical and Surgical

Staffed Beds: 298

### SOUTH BOSTON—Halifax County

✠ **HALIFAX REGIONAL HEALTH SYSTEM (490013)**, 2204 Wilborn Avenue, Zip 24592–1638; tel. 434/517–3100, (Total facility includes 300 beds in nursing home–type unit) **A**1 9 10 **F**3 13 14 15 17 18 20 28 29 30 31 35 36 38 40 44 45 46 47 48 57 60 62 63 64 65 66 67 68 70 74 75 76 77 78 79 81 82 84 85 86 87 89 92 93 94 96 97 100 101 102 103 104 107 108 110 111 113 114 115 116 117 118 126 127 128 129 130 131 134 145 146 147 **P**1 7
Primary Contact: Chris A. Lumsden, Chief Executive Officer
COO: Thomas S. Kluge, Chief Operating Officer
CFO: Stewart R. Nelson, Chief Financial Officer
CMO: James F. Witko, M.D., Chief Medical Officer
CIO: William Zirkle, Manager Information Systems
CHR: Catherine Howard, Director Human Resources
Web address: www.hrhs.org
**Control:** Other not–for–profit (including NFP Corporation) **Service:** General Medical and Surgical

Staffed Beds: 390 Admissions: 4411 Census: 378 Outpatient Visits: 64092 Births: 375 Total Expense ($000): 85114 Payroll Expense ($000): 33331 Personnel: 684

### SOUTH HILL—Mecklenburg County

✠ **COMMUNITY MEMORIAL HEALTHCENTER (490098)**, 125 Buena Vista Circle, Zip 23970–0090, Mailing Address: P.O. Box 90, Zip 23970–0090; tel. 434/447–3151, (Total facility includes 161 beds in nursing home–type unit) **A**1 9 10 20 **F**3 4 11 13 15 18 28 29 30 31 32 34 35 38 39 40 45 46 49 50 53 54 56 57 59 60 61 62 63 64 65 70 74 75 76 77 78 79 81 82 84 85 86 87 93 96 97 98 100 101 102 103 107 108 110 111 113 117 118 126 129 130 131 132 134 142 145 146 147 **P**8
Primary Contact: W. Scott Burnette, President and Chief Executive Officer
COO: Edward M. Brandenburg, FACHE, Vice President Professional Services
CFO: Kenneth Libby, Chief Financial Officer
CIO: Mark Clemmons, Director Information Systems
CHR: Barry A. Nateman, Director Human Resources
Web address: www.cmh–sh.org
**Control:** Other not–for–profit (including NFP Corporation) **Service:** General Medical and Surgical

Staffed Beds: 284 Admissions: 5290 Census: 184 Outpatient Visits: 129776 Births: 266 Total Expense ($000): 76622 Payroll Expense ($000): 30734 Personnel: 720

### STAFFORD—Stafford County

✠ **STAFFORD HOSPITAL (490140)**, 101 Hospital Center Boulevard, Zip 22554–6200; tel. 540/741–9000 **A**1 9 10 **F**3 5 13 15 18 20 22 24 29 30 31 34 35 40 48 49 50 57 59 60 64 68 70 74 76 77 78 79 81 82 85 86 87 91 93 107 108 109 110 111 114 117 118 119 120 131 134 145 **P**6 **S** Mary Washington Healthcare, Fredericksburg, VA
Primary Contact: Fred M. Rankin, III, President and Chief Executive Officer
COO: Walter J. Kiwall, Executive Vice President and Chief Operating Officer
CFO: Sean Barden, Executive Vice President and Chief Financial Officer
CMO: J. Thomas Ryan, M.D., Executive Vice President and Chief Medical Officer
CHR: Kathryn S. Wall, Executive Vice President Human Resources and Organizational Development
Web address: www.marywashingtonhealthcare.com
**Control:** Other not–for–profit (including NFP Corporation) **Service:** General Medical and Surgical

Staffed Beds: 70 Admissions: 3422 Census: 33 Outpatient Visits: 65731 Births: 504 Total Expense ($000): 76095 Payroll Expense ($000): 25005 Personnel: 412

### STAUNTON—Staunton City County

**COMMONWEALTH CENTER FOR CHILDREN AND ADOLESCENTS**, 1355 Richmond Road, Zip 24401–1091, Mailing Address: Box 4000, Zip 24402–4000; tel. 540/332–2100, (Nonreporting) **A**3 5 9 **S** Virginia Department of Mental Health, Richmond, VA
Primary Contact: William J. Tuell, MSN, Facility Director
Web address: www.ccca.dbhds.virginia.gov
**Control:** State–Government, nonfederal **Service:** Children's other specialty

Staffed Beds: 60

☐ **WESTERN STATE HOSPITAL (490106)**, 1301 Richmond Avenue, Zip 24401, Mailing Address: P.O. Box 2500, Zip 24402–2500; tel. 540/332–8000, (Nonreporting) **A**1 3 5 9 10 **S** Virginia Department of Mental Health, Richmond, VA
Primary Contact: Jack W. Barber, M.D., Director
CFO: David Mawyer, Chief Financial Officer
CMO: Mary Clare Smith, M.D., Medical Director
CIO: Sharon Johnson, Director Health Information Management
CHR: Kimberly Harman, Regional Manager Human Resources
Web address: www.dbhds.virginia.gov
**Control:** State–Government, nonfederal **Service:** Psychiatric

Staffed Beds: 260

### STUART—Patrick County

★ **PIONEER COMMUNITY HOSPITAL OF PATRICK COUNTY (491306)**, 18688 Jeb Stuart Highway, Zip 24171–1559; tel. 276/694–3151, (Nonreporting) **A**9 10 18 21 **S** Pioneer Health Services, Magee, MS
Primary Contact: Jeanette Filpi, Chief Executive Officer
CFO: Julie Gieger, Chief Financial Officer
CMO: Nicholas Kipreos, M.D., Chief Medical Staff
CIO: Eddie Pope, Director Information Systems
CHR: Donn Paul, Vice President Human Resources
Web address: www.phscorporate.com
**Control:** Corporation, Investor–owned, for–profit **Service:** General Medical and Surgical

Staffed Beds: 25

### SUFFOLK—Suffolk City County

✠ **SENTARA OBICI HOSPITAL (490044)**, 2800 Godwin Boulevard, Zip 23434–4323; tel. 757/934–4000 **A**1 3 5 9 10 **F**3 11 15 18 20 22 26 28 29 30 31 34 35 36 37 40 41 42 45 47 48 49 50 51 54 56 57 58 59 64 68 70 74 75 76 77 78 79 81 85 86 87 92 93 94 96 98 99 102 107 108 110 111 113 115 116 117 118 120 128 129 130 131 145 146 147 **S** Sentara Healthcare, Norfolk, VA
Primary Contact: Kurt T. Hofelich, Vice President and Administrator
CFO: Mike Mounie, Director Finance
CMO: Lindsey Vaughn, M.D., President Medical Staff
CIO: Chip Mills, Director Information Technology
CHR: Deborah Ferguson, Human Resources Consultant
Web address: www.sentara.com
**Control:** Other not–for–profit (including NFP Corporation) **Service:** General Medical and Surgical

Staffed Beds: 168 Admissions: 8825 Census: 99 Outpatient Visits: 300923 Births: 1309 Total Expense ($000): 145477 Payroll Expense ($000): 59188 Personnel: 968

### TAPPAHANNOCK—Essex County

☐ **RIVERSIDE TAPPAHANNOCK HOSPITAL (490084)**, 618 Hospital Road, Zip 22560–5000; tel. 804/443–3311 **A**1 9 10 20 **F**3 11 15 29 31 34 35 38 40 43 44 45 49 50 51 56 57 59 62 63 64 70 75 77 78 79 81 82 85 86 87 92 93 97 107 108 111 113 115 116 117 118 129 130 131 132 134 145 147 **P**6 **S** Riverside Health System, Newport News, VA
Primary Contact: Elizabeth J. Martin, Vice President and Administrator
COO: Elizabeth J. Martin, Vice President and Administrator
CFO: Jeri Sibley, Director Revenue Cycle
CMO: Reginald Mason, M.D., President Medical Staff
CHR: Jaime Cook, Director Human Resources
Web address: www.riverside–online.com
**Control:** Other not–for–profit (including NFP Corporation) **Service:** General Medical and Surgical

Staffed Beds: 17 Admissions: 1874 Census: 16 Outpatient Visits: 56896 Births: 0 Total Expense ($000): 34236 Payroll Expense ($000): 11593 Personnel: 174

### TAZEWELL—Tazewell County

✠ **CARILION TAZEWELL COMMUNITY HOSPITAL (490117)**, 141 Ben Bolt Avenue, Zip 24651–9700; tel. 276/988–8700 **A**1 9 10 **F**3 11 15 28 29 30 34 39 40 45 50 59 62 64 68 75 79 81 84 85 87 107 111 113 118 132 134 145 **S** Carilion Clinic, Roanoke, VA
Primary Contact: John S. Piatkowski, M.D., Chief Executive Officer
CMO: Kerry Moore, M.D., Chief of Staff
CHR: Carrie Boggess, Human Resources Generalist
Web address: www.carilionclinic.org
**Control:** Other not–for–profit (including NFP Corporation) **Service:** General Medical and Surgical

Staffed Beds: 7 Admissions: 639 Census: 5 Outpatient Visits: 14160 Births: 0 Total Expense ($000): 11329 Payroll Expense ($000): 3256 Personnel: 83

**VA**

*Many Facility Codes have changed. Please refer to the AHA Guide Code Chart.*
© 2012 AHA Guide

## VIRGINIA BEACH—Virginia Beach City County

☒ **SENTARA PRINCESS ANNE HOSPITAL (490119)**, 2025 Glenn Mitchell Drive, Zip 23456–0178; tel. 757/363–6100, (Data for 150 days) **A**1 3 5 9 10 **F**3 11 13 15 18 20 22 26 28 29 30 31 34 35 36 38 40 41 43 44 45 46 47 49 50 54 57 58 59 60 61 64 65 68 70 71 73 74 75 76 77 78 79 81 82 84 85 86 87 92 93 94 96 100 102 107 108 110 111 113 114 117 118 128 129 130 131 144 145 146 147 **S** Sentara Healthcare, Norfolk, VA
Primary Contact: Stephen D. Porter, President
COO: Howard P. Kern, Chief Operating Officer
CFO: Robert Broermann, Senior Vice President and Chief Financial Officer
CMO: Thomas B. Thames, M.D., Vice President Medical Affairs
CIO: Bert Reese, Chief Information Officer
CHR: Michael V. Taylor, Vice President Human Resources
Web address: www.sentara.com
**Control:** Other not–for–profit (including NFP Corporation) **Service:** General Medical and Surgical

**Staffed Beds:** 160 **Admissions:** 3505 **Census:** 97 **Outpatient Visits:** 85016 **Births:** 873 **Total Expense ($000):** 58635 **Payroll Expense ($000):** 20645 **Personnel:** 914

☒ **SENTARA VIRGINIA BEACH GENERAL HOSPITAL (490057)**, 1060 First Colonial Road, Zip 23454–3002; tel. 757/395–8000 **A**1 2 3 5 9 10 **F**2 3 11 13 15 17 18 20 22 24 26 28 29 30 31 34 35 36 37 38 39 40 41 42 43 44 45 46 47 49 50 51 53 57 58 59 60 61 63 64 65 68 70 71 74 75 77 78 79 81 82 84 85 86 87 90 92 93 94 95 100 102 107 108 109 110 111 113 114 117 118 119 120 128 129 130 131 140 141 143 144 145 146 147 **S** Sentara Healthcare, Norfolk, VA
Primary Contact: Thomas B. Thames, M.D., Interim President
CFO: Leo DeLeon, Vice President Finance
CMO: Thomas B. Thames, M.D., Vice President Medical Affairs
CHR: Michelle Meekins, Manager Human Resources
Web address: www.sentara.com
**Control:** Other not–for–profit (including NFP Corporation) **Service:** General Medical and Surgical

**Staffed Beds:** 234 **Admissions:** 13942 **Census:** 207 **Outpatient Visits:** 306187 **Births:** 1174 **Total Expense ($000):** 231619 **Payroll Expense ($000):** 91520 **Personnel:** 1399

☐ **VIRGINIA BEACH PSYCHIATRIC CENTER (494025)**, 1100 First Colonial Road, Zip 23454; tel. 757/496–6000, (Nonreporting) **A**1 9 10 **S** Universal Health Services, Inc., King of Prussia, PA
Primary Contact: Denise Webb, Administrator
Web address: www.absfirst.com
**Control:** Corporation, Investor–owned, for–profit **Service:** Psychiatric

**Staffed Beds:** 100

## WARRENTON—Fauquier County

☒ **FAUQUIER HOSPITAL (490023)**, 500 Hospital Drive, Zip 20186–3099; tel. 540/316–5000 **A**1 9 10 **F**3 11 13 15 18 28 29 30 31 34 35 36 37 40 45 47 48 49 53 57 59 62 64 70 74 75 76 77 78 79 81 85 86 87 93 107 108 110 111 113 118 128 129 130 131 134 145 147
Primary Contact: Rodger H. Baker, President and Chief Executive Officer
CFO: Lionel J. Phillips, Vice President Financial Services
CMO: Nasser Sitta, M.D., President Medical Staff
CIO: Donna Staton, Chief Information Officer
CHR: Katy Reeves, Vice President Human Resources
Web address: www.fauquierhospital.org
**Control:** Other not–for–profit (including NFP Corporation) **Service:** General Medical and Surgical

**Staffed Beds:** 86 **Admissions:** 5595 **Census:** 62 **Outpatient Visits:** 109958 **Births:** 849 **Total Expense ($000):** 116546 **Payroll Expense ($000):** 48398 **Personnel:** 717

## WILLIAMSBURG—James City County

☐ **EASTERN STATE HOSPITAL (490109)**, 4601 Ironbound Road, Zip 23188–2652; tel. 757/253–5161, (Nonreporting) **A**1 3 5 9 10 **S** Virginia Department of Mental Health, Richmond, VA
Primary Contact: John M. Favret, Director
CFO: E. Clifford Love, Director Fiscal Services
CMO: Guillermo Schrader, M.D., Acting Medical Director
CIO: Barbara Lambert, Director Healthcare Compliance
CHR: Edie Rogan, Manager Human Resources
Web address: www.esh.dmhmrsas.virginia.gov/
**Control:** State–Government, nonfederal **Service:** Psychiatric

**Staffed Beds:** 334

★ **SENTARA WILLIAMSBURG REGIONAL MEDICAL CENTER (490066)**, 100 Sentara Circle, Zip 23188–5713; tel. 757/984–6000 **A**2 9 10 21 **F**3 8 11 13 15 18 20 22 26 28 29 30 31 34 35 36 37 38 39 40 41 43 44 45 46 48 49 50 51 54 56 57 58 59 60 64 70 74 75 76 77 78 79 81 82 83 84 85 86 87 89 90 92 93 94 96 100 102 107 108 110 111 113 115 116 117 118 128 129 130 131 134 143 145 146 147 **S** Sentara Healthcare, Norfolk, VA
Primary Contact: Robert L. Graves, Vice President and Administrator
CFO: Andreas Roehrle, Director Finance
CMO: James Sammons, M.D., Vice President Medical Affairs
CIO: Thomas Ewing, Director Information Technology
CHR: Brett Willsie, Manager Human Resources
Web address: www.sentara.com
**Control:** Other not–for–profit (including NFP Corporation) **Service:** General Medical and Surgical

**Staffed Beds:** 145 **Admissions:** 8150 **Census:** 89 **Outpatient Visits:** 214236 **Births:** 1015 **Total Expense ($000):** 131276 **Payroll Expense ($000):** 50111 **Personnel:** 740

## WINCHESTER—Winchester City County

☒ **WINCHESTER MEDICAL CENTER (490005)**, 1840 Amherst Street, Zip 22601–2540, Mailing Address: P.O. Box 3340, Zip 22604–3340; tel. 540/536–8000 **A**1 2 9 10 19 **F**3 5 11 12 13 15 17 18 20 22 24 26 28 29 30 31 32 34 35 38 39 40 41 43 44 45 47 49 50 51 54 56 57 58 59 61 62 64 68 70 71 72 74 75 76 77 78 79 81 82 84 85 86 87 89 90 91 92 93 97 98 100 101 102 103 107 108 110 111 113 114 115 116 117 118 119 120 122 123 128 129 130 131 134 135 145 146 147 **P**5 **S** Valley Health System, Winchester, VA
Primary Contact: Alfred E. Pilong, President and Chief Executive Officer
CFO: Robert Amos, Vice President and Chief Financial Officer
CMO: Nicolas Restrepo, M.D., Vice President Medical Affairs
CIO: Joan Roscoe, Chief Information Officer
CHR: Elizabeth Savage–Tracy, Vice President and Human Resources Officer
Web address: www.valleyhealthlink.com
**Control:** Other not–for–profit (including NFP Corporation) **Service:** General Medical and Surgical

**Staffed Beds:** 459 **Admissions:** 25001 **Census:** 320 **Outpatient Visits:** 369971 **Births:** 2323 **Total Expense ($000):** 412156 **Payroll Expense ($000):** 143520 **Personnel:** 2661

## WOODBRIDGE—Prince William County

☒ **SENTARA NORTHERN VIRGINIA MEDICAL CENTER (490113)**, 2300 Opitz Boulevard, Zip 22191–3399; tel. 703/670–1313 **A**1 2 9 10 **F**3 7 8 11 12 13 15 18 20 22 28 29 30 31 34 35 40 41 45 49 51 57 59 60 63 65 68 70 71 74 75 76 78 79 80 81 82 84 85 87 89 102 107 108 110 111 113 114 118 120 125 128 129 131 134 145 146 147 **S** Sentara Healthcare, Norfolk, VA
Primary Contact: Megan R. Perry, Vice President and Administrator
CFO: Paula Brown, Senior Vice President Corporate Finance
CMO: Denis J. Halmi, M.D., President Medical Staff
CIO: Khali Bouharoun, Vice President and Director Management Information Systems
CHR: Charles W. Ramey, Vice President
Web address: www.potomachospital.com
**Control:** Other not–for–profit (including NFP Corporation) **Service:** General Medical and Surgical

**Staffed Beds:** 169 **Admissions:** 10251 **Census:** 109 **Outpatient Visits:** 113196 **Births:** 1877 **Total Expense ($000):** 159541 **Payroll Expense ($000):** 66285 **Personnel:** 1307

## WOODSTOCK—Shenandoah County

☒ **SHENANDOAH MEMORIAL HOSPITAL (491305)**, 759 South Main Street, Zip 22664–1127; tel. 540/459–1100 **A**1 9 10 18 **F**3 11 15 28 29 30 35 40 45 50 53 57 59 64 65 68 69 70 75 77 79 81 82 87 92 93 97 107 108 110 113 117 118 129 131 132 134 145 147 **S** Valley Health System, Winchester, VA
Primary Contact: Floyd Heater, President
CFO: Virginia Kilmer, Chief Financial Officer
CMO: Donald Jansen, M.D., Vice President Medical Affairs
CIO: Joan Roscoe, Chief Information Officer
CHR: Charles Walton, Corporate Director Human Resources
Web address: www.valleyhealthlink.com
**Control:** Other not–for–profit (including NFP Corporation) **Service:** General Medical and Surgical

**Staffed Beds:** 18 **Admissions:** 1759 **Census:** 16 **Outpatient Visits:** 81442 **Births:** 0 **Total Expense ($000):** 45909 **Payroll Expense ($000):** 15024 **Personnel:** 282

**VA**

---

**Hospital, Medicare Provider Number, Address, Telephone, Approval, Facility, and Physician Codes, Health Care System**

★ American Hospital Association (AHA) membership
☐ The Joint Commission accreditation ◇ DNV Healthcare Inc. accreditation
○ American Osteopathic Association (AOA) accreditation
△ Commission on Accreditation of Rehabilitation Facilities (CARF) accreditation

☒ **WYTHE COUNTY COMMUNITY HOSPITAL (490111)**, 600 West Ridge Road,
Zip 24382–1099; tel. 276/228–0200, (Total facility includes 8 beds in nursing
home–type unit) **A**1 9 10 20 **F**3 11 13 15 17 18 19 28 29 30 32 34 35 40 45
49 50 51 54 56 57 59 61 62 63 64 65 68 70 75 76 77 78 79 81 84 86 87
89 90 93 94 97 100 102 107 108 110 111 113 117 118 127 128 129 130
131 132 134 145 146 147 **S** LifePoint Hospitals, Inc., Brentwood, TN
Primary Contact: Timothy A. Bess, Chief Executive Officer
CFO: John D. White, Chief Financial Officer
CMO: George Farrell, M.D., Chief of Staff
CIO: Andrea Harless, Director Information Services
CHR: Dale Clark, Assistant Administrator and Director Human Resources
Web address: www.wcchcares.com
**Control:** Corporation, Investor–owned, for–profit **Service:** General Medical and
Surgical

**Staffed Beds:** 90 **Admissions:** 2412 **Census:** 20 **Outpatient Visits:** 60094
**Births:** 324 **Total Expense ($000):** 37607 **Payroll Expense ($000):** 13938
**Personnel:** 292

VA

*Many Facility Codes have changed. Please refer to the AHA Guide Code Chart.* © 2012 AHA Guide

# WASHINGTON

## ABERDEEN—Grays Harbor County

☐ **GRAYS HARBOR COMMUNITY HOSPITAL (500031)**, 915 Anderson Drive, Zip 98520–1097; tel. 360/532–8330, (Nonreporting) **A**1 9 10 20
Primary Contact: Tom Jensen, Chief Executive Officer
COO: Thomas Hightower, Chief Operating Officer
CFO: Tim Howden, Interim Chief Financial Officer
CMO: Bill Hofmann, M.D., Chief Medical Staff
CIO: Scott Quigley, Director Information Services
CHR: Julie Feller, Director Human Resources
Web address: www.ghchwa.org
**Control:** Other not–for–profit (including NFP Corporation) **Service:** General Medical and Surgical

**Staffed Beds:** 200

## ANACORTES—Skagit County

★ **ISLAND HOSPITAL (500007)**, 1211 24th Street, Zip 98221–2590; tel. 360/299–1300 **A**2 5 9 10 21 **F**3 7 8 11 13 15 28 29 30 31 34 35 40 43 45 50 53 57 59 62 64 70 75 76 77 78 79 81 82 85 86 89 93 99 100 102 104 107 108 110 111 113 114 115 118 126 128 129 131 133 134 145 146 147 **P**6 8
Primary Contact: Vincent Oliver, Administrator
CFO: Peter Swanson, Assistant Administrator Fiscal Services
CMO: Linda Brown, M.D., Chief of Staff
CIO: Tom Bluhm, Director Information Systems
CHR: Carolyn Tucker, Director Human Resources
Web address: www.islandhospital.org
**Control:** Hospital district or authority, Government, nonfederal **Service:** General Medical and Surgical

**Staffed Beds:** 43 **Admissions:** 2995 **Census:** 26 **Outpatient Visits:** 184970 **Births:** 362 **Total Expense ($000):** 74958 **Payroll Expense ($000):** 32603 **Personnel:** 402

## ARLINGTON—Snohomish County

**CASCADE VALLEY HOSPITAL AND CLINICS (500060)**, 330 South Stillaguamish Avenue, Zip 98223–1642; tel. 360/435–2133, (Nonreporting) **A**9 10 21
Primary Contact: W. Clark Jones, Administrator
CFO: Ardis Schmiege, Chief Financial Officer
CMO: Ross Hartling, M.D., President Medical Staff
CIO: Heather Logan, Assistant Administrator Diagnostic and Support Services
CHR: Connie L. DiGregorio, Assistant Administrator
Web address: www.cascadevalley.org
**Control:** Hospital district or authority, Government, nonfederal **Service:** General Medical and Surgical

**Staffed Beds:** 48

## AUBURN—King County

☐ △ **AUBURN REGIONAL MEDICAL CENTER (500015)**, 202 North Division, Plaza One, Zip 98001–4908; tel. 253/833–7711, (Nonreporting) **A**1 2 7 9 10 **S** Universal Health Services, Inc., King of Prussia, PA
Primary Contact: Robert Dickens, Interim Chief Executive Officer
CIO: Denis Uhler, Manager Information Systems
Web address: www.auburnregional.com
**Control:** Corporation, Investor–owned, for–profit **Service:** General Medical and Surgical

**Staffed Beds:** 120

## BELLEVUE—King County

⊞ **OVERLAKE HOSPITAL MEDICAL CENTER (500051)**, 1035 116th Avenue N.E., Zip 98004–4604; tel. 425/688–5000 **A**1 2 9 10 **F**3 11 12 13 15 17 18 20 22 24 26 29 30 31 34 35 40 43 44 45 46 48 49 56 57 58 59 64 68 70 72 74 75 76 77 78 79 81 84 85 86 87 91 92 93 97 98 99 100 101 102 103 104 105 107 108 110 111 113 114 115 116 117 118 119 120 122 123 125 129 131 133 143 144 145 146 147 **P**6
Primary Contact: Craig L. Hendrickson, President and Chief Executive Officer
COO: David W. Schultz, FACHE, Executive Vice President and Chief Operating Officer
CFO: Gary McLaughlin, Vice President Finance and Chief Financial Officer
CIO: Jody Albright, Vice President Information Services and Chief Information Officer
CHR: Lisa Brock, Vice President Human Resources
Web address: www.overlakehospital.org
**Control:** Other not–for–profit (including NFP Corporation) **Service:** General Medical and Surgical

**Staffed Beds:** 307 **Admissions:** 21235 **Census:** 196 **Outpatient Visits:** 237927 **Births:** 4029 **Total Expense ($000):** 372469 **Payroll Expense ($000):** 158069 **Personnel:** 1849

## BELLINGHAM—Whatcom County

⊞ △ **PEACEHEALTH ST. JOSEPH MEDICAL CENTER (500030)**, 2901 Squalicum Parkway, Zip 98225–1851; tel. 360/734–5400 **A**1 2 7 9 10 **F**2 3 13 17 18 20 22 24 26 28 29 30 31 34 35 40 41 43 45 46 47 48 49 50 51 56 57 58 59 63 64 65 70 74 75 76 77 78 79 81 84 85 86 87 89 90 92 93 94 96 97 98 106 107 108 109 113 114 117 118 119 120 122 128 129 130 131 134 140 145 147 **S** PeaceHealth, Bellevue, WA
Primary Contact: Nancy Steiger, R.N., Chief Executive Officer and Chief Mission Officer
COO: Stephen R. Omta, Chief Operating Officer
CFO: Dale Zender, Regional Vice President Finance and Chief Financial Officer
CMO: Chris Sprowl, M.D., Vice President
CIO: Marc Pierson, M.D., Vice President Clinical Information and Quality
CHR: Cindy C. Klein, Vice President Human Resources
Web address: www.peacehealth.org
**Control:** Church–operated, Nongovernment, not–for profit **Service:** General Medical and Surgical

**Staffed Beds:** 253 **Admissions:** 15691 **Census:** 164 **Outpatient Visits:** 90477 **Births:** 2036 **Total Expense ($000):** 373287 **Payroll Expense ($000):** 149368

**ST. JOSEPH HOSPITAL** See PeaceHealth St. Joseph Medical Center

## BREMERTON—Kitsap County

⊞ **HARRISON MEDICAL CENTER (500039)**, 2520 Cherry Avenue, Zip 98310–4229; tel. 360/377–3911, (Nonreporting) **A**1 2 9 10
Primary Contact: Scott W. Bosch, President and Chief Executive Officer
COO: Patricia Cochrell, R.N., Executive Vice President and Chief Operating Officer
CFO: Forrest Ehlinger, Vice President and Chief Financial Officer
CIO: Adar Palis, Executive Vice President and Chief Administrative Officer
CHR: Marie LaMarche, Director Human Resources
Web address: www.harrisonmedical.org
**Control:** Other not–for–profit (including NFP Corporation) **Service:** General Medical and Surgical

**Staffed Beds:** 273

⊞ **NAVAL HOSPITAL BREMERTON**, One Boone Road, Zip 98312–1898; tel. 360/475–4000 **A**1 3 5 9 **F**3 5 8 13 15 18 20 29 30 32 33 34 35 38 39 40 43 45 46 50 53 54 57 58 59 64 65 70 74 75 76 77 79 81 82 85 86 87 92 93 97 99 100 101 104 107 108 110 111 113 114 117 118 129 131 133 134 145 146 **S** Bureau of Medicine and Surgery, Department of the Navy, Washington, DC
Primary Contact: Captain Christopher M. Culp, Commanding Officer
COO: Lieutenant Kirk Houser, Director Administration
CFO: Judith Hogan, Comptroller and Director Resources and Logistics
CIO: Patrick Flaherty, Director Management Information
Web address: www.med.navy.mil/sites/nhbrem
**Control:** Navy, Government, federal **Service:** General Medical and Surgical

**Staffed Beds:** 40 **Admissions:** 1947 **Census:** 11 **Outpatient Visits:** 293664 **Births:** 795 **Total Expense ($000):** 101167 **Personnel:** 1221

**WA**

---

**Hospital, Medicare Provider Number, Address, Telephone, Approval, Facility, and Physician Codes, Health Care System**

★ American Hospital Association (AHA) membership
☐ The Joint Commission accreditation          ◇ DNV Healthcare Inc. accreditation
○ American Osteopathic Association (AOA) accreditation
△ Commission on Accreditation of Rehabilitation Facilities (CARF) accreditation

## BREWSTER—Okanogan County

**OKANOGAN DOUGLAS DISTRICT HOSPITAL (501324)**, 507 Hospital Way, Zip 98812–0577, Mailing Address: P.O. Box 577, Zip 98812–0577; tel. 509/689–2517, (Nonreporting) **A**9 10 18
Primary Contact: O. E. Hufnagel, Chief Executive Officer
COO: Sandy Sylvester, Chief Operating Officer
CFO: Jennifer Munson, Chief Financial Officer
CMO: Eric Haeger, M.D., President Medical Staff
CIO: Christopher Freel, Chief Information Technologist
CHR: Anita Fisk, Director Human Resources
Web address: www.oddh.org
**Control:** Hospital district or authority, Government, nonfederal **Service:** General Medical and Surgical

| Staffed Beds: 20 |
|---|

## BURIEN—King County

☒ **HIGHLINE MEDICAL CENTER (500011)**, 16251 Sylvester Road S.W., Zip 98166–3052; tel. 206/244–9970, (Includes HIGHLINE SPECIALTY CENTER, 12844 MILITARY ROAD FORK, TUKWILA, ZIP 98168; MARK BENEDUM, ADMINISTRATOR ), (Nonreporting) **A**1 2 9 10
Primary Contact: Mark Benedum, Chief Executive Officer
COO: Bud Musselman, Chief Operating Officer and Chief Financial Officer
CFO: Bud Musselman, Chief Operating Officer and Chief Financial Officer
CIO: Matt Crockett, Assistant Administrator and Chief Information Officer
CHR: Rozanne Martin, Assistant Administrator Human Resources
Web address: www.hchnet.org
**Control:** Other not–for–profit (including NFP Corporation) **Service:** General Medical and Surgical

| Staffed Beds: 179 |
|---|

## CENTRALIA—Lewis County

☒ **PROVIDENCE CENTRALIA HOSPITAL (500019)**, 914 South Scheuber Road, Zip 98531–9027; tel. 360/736–2803 **A**1 9 10 20 **F**5 8 11 13 15 30 31 32 34 35 40 43 48 57 58 59 64 68 70 75 76 77 78 79 80 81 86 87 90 93 102 107 108 111 113 116 118 128 129 130 131 145 146 147 **S** Providence Health & Services, Renton, WA
Primary Contact: Cindy Mayo, Chief Executive
COO: Dennis Mesaros, Chief Operating Officer
CFO: Denise Marroni, Chief Financial Officer
CMO: Kevin Caserta, M.D., Chief Medical Officer
CIO: Kerry Miles, Site Director
CHR: Susan Meenk, Vice President Service Area
Web address: www.providence.org
**Control:** Church–operated, Nongovernment, not–for profit **Service:** General Medical and Surgical

| Staffed Beds: 100 Admissions: 5357 Census: 46 Outpatient Visits: 268593 Births: 611 Total Expense ($000): 133717 Payroll Expense ($000): 46030 Personnel: 636 |
|---|

## CHELAN—Chelan County

★ **LAKE CHELAN COMMUNITY HOSPITAL (501334)**, 503 East Highland Avenue, Zip 98816–0908, Mailing Address: P.O. Box 908, Zip 98816–0908; tel. 509/682–3300 **A**9 10 18 **F**4 5 7 8 11 13 15 18 29 30 34 35 36 38 39 40 41 43 44 45 50 56 57 59 62 63 64 65 66 68 71 75 76 77 79 81 84 85 86 87 91 92 93 94 96 100 101 102 103 104 106 107 108 110 111 118 124 129 130 131 132 134 142 145 146 147 **P**6
Primary Contact: Kevin Abel, Chief Executive Officer
CFO: Karen Spurgeon, Chief Financial Officer
CMO: John Kremer, M.D., Chief Medical Officer
CIO: Ross Hurd, Chief Information Officer
CHR: Nancy Young, Director Human Resources
Web address: www.lakechelancommunityhospital.com
**Control:** Hospital district or authority, Government, nonfederal **Service:** General Medical and Surgical

| Staffed Beds: 25 Admissions: 811 Census: 16 Outpatient Visits: 19828 Births: 98 Total Expense ($000): 18346 Payroll Expense ($000): 11352 Personnel: 189 |
|---|

## CHEWELAH—Stevens County

☒ **PROVIDENCE ST. JOSEPH'S HOSPITAL (501309)**, 500 East Webster Street, Zip 99109–9523; tel. 509/935–8211, (Total facility includes 40 beds in nursing home–type unit) **A**1 9 10 18 **F**3 8 10 11 13 15 29 30 34 35 40 43 44 45 57 59 65 75 79 81 82 84 87 91 93 107 113 118 127 132 145 147 **P**6 **S** Providence Health & Services, Renton, WA
Primary Contact: Robert D. Campbell, Jr., President and Chief Executive
CFO: Chris Hargis, Chief Financial Officer
CHR: Linda Grittner, Director Human Resources
Web address: www.sjhospital.org
**Control:** Church–operated, Nongovernment, not–for profit **Service:** General Medical and Surgical

| Staffed Beds: 65 Admissions: 632 Census: 48 Outpatient Visits: 19248 Births: 75 Total Expense ($000): 20384 Payroll Expense ($000): 9960 Personnel: 129 |
|---|

## CLARKSTON—Asotin County

☒ **TRI–STATE MEMORIAL HOSPITAL (501332)**, 1221 Highland Avenue, Zip 99403–0189, Mailing Address: P.O. Box 189, Zip 99403–0189; tel. 509/758–5511, (Nonreporting) **A**1 9 10 18
Primary Contact: Donald Wee, Chief Executive Officer
CFO: Alex Town, Chief Financial Officer
CMO: Kim Wilson, M.D., Chief of Staff
CIO: Joleen Carper, Director Quality and Risk
CHR: Muriel R. Uhlenkott, Human Resources Officer
Web address: www.tristatehospital.org
**Control:** Other not–for–profit (including NFP Corporation) **Service:** General Medical and Surgical

| Staffed Beds: 25 |
|---|

## COLFAX—Whitman County

★ **WHITMAN HOSPITAL AND MEDICAL CENTER (501327)**, 1200 West Fairview Street, Zip 99111–9579; tel. 509/397–3435 **A**9 10 18 **F**29 30 34 35 40 45 59 64 65 68 69 76 77 79 81 85 93 107 110 111 118 129 132 134 147 **S** Providence Health & Services, Renton, WA
Primary Contact: Deborah Glass, MS, R.N., Chief Executive Officer
COO: Jim Heilsberg, Chief Financial Officer and Chief Information Officer
CFO: Jim Heilsberg, Chief Financial Officer and Chief Information Officer
CMO: Nathan Ullrich, M.D., Chief Medical Officer
CIO: Jim Heilsberg, Chief Financial Officer and Chief Information Officer
CHR: Linda Ledgerwood, Director Human Resources
Web address: www.whitmanhospital.com
**Control:** Hospital district or authority, Government, nonfederal **Service:** General Medical and Surgical

| Staffed Beds: 25 Admissions: 562 Census: 6 Outpatient Visits: 16042 Births: 53 Total Expense ($000): 22235 Payroll Expense ($000): 8928 Personnel: 174 |
|---|

## COLVILLE—Stevens County

☒ **PROVIDENCE MOUNT CARMEL HOSPITAL (501326)**, 982 East Columbia Avenue, Zip 99114–3352; tel. 509/685–5100 **A**1 9 10 18 **F**3 11 13 15 29 30 34 40 43 44 45 57 59 64 70 75 76 77 79 81 82 84 85 86 87 93 107 108 114 117 118 122 128 130 131 132 134 145 147 **P**6 **S** Providence Health & Services, Renton, WA
Primary Contact: Robert D. Campbell, Jr., President and Chief Executive
COO: Gary V. Peck, Chief Operating Officer
CFO: Chris Hargis, Chief Financial Officer
CMO: Bernie Currigan, M.D., Chief Medical Officer
CIO: Theron DePaulo, Manager Information Systems
CHR: Linda Grittner, Vice President Human Resources
Web address: www.mtcarmelhospital.org
**Control:** Church–operated, Nongovernment, not–for profit **Service:** General Medical and Surgical

| Staffed Beds: 25 Admissions: 1149 Census: 10 Outpatient Visits: 31169 Births: 190 Total Expense ($000): 34202 Payroll Expense ($000): 13820 Personnel: 172 |
|---|

## COUPEVILLE—Island County

★ **WHIDBEY GENERAL HOSPITAL (501339)**, 101 North Main Street, Zip 98239–3413; tel. 360/678–5151, (Nonreporting) **A**2 9 10 18
Primary Contact: Tom Tomasino, Administrator and Chief Executive Officer
COO: Hank Hanigan, Chief Operating Officer
CMO: Doug Langrock, M.D., Chief of Staff
CIO: Tom Tomasino, Administrator and Chief Executive Officer
CHR: Carolyn Pape, Director Human Resources
Web address: www.whidbeygen.org
**Control:** Hospital district or authority, Government, nonfederal **Service:** General Medical and Surgical

| Staffed Beds: 25 |
|---|

## DAVENPORT—Lincoln County

★ **LINCOLN HOSPITAL (501305)**, 10 Nichols Street, Zip 99122–9729; tel. 509/725–7101, (Nonreporting) **A**9 10 18
Primary Contact: Thomas J. Martin, Chief Executive Officer
CFO: Tyson Lacy, Chief Financial Officer
CMO: Fred Reed, M.D., Chief of Staff
CIO: Elliott Donson, Chief Information Specialist
CHR: Janelle Hiccox, Director Human Resources
Web address: www.lincolnhospital.org
**Control:** Hospital district or authority, Government, nonfederal **Service:** General Medical and Surgical

| Staffed Beds: 60 |
|---|

**WA**

*Many Facility Codes have changed. Please refer to the AHA Guide Code Chart.* © 2012 AHA Guide

## DAYTON—Columbia County

**DAYTON GENERAL HOSPITAL (501302)**, 1012 South Third Street, Zip 99328–1696; tel. 509/382–2531, (Total facility includes 34 beds in nursing home–type unit) **A**9 10 18 **F**34 35 40 67 93 97 107 111 113 126 127 **P**6
Primary Contact: Charles A. Button, Chief Executive Officer
CFO: Gary Schroeder, Chief Financial Officer
CHR: Kari Newman, Director Human Resources
Web address: www.cchd–wa.org
**Control:** County–Government, nonfederal **Service:** Long–Term Acute Care hospital

**Staffed Beds:** 59 **Admissions:** 186 **Census:** 41 **Outpatient Visits:** 57996
**Births:** 0 **Total Expense ($000):** 10059 **Payroll Expense ($000):** 5113

## EDMONDS—Snohomish County

**STEVENS HEALTHCARE** See Swedish/Edmonds

✠ **SWEDISH/EDMONDS (500026)**, 21601 76th Avenue West, Zip 98026–7506; tel. 425/640–4000 **A**1 2 9 10 **F**3 11 12 13 15 18 20 22 28 29 30 31 34 35 40 43 45 49 59 65 68 70 72 74 75 76 77 78 79 80 81 82 84 85 86 87 92 93 94 96 98 100 101 102 105 107 108 110 111 112 113 115 116 117 118 119 123 128 129 130 131 134 145 146 147 **P**6 7 **S** Swedish Health Services, Seattle, WA
Primary Contact: David E. Jaffe, Chief Administrative Officer
CMO: Tim Roddy, M.D., Vice President Medical Affairs
CIO: Robert Pageler, Director Information Services
CHR: Steven Losleben, Vice President Human Resources
Web address: www.swedish.org
**Control:** Other not–for–profit (including NFP Corporation) **Service:** General Medical and Surgical

**Staffed Beds:** 161 **Admissions:** 9042 **Census:** 109 **Outpatient Visits:** 109510 **Births:** 1054 **Total Expense ($000):** 173030 **Payroll Expense ($000):** 89956 **Personnel:** 1240

## ELLENSBURG—Kittitas County

★ **KITTITAS VALLEY COMMUNITY HOSPITAL (501333)**, 603 South Chestnut Street, Zip 98926–3875; tel. 509/962–7302, (Nonreporting) **A**9 10 18
Primary Contact: Paul E. Nurick, Chief Executive Officer
CFO: Libby Allgood, Chief Financial Officer
CHR: Lisa McDaniel, Assistant Administrator Human Resources
Web address: www.kvch.com
**Control:** Hospital district or authority, Government, nonfederal **Service:** General Medical and Surgical

**Staffed Beds:** 25

## ENUMCLAW—King County

★ **ST. ELIZABETH HOSPITAL (501335)**, 1450 Battersby Avenue, Zip 98022–0218, Mailing Address: P.O. Box 218, Zip 98022–0218; tel. 360/825–2505, (Nonreporting) **A**9 10 18 **S** Catholic Health Initiatives, Englewood, CO
Primary Contact: Donna Russell–Cook, President
COO: Joseph Wilczek, Chief Executive Officer
CFO: Philip Hjembo, Chief Financial Officer
CHR: Jerilyn Ray, Manager Human Resources
Web address: www.fhshealth.org
**Control:** Other not–for–profit (including NFP Corporation) **Service:** General Medical and Surgical

**Staffed Beds:** 25

## EPHRATA—Grant County

★ **COLUMBIA BASIN HOSPITAL (501317)**, 200 Nat Washington Way, Zip 98823–1973; tel. 509/754–4631, (Nonreporting) **A**9 10 18
Primary Contact: Robert Reeder, FACHE, Chief Executive Officer
CFO: Rhonda Handley, Chief Financial Officer
CMO: Lowell C. Allred, M.D., Chief of Staff
CHR: Suzanne Little, Human Resources Specialist
Web address: www.columbiabasinhospital.org
**Control:** Hospital district or authority, Government, nonfederal **Service:** General Medical and Surgical

**Staffed Beds:** 25

## EVERETT—Snohomish County

✠ △ **PROVIDENCE REGIONAL MEDICAL CENTER EVERETT (500014)**, 1321 Colby Avenue, Zip 98206–1147, Mailing Address: P.O. Box 1147, Zip 98206–1147; tel. 425/261–2000, (Includes PROVIDENCE EVERETT MEDICAL CENTER – COLBY CAMPUS, 1321 Colby Avenue, Zip 98206, Mailing Address: P.O. Box 1147, Zip 98206; tel. 425/261–2000; PROVIDENCE EVERETT MEDICAL CENTER – PACIFIC CAMPUS, Pacific and Nassau Streets, Zip 98201, Mailing Address: P.O. Box 1067, Zip 98206–1067; tel. 206/258–7123) **A**1 2 5 7 9 10 **F**3 4 5 8 11 13 15 17 18 20 22 24 26 28 29 30 31 32 34 35 36 38 40 43 44 46 47 48 49 50 53 54 55 56 57 58 59 60 61 64 65 66 68 70 72 73 74 75 76 77 78 79 80 81 82 83 84 85 86 87 89 90 93 97 107 108 109 111 113 114 115 116 117 118 119 120 122 123 125 128 129 130 131 134 143 145 146 147 **P**6 8 **S** Providence Health & Services, Renton, WA
Primary Contact: David Brooks, Chief Executive Officer
COO: Preston M. Simmons, Chief Operating Officer
CFO: Todd Hofheins, Chief Financial Officer
CMO: Lawrence Schecter, M.D., Chief Medical Officer
CHR: Bob Sampson, Vice President Human Resources
Web address: www.providence.org
**Control:** Church–operated, Nongovernment, not–for profit **Service:** General Medical and Surgical

**Staffed Beds:** 491 **Admissions:** 26580 **Census:** 296 **Outpatient Visits:** 566733 **Births:** 3973 **Total Expense ($000):** 590163 **Payroll Expense ($000):** 224225

## FEDERAL WAY—King County

✠ **ST. FRANCIS HOSPITAL (500141)**, 34515 Ninth Avenue South, Zip 98003–6799; tel. 253/944–8100, (Nonreporting) **A**1 2 9 10 **S** Catholic Health Initiatives, Englewood, CO
Primary Contact: Anthony McLean, President
CFO: Mike Fitzgerald, Chief Financial Officer
CMO: Mark C. Adams, M.D., Associate Chief Medical Officer
CIO: Bruce Elkington, Regional Chief Information Officer
CHR: David Lawson, Senior Vice President Human Resources
Web address: www.fhshealth.org
**Control:** Church–operated, Nongovernment, not–for profit **Service:** General Medical and Surgical

**Staffed Beds:** 110

## FORKS—Clallam County

**FORKS COMMUNITY HOSPITAL (501325)**, 530 Bogachiel Way, Zip 98331–9120; tel. 360/374–6271, (Nonreporting) **A**9 10 18
Primary Contact: Camille Scott, Administrator
COO: John Sherrett, Chief Financial Officer and Chief Operating Officer
CFO: John Sherrett, Chief Financial Officer and Chief Operating Officer
CIO: Andrea Perkins–Peppers, Manager Information Services
CHR: Geoff Roach, Director Human Resources
Web address: www.forkshospital.org
**Control:** Hospital district or authority, Government, nonfederal **Service:** General Medical and Surgical

**Staffed Beds:** 45

## GIG HARBOR—Pierce County

✠ **ST. ANTHONY HOSPITAL (500151)**, 11567 Canterwood Boulevard N.W., Zip 98332–5812; tel. 253/530–2000, (Nonreporting) **A**1 9 10 **S** Catholic Health Initiatives, Englewood, CO
Primary Contact: Kurt Schley, President
Web address: www.fhshealth.org/
**Control:** Other not–for–profit (including NFP Corporation) **Service:** General Medical and Surgical

**Staffed Beds:** 80

## GOLDENDALE—Klickitat County

★ **KLICKITAT VALLEY HEALTH (501316)**, 310 South Roosevelt Avenue, Zip 98620–9201; tel. 509/773–4022 **A**9 10 18 **F**3 7 8 10 15 18 29 30 34 35 40 43 45 57 59 62 63 64 65 68 75 77 81 83 84 85 97 107 111 118 126 127 129 132 134 143 145 147
Primary Contact: John R. White, Chief Executive Officer
CFO: Leslie Hiebert, Chief Financial Officer
CMO: Dagmar Crosby, M.D., Chief of Staff
CIO: Jonathan Hatfield, Supervisor Information Technology
CHR: Gwyn Miller, Director Human Resources
Web address: www.kvhealth.net
**Control:** Hospital district or authority, Government, nonfederal **Service:** General Medical and Surgical

**Staffed Beds:** 17 **Admissions:** 236 **Census:** 5 **Outpatient Visits:** 4879
**Births:** 0 **Total Expense ($000):** 18949 **Payroll Expense ($000):** 8858
**Personnel:** 176

**WA**

---

**Hospital, Medicare Provider Number, Address, Telephone, Approval, Facility, and Physician Codes, Health Care System**

★ American Hospital Association (AHA) membership
□ The Joint Commission accreditation
◇ DNV Healthcare Inc. accreditation
○ American Osteopathic Association (AOA) accreditation
△ Commission on Accreditation of Rehabilitation Facilities (CARF) accreditation

## GRAND COULEE—Grant County

**COULEE COMMUNITY HOSPITAL** See Coulee Medical Center

**COULEE MEDICAL CENTER (501308)**, 411 Fortuyn Road, Zip 99133–8718; tel. 509/633–1753, (Nonreporting) **A**9 10 18
Primary Contact: J. Scott Graham, Chief Executive Officer
COO: Alan Wagner, Chief Operating Officer
CFO: Debbie Bigelow, Chief Financial Officer
CMO: Jacob Chaffee, M.D., Chief Medical Officer
CHR: Julie D. Bjorklund, Director Human Resources
Web address: www.cmccares.org
**Control:** Hospital district or authority, Government, nonfederal **Service:** General Medical and Surgical

**Staffed Beds:** 25

## ILWACO—Pacific County

★ **OCEAN BEACH HOSPITAL (501314)**, 174 First Avenue North, Zip 98624–0258, Mailing Address: P.O. Box H., Zip 98624–0258; tel. 360/642–3181 **A**9 10 18 **F**3 11 15 28 29 30 31 34 35 40 43 45 57 59 68 75 77 78 79 81 85 86 87 97 107 111 113 118 126 129 131 132 134 146
Primary Contact: Joe Devin, Chief Executive Officer
CMO: Randy Ensminger, M.D., Chief Medical Officer
CIO: Julie P. Oakes, R.N., Manager Risk and Quality
CHR: Kary Holloway, Director Human Resources
Web address: www.oceanbeachhospital.net
**Control:** Hospital district or authority, Government, nonfederal **Service:** General Medical and Surgical

**Staffed Beds:** 15 **Admissions:** 474 **Census:** 5 **Outpatient Visits:** 30440
**Births:** 0 **Total Expense ($000):** 23960 **Payroll Expense ($000):** 10784

## ISSAQUAH—King County

**SWEDISH/ISSAQUAH (500152)**, 751 N.E. Blakely Drive, Zip 98029–6201; tel. 425/313–4000, (Data for 61 days) **A**10 21 **F**3 8 13 15 18 19 22 29 30 31 35 37 40 41 43 45 49 60 64 65 70 74 75 78 79 81 82 83 84 85 86 87 89 107 108 110 111 114 116 117 118 125 128 129 130 131 145 146 **P**6 **S** Swedish Health Services, Seattle, WA
Primary Contact: Chuck Salmon, Chief Executive
Web address: www.swedish.org/issaquah
**Control:** Other not–for–profit (including NFP Corporation) **Service:** General Medical and Surgical

**Staffed Beds:** 49 **Admissions:** 385 **Census:** 17 **Outpatient Visits:** 28321
**Births:** 47 **Total Expense ($000):** 20232 **Payroll Expense ($000):** 5680
**Personnel:** 354

## KENNEWICK—Benton County

✠ **KENNEWICK GENERAL HOSPITAL (500053)**, 900 South Auburn Street, Zip 99336–6128, Mailing Address: P.O. Box 6128, Zip 99336–0128; tel. 509/586–6111, (Nonreporting) **A**1 2 9 10
Primary Contact: Glen Marshall, Chief Executive Officer
CFO: Gerald Paule, Chief Financial Officer
CFO: Gerald Paule, Chief Financial Officer
CMO: James Newman, M.D., President Medical Staff
CIO: Michael Cloutier, Director Information Services
CHR: Russ Keefer, Chief Human Resources Officer
Web address: www.kennewickgeneral.com
**Control:** Hospital district or authority, Government, nonfederal **Service:** General Medical and Surgical

**Staffed Beds:** 101

## KIRKLAND—King County

**EVERGREEN HEALTHCARE** See Evergreen Hospital Medical Center

✠ **EVERGREEN HOSPITAL MEDICAL CENTER (500124)**, 12040 N.E. 128th Street, Zip 98034–9917; tel. 425/899–1000 **A**1 2 5 9 10 **F**3 11 12 13 15 18 20 22 28 29 30 31 34 35 37 38 40 42 43 44 46 49 50 51 53 54 55 56 57 58 59 62 63 64 68 70 71 72 73 74 75 76 78 79 81 82 84 85 86 87 89 90 92 93 96 97 103 107 108 110 111 113 114 118 119 120 122 123 125 128 129 130 131 134 143 145 146 147 **P**4 6
Primary Contact: Robert H. Malte, Chief Executive Officer
COO: David S. Danielson, Senior Vice President Operations
CFO: Chrissy Yamada, CPA, Senior Vice President Finance
CMO: Mitch Weinberg, M.D., Chief of Staff
CIO: Tom Martin, Vice President and Chief Information Officer
Web address: www.evergreenhealthcare.org
**Control:** Hospital district or authority, Government, nonfederal **Service:** General Medical and Surgical

**Staffed Beds:** 274 **Admissions:** 16029 **Census:** 147 **Outpatient Visits:** 493483 **Births:** 4555 **Total Expense ($000):** 413378 **Payroll Expense ($000):** 205869 **Personnel:** 2630

## FAIRFAX HOSPITAL (504002)

☐ **FAIRFAX HOSPITAL (504002)**, 10200 N.E. 132nd Street, Zip 98034–2899; tel. 425/821–2000 **A**1 9 10 **F**4 29 35 38 54 98 99 100 101 102 105 129 131 **P**6 **S** Universal Health Services, Inc., King of Prussia, PA
Primary Contact: Ron Escarda, Chief Executive Officer
COO: Michael Uradnik, Chief Operating Officer
CFO: Pam Rhoads, Chief Financial Officer
CMO: William Adams, M.D., Medical Director
CHR: Anne Schreiber, Manager Human Resources
Web address: www.fairfaxhospital.com
**Control:** Corporation, Investor–owned, for–profit **Service:** Psychiatric

**Staffed Beds:** 95 **Admissions:** 2903 **Census:** 81 **Outpatient Visits:** 1857
**Births:** 0 **Total Expense ($000):** 19649 **Payroll Expense ($000):** 10998
**Personnel:** 172

## LAKEWOOD—Pierce County

✠ △ **ST. CLARE HOSPITAL (500021)**, 11315 Bridgeport Way S.W., Zip 98499–3004; tel. 253/588–1711, (Nonreporting) **A**1 2 7 9 10 **S** Catholic Health Initiatives, Englewood, CO
Primary Contact: Kathy Bressler, President
COO: Kathy Bressler, President
CFO: Mike Fitzgerald, Chief Financial Officer
CIO: Bruce Elkington, Regional Chief Information Officer
CHR: David Lawson, Senior Vice President Human Resources
Web address: www.fhshealth.org
**Control:** Church–operated, Nongovernment, not–for profit **Service:** General Medical and Surgical

**Staffed Beds:** 98

## LEAVENWORTH—Chelan County

★ **CASCADE MEDICAL CENTER (501313)**, 817 Commercial Street, Zip 98826–1316, Mailing Address: P.O. Box 330, Zip 98826–0330; tel. 509/548–3423 **A**9 10 18 **F**3 7 15 30 34 40 43 45 59 63 64 65 68 77 93 97 104 107 110 113 126 129 130 132 147 **P**6
Primary Contact: Jon R. Davis, FACHE, Administrator
CFO: Alan MacPhee, Chief Financial Officer
CMO: John Deliduka, M.D., Chief Medical Officer
CHR: Lance Heise, Director Human Resources
Web address: www.cascademedicalcenter.org
**Control:** Hospital district or authority, Government, nonfederal **Service:** General Medical and Surgical

**Staffed Beds:** 9 **Admissions:** 300 **Census:** 3 **Outpatient Visits:** 48949
**Births:** 0 **Total Expense ($000):** 11880 **Payroll Expense ($000):** 6388
**Personnel:** 93

## LONGVIEW—Cowlitz County

✠ **PEACEHEALTH ST. JOHN MEDICAL CENTER (500041)**, 1615 Delaware Street, Zip 98632–2310, Mailing Address: P.O. Box 3002, Zip 98632–3002; tel. 360/414–2000, (Nonreporting) **A**1 2 9 10 **S** PeaceHealth, Bellevue, WA
Primary Contact: Sy Johnson, Chief Executive Officer
Web address: www.peacehealth.org
**Control:** Church–operated, Nongovernment, not–for profit **Service:** General Medical and Surgical

**Staffed Beds:** 202

## MCCLEARY—Grays Harbor County

**MARK REED HEALTH CARE DISTRICT (501304)**, 322 South Birch Street, Zip 98557–9522; tel. 360/495–3244, (Nonreporting) **A**9 10 18
Primary Contact: Renee K. Jensen, Chief Executive Officer
CFO: Ronald Hulscher, Chief Financial Officer
CMO: Patrick Ogilvie, M.D., Chief Medical Officer
CIO: Chayne King, Contracted Manager Information Technology
CHR: Mindy Portchy, Manager Human Resources
Web address: www.markreed.org
**Control:** Corporation, Investor–owned, for–profit **Service:** General Medical and Surgical

**Staffed Beds:** 6

## MEDICAL LAKE—Spokane County

☐ **EASTERN STATE HOSPITAL (504004)**, Maple Street, Zip 99022–0045, Mailing Address: P.O. Box 800, Zip 99022–0800; tel. 509/299–3121, (Nonreporting) **A**1 9 10
Primary Contact: Harold E. Wilson, Chief Executive Officer
Web address: www.www1.dsgs.wa.gov/mentalhealth/eshfaqs.shtml
**Control:** State–Government, nonfederal **Service:** Psychiatric

**Staffed Beds:** 319

**WA**

## MONROE—Snohomish County

✠ **VALLEY GENERAL HOSPITAL (500084)**, 14701 179th S.E., Zip 98272–1108,
Mailing Address: P.O. Box 646, Zip 98272–0646; tel. 360/794–7497,
(Nonreporting) **A**1 2 9 10 21
Primary Contact: Michael T. Liepman, Chief Executive Officer
CFO: John Beltz, Chief Financial Officer
CIO: Kathy Nelson, Director Marketing and Strategic Planning
CHR: Joan Catlett, Director Human Resources
Web address: www.valleygeneral.com
**Control:** Hospital district or authority, Government, nonfederal **Service:** General
Medical and Surgical

**Staffed Beds:** 68

## MORTON—Lewis County

★ **MORTON GENERAL HOSPITAL (501319)**, 521 Adams Avenue, Zip 98356,
Mailing Address: P.O. Box 1138, Zip 98356–0019; tel. 360/496–5112 **A**9 10 18
**F**3 8 13 40 45 81 85 93 107 111 113 118 126 128 129 132 147
Primary Contact: Ron DeArth, Superintendent
CFO: Tim Cournyer, Chief Financial Officer
CHR: Shannon Kelly, Director Human Resources
Web address: www.mortongeneral.org
**Control:** Hospital district or authority, Government, nonfederal **Service:** General
Medical and Surgical

**Staffed Beds:** 25 **Admissions:** 377 **Census:** 18

## MOSES LAKE—Grant County

★ **SAMARITAN HEALTHCARE (500033)**, 801 East Wheeler Road,
Zip 98837–1899; tel. 509/765–5606, (Nonreporting) **A**5 9 10 20
Primary Contact: Andrew P. Bair, President and Chief Executive Officer
CIO: Marlin Howell, Director Information Systems
CHR: Kim Garza, Vice President Human Resources
Web address: www.samaritanhealthcare.com
**Control:** Hospital district or authority, Government, nonfederal **Service:** General
Medical and Surgical

**Staffed Beds:** 47

## MOUNT VERNON—Skagit County

★ **SKAGIT VALLEY HOSPITAL (500003)**, 1415 East Kincaid Street, Zip 98273,
Mailing Address: P.O. Box 1376, Zip 98273–1376; tel. 360/424–4111 **A**2 5 9
10 19 21 **F**3 11 13 15 18 20 22 26 28 29 30 31 34 35 36 40 43 44 45 49
50 54 57 59 60 64 65 68 70 73 74 75 76 77 78 79 80 81 84 85 86 87 89
93 97 98 99 100 101 102 107 115 119 120 122 126 128 129 131 143 145
146 147 **P**6
Primary Contact: Gregg A. Davidson, FACHE, Chief Executive Officer
COO: Lori Harlow, Chief Operating Officer
CFO: Thomas Litaker, Chief Financial Officer
CMO: Richard Abbott, M.D., Medical Advisor Quality Improvement
CIO: Doug Riley, Director Information Services
CHR: Deborah Martin, Assistant Administrator
Web address: www.skagitvalleyhospital.org
**Control:** Hospital district or authority, Government, nonfederal **Service:** General
Medical and Surgical

**Staffed Beds:** 137 **Admissions:** 8845 **Census:** 88 **Outpatient Visits:** 370226
**Births:** 1303 **Total Expense ($000):** 201837 **Payroll Expense ($000):**
90929 **Personnel:** 1455

## NEWPORT—Pend Oreille County

**NEWPORT HOSPITAL AND HEALTH SERVICES (501310)**, 714 West Pine
Street, Zip 99156–9046; tel. 509/447–2441, (Total facility includes 50 beds in
nursing home–type unit) **A**9 10 18 **F**8 10 11 13 15 32 34 40 41 50 57 59 64
65 75 76 81 87 89 93 97 107 113 118 126 127 129 132 145 146 147
Primary Contact: Thomas W. Wilbur, Chief Executive Officer and Superintendent
COO: Ginny Monroe, Chief Operating Officer
CFO: Kim Manus, Chief Financial Officer
CMO: Sara Ragsdale, D.O., Chief Medical Staff
CIO: Kim Manus, Chief Financial Officer
CHR: Roger Rasmussen, Chief Administrative Officer
Web address: www.phd1.org
**Control:** Hospital district or authority, Government, nonfederal **Service:** General
Medical and Surgical

**Staffed Beds:** 70 **Admissions:** 548 **Census:** 44 **Outpatient Visits:** 35000
**Births:** 86 **Total Expense ($000):** 22757 **Payroll Expense ($000):** 13138
**Personnel:** 267

## OAK HARBOR—Island County

✠ **NAVAL HOSPITAL**, 3475 North Saratoga Street, Zip 98278–8800;
tel. 360/257–9500, (Nonreporting) **A**1 9 **S** Bureau of Medicine and Surgery,
Department of the Navy, Washington, DC
Primary Contact: Captain Susan Lickenstein, Commander
CFO: Lieutenant Gerald Hall, Director Resource Management
CMO: Commander Stephen Cooley, M.D., Chairman Executive Committee Medical
Staff
CIO: Gregory Carruth, Head Information Management
CHR: Kathy Vass, Head Human Resources
Web address: www.med.navy.mil/sites/nhoh/Pages/default.aspx
**Control:** Navy, Government, federal **Service:** General Medical and Surgical

**Staffed Beds:** 29

## ODESSA—Lincoln County

**ODESSA MEMORIAL HEALTHCARE CENTER (501307)**, 502 East Amende
Drive, Zip 99159–0368, Mailing Address: P.O. Box 368, Zip 99159–0368;
tel. 509/982–2611 **A**9 10 18 **F**3 7 10 11 29 30 34 40 43 45 50 57 59 65 77
81 93 126 129 131 132 **P**6
Primary Contact: Gary L. DelForge, Administrator
COO: Alyssa Oestreich, Chief Operating Officer
CFO: Annette Edwards, Chief Financial Officer
CMO: Linda J. Powel, M.D., Medical Director
CHR: Julie Wehr, Director Human Resources
Web address: www.omhc.org
**Control:** Hospital district or authority, Government, nonfederal **Service:** General
Medical and Surgical

**Staffed Beds:** 25 **Admissions:** 64 **Census:** 21 **Outpatient Visits:** 8323 **Total
Expense ($000):** 5693 **Payroll Expense ($000):** 2839 **Personnel:** 75

## OLYMPIA—Thurston County

☐ **CAPITAL MEDICAL CENTER (500139)**, 3900 Capital Mall Drive S.W.,
Zip 98502–5026, Mailing Address: P.O. Box 19002, Zip 98507–9002;
tel. 360/754–5858, (Nonreporting) **A**1 9 10 **S** Capella Healthcare, Franklin, TN
Primary Contact: Jim Geist, Chief Executive Officer
CFO: Brian Anderson, Chief Financial Officer
CMO: Rojesh Sharangpani, M.D., Chief of Staff
CIO: Renee Crotty, Coordinator Marketing and Public Relations
CHR: Dana Vandewege, Director Human Resources
Web address: www.capitalmedical.com
**Control:** Partnership, Investor–owned, for–profit **Service:** General Medical and
Surgical

**Staffed Beds:** 110

✠ △ **PROVIDENCE ST. PETER HOSPITAL (500024)**, 413 Lilly Road N.E.,
Zip 98506–5166; tel. 360/491–9480 **A**1 7 9 10 **F**3 4 5 11 12 13 15 18 20 22
24 26 28 29 30 34 35 36 38 40 43 44 45 46 48 49 51 53 56 57 58 59 60
61 64 66 70 73 74 75 76 77 78 79 80 81 83 84 85 86 87 89 90 91 92 93
94 97 98 99 100 101 102 104 105 107 108 111 113 114 117 118 128 129
130 131 133 134 142 145 146 147 **P**6 **S** Providence Health & Services,
Renton, WA
Primary Contact: Medrice Coluccio, R.N., Chief Executive Officer
COO: Paul G. Wilkinson, Chief Operating Officer
CFO: Thomas Risse, Chief Financial Officer
CMO: Mike Matlock, M.D., Chief Medical Officer
CIO: Kerry Miles, Chief Information Officer
CHR: Susan Meenk, Vice President Service Area
Web address: www.providence.org/swsa/facilities/st_peter_hospital
**Control:** Church–operated, Nongovernment, not–for profit **Service:** General
Medical and Surgical

**Staffed Beds:** 378 **Admissions:** 21332 **Census:** 261 **Outpatient Visits:**
310888 **Births:** 2173 **Total Expense ($000):** 369683 **Payroll Expense
($000):** 134992 **Personnel:** 1791

## OMAK—Okanogan County

**MID–VALLEY HOSPITAL (501328)**, 810 Jasmine, Zip 98841–0793, Mailing
Address: P.O. Box 793, Zip 98841–0793; tel. 509/826–1760 **A**5 9 10 18 **F**11
13 15 29 34 40 43 45 57 59 64 65 68 70 76 81 82 87 89 93 107 114 118
126 132 134 **P**6
Primary Contact: Michael D. Billing, Administrator
CFO: Scott Attridge, Controller
CMO: David Bradford, M.D., Chief Medical Officer
CIO: Kelly Cariker, Manager
CHR: Randy Coffell, Manager Human Resources
Web address: www.mvhealth.org
**Control:** Hospital district or authority, Government, nonfederal **Service:** General
Medical and Surgical

**Staffed Beds:** 30 **Admissions:** 1068 **Census:** 8 **Outpatient Visits:** 44331
**Births:** 263 **Total Expense ($000):** 28219 **Payroll Expense ($000):** 13592
**Personnel:** 197

**WA**

**Hospital, Medicare Provider Number, Address, Telephone, Approval, Facility, and Physician Codes, Health Care System**

★ American Hospital Association (AHA) membership
☐ The Joint Commission accreditation    ◇ DNV Healthcare Inc. accreditation
○ American Osteopathic Association (AOA) accreditation
△ Commission on Accreditation of Rehabilitation Facilities (CARF) accreditation

© 2012 AHA Guide    *Many Facility Codes have changed. Please refer to the AHA Guide Code Chart.*    Hospitals **A663**

## OTHELLO—Adams County

★ **OTHELLO COMMUNITY HOSPITAL (501318)**, 315 North 14th Avenue, Zip 99344–1297; tel. 509/488–2636, (Nonreporting) **A**9 10 18
Primary Contact: Harold S. Geller, Administrator
CFO: Mark Bunch, Director Finance
CHR: Cheryl Olson, Chief Human Resources Officer
Web address: www.othellocommunityhospital.org
**Control:** Hospital district or authority, Government, nonfederal **Service:** General Medical and Surgical

Staffed Beds: 25

## PASCO—Franklin County

⊠ △ **LOURDES MEDICAL CENTER (501337)**, 520 North Fourth Avenue, Zip 99301–2568, Mailing Address: P.O. Box 2568, Zip 99302–2568; tel. 509/547–7704, (Nonreporting) **A**1 7 9 10 18 **S** Ascension Health, Saint Louis, MO
Primary Contact: John Serle, President and Chief Executive Officer
COO: Janet Wright, R.N., Vice President Patient Care Executive
CFO: Frank Becker, Chief Financial Officer
CIO: Vern Turney, Director Information Technology
Web address: www.lourdeshealth.net
**Control:** Church–operated, Nongovernment, not–for profit **Service:** General Medical and Surgical

Staffed Beds: 35

## POMEROY—Garfield County

★ **GARFIELD COUNTY PUBLIC HOSPITAL DISTRICT (501301)**, (Critical Access Hospital), 66 North 6th Street, Zip 99347–9705; tel. 509/843–1591 **A**9 10 18 **F**7 11 29 34 35 40 50 54 56 57 59 64 65 126 127 129 132 **P**6
Primary Contact: Andrew Craigie, Chief Executive Officer
CFO: Shannon Jones, Chief Financial Officer
CMO: Elizabeth Black, M.D., Chief Medical Officer
CIO: Jorie Gaines, Manager Information
CHR: Michele Beehler, Human Resources and Executive Assistant
Web address: www.garfieldcountyphd.org
**Control:** Hospital district or authority, Government, nonfederal **Service:** General Medical and Surgical

Staffed Beds: 40 Admissions: 117 Census: 25 Outpatient Visits: 8687
Births: 0 Total Expense ($000): 6541 Payroll Expense ($000): 3732
Personnel: 82

## PORT ANGELES—Clallam County

⊠ **OLYMPIC MEDICAL CENTER (500072)**, 939 Caroline Street, Zip 98362–3997; tel. 360/417–7000 **A**1 2 5 9 10 **F**3 8 11 13 15 17 18 24 26 28 29 31 34 36 40 43 49 54 57 59 62 64 65 70 75 76 77 78 79 81 82 84 85 86 87 89 93 94 97 107 108 110 111 113 114 115 116 118 119 120 122 123 126 128 129 130 134 145 146 147 **P**6
Primary Contact: Eric Lewis, Chief Executive Officer
CFO: Julie Rukstad, Chief Financial Officer
CMO: R. Scott Kennedy, M.D., Assistant Administrator and Chief Medical Officer
CIO: Linda Brown, Chief Information Officer
CHR: Richard Neuman, Assistant Administrator and Chief Human Resources Officer
Web address: www.olympicmedical.org
**Control:** Hospital district or authority, Government, nonfederal **Service:** General Medical and Surgical

Staffed Beds: 78 Admissions: 4753 Census: 44 Outpatient Visits: 272006
Births: 488 Total Expense ($000): 134711 Payroll Expense ($000): 61498
Personnel: 902

## PORT TOWNSEND—Jefferson County

★ **JEFFERSON HEALTHCARE (501323)**, 834 Sheridan Street, Zip 98368–2443; tel. 360/385–2200, (Nonreporting) **A**9 10 18 21
Primary Contact: Mike Glenn, Administrator and Chief Executive Officer
COO: Paula Dowdle, Chief Operating Officer
CFO: Hilary Whittington, Chief Financial Officer
CMO: Todd Carlson, M.D., Chief Medical Officer
CHR: Beki Lischalk, Director Human Resources
Web address: www.jeffersonhealthcare.org
**Control:** Hospital district or authority, Government, nonfederal **Service:** General Medical and Surgical

Staffed Beds: 42

## PROSSER—Benton County

★ **PROSSER MEMORIAL HOSPITAL (501312)**, 723 Memorial Street, Zip 99350–1593; tel. 509/786–2222 **A**9 10 18 **F**7 11 13 15 29 34 35 37 40 43 45 54 56 57 59 62 64 68 75 76 77 79 81 85 89 97 107 108 110 113 118 126 129 130 132 134 142 145 147 **P**6
Primary Contact: Julie Petersen, Chief Executive Officer
CFO: Tim Cooper, Chief Financial Officer
CIO: Dan Harter, Manager Information Systems
Web address: www.prossermemorial.com
**Control:** Hospital district or authority, Government, nonfederal **Service:** General Medical and Surgical

Staffed Beds: 25 Admissions: 768 Census: 8 Outpatient Visits: 22550
Births: 344 Total Expense ($000): 30038 Payroll Expense ($000): 15582
Personnel: 188

## PULLMAN—Whitman County

☐ **PULLMAN REGIONAL HOSPITAL (501331)**, 835 S.E. Bishop Boulevard, Zip 99163–5512; tel. 509/332–2541 **A**1 9 10 18 **F**3 13 15 28 29 30 34 35 36 38 40 43 44 45 47 51 53 55 57 59 64 68 70 74 75 76 77 78 79 81 86 87 89 93 98 101 102 104 105 107 108 110 111 113 117 118 125 128 129 130 131 132 143 145 **P**4 6
Primary Contact: Scott K. Adams, Chief Executive Officer
CFO: Steven Febus, Chief Financial Officer
CMO: Richard Caggiano, M.D., Chief Medical Officer
CHR: Bernadette Berney, Director Human Resources
Web address: www.pullmanhospital.org
**Control:** Hospital district or authority, Government, nonfederal **Service:** General Medical and Surgical

Staffed Beds: 25 Admissions: 1290 Census: 11 Outpatient Visits: 60347
Births: 392 Total Expense ($000): 44130 Payroll Expense ($000): 21670
Personnel: 329

## PUYALLUP—Pierce County

**GOOD SAMARITAN COMMUNITY HEALTHCARE** See MultiCare Good Samaritan Hospital

☐ △ **MULTICARE GOOD SAMARITAN HOSPITAL (500079)**, 407 14th Avenue S.E., Zip 98372–0118, Mailing Address: P.O. Box 1247, Zip 98371–1247; tel. 253/697–4000 **A**1 2 7 9 10 **F**3 11 13 17 18 20 22 24 28 29 30 31 34 38 40 42 43 50 54 56 59 64 65 70 71 74 75 76 77 78 79 81 84 85 86 87 89 90 91 92 93 94 96 99 100 102 103 104 106 107 108 111 113 114 116 118 125 128 129 131 133 145 147 **S** MultiCare Health System, Tacoma, WA
Primary Contact: Glenn Kasman, President and Chief Executive Officer
CFO: Kim Lintott, Vice President
CMO: J. D. Fitz, M.D., Vice President Medical Affairs
CIO: Florence Chang, Senior Vice President, Clinical Support Services and Chief Information Officer
CHR: Sarah Horsman, Vice President Human Resources
Web address: www.goodsamhealth.org
**Control:** Other not–for–profit (including NFP Corporation) **Service:** General Medical and Surgical

Staffed Beds: 256 Admissions: 16898 Census: 173 Outpatient Visits: 112468 Births: 2153 Total Expense ($000): 275207 Payroll Expense ($000): 108173 Personnel: 1478

## QUINCY—Grant County

★ **QUINCY VALLEY MEDICAL CENTER (501320)**, 908 10th Avenue S.W., Zip 98848–1376; tel. 509/787–3531, (Nonreporting) **A**9 10 18
Primary Contact: Mehdi Merred, Chief Executive Officer
CFO: Dean Taplett, Controller
CMO: Mark Vance, M.D., Chief Medical Officer
CIO: Ruth Vance, Director Information Systems
CHR: Alene Walker, Director Human Resources
Web address: www.quincyhospital.org
**Control:** County–Government, nonfederal **Service:** General Medical and Surgical

Staffed Beds: 47

## RENTON—King County

⊠ **VALLEY MEDICAL CENTER (500088)**, 400 South 43rd Street, Zip 98055–5714; tel. 425/228–3450 **A**1 2 3 5 9 10 **F**3 8 11 13 15 18 19 20 22 26 28 29 30 31 32 34 35 36 37 38 40 43 44 46 47 49 50 51 53 54 55 57 58 59 60 64 65 66 68 70 72 74 76 77 78 79 81 82 84 85 86 87 89 91 92 93 94 97 100 101 104 107 110 113 114 117 118 119 120 122 123 125 128 129 130 131 134 143 145 146 147 **P**8 **S** UW Medicine, Seattle, WA
Primary Contact: Richard D. Roodman, Chief Executive Officer
COO: Paul Hayes, Executive Vice President and Chief Operating Officer
CFO: Larry Smith, Senior Vice President and Chief Financial Officer
CMO: Kathryn Beattie, M.D., Senior Vice President and Chief Medical Officer
CIO: Rand Strobel, Vice President Information Technology
CHR: Barbara Mitchell, Senior Vice President Marketing and Human Resources
Web address: www.valleymed.org
**Control:** Hospital district or authority, Government, nonfederal **Service:** General Medical and Surgical

Staffed Beds: 176 Admissions: 16811 Census: 174 Outpatient Visits: 609847 Births: 3822 Total Expense ($000): 380903 Payroll Expense ($000): 184010 Personnel: 2381

*Many Facility Codes have changed. Please refer to the AHA Guide Code Chart.* © 2012 AHA Guide

WA

## REPUBLIC—Ferry County

★ **FERRY COUNTY MEMORIAL HOSPITAL (501322)**, 36 Klondike Road, Zip 99166–9701; tel. 509/775–3333, (Nonreporting) **A**9 10 18
Primary Contact: Gary W. Robertson, Chief Executive Officer
CFO: Kelly Leslie, Chief Financial Officer
CHR: Sharon Sattler, Human Resources Officer
Web address: www.fcphd.org
**Control:** Hospital district or authority, Government, nonfederal **Service:** General Medical and Surgical

**Staffed Beds: 25**

## RICHLAND—Benton County

✠ △ **KADLEC MEDICAL CENTER (500058)**, 888 Swift Boulevard, Zip 99352–3514; tel. 509/946–4611 **A**1 2 7 9 10 **F**3 5 11 13 15 18 20 22 24 26 28 29 30 31 34 36 40 43 46 47 48 49 50 56 57 59 64 68 70 72 75 76 77 78 79 81 82 85 86 87 89 90 93 96 97 107 108 110 111 113 114 115 116 117 118 129 145 147 **S** QHR, Brentwood, TN
Primary Contact: Rand J. Wortman, Chief Executive Officer
COO: Lane A. Savitch, President
CFO: Julie Meek, Vice President Finance
CMO: Wassim Khawandi, M.D., Chief of Staff
CIO: David Roach, Vice President Information Systems
CHR: Jeff Clark, Vice President Human Resources
Web address: www.kadlecmed.org
**Control:** Other not–for–profit (including NFP Corporation) **Service:** General Medical and Surgical

**Staffed Beds: 249 Admissions: 13372 Census: 154 Outpatient Visits:** 193990 **Births:** 2614 **Total Expense ($000):** 278030 **Payroll Expense ($000):** 105134 **Personnel:** 1545

★ **LOURDES COUNSELING CENTER (504008)**, 1175 Carondelet Drive, Zip 99354–3300; tel. 509/943–9104 **A**9 10 **F**3 29 30 38 50 64 98 99 100 101 103 104 106 **P**6 **S** Ascension Health, Saint Louis, MO
Primary Contact: Barbara Mead, Executive Director
CFO: Frank Becker, Chief Financial Officer
CIO: Vern Turney, Director Information Services
CHR: Craig K. Pearsall, Director Human Resources
Web address: www.lourdeshealth.net
**Control:** Church–operated, Nongovernment, not–for profit **Service:** Psychiatric

**Staffed Beds: 20 Admissions: 626 Census: 16 Outpatient Visits:** 65299 **Births:** 0 **Personnel:** 114

## RITZVILLE—Adams County

★ **EAST ADAMS RURAL HOSPITAL (501311)**, 903 South Adams Street, Zip 99169–2298; tel. 509/659–1200, (Nonreporting) **A**9 10 18
Primary Contact: Gary V. Peck, Interim Chief Executive Officer
CFO: Jennifer Wilbur, Interim Chief Financial Officer
CMO: Charles Sackman, M.D., Chief of Staff
CIO: Kellie Ottmar, Manager Information Services
CHR: Leslie Lzicar, Director Human Resources
Web address: www.earh.com
**Control:** Hospital district or authority, Government, nonfederal **Service:** General Medical and Surgical

**Staffed Beds: 10**

## SEATTLE—King County

**GROUP HEALTH COOPERATIVE CENTRAL HOSPITAL (500052)**, 201 16th Avenue East, Zip 98112; tel. 206/326–6300, (Nonreporting) **A**3 5 9 10 21
Primary Contact: Jane Hutcheson, Administrator
**Control:** Corporation, Investor–owned, for–profit **Service:** General Medical and Surgical

**Staffed Beds: 306**

✠ △ **HARBORVIEW MEDICAL CENTER (500064)**, 325 Ninth Avenue, Zip 98104–2499, Mailing Address: P.O. Box 359717, Zip 98195–9717; tel. 206/744–3000 **A**1 3 5 7 8 9 10 **F**3 5 8 16 17 18 20 22 29 30 31 34 35 36 37 38 40 43 45 46 49 50 56 57 58 59 61 64 65 66 68 70 72 73 74 75 77 78 79 80 81 82 84 85 86 87 88 89 90 91 93 94 96 97 98 100 101 102 104 105 107 108 111 113 114 116 117 118 123 125 128 129 130 131 134 143 145 146 147 **P**6 **S** UW Medicine, Seattle, WA
Primary Contact: Eileen Whalen, R.N., Executive Director
COO: Cynthia Hecker, Chief Nursing Officer and Senior Associate Administrator Patient Care Operations
CFO: Lori J. Mitchell, Chief Financial Officer
CMO: Richard Goss, M.D., Medical Director
CIO: James Fine, M.D., Executive Director Clinical Computing
CHR: Nicki McCraw, Assistant Vice President Human Resources
Web address: www.uwmedicine.washington.edu/pages/default.aspx
**Control:** County–Government, nonfederal **Service:** General Medical and Surgical

**Staffed Beds: 413 Admissions: 19879 Census: 374 Outpatient Visits:** 340036 **Births:** 0 **Total Expense ($000):** 692772 **Payroll Expense ($000):** 342689 **Personnel:** 4930

✠ **KINDRED HOSPITAL SEATTLE–NORTHGATE (502002)**, 10631 8th Avenue N.E., Zip 98125–0716; tel. 206/364–2050, (Includes KINDRED HOSPITAL SEATTLE–FIRST HILL, 1334 Terry Avenue, Zip 98101–2747; tel. 206/682–2661; Gregory Davis, Chief Executive Officer), (Nonreporting) **A**1 9 10 **S** Kindred Healthcare, Louisville, KY
Primary Contact: Lauren Suarez, Chief Executive Officer
CFO: David Stob, Chief Financial Officer
Web address: www.kindredhospitalseattle.com/
**Control:** Corporation, Investor–owned, for–profit **Service:** Long–Term Acute Care hospital

**Staffed Beds: 42**

☐ **NAVOS (504009)**, 2600 S.W. Holden Street, Zip 98126–3505; tel. 206/933–7199 **A**1 9 10 **F**29 97 98 99 100 101 102 103 104
Primary Contact: David Johnson, Chief Executive Officer
COO: Jerry Scott, Chief Operating Officer
CFO: Jerry Scott, Chief Operating Officer
CMO: Samir Aziz, M.D., Inpatient Medical Director
CIO: Jeff Coleman, Manager Information Systems
CHR: Judi Mitchell, Vice President Human Resources
Web address: www.navos.org
**Control:** Other not–for–profit (including NFP Corporation) **Service:** Psychiatric

**Staffed Beds: 69 Admissions: 1687 Census: 65 Outpatient Visits:** 0 **Births:** 0

✠ △ **NORTHWEST HOSPITAL & MEDICAL CENTER (500001)**, 1550 North 115th Street, Zip 98133–8401; tel. 206/364–0500 **A**1 2 3 5 7 9 10 **F**2 3 8 9 11 12 13 15 17 18 20 22 24 26 28 29 30 31 34 35 40 41 43 45 46 47 48 49 53 54 56 70 73 74 75 76 77 78 79 81 82 84 85 86 90 91 93 94 96 97 98 100 102 103 104 107 108 110 111 113 114 118 119 125 128 129 130 131 132 134 145 146 147 **P**1 8 **S** UW Medicine, Seattle, WA
Primary Contact: C. W. Schneider, President and Chief Executive Officer
COO: Annika Andrews, Senior Vice President and Chief Operating Officer
CFO: Bruce Ferguson, Chief Financial Officer
CMO: Greg Schroedl, M.D., Vice President Medical and Chief Quality Officer
CIO: Morton Latta, Chief Information Officer
CHR: Linda Olmstead, Director Human Resources
Web address: www.nwhospital.org
**Control:** Other not–for–profit (including NFP Corporation) **Service:** General Medical and Surgical

**Staffed Beds: 176 Admissions: 9576 Census: 123 Outpatient Visits:** 418442 **Births:** 1167 **Total Expense ($000):** 252110 **Payroll Expense ($000):** 100453 **Personnel:** 1290

✠ **REGIONAL HOSPITAL FOR RESPIRATORY AND COMPLEX CARE (502001)**, 12844 Military Road South, Zip 98168–3045; tel. 206/248–4548 **A**1 9 10 **F**1 29 30 50 85 87 129 147 **P**1 5
Primary Contact: Eric Jensen, Chief Executive Officer
COO: Barbara Hostetler, Chief Operating Officer and Chief Nursing Officer
CFO: Anne McBride, Chief Financial Officer
CMO: Robert L. Clark, M.D., Medical Director
CHR: Valerie Albano, Manager Human Resources
Web address: www.regionalhospital.org
**Control:** Other not–for–profit (including NFP Corporation) **Service:** Long–Term Acute Care hospital

**Staffed Beds: 31 Admissions: 191 Census: 23 Outpatient Visits:** 0 **Births:** 0 **Total Expense ($000):** 13558 **Payroll Expense ($000):** 8383 **Personnel:** 78

**WA**

**SCHICK SHADEL HOSPITAL**, 12101 Ambaum Boulevard S.W., Zip 98146–2699, Mailing Address: P.O. Box 48149, Zip 98148–0149; tel. 206/244–8100, (Nonreporting) **A**9
Primary Contact: Elaine Oksendahl, Administrator
CFO: Scott Miller, Chief Financial Officer
CMO: Ron Merchant, M.D., Medical Director
CIO: Henry Brown, Director Plant Operations and Information Technology
CHR: Janet Sill–Leahy, Manager Human Resources
Web address: www.schickshadel.com
**Control:** Corporation, Investor–owned, for–profit **Service:** Alcoholism and other chemical dependency

**Staffed Beds:** 48

☐ **SEATTLE CANCER CARE ALLIANCE (500138)**, 825 Eastlake Avenue East, Zip 98109, Mailing Address: P.O. Box 19023, Zip 98109–1023; tel. 206/288–1400 **A**1 2 9 10 **F**3 8 15 30 31 34 39 45 46 47 55 58 59 68 71 75 78 80 84 86 87 107 108 110 111 113 114 116 117 118 119 120 122 129 131 134 135 142 145 146
Primary Contact: Norm Hubbard, Executive Vice President
COO: Madeline Buelt, Vice President Operations
CFO: Jonathan Tingstad, Vice President and Chief Financial Officer
CMO: Marc Stewart, M.D., Vice President and Medical Director
CIO: David Ackerson, Chief Information Officer
CHR: Han Nachtrieb, Vice President Human Resources
Web address: www.seattlecca.org
**Control:** Other not–for–profit (including NFP Corporation) **Service:** Cancer

**Staffed Beds:** 18 **Admissions:** 654 **Census:** 16 **Outpatient Visits:** 72217 **Births:** 0 **Total Expense ($000):** 302539 **Payroll Expense ($000):** 61257

☐ △ **SEATTLE CHILDREN'S HOSPITAL (503300)**, 4800 Sand Point Way N.E., Zip 98105–3901, Mailing Address: P.O. Box 5371, Zip 98145–5005; tel. 206/987–2000, (Nonreporting) **A**1 2 3 5 7 8 9 10
Primary Contact: Thomas N. Hansen, M.D., Chief Executive Officer
COO: Patrick J. Hagan, President and Chief Operating Officer
CFO: Kelly Wallace, Senior Vice President and Chief Financial Officer
CMO: David Fisher, M.D., Senior Vice President and Medical Director
CIO: Drexel DeFord, Vice President and Chief Information Officer
CHR: Steven Hurwitz, Vice President Human Resources
Web address: www.seattlechildrens.org
**Control:** Other not–for–profit (including NFP Corporation) **Service:** Children's general

**Staffed Beds:** 250

✳ △ **SWEDISH MEDICAL CENTER–CHERRY HILL CAMPUS (500025)**, 500 17th Avenue, Zip 98122–5711; tel. 206/320–2000 **A**1 2 3 5 7 9 10 **F**3 11 15 17 18 20 22 24 26 28 29 30 31 34 35 39 40 42 44 45 46 48 49 50 53 54 57 58 59 60 61 64 65 66 68 71 74 75 77 78 79 81 82 84 85 86 87 90 92 93 94 96 97 98 99 100 101 102 103 104 106 107 108 109 110 111 112 114 118 119 120 122 123 128 129 131 134 145 146 147 **P**6 **S** Swedish Health Services, Seattle, WA
Primary Contact: Rayburn Lewis, M.D., Executive
CFO: Jeffrey Veilleux, Senior Vice President and Chief Financial Officer
CMO: John Vassall, M.D., Chief Medical Officer
CIO: Janice Newell, Chief Information Officer
CHR: Joanne Suffis, Vice President Human Resources
Web address: www.swedish.org
**Control:** Other not–for–profit (including NFP Corporation) **Service:** General Medical and Surgical

**Staffed Beds:** 198 **Admissions:** 8263 **Census:** 119 **Outpatient Visits:** 129154 **Births:** 0 **Total Expense ($000):** 365573 **Payroll Expense ($000):** 135802 **Personnel:** 1167

✳ **SWEDISH MEDICAL CENTER–FIRST HILL (500027)**, 747 Broadway, Zip 98122–4307; tel. 206/386–6000, (Includes SWEDISH MEDICAL CENTER–BALLARD, 5300 Tallman Avenue N.W., Zip 98107–3932; tel. 206/782–2700; Jennifer Graves, R.N., MS, Chief Executive) **A**1 2 3 5 9 10 **F**3 4 5 8 11 12 13 15 17 18 19 20 22 29 30 31 32 33 34 35 36 37 38 39 40 43 44 45 46 47 48 49 50 51 54 55 56 57 58 59 60 61 62 63 64 65 66 68 70 71 72 74 75 76 77 78 79 81 82 83 84 85 86 87 88 89 93 94 96 97 99 100 101 102 103 104 106 107 108 110 111 113 115 116 117 118 119 120 122 123 125 128 129 130 131 133 134 135 137 138 140 141 145 146 147 **P**6 **S** Swedish Health Services, Seattle, WA
Primary Contact: Todd Strumwasser, M.D., Chief Executive
CFO: Jeffrey Veilleux, Executive Vice President and Chief Financial Officer
CMO: John Vassall, M.D., Chief Medical Officer
CIO: Janice Newell, Chief Information Officer
CHR: Joanne Suffis, Vice President Human Resources
Web address: www.swedish.org
**Control:** Other not–for–profit (including NFP Corporation) **Service:** General Medical and Surgical

**Staffed Beds:** 620 **Admissions:** 32236 **Census:** 386 **Outpatient Visits:** 594925 **Births:** 7211 **Total Expense ($000):** 1003968 **Payroll Expense ($000):** 405298 **Personnel:** 4728

✳ △ **UNIVERSITY OF WASHINGTON MEDICAL CENTER (500008)**, 1959 N.E. Pacific Street, Zip 98195–6151; tel. 206/598–3300 **A**1 2 3 5 7 8 9 10 **F**3 8 9 11 12 13 15 17 18 20 22 24 25 26 28 29 30 31 34 35 36 39 40 44 45 46 47 48 49 50 51 52 54 55 56 57 58 59 60 61 64 65 68 70 72 74 75 76 77 78 79 80 81 82 84 85 86 87 90 91 92 93 94 95 96 97 98 100 101 102 103 104 106 107 108 110 111 113 114 115 116 117 118 119 120 122 123 125 129 130 131 135 136 137 138 139 140 141 143 144 145 146 147 **P**6 **S** UW Medicine, Seattle, WA
Primary Contact: Stephen P. Zieniewicz, FACHE, Executive Director
CFO: Paul Ishizuka, Chief Financial Officer
CMO: Tom Staiger, M.D., Medical Director
CHR: Jennifer J. Petritz, Director Human Resources
Web address: www.uwmedicine.washington.edu/pages/default.aspx
**Control:** State–Government, nonfederal **Service:** General Medical and Surgical

**Staffed Beds:** 396 **Admissions:** 18919 **Census:** 316 **Outpatient Visits:** 470998 **Births:** 1948 **Total Expense ($000):** 785115 **Payroll Expense ($000):** 297351 **Personnel:** 4749

✳ △ **VETERANS AFFAIRS PUGET SOUND HEALTH CARE SYSTEM**, 1660 South Columbian Way, Zip 98108–1597; tel. 206/762–1010, (Includes VETERANS AFFAIRS PUGET SOUND HEALTH CARE SYSTEM–AMERICAN LAKE DIVISION, Tacoma, Zip 98493; tel. 253/582–8440), (Nonreporting) **A**1 2 3 5 7 8 9 **S** Department of Veterans Affairs, Washington, DC
Primary Contact: David A. Elizalde, Director
CFO: Kenneth J. Hudson, Chief Financial Officer
CMO: Gordon Starkebaum, M.D., Chief of Staff
CIO: Glenn Zwinger, Manager Information Systems Services
Web address: www.va.gov/sta/guide/home.asp
**Control:** Veterans Affairs, Government, federal **Service:** General Medical and Surgical

**Staffed Beds:** 358

✳ △ **VIRGINIA MASON MEDICAL CENTER (500005)**, 1100 Ninth Avenue, Zip 98101–2756, Mailing Address: P.O. Box 900, Zip 98111–0900; tel. 206/223–6600, (Total facility includes 35 beds in nursing home–type unit) **A**1 2 3 5 7 9 10 **F**2 3 5 6 8 9 12 15 17 18 20 22 24 26 28 29 30 31 32 34 35 36 37 38 39 40 44 45 46 47 48 49 50 51 54 55 56 57 58 59 60 61 63 64 65 66 68 70 71 74 75 77 78 79 81 82 83 84 85 86 87 90 91 92 93 94 96 97 100 101 102 103 104 105 107 108 110 111 113 114 115 116 117 118 119 120 122 125 127 128 129 130 131 134 135 137 140 141 142 144 145 146 147 **P**6
Primary Contact: Gary Kaplan, M.D., Chairman and Chief Executive Officer
COO: Sarah Patterson, Executive Vice President and Chief Operating Officer
CFO: Sue Anderson, Senior Vice President, Chief Financial Officer and Chief Information Officer
CMO: Andrew Jacobs, M.D., Chief Medical Officer
CIO: Sue Anderson, Senior Vice President, Chief Financial Officer and Chief Information Officer
Web address: www.vmmc.org
**Control:** Other not–for–profit (including NFP Corporation) **Service:** General Medical and Surgical

**Staffed Beds:** 292 **Admissions:** 16542 **Census:** 238 **Outpatient Visits:** 864645 **Births:** 0 **Total Expense ($000):** 843454 **Payroll Expense ($000):** 428396 **Personnel:** 4868

**SEDRO WOOLLEY—Skagit County**

✳ **UNITED GENERAL HOSPITAL (501329)**, 2000 Hospital Drive, Zip 98284–4327; tel. 360/856–6021, (Nonreporting) **A**1 2 9 10 18
Primary Contact: Gregory C. Reed, FACHE, Chief Executive Officer
CFO: Michael W. Bonthuis, Chief Financial Officer
CMO: Edwin Stickle, M.D., Chief Medical Officer
CHR: Tracie Skrinde, Director Human Resources
Web address: www.unitedgeneral.org
**Control:** Hospital district or authority, Government, nonfederal **Service:** General Medical and Surgical

**Staffed Beds:** 25

**SHELTON—Mason County**

✳ **MASON GENERAL HOSPITAL (501336)**, 901 Mountain View Drive, Zip 98584–1668, Mailing Address: P.O. Box 1668, Zip 98584–5001; tel. 360/426–1611 **A**1 9 10 18 **F**11 13 15 29 30 40 57 68 70 75 79 81 83 85 107 110 129 131 146
Primary Contact: G. Robert Appel, Chief Executive Officer
COO: Eileen Branscome, Chief Operating Officer
CFO: Merle Brandt, Chief Financial Officer
CMO: Dean Gushee, M.D., Medical Director
CIO: Tom Hornburg, Director Information Systems
CHR: Claudia Hawley, Director Human Resources
Web address: www.masongeneral.com
**Control:** Hospital district or authority, Government, nonfederal **Service:** General Medical and Surgical

**Staffed Beds:** 25 **Admissions:** 1648 **Census:** 13 **Outpatient Visits:** 72560 **Births:** 241 **Total Expense ($000):** 59658 **Payroll Expense ($000):** 30459 **Personnel:** 414

WA

*Many Facility Codes have changed. Please refer to the AHA Guide Code Chart.* © 2012 AHA Guide

## SNOQUALMIE—King County

**SNOQUALMIE VALLEY HOSPITAL (501338)**, 9575 Ethan Wade Way S.E.,
Zip 98065–9577, Mailing Address: P.O. Box 2021, Zip 98065–2021;
tel. 425/831–2300, (Nonreporting) **A**9 10 18
Primary Contact: Rodger McCollum, Chief Executive Officer
Web address: www.snoqualmiehospital.org/
**Control:** Hospital district or authority, Government, nonfederal **Service:** General
Medical and Surgical

**Staffed Beds:** 18

## SOUTH BEND—Pacific County

**WILLAPA HARBOR HOSPITAL (501303)**, 800 Alder Street, Zip 98586–0438,
Mailing Address: P.O. Box 438, Zip 98586–0438; tel. 360/875–5526 **A**9 10 18
**F**3 8 11 15 34 35 40 41 45 46 50 81 85 87 92 97 107 110 113 118 126
132 144
Primary Contact: Carole Halsan, R.N., Chief Executive Officer
CFO: Terry Stone, Chief Financial Officer and Chief Information Officer
CIO: Terry Stone, Chief Financial Officer and Chief Information Officer
CHR: Krisy L. Funkhouser, Manager Human Resources
Web address: www.willapaharborhospital.com
**Control:** Hospital district or authority, Government, nonfederal **Service:** General
Medical and Surgical

**Staffed Beds:** 15 **Admissions:** 263 **Census:** 2 **Outpatient Visits:** 17154
**Births:** 0 **Total Expense ($000):** 13505 **Payroll Expense ($000):** 6497
**Personnel:** 98

## SPOKANE—Spokane County

✠ **DEACONESS MEDICAL CENTER (500044)**, 800 West Fifth Avenue,
Zip 99204–2803, Mailing Address: P.O. Box 248, Zip 99210–0248;
tel. 509/458–5800, (Nonreporting) **A**1 2 3 5 9 10 **S** Community Health Systems,
Inc., Franklin, TN
Primary Contact: William L. Gilbert, Chief Executive Officer
CFO: Garman E. Lutz, Chief Financial Officer
CIO: Paul Fitzpatrick, Manager Information Technology
Web address: www.deaconess–spokane.org
**Control:** Other not–for–profit (including NFP Corporation) **Service:** General
Medical and Surgical

**Staffed Beds:** 388

✠ **PROVIDENCE HOLY FAMILY HOSPITAL (500077)**, 5633 North Lidgerwood
Street, Zip 99208–1224; tel. 509/482–0111 **A**1 2 5 9 10 **F**3 4 8 11 12 13 15
18 20 22 29 30 31 34 35 37 38 39 40 41 43 45 46 47 48 49 50 53 56 57
58 59 60 61 64 68 70 73 74 75 76 77 78 79 81 82 84 85 86 87 89 92 93
100 107 108 120 122 128 129 130 131 134 142 144 145 146 147 **P**4 6
**S** Providence Health & Services, Renton, WA
Primary Contact: Elaine Couture, R.N., Chief Executive Officer
COO: Cathy J. Simchuk, Chief Operating Officer
CMO: Jeff Collins, M.D., Chief Medical Officer
CIO: Mark Vogelsang, Director Information Services
CHR: Patrick M. Clarry, Vice President Human Resources
Web address: www.providence.org
**Control:** Church–operated, Nongovernment, not–for profit **Service:** General
Medical and Surgical

**Staffed Beds:** 182 **Admissions:** 8910 **Census:** 93 **Outpatient Visits:** 115367
**Births:** 1226 **Total Expense ($000):** 172718 **Payroll Expense ($000):**
63993 **Personnel:** 797

✠ **PROVIDENCE SACRED HEART MEDICAL CENTER & CHILDREN'S HOSPITAL
(500054)**, 101 West Eighth Avenue, Zip 99204–2364, Mailing Address: P.O. Box
2555, Zip 99220–2555; tel. 509/474–3131, (Includes SACRED HEART
CHILDREN'S HOSPITAL, 101 West Eight Avenue, Zip 99204–2307, Mailing
Address: PO Box 2555, Zip 99220–2555, tel. 509/474–4841) **A**1 2 3 5 9 10
**F**3 8 11 12 13 15 16 17 18 19 20 21 22 23 24 25 26 27 28 29 30 31 35 36
37 40 43 45 46 47 48 49 50 56 57 58 60 64 68 70 72 74 75 76 78 79 81
82 83 84 85 86 87 88 89 92 98 99 100 102 103 104 105 106 107 108 110
111 113 114 117 118 119 120 122 123 125 129 131 136 137 140 144 145
146 147 **P**6 **S** Providence Health & Services, Renton, WA
Primary Contact: Elaine Couture, R.N., Chief Executive Officer
COO: Elaine Couture, R.N., Chief Executive Officer
CMO: Jeff Collins, M.D., Chief Medical Officer
CHR: Patrick Clary, Vice President Human Resources
Web address: www.shmc.org
**Control:** Church–operated, Nongovernment, not–for profit **Service:** General
Medical and Surgical

**Staffed Beds:** 628 **Admissions:** 28699 **Census:** 407 **Outpatient Visits:**
138522 **Births:** 2867 **Total Expense ($000):** 668587 **Payroll Expense
($000):** 243755 **Personnel:** 3089

☐ **SHRINERS HOSPITALS FOR CHILDREN (503302)**, 911 West Fifth Avenue,
Zip 99204, Mailing Address: P.O. Box 2472, Zip 99210–2472;
tel. 509/455–7844, (Nonreporting) **A**1 10 **S** Shriners Hospitals for Children,
Tampa, FL
Primary Contact: Eugene Raynaud, Administrator
CFO: Margreta Kilgore, Director Fiscal Services
CMO: Paul Caskey, M.D., Chief of Staff
CIO: Jeremy Long, Manager Information Systems
CHR: Odetta Webster, Director Human Resources
Web address: www.shrinershospital.org
**Control:** Other not–for–profit (including NFP Corporation) **Service:** Children's
orthopedic

**Staffed Beds:** 30

✠ △ **ST. LUKE'S REHABILITATION INSTITUTE (503025)**, 711 South Cowley
Street, Zip 99202–1388; tel. 509/473–6000 **A**1 7 9 10 **F**28 29 30 43 50 58
64 68 74 75 77 79 82 86 87 90 91 92 93 94 95 96 129 130 131 145 **P**6
Primary Contact: Thomas M. Fritz, Chief Executive Officer
COO: Ulrike Bersau, Administrator
CFO: John D. Craig, Chief Financial Officer
CMO: Stefan Humphries, M.D., Medical Director
CIO: Fred Galusha, Chief Information Officer
CHR: Phyllis Gabel, Chief Human Resource Officer
CNO: Ginger Cohen, Chief Nurse Executive
Web address: www.st–lukes.org
**Control:** Other not–for–profit (including NFP Corporation) **Service:** Rehabilitation

**Staffed Beds:** 102 **Admissions:** 1675 **Census:** 61 **Outpatient Visits:** 71458
**Births:** 0 **Total Expense ($000):** 35086 **Payroll Expense ($000):** 20554
**Personnel:** 446

✠ **VETERANS AFFAIRS MEDICAL CENTER**, 4815 North Assembly Street,
Zip 99205–6197; tel. 509/434–7200, (Total facility includes 34 beds in nursing
home–type unit) **A**1 5 9 **F**1 3 5 8 10 12 15 17 18 29 30 31 34 35 38 39 40
45 46 47 48 49 54 56 57 59 63 64 65 68 70 71 75 77 78 79 81 82 83 84
86 87 93 94 97 98 101 102 103 104 105 107 108 111 114 118 128 129
131 134 142 143 144 145 146 147 **S** Department of Veterans Affairs,
Washington, DC
Primary Contact: Sandy J. Nielsen, Director
COO: Cheryl L. Wood, Chief Engineering and Technology
CFO: Michael Gathman, Chief Financial Officer
CMO: Nirmala Rozario, M.D., Chief of Staff
CIO: Rob Fortenberry, Chief Information Officer
CHR: Jacqueline Ross, Chief Human Resources Officer
Web address: www.va.gov/sta/guide/home.asp
**Control:** Veterans Affairs, Government, federal **Service:** General Medical and
Surgical

**Staffed Beds:** 70 **Admissions:** 1637 **Census:** 25 **Outpatient Visits:** 305133
**Births:** 0 **Total Expense ($000):** 153967 **Payroll Expense ($000):** 79778

## SPOKANE VALLEY—Spokane County

✠ **VALLEY HOSPITAL AND MEDICAL CENTER (500119)**, 12606 East Mission
Avenue, Zip 99216–1090; tel. 509/924–6650 **A**1 2 9 10 **F**15 29 30 31 34 40
50 64 70 76 77 81 107 111 113 118 146 147 **S** Community Health Systems,
Inc., Franklin, TN
Primary Contact: Dennis Barts, Chief Executive Officer
COO: David Martin, Chief Operating Officer
CFO: Justin Voelker, Chief Financial Officer
CMO: Robert Hartman, M.D., Vice President Medical Affairs
Web address: www.valleyhospital.org
**Control:** Corporation, Investor–owned, for–profit **Service:** General Medical and
Surgical

**Staffed Beds:** 123 **Admissions:** 6164 **Census:** 60 **Outpatient Visits:** 54896
**Births:** 629 **Total Expense ($000):** 82837 **Payroll Expense ($000):** 37744
**Personnel:** 546

## SUNNYSIDE—Yakima County

★ **SUNNYSIDE COMMUNITY HOSPITAL (501330)**, 1016 Tacoma Avenue,
Zip 98944–0719, Mailing Address: P.O. Box 719, Zip 98944–0719;
tel. 509/837–1500 **A**9 10 18 **F**3 8 11 13 15 30 34 35 40 41 43 45 50 59 64
65 70 75 76 77 79 81 85 87 97 107 110 118 126 129 145 146 147
**S** HealthTech Management Services, Franklin, TN
Primary Contact: Robert L. Brendgard, Interim Chief Executive Officer
CFO: Martha Rodriguez, Chief Financial Officer
CMO: Coke R. Smith, M.D., Medical Director
CIO: Salvador Betancourt, Manager Information Systems
CHR: Lisa Garcia, Director Human Resources
Web address: www.sunnysidehospital.com
**Control:** Other not–for–profit (including NFP Corporation) **Service:** General
Medical and Surgical

**Staffed Beds:** 25 **Admissions:** 1363 **Census:** 10 **Outpatient Visits:** 61945
**Births:** 512 **Total Expense ($000):** 48694 **Payroll Expense ($000):** 24429

**WA**

---

**Hospital, Medicare Provider Number, Address, Telephone, Approval, Facility, and Physician Codes, Health Care System**

★ American Hospital Association (AHA) membership
☐ The Joint Commission accreditation
◇ DNV Healthcare Inc. accreditation
◯ American Osteopathic Association (AOA) accreditation
△ Commission on Accreditation of Rehabilitation Facilities (CARF) accreditation

## TACOMA—Pierce County

**ALLENMORE HOSPITAL** See MultiCare Tacoma General Hospital

✠ **MADIGAN HEALTHCARE SYSTEM**, Fitzsimmons Drive, Building 9040, Zip 98431–1100; tel. 253/968–1110 **A**1 2 3 5 9 **F**3 5 7 8 11 12 14 15 17 18 19 20 21 22 24 26 27 28 29 30 31 32 33 34 35 36 38 39 40 41 43 44 45 46 48 49 50 51 52 53 54 55 56 57 58 59 60 61 65 68 70 72 73 74 75 76 77 78 79 80 81 82 84 85 86 87 88 89 91 92 93 94 96 97 98 99 100 101 102 103 104 105 107 108 110 111 113 116 117 118 119 120 122 125 126 128 129 130 131 133 134 143 145 146 147 **S** Department of the Army, Office of the Surgeon General, Falls Church, VA
Primary Contact: Colonel Dallas Homas, Commander
COO: Colonel R. Neal David, Administrator and Chief of Staff
CFO: Lieutenant Colonel Bryan Longmuir, Chief Resource Management
CIO: Lieutenant Colonel Andrew Smith, Chief Information Management
CHR: David Aiken, Chief Human Resources Officer
Web address: www.mamc.amedd.army.mil
**Control:** Army, Government, federal **Service:** General Medical and Surgical

Staffed Beds: 235 Admissions: 15330 Census: 130 Outpatient Visits: 1264402 Births: 2555 Total Expense ($000): 540000 Payroll Expense ($000): 300000 Personnel: 4078

☐ **MULTICARE MARY BRIDGE CHILDREN'S HOSPITAL AND HEALTH CENTER (503301)**, 317 Martin Luther King Jr. Way, Zip 98405–0299, Mailing Address: P.O. Box 5299, Zip 98415–0299; tel. 253/403–1400 **A**1 3 5 9 10 **F**3 7 8 12 19 21 23 25 27 29 30 31 32 34 35 38 40 43 48 50 54 55 57 59 64 65 66 71 74 75 78 79 81 82 84 85 86 87 88 89 99 102 104 107 108 110 111 113 114 115 116 118 128 129 130 131 133 134 142 143 145 147 **S** MultiCare Health System, Tacoma, WA
Primary Contact: Mady Murrey, R.N., Vice President and Administrator
CFO: Vince Schmitz, Senior Vice President and Chief Financial Officer
CMO: Lester Reed, M.D., Vice President Medical Affairs and Acute Care
CIO: Florence Chang, Senior Vice President, Clinical Support Services and Chief Information Officer
CHR: Sarah Horsman, Senior Vice President Human Potential
Web address: www.multicare.org/marybridge
**Control:** Other not–for–profit (including NFP Corporation) **Service:** Children's general

Staffed Beds: 72 Admissions: 4366 Census: 38 Outpatient Visits: 36510 Births: 0 Total Expense ($000): 170511 Payroll Expense ($000): 56585 Personnel: 473

✠ **MULTICARE TACOMA GENERAL HOSPITAL (500129)**, 315 Martin Luther King Jr. Way, Zip 98405–0299, Mailing Address: P.O. Box 5299, Zip 98415–0299; tel. 253/403–1000, (Includes ALLENMORE HOSPITAL, South 19th and Union Avenue, Zip 98405, Mailing Address: P.O. Box 11414, Zip 98411–0414; tel. 253/403–2323) **A**1 2 3 5 9 10 **F**3 8 13 17 18 19 20 21 22 23 24 25 26 27 28 29 30 31 34 36 40 41 42 43 45 46 47 48 49 50 54 55 57 59 62 63 64 65 66 70 71 72 73 74 75 76 77 78 79 80 81 82 84 85 86 87 91 92 93 94 96 97 99 102 107 108 110 111 113 114 115 116 118 119 120 122 123 125 126 128 129 130 131 134 143 145 146 147 **S** MultiCare Health System, Tacoma, WA
Primary Contact: Diane E. Cecchettini, R.N., President and Chief Executive Officer
CFO: Vince Schmitz, Senior Vice President and Chief Financial Officer
CMO: Lester Reed, M.D., Vice President Medical Affairs and Acute Care
CIO: Florence Chang, Senior Vice President, Clinical Support Services and Chief Information Officer
CHR: Sarah Horsman, Senior Vice President Human Potential
Web address: www.multicare.org
**Control:** Other not–for–profit (including NFP Corporation) **Service:** General Medical and Surgical

Staffed Beds: 420 Admissions: 18302 Census: 223 Outpatient Visits: 221668 Births: 3000 Total Expense ($000): 592270 Payroll Expense ($000): 204030 Personnel: 2080

✠ △ **ST. JOSEPH MEDICAL CENTER (500108)**, 1717 South J Street, Zip 98405–3004, Mailing Address: P.O. Box 2197, Zip 98401–2197; tel. 253/426–4101, (Nonreporting) **A**1 2 5 7 9 10 **S** Catholic Health Initiatives, Englewood, CO
Primary Contact: Syd Bersante, President
COO: Syd Bersante, President
CFO: Mike Fitzgerald, Chief Financial Officer
CMO: Gregory Semerdjian, M.D., Senior Vice President Medical Affairs
CIO: Bruce Elkington, Vice President Information Technology
CHR: David Lawson, Senior Vice President Human Resources
Web address: www.fhshealth.org
**Control:** Church–operated, Nongovernment, not–for profit **Service:** General Medical and Surgical

Staffed Beds: 299

**VETERANS AFFAIRS PUGET SOUND HEALTH CARE SYSTEM–AMERICAN LAKE DIVISION** See Veterans Affairs Puget Sound Health Care System, Seattle

**WESTERN STATE HOSPITAL (504003)**, 9601 Steilacom Boulevard S.W., Zip 98498–7213; tel. 253/582–8900, (Nonreporting) **A**9 10
Primary Contact: Jess Jamieson, Chief Executive Officer
COO: Dale Thompson, Chief Operating Officer
CFO: Charm Reimer, Chief Financial Officer
CMO: John Chiles, M.D., Medical Director
CHR: Lori Manning, Administrator Human Resources
Web address: www.dshs.wa.gov/mentalhealth/wsh.shtml
**Control:** State–Government, nonfederal **Service:** Psychiatric

Staffed Beds: 867

## TONASKET—Okanogan County

★ **NORTH VALLEY HOSPITAL (501321)**, 203 South Western Avenue, Zip 98855; tel. 509/486–2151, (Nonreporting) **A**9 10 18
Primary Contact: Linda Michel, Administrator
COO: Marcia Naillon, Chief Operating Officer and Administrative Registered Nurse
CFO: Bomi Bharucha, Chief Financial Officer
CMO: Theresa M. DiCroce, M.D., Chief Medical Staff
CIO: John Boyd, Manager Information Systems
CHR: Jan Gonzales, Director Human Resources
Web address: www.nvhospital.org
**Control:** Hospital district or authority, Government, nonfederal **Service:** General Medical and Surgical

Staffed Beds: 85

## TOPPENISH—Yakima County

☐ **TOPPENISH COMMUNITY HOSPITAL (500037)**, 502 West Fourth Avenue, Zip 98948–0672, Mailing Address: P.O. Box 672, Zip 98948–0672; tel. 509/865–3105, (Nonreporting) **A**1 9 10 **S** Health Management Associates, Naples, FL
Primary Contact: Derrick Yu, Administrator
CFO: Curtis Herrin, Chief Financial Officer
CHR: Rosa Solorzano, Interim Director Human Resources
Web address: www.hma–corp.com
**Control:** Corporation, Investor–owned, for–profit **Service:** General Medical and Surgical

Staffed Beds: 63

## VANCOUVER—Clark County

**LEGACY SALMON CREEK HOSPITAL** See Legacy Salmon Creek Medical Center

✠ **LEGACY SALMON CREEK MEDICAL CENTER (500150)**, 2211 N.E. 139th Street, Zip 98686–2742; tel. 360/487–1000 **A**1 2 9 10 **F**3 11 13 15 18 20 26 28 29 30 31 32 33 38 39 40 44 45 47 49 50 51 57 59 60 64 65 68 70 72 74 75 76 77 78 79 80 81 82 84 85 87 89 93 96 97 102 105 107 108 110 111 113 115 116 117 118 119 120 125 128 129 131 145 146 147 **P**8 **S** Legacy Health, Portland, OR
Primary Contact: Jonathan Avery, Chief Administrative Officer
CFO: Pamela S. Vukovich, Senior Vice President and Chief Financial Officer
CMO: Jack Cioffi, M.D., Senior Vice President and Chief Medical Officer
CHR: Sonja Steves, Vice President Human Resources
Web address: www.legacyhealth.org
**Control:** Other not–for–profit (including NFP Corporation) **Service:** General Medical and Surgical

Staffed Beds: 194 Admissions: 10796 Census: 102 Outpatient Visits: 173654 Births: 2046 Total Expense ($000): 165675 Payroll Expense ($000): 82044 Personnel: 958

✠ △ **PEACEHEALTH SOUTHWEST MEDICAL CENTER (500050)**, 400 N.E. Mother Joseph Place, Zip 98664–3200, Mailing Address: P.O. Box 1600, Zip 98668–1600; tel. 360/256–2000, (Includes VANCOUVER MEMORIAL CAMPUS, 3400 Main Street, Zip 98663; tel. 206/696–5000), (Data for 183 days) **A**1 2 5 7 9 10 **F**3 11 12 13 15 17 18 20 22 24 26 28 29 30 31 34 35 40 42 43 44 45 46 49 50 51 54 57 58 59 60 61 62 63 64 65 68 70 72 73 74 75 76 77 78 79 81 82 84 85 86 87 89 90 92 93 94 97 98 100 101 102 103 104 105 107 108 109 110 111 113 114 115 116 118 119 120 121 123 125 128 129 130 131 134 143 144 145 146 147 **P**6 **S** PeaceHealth, Bellevue, WA
Primary Contact: Joseph M. Kortum, President and Chief Mission Officer
COO: Rainy Atkins, Chief Operating Officer and Administrator
CFO: David Willie, Chief Financial Officer
CMO: Alden Roberts, M.D., Chief Medical Officer
CIO: Petra Knowles, Chief Information Officer
CHR: Cheri Meyerhofer, Vice President Human Resources
Web address: www.swmedicalcenter.org
**Control:** Other not–for–profit (including NFP Corporation) **Service:** General Medical and Surgical

Staffed Beds: 450 Admissions: 12783 Census: 266 Outpatient Visits: 163181 Births: 1589 Total Expense ($000): 247355 Payroll Expense ($000): 103506 Personnel: 2788

**SOUTHWEST WASHINGTON MEDICAL CENTER** See PeaceHealth Southwest Medical Center

**WA**

## WALLA WALLA—Walla Walla County

★ **JONATHAN M. WAINWRIGHT MEMORIAL VA MEDICAL CENTER**, 77 Wainwright Drive, Zip 99362–3994; tel. 509/525–5200, (Nonreporting) **A**9 **S** Department of Veterans Affairs, Washington, DC
Primary Contact: Brian W. Westfield, MSN, Director
COO: Brian W. Westfield, MSN, Director
CIO: Gary Ramer, Manager Information Management
CHR: Mary C. Lee, Manager Human Resources
Web address: www.va.gov/sta/guide/home.asp
**Control:** Veterans Affairs, Government, federal **Service:** General Medical and Surgical

**Staffed Beds:** 14

🅐 △ **PROVIDENCE ST. MARY MEDICAL CENTER (500002)**, 401 West Poplar Street, Zip 99362, Mailing Address: P.O. Box 1477, Zip 99362–0312; tel. 509/525–3320 **A**1 2 7 9 10 19 **F**3 8 11 13 15 17 18 20 28 29 30 31 34 35 40 43 45 46 49 51 57 58 59 60 62 64 65 68 70 73 74 75 76 77 78 79 81 84 85 87 89 90 93 94 96 107 108 109 110 111 112 113 114 115 117 118 120 122 128 129 131 134 142 143 145 146 147 **P**6 **S** Providence Health & Services, Renton, WA
Primary Contact: Steven A. Burdick, Chief Executive Officer
CFO: Michael Parenteau, Vice President and Chief Financial Officer
CMO: Tim Davidson, M.D., Chief Executive Physician Services
CIO: Kathleen Obenland, Director Public Affairs
CHR: Susan Blackburn, Vice President Human Resources and Support Services
Web address: www.smmc.com
**Control:** Church–operated, Nongovernment, not–for profit **Service:** General Medical and Surgical

**Staffed Beds:** 76 **Admissions:** 3986 **Census:** 36 **Outpatient Visits:** 122595 **Births:** 573 **Total Expense ($000):** 144025 **Payroll Expense ($000):** 58924 **Personnel:** 799

**STATE PENITENTIARY HOSPITAL**, 1313 North 13th Street, Zip 99362–8817; tel. 509/525–3610, (Nonreporting)
Primary Contact: Pat Rima, Health Care Manager
**Control:** State–Government, nonfederal **Service:** Hospital unit of an institution (prison hospital, college infirmary, etc.)

**Staffed Beds:** 36

🅐 **WALLA WALLA GENERAL HOSPITAL (500049)**, 1025 South Second Avenue, Zip 99362–1398, Mailing Address: P.O. Box 1398, Zip 99362–0309; tel. 509/525–0480 **A**1 9 10 **F**13 15 20 28 29 30 34 35 40 43 45 49 52 56 57 59 62 64 68 69 70 73 74 75 76 79 81 82 83 85 87 89 93 97 107 110 111 114 118 126 128 129 131 132 134 145 146 147 **S** Adventist Health, Roseville, CA
Primary Contact: Monty E. Knittel, President and Chief Executive Officer
CFO: Duane Meidinger, Vice President Finance
CIO: Gary Dietz, Director Information Technology Services
CHR: Barbara Blood, Director Human Resources
Web address: www.wwgh.com
**Control:** Church–operated, Nongovernment, not–for profit **Service:** General Medical and Surgical

**Staffed Beds:** 37 **Admissions:** 1517 **Census:** 12 **Outpatient Visits:** 57003 **Births:** 270 **Total Expense ($000):** 49978 **Payroll Expense ($000):** 23187 **Personnel:** 439

## WENATCHEE—Chelan County

🅐 **CENTRAL WASHINGTON HOSPITAL (500016)**, 1201 South Miller Street, Zip 98801–1948, Mailing Address: P.O. Box 1887, Zip 98807–1887; tel. 509/662–1511, (Nonreporting) **A**1 9 10 13 19
Primary Contact: John B. Hamilton, FACHE, Interim President and Chief Executive Officer
COO: John B. Hamilton, FACHE, Executive Vice President and Chief Operating Officer
CFO: Steven R. Jacobs, Chief Financial Officer
CHR: Jack Powers, Director Human Resources
Web address: www.cwhs.com
**Control:** Other not–for–profit (including NFP Corporation) **Service:** General Medical and Surgical

**Staffed Beds:** 128

△ **WENATCHEE VALLEY HOSPITAL (500148)**, 820 North Chelan Avenue, Zip 98801–2028; tel. 509/663–8711 **A**2 5 7 9 10 **F**29 31 34 40 45 46 58 59 64 65 68 75 77 78 79 81 82 84 85 87 90 93 96 97 100 107 108 110 111 113 116 118 119 120 125 126 128 129 130 131 134 142 143 144 146 147 **P**8
Primary Contact: Shaun Koos, Administrator
COO: Kevin Gilbert, R.N., Director Surgical and Operations
CFO: John Doyle, Chief Financial Officer
CMO: Stuart Freed, M.D., Medical Director
CIO: Joe Janda, Chief Information Officer
CHR: Alan Patterson, Director Human Resources
Web address: www.wvmedical.com
**Control:** Corporation, Investor–owned, for–profit **Service:** Surgical

**Staffed Beds:** 20 **Admissions:** 1449 **Census:** 9 **Outpatient Visits:** 38809 **Total Expense ($000):** 78619 **Payroll Expense ($000):** 41328

## WHITE SALMON—Klickitat County

**SKYLINE HOSPITAL (501315)**, 211 Skyline Drive, Zip 98672–0099, Mailing Address: P.O. Box 99, Zip 98672–0099; tel. 509/493–1101 **A**9 10 18 **F**17 34 40 43 57 64 67 76 81 89 93 97 107 118 127 132 144 145 **P**5
Primary Contact: Michael J. Madden, Superintendent and Chief Executive Officer
CFO: Brenda Schneider, Chief Financial Officer
CMO: Cynthia Horton, M.D., Chief Medical Officer
CHR: Robin Loomis, Manager Human Resources
Web address: www.skylinehospital.com
**Control:** Hospital district or authority, Government, nonfederal **Service:** General Medical and Surgical

**Staffed Beds:** 25 **Admissions:** 513 **Census:** 4 **Outpatient Visits:** 21048 **Births:** 61 **Total Expense ($000):** 17049 **Payroll Expense ($000):** 9136 **Personnel:** 199

## YAKIMA—Yakima County

☐ △ **YAKIMA REGIONAL MEDICAL AND CARDIAC CENTER (500012)**, 110 South Ninth Avenue, Zip 98902–3397; tel. 509/575–5000, (Nonreporting) **A**1 2 3 5 7 9 10 **S** Health Management Associates, Naples, FL
Primary Contact: Richard H. Robinson, Chief Executive Officer
CFO: Curtis Herrin, Chief Financial Officer
CMO: Albert Brady, M.D., Chief of Staff
Web address: www.yakimaregional.net
**Control:** Corporation, Investor–owned, for–profit **Service:** General Medical and Surgical

**Staffed Beds:** 214

🅐 **YAKIMA VALLEY MEMORIAL HOSPITAL (500036)**, 2811 Tieton Drive, Zip 98902–3761; tel. 509/575–8000 **A**1 2 3 5 9 10 **F**3 8 11 13 15 18 20 22 28 29 30 31 32 34 35 40 43 44 45 46 47 49 50 51 55 57 59 60 62 63 64 68 70 72 73 74 75 76 77 78 79 81 82 84 85 86 87 89 92 98 100 102 104 107 108 111 113 115 116 118 119 120 122 123 128 129 130 131 134 143 145 146 147 **P**4 6 7
Primary Contact: Richard W. Linneweh, Jr., President and Chief Executive Officer
COO: Russ Myers, Senior Vice President and Chief Operating Officer
CFO: Scott Olander, Vice President and Chief Financial Officer
CMO: Gregory D. Sawyer, M.D., Vice President Physician Practices
CIO: Jeff Yamada, Assistant Vice President
CHR: Teresa Pritchard, Vice President
Web address: www.yakimamemorial.org
**Control:** Other not–for–profit (including NFP Corporation) **Service:** General Medical and Surgical

**Staffed Beds:** 222 **Admissions:** 14467 **Census:** 151 **Outpatient Visits:** 440612 **Births:** 3060 **Total Expense ($000):** 281731 **Payroll Expense ($000):** 108449 **Personnel:** 2194

**WA**

# WEST VIRGINIA

## BECKLEY—Raleigh County

☐ **BECKLEY ARH HOSPITAL (510062)**, 306 Stanaford Road, Zip 25801–3142; tel. 304/255–3000 **A**1 9 10 **F**3 11 15 17 18 20 28 29 30 31 34 35 38 39 40 43 44 45 46 47 48 49 50 54 57 59 60 61 62 64 65 70 74 75 77 78 79 81 82 85 86 87 89 90 93 97 98 99 100 101 102 103 107 108 110 111 114 115 117 118 128 129 145 **P**6 **S** Appalachian Regional Healthcare, Inc., Lexington, KY
Primary Contact: Rocco K. Massey, Community Chief Executive Officer
CMO: Prakash Puranik, M.D., Chief of Staff
CHR: Sue Thomas, Manager Human Resources
Web address: www.arh.org
**Control:** Other not–for–profit (including NFP Corporation) **Service:** General Medical and Surgical

| | |
|---|---|
| **Staffed Beds:** 167 **Admissions:** 7511 **Census:** 118 **Outpatient Visits:** 78567 **Births:** 0 **Total Expense ($000):** 72514 **Payroll Expense ($000):** 26623 **Personnel:** 480 | |

☒ **RALEIGH GENERAL HOSPITAL (510070)**, 1710 Harper Road, Zip 25801–3397; tel. 304/256–4100 **A**1 9 10 19 **F**3 13 15 17 18 20 22 29 30 34 35 40 43 49 57 59 60 64 70 75 76 78 79 81 85 87 89 93 107 110 111 113 114 116 118 129 130 131 145 146 **S** LifePoint Hospitals, Inc., Brentwood, TN
Primary Contact: Allen Peters, President and Chief Executive Officer
COO: Jim Bills, Chief Operating Officer
CFO: Tom Thompson, Vice President and Chief Financial Officer
CMO: Michael Kelly, M.D., President Medical Staff
CIO: Kevin Sexton, Director Information Systems
CHR: Matthew Hess, Director Human Resources
Web address: www.raleighgeneral.com
**Control:** Corporation, Investor–owned, for–profit **Service:** General Medical and Surgical

| | |
|---|---|
| **Staffed Beds:** 229 **Admissions:** 12461 **Census:** 159 **Outpatient Visits:** 106909 **Births:** 1447 **Total Expense ($000):** 121163 **Payroll Expense ($000):** 47830 **Personnel:** 929 | |

☒ **VETERANS AFFAIRS MEDICAL CENTER**, 200 Veterans Avenue, Zip 25801–6499; tel. 304/255–2121, (Nonreporting) **A**1 9 **S** Department of Veterans Affairs, Washington, DC
Primary Contact: Karin McGraw, Director
CFO: Chris Raines, Chief Fiscal Services
Web address: www.va.gov/sta/guide/home.asp
**Control:** Veterans Affairs, Government, federal **Service:** General Medical and Surgical

| | |
|---|---|
| **Staffed Beds:** 40 | |

## BERKELEY SPRINGS— County

★ **WAR MEMORIAL HOSPITAL (511309)**, One Healthy Way, Zip 25411; tel. 304/258–1234, (Total facility includes 16 beds in nursing home–type unit) **A**9 10 18 **F**3 11 15 28 29 34 35 40 45 50 53 54 57 59 65 77 81 85 86 93 97 107 118 129 132 **P**6 **S** Valley Health System, Winchester, VA
Primary Contact: Neil R. McLaughlin, R.N., President
CFO: Christine Lowman, Vice President Finance
CHR: Helen M. Miller, Director Human Resources
Web address: www.warmemorialhospital.com
**Control:** Other not–for–profit (including NFP Corporation) **Service:** General Medical and Surgical

| | |
|---|---|
| **Staffed Beds:** 41 **Admissions:** 494 **Census:** 24 **Outpatient Visits:** 37414 **Births:** 0 **Total Expense ($000):** 17755 **Payroll Expense ($000):** 7678 **Personnel:** 132 | |

## BLUEFIELD—Mercer County

☒ **BLUEFIELD REGIONAL MEDICAL CENTER (510071)**, 500 Cherry Street, Zip 24701–3390; tel. 304/327–1100 **A**1 9 10 12 13 19 **F**3 8 13 15 17 18 20 28 29 30 31 34 40 43 45 46 47 49 50 56 57 59 60 64 68 70 74 75 76 77 78 79 81 85 86 89 96 107 108 110 114 117 118 120 123 126 128 129 131 143 145 146 147 **P**8 **S** Community Health Systems, Inc., Franklin, TN
Primary Contact: William Hawley, Chief Executive Officer
CMO: Joel Shor, M.D., Chief of Staff
CIO: Rose Lasker, Director Information Services
CHR: Sandee Cheynet, Vice President Administrative Services
Web address: www.bluefield.org
**Control:** Corporation, Investor–owned, for–profit **Service:** General Medical and Surgical

| | |
|---|---|
| **Staffed Beds:** 240 **Admissions:** 5813 **Census:** 63 **Outpatient Visits:** 83195 **Births:** 620 **Total Expense ($000):** 75307 **Payroll Expense ($000):** 26659 **Personnel:** 613 | |

## BRIDGEPORT—Harrison County

☒ **UNITED HOSPITAL CENTER (510006)**, 327 Medical Park Drive, Zip 26330–9006; tel. 681/342–1000 **A**1 2 3 5 9 10 12 13 **F**3 5 11 13 15 17 18 20 22 28 29 30 31 34 36 38 39 40 45 46 48 49 51 54 57 58 59 60 62 63 64 65 68 70 74 75 76 77 78 79 81 82 84 85 86 87 89 93 97 98 99 100 101 102 103 104 107 108 109 110 111 113 114 115 116 117 118 119 120 122 127 128 129 131 145 147 **P**6 8 **S** West Virginia United Health System, Fairmont, WV
Primary Contact: Bruce C. Carter, President
COO: Michael Tillman, Vice President Patient Services and Chief Operating Officer
CFO: Douglas Coffman, Vice President and Chief Financial Officer
CMO: Eric Radcliffe, M.D., Medical Director
CIO: Brian Cottrill, Chief Information Officer
CHR: Timothy M. Allen, Vice President Human Resources
Web address: www.uhcwv.org
**Control:** Other not–for–profit (including NFP Corporation) **Service:** General Medical and Surgical

| | |
|---|---|
| **Staffed Beds:** 264 **Admissions:** 13108 **Census:** 197 **Outpatient Visits:** 413367 **Births:** 902 **Total Expense ($000):** 218173 **Payroll Expense ($000):** 85692 **Personnel:** 1685 | |

## BUCKEYE—Pocahontas County

★ **POCAHONTAS MEMORIAL HOSPITAL (511314)**, RR2, Box 52W, Zip 24924; tel. 304/799–7400 **A**9 10 18 **F**2 3 7 11 29 30 34 35 40 56 57 59 64 65 86 87 93 97 107 108 118 127 129 131 132 134 143
Primary Contact: Barbara Lay, Chief Executive Officer
CFO: Marvina Irvine, Chief Financial Officer
CMO: Luis Soriano, M.D., Chief of Staff
CIO: Marvina Irvine, Chief Financial Officer
CHR: Sara Casto, Executive Secretary
Web address: www.wvha.com/web/pmh/index.htm
**Control:** County–Government, nonfederal **Service:** General Medical and Surgical

| | |
|---|---|
| **Staffed Beds:** 25 **Admissions:** 269 **Census:** 3 **Outpatient Visits:** 15896 **Births:** 0 **Total Expense ($000):** 6612 **Payroll Expense ($000):** 3946 **Personnel:** 107 | |

## BUCKHANNON—Upshur County

☒ **ST. JOSEPH'S HOSPITAL OF BUCKHANNON (510053)**, 1 Amalia Drive, Zip 26201–2222; tel. 304/473–2000, (Total facility includes 16 beds in nursing home–type unit) **A**1 9 10 **F**3 11 13 15 18 28 29 30 31 34 35 40 43 44 50 57 59 62 63 64 65 70 75 76 79 81 84 85 87 89 107 110 113 118 127 128 129 131 132 134 143 145 **P**6 **S** Pallottine Health Services, Huntington, WV
Primary Contact: Sue E. Johnson–Phillippe, President and Chief Executive Officer
CFO: Renee Hofer, Senior Vice President Fiscal Services
CMO: Robert Blake, M.D., Chief of Staff
CIO: Brian Williams, Director Information Systems
CHR: Anissa Hite–Davis, Vice President Human Resources
Web address: www.stj.net
**Control:** Other not–for–profit (including NFP Corporation) **Service:** General Medical and Surgical

| | |
|---|---|
| **Staffed Beds:** 69 **Admissions:** 1403 **Census:** 29 **Outpatient Visits:** 99586 **Births:** 304 **Total Expense ($000):** 39120 **Payroll Expense ($000):** 18445 **Personnel:** 377 | |

**WV**

*Many Facility Codes have changed. Please refer to the AHA Guide Code Chart.* © 2012 AHA Guide

## CHARLESTON—Kanawha County

☒ △ **CHARLESTON AREA MEDICAL CENTER (510022)**, 501 Morris Street, Zip 25301–1300, Mailing Address: P.O. Box 1547, Zip 25326–1547; tel. 304/388–5432, (Includes GENERAL HOSPITAL, 501 Morris Street, Zip 25301, Mailing Address: Box 1393, Zip 25325; tel. 304/388–5432; Michael D. Williams, Vice President and Administrator; MEMORIAL HOSPITAL, 3200 MacCorkle Avenue S.E., Zip 25304; tel. 304/388–5973; WOMEN AND CHILDREN'S HOSPITAL, 800 Pennsylvania Avenue, Zip 25302, Mailing Address: P.O. Box 6669, Zip 25362; tel. 304/388–5432; Andrew Weber, Vice President and Administrator) **A**1 2 3 5 7 8 9 10 12 13 **F**3 8 11 12 13 15 17 18 19 20 22 24 26 28 29 30 31 32 34 35 38 40 41 43 44 45 46 47 48 49 50 51 52 54 55 56 57 59 60 61 64 65 68 70 72 74 75 76 77 78 79 81 82 84 85 86 88 89 90 92 93 94 96 97 98 99 100 101 102 103 104 107 108 110 111 113 114 115 116 117 118 123 125 128 129 130 131 133 134 137 140 142 143 144 145 146 147 **P**6 **S** Charleston Area Medical Center Health System, Inc., Charleston, WV
Primary Contact: David L. Ramsey, President and Chief Executive Officer
COO: Glenn Crotty, Jr., M.D., Executive Vice President and Chief Operating Officer
CFO: Larry C. Hudson, Executive Vice President and Chief Financial Officer
CMO: Elizabeth L. Spangler, M.D., Vice President Medical Affairs
CIO: Lynn Brookshire, Vice President Information Services and Chief Information Officer
CHR: Beth A. Samples, Vice President Human Resources
Web address: www.camc.org
**Control:** Other not–for–profit (including NFP Corporation) **Service:** General Medical and Surgical

**Staffed Beds:** 795 **Admissions:** 37605 **Census:** 556 **Outpatient Visits:** 562854 **Births:** 2910 **Total Expense ($000):** 660499 **Payroll Expense ($000):** 259666 **Personnel:** 5562

☐ **EYE AND EAR CLINIC OF CHARLESTON (510059)**, 1306 Kanawha Boulevard East, Zip 25301–3001, Mailing Address: P.O. Box 2271, Zip 25328–2271; tel. 304/343–4371 **A**1 10 **F**39 45 57 64 79 81 89 111 118 140
Primary Contact: Christina Arvon, Administrator and Chief Executive Officer
CMO: James W. Candill, M.D., President Medical Staff
Web address: www.eyeandearclinicwv.org
**Control:** Corporation, Investor–owned, for–profit **Service:** General Medical and Surgical

**Staffed Beds:** 21 **Admissions:** 3 **Census:** 1 **Outpatient Visits:** 11357 **Births:** 0 **Total Expense ($000):** 10440 **Payroll Expense ($000):** 3932 **Personnel:** 103

**GENERAL HOSPITAL** See Charleston Area Medical Center

☒ **HIGHLAND HOSPITAL (514001)**, 300 56th Street S.E., Zip 25304–2361, Mailing Address: P.O. Box 4107, Zip 25364–4107; tel. 304/926–1600 **A**1 9 10 **F**29 35 57 75 92 98 99 101 105 129 **P**6
Primary Contact: David M. McWatters, III, President and Chief Executive Officer
CFO: Lisa Layden, Director of Finance
CMO: Charles Weise, M.D., Medical Director
CIO: Pearl McWatters, Director Information Services
Web address: www.highlandhosp.com
**Control:** Other not–for–profit (including NFP Corporation) **Service:** Psychiatric

**Staffed Beds:** 58 **Admissions:** 1300 **Census:** 36 **Outpatient Visits:** 1924 **Births:** 0 **Total Expense ($000):** 10035 **Payroll Expense ($000):** 5959 **Personnel:** 235

**MEMORIAL HOSPITAL** See Charleston Area Medical Center

☒ **SAINT FRANCIS HOSPITAL (510031)**, 333 Laidley Street, Zip 25301–1628, Mailing Address: P.O. Box 471, Zip 25322–0471; tel. 304/347–6500, (Total facility includes 29 beds in nursing home–type unit) **A**1 9 10 **F**3 11 19 20 22 29 30 34 40 46 48 49 51 57 59 60 64 68 69 70 74 75 79 81 82 84 86 87 93 97 107 108 110 111 114 115 118 127 129 130 134 142 144 145 146 147 **P**5 **S** Thomas Health System, Inc., South Charleston, WV
Primary Contact: Stephen P. Dexter, President and Chief Executive Officer
COO: Daniel Lauffer, FACHE, Executive Vice President and Chief Operating Officer
CFO: Charles O. Covert, Chief Financial Officer
CMO: Dionisio Policarpio, M.D., President Medical Staff
CIO: Jane Harless, Director Information Services
CHR: Marybeth Smith, Director Human Resources
Web address: www.stfrancishospital.com
**Control:** Other not–for–profit (including NFP Corporation) **Service:** General Medical and Surgical

**Staffed Beds:** 142 **Admissions:** 3775 **Census:** 57 **Outpatient Visits:** 87521 **Births:** 0 **Total Expense ($000):** 95481 **Payroll Expense ($000):** 29748 **Personnel:** 659

☒ **SELECT SPECIALTY HOSPITAL–CHARLESTON (512002)**, 333 Laidley Street, Zip 25322; tel. 304/720–7234 **A**1 9 10 **F**1 29 74 75 79 85 129 147 **S** Select Medical Corporation, Mechanicsburg, PA
Primary Contact: Frank Weber, Chief Executive Officer
CHR: Sabrina White, Coordinator Human Resources
Web address: www.selectmedical.com
**Control:** Corporation, Investor–owned, for–profit **Service:** Long–Term Acute Care hospital

**Staffed Beds:** 32 **Admissions:** 409 **Census:** 30 **Outpatient Visits:** 0 **Births:** 0 **Total Expense ($000):** 15216 **Payroll Expense ($000):** 5319 **Personnel:** 108

**WOMEN AND CHILDREN'S HOSPITAL** See Charleston Area Medical Center

## CLARKSBURG—Harrison County

☒ **LOUIS A. JOHNSON VETERANS AFFAIRS MEDICAL CENTER**, 1 Medical Center Drive, Zip 26301–4199; tel. 304/623–3461, (Nonreporting) **A**1 3 5 9 **S** Department of Veterans Affairs, Washington, DC
Primary Contact: Beth Brown, Director
CMO: Glenn R. Snider, M.D., Chief of Staff
CIO: Michael Matthey, Facility Chief Information Officer
CHR: Ian Jacobs, Chief, Human Resource Management Service
Web address: www.clarksburg.va.gov
**Control:** Veterans Affairs, Government, federal **Service:** General Medical and Surgical

**Staffed Beds:** 71

## ELKINS—Randolph County

☒ **DAVIS MEMORIAL HOSPITAL (510030)**, Gorman Avenue and Reed Street, Zip 26241, Mailing Address: P.O. Box 1484, Zip 26241–1484; tel. 304/636–3300 **A**1 2 9 10 20 **F**11 13 15 20 28 29 30 31 34 35 40 49 50 51 54 57 59 64 68 69 70 71 74 75 76 77 78 79 81 82 85 86 87 89 92 93 107 108 109 110 111 114 115 116 117 118 120 122 128 129 131 134 145 146 147 **P**8 **S** Davis Health System, Elkins, WV
Primary Contact: Mark Doak, President and Chief Executive Officer
COO: D. Parker Haddix, Chief Operating Officer
CFO: Rebecca J. Hammer, Chief Financial Officer
CMO: Nitesh Ratnakar, M.D., Chief Medical Officer
CHR: Judith L. Williams, Director Human Resources
Web address: www.davishealthsystem.com
**Control:** Other not–for–profit (including NFP Corporation) **Service:** General Medical and Surgical

**Staffed Beds:** 90 **Admissions:** 4791 **Census:** 46 **Outpatient Visits:** 136176 **Births:** 334 **Total Expense ($000):** 73558 **Payroll Expense ($000):** 31139 **Personnel:** 567

## FAIRMONT—Marion County

☒ **FAIRMONT GENERAL HOSPITAL (510047)**, 1325 Locust Avenue, Zip 26554–1435; tel. 304/367–7100 **A**1 2 9 10 19 **F**3 5 11 13 15 18 20 28 29 30 31 34 35 38 40 43 44 45 48 49 50 51 54 55 57 59 61 62 65 68 69 70 74 75 76 78 79 81 84 85 86 87 89 92 96 98 99 100 101 102 103 104 107 108 111 113 114 115 116 117 118 128 129 130 131 133 134 145 146 147 **P**6 7
Primary Contact: Robert C. Marquardt, FACHE, President and Chief Executive Officer
CFO: Daniel Honerbrink, Vice President Finance and Chief Financial Officer
CMO: Richard Simpson, M.D., Chief of Staff
CIO: John Stone, Director Information Services and Chief Information Officer
CHR: John R. Petrov, Vice President Human Resources
Web address: www.fghi.com
**Control:** Other not–for–profit (including NFP Corporation) **Service:** General Medical and Surgical

**Staffed Beds:** 116 **Admissions:** 5010 **Census:** 81 **Outpatient Visits:** 187516 **Births:** 444 **Total Expense ($000):** 81802 **Payroll Expense ($000):** 27747 **Personnel:** 636

## GASSAWAY—Braxton County

★ **BRAXTON COUNTY MEMORIAL HOSPITAL (511308)**, 100 Hoylman Drive, Zip 26624–9320; tel. 304/364–5156 **A**9 10 18 **F**3 8 11 15 30 32 34 35 40 43 45 57 59 62 64 75 81 97 107 108 113 115 126 129 132 145 146 **P**6
Primary Contact: Ben Vincent, FACHE, Chief Executive Officer
CFO: Kimber Knight, Chief Financial Officer
CMO: Russell L. Stewart, M.D., Chief Medical Officer
Web address: www.braxtonmemorial.org
**Control:** Other not–for–profit (including NFP Corporation) **Service:** General Medical and Surgical

**Staffed Beds:** 25 **Admissions:** 346 **Census:** 3 **Outpatient Visits:** 41457 **Births:** 0 **Total Expense ($000):** 14441 **Payroll Expense ($000):** 6528 **Personnel:** 156

**WV**

---

**Hospital, Medicare Provider Number, Address, Telephone, Approval, Facility, and Physician Codes, Health Care System**

★ American Hospital Association (AHA) membership
☐ The Joint Commission accreditation
◇ DNV Healthcare Inc. accreditation
○ American Osteopathic Association (AOA) accreditation
△ Commission on Accreditation of Rehabilitation Facilities (CARF) accreditation

## GLEN DALE—Marshall County

✠ **REYNOLDS MEMORIAL HOSPITAL (510013)**, 800 Wheeling Avenue, Zip 26038–1697; tel. 304/845–3211, (Total facility includes 20 beds in nursing home–type unit) **A**1 9 10 **F**3 11 13 15 18 20 28 30 34 39 40 43 53 56 57 59 62 64 65 70 74 75 76 77 78 79 80 81 84 85 86 89 92 93 107 108 110 111 113 117 118 127 129 131 134 145 147 **P**8
Primary Contact: Jay E. Prager, Chief Executive Officer
CFO: William Robert Hunt, Chief Financial Officer
CMO: David F. Hess, M.D., President Medical Staff
CIO: Warren Kelley, Chief Information Officer
CHR: R. Craig Madden, Director Employee Relations
Web address: www.reynoldsmemorial.com
**Control:** Other not–for–profit (including NFP Corporation) **Service:** General Medical and Surgical

**Staffed Beds:** 127 **Admissions:** 2820 **Census:** 47 **Outpatient Visits:** 77439 **Births:** 103 **Total Expense ($000):** 35768 **Payroll Expense ($000):** 17224 **Personnel:** 355

## GRAFTON—Taylor County

**GRAFTON CITY HOSPITAL (511307)**, 500 Market Street, Zip 26354–1187; tel. 304/265–0400, (Nonreporting) **A**9 10 18
Primary Contact: Patrick Shaw, Chief Executive Officer
CFO: Susie Higgins, Chief Financial Officer
CFO: Brian Kelbaugh, Chief Financial Officer
CMO: Christopher Villaraza, II, M.D., Chief Medical Staff
CIO: Ann Rexroad, Director Information Technology
CHR: Missey Kimbrew, Director Human Resources
CNO: Violet Shaw, R.N., Director of Nursing
Web address: www.graftonhospital.com
**Control:** City–Government, nonfederal **Service:** General Medical and Surgical

**Staffed Beds:** 101

## GRANTSVILLE—Calhoun County

★ **MINNIE HAMILTON HEALTHCARE CENTER (511303)**, 186 Hospital Drive, Zip 26147; tel. 304/354–9244, (Total facility includes 24 beds in nursing home–type unit) **A**9 10 18 **F**3 7 11 15 29 30 32 34 35 36 39 40 41 44 50 53 56 57 59 61 64 65 66 68 75 82 84 86 87 93 97 99 101 107 108 118 126 128 129 131 132 133 134 142 143 145 146 147 **P**6
Primary Contact: Steve Whited, Chief Executive Officer
COO: Steve Whited, Chief Operating Officer
CFO: Steve Whited, Chief Operating Officer
CMO: Vishwanath Hande, M.D., Chief Medical Officer
CIO: Brent Barr, Chief Information Officer
CHR: Sheila Gherke, Director Human Resources
Web address: www.mhhcc.com
**Control:** Other not–for–profit (including NFP Corporation) **Service:** General Medical and Surgical

**Staffed Beds:** 42 **Admissions:** 332 **Census:** 26 **Outpatient Visits:** 62151 **Births:** 0 **Total Expense ($000):** 16071 **Payroll Expense ($000):** 9820 **Personnel:** 245

## HINTON—Summers County

☐ **SUMMERS COUNTY ARH HOSPITAL (511310)**, Terrace Street, Zip 25951–2407, Mailing Address: Drawer 940, Zip 25951–0940; tel. 304/466–1000, (Total facility includes 36 beds in nursing home–type unit) **A**1 9 10 18 **F**11 15 29 30 32 34 35 40 43 44 50 54 57 59 62 64 65 67 71 81 82 86 87 90 93 97 107 113 118 126 127 129 132 145 146 147 **P**6
**S** Appalachian Regional Healthcare, Inc., Lexington, KY
Primary Contact: Wesley Dangerfield, Community Chief Executive Officer
CFO: Ryan St. John, Assistant Administrator
CMO: Ajay Anand, M.D., President Medical Staff
CIO: Polly Bentley, Chief Information Officer
CHR: Nancy Whitlock, Manager Human Resources
Web address: www.arh.org
**Control:** Other not–for–profit (including NFP Corporation) **Service:** General Medical and Surgical

**Staffed Beds:** 61 **Admissions:** 730 **Census:** 20 **Outpatient Visits:** 26048 **Births:** 0 **Total Expense ($000):** 13356 **Payroll Expense ($000):** 5235 **Personnel:** 107

## HUNTINGTON—Cabell County

✠ **CABELL HUNTINGTON HOSPITAL (510055)**, 1340 Hal Greer Boulevard, Zip 25701–0195; tel. 304/526–2000, (Total facility includes 15 beds in nursing home–type unit) **A**1 2 3 5 9 10 12 13 **F**3 7 11 12 13 15 16 17 18 19 20 26 28 29 30 31 32 34 35 37 38 39 40 41 43 44 45 46 49 50 51 52 54 55 56 57 58 59 60 61 62 64 65 66 70 72 73 74 75 76 77 78 79 81 82 84 85 86 87 88 89 92 93 96 97 107 108 110 111 113 114 116 117 118 119 120 122 125 127 128 129 130 131 134 143 144 145 146 147 **P**8
Primary Contact: Brent A. Marsteller, President and Chief Executive Officer
COO: Glen A. Washington, Senior Vice President and Chief Operating Officer
CFO: David M. Ward, Senior Vice President and Chief Financial Officer
CMO: Hoyt J. Burdick, M.D., Vice President Medical Affairs
CHR: Barry Tourigny, Vice President Human Resources and Organizational Development
Web address: www.cabellhuntington.org
**Control:** Other not–for–profit (including NFP Corporation) **Service:** General Medical and Surgical

**Staffed Beds:** 303 **Admissions:** 24942 **Census:** 220 **Outpatient Visits:** 472092 **Births:** 2468 **Total Expense ($000):** 345104 **Payroll Expense ($000):** 121718 **Personnel:** 2022

☐ **CORNERSTONE HOSPITAL OF HUNTINGTON (512003)**, 2900 First Avenue, Two East, Zip 25702; tel. 304/399–2600, (Nonreporting) **A**1 9 10 **S** Cornerstone Healthcare Group, Dallas, TX
Primary Contact: Cynthia Isaacs, Chief Executive Officer
CFO: Frank Carter, Chief Financial Officer
CMO: William Beam, M.D., Chief of Staff
Web address: www.chghospitals.com
**Control:** Corporation, Investor–owned, for–profit **Service:** Long–Term Acute Care hospital

**Staffed Beds:** 28

✠ **HEALTHSOUTH HUNTINGTON REHABILITATION HOSPITAL (513028)**, 6900 West Country Club Drive, Zip 25705–2000; tel. 304/733–1060 **A**1 10 **F**29 59 90 95 96 131 145 **S** HEALTHSOUTH Corporation, Birmingham, AL
Primary Contact: Michael E. Zuliani, Chief Executive Officer
CHR: Chad Bailey, Director of Human Resources
Web address: www.healthsouthhuntington.com
**Control:** Corporation, Investor–owned, for–profit **Service:** Rehabilitation

**Staffed Beds:** 52 **Admissions:** 1121 **Census:** 45 **Outpatient Visits:** 0 **Births:** 0 **Total Expense ($000):** 11578 **Payroll Expense ($000):** 6505 **Personnel:** 153

☐ **MILDRED MITCHELL–BATEMAN HOSPITAL (514009)**, 1530 Norway Avenue, Zip 25705–1358, Mailing Address: P.O. Box 448, Zip 25709–0448; tel. 304/525–7801 **A**1 9 10 **F**11 29 30 86 87 98 99 105 129 134 145 **P**6
Primary Contact: Mary Beth Carlisle, Chief Executive Officer
COO: Mary Beth Carlisle, Chief Executive Officer
CFO: James Spencer, Chief Financial Officer
CMO: Shahid Masood, M.D., Clinical Director
CIO: Elias Majdalani, Director Management Information Systems
CHR: Kieth Anne Worden, Director Human Resources
Web address: www.batemanhospital.org
**Control:** State–Government, nonfederal **Service:** Psychiatric

**Staffed Beds:** 110 **Admissions:** 563 **Census:** 104 **Outpatient Visits:** 0 **Births:** 0

☐ **RIVER PARK HOSPITAL (514008)**, 1230 Sixth Avenue, Zip 25701–2312, Mailing Address: P.O. Box 1875, Zip 25719–1875; tel. 304/526–9111 **A**1 9 10 **F**29 34 35 38 40 98 99 100 101 102 103 106 129 142 **S** Universal Health Services, Inc., King of Prussia, PA
Primary Contact: Terry A. Stephens, Chief Executive Officer
CFO: Steve Kuhn, Chief Financial Officer
CMO: David J. Humphreys, M.D., Medical Director
CIO: Tony Radenheimer, Network Administrator
CHR: Mary Stratton, Director Human Resources
CNO: Charles Christopher Whitt, Chief Nursing Officer
Web address: www.riverparkhospital.net
**Control:** Corporation, Investor–owned, for–profit **Service:** Psychiatric

**Staffed Beds:** 147 **Admissions:** 1452 **Census:** 132 **Outpatient Visits:** 0 **Births:** 0 **Total Expense ($000):** 18914 **Payroll Expense ($000):** 10321 **Personnel:** 306

**WV**

*Many Facility Codes have changed. Please refer to the AHA Guide Code Chart.* © 2012 AHA Guide

✖ **ST. MARY'S MEDICAL CENTER (510007)**, 2900 First Avenue,
Zip 25702–1272; tel. 304/526–1234, (Total facility includes 19 beds in nursing home–type unit) **A**1 2 3 5 9 10 **F**3 9 11 12 13 15 17 18 20 22 24 26 28 29 30 31 32 34 35 36 40 43 44 45 46 47 48 49 50 53 55 57 58 59 60 62 64 65 66 67 68 70 73 74 75 76 77 78 79 81 82 84 85 86 87 89 92 93 96 97 98 100 101 102 103 107 108 110 111 113 114 117 118 119 120 122 123 125 127 128 129 131 132 134 144 145 146 147 **P**8 **S** Pallottine Health Services, Huntington, WV
Primary Contact: Michael G. Sellards, President and Chief Executive Officer
COO: Todd Campbell, Senior Vice President and Chief Operating Officer
CMO: Tyson Smith, M.D., Vice President Medical Affairs
CIO: Charles Wilson, Director Information Systems
CHR: Susan Beth McKenzie, Vice President Human Resources
Web address: www.st-marys.org
**Control:** Church–operated, Nongovernment, not–for profit **Service:** General Medical and Surgical

**Staffed Beds:** 375 **Admissions:** 17440 **Census:** 259 **Outpatient Visits:** 260612 **Births:** 435 **Total Expense ($000):** 318683 **Payroll Expense ($000):** 108551 **Personnel:** 2146

✖ **VETERANS AFFAIRS MEDICAL CENTER**, 1540 Spring Valley Drive,
Zip 25704–9300; tel. 304/429–6741, (Nonreporting) **A**1 3 5 9 **S** Department of Veterans Affairs, Washington, DC
Primary Contact: Edward H. Seiler, Director
CIO: Gary Henderson, Chief Information Resources Management Services
Web address: www.huntington.va.gov/
**Control:** Veterans Affairs, Government, federal **Service:** General Medical and Surgical

**Staffed Beds:** 80

### HURRICANE—Putnam County

✖ **CAMC TEAYS VALLEY HOSPITAL (510085)**, 1400 Hospital Drive,
Zip 25526–9202; tel. 304/757–1700 **A**1 9 10 **F**3 11 15 28 29 34 35 39 40 45 46 47 50 54 56 57 59 64 65 70 74 75 77 79 81 82 85 87 93 97 100 102 107 108 110 111 114 117 118 129 130 131 134 144 145 147 **S** Charleston Area Medical Center Health System, Inc., Charleston, WV
Primary Contact: Randall H. Hodges, President and Chief Executive Officer
CFO: Larry C. Hudson, Executive Vice President and Chief Financial Officer
CMO: Elizabeth L. Spangler, M.D., Vice President Medical Affairs and Chief Medical Officer
CIO: Lynn Brookshire, Vice President Information Services and Chief Information Officer
CHR: Beth A. Samples, Vice President Human Resources
Web address: www.camc.org
**Control:** Other not–for–profit (including NFP Corporation) **Service:** General Medical and Surgical

**Staffed Beds:** 70 **Admissions:** 2728 **Census:** 38 **Outpatient Visits:** 80215 **Births:** 0 **Total Expense ($000):** 41306 **Payroll Expense ($000):** 16560 **Personnel:** 319

### KEYSER—Mineral County

☐ **POTOMAC VALLEY HOSPITAL (511315)**, 100 Pin Oak Lane, Zip 26726–2699; tel. 304/597–3500 **A**1 9 10 18 **F**3 15 18 28 29 30 34 40 45 57 59 63 70 75 79 81 85 87 93 107 108 110 111 113 118 126 127 129 131 132 134 145 **S** Mid Atlantic Health Management, Inc., Stevensville, MD
Primary Contact: Linda K. Shroyer, Administrator
CFO: Marian Cardwell, Chief Financial Officer
Web address: www.potomacvalleyhospital.com
**Control:** Corporation, Investor–owned, for–profit **Service:** General Medical and Surgical

**Staffed Beds:** 25 **Admissions:** 804 **Census:** 9 **Outpatient Visits:** 55577 **Births:** 0 **Total Expense ($000):** 19906 **Payroll Expense ($000):** 6901 **Personnel:** 193

### KINGWOOD—Preston County

★ **PRESTON MEMORIAL HOSPITAL (511312)**, 300 South Price Street,
Zip 26537–1495; tel. 304/329–1400 **A**9 10 18 **F**3 11 12 13 15 18 29 30 34 35 40 43 45 47 48 53 57 59 64 65 74 75 76 77 79 81 93 107 108 111 113 118 128 129 131 132 134 145 146
Primary Contact: Melissa Lockwood, Chief Executive Officer
CFO: Robert W. Milvet, Jr., Chief Financial Officer
CIO: Beth Horne, System Administrator Information Technology
CHR: Michele Batiste, Director Human Resources
Web address: www.prestonmemorial.org
**Control:** Other not–for–profit (including NFP Corporation) **Service:** General Medical and Surgical

**Staffed Beds:** 25 **Admissions:** 790 **Census:** 10 **Outpatient Visits:** 50076 **Births:** 29 **Total Expense ($000):** 20038 **Payroll Expense ($000):** 10342 **Personnel:** 255

### LOGAN—Logan County

✖ **LOGAN REGIONAL MEDICAL CENTER (510048)**, 20 Hospital Drive,
Zip 25601–3473; tel. 304/831–1101 **A**1 9 10 20 **F**3 11 13 15 18 20 28 29 31 34 35 40 43 45 49 51 54 57 59 64 65 70 74 75 76 77 78 79 81 86 87 89 90 92 93 97 107 108 110 111 113 114 116 117 118 128 129 132 134 145 146 **P**6 **S** LifePoint Hospitals, Inc., Brentwood, TN
Primary Contact: John E. Walker, FACHE, Chief Executive Officer
CFO: Tim Matney, Chief Financial Officer
Web address: www.loganregionalmedicalcenter.com
**Control:** Corporation, Investor–owned, for–profit **Service:** General Medical and Surgical

**Staffed Beds:** 129 **Admissions:** 6461 **Census:** 83 **Outpatient Visits:** 96978 **Births:** 321 **Total Expense ($000):** 77000 **Payroll Expense ($000):** 25943 **Personnel:** 611

### MADISON—Boone County

✖ **BOONE MEMORIAL HOSPITAL (511313)**, 701 Madison Avenue,
Zip 25130–1699; tel. 304/369–1230 **A**1 9 10 18 **F**3 11 15 28 34 35 40 43 45 50 53 54 57 59 64 65 75 77 81 87 97 107 108 111 118 126 127 128 129 130 132 134 145 146
Primary Contact: Tommy H. Mullins, Administrator
COO: Tommy H. Mullins, Administrator
CFO: Randy Foxx, Chief Financial Officer
CMO: Ziad Chanaa, M.D., Chief of Staff
CIO: Susan Shreve, Executive Director Information Technology
CHR: Sheliah Cook, Director Human Resources
Web address: www.bmh.org
**Control:** County–Government, nonfederal **Service:** General Medical and Surgical

**Staffed Beds:** 25 **Admissions:** 517 **Census:** 10 **Outpatient Visits:** 53626 **Births:** 0 **Total Expense ($000):** 13988 **Payroll Expense ($000):** 6180 **Personnel:** 197

### MARTINSBURG—Berkeley County

✖ **CITY HOSPITAL (510008)**, 2500 Hospital Drive, Zip 25401–3402, Mailing Address: P.O. Box 1418, Zip 25402–1418; tel. 304/264–1000 **A**1 2 3 5 9 10 **F**3 11 12 13 15 20 21 28 29 30 31 34 35 38 40 43 45 47 49 51 53 57 59 62 64 70 74 75 76 77 78 79 81 82 85 86 87 89 93 98 102 103 107 108 110 111 114 117 118 128 129 130 131 134 144 145 146 147 **P**8 **S** West Virginia United Health System, Fairmont, WV
Primary Contact: Anthony Zelenka, Chief Administrative Officer
CFO: Christopher D. Knight, Chief Financial Officer
Web address: www.cityhospital.org
**Control:** Other not–for–profit (including NFP Corporation) **Service:** General Medical and Surgical

**Staffed Beds:** 171 **Admissions:** 8002 **Census:** 94 **Outpatient Visits:** 189579 **Births:** 914 **Total Expense ($000):** 122863 **Payroll Expense ($000):** 48461 **Personnel:** 789

✖ △ **VETERANS AFFAIRS MEDICAL CENTER**, 510 Butler Avenue,
Zip 25401–0205; tel. 304/263–0811, (Nonreporting) **A**1 3 5 7 9 **S** Department of Veterans Affairs, Washington, DC
Primary Contact: Ann Brown, Director
CFO: Jody Slonaker, Chief Fiscal Section
CIO: Debe Gantt, Chief Information Resource Management
CHR: Steve Childs, Chief Business Programs and Operations
Web address: www.va.gov/sta/guide/home.asp
**Control:** Veterans Affairs, Government, federal **Service:** General Medical and Surgical

**Staffed Beds:** 246

### MONTGOMERY—Fayette County

✖ **MONTGOMERY GENERAL HOSPITAL (511318)**, 401 Sixth Avenue,
Zip 25136–0270, Mailing Address: P.O. Box 270, Zip 25136–0270; tel. 304/442–5151, (Total facility includes 44 beds in nursing home–type unit) **A**1 9 10 18 **F**11 15 29 30 35 40 45 49 53 57 59 64 67 77 81 87 93 97 107 111 113 118 127 128 129 130 132 134 145 147 **P**6 8
Primary Contact: Vickie Gay, Chief Executive Officer
CFO: Sherri Murray, Chief Financial Officer
CMO: Traci Acklin, M.D., Chief of Staff
CIO: Denzil Blevins, Director Information Systems
CHR: Kelly D. Frye, Director Human Resources
Web address: www.mghwv.com
**Control:** Other not–for–profit (including NFP Corporation) **Service:** General Medical and Surgical

**Staffed Beds:** 69 **Admissions:** 820 **Census:** 42 **Outpatient Visits:** 61832 **Births:** 0 **Total Expense ($000):** 18614 **Payroll Expense ($000):** 9864 **Personnel:** 203

**WV**

---

**Hospital, Medicare Provider Number, Address, Telephone, Approval, Facility, and Physician Codes, Health Care System**

★ American Hospital Association (AHA) membership
☐ The Joint Commission accreditation
◇ DNV Healthcare Inc. accreditation
○ American Osteopathic Association (AOA) accreditation
△ Commission on Accreditation of Rehabilitation Facilities (CARF) accreditation

## MORGANTOWN—Monongalia County

**CHESTNUT RIDGE HOSPITAL** See West Virginia University Hospitals

☒ **HEALTHSOUTH MOUNTAINVIEW REGIONAL REHABILITATION HOSPITAL (513030)**, 1160 Van Voorhis Road, Zip 26505–3437; tel. 304/598–1100 **A**1 3 5 10 **F**3 9 29 64 74 75 77 79 86 90 93 94 95 96 129 130 131 134 147 **S** HEALTHSOUTH Corporation, Birmingham, AL
Primary Contact: Vickie Demers, Chief Executive Officer
CFO: Jason Gizzi, Controller
CMO: Russell Biundo, M.D., Medical Director
CIO: Robin Wherry, Risk Manager and Director Quality Assurance and Health Information Management
CHR: Joseph Huffman, Director Human Resources
Web address: www.healthsouthmountainview.com
**Control:** Corporation, Investor–owned, for–profit **Service:** Rehabilitation

**Staffed Beds:** 80 **Admissions:** 1602 **Census:** 66 **Outpatient Visits:** 8345 **Births:** 0 **Total Expense ($000):** 20805 **Payroll Expense ($000):** 10902 **Personnel:** 268

☒ **MONONGALIA GENERAL HOSPITAL (510024)**, 1200 J. D. Anderson Drive, Zip 26505–3486; tel. 304/598–1200 **A**1 9 10 19 **F**3 13 15 17 18 20 22 24 26 28 29 30 31 32 34 35 36 40 43 45 50 51 54 57 59 60 63 64 65 68 70 74 75 76 77 78 79 81 82 84 85 86 87 89 107 108 111 113 114 115 117 118 128 129 131 134 143 144 145 146 147 **P**6 8
Primary Contact: Darryl L. Duncan, President and Chief Executive Officer
COO: Linda Neu Ollis, FACHE, Chief Operating Officer
CFO: Daris Rosencrance, Chief Financial Officer
CMO: Mike Ferrebee, M.D., Vice President Medical Affairs
CIO: Linda Allen, Vice President Quality and Information Systems
CHR: Melissa Shreves, Director Human Resources
Web address: www.mongeneral.com
**Control:** Other not–for–profit (including NFP Corporation) **Service:** General Medical and Surgical

**Staffed Beds:** 175 **Admissions:** 9853 **Census:** 115 **Outpatient Visits:** 159449 **Births:** 1002 **Total Expense ($000):** 196174 **Payroll Expense ($000):** 64929 **Personnel:** 1302

☒ **WEST VIRGINIA UNIVERSITY HOSPITALS (510001)**, 1 Medical Center Drive, Zip 26506–4749; tel. 304/598–4000, (Includes CHESTNUT RIDGE HOSPITAL, 930 Chestnut Ridge Road, Zip 26505–2854; tel. 304/293–4000; WEST VIRGINIA UNIVERSITY CHILDREN'S HOSPITAL, Medical Center Drive, Zip 26506–8111; tel. 800/982–6277), (Total facility includes 20 beds in nursing home–type unit) **A**1 3 5 8 9 10 12 13 19 **F**3 4 5 11 13 15 17 18 19 20 21 22 23 24 25 26 27 28 29 30 31 35 36 37 38 39 40 43 45 46 47 48 49 50 51 57 59 60 61 64 68 70 72 74 75 76 77 78 79 80 81 82 84 85 86 87 88 89 92 98 99 100 101 102 103 105 106 107 108 110 113 114 117 118 119 120 122 123 125 127 128 129 131 135 140 144 145 146 **P**6 **S** West Virginia United Health System, Fairmont, WV
Primary Contact: Bruce McClymonds, President and Chief Executive Officer
CFO: Mary Jo Shahan, Vice President and Chief Financial Officer
CMO: Michelle Nuss, M.D., Chief Medical Officer
CIO: Rich King, Vice President Information Technology
CHR: Charlotte Bennett, Vice President Human Resources
Web address: www.health.wvu.edu
**Control:** Other not–for–profit (including NFP Corporation) **Service:** General Medical and Surgical

**Staffed Beds:** 509 **Admissions:** 25709 **Census:** 421 **Outpatient Visits:** 598526 **Births:** 1367 **Total Expense ($000):** 574338 **Payroll Expense ($000):** 201155 **Personnel:** 4065

## NEW MARTINSVILLE—Wetzel County

☒ **WETZEL COUNTY HOSPITAL (510072)**, 3 East Benjamin Drive, Zip 26155–2758; tel. 304/455–8000 **A**1 9 10 20 **F**3 15 28 30 31 34 40 43 45 57 59 64 65 70 75 77 81 85 93 94 107 108 113 117 118 126 129 131 132 134 145 147 **P**6
Primary Contact: Brian K. Felici, Chief Executive Officer
CFO: John May, Chief Financial Officer
CIO: Amy Frazier, Supervisor Management Information Systems
CHR: Sarah Boley, Director Human Resources
Web address: www.wetzelcountyhospital.com
**Control:** County–Government, nonfederal **Service:** General Medical and Surgical

**Staffed Beds:** 44 **Admissions:** 1202 **Census:** 17 **Outpatient Visits:** 97716 **Births:** 0 **Total Expense ($000):** 20165 **Payroll Expense ($000):** 9727 **Personnel:** 226

## OAK HILL—Fayette County

☒ **PLATEAU MEDICAL CENTER (511317)**, 430 Main Street, Zip 25901–3455; tel. 304/469–8600 **A**1 9 10 18 **F**3 8 15 29 30 34 35 40 45 46 50 57 59 64 68 70 75 77 79 81 87 91 93 97 107 108 110 111 113 118 145 **S** Community Health Systems, Inc., Franklin, TN
Primary Contact: Chad Hatfield, Chief Executive Officer
CFO: Heather Hylton, Chief Financial Officer
CMO: Ryan Newell, M.D., Chief of Staff
CIO: Steve Bowen, Director Information Systems
CHR: Tammie Miller, Director Marketing and Public Relations
Web address: www.plateaumedicalcenter.com
**Control:** Corporation, Investor–owned, for–profit **Service:** General Medical and Surgical

**Staffed Beds:** 25 **Admissions:** 1517 **Census:** 16 **Outpatient Visits:** 46291 **Births:** 0 **Total Expense ($000):** 29297 **Payroll Expense ($000):** 11724 **Personnel:** 216

## PARKERSBURG—Wood County

☒ **CAMDEN–CLARK MEDICAL CENTER (510058)**, 800 Garfield Avenue, Zip 26101–5378, Mailing Address: P.O. Box 718, Zip 26102–0718; tel. 304/424–2111, (Includes ST. JOSEPH'S HOSPITAL, 1824 Murdoch Avenue, Zip 26101–3246, Mailing Address: P.O. Box 327, Zip 26102–0327; tel. 304/424–4111), (Total facility includes 25 beds in nursing home–type unit) **A**1 9 10 13 **F**3 7 11 12 13 15 17 18 20 22 24 28 29 30 31 34 35 40 43 45 49 50 51 53 57 58 59 64 65 68 70 71 74 75 76 78 79 81 82 84 85 86 87 89 92 98 100 101 102 107 108 110 111 113 114 115 116 117 118 119 120 122 123 127 129 131 134 144 145 146 147 **P**6 8 **S** West Virginia United Health System, Fairmont, WV
Primary Contact: Michael A. King, FACHE, President and Chief Executive Officer
COO: Michael A. King, FACHE, President and Chief Executive Officer
CFO: Allen R. Butcher, Vice President Finance
CMO: Gregory Moses, M.D., President Medical Staff
CIO: Josh Woods, Director Information Systems
CHR: Tom Heller, Vice President Human Resources
Web address: www.ccmh.org
**Control:** Other not–for–profit (including NFP Corporation) **Service:** General Medical and Surgical

**Staffed Beds:** 435 **Admissions:** 15862 **Census:** 210 **Outpatient Visits:** 336953 **Births:** 1542 **Total Expense ($000):** 231029 **Payroll Expense ($000):** 80237 **Personnel:** 1818

☒ **HEALTHSOUTH WESTERN HILLS REHABILITATION HOSPITAL (513027)**, 3 Western Hills Drive, Zip 26101–8122; tel. 304/420–1300 **A**1 10 **F**29 54 57 64 90 93 94 95 96 129 145 **S** HEALTHSOUTH Corporation, Birmingham, AL
Primary Contact: Alvin R. Lawson, JD, FACHE, Chief Executive Officer
CFO: Daniel Hungerford, Controller
CMO: Kalapala Rao, M.D., Medical Director
CHR: Candace Ross, Coordinator Human Resources
Web address: www.healthsouthwesternhills.com
**Control:** Corporation, Investor–owned, for–profit **Service:** Rehabilitation

**Staffed Beds:** 50 **Admissions:** 1258 **Census:** 43 **Outpatient Visits:** 16590 **Births:** 0 **Total Expense ($000):** 14375 **Payroll Expense ($000):** 6872 **Personnel:** 150

## PETERSBURG—Grant County

★ **GRANT MEMORIAL HOSPITAL (511316)**, Route 55 West, Zip 26847, Mailing Address: P.O. Box 1019, Zip 26847–1019; tel. 304/257–1026, (Total facility includes 20 beds in nursing home–type unit) **A**9 10 18 **F**3 11 13 15 28 29 30 31 34 35 40 45 50 53 57 59 62 63 64 65 67 68 70 75 76 77 79 81 84 85 86 87 91 93 107 108 113 117 118 127 129 131 132 145 146 **P**6
Primary Contact: Mary Beth Barr, R.N., Chief Executive Officer
COO: Mary Beth Barr, R.N., Chief Executive Officer
CMO: Bruce Leslie, M.D., Chief of Staff
CIO: Jenny McKinney, Director Information Systems
CHR: Roanie Arbaugh, Director Human Resources
Web address: www.grantmemorial.com
**Control:** County–Government, nonfederal **Service:** General Medical and Surgical

**Staffed Beds:** 41 **Admissions:** 1758 **Census:** 25 **Outpatient Visits:** 70625 **Births:** 217 **Total Expense ($000):** 28478 **Payroll Expense ($000):** 9664 **Personnel:** 297

## PHILIPPI—Barbour County

★ **BROADDUS HOSPITAL (511300)**, 1 Healthcare Drive, Zip 26416–1051, Mailing Address: P.O. Box 930, Zip 26416–1051; tel. 304/457–1760, (Total facility includes 60 beds in nursing home–type unit) **A**9 10 18 **F**3 15 29 30 34 35 40 57 59 64 65 67 75 85 107 110 113 118 127 129 132 142 145 **S** Davis Health System, Elkins, WV
Primary Contact: Jeffrey A. Powelson, Chief Executive Officer
CFO: Cathy Kalar, Chief Financial Officer
CHR: Penny Brown, Human Resource Representative
Web address: www.davishealthsystem.org/
**Control:** Other not–for–profit (including NFP Corporation) **Service:** General Medical and Surgical

**Staffed Beds:** 72 **Admissions:** 403 **Census:** 64 **Outpatient Visits:** 23513 **Births:** 0 **Total Expense ($000):** 13900 **Payroll Expense ($000):** 4911 **Personnel:** 156

**WV**

*Many Facility Codes have changed. Please refer to the AHA Guide Code Chart.*    © 2012 AHA Guide

## POINT PLEASANT—Mason County

☒ **PLEASANT VALLEY HOSPITAL (510012)**, 2520 Valley Drive, Zip 25550–2083; tel. 304/675–4340, (Total facility includes 100 beds in nursing home–type unit) **A**1 9 10 **F**3 11 13 15 17 18 28 29 33 34 35 36 39 40 43 50 53 56 57 59 62 63 68 70 74 75 76 77 78 79 81 85 86 87 89 93 107 108 111 113 114 117 118 127 128 129 130 131 142 143 145 146 147
Primary Contact: Thomas Schauer, Chief Executive Officer
COO: Sandy Wood, Vice President Patient Services
CMO: Stephen Rerych, M.D., President Medical Staff
CIO: Paula Brooker, Director Information Services
CHR: Terri Hill, Director Human Resources
Web address: www.pvalley.org
**Control:** Other not–for–profit (including NFP Corporation) **Service:** General Medical and Surgical

**Staffed Beds:** 201 **Admissions:** 3050 **Census:** 120 **Outpatient Visits:** 205191 **Births:** 215 **Total Expense ($000):** 63340 **Payroll Expense ($000):** 29025 **Personnel:** 669

## PRINCETON—Mercer County

☒ **HEALTHSOUTH SOUTHERN HILLS REHABILITATION HOSPITAL (513026)**, 120 Twelfth Street, Zip 24740–2312; tel. 304/487–8000 **A**1 10 **F**29 56 57 59 60 64 74 75 77 79 87 90 93 94 129 131 147 **S** HEALTHSOUTH Corporation, Birmingham, AL
Primary Contact: Deborah S. Guthrie, Chief Executive Officer
CFO: Melinda Fanning, Chief Financial Officer and Controller
CMO: Carl Shelton, M.D., Medical Director
CIO: Bruce D. Bales, Regional Director Plant Operations
CHR: Jan Thibodeau, Director Human Resources
Web address: www.healthsouthsouthernhills.com
**Control:** Corporation, Investor–owned, for–profit **Service:** Rehabilitation

**Staffed Beds:** 42 **Admissions:** 804 **Census:** 27 **Outpatient Visits:** 4196 **Births:** 0 **Personnel:** 116

☒ **PRINCETON COMMUNITY HOSPITAL (510046)**, 122 12th Street, Zip 24740–2352, Mailing Address: P.O. Box 1369, Zip 24740–1369; tel. 304/487–7000 **A**1 2 9 10 19 **F**3 11 12 13 15 17 29 30 31 32 34 35 39 40 44 45 46 48 49 50 51 53 57 59 64 65 70 74 75 76 77 78 79 81 85 86 87 89 93 98 100 101 102 103 104 107 108 110 111 113 114 117 118 126 128 129 130 131 134 140 141 143 145 146 **P**1
Primary Contact: Wayne B. Griffith, FACHE, Chief Executive Officer
COO: Richard W. Zborowski, Vice President Administration
CFO: Frank J. Sinicrope, Jr., Vice President Financial Services
CMO: Phil Branson, M.D., President Medical Staff
CIO: Stephen A. Curry, Director Information Services
CHR: D Darlene Huffman, Director Human Resources
Web address: www.pchonline.org
**Control:** City–Government, nonfederal **Service:** General Medical and Surgical

**Staffed Beds:** 230 **Admissions:** 8898 **Census:** 112 **Outpatient Visits:** 196751 **Births:** 600 **Total Expense ($000):** 102678 **Payroll Expense ($000):** 41795 **Personnel:** 1018

## RANSON—Jefferson County

☒ **JEFFERSON MEMORIAL HOSPITAL (511319)**, 300 South Preston Street, Zip 25438–1699; tel. 304/728–1600 **A**1 3 5 9 10 18 **F**3 11 13 15 29 30 34 35 38 40 43 45 51 57 59 64 70 74 75 76 77 81 85 86 87 93 107 108 110 111 114 117 118 128 129 131 134 145 146 **P**8 **S** West Virginia United Health System, Fairmont, WV
Primary Contact: Christina D. Coad, Ph.D., Chief Administrative Officer
CFO: Christopher D. Knight, Vice President Finance
CMO: Robert Jones, III, M.D., President Medical Staff
CIO: Todd Smoot, Chief Information Officer
CHR: Christina D. Coad, Ph.D., Interim Vice President Human Resources
Web address: www.jeffmem.com
**Control:** Other not–for–profit (including NFP Corporation) **Service:** General Medical and Surgical

**Staffed Beds:** 25 **Admissions:** 1793 **Census:** 15 **Outpatient Visits:** 72361 **Births:** 294 **Total Expense ($000):** 37822 **Payroll Expense ($000):** 16773 **Personnel:** 295

## RIPLEY—Jackson County

☐ **JACKSON GENERAL HOSPITAL (510018)**, 122 Pinnell Street, Zip 25271–9101, Mailing Address: P.O. Box 720, Zip 25271–0720; tel. 304/372–2731 **A**1 9 10 **F**3 11 15 17 29 30 34 35 40 50 57 59 64 68 75 79 81 85 93 107 113 118 126 127 131 132 **P**6
Primary Contact: Stephanie McCoy, President and Chief Executive Officer
CFO: Angela Frame, Chief Financial Officer
CMO: James G. Gaal, M.D., Chief of Medical Staff
CIO: John Manley, Director Information Systems
CHR: Jeffrey Tabor, Director Human Resources
Web address: www.jacksongeneral.com
**Control:** Other not–for–profit (including NFP Corporation) **Service:** General Medical and Surgical

**Staffed Beds:** 36 **Admissions:** 1279 **Census:** 17 **Outpatient Visits:** 45631 **Births:** 0 **Total Expense ($000):** 23990 **Payroll Expense ($000):** 10953 **Personnel:** 273

## ROMNEY—Hampshire County

☒ **HAMPSHIRE MEMORIAL HOSPITAL (511311)**, 363 Sunrise Boulevard, Zip 26757; tel. 304/822–4561, (Total facility includes 30 beds in nursing home–type unit) **A**1 9 10 18 **F**3 15 29 40 45 59 65 77 81 85 93 107 118 126 127 128 129 132 **P**6 **S** Valley Health System, Winchester, VA
Primary Contact: Neil R. McLaughlin, R.N., Interim President
CFO: Christine Lowman, Vice President Finance
CMO: Vijay K. Chowdhary, M.D., Medical Director
CHR: Cindy Combs, Supervisor Human Resources
CNO: Gena Swisher, Vice President Nursing
Web address: www.valleyhealthlink.com/hampshire
**Control:** Other not–for–profit (including NFP Corporation) **Service:** General Medical and Surgical

**Staffed Beds:** 44 **Admissions:** 440 **Census:** 36 **Outpatient Visits:** 37909 **Births:** 0 **Total Expense ($000):** 17026 **Payroll Expense ($000):** 6206 **Personnel:** 152

## RONCEVERTE—Greenbrier County

★ ○ **GREENBRIER VALLEY MEDICAL CENTER (510002)**, 202 Maplewood Avenue, Zip 24970–0497, Mailing Address: P.O. Box 497, Zip 24970–0497; tel. 304/647–4411 **A**9 10 11 12 13 **F**8 13 15 18 20 29 31 34 40 45 49 51 57 59 60 68 70 74 75 76 78 79 81 85 86 87 89 107 108 110 111 113 115 118 119 128 132 134 145 147 **P**6 **S** Community Health Systems, Inc., Franklin, TN
Primary Contact: Paul Storey, Chief Executive Officer
CFO: Joy Fergie, Chief Financial Officer
CMO: Connie Perkins, M.D., Chief of Staff
CIO: Kevin Sexton, Director Information Systems
CHR: Melissa Wickline, Director Marketing
Web address: www.gvmc.com
**Control:** Corporation, Investor–owned, for–profit **Service:** General Medical and Surgical

**Staffed Beds:** 113 **Admissions:** 4152 **Census:** 47 **Outpatient Visits:** 57067 **Births:** 580 **Total Expense ($000):** 45966 **Payroll Expense ($000):** 19033 **Personnel:** 467

## SISTERSVILLE—Tyler County

★ **SISTERSVILLE GENERAL HOSPITAL (511304)**, 314 South Wells Street, Zip 26175–1098; tel. 304/652–2611 **A**9 10 18 **F**3 7 11 15 28 29 30 32 35 40 43 50 53 57 59 63 64 65 79 83 84 87 93 97 107 118 126 128 129 131 132 134 145 146 147 **P**6
Primary Contact: Brian K. Lowther, Chief Executive Officer
COO: Mike Hall, Risk Manager
CFO: Pat Burdette, Chief Financial Officer
CMO: Ramon Fagundo, M.D., Chief of Staff
CHR: Mary Beth Neff, Director Human Resources
Web address: www.sistersvillehospital.com
**Control:** City–Government, nonfederal **Service:** General Medical and Surgical

**Staffed Beds:** 12 **Admissions:** 212 **Census:** 2 **Outpatient Visits:** 22287 **Births:** 0 **Total Expense ($000):** 9423 **Payroll Expense ($000):** 5599 **Personnel:** 157

**WV**

---

**Hospital, Medicare Provider Number, Address, Telephone, Approval, Facility, and Physician Codes, Health Care System**

★ American Hospital Association (AHA) membership
☐ The Joint Commission accreditation   ◇ DNV Healthcare Inc. accreditation

○ American Osteopathic Association (AOA) accreditation
△ Commission on Accreditation of Rehabilitation Facilities (CARF) accreditation

## SOUTH CHARLESTON—Kanawha County

✠ **THOMAS MEMORIAL HOSPITAL (510029)**, 4605 MacCorkle Avenue S.W., Zip 25309–1398; tel. 304/766–3600 **A**1 5 9 10 **F**3 5 8 11 13 15 17 18 20 22 29 30 31 32 34 35 37 38 40 43 45 46 47 48 49 50 53 54 57 59 60 62 64 65 68 69 70 72 74 75 76 77 78 79 81 84 85 86 87 89 92 93 98 99 100 101 102 103 104 105 107 108 110 111 113 114 117 118 119 120 122 123 125 128 129 130 131 143 145 146 **S** Thomas Health System, Inc., South Charleston, WV
Primary Contact: Stephen P. Dexter, President and Chief Executive Officer
COO: Daniel Lauffer, FACHE, Senior Vice President and Chief Operating Officer
CFO: Charles O. Covert, Vice President Finance
CHR: Marybeth Smith, Director Human Resources
Web address: www.thomaswv.org
**Control:** Other not–for–profit (including NFP Corporation) **Service:** General Medical and Surgical

**Staffed Beds:** 241 **Admissions:** 9566 **Census:** 135 **Outpatient Visits:** 178585 **Births:** 985 **Total Expense ($000):** 152796 **Payroll Expense ($000):** 52458 **Personnel:** 1001

## SPENCER—Roane County

✠ **ROANE GENERAL HOSPITAL (511306)**, 200 Hospital Drive, Zip 25276–1060; tel. 304/927–4444, (Total facility includes 35 beds in nursing home–type unit) **A**1 9 10 18 **F**3 15 28 29 34 40 43 45 53 57 59 64 65 81 93 97 107 108 118 126 127 129 132 143 **P**6
Primary Contact: Douglas E. Bentz, Chief Executive Officer
CFO: Louise Ward, Vice President Financial and Support Services
CMO: Brent Watson, M.D., Chief Medical Staff
CIO: Tony Keaton, Director Information Systems
CHR: Jeff Beane, Director Human Resources
Web address: www.roanegeneralhospital.com
**Control:** Other not–for–profit (including NFP Corporation) **Service:** General Medical and Surgical

**Staffed Beds:** 60 **Admissions:** 551 **Census:** 42 **Outpatient Visits:** 59318 **Births:** 0 **Total Expense ($000):** 22503 **Payroll Expense ($000):** 10807 **Personnel:** 255

## SUMMERSVILLE—Nicholas County

★ **SUMMERSVILLE REGIONAL MEDICAL CENTER (510082)**, 400 Fairview Heights Road, Zip 26651–0400; tel. 304/872–2891, (Total facility includes 52 beds in nursing home–type unit) **A**9 10 **F**1 3 13 15 28 30 34 35 40 43 57 67 70 75 76 79 81 83 84 85 89 93 97 107 108 110 111 114 118 126 127 128 129 130 132 134 145 146 147
Primary Contact: Deborah A. Hill, R.N., FACHE, Chief Executive Officer
CFO: Dora Douglas, Chief Financial Officer
CMO: Robert Fleer, M.D., Chief of Staff
CIO: Mike Ellison, Information Systems Lead
CHR: David M. Henderson, Director Human Resources
Web address: www.summersvillememorial.org
**Control:** City–Government, nonfederal **Service:** General Medical and Surgical

**Staffed Beds:** 93 **Admissions:** 1008 **Census:** 65 **Outpatient Visits:** 73029 **Births:** 445 **Total Expense ($000):** 45234 **Payroll Expense ($000):** 22698 **Personnel:** 478

## WEBSTER SPRINGS—Webster County

★ **WEBSTER COUNTY MEMORIAL HOSPITAL (511301)**, 324 Miller Mountain Drive, Zip 26288–1087, Mailing Address: P.O. Box 312, Zip 26288–0312; tel. 304/847–5682 **A**9 10 18 **F**7 11 15 28 30 34 35 40 50 57 59 65 66 75 87 89 93 97 107 111 113 118 126 127 129 132 134 146 147 **P**6
Primary Contact: Annette M. Keenan, Chief Executive Officer
CMO: Robert Mace, M.D., Chief of Staff
CIO: Margaret W. Short, Coordinator Information Technology
CHR: Deborah Bragg, Director Human Resources
Web address: www.wcmhwv.com
**Control:** Other not–for–profit (including NFP Corporation) **Service:** General Medical and Surgical

**Staffed Beds:** 15 **Admissions:** 264 **Census:** 2 **Outpatient Visits:** 42162 **Total Expense ($000):** 7745 **Payroll Expense ($000):** 5622 **Personnel:** 123

## WEIRTON—Brooke County

✠ **WEIRTON MEDICAL CENTER (510023)**, 601 Colliers Way, Zip 26062–5091; tel. 304/797–6000, (Nonreporting) **A**1 9 10
Primary Contact: Joseph Endrich, M.D., President and Chief Executive Officer
CFO: Robert A. Frank, Chief Financial Officer
CIO: Richard Lucas, Director Information Services
CHR: Jennifer Anderson, Director Human Resources
Web address: www.weirtonmedical.com
**Control:** Other not–for–profit (including NFP Corporation) **Service:** General Medical and Surgical

**Staffed Beds:** 238

## WELCH—Mcdowell County

**WELCH COMMUNITY HOSPITAL (510086)**, 454 McDowell Street, Zip 24801–2097; tel. 304/436–8461, (Total facility includes 59 beds in nursing home–type unit) **A**9 10 20 **F**3 13 15 29 35 40 45 50 57 59 64 65 66 67 68 70 75 76 81 86 87 97 107 110 113 118 126 129 134 145 146 147 **P**6
Primary Contact: Walter J. Garrett, Chief Executive Officer
CFO: Johnny Brant, Chief Financial Officer
CMO: Chandra Sharma, M.D., Chief of Staff
CIO: Thaddeus Robinson, Chief Information Officer
CHR: Diana Blankenship, Director Human Resources
**Control:** State–Government, nonfederal **Service:** General Medical and Surgical

**Staffed Beds:** 108 **Admissions:** 665 **Census:** 53 **Outpatient Visits:** 34156 **Births:** 50 **Total Expense ($000):** 26349 **Payroll Expense ($000):** 9384 **Personnel:** 312

## WESTON—Lewis County

✠ **STONEWALL JACKSON MEMORIAL HOSPITAL (510038)**, 230 Hospital Plaza, Zip 26452–8558; tel. 304/269–8000 **A**1 9 10 **F**3 11 13 15 28 29 30 35 40 43 45 48 50 56 57 59 62 64 68 70 75 76 79 81 85 86 87 93 94 97 107 108 111 113 117 118 128 129 130 131 132 134 144 145 146 147 **P**8
Primary Contact: Avah Stalnaker, Chief Executive Officer
CFO: Dodie Arbogest, Controller
CIO: Kay Butcher, Director Management Information
CHR: Aimee Green, Director Human Resources
Web address: www.stonewallhospital.com
**Control:** Other not–for–profit (including NFP Corporation) **Service:** General Medical and Surgical

**Staffed Beds:** 70 **Admissions:** 2943 **Census:** 29 **Outpatient Visits:** 81702 **Births:** 337 **Total Expense ($000):** 33559 **Payroll Expense ($000):** 20634 **Personnel:** 407

☐ **WILLIAM R. SHARPE, JR. HOSPITAL (514010)**, 936 Sharpe Hospital Road, Zip 26452–8550; tel. 304/269–1210 **A**1 5 9 10 **F**11 30 56 86 87 98 100 101 103 129 131 142 145 **P**6
Primary Contact: Parker Haddix, Chief Executive Officer
COO: Terry L. Small, Assistant Chief Executive Officer
CFO: Tammy Keough, Chief Financial Officer
CMO: Robert Keefover, M.D., Chief Medical Officer
CIO: Pam Lewis, Chief Compliance Officer
Web address: www.wvdhhr.org/sharpe
**Control:** State–Government, nonfederal **Service:** Psychiatric

**Staffed Beds:** 150 **Admissions:** 732 **Census:** 157 **Outpatient Visits:** 0 **Births:** 0 **Total Expense ($000):** 40316 **Payroll Expense ($000):** 13288 **Personnel:** 454

## WHEELING—Ohio County

☐ **OHIO VALLEY MEDICAL CENTER (510039)**, 2000 Eoff Street, Zip 26003–3870; tel. 304/234–0123 **A**1 2 5 9 10 12 13 **F**3 5 9 11 13 15 17 18 20 28 29 30 31 34 35 38 39 40 43 44 48 49 50 51 53 55 56 57 58 59 60 61 64 65 68 70 74 75 76 77 78 79 81 82 84 85 86 87 89 93 97 98 99 100 101 102 103 104 105 107 108 111 113 114 115 116 118 120 122 128 129 130 131 133 134 145 146 147 **P**6 **S** Ohio Valley Health Services and Education Corporation, Wheeling, WV
Primary Contact: Bernie Albertini, Chief Administrative Officer
COO: Michael J. Caruso, Chief Operating Officer
CFO: David T. Baranik, Senior Vice President and Chief Financial Officer
CIO: Robert Panichi, Chief Information Officer
CHR: James R. Stultz, Senior Vice President Human Resources
Web address: www.ohiovalleymedicalcenter.com
**Control:** Other not–for–profit (including NFP Corporation) **Service:** General Medical and Surgical

**Staffed Beds:** 159 **Admissions:** 6177 **Census:** 90 **Outpatient Visits:** 146087 **Births:** 268 **Total Expense ($000):** 72602 **Payroll Expense ($000):** 34507 **Personnel:** 816

★ **PETERSON REHABILITATION HOSPITAL (513025)**, Homestead Avenue, Zip 26003; tel. 304/234–0500, (Total facility includes 150 beds in nursing home–type unit) **A**10 **F**29 34 56 57 59 75 77 86 87 90 93 96 127 129 130 131 142 147
Primary Contact: Barbara Sisarcick, Administrator
COO: Tom Barr, Director Operational Support Services
CFO: Tammy Parasida, Manager Business Office
CMO: William Mercer, M.D., Director
CIO: Jolene Nagle, Director Medical Records
CHR: Annie Barton, Director Human Resources
Web address: www.weat.com/site6/
**Control:** Corporation, Investor–owned, for–profit **Service:** Rehabilitation

**Staffed Beds:** 172 **Admissions:** 873 **Census:** 152 **Outpatient Visits:** 3330 **Births:** 0 **Total Expense ($000):** 18462 **Payroll Expense ($000):** 5827 **Personnel:** 161

**WV**

*Many Facility Codes have changed. Please refer to the AHA Guide Code Chart.* © 2012 AHA Guide

☐ **WHEELING HOSPITAL (510050)**, 1 Medical Park, Zip 26003–0708;
tel. 304/243–3000, (Total facility includes 24 beds in nursing home–type unit) **A**1
2 9 10 13 **F**3 11 13 15 17 18 20 22 24 26 28 29 30 31 32 34 35 36 40 43
44 45 49 50 53 54 57 58 59 61 62 64 65 66 70 74 75 76 77 78 79 81 82
85 86 87 89 92 93 94 96 97 99 107 108 110 113 114 116 117 118 119
120 122 127 128 129 130 131 134 142 145 146 147 **P**5
Primary Contact: Ronald L. Violi, Chief Executive Officer
COO: Scott McKee, Chief Operating Officer
CMO: Angelo Georges, M.D., President Medical and Dental Staff
CIO: David Rapp, Chief Information Officer
CHR: Susan Falbo, Vice President Human Resources
Web address: www.wheelinghospital.org
**Control:** Other not–for–profit (including NFP Corporation) **Service:** General
Medical and Surgical

**Staffed Beds:** 276 **Admissions:** 10643 **Census:** 130 **Outpatient Visits:**
551883 **Births:** 1163 **Total Expense ($000):** 238947 **Payroll Expense
($000):** 102126 **Personnel:** 2159

**WILLIAMSON—Mingo County**

☐ **WILLIAMSON MEMORIAL HOSPITAL (510077)**, 859 Alderson Street,
Zip 25661–3215, Mailing Address: P.O. Box 1980, Zip 25661–1980;
tel. 304/235–2500 **A**1 9 10 **F**3 13 15 18 20 26 28 29 30 34 40 45 49 50 51
57 59 61 65 70 74 75 76 77 79 81 87 91 93 107 108 113 118 128 129 130
134 145 **P**6 **S** Health Management Associates, Naples, FL
Primary Contact: Todd C. Hubler, Chief Executive Officer
CFO: Todd C. Hubler, Controller
CMO: Manuel Angco, M.D., Chief of Staff
CHR: Tina Jackson, Manager Human Resources
Web address: www.hmawmh.com
**Control:** Corporation, Investor–owned, for–profit **Service:** General Medical and
Surgical

**Staffed Beds:** 76 **Admissions:** 2479 **Census:** 20 **Outpatient Visits:** 34988
**Births:** 104 **Total Expense ($000):** 27259 **Payroll Expense ($000):** 9777
**Personnel:** 199

WV

---

**Hospital, Medicare Provider Number, Address, Telephone, Approval, Facility, and Physician Codes, Health Care System**

★ American Hospital Association (AHA) membership
☐ The Joint Commission accreditation
◇ DNV Healthcare Inc. accreditation
○ American Osteopathic Association (AOA) accreditation
△ Commission on Accreditation of Rehabilitation Facilities (CARF) accreditation

# WISCONSIN

## AMERY—Polk County

★ **AMERY REGIONAL MEDICAL CENTER (521308)**, 265 Griffin Street East, Zip 54001–1439; tel. 715/268–8000 **A**9 10 18 **F**11 13 15 28 29 34 36 40 43 53 54 56 64 75 76 77 78 81 82 86 87 93 98 100 101 102 103 104 105 107 108 111 118 129 130 143 **P**6 **S** QHR, Brentwood, TN
Primary Contact: Michael Karuschak, Jr., Chief Executive Officer
CFO: Scott D. Edin, Chief Financial Officer
CMO: James Quenan, M.D., Chief Medical Officer
CIO: Bill Lehner, Director Management Information Systems
CHR: Joanne Jackson, Administrator Human Resources, Community Relations and Quality Improvement
Web address: www.amerymedicalcenter.org
**Control:** Other not–for–profit (including NFP Corporation) **Service:** General Medical and Surgical

**Staffed Beds:** 35 **Admissions:** 1311 **Census:** 17 **Outpatient Visits:** 111485 **Births:** 145 **Total Expense ($000):** 48983 **Payroll Expense ($000):** 16834 **Personnel:** 343

## ANTIGO—Langlade County

☐ **LANGLADE MEMORIAL HOSPITAL (521350)**, 112 East Fifth Avenue, Zip 54409–2796; tel. 715/623–2331 **A**1 5 9 10 18 **F**2 3 10 11 13 15 28 29 30 31 34 40 43 44 45 53 54 56 57 59 60 63 64 68 69 70 74 75 76 77 78 81 82 86 87 89 92 93 96 107 108 109 110 111 113 115 117 118 119 120 122 123 128 129 130 131 132 143
Primary Contact: David R. Schneider, Executive Director
CFO: Pat Tincher, Director Finance
CMO: Noel Deep, M.D., Chief Medical Staff
CHR: Janelle Markgraf, Director Human Resources
Web address: www.langladehospital.org
**Control:** Church–operated, Nongovernment, not–for profit **Service:** General Medical and Surgical

**Staffed Beds:** 25 **Admissions:** 1166 **Census:** 11 **Outpatient Visits:** 112628 **Births:** 165 **Total Expense ($000):** 63514 **Payroll Expense ($000):** 23069 **Personnel:** 390

## APPLETON—Outagamie County

☐ **APPLETON MEDICAL CENTER (520160)**, 1818 North Meade Street, Zip 54911–3496; tel. 920/731–4101 **A**1 3 5 9 10 **F**3 4 8 9 11 13 15 17 18 19 20 21 22 23 24 25 26 28 29 30 31 32 34 35 36 37 39 40 41 43 44 45 46 49 50 51 53 55 56 59 60 64 68 69 70 74 75 76 78 79 80 81 82 84 85 86 87 88 89 93 107 108 110 111 113 115 116 117 118 119 120 122 123 129 131 134 142 143 145 146 147 **P**1 6 **S** ThedaCare, Inc., Appleton, WI
Primary Contact: Kim Barnas, Senior Vice President
COO: Matthew Furlan, Chief Operating Officer
CFO: Tim Olson, Senior Vice President Finance
CMO: Gregory L. Long, M.D., Chief Medical Officer
CIO: Keith Livingston, Senior Vice President and Chief Information Officer
CHR: Roberta Chapman, Manager Human Resources
Web address: www.thedacare.org
**Control:** Other not–for–profit (including NFP Corporation) **Service:** General Medical and Surgical

**Staffed Beds:** 147 **Admissions:** 8448 **Census:** 89 **Outpatient Visits:** 121429 **Births:** 1282 **Total Expense ($000):** 209030 **Payroll Expense ($000):** 81892 **Personnel:** 1166

✠ **ST. ELIZABETH HOSPITAL (520009)**, 1506 South Oneida Street, Zip 54915–1397; tel. 920/730–2000 **A**1 2 3 5 9 10 **F**4 5 6 8 9 11 13 15 17 18 20 22 24 26 27 28 29 30 31 32 34 35 36 39 40 43 44 45 46 47 48 49 50 56 57 59 66 68 69 70 72 74 75 76 77 78 79 80 81 82 84 85 86 87 88 89 93 94 97 98 99 100 102 103 104 105 107 108 110 111 113 114 116 117 118 119 120 122 123 125 128 129 130 131 134 143 144 145 146 147 **S** Wheaton Franciscan Healthcare, Wheaton, IL
Primary Contact: Travis Andersen, President
COO: Travis Andersen, President
CFO: Jeff Badger, Chief Financial Officer
CMO: Lawrence Donatelle, M.D., Vice President Medical Affairs
CIO: Will Weider, Chief Information Officer
CHR: Vince Gallucci, Senior Vice President Human Resources
Web address: www.affinityhealth.org
**Control:** Church–operated, Nongovernment, not–for profit **Service:** General Medical and Surgical

**Staffed Beds:** 206 **Admissions:** 7812 **Census:** 95 **Outpatient Visits:** 143422 **Births:** 1092 **Total Expense ($000):** 142777 **Payroll Expense ($000):** 56350 **Personnel:** 836

## ASHLAND—Ashland County

✠ **MEMORIAL MEDICAL CENTER – ASHLAND (521359)**, 1615 Maple Lane, Zip 54806–3689; tel. 715/685–5500 **A**1 9 10 18 **F**3 5 13 15 28 30 31 34 40 43 45 48 49 56 57 59 64 68 76 79 81 85 86 93 94 96 98 99 100 102 103 104 105 107 108 110 111 114 117 118 129 131 134 143 147
Primary Contact: Daniel J. Hymans, President
COO: Daniel H. Adams, Vice President and Chief Operating Officer
CFO: Les Whiteaker, Vice President and Chief Financial Officer
CMO: F. Daniel Rochman, M.D., President Medical Staff
CIO: Todd Reynolds, Chief Information Officer
CHR: Diane Lulich, Director Human Resources
Web address: www.ashlandmmc.com
**Control:** Other not–for–profit (including NFP Corporation) **Service:** General Medical and Surgical

**Staffed Beds:** 35 **Admissions:** 2336 **Census:** 18 **Outpatient Visits:** 12838 **Births:** 240 **Total Expense ($000):** 49375 **Payroll Expense ($000):** 21563 **Personnel:** 371

## BALDWIN—St. Croix County

★ **BALDWIN AREA MEDICAL CENTER (521347)**, 730 10th Avenue, Zip 54002; tel. 715/684–3311 **A**9 10 18 **F**3 11 13 15 17 28 29 31 34 36 40 43 45 48 50 53 64 65 68 70 75 76 77 78 80 81 86 87 89 90 93 97 107 108 111 114 118 126 129 130 132 134 142 145 147
Primary Contact: Alison Page, Chief Executive Officer
CFO: Brian A. Lovdahl, Chief Financial Officer
CMO: Joel Stoeckeler, M.D., Chief of Staff
CIO: Scott Swedien, Director Information Services
CHR: Trudy Acterhof, Director Human Resources
Web address: www.baldwinhospital.com
**Control:** Other not–for–profit (including NFP Corporation) **Service:** General Medical and Surgical

**Staffed Beds:** 25 **Admissions:** 788 **Census:** 6 **Outpatient Visits:** 29523 **Births:** 75 **Total Expense ($000):** 26949 **Payroll Expense ($000):** 11205 **Personnel:** 199

## BARABOO—Sauk County

✠ **ST. CLARE HOSPITAL AND HEALTH SERVICES (520057)**, 707 14th Street, Zip 53913–1597; tel. 608/356–1400 **A**1 3 5 10 **F**5 11 12 13 15 28 29 34 36 38 40 56 60 64 69 70 75 76 77 78 81 82 86 93 107 108 115 117 118 129 130 143 146 **S** SSM Health Care, Saint Louis, MO
Primary Contact: Sandra L. Anderson, President
CFO: Troy Walker, Director Finance
CIO: Alan Steevens, Director Information Management
CHR: Jason Stelzer, Director Human Resources
Web address: www.stclare.com
**Control:** Church–operated, Nongovernment, not–for profit **Service:** General Medical and Surgical

**Staffed Beds:** 54 **Admissions:** 2322 **Census:** 20 **Outpatient Visits:** 82787 **Births:** 296 **Total Expense ($000):** 51979 **Payroll Expense ($000):** 21220 **Personnel:** 327

## BARRON—Barron County

☐ **MAYO CLINIC HEALTH SYSTEM – NORTHLAND IN BARRON (521315)**, 1222 Woodland Avenue, Zip 54812–1798; tel. 715/537–3186, (Total facility includes 20 beds in nursing home–type unit) **A**1 9 10 18 **F**3 7 10 13 15 18 28 29 30 31 34 35 36 40 43 44 45 56 57 59 60 64 65 67 68 69 74 75 76 77 78 79 80 81 84 85 86 87 89 93 97 102 107 108 110 113 117 118 124 126 127 129 130 131 132 134 142 143 144 145 147 **P**6 **S** Mayo Clinic Health System, Rochester, MN
Primary Contact: Maurita Sullivan, Administrator
COO: Karolyn Bartlett, Assistant Administrator
CFO: Kristy Hanson, Chief Financial Officer
CMO: Richard Nagler, M.D., Chief of Staff
CIO: Brian Foster, Vice President
Web address: www.luthermidelfortnorthland.org
**Control:** Other not–for–profit (including NFP Corporation) **Service:** General Medical and Surgical

**Staffed Beds:** 45 **Admissions:** 966 **Census:** 29 **Outpatient Visits:** 145897 **Births:** 104 **Total Expense ($000):** 43115 **Payroll Expense ($000):** 21579 **Personnel:** 360

*Many Facility Codes have changed. Please refer to the AHA Guide Code Chart.* © 2012 AHA Guide

WI

## BEAVER DAM—Dodge County

⊞ **BEAVER DAM COMMUNITY HOSPITALS (520076)**, 707 South University Avenue, Zip 53916–3089; tel. 920/887–7181, (Total facility includes 123 beds in nursing home–type unit) **A**1 9 10 19 **F**3 6 8 10 15 17 28 29 31 34 36 40 43 44 50 53 56 57 59 62 63 64 65 69 70 74 75 76 77 78 79 80 81 82 84 85 86 87 89 93 94 96 107 108 110 113 114 117 118 127 128 129 130 131 132 134 142 143 145 146 147 **P**6
Primary Contact: Kimberly J. Miller, FACHE, Chief Executive Officer
COO: Mark Monson, Chief Operating Officer
CFO: Donna Hutchinson, Chief Financial Officer
CMO: Eric Miller, M.D., Chief of Staff
CIO: Amy Nyberg, Chief Strategy Officer
CHR: Bridget Sheridan, Chief Human Resources Officer
Web address: www.bdch.com
**Control:** Other not–for–profit (including NFP Corporation) **Service:** General Medical and Surgical

**Staffed Beds:** 172 **Admissions:** 2624 **Census:** 136 **Outpatient Visits:** 99667 **Births:** 375 **Total Expense ($000):** 78327 **Payroll Expense ($000):** 24366 **Personnel:** 532

## BELOIT—Rock County

☐ **BELOIT HEALTH SYSTEM (520100)**, 1969 West Hart Road, Zip 53511–2299; tel. 608/364–5011 **A**1 9 10 **F**5 6 8 9 10 11 12 13 15 17 18 20 22 24 26 28 29 31 34 35 36 40 43 47 49 50 51 53 54 56 57 59 60 62 68 70 74 75 76 77 78 79 80 81 82 85 86 87 89 93 97 99 100 101 102 103 104 107 108 110 111 113 114 115 116 117 118 128 129 130 131 143 145 146 147 **P**1
Primary Contact: Gregory K. Britton, President and Chief Executive Officer
CFO: William E. Groeper, Vice President Finance
CMO: Leland From, M.D., Vice President Medical Affairs
CHR: Kristinn P. Armann, Vice President Human Resources
Web address: www.beloithealthsystem.org
**Control:** Other not–for–profit (including NFP Corporation) **Service:** General Medical and Surgical

**Staffed Beds:** 101 **Admissions:** 4404 **Census:** 47 **Outpatient Visits:** 370750 **Births:** 610 **Total Expense ($000):** 179779 **Payroll Expense ($000):** 79072 **Personnel:** 1158

## BERLIN—Green Lake County

☐ **BERLIN MEMORIAL HOSPITAL (521355)**, 225 Memorial Drive, Zip 54923–1295; tel. 920/361–1313, (Includes JULIETTE MANOR NURSING HOME, COMMUNITY CLINICS ), (Total facility includes 76 beds in nursing home–type unit) **A**1 9 10 18 **F**10 11 13 15 17 28 29 34 40 43 51 54 56 62 64 69 70 75 76 77 78 80 81 82 86 88 89 93 107 108 111 118 124 127 129 130 143 146
Primary Contact: John Feeney, President and Chief Executive Officer
CFO: Thomas P. Krystowiak, Vice President Finance
CIO: Greg Beltran, Director Information Technology
Web address: www.chnwi.org
**Control:** Other not–for–profit (including NFP Corporation) **Service:** General Medical and Surgical

**Staffed Beds:** 97 **Admissions:** 1957 **Census:** 76 **Outpatient Visits:** 61903 **Births:** 184 **Total Expense ($000):** 61795 **Payroll Expense ($000):** 28781 **Personnel:** 316

## BLACK RIVER FALLS—Jackson County

☐ **BLACK RIVER MEMORIAL HOSPITAL (521333)**, 711 West Adams Street, Zip 54615–9113; tel. 715/284–5361 **A**1 9 10 18 **F**3 8 11 13 18 29 30 40 48 53 56 57 62 63 65 69 75 76 77 79 80 81 85 86 89 90 93 107 111 112 114 115 116 117 118 128 129 130 131 132 134 143 145 147
Primary Contact: Stanley J. Gaynor, FACHE, President and Chief Executive Officer
CFO: Robert Daley, Vice President Fiscal and Information Technology Services
CMO: Jerome Kitowski, M.D., Chief of Staff
CIO: Robert Daley, Vice President Fiscal and Information Technology Services
CHR: Holly Winn, Vice President Human Resources and Ancillary Services
CNO: Mary Beth White–Jacobs, R.N., Vice President Patient Care Services
Web address: www.brmh.net
**Control:** Other not–for–profit (including NFP Corporation) **Service:** General Medical and Surgical

**Staffed Beds:** 25 **Admissions:** 881 **Census:** 7 **Outpatient Visits:** 17375 **Births:** 157 **Total Expense ($000):** 33808 **Payroll Expense ($000):** 14741 **Personnel:** 259

## BLOOMER—Chippewa County

☐ **MAYO CLINIC HEALTH SYSTEM – CHIPPEWA VALLEY IN BLOOMER (521314)**, 1501 Thompson Street, Zip 54724–1299; tel. 715/568–2000, (Total facility includes 30 beds in nursing home–type unit) **A**1 9 10 18 **F**3 15 18 28 29 30 31 32 34 35 40 43 44 54 56 57 59 64 65 67 75 77 78 81 84 85 86 87 93 96 97 102 107 108 110 113 118 127 129 131 132 143 145 147 **P**6 **S** Mayo Clinic Health System, Rochester, MN
Primary Contact: Edward A. Wittrock, Vice President Regional System
COO: Jennifer Abernathy, Assistant Administrator
CFO: Michele Eberle, Assistant Administrator
CHR: Sandra Moore, Director Human Resources
Web address: www.bloomermedicalcenter.org
**Control:** Other not–for–profit (including NFP Corporation) **Service:** General Medical and Surgical

**Staffed Beds:** 55 **Admissions:** 535 **Census:** 41 **Outpatient Visits:** 70616 **Births:** 0 **Total Expense ($000):** 28035 **Payroll Expense ($000):** 15465 **Personnel:** 248

## BOSCOBEL—Grant County

**BOSCOBEL AREA HEALTH CARE (521344)**, 205 Parker Street, Zip 53805–1698; tel. 608/375–4112 **A**9 10 18 **F**11 13 15 28 29 34 38 40 43 54 56 64 70 75 76 77 78 80 81 82 86 87 89 90 93 101 102 107 111 118 129 130 143 **P**6
Primary Contact: Richard Rogers, Administrator
CFO: Rita Moore, Director Finance
CMO: Thomas Pelz, M.D., Chief of Staff
CIO: Mathew Young, Manager Information Systems
CHR: Dennis Carpenter, Director Human Resources
Web address: www.boscobelhealth.com
**Control:** Other not–for–profit (including NFP Corporation) **Service:** General Medical and Surgical

**Staffed Beds:** 25 **Admissions:** 404 **Census:** 4 **Outpatient Visits:** 11846 **Births:** 57 **Total Expense ($000):** 13711 **Payroll Expense ($000):** 5171 **Personnel:** 97

## BROOKFIELD—Waukesha County

⊞ **WHEATON FRANCISCAN HEALTHCARE – ELMBROOK MEMORIAL (520170)**, 19333 West North Avenue, Zip 53045–4198; tel. 262/785–2000 **A**1 2 9 10 **F**3 4 8 11 12 13 15 17 29 30 31 34 35 36 40 43 44 47 49 50 54 56 58 59 64 68 70 72 74 75 76 77 78 79 80 81 82 84 85 86 87 89 90 91 93 96 97 99 100 107 108 109 110 111 112 113 114 116 117 118 119 120 122 125 129 130 131 132 134 142 143 144 145 146 147 **S** Wheaton Franciscan Healthcare, Wheaton, IL
Primary Contact: Debra K. Standridge, President
CFO: Annette Schiebel, Controller
CHR: Christopher Morris, Director Human Resources
Web address: www.wfhealthcare.org
**Control:** Church–operated, Nongovernment, not–for profit **Service:** General Medical and Surgical

**Staffed Beds:** 100 **Admissions:** 5029 **Census:** 55 **Outpatient Visits:** 73371 **Births:** 431 **Total Expense ($000):** 110897 **Payroll Expense ($000):** 32506 **Personnel:** 431

## BURLINGTON—Racine County

⊞ **AURORA MEMORIAL HOSPITAL OF BURLINGTON (520059)**, 252 McHenry Street, Zip 53105–1828; tel. 262/767–6000 **A**1 2 9 10 **F**3 11 13 15 17 18 20 26 29 30 34 35 36 39 40 41 44 45 46 47 48 49 50 51 53 56 57 58 59 64 65 68 70 74 75 76 79 80 81 82 84 85 86 87 89 93 94 96 100 107 108 109 110 111 113 115 117 118 129 130 131 133 134 145 147 **P**6 **S** Aurora Health Care, Milwaukee, WI
Primary Contact: Vicki Lewis, R.N., MS, FACHE, Vice President and Chief Administrative Officer
CFO: Stuart Arnett, Vice President Finance and Chief Financial Officer
CMO: David Farkas, M.D., President Medical Staff
CIO: Jean Chase, Regional Manager Information Services
CHR: Gene Krauklis, Regional Vice President Human Resources
Web address: www.aurorahealthcare.org
**Control:** Other not–for–profit (including NFP Corporation) **Service:** General Medical and Surgical

**Staffed Beds:** 65 **Admissions:** 2893 **Census:** 26 **Outpatient Visits:** 69616 **Births:** 289 **Total Expense ($000):** 64647 **Payroll Expense ($000):** 24759 **Personnel:** 475

**WI**

---

**Hospital, Medicare Provider Number, Address, Telephone, Approval, Facility, and Physician Codes, Health Care System**

★ American Hospital Association (AHA) membership
☐ The Joint Commission accreditation          ◇ DNV Healthcare Inc. accreditation
◯ American Osteopathic Association (AOA) accreditation
△ Commission on Accreditation of Rehabilitation Facilities (CARF) accreditation

### CHILTON—Calumet County

☐ **CALUMET MEDICAL CENTER (521317)**, 614 Memorial Drive,
Zip 53014–1597; tel. 920/849–2386 **A**1 9 10 18 **F**3 7 11 15 28 29 34 35 36
40 43 45 56 57 59 64 65 75 77 78 79 80 81 82 85 86 87 89 92 93 97 102
107 108 110 113 118 125 126 128 129 130 131 132 143 144 145 146 147
Primary Contact: Timothy Richman, President
CFO: Jeff Badger, Chief Financial Officer
CMO: Mark Kehrberg, M.D., Chief Medical Officer
CIO: Will Weider, Chief Information Officer
Web address: www.affinityhealth.org
**Control:** Other not–for–profit (including NFP Corporation) **Service:** General
Medical and Surgical

> **Staffed Beds:** 15 **Admissions:** 633 **Census:** 7 **Outpatient Visits:** 33629
> **Births:** 0 **Total Expense ($000):** 21109 **Payroll Expense ($000):** 9114
> **Personnel:** 134

### CHIPPEWA FALLS—Chippewa County

✠ **ST. JOSEPH'S HOSPITAL (520017)**, 2661 County Highway I, Zip 54729–1498;
tel. 715/723–1811 **A**1 9 10 **F**3 4 5 13 15 17 28 29 30 34 35 38 39 40 41 43
45 50 56 57 59 62 63 64 65 68 70 71 75 76 77 79 80 81 82 84 86 87 88
89 92 93 97 100 101 102 104 105 106 107 110 111 113 116 118 128 129
131 134 143 145 146 147 **S** Hospital Sisters Health System, Springfield, IL
Primary Contact: Joan Coffman, President and Chief Executive Officer
CFO: Kenneth Venuto, Chief Financial Officer
CMO: Stephen Carlson, M.D., President Medical Staff
CIO: Kevin Groskreutz, Director Information Systems
CHR: Kim Entenmann, Director People Services
Web address: www.stjoeschipfalls.com
**Control:** Other not–for–profit (including NFP Corporation) **Service:** General
Medical and Surgical

> **Staffed Beds:** 102 **Admissions:** 3291 **Census:** 38 **Outpatient Visits:** 68441
> **Births:** 453 **Total Expense ($000):** 60370 **Payroll Expense ($000):** 26134
> **Personnel:** 426

### COLUMBUS—Columbia County

✠ **COLUMBUS COMMUNITY HOSPITAL (521338)**, 1515 Park Avenue,
Zip 53925–2402; tel. 920/623–2200 **A**1 9 10 18 **F**3 8 13 15 16 17 18 28 29
34 40 45 51 56 57 64 70 75 76 77 78 79 80 81 85 86 88 89 91 93 94 96
107 108 110 113 117 118 128 129 131 132 134 143 145 146
Primary Contact: John D. Russell, President and Chief Executive Officer
CFO: Phillip Roberts, Vice President Finance and Chief Financial Officer
CMO: Gary Galvin, M.D., Chief of Staff
CIO: Phillip Roberts, Vice President Finance and Chief Financial Officer
CHR: Ann Roundy, Vice President Employee Services
Web address: www.cch–inc.com
**Control:** Other not–for–profit (including NFP Corporation) **Service:** General
Medical and Surgical

> **Staffed Beds:** 25 **Admissions:** 846 **Census:** 9 **Outpatient Visits:** 40513
> **Births:** 56 **Total Expense ($000):** 25927 **Payroll Expense ($000):** 10194
> **Personnel:** 155

### CUBA CITY—Grant County

**SOUTHWEST HEALTH CENTER NURSING HOME** See Southwest Health Center,
Platteville

### CUDAHY—Milwaukee County

**AURORA ST. LUKE'S SOUTH SHORE** See Aurora St. Luke's Medical Center,
Milwaukee

### CUMBERLAND—Barron County

☐ **CUMBERLAND MEMORIAL HOSPITAL (521353)**, 1110 Seventh Avenue,
Zip 54829–9133; tel. 715/822–2741, (Total facility includes 50 beds in nursing
home–type unit) **A**1 9 10 18 **F**11 13 28 29 34 40 43 53 56 75 76 77 81 82 86
87 89 93 98 102 103 104 107 124 127 129 130 143
Primary Contact: Debora A. Kunferman, Administrator and Chief Executive Officer
COO: Debora A. Kunferman, Administrator and Chief Executive Officer
CFO: Angela Martens, Controller
CMO: Kenneth Garrison, M.D., Chief of Staff
CHR: Hilary Butzler, Director Human Resources
Web address: www.cumberlandhealthcare.com
**Control:** Other not–for–profit (including NFP Corporation) **Service:** General
Medical and Surgical

> **Staffed Beds:** 85 **Admissions:** 1230 **Census:** 55 **Outpatient Visits:** 10066
> **Births:** 58 **Total Expense ($000):** 15962 **Payroll Expense ($000):** 7884
> **Personnel:** 137

### DARLINGTON—Lafayette County

**MEMORIAL HOSPITAL OF LAFAYETTE COUNTY (521312)**, 800 Clay Street,
Zip 53530–1228, Mailing Address: P.O. Box 70, Zip 53530–0070;
tel. 608/776–4466 **A**9 10 18 **F**1 3 11 13 15 18 26 28 29 32 35 40 43 45 46
47 48 56 57 60 64 68 74 75 76 79 80 81 82 86 89 90 93 102 105 107 111
115 116 118 129 130 132 143
Primary Contact: Sherry Kudronowicz, Administrator
CFO: Marie Wamsley, Chief Financial Officer
Web address: www.memorialhospitaloflafayettecounty.org
**Control:** County–Government, nonfederal **Service:** General Medical and Surgical

> **Staffed Beds:** 23 **Admissions:** 428 **Census:** 4 **Outpatient Visits:** 18594
> **Births:** 41 **Total Expense ($000):** 11708 **Payroll Expense ($000):** 3408
> **Personnel:** 90

### DODGEVILLE—Iowa County

✠ **UPLAND HILLS HEALTH (521352)**, 800 Compassion Way, Zip 53533–0800,
Mailing Address: P.O. Box 800, Zip 53533–0800; tel. 608/930–8000, (Total
facility includes 44 beds in nursing home–type unit) **A**1 9 10 18 **F**3 11 13 15 17
28 29 34 36 40 41 43 45 47 53 54 56 57 59 60 62 63 64 67 70 75 76 77
78 79 80 81 82 84 85 86 87 88 89 90 92 93 96 97 107 110 113 118 127
128 129 130 132 143 145 146 147 **P**6
Primary Contact: Phyllis Fritsch, Administrator
COO: Steve McCarthy, Assistant Administrator Business Operations
CFO: Karl Pustina, Assistant Administrator Finance
CIO: Karen Thuli, Coordinator Information Systems
CHR: Troy Marx, Director Human Resources
Web address: www.uplandhillshealth.org
**Control:** Other not–for–profit (including NFP Corporation) **Service:** General
Medical and Surgical

> **Staffed Beds:** 69 **Admissions:** 1227 **Census:** 52 **Outpatient Visits:** 49829
> **Births:** 254 **Total Expense ($000):** 35587 **Payroll Expense ($000):** 14535
> **Personnel:** 257

### DURAND—Pepin County

★ **CHIPPEWA VALLEY HOSPITAL AND OAKVIEW CARE CENTER (521307)**,
1220 Third Avenue West, Zip 54736–1600, Mailing Address: P.O. Box 224,
Zip 54736–0224; tel. 715/672–4211, (Total facility includes 50 beds in nursing
home–type unit) **A**9 10 18 **F**3 15 28 29 30 40 56 69 75 81 85 86 87 97 107
108 114 127 129 132 **S** Adventist Health System Sunbelt Health Care
Corporation, Altamonte Springs, FL
Primary Contact: Douglas R. Peterson, President and Chief Executive Officer
Web address: www.keepingyouwell.com
**Control:** Church–operated, Nongovernment, not–for profit **Service:** General
Medical and Surgical

> **Staffed Beds:** 75 **Admissions:** 432 **Census:** 52 **Outpatient Visits:** 14974
> **Births:** 0 **Total Expense ($000):** 14751 **Payroll Expense ($000):** 5793
> **Personnel:** 85

### EAGLE RIVER—Vilas County

★ **EAGLE RIVER MEMORIAL HOSPITAL (521300)**, 201 Hospital Road,
Zip 54521–8835; tel. 715/479–7411 **A**9 10 18 **F**3 11 15 28 29 30 35 40 41
45 47 50 59 68 69 75 80 81 82 84 85 86 89 93 107 108 110 113 118 129
132 145 147 **S** Marian Health System, Tulsa, OK
Primary Contact: Sheila Clough, President
COO: Sheila Clough, President
CFO: Cathy Bukowski, Regional Chief Financial Officer
CMO: Terrance D. Moe, M.D., President Medical Staff
CIO: Will Weider, Chief Information Officer
CHR: Michelle Cornelius, Director Human Resources for Northern Region
Web address: www.ministryhealth.org
**Control:** Church–operated, Nongovernment, not–for profit **Service:** General
Medical and Surgical

> **Staffed Beds:** 9 **Admissions:** 481 **Census:** 6 **Outpatient Visits:** 22007
> **Births:** 0 **Total Expense ($000):** 13857 **Payroll Expense ($000):** 5573
> **Personnel:** 103

**WI**

*Many Facility Codes have changed. Please refer to the AHA Guide Code Chart.*

## EAU CLAIRE—Eau Claire County

☐ **MAYO CLINIC HEALTH SYSTEM IN EAU CLAIRE (520070)**, 1221 Whipple Street, Zip 54702–4105, Mailing Address: P.O. Box 5, Zip 54702–0005; tel. 715/838–3311 **A**1 2 3 5 7 9 10 **F**3 4 5 8 11 12 13 15 17 18 20 22 24 26 28 29 30 31 32 34 35 37 40 43 44 45 46 48 49 50 51 53 57 58 59 60 64 65 68 70 71 72 74 75 76 77 78 79 80 81 82 83 84 85 86 87 89 90 92 93 96 98 99 100 101 102 103 104 105 107 108 110 111 114 117 118 119 120 123 125 128 129 131 134 144 145 146 147 **P**6 **S** Mayo Clinic Health System, Rochester, MN
Primary Contact: Randall L. Linton, M.D., President and Chief Executive Officer
COO: John M. Dickey, Chief Administrative Officer
CFO: Paul Bammel, Vice President
CMO: Terrance Borman, M.D., Medical Director
CIO: Brian Foster, Chief Information Officer
CHR: Blythe Loyd, Vice President
Web address: www.mhs.mayo.edu
**Control:** Other not–for–profit (including NFP Corporation) **Service:** General Medical and Surgical

> **Staffed Beds:** 204 **Admissions:** 11207 **Census:** 124 **Outpatient Visits:** 160792 **Births:** 1053 **Total Expense ($000):** 222152 **Payroll Expense ($000):** 86465 **Personnel:** 1666

☐ **OAKLEAF SURGICAL HOSPITAL (520196)**, 3802 West Oakwood Mall Drive, Zip 54701; tel. 715/831–8130 **A**1 9 10 **F**3 37 45 47 48 51 64 75 79 80 81 82 85 108 118 129 141 144 **S** National Surgical Hospitals, Chicago, IL
Primary Contact: Anne Hargrave–Thomas, Chief Executive Officer
Web address: www.oakleafmedical.com
**Control:** Corporation, Investor–owned, for–profit **Service:** General Medical and Surgical

> **Staffed Beds:** 13 **Admissions:** 493 **Census:** 4 **Outpatient Visits:** 8658 **Births:** 0 **Total Expense ($000):** 27477 **Payroll Expense ($000):** 7821 **Personnel:** 114

☒ △ **SACRED HEART HOSPITAL (520013)**, 900 West Clairemont Avenue, Zip 54701–6122; tel. 715/717–4121 **A**1 2 3 5 7 9 10 **F**3 6 8 11 12 13 15 17 18 20 22 24 28 29 30 31 32 34 35 38 39 40 41 43 45 46 48 49 50 53 56 57 59 60 64 65 68 69 70 71 72 74 75 76 77 78 79 80 81 82 84 85 86 87 88 89 90 91 92 93 94 97 98 99 100 101 103 107 108 109 110 111 112 113 114 115 116 117 118 119 120 123 125 128 129 131 133 134 140 143 144 145 146 147 **S** Hospital Sisters Health System, Springfield, IL
Primary Contact: Julie Manas, President and Chief Executive Officer
COO: Faye L. Deich, R.N., Chief Operating Officer
CMO: Melissa Emmerich, M.D., President Medical Staff
CIO: Pete Nohelty, Chief Information Officer
CHR: Robert J. Hassemer, Division Director Human Resources
Web address: www.sacredhearthospital–ec.org
**Control:** Other not–for–profit (including NFP Corporation) **Service:** General Medical and Surgical

> **Staffed Beds:** 212 **Admissions:** 9843 **Census:** 127 **Outpatient Visits:** 106675 **Births:** 893 **Total Expense ($000):** 188519 **Payroll Expense ($000):** 65930 **Personnel:** 1051

## EDGERTON—Rock County

★ **EDGERTON HOSPITAL AND HEALTH SERVICES (521319)**, 11101 North Sherman Road, Zip 53534–9002; tel. 608/884–3441 **A**9 10 18 **F**11 15 28 34 40 43 64 75 77 81 86 90 93 107 108 111 118 129 143 **P**6
Primary Contact: James O. Pernau, Chief Executive Officer
CFO: Charles Roader, Vice President Finance
CMO: William West, M.D., Chief of Staff
CIO: Sheryl Rucker, Chief Information Officer
CHR: Brad Olm, Director Human Resources
Web address: www.edgertonhospital.com
**Control:** Other not–for–profit (including NFP Corporation) **Service:** General Medical and Surgical

> **Staffed Beds:** 18 **Admissions:** 349 **Census:** 6 **Outpatient Visits:** 17927 **Births:** 0 **Total Expense ($000):** 16350 **Payroll Expense ($000):** 6745 **Personnel:** 117

## ELKHORN—Walworth County

☒ △ **AURORA LAKELAND MEDICAL CENTER (520102)**, W3985 County Road NN, Zip 53121–4389; tel. 262/741–2000 **A**1 2 7 9 10 **F**3 11 13 15 17 18 29 30 31 34 35 36 40 41 44 45 46 47 48 49 50 51 56 57 58 59 64 65 68 70 74 75 76 78 79 80 81 82 84 85 86 87 89 90 93 94 96 100 107 108 110 111 113 115 117 118 128 129 130 131 134 145 147 **P**6 **S** Aurora Health Care, Milwaukee, WI
Primary Contact: Vicki Lewis, R.N., MS, FACHE, Vice President and Chief Administrative Officer
CFO: Stuart Arnett, Regional Vice President Finance
CMO: Greg Gerber, M.D., Chief Medical Officer
CIO: Jean Chase, Regional Manager Information Services
CHR: Gene Krauklis, Regional Vice President Human Resources
Web address: www.aurorahealthcare.org
**Control:** Other not–for–profit (including NFP Corporation) **Service:** General Medical and Surgical

> **Staffed Beds:** 75 **Admissions:** 3142 **Census:** 33 **Outpatient Visits:** 76195 **Births:** 670 **Total Expense ($000):** 67042 **Payroll Expense ($000):** 22418 **Personnel:** 427

## FOND DU LAC—Fond Du Lac County

★ △ **AGNESIAN HEALTHCARE (520088)**, 430 East Division Street, Zip 54935–0385, Mailing Address: P.O. Box 385, Zip 54936–0385; tel. 920/929–2300 **A**2 7 9 10 20 **F**2 3 4 5 6 11 13 15 17 18 20 22 24 26 28 29 30 31 34 35 38 40 43 44 45 46 47 48 49 50 51 53 54 55 56 57 59 60 62 63 64 66 67 68 69 70 71 74 75 76 77 78 79 80 81 82 83 86 87 88 89 90 93 97 98 99 100 101 102 103 104 105 107 108 110 111 113 114 116 117 118 119 120 122 128 129 130 131 133 134 142 143 145 146 147 **P**3 6
Primary Contact: Steven N. Little, President and Chief Executive Officer
CIO: Nancy Birschbach, Vice President Information Services
Web address: www.agnesian.com
**Control:** Church–operated, Nongovernment, not–for profit **Service:** General Medical and Surgical

> **Staffed Beds:** 167 **Admissions:** 6572 **Census:** 76 **Outpatient Visits:** 662445 **Births:** 870 **Total Expense ($000):** 275670 **Payroll Expense ($000):** 91082 **Personnel:** 1168

**FOND DU LAC COUNTY MENTAL HEALTH CENTER (524025)**, 459 East First Street, Zip 54935–4599; tel. 920/929–3571 **A**9 10 **F**4 38 98 99 102 103 129 **P**6
Primary Contact: Don Stout, Administrator
Web address: www.fdlco.wi.gov
**Control:** County–Government, nonfederal **Service:** Psychiatric

> **Staffed Beds:** 25 **Admissions:** 1025 **Census:** 14 **Outpatient Visits:** 449 **Births:** 0 **Total Expense ($000):** 3779 **Payroll Expense ($000):** 2090 **Personnel:** 44

## FORT ATKINSON—Jefferson County

☒ **FORT HEALTHCARE (520071)**, 611 East Sherman Avenue, Zip 53538–1998; tel. 920/568–5000, (Total facility includes 28 beds in nursing home–type unit) **A**1 9 10 **F**3 11 12 13 15 28 29 34 35 40 53 56 57 59 62 68 75 76 77 79 80 81 82 85 86 87 89 90 93 94 96 107 108 110 111 113 114 117 118 126 127 128 129 131 134 143 144 145 146 **P**1 5
Primary Contact: Michael S. Wallace, President and Chief Executive Officer
CFO: James J. Nelson, Senior Vice President Finance and Strategic Planning
CIO: James E. Dahl, Chief Information Officer
CHR: Nancy Alstad, Director Human Resources
Web address: www.forthealthcare.com
**Control:** Other not–for–profit (including NFP Corporation) **Service:** General Medical and Surgical

> **Staffed Beds:** 100 **Admissions:** 3114 **Census:** 34 **Outpatient Visits:** 192674 **Births:** 450 **Total Expense ($000):** 124959 **Payroll Expense ($000):** 40813 **Personnel:** 698

## FRANKLIN—Milwaukee County

☒ **MIDWEST ORTHOPEDIC SPECIALTY HOSPITAL (520205)**, 10101 South 27th Street, 2nd Floor, Zip 53132–7209; tel. 414/817–5800 **A**1 9 10 **F**29 34 81 86 129 130 **S** Wheaton Franciscan Healthcare, Wheaton, IL
Primary Contact: Daniel Mattes, Chief Executive Officer
Web address: www.mymosh.com/
**Control:** Partnership, Investor–owned, for–profit **Service:** General Medical and Surgical

> **Staffed Beds:** 16 **Admissions:** 1288 **Census:** 10 **Outpatient Visits:** 7666 **Births:** 0 **Total Expense ($000):** 33141 **Payroll Expense ($000):** 5150 **Personnel:** 93

**WI**

---

**Hospital, Medicare Provider Number, Address, Telephone, Approval, Facility, and Physician Codes, Health Care System**

★ American Hospital Association (AHA) membership
☐ The Joint Commission accreditation ◇ DNV Healthcare Inc. accreditation
○ American Osteopathic Association (AOA) accreditation
△ Commission on Accreditation of Rehabilitation Facilities (CARF) accreditation

⊠ **WHEATON FRANCISCAN HEALTHCARE – FRANKLIN (520204)**, 10101 South 27th Street, Zip 53132–7209; tel. 414/325–4700 **A**1 9 10 **F**15 29 34 40 64 70 75 77 82 86 87 93 107 108 111 118 129 130 143 146 **S** Wheaton Franciscan Healthcare, Wheaton, IL
Primary Contact: Daniel Mattes, President
Web address: www.mywheaton.org/
**Control:** Church–operated, Nongovernment, not–for profit **Service:** General Medical and Surgical

**Staffed Beds:** 19 **Admissions:** 1145 **Census:** 11 **Outpatient Visits:** 58900 **Births:** 0 **Total Expense ($000):** 40224 **Payroll Expense ($000):** 14984 **Personnel:** 268

**FRIENDSHIP—Adams County**

**MOUNDVIEW MEMORIAL HOSPITAL & CLINICS (521309)**, 402 West Lake Street, Zip 53934–0040, Mailing Address: P.O. Box 40, Zip 53934–0040; tel. 608/339–3331 **A**9 10 18 **F**6 11 15 28 29 34 36 40 43 56 64 77 81 82 86 87 93 107 111 117 118 129 143 **P**5 6
Primary Contact: Jeremy Normington–Slay, FACHE, Chief Executive Officer
Web address: www.moundview.org
**Control:** Other not–for–profit (including NFP Corporation) **Service:** General Medical and Surgical

**Staffed Beds:** 25 **Admissions:** 265 **Census:** 4 **Outpatient Visits:** 23833 **Births:** 0 **Total Expense ($000):** 14105 **Payroll Expense ($000):** 5948 **Personnel:** 104

**GRAFTON—Ozaukee County**

⊠ **AURORA MEDICAL CENTER GRAFTON (520207)**, 975 Port Washington Road, Zip 53024–9201; tel. 262/329–1000 **A**1 9 10 **F**3 6 8 13 15 17 18 20 22 24 26 28 29 30 36 40 41 43 44 45 46 48 49 50 51 53 56 65 68 69 70 72 74 75 76 79 80 81 85 86 87 89 91 93 96 107 108 109 110 111 112 113 114 117 118 125 129 130 145 147 **P**6 **S** Aurora Health Care, Milwaukee, WI
Primary Contact: Leonard E. Wilk, Vice President and Chief Administrative Officer
CMO: William Ebinger, M.D., President and Chief of Staff
Web address: www.aurorahealthcare.org
**Control:** Other not–for–profit (including NFP Corporation) **Service:** General Medical and Surgical

**Staffed Beds:** 81 **Admissions:** 4440 **Census:** 43 **Outpatient Visits:** 29329 **Births:** 497 **Total Expense ($000):** 107707 **Payroll Expense ($000):** 36115 **Personnel:** 691

**GRANTSBURG—Burnett County**

★ **BURNETT MEDICAL CENTER (521331)**, 257 West St. George Avenue, Zip 54840–7827; tel. 715/463–5353, (Total facility includes 50 beds in nursing home–type unit) **A**9 10 18 **F**2 3 13 15 28 29 31 35 40 45 56 57 59 64 67 68 75 76 77 78 80 81 85 86 87 89 90 93 97 107 113 126 127 129 130 131 132 134 143 147 **P**6
Primary Contact: Gordon Lewis, Chief Executive Officer
CFO: Charles J. Faught, Chief Financial Officer
CMO: Hans Rechsteiner, M.D., Chief of Staff
CIO: Andy Douglas, Manager Information Technology
CHR: Sandy Hinrichs, Director Human Resources
Web address: www.burnettmedicalcenter.com
**Control:** Other not–for–profit (including NFP Corporation) **Service:** General Medical and Surgical

**Staffed Beds:** 67 **Admissions:** 582 **Census:** 54 **Outpatient Visits:** 35121 **Births:** 44 **Total Expense ($000):** 16228 **Payroll Expense ($000):** 6916 **Personnel:** 128

**GREEN BAY—Brown County**

⊠ △ **AURORA BAYCARE MEDICAL CENTER (520193)**, 2845 Greenbrier Road, Zip 54311, Mailing Address: P.O. Box 8900, Zip 54308; tel. 920/288–8000 **A**1 2 7 9 10 **F**3 8 12 13 15 17 18 20 22 24 26 28 29 30 31 34 35 36 40 41 43 44 45 46 47 48 49 50 53 54 57 58 59 64 65 70 72 74 75 76 78 79 80 81 82 85 86 87 89 90 93 94 96 107 109 110 111 113 114 115 116 117 118 119 120 122 123 125 128 129 130 131 134 143 145 146 147 **P**6 **S** Aurora Health Care, Milwaukee, WI
Primary Contact: Daniel T. Meyer, Chief Administrative Officer
COO: Daniel T. Meyer, Chief Administrative Officer
CFO: Sandra Ewald, Vice President Finance
CMO: Corey Vogel, M.D., Chief of Staff
CIO: Chuck Geurts, Manager Management Information Services
CHR: Elizabeth A. Kirby, Director Human Resources
Web address: www.aurorabaycare.com
**Control:** Partnership, Investor–owned, for–profit **Service:** General Medical and Surgical

**Staffed Beds:** 159 **Admissions:** 7788 **Census:** 92 **Outpatient Visits:** 172654 **Births:** 1724 **Total Expense ($000):** 203097 **Payroll Expense ($000):** 63166 **Personnel:** 1191

⊠ **BELLIN MEMORIAL HOSPITAL (520049)**, 744 South Webster Avenue, Zip 54301–3581, Mailing Address: P.O. Box 23400, Zip 54305–3400; tel. 920/433–3500 **A**1 9 10 21 **F**12 13 15 17 20 22 24 28 29 34 36 40 43 51 53 54 56 62 64 75 76 77 78 80 81 82 86 87 89 90 108 111 115 117 118 129 130 143 **P**2 6 8
Primary Contact: George Kerwin, President
CFO: Jim Dietsche, Chief Financial Officer
CMO: Christopher Watson, M.D., Chief Medical Officer
CIO: Jacquelyn Hunt, Vice President Clinical Support and Information Services
CHR: Ken Peters, Director Human Resources Management
Web address: www.bellin.org
**Control:** Church–operated, Nongovernment, not–for profit **Service:** General Medical and Surgical

**Staffed Beds:** 238 **Admissions:** 8556 **Census:** 91 **Outpatient Visits:** 611705 **Births:** 1263 **Total Expense ($000):** 319540 **Payroll Expense ($000):** 144094 **Personnel:** 2017

☐ **BELLIN PSYCHIATRIC CENTER (524038)**, 301 East St. Joseph Street, Zip 54305–3725, Mailing Address: P.O. Box 23725, Zip 54305–3725; tel. 920/433–3630 **A**1 9 10 21 **F**4 5 6 29 34 36 38 53 54 56 64 75 86 87 98 99 100 101 102 103 104 105 129 **P**6
Primary Contact: Sharla Baenen, President
CFO: Kevin McGurk, Controller
CMO: Anthony Marchlewski, M.D., President Medical and Psychological Staff
CIO: Randy Ronsman, Director Information Services
CHR: Ken Peters, Director Human Resources
Web address: www.bellin.org
**Control:** Church–operated, Nongovernment, not–for profit **Service:** Psychiatric

**Staffed Beds:** 53 **Admissions:** 1889 **Census:** 21 **Outpatient Visits:** 60600 **Births:** 0 **Total Expense ($000):** 16893 **Payroll Expense ($000):** 10625 **Personnel:** 141

**BROWN COUNTY COMMUNITY TREATMENT CENTER (524014)**, 3150 Gershwin Drive, Zip 54311–5899; tel. 920/391–4700 **A**10 **F**4 5 75 98 101 102 103 104 129
Primary Contact: Mary Johnson, Administrator
CFO: Margaret Hoff, Account Manager
CMO: Yogesh Pareek, M.D., Clinical Director
CIO: Linda Turner, Manager Health Information Management
CHR: Debbie Klarkowski, Manager Human Resources
Web address: www.co.brown.wi.us/
**Control:** County–Government, nonfederal **Service:** Psychiatric

**Staffed Beds:** 22 **Admissions:** 1800 **Census:** 20 **Outpatient Visits:** 1188 **Births:** 0 **Total Expense ($000):** 5827 **Payroll Expense ($000):** 3118 **Personnel:** 84

**BROWN COUNTY HUMAN SERVICES MENTAL HEALTH CENTER** See Brown County Community Treatment Center

⊠ **ST. MARY'S HOSPITAL MEDICAL CENTER (520097)**, 1726 Shawano Avenue, Zip 54303–3282; tel. 920/498–4200 **A**1 9 10 **F**3 13 15 17 18 20 22 28 29 30 31 34 35 40 43 44 45 46 47 48 49 50 51 53 55 57 59 64 65 68 69 70 74 75 76 77 78 79 80 81 82 84 85 86 87 88 89 93 94 96 102 107 108 110 113 114 115 116 117 118 129 131 142 143 144 145 146 147 **P**2 **S** Hospital Sisters Health System, Springfield, IL
Primary Contact: Therese B. Pandl, President and Chief Executive Officer
COO: Lawrence J. Connors, Chief Operating Officer
CFO: John Miller, Chief Financial Officer
CMO: Timothy Jahn, M.D., Medical Director and Liaison
CIO: Tanya Townsend, Chief Information Officer
CHR: Amy Unrath, Administrator Human Resources
Web address: www.stmgb.org
**Control:** Church–operated, Nongovernment, not–for profit **Service:** General Medical and Surgical

**Staffed Beds:** 83 **Admissions:** 4661 **Census:** 45 **Outpatient Visits:** 101372 **Births:** 665 **Total Expense ($000):** 109526 **Payroll Expense ($000):** 34400 **Personnel:** 410

⊠ **ST. VINCENT HOSPITAL (520075)**, 835 South Van Buren Street, Zip 54301–3526, Mailing Address: P.O. Box 13508, Zip 54307–3508; tel. 920/433–0111 **A**1 2 9 10 **F**3 9 11 12 13 15 17 18 20 22 24 29 30 31 32 34 35 36 40 43 44 45 49 50 51 56 57 58 59 60 62 64 65 68 69 70 72 74 75 76 77 78 79 80 81 83 84 85 86 88 89 90 91 92 93 94 96 107 108 110 111 113 114 115 116 117 118 119 120 122 123 125 128 129 131 134 142 143 145 146 147 **P**6 **S** Hospital Sisters Health System, Springfield, IL
Primary Contact: Therese B. Pandl, President and Chief Executive Officer
COO: Thomas R. Bayer, Chief Operating Officer
CFO: Kelly Gigot, Assistant Administrator and Chief Financial Officer
CMO: Kenneth Johnson, M.D., President Medical Staff
CIO: Tanya Townsend, Chief Information Officer
CHR: Jean Marsch, Director Human Resources
Web address: www.stvgh.org
**Control:** Church–operated, Nongovernment, not–for profit **Service:** General Medical and Surgical

**Staffed Beds:** 255 **Admissions:** 9481 **Census:** 137 **Outpatient Visits:** 177372 **Births:** 837 **Total Expense ($000):** 247780 **Payroll Expense ($000):** 85193 **Personnel:** 1606

*Many Facility Codes have changed. Please refer to the AHA Guide Code Chart.* © 2012 AHA Guide

**GREENFIELD—Milwaukee County**

⊠ **KINDRED HOSPITAL–MILWAUKEE (522004)**, 5017 South 110Th Stret, Zip 53228–3131; tel. 414/427–8282 **A**1 9 10 **F**1 3 29 56 75 80 85 86 87 90 96 97 100 129 147 **S** Kindred Healthcare, Louisville, KY
Primary Contact: Linda Newberry-Ferguson, Chief Executive Officer
COO: Christine Ninu, Chief Operating Officer
CMO: Alok Goyal, M.D., Medical Director
Web address: www.khmilwaukee.com/
**Control:** Corporation, Investor–owned, for-profit **Service:** Long–Term Acute Care hospital

**Staffed Beds:** 56 **Admissions:** 436 **Census:** 32 **Outpatient Visits:** 0 **Births:** 0 **Total Expense ($000):** 17898 **Payroll Expense ($000):** 6452 **Personnel:** 135

**HARTFORD—Washington County**

⊠ **AURORA MEDICAL CENTER OF WASHINGTON COUNTY (520038)**, 1032 East Sumner Street, Zip 53027–1698; tel. 262/673–2300 **A**1 2 9 10 **F**2 3 8 11 13 15 17 28 29 30 32 34 35 37 39 40 41 43 44 46 47 48 49 50 53 54 56 57 58 59 60 64 65 68 70 74 75 76 79 80 81 82 84 85 87 89 90 93 97 107 108 111 117 118 128 129 130 131 132 133 134 142 145 147 **P**6 **S** Aurora Health Care, Milwaukee, WI
Primary Contact: Lisa Just, Vice President and Chief Administrative Officer
CMO: Steven Holcomb, M.D., Chief of Staff
CIO: John Sipek, Supervisor Client Services
CHR: Tom TerHorst, Director Human Resources
Web address: www.aurorahealthcare.org
**Control:** Other not–for–profit (including NFP Corporation) **Service:** General Medical and Surgical

**Staffed Beds:** 45 **Admissions:** 1857 **Census:** 17 **Outpatient Visits:** 60373 **Births:** 213 **Total Expense ($000):** 45932 **Payroll Expense ($000):** 17756 **Personnel:** 327

**HAYWARD—Sawyer County**

★ **HAYWARD AREA MEMORIAL HOSPITAL AND NURSING HOME (521336)**, 11040 North State Road 77, Zip 54843–6391; tei. 715/934–4321, (Total facility includes 57 beds in nursing home–type unit) **A**9 10 18 **F**10 11 13 15 34 40 43 51 56 64 75 76 78 81 82 86 93 107 118 127 129
Primary Contact: Timothy M. Gullingsrud, Chief Executive Officer
CHR: Rose Gates, Director Human Resources
Web address: www.hamhnh.com
**Control:** Other not–for–profit (including NFP Corporation) **Service:** General Medical and Surgical

**Staffed Beds:** 75 **Admissions:** 1062 **Census:** 66 **Outpatient Visits:** 22160 **Births:** 149 **Total Expense ($000):** 27021 **Payroll Expense ($000):** 12024 **Personnel:** 148

**HILLSBORO—Vernon County**

★ **ST. JOSEPH'S HEALTH SERVICES (521304)**, 400 Water Avenue, Zip 54634–0527, Mailing Address: P.O. Box 527, Zip 54634–0527; tel. 608/489–8000 **A**9 10 18 **F**11 15 28 29 34 40 43 53 54 56 64 69 75 77 80 81 82 86 87 89 90 93 107 129 130 143 146 **P**6
Primary Contact: Debra Smith, Chief Executive Officer
CFO: Tom Jones, Interim Chief Financial Officer
CMO: Sheila A. Patel, M.D., Chief of Staff
CHR: Kristie McCoic, Director Human Resources
Web address: www.stjhealthcare.org
**Control:** Other not–for–profit (including NFP Corporation) **Service:** General Medical and Surgical

**Staffed Beds:** 18 **Admissions:** 307 **Census:** 3 **Outpatient Visits:** 20601 **Births:** 0 **Total Expense ($000):** 14657 **Payroll Expense ($000):** 6528 **Personnel:** 130

**HUDSON—St. Croix County**

☐ **HUDSON HOSPITAL (521335)**, 405 Stageline Road, Zip 54016–1600; tel. 715/531–6000 **A**1 9 10 18 **F**3 5 13 15 22 28 29 30 31 34 35 36 37 40 44 45 46 50 53 56 59 64 68 69 74 75 76 78 79 80 81 85 86 87 89 93 94 96 97 107 108 110 111 114 116 118 128 129 130 131 132 134 145 147
Primary Contact: Marian M. Furlong, R.N., Chief Executive Officer
CFO: Sheila R. Proehl, Chief Financial Officer
CMO: Mark Stannard, M.D., Chief of Staff
CIO: Sheila R. Proehl, Chief Financial Officer
CHR: Brenda L. Creighton, Director Human Resources
Web address: www.hudsonhospital.org
**Control:** Other not–for–profit (including NFP Corporation) **Service:** General Medical and Surgical

**Staffed Beds:** 23 **Admissions:** 1653 **Census:** 14 **Outpatient Visits:** 41980 **Births:** 624 **Total Expense ($000):** 47976 **Payroll Expense ($000):** 17302 **Personnel:** 323

**JANESVILLE—Rock County**

⊠ **MERCY HOSPITAL AND TRAUMA CENTER (520066)**, 1000 Mineral Point Avenue, Zip 53547–2982, Mailing Address: P.O. Box 5003, Zip 53547–5003; tel. 608/756–6000, (Total facility includes 27 beds in nursing home–type unit) **A**1 2 9 10 **F**4 5 6 9 11 12 13 15 17 20 22 24 28 29 34 38 40 43 54 55 56 60 61 64 69 70 75 76 77 78 80 81 82 86 87 88 89 90 93 98 100 101 102 103 104 105 107 108 111 115 117 118 127 129 130 146 **P**5 6 **S** Mercy Health System, Janesville, WI
Primary Contact: Javon R. Bea, President and Chief Executive Officer
CFO: John Cook, Vice President and Chief Financial Officer
CHR: Kathy Harris, Vice President
Web address: www.mercyhealthsystem.org
**Control:** Other not–for–profit (including NFP Corporation) **Service:** General Medical and Surgical

**Staffed Beds:** 148 **Admissions:** 9677 **Census:** 114 **Outpatient Visits:** 984114 **Births:** 1152 **Total Expense ($000):** 367302 **Payroll Expense ($000):** 91191 **Personnel:** 2110

**KENOSHA—Kenosha County**

⊠ **AURORA MEDICAL CENTER (520189)**, 10400 South 75th Street, Zip 53142; tel. 262/948–5600 **A**1 2 9 10 **F**3 8 11 13 15 17 18 20 28 29 30 34 35 36 39 40 41 44 45 46 47 48 49 50 51 54 57 58 59 64 65 68 70 74 75 76 79 80 81 82 85 86 87 89 93 94 96 107 108 110 111 113 114 115 116 117 118 119 120 122 128 129 130 131 134 145 147 **P**6 **S** Aurora Health Care, Milwaukee, WI
Primary Contact: Christine K. Olson, R.N., MSN, Chief Administrative Officer and Chief Nursing Executive
COO: Christine K. Olson, R.N., Chief Administrative Officer and Chief Nursing Executive
CFO: Stuart Arnett, Vice President Finance
CMO: David Farkas, M.D., President Medical Staff
CIO: Jean Chase, Regional Manager Information Services
CHR: Gene Krauklis, Regional Vice President Human Resources
Web address: www.aurorahealthcare.org
**Control:** Other not–for–profit (including NFP Corporation) **Service:** General Medical and Surgical

**Staffed Beds:** 73 **Admissions:** 4419 **Census:** 44 **Outpatient Visits:** 143242 **Births:** 827 **Total Expense ($000):** 100728 **Payroll Expense ($000):** 30895 **Personnel:** 597

☐ **UNITED HEALTH SYSTEM–KENOSHA CAMPUS (520021)**, 6308 Eighth Avenue, Zip 53143–5082; tel. 262/656–2011 **A**1 9 10 **F**1 11 12 13 15 17 20 22 24 28 29 34 40 43 51 53 60 64 70 72 75 76 77 78 80 81 86 87 89 90 93 100 102 107 108 111 117 118 129 130 143 146 **P**6
Primary Contact: Richard O. Schmidt, Jr., President and Chief Executive Officer
Web address: www.unitedhospitalsystem.org/
**Control:** Other not–for–profit (including NFP Corporation) **Service:** General Medical and Surgical

**Staffed Beds:** 213 **Admissions:** 10405 **Census:** 116 **Outpatient Visits:** 425998 **Births:** 1025 **Total Expense ($000):** 249642 **Payroll Expense ($000):** 109089 **Personnel:** 1664

**LA CROSSE—La Crosse County**

⊠ △ **GUNDERSEN LUTHERAN MEDICAL CENTER (520087)**, 1900 South Avenue, Zip 54601–9980; tel. 608/782–7300 **A**1 2 3 5 7 8 9 10 **F**3 4 5 9 11 13 16 18 19 20 22 24 28 29 30 31 36 38 40 43 51 56 60 61 62 63 69 72 76 78 80 81 82 83 85 86 87 88 89 90 91 93 94 97 98 99 100 101 102 103 104 105 108 110 113 114 116 119 120 122 123 125 128 129 143 145 146 147
Primary Contact: Jeffrey E. Thompson, M.D., Chief Executive Officer
COO: Kathy Klock, R.N., Senior Vice President Clinical Operations and Human Resources
CFO: Gordon Edwards, Chief Financial Officer
CMO: Julio J. Bird, M.D., Chief Medical Officer
CIO: Deb Rislow, Chief Information Officer
CHR: Kathy Klock, R.N., Senior Vice President Clinical Operations and Human Resources
Web address: www.gundluth.org
**Control:** Other not–for–profit (including NFP Corporation) **Service:** General Medical and Surgical

**Staffed Beds:** 257 **Admissions:** 12955 **Census:** 147 **Outpatient Visits:** 231446 **Births:** 1378 **Total Expense ($000):** 349483 **Payroll Expense ($000):** 95826 **Personnel:** 1481

WI

**Hospital, Medicare Provider Number, Address, Telephone, Approval, Facility, and Physician Codes, Health Care System**

★ American Hospital Association (AHA) membership
☐ The Joint Commission accreditation    ◇ DNV Healthcare Inc. accreditation
○ American Osteopathic Association (AOA) accreditation
△ Commission on Accreditation of Rehabilitation Facilities (CARF) accreditation

☐ **MAYO CLINIC HEALTH SYSTEM – FRANCISCAN HEALTHCARE IN LA CROSSE (520004)**, 700 West Avenue South, Zip 54601–4783; tel. 608/785–0940 **A**1 2 3 5 9 10 **F**1 3 4 5 6 8 9 11 13 15 16 17 18 19 20 21 22 23 25 26 27 28 29 30 31 32 34 35 36 40 41 42 43 50 52 53 54 55 56 57 58 59 61 64 65 66 68 69 70 71 72 74 75 76 77 78 79 80 81 82 84 86 87 88 89 90 93 94 97 98 99 100 101 102 103 104 105 106 107 110 111 113 114 116 117 118 119 120 122 123 126 128 129 130 131 133 134 142 143 144 145 146 147 **S** Mayo Clinic Health System, Rochester, MN
Primary Contact: Timothy J. Johnson, President and Chief Executive Officer
COO: Ronald R. Paczkowski, Executive Vice President
CFO: Tom Tiggelaar, Vice President Finance
CMO: P. Stephen Shultz, M.D., Vice President Medical Affairs
CIO: Daniel Schaefer, Vice President Information Services
Web address: www.franciscanskemp.org
**Control:** Church–operated, Nongovernment, not–for profit **Service:** General Medical and Surgical

**Staffed Beds:** 155 **Admissions:** 7401 **Census:** 74 **Outpatient Visits:** 78214 **Births:** 933 **Total Expense ($000):** 169689 **Payroll Expense ($000):** 71715 **Personnel:** 1633

**LADYSMITH—Rusk County**

★ **RUSK COUNTY MEMORIAL HOSPITAL AND NURSING HOME (521328)**, 900 College Avenue West, Zip 54848–2116; tel. 715/532–5561, (Total facility includes 50 beds in nursing home–type unit) **A**9 10 18 **F**3 13 15 28 29 30 34 40 41 43 45 53 56 59 64 70 76 77 81 84 85 89 90 93 97 107 110 111 113 116 127 129 132 143 147
Primary Contact: J. Michael Shaw, Chief Executive Officer
CFO: Judith Strop, Director Finance
CMO: John Ziemer, M.D., Chief of Staff
CHR: Rita Telitz, Director Human Resources
Web address: www.ruskhospital.org
**Control:** County–Government, nonfederal **Service:** General Medical and Surgical

**Staffed Beds:** 75 **Admissions:** 602 **Census:** 55 **Outpatient Visits:** 32320 **Births:** 62 **Total Expense ($000):** 17296 **Payroll Expense ($000):** 6467 **Personnel:** 110

**LAKE GENEVA—Walworth County**

**MERCY WALWORTH HOSPITAL AND MEDICAL CENTER (521357)**, N2950 State Road 67, Zip 53147; tel. 262/245–0535 **A**9 10 18 **F**3 5 9 15 18 26 30 31 34 35 36 40 41 44 45 50 54 55 57 59 64 65 74 75 77 78 79 81 82 85 86 92 93 94 97 100 101 103 104 107 108 111 113 118 129 130 131 134 143 145 147 **P**5 6 **S** Mercy Health System, Janesville, WI
Primary Contact: Jennifer Hallatt, Administrator
Web address: www.mercyhealthsystem.org
**Control:** Other not–for–profit (including NFP Corporation) **Service:** General Medical and Surgical

**Staffed Beds:** 6 **Admissions:** 420 **Census:** 4 **Outpatient Visits:** 116019 **Births:** 0 **Total Expense ($000):** 45510 **Payroll Expense ($000):** 8783 **Personnel:** 217

**LANCASTER—Grant County**

✠ **GRANT REGIONAL HEALTH CENTER (521322)**, 507 South Monroe Street, Zip 53813–2054; tel. 608/723–2143 **A**1 9 10 18 **F**3 8 11 13 15 20 22 28 29 34 35 36 40 43 53 56 57 59 64 68 69 70 75 76 77 78 80 81 82 84 85 86 89 90 93 107 108 113 118 128 129 130 131 132 134 143 145 147 **S** HealthTech Management Services, Franklin, TN
Primary Contact: Nicole Clapp, R.N., MSN, FACHE, President and Chief Executive Officer
CMO: Eric Slane, M.D., Chief of Staff
CIO: Kevin Ruchti, Coordinator Information Systems
CHR: Sheri Fischer, Manager Human Resources
Web address: www.grantregional.com
**Control:** Other not–for–profit (including NFP Corporation) **Service:** General Medical and Surgical

**Staffed Beds:** 25 **Admissions:** 608 **Census:** 4 **Outpatient Visits:** 26616 **Births:** 122 **Total Expense ($000):** 17158 **Payroll Expense ($000):** 7596 **Personnel:** 120

**MADISON—Dane County**

☐ **MENDOTA MENTAL HEALTH INSTITUTE (524008)**, 301 Troy Drive, Zip 53704–1599; tel. 608/301–1000 **A**1 3 5 9 10 **F**6 29 30 38 39 56 68 75 82 86 87 98 99 100 101 103 104 105 129 **P**6
Primary Contact: Greg Van Rybroek, Chief Executive Officer
CFO: Stacie Schiereck, Manager Business Office
CMO: Kenneth Casimir, M.D., Medical Director
Web address: www.dhfs.state.wi.us
**Control:** State–Government, nonfederal **Service:** Psychiatric

**Staffed Beds:** 234 **Admissions:** 820 **Census:** 224 **Outpatient Visits:** 19500 **Births:** 0 **Total Expense ($000):** 52317 **Payroll Expense ($000):** 21116 **Personnel:** 640

✠ △ **MERITER HOSPITAL (520089)**, 202 South Park Street, Zip 53715–1599; tel. 608/417–6000 **A**1 3 5 7 9 10 **F**3 4 5 9 11 12 13 15 17 18 20 22 24 26 28 29 30 31 32 34 35 36 37 39 40 41 43 45 48 49 50 53 56 57 58 59 64 65 66 68 70 71 72 74 75 76 78 79 80 81 84 85 86 87 89 90 92 93 97 98 99 100 101 102 103 104 105 106 107 108 111 114 116 117 118 125 129 131 134 144 145 146 147 **P**6
Primary Contact: James L. Woodward, President and Chief Executive Officer
COO: Lynne L. Myers, Executive Vice President and Chief Operating Officer
CFO: Linda Hoff, Chief Financial Officer
CMO: Geoff Priest, M.D., Chief Medical Officer
CIO: Kerra Guffey, Chief Information Officer
CHR: Tammy Saunaitis, Chief Human Resources Officer
Web address: www.meriter.com
**Control:** Other not–for–profit (including NFP Corporation) **Service:** General Medical and Surgical

**Staffed Beds:** 301 **Admissions:** 17972 **Census:** 197 **Outpatient Visits:** 180352 **Births:** 3770 **Total Expense ($000):** 372553 **Payroll Expense ($000):** 162862 **Personnel:** 2096

✠ **SELECT SPECIALTY HOSPITAL–MADISON (522008)**, 801 Braxton Place, Zip 53715; tel. 608/260–2703 **A**1 10 **F**1 3 18 29 74 75 77 79 82 83 85 86 87 91 97 107 108 113 129 147 **P**4 **S** Select Medical Corporation, Mechanicsburg, PA
Primary Contact: Patrice L. Komoroski, Ph.D., R.N., Chief Executive Officer
Web address: www.selectmedicalcorp.com
**Control:** Corporation, Investor–owned, for–profit **Service:** Long–Term Acute Care hospital

**Staffed Beds:** 58 **Admissions:** 488 **Census:** 42 **Outpatient Visits:** 0 **Births:** 0 **Total Expense ($000):** 25512 **Payroll Expense ($000):** 8959 **Personnel:** 94

✠ **ST. MARY'S HOSPITAL (520083)**, 700 South Park Street, Zip 53715–0450; tel. 608/251–6100 **A**1 3 5 10 **F**7 11 12 13 17 20 22 24 28 29 34 38 40 43 60 70 72 75 76 77 78 80 81 86 87 88 89 93 98 100 101 103 107 108 118 129 143 **S** SSM Health Care, Saint Louis, MO
Primary Contact: Frank D. Byrne, M.D., President
COO: Jon Rozenfeld, Executive Vice President and Chief Operating Officer
CFO: Charlie Johnson, Vice President Finance and Chief Financial Officer
CMO: John Butler, M.D., Vice President Medical Affairs
CIO: Major Dave Lundal, Vice President and Regional Chief Information Officer
CHR: Craig Brenholt, Director Human Resources
Web address: www.stmarysmadison.com
**Control:** Other not–for–profit (including NFP Corporation) **Service:** General Medical and Surgical

**Staffed Beds:** 361 **Admissions:** 21301 **Census:** 255 **Outpatient Visits:** 132542 **Births:** 3320 **Total Expense ($000):** 368104 **Payroll Expense ($000):** 138589 **Personnel:** 1928

✠ △ **UNIVERSITY OF WISCONSIN HOSPITAL AND CLINICS (520098)**, 600 Highland Avenue, Zip 53792–0002; tel. 608/263–6400, (Includes UNIVERSITY OF WISCONSIN CHILDREN'S HOSPITAL ; AMERICAN FAMILY CHILDREN'S HOSPITAL, 1675 Highland Avenue, Zip 53705; tel. 608/890–5437) **A**1 3 5 7 8 9 10 13 **F**3 5 6 7 8 9 12 15 16 17 18 19 20 21 22 23 24 25 26 27 28 29 30 31 32 34 35 36 37 39 40 43 44 45 46 47 48 49 50 51 52 54 55 56 57 58 59 60 61 62 64 68 70 71 74 75 77 78 79 80 81 82 83 84 85 86 87 88 90 92 93 94 96 97 98 100 102 103 104 107 108 109 110 111 112 113 114 115 116 117 118 119 120 122 123 125 128 129 131 133 134 135 136 137 138 139 141 142 143 144 145 146 147 **P**3
Primary Contact: Donna Katen–Bahensky, President and Chief Executive Officer
COO: Ron Sliwinski, Chief Operations Officer
CFO: Michael D. Buhl, Senior Vice President and Chief Financial Officer
CMO: Carl J. Getto, M.D., Senior Vice President Medical Affairs and Associate Dean Hospital Affairs
CIO: Michael Sauk, Chief Information Officer
CHR: Janice K. Bultema, MSN, Senior Vice President Human Resources
Web address: www.uwhospital.org
**Control:** Other not–for–profit (including NFP Corporation) **Service:** General Medical and Surgical

**Staffed Beds:** 504 **Admissions:** 26767 **Census:** 380 **Outpatient Visits:** 906549 **Births:** 0 **Total Expense ($000):** 1018029 **Payroll Expense ($000):** 376302 **Personnel:** 6372

✠ △ **WILLIAM S. MIDDLETON MEMORIAL VETERANS HOSPITAL**, 2500 Overlook Terrace, Zip 53705–2286; tel. 608/256–1901, (Nonreporting) **A**1 3 5 7 **S** Department of Veterans Affairs, Washington, DC
Primary Contact: Deborah A. Thompson, Director
COO: Allen R. Ackers, Associate Director
CFO: Abraham Rabinowitz, Assistant Finance Officer
CMO: Alan J. Bridges, M.D., Chief of Staff
CIO: Randall Margenau, Chief Information Officer
CHR: Stuart Souders, Coordinator Human Resources
Web address: www.madison.va.gov
**Control:** Veterans Affairs, Government, federal **Service:** General Medical and Surgical

**Staffed Beds:** 86

## MANITOWOC—Manitowoc County

✠ **HOLY FAMILY MEMORIAL MEDICAL CENTER (520107)**, 2300 Western Avenue, Zip 54220, Mailing Address: P.O. Box 1450, Zip 54221–1450; tel. 920/320–2011 **A**1 2 9 10 **F**3 4 5 8 11 13 15 17 20 22 28 29 30 31 34 36 40 43 45 46 47 48 49 50 51 53 54 56 57 58 59 62 63 64 65 68 70 71 74 75 76 77 78 79 80 81 82 84 85 86 89 93 97 99 100 101 102 103 104 107 108 110 111 114 115 117 118 120 128 129 130 131 134 143 145 146 147 **P**6 8 **S** Franciscan Sisters of Christian Charity Sponsored Ministries, Inc., Manitowoc, WI
Primary Contact: Mark P. Herzog, President and Chief Executive Officer
CFO: Patricia Huettl, Vice President Finance and Chief Financial Officer
CMO: Steve Driggers, M.D., Chief Medical Officer
CIO: Ed Bauknecht, Director Management Information Systems
CHR: Laura M. Fielding, Administrative Director Organizational Development
Web address: www.hfmhealth.org
**Control:** Church–operated, Nongovernment, not–for profit **Service:** General Medical and Surgical

**Staffed Beds:** 62 **Admissions:** 3078 **Census:** 29 **Outpatient Visits:** 288707 **Births:** 242 **Total Expense ($000):** 126931 **Payroll Expense ($000):** 64035 **Personnel:** 788

## MARINETTE—Marinette County

✠ **BAY AREA MEDICAL CENTER (520113)**, 3100 Shore Drive, Zip 54143–4242; tel. 715/735–6621 **A**1 9 10 20 **F**3 7 8 11 13 15 17 18 20 22 28 29 30 31 34 40 43 45 48 50 55 57 60 64 68 70 74 75 76 77 78 79 80 81 85 86 87 89 93 107 110 111 118 128 129 130 145 146
Primary Contact: Edward A. Harding, FACHE, President and Chief Executive Officer
COO: Bernie VanCourt, Chief Operating Officer
CFO: Dan Carlson, Chief Financial Officer
CMO: Richard Stein, M.D., Chief of Staff
CIO: Pete Eisenzoph, Director Information Technology
CHR: Curt Oberholtzer, Assistant Administrator Human Resources and Organizational Development
Web address: www.bamc.org
**Control:** Other not–for–profit (including NFP Corporation) **Service:** General Medical and Surgical

**Staffed Beds:** 46 **Admissions:** 4405 **Census:** 46 **Outpatient Visits:** 65375 **Births:** 297 **Total Expense ($000):** 115811 **Payroll Expense ($000):** 46470 **Personnel:** 585

## MARSHFIELD—Wood County

**NORWOOD HEALTH CENTER (524019)**, 1600 North Chestnut Avenue, Zip 54449–1499; tel. 715/384–2188, (Total facility includes 33 beds in nursing home–type unit) **A**9 10 **F**1 3 4 30 34 67 98 99 100 101 102 105 127 129 142 145 147 **P**6
Primary Contact: Rhonda Kozik, Administrator
CFO: Jo Timmerman, Manager Accounting
CHR: Larry Shear, Administrative Assistant
Web address: www.co.wood.wi.us/norwood/index.htm
**Control:** County–Government, nonfederal **Service:** Psychiatric

**Staffed Beds:** 49 **Admissions:** 728 **Census:** 35 **Outpatient Visits:** 0 **Births:** 0 **Total Expense ($000):** 3301 **Payroll Expense ($000):** 1500 **Personnel:** 43

✠ △ **SAINT JOSEPH'S HOSPITAL (520037)**, 611 St. Joseph Avenue, Zip 54449–1898; tel. 715/387–1713, (Includes SAINT JOSEPH'S CHILDEN'S HOSPITAL, 611 Saint Joseph Avenue, Zip 54449–1832; tel. 715/387–1713) **A**1 2 3 5 7 9 10 20 **F**3 4 5 6 7 9 11 12 13 16 17 18 19 20 22 24 26 27 28 29 30 31 34 35 36 38 39 40 41 43 44 49 50 53 56 57 59 61 64 68 69 70 72 74 75 76 77 78 79 80 81 82 83 84 85 86 87 88 89 90 93 96 98 100 101 102 103 108 111 112 115 116 117 118 119 120 122 123 125 129 131 134 135 143 145 146 147 **S** Marian Health System, Tulsa, OK
Primary Contact: Brian Kief, President and Chief Executive Officer
CFO: John Skaden, Chief Financial Officer
CMO: Peter Stamas, M.D., Vice President Medical Affairs
CIO: Will Weider, Chief Information Officer
CHR: Layton Anderson, Regional Director Human Resources
Web address: www.stjosephs–marshfield.org
**Control:** Church–operated, Nongovernment, not–for profit **Service:** General Medical and Surgical

**Staffed Beds:** 319 **Admissions:** 17817 **Census:** 248 **Outpatient Visits:** 67094 **Births:** 996 **Total Expense ($000):** 304502 **Payroll Expense ($000):** 101056 **Personnel:** 1622

## MAUSTON—Juneau County

☐ **MILE BLUFF MEDICAL CENTER (520109)**, 1050 Division Street, Zip 53948–1997; tel. 608/847–6161, (Total facility includes 132 beds in nursing home–type unit) **A**1 9 10 20 **F**3 10 11 13 15 28 29 30 31 34 35 36 40 43 44 45 46 50 56 57 59 60 62 64 65 68 69 71 75 76 77 78 79 80 81 82 85 86 87 89 92 93 94 96 97 99 100 101 103 104 107 108 111 112 113 116 117 118 124 126 127 129 130 131 134 142 143 144 145 147
Primary Contact: James M. O'Keefe, President and Chief Executive Officer
Web address: www.milebluff.com
**Control:** Other not–for–profit (including NFP Corporation) **Service:** General Medical and Surgical

**Staffed Beds:** 157 **Admissions:** 1698 **Census:** 138 **Outpatient Visits:** 126195 **Births:** 171 **Total Expense ($000):** 51057 **Payroll Expense ($000):** 26817 **Personnel:** 345

## MEDFORD—Taylor County

✠ **MEMORIAL HEALTH CENTER (521324)**, 135 South Gibson Street, Zip 54451–1696; tel. 715/748–8100, (Includes MEMORIAL NURSING HOME ), (Total facility includes 109 beds in nursing home–type unit) **A**1 9 10 18 **F**1 3 10 11 13 15 28 29 31 34 35 36 40 43 50 53 54 57 59 60 62 68 75 76 77 78 81 82 86 87 89 90 93 97 100 107 108 110 111 112 114 115 116 117 118 124 126 127 128 129 130 131 132 143 145 146 **S** Aspirus, Inc., Wausau, WI
Primary Contact: Gregory A. Olson, President and Chief Executive Officer
COO: Kaaron Keene, Vice President Patient Care Services
CFO: Lori Peck, Vice President Finance
CMO: Mark Reuter, M.D., Medical Director and Chief of Staff
CHR: Angela Hupf, Vice President Human Resources and Community Relations
Web address: www.memhc.com
**Control:** Other not–for–profit (including NFP Corporation) **Service:** General Medical and Surgical

**Staffed Beds:** 124 **Admissions:** 872 **Census:** 103 **Outpatient Visits:** 62472 **Births:** 195 **Total Expense ($000):** 42394 **Payroll Expense ($000):** 20188 **Personnel:** 380

## MENOMONEE FALLS—Waukesha County

✠ △ **COMMUNITY MEMORIAL HOSPITAL (520103)**, W180 N8085 Town Hall Road, Zip 53051–3518, Mailing Address: P.O. Box 408, Zip 53052–0408; tel. 262/251–1000 **A**1 2 3 5 7 9 10 **F**3 4 5 11 12 13 15 17 18 20 24 26 28 29 30 31 34 35 36 38 39 40 43 44 45 46 47 48 49 50 51 55 56 57 58 59 60 64 65 66 70 72 74 75 76 77 78 79 80 81 82 83 84 85 86 88 89 90 92 93 94 96 98 100 101 102 103 104 105 107 108 109 111 114 115 116 117 118 119 120 122 126 128 129 130 131 134 144 145 146 147 **P**5 6
Primary Contact: Dennis Pollard, President
CFO: Thomas Knoll, Site Director Finance
CMO: David Goldberg, M.D., Vice President Medical Affairs
CIO: Robert DeGrand, Chief Information Officer
Web address: www.communitymemorial.com
**Control:** Other not–for–profit (including NFP Corporation) **Service:** General Medical and Surgical

**Staffed Beds:** 194 **Admissions:** 9449 **Census:** 118 **Outpatient Visits:** 92249 **Births:** 987 **Total Expense ($000):** 179202 **Payroll Expense ($000):** 62746 **Personnel:** 949

## MENOMONIE—Dunn County

☐ **MAYO CLINIC HEALTH SYSTEM – RED CEDAR IN MENOMONIE (521340)**, 2321 Stout Road, Zip 54751–2397; tel. 715/235–5531 **A**1 5 9 10 18 **F**6 11 13 15 17 28 34 36 40 41 43 52 54 55 64 70 75 76 77 80 81 82 86 87 89 90 93 99 100 101 102 103 104 107 108 111 118 124 129 130 143 146 **S** Mayo Clinic Health System, Rochester, MN
Primary Contact: Steven Lindberg, Chief Administrative Officer
CFO: Jeanie Lubinsky, Chief Financial Officer
CMO: Mark Deyo Svendsen, M.D., Medical Director
CIO: Frank Wrogg, Director Information Technology
CHR: Leann Wurtzel, Director Human Resources
Web address: www.rcmc–mhs.org
**Control:** Other not–for–profit (including NFP Corporation) **Service:** General Medical and Surgical

**Staffed Beds:** 25 **Admissions:** 1529 **Census:** 14 **Outpatient Visits:** 37548 **Births:** 343 **Total Expense ($000):** 74378 **Payroll Expense ($000):** 37359 **Personnel:** 608

**RED CEDAR MEDICAL CENTER–MAYO HEALTH SYSTEM** See Mayo Clinic Health System – Red Cedar in Menomonie

**WI**

---

**Hospital, Medicare Provider Number, Address, Telephone, Approval, Facility, and Physician Codes, Health Care System**

★ American Hospital Association (AHA) membership
☐ The Joint Commission accreditation ◇ DNV Healthcare Inc. accreditation
○ American Osteopathic Association (AOA) accreditation
△ Commission on Accreditation of Rehabilitation Facilities (CARF) accreditation

## MEQUON—Ozaukee County

★ ⬩COLUMBIA CENTER (520195), 13125 North Port Washington Road, Zip 53097; tel. 262/243–7408 A9 10 F3 8 13 34 64 65 68 76 81 85 86 87 104 131
Primary Contact: Karen J. Casey, R.N., MS, President and Chief Executive Officer
CMO: Robert Stumpf, M.D., President Medical Staff
Web address: www.columbiacenter.org
**Control:** Other not–for–profit (including NFP Corporation) **Service:** General Medical and Surgical

**Staffed Beds:** 17 **Admissions:** 731 **Census:** 5 **Outpatient Visits:** 482 **Births:** 728 **Total Expense ($000):** 7997 **Payroll Expense ($000):** 3490 **Personnel:** 32

⊞ COLUMBIA ST. MARY'S OZAUKEE HOSPITAL (520027), 13111 North Port Washington Road, Zip 53097–2416; tel. 262/243–7300 A1 2 9 10 F3 4 5 9 15 17 18 20 22 24 26 28 29 30 31 34 35 36 37 38 39 40 43 48 49 50 51 53 54 56 57 58 59 64 65 66 68 70 71 74 75 77 78 79 80 81 85 86 89 90 93 98 99 100 101 102 103 104 105 107 108 110 111 112 113 115 117 118 119 120 122 125 128 129 131 133 134 142 143 144 145 146 147 P6 S Ascension Health, Saint Louis, MO
Primary Contact: Deborah G. Friberg, President
CFO: Rhonda Anderson, Executive Vice President Finance and Chief Financial Officer
CMO: David Shapiro, M.D., Vice President Medical Affairs and Chief Medical Officer
CIO: Mary Paul, Chief Information Officer
CHR: Cheryl Hill, Vice President Human Resources
Web address: www.columbia–stmarys.org
**Control:** Church–operated, Nongovernment, not–for profit **Service:** General Medical and Surgical

**Staffed Beds:** 152 **Admissions:** 6260 **Census:** 75 **Outpatient Visits:** 153594 **Births:** 0 **Total Expense ($000):** 181434 **Payroll Expense ($000):** 60186 **Personnel:** 506

## MERRILL—Lincoln County

GOOD SAMARITAN HEALTH CENTER OF MERRILL See Ministry Good Samaritan Health

⊞ MINISTRY GOOD SAMARITAN HEALTH CENTER (521339), 601 South Center Avenue, Zip 54452–3404; tel. 715/536–5511 A1 9 10 18 F3 15 28 30 31 34 40 43 45 50 56 64 75 77 78 79 80 81 82 85 86 87 89 93 107 108 110 111 113 117 118 129 131 132 143 145 146 S Marian Health System, Tulsa, OK
Primary Contact: Kristine McGarigle, President
CFO: David Jirovec, Director Finance
CHR: Nancy Kwiesielewicz, Human Resources Business Partner
Web address: www.ministryhealth.org
**Control:** Church–operated, Nongovernment, not–for profit **Service:** General Medical and Surgical

**Staffed Beds:** 16 **Admissions:** 606 **Census:** 6 **Outpatient Visits:** 29380 **Births:** 0 **Total Expense ($000):** 23888 **Payroll Expense ($000):** 11517 **Personnel:** 158

## MILWAUKEE—Milwaukee County

★ △ AURORA SINAI MEDICAL CENTER (520064), 945 North 12th Street, Zip 53233–1337, Mailing Address: P.O. Box 342, Zip 53201–0342; tel. 414/219–2000 A2 3 5 7 8 9 10 F1 3 5 6 8 11 12 13 15 17 18 20 22 24 26 28 29 30 31 34 35 36 38 39 40 41 42 43 44 49 50 54 55 56 57 59 64 65 68 69 70 72 75 76 77 78 79 80 81 82 84 85 86 87 89 90 93 96 100 102 103 104 107 108 110 111 113 115 116 117 118 122 128 129 130 131 134 142 143 145 146 147 P6 S Aurora Health Care, Milwaukee, WI
Primary Contact: George Hinton, Administrator
CFO: Kevin Jones, Director Finance
Web address: www.aurorahealthcare.org
**Control:** Other not–for–profit (including NFP Corporation) **Service:** General Medical and Surgical

**Staffed Beds:** 188 **Admissions:** 7876 **Census:** 105 **Outpatient Visits:** 252191 **Births:** 2481 **Total Expense ($000):** 224393 **Payroll Expense ($000):** 67493 **Personnel:** 1235

⊞ △ AURORA ST. LUKE'S MEDICAL CENTER (520138), 2900 West Oklahoma Avenue, Zip 53215–4330, Mailing Address: P.O. Box 2901, Zip 53201–2901; tel. 414/649–6000, (Includes AURORA ST. LUKE'S SOUTH SHORE, 5900 South Lake Drive, Cudahy, Zip 53110–8903; tel. 414/769–9000) A1 2 3 5 7 8 9 10 F1 2 4 5 6 11 12 15 17 20 22 24 28 29 34 36 38 40 41 43 51 54 56 64 69 70 72 75 78 80 81 82 86 87 89 90 93 98 100 101 102 103 104 105 107 108 111 115 117 118 129 135 136 137 139 140 143 P6 S Aurora Health Care, Milwaukee, WI
Primary Contact: Mary O'Brien, Administrator
COO: Sue Ela, Executive Vice President and Chief Operating Officer
CMO: Bruce L. Van Cleave, M.D., Senior Vice President and Chief Medical Officer
CIO: Philip Loftus, Ph.D., Vice President and Chief Information Officer
CHR: Dwight Morgan, Vice President Human Resources
Web address: www.aurorahealthcare.org
**Control:** Other not–for–profit (including NFP Corporation) **Service:** General Medical and Surgical

**Staffed Beds:** 710 **Admissions:** 33016 **Census:** 516 **Outpatient Visits:** 438300 **Births:** 0 **Total Expense ($000):** 836600 **Payroll Expense ($000):** 251520 **Personnel:** 4701

⊞ CHILDREN'S HOSPITAL OF WISCONSIN (523300), 9000 West Wisconsin Avenue, Zip 53226–4810, Mailing Address: P.O. Box 1997, Zip 53201–1997; tel. 414/266–2000 A1 3 5 8 9 10 F7 9 12 16 17 20 22 24 28 29 34 36 38 40 43 51 60 61 64 72 75 77 78 80 81 82 87 88 89 90 93 99 100 104 107 108 111 115 117 118 129 130 135 136 137 139 140 143 S Children's Hospital and Health System, Milwaukee, WI
Primary Contact: Peggy N. Troy, President and Chief Executive Officer
COO: Cinthia S. Christensen, JD, Executive Vice President and Chief Operating Officer
CMO: Michael Gutzeit, M.D., Chief Medical Officer
CIO: Michael Jones, Vice President and Chief Information Officer
CHR: Peggy Niemer, Vice President Human Resources
Web address: www.chw.org
**Control:** Other not–for–profit (including NFP Corporation) **Service:** Children's general

**Staffed Beds:** 296 **Admissions:** 24207 **Census:** 231 **Outpatient Visits:** 372507 **Births:** 0 **Total Expense ($000):** 495293 **Payroll Expense ($000):** 149248 **Personnel:** 2433

⊞ △ CLEMENT J. ZABLOCKI VETERANS AFFAIRS MEDICAL CENTER, 5000 West National Avenue, Zip 53295; tel. 414/384–2000, (Nonreporting) A1 2 3 5 7 S Department of Veterans Affairs, Washington, DC
Primary Contact: Robert H. Beller, FACHE, Director
COO: Larry L. Berkeley, Associate Director
CFO: John La Sota, Assistant Finance Officer
CMO: Michael Erdmann, M.D., Chief of Staff
CIO: Bryan Vail, Chief Information Officer
CHR: Wayne Davis, Chief Human Resources
Web address: www.va.gov/sta/guide/home.asp
**Control:** Veterans Affairs, Government, federal **Service:** General Medical and Surgical

**Staffed Beds:** 370

⊞ COLUMBIA ST. MARY'S HOSPITAL MILWAUKEE (520051), 2301 North Lake Drive, Zip 53211–4508; tel. 414/291–1000, (Includes COLUMBIA ST. MARY'S COLUMBIA HOSPITAL, 2025 East Newport Avenue, Zip 53211–2990; tel. 414/961–3300; COLUMBIA ST. MARY'S MILWAUKEE HOSPITAL, 2323 North Lake Drive, Zip 53211–9682, Mailing Address: P.O. Box 503, Zip 53201–0503; tel. 414/291–1000) A1 2 9 10 F3 4 9 13 15 16 17 18 20 22 24 26 28 29 30 31 32 33 34 35 36 37 38 39 40 43 45 46 47 48 49 50 51 53 54 56 57 58 59 60 64 65 66 68 70 72 74 75 76 77 78 79 80 81 84 85 86 87 89 91 92 94 98 104 107 108 110 111 113 114 115 116 117 118 119 120 121 122 123 125 126 128 129 131 134 140 142 143 144 145 146 147 P6 S Ascension Health, Saint Louis, MO
Primary Contact: Mark R. Taylor, FACHE, President and Chief Executive Officer
CFO: Rhonda Anderson, Executive Vice President Finance and Chief Financial Officer
CMO: David Shapiro, M.D., Vice President Medical Affairs and Chief Medical Officer
CIO: Mary Paul, Chief Information Officer
CHR: Cheryl Hill, Vice President Human Resources
Web address: www.columbia–stmarys.org
**Control:** Church–operated, Nongovernment, not–for profit **Service:** General Medical and Surgical

**Staffed Beds:** 306 **Admissions:** 12012 **Census:** 150 **Outpatient Visits:** 272290 **Births:** 3245 **Total Expense ($000):** 514212 **Payroll Expense ($000):** 186706 **Personnel:** 1437

⊞ △ FROEDTERT MEMORIAL LUTHERAN HOSPITAL (520177), 9200 West Wisconsin Avenue, Zip 53226–3596, Mailing Address: P.O. Box 26099, Zip 53226–3596; tel. 414/805–3000 A1 2 3 5 7 8 9 10 F3 6 11 12 13 15 17 18 20 22 24 26 29 30 31 34 35 38 40 43 44 45 46 47 48 49 50 51 52 55 56 57 58 59 60 64 68 70 74 75 76 77 78 79 80 81 84 85 86 87 90 91 92 93 94 95 97 98 100 107 108 110 111 113 114 115 116 117 118 119 120 122 123 125 128 129 130 131 133 134 135 136 137 138 139 140 143 144 145 146 147 P5 6
Primary Contact: Catherine A. Jacobson, President and Chief Executive Officer
COO: Catherine Buck, Executive Vice President Operations
CFO: Jeffrey Van De Kreeke, Senior Vice President Finance
CMO: Andrew J. Norton, M.D., Senior Vice President Medical Affairs
CIO: Robert DeGrand, Chief Information Officer
Web address: www.froedtert.com
**Control:** Other not–for–profit (including NFP Corporation) **Service:** General Medical and Surgical

**Staffed Beds:** 499 **Admissions:** 28439 **Census:** 394 **Outpatient Visits:** 630507 **Births:** 1929 **Total Expense ($000):** 845614 **Payroll Expense ($000):** 233212 **Personnel:** 4239

WI

*Many Facility Codes have changed. Please refer to the AHA Guide Code Chart.* © 2012 AHA Guide

★ **MILWAUKEE COUNTY BEHAVIORAL HEALTH DIVISION (524001)**, 9455 Watertown Plank Road, Zip 53226–3559; tel. 414/257–6995, (Total facility includes 72 beds in nursing home–type unit) **A**3 5 10 **F**30 42 44 66 67 71 75 77 79 87 104 105 106 127 129 145 **P**3 6
Primary Contact: Paula A. Lucey, MSN, R.N., Administrator
CFO: Michael Kreuser, Director Fiscal Services
CMO: Thomas Harding, M.D., Medical Director
CIO: William Borja, Chief Information Officer
Web address: www.milwaukeecounty.org
**Control:** County–Government, nonfederal **Service:** Psychiatric

**Staffed Beds:** 216 **Admissions:** 3220 **Census:** 216 **Outpatient Visits:** 15259 **Births:** 0 **Total Expense ($000):** 161052 **Payroll Expense ($000):** 32997 **Personnel:** 604

**ORTHOPAEDIC HOSPITAL OF WISCONSIN – GLENDALE (520194)**, 475 West River Woods Parkway, Zip 53212–1081; tel. 414/961–6800 **A**9 10 **F**29 34 38 53 64 80 81 82 86 93 107 111 118 129 130
Primary Contact: Brian J. Cramer, Chief Executive Officer
CFO: Tom Swiderski, Chief Financial Officer
CMO: Rory Wright, M.D., President Medical Staff
CIO: Todd Heikkinen, Director Rehabilitation Services
Web address: www.ohow.org
**Control:** Partnership, Investor–owned, for–profit **Service:** General Medical and Surgical

**Staffed Beds:** 30 **Admissions:** 1016 **Census:** 8 **Outpatient Visits:** 29750 **Births:** 0 **Total Expense ($000):** 33730 **Payroll Expense ($000):** 9116 **Personnel:** 153

⊠ △ **SACRED HEART REHABILITATION INSTITUTE (523025)**, 2025 East Newport Avenue, Zip 53211–2906; tel. 414/298–6700 **A**1 7 9 10 **F**9 29 34 54 56 64 75 77 86 90 93 129 130 131 **P**6 **S** Ascension Health, Saint Louis, MO
Primary Contact: Deborah G. Friberg, President
CFO: Rhonda Anderson, Executive Vice President Finance and Chief Financial Officer
CMO: David Shapiro, M.D., Vice President Medical Affairs and Chief Medical Officer
CIO: Mary Paul, Vice President and Chief Information Officer
CHR: Cheryl Hill, Vice President Human Resources
Web address: www.columbia–stmarys.com
**Control:** Church–operated, Nongovernment, not–for profit **Service:** Rehabilitation

**Staffed Beds:** 20 **Admissions:** 381 **Census:** 17 **Outpatient Visits:** 10698 **Births:** 0 **Total Expense ($000):** 12015 **Payroll Expense ($000):** 5551 **Personnel:** 72

⊠ **SELECT SPECIALTY HOSPITAL–MILWAUKEE (522006)**, 8901 West Lincoln Avenue, 6th Floor, Zip 53227; tel. 414/328–7700 **A**1 9 10 **F**1 3 17 29 30 36 38 39 56 70 74 75 77 78 79 80 82 84 87 90 100 103 129 147 **S** Select Medical Corporation, Mechanicsburg, PA
Primary Contact: Richard Keddington, Chief Executive Officer
COO: Mary Puetzer, MS, Chief Operating Officer
CMO: Matt Mathai, M.D., Medical Director
CHR: Chris Froh, Senior Coordinator Human Resources
Web address: www.selectmedicalcorp.com
**Control:** Corporation, Investor–owned, for–profit **Service:** Long–Term Acute Care hospital

**Staffed Beds:** 34 **Admissions:** 409 **Census:** 30 **Outpatient Visits:** 0 **Births:** 0 **Total Expense ($000):** 17114 **Payroll Expense ($000):** 4887 **Personnel:** 94

⊠ **WHEATON FRANCISCAN HEALTHCARE – ST. FRANCIS (520078)**, 3237 South 16th Street, Zip 53215–4592; tel. 414/647–5000 **A**1 2 9 10 **F**3 4 9 13 15 17 18 20 22 24 26 28 29 30 31 34 35 36 38 40 46 47 48 49 54 56 57 59 64 68 70 72 74 75 76 77 78 79 80 81 82 83 84 85 86 87 89 93 97 98 99 100 101 102 103 104 105 107 108 109 110 111 112 113 114 117 118 119 120 121 122 123 128 129 130 131 134 143 145 146 147 **S** Wheaton Franciscan Healthcare, Wheaton, IL
Primary Contact: Daniel Mattes, President
CFO: Aaron Bridgeland, Director Finance
CIO: Gregory Smith, Senior Vice President and Chief Information Officer
CHR: Robert Bauer, Director Human Resources
Web address: www.mywheaton.org
**Control:** Church–operated, Nongovernment, not–for profit **Service:** General Medical and Surgical

**Staffed Beds:** 164 **Admissions:** 7494 **Census:** 103 **Outpatient Visits:** 151625 **Births:** 829 **Total Expense ($000):** 149486 **Payroll Expense ($000):** 54356 **Personnel:** 833

⊠ **WHEATON FRANCISCAN HEALTHCARE – ST. JOSEPH'S (520136)**, 5000 West Chambers Street, Zip 53210–9988; tel. 414/447–2000 **A**1 2 3 5 9 10 **F**11 13 15 17 20 22 24 28 29 40 43 53 54 56 64 70 72 75 76 77 78 80 81 82 87 89 90 93 107 108 111 115 117 118 129 130 143 146 **P**6 **S** Wheaton Franciscan Healthcare, Wheaton, IL
Primary Contact: Debra K. Standridge, President
COO: Norma J. McCutcheon, R.N., Senior Vice President Operations
CMO: Rita Hanson, M.D., Vice President Medical Affairs
CIO: Dawn Hansen, Regional Director Information Services
CHR: Christopher Morris, Director Human Resources
Web address: www.whfc.org
**Control:** Church–operated, Nongovernment, not–for profit **Service:** General Medical and Surgical

**Staffed Beds:** 317 **Admissions:** 11454 **Census:** 144 **Outpatient Visits:** 387385 **Births:** 2761 **Total Expense ($000):** 267299 **Payroll Expense ($000):** 90434 **Personnel:** 1503

## MONROE—Green County

☐ **MONROE CLINIC (520028)**, 515 22nd Avenue, Zip 53566–1598; tel. 608/324–1000 **A**1 9 10 **F**3 5 6 8 9 11 13 15 17 18 20 26 28 30 31 32 34 35 36 37 38 40 43 44 46 49 50 55 56 57 59 62 63 65 68 70 74 75 76 77 79 80 81 84 85 86 87 89 90 93 97 99 100 101 102 103 104 107 108 110 111 112 114 116 118 125 128 129 130 131 134 143 144 145 146 147 **P**6
Primary Contact: Michael B. Sanders, President and Chief Executive Officer
CFO: Julie Wilke, Vice President and Chief Financial Officer
CMO: Mark Thompson, M.D., Chief Medical Officer
CIO: Carrie Blum, Director Information Systems
CHR: Jane Monahan, Director Human Resources
Web address: www.monroeclinic.org
**Control:** Other not–for–profit (including NFP Corporation) **Service:** General Medical and Surgical

**Staffed Beds:** 51 **Admissions:** 2814 **Census:** 25 **Outpatient Visits:** 251787 **Births:** 461 **Total Expense ($000):** 141783 **Payroll Expense ($000):** 71666 **Personnel:** 969

## NEENAH—Winnebago County

☐ **CHILDREN'S HOSPITAL OF WISCONSIN–FOX VALLEY (523302)**, 130 Second Avenue, 3rd Floor South, Zip 54956; tel. 920/969–7900 **A**1 9 10 **F**7 29 34 38 72 75 80 81 86 89 90 93 99 100 101 104 129 **P**6 **S** Children's Hospital and Health System, Milwaukee, WI
Primary Contact: Peggy N. Troy, President and Chief Executive Officer
COO: Tim Klunk, Executive Director
CMO: Paul Myers, M.D., Neonatologist and Chief Medical Officer
Web address: www.chw.org
**Control:** Other not–for–profit (including NFP Corporation) **Service:** Children's general

**Staffed Beds:** 42 **Admissions:** 1202 **Census:** 17 **Outpatient Visits:** 14017 **Births:** 0 **Total Expense ($000):** 21963 **Payroll Expense ($000):** 7988 **Personnel:** 108

☐ △ **THEDA CLARK MEDICAL CENTER (520045)**, 130 Second Street, Zip 54956–2883, Mailing Address: P.O. Box 2021, Zip 54957–2021; tel. 920/729–3100 **A**1 2 7 9 10 **F**3 4 5 7 9 10 11 12 13 15 17 18 19 20 21 22 23 25 28 29 30 31 32 34 35 36 39 40 41 43 44 45 46 47 48 49 50 51 53 55 56 59 60 64 68 69 70 74 75 76 78 79 80 82 84 85 86 87 88 90 93 98 99 101 102 103 104 105 107 108 110 111 112 113 114 117 118 125 129 131 133 134 143 145 146 147 **P**1 6 **S** ThedaCare, Inc., Appleton, WI
Primary Contact: Kim Barnas, Senior Vice President
COO: Matthew Furlan, Chief Operating Officer
CFO: Tim Olson, Senior Vice President Finance
CIO: Keith Livingston, Senior Vice President and Chief Information Officer
CHR: Maureen Pistone, Senior Vice President Human Resources
CNO: Jill Case–Wirth, Vice President and Chief Nursing Officer
Web address: www.thedacare.org
**Control:** Other not–for–profit (including NFP Corporation) **Service:** General Medical and Surgical

**Staffed Beds:** 147 **Admissions:** 8280 **Census:** 87 **Outpatient Visits:** 91207 **Births:** 1372 **Total Expense ($000):** 160757 **Payroll Expense ($000):** 60190 **Personnel:** 911

**WI**

---

**Hospital, Medicare Provider Number, Address, Telephone, Approval, Facility, and Physician Codes, Health Care System**

★ American Hospital Association (AHA) membership
☐ The Joint Commission accreditation
◇ DNV Healthcare Inc. accreditation
○ American Osteopathic Association (AOA) accreditation
△ Commission on Accreditation of Rehabilitation Facilities (CARF) accreditation

---

## NEILLSVILLE—Clark County

**MEMORIAL MEDICAL CENTER – NEILLSVILLE (521323)**, 216 Sunset Place,
Zip 54456–1799; tel. 715/743–3101, (Includes NEILLSVILLE MEMORIAL HOME )
**A**9 10 18 **F**3 6 10 11 13 15 28 34 35 40 43 45 50 56 57 59 62 64 65 68 75
76 77 79 80 81 82 85 86 89 97 107 108 110 113 118 119 126 129 130
132 134 143 145 146 **P**6
Primary Contact: Kelly Moen, Interim Chief Executive Officer
CFO: Kelly Moen, Chief Financial Officer
CMO: Timothy Meyer, M.D., Chief of Staff
CIO: Travis Obrycki, Director Information Systems
CHR: Tamie Zarak, Director Human Resources
Web address: www.mmcneillsville.com
**Control:** Other not–for–profit (including NFP Corporation) **Service:** General
Medical and Surgical

**Staffed Beds:** 25 **Admissions:** 459 **Census:** 5 **Outpatient Visits:** 20703
**Births:** 54 **Total Expense ($000):** 20132 **Payroll Expense ($000):** 11073
**Personnel:** 212

## NEW LONDON—Outagamie County

☐ **NEW LONDON FAMILY MEDICAL CENTER (521326)**, 1405 Mill Street,
Zip 54961–2155, Mailing Address: P.O. Box 307, Zip 54961–0307;
tel. 920/531–2000 **A**1 9 10 18 **F**3 7 8 11 13 15 28 29 30 34 35 40 43 45 47
56 57 59 64 65 66 75 76 79 80 81 82 85 86 87 89 90 91 92 93 96 97 107
108 109 110 113 116 118 130 131 132 140 142 145 **S** ThedaCare, Inc.,
Appleton, WI
Primary Contact: William Schmidt, President and Chief Executive Officer
CFO: Gina Moon, Vice President Finance
CMO: Paul Hoell, M.D., President Medical Staff
Web address: www.thedacare.org
**Control:** Other not–for–profit (including NFP Corporation) **Service:** General
Medical and Surgical

**Staffed Beds:** 25 **Admissions:** 1003 **Census:** 13 **Outpatient Visits:** 30703
**Births:** 127 **Total Expense ($000):** 24898 **Payroll Expense ($000):** 11502
**Personnel:** 170

## NEW RICHMOND—St. Croix County

★ **WESTFIELDS HOSPITAL (521345)**, 535 Hospital Road, Zip 54017–1495;
tel. 715/243–2600 **A**9 10 18 **F**1 3 13 15 18 27 28 29 30 31 34 35 38 40 42
43 45 46 50 56 57 59 64 65 66 69 70 71 74 75 76 77 78 79 80 81 82 86
87 89 90 93 107 110 111 112 113 116 118 128 129 130 131 132 145 147
**P**5 **S** HealthPartners, Bloomington, MN
Primary Contact: Steven Massey, President and Chief Executive Officer
CFO: Jason J. Luhrs, Vice President Fiscal Services
CMO: David O. DeGear, M.D., Vice President Medical Affairs
CIO: Patrice P. Wolff, Director Information Services
CHR: Chad P. Engstrom, Director Human Resources
Web address: www.westfieldshospital.com
**Control:** Other not–for–profit (including NFP Corporation) **Service:** General
Medical and Surgical

**Staffed Beds:** 25 **Admissions:** 1112 **Census:** 10 **Outpatient Visits:** 28240
**Births:** 129 **Total Expense ($000):** 29620 **Payroll Expense ($000):** 10584
**Personnel:** 185

## OCONOMOWOC—Waukesha County

⊞ **OCONOMOWOC MEMORIAL HOSPITAL (520062)**, 791 Summit Avenue,
Zip 53066–3896; tel. 262/569–9400 **A**1 2 9 10 **F**3 11 13 15 18 20 22 28 29
30 31 35 40 45 46 47 48 49 64 74 75 79 80 81 82 84 85 87 89 93
107 108 110 111 113 114 117 118 119 120 125 129 131 145 146 147
**S** ProHealth Care, Inc., Waukesha, WI
Primary Contact: John R. Robertstad, FACHE, President
COO: Mary Jo O'Malley, R.N., Vice President Diagnostics and Support Services
CFO: Nan Nelson, Chief Financial Officer
CMO: Brian Lipman, M.D., Vice President Medical Affairs
CIO: Rodney Dykehouse, Vice President Information Services
CHR: Nadine T. Guirl, Senior Vice President Human Resources
Web address: www.oconomowocmemorial.org
**Control:** Other not–for–profit (including NFP Corporation) **Service:** General
Medical and Surgical

**Staffed Beds:** 76 **Admissions:** 2962 **Census:** 25 **Outpatient Visits:** 72696
**Births:** 437 **Total Expense ($000):** 88350 **Payroll Expense ($000):** 23185
**Personnel:** 343

⊞ **ROGERS MEMORIAL HOSPITAL (524018)**, 34700 Valley Road,
Zip 53066–4599; tel. 262/646–4411 **A**1 3 5 9 10 **F**5 29 34 38 75 86 87 98
99 100 101 102 103 104 105 129
Primary Contact: David L. Moulthrop, Ph.D., President and Chief Executive Officer
COO: Paul A. Mueller, Chief Operating Officer
CFO: Gerald A. Noll, Chief Financial Officer
CMO: Peter M. Lake, M.D., Chief Medical Officer
CIO: Wayne Mattson, Management Information Systems Specialist
CHR: Renee A. Patterson, Vice President Employment and Training Services
Web address: www.rogershospital.org
**Control:** Other not–for–profit (including NFP Corporation) **Service:** Psychiatric

**Staffed Beds:** 90 **Admissions:** 1843 **Census:** 30 **Outpatient Visits:** 39845
**Births:** 0 **Total Expense ($000):** 35615 **Payroll Expense ($000):** 19897
**Personnel:** 465

## OCONTO—Oconto County

**OCONTO HOSPITAL & MEDICAL CENTER (521356)**, 820 Arbutus Avenue,
Zip 54153, Mailing Address: P.O. Box 357, Zip 54153–0357; tel. 920/835–1100
**A**9 10 18 21 **F**3 34 35 40 43 59 62 65 85 97 107 108 113 118 126 128 132
143 **P**8
Primary Contact: Laura Cormier, Director
Web address: www.ocontohospital.org
**Control:** Other not–for–profit (including NFP Corporation) **Service:** General
Medical and Surgical

**Staffed Beds:** 4 **Admissions:** 34 **Census:** 1 **Outpatient Visits:** 6899 **Births:**
0 **Total Expense ($000):** 4101 **Payroll Expense ($000):** 1968 **Personnel:**
29

## OCONTO FALLS—Oconto County

★ **COMMUNITY MEMORIAL HOSPITAL (521310)**, 855 South Main Street,
Zip 54154–1296; tel. 920/846–3444 **A**9 10 18 **F**3 11 13 15 18 28 29 30 40
43 55 56 57 59 64 65 75 76 77 80 81 85 86 87 89 90 93 97 107 111 113
118 132 145 146 **P**2 4 6
Primary Contact: Daniel DeGroot, Chief Executive Officer
CFO: Michele Miller, Chief Financial Officer
CMO: Judith Bowers, D.O., Chief of Staff
CIO: Jared Alfson, Chief Information Officer
CHR: Trisha Brown, Manager Human Resources
Web address: www.cmhospital.org
**Control:** Other not–for–profit (including NFP Corporation) **Service:** General
Medical and Surgical

**Staffed Beds:** 12 **Admissions:** 951 **Census:** 11 **Outpatient Visits:** 68344
**Births:** 91 **Total Expense ($000):** 37074 **Payroll Expense ($000):** 16269
**Personnel:** 245

## OSCEOLA—Polk County

**OSCEOLA MEDICAL CENTER (521318)**, 2600 65th Avenue, Zip 54020,
Mailing Address: P.O. Box 218, Zip 54020–0218; tel. 715/294–2111 **A**9 10 18
**F**11 13 15 28 29 40 43 53 56 64 70 75 76 77 78 81 86 87 89 93 107 118
126 143 **P**6
Primary Contact: Jeffrey K. Meyer, Chief Executive Officer
CMO: Rob Dybvig, M.D., Chief Medical Officer
CIO: Shawn Kammerud, Manager Information Services
CHR: Margie Evenson, Manager Human Resources
Web address: www.osceolamedicalcenter.com
**Control:** Other not–for–profit (including NFP Corporation) **Service:** General
Medical and Surgical

**Staffed Beds:** 18 **Admissions:** 705 **Census:** 6 **Outpatient Visits:** 45386
**Births:** 84 **Total Expense ($000):** 26991 **Payroll Expense ($000):** 9806
**Personnel:** 213

## OSHKOSH—Winnebago County

⊞ **AURORA MEDICAL CENTER OF OSHKOSH (520198)**, 855 North Westhaven
Drive, Zip 54904; tel. 920/456–6000 **A**1 2 9 10 **F**3 8 11 12 13 15 17 18 20
22 26 29 30 34 37 40 41 47 49 53 54 56 64 68 70 71 74 75 76 79 80
81 82 85 86 87 89 92 93 94 107 108 109 110 111 113 114 116 117 118
119 120 121 122 128 129 130 144 145 146 147 **P**6 **S** Aurora Health Care,
Milwaukee, WI
Primary Contact: Jeffrey Bard, Vice President Operations
COO: Sue Ela, Executive Vice President and Chief Operating Officer
CFO: Sandra Ewald, Vice President Finance
CMO: Bruce L. Van Cleave, M.D., Senior Vice President and Chief Medical Officer
CIO: Philip Loftus, Ph.D., Vice President and Chief Information Officer
CHR: Linda Mingus, Director Human Resources
Web address: www.aurorahealthcare.com
**Control:** Other not–for–profit (including NFP Corporation) **Service:** General
Medical and Surgical

**Staffed Beds:** 61 **Admissions:** 2985 **Census:** 28 **Outpatient Visits:** 97924
**Births:** 687 **Total Expense ($000):** 81156 **Payroll Expense ($000):** 25297
**Personnel:** 491

☐ △ **MERCY MEDICAL CENTER (520048)**, 500 South Oakwood Road,
Zip 54904–7944, Mailing Address: P.O. Box 3370, Zip 54903–3370;
tel. 920/223–2000 **A**1 2 7 9 10 **F**3 4 5 10 11 16 17 18 20 22 26 28 29
30 31 34 35 38 39 40 41 43 44 46 47 48 49 50 51 53 56 57 59 64 65 67
68 70 75 76 78 80 81 82 86 87 88 89 90 92 93 96 98 103 104 107 108
110 111 112 113 116 117 118 119 120 121 122 128 129 130 131 133 143
145 146 147
Primary Contact: William Calhoun, President
CFO: Jeff Badger, Chief Financial Officer
CMO: Mark W. Kehrberg, M.D., Senior Vice President and Chief Medical Officer
CIO: Will Weider, Chief Information Officer
CHR: Vince Gallucci, Senior Vice President Human Resources
Web address: www.affinityhealth.org
**Control:** Church–operated, Nongovernment, not–for profit **Service:** General
Medical and Surgical

**Staffed Beds:** 172 **Admissions:** 5872 **Census:** 69 **Outpatient Visits:** 88330
**Births:** 621 **Total Expense ($000):** 108188 **Payroll Expense ($000):** 40869
**Personnel:** 588

**WI**

*Many Facility Codes have changed. Please refer to the AHA Guide Code Chart.* © 2012 AHA Guide

## OSSEO—Trempealeau County

☐ **MAYO CLINIC HEALTH SYSTEM – OAKRIDGE IN OSSEO (521302)**, 13025 Eighth Street, Zip 54758–7673, Mailing Address: P.O. Box 70, Zip 54758–0070; tel. 715/597–3121, (Total facility includes 35 beds in nursing home–type unit) **A**1 9 10 18 **F**2 3 7 10 15 18 26 28 29 34 35 40 43 44 56 59 65 69 75 79 80 84 85 86 87 89 90 93 97 107 108 110 113 124 127 129 132 134 142 143 145 147 **P**6 **S** Mayo Clinic Health System, Rochester, MN
Primary Contact: Michael Ryan, Administrator
COO: Michael Ryan, Administrator
CFO: Nancy Steig, Director Fiscal Services
CHR: Rhonda Wilson, Director Human Resources
Web address: www.luthermidelfortoakridge.com
**Control:** Other not–for–profit (including NFP Corporation) **Service:** General Medical and Surgical

**Staffed Beds:** 39 **Admissions:** 382 **Census:** 39 **Outpatient Visits:** 38965 **Births:** 0 **Total Expense ($000):** 16773 **Payroll Expense ($000):** 9574 **Personnel:** 174

## PARK FALLS—Price County

★ **FLAMBEAU HOSPITAL (521325)**, 98 Sherry Avenue, Zip 54552–1467, Mailing Address: P.O. Box 310, Zip 54552–0310; tel. 715/762–2484 **A**9 10 18 **F**8 11 14 15 17 28 29 30 31 34 35 40 45 50 53 56 57 59 62 63 64 65 68 69 70 75 77 79 80 81 82 84 85 86 87 89 90 93 96 97 107 110 113 118 129 130 131 132 142 143 145 147 **S** Marian Health System, Tulsa, OK
Primary Contact: David A. Grundstrom, Chief Administrative Officer
CFO: James R. Braun, Chief Financial Officer
CHR: Barb Michalski, Manager Human Resources
Web address: www.flambeauhospital.org
**Control:** Other not–for–profit (including NFP Corporation) **Service:** General Medical and Surgical

**Staffed Beds:** 25 **Admissions:** 772 **Census:** 6 **Outpatient Visits:** 28790 **Births:** 0 **Total Expense ($000):** 18679 **Payroll Expense ($000):** 7944 **Personnel:** 171

## PEWAUKEE—Waukesha County

⊞ **LIFECARE HOSPITALS OF WISCONSIN (522007)**, 2400 Golf Road, Zip 53072; tel. 262/524–2600 **A**1 9 10 **F**1 29 34 86 129 **S** LifeCare Management Services, Plano, TX
Primary Contact: Jevne Conover, Administrator
COO: Jennifer Groeneweg, R.N., Director Nursing
CFO: Susan Stermer, Director Finance
CMO: John Daniels, M.D., Medical Director
CHR: Jill Schuetz, Manager Human Resources
Web address: www.lifecare–hospitals.com
**Control:** Corporation, Investor–owned, for–profit **Service:** Long–Term Acute Care hospital

**Staffed Beds:** 35 **Admissions:** 329 **Census:** 31 **Outpatient Visits:** 0 **Births:** 0 **Total Expense ($000):** 22446 **Payroll Expense ($000):** 8858 **Personnel:** 153

## PLATTEVILLE—Grant County

⊞ **SOUTHWEST HEALTH CENTER (521354)**, 1400 Eastside Road, Zip 53818–9800; tel. 608/348–2331, (Includes SOUTHWEST HEALTH CENTER NURSING HOME, 808 South Washington Street, Cuba City, Zip 53807; tel. 608/744–2161), (Total facility includes 84 beds in nursing home–type unit) **A**1 9 10 18 **F**2 3 6 8 13 15 28 29 31 34 35 40 43 50 56 57 59 64 68 74 75 76 77 79 81 82 83 84 85 86 87 93 96 97 98 100 101 102 103 104 105 107 108 110 113 116 118 127 128 129 131 132 142 143 145 147 **P**2 **S** HealthTech Management Services, Franklin, TN
Primary Contact: Dan D. Rohrbach, President and Chief Executive Officer
CFO: Michael Gutsch, Chief Financial Officer
CMO: Kevin Carr, M.D., Chief of Staff
CHR: Tammy Nelson, Manager Human Resources
Web address: www.southwesthealth.org
**Control:** Other not–for–profit (including NFP Corporation) **Service:** General Medical and Surgical

**Staffed Beds:** 119 **Admissions:** 952 **Census:** 87 **Outpatient Visits:** 38097 **Births:** 132 **Total Expense ($000):** 25870 **Payroll Expense ($000):** 8466 **Personnel:** 180

## PLEASANT PRAIRIE—Kenosha County

★ **UNITED HOSPITAL SYSTEM, ST. CATHERINE'S MEDICAL CENTER CAMPUS**, 9555 76th Street, Zip 53158; tel. 262/656–2011, (Nonreporting) **A**2 9 10 **S** Wheaton Franciscan Healthcare, Wheaton, IL
Primary Contact: Richard O. Schmidt, Jr., President and Chief Executive Officer
Web address: www.uhsi.org
**Control:** Other not–for–profit (including NFP Corporation) **Service:** General Medical and Surgical

**Staffed Beds:** 202

## PORTAGE—Columbia County

☐ **DIVINE SAVIOR HEALTHCARE (520041)**, 2817 New Pinery Road, Zip 53901–0387, Mailing Address: P.O. Box 387, Zip 53901–0387; tel. 608/742–4131, (Total facility includes 123 beds in nursing home–type unit) **A**1 9 10 **F**3 4 7 11 12 13 15 28 30 31 34 35 36 40 43 44 45 50 54 55 57 59 60 62 64 68 69 70 74 75 76 77 78 79 80 81 82 85 86 87 89 90 92 93 96 97 107 108 110 111 114 116 117 118 127 128 129 130 131 132 142 143 144 145 146 147 **P**6
Primary Contact: Michael Decker, President and Chief Executive Officer
CFO: Marlin Pete Nelson, Vice President Fiscal Services
CMO: Elizabeth Strabel, M.D., Chief Medical Staff
CHR: Carol J. Bank, Vice President Human Resources
Web address: www.dshealthcare.com
**Control:** Church–operated, Nongovernment, not–for profit **Service:** General Medical and Surgical

**Staffed Beds:** 167 **Admissions:** 2355 **Census:** 101 **Outpatient Visits:** 146437 **Births:** 267 **Total Expense ($000):** 62682 **Payroll Expense ($000):** 30146 **Personnel:** 525

## PRAIRIE DU CHIEN—Crawford County

⊞ **PRAIRIE DU CHIEN MEMORIAL HOSPITAL (521330)**, 705 East Taylor Street, Zip 53821–2196; tel. 608/357–2000 **A**1 9 10 18 **F**10 11 13 15 17 28 29 34 36 40 53 56 62 63 64 69 70 75 76 80 81 82 86 87 93 107 108 111 118 129 130 143 146
Primary Contact: William P. Sexton, Chief Executive Officer
CFO: Dave Breitbach, Chief Financial Officer
CIO: John Daane, Information Systems Officer
CHR: Laurie Hampton, Director Human Resources
Web address: www.pdcmemorialhospital.org
**Control:** Other not–for–profit (including NFP Corporation) **Service:** General Medical and Surgical

**Staffed Beds:** 15 **Admissions:** 1116 **Census:** 12 **Outpatient Visits:** 11243 **Births:** 119 **Total Expense ($000):** 29586 **Payroll Expense ($000):** 14087 **Personnel:** 252

## PRAIRIE DU SAC—Sauk County

★ ◯ **SAUK PRAIRIE MEMORIAL HOSPITAL & CLINICS (520095)**, 80 First Street, Zip 53578–1599; tel. 608/643–3311 **A**9 10 11 **F**3 11 13 15 29 32 34 35 36 40 43 45 47 48 53 54 56 57 59 64 68 69 75 76 78 79 81 82 84 85 86 93 97 107 108 114 117 118 126 128 129 130 131 132 143 145 147 **P**7
Primary Contact: Larry Schroeder, Chief Executive Officer
CFO: Carol May, Chief Financial Officer, Vice President Finance and Operations
CMO: John McAuliffe, M.D., Medical Director
CIO: Marybeth Bay, Director Information Technology
CHR: Robbi Eccher, Vice President Human Resources
Web address: www.spmh.org
**Control:** Other not–for–profit (including NFP Corporation) **Service:** General Medical and Surgical

**Staffed Beds:** 36 **Admissions:** 1769 **Census:** 13 **Outpatient Visits:** 69653 **Births:** 269 **Total Expense ($000):** 53691 **Payroll Expense ($000):** 24341 **Personnel:** 385

## RACINE—Racine County

⊞ △ **WHEATON FRANCISCAN HEALTHCARE – ALL SAINTS (520096)**, 3801 Spring Street, Zip 53405–1690; tel. 262/687–4011, (Total facility includes 50 beds in nursing home–type unit) **A**1 2 7 9 10 **F**3 4 5 6 13 15 17 18 20 22 24 26 28 29 30 31 34 35 38 40 41 43 44 45 48 49 50 51 53 55 56 57 58 59 64 65 68 70 72 75 76 77 78 79 80 81 85 86 87 89 90 91 93 94 95 97 98 99 100 101 102 103 104 105 107 110 111 112 114 115 117 118 119 120 122 123 127 128 129 130 131 133 134 145 146 147 **P**6 **S** Wheaton Franciscan Healthcare, Wheaton, IL
Primary Contact: Kenneth R. Buser, President and Chief Executive Officer
COO: Susan Boland, Senior Vice President and Chief Operating Officer
CFO: Lynn Lile, Director Finance
CIO: Joanne Bisterfeldt, Chief Information Officer
CHR: Mary Jo Wodicka, Director Human Resources
Web address: www.allsaintshealth.com
**Control:** Church–operated, Nongovernment, not–for profit **Service:** General Medical and Surgical

**Staffed Beds:** 356 **Admissions:** 15624 **Census:** 247 **Outpatient Visits:** 460119 **Births:** 1795 **Total Expense ($000):** 337082 **Payroll Expense ($000):** 119809 **Personnel:** 2420

**WI**

---

**Hospital, Medicare Provider Number, Address, Telephone, Approval, Facility, and Physician Codes, Health Care System**

★ American Hospital Association (AHA) membership
☐ The Joint Commission accreditation ◇ DNV Healthcare Inc. accreditation
◯ American Osteopathic Association (AOA) accreditation
△ Commission on Accreditation of Rehabilitation Facilities (CARF) accreditation

## REEDSBURG—Sauk County

✠ **REEDSBURG AREA MEDICAL CENTER (521351)**, 2000 North Dewey Street, Zip 53959–1097; tel. 608/524–6487 **A**1 9 10 18 **F**3 8 10 11 12 13 15 17 26 28 30 31 34 35 40 43 45 50 53 54 57 64 66 68 70 75 76 77 78 79 80 81 82 83 84 85 86 87 88 89 91 92 93 96 107 108 110 111 112 114 128 129 130 131 132 134 143 145 146 147
Primary Contact: Robert Van Meeteren, President and Chief Executive Officer
CFO: Joe Svetlik, Vice President Finance
CHR: Dale Turner, Vice President Human Resources
Web address: www.ramchealth.com
**Control:** Other not–for–profit (including NFP Corporation) **Service:** General Medical and Surgical

**Staffed Beds:** 25 **Admissions:** 1418 **Census:** 14 **Outpatient Visits:** 56410 **Births:** 289 **Total Expense ($000):** 42642 **Payroll Expense ($000):** 17498 **Personnel:** 355

## RHINELANDER—Oneida County

✠ **SACRED HEART–ST. MARY'S HOSPITALS (520019)**, 2251 North Shore Drive, Zip 54501–3998; tel. 715/361–2000, (Includes ST. MARY'S HOSPITAL, 1044 Kabel Avenue, Zip 54501; tel. 715/369–6600) **A**1 9 10 20 **F**3 4 5 13 15 28 29 30 31 34 35 36 40 44 45 49 50 54 57 59 64 65 68 69 74 75 76 77 78 79 80 81 82 84 85 86 87 89 91 92 93 94 96 98 99 100 101 103 104 107 108 109 110 111 112 113 115 116 118 120 129 130 131 132 143 145 147 **S** Marian Health System, Tulsa, OK
Primary Contact: Monica Hilt, President and Chief Operating Officer
COO: William A. Erickson, Vice President and Chief Operating Officer
CFO: Cathy Bukowski, Regional Chief Financial Officer
CMO: Shishir Sheth, M.D., President Medical Staff
CIO: Howard Dobizl, Director Information Services for the Northern Region
CHR: Michelle Cornelius, Director Human Resources for the Northern Region
Web address: www.ministryhealth.org
**Control:** Church–operated, Nongovernment, not–for profit **Service:** General Medical and Surgical

**Staffed Beds:** 58 **Admissions:** 3153 **Census:** 30 **Outpatient Visits:** 94411 **Births:** 357 **Total Expense ($000):** 112234 **Payroll Expense ($000):** 57174 **Personnel:** 623

## RICE LAKE—Barron County

✠ **LAKEVIEW MEDICAL CENTER (520011)**, 1700 West Stout Street, Zip 54868–5000; tel. 715/234–1515 **A**1 9 10 20 **F**7 11 13 15 28 29 34 36 40 43 51 53 54 56 60 62 63 64 69 75 76 77 78 80 81 82 86 87 89 93 107 111 118 129 143 146
Primary Contact: Edward H. Wolf, President and Chief Executive Officer
COO: Cindy Arts–Strenke, Chief Operating Officer and Chief Nursing Officer
CFO: Jacqueline Klein, Vice President Finance
CMO: John L. Olson, M.D., Medical Director
CIO: Brad Gerrits, Director Information Systems
CHR: Kathy Mitchell, Director Human Resources
Web address: www.lakeviewmedical.com
**Control:** Other not–for–profit (including NFP Corporation) **Service:** General Medical and Surgical

**Staffed Beds:** 40 **Admissions:** 2413 **Census:** 19 **Outpatient Visits:** 65802 **Births:** 415 **Total Expense ($000):** 58619 **Payroll Expense ($000):** 22753 **Personnel:** 427

## RICHLAND CENTER—Richland County

☐ **RICHLAND HOSPITAL (521341)**, 333 East Second Street, Zip 53581–1899; tel. 608/647–6321 **A**1 9 10 18 **F**2 12 13 15 28 34 40 43 56 64 70 76 78 80 81 86 89 93 107 118 129 130 143
Primary Contact: Steven R. Nockerts, Chief Executive Officer
CFO: Karen Traynor, Chief Financial Officer
CMO: Kay M. Balink, M.D., Chief of Staff
CIO: Jerry Cooper, Manager Data Processing
CHR: Rhonda Sutton, Director Human Resources
Web address: www.richlandhospital.com
**Control:** Other not–for–profit (including NFP Corporation) **Service:** General Medical and Surgical

**Staffed Beds:** 25 **Admissions:** 1179 **Census:** 11 **Outpatient Visits:** 32509 **Births:** 153 **Total Expense ($000):** 34293 **Payroll Expense ($000):** 14880 **Personnel:** 257

## RIPON—Fond Du Lac County

✠ **RIPON MEDICAL CENTER (521321)**, 933 Newbury Street, Zip 54971–1798, Mailing Address: P.O. Box 390, Zip 54971–0390; tel. 920/748–3101 **A**1 9 10 18 **F**3 11 15 17 18 26 27 28 29 34 35 37 40 43 45 46 48 53 56 57 59 64 68 69 70 74 75 77 78 79 80 81 85 86 87 88 89 93 94 96 97 100 104 107 108 110 113 118 129 130 131 132 143 145 147 **P**6
Primary Contact: Katherine Vergos, Chief Operating Officer
CFO: Bobbie Pollesch, Chief Financial Officer
CIO: Wayne Johnston, Director Information Systems
CHR: Sarah Brus, Director Human Resources
Web address: www.riponmedicalcenter.org
**Control:** Other not–for–profit (including NFP Corporation) **Service:** General Medical and Surgical

**Staffed Beds:** 25 **Admissions:** 484 **Census:** 5 **Outpatient Visits:** 26034 **Births:** 0 **Total Expense ($000):** 17295 **Payroll Expense ($000):** 7558 **Personnel:** 158

## RIVER FALLS—St. Croix County

✠ **RIVER FALLS AREA HOSPITAL (521349)**, 1629 East Division Street, Zip 54022–1571; tel. 715/425–6155 **A**1 2 9 10 18 **F**8 13 14 15 18 28 29 31 34 35 40 43 44 45 50 53 57 59 64 65 68 74 76 77 78 79 80 81 82 83 85 86 87 89 90 91 93 94 96 107 108 110 113 118 125 128 129 130 131 132 134 146 147 **S** Allina Health, Minneapolis, MN
Primary Contact: David R. Miller, President
COO: William Frommelt, Director Operations and Finance
CFO: William Frommelt, Director Operations and Finance
CHR: Kristen Novak, Manager Human Resources
Web address: www.allina.com
**Control:** Other not–for–profit (including NFP Corporation) **Service:** General Medical and Surgical

**Staffed Beds:** 25 **Admissions:** 1312 **Census:** 10 **Outpatient Visits:** 21047 **Births:** 198 **Total Expense ($000):** 34338 **Payroll Expense ($000):** 12501 **Personnel:** 164

## SHAWANO—Shawano County

✠ **SHAWANO MEDICAL CENTER (521346)**, 309 North Bartlette Street, Zip 54166; tel. 715/526–2111 **A**1 9 10 18 **F**3 11 13 15 28 29 30 40 53 56 57 59 63 64 75 76 77 79 80 81 82 85 86 87 90 93 102 107 111 118 128 130 131 134 145 **P**5 **S** ThedaCare, Inc., Appleton, WI
Primary Contact: Dorothy Erdmann, Chief Executive Officer
CFO: Kenneth Monger, Chief Financial Officer
CMO: Amy Slagle, M.D., President Medical Staff, Menominee Tribal Clinic
CIO: Jennifer Quinn, Quality and Safety Coordinator
CHR: Mark Gabavics, Director Human Resources
Web address: www.shawanomed.org
**Control:** Other not–for–profit (including NFP Corporation) **Service:** General Medical and Surgical

**Staffed Beds:** 25 **Admissions:** 1896 **Census:** 14 **Outpatient Visits:** 73513 **Births:** 315 **Total Expense ($000):** 41037 **Payroll Expense ($000):** 16956 **Personnel:** 238

## SHEBOYGAN—Sheboygan County

✠ **AURORA SHEBOYGAN MEMORIAL MEDICAL CENTER (520035)**, 2629 North Seventh Street, Zip 53083–4998; tel. 920/451–5000 **A**1 2 9 10 **F**3 4 8 13 17 18 20 22 26 28 29 31 34 35 36 40 41 43 44 45 49 50 53 54 56 57 59 64 65 68 70 74 75 76 78 79 80 81 82 85 86 87 89 93 94 96 98 99 100 102 103 107 108 111 112 113 114 117 118 119 120 122 128 129 130 131 134 145 146 147 **P**6 **S** Aurora Health Care, Milwaukee, WI
Primary Contact: David Graebner, Chief Administrative Officer
CFO: Connie Debbink, Director Finance
CMO: Jeffrey C. Lynds, M.D., President Medical Staff
CIO: Steve Serketich, Manager Information Services
Web address: www.aurorahealthcare.org
**Control:** Other not–for–profit (including NFP Corporation) **Service:** General Medical and Surgical

**Staffed Beds:** 130 **Admissions:** 4983 **Census:** 47 **Outpatient Visits:** 60486 **Births:** 978 **Total Expense ($000):** 87722 **Payroll Expense ($000):** 27863 **Personnel:** 596

✠ **ST. NICHOLAS HOSPITAL (520044)**, 3100 Superior Avenue, Zip 53081; tel. 920/459–8300 **A**1 2 9 10 **F**11 13 15 17 20 28 29 34 36 38 40 43 53 54 56 60 62 63 64 70 75 76 78 80 81 82 86 87 89 90 93 107 108 111 117 118 129 **P**5 **S** Hospital Sisters Health System, Springfield, IL
Primary Contact: Andrew Bagnall, Chief Executive Officer
CMO: Clifford G. Martin, M.D., President Medical Staff
CIO: Karen Held, Site Coordinator Information Technology
CHR: Barbara Hamann, Manager People Services
Web address: www.stnicholashospital.org
**Control:** Church–operated, Nongovernment, not–for profit **Service:** General Medical and Surgical

**Staffed Beds:** 78 **Admissions:** 2795 **Census:** 27 **Outpatient Visits:** 92081 **Births:** 330 **Total Expense ($000):** 73130 **Payroll Expense ($000):** 19993 **Personnel:** 279

WI

*Many Facility Codes have changed. Please refer to the AHA Guide Code Chart.* © 2012 AHA Guide

## SHELL LAKE—Washburn County

☐ **INDIANHEAD MEDICAL CENTER (521342)**, 113 Fourth Avenue, Zip 54871, Mailing Address: P.O. Box 300, Zip 54871–0300; tel. 715/468–7833 **A**1 9 10 18 **F**11 13 15 17 28 31 34 40 45 56 59 62 64 68 70 76 77 78 80 81 86 87 89 107 113 118 126 129 130 132 **P**5 **S** Mid Atlantic Health Management, inc., Stevensville, MD
Primary Contact: Paul Naglosky, Administrator
CFO: Michael Elliott, Controller
CMO: Allan Haesemeyer, M.D., Chief of Staff
CHR: Gwen Nielsen, Manager Human Resources
Web address: www.indianheadmedicalcenter.com
**Control:** Corporation, Investor–owned, for–profit **Service:** General Medical and Surgical

**Staffed Beds:** 25 **Admissions:** 391 **Census:** 3 **Outpatient Visits:** 9319
**Births:** 5 **Total Expense ($000):** 6500 **Payroll Expense ($000):** 2739
**Personnel:** 69

## SPARTA—Monroe County

☐ **MAYO CLINIC HEALTH SYSTEM – FRANCISCAN HEALTHCARE IN SPARTA (521305)**, 310 West Main Street, Zip 54656–2171; tel. 608/269–2132 **A**1 9 10 18 **F**5 11 15 28 29 30 34 35 40 42 43 53 56 57 59 64 65 66 68 75 77 80 81 86 87 93 97 107 118 126 129 131 132 142 143 145 **S** Mayo Clinic Health System, Rochester, MN
Primary Contact: Kimberly Hawthorne, Administrator
CMO: Tracy Warsing, M.D., Site Leader Chief of Staff
Web address: www.mayohealthsystem.com
**Control:** Church–operated, Nongovernment, not–for profit **Service:** General Medical and Surgical

**Staffed Beds:** 14 **Admissions:** 306 **Census:** 6 **Outpatient Visits:** 20756
**Births:** 0 **Total Expense ($000):** 12517 **Payroll Expense ($000):** 6508
**Personnel:** 158

## SPOONER—Washburn County

★ **SPOONER HEALTH SYSTEM (521332)**, 819 Ash Street, Zip 54801–1299; tel. 715/635–2111, (Total facility includes 90 beds in nursing home–type unit) **A**9 10 18 **F**3 13 15 17 29 31 34 35 40 41 50 56 57 59 62 63 64 65 68 69 70 75 76 78 80 81 85 86 87 89 90 93 107 108 111 114 118 127 129 131 132 134 145 147 **S** HealthTech Management Services, Franklin, TN
Primary Contact: Michael Schafer, Chief Executive Officer and Administrator
CFO: Rebecca Busch, Chief Financial Officer
CHR: Cindy Rouzer, Director Human Resources
Web address: www.spoonerhealthsystem.com
**Control:** Other not–for–profit (including NFP Corporation) **Service:** General Medical and Surgical

**Staffed Beds:** 115 **Admissions:** 786 **Census:** 92 **Outpatient Visits:** 16461
**Births:** 79 **Total Expense ($000):** 14706 **Payroll Expense ($000):** 7177
**Personnel:** 103

## ST. CROIX FALLS—Polk County

**ST. CROIX REGIONAL MEDICAL CENTER (521337)**, 235 State Street, Zip 54024–9400; tel. 715/483–3261 **A**9 10 18 **F**6 11 13 15 28 29 34 36 40 43 51 53 55 56 64 70 75 76 77 78 80 81 82 86 87 93 99 100 101 103 104 107 108 111 115 117 118 130 143 146 **P**5 6
Primary Contact: Dave Dobosenski, Chief Executive Officer
CFO: John Tremble, Chief Financial Officer
CMO: William Beyer, M.D., Chief Medical Officer
CIO: Brent McCurdy, Director Management Information
CHR: Lee Ann Vitalis, Executive Director Human Resources
Web address: www.scrmc.org
**Control:** Other not–for–profit (including NFP Corporation) **Service:** General Medical and Surgical

**Staffed Beds:** 25 **Admissions:** 1848 **Census:** 14 **Outpatient Visits:** 169050
**Births:** 308 **Total Expense ($000):** 58071 **Payroll Expense ($000):** 18584
**Personnel:** 391

## STANLEY—Chippewa County

★ **OUR LADY OF VICTORY HOSPITAL (521311)**, 1120 Pine Street, Zip 54768–0220; tel. 715/644–5571 **A**9 10 18 **F**3 15 28 29 30 34 37 40 43 45 50 57 59 65 75 77 80 81 84 86 87 89 90 93 94 96 97 107 108 110 113 126 129 130 131 132 143 145 147 **P**6 **S** Marian Health System, Tulsa, OK
Primary Contact: Cynthia Eichman, President
CFO: Terri Lewandowski, Director Financial Services
Web address: www.ministryhealth.org
**Control:** Other not–for–profit (including NFP Corporation) **Service:** General Medical and Surgical

**Staffed Beds:** 7 **Admissions:** 387 **Census:** 7 **Outpatient Visits:** 28627
**Births:** 0 **Total Expense ($000):** 19994 **Payroll Expense ($000):** 8235
**Personnel:** 147

## STEVENS POINT—Portage County

★ **MINISTRY SAINT MICHAEL'S HOSPITAL (520002)**, 900 Illinois Avenue, Zip 54481–3196; tel. 715/346–5000 **A**9 10 19 **F**3 4 5 12 13 15 17 20 28 29 30 34 35 40 43 44 45 47 48 50 51 56 59 64 65 68 70 72 74 75 76 77 79 80 81 82 84 85 86 87 88 89 93 94 98 99 100 101 102 103 104 105 106 107 108 110 111 113 115 117 118 120 128 129 130 131 134 143 145 146 147 **P**2 **S** Marian Health System, Tulsa, OK
Primary Contact: Jeffrey L. Martin, President
CFO: William J. Hinner, Vice President Fiscal Services and Chief Financial Officer
CIO: Will Weider, Chief Information Officer
CHR: Cheryl F. Zima, Vice President Human Resources
Web address: www.ministryhealth.org/SMH/home.nws
**Control:** Church–operated, Nongovernment, not–for profit **Service:** General Medical and Surgical

**Staffed Beds:** 50 **Admissions:** 4422 **Census:** 41 **Outpatient Visits:** 367409
**Births:** 521 **Total Expense ($000):** 154800 **Payroll Expense ($000):** 80787
**Personnel:** 771

**SAINT MICHAEL'S HOSPITAL** See Ministry Saint Michael's Hospital

## STOUGHTON—Dane County

☐ **STOUGHTON HOSPITAL ASSOCIATION (521343)**, 900 Ridge Street, Zip 53589–1896; tel. 608/873–6611 **A**1 9 10 18 **F**3 4 6 8 14 15 28 29 34 35 36 40 41 43 45 53 54 56 57 59 62 64 65 70 75 77 80 81 85 86 89 90 91 93 96 97 98 100 103 107 108 110 113 114 116 128 129 130 131 132 134 143 145 146 147
Primary Contact: Terrence Brenny, President and Chief Executive Officer
CFO: Karen Myers, Vice President Financial Services
CMO: Guirish Agni, M.D., Chief of Staff
CIO: Karen Myers, Vice President Financial Services
CHR: Christopher Schmitz, Director Human Resources
Web address: www.stoughtonhospital.com
**Control:** Other not–for–profit (including NFP Corporation) **Service:** General Medical and Surgical

**Staffed Beds:** 32 **Admissions:** 1103 **Census:** 14 **Outpatient Visits:** 36799
**Births:** 0 **Total Expense ($000):** 36309 **Payroll Expense ($000):** 15265
**Personnel:** 280

## STURGEON BAY—Door County

**DOOR COUNTY MEMORIAL HOSPITAL** See Ministry Door County Medical Center

✠ **MINISTRY DOOR COUNTY MEDICAL CENTER (521358)**, 323 South 18th Avenue, Zip 54235–1495; tel. 920/743–5566, (Total facility includes 30 beds in nursing home–type unit) **A**1 9 10 18 **F**2 3 11 13 15 17 28 29 30 31 32 34 35 39 40 41 43 55 56 57 59 61 64 65 66 68 70 75 76 77 78 79 80 81 82 84 85 86 87 89 90 93 107 110 111 113 116 117 118 126 127 128 129 131 132 134 143 144 147 **P**6 **S** Marian Health System, Tulsa, OK
Primary Contact: Gerald M. Worrick, President and Chief Executive Officer
CFO: Robert C. Scieszinski, Vice President Finance
CIO: Mary Lopas, Chief Information Officer
CHR: Kelli Bowling, Chief Culture Officer
Web address: www.dcmh.org
**Control:** Church–operated, Nongovernment, not–for profit **Service:** General Medical and Surgical

**Staffed Beds:** 55 **Admissions:** 1791 **Census:** 40 **Outpatient Visits:** 79310
**Births:** 142 **Total Expense ($000):** 62235 **Payroll Expense ($000):** 31457
**Personnel:** 474

## SUMMIT—Waukesha County

✠ **AURORA MEDICAL CENTER SUMMIT (520206)**, 36500 Aurora Drive, Zip 53066–4899; tel. 262/434–1000 **A**1 9 10 **F**3 8 11 12 13 15 17 18 20 22 24 26 28 29 30 34 36 37 39 40 41 44 45 46 47 48 49 53 54 59 64 68 70 72 75 76 77 79 80 81 82 85 86 89 90 93 96 107 108 110 111 112 114 115 116 117 118 120 122 123 125 128 129 130 145 146 147 **P**6 **S** Aurora Health Care, Milwaukee, WI
Primary Contact: Daniel J. Bonk, Chief Executive Officer
Web address: www.aurorahealthcare.org
**Control:** Other not–for–profit (including NFP Corporation) **Service:** General Medical and Surgical

**Staffed Beds:** 71 **Admissions:** 2437 **Census:** 24 **Outpatient Visits:** 77272
**Births:** 420 **Total Expense ($000):** 91726 **Payroll Expense ($000):** 28490
**Personnel:** 537

**WI**

## SUPERIOR—Douglas County

✠ **ESSENTIA HEALTH ST. MARY'S HOSPITAL OF SUPERIOR (521329)**, 3500 Tower Avenue, Zip 54880–5395; tel. 715/395–5400 **A**1 9 10 18 **F**3 11 15 28 29 30 40 56 59 64 65 75 77 78 80 81 82 86 87 90 93 96 97 107 108 110 118 129 132 134 141 145 147 **S** Essentia Health, Duluth, MN
Primary Contact: Mary Shaw, Chief Operating Officer
Web address: www.smdc.org
**Control:** Other not–for–profit (including NFP Corporation) **Service:** General Medical and Surgical

| Staffed Beds: 25 Admissions: 579 Census: 12 Outpatient Visits: 47301 Births: 0 Total Expense ($000): 34340 Payroll Expense ($000): 17139 Personnel: 201 |

## TOMAH—Monroe County

✠ **TOMAH MEMORIAL HOSPITAL (521320)**, 321 Butts Avenue, Zip 54660–1412; tel. 608/372–2181 **A**1 9 10 18 **F**3 11 12 13 28 30 31 34 35 40 42 43 50 57 59 63 64 76 77 79 80 81 82 84 85 86 87 89 90 93 96 107 108 111 118 128 129 131 132 134 143 145 147 **P**5 **S** HealthTech Management Services, Franklin, TN
Primary Contact: Philip J. Stuart, Administrator and Chief Executive Officer
CFO: Joseph Zeps, Vice President Finance
Web address: www.tomahhospital.org
**Control:** Other not–for–profit (including NFP Corporation) **Service:** General Medical and Surgical

| Staffed Beds: 25 Admissions: 970 Census: 8 Outpatient Visits: 22689 Births: 329 Total Expense ($000): 32215 Payroll Expense ($000): 13023 Personnel: 217 |

✠ △ **VETERANS AFFAIRS MEDICAL CENTER**, 500 East Veterans Street, Zip 54660; tel. 608/372–3971, (Nonreporting) **A**1 7 **S** Department of Veterans Affairs, Washington, DC
Primary Contact: Mario DeSanctis, FACHE, Director
CFO: Jane Mashak–Ekern, Fiscal Officer
CMO: David Houlihan, M.D., Chief of Staff
CIO: Mary Monroe, Chief Information Officer
Web address: www.tomah.va.gov
**Control:** Veterans Affairs, Government, federal **Service:** General Medical and Surgical

| Staffed Beds: 71 |

## TOMAHAWK—Lincoln County

**SACRED HEART HOSPITAL (521313)**, 401 West Mohawk Drive, Zip 54487; tel. 715/453–7700 **A**9 10 18 **F**15 28 29 34 36 40 56 64 75 77 80 81 86 87 89 93 100 101 104 107 118 129 130
Primary Contact: Monica Hilt, President
Web address: www.ministryhealth.org
**Control:** Church–operated, Nongovernment, not–for profit **Service:** General Medical and Surgical

| Staffed Beds: 8 Admissions: 429 Census: 4 Outpatient Visits: 9588 Births: 0 Total Expense ($000): 12281 Payroll Expense ($000): 6945 Personnel: 85 |

## TWO RIVERS—Manitowoc County

✠ **AURORA MEDICAL CENTER – MANITOWOC COUNTY (520034)**, 5000 Memorial Drive, Zip 54241–2399; tel. 920/794–5000 **A**1 2 9 10 **F**3 11 13 28 29 30 31 34 35 36 37 40 41 43 44 45 47 48 49 50 54 56 57 59 75 76 78 79 80 81 82 85 86 87 89 93 94 107 108 111 113 118 120 122 128 129 131 132 133 134 142 145 146 147 **P**6 **S** Aurora Health Care, Milwaukee, WI
Primary Contact: Cathie A. Kocourek, Chief Administrative Officer
COO: Carrie L. Penovich, Director Clinical and Support Services
CFO: Sandra Ewald, Vice President Finance
CHR: Stacie A. Schneider, Manager Human Resources
Web address: www.aurorahealthcare.org
**Control:** Other not–for–profit (including NFP Corporation) **Service:** General Medical and Surgical

| Staffed Beds: 66 Admissions: 2264 Census: 20 Outpatient Visits: 54811 Births: 422 Total Expense ($000): 50074 Payroll Expense ($000): 16318 Personnel: 336 |

## VIROQUA—Vernon County

**VERNON MEMORIAL HEALTHCARE (521348)**, 507 South Main Street, Zip 54665–2096; tel. 608/637–2101 **A**9 10 18 **F**3 8 11 13 17 28 29 34 35 36 37 40 43 45 53 56 57 59 62 63 75 76 77 80 81 82 86 87 89 93 107 108 110 114 126 129 130 131 132 134 143 145 147 **P**6
Primary Contact: Garith W. Steiner, Chief Executive Officer and Administrator
COO: Kyle Bakkum, Chief Operating Officer
CFO: Mary Koenig, Chief Financial Officer
CIO: Julie Steiner, Manager Marketing and Public Relations
CHR: Kay Starr, Manager Human Resources
Web address: www.vmh.org
**Control:** Other not–for–profit (including NFP Corporation) **Service:** General Medical and Surgical

| Staffed Beds: 11 Admissions: 1409 Census: 11 Outpatient Visits: 87602 Births: 155 Total Expense ($000): 58795 Payroll Expense ($000): 23470 Personnel: 275 |

## WATERFORD—Racine County

☐ **LAKEVIEW SPECIALTY HOSPITAL AND REHABILITATION CENTER (522005)**, 1701 Sharp Road, Zip 53185; tel. 262/534–7297 **A**1 9 10 **F**1 12 28 29 34 36 38 53 62 64 75 82 86 87 90 93 99 100 101 104 129 **P**6
Primary Contact: Robyn Rushing, Administrator
Web address: www.lakeviewsystem.com
**Control:** Corporation, Investor–owned, for–profit **Service:** Long–Term Acute Care hospital

| Staffed Beds: 39 Admissions: 236 Census: 20 Outpatient Visits: 4022 Births: 0 Total Expense ($000): 14194 Payroll Expense ($000): 5950 Personnel: 169 |

## WATERTOWN—Dodge County

★ **WATERTOWN REGIONAL MEDICAL CENTER (520116)**, 125 Hospital Drive, Zip 53098–3303; tel. 920/261–4210 **A**9 10 **F**3 10 11 13 15 18 20 26 28 29 34 35 36 40 53 54 56 57 59 62 64 65 68 69 71 74 75 76 77 78 79 80 81 82 86 87 89 90 93 104 107 108 111 112 113 117 118 124 128 129 130 131 134 143 145 146 147 **P**8
Primary Contact: John P. Kosanovich, President
CFO: John Graf, Senior Vice President
CMO: Jeff Meade, M.D., Chief Medical Officer
CIO: Jennifer Laughlin, Vice President and Chief Information Officer
CHR: Duane Floyd, Vice President Human Resources and Professional Services
Web address: www.uwphwatertown.com
**Control:** Other not–for–profit (including NFP Corporation) **Service:** General Medical and Surgical

| Staffed Beds: 55 Admissions: 1801 Census: 16 Outpatient Visits: 200308 Births: 287 Total Expense ($000): 88913 Payroll Expense ($000): 37651 Personnel: 596 |

## WAUKESHA—Waukesha County

✠ **REHABILITATION HOSPITAL OF WISCONSIN (523027)**, 1625 Coldwater Creek Drive, Zip 53188–8028; tel. 262/521–8800 **A**1 9 10 **F**3 29 64 68 74 75 79 86 90 93 96 99 103 129 **S** ProHealth Care, Inc., Waukesha, WI
Primary Contact: Anne E. Jurenec, Chief Executive Officer
CFO: Robert Koehne, Controller
CMO: Yachiel Kleen, M.D., Medical Director
CHR: Annette Hahn, Director Human Resources
Web address: www.rehabhospitalwi.com
**Control:** Partnership, Investor–owned, for–profit **Service:** Rehabilitation

| Staffed Beds: 40 Admissions: 726 Census: 29 Outpatient Visits: 5670 Births: 0 Total Expense ($000): 12282 Payroll Expense ($000): 5953 Personnel: 101 |

**WAUKESHA COUNTY MENTAL HEALTH CENTER (524026)**, 2501 Airport Road, Zip 53188; tel. 262/548–7950 **A**10 **F**4 98 129 **P**2
Primary Contact: Michele A. Cusatis, Ph.D., Administrator
Web address: www.waukeshacounty.gov/
**Control:** County–Government, nonfederal **Service:** Psychiatric

| Staffed Beds: 28 Admissions: 998 Census: 18 Outpatient Visits: 0 Births: 0 Total Expense ($000): 6047 Payroll Expense ($000): 3084 Personnel: 55 |

✠ **WAUKESHA MEMORIAL HOSPITAL (520008)**, 725 American Avenue, Zip 53188–5099; tel. 262/928–1000 **A**1 2 3 5 9 10 **F**3 4 5 6 11 12 13 15 18 20 22 24 26 28 29 30 31 32 34 35 40 44 45 46 48 49 50 56 57 58 59 64 68 72 74 75 76 78 79 80 81 82 84 85 87 89 93 97 98 100 101 102 103 105 107 108 110 111 113 114 115 116 117 118 119 120 122 123 125 128 129 131 134 142 145 146 147 **S** ProHealth Care, Inc., Waukesha, WI
Primary Contact: John R. Robertstad, FACHE, President
CFO: Nan Nelson, Vice President Finance
CMO: James D. Gardner, M.D., Vice President and Chief Medical Officer
CIO: Rodney Dykehouse, Senior Vice President Information Services
CHR: Nadine T. Guirl, Senior Vice President Human Resources
Web address: www.waukeshamemorial.org
**Control:** Other not–for–profit (including NFP Corporation) **Service:** General Medical and Surgical

| Staffed Beds: 317 Admissions: 15604 Census: 187 Outpatient Visits: 289915 Births: 1884 Total Expense ($000): 379053 Payroll Expense ($000): 107879 Personnel: 1760 |

## WAUPACA—Waupaca County

☐ **RIVERSIDE MEDICAL CENTER (521334)**, 800 Riverside Drive, Zip 54981–1999; tel. 715/258–1000 **A**1 9 10 18 **F**3 8 11 13 17 28 29 34 35 40 41 45 57 59 64 68 70 76 78 80 81 82 85 86 87 88 89 90 97 107 108 111 112 114 118 129 131 143 145 146 147 **S** ThedaCare, Inc., Appleton, WI
Primary Contact: Craig A. Kantos, Chief Executive Officer
CFO: Kerry Lee Blanke, Director Financial Services
CMO: James Williams, M.D., Chief of Staff
CHR: Kevin Gossens, Director Human Resources
Web address: www.riversidemedical.org
**Control:** Other not–for–profit (including NFP Corporation) **Service:** General Medical and Surgical

| Staffed Beds: 25 Admissions: 1158 Census: 10 Outpatient Visits: 53149 Births: 166 Total Expense ($000): 31687 Payroll Expense ($000): 15705 Personnel: 239 |

**WI**

*Many Facility Codes have changed. Please refer to the AHA Guide Code Chart.* © 2012 AHA Guide

## WAUPUN—Dodge County

☐ **WAUPUN MEMORIAL HOSPITAL (521327)**, 620 West Brown Street, Zip 53963–1799; tel. 920/324–5581 **A**1 9 10 18 **F**3 11 13 15 25 28 29 30 31 34 35 36 40 44 50 51 54 57 59 60 64 66 68 69 70 71 74 75 76 77 79 81 82 84 85 86 97 107 111 114 117 118 129 131 132 133 142 143 145 147 **P**6
Primary Contact: DeAnn Thurmer, Chief Operating Officer
CFO: Bonnie Schmitz, Chief Financial Officer
Web address: www.agnesian.com
**Control:** Church–operated, Nongovernment, not–for profit **Service:** General Medical and Surgical

**Staffed Beds:** 25 **Admissions:** 1063 **Census:** 10 **Outpatient Visits:** 51948 **Births:** 143 **Total Expense ($000):** 29333 **Payroll Expense ($000):** 11536 **Personnel:** 191

## WAUSAU—Marathon County

✠ △ **ASPIRUS WAUSAU HOSPITAL (520030)**, 333 Pine Ridge Boulevard, Zip 54401–4187; tel. 715/847–2121 **A**1 2 3 5 7 9 10 **F**3 4 5 7 8 11 12 13 15 17 18 20 22 24 26 28 29 30 31 34 35 40 44 45 46 47 48 49 50 51 54 55 56 58 59 60 62 63 64 65 68 69 70 71 72 74 75 76 78 79 80 81 82 83 84 85 86 87 89 90 92 93 96 97 98 100 102 103 104 107 108 110 111 113 114 115 116 117 118 119 120 122 123 125 128 129 131 134 142 145 146 147 **P**8 **S** Aspirus, Inc., Wausau, WI
Primary Contact: Diane Postler–Slattery, Ph.D., President and Chief Operating Officer
COO: Diane Postler–Slattery, Ph.D., President and Chief Operating Officer
CFO: Sidney C. Sczygelski, Senior Vice President Finance and Chief Financial Officer
CIO: Jerry Mourey, Vice President Information Technology and Chief Information Officer
CHR: Roger Lucas, Vice President Human Resources
Web address: www.aspirus.org
**Control:** Other not–for–profit (including NFP Corporation) **Service:** General Medical and Surgical

**Staffed Beds:** 262 **Admissions:** 13550 **Census:** 152 **Outpatient Visits:** 106599 **Births:** 1268 **Total Expense ($000):** 308499 **Payroll Expense ($000):** 105067 **Personnel:** 1911

**NORTH CENTRAL HEALTH CARE (524017)**, 1100 Lake View Drive, Zip 54403–6785; tel. 715/848–4600, (Total facility includes 247 beds in nursing home–type unit) **A**9 10 **F**4 5 6 29 34 38 56 75 86 93 98 99 100 101 102 103 104 105 127
Primary Contact: Gary Bezucha, FACHE, Chief Executive Officer
CFO: Brenda Glodowski, Chief Financial Officer
CHR: Chad Bastable, Director Human Resources
Web address: www.norcen.org
**Control:** County–Government, nonfederal **Service:** Psychiatric

**Staffed Beds:** 260 **Admissions:** 1207 **Census:** 256 **Outpatient Visits:** 274471 **Births:** 0 **Total Expense ($000):** 26218 **Payroll Expense ($000):** 15281 **Personnel:** 230

**NORTH CENTRAL HEALTH CARE FACILITIES** See North Central Health Care

## WAUWATOSA—Milwaukee County

✠ **AURORA PSYCHIATRIC HOSPITAL (524000)**, 1220 Dewey Avenue, Zip 53213–2598; tel. 414/454–6600 **A**1 9 10 **F**4 5 30 35 38 44 50 54 59 64 68 75 86 87 98 99 100 101 102 104 105 106 129 131 134 **P**6 **S** Aurora Health Care, Milwaukee, WI
Primary Contact: Peter Carlson, Administrator
CMO: Anthony Meyer, M.D., Medical Director
CIO: Philip Loftus, Ph.D., Vice President and Chief Information Officer
CHR: Barbara Molthen, Director Human Resources
Web address: www.aurorahealthcare.org
**Control:** Other not–for–profit (including NFP Corporation) **Service:** Psychiatric

**Staffed Beds:** 65 **Admissions:** 3191 **Census:** 41 **Outpatient Visits:** 13776 **Births:** 0 **Total Expense ($000):** 21822 **Payroll Expense ($000):** 10884 **Personnel:** 216

★ **WHEATON FRANCISCAN HEALTHCARE – THE WISCONSIN HEART HOSPITAL (520199)**, 10000 West Bluemound Road, Zip 53226; tel. 414/778–7800 **A**9 10 **F**3 8 17 18 20 22 24 26 29 37 39 40 42 43 44 45 46 47 50 64 68 74 75 77 79 81 85 86 97 107 108 114 117 118 123 125 129 145 147 **P**6 **S** Wheaton Franciscan Healthcare, Wheaton, IL
Primary Contact: Debra K. Standridge, President
COO: Norma J. McCutcheon, R.N., Senior Vice President Operations
CMO: Stephen Cardamone, D.O., Senior Vice President and Chief Medical Officer
CIO: Gregory Smith, Senior Vice President and Chief Information Officer
CHR: Christopher Morris, Director Human Resources
Web address: www.twhh.org
**Control:** Church–operated, Nongovernment, not–for profit **Service:** General Medical and Surgical

**Staffed Beds:** 30 **Admissions:** 1293 **Census:** 13 **Outpatient Visits:** 12646 **Births:** 0 **Total Expense ($000):** 44519 **Payroll Expense ($000):** 10561 **Personnel:** 140

## WEST ALLIS—Milwaukee County

✠ △ **AURORA WEST ALLIS MEDICAL CENTER (520139)**, 8901 West Lincoln Avenue, Zip 53227–2409, Mailing Address: P.O. Box 27901, Zip 53227–0901; tel. 414/328–6000 **A**1 2 7 9 10 **F**2 3 11 12 13 15 28 29 30 31 34 35 37 38 40 41 43 44 45 49 50 51 52 54 55 56 57 59 64 65 68 70 72 74 75 76 78 79 80 81 82 84 85 86 87 91 93 94 95 96 97 100 107 108 110 111 113 114 115 117 118 119 120 122 125 129 131 133 134 145 146 147 **P**6 **S** Aurora Health Care, Milwaukee, WI
Primary Contact: Richard A. Kellar, Administrator
CHR: Mindy Necci, Director Human Resources
Web address: www.aurorahealthcare.org
**Control:** Other not–for–profit (including NFP Corporation) **Service:** General Medical and Surgical

**Staffed Beds:** 220 **Admissions:** 12752 **Census:** 142 **Outpatient Visits:** 143548 **Births:** 3562 **Total Expense ($000):** 192687 **Payroll Expense ($000):** 60327 **Personnel:** 1161

## WEST BEND—Washington County

✠ **ST. JOSEPH'S COMMUNITY HOSPITAL OF WEST BEND (520063)**, 3200 Pleasant Valley Road, Zip 53095; tel. 262/334–5533 **A**1 9 10 **F**3 4 13 15 17 28 29 30 31 34 35 40 43 44 46 47 49 50 51 54 57 59 68 70 74 75 76 77 78 79 80 81 85 86 87 89 100 101 107 108 110 111 113 114 117 118 119 120 128 129 134 145 146 147 **P**6
Primary Contact: David Olson, Interim President
CFO: Mike Malzewski, Chief Financial Officer
CMO: Patrick Gardner, M.D., Vice President Medical Affairs
CHR: Deb Lauenstein, Director Human Resources and Marketing
Web address: www.stjosephswbclinic.com
**Control:** Other not–for–profit (including NFP Corporation) **Service:** General Medical and Surgical

**Staffed Beds:** 78 **Admissions:** 3871 **Census:** 40 **Outpatient Visits:** 76207 **Births:** 698 **Total Expense ($000):** 74449 **Payroll Expense ($000):** 25727 **Personnel:** 403

## WESTON—Marathon County

✠ **SAINT CLARE'S HOSPITAL (520202)**, 3400 Ministry Parkway, Zip 54476; tel. 715/393–3000 **A**1 9 10 **F**3 11 13 17 18 20 22 24 26 29 30 31 34 35 37 40 43 44 50 51 57 59 64 68 70 72 74 75 76 78 79 80 81 82 85 86 87 89 129 131 134 142 145 147 **P**6 **S** Marian Health System, Tulsa, OK
Primary Contact: Mary T. Krueger, President
CFO: William J. Hinner, Vice President Finance and Chief Financial Officer
CMO: Larry T. Hegland, M.D., Chief Medical Officer
CIO: Stacy Marver, Director Information Technology
CHR: Nancy Kwiesielewicz, Human Resources Representative
Web address: www.ministryhealth.org
**Control:** Church–operated, Nongovernment, not–for profit **Service:** General Medical and Surgical

**Staffed Beds:** 60 **Admissions:** 4936 **Census:** 43 **Outpatient Visits:** 17126 **Births:** 681 **Total Expense ($000):** 89752 **Payroll Expense ($000):** 28647 **Personnel:** 389

**WI**

**WHITEHALL—Trempealeau County**

★ **TRI–COUNTY MEMORIAL HOSPITAL (521316)**, 18601 Lincoln Street, Zip 54773–8605; tel. 715/538–4361, (Total facility includes 62 beds in nursing home–type unit) **A**9 10 18 **F**7 10 11 28 34 40 43 53 56 64 69 75 78 81 86 90 93 107 108 127 129 143
Primary Contact: Brian Theiler, President and Chief Executive Officer
COO: Brian Theiler, President and Chief Executive Officer
CFO: Patti Dockendorff, Director Finance
CMO: Jesse Leahy, M.D., Chief Medical Officer
CIO: John Rohland, Director Information Technology
CHR: Jill Wesener Dieck, Director Human Resources
Web address: www.tricountymemorial.org/index.html
**Control:** Other not–for–profit (including NFP Corporation) **Service:** General Medical and Surgical

**Staffed Beds:** 77 **Admissions:** 456 **Census:** 60 **Outpatient Visits:** 12238 **Births:** 0 **Total Expense ($000):** 10672 **Payroll Expense ($000):** 4362 **Personnel:** 109

**WILD ROSE—Waushara County**

**WILD ROSE COMMUNITY MEMORIAL HOSPITAL (521303)**, 601 Grove Avenue, Zip 54984, Mailing Address: P.O. Box 243, Zip 54984–0243; tel. 920/622–3257 **A**9 10 18 **F**3 8 10 11 15 18 29 34 35 40 43 45 56 59 64 65 68 75 77 79 80 81 82 84 86 87 89 90 93 97 99 100 101 102 103 104 107 108 111 113 118 130 131 132 143 145 146 147 **P**7
Primary Contact: Donald Caves, President
CFO: Thomas P. Krystowiak, Vice President Finance
CMO: Reginaldo Arboleda, M.D., Chief of Staff
CHR: Karen M. West, Administrator Support Services
Web address: www.wildrosehospital.org
**Control:** Other not–for–profit (including NFP Corporation) **Service:** General Medical and Surgical

**Staffed Beds:** 25 **Admissions:** 515 **Census:** 11 **Outpatient Visits:** 17119 **Births:** 0 **Total Expense ($000):** 12514 **Payroll Expense ($000):** 4622 **Personnel:** 116

**WINNEBAGO—Winnebago County**

☐ **WINNEBAGO MENTAL HEALTH INSTITUTE (524002)**, 1300 South Drive, Zip 54985, Mailing Address: Box 9, Zip 54985–0009; tel. 920/235–4910 **A**1 9 10 **F**4 5 29 30 39 75 82 87 92 98 99 100 101 103 129 **P**6
Primary Contact: Thomas Speech, M.D., Director
CMO: Randy Kerswill, M.D., Medical Director
CIO: Greg Schneider, Director Information Technology
CHR: Frances Dujon–Reynolds, Director Human Resources
Web address: www.dhfs.state.wi.us/mh_winnebago
**Control:** State–Government, nonfederal **Service:** Psychiatric

**Staffed Beds:** 183 **Admissions:** 1363 **Census:** 176 **Outpatient Visits:** 0 **Births:** 0 **Total Expense ($000):** 54878 **Payroll Expense ($000):** 28740 **Personnel:** 550

**WISCONSIN RAPIDS—Wood County**

⊡ **RIVERVIEW HOSPITAL ASSOCIATION (520033)**, 410 Dewey Street, Zip 54494–4715, Mailing Address: P.O. Box 8080, Zip 54495–8080; tel. 715/423–6060 **A**1 9 10 **F**3 4 8 13 14 15 17 28 30 31 34 35 39 40 41 43 56 59 64 65 68 69 70 75 76 77 78 79 80 81 84 85 86 88 89 90 93 97 98 100 107 108 110 111 114 116 117 118 119 120 123 128 129 130 131 134 145 147
Primary Contact: Celse A. Berard, President
CFO: Michael Bovee, Vice President Finance
CMO: Timothy K. Huebner, M.D., President Medical Affairs
CIO: Marjorie Tell, Vice President Information Technology
CHR: Tom Hunsberger, Vice President Human Resources
Web address: www.riverviewhospital.org
**Control:** Other not–for–profit (including NFP Corporation) **Service:** General Medical and Surgical

**Staffed Beds:** 69 **Admissions:** 2687 **Census:** 24 **Outpatient Visits:** 59335 **Births:** 464 **Total Expense ($000):** 70833 **Payroll Expense ($000):** 26791 **Personnel:** 483

**WOODRUFF—Oneida County**

⊡ **HOWARD YOUNG MEDICAL CENTER (520091)**, 240 Maple Street, Zip 54568, Mailing Address: P.O. Box 470, Zip 54568–0470; tel. 715/356–8000 **A**1 9 10 20 **F**3 8 11 13 15 18 28 29 30 35 40 41 43 45 47 48 49 50 57 68 75 76 77 80 81 82 84 85 86 87 88 89 93 96 107 108 110 114 118 128 129 132 145 147 **S** Marian Health System, Tulsa, OK
Primary Contact: Sheila Clough, President
CFO: Cathy Bukowski, Chief Financial Officer
CIO: Howard Dobizl, Director Information Technology Services
CHR: Michelle Cornelius, Director Human Resources
Web address: www.ministryhealth.org
**Control:** Church–operated, Nongovernment, not–for profit **Service:** General Medical and Surgical

**Staffed Beds:** 52 **Admissions:** 2888 **Census:** 30 **Outpatient Visits:** 48494 **Births:** 320 **Total Expense ($000):** 53243 **Payroll Expense ($000):** 20315 **Personnel:** 330




*Many Facility Codes have changed. Please refer to the AHA Guide Code Chart.*

# WYOMING

## AFTON—Lincoln County

★ **STAR VALLEY MEDICAL CENTER (531313)**, 901 Adams Street, Zip 83110–0579, Mailing Address: P.O. Box 579, Zip 83110–0579; tel. 307/885–5800, (Total facility includes 24 beds in nursing home–type unit) **A**9 10 18 **F**3 7 11 13 15 29 31 34 40 43 45 57 59 64 65 67 74 75 76 77 78 79 81 82 85 86 87 89 97 102 107 110 111 113 117 118 127 128 129 130 131 132 134 143 145 146 147 **P**6
Primary Contact: Don Herbert, Interim Chief Executive Officer
CFO: Ken Brough, Chief Financial Officer
CMO: David Shrader, M.D., Chief of Staff
CIO: Marty Ashton, Chief Information Officer
CHR: Joel Johnson, Director Human Resources
Web address: www.svmcwy.org
**Control:** Hospital district or authority, Government, nonfederal **Service:** General Medical and Surgical

**Staffed Beds:** 44 **Admissions:** 690 **Census:** 29 **Outpatient Visits:** 17796 **Births:** 96 **Total Expense ($000):** 22837 **Payroll Expense ($000):** 10192 **Personnel:** 170

## BASIN—Big Horn County

**SOUTH BIG HORN COUNTY HOSPITAL (531301)**, 388 South U.S. Highway 20, Zip 82410; tel. 307/568–3311, (Total facility includes 37 beds in nursing home–type unit) **A**9 10 18 **F**1 32 34 35 40 56 57 59 64 82 93 97 107 110 118 126 127 129 132 **P**4
Primary Contact: Jackie Claudson, Administrator
Web address: www.midwayclinic.com
**Control:** Hospital district or authority, Government, nonfederal **Service:** General Medical and Surgical

**Staffed Beds:** 43 **Admissions:** 106 **Census:** 32 **Outpatient Visits:** 1274 **Births:** 1 **Total Expense ($000):** 4036 **Payroll Expense ($000):** 2863 **Personnel:** 91

## BUFFALO—Johnson County

★ **JOHNSON COUNTY HEALTHCARE CENTER (531308)**, 497 West Lott Street, Zip 82834–1691; tel. 307/684–5521, (Total facility includes 50 beds in nursing home–type unit) **A**9 10 18 **F**6 11 13 15 28 31 40 57 62 63 67 70 76 78 79 81 89 93 107 118 129 132
Primary Contact: Sandy Ward, Administrator
CMO: Grace Gosar, M.D., Chief of Staff
CIO: Laurie Hansen, Director Administrative Services
CHR: Karen Ferguson, Director Human Resources
Web address: www.buffalowyoming.com/hospital/
**Control:** Hospital district or authority, Government, nonfederal **Service:** General Medical and Surgical

**Staffed Beds:** 75 **Admissions:** 482 **Census:** 48 **Outpatient Visits:** 9785 **Births:** 50 **Total Expense ($000):** 15364 **Payroll Expense ($000):** 8058 **Personnel:** 171

## CASPER—Natrona County

☐ **ELKHORN VALLEY REHABILITATION HOSPITAL (533027)**, 5715 East 2nd Street, Zip 82609; tel. 307/265–0005, (Nonreporting) **A**1 10 **S** Ernest Health, Inc., Albuquerque, NM
Primary Contact: Michael Phillips, Chief Executive Officer
Web address: www.evrh.ernesthealth.com/
**Control:** Corporation, Investor–owned, for–profit **Service:** Rehabilitation

**Staffed Beds:** 40

○ **MOUNTAIN VIEW REGIONAL HOSPITAL (530033)**, 6550 East Second Street, Zip 82609–4321, Mailing Address: P.O. Box 51888, Zip 82605–1888; tel. 307/995–8100, (Nonreporting) **A**10 11
Primary Contact: William Stangl, Chief Executive Officer
Web address: www.mountainviewregionalhospital.com
**Control:** Partnership, Investor–owned, for–profit **Service:** Surgical

**Staffed Beds:** 23

☐ **WYOMING BEHAVIORAL INSTITUTE (534004)**, 2521 East 15th Street, Zip 82609–4126; tel. 307/237–7444, (Nonreporting) **A**1 9 10 **S** Universal Health Services, Inc., King of Prussia, PA
Primary Contact: Joseph Gallagher, Chief Executive Officer
CFO: Carmel Bickford, Chief Financial Officer
CMO: Steven Brown, M.D., Medical Director
CHR: Jon Barra, Director Human Resources
Web address: www.wbihelp.com
**Control:** Corporation, Investor–owned, for–profit **Service:** Psychiatric

**Staffed Beds:** 124

⊡ **WYOMING MEDICAL CENTER (530012)**, 1233 East Second Street, Zip 82601–2988; tel. 307/577–7201, (Total facility includes 15 beds in nursing home–type unit) **A**1 9 10 20 **F**3 7 11 12 13 18 20 22 24 28 29 30 31 34 35 40 41 43 45 46 49 50 51 57 59 60 61 68 70 74 76 79 81 82 85 86 87 89 97 102 107 108 111 113 117 118 119 120 122 123 125 127 128 129 131 134 143 145 146 147 **P**6
Primary Contact: Vickie L. Diamond, R.N., MS, President and Chief Executive Officer
COO: Julie Cann–Taylor, R.N., Chief Operating Officer, Senior Vice President Patient Care Services and Chief Nursing Officer
CFO: Don Claunch, Senior Vice President, Chief Financial Officer and Chief Information Officer
CMO: Carol M. Solie, M.D., Chief Medical Officer
CIO: Don Claunch, Senior Vice President, Chief Financial Officer and Chief Information Officer
CHR: Matt Kaiser, Director Human Resources
CNO: Julie Cann–Taylor, R.N., Senior Vice President Patient care and Chief Nursing Officer
Web address: www.wmcnet.org
**Control:** Other not–for–profit (including NFP Corporation) **Service:** General Medical and Surgical

**Staffed Beds:** 207 **Admissions:** 8423 **Census:** 97 **Outpatient Visits:** 80463 **Births:** 1041 **Total Expense ($000):** 180239 **Payroll Expense ($000):** 68203 **Personnel:** 1139

## CHEYENNE—Laramie County

⊡ △ **CHEYENNE REGIONAL MEDICAL CENTER (530014)**, 214 East 23rd Street, Zip 82001–3790; tel. 307/634–2273, (Total facility includes 16 beds in nursing home–type unit) **A**1 2 5 7 9 10 20 **F**3 4 5 11 12 13 15 18 20 22 24 26 28 29 30 31 34 35 38 40 43 46 47 48 49 51 53 57 59 60 62 63 65 68 70 72 73 74 75 76 77 78 79 81 82 83 84 85 86 87 89 90 93 94 98 99 100 101 102 103 104 105 107 108 110 111 113 117 118 119 120 122 123 127 128 129 131 134 142 145 146 147 **P**6 7
Primary Contact: John Lucas, M.D., Chief Executive Officer
COO: Paul Panico, Chief Operating Officer
CFO: Kimberly Webb, Chief Financial Officer
CMO: David Lind, M.D., Interim Chief Medical Officer
CIO: David Squires, Senior Vice President
CHR: Sandra Colman, Director Human Resources
Web address: www.crmcwy.org
**Control:** County–Government, nonfederal **Service:** General Medical and Surgical

**Staffed Beds:** 222 **Admissions:** 10295 **Census:** 128 **Outpatient Visits:** 149599 **Births:** 1197 **Total Expense ($000):** 187693 **Payroll Expense ($000):** 95261 **Personnel:** 1699

⊡ **VETERANS AFFAIRS MEDICAL CENTER**, 2360 East Pershing Boulevard, Zip 82001–5392; tel. 307/778–7550, (Nonreporting) **A**1 9 **S** Department of Veterans Affairs, Washington, DC
Primary Contact: Cynthia McCormack, MS, Director
CFO: Melvin Cranford, Chief Fiscal Services
CMO: Roger Johnson, M.D., Chief of Staff
CIO: Liz McCulloch, Chief Information Resource Management Systems
CHR: Ron Lester, Chief Human Resources
Web address: www.cheyenne.va.gov/
**Control:** Veterans Affairs, Government, federal **Service:** General Medical and Surgical

**Staffed Beds:** 21

---

**Hospital, Medicare Provider Number, Address, Telephone, Approval, Facility, and Physician Codes, Health Care System**

★ American Hospital Association (AHA) membership
☐ The Joint Commission accreditation    ◇ DNV Healthcare Inc. accreditation
○ American Osteopathic Association (AOA) accreditation
△ Commission on Accreditation of Rehabilitation Facilities (CARF) accreditation

## CODY—Park County

★ **WEST PARK HOSPITAL (531312)**, 707 Sheridan Avenue, Zip 82414–3409;
tel. 307/527–7501, (Total facility includes 97 beds in nursing home–type unit) **A**9
10 18 **F**3 4 5 6 7 11 13 15 18 24 26 28 29 30 31 34 35 36 38 40 42 43 45
46 56 57 59 60 62 63 64 65 68 70 75 76 78 79 81 82 84 85 86 89 93 97
99 102 103 104 105 107 108 110 111 113 118 119 127 129 130 131 132
133 134 143 144 145 146 147 **S** QHR, Brentwood, TN
Primary Contact: Douglas A. McMillan, Administrator and Chief Executive Officer
CFO: Patrick G. McConnell, Chief Financial Officer
CHR: Dick Smith, Director Human Resources
Web address: www.westparkhospital.org
**Control:** Hospital district or authority, Government, nonfederal **Service:** General
Medical and Surgical

**Staffed Beds:** 140 **Admissions:** 1954 **Census:** 88 **Outpatient Visits:** 62046
**Births:** 265 **Total Expense ($000):** 52511 **Payroll Expense ($000):** 24215
**Personnel:** 359

## DOUGLAS—Converse County

★ **MEMORIAL HOSPITAL OF CONVERSE COUNTY (531302)**, 111 South Fifth
Street, Zip 82633–1450, Mailing Address: P.O. Box 1450, Zip 82633–1450;
tel. 307/358–2122 **A**9 10 18 **F**3 7 8 13 15 28 29 32 34 35 40 43 45 46 50
57 59 64 68 70 75 76 79 81 85 86 87 107 110 114 118 126 128 132 134
145 146 147 **P**6
Primary Contact: Ryan K. Smith, Chief Executive Officer
CMO: Jonathan L. Grosdidier, M.D., Chief of Staff
CIO: Dave Patterson, Director
CHR: Linda York, Manager Human Resources
Web address: www.conversehospital.com
**Control:** County–Government, nonfederal **Service:** General Medical and Surgical

**Staffed Beds:** 25 **Admissions:** 678 **Census:** 6 **Outpatient Visits:** 24582
**Births:** 112 **Total Expense ($000):** 31763 **Payroll Expense ($000):** 14088
**Personnel:** 305

## EVANSTON—Uinta County

⊞ **EVANSTON REGIONAL HOSPITAL (530032)**, 190 Arrowhead Drive,
Zip 82930–9266; tel. 307/789–3636 **A**1 9 10 20 **F**3 11 15 29 34 35 40 43
45 48 60 65 70 74 75 76 77 79 81 82 85 86 87 89 93 107 108 111 113
118 127 128 132 133 145 **P**6 **S** Community Health Systems, Inc., Franklin, TN
Primary Contact: George Winn, Chief Executive Officer
CFO: Jared Stimpson, Chief Financial Officer
CHR: Laura Elliott, Director Marketing and Human Resources
Web address: www.evanstonregionalhospital.com
**Control:** Corporation, Investor–owned, for–profit **Service:** General Medical and
Surgical

**Staffed Beds:** 42 **Admissions:** 987 **Census:** 6 **Outpatient Visits:** 18850
**Births:** 303 **Total Expense ($000):** 18758 **Payroll Expense ($000):** 8278
**Personnel:** 159

△ **WYOMING STATE HOSPITAL (534001)**, 830 Highway 150 South,
Zip 82931–5341, Mailing Address: P.O. Box 177, Zip 82931–0177;
tel. 307/789–3464 **A**7 9 10 **F**29 30 50 75 77 87 98 100 101 102 103 129
134 142 **P**6
Primary Contact: William J. Sexton, Administrator
CFO: Paul Mullenax, Business Manager
CIO: Steve Baldwin, Manager Information Technology
Web address: www.mentalhealth.state.wy.us/hospital/index.html
**Control:** State–Government, nonfederal **Service:** Psychiatric

**Staffed Beds:** 183 **Admissions:** 208 **Census:** 73 **Outpatient Visits:** 0 **Births:**
0 **Total Expense ($000):** 32704 **Payroll Expense ($000):** 16040
**Personnel:** 401

## GILLETTE—Campbell County

★ **CAMPBELL COUNTY MEMORIAL HOSPITAL (530002)**, 501 South Burma
Avenue, Zip 82716–3426, Mailing Address: P.O. Box 3011, Zip 82717–3011;
tel. 307/682–8811, (Total facility includes 143 beds in nursing home–type unit)
**A**9 10 20 21 **F**3 5 6 7 11 13 15 28 31 34 35 38 40 43 45 51 53 54
56 59 60 62 63 64 65 66 68 69 70 71 73 75 76 77 78 79 81 82 84 85 86
87 88 93 94 96 97 98 99 100 101 102 103 104 105 107 108 109 110 111
113 114 115 117 118 119 120 124 128 129 130 131 132 133 134 142 143
145 146 147 **P**6
Primary Contact: Robert A. Morasko, Chief Executive Officer
COO: Andy Fitzgerald, Executive Vice President
CFO: Andy Fitzgerald, Executive Vice President
CIO: Stevan Bailey, Manager Information Systems
CHR: John A. Fitch, Vice President Human Resources
Web address: www.ccmh.net
**Control:** Hospital district or authority, Government, nonfederal **Service:** General
Medical and Surgical

**Staffed Beds:** 215 **Admissions:** 3453 **Census:** 143 **Outpatient Visits:**
222314 **Births:** 737 **Total Expense ($000):** 113572 **Payroll Expense
($000):** 60541 **Personnel:** 907

## JACKSON—Teton County

⊞ **ST. JOHN'S MEDICAL CENTER AND LIVING CENTER (530015)**, 625 East
Broadway Street, Zip 83001, Mailing Address: P.O. Box 428, Zip 83001–0428;
tel. 307/733–3636, (Total facility includes 60 beds in nursing home–type unit) **A**1
9 10 20 **F**3 11 13 15 29 30 31 34 35 40 43 44 45 46 51 53 54 57 59 62 63
67 68 70 74 75 76 77 78 81 82 84 86 87 97 107 108 110 111 114 118 128
129 131 132 134 143 144 145 147 **P**5
Primary Contact: John Kren, Acting Chief Executive Officer
COO: Gary Tauner, Chief Operating Officer
CFO: John Kren, Chief Financial Officer
CIO: David Witton, Manager Information Systems
Web address: www.tetonhospital.org
**Control:** Hospital district or authority, Government, nonfederal **Service:** General
Medical and Surgical

**Staffed Beds:** 108 **Admissions:** 2154 **Census:** 63 **Outpatient Visits:** 70621
**Births:** 470 **Total Expense ($000):** 67821 **Payroll Expense ($000):** 27350
**Personnel:** 422

## KEMMERER—Lincoln County

★ **SOUTH LINCOLN MEDICAL CENTER (531315)**, 711 Onyx Street,
Zip 83101–3214; tel. 307/877–4401, (Total facility includes 24 beds in nursing
home–type unit) **A**9 10 18 **F**3 7 13 15 32 34 39 40 43 57 59 65 68 75 76 77
79 81 93 97 107 111 113 118 127 128 129 132 145 147 **P**6
Primary Contact: Eric Boley, Administrator and Chief Executive Officer
COO: Lou Ann Carmichael, Director Operations
CFO: Curtis Nielson, Director Finance
CMO: G. Christopher Krell, M.D., Chief of Staff
CIO: Kristin Housley, Chief Management Information Systems
CHR: Armand Drummond, Manager Human Resources
Web address: www.southlincolnmedical.com
**Control:** Hospital district or authority, Government, nonfederal **Service:** General
Medical and Surgical

**Staffed Beds:** 40 **Admissions:** 126 **Census:** 23 **Outpatient Visits:** 27413
**Births:** 37 **Total Expense ($000):** 11490 **Payroll Expense ($000):** 6673
**Personnel:** 138

## LANDER—Fremont County

⊞ **LANDER REGIONAL HOSPITAL (530010)**, 1320 Bishop Randall Drive,
Zip 82520–3996; tel. 307/332–4420 **A**1 9 10 20 **F**3 11 13 15 28 29 30 34
35 39 40 43 57 59 70 74 76 77 79 80 81 85 87 90 91 93 96 98 103 106
107 108 110 111 113 118 127 129 132 134 146 **P**5 **S** LifePoint Hospitals,
Inc., Brentwood, TN
Primary Contact: Ben Quinton, Chief Executive Officer
CFO: Ann Huhnke, Chief Financial Officer
CMO: Brian Gee, M.D., Director Emergency Services
CIO: Keith Blair, M.D., Manager Information Systems
CHR: Janet Morgan, Manager Human Resources
Web address: www.landerhospital.com
**Control:** Corporation, Investor–owned, for–profit **Service:** General Medical and
Surgical

**Staffed Beds:** 89 **Admissions:** 2108 **Census:** 25 **Outpatient Visits:** 34235
**Births:** 251 **Total Expense ($000):** 22512 **Payroll Expense ($000):** 10752
**Personnel:** 214

## LARAMIE—Albany County

⊞ **IVINSON MEMORIAL HOSPITAL (530025)**, 255 North 30th Street, Zip 82072;
tel. 307/742–2141, (Total facility includes 9 beds in nursing home–type unit) **A**1
9 10 20 **F**11 13 15 28 29 30 31 34 38 40 45 50 56 57 59 60 64 70 73 75
76 77 78 79 81 85 89 98 99 102 107 108 111 114 118 120 127 128 129
131 132 145 146 **P**8
Primary Contact: Carol Dozier, Chief Executive Officer
COO: Linda Mink, R.N., Vice President Clinical Service Line Development
CFO: Karl Vilums, Chief Financial Officer
CMO: Jim Martinchick, M.D., Chief of Staff
CIO: Bill Winn, Chief Information Officer
CHR: Holly Zajic, Vice President Human Resources and Physician Services
Web address: www.ivinsonhospital.org
**Control:** Hospital district or authority, Government, nonfederal **Service:** General
Medical and Surgical

**Staffed Beds:** 99 **Admissions:** 2448 **Census:** 22 **Outpatient Visits:** 42186
**Births:** 414 **Total Expense ($000):** 60577 **Payroll Expense ($000):** 22625
**Personnel:** 372

*Many Facility Codes have changed. Please refer to the AHA Guide Code Chart.*

## LOVELL—Big Horn County

★ **NORTH BIG HORN HOSPITAL DISTRICT (531309)**, 1115 Lane 12,
Zip 82431–9537; tel. 307/548–5200, (Total facility includes 85 beds in nursing
home–type unit) **A**9 10 18 **F**3 6 7 10 15 28 29 34 40 41 45 56 57 59 64 65
66 68 75 77 81 85 86 87 93 97 107 113 118 126 129 130 131 132 142
145 146 **P**6
Primary Contact: Rick Schroeder, Chief Executive Officer
CFO: Daphne Hartman, Chief Financial Officer
CMO: David E. Hoffman, M.D., Chief of Staff
CIO: Eileen Fink, Health Information Officer
CHR: Barbara Shumway, Director Human Resources
Web address: www.nbhh.com
**Control:** Hospital district or authority, Government, nonfederal **Service:** General
Medical and Surgical

**Staffed Beds:** 100 **Admissions:** 484 **Census:** 82 **Outpatient Visits:** 14550
**Total Expense ($000):** 13614 **Payroll Expense ($000):** 8035 **Personnel:**
171

## LUSK—Niobrara County

**NIOBRARA HEALTH AND LIFE CENTER (531314)**, 921 Ballencee Avenue,
Zip 82225, Mailing Address: P.O. Box 780, Zip 82225–0780;
tel. 307/334–4000, (Nonreporting) **A**9 10 18
Primary Contact: Gary R. Poquette, FACHE, Chief Executive Officer
Web address: www.niobrarahospital.com
**Control:** Hospital district or authority, Government, nonfederal **Service:** General
Medical and Surgical

**Staffed Beds:** 24

## NEWCASTLE—Weston County

★ **WESTON COUNTY HEALTH SERVICES (531303)**, 1124 Washington
Boulevard, Zip 82701–2996; tel. 307/746–4491, (Total facility includes 54 beds
in nursing home–type unit) **A**9 10 18 **F**28 29 40 41 56 57 59 62 64 77 91 93
107 118 129 132 **S** Regional Health, Rapid City, SD
Primary Contact: Gary Bieganski, FACHE, Interim Chief Executive Officer
CFO: Linda Holland, Controller
CMO: Lanny Reimer, M.D., Chief Medical Staff
CIO: Terri Frye, Manager Information Systems
CHR: Shirley Parks, Manager Human Resources
Web address: www.wchs–wy.org
**Control:** Hospital district or authority, Government, nonfederal **Service:** General
Medical and Surgical

**Staffed Beds:** 75 **Admissions:** 268 **Census:** 57 **Outpatient Visits:** 9184
**Births:** 0 **Personnel:** 129

## POWELL—Park County

★ **POWELL VALLEY HEALTHCARE (531310)**, 777 Avenue H, Zip 82435–2296;
tel. 307/754–2267, (Total facility includes 100 beds in nursing home–type unit)
**A**9 10 18 **F**7 10 11 13 15 28 29 34 35 36 40 43 56 57 59 62 63 64 70 76
79 81 82 85 107 108 111 114 118 127 129 130 131 132 134 143 145 146
147 **P**1 **S** HealthTech Management Services, Franklin, TN
Primary Contact: Bill D. Patten, Chief Executive Officer
CFO: Steve Ramsey, Chief Financial Officer
CMO: Robert Chandler, M.D., Chief of Staff
CIO: Greg Platko, Director Information Systems
CHR: Kara Beech, Director Human Resource
Web address: www.pvhc.org
**Control:** Other not–for–profit (including NFP Corporation) **Service:** General
Medical and Surgical

**Staffed Beds:** 125 **Admissions:** 918 **Census:** 100 **Outpatient Visits:** 28434
**Births:** 165 **Total Expense ($000):** 40171 **Payroll Expense ($000):** 22976
**Personnel:** 315

## RAWLINS—Carbon County

★ **MEMORIAL HOSPITAL OF CARBON COUNTY (531316)**, 2221 West Elm
Street, Zip 82301–0460, Mailing Address: P.O. Box 460, Zip 82301–0460;
tel. 307/324–2221 **A**9 10 18 **F**3 7 8 11 13 15 29 30 31 38 40 43 45 57 59
64 68 70 76 79 81 87 90 93 107 110 111 113 118 129 132 134 145
**S** QHR, Brentwood, TN
Primary Contact: Daniel E. Jessop, CPA, Chief Executive Officer
CFO: Brenda Rees, Chief Financial Officer
CMO: Duane E. Abels, M.D., Chief of Staff
CHR: Beverly Young, Director Human Resources
Web address: www.imhcc.com
**Control:** County–Government, nonfederal **Service:** General Medical and Surgical

**Staffed Beds:** 25 **Admissions:** 1097 **Census:** 5 **Outpatient Visits:** 13036
**Births:** 100 **Total Expense ($000):** 17740 **Payroll Expense ($000):** 10612
**Personnel:** 185

## RIVERTON—Fremont County

✠ **RIVERTON MEMORIAL HOSPITAL (530008)**, 2100 West Sunset Drive,
Zip 82501–2274; tel. 307/856–4161, (Nonreporting) **A**1 9 10 20 **S** LifePoint
Hospitals, Inc., Brentwood, TN
Primary Contact: James Christian Smolik, Chief Executive Officer
CFO: Susan Goetzinger, Chief Financial Officer
CMO: James White, M.D., Chief of Staff
CIO: Linda Tice, Director Information Systems
CHR: Norma Atwood, Director Human Resources
Web address: www.riverton–hospital.com
**Control:** Corporation, Investor–owned, for–profit **Service:** General Medical and
Surgical

**Staffed Beds:** 49

## ROCK SPRINGS—Sweetwater County

✠ **MEMORIAL HOSPITAL OF SWEETWATER COUNTY (530011)**, 1200 College
Drive, Zip 82901–5868, Mailing Address: P.O. Box 1359, Zip 82902–1359;
tel. 307/362–3711 **A**1 9 10 20 **F**3 8 11 13 15 28 29 30 31 34 35 40 43 48
57 59 60 70 75 76 78 79 81 82 87 93 97 100 102 103 104 105 107 110
111 114 115 118 128 129 134 145
Primary Contact: Gerard D. Klein, Chief Executive Officer
CFO: Irene Richardson, Chief Financial Officer
CMO: Richard Clark, M.D., President, Medical Staff
CHR: Charles Frye, Director Human Resources
CNO: Deborah L. Gaspar, R.N., Chief Nursing Officer
Web address: www.sweetwatermedicalcenter.com
**Control:** County–Government, nonfederal **Service:** General Medical and Surgical

**Staffed Beds:** 58 **Admissions:** 2200 **Census:** 15 **Outpatient Visits:** 97638
**Births:** 490 **Total Expense ($000):** 41179 **Payroll Expense ($000):** 19892
**Personnel:** 391

## SHERIDAN—Sheridan County

☐ **SHERIDAN MEMORIAL HOSPITAL (530006)**, 1401 West Fifth Street,
Zip 82801–2799; tel. 307/672–1000, (Nonreporting) **A**1 9 10 20
Primary Contact: Michael McCafferty, Chief Executive Officer
CFO: Ed Johlman, Chief Financial Officer
CMO: Brad Hanebrink, D.O., Chief of Staff
CIO: Nyle Morgan, Chief Information Officer
CHR: Len Gross, Director Human Resources
Web address: www.sheridanhospital.org
**Control:** County–Government, nonfederal **Service:** General Medical and Surgical

**Staffed Beds:** 72

✠ △ **VETERANS AFFAIRS MEDICAL CENTER**, 1898 Fort Road,
Zip 82801–8320; tel. 307/672–3473, (Total facility includes 38 beds in nursing
home–type unit) **A**1 5 7 9 **F**1 3 4 5 7 30 31 34 35 38 39 45 48 53 56 57 59
61 62 63 64 65 71 74 75 77 78 82 83 84 85 86 87 93 94 96 97 98 100
101 102 103 104 105 106 107 111 114 118 126 128 129 131 134 142 143
145 146 147 **S** Department of Veterans Affairs, Washington, DC
Primary Contact: Debra L. Hirschman, R.N., MSN, Director
COO: Michele Beach, Associate Director
CFO: Donna Fuerstenberg, Fiscal Chief
CMO: Wendell Robison, M.D., Chief of Staff
CIO: Cynthia Sostrom, Chief Information Officer
CHR: James Hardin, Human Resources Officer
Web address: www.va.gov/sta/guide/home.asp
**Control:** Veterans Affairs, Government, federal **Service:** Psychiatric

**Staffed Beds:** 185 **Admissions:** 1527 **Census:** 158 **Outpatient Visits:**
126826 **Births:** 0 **Personnel:** 544

## SUNDANCE—Crook County

★ **CROOK COUNTY MEDICAL SERVICES DISTRICT (531311)**, 713 Oak Street,
Zip 82729, Mailing Address: P.O. Box 517, Zip 82729–0517;
tel. 307/283–3501, (Nonreporting) **A**9 10 18 **S** Regional Health, Rapid City, SD
Primary Contact: Jan VanBeek, Chief Executive Officer
CFO: Betty Meyers, Chief Financial Officer
CMO: Jeremi Villano, M.D., Chief of Staff
CHR: Patricia Feist, Manager Human Resources
Web address: www.crookcountymedical.com
**Control:** Hospital district or authority, Government, nonfederal **Service:** General
Medical and Surgical

**Staffed Beds:** 48

---

**Hospital, Medicare Provider Number, Address, Telephone, Approval, Facility, and Physician Codes, Health Care System**

★ American Hospital Association (AHA) membership
☐ The Joint Commission accreditation ◇ DNV Healthcare Inc. accreditation
○ American Osteopathic Association (AOA) accreditation
△ Commission on Accreditation of Rehabilitation Facilities (CARF) accreditation

**WY**

**THERMOPOLIS—Hot Springs County**

★ **HOT SPRINGS COUNTY MEMORIAL HOSPITAL (531304)**, 150 East Arapahoe Street, Zip 82443–2498; tel. 307/864–3121 **A**9 10 18 **F**3 11 13 15 28 29 31 34 40 43 45 64 75 76 78 79 81 82 85 86 89 107 108 110 111 114 118 126 128 129 132 144 145 **S** HealthTech Management Services, Franklin, TN
Primary Contact: Robin Roling, President and Chief Executive Officer
CFO: Shelly Larson, Chief Financial Officer
CIO: Tim Knight, Director Information Technology
CHR: Patti Jeunehomme, Director Human Resources
Web address: www.hscmh.org
**Control:** County–Government, nonfederal **Service:** General Medical and Surgical

> **Staffed Beds:** 25 **Admissions:** 513 **Census:** 5 **Outpatient Visits:** 18575
> **Births:** 78 **Total Expense ($000):** 12685 **Payroll Expense ($000):** 5004
> **Personnel:** 98

**TORRINGTON—Goshen County**

★ **COMMUNITY HOSPITAL (531307)**, 2000 Campbell Drive, Zip 82240–1597; tel. 307/532–4181 **A**9 10 18 **F**3 8 11 13 15 29 30 35 36 40 42 43 45 46 57 59 64 68 70 75 77 79 81 84 87 107 118 127 128 129 130 131 132 134 144 145 **S** Banner Health, Phoenix, AZ
Primary Contact: Vincent B. DiFranco, Chief Executive Officer
CFO: C. Dale Spencer, Chief Financial Officer
CMO: Richard Campbell, D.O., Chief of Staff
CIO: Rod Miller, Chief Information Technology
CHR: Sandy Dugger, Director Human Resources
Web address: www.bannerhealth.com
**Control:** Other not–for–profit (including NFP Corporation) **Service:** General Medical and Surgical

> **Staffed Beds:** 25 **Admissions:** 599 **Census:** 7 **Outpatient Visits:** 32937
> **Births:** 67 **Total Expense ($000):** 16059 **Payroll Expense ($000):** 7036
> **Personnel:** 170

**WHEATLAND—Platte County**

⊠ **PLATTE COUNTY MEMORIAL HOSPITAL (531305)**, 201 14th Street, Zip 82201–3201, Mailing Address: P.O. Box 848, Zip 82201–0848; tel. 307/322–3636 **A**1 9 10 18 **F**3 13 15 29 30 40 43 46 47 48 49 59 64 70 75 76 81 107 110 113 118 127 128 129 131 132 **S** Banner Health, Phoenix, AZ
Primary Contact: Shelby Nelson, Chief Executive Officer
CFO: Stephanie Kaul, Chief Financial Officer
CMO: Jeffrey Cecil, M.D., Chief of Staff
CIO: Robin Wood, Director Information Systems
CHR: Michele Nevarez, Chief Human Resources Officer
Web address: www.bannerhealth.com
**Control:** Other not–for–profit (including NFP Corporation) **Service:** General Medical and Surgical

> **Staffed Beds:** 25 **Admissions:** 577 **Census:** 5 **Outpatient Visits:** 19713
> **Births:** 61 **Total Expense ($000):** 13810 **Payroll Expense ($000):** 6267
> **Personnel:** 116

**WORLAND—Washakie County**

★ **WASHAKIE MEDICAL CENTER (531306)**, 400 South 15th Street, Zip 82401–3531, Mailing Address: P.O. Box 700, Zip 82401–0700; tel. 307/347–3221 **A**9 10 18 **F**3 11 13 15 28 29 34 35 40 43 45 57 59 64 68 70 75 76 77 79 81 82 85 87 89 93 97 107 110 111 113 118 128 129 130 132 134 144 145 147 **P**6 **S** Banner Health, Phoenix, AZ
Primary Contact: Margie Molitor, R.N., Chief Executive Officer
CFO: Jennifer Montgomery, Chief Financial Officer
CMO: Ryan Clifford, M.D., Chief of Staff
CHR: Jerry Clipp, Manager Human Resources
Web address: www.washakiemedicalcenter.com
**Control:** Other not–for–profit (including NFP Corporation) **Service:** General Medical and Surgical

> **Staffed Beds:** 25 **Admissions:** 956 **Census:** 9 **Outpatient Visits:** 33710
> **Births:** 59 **Total Expense ($000):** 16582 **Payroll Expense ($000):** 7203
> **Personnel:** 136

## AMERICAN SAMOA

### PAGO PAGO— County

**LYNDON B. JOHNSON TROPICAL MEDICAL CENTER (640001)**, Faga'alu Village, Zip 96799, Mailing Address: P.O. Box LBJ, Zip 96799; tel. 684/633–1222, (Nonreporting) **A**10
Primary Contact: Patricia Tindall, Chief Executive Officer
Web address: www.asmca.org
**Control:** State–Government, nonfederal **Service:** General Medical and Surgical

**Staffed Beds:** 125

## GUAM

### AGANA—Guam County

★ **U. S. NAVAL HOSPITAL**, Zip 96910; Mailing Address: FPO, AP, tel. 671/344–9340, (Nonreporting) **S** Bureau of Medicine and Surgery, Department of the Navy, Washington, DC
Primary Contact: Captain Kevin W. Haws, USN, Commanding Officer
Web address: www.med.navy.mil/sites/nmw/commands
**Control:** Navy, Government, federal **Service:** General Medical and Surgical

**Staffed Beds:** 55

### TAMUNING—Guam County

★ **GUAM MEMORIAL HOSPITAL AUTHORITY (650001)**, 850 Governor Carlos G. Camacho Road, Zip 96913; tel. 671/647–2108, (Nonreporting) **A**10
Primary Contact: Peter John Diaz Camacho, M.P.H., Administrator and Chief Executive Officer
CFO: Wilfred Aflague, Chief Financial Officer
CMO: James J. Stadler, M.D., Associate Administrator Medical Services
CIO: Vince Quichocho, Manager Information Systems
CHR: Elizabeth Claros, Administrator Personnel Services
Web address: www.gmha.org
**Control:** Hospital district or authority, Government, nonfederal **Service:** General Medical and Surgical

**Staffed Beds:** 104

## MARSHALL ISLANDS

### KWAJALEIN ISLAND— County

**KWAJALEIN HOSPITAL**, U.S. Army Kwajalein Atoll, Zip 96960, Mailing Address: Box 1702, APO, AP, Zip 96555–5000; tel. 805/355–2225, (Nonreporting) **S** Department of the Army, Office of the Surgeon General, Falls Church, VA
Primary Contact: Elaine McMahon, Administrator
**Control:** Army, Government, federal **Service:** General Medical and Surgical

**Staffed Beds:** 14

## NORTHERN MARIANA ISLANDS

### SAIPAN— County

**COMMONWEALTH HEALTH CENTER (660001)**, Navy Hill Road, Zip 96950, Mailing Address: P.O. Box 409, Zip 96950; tel. 670/234–8950, (Nonreporting) **A**10
Primary Contact: Joseph C. Santos, M.P.H., Deputy Secretary for Hospital Administration
Web address: www.dphsaipan.com
**Control:** Corporation, Investor–owned, for–profit **Service:** Other specialty

**Staffed Beds:** 86

## PUERTO RICO

### AGUADILLA—Aguadilla County

★ **HOSPITAL BUEN SAMARITANO (400079)**, Carr #2 Km 141–1 Avenue Severiano Cuevas, Zip 603, Mailing Address: P.O. Box 4055, Zip 00605–4055; tel. 787/658–0000 **A**9 10 **F**3 29 30 34 35 40 41 45 46 59 70 74 75 76 77 79 81 82 87 89 107 111 118 128 129 145 147 **P**8
Primary Contact: Elyonel Ponton Cruz, Executive Director
CFO: Taira Valentin, Interim Director Finance
CMO: Arturo Cedeno, M.D., Medical Director
CIO: Carmen E. Rivera–Jimenez, Director Information Management
CHR: Jose Garcia Rivera, Director Human Resources
Web address: www.hbspr.org
**Control:** Other not–for–profit (including NFP Corporation) **Service:** General Medical and Surgical

**Staffed Beds:** 154 **Admissions:** 8300 **Census:** 112 **Outpatient Visits:** 28711 **Births:** 472 **Total Expense ($000):** 34251 **Payroll Expense ($000):** 12835 **Personnel:** 536

### AIBONITO—Aibonito County

★ **CENTRO DE SALUD CONDUCTUAL MENONITA–CIMA (404009)**, Carretera Estatal 14 Interior, Zip 705, Mailing Address: CIMA Calle Sargento Gerardo Santiago, Zip 705; tel. 787/714–2462, (Nonreporting)
Primary Contact: Pedro Melendez, Administrator
**Control:** Other not–for–profit (including NFP Corporation) **Service:** Psychiatric

**Staffed Beds:** 32

⊞ **MENNONITE GENERAL HOSPITAL (400018)**, Calle Jose C. Vasquez, Zip 705, Mailing Address: P.O. Box 373130, Cayey, Zip 00737–3130; tel. 787/535–1001, (Nonreporting) **A**1 9 10
Primary Contact: Pedro Melendez, Administrator
COO: Marta R Mercado Suro, Chief Operating Officer
CFO: Jose E. Solivan, Chief Financial Officer
CMO: Victor Hernandez Miranda, M.D., Chief of Staff
CIO: Daniza Morales, Manager Information System
CHR: Evelyn Padilla Ortiz, Director Human Resources
Web address: www.hospitalmenonita.com
**Control:** Other not–for–profit (including NFP Corporation) **Service:** General Medical and Surgical

**Staffed Beds:** 131

**Hospital, Medicare Provider Number, Address, Telephone, Approval, Facility, and Physician Codes, Health Care System**

★ American Hospital Association (AHA) membership
☐ The Joint Commission accreditation
○ American Osteopathic Association (AOA) accreditation
△ Commission on Accreditation of Rehabilitation Facilities (CARF) accreditation

## ARECIBO—Arecibo County

✠ **HOSPITAL DR. CAYETANO COLL Y TOSTE (400087)**, 129 San Luis Avenue, Zip 612, Mailing Address: P.O. Box 659, Zip 613; tel. 787/650-7272, (Nonreporting) **A**1 9 10
Primary Contact: Homar Perez, Chief Executive Officer and Vice President Administration
COO: Maritza Rodriguez, Chief Financial Officer
CFO: Luis Curbelo, Director Finance
CMO: Ada S. Miranda, M.D., Medical Director
CIO: Vicent Ortiz, Chief Information Officer
CHR: Carmen Sanchez, Director Human Resources
Web address: www.cayetano@xsn.net
**Control:** Corporation, Investor-owned, for-profit **Service:** General Medical and Surgical

**Staffed Beds:** 188

★ **HOSPITAL METROPOLITANO DR. SUSONI (400117)**, 55 Nicomedes Rivera Street, Zip 612, Mailing Address: P.O. Box 145200, Zip 614; tel. 787/650-1030 **A**9 10 **F**39 40 41 70 81 89 107 110 111 129
Primary Contact: Luis Z. Allende Ruiz, Executive Director
CFO: Vivian Aceuedo, CPA, Chief Financial Director
CMO: Ada S. Miranda, M.D., Medical Director
CIO: Mayra Montano, Director Information Systems
CHR: Patria Nieves, Director
**Control:** Corporation, Investor-owned, for-profit **Service:** General Medical and Surgical

**Staffed Beds:** 138 **Admissions:** 7310 **Census:** 100 **Outpatient Visits:** 31217 **Births:** 84 **Total Expense ($000):** 31690 **Payroll Expense ($000):** 12182 **Personnel:** 433

## ARROYO—Arroyo County

★ **LAFAYETTE HOSPITAL (400026)**, Central Lafayette, Zip 714, Mailing Address: P.O. Box 207, Zip 714; tel. 787/839-3232, (Nonreporting) **A**9 10
Primary Contact: Ruth M. Ortiz Vargas, Administrator
CMO: Jose L. Pimentel Fernandez, Medical Director
**Control:** Corporation, Investor-owned, for-profit **Service:** General Medical and Surgical

**Staffed Beds:** 38

## BAYAMON—Bayamon County

★ **DOCTOR'S CENTER OF BAYAMON (400102)**, Extension Hermanas Davila, Zip 960, Mailing Address: P.O. Box 2957, Zip 960; tel. 787/622-5420, (Nonreporting) **A**10
Primary Contact: Carlos Blanco, M.D., Administrator
**Control:** Corporation, Investor-owned, for-profit **Service:** General Medical and Surgical

**Staffed Beds:** 91

✠ **HOSPITAL HERMANOS MELENDEZ (400032)**, Route 2, KM 11-7, Zip 960, Mailing Address: P.O. Box 306, Zip 960; tel. 787/620-8181, (Nonreporting) **A**1 9 10
Primary Contact: Waleska Crespo, Administrator
CFO: Luz D. Medina, Controller
CMO: Norma Ortiz, M.D., Medical Director
CIO: Leticia Santana, Administrator Medical Records
Web address: www.hospitalhermanosmelendez.net
**Control:** Corporation, Investor-owned, for-profit **Service:** General Medical and Surgical

**Staffed Beds:** 211

✠ **HOSPITAL SAN PABLO (400109)**, Calle Santa Cruz 70, Zip 00961-7020, Mailing Address: P.O. Box 236, Zip 00960-0236; tel. 787/740-4747, (Nonreporting) **A**1 3 5 9 10
Primary Contact: Jose E. Carballo, Chief Executive Officer and Managing Director
Web address: www.sanpablo.com
**Control:** Corporation, Investor-owned, for-profit **Service:** General Medical and Surgical

**Staffed Beds:** 410

✠ **HOSPITAL UNIVERSITARIO DR. RAMON RUIZ ARNAU (400105)**, Avenue Laurel, Santa Juanita, Zip 956; tel. 787/787-5151 **A**1 3 5 9 10 **F**3 7 8 11 29 30 40 46 65 66 68 70 75 79 81 86 87 89 97 107 118 129 144 145 146 **S** Puerto Rico Department of Health, San Juan, PR
Primary Contact: Rafael Garcia Alvarez, Chief Executive Officer
CFO: Elsie Morales, Chief Financial Officer
CMO: Hector Cintron Principe, M.D., Director
CIO: Irma Duprey, Administrator Medical Records
CHR: Aurea De Leon, Chief Human Resources Officer
**Control:** State-Government, nonfederal **Service:** General Medical and Surgical

**Staffed Beds:** 102 **Admissions:** 2545 **Census:** 45 **Outpatient Visits:** 58489 **Births:** 0

## CABO ROJO—Cabo Rojo County

★ **HOSPITAL PSIQUIATRICO METROPOLITANO (404007)**, 108 Munoz Rivera Street, Zip 00623-4060, Mailing Address: P.O. Box 910, Zip 00623-0910; tel. 787/851-2025, (Nonreporting)
Primary Contact: Elizabeth De Santiago, Director
**Control:** Other not-for-profit (including NFP Corporation) **Service:** General Medical and Surgical

**Staffed Beds:** 39

## CAGUAS—Caguas County

✠ **HOSPITAL INTERAMERICANO DE MEDICINA AVANZADA (400120)**, Avenida Luis Munoz Marin, Zip 726, Mailing Address: P.O. Box 4980, Zip 726; tel. 787/653-3434, (Nonreporting) **A**1 9 10
Primary Contact: Carlos M. Pineiro, President
CFO: Luis A. Arroyo, Chief Financial Officer
CIO: Fernando Mora, Vice President Management Information Systems
**Control:** Partnership, Investor-owned, for-profit **Service:** General Medical and Surgical

**Staffed Beds:** 300

## CAROLINA—Carolina County

✠ **HOSPITAL DE LA UNIVERSIDAD DE PUERTO RICO/DR. FEDERICO TRILLA (400112)**, 65th Infanteria, KM 8 3, Zip 984, Mailing Address: P.O. Box 6021, Zip 984; tel. 787/757-1800 **A**1 3 5 9 10 **F**3 8 11 12 15 29 30 34 39 40 45 50 56 64 70 72 73 74 75 76 78 79 80 81 87 89 91 93 94 96 97 98 99 100 101 102 103 104 105 107 108 110 111 118 129 144 145 147
Primary Contact: Domingo Nevarez, Chief Executive Officer
COO: Diraida Maldonado, Administrator
CFO: Yolanda Quinonez, Chief Financial Officer
CMO: Marina Roman, M.D., Medical Director
CIO: Francisco Perez, Manager Management Information Systems
CHR: Betzaida Jimenez, Director Human Resources
Web address: www.hospitalupr.org
**Control:** State-Government, nonfederal **Service:** General Medical and Surgical

**Staffed Beds:** 250 **Admissions:** 10337 **Census:** 166 **Outpatient Visits:** 58317 **Births:** 1130 **Total Expense ($000):** 42590 **Payroll Expense ($000):** 12854 **Personnel:** 520

## CASTANER—Lares County

★ **CASTANER GENERAL HOSPITAL (400010)**, KM 64-2, Route 135, Zip 631, Mailing Address: P.O. Box 1003, Zip 631; tel. 787/829-5010, (Nonreporting) **A**5 10
Primary Contact: Domingo Monroig, Administrator
COO: Agustin Ponce, Supervisor Maintenance
CFO: Ernesto Montes, Director Finance
CMO: Jose O. Rodriguez, M.D., Medical Director
CIO: Domingo Monroig, Administrator
CHR: Nydimar Salcedo, Chief Human Resources Officer
**Control:** Other not-for-profit (including NFP Corporation) **Service:** General Medical and Surgical

**Staffed Beds:** 24

## CAYEY—Cayey County

✠ **HOSPITAL MENONITA DE CAYEY (400013)**, 4 H. Mendoza Street, Zip 00736-3801, Mailing Address: P.O. Box 373130, Zip 00737-3130; tel. 787/263-1001, (Nonreporting) **A**1 9 10
Primary Contact: Pedro Melender, Administrator
COO: Leda Marta R Mercado, Chief Operating Officer
CFO: Jose E. Solivan, Chief Financial Officer
CMO: Luis J Rodriquez Saenz, M.D., Medical Director
CIO: Daniza Morales, Chief Information Officer
CHR: Evelyn Padilla Ortiz, Director Human Resources
Web address: www.hospitalmenonita.com
**Control:** Other not-for-profit (including NFP Corporation) **Service:** General Medical and Surgical

**Staffed Beds:** 145

## CIDRA—Cidra County

✠ **FIRST HOSPITAL PANAMERICANO (404004)**, State Road 787 KM 1 5, Zip 739, Mailing Address: P.O. Box 1400, Zip 739; tel. 787/739-5555, (Nonreporting) **A**1 3 5 9 10 **S** Universal Health Services, Inc., King of Prussia, PA
Primary Contact: Marta Rivera, Executive Director
COO: Tim McCarthy, President Puerto Rico Division
CFO: Gabriel Rivera, Controller
CMO: Ramon Parrilla, M.D., Chief Medical Officer
CIO: Carlos Nunez, Director Management Information Systems
CHR: Shirley Ayala, Director Human Resources
Web address: www.hospitalpanamericano.com
**Control:** Corporation, Investor-owned, for-profit **Service:** Psychiatric

**Staffed Beds:** 153

**COTO LAUREL—Ponce County**

★ **HOSPITAL SAN CRISTOBAL (400113)**, 506 Carr Road, Zip 780;
tel. 787/848–2100, (Nonreporting) **A**3 5 10
Primary Contact: Pedro L. Benetti–Loyola, Administrator
COO: Pedro L. Benetti–Loyola, Senior Executive and Vice President
CFO: Marian Collazo, Director Finance
CMO: Ramon Rodriguez Rivas, M.D., Medical Director
CIO: Ramon Acevedo, Supervisor Information Systems
CHR: Candie Rodriguez, Director Human Resources
Web address: www.hospitalsancristobal.com
**Control:** Corporation, Investor–owned, for–profit **Service:** Other specialty

Staffed Beds: 103

**FAJARDO—Fajardo County**

★ **CARIBBEAN MEDICAL CENTER (400131)**, 151 Avenue Osvaldo Molina,
Zip 00738–4013, Mailing Address: Call Box 70006, Zip 00738–7006;
tel. 787/801–0081, (Nonreporting)
Primary Contact: Eduardo Sotomayor, Director
**Control:** Other not–for–profit (including NFP Corporation) **Service:** General
Medical and Surgical

Staffed Beds: 10

⊞ **HOSPITAL SAN PABLO DEL ESTE (400125)**, Avenida General Valero, 404,
Zip 738, Mailing Address: P.O. Box 1028, Zip 00738–1028; tel. 787/863–0505,
(Nonreporting) **A**1 9 10
Primary Contact: Aixa Irizarry, Executive Director
CFO: Luis A. Arroyo, Chief Financial Officer
CMO: Manuel Navas, M.D., Medical Director
CHR: Vilma Rodriguez, Director Human Resources
Web address: www.sanpablo.com
**Control:** Corporation, Investor–owned, for–profit **Service:** General Medical and
Surgical

Staffed Beds: 136

**GUAYAMA—Guayama County**

⊞ **HOSPITAL EPISCOPAL SAN LUCAS GUAYAMA (400048)**, Avenue Pedro
Albesus, Zip 784, Mailing Address: PO Box 10011, Zip 00785–1006;
tel. 787/864–4300, (Nonreporting) **A**1 5 9 10
Primary Contact: Juan Carlos Latorre, President and Chief Executive Officer
COO: Wilfredo Rabelo, Chief Operating Officer
CFO: Carlos Porrata, CPA, Chief Financial Officer
CMO: Gerson Jimenez, M.D., Medical Director
CHR: Ivette Lacot, Director Human Resources
**Control:** Church–operated, Nongovernment, not–for profit **Service:** General
Medical and Surgical

Staffed Beds: 115

★ **HOSPITAL SANTA ROSA (400009)**, Veterans Avenue, Zip 784, Mailing
Address: P.O. Box 10008, Zip 785; tel. 787/864–0101 **A**9 10 **F**7 20 40 45 46
70 76 81 89 91 92 93 94 107 110 111 118 129
Primary Contact: Gloria Diaz, Executive Director
CFO: Edwin De Jesus, Comptroller
CMO: Joaquin Pales, President
CIO: Waleska Rolon, Manager
**Control:** Other not–for–profit (including NFP Corporation) **Service:** General
Medical and Surgical

Staffed Beds: 86 Admissions: 3601 Census: 36 Outpatient Visits: 48613
Births: 89 Total Expense ($000): 15316 Payroll Expense ($000): 3682
Personnel: 169

**HATO REY—San Juan County, See San Juan**

**HUMACAO—Humacao County**

**HOSPITAL DR. DOMINGUEZ** See Hospital Oriente

⊞ **HOSPITAL HMA DE HUMACAO (400005)**, 3 Font Martelo Street,
Zip 00791–3342, Mailing Address: P.O. Box 639, Zip 00792–0639;
tel. 787/656–2424, (Nonreporting) **A**1 9 10
Primary Contact: Aixa Irizarry, Executive Director
COO: Carlos M. Pineiro, President
CFO: Luis A. Arroyo, Chief Financial Officer
CMO: Francisco R. Carballo, M.D., Medical Director
CIO: Giovanni Piereschi, Vice President Management Information Systems
CHR: Iris Abreu, Supervisor Human Resources
**Control:** Corporation, Investor–owned, for–profit **Service:** General Medical and
Surgical

Staffed Beds: 64

★ **HOSPITAL ORIENTE (400011)**, 300 Font Martelo Street, Zip 00791–3230,
Mailing Address: P.O. Box 699, Zip 00792–0699; tel. 787/852–0505 **A**9 10 **F**17
40 75 81 89 129
Primary Contact: Miguel A. Solivan, Administrator
CFO: Ivonne Rivera, Director Finance
CMO: Carmelo Herrero, M.D., Medical Director
CHR: Ivonne Lopez, Director Human Resources
**Control:** Corporation, Investor–owned, for–profit **Service:** General Medical and
Surgical

Staffed Beds: 71 Admissions: 3553 Census: 45 Births: 0 Personnel: 228

★ **RYDER MEMORIAL HOSPITAL (400007)**, 355 Font Martelo Street,
Zip 00791–3249, Mailing Address: P.O. Box 859, Zip 00792–0859;
tel. 787/852–0768, (Total facility includes 62 beds in nursing home–type unit) **A**9
10 **F**3 6 8 10 11 13 15 18 19 20 26 30 31 34 35 39 40 41 42 45 48 54 56
57 59 61 62 63 65 70 72 73 75 76 77 78 79 81 82 84 86 87 89 93 104
107 108 111 114 117 118 124 127 129 142 144 145 146 147
Primary Contact: Jose R. Feliciano, Chief Executive Officer
COO: Nemuel O. Artiles, FACHE, Administrator
CFO: Jose O. Ortiz, Chief Financial Officer
CMO: Raul Ramos Pereira, M.D., Medical Director
CIO: Joseph V. Cruz, Chief Information Officer
CHR: Maria Figueroa, Director Human Resources
Web address: www.hryder@prtc.net
**Control:** Other not–for–profit (including NFP Corporation) **Service:** General
Medical and Surgical

Staffed Beds: 227 Admissions: 9024 Census: 149 Outpatient Visits:
145335 Births: 1201 Total Expense ($000): 58903 Payroll Expense
($000): 22745 Personnel: 943

**MANATI—Manati County**

★ **DOCTORS CENTER (400118)**, KM 47–7, Zip 674, Mailing Address: P.O. Box
30532, Zip 674; tel. 787/854–3322, (Nonreporting) **A**10
Primary Contact: Carlos Blanco, M.D., Administrator
**Control:** Corporation, Investor–owned, for–profit **Service:** General Medical and
Surgical

Staffed Beds: 150

**HEALTHSOUTH HOSPITAL OF MANATI**, Carretera, 2 Kilometro 47 7,
Zip 00674; tel. 787/621–3800 **S** HEALTHSOUTH Corporation, Birmingham, AL
Primary Contact: Enrique A. Vicens–Rivera, Jr., J.D., Chief Executive Officer
CFO: Jesus Corazon, Controller
CMO: Jamie Marrero, Chief Medical Officer
CHR: Erika Landrau, Human Resources Coordinator
CNO: Evelyn Diaz, Chief Nursing Officer
Web address: http://healthsouth.com
**Control:** Investor–owned, for–profit **Service:** Rehabilitation

Staffed Beds: 40

⊞ **HOSPITAL MANATI MEDICAL CENTER (400114)**, Calle Hernandez, Carrion
668, Zip 674, Mailing Address: P.O. Box 1142, Zip 00674–1142;
tel. 787/621–3700, (Nonreporting) **A**1 5 9 10
Primary Contact: Jorge Galva, Executive Director
CFO: Noriselle Rivera–Pol, Vice President Finance
CMO: Luis R. Rosa–Toledo, M.D., Medical Director
CIO: Alberto Medina, Information Technology Senior Consultant
CHR: Nilda Paravisini, Director Human Resources
Web address: www.manatimedical.com
**Control:** Corporation, Investor–owned, for–profit **Service:** General Medical and
Surgical

Staffed Beds: 215

**MAYAGUEZ—Mayaguez County**

⊞ **BELLA VISTA HOSPITAL (400014)**, State Road 349, Zip 680, Mailing Address:
P.O. Box 1750, Zip 681; tel. 787/834–6000, (Nonreporting) **A**1 9 10
Primary Contact: Jesus Nieves, Chief Executive Officer
CFO: Enrique Rivera, Chief Financial Officer
CMO: Miguel Cruz, M.D., Medical Director
CHR: Benjamin Astacio, Director Human Resources
Web address: www.bvhpr.org
**Control:** Church–operated, Nongovernment, not–for profit **Service:** General
Medical and Surgical

Staffed Beds: 157

---

**Hospital, Medicare Provider Number, Address, Telephone, Approval, Facility, and Physician Codes, Health Care System**

★ American Hospital Association (AHA) membership
□ The Joint Commission accreditation ◇ DNV Healthcare Inc. accreditation
○ American Osteopathic Association (AOA) accreditation
△ Commission on Accreditation of Rehabilitation Facilities (CARF) accreditation

**CLINICA ESPANOLA (400024)**, Barrio La Quinta, Zip 680, Mailing Address: P.O. Box 490, Zip 00681–0490; tel. 787/832–0442, (Nonreporting) **A**10
Primary Contact: Emigdio Inigo–Agostini, M.D., Board President
**Control:** Corporation, Investor–owned, for–profit **Service:** General Medical and Surgical

**Staffed Beds:** 89

✠ **DR. RAMON E. BETANCES HOSPITAL–MAYAGUEZ MEDICAL CENTER BRANCH (400103)**, 410 Hostos Avenue, Zip 00680–1501, Mailing Address: P.O. Box 600, Zip 00681–0600; tel. 787/652–9200 **A**1 3 5 9 10 **F**3 14 17 18 20 22 24 26 29 30 40 41 49 70 75 79 81 87 89 107 111 114 118 129 147
Primary Contact: Jaime Maestre, Chief Executive Officer
CMO: Milton D. Carrero, M.D., Medical Director
CIO: Ivette Roman, Chief Information Officer
CHR: Betsmari Medina, Director Human Resources
**Control:** State–Government, nonfederal **Service:** General Medical and Surgical

**Staffed Beds:** 181 **Admissions:** 7380 **Census:** 141 **Outpatient Visits:** 65837 **Total Expense ($000):** 51064 **Payroll Expense ($000):** 14698 **Personnel:** 700

★ **HOSPITAL PEREA (400123)**, 15 Basora Street, Zip 681, Mailing Address: P.O. Box 170, Zip 681; tel. 787/834–0101, (Nonreporting) **A**9 10 **S** United Medical Corporation, Windermere, FL
Primary Contact: Marco Reyes Concepcion, Executive Director
CFO: Joannie Garcia, CPA, Director Finance
CMO: Humberto Olivencia, M.D., Medical Director
Web address: www.paviahealth.com/perea_hospital.htm
**Control:** Corporation, Investor–owned, for–profit **Service:** General Medical and Surgical

**Staffed Beds:** 103

**MOCA—Moca County**

★ **HOSPITAL SAN CARLOS BORROMEO (400111)**, 550 Concepcion Vera Ayala, Zip 676; tel. 787/877–8000 **A**9 10 **F**8 15 17 29 30 34 40 45 65 70 73 74 75 76 79 81 89 107 111 114 118 129 132 144 145 147 **P**8
Primary Contact: Rosaida M. Crespo, Executive Director
CFO: Irma Cabrera, Finance Director
CMO: Erick Nieves, M.D., Medical Director
CIO: Jose Nieves, Director Information Systems
CHR: Migdalia Ortiz, Director Human Resources
Web address: www.hospitalsancarlos.org
**Control:** Other not–for–profit (including NFP Corporation) **Service:** General Medical and Surgical

**Staffed Beds:** 106 **Admissions:** 4981 **Census:** 69 **Outpatient Visits:** 34057 **Births:** 817 **Total Expense ($000):** 23648 **Payroll Expense ($000):** 8083 **Personnel:** 381

**PONCE—Ponce County**

✠ **DR. PILA'S HOSPITAL (400003)**, Avenida Las Americas, Zip 731, Mailing Address: P.O. Box 1910, Zip 00733–1910; tel. 787/848–5600, (Nonreporting) **A**1 3 5 9 10
Primary Contact: Rafael Alvarado, Chief Executive Officer
Web address: www.drpila.com
**Control:** Other not–for–profit (including NFP Corporation) **Service:** General Medical and Surgical

**Staffed Beds:** 115

✠ **HOSPITAL DE DAMAS (400022)**, Ponce by Pass, Zip 731; tel. 787/840–8686, (Total facility includes 22 beds in nursing home–type unit) **A**1 3 5 9 10 **F**3 13 14 17 18 20 22 24 29 30 40 45 47 49 62 67 70 72 76 80 81 88 89 107 113 118 127 128 129 145
Primary Contact: Edwin Sueiro, Administrator
CMO: Pedro Benitez, M.D., Medical Director
CIO: Bienvenido Ortiz, Coordinator Information Systems
CHR: Gilberto Cuevas, Director Human Resources
Web address: www.hospitaldamas.com
**Control:** Other not–for–profit (including NFP Corporation) **Service:** General Medical and Surgical

**Staffed Beds:** 251 **Admissions:** 12693 **Census:** 177 **Outpatient Visits:** 45501 **Total Expense ($000):** 70708 **Payroll Expense ($000):** 24539 **Personnel:** 818

✠ **HOSPITAL ONCOLOGICO ANDRES GRILLASCA (400028)**, Centro Medico De Ponce, Zip 733, Mailing Address: P.O. Box 331324, Zip 00733–1324; tel. 787/848–0800, (Nonreporting) **A**1 5 9 10
Primary Contact: Manuel J. Vazquez, Executive Administrator
CMO: Roberto Velasquez, M.D., Medical Director
CIO: Maria T. Teissonniere, Director Public Relations
CHR: Carlos T. Santiago, Director Human Resources
**Control:** Other not–for–profit (including NFP Corporation) **Service:** Cancer

**Staffed Beds:** 49

✠ **ST. LUKE'S EPISCOPAL HOSPITAL (400044)**, 917 Tito Castro Avenue, Zip 00731–4717, Mailing Address: P.O. Box 336810, Zip 00733–6810; tel. 787/844–2080 **A**1 9 10 **F**3 7 13 14 15 17 18 20 22 24 26 30 40 41 42 45 46 49 51 57 67 70 72 73 76 79 81 82 85 88 89 91 92 93 107 111 113 114 118 129 130 131 143 144 147
Primary Contact: Julio Colon, Interim President and Chief Executive Officer
CFO: Julio Colon, Chief Financial Officer
CMO: Jenaro Scarano, M.D., Medical Director
CHR: Juan Salazar, Director Human Resources
Web address: www.sanlucaspr.com
**Control:** Church–operated, Nongovernment, not–for profit **Service:** General Medical and Surgical

**Staffed Beds:** 385 **Admissions:** 16137 **Census:** 263 **Outpatient Visits:** 81809 **Births:** 1785 **Total Expense ($000):** 114551 **Payroll Expense ($000):** 32478 **Personnel:** 1118

**RIO PIEDRAS—San Juan County, See San Juan**

**SAN GERMAN—San German County**

✠ **HOSPITAL DE LA CONCEPCION (400021)**, Carr 2, Km 173, Bo Cain Alto, Zip 00683–3920, Mailing Address: P.O. Box 285, Zip 00683–0285; tel. 787/892–1860, (Nonreporting) **A**1 3 5 9 10
Primary Contact: Felicita Bonilla, Administrator
CFO: Lizmari Calderon, Director Finance
CMO: Ivan Acosta, M.D., Medical Director
CIO: Aaron Mendez, Director Management Information Systems
CHR: Jorge Rodriguez Diaz, Director Human Resources
Web address: www.hospitalconcepcion.org
**Control:** Church–operated, Nongovernment, not–for profit **Service:** General Medical and Surgical

**Staffed Beds:** 167

★ **HOSPITAL METROPOLITANO SAN GERMAN (400126)**, Calle Javilla Al Costado Parque de Bombas, Zip 683; tel. 787/892–5300, (Nonreporting) **A**9 10
Primary Contact: Ramon E. Lopez–Maldonado, Chief Executive Officer
**Control:** Corporation, Investor–owned, for–profit **Service:** Other specialty

**Staffed Beds:** 40

**SAN JUAN—San Juan County**
**(Mailing Addresses - Hato Rey, Rio Piedras)**

✠ **ASHFORD PRESBYTERIAN COMMUNITY HOSPITAL (400001)**, 1451 Avenue Ashford, Zip 00907–1511, Mailing Address: P.O. Box 9020032, Zip 00902–0032; tel. 787/721–2160, (Nonreporting) **A**1 9 10
Primary Contact: Pedro J. Gonzalez, Executive Director
COO: Marilyn Morales, Assistant Administrator and Chief Operating Officer
CFO: Milagros Ortiz, CPA, Chief Financial Officer
CMO: Francisco de Torres, M.D., Medical Director
CIO: Arnaldo Quinones, Chief Information Officer
CHR: Irma Carrillo, Director Human Resources
Web address: www.presbypr.com
**Control:** Other not–for–profit (including NFP Corporation) **Service:** General Medical and Surgical

**Staffed Beds:** 199

✠ **AUXILIO MUTUO HOSPITAL (400016)**, Ponce De Leon Avenue, Zip 00918–1000, Mailing Address: P.O. Box 191227, Zip 00919–1227; tel. 787/758–2000, (Nonreporting) **A**1 5 9 10
Primary Contact: Jorge L. Matta Serrano, Administrator
COO: Carmen Martin, Associate Administrator
CFO: Maria L. Marti, Director Fiscal Services
CMO: Jose Isado, M.D., Medical Director
CIO: Edgardo Rodriguez, Director Management Information Systems
CHR: Maria Vega, Director Human Resources
Web address: www.auxiliomutuo.com
**Control:** Other not–for–profit (including NFP Corporation) **Service:** General Medical and Surgical

**Staffed Beds:** 483

✠ **CARDIOVASCULAR CENTER OF PUERTO RICO AND THE CARIBBEAN (400124)**, Americo Miranda Centro Medico, Zip 936, Mailing Address: P.O. Box 366528, Zip 00936–6528; tel. 787/754–8500, (Nonreporting) **A**1 3 5 9 10 **S** Puerto Rico Department of Health, San Juan, PR
Primary Contact: Javier E. Malave Rosario, Executive Director
COO: Ivette Nunez Lopez, Executive Subdirector
CFO: Maria de Lourdes Alegria, Comptroller
CMO: Jose E. Novoa, M.D., Medical Director
CIO: Eugenio Torres Ayala, Director Information Systems
CHR: Hector Troche Garcia, Director Human Resources
Web address: www.cardiovascular.gobierno.pr
**Control:** State–Government, nonfederal **Service:** General Medical and Surgical

**Staffed Beds:** 146

*Many Facility Codes have changed. Please refer to the AHA Guide Code Chart.* © 2012 AHA Guide

★ **DOCTORS' CENTER HOSPITAL SAN JUAN (400006)**, 1395 San Rafael Street, Zip 00909–2518, Mailing Address: Box 11338, Santurce Station, Zip 00910–1338; tel. 787/723–2950 **A**9 10 **F**40 45 46 70 74 76 81 89 107 108 118 129 147 **P**4 5 7 8
Primary Contact: Norma Marrero, Executive Administrator
COO: Norma Marrero, Executive Administrator
CFO: Alejandro Santiago, Director Finance
CMO: Lourdes Feliciano, M.D., Chairman
CIO: Ismael Ruiz, Chief Information Officer
CHR: Carmen Perez, Director Human Resources
Web address: www.tuhospitalfamiliar.com
**Control:** Corporation, Investor–owned, for–profit **Service:** General Medical and Surgical

**Staffed Beds:** 125 **Admissions:** 5295 **Census:** 81 **Outpatient Visits:** 16451 **Births:** 557 **Total Expense ($000):** 21032 **Payroll Expense ($000):** 7507 **Personnel:** 330

★ **HEALTHSOUTH REHABILITATION HOSPITAL (403025)**, University Hospital, 3rd Floor, Zip 923, Mailing Address: P.O. Box 70344, Zip 923; tel. 787/274–5100, (Nonreporting) **A**3 5 10 **S** HEALTHSOUTH Corporation, Birmingham, AL
Primary Contact: Daniel Del Castillo, Chief Executive Officer
CMO: Eduardo Ramos, M.D., Medical Director
CHR: Frances Fuentes, Coordinator Human Resources
Web address: www.healthsouth.com
**Control:** Corporation, Investor–owned, for–profit **Service:** Rehabilitation

**Staffed Beds:** 32

⊞ **HOSPITAL DEL MAESTRO (400004)**, 550 Sergio Cuevas, Zip 00918–3741, Mailing Address: P.O. Box 364708, Zip 00936–4708; tel. 787/758–8383, (Nonreporting) **A**1 9 10
Primary Contact: Tania Conde–Sterling, Executive Director
CFO: Marisol Vargas, Director Finance
CMO: Jose Montalvo, M.D., Medical Director
CIO: Laura Rodriguez, Director Medical Records
CHR: Orlando Santiago, Human Resources Officer
**Control:** Corporation, Investor–owned, for–profit **Service:** General Medical and Surgical

**Staffed Beds:** 250

⊞ **HOSPITAL METROPOLITAN (400106)**, 1785 Carr 21, Zip 00921–3399, Mailing Address: P.O. Box 11981, Zip 922; tel. 787/782–9999, (Nonreporting) **A**1 9 10
Primary Contact: Gilberto Gonzalez, Chief Executive Officer
CFO: Maritza Rodriguez, Chief Financial Officer
CMO: Maria de los Angeles Correa, M.D., Medical Director
CIO: Manuel Santiago, Chief Information Officer
**Control:** Corporation, Investor–owned, for–profit **Service:** General Medical and Surgical

**Staffed Beds:** 122

⊞ **HOSPITAL PAVIA–HATO REY (400128)**, 435 Ponce De Leon Avenue, Zip 00917–3428; tel. 787/754–0909, (Nonreporting) **A**1 3 5 9 10 **S** United Medical Corporation, Windermere, FL
Primary Contact: Astro Munoz, Chief Executive Officer
Web address: www.paviahealth.com
**Control:** Corporation, Investor–owned, for–profit **Service:** General Medical and Surgical

**Staffed Beds:** 180

⊞ **HOSPITAL PAVIA–SANTURCE (400019)**, 1462 Asia Street, Zip 00909–2143, Mailing Address: Box 11137, Santurce Station, Zip 00910–1137; tel. 787/727–6060, (Nonreporting) **A**1 9 10 **S** United Medical Corporation, Windermere, FL
Primary Contact: Jose Luis Rodriguez, Chief Executive Officer
CFO: Francisco Espina, Director Finance
Web address: www.paviahealth.com
**Control:** Corporation, Investor–owned, for–profit **Service:** General Medical and Surgical

**Staffed Beds:** 215

★ **HOSPITAL SAN FRANCISCO (400098)**, 371 Avenida De Diego, Zip 00923–1711, Mailing Address: P.O. Box 29025, Zip 00929–0025; tel. 787/767–5100, (Nonreporting) **A**9 10
Primary Contact: Hector L. Boria, Chief Executive Officer
CFO: Lizzette Rodriguez, Director Finance
CMO: Hector L. Cotto, M.D., Medical Director
CIO: Deborah Nieves, Director Management Information Systems
CHR: Sugehi Santiago, Director
Web address: www.sanpablo.com
**Control:** Corporation, Investor–owned, for–profit **Service:** General Medical and Surgical

**Staffed Beds:** 150

★ **HOSPITAL SAN GERARDO (400121)**, 138 Avenue Winston Churchill, Zip 00926–6013; tel. 787/761–8383, (Nonreporting) **A**9 10
Primary Contact: Henry Ruberte, Administrator
**Control:** Other not–for–profit (including NFP Corporation) **Service:** Chronic disease

**Staffed Beds:** 60

⊞ **I. GONZALEZ MARTINEZ ONCOLOGIC HOSPITAL (400012)**, Puerto Rico Medical Center, Hato Rey, Zip 935, Mailing Address: P.O. Box 191811, Zip 00919–1811; tel. 787/765–2382, (Nonreporting) **A**1 2 3 5 10
Primary Contact: Carlos Cabrera, Executive Director
COO: Felix Ortiz, Administrator
CFO: Yolanda Quinones, Director Finance
CMO: Carlos Chevere, M.D., Medical Director
CHR: Luz Maria Hernandez, Director Human Resources
**Control:** Other not–for–profit (including NFP Corporation) **Service:** General Medical and Surgical

**Staffed Beds:** 47

★ **INDUSTRIAL HOSPITAL**, Puerto Rico Medical Center, Zip 936, Mailing Address: P.O. Box 365028, Zip 936; tel. 787/764–3660 **A**9 **F**3 8 16 18 36 40 64 70 74 75 77 79 81 82 90 93 94 104 129 147
Primary Contact: Jorge Garcia Ortiz, Executive Director
CFO: Robert Bernier Casanova, Chief Financial Officer
CMO: Carmen Carrasquillo, M.D., Medical Director
CHR: Sonia M. Lebron, Human Resources Specialist
**Control:** State–Government, nonfederal **Service:** General Medical and Surgical

**Staffed Beds:** 108 **Admissions:** 2308 **Census:** 57 **Outpatient Visits:** 40120 **Births:** 0 **Total Expense ($000):** 66250 **Personnel:** 544

⊞ **SAN JORGE CHILDREN'S HOSPITAL**, 252 San Jorge Street, Santurce, Zip 00912–3310; tel. 787/727–1000, (Nonreporting) **A**1 3 5 9 **S** United Medical Corporation, Windermere, FL
Primary Contact: Domingo Cruz, Senior Vice President Operations
CFO: Jose Marrero, Director Finance
CMO: Luis Clavell, M.D., Medical Director
CIO: Rogelio Caballero, Chief Information Systems
CHR: Ana Acevedo, Supervisor Human Resources
Web address: www.sanjorgechildrenshospital.com
**Control:** Corporation, Investor–owned, for–profit **Service:** Children's general

**Staffed Beds:** 125

⊞ **SAN JUAN CAPESTRANO HOSPITAL (404005)**, Rural Route 2, Box 11, Zip 926; tel. 787/625–2900 **A**1 10 **F**2 4 5 29 30 38 75 98 99 100 101 102 103 104 105 106 129 131
Primary Contact: Laura Vargas, Chief Executive Officer and Managing Director
CFO: Julia Cruz, Chief Financial Officer
CMO: Jose' Alonso, M.D., Medical Director
CIO: Ana Morandeira, Director Marketing
CHR: Luis Rivera, Director Human Resources
Web address: www.sjcapestrano.com
**Control:** Corporation, Investor–owned, for–profit **Service:** Psychiatric

**Staffed Beds:** 108 **Admissions:** 4750 **Census:** 89 **Outpatient Visits:** 46386 **Births:** 0 **Total Expense ($000):** 19482 **Payroll Expense ($000):** 6630

⊞ **SAN JUAN CITY HOSPITAL (400015)**, Puerto Rico Medical Center, Zip 928, Mailing Address: PMB 79, P.O. Box 70344, Zip 00936–8344; tel. 787/766–2222, (Nonreporting) **A**1 3 5 10
Primary Contact: Myrna Boissen, Executive Director
COO: Norma Marcano, Chief Operating Officer
CFO: Jaime Rodriguez, Chief Financial Officer
CMO: Raul Reyes, M.D., Medical Director
CIO: Gustavo Mesa, Chief Information Officer
CHR: Jose Garcia, Chief Human Resources Officer
Web address: www.massalud.com
**Control:** City–Government, nonfederal **Service:** General Medical and Surgical

**Staffed Beds:** 267

★ **STATE PSYCHIATRIC HOSPITAL (404006)**, Monacillos Avenue, Zip 936,
Mailing Address: Call Box 2100, Caparra Heights Station, Zip 00922–2100;
tel. 787/766–4646, (Nonreporting) **A**5 10
Primary Contact: Marcos Aguila, Executive Director
CMO: Brunilda Vazquez, Medical Director
CHR: Idalia Garcia, Chief Human Resources Officer
**Control:** State–Government, nonfederal **Service:** Psychiatric

**Staffed Beds: 153**

★ **UNIVERSITY HOSPITAL (400061)**, Nineyas 869 Rio Piedras, Zip 922, Mailing
Address: P.O. Box 2116, Zip 922; tel. 787/754–0101, (Nonreporting) **A**3 5 10
**S** Puerto Rico Department of Health, San Juan, PR
Primary Contact: Jorge Matta Gonzalez, Executive Director
CFO: Janet Baez, Director
CMO: Ricardo Moscoso, M.D., Medical Director
CIO: Josue Martinez, Coordinator Information Systems
CHR: Wanda Maldonado, Director Human Resources
**Control:** State–Government, nonfederal **Service:** General Medical and Surgical

**Staffed Beds: 262**

★ **UNIVERSITY PEDIATRIC HOSPITAL (403301)**, Barrio Monacenno, Carretera
22, Rio Piedras, Zip 935, Mailing Address: P.O. Box 2129, San Juan,
Zip 00922–2129; tel. 787/777–3535, (Nonreporting) **A**3 5 10 **S** Puerto Rico
Department of Health, San Juan, PR
Primary Contact: Sylvia Mercado, Executive Director
CFO: Blanca Olmo, Director Finance
CMO: Concepcion Quinones De Longo, M.D., Medical Director
**Control:** State–Government, nonfederal **Service:** Children's general

**Staffed Beds: 145**

⊠ △ **VETERANS AFFAIRS MEDICAL CENTER**, 10 Casia Street,
Zip 00921–3201; tel. 787/641–7582, (Nonreporting) **A**1 2 3 5 7 8 9
**S** Department of Veterans Affairs, Washington, DC
Primary Contact: Wanda Mims, Director
CFO: Ricardo Ochoa, Chief Fiscal Officer
CMO: Sandra C. Gracia, M.D., Chief of Staff
CIO: Manuel Negron, Chief Information Technology Service
CHR: Damaris Tosado, Manager Human Resources
Web address: www.va.gov/visn8/sanjuan
**Control:** Veterans Affairs, Government, federal **Service:** General Medical and Surgical

**Staffed Beds: 330**

**VEGA BAJA—Vega Alta County**

★ **WILMA N. VAZQUEZ MEDICAL CENTER (400115)**, KM 39 1/2 Road 2, Call
Box 7001, Zip 694; tel. 787/858–1580, (Nonreporting) **A**9 10
Primary Contact: Ramon J. Vilar, Administrator
COO: Jose O. Pabon, Director Operations
CFO: Youdie Reynolds–Gossette, Controller
CMO: Jorge Feria, M.D., President Medical Staff
CIO: Miguel Aponte, Supervisor Management Information Systems
CHR: Aymette Garcia, Manager Human Resources
**Control:** Corporation, Investor–owned, for–profit **Service:** General Medical and Surgical

**Staffed Beds: 110**

**YAUCO—Yauco County**

⊠ **HOSPITAL METROPOLITANO DR. TITO MATTEI (400110)**, Carretera 128 KM
1, Zip 698, Mailing Address: P.O. Box 5643, Zip 698; tel. 787/856–1000 **A**1 5
9 10 **F**8 17 40 41 45 46 49 70 76 79 80 89 93 98 99 102 103 104 107 110
111 112 113 118 129 147 **P**8
Primary Contact: Astrid J. Abreu, Chief Executive Officer
CFO: Elizabeth Gonzalez, Chief Financial Officer
CMO: Manuel Ramirez Soto, M.D., Medical Director
CIO: Edson Ortiz, Chief Information Officer
CHR: Nannete Acosta, Director Human Resources
Web address: www.hmyauco.com
**Control:** Corporation, Investor–owned, for–profit **Service:** General Medical and Surgical

**Staffed Beds: 105 Admissions: 1271 Census: 99 Outpatient Visits: 44382
Births: 981 Total Expense ($000): 12677 Payroll Expense ($000): 8407
Personnel: 318**

# VIRGIN ISLANDS

**CHRISTIANSTED—St. Croix County**

⊠ **GOVERNOR JUAN F. LOUIS HOSPITAL (480002)**, 4007 Estate Diamond Ruby,
Zip 00820–4421; tel. 340/778–6311 **A**1 9 10 **F**3 5 13 14 17 18 20 22 24 28
32 35 40 44 45 46 48 49 57 59 60 61 64 65 70 72 73 75 76 77 79 80 81
82 85 87 89 90 93 97 98 100 101 105 107 108 111 118 129 131 143
145 147
Primary Contact: Darice S. Plaskett, R.N., FACHE, Interim Chief Executive Officer
CFO: Rosalie Javois, Chief Financial Officer
CMO: Robert Centeno, M.D., Chief Medical Officer
CIO: Reuben D. Molloy, Chief Information Officer
CHR: Joan Jean–Baptiste, Vice President Human Resources
Web address: www.jflusvi.org
**Control:** State–Government, nonfederal **Service:** General Medical and Surgical

**Staffed Beds: 108 Admissions: 3810 Census: 66 Outpatient Visits: 50683
Births: 732 Total Expense ($000): 45009 Payroll Expense ($000): 32517
Personnel: 635**

**SAINT THOMAS—St. Thomas County**

⊠ **SCHNEIDER REGIONAL MEDICAL CENTER (480001)**, 9048 Sugar Estate,
Charlotte Amalie, Zip 802; tel. 340/776–8311, (Nonreporting) **A**1 9 10
Primary Contact: Angela Rennalls–Atkinson, MS, R.N., Interim Chief Executive Officer
CMO: Thelma Ruth Watson, M.D., Medical Director
CIO: J. C. Creque, Director Management Information Systems
CHR: Marlene J. Adams, Director Human Resources
Web address: www.rlshospital.org
**Control:** State–Government, nonfederal **Service:** General Medical and Surgical

**Staffed Beds: 123**

# U.S. Government Hospitals
## Outside the United States, by Area

**GERMANY**

**Heidelberg:** ★ Heidelberg Army Community Hospital, APO, CMR 242, AE 09042

**Landstuhl:** ★ Landstuhl Army Regional Medical Center, APO, CMR 402, AE 09180

**Wuerzburg:** ★ Wuerzburg Army Community Hospital, APO, USAMEDDAC Wuerzburg, Ut 26610, AE 09244

**ITALY**

**Naples:** ★ U. S. Naval Hospital, FPO, AE 09619

**JAPAN**

**Yokosuka:** ★ U. S. Naval Hospital, FPO, Box 1487, AP 96350

**SOUTH KOREA**

**Seoul:** ★ Brian Allgood Army Community Hospital, APO, 121st General Hospital, AP 96205

**SPAIN**

**Rota:** ★ U. S. Naval Hospital, Rota, FPO, PSC 819, Box 18, AE 09645–2500

**Yongsan:** ★ Medcom 18th Commander, Facilities Division Eamc L EM, APO, AP 96205

**TAIWAN**

**Taipei:** ★ U. S. Naval Hospital Taipei, No 300 Shin–Pai Road, Sec 2

# Notes

# Notes

# Notes

# Notes

# Index of Hospitals

This section is an index of all hospitals in alphabetical order by hospital name, followed by the city, state, and page reference to the hospital's listing in Section A.

ANDERSON COUNTY HOSPITAL, GARNETT, KS, p. A233
ANDERSON HOSPITAL, MARYVILLE, IL, p. A187
ANDERSON REGIONAL MEDICAL CENTER, MERIDIAN, MS, p. A350
ANDERSON REGIONAL MEDICAL CENTER–SOUTH CAMPUS, MERIDIAN, MS, p. A350
ANDREW MCFARLAND MENTAL HEALTH CENTER, SPRINGFIELD, IL, p. A194
ANDROSCOGGIN VALLEY HOSPITAL, BERLIN, NH, p. A397
ANDRUS PAVILION, YONKERS, NEW YORK (see ST. JOHN'S RIVERSIDE HOSPITAL), p. A447
ANGEL MEDICAL CENTER, FRANKLIN, NC, p. A453
ANGLETON DANBURY MEDICAL CENTER, ANGLETON, TX, p. A579
ANIMAS SURGICAL HOSPITAL, DURANGO, CO, p. A100
ANMED HEALTH MEDICAL CENTER, ANDERSON, SC, p. A546
ANMED HEALTH REHABILITATION HOSPITAL, ANDERSON, SC, p. A546
ANMED HEALTH WOMEN'S AND CHILDREN'S HOSPITAL, ANDERSON, SOUTH CAROLINA (see ANMED HEALTH MEDICAL CENTER), p. A546
ANN & ROBERT H. LURIE CHILDREN'S HOSPITAL OF CHICAGO, CHICAGO, IL, p. A175
ANNA JAQUES HOSPITAL, NEWBURYPORT, MA, p. A302
ANNE ARUNDEL MEDICAL CENTER, ANNAPOLIS, MD, p. A287
ANNIE JEFFREY MEMORIAL COUNTY HEALTH CENTER, OSCEOLA, NE, p. A388
ANNIE PENN HOSPITAL, REIDSVILLE, NORTH CAROLINA (see CONE HEALTH), p. A454
ANOKA–METROPOLITAN REGIONAL TREATMENT CENTER, ANOKA, MN, p. A327
ANSON COMMUNITY HOSPITAL, WADESBORO, NC, p. A462
ANSON GENERAL HOSPITAL, ANSON, TX, p. A579
ANTELOPE MEMORIAL HOSPITAL, NELIGH, NE, p. A386
ANTELOPE VALLEY HOSPITAL, LANCASTER, CA, p. A67
ANTHONY MEDICAL CENTER, ANTHONY, KS, p. A230
ANTIOCH MEDICAL CENTER, ANTIOCH, CA, p. A53
APACHE JUNCTION HOSPITAL, APACHE JUNCTION, ARIZONA (see ARIZONA REGIONAL MEDICAL CENTER), p. A33
APPALACHIAN BEHAVIORAL HEALTHCARE, ATHENS, OH, p. A470
APPLETON AREA HEALTH SERVICES, APPLETON, MN, p. A327
APPLETON MEDICAL CENTER, APPLETON, WI, p. A678
APPLING HEALTHCARE SYSTEM, BAXLEY, GA, p. A147
ARBOUR H. R. I. HOSPITAL, BROOKLINE, MA, p. A298
ARBOUR HOSPITAL, BOSTON, MA, p. A295
ARBOUR–FULLER HOSPITAL, ATTLEBORO, MA, p. A295
ARBUCKLE MEMORIAL HOSPITAL, SULPHUR, OK, p. A505
ARCHBOLD HOSPITAL, ARCHBOLD, OHIO (see COMMUNITY HOSPITALS AND WELLNESS CENTERS), p. A471
ARIA HEALTH, PHILADELPHIA, PA, p. A531
ARIZONA CHILDREN'S CENTER, PHOENIX, ARIZONA (see MARICOPA INTEGRATED HEALTH SYSTEM), p. A36
ARIZONA HEART HOSPITAL, PHOENIX, ARIZONA (see PHOENIX BAPTIST HOSPITAL), p. A36
ARIZONA ORTHOPEDIC SURGICAL HOSPITAL, CHANDLER, AZ, p. A31
ARIZONA REGIONAL MEDICAL CENTER, MESA, AZ, p. A33
ARIZONA SPINE AND JOINT HOSPITAL, MESA, AZ, p. A33
ARIZONA STATE HOSPITAL, PHOENIX, AZ, p. A35
ARKANSAS CHILDREN'S HOSPITAL, LITTLE ROCK, AR, p. A47
ARKANSAS DEPARTMENT OF CORRECTION HOSPITAL, PINE BLUFF, AR, p. A50
ARKANSAS HEART HOSPITAL, LITTLE ROCK, AR, p. A47
ARKANSAS METHODIST MEDICAL CENTER, PARAGOULD, AR, p. A50
ARKANSAS STATE HOSPITAL, LITTLE ROCK, AR, p. A47
ARKANSAS SURGICAL HOSPITAL, NORTH LITTLE ROCK, AR, p. A49
ARKANSAS VALLEY REGIONAL MEDICAL CENTER, LA JUNTA, CO, p. A103
ARMS ACRES, CARMEL, NY, p. A423
ARNOLD PALMER CHILDREN'S HOSPITAL, ORLANDO, FLORIDA (see ORLANDO REGIONAL MEDICAL CENTER), p. A134
ARNOT OGDEN MEDICAL CENTER, ELMIRA, NY, p. A425
AROOSTOOK HEALTH CENTER, MARS HILL, MAINE (see THE AROOSTOOK MEDICAL CENTER), p. A285
ARROWHEAD BEHAVIORAL HEALTH HOSPITAL, MAUMEE, OH, p. A484
ARROWHEAD HOSPITAL, GLENDALE, AZ, p. A32
ARROWHEAD REGIONAL MEDICAL CENTER, COLTON, CA, p. A58
ARROYO GRANDE COMMUNITY HOSPITAL, ARROYO GRANDE, CA, p. A54
ARTESIA GENERAL HOSPITAL, ARTESIA, NM, p. A415
ARTHUR R. GOULD MEMORIAL HOSPITAL, PRESQUE ISLE, MAINE (see THE AROOSTOOK MEDICAL CENTER), p. A285
ASCENSION GONZALES REHABILITATION HOSPITAL, GONZALES, LA, p. A266
ASHE MEMORIAL HOSPITAL, JEFFERSON, NC, p. A455

ASHEVILLE SPECIALTY HOSPITAL, ASHEVILLE, NC, p. A448
ASHFORD PRESBYTERIAN COMMUNITY HOSPITAL, SAN JUAN, PR, p. A702
ASHLAND COMMUNITY HOSPITAL, ASHLAND, OR, p. A509
ASHLAND HEALTH CENTER, ASHLAND, KS, p. A230
ASHLEY COUNTY MEDICAL CENTER, CROSSETT, AR, p. A43
ASHLEY MEDICAL CENTER, ASHLEY, ND, p. A464
ASHLEY REGIONAL MEDICAL CENTER, VERNAL, UT, p. A642
ASHTABULA COUNTY MEDICAL CENTER, ASHTABULA, OH, p. A469
ASPEN VALLEY HOSPITAL DISTRICT, ASPEN, CO, p. A97
ASPIRE BEHAVIORAL HEALTH OF CONROE, CONROE, TX, p. A588
ASPIRUS GRAND VIEW HOSPITAL, IRONWOOD, MI, p. A316
ASPIRUS KEWEENAW HOSPITAL, LAURIUM, MI, p. A317
ASPIRUS ONTONAGON HOSPITAL, ONTONAGON, MI, p. A320
ASPIRUS WAUSAU HOSPITAL, WAUSAU, WI, p. A693
ASSUMPTION COMMUNITY HOSPITAL, NAPOLEONVILLE, LA, p. A274
ATASCADERO STATE HOSPITAL, ATASCADERO, CA, p. A54
ATCHISON HOSPITAL, ATCHISON, KS, p. A230
ATHENS REGIONAL MEDICAL CENTER, ATHENS, GA, p. A144
ATHENS REGIONAL MEDICAL CENTER, ATHENS, TN, p. A562
ATHENS–LIMESTONE HOSPITAL, ATHENS, AL, p. A16
ATHOL MEMORIAL HOSPITAL, ATHOL, MA, p. A295
ATLANTA MEDICAL CENTER, ATLANTA, GA, p. A145
ATLANTA MEMORIAL HOSPITAL, ATLANTA, TX, p. A580
ATLANTIC GENERAL HOSPITAL, BERLIN, MD, p. A289
ATLANTIC SHORES HOSPITAL, FORT LAUDERDALE, FL, p. A123
ATLANTICARE REGIONAL MEDICAL CENTER, ATLANTIC CITY, NJ, p. A401
ATLANTICARE REGIONAL MEDICAL CENTER–MAINLAND DIVISION, POMONA, NEW JERSEY (see ATLANTICARE REGIONAL MEDICAL CENTER), p. A401
ATMORE COMMUNITY HOSPITAL, ATMORE, AL, p. A16
ATOKA COUNTY MEDICAL CENTER, ATOKA, OK, p. A493
ATRIUM MEDICAL CENTER, MIDDLETOWN, OH, p. A485
ATRIUM MEDICAL CENTER, STAFFORD, TX, p. A628
ATRIUM MEDICAL CENTER OF CORINTH, CORINTH, TX, p. A588
AUBURN COMMUNITY HOSPITAL, AUBURN, NY, p. A421
AUBURN REGIONAL MEDICAL CENTER, AUBURN, WA, p. A659
AUDRAIN MEDICAL CENTER, MEXICO, MO, p. A365
AUDUBON COUNTY MEMORIAL HOSPITAL, AUDUBON, IA, p. A214
AUGUSTA HEALTH, FISHERSVILLE, VA, p. A648
AULTMAN HOSPITAL, CANTON, OH, p. A472
AULTMAN HOSPITAL PEDIATRIC SERVICES, CANTON, OHIO (see AULTMAN HOSPITAL), p. A472
AULTMAN ORRVILLE HOSPITAL, ORRVILLE, OH, p. A487
AURELIA OSBORN FOX MEMORIAL HOSPITAL, ONEONTA, NY, p. A439
AURORA BAYCARE MEDICAL CENTER, GREEN BAY, WI, p. A682
AURORA BEHAVIORAL HEALTH CARE, SAN DIEGO, CA, p. A85
AURORA BEHAVIORAL HEALTH SYSTEM–GLENDALE, GLENDALE, AZ, p. A32
AURORA CHARTER OAK HOSPITAL, COVINA, CA, p. A58
AURORA CHICAGO LAKESHORE HOSPITAL, CHICAGO, IL, p. A175
AURORA LAKELAND MEDICAL CENTER, ELKHORN, WI, p. A681
AURORA LAS ENCINAS HOSPITAL, PASADENA, CA, p. A79
AURORA MEDICAL CENTER, KENOSHA, WI, p. A683
AURORA MEDICAL CENTER – MANITOWOC COUNTY, TWO RIVERS, WI, p. A692
AURORA MEDICAL CENTER GRAFTON, GRAFTON, WI, p. A682
AURORA MEDICAL CENTER OF OSHKOSH, OSHKOSH, WI, p. A688
AURORA MEDICAL CENTER OF WASHINGTON COUNTY, HARTFORD, WI, p. A683
AURORA MEDICAL CENTER SUMMIT, SUMMIT, WI, p. A691
AURORA MEMORIAL HOSPITAL OF BURLINGTON, BURLINGTON, WI, p. A679
AURORA PAVILION, AIKEN, SOUTH CAROLINA (see AIKEN REGIONAL MEDICAL CENTERS), p. A546
AURORA PSYCHIATRIC HOSPITAL, WAUWATOSA, WI, p. A693
AURORA SHEBOYGAN MEMORIAL MEDICAL CENTER, SHEBOYGAN, WI, p. A690
AURORA SINAI MEDICAL CENTER, MILWAUKEE, WI, p. A686
AURORA ST. LUKE'S MEDICAL CENTER, MILWAUKEE, WI, p. A686
AURORA ST. LUKE'S SOUTH SHORE, CUDAHY, WISCONSIN (see AURORA ST. LUKE'S MEDICAL CENTER), p. A686
AURORA VISTA DEL MAR HOSPITAL, VENTURA, CA, p. A94
AURORA WEST ALLIS MEDICAL CENTER, WEST ALLIS, WI, p. A693
AUSTEN RIGGS CENTER, STOCKBRIDGE, MA, p. A305
AUSTIN LAKES HOSPITAL, AUSTIN, TX, p. A580
AUSTIN STATE HOSPITAL, AUSTIN, TX, p. A580
AUSTIN SURGICAL HOSPITAL, AUSTIN, TX, p. A580
AUXILIO MUTUO HOSPITAL, SAN JUAN, PR, p. A702

AVENTURA HOSPITAL AND MEDICAL CENTER, AVENTURA, FL, p. A118
AVERA CHILDREN'S HOSPITAL, SIOUX FALLS, SOUTH DAKOTA (see AVERA MCKENNAN HOSPITAL AND UNIVERSITY HEALTH CENTER), p. A559
AVERA CREIGHTON HOSPITAL, CREIGHTON, NE, p. A383
AVERA DE SMET MEMORIAL HOSPITAL, DE SMET, SD, p. A556
AVERA DELLS AREA HOSPITAL, DELL RAPIDS, SD, p. A556
AVERA FLANDREAU HOSPITAL, FLANDREAU, SD, p. A556
AVERA GREGORY HOSPITAL, GREGORY, SD, p. A557
AVERA HAND COUNTY MEMORIAL HOSPITAL & CLINIC, MILLER, SD, p. A557
AVERA HEART HOSPITAL OF SOUTH DAKOTA, SIOUX FALLS, SD, p. A559
AVERA HOLY FAMILY HOSPITAL, ESTHERVILLE, IA, p. A219
AVERA MARSHALL REGIONAL MEDICAL CENTER, MARSHALL, MN, p. A334
AVERA MCKENNAN HOSPITAL AND UNIVERSITY HEALTH CENTER, SIOUX FALLS, SD, p. A559
AVERA QUEEN OF PEACE HOSPITAL, MITCHELL, SD, p. A558
AVERA SACRED HEART HOSPITAL, YANKTON, SD, p. A561
AVERA ST. ANTHONY'S HOSPITAL, O'NEILL, NE, p. A386
AVERA ST. BENEDICT HOSPITAL, PARKSTON, SD, p. A558
AVERA ST. LUKE'S HOSPITAL, ABERDEEN, SD, p. A555
AVERA WESKOTA MEMORIAL HOSPITAL, WESSINGTON SPRINGS, SD, p. A561
AVISTA ADVENTIST HOSPITAL, LOUISVILLE, CO, p. A104
AVOYELLES HOSPITAL, MARKSVILLE, LA, p. A272

# B

BACHARACH INSTITUTE FOR REHABILITATION, POMONA, NJ, p. A409
BACON COUNTY HOSPITAL AND HEALTH SYSTEM, ALMA, GA, p. A144
BAILEY MEDICAL CENTER, OWASSO, OK, p. A502
BAKERSFIELD HEART HOSPITAL, BAKERSFIELD, CA, p. A54
BAKERSFIELD MEMORIAL HOSPITAL, BAKERSFIELD, CA, p. A54
BALDPATE HOSPITAL, HAVERHILL, MA, p. A300
BALDWIN AREA MEDICAL CENTER, BALDWIN, WI, p. A678
BALDWIN PARK MEDICAL CENTER, BALDWIN PARK, CA, p. A55
BALLINGER MEMORIAL HOSPITAL, BALLINGER, TX, p. A582
BALTIMORE WASHINGTON MEDICAL CENTER, GLEN BURNIE, MD, p. A292
BANNER BAYWOOD MEDICAL CENTER, MESA, AZ, p. A34
BANNER BEHAVIORAL HEALTH CENTER–THUNDERBIRD CAMPUS, GLENDALE, ARIZONA (see BANNER THUNDERBIRD MEDICAL CENTER), p. A33
BANNER BEHAVIORAL HEALTH HOSPITAL – SCOTTSDALE, SCOTTSDALE, AZ, p. A38
BANNER BOSWELL MEDICAL CENTER, SUN CITY, AZ, p. A39
BANNER CHURCHILL COMMUNITY HOSPITAL, FALLON, NV, p. A391
BANNER DEL E. WEBB MEDICAL CENTER, SUN CITY WEST, AZ, p. A39
BANNER DESERT MEDICAL CENTER, MESA, AZ, p. A34
BANNER ESTRELLA MEDICAL CENTER, PHOENIX, AZ, p. A35
BANNER GATEWAY MEDICAL CENTER, GILBERT, AZ, p. A32
BANNER GOOD SAMARITAN MEDICAL CENTER, PHOENIX, AZ, p. A35
BANNER HEART HOSPITAL, MESA, AZ, p. A34
BANNER IRONWOOD MEDICAL CENTER, SAN TAN VALLEY, AZ, p. A38
BANNER LASSEN MEDICAL CENTER, SUSANVILLE, CA, p. A92
BANNER THUNDERBIRD MEDICAL CENTER, GLENDALE, AZ, p. A33
BAPTIST CHILDREN'S HOSPITAL, MIAMI, FLORIDA (see BAPTIST HEALTH SOUTH FLORIDA, BAPTIST HOSPITAL OF MIAMI), p. A130
BAPTIST EASLEY HOSPITAL, EASLEY, SC, p. A549
BAPTIST HEALTH EXTENDED CARE HOSPITAL, LITTLE ROCK, AR, p. A47
BAPTIST HEALTH MEDICAL CENTER – NORTH LITTLE ROCK, NORTH LITTLE ROCK, AR, p. A50
BAPTIST HEALTH MEDICAL CENTER–ARKADELPHIA, ARKADELPHIA, AR, p. A42
BAPTIST HEALTH MEDICAL CENTER–HEBER SPRINGS, HEBER SPRINGS, AR, p. A45
BAPTIST HEALTH MEDICAL CENTER–LITTLE ROCK, LITTLE ROCK, AR, p. A47
BAPTIST HEALTH MEDICAL CENTER–STUTTGART, STUTTGART, AR, p. A51
BAPTIST HEALTH REHABILITATION INSTITUTE, LITTLE ROCK, AR, p. A48
BAPTIST HEALTH SOUTH FLORIDA, BAPTIST HOSPITAL OF MIAMI, MIAMI, FL, p. A130

BAPTIST HEALTH SOUTH FLORIDA, DOCTORS HOSPITAL, CORAL GABLES, FL, p. A121
BAPTIST HEALTH SOUTH FLORIDA, HOMESTEAD HOSPITAL, HOMESTEAD, FL, p. A125
BAPTIST HEALTH SOUTH FLORIDA, MARINERS HOSPITAL, TAVERNIER, FL, p. A142
BAPTIST HEALTH SOUTH FLORIDA, SOUTH MIAMI HOSPITAL, MIAMI, FL, p. A130
BAPTIST HEALTH SOUTH FLORIDA, WEST KENDALL BAPTIST HOSPITAL, MIAMI, FL, p. A131
BAPTIST HEALTH SYSTEM, SAN ANTONIO, TX, p. A624
BAPTIST HOSPITAL, PENSACOLA, FL, p. A136
BAPTIST HOSPITAL, NASHVILLE, TN, p. A573
BAPTIST HOSPITAL EAST, LOUISVILLE, KY, p. A254
BAPTIST HOSPITAL NORTHEAST, LA GRANGE, KY, p. A252
BAPTIST HOSPITALS OF SOUTHEAST TEXAS, BEAUMONT, TX, p. A582
BAPTIST HOSPITALS OF SOUTHEAST TEXAS FANNIN BEHAVIORAL HEALTH CENTER, BEAUMONT, TEXAS (see BAPTIST HOSPITALS OF SOUTHEAST TEXAS), p. A582
BAPTIST MEDICAL CENTER, JACKSONVILLE, FL, p. A126
BAPTIST MEDICAL CENTER BEACHES, JACKSONVILLE BEACH, FL, p. A127
BAPTIST MEDICAL CENTER EAST, MONTGOMERY, AL, p. A23
BAPTIST MEDICAL CENTER LEAKE, CARTHAGE, MS, p. A344
BAPTIST MEDICAL CENTER NASSAU, FERNANDINA BEACH, FL, p. A123
BAPTIST MEDICAL CENTER SOUTH, JACKSONVILLE, FLORIDA (see BAPTIST MEDICAL CENTER), p. A126
BAPTIST MEDICAL CENTER SOUTH, MONTGOMERY, AL, p. A23
BAPTIST MEMORIAL HOSPITAL – MEMPHIS, MEMPHIS, TN, p. A571
BAPTIST MEMORIAL HOSPITAL FOR WOMEN, MEMPHIS, TN, p. A571
BAPTIST MEMORIAL HOSPITAL-BOONEVILLE, BOONEVILLE, MS, p. A344
BAPTIST MEMORIAL HOSPITAL-COLLIERVILLE, COLLIERVILLE, TN, p. A564
BAPTIST MEMORIAL HOSPITAL-DESOTO, SOUTHAVEN, MS, p. A352
BAPTIST MEMORIAL HOSPITAL-GOLDEN TRIANGLE, COLUMBUS, MS, p. A345
BAPTIST MEMORIAL HOSPITAL-HUNTINGDON, HUNTINGDON, TN, p. A566
BAPTIST MEMORIAL HOSPITAL-NORTH MISSISSIPPI, OXFORD, MS, p. A351
BAPTIST MEMORIAL HOSPITAL-TIPTON, COVINGTON, TN, p. A564
BAPTIST MEMORIAL HOSPITAL-UNION CITY, UNION CITY, TN, p. A576
BAPTIST MEMORIAL HOSPITAL-UNION COUNTY, NEW ALBANY, MS, p. A351
BAPTIST MEMORIAL RESTORATIVE CARE HOSPITAL, MEMPHIS, TN, p. A571
BAPTIST ORANGE HOSPITAL, ORANGE, TX, p. A619
BAPTIST REGIONAL MEDICAL CENTER, CORBIN, KY, p. A248
BAPTIST REHABILITATION-GERMANTOWN, GERMANTOWN, TN, p. A566
BAPTIST ST. ANTHONY HEALTH SYSTEM, AMARILLO, TX, p. A578
BARAGA COUNTY MEMORIAL HOSPITAL, L'ANSE, MI, p. A317
BARBARA BUSH CHILDREN'S HOSPITAL, PORTLAND, MAINE (see MAINE MEDICAL CENTER), p. A284
BARIX CLINICS OF OHIO, GROVEPORT, OH, p. A481
BARLOW RESPIRATORY HOSPITAL, LOS ANGELES, CA, p. A68
BARNES-JEWISH HOSPITAL, SAINT LOUIS, MO, p. A368
BARNES-JEWISH ST. PETERS HOSPITAL, SAINT PETERS, MO, p. A370
BARNES-JEWISH WEST COUNTY HOSPITAL, SAINT LOUIS, MO, p. A368
BARNES-KASSON COUNTY HOSPITAL, SUSQUEHANNA, PA, p. A539
BARNESVILLE HOSPITAL, BARNESVILLE, OH, p. A470
BARNWELL COUNTY HOSPITAL, BARNWELL, SC, p. A546
BARRETT HOSPITAL & HEALTHCARE, DILLON, MT, p. A375
BARROW REGIONAL MEDICAL CENTER, WINDER, GA, p. A162
BARSTOW COMMUNITY HOSPITAL, BARSTOW, CA, p. A55
BARTLETT REGIONAL HOSPITAL, JUNEAU, AK, p. A29
BARTON COUNTY MEMORIAL HOSPITAL, LAMAR, MO, p. A363
BARTON HEALTHCARE SYSTEM, SOUTH LAKE TAHOE, CA, p. A91
BARTOW REGIONAL MEDICAL CENTER, BARTOW, FL, p. A118
BASCOM PALMER EYE INSTITUTE-ANNE BATES LEACH EYE HOSPITAL, MIAMI, FL, p. A131
BASIN HEALTHCARE CENTER, ODESSA, TX, p. A619
BASSETT ARMY COMMUNITY HOSPITAL, FORT WAINWRIGHT, AK, p. A29
BASSETT MEDICAL CENTER, COOPERSTOWN, NY, p. A424
BASTROP REHABILITATION HOSPITAL, BASTROP, LA, p. A262
BATES COUNTY MEMORIAL HOSPITAL, BUTLER, MO, p. A356

BATESVILLE SPECIALTY HOSPITAL, BATESVILLE, MS, p. A343
BATH COMMUNITY HOSPITAL, HOT SPRINGS, VA, p. A650
BATON ROUGE GENERAL MEDICAL CENTER, BATON ROUGE, LA, p. A262
BATON ROUGE GENERAL MEDICAL CENTER-BLUEBONNET, BATON ROUGE, LOUISIANA (see BATON ROUGE GENERAL MEDICAL CENTER), p. A262
BATON ROUGE REHABILITATION HOSPITAL, BATON ROUGE, LA, p. A262
BATTLE MOUNTAIN GENERAL HOSPITAL, BATTLE MOUNTAIN, NV, p. A391
BAUM HARMON MERCY HOSPITAL, PRIMGHAR, IA, p. A225
BAXTER REGIONAL MEDICAL CENTER, MOUNTAIN HOME, AR, p. A49
BAY AREA HOSPITAL, COOS BAY, OR, p. A510
BAY AREA MEDICAL CENTER, MARINETTE, WI, p. A685
BAY MEDICAL CENTER, PANAMA CITY, FL, p. A135
BAY REGIONAL MEDICAL CENTER-WEST CAMPUS, BAY CITY, MICHIGAN (see MCLAREN BAY REGION), p. A308
BAYCARE ALLIANT HOSPITAL, DUNEDIN, FL, p. A122
BAYFRONT MEDICAL CENTER, SAINT PETERSBURG, FL, p. A138
BAYHEALTH MEDICAL CENTER, DOVER, DE, p. A114
BAYHEALTH MEDICAL CENTER AT KENT GENERAL, DOVER, DELAWARE (see BAYHEALTH MEDICAL CENTER), p. A114
BAYHEALTH MEDICAL CENTER, MILFORD MEMORIAL HOSPITAL, MILFORD, DELAWARE (see BAYHEALTH MEDICAL CENTER), p. A114
BAYLOR ALL SAINTS MEDICAL CENTER AT FORT WORTH, FORT WORTH, TX, p. A598
BAYLOR INSTITUTE FOR REHABILITATION, DALLAS, TX, p. A590
BAYLOR INSTITUTE FOR REHABILITATION AT FRISCO, FRISCO, TX, p. A600
BAYLOR JACK AND JANE HAMILTON HEART AND VASCULAR HOSPITAL, DALLAS, TX, p. A590
BAYLOR MEDICAL CENTER AT CARROLLTON, CARROLLTON, TX, p. A586
BAYLOR MEDICAL CENTER AT FRISCO, FRISCO, TX, p. A600
BAYLOR MEDICAL CENTER AT GARLAND, GARLAND, TX, p. A600
BAYLOR MEDICAL CENTER AT IRVING, IRVING, TX, p. A609
BAYLOR MEDICAL CENTER AT TROPHY CLUB, TROPHY CLUB, TX, p. A631
BAYLOR MEDICAL CENTER AT UPTOWN, DALLAS, TX, p. A590
BAYLOR MEDICAL CENTER AT WAXAHACHIE, WAXAHACHIE, TX, p. A633
BAYLOR ORTHOPEDIC AND SPINE HOSPITAL AT ARLINGTON, ARLINGTON, TX, p. A579
BAYLOR REGIONAL MEDICAL CENTER AT GRAPEVINE, GRAPEVINE, TX, p. A601
BAYLOR REGIONAL MEDICAL CENTER AT PLANO, PLANO, TX, p. A621
BAYLOR SPECIALTY HOSPITAL, DALLAS, TX, p. A590
BAYLOR SURGICAL HOSPITAL AT FORT WORTH, FORT WORTH, TX, p. A598
BAYLOR UNIVERSITY MEDICAL CENTER, DALLAS, TX, p. A590
BAYNE-JONES ARMY COMMUNITY HOSPITAL, FORT POLK, LA, p. A266
BAYONNE MEDICAL CENTER, BAYONNE, NJ, p. A401
BAYPOINTE BEHAVIORAL HEALTH, MOBILE, AL, p. A22
BAYSHORE COMMUNITY HOSPITAL, HOLMDEL, NJ, p. A405
BAYSHORE MEDICAL CENTER, PASADENA, TX, p. A620
BAYSTATE CHILDREN'S HOSPITAL, SPRINGFIELD, MASSACHUSETTS (see BAYSTATE MEDICAL CENTER), p. A304
BAYSTATE FRANKLIN MEDICAL CENTER, GREENFIELD, MA, p. A300
BAYSTATE MARY LANE HOSPITAL, WARE, MA, p. A305
BAYSTATE MEDICAL CENTER, SPRINGFIELD, MA, p. A304
BAYVIEW BEHAVIORAL HEALTH CAMPUS, CHULA VISTA, CA, p. A57
BAYVIEW BEHAVIORAL HOSPITAL, CORPUS CHRISTI, TEXAS (see CORPUS CHRISTI MEDICAL CENTER), p. A589
BCA PERMIAN BASIN, MIDLAND, TX, p. A616
BCA STONECREST HOSPITAL, DETROIT, MI, p. A310
BEACHAM MEMORIAL HOSPITAL, MAGNOLIA, MS, p. A349
BEACON BEHAVIORAL HOSPITAL – NEW ORLEANS, NEW ORLEANS, LA, p. A274
BEACON CHILDREN'S HOSPITAL, LUVERNE, AL, p. A22
BEAR LAKE MEMORIAL HOSPITAL, MONTPELIER, ID, p. A169
BEAR RIVER VALLEY HOSPITAL, TREMONTON, UT, p. A642
BEAR VALLEY COMMUNITY HOSPITAL, BIG BEAR LAKE, CA, p. A55
BEARTOOTH BILLINGS CLINIC, RED LODGE, MT, p. A378
BEATRICE COMMUNITY HOSPITAL AND HEALTH CENTER, BEATRICE, NE, p. A382
BEAUFORT MEMORIAL HOSPITAL, BEAUFORT, SC, p. A546
BEAUMONT BONE AND JOINT INSTITUTE, BEAUMONT, TX, p. A582

BEAUMONT CHILDREN'S HOSPITAL, ROYAL OAK, MICHIGAN (see BEAUMONT HOSPITAL – ROYAL OAK), p. A322
BEAUMONT HOSPITAL – ROYAL OAK, ROYAL OAK, MI, p. A322
BEAUMONT HOSPITAL – TROY, TROY, MI, p. A324
BEAUMONT HOSPITAL GROSSE POINTE, GROSSE POINTE, MI, p. A314
BEAUREGARD MEMORIAL HOSPITAL, DE RIDDER, LA, p. A265
BEAVER COUNTY MEMORIAL HOSPITAL, BEAVER, OK, p. A494
BEAVER DAM COMMUNITY HOSPITALS, BEAVER DAM, WI, p. A679
BEAVER VALLEY HOSPITAL, BEAVER, UT, p. A637
BECK BEHAVIORAL HOSPITAL, BATON ROUGE, LA, p. A262
BECKLEY ARH HOSPITAL, BECKLEY, WV, p. A670
BEDFORD MEMORIAL HOSPITAL, BEDFORD, VA, p. A645
BEEBE MEDICAL CENTER, LEWES, DE, p. A114
BEHAVIORAL CENTER OF MICHIGAN, WARREN, MI, p. A324
BEHAVIORAL HEALTH CENTER, WINFIELD, ILLINOIS (see CENTRAL DUPAGE HOSPITAL), p. A196
BEHAVIORAL HEALTH CENTER, GREENSBORO, NORTH CAROLINA (see CONE HEALTH), p. A454
BEHAVIORAL HOSPITAL OF BELLAIRE, HOUSTON, TX, p. A603
BEHAVIORAL HOSPITAL OF LONGVIEW, LONGVIEW, TX, p. A613
BEHAVIORAL HOSPITAL OF SOUTHEAST LOUISIANA, BATON ROUGE, LA, p. A262
BELL HOSPITAL, ISHPEMING, MI, p. A316
BELLA VISTA HOSPITAL, MAYAGUEZ, PR, p. A701
BELLEVUE HOSPITAL, BELLEVUE, OH, p. A470
BELLEVUE HOSPITAL CENTER, NEW YORK, NY, p. A431
BELLEVUE MEDICAL CENTER, BELLEVUE, NE, p. A382
BELLEVUE WOMAN'S CARE CENTER, SCHENECTADY, NEW YORK (see ELLIS HOSPITAL), p. A443
BELLFLOWER MEDICAL CENTER, BELLFLOWER, CA, p. A55
BELLIN MEMORIAL HOSPITAL, GREEN BAY, WI, p. A682
BELLIN PSYCHIATRIC CENTER, GREEN BAY, WI, p. A682
BELLVILLE GENERAL HOSPITAL, BELLVILLE, TX, p. A583
BELMONT CENTER FOR COMPREHENSIVE TREATMENT, PHILADELPHIA, PA, p. A531
BELMONT COMMUNITY HOSPITAL, BELLAIRE, OH, p. A470
BELMONT PINES HOSPITAL, YOUNGSTOWN, OH, p. A492
BELOIT HEALTH SYSTEM, BELOIT, WI, p. A679
BELTON REGIONAL MEDICAL CENTER, BELTON, MO, p. A355
BEN TAUB GENERAL HOSPITAL, HOUSTON, TEXAS (see HARRIS COUNTY HOSPITAL DISTRICT), p. A604
BENEDICTINE HOSPITAL, KINGSTON, NY, p. A428
BENEFIS HEALTH CARE-EAST CAMPUS, GREAT FALLS, MONTANA (see BENEFIS HOSPITALS), p. A376
BENEFIS HEALTH CARE-WEST CAMPUS, GREAT FALLS, MONTANA (see BENEFIS HOSPITALS), p. A376
BENEFIS HOSPITALS, GREAT FALLS, MT, p. A376
BENEWAH COMMUNITY HOSPITAL, SAINT MARIES, ID, p. A170
BENNETT COUNTY HOSPITAL AND NURSING HOME, MARTIN, SD, p. A557
BENSON HOSPITAL, BENSON, AZ, p. A31
BERGEN REGIONAL MEDICAL CENTER, PARAMUS, NJ, p. A408
BERGER HEALTH SYSTEM, CIRCLEVILLE, OH, p. A474
BERKSHIRE MEDICAL CENTER, PITTSFIELD, MA, p. A303
BERLIN MEMORIAL HOSPITAL, BERLIN, WI, p. A679
BERNARD MITCHELL HOSPITAL, CHICAGO, ILLINOIS (see UNIVERSITY OF CHICAGO MEDICAL CENTER), p. A179
BERRIEN COUNTY HOSPITAL, NASHVILLE, GA, p. A157
BERT FISH MEDICAL CENTER, NEW SMYRNA BEACH, FL, p. A133
BERTRAND CHAFFEE HOSPITAL, SPRINGVILLE, NY, p. A443
BERWICK HOSPITAL CENTER, BERWICK, PA, p. A518
BETH ISRAEL DEACONESS HOSPITAL-NEEDHAM CAMPUS, NEEDHAM, MASSACHUSETTS (see BETH ISRAEL DEACONESS MEDICAL CENTER), p. A296
BETH ISRAEL DEACONESS MEDICAL CENTER, BOSTON, MA, p. A296
BETH ISRAEL MEDICAL CENTER, NEW YORK, NY, p. A431
BETH ISRAEL MEDICAL CENTER-KINGS HIGHWAY DIVISION,, NEW YORK (see BETH ISRAEL MEDICAL CENTER), p. A431
BETHESDA HOSPITAL, ZANESVILLE, OHIO (see GENESIS HEALTHCARE SYSTEM), p. A492
BETHESDA MEMORIAL HOSPITAL, BOYNTON BEACH, FL, p. A119
BETHESDA NORTH HOSPITAL, CINCINNATI, OH, p. A472
BETHESDA REHABILITATION HOSPITAL, BATON ROUGE, LA, p. A262
BETSY JOHNSON REGIONAL HOSPITAL, DUNN, NC, p. A452
BEVERLY HOSPITAL, MONTEBELLO, CA, p. A75
BEVERLY HOSPITAL, BEVERLY, MA, p. A295
BHC ALHAMBRA HOSPITAL, ROSEMEAD, CA, p. A83
BIBB MEDICAL CENTER, CENTREVILLE, AL, p. A18
BIENVILLE MEDICAL CENTER, ARCADIA, LA, p. A261
BIG BEND REGIONAL MEDICAL CENTER, ALPINE, TX, p. A577
BIG HORN COUNTY MEMORIAL HOSPITAL, HARDIN, MT, p. A376
BIG SANDY MEDICAL CENTER, BIG SANDY, MT, p. A373
BIG SPRING STATE HOSPITAL, BIG SPRING, TX, p. A584

BIGFORK VALLEY HOSPITAL, BIGFORK, MN, p. A328
BIGGS–GRIDLEY MEMORIAL HOSPITAL, GRIDLEY, CA, p. A64
BILLINGS CLINIC, BILLINGS, MT, p. A373
BILOXI REGIONAL MEDICAL CENTER, BILOXI, MS, p. A343
BINGHAM MEMORIAL HOSPITAL, BLACKFOOT, ID, p. A166
BINGHAMTON GENERAL HOSPITAL, BINGHAMTON, NEW YORK
(see UNITED HEALTH SERVICES HOSPITALS–BINGHAMTON),
p. A422
BLACK HILLS SURGERY CENTER, RAPID CITY, SD, p. A558
BLACK RIVER MEDICAL CENTER, POPLAR BLUFF, MO, p. A366
BLACK RIVER MEMORIAL HOSPITAL, BLACK RIVER FALLS, WI,
p. A679
BLAIR E. BATSON HOSPITAL FOR CHILDREN, JACKSON,
MISSISSIPPI (see UNIVERSITY HOSPITALS AND HEALTH
SYSTEM, UNIVERSITY OF MISSISSIPPI MEDICAL CENTER),
p. A348
BLAKE MEDICAL CENTER, BRADENTON, FL, p. A119
BLANCHARD VALLEY HOSPITAL, FINDLAY, OH, p. A480
BLANCHARD VALLEY HOSPITAL, FINDLAY, OHIO (see
BLANCHARD VALLEY HOSPITAL), p. A480
BLANK CHILDREN'S HOSPITAL, DES MOINES, IOWA (see IOWA
METHODIST MEDICAL CENTER), p. A218
BLECKLEY MEMORIAL HOSPITAL, COCHRAN, GA, p. A149
BLESSING HOSPITAL, QUINCY, IL, p. A192
BLESSING HOSPITAL, QUINCY, ILLINOIS (see BLESSING
HOSPITAL), p. A192
BLOOMINGTON MEADOWS HOSPITAL, BLOOMINGTON, IN,
p. A198
BLOUNT MEMORIAL HOSPITAL, MARYVILLE, TN, p. A570
BLOWING ROCK HOSPITAL, BLOWING ROCK, NC, p. A449
BLUE HILL MEMORIAL HOSPITAL, BLUE HILL, ME, p. A282
BLUE MOUNTAIN HOSPITAL, JOHN DAY, OR, p. A511
BLUE MOUNTAIN HOSPITAL, BLANDING, UT, p. A637
BLUE MOUNTAIN RECOVERY CENTER, PENDLETON, OR,
p. A513
BLUE RIDGE REGIONAL HOSPITAL, SPRUCE PINE, NC, p. A461
BLUEFIELD REGIONAL MEDICAL CENTER, BLUEFIELD, WV,
p. A670
BLUEGRASS COMMUNITY HOSPITAL, VERSAILLES, KY, p. A259
BLUFFTON HOSPITAL, BLUFFTON, OH, p. A471
BLUFFTON REGIONAL MEDICAL CENTER, BLUFFTON, IN,
p. A198
BLYTHEDALE CHILDREN'S HOSPITAL, VALHALLA, NY, p. A445
BOB WILSON MEMORIAL GRANT COUNTY HOSPITAL, ULYSSES,
KS, p. A244
BOCA RATON REGIONAL HOSPITAL, BOCA RATON, FL, p. A118
BOGALUSA COMMUNITY MEDICAL CENTER, BOGALUSA,
LOUISIANA (see LSU BOGALUSA MEDICAL CENTER), p. A263
BOISE BEHAVIORAL HEALTH HOSPITAL, BOISE, ID, p. A166
BOLIVAR GENERAL HOSPITAL, BOLIVAR, TN, p. A562
BOLIVAR MEDICAL CENTER, CLEVELAND, MS, p. A345
BON SECOURS BALTIMORE HEALTH SYSTEM, BALTIMORE, MD,
p. A287
BON SECOURS COMMUNITY HOSPITAL, PORT JERVIS, NY,
p. A440
BON SECOURS MARYVIEW MEDICAL CENTER, PORTSMOUTH,
VA, p. A654
BON SECOURS MEMORIAL REGIONAL MEDICAL CENTER,
MECHANICSVILLE, VA, p. A651
BON SECOURS ST. FRANCIS HOSPITAL, CHARLESTON, SC,
p. A547
BON SECOURS ST. FRANCIS EASTSIDE, GREENVILLE, SOUTH
CAROLINA (see BON SECOURS ST. FRANCIS HEALTH
SYSTEM), p. A550
BON SECOURS ST. FRANCIS HEALTH SYSTEM, GREENVILLE,
SC, p. A550
BON SECOURS ST. FRANCIS MEDICAL CENTER, MIDLOTHIAN,
VA, p. A651
BON SECOURS ST. MARY'S CHILDREN'S SERVICES, RICHMOND,
VIRGINIA (see BON SECOURS ST. MARY'S HOSPITAL),
p. A654
BON SECOURS ST. MARY'S HOSPITAL, RICHMOND, VA, p. A654
BON SECOURS–DEPAUL MEDICAL CENTER, NORFOLK, VA,
p. A652
BON SECOURS–RICHMOND COMMUNITY HOSPITAL,
RICHMOND, VA, p. A654
BONE AND JOINT HOSPITAL, OKLAHOMA CITY, OKLAHOMA (see
ST. ANTHONY HOSPITAL), p. A502
BONNER GENERAL HOSPITAL, SANDPOINT, ID, p. A170
BOONE COUNTY HEALTH CENTER, ALBION, NE, p. A381
BOONE COUNTY HOSPITAL, BOONE, IA, p. A215
BOONE HOSPITAL CENTER, COLUMBIA, MO, p. A358
BOONE MEMORIAL HOSPITAL, MADISON, WV, p. A673
BOONEVILLE COMMUNITY HOSPITAL, BOONEVILLE, AR, p. A42
BORGESS MEDICAL CENTER, KALAMAZOO, MI, p. A316
BORGESS–LEE MEMORIAL HOSPITAL, DOWAGIAC, MI, p. A311
BORGESS–PIPP HOSPITAL, PLAINWELL, MI, p. A320
BOSCOBEL AREA HEALTH CARE, BOSCOBEL, WI, p. A679
BOSTON MEDICAL CENTER, BOSTON, MA, p. A296
BOTHWELL REGIONAL HEALTH CENTER, SEDALIA, MO, p. A370

BOTSFORD HOSPITAL, FARMINGTON HILLS, MI, p. A312
BOULDER CITY HOSPITAL, BOULDER CITY, NV, p. A391
BOULDER COMMUNITY FOOTHILLS HOSPITAL, BOULDER,
COLORADO (see BOULDER COMMUNITY HOSPITAL), p. A97
BOULDER COMMUNITY HOSPITAL, BOULDER, CO, p. A97
BOUNDARY COMMUNITY HOSPITAL, BONNERS FERRY, ID,
p. A167
BOUNDARY COUNTY NURSING HOME (see BOUNDARY
COMMUNITY HOSPITAL), p. A167
BOURBON COMMUNITY HOSPITAL, PARIS, KY, p. A258
BOURNEWOOD HEALTH SYSTEMS, BROOKLINE, MA, p. A298
BOWDLE HOSPITAL, BOWDLE, SD, p. A555
BOWIE MEMORIAL HOSPITAL, BOWIE, TX, p. A584
BOX BUTTE GENERAL HOSPITAL, ALLIANCE, NE, p. A381
BOYS TOWN NATIONAL RESEARCH HOSPITAL, OMAHA, NE,
p. A387
BOZEMAN DEACONESS HOSPITAL, BOZEMAN, MT, p. A373
BRADFORD HEALTH SERVICES AT HUNTSVILLE, MADISON, AL,
p. A22
BRADFORD HEALTH SERVICES AT WARRIOR LODGE, WARRIOR,
AL, p. A26
BRADFORD REGIONAL MEDICAL CENTER, BRADFORD, PA,
p. A519
BRADLEY CENTER OF ST. FRANCIS, COLUMBUS, GEORGIA (see
ST. FRANCIS HOSPITAL), p. A149
BRADLEY COUNTY MEDICAL CENTER, WARREN, AR, p. A52
BRADLEY MEMORIAL, SOUTHINGTON, CONNECTICUT (see THE
HOSPITAL OF CENTRAL CONNECTICUT), p. A110
BRAINERD REGIONAL HUMAN SERVICES CENTER, BRAINERD,
MN, p. A328
BRAINTREE REHABILITATION HOSPITAL, BRAINTREE, MA,
p. A298
BRANDON REGIONAL HOSPITAL, BRANDON, FL, p. A119
BRANDYWINE HOSPITAL, COATESVILLE, PA, p. A520
BRATTLEBORO MEMORIAL HOSPITAL, BRATTLEBORO, VT,
p. A643
BRATTLEBORO RETREAT, BRATTLEBORO, VT, p. A643
BRAXTON COUNTY MEMORIAL HOSPITAL, GASSAWAY, WV,
p. A671
BRAZOSPORT REGIONAL HEALTH SYSTEM, LAKE JACKSON, TX,
p. A611
BRECKINRIDGE MEMORIAL HOSPITAL, HARDINSBURG, KY,
p. A251
BRENNER CHILDREN'S HOSPITAL & HEALTH SERVICES,
WINSTON SALEM, NORTH CAROLINA (see WAKE FOREST
BAPTIST MEDICAL CENTER), p. A463
BRENTWOOD BEHAVIORAL HEALTHCARE OF MISSISSIPPI,
JACKSON, MS, p. A347
BRENTWOOD HOSPITAL, SHREVEPORT, LA, p. A277
BRIDGEPORT HOSPITAL, BRIDGEPORT, CT, p. A108
BRIDGETON HEALTH CENTER, BRIDGETON, NEW JERSEY (see
SOUTH JERSEY HEALTHCARE – REGIONAL MEDICAL
CENTER), p. A411
BRIDGEWATER STATE HOSPITAL, BRIDGEWATER, MA, p. A298
BRIDGTON HOSPITAL, BRIDGTON, ME, p. A282
BRIGHAM AND WOMEN'S HOSPITAL, BOSTON, MA, p. A296
BRIGHAM CITY COMMUNITY HOSPITAL, BRIGHAM CITY, UT,
p. A637
BRIGHTON CENTER FOR RECOVERY, BRIGHTON, MI, p. A308
BRISTOL BAY AREA HEALTH CORPORATION, DILLINGHAM, AK,
p. A28
BRISTOL HOSPITAL, BRISTOL, CT, p. A108
BRISTOL–MYERS SQUIBB CHILDREN'S HOSPITAL, NEW
BRUNSWICK, NEW JERSEY (see ROBERT WOOD JOHNSON
UNIVERSITY HOSPITAL), p. A407
BRISTOW MEDICAL CENTER, BRISTOW, OK, p. A494
BROADDUS HOSPITAL, PHILIPPI, WV, p. A674
BROADLAWNS MEDICAL CENTER, DES MOINES, IA, p. A218
BROADWATER HEALTH CENTER, TOWNSEND, MT, p. A379
BROCKTON VETERANS AFFAIRS MEDICAL CENTER, BROCKTON,
MA, p. A298
BRODSTONE MEMORIAL HOSPITAL, SUPERIOR, NE, p. A390
BROMENN REGIONAL MEDICAL CENTER, NORMAL, ILLINOIS
(see ADVOCATE BROMENN MEDICAL CENTER), p. A189
BRONSON BATTLE CREEK, BATTLE CREEK, MI, p. A308
BRONSON LAKEVIEW HOSPITAL, PAW PAW, MI, p. A320
BRONSON METHODIST HOSPITAL, KALAMAZOO, MI, p. A316
BRONSON VICKSBURG HOSPITAL, VICKSBURG, MICHIGAN (see
BRONSON METHODIST HOSPITAL), p. A316
BRONX CHILDREN'S PSYCHIATRIC CENTER,, NY, p. A431
BRONX PSYCHIATRIC CENTER,, NY, p. A431
BRONX–LEBANON HOSPITAL CENTER HEALTH CARE SYSTEM,,
NY, p. A431
BRONX–LEBANON SPECIAL CARE CENTER,, NEW YORK (see
BRONX–LEBANON HOSPITAL CENTER HEALTH CARE
SYSTEM), p. A431
BROOK LANE HEALTH SERVICES, HAGERSTOWN, MD, p. A292
BROOKDALE HOSPITAL MEDICAL CENTER,, NY, p. A431
BROOKE GLEN BEHAVIORAL HOSPITAL, FORT WASHINGTON,
PA, p. A523

BROOKHAVEN HOSPITAL, TULSA, OK, p. A505
BROOKHAVEN MEMORIAL HOSPITAL MEDICAL CENTER,
PATCHOGUE, NY, p. A440
BROOKINGS HEALTH SYSTEM, BROOKINGS, SD, p. A555
BROOKLYN CHILDREN'S PSYCHIATRIC CENTER,, NY, p. A431
BROOKLYN HOSPITAL CENTER,, NY, p. A431
BROOKS COUNTY HOSPITAL, QUITMAN, GA, p. A157
BROOKS MEMORIAL HOSPITAL, DUNKIRK, NY, p. A425
BROOKS REHABILITATION HOSPITAL, JACKSONVILLE, FL,
p. A126
BROOKSVILLE REGIONAL HOSPITAL, BROOKSVILLE, FL,
p. A119
BROOKVILLE HOSPITAL, BROOKVILLE, PA, p. A519
BROOKWOOD MEDICAL CENTER, BIRMINGHAM, AL, p. A16
BROTMAN MEDICAL CENTER, CULVER CITY, CA, p. A59
BROUGHTON HOSPITAL, MORGANTON, NC, p. A457
BROWARD HEALTH CORAL SPRINGS, CORAL SPRINGS, FL,
p. A121
BROWARD HEALTH IMPERIAL POINT, FORT LAUDERDALE, FL,
p. A123
BROWARD HEALTH MEDICAL CENTER, FORT LAUDERDALE, FL,
p. A123
BROWARD HEALTH NORTH, DEERFIELD BEACH, FL, p. A122
BROWN COUNTY COMMUNITY TREATMENT CENTER, GREEN
BAY, WI, p. A682
BROWN COUNTY HOSPITAL, AINSWORTH, NE, p. A381
BROWN MEMORIAL CONVALESCENT CENTER, COBB HEALTH
CARE CENTER AND THE GABLES (see COBB MEMORIAL
HOSPITAL), p. A158
BROWNFIELD REGIONAL MEDICAL CENTER, BROWNFIELD, TX,
p. A585
BROWNSVILLE DOCTORS HOSPITAL, BROWNSVILLE, TX,
p. A585
BROWNWOOD REGIONAL MEDICAL CENTER, BROWNWOOD, TX,
p. A585
BRUNSWICK NOVANT MEDICAL CENTER, BOLIVIA, NC, p. A449
BRYAN HOSPITAL, BRYAN, OHIO (see COMMUNITY HOSPITALS
AND WELLNESS CENTERS), p. A471
BRYAN W. WHITFIELD MEMORIAL HOSPITAL, DEMOPOLIS, AL,
p. A19
BRYANLGH MEDICAL CENTER, LINCOLN, NE, p. A385
BRYANLGH MEDICAL CENTER–EAST, LINCOLN, NEBRASKA (see
BRYANLGH MEDICAL CENTER), p. A385
BRYANLGH MEDICAL CENTER–WEST, LINCOLN, NEBRASKA
(see BRYANLGH MEDICAL CENTER), p. A385
BRYCE HOSPITAL, TUSCALOOSA, AL, p. A26
BRYLIN HOSPITALS, BUFFALO, NY, p. A422
BRYN MAWR HOSPITAL, BRYN MAWR, PA, p. A519
BRYN MAWR REHABILITATION HOSPITAL, MALVERN, PA,
p. A528
BRYNN MARR HOSPITAL, JACKSONVILLE, NC, p. A455
BUCHANAN COUNTY HEALTH CENTER, INDEPENDENCE, IA,
p. A221
BUCHANAN GENERAL HOSPITAL, GRUNDY, VA, p. A649
BUCKS COUNTY CAMPUS, LANGHORNE, PENNSYLVANIA (see
ARIA HEALTH), p. A531
BUCKTAIL MEDICAL CENTER, RENOVO, PA, p. A537
BUCYRUS COMMUNITY HOSPITAL, BUCYRUS, OH, p. A471
BUENA VISTA REGIONAL MEDICAL CENTER, STORM LAKE, IA,
p. A227
BUFFALO HOSPITAL, BUFFALO, MN, p. A329
BUFFALO PSYCHIATRIC CENTER, BUFFALO, NY, p. A422
BULLOCK COUNTY HOSPITAL, UNION SPRINGS, AL, p. A26
BUNKIE GENERAL HOSPITAL, BUNKIE, LA, p. A264
BURGESS HEALTH CENTER, ONAWA, IA, p. A224
BURKE MEDICAL CENTER, WAYNESBORO, GA, p. A162
BURKE REHABILITATION HOSPITAL, WHITE PLAINS, NY, p. A447
BURLESON ST. JOSEPH HEALTH CENTER, CALDWELL, TX,
p. A586
BURNETT MEDICAL CENTER, GRANTSBURG, WI, p. A682
BUTLER COUNTY HEALTH CARE CENTER, DAVID CITY, NE,
p. A383
BUTLER COUNTY MEDICAL CENTER, HAMILTON, OH, p. A481
BUTLER HEALTH SYSTEM, BUTLER, PA, p. A519
BUTLER HOSPITAL, PROVIDENCE, RI, p. A544
BYRD REGIONAL HOSPITAL, LEESVILLE, LA, p. A271

## C

C.S. MOTT CHILDREN'S HOSPITAL, ANN ARBOR, MICHIGAN (see
UNIVERSITY OF MICHIGAN HOSPITALS AND HEALTH
CENTERS), p. A307
CABELL HUNTINGTON HOSPITAL, HUNTINGTON, WV, p. A672
CACHE VALLEY SPECIALTY HOSPITAL, NORTH LOGAN, UT,
p. A639
CALAIS REGIONAL HOSPITAL, CALAIS, ME, p. A282

CHRISTUS ST. PATRICK HOSPITAL OF LAKE CHARLES, LAKE CHARLES, LA, p. A271

CHRISTUS ST. VINCENT REGIONAL MEDICAL CENTER, SANTA FE, NM, p. A418

CIBOLA GENERAL HOSPITAL, GRANTS, NM, p. A416

CIMARRON MEMORIAL HOSPITAL, BOISE CITY, OK, p. A494

CINCINNATI CHILDREN'S HOSPITAL MEDICAL CENTER, CINCINNATI, OH, p. A473

CIRCLES OF CARE, MELBOURNE, FL, p. A130

CITIZENS BAPTIST MEDICAL CENTER, TALLADEGA, AL, p. A26

CITIZENS MEDICAL CENTER, COLBY, KS, p. A231

CITIZENS MEDICAL CENTER, COLUMBIA, LA, p. A264

CITIZENS MEDICAL CENTER, VICTORIA, TX, p. A633

CITIZENS MEMORIAL HOSPITAL, BOLIVAR, MO, p. A355

CITRUS MEMORIAL HEALTH SYSTEM, INVERNESS, FL, p. A126

CITRUS VALLEY MEDICAL CENTER–INTER–COMMUNITY CAMPUS, COVINA, CA, p. A59

CITRUS VALLEY MEDICAL CENTER–QUEEN OF THE VALLEY CAMPUS, WEST COVINA, CA, p. A95

CITY HOSPITAL, MARTINSBURG, WV, p. A673

CITY OF HOPE'S HELFORD CLINICAL RESEARCH HOSPITAL, DUARTE, CA, p. A59

CIVISTA HEALTH, LA PLATA, MD, p. A292

CJW MEDICAL CENTER, RICHMOND, VA, p. A654

CLAIBORNE COUNTY HOSPITAL, TAZEWELL, TN, p. A576

CLARA BARTON HOSPITAL, HOISINGTON, KS, p. A234

CLARA MAASS MEDICAL CENTER, BELLEVILLE, NJ, p. A401

CLAREMORE INDIAN HOSPITAL, CLAREMORE, OK, p. A494

CLARENDON MEMORIAL HOSPITAL, MANNING, SC, p. A552

CLARINDA REGIONAL HEALTH CENTER, CLARINDA, IA, p. A216

CLARION HOSPITAL, CLARION, PA, p. A520

CLARION PSYCHIATRIC CENTER, CLARION, PA, p. A520

CLARITY CHILD GUIDANCE CENTER, SAN ANTONIO, TX, p. A624

CLARK FORK VALLEY HOSPITAL, PLAINS, MT, p. A378

CLARK MEMORIAL HOSPITAL, JEFFERSONVILLE, IN, p. A205

CLARK REGIONAL MEDICAL CENTER, WINCHESTER, KY, p. A260

CLARKE COUNTY HOSPITAL, OSCEOLA, IA, p. A225

CLARKS SUMMIT STATE HOSPITAL, CLARKS SUMMIT, PA, p. A520

CLAXTON–HEPBURN MEDICAL CENTER, OGDENSBURG, NY, p. A439

CLAY COUNTY HOSPITAL, ASHLAND, AL, p. A15

CLAY COUNTY HOSPITAL, FLORA, IL, p. A182

CLAY COUNTY MEDICAL CENTER, CLAY CENTER, KS, p. A231

CLAY COUNTY MEMORIAL HOSPITAL, HENRIETTA, TX, p. A603

CLEAR BROOK LODGE, SHICKSHINNY, PA, p. A538

CLEAR BROOK MANOR, WILKES–BARRE, PA, p. A541

CLEAR LAKE REGIONAL MEDICAL CENTER, WEBSTER, TX, p. A634

CLEARFIELD HOSPITAL, CLEARFIELD, PA, p. A520

CLEARWATER VALLEY HOSPITAL AND CLINICS, OROFINO, ID, p. A169

CLEMENT J. ZABLOCKI VETERANS AFFAIRS MEDICAL CENTER, MILWAUKEE, WI, p. A686

CLEO WALLACE CENTERS HOSPITAL, WESTMINSTER, CO, p. A106

CLEVELAND AREA HOSPITAL, CLEVELAND, OK, p. A495

CLEVELAND CAMPUS, CLEVELAND, OHIO (see NORTHCOAST BEHAVIORAL HEALTHCARE SYSTEM), p. A486

CLEVELAND CLINIC CHILDREN'S HOSPITAL, CLEVELAND, OHIO (see CLEVELAND CLINIC FOUNDATION), p. A474

CLEVELAND CLINIC CHILDREN'S HOSPITAL FOR REHABILITATION, CLEVELAND, OH, p. A474

CLEVELAND CLINIC FLORIDA, WESTON, FL, p. A143

CLEVELAND CLINIC FOUNDATION, CLEVELAND, OH, p. A474

CLEVELAND REGIONAL MEDICAL CENTER, SHELBY, NC, p. A460

CLEVELAND REGIONAL MEDICAL CENTER, CLEVELAND, TX, p. A587

CLIFTON SPRINGS HOSPITAL AND CLINIC, CLIFTON SPRINGS, NY, p. A424

CLIFTON T. PERKINS HOSPITAL CENTER, JESSUP, MD, p. A292

CLIFTON–FINE HOSPITAL, STAR LAKE, NY, p. A443

CLINCH MEMORIAL HOSPITAL, HOMERVILLE, GA, p. A154

CLINCH VALLEY MEDICAL CENTER, RICHLANDS, VA, p. A654

CLINICA ESPANOLA, MAYAGUEZ, PR, p. A702

CLINTON COUNTY HOSPITAL, ALBANY, KY, p. A247

CLINTON HOSPITAL, CLINTON, MA, p. A299

CLINTON MEMORIAL HOSPITAL, WILMINGTON, OH, p. A491

CLOUD COUNTY HEALTH CENTER, CONCORDIA, KS, p. A232

CLOVIS COMMUNITY MEDICAL CENTER, CLOVIS, CA, p. A57

COAL COUNTY GENERAL HOSPITAL, COALGATE, OK, p. A495

COALINGA REGIONAL MEDICAL CENTER, COALINGA, CA, p. A58

COAST PLAZA HOSPITAL, NORWALK, CA, p. A77

COASTAL CAROLINA HOSPITAL, HARDEEVILLE, SC, p. A551

COASTAL COMMUNITIES HOSPITAL, SANTA ANA, CA, p. A89

COASTAL HARBOR TREATMENT CENTER, SAVANNAH, GA, p. A159

COBB MEMORIAL HOSPITAL, ROYSTON, GA, p. A158

COBLESKILL REGIONAL HOSPITAL, COBLESKILL, NY, p. A424

COBRE VALLEY REGIONAL MEDICAL CENTER, GLOBE, AZ, p. A33

COCHRAN MEMORIAL HOSPITAL, MORTON, TX, p. A617

COFFEE REGIONAL MEDICAL CENTER, DOUGLAS, GA, p. A151

COFFEY COUNTY HOSPITAL, BURLINGTON, KS, p. A231

COFFEYVILLE REGIONAL MEDICAL CENTER, COFFEYVILLE, KS, p. A231

COGDELL MEMORIAL HOSPITAL, SNYDER, TX, p. A628

COLEMAN COUNTY MEDICAL CENTER, COLEMAN, TX, p. A588

COLER MEMORIAL HOSPITAL, NEW YORK, NEW YORK (see COLER–GOLDWATER SPECIALTY HOSPITAL AND NURSING FACILITY), p. A432

COLER–GOLDWATER SPECIALTY HOSPITAL AND NURSING FACILITY, NEW YORK, NY, p. A432

COLISEUM MEDICAL CENTERS, MACON, GA, p. A155

COLISEUM NORTHSIDE HOSPITAL, MACON, GA, p. A155

COLISEUM PSYCHIATRIC CENTER, MACON, GA, p. A155

COLLEGE HOSPITAL, CERRITOS, CA, p. A57

COLLEGE HOSPITAL COSTA MESA, COSTA MESA, CA, p. A58

COLLEGE STATION MEDICAL CENTER, COLLEGE STATION, TX, p. A588

COLLETON MEDICAL CENTER, WALTERBORO, SC, p. A554

COLLINGSWORTH GENERAL HOSPITAL, WELLINGTON, TX, p. A634

COLMERY–O'NEIL VETERANS AFFAIRS MEDICAL CENTER, TOPEKA, KANSAS (see VETERANS AFFAIRS EASTERN KANSAS HEALTH CARE SYSTEM), p. A244

COLONEL FLORENCE A. BLANCHFIELD ARMY COMMUNITY HOSPITAL, FORT CAMPBELL, KY, p. A250

COLORADO ACUTE LONG TERM HOSPITAL, DENVER, CO, p. A99

COLORADO MENTAL HEALTH INSTITUTE AT FORT LOGAN, DENVER, CO, p. A99

COLORADO MENTAL HEALTH INSTITUTE AT PUEBLO, PUEBLO, CO, p. A105

COLORADO PLAINS MEDICAL CENTER, FORT MORGAN, CO, p. A101

COLORADO RIVER MEDICAL CENTER, NEEDLES, CA, p. A76

COLORADO WEST PSYCHIATRIC HOSPITAL, GRAND JUNCTION, CO, p. A101

COLORADO–FAYETTE MEDICAL CENTER, WEIMAR, TX, p. A634

COLQUITT REGIONAL MEDICAL CENTER, MOULTRIE, GA, p. A157

COLUMBIA BASIN HOSPITAL, EPHRATA, WA, p. A661

COLUMBIA CENTER, MEQUON, WI, p. A686

COLUMBIA HOSPITAL, WEST PALM BEACH, FL, p. A142

COLUMBIA MEMORIAL HOSPITAL, HUDSON, NY, p. A427

COLUMBIA MEMORIAL HOSPITAL, ASTORIA, OR, p. A509

COLUMBIA ST. MARY'S COLUMBIA HOSPITAL, MILWAUKEE, WISCONSIN (see COLUMBIA ST. MARY'S HOSPITAL MILWAUKEE), p. A686

COLUMBIA ST. MARY'S HOSPITAL MILWAUKEE, MILWAUKEE, WI, p. A686

COLUMBIA ST. MARY'S MILWAUKEE HOSPITAL, MILWAUKEE, WISCONSIN (see COLUMBIA ST. MARY'S HOSPITAL MILWAUKEE), p. A686

COLUMBIA ST. MARY'S OZAUKEE HOSPITAL, MEQUON, WI, p. A686

COLUMBUS COMMUNITY HOSPITAL, COLUMBUS, NE, p. A382

COLUMBUS COMMUNITY HOSPITAL, COLUMBUS, TX, p. A588

COLUMBUS COMMUNITY HOSPITAL, COLUMBUS, WI, p. A680

COLUMBUS REGIONAL HEALTHCARE SYSTEM, WHITEVILLE, NC, p. A462

COLUMBUS REGIONAL HOSPITAL, COLUMBUS, IN, p. A199

COLUMBUS SPECIALTY HOSPITAL, COLUMBUS, GA, p. A149

COLUSA REGIONAL MEDICAL CENTER, COLUSA, CA, p. A58

COMANCHE COUNTY HOSPITAL, COLDWATER, KS, p. A231

COMANCHE COUNTY MEDICAL CENTER, COMANCHE, TX, p. A588

COMANCHE COUNTY MEMORIAL HOSPITAL, LAWTON, OK, p. A498

COMMONWEALTH CENTER FOR CHILDREN AND ADOLESCENTS, STAUNTON, VA, p. A656

COMMONWEALTH HEALTH CENTER, SAIPAN, MP, p. A699

COMMONWEALTH REGIONAL SPECIALTY HOSPITAL, BOWLING GREEN, KY, p. A247

COMMUNITY BEHAVIORAL HEALTH CENTER, FRESNO, CA, p. A62

COMMUNITY BEHAVIORAL HEALTH HOSPITAL – ALEXANDRIA, ALEXANDRIA, MN, p. A327

COMMUNITY BEHAVIORAL HEALTH HOSPITAL – ANNANDALE, ANNANDALE, MN, p. A327

COMMUNITY BEHAVIORAL HEALTH HOSPITAL – BAXTER, BAXTER, MN, p. A328

COMMUNITY BEHAVIORAL HEALTH HOSPITAL – BEMIDJI, BEMIDJI, MN, p. A328

COMMUNITY BEHAVIORAL HEALTH HOSPITAL – FERGUS FALLS, FERGUS FALLS, MN, p. A331

COMMUNITY BEHAVIORAL HEALTH HOSPITAL – ROCHESTER, ROCHESTER, MN, p. A338

COMMUNITY BEHAVIORAL HEALTH HOSPITAL – ST. PETER, SAINT PETER, MN, p. A339

COMMUNITY CARE HOSPITAL, NEW ORLEANS, LA, p. A274

COMMUNITY GENERAL HEALTH CENTER, FORT FAIRFIELD, MAINE (see THE AROOSTOOK MEDICAL CENTER), p. A285

COMMUNITY GENERAL HOSPITAL, DILLEY, TX, p. A594

COMMUNITY HEALTH CARE SYSTEM, ONAGA, KS, p. A240

COMMUNITY HEALTH CENTER OF BRANCH COUNTY, COLDWATER, MI, p. A310

COMMUNITY HOSPITAL, TALLASSEE, AL, p. A26

COMMUNITY HOSPITAL, GRAND JUNCTION, CO, p. A101

COMMUNITY HOSPITAL, MUNSTER, IN, p. A209

COMMUNITY HOSPITAL, MCCOOK, NE, p. A386

COMMUNITY HOSPITAL, OKLAHOMA CITY, OK, p. A500

COMMUNITY HOSPITAL, TORRINGTON, WY, p. A698

COMMUNITY HOSPITAL, HARRISBURG, PENNSYLVANIA (see PINNACLE HEALTH SYSTEM), p. A524

COMMUNITY HOSPITAL AT DOBBS FERRY, DOBBS FERRY, NY, p. A425

COMMUNITY HOSPITAL EAST, INDIANAPOLIS, IN, p. A204

COMMUNITY HOSPITAL NORTH, INDIANAPOLIS, IN, p. A204

COMMUNITY HOSPITAL OF ANACONDA, ANACONDA, MT, p. A373

COMMUNITY HOSPITAL OF ANDERSON AND MADISON COUNTY, ANDERSON, IN, p. A197

COMMUNITY HOSPITAL OF BREMEN, BREMEN, IN, p. A198

COMMUNITY HOSPITAL OF HUNTINGTON PARK, HUNTINGTON PARK, CA, p. A65

COMMUNITY HOSPITAL OF LONG BEACH, LONG BEACH, CA, p. A68

COMMUNITY HOSPITAL OF SAN BERNARDINO, SAN BERNARDINO, CA, p. A84

COMMUNITY HOSPITAL OF THE MONTEREY PENINSULA, MONTEREY, CA, p. A75

COMMUNITY HOSPITAL SOUTH, INDIANAPOLIS, IN, p. A204

COMMUNITY HOSPITAL–FAIRFAX, FAIRFAX, MO, p. A359

COMMUNITY HOSPITALS AND WELLNESS CENTERS, BRYAN, OH, p. A471

COMMUNITY HOSPITALS AND WELLNESS CENTERS–MONTPELIER, MONTPELIER, OH, p. A485

COMMUNITY HOWARD REGIONAL HOSPITAL, KOKOMO, IN, p. A206

COMMUNITY HOWARD SPECIALTY HOSPITAL, KOKOMO, IN, p. A206

COMMUNITY MEDICAL CENTER, MISSOULA, MT, p. A377

COMMUNITY MEDICAL CENTER, FALLS CITY, NE, p. A383

COMMUNITY MEDICAL CENTER, TOMS RIVER, NJ, p. A411

COMMUNITY MEDICAL CENTER OF IZARD COUNTY, CALICO ROCK, AR, p. A42

COMMUNITY MEMORIAL HEALTH SYSTEM, VENTURA, CA, p. A94

COMMUNITY MEMORIAL HEALTHCARE, MARYSVILLE, KS, p. A238

COMMUNITY MEMORIAL HEALTHCENTER, SOUTH HILL, VA, p. A656

COMMUNITY MEMORIAL HOSPITAL, VENTURA, CALIFORNIA (see COMMUNITY MEMORIAL HEALTH SYSTEM), p. A94

COMMUNITY MEMORIAL HOSPITAL, STAUNTON, IL, p. A194

COMMUNITY MEMORIAL HOSPITAL, SUMNER, IA, p. A227

COMMUNITY MEMORIAL HOSPITAL, CLOQUET, MN, p. A329

COMMUNITY MEMORIAL HOSPITAL, SYRACUSE, NE, p. A390

COMMUNITY MEMORIAL HOSPITAL, HAMILTON, NY, p. A427

COMMUNITY MEMORIAL HOSPITAL, TURTLE LAKE, ND, p. A468

COMMUNITY MEMORIAL HOSPITAL, HICKSVILLE, OH, p. A481

COMMUNITY MEMORIAL HOSPITAL, BURKE, SD, p. A555

COMMUNITY MEMORIAL HOSPITAL, REDFIELD, SD, p. A559

COMMUNITY MEMORIAL HOSPITAL, MENOMONEE FALLS, WI, p. A685

COMMUNITY MEMORIAL HOSPITAL, OCONTO FALLS, WI, p. A688

COMMUNITY MENTAL HEALTH CENTER, LAWRENCEBURG, IN, p. A207

COMMUNITY REGIONAL MEDICAL CENTER, FRESNO, CA, p. A62

COMMUNITY SPECIALTY HOSPITAL, LAFAYETTE, LA, p. A270

COMMUNITY WESTVIEW HOSPITAL, INDIANAPOLIS, IN, p. A204

COMPASS BEHAVIORAL CENTER OF CROWLEY, CROWLEY, LA, p. A265

COMPLEX CARE HOSPITAL AT RIDGELAKE, SARASOTA, FL, p. A138

COMPLEX CARE HOSPITAL AT TENAYA, LAS VEGAS, NV, p. A392

COMPLEX CARE HOSPITAL OF IDAHO, MERIDIAN, ID, p. A169

CONCHO COUNTY HOSPITAL, EDEN, TX, p. A595

CONCORD HOSPITAL, CONCORD, NH, p. A397

CONCOURSE DIVISION, NEW YORK (see BRONX–LEBANON HOSPITAL CENTER HEALTH CARE SYSTEM), p. A431

CONE HEALTH, GREENSBORO, NC, p. A454

CONEJOS COUNTY HOSPITAL, LA JARA, CO, p. A103

DELTA COUNTY MEMORIAL HOSPITAL, DELTA, CO, p. A99
DELTA MEDICAL CENTER, MEMPHIS, TN, p. A571
DELTA MEMORIAL HOSPITAL, DUMAS, AR, p. A44
DELTA REGIONAL MEDICAL CENTER, GREENVILLE, MS, p. A346
DENTON REGIONAL MEDICAL CENTER, DENTON, TX, p. A593
DENVER HEALTH MEDICAL CENTER, DENVER, CO, p. A99
DEPAUL CENTER, WACO, TEXAS (see PROVIDENCE HEALTH CENTER), p. A633
DEQUINCY MEMORIAL HOSPITAL, DEQUINCY, LA, p. A266
DES MOINES DIVISION, DES MOINES, IOWA (see VETERANS AFFAIRS CENTRAL IOWA HEALTH CARE SYSTEM), p. A218
DES PERES HOSPITAL, SAINT LOUIS, MO, p. A368
DESERT REGIONAL MEDICAL CENTER, PALM SPRINGS, CA, p. A78
DESERT SPRINGS HOSPITAL MEDICAL CENTER, LAS VEGAS, NV, p. A392
DESERT VALLEY HOSPITAL, VICTORVILLE, CA, p. A95
DESERT VIEW HOSPITAL, PAHRUMP, NV, p. A395
DESERT WILLOW TREATMENT CENTER, LAS VEGAS, NV, p. A392
DESOTO MEMORIAL HOSPITAL, ARCADIA, FL, p. A118
DETAR HEALTHCARE SYSTEM, VICTORIA, TX, p. A633
DETAR HOSPITAL NORTH, VICTORIA, TEXAS (see DETAR HEALTHCARE SYSTEM), p. A633
DETROIT RECEIVING HOSPITAL/UNIVERSITY HEALTH CENTER, DETROIT, MI, p. A310
DETTMER HOSPITAL, TROY, OHIO (see UPPER VALLEY MEDICAL CENTER), p. A490
DEVEREUX CHILDREN'S BEHAVIORAL HEALTH CENTER, MALVERN, PA, p. A528
DEVEREUX GEORGIA TREATMENT NETWORK, KENNESAW, GA, p. A154
DEVEREUX HOSPITAL AND CHILDREN'S CENTER OF FLORIDA, MELBOURNE, FL, p. A130
DEVEREUX TEXAS TREATMENT NETWORK, LEAGUE CITY, TX, p. A612
DEWITT ARMY COMMUNITY HOSPITAL, FORT BELVOIR, VA, p. A648
DEWITT HOSPITAL, DE WITT, AR, p. A44
DIAMOND GROVE CENTER FOR CHILDREN AND ADOLESCENTS, LOUISVILLE, MS, p. A349
DICKENSON COMMUNITY HOSPITAL, CLINTWOOD, VA, p. A647
DICKINSON COUNTY HEALTHCARE SYSTEM, IRON MOUNTAIN, MI, p. A315
DILEY RIDGE MEDICAL CENTER, CANAL WINCHESTER, OH, p. A472
DIMMIT COUNTY MEMORIAL HOSPITAL, CARRIZO SPRINGS, TX, p. A586
DISNEY CHILDREN'S HOSPITAL, ORLANDO, FLORIDA (see FLORIDA HOSPITAL), p. A134
DISTRICT ONE HOSPITAL, FARIBAULT, MN, p. A331
DIVINE PROVIDENCE HOSPITAL, WILLIAMSPORT, PA, p. A542
DIVINE SAVIOR HEALTHCARE, PORTAGE, WI, p. A689
DIVISION OF ADOLESCENT MEDICINE, CINCINNATI CENTER FOR DEVELOPMENTAL DISORDERS, AND CONVALESCENT HOSPITAL FOR CHILDREN, CHILDREN'S HOSPITAL, CINCINNATI, OHIO (see CINCINNATI CHILDREN'S HOSPITAL MEDICAL CENTER), p. A473
DIXIE REGIONAL MEDICAL CENTER, SAINT GEORGE, UT, p. A640
DIXIE REGIONAL MEDICAL CENTER, ST. GEORGE, UTAH (see DIXIE REGIONAL MEDICAL CENTER), p. A640
DMC SURGERY HOSPITAL, MADISON HEIGHTS, MICHIGAN (see HARPER UNIVERSITY HOSPITAL/HUTZEL WOMEN'S HOSPITAL), p. A310
DOCTOR'S CENTER OF BAYAMON, BAYAMON, PR, p. A700
DOCTOR'S HOSPITAL, LEAWOOD, KS, p. A237
DOCTOR'S HOSPITAL – TIDWELL, HOUSTON, TX, p. A604
DOCTOR'S HOSPITAL AND NEUROMUSCULAR CENTER, BREMEN, IN, p. A198
DOCTOR'S HOSPITAL AT RENAISSANCE, EDINBURG, TX, p. A595
DOCTOR'S HOSPITAL OF DEER CREEK, LEESVILLE, LA, p. A271
DOCTOR'S MEMORIAL HOSPITAL, PERRY, FL, p. A136
DOCTORS CENTER, MANATI, PR, p. A701
DOCTORS COMMUNITY HOSPITAL, LANHAM, MD, p. A292
DOCTORS DIAGNOSTIC HOSPITAL, CLEVELAND, TX, p. A587
DOCTORS HOSPITAL, AUGUSTA, GA, p. A146
DOCTORS HOSPITAL, COLUMBUS, OH, p. A476
DOCTORS HOSPITAL AT WHITE ROCK LAKE, DALLAS, TX, p. A591
DOCTORS HOSPITAL NELSONVILLE, NELSONVILLE, OH, p. A486
DOCTORS HOSPITAL OF COLUMBUS, COLUMBUS, GA, p. A149
DOCTORS HOSPITAL OF JEFFERSON, METAIRIE, LOUISIANA (see EAST JEFFERSON GENERAL HOSPITAL), p. A273
DOCTORS HOSPITAL OF LAREDO, LAREDO, TX, p. A612
DOCTORS HOSPITAL OF MANTECA, MANTECA, CA, p. A73
DOCTORS HOSPITAL OF SARASOTA, SARASOTA, FL, p. A138
DOCTORS HOSPITAL OF TATTNALL, REIDSVILLE, GA, p. A157

DOCTORS HOSPITAL OF WEST COVINA, WEST COVINA, CA, p. A95
DOCTORS HOSPITAL PARKWAY, HOUSTON, TEXAS (see DOCTOR'S HOSPITAL – TIDWELL), p. A604
DOCTORS MEDICAL CENTER, MODESTO, CA, p. A75
DOCTORS MEDICAL CENTER–SAN PABLO CAMPUS, SAN PABLO, CA, p. A89
DOCTORS MEMORIAL HOSPITAL, BONIFAY, FL, p. A119
DOCTORS' CENTER HOSPITAL SAN JUAN, SAN JUAN, PR, p. A703
DOCTORS' HOSPITAL OF MICHIGAN, PONTIAC, MI, p. A320
DODGE COUNTY HOSPITAL, EASTMAN, GA, p. A152
DOERNBECHER CHILDREN'S HOSPITAL, PORTLAND, OREGON (see OHSU HOSPITAL), p. A514
DOMINICAN HOSPITAL, SANTA CRUZ, CA, p. A90
DOMINION HOSPITAL, FALLS CHURCH, VA, p. A647
DONALSONVILLE HOSPITAL, DONALSONVILLE, GA, p. A151
DORCHESTER GENERAL HOSPITAL, CAMBRIDGE, MD, p. A290
DORMINY MEDICAL CENTER, FITZGERALD, GA, p. A152
DOROTHEA DIX HOSPITAL, RALEIGH, NC, p. A459
DOROTHEA DIX PSYCHIATRIC CENTER, BANGOR, ME, p. A281
DOUGLAS COUNTY COMMUNITY MENTAL HEALTH CENTER, OMAHA, NE, p. A388
DOUGLAS COUNTY HOSPITAL, ALEXANDRIA, MN, p. A327
DOUGLAS COUNTY MEMORIAL HOSPITAL, ARMOUR, SD, p. A555
DOVER BEHAVIORAL HEALTH SYSTEM, DOVER, DE, p. A114
DOWN EAST COMMUNITY HOSPITAL, MACHIAS, ME, p. A284
DOWNEY REGIONAL MEDICAL CENTER, DOWNEY, CA, p. A59
DOYLESTOWN HOSPITAL, DOYLESTOWN, PA, p. A522
DR. DAN C. TRIGG MEMORIAL HOSPITAL, TUCUMCARI, NM, p. A418
DR. J. CORRIGAN MENTAL HEALTH CENTER, FALL RIVER, MA, p. A299
DR. JOHN WARNER HOSPITAL, CLINTON, IL, p. A179
DR. PILA'S HOSPITAL, PONCE, PR, p. A702
DR. RAMON E. BETANCES HOSPITAL–MAYAGUEZ MEDICAL CENTER BRANCH, MAYAGUEZ, PR, p. A702
DR. SOLOMON CARTER FULLER MENTAL HEALTH CENTER, BOSTON, MA, p. A296
DRAKE CENTER, CINCINNATI, OH, p. A473
DREW MEMORIAL HOSPITAL, MONTICELLO, AR, p. A49
DRISCOLL CHILDREN'S HOSPITAL, CORPUS CHRISTI, TX, p. A589
DRUMRIGHT REGIONAL HOSPITAL, DRUMRIGHT, OK, p. A495
DUANE L. WATERS HOSPITAL, JACKSON, MI, p. A316
DUBLIN METHODIST HOSPITAL, DUBLIN, OH, p. A479
DUBOIS REGIONAL MEDICAL CENTER, DU BOIS, PA, p. A522
DUBUIS HOSPITAL OF ALEXANDRIA, ALEXANDRIA, LA, p. A261
DUBUIS HOSPITAL OF BEAUMONT, BEAUMONT, TX, p. A583
DUBUIS HOSPITAL OF CORPUS CHRISTI, CORPUS CHRISTI, TX, p. A589
DUBUIS HOSPITAL OF LAKE CHARLES, LAKE CHARLES, LA, p. A271
DUBUIS HOSPITAL OF PARIS, PARIS, TX, p. A620
DUBUIS HOSPITAL OF SHREVEPORT, SHREVEPORT, LA, p. A277
DUBUIS HOSPITAL OF TEXARKANA, TEXARKANA, TX, p. A631
DUKE CHILDREN'S HOSPITAL & HEALTH CENTER, DURHAM, NORTH CAROLINA (see DUKE UNIVERSITY HOSPITAL), p. A452
DUKE RALEIGH HOSPITAL, RALEIGH, NC, p. A459
DUKE UNIVERSITY HOSPITAL, DURHAM, NC, p. A452
DUKES MEMORIAL HOSPITAL, PERU, IN, p. A210
DUNCAN REGIONAL HOSPITAL, DUNCAN, OK, p. A495
DUNDY COUNTY HOSPITAL, BENKELMAN, NE, p. A382
DUPONT HOSPITAL, FORT WAYNE, IN, p. A201
DURHAM REGIONAL HOSPITAL, DURHAM, NC, p. A452
DURHAM VETERANS AFFAIRS MEDICAL CENTER, DURHAM, NC, p. A452
DWIGHT D. EISENHOWER VETERANS AFFAIRS MEDICAL CENTER, LEAVENWORTH, KANSAS (see VETERANS AFFAIRS EASTERN KANSAS HEALTH CARE SYSTEM), p. A244
DWIGHT DAVID EISENHOWER ARMY MEDICAL CENTER, FORT GORDON, GA, p. A153
DYERSBURG REGIONAL MEDICAL CENTER, DYERSBURG, TN, p. A565

# E

E. A. CONWAY MEDICAL CENTER, MONROE, LA, p. A273
EAGLE RIVER MEMORIAL HOSPITAL, EAGLE RIVER, WI, p. A680
EAGLEVILLE HOSPITAL, EAGLEVILLE, PA, p. A522
EARL K. LONG MEDICAL CENTER, BATON ROUGE, LA, p. A262
EARLE E. MORRIS ALCOHOL AND DRUG TREATMENT CENTER, COLUMBIA, SC, p. A548
EAST ADAMS RURAL HOSPITAL, RITZVILLE, WA, p. A665

EAST ALABAMA MEDICAL CENTER, OPELIKA, AL, p. A24
EAST CAMPUS, NORFOLK, NEBRASKA (see FAITH REGIONAL HEALTH SERVICES), p. A386
EAST CARROLL PARISH HOSPITAL, LAKE PROVIDENCE, LA, p. A271
EAST CENTRAL REGIONAL HOSPITAL, AUGUSTA, GA, p. A146
EAST CENTRAL REGIONAL HOSPITAL, GRACEWOOD, GEORGIA (see EAST CENTRAL REGIONAL HOSPITAL), p. A146
EAST COOPER MEDICAL CENTER, MOUNT PLEASANT, SC, p. A552
EAST EL PASO PHYSICIANS MEDICAL CENTER, EL PASO, TX, p. A596
EAST GEORGIA REGIONAL MEDICAL CENTER, STATESBORO, GA, p. A160
EAST HOUSTON REGIONAL MEDICAL CENTER, HOUSTON, TEXAS (see BAYSHORE MEDICAL CENTER), p. A620
EAST JEFFERSON GENERAL HOSPITAL, METAIRIE, LA, p. A273
EAST LIVERPOOL CITY HOSPITAL, EAST LIVERPOOL, OH, p. A479
EAST LOS ANGELES DOCTORS HOSPITAL, LOS ANGELES, CA, p. A69
EAST MISSISSIPPI STATE HOSPITAL, MERIDIAN, MS, p. A350
EAST MORGAN COUNTY HOSPITAL, BRUSH, CO, p. A98
EAST MOUNTAIN HOSPITAL, BELLE MEAD, NJ, p. A401
EAST OHIO REGIONAL HOSPITAL, MARTINS FERRY, OH, p. A484
EAST ORANGE DIVISION, EAST ORANGE, NEW JERSEY (see VETERANS AFFAIRS NEW JERSEY HEALTH CARE SYSTEM), p. A403
EAST ORANGE GENERAL HOSPITAL, EAST ORANGE, NJ, p. A403
EAST RIDGE HOSPITAL, EAST RIDGE, TENNESSEE (see PARKRIDGE MEDICAL CENTER), p. A563
EAST TENNESSEE CHILDREN'S HOSPITAL, KNOXVILLE, TN, p. A568
EAST TEXAS MEDICAL CENTER ATHENS, ATHENS, TX, p. A580
EAST TEXAS MEDICAL CENTER BEHAVIORAL HEALTH CENTER, TYLER, TEXAS (see EAST TEXAS MEDICAL CENTER TYLER), p. A632
EAST TEXAS MEDICAL CENTER CARTHAGE, CARTHAGE, TX, p. A586
EAST TEXAS MEDICAL CENTER CLARKSVILLE, CLARKSVILLE, TX, p. A587
EAST TEXAS MEDICAL CENTER CROCKETT, CROCKETT, TX, p. A589
EAST TEXAS MEDICAL CENTER FAIRFIELD, FAIRFIELD, TX, p. A597
EAST TEXAS MEDICAL CENTER HENDERSON, HENDERSON, TX, p. A603
EAST TEXAS MEDICAL CENTER JACKSONVILLE, JACKSONVILLE, TX, p. A609
EAST TEXAS MEDICAL CENTER PITTSBURG, PITTSBURG, TX, p. A620
EAST TEXAS MEDICAL CENTER REHABILITATION CENTER, TYLER, TX, p. A632
EAST TEXAS MEDICAL CENTER SPECIALTY HOSPITAL, TYLER, TX, p. A632
EAST TEXAS MEDICAL CENTER TRINITY, TRINITY, TX, p. A631
EAST TEXAS MEDICAL CENTER TYLER, TYLER, TX, p. A632
EAST TEXAS MEDICAL CENTER–GILMER, GILMER, TX, p. A601
EAST TEXAS MEDICAL CENTER–MOUNT VERNON, MOUNT VERNON, TX, p. A617
EAST TEXAS MEDICAL CENTER–QUITMAN, QUITMAN, TX, p. A622
EAST VALLEY HOSPITAL MEDICAL CENTER, GLENDORA, CA, p. A63
EASTERN IDAHO REGIONAL MEDICAL CENTER, IDAHO FALLS, ID, p. A168
EASTERN LONG ISLAND HOSPITAL, GREENPORT, NY, p. A427
EASTERN LOUISIANA MENTAL HEALTH SYSTEM, JACKSON, LA, p. A268
EASTERN MAINE MEDICAL CENTER, BANGOR, ME, p. A281
EASTERN NEW MEXICO MEDICAL CENTER, ROSWELL, NM, p. A417
EASTERN NIAGARA HEALTH SYSTEM, LOCKPORT, NY, p. A429
EASTERN NIAGARA HOSPITAL INTER–COMMUNITY, NEWFANE, NEW YORK (see EASTERN NIAGARA HEALTH SYSTEM), p. A429
EASTERN NIAGARA HOSPITAL LOCKPORT, LOCKPORT, NEW YORK (see EASTERN NIAGARA HEALTH SYSTEM), p. A429
EASTERN OKLAHOMA MEDICAL CENTER, POTEAU, OK, p. A503
EASTERN PLUMAS HEALTH CARE DISTRICT, PORTOLA, CA, p. A81
EASTERN REGIONAL MEDICAL CENTER, PHILADELPHIA, PA, p. A532
EASTERN SHORE HOSPITAL CENTER, CAMBRIDGE, MD, p. A290
EASTERN STATE HOSPITAL, LEXINGTON, KY, p. A253
EASTERN STATE HOSPITAL, WILLIAMSBURG, VA, p. A657
EASTERN STATE HOSPITAL, MEDICAL LAKE, WA, p. A662
EASTLAND MEMORIAL HOSPITAL, EASTLAND, TX, p. A595

EASTON HOSPITAL, EASTON, PA, p. A522

EASTSIDE MEDICAL CENTER, SNELLVILLE, GA, p. A159

EASTSIDE PSYCHIATRIC HOSPITAL, TALLAHASSEE, FL, p. A140

EATON RAPIDS MEDICAL CENTER, EATON RAPIDS, MI, p. A312

ED FRASER MEMORIAL HOSPITAL AND BAKER COMMUNITY HEALTH CENTER, MACCLENNY, FL, p. A129

EDDY COHOES REHABILITATION CENTER, COHOES, NY, p. A424

EDEN MEDICAL CENTER, CASTRO VALLEY, CA, p. A56

EDGEFIELD COUNTY HOSPITAL, EDGEFIELD, SC, p. A549

EDGERTON HOSPITAL AND HEALTH SERVICES, EDGERTON, WI, p. A681

EDGEWOOD SURGICAL HOSPITAL, TRANSFER, PA, p. A539

EDINBURG CHILDREN'S HOSPITAL, EDINBURG, TEXAS (see SOUTH TEXAS HEALTH SYSTEM), p. A595

EDINBURG REGIONAL MEDICAL CENTER, EDINBURG, TEXAS (see SOUTH TEXAS HEALTH SYSTEM), p. A595

EDITH NOURSE ROGERS MEMORIAL VETERANS HOSPITAL, BEDFORD, MA, p. A295

EDWARD HOSPITAL, NAPERVILLE, IL, p. A189

EDWARD JOHN NOBLE HOSPITAL OF GOUVERNEUR, GOUVERNEUR, NY, p. A427

EDWARD WHITE HOSPITAL, SAINT PETERSBURG, FL, p. A138

EDWARDS COUNTY HOSPITAL AND HEALTHCARE CENTER, KINSLEY, KS, p. A236

EDWIN SHAW REHAB, CUYAHOGA FALLS, OH, p. A478

EFFINGHAM HOSPITAL, SPRINGFIELD, GA, p. A159

EINSTEIN MEDICAL CENTER ELKINS PARK, ELKINS PARK, PENNSYLVANIA (see EINSTEIN MEDICAL CENTER PHILADELPHIA), A532

EINSTEIN MEDICAL CENTER PHILADELPHIA, PHILADELPHIA, PA, p. A532

EISENHOWER MEDICAL CENTER, RANCHO MIRAGE, CA, p. A81

EL CAMINO HOSPITAL, MOUNTAIN VIEW, CA, p. A76

EL CAMINO HOSPITAL LOS GATOS, LOS GATOS, CALIFORNIA (see EL CAMINO HOSPITAL), p. A76

EL CAMPO MEMORIAL HOSPITAL, EL CAMPO, TX, p. A595

EL CENTRO REGIONAL MEDICAL CENTER, EL CENTRO, CA, p. A60

EL PASO CHILDREN'S HOSPITAL, EL PASO, TX, p. A596

EL PASO LTAC HOSPITAL, EL PASO, TX, p. A596

EL PASO PSYCHIATRIC CENTER, EL PASO, TX, p. A596

EL PASO SPECIALTY HOSPITAL, EL PASO, TX, p. A596

ELBA GENERAL HOSPITAL, ELBA, AL, p. A19

ELBERT MEMORIAL HOSPITAL, ELBERTON, GA, p. A152

ELEANOR SLATER HOSPITAL, CRANSTON, RI, p. A544

ELECTRA MEMORIAL HOSPITAL, ELECTRA, TX, p. A597

ELGIN MENTAL HEALTH CENTER, ELGIN, IL, p. A180

ELIZA COFFEE MEMORIAL HOSPITAL, FLORENCE, AL, p. A20

ELIZABETHTOWN COMMUNITY HOSPITAL, ELIZABETHTOWN, NY, p. A425

ELK REGIONAL HEALTH CENTER, SAINT MARYS, PA, p. A537

ELKHART GENERAL HEALTHCARE SYSTEM, ELKHART, IN, p. A200

ELKHORN VALLEY REHABILITATION HOSPITAL, CASPER, WY, p. A695

ELKS REHAB HOSPITAL, BOISE, ID, p. A166

ELKVIEW GENERAL HOSPITAL, HOBART, OK, p. A497

ELLENVILLE REGIONAL HOSPITAL, ELLENVILLE, NY, p. A425

ELLETT MEMORIAL HOSPITAL, APPLETON CITY, MO, p. A355

ELLINWOOD DISTRICT HOSPITAL, ELLINWOOD, KS, p. A232

ELLIOT HOSPITAL, MANCHESTER, NH, p. A399

ELLIS FISCHEL CANCER CENTER, COLUMBIA, MISSOURI (see UNIVERSITY OF MISSOURI HOSPITALS AND CLINICS), p. A358

ELLIS HOSPITAL, SCHENECTADY, NY, p. A443

ELLIS HOSPITAL HEALTH CENTER, SCHENECTADY, NEW YORK (see ELLIS HOSPITAL), p. A443

ELLSWORTH COUNTY MEDICAL CENTER, ELLSWORTH, KS, p. A232

ELLSWORTH MUNICIPAL HOSPITAL, IOWA FALLS, IA, p. A222

ELLWOOD CITY HOSPITAL, ELLWOOD CITY, PA, p. A522

ELMHURST HOSPITAL CENTER,, NY, p. A432

ELMHURST MEMORIAL HOSPITAL,, IL, p. A181

ELMIRA PSYCHIATRIC CENTER, ELMIRA, NY, p. A426

ELMORE COMMUNITY HOSPITAL, WETUMPKA, AL, p. A27

ELMORE MEDICAL CENTER, MOUNTAIN HOME, ID, p. A169

ELY–BLOOMENSON COMMUNITY HOSPITAL, ELY, MN, p. A331

EMANUEL MEDICAL CENTER, TURLOCK, CA, p. A93

EMANUEL MEDICAL CENTER, SWAINSBORO, GA, p. A160

EMERALD COAST BEHAVIORAL HOSPITAL, PANAMA CITY, FL, p. A135

EMERALD–HODGSON HOSPITAL, SEWANEE, TENNESSEE (see SOUTHERN TENNESSEE MEDICAL CENTER), p. A576

EMERSON HOSPITAL, CONCORD, MA, p. A299

EMH ELYRIA MEDICAL CENTER, ELYRIA, OH, p. A480

EMMA PENDLETON BRADLEY HOSPITAL, EAST PROVIDENCE, RI, p. A544

EMORY JOHNS CREEK HOSPITAL, JOHNS CREEK, GA, p. A154

EMORY UNIVERSITY HOSPITAL, ATLANTA, GA, p. A145

EMORY UNIVERSITY HOSPITAL MIDTOWN, ATLANTA, GA, p. A145

EMORY UNIVERSITY ORTHOPAEDIC AND SPINE HOSPITAL, TUCKER, GEORGIA (see EMORY UNIVERSITY HOSPITAL), p. A145

EMORY–ADVENTIST HOSPITAL, SMYRNA, GA, p. A159

ENCINO HOSPITAL MEDICAL CENTER, CA, p. A69

ENDLESS MOUNTAIN HEALTH SYSTEMS, MONTROSE, PA, p. A529

ENGLEWOOD COMMUNITY HOSPITAL, ENGLEWOOD, FL, p. A122

ENGLEWOOD HOSPITAL AND MEDICAL CENTER, ENGLEWOOD, NJ, p. A404

ENLOE MEDICAL CENTER, CHICO, CA, p. A57

ENLOE MEDICAL CENTER–COHASSET, CHICO, CALIFORNIA (see ENLOE MEDICAL CENTER), p. A57

ENNIS REGIONAL MEDICAL CENTER, ENNIS, TX, p. A597

EPHRAIM MCDOWELL FORT LOGAN HOSPITAL, STANFORD, KY, p. A259

EPHRAIM MCDOWELL REGIONAL MEDICAL CENTER, DANVILLE, KY, p. A249

EPHRATA COMMUNITY HOSPITAL, EPHRATA, PA, p. A523

EPIC MEDICAL CENTER, EUFAULA, OK, p. A496

ERIE COUNTY MEDICAL CENTER, BUFFALO, NY, p. A422

ERIK AND MARGARET JONSSON HOSPITAL, DALLAS, TEXAS (see BAYLOR UNIVERSITY MEDICAL CENTER), p. A590

ERLANGER AT HUTCHESON, FORT OGLETHORPE, GA, p. A153

ERLANGER BLEDSOE HOSPITAL, PIKEVILLE, TN, p. A574

ERLANGER EAST HOSPITAL, CHATTANOOGA, TENNESSEE (see ERLANGER MEDICAL CENTER), p. A563

ERLANGER MEDICAL CENTER, CHATTANOOGA, TN, p. A563

ERLANGER NORTH HOSPITAL, CHATTANOOGA, TENNESSEE (see ERLANGER MEDICAL CENTER), p. A563

ESPANOLA HOSPITAL, ESPANOLA, NM, p. A416

ESSENTIA HEALTH ADA, ADA, MN, p. A327

ESSENTIA HEALTH DULUTH, DULUTH, MN, p. A330

ESSENTIA HEALTH FARGO, FARGO, ND, p. A465

ESSENTIA HEALTH FOSSTON, FOSSTON, MN, p. A331

ESSENTIA HEALTH NORTHERN PINES, AURORA, MN, p. A328

ESSENTIA HEALTH SANDSTONE, SANDSTONE, MN, p. A339

ESSENTIA HEALTH ST. JOSEPH'S MEDICAL CENTER, BRAINERD, MN, p. A328

ESSENTIA HEALTH ST. MARY'S HOSPITAL – DETROIT LAKES, DETROIT LAKES, MN, p. A330

ESSENTIA HEALTH ST. MARY'S HOSPITAL OF SUPERIOR, SUPERIOR, WI, p. A692

ESSENTIA HEALTH ST. MARY'S MEDICAL CENTER, DULUTH, MN, p. A330

ESSENTIA HEALTH–HOLY TRINITY HOSPITAL, GRACEVILLE, MN, p. A332

ESSEX COUNTY HOSPITAL CENTER, CEDAR GROVE, NJ, p. A402

ESTES PARK MEDICAL CENTER, ESTES PARK, CO, p. A101

ETHICUS HOSPITAL – GRAPEVINE, GRAPEVINE, TX, p. A601

EUCLID HOSPITAL, EUCLID, OH, p. A480

EUNICE EXTENDED CARE HOSPITAL, EUNICE, LA, p. A266

EUREKA COMMUNITY HEALTH SERVICES AVERA, EUREKA, SD, p. A556

EUREKA SPRINGS HOSPITAL, EUREKA SPRINGS, AR, p. A44

EVANGELICAL COMMUNITY HOSPITAL, LEWISBURG, PA, p. A527

EVANGELINE EXTENDED CARE HOSPITAL–MAMOU, MAMOU, LA, p. A272

EVANS MEMORIAL HOSPITAL, CLAXTON, GA, p. A149

EVANS U. S. ARMY COMMUNITY HOSPITAL, FORT CARSON, CO, p. A101

EVANSTON REGIONAL HOSPITAL, EVANSTON, WY, p. A696

EVANSVILLE PSYCHIATRIC CHILDREN CENTER, EVANSVILLE, IN, p. A201

EVANSVILLE STATE HOSPITAL, EVANSVILLE, IN, p. A201

EVENDALE MEDICAL CENTER, CINCINNATI, OH, p. A473

EVERETT TOWER, OKLAHOMA CITY, OKLAHOMA (see OU MEDICAL CENTER), p. A502

EVERGREEN HOSPITAL MEDICAL CENTER, KIRKLAND, WA, p. A662

EVERGREEN MEDICAL CENTER, EVERGREEN, AL, p. A20

EXCELA FRICK HOSPITAL, MOUNT PLEASANT, PA, p. A530

EXCELA HEALTH WESTMORELAND HOSPITAL, GREENSBURG, PA, p. A524

EXCELA LATROBE AREA HOSPITAL, LATROBE, PA, p. A527

EXCELSIOR SPRINGS HOSPITAL, EXCELSIOR SPRINGS, MO, p. A359

EXEMPLA GOOD SAMARITAN MEDICAL CENTER, LAFAYETTE, CO, p. A103

EXEMPLA LUTHERAN MEDICAL CENTER, WHEAT RIDGE, CO, p. A107

EXEMPLA SAINT JOSEPH HOSPITAL, DENVER, CO, p. A99

EXEMPLA WEST PINES, WHEAT RIDGE, COLORADO (see EXEMPLA LUTHERAN MEDICAL CENTER), p. A107

EXETER HOSPITAL, EXETER, NH, p. A398

EXTENDED CARE OF SOUTHWEST LOUISIANA, LAKE CHARLES, LA, p. A271

EYE AND EAR CLINIC OF CHARLESTON, CHARLESTON, WV, p. A671

EYE AND EAR HOSPITAL OF PITTSBURGH, PITTSBURGH, PENNSYLVANIA (see UPMC PRESBYTERIAN SHADYSIDE), p. A535

# F

F. F. THOMPSON HOSPITAL, CANANDAIGUA, NY, p. A423

F. W. HUSTON MEDICAL CENTER, WINCHESTER, KS, p. A246

FAIR OAKS (see GREENVILLE REGIONAL HOSPITAL), p. A183

FAIR OAKS PAVILION, DELRAY BEACH, FLORIDA (see DELRAY MEDICAL CENTER), p. A122

FAIRBANKS, INDIANAPOLIS, IN, p. A204

FAIRBANKS MEMORIAL HOSPITAL, FAIRBANKS, AK, p. A29

FAIRCHILD MEDICAL CENTER, YREKA, CA, p. A96

FAIRFAX COMMUNITY HOSPITAL, FAIRFAX, OK, p. A496

FAIRFAX HOSPITAL, KIRKLAND, WA, p. A662

FAIRFIELD MEDICAL CENTER, LANCASTER, OH, p. A482

FAIRFIELD MEMORIAL HOSPITAL, FAIRFIELD, IL, p. A182

FAIRFIELD MEMORIAL HOSPITAL, WINNSBORO, SC, p. A554

FAIRLAWN REHABILITATION HOSPITAL, WORCESTER, MA, p. A306

FAIRMONT GENERAL HOSPITAL, FAIRMONT, WV, p. A671

FAIRMOUNT BEHAVIORAL HEALTH SYSTEM, PHILADELPHIA, PA, p. A532

FAIRVIEW HOSPITAL, GREAT BARRINGTON, MA, p. A300

FAIRVIEW HOSPITAL, CLEVELAND, OH, p. A475

FAIRVIEW LAKES HEALTH SERVICES, WYOMING, MN, p. A342

FAIRVIEW NORTHLAND MEDICAL CENTER, PRINCETON, MN, p. A337

FAIRVIEW PARK HOSPITAL, DUBLIN, GA, p. A152

FAIRVIEW REGIONAL MEDICAL CENTER, FAIRVIEW, OK, p. A496

FAIRVIEW RIDGES HOSPITAL, BURNSVILLE, MN, p. A329

FAIRVIEW RIVERSIDE HOSPITAL, MINNEAPOLIS, MINNESOTA (see UNIVERSITY OF MINNESOTA MEDICAL CENTER, FAIRVIEW), p. A335

FAIRVIEW SOUTHDALE HOSPITAL, EDINA, MN, p. A331

FAIRWAY MEDICAL CENTER, COVINGTON, LA, p. A265

FAITH COMMUNITY HOSPITAL, JACKSBORO, TX, p. A609

FAITH REGIONAL HEALTH SERVICES, NORFOLK, NE, p. A386

FALL RIVER HOSPITAL, HOT SPRINGS, SD, p. A557

FALLBROOK HOSPITAL, FALLBROOK, CA, p. A60

FALLON MEDICAL COMPLEX, BAKER, MT, p. A373

FALLS COMMUNITY HOSPITAL AND CLINIC, MARLIN, TX, p. A615

FALMOUTH HOSPITAL, FALMOUTH, MA, p. A300

FAMILY HEALTH WEST, FRUITA, CO, p. A101

FANNIN REGIONAL HOSPITAL, BLUE RIDGE, GA, p. A148

FANNY ALLEN CAMPUS, COLCHESTER, VERMONT (see FLETCHER ALLEN HEALTH CARE), p. A643

FAULKNER HOSPITAL, BOSTON, MA, p. A296

FAULKTON AREA MEDICAL CENTER, FAULKTON, SD, p. A556

FAUQUIER HOSPITAL, WARRENTON, VA, p. A657

FAWCETT MEMORIAL HOSPITAL, PORT CHARLOTTE, FL, p. A136

FAXTON CAMPUS, UTICA, NEW YORK (see FAXTON–ST. LUKE'S HEALTHCARE), p. A445

FAXTON–ST. LUKE'S HEALTHCARE, UTICA, NY, p. A445

FAYETTE COUNTY HOSPITAL, VANDALIA, IL, p. A195

FAYETTE COUNTY MEMORIAL HOSPITAL, WASHINGTON COURT HOUSE, OH, p. A490

FAYETTE MEDICAL CENTER, FAYETTE, AL, p. A20

FAYETTE REGIONAL HEALTH SYSTEM, CONNERSVILLE, IN, p. A199

FEATHER RIVER HOSPITAL, PARADISE, CA, p. A79

FEDERAL CORRECTIONAL INSTITUTE HOSPITAL, LITTLETON, CO, p. A103

FEDERAL MEDICAL CENTER, LEXINGTON, KY, p. A253

FERRELL HOSPITAL, ELDORADO, IL, p. A180

FERRY COUNTY MEMORIAL HOSPITAL, REPUBLIC, WA, p. A665

FHN MEMORIAL HOSPITAL, FREEPORT, IL, p. A182

FIELD MEMORIAL COMMUNITY HOSPITAL, CENTREVILLE, MS, p. A344

FIELDSTONE CENTER, BATTLE CREEK, MICHIGAN (see BRONSON BATTLE CREEK), p. A308

FILLMORE COMMUNITY MEDICAL CENTER, FILLMORE, UT, p. A637

FILLMORE COUNTY HOSPITAL, GENEVA, NE, p. A383

FINLEY HOSPITAL, DUBUQUE, IA, p. A219

FIRELANDS REGIONAL HEALTH SYSTEM, SANDUSKY, OH, p. A488

FIRELANDS REGIONAL MEDICAL CENTER – MAIN CAMPUS, SANDUSKY, OHIO (see FIRELANDS REGIONAL HEALTH SYSTEM), p. A488

FIRELANDS REGIONAL MEDICAL CENTER SOUTH CAMPUS, SANDUSKY, OHIO (see FIRELANDS REGIONAL HEALTH SYSTEM), p. A488
FIRST CARE HEALTH CENTER, PARK RIVER, ND, p. A468
FIRST HOSPITAL PANAMERICANO, CIDRA, PR, p. A700
FIRST HOSPITAL WYOMING VALLEY, WILKES–BARRE, PA, p. A541
FIRST STREET HOSPITAL, BELLAIRE, TX, p. A583
FIRSTHEALTH MONTGOMERY MEMORIAL HOSPITAL, TROY, NC, p. A462
FIRSTHEALTH MOORE REGIONAL HOSPITAL, PINEHURST, NC, p. A458
FIRSTHEALTH RICHMOND MEMORIAL HOSPITAL, ROCKINGHAM, NC, p. A459
FIRSTLIGHT HEALTH SYSTEM, MORA, MN, p. A336
FISHER COUNTY HOSPITAL DISTRICT, ROTAN, TX, p. A623
FISHER–TITUS MEDICAL CENTER, NORWALK, OH, p. A486
FISHERMEN'S HOSPITAL, MARATHON, FL, p. A129
FITZGIBBON HOSPITAL, MARSHALL, MO, p. A364
FIVE RIVERS MEDICAL CENTER, POCAHONTAS, AR, p. A50
FLAGET MEMORIAL HOSPITAL, BARDSTOWN, KY, p. A247
FLAGLER HOSPITAL, SAINT AUGUSTINE, FL, p. A137
FLAGSTAFF MEDICAL CENTER, FLAGSTAFF, AZ, p. A32
FLAMBEAU HOSPITAL, PARK FALLS, WI, p. A689
FLEMING COUNTY HOSPITAL, FLEMINGSBURG, KY, p. A249
FLETCHER ALLEN HEALTH CARE, BURLINGTON, VT, p. A643
FLINT RIVER COMMUNITY HOSPITAL, MONTEZUMA, GA, p. A156
FLORALA MEMORIAL HOSPITAL, FLORALA, AL, p. A20
FLORENCE COMMUNITY HEALTHCARE, FLORENCE, AZ, p. A32
FLORENCE HOSPITAL AT ANTHEM, FLORENCE, AZ, p. A32
FLORIDA HOSPITAL, ORLANDO, FL, p. A134
FLORIDA HOSPITAL AT CONNERTON LONG TERM ACUTE CARE, LAND O'LAKES, FL, p. A128
FLORIDA HOSPITAL CELEBRATION HEALTH, CELEBRATION, FLORIDA (see FLORIDA HOSPITAL), p. A134
FLORIDA HOSPITAL DELAND, DELAND, FL, p. A122
FLORIDA HOSPITAL EAST ORLANDO, ORLANDO, FLORIDA (see FLORIDA HOSPITAL), p. A134
FLORIDA HOSPITAL FISH MEMORIAL, ORANGE CITY, FL, p. A134
FLORIDA HOSPITAL HEARTLAND MEDICAL CENTER, SEBRING, FL, p. A139
FLORIDA HOSPITAL KISSIMMEE, KISSIMMEE, FLORIDA (see FLORIDA HOSPITAL), p. A134
FLORIDA HOSPITAL MEMORIAL MEDICAL CENTER, DAYTONA BEACH, FL, p. A121
FLORIDA HOSPITAL NORTH PINELLAS, TARPON SPRINGS, FL, p. A141
FLORIDA HOSPITAL TAMPA, TAMPA, FL, p. A140
FLORIDA HOSPITAL WATERMAN, TAVARES, FL, p. A141
FLORIDA HOSPITAL WAUCHULA, WAUCHULA, FL, p. A142
FLORIDA HOSPITAL ZEPHYRHILLS, ZEPHYRHILLS, FL, p. A143
FLORIDA HOSPITAL–ALTAMONTE, ALTAMONTE SPRINGS, FLORIDA (see FLORIDA HOSPITAL), p. A134
FLORIDA HOSPITAL–APOPKA, APOPKA, FLORIDA (see FLORIDA HOSPITAL), p. A134
FLORIDA HOSPITAL–CARROLLWOOD, TAMPA, FL, p. A140
FLORIDA HOSPITAL–FLAGLER, PALM COAST, FL, p. A135
FLORIDA HOSPITAL–OCEANSIDE, ORMOND BEACH, FLORIDA (see FLORIDA HOSPITAL MEMORIAL MEDICAL CENTER), p. A121
FLORIDA MEDICAL CENTER, FORT LAUDERDALE, FL, p. A123
FLORIDA STATE HOSPITAL, CHATTAHOOCHEE, FL, p. A120
FLOWERS HOSPITAL, DOTHAN, AL, p. A19
FLOYD COUNTY MEDICAL CENTER, CHARLES CITY, IA, p. A216
FLOYD MEDICAL CENTER, ROME, GA, p. A158
FLOYD MEMORIAL HOSPITAL AND HEALTH SERVICES, NEW ALBANY, IN, p. A209
FLOYD VALLEY HOSPITAL, LE MARS, IA, p. A222
FLUSHING HOSPITAL MEDICAL CENTER,, NY, p. A432
FOCUS HEALTHCARE OF FLORIDA, COOPER CITY, FL, p. A121
FOND DU LAC COUNTY MENTAL HEALTH CENTER, FOND DU LAC, WI, p. A681
FONTANA MEDICAL CENTER, FONTANA, CA, p. A61
FOOTHILL PRESBYTERIAN HOSPITAL, GLENDORA, CA, p. A63
FORBES REGIONAL HOSPITAL, MONROEVILLE, PA, p. A529
FOREST HEALTH MEDICAL CENTER, YPSILANTI, MI, p. A326
FOREST HILLS HOSPITAL,, NY, p. A432
FOREST PARK MEDICAL CENTER, DALLAS, TX, p. A591
FOREST PARK MEDICAL CENTER FRISCO, FRISCO, TX, p. A600
FOREST VIEW PSYCHIATRIC HOSPITAL, GRAND RAPIDS, MI, p. A313
FORKS COMMUNITY HOSPITAL, FORKS, WA, p. A661
FORREST CITY MEDICAL CENTER, FORREST CITY, AR, p. A45
FORREST GENERAL HOSPITAL, HATTIESBURG, MS, p. A346
FORSYTH MEDICAL CENTER, WINSTON–SALEM, NC, p. A463
FORT BELKNAP U. S. PUBLIC HEALTH SERVICE INDIAN HOSPITAL, HARLEM, MT, p. A376
FORT DEFIANCE INDIAN HEALTH SERVICE HOSPITAL, FORT DEFIANCE, AZ, p. A32

FORT DUNCAN REGIONAL MEDICAL CENTER, EAGLE PASS, TX, p. A595
FORT HAMILTON HOSPITAL, HAMILTON, OH, p. A481
FORT HEALTHCARE, FORT ATKINSON, WI, p. A681
FORT LAUDERDALE HOSPITAL, FORT LAUDERDALE, FL, p. A123
FORT LOUDOUN MEDICAL CENTER, LENOIR CITY, TN, p. A569
FORT MADISON COMMUNITY HOSPITAL, FORT MADISON, IA, p. A220
FORT SANDERS REGIONAL MEDICAL CENTER, KNOXVILLE, TN, p. A568
FORT WALTON BEACH MEDICAL CENTER, FORT WALTON BEACH, FL, p. A124
FORT WASHINGTON MEDICAL CENTER, FORT WASHINGTON, MD, p. A291
FOUNDATION SURGICAL HOSPITAL OF SAN ANTONIO, SAN ANTONIO, TX, p. A624
FOUNDATIONS BEHAVIORAL HEALTH, DOYLESTOWN, PA, p. A522
FOUNTAIN VALLEY REGIONAL HOSPITAL AND MEDICAL CENTER, FOUNTAIN VALLEY, CA, p. A61
FOUR WINDS HOSPITAL, KATONAH, NY, p. A428
FOUR WINDS HOSPITAL, SARATOGA SPRINGS, NY, p. A442
FOX CHASE CANCER CENTER–AMERICAN ONCOLOGIC HOSPITAL, PHILADELPHIA, PA, p. A532
FRAMINGHAM UNION HOSPITAL, FRAMINGHAM, MASSACHUSETTS (see METROWEST MEDICAL CENTER), p. A300
FRANCES MAHON DEACONESS HOSPITAL, GLASGOW, MT, p. A375
FRANCISCAN HOSPITAL FOR CHILDREN, BOSTON, MA, p. A296
FRANCISCAN PHYSICIANS HOSPITAL, MUNSTER, IN, p. A209
FRANCISCAN ST. ANTHONY HEALTH – CROWN POINT, CROWN POINT, IN, p. A200
FRANCISCAN ST. ANTHONY HEALTH – MICHIGAN CITY, MICHIGAN CITY, IN, p. A208
FRANCISCAN ST. ELIZABETH HEALTH – CRAWFORDSVILLE, CRAWFORDSVILLE, IN, p. A199
FRANCISCAN ST. ELIZABETH HEALTH – LAFAYETTE CENTRAL, LAFAYETTE, IN, p. A206
FRANCISCAN ST. FRANCIS HEALTH – BEECH GROVE, BEECH GROVE, IN, p. A
FRANCISCAN ST. FRANCIS HEALTH – INDIANAPOLIS, INDIANAPOLIS, IN, p. A204
FRANCISCAN ST. FRANCIS HEALTH – MOORESVILLE, MOORESVILLE, IN, p. A209
FRANCISCAN ST. FRANCIS HEALTH–CARMEL, CARMEL, IN, p. A198
FRANCISCAN ST. JAMES HOSPITAL AND HEALTH CENTERS, OLYMPIA FIELDS, IL, p. A190
FRANCISCAN ST. MARGARET HEALTH – DYER, DYER, INDIANA (see FRANCISCAN ST. MARGARET HEALTH – HAMMOND), p. A203
FRANCISCAN ST. MARGARET HEALTH – HAMMOND, HAMMOND, IN, p. A203
FRANK R. HOWARD MEMORIAL HOSPITAL, WILLITS, CA, p. A96
FRANKFORD CAMPUS, PHILADELPHIA, PENNSYLVANIA (see ARIA HEALTH), p. A531
FRANKFORT REGIONAL MEDICAL CENTER, FRANKFORT, KY, p. A250
FRANKLIN COUNTY MEDICAL CENTER, PRESTON, ID, p. A170
FRANKLIN COUNTY MEMORIAL HOSPITAL, MEADVILLE, MS, p. A350
FRANKLIN COUNTY MEMORIAL HOSPITAL, FRANKLIN, NE, p. A383
FRANKLIN FOUNDATION HOSPITAL, FRANKLIN, LA, p. A266
FRANKLIN GENERAL HOSPITAL, HAMPTON, IA, p. A220
FRANKLIN HOSPITAL, VALLEY STREAM, NY, p. A445
FRANKLIN HOSPITAL DISTRICT, BENTON, IL, p. A173
FRANKLIN MEDICAL CENTER, WINNSBORO, LA, p. A279
FRANKLIN MEMORIAL HOSPITAL, FARMINGTON, ME, p. A283
FRANKLIN REGIONAL HOSPITAL, FRANKLIN, NH, p. A398
FRANKLIN REGIONAL MEDICAL CENTER, LOUISBURG, NC, p. A457
FRANKLIN WOODS COMMUNITY HOSPITAL, JOHNSON CITY, TN, p. A567
FRAZIER REHAB INSTITUTE, LOUISVILLE, KY, p. A254
FREDERICK MEMORIAL HOSPITAL, FREDERICK, MD, p. A291
FREDONIA REGIONAL HOSPITAL, FREDONIA, KS, p. A233
FREEMAN HOSPITAL EAST, JOPLIN, MISSOURI (see FREEMAN HOSPITAL WEST), p. A361
FREEMAN HOSPITAL WEST, JOPLIN, MO, p. A361
FREEMAN NEOSHO HOSPITAL, NEOSHO, MO, p. A366
FREEMAN REGIONAL HEALTH SERVICES, FREEMAN, SD, p. A557
FREMONT AREA MEDICAL CENTER, FREMONT, NE, p. A383
FREMONT HOSPITAL, FREMONT, CA, p. A61
FREMONT MEDICAL CENTER, YUBA CITY, CALIFORNIA (see FREMONT–RIDEOUT HEALTH GROUP), p. A74
FREMONT MEDICAL CENTER, FREMONT, CALIFORNIA (see HAYWARD MEDICAL CENTER), p. A64

FREMONT–RIDEOUT HEALTH GROUP, MARYSVILLE, CA, p. A74
FRENCH HOSPITAL MEDICAL CENTER, SAN LUIS OBISPO, CA, p. A88
FRESNO HEART AND SURGICAL HOSPITAL, FRESNO, CA, p. A62
FRESNO MEDICAL CENTER, FRESNO, CA, p. A62
FRESNO SURGICAL HOSPITAL, FRESNO, CA, p. A62
FRIENDS HOSPITAL, PHILADELPHIA, PA, p. A532
FRIO REGIONAL HOSPITAL, PEARSALL, TX, p. A620
FRISBIE MEMORIAL HOSPITAL, ROCHESTER, NH, p. A400
FROEDTERT MEMORIAL LUTHERAN HOSPITAL, MILWAUKEE, WI, p. A686
FRYE REGIONAL MEDICAL CENTER, HICKORY, NC, p. A455
FRYE REGIONAL MEDICAL CENTER–SOUTH CAMPUS, HICKORY, NORTH CAROLINA (see FRYE REGIONAL MEDICAL CENTER), p. A455
FULTON COUNTY HEALTH CENTER, WAUSEON, OH, p. A491
FULTON COUNTY HOSPITAL, SALEM, AR, p. A51
FULTON COUNTY MEDICAL CENTER, MC CONNELLSBURG, PA, p. A528
FULTON DIVISION,, NEW YORK (see BRONX–LEBANON HOSPITAL CENTER HEALTH CARE SYSTEM), p. A431
FULTON STATE HOSPITAL, FULTON, MO, p. A360

# G

G. WERBER BRYAN PSYCHIATRIC HOSPITAL, COLUMBIA, SC, p. A548
G.V. MONTGOMERY VETERANS AFFAIRS MEDICAL CENTER, JACKSON, MS, p. A347
GADSDEN REGIONAL MEDICAL CENTER, GADSDEN, AL, p. A20
GALESBURG COTTAGE HOSPITAL, GALESBURG, IL, p. A182
GALICHIA HEART HOSPITAL, WICHITA, KANSAS (see WESLEY MEDICAL CENTER), p. A246
GALION COMMUNITY HOSPITAL, GALION, OH, p. A480
GALLUP INDIAN MEDICAL CENTER, GALLUP, NM, p. A416
GARDEN CITY HOSPITAL, GARDEN CITY, MI, p. A313
GARDEN COUNTY HEALTH SERVICES, OSHKOSH, NE, p. A388
GARDEN GROVE HOSPITAL AND MEDICAL CENTER, GARDEN GROVE, CA, p. A63
GARDEN PARK MEDICAL CENTER, GULFPORT, MS, p. A346
GARDENVIEW NURSING HOME (see MINNESOTA VALLEY HEALTH CENTER), p. A333
GARFIELD COUNTY HEALTH CENTER, JORDAN, MT, p. A376
GARFIELD COUNTY PUBLIC HOSPITAL DISTRICT, POMEROY, WA, p. A664
GARFIELD MEDICAL CENTER, MONTEREY PARK, CA, p. A75
GARFIELD MEMORIAL HOSPITAL AND CLINICS, PANGUITCH, UT, p. A639
GARRETT COUNTY MEMORIAL HOSPITAL, OAKLAND, MD, p. A293
GARRISON MEMORIAL HOSPITAL, GARRISON, ND, p. A466
GASTON MEMORIAL HOSPITAL, GASTONIA, NC, p. A453
GATEWAY MEDICAL CENTER, CLARKSVILLE, TN, p. A564
GATEWAY REGIONAL MEDICAL CENTER, GRANITE CITY, IL, p. A183
GATEWAY REHABILITATION HOSPITAL, FLORENCE, KY, p. A249
GATEWAYS HOSPITAL AND MENTAL HEALTH CENTER, LOS ANGELES, CA, p. A69
GAYLORD HOSPITAL, WALLINGFORD, CT, p. A112
GEARY COMMUNITY HOSPITAL, JUNCTION CITY, KS, p. A235
GEISINGER HEALTHSOUTH REHABILITATION HOSPITAL, DANVILLE, PA, p. A521
GEISINGER MEDICAL CENTER, DANVILLE, PA, p. A521
GEISINGER WYOMING VALLEY MEDICAL CENTER, WILKES BARRE, PA, p. A541
GEISINGER–BLOOMSBURG HOSPITAL, BLOOMSBURG, PA, p. A519
GEISINGER–COMMUNITY MEDICAL CENTER, SCRANTON, PA, p. A537
GEISINGER–SHAMOKIN AREA COMMUNITY HOSPITAL, COAL TOWNSHIP, PENNSYLVANIA (see GEISINGER MEDICAL CENTER), p. A521
GENERAL HOSPITAL, CHARLESTON, WEST VIRGINIA (see CHARLESTON AREA MEDICAL CENTER), p. A671
GENERAL HOSPITAL, LOS ANGELES, CALIFORNIA (see LAC/UNIVERSITY OF SOUTHERN CALIFORNIA MEDICAL CENTER), p. A70
GENERAL HOSPITAL, EUREKA, CALIFORNIA (see ST. JOSEPH HOSPITAL), p. A60
GENERAL JOHN J. PERSHING MEMORIAL HOSPITAL, BROOKFIELD, MO, p. A356
GENERAL LEONARD WOOD ARMY COMMUNITY HOSPITAL, FORT LEONARD WOOD, MO, p. A360
GENESIS BEHAVIORAL HOSPITAL, BREAUX BRIDGE, LA, p. A264
GENESIS HEALTHCARE SYSTEM, ZANESVILLE, OH, p. A492
GENESIS MEDICAL CENTER, DEWITT, DE WITT, IA, p. A217

GENESIS MEDICAL CENTER, ILLINI CAMPUS, SILVIS, IL, p. A193

GENESIS MEDICAL CENTER–DAVENPORT, DAVENPORT, IA, p. A217

GENESIS MEDICAL CENTER–EAST CAMPUS, DAVENPORT, IOWA (see GENESIS MEDICAL CENTER–DAVENPORT), p. A217

GENESIS MEDICAL CENTER–WEST CAMPUS, DAVENPORT, IOWA (see GENESIS MEDICAL CENTER–DAVENPORT), p. A217

GENESYS REGIONAL MEDICAL CENTER, GRAND BLANC, MI, p. A313

GENEVA GENERAL HOSPITAL, GENEVA, NY, p. A426

GENOA COMMUNITY HOSPITAL, GENOA, NE, p. A384

GEORGE C GRAPE COMMUNITY HOSPITAL, HAMBURG, IA, p. A220

GEORGE COUNTY HOSPITAL, LUCEDALE, MS, p. A349

GEORGE E. WEEMS MEMORIAL HOSPITAL, APALACHICOLA, FL, p. A118

GEORGE L. MEE MEMORIAL HOSPITAL, KING CITY, CA, p. A65

GEORGE NIGH REHABILITATION INSTITUTE, OKMULGEE, OK, p. A502

GEORGE W. TRUETT MEMORIAL HOSPITAL, DALLAS, TEXAS (see BAYLOR UNIVERSITY MEDICAL CENTER), p. A590

GEORGE WASHINGTON UNIVERSITY HOSPITAL, WASHINGTON, DC, p. A116

GEORGETOWN COMMUNITY HOSPITAL, GEORGETOWN, KY, p. A250

GEORGETOWN MEMORIAL HOSPITAL, GEORGETOWN, SC, p. A550

GEORGIA HEALTH SCIENCES MEDICAL CENTER, AUGUSTA, GA, p. A146

GEORGIA REGIONAL HOSPITAL AT ATLANTA, DECATUR, GA, p. A151

GEORGIA REGIONAL HOSPITAL AT SAVANNAH, SAVANNAH, GA, p. A159

GEORGIANA HOSPITAL, GEORGIANA, AL, p. A21

GERALD CHAMPION REGIONAL MEDICAL CENTER, ALAMOGORDO, NM, p. A414

GETTYSBURG HOSPITAL, GETTYSBURG, PA, p. A524

GETTYSBURG MEMORIAL HOSPITAL, GETTYSBURG, SD, p. A557

GIBSON AREA HOSPITAL AND HEALTH SERVICES, GIBSON CITY, IL, p. A183

GIBSON COMMUNITY HOSPITAL NURSING HOME (see GIBSON AREA HOSPITAL AND HEALTH SERVICES), p. A183

GIBSON GENERAL HOSPITAL, PRINCETON, IN, p. A210

GIBSON GENERAL HOSPITAL, TRENTON, TN, p. A576

GIFFORD MEDICAL CENTER, RANDOLPH, VT, p. A644

GILA REGIONAL MEDICAL CENTER, SILVER CITY, NM, p. A418

GILBERT HOSPITAL, GILBERT, AZ, p. A32

GILLETTE CHILDREN'S SPECIALTY HEALTHCARE, SAINT PAUL, MN, p. A339

GILMORE MEMORIAL REGIONAL MEDICAL CENTER, AMORY, MS, p. A343

GIRARD MEDICAL CENTER, GIRARD, KS, p. A233

GIRARD MEDICAL CENTER, PHILADELPHIA, PA, p. A532

GLACIAL RIDGE HEALTH SYSTEM, GLENWOOD, MN, p. A332

GLADYS SPELLMAN SPECIALTY HOSPITAL AND NURSING CENTER, CHEVERLY, MD, p. A290

GLEN COVE HOSPITAL, GLEN COVE, NY, p. A426

GLEN OAKS HOSPITAL, GREENVILLE, TX, p. A601

GLEN ROSE MEDICAL CENTER, GLEN ROSE, TX, p. A601

GLENBEIGH HOSPITAL AND OUTPATIENT CENTERS, ROCK CREEK, OH, p. A487

GLENCOE REGIONAL HEALTH SERVICES, GLENCOE, MN, p. A332

GLENDALE ADVENTIST MEDICAL CENTER, GLENDALE, CA, p. A63

GLENDALE MEMORIAL HOSPITAL AND HEALTH CENTER, GLENDALE, CA, p. A63

GLENDIVE MEDICAL CENTER, GLENDIVE, MT, p. A375

GLENN MEDICAL CENTER, WILLOWS, CA, p. A96

GLENS FALLS HOSPITAL, GLENS FALLS, NY, p. A426

GLENWOOD REGIONAL MEDICAL CENTER, WEST MONROE, LA, p. A279

GLOBALREHAB HOSPITAL – DALLAS, DALLAS, TX, p. A591

GLOBALREHAB HOSPITAL – FORT WORTH, FORT WORTH, TX, p. A598

GLOBALREHAB HOSPITAL – SAN ANTONIO, SAN ANTONIO, TX, p. A624

GNADEN HUETTEN MEMORIAL HOSPITAL, LEHIGHTON, PA, p. A527

GOLDEN OURS CONVALESCENT HOME (see PERKINS COUNTY HEALTH SERVICES), p. A384

GOLDEN PLAINS COMMUNITY HOSPITAL, BORGER, TX, p. A584

GOLDEN VALLEY MEMORIAL HEALTHCARE, CLINTON, MO, p. A358

GOLDWATER MEMORIAL HOSPITAL, NEW YORK, NEW YORK (see COLER–GOLDWATER SPECIALTY HOSPITAL AND NURSING FACILITY), p. A432

GOLETA VALLEY COTTAGE HOSPITAL, SANTA BARBARA, CA, p. A89

GOLISANO CHILDREN'S HOSPITAL, ROCHESTER, NEW YORK (see STRONG MEMORIAL HOSPITAL OF THE UNIVERSITY OF ROCHESTER), p. A442

GOOD SAMARITAN HOSPITAL, BAKERSFIELD, CA, p. A54

GOOD SAMARITAN HOSPITAL, LOS ANGELES, CA, p. A69

GOOD SAMARITAN HOSPITAL, SAN JOSE, CA, p. A88

GOOD SAMARITAN HOSPITAL, GREENSBORO, GA, p. A153

GOOD SAMARITAN HOSPITAL, VINCENNES, IN, p. A212

GOOD SAMARITAN HOSPITAL, KEARNEY, NE, p. A385

GOOD SAMARITAN HOSPITAL, SUFFERN, NY, p. A444

GOOD SAMARITAN HOSPITAL, CINCINNATI, OH, p. A473

GOOD SAMARITAN HOSPITAL, DAYTON, OH, p. A478

GOOD SAMARITAN HOSPITAL AND MEDICAL CENTER, PORTLAND, OREGON (see LEGACY GOOD SAMARITAN HOSPITAL AND MEDICAL CENTER), p. A514

GOOD SAMARITAN HOSPITAL MEDICAL CENTER, WEST ISLIP, NY, p. A446

GOOD SAMARITAN MEDICAL AND REHABILITATION CENTER, ZANESVILLE, OHIO (see GENESIS HEALTHCARE SYSTEM), p. A492

GOOD SAMARITAN MEDICAL CENTER, WEST PALM BEACH, FL, p. A142

GOOD SAMARITAN MEDICAL CENTER, BROCKTON, MA, p. A298

GOOD SAMARITAN MEDICAL CENTER, JOHNSTOWN, PENNSYLVANIA (see MEMORIAL MEDICAL CENTER), p. A526

GOOD SAMARITAN MEDICAL CENTER – CUSHING CAMPUS, BROCKTON, MASSACHUSETTS (see GOOD SAMARITAN MEDICAL CENTER), p. A298

GOOD SAMARITAN REGIONAL HEALTH CENTER, MOUNT VERNON, IL, p. A188

GOOD SAMARITAN REGIONAL MEDICAL CENTER, CORVALLIS, OR, p. A510

GOOD SHEPHERD CAMPUS, WICHITA, KANSAS (see VIA CHRISTI HOSPITALS WICHITA), p. A245

GOOD SHEPHERD HEALTH CARE SYSTEM, HERMISTON, OR, p. A511

GOOD SHEPHERD MEDICAL CENTER, LONGVIEW, TX, p. A613

GOOD SHEPHERD MEDICAL CENTER–LINDEN, LINDEN, TX, p. A612

GOOD SHEPHERD MEDICAL CENTER–MARSHALL, MARSHALL, TX, p. A615

GOOD SHEPHERD PENN PARTNERS SPECIALTY HOSPITAL AT RITTENHOUSE, PHILADELPHIA, PA, p. A532

GOOD SHEPHERD REHABILITATION HOSPITAL, ALLENTOWN, PA, p. A517

GOOD SHEPHERD SPECIALTY HOSPITAL, BETHLEHEM, PA, p. A518

GOODALL–WITCHER HEALTHCARE, CLIFTON, TX, p. A587

GOODLAND REGIONAL MEDICAL CENTER, GOODLAND, KS, p. A233

GORDON HOSPITAL, CALHOUN, GA, p. A148

GORDON MEMORIAL HOSPITAL, GORDON, NE, p. A384

GOTHENBURG MEMORIAL HOSPITAL, GOTHENBURG, NE, p. A384

GOTTLIEB MEMORIAL HOSPITAL, MELROSE PARK, IL, p. A187

GOVE COUNTY MEDICAL CENTER, QUINTER, KS, p. A242

GOVERNOR JUAN F. LOUIS HOSPITAL, CHRISTIANSTED, VI, p. A704

GRACE COTTAGE HOSPITAL, TOWNSHEND, VT, p. A644

GRACE HOSPITAL, MORGANTON, NC, p. A458

GRACE HOSPITAL, CLEVELAND, OH, p. A475

GRACE MEDICAL CENTER, LUBBOCK, TX, p. A614

GRACIE SQUARE HOSPITAL, NEW YORK, NY, p. A432

GRADY GENERAL HOSPITAL, CAIRO, GA, p. A148

GRADY MEMORIAL HOSPITAL, ATLANTA, GA, p. A145

GRADY MEMORIAL HOSPITAL, DELAWARE, OH, p. A479

GRADY MEMORIAL HOSPITAL, CHICKASHA, OK, p. A494

GRAFTON CITY HOSPITAL, GRAFTON, WV, p. A672

GRAHAM COUNTY HOSPITAL, HILL CITY, KS, p. A234

GRAHAM HOSPITAL, CANTON, IL, p. A174

GRAHAM REGIONAL MEDICAL CENTER, GRAHAM, TX, p. A601

GRAND ITASCA CLINIC AND HOSPITAL, GRAND RAPIDS, MN, p. A332

GRAND RIVER HOSPITAL DISTRICT, RIFLE, CO, p. A105

GRAND STRAND REGIONAL MEDICAL CENTER, MYRTLE BEACH, SC, p. A552

GRAND VIEW HOSPITAL, SELLERSVILLE, PA, p. A538

GRANDE RONDE HOSPITAL, LA GRANDE, OR, p. A512

GRANDVIEW MEDICAL CENTER, DAYTON, OH, p. A478

GRANDVIEW MEDICAL CENTER, JASPER, TN, p. A567

GRANITE COUNTY MEDICAL CENTER, PHILIPSBURG, MT, p. A378

GRANITE FALLS MUNICIPAL HOSPITAL AND MANOR, GRANITE FALLS, MN, p. A332

GRANT MEDICAL CENTER, COLUMBUS, OH, p. A476

GRANT MEMORIAL HOSPITAL, PETERSBURG, WV, p. A674

GRANT REGIONAL HEALTH CENTER, LANCASTER, WI, p. A684

GRANT–BLACKFORD MENTAL HEALTH CENTER, MARION, IN, p. A208

GRANVILLE HEALTH SYSTEM, OXFORD, NC, p. A458

GRAYS HARBOR COMMUNITY HOSPITAL, ABERDEEN, WA, p. A659

GREAT BEND REGIONAL HOSPITAL, GREAT BEND, KS, p. A233

GREAT FALLS CLINIC MEDICAL CENTER, GREAT FALLS, MT, p. A376

GREAT LAKES SPECIALTY HOSPITAL–HACKLEY CAMPUS, MUSKEGON, MI, p. A319

GREAT LAKES SPECIALTY HOSPITAL–OAK CAMPUS, GRAND RAPIDS, MI, p. A313

GREAT PLAINS REGIONAL MEDICAL CENTER, NORTH PLATTE, NE, p. A386

GREAT PLAINS REGIONAL MEDICAL CENTER, ELK CITY, OK, p. A496

GREAT RIVER MEDICAL CENTER, BLYTHEVILLE, AR, p. A42

GREAT RIVER MEDICAL CENTER, WEST BURLINGTON, IA, p. A228

GREATER BALTIMORE MEDICAL CENTER, BALTIMORE, MD, p. A287

GREATER BATON ROUGE SURGICAL HOSPITAL, BATON ROUGE, LA, p. A262

GREATER BINGHAMTON HEALTH CENTER, BINGHAMTON, NY, p. A421

GREATER EL MONTE COMMUNITY HOSPITAL, SOUTH EL MONTE, CA, p. A91

GREATER REGIONAL MEDICAL CENTER, CRESTON, IA, p. A217

GREELEY COUNTY HEALTH SERVICES, TRIBUNE, KS, p. A244

GREEN CLINIC SURGICAL HOSPITAL, RUSTON, LA, p. A276

GREEN OAKS HOSPITAL, DALLAS, TX, p. A591

GREENBRIAR REHABILITATION HOSPITAL, BOARDMAN, OH, p. A471

GREENBRIER HOSPITAL, COVINGTON, LA, p. A265

GREENBRIER VALLEY MEDICAL CENTER, RONCEVERTE, WV, p. A675

GREENE COUNTY GENERAL HOSPITAL, LINTON, IN, p. A207

GREENE COUNTY HOSPITAL, EUTAW, AL, p. A19

GREENE COUNTY HOSPITAL, LEAKESVILLE, MS, p. A349

GREENE COUNTY MEDICAL CENTER, JEFFERSON, IA, p. A222

GREENE MEMORIAL HOSPITAL, XENIA, OH, p. A492

GREENLEAF CENTER, VALDOSTA, GEORGIA (see SOUTH GEORGIA MEDICAL CENTER), p. A161

GREENVIEW REGIONAL HOSPITAL, BOWLING GREEN, KY, p. A248

GREENVILLE CAMPUS, GREENVILLE, PENNSYLVANIA (see UPMC HORIZON), p. A524

GREENVILLE MEMORIAL HOSPITAL, GREENVILLE, SC, p. A550

GREENVILLE REGIONAL HOSPITAL, GREENVILLE, IL, p. A183

GREENWICH HOSPITAL, GREENWICH, CT, p. A109

GREENWOOD COUNTY HOSPITAL, EUREKA, KS, p. A233

GREENWOOD LEFLORE HOSPITAL, GREENWOOD, MS, p. A346

GREENWOOD REGIONAL REHABILITATION HOSPITAL, GREENWOOD, SC, p. A551

GREER MEMORIAL HOSPITAL, GREER, SC, p. A551

GREIL MEMORIAL PSYCHIATRIC HOSPITAL, MONTGOMERY, AL, p. A23

GRENADA LAKE MEDICAL CENTER, GRENADA, MS, p. A346

GREYSTONE PARK PSYCHIATRIC HOSPITAL, MORRIS PLAINS, NJ, p. A406

GRIFFIN HOSPITAL, DERBY, CT, p. A108

GRIFFIN MEMORIAL HOSPITAL, NORMAN, OK, p. A500

GRIMES ST. JOSEPH HEALTH CENTER, NAVASOTA, TX, p. A618

GRINNELL REGIONAL MEDICAL CENTER, GRINNELL, IA, p. A220

GRISELL MEMORIAL HOSPITAL DISTRICT ONE, RANSOM, KS, p. A242

GRITMAN MEDICAL CENTER, MOSCOW, ID, p. A169

GROUP HEALTH COOPERATIVE CENTRAL HOSPITAL, SEATTLE, WA, p. A665

GROVE CITY MEDICAL CENTER, GROVE CITY, PA, p. A524

GROVE HILL MEMORIAL HOSPITAL, GROVE HILL, AL, p. A21

GROVER C. DILS MEDICAL CENTER, CALIENTE, NV, p. A391

GRUNDY COUNTY MEMORIAL HOSPITAL, GRUNDY CENTER, IA, p. A220

GUADALUPE COUNTY HOSPITAL, SANTA ROSA, NM, p. A418

GUADALUPE REGIONAL MEDICAL CENTER, SEGUIN, TX, p. A627

GUAM MEMORIAL HOSPITAL AUTHORITY, TAMUNING, GU, p. A699

GULF BREEZE HOSPITAL, GULF BREEZE, FL, p. A124

GULF COAST MEDICAL CENTER, FORT MYERS, FL, p. A123

GULF COAST MEDICAL CENTER, PANAMA CITY, FL, p. A135

GULF COAST MEDICAL CENTER, WHARTON, TX, p. A634

GUNDERSEN LUTHERAN MEDICAL CENTER, LA CROSSE, WI, p. A683

GUNNISON VALLEY HOSPITAL, GUNNISON, CO, p. A102

GUNNISON VALLEY HOSPITAL, GUNNISON, UT, p. A637

GUTHRIE COUNTY HOSPITAL, GUTHRIE CENTER, IA, p. A220

GUTTENBERG MUNICIPAL HOSPITAL, GUTTENBERG, IA, p. A220

GWINNETT HOSPITAL SYSTEM, LAWRENCEVILLE, GA, p. A155

GWINNETT MEDICAL CENTER, LAWRENCEVILLE, GEORGIA (see GWINNETT HOSPITAL SYSTEM), p. A155
GWINNETT MEDICAL CENTER–DULUTH, DULUTH, GEORGIA (see GWINNETT HOSPITAL SYSTEM), p. A155

# H

H. B. MAGRUDER MEMORIAL HOSPITAL, PORT CLINTON, OH, p. A487
H. C. WATKINS MEMORIAL HOSPITAL, QUITMAN, MS, p. A352
H. DOUGLAS SINGER MENTAL HEALTH AND DEVELOPMENTAL CENTER, ROCKFORD, IL, p. A192
H. LEE MOFFITT CANCER CENTER AND RESEARCH INSTITUTE, TAMPA, FL, p. A140
H.S.C. MEDICAL CENTER, MALVERN, AR, p. A48
HABERSHAM MEDICAL CENTER, DEMOREST, GA, p. A151
HACKENSACK UNIVERSITY MEDICAL CENTER, HACKENSACK, NJ, p. A404
HACKENSACK UNIVERSITY MEDICAL CENTER MOUNTAINSIDE, MONTCLAIR, NJ, p. A406
HACKETTSTOWN REGIONAL MEDICAL CENTER, HACKETTSTOWN, NJ, p. A404
HAHNEMANN CAMPUS, WORCESTER, MASSACHUSETTS (see UMASS MEMORIAL MEDICAL CENTER), p. A306
HAHNEMANN UNIVERSITY HOSPITAL, PHILADELPHIA, PA, p. A532
HALE COUNTY HOSPITAL, GREENSBORO, AL, p. A21
HALE HO'OLA HAMAKUA, HONOKAA, HI, p. A163
HALIFAX BEHAVIORAL SERVICES, DAYTONA BEACH, FLORIDA (see HALIFAX HEALTH MEDICAL CENTER OF DAYTONA BEACH), p. A122
HALIFAX HEALTH MEDICAL CENTER OF DAYTONA BEACH, DAYTONA BEACH, FL, p. A122
HALIFAX HEALTH MEDICAL CENTER OF PORT ORANGE, PORT ORANGE, FLORIDA (see HALIFAX HEALTH MEDICAL CENTER OF DAYTONA BEACH), p. A122
HALIFAX REGIONAL HEALTH SYSTEM, SOUTH BOSTON, VA, p. A656
HALIFAX REGIONAL MEDICAL CENTER, ROANOKE RAPIDS, NC, p. A459
HALLMARK HEALTH SYSTEM, MELROSE, MA, p. A302
HALLMARK YOUTHCARE – RICHMOND, RICHMOND, VA, p. A655
HAMILTON CENTER, TERRE HAUTE, IN, p. A212
HAMILTON COUNTY HOSPITAL, SYRACUSE, KS, p. A243
HAMILTON GENERAL HOSPITAL, HAMILTON, TX, p. A602
HAMILTON HOSPITAL, OLNEY, TX, p. A619
HAMILTON MEDICAL CENTER, DALTON, GA, p. A151
HAMILTON MEMORIAL HOSPITAL DISTRICT, MCLEANSBORO, IL, p. A187
HAMLIN MEMORIAL HOSPITAL, HAMLIN, TX, p. A602
HAMMOND–HENRY HOSPITAL, GENESEO, IL, p. A182
HAMPSHIRE MEMORIAL HOSPITAL, ROMNEY, WV, p. A675
HAMPSTEAD HOSPITAL, HAMPSTEAD, NH, p. A398
HAMPTON BEHAVIORAL HEALTH CENTER, WESTAMPTON TOWNSHIP, NJ, p. A412
HAMPTON REGIONAL MEDICAL CENTER, VARNVILLE, SC, p. A554
HAMPTON ROADS SPECIALTY HOSPITAL, NEWPORT NEWS, VA, p. A652
HANCOCK COUNTY MEMORIAL HOSPITAL, BRITT, IA, p. A215
HANCOCK MEDICAL CENTER, BAY SAINT LOUIS, MS, p. A343
HANCOCK REGIONAL HOSPITAL, GREENFIELD, IN, p. A203
HANFORD COMMUNITY MEDICAL CENTER, HANFORD, CA, p. A64
HANNIBAL REGIONAL HOSPITAL, HANNIBAL, MO, p. A360
HANOVER HOSPITAL, HANOVER, KS, p. A234
HANOVER HOSPITAL, HANOVER, PA, p. A524
HANSFORD HOSPITAL, SPEARMAN, TX, p. A628
HARBOR BEACH COMMUNITY HOSPITAL, HARBOR BEACH, MI, p. A315
HARBOR HOSPITAL OF SOUTHEAST TEXAS, BEAUMONT, TX, p. A583
HARBOR OAKS HOSPITAL, NEW BALTIMORE, MI, p. A320
HARBORVIEW MEDICAL CENTER, SEATTLE, WA, p. A665
HARDEMAN COUNTY MEMORIAL HOSPITAL, QUANAH, TX, p. A622
HARDIN COUNTY GENERAL HOSPITAL, ROSICLARE, IL, p. A193
HARDIN MEDICAL CENTER, SAVANNAH, TN, p. A575
HARDIN MEMORIAL HOSPITAL, ELIZABETHTOWN, KY, p. A249
HARDIN MEMORIAL HOSPITAL, KENTON, OH, p. A482
HARDTNER MEDICAL CENTER, OLLA, LA, p. A275
HARDY WILSON MEMORIAL HOSPITAL, HAZLEHURST, MS, p. A347
HARFORD MEMORIAL HOSPITAL, HAVRE DE GRACE, MD, p. A292
HARLAN ARH HOSPITAL, HARLAN, KY, p. A251
HARLAN COUNTY HEALTH SYSTEM, ALMA, NE, p. A381

HARLEM GENERAL CARE UNIT AND HARLEM PSYCHIATRIC UNIT (see HARLEM HOSPITAL CENTER), p. A432
HARLEM HOSPITAL CENTER, NEW YORK, NY, p. A432
HARLINGEN MEDICAL CENTER, HARLINGEN, TX, p. A602
HARMON MEDICAL AND REHABILITATION HOSPITAL, LAS VEGAS, NV, p. A392
HARMON MEMORIAL HOSPITAL, HOLLIS, OK, p. A498
HARNEY DISTRICT HOSPITAL, BURNS, OR, p. A509
HARPER COUNTY COMMUNITY HOSPITAL, BUFFALO, OK, p. A494
HARPER HOSPITAL DISTRICT FIVE, HARPER, KS, p. A234
HARPER UNIVERSITY HOSPITAL/HUTZEL WOMEN'S HOSPITAL, DETROIT, MI, p. A310
HARRINGTON MEMORIAL HOSPITAL, SOUTHBRIDGE, MA, p. A304
HARRIS COUNTY HOSPITAL DISTRICT, HOUSTON, TX, p. A604
HARRIS HOSPITAL, NEWPORT, AR, p. A49
HARRIS METHODIST–SPRINGWOOD, BEDFORD, TEXAS (see TEXAS HEALTH HARRIS METHODIST HOSPITAL HURST–EULESS–BEDFORD), p. A583
HARRISBURG HOSPITAL, HARRISBURG, PENNSYLVANIA (see PINNACLE HEALTH SYSTEM), p. A524
HARRISBURG MEDICAL CENTER, HARRISBURG, IL, p. A183
HARRISON COMMUNITY HOSPITAL, CADIZ, OH, p. A471
HARRISON COUNTY COMMUNITY HOSPITAL, BETHANY, MO, p. A355
HARRISON COUNTY HOSPITAL, CORYDON, IN, p. A199
HARRISON MEDICAL CENTER, BREMERTON, WA, p. A659
HARRISON MEMORIAL HOSPITAL, CYNTHIANA, KY, p. A249
HARRY S. TRUMAN MEMORIAL VETERANS HOSPITAL, COLUMBIA, MO, p. A358
HARSHA BEHAVIORAL CENTER, TERRE HAUTE, IN, p. A212
HART COUNTY HOSPITAL, HARTWELL, GA, p. A153
HARTFORD HOSPITAL, HARTFORD, CT, p. A109
HARTGROVE HOSPITAL, CHICAGO, IL, p. A175
HARTON REGIONAL MEDICAL CENTER, TULLAHOMA, TN, p. A576
HASBRO CHILDREN'S HOSPITAL, PROVIDENCE, RHODE ISLAND (see RHODE ISLAND HOSPITAL), p. A544
HASKELL COUNTY COMMUNITY HOSPITAL, STIGLER, OK, p. A504
HASKELL MEMORIAL HOSPITAL, HASKELL, TX, p. A603
HASTINGS REGIONAL CENTER, HASTINGS, NE, p. A384
HAVASU REGIONAL MEDICAL CENTER, LAKE HAVASU CITY, AZ, p. A33
HAVEN BEHAVIORAL HEALTH OF EASTERN PENNSYLVANIA, READING, PA, p. A536
HAVEN BEHAVIORAL SENIOR CARE OF NORTH DENVER, THORNTON, CO, p. A106
HAVEN BEHAVIORAL WAR HEROES HOSPITAL, PUEBLO, CO, p. A105
HAVEN SENIOR HORIZONS, PHOENIX, AZ, p. A35
HAVENWYCK HOSPITAL, AUBURN HILLS, MI, p. A307
HAWAII STATE HOSPITAL, KANEOHE, HI, p. A164
HAWARDEN COMMUNITY HOSPITAL, HAWARDEN, IA, p. A221
HAWTHORN CENTER, NORTHVILLE, MI, p. A320
HAWTHORN CHILDREN PSYCHIATRIC HOSPITAL, SAINT LOUIS, MO, p. A368
HAWTHORNE HOSPITAL, HAWTHORNE, CALIFORNIA (see LOS ANGELES METROPOLITAN MEDICAL CENTER), p. A70
HAXTUN HOSPITAL DISTRICT, HAXTUN, CO, p. A102
HAYES GREEN BEACH MEMORIAL HOSPITAL, CHARLOTTE, MI, p. A309
HAYS MEDICAL CENTER, HAYS, KS, p. A234
HAYWARD AREA MEMORIAL HOSPITAL AND NURSING HOME, HAYWARD, WI, p. A683
HAYWARD MEDICAL CENTER, HAYWARD, CA, p. A64
HAYWOOD PARK COMMUNITY HOSPITAL, BROWNSVILLE, TN, p. A562
HAZARD ARH REGIONAL MEDICAL CENTER, HAZARD, KY, p. A251
HAZEL HAWKINS MEMORIAL HOSPITAL, HOLLISTER, CA, p. A64
HAZLETON GENERAL HOSPITAL, HAZLETON, PA, p. A525
HCMC DEPARTMENT OF PEDIATRICS, MINNEAPOLIS, MINNESOTA (see HENNEPIN COUNTY MEDICAL CENTER), p. A335
HEALDSBURG DISTRICT HOSPITAL, HEALDSBURG, CA, p. A64
HEALTH ALLIANCE HOSPITALS, LEOMINSTER, MA, p. A301
HEALTH CENTRAL, OCOEE, FL, p. A134
HEALTHBRIDGE CHILDREN'S HOSPITAL OF HOUSTON, HOUSTON, TX, p. A604
HEALTHBRIDGE CHILDRENS REHABILITATION HOSPITAL, ORANGE, CA, p. A78
HEALTHEAST BETHESDA HOSPITAL, SAINT PAUL, MN, p. A339
HEALTHMARK REGIONAL MEDICAL CENTER, DEFUNIAK SPRINGS, FL, p. A122
HEALTHPARK, OWENSBORO, KENTUCKY (see OWENSBORO MEDICAL HEALTH SYSTEM), p. A257
HEALTHPARK HOSPITAL, HOT SPRINGS NATIONAL PARK, ARKANSAS (see MERCY HOSPITAL HOT SPRINGS), p. A46

HEALTHPARK MEDICAL CENTER, FORT MYERS, FLORIDA (see LEE MEMORIAL HOSPITAL), p. A124
HEALTHSOURCE SAGINAW, SAGINAW, MI, p. A322
HEALTHSOUTH BAKERSFIELD REHABILITATION HOSPITAL, BAKERSFIELD, CA, p. A54
HEALTHSOUTH CANE CREEK REHABILITATION HOSPITAL, MARTIN, TN, p. A570
HEALTHSOUTH CHATTANOOGA REHABILITATION HOSPITAL, CHATTANOOGA, TN, p. A563
HEALTHSOUTH CHESAPEAKE REHABILITATION HOSPITAL, SALISBURY, MD, p. A294
HEALTHSOUTH DEACONESS REHABILITATION HOSPITAL, EVANSVILLE, IN, p. A201
HEALTHSOUTH DESERT CANYON REHABILITATION HOSPITAL, LAS VEGAS, NV, p. A392
HEALTHSOUTH EAST VALLEY REHABILITATION HOSPITAL, MESA, AZ, p. A34
HEALTHSOUTH EMERALD COAST REHABILITATION HOSPITAL, PANAMA CITY, FL, p. A135
HEALTHSOUTH HARMARVILLE REHABILITATION HOSPITAL, PITTSBURGH, PA, p. A534
HEALTHSOUTH HUNTINGTON REHABILITATION HOSPITAL, HUNTINGTON, WV, p. A672
HEALTHSOUTH LAKESHORE REHABILITATION HOSPITAL, BIRMINGHAM, AL, p. A16
HEALTHSOUTH LAKEVIEW REHABILITATION HOSPITAL, ELIZABETHTOWN, KY, p. A249
HEALTHSOUTH MOUNTAINVIEW REGIONAL REHABILITATION HOSPITAL, MORGANTOWN, WV, p. A674
HEALTHSOUTH NITTANY VALLEY REHABILITATION HOSPITAL, PLEASANT GAP, PA, p. A536
HEALTHSOUTH NORTHERN KENTUCKY REHABILITATION HOSPITAL, EDGEWOOD, KY, p. A249
HEALTHSOUTH PLANO REHABILITATION HOSPITAL, PLANO, TX, p. A621
HEALTHSOUTH READING REHABILITATION HOSPITAL, READING, PA, p. A537
HEALTHSOUTH REHABILITATION HOSPITAL, DOTHAN, AL, p. A19
HEALTHSOUTH REHABILITATION HOSPITAL, FAYETTEVILLE, AR, p. A44
HEALTHSOUTH REHABILITATION HOSPITAL, LARGO, FL, p. A128
HEALTHSOUTH REHABILITATION HOSPITAL, CONCORD, NH, p. A397
HEALTHSOUTH REHABILITATION HOSPITAL, ALBUQUERQUE, NM, p. A414
HEALTHSOUTH REHABILITATION HOSPITAL, SEWICKLEY, PA, p. A538
HEALTHSOUTH REHABILITATION HOSPITAL, SAN JUAN, PR, p. A703
HEALTHSOUTH REHABILITATION HOSPITAL, COLUMBIA, SC, p. A548
HEALTHSOUTH REHABILITATION HOSPITAL, FLORENCE, SC, p. A549
HEALTHSOUTH REHABILITATION HOSPITAL, ROCK HILL, SC, p. A553
HEALTHSOUTH REHABILITATION HOSPITAL, KINGSPORT, TN, p. A568
HEALTHSOUTH REHABILITATION HOSPITAL, MEMPHIS, TN, p. A571
HEALTHSOUTH REHABILITATION HOSPITAL, FORT WORTH, TX, p. A598
HEALTHSOUTH REHABILITATION HOSPITAL, HUMBLE, TX, p. A608
HEALTHSOUTH REHABILITATION HOSPITAL – HENDERSON, HENDERSON, NV, p. A392
HEALTHSOUTH REHABILITATION HOSPITAL AT DRAKE, CINCINNATI, OH, p. A473
HEALTHSOUTH REHABILITATION HOSPITAL MIDLAND–ODESSA, MIDLAND, TX, p. A616
HEALTHSOUTH REHABILITATION HOSPITAL OF ALEXANDRIA, ALEXANDRIA, LA, p. A261
HEALTHSOUTH REHABILITATION HOSPITAL OF ALTOONA, ALTOONA, PA, p. A517
HEALTHSOUTH REHABILITATION HOSPITAL OF ARLINGTON, ARLINGTON, TX, p. A579
HEALTHSOUTH REHABILITATION HOSPITAL OF AUSTIN, AUSTIN, TX, p. A580
HEALTHSOUTH REHABILITATION HOSPITAL OF BEAUMONT, BEAUMONT, TX, p. A583
HEALTHSOUTH REHABILITATION HOSPITAL OF CHARLESTON, CHARLESTON, SC, p. A547
HEALTHSOUTH REHABILITATION HOSPITAL OF COLORADO SPRINGS, COLORADO SPRINGS, CO, p. A98
HEALTHSOUTH REHABILITATION HOSPITAL OF CYPRESS, HOUSTON, TX, p. A604
HEALTHSOUTH REHABILITATION HOSPITAL OF ERIE, ERIE, PA, p. A523

HEALTHSOUTH REHABILITATION HOSPITAL OF FORT SMITH, FORT SMITH, AR, p. A45

HEALTHSOUTH REHABILITATION HOSPITAL OF FREDERICKSBURG, FREDERICKSBURG, VA, p. A648

HEALTHSOUTH REHABILITATION HOSPITAL OF JONESBORO, JONESBORO, AR, p. A46

HEALTHSOUTH REHABILITATION HOSPITAL OF MECHANICSBURG, MECHANICSBURG, PA, p. A529

HEALTHSOUTH REHABILITATION HOSPITAL OF MEMPHIS, MEMPHIS, TN, p. A571

HEALTHSOUTH REHABILITATION HOSPITAL OF MIAMI, MIAMI, FL, p. A131

HEALTHSOUTH REHABILITATION HOSPITAL OF MONTGOMERY, MONTGOMERY, AL, p. A24

HEALTHSOUTH REHABILITATION HOSPITAL OF NORTH ALABAMA, HUNTSVILLE, AL, p. A21

HEALTHSOUTH REHABILITATION HOSPITAL OF NORTH HOUSTON, CONROE, TX, p. A588

HEALTHSOUTH REHABILITATION HOSPITAL OF NORTHERN VIRGINIA, ALDIE, VA, p. A645

HEALTHSOUTH REHABILITATION HOSPITAL OF PETERSBURG, PETERSBURG, VA, p. A653

HEALTHSOUTH REHABILITATION HOSPITAL OF SARASOTA, SARASOTA, FL, p. A139

HEALTHSOUTH REHABILITATION HOSPITAL OF SOUTHERN ARIZONA, TUCSON, AZ, p. A39

HEALTHSOUTH REHABILITATION HOSPITAL OF SPRING HILL, BROOKSVILLE, FL, p. A120

HEALTHSOUTH REHABILITATION HOSPITAL OF TALLAHASSEE, TALLAHASSEE, FL, p. A140

HEALTHSOUTH REHABILITATION HOSPITAL OF TEXARKANA, TEXARKANA, TX, p. A631

HEALTHSOUTH REHABILITATION HOSPITAL OF TOMS RIVER, TOMS RIVER, NJ, p. A411

HEALTHSOUTH REHABILITATION HOSPITAL OF UTAH, SANDY, UT, p. A641

HEALTHSOUTH REHABILITATION HOSPITAL OF VINELAND, VINELAND, NJ, p. A411

HEALTHSOUTH REHABILITATION HOSPITAL OF VIRGINIA, RICHMOND, VA, p. A655

HEALTHSOUTH REHABILITATION HOSPITAL OF WESTERN MASSACHUSETTS, LUDLOW, MA, p. A302

HEALTHSOUTH REHABILITATION HOSPITAL OF YORK, YORK, PA, p. A542

HEALTHSOUTH REHABILITATION HOSPITAL–CITYVIEW, FORT WORTH, TX, p. A598

HEALTHSOUTH REHABILITATION HOSPITAL–LAS VEGAS, LAS VEGAS, NV, p. A393

HEALTHSOUTH REHABILITATION HOSPITAL–WICHITA FALLS, WICHITA FALLS, TX, p. A635

HEALTHSOUTH REHABILITATION INSTITUTE OF SAN ANTONIO, SAN ANTONIO, TX, p. A625

HEALTHSOUTH REHABILITATION INSTITUTE OF TUCSON, TUCSON, AZ, p. A40

HEALTHSOUTH REHABILITATION OF GADSDEN, GADSDEN, AL, p. A20

HEALTHSOUTH SCOTTSDALE REHABILITATION HOSPITAL, SCOTTSDALE, AZ, p. A38

HEALTHSOUTH SEA PINES REHABILITATION HOSPITAL, MELBOURNE, FL, p. A130

HEALTHSOUTH SOUTHERN HILLS REHABILITATION HOSPITAL, PRINCETON, WV, p. A675

HEALTHSOUTH SUGAR LAND REHABILITATION HOSPITAL, SUGAR LAND, TX, p. A629

HEALTHSOUTH SUNRISE REHABILITATION HOSPITAL, FORT LAUDERDALE, FL, p. A123

HEALTHSOUTH TREASURE COAST REHABILITATION HOSPITAL, VERO BEACH, FL, p. A142

HEALTHSOUTH TUSTIN REHABILITATION HOSPITAL, TUSTIN, CA, p. A93

HEALTHSOUTH VALLEY OF THE SUN REHABILITATION HOSPITAL, GLENDALE, AZ, p. A33

HEALTHSOUTH WESTERN HILLS REHABILITATION HOSPITAL, PARKERSBURG, WV, p. A674

HEART HOSPITAL OF AUSTIN, AUSTIN, TEXAS (see ST. DAVID'S MEDICAL CENTER), p. A581

HEART HOSPITAL OF LAFAYETTE, LAFAYETTE, LA, p. A270

HEART HOSPITAL OF NEW MEXICO, ALBUQUERQUE, NEW MEXICO (see LOVELACE MEDICAL CENTER), p. A414

HEART OF AMERICA MEDICAL CENTER, RUGBY, ND, p. A468

HEART OF FLORIDA REGIONAL MEDICAL CENTER, DAVENPORT, FL, p. A121

HEART OF LANCASTER REGIONAL MEDICAL CENTER, LITITZ, PA, p. A528

HEART OF TEXAS MEMORIAL HOSPITAL, BRADY, TX, p. A584

HEART OF THE ROCKIES REGIONAL MEDICAL CENTER, SALIDA, CO, p. A105

HEARTLAND BEHAVIORAL HEALTH SERVICES, NEVADA, MO, p. A366

HEARTLAND BEHAVIORAL HEALTHCARE, MASSILLON, OH, p. A484

HEARTLAND LONG TERM ACUTE CARE HOSPITAL, SAINT JOSEPH, MO, p. A368

HEARTLAND REGIONAL MEDICAL CENTER, MARION, IL, p. A186

HEARTLAND REGIONAL MEDICAL CENTER, SAINT JOSEPH, MO, p. A368

HEARTLAND SURGICAL SPECIALTY HOSPITAL, OVERLAND PARK, KS, p. A240

HEATHERHILL CARE COMMUNITIES, CHARDON, OH, p. A472

HEBER VALLEY MEDICAL CENTER, HEBER CITY, UT, p. A638

HEBREW REHABILITATION CENTER, BOSTON, MA, p. A297

HEDRICK MEDICAL CENTER, CHILLICOTHE, MO, p. A357

HEGG MEMORIAL HEALTH CENTER AVERA, ROCK VALLEY, IA, p. A226

HELEN DEVOS CHILDREN'S HOSPITAL, GRAND RAPIDS, MICHIGAN (see SPECTRUM HEALTH BUTTERWORTH HOSPITAL), p. A314

HELEN HAYES HOSPITAL, WEST HAVERSTRAW, NY, p. A446

HELEN KELLER HOSPITAL, SHEFFIELD, AL, p. A25

HELEN NEWBERRY JOY HOSPITAL, NEWBERRY, MI, p. A320

HELEN NEWBERRY JOY HOSPITAL ANNEX (see HELEN NEWBERRY JOY HOSPITAL), p. A320

HELENA REGIONAL MEDICAL CENTER, HELENA, AR, p. A46

HEMET VALLEY MEDICAL CENTER, HEMET, CA, p. A64

HEMPHILL COUNTY HOSPITAL, CANADIAN, TX, p. A586

HENDERSON COUNTY COMMUNITY HOSPITAL, LEXINGTON, TN, p. A569

HENDERSON HEALTH CARE SERVICES, HENDERSON, NE, p. A384

HENDERSONVILLE MEDICAL CENTER, HENDERSONVILLE, TN, p. A566

HENDRICK CENTER FOR EXTENDED CARE, ABILENE, TX, p. A577

HENDRICK HEALTH SYSTEM, ABILENE, TX, p. A577

HENDRICKS COMMUNITY HOSPITAL, HENDRICKS, MN, p. A332

HENDRICKS REGIONAL HEALTH, DANVILLE, IN, p. A200

HENDRY REGIONAL MEDICAL CENTER, CLEWISTON, FL, p. A120

HENNEPIN COUNTY MEDICAL CENTER, MINNEAPOLIS, MN, p. A335

HENRICO DOCTORS' HOSPITAL, RICHMOND, VA, p. A655

HENRICO DOCTORS' HOSPITAL – FOREST, RICHMOND, VIRGINIA (see HENRICO DOCTORS' HOSPITAL), p. A655

HENRICO DOCTORS' HOSPITAL – PARHAM, RICHMOND, VIRGINIA (see HENRICO DOCTORS' HOSPITAL), p. A655

HENRICO DOCTORS' HOSPITAL – RETREAT CAMPUS, RICHMOND, VIRGINIA (see HENRICO DOCTORS' HOSPITAL), p. A655

HENRIETTA D. GOODALL HOSPITAL, SANFORD, ME, p. A285

HENRY COUNTY HEALTH CENTER, MOUNT PLEASANT, IA, p. A223

HENRY COUNTY HOSPITAL, NEW CASTLE, IN, p. A209

HENRY COUNTY HOSPITAL, NAPOLEON, OH, p. A485

HENRY COUNTY MEDICAL CENTER, PARIS, TN, p. A574

HENRY FORD HOSPITAL, DETROIT, MI, p. A310

HENRY FORD KINGSWOOD HOSPITAL, FERNDALE, MI, p. A312

HENRY FORD MACOMB HOSPITAL – MOUNT CLEMENS CAMPUS, MOUNT CLEMENS, MICHIGAN (see HENRY FORD MACOMB HOSPITALS), p. A309

HENRY FORD MACOMB HOSPITALS, CLINTON TOWNSHIP, MI, p. A309

HENRY FORD WEST BLOOMFIELD HOSPITAL, WEST BLOOMFIELD, MI, p. A325

HENRY FORD WYANDOTTE HOSPITAL, WYANDOTTE, MI, p. A325

HENRY MAYO NEWHALL MEMORIAL HOSPITAL, VALENCIA, CA, p. A94

HENRY MEDICAL CENTER, STOCKBRIDGE, GA, p. A160

HENRYETTA MEDICAL CENTER, HENRYETTA, OK, p. A497

HEREFORD REGIONAL MEDICAL CENTER, HEREFORD, TX, p. A603

HERINGTON MUNICIPAL HOSPITAL, HERINGTON, KS, p. A234

HERITAGE MEDICAL CENTER, SHELBYVILLE, TN, p. A575

HERITAGE OAKS HOSPITAL, SACRAMENTO, CA, p. A83

HERITAGE PARK SURGICAL HOSPITAL, SHERMAN, TX, p. A627

HERITAGE VALLEY BEAVER, BEAVER, PA, p. A518

HERMANN AREA DISTRICT HOSPITAL, HERMANN, MO, p. A360

HERRIN HOSPITAL, HERRIN, IL, p. A184

HEYWOOD HOSPITAL, GARDNER, MA, p. A300

HI-DESERT MEDICAL CENTER, JOSHUA TREE, CA, p. A65

HIALEAH HOSPITAL, HIALEAH, FL, p. A125

HIAWATHA COMMUNITY HOSPITAL, HIAWATHA, KS, p. A234

HICKMAN COMMUNITY HOSPITAL, CENTERVILLE, TN, p. A563

HICKORY TRAIL HOSPITAL, DESOTO, TX, p. A594

HIGGINS GENERAL HOSPITAL, BREMEN, GA, p. A148

HIGH POINT REGIONAL HEALTH SYSTEM, HIGH POINT, NC, p. A455

HIGHBRIDGE WOODYCREST CENTER,, NEW YORK (see BRONX–LEBANON HOSPITAL CENTER HEALTH CARE SYSTEM), p. A431

HIGHLAND COMMUNITY HOSPITAL, PICAYUNE, MS, p. A351

HIGHLAND DISTRICT HOSPITAL, HILLSBORO, OH, p. A482

HIGHLAND HOSPITAL, CHARLESTON, WV, p. A671

HIGHLAND HOSPITAL OF ROCHESTER, ROCHESTER, NY, p. A441

HIGHLAND PARK HOSPITAL, MIAMI, FLORIDA (see JACKSON HEALTH SYSTEM), p. A131

HIGHLANDS BEHAVIORAL HEALTH SYSTEM, LITTLETON, CO, p. A103

HIGHLANDS HOSPITAL, CONNELLSVILLE, PA, p. A521

HIGHLANDS MEDICAL CENTER, SCOTTSBORO, AL, p. A25

HIGHLANDS MEDICAL CENTER, SPARTA, TN, p. A576

HIGHLANDS REGIONAL MEDICAL CENTER, SEBRING, FL, p. A139

HIGHLANDS REGIONAL MEDICAL CENTER, PRESTONSBURG, KY, p. A258

HIGHLANDS REGIONAL REHABILITATION HOSPITAL, EL PASO, TX, p. A596

HIGHLANDS–CASHIERS HOSPITAL, HIGHLANDS, NC, p. A455

HIGHLINE MEDICAL CENTER, BURIEN, WA, p. A660

HIGHLINE SPECIALTY CENTER, 12844 MILITARY ROAD FORK, TUKWILA, ZIP 98168; MARK BENEDUM, ADMINISTRATOR (see HIGHLINE MEDICAL CENTER), p. A660

HIGHSMITH–RAINEY SPECIALTY HOSPITAL, FAYETTEVILLE, NC, p. A453

HILL COUNTRY MEMORIAL HOSPITAL, FREDERICKSBURG, TX, p. A600

HILL COUNTRY SPECIALTY HOSPITAL, NEW BRAUNFELS, TX, p. A618

HILL CREST BEHAVIORAL HEALTH SERVICES, BIRMINGHAM, AL, p. A16

HILL HOSPITAL OF SUMTER COUNTY, YORK, AL, p. A27

HILL REGIONAL HOSPITAL, HILLSBORO, TX, p. A603

HILLCREST BAPTIST MEDICAL CENTER, WACO, TX, p. A633

HILLCREST BAPTIST MEDICAL CENTER – HERRING AVENUE CAMPUS, 3000 HERRING AVENUE, ZIP 76708 (see HILLCREST BAPTIST MEDICAL CENTER), p. A633

HILLCREST HOSPITAL, PITTSFIELD, MASSACHUSETTS (see BERKSHIRE MEDICAL CENTER), p. A303

HILLCREST HOSPITAL, CLEVELAND, OH, p. A475

HILLCREST HOSPITAL CLAREMORE, CLAREMORE, OK, p. A495

HILLCREST MEDICAL CENTER, TULSA, OK, p. A506

HILLCREST MEMORIAL HOSPITAL, SIMPSONVILLE, SC, p. A553

HILLS & DALES GENERAL HOSPITAL, CASS CITY, MI, p. A309

HILLSBORO AREA HOSPITAL, HILLSBORO, IL, p. A184

HILLSBORO COMMUNITY HOSPITAL, HILLSBORO, KS, p. A234

HILLSBORO MEDICAL CENTER, HILLSBORO, ND, p. A466

HILLSDALE COMMUNITY HEALTH CENTER, HILLSDALE, MI, p. A315

HILLSIDE HOSPITAL, PULASKI, TN, p. A574

HILLSIDE REHABILITATION HOSPITAL, WARREN, OH, p. A490

HILO MEDICAL CENTER, HILO, HI, p. A163

HILTON HEAD HOSPITAL, HILTON HEAD ISLAND, SC, p. A551

HIND GENERAL HOSPITAL, HOBART, IN, p. A203

HIRAM W. DAVIS MEDICAL CENTER, PETERSBURG, VA, p. A653

HOAG HOSPITAL IRVINE, IRVINE, CA, p. A65

HOAG MEMORIAL HOSPITAL PRESBYTERIAN, NEWPORT BEACH, CA, p. A76

HOBOKEN UNIVERSITY MEDICAL CENTER, HOBOKEN, NJ, p. A404

HOCKING VALLEY COMMUNITY HOSPITAL, LOGAN, OH, p. A483

HODGEMAN COUNTY HEALTH CENTER, JETMORE, KS, p. A235

HOLDENVILLE GENERAL HOSPITAL, HOLDENVILLE, OK, p. A497

HOLLAND HOSPITAL, HOLLAND, MI, p. A315

HOLLISWOOD HOSPITAL,, NY, p. A432

HOLLY HILL HOSPITAL, RALEIGH, NC, p. A459

HOLLYWOOD COMMUNITY HOSPITAL, LOS ANGELES, CA, p. A69

HOLLYWOOD COMMUNITY HOSPITAL OF VAN NUYS,, CALIFORNIA (see HOLLYWOOD COMMUNITY HOSPITAL), p. A69

HOLLYWOOD PAVILION,, FL, p. A125

HOLLYWOOD PRESBYTERIAN MEDICAL CENTER, LOS ANGELES, CA, p. A69

HOLMES COUNTY HOSPITAL AND CLINICS, LEXINGTON, MS, p. A349

HOLMES REGIONAL MEDICAL CENTER, MELBOURNE, FL, p. A130

HOLTON COMMUNITY HOSPITAL, HOLTON, KS, p. A234

HOLTZ CHILDREN'S HOSPITAL, MIAMI, FLORIDA (see JACKSON HEALTH SYSTEM), p. A131

HOLY CROSS HOSPITAL, FORT LAUDERDALE, FL, p. A123

HOLY CROSS HOSPITAL, CHICAGO, IL, p. A176

HOLY CROSS HOSPITAL, SILVER SPRING, MD, p. A294

HOLY CROSS HOSPITAL, TAOS, NM, p. A418

HOLY FAMILY HOSPITAL AND MEDICAL CENTER, METHUEN, MA, p. A302

HOLY FAMILY MEDICAL CENTER, DES PLAINES, IL, p. A180
HOLY FAMILY MEMORIAL MEDICAL CENTER, MANITOWOC, WI, p. A685
HOLY NAME MEDICAL CENTER, TEANECK, NJ, p. A410
HOLY REDEEMER HOSPITAL AND MEDICAL CENTER, MEADOWBROOK, PA, p. A528
HOLY ROSARY HEALTHCARE, MILES CITY, MT, p. A377
HOLY SPIRIT HOSPITAL, CAMP HILL, PA, p. A519
HOLYOKE MEDICAL CENTER, HOLYOKE, MA, p. A300
HOLZER MEDICAL CENTER, GALLIPOLIS, OH, p. A480
HOLZER MEDICAL CENTER – JACKSON, JACKSON, OH, p. A482
HOMER MEMORIAL HOSPITAL, HOMER, LA, p. A267
HOOD MEMORIAL HOSPITAL, AMITE, LA, p. A261
HOOPESTON REGIONAL HEALTH CENTER, HOOPESTON, IL, p. A185
HOPEDALE MEDICAL COMPLEX, HOPEDALE, IL, p. A185
HOPI HEALTH CARE CENTER, KEAMS CANYON, AZ, p. A33
HOPKINS COUNTY MEMORIAL HOSPITAL, SULPHUR SPRINGS, TX, p. A629
HORIZON MEDICAL CENTER, DICKSON, TN, p. A565
HORIZON SPECIALTY HOSPITAL, LAS VEGAS, NV, p. A393
HORN MEMORIAL HOSPITAL, IDA GROVE, IA, p. A221
HORSHAM CLINIC, AMBLER, PA, p. A518
HORTON COMMUNITY HOSPITAL, HORTON, KS, p. A235
HOSPITAL BUEN SAMARITANO, AGUADILLA, PR, p. A699
HOSPITAL DE DAMAS, PONCE, PR, p. A702
HOSPITAL DE LA CONCEPCION, SAN GERMAN, PR, p. A702
HOSPITAL DE LA UNIVERSIDAD DE PUERTO RICO/DR. FEDERICO TRILLA, CAROLINA, PR, p. A700
HOSPITAL DEL MAESTRO, SAN JUAN, PR, p. A703
HOSPITAL DR. CAYETANO COLL Y TOSTE, ARECIBO, PR, p. A700
HOSPITAL EPISCOPAL SAN LUCAS GUAYAMA, GUAYAMA, PR, p. A701
HOSPITAL FOR EXTENDED RECOVERY, NORFOLK, VA, p. A652
HOSPITAL FOR SPECIAL CARE, NEW BRITAIN, CT, p. A110
HOSPITAL FOR SPECIAL SURGERY, NEW YORK, NY, p. A433
HOSPITAL HERMANOS MELENDEZ, BAYAMON, PR, p. A700
HOSPITAL HMA DE HUMACAO, HUMACAO, PR, p. A701
HOSPITAL INTERAMERICANO DE MEDICINA AVANZADA, CAGUAS, PR, p. A700
HOSPITAL MANATI MEDICAL CENTER, MANATI, PR, p. A701
HOSPITAL MENONITA DE CAYEY, CAYEY, PR, p. A700
HOSPITAL METROPOLITAN, SAN JUAN, PR, p. A703
HOSPITAL METROPOLITANO DR. SUSONI, ARECIBO, PR, p. A700
HOSPITAL METROPOLITANO DR. TITO MATTEI, YAUCO, PR, p. A704
HOSPITAL METROPOLITANO SAN GERMAN, SAN GERMAN, PR, p. A702
HOSPITAL OF SAINT RAPHAEL, NEW HAVEN, CT, p. A110
HOSPITAL OF THE UNIVERSITY OF PENNSYLVANIA, PHILADELPHIA, PA, p. A532
HOSPITAL ONCOLOGICO ANDRES GRILLASCA, PONCE, PR, p. A702
HOSPITAL ORIENTE, HUMACAO, PR, p. A701
HOSPITAL PAVIA-HATO REY, SAN JUAN, PR, p. A703
HOSPITAL PAVIA-SANTURCE, SAN JUAN, PR, p. A703
HOSPITAL PEREA, MAYAGUEZ, PR, p. A702
HOSPITAL PSIQUIATRICO METROPOLITANO, CABO ROJO, PR, p. A700
HOSPITAL SAN CARLOS BORROMEO, MOCA, PR, p. A702
HOSPITAL SAN CRISTOBAL, COTO LAUREL, PR, p. A701
HOSPITAL SAN FRANCISCO, SAN JUAN, PR, p. A703
HOSPITAL SAN GERARDO, SAN JUAN, PR, p. A703
HOSPITAL SAN PABLO, BAYAMON, PR, p. A700
HOSPITAL SAN PABLO DEL ESTE, FAJARDO, PR, p. A701
HOSPITAL SANTA ROSA, GUAYAMA, PR, p. A701
HOSPITAL UNIVERSITARIO DR. RAMON RUIZ ARNAU, BAYAMON, PR, p. A700
HOT SPRINGS COUNTY MEMORIAL HOSPITAL, THERMOPOLIS, WY, p. A698
HOT SPRINGS REHABILITATION CENTER, HOT SPRINGS NATIONAL PARK, AR, p. A46
HOULTON REGIONAL HOSPITAL, HOULTON, ME, p. A283
HOUSTON HOSPITAL FOR SPECIALIZED SURGERY, HOUSTON, TX, p. A604
HOUSTON MEDICAL CENTER, WARNER ROBINS, GA, p. A161
HOUSTON NORTHWEST MEDICAL CENTER, HOUSTON, TX, p. A604
HOUSTON ORTHOPEDIC AND SPINE HOSPITAL, BELLAIRE, TX, p. A583
HOUSTON PHYSICIANS HOSPITAL, WEBSTER, TX, p. A634
HOWARD A. RUSK REHABILITATION CENTER, COLUMBIA, MO, p. A358
HOWARD COUNTY GENERAL HOSPITAL, COLUMBIA, MD, p. A290
HOWARD COUNTY MEDICAL CENTER, SAINT PAUL, NE, p. A389
HOWARD MEMORIAL HOSPITAL, NASHVILLE, AR, p. A49
HOWARD UNIVERSITY HOSPITAL, WASHINGTON, DC, p. A116

HOWARD YOUNG MEDICAL CENTER, WOODRUFF, WI, p. A694
HUDSON HOSPITAL, HUDSON, WI, p. A683
HUDSON VALLEY HOSPITAL CENTER, CORTLANDT MANOR, NY, p. A424
HUEY P. LONG MEDICAL CENTER, PINEVILLE, LA, p. A276
HUGGINS HOSPITAL, WOLFEBORO, NH, p. A400
HUGH CHATHAM MEMORIAL HOSPITAL, ELKIN, NC, p. A453
HUGHSTON HOSPITAL, COLUMBUS, GA, p. A149
HUGULEY MEMORIAL MEDICAL CENTER, FORT WORTH, TX, p. A598
HUHUKAM MEMORIAL HOSPITAL, SACATON, AZ, p. A37
HUMBOLDT COUNTY MEMORIAL HOSPITAL, HUMBOLDT, IA, p. A221
HUMBOLDT GENERAL HOSPITAL, WINNEMUCCA, NV, p. A396
HUMBOLDT GENERAL HOSPITAL, HUMBOLDT, TN, p. A566
HUNT MEMORIAL HOSPITAL DISTRICT, GREENVILLE, TX, p. A602
HUNT MEMORIAL HOSPITAL DISTRICT, GREENVILLE, TEXAS (see HUNT MEMORIAL HOSPITAL DISTRICT), p. A602
HUNT REGIONAL COMMUNITY HOSPITAL, COMMERCE, TX, p. A588
HUNTER HOLMES MCGUIRE VETERANS AFFAIRS MEDICAL CENTER, RICHMOND, VA, p. A655
HUNTERDON MEDICAL CENTER, FLEMINGTON, NJ, p. A404
HUNTINGTON BEACH HOSPITAL, HUNTINGTON BEACH, CA, p. A65
HUNTINGTON HOSPITAL, HUNTINGTON, NY, p. A427
HUNTINGTON MEMORIAL HOSPITAL, PASADENA, CA, p. A80
HUNTSVILLE HOSPITAL, HUNTSVILLE, AL, p. A22
HUNTSVILLE HOSPITAL FOR WOMEN AND CHILDREN, HUNTSVILLE, ALABAMA (see HUNTSVILLE HOSPITAL), p. A22
HUNTSVILLE MEMORIAL HOSPITAL, HUNTSVILLE, TX, p. A608
HURLEY MEDICAL CENTER, FLINT, MI, p. A312
HURON MEDICAL CENTER, BAD AXE, MI, p. A307
HURON REGIONAL MEDICAL CENTER, HURON, SD, p. A557
HURON VALLEY-SINAI HOSPITAL, COMMERCE TOWNSHIP, MI, p. A310
HUTCHINSON AREA HEALTH CARE, HUTCHINSON, MN, p. A333
HUTCHINSON REGIONAL MEDICAL CENTER, HUTCHINSON, KS, p. A235
HUTZEL HOSPITAL, DETROIT, MICHIGAN (see HARPER UNIVERSITY HOSPITAL/HUTZEL WOMEN'S HOSPITAL), p. A310

# I

I-70 COMMUNITY HOSPITAL, SWEET SPRINGS, MO, p. A371
I. GONZALEZ MARTINEZ ONCOLOGIC HOSPITAL,, PR, p. A703
IBERIA EXTENDED CARE HOSPITAL, NEW IBERIA, LA, p. A274
IBERIA MEDICAL CENTER, NEW IBERIA, LA, p. A274
IBERIA REHABILITATION HOSPITAL, NEW IBERIA, LA, p. A274
ICON HOSPITAL, HUMBLE, TX, p. A608
IDAHO FALLS RECOVERY CENTER, IDAHO FALLS, ID, p. A168
ILLINI COMMUNITY HOSPITAL, PITTSFIELD, IL, p. A192
ILLINOIS VALLEY COMMUNITY HOSPITAL, PERU, IL, p. A191
INCLINE VILLAGE COMMUNITY HOSPITAL, INCLINE VILLAGE, NV, p. A392
INDIAN HEALTH SERVICE HOSPITAL, RAPID CITY, SD, p. A558
INDIAN PATH MEDICAL CENTER, KINGSPORT, TN, p. A568
INDIAN RIVER MEDICAL CENTER, VERO BEACH, FL, p. A142
INDIANA HEART HOSPITAL, INDIANAPOLIS, IN, p. A204
INDIANA ORTHOPAEDIC HOSPITAL, INDIANAPOLIS, IN, p. A204
INDIANA REGIONAL MEDICAL CENTER, INDIANA, PA, p. A525
INDIANA UNIVERSITY HEALTH ARNETT HOSPITAL, LAFAYETTE, IN, p. A206
INDIANA UNIVERSITY HEALTH BALL MEMORIAL HOSPITAL, MUNCIE, IN, p. A209
INDIANA UNIVERSITY HEALTH BEDFORD HOSPITAL, BEDFORD, IN, p. A197
INDIANA UNIVERSITY HEALTH BLACKFORD HOSPITAL, HARTFORD CITY, IN, p. A203
INDIANA UNIVERSITY HEALTH BLOOMINGTON HOSPITAL, BLOOMINGTON, IN, p. A198
INDIANA UNIVERSITY HEALTH GOSHEN HOSPITAL, GOSHEN, IN, p. A202
INDIANA UNIVERSITY HEALTH LA PORTE HOSPITAL, LA PORTE, IN, p. A206
INDIANA UNIVERSITY HEALTH METHODIST HOSPITAL, INDIANAPOLIS, INDIANA (see INDIANA UNIVERSITY HEALTH UNIVERSITY HOSPITAL), p. A204
INDIANA UNIVERSITY HEALTH MORGAN HOSPITAL, MARTINSVILLE, IN, p. A208
INDIANA UNIVERSITY HEALTH NORTH HOSPITAL, CARMEL, IN, p. A199
INDIANA UNIVERSITY HEALTH PAOLI HOSPITAL, PAOLI, IN, p. A210

INDIANA UNIVERSITY HEALTH STARKE HOSPITAL, KNOX, IN, p. A206
INDIANA UNIVERSITY HEALTH TIPTON HOSPITAL, TIPTON, IN, p. A212
INDIANA UNIVERSITY HEALTH UNIVERSITY HOSPITAL, INDIANAPOLIS, IN, p. A204
INDIANA UNIVERSITY HEALTH WEST HOSPITAL, AVON, IN, p. A197
INDIANA UNIVERSITY HEALTH WHITE MEMORIAL HOSPITAL, MONTICELLO, IN, p. A208
INDIANA UNIVERSITY HOSPITAL, INDIANAPOLIS, INDIANA (see INDIANA UNIVERSITY HEALTH UNIVERSITY HOSPITAL), p. A204
INDIANHEAD MEDICAL CENTER, SHELL LAKE, WI, p. A691
INDUSTRIAL HOSPITAL, SAN JUAN, PR, p. A703
INFIRMARY LONG TERM ACUTE CARE HOSPITAL, MOBILE, AL, p. A22
INFIRMARY WEST, MOBILE, AL, p. A22
INGALLS MEMORIAL HOSPITAL, HARVEY, IL, p. A183
INGHAM REGIONAL MEDICAL CENTER, GREENLAWN CAMPUS, LANSING, MICHIGAN (see MCLAREN GREATER LANSING), p. A317
INLAND HOSPITAL, WATERVILLE, ME, p. A285
INLAND VALLEY MEDICAL CENTER, WILDOMAR, CA, p. A96
INOVA ALEXANDRIA HOSPITAL, ALEXANDRIA, VA, p. A645
INOVA FAIR OAKS HOSPITAL, FAIRFAX, VA, p. A647
INOVA FAIRFAX HOSPITAL, FALLS CHURCH, VA, p. A647
INOVA FAIRFAX HOSPITAL FOR CHILDREN, FALLS CHURCH, VIRGINIA (see INOVA FAIRFAX HOSPITAL), p. A647
INOVA LOUDOUN HOSPITAL, LEESBURG, VA, p. A650
INOVA MOUNT VERNON HOSPITAL, ALEXANDRIA, VA, p. A645
INSTITUTE FOR ORTHOPAEDIC SURGERY, LIMA, OH, p. A482
INSTITUTE OF LIVING, HARTFORD, CONNECTICUT (see HARTFORD HOSPITAL), p. A109
INTEGRA SPECIALTY HOSPITAL, MUNCIE, IN, p. A209
INTEGRIS BAPTIST MEDICAL CENTER, OKLAHOMA CITY, OK, p. A501
INTEGRIS BAPTIST REGIONAL HEALTH CENTER, MIAMI, OK, p. A499
INTEGRIS BASS BAPTIST HEALTH CENTER, ENID, OK, p. A496
INTEGRIS BASS PAVILION, ENID, OK, p. A496
INTEGRIS BLACKWELL REGIONAL HOSPITAL, BLACKWELL, OK, p. A494
INTEGRIS CANADIAN VALLEY HOSPITAL, YUKON, OK, p. A508
INTEGRIS CLINTON REGIONAL HOSPITAL, CLINTON, OK, p. A495
INTEGRIS GROVE GENERAL HOSPITAL, GROVE, OK, p. A497
INTEGRIS HEALTH EDMOND, EDMOND, OK, p. A495
INTEGRIS MARSHALL COUNTY MEDICAL CENTER, MADILL, OK, p. A498
INTEGRIS MAYES COUNTY MEDICAL CENTER, PRYOR, OK, p. A503
INTEGRIS MENTAL HEALTH SYSTEM–SPENCER, SPENCER, OKLAHOMA (see INTEGRIS BAPTIST MEDICAL CENTER), p. A501
INTEGRIS SEMINOLE MEDICAL CENTER, SEMINOLE, OK, p. A504
INTEGRIS SOUTHWEST MEDICAL CENTER, OKLAHOMA CITY, OK, p. A501
INTEGRITY TRANSITIONAL HOSPITAL, DENTON, TX, p. A593
INTERFAITH MEDICAL CENTER,, NY, p. A433
INTERIM LSU PUBLIC HOSPITAL, NEW ORLEANS, LA, p. A274
INTERMEDICAL HOSPITAL OF SOUTH CAROLINA, COLUMBIA, SC, p. A548
INTERMOUNTAIN HOSPITAL, BOISE, ID, p. A166
INTERMOUNTAIN MEDICAL CENTER, MURRAY, UT, p. A638
INTRACARE NORTH HOSPITAL, HOUSTON, TX, p. A604
IOWA CITY VETERANS AFFAIRS HEALTH CARE SYSTEM, IOWA CITY, IA, p. A221
IOWA LUTHERAN HOSPITAL, DES MOINES, IA, p. A218
IOWA MEDICAL AND CLASSIFICATION CENTER, OAKDALE, IA, p. A224
IOWA METHODIST MEDICAL CENTER, DES MOINES, IA, p. A218
IOWA SPECIALTY HOSPITAL–BELMOND, BELMOND, IA, p. A214
IOWA SPECIALTY HOSPITAL–CLARION, CLARION, IA, p. A216
IRA DAVENPORT MEMORIAL HOSPITAL, BATH, NY, p. A421
IRAAN GENERAL HOSPITAL, IRAAN, TX, p. A608
IREDELL MEMORIAL HOSPITAL, STATESVILLE, NC, p. A461
IRELAND ARMY COMMUNITY HOSPITAL, FORT KNOX, KY, p. A250
IRON COUNTY HOSPITAL, PILOT KNOB, MO, p. A366
IROQUOIS MEMORIAL HOSPITAL AND RESIDENT HOME, WATSEKA, IL, p. A195
IRVING COPPELL SURGICAL HOSPITAL, IRVING, TX, p. A609
IRWIN ARMY COMMUNITY HOSPITAL, JUNCTION CITY, KS, p. A236
IRWIN COUNTY HOSPITAL, OCILLA, GA, p. A157
ISHAM HEALTH CENTER, ANDOVER, MA, p. A295
ISLAND HOSPITAL, ANACORTES, WA, p. A659
IVINSON MEMORIAL HOSPITAL, LARAMIE, WY, p. A696

## J

J. ARTHUR DOSHER MEMORIAL HOSPITAL, SOUTHPORT, NC, p. A461
J. C. BLAIR MEMORIAL HOSPITAL, HUNTINGDON, PA, p. A525
J. D. MCCARTY CENTER FOR CHILDREN WITH DEVELOPMENTAL DISABILITIES, NORMAN, OK, p. A500
J. F. K. MEDICAL CENTER, ATLANTIS, FL, p. A118
J. PAUL JONES HOSPITAL, CAMDEN, AL, p. A18
JACK C. MONTGOMERY VETERANS AFFAIRS MEDICAL CENTER, MUSKOGEE, OK, p. A499
JACK D WEILER HOSPITAL OF ALBERT EINSTEIN COLLEGE OF MEDICINE,, NEW YORK (see MONTEFIORE MEDICAL CENTER), p. A434
JACK HUGHSTON MEMORIAL HOSPITAL, PHENIX CITY, AL, p. A25
JACKSON COUNTY HOSPITAL DISTRICT, EDNA, TX, p. A595
JACKSON COUNTY MEMORIAL HOSPITAL, ALTUS, OK, p. A493
JACKSON COUNTY REGIONAL HEALTH CENTER, MAQUOKETA, IA, p. A223
JACKSON GENERAL HOSPITAL, RIPLEY, WV, p. A675
JACKSON HEALTH SYSTEM, MIAMI, FL, p. A131
JACKSON HOSPITAL, MARIANNA, FL, p. A130
JACKSON HOSPITAL AND CLINIC, MONTGOMERY, AL, p. A24
JACKSON MEDICAL CENTER, JACKSON, AL, p. A22
JACKSON MEMORIAL HOSPITAL, MIAMI, FLORIDA (see JACKSON HEALTH SYSTEM), p. A131
JACKSON NORTH MEDICAL CENTER, NORTH MIAMI BEACH, FLORIDA (see JACKSON HEALTH SYSTEM), p. A131
JACKSON PARISH HOSPITAL, JONESBORO, LA, p. A268
JACKSON PARK HOSPITAL AND MEDICAL CENTER, CHICAGO, IL, p. A176
JACKSON PURCHASE MEDICAL CENTER, MAYFIELD, KY, p. A256
JACKSON SOUTH COMMUNITY HOSPITAL, MIAMI, FLORIDA (see JACKSON HEALTH SYSTEM), p. A131
JACKSON–MADISON COUNTY GENERAL HOSPITAL, JACKSON, TN, p. A567
JACKSONVILLE MEDICAL CENTER, JACKSONVILLE, AL, p. A22
JACOBI MEDICAL CENTER,, NY, p. A433
JACOBSON MEMORIAL HOSPITAL CARE CENTER, ELGIN, ND, p. A465
JAMAICA HOSPITAL MEDICAL CENTER,, NY, p. A433
JAMES A. HALEY VETERANS HOSPITAL, TAMPA, FL, p. A140
JAMES B. HAGGIN MEMORIAL HOSPITAL, HARRODSBURG, KY, p. A251
JAMES CANCER HOSPITAL AND SOLOVE RESEARCH INSTITUTE, COLUMBUS, OH, p. A476
JAMES E. VAN ZANDT VETERANS AFFAIRS MEDICAL CENTER, ALTOONA, PA, p. A517
JAMES H. QUILLEN VETERANS AFFAIRS MEDICAL CENTER, MOUNTAIN HOME, TN, p. A572
JAMESON HOSPITAL, NEW CASTLE, PA, p. A530
JAMESTOWN REGIONAL MEDICAL CENTER, JAMESTOWN, ND, p. A466
JAMESTOWN REGIONAL MEDICAL CENTER, JAMESTOWN, TN, p. A567
JANE PHILLIPS MEDICAL CENTER, BARTLESVILLE, OK, p. A494
JANE PHILLIPS NOWATA HEALTH CENTER, NOWATA, OK, p. A500
JANE TODD CRAWFORD HOSPITAL, GREENSBURG, KY, p. A251
JASPER COUNTY HOSPITAL, RENSSELAER, IN, p. A211
JASPER COUNTY NURSING HOME (see JASPER GENERAL HOSPITAL), p. A343
JASPER GENERAL HOSPITAL, BAY SPRINGS, MS, p. A343
JASPER MEMORIAL HOSPITAL, MONTICELLO, GA, p. A156
JAY COUNTY HOSPITAL, PORTLAND, IN, p. A210
JAY HOSPITAL, JAY, FL, p. A127
JEANES HOSPITAL, PHILADELPHIA, PA, p. A532
JEFF DAVIS HOSPITAL, HAZLEHURST, GA, p. A154
JEFFERSON COMMUNITY HEALTH CENTER, FAIRBURY, NE, p. A383
JEFFERSON COUNTY HEALTH CENTER, FAIRFIELD, IA, p. A219
JEFFERSON COUNTY HOSPITAL, FAYETTE, MS, p. A345
JEFFERSON COUNTY HOSPITAL, WAURIKA, OK, p. A507
JEFFERSON DAVIS COMMUNITY HOSPITAL, PRENTISS, MS, p. A352
JEFFERSON HEALTHCARE, PORT TOWNSEND, WA, p. A664
JEFFERSON HOSPITAL, LOUISVILLE, GA, p. A155
JEFFERSON MEMORIAL HOSPITAL, JEFFERSON CITY, TN, p. A567
JEFFERSON MEMORIAL HOSPITAL, RANSON, WV, p. A675
JEFFERSON REGIONAL MEDICAL CENTER, PINE BLUFF, AR, p. A50
JEFFERSON REGIONAL MEDICAL CENTER, CRYSTAL CITY, MO, p. A358

JEFFERSON REGIONAL MEDICAL CENTER, JEFFERSON HILLS, PA, p. A525
JELLICO COMMUNITY HOSPITAL, JELLICO, TN, p. A567
JENKINS COUNTY HOSPITAL, MILLEN, GA, p. A156
JENNERSVILLE REGIONAL HOSPITAL, WEST GROVE, PA, p. A541
JENNIE EDMUNDSON HOSPITAL, COUNCIL BLUFFS, IA, p. A217
JENNIE M. MELHAM MEMORIAL MEDICAL CENTER, BROKEN BOW, NE, p. A382
JENNIE STUART MEDICAL CENTER, HOPKINSVILLE, KY, p. A251
JENNINGS AMERICAN LEGION HOSPITAL, JENNINGS, LA, p. A268
JENNINGS SENIOR CARE HOSPITAL, JENNINGS, LA, p. A268
JEROLD PHELPS COMMUNITY HOSPITAL, GARBERVILLE, CA, p. A62
JEROME GOLDEN CENTER FOR BEHAVIORAL HEALTH, INC., WEST PALM BEACH, FL, p. A142
JERRY L. PETTIS MEMORIAL VETERANS MEDICAL CENTER, LOMA LINDA, CA, p. A67
JERSEY COMMUNITY HOSPITAL, JERSEYVILLE, IL, p. A185
JERSEY SHORE HOSPITAL, JERSEY SHORE, PA, p. A525
JERSEY SHORE UNIVERSITY MEDICAL CENTER, NEPTUNE, NJ, p. A406
JESSE BROWN VETERANS AFFAIRS CHICAGO HEALTH CARE SYSTEM, CHICAGO, IL, p. A176
JEWELL COUNTY HOSPITAL, MANKATO, KS, p. A238
JEWISH HOSPITAL, LOUISVILLE, KY, p. A254
JEWISH HOSPITAL–SHELBYVILLE, SHELBYVILLE, KY, p. A259
JFK JOHNSON REHABILITATION INSTITUTE, EDISON, NJ, p. A403
JFK MEDICAL CENTER, EDISON, NJ, p. A403
JIM TALIAFERRO COMMUNITY MENTAL HEALTH, LAWTON, OK, p. A498
JOE DIMAGGIO CHILDREN'S HOSPITAL,, FLORIDA (see MEMORIAL REGIONAL HOSPITAL SOUTH), p. A125
JOHN C. FREMONT HEALTHCARE DISTRICT, MARIPOSA, CA, p. A74
JOHN C. LINCOLN DEER VALLEY HOSPITAL, PHOENIX, AZ, p. A35
JOHN C. LINCOLN NORTH MOUNTAIN HOSPITAL, PHOENIX, AZ, p. A35
JOHN C. STENNIS MEMORIAL HOSPITAL, DE KALB, MS, p. A345
JOHN D. ARCHBOLD MEMORIAL HOSPITAL, THOMASVILLE, GA, p. A160
JOHN D. DINGELL VETERANS AFFAIRS MEDICAL CENTER, DETROIT, MI, p. A311
JOHN F. KENNEDY MEMORIAL HOSPITAL, INDIO, CA, p. A65
JOHN H. STROGER JR. HOSPITAL OF COOK COUNTY, CHICAGO, IL, p. A176
JOHN HEINZ INSTITUTE OF REHABILITATION MEDICINE, WILKES-BARRE, PA, p. A541
JOHN J. MADDEN MENTAL HEALTH CENTER, HINES, IL, p. A184
JOHN J. PERSHING VETERANS AFFAIRS MEDICAL CENTER, POPLAR BLUFF, MO, p. A367
JOHN MUIR BEHAVIORAL HEALTH CENTER, CONCORD, CA, p. A58
JOHN MUIR MEDICAL CENTER, CONCORD, CONCORD, CA, p. A58
JOHN MUIR MEDICAL CENTER, WALNUT CREEK, WALNUT CREEK, CA, p. A95
JOHN PETER SMITH HOSPITAL, FORT WORTH, TEXAS (see JPS HEALTH NETWORK), p. A599
JOHN RANDOLPH MEDICAL CENTER, HOPEWELL, VA, p. A649
JOHN STODDARD CANCER CENTER, DES MOINES, IOWA (see IOWA METHODIST MEDICAL CENTER), p. A218
JOHN T. MATHER MEMORIAL HOSPITAL, PORT JEFFERSON, NY, p. A440
JOHN UMSTEAD HOSPITAL, BUTNER, NC, p. A450
JOHNS HOPKINS BAYVIEW MEDICAL CENTER, BALTIMORE, MD, p. A287
JOHNS HOPKINS CHILDREN'S CENTER, BALTIMORE, MARYLAND (see JOHNS HOPKINS HOSPITAL), p. A287
JOHNS HOPKINS HOSPITAL, BALTIMORE, MD, p. A287
JOHNSON CITY MEDICAL CENTER, JOHNSON CITY, TN, p. A567
JOHNSON COUNTY COMMUNITY HOSPITAL, MOUNTAIN CITY, TN, p. A572
JOHNSON COUNTY HEALTHCARE CENTER, BUFFALO, WY, p. A695
JOHNSON COUNTY HOSPITAL, TECUMSEH, NE, p. A390
JOHNSON MEMORIAL HEALTH SERVICES, DAWSON, MN, p. A330
JOHNSON MEMORIAL HOSPITAL, STAFFORD SPRINGS, CT, p. A112
JOHNSON MEMORIAL HOSPITAL, FRANKLIN, IN, p. A202
JOHNSON REGIONAL MEDICAL CENTER, CLARKSVILLE, AR, p. A43
JOHNSON–MATHERS NURSING HOME (see NICHOLAS COUNTY HOSPITAL), p. A248

JOHNSTON HEALTH, SMITHFIELD, NC, p. A461
JOHNSTON MEMORIAL HOSPITAL, ABINGDON, VA, p. A645
JOHNSTON R. BOWMAN HEALTH CENTER, CHICAGO, ILLINOIS (see RUSH UNIVERSITY MEDICAL CENTER), p. A178
JOHNSTON–WILLIS HOSPITAL, RICHMOND, VIRGINIA (see CJW MEDICAL CENTER), p. A654
JOINT TOWNSHIP DISTRICT MEMORIAL HOSPITAL, SAINT MARYS, OH, p. A488
JONATHAN M. WAINWRIGHT MEMORIAL VA MEDICAL CENTER, WALLA WALLA, WA, p. A669
JONES MEMORIAL HOSPITAL, WELLSVILLE, NY, p. A446
JONES REGIONAL MEDICAL CENTER, ANAMOSA, IA, p. A214
JORDAN HOSPITAL, PLYMOUTH, MA, p. A304
JORDAN VALLEY MEDICAL CENTER, WEST JORDAN, UT, p. A642
JPS HEALTH NETWORK, FORT WORTH, TX, p. A599
JULIAN F. KEITH ALCOHOL AND DRUG ABUSE TREATMENT CENTER, BLACK MOUNTAIN, NC, p. A448
JULIETTE MANOR NURSING HOME, COMMUNITY CLINICS (see BERLIN MEMORIAL HOSPITAL), p. A679
JUPITER MEDICAL CENTER, JUPITER, FL, p. A127

## K

K. HOVNANIAN CHILDREN'S HOSPITAL, NEPTUNE, NEW JERSEY (see JERSEY SHORE UNIVERSITY MEDICAL CENTER), p. A406
KAATERSKILL CARE, CATSKILL, NEW YORK (see COLUMBIA MEMORIAL HOSPITAL), p. A427
KADLEC MEDICAL CENTER, RICHLAND, WA, p. A665
KAHI MOHALA BEHAVIORAL HEALTH, EWA BEACH, HI, p. A163
KAHUKU MEDICAL CENTER, KAHUKU, HI, p. A164
KAISER FOUNDATION HOSPITAL, MARTINEZ, CALIFORNIA (see WALNUT CREEK MEDICAL CENTER), p. A95
KAISER FOUNDATION MENTAL HEALTH CENTER, LOS ANGELES, CALIFORNIA (see LOS ANGELES MEDICAL CENTER), p. A70
KAISER PERMANENTE DOWNEY MEDICAL CENTER, DOWNEY,, p. A59
KAISER PERMANENTE MEDICAL CENTER, HONOLULU, HI, p. A163
KALAMAZOO PSYCHIATRIC HOSPITAL, KALAMAZOO, MI, p. A316
KALEIDA HEALTH, BUFFALO, NY, p. A422
KALISPELL REGIONAL MEDICAL CENTER, KALISPELL, MT, p. A377
KALKASKA MEMORIAL HEALTH CENTER, KALKASKA, MI, p. A317
KANE COMMUNITY HOSPITAL, KANE, PA, p. A526
KANE COUNTY HOSPITAL, KANAB, UT, p. A638
KANSAS CITY ORTHOPAEDIC INSTITUTE, LEAWOOD, KS, p. A237
KANSAS HEART HOSPITAL, WICHITA, KS, p. A245
KANSAS MEDICAL CENTER, ANDOVER, KS, p. A230
KANSAS NEUROLOGICAL INSTITUTE, TOPEKA, KS, p. A244
KANSAS REHABILITATION HOSPITAL, TOPEKA, KS, p. A244
KANSAS SPINE HOSPITAL, WICHITA, KS, p. A245
KANSAS SURGERY AND RECOVERY CENTER, WICHITA, KS, p. A245
KAPIOLANI MEDICAL CENTER FOR WOMEN & CHILDREN, HONOLULU, HI, p. A163
KARL AND ESTHER HOBLITZELLE MEMORIAL HOSPITAL, DALLAS, TEXAS (see BAYLOR UNIVERSITY MEDICAL CENTER), p. A590
KARMANOS CANCER CENTER, DETROIT, MI, p. A311
KATHERINE SHAW BETHEA HOSPITAL, DIXON, IL, p. A180
KAU HOSPITAL, PAHALA, HI, p. A165
KAUAI VETERANS MEMORIAL HOSPITAL, WAIMEA, HI, p. A165
KAWEAH DELTA MEDICAL CENTER, VISALIA, CA, p. A95
KEARNEY COUNTY HEALTH SERVICES, MINDEN, NE, p. A386
KEARNY COUNTY HOSPITAL, LAKIN, KS, p. A237
KECK HOSPITAL OF USC, LOS ANGELES, CA, p. A70
KEEFE MEMORIAL HOSPITAL, CHEYENNE WELLS, CO, p. A98
KELL WEST REGIONAL HOSPITAL, WICHITA FALLS, TX, p. A635
KELLER ARMY COMMUNITY HOSPITAL, WEST POINT, NY, p. A446
KENDALL REGIONAL MEDICAL CENTER, MIAMI, FL, p. A131
KENMARE COMMUNITY HOSPITAL, KENMARE, ND, p. A467
KENMORE MERCY HOSPITAL, KENMORE, NY, p. A428
KENNEDY KRIEGER INSTITUTE, BALTIMORE, MD, p. A287
KENNEDY MEMORIAL HOSPITAL, STRATFORD, NEW JERSEY (see KENNEDY MEMORIAL HOSPITALS–UNIVERSITY MEDICAL CENTER), p. A403
KENNEDY MEMORIAL HOSPITAL, TURNERSVILLE, NEW JERSEY (see KENNEDY MEMORIAL HOSPITALS–UNIVERSITY MEDICAL CENTER), p. A403
KENNEDY MEMORIAL HOSPITALS–UNIVERSITY MEDICAL CENTER, CHERRY HILL, NJ, p. A403

KENNEWICK GENERAL HOSPITAL, KENNEWICK, WA, p. A662
KENSINGTON MEDICAL CENTER, PHILADELPHIA, PA, p. A533
KENT COUNTY MEMORIAL HOSPITAL, WARWICK, RI, p. A545
KENTFIELD REHABILITATION AND SPECIALTY HOSPITAL, KENTFIELD, CA, p. A65
KENTUCKIANA MEDICAL CENTER, CLARKSVILLE, IN, p. A199
KENTUCKY CHILDREN'S HOSPITAL, LEXINGTON, KENTUCKY (see UNIVERSITY OF KENTUCKY ALBERT B. CHANDLER HOSPITAL), p. A253
KENTUCKY RIVER MEDICAL CENTER, JACKSON, KY, p. A252
KEOKUK AREA HOSPITAL, KEOKUK, IA, p. A222
KEOKUK COUNTY HEALTH CENTER, SIGOURNEY, IA, p. A226
KERN MEDICAL CENTER, BAKERSFIELD, CA, p. A55
KERN VALLEY HEALTHCARE DISTRICT, LAKE ISABELLA, CA, p. A66
KERNAN ORTHOPAEDICS AND REHABILITATION, BALTIMORE, MD, p. A287
KERNERSVILLE MEDICAL CENTER, KERNERSVILLE, NORTH CAROLINA (see FORSYTH MEDICAL CENTER), p. A463
KERRVILLE DIVISION, KERRVILLE, TEXAS (see SOUTH TEXAS VETERANS HEALTH CARE SYSTEM), p. A626
KERRVILLE STATE HOSPITAL, KERRVILLE, TX, p. A610
KERSHAWHEALTH, CAMDEN, SC, p. A546
KESSLER INSTITUTE FOR REHABILITATION, WEST ORANGE, NJ, p. A412
KESSLER INSTITUTE FOR REHABILITATION, CHESTER, NEW JERSEY (see KESSLER INSTITUTE FOR REHABILITATION), p. A412
KESSLER INSTITUTE FOR REHABILITATION, SADDLE BROOK, NEW JERSEY (see KESSLER INSTITUTE FOR REHABILITATION), p. A412
KESSLER INSTITUTE FOR REHABILITATION, WEST ORANGE, NEW JERSEY (see KESSLER INSTITUTE FOR REHABILITATION), p. A412
KETTERING MEDICAL CENTER, KETTERING, OH, p. A482
KEWANEE HOSPITAL, KEWANEE, IL, p. A186
KEYSTONE NEWPORT NEWS, NEWPORT NEWS, VA, p. A652
KIDSPEACE CHILDREN'S HOSPITAL, OREFIELD, PA, p. A531
KILMICHAEL HOSPITAL, KILMICHAEL, MS, p. A348
KIMBALL HEALTH SERVICES, KIMBALL, NE, p. A385
KIMBALL MEDICAL CENTER, LAKEWOOD, NJ, p. A405
KIMBALL-RIDGE CENTER, WATERLOO, IOWA (see COVENANT MEDICAL CENTER), p. A228
KIMBLE HOSPITAL, JUNCTION, TX, p. A609
KINDRED CHICAGO LAKESHORE, CHICAGO, ILLINOIS (see KINDRED CHICAGO-CENTRAL HOSPITAL), p. A176
KINDRED CHICAGO-CENTRAL HOSPITAL, CHICAGO, IL, p. A176
KINDRED HOSPITAL ARIZONA-NORTHWEST PHOENIX, PEORIA, ARIZONA (see KINDRED HOSPITAL ARIZONA-PHOENIX), p. A35
KINDRED HOSPITAL ARIZONA-PHOENIX, PHOENIX, AZ, p. A35
KINDRED HOSPITAL ARIZONA-SCOTTSDALE, SCOTTSDALE, ARIZONA (see KINDRED HOSPITAL ARIZONA-PHOENIX), p. A35
KINDRED HOSPITAL BAY AREA-TAMPA, TAMPA, FL, p. A141
KINDRED HOSPITAL BAYTOWN, BAYTOWN, TEXAS (see KINDRED HOSPITAL EAST HOUSTON), p. A587
KINDRED HOSPITAL BOSTON-NORTH SHORE, PEABODY, MA, p. A303
KINDRED HOSPITAL CHICAGO NORTH, CHICAGO, ILLINOIS (see KINDRED CHICAGO-CENTRAL HOSPITAL), p. A176
KINDRED HOSPITAL CHICAGO-NORTHLAKE, NORTHLAKE, IL, p. A189
KINDRED HOSPITAL CLEVELAND-GATEWAY, CLEVELAND, OH, p. A475
KINDRED HOSPITAL DALLAS CENTRAL, DALLAS, TX, p. A591
KINDRED HOSPITAL DALLAS-WALNUT HILL, DALLAS, TEXAS (see KINDRED HOSPITAL-DALLAS), p. A591
KINDRED HOSPITAL DETROIT, DETROIT, MI, p. A311
KINDRED HOSPITAL EAST HOUSTON, CHANNELVIEW, TX, p. A587
KINDRED HOSPITAL EASTON, EASTON, PA, p. A522
KINDRED HOSPITAL EL PASO, EL PASO, TX, p. A596
KINDRED HOSPITAL FARGO, FARGO, ND, p. A465
KINDRED HOSPITAL INDIANAPOLIS SOUTH, GREENWOOD, IN, p. A203
KINDRED HOSPITAL KANSAS CITY, KANSAS CITY, MO, p. A362
KINDRED HOSPITAL LAFAYETTE, LAFAYETTE, LA, p. A270
KINDRED HOSPITAL LAS VEGAS, DESERT SPRINGS CAMPUS, LAS VEGAS, NEVADA (see KINDRED HOSPITAL LAS VEGAS-SAHARA), p. A393
KINDRED HOSPITAL LAS VEGAS-SAHARA, LAS VEGAS, NV, p. A393
KINDRED HOSPITAL LIMA, LIMA, OH, p. A482
KINDRED HOSPITAL LOUISVILLE AT JEWISH HOSPITAL, LOUISVILLE, KENTUCKY (see KINDRED HOSPITAL-LOUISVILLE), p. A254
KINDRED HOSPITAL MELBOURNE, MELBOURNE, FL, p. A130
KINDRED HOSPITAL MIDTOWN, HOUSTON, TX, p. A604

KINDRED HOSPITAL NEW JERSEY - RAHWAY, RAHWAY, NEW JERSEY (see KINDRED HOSPITAL-NEW JERSEY MORRIS COUNTY), p. A403
KINDRED HOSPITAL NEW JERSEY - WAYNE, WAYNE, NEW JERSEY (see KINDRED HOSPITAL-NEW JERSEY MORRIS COUNTY), p. A403
KINDRED HOSPITAL NORTH FLORIDA, GREEN COVE SPRINGS, FL, p. A124
KINDRED HOSPITAL NORTH HOUSTON, HOUSTON, TX, p. A604
KINDRED HOSPITAL NORTHEAST-STOUGHTON, STOUGHTON, MA, p. A305
KINDRED HOSPITAL NORTHLAND, KANSAS CITY, MO, p. A362
KINDRED HOSPITAL NORTHWEST INDIANA, HAMMOND, IN, p. A203
KINDRED HOSPITAL OCALA, OCALA, FL, p. A133
KINDRED HOSPITAL OF CENTRAL OHIO, MANSFIELD, OH, p. A483
KINDRED HOSPITAL OF CLEVELAND, CLEVELAND, OHIO (see KINDRED HOSPITAL CLEVELAND-GATEWAY), p. A475
KINDRED HOSPITAL OF NORTHERN INDIANA, MISHAWAKA, IN, p. A208
KINDRED HOSPITAL OF RIVERSIDE, PERRIS, CA, p. A80
KINDRED HOSPITAL OF SOUTH BAY, GARDENA, CA, p. A63
KINDRED HOSPITAL PARK VIEW, SPRINGFIELD, MA, p. A304
KINDRED HOSPITAL PARK VIEW-CENTRAL MASSACHUSETTS, ROCHDALE, MASSACHUSETTS (see KINDRED HOSPITAL PARK VIEW), p. A304
KINDRED HOSPITAL PEORIA, PEORIA, IL, p. A191
KINDRED HOSPITAL PITTSBURGH-NORTH SHORE, PITTSBURGH, PA, p. A534
KINDRED HOSPITAL RANCHO, RANCHO CUCAMONGA, CA, p. A81
KINDRED HOSPITAL RICHMOND, RICHMOND, VA, p. A655
KINDRED HOSPITAL ROME, ROME, GA, p. A158
KINDRED HOSPITAL SAN GABRIEL VALLEY, WEST COVINA, CALIFORNIA (see KINDRED HOSPITAL-LA MIRADA), p. A66
KINDRED HOSPITAL SANTA ANA, SANTA ANA, CALIFORNIA (see KINDRED HOSPITAL-LA MIRADA), p. A66
KINDRED HOSPITAL SEATTLE-FIRST HILL, SEATTLE, WASHINGTON (see KINDRED HOSPITAL SEATTLE-NORTHGATE), p. A665
KINDRED HOSPITAL SEATTLE-NORTHGATE, SEATTLE, WA, p. A665
KINDRED HOSPITAL SOUTH FLORIDA-CORAL GABLES, CORAL GABLES, FLORIDA (see KINDRED HOSPITAL SOUTH FLORIDA-FORT LAUDERDALE), p. A123
KINDRED HOSPITAL SOUTH FLORIDA-FORT LAUDERDALE, FORT LAUDERDALE, FL, p. A123
KINDRED HOSPITAL SOUTH FLORIDA-HOLLYWOOD,, FL, p. A125
KINDRED HOSPITAL SOUTH PHILADELPHIA, PHILADELPHIA, PA, p. A533
KINDRED HOSPITAL SPRING, HOUSTON, TEXAS (see KINDRED HOSPITAL NORTH HOUSTON), p. A604
KINDRED HOSPITAL SPRINGFIELD, SPRINGFIELD, IL, p. A194
KINDRED HOSPITAL ST. LOUIS-ST. ANTHONY'S, SAINT LOUIS, MISSOURI (see KINDRED HOSPITAL-ST. LOUIS), p. A368
KINDRED HOSPITAL SUGAR LAND, SUGAR LAND, TX, p. A629
KINDRED HOSPITAL TARRANT COUNTY-ARLINGTON, ARLINGTON, TX, p. A579
KINDRED HOSPITAL TARRANT COUNTY-FORT WORTH SOUTHWEST, FORT WORTH, TX, p. A599
KINDRED HOSPITAL THE PALM BEACHES, RIVIERA BEACH, FL, p. A137
KINDRED HOSPITAL TULSA, TULSA, OK, p. A506
KINDRED HOSPITAL VICTORIA, VICTORIA, TX, p. A633
KINDRED HOSPITAL WEST-JEFFERSON, MARRERO, LA, p. A272
KINDRED HOSPITAL- OKLAHOMA CITY, OKLAHOMA CITY, OK, p. A501
KINDRED HOSPITAL-ALBUQUERQUE, ALBUQUERQUE, NM, p. A414
KINDRED HOSPITAL-AMARILLO, AMARILLO, TX, p. A578
KINDRED HOSPITAL-ATLANTA, ATLANTA, GA, p. A145
KINDRED HOSPITAL-AURORA, AURORA, CO, p. A97
KINDRED HOSPITAL-BALDWIN PARK, BALDWIN PARK, CA, p. A55
KINDRED HOSPITAL-BAY AREA, PASADENA, TX, p. A620
KINDRED HOSPITAL-BAY AREA ST. PETERSBURG, SAINT PETERSBURG, FL, p. A138
KINDRED HOSPITAL-BOSTON, BRIGHTON, MA, p. A298
KINDRED HOSPITAL-BREA, BREA, CA, p. A56
KINDRED HOSPITAL-CENTRAL DAKOTAS, MANDAN, ND, p. A467
KINDRED HOSPITAL-CENTRAL TAMPA, TAMPA, FL, p. A141
KINDRED HOSPITAL-CHARLESTON, CHARLESTON, SC, p. A547
KINDRED HOSPITAL-CHATTANOOGA, CHATTANOOGA, TN, p. A563
KINDRED HOSPITAL-CORPUS CHRISTI, CORPUS CHRISTI, TX, p. A589
KINDRED HOSPITAL-DALLAS, DALLAS, TX, p. A591

KINDRED HOSPITAL-DAYTON, DAYTON, OH, p. A478
KINDRED HOSPITAL-DELAWARE COUNTY, DARBY, PA, p. A521
KINDRED HOSPITAL-DENVER, DENVER, CO, p. A99
KINDRED HOSPITAL-FLAMINGO, LAS VEGAS, NEVADA (see KINDRED HOSPITAL LAS VEGAS-SAHARA), p. A393
KINDRED HOSPITAL-FORT WORTH, FORT WORTH, TX, p. A599
KINDRED HOSPITAL-GREENSBORO, GREENSBORO, NC, p. A454
KINDRED HOSPITAL-HERITAGE VALLEY, BEAVER, PA, p. A518
KINDRED HOSPITAL-HOUSTON, HOUSTON, TX, p. A605
KINDRED HOSPITAL-HOUSTON NORTHWEST, HOUSTON, TX, p. A605
KINDRED HOSPITAL-INDIANAPOLIS, INDIANAPOLIS, IN, p. A204
KINDRED HOSPITAL-LA MIRADA, LA MIRADA, CA, p. A66
KINDRED HOSPITAL-LOS ANGELES, LOS ANGELES, CA, p. A70
KINDRED HOSPITAL-LOUISVILLE, LOUISVILLE, KY, p. A254
KINDRED HOSPITAL-MANSFIELD, MANSFIELD, TX, p. A615
KINDRED HOSPITAL-MILWAUKEE, GREENFIELD, WI, p. A683
KINDRED HOSPITAL-NASHVILLE, NASHVILLE, TN, p. A573
KINDRED HOSPITAL-NEW JERSEY MORRIS COUNTY, DOVER, NJ, p. A403
KINDRED HOSPITAL-NEW ORLEANS, NEW ORLEANS, LA, p. A274
KINDRED HOSPITAL-OKLAHOMA CITY SOUTH, OKLAHOMA CITY, OKLAHOMA (see KINDRED HOSPITAL- OKLAHOMA CITY), p. A501
KINDRED HOSPITAL-ONTARIO, ONTARIO, CA, p. A78
KINDRED HOSPITAL-PHILADELPHIA, PHILADELPHIA, PA, p. A533
KINDRED HOSPITAL-PITTSBURGH, OAKDALE, PA, p. A531
KINDRED HOSPITAL-SACRAMENTO, FOLSOM, CA, p. A60
KINDRED HOSPITAL-SAN ANTONIO, SAN ANTONIO, TX, p. A625
KINDRED HOSPITAL-SAN DIEGO, SAN DIEGO, CA, p. A85
KINDRED HOSPITAL-SAN FRANCISCO BAY AREA, SAN LEANDRO, CA, p. A88
KINDRED HOSPITAL-ST. LOUIS, SAINT LOUIS, MO, p. A368
KINDRED HOSPITAL-SYCAMORE, SYCAMORE, IL, p. A195
KINDRED HOSPITAL-TUCSON, TUCSON, AZ, p. A40
KINDRED HOSPITAL-WESTMINSTER, WESTMINSTER, CA, p. A96
KINDRED HOSPITAL-WHITE ROCK, DALLAS, TX, p. A591
KINDRED HOSPITAL-WYOMING VALLEY, WILKES BARRE, PA, p. A541
KINDRED REHABILITATION HOSPITAL, AMARILLO, TX, p. A578
KINDRED REHABILITATION HOSPITAL ARLINGTON, ARLINGTON, TX, p. A579
KINDRED REHABILITATION HOSPITAL CLEAR LAKE, WEBSTER, TX, p. A634
KINDRED REHABILITATION HOSPITAL NORTHEAST HOUSTON, HUMBLE, TX, p. A608
KING'S DAUGHTERS HOSPITAL, YAZOO CITY, MS, p. A354
KING'S DAUGHTERS HOSPITAL, TEMPLE, TEXAS (see SCOTT AND WHITE MEMORIAL HOSPITAL), p. A630
KING'S DAUGHTERS MEDICAL CENTER, ASHLAND, KY, p. A247
KING'S DAUGHTERS MEDICAL CENTER, BROOKHAVEN, MS, p. A344
KING'S DAUGHTERS' HOSPITAL AND HEALTH SERVICES, MADISON, IN, p. A208
KINGFISHER REGIONAL HOSPITAL, KINGFISHER, OK, p. A498
KINGMAN REGIONAL MEDICAL CENTER, KINGMAN, AZ, p. A33
KINGS COUNTY HOSPITAL CENTER,, NY, p. A433
KINGS MOUNTAIN HOSPITAL, KINGS MOUNTAIN, NC, p. A456
KINGSBORO PSYCHIATRIC CENTER,, NY, p. A433
KINGSBROOK JEWISH MEDICAL CENTER,, NY, p. A433
KINGSTON HOSPITAL, KINGSTON, NY, p. A428
KINGWOOD MEDICAL CENTER, KINGWOOD, TX, p. A611
KINGWOOD PINES HOSPITAL, KINGWOOD, TX, p. A611
KIOWA COUNTY MEMORIAL HOSPITAL, GREENSBURG, KS, p. A234
KIOWA DISTRICT HOSPITAL AND MANOR, KIOWA, KS, p. A236
KIRBY MEDICAL CENTER, MONTICELLO, IL, p. A188
KISHWAUKEE COMMUNITY HOSPITAL, DEKALB, IL, p. A180
KIT CARSON COUNTY MEMORIAL HOSPITAL, BURLINGTON, CO, p. A98
KITTITAS VALLEY COMMUNITY HOSPITAL, ELLENSBURG, WA, p. A661
KITTSON MEMORIAL HEALTHCARE CENTER, HALLOCK, MN, p. A332
KLICKITAT VALLEY HEALTH, GOLDENDALE, WA, p. A661
KNAPP MEDICAL CENTER, WESLACO, TX, p. A634
KNOX COMMUNITY HOSPITAL, MOUNT VERNON, OH, p. A485
KNOX COUNTY HOSPITAL, BARBOURVILLE, KY, p. A247
KNOX COUNTY HOSPITAL, KNOX CITY, TX, p. A611
KNOXVILLE DIVISION, KNOXVILLE, IOWA (see VETERANS AFFAIRS CENTRAL IOWA HEALTH CARE SYSTEM), p. A218
KNOXVILLE HOSPITAL & CLINICS, KNOXVILLE, IA, p. A222
KOHALA HOSPITAL, KOHALA, HI, p. A165
KONA COMMUNITY HOSPITAL, KEALAKEKUA, HI, p. A165
KOOTENAI MEDICAL CENTER, COEUR D'ALENE, ID, p. A167
KOSAIR CHILDREN'S HOSPITAL, LOUISVILLE, KY, p. A254
KOSCIUSKO COMMUNITY HOSPITAL, WARSAW, IN, p. A213

LIFECARE HOSPITALS OF NORTH CAROLINA, ROCKY MOUNT, NC, p. A459
LIFECARE HOSPITALS OF PITTSBURGH, PITTSBURGH, PA, p. A534
LIFECARE HOSPITALS OF PITTSBURGH – MONROEVILLE, MONROEVILLE, PA, p. A529
LIFECARE HOSPITALS OF PITTSBURGH – SUBURBAN CAMPUS, PITTSBURGH, PENNSYLVANIA (see LIFECARE HOSPITALS OF PITTSBURGH), p. A534
LIFECARE HOSPITALS OF SAN ANTONIO, SAN ANTONIO, TX, p. A625
LIFECARE HOSPITALS OF SHREVEPORT, SHREVEPORT, LA, p. A277
LIFECARE HOSPITALS OF SHREVEPORT–WILLIS KNIGHTON, SHREVEPORT, LOUISIANA (see LIFECARE HOSPITALS OF SHREVEPORT), p. A277
LIFECARE HOSPITALS OF SOUTH SHREVEPORT–WILLIS KNIGHTON NORTH, SHREVEPORT, LOUISIANA (see LIFECARE HOSPITALS OF SHREVEPORT), p. A277
LIFECARE HOSPITALS OF SOUTH TEXAS–MCALLEN, MCALLEN, TEXAS (see LIFECARE HOSPITALS OF SOUTH TEXAS–NORTH MCALLEN), p. A615
LIFECARE HOSPITALS OF SOUTH TEXAS–NORTH MCALLEN, MCALLEN, TX, p. A615
LIFECARE HOSPITALS OF WISCONSIN, PEWAUKEE, WI, p. A689
LIFECARE MEDICAL CENTER, ROSEAU, MN, p. A338
LIFECARE SPECIALTY HOSPITAL OF NORTH LOUISIANA, RUSTON, LA, p. A276
LIGHTHOUSE CARE CENTER OF CONWAY, CONWAY, SC, p. A549
LILA DOYLE NURSING CARE FACILITY (see OCONEE MEDICAL CENTER), p. A553
LILLIAN M. HUDSPETH MEMORIAL HOSPITAL, SONORA, TX, p. A628
LIMA MEMORIAL HEALTH SYSTEM, LIMA, OH, p. A482
LIMESTONE MEDICAL CENTER, GROESBECK, TX, p. A602
LINCOLN COMMUNITY HOSPITAL AND NURSING HOME, HUGO, CO, p. A102
LINCOLN COUNTY HEALTH SYSTEM, FAYETTEVILLE, TN, p. A565
LINCOLN COUNTY HOSPITAL, LINCOLN, KS, p. A238
LINCOLN COUNTY MEDICAL CENTER, TROY, MO, p. A372
LINCOLN COUNTY MEDICAL CENTER, RUIDOSO, NM, p. A417
LINCOLN DIVISION, LINCOLN, NEBRASKA (see VETERANS AFFAIRS NEBRASKA–WESTERN IOWA HEALTH CARE SYSTEM), p. A386
LINCOLN HOSPITAL, DAVENPORT, WA, p. A660
LINCOLN MEDICAL AND MENTAL HEALTH CENTER,, NY, p. A434
LINCOLN PRAIRIE BEHAVIORAL HEALTH CENTER, SPRINGFIELD, IL, p. A194
LINCOLN REGIONAL CENTER, LINCOLN, NE, p. A385
LINCOLN SURGICAL HOSPITAL, LINCOLN, NE, p. A385
LINCOLN TRAIL BEHAVIORAL HEALTH SYSTEM, RADCLIFF, KY, p. A258
LINDEN OAKS HOSPITAL AT EDWARD, NAPERVILLE, IL, p. A189
LINDNER CENTER OF HOPE, MASON, OH, p. A484
LINDSAY MUNICIPAL HOSPITAL, LINDSAY, OK, p. A498
LINDSBORG COMMUNITY HOSPITAL, LINDSBORG, KS, p. A238
LINTON HOSPITAL, LINTON, ND, p. A467
LISBON AREA HEALTH SERVICES, LISBON, ND, p. A467
LITTLE COLORADO MEDICAL CENTER, WINSLOW, AZ, p. A41
LITTLE COMPANY OF MARY HOSPITAL AND HEALTH CARE CENTERS, EVERGREEN PARK, IL, p. A181
LITTLE FALLS HOSPITAL, LITTLE FALLS, NY, p. A428
LITTLE RIVER MEDICAL CENTER, ROCKDALE, TX, p. A623
LITTLE RIVER MEMORIAL HOSPITAL, ASHDOWN, AR, p. A42
LITTLETON ADVENTIST HOSPITAL, LITTLETON, CO, p. A103
LITTLETON REGIONAL HOSPITAL, LITTLETON, NH, p. A399
LITZENBERG MEMORIAL COUNTY HOSPITAL, CENTRAL CITY, NE, p. A382
LIVENGRIN FOUNDATION, BENSALEM, PA, p. A518
LIVINGSTON HOSPITAL AND HEALTHCARE SERVICES, SALEM, KY, p. A258
LIVINGSTON MEMORIAL HOSPITAL, LIVINGSTON, MT, p. A377
LIVINGSTON REGIONAL HOSPITAL, LIVINGSTON, TN, p. A570
LLANO SPECIALTY HOSPITAL OF LUBBOCK, LUBBOCK, TX, p. A614
LOCK HAVEN HOSPITAL, LOCK HAVEN, PA, p. A528
LODI COMMUNITY HOSPITAL, LODI, OH, p. A483
LODI MEMORIAL HOSPITAL, LODI, CA, p. A67
LODI MEMORIAL HOSPITAL WEST, LODI, CALIFORNIA (see LODI MEMORIAL HOSPITAL), p. A67
LOGAN COUNTY HOSPITAL, OAKLEY, KS, p. A240
LOGAN MEMORIAL HOSPITAL, RUSSELLVILLE, KY, p. A258
LOGAN REGIONAL HOSPITAL, LOGAN, UT, p. A638
LOGAN REGIONAL MEDICAL CENTER, LOGAN, WV, p. A673
LOGANSPORT MEMORIAL HOSPITAL, LOGANSPORT, IN, p. A207
LOGANSPORT STATE HOSPITAL, LOGANSPORT, IN, p. A207

LOMA LINDA UNIVERSITY BEHAVIORAL MEDICINE CENTER, REDLANDS, CA, p. A82
LOMA LINDA UNIVERSITY CHILDREN'S HOSPITAL, LOMA LINDA, CALIFORNIA (see LOMA LINDA UNIVERSITY MEDICAL CENTER), p. A67
LOMA LINDA UNIVERSITY EAST CAMPUS HOSPITAL, LOMA LINDA, CALIFORNIA (see LOMA LINDA UNIVERSITY MEDICAL CENTER), p. A67
LOMA LINDA UNIVERSITY HEART & SURGICAL HOSPITAL, LOMA LINDA, CALIFORNIA (see LOMA LINDA UNIVERSITY MEDICAL CENTER), p. A67
LOMA LINDA UNIVERSITY MEDICAL CENTER, LOMA LINDA, CA, p. A67
LOMA LINDA UNIVERSITY MEDICAL CENTER–MURRIETA, MURRIETA, CA, p. A76
LOMPOC VALLEY MEDICAL CENTER, LOMPOC, CA, p. A67
LONG BEACH MEDICAL CENTER, LONG BEACH, NY, p. A429
LONG BEACH MEMORIAL MEDICAL CENTER, LONG BEACH, CA, p. A68
LONG ISLAND JEWISH MEDICAL CENTER,, NY, p. A434
LONG TERM CARE CENTER (see NORTHFIELD HOSPITAL), p. A336
LONGMONT UNITED HOSPITAL, LONGMONT, CO, p. A104
LONGVIEW REGIONAL MEDICAL CENTER, LONGVIEW, TX, p. A613
LORETTO HOSPITAL, CHICAGO, IL, p. A176
LORING HOSPITAL, SAC CITY, IA, p. A226
LOS ALAMITOS MEDICAL CENTER, LOS ALAMITOS, CA, p. A68
LOS ALAMOS MEDICAL CENTER, LOS ALAMOS, NM, p. A417
LOS ANGELES COMMUNITY HOSPITAL, LOS ANGELES, CA, p. A70
LOS ANGELES COMMUNITY HOSPITAL OF NORWALK, NORWALK, CALIFORNIA (see LOS ANGELES COMMUNITY HOSPITAL), p. A70
LOS ANGELES COUNTY CENTRAL JAIL HOSPITAL, LOS ANGELES, CA, p. A70
LOS ANGELES MEDICAL CENTER, LOS ANGELES, CA, p. A70
LOS ANGELES METROPOLITAN MEDICAL CENTER, LOS ANGELES, CA, p. A70
LOS NINOS HOSPITAL, PHOENIX, AZ, p. A36
LOS ROBLES HOSPITAL AND MEDICAL CENTER, THOUSAND OAKS, CA, p. A92
LOST RIVERS DISTRICT HOSPITAL, ARCO, ID, p. A166
LOUIS A. JOHNSON VETERANS AFFAIRS MEDICAL CENTER, CLARKSBURG, WV, p. A671
LOUIS A. WEISS MEMORIAL HOSPITAL, CHICAGO, IL, p. A176
LOUIS SMITH MEMORIAL HOSPITAL, LAKELAND, GA, p. A155
LOUISIANA EXTENDED CARE HOSPITAL OF LAFAYETTE, LAFAYETTE, LA, p. A270
LOUISIANA EXTENDED CARE HOSPITAL OF NATCHITOCHES, NATCHITOCHES, LA, p. A274
LOUISIANA EXTENDED CARE HOSPITAL WEST MONROE, WEST MONROE, LA, p. A279
LOUISIANA MEDICAL CENTER AND HEART HOSPITAL, LACOMBE, LA, p. A269
LOURDES COUNSELING CENTER, RICHLAND, WA, p. A665
LOURDES HOSPITAL, PADUCAH, KY, p. A257
LOURDES MEDICAL CENTER, PASCO, WA, p. A664
LOURDES MEDICAL CENTER OF BURLINGTON COUNTY, WILLINGBORO, NJ, p. A412
LOURDES SPECIALTY HOSPITAL OF SOUTHERN NEW JERSEY, WILLINGBORO, NJ, p. A412
LOVELACE MEDICAL CENTER, ALBUQUERQUE, NM, p. A414
LOVELACE REHABILITATION HOSPITAL, ALBUQUERQUE, NM, p. A414
LOVELACE WESTSIDE HOSPITAL, ALBUQUERQUE, NM, p. A414
LOVELACE WOMEN'S HOSPITAL, ALBUQUERQUE, NM, p. A414
LOWELL GENERAL HOSPITAL, LOWELL, MA, p. A301
LOWER BUCKS HOSPITAL, BRISTOL, PA, p. A519
LOWER KEYS MEDICAL CENTER, KEY WEST, FL, p. A127
LOWER OCONEE COMMUNITY HOSPITAL, GLENWOOD, GA, p. A153
LOWER UMPQUA HOSPITAL DISTRICT, REEDSPORT, OR, p. A515
LOYOLA UNIVERSITY MEDICAL CENTER, MAYWOOD, IL, p. A187
LSU BOGALUSA MEDICAL CENTER, BOGALUSA, LA, p. A263
LSU MEDICAL CENTER–UNIVERSITY HOSPITAL, SHREVEPORT, LA, p. A277
LTAC HOSPITAL OF GREENWOOD, GREENWOOD, MS, p. A346
LTAC OF EDMOND, EDMOND, OK, p. A496
LTAC OF WICHITA, WICHITA, KS, p. A245
LUBBOCK HEART HOSPITAL, LUBBOCK, TX, p. A614
LUCAS COUNTY HEALTH CENTER, CHARITON, IA, p. A216
LUCILE SALTER PACKARD CHILDREN'S HOSPITAL AT STANFORD, PALO ALTO, CA, p. A79
LUTHERAN HOSPITAL, CLEVELAND, OH, p. A475
LUTHERAN HOSPITAL OF INDIANA, FORT WAYNE, IN, p. A201
LUTHERAN MEDICAL CENTER,, NY, p. A434
LUTZ WING CONVALESCENT AND NURSING CARE UNIT (see MAYO CLINIC HEALTH SYSTEM IN FAIRMONT), p. A331

LYNCHBURG GENERAL HOSPITAL, LYNCHBURG, VIRGINIA (see CENTRA LYNCHBURG GENERAL HOSPITAL), p. A650
LYNDON B JOHNSON GENERAL HOSPITAL, HOUSTON, TEXAS (see HARRIS COUNTY HOSPITAL DISTRICT), p. A604
LYNDON B. JOHNSON TROPICAL MEDICAL CENTER, PAGO PAGO, AS, p. A699
LYNN COUNTY HOSPITAL DISTRICT, TAHOKA, TX, p. A630
LYONS DIVISION, LYONS, NEW JERSEY (see VETERANS AFFAIRS NEW JERSEY HEALTH CARE SYSTEM), p. A403

# M

MACKINAC STRAITS HEALTH SYSTEM, SAINT IGNACE, MI, p. A322
MACNEAL HOSPITAL, BERWYN, IL, p. A173
MACON COUNTY GENERAL HOSPITAL, LAFAYETTE, TN, p. A569
MAD RIVER COMMUNITY HOSPITAL, ARCATA, CA, p. A54
MADELIA COMMUNITY HOSPITAL, MADELIA, MN, p. A334
MADERA COMMUNITY HOSPITAL, MADERA, CA, p. A73
MADIGAN HEALTHCARE SYSTEM, TACOMA, WA, p. A668
MADISON CENTER AND HOSPITAL, SOUTH BEND, IN, p. A211
MADISON COMMUNITY HOSPITAL, MADISON, SD, p. A557
MADISON COUNTY HEALTH CARE SYSTEM, WINTERSET, IA, p. A228
MADISON COUNTY HOSPITAL, LONDON, OH, p. A483
MADISON COUNTY MEMORIAL HOSPITAL, MADISON, FL, p. A129
MADISON HOSPITAL, MADISON, AL, p. A22
MADISON HOSPITAL, MADISON, MN, p. A334
MADISON MEDICAL CENTER, FREDERICKTOWN, MO, p. A360
MADISON MEMORIAL HOSPITAL, REXBURG, ID, p. A170
MADISON PARISH HOSPITAL, TALLULAH, LA, p. A278
MADISON RIVER OAKS MEDICAL CENTER, CANTON, MS, p. A344
MADISON ST. JOSEPH HEALTH CENTER, MADISONVILLE, TX, p. A615
MADISON STATE HOSPITAL, MADISON, IN, p. A208
MADISON VALLEY MEDICAL CENTER, ENNIS, MT, p. A375
MADONNA REHABILITATION HOSPITAL, LINCOLN, NE, p. A385
MAGEE GENERAL HOSPITAL, MAGEE, MS, p. A349
MAGEE REHABILITATION HOSPITAL, PHILADELPHIA, PA, p. A533
MAGEE–WOMENS HOSPITAL OF UPMC, PITTSBURGH, PA, p. A535
MAGNOLIA BEHAVIORAL HEALTHCARE, LACOMBE, LA, p. A269
MAGNOLIA REGIONAL HEALTH CENTER, CORINTH, MS, p. A345
MAGNOLIA REGIONAL MEDICAL CENTER, MAGNOLIA, AR, p. A48
MAHASKA HEALTH PARTNERSHIP, OSKALOOSA, IA, p. A225
MAHNOMEN HEALTH CENTER, MAHNOMEN, MN, p. A334
MAIMONIDES INFANTS AND CHILDREN'S HOSPITAL OF BROOKLYN,, NEW YORK (see MAIMONIDES MEDICAL CENTER), p. A434
MAIMONIDES MEDICAL CENTER,, NY, p. A434
MAIN CAMPUS, BATTLE CREEK, MICHIGAN (see BRONSON BATTLE CREEK), p. A308
MAINE COAST MEMORIAL HOSPITAL, ELLSWORTH, ME, p. A283
MAINE MEDICAL CENTER, PORTLAND, ME, p. A284
MAINE MEDICAL CENTER, BRIGHTON CAMPUS, PORTLAND, MAINE (see MAINE MEDICAL CENTER), p. A284
MAINEGENERAL MEDICAL CENTER–AUGUSTA CAMPUS, AUGUSTA, MAINE (see MAINEGENERAL MEDICAL CENTER–WATERVILLE CAMPUS), p. A286
MAINEGENERAL MEDICAL CENTER–WATERVILLE CAMPUS, WATERVILLE, ME, p. A286
MAINLAND MEDICAL CENTER, TEXAS CITY, TEXAS (see CLEAR LAKE REGIONAL MEDICAL CENTER), p. A634
MAJOR HOSPITAL, SHELBYVILLE, IN, p. A211
MALCOM RANDALL VETERANS AFFAIRS MEDICAL CENTER, GAINESVILLE, FL, p. A124
MALVERN INSTITUTE, MALVERN, PA, p. A528
MAMMOTH HOSPITAL, MAMMOTH LAKES, CA, p. A73
MANATEE GLENS HOSPITAL AND ADDICTION CENTER, BRADENTON, FL, p. A119
MANATEE MEMORIAL HOSPITAL, BRADENTON, FL, p. A119
MANATEE PALMS YOUTH SERVICES, BRADENTON, FL, p. A119
MANCHESTER MEMORIAL HOSPITAL, MANCHESTER, CT, p. A109
MANCHESTER MEMORIAL HOSPITAL, MANCHESTER, KY, p. A256
MANHASSET AMBULATORY CARE PAVILION, MANHASSET, NEW YORK (see LONG ISLAND JEWISH MEDICAL CENTER), p. A434
MANHATTAN EYE, EAR AND THROAT HOSPITAL, NEW YORK, NEW YORK (see LENOX HILL HOSPITAL), p. A433
MANHATTAN PSYCHIATRIC CENTER–WARD'S ISLAND, NEW YORK, NY, p. A434
MANHATTAN SURGICAL CENTER,, KS, p. A238

MOBERLY REGIONAL MEDICAL CENTER, MOBERLY, MO, p. A365
MOBILE INFIRMARY MEDICAL CENTER, MOBILE, AL, p. A22
MOBRIDGE REGIONAL HOSPITAL, MOBRIDGE, SD, p. A558
MOCCASIN BEND MENTAL HEALTH INSTITUTE, CHATTANOOGA, TN, p. A563
MODESTO MEDICAL CENTER, MODESTO, CALIFORNIA (see MANTECA MEDICAL CENTER), p. A74
MODOC MEDICAL CENTER, ALTURAS, CA, p. A53
MOHAWK VALLEY PSYCHIATRIC CENTER, UTICA, NY, p. A445
MOLOKAI GENERAL HOSPITAL, KAUNAKAKAI, HI, p. A165
MONADNOCK COMMUNITY HOSPITAL, PETERBOROUGH, NH, p. A400
MONCKS CORNER MEDICAL CENTER, MONCKS CORNER, SOUTH CAROLINA (see TRIDENT MEDICAL CENTER), p. A547
MONCRIEF ARMY COMMUNITY HOSPITAL, FORT JACKSON, SC, p. A550
MONMOUTH MEDICAL CENTER, LONG BRANCH, NJ, p. A405
MONONGAHELA VALLEY HOSPITAL, MONONGAHELA, PA, p. A529
MONONGALIA GENERAL HOSPITAL, MORGANTOWN, WV, p. A674
MONROE CARELL JR. CHILDREN'S HOSPITAL AT VANDERBILT, NASHVILLE, TENNESSEE (see VANDERBILT HOSPITAL AND CLINICS), p. A574
MONROE CLINIC, MONROE, WI, p. A687
MONROE COUNTY HOSPITAL, MONROEVILLE, AL, p. A23
MONROE COUNTY HOSPITAL, FORSYTH, GA, p. A153
MONROE COUNTY HOSPITAL, ALBIA, IA, p. A214
MONROE COUNTY MEDICAL CENTER, TOMPKINSVILLE, KY, p. A259
MONROE HOSPITAL, BLOOMINGTON, IN, p. A198
MONROE SURGICAL HOSPITAL, MONROE, LA, p. A273
MONROVIA MEMORIAL HOSPITAL, MONROVIA, CA, p. A75
MONTANA STATE HOSPITAL, WARM SPRINGS, MT, p. A379
MONTCLAIR HOSPITAL MEDICAL CENTER, MONTCLAIR, CA, p. A75
MONTEFIORE MEDICAL CENTER,, NY, p. A434
MONTEFIORE MEDICAL CENTER – NORTH DIVISION,, NEW YORK (see MONTEFIORE MEDICAL CENTER), p. A434
MONTEREY PARK HOSPITAL, MONTEREY PARK, CA, p. A75
MONTEVISTA HOSPITAL, LAS VEGAS, NV, p. A393
MONTFORT JONES MEMORIAL HOSPITAL, KOSCIUSKO, MS, p. A348
MONTGOMERY COUNTY EMERGENCY SERVICE, NORRISTOWN, PA, p. A530
MONTGOMERY COUNTY MEMORIAL HOSPITAL, RED OAK, IA, p. A225
MONTGOMERY DIVISION, MONTGOMERY, ALABAMA (see CENTRAL ALABAMA VETERANS HEALTH CARE SYSTEM), p. A23
MONTGOMERY GENERAL HOSPITAL, MONTGOMERY, WV, p. A673
MONTGOMERY HOSPITAL MEDICAL CENTER, NORRISTOWN, PA, p. A530
MONTGOMERY REGIONAL HOSPITAL, BLACKSBURG, VA, p. A646
MONTPELIER HOSPITAL, MONTPELIER, OHIO (see COMMUNITY HOSPITALS AND WELLNESS CENTERS), p. A471
MONTROSE MEMORIAL HOSPITAL, MONTROSE, CO, p. A104
MOORE COUNTY HOSPITAL DISTRICT, DUMAS, TX, p. A594
MOORE MEDICAL CENTER, MOORE, OKLAHOMA (see NORMAN REGIONAL HEALTH SYSTEM), p. A500
MOREHEAD MEMORIAL HOSPITAL, EDEN, NC, p. A452
MOREHOUSE GENERAL HOSPITAL, BASTROP, LA, p. A262
MORENO VALLEY COMMUNITY HOSPITAL, MORENO VALLEY, CA, p. A75
MORGAN COUNTY ARH HOSPITAL, WEST LIBERTY, KY, p. A259
MORGAN MEMORIAL HOSPITAL, MADISON, GA, p. A156
MORGAN STANLEY CHILDREN'S HOSPITAL OF NEW YORK–PRESBYTERIAN, NEW YORK, NEW YORK (see NEW YORK–PRESBYTERIAN HOSPITAL), p. A436
MORRILL COUNTY COMMUNITY HOSPITAL, BRIDGEPORT, NE, p. A382
MORRIS COUNTY HOSPITAL, COUNCIL GROVE, KS, p. A232
MORRIS HOSPITAL & HEALTHCARE CENTERS, MORRIS, IL, p. A188
MORRISON COMMUNITY HOSPITAL, MORRISON, IL, p. A188
MORRISTOWN MEDICAL CENTER, MORRISTOWN, NJ, p. A406
MORRISTOWN–HAMBLEN HEALTHCARE SYSTEM, MORRISTOWN, TN, p. A572
MORROW COUNTY HOSPITAL, MOUNT GILEAD, OH, p. A485
MORTON COUNTY HEALTH SYSTEM, ELKHART, KS, p. A232
MORTON GENERAL HOSPITAL, MORTON, WA, p. A663
MORTON HOSPITAL AND MEDICAL CENTER, TAUNTON, MA, p. A305
MORTON PLANT HOSPITAL, CLEARWATER, FL, p. A120
MORTON PLANT NORTH BAY HOSPITAL, NEW PORT RICHEY, FL, p. A133

MOSES H. CONE MEMORIAL HOSPITAL, GREENSBORO, NORTH CAROLINA (see CONE HEALTH), p. A454
MOSES LUDINGTON HOSPITAL, TICONDEROGA, NY, p. A444
MOSES TAYLOR HOSPITAL, SCRANTON, PA, p. A538
MOTHER FRANCES HOSPITAL – JACKSONVILLE, JACKSONVILLE, TX, p. A609
MOTHER FRANCES HOSPITAL – TYLER, TYLER, TX, p. A632
MOTHER FRANCES HOSPITAL – WINNSBORO, WINNSBORO, TX, p. A635
MOTION PICTURE AND TELEVISION FUND HOSPITAL AND RESIDENTIAL SERVICES,, CA, p. A70
MOUNDVIEW MEMORIAL HOSPITAL & CLINICS, FRIENDSHIP, WI, p. A682
MOUNT AUBURN HOSPITAL, CAMBRIDGE, MA, p. A299
MOUNT CARMEL, COLUMBUS, OH, p. A476
MOUNT CARMEL EAST HOSPITAL, COLUMBUS, OHIO (see MOUNT CARMEL), p. A476
MOUNT CARMEL NEW ALBANY SURGICAL HOSPITAL, NEW ALBANY, OH, p. A486
MOUNT CARMEL ST. ANN'S, WESTERVILLE, OH, p. A491
MOUNT CARMEL WEST HOSPITAL, COLUMBUS, OHIO (see MOUNT CARMEL), p. A476
MOUNT DESERT ISLAND HOSPITAL, BAR HARBOR, ME, p. A281
MOUNT GRANT GENERAL HOSPITAL, HAWTHORNE, NV, p. A392
MOUNT NITTANY MEDICAL CENTER, STATE COLLEGE, PA, p. A539
MOUNT PLEASANT HOSPITAL, MOUNT PLEASANT, SC, p. A552
MOUNT SINAI HOSPITAL, CHICAGO, IL, p. A177
MOUNT SINAI HOSPITAL, NEW YORK, NY, p. A435
MOUNT SINAI MEDICAL CENTER, MIAMI BEACH, FL, p. A132
MOUNT SINAI REHABILITATION HOSPITAL, HARTFORD, CT, p. A109
MOUNT ST. MARY'S HOSPITAL AND HEALTH CENTER, LEWISTON, NY, p. A428
MOUNT VERNON HOSPITAL, MOUNT VERNON, NY, p. A430
MOUNTAIN CREST HOSPITAL, FORT COLLINS, COLORADO (see POUDRE VALLEY HOSPITAL), p. A101
MOUNTAIN LAKES MEDICAL CENTER, CLAYTON, GA, p. A149
MOUNTAIN MANOR TREATMENT CENTER, EMMITSBURG, MD, p. A291
MOUNTAIN RIVER BIRTHING AND SURGERY CENTER, BLACKFOOT, ID, p. A166
MOUNTAIN VALLEY REGIONAL REHABILITATION HOSPITAL, PRESCOTT VALLEY, AZ, p. A37
MOUNTAIN VIEW HOSPITAL, GADSDEN, AL, p. A20
MOUNTAIN VIEW HOSPITAL, IDAHO FALLS, ID, p. A168
MOUNTAIN VIEW HOSPITAL, PAYSON, UT, p. A639
MOUNTAIN VIEW HOSPITAL DISTRICT, MADRAS, OR, p. A512
MOUNTAIN VIEW REGIONAL HOSPITAL, CASPER, WY, p. A695
MOUNTAIN VIEW REGIONAL MEDICAL CENTER, NORTON, VA, p. A653
MOUNTAIN VISTA MEDICAL CENTER, MESA, AZ, p. A34
MOUNTAIN WEST MEDICAL CENTER, TOOELE, UT, p. A641
MOUNTAINVIEW HOSPITAL, LAS VEGAS, NV, p. A393
MOUNTAINVIEW MEDICAL CENTER, WHITE SULPHUR SPRINGS, MT, p. A379
MOUNTAINVIEW REGIONAL MEDICAL CENTER, LAS CRUCES, NM, p. A416
MOUNTRAIL COUNTY MEDICAL CENTER, STANLEY, ND, p. A468
MT. ASCUTNEY HOSPITAL AND HEALTH CENTER, WINDSOR, VT, p. A644
MT. GRAHAM REGIONAL MEDICAL CENTER, SAFFORD, AZ, p. A37
MT. SAN RAFAEL HOSPITAL, TRINIDAD, CO, p. A106
MT. WASHINGTON PEDIATRIC HOSPITAL, BALTIMORE, MD, p. A288
MUENSTER MEMORIAL HOSPITAL, MUENSTER, TX, p. A617
MUHLENBERG COMMUNITY HOSPITAL, GREENVILLE, KY, p. A251
MULESHOE AREA MEDICAL CENTER, MULESHOE, TX, p. A618
MULTICARE GOOD SAMARITAN HOSPITAL, PUYALLUP, WA, p. A664
MULTICARE MARY BRIDGE CHILDREN'S HOSPITAL AND HEALTH CENTER, TACOMA, WA, p. A668
MULTICARE TACOMA GENERAL HOSPITAL, TACOMA, WA, p. A668
MUNCY VALLEY HOSPITAL, MUNCY, PA, p. A530
MUNISING MEMORIAL HOSPITAL, MUNISING, MI, p. A319
MUNROE REGIONAL MEDICAL CENTER, OCALA, FL, p. A133
MUNSON MEDICAL CENTER, TRAVERSE CITY, MI, p. A324
MURPHY MEDICAL CENTER, MURPHY, NC, p. A458
MURRAY COUNTY MEDICAL CENTER, SLAYTON, MN, p. A340
MURRAY MEDICAL CENTER, CHATSWORTH, GA, p. A149
MURRAY–CALLOWAY COUNTY HOSPITAL, MURRAY, KY, p. A257
MUSC CHILDREN'S HOSPITAL, CHARLESTON, SOUTH CAROLINA (see MUSC MEDICAL CENTER OF MEDICAL UNIVERSITY OF SOUTH CAROLINA), p. A547
MUSC MEDICAL CENTER OF MEDICAL UNIVERSITY OF SOUTH CAROLINA, CHARLESTON, SC, p. A547

MUSKOGEE COMMUNITY HOSPITAL, MUSKOGEE, OK, p. A499
MUSKOGEE REGIONAL MEDICAL CENTER, MUSKOGEE, OK, p. A499
MYRTUE MEDICAL CENTER, HARLAN, IA, p. A220

# N

NACOGDOCHES MEDICAL CENTER, NACOGDOCHES, TX, p. A618
NACOGDOCHES MEMORIAL HOSPITAL, NACOGDOCHES, TX, p. A618
NANTICOKE MEMORIAL HOSPITAL, SEAFORD, DE, p. A114
NANTUCKET COTTAGE HOSPITAL, NANTUCKET, MA, p. A302
NAPA STATE HOSPITAL, NAPA, CA, p. A76
NASH HEALTH CARE SYSTEMS, ROCKY MOUNT, NC, p. A460
NASHOBA VALLEY MEDICAL CENTER, AYER, MA, p. A295
NASHVILLE CAMPUS, NASHVILLE, TENNESSEE (see VETERANS AFFAIRS TENNESSEE VALLEY HEALTHCARE SYSTEM), p. A574
NASHVILLE GENERAL HOSPITAL, NASHVILLE, TN, p. A573
NASON HOSPITAL, ROARING SPRING, PA, p. A537
NASSAU UNIVERSITY MEDICAL CENTER, EAST MEADOW, NY, p. A425
NATCHAUG HOSPITAL, MANSFIELD CENTER, CT, p. A109
NATCHEZ COMMUNITY HOSPITAL, NATCHEZ, MS, p. A350
NATCHEZ REGIONAL MEDICAL CENTER, NATCHEZ, MS, p. A351
NATCHITOCHES REGIONAL MEDICAL CENTER, NATCHITOCHES, LA, p. A274
NATHAN LITTAUER HOSPITAL AND NURSING HOME, GLOVERSVILLE, NY, p. A426
NATIONAL INSTITUTES OF HEALTH CLINICAL CENTER, BETHESDA, MD, p. A289
NATIONAL JEWISH HEALTH, DENVER, CO, p. A99
NATIONAL PARK MEDICAL CENTER, HOT SPRINGS, AR, p. A46
NATIONWIDE CHILDREN'S HOSPITAL, COLUMBUS, OH, p. A477
NATIVIDAD MEDICAL CENTER, SALINAS, CA, p. A84
NAVAL HOSPITAL, CAMP PENDLETON, CA, p. A56
NAVAL HOSPITAL, LEMOORE, CA, p. A67
NAVAL HOSPITAL, TWENTYNINE PALMS, CA, p. A93
NAVAL HOSPITAL, JACKSONVILLE, FL, p. A126
NAVAL HOSPITAL, PENSACOLA, FL, p. A136
NAVAL HOSPITAL, CAMP LEJEUNE, NC, p. A450
NAVAL HOSPITAL, OAK HARBOR, WA, p. A663
NAVAL HOSPITAL BEAUFORT, BEAUFORT, SC, p. A546
NAVAL HOSPITAL BREMERTON, BREMERTON, WA, p. A659
NAVAL MEDICAL CENTER, SAN DIEGO, CA, p. A85
NAVAL MEDICAL CENTER, PORTSMOUTH, VA, p. A654
NAVARRO REGIONAL HOSPITAL, CORSICANA, TX, p. A589
NAVOS, SEATTLE, WA, p. A665
NAZARETH HOSPITAL, PHILADELPHIA, PA, p. A533
NCH DOWNTOWN NAPLES HOSPITAL, NAPLES, FL, p. A133
NCH NORTH NAPLES HOSPITAL, NAPLES, FLORIDA (see NCH DOWNTOWN NAPLES HOSPITAL), p. A133
NEA BAPTIST MEMORIAL HOSPITAL, JONESBORO, AR, p. A47
NEBRASKA HEART INSTITUTE AND HEART HOSPITAL, LINCOLN, NE, p. A385
NEBRASKA MEDICAL CENTER, OMAHA, NE, p. A388
NEBRASKA METHODIST HOSPITAL, OMAHA, NE, p. A388
NEBRASKA ORTHOPAEDIC HOSPITAL, OMAHA, NE, p. A388
NEBRASKA PENAL AND CORRECTIONAL HOSPITAL, LINCOLN, NE, p. A385
NEILLSVILLE MEMORIAL HOME (see MEMORIAL MEDICAL CENTER – NEILLSVILLE), p. A688
NELSON COUNTY HEALTH SYSTEM, MCVILLE, ND, p. A467
NEMAHA COUNTY HOSPITAL, AUBURN, NE, p. A381
NEMAHA VALLEY COMMUNITY HOSPITAL, SENECA, KS, p. A243
NEOSHO MEMORIAL REGIONAL MEDICAL CENTER, CHANUTE, KS, p. A231
NESHOBA COUNTY GENERAL HOSPITAL, PHILADELPHIA, MS, p. A351
NESS COUNTY HOSPITAL, NESS CITY, KS, p. A239
NEUROMEDICAL CENTER REHABILITATION HOSPITAL, BATON ROUGE, LA, p. A262
NEVADA REGIONAL MEDICAL CENTER, NEVADA, MO, p. A366
NEW BEDFORD REHABILITATION HOSPITAL, NEW BEDFORD, MA, p. A302
NEW BRAUNFELS REGIONAL REHABILITATION HOSPITAL, NEW BRAUNFELS, TX, p. A618
NEW BRITAIN GENERAL, NEW BRITAIN, CONNECTICUT (see THE HOSPITAL OF CENTRAL CONNECTICUT), p. A110
NEW ENGLAND BAPTIST HOSPITAL, BOSTON, MA, p. A297
NEW ENGLAND REHABILITATION HOSPITAL, WOBURN, MA, p. A306
NEW ENGLAND REHABILITATION HOSPITAL OF PORTLAND, PORTLAND, ME, p. A285
NEW ENGLAND SINAI HOSPITAL AND REHABILITATION CENTER, STOUGHTON, MA, p. A305

NEW HAMPSHIRE HOSPITAL, CONCORD, NH, p. A397
NEW HANOVER REGIONAL MEDICAL CENTER, WILMINGTON, NC, p. A462
NEW HORIZONS HEALTH SYSTEMS, OWENTON, KY, p. A257
NEW LONDON FAMILY MEDICAL CENTER, NEW LONDON, WI, p. A688
NEW LONDON HOSPITAL, NEW LONDON, NH, p. A399
NEW MEXICO BEHAVIORAL HEALTH INSTITUTE AT LAS VEGAS, LAS VEGAS, NM, p. A417
NEW MEXICO REHABILITATION CENTER, ROSWELL, NM, p. A417
NEW MILFORD HOSPITAL, NEW MILFORD, CT, p. A111
NEW RIVER MEDICAL CENTER, MONTICELLO, MN, p. A335
NEW ULM MEDICAL CENTER, NEW ULM, MN, p. A336
NEW YORK COMMUNITY HOSPITAL,, NY, p. A435
NEW YORK DOWNTOWN HOSPITAL, NEW YORK, NY, p. A435
NEW YORK EYE AND EAR INFIRMARY, NEW YORK, NY, p. A435
NEW YORK HOSPITAL QUEENS,, NY, p. A435
NEW YORK METHODIST HOSPITAL,, NY, p. A435
NEW YORK STATE PSYCHIATRIC INSTITUTE, NEW YORK, NY, p. A435
NEW YORK WESTCHESTER SQUARE MEDICAL CENTER,, NY, p. A435
NEW YORK–PRESBYTERIAN HOSPITAL, NEW YORK, NY, p. A436
NEW YORK–PRESBYTERIAN HOSPITAL, WESTCHESTER DIVISION, WHITE PLAINS, NEW YORK (see NEW YORK–PRESBYTERIAN HOSPITAL), p. A436
NEW YORK–PRESBYTERIAN HOSPITAL/WEILL CORNELL MEDICAL CENTER, NEW YORK, NEW YORK (see NEW YORK–PRESBYTERIAN HOSPITAL), p. A436
NEW YORK–PRESBYTERIAN/COLUMBIA UNIVERSITY MEDICAL CENTER, NEW YORK, NEW YORK (see NEW YORK–PRESBYTERIAN HOSPITAL), p. A436
NEWARK BETH ISRAEL MEDICAL CENTER, NEWARK, NJ, p. A407
NEWARK–WAYNE COMMUNITY HOSPITAL, NEWARK, NY, p. A438
NEWBERRY COUNTY MEMORIAL HOSPITAL, NEWBERRY, SC, p. A553
NEWMAN MEMORIAL HOSPITAL, SHATTUCK, OK, p. A504
NEWMAN REGIONAL HEALTH, EMPORIA, KS, p. A232
NEWPORT BAY HOSPITAL, NEWPORT BEACH, CA, p. A77
NEWPORT HOSPITAL, NEWPORT, RI, p. A544
NEWPORT HOSPITAL AND HEALTH SERVICES, NEWPORT, WA, p. A663
NEWPORT MEDICAL CENTER, NEWPORT, TN, p. A574
NEWPORT SPECIALTY HOSPITAL, TUSTIN, CA, p. A93
NEWTON MEDICAL CENTER, COVINGTON, GA, p. A150
NEWTON MEDICAL CENTER, NEWTON, KS, p. A239
NEWTON MEDICAL CENTER, NEWTON, NJ, p. A407
NEWTON–WELLESLEY HOSPITAL, NEWTON LOWER FALLS, MA, p. A303
NEXUS SPECIALTY HOSPITAL, SHENANDOAH, TX, p. A627
NEXUS SPECIALTY HOSPITAL THE WOODLANDS, SPRING, TX, p. A628
NIAGARA FALLS MEMORIAL MEDICAL CENTER, NIAGARA FALLS, NY, p. A438
NICHOLAS COUNTY HOSPITAL, CARLISLE, KY, p. A248
NICHOLAS H. NOYES MEMORIAL HOSPITAL, DANSVILLE, NY, p. A425
NINNESCAH VALLEY HEALTH SYSTEM, KINGMAN, KS, p. A236
NIOBRARA HEALTH AND LIFE CENTER, LUSK, WY, p. A697
NIOBRARA VALLEY HOSPITAL, LYNCH, NE, p. A386
NISWONGER CHILDREN'S HOSPITAL, JOHNSON CITY, TENNESSEE (see JOHNSON CITY MEDICAL CENTER), p. A567
NIX HEALTH CARE SYSTEM, SAN ANTONIO, TX, p. A625
NOBLE HOSPITAL, WESTFIELD, MA, p. A306
NOCONA GENERAL HOSPITAL, NOCONA, TX, p. A618
NOLAND HOSPITAL ANNISTON, ANNISTON, AL, p. A15
NOLAND HOSPITAL BIRMINGHAM, BIRMINGHAM, AL, p. A16
NOLAND HOSPITAL DOTHAN, DOTHAN, AL, p. A19
NOLAND HOSPITAL MONTGOMERY, MONTGOMERY, AL, p. A24
NOLAND HOSPITAL SHELBY, ALABASTER, AL, p. A15
NOLAND HOSPITAL TUSCALOOSA, TUSCALOOSA, AL, p. A26
NOR–LEA GENERAL HOSPITAL, LOVINGTON, NM, p. A417
NORFOLK PSYCHIATRIC CENTER, NORFOLK, VA, p. A652
NORFOLK REGIONAL CENTER, NORFOLK, NE, p. A386
NORMAN REGIONAL HEALTH SYSTEM, NORMAN, OK, p. A500
NORMAN REGIONAL HOSPITAL, NORMAN, OKLAHOMA (see NORMAN REGIONAL HEALTH SYSTEM), p. A500
NORMAN SPECIALTY HOSPITAL, NORMAN, OK, p. A500
NORRISTOWN STATE HOSPITAL, NORRISTOWN, PA, p. A530
NORTH ADAMS REGIONAL HOSPITAL, NORTH ADAMS, MA, p. A303
NORTH ALABAMA REGIONAL HOSPITAL, DECATUR, AL, p. A18
NORTH ARKANSAS REGIONAL MEDICAL CENTER, HARRISON, AR, p. A45
NORTH BALDWIN INFIRMARY, BAY MINETTE, AL, p. A16
NORTH BIG HORN HOSPITAL DISTRICT, LOVELL, WY, p. A697

NORTH CADDO MEDICAL CENTER, VIVIAN, LA, p. A279
NORTH CANYON MEDICAL CENTER, GOODING, ID, p. A168
NORTH CAROLINA CHILDREN'S AND WOMEN'S HOSPITAL, NORTH CAROLINA CHILDREN'S HOSPITAL, CHAPEL HILL, NORTH CAROLINA (see UNIVERSITY OF NORTH CAROLINA HOSPITALS), p. A450
NORTH CAROLINA NEUROSCIENCES HOSPITAL, CHAPEL HILL, NORTH CAROLINA (see UNIVERSITY OF NORTH CAROLINA HOSPITALS), p. A450
NORTH CAROLINA SPECIALTY HOSPITAL, DURHAM, NC, p. A452
NORTH CENTRAL BAPTIST HOSPITAL, SAN ANTONIO, TEXAS (see BAPTIST HEALTH SYSTEM), p. A624
NORTH CENTRAL BRONX HOSPITAL,, NY, p. A436
NORTH CENTRAL HEALTH CARE, WAUSAU, WI, p. A693
NORTH CENTRAL SURGICAL CENTER, DALLAS, TX, p. A592
NORTH COLORADO MEDICAL CENTER, GREELEY, CO, p. A102
NORTH COUNTRY HOSPITAL AND HEALTH CENTER, NEWPORT, VT, p. A644
NORTH CYPRESS MEDICAL CENTER, CYPRESS, TX, p. A590
NORTH DAKOTA STATE HOSPITAL, JAMESTOWN, ND, p. A467
NORTH FLORIDA REGIONAL MEDICAL CENTER, GAINESVILLE, FL, p. A124
NORTH FULTON REGIONAL MEDICAL CENTER, ROSWELL, GA, p. A158
NORTH GEORGIA MEDICAL CENTER, ELLIJAY, GA, p. A152
NORTH GREENVILLE HOSPITAL, TRAVELERS REST, SC, p. A554
NORTH HAWAII COMMUNITY HOSPITAL, KAMUELA, HI, p. A164
NORTH HILLS HOSPITAL, NORTH RICHLAND HILLS, TX, p. A618
NORTH IDAHO BEHAVIORAL HEALTH, DIVISION OF KOOTENAI MEDICAL CENTER, COEUR D'ALENE, IDAHO (see KOOTENAI MEDICAL CENTER), p. A167
NORTH KANSAS CITY HOSPITAL, NORTH KANSAS CITY, MO, p. A366
NORTH KNOXVILLE MEDICAL CENTER, POWELL, TENNESSEE (see PHYSICIANS REGIONAL MEDICAL CENTER), p. A568
NORTH LITTLE ROCK DIVISION, NORTH LITTLE ROCK, ARKANSAS (see CENTRAL ARKANSAS VETERANS HEALTHCARE SYSTEM), p. A48
NORTH MEMORIAL HEALTH CARE, ROBBINSDALE, MN, p. A338
NORTH METRO MEDICAL CENTER, JACKSONVILLE, AR, p. A46
NORTH MISSISSIPPI MEDICAL CENTER – TUPELO, TUPELO, MS, p. A353
NORTH MISSISSIPPI MEDICAL CENTER–EUPORA, EUPORA, MS, p. A345
NORTH MISSISSIPPI MEDICAL CENTER–HAMILTON, HAMILTON, AL, p. A21
NORTH MISSISSIPPI MEDICAL CENTER–IUKA, IUKA, MS, p. A347
NORTH MISSISSIPPI MEDICAL CENTER–PONTOTOC HOSPITAL AND NURSING HOME, PONTOTOC, MS, p. A352
NORTH MISSISSIPPI MEDICAL CENTER–WEST POINT, WEST POINT, MS, p. A353
NORTH MISSISSIPPI STATE HOSPITAL, TUPELO, MS, p. A353
NORTH OAK REGIONAL MEDICAL CENTER, SENATOBIA, MS, p. A352
NORTH OAKS MEDICAL CENTER, HAMMOND, LA, p. A267
NORTH OAKS REHABILITATION HOSPITAL, HAMMOND, LA, p. A267
NORTH OKALOOSA MEDICAL CENTER, CRESTVIEW, FL, p. A121
NORTH OTTAWA COMMUNITY HOSPITAL, GRAND HAVEN, MI, p. A313
NORTH PHILADELPHIA HEALTH SYSTEM, PHILADELPHIA, PA, p. A533
NORTH RUNNELS HOSPITAL, WINTERS, TX, p. A636
NORTH SHORE MEDICAL CENTER, MIAMI, FL, p. A131
NORTH SHORE MEDICAL CENTER, SALEM, MA, p. A304
NORTH SHORE UNIVERSITY HOSPITAL, MANHASSET, NY, p. A429
NORTH STAR BEHAVIORAL HEALTH, ANCHORAGE, ALASKA (see NORTH STAR BEHAVIORAL HEALTH SYSTEM), p. A28
NORTH STAR BEHAVIORAL HEALTH SYSTEM, ANCHORAGE, AK, p. A28
NORTH SUBURBAN MEDICAL CENTER, THORNTON, CO, p. A106
NORTH SUNFLOWER MEDICAL CENTER, RULEVILLE, MS, p. A352
NORTH TEXAS COMMUNITY HOSPITAL, BRIDGEPORT, TX, p. A585
NORTH TEXAS HOSPITAL, DENTON, TX, p. A594
NORTH TEXAS MEDICAL CENTER, GAINESVILLE, TX, p. A600
NORTH TEXAS STATE HOSPITAL, VERNON, TX, p. A633
NORTH TEXAS STATE HOSPITAL, WICHITA FALLS CAMPUS, WICHITA FALLS, TX, p. A635
NORTH VALLEY HEALTH CENTER, WARREN, MN, p. A341
NORTH VALLEY HOSPITAL, WHITEFISH, MT, p. A380
NORTH VALLEY HOSPITAL, TONASKET, WA, p. A668
NORTH VISTA HOSPITAL, NORTH LAS VEGAS, NV, p. A394
NORTHBAY MEDICAL CENTER, FAIRFIELD, CA, p. A60
NORTHBAY VACAVALLEY HOSPITAL, VACAVILLE, CALIFORNIA (see NORTHBAY MEDICAL CENTER), p. A60

NORTHCOAST BEHAVIORAL HEALTHCARE SYSTEM, NORTHFIELD, OH, p. A486
NORTHCREST MEDICAL CENTER, SPRINGFIELD, TN, p. A576
NORTHEAST ALABAMA REGIONAL MEDICAL CENTER, ANNISTON, AL, p. A15
NORTHEAST BAPTIST HOSPITAL, SAN ANTONIO, TEXAS (see BAPTIST HEALTH SYSTEM), p. A624
NORTHEAST GEORGIA MEDICAL CENTER, GAINESVILLE, GA, p. A153
NORTHEAST METHODIST HOSPITAL, LIVE OAK, TEXAS (see METHODIST HOSPITAL), p. A625
NORTHEAST REGIONAL MEDICAL CENTER, KIRKSVILLE, MO, p. A363
NORTHEAST REHABILITATION HOSPITAL, SALEM, NH, p. A400
NORTHEASTERN NEVADA REGIONAL HOSPITAL, ELKO, NV, p. A391
NORTHEASTERN VERMONT REGIONAL HOSPITAL, SAINT JOHNSBURY, VT, p. A644
NORTHERN ARIZONA VA HEALTH CARE SYSTEM, PRESCOTT, AZ, p. A37
NORTHERN CALIFORNIA REHABILITATION HOSPITAL, REDDING, CA, p. A82
NORTHERN COCHISE COMMUNITY HOSPITAL, WILLCOX, AZ, p. A41
NORTHERN COLORADO LONG TERM ACUTE HOSPITAL, JOHNSTOWN, CO, p. A102
NORTHERN COLORADO REHABILITATION HOSPITAL, JOHNSTOWN, CO, p. A102
NORTHERN DUTCHESS HOSPITAL, RHINEBECK, NY, p. A441
NORTHERN HOSPITAL OF SURRY COUNTY, MOUNT AIRY, NC, p. A458
NORTHERN IDAHO ADVANCED CARE HOSPITAL, POST FALLS, ID, p. A170
NORTHERN INYO HOSPITAL, BISHOP, CA, p. A56
NORTHERN LOUISIANA MEDICAL CENTER, RUSTON, LA, p. A276
NORTHERN MAINE MEDICAL CENTER, FORT KENT, ME, p. A283
NORTHERN MONTANA HOSPITAL, HAVRE, MT, p. A376
NORTHERN NAVAJO MEDICAL CENTER, SHIPROCK, NM, p. A418
NORTHERN NEVADA ADULT MENTAL HEALTH SERVICES, SPARKS, NV, p. A395
NORTHERN NEVADA MEDICAL CENTER, SPARKS, NV, p. A396
NORTHERN ROCKIES MEDICAL CENTER, CUT BANK, MT, p. A374
NORTHERN VIRGINIA MENTAL HEALTH INSTITUTE, FALLS CHURCH, VA, p. A648
NORTHERN WESTCHESTER HOSPITAL, MOUNT KISCO, NY, p. A430
NORTHFIELD CAMPUS, NORTHFIELD, OHIO (see NORTHCOAST BEHAVIORAL HEALTHCARE SYSTEM), p. A486
NORTHFIELD HOSPITAL, NORTHFIELD, MN, p. A336
NORTHKEY COMMUNITY CARE, COVINGTON, KY, p. A249
NORTHPORT MEDICAL CENTER, NORTHPORT, AL, p. A24
NORTHRIDGE HOSPITAL MEDICAL CENTER–ROSCOE BOULEVARD CAMPUS,, CA, p. A70
NORTHRIDGE MEDICAL CENTER, COMMERCE, GA, p. A150
NORTHSHORE GLENBROOK HOSPITAL, GLENVIEW, ILLINOIS (see NORTHSHORE UNIVERSITY HEALTH SYSTEM EVANSTON HOSPITAL), p. A181
NORTHSHORE HIGHLAND PARK HOSPITAL, HIGHLAND PARK, ILLINOIS (see NORTHSHORE UNIVERSITY HEALTH SYSTEM EVANSTON HOSPITAL), p. A181
NORTHSHORE SPECIALTY HOSPITAL, COVINGTON, LA, p. A265
NORTHSHORE UNIVERSITY HEALTH SYSTEM EVANSTON HOSPITAL, EVANSTON, IL, p. A181
NORTHSHORE UNIVERSITY HEALTH SYSTEM SKOKIE HOSPITAL, SKOKIE, IL, p. A194
NORTHSIDE HOSPITAL, ATLANTA, GA, p. A145
NORTHSIDE HOSPITAL – CHEROKEE, CANTON, GA, p. A148
NORTHSIDE HOSPITAL AND HEART INSTITUTE, SAINT PETERSBURG, FL, p. A138
NORTHSIDE HOSPITAL FORSYTH, CUMMING, GA, p. A150
NORTHSIDE MEDICAL CENTER, YOUNGSTOWN, OH, p. A492
NORTHSIDE MEDICAL CENTER, YOUNGSTOWN, OHIO (see NORTHSIDE HOSPITAL MEDICAL CENTER), p. A492
NORTHSTAR HEALTH SYSTEM, IRON RIVER, MI, p. A316
NORTHWEST CENTER FOR BEHAVIORAL HEALTH, FORT SUPPLY, OK, p. A497
NORTHWEST COMMUNITY HOSPITAL, ARLINGTON HEIGHTS, IL, p. A172
NORTHWEST FLORIDA COMMUNITY HOSPITAL, CHIPLEY, FL, p. A120
NORTHWEST HILLS SURGICAL HOSPITAL, AUSTIN, TX, p. A581
NORTHWEST HOSPITAL, RANDALLSTOWN, MD, p. A293
NORTHWEST HOSPITAL & MEDICAL CENTER, SEATTLE, WA, p. A665
NORTHWEST MEDICAL CENTER, WINFIELD, AL, p. A27
NORTHWEST MEDICAL CENTER, TUCSON, AZ, p. A40
NORTHWEST MEDICAL CENTER, SPRINGDALE, AR, p. A51

NORTHWEST MEDICAL CENTER, MARGATE, FL, p. A129
NORTHWEST MEDICAL CENTER, ALBANY, MO, p. A355
NORTHWEST MEDICAL CENTER – BENTONVILLE, BENTONVILLE, ARKANSAS (see NORTHWEST MEDICAL CENTER), p. A51
NORTHWEST MISSISSIPPI REGIONAL MEDICAL CENTER, CLARKSDALE, MS, p. A344
NORTHWEST MISSOURI PSYCHIATRIC REHABILITATION CENTER, SAINT JOSEPH, MO, p. A368
NORTHWEST OHIO PSYCHIATRIC HOSPITAL, TOLEDO, OH, p. A489
NORTHWEST SPECIALTY HOSPITAL, POST FALLS, ID, p. A170
NORTHWEST SURGICAL HOSPITAL, OKLAHOMA CITY, OK, p. A501
NORTHWEST TEXAS HEALTHCARE SYSTEM, AMARILLO, TX, p. A578
NORTHWEST TEXAS SURGERY CENTER, AMARILLO, TX, p. A578
NORTHWESTERN LAKE FOREST HOSPITAL, LAKE FOREST, IL, p. A186
NORTHWESTERN MEDICAL CENTER, SAINT ALBANS, VT, p. A644
NORTHWESTERN MEMORIAL HOSPITAL, CHICAGO, IL, p. A177
NORTON AUDUBON HOSPITAL, LOUISVILLE, KY, p. A254
NORTON BROWNSBORO HOSPITAL, LOUISVILLE, KY, p. A255
NORTON COMMUNITY HOSPITAL, NORTON, VA, p. A653
NORTON COUNTY HOSPITAL, NORTON, KS, p. A239
NORTON HEALTHCARE PAVILION, LOUISVILLE, KENTUCKY (see NORTON HOSPITAL), p. A255
NORTON HOSPITAL, LOUISVILLE, KY, p. A255
NORTON SOUND REGIONAL HOSPITAL, NOME, AK, p. A29
NORTON SUBURBAN HOSPITAL, LOUISVILLE, KY, p. A255
NORWALK HOSPITAL, NORWALK, CT, p. A111
NORWEGIAN AMERICAN HOSPITAL, CHICAGO, IL, p. A177
NORWOOD HEALTH CENTER, MARSHFIELD, WI, p. A685
NORWOOD HOSPITAL, NORWOOD, MA, p. A303
NOVATO COMMUNITY HOSPITAL, NOVATO, CA, p. A77
NOXUBEE GENERAL HOSPITAL, MACON, MS, p. A349
NYACK HOSPITAL, NYACK, NY, p. A438
NYE REGIONAL MEDICAL CENTER, TONOPAH, NV, p. A396
NYU CHILDREN'S HOSPITAL, NEW YORK, NEW YORK (see NYU LANGONE MEDICAL CENTER), p. A436
NYU LANGONE MEDICAL CENTER, NEW YORK, NY, p. A436
NYU LANGONE MEDICAL CENTER'S HOSPITAL FOR JOINT DISEASES, NEW YORK, NEW YORK (see NYU LANGONE MEDICAL CENTER), p. A436

# O

O'BLENESS MEMORIAL HOSPITAL, ATHENS, OH, p. A470
O'CONNOR HOSPITAL, SAN JOSE, CA, p. A88
O'CONNOR HOSPITAL, DELHI, NY, p. A425
OAK HILL HOSPITAL, BROOKSVILLE, FL, p. A120
OAK TREE HOSPITAL, CORBIN, KY, p. A249
OAK VALLEY HOSPITAL DISTRICT, OAKDALE, CA, p. A77
OAKBEND MEDICAL CENTER, RICHMOND, TX, p. A622
OAKDALE COMMUNITY HOSPITAL, OAKDALE, LA, p. A275
OAKES COMMUNITY HOSPITAL, OAKES, ND, p. A467
OAKLAND MEDICAL CENTER, OAKLAND, CA, p. A77
OAKLAND MERCY HOSPITAL, OAKLAND, NE, p. A387
OAKLAND REGIONAL HOSPITAL, SOUTHFIELD, MI, p. A323
OAKLAWN HOSPITAL, MARSHALL, MI, p. A318
OAKLAWN PSYCHIATRIC CENTER, GOSHEN, IN, p. A202
OAKLEAF SURGICAL HOSPITAL, EAU CLAIRE, WI, p. A681
OAKWOOD ANNAPOLIS HOSPITAL, WAYNE, MI, p. A325
OAKWOOD CORRECTIONAL FACILITY, LIMA, OH, p. A483
OAKWOOD HERITAGE HOSPITAL, TAYLOR, MI, p. A324
OAKWOOD HOSPITAL & MEDICAL CENTER–DEARBORN, DEARBORN, MI, p. A310
OAKWOOD SOUTHSHORE MEDICAL CENTER, TRENTON, MI, p. A324
OCALA REGIONAL MEDICAL CENTER, OCALA, FL, p. A133
OCEAN BEACH HOSPITAL, ILWACO, WA, p. A662
OCEAN MEDICAL CENTER, BRICK TOWNSHIP, NJ, p. A402
OCEAN SPRINGS HOSPITAL, OCEAN SPRINGS, MISSISSIPPI (see SINGING RIVER HEALTH SYSTEM), p. A351
OCEANS BEHAVIORAL HOSPITAL OF ALEXANDRIA, ALEXANDRIA, LA, p. A261
OCEANS BEHAVIORAL HOSPITAL OF BATON ROUGE, BATON ROUGE, LA, p. A262
OCEANS BEHAVIORAL HOSPITAL OF BROUSSARD, BROUSSARD, LA, p. A264
OCEANS BEHAVIORAL HOSPITAL OF DE RIDDER, DERIDDER, LA, p. A266
OCEANS BEHAVIORAL HOSPITAL OF GREATER NEW ORLEANS, KENNER, LA, p. A269

OCEANS BEHAVIORAL HOSPITAL OF KENTWOOD, KENTWOOD, LA, p. A269
OCEANS BEHAVIORAL HOSPITAL OF LAKE CHARLES, LAKE CHARLES, LA, p. A271
OCEANS BEHAVIORAL HOSPITAL OF OPELOUSAS, OPELOUSAS, LA, p. A275
OCEANS SPECIALTY HOSPITAL OF GRETNA, GRETNA, LA, p. A267
OCH REGIONAL MEDICAL CENTER, STARKVILLE, MS, p. A353
OCHILTREE GENERAL HOSPITAL, PERRYTON, TX, p. A620
OCHSNER BAPTIST MEDICAL CENTER, NEW ORLEANS, LA, p. A274
OCHSNER EXTENDED CARE HOSPITAL OF KENNER, KENNER, LA, p. A269
OCHSNER MEDICAL CENTER, NEW ORLEANS, LA, p. A275
OCHSNER MEDICAL CENTER – KENNER, KENNER, LA, p. A269
OCHSNER MEDICAL CENTER – NORTH SHORE, SLIDELL, LA, p. A278
OCHSNER MEDICAL CENTER – WEST BANK, GRETNA, LOUISIANA (see OCHSNER MEDICAL CENTER), p. A275
OCHSNER MEDICAL CENTER–BATON ROUGE, BATON ROUGE, LA, p. A262
OCHSNER ST. ANNE GENERAL HOSPITAL, RACELAND, LA, p. A276
OCONEE MEDICAL CENTER, SENECA, SC, p. A553
OCONEE REGIONAL MEDICAL CENTER, MILLEDGEVILLE, GA, p. A156
OCONOMOWOC MEMORIAL HOSPITAL, OCONOMOWOC, WI, p. A688
OCONTO HOSPITAL & MEDICAL CENTER, OCONTO, WI, p. A688
ODESSA MEMORIAL HEALTHCARE CENTER, ODESSA, WA, p. A663
ODESSA REGIONAL MEDICAL CENTER, ODESSA, TX, p. A619
OGALLALA COMMUNITY HOSPITAL, OGALLALA, NE, p. A387
OGDEN REGIONAL MEDICAL CENTER, OGDEN, UT, p. A639
OHIO COUNTY HOSPITAL, HARTFORD, KY, p. A251
OHIO HOSPITAL FOR CHILD AND ADOLESCENT PSYCHIATRY, COLUMBUS, OH, p. A477
OHIO STATE UNIVERSITY HOSPITALS EAST, COLUMBUS, OHIO (see OHIO STATE UNIVERSITY MEDICAL CENTER), p. A477
OHIO STATE UNIVERSITY MEDICAL CENTER, COLUMBUS, OH, p. A477
OHIO VALLEY GENERAL HOSPITAL, MCKEES ROCKS, PA, p. A528
OHIO VALLEY MEDICAL CENTER, SPRINGFIELD, OH, p. A488
OHIO VALLEY MEDICAL CENTER, WHEELING, WV, p. A676
OHIOHEALTH MARION GENERAL HOSPITAL, MARION, OH, p. A484
OHSU HOSPITAL, PORTLAND, OR, p. A514
OJAI VALLEY COMMUNITY HOSPITAL, OJAI, CALIFORNIA (see COMMUNITY MEMORIAL HEALTH SYSTEM), p. A94
OKANOGAN DOUGLAS DISTRICT HOSPITAL, BREWSTER, WA, p. A660
OKEENE MUNICIPAL HOSPITAL, OKEENE, OK, p. A500
OKLAHOMA CENTER FOR ORTHOPEDIC AND MULTI-SPECIALTY SURGERY, OKLAHOMA CITY, OK, p. A501
OKLAHOMA FORENSIC CENTER, VINITA, OK, p. A507
OKLAHOMA HEART HOSPITAL, OKLAHOMA CITY, OK, p. A501
OKLAHOMA HEART HOSPITAL SOUTH CAMPUS, OKLAHOMA CITY, OK, p. A501
OKLAHOMA NEUROSPECIALTY CENTER, TULSA, OK, p. A506
OKLAHOMA SPINE HOSPITAL, OKLAHOMA CITY, OK, p. A501
OKLAHOMA STATE UNIVERSITY MEDICAL CENTER, TULSA, OK, p. A506
OKLAHOMA SURGICAL HOSPITAL, TULSA, OK, p. A506
OKMULGEE MEMORIAL HOSPITAL, OKMULGEE, OK, p. A502
OLATHE MEDICAL CENTER, OLATHE, KS, p. A240
OLD BRIDGE DIVISION, OLD BRIDGE, NEW JERSEY (see RARITAN BAY MEDICAL CENTER), p. A408
OLD VINEYARD BEHAVIORAL HEALTH SERVICES, WINSTON–SALEM, NC, p. A463
OLEAN GENERAL HOSPITAL, OLEAN, NY, p. A439
OLIN E. TEAGUE VETERANS' CENTER, TEMPLE, TEXAS (see CENTRAL TEXAS VETERANS HEALTHCARE SYSTEM), p. A630
OLMSTED MEDICAL CENTER, ROCHESTER, MN, p. A338
OLYMPIA MEDICAL CENTER, LOS ANGELES, CA, p. A71
OLYMPIC MEDICAL CENTER, PORT ANGELES, WA, p. A664
OMEGA HOSPITAL, METAIRIE, LA, p. A273
ONEIDA COUNTY HOSPITAL, MALAD CITY, ID, p. A169
ONEIDA HEALTHCARE, ONEIDA, NY, p. A439
ONSLOW MEMORIAL HOSPITAL, JACKSONVILLE, NC, p. A455
OPELOUSAS GENERAL HEALTH SYSTEM, OPELOUSAS, LA, p. A276
OPELOUSAS GENERAL HEALTH SYSTEM–SOUTH CAMPUS, OPELOUSAS, LOUISIANA (see OPELOUSAS GENERAL HEALTH SYSTEM), p. A276
OPTIMA SPECIALTY HOSPITAL, LAFAYETTE, LA, p. A270
ORANGE CITY AREA HEALTH SYSTEM, ORANGE CITY, IA, p. A224

ORANGE COAST MEMORIAL MEDICAL CENTER, FOUNTAIN VALLEY, CA, p. A61
ORANGE COUNTY IRVINE MEDICAL CENTER, IRVINE, CALIFORNIA (see ANAHEIM MEDICAL CENTER), p. A53
ORANGE PARK MEDICAL CENTER, ORANGE PARK, FL, p. A134
ORANGE REGIONAL MEDICAL CENTER, MIDDLETOWN, NY, p. A430
OREGON STATE HOSPITAL, SALEM, OR, p. A515
OREM COMMUNITY HOSPITAL, OREM, UT, p. A639
ORLANDO REGIONAL MEDICAL CENTER, ORLANDO, FL, p. A134
ORLANDO REGIONAL SOUTH SEMINOLE HOSPITAL, LONGWOOD, FL, p. A129
ORLANDO REGIONAL–LUCERNE, ORLANDO, FLORIDA (see ORLANDO REGIONAL MEDICAL CENTER), p. A134
ORO VALLEY HOSPITAL, ORO VALLEY, AZ, p. A34
OROVILLE HOSPITAL, OROVILLE, CA, p. A78
ORTHOCOLORADO HOSPITAL, LAKEWOOD, CO, p. A103
ORTHOPAEDIC HOSPITAL OF LUTHERAN HEALTH, FORT WAYNE, IN, p. A201
ORTHOPAEDIC HOSPITAL OF WISCONSIN – GLENDALE, MILWAUKEE, WI, p. A687
ORTHOPEDIC HOSPITAL, OKLAHOMA CITY, OK, p. A502
ORTONVILLE AREA HEALTH SERVICES, ORTONVILLE, MN, p. A336
OSAWATOMIE STATE HOSPITAL, OSAWATOMIE, KS, p. A240
OSBORNE COUNTY MEMORIAL HOSPITAL, OSBORNE, KS, p. A240
OSCEOLA COMMUNITY HOSPITAL, SIBLEY, IA, p. A226
OSCEOLA MEDICAL CENTER, OSCEOLA, WI, p. A688
OSCEOLA REGIONAL MEDICAL CENTER, KISSIMMEE, FL, p. A127
OSF HOLY FAMILY MEDICAL CENTER, MONMOUTH, IL, p. A188
OSF SAINT ANTHONY MEDICAL CENTER, ROCKFORD, IL, p. A192
OSF SAINT FRANCIS MEDICAL CENTER, PEORIA, IL, p. A191
OSF SAINT JAMES – JOHN W. ALBRECHT MEDICAL CENTER, PONTIAC, IL, p. A192
OSF ST. FRANCIS HOSPITAL, ESCANABA, MI, p. A312
OSF ST. JOSEPH MEDICAL CENTER, BLOOMINGTON, IL, p. A173
OSF ST. MARY MEDICAL CENTER, GALESBURG, IL, p. A182
OSMOND GENERAL HOSPITAL, OSMOND, NE, p. A388
OSS ORTHOPAEDIC SPECIALTY HOSPITAL, YORK, PA, p. A543
OSSINING CORRECTIONAL FACILITIES HOSPITAL, OSSINING, NY, p. A439
OSWEGO COMMUNITY HOSPITAL, OSWEGO, KS, p. A240
OSWEGO HOSPITAL, OSWEGO, NY, p. A440
OTHELLO COMMUNITY HOSPITAL, OTHELLO, WA, p. A664
OTIS R BOWEN CENTER FOR HUMAN SERVICES, WARSAW, IN, p. A213
OTSEGO MEMORIAL HOSPITAL, GAYLORD, MI, p. A313
OTTAWA COUNTY HEALTH CENTER, MINNEAPOLIS, KS, p. A239
OTTAWA REGIONAL HOSPITAL AND HEALTHCARE CENTER, OTTAWA, IL, p. A190
OTTO KAISER MEMORIAL HOSPITAL, KENEDY, TX, p. A610
OTTUMWA REGIONAL HEALTH CENTER, OTTUMWA, IA, p. A225
OU MEDICAL CENTER, OKLAHOMA CITY, OK, p. A502
OU MEDICAL CENTER EDMOND, EDMOND, OKLAHOMA (see OU MEDICAL CENTER), p. A502
OUACHITA COMMUNITY HOSPITAL, WEST MONROE, LA, p. A279
OUACHITA COUNTY MEDICAL CENTER, CAMDEN, AR, p. A43
OUR CHILDREN'S HOUSE AT BAYLOR, DALLAS, TX, p. A592
OUR COMMUNITY HOSPITAL, SCOTLAND NECK, NC, p. A460
OUR LADY OF BELLEFONTE HOSPITAL, ASHLAND, KY, p. A247
OUR LADY OF FATIMA HOSPITAL, NORTH PROVIDENCE, RHODE ISLAND (see ST. JOSEPH HEALTH SERVICES OF RHODE ISLAND), p. A544
OUR LADY OF LOURDES MEDICAL CENTER, CAMDEN, NJ, p. A402
OUR LADY OF LOURDES MEMORIAL HOSPITAL, BINGHAMTON, NY, p. A422
OUR LADY OF LOURDES REGIONAL MEDICAL CENTER, LAFAYETTE, LA, p. A270
OUR LADY OF PEACE, LOUISVILLE, KY, p. A255
OUR LADY OF THE LAKE CHILDREN'S HOSPITAL, BATON ROUGE, LOUISIANA (see OUR LADY OF THE LAKE REGIONAL MEDICAL CENTER), p. A262
OUR LADY OF THE LAKE REGIONAL MEDICAL CENTER, BATON ROUGE, LA, p. A262
OUR LADY OF THE RESURRECTION MEDICAL CENTER, CHICAGO, IL, p. A177
OUR LADY OF VICTORY HOSPITAL, STANLEY, WI, p. A691
OVERLAKE HOSPITAL MEDICAL CENTER, BELLEVUE, WA, p. A659
OVERLAND PARK REGIONAL MEDICAL CENTER, OVERLAND PARK, KS, p. A241
OVERLOOK MEDICAL CENTER, SUMMIT, NJ, p. A410

OVERTON BROOKS VETERANS AFFAIRS MEDICAL CENTER, SHREVEPORT, LA, p. A277
OWATONNA HOSPITAL, OWATONNA, MN, p. A336
OWENSBORO MEDICAL HEALTH SYSTEM, OWENSBORO, KY, p. A257
OZARK HEALTH MEDICAL CENTER, CLINTON, AR, p. A43
OZARKS COMMUNITY HOSPITAL, GRAVETTE, AR, p. A45
OZARKS COMMUNITY HOSPITAL, SPRINGFIELD, MO, p. A371
OZARKS MEDICAL CENTER, WEST PLAINS, MO, p. A372

# P

P & S SURGICAL HOSPITAL, MONROE, LA, p. A273
PACIFIC ALLIANCE MEDICAL CENTER, LOS ANGELES, CA, p. A71
PACIFIC HOSPITAL OF LONG BEACH, LONG BEACH, CA, p. A68
PACIFICA HOSPITAL OF THE VALLEY,, CA, p. A71
PAGE HOSPITAL, PAGE, AZ, p. A34
PAGE MEMORIAL HOSPITAL, LURAY, VA, p. A650
PAGOSA SPRINGS MEDICAL CENTER, PAGOSA SPRINGS, CO, p. A104
PALACIOS COMMUNITY MEDICAL CENTER, PALACIOS, TX, p. A619
PALESTINE REGIONAL MEDICAL CENTER–EAST, PALESTINE, TX, p. A619
PALESTINE REGIONAL REHABILITATION CENTER, PALESTINE, TX, p. A619
PALI MOMI MEDICAL CENTER, AIEA, HI, p. A163
PALISADES MEDICAL CENTER, NORTH BERGEN, NJ, p. A407
PALM BAY HOSPITAL, MELBOURNE, FL, p. A130
PALM BEACH CHILDREN'S HOSPITAL, WEST PALM BEACH, FLORIDA (see ST. MARY'S MEDICAL CENTER), p. A143
PALM BEACH GARDENS MEDICAL CENTER, PALM BEACH GARDENS, FL, p. A135
PALM DRIVE HOSPITAL, SEBASTOPOL, CA, p. A90
PALM SPRINGS GENERAL HOSPITAL, HIALEAH, FL, p. A125
PALMDALE REGIONAL MEDICAL CENTER, PALMDALE, CA, p. A79
PALMER LUTHERAN HEALTH CENTER, WEST UNION, IA, p. A228
PALMERTON HOSPITAL, PALMERTON, PA, p. A531
PALMETTO GENERAL HOSPITAL, HIALEAH, FL, p. A125
PALMETTO HEALTH BAPTIST, COLUMBIA, SC, p. A548
PALMETTO HEALTH CHILDREN'S HOSPITAL, COLUMBIA, SOUTH CAROLINA (see PALMETTO HEALTH RICHLAND), p. A548
PALMETTO HEALTH RICHLAND, COLUMBIA, SC, p. A548
PALMETTO LOWCOUNTRY BEHAVIORAL HEALTH, CHARLESTON, SC, p. A547
PALMS OF PASADENA HOSPITAL, SAINT PETERSBURG, FL, p. A138
PALMS WEST HOSPITAL, LOXAHATCHEE, FL, p. A129
PALO ALTO COUNTY HEALTH SYSTEM, EMMETSBURG, IA, p. A219
PALO ALTO DIVISION, PALO ALTO, CALIFORNIA (see VETERANS AFFAIRS PALO ALTO HEALTH CARE SYSTEM), p. A79
PALO PINTO GENERAL HOSPITAL, MINERAL WELLS, TX, p. A617
PALO VERDE HOSPITAL, BLYTHE, CA, p. A56
PALO VERDE MENTAL HEALTH SERVICES, TUCSON, ARIZONA (see TMC HEALTHCARE), p. A40
PALOMAR MEDICAL CENTER, ESCONDIDO, CA, p. A60
PALOS COMMUNITY HOSPITAL, PALOS HEIGHTS, IL, p. A190
PAMPA REGIONAL MEDICAL CENTER, PAMPA, TX, p. A620
PANA COMMUNITY HOSPITAL, PANA, IL, p. A190
PANORAMA CITY MEDICAL CENTER,, CA, p. A71
PAOLI HOSPITAL, PAOLI, PA, p. A531
PARADISE VALLEY HOSPITAL, PHOENIX, AZ, p. A36
PARADISE VALLEY HOSPITAL, NATIONAL CITY, CA, p. A76
PARIS COMMUNITY HOSPITAL, PARIS, IL, p. A190
PARIS REGIONAL MEDICAL CENTER, PARIS, TX, p. A620
PARIS REGIONAL MEDICAL CENTER, PARIS, TEXAS (see PARIS REGIONAL MEDICAL CENTER), p. A620
PARIS REGIONAL MEDICAL CENTER–SOUTH CAMPUS, PARIS, TEXAS (see PARIS REGIONAL MEDICAL CENTER), p. A620
PARK CITY MEDICAL CENTER, PARK CITY, UT, p. A639
PARK NICOLLET METHODIST HOSPITAL, SAINT LOUIS PARK, MN, p. A339
PARK PLACE SURGICAL HOSPITAL, LAFAYETTE, LA, p. A270
PARK PLAZA HOSPITAL, HOUSTON, TX, p. A606
PARK RIDGE HEALTH, HENDERSONVILLE, NC, p. A454
PARKCARE PAVILION, YONKERS, NEW YORK (see ST. JOHN'S RIVERSIDE HOSPITAL), p. A447
PARKER ADVENTIST HOSPITAL, PARKER, CO, p. A105
PARKLAND HEALTH & HOSPITAL SYSTEM, DALLAS, TX, p. A592
PARKLAND HEALTH CENTER, FARMINGTON, MO, p. A359

PARKLAND HEALTH CENTER–BONNE TERRE, BONNE TERRE, MO, p. A355
PARKLAND MEDICAL CENTER, DERRY, NH, p. A397
PARKRIDGE MEDICAL CENTER, CHATTANOOGA, TN, p. A563
PARKRIDGE VALLEY HOSPTIAL, CHATTANOOGA, TENNESSEE (see PARKRIDGE MEDICAL CENTER), p. A563
PARKSIDE HOSPITAL, TULSA, OK, p. A506
PARKVIEW ADVENTIST MEDICAL CENTER, BRUNSWICK, ME, p. A282
PARKVIEW COMMUNITY HOSPITAL MEDICAL CENTER, RIVERSIDE, CA, p. A82
PARKVIEW HOSPITAL, FORT WAYNE, IN, p. A201
PARKVIEW HOSPITAL, WHEELER, TX, p. A634
PARKVIEW HUNTINGTON HOSPITAL, HUNTINGTON, IN, p. A203
PARKVIEW LAGRANGE HOSPITAL, LAGRANGE, IN, p. A207
PARKVIEW MEDICAL CENTER, PUEBLO, CO, p. A105
PARKVIEW NOBLE HOSPITAL, KENDALLVILLE, IN, p. A206
PARKVIEW NORTH HOSPITAL, FORT WAYNE, INDIANA (see PARKVIEW HOSPITAL), p. A201
PARKVIEW REGIONAL HOSPITAL, MEXIA, TX, p. A616
PARKVIEW WHITLEY HOSPITAL, COLUMBIA CITY, IN, p. A199
PARKWAY MEDICAL CENTER, DECATUR, AL, p. A18
PARKWAY REGIONAL HOSPITAL, FULTON, KY, p. A250
PARKWEST MEDICAL CENTER, KNOXVILLE, TN, p. A568
PARKWOOD BEHAVIORAL HEALTH SYSTEM, OLIVE BRANCH, MS, p. A351
PARMA COMMUNITY GENERAL HOSPITAL, PARMA, OH, p. A487
PARMER MEDICAL CENTER, FRIONA, TX, p. A600
PARRISH MEDICAL CENTER, TITUSVILLE, FL, p. A142
PARSONS STATE HOSPITAL AND TRAINING CENTER, PARSONS, KS, p. A241
PASCO REGIONAL MEDICAL CENTER, DADE CITY, FL, p. A121
PASSAVANT AREA HOSPITAL, JACKSONVILLE, IL, p. A185
PATEWOOD MEMORIAL HOSPITAL, GREENVILLE, SC, p. A550
PATHWAY REHABILITATION HOSPITAL, BOSSIER CITY, LA, p. A263
PATHWAYS OF TENNESSEE, JACKSON, TN, p. A567
PATHWAYS TREATMENT CENTER, KALISPELL, MONTANA (see KALISPELL REGIONAL MEDICAL CENTER), p. A377
PATIENT'S CHOICE MEDICAL CENTER, BELZONI, MS, p. A343
PATIENT'S CHOICE MEDICAL CENTER OF CLAIBORNE COUNTY, PORT GIBSON, MS, p. A352
PATIENTS' CHOICE MEDICAL CENTER OF ERIN, ERIN, TN, p. A565
PATIENTS' HOSPITAL OF REDDING, REDDING, CA, p. A82
PATRICK B. HARRIS PSYCHIATRIC HOSPITAL, ANDERSON, SC, p. A546
PATTIE A. CLAY REGIONAL MEDICAL CENTER, RICHMOND, KY, p. A258
PATTON STATE HOSPITAL, PATTON, CA, p. A80
PAUL B. HALL REGIONAL MEDICAL CENTER, PAINTSVILLE, KY, p. A257
PAUL OLIVER MEMORIAL HOSPITAL, FRANKFORT, MI, p. A312
PAULDING COUNTY HOSPITAL, PAULDING, OH, p. A487
PAULS VALLEY GENERAL HOSPITAL, PAULS VALLEY, OK, p. A503
PAWHUSKA HOSPITAL, PAWHUSKA, OK, p. A503
PAWNEE COUNTY MEMORIAL HOSPITAL, PAWNEE CITY, NE, p. A389
PAWNEE VALLEY COMMUNITY HOSPITAL, LARNED, KS, p. A237
PAYNE WHITNEY PSYCHIATRIC CLINIC, NEW YORK, NEW YORK (see NEW YORK–PRESBYTERIAN HOSPITAL), p. A436
PAYNESVILLE AREA HEALTH CARE SYSTEM, PAYNESVILLE, MN, p. A337
PAYSON REGIONAL MEDICAL CENTER, PAYSON, AZ, p. A35
PEACE HARBOR HOSPITAL, FLORENCE, OR, p. A510
PEACE RIVER REGIONAL MEDICAL CENTER, PORT CHARLOTTE, FL, p. A137
PEACEHEALTH KETCHIKAN MEDICAL CENTER, KETCHIKAN, AK, p. A29
PEACEHEALTH SOUTHWEST MEDICAL CENTER, VANCOUVER, WA, p. A668
PEACEHEALTH ST. JOHN MEDICAL CENTER, LONGVIEW, WA, p. A662
PEACEHEALTH ST. JOSEPH MEDICAL CENTER, BELLINGHAM, WA, p. A659
PEACH REGIONAL MEDICAL CENTER, FORT VALLEY, GA, p. A153
PEACHFORD BEHAVIORAL HEALTH SYSTEM, ATLANTA, GA, p. A145
PEAK BEHAVIORAL HEALTH SERVICES, SANTA TERESA, NM, p. A418
PEAK VIEW BEHAVIORAL HEALTH, COLORADO SPRINGS, CO, p. A98
PEARL RIVER COUNTY HOSPITAL, POPLARVILLE, MS, p. A352
PECONIC BAY MEDICAL CENTER, RIVERHEAD, NY, p. A441
PECOS COUNTY MEMORIAL HOSPITAL, FORT STOCKTON, TX, p. A598
PECOS VALLEY LODGE, ROSWELL, NEW MEXICO (see NEW MEXICO REHABILITATION CENTER), p. A417

PEKIN HOSPITAL, PEKIN, IL, p. A191
PELLA REGIONAL HEALTH CENTER, PELLA, IA, p. A225
PEMBINA COUNTY MEMORIAL HOSPITAL AND WEDGEWOOD MANOR, CAVALIER, ND, p. A464
PEMBROKE HOSPITAL, PEMBROKE, MA, p. A303
PEMISCOT MEMORIAL HEALTH SYSTEM, HAYTI, MO, p. A360
PEN BAY MEDICAL CENTER, ROCKPORT, ME, p. A285
PENDER COMMUNITY HOSPITAL, PENDER, NE, p. A389
PENDER MEMORIAL HOSPITAL, BURGAW, NC, p. A449
PENINSULA HOSPITAL, BURLINGAME, CALIFORNIA (see MILLS–PENINSULA HEALTH SERVICES), p. A56
PENINSULA HOSPITAL, LOUISVILLE, TN, p. A570
PENINSULA REGIONAL HEALTH SYSTEM, SALISBURY, MD, p. A294
PENN PRESBYTERIAN MEDICAL CENTER, PHILADELPHIA, PA, p. A533
PENN STATE CHILDREN'S HOSPITAL, HERSHEY, PENNSYLVANIA (see PENN STATE MILTON S. HERSHEY MEDICAL CENTER), p. A525
PENN STATE HERSHEY REHABILITATION HOSPITAL, HUMMELSTOWN, PA, p. A525
PENN STATE MILTON S. HERSHEY MEDICAL CENTER, HERSHEY, PA, p. A525
PENNOCK HOSPITAL, HASTINGS, MI, p. A315
PENNSYLVANIA HOSPITAL, PHILADELPHIA, PA, p. A533
PENNSYLVANIA PSYCHIATRIC HOSPITAL, HARRISBURG, PA, p. A524
PENOBSCOT VALLEY HOSPITAL, LINCOLN, ME, p. A284
PENROSE HOSPITAL, COLORADO SPRINGS, COLORADO (see PENROSE–ST. FRANCIS HEALTH SERVICES), p. A98
PENROSE–ST. FRANCIS HEALTH SERVICES, COLORADO SPRINGS, CO, p. A98
PERHAM HEALTH, PERHAM, MN, p. A337
PERKINS COUNTY HEALTH SERVICES, GRANT, NE, p. A384
PERMIAN REGIONAL MEDICAL CENTER, ANDREWS, TX, p. A578
PERRY COMMUNITY HOSPITAL, LINDEN, TN, p. A569
PERRY COUNTY GENERAL HOSPITAL, RICHTON, MS, p. A352
PERRY COUNTY MEMORIAL HOSPITAL, TELL CITY, IN, p. A212
PERRY COUNTY MEMORIAL HOSPITAL, PERRYVILLE, MO, p. A366
PERRY HOSPITAL, PERRY, GA, p. A157
PERRY MEMORIAL HOSPITAL, PRINCETON, IL, p. A192
PERRY MEMORIAL HOSPITAL, PERRY, OK, p. A503
PERSHING GENERAL HOSPITAL, LOVELOCK, NV, p. A394
PERSON MEMORIAL HOSPITAL, ROXBORO, NC, p. A460
PERTH AMBOY DIVISION, PERTH AMBOY, NEW JERSEY (see RARITAN BAY MEDICAL CENTER), p. A408
PETALUMA VALLEY HOSPITAL, PETALUMA, CA, p. A80
PETERSBURG MEDICAL CENTER, PETERSBURG, AK, p. A30
PETERSON REGIONAL MEDICAL CENTER, KERRVILLE, TX, p. A610
PETERSON REHABILITATION HOSPITAL, WHEELING, WV, p. A676
PEYTON MANNING CHILDREN'S HOSPITAL, INDIANAPOLIS, INDIANA (see ST. VINCENT INDIANAPOLIS HOSPITAL), p. A205
PEYTON MANNING CHILDREN'S HOSPITAL AT ST. VINCENT, INDIANAPOLIS, INDIANA (see ST. VINCENT INDIANAPOLIS HOSPITAL), p. A205
PHELPS COUNTY REGIONAL MEDICAL CENTER, ROLLA, MO, p. A367
PHELPS MEMORIAL HEALTH CENTER, HOLDREGE, NE, p. A384
PHELPS MEMORIAL HOSPITAL CENTER, SLEEPY HOLLOW, NY, p. A443
PHILHAVEN, MOUNT GRETNA, PA, p. A529
PHILIP HEALTH SERVICES, PHILIP, SD, p. A558
PHILLIPS COUNTY HOSPITAL, PHILLIPSBURG, KS, p. A241
PHILLIPS COUNTY HOSPITAL, MALTA, MT, p. A377
PHILLIPS EYE INSTITUTE, MINNEAPOLIS, MN, p. A335
PHOEBE NORTH, ALBANY, GA, p. A144
PHOEBE PUTNEY MEMORIAL HOSPITAL, ALBANY, GA, p. A144
PHOEBE SUMTER MEDICAL CENTER, AMERICUS, GA, p. A144
PHOEBE WORTH MEDICAL CENTER, SYLVESTER, GA, p. A160
PHOENIX BAPTIST HOSPITAL, PHOENIX, AZ, p. A36
PHOENIX BEHAVIORAL HOSPITAL, RAYNE, LA, p. A276
PHOENIX CHILDREN'S HOSPITAL, PHOENIX, AZ, p. A36
PHOENIX VETERANS AFFAIRS HEALTH CARE SYSTEM, PHOENIX, AZ, p. A36
PHOENIXVILLE HOSPITAL, PHOENIXVILLE, PA, p. A534
PHS SANTA FE INDIAN HOSPITAL, SANTA FE, NM, p. A418
PHYSICIAN'S CHOICE HOSPITAL – FREMONT, FREMONT, OH, p. A480
PHYSICIANS BEHAVIORAL HOSPITAL, SHREVEPORT, LA, p. A277
PHYSICIANS CARE SURGICAL HOSPITAL, ROYERSFORD, PA, p. A537
PHYSICIANS MEDICAL CENTER, HOUMA, LA, p. A268
PHYSICIANS MEDICAL CENTER OF SANTA FE HOSPITAL, SANTA FE, NM, p. A418

PHYSICIANS REGIONAL MEDICAL CENTER, KNOXVILLE, TN, p. A568

PHYSICIANS REGIONAL MEDICAL CENTER, NAPLES, FLORIDA (*see* PHYSICIANS REGIONAL MEDICAL CENTER – PINE RIDGE), p. A133

PHYSICIANS REGIONAL MEDICAL CENTER – PINE RIDGE, NAPLES, FL, p. A133

PHYSICIANS SURGICAL HOSPITAL – PANHANDLE CAMPUS, AMARILLO, TX, p. A578

PHYSICIANS SURGICAL HOSPITAL – QUAIL CREEK, AMARILLO, TX, p. A578

PHYSICIANS' HOSPITAL IN ANADARKO, ANADARKO, OK, p. A493

PHYSICIANS' MEDICAL CENTER, NEW ALBANY, IN, p. A209

PHYSICIANS' SPECIALTY HOSPITAL, FAYETTEVILLE, AR, p. A44

PICKENS COUNTY MEDICAL CENTER, CARROLLTON, AL, p. A18

PIEDMONT FAYETTE HOSPITAL, FAYETTEVILLE, GA, p. A152

PIEDMONT GERIATRIC HOSPITAL, BURKEVILLE, VA, p. A646

PIEDMONT HOSPITAL, ATLANTA, GA, p. A146

PIEDMONT MEDICAL CENTER, ROCK HILL, SC, p. A553

PIEDMONT MOUNTAINSIDE HOSPITAL, JASPER, GA, p. A154

PIEDMONT NEWNAN HOSPITAL, NEWNAN, GA, p. A157

PIGGOTT COMMUNITY HOSPITAL, PIGGOTT, AR, p. A50

PIKE COMMUNITY HOSPITAL, WAVERLY, OH, p. A491

PIKE COUNTY MEMORIAL HOSPITAL, LOUISIANA, MO, p. A364

PIKES PEAK REGIONAL HOSPITAL, WOODLAND PARK, CO, p. A107

PIKEVILLE MEDICAL CENTER, PIKEVILLE, KY, p. A258

PILGRIM PSYCHIATRIC CENTER, BRENTWOOD, NY, p. A422

PINCKNEYVILLE COMMUNITY HOSPITAL, PINCKNEYVILLE, IL, p. A191

PINE CREEK MEDICAL CENTER, DALLAS, TX, p. A592

PINE REST CHRISTIAN MENTAL HEALTH SERVICES, GRAND RAPIDS, MI, p. A313

PINECREST REHABILITATION HOSPITAL, DELRAY BEACH, FLORIDA (*see* DELRAY MEDICAL CENTER), p. A122

PINEVILLE COMMUNITY HOSPITAL ASSOCIATION, PINEVILLE, KY, p. A258

PINNACLE HEALTH SYSTEM, HARRISBURG, PA, p. A524

PINNACLE HOSPITAL, CROWN POINT, IN, p. A200

PINNACLE POINTE HOSPITAL, LITTLE ROCK, AR, p. A48

PINNACLE SPECIALTY HOSPITAL, TULSA, OK, p. A506

PIONEER COMMUNITY HOSPITAL OF ABERDEEN, ABERDEEN, MS, p. A343

PIONEER COMMUNITY HOSPITAL OF CHOCTAW, ACKERMAN, MS, p. A343

PIONEER COMMUNITY HOSPITAL OF EARLY, BLAKELY, GA, p. A147

PIONEER COMMUNITY HOSPITAL OF NEWTON, NEWTON, MS, p. A351

PIONEER COMMUNITY HOSPITAL OF PATRICK COUNTY, STUART, VA, p. A656

PIONEER COMMUNITY HOSPITAL OF STOKES, DANBURY, NC, p. A451

PIONEER MEDICAL CENTER, BIG TIMBER, MT, p. A373

PIONEER MEMORIAL HOSPITAL, HEPPNER, OR, p. A511

PIONEER MEMORIAL HOSPITAL, PRINEVILLE, OR, p. A514

PIONEER MEMORIAL HOSPITAL AND HEALTH SERVICES, VIBORG, SD, p. A560

PIONEER VALLEY HOSPITAL, WEST VALLEY CITY, UT, p. A642

PIONEERS MEDICAL CENTER, MEEKER, CO, p. A104

PIONEERS MEMORIAL HEALTHCARE DISTRICT, BRAWLEY, CA, p. A56

PIPESTONE COUNTY MEDICAL CENTER AVERA, PIPESTONE, MN, p. A337

PLACENTIA–LINDA HOSPITAL, PLACENTIA, CA, p. A80

PLAINS MEMORIAL HOSPITAL, DIMMITT, TX, p. A594

PLAINS REGIONAL MEDICAL CENTER, CLOVIS, NM, p. A415

PLAINVIEW HOSPITAL, PLAINVIEW, NY, p. A440

PLANO SPECIALTY HOSPITAL, PLANO, TX, p. A621

PLANTATION GENERAL HOSPITAL, PLANTATION, FL, p. A136

PLATEAU MEDICAL CENTER, OAK HILL, WV, p. A674

PLATTE COUNTY MEMORIAL HOSPITAL, WHEATLAND, WY, p. A698

PLATTE HEALTH CENTER AVERA, PLATTE, SD, p. A558

PLATTE VALLEY MEDICAL CENTER, BRIGHTON, CO, p. A98

PLAZA MEDICAL CENTER OF FORT WORTH, FORT WORTH, TX, p. A599

PLAZA SPECIALTY HOSPITAL, HOUSTON, TX, p. A606

PLEASANT VALLEY HOSPITAL, POINT PLEASANT, WV, p. A675

PLUM CREEK SPECIALTY HOSPITAL, AMARILLO, TX, p. A578

PLUMAS DISTRICT HOSPITAL, QUINCY, CA, p. A81

POCAHONTAS COMMUNITY HOSPITAL, POCAHONTAS, IA, p. A225

POCAHONTAS MEMORIAL HOSPITAL, BUCKEYE, WV, p. A670

POCONO MEDICAL CENTER, EAST STROUDSBURG, PA, p. A522

POINTE COUPEE GENERAL HOSPITAL, NEW ROADS, LA, p. A275

POLK MEDICAL CENTER, CEDARTOWN, GA, p. A149

POLYCLINIC HOSPITAL, HARRISBURG, PENNSYLVANIA (*see* PINNACLE HEALTH SYSTEM), p. A524

POMERADO HOSPITAL, POWAY, CA, p. A81

POMERENE HOSPITAL, MILLERSBURG, OH, p. A485

POMONA VALLEY HOSPITAL MEDICAL CENTER, POMONA, CA, p. A80

PONCA CITY MEDICAL CENTER, PONCA CITY, OK, p. A503

PONDERA MEDICAL CENTER, CONRAD, MT, p. A374

POPLAR BLUFF REGIONAL MEDICAL CENTER, POPLAR BLUFF, MO, p. A367

POPLAR BLUFF REGIONAL MEDICAL CENTER–NORTH CAMPUS, POPLAR BLUFF, MISSOURI (*see* POPLAR BLUFF REGIONAL MEDICAL CENTER), p. A367

POPLAR BLUFF REGIONAL MEDICAL CENTER–SOUTH CAMPUS, POPLAR BLUFF, MISSOURI (*see* POPLAR BLUFF REGIONAL MEDICAL CENTER), p. A367

POPLAR COMMUNITY HOSPITAL, POPLAR, MT, p. A378

POPLAR SPRINGS HOSPITAL, PETERSBURG, VA, p. A653

PORT HURON HOSPITAL, PORT HURON, MI, p. A321

PORT ST. LUCIE HOSPITAL, PORT ST. LUCIE, FL, p. A137

PORTAGE HEALTH, HANCOCK, MI, p. A314

PORTER ADVENTIST HOSPITAL, DENVER, CO, p. A100

PORTER MEDICAL CENTER, MIDDLEBURY, VT, p. A643

PORTER–VALPARAISO HOSPITAL CAMPUS, VALPARAISO, IN, p. A212

PORTERVILLE DEVELOPMENTAL CENTER, PORTERVILLE, CA, p. A81

PORTNEUF MEDICAL CENTER, POCATELLO, ID, p. A170

PORTSMOUTH REGIONAL HOSPITAL, PORTSMOUTH, NH, p. A400

POTOMAC VALLEY HOSPITAL, KEYSER, WV, p. A673

POTTSTOWN MEMORIAL MEDICAL CENTER, POTTSTOWN, PA, p. A536

POUDRE VALLEY HOSPITAL, FORT COLLINS, CO, p. A101

POWELL CONVALESCENT CENTER, DES MOINES, IOWA (*see* IOWA METHODIST MEDICAL CENTER), p. A218

POWELL COUNTY MEDICAL CENTER, DEER LODGE, MT, p. A374

POWELL VALLEY HEALTHCARE, POWELL, WY, p. A697

POWER COUNTY HOSPITAL DISTRICT, AMERICAN FALLS, ID, p. A166

PRAGUE COMMUNITY HOSPITAL, PRAGUE, OK, p. A503

PRAIRIE COMMUNITY HOSPITAL, TERRY, MT, p. A379

PRAIRIE DU CHIEN MEMORIAL HOSPITAL, PRAIRIE DU CHIEN, WI, p. A689

PRAIRIE LAKES HEALTHCARE SYSTEM, WATERTOWN, SD, p. A560

PRAIRIE RIDGE HOSPITAL AND HEALTH SERVICES, ELBOW LAKE, MN, p. A331

PRAIRIE ST. JOHN'S, FARGO, ND, p. A465

PRAIRIE VIEW, NEWTON, KS, p. A239

PRATT REGIONAL MEDICAL CENTER, PRATT, KS, p. A242

PRATTVILLE BAPTIST HOSPITAL, PRATTVILLE, AL, p. A25

PRENTICE WOMEN'S HOSPITAL, CHICAGO, ILLINOIS (*see* NORTHWESTERN MEMORIAL HOSPITAL), p. A177

PRESBYTERIAN HEMBY CHILDREN'S HOSPITAL, CHARLOTTE, NORTH CAROLINA (*see* PRESBYTERIAN HOSPITAL), p. A451

PRESBYTERIAN HOSPITAL, ALBUQUERQUE, NM, p. A414

PRESBYTERIAN HOSPITAL, CHARLOTTE, NC, p. A451

PRESBYTERIAN HOSPITAL HUNTERSVILLE, HUNTERSVILLE, NC, p. A455

PRESBYTERIAN HOSPITAL MATTHEWS, MATTHEWS, NC, p. A457

PRESBYTERIAN HOSPITAL OF ROCKWALL, ROCKWALL, TX, p. A623

PRESBYTERIAN INTERCOMMUNITY HOSPITAL, WHITTIER, CA, p. A96

PRESBYTERIAN KASEMAN HOSPITAL, ALBUQUERQUE, NM, p. A414

PRESBYTERIAN TOWER, OKLAHOMA CITY, OKLAHOMA (*see* OU MEDICAL CENTER), p. A502

PRESBYTERIAN–ORTHOPAEDIC HOSPITAL, CHARLOTTE, NC, p. A451

PRESBYTERIAN–ST. LUKE'S MEDICAL CENTER, DENVER, CO, p. A100

PRESENTATION MEDICAL CENTER, ROLLA, ND, p. A468

PRESTON MEMORIAL HOSPITAL, KINGWOOD, WV, p. A673

PREVOST MEMORIAL HOSPITAL, DONALDSONVILLE, LA, p. A266

PRIMARY CHILDREN'S MEDICAL CENTER, SALT LAKE CITY, UT, p. A640

PRINCE GEORGE'S HOSPITAL CENTER, CHEVERLY, MD, p. A290

PRINCE WILLIAM HOSPITAL, MANASSAS, VA, p. A651

PRINCETON BAPTIST MEDICAL CENTER, BIRMINGHAM, AL, p. A16

PRINCETON COMMUNITY HOSPITAL, PRINCETON, WV, p. A675

PROCTOR HOSPITAL, PEORIA, IL, p. A191

PROGRESS WEST HEALTHCARE CENTER, SAINT CHARLES, MO, p. A367

PROGRESSIVE HOSPITAL, LAS VEGAS, NV, p. A393

PROMEDICA BAY PARK HOSPITAL, OREGON, OH, p. A486

PROMEDICA BIXBY HOSPITAL, ADRIAN, MI, p. A307

PROMEDICA DEFIANCE REGIONAL HOSPITAL, DEFIANCE, OH, p. A479

PROMEDICA FLOWER HOSPITAL, SYLVANIA, OH, p. A489

PROMEDICA FOSTORIA COMMUNITY HOSPITAL, FOSTORIA, OH, p. A480

PROMEDICA HERRICK HOSPITAL, TECUMSEH, MI, p. A324

PROMEDICA ST. LUKE'S HOSPITAL, MAUMEE, OH, p. A484

PROMEDICA TOLEDO HOSPITAL, TOLEDO, OH, p. A489

PROMEDICA WILDWOOD ORTHOPAEDIC AND SPINE HOSPITAL, TOLEDO, OHIO (*see* PROMEDICA TOLEDO HOSPITAL), p. A489

PROMISE HOSPITAL BATON ROUGE, BATON ROUGE, LA, p. A263

PROMISE HOSPITAL OF BATON ROUGE, BATON ROUGE, LA, p. A263

PROMISE HOSPITAL OF BATON ROUGE, BATON ROUGE, LA, p. A263

PROMISE HOSPITAL OF BOSSIER CITY, BOSSIER CITY, LA, p. A264

PROMISE HOSPITAL OF EAST LOS ANGELES, LOS ANGELES, CA, p. A71

PROMISE HOSPITAL OF EAST LOS ANGELES, SUBURBAN MEDICAL CENTER CAMPUS, PARAMOUNT, CA, p. A79

PROMISE HOSPITAL OF LOUISIANA – SHREVEPORT CAMPUS, SHREVEPORT, LA, p. A277

PROMISE HOSPITAL OF MISS LOU, VIDALIA, LA, p. A279

PROMISE HOSPITAL OF PHOENIX, MESA, AZ, p. A34

PROMISE HOSPITAL OF SAN ANTONIO, SAN ANTONIO, TX, p. A625

PROMISE HOSPITAL OF SAN DIEGO, SAN DIEGO, CA, p. A85

PROMISE HOSPITAL OF VICKSBURG, VICKSBURG, MS, p. A353

PROMISE SPECIALTY HOSPITAL OF SALT LAKE, SALT LAKE CITY, UT, p. A640

PROMISE SPECIALTY HOSPITAL OF SOUTHEAST TEXAS, NEDERLAND, TX, p. A618

PROSSER MEMORIAL HOSPITAL, PROSSER, WA, p. A664

PROVENA COVENANT MEDICAL CENTER, URBANA, IL, p. A195

PROVENA MERCY MEDICAL CENTER, AURORA, IL, p. A172

PROVENA SAINT JOSEPH HOSPITAL, ELGIN, IL, p. A181

PROVENA SAINT JOSEPH MEDICAL CENTER, JOLIET, IL, p. A185

PROVENA ST. MARY'S HOSPITAL, KANKAKEE, IL, p. A185

PROVENA UNITED SAMARITANS MEDICAL CENTER, DANVILLE, IL, p. A179

PROVIDENCE ALASKA MEDICAL CENTER, ANCHORAGE, AK, p. A28

PROVIDENCE CENTRALIA HOSPITAL, CENTRALIA, WA, p. A660

PROVIDENCE EVERETT MEDICAL CENTER – COLBY CAMPUS, EVERETT, WASHINGTON (*see* PROVIDENCE REGIONAL MEDICAL CENTER EVERETT), p. A661

PROVIDENCE EVERETT MEDICAL CENTER – PACIFIC CAMPUS, EVERETT, WASHINGTON (*see* PROVIDENCE REGIONAL MEDICAL CENTER EVERETT), p. A661

PROVIDENCE HEALTH CENTER, WACO, TX, p. A633

PROVIDENCE HOLY CROSS MEDICAL CENTER,, CA, p. A71

PROVIDENCE HOLY FAMILY HOSPITAL, SPOKANE, WA, p. A667

PROVIDENCE HOOD RIVER MEMORIAL HOSPITAL, HOOD RIVER, OR, p. A511

PROVIDENCE HOSPITAL, MOBILE, AL, p. A23

PROVIDENCE HOSPITAL, WASHINGTON, DC, p. A116

PROVIDENCE HOSPITAL, SOUTHFIELD, MI, p. A323

PROVIDENCE HOSPITAL, COLUMBIA, SC, p. A548

PROVIDENCE HOSPITAL NORTHEAST, COLUMBIA, SOUTH CAROLINA (*see* PROVIDENCE HOSPITAL), p. A548

PROVIDENCE KODIAK ISLAND MEDICAL CENTER, KODIAK, AK, p. A29

PROVIDENCE LITTLE COMPANY OF MARY MEDICAL CENTER, TORRANCE, CA, p. A92

PROVIDENCE LITTLE COMPANY OF MARY MEDICAL CENTER SAN PEDRO,, CA, p. A71

PROVIDENCE MEDFORD MEDICAL CENTER, MEDFORD, OR, p. A512

PROVIDENCE MEDICAL CENTER, KANSAS CITY, KS, p. A236

PROVIDENCE MEDICAL CENTER, WAYNE, NE, p. A390

PROVIDENCE MEMORIAL HOSPITAL, EL PASO, TX, p. A596

PROVIDENCE MILWAUKIE HOSPITAL, MILWAUKIE, OR, p. A513

PROVIDENCE MOUNT CARMEL HOSPITAL, COLVILLE, WA, p. A660

PROVIDENCE NEWBERG MEDICAL CENTER, NEWBERG, OR, p. A513

PROVIDENCE PARK HOSPITAL, NOVI, MICHIGAN (*see* PROVIDENCE HOSPITAL), p. A323

PROVIDENCE PORTLAND MEDICAL CENTER, PORTLAND, OR, p. A514

PROVIDENCE REGIONAL MEDICAL CENTER EVERETT, EVERETT, WA, p. A661

PROVIDENCE SACRED HEART MEDICAL CENTER & CHILDREN'S HOSPITAL, SPOKANE, WA, p. A667
PROVIDENCE SAINT JOSEPH MEDICAL CENTER, BURBANK, CA, p. A56
PROVIDENCE SEASIDE HOSPITAL, SEASIDE, OR, p. A515
PROVIDENCE SEWARD MEDICAL CENTER, SEWARD, AK, p. A30
PROVIDENCE ST. JOSEPH'S HOSPITAL, CHEWELAH, WA, p. A660
PROVIDENCE ST. MARY MEDICAL CENTER, WALLA WALLA, WA, p. A669
PROVIDENCE ST. PETER HOSPITAL, OLYMPIA, WA, p. A663
PROVIDENCE ST. VINCENT MEDICAL CENTER, PORTLAND, OR, p. A514
PROVIDENCE TARZANA MEDICAL CENTER,, CA, p. A71
PROVIDENCE VALDEZ MEDICAL CENTER, VALDEZ, AK, p. A30
PROVIDENCE WILLAMETTE FALLS MEDICAL CENTER, OREGON CITY, OR, p. A513
PROVIDENT HOSPITAL OF COOK COUNTY, CHICAGO, IL, p. A177
PROWERS MEDICAL CENTER, LAMAR, CO, p. A103
PSYCHIATRIC HOSPITAL AT VANDERBILT, NASHVILLE, TENNESSEE (see VANDERBILT HOSPITAL AND CLINICS), p. A574
PSYCHIATRIC INSTITUTE OF WASHINGTON, WASHINGTON, DC, p. A117
PSYCHIATRIC MEDICINE CENTER, SALEM, OREGON (see SALEM HOSPITAL), p. A515
PSYCHIATRIC PAVILION, AMARILLO, TEXAS (see NORTHWEST TEXAS HEALTHCARE SYSTEM), p. A578
PUBLIC HEALTH SERVICE INDIAN HOSPITAL – QUENTIN N. BURDICK MEMORIAL HEALTH FACILITY, BELCOURT, ND, p. A464
PULASKI MEMORIAL HOSPITAL, WINAMAC, IN, p. A213
PULLMAN REGIONAL HOSPITAL, PULLMAN, WA, p. A664
PUNXSUTAWNEY AREA HOSPITAL, PUNXSUTAWNEY, PA, p. A536
PURCELL MUNICIPAL HOSPITAL, PURCELL, OK, p. A503
PUSHMATAHA HOSPITAL & HOME HEALTH, ANTLERS, OK, p. A493
PUTNAM COMMUNITY MEDICAL CENTER, PALATKA, FL, p. A135
PUTNAM COUNTY HOSPITAL, GREENCASTLE, IN, p. A202
PUTNAM COUNTY MEMORIAL HOSPITAL, UNIONVILLE, MO, p. A372
PUTNAM GENERAL HOSPITAL, EATONTON, GA, p. A152
PUTNAM HOSPITAL CENTER, CARMEL, NY, p. A423

# Q

QUARTZ MOUNTAIN MEDICAL CENTER, MANGUM, OK, p. A498
QUEEN OF THE VALLEY MEDICAL CENTER, NAPA, CA, p. A76
QUEEN'S MEDICAL CENTER, HONOLULU, HI, p. A164
QUEENS CHILDREN'S PSYCHIATRIC CENTER,, NY, p. A436
QUEENS HOSPITAL CENTER,, NY, p. A436
QUENTIN MEASE HOSPITAL, HOUSTON, TEXAS (see HARRIS COUNTY HOSPITAL DISTRICT), p. A604
QUILLEN REHABILITATION HOSPITAL, JOHNSON CITY, TN, p. A567
QUINCY MEDICAL CENTER, QUINCY, MA, p. A304
QUINCY VALLEY MEDICAL CENTER, QUINCY, WA, p. A664
QUITMAN COUNTY HOSPITAL, MARKS, MS, p. A349

# R

R M L SPECIALTY HOSPITAL, HINSDALE, IL, p. A184
RADIUS SPECIALTY HOSPITAL BOSTON, BOSTON, MA, p. A297
RADY CHILDREN'S HOSPITAL – SAN DIEGO, SAN DIEGO, CA, p. A85
RAINBOW MENTAL HEALTH FACILITY, KANSAS CITY, KS, p. A236
RAINY LAKE MEDICAL CENTER, INTERNATIONAL FALLS, MN, p. A333
RALEIGH GENERAL HOSPITAL, BECKLEY, WV, p. A670
RALPH H. JOHNSON VETERANS AFFAIRS MEDICAL CENTER, CHARLESTON, SC, p. A547
RANCHO LOS AMIGOS NATIONAL REHABILITATION CENTER, DOWNEY, CA, p. A59
RANCHO SPRINGS MEDICAL CENTER, MURRIETA, CA, p. A76
RANDALL CHILDREN'S HOSPITAL, PORTLAND, OREGON (see LEGACY EMANUEL HOSPITAL AND HEALTH CENTER), p. A514
RANDOLPH HOSPITAL, ASHEBORO, NC, p. A448
RANGE REGIONAL HEALTH SERVICES, HIBBING, MN, p. A333
RANGELY DISTRICT HOSPITAL, RANGELY, CO, p. A105

RANKEN JORDAN – A PEDIATRIC SPECIALTY HOSPITAL, MARYLAND HEIGHTS, MO, p. A364
RANKIN HOSPITAL DISTRICT, RANKIN, TX, p. A622
RANSOM MEMORIAL HOSPITAL, OTTAWA, KS, p. A240
RAPID CITY REGIONAL HOSPITAL, RAPID CITY, SD, p. A559
RAPIDES REGIONAL MEDICAL CENTER, ALEXANDRIA, LA, p. A261
RAPPAHANNOCK GENERAL HOSPITAL, KILMARNOCK, VA, p. A650
RARITAN BAY MEDICAL CENTER, PERTH AMBOY, NJ, p. A408
RAULERSON HOSPITAL, OKEECHOBEE, FL, p. A134
RAWLINS COUNTY HEALTH CENTER, ATWOOD, KS, p. A230
RAY COUNTY MEMORIAL HOSPITAL, RICHMOND, MO, p. A367
RAYMOND BLANK MEMORIAL HOSPITAL FOR CHILDREN, DES MOINES, IOWA (see IOWA METHODIST MEDICAL CENTER), p. A218
RC HOSPITAL AND CLINICS, OLIVIA, MN, p. A336
READING HOSPITAL AND MEDICAL CENTER, WEST READING, PA, p. A541
REAGAN MEMORIAL HOSPITAL, BIG LAKE, TX, p. A584
RECEPTION AND MEDICAL CENTER, LAKE BUTLER, FL, p. A128
RED BAY HOSPITAL, RED BAY, AL, p. A25
RED BUD REGIONAL HOSPITAL, RED BUD, IL, p. A192
RED RIVER BEHAVIORAL CENTER, BOSSIER CITY, LA, p. A264
RED RIVER HOSPITAL, WICHITA FALLS, TX, p. A635
RED RIVER REGIONAL HOSPITAL, BONHAM, TX, p. A584
RED ROCK BEHAVIORAL HOSPITAL, LAS VEGAS, NV, p. A393
REDGATE MEMORIAL RECOVERY CENTER, LONG BEACH, CA, p. A68
REDINGTON–FAIRVIEW GENERAL HOSPITAL, SKOWHEGAN, ME, p. A285
REDLANDS COMMUNITY HOSPITAL, REDLANDS, CA, p. A82
REDMOND REGIONAL MEDICAL CENTER, ROME, GA, p. A158
REDWOOD AREA HOSPITAL, REDWOOD FALLS, MN, p. A337
REDWOOD CITY MEDICAL CENTER, REDWOOD CITY, CA, p. A82
REDWOOD MEMORIAL HOSPITAL, FORTUNA, CA, p. A61
REEDSBURG AREA MEDICAL CENTER, REEDSBURG, WI, p. A690
REEVES COUNTY HOSPITAL, PECOS, TX, p. A620
REEVES MEMORIAL MEDICAL CENTER, BERNICE, LA, p. A263
REFUGIO COUNTY MEMORIAL HOSPITAL, REFUGIO, TX, p. A622
REGENCY HOSPITAL CLEVELAND EAST, CLEVELAND, OH, p. A475
REGENCY HOSPITAL OF AKRON, BARBERTON, OHIO (see REGENCY HOSPITAL CLEVELAND EAST), p. A475
REGENCY HOSPITAL OF CENTRAL GEORGIA, MACON, GA, p. A156
REGENCY HOSPITAL OF CINCINNATI, CINCINNATI, OH, p. A474
REGENCY HOSPITAL OF CLEVELAND – WEST, MIDDLEBURG HEIGHTS, OHIO (see REGENCY HOSPITAL CLEVELAND EAST), p. A475
REGENCY HOSPITAL OF COLUMBUS, COLUMBUS, OH, p. A477
REGENCY HOSPITAL OF COVINGTON, COVINGTON, LA, p. A265
REGENCY HOSPITAL OF FLORENCE, FLORENCE, SC, p. A550
REGENCY HOSPITAL OF FORT WORTH, FORT WORTH, TX, p. A599
REGENCY HOSPITAL OF GREENVILLE, GREENVILLE, SC, p. A550
REGENCY HOSPITAL OF HATTIESBURG, HATTIESBURG, MS, p. A347
REGENCY HOSPITAL OF JACKSON, JACKSON, MS, p. A348
REGENCY HOSPITAL OF MERIDIAN, MERIDIAN, MS, p. A350
REGENCY HOSPITAL OF MINNEAPOLIS, GOLDEN VALLEY, MN, p. A332
REGENCY HOSPITAL OF NORTHWEST ARKANSAS, FAYETTEVILLE, AR, p. A44
REGENCY HOSPITAL OF NORTHWEST ARKANSAS – SPRINGDALE, SPRINGDALE, ARKANSAS (see REGENCY HOSPITAL OF NORTHWEST ARKANSAS), p. A44
REGENCY HOSPITAL OF NORTHWEST INDIANA, EAST CHICAGO, IN, p. A200
REGENCY HOSPITAL OF ODESSA, ODESSA, TX, p. A619
REGENCY HOSPITAL OF PORTER COUNTY, PORTAGE, INDIANA (see REGENCY HOSPITAL OF NORTHWEST INDIANA), p. A200
REGENCY HOSPITAL OF RAVENNA, RAVENNA, OHIO (see REGENCY HOSPITAL CLEVELAND EAST), p. A475
REGENCY HOSPITAL OF SOUTH ATLANTA, EAST POINT, GA, p. A152
REGENCY HOSPITAL OF TOLEDO, SYLVANIA, OH, p. A489
REGINA MEDICAL CENTER, HASTINGS, MN, p. A332
REGIONAL HEALTH SERVICES OF HOWARD COUNTY, CRESCO, IA, p. A217
REGIONAL HOSPITAL FOR RESPIRATORY AND COMPLEX CARE, SEATTLE, WA, p. A665
REGIONAL HOSPITAL OF JACKSON, JACKSON, TN, p. A567
REGIONAL HOSPITAL OF SCRANTON, SCRANTON, PA, p. A538
REGIONAL MEDICAL CENTER, MANCHESTER, IA, p. A222
REGIONAL MEDICAL CENTER, ORANGEBURG, SC, p. A553
REGIONAL MEDICAL CENTER AT MEMPHIS, MEMPHIS, TN, p. A572

REGIONAL MEDICAL CENTER OF HOPKINS COUNTY, MADISONVILLE, KY, p. A255
REGIONAL MEDICAL CENTER OF SAN JOSE, SAN JOSE, CA, p. A88
REGIONAL MEDICAL CENTER–BAYONET POINT, HUDSON, FL, p. A125
REGIONAL MENTAL HEALTH CENTER, MERRILLVILLE, IN, p. A208
REGIONAL REHABILITATION CENTER, SALEM, OREGON (see SALEM HOSPITAL), p. A515
REGIONAL REHABILITATION HOSPITAL, PHENIX CITY, AL, p. A25
REGIONAL WEST MEDICAL CENTER, SCOTTSBLUFF, NE, p. A389
REGIONS HOSPITAL, SAINT PAUL, MN, p. A339
REHABILITATION HOSPITAL OF DEQUINCY, DEQUINCY, LA, p. A266
REHABILITATION HOSPITAL OF FORT WAYNE, FORT WAYNE, IN, p. A202
REHABILITATION HOSPITAL OF INDIANA, INDIANAPOLIS, IN, p. A205
REHABILITATION HOSPITAL OF JENNINGS, JENNINGS, LA, p. A268
REHABILITATION HOSPITAL OF RHODE ISLAND, NORTH SMITHFIELD, RI, p. A544
REHABILITATION HOSPITAL OF SOUTHERN NEW MEXICO, LAS CRUCES, NM, p. A416
REHABILITATION HOSPITAL OF SOUTHWEST VIRGINIA, BRISTOL, VA, p. A646
REHABILITATION HOSPITAL OF THE PACIFIC, HONOLULU, HI, p. A164
REHABILITATION HOSPITAL OF TINTON FALLS, TINTON FALLS, NJ, p. A410
REHABILITATION HOSPITAL OF WISCONSIN, WAUKESHA, WI, p. A692
REHABILITATION INSTITUTE AT THE MOUNT KEMBLE DIVISION, GORYEB CHILDREN'S HOSPITAL, MORRISTOWN, NEW JERSEY (see MORRISTOWN MEDICAL CENTER), p. A406
REHABILITATION INSTITUTE OF CHICAGO, CHICAGO, IL, p. A177
REHABILITATION INSTITUTE OF MICHIGAN, DETROIT, MI, p. A311
REHABILITATION INSTITUTE OF OREGON, PORTLAND, OREGON (see LEGACY GOOD SAMARITAN HOSPITAL AND MEDICAL CENTER), p. A514
REHABILITATION INSTITUTE OF WEST FLORIDA, PENSACOLA, FLORIDA (see WEST FLORIDA HOSPITAL), p. A136
REHABILITATION INSTITUTES OF NEVADA, LAS VEGAS, NV, p. A393 *
REHOBOTH MCKINLEY CHRISTIAN HEALTH CARE SERVICES, GALLUP, NM, p. A416
REID HOSPITAL AND HEALTH CARE SERVICES, RICHMOND, IN, p. A211
REISCH MEMORIAL NURSING HOME (see THOMAS H. BOYD MEMORIAL HOSPITAL), p. A174
RELIANT REHABILITATION HOSPITAL ABILENE, ABILENE, TX, p. A577
RELIANT REHABILITATION HOSPITAL CENTRAL TEXAS, ROUND ROCK, TX, p. A623
RELIANT REHABILITATION HOSPITAL DALLAS, DALLAS, TX, p. A592
RELIANT REHABILITATION HOSPITAL MID–CITIES, BEDFORD, TX, p. A583
RELIANT REHABILITATION HOSPITAL NORTH HOUSTON, SHENANDOAH, TX, p. A627
RELIANT REHABILITATION HOSPITAL NORTH TEXAS, RICHARDSON, TX, p. A622
RENAISSANCE HOSPITAL, GROVES, TX, p. A602
RENAISSANCE HOSPITAL TERRELL, TERRELL, TX, p. A630
RENOWN REGIONAL MEDICAL CENTER, RENO, NV, p. A395
RENOWN REHABILITATION HOSPITAL, RENO, NV, p. A395
RENOWN SOUTH MEADOWS MEDICAL CENTER, RENO, NV, p. A395
REPUBLIC COUNTY HOSPITAL, BELLEVILLE, KS, p. A230
RESEARCH MEDICAL CENTER, KANSAS CITY, MO, p. A362
RESEARCH PSYCHIATRIC CENTER, KANSAS CITY, MO, p. A362
RESTON HOSPITAL CENTER, RESTON, VA, p. A654
RESURRECTION MEDICAL CENTER, CHICAGO, IL, p. A177
REX HEALTHCARE, RALEIGH, NC, p. A459
REYNOLDS ARMY COMMUNITY HOSPITAL, FORT SILL, OK, p. A497
REYNOLDS MEMORIAL HOSPITAL, GLEN DALE, WV, p. A672
RHEA MEDICAL CENTER, DAYTON, TN, p. A565
RHODE ISLAND HOSPITAL, PROVIDENCE, RI, p. A544
RICE COUNTY DISTRICT HOSPITAL, LYONS, KS, p. A238
RICE MEDICAL CENTER, EAGLE LAKE, TX, p. A595
RICE MEMORIAL HOSPITAL, WILLMAR, MN, p. A342
RICHARD H. HUTCHINGS PSYCHIATRIC CENTER, SYRACUSE, NY, p. A444
RICHARD H. YOUNG HOSPITAL, KEARNEY, NEBRASKA (see GOOD SAMARITAN HOSPITAL), p. A385

RICHARD L. ROUDEBUSH VETERANS AFFAIRS MEDICAL CENTER, INDIANAPOLIS, IN, p. A205
RICHARD P. STADTER PSYCHIATRIC CENTER, GRAND FORKS, ND, p. A466
RICHARDSON MEDICAL CENTER, RAYVILLE, LA, p. A276
RICHLAND HOSPITAL, RICHLAND CENTER, WI, p. A690
RICHLAND MEMORIAL HOSPITAL, OLNEY, IL, p. A190
RICHLAND PARISH HOSPITAL, DELHI, LA, p. A265
RICHMOND MEDICAL CENTER, RICHMOND, CALIFORNIA (see OAKLAND MEDICAL CENTER), p. A77
RICHMOND STATE HOSPITAL, RICHMOND, IN, p. A211
RICHMOND UNIVERSITY MEDICAL CENTER,, NY, p. A436
RIDDLE HOSPITAL, MEDIA, PA, p. A529
RIDGE BEHAVIORAL HEALTH SYSTEM, LEXINGTON, KY, p. A253
RIDGECREST REGIONAL HOSPITAL, RIDGECREST, CA, p. A82
RIDGEVIEW INSTITUTE, SMYRNA, GA, p. A159
RIDGEVIEW MEDICAL CENTER, WACONIA, MN, p. A341
RIDGEVIEW PSYCHIATRIC HOSPITAL AND CENTER, OAK RIDGE, TN, p. A574
RILEY HOSPITAL FOR CHILDREN AT INDIANA UNIVERSITY HEALTH, INDIANAPOLIS, INDIANA (see INDIANA UNIVERSITY HEALTH UNIVERSITY HOSPITAL), p. A204
RINGGOLD COUNTY HOSPITAL, MOUNT AYR, IA, p. A223
RIO GRANDE HOSPITAL, DEL NORTE, CO, p. A99
RIO GRANDE REGIONAL HOSPITAL, MCALLEN, TX, p. A615
RIO GRANDE STATE CENTER, HARLINGEN, TEXAS (see RIO GRANDE STATE CENTER/SOUTH TEXAS HEALTH CARE SYSTEM), p. A602
RIO GRANDE STATE CENTER/SOUTH TEXAS HEALTH CARE SYSTEM, HARLINGEN, TX, p. A602
RIPON MEDICAL CENTER, RIPON, WI, p. A690
RIVENDELL BEHAVIORAL HEALTH, BOWLING GREEN, KY, p. A248
RIVENDELL BEHAVIORAL HEALTH SERVICES OF ARKANSAS, BENTON, AR, p. A42
RIVER BEND HOSPITAL, WEST LAFAYETTE, IN, p. A213
RIVER CREST HOSPITAL, SAN ANGELO, TX, p. A624
RIVER FALLS AREA HOSPITAL, RIVER FALLS, WI, p. A690
RIVER HOSPITAL, ALEXANDRIA BAY, NY, p. A420
RIVER OAKS CHILD AND ADOLESCENT HOSPITAL, NEW ORLEANS, LOUISIANA (see RIVER OAKS HOSPITAL), p. A275
RIVER OAKS HOSPITAL, NEW ORLEANS, LA, p. A275
RIVER OAKS HOSPITAL, FLOWOOD, MS, p. A345
RIVER PARISHES HOSPITAL, LA PLACE, LA, p. A269
RIVER PARK HOSPITAL, MC MINNVILLE, TN, p. A570
RIVER PARK HOSPITAL, HUNTINGTON, WV, p. A672
RIVER POINT BEHAVIORAL HEALTH, JACKSONVILLE, FL, p. A126
RIVER REGION MEDICAL CENTER, VICKSBURG, MS, p. A353
RIVER REGION WEST CAMPUS, VICKSBURG, MISSISSIPPI (see RIVER REGION MEDICAL CENTER), p. A353
RIVER VALLEY MEDICAL CENTER, DARDANELLE, AR, p. A43
RIVER'S EDGE HOSPITAL AND CLINIC, SAINT PETER, MN, p. A339
RIVERCREST SPECIALTY HOSPITAL, MISHAWAKA, IN, p. A208
RIVEREDGE HOSPITAL, FOREST PARK, IL, p. A182
RIVERLAND MEDICAL CENTER, FERRIDAY, LA, p. A266
RIVERSIDE BEHAVIORAL HEALTH CENTER, HAMPTON, VA, p. A649
RIVERSIDE CENTER FOR BEHAVIORAL MEDICINE, RIVERSIDE, CA, p. A83
RIVERSIDE COMMUNITY HOSPITAL, RIVERSIDE, CA, p. A83
RIVERSIDE COUNTY REGIONAL MEDICAL CENTER, MORENO VALLEY, CA, p. A76
RIVERSIDE GENERAL HOSPITAL, HOUSTON, TX, p. A606
RIVERSIDE HOSPITAL, SOUTH BEND, IN, p. A212
RIVERSIDE HOSPITAL OF LOUISIANA, ALEXANDRIA, LA, p. A261
RIVERSIDE MEDICAL CENTER, RIVERSIDE, CA, p. A83
RIVERSIDE MEDICAL CENTER, KANKAKEE, IL, p. A185
RIVERSIDE MEDICAL CENTER, FRANKLINTON, LA, p. A266
RIVERSIDE MEDICAL CENTER, WAUPACA, WI, p. A692
RIVERSIDE METHODIST HOSPITAL, COLUMBUS, OH, p. A477
RIVERSIDE PSYCHIATRIC INSTITUTE (see RIVERSIDE REGIONAL MEDICAL CENTER), p. A652
RIVERSIDE REGIONAL MEDICAL CENTER, NEWPORT NEWS, VA, p. A652
RIVERSIDE REHABILITATION INSTITUTE, NEWPORT NEWS, VA, p. A652
RIVERSIDE SHORE MEMORIAL HOSPITAL, NASSAWADOX, VA, p. A651
RIVERSIDE TAPPAHANNOCK HOSPITAL, TAPPAHANNOCK, VA, p. A656
RIVERSIDE WALTER REED HOSPITAL, GLOUCESTER, VA, p. A649
RIVERTON HOSPITAL, RIVERTON, UT, p. A640
RIVERTON MEMORIAL HOSPITAL, RIVERTON, WY, p. A697
RIVERVALLEY BEHAVIORAL HEALTH HOSPITAL, OWENSBORO, KY, p. A257
RIVERVIEW HEALTH, CROOKSTON, MN, p. A330
RIVERVIEW HOSPITAL, NOBLESVILLE, IN, p. A210

RIVERVIEW HOSPITAL ASSOCIATION, WISCONSIN RAPIDS, WI, p. A694
RIVERVIEW HOSPITAL FOR CHILDREN AND YOUTH, MIDDLETOWN, CT, p. A110
RIVERVIEW MEDICAL CENTER, RED BANK, NJ, p. A409
RIVERVIEW PSYCHIATRIC CENTER, AUGUSTA, ME, p. A281
RIVERVIEW REGIONAL MEDICAL CENTER, GADSDEN, AL, p. A20
RIVERVIEW REGIONAL MEDICAL CENTER NORTH, CARTHAGE, TN, p. A562
RIVERVIEW REGIONAL MEDICAL CENTER SOUTH, CARTHAGE, TN, p. A563
RIVERWOOD HEALTHCARE CENTER, AITKIN, MN, p. A327
RIVERWOODS BEHAVIORAL HEALTH SYSTEM, RIVERDALE, GA, p. A157
RML SPECIALTY HOSPITAL, CHICAGO, IL, p. A177
ROANE GENERAL HOSPITAL, SPENCER, WV, p. A676
ROANE MEDICAL CENTER, HARRIMAN, TN, p. A566
ROANOKE MEMORIAL REHABILITATION CENTER, ROANOKE, VIRGINIA (see CARILION MEDICAL CENTER), p. A655
ROBERT H. BALLARD REHABILITATION HOSPITAL, SAN BERNARDINO, CA, p. A84
ROBERT J. DOLE VETERANS AFFAIRS MEDICAL CENTER, WICHITA, KS, p. A245
ROBERT PACKER HOSPITAL, SAYRE, PA, p. A537
ROBERT WOOD JOHNSON UNIVERSITY HOSPITAL, NEW BRUNSWICK, NJ, p. A407
ROBERT WOOD JOHNSON UNIVERSITY HOSPITAL AT HAMILTON, HAMILTON, NJ, p. A404
ROBERT WOOD JOHNSON UNIVERSITY HOSPITAL RAHWAY, RAHWAY, NJ, p. A409
ROBINSON MEMORIAL HOSPITAL, RAVENNA, OH, p. A487
ROCHELLE COMMUNITY HOSPITAL, ROCHELLE, IL, p. A192
ROCHESTER GENERAL HOSPITAL, ROCHESTER, NY, p. A441
ROCHESTER PSYCHIATRIC CENTER, ROCHESTER, NY, p. A442
ROCK COUNTY HOSPITAL, BASSETT, NE, p. A381
ROCKCASTLE REGIONAL HOSPITAL AND RESPIRATORY CARE CENTER, MOUNT VERNON, KY, p. A257
ROCKDALE MEDICAL CENTER, CONYERS, GA, p. A150
ROCKEFELLER UNIVERSITY HOSPITAL, NEW YORK, NY, p. A436
ROCKFORD CENTER, NEWARK, DE, p. A114
ROCKFORD MEMORIAL HOSPITAL, ROCKFORD, IL, p. A193
ROCKINGHAM MEMORIAL HOSPITAL, HARRISONBURG, VA, p. A649
ROCKLAND CHILDREN'S PSYCHIATRIC CENTER, ORANGEBURG, NY, p. A439
ROCKLAND PSYCHIATRIC CENTER, ORANGEBURG, NY, p. A439
ROCKVILLE GENERAL HOSPITAL, VERNON ROCKVILLE, CT, p. A112
ROCKY MOUNTAIN HOSPITAL FOR CHILDREN, DENVER, COLORADO (see PRESBYTERIAN–ST. LUKE'S MEDICAL CENTER), p. A100
ROGER C. PEACE REHABILITATION HOSPITAL, GREENVILLE, SOUTH CAROLINA (see GREENVILLE MEMORIAL HOSPITAL), p. A550
ROGER HUNTINGTON NURSING CENTER (see GREER MEMORIAL HOSPITAL), p. A551
ROGER MILLS MEMORIAL HOSPITAL, CHEYENNE, OK, p. A494
ROGER WILLIAMS MEDICAL CENTER, PROVIDENCE, RI, p. A545
ROGERS CITY REHABILITATION HOSPITAL, ROGERS CITY, MI, p. A321
ROGERS MEMORIAL HOSPITAL, OCONOMOWOC, WI, p. A688
ROGUE VALLEY MEDICAL CENTER, MEDFORD, OR, p. A512
ROLLING HILLS HOSPITAL, ADA, OK, p. A493
ROLLING HILLS HOSPITAL, FRANKLIN, TN, p. A565
ROLLING PLAINS MEMORIAL HOSPITAL, SWEETWATER, TX, p. A630
ROLLINS–BROOK COMMUNITY HOSPITAL, LAMPASAS, TX, p. A611
ROME MEMORIAL HOSPITAL, ROME, NY, p. A442
RONALD REAGAN UNIVERSITY OF CALIFORNIA LOS ANGELES MEDICAL CENTER, LOS ANGELES, CA, p. A71
ROOKS COUNTY HEALTH CENTER, PLAINVILLE, KS, p. A242
ROOSEVELT GENERAL HOSPITAL, PORTALES, NM, p. A417
ROOSEVELT HOSPITAL, NEW YORK, NEW YORK (see ST. LUKE'S–ROOSEVELT HOSPITAL CENTER), p. A437
ROOSEVELT MEDICAL CENTER, CULBERTSON, MT, p. A374
ROOSEVELT WARM SPRINGS INSTITUTE FOR REHABILITATION, WARM SPRINGS, GA, p. A161
ROOSEVELT WARM SPRINGS LTAC HOSPITAL, WARM SPRINGS, GA, p. A161
ROPER HOSPITAL, CHARLESTON, SC, p. A547
ROSE MEDICAL CENTER, DENVER, CO, p. A100
ROSEBUD HEALTH CARE CENTER, FORSYTH, MT, p. A375
ROSELAND COMMUNITY HOSPITAL, CHICAGO, IL, p. A177
ROSEVILLE MEDICAL CENTER, ROSEVILLE, CA, p. A83
ROSS SKILLED NURSING FACILITY (see EASTERN MAINE MEDICAL CENTER), p. A281
ROSWELL PARK CANCER INSTITUTE, BUFFALO, NY, p. A423
ROSWELL REGIONAL HOSPITAL, ROSWELL, NM, p. A417

ROTARY REHABILITATION HOSPITAL, MOBILE, ALABAMA (see MOBILE INFIRMARY MEDICAL CENTER), p. A22
ROTHMAN SPECIALTY HOSPITAL, BENSALEM, PA, p. A518
ROUNDUP MEMORIAL HEALTHCARE, ROUNDUP, MT, p. A378
ROWAN REGIONAL MEDICAL CENTER, SALISBURY, NC, p. A460
ROXBOROUGH MEMORIAL HOSPITAL, PHILADELPHIA, PA, p. A533
ROXBURY TREATMENT CENTER, SHIPPENSBURG, PA, p. A538
ROYAL OAKS HOSPITAL, WINDSOR, MO, p. A372
RUBY VALLEY HOSPITAL, SHERIDAN, MT, p. A379
RUMFORD HOSPITAL, RUMFORD, ME, p. A285
RUNNELLS SPECIALIZED HOSPITAL OF UNION COUNTY, BERKELEY HEIGHTS, NJ, p. A401
RUSH COUNTY MEMORIAL HOSPITAL, LA CROSSE, KS, p. A237
RUSH FOUNDATION HOSPITAL, MERIDIAN, MS, p. A350
RUSH MEMORIAL HOSPITAL, RUSHVILLE, IN, p. A211
RUSH OAK PARK HOSPITAL, OAK PARK, IL, p. A190
RUSH UNIVERSITY MEDICAL CENTER, CHICAGO, IL, p. A178
RUSH–COPLEY MEDICAL CENTER, AURORA, IL, p. A173
RUSK COUNTY MEMORIAL HOSPITAL AND NURSING HOME, LADYSMITH, WI, p. A684
RUSK INSTITUTE, NEW YORK, NEW YORK (see NYU LANGONE MEDICAL CENTER), p. A436
RUSK STATE HOSPITAL, RUSK, TX, p. A623
RUSSELL COUNTY HOSPITAL, RUSSELL SPRINGS, KY, p. A258
RUSSELL COUNTY MEDICAL CENTER, LEBANON, VA, p. A650
RUSSELL MEDICAL CENTER, ALEXANDER CITY, AL, p. A15
RUSSELL REGIONAL HOSPITAL, RUSSELL, KS, p. A242
RUSSELLVILLE HOSPITAL, RUSSELLVILLE, AL, p. A25
RUTHERFORD REGIONAL MEDICAL CENTER, RUTHERFORDTON, NC, p. A460
RUTLAND REGIONAL MEDICAL CENTER, RUTLAND, VT, p. A644
RYDER MEMORIAL HOSPITAL, HUMACAO, PR, p. A701
RYE HOSPITAL CENTER, RYE, NY, p. A442

# S

S. E. LACKEY MEMORIAL HOSPITAL, FOREST, MS, p. A346
SABETHA COMMUNITY HOSPITAL, SABETHA, KS, p. A242
SABINE COUNTY HOSPITAL, HEMPHILL, TX, p. A603
SABINE MEDICAL CENTER, MANY, LA, p. A272
SAC–OSAGE HOSPITAL, OSCEOLA, MO, p. A366
SACRAMENTO MEDICAL CENTER, SACRAMENTO, CA, p. A83
SACRED HEART CHILDREN'S HOSPITAL, SPOKANE, WASHINGTON (see PROVIDENCE SACRED HEART MEDICAL CENTER & CHILDREN'S HOSPITAL), p. A667
SACRED HEART HOSPITAL, CHICAGO, IL, p. A178
SACRED HEART HOSPITAL, ALLENTOWN, PA, p. A517
SACRED HEART HOSPITAL, EAU CLAIRE, WI, p. A681
SACRED HEART HOSPITAL, TOMAHAWK, WI, p. A692
SACRED HEART HOSPITAL OF PENSACOLA, PENSACOLA, FL, p. A136
SACRED HEART HOSPITAL ON THE EMERALD COAST, MIRAMAR BEACH, FL, p. A132
SACRED HEART HOSPITAL ON THE GULF, PORT ST. JOE, FL, p. A137
SACRED HEART MEDICAL CENTER, EUGENE, OR, p. A510
SACRED HEART MEDICAL CENTER AT RIVERBEND, SPRINGFIELD, OR, p. A516
SACRED HEART REHABILITATION INSTITUTE, MILWAUKEE, WI, p. A687
SACRED HEART–ST. MARY'S HOSPITALS, RHINELANDER, WI, p. A690
SADDLEBACK MEMORIAL MEDICAL CENTER, LAGUNA HILLS, CA, p. A66
SADDLEBACK MEMORIAL MEDICAL CENTER – SAN CLEMENTE CAMPUS, SAN CLEMENTE, CALIFORNIA (see SADDLEBACK MEMORIAL MEDICAL CENTER), p. A66
SAFE HAVEN HOSPITAL OF POCATELLO, POCATELLO, ID, p. A170
SAGAMORE CHILDREN'S PSYCHIATRIC CENTER, DIX HILLS, NY, p. A425
SAGE MEMORIAL HOSPITAL, GANADO, AZ, p. A32
SAGE REHABILITATION HOSPITAL, BATON ROUGE, LA, p. A263
SAINT AGNES HOSPITAL, BALTIMORE, MD, p. A288
SAINT AGNES MEDICAL CENTER, FRESNO, CA, p. A62
SAINT ALPHONSUS MEDICAL CENTER – BAKER CITY, BAKER CITY, OR, p. A509
SAINT ALPHONSUS MEDICAL CENTER – NAMPA, NAMPA, ID, p. A169
SAINT ALPHONSUS MEDICAL CENTER – ONTARIO, ONTARIO, OR, p. A513
SAINT ALPHONSUS REGIONAL MEDICAL CENTER, BOISE, ID, p. A166
SAINT ANNE'S HOSPITAL, FALL RIVER, MA, p. A299
SAINT ANTHONY HOSPITAL, CHICAGO, IL, p. A178
SAINT ANTHONY'S HEALTH CENTER, ALTON, IL, p. A172

SAINT BARNABAS BEHAVIORAL HEALTH CENTER, TOMS RIVER, NJ, p. A411
SAINT BARNABAS MEDICAL CENTER, LIVINGSTON, NJ, p. A405
SAINT CATHERINE MEDICAL CENTER FOUNTAIN SPRINGS, ASHLAND, PA, p. A518
SAINT CATHERINE REGIONAL HOSPITAL, CHARLESTOWN, IN, p. A199
SAINT CLARE'S HEALTH SYSTEM, DENVILLE, NJ, p. A403
SAINT CLARE'S HOSPITAL, ALTON, ILLINOIS (see SAINT ANTHONY'S HEALTH CENTER), p. A172
SAINT CLARE'S HOSPITAL, WESTON, WI, p. A693
SAINT CLARE'S HOSPITAL/BOONTON TOWNSHIP, BOONTON TOWNSHIP, NEW JERSEY (see SAINT CLARE'S HEALTH SYSTEM), p. A403
SAINT CLARE'S HOSPITAL/DENVILLE, DENVILLE, NEW JERSEY (see SAINT CLARE'S HEALTH SYSTEM), p. A403
SAINT CLARE'S HOSPITAL/SUSSEX, SUSSEX, NEW JERSEY (see SAINT CLARE'S HEALTH SYSTEM), p. A403
SAINT ELIZABETH REGIONAL MEDICAL CENTER, LINCOLN, NE, p. A385
SAINT ELIZABETH'S MEDICAL CENTER, WABASHA, MN, p. A341
SAINT FRANCIS HEART HOSPITAL, TULSA, OKLAHOMA (see SAINT FRANCIS HOSPITAL), p. A506
SAINT FRANCIS HOSPITAL, EVANSTON, IL, p. A181
SAINT FRANCIS HOSPITAL, TULSA, OK, p. A506
SAINT FRANCIS HOSPITAL, MEMPHIS, TN, p. A572
SAINT FRANCIS HOSPITAL, CHARLESTON, WV, p. A671
SAINT FRANCIS HOSPITAL AND HEALTH CENTERS, POUGHKEEPSIE, NY, p. A441
SAINT FRANCIS HOSPITAL AND MEDICAL CENTER, HARTFORD, CT, p. A109
SAINT FRANCIS HOSPITAL SOUTH, TULSA, OK, p. A506
SAINT FRANCIS HOSPITAL–BARTLETT, BARTLETT, TN, p. A562
SAINT FRANCIS MEDICAL CENTER, CAPE GIRARDEAU, MO, p. A356
SAINT FRANCIS MEDICAL CENTER, GRAND ISLAND, NE, p. A384
SAINT FRANCIS MEMORIAL HEALTH CENTER, GRAND ISLAND, NEBRASKA (see SAINT FRANCIS MEDICAL CENTER), p. A384
SAINT FRANCIS MEMORIAL HOSPITAL, SAN FRANCISCO, CA, p. A87
SAINT JOHN HOSPITAL, LEAVENWORTH, KS, p. A237
SAINT JOHN'S HEALTH CENTER, SANTA MONICA, CA, p. A90
SAINT JOHN'S HEALTH SYSTEM, ANDERSON, IN, p. A197
SAINT JOSEPH – LONDON, LONDON, KY, p. A254
SAINT JOSEPH – MARTIN, MARTIN, KY, p. A256
SAINT JOSEPH BEREA, BEREA, KY, p. A247
SAINT JOSEPH EAST, LEXINGTON, KY, p. A253
SAINT JOSEPH HOSPITAL, CHICAGO, IL, p. A178
SAINT JOSEPH HOSPITAL, LEXINGTON, KY, p. A253
SAINT JOSEPH MOUNT STERLING, MOUNT STERLING, KY, p. A257
SAINT JOSEPH REGIONAL MEDICAL CENTER, MISHAWAKA, IN, p. A208
SAINT JOSEPH REGIONAL MEDICAL CENTER–PLYMOUTH CAMPUS, PLYMOUTH, IN, p. A210
SAINT JOSEPH'S CHILDEN'S HOSPITAL, MARSHFIELD, WISCONSIN (see SAINT JOSEPH'S HOSPITAL), p. A685
SAINT JOSEPH'S HOSPITAL, MARSHFIELD, WI, p. A685
SAINT JOSEPH'S HOSPITAL OF ATLANTA, ATLANTA, GA, p. A146
SAINT LOUIS UNIVERSITY HOSPITAL, SAINT LOUIS, MO, p. A369
SAINT LOUISE REGIONAL HOSPITAL, GILROY, CA, p. A63
SAINT LUKE INSTITUTE, SILVER SPRING, MD, p. A294
SAINT LUKE'S CANCER INSTITUTE, KANSAS CITY, MO, p. A362
SAINT LUKE'S EAST HOSPITAL, LEE'S SUMMIT, MO, p. A364
SAINT LUKE'S HOSPITAL OF KANSAS CITY, KANSAS CITY, MO, p. A362
SAINT LUKE'S MEDICAL CENTER, CLEVELAND, OHIO (see ST. VINCENT CHARITY MEDICAL CENTER), p. A475
SAINT LUKE'S NORTH HOSPITAL – BARRY ROAD, KANSAS CITY, MO, p. A362
SAINT LUKE'S NORTH HOSPITAL–SMITHVILLE CAMPUS, SMITHVILLE, MISSOURI (see SAINT LUKE'S NORTH HOSPITAL – BARRY ROAD), p. A362
SAINT LUKE'S SOUTH HOSPITAL, OVERLAND PARK, KS, p. A241
SAINT MARGARET MERCY HEALTHCARE CENTERS–NORTH CAMPUS, HAMMOND, INDIANA (see FRANCISCAN ST. MARGARET HEALTH – HAMMOND), p. A203
SAINT MARY'S HEALTH CARE, GRAND RAPIDS, MI, p. A314
SAINT MARY'S HOSPITAL, WATERBURY, CT, p. A112
SAINT MARY'S REGIONAL MEDICAL CENTER, RUSSELLVILLE, AR, p. A51
SAINT MARY'S REGIONAL MEDICAL CENTER, RENO, NV, p. A395
SAINT MICHAEL'S MEDICAL CENTER, NEWARK, NJ, p. A407
SAINT PETER'S UNIVERSITY HOSPITAL, NEW BRUNSWICK, NJ, p. A407

SAINT SIMONS BY–THE–SEA HOSPITAL, SAINT SIMONS ISLAND, GA, p. A158
SAINT THOMAS HOSPITAL, NASHVILLE, TN, p. A573
SAINT VINCENT HEALTH CENTER, ERIE, PA, p. A523
SAINT VINCENT HOSPITAL, WORCESTER, MA, p. A306
SAINTS MARY & ELIZABETH MEDICAL CENTER, CHICAGO, IL, p. A178
SAINTS MARY & ELIZABETH MEDICAL CENTER, CLAREMONT AVENUE, CHICAGO, ILLINOIS (see SAINTS MARY & ELIZABETH MEDICAL CENTER), p. A178
SAINTS MEDICAL CENTER, LOWELL, MA, p. A301
SAKAKAWEA MEDICAL CENTER, HAZEN, ND, p. A466
SALEM CAMPUS, SALEM, MASSACHUSETTS (see NORTH SHORE MEDICAL CENTER), p. A304
SALEM COMMUNITY HOSPITAL, SALEM, OH, p. A488
SALEM HOSPITAL, SALEM, OR, p. A515
SALEM MEMORIAL DISTRICT HOSPITAL, SALEM, MO, p. A370
SALEM TOWNSHIP HOSPITAL, SALEM, IL, p. A193
SALINA REGIONAL HEALTH CENTER, SALINA, KS, p. A242
SALINA REGIONAL HEALTH CENTER– PENN CAMPUS, SALINA, KANSAS (see SALINA REGIONAL HEALTH CENTER), p. A242
SALINA REGIONAL HEALTH CENTER–SANTA FE CAMPUS, SALINA, KANSAS (see SALINA REGIONAL HEALTH CENTER), p. A242
SALINA SURGICAL HOSPITAL, SALINA, KS, p. A243
SALINAS VALLEY MEMORIAL HEALTHCARE SYSTEM, SALINAS, CA, p. A84
SALINE MEMORIAL HOSPITAL, BENTON, AR, p. A42
SALT LAKE BEHAVIORAL HEALTH, SALT LAKE CITY, UT, p. A641
SALT LAKE REGIONAL MEDICAL CENTER, SALT LAKE CITY, UT, p. A641
SAM RAYBURN MEMORIAL VETERANS CENTER, BONHAM, TEXAS (see VETERANS AFFAIRS NORTH TEXAS HEALTH CARE SYSTEM), p. A593
SAMARITAN ALBANY GENERAL HOSPITAL, ALBANY, OR, p. A509
SAMARITAN BEHAVIORAL HEALTH CENTER–DESERT SAMARITAN MEDICAL CENTER, MESA, ARIZONA (see BANNER DESERT MEDICAL CENTER), p. A34
SAMARITAN HEALTHCARE, MOSES LAKE, WA, p. A663
SAMARITAN HOSPITAL, TROY, NY, p. A445
SAMARITAN LEBANON COMMUNITY HOSPITAL, LEBANON, OR, p. A512
SAMARITAN MEDICAL CENTER, WATERTOWN, NY, p. A446
SAMARITAN MEMORIAL HOSPITAL, MACON, MO, p. A364
SAMARITAN NORTH LINCOLN HOSPITAL, LINCOLN CITY, OR, p. A512
SAMARITAN PACIFIC COMMUNITIES HOSPITAL, NEWPORT, OR, p. A513
SAMARITAN REGIONAL HEALTH SYSTEM, ASHLAND, OH, p. A469
SAME DAY SURGERY CENTER, RAPID CITY, SD, p. A559
SAMPSON REGIONAL MEDICAL CENTER, CLINTON, NC, p. A451
SAMUEL MAHELONA MEMORIAL HOSPITAL, KAPAA, HI, p. A164
SAMUEL SIMMONDS MEMORIAL HOSPITAL, BARROW, AK, p. A28
SAN ANGELO COMMUNITY MEDICAL CENTER, SAN ANGELO, TX, p. A624
SAN ANTONIO COMMUNITY HOSPITAL, UPLAND, CA, p. A94
SAN ANTONIO DIVISION, SAN ANTONIO, TEXAS (see SOUTH TEXAS VETERANS HEALTH CARE SYSTEM), p. A626
SAN ANTONIO MILITARY MEDICAL CENTER, FORT SAM HOUSTON, TX, p. A598
SAN ANTONIO STATE HOSPITAL, SAN ANTONIO, TX, p. A626
SAN BERNARDINO MOUNTAINS COMMUNITY HOSPITAL DISTRICT, LAKE ARROWHEAD, CA, p. A66
SAN DIEGO COUNTY PSYCHIATRIC HOSPITAL, SAN DIEGO, CA, p. A85
SAN DIEGO HOSPICE & THE INSTITUTE OF PALLIATIVE MEDICINE, SAN DIEGO, CA, p. A85
SAN DIEGO MEDICAL CENTER, SAN DIEGO, CA, p. A85
SAN DIMAS COMMUNITY HOSPITAL, SAN DIMAS, CA, p. A86
SAN FRANCISCO GENERAL HOSPITAL MEDICAL CENTER, SAN FRANCISCO, CA, p. A87
SAN FRANCISCO MEDICAL CENTER, SAN FRANCISCO, CA, p. A87
SAN GABRIEL VALLEY MEDICAL CENTER, SAN GABRIEL, CA, p. A87
SAN GORGONIO MEMORIAL HOSPITAL, BANNING, CA, p. A55
SAN JACINTO METHODIST HOSPITAL, BAYTOWN, TX, p. A582
SAN JACINTO METHODIST HOSPITAL – ALEXANDER, BAYTOWN, TEXAS (see SAN JACINTO METHODIST HOSPITAL), p. A582
SAN JOAQUIN COMMUNITY HOSPITAL, BAKERSFIELD, CA, p. A55
SAN JOAQUIN GENERAL HOSPITAL, FRENCH CAMP, CA, p. A61
SAN JOAQUIN VALLEY REHABILITATION HOSPITAL, FRESNO, CA, p. A62
SAN JORGE CHILDREN'S HOSPITAL, SAN JUAN, PR, p. A703
SAN JOSE MEDICAL CENTER, SAN JOSE, CA, p. A88

SAN JUAN CAPESTRANO HOSPITAL, SAN JUAN, PR, p. A703
SAN JUAN CITY HOSPITAL, SAN JUAN, PR, p. A703
SAN JUAN HOSPITAL, MONTICELLO, UT, p. A638
SAN JUAN REGIONAL MEDICAL CENTER, FARMINGTON, NM, p. A416
SAN JUAN REGIONAL MEDICAL CENTER REHABILITATION HOSPITAL, FARMINGTON, NEW MEXICO (see SAN JUAN REGIONAL MEDICAL CENTER), p. A416
SAN LEANDRO HOSPITAL, SAN LEANDRO, CALIFORNIA (see EDEN MEDICAL CENTER), p. A56
SAN LUIS VALLEY REGIONAL MEDICAL CENTER, ALAMOSA, CO, p. A97
SAN MATEO MEDICAL CENTER, SAN MATEO, CA, p. A89
SAN RAFAEL MEDICAL CENTER, SAN RAFAEL, CA, p. A89
SAN RAMON REGIONAL MEDICAL CENTER, SAN RAMON, CA, p. A89
SANDHILLS REGIONAL MEDICAL CENTER, HAMLET, NC, p. A454
SANFORD BAGLEY MEDICAL CENTER, BAGLEY, MN, p. A328
SANFORD BEMIDJI MEDICAL CENTER, BEMIDJI, MN, p. A328
SANFORD CANTON–INWOOD MEDICAL CENTER, CANTON, SD, p. A555
SANFORD CHILDREN'S HOSPITAL, SIOUX FALLS, SOUTH DAKOTA (see SANFORD UNIVERSITY OF SOUTH DAKOTA MEDICAL CENTER), p. A559
SANFORD DEUEL COUNTY MEDICAL CENTER, CLEAR LAKE, SD, p. A556
SANFORD JACKSON MEDICAL CENTER, JACKSON, MN, p. A333
SANFORD LUVERNE MEDICAL CENTER, LUVERNE, MN, p. A334
SANFORD MEDICAL CENTER CANBY, CANBY, MN, p. A329
SANFORD MEDICAL CENTER CHAMBERLAIN, CHAMBERLAIN, SD, p. A555
SANFORD MEDICAL CENTER FARGO, FARGO, ND, p. A465
SANFORD MEDICAL CENTER MAYVILLE, MAYVILLE, ND, p. A467
SANFORD MEDICAL CENTER ROCK RAPIDS, ROCK RAPIDS, IA, p. A225
SANFORD MEDICAL CENTER THIEF RIVER FALLS, THIEF RIVER FALLS, MN, p. A340
SANFORD MEDICAL CENTER WEBSTER, WEBSTER, SD, p. A561
SANFORD NORTHWOOD DEACONESS HEALTH CENTER, NORTHWOOD, ND, p. A467
SANFORD SHELDON MEDICAL CENTER, SHELDON, IA, p. A226
SANFORD TRACY MEDICAL CENTER, TRACY, MN, p. A340
SANFORD UNIVERSITY OF SOUTH DAKOTA MEDICAL CENTER, SIOUX FALLS, SD, p. A559
SANFORD VERMILLION MEDICAL CENTER, VERMILLION, SD, p. A560
SANFORD WESTBROOK MEDICAL CENTER, WESTBROOK, MN, p. A341
SANFORD WHEATON MEDICAL CENTER, WHEATON, MN, p. A341
SANFORD WORTHINGTON MEDICAL CENTER, WORTHINGTON, MN, p. A342
SANPETE VALLEY HOSPITAL, MOUNT PLEASANT, UT, p. A638
SANTA BARBARA COTTAGE HOSPITAL, SANTA BARBARA, CA, p. A89
SANTA CLARA MEDICAL CENTER, SANTA CLARA, CA, p. A90
SANTA CLARA VALLEY MEDICAL CENTER, SAN JOSE, CA, p. A88
SANTA MONICA–UCLA MEDICAL CENTER AND ORTHOPAEDIC HOSPITAL, SANTA MONICA, CA, p. A90
SANTA ROSA MEDICAL CENTER, SANTA ROSA, CA, p. A90
SANTA ROSA MEDICAL CENTER, MILTON, FL, p. A132
SANTA ROSA MEMORIAL HOSPITAL, SANTA ROSA, CA, p. A90
SANTA YNEZ VALLEY COTTAGE HOSPITAL, SOLVANG, CA, p. A91
SANTIAM MEMORIAL HOSPITAL, STAYTON, OR, p. A516
SARAH BUSH LINCOLN HEALTH CENTER, MATTOON, IL, p. A187
SARAH D. CULBERTSON MEMORIAL HOSPITAL, RUSHVILLE, IL, p. A193
SARASOTA MEMORIAL HOSPITAL, SARASOTA, FL, p. A139
SARATOGA HOSPITAL, SARATOGA SPRINGS, NY, p. A443
SARTORI MEMORIAL HOSPITAL, CEDAR FALLS, IA, p. A215
SATANTA DISTRICT HOSPITAL, SATANTA, KS, p. A243
SAUK PRAIRIE MEMORIAL HOSPITAL & CLINICS, PRAIRIE DU SAC, WI, p. A689
SAUNDERS MEDICAL CENTER, WAHOO, NE, p. A390
SAVOY MEDICAL CENTER, MAMOU, LA, p. A272
SAYRE MEMORIAL HOSPITAL, SAYRE, OK, p. A504
SCENIC MOUNTAIN MEDICAL CENTER, BIG SPRING, TX, p. A584
SCHEURER HOSPITAL, PIGEON, MI, p. A320
SCHICK SHADEL HOSPITAL, SEATTLE, WA, p. A666
SCHLEICHER COUNTY MEDICAL CENTER, ELDORADO, TX, p. A597
SCHNECK MEDICAL CENTER, SEYMOUR, IN, p. A211
SCHNEIDER REGIONAL MEDICAL CENTER, SAINT THOMAS, VI, p. A704
SCHOOLCRAFT MEMORIAL HOSPITAL, MANISTIQUE, MI, p. A318

SCHUYLER HOSPITAL, MONTOUR FALLS, NY, p. A430
SCHUYLKILL MEDICAL CENTER – EAST NORWEGIAN STREET, POTTSVILLE, PA, p. A536
SCHUYLKILL MEDICAL CENTER – SOUTH JACKSON STREET, POTTSVILLE, PA, p. A536
SCHWAB REHABILITATION HOSPITAL, CHICAGO, IL, p. A178
SCOTLAND COUNTY HOSPITAL, MEMPHIS, MO, p. A365
SCOTLAND HEALTH CARE SYSTEM, LAURINBURG, NC, p. A456
SCOTT & WHITE HOSPITAL – BRENHAM, BRENHAM, TX, p. A585
SCOTT & WHITE HOSPITAL – LLANO, LLANO, TX, p. A613
SCOTT & WHITE HOSPITAL – TAYLOR, TAYLOR, TX, p. A630
SCOTT & WHITE HOSPITAL AT ROUND ROCK, ROUND ROCK, TX, p. A623
SCOTT AND WHITE CONTINUING CARE HOSPITAL, TEMPLE, TX, p. A630
SCOTT AND WHITE MEMORIAL HOSPITAL, TEMPLE, TX, p. A630
SCOTT COUNTY HOSPITAL, SCOTT CITY, KS, p. A243
SCOTT MEMORIAL HOSPITAL, SCOTTSBURG, IN, p. A211
SCOTT REGIONAL HOSPITAL, MORTON, MS, p. A350
SCOTTSDALE HEALTHCARE SHEA MEDICAL CENTER, SCOTTSDALE, AZ, p. A38
SCOTTSDALE HEALTHCARE THOMPSON PEAK HOSPITAL, SCOTTSDALE, AZ, p. A38
SCOTTSDALE HEALTHCARE–OSBORN MEDICAL CENTER, SCOTTSDALE, AZ, p. A38
SCREVEN COUNTY HOSPITAL, SYLVANIA, GA, p. A160
SCRIPPS GREEN HOSPITAL, LA JOLLA, CA, p. A65
SCRIPPS MEMORIAL HOSPITAL–ENCINITAS, ENCINITAS, CA, p. A60
SCRIPPS MEMORIAL HOSPITAL–LA JOLLA, LA JOLLA, CA, p. A66
SCRIPPS MERCY HOSPITAL, SAN DIEGO, CA, p. A86
SCRIPPS MERCY HOSPITAL CHULA VISTA, CHULA VISTA, CALIFORNIA (see SCRIPPS MERCY HOSPITAL), p. A86
SEARCY HOSPITAL, MOUNT VERNON, AL, p. A24
SEARHC MT. EDGECUMBE HOSPITAL, SITKA, AK, p. A30
SEATTLE CANCER CARE ALLIANCE, SEATTLE, WA, p. A666
SEATTLE CHILDREN'S HOSPITAL, SEATTLE, WA, p. A666
SEBASTIAN RIVER MEDICAL CENTER, SEBASTIAN, FL, p. A139
SEBASTICOOK VALLEY HEALTH, PITTSFIELD, ME, p. A284
SEDAN CITY HOSPITAL, SEDAN, KS, p. A243
SEDGWICK COUNTY HEALTH CENTER, JULESBURG, CO, p. A102
SEILING COMMUNITY HOSPITAL, SEILING, OK, p. A504
SELBY GENERAL HOSPITAL, MARIETTA, OH, p. A484
SELECT LONG TERM CARE HOSPITAL – COLORADO SPRINGS, COLORADO SPRINGS, CO, p. A98
SELECT REHABILITATION HOSPITAL OF DENTON, DENTON, TX, p. A594
SELECT SPECIALTY HOSPITAL DENVER SOUTH, DENVER, COLORADO (see SELECT SPECIALTY HOSPITAL–DENVER), p. A100
SELECT SPECIALTY HOSPITAL–AKRON, AKRON, OH, p. A469
SELECT SPECIALTY HOSPITAL–ANN ARBOR, YPSILANTI, MI, p. A326
SELECT SPECIALTY HOSPITAL–ATLANTA, ATLANTA, GA, p. A146
SELECT SPECIALTY HOSPITAL–AUGUSTA, AUGUSTA, GA, p. A147
SELECT SPECIALTY HOSPITAL–BATTLE CREEK, BATTLE CREEK, MI, p. A308
SELECT SPECIALTY HOSPITAL–BEECH GROVE, BEECH GROVE, IN, p. A198
SELECT SPECIALTY HOSPITAL–BIRMINGHAM, BIRMINGHAM, AL, p. A16
SELECT SPECIALTY HOSPITAL–CANTON, CANTON, OH, p. A472
SELECT SPECIALTY HOSPITAL–CENTRAL PENNSYLVANIA, CAMP HILL, PA, p. A520
SELECT SPECIALTY HOSPITAL–CHARLESTON, CHARLESTON, WV, p. A671
SELECT SPECIALTY HOSPITAL–CINCINNATI, CINCINNATI, OH, p. A474
SELECT SPECIALTY HOSPITAL–COLUMBUS, COLUMBUS, OH, p. A477
SELECT SPECIALTY HOSPITAL–COLUMBUS, MOUNT CARMEL CAMPUS, COLUMBUS, OHIO (see SELECT SPECIALTY HOSPITAL–COLUMBUS), p. A477
SELECT SPECIALTY HOSPITAL–DALLAS, CARROLLTON, TX, p. A586
SELECT SPECIALTY HOSPITAL–DANVILLE, DANVILLE, PA, p. A521
SELECT SPECIALTY HOSPITAL–DENVER, DENVER, CO, p. A100
SELECT SPECIALTY HOSPITAL–DOWNRIVER, TAYLOR, MI, p. A324
SELECT SPECIALTY HOSPITAL–DURHAM, DURHAM, NC, p. A452
SELECT SPECIALTY HOSPITAL–ERIE, ERIE, PA, p. A523
SELECT SPECIALTY HOSPITAL–EVANSVILLE, EVANSVILLE, IN, p. A201

SELECT SPECIALTY HOSPITAL–FLINT, FLINT, MI, p. A312
SELECT SPECIALTY HOSPITAL–FORT SMITH, FORT SMITH, AR, p. A45
SELECT SPECIALTY HOSPITAL–FORT WAYNE, FORT WAYNE, IN, p. A202
SELECT SPECIALTY HOSPITAL–GAINESVILLE, GAINESVILLE, FL, p. A124
SELECT SPECIALTY HOSPITAL–GREENSBORO, GREENSBORO, NC, p. A454
SELECT SPECIALTY HOSPITAL–GROSSE POINTE, GROSSE POINTE FARMS, MI, p. A314
SELECT SPECIALTY HOSPITAL–GULF COAST, GULFPORT, MS, p. A346
SELECT SPECIALTY HOSPITAL–HARRISBURG, HARRISBURG, PENNSYLVANIA (see SELECT SPECIALTY HOSPITAL–CENTRAL PENNSYLVANIA), p. A520
SELECT SPECIALTY HOSPITAL–HOUSTON, HOUSTON, TX, p. A606
SELECT SPECIALTY HOSPITAL–HOUSTON MEDICAL CENTER, HOUSTON, TEXAS (see SELECT SPECIALTY HOSPITAL–HOUSTON), p. A606
SELECT SPECIALTY HOSPITAL–HOUSTON WEST, HOUSTON, TEXAS (see SELECT SPECIALTY HOSPITAL–HOUSTON), p. A606
SELECT SPECIALTY HOSPITAL–JACKSON, JACKSON, MS, p. A348
SELECT SPECIALTY HOSPITAL–JOHNSTOWN, JOHNSTOWN, PA, p. A526
SELECT SPECIALTY HOSPITAL–KANSAS CITY, KANSAS CITY, KS, p. A236
SELECT SPECIALTY HOSPITAL–KNOXVILLE, KNOXVILLE, TN, p. A568
SELECT SPECIALTY HOSPITAL–LAUREL HIGHLANDS, LATROBE, PA, p. A527
SELECT SPECIALTY HOSPITAL–LEXINGTON, LEXINGTON, KY, p. A253
SELECT SPECIALTY HOSPITAL–LITTLE ROCK, LITTLE ROCK, AR, p. A48
SELECT SPECIALTY HOSPITAL–LONGVIEW, LONGVIEW, TX, p. A613
SELECT SPECIALTY HOSPITAL–MACOMB COUNTY, MOUNT CLEMENS, MI, p. A319
SELECT SPECIALTY HOSPITAL–MADISON, MADISON, WI, p. A684
SELECT SPECIALTY HOSPITAL–MCKEESPORT, MCKEESPORT, PA, p. A528
SELECT SPECIALTY HOSPITAL–MEMPHIS, MEMPHIS, TN, p. A572
SELECT SPECIALTY HOSPITAL–MIAMI, MIAMI, FL, p. A131
SELECT SPECIALTY HOSPITAL–MIDLAND, MIDLAND, TX, p. A617
SELECT SPECIALTY HOSPITAL–MILWAUKEE, MILWAUKEE, WI, p. A687
SELECT SPECIALTY HOSPITAL–NASHVILLE, NASHVILLE, TN, p. A573
SELECT SPECIALTY HOSPITAL–NORTH KNOXVILLE, KNOXVILLE, TN, p. A568
SELECT SPECIALTY HOSPITAL–NORTHEAST NEW JERSEY, ROCHELLE PARK, NJ, p. A409
SELECT SPECIALTY HOSPITAL–NORTHWEST DETROIT, DETROIT, MI, p. A311
SELECT SPECIALTY HOSPITAL–OKLAHOMA CITY, OKLAHOMA CITY, OK, p. A502
SELECT SPECIALTY HOSPITAL–OMAHA, OMAHA, NE, p. A388
SELECT SPECIALTY HOSPITAL–ORLANDO, ORLANDO, FL, p. A134
SELECT SPECIALTY HOSPITAL–ORLANDO SOUTH, ORLANDO, FLORIDA (see SELECT SPECIALTY HOSPITAL–ORLANDO), p. A134
SELECT SPECIALTY HOSPITAL–PALM BEACH, LAKE WORTH, FL, p. A128
SELECT SPECIALTY HOSPITAL–PANAMA CITY, PANAMA CITY, FL, p. A135
SELECT SPECIALTY HOSPITAL–PENSACOLA, PENSACOLA, FL, p. A136
SELECT SPECIALTY HOSPITAL–PHOENIX, PHOENIX, AZ, p. A36
SELECT SPECIALTY HOSPITAL–PHOENIX DOWNTOWN, PHOENIX, ARIZONA (see SELECT SPECIALTY HOSPITAL–SCOTTSDALE), p. A38
SELECT SPECIALTY HOSPITAL–PITTSBURGH/UPMC, PITTSBURGH, PA, p. A535
SELECT SPECIALTY HOSPITAL–PONTIAC, PONTIAC, MI, p. A321
SELECT SPECIALTY HOSPITAL–QUAD CITIES, DAVENPORT, IA, p. A217
SELECT SPECIALTY HOSPITAL–SAGINAW, SAGINAW, MI, p. A322
SELECT SPECIALTY HOSPITAL–SAN ANTONIO, SAN ANTONIO, TX, p. A626
SELECT SPECIALTY HOSPITAL–SAVANNAH, SAVANNAH, GA, p. A159

SELECT SPECIALTY HOSPITAL–SCOTTSDALE, SCOTTSDALE, AZ, p. A38
SELECT SPECIALTY HOSPITAL–SIOUX FALLS, SIOUX FALLS, SD, p. A559
SELECT SPECIALTY HOSPITAL–SOUTH DALLAS, DE SOTO, TX, p. A593
SELECT SPECIALTY HOSPITAL–SPRINGFIELD, SPRINGFIELD, MO, p. A371
SELECT SPECIALTY HOSPITAL–ST. LOUIS, SAINT CHARLES, MO, p. A367
SELECT SPECIALTY HOSPITAL–TALLAHASSEE, TALLAHASSEE, FL, p. A140
SELECT SPECIALTY HOSPITAL–TOPEKA, TOPEKA, KS, p. A244
SELECT SPECIALTY HOSPITAL–TRICITIES, BRISTOL, TN, p. A562
SELECT SPECIALTY HOSPITAL–TULSA MIDTOWN, TULSA, OK, p. A506
SELECT SPECIALTY HOSPITAL–WESTERN MISSOURI, KANSAS CITY, MO, p. A362
SELECT SPECIALTY HOSPITAL–WICHITA, WICHITA, KS, p. A245
SELECT SPECIALTY HOSPITAL–WILMINGTON, WILMINGTON, DE, p. A115
SELECT SPECIALTY HOSPITAL–WINSTON-SALEM, WINSTON-SALEM, NC, p. A463
SELECT SPECIALTY HOSPITAL–YORK, YORK, PENNSYLVANIA (see SELECT SPECIALTY HOSPITAL–CENTRAL PENNSYLVANIA), p. A520
SELECT SPECIALTY HOSPITAL–YOUNGSTOWN, YOUNGSTOWN, OH, p. A492
SELECT SPECIALTY HOSPITAL–YOUNGSTOWN, BOARDMAN CAMPUS, BORDMAN, OHIO (see SELECT SPECIALTY HOSPITAL–YOUNGSTOWN), p. A492
SELECT SPECIALTY HOSPITAL–ZANESVILLE, ZANESVILLE, OH, p. A492
SELF REGIONAL HEALTHCARE, GREENWOOD, SC, p. A551
SENECA HEALTHCARE DISTRICT, CHESTER, CA, p. A57
SENIOR HAVEN CONVALESCENT NURSING CENTER (see SANFORD MEDICAL CENTER CANBY), p. A329
SENTARA CAREPLEX HOSPITAL, HAMPTON, VA, p. A649
SENTARA LEIGH HOSPITAL, NORFOLK, VA, p. A652
SENTARA NORFOLK GENERAL HOSPITAL, NORFOLK, VA, p. A653
SENTARA NORTHERN VIRGINIA MEDICAL CENTER, WOODBRIDGE, VA, p. A657
SENTARA OBICI HOSPITAL, SUFFOLK, VA, p. A656
SENTARA PRINCESS ANNE HOSPITAL, VIRGINIA BEACH, VA, p. A657
SENTARA VIRGINIA BEACH GENERAL HOSPITAL, VIRGINIA BEACH, VA, p. A657
SENTARA WILLIAMSBURG REGIONAL MEDICAL CENTER, WILLIAMSBURG, VA, p. A657
SEQUOIA HOSPITAL, REDWOOD CITY, CA, p. A82
SEQUOYAH MEMORIAL HOSPITAL, SALLISAW, OK, p. A504
SERENITY LANE, EUGENE, OR, p. A510
SERENITY SPRINGS SPECIALTY HOSPITAL, FARMERVILLE, LA, p. A266
SETON EDGAR B. DAVIS HOSPITAL, LULING, TX, p. A614
SETON HEALTH SYSTEM–ST. MARY'S HOSPITAL, TROY, NEW YORK (see ST. MARY'S HOSPITAL), p. A445
SETON HIGHLAND LAKES, BURNET, TX, p. A586
SETON MEDICAL CENTER, DALY CITY, CA, p. A59
SETON MEDICAL CENTER AUSTIN, AUSTIN, TX, p. A581
SETON MEDICAL CENTER HAYS, KYLE, TX, p. A611
SETON MEDICAL CENTER WILLIAMSON, ROUND ROCK, TX, p. A623
SETON NORTHWEST HOSPITAL, AUSTIN, TX, p. A581
SETON SHOAL CREEK HOSPITAL, AUSTIN, TX, p. A581
SETON SMITHVILLE REGIONAL HOSPITAL, SMITHVILLE, TX, p. A628
SETON SOUTHWEST HEALTHCARE CENTER, AUSTIN, TX, p. A581
SEVEN HILLS BEHAVIORAL INSTITUTE, HENDERSON, NV, p. A392
SEVEN RIVERS REGIONAL MEDICAL CENTER, CRYSTAL RIVER, FL, p. A121
SEVIER VALLEY MEDICAL CENTER, RICHFIELD, UT, p. A640
SEWICKLEY VALLEY HOSPITAL, (A DIVISION OF VALLEY MEDICAL FACILITIES), SEWICKLEY, PA, p. A538
SEYMOUR HOSPITAL, SEYMOUR, TX, p. A627
SHADOW MOUNTAIN BEHAVIORAL HEALTH SYSTEM, TULSA, OK, p. A506
SHADY GROVE ADVENTIST HOSPITAL, ROCKVILLE, MD, p. A294
SHAMROCK GENERAL HOSPITAL, SHAMROCK, TX, p. A627
SHANDS AGH, GAINESVILLE, FLORIDA (see SHANDS AT THE UNIVERSITY OF FLORIDA), p. A124
SHANDS AT THE UNIVERSITY OF FLORIDA, GAINESVILLE, FL, p. A124
SHANDS CHILDRENS HOSPITAL, GAINESVILLE, FLORIDA (see SHANDS AT THE UNIVERSITY OF FLORIDA), p. A124

© 2012 AHA Guide

SUMNER REGIONAL MEDICAL CENTER, WELLINGTON, KS, p. A245

SUMNER REGIONAL MEDICAL CENTER, GALLATIN, TN, p. A566

SUN COAST HOSPITAL, LARGO, FL, p. A128

SUNBURY COMMUNITY HOSPITAL, SUNBURY, PA, p. A539

SUNDANCE HOSPITAL, ARLINGTON, TX, p. A579

SUNNYSIDE COMMUNITY HOSPITAL, SUNNYSIDE, WA, p. A667

SUNNYSIDE MEDICAL CENTER, CLACKAMAS, OR, p. A509

SUNNYVIEW REHABILITATION HOSPITAL, SCHENECTADY, NY, p. A443

SUNRISE CANYON HOSPITAL, LUBBOCK, TX, p. A614

SUNRISE CHILDREN'S HOSPITAL (see SUNRISE HOSPITAL AND MEDICAL CENTER), p. A394

SUNRISE HOSPITAL AND MEDICAL CENTER, LAS VEGAS, NV, p. A394

SUNY DOWNSTATE MEDICAL CENTER UNIVERSITY HOSPITAL OF BROOKLYN,, NY, p. A437

SURGERY SPECIALTY HOSPITALS OF AMERICA, PASADENA, TX, p. A620

SURGICAL HOSPITAL AT SOUTHWOODS, YOUNGSTOWN, OH, p. A492

SURGICAL HOSPITAL OF JONESBORO, JONESBORO, AR, p. A47

SURGICAL HOSPITAL OF OKLAHOMA, OKLAHOMA CITY, OK, p. A502

SURGICAL INSTITUTE OF READING, WYOMISSING, PA, p. A542

SURGICAL SPECIALTY CENTER AT COORDINATED HEALTH, ALLENTOWN, PA, p. A517

SURGICAL SPECIALTY CENTER OF BATON ROUGE, BATON ROUGE, LA, p. A263

SURGICAL SPECIALTY HOSPITAL OF ARIZONA, PHOENIX, AZ, p. A37

SURPRISE VALLEY HEALTHCARE DISTRICT, CEDARVILLE, CA, p. A57

SUSAN B. ALLEN MEMORIAL HOSPITAL, EL DORADO, KS, p. A232

SUTTER AMADOR HOSPITAL, JACKSON, CA, p. A65

SUTTER AUBURN FAITH HOSPITAL, AUBURN, CA, p. A54

SUTTER CENTER FOR PSYCHIATRY, SACRAMENTO, CA, p. A84

SUTTER CHILDREN'S CENTER, SACRAMENTO, CALIFORNIA (see SUTTER MEDICAL CENTER, SACRAMENTO), p. A84

SUTTER COAST HOSPITAL, CRESCENT CITY, CA, p. A59

SUTTER DAVIS HOSPITAL, DAVIS, CA, p. A59

SUTTER DELTA MEDICAL CENTER, ANTIOCH, CA, p. A53

SUTTER GENERAL HOSPITAL, SACRAMENTO, CALIFORNIA (see SUTTER MEDICAL CENTER, SACRAMENTO), p. A84

SUTTER LAKESIDE HOSPITAL, LAKEPORT, CA, p. A66

SUTTER MATERNITY AND SURGERY CENTER OF SANTA CRUZ, SANTA CRUZ, CA, p. A90

SUTTER MEDICAL CENTER OF SANTA ROSA, CHANATE CAMPUS, SANTA ROSA, CA, p. A90

SUTTER MEDICAL CENTER, SACRAMENTO, SACRAMENTO, CA, p. A84

SUTTER ROSEVILLE MEDICAL CENTER, ROSEVILLE, CA, p. A83

SUTTER SOLANO MEDICAL CENTER, VALLEJO, CA, p. A94

SUTTER SURGICAL HOSPITAL – NORTH VALLEY, YUBA CITY, CA, p. A96

SUTTER TRACY COMMUNITY HOSPITAL, TRACY, CA, p. A93

SWEDISH COVENANT HOSPITAL, CHICAGO, IL, p. A178

SWEDISH MEDICAL CENTER, ENGLEWOOD, CO, p. A100

SWEDISH MEDICAL CENTER-BALLARD, SEATTLE, WASHINGTON (see SWEDISH MEDICAL CENTER-FIRST HILL), p. A666

SWEDISH MEDICAL CENTER-CHERRY HILL CAMPUS, SEATTLE, WA, p. A666

SWEDISH MEDICAL CENTER-FIRST HILL, SEATTLE, WA, p. A666

SWEDISH/EDMONDS, EDMONDS, WA, p. A661

SWEDISH/ISSAQUAH, ISSAQUAH, WA, p. A662

SWEDISHAMERICAN HOSPITAL, ROCKFORD, IL, p. A193

SWEENY COMMUNITY HOSPITAL, SWEENY, TX, p. A629

SWEETWATER HOSPITAL, SWEETWATER, TN, p. A576

SWIFT COUNTY-BENSON HOSPITAL, BENSON, MN, p. A328

SWISHER MEMORIAL HOSPITAL DISTRICT, TULIA, TX, p. A632

SYCAMORE MEDICAL CENTER, MIAMISBURG, OH, p. A485

SYCAMORE SHOALS HOSPITAL, ELIZABETHTON, TN, p. A565

SYLVAN GROVE HOSPITAL, JACKSON, GA, p. A154

SYOSSET HOSPITAL, SYOSSET, NY, p. A444

SYRINGA HOSPITAL AND CLINICS, GRANGEVILLE, ID, p. A168

# T

T. C. THOMPSON CHILDREN'S HOSPITAL, CHATTANOOGA, TENNESSEE (see ERLANGER MEDICAL CENTER), p. A563

T. J. SAMSON COMMUNITY HOSPITAL, GLASGOW, KY, p. A250

TAHLEQUAH CITY HOSPITAL, TAHLEQUAH, OK, p. A505

TAHOE FOREST HOSPITAL DISTRICT, TRUCKEE, CA, p. A93

TAHOE PACIFIC HOSPITALS, RENO, NV, p. A395

TAHOE PACIFIC HOSPITALS – WEST, RENO, NEVADA (see TAHOE PACIFIC HOSPITALS), p. A395

TAKOMA REGIONAL HOSPITAL, GREENEVILLE, TN, p. A566

TALLAHASSEE MEMORIAL HEALTHCARE, TALLAHASSEE, FL, p. A140

TALLAHATCHIE GENERAL HOSPITAL, CHARLESTON, MS, p. A344

TAMPA GENERAL HOSPITAL, TAMPA, FL, p. A141

TAMPA GENERAL HOSPITAL CHILDREN'S MEDICAL CENTER, TAMPA, FLORIDA (see TAMPA GENERAL HOSPITAL), p. A141

TANNER MEDICAL CENTER, CARROLLTON, GA, p. A148

TANNER MEDICAL CENTER-VILLA RICA, VILLA RICA, GA, p. A161

TAUNTON STATE HOSPITAL, TAUNTON, MA, p. A305

TAYLOR HARDIN SECURE MEDICAL FACILITY, TUSCALOOSA, AL, p. A26

TAYLOR HOSPITAL, RIDLEY PARK, PENNSYLVANIA (see CROZER-CHESTER MEDICAL CENTER), p. A540

TAYLOR REGIONAL HOSPITAL, HAWKINSVILLE, GA, p. A154

TAYLOR REGIONAL HOSPITAL, CAMPBELLSVILLE, KY, p. A248

TAYLORVILLE MEMORIAL HOSPITAL, TAYLORVILLE, IL, p. A195

TECHE REGIONAL MEDICAL CENTER, MORGAN CITY, LA, p. A273

TEHACHAPI VALLEY HEALTHCARE DISTRICT, TEHACHAPI, CA, p. A92

TELECARE HERITAGE PSYCHIATRIC HEALTH CENTER, OAKLAND, CA, p. A77

TEMPE ST. LUKE'S HOSPITAL, TEMPE, ARIZONA (see ST. LUKE'S MEDICAL CENTER), p. A36

TEMPLE COMMUNITY HOSPITAL, LOS ANGELES, CA, p. A72

TEMPLE UNIVERSITY HOSPITAL, PHILADELPHIA, PA, p. A534

TEMPLE UNIVERSITY HOSPITAL – EPISCOPAL DIVISION, PHILADELPHIA, PENNSYLVANIA (see TEMPLE UNIVERSITY HOSPITAL), p. A534

TEN LAKES CENTER, DENNISON, OH, p. A479

TERENCE CARDINAL COOKE HEALTH CARE CENTER, NEW YORK, NY, p. A437

TERRE HAUTE REGIONAL HOSPITAL, TERRE HAUTE, IN, p. A212

TERREBONNE GENERAL MEDICAL CENTER, HOUMA, LA, p. A268

TERRELL STATE HOSPITAL, TERRELL, TX, p. A630

TETON MEDICAL CENTER, CHOTEAU, MT, p. A374

TETON VALLEY HOSPITAL AND SURGICENTER, DRIGGS, ID, p. A168

TEWKSBURY HOSPITAL, TEWKSBURY, MA, p. A305

TEXAS CENTER FOR INFECTIOUS DISEASE, SAN ANTONIO, TX, p. A626

TEXAS CHILDREN'S HOSPITAL, HOUSTON, TX, p. A607

TEXAS COUNTY MEMORIAL HOSPITAL, HOUSTON, MO, p. A360

TEXAS HEALTH ARLINGTON MEMORIAL HOSPITAL, ARLINGTON, TX, p. A579

TEXAS HEALTH CENTER FOR DIAGNOSTIC & SURGERY, PLANO, TX, p. A621

TEXAS HEALTH HARRIS METHODIST HOSPITAL AZLE, AZLE, TX, p. A582

TEXAS HEALTH HARRIS METHODIST HOSPITAL CLEBURNE, CLEBURNE, TX, p. A587

TEXAS HEALTH HARRIS METHODIST HOSPITAL FORT WORTH, FORT WORTH, TX, p. A599

TEXAS HEALTH HARRIS METHODIST HOSPITAL HURST-EULESS-BEDFORD, BEDFORD, TX, p. A583

TEXAS HEALTH HARRIS METHODIST HOSPITAL SOUTHLAKE, SOUTHLAKE, TX, p. A628

TEXAS HEALTH HARRIS METHODIST HOSPITAL SOUTHWEST FORT WORTH, FORT WORTH, TX, p. A599

TEXAS HEALTH HARRIS METHODIST HOSPITAL STEPHENVILLE, STEPHENVILLE, TX, p. A629

TEXAS HEALTH HEART & VASCULAR HOSPITAL ARLINGTON, ARLINGTON, TX, p. A580

TEXAS HEALTH PRESBYTERIAN HOSPITAL ALLEN, ALLEN, TX, p. A577

TEXAS HEALTH PRESBYTERIAN HOSPITAL DALLAS, DALLAS, TX, p. A592

TEXAS HEALTH PRESBYTERIAN HOSPITAL DENTON, DENTON, TX, p. A594

TEXAS HEALTH PRESBYTERIAN HOSPITAL FLOWER MOUND, FLOWER MOUND, TX, p. A597

TEXAS HEALTH PRESBYTERIAN HOSPITAL KAUFMAN, KAUFMAN, TX, p. A610

TEXAS HEALTH PRESBYTERIAN HOSPITAL PLANO, PLANO, TX, p. A621

TEXAS HEALTH PRESBYTERIAN HOSPITAL-WNJ, SHERMAN, TX, p. A628

TEXAS HEALTH SPECIALTY HOSPITAL, FORT WORTH, TX, p. A599

TEXAS INSTITUTE FOR SURGERY AT TEXAS HEALTH PRESBYTERIAN DALLAS, DALLAS, TX, p. A592

TEXAS NEUROREHAB CENTER, AUSTIN, TX, p. A582

TEXAS ORTHOPEDIC HOSPITAL, HOUSTON, TX, p. A607

TEXAS REGIONAL MEDICAL CENTER, SUNNYVALE, TX, p. A629

TEXAS REHABILITATION HOSPITAL OF FORT WORTH, FORT WORTH, TX, p. A599

TEXAS SCOTTISH RITE HOSPITAL FOR CHILDREN, DALLAS, TX, p. A592

TEXAS SPECIALTY HOSPITAL AT DALLAS, DALLAS, TX, p. A593

TEXAS SPECIALTY HOSPITAL AT HOUSTON, HOUSTON, TX, p. A607

TEXAS SPECIALTY HOSPITAL AT LUBBOCK, LUBBOCK, TX, p. A614

TEXAS SPECIALTY HOSPITAL AT WICHITA FALLS, WICHITA FALLS, TX, p. A635

TEXAS SPINE & JOINT HOSPITAL, TYLER, TX, p. A632

TEXOMA MEDICAL CENTER, DENISON, TX, p. A593

THAYER COUNTY HEALTH SERVICES, HEBRON, NE, p. A384

THE ACADIA HOSPITAL, BANGOR, ME, p. A281

THE ALLEN PAVILION, NEW YORK, NEW YORK (see NEW YORK-PRESBYTERIAN HOSPITAL), p. A436

THE AROOSTOOK MEDICAL CENTER, PRESQUE ISLE, ME, p. A285

THE BRIDGEWAY, NORTH LITTLE ROCK, AR, p. A50

THE BROOK AT DUPONT, LOUISVILLE, KY, p. A255

THE BROOK HOSPITAL – KMI, LOUISVILLE, KY, p. A255

THE CENTER FOR SPINAL SURGERY, NASHVILLE, TN, p. A573

THE CHARLOTTE HUNGERFORD HOSPITAL, TORRINGTON, CT, p. A112

THE CHILDREN'S CENTER, BETHANY, OK, p. A494

THE CHILDREN'S HOME OF PITTSBURGH, PITTSBURGH, PA, p. A535

THE CHILDREN'S HOSPITAL OF ALABAMA, BIRMINGHAM, AL, p. A17

THE CHILDREN'S INSTITUTE OF PITTSBURGH, PITTSBURGH, PA, p. A535

THE CONNECTICUT HOSPICE, BRANFORD, CT, p. A108

THE GOOD SAMARITAN HOSPITAL, LEBANON, PA, p. A527

THE HEALTHCENTER, KALISPELL, MT, p. A377

THE HEART HOSPITAL AT DEACONESS GATEWAY, NEWBURGH, IN, p. A210

THE HEART HOSPITAL BAYLOR PLANO, PLANO, TX, p. A621

THE HOSPITAL AT CRAIG RANCH, MCKINNEY, TX, p. A616

THE HOSPITAL AT HEBREW HEALTH CARE, WEST HARTFORD, CT, p. A113

THE HOSPITAL AT WESTLAKE MEDICAL CENTER, AUSTIN, TX, p. A582

THE HOSPITAL OF CENTRAL CONNECTICUT, NEW BRITAIN, CT, p. A110

THE HSC PEDIATRIC CENTER, WASHINGTON, DC, p. A117

THE JEWISH HOSPITAL, CINCINNATI, OH, p. A474

THE JOSEPH M. SANZARI CHILDREN'S HOSPITAL, HACKENSACK, NEW JERSEY (see HACKENSACK UNIVERSITY MEDICAL CENTER), p. A404

THE KING'S DAUGHTERS HOSPITAL, GREENVILLE, MISSISSIPPI (see DELTA REGIONAL MEDICAL CENTER), p. A346

THE MEDICAL CENTER, COLUMBUS, GA, p. A150

THE MEDICAL CENTER AT ELIZABETH PLACE, DAYTON, OH, p. A478

THE MEDICAL CENTER OF SOUTHEAST TEXAS, PORT ARTHUR, TX, p. A622

THE METHODIST HOSPITAL, HOUSTON, TX, p. A607

THE MOUNT SINAI HOSPITAL OF QUEENS,, NY, p. A437

THE NEUROMEDICAL CENTER SURGICAL HOSPITAL, BATON ROUGE, LA, p. A263

THE ORTHOPEDIC SPECIALTY HOSPITAL, MURRAY, UT, p. A638

THE OUTER BANKS HOSPITAL, NAGS HEAD, NC, p. A458

THE PAVILION, CHAMPAIGN, IL, p. A175

THE PAVILION, PENSACOLA, FLORIDA (see WEST FLORIDA HOSPITAL), p. A136

THE PHYSICIANS CENTRE HOSPITAL, BRYAN, TX, p. A586

THE REHABILITATION HOSPITAL, FORT MYERS, FLORIDA (see LEE MEMORIAL HOSPITAL), p. A124

THE REHABILITATION INSTITUTE OF ST. LOUIS, SAINT LOUIS, MO, p. A370

THE UNIVERSITY OF KANSAS HOSPITAL, KANSAS CITY, KS, p. A236

THE UNIVERSITY OF TENNESSEE MEDICAL CENTER, KNOXVILLE, TN, p. A569

THE UNIVERSITY OF TOLEDO MEDICAL CENTER, TOLEDO, OH, p. A489

THE VILLAGES HEALTH SYSTEM, THE VILLAGES, FL, p. A142

THE VINES, OCALA, FL, p. A134

THE WILLIAM W. BACKUS HOSPITAL, NORWICH, CT, p. A111

THE WOMAN'S HOSPITAL OF TEXAS, HOUSTON, TX, p. A607

THE WOMEN'S HOSPITAL, NEWBURGH, IN, p. A210

THEDA CLARK MEDICAL CENTER, NEENAH, WI, p. A687

THIBODAUX REGIONAL MEDICAL CENTER, THIBODAUX, LA, p. A278

THOMAS B. FINAN CENTER, CUMBERLAND, MD, p. A291

THOMAS H. BOYD MEMORIAL HOSPITAL, CARROLLTON, IL, p. A174

THOMAS HOSPITAL, FAIRHOPE, AL, p. A20

## U

# V

# W

WADLEY REGIONAL MEDICAL CENTER, TEXARKANA, TX, p. A631

WAGNER COMMUNITY MEMORIAL HOSPITAL AVERA, WAGNER, SD, p. A560

WAGONER COMMUNITY HOSPITAL, WAGONER, OK, p. A507

WAHIAWA GENERAL HOSPITAL, WAHIAWA, HI, p. A165

WAKE FOREST BAPTIST HEALTH–DAVIE HOSPITAL, MOCKSVILLE, NC, p. A457

WAKE FOREST BAPTIST HEALTH–LEXINGTON MEDICAL CENTER, LEXINGTON, NC, p. A456

WAKE FOREST BAPTIST MEDICAL CENTER, WINSTON–SALEM, NC, p. A463

WAKE FOREST UNIVERSITY HEALTH SERVICE, WINSTON–SALEM, NC, p. A463

WAKEMED CARY HOSPITAL, CARY, NC, p. A450

WAKEMED RALEIGH CAMPUS, RALEIGH, NC, p. A459

WALBRIDGE MEMORIAL CONVALESCENT WING (see PIONEERS MEDICAL CENTER), p. A104

WALDEN PSYCHIATRIC CARE, WALTHAM, MA, p. A305

WALDO COUNTY GENERAL HOSPITAL, BELFAST, ME, p. A281

WALKER BAPTIST MEDICAL CENTER, JASPER, AL, p. A22

WALLA WALLA GENERAL HOSPITAL, WALLA WALLA, WA, p. A669

WALLACE THOMSON HOSPITAL, UNION, SC, p. A554

WALLOWA MEMORIAL HOSPITAL, ENTERPRISE, OR, p. A510

WALNUT CREEK MEDICAL CENTER, WALNUT CREEK, CA, p. A95

WALTER B. JONES ALCOHOL AND DRUG ABUSE TREATMENT CENTER, GREENVILLE, NC, p. A454

WALTER KNOX MEMORIAL HOSPITAL, EMMETT, ID, p. A168

WALTER OLIN MOSS REGIONAL MEDICAL CENTER, LAKE CHARLES, LA, p. A271

WALTER P. REUTHER PSYCHIATRIC HOSPITAL, WESTLAND, MI, p. A325

WALTER REED NATIONAL MILITARY MEDICAL CENTER, BETHESDA, MD, p. A290

WALTHALL COUNTY GENERAL HOSPITAL, TYLERTOWN, MS, p. A353

WALTON REGIONAL MEDICAL CENTER, MONROE, GA, p. A156

WALTON REHABILITATION HOSPITAL, AUGUSTA, GA, p. A147

WAMEGO CITY HOSPITAL, WAMEGO, KS, p. A244

WAR MEMORIAL HOSPITAL, SAULT SAINTE MARIE, MI, p. A323

WAR MEMORIAL HOSPITAL, BERKELEY SPRINGS, WV, p. A670

WARD MEMORIAL HOSPITAL, MONAHANS, TX, p. A617

WARM SPRINGS MEDICAL CENTER, WARM SPRINGS, GA, p. A161

WARM SPRINGS REHABILITATION HOSPITAL, SAN ANTONIO, TX, p. A626

WARM SPRINGS SPECIALTY HOSPITAL, LULING, TX, p. A615

WARM SPRINGS SPECIALTY HOSPITAL OF VICTORIA, VICTORIA, TX, p. A633

WARRACK CAMPUS, SANTA ROSA, CALIFORNIA (see SUTTER MEDICAL CENTER OF SANTA ROSA, CHANATE CAMPUS), p. A90

WARREN GENERAL HOSPITAL, WARREN, PA, p. A540

WARREN MEMORIAL HOSPITAL, FRIEND, NE, p. A383

WARREN MEMORIAL HOSPITAL, FRONT ROYAL, VA, p. A648

WARREN STATE HOSPITAL, WARREN, PA, p. A540

WARWICK MANOR BEHAVIORAL HEALTH, EAST NEW MARKET, MD, p. A291

WASHAKIE MEDICAL CENTER, WORLAND, WY, p. A698

WASHINGTON ADVENTIST HOSPITAL, TAKOMA PARK, MD, p. A294

WASHINGTON COUNTY HOSPITAL, NASHVILLE, IL, p. A189

WASHINGTON COUNTY HOSPITAL, WASHINGTON, KS, p. A245

WASHINGTON COUNTY HOSPITAL, PLYMOUTH, NC, p. A458

WASHINGTON COUNTY HOSPITAL AND CLINICS, WASHINGTON, IA, p. A227

WASHINGTON COUNTY HOSPITAL AND NURSING HOME, CHATOM, AL, p. A18

WASHINGTON COUNTY MEMORIAL HOSPITAL, POTOSI, MO, p. A367

WASHINGTON COUNTY REGIONAL MEDICAL CENTER, SANDERSVILLE, GA, p. A158

WASHINGTON HOSPITAL, WASHINGTON, PA, p. A540

WASHINGTON HOSPITAL HEALTHCARE SYSTEM, FREMONT, CA, p. A61

WASHINGTON REGIONAL MEDICAL CENTER, FAYETTEVILLE, AR, p. A44

WATAUGA MEDICAL CENTER, BOONE, NC, p. A449

WATERBURY HOSPITAL, WATERBURY, CT, p. A112

WATERTOWN REGIONAL MEDICAL CENTER, WATERTOWN, WI, p. A692

WATONGA MUNICIPAL HOSPITAL, WATONGA, OK, p. A507

WATSONVILLE COMMUNITY HOSPITAL, WATSONVILLE, CA, p. A95

WAUKESHA COUNTY MENTAL HEALTH CENTER, WAUKESHA, WI, p. A692

WAUKESHA MEMORIAL HOSPITAL, WAUKESHA, WI, p. A692

WAUPUN MEMORIAL HOSPITAL, WAUPUN, WI, p. A693

WAVERLY HEALTH CENTER, WAVERLY, IA, p. A228

WAYNE COUNTY HOSPITAL, CORYDON, IA, p. A217

WAYNE COUNTY HOSPITAL, MONTICELLO, KY, p. A256

WAYNE GENERAL HOSPITAL, WAYNESBORO, MS, p. A353

WAYNE HOSPITAL, GREENVILLE, OH, p. A481

WAYNE MEDICAL CENTER, WAYNESBORO, TN, p. A576

WAYNE MEMORIAL HOSPITAL, JESUP, GA, p. A154

WAYNE MEMORIAL HOSPITAL, GOLDSBORO, NC, p. A453

WAYNE MEMORIAL HOSPITAL, HONESDALE, PA, p. A525

WAYNESBORO HOSPITAL, WAYNESBORO, PA, p. A540

WEATHERFORD REGIONAL HOSPITAL, WEATHERFORD, OK, p. A507

WEATHERFORD REGIONAL MEDICAL CENTER, WEATHERFORD, TX, p. A634

WEBSTER COUNTY COMMUNITY HOSPITAL, RED CLOUD, NE, p. A389

WEBSTER COUNTY MEMORIAL HOSPITAL, WEBSTER SPRINGS, WV, p. A676

WEDOWEE HOSPITAL, WEDOWEE, AL, p. A26

WEED ARMY COMMUNITY HOSPITAL, FORT IRWIN, CA, p. A61

WEEKS MEDICAL CENTER, LANCASTER, NH, p. A398

WEIRTON MEDICAL CENTER, WEIRTON, WV, p. A676

WEISBROD MEMORIAL COUNTY HOSPITAL, EADS, CO, p. A100

WEISER MEMORIAL HOSPITAL, WEISER, ID, p. A171

WEISMAN CHILDREN'S REHABILITATION HOSPITAL, MARLTON, NJ, p. A406

WEKIVA SPRINGS CENTER FOR WOMEN, JACKSONVILLE, FL, p. A127

WELCH COMMUNITY HOSPITAL, WELCH, WV, p. A676

WELLINGTON REGIONAL MEDICAL CENTER, WEST PALM BEACH, FL, p. A143

WELLMONT BRISTOL REGIONAL MEDICAL CENTER, BRISTOL, TN, p. A562

WELLMONT HANCOCK COUNTY HOSPITAL, SNEEDVILLE, TN, p. A575

WELLMONT HAWKINS COUNTY MEMORIAL HOSPITAL, ROGERSVILLE, TN, p. A575

WELLMONT HOLSTON VALLEY MEDICAL CENTER, KINGSPORT, TN, p. A568

WELLMONT LONESOME PINE HOSPITAL, BIG STONE GAP, VA, p. A645

WELLSPAN SURGERY AND REHABILLITATION HOSPITAL, YORK, PENNSYLVANIA (see YORK HOSPITAL), p. A543

WELLSPRING FOUNDATION, BETHLEHEM, CT, p. A108

WELLSTAR COBB HOSPITAL, AUSTELL, GA, p. A147

WELLSTAR DOUGLAS HOSPITAL, DOUGLASVILLE, GA, p. A151

WELLSTAR KENNESTONE HOSPITAL, MARIETTA, GA, p. A156

WELLSTAR PAULDING HOSPITAL, DALLAS, GA, p. A150

WELLSTAR WINDY HILL HOSPITAL, MARIETTA, GA, p. A156

WELLSTONE REGIONAL HOSPITAL, JEFFERSONVILLE, IN, p. A205

WENATCHEE VALLEY HOSPITAL, WENATCHEE, WA, p. A669

WENTWORTH–DOUGLASS HOSPITAL, DOVER, NH, p. A397

WERNERSVILLE STATE HOSPITAL, WERNERSVILLE, PA, p. A540

WESLACO REHABILITATION HOSPITAL, WESLACO, TX, p. A634

WESLEY LONG COMMUNITY HOSPITAL, GREENSBORO, NORTH CAROLINA (see CONE HEALTH), p. A454

WESLEY MEDICAL CENTER, WICHITA, KS, p. A246

WESLEY MEDICAL CENTER, HATTIESBURG, MS, p. A347

WESLEY REHABILITATION HOSPITAL, WICHITA, KS, p. A246

WESLEY WOODS GERIATRIC HOSPITAL OF EMORY UNIVERSITY, ATLANTA, GA, p. A146

WESLEY WOODS LONG TERM CARE HOSPITAL, ATLANTA, GA, p. A146

WEST ANAHEIM MEDICAL CENTER, ANAHEIM, CA, p. A53

WEST BOCA MEDICAL CENTER, BOCA RATON, FL, p. A119

WEST BRANCH REGIONAL MEDICAL CENTER, WEST BRANCH, MI, p. A325

WEST CALCASIEU CAMERON HOSPITAL, SULPHUR, LA, p. A278

WEST CAMPUS, NORFOLK, NEBRASKA (see FAITH REGIONAL HEALTH SERVICES), p. A386

WEST CARROLL MEMORIAL HOSPITAL, OAK GROVE, LA, p. A275

WEST CENTRAL GEORGIA REGIONAL HOSPITAL, COLUMBUS, GA, p. A150

WEST CHESTER HOSPITAL, WEST CHESTER, OH, p. A491

WEST FELICIANA PARISH HOSPITAL, SAINT FRANCISVILLE, LA, p. A276

WEST FLORIDA COMMUNITY CARE CENTER, MILTON, FL, p. A132

WEST FLORIDA HOSPITAL, PENSACOLA, FL, p. A136

WEST GABLES REHABILITATION HOSPITAL, MIAMI, FL, p. A132

WEST GEORGIA HEALTH, LA GRANGE, GA, p. A155

WEST HAVEN DIVISION, WEST HAVEN, CONNECTICUT (see VETERANS AFFAIRS CONNECTICUT HEALTHCARE SYSTEM), p. A113

WEST HILLS HOSPITAL, RENO, NV, p. A395

WEST HILLS HOSPITAL AND MEDICAL CENTER,, CA, p. A72

WEST HOLT MEMORIAL HOSPITAL, ATKINSON, NE, p. A381

WEST HOUSTON MEDICAL CENTER, HOUSTON, TX, p. A608

WEST JEFFERSON MEDICAL CENTER, MARRERO, LA, p. A272

WEST LOS ANGELES MEDICAL CENTER, LOS ANGELES, CA, p. A72

WEST MARION COMMUNITY HOSPITAL, OCALA, FLORIDA (see OCALA REGIONAL MEDICAL CENTER), p. A133

WEST OAKS HOSPITAL, HOUSTON, TX, p. A608

WEST PARK HOSPITAL, CODY, WY, p. A696

WEST RIVER REGIONAL MEDICAL CENTER, HETTINGER, ND, p. A466

WEST SHORE MEDICAL CENTER, MANISTEE, MI, p. A318

WEST SUBURBAN MEDICAL CENTER, OAK PARK, IL, p. A190

WEST TEXAS VA HEALTH CARE SYSTEM, BIG SPRING, TX, p. A584

WEST VALLEY HOSPITAL, GOODYEAR, AZ, p. A33

WEST VALLEY HOSPITAL, DALLAS, OR, p. A510

WEST VALLEY MEDICAL CENTER, CALDWELL, ID, p. A167

WEST VIRGINIA UNIVERSITY CHILDREN'S HOSPITAL, MORGANTOWN, WEST VIRGINIA (see WEST VIRGINIA UNIVERSITY HOSPITALS), p. A674

WEST VIRGINIA UNIVERSITY HOSPITALS, MORGANTOWN, WV, p. A674

WESTBURY COMMUNITY HOSPITAL, HOUSTON, TX, p. A608

WESTCHESTER GENERAL HOSPITAL, MIAMI, FL, p. A132

WESTCHESTER MEDICAL CENTER, VALHALLA, NY, p. A445

WESTEND HOSPITAL, JENNINGS, LA, p. A268

WESTERLY HOSPITAL, WESTERLY, RI, p. A545

WESTERN ARIZONA REGIONAL MEDICAL CENTER, BULLHEAD CITY, AZ, p. A31

WESTERN BAPTIST HOSPITAL, PADUCAH, KY, p. A257

WESTERN MARYLAND HOSPITAL CENTER, HAGERSTOWN, MD, p. A292

WESTERN MARYLAND REGIONAL MEDICAL CENTER, CUMBERLAND, MD, p. A291

WESTERN MASSACHUSETTS HOSPITAL, WESTFIELD, MA, p. A306

WESTERN MEDICAL CENTER ANAHEIM, ANAHEIM, CA, p. A53

WESTERN MEDICAL CENTER–SANTA ANA, SANTA ANA, CA, p. A89

WESTERN MENTAL HEALTH INSTITUTE, BOLIVAR, TN, p. A562

WESTERN MISSOURI MEDICAL CENTER, WARRENSBURG, MO, p. A372

WESTERN NEW YORK CHILDREN'S PSYCHIATRIC CENTER, WEST SENECA, NY, p. A446

WESTERN PENNSYLVANIA HOSPITAL, PITTSBURGH, PA, p. A536

WESTERN PLAINS MEDICAL COMPLEX, DODGE CITY, KS, p. A232

WESTERN PSYCHIATRIC INSTITUTE AND CLINIC, PITTSBURGH, PENNSYLVANIA (see UPMC PRESBYTERIAN SHADYSIDE), p. A535

WESTERN REGIONAL MEDICAL CENTER, GOODYEAR, AZ, p. A33

WESTERN STATE HOSPITAL, HOPKINSVILLE, KY, p. A252

WESTERN STATE HOSPITAL, STAUNTON, VA, p. A656

WESTERN STATE HOSPITAL, TACOMA, WA, p. A668

WESTFIELD HOSPITAL, ALLENTOWN, PA, p. A517

WESTFIELD MEMORIAL HOSPITAL, WESTFIELD, NY, p. A446

WESTFIELDS HOSPITAL, NEW RICHMOND, WI, p. A688

WESTLAKE HOSPITAL, MELROSE PARK, IL, p. A187

WESTLAKE REGIONAL HOSPITAL, COLUMBIA, KY, p. A248

WESTON COUNTY HEALTH SERVICES, NEWCASTLE, WY, p. A697

WESTSIDE REGIONAL MEDICAL CENTER, PLANTATION, FL, p. A136

WESTWOOD LODGE HOSPITAL, WESTWOOD, MA, p. A306

WETZEL COUNTY HOSPITAL, NEW MARTINSVILLE, WV, p. A674

WHEATLAND MEMORIAL HEALTHCARE, HARLOWTON, MT, p. A376

WHEATON FRANCISCAN HEALTHCARE – ALL SAINTS, RACINE, WI, p. A689

WHEATON FRANCISCAN HEALTHCARE – ELMBROOK MEMORIAL, BROOKFIELD, WI, p. A679

WHEATON FRANCISCAN HEALTHCARE – FRANKLIN, FRANKLIN, WI, p. A682

WHEATON FRANCISCAN HEALTHCARE – ST. FRANCIS, MILWAUKEE, WI, p. A687

WHEATON FRANCISCAN HEALTHCARE – ST. JOSEPH'S, MILWAUKEE, WI, p. A687

WHEATON FRANCISCAN HEALTHCARE – THE WISCONSIN HEART HOSPITAL, WAUWATOSA, WI, p. A693

WHEELING HOSPITAL, WHEELING, WV, p. A677

WHIDBEY GENERAL HOSPITAL, COUPEVILLE, WA, p. A660

WHIDDEN MEMORIAL HOSPITAL, EVERETT, MASSACHUSETTS (see CAMBRIDGE HEALTH ALLIANCE), p. A299

WHITE COUNTY MEDICAL CENTER, SEARCY, AR, p. A51

WHITE MEMORIAL MEDICAL CENTER, LOS ANGELES, CA, p. A73

WHITE MOUNTAIN REGIONAL MEDICAL CENTER, SPRINGERVILLE, AZ, p. A38

WHITE PLAINS HOSPITAL CENTER, WHITE PLAINS, NY, p. A447

# Y

# Z

This section is an index of the key health care professionals for the hospitals and/or health care systems listed in this publication. The index is in alphabetical order, by individual, followed by the title, institutional affiliation, city, state and page reference to the hospital and/or health care system listing in section A and/or B.

## A

AAFEDT, Karen, Assistant Administrator and Controller, Community Memorial Hospital, Turtle Lake, ND, p. A468

AAGARD, Kim, Chief Financial Officer, Tri–County Hospital, Wadena, MN, p. A341

AARON, Michael, M.D. Chief of Staff, Weatherford Regional Hospital, Weatherford, OK, p. A507

AASVED, Craig E., Chief Operating Officer, St. Patrick Hospital, Missoula, MT, p. A378

ABAD, Ann, Vice President Operations, Barnes–Jewish St. Peters Hospital, Saint Peters, MO, p. A370

ABADIER, Ralph, M.D. Chief of Staff, Citrus Memorial Health System, Inverness, FL, p. A126

ABAIR, Cynthia, Associate Director, Veterans Affairs San Diego Healthcare System, San Diego, CA, p. A86

ABARICIA, Eduardo, Director Information Technology, Northwest Missouri Psychiatric Rehabilitation Center, Saint Joseph, MO, p. A368

ABBATE, Richard, Director Human Resources, Sutter Lakeside Hospital, Lakeport, CA, p. A66

ABBEN, Richard, M.D. Chief of Staff, Terrebonne General Medical Center, Houma, LA, p. A268

ABBOTT, Jody, Senior Vice President and Chief Operating Officer, North Kansas City Hospital, North Kansas City, MO, p. A366

ABBOTT, Keith, Chief Executive Officer, Basin Healthcare Center, Odessa, TX, p. A619

ABBOTT, Peggy, Vice President, Ouachita County Medical Center, Camden, AR, p. A43

ABBOTT, Richard, M.D. Medical Advisor Quality Improvement, Skagit Valley Hospital, Mount Vernon, WA, p. A663

ABBOUD, Della, Chief Executive Officer, St. Luke's Rehabilitation Hospital, Chesterfield, MO, p. A357

ABDA, William, Chief Human Resources Officer, Clarks Summit State Hospital, Clarks Summit, PA, p. A520

ABE, John, M.D. Chief of Staff, Saint Joseph – London, London, KY, p. A254

ABEL, Barbara J., Vice President Human Resources, Heart of the Rockies Regional Medical Center, Salida, CO, p. A105

ABEL, Douglas A., Chief Information Officer, Anne Arundel Medical Center, Annapolis, MD, p. A287

ABEL, Kevin, Chief Executive Officer, Lake Chelan Community Hospital, Chelan, WA, p. A660

ABEL, Stacy L., Director Human Resources, Craig Hospital, Englewood, CO, p. A100

ABELS, Duane E., M.D. Chief of Staff, Memorial Hospital of Carbon County, Rawlins, WY, p. A697

ABELSON, David, M.D. Chief Executive Officer, Park Nicollet Health Services, Saint Louis Park, MN, p. B100

ABELSON, David, M.D. President and Chief Executive Officer, Park Nicollet Methodist Hospital, Saint Louis Park, MN, p. A339

ABELY, Susan Cerrone, Vice President and Chief Information Officer, Roger Williams Medical Center, Providence, RI, p. A545

ABENDROTH, Thomas, M.D. Chief Information Officer, Penn State Milton S. Hershey Medical Center, Hershey, PA, p. A525

ABERCROMBIE, David, Chief Executive Officer, Madison County Memorial Hospital, Madison, FL, p. A129

ABERNATHY, Jennifer, Assistant Administrator, Mayo Clinic Health System – Chippewa Valley in Bloomer, Bloomer, WI, p. A679

ABERNETHY, Linda O., R.N. Superintendent, Dorothea Dix Psychiatric Center, Bangor, ME, p. A281

ABERNETHY, Robert, Chief Financial Officer, Medical Center Health System, Odessa, TX, p. A619

ABEYTA, Mary Anna, R.N. Chief Nursing/Clinical Services Officer, Holy Cross Hospital, Taos, NM, p. A418

ABINSAY, Alvin, M.D. Chief Medical Staff, Marion Regional Hospital, Mullins, SC, p. A552

ABNEY, Stuart, Controller, Jasper Memorial Hospital, Monticello, GA, p. A156

ABOUD, Al, Chief Financial Officer, East Orange General Hospital, East Orange, NJ, p. A403

ABRAHAM, Akram, M.D. Chief of Staff, Harmon Memorial Hospital, Hollis, OK, p. A498

ABRAHAM, Paul, Chief Operating Officer, Centennial Medical Center, Frisco, TX, p. A600

ABRAHAMY, Ran, M.D. Chief of Staff, University Hospital and Medical Center, Tamarac, FL, p. A140

ABRAMOVICH, Mark, M.D. Chief of Staff, Flaget Memorial Hospital, Bardstown, KY, p. A247

ABRAMOVITZ, Alan L., Director Human Resources, Saint Luke's North Hospital – Barry Road, Kansas City, MO, p. A362

ABRAMS, David, Vice President Human Resources, North Memorial Health Care, Robbinsdale, MN, p. A338

ABREU, Astrid J., Chief Executive Officer, Hospital Metropolitano Dr. Tito Mattei, Yauco, PR, p. A704

ABREU, Iris, Supervisor Human Resources, Hospital HMA de Humacao, Humacao, PR, p. A701

ABREU, John, Vice President and Chief Financial Officer, Portneuf Medical Center, Pocatello, ID, p. A170

ABRINA, Sofia
Administrator and Chief Nursing Officer, Garden Grove Hospital and Medical Center, Garden Grove, CA, p. A63
Administrator and Chief Nursing Officer, Huntington Beach Hospital, Huntington Beach, CA, p. A65

ABROMOVICH, Sari, Chief Executive Officer, Harbor Oaks Hospital, New Baltimore, MI, p. A320

ABRUTZ Jr., Joseph F., Administrator, Cameron Regional Medical Center, Cameron, MO, p. A356

ABSHIRE, Allen, Director Information Services, CHRISTUS St. Patrick Hospital of Lake Charles, Lake Charles, LA, p. A271

ABUIN, Jack, Director Management Information Systems, The Mount Sinai Hospital of Queens, NY, p. A437

ACEBO, Raymond, M.D. Director Medical Staff, Corpus Christi Specialty Hospital, Corpus Christi, TX, p. A589

ACETO, Anthony, Vice President Human Resources, Norwalk Hospital, Norwalk, CT, p. A111

ACEUEDO, Vivian, CPA Chief Financial Director, Hospital Metropolitano Dr. Susoni, Arecibo, PR, p. A700

ACEVEDO, Ana, Supervisor Human Resources, San Jorge Children's Hospital, San Juan, PR, p. A703

ACEVEDO, Jose, M.D. President and Chief Executive Officer, Finger Lakes Health, Geneva, NY, p. B52

ACEVEDO, Jose, M.D
President and Chief Executive Officer, Geneva General Hospital, Geneva, NY, p. A426
President and Chief Executive Officer, Soldiers and Sailors Memorial Hospital of Yates County, Penn Yan, NY, p. A440

ACEVEDO, Ramon, Supervisor Information Systems, Hospital San Cristobal, Coto Laurel, PR, p. A701

ACEVEDO, Vivian, Chief Financial Officer, Metropolitan Hospital of Miami, Miami, FL, p. A131

ACHAMALLAH, Nagui, M.D. Chief of Staff, John Muir Behavioral Health Center, Concord, CA, p. A58

ACHBER, Linda, Director Clinical Services, Aurora Behavioral Health Care, San Diego, CA, p. A85

ACHTER, Dick, Chief Financial Officer, Barrett Hospital & HealthCare, Dillon, MT, p. A375

ACHTERHOFF, Shari, R.N. Chief Nursing Officer, Murray County Medical Center, Slayton, MN, p. A340

ACKELSON, Rocky, Director Information Services, Arkansas Valley Regional Medical Center, La Junta, CO, p. A103

ACKER, Carmen
Chief Financial Officer, Fishermen's Hospital, Marathon, FL, p. A129
Chief Financial Officer, St. Cloud Regional Medical Center, Saint Cloud, FL, p. A137

ACKER, David B., FACHE President and Chief Executive Officer, Canton–Potsdam Hospital, Potsdam, NY, p. A441

ACKER, Peter W., President, Carolinas Medical Center–Lincoln, Lincolnton, NC, p. A456

ACKERMAN, S. Jeffrey, M.D. Chief Executive Officer, Doctors Diagnostic Hospital, Cleveland, TX, p. A587

ACKERMAN, Sigurd H., M.D. President and Chief Executive Officer, Silver Hill Hospital, New Canaan, CT, p. A110

ACKERS, Allen R., Associate Director, William S. Middleton Memorial Veterans Hospital, Madison, WI, p. A684

ACKERSON, David, Chief Information Officer, Seattle Cancer Care Alliance, Seattle, WA, p. A666

ACKERT, Sara, Associate Director, Sioux Falls VA Health Care System, Sioux Falls, SD, p. A560

ACKISS, Jane, Site Manager Human Resources, Naval Medical Center, Portsmouth, VA, p. A654

ACKLAND, Jeanne, Manager Accounting and Acting Chief Financial Officer, Fillmore County Hospital, Geneva, NE, p. A383

ACKLEY, Michael, Chief Financial Officer, Kentucky River Medical Center, Jackson, KY, p. A252

ACKLIN, Traci, M.D. Chief of Staff, Montgomery General Hospital, Montgomery, WV, p. A673

ACKMAN, Jeffrey D., M.D. Chief of Staff, Shriners Hospitals for Children–Chicago, Chicago, IL, p. A178

ACKMAN, Laura, Administrator, Essentia Health Northern Pines, Aurora, MN, p. A328

ACOSTA, Ivan, M.D. Medical Director, Hospital De La Concepcion, San German, PR, p. A702

ACOSTA, Louis, M.D. Chief of Staff, Silver Lake Medical Center, Los Angeles, CA, p. A72

ACOSTA, Maridel, Chief Executive Officer, Alta Vista Regional Hospital, Las Vegas, NM, p. A417

ACOSTA, Nannete, Director Human Resources, Hospital Metropolitano Dr. Tito Mattei, Yauco, PR, p. A704

ACOSTA–CARLSON, Francisca, M.D. Chief of Staff, Lexington Regional Health Center, Lexington, NE, p. A385

ACREE, Charis, Senior Vice President, West Georgia Health, La Grange, GA, p. A155

ACTERHOF, Trudy, Director Human Resources, Baldwin Area Medical Center, Baldwin, WI, p. A678

ADAIR, Dale K., M.D. Chief Medical Officer, Wernersville State Hospital, Wernersville, PA, p. A540

ADAM, Sheryl, Chief Financial Officer, Hanover Hospital, Hanover, KS, p. A234

ADAMO, James S., M.D. Medical Director, Harbor Oaks Hospital, New Baltimore, MI, p. A320

ADAMO, Peter J., Chief Executive Officer, Roxborough Memorial Hospital, Philadelphia, PA, p. A533

ADAMS, Alan L., President, Memorial Hospital, Stilwell, OK, p. A505

ADAMS, Amy B.
Executive Director Human Resources, Laureate Psychiatric Clinic and Hospital, Tulsa, OK, p. A506
Executive Director Human Resources, Saint Francis Hospital, Tulsa, OK, p. A506

ADAMS, Angela C., Director Human Resources, Good Samaritan Hospital, Greensboro, GA, p. A153

ADAMS, Bob, Director Information Services, Bay Area Hospital, Coos Bay, OR, p. A510

ADAMS, Carolyn L., Director, Ralph H. Johnson Veterans Affairs Medical Center, Charleston, SC, p. A547

ADAMS, Charles T., President and Chief Executive Officer, Ty Cobb Healthcare System, Inc., Royston, GA, p. B131

ADAMS, Charlotte, Director Associate Resources, Carolina Pines Regional Medical Center, Hartsville, SC, p. A551

ADAMS, Chris, Vice President Operations, Good Samaritan Regional Health Center, Mount Vernon, IL, p. A188

ADAMS, Chris, M.D. Physician, Rangely District Hospital, Rangely, CO, p. A105

ADAMS, Cynthia, Vice President Human Resources, StoneCrest Medical Center, Smyrna, TN, p. A575

ADAMS, Daniel H., Vice President and Chief Operating Officer, Memorial Medical Center – Ashland, Ashland, WI, p. A678

ADAMS, Dian, R.N. Chief Nursing Officer, Good Samaritan Hospital, San Jose, CA, p. A88

ADAMS, Diane, Director Business Services, Temple Community Hospital, Los Angeles, CA, p. A72

ADAMS, Earl, Chief Information Officer, Indiana University Health La Porte Hospital, La Porte, IN, p. A206

ADAMS, Gini, Director Employee and Public Relations, Yuma District Hospital, Yuma, CO, p. A107

ADAMS, Jason M., Chief Operating Officer, Cape Cod Hospital, Hyannis, MA, p. A301

ADAMS, Jennifer B., Chief Operating Officer and Chief Financial Officer, Lake City Medical Center, Lake City, FL, p. A128

ADAMS, Jo, Director Human Resources, Donalsonville Hospital, Donalsonville, GA, p. A151

ADAMS, Karen, Director Human Resources, Baxter Regional Medical Center, Mountain Home, AR, p. A49

ADAMS, Liz, Manager Informatics, The Women's Hospital, Newburgh, IN, p. A210

Index of Health Care Professionals

Index of Health Care Professionals / Albaugh


ALBAUGH, Jolene, R.N. Vice President and Chief Nursing Officer, Adventist Bolingbrook Hospital, Bolingbrook, IL, p. A174

ALBAUGH, Rick, Manager Information Services, Southwest Regional Rehabilitation Center, Battle Creek, MI, p. A308

ALBERG, Ellen, Director Human Resources, Johnson Memorial Health Services, Dawson, MN, p. A330

ALBERT, Debra, MSN Chief Nursing Officer, MacNeal Hospital, Berwyn, IL, p. A173

ALBERT, James, Chief Information Officer, Jordan Hospital, Plymouth, MA, p. A304

ALBERT, Kristine, Personnel Officer, Riverview Psychiatric Center, Augusta, ME, p. A281

ALBERT, Waleed, M.D. Chief Medical Officer, Rome Memorial Hospital, Rome, NY, p. A442

ALBERTI, Harry, M.D. Chief Medical Officer and Vice President Medical Affairs, Verde Valley Medical Center, Cottonwood, AZ, p. A31

ALBERTINI, Bernie, Chief Administrative Officer, Ohio Valley Medical Center, Wheeling, WV, p. A676

ALBERTO, Carl M., Vice President Finance and Chief Financial Officer, St. Luke's Hospital – Warren Campus, Phillipsburg, NJ, p. A408

ALBERTS, Patrick J., Senior Vice President and Chief Operating Officer, Monongahela Valley Hospital, Monongahela, PA, p. A529

ALBERTS, W. Michael, M.D. Vice President Medical Affairs, H. Lee Moffitt Cancer Center and Research Institute, Tampa, FL, p. A140

ALBIN, James, Interim Chief Information Officer, St. Luke's Episcopal Hospital, Houston, TX, p. A606

ALBRECHT, David L., President, Owatonna Hospital, Owatonna, MN, p. A336

ALBRIGHT, Aaron, Chief Information Officer, Booneville Community Hospital, Booneville, AR, p. A42

ALBRIGHT, Bill, Director Human Resources, Stewart Memorial Community Hospital, Lake City, IA, p. A222

ALBRIGHT, David, M.D. Chief Medical Officer, Brattleboro Memorial Hospital, Brattleboro, VT, p. A643

ALBRIGHT, Jody, Vice President Information Services and Chief Information Officer, Overlake Hospital Medical Center, Bellevue, WA, p. A659

ALBRIGHT, Mark, Director of Information Services, Yampa Valley Medical Center, Steamboat Springs, CO, p. A106

ALBRIGHT, Tina, Vice President Human Resources and Consumer Advocacy, Arkansas Surgical Hospital, North Little Rock, AR, p. A49

ALBRITTON, Kathy, Director Human Resources, Roosevelt Warm Springs LTAC Hospital, Warm Springs, GA, p. A161

ALBUS, Nicole, Chief Human Resources, James E. Van Zandt Veterans Affairs Medical Center, Altoona, PA, p. A517

ALCALA, Paul, Vice President and Chief Information Officer, NorthBay Medical Center, Fairfield, CA, p. A60

ALCOCER, Deborah, Chief Information Officer, South Texas Rehabilitation Hospital, Brownsville, TX, p. A585

ALDERFER, Jennifer, Chief Executive Officer, North Suburban Medical Center, Thornton, CO, p. A106

ALDERSON, Charles
- Chief Financial Officer, Summa Barberton Citizens Hospital, Barberton, OH, p. A470
- Chief Financial Officer, Summa Wadsworth–Rittman Hospital, Wadsworth, OH, p. A490

ALDIS, Karen, Director of Nursing, Harper Hospital District Five, Harper, KS, p. A234

ALDRED, Linda W., Senior Vice President, Texas Children's Hospital, Houston, TX, p. A607

ALDREDGE, Sarah, M.D. Chief Medical Officer, Essentia Health Sandstone, Sandstone, MN, p. A339

ALDRICH, Alan, Chief Financial Officer, Central Montana Medical Center, Lewistown, MT, p. A377

ALDRIDGE, Kenneth, M.D. Vice President Medical Affairs, DCH Regional Medical Center, Tuscaloosa, AL, p. A26

ALEEM, Asaf, M.D. Medical Director, Peachford Behavioral Health System, Atlanta, GA, p. A145

ALEMAN, Ralph A., Chief Executive Officer, Hialeah Hospital, Hialeah, FL, p. A125

ALENDER, James P., President and Chief Executive Officer, Community Howard Regional Hospital, Kokomo, IN, p. A206

ALESI, Linda, Director Human Resources, OhioHealth Marion General Hospital, Marion, OH, p. A484

ALEXANDA, Lisa, M.D. Vice President Medical Affairs, Parrish Medical Center, Titusville, FL, p. A142

ALEXANDER, Alan B., Chief Executive Officer, Caverna Memorial Hospital, Horse Cave, KY, p. A252

ALEXANDER, Albert L., Chief Human Resources Officer, Halifax Health Medical Center of Daytona Beach, Daytona Beach, FL, p. A122

ALEXANDER, April, Director Human Resources, Metropolitan Hospital Center, New York, NY, p. A434

ALEXANDER, Craig, Fiscal Specialist, Thomas B. Finan Center, Cumberland, MD, p. A291

ALEXANDER, Dean M., Chief Executive Officer, Methodist Stone Oak Hospital, San Antonio, TX, p. A625

ALEXANDER, Debra, Chief Information Officer, Boise Behavioral Health Hospital, Boise, ID, p. A166

ALEXANDER, Fred, M.D. Medical Director, West Los Angeles Medical Center, Los Angeles, CA, p. A72

ALEXANDER, Gene, Chief Financial Officer, MountainView Regional Medical Center, Las Cruces, NM, p. A416

ALEXANDER, Jack, M.D. Chief Medical Officer, Mayo Clinic Health System in Red Wing, Red Wing, MN, p. A337

ALEXANDER, Jason P., FACHE Chief Executive Officer, East Cooper Medical Center, Mount Pleasant, SC, p. A552

ALEXANDER, Jr., John, M.D. Chief of Staff, Magnolia Regional Medical Center, Magnolia, AR, p. A48

ALEXANDER, Keith N., Chief Executive Officer, Memorial Hermann Memorial City Medical Center, Houston, TX, p. A605

ALEXANDER, Michael, Administrator, Higgins General Hospital, Bremen, GA, p. A148

ALEXANDER, Peter H.
- Administrator, St. Vincent Seton Specialty Hospital, Indianapolis, IN, p. A205
- Administrator, St. Vincent Seton Specialty Hospital, Lafayette, IN, p. A207

ALEXANDER, Richmond, M.D. President Medical Staff, Specialty Hospital of Meridian, Meridian, MS, p. A350

ALEXANDER, Steven, Chief Operating Officer, Bellevue Hospital Center, New York, NY, p. A431

ALEXANDER, Thomas G., Chief Executive Officer, Kindred Hospital–New Orleans, New Orleans, LA, p. A274

ALEXANDER, Trudi, Director Human Resources, Jersey Shore Hospital, Jersey Shore, PA, p. A525

ALEXANDER–HINES, Joyce, R.N. Associate Director, Patient Care Services, Veterans Affairs Medical Center, Fayetteville, NC, p. A453

ALEXANDER–LANE, Victoria, President and Chief Executive Officer, Sebasticook Valley Health, Pittsfield, ME, p. A284

ALFANO, Anthony, Senior Vice President and Chief Operating Officer, New York Downtown Hospital, New York, NY, p. A435

ALFANO, Samuel, D.O. Vice President Medical Affairs, St. Joseph Medical Center, Reading, PA, p. A537

ALFARO, Pedro, Vice President and Chief Financial Officer, Miami Children's Hospital, Miami, FL, p. A131

ALFONSO, Eduardo, M.D. Chairman Ophthalmology, Bascom Palmer Eye Institute–Anne Bates Leach Eye Hospital, Miami, FL, p. A131

ALFORD, Charles, Vice President Financial Services, Vidant Edgecombe Hospital, Tarboro, NC, p. A461

ALFORD, Larry Don, Chief Financial Officer, Saline Memorial Hospital, Benton, AR, p. A42

ALFORD, Wendell, Administrator, Madison Parish Hospital, Tallulah, LA, p. A278

ALFRED, Lorrie, Director Human Resources, Southern Surgical Hospital, Slidell, LA, p. A278

ALFSON, Jared, Chief Information Officer, Community Memorial Hospital, Oconto Falls, WI, p. A688

ALGER, Steve, Senior Vice President and Chief Financial Officer, Lakes Regional Healthcare, Spirit Lake, IA, p. A227

ALI, Irfan, Director Information Services, Saint Agnes Medical Center, Fresno, CA, p. A62

ALI, Juzar, M.D. Chief of Staff, Kindred Hospital–New Orleans, New Orleans, LA, p. A274

ALI, Mirza Z., M.D. Chief of Staff, Veterans Affairs Medical Center, Wilkes–Barre, PA, p. A542

ALI, Mohammad, M.D. President Medical Staff, Jameson Hospital, New Castle, PA, p. A530

ALI, Solomon, M.D. Chief of Staff, Fairview Regional Medical Center, Fairview, OK, p. A496

ALI–KHAN, Mir, M.D. Medical Director, Canyon Ridge Hospital, Chino, CA, p. A57

ALKHOULI, Hassan, M.D
- Chief Medical Officer, Garden Grove Hospital and Medical Center, Garden Grove, CA, p. A63
- Medical Director, Huntington Beach Hospital, Huntington Beach, CA, p. A65
- Chief Medical Officer, West Anaheim Medical Center, Anaheim, CA, p. A53

ALLARD, Joan, Director Human Resources, Heart of Florida Regional Medical Center, Davenport, FL, p. A121

ALLARD, Rebecca, M.D. Chief of Staff, Cheyenne County Hospital, Saint Francis, KS, p. A242

ALLATT, Richard, M.D. Medical Director, HEALTHSOUTH Nittany Valley Rehabilitation Hospital, Pleasant Gap, PA, p. A536

ALLBRITTON, James, Chief Financial Officer, Morehouse General Hospital, Bastrop, LA, p. A262

ALLEN, Audrey, Coordinator Benefits, Dallas County Medical Center, Fordyce, AR, p. A45

ALLEN, Brian, M.D. President Medical Staff, Georgetown Community Hospital, Georgetown, KY, p. A250

ALLEN, Carolyn, Chief Financial Officer, Sharon Hospital, Sharon, CT, p. A111

ALLEN, Claudia, Chief Information Officer, St. John Hospital and Medical Center, Detroit, MI, p. A311

ALLEN, Cyril, M.D. Chief Medical Officer, United Medical Center, Washington, DC, p. A117

ALLEN, David B., Chief Executive Officer, Richland Memorial Hospital, Olney, IL, p. A190

ALLEN, Dawn, R.N. Chief Clinical Officer, Redwood Area Hospital, Redwood Falls, MN, p. A337

ALLEN, Denise, Administrator, Behavioral Hospital of Longview, Longview, TX, p. A613

ALLEN, Douglas, Vice President Human Resources, Cooper Health System, Camden, NJ, p. A402

ALLEN, Elizabeth, Vice President Finance, Trinity Health System, Steubenville, OH, p. A489

ALLEN, Elms, M.D
- Senior Vice President Medical Affairs, Forsyth Medical Center, Winston–Salem, NC, p. A463
- Senior Vice President Medical Affairs, Medical Park Hospital, Winston–Salem, NC, p. A463

ALLEN, Jane, Director Human Resources and Payroll, Liberty Medical Center, Chester, MT, p. A374

ALLEN, Joanne E., President and Chief Executive Officer, Saint Louise Regional Hospital, Gilroy, CA, p. A63

ALLEN, John
- Chief Information Officer, Holzer Medical Center, Gallipolis, OH, p. A480
- Chief Executive Officer, Regency Hospital of Minneapolis, Golden Valley, MN, p. A332

ALLEN, Judy, Human Resource Specialist, Carl Albert Community Mental Health Center, McAlester, OK, p. A499

ALLEN, Kandice K., R.N. Interim Chief Executive Officer, Share Medical Center, Alva, OK, p. A493

ALLEN, Laura, Chief Financial Officer, Dauterive Hospital, New Iberia, LA, p. A274

ALLEN, Linda, Vice President Quality and Information Systems, Monongalia General Hospital, Morgantown, WV, p. A674

ALLEN, Lori, Chief Financial Officer, Anthony Medical Center, Anthony, KS, p. A230

ALLEN, Maria, Chief Financial Officer, Ed Fraser Memorial Hospital and Baker Community Health Center, MacClenny, FL, p. A129

ALLEN, Mark L., FACHE Administrator, Sanpete Valley Hospital, Mount Pleasant, UT, p. A638

ALLEN, Marsha, Director Human Resources, W. J. Mangold Memorial Hospital, Lockney, TX, p. A613

ALLEN, Michael, Chief Financial Officer, Winona Health, Winona, MN, p. A342

ALLEN, Mike
- Director Information Technology, McKenzie–Willamette Medical Center, Springfield, OR, p. A515
- Director Information Services, Shawnee Mission Medical Center, Shawnee Mission, KS, p. A243
- Director Information Technology, Shriners Hospitals for Children–Intermountain, Salt Lake City, UT, p. A641

ALLEN, Nancy, R.N. Director, Patient Services/CNE, Advocate Eureka Hospital, Eureka, IL, p. A181

ALLEN, Nikki, Patient Care Executive, Sutter Amador Hospital, Jackson, CA, p. A65

ALLEN, Paul, M.D. Vice President Medical Affairs, Holy Family Hospital and Medical Center, Methuen, MA, p. A302

ALLEN, R. Keith, Senior Vice President Human Resources, University of Maryland Medical Center, Baltimore, MD, p. A289

ALLEN, Robert
- Chief Financial Officer, California Hospital Medical Center, Los Angeles, CA, p. A68
- Vice President and Chief Financial Officer, Glendale Memorial Hospital and Health Center, Glendale, CA, p. A63

ALLEN, Robert, M.D. Vice President Medical Affairs, Rapid City Regional Hospital, Rapid City, SD, p. A559

ALLEN, Robert W., Chief Executive Officer, Park City Medical Center, Park City, UT, p. A639

ALLEN, Steve, M.D. Chief Executive Officer, Nationwide Children's Hospital, Columbus, OH, p. A477

ALLEN, Timothy, Senior Vice President and Chief Operating Officer, Parkview Medical Center, Pueblo, CO, p. A105

ALLEN, Timothy M., Vice President Human Resources, United Hospital Center, Bridgeport, WV, p. A670

ALLEN, Tracey, Chief Financial Officer, HEALTHSOUTH Rehabilitation Hospital of Beaumont, Beaumont, TX, p. A583

ALLEN, Vicki, R.N. Chief Nursing Officer & Vice President Patient Care Services, Betsy Johnson Regional Hospital, Dunn, NC, p. A452

ALLEN, Vicki, Chief Financial Officer, Chicot Memorial Medical Center, Lake Village, AR, p. A47

ALLEN, Wayne, Chief Financial Officer, Mendocino Coast District Hospital, Fort Bragg, CA, p. A61


**A750** Index of Health Care Professionals 

Index of Health Care Professionals / Anderson

Index of Health Care Professionals


ALLEN, Zac, CPA Chief Financial Officer, Cherokee Medical Center, Centre, AL, p. A18
ALLENDE RUIZ, Luis Z., Executive Director, Hospital Metropolitano Dr. Susoni, Arecibo, PR, p. A700
ALLENSWORTH, Ed, M.D. Medical Director, Craig General Hospital, Vinita, OK, p. A507
ALLEY, Anne, Director Human Resources, Stony Lodge Hospital, Ossining, NY, p. A440
ALLEY, David, Chief Financial Officer, Athens Regional Medical Center, Athens, TN, p. A562
ALLEY, John L., Chief Executive Officer, Woodlawn Hospital, Rochester, IN, p. A211
ALLEY, Steve B., M.D. Chief of Staff, Crosbyton Clinic Hospital, Crosbyton, TX, p. A590
ALLGOOD, Libby, Chief Financial Officer, Kittitas Valley Community Hospital, Ellensburg, WA, p. A661
ALLICON, Keary T., Vice President Finance and Chief Financial Officer, Wing Memorial Hospital and Medical Centers, Palmer, MA, p. A303
ALLIES, Karla, Director Human Resources, Rosebud Health Care Center, Forsyth, MT, p. A375
ALLISON, David G., President and Chief Executive Officer, University Medical Center, Lubbock, TX, p. A614
ALLISON, Joel T., President and Chief Executive Officer, Baylor Health Care System, Dallas, TX, p. B20
ALLISON, Russell, Human Resources Representative, University Behavioral Health of Denton, Denton, TX, p. A594
ALLISON, Shannon, Chief Financial Officer, Patients' Choice Medical Center of Erin, Erin, TN, p. A565
ALLISON, Steve, Director Human Resources, Logan County Hospital, Oakley, KS, p. A240
ALLMAN, Rex, M.D. President Medical Staff, Pulaski Memorial Hospital, Winamac, IN, p. A213
ALLMAN, Roger J., Chief Executive Officer, King's Daughters' Hospital and Health Services, Madison, IN, p. A208
ALLORE, Gary
Chief Financial Officer, Mercy Health Partners, Hackley Campus, Muskegon, MI, p. A319
Chief Financial Officer, Mercy Health Partners, Mercy Campus, Muskegon, MI, p. A319
ALLOWAY, Cindy, Vice President and Chief Operating Officer, Alegent Health–Lakeside Hospital, Omaha, NE, p. A387
ALLPHIN, Allan, M.D. Chief of Staff, Mercy Hospital Springfield, Springfield, MO, p. A371
ALLRED, Al W., Chief Financial Officer, Bert Fish Medical Center, New Smyrna Beach, FL, p. A133
ALLRED, B. Dee, M.D
President Medical Staff, Jordan Valley Medical Center, West Jordan, UT, p. A642
President Medical Staff, Pioneer Valley Hospital, West Valley City, UT, p. A642
ALLRED, Kyla, Manager Human Resources, Bartlett Regional Hospital, Juneau, AK, p. A29
ALLRED, Lowell C., M.D. Chief of Staff, Columbia Basin Hospital, Ephrata, WA, p. A661
ALLRED, Russ, Manager Information Systems, Shoshone Medical Center, Kellogg, ID, p. A168
ALLRED, William, M.D. Vice President Medical Affairs, St. John Medical Center, Tulsa, OK, p. A507
ALLSOP, Brian, Director Human Resources, Central Valley Medical Center, Nephi, UT, p. A639
ALLSTOTT, Patti, Administrative Coordinator Human Resources and Grant Writer, Pioneer Memorial Hospital, Heppner, OR, p. A511
ALLUMS, Allyson, Director Medical Records, North Caddo Medical Center, Vivian, LA, p. A279
ALLVIN, Patricia, Account Executive Information Technology, San Luis Valley Regional Medical Center, Alamosa, CO, p. A97
ALMAUHY, Deborah, R.N. Chief Nursing Officer, Rockdale Medical Center, Conyers, GA, p. A150
ALMEIDA, Sergio, Director Information Systems, West Houston Medical Center, Houston, TX, p. A608
ALMENDINGER, J. Todd, Vice President Finance and Chief Financial Officer, H. B. Magruder Memorial Hospital, Port Clinton, OH, p. A487
ALO, Kathleen, R.N. Chief Nursing Officer, Mammoth Hospital, Mammoth Lakes, CA, p. A73
ALONSO, Jose', M.D. Medical Director, San Juan Capestrano Hospital, San Juan, PR, p. A703
ALONSO, Nancy, Vice President Human Resources, Vista Medical Center East, Waukegan, IL, p. A196
ALONZO, Patti, Manager Human Resources, Pacifica Hospital of the Valley,, CA, p. A71
ALOUISE, Tony, Chief Executive Officer, Three Gables Surgery Center, Proctorville, OH, p. A487
ALPERT, Jeffrey, M.D. Medical Director, Wichita County Health Center, Leoti, KS, p. A238
ALPERT, Len, Director Human Resources, Hollywood Pavilion,, FL, p. A125
ALREDGE, Will, Administrator, Genesis Behavioral Hospital, Breaux Bridge, LA, p. A264
ALSLEBEN, Tony, Director Information Technology, Glencoe Regional Health Services, Glencoe, MN, p. A332
ALSTAD, Nancy, Director Human Resources, Fort HealthCare, Fort Atkinson, WI, p. A681
ALSTER, Howard, M.D. President Medical Staff, Carlisle Regional Medical Center, Carlisle, PA, p. A520
ALSTON, Shawanza L., Administrator, Ascension Gonzales Rehabilitation Hospital, Gonzales, LA, p. A266
ALT, Melinda, Chief Financial Officer, Guthrie County Hospital, Guthrie Center, IA, p. A220
ALTEBARMAKIAN, Varouj, M.D. Physician in Chief, Fresno Medical Center, Fresno, CA, p. A62
ALTENBURGER, Andy, Chief Information Officer, Marietta Memorial Hospital, Marietta, OH, p. A483
ALTMAN, III, Alexander B., Chief Executive Officer and Chief Financial Officer, Copper Basin Medical Center, Copperhill, TN, p. A564
ALTMAN, Brett, Clinical Operations Officer, Skiff Medical Center, Newton, IA, p. A224
ALTMAN, Harold, M.D. Chief Medical Officer, ACMH Hospital, Kittanning, PA, p. A526
ALTMILLER, Steve, President and Chief Executive Officer, North Mississippi Medical Center – Tupelo, Tupelo, MS, p. A353
ALTOE, Ann, Senior Director Information Systems and Security Officer, Alfred I. duPont Hospital for Children, Wilmington, DE, p. A114
ALTON, Aaron K., President and Chief Executive Officer, Sisters of Mary of the Presentation Health System, Fargo, ND, p. B119
ALTON, Andy, Chief Executive Officer, Methodist Behavioral Hospital of Arkansas, Maumelle, AR, p. A48
ALTON, Guy, Chief Financial Officer, St. Bernard Hospital and Health Care Center, Chicago, IL, p. A178
ALTOSE, Murray, M.D. Chief of Staff, Veterans Affairs Medical Center, Cleveland, OH, p. A476
ALTSCHULER, Steven M., M.D. President and Chief Executive Officer, Children's Hospital of Philadelphia, Philadelphia, PA, p. A532
ALTSHULER, Keith, President and Chief Administrative Officer, Fort Sanders Regional Medical Center, Knoxville, TN, p. A568
ALVARADO, Rafael, Chief Executive Officer, Dr. Pila's Hospital, Ponce, PR, p. A702
ALVARADO, Ramona, Interim Manager Human Resources, Adventist Medical Center–Reedley, Reedley, CA, p. A82
ALVAREZ, Dena C., R.N. COO & Chief Compliance Officer, Brodstone Memorial Hospital, Superior, NE, p. A390
ALVAREZ, Jose, M.D. Chief Medical Staff, Circles of Care, Melbourne, FL, p. A130
ALVAREZ, Maria Charlotte, M.D. Chief of Staff, Sheridan Community Hospital, Sheridan, MI, p. A323
ALVAREZ, Mike, M.D. Chief Medical Officer, Dauterive Hospital, New Iberia, LA, p. A274
ALVAREZ, Rafael Garcia, Chief Executive Officer, Hospital Universitario Dr. Ramon Ruiz Arnau, Bayamon, PR, p. A700
ALVAREZ, Valerie, Executive Assistant, Adventist Medical Center–Reedley, Reedley, CA, p. A82
ALVERSON, Tammy S., M.D. Chief of Staff, Coshocton County Memorial Hospital, Coshocton, OH, p. A478
ALVES, Richard, Chief Financial Officer, Fresno Medical Center, Fresno, CA, p. A62
ALVEY, Raymond, Chief Financial Officer, Saint Louis University Hospital, Saint Louis, MO, p. A369
ALVIS, Darlene, Chief Human Resources Officer, McKee Medical Center, Loveland, CO, p. A104
ALWELL, James, Interim Vice President and Chief Financial Officer, Morristown–Hamblen Healthcare System, Morristown, TN, p. A572
ALWINE, Steven, Chief Executive Officer, HEALTHSOUTH Rehabilitation Hospital of York, York, PA, p. A542
AMADO, Mitchell, Chief Financial Officer, Catskill Regional Medical Center, Harris, NY, p. A427
AMAN, Diane, Acting Executive Director, Brooklyn Children's Psychiatric Center,, NY, p. A431
AMANTEA, Paul, Director Finance, University Hospitals Geauga Medical Center, Chardon, OH, p. A472
AMAR Jr., Eugene, Administrator, Kohala Hospital, Kohala, HI, p. A165
AMARO, Wanda, Director Human Resources, Shriners Hospitals for Children, Philadelphia, Philadelphia, PA, p. A533
AMATO, Jerry, Chief Executive Officer, Plano Specialty Hospital, Plano, TX, p. A621
AMATO, Joe, Interim Chief Financial Officer, DeSoto Memorial Hospital, Arcadia, FL, p. A118
AMBACHER, Linda, Interim Chief Nursing Officer, Hackettstown Regional Medical Center, Hackettstown, NJ, p. A404
AMBROSIANI, Michael, Chief Financial Officer, Knox Community Hospital, Mount Vernon, OH, p. A485
AMEEN, David J., President and Chief Executive Officer, Logansport Memorial Hospital, Logansport, IN, p. A207
AMEND, Jeff, Chief Operating Officer, Summit Behavioral Healthcare, Cincinnati, OH, p. A474
AMERSON, Jeff, Director Information System, West Florida Hospital, Pensacola, FL, p. A136
AMES, Julie
Chief Information Officer, R M L Specialty Hospital, Hinsdale, IL, p. A184
Chief Information Officer, RML Specialty Hospital, Chicago, IL, p. A177
AMEY, Mark, Chief Information Officer, Keck Hospital of USC, Los Angeles, CA, p. A70
AMIN, Yogesh, M.D. Medical Director, Select Specialty Hospital–Fort Wayne, Fort Wayne, IN, p. A202
AMIR, Adel, Interim Chief Executive Officer, Carthage Area Hospital, Carthage, NY, p. A424
AMIZICH, Tammy, Chief Nursing Executive, Washington County Hospital, Nashville, IL, p. A189
AMMONS, Brandon, Director Human Resources, Kindred Hospital–Amarillo, Amarillo, TX, p. A578
AMMONS, Donna, Director Human Resources, East Jefferson General Hospital, Metairie, LA, p. A273
AMMONS, Eric, President and Chief Executive Officer, Mercy Hospital Independence, Independence, KS, p. A235
AMODO, Mitch, Vice President and Chief Financial Officer, Orange Regional Medical Center, Middletown, NY, p. A430
AMONS, Gene, Administrator, Oceans Behavioral Hospital of Alexandria, Alexandria, LA, p. A261
AMOROSE, Carl, Vice President Finance, Norton Hospital, Louisville, KY, p. A255
AMOS, Gene, Administrator, Oceans Behavioral Hospital of Baton Rouge, Baton Rouge, LA, p. A262
AMOS, John, COO East Campus, Yavapai Regional Medical Center – East, Prescott Valley, AZ, p. A37
AMOS, Robert, Vice President and Chief Financial Officer, Winchester Medical Center, Winchester, VA, p. A657
AMROM, George, M.D. Vice President Medical Affairs, Hahnemann University Hospital, Philadelphia, PA, p. A532
AMUNDSON, David H., Chief Financial Officer, FirstLight Health System, Mora, MN, p. A336
AMY, Christy, Chief Financial Officer, West Oaks Hospital, Houston, TX, p. A608
AMYX, Maleigha, Chief Information Officer, Rockcastle Regional Hospital and Respiratory Care Center, Mount Vernon, KY, p. A257
ANAND, Ajay, M.D. President Medical Staff, Summers County ARH Hospital, Hinton, WV, p. A672
ANASTASI, Frank, Chief Financial Officer, Pennsylvania Hospital, Philadelphia, PA, p. A533
ANASTASIO, Lance W., President, Winter Haven Hospital, Winter Haven, FL, p. A143
ANAYA Sr., Michael A., FACHE Medical Center Director, Jesse Brown Veterans Affairs Chicago Health Care System, Chicago, IL, p. A176
ANCHONDO, Laura, Administrator Human Resources, Kindred Hospital El Paso, El Paso, TX, p. A596
ANDERMAN, Steven, Chief Operating Officer, Bronx–Lebanon Hospital Center Health Care System,, NY, p. A431
ANDERS, Jr., James M., Administrator and Chief Operating Officer, Kennedy Krieger Institute, Baltimore, MD, p. A287
ANDERS, Robert, Chief Financial Officer, Ouachita County Medical Center, Camden, AR, p. A43
ANDERSEN, Edward, President and Chief Executive Officer, CGH Medical Center, Sterling, IL, p. A194
ANDERSEN, Mark, Senior Vice President Information Systems and Chief Information Officer, Yale–New Haven Hospital, New Haven, CT, p. A111
ANDERSEN, Sue
Chief Financial Officer, French Hospital Medical Center, San Luis Obispo, CA, p. A88
Chief Financial Officer, Marian Medical Center, Santa Maria, CA, p. A90
ANDERSEN, Travis, President, St. Elizabeth Hospital, Appleton, WI, p. A678
ANDERSEN, Wendy, Director Human Resources, Eastern Idaho Regional Medical Center, Idaho Falls, ID, p. A168
ANDERSON, A. Elizabeth, Administrator, University of South Alabama Medical Center, Mobile, AL, p. A23
ANDERSON, Allyson, Chief Administrative Officer, Legacy Meridian Park Hospital, Tualatin, OR, p. A516
ANDERSON, Angie, Director Information Technology, Crawford County Memorial Hospital, Denison, IA, p. A218
ANDERSON, Barbara, Chief Financial Officer, Stanton County Hospital, Johnson, KS, p. A235
ANDERSON, Benjamin, Chief Executive Officer, Ashland Health Center, Ashland, KS, p. A230
ANDERSON, Brad, Chief Financial Officer, Community Memorial Hospital, Cloquet, MN, p. A329


© 2012 AHA Guide Index of Health Care Professionals **A751**

ANDERSON, Brian, Chief Financial Officer, Capital Medical Center, Olympia, WA, p. A663

ANDERSON, Bruce S., Ph.D. President and Chief Executive Officer, Hawaii Health Systems Corporation, Honolulu, HI, p. B57

ANDERSON, C. Lynn, M.D. Interim Chief Executive Officer, Brownsville Doctors Hospital, Brownsville, TX, p. A585

ANDERSON, Cherri, Chief Nursing Officer, Banner Behavioral Health Hospital – Scottsdale, Scottsdale, AZ, p. A38

ANDERSON, Chris, Chief Executive Officer, Singing River Health System, Pascagoula, MS, p. A351

ANDERSON, Colette, Manager Finance, McKenzie County Healthcare System, Watford City, ND, p. A468

ANDERSON, Craig, Director Management Information Systems, River Bend Hospital, West Lafayette, IN, p. A213

ANDERSON, Cy, M.D. Chief of Staff, Newman Regional Health, Emporia, KS, p. A232

ANDERSON, Darla, Chief Financial Officer, Sibley Medical Center, Arlington, MN, p. A327

ANDERSON, David, Chief Executive Officer, Ennis Regional Medical Center, Ennis, TX, p. A597

ANDERSON, David, M.D. Medical Director, Heartland Surgical Specialty Hospital, Overland Park, KS, p. A240

ANDERSON, David W., Executive Vice President Human Resources and Chief Compliance Officer, WellStar Kennestone Hospital, Marietta, GA, p. A156

ANDERSON, Dianne J., R.N. President and Chief Executive Officer, Lawrence General Hospital, Lawrence, MA, p. A301

ANDERSON, Donna C., Director Human Resources, HEALTHSOUTH Sea Pines Rehabilitation Hospital, Melbourne, FL, p. A130

ANDERSON, Duke, President and Chief Executive Officer, Hillsdale Community Health Center, Hillsdale, MI, p. A315

ANDERSON, Edward, Chief Financial Officer, Johnson Regional Medical Center, Clarksville, AR, p. A43

ANDERSON, Jr., Gail, M.D. Chief Medical Officer, LAC–Harbor–University of California at Los Angeles Medical Center, Torrance, CA, p. A92

ANDERSON, Gaynell, M.D. Medical Director, St. Anthony Shawnee Hospital, Shawnee, OK, p. A504

ANDERSON, Gina
Chief Financial Officer, Lovelace Medical Center, Albuquerque, NM, p. A414
Human Resources Officer, Riverview Regional Medical Center North, Carthage, TN, p. A562

ANDERSON, Gladys, Interim CEO, Patients' Choice Medical Center of Erin, Erin, TN, p. A565

ANDERSON, Greg E.
Chief Financial Officer, Emory University Hospital Midtown, Atlanta, GA, p. A145
Chief Financial Officer, Wesley Woods Geriatric Hospital of Emory University, Atlanta, GA, p. A146

ANDERSON, Heidi, Human Resources Specialist, State Hospital South, Blackfoot, ID, p. A166

ANDERSON, J. Bryant, Administrator and Chief Executive Officer, Anthony Medical Center, Anthony, KS, p. A230

ANDERSON, J. Mark, Acting Director, Carl Vinson Veterans Affairs Medical Center, Dublin, GA, p. A152

ANDERSON, JaNelle, Director, Mary Greeley Medical Center, Ames, IA, p. A214

ANDERSON, Jason, Chief Financial Officer, Mackinac Straits Health System, Saint Ignace, MI, p. A322

ANDERSON, Jennifer, Director Human Resources, Weirton Medical Center, Weirton, WV, p. A676

ANDERSON, Jim, Chief Information Officer, Great Plains Regional Medical Center, North Platte, NE, p. A386

ANDERSON, Joann, President and Chief Executive Officer, Southeastern Regional Medical Center, Lumberton, NC, p. A457

ANDERSON, John D., FACHE Administrator, Marshall Medical Center South, Boaz, AL, p. A17

ANDERSON, Jon P., CPA, Chief Executive Officer, Community Westview Hospital, Indianapolis, IN, p. A204

ANDERSON, Jonathon, Director Information Technology and Telecommunications, Fresno Heart and Surgical Hospital, Fresno, CA, p. A62

ANDERSON, Kimball, FACH
Chief Operating Officer, Mountain View Hospital, Payson, UT, p. A639
Chief Executive Officer, Southern Hills Hospital and Medical Center, Las Vegas, NV, p. A393

ANDERSON, Larry B., Chief Executive Officer, Tri-City Medical Center, Oceanside, CA, p. A77

ANDERSON, Layton, Regional Director Human Resources, Saint Joseph's Hospital, Marshfield, WI, p. A685

ANDERSON, Lex S.
Chief Financial Officer, St. John Broken Arrow, Broken Arrow, OK, p. A494
Chief Financial Officer, St. John Medical Center, Tulsa, OK, p. A507
Chief Financial Officer, St. John Owasso, Owasso, OK, p. A503

ANDERSON, Libby, Chief Financial Officer, Satanta District Hospital, Satanta, KS, p. A243

ANDERSON, Lisa K., Vice President Finance, Unity Hospital, Fridley, MN, p. A331

ANDERSON, Lucia E., Senior Vice President Nursing and Chief Nurse Executive, Lake Region Healthcare Corporation, Fergus Falls, MN, p. A331

ANDERSON, Mark, Chief Financial Officer, Lane Regional Medical Center, Zachary, LA, p. A280

ANDERSON, Mark T., Chief Financial Officer, Danville Regional Medical Center, Danville, VA, p. A647

ANDERSON, Mary, R.N. Chief Nursing Officer, East Georgia Regional Medical Center, Statesboro, GA, p. A160

ANDERSON, Mary Ann, R.N. Chief Nursing Officer, Nyack Hospital, Nyack, NY, p. A438

ANDERSON, Matthew, Director Human Resources, Mesa View Regional Hospital, Mesquite, NV, p. A394

ANDERSON, Michael, M.D. Chief Medical Officer, University Hospitals Case Medical Center, Cleveland, OH, p. A476

ANDERSON, Michael S., M.D. Chief of Staff, Southern Virginia Regional Medical Center, Emporia, VA, p. A647

ANDERSON, Mike, Chief Financial Officer, Skiff Medical Center, Newton, IA, p. A224

ANDERSON, Noble, Director Patient Financial Services, Rice Medical Center, Eagle Lake, TX, p. A595

ANDERSON, Patrick, Chief Information Officer, Memorial Medical Center, Modesto, CA, p. A75

ANDERSON, Paula, Administrative Director Human Resources, Endless Mountain Health Systems, Montrose, PA, p. A529

ANDERSON, Rhonda
Executive Vice President Finance and Chief Financial Officer, Columbia St. Mary's Hospital Milwaukee, Milwaukee, WI, p. A686
Executive Vice President Finance and Chief Financial Officer, Columbia St. Mary's Ozaukee Hospital, Mequon, WI, p. A686
Executive Vice President Finance and Chief Financial Officer, Sacred Heart Rehabilitation Institute, Milwaukee, WI, p. A687

ANDERSON, Richard A., President and Chief Executive Officer, St. Luke's University Health Network, Bethlehem, PA, p. B123

ANDERSON, Richard A., President and Chief Executive Officer, St. Luke's University Hospital – Bethlehem Campus, Bethlehem, PA, p. A518

ANDERSON, Rick, M.D. Senior Vice President Medical Affairs and Chief Medical Officer, Methodist Medical Center of Illinois, Peoria, IL, p. A191

ANDERSON, Robert C., Interim Chief Financial Officer, Alameda Hospital, Alameda, CA, p. A53

ANDERSON, Roland, M.D. Medical Director, Arkansas Department of Correction Hospital, Pine Bluff, AR, p. A50

ANDERSON, S. Charles, President and Chief Executive Officer, St. John Medical Center, Tulsa, OK, p. A507

ANDERSON, Sandra L., President, St. Clare Hospital and Health Services, Baraboo, WI, p. A678

ANDERSON, Sharla, Chief Executive Officer, Trinity Mother Frances Rehabilitation Hospital, Tyler, TX, p. A632

ANDERSON, Shawn, Chief Operating Officer, Cary Medical Center, Caribou, ME, p. A282

ANDERSON, Stephanie, Senior Vice President, Finance and Administration, Woman's Hospital, Baton Rouge, LA, p. A263

ANDERSON, Steve
Chief Financial Officer, Community Health Center of Branch County, Coldwater, MI, p. A310
Administrator, Heber Valley Medical Center, Heber City, UT, p. A638
Interim Chief Financial Officer, Newberry County Memorial Hospital, Newberry, SC, p. A553
Chief Operating Officer, Park City Medical Center, Park City, UT, p. A639

ANDERSON, Sue, Senior Vice President, Chief Financial Officer and Chief Information Officer, Virginia Mason Medical Center, Seattle, WA, p. A666

ANDERSON, Susan, Director Information Systems, Texas Health Presbyterian Hospital Plano, Plano, TX, p. A621

ANDERSON, Thomas, M.D
Vice President Medical Affairs, Chambersburg Hospital, Chambersburg, PA, p. A520
Chief of Staff, Veterans Affairs Medical Center, Portland, OR, p. A514
Vice President Medical Affairs, Waynesboro Hospital, Waynesboro, PA, p. A540

ANDERSON, Todd, Chief Financial Officer, Grandview Medical Center, Dayton, OH, p. A478

ANDERSON, Traci, Chief Financial Officer, Memorial Hospital, Seminole, TX, p. A627

ANDERSON, William, M.D. Medical Director, Rosebud Health Care Center, Forsyth, MT, p. A375

ANDERT, Nancy, Director Human Resources, Murray County Medical Center, Slayton, MN, p. A340

ANDERTON, Beth, Vice President Human Resources, Ferrell Hospital, Eldorado, IL, p. A180

ANDRADA, Sally, Chief Information Officer, Los Alamitos Medical Center, Los Alamitos, CA, p. A68

ANDRAE, Andrea, Chief Financial Officer, Palmerton Hospital, Palmerton, PA, p. A531

ANDREASEN, Raymond, M.D. Chief Medical Officer–Inpatient, California Medical Facility, Vacaville, CA, p. A94

ANDRES, Dale, D.O. Senior Vice President Medical Affairs, Mercy Medical Center–Des Moines, Des Moines, IA, p. A218

ANDRES, Leonidas, M.D
Chief of Staff, Chambers County Public Hospital District 1, Anahuac, TX, p. A578
Chief of Staff, Winnie Community Hospital, Winnie, TX, p. A635

ANDRES, Priscilla B., Director Human Resources, OHSU Hospital, Portland, OR, p. A514

ANDRESEN, Daniel, Director Information Services, Conroe Regional Medical Center, Conroe, TX, p. A588

ANDREW, Larry, M.D. Deputy Commander Clinical Services, Moncrief Army Community Hospital, Fort Jackson, SC, p. A550

ANDREW, Mark, M.D. Chief of Staff, Van Diest Medical Center, Webster City, IA, p. A228

ANDREWS, Annika, Senior Vice President and Chief Operating Officer, Northwest Hospital & Medical Center, Seattle, WA, p. A665

ANDREWS, Ashleigh, Manager Human Resources, Riverside Rehabilitation Institute, Newport News, VA, p. A652

ANDREWS, Carolle, Interim Chief Human Resources Officer, University of Connecticut Health Center, John Dempsey Hospital, Farmington, CT, p. A109

ANDREWS, David, Manager Information Systems, Chicot Memorial Medical Center, Lake Village, AR, p. A47

ANDREWS, Jade, Chief Financial Officer, Methodist Hospital for Surgery, Addison, TX, p. A577

ANDREWS, Jim, Chief Financial Officer, North Okaloosa Medical Center, Crestview, FL, p. A121

ANDREWS, John, M.D. Chief of Staff, East Texas Medical Center Tyler, Tyler, TX, p. A632

ANDREWS, Laurie, Chief Human Resources Officer, Memorial Community Health, Aurora, NE, p. A381

ANDREWS, Lawrence, Chief Fiscal Services, Veterans Affairs Medical Center, Dayton, OH, p. A479

ANDREWS, Lisa, Director Human Resources, Lancaster Rehabilitation Hospital, Lancaster, PA, p. A526

ANDREWS, Mike, Assistant Administrator and Chief Operating Officer, OCH Regional Medical Center, Starkville, MS, p. A353

ANDREWS, Paul
Chief Executive Officer, The Brook at Dupont, Louisville, KY, p. A255
Chief Executive Officer, The Brook Hospital – KMI, Louisville, KY, p. A255

ANDREWS, Rebecca, Chief Financial Officer, Northern California Rehabilitation Hospital, Redding, CA, p. A82

ANDREWS, Steve, Chief Financial Officer, Three Rivers Health, Three Rivers, MI, p. A324

ANDREWS, Susan, Chief Executive Officer, Valley Regional Medical Center, Brownsville, TX, p. A585

ANDRITSCH, Scott, Vice President and Chief Financial Officer, Indiana University Health Morgan Hospital, Martinsville, IN, p. A208

ANDRO, Ronald J., Senior Vice President and Chief Operating Officer, Baltimore Washington Medical Center, Glen Burnie, MD, p. A292

ANDRUS, Jonathon, Chief Executive Officer, Fairchild Medical Center, Yreka, CA, p. A96

ANDRUS, Michael G., Administrator and Chief Executive Officer, Franklin County Medical Center, Preston, ID, p. A170

ANDRUS, Terry W., President, East Alabama Medical Center, Opelika, AL, p. A24

ANDURSKY, John, Chief Financial Officer, Highlands Hospital, Connellsville, PA, p. A521

ANFINSON, Julie, Director Human Resources, Mercy Medical Center–Sioux City, Sioux City, IA, p. A226

ANGCO, Manuel, M.D. Chief of Staff, Williamson Memorial Hospital, Williamson, WV, p. A677

ANGELL, Marlin, Associate Director, Veterans Affairs Medical Center, Memphis, TN, p. A572

ANGELL, Troy, Director Human Resources, Two Rivers Behavioral Health System, Kansas City, MO, p. A363

Index of Health Care Professionals / Arledge

ANGELO, Gregory, Chief Fiscal Program, Veterans Affairs Medical Center,, NY, p. A437
ANGLE, Gregory R., President and Chief Executive Officer, Los Robles Hospital and Medical Center, Thousand Oaks, CA, p. A92
ANGLE, James L., FACH
Chief Executive Officer, St. Luke's Jerome Family Medical Center, Jerome, ID, p. A168
Chief Executive Officer, St. Luke's Magic Valley Medical Center, Twin Falls, ID, p. A171
ANGLIN, Jason, Chief Executive Officer, Memorial Medical Center, Port Lavaca, TX, p. A622
ANGUEIRA, Carlos, Deputy Commander Clinical Services, San Antonio Military Medical Center, Fort Sam Houston, TX, p. A598
ANGUIANO, Francisco, M.D. Chief of Staff, Sharp Chula Vista Medical Center, Chula Vista, CA, p. A57
ANKIN, Michael G., M.D
Vice President Medical Affairs & Chief Medical Officer, Northwestern Lake Forest Hospital, Lake Forest, IL, p. A186
Vice President Medical Affairs & Chief Medical Officer, Northwestern Memorial Hospital, Chicago, IL, p. A177
ANMUTH, Craig, M.D. Medical Director, Bacharach Institute for Rehabilitation, Pomona, NJ, p. A409
ANNARINO, Phillip, Vice President Human Resources, Fisher–Titus Medical Center, Norwalk, OH, p. A486
ANNECHARICO, Mary Alice
Chief Information Officer, Henry Ford Hospital, Detroit, MI, p. A310
Senior VP and CIO, Henry Ford Health System, Henry Ford Wyandotte Hospital, Wyandotte, MI, p. A325
ANNESSER, Sue
Director Information Technology, Freeman Hospital West, Joplin, MO, p. A361
Director Information Systems, Freeman Neosho Hospital, Neosho, MO, p. A366
ANNICELLI, Susan, Commander, DeWitt Army Community Hospital, Fort Belvoir, VA, p. A648
ANNIS, Donald E., Chief Executive Officer, Crawford Memorial Hospital, Robinson, IL, p. A192
ANOTHAYANONTHA, Aaron, Chief Executive Officer, Kindred Hospital Kansas City, Kansas City, MO, p. A362
ANSEDE, Scott, Chief Operating Officer, Aiken Regional Medical Centers, Aiken, SC, p. A546
ANSELL, David A., M.D. Vice President and Chief Medical Officer, Rush University Medical Center, Chicago, IL, p. A178
ANSELL, L. V., M.D. Medical Director, Houston Orthopedic and Spine Hospital, Bellaire, TX, p. A583
ANSI, Azena, Manager Health Information Management, Horizon Specialty Hospital, Las Vegas, NV, p. A393
ANSLEY, Pamela, Director Finance, Sutter Center for Psychiatry, Sacramento, CA, p. A84
ANTANGAN, Cesar, Director Information Systems, Bellflower Medical Center, Bellflower, CA, p. A55
ANTCZAK, Kenneth
Vice President Human Resources, St. Joseph Mercy Livingston Hospital, Howell, MI, p. A315
Vice President Human Resources, St. Mary Mercy Hospital, Livonia, MI, p. A318
ANTES, John
President, Barnes–Jewish St. Peters Hospital, Saint Peters, MO, p. A370
President, Progress West HealthCare Center, Saint Charles, MO, p. A367
ANTHONY, Anne G., FACHE President and Chief Executive Officer, Willow Crest Hospital, Miami, OK, p. A499
ANTHONY, Jean, Chief Operating Officer and Vice President Patient Services, Hills & Dales General Hospital, Cass City, MI, p. A309
ANTHONY, Kenneth J., Chief Executive Officer, HEALTHSOUTH Harmarville Rehabilitation Hospital, Pittsburgh, PA, p. A534
ANTHONY, Kimberly L., Chief Executive Officer, Jamestown Regional Medical Center, Jamestown, TN, p. A567
ANTHONY, Mark, Executive Vice President and Chief Operating Officer, Borgess Medical Center, Kalamazoo, MI, p. A316
ANTHONY, Paula
Vice President Information Services, East Texas Medical Center Pittsburg, Pittsburg, TX, p. A620
Vice President Information Services, East Texas Medical Center Rehabilitation Center, Tyler, TX, p. A632
Vice President Information Services, East Texas Medical Center Specialty Hospital, Tyler, TX, p. A632
Vice President Information Services, East Texas Medical Center Tyler, Tyler, TX, p. A632
ANTINELLI, Mark, Manager Human Resources, Veterans Affairs Medical Center, Syracuse, NY, p. A444
ANTINORI, James, M.D. Chief of Staff, Mountain West Medical Center, Tooele, UT, p. A641
ANTON, Lourdes, Director Human Resources, Palm Springs General Hospital, Hialeah, FL, p. A125
ANTONACCI, Amy, Vice President Nursing Services, Alliance Community Hospital, Alliance, OH, p. A469
ANTONECCHIA, Paul, M.D. Vice President Medical Affairs, St. John's Riverside Hospital, Yonkers, NY, p. A447
ANTONSON, Pete, Chief Executive Officer, Sanford Northwood Deaconess Health Center, Northwood, ND, p. A467
ANTONUCCI, Lawrence, M.D
Chief Operating Officer, Cape Coral Hospital, Cape Coral, FL, p. A120
Chief Operating Officer, Gulf Coast Medical Center, Fort Myers, FL, p. A123
Chief Operating Officer, Lee Memorial Hospital, Fort Myers, FL, p. A124
ANTWINE, Brenda M.
Chief Executive Officer, Mesquite Rehabilitation Hospital, Mesquite, TX, p. A616
Chief Executive Officer, Mesquite Specialty Hospital, Mesquite, TX, p. A616
ANUSZKIEWICZ, Dawn, Chief Operating Officer, Saint Louis University Hospital, Saint Louis, MO, p. A369
ANWAR, Muhammad, M.D. Chief Medical Officer, Encino Hospital Medical Center,, CA, p. A69
ANZEVENO, Jim, Chief Information Officer, Faulkner Hospital, Boston, MA, p. A296
APKON, Michael, M.D. Senior Vice President and Chief Medical Officer, Children's Hospital of Philadelphia, Philadelphia, PA, p. A532
APLAND, Wendy
Interim Chief Financial Officer, Sacred Heart Medical Center, Eugene, OR, p. A510
Regional Vice President of Finance/Chief Financial Officer, Sacred Heart Medical Center at RiverBend, Springfield, OR, p. A516
APODACA, Mark, Chief Financial Officer, Anaheim General Hospital, Anaheim, CA, p. A53
APOLIONA, Nicole, M.D. Medical Director, Kula Hospital, Kula, HI, p. A165
APONTE, Miguel, Supervisor Management Information Systems, Wilma N. Vazquez Medical Center, Vega Baja, PR, p. A704
APPEL, G. Robert, Chief Executive Officer, Mason General Hospital, Shelton, WA, p. A666
APPENHEIMER, Tim, M.D. Vice President and Chief Medical Officer, Katherine Shaw Bethea Hospital, Dixon, IL, p. A180
APPENZELLER, George, Commander, Bassett Army Community Hospital, Fort Wainwright, AK, p. A29
APPLE, Donald L., Chief Financial Officer, Saint John's Health System, Anderson, IN, p. A197
APPLEBAUM, Jon D., President and Chief Executive Officer, Twin County Regional Hospital, Galax, VA, p. A649
APPLEGATE, Mary Jane, Chief Nursing Officer, Knoxville Hospital & Clinics, Knoxville, IA, p. A222
APPLING, J. Scott, M.D. Chief of Staff, Rush County Memorial Hospital, La Crosse, KS, p. A237
APRILE, Patricia, Chief Executive Officer, Henrietta D. Goodall Hospital, Sanford, ME, p. A285
AQUILINA, Joanne, Vice President Finance and Chief Financial Officer, Bethesda Memorial Hospital, Boynton Beach, FL, p. A119
ARABIT, Aleen D., Chief Executive Officer, Kindred Hospital El Paso, El Paso, TX, p. A596
ARAD, Lana, Chief Financial Officer, MountainView Hospital, Las Vegas, NV, p. A393
ARAIR, Sohaib, M.D. Chairman of Medical Staff, Pioneer Community Hospital of Newton, Newton, MS, p. A351
ARAKELIAN, Armen, Chief Information Officer, Nashoba Valley Medical Center, Ayer, MA, p. A295
ARAMBULA, Frank, Chief Financial Officer, Arrowhead Regional Medical Center, Colton, CA, p. A58
ARAN, Lana, Chief Financial Officer, Good Samaritan Hospital, San Jose, CA, p. A88
ARAN, Peter, M.D
Senior Vice President and Chief Medical Officer, Laureate Psychiatric Clinic and Hospital, Tulsa, OK, p. A506
Senior Vice President and Chief Medical Officer, Saint Francis Hospital, Tulsa, OK, p. A506
ARANDA, Brenda, Director Communications and Government Relations, Advocate Trinity Hospital, Chicago, IL, p. A175
ARANDA, Daniel, Chief Executive Officer, Windsor–Laurelwood Center for Behavioral Medicine, Willoughby, OH, p. A491
ARANIO, Lani, Regional Director Human Resources, Samuel Mahelona Memorial Hospital, Kapaa, HI, p. A164
ARATOW, Michael, M.D. Chief Information Officer, San Mateo Medical Center, San Mateo, CA, p. A89
ARBACH, Joan M., Interim President, Phillips Eye Institute, Minneapolis, MN, p. A335
ARBAUGH, Roanie, Director Human Resources, Grant Memorial Hospital, Petersburg, WV, p. A674
ARBOGAST, Richard, M.D. Chief Medical Officer, McKay–Dee Hospital Center, Ogden, UT, p. A639
ARBOGEST, Dodie, Controller, Stonewall Jackson Memorial Hospital, Weston, WV, p. A676
ARBOLEDA, Reginaldo, M.D. Chief of Staff, Wild Rose Community Memorial Hospital, Wild Rose, WI, p. A694
ARBON, Don, Vice President Finance, Mid–Columbia Medical Center, The Dalles, OR, p. A516
ARBONEAUX, Jane, Chief Financial Officer, Prevost Memorial Hospital, Donaldsonville, LA, p. A266
ARBONEAUX, Wayne M., Chief Executive Officer, Assumption Community Hospital, Napoleonville, LA, p. A274
ARBOUR, Douglas T., Chief Executive Officer, Springs Memorial Hospital, Lancaster, SC, p. A552
ARBUCKLE, Barry S., Ph.D. President and Chief Executive Officer, MemorialCare, Fountain Valley, CA, p. B87
ARBUTHNOT, Rena, Director Human Resources, Shriners Hospitals for Children, Shreveport, Shreveport, LA, p. A277
ARCANGELI, Barbara J., Vice President Human Resources, Newport Hospital, Newport, RI, p. A544
ARCENEAUX, Susan, R.N. Coordinator Information Technology, Leonard J. Chabert Medical Center, Houma, LA, p. A268
ARCEO, Richard, Director Information Technology, Maryville Scott Nolan Center, Des Plaines, IL, p. A180
ARCH, Chrissy, Chief Financial Officer, Cherokee Indian Hospital, Cherokee, NC, p. A451
ARCH, John K., FACHE Administrator, Boys Town National Research Hospital, Omaha, NE, p. A387
ARCHAMBEAULT, Shirley, Chief Information Officer, Medical Center of Lewisville, Lewisville, TX, p. A612
ARCHER, David, Director Information Systems, Tristar Ashland City Medical Center, Ashland City, TN, p. A562
ARCHER, David L., Chief Executive Officer, Saint Francis Hospital, Memphis, TN, p. A572
ARCHER, Doug, Assistant Administrator, Sutter Tracy Community Hospital, Tracy, CA, p. A93
ARCHER, Joe, Chief Information Officer, Victor Valley Community Hospital, Victorville, CA, p. A95
ARCHER, Kenneth W., Chief Executive Officer, Saunders Medical Center, Wahoo, NE, p. A390
ARCHER, Martha, Director Human Resources, St. Francis Hospital and Health Services, Maryville, MO, p. A365
ARCHER–DUSTE, Helen, Chief Operating Officer, San Francisco Medical Center, San Francisco, CA, p. A87
ARCHEY, Eugene, Chief Information Technology, Veterans Affairs Greater Los Angeles Healthcare System, Los Angeles, CA, p. A72
ARCHIBOLD, Robert, Director, Human Resources, St. Anthony North Hospital, Westminster, CO, p. A106
ARCIDI, Alfred J., M.D
Senior Vice President, Whittier Rehabilitation Hospital, Bradford, MA, p. A297
Senior Vice President, Whittier Rehabilitation Hospital, Westborough, MA, p. A305
ARCIDI, Alfred L., M.D. President, Whittier Health Network, Haverhill, MA, p. B146
ARD, Jana, R.N. Director Clinical Resource Management, Madison St. Joseph Health Center, Madisonville, TX, p. A615
ARDABELL, Toni R., R.N. Chief Executive Officer, Bon Secours St. Mary's Hospital, Richmond, VA, p. A654
ARDEMAGNI, Jeff, Chief Financial Officer, Medical Center of Arlington, Arlington, TX, p. A579
ARDOIN, Candice, Director Human Resources, Dauterive Hospital, New Iberia, LA, p. A274
ARDOIN, Stan, M.D. Medical Director, Griffin Memorial Hospital, Norman, OK, p. A500
ARGIRO, Don
Regional Director Human Resources, Summa Barberton Citizens Hospital, Barberton, OH, p. A470
Regional Director Human Resources, Summa Wadsworth–Rittman Hospital, Wadsworth, OH, p. A490
ARIGLIO, Basil, President and Chief Executive Officer, Rome Memorial Hospital, Rome, NY, p. A442
ARISMENDI, Christopher, M.D. Chief Executive Officer, Dameron Hospital, Stockton, CA, p. A91
ARISPIE, Joe, Director Information Systems, Wise Regional Health System, Decatur, TX, p. A593
ARIZMENDEZ, Elena, M.D. Executive Medical Director, HEALTHSOUTH Rehabilitation Hospital of Austin, Austin, TX, p. A580
ARIZPE, Robert C., Superintendent, San Antonio State Hospital, San Antonio, TX, p. A626
ARKFELD, Diane, R.N. Director of Nursing, Crawford County Memorial Hospital, Denison, IA, p. A218
ARLEDGE, Amy, Vice President Support Services, St. Luke's Hospital, Columbus, NC, p. A451



Index of Health Care Professionals

Index of Health Care Professionals / Babakanian
Index of Health Care Professionals

ASKIE, Charity L., Director Finance, Sage Memorial Hospital, Ganado, AZ, p. A32
ASKINAZI, Murray, Senior Vice President and Chief Financial Officer, Lawrence Hospital Center, Bronxville, NY, p. A422
ASMUTH, Peter J., Executive Director and Administrator, Serenity Lane, Eugene, OR, p. A510
ASPAAS, Ken, M.D. Chief Medical Officer, Sanford University of South Dakota Medical Center, Sioux Falls, SD, p. A559
ASPER, Mirelis, Human Resources Generalist, Metropolitan Hospital of Miami, Miami, FL, p. A131
ASSAAD, Haney, Chief of Staff, North Ottawa Community Hospital, Grand Haven, MI, p. A313
ASTACIO, Benjamin, Director Human Resources, Bella Vista Hospital, Mayaguez, PR, p. A701
ASTOLFO, Sean, Administrator, Renaissance Hospital Terrell, Terrell, TX, p. A630
ASTON, Brian W., Chief Operating Officer, Mission Hospital, Asheville, NC, p. A448
ASTRAN, Melinda, M.D. Chief of Staff, La Paz Regional Hospital, Parker, AZ, p. A34
ATCHLEY, Mark, Vice President and Chief Financial Officer, Medical City Dallas Hospital, Dallas, TX, p. A591
ATEIA, Nashat, M.D. Chief of Staff, Doctors Hospital of West Covina, West Covina, CA, p. A95
ATEN, Byron, Controller, HEALTHSOUTH Rehabilitation Hospital, Albuquerque, NM, p. A414
ATHA, Shannon M., Director Finance, Doctors Hospital Nelsonville, Nelsonville, OH, p. A486
ATHENAIS, Dierdre, Director Human Resources, Colusa Regional Medical Center, Colusa, CA, p. A58
ATIENZA, Terry S., Associate Director, Veterans Affairs Eastern Colorado Health Care System, Denver, CO, p. A100
ATKIN, Suzanne, M.D. Chief of Staff and Associate Dean Clinical Affairs, University of Medicine and Dentistry of New Jersey–University Hospital, Newark, NJ, p. A407
ATKINS, James, Chief Operating Officer, Rockdale Medical Center, Conyers, GA, p. A150
ATKINS, Jim, Director Employee Services, Elks Rehab Hospital, Boise, ID, p. A166
ATKINS, Melissa, CPA, Chief Executive Officer, Graham County Hospital, Hill City, KS, p. A234
ATKINS, Rainy, Chief Operating Officer and Administrator, PeaceHealth Southwest Medical Center, Vancouver, WA, p. A668
ATKINS, Stephen R., M.D. Medical Director, Southwest Connecticut Mental Health System, Bridgeport, CT, p. A108
ATKINS, Tracy, Interim Chief Executive Officer, Biggs–Gridley Memorial Hospital, Gridley, CA, p. A64
ATKINS–GUIDRY, Stephanie, Administrator, USMD Hospital at Fort Worth, Fort Worth, TX, p. A599
ATKINSON, Chris, Director of Human Resources, Ochsner Medical Center–Baton Rouge, Baton Rouge, LA, p. A262
ATKINSON, James, M.D. Medical Director, Santa Monica–UCLA Medical Center and Orthopaedic Hospital, Santa Monica, CA, p. A90
ATKINSON, Jodi, President and Chief Executive Officer, St. Andrew's Health Center, Bottineau, ND, p. A464
ATKINSON, Mike, Director Administrative Services, Brookhaven Hospital, Tulsa, OK, p. A505
ATKINSON II, William K., Ph.D. President and Chief Executive Officer, WakeMed Raleigh Campus, Raleigh, NC, p. A459
ATKINSON II,, William K., Ph.D. President and Chief Executive Officer, WakeMed Health & Hospitals, Raleigh, NC, p. B143
ATTEBURY, Mary, Chief Operating Officer, Northwest Missouri Psychiatric Rehabilitation Center, Saint Joseph, MO, p. A368
ATTI, Lucretia, Interim Chief Executive Officer, HEALTHSOUTH Rehabilitation Hospital of Erie, Erie, PA, p. A523
ATTRIDGE, Scott, Controller, Mid–Valley Hospital, Omak, WA, p. A663
ATTY, James, Chief Executive Officer, Humboldt County Memorial Hospital, Humboldt, IA, p. A221
ATWAL, Money, Chief Financial Officer, Hilo Medical Center, Hilo, HI, p. A163
ATWATER, Gregory, Chief Operating Officer, Metropolitan Hospital Center, New York, NY, p. A434
ATWELL, Denaye, Manager Human Resources, George Nigh Rehabilitation Institute, Okmulgee, OK, p. A502
ATWOOD, Julie, Director Human Resources, San Bernardino Mountains Community Hospital District, Lake Arrowhead, CA, p. A66
ATWOOD, Norma, Director Human Resources, Riverton Memorial Hospital, Riverton, WY, p. A697
ATWOOD, Sheila, R.N. Chief Operating Officer, Kalkaska Memorial Health Center, Kalkaska, MI, p. A317
ATZROTT, Allan E., FACHE President and Chief Executive Officer, St. Luke's Cornwall Hospital, Newburgh, NY, p. A438
AUBEL, Eugenia, President, St. Elizabeth Boardman Health Center, Boardman, OH, p. A471
AUBEL, James, Chief Financial Officer, Jameson Hospital, New Castle, PA, p. A530
AUBRY, Michael, Director Information Systems, Hanford Community Medical Center, Hanford, CA, p. A64
AUBUT, Richard H., R.N. President and Chief Executive Officer, South Shore Hospital, South Weymouth, MA, p. A304
AUCKER, Kendra A., Vice President Operations, Evangelical Community Hospital, Lewisburg, PA, p. A527
AUDETT, John R., M.D. Chief Medical Officer, Inova Alexandria Hospital, Alexandria, VA, p. A645
AUDIRSCH, Lanell, Administrative Assistant, North Caddo Medical Center, Vivian, LA, p. A279
AUER, Kenneth E., Director Human Resources, Unity Hospital, Fridley, MN, p. A331
AUERBACH, Jeffrey, D.O. Medical Director, Bon Secours Community Hospital, Port Jervis, NY, p. A440
AUERBACH, John, Commissioner, Massachusetts Department of Public Health, Boston, MA, p. B85
AUERBACH, Lorraine P., President and Chief Executive Officer, Seton Medical Center, Daly City, CA, p. A59
AUFDENGARTEN, John E., R.N. Vice President, Administration, Alice Hyde Medical Center, Malone, NY, p. A429
AUFDERHEIDE, Allen D., Chief Executive Officer, Callaway Community Hospital, Fulton, MO, p. A360
AUGSBURGER, Marc, President and Chief Executive Officer, Horn Memorial Hospital, Ida Grove, IA, p. A221
AUGSBURGER, Tod, Senior Vice President and Chief Operating Officer, Lexington Medical Center, West Columbia, SC, p. A554
AUGUSTIN, Robert, Director Human Resources, Crockett Hospital, Lawrenceburg, TN, p. A569
AUGUSTIN, III, W. Walter, CPA Vice President Financial Services and Chief Financial Officer, Kernan Orthopaedics and Rehabilitation, Baltimore, MD, p. A287
AUGUSTYNIAK, Becky, Director Human Resources, Hughston Hospital, Columbus, GA, p. A149
AUJERO, Moftia, Chief Nurse Executive, Bellevue Hospital Center, New York, NY, p. A431
AUMER, Lynn, Director Information Management, Ohio Valley General Hospital, McKees Rocks, PA, p. A528
AUNAN, II, Milton E., CPA Vice President and Chief Financial Officer, St. Luke's Hospital, Cedar Rapids, IA, p. A215
AURILIO, Lisa, R.N. Vice President Patient Services and Chief Nursing Officer, Akron Children's Hospital, Akron, OH, p. A469
AUSMAN, Dan F., President and Chief Executive Officer, Methodist Hospital of Southern California, Arcadia, CA, p. A54
AUSTELLI, Oscar, Chief Information Officer, LAC/University of Southern California Medical Center, Los Angeles, CA, p. A70
AUSTEN, Terry L., Senior Vice President and Area Manager, San Jose Medical Center, San Jose, CA, p. A88
AUSTIN, Aaron
Vice President Human Resources, Saint Joseph Regional Medical Center, Mishawaka, IN, p. A208
Vice President Human Resources, Saint Joseph Regional Medical Center–Plymouth Campus, Plymouth, IN, p. A210
AUSTIN, Arthur, M.D. Vice President Medical Affairs, Gerald Champion Regional Medical Center, Alamogordo, NM, p. A414
AUSTIN, Cheryse, Vice President Patient Care Services and Chief Nursing Officer, Casa Grande Regional Medical Center, Casa Grande, AZ, p. A31
AUSTIN, Cynthia, Manager Health Information Management, Murray Medical Center, Chatsworth, GA, p. A149
AUSTIN, Dan, Manager Data Processing, Ashley County Medical Center, Crossett, AR, p. A43
AUSTIN, Debbie W., R.N. Vice President Patient Care Services, P & S Surgical Hospital, Monroe, LA, p. A273
AUSTIN, James D., FACH
Administrator, Kalkaska Memorial Health Center, Kalkaska, MI, p. A317
Administrator, Paul Oliver Memorial Hospital, Frankfort, MI, p. A312
AUSTIN, John, M.D. Director Medical Staff, Aspirus Ontonagon Hospital, Ontonagon, MI, p. A320
AUSTIN, Judy, Director Human Resources, Campbellton Graceville Hospital, Graceville, FL, p. A124
AUSTIN, Laura, Chief Financial Officer and Chief Operating Officer, Community Hospital of Anaconda, Anaconda, MT, p. A373
AUSTIN, Lori, Director Human Resources, Troy Regional Medical Center, Troy, AL, p. A26
AUSTIN, Robert S., FACHE Chief Executive Officer, Estes Park Medical Center, Estes Park, CO, p. A101
AUSTIN, Warren, M.D. Vice President Medical Affairs, Bon Secours Maryview Medical Center, Portsmouth, VA, p. A654
AUSTIN–MOORE, Gale, Director Area Technology, Vallejo Medical Center, Vallejo, CA, p. A94
AUTRY, Randall, Administrator, Maryville Scott Nolan Center, Des Plaines, IL, p. A180
AVANT, Andre, Facility Automation Manager, Texas Center for Infectious Disease, San Antonio, TX, p. A626
AVANT, Donna, Chief Financial Officer, Oklahoma Center for Orthopedic and Multi–Specialty Surgery, Oklahoma City, OK, p. A501
AVATO, Rich, Director, St. Mary's Medical Center, West Palm Beach, FL, p. A143
AVENEL, William, Assistant Vice President Information Services, Medical Center of Central Georgia, Macon, GA, p. A155
AVERETT, Elaine, Chief Financial Officer, Grove Hill Memorial Hospital, Grove Hill, AL, p. A21
AVERILL, Clark, Director Information Technology, St. Luke's Hospital, Duluth, MN, p. A330
AVERNA, Russell, Director Human Resources, Spaulding Rehabilitation Hospital, Boston, MA, p. A297
AVERY, Danny, Chief Financial Officer and Chief Operating Officer, Quartz Mountain Medical Center, Mangum, OK, p. A498
AVERY, Donald R., FACHE President and Chief Executive Officer, Fairview Park Hospital, Dublin, GA, p. A152
AVERY III, John B., Administrator, Perry Community Hospital, Linden, TN, p. A569
AVERY, Jonathan, Chief Administrative Officer, Legacy Salmon Creek Medical Center, Vancouver, WA, p. A668
AVILA, Daniel, Director Human Resources, St. Cloud Regional Medical Center, Saint Cloud, FL, p. A137
AVILES, Alan D., President, New York City Health and Hospitals Corporation, New York, NY, p. B93
AVRIETT, David E., Assistant Administrator, Blount Memorial Hospital, Maryville, TN, p. A570
AVVISATO, Michael, Senior Vice President and Chief Financial Officer, Allied Services Rehabilitation Hospital, Scranton, PA, p. A537
AVVISATO, Mike, Vice President and Chief Financial Officer, John Heinz Institute of Rehabilitation Medicine, Wilkes–Barre, PA, p. A541
AWAN, Naveed, FACHE Chief Executive Officer, St. Helena Parish Hospital, Greensburg, LA, p. A267
AWOLOWO, Yinusa, Business Officer, Kingsboro Psychiatric Center,, NY, p. A433
AXTMAN, Cheryl, Administrative Assistant, Sakakawea Medical Center, Hazen, ND, p. A466
AYALA, Lisa, R.N. Director Human Resources, Specialty Hospital Jacksonville, Jacksonville, FL, p. A126
AYALA, Mercedes, Business Manager, Senator Garrett W. Hagedorn Psychiatric Hospital, Glen Gardner, NJ, p. A
AYALA, Raquel, Deputy Executive Director Network and Human Resources, Kings County Hospital Center,, NY, p. A433
AYALA, Shirley, Director Human Resources, First Hospital Panamericano, Cidra, PR, p. A700
AYCOCK, Jean, President and Chief Executive Officer, Oconee Regional Health Systems, Milledgeville, GA, p. B97
AYCOCK, Jean, President and Chief Executive Officer, Oconee Regional Medical Center, Milledgeville, GA, p. A156
AYERS, James G., Chief Financial Officer, Piedmont Geriatric Hospital, Burkeville, VA, p. A646
AYERS, James L., Director Resource Management, Naval Hospital, Pensacola, FL, p. A136
AYKUL, Nikki, Manager Business Office, LifeCare Hospitals of Pittsburgh, Pittsburgh, PA, p. A534
AYOUB, John J., FACHE Chief Executive Officer, Melissa Memorial Hospital, Holyoke, CO, p. A102
AYRES, Daniel M., Chief Executive Officer, O'Connor Hospital, Delhi, NY, p. A425
AYRES, Robert, Director Information Systems, Firelands Regional Health System, Sandusky, OH, p. A488
AYRES, Shane, Chief Financial Officer, Sanford Wheaton Medical Center, Wheaton, MN, p. A341
AYSCUE, Charles F., Senior Vice President Finance and Chief Financial Officer, Mission Hospital, Asheville, NC, p. A448
AYYASH, Maher, M.D. Chief Medical Officer, Clarion Psychiatric Center, Clarion, PA, p. A520
AZCONA, Alain, Director Business Development, Aurora Behavioral Health Care, San Diego, CA, p. A85
AZEVEDO, Michael, M.D. Medical Director, San Joaquin Valley Rehabilitation Hospital, Fresno, CA, p. A62
AZIZ, Samir, M.D. Inpatient Medical Director, Navos, Seattle, WA, p. A665

## B

BAADE, Leigh, Director Human Resources, New England Rehabilitation Hospital of Portland, Portland, ME, p. A285
BAARSON, Gerrie, Chief Executive Officer, Select Specialty Hospital–Battle Creek, Battle Creek, MI, p. A308
BAAS, Dina, Director Financial Services, Orange City Area Health System, Orange City, IA, p. A224
BABAKANIAN, Ed, Chief Information Officer, UC San Diego Health System, San Diego, CA, p. A86

BABAT, L. Brett, M.D
  Chief Medical Officer, Skyline Madison Campus, Madison, TN, p. A570
  Chief Medical Officer, Skyline Medical Center, Nashville, TN, p. A573
BABB, Cindy, Executive Director Human Resources and Organizational Effectiveness, St. Joseph Hospital and Health Center, Kokomo, IN, p. A206
BABB, Daniel R., Chief Executive Officer, Oakland Regional Hospital, Southfield, MI, p. A323
BABB, Donald J., Chief Executive Officer, Citizens Memorial Hospital, Bolivar, MO, p. A355
BABB, Kathy, Manager Human Resources, Clifton Springs Hospital and Clinic, Clifton Springs, NY, p. A424
BABB, Merri Lynn, Chief Human Resources, Stewart–Webster Hospital, Richland, GA, p. A157
BABCOCK, Daniel, Chief Executive Officer, Marlette Regional Hospital, Marlette, MI, p. A318
BABCOCK, Kimberly, Administrator Human Resources, Kalkaska Memorial Health Center, Kalkaska, MI, p. A317
BABCOCK, Robert, M.D. Chief of Staff, Veterans Affairs Medical Center, Canandaigua, NY, p. A423
BABIN, Beth, Vice President Human Resources, Tulane Medical Center, New Orleans, LA, p. A275
BABINEAU, Timothy J., M.D. President and Chief Executive Officer, Rhode Island Hospital, Providence, RI, p. A544
BABUSCIO, Cathy, Director Human Resources, Mat–Su Regional Medical Center, Palmer, AK, p. A30
BACA, Modesto, Chief Information Officer, Amarillo Veterans Affairs Health Care System, Amarillo, TX, p. A578
BACH, Dawn M., MS Chief Clinical Officer, Buena Vista Regional Medical Center, Storm Lake, IA, p. A227
BACHARACH, Paul, President and Chief Executive Officer, Uniontown Hospital, Uniontown, PA, p. A540
BACHE–WIIG, Ben, M.D. President, Abbott Northwestern Hospital, Minneapolis, MN, p. A334
BACHELDOR, H. Lee, D.O. Medical Director, St. John River District Hospital, East China, MI, p. A311
BACHENBERG, Timothy, M.D. Chief Medical Officer, Madelia Community Hospital, Madelia, MN, p. A334
BACHER, Beth, Chief Executive Officer, HEALTHSOUTH Valley of the Sun Rehabilitation Hospital, Glendale, AZ, p. A33
BACHETTI, Kathleen, Director Human Resources, Shriners Hospitals for Children, Springfield, Springfield, MA, p. A305
BACHMAN, Page, Corporate Vice President, St. John Medical Center, Tulsa, OK, p. A507
BACHMAN, Robert J., Chief Operating Officer, Emory University Hospital, Atlanta, GA, p. A145
BACHUS KEITH, Beryl, M.D. Chief of Staff, Clarendon Memorial Hospital, Manning, SC, p. A552
BACIARELLI, Val, Chief Operating Officer, CHRISTUS Santa Rosa Health Care, San Antonio, TX, p. A624
BACK, Barbara, Manager Human Resources, Encino Hospital Medical Center,, CA, p. A69
BACK, Bill, M.D. Chief of Staff, Mercy Willard Hospital, Willard, OH, p. A491
BACKS, Craig, M.D. Medical Director, St. John's Hospital, Springfield, IL, p. A194
BACKSTROM, Dean, M.D. Vice President Medical Affairs, Rutherford Regional Medical Center, Rutherfordton, NC, p. A460
BACON, Jim, Director Team Resources, St. Anthony's Hospital, Saint Petersburg, FL, p. A138
BACON, Ken J., President and Chief Executive Officer, Shawnee Mission Medical Center, Shawnee Mission, KS, p. A243
BACON, William, M.D. Chief of Staff, Fleming County Hospital, Flemingsburg, KY, p. A249
BACUS, Randy B., FACHE Chief Executive Officer, North Texas Medical Center, Gainesville, TX, p. A600
BADALIAN, B. Joseph, President and Chief Executive Officer, Lakewood Regional Medical Center, Lakewood, CA, p. A67
BADEN, Robert M., Chief Financial Officer, Lompoc Valley Medical Center, Lompoc, CA, p. A67
BADGER, Jeff
  Chief Financial Officer, Calumet Medical Center, Chilton, WI, p. A680
  Chief Financial Officer, Mercy Medical Center, Oshkosh, WI, p. A688
  Chief Financial Officer, St. Elizabeth Hospital, Appleton, WI, p. A678
BADGER, Steven, R.N. Administrator, Orem Community Hospital, Orem, UT, p. A639
BADGER Jr., Theodore J., FACHE Chief Executive Officer, Beauregard Memorial Hospital, De Ridder, LA, p. A265
BADILLO, Linda, M.D. Chief of Medical Staff, Medical Center of Trinity, Trinity, FL, p. A142
BADINGER, Sandy, Chief Financial Officer, Fairway Medical Center, Covington, LA, p. A265

BADR, Safwan, M.D. Executive Vice President and Chief Medical Officer, Detroit Receiving Hospital/University Health Center, Detroit, MI, p. A310
BAENEN, Sharla, President, Bellin Psychiatric Center, Green Bay, WI, p. A682
BAER, Douglas, Chief Executive Officer, Brooks Rehabilitation Hospital, Jacksonville, FL, p. A126
BAER, James E., FACHE President and Chief Executive Officer, Highland District Hospital, Hillsboro, OH, p. A482
BAEZ, Janet, Director, University Hospital, San Juan, PR, p. A704
BAGGETT, Al, M.D. Interim Chief of Staff, Taylor Regional Hospital, Hawkinsville, GA, p. A154
BAGGETT, Margarita, MSN Interim Chief Operating Officer, UC San Diego Health System, San Diego, CA, p. A86
BAGLEY, Brenda, Director Human Resources, Red River Regional Hospital, Bonham, TX, p. A584
BAGLEY, Douglas D., Chief Executive Officer, Riverside County Regional Medical Center, Moreno Valley, CA, p. A76
BAGLEY, Peter, M.D. Medical Director, Fairlawn Rehabilitation Hospital, Worcester, MA, p. A306
BAGNALL, Andrew, Chief Executive Officer, St. Nicholas Hospital, Sheboygan, WI, p. A690
BAGNELL, Kelly, M.D. Chief of Staff, St. Joseph Hospital, Polson, MT, p. A378
BAHKTAVAR, Mohommad, M.D. Chief of Staff, Palo Verde Hospital, Blythe, CA, p. A56
BAHL, Barry I., Director, St. Cloud Veterans Affairs Health Care System, Saint Cloud, MN, p. A338
BAHLS, Fredrick, M.D. Chief of Staff, Veterans Affairs Central Iowa Health Care System, Des Moines, IA, p. A218
BAHNLEIN, Carl, Executive Vice President and Chief Operating Officer, Virginia Hospital Center – Arlington, Arlington, VA, p. A645
BAICKER, Martin W., Senior Vice President and Administrator, Meadowlands Hospital Medical Center, Secaucus, NJ, p. A410
BAIDA–FRAGOSO, Nicolas, M.D. Clinical Director, El Paso Psychiatric Center, El Paso, TX, p. A596
BAIER, Roger, Chief Executive Officer, Sanford Medical Center Mayville, Mayville, ND, p. A467
BAIG, Mirza, M.D. Chief of Staff, RiverView Health, Crookston, MN, p. A330
BAILEY, Becky, R.N. Director of Nursing, Kansas Surgery and Recovery Center, Wichita, KS, p. A245
BAILEY, Brian, Chief Administrative and Financial Officer, Maryland General Hospital, Baltimore, MD, p. A288
BAILEY, Bruce P., President and Chief Executive Officer, Georgetown Hospital System, Georgetown, SC, p. B54
BAILEY, Bruce P., Chief Executive Officer, Georgetown Memorial Hospital, Georgetown, SC, p. A550
BAILEY, Chad, Director of Human Resources, HEALTHSOUTH Huntington Rehabilitation Hospital, Huntington, WV, p. A672
BAILEY, Cindy, R.N. Chief Nursing Officer, Richland Memorial Hospital, Olney, IL, p. A190
BAILEY, Cori, Accountant, Tyler Holmes Memorial Hospital, Winona, MS, p. A354
BAILEY, Craig, MS Chief Operating Officer, Boulder City Hospital, Boulder City, NV, p. A391
BAILEY, Dan, Director Information Systems, Norton Sound Regional Hospital, Nome, AK, p. A29
BAILEY, Dan, M.D. Vice President Medical Affairs and Chief Medical Officer, Upper Valley Medical Center, Troy, OH, p. A490
BAILEY, David, Administrator, East Texas Medical Center–Mount Vernon, Mount Vernon, TX, p. A617
BAILEY, Dianne, Coordinator Information Systems, Pana Community Hospital, Pana, IL, p. A190
BAILEY, Jim, M.D. Chief Medical Officer, Northeast Georgia Medical Center, Gainesville, GA, p. A153
BAILEY, John, D.O. Chief of Staff, Northeast Regional Medical Center, Kirksville, MO, p. A363
BAILEY, John E., Chief Financial Officer, Moore County Hospital District, Dumas, TX, p. A594
BAILEY, Jonathan D., Chief Executive Officer, Hansford Hospital, Spearman, TX, p. A628
BAILEY, Kathy C., Ph.D
  Sr. Vice President, Chief Operating Officer, Grace Hospital, Morganton, NC, p. A458
  Sr. Vice President, Chief Operating Officer, Valdese General Hospital, Valdese, NC, p. A462
BAILEY, Larry, Chief Executive Officer, Indiana University Health Paoli Hospital, Paoli, IN, p. A210
BAILEY, Leisa, M.D. Chief of Staff, Doctors Memorial Hospital, Bonifay, FL, p. A119
BAILEY, Lynn, M.D. Director Primary Care and Medical Services, Naval Hospital, Camp Pendleton, CA, p. A56
BAILEY, Marquita, Chief Nursing Officer, DeKalb Regional Medical Center, Fort Payne, AL, p. A20

BAILEY, Matthew D., FACHE President and Chief Executive Officer, Indiana University Health West Hospital, Avon, IN, p. A197
BAILEY, Mikeana, Director Human Resources, Brownwood Regional Medical Center, Brownwood, TX, p. A585
BAILEY, Owen, Administrator, University of South Alabama Children's and Women's Hospital, Mobile, AL, p. A23
BAILEY, Peggy, Chief Nursing Officer, Alvarado Hospital, San Diego, CA, p. A85
BAILEY, Robert W., Chief Information Officer, Hawthorn Center, Northville, MI, p. A320
BAILEY, Ron, Chief Financial Officer, Franklin Foundation Hospital, Franklin, LA, p. A266
BAILEY, Russell, Chief Executive Officer, Texas Rehabilitation Hospital of Fort Worth, Fort Worth, TX, p. A599
BAILEY, Scott, Chief Financial Officer, Mat–Su Regional Medical Center, Palmer, AK, p. A30
BAILEY, Stevan, Manager Information Systems, Campbell County Memorial Hospital, Gillette, WY, p. A696
BAILEY, Susan P., R.N. Chief Executive Officer, Specialty Hospital of Washington, Washington, DC, p. A117
BAILEY, Ted, Vice President Information Systems, Peace River Regional Medical Center, Port Charlotte, FL, p. A137
BAILEY, Travis A., Vice President Administration, St. Claire Regional Medical Center, Morehead, KY, p. A256
BAILEY–DELEEUW, Sandra, Administrator, Methodist Extended Care Hospital, Memphis, TN, p. A571
BAILON, Amy R., M.D. Medical Director, Woodbridge Development Center, Woodbridge, NJ, p. A412
BAIN, Brad, Information Systems Leader, Fresno Medical Center, Fresno, CA, p. A62
BAIN, Holly, Chief Nursing Officer, Integris Marshall County Medical Center, Madill, OK, p. A498
BAIN, Mark, Chief Human Resources, Veterans Affairs Connecticut Healthcare System, West Haven, CT, p. A113
BAINBRIDGE, Deb, Chief Financial Officer, Via Christi Hospital, Pittsburg, KS, p. A241
BAINE, Rodney, M.D. Chief of Staff, Northwest Mississippi Regional Medical Center, Clarksdale, MS, p. A344
BAIOCCO, Jeffrey D., Chief Financial Officer, Eastern Idaho Regional Medical Center, Idaho Falls, ID, p. A168
BAIR, Ada, Chief Executive Officer, Memorial Hospital, Carthage, IL, p. A174
BAIR, Andrew P., President and Chief Executive Officer, Samaritan Healthcare, Moses Lake, WA, p. A663
BAIR, Betsy, Chief Operating Officer, Gunnison Valley Hospital, Gunnison, CO, p. A102
BAIRD, David
  Chief Information Officer, LDS Hospital, Salt Lake City, UT, p. A640
  Chief Information Officer, The Orthopedic Specialty Hospital, Murray, UT, p. A638
BAIRD, Donna, Vice President Corporate Services, Bay Medical Center, Panama City, FL, p. A135
BAIRD, John D., Chief Executive Officer, Resurrection Medical Center, Chicago, IL, p. A177
BAIRD, Nancy, Director Human Resources, Galesburg Cottage Hospital, Galesburg, IL, p. A182
BAJARI, Pamela R., R.N. Interim Administrator, Community Behavioral Health Hospital – Annandale, Annandale, MN, p. A327
BAJGROWICZ, Maryanne, Vice President, Patient Care Services/Chief Nursing Officer, Our Lady of the Resurrection Medical Center, Chicago, IL, p. A177
BAKER, Amy, Associate Director Finance Services, Missouri Rehabilitation Center, Mount Vernon, MO, p. A365
BAKER, Bonnie, Vice President Finance and Chief Financial Officer, Butler Hospital, Providence, RI, p. A544
BAKER, Bonnie, M.D. Chief Medical Services, Veterans Health Care System of the Ozarks, Fayetteville, AR, p. A44
BAKER, Cambrea, Coordinator Human Resources, Select Specialty Hospital–Ann Arbor, Ypsilanti, MI, p. A326
BAKER, Chuck, R.N. Chief Operating Officer and Chief Nursing Officer, Callaway Community Hospital, Fulton, MO, p. A360
BAKER, Damon, D.O. Chief Medical Officer, Oklahoma State University Medical Center, Tulsa, OK, p. A506
BAKER, Denis, Chief Information Officer, Sarasota Memorial Hospital, Sarasota, FL, p. A139
BAKER, Denise, Interim Chief Financial Officer, Erlanger at Hutcheson, Fort Oglethorpe, GA, p. A153
BAKER, Frank, Chief Information Officer, Mary Breckinridge ARH Hospital, Hyden, KY, p. A252
BAKER, Gary A., President, Memorial Hospital, Towanda, PA, p. A539
BAKER, Gary E., Senior Vice President and Administrator, Scottsdale Healthcare–Osborn Medical Center, Scottsdale, AZ, p. A38
BAKER, Harlan T., Department Leader Information Systems, McDonough District Hospital, Macomb, IL, p. A186

Index of Health Care Professionals / Barber

Index of Health Care Professionals

BAKER, Holli, Chief Executive Officer, Vista Health of Fort Smith, Barling, AR, p. A42
BAKER, J. Matthew, M.D. President Medical Staff, Bertrand Chaffee Hospital, Springville, NY, p. A443
BAKER, James, Vice President Business Support Services, Veterans Affairs Pittsburgh Healthcare System, Pittsburgh, PA, p. A536
BAKER, Joann, Administrator, Doctors Memorial Hospital, Bonifay, FL, p. A119
BAKER, Joel, D.O. Chief Medical Officer, Wayne County Hospital, Corydon, IA, p. A217
BAKER, John
Interim Chief Executive Officer, Haven Behavioral Health of Eastern Pennsylvania, Reading, PA, p. A536
Chief Executive Officer, Rolling Hills Hospital, Ada, OK, p. A493
BAKER, Judy, Chief Financial Officer, Kindred Hospital–Mansfield, Mansfield, TX, p. A615
BAKER, Ken, Administrative Director Human Resources, Grenada Lake Medical Center, Grenada, MS, p. A346
BAKER, Leslie, R.N. Chief Nursing Officer, Walton Rehabilitation Hospital, Augusta, GA, p. A147
BAKER, Linda, Director Human Resources, St. Alexius Medical Center, Hoffman Estates, IL, p. A185
BAKER, Maribel, Director Human Resources, Johnson Regional Medical Center, Clarksville, AR, p. A43
BAKER, Mark A., Chief Executive Officer, Jack Hughston Memorial Hospital, Phenix City, AL, p. A25
BAKER, Michael, D.O. Chief of Staff, Daviess Community Hospital, Washington, IN, p. A213
BAKER, Michelle, Director Information Systems, Indiana University Health White Memorial Hospital, Monticello, IN, p. A208
BAKER, Nathan, Manager Information Technology, Central Community Hospital, Elkader, IA, p. A219
BAKER, Paula F., President and Chief Executive Officer, Freeman Health System, Joplin, MO, p. B53
BAKER, Paula F., President and Chief Executive Officer, Freeman Hospital West, Joplin, MO, p. A361
BAKER, R. Hai, M.D. Vice President and Chief Information Officer, York Hospital, York, PA, p. A543
BAKER, Reese, Director Information Systems, Crittenden County Hospital, Marion, KY, p. A256
BAKER, Reta K., President, Mercy Hospital Fort Scott, Fort Scott, KS, p. A233
BAKER, Rodger H., President and Chief Executive Officer, Fauquier Hospital, Warrenton, VA, p. A657
BAKER, Ron, Administrator, Satanta District Hospital, Satanta, KS, p. A243
BAKER, Ronald L., Chief Executive Officer, Saint Luke's East Hospital, Lee's Summit, MO, p. A364
BAKER, Shari, Director Human Resources, Orange City Area Health System, Orange City, IA, p. A224
BAKER, Sharon, Director Support Services, Fairbanks, Indianapolis, IN, p. A204
BAKER, Shawna, M.D. Chief of Staff, Community Hospital of Anaconda, Anaconda, MT, p. A373
BAKER, Susan, M.D. Chief of Staff, North Shore Medical Center, Miami, FL, p. A131
BAKER, Terrence, Manager Information Services, Indiana University Health North Hospital, Carmel, IN, p. A199
BAKER, Thomas, Chief Information Management Division, Bayne–Jones Army Community Hospital, Fort Polk, LA, p. A266
BAKER, Vanya, Director, Wilkes Regional Medical Center, North Wilkesboro, NC, p. A458
BAKER, W. Douglas, Director, Julian F. Keith Alcohol and Drug Abuse Treatment Center, Black Mountain, NC, p. A448
BAKER Jr., Wendell H., President, Vidant Edgecombe Hospital, Tarboro, NC, p. A461
BAKICH, Sandy, Director Information Management, Delano Regional Medical Center, Delano, CA, p. A59
BAKKEN, Mary, Executive Vice President and Chief Operating Officer, Silver Cross Hospital, New Lenox, IL, p. A189
BAKKUM, Kyle, Chief Operating Officer, Vernon Memorial Healthcare, Viroqua, WI, p. A692
BALAY Jr., William, Chief Executive Officer, Mesa Hills Specialty Hospital, El Paso, TX, p. A596
BALAZY, Thomas E., M.D. Medical Director, Craig Hospital, Englewood, CO, p. A100
BALCAVAGE, Thomas, Vice President Information Systems and Chief Information Officer, Kennedy Memorial Hospitals–University Medical Center, Cherry Hill, NJ, p. A403
BALCH, Jackson, IT Director, Garden Park Medical Center, Gulfport, MS, p. A346
BALCITIS, Judith, MS Vice President, Nursing and Chief Nursing Officer, Sherman Hospital, Elgin, IL, p. A181
BALDAUF, Robb, Coordinator Information Systems, Lodi Community Hospital, Lodi, OH, p. A483
BALDERRAMA, Jose, Vice President Human Resources, Nationwide Children's Hospital, Columbus, OH, p. A477
BALDRIDGE, Casey, Supervisor Information Technology, Red Bud Regional Hospital, Red Bud, IL, p. A192
BALDRIDGE, Dava, Chief Nursing Officer, Hillcrest Hospital Claremore, Claremore, OK, p. A495
BALDWIN, Barbara, Chief Information Officer, University of Virginia Medical Center, Charlottesville, VA, p. A646
BALDWIN, Bruce A., Chief Executive Officer, Grandview Medical Center, Jasper, TN, p. A567
BALDWIN, Christopher, Vice President Information Systems, Southcoast Hospitals Group, Fall River, MA, p. A300
BALDWIN, David, Chief Information Officer, Robinson Memorial Hospital, Ravenna, OH, p. A487
BALDWIN, Ellen, R.N. Chief Nursing Officer, Texas Health Center for Diagnostic & Surgery, Plano, TX, p. A621
BALDWIN, Gilda, Chief Executive Officer, Westchester General Hospital, Miami, FL, p. A132
BALDWIN, Lee, Administrator and Chief Executive Officer, Landmann–Jungman Memorial Hospital Avera, Scotland, SD, p. A559
BALDWIN, Nathan, M.D. President Medical Staff, Baptist Memorial Hospital–Booneville, Booneville, MS, p. A344
BALDWIN, Steve
Vice President Finance, Willough Healthcare System, Naples, FL, p. A133
Manager Information Technology, Wyoming State Hospital, Evanston, WY, p. A696
BALDWIN, Susan Louise, FACHE President and Chief Nursing Officer, Texas Health Specialty Hospital, Fort Worth, TX, p. A599
BALDWIN, William, Chief Information Officer, Ashe Memorial Hospital, Jefferson, NC, p. A455
BALENTINE, Jerry, D.O. Executive Vice President and Chief Medical Director, St. Barnabas Hospital,, NY, p. A436
BALES, Bruce D., Regional Director Plant Operations, HEALTHSOUTH Southern Hills Rehabilitation Hospital, Princeton, WV, p. A675
BALFOUR, Ann M., R.N. Administrator, St. Joseph Health System, Tawas City, MI, p. A324
BALINK, Kay M., M.D. Chief of Staff, Richland Hospital, Richland Center, WI, p. A690
BALKO, Tom, Manager Information Systems, Redwood Area Hospital, Redwood Falls, MN, p. A337
BALL, Cassie, Chief Financial Officer, Hilton Head Hospital, Hilton Head Island, SC, p. A551
BALL, Charles, Administrator, Specialty Long Term Acute Care Hospital of Hammond, Hammond, LA, p. A267
BALL, Charles A., M.D. Chief Medical Officer, Maury Regional Hospital, Columbia, TN, p. A564
BALL, Charlie, Chief Operating Officer, Specialty Rehabilitation Hospital, Coushatta, LA, p. A264
BALL, Craig, Chairman and Chief Executive Officer, Specialty Healthcare, LLC, Leesville, LA, p. B121
BALL, Craig, Chief Executive Officer, Specialty Rehabilitation Hospital, Coushatta, LA, p. A264
BALL, Jim, Chief Operating Officer, St. Catherine's Rehabilitation Hospital, North Miami, FL, p. A133
BALL, Kristie, Director of Nursing, William Newton Hospital, Winfield, KS, p. A246
BALLANCE, William, M.D. Chief of Medical Staff, Vidant Bertie Hospital, Windsor, NC, p. A463
BALLARD, Bryan M., FACHE Chief Executive Officer, Catalina Island Medical Center, Avalon, CA, p. A54
BALLARD, Lorraine L., Director Human Resources, St. Helena Parish Hospital, Greensburg, LA, p. A267
BALLARD, Paul H., Chief Executive Officer, Victory Medical Center – San Antonio, San Antonio, TX, p. A626
BALLARD, Richard R., Administrator, University of Miami Hospital and Clinics, Miami, FL, p. A132
BALLESTERO, Susan, Vice President Human Resources, Saint Peter's University Hospital, New Brunswick, NJ, p. A407
BALLOCK, Steve, Chief Financial Officer, St. Vincent Healthcare, Billings, MT, p. A373
BALON, Stanley, M.D. President Medical Staff, Landmark Medical Center, Woonsocket, RI, p. A545
BALSANO, Tony, Vice President Finance, Saint Francis Medical Center, Cape Girardeau, MO, p. A356
BALTZ, Phyllis, Interim President, Mercy General Hospital, Sacramento, CA, p. A83
BALZANO, Janice, Chief Operating Officer, Brandon Regional Hospital, Brandon, FL, p. A119
BAMMEL, Paul, Vice President, Mayo Clinic Health System in Eau Claire, Eau Claire, WI, p. A681
BANAS, Thomas, Chief Medical Officer, Rehabilitation Hospital of Fort Wayne, Fort Wayne, IN, p. A202
BANBURY, Brian, Director Site Information Systems, Advocate Christ Medical Center, Oak Lawn, IL, p. A189
BANCO, Leonard, M.D. Senior Vice President and Chief Medical Officer, Bristol Hospital, Bristol, CT, p. A108
BANDA, Venkat, M.D
President of the Medical Staff, Promise Hospital of Baton Rouge, Baton Rouge, LA, p. A263
President Medical Staff, Promise Hospital of Baton Rouge, Baton Rouge, LA, p. A263
BANDY, Don, Director Information Technology, Deaconess Hospital, Oklahoma City, OK, p. A500
BANDY, P. Ross, M.D. Chief Medical Officer and Chief of Staff, Levi Hospital, Hot Springs National Park, AR, p. A46
BANE, Bill, Assistant Vice President and Chief Financial Officer, Inova Fair Oaks Hospital, Fairfax, VA, p. A647
BANG, W. J., M.D. Chief of Staff, Reeves County Hospital, Pecos, TX, p. A620
BANGERT, Richard A., Chief Executive Officer, Rolling Hills Hospital, Franklin, TN, p. A565
BANIGAN, Elisa, Chief Financial Officer, Huhukam Memorial Hospital, Sacaton, AZ, p. A37
BANK, Carol J., Vice President Human Resources, Divine Savior Healthcare, Portage, WI, p. A689
BANKO, Peter D., FACHE President and Chief Executive Officer, St. Vincent Infirmary Medical Center, Little Rock, AR, p. A48
BANKS, Chester, Director Human Resources, East Orange General Hospital, East Orange, NJ, p. A403
BANKS, Elizabeth, Chief Executive Officer, Summit Behavioral Healthcare, Cincinnati, OH, p. A474
BANKS, Maureen, MS,
President, Spaulding Hospital for Continuing Medical Care North Shore, Salem, MA, p. A304
President, Spaulding Hospital for Continuing Medical Care Cambridge, Cambridge, MA, p. A299
BANKS, Maureen, R.N. Chief Operating Officer, Spaulding Rehabilitation Hospital, Boston, MA, p. A297
BANKS, Maureen, MS, President and Chief Executive Officer, Spaulding Rehabilitation Hospital Cape Cod, East Sandwich, MA, p. A299
BANKS, Ronni, Administrator, RiverCrest Specialty Hospital, Mishawaka, IN, p. A208
BANKS, Scott, Chief Financial Officer, Mountain West Medical Center, Tooele, UT, p. A641
BANKS, Walter, Director Human Resources, Baptist Memorial Hospital–Desoto, Southaven, MS, p. A352
BANKTSON, Julie, Manager Human Resources, Paul Oliver Memorial Hospital, Frankfort, MI, p. A312
BANNER, Fred, Chief Information Officer, Shore Medical Center, Somers Point, NJ, p. A410
BANOS, Edward D., President and Chief Executive Officer, Good Shepherd Health System, Longview, TX, p. B55
BANOS, Edward D., President and Chief Executive Officer, Good Shepherd Medical Center, Longview, TX, p. A613
BANSBACH, Steven, M.D. Medical Director, Thousand Oaks Surgical Hospital, Thousand Oaks, CA, p. A92
BANTA, Mary, Director Human Resources, Mercy Medical Center, Williston, ND, p. A468
BANUELOS, Jr., Alfonso F., M.D. Chief Medical Officer, Santa Clara Valley Medical Center, San Jose, CA, p. A88
BAPTISTE, Ernest, Executive Vice President and Chief Operating Officer, St. Francis Hospital, Wilmington, DE, p. A115
BARABANI, Paul, Superintendent, Soldiers' Home in Holyoke, Holyoke, MA, p. A301
BARABAS, Mark C., President and Chief Operating Officer, Erie County Medical Center, Buffalo, NY, p. A422
BARAN, John, Chief Financial Officer, Auburn Community Hospital, Auburn, NY, p. A421
BARANIK, David T., Senior Vice President and Chief Financial Officer, Ohio Valley Medical Center, Wheeling, WV, p. A676
BARANSKI, David J., Vice President Human Resources, Phoebe Putney Memorial Hospital, Albany, GA, p. A144
BARANSKI, Kenneth, Chief Financial Officer, Hills & Dales General Hospital, Cass City, MI, p. A309
BARBA, James J., President and Chief Executive Officer, Albany Medical Center, Albany, NY, p. A420
BARBADIAN, John, Vice President Human Resources, Tulare Regional Medical Center, Tulare, CA, p. A93
BARBAGLIA, J. Joseph, Vice President Financial Services, Columbus Community Hospital, Columbus, NE, p. A382
BARBAGLIA, Jim, Chief Information Officer, Valley Baptist Medical Center–Harlingen, Harlingen, TX, p. A602
BARBAREE, Jerry, Director Human Resources, Baptist Memorial Hospital – Memphis, Memphis, TN, p. A571
BARBARIN, LaSharndra, Chief Operating Officer, Medical Center of McKinney, McKinney, TX, p. A616
BARBE, Brian S., Chief Executive Officer, Memorial Hermann Katy Hospital, Katy, TX, p. A610
BARBEN, Tammy, Chief Executive Officer, Kindred Hospital Victoria, Victoria, TX, p. A633
BARBER, Chris B., FACHE President and Chief Executive Officer, St. Bernards Medical Center, Jonesboro, AR, p. A47
BARBER, Eric A., Chief Executive Officer, Northeast Regional Medical Center, Kirksville, MO, p. A363


Index of Health Care Professionals A757

BARBER, Jack W., M.D. Director, Western State Hospital, Staunton, VA, p. A656

BARBER, Jeffrey B., FACHE President and Chief Executive Officer, Owensboro Medical Health System, Owensboro, KY, p. A257

BARBER, Karen, Chief Executive Officer, Yoakum Community Hospital, Yoakum, TX, p. A636

BARBER, Keith, CPA Chief Operating Officer and Chief Financial Officer, Tomball Regional Medical Center, Tomball, TX, p. A631

BARBER, Laurie, Director Human Resources, Trumbull Memorial Hospital, Warren, OH, p. A490

BARBER, Michael, System Chief Operating Officer, Chester County Hospital, West Chester, PA, p. A541

BARBER, Teresa Rini, Vice President Support Services, Southwest General Health Center, Middleburg Heights, OH, p. A485

BARBERA, Sal A., FACHE Administrator, South Florida State Hospital,, FL, p. A125

BARBIER, Robert P., Senior Vice President and Chief Financial Officer, University of Louisville Hospital, Louisville, KY, p. A255

BARBINI, Gerald J., President and Chief Executive Officer, Allegan General Hospital, Allegan, MI, p. A307

BARBO, Steve, R.N. Administrator, Citizens Medical Center, Columbia, LA, p. A264

BARBOSA, Robert, D.O. Chief Medical Officer, Oakland Regional Hospital, Southfield, MI, p. A323

BARBUAT, James P., Chief Financial Officer, Heart Hospital of Lafayette, Lafayette, LA, p. A270

BARCA, Robin
　Chief Operating Officer, Baptist Medical Center East, Montgomery, AL, p. A23
　Chief Executive Officer, Baptist Medical Center South, Montgomery, AL, p. A23
　Chief Executive Officer, Baptist Medical Center South, Montgomery, AL, p. A23

BARCHI, Daniel
　Senior Vice President, Technical Services and Chief Information Officer, Bridgeport Hospital, Bridgeport, CT, p. A108
　Senior Vice President and Chief Information Officer, Carilion Medical Center, Roanoke, VA, p. A655

BARCLAY, Duane, D.O
　Chief Medical Officer, DeKalb Medical at Hillandale, Lithonia, GA, p. A155
　Vice President Physician Support Services, DeKalb Medical at North Decatur, Decatur, GA, p. A151

BARCLAY, Emily, Vice President Human Resources, Dana–Farber Cancer Institute, Boston, MA, p. A296

BARCLAY, Jeremy, Chief Operating Officer, Cedar Park Regional Medical Center, Cedar Park, TX, p. A587

BARCLAY, Rick, Vice President Support Services, Mercy Hospital Rogers, Rogers, AR, p. A50

BARCLIFT, Larry, Interim Chief Executive Officer, Yuma Rehabilitation Hospital, Yuma, AZ, p. A41

BARD, Jeffrey, Vice President Operations, Aurora Medical Center of Oshkosh, Oshkosh, WI, p. A688

BARDEN, Sean
　Executive Vice President and Chief Financial Officer, Mary Washington Hospital, Fredericksburg, VA, p. A648
　Executive Vice President and Chief Financial Officer, Stafford Hospital, Stafford, VA, p. A656

BARDIER, Catherine, Senior Director Human Resources, New London Hospital, New London, NH, p. A399

BARDILL, Janice, Chief Financial Officer, Roane Medical Center, Harriman, TN, p. A566

BARDWELL, Carol A., R.N. Chief Nurse Executive, Martha's Vineyard Hospital, Oak Bluffs, MA, p. A303

BARDWELL, Jean, Vice President and Chief Financial Officer, Ranken Jordan – A Pediatric Specialty Hospital, Maryland Heights, MO, p. A364

BARDWELL, Sheila, Director Information Systems, Baptist Memorial Hospital–Golden Triangle, Columbus, MS, p. A345

BARDWELL, Tom, Vice President Human Resources, Hills & Dales General Hospital, Cass City, MI, p. A309

BAREFOOT, Denise, Director Health Information Systems, Carolina Pines Regional Medical Center, Hartsville, SC, p. A551

BAREIS, Charles, M.D. Medical Director, MacNeal Hospital, Berwyn, IL, p. A173

BARELA, Barbara, Director Human Resources, Gila Regional Medical Center, Silver City, NM, p. A418

BARELA, Chris, Controller, East El Paso Physicians Medical Center, El Paso, TX, p. A596

BARFIELD, Deirdre, M.D. Vice President Medical Affairs and Chief Medical Officer, CHRISTUS Health Shreveport–Bossier, Shreveport, LA, p. A277

BARGINERE, Cynthia, MSN Vice President Clinical Nursing and Chief Nursing Officer, Rush University Medical Center, Chicago, IL, p. A178

BARHAM, Martha, Vice President and Chief Operating Officer, High Point Regional Health System, High Point, NC, p. A455

BARISANO, Nancy, Chief Information Officer, Westerly Hospital, Westerly, RI, p. A545

BARKASY, Michael, M.D. Chief of Staff, Jennersville Regional Hospital, West Grove, PA, p. A541

BARKEMA, Annette, Chief Financial Officer, Veterans Affairs Medical Center, Portland, OR, p. A514

BARKER, Alanna, Director Human Resources, Washington County Hospital, Nashville, IL, p. A189

BARKER, Jaime, M.D. Medical Director, Manatee Palms Youth Services, Bradenton, FL, p. A119

BARKER, James, President, West Shore Medical Center, Manistee, MI, p. A318

BARKER, Jason, Chief Executive Officer, St. Vincent Healthcare, Billings, MT, p. A373

BARKER, Karen
　Vice President and Chief Information Officer, Levindale Hebrew Geriatric Center and Hospital, Baltimore, MD, p. A288
　Vice President and Chief Information Officer, Northwest Hospital, Randallstown, MD, p. A293
　Vice President and Chief Information Officer, Sinai Hospital of Baltimore, Baltimore, MD, p. A289

BARKER, Kathryn L., Chief Human Resources Management, Veterans Health Care System of the Ozarks, Fayetteville, AR, p. A44

BARKER, Larry
　Chief Operating Officer, Clearwater Valley Hospital and Clinics, Orofino, ID, p. A169
　Chief Operating Officer, St. Mary's Hospital, Cottonwood, ID, p. A168

BARKER, Louise, R.N. Chief Executive Officer, Central Louisiana Surgical Hospital, Alexandria, LA, p. A261

BARKER, M. Debby, Director Human Resources, Siskin Hospital for Physical Rehabilitation, Chattanooga, TN, p. A564

BARKER, Richard
　Administrator, Mercy Health Love County, Marietta, OK, p. A499
　Interim Chief Executive Officer, Mercy Hospital Tishomingo, Tishomingo, OK, p. A505

BARKER, Russell
　Community Chief Executive Officer, McDowell ARH Hospital, McDowell, KY, p. A256
　Chief Information Officer, U. S. Public Health Service Indian Hospital–Whiteriver, Whiteriver, AZ, p. A40

BARKER, Thomas, Director Information, Advanced Healthcare Medical Center, Ellington, MO, p. A359

BARKHYMER, Mary C., R.N. Vice President Patient Care Services and Chief Nursing Officer, UPMC St. Margaret, Pittsburgh, PA, p. A536

BARKMAN, H. William, M.D. Chief of Staff, The University of Kansas Hospital, Kansas City, KS, p. A236

BARKMAN, Sam D., Vice President Operations, Cornerstone Hospital of South Houston, Houston, TX, p. A603

BARKSDALE, Kimberly, M.D. President Medical Staff, Texas Health Presbyterian Hospital Allen, Allen, TX, p. A577

BARKSDALE, Vickie, Manager Human Resources, North Oak Regional Medical Center, Senatobia, MS, p. A352

BARLEY, Leonard, M.D. Chief Medical Officer, Windsor–Laurelwood Center for Behavioral Medicine, Willoughby, OH, p. A491

BARLEY, Tammy, Director Human Resources, HEALTHSOUTH Rehabilitation Hospital of Jonesboro, Jonesboro, AR, p. A46

BARLOW, Mark, M.D. Chief Medical Officer and President Medical Staff, Cornerstone Hospital of Houston – Bellaire, Houston, TX, p. A603

BARNARD, David, M.D. Medical Director, Huey P. Long Medical Center, Pineville, LA, p. A276

BARNARD, Dawn, Administrator, Minnesota Neurorehabilitation Hospital, Brainerd, MN, p. A329

BARNARD, Jeanna, Chief Operating Officer, Bayshore Medical Center, Pasadena, TX, p. A620

BARNARD, Ryan, Chief Operating Officer, Mercy Hospital Ardmore, Ardmore, OK, p. A493

BARNAS, Kim
　Senior Vice President, Appleton Medical Center, Appleton, WI, p. A678
　Senior Vice President, Theda Clark Medical Center, Neenah, WI, p. A687

BARNCORD, Sharon
　Business Partner Human Resources, Redwood City Medical Center, Redwood City, CA, p. A82
　Human Resource Business Partner, South San Francisco Medical Center, South San Francisco, CA, p. A91

BARNES, Betty, Director Human Resources, Maryville Scott Nolan Center, Des Plaines, IL, p. A180

BARNES, Deborah, Vice President and Chief Information Officer, Children's Hospital of The King's Daughters, Norfolk, VA, p. A652

BARNES, Don, Chief Human Resources Officer, Duke Raleigh Hospital, Raleigh, NC, p. A459

BARNES, Douglas A., M.D. Chief of Staff, Shriners Hospitals for Children, Houston, Houston, TX, p. A606

BARNES, Gary, Chief Information Officer, Medical Center Health System, Odessa, TX, p. A619

BARNES, George, M.D. Medical Director, Lakeview Regional Medical Center, Covington, LA, p. A265

BARNES, Jacqueline, Manager Health Information, Select Specialty Hospital–Jackson, Jackson, MS, p. A348

BARNES, Jeff, Director of Information Technology, Girard Medical Center, Girard, KS, p. A233

BARNES, Larry, Vice President Information Technology, Salina Regional Health Center, Salina, KS, p. A242

BARNES, Laura P., MSN Vice President Patient Care Services and Chief Nursing Officer, East Tennessee Children's Hospital, Knoxville, TN, p. A568

BARNES, Mary Ann, Senior Vice President and Executive Director, San Diego Medical Center, San Diego, CA, p. A85

BARNES, Michael, Chief Information Officer, North Valley Hospital, Whitefish, MT, p. A380

BARNES, P. Marie, Director, Human Resources, North Mississippi Medical Center–Pontotoc Hospital and Nursing Home, Pontotoc, MS, p. A352

BARNES, Ronald W., Chief Executive Officer, Garfield County Health Center, Jordan, MT, p. A376

BARNES, Sherry, Director Health Information and Quality Management, Rolling Hills Hospital, Ada, OK, p. A493

BARNES, Sheryl L., MSN Senior Director Clinical Services, Mercy Medical Center – West Lakes, West Des Moines, IA, p. A228

BARNES, Shirley A., Senior Vice President and Chief Human Resources Officer, Mission Hospital, Mission Viejo, CA, p. A74

BARNES, William H., Administrator, Sweeny Community Hospital, Sweeny, TX, p. A629

BARNETT, Frederick, M.D. Chief of Staff, Metroplex Adventist Hospital, Killeen, TX, p. A610

BARNETT, Jeffrey, Chief Executive Officer, Three Rivers Behavioral Health, West Columbia, SC, p. A554

BARNETT, Julia, Chief Nursing Officer, Fannin Regional Hospital, Blue Ridge, GA, p. A148

BARNETT, Marcus, M.D. Chief of Staff, Cypress Fairbanks Medical Center, Houston, TX, p. A604

BARNETT, Patricia, Chief Executive Officer, Hamlin Memorial Hospital, Hamlin, TX, p. A602

BARNETT, Shawn
　Vice President and Chief Financial Officer, CHRISTUS Santa Rosa Health Care, San Antonio, TX, p. A624
　Vice President and Chief Financial Officer, CHRISTUS St. Michael Health System, Texarkana, TX, p. A630
　Vice President and Chief Financial Officer, CHRISTUS St. Michael Rehabilitation Hospital, Texarkana, TX, p. A630

BARNETT, Steve, MS, President and Chief Executive Officer, McKenzie Health System, Sandusky, MI, p. A322

BARNETT, Timothy
　Chief Executive Officer, Yavapai Regional Medical Center – East, Prescott Valley, AZ, p. A37
　President and Chief Executive Officer, Yavapai Regional Medical Center, Prescott, AZ, p. A37

BARNHARDT, Bonnie, Executive Director Human Resources, Minnesota Valley Health Center, Le Sueur, MN, p. A333

BARNHART, David, Director Information Systems, Wuesthoff Medical Center – Rockledge, Rockledge, FL, p. A137

BARNHART, J. T., Chief Executive Officer, Walton Regional Medical Center, Monroe, GA, p. A156

BARNHART, Jeff, Chief Executive Officer, Ochiltree General Hospital, Perryton, TX, p. A620

BARNHILL–KEENER, Vickie, Director Human Resources, Medical Park Hospital, Hope, AR, p. A46

BAROCO, Paul T., M.D. Chief Medical Officer, Sacred Heart Hospital of Pensacola, Pensacola, FL, p. A136

BARONE, Charles, M.D. Vice President Medical Affairs, Children's Hospital of Michigan, Detroit, MI, p. A310

BARONE, Nancy, Vice President and Executive Director Operations and Strategic Planning, University Hospital, Cincinnati, OH, p. A474

BARONE, Richard, M.D. Medical Director, Sound Shore Medical Center of Westchester, New Rochelle, NY, p. A431

BARONOFF, Peter R., President and Chief Executive Officer, Success Healthcare, Boca Raton, FL, p. B124

BARR, Brant, M.D. Chief Medical Officer, District One Hospital, Faribault, MN, p. A331

BARR, Brent, Chief Information Officer, Minnie Hamilton HealthCare Center, Grantsville, WV, p. A672

BARR, Bret, Vice President Fiscal Services, Conway Medical Center, Conway, SC, p. A549

Index of Health Care Professionals / Batey

Index of Health Care Professionals

BARR, Catherine, President, HealthEast Bethesda Hospital, Saint Paul, MN, p. A339
BARR, Kristine, Vice President Communication Services, O'Bleness Memorial Hospital, Athens, OH, p. A470
BARR, Mary Beth, R.N. Chief Executive Officer, Grant Memorial Hospital, Petersburg, WV, p. A674
BARR, Steven, MSN, Chief Executive Officer, Plaza Specialty Hospital, Houston, TX, p. A606
BARR, Tamara, Human Resources Generalist, St. Vincent's St. Clair, Pell City, AL, p. A25
BARR, Tom, Director Operational Support Services, Peterson Rehabilitation Hospital, Wheeling, WV, p. A676
BARR, Vivian C.
Director Human Resources, Higgins General Hospital, Bremen, GA, p. A148
Director Human Resources, Tanner Medical Center, Carrollton, GA, p. A148
BARRA, Jon, Director Human Resources, Wyoming Behavioral Institute, Casper, WY, p. A695
BARRA, Peter, M.D. Chief Medical Officer, Flushing Hospital Medical Center,, NY, p. A432
BARRACK, Amy, Director Human Resources, Riverside Behavioral Health Center, Hampton, VA, p. A649
BARRACLOUGH, Roy E., Administrator and Chief Executive Officer, Moab Regional Hospital, Moab, UT, p. A638
BARRACO, Dennis, D.O. Medical Director, Wickenburg Community Hospital, Wickenburg, AZ, p. A41
BARRAMEDA, Maricar, Chief Information Officer, Lincoln Medical and Mental Health Center,, NY, p. A434
BARRAN, Peter, M.D. Chief of Staff, Pondera Medical Center, Conrad, MT, p. A374
BARREIRO, Maggie E., Administrator, Weslaco Rehabilitation Hospital, Weslaco, TX, p. A634
BARRERA, Celia, Administrator, Surgery Specialty Hospitals of America, Pasadena, TX, p. A620
BARRERA, Diahann, Chief Financial Officer, Willow Springs Center, Reno, NV, p. A395
BARRERA, Edward, Director Communications, Encino Hospital Medical Center,, CA, p. A69
BARRETO, Marcelino, M.D. Chief Medical Staff, MidMichigan Medical Center–Gladwin, Gladwin, MI, p. A313
BARRETT, A. R., D.O. Chief of Staff, East Texas Medical Center Carthage, Carthage, TX, p. A586
BARRETT, Anne J., Associate Executive Director Human Resources, Southside Hospital, Bay Shore, NY, p. A421
BARRETT, Bob, Chief Financial Officer, Clinch Valley Medical Center, Richlands, VA, p. A654
BARRETT, Cindy, Administrative Assistant, Patton State Hospital, Patton, CA, p. A80
BARRETT, Debbie, Director Human Resources, J. D. McCarty Center for Children With Developmental Disabilities, Norman, OK, p. A500
BARRETT, Douglas T., Senior Vice President Human Resources, Masonicare Health Center, Wallingford, CT, p. A112
BARRETT Jr., James W., Chief Executive Officer, Richardson Medical Center, Rayville, LA, p. A276
BARRETT, Janet, R.N. Chief Nurse Executive, Massac Memorial Hospital, Metropolis, IL, p. A188
BARRETT, Jason P., Chief Operating Officer, Flagler Hospital, Saint Augustine, FL, p. A137
BARRETT III, John E., Chief Executive Officer, Bon Secours–DePaul Medical Center, Norfolk, VA, p. A652
BARRETT, Kerry Flynn, Vice President Human Resources, Northern Westchester Hospital, Mount Kisco, NY, p. A430
BARRETT, Linda, Vice President of Information Services, Community Hospital of Bremen, Bremen, IN, p. A198
BARRETT, Peggy, R.N. Chief Executive Officer, Central Texas Rehabilitation Hospital, Austin, TX, p. A580
BARRETT, T. Marc, M.D. Senior Vice President Medical Affairs, Providence Health Center, Waco, TX, p. A633
BARRETTO, Shirley, M.D. Chief of Staff, Knox County Hospital, Knox City, TX, p. A611
BARRICK, Lisa, Controller, HEALTHSOUTH Scottsdale Rehabilitation Hospital, Scottsdale, AZ, p. A38
BARRILLEAUX, Scott G., FACHE Chief Executive Officer, Homer Memorial Hospital, Homer, LA, p. A267
BARROCAS, Albert, M.D. Chief Medical Officer, South Fulton Medical Center, Atlanta, GA, p. A146
BARROETA, Jennifer
Chief Human Resources Officer, Baptist Hospitals of Southeast Texas, Beaumont, TX, p. A582
Manager Human Resources, Baptist Orange Hospital, Orange, TX, p. A619
BARRON, Bill, M.D. Chief Medical Officer, University of California, Irvine Healthcare, Orange, CA, p. A78
BARRON, Cynthia, Manager Business Office, Corpus Christi Specialty Hospital, Corpus Christi, TX, p. A589
BARRON, Lee, Chief Executive Officer, Southern Inyo Healthcare District, Lone Pine, CA, p. A67
BARRON, Steven R., President, St. Bernardine Medical Center, San Bernardino, CA, p. A85
BARROW, Stella, Director Human Resources, Longview Regional Medical Center, Longview, TX, p. A613
BARROW II, William F., President and Chief Executive Officer, Our Lady of Lourdes Regional Medical Center, Lafayette, LA, p. A270
BARROWS, Cheryl, Vice President Human Resources, Sturdy Memorial Hospital, Attleboro, MA, p. A295
BARRY, Amy, Vice President and Chief Human Resources Officer, Martin Health System, Stuart, FL, p. A139
BARRY, Tom, President and Chief Executive Officer, Ferrell Hospital, Eldorado, IL, p. A180
BARSE, Steve, Chief Information Officer, Lawton Indian Hospital, Lawton, OK, p. A498
BARSOM, Michael, M.D. Medical Director, Metropolitan State Hospital, Norwalk, CA, p. A77
BARSTAD, Stacy
Chief Executive Officer, Sanford Tracy Medical Center, Tracy, MN, p. A340
Chief Executive Officer, Sanford Westbrook Medical Center, Westbrook, MN, p. A341
BARTAL, Ely, M.D. Chief Executive Officer, Kansas Surgery and Recovery Center, Wichita, KS, p. A245
BARTELS, Bruce M., President, WellSpan Health, York, PA, p. B144
BARTELS, Jennifer, HR Director, Pawnee County Memorial Hospital, Pawnee City, NE, p. A389
BARTH, Tara, Chief Nursing Officer, Palo Verde Hospital, Blythe, CA, p. A56
BARTHEL, Gayle, Coordinator Human Resources, Select Specialty Hospital–Flint, Flint, MI, p. A312
BARTHOLOMEW, K. A., M.D. Medical Director, Faulkton Area Medical Center, Faulkton, SD, p. A556
BARTHOLOMEW, Shelley, Director Human Resources, Decatur County General Hospital, Parsons, TN, p. A574
BARTILSON, Jim, Manager Information Systems, South Peninsula Hospital, Homer, AK, p. A29
BARTINGALE, Robert, Chief Administrative Officer, Mayo Clinic Health System in Fairmont, Fairmont, MN, p. A331
BARTLE, James W., Vice President Finance, Beebe Medical Center, Lewes, DE, p. A114
BARTLETT, James, Chief Financial Officer, Faith Community Hospital, Jacksboro, TX, p. A609
BARTLETT, Karolyn, Assistant Administrator, Mayo Clinic Health System – Northland in Barron, Barron, WI, p. A678
BARTLETT, Regina, Chief Executive Officer, Hendersonville Medical Center, Hendersonville, TN, p. A566
BARTLETT, Richard, M.D. Chief Medical Officer, Basin Healthcare Center, Odessa, TX, p. A619
BARTLETT, Roderick, M.D. President Medical Staff, Hannibal Regional Hospital, Hannibal, MO, p. A360
BARTLETT, Ronald E., Chief Financial Officer, Boston Medical Center, Boston, MA, p. A296
BARTLETT, Taci, Chief Financial Officer, Gothenburg Memorial Hospital, Gothenburg, NE, p. A384
BARTLETT III, Thomas G., M.D. Administrator, Laird Hospital, Union, MS, p. A353
BARTLEY, Tracy, Manager Information Technology, Bath Community Hospital, Hot Springs, VA, p. A650
BARTO Jr., John K., President and Chief Executive Officer, New Hanover Regional Medical Center, Wilmington, NC, p. A462
BARTO Jr.,, John K., President and Chief Executive Officer, New Hanover Regional Medical Center, Wilmington, NC, p. B92
BARTON, Annie, Director Human Resources, Peterson Rehabilitation Hospital, Wheeling, WV, p. A676
BARTON, Brent, Director Information Technology, Lakeview Hospital, Bountiful, UT, p. A637
BARTON, Charles, Business Manager, Southwestern State Hospital, Thomasville, GA, p. A160
BARTON, Gratia, Chief Financial Officer, Sequoia Hospital, Redwood City, CA, p. A82
BARTON, Larry O., FACHE President, Western Baptist Hospital, Paducah, KY, p. A257
BARTON, Rod, Administrator, Cassia Regional Medical Center, Burley, ID, p. A167
BARTON, Thomas, M.D. Medical Director, TOPS Surgical Specialty Hospital, Houston, TX, p. A607
BARTON, Wendy, Manager Business Office, Fredonia Regional Hospital, Fredonia, KS, p. A233
BARTOS, John M., Chief Executive Officer, Marcus Daly Memorial Hospital, Hamilton, MT, p. A376
BARTRUFF, Craig, M.D. Medical Director, Gothenburg Memorial Hospital, Gothenburg, NE, p. A384
BARTS, Dennis, Chief Executive Officer, Valley Hospital and Medical Center, Spokane Valley, WA, p. A667
BARTZ, Daniel R., CPA Chief Financial Officer, Warren Memorial Hospital, Friend, NE, p. A383
BARTZ, Ryan, D.O. Chief of Staff, McNairy Regional Hospital, Selmer, TN, p. A575
BARWICK, Kim, Vice President Human Resources, Anthony Medical Center, Anthony, KS, p. A230
BARWIS, Kurt A., FACHE President and Chief Executive Officer, Bristol Hospital, Bristol, CT, p. A108
BASCOM, Steven, M.D. Chief Medical Officer, Guthrie County Hospital, Guthrie Center, IA, p. A220
BASEY, Marjorie, Chief Financial Officer, Rehabilitation Hospital of Indiana, Indianapolis, IN, p. A205
BASH, Robert R., FACHE Chief Executive Officer and Administrator, Doctor's Hospital of Deer Creek, Leesville, LA, p. A271
BASLER, Cyndi, Interim Chief Executive Officer, Iron County Hospital, Pilot Knob, MO, p. A366
BASNIGHT, Tom, Chief Financial Officer, Walter B. Jones Alcohol and Drug Abuse Treatment Center, Greenville, NC, p. A454
BASS, Anne, Chief Financial Officer, Fairfield Memorial Hospital, Winnsboro, SC, p. A554
BASS, G. Michael, President and Chief Executive Officer, Piedmont Newnan Hospital, Newnan, GA, p. A157
BASS, Gordon B., Chief Operating Officer, Ann & Robert H. Lurie Children's Hospital of Chicago, Chicago, IL, p. A175
BASS, Louis A., Vice President Finance, Northeast Alabama Regional Medical Center, Anniston, AL, p. A15
BASS, Sonya, MS Chief Nursing Officer, Colorado Plains Medical Center, Fort Morgan, CO, p. A101
BASS, Jr., William L., Vice President Finance and Chief Financial Officer, Centra Southside Community Hospital, Farmville, VA, p. A648
BASSETT, Annie, Director Finance, McBride Clinic Orthopedic Hospital, Oklahoma City, OK, p. A501
BASSETT, Christine, Chief Executive Officer, Radius Specialty Hospital Boston, Boston, MA, p. A297
BASSETT, Eugene, Interim President and Chief Executive Officer, Methodist Hospital of Sacramento, Sacramento, CA, p. A83
BASSO, James, Chief Human Resources Officer, Central Texas Veterans Healthcare System, Temple, TX, p. A630
BASSO, Marty, Senior Vice President Finance, Suburban Hospital, Bethesda, MD, p. A290
BASTABLE, Chad, Director Human Resources, North Central Health Care, Wausau, WI, p. A693
BASTIANELLO, Carol, Director Employee Services, NORTHSTAR Health System, Iron River, MI, p. A316
BASTIEN IV, Samua A., Ph.D. Executive Director, St. Lawrence Psychiatric Center, Ogdensburg, NY, p. A439
BASTING, Gregory, M.D
Vice President Medical Affairs, Allied Services Rehabilitation Hospital, Scranton, PA, p. A537
Vice President Medical Affairs, John Heinz Institute of Rehabilitation Medicine, Wilkes–Barre, PA, p. A541
BATA, Katie, Vice President Human Resources, Sherman Hospital, Elgin, IL, p. A181
BATAL, Lucille M., Administrator, Baldpate Hospital, Haverhill, MA, p. A300
BATCHELOR, Dale, M.D. Chief Medical Officer, Saint Thomas Hospital, Nashville, TN, p. A573
BATCHELOR, Daniela, Director Human Resources, Springhill Memorial Hospital, Mobile, AL, p. A23
BATCHELOR, Diana, Chief Nursing Officer, Finley Hospital, Dubuque, IA, p. A219
BATCHELOR, Michael, President, North Greenville Hospital, Travelers Rest, SC, p. A554
BATEMAN, Bryan S., Chief Executive Officer, Women and Children's Hospital, Lake Charles, LA, p. A271
BATEMAN, Kenneth, CPA, President and Chief Executive Officer, Somerset Medical Center, Somerville, NJ, p. A410
BATEMAN, Mark T., Interim Chief Operating Officer, Saint Agnes Medical Center, Fresno, CA, p. A62
BATEMAN, Steven B., Chief Executive Officer, St. Mark's Hospital, Salt Lake City, UT, p. A641
BATES, Don, Chief Executive Officer, Palacios Community Medical Center, Palacios, TX, p. A619
BATES, Earl, Director Information Technology, Western Mental Health Institute, Bolivar, TN, p. A562
BATES, Jonathan R., M.D. President and Chief Executive Officer, Arkansas Children's Hospital, Little Rock, AR, p. A47
BATES, Juanita Ann, Administrator, St. Charles Specialty Rehabilitation Hospital, Luling, LA, p. A272
BATES, Mary, Director Human Resources, Bowie Memorial Hospital, Bowie, TX, p. A584
BATES, Peter, M.D. Vice President Medical Affairs and Chief Medical Officer, Maine Medical Center, Portland, ME, p. A284
BATES, Robert A., Executive Director Finance and Chief Financial Officer, St. Vincent Carmel Hospital, Carmel, IN, p. A199
BATEY, James, M.D. President Medical Staff, Baptist Memorial Hospital–Union City, Union City, TN, p. A576

BATH, Jeffrey, M.D. President Medical Staff, North Adams Regional Hospital, North Adams, MA, p. A303

BATISTA, David J., Chief Executive Officer, Garfield Medical Center, Monterey Park, CA, p. A75

BATISTE, Michele, Director Human Resources, Preston Memorial Hospital, Kingwood, WV, p. A673

BATORY, Robert J., Vice President Human Resources, York Hospital, York, PA, p. A543

BATSHAW, Mark L., M.D. Interim Chief Medical Officer and Chief Academic Officer, Children's National Medical Center, Washington, DC, p. A116

BATTERTON, Owen A., M.D. Chief of Staff, Greene County General Hospital, Linton, IN, p. A207

BATTISTA, Donald P., President and Chief Executive Officer, Garrett County Memorial Hospital, Oakland, MD, p. A293

BATTISTA, Edward, Vice President Human Resources, West Hills Hospital and Medical Center,, CA, p. A72

BATTLES, Ruth, Administrative Director Human Resources, Corona Regional Medical Center, Corona, CA, p. A58

BATTY, Jill I., Chief Financial Officer, Cheshire Medical Center, Keene, NH, p. A398

BATTY, Mark, Chief Executive Officer, Rochelle Community Hospital, Rochelle, IL, p. A192

BATULIS, Scott, Chief Executive Officer, Orange Regional Medical Center, Middletown, NY, p. A430

BATY, Grace, Director Human Resources, Sweeny Community Hospital, Sweeny, TX, p. A629

BAUER, Brian, Chief Executive Officer, Lutheran Hospital of Indiana, Fort Wayne, IN, p. A201

BAUER, Gregory P., President and Chief Executive Officer, Elk Regional Health Center, Saint Marys, PA, p. A537

BAUER, Janice, Administrator, Cardinal Hill Specialty Hospital, Fort Thomas, KY, p. A250

BAUER, Jonathan, Director Information Services, Somerset Hospital, Somerset, PA, p. A538

BAUER, Kyle, Chief Financial Officer, Cuyuna Regional Medical Center, Crosby, MN, p. A330

BAUER, Richard, M.D. Chief of Staff, South Texas Veterans Health Care System, San Antonio, TX, p. A626

BAUER, Robert, Director Human Resources, Wheaton Franciscan Healthcare – St. Francis, Milwaukee, WI, p. A687

BAUER, Roberta, M.D. Acting Chair Medical Staff, Cleveland Clinic Children's Hospital for Rehabilitation, Cleveland, OH, p. A474

BAUER, Roger, M.D. Chief Medical Officer, Swift County–Benson Hospital, Benson, MN, p. A328

BAUER, Sandra A., Director Human Resources, Jefferson Community Health Center, Fairbury, NE, p. A383

BAUER, Shar, Executive Secretary, Wishek Community Hospital and Clinics, Wishek, ND, p. A468

BAUER, Tracy, Chief Executive Officer, Midwest Medical Center, Galena, IL, p. A182

BAUER, William, Vice President Finance and Chief Financial Officer, Hazleton General Hospital, Hazleton, PA, p. A525

BAUER, William, M.D. Medical Director, Montevista Hospital, Las Vegas, NV, p. A393

BAUKNECHT, Ed, Director Management Information Systems, Holy Family Memorial Medical Center, Manitowoc, WI, p. A685

BAUMAN, Jonathan, M.D. Chief Medical Officer, Four Winds Hospital, Katonah, NY, p. A428

BAUMCHEN, Sandra, Chief Executive Officer, Select Specialty Hospital–Northwest Detroit, Detroit, MI, p. A311

BAUMEIER, Mark, M.D. Chief of Staff, St. Joseph Mercy Livingston Hospital, Howell, MI, p. A315

BAUMERT, Steven P., President and Chief Executive Officer, Jennie Edmundson Hospital, Council Bluffs, IA, p. A217

BAUMGARDNER, Brian, Chief Executive Officer, West Florida Hospital, Pensacola, FL, p. A136

BAUMGARDNER, Charles J., Vice President Corporate Operations, Psychiatric Institute of Washington, Washington, DC, p. A117

BAUMGARDNER, David, Director Information Management, Union Hospital, Dover, OH, p. A479

BAUMGARTEN, Alan, M.D. Chief of Staff, Mission Hospital, Asheville, NC, p. A448

BAUMGARTNER, David, M.D. Vice President Medical Affairs, Saint Mary's Health Care, Grand Rapids, MI, p. A314

BAUMGARTNER, Jennifer, Chief Information Officer, Perkins County Health Services, Grant, NE, p. A384

BAUMGARTNER, Michael A., President, St. Francis Regional Medical Center, Shakopee, MN, p. A340

BAUNCHALK, James M., Deputy Chief Clinical Services, Dwight David Eisenhower Army Medical Center, Fort Gordon, GA, p. A153

BAUTE, Corey, Chief Human Resources Management Services, Richard L. Roudebush Veterans Affairs Medical Center, Indianapolis, IN, p. A205

BAUTISTA, Veronica, Chief Financial Officer, Memorial Regional Hospital South,, FL, p. A125

BAVERSO, Lou, Chief Information Officer, Magee–Womens Hospital of UPMC, Pittsburgh, PA, p. A535

BAW, Joseph, Director Human Resources, Riveredge Hospital, Forest Park, IL, p. A182

BAWA, Balraj, M.D. Assistant Director Medical Services, Central Virginia Training Center, Madison Heights, VA, p. A650

BAXTER, Anne, Director Fiscal Services, Northern Virginia Mental Health Institute, Falls Church, VA, p. A648

BAXTER, Greg, M.D. Vice President Medical Affairs, Elliot Hospital, Manchester, NH, p. A399

BAXTER, Michael T., Chief Executive Officer, Parkview Medical Center, Pueblo, CO, p. A105

BAXTER, Robert, Chief Operating Officer, Rapid City Regional Hospital, Rapid City, SD, p. A559

BAXTER, Robert O., President, St. Rita's Medical Center, Lima, OH, p. A483

BAY, Marybeth, Director Information Technology, Sauk Prairie Memorial Hospital & Clinics, Prairie Du Sac, WI, p. A689

BAY, Shelley, Chief Financial Officer, Fayette County Hospital, Vandalia, IL, p. A195

BAYER, Allison, Executive Vice President and Chief Operating Officer, Cambridge Health Alliance, Cambridge, MA, p. A299

BAYER, Thomas R., Chief Operating Officer, St. Vincent Hospital, Green Bay, WI, p. A682

BAYLESS, Betsey, President and Chief Executive Officer, Maricopa Integrated Health System, Phoenix, AZ, p. A36

BAYLESS, Victoria, President and Chief Executive Officer, Anne Arundel Medical Center, Annapolis, MD, p. A287

BAYLESS–BERNEY, Jill, MSN Chief Operating Officer, Longview Regional Medical Center, Longview, TX, p. A613

BAYTOS, David G., Interim Chief Executive Officer, Crittenden Regional Hospital, West Memphis, AR, p. A52

BAYUS, Robin, Chief Financial Officer, Rancho Los Amigos National Rehabilitation Center, Downey, CA, p. A59

BAZELEY, Stephen, M.D. Vice President Medical Affairs, ProMedica St. Luke's Hospital, Maumee, OH, p. A484

BEA, Javon R., President and Chief Executive Officer, Mercy Health System, Janesville, WI, p. B89

BEA, Javon R., President and Chief Executive Officer, Mercy Hospital and Trauma Center, Janesville, WI, p. A683

BEACH, Karrie, Director Human Resources, Community Memorial Hospital, Syracuse, NE, p. A390

BEACH, Michele, Associate Director, Veterans Affairs Medical Center, Sheridan, WY, p. A697

BEADMAN, Cindi, Director Medical Records, Harper Hospital District Five, Harper, KS, p. A234

BEALE, George L., M.D. Director Medical Staff, Clay County Hospital, Ashland, AL, p. A15

BEALER, Ruth, Director Human Resources, Great Bend Regional Hospital, Great Bend, KS, p. A233

BEALER, Shirley, Director, Overton Brooks Veterans Affairs Medical Center, Shreveport, LA, p. A277

BEAM, William, M.D. Chief of Staff, Cornerstone Hospital of Huntington, Huntington, WV, p. A672

BEAMAN Jr.,, Charles D., Chief Executive Officer, Palmetto Health, Columbia, SC, p. B99

BEAMAN, Frank, Administrator, Faith Community Hospital, Jacksboro, TX, p. A609

BEAMAN, John, Senior Vice President and Chief Financial Officer, Simi Valley Hospital and Health Care Services, Simi Valley, CA, p. A91

BEAMES, Bo, Administrator, Socorro General Hospital, Socorro, NM, p. A418

BEAN, Robert H., Ph.D. President and Chief Executive Officer, Sumner Regional Medical Center, Wellington, KS, p. A245

BEANE, Jeff, Director Human Resources, Roane General Hospital, Spencer, WV, p. A676

BEAR, Lawrence P., Administrator and Chief Executive Officer, Jersey Community Hospital, Jerseyville, IL, p. A185

BEARB, April, Administrator, Jennings Senior Care Hospital, Jennings, LA, p. A268

BEARD, Bradley, President, Fairview Southdale Hospital, Edina, MN, p. A331

BEARD, Dewaine, Chief Information Officer, Veterans Affairs Pittsburgh Healthcare System, Pittsburgh, PA, p. A536

BEARD, Edward L., MSN Senior Vice President, Patient Care Services & CNO, Catawba Valley Medical Center, Hickory, NC, p. A455

BEARD, Gerald C., Chief Operating Officer, Healthmark Regional Medical Center, DeFuniak Springs, FL, p. A122

BEARD, Joan, Chief Nursing Officer, Northwest Florida Community Hospital, Chipley, FL, p. A120

BEARD, Pat, Director Human Resources, Clinton County Hospital, Albany, KY, p. A247

BEARD, Raleigh, Chief Fiscal Services, Veterans Affairs Edward Hines, Jr. Hospital, Hines, IL, p. A184

BEARD, Rhonda
Director Human Resources, Palestine Regional Medical Center–East, Palestine, TX, p. A619
Director Human Resources, Palestine Regional Rehabilitation Center, Palestine, TX, p. A619

BEARD, Scott, M.D. Chief of Staff, Nevada Regional Medical Center, Nevada, MO, p. A366

BEASLEY, Christina, Director Human Resources, Carlsbad Medical Center, Carlsbad, NM, p. A415

BEASLEY, Craig, M.D. Chief of Staff and Medical Officer, Throckmorton County Memorial Hospital, Throckmorton, TX, p. A631

BEASLEY, Leslie, Director Human Resources, Temple Community Hospital, Los Angeles, CA, p. A72

BEASLEY, Lynn W., FACHE Chief Executive Officer, Hendry Regional Medical Center, Clewiston, FL, p. A120

BEASLEY, Ruth, Director Human Resources, Vanderbilt Stallworth Rehabilitation Hospital, Nashville, TN, p. A574

BEASLEY, Tareka, Director Human Resources, RiverWoods Behavioral Health System, Riverdale, GA, p. A157

BEATTIE, Kathryn, M.D. Senior Vice President and Chief Medical Officer, Valley Medical Center, Renton, WA, p. A664

BEATTIE, Mac, Computer Network Specialist, Deer's Head Hospital Center, Salisbury, MD, p. A294

BEATTY, Alan, Vice President Human Resources, Shore Medical Center, Somers Point, NJ, p. A410

BEATTY, Ann, Director Human Resources, Fairview Hospital, Cleveland, OH, p. A475

BEATTY, James R., Chief Operating Officer, Lawnwood Regional Medical Center, Fort Pierce, FL, p. A124

BEATTY, John, Vice President Human Resources, Barnes–Jewish Hospital, Saint Louis, MO, p. A368

BEATTY, Kemp, Director Information Management, Carlisle Regional Medical Center, Carlisle, PA, p. A520

BEATTY, Talia, Director Human Resources, Sunbury Community Hospital, Sunbury, PA, p. A539

BEATY, Holly, Chief Financial Officer, South Central Kansas Medical Center, Arkansas City, KS, p. A230

BEATY, Ralph E., Chief Executive Officer, Great River Medical Center, Blytheville, AR, p. A42

BEATY, Ralph E., Chief Executive Officer, Mississippi County Hospital System, Blytheville, AR, p. B91

BEATY, Ralph E., Chief Executive Officer, South Mississippi County Regional Medical Center, Osceola, AR, p. A50

BEATY, Ryan D., President and Chief Executive Officer, Citrus Memorial Health System, Inverness, FL, p. A126

BEAUBIEN, Troy, Director Information Services, Manatee Memorial Hospital, Bradenton, FL, p. A119

BEAUDOIN, Dale, Vice President Human Resources, Lewis–Gale Medical Center, Salem, VA, p. A655

BEAUDOIN, Paul, Senior Vice President Finance and Chief Financial Officer, Kent County Memorial Hospital, Warwick, RI, p. A545

BEAUDRY, Lisa, M.P.H. Director, Patient Care, Baystate Mary Lane Hospital, Ware, MA, p. A305

BEAULAC, Gary, Chief Operating Officer, Henry Ford Macomb Hospitals, Clinton Township, MI, p. A309

BEAULIEU, Mary Lou, Director Human Resources and Compliance Officer, Northwestern Medical Center, Saint Albans, VT, p. A644

BEAULIEU, Sue, Chief Nurse Executive, Massena Memorial Hospital, Massena, NY, p. A429

BEAUPRE, Paul, M.D. Chief Executive Officer, Good Samaritan Hospital, San Jose, CA, p. A88

BEAUREGARD, Jodi, Chief Executive Officer, Martin General Hospital, Williamston, NC, p. A462

BEAUVAIS, Richard E., Ph.D. Chief Executive Officer, Wellspring Foundation, Bethlehem, CT, p. A108

BEAVER, Michael E., Chief Operating Officer, Methodist Hospital, San Antonio, TX, p. A625

BEAVER, Patrick, R.N. Vice President Patient Care and Chief Nursing Officer, East Liverpool City Hospital, East Liverpool, OH, p. A479

BEAVER, Randy, Chief Information Officer, Palo Alto County Health System, Emmetsburg, IA, p. A219

BEAZLEY, Gary, Coordinator Information Systems, Baylor Medical Center at Waxahachie, Waxahachie, TX, p. A633

BEBEE, Beldia, Acting Chief Financial Officer, Huey P. Long Medical Center, Pineville, LA, p. A276

BEBOW, Gary, FACHE Administrator and Chief Executive Officer, White River Health System, Batesville, AR, p. B146

BEBOW, Gary, FACHE Administrator and Chief Executive Officer, White River Medical Center, Batesville, AR, p. A42

BECHTLE, Mavis, MSN Vice President and Chief Nursing Officer, MetroHealth Medical Center, Cleveland, OH, p. A475

BECK, Allan, Chief Executive Officer, Baylor Orthopedic and Spine Hospital at Arlington, Arlington, TX, p. A579

BECK, Ann, Vice President Finance, Carson Tahoe Regional Healthcare, Carson City, NV, p. A391

Index of Health Care Professionals / Bides

Index of Health Care Professionals

BERGLIN, Sally L., Vice President, Bronson LakeView Hospital, Paw Paw, MI, p. A320
BERGLING, Richard Q., Chief Executive Officer, Gove County Medical Center, Quinter, KS, p. A242
BERGMAN, Chris, Chief Financial Officer, Christ Hospital, Cincinnati, OH, p. A473
BERGMAN, Jim, Director Human Resources, Northeast Regional Medical Center, Kirksville, MO, p. A363
BERGMANN, Dan, M.D. Chief Medical Officer, Barnes–Jewish St. Peters Hospital, Saint Peters, MO, p. A370
BERGMANN, Peter U., President and Chief Executive Officer, Sisters of Charity Hospital of Buffalo, Buffalo, NY, p. A423
BERGSENG, John H., D.O. Vice President Medical Affairs, Glencoe Regional Health Services, Glencoe, MN, p. A332
BERKELEY, Larry L., Associate Director, Clement J. Zablocki Veterans Affairs Medical Center, Milwaukee, WI, p. A686
BERKHOUSE, Steve, Chief Financial Officer, Hocking Valley Community Hospital, Logan, OH, p. A483
BERKOWITZ, David J., Vice President and Chief Operating Officer, Palisades Medical Center, North Bergen, NJ, p. A407
BERKRAM, Treasure, Chief Financial Officer, Northern Rockies Medical Center, Cut Bank, MT, p. A374
BERLINGHOFF, Kathleen, Director Human Resources, Sharon Hospital, Sharon, CT, p. A111
BERLOT, Alvin, M.D. Medical Director, Bucktail Medical Center, Renovo, PA, p. A537
BERLUCCHI, Scott A., FACHE President and Chief Executive Officer, Auburn Community Hospital, Auburn, NY, p. A421
BERMAN, Manuel S., Administrator and Chief Operating Officer, Tuality Healthcare, Hillsboro, OR, p. A511
BERNAL, Enrique, Chief Financial Officer, Sierra Medical Center, El Paso, TX, p. A596
BERNARD, David, M.D. Chief Medical Officer, Beth Israel Medical Center, New York, NY, p. A431
BERNARD, Donald P., Chief Financial Officer, Fontana Medical Center, Fontana, CA, p. A61
BERNARD, Lorrie, Manager Patient Accounts and Information Systems, Athol Memorial Hospital, Athol, MA, p. A295
BERNARD, Peter J., Chief Executive Officer, Bon Secours St. Francis Medical Center, Midlothian, VA, p. A651
BERNARD, Traci, President, Texas Health Harris Methodist Hospital Southlake, Southlake, TX, p. A628
BERNARDO, Maria, M.D. Chief of Staff, Bullock County Hospital, Union Springs, AL, p. A26
BERNATIS, Terry, Manager Human Resources, Community Health Care System, Onaga, KS, p. A240
BERND, David L., Chief Executive Officer, Sentara Healthcare, Norfolk, VA, p. B117
BERNDT, Julia L., Chief Financial Officer, Logansport Memorial Hospital, Logansport, IN, p. A207
BERNER, Tom, Vice President and Chief Financial Officer, Bristol Bay Area Health Corporation, Dillingham, AK, p. A28
BERNEY, Bernadette, Director Human Resources, Pullman Regional Hospital, Pullman, WA, p. A664
BERNICK, Michael, Vice President Finance, Clarity Child Guidance Center, San Antonio, TX, p. A624
BERNINI, A. Susan, Chief Operating Officer, Einstein Medical Center Philadelphia, Philadelphia, PA, p. A532
BERNS, Erin, Director Human Resources, Veterans Memorial Hospital, Waukon, IA, p. A228
BERNSTEIN, Lee, Executive Vice President and Chief Operating Officer, SSM St. Joseph Health Center, Saint Charles, MO, p. A368
BERNSTEIN, Les, Director Information Systems, Cookeville Regional Medical Center, Cookeville, TN, p. A564
BERNSTEIN, Michael, Chief Financial Officer, Tulare Regional Medical Center, Tulare, CA, p. A93
BERNSTEIN, Paul E., M.D. Area Medical Director, San Diego Medical Center, San Diego, CA, p. A85
BERRETT, Britt, President and Chief Executive Officer, Texas Health Presbyterian Hospital Dallas, Dallas, TX, p. A592
BERRIGAN, Mary, Chief Operating Officer, Medical Center of Aurora, Aurora, CO, p. A97
BERRY, David, Senior Vice President and Chief Operating Officer, Arkansas Children's Hospital, Little Rock, AR, p. A47
BERRY, Deborah, Director of Operations, Greene County Hospital, Leakesville, MS, p. A349
BERRY, Eilleen, Manager Information Technology, Webster County Community Hospital, Red Cloud, NE, p. A389
BERRY, Greg, Chief Financial Officer, Doctors Medical Center, Modesto, CA, p. A75
BERRY, James T., Chief Executive Officer, Purcell Municipal Hospital, Purcell, OK, p. A503
BERRY, Jonathan, Chief Support Services and Chief Financial Officer, Broughton Hospital, Morganton, NC, p. A457
BERRY, Linda, Vice President Human Resources, Memorial Hospital, Towanda, PA, p. A539
BERRY, Lisa, Director, Saint Anne's Hospital, Fall River, MA, p. A299
BERRY, Robert F., Chief Executive Officer, Lane Frost Health and Rehabilitation Center, Hugo, OK, p. A498
BERRY, Roberta, Manager Human Resources, Southeast Arizona Medical Center, Douglas, AZ, p. A31
BERRY, Ross, Chief Executive Officer, Shoals Hospital, Muscle Shoals, AL, p. A24
BERRY, Stanley B., FACHE Administrator, Shriners Hospitals for Children, Honolulu, Honolulu, HI, p. A164
BERRY, Tiffany, Chief Financial Officer, Twin Rivers Regional Medical Center, Kennett, MO, p. A363
BERRY, Wesley, Chief Financial Officer, Nicholas County Hospital, Carlisle, KY, p. A248
BERRYMAN, William R., M.D. Acting Director, Veterans Affairs Medical Center, Grand Junction, CO, p. A102
BERSANTE, Syd, President, St. Joseph Medical Center, Tacoma, WA, p. A668
BERSAU, Ulrike, Administrator, St. Luke's Rehabilitation Institute, Spokane, WA, p. A667
BERSHAD, Joshua M., M.D. Senior Vice President Medical Affairs and Chief Medical Officer, Robert Wood Johnson University Hospital, New Brunswick, NJ, p. A407
BERSINGER, David, M.D. Chief of Staff, Chesterfield General Hospital, Cheraw, SC, p. A547
BERT, Alisa, Chief Financial Officer, Aventura Hospital and Medical Center, Aventura, FL, p. A118
BERTKE, Bradley J., President and Chief Executive Officer, Mercy St. Anne Hospital, Toledo, OH, p. A489
BERTRAM, Jo, Vice President Finance, SSM St. Mary's Health Center, Saint Louis, MO, p. A369
BERTRAND, Joan L., Vice President Human Resources, Adcare Hospital of Worcester, Worcester, MA, p. A306
BERTRAND, Neil W., Chief Financial Officer, Longmont United Hospital, Longmont, CO, p. A104
BERTSCH, Darrold, Chief Executive Officer, Sakakawea Medical Center, Hazen, ND, p. A466
BESHARAT, Fred, M.D. Chief of Staff, Los Angeles Metropolitan Medical Center, Los Angeles, CA, p. A70
BESS, Amy, Chief Financial Officer, Mizell Memorial Hospital, Opp, AL, p. A24
BESS, Timothy A., Chief Executive Officer, Wythe County Community Hospital, Wytheville, VA, p. A658
BESSEL, Marjorie, M.D. Chief Medical Officer, Banner Desert Medical Center, Mesa, AZ, p. A34
BESSER, Sherry L., R.N. Vice President Quality, Risk Management and Chief Nursing Officer, Pratt Regional Medical Center, Pratt, KS, p. A242
BESSLER, September, Manager Human Resources, Brookings Health System, Brookings, SD, p. A555
BESST, Kara, President and Chief Executive Officer, Gritman Medical Center, Moscow, ID, p. A169
BESTEN, Robert, Chief Financial Officer, Mary Breckinridge ARH Hospital, Hyden, KY, p. A252
BESTGEN, Pat, Manager Human Resources, Cameron Regional Medical Center, Cameron, MO, p. A356
BESWICK, Elizabeth, Vice President Human Resources and Public Relations, Carteret General Hospital, Morehead City, NC, p. A457
BETANCOURT, Erika, Coordinator Human Resources, Cornerstone Regional Hospital, Edinburg, TX, p. A595
BETANCOURT, Salvador, Manager Information Systems, Sunnyside Community Hospital, Sunnyside, WA, p. A667
BETHALA, Vasanth, M.D. Medical Director, Louisiana Medical Center and Heart Hospital, Lacombe, LA, p. A269
BETHELL, Mark, Chief Executive Officer, Gateway Regional Medical Center, Granite City, IL, p. A183
BETKE, Bryce, Chief Financial Officer, Crete Area Medical Center, Crete, NE, p. A383
BETKE–MENA, Rachel, Director Health Information Management, Colusa Regional Medical Center, Colusa, CA, p. A58
BETTEM, Kelly, Assistant Chief Operating Officer, East Ohio Regional Hospital, Martins Ferry, OH, p. A484
BETTS, Brooks
Vice President and Chief Information Officer, Miles Memorial Hospital, Damariscotta, ME, p. A283
Director Information Systems and Chief Information Officer, Pen Bay Medical Center, Rockport, ME, p. A285
Vice President and Chief Information Officer, St. Andrews Hospital and Healthcare Center, Boothbay Harbor, ME, p. A282
BETTS, Crystal
Chief Financial Officer, Incline Village Community Hospital, Incline Village, NV, p. A392
Chief Financial Officer, Tahoe Forest Hospital District, Truckee, CA, p. A93
BETTS, Nicholas, Director Information Technology, Grundy County Memorial Hospital, Grundy Center, IA, p. A220
BETZ, Randal, M.D. Chief of Staff, Shriners Hospitals for Children, Philadelphia, Philadelphia, PA, p. A533
BEUTKE, Kenneth, Vice President Organization Development and Planning, OSF Saint James – John W. Albrecht Medical Center, Pontiac, IL, p. A192
BEVEL, John, Manager Information Systems, Shriners Hospitals for Children, Northern California, Sacramento, CA, p. A84
BEVERLY, DeAnna, Chief Operating Officer, Seven Rivers Regional Medical Center, Crystal River, FL, p. A121
BEVERLY, Douglas H., Chief Executive Officer, HEALTHSOUTH Rehabilitation Hospital of North Alabama, Huntsville, AL, p. A21
BEVERS, Donald, Chief Financial Officer, Memorial Hospital of Salem County, Salem, NJ, p. A410
BEVERS, Jonathan, M.D. Medical Director, Bloomington Meadows Hospital, Bloomington, IN, p. A198
BEWLEY, Lisa, Vice President and Chief Information Officer, Regional West Medical Center, Scottsbluff, NE, p. A389
BEWLEY, Martha, Chief Financial Officer, Mountain View Hospital District, Madras, OR, p. A512
BEYER, Eric J., President and Chief Executive Officer, Tufts Medical Center, Boston, MA, p. A297
BEYER, Jim, Director Human Resources, Norman Regional Health System, Norman, OK, p. A500
BEYER, Laura, Director Patient Care, Guttenberg Municipal Hospital, Guttenberg, IA, p. A220
BEYER, Laurie, Senior Vice President and Chief Financial Officer, Union Hospital, Elkton, MD, p. A291
BEYER, Teri, Chief Information Officer, Rice Memorial Hospital, Willmar, MN, p. A342
BEYER, William, M.D. Chief Medical Officer, St. Croix Regional Medical Center, St. Croix Falls, WI, p. A691
BEZUCHA, Gary, FACHE Chief Executive Officer, North Central Health Care, Wausau, WI, p. A693
BHAMBRA, Jody, Chief Nursing Officer, Hartgrove Hospital, Chicago, IL, p. A175
BHANDARI, Raj, M.D. Physician–in–Chief, San Jose Medical Center, San Jose, CA, p. A88
BHARGAVA, Mukesh, M.D. Vice President Medical Affairs, Henrietta D. Goodall Hospital, Sanford, ME, p. A285
BHARUCHA, Bomi, Chief Financial Officer, North Valley Hospital, Tonasket, WA, p. A668
BHASIN, Chetan, Chief Executive Officer, Kindred Rehabilitation Hospital Arlington, Arlington, TX, p. A579
BHATEJA, Renu, M.D. President Medical Staff, Ridgeview Psychiatric Hospital and Center, Oak Ridge, TN, p. A574
BHAYANI, Sam B., Chief Medical Officer, Barnes–Jewish West County Hospital, Saint Louis, MO, p. A368
BHOORASINGH, Merlene, Chief Clinical Officer, Kindred Hospital Ocala, Ocala, FL, p. A133
BHUCHAR, Subodh, M.D. Chief of Staff, Kindred Hospital Sugar Land, Sugar Land, TX, p. A629
BIALORVCKI, Tom, Chief Information Officer, Bay Medical Center, Panama City, FL, p. A135
BIANCAMANO, John, Chief Financial Officer, University of Connecticut Health Center, John Dempsey Hospital, Farmington, CT, p. A109
BIANCHI, Cynthia, Chief Information Officer, Woodhull Medical and Mental Health Center,, NY, p. A438
BIAS, Richard R., Acting Vice President Information Systems and Chief Information Officer, Georgia Health Sciences Medical Center, Augusta, GA, p. A146
BIBAL, Antoinette, Director Human Resources, Kindred Hospital–Baldwin Park, Baldwin Park, CA, p. A55
BIBB, Lisa, Director Human Resources, San Angelo Community Medical Center, San Angelo, TX, p. A624
BIBEAU, Roland R., President, Presbyterian Hospital Matthews, Matthews, NC, p. A457
BIBER, Carl, Chief Financial Officer, Columbus Regional Healthcare System, Whiteville, NC, p. A462
BIBY, Thom, Chief Financial Officer, Tulsa Spine and Specialty Hospital, Tulsa, OK, p. A507
BICHIMER, Michael, Director Financial Operations, Dublin Methodist Hospital, Dublin, OH, p. A479
BICKEL, Brian E., President and Chief Executive Officer, Southeast Arizona Medical Center, Douglas, AZ, p. A31
BICKEL, James, Chief Executive Officer, Columbus Regional Hospital, Columbus, IN, p. A199
BICKERSTAFF, Detra, Chief Human Resources Officer, South Fulton Medical Center, Atlanta, GA, p. A146
BICKFORD, Carmel, Chief Financial Officer, Wyoming Behavioral Institute, Casper, WY, p. A695
BICKINGS, John, Chief Operating Officer and Vice President Support Services, South Jersey Healthcare – Elmer Hospital, Elmer, NJ, p. A404
BICKNELL, James, M.D. Medical Director, MidMichigan Medical Center–Midland, Midland, MI, p. A319
BIDDLE, Kenneth, Controller, Kensington Hospital, Philadelphia, PA, p. A533
BIDES, Adrienne, Assistant Chief Financial Officer and Budget Analyst, Big Spring State Hospital, Big Spring, TX, p. A584



Index of Health Care Professionals A763

Index of Health Care Professionals

Index of Health Care Professionals / Bidleman


BIDLEMAN, Angela, R.N. Chief Nursing Officer, Integris Grove General Hospital, Grove, OK, p. A497
BIE, Gary E., Chief Financial Officer, Stony Brook University Medical Center, Stony Brook, NY, p. A444
BIEBER, Courtney, Director Information Systems, Mercy Regional Medical Center, Ville Platte, LA, p. A279
BIEBER, Martin A., President and Chief Executive Officer, Kennedy Memorial Hospitals–University Medical Center, Cherry Hill, NJ, p. A403
BIEDIGER, Dan, Vice President Human Resources, FirstHealth Moore Regional Hospital, Pinehurst, NC, p. A458
BIEDIGER, Michael J., FACHE President and Chief Executive Officer, Lexington Medical Center, West Columbia, SC, p. A554
BIEDRON, Janet, R.N. Chief Executive Officer, Kindred Hospital–Sacramento, Folsom, CA, p. A60
BIEGANSKI, Gary, FACHE Interim Chief Executive Officer, Weston County Health Services, Newcastle, WY, p. A697
BIEGERT, Dara, Assistant Vice President Human Resources, Medical Center of Lewisville, Lewisville, TX, p. A612
BIEGLER, Elizabeth A., R.N
Chief Nursing Officer, Dublin Methodist Hospital, Dublin, OH, p. A479
Chief Nursing Officer, Grady Memorial Hospital, Delaware, OH, p. A479
BIEHL, Albert, M.D. Vice President Medical Affairs, Bethesda Memorial Hospital, Boynton Beach, FL, p. A119
BIELECKI, Thomas A., Chief Financial Officer, Geisinger Wyoming Valley Medical Center, Wilkes Barre, PA, p. A541
BIEN, Jim, M.D. Vice President Quality and Patient Safety, Indiana University Health Arnett Hospital, Lafayette, IN, p. A206
BIEN, John, Vice President Finance, United Hospital, Saint Paul, MN, p. A339
BIER, Alan, M.D. Executive Vice President and Chief Medical Officer, Gwinnett Hospital System, Lawrenceville, GA, p. A155
BIERIG, Kirt, D.O. Chief of Staff, Share Medical Center, Alva, OK, p. A493
BIERMAN, Joan, Vice President Finance, Cherokee Regional Medical Center, Cherokee, IA, p. A216
BIERMAN, Ronald L., Chief Executive Officer, Affinity Medical Center, Massillon, OH, p. A484
BIERSCHENK, Kevin, Chief Executive Officer, Dodge County Hospital, Eastman, GA, p. A152
BIERUT, Barbara, Chief Financial Officer, HEALTHSOUTH Rehabilitation Hospital of Sarasota, Sarasota, FL, p. A139
BIFFLE, Sandra, Personnel Clerk, Quitman County Hospital, Marks, MS, p. A349
BIFULCO, William, Vice President/Chief Information Officer, Southampton Hospital, Southampton, NY, p. A443
BIGELOW, David C., PharmD, Chief Executive Officer, Samaritan Pacific Communities Hospital, Newport, OR, p. A513
BIGELOW, Debbie, Chief Financial Officer, Coulee Medical Center, Grand Coulee, WA, p. A662
BIGELOW, Timothy, Director Human Resources, Butler Hospital, Providence, RI, p. A544
BIGGINS, Lillie, R.N. President, Texas Health Harris Methodist Hospital Fort Worth, Fort Worth, TX, p. A599
BIGGS, Alan W., Vice President Financial Services, Community Howard Regional Hospital, Kokomo, IN, p. A206
BIGGS, Daniel, Director Human Resources, Valley View Hospital, Glenwood Springs, CO, p. A101
BIGHAM, Bryon, M.D. Chief of Staff, Hiawatha Community Hospital, Hiawatha, KS, p. A234
BIGHAM, Laurie S., R.N. Chief Nursing Officer, Lovelace Medical Center, Albuquerque, NM, p. A414
BIGLER, Nate, Director Human Resource, American Fork Hospital, American Fork, UT, p. A637
BIGLEY, John, M.D. Medical Director, Baldwin Park Medical Center, Baldwin Park, CA, p. A55
BIGLEY, Robert F., President and Chief Executive Officer, East Georgia Regional Medical Center, Statesboro, GA, p. A160
BIGNAULT, Jon, M.D. Chief of Staff, Athens–Limestone Hospital, Athens, AL, p. A16
BIGNOTTI, Donald, M.D. Vice President Medical Affairs, St. Joseph Mercy Oakland, Pontiac, MI, p. A321
BIHUNIAK, Peter, Vice President Finance, Robert Wood Johnson University Hospital Rahway, Rahway, NJ, p. A409
BIK, Lymar, M.D. Medical Director, Coalinga Regional Medical Center, Coalinga, CA, p. A58
BILES, Don, Chief Financial Officer, Manatee Glens Hospital and Addiction Center, Bradenton, FL, p. A119
BILLERBECK, Robert, M.D. Vice President and Chief Medical Officer, Exempla Good Samaritan Medical Center, Lafayette, CO, p. A103
BILLING, Michael D., Administrator, Mid–Valley Hospital, Omak, WA, p. A663
BILLING, Tommye, Vice President and Chief Information Officer, St. Vincent Medical Center–North, Sherwood, AR, p. A51
BILLINGS, Derrick Mark, President, Presbyterian Hospital, Charlotte, NC, p. A451
BILLINGS, Robert E., Chief Financial Officer, Largo Medical Center, Largo, FL, p. A128
BILLINGSLEY, Angela, Director Human Resources, Intermountain Hospital, Boise, ID, p. A166
BILLINGSLEY, Annette, Director Human Resources, Hill Hospital of Sumter County, York, AL, p. A27
BILLINGSLEY, Richard A., MSN Chief Operating Officer and Chief Nursing Officer, Mena Regional Health System, Mena, AR, p. A49
BILLINGTON, Carole, R.N. Vice President Patient Care Services, Saint Anne's Hospital, Fall River, MA, p. A299
BILLS, Jim, Chief Operating Officer, Raleigh General Hospital, Beckley, WV, p. A670
BILLS, Robert C.
Chief Executive Officer, Encino Hospital Medical Center,, CA, p. A69
Chief Executive Officer, Sherman Oaks Hospital,, CA, p. A71
BILLY, Frank, Chief Financial Officer, Kindred Hospital Bay Area–Tampa, Tampa, FL, p. A141
BILMER, Janice, Director, Information Services, Skiff Medical Center, Newton, IA, p. A224
BILUNKA, Dianne C., Director Human Resources, Clarion Psychiatric Center, Clarion, PA, p. A520
BINDER, Forest, Vice President Finance, St. Mary's Hospital and Medical Center, Grand Junction, CO, p. A102
BINDRA, Pavel, M.D. Chief Information Officer and Chief Medical Officer, Citrus Valley Medical Center–Queen of the Valley Campus, West Covina, CA, p. A95
BING, William W., Chief Executive Officer, Liberty Healthcare Systems, Bastrop, LA, p. A262
BINGHAM, Leslie, Senior Vice President and Chief Executive Officer, Valley Baptist Medical Center–Brownsville, Brownsville, TX, p. A585
BINGHAM, Roxane, Director Marketing, Baton Rouge Rehabilitation Hospital, Baton Rouge, LA, p. A262
BINGMAN, Ryan, Director Operations, Grundy County Memorial Hospital, Grundy Center, IA, p. A220
BINKLEY, Jr., Leonard, Interim Chief Financial Officer, Henderson County Community Hospital, Lexington, TN, p. A569
BINKLEY, Sharon, Director Human Resources, Fairfax Community Hospital, Fairfax, OK, p. A496
BIRA, Patrick G., FACHE Chief Executive Officer, Lincoln County Medical Center, Troy, MO, p. A372
BIRCH, Misty, Director Human Resources, Pioneer Valley Hospital, West Valley City, UT, p. A642
BIRCHLER, James, Vice President Finance, Chelsea Community Hospital, Chelsea, MI, p. A309
BIRD, Alan, Chief Executive Officer, Powell County Medical Center, Deer Lodge, MT, p. A374
BIRD, Jeffrey C., M.D. Chief Medical Officer, Indiana University Health Ball Memorial Hospital, Muncie, IN, p. A209
BIRD, Julio J., M.D. Chief Medical Officer, Gundersen Lutheran Medical Center, La Crosse, WI, p. A683
BIRD, Kim B., President and Chief Executive Officer, Cypress Health Systems, Benton, LA, p. B40
BIRD, Lindsay, Director Finance, South Pointe Hospital, Warrensville Heights, OH, p. A490
BIRD, Michael, M.D. Vice President Medical Services, Akron Children's Hospital, Akron, OH, p. A469
BIRD, Michele
Chief Human Resources Officer, Hemet Valley Medical Center, Hemet, CA, p. A64
Chief Human Resources Officer, Menifee Valley Medical Center, Sun City, CA, p. A92
BIRDSONG, Jill, Chief Financial Officer, Texas Orthopedic Hospital, Houston, TX, p. A607
BIRDZELL, JoAnn, Chief Executive Officer and Administrator, St. Catherine Hospital, East Chicago, IN, p. A200
BIREN, David, Chief Financial Officer, Mayo Clinic Health System in Lake City, Lake City, MN, p. A333
BIRENBERG, Allan, Vice President Medical Affairs, Medstar Harbor Hospital, Baltimore, MD, p. A288
BIRKEL, Sue M., R.N. Director of Nursing, Butler County Health Care Center, David City, NE, p. A383
BIRKHOFER, Colleen, Chief Nursing Officer, Trenton Psychiatric Hospital, Trenton, NJ, p. A411
BIRLEW, Ron, Director Human Resources, Des Peres Hospital, Saint Louis, MO, p. A368
BIRMINGHAM, Roy, Controller, Oakwood Annapolis Hospital, Wayne, MI, p. A325
BIRNBAUM, Bernard, M.D. Senior Vice President, Vice Dean and Chief Hospital Operations, NYU Langone Medical Center, New York, NY, p. A436
BIRSCHBACH, Nancy, Vice President Information Services, Agnesian HealthCare, Fond Du Lac, WI, p. A681
BISCHALANEY, George, President and Chief Executive Officer, Eden Medical Center, Castro Valley, CA, p. A56
BISCONE, Mark A., Executive Director, Waldo County General Hospital, Belfast, ME, p. A281
BISGROVE, Michele, Manager Human Resources, Mad River Community Hospital, Arcata, CA, p. A54
BISHKU, Dilek, M.D. Vice President Medical Affairs, La Rabida Children's Hospital, Chicago, IL, p. A176
BISHOP, April, Chief Executive Officer, Kindred Hospital–Central Dakotas, Mandan, ND, p. A467
BISHOP, Clint, Program Manager, Veterans Affairs Medical Center, Marion, IL, p. A187
BISHOP, Jim, Chief Executive Officer, Harney District Hospital, Burns, OR, p. A509
BISHOP, John
Chief Financial Officer, Long Beach Memorial Medical Center, Long Beach, CA, p. A68
Chief Financial Officer, Madison Valley Medical Center, Ennis, MT, p. A375
Chief Financial Officer, Madison Valley Medical Center, Ennis, MT, p. A375
BISSEL, Jane, Chief Financial Officer, Wabash County Hospital, Wabash, IN, p. A213
BISSENDEN, Chris, Director Human Resources, Ogden Regional Medical Center, Ogden, UT, p. A639
BISSON, Ellen, Chief Operating Officer, Cameron Memorial Community Hospital, Angola, IN, p. A197
BISSONETTE, Christine, R.N. Chief Nursing Officer, Kalkaska Memorial Health Center, Kalkaska, MI, p. A317
BISSONNETTE, Andre, Vice President Finance, North Country Hospital and Health Center, Newport, VT, p. A644
BISTERFELDT, Joanne, Chief Information Officer, Wheaton Franciscan Healthcare – All Saints, Racine, WI, p. A689
BISTON, Jody, Director Risk Management and Physician Clinic, Sullivan County Memorial Hospital, Milan, MO, p. A365
BITAR, Adib, M.D. Medical Director, Aurora Charter Oak Hospital, Covina, CA, p. A58
BITAR, Ali, M.D. Vice President Medical Affairs, Rehabilitation Institute of Michigan, Detroit, MI, p. A311
BITHER, Dean, Chief Financial Officer, Inland Hospital, Waterville, ME, p. A285
BITHONEY, William, M.D. Chief Operating Officer, Mercy Medical Center, Springfield, MA, p. A305
BITSOLI, Deborah, Chief Operating Officer, Saint Vincent Hospital, Worcester, MA, p. A306
BITTNER, Augustine, Chief Information Officer, Veterans Affairs Medical Center–Louisville, Louisville, KY, p. A255
BITTNER, Mary J., R.N. Vice President Nursing, Barton Healthcare System, South Lake Tahoe, CA, p. A91
BIUNDO, Russell, M.D. Medical Director, HEALTHSOUTH MountainView Regional Rehabilitation Hospital, Morgantown, WV, p. A674
BIXEL, Kenneth, Vice President and Chief Information Officer, Mount Nittany Medical Center, State College, PA, p. A539
BIXLER, Jacquelyn, Vice President Human Resources, BryLin Hospitals, Buffalo, NY, p. A422
BJELICH, Steven C., President and Chief Executive Officer, Saint Francis Medical Center, Cape Girardeau, MO, p. A356
BJELLA, Karmon T., Chief Executive Officer, Alpena Regional Medical Center, Alpena, MI, p. A307
BJERKE, Carolyn, Director Human Resources, Kingfisher Regional Hospital, Kingfisher, OK, p. A498
BJERKNES, Dan, Director Human Resources, Richard P. Stadter Psychiatric Center, Grand Forks, ND, p. A466
BJORDAHL, Kevin, M.D. Chief Medical Officer, Milbank Area Hospital Avera, Milbank, SD, p. A557
BJORGUM, Deb, Manager Data Processing, Johnson Regional Medical Center, Clarksville, AR, p. A43
BJORKLUND, Julie D., Director Human Resources, Coulee Medical Center, Grand Coulee, WA, p. A662
BJORNDAL, Judith, M.D. Medical Director, Sonoma Developmental Center, Eldridge, CA, p. A60
BJORNSTAD, Brad, M.D. Vice President and Chief Medical Officer, Florida Hospital Tampa, Tampa, FL, p. A140
BLACK, Jr., Albert P., Chief Operating Officer, Hospital of the University of Pennsylvania, Philadelphia, PA, p. A532
BLACK, Jr., Charles, Chief Financial Officer, Rockcastle Regional Hospital and Respiratory Care Center, Mount Vernon, KY, p. A257
BLACK, Doug, Vice President Operations, Missouri Baptist Medical Center, Saint Louis, MO, p. A369
BLACK, Elizabeth, M.D. Chief Medical Officer, Garfield County Public Hospital District, Pomeroy, WA, p. A664
BLACK, Ethel, Director Human Resources, HEALTHSOUTH Harmarville Rehabilitation Hospital, Pittsburgh, PA, p. A534
BLACK, Gary E., President and Chief Executive Officer, Lenoir Memorial Hospital, Kinston, NC, p. A456
BLACK, James M., Director Administration, Soldiers' Home in Holyoke, Holyoke, MA, p. A301
BLACK, Kim, Manager Human Resources, Dukes Memorial Hospital, Peru, IN, p. A210


A764 Index of Health Care Professionals

Index of Health Care Professionals / Blood

Index of Health Care Professionals


BLACK, Marcey, Chief Financial Officer, Northwest Florida Community Hospital, Chipley, FL, p. A120
BLACK, Marilynn, Chief Information Officer, Verde Valley Medical Center, Cottonwood, AZ, p. A31
BLACK, Michael, Director Human Resources, East Georgia Regional Medical Center, Statesboro, GA, p. A160
BLACK, Paul S.
Controller, H. C. Watkins Memorial Hospital, Quitman, MS, p. A352
Chief Financial Officer, Jefferson Davis Community Hospital, Prentiss, MS, p. A352
Chief Financial Officer, Scott Regional Hospital, Morton, MS, p. A350
BLACK, Sharon, Chief Executive Officer, Kindred Hospital Lafayette, Lafayette, LA, p. A270
BLACK, Tim, Director Human Resources, Southern Hills Hospital and Medical Center, Las Vegas, NV, p. A393
BLACKBEAR, Annabelle, Human Resources Specialist, U. S. Public Health Service Indian Hospital, Pine Ridge, SD, p. A558
BLACKBURN, Gloria C., Executive Director, West Los Angeles Medical Center, Los Angeles, CA, p. A72
BLACKBURN, Laura, Administrator, Ten Lakes Center, Dennison, OH, p. A479
BLACKBURN, Michael R., Chief Executive Officer, Frye Regional Medical Center, Hickory, NC, p. A455
BLACKBURN, Susan, Vice President Human Resources and Support Services, Providence St. Mary Medical Center, Walla Walla, WA, p. A669
BLACKMAN, Elliot, Chief Information Management and Technology, U. S. Air Force Hospital, Hampton, VA, p. A649
BLACKMAN, Jay H., Senior Vice President and Chief Operating Officer, Howard County General Hospital, Columbia, MD, p. A290
BLACKMON, Brian, Director Information Systems, Troy Regional Medical Center, Troy, AL, p. A26
BLACKMON, David, Chief Financial Officer, Comanche County Memorial Hospital, Lawton, OK, p. A498
BLACKMON, Edward, M.D. Chief of Staff, South Texas Regional Medical Center, Jourdanton, TX, p. A609
BLACKMON, Jenean
Assistant Vice President and Chief Information Officer, McLeod Medical Center Dillon, Dillon, SC, p. A549
Associate Vice President and Chief Information Officer, McLeod Regional Medical Center, Florence, SC, p. A550
BLACKMON, Tanya S., President, Presbyterian Hospital Huntersville, Huntersville, NC, p. A455
BLACKWELL, David, Vice President Human Resources, Vail Valley Medical Center, Vail, CO, p. A106
BLACKWELL, Dawn, R.N. VP of Patient Care Services, Memorial Healthcare, Owosso, MI, p. A320
BLACKWELL, Jack, Chief Financial Officer, Highlands Regional Medical Center, Prestonsburg, KY, p. A258
BLACKWELL, James
Vice President and Chief Financial Officer, Clara Barton Hospital, Hoisington, KS, p. A234
Director Information Systems, Decatur Memorial Hospital, Decatur, IL, p. A179
BLACKWELL, Kim, Chief Financial Officer, Arrowhead Behavioral Health Hospital, Maumee, OH, p. A484
BLACKWELL, Lenore, Director Human Resources, Harton Regional Medical Center, Tullahoma, TN, p. A576
BLACKWELL, Timothy, Manager Human Resources, Rolling Hills Hospital, Ada, OK, p. A493
BLACKWOOD, Jim, Chief Executive Officer, Tallahatchie General Hospital, Charleston, MS, p. A344
BLAD, Nate, Chief Financial Officer, RC Hospital and Clinics, Olivia, MN, p. A336
BLADEN, Anthony M., Vice President Human Resources, Calvert Memorial Hospital, Prince Frederick, MD, p. A293
BLADERGROEN, Mark, M.D. Vice President Medical Affairs, Bon Secours St. Mary's Hospital, Richmond, VA, p. A654
BLAHA, Bill, Manager Information Technology, Tri–County Hospital, Wadena, MN, p. A341
BLAHA, John E., Vice President Finance and Chief Financial Officer, Brattleboro Retreat, Brattleboro, VT, p. A643
BLAHNIK, David, Chief Operating Officer, Twin Valley Behavioral Healthcare, Columbus, OH, p. A477
BLAIN, Brenda K., MSN Chief Nursing Officer and Chief Operating Officer, Baylor Medical Center at Irving, Irving, TX, p. A609
BLAIR, Betsy, R.N. Chief Operating Officer, CJW Medical Center, Richmond, VA, p. A654
BLAIR, Brenda, Association Vice President Human Resources and Organizational Learning, Alice Peck Day Memorial Hospital, Lebanon, NH, p. A398
BLAIR, Diane, Director Human Resources and Admissions, Alegent Health Plainview Hospital, Plainview, NE, p. A389
BLAIR, Judy, Senior Vice President Clinical Services and Chief Nursing Officer, Glendale Adventist Medical Center, Glendale, CA, p. A63
BLAIR, Keith, M.D. Manager Information Systems, Lander Regional Hospital, Lander, WY, p. A696
BLAIR, Jr., Ralph W., M.D. Chief of Staff, Ennis Regional Medical Center, Ennis, TX, p. A597
BLAIR, Rebecca, Vice President Human Resources and Service Excellence, Faulkner Hospital, Boston, MA, p. A296
BLAIR, Robert D., Chief Executive Officer, The NeuroMedical Center Surgical Hospital, Baton Rouge, LA, p. A263
BLAKE, Hugo, M.D. Chief Medical Staff, Harlingen Medical Center, Harlingen, TX, p. A602
BLAKE, Kelly, Chief Executive Officer, Select Specialty Hospital–Johnstown, Johnstown, PA, p. A526
BLAKE, Robert, Chief Human Resources Officer Southwest Market, Memorial Hermann Sugar Land Hospital, Sugar Land, TX, p. A629
BLAKE, Robert, M.D. Chief of Staff, St. Joseph's Hospital of Buckhannon, Buckhannon, WV, p. A670
BLAKE, Sheryl Lewis, FACHE Chief Executive Officer, Pennock Hospital, Hastings, MI, p. A315
BLAKE, Sue, Chief Financial Officer, Myrtue Medical Center, Harlan, IA, p. A220
BLAKELY, Amy, Assistant Executive Director Operations, Devereux Hospital and Children's Center of Florida, Melbourne, FL, p. A130
BLAKELY, Michelle, Associate Director, Jesse Brown Veterans Affairs Chicago Health Care System, Chicago, IL, p. A176
BLAKEY GORMAN, Mary, Director Human Resources, Northwest Missouri Psychiatric Rehabilitation Center, Saint Joseph, MO, p. A368
BLALOCK, Andy, M.D. Physician Executive, Our Lady of Lourdes Regional Medical Center, Lafayette, LA, p. A270
BLALOCK, Cam, Senior Vice President Corporate Services, Nash Health Care Systems, Rocky Mount, NC, p. A460
BLANCAS, Gilbert, Director Human Resources, University Medical Center of El Paso, El Paso, TX, p. A597
BLANCHARD, Timothy D., Chief Financial Officer, Kingman Regional Medical Center, Kingman, AZ, p. A33
BLANCHARD, Wayne D., Chief Executive Officer, Kindred Hospital–New Jersey Morris County, Dover, NJ, p. A403
BLANCHARD, William R., Chief Executive Officer, DeTar Healthcare System, Victoria, TX, p. A633
BLANCHET, Jacques, M.D. Director Medical Affairs, Baystate Franklin Medical Center, Greenfield, MA, p. A300
BLANCHET, Mike, President, CHI, Community Hospital North, Indianapolis, IN, p. A204
BLANCHETTE, Edward A., M.D. Director, Connecticut Department of Correction's Hospital, Somers, CT, p. A112
BLANCO, Andres, Director Management Information Systems, Westside Regional Medical Center, Plantation, FL, p. A136
BLANCO, Carlos, M.D
Administrator, Doctor's Center of Bayamon, Bayamon, PR, p. A700
Administrator, Doctors Center, Manati, PR, p. A701
BLAND, Douglas, Manager Information Services, Spring View Hospital, Lebanon, KY, p. A252
BLAND, James G., M.D. Chief of Staff, Jane Todd Crawford Hospital, Greensburg, KY, p. A251
BLANFORD, Donald, M.D. Chief Medical Officer, Mercy Regional Medical Center, Lorain, OH, p. A483
BLANK, Arthur J., President and Chief Executive Officer, Mount Desert Island Hospital, Bar Harbor, ME, p. A281
BLANKE, Kerry Lee, Director Financial Services, Riverside Medical Center, Waupaca, WI, p. A692
BLANKENSHIP, Diana, Director Human Resources, Welch Community Hospital, Welch, WV, p. A676
BLANKENSHIP, Jeff, CPA Vice President and Chief Financial Officer, Jackson–Madison County General Hospital, Jackson, TN, p. A567
BLANTON, Forest
Senior VP and Chief Information Officer, Memorial Hospital Miramar, Miramar, FL, p. A132
Chief Information Officer, Memorial Hospital Pembroke, Pembroke Pines, FL, p. A135
Chief Information Officer, Memorial Hospital West, Pembroke Pines, FL, p. A135
Administrator Process Engineering, Memorial Regional Hospital,, FL, p. A125
BLANTON, James
Chief Financial Officer, East Texas Medical Center Rehabilitation Center, Tyler, TX, p. A632
Chief Financial Officer, East Texas Medical Center Specialty Hospital, Tyler, TX, p. A632
BLANTON, Karen, Chief Financial Officer, Warm Springs Medical Center, Warm Springs, GA, p. A161
BLANTON, Marion, Chief Financial Officer, Minneola District Hospital, Minneola, KS, p. A239
BLANTON, Ron, Chief Fiscal Services, Veterans Affairs Medical Center, Boise, ID, p. A167
BLAPPERT, Bradley, M.D. Chief Medical Officer, AMG Specialty Hospital – Lafayette, Lafayette, LA, p. A269
BLASER, Karla, Director Human Resources, Trinity Muscatine, Muscatine, IA, p. A224
BLASINGAME, Billy, Chief Executive Officer, Plum Creek Specialty Hospital, Amarillo, TX, p. A578
BLASIUS, Rita, Assistant Administrator and Chief Financial Officer, Avera St. Benedict Hospital, Parkston, SD, p. A558
BLAUER, Michael, Administrator, Pioneer Memorial Hospital, Heppner, OR, p. A511
BLAUFUSS, Max, Administrator and Chief Executive Officer, Lakeside Medical Center, Pine City, MN, p. A337
BLAUWET, Judy, M.P.H. Senior Vice President Operations and Chief Nursing Officer, Avera McKennan Hospital and University Health Center, Sioux Falls, SD, p. A559
BLAYLOCK, Darrell, Chief Executive Officer, McKenzie Regional Hospital, McKenzie, TN, p. A570
BLAYLOCK, Kevin, Chief Executive Officer, Oklahoma Spine Hospital, Oklahoma City, OK, p. A501
BLAYLOCK, L. Dwayne, Chief Executive Officer, Gilmore Memorial Regional Medical Center, Amory, MS, p. A343
BLAZEK, Dennis, Chief Information Officer, Clarke County Hospital, Osceola, IA, p. A225
BLAZEK, Lisa, Chief Financial Officer, Adair County Memorial Hospital, Greenfield, IA, p. A220
BLAZIER, Patty, Chief Nursing Officer, Hamilton Memorial Hospital District, McLeansboro, IL, p. A187
BLEAK, Jason, Administrator and Chief Executive Officer, Grover C. Dils Medical Center, Caliente, NV, p. A391
BLEAKNEY, David A., Administrator, Angleton Danbury Medical Center, Angleton, TX, p. A579
BLECHA, Timothy, M.D. Medical Director, Brodstone Memorial Hospital, Superior, NE, p. A390
BLEDSOE, Richard, Director Information Systems, Upstate Carolina Medical Center, Gaffney, SC, p. A550
BLEICHER, James J., M.D. President and Chief Executive Officer, Verde Valley Medical Center, Cottonwood, AZ, p. A31
BLESI, Michael, Director Information Technology, Rainy Lake Medical Center, International Falls, MN, p. A333
BLESSING, Brian, Chief Financial Officer, Texas Health Harris Methodist Hospital Azle, Azle, TX, p. A582
BLESSITT, Harold J., Administrator, South Sunflower County Hospital, Indianola, MS, p. A347
BLEVINS, Bonnie, Chief Financial Officer, Graham Regional Medical Center, Graham, TX, p. A601
BLEVINS, Denzil, Director Information Systems, Montgomery General Hospital, Montgomery, WV, p. A673
BLEVINS, Gary, Director Human Resources, Mercy Medical Center Mount Shasta, Mount Shasta, CA, p. A76
BLEVINS, Heather, Director Human Resources, HEALTHSOUTH Rehabilitation of Gadsden, Gadsden, AL, p. A20
BLEVINS, Matthew H., Chief Executive Officer, Select Specialty Hospital–Kansas City, Kansas City, KS, p. A236
BLEVINS, Pam, R.N. Director, Clinical Informatics, Blue Ridge Regional Hospital, Spruce Pine, NC, p. A461
BLIGHTON, Gordon, Director Resource Management, Naval Hospital, Camp Pendleton, CA, p. A56
BLIK, Lior, Chief Information Officer, Hoboken University Medical Center, Hoboken, NJ, p. A404
BLISE, Cathi, Interim Chief Nursing Officer, St. Anthony's Medical Center, Saint Louis, MO, p. A370
BLISS, Ann, Manager Computer Services, Southeast Arizona Medical Center, Douglas, AZ, p. A31
BLIVEN, Donna, Vice President Patient Management Services, Jones Memorial Hospital, Wellsville, NY, p. A446
BLOB, Burchkhard, Manager Human Resources, Central Virginia Training Center, Madison Heights, VA, p. A650
BLOCK, Annie, Director Human Resources, Poplar Community Hospital, Poplar, MT, p. A378
BLOCK, George, M.D. Chief Medical Officer, O'Connor Hospital, San Jose, CA, p. A88
BLOCK, Marian R., M.D. Chief Quality Officer, Western Pennsylvania Hospital, Pittsburgh, PA, p. A536
BLOCK, Sherri, Chief Operating Officer, Aurora Vista Del Mar Hospital, Ventura, CA, p. A94
BLOEMER, Brad, Vice President Finance and Chief Financial Officer, Arkansas Methodist Medical Center, Paragould, AR, p. A50
BLOM, Clara
Chief Financial Officer, Bellflower Medical Center, Bellflower, CA, p. A55
Chief Financial Officer, Los Angeles Metropolitan Medical Center, Los Angeles, CA, p. A70
BLOM, David P., President and Chief Executive Officer, OhioHealth, Columbus, OH, p. B98
BLOMELEY, Geoff, Interim Chief Financial Officer, Ponca City Medical Center, Ponca City, OK, p. A503
BLOOD, Barbara, Director Human Resources, Walla Walla General Hospital, Walla Walla, WA, p. A669
BLOOD, Dana, Director Human Resources, Oakdale Community Hospital, Oakdale, LA, p. A275




Index of Health Care Professionals A765

Index of Health Care Professionals

Index of Health Care Professionals / Blood

BLOOD, Michael, VP Human Resources, Monadnock Community Hospital, Peterborough, NH, p. A400
BLOOM, Kerry, Director Human Resources, Kalamazoo Psychiatric Hospital, Kalamazoo, MI, p. A316
BLOOM, Laura, Director Human Resources, Coffee Regional Medical Center, Douglas, GA, p. A151
BLOOM, Sarah, Director Information Systems, Belton Regional Medical Center, Belton, MO, p. A355
BLOOM, Stephanie L., FACHE President and Chief Executive Officer, Community Medical Center, Toms River, NJ, p. A411
BLOOMFIELD, Deborah, Chief Financial Officer, Mercy Hospital Anderson, Cincinnati, OH, p. A473
BLOOMQUIST, Margaret A., Assistant Administrator Human Resources, Emory University Hospital, Atlanta, GA, p. A145
BLOOMQUIST, Trudy, Director of Nursing, Warren General Hospital, Warren, PA, p. A540
BLOUGH Jr., Daniel D., Chief Executive Officer, Punxsutawney Area Hospital, Punxsutawney, PA, p. A536
BLOUGH, David, Chief Information Officer, University of South Alabama Children's and Women's Hospital, Mobile, AL, p. A23
BLUE, Gaea, Administrator and Chief Executive Officer, Avera Weskota Memorial Hospital, Wessington Springs, SD, p. A561
BLUE, Jan L.
Senior Vice President Human Resources, Hoag Hospital Irvine, Irvine, CA, p. A65
Vice President Human Resources, Hoag Memorial Hospital Presbyterian, Newport Beach, CA, p. A76
BLUE, Lawrence, Administrator and Chief Executive Officer, Cavalier County Memorial Hospital, Langdon, ND, p. A467
BLUE, Yvonne, Chief Operations Officer, Moore County Hospital District, Dumas, TX, p. A594
BLUFORD, John W.
President and Chief Executive Officer, Truman Medical Center–Hospital Hill, Kansas City, MO, p. A363
President and Chief Executive Officer, Truman Medical Center–Lakewood, Kansas City, MO, p. A363
BLUFORD, John W., President and Chief Executive Officer, Truman Medical Centers, Kansas City, MO, p. B131
BLUHM, Tom, Director Information Systems, Island Hospital, Anacortes, WA, p. A659
BLUM, Carrie, Director Information Systems, Monroe Clinic, Monroe, WI, p. A687
BLUM, Walter B., M.D. Chief of Staff, McLeod Medical Center Dillon, Dillon, SC, p. A549
BLUMENFELD, Barry, M.D. Chief Information Officer, Maine Medical Center, Portland, ME, p. A284
BLUNCK, Marilyn, Director Health Information Management, Norfolk Regional Center, Norfolk, NE, p. A386
BLUNK, Jim, D.O. Chief Medical Officer, Sumner County Hospital District One, Caldwell, KS, p. A231
BLUNT, Margaret, Director Human Resources, Cornerstone Hospital of Houston – Bellaire, Houston, TX, p. A603
BLUNT, Mary L., Corporate Vice President and Administrator, Sentara Norfolk General Hospital, Norfolk, VA, p. A653
BLURTON, Cheri, Director Human Resources, Great River Medical Center, Blytheville, AR, p. A42
BLUTE, III, James, M.D. Chief Medical Officer, Nazareth Hospital, Philadelphia, PA, p. A533
BLYTHE, Sheryl, Director Human Resources, St. Anthony Hospital, Lakewood, CO, p. A103
BLYTHE, Thomas W.
Vice President Human Resources, Good Samaritan Regional Health Center, Mount Vernon, IL, p. A188
Vice President Human Resources, St. Mary's Hospital, Centralia, IL, p. A174
BOAL, Jeremy, M.D. Medical Director, Long Island Jewish Medical Center,, NY, p. A434
BOARD, Patricia, Vice President Human Resources, Community Hospital of Bremen, Bremen, IN, p. A198
BOARDMAN, Debra K., FACHE President and Chief Executive Officer, Range Regional Health Services, Hibbing, MN, p. A333
BOAS, Erik, Vice President Finance, Civista Health, La Plata, MD, p. A292
BOATMAN, James, Chief Financial Officer, Doctors Medical Center–San Pablo Campus, San Pablo, CA, p. A89
BOATMAN, Robert, Director Information Technology, Richmond State Hospital, Richmond, IN, p. A211
BOATRIGHT, Donna, MSN, Administrator, Rolling Plains Memorial Hospital, Sweetwater, TX, p. A630
BOATWRIGHT, Damond, Chief Executive Officer, Overland Park Regional Medical Center, Overland Park, KS, p. A241
BOBBITT, Gina, Director Human Resources, Salem Memorial District Hospital, Salem, MO, p. A370
BOBBITT, James, Vice President Human Resources, Saint Agnes Hospital, Baltimore, MD, p. A288
BOBBS, Kathy J., FACHE Interim Chief Executive Officer, AMG Specialty Hospital–Lafayette Regional Campus, Lafayette, LA, p. A270
BOCKELMAN, Paul, Director, Veterans Affairs Medical Center, Marion, IL, p. A187
BOCKENEK, William, M.D. Medical Director, Carolinas Rehabilitation, Charlotte, NC, p. A450
BOCKMANN, Rick, Chief Executive Officer, Frank R. Howard Memorial Hospital, Willits, CA, p. A96
BOCKNEK, Marc, D.O. Vice President Medical Affairs, Huron Valley–Sinai Hospital, Commerce Township, MI, p. A310
BODE, Patti, Chief Financial Officer, Orthopedic Hospital, Oklahoma City, OK, p. A502
BODEN, DeShawna, Director Human Resources, Harbor Oaks Hospital, New Baltimore, MI, p. A320
BODEN, Shelley, Administrator and Chief Executive Officer, Russell Regional Hospital, Russell, KS, p. A242
BODENMANN, Linda, Chief Operating Officer, Southcoast Hospitals Group, Fall River, MA, p. A300
BODENNER, Nancy, Director Human Resources, St. Joseph Health System, Tawas City, MI, p. A324
BODENSTEINER, Kim, Chief Financial Officer, Essentia Health Fosston, Fosston, MN, p. A331
BODIN, Donna L., Vice President, Woman's Hospital, Baton Rouge, LA, p. A263
BODLOVIC, Kirk, Vice President and Chief Financial Officer, St. Joseph Hospital, Polson, MT, p. A378
BODME, Maureen, Chief Clinical Officer, Kindred Hospital–San Diego, San Diego, CA, p. A85
BODNAR, Darrell, Director Information, Weeks Medical Center, Lancaster, NH, p. A398
BOE, Kim, Administrator, Colorado West Psychiatric Hospital, Grand Junction, CO, p. A101
BOECKER, Thomas J., President and Chief Executive Officer, Wilson Memorial Hospital, Sidney, OH, p. A488
BOEHLER, Richard, M.D. Senior Vice President Medical Affairs and Chief Medical Officer, Kennedy Memorial Hospitals–University Medical Center, Cherry Hill, NJ, p. A403
BOEHM, Scott D., Vice President Human Resources, Medcenter One, Bismarck, ND, p. A464
BOEHNKE, Winnie, Director Human Resources, Timberlawn Mental Health System, Dallas, TX, p. A593
BOEHRER, Mark, Director Human Resources, St. Charles Hospital, Port Jefferson, NY, p. A440
BOEMER, Sally Mason
Senior Vice President Finance, Massachusetts General Hospital, Boston, MA, p. A297
Chief Financial Officer, North Shore Medical Center, Salem, MA, p. A304
BOEMMEL, Michael, Vice President and Chief Financial Officer, Medstar National Rehabilitation Network, Washington, DC, p. A116
BOER, Jeff, Director Information Technology, Pulaski Memorial Hospital, Winamac, IN, p. A213
BOERNER, Carol F., M.D. President Medical Staff, Valley Regional Hospital, Claremont, NH, p. A397
BOGAN, James, FACHE President and Chief Executive Officer, Portage Health, Hancock, MI, p. A314
BOGEDAIN, Carol, FACHE Director, Veterans Affairs Roseburg Healthcare System, Roseburg, OR, p. A515
BOGEN, Mark A., Senior Vice President and Chief Financial Officer, South Nassau Communities Hospital, Oceanside, NY, p. A439
BOGGESS, Carrie
Human Resource Generalist, Carilion Giles Community Hospital, Pearisburg, VA, p. A653
Human Resources Generalist, Carilion Tazewell Community Hospital, Tazewell, VA, p. A656
BOGGESS, Jack, Chief Executive Officer, Solara Hospital McAllen, McAllen, TX, p. A615
BOGGESS, Richard, Chief Financial Officer, Central Texas Medical Center, San Marcos, TX, p. A627
BOGGS, Danny L., President and Chief Executive Officer, Samaritan Regional Health System, Ashland, OH, p. A469
BOGGS, Lynn Ingram, President and Chief Executive Officer, McDowell Hospital, Marion, NC, p. A457
BOGGS, Michael S., Chief Executive Officer, Regency Hospital of Central Georgia, Macon, GA, p. A156
BOGLE, Bryan, Interim Chief Executive Officer, Winn Parish Medical Center, Winnfield, LA, p. A279
BOHALL, Karen, Director Human Resources, Woman's Christian Association Hospital, Jamestown, NY, p. A428
BOHANNON, Michelle, Director of Nursing Operations and Risk, Compliance, Quality and Safety, Wilson Medical Center, Neodesha, KS, p. A239
BOHATY, Richard, Director Information Technology, Saint Elizabeth Regional Medical Center, Lincoln, NE, p. A385
BOHLMANN, Chuck, Chief Information Officer, Community Memorial Hospital, Hicksville, OH, p. A481
BOHNENKAMP, Russ, Director Finance, Chadron Community Hospital and Health Services, Chadron, NE, p. A382
BOHNSACK, Michael, M.D. Chief of Staff, Stanly Regional Medical Center, Albemarle, NC, p. A448
BOHON, Cindy, Director Human Resources, Fayette Medical Center, Fayette, AL, p. A20
BOICE, Sheila, Director Human Resources, Barton County Memorial Hospital, Lamar, MO, p. A363
BOIKE, Darlene, Chief Financial Officer, Chippewa County–Montevideo Hospital, Montevideo, MN, p. A335
BOILEAU, Michel, M.D
Chief Clinical Officer, Pioneer Memorial Hospital, Prineville, OR, p. A514
Chief Clinical Officer, St. Charles Medical Center – Bend, Bend, OR, p. A509
Chief Clinical Officer, St. Charles Medical Center – Redmond, Redmond, OR, p. A515
BOISSEN, Myrna, Executive Director, San Juan City Hospital, San Juan, PR, p. A703
BOISVERT, Gerald J., Executive Vice President and Chief Financial Officer, Connecticut Children's Medical Center, Hartford, CT, p. A109
BOK, Duard, M.D. Clinical Director, North Alabama Regional Hospital, Decatur, AL, p. A18
BOKERN, Bob, Director Human Resources, St. Mary Medical Center, Long Beach, CA, p. A68
BOKOVITZ, Beverly, R.N
Senior Vice President and Chief Nursing Officer, Akron General Medical Center, Akron, OH, p. A469
Senior Vice President and Chief Nursing Officer, Lodi Community Hospital, Lodi, OH, p. A483
BOLAND, Susan, Senior Vice President and Chief Operating Officer, Wheaton Franciscan Healthcare – All Saints, Racine, WI, p. A689
BOLANDER, Patrick C., Chief Financial Officer, Georgetown Community Hospital, Georgetown, KY, p. A250
BOLCAVAGE, Ted, Vice President and Division Controller, Baylor Institute for Rehabilitation, Dallas, TX, p. A590
BOLD, Harry, Administrator, Big Sandy Medical Center, Big Sandy, MT, p. A373
BOLDA, Craig, Chief Operating Officer, St. Catherine Hospital, East Chicago, IN, p. A200
BOLDING, Kay, R.N. Vice President Patient Care Services and Chief Nursing Officer, Jackson County Memorial Hospital, Altus, OK, p. A493
BOLDS, Kevin, Director Information Technology, Earl K. Long Medical Center, Baton Rouge, LA, p. A262
BOLDUC, Tiana, Chief Information Officer, Mercy Hospital Ozark, Ozark, AR, p. A50
BOLEN, David, Vice President and Chief Financial Officer, Passavant Area Hospital, Jacksonville, IL, p. A185
BOLEN, Shannon, Director Human Resources, Baptist Memorial Hospital–Booneville, Booneville, MS, p. A344
BOLES, Glen, Chief Financial Officer, Valley Baptist Medical Center–Brownsville, Brownsville, TX, p. A585
BOLES, Mark D., Chief Executive Officer, Baylor Institute for Rehabilitation at Frisco, Frisco, TX, p. A600
BOLEWARE, Mike, Administrator, Pearl River County Hospital, Poplarville, MS, p. A352
BOLEY, Eric, Administrator and Chief Executive Officer, South Lincoln Medical Center, Kemmerer, WY, p. A696
BOLEY, Sarah, Director Human Resources, Wetzel County Hospital, New Martinsville, WV, p. A674
BOLGER, Thomas, Chief Financial Officer, Chinese Hospital, San Francisco, CA, p. A86
BOLICK, Diann, Chief Financial Officer, CarePartners Health Services, Asheville, NC, p. A448
BOLIN, Cris, Chief Executive Officer, Delta Memorial Hospital, Dumas, AR, p. A44
BOLIN, Kari, R.N. Chief Nursing Officer, Highlands Regional Medical Center, Sebring, FL, p. A139
BOLINGER, John, M.D. Vice President Medical Affairs, Union Hospital, Terre Haute, IN, p. A212
BOLLARD, Robert, Interim Chief Executive Officer, HEALTHSOUTH Rehabilitation Hospital – Henderson, Henderson, NV, p. A392
BOLLICH, Mary, Director of Nurses, AMG Specialty Hospital – Lafayette, Lafayette, LA, p. A269
BOLLONE, Ann M., Vice President Human Resources, St. Anthony's Medical Center, Saint Louis, MO, p. A370
BOLOGNANI, Laurie, Human Resources Officer, Speare Memorial Hospital, Plymouth, NH, p. A400
BOLOUKI, Shawn, Chief Executive Officer, Tulare Regional Medical Center, Tulare, CA, p. A93
BOLTON, Christopher, Administrator, Providence Seward Medical Center, Seward, AK, p. A30
BOLTON, Josh, Chief Information Officer, Serenity Lane, Eugene, OR, p. A510
BOLTON, Lauri, Director Human Resources, Samaritan North Lincoln Hospital, Lincoln City, OR, p. A512
BOLTON, Neal, Chief Financial Officer, Person Memorial Hospital, Roxboro, NC, p. A460
BOMAR, Betsy, Chief Operating Officer, Northside Hospital and Heart Institute, Saint Petersburg, FL, p. A138

A766 Index of Health Care Professionals

Index of Health Care Professionals

Index of Health Care Professionals / Boula

BOULA, Rodney C., Administrator and Chief Executive Officer, Elizabethtown Community Hospital, Elizabethtown, NY, p. A425
BOULENGER, Bo, Chief Executive Officer, Baptist Health South Florida, Baptist Hospital of Miami, Miami, FL, p. A130
BOUQUIO, George, Director Human Resources, South Beach Psychiatric Center,, NY, p. A436
BOUR, Eric, M.D. President, Hillcrest Memorial Hospital, Simpsonville, SC, p. A553
BOURDEAU, Patricia, Director Human Resources, Brook Lane Health Services, Hagerstown, MD, p. A292
BOURGASSER, Gene, M.D. Chief of Staff, Sullivan County Community Hospital, Sullivan, IN, p. A212
BOURGAULT, Catherine, Director Human Resources, Providence Hood River Memorial Hospital, Hood River, OR, p. A511
BOURGEOIS Jr., Milton D., Chief Executive Officer, Ochsner St. Anne General Hospital, Raceland, LA, p. A276
BOURGHLI, Mahmoud, M.D. Chief of Staff, Spring Hill Regional Hospital, Spring Hill, FL, p. A139
BOURLAND, Don, Vice President Human Resources, Peace Harbor Hospital, Florence, OR, p. A510
BOURLAND, Renee, Human Resources Specialist, San Antonio State Hospital, San Antonio, TX, p. A626
BOURN, Jennifer, Coordinator Health Information Systems, CenterPointe Hospital, Saint Charles, MO, p. A367
BOURNE, Kara, R.N. Chief Nursing Officer and Chief Operating Officer, Newport Specialty Hospital, Tustin, CA, p. A93
BOURQUE, Nancy, Administrator, Phoenix Behavioral Hospital, Rayne, LA, p. A276
BOURQUE, Teresa, Sr. Administrator for Nursing/Chief Nurse, Hurley Medical Center, Flint, MI, p. A312
BOURSEAU, Robert, Chief Financial Officer, Bayview Behavioral Health Campus, Chula Vista, CA, p. A57
BOUYEA, Janine, Director Human Resources, Natividad Medical Center, Salinas, CA, p. A84
BOVEE, Michael, Vice President Finance, Riverview Hospital Association, Wisconsin Rapids, WI, p. A694
BOVIO Jr., Ernest L., Chief Executive Officer, Scott & White Hospital at Round Rock, Round Rock, TX, p. A623
BOW, Beverly
Vice President Human Resources, Salem Hospital, Salem, OR, p. A515
Vice President Human Resources, West Valley Hospital, Dallas, OR, p. A510
BOWCUTT, Marilyn A., R.N. Senior Vice President and Chief Operating Officer, University Health Care System, Augusta, GA, p. A147
BOWE, Larry, Chief Executive, Providence Holy Cross Medical Center,, CA, p. A71
BOWEN, Claire L., Chief Executive Officer, Valley Regional Hospital, Claremont, NH, p. A397
BOWEN, Jill Berry, President and Chief Executive Officer, Northwestern Medical Center, Saint Albans, VT, p. A644
BOWEN, Sandra, Chief Financial Officer, Shasta Regional Medical Center, Redding, CA, p. A82
BOWEN, Steve
Chief Executive Officer, Kimble Hospital, Junction, TX, p. A609
Director Information Systems, Plateau Medical Center, Oak Hill, WV, p. A674
BOWEN, Tim, Chief Executive Officer, Mena Regional Health System, Mena, AR, p. A49
BOWER, David, M.D. Chief of Staff, Veterans Affairs Medical Center, Decatur, GA, p. A151
BOWER, Kay, Associate Director for Patient Care Services, Veterans Affairs Medical Center, Battle Creek, MI, p. A308
BOWERMAN, Joeann, Director of Nursing Services, Chambers Memorial Hospital, Danville, AR, p. A43
BOWERMAN, Stephen, Chief Financial Officer, Midland Memorial Hospital, Midland, TX, p. A617
BOWERS, Daniel, Chief Executive Officer, John F. Kennedy Memorial Hospital, Indio, CA, p. A65
BOWERS, David, Vice President Human Resources and Support Services, Children's Hospital of The King's Daughters, Norfolk, VA, p. A652
BOWERS, David N., M.D. Medical Director, Siskin Hospital for Physical Rehabilitation, Chattanooga, TN, p. A564
BOWERS, Gary, Chief Operating Officer, CarePartners Health Services, Asheville, NC, p. A448
BOWERS, Gregory, Chief Financial Officer, Spring Harbor Hospital, Westbrook, ME, p. A286
BOWERS, Judith, D.O. Chief of Staff, Community Memorial Hospital, Oconto Falls, WI, p. A688
BOWERS, Maria, M.D. Chief of Staff, Erlanger at Hutcheson, Fort Oglethorpe, GA, p. A153
BOWERS, Sharon, R.N. Manager of Community, Public and Employee Relations, Sheridan Community Hospital, Sheridan, MI, p. A323
BOWERS, Stephen, M.D. Clinical Director, Northern Navajo Medical Center, Shiprock, NM, p. A418
BOWERS, Susan, R.N. President and Chief Nursing Officer, Mercy Allen Hospital, Oberlin, OH, p. A486
BOWES, Arthur, Senior Vice President Human Resources, North Shore Medical Center, Salem, MA, p. A304
BOWIE, Craig, Information Technology Manager, Pauls Valley General Hospital, Pauls Valley, OK, p. A503
BOWLBY, Debbie, Director Information Systems, St. Luke's Hospital – Warren Campus, Phillipsburg, NJ, p. A408
BOWLEG, Teresa, R.N. Chief Nursing Officer, Murphy Medical Center, Murphy, NC, p. A458
BOWLING, Judy, Director Human Resources, Missouri Southern Healthcare, Dexter, MO, p. A358
BOWLING, Karen, Chief Information Officer, St. Joseph Hospital, Bangor, ME, p. A281
BOWLING, Kay, Chief Executive Officer, Center for Restorative Care and Rehabilitation, Lynchburg, VA, p. A650
BOWLING, Kelli, Chief Culture Officer, Ministry Door County Medical Center, Sturgeon Bay, WI, p. A691
BOWMAN, Barbara, Chief Human Resource Officer, Ann & Robert H. Lurie Children's Hospital of Chicago, Chicago, IL, p. A175
BOWMAN, Dyan, Director Human Resources, Newberry County Memorial Hospital, Newberry, SC, p. A553
BOWMAN, Joseph E., Chief Financial Officer, StoneCrest Medical Center, Smyrna, TN, p. A575
BOWMAN, Julie, Chief Nursing Officer, Havasu Regional Medical Center, Lake Havasu City, AZ, p. A33
BOWMAN, Ken, Chief Executive Officer, Van Matre HEALTHSOUTH Rehabilitation Hospital, Rockford, IL, p. A193
BOWMAN, Scott, Administrator, Sweetwater Hospital, Sweetwater, TN, p. A576
BOWMAN, Terry R., Chief Financial Officer, Wake Forest Baptist Health–Davie Hospital, Mocksville, NC, p. A457
BOWMAN, Wayne, Interim Chief Nursing Officer, Parkway Medical Center, Decatur, AL, p. A18
BOWMAN, William, M.D. Vice President Medical Affairs, Cone Health, Greensboro, NC, p. A454
BOX, Darrel, VP of Operations, Lafayette Regional Health Center, Lexington, MO, p. A364
BOX, Lynette, Director Medical Records, Arrowhead Behavioral Health Hospital, Maumee, OH, p. A484
BOX, Tom, CPA Chief Financial Officer, HEALTHSOUTH Rehabilitation Hospital–Wichita Falls, Wichita Falls, TX, p. A635
BOXELL, Shelley, R.N. Chief Nursing Officer and Quality Coordinator, Rehabilitation Hospital of Fort Wayne, Fort Wayne, IN, p. A202
BOYCE, Carol
Administrative Director Support Services, ProMedica Bixby Hospital, Adrian, MI, p. A307
Administrative Director Support Services, ProMedica Herrick Hospital, Tecumseh, MI, p. A324
BOYCE, Joe, M.D. Chief Information Officer, Heartland Regional Medical Center, Saint Joseph, MO, p. A368
BOYD, Amber, Nurse Practitioner and Director of Nursing, Devereux Georgia Treatment Network, Kennesaw, GA, p. A154
BOYD, Amy, Information Systems Manager, Vidant Beaufort Hospital, Washington, NC, p. A462
BOYD, Christopher L., Senior Vice President and Area Manager, Santa Clara Medical Center, Santa Clara, CA, p. A90
BOYD, Dennis, Chief Financial Officer, St. Mark's Medical Center, La Grange, TX, p. A611
BOYD, Diana, Vice President Nursing, Union Hospital, Dover, OH, p. A479
BOYD, Ellen, Director Human Resources, Emanuel Medical Center, Swainsboro, GA, p. A160
BOYD, Fred, Interim Vice President Human Resources, Regional Medical Center at Memphis, Memphis, TN, p. A572
BOYD, Gary, M.P.H. Chief Executive Officer, Mammoth Hospital, Mammoth Lakes, CA, p. A73
BOYD, Jason E., FACHE Interim Chief Executive Officer, Nashville General Hospital, Nashville, TN, p. A573
BOYD, JoAnn, Administrative Assistant, Jasper General Hospital, Bay Springs, MS, p. A343
BOYD, John, Manager Information Systems, North Valley Hospital, Tonasket, WA, p. A668
BOYD, John A K, M.D. Vice President Mission and Medical Affairs and Chief Medical Officer, Mercy Regional Medical Center, Durango, CO, p. A100
BOYD, John W., PsyD, Chief Administrative Officer, Sutter Center for Psychiatry, Sacramento, CA, p. A84
BOYD Jr., Kenneth, President and Chief Executive Officer, McDonough District Hospital, Macomb, IL, p. A186
BOYD, Kim, Chief Financial Officer, Buchanan General Hospital, Grundy, VA, p. A649
BOYD, Steven, R.N. Nurse Executive, Levi Hospital, Hot Springs National Park, AR, p. A46
BOYD, Travis, Manager Information Technology, Lincoln County Medical Center, Troy, MO, p. A372
BOYD, Wallace N., Chief Executive Officer, Sayre Memorial Hospital, Sayre, OK, p. A504
BOYDEN, Jenny, Chief Financial Officer, Riverview Psychiatric Center, Augusta, ME, p. A281
BOYER, Allan, Chief Executive Officer, Ancora Psychiatric Hospital, Ancora, NJ, p. A401
BOYER, Aurelia, Senior Vice President and Chief Information Officer, New York–Presbyterian Hospital, New York, NY, p. A436
BOYER, Charlene, Chief Nursing Officer, Oakland Medical Center, Oakland, CA, p. A77
BOYER, Cheryl T., Vice President Human Resources, Levindale Hebrew Geriatric Center and Hospital, Baltimore, MD, p. A288
BOYER, Craig, Vice President Finance, Sanford Bemidji Medical Center, Bemidji, MN, p. A328
BOYER, David, Chief Financial Officer, Mercy Hospital Grayling, Grayling, MI, p. A314
BOYER, Diana, Chief Information Officer, Columbus Regional Hospital, Columbus, IN, p. A199
BOYER, Gregory E., Chief Executive Officer, Renown Regional Medical Center, Reno, NV, p. A395
BOYER, Jim, Vice President Information Technology and Chief Information Officer, Rush Memorial Hospital, Rushville, IN, p. A211
BOYER, Marta, Vice President Human Resources, Children's Hospital Central California, Madera, CA, p. A73
BOYER, Roderick, M.D. Medical Director, Select Specialty Hospital–Downriver, Taylor, MI, p. A324
BOYKIN, Alfred, M.D. Chief of Staff, Wm. Jennings Bryan Dorn Veterans Affairs Medical Center, Columbia, SC, p. A549
BOYKIN, Doyle, MSN, Administrator, Presbyterian Kaseman Hospital, Albuquerque, NM, p. A414
BOYLE, Donna, Director, Columbia Hospital, West Palm Beach, FL, p. A142
BOYLE, James W., M.D. Chief Medical Officer, UPMC Passavant, Pittsburgh, PA, p. A535
BOYLE, Kathy, R.N. Chief Nursing Officer, Denver Health Medical Center, Denver, CO, p. A99
BOYLE, Patrick R.
Vice President Human Resources, Geneva General Hospital, Geneva, NY, p. A426
Vice President Human Resources, Soldiers and Sailors Memorial Hospital of Yates County, Penn Yan, NY, p. A440
BOYLE, Steven P.
Executive Vice President, Albany Memorial Hospital, Albany, NY, p. A420
Executive Vice President, St. Peter's Hospital, Albany, NY, p. A420
BOYLE, Thomas W., Chief Financial Officer, St. Lawrence Rehabilitation Center, Lawrenceville, NJ, p. A405
BOYLES, Clay, Director Human Resources, Peachford Behavioral Health System, Atlanta, GA, p. A145
BOYLES, George, Vice President Finance and Chief Financial Officer, Mercer County Joint Township Community Hospital, Coldwater, OH, p. A476
BOYLES, Larry, Senior Vice President, Riverside Regional Medical Center, Newport News, VA, p. A652
BOYLES, Laura, Director Human Resources, Stanislaus Surgical Hospital, Modesto, CA, p. A75
BOYLES, Lee, Chief Executive Officer, Oakes Community Hospital, Oakes, ND, p. A467
BOYNE, Diane, Chief Nursing Officer, Baylor Medical Center at Uptown, Dallas, TX, p. A590
BOYNTON, Kimberly, Chief Financial Officer, Crouse Hospital, Syracuse, NY, p. A444
BOYNTON, Stephanie, Administrator, Erlanger Bledsoe Hospital, Pikeville, TN, p. A574
BOYS, Edward, Chief Information Officer, Ozarks Medical Center, West Plains, MO, p. A372
BOYSEN, James, M.D. Executive Medical Director, Texas NeuroRehab Center, Austin, TX, p. A582
BOYSEN, Joan, Chief Operating Officer, District One Hospital, Faribault, MN, p. A331
BOZELL, Jerry, Administrative Director Human Resources, Jay County Hospital, Portland, IN, p. A210
BOZEMAN, Tom, Chief Information Officer, North Mississippi Medical Center – Tupelo, Tupelo, MS, p. A353
BOZZUTO, Elizabeth, R.N. Interim Chief Nursing Officer and Vice President Surgical Services, Saint Mary's Hospital, Waterbury, CT, p. A112
BRAAM, Richard, Vice President Finance, Medstar St. Mary's Hospital, Leonardtown, MD, p. A293
BRAASCH, David A., President, Alton Memorial Hospital, Alton, IL, p. A172
BRAASCH, Robert, Administrator Human Resources, Andrew McFarland Mental Health Center, Springfield, IL, p. A194
BRABAND, Jon D., FACHE President and Chief Executive Officer, Glencoe Regional Health Services, Glencoe, MN, p. A332

**A768** Index of Health Care Professionals

Index of Health Care Professionals / Braun

Index of Health Care Professionals

BRABSON, Amanda, Director Marketing and Public Relations, LeConte Medical Center, Sevierville, TN, p. A575
BRACE, Bob, Director Human Resources, Hillcrest Baptist Medical Center, Waco, TX, p. A633
BRACEY, Donny, Director Information Services, Marion General Hospital, Columbia, MS, p. A345
BRACHT, Gerald E., Chief Administrative Officer, Palomar Medical Center, Escondido, CA, p. A60
BRACKEN, Richard M., Chairman and Chief Executive Officer, HCA, Nashville, TN, p. B57
BRACKEN, Thomas H., M.D. Vice President Medical Affairs, Mille Lacs Health System, Onamia, MN, p. A336
BRACKLEY, Donna, Senior Vice President Patient Care Services, John Muir Medical Center, Concord, Concord, CA, p. A58
BRACY, Dale, Chief Financial Officer, College Hospital Costa Mesa, Costa Mesa, CA, p. A58
BRADDY, Rufus, Director Management Information Systems, Roosevelt Warm Springs LTAC Hospital, Warm Springs, GA, p. A161
BRADEL, William T.
President, Flagstaff Medical Center, Flagstaff, AZ, p. A32
President, Flagstaff Medical Center, Flagstaff, AZ, p. A32
BRADEL, William T., President and Co–Chief Executive Officer, Northern Arizona Healthcare, Flagstaff, AZ, p. B95
BRADEN, III, Terence, D.O. Medical Director, HEALTHSOUTH Rehabilitation Hospital of Jonesboro, Jonesboro, AR, p. A46
BRADEY, Sarah, Vice President Finance, Mercy Hospital Hot Springs, Hot Springs National Park, AR, p. A46
BRADFORD, Anna, R.N. Chief Nursing Officer, Crosbyton Clinic Hospital, Crosbyton, TX, p. A590
BRADFORD, Beth, Director Human Resources, Floyd Medical Center, Rome, GA, p. A158
BRADFORD, David, M.D. Chief Medical Officer, Mid–Valley Hospital, Omak, WA, p. A663
BRADFORD, James, M.D. President Medical Staff, Iredell Memorial Hospital, Statesville, NC, p. A461
BRADFORD, John, Vice President Finance, Flaget Memorial Hospital, Bardstown, KY, p. A247
BRADFORD, Karin, Chief Financial Officer, LifeCare Hospitals of Dallas, Dallas, TX, p. A591
BRADFORD, Randy L., Assistant Superintendent, Eastern Shore Hospital Center, Cambridge, MD, p. A290
BRADFORD, Scot, Chief Information Officer, Baylor Medical Center at Trophy Club, Trophy Club, TX, p. A631
BRADFORD, Sue E., R.N. Chief Nursing Officer, Memorial Hospital West, Pembroke Pines, FL, p. A135
BRADLEY, Betsy, Coordinator Performance Improvement, Central State Hospital, Milledgeville, GA, p. A156
BRADLEY, Carol, MSN Senior Vice President and Chief Nursing Officer, Legacy Meridian Park Hospital, Tualatin, OR, p. A516
BRADLEY, David
Chief Executive Officer, Alta Bates Summit Medical Center, Berkeley, CA, p. A55
Chief Executive Officer, Alta Bates Summit Medical Center – Summit Campus, Oakland, CA, p. A77
BRADLEY, David K., FACHE Chief Executive Officer, Geary Community Hospital, Junction City, KS, p. A235
BRADLEY, Douglas, M.D. Vice President Medical Affairs, Belton Regional Medical Center, Belton, MO, p. A355
BRADLEY, Eric, Director Computer Information Services, Summit Behavioral Healthcare, Cincinnati, OH, p. A474
BRADLEY Jr.,, J. Lindsey, FACHE President, Trinity Mother Frances Hospitals and Clinics, Tyler, TX, p. B131
BRADLEY, Joel, Director Information Systems, Laurens County Health Care System, Clinton, SC, p. A548
BRADLEY, John, M.D. Chief of Staff, Longmont United Hospital, Longmont, CO, p. A104
BRADLEY, Linda, Chief Executive Officer, Centinela Hospital Medical Center, Inglewood, CA, p. A65
BRADLEY, Louis, Chief Executive Officer, Life Center Specialty Hospital, Sherman, TX, p. A627
BRADLEY, Michelle, Director Health Information Management, LTAC of Wichita, Wichita, KS, p. A245
BRADLEY, Peggy A., Chief Operating Officer, Plains Memorial Hospital, Dimmitt, TX, p. A594
BRADLEY, Stacye, R.N. Chief Nursing Officer, Union County General Hospital, Clayton, NM, p. A415
BRADLEY, Teresa, M.D. Vice President Medical Affairs, St. Anthony's Hospital, Saint Petersburg, FL, p. A138
BRADLEY, Terri, CPA Vice President Financial Services and Chief Financial Officer, Western Missouri Medical Center, Warrensburg, MO, p. A372
BRADLEY, Virginia D., Chief Information Officer, Breckinridge Memorial Hospital, Hardinsburg, KY, p. A251
BRADLEY, William L., President and Chief Executive Officer, Washington Regional Medical Center, Fayetteville, AR, p. A44
BRADSHAW, David
Chief Information Officer, Memorial Hermann – Texas Medical Center, Houston, TX, p. A605
Chief Information, Planning and Marketing Officer, Memorial Hermann Memorial City Medical Center, Houston, TX, p. A605
Chief Information Officer, Memorial Hermann Northwest Hospital, Houston, TX, p. A605
BRADSHAW, Deborah, Director Human Resources, Holy Family Hospital and Medical Center, Methuen, MA, p. A302
BRADSHAW, Rita, Director Human Resources, Chatuge Regional Hospital and Nursing Home, Hiawassee, GA, p. A154
BRADSHAW, Thomas A., Vice President Operations, Wayne Memorial Hospital, Goldsboro, NC, p. A453
BRADSHAW, William, M.D. Chief of Staff, St. Vincent General Hospital District, Leadville, CO, p. A103
BRADY, Albert, M.D. Chief of Staff, Yakima Regional Medical and Cardiac Center, Yakima, WA, p. A669
BRADY, Jeff
Director Information Systems, Hazard ARH Regional Medical Center, Hazard, KY, p. A251
Director Information Systems, McDowell ARH Hospital, McDowell, KY, p. A256
Director Information Systems, Morgan County ARH Hospital, West Liberty, KY, p. A259
Chief Information Officer, Williamson ARH Hospital, South Williamson, KY, p. A259
BRADY, John, Vice President Physician Services and Organizational Planning, Marianjoy Rehabilitation Hospital, Wheaton, IL, p. A196
BRADY, Linda, M.D. President and Chief Executive Officer, Kingsbrook Jewish Medical Center,, NY, p. A433
BRADY, Patrick R., Chief Executive Officer, Sutter Roseville Medical Center, Roseville, CA, p. A83
BRADY, Reta, Administrative Assistant and Manager Human Resources, Patients' Choice Medical Center of Erin, Erin, TN, p. A565
BRADY, Tim, Director Information Systems, Mt. Washington Pediatric Hospital, Baltimore, MD, p. A288
BRAESE, Nancy, D.O. President Medical Staff, Exeter Hospital, Exeter, NH, p. A398
BRAGDON, Carol, Director Human Resources, Middle Tennessee Medical Center, Murfreesboro, TN, p. A573
BRAGG, Craig, Chief Executive Officer, TrustPoint Hospital, Lubbock, TX, p. A614
BRAGG, Deborah, Director Human Resources, Webster County Memorial Hospital, Webster Springs, WV, p. A676
BRAGG, Lisa, Vice President Human Resources, Knox Community Hospital, Mount Vernon, OH, p. A485
BRAGG, Melissa, Chief Human Resources Management, Charles George Veterans Affairs Medical Center, Asheville, NC, p. A448
BRAINERD, Mary K., President and Chief Executive Officer, HealthPartners, Bloomington, MN, p. B64
BRAITHWAITE, Robert
Chief Operating Officer, Hoag Hospital Irvine, Irvine, CA, p. A65
Senior Vice President and Chief Operating Officer, Hoag Memorial Hospital Presbyterian, Newport Beach, CA, p. A76
BRAKE, Joe, Director Information Services, Fishermen's Hospital, Marathon, FL, p. A129
BRAMBLE, Steve, Director Human Resources, LeConte Medical Center, Sevierville, TN, p. A575
BRAMLETT, Larry, Chief Information Officer, LTAC Hospital of Greenwood, Greenwood, MS, p. A346
BRAMLIET, Charles, M.D. Medical Director, WestEnd Hospital, Jennings, LA, p. A268
BRANCATO, Joyce A., Chief Executive Officer, Seven Rivers Regional Medical Center, Crystal River, FL, p. A121
BRANCEL, Dale, D.O. Chief of Staff, Southwest Surgical Hospital, Hurst, TX, p. A608
BRANCH, Terrance, Chief Information Management, DeWitt Army Community Hospital, Fort Belvoir, VA, p. A648
BRANCH, Tim, Manager Information Technology, Covenant Hospital Plainview, Plainview, TX, p. A621
BRANCHICK, Jim, R.N. Chief Operating Officer, Kaiser Permanente Downey Medical Center, Downey,, p. A59
BRANCO, Patrick J., Chief Executive Officer, PeaceHealth Ketchikan Medical Center, Ketchikan, AK, p. A29
BRAND, James R., M.D. Chief of Staff, DeTar Healthcare System, Victoria, TX, p. A633
BRAND, Lamar, M.D. Chief of Staff, Miller County Hospital, Colquitt, GA, p. A149
BRANDENBURG, Edward M., FACHE Vice President Professional Services, Community Memorial Healthcenter, South Hill, VA, p. A656
BRANDENBURG, Valerie, Director Human Resources, Northwest Hospital, Randallstown, MD, p. A293
BRANDIS, Destin, Chief Information Officer, William Bee Ririe Hospital, Ely, NV, p. A391
BRANDNER, Nicholas R., Chief Executive Officer, Community Memorial Hospital, Redfield, SD, p. A559
BRANDON, David R., President and Chief Executive Officer, Finley Hospital, Dubuque, IA, p. A219
BRANDON, Deborah, Director Total Quality Management, Eastern Louisiana Mental Health System, Jackson, LA, p. A268
BRANDON, Paula, MSN Vice President Patient Care Services, Good Shepherd Medical Center–Marshall, Marshall, TX, p. A615
BRANDON, Wendy H., Chief Executive Officer, Central Florida Regional Hospital, Sanford, FL, p. A138
BRANDT, Cynthia, Interim Chief Financial Officer, Norton Sound Regional Hospital, Nome, AK, p. A29
BRANDT, Jason, M.D. Medical Director, Surgical Hospital of Jonesboro, Jonesboro, AR, p. A47
BRANDT, Matthew, Chief Financial Officer, St. Alexius Hospital – Broadway Campus, Saint Louis, MO, p. A369
BRANDT, Merle, Chief Financial Officer, Mason General Hospital, Shelton, WA, p. A666
BRANDT, Steve, M.D. Chief of Staff, Dale Medical Center, Ozark, AL, p. A24
BRANNAN, Debbie
Chief Financial Officer, George County Hospital, Lucedale, MS, p. A349
Chief Financial Officer, Greene County Hospital, Leakesville, MS, p. A349
BRANNEN, Charles C., Senior Vice President and Chief Operating Officer, Southeast Alabama Medical Center, Dothan, AL, p. A19
BRANNEN, Judy, M.D. Interim Chief of Staff, Hunter Holmes McGuire Veterans Affairs Medical Center, Richmond, VA, p. A655
BRANNIGAN, Robert C., Administrator, West Valley Hospital, Dallas, OR, p. A510
BRANNMAN, Brian G., Chief Executive Officer, University Medical Center, Las Vegas, NV, p. A394
BRANNON, Jeffrey M., Chief Executive Officer, Medical Center Enterprise, Enterprise, AL, p. A19
BRANNON, Jim, Vice President Human Resources, Atlantic General Hospital, Berlin, MD, p. A289
BRANNON, Linda, Vice President Human Resources, Circles of Care, Melbourne, FL, p. A130
BRANSCOME, Eileen, Chief Operating Officer, Mason General Hospital, Shelton, WA, p. A666
BRANSCUM, Patsy, Director Human Resources, Renaissance Hospital Terrell, Terrell, TX, p. A630
BRANSFORD, Charles, M.D. Medical Director, Lakeview Hospital, Stillwater, MN, p. A340
BRANSKY, Shawn, Flight Commander Resources Management, U. S. Air Force Regional Hospital, Elmendorf AFB, AK, p. A28
BRANSON, Jason, Chief Executive Officer, AMG Specialty Hospital – Lafayette, Lafayette, LA, p. A269
BRANSON, Phil, M.D. President Medical Staff, Princeton Community Hospital, Princeton, WV, p. A675
BRANSTETTER, Jon, Vice President Finance, Missouri Delta Medical Center, Sikeston, MO, p. A371
BRANT, James R., Senior Vice President Finance and Chief Financial Officer, Underwood–Memorial Hospital, Woodbury, NJ, p. A412
BRANT, Johnny, Chief Financial Officer, Welch Community Hospital, Welch, WV, p. A676
BRANT, Mick, Chief Executive Officer, Grace Cottage Hospital, Townshend, VT, p. A644
BRANTZ, Jerry, Chief Financial Officer, Shoshone Medical Center, Kellogg, ID, p. A168
BRASEL, James, Chief Financial Officer, Craig General Hospital, Vinita, OK, p. A507
BRASH, David L.
System Regional Vice President and President, Mountain View Regional Medical Center, Norton, VA, p. A653
Interim President, Wellmont Lonesome Pine Hospital, Big Stone Gap, VA, p. A645
BRASHER, Tanya, Director of Nursing, North Mississippi Medical Center–Hamilton, Hamilton, AL, p. A21
BRASSER, Bruce A., R.N. VP of Inpatient and Network Operations, Mary Free Bed Rehabilitation Hospital, Grand Rapids, MI, p. A313
BRASSINGER, Cindy, Chief Operating Officer, Vibra Hospital of Southeastern Michigan, Lincoln Park, MI, p. A318
BRASWELL, Gingie, Director Human Resources, DeKalb Community Hospital, Smithville, TN, p. A575
BRAUN, James R., Chief Financial Officer, Flambeau Hospital, Park Falls, WI, p. A689
BRAUN, Norma, Vice President Human Resources, Hollywood Presbyterian Medical Center, Los Angeles, CA, p. A69


Index of Health Care Professionals A769

Index of Health Care Professionals
Index of Health Care Professionals / Braun

BRAUN, Jr., Richard G., CP
Senior Vice President and Chief Financial Officer, Bradford Regional Medical Center, Bradford, PA, p. A519
Senior Vice President and Chief Financial Officer, Olean General Hospital, Olean, NY, p. A439
BRAUN, Sahlenia, Chief Financial Officer, Wishek Community Hospital and Clinics, Wishek, ND, p. A468
BRAVO, Chebon, Director Information Systems, Green Oaks Hospital, Dallas, TX, p. A591
BRAXTON, Edwin R., Director Human Resources, Lompoc Valley Medical Center, Lompoc, CA, p. A67
BRAY, Bob, Chief Information Officer, Jersey Community Hospital, Jerseyville, IL, p. A185
BRAY, Delnita, Administrator, Texas Specialty Hospital at Wichita Falls, Wichita Falls, TX, p. A635
BRAY, John, M.D. Medical Director, Select Specialty Hospital–Pensacola, Pensacola, FL, p. A136
BRAY, Pam, Director of Nursing and Director Inpatient Services, Kane Community Hospital, Kane, PA, p. A526
BRAYTON, Jackie, Vice President Human Resources, Portsmouth Regional Hospital, Portsmouth, NH, p. A400
BRAYTON, Ranee C., R.N. Associate Chief Executive Officer, Northeast Regional Medical Center, Kirksville, MO, p. A363
BRAZ, Marcus, Chief Executive Officer, HEALTHSOUTH Rehabilitation Hospital of Sarasota, Sarasota, FL, p. A139
BRAZASKI, Karrie, Chief Operating Officer and Chief Nursing Officer, Lovelace Westside Hospital, Albuquerque, NM, p. A414
BRAZEL, Gary, M.D. Chief Medical Officer, Saint John's Health System, Anderson, IN, p. A197
BRAZIL, Robert, Chief Operating Officer, Memorial Health System, Abilene, KS, p. A230
BREA, Christie, Manager Human Resources, Promise Hospital of Phoenix, Mesa, AZ, p. A34
BREADY, Sharon, R.N. Chief Executive Officer, Care One at Raritan Bay Medical Center, Perth Amboy, NJ, p. A408
BREAKWELL, Michael, R.N. Nurse Executive, Twin Valley Behavioral Healthcare, Columbus, OH, p. A477
BRECHBILL, Alan L., Executive Director, Penn State Milton S. Hershey Medical Center, Hershey, PA, p. A525
BRECKLIN, Mary Jane, Network Vice President, South Operating Group, SSM Cardinal Glennon Children's Medical Center, Saint Louis, MO, p. A369
BREEDEN, Susan M., Administrator and Chief Executive Officer, Baptist Memorial Hospital–Huntingdon, Huntingdon, TN, p. A566
BREEDING, Donnie, Chief Executive Officer, Heart of Florida Regional Medical Center, Davenport, FL, p. A121
BREEDLOVE, Jean Ann
Chief Information Officer, Children's Mercy Hospitals and Clinics, Kansas City, MO, p. A361
Chief Information Officer, Children's Mercy South, Overland Park, KS, p. A240
BREEDVELD, Stacey, R.N. Associate Director for Patient Care, Veterans Affairs Ann Arbor Healthcare System, Ann Arbor, MI, p. A307
BREEN, Charles J., M.D. Medical Director, Hillsboro Medical Center, Hillsboro, ND, p. A466
BREEN, Thomas, Vice President and Chief Financial Officer, South County Hospital, Wakefield, RI, p. A545
BREHM, Jay R., Executive Vice President and Chief Financial Officer, Franciscan St. Francis Health – Indianapolis, Indianapolis, IN, p. A204
BREHM, Robert, Division President, Kessler Institute for Rehabilitation, West Orange, NJ, p. A412
BREILAND, Keith, M.D. Medical Director, Seven Hills Behavioral Institute, Henderson, NV, p. A392
BREITBACH, Dave, Chief Financial Officer, Prairie du Chien Memorial Hospital, Prairie Du Chien, WI, p. A689
BREITENBACH, Ray, M.D. Chief of Staff, Doctors' Hospital of Michigan, Pontiac, MI, p. A320
BREITFELDER, Michelle, Chief Operating Officer, Hughston Hospital, Columbus, GA, p. A149
BREITLING, Bryan, Administrator, Avera Hand County Memorial Hospital & Clinic, Miller, SD, p. A557
BRELAND, Kelly R., CPA Director Support Services, Mississippi State Hospital, Whitfield, MS, p. A354
BRELSFORD, George W., M.D. Chief Medical Staff, Effingham Hospital, Springfield, GA, p. A159
BREMER, David, D.O. Chief of Staff, MidMichigan Medical Center–Clare, Clare, MI, p. A309
BREMER Jr., Louis H., President and Chief Executive Officer, St. Francis Medical Center, Monroe, LA, p. A273
BRENAN, Kevin, Chief Financial Officer, Saint Joseph's Hospital of Atlanta, Atlanta, GA, p. A146
BRENDGARD, Robert L., Interim Chief Executive Officer, Sunnyside Community Hospital, Sunnyside, WA, p. A667
BRENDLER, Stephen, Director Information Systems, Hilton Head Hospital, Hilton Head Island, SC, p. A551
BRENHOLT, Craig, Director Human Resources, St. Mary's Hospital, Madison, WI, p. A684
BRENKLE, George, Chief Information Officer, UMass Memorial Medical Center, Worcester, MA, p. A306
BRENN, Jonathan, Chief Executive Officer, Corcoran District Hospital, Corcoran, CA, p. A58
BRENNAN, James, M.D. Chief of Staff, Carolinas Hospital System, Florence, SC, p. A549
BRENNAN, John A., M.P.H. President and Chief Executive Officer, Newark Beth Israel Medical Center, Newark, NJ, p. A407
BRENNAN, Kevin F., CPA Executive Vice President and Chief Financial Officer, Geisinger Medical Center, Danville, PA, p. A521
BRENNAN, Patrick, Director Information System Technology, Saint Louis University Hospital, Saint Louis, MO, p. A369
BRENNAN, Patrick J., M.D. Senior Vice President and Chief Medical Officer, Hospital of the University of Pennsylvania, Philadelphia, PA, p. A532
BRENNAN, Theresa, M.D. Chief Medical Officer, University of Iowa Hospitals and Clinics, Iowa City, IA, p. A221
BRENNER, Pattie, R.N. Chief Nursing Officer, HEALTHSOUTH Rehabilitation Hospital, Largo, FL, p. A128
BRENNER, William
Chief Financial Officer, Kindred Hospital Indianapolis South, Greenwood, IN, p. A203
Chief Financial Officer, Kindred Hospital–Indianapolis, Indianapolis, IN, p. A204
BRENNY, Terrence, President and Chief Executive Officer, Stoughton Hospital Association, Stoughton, WI, p. A691
BRENTANO, Gregory
Chief Financial Officer, Chino Valley Medical Center, Chino, CA, p. A57
Chief Executive Officer, Montclair Hospital Medical Center, Montclair, CA, p. A75
Chief Executive Officer, San Dimas Community Hospital, San Dimas, CA, p. A86
BRENZEL, Mark T., Chief Executive Officer, Lake Cumberland Regional Hospital, Somerset, KY, p. A259
BREON, Richard C., President and Chief Executive Officer, Spectrum Health, Grand Rapids, MI, p. B121
BRES, Thomas, Vice President and Chief Information Officer, Sparrow Hospital, Lansing, MI, p. A317
BRESCIA, Michael J., M.D. Executive Medical Director, Calvary Hospital,, NY, p. A432
BRESLIN, Michael P., Executive Vice President and Chief Financial Officer, Lenox Hill Hospital, New York, NY, p. A433
BRESLIN, Susan E., Vice President and Chief Nursing Officer, Providence Hospital, Mobile, AL, p. A23
BRESLIN, Tim, Chief Financial Officer, Lakeview Regional Medical Center, Covington, LA, p. A265
BRESNAHAN, Christine, Manager Human Resources, Radius Specialty Hospital Boston, Boston, MA, p. A297
BRESNAHAN, Jacky, Director Human Resources, Mahaska Health Partnership, Oskaloosa, IA, p. A225
BRESSLER, Kathy, President, St. Clare Hospital, Lakewood, WA, p. A662
BRETTNER, Eric, Vice President and Chief Financial Officer, St. Mary's Medical Center, San Francisco, CA, p. A87
BRETZ, Joseph W., Director Human Resources, St. John's Hospital, Springfield, IL, p. A194
BRETZ, Joy, Chief Financial Officer, Gove County Medical Center, Quinter, KS, p. A242
BREUDER, Andrew, M.D. Chief of Staff, Veterans Affairs Medical Center, Manchester, NH, p. A399
BREUER, Jason, Administrator, LakeWood Health Center, Baudette, MN, p. A328
BREUER, Rick, Chief Executive Officer and Administrator, Community Memorial Hospital, Cloquet, MN, p. A329
BREUM, Linda, R.N. Chief Nursing Officer, Bert Fish Medical Center, New Smyrna Beach, FL, p. A133
BREWER, David, Director Finance, ProMedica Bay Park Hospital, Oregon, OH, p. A486
BREWER, Gary L., Chief Executive Officer, Valley View Hospital, Glenwood Springs, CO, p. A101
BREWER, Jennifer, R.N. Chief Nursing Officer and Vice President Nursing Services, Verde Valley Medical Center, Cottonwood, AZ, p. A31
BREWER, Jennifer Lynn, Chief Executive Officer, HEALTHSOUTH Plano Rehabilitation Hospital, Plano, TX, p. A621
BREWER, Jim, M.P.H. Chief Financial Officer, Healthmark Regional Medical Center, DeFuniak Springs, FL, p. A122
BREWER, Kaye, Director Human Resources, Maury Regional Hospital, Columbia, TN, p. A564
BREWER, Kelley, MSN, Chief Executive Officer, Lakeside Women's Hospital, Oklahoma City, OK, p. A501
BREWER, Patricia, Chief Nursing Officer, University Behavioral Health of Denton, Denton, TX, p. A594
BREWINGTON, Kenneth, M.D. Vice President Administrator and Chief Marketing Officer, Infirmary West, Mobile, AL, p. A22
BREWINGTON, Yvonne, Director Human Resources, Belton Regional Medical Center, Belton, MO, p. A355
BREWIS, Laurie, Vice President Human Resources, McLaren Greater Lansing, Lansing, MI, p. A317
BREWSTER, Joseph, M.D. Chief of Staff, Bates County Memorial Hospital, Butler, MO, p. A356
BREWSTER, Melvin, Chief Information Officer, LAC–Olive View–UCLA Medical Center,, CA, p. A70
BREYFOGLE, Cynthia, Director, Charles George Veterans Affairs Medical Center, Asheville, NC, p. A448
BREZA, Lisa, R.N. Vice President and Chief Nursing Officer, Robert Wood Johnson University Hospital at Hamilton, Hamilton, NJ, p. A404
BREZENOFF, Stanley, President and Chief Executive Officer, Continuum Health Partners, New York, NY, p. B38
BREZNY, Angie, Director Human Resources, Prague Community Hospital, Prague, OK, p. A503
BREZOVSKY, Patricia, Director Human Resources, St. Joseph Hospital, Bangor, ME, p. A281
BRIAN, David, Director Information Services, Shriners Hospitals for Children–Lexington, Lexington, KY, p. A253
BRIAN, Francis, M.D. Senior Vice President Medical Affairs, Rapides Regional Medical Center, Alexandria, LA, p. A261
BRICHER, Joan
Senior Vice President Finance and Chief Financial Officer, Goleta Valley Cottage Hospital, Santa Barbara, CA, p. A89
Senior Vice President Finance and Chief Financial Officer, Santa Barbara Cottage Hospital, Santa Barbara, CA, p. A89
Senior Vice President Finance and Chief Financial Officer, Santa Ynez Valley Cottage Hospital, Solvang, CA, p. A91
BRICKER, Steven A., Chief Financial Officer, Sparta Community Hospital, Sparta, IL, p. A194
BRICKER, Tim
President and Chief Executive Officer, Chandler Regional Medical Center, Chandler, AZ, p. A31
President and Chief Executive Officer, Mercy Gilbert Medical Center, Gilbert, AZ, p. A32
BRICKMAN, Jeffrey, FACHE President and Chief Executive Officer, St. Anthony Hospital, Lakewood, CO, p. A103
BRIDEN, David, Chief Information Officer, Exeter Hospital, Exeter, NH, p. A398
BRIDGE, Lauren M., R.N. Chief Nurse Executive, Providence Milwaukie Hospital, Milwaukie, OR, p. A513
BRIDGELAND, Aaron, Director Finance, Wheaton Franciscan Healthcare – St. Francis, Milwaukee, WI, p. A687
BRIDGES, Alan J., M.D. Chief of Staff, William S. Middleton Memorial Veterans Hospital, Madison, WI, p. A684
BRIDGES, James M., Executive Vice President and Chief Operating Officer, Palmetto Health Baptist, Columbia, SC, p. A548
BRIDGES, Jane Ann, Chief Financial Officer, Nacogdoches Memorial Hospital, Nacogdoches, TX, p. A618
BRIDGES, Mary, Director Human Resources, Ouachita County Medical Center, Camden, AR, p. A43
BRIDGES, Theresa, Chief Information Officer, Crawley Memorial Hospital, Boiling Springs, NC, p. A449
BRIDGES KEE, Lorinnsa, Director Human Resource, Cypress Fairbanks Medical Center, Houston, TX, p. A604
BRIER, Pamela S., President and Chief Executive Officer, Maimonides Medical Center,, NY, p. A434
BRIESEMEISTER, Eric, Chief Executive Officer, Jones Regional Medical Center, Anamosa, IA, p. A214
BRIETE, Mark, M.D. Vice President Medical Affairs, Jefferson Regional Medical Center, Crystal City, MO, p. A358
BRIGGS, Bryon, Assistant Chief Financial Officer, Select Specialty Hospital–Tulsa Midtown, Tulsa, OK, p. A506
BRIGGS, Deborah, Director Human Resources, Ellenville Regional Hospital, Ellenville, NY, p. A425
BRIGGS, Gary, Director Human Resources, Southern Hills Medical Center, Nashville, TN, p. A573
BRIGGS, Michael, M.D. Chief Medical Officer, Essentia Health Fargo, Fargo, ND, p. A465
BRIGGS, Paul
Executive Vice President and Chief Financial Officer, Presbyterian Hospital, Albuquerque, NM, p. A414
Executive VP/Chief Operating Officer, Presbyterian Kaseman Hospital, Albuquerque, NM, p. A414
BRIGGS, Ronald O., FACHE President and Chief Executive Officer, St. Francis Memorial Hospital, West Point, NE, p. A390
BRIGGS, Thomas, Chief Financial Officer, Integris Marshall County Medical Center, Madill, OK, p. A498
BRIGHAM, Randy, Chief Human Resource Officer, Sterling Regional MedCenter, Sterling, CO, p. A106
BRIGHT, Cheryl, Executive Director, Lanterman Developmental Center, Pomona, CA, p. A80
BRIGHT, John, Director, Veterans Affairs Southern Nevada Healthcare System, North Las Vegas, NV, p. A394

A770 Index of Health Care Professionals

Index of Health Care Professionals / Broughman

BRIGHT, Tony, M.D. Administrator Medical Services, Caswell Center, Kinston, NC, p. A456
BRILEY, Ellen C., Administrator and Chief Executive Officer, Elba General Hospital, Elba, AL, p. A19
BRILEY, Jana, Director Financial Services, Murray Medical Center, Chatsworth, GA, p. A149
BRILEY, Jay, Chief Executive Officer, Vidant Duplin Hospital, Kenansville, NC, p. A456
BRILL, Beth K., Director Human Resources, Barnesville Hospital, Barnesville, OH, p. A470
BRILLANTES, Dorothy, Senior Vice President Human Resources, Howard County General Hospital, Columbia, MD, p. A290
BRILLI, Richard, M.D. Chief Medical Officer, Nationwide Children's Hospital, Columbus, OH, p. A477
BRILLIANT, Patrick D., President and Chief Executive Officer, Riverside Community Hospital, Riverside, CA, p. A83
BRILLIANT, Steven, M.D. Chief of Staff, Veterans Affairs Sierra Nevada Health Care System, Reno, NV, p. A395
BRINDLE, Charles B., M.D. Chief Medical Staff, Iowa Specialty Hospital–Belmond, Belmond, IA, p. A214
BRINGLE, Dottie, R.N. Chief Operating Officer and Chief Nursing Officer, Mercy Hospital Joplin, Joplin, MO, p. A361
BRINK, Greg, Chief Financial Officer, Surgical Specialty Hospital of Arizona, Phoenix, AZ, p. A37
BRINKERHOFF, Cindy H., Director Human Resources, South Peninsula Hospital, Homer, AK, p. A29
BRINKHAUS, Theresa, Chief Financial Officer and Compliance, Sage Rehabilitation Hospital, Baton Rouge, LA, p. A263
BRINKLEY, Terry, Vice President Finance, Paris Community Hospital, Paris, IL, p. A190
BRINKMAN, Dan, Chief Nurse Executive, Hilo Medical Center, Hilo, HI, p. A163
BRINKMAN, Janet, Director Human Resources, Colorado Plains Medical Center, Fort Morgan, CO, p. A101
BRINKMAN, Jim, Chief Financial Officer, Clay County Medical Center, Clay Center, KS, p. A231
BRINKMAN, Larry, Chief Human Resources, Veterans Affairs Medical Center, Miami, FL, p. A132
BRINSON, David, Director Information Technology, Wabash County Hospital, Wabash, IN, p. A213
BRIONES, Melba, M.D. Medical Director, Evansville State Hospital, Evansville, IN, p. A201
BRISBOE, Mark
Vice President & CFO, Sparrow Clinton Hospital, Saint Johns, MI, p. A322
Vice President and Chief Financial Officer, Sparrow Ionia Hospital, Ionia, MI, p. A315
BRISCOE, Betsy, Chief Executive Officer, Memorial Hospital, Seminole, TX, p. A627
BRISCOE, Charles, Chief Executive Officer, Coliseum Medical Centers, Macon, GA, p. A155
BRISCOE, Mary Beth, Chief Financial Officer, University of Alabama Hospital, Birmingham, AL, p. A17
BRISENDINE, Chad
Vice President and Chief Information Officer, St. Luke's Hospital – Miners Campus, Coaldale, PA, p. A520
Chief Information Officer, St. Luke's Hospital – Quakertown Campus, Quakertown, PA, p. A536
Chief Information Officer, St. Luke's University Hospital – Bethlehem Campus, Bethlehem, PA, p. A518
BRISTER, Kim, Director Human Resources, Gettysburg Hospital, Gettysburg, PA, p. A524
BRISTO, Cathie, Director Human Resources, Wilbarger General Hospital, Vernon, TX, p. A633
BRISTOL, Michelle, Director of Nursing, Clifton–Fine Hospital, Star Lake, NY, p. A443
BRISTOLL, Holly L., President, ProMedica Bay Park Hospital, Oregon, OH, p. A486
BRITT, Key, Associate Director, Greenwood Leflore Hospital, Greenwood, MS, p. A346
BRITT, Linda, Director Information Systems, Baptist Memorial Hospital–North Mississippi, Oxford, MS, p. A351
BRITT, Suzanne, Director Human Resources, Samaritan Memorial Hospital, Macon, MO, p. A364
BRITT, Tommy, Director Human Resources, West Georgia Health, La Grange, GA, p. A155
BRITTAIN, James G., Chief Financial Officer, Mid–Valley Hospital, Peckville, PA, p. A531
BRITTEN, Gary L., Chief Financial Officer, Stone County Medical Center, Mountain View, AR, p. A49
BRITTON, Gregory K., President and Chief Executive Officer, Beloit Health System, Beloit, WI, p. A679
BRITTON, John, Director Information Services, Fisher–Titus Medical Center, Norwalk, OH, p. A486
BRITTON, Lynn, President and Chief Executive Officer, Mercy Health, Chesterfield, MO, p. B88
BRITTON, William N., Associate Administrator Finance, Alfred I. duPont Hospital for Children, Wilmington, DE, p. A114
BRIZZEE, Celeste, Chief Nursing Officer, Connally Medical Center, Floresville, TX, p. A597
BROADDUS, Jackie, Business Partner, Taylorville Memorial Hospital, Taylorville, IL, p. A195
BROADHEAD, Susie, Director Public Information, East Mississippi State Hospital, Meridian, MS, p. A350
BROADHURST, Laura, R.N. Chief Executive Officer, Greater Baton Rouge Surgical Hospital, Baton Rouge, LA, p. A262
BROADUS, Ronald, Assistant Administrator Human Resources, Interim LSU Public Hospital, New Orleans, LA, p. A274
BROADWATER, Gary W., Chief Financial Officer, McCready Health Services Foundation, Crisfield, MD, p. A290
BROBERG, John R., FACHE President and Chief Executive Officer, Mercy Regional Health Center,, KS, p. A238
BROBST, Charles R., Senior Vice President and Chief Financial Officer, Saint Anthony Hospital, Chicago, IL, p. A178
BROBST, Mary, R.N. Vice President of Nursing, SSM St. Clare Health Center, Fenton, MO, p. A359
BROCCOLINO, Victor A., President and Chief Executive Officer, Howard County General Hospital, Columbia, MD, p. A290
BROCK, Berna, Vice President Human Resources, Pike Community Hospital, Waverly, OH, p. A491
BROCK, Jamie, Director Human Resources, Windber Medical Center, Windber, PA, p. A542
BROCK, Lisa, Vice President Human Resources, Overlake Hospital Medical Center, Bellevue, WA, p. A659
BROCK, Nancy, Chief Financial Officer, CHRISTUS St. Catherine Hospital, Katy, TX, p. A610
BROCK, Robert
Vice President Finance and Business Development, Saint Joseph – London, London, KY, p. A254
Vice President Finance, Saint Joseph – Martin, Martin, KY, p. A256
BROCK, Steve, Chief Financial Officer, Medical Arts Hospital, Lamesa, TX, p. A611
BROCK, Sue, Chief Financial Officer, Indiana University Health Paoli Hospital, Paoli, IN, p. A210
BROCK, Theresa, Vice President Nursing, Good Shepherd Health Care System, Hermiston, OR, p. A511
BROCK, William, Chief Information Officer, Veterans Affairs Medical Center, Decatur, GA, p. A151
BROCKETTE, Darby, Chief Executive Officer, Ernest Health, Inc., Albuquerque, NM, p. B50
BROCKMEYER, JoEllyn, Director Human Resources, Indiana University Health White Memorial Hospital, Monticello, IN, p. A208
BROCKUS, Harry, Chief Executive Officer, Hoopeston Regional Health Center, Hoopeston, IL, p. A185
BROCKWELL, Linda, R.N. Chief Nursing Officer, Wickenburg Community Hospital, Wickenburg, AZ, p. A41
BRODALE, Sean, D.O. Chief Medical Staff, Davis County Hospital, Bloomfield, IA, p. A215
BRODBECK, Lisa, Chief Financial Officer, Medical Center of Lewisville, Lewisville, TX, p. A612
BRODEUR, Mark S., FACHE Chief Executive Officer, HEALTHSOUTH Rehabilitation Hospital at Drake, Cincinnati, OH, p. A473
BRODHEAD, Ross, Human Resource Assistant, St. Vincent Randolph Hospital, Winchester, IN, p. A213
BRODIAN, Craig, Vice President Human Resources, Johns Hopkins Bayview Medical Center, Baltimore, MD, p. A287
BRODY, Robert J., President and Chief Executive Officer, Franciscan St. Francis Health – Indianapolis, Indianapolis, IN, p. A204
BRODY, Sue G., President and Chief Executive Officer, Bayfront Medical Center, Saint Petersburg, FL, p. A138
BROEKHUIS, Arlyn, Vice President and Chief Information Officer, Sanford University of South Dakota Medical Center, Sioux Falls, SD, p. A559
BROEMELING, Richard, Information Systems Flight Commander, U. S. Air Force Clinic, Mountain Home AFB, ID, p. A169
BROERMANN, Robert
Senior Vice President and Chief Financial Officer, Sentara Leigh Hospital, Norfolk, VA, p. A652
Senior Vice President and Chief Financial Officer, Sentara Norfolk General Hospital, Norfolk, VA, p. A653
Senior Vice President and Chief Financial Officer, Sentara Princess Anne Hospital, Virginia Beach, VA, p. A657
BROFMAN, John, M.D. Medical Director, R M L Specialty Hospital, Hinsdale, IL, p. A184
BROHM, Michael, President and Chief Executive Officer, Solara Healthcare, Dallas, TX, p. B119
BROKKE, James, M.D. Chief of Staff, Audubon County Memorial Hospital, Audubon, IA, p. A214
BROMAN, Craig J., FACHE President, St. Cloud Hospital, St. Cloud Hospital, Saint Cloud, MN, p. A338
BROMLEY, Trudy, Vice President Human Resources, J. F. K. Medical Center, Atlantis, FL, p. A118
BRONER, Eloise, President and Chief Executive Officer, Good Samaritan Hospital, Dayton, OH, p. A478
BROOKE, William R., M.D. President Medical Staff, Pickens County Medical Center, Carrollton, AL, p. A18
BROOKER, Brian, Chief Executive Officer, Cypress Creek Hospital, Houston, TX, p. A604
BROOKER, Paula, Director Information Services, Pleasant Valley Hospital, Point Pleasant, WV, p. A675
BROOKES, Jeffrey, M.D
Chief Medical Officer, Parkview LaGrange Hospital, LaGrange, IN, p. A207
Medical Director, Parkview Whitley Hospital, Columbia City, IN, p. A199
BROOKHOUSER, Patrick E., M.D. Director and Chief Medical Officer, Boys Town National Research Hospital, Omaha, NE, p. A387
BROOKMAN, Mark, Director Information Technology, Hardin Memorial Hospital, Elizabethtown, KY, p. A249
BROOKS, Albert, M.D. Chief Medical Staff Services, Washington Hospital Healthcare System, Fremont, CA, p. A61
BROOKS, Christopher
Vice President Finance, Bay Medical Center, Panama City, FL, p. A135
Chief Executive Officer, Port St. Lucie Hospital, Port St. Lucie, FL, p. A137
BROOKS, David, Chief Executive Officer, Providence Regional Medical Center Everett, Everett, WA, p. A661
BROOKS, Harris W., Administrator and Chief Executive Officer, Palo Pinto General Hospital, Mineral Wells, TX, p. A617
BROOKS III, J. Milton, Administrator, Pineville Community Hospital Association, Pineville, KY, p. A258
BROOKS, Janet, R.N. Vice President and Chief Nursing Officer, West Hills Hospital and Medical Center,, CA, p. A72
BROOKS, Jerome M., Chief Executive Officer, Connally Medical Center, Floresville, TX, p. A597
BROOKS, Karen, M.D. Medical Director, Cedar Crest Hospital, Belton, TX, p. A584
BROOKS, Kathleen, Director Human Resources, Brattleboro Retreat, Brattleboro, VT, p. A643
BROOKS, Lisa, Chief Financial Officer, Comanche County Hospital, Coldwater, KS, p. A231
BROOKS, Lori, Director Human Resources, Red Bud Regional Hospital, Red Bud, IL, p. A192
BROOKS, Patrice Gay, Chief Executive Officer, Cumberland Hospital, New Kent, VA, p. A651
BROOKS, Patti, Director Information Systems, Avera Queen of Peace Hospital, Mitchell, SD, p. A558
BROOKS, Robert L., M.D. Vice President Medical Affairs, Meritus Medical Center, Hagerstown, MD, p. A292
BROOKS, Scott, Manager Information Technology, Boulder City Hospital, Boulder City, NV, p. A391
BROOKS, Steven, Vice President Human Resources, McAlester Regional Health Center, McAlester, OK, p. A499
BROOKS, Troy, Assistant Administrator Fiscal Services, Newton Medical Center, Covington, GA, p. A150
BROOKS–WILLIAMS, Denise, President and Chief Executive Officer, Bronson Battle Creek, Battle Creek, MI, p. A308
BROOKSBY, Nolan, M.D. Chief of Staff, Ashley Regional Medical Center, Vernal, UT, p. A642
BROOKSHIRE, Lynn
Vice President Information Services and Chief Information Officer, CAMC Teays Valley Hospital, Hurricane, WV, p. A673
Vice President Information Services and Chief Information Officer, Charleston Area Medical Center, Charleston, WV, p. A671
BROOS, Timothy W., Vice President and Chief Information Officer, Katherine Shaw Bethea Hospital, Dixon, IL, p. A180
BROPHY, Beth, Interim VP for Human Resources, Hurley Medical Center, Flint, MI, p. A312
BROSIUS, William, Vice President and Chief Financial Officer, St. Luke's Episcopal Hospital, Houston, TX, p. A606
BROSNAN, Kimberly, Director Human Resources, Norwood Hospital, Norwood, MA, p. A303
BROSS, Mary Ann, Vice President Human Resources, Somerset Medical Center, Somerville, NJ, p. A410
BROST, Michelle, Financial Officer, Southwest Surgical Hospital, Hurst, TX, p. A608
BROTEN, Kurt, Chief Financial Officer, Palmdale Regional Medical Center, Palmdale, CA, p. A79
BROTHMAN, Daniel, Chief Executive Officer, Western Medical Center–Santa Ana, Santa Ana, CA, p. A89
BROTHMAN, Joe, Vice President Information Systems, Medstar Washington Hospital Center, Washington, DC, p. A116
BROUGH, Ken, Chief Financial Officer, Star Valley Medical Center, Afton, WY, p. A695
BROUGHMAN, Wade
Executive Vice President and Chief Financial Officer, Riverside Regional Medical Center, Newport News, VA, p. A652
Executive Vice President and Chief Financial Officer, Riverside Rehabilitation Institute, Newport News, VA, p. A652
Chief Financial Officer, Riverside Shore Memorial Hospital, Nassawadox, VA, p. A651

Index of Health Care Professionals

Index of Health Care Professionals

Index of Health Care Professionals / Brouillette


BROUILLETTE, Cindy
Chief Financial Officer, St. David's Medical Center, Austin, TX, p. A581
Chief Financial Officer, St. David's Rehabilitation Center, Austin, TX, p. A581
BROUSSARD, Clifford M., FACHE Administrator, WK Bossier Health Center, Bossier City, LA, p. A264
BROUSSARD, Tammy, Chief Financial Officer, West Calcasieu Cameron Hospital, Sulphur, LA, p. A278
BROUWER, Heath, Administrator, Douglas County Memorial Hospital, Armour, SD, p. A555
BROWER, Fred B., President and Chief Executive Officer, Trinity Health System, Steubenville, OH, p. A489
BROWN, Allen, M.D. Vice President Medical Affairs, Ochsner Baptist Medical Center, New Orleans, LA, p. A274
BROWN, Andy, M.D. Vice President Medical Affairs, Middle Tennessee Medical Center, Murfreesboro, TN, p. A573
BROWN, Ann, Director, Veterans Affairs Medical Center, Martinsburg, WV, p. A673
BROWN, B. Blaine, Vice President and General Counsel, Prattville Baptist Hospital, Prattville, AL, p. A25
BROWN, Barbara, D.O. Chief of Staff, Osborne County Memorial Hospital, Osborne, KS, p. A240
BROWN, Beth, Director, Louis A. Johnson Veterans Affairs Medical Center, Clarksburg, WV, p. A671
BROWN, Bill, Vice President Human Resources, North Hawaii Community Hospital, Kamuela, HI, p. A164
BROWN, Bob, Director Human Resources, The Children's Institute of Pittsburgh, Pittsburgh, PA, p. A535
BROWN, Chad, M.P.H. Chief Executive Officer, Person Memorial Hospital, Roxboro, NC, p. A460
BROWN, Cheryl, Administrator, Henderson Health Care Services, Henderson, NE, p. A384
BROWN, Christi, Director Human Resources, LSU Bogalusa Medical Center, Bogalusa, LA, p. A263
BROWN, Crystal, M.D. Medical Director, Peach Regional Medical Center, Fort Valley, GA, p. A153
BROWN, David P., Administrator, Citizens Medical Center, Victoria, TX, p. A633
BROWN, Deana, Director Administrative Services, Jasper County Hospital, Rensselaer, IN, p. A211
BROWN, Debra L., Area Financial Officer, Manteca Medical Center, Manteca, CA, p. A74
BROWN, Denise, Vice President Human Resources, Saint Joseph Hospital, Chicago, IL, p. A178
BROWN, Derek, Chief Information Officer, Jellico Community Hospital, Jellico, TN, p. A567
BROWN, Donald L., Director Human Resources, Western Baptist Hospital, Paducah, KY, p. A257
BROWN, Ed
Chief Financial Officer, Effingham Hospital, Springfield, GA, p. A159
Senior Vice President and Chief Information Officer, Gwinnett Hospital System, Lawrenceville, GA, p. A155
BROWN, Eric, Senior Business Partner, Shady Grove Adventist Hospital, Rockville, MD, p. A294
BROWN, Frank, M.D. Chief Medical Officer, Wesley Woods Geriatric Hospital of Emory University, Atlanta, GA, p. A146
BROWN, Geoffrey
Senior Vice President Information Services, Inova Alexandria Hospital, Alexandria, VA, p. A645
Chief Information Officer, Inova Fair Oaks Hospital, Fairfax, VA, p. A647
Vice President Information Systems, Inova Fairfax Hospital, Falls Church, VA, p. A647
BROWN, George J., M.D. President and Chief Executive Officer, Legacy Health, Portland, OR, p. B79
BROWN, Gordon, Chief Information Resources Management, Veterans Affairs Edward Hines, Jr. Hospital, Hines, IL, p. A184
BROWN, Henry
Director Plant Operations and Information Technology, Schick Shadel Hospital, Seattle, WA, p. A666
Chief Financial Officer, Westchester General Hospital, Miami, FL, p. A132
BROWN, James, M.D. President, Tyler County Hospital, Woodville, TX, p. A636
BROWN, James H., Chief Financial Officer, Centerpoint Medical Center, Independence, MO, p. A360
BROWN, James T., M.D. President of Medical Staff, Mason District Hospital, Havana, IL, p. A183
BROWN, Janice, Chief Financial Officer, Coosa Valley Medical Center, Sylacauga, AL, p. A25
BROWN, Jay, Vice President and Chief Information Officer, University Hospital, Cincinnati, OH, p. A474
BROWN, Jeff, Interim Director Information Systems, Simi Valley Hospital and Health Care Services, Simi Valley, CA, p. A91
BROWN, Jeffrey L., Director Information Systems, Lawrence General Hospital, Lawrence, MA, p. A301
BROWN, Jenny, Director Human Resources and Public Relations, Vidant Pungo Hospital, Belhaven, NC, p. A448
BROWN, Jill, Chief Financial Officer, Miller County Hospital, Colquitt, GA, p. A149
BROWN, Jim, Chief Executive Officer, Memorial Hermann Sugar Land Hospital, Sugar Land, TX, p. A629
BROWN, John D., Director Information Systems, Pacific Alliance Medical Center, Los Angeles, CA, p. A71
BROWN, Joni, Director Human Resources, Rehabilitation Hospital of Indiana, Indianapolis, IN, p. A205
BROWN, Joseph, M.D. Chief Medical Staff, Alta Vista Regional Hospital, Las Vegas, NM, p. A417
BROWN, Julie, Human Resources Specialist, Alegent Health–Community Memorial Hospital, Missouri Valley, IA, p. A223
BROWN, Karen, Director Health Information, Community Medical Center, Falls City, NE, p. A383
BROWN, Karen C., Vice President Strategic Human Resources, OSF Saint Anthony Medical Center, Rockford, IL, p. A192
BROWN, Karla, Interim Chief Nursing Officer, Pauls Valley General Hospital, Pauls Valley, OK, p. A503
BROWN, Ken, Vice President and Chief Human Resource Officer, Pratt Regional Medical Center, Pratt, KS, p. A242
BROWN, Kenneth, M.D. Medical Director, Woman's Hospital, Baton Rouge, LA, p. A263
BROWN, Kevin, Chief Executive, Swedish Health Services, Seattle, WA, p. B126
BROWN, Kevin F., D.O. Medical Director, Wesley Rehabilitation Hospital, Wichita, KS, p. A246
BROWN, Kimberly, Human Resources Recruiter Generalist, INTEGRIS Canadian Valley Hospital, Yukon, OK, p. A508
BROWN, Kris, Associate Director, Veterans Affairs Medical Center, Bay Pines, FL, p. A118
BROWN, Larry, Chief Financial Officer, Lucas County Health Center, Chariton, IA, p. A216
BROWN, Laura, Chief Financial Officer, Laurel Ridge Treatment Center, San Antonio, TX, p. A625
BROWN, Linda, M.D. Chief of Staff, Island Hospital, Anacortes, WA, p. A659
BROWN, Linda, Chief Information Officer, Olympic Medical Center, Port Angeles, WA, p. A664
BROWN, Linda E., Vice President of Support Services, St. Anthony Shawnee Hospital, Shawnee, OK, p. A504
BROWN, Lori J., MSN Senior Vice President and Chief Nursing Officer, Arkansas Children's Hospital, Little Rock, AR, p. A47
BROWN, Marci, Director Information Technology, Blue Mountain Hospital, John Day, OR, p. A511
BROWN, Margaret, Director Medical Records, Vista Health, Fayetteville, AR, p. A44
BROWN, Markham, M.D. Chief Medical Staff, Mike O'Callaghan Federal Hospital, Nellis AFB, NV, p. A394
BROWN, Martin, Vice President Information Services and Chief Information Officer, Nathan Littauer Hospital and Nursing Home, Gloversville, NY, p. A426
BROWN, Mary, Chief Nursing Officer, UMass Memorial–Marlborough Hospital, Marlborough, MA, p. A302
BROWN, Mary Beth, Director Human Resources, Bertrand Chaffee Hospital, Springville, NY, p. A443
BROWN, Mary W., Senior Vice President Operations, St. Joseph's Hospital Health Center, Syracuse, NY, p. A444
BROWN, Michael, Senior Vice President Finance and Chief Financial Officer, Children's Hospital and Medical Center, Omaha, NE, p. A387
BROWN, Michael, D.O. Chief of Staff, Red River Regional Hospital, Bonham, TX, p. A584
BROWN, Michael J., Chief Financial Officer, Fairfield Memorial Hospital, Fairfield, IL, p. A182
BROWN, Michael L.
President and Chief Executive Officer, Provena Covenant Medical Center, Urbana, IL, p. A195
President and Chief Executive Officer, Provena United Samaritans Medical Center, Danville, IL, p. A179
BROWN, Mike, IT Manager, Highlands–Cashiers Hospital, Highlands, NC, p. A455
BROWN, Pat, R.N. Chief Nursing Officer, San Gorgonio Memorial Hospital, Banning, CA, p. A55
BROWN, Patsy, Site Coordinator Human Resources, Erlanger Bledsoe Hospital, Pikeville, TN, p. A574
BROWN, Patti, M.D. Medical Director, HEALTHSOUTH Reading Rehabilitation Hospital, Reading, PA, p. A537
BROWN, Paula, Senior Vice President Corporate Finance, Sentara Northern Virginia Medical Center, Woodbridge, VA, p. A657
BROWN, Paulette, Chief Operating Officer, Indiana University Health Goshen Hospital, Goshen, IN, p. A202
BROWN, Penny, Human Resource Representative, Broaddus Hospital, Philippi, WV, p. A674
BROWN, Philip, D.O. Vice President Medical Affairs, Central Vermont Medical Center, Berlin, VT, p. A643
BROWN, Phyllis, Chief Executive Officer, Marshall Medical Center, Lewisburg, TN, p. A569
BROWN, Randal, M.D. Chief of Staff, Guadalupe County Hospital, Santa Rosa, NM, p. A418
BROWN, Regenia, Vice President Human Resources, Magnolia Regional Health Center, Corinth, MS, p. A345
BROWN, Rex H., Chief Executive Officer, Hillsboro Area Hospital, Hillsboro, IL, p. A184
BROWN, Rickie F., Chief Financial Officer, Monroe County Medical Center, Tompkinsville, KY, p. A259
BROWN, Rita, Director Human Resources, Richardson Medical Center, Rayville, LA, p. A276
BROWN, Robin
Senior Vice President and Chief Executive, Scripps Green Hospital, La Jolla, CA, p. A65
Chief Information Officer and Compliance Officer, St. Joseph Medical Center, Houston, TX, p. A606
BROWN, Rodger, Vice President Human Resources, North Mississippi Medical Center – Tupelo, Tupelo, MS, p. A353
BROWN, Rodney, Chief Executive Officer, Landmark Hospital, Cape Girardeau, MO, p. A356
BROWN, Samuel L., CPA Vice President Financial Services, Jennie Stuart Medical Center, Hopkinsville, KY, p. A251
BROWN, Scott, Interim Chief Executive Officer, Valir Rehabilitation Hospital, Oklahoma City, OK, p. A502
BROWN, Sharon
Director Human Resources, Sierra View District Hospital, Porterville, CA, p. A81
Deputy Commander Nursing, Winn Army Community Hospital, Hinesville, GA, p. A154
BROWN, Shelia, Director Human Resources, LTAC Hospital of Greenwood, Greenwood, MS, p. A346
BROWN, Sherri, Director Human Resources, Lawrence Memorial Hospital, Walnut Ridge, AR, p. A52
BROWN, Sherry
Director Information Services, Chelsea Community Hospital, Chelsea, MI, p. A309
Director Human Resources, Cleveland Area Hospital, Cleveland, OK, p. A495
BROWN, Stephen, M.D. Chief Medical Officer, St. Mary–Corwin Medical Center, Pueblo, CO, p. A105
BROWN, Stephen A., Chief Financial Officer, Grace Cottage Hospital, Townshend, VT, p. A644
BROWN, Steve, M.D. Chief Quality Officer, Saint Alphonsus Regional Medical Center, Boise, ID, p. A166
BROWN, Steve
Director Information Systems, Spalding Regional Medical Center, Griffin, GA, p. A153
Chief Information Officer, Sylvan Grove Hospital, Jackson, GA, p. A154
BROWN, Steven, Vice President Finance, OhioHealth Marion General Hospital, Marion, OH, p. A484
BROWN, Steven, M.D. Medical Director, Wyoming Behavioral Institute, Casper, WY, p. A695
BROWN, Steven E., FACHE President and Chief Executive Officer, Mount Nittany Medical Center, State College, PA, p. A539
BROWN, Steven J., Senior Vice President and Chief Operating Officer, Faxton–St. Luke's Healthcare, Utica, NY, p. A445
BROWN, Sue, Administrator Human Resources, South Lake Hospital, Clermont, FL, p. A120
BROWN, Susan, R.N. Sr. Vice President, Chief Nursing Officer, Grace Hospital, Morganton, NC, p. A458
BROWN, Susan, Chief Human Resources Officer, North Fulton Regional Hospital, Roswell, GA, p. A158
BROWN, Susan, R.N. Sr. Vice President, Chief Nursing Officer, Valdese General Hospital, Valdese, NC, p. A462
BROWN, Terrence E., Chief Executive Officer, HEALTHSOUTH Lakeshore Rehabilitation Hospital, Birmingham, AL, p. A16
BROWN, Theodore, Chief Operating Officer, Community Howard Regional Hospital, Kokomo, IN, p. A206
BROWN, Tim S., Chief Executive Officer, Claiborne County Hospital, Tazewell, TN, p. A576
BROWN, Todd A., M.D. Medical Director, Logan Regional Hospital, Logan, UT, p. A638
BROWN, Tom, Senior Vice President, Nanticoke Memorial Hospital, Seaford, DE, p. A114
BROWN, Towanda, Director Standards and Regulatory Compliance, Cumberland Hospital, New Kent, VA, p. A651
BROWN, Trisha, Manager Human Resources, Community Memorial Hospital, Oconto Falls, WI, p. A688
BROWN, Wendy W., M.D. Chief of Staff, Jesse Brown Veterans Affairs Chicago Health Care System, Chicago, IL, p. A176
BROWN, William A., FACHE Chief Executive Officer, Westlake Hospital, Melrose Park, IL, p. A187
BROWN, Winfield S., President and Chief Executive Officer, Heywood Hospital, Gardner, MA, p. A300
BROWN–OLDS, Connie A., R.N. Chief Nursing Officer, Mary Free Bed Rehabilitation Hospital, Grand Rapids, MI, p. A313


**A772** Index of Health Care Professionals

Index of Health Care Professionals / Buck

Index of Health Care Professionals

BROWNE, Fred, M.D. Chief Medical Officer and Vice President Medical Affairs, New Milford Hospital, New Milford, CT, p. A111
BROWNE, J. Timothy, FACHE Chief Executive Officer, Carolina Pines Regional Medical Center, Hartsville, SC, p. A551
BROWNE, John, Assistant Administrator Finance, Kindred Hospital–Brea, Brea, CA, p. A56
BROWNER, Warren S., M.P.H
Chief Executive Officer, California Pacific Medical Center, San Francisco, CA, p. A86
Chief Executive Officer, St. Luke's Hospital, San Francisco, CA, p. A87
BROWNING, Douglas, Chief Financial Officer, Texas Health Center for Diagnostic & Surgery, Plano, TX, p. A621
BROWNING, Michael, Chief Financial Officer, Madison County Hospital, London, OH, p. A483
BROWNING, Michael P., Chief Financial Officer, Parkview Noble Hospital, Kendallville, IN, p. A206
BROWNLEE, Ernest, M.D. Medical Director, Millwood Hospital, Arlington, TX, p. A579
BROWNLOW, William R., Senior Vice President Finance, Silver Cross Hospital, New Lenox, IL, p. A189
BROWNSTEIN, Gregory, Chief Executive Officer, Westwood Lodge Hospital, Westwood, MA, p. A306
BROYLES, Susan, Director Human Resources and Safety, Unicoi County Memorial Hospital, Erwin, TN, p. A565
BRUCE, Bill, FACHE Chief Executive Officer, Crawford County Memorial Hospital, Denison, IA, p. A218
BRUCE, Glenda, Director Community Relations, Rusk State Hospital, Rusk, TX, p. A623
BRUCE, Michael D., Chief Executive Officer, Lake Martin Community Hospital, Dadeville, AL, p. A18
BRUCE, Mike, Chief Financial Officer, Elmore Community Hospital, Wetumpka, AL, p. A27
BRUCE, Sandra B., FACHE President and Chief Executive Officer, Presence Health, Chicago, IL, p. B103
BRUCE, Scott, Vice President Operations, St. Mary's Healthcare, Amsterdam, NY, p. A420
BRUCE, Sheila, Director Information System, Regional Medical Center of Hopkins County, Madisonville, KY, p. A255
BRUCHHOF, Lynn
Vice President Human Resources, MidMichigan Medical Center–Clare, Clare, MI, p. A309
Vice President, MidMichigan Medical Center–Gladwin, Gladwin, MI, p. A313
Vice President, MidMichigan Medical Center–Midland, Midland, MI, p. A319
BRUDNICKI, Gary F., Senior Executive Vice President, Chief Operating Officer and Chief Financial Officer, Westchester Medical Center, Valhalla, NY, p. A445
BRUEGGEMAN, Mary Jo, R.N. Vice President Patient Care, Fairview Lakes Health Services, Wyoming, MN, p. A342
BRUFF, Edward, Executive Vice President and Chief Operating Officer, Covenant Medical Center, Saginaw, MI, p. A322
BRUGGEMAN, Chris, Chief Information Officer, RiverView Health, Crookston, MN, p. A330
BRUGGER, John, Director Information Systems, Gifford Medical Center, Randolph, VT, p. A644
BRUHL, Lisa G., Chief Operating Officer, Lallie Kemp Medical Center, Independence, LA, p. A268
BRUHN, Julie, R.N. Associate Director Patient Care and Nurse Executive, Veterans Affairs Health Care System, Fargo, ND, p. A466
BRUI, Thomas M., Director Resource Management, Naval Hospital, Lemoore, CA, p. A67
BRUMBAUGH, David
Vice President Human Resources, Children's Hospitals and Clinics of Minnesota, Minneapolis, MN, p. A335
Vice President Human Resources, Children's Hospitals and Clinics of Minnesota, Saint Paul, MN, p. A339
BRUMFIELD, Cynthia, M.D. Chief of Staff, University of Alabama Hospital, Birmingham, AL, p. A17
BRUMMETT, Vince, Director Administrative Services, Tri–Lakes Medical Center, Batesville, MS, p. A343
BRUMMUND, Calvin J., Interim Chief Financial Officer, Neshoba County General Hospital, Philadelphia, MS, p. A351
BRUMSTED, John R., M.D. President and Chief Executive Officer, Fletcher Allen Health Care, Burlington, VT, p. A643
BRUNDISE, Cynthia, Vice President Human Resources, St. Anthony Hospital, Oklahoma City, OK, p. A502
BRUNELLE, Diane, MSN Vice President of Patient Care Services and Chief Nursing Officer, Noble Hospital, Westfield, MA, p. A306
BRUNER, Deborah, Chief Executive Officer, St. Vincent Dunn Hospital, Bedford, IN, p. A197
BRUNING, Gary, M.D. President Medical Staff, Avera Flandreau Hospital, Flandreau, SD, p. A556
BRUNKE, Renea
Vice President Human Resources, Chandler Regional Medical Center, Chandler, AZ, p. A31
Vice President Human Resources, Mercy Gilbert Medical Center, Gilbert, AZ, p. A32
BRUNNQUELL, Stephen, M.D. President Medical Staff, Englewood Hospital and Medical Center, Englewood, NJ, p. A404
BRUNNWORTH, Donald, Chief Financial Officer, Community Memorial Hospital, Staunton, IL, p. A194
BRUNO, Catherine, FACH
Chief Information Officer, Eastern Maine Medical Center, Bangor, ME, p. A281
Chief Information Officer, The Aroostook Medical Center, Presque Isle, ME, p. A285
BRUNO, Frank, Chief Executive Officer, Gracie Square Hospital, New York, NY, p. A432
BRUNO, John, Vice President Human Resources, St. Joseph's Regional Medical Center, Paterson, NJ, p. A408
BRUNO, Judy, R.N. Vice President, Clinical Operations, The Outer Banks Hospital, Nags Head, NC, p. A458
BRUNO, Yolanda, M.D. Medical Director, Coler–Goldwater Specialty Hospital and Nursing Facility, New York, NY, p. A432
BRUNS, Dennis R., Chief Executive Officer, River Oaks Hospital, Flowood, MS, p. A345
BRUNSMAN, William, M.D. Chief of Staff, Mercy Medical Center, Williston, ND, p. A468
BRUNSON, Brian, Chief Executive Officer, Crossroads Regional Hospital, Alexandria, LA, p. A261
BRUNSON, Pam, Director Human Resources, South Baldwin Regional Medical Center, Foley, AL, p. A20
BRUNT, C. Hal, M.D. Medical Director, Lakeside Behavioral Health System, Memphis, TN, p. A571
BRUNTLETT, Melissa, Chief Financial Officer, Magee General Hospital, Magee, MS, p. A349
BRUNTZ, Troy, Vice President Finance and Chief Financial Officer, Community Hospital, McCook, NE, p. A386
BRUS, Sarah, Director Human Resources, Ripon Medical Center, Ripon, WI, p. A690
BRUSKI, Gayle, R.N. Chief Nursing Officer, Alpena Regional Medical Center, Alpena, MI, p. A307
BRUSS, Jonathan R., President, Advocate Trinity Hospital, Chicago, IL, p. A175
BRUTON, Jeff, Director Human Resources, Fairview Park Hospital, Dublin, GA, p. A152
BRUTSCHEA, Christine, Chief Information Technology, Nazareth Hospital, Philadelphia, PA, p. A533
BRUUN, Edward, President and Chief Executive Officer, Sparrow Clinton Hospital, Saint Johns, MI, p. A322
BRVENIK, Richard A., FACHE President, Carteret General Hospital, Morehead City, NC, p. A457
BRYAN, Jay, President and Chief Executive Officer, Mercy Health Partners, Lakeshore Campus, Shelby, MI, p. A323
BRYAN, Kenneth E., President and Chief Executive Officer, Betsy Johnson Regional Hospital, Dunn, NC, p. A452
BRYAN, Linda, Vice President Human Resources, Plantation General Hospital, Plantation, FL, p. A136
BRYAN, Margaret, Administrator, Shriners Hospitals for Children, Northern California, Sacramento, CA, p. A84
BRYAN, Marilyn, Administrator, Roger Mills Memorial Hospital, Cheyenne, OK, p. A494
BRYAN, Mark, Chief Executive Officer, Delray Medical Center, Delray Beach, FL, p. A122
BRYAN, Steven, Chief Financial Officer, Kindred Hospital Sugar Land, Sugar Land, TX, p. A629
BRYAN–SMITH, Lissa, Chief Administrative Officer, Geisinger–Bloomsburg Hospital, Bloomsburg, PA, p. A519
BRYANT, Amy, Chief Financial Officer, Cornerstone Hospital of Southwest Louisiana, Sulphur, LA, p. A278
BRYANT, Dawn, Vice President Organizational Development, St. Joseph Medical Center, Kansas City, MO, p. A362
BRYANT, Dawn L.
Senior Vice President and Chief Human Resource Officer, Saint Francis Hospital and Medical Center, Hartford, CT, p. A109
Vice President Organizational Development, St. Joseph Medical Center, Kansas City, MO, p. A362
BRYANT, Gary, M.D. Chief of Staff, United Regional Medical Center, Manchester, TN, p. A570
BRYANT, Karen, Chief Support Services Officer, Prowers Medical Center, Lamar, CO, p. A103
BRYANT, Kim, Chief Executive Officer, Highlands Medical Center, Scottsboro, AL, p. A25
BRYANT, Lisa G., Director Human Resources, Cannon Memorial Hospital, Pickens, SC, p. A553
BRYANT, Mandy, Chief Information Officer, Twin Lakes Regional Medical Center, Leitchfield, KY, p. A252
BRYANT, Maureen A., FACHE President and Chief Executive Officer, Provena Mercy Medical Center, Aurora, IL, p. A172
BRYANT, Pam
Director Human Resources, Helen Keller Hospital, Sheffield, AL, p. A25
Director Human Resources, Red Bay Hospital, Red Bay, AL, p. A25
BRYANT, Ron, President and Chief Executive Officer, Noble Hospital, Westfield, MA, p. A306
BRYANT, Rusty, Director Information Technology, Drew Memorial Hospital, Monticello, AR, p. A49
BRYANT, Stephanie, Chief Financial Officer, Twin County Regional Hospital, Galax, VA, p. A649
BRYANT, Tracy, Coordinator Information Technology, Marcum and Wallace Memorial Hospital, Irvine, KY, p. A252
BRYANT, W. Michael, President and Chief Executive Officer, Centra Health, Inc., Lynchburg, VA, p. B30
BRYANT, W. Michael, President and Chief Executive Officer, Centra Lynchburg General Hospital, Lynchburg, VA, p. A650
BRYANT, William J., Chief Executive Officer, Kindred Hospital–Chattanooga, Chattanooga, TN, p. A563
BRYANT–MOBLEY, Phyllis, M.D. Director Medical Services, William S. Hall Psychiatric Institute, Columbia, SC, p. A548
BRYCE, Keith, Chief Financial Officer, Mt. Graham Regional Medical Center, Safford, AZ, p. A37
BRYDON, Paul, Chief Financial Officer, Tri–City Regional Medical Center, Hawaiian Gardens, CA, p. A64
BRYNER, Jennifer, Chief Nursing Officer, Petersburg Medical Center, Petersburg, AK, p. A30
BRYSON, Brent J., Chief Executive Officer, Intermountain Hospital, Boise, ID, p. A166
BRYSON, Kellie, Director Human Resources, The Hospital at Westlake Medical Center, Austin, TX, p. A582
BUBACZ, Joe, Chief Information Officer, Soldiers and Sailors Memorial Hospital, Wellsboro, PA, p. A540
BUBRIG, Destini, Director Health Information Management, Hardtner Medical Center, Olla, LA, p. A275
BUCCI, Annette, Senior Administrator Human Resources, Burke Rehabilitation Hospital, White Plains, NY, p. A447
BUCCI, Domenick, M.D. Medical Director, Aria Health, Philadelphia, PA, p. A531
BUCCOLO, Martin A., Ph.D. Chief Executive Officer, Four Winds Hospital, Katonah, NY, p. A428
BUCH, Naishadh, Director Pharmacy and Chief Operating Officer, Lompoc Valley Medical Center, Lompoc, CA, p. A67
BUCHANAN, Dennis, Vice President Human Resources, New York Methodist Hospital,, NY, p. A435
BUCHANAN, Donna, Director Nursing, Stroud Regional Medical Center, Stroud, OK, p. A505
BUCHANAN, Herbert, Senior Vice President and Chief Operating Officer, University of Maryland Medical Center, Baltimore, MD, p. A289
BUCHANAN, Kevin, Chief Information Officer, Wake Forest Baptist Health–Lexington Medical Center, Lexington, NC, p. A456
BUCHANAN, Richard, Interim Chief Executive Officer, Warm Springs Medical Center, Warm Springs, GA, p. A161
BUCHANAN, Robert, Chief Information Officer, Anna Jaques Hospital, Newburyport, MA, p. A302
BUCHANAN, Ron, Director Information Services, West Central Georgia Regional Hospital, Columbus, GA, p. A150
BUCHANAN, Toni, Chief Financial Officer, Unicoi County Memorial Hospital, Erwin, TN, p. A565
BUCHANAN, Tracy, Chief Executive Officer, CarePartners Health Services, Asheville, NC, p. A448
BUCHART, Phyllis, Chief Operating Officer, Marina Del Rey Hospital, Marina Del Rey, CA, p. A74
BUCHE, Daniel L., Chief Executive Officer, Brazosport Regional Health System, Lake Jackson, TX, p. A611
BUCHELE, Paula, Chief Human Resources, Veterans Affairs Medical Center, Bay Pines, FL, p. A118
BUCHERT, Charles, Director Human Resources, Women and Children's Hospital, Lake Charles, LA, p. A271
BUCHHEIT, Anne, Coordinator Mental Health Local Information Systems, Buffalo Psychiatric Center, Buffalo, NY, p. A422
BUCHHEIT, Joe, Chief Financial Officer, Our Lady of Bellefonte Hospital, Ashland, KY, p. A247
BUCHHOLZ, Kari, Director Health Information Management, Wishek Community Hospital and Clinics, Wishek, ND, p. A468
BUCHHOLZ, Troy, M.D. Chief Medical Staff, Community Memorial Hospital, Sumner, IA, p. A227
BUCIENSKI, Jennifer, Director Human Resources, Hayes Green Beach Memorial Hospital, Charlotte, MI, p. A309
BUCK, Catherine, Executive Vice President Operations, Froedtert Memorial Lutheran Hospital, Milwaukee, WI, p. A686
BUCK, Cheryl, Vice President Human Resources, Lake Region Healthcare Corporation, Fergus Falls, MN, p. A331
BUCK, Cindy D., Interim Chief Executive Officer, Rutherford Regional Medical Center, Rutherfordton, NC, p. A460
BUCK, Jack S., Chief Executive Officer, Henderson County Community Hospital, Lexington, TN, p. A569

BUCK, Jeffrey W., Interim Chief Executive Officer, Jefferson Regional Medical Center, Crystal City, MO, p. A358

BUCK, Linda K., Vice President Human Resources, Proctor Hospital, Peoria, IL, p. A191

BUCK, Phylis, Controller, HEALTHSOUTH Rehabilitation Hospital of Texarkana, Texarkana, TX, p. A631

BUCKHOY, Sandra, Chief Clinical Officer, Kindred Hospital Chicago–Northlake, Northlake, IL, p. A189

BUCKINGHAM, Deborah, R.N. Director Human Resources, Redington–Fairview General Hospital, Skowhegan, ME, p. A285

BUCKINGHAM, Maura, D.O. Chief of Staff, South Haven Health System, South Haven, MI, p. A323

BUCKLEY, John J., Chief Administrative Officer, Geisinger Wyoming Valley Medical Center, Wilkes Barre, PA, p. A541

BUCKLEY, Patrick, Vice President Human Resources, St. Elizabeth Medical Center, Utica, NY, p. A445

BUCKLEY, R. Michael, M.D. Executive Director, Pennsylvania Hospital, Philadelphia, PA, p. A533

BUCKNER, Daniel, Interim Chief Executive Officer, Heritage Medical Center, Shelbyville, TN, p. A575

BUCKNER Jr., James E., FACHE Administrator, Uvalde County Hospital Authority, Uvalde, TX, p. A632

BUCKNER, Terry, Chief Executive Officer, Eastern Oklahoma Medical Center, Poteau, OK, p. A503

BUCKWORTH, Albert Bennett, Director Human Resources, Primary Children's Medical Center, Salt Lake City, UT, p. A640

BUDD, Edward, President and Chief Executive Officer, Thorek Memorial Hospital, Chicago, IL, p. A178

BUDDA, Jeff, Chief Information Officer, Floyd Medical Center, Rome, GA, p. A158

BUDDE, Rex P., President and Chief Executive Officer, Southern Illinois Hospital Services, Carbondale, IL, p. B120

BUDIG, Aletha, R.N. Director of Nursing, Ellinwood District Hospital, Ellinwood, KS, p. A232

BUDIN, Kirsten, Director Human Resources, Northfield Hospital, Northfield, MN, p. A336

BUDINGER, David P., Associate Director, Hunter Holmes McGuire Veterans Affairs Medical Center, Richmond, VA, p. A655

BUDNICK, Michael J., FACHE Chief Operating Officer and Clinic Manager, Franklin Hospital District, Benton, IL, p. A173

BUDZINSKI, A. James, Vice President and Chief Financial Officer, WellStar Kennestone Hospital, Marietta, GA, p. A156

BUDZINSKI, William, Vice President Human Resources, Methodist Hospital of Southern California, Arcadia, CA, p. A54

BUDZINSKY, Chris, R.N. Vice President Nursing/CNO Alexian Brothers Acute Care Ministries, St. Alexius Medical Center, Hoffman Estates, IL, p. A185

BUELL, Jack, Director Information Services, Sutter Lakeside Hospital, Lakeport, CA, p. A66

BUELL, Lindsay, Chief Information Management Services, Veterans Affairs Medical Center, Oklahoma City, OK, p. A502

BUELT, Madeline, Vice President Operations, Seattle Cancer Care Alliance, Seattle, WA, p. A666

BUENVENIDA, Brenda, Facility Administrator, Hiram W. Davis Medical Center, Petersburg, VA, p. A653

BUER, Shane, Director Human Resources, Presbyterian–St. Luke's Medical Center, Denver, CO, p. A100

BUFFINGTON, John, Chief Operating Officer, San Juan Regional Medical Center, Farmington, NM, p. A416

BUGG, Robert, Chief Financial Officer, Broward Health North, Deerfield Beach, FL, p. A122

BUGNA, Eric, M.D. Chief of Staff, Eastern Plumas Health Care District, Portola, CA, p. A81

BUHEIS, Nidal, M.D. Chief of Staff, The Medical Center of Southeast Texas, Port Arthur, TX, p. A622

BUHL, Michael D., Senior Vice President and Chief Financial Officer, University of Wisconsin Hospital and Clinics, Madison, WI, p. A684

BUHLKE, Brian, M.D. Medical Director, Genoa Community Hospital, Genoa, NE, p. A384

BUHOWSKI, Richard, Chief Financial Officer, Helen Hayes Hospital, West Haverstraw, NY, p. A446

BUI, Kim, Director Human Resources, East Valley Hospital Medical Center, Glendora, CA, p. A63

BUIE, Rhonda, Chief Civilian Personnel, Wright Patterson Medical Center, Wright–Patterson AFB, OH, p. A492

BUIT, Timothy, Vice President of Finance and Chief Financial Officer, Bellevue Hospital, Bellevue, OH, p. A470

BUJAK, Joseph, M.D. Vice President Medical Affairs, Kootenai Medical Center, Coeur D'Alene, ID, p. A167

BUKHARI, Kim, Manager Human Resources, Oak Valley Hospital District, Oakdale, CA, p. A77

BUKOWSKI, Cathy
Regional Chief Financial Officer, Eagle River Memorial Hospital, Eagle River, WI, p. A680
Chief Financial Officer, Howard Young Medical Center, Woodruff, WI, p. A694
Regional Chief Financial Officer, Sacred Heart–St. Mary's Hospitals, Rhinelander, WI, p. A690

BULAU, Chris, Manager Information Technology, Sibley Medical Center, Arlington, MN, p. A327

BULEN, Susan, M.D. Medical Director, HEALTHSOUTH Rehabilitation Hospital of Southern Arizona, Tucson, AZ, p. A39

BULLARD, Brandon
Chief Financial Officer, Cushing Regional Hospital, Cushing, OK, p. A495
Chief Financial Officer, Henryetta Medical Center, Henryetta, OK, p. A497

BULLARD, Michael R., Chief Executive Officer, Doctor's Hospital – Tidwell, Houston, TX, p. A604

BULLARD, Patrick, Chief Financial Officer, Veterans Affairs Medical Center, Fayetteville, NC, p. A453

BULLARD, Timothy, M.D. Chief of Staff, Orlando Regional Medical Center, Orlando, FL, p. A134

BULLINGTON, Benjamin P., M.D. Chief of Staff, Pioneer Medical Center, Big Timber, MT, p. A373

BULLITT, Michael L., Chief Executive Officer, HEALTHSOUTH Rehabilitation Hospital–Wichita Falls, Wichita Falls, TX, p. A635

BULLOCH, Bill, Director Human Resources, Roosevelt Warm Springs Institute for Rehabilitation, Warm Springs, GA, p. A161

BULLOCK, David, Director Information Services, Northwest Medical Center, Tucson, AZ, p. A40

BULLOCK, Lance, M.D. Medical Director, St. James Behavioral Health Hospital, Gonzales, LA, p. A267

BULLOCK, Renee, Vice President Human Resources, Saint Joseph Berea, Berea, KY, p. A247

BULLOCK, Tracy, Director Management Information Systems, Southern Virginia Regional Medical Center, Emporia, VA, p. A647

BULMAN, Laurie, Director Human Resources, Winneshiek Medical Center, Decorah, IA, p. A218

BULTEMA, Janice K., MSN Senior Vice President Human Resources, University of Wisconsin Hospital and Clinics, Madison, WI, p. A684

BULUSU, Somayaji, Chief Information Officer, Marin General Hospital, Greenbrae, CA, p. A64

BUMAN, Karen, Chief Nurse Executive, Myrtue Medical Center, Harlan, IA, p. A220

BUMATAY, Susan C., R.N. Assistant Administrator, Sutter Delta Medical Center, Antioch, CA, p. A53

BUMGARDNER, Chuck, Director Information Systems, Southeast Georgia Health System Brunswick Campus, Brunswick, GA, p. A148

BUMGARNER, William J., President, Spencer Hospital, Spencer, IA, p. A227

BUMPUS, Joe, Director Information Technology, St. Elizabeth Hospital, Gonzales, LA, p. A267

BUNCH, David V., President, Jefferson Memorial Hospital, Jefferson City, TN, p. A567

BUNCH, Elicia, Chief Executive Officer, Centennial Peaks Hospital, Louisville, CO, p. A104

BUNCH, Jimm, President and Chief Executive Officer, Park Ridge Health, Hendersonville, NC, p. A454

BUNCH, Kim, Director Information Technology, Marshall Medical Center North, Guntersville, AL, p. A21

BUNCH, Mark, Director Finance, Othello Community Hospital, Othello, WA, p. A664

BUNCH, Mike, Executive Vice President, Chief Operating Officer and Chief Financial Officer, KershawHealth, Camden, SC, p. A546

BUND, Linda, Chief Information Officer and Director Education, Veterans Affairs Medical Center,, NY, p. A437

BUNDGARD, Susan, Vice President Human Resources, Saint Alphonsus Regional Medical Center, Boise, ID, p. A166

BUNDICK, Ida, Chief Financial Officer, Eastern Shore Hospital Center, Cambridge, MD, p. A290

BUNKER, Marla, Vice President of Operations, War Memorial Hospital, Sault Sainte Marie, MI, p. A323

BUNN, Barry, M.D. Chief of Staff, Vidant Edgecombe Hospital, Tarboro, NC, p. A461

BUNNER, Blake, Director Human Resources, HEALTHSOUTH Deaconess Rehabilitation Hospital, Evansville, IN, p. A201

BUNSELMEYER, Becky, Director Information Services, Memorial Hospital, Chester, IL, p. A175

BUNTING, Katherine, Chief Executive Officer, Fairfield Memorial Hospital, Fairfield, IL, p. A182

BUNTYN, Diane, MSN Vice President Patient Care Services, Southeast Alabama Medical Center, Dothan, AL, p. A19

BUNYARD, Steve, Chief Operating Officer, Dublin Methodist Hospital, Dublin, OH, p. A479

BUONGIORNO, Michael J.
Executive Vice President Finance and Chief Financial Officer, Bryn Mawr Hospital, Bryn Mawr, PA, p. A519
Vice President Finance and Treasurer, Bryn Mawr Rehabilitation Hospital, Malvern, PA, p. A528
Vice President Finance, Lankenau Medical Center, Wynnewood, PA, p. A542

BURASCO, Carmen, Director Human Resources, Siloam Springs Memorial Hospital, Siloam Springs, AR, p. A51

BURBANK, Jimmy, Chief Information Officer, U. S. Public Health Service Indian Hospital, Crownpoint, NM, p. A415

BURBULES, Kevin, Chief Information Officer, Civista Health, La Plata, MD, p. A292

BURCH, Eric, Chief Executive Officer, Lewis County General Hospital, Lowville, NY, p. A429

BURCH, Janel, Chief Financial Officer, Russell Regional Hospital, Russell, KS, p. A242

BURCH, Larry, M.D. Vice President Medical Affairs, Saint Anthony's Health Center, Alton, IL, p. A172

BURCH, Lee, Director Management Information Systems, Brooksville Regional Hospital, Brooksville, FL, p. A119

BURCHAM, Jim, Chief Executive Officer, Gateway Rehabilitation Hospital, Florence, KY, p. A249

BURCHAM Sr., Michael G., President and CEO, Black River Medical Center, Poplar Bluff, MO, p. A366

BURCHELL, Pam, Director Human Resources, Lawnwood Regional Medical Center, Fort Pierce, FL, p. A124

BURCHETT, Claudia L., R.N. Vice President Patient Services, Southern Ohio Medical Center, Portsmouth, OH, p. A487

BURCHETT, Travis, Troop Commander Human Resources, Colonel Florence A. Blanchfield Army Community Hospital, Fort Campbell, KY, p. A250

BURCHFIELD, Charla, Manager Human Resources, St. James Behavioral Health Hospital, Gonzales, LA, p. A267

BURCZEUSKI, Jason, Controller, Conifer Park, Glenville, NY, p. A426

BURD, Vanessa, R.N. Chief Nursing Officer, Caverna Memorial Hospital, Horse Cave, KY, p. A252

BURDEN, Jennifer, Vice President Human Resources, Hendersonville Medical Center, Hendersonville, TN, p. A566

BURDETT, Gregg, Vice President Administration and Physician Services, Valley Regional Hospital, Claremont, NH, p. A397

BURDETTE, Pat, Chief Financial Officer, Sistersville General Hospital, Sistersville, WV, p. A675

BURDICK, Ginny
Senior Vice President and Chief Human Resources Officer, Clovis Community Medical Center, Clovis, CA, p. A57
Vice President Human Resources, Community Behavioral Health Center, Fresno, CA, p. A62
Vice President Human Resources, Community Regional Medical Center, Fresno, CA, p. A62

BURDICK, Hoyt J., M.D. Vice President Medical Affairs, Cabell Huntington Hospital, Huntington, WV, p. A672

BURDICK, Mindy, FACHE President, Mercy Hospital Ardmore, Ardmore, OK, p. A493

BURDICK, Steven A., Chief Executive Officer, Providence St. Mary Medical Center, Walla Walla, WA, p. A669

BURGER, Janice, Administrator, Providence St. Vincent Medical Center, Portland, OR, p. A514

BURGESS, Alan J., FACHE Chief Executive Officer, Tehachapi Valley Healthcare District, Tehachapi, CA, p. A92

BURGESS, Angela, Chief Information Officer, Randolph Hospital, Asheboro, NC, p. A448

BURGESS, Carolyn, Director Human Resources, Henrietta D. Goodall Hospital, Sanford, ME, p. A285

BURGESS, Daniel, Chief Information Officer, MaineGeneral Medical Center–Waterville Campus, Waterville, ME, p. A286

BURGESS, Debbie, Director Information Services, Bert Fish Medical Center, New Smyrna Beach, FL, p. A133

BURGESS, John, Director Information Services, Hocking Valley Community Hospital, Logan, OH, p. A483

BURGESS, Mike, Chief Financial Officer, The Children's Hospital of Alabama, Birmingham, AL, p. A17

BURGESS, Steven, Administrator Human Resources, Henrico Doctors' Hospital, Richmond, VA, p. A655

BURGHART, Steven, Chief Operating Officer, Hialeah Hospital, Hialeah, FL, p. A125

BURGIN, Kelli, Director Information Technology, Audubon County Memorial Hospital, Audubon, IA, p. A214

BURGUILLOS, Richard, Chief Financial Officer, Care One at Raritan Bay Medical Center, Perth Amboy, NJ, p. A408

BURIANEK, Amy, Director Nurses, First Care Health Center, Park River, ND, p. A468

BURINGRUD, Duane, M.D. Chief Medical and Quality Officer, Palomar Medical Center, Escondido, CA, p. A60

Index of Health Care Professionals / Burton

Index of Health Care Professionals


BURISH, Brent
Chief Operating Officer, Heart of Florida Regional Medical Center, Davenport, FL, p. A121
Chief Executive Officer, Shands Starke Regional Medical Center, Starke, FL, p. A139
BURK, Jackie, Director Human Resources, Cedar Crest Hospital, Belton, TX, p. A584
BURK, Thomas J., Chief Operating Officer, Danville State Hospital, Danville, PA, p. A521
BURKE, Aron, M.D. Chief Medical Officer, Community Hospital–Fairfax, Fairfax, MO, p. A359
BURKE, Brian, M.D. President Medical Staff, Fairview Hospital, Great Barrington, MA, p. A300
BURKE, Curtis, M.D. Chief of Staff, LeConte Medical Center, Sevierville, TN, p. A575
BURKE, David, Administrator and Chief Executive Officer, Muleshoe Area Medical Center, Muleshoe, TX, p. A618
BURKE, David J., Director Finance and Chief Financial Officer, Nantucket Cottage Hospital, Nantucket, MA, p. A302
BURKE, Dennis E., President and Chief Executive Officer, Good Shepherd Health Care System, Hermiston, OR, p. A511
BURKE, Drew, Director Human Resources, Willamette Valley Medical Center, McMinnville, OR, p. A512
BURKE, Ed, Chief Financial Officer, Interim LSU Public Hospital, New Orleans, LA, p. A274
BURKE, Greg, M.D. Medical Director, Geisinger HEALTHSOUTH Rehabilitation Hospital, Danville, PA, p. A521
BURKE, James, M.D
Senior Vice President and Chief Medical Officer, Scottsdale Healthcare Shea Medical Center, Scottsdale, AZ, p. A38
Senior Vice President and Chief Medical Officer, Scottsdale Healthcare Thompson Peak Hospital, Scottsdale, AZ, p. A38
Senior Vice President and Chief Medical Officer, Scottsdale Healthcare–Osborn Medical Center, Scottsdale, AZ, p. A38
BURKE, James B., Chief Operating Officer, Hahnemann University Hospital, Philadelphia, PA, p. A532
BURKE, Jeff
Chief Information Officer, Bon Secours St. Mary's Hospital, Richmond, VA, p. A654
Chief Information Officer, Bon Secours–Richmond Community Hospital, Richmond, VA, p. A654
BURKE, Jo–Ann, R.N. Vice President Patient Care Services, Children's Hospital of The King's Daughters, Norfolk, VA, p. A652
BURKE, John, Chief Financial Officer, Nyack Hospital, Nyack, NY, p. A438
BURKE, Kaye, Administrator, Noland Hospital Dothan, Dothan, AL, p. A19
BURKE, Marsha
Senior Vice President Financial Services, WellStar Paulding Hospital, Dallas, GA, p. A150
Senior Vice President and Chief Financial Officer, WellStar Windy Hill Hospital, Marietta, GA, p. A156
BURKE, Michael, Senior Vice President and Corporate Chief Financial Officer, NYU Langone Medical Center, New York, NY, p. A436
BURKE, Paul, Administrator, Schleicher County Medical Center, Eldorado, TX, p. A597
BURKE, Rebecca, R.N. Senior Vice President, Patient Care and Clinical Services and Chief Nursing Officer, Saint Francis Hospital and Medical Center, Hartford, CT, p. A109
BURKE, Thomas, M.D. Executive Vice President and Physician–in–Chief, University of Texas M.D. Anderson Cancer Center, Houston, TX, p. A608
BURKE, Timothy, M.D. Medical Director, The Brook Hospital – KMI, Louisville, KY, p. A255
BURKE, Timothy R., M.D. Chief of Staff, VA Butler Healthcare, Butler, PA, p. A519
BURKEL, Gregory, Chief Financial Officer, Alaska Native Medical Center, Anchorage, AK, p. A28
BURKET, Mark, Chief Executive Officer, Platte Health Center Avera, Platte, SD, p. A558
BURKETT, Eric, M.D. Vice President Medical Affairs, Monmouth Medical Center, Long Branch, NJ, p. A405
BURKETT, Evan, Chief Human Resource Officer, Sanford University of South Dakota Medical Center, Sioux Falls, SD, p. A559
BURKETT, William T., Chief Executive Officer, Oklahoma Forensic Center, Vinita, OK, p. A507
BURKHARDT, Minnie, Associate Administrator, Texoma Medical Center, Denison, TX, p. A593
BURKHARDT, Raye, Chief Nursing Officer, St. John's Pleasant Valley Hospital, Camarillo, CA, p. A56
BURKHART, Brad, Assistant Administrator, Harlan ARH Hospital, Harlan, KY, p. A251
BURKHART, James R., FACHE President and Chief Executive Officer, Shands Jacksonville Medical Center, Jacksonville, FL, p. A126
BURKHART, Steven, M.D. Chief Medical Officer, Crittenden County Hospital, Marion, KY, p. A256
BURKHART, Tracy, Vice President Information Services, Sacred Heart Hospital, Allentown, PA, p. A517
BURKHOLDER, Adrienne, Director Human Resources, LTAC of Wichita, Wichita, KS, p. A245
BURKITT, David, Director Fiscal Services, Shriners Hospitals for Children, Los Angeles, Los Angeles, CA, p. A72
BURKLOW, Bryan, Chief Executive Officer, Brandywine Hospital, Coatesville, PA, p. A520
BURKS, Matt, Director Information Technology, United Regional Medical Center, Manchester, TN, p. A570
BURKS, Mel, Executive Director Administrative Services, Hamilton·Center, Terre Haute, IN, p. A212
BURKS, Tami
Chief Fiscal Services, Iraan General Hospital, Iraan, TX, p. A608
Comptroller, Rankin Hospital District, Rankin, TX, p. A622
BURLESON, Linda, Administrative Secretary, Clay County Memorial Hospital, Henrietta, TX, p. A603
BURLESON, Scott D., Executive Vice President, Chester River Health System, Chestertown, MD, p. A290
BURLESON, Stan, M.D. Chief Medical Staff, DeWitt Hospital, De Witt, AR, p. A44
BURMAN, Don, Chief Executive Officer, Heartland Surgical Specialty Hospital, Overland Park, KS, p. A240
BURMEISTER, Geraldine F., FACHE Chief Executive Officer, Windom Area Hospital, Windom, MN, p. A342
BURMESTER, Mark A., Vice President Strategy and Communications, Sunnyside Medical Center, Clackamas, OR, p. A509
BURNAM, Gregg, Chief Information Officer and Manager Business Office, Quartz Mountain Medical Center, Mangum, OK, p. A498
BURNELL, Thomas, Chief Executive Officer, Nebraska Heart Institute and Heart Hospital, Lincoln, NE, p. A385
BURNETT, Anthony, M.D. Medical Director, Julian F. Keith Alcohol and Drug Abuse Treatment Center, Black Mountain, NC, p. A448
BURNETT, Brad, Chief Financial Officer, Heart of Texas Memorial Hospital, Brady, TX, p. A584
BURNETT, Cindi, Chief Human Resources Officer, Madison County Memorial Hospital, Madison, FL, p. A129
BURNETT, Karen, Regional Director Human Resources, McKay–Dee Hospital Center, Ogden, UT, p. A639
BURNETT, Mark, President and Chief Executive Officer, Scott County Hospital, Scott City, KS, p. A243
BURNETT, Michael, Chief Operating Officer, Piedmont Fayette Hospital, Fayetteville, GA, p. A152
BURNETTE, Peg, Chief Financial Officer, Denver Health Medical Center, Denver, CO, p. A99
BURNETTE, Sheri, R.N. Chief Executive Officer and Administrator, Cornerstone Hospital of Bossier City, Bossier City, LA, p. A263
BURNETTE, W. Scott, President and Chief Executive Officer, Community Memorial Healthcenter, South Hill, VA, p. A656
BURNEY, Sibte, M.D. Senior Vice President Medical Affairs and Chief Medical Officer, Kingsbrook Jewish Medical Center,, NY, p. A433
BURNHAM, David, M.D. Chief of Staff, Longmont United Hospital, Longmont, CO, p. A104
BURNHAM, Sharon, Director of Nursing, Simpson General Hospital, Mendenhall, MS, p. A350
BURNS, Becky L., Manager Health Information Management, Ellinwood District Hospital, Ellinwood, KS, p. A232
BURNS, Brantly, M.D. Medical Director, Select Specialty Hospital–Knoxville, Knoxville, TN, p. A568
BURNS, Bruce R., Chief Financial Officer, Concord Hospital, Concord, NH, p. A397
BURNS, Charlotte, Administrator and Chief Executive Officer, Hardin Medical Center, Savannah, TN, p. A575
BURNS, Coreg, Human Resources Lead, West Central Georgia Regional Hospital, Columbus, GA, p. A150
BURNS, Gregory T., President and Chief Executive Officer, Cameron Memorial Community Hospital, Angola, IN, p. A197
BURNS, James P., Vice President and Chief Financial Officer, Fawcett Memorial Hospital, Port Charlotte, FL, p. A136
BURNS, Jared, Coordinator Human Resources, Regency Hospital of Hattiesburg, Hattiesburg, MS, p. A347
BURNS, Jeff, Manager of Information Technology, Mary Free Bed Rehabilitation Hospital, Grand Rapids, MI, p. A313
BURNS, Joanne, Chief Information Officer, Women's and Children's Hospital, Columbia, MO, p. A358
BURNS, Jon P.
Senior Vice President and Chief Information Officer, Maryland General Hospital, Baltimore, MD, p. A288
Chief Information Officer, University of Maryland Medical Center, Baltimore, MD, p. A289
BURNS, Katherine, Vice President Human Resources, High Point Regional Health System, High Point, NC, p. A455
BURNS, Kathryn I., R.N. Director of Nursing, Medicine Lodge Memorial Hospital, Medicine Lodge, KS, p. A239
BURNS, Kay, Chief Financial Officer, Santa Rosa Medical Center, Milton, FL, p. A132
BURNS, Jr., Larry P., Chief Operating Officer, Yavapai Regional Medical Center, Prescott, AZ, p. A37
BURNS, Lawrence, Vice President Institutional Advancement, The University of Toledo Medical Center, Toledo, OH, p. A489
BURNS, Patrick, Vice President Finance, ACMH Hospital, Kittanning, PA, p. A526
BURNS, Steven, Director Fiscal Services, Summit Behavioral Healthcare, Cincinnati, OH, p. A474
BURNS, Terry M.
President, Greene Memorial Hospital, Xenia, OH, p. A492
President, Soin Medical Center, Beavercreek, OH, p. A470
BURNS, Tom, M.D. Chief of Staff, The Hospital at Westlake Medical Center, Austin, TX, p. A582
BURNS, Wes, Director Human Resources, Vibra Hospital of San Diego, San Diego, CA, p. A86
BURNS–TISDALE, Susan, Senior Vice President Clinical Operations, Exeter Hospital, Exeter, NH, p. A398
BURNSIDE, Brian D., FACHE Chief Executive Officer, Marshalltown Medical & Surgical Center, Marshalltown, IA, p. A223
BURNSIDE, David, M.D. Chief Medical Officer, Alton Memorial Hospital, Alton, IL, p. A172
BURRELL, Carol H., President and Chief Executive Officer, Northeast Georgia Medical Center, Gainesville, GA, p. A153
BURRIS, Bradley D., Chief Executive Officer, Pipestone County Medical Center Avera, Pipestone, MN, p. A337
BURRIS, Don, Chief Executive Officer, Haxtun Hospital District, Haxtun, CO, p. A102
BURRIS, J. Michael, Vice President Corporate Services and Chief Financial Officer, Martha Jefferson Hospital, Charlottesville, VA, p. A646
BURRIS, Lisa
Manager Human Resources, Frazier Rehab Institute, Louisville, KY, p. A254
Director Human Resources, Southern Indiana Rehabilitation Hospital, New Albany, IN, p. A209
BURRISS, Jessica, Chief Financial Officer, HEALTHSOUTH Rehabilitation Hospital, Columbia, SC, p. A548
BURRISS, Steve W., Chief Operating Officer, Rex Healthcare, Raleigh, NC, p. A459
BURRITT, Joan, R.N. Chief Operating Officer, San Diego Medical Center, San Diego, CA, p. A85
BURROUGHS, James, Chief Executive Officer, Kingwood Pines Hospital, Kingwood, TX, p. A611
BURROUGHS, Michael R., FACHE Chief Executive Officer, Western Plains Medical Complex, Dodge City, KS, p. A232
BURROUGHS, Valentine, M.D. Chief Medical Officer, East Orange General Hospital, East Orange, NJ, p. A403
BURROWS, Randy, Director Administrative Services, McKenzie–Willamette Medical Center, Springfield, OR, p. A515
BURROWS, Susan M.
Vice President Human Resources, Children's Hospital at Mission, Mission Viejo, CA, p. A74
Vice President Human Resources, Children's Hospital of Orange County, Orange, CA, p. A78
BURRY, V. Fred, M.D. Executive Medical Director, Children's Mercy Hospitals and Clinics, Kansas City, MO, p. A361
BURSCH, Lowell, M.D. Executive Vice President Medical Affairs, Spectrum Health Butterworth Hospital, Grand Rapids, MI, p. A314
BURT, Alan, Director Information Services, Sunrise Hospital and Medical Center, Las Vegas, NV, p. A394
BURT, Keith, Director Marketing, Woodrow Wilson Rehabilitation Center, Fishersville, VA, p. A648
BURT, Linda K.
Corporate Vice President Finance, Jennie Edmundson Hospital, Council Bluffs, IA, p. A217
Corporate Vice President Finance, Nebraska Methodist Hospital, Omaha, NE, p. A388
BURT, Noel F., Ph.D. Chief Human Resources Officer, Cone Health, Greensboro, NC, p. A454
BURTCH, Gloria, Director Human Resources, Cornerstone of Medical Arts Center Hospital, Fresh Meadows, NY, p. A426
BURTHAY, Darcy, MSN Chief Nursing Officer and Chief Operating Officer, St. Vincent Indianapolis Hospital, Indianapolis, IN, p. A205
BURTON, Charles, Chief Human Resources, Carl R. Darnall Army Medical Center, Fort Hood, TX, p. A598
BURTON, Cynthia, R.N. Chief Nursing Officer, Rockcastle Regional Hospital and Respiratory Care Center, Mount Vernon, KY, p. A257
BURTON, Faye, Director Health Information Management, Edgefield County Hospital, Edgefield, SC, p. A549
BURTON, John T., Administrator, Kindred Hospital–Pittsburgh, Oakdale, PA, p. A531

BURTON, Luanne, Director Human Resources, HEALTHSOUTH Rehabilitation Hospital, Columbia, SC, p. A548

BURTON, Nancy L.
Chief Executive Officer, Select Specialty Hospital–Phoenix, Phoenix, AZ, p. A36
Chief Executive Officer, Select Specialty Hospital–Scottsdale, Scottsdale, AZ, p. A38

BURTON, Robert, Manager Finance, Utah State Hospital, Provo, UT, p. A640

BURTON, Stacey R., Director Human Resources, Okmulgee Memorial Hospital, Okmulgee, OK, p. A502

BURTRON, Sandra, MS Chief Nursing Officer, Crawford Memorial Hospital, Robinson, IL, p. A192

BURY, Peter, Vice President Finance, Riverside Methodist Hospital, Columbus, OH, p. A477

BURY, Randy, Chief Operating Officer, Sanford University of South Dakota Medical Center, Sioux Falls, SD, p. A559

BURZYNSKI, Cheryl A., President, McLaren Bay Special Care, Bay City, MI, p. A308

BUSATTI, David A., Vice President Finance, Hutchinson Regional Medical Center, Hutchinson, KS, p. A235

BUSBEE, Lara, Chief Financial Officer, Flint River Community Hospital, Montezuma, GA, p. A156

BUSBY, Billie, Assistant Director, Colorado Mental Health Institute at Fort Logan, Denver, CO, p. A99

BUSBY, Jay, M.D. President Medical Staff, Franklin Medical Center, Winnsboro, LA, p. A279

BUSBY, Kathy, Medical Record Technician, Chillicothe Hospital District, Chillicothe, TX, p. A587

BUSBY, Lisa, Manager Information Systems, Moses Ludington Hospital, Ticonderoga, NY, p. A444

BUSCH, Michael D., Executive Vice President and Chief Operating Officer, Excela Latrobe Area Hospital, Latrobe, PA, p. A527

BUSCH, Rebecca, Chief Financial Officer, Spooner Health System, Spooner, WI, p. A691

BUSCH, Steve, Chief Operating Officer, Midwest Medical Center, Galena, IL, p. A182

BUSER, Kenneth R., President and Chief Executive Officer, Wheaton Franciscan Healthcare – All Saints, Racine, WI, p. A689

BUSH, Bruce A., M.D. Senior Vice President Medical Affairs, Indiana Regional Medical Center, Indiana, PA, p. A525

BUSH, Deborah, Director Information Services, North Florida Regional Medical Center, Gainesville, FL, p. A124

BUSH, Linda, Chief Executive Officer, Franklin County Memorial Hospital, Franklin, NE, p. A383

BUSH, Stephen, Chief Financial Officer, TMC Healthcare, Tucson, AZ, p. A40

BUSH, William, Chief Executive Officer, HEALTHSOUTH Rehabilitation Hospital of Alexandria, Alexandria, LA, p. A261

BUSH, William B., CP
Chief Financial Officer, University of South Alabama Children's and Women's Hospital, Mobile, AL, p. A23
Chief Financial Officer, University of South Alabama Medical Center, Mobile, AL, p. A23

BUSHAW, Darlene, Information Technology Systems Site Lead, LakeWood Health Center, Baudette, MN, p. A328

BUSHELL, Michael, Vice President Finance, Business Development and Support Services, Saint Anne's Hospital, Fall River, MA, p. A299

BUSINELLE, Denise, Account Administrator, Southeast Louisiana Hospital, Mandeville, LA, p. A272

BUSKEY, Irene, Director Human Resources, Southside Regional Medical Center, Petersburg, VA, p. A653

BUSS, Georganna, Chief Financial Officer, Harper County Community Hospital, Buffalo, OK, p. A494

BUSS, Theresa L., Vice President, Human Resources and Organizational Development, The William W. Backus Hospital, Norwich, CT, p. A111

BUSSELL, Walter, Chief Financial Officer, Memorial Hospital West, Pembroke Pines, FL, p. A135

BUSSEY, George, M.D. Chief Medical Officer, FirstHealth Richmond Memorial Hospital, Rockingham, NC, p. A459

BUSSIERE, Mark, Administrator Human Resources, New Hampshire Hospital, Concord, NH, p. A397

BUSSLER, David, Chief Information Officer, Sheridan Community Hospital, Sheridan, MI, p. A323

BUSTIN, Sherry, Chief Executive Officer, Allegiance Specialty Hospital of Kilgore, Kilgore, TX, p. A610

BUTCHER, Allen R., Vice President Finance, Camden–Clark Medical Center, Parkersburg, WV, p. A674

BUTCHER, Cindi, Chief Operating Officer, East Georgia Regional Medical Center, Statesboro, GA, p. A160

BUTCHER, Gina, Chief Financial Officer, St. Mary's of Michigan, Saginaw, MI, p. A322

BUTCHER, Kay, Director Management Information, Stonewall Jackson Memorial Hospital, Weston, WV, p. A676

BUTCHER, Scott, Chief Executive Officer, HEALTHSOUTH Rehabilitation Institute of San Antonio, San Antonio, TX, p. A625

BUTCHER, Steven, D.O. Director Medical Affairs, Citizens Memorial Hospital, Bolivar, MO, p. A355

BUTERBAUGH, William, Director Support Services, Fulton County Medical Center, Mc Connellsburg, PA, p. A528

BUTIKOFER, Lon D., Ph.D. Chief Executive Officer, Regional Medical Center, Manchester, IA, p. A222

BUTKER, Jeff, Chief Information Officer, Memorial Hospital, Martinsville, VA, p. A651

BUTLER, Anita M., Chief Executive Officer, Spartanburg Hospital for Restorative Care, Spartanburg, SC, p. A553

BUTLER, Barbara, Chief Executive Officer, HEALTHSOUTH Deaconess Rehabilitation Hospital, Evansville, IN, p. A201

BUTLER, Brad, Network Administrator, Barton County Memorial Hospital, Lamar, MO, p. A363

BUTLER, Carol A., R.N. VP Patient Care Services & Operations, St. Anthony North Hospital, Westminster, CO, p. A106

BUTLER, Catherine, M.D. Chief Medical Staff, Hancock County Memorial Hospital, Britt, IA, p. A215

BUTLER, Chris, Deputy CIO/System Vice President, Kimball Medical Center, Lakewood, NJ, p. A405

BUTLER, David, Chief Executive Officer, North Canyon Medical Center, Gooding, ID, p. A168

BUTLER, Debby, Director Human Resources, Wadley Regional Medical Center, Texarkana, TX, p. A631

BUTLER, Everett A.
Chief Executive Officer, Pembina County Memorial Hospital and Wedgewood Manor, Cavalier, ND, p. A464
Chief Executive Officer, Unity Medical Center, Grafton, ND, p. A466

BUTLER, Jeffrey, Superintendent, Richmond State Hospital, Richmond, IN, p. A211

BUTLER, John, M.D
Director Medical Staff, Mayo Clinic Health System in Waycross, Waycross, GA, p. A162
Vice President Medical Affairs, St. Mary's Hospital, Madison, WI, p. A684

BUTLER, Joseph, Vice President and Chief Information Officer, UPMC Hamot, Erie, PA, p. A523

BUTLER, Keith L., Chief Executive Officer, Lillian M. Hudspeth Memorial Hospital, Sonora, TX, p. A628

BUTLER, Linda H., M.D. Chief Medical Officer, Rex Healthcare, Raleigh, NC, p. A459

BUTLER, Margaret, Vice President Human Resources, Abbott Northwestern Hospital, Minneapolis, MN, p. A334

BUTLER, Michael K., M.D. Executive Vice President and Chief Medical Officer, Jackson Health System, Miami, FL, p. A131

BUTLER, Peter W., President and Chief Operating Officer, Rush University Medical Center, Chicago, IL, p. A178

BUTLER, Randy, Chief Financial Officer, West Florida Hospital, Pensacola, FL, p. A136

BUTLER, Stuart, Director Information Technology, Sweeny Community Hospital, Sweeny, TX, p. A629

BUTT, Shiraz, M.D. Medical Director, Maryville Scott Nolan Center, Des Plaines, IL, p. A180

BUTTELL, Christine, Chief Operating Officer, Knoxville Hospital & Clinics, Knoxville, IA, p. A222

BUTTELL, Phil, Chief Operating Officer, Centerpoint Medical Center, Independence, MO, p. A360

BUTTERFIELD, Jon
Chief Operating Officer, Jordan Valley Medical Center, West Jordan, UT, p. A642
Chief Operating Officer, Pioneer Valley Hospital, West Valley City, UT, p. A642

BUTTERICK, James D., M.D. Chief Medical Officer, Cape Cod Hospital, Hyannis, MA, p. A301

BUTTERLY, John R., M.D. Medical Director, Dartmouth–Hitchcock Medical Center, Lebanon, NH, p. A398

BUTTERWORTH, Jack, M.D. Vice President Medical Affairs, Wellmont Bristol Regional Medical Center, Bristol, TN, p. A562

BUTTNER, Murray, M.D. Medical Director, Cordova Community Medical Center, Cordova, AK, p. A28

BUTTON, Charles A., Chief Executive Officer, Dayton General Hospital, Dayton, WA, p. A661

BUTZER, John, M.D. Medical Director, Mary Free Bed Rehabilitation Hospital, Grand Rapids, MI, p. A313

BUTZLER, Hilary, Director Human Resources, Cumberland Memorial Hospital, Cumberland, WI, p. A680

BUUCK, Brian, Chief Operating Officer, Ridgeview Psychiatric Hospital and Center, Oak Ridge, TN, p. A574

BUXTON, Barton, Ed.D. President and Chief Executive Officer, McLaren Lapeer Region, Lapeer, MI, p. A317

BUYOK, Tammy K., Vice President Support Services, St. Peter's Hospital, Helena, MT, p. A376

BUZACHERO, Victor, Corporate Senior Vice President for Innovation, Human Resources and Performance Management, Scripps Green Hospital, La Jolla, CA, p. A65

BYBERG, Jeff, Manager Human Resources, Mammoth Hospital, Mammoth Lakes, CA, p. A73

BYCROFT, Victor, R.N. Chief Nursing Officer, Shenandoah Medical Center, Shenandoah, IA, p. A226

BYDA, Jeff, Vice President Information Technology, Mercy Fitzgerald Hospital, Darby, PA, p. A521

BYERLY, Carolyn, Chief Information Officer, Stanford Hospital and Clinics, Palo Alto, CA, p. A79

BYERS, Suzann, Director of Nursing, Southern Indiana Rehabilitation Hospital, New Albany, IN, p. A209

BYERS, Tracy, Chief Operating Officer, Harton Regional Medical Center, Tullahoma, TN, p. A576

BYERS, William, Vice President and Chief Information Officer, Western Maryland Regional Medical Center, Cumberland, MD, p. A291

BYLAND, Mark, M.D. Chief of Staff, Spectrum Health Gerber Memorial, Fremont, MI, p. A312

BYLER, Karen, Information Technician, Warren State Hospital, Warren, PA, p. A540

BYNUM, Chigger, Chief Financial Officer, John Randolph Medical Center, Hopewell, VA, p. A649

BYNUM, Dennis T., Interim Chief Financial Officer, Watsonville Community Hospital, Watsonville, CA, p. A95

BYORICK, F. Joseph, Senior Vice President Finance and Chief Financial Officer, Lancaster General Health, Lancaster, PA, p. A526

BYRD, David, Chief Financial Officer, Des Peres Hospital, Saint Louis, MO, p. A368

BYRD, O. Wayne, M.D. Chief of Staff, H. C. Watkins Memorial Hospital, Quitman, MS, p. A352

BYRD, Sue, Coordinator Human Resources, Northwest Florida Community Hospital, Chipley, FL, p. A120

BYRNE, Bobbie, M.D. Vice President Chief Information Officer, Edward Hospital, Naperville, IL, p. A189

BYRNE, Frank D., M.D. President, St. Mary's Hospital, Madison, WI, p. A684

BYRNE, Frank J., Director Finance and Treasurer, Newport Hospital, Newport, RI, p. A544

BYRNE, John, Executive Vice President and Chief Operating Officer, University Hospital of Brooklyn at Long Island College Hospital,, NY, p. A437

BYRNS, David, Chief Executive Officer, South Cameron Memorial Hospital, Cameron, LA, p. A264

BYROM, David, Chief Executive Officer, Coryell Memorial Hospital, Gatesville, TX, p. A601

# C

CAAMANO, Tero, Director Information Technology, Saint Clare's Health System, Denville, NJ, p. A403

CABALLERO, Mechi R., Assistant Administrator, Panorama City Medical Center,, CA, p. A71

CABALLERO, Rogelio, Chief Information Systems, San Jorge Children's Hospital, San Juan, PR, p. A703

CABANA, David, Director Management Information Systems, Southwest Memorial Hospital, Cortez, CO, p. A99

CABANAS, Deborah, R.N. Chief Nursing Officer, HEALTHSOUTH Rehabilitation Hospital of Western Massachusetts, Ludlow, MA, p. A302

CABELL–MAINS, Susan M., Vice President Administration, Martha Jefferson Hospital, Charlottesville, VA, p. A646

CABEZZAS, Noel, Chief Operating Officer, Good Samaritan Hospital, Bakersfield, CA, p. A54

CABRAL, Joseph, Vice President and Chief Human Resources Officer, Forest Hills Hospital,, NY, p. A432

CABRERA, Carlos, Executive Director, I. Gonzalez Martinez Oncologic Hospital,, PR, p. A703

CABRERA, Irma, Finance Director, Hospital San Carlos Borromeo, Moca, PR, p. A702

CABUNOC, Brenda, Chief Human Resource Management Services, Veterans Affairs Medical Center, Memphis, TN, p. A572

CACCIAMANI, John D., Chief Executive Officer, Chestnut Hill Hospital, Philadelphia, PA, p. A531

CACERES, Janet L., Chief Financial Officer, Paradise Valley Hospital, National City, CA, p. A76

CADE, Paul, Administrator and Chief Executive Officer, Baptist Memorial Hospital–Golden Triangle, Columbus, MS, p. A345

CADWELL, Maureen K., Chief Executive Officer, Sanford Medical Center Chamberlain, Chamberlain, SD, p. A555

CADY, Kathy, Coordinator Human Resources, Accounts Payable and Payroll, Boise Behavioral Health Hospital, Boise, ID, p. A166

CADY, Thomas, Vice President Human Resources, Heywood Hospital, Gardner, MA, p. A300

CADY, Tina, Controller, The Women's Hospital, Newburgh, IN, p. A210

Index of Health Care Professionals / Campbell

Index of Health Care Professionals


CAFASSO, Michael, Vice President Operations, St. Mary–Corwin Medical Center, Pueblo, CO, p. A105
CAFFREY, Richard, Interim Assistant Chief Financial Officer, Saint Alphonsus Medical Center – Nampa, Nampa, ID, p. A169
CAGEN, Richard M., Administrator, Silverton Hospital, Silverton, OR, p. A515
CAGGIANO, Richard, M.D. Chief Medical Officer, Pullman Regional Hospital, Pullman, WA, p. A664
CAGLE, Cleo, Chief Financial Officer, Comanche County Medical Center, Comanche, TX, p. A588
CAGLE, Mary Jo, M.D. Chief Medical Officer, Bon Secours St. Francis Health System, Greenville, SC, p. A550
CAGNA, Ralph A.
Director Information Technology Operations, Cleveland Clinic Health System South Market, Marymount Hospital, Garfield Heights, OH, p. A481
Director Information Technology, South Pointe Hospital, Warrensville Heights, OH, p. A490
CAHALAN, Jay P., Chief Operating Officer, Columbia Memorial Hospital, Hudson, NY, p. A427
CAHILL, Donna, Vice President Human Resources, Palisades Medical Center, North Bergen, NJ, p. A407
CAHILL, Holly, Director Human Resources, Presentation Medical Center, Rolla, ND, p. A468
CAHILL, Joseph, Executive Vice President and Chief Operating Officer, South Shore Hospital, South Weymouth, MA, p. A304
CAHILL, Kathleen, Chief Operations Officer, MountainView Regional Medical Center, Las Cruces, NM, p. A416
CAHILL, Marty, Chief Executive Officer, Samaritan North Lincoln Hospital, Lincoln City, OR, p. A512
CAHILL, Peter, M.D. President Medical Staff, Vibra Hospital of Denver, Thornton, CO, p. A106
CAHN, Jack, M.D. Chief Medical Staff, Alleghany Memorial Hospital, Sparta, NC, p. A461
CAHO–MOONEY, Linda, Chief Financial Officer, Patient's Choice Medical Center of Claiborne County, Port Gibson, MS, p. A352
CAIN, Donna, Director Information Systems Department, Cypress Fairbanks Medical Center, Houston, TX, p. A604
CAIN, Julie, Administrator, Stone County Hospital, Wiggins, MS, p. A354
CAIN, Mark, Chief Executive Officer, LaFollette Medical Center, La Follette, TN, p. A569
CAIN, Roxie, Chief Financial Officer, Big Horn County Memorial Hospital, Hardin, MT, p. A376
CAINE, Claudia, Executive Vice President and Chief Operating Officer, Lutheran Medical Center,, NY, p. A434
CAINE, Kirsten, M.D. Chief Medical Staff, Wallowa Memorial Hospital, Enterprise, OR, p. A510
CAIRNS, Craig, M.D. Vice President Medical Affairs, Licking Memorial Hospital, Newark, OH, p. A486
CALABRESE, Joan L., Director Human Resources, Putnam Hospital Center, Carmel, NY, p. A423
CALABRESE, Susan, Director of Nursing, Bloomington Meadows Hospital, Bloomington, IN, p. A198
CALABRESI, Joseph, Chief Information Service, Edith Nourse Rogers Memorial Veterans Hospital, Bedford, MA, p. A295
CALAIS, C. Matthew, Senior Vice President and Chief Information Officer, Legacy Good Samaritan Hospital and Medical Center, Portland, OR, p. A514
CALAMARI, Frank A., President and Chief Executive Officer, Calvary Hospital,, NY, p. A432
CALAMARI, Jacquelyn, MSN Vice President and Chief Nursing Officer, Middlesex Hospital, Middletown, CT, p. A110
CALAME, Norma, Director Human Resources, The Mount Sinai Hospital of Queens,, NY, p. A437
CALANDRIELLO, John, Vice President and Chief Financial Officer, Palisades Medical Center, North Bergen, NJ, p. A407
CALAWAY, Shearmaine, Director Human Resources, East Mississippi State Hospital, Meridian, MS, p. A350
CALBONE, Angelo G., President and Chief Executive Officer, Saratoga Hospital, Saratoga Springs, NY, p. A443
CALBY, Elizabeth, Vice President Human Resources, Advocate Good Samaritan Hospital, Downers Grove, IL, p. A180
CALDARI, Patricia, Vice President, Richmond University Medical Center,, NY, p. A436
CALDERA, Ken, Director Human Resources, Kessler Institute for Rehabilitation, West Orange, NJ, p. A412
CALDERON, Lizmari, Director Finance, Hospital De La Concepcion, San German, PR, p. A702
CALDERONE, John A., Ph.D. Chief Executive Officer, Olympia Medical Center, Los Angeles, CA, p. A71
CALDWELL, Carolyn W., President and Chief Executive Officer, Centerpoint Medical Center, Independence, MO, p. A360
CALDWELL, Dari, President, Rowan Regional Medical Center, Salisbury, NC, p. A460
CALDWELL, Darren, Chief Executive Officer, DeWitt Hospital, De Witt, AR, p. A44
CALDWELL, Janice, Director Human Resources, Oak Tree Hospital, Corbin, KY, p. A249
CALDWELL, Matthew T., Chief Executive Officer, Dallas Regional Medical Center, Mesquite, TX, p. A616
CALDWELL, Noah, Senior Vice President and Chief Information Officer, St. Barnabas Hospital,, NY, p. A436
CALDWELL, R. D., M.D. Chief of Staff, Childress Regional Medical Center, Childress, TX, p. A587
CALDWELL, Richard E., Vice President Support Services, Jackson Hospital and Clinic, Montgomery, AL, p. A24
CALHOUN, Cathy, Director Human Resources, River Point Behavioral Health, Jacksonville, FL, p. A126
CALHOUN, Joshua, M.D. Medical Director, Hawthorn Children Psychiatric Hospital, Saint Louis, MO, p. A368
CALHOUN, Kevin P., Chief Executive Officer, Munising Memorial Hospital, Munising, MI, p. A319
CALHOUN, Kirk A., M.D. President, University of Texas Health Science Center at Tyler, Tyler, TX, p. A632
CALHOUN, Royce
Assistant Director, Veterans Affairs Western New York Healthcare System–Batavia Division, Batavia, NY, p. A421
Business Manager, Veterans Affairs Western New York Healthcare System–Buffalo Division, Buffalo, NY, p. A423
CALHOUN, Sharon, R.N. Director Human Resources, Miller County Hospital, Colquitt, GA, p. A149
CALHOUN, Timothy, Vice President Finance and Chief Financial Officer, Lakeland Regional Medical Center–St. Joseph, Saint Joseph, MI, p. A322
CALHOUN, William, President, Mercy Medical Center, Oshkosh, WI, p. A688
CALIA, Christopher, Director Human Resources, Brazosport Regional Health System, Lake Jackson, TX, p. A611
CALIFORNIA, Randy, Chief Operating Officer, Warren General Hospital, Warren, PA, p. A540
CALIGIURI, Michael, Chief Executive Officer, James Cancer Hospital and Solove Research Institute, Columbus, OH, p. A476
CALIVA, Todd, Chief Executive Officer, West Houston Medical Center, Houston, TX, p. A608
CALKIN, Pitt, Interim Chief Financial Officer, St. Mary Medical Center, Apple Valley, CA, p. A54
CALKIN, Steven, D.O. Vice President Medical Affairs, McLaren Oakland, Pontiac, MI, p. A321
CALL, Brett, D.O. Chief of Staff, Berger Health System, Circleville, OH, p. A474
CALL, Carie, Director Computer Support, Cassia Regional Medical Center, Burley, ID, p. A167
CALL, Dave, M.D. Medical Director, Select Long Term Care Hospital – Colorado Springs, Colorado Springs, CO, p. A98
CALL, Gary, M.D. Chief Medical Officer, Bingham Memorial Hospital, Blackfoot, ID, p. A166
CALLAGHAN III, James, M.D. President, Franciscan St. Anthony Health – Michigan City, Michigan City, IN, p. A208
CALLAHAN, Ame, Acting Manager Resource Management Service, Northern Arizona VA Health Care System, Prescott, AZ, p. A37
CALLAHAN, Christopher, Vice President Human Resources, Exeter Hospital, Exeter, NH, p. A398
CALLAHAN, Deanna, Director Information Systems, Titusville Area Hospital, Titusville, PA, p. A539
CALLAHAN, Jean, Manager Human Resources, Thousand Oaks Surgical Hospital, Thousand Oaks, CA, p. A92
CALLAHAN, John, Acting Director, Veterans Affairs Connecticut Healthcare System, West Haven, CT, p. A113
CALLAHAN, Kelly, Public Information Officer, Elgin Mental Health Center, Elgin, IL, p. A180
CALLAHAN, Kevin J., President and Chief Executive Officer, Exeter Hospital, Exeter, NH, p. A398
CALLAHAN, Larry, Interim Vice President and Chief Human Resources Officer, University of Chicago Medical Center, Chicago, IL, p. A179
CALLAHAN, Mary Beth, Chief Financial Officer, McLaren Lapeer Region, Lapeer, MI, p. A317
CALLAHAN, Michael E., M.D. President Medical Staff, Charles Cole Memorial Hospital, Coudersport, PA, p. A521
CALLAHAN, Neil, Chief Executive Officer, Brooke Glen Behavioral Hospital, Fort Washington, PA, p. A523
CALLAHAN Jr., Robert W., Director, Veterans Affairs Medical Center, Lebanon, PA, p. A527
CALLAHAN, Teresa, MSN, Chief Executive Officer, Iraan General Hospital, Iraan, TX, p. A608
CALLAIS, Elizabeth, Chief Fiscal Officer, Leonard J. Chabert Medical Center, Houma, LA, p. A268
CALLAIS, Ronnie, Chief Financial Officer, WestEnd Hospital, Jennings, LA, p. A268
CALLAN, C. M., M.D. Chief of Staff, Fisher County Hospital District, Rotan, TX, p. A623
CALLAS, Robin, Director Human Resources, Laurens County Health Care System, Clinton, SC, p. A548
CALLECOD, David L., FACHE President and Chief Executive Officer, Lafayette General Medical Center, Lafayette, LA, p. A270
CALLENS, Don, M.D. Chief Medical Officer, Liberty Dayton Regional Medical Center, Liberty, TX, p. A612
CALLENS, Paul A., Ph.D. Director, North Mississippi State Hospital, Tupelo, MS, p. A353
CALLISTER, T. Brian, M.D. Chief Medical Officer, Tahoe Pacific Hospitals, Reno, NV, p. A395
CALLOWAY, Jennifer, Human Resources Coordinator, Asheville Specialty Hospital, Asheville, NC, p. A448
CALLOWAY, Maria, R.N. Chief Nursing Officer, Granville Health System, Oxford, NC, p. A458
CALTRIDER, Joyce, Chief Financial Officer, Kindred Hospital Ocala, Ocala, FL, p. A133
CALVARUSO, Gaspare, President, SSM St. Joseph Health Center, Saint Charles, MO, p. A368
CALVERT, Randy, Chief Financial Officer, Gilbert Hospital, Gilbert, AZ, p. A32
CALVERT, Sarah, Chief Nursing Officer, McGehee–Desha County Hospital, McGehee, AR, p. A48
CALVIN, Jeff, Chief Financial Officer, Michiana Behavioral Health Center, Plymouth, IN, p. A210
CALVIN, Jr., Travis, M.D. Chief of Staff, Pioneers Memorial Healthcare District, Brawley, CA, p. A56
CAMACHO, Peter John Diaz, M.P.H. Administrator and Chief Executive Officer, Guam Memorial Hospital Authority, Tamuning, GU, p. A699
CAMARATA, Chris, M.D. Chief of Staff, Mayers Memorial Hospital District, Fall River Mills, CA, p. A60
CAMERON, Carl, Director Information Systems, Holyoke Medical Center, Holyoke, MA, p. A300
CAMERON, Don, Chief Operating Officer, Allegiance Behavioral Health Center of Plainview, Plainview, TX, p. A621
CAMERON, Kim, Manager Health Information Services, Patients' Hospital of Redding, Redding, CA, p. A82
CAMIRE, Patricia M., MS Chief Nursing Officer, Southern Maine Medical Center, Biddeford, ME, p. A282
CAMMACK Jr., Thomas N., Chief Administrative Officer, Mother Frances Hospital – Jacksonville, Jacksonville, TX, p. A609
CAMMENGA, Randall, M.D. Vice President Medical Affairs, Indiana University Health Goshen Hospital, Goshen, IN, p. A202
CAMP III, Claude E., Chief Executive Officer, Brownwood Regional Medical Center, Brownwood, TX, p. A585
CAMP, James, R.N. Chief Executive Officer, Cornerstone Hospital of Houston – Bellaire, Houston, TX, p. A603
CAMP, Julie A., R.N. Chief Executive Officer, Forest Park Medical Center Frisco, Frisco, TX, p. A600
CAMP, Lea Ann, R.N. Chief Nursing Officer, Greene County General Hospital, Linton, IN, p. A207
CAMPANELLA, Alfred
Vice President and Chief Information Officer, Virtua Berlin, Berlin, NJ, p. A402
Chief Information Officer, Virtua Marlton, Marlton, NJ, p. A406
Chief Information Officer, Virtua Voorhees, Voorhees, NJ, p. A412
CAMPAS, Janice, Chief Financial Officer, Wichita County Health Center, Leoti, KS, p. A238
CAMPBELL, Ann, Chief Nursing Officer, Virtua Marlton, Marlton, NJ, p. A406
CAMPBELL, Belinda H., Director Human Resources, Legal Compliance and Risk Management, University Hospital McDuffie, Thomson, GA, p. A160
CAMPBELL, Bob, Vice President Business Development and Chief Strategy Officer, Mercy Gilbert Medical Center, Gilbert, AZ, p. A32
CAMPBELL, Chad, Chief Executive Officer, Carlsbad Medical Center, Carlsbad, NM, p. A415
CAMPBELL, Charlotte, Chief Human Resources Officer, Beatrice Community Hospital and Health Center, Beatrice, NE, p. A382
CAMPBELL, Christopher, M.D. Chief of Staff, Ashe Memorial Hospital, Jefferson, NC, p. A455
CAMPBELL, Darrell, M.D. Chief Clinical Affairs, University of Michigan Hospitals and Health Centers, Ann Arbor, MI, p. A307
CAMPBELL, David, Administrator, Perry Hospital, Perry, GA, p. A157
CAMPBELL, Dean, Vice President Information Services and Chief Information Officer, Good Samaritan Hospital, Los Angeles, CA, p. A69
CAMPBELL, Deborah, Administrator, Thomas H. Boyd Memorial Hospital, Carrollton, IL, p. A174
CAMPBELL, Don, M.D. Senior Vice President and Chief Medical Officer, WellStar Cobb Hospital, Austell, GA, p. A147
CAMPBELL, Emily, Director Human Resources, Alice Hyde Medical Center, Malone, NY, p. A429
CAMPBELL, Eric, Chief Financial Officer, Oswego Hospital, Oswego, NY, p. A440

Index of Health Care Professionals
Index of Health Care Professionals / Campbell

CAMPBELL, Fritz, Director Information Systems, Olympia Medical Center, Los Angeles, CA, p. A71
CAMPBELL, Gayla, Chief Executive Officer, Kindred Hospital–Oklahoma City, Oklahoma City, OK, p. A501
CAMPBELL, Ginger, Senior Vice President and Area Manager, Walnut Creek Medical Center, Walnut Creek, CA, p. A95
CAMPBELL, John
Director Management Information Systems, Spaulding Rehabilitation Hospital, Boston, MA, p. A297
Chief Information Officer, Spaulding Rehabilitation Hospital Cape Cod, East Sandwich, MA, p. A299
CAMPBELL, Karen M., Director Finance, Bigfork Valley Hospital, Bigfork, MN, p. A328
CAMPBELL, Kevin, Administrator Compliance and Mission, Hickman Community Hospital, Centerville, TN, p. A563
CAMPBELL, Lewis, Executive Director, Capital District Psychiatric Center, Albany, NY, p. A420
CAMPBELL, Margaret, Vice President, Associate Chief Information Officer, Health Alliance Hospitals, Leominster, MA, p. A301
CAMPBELL, Patricia
Director Employee Relations, SSM DePaul Health Center, Bridgeton, MO, p. A356
Vice President Human Resources, SSM St. Clare Health Center, Fenton, MO, p. A359
CAMPBELL, Phil, Chief Operating Officer, King's Daughters Medical Center, Brookhaven, MS, p. A344
CAMPBELL, Richard, M.D. President Medical Staff, Comanche County Memorial Hospital, Lawton, OK, p. A498
CAMPBELL, Richard, D.O. Chief of Staff, Community Hospital, Torrington, WY, p. A698
CAMPBELL Jr., Robert D.
President and Chief Executive, Providence Mount Carmel Hospital, Colville, WA, p. A660
President and Chief Executive, Providence St. Joseph's Hospital, Chewelah, WA, p. A660
CAMPBELL, Rose, R.N. President, Brookville Hospital, Brookville, PA, p. A519
CAMPBELL, Sandra M., R.N. Chief Nursing Officer, Dodge County Hospital, Eastman, GA, p. A152
CAMPBELL, Stephen J., Chief Operating Officer, Pioneers Memorial Healthcare District, Brawley, CA, p. A56
CAMPBELL, Susie, Chief Executive Officer, Community Memorial Hospital, Staunton, IL, p. A194
CAMPBELL, Teresa L., Chief Nurse Executive, Sutter Lakeside Hospital, Lakeport, CA, p. A66
CAMPBELL, Todd, Senior Vice President and Chief Operating Officer, St. Mary's Medical Center, Huntington, WV, p. A673
CAMPION, John, Chief Financial Officer, Essentia Health–Holy Trinity Hospital, Graceville, MN, p. A332
CAMPO, Linda, Director Human Resources, Spring Hill Regional Hospital, Spring Hill, FL, p. A139
CAMPOS, Christina, Administrator, Guadalupe County Hospital, Santa Rosa, NM, p. A418
CAMPOS–DIAZ, Evelyn, Director Human Resources, Medstar St. Mary's Hospital, Leonardtown, MD, p. A293
CANADY, Carolyn, Chief Financial Officer, Sierra Nevada Memorial Hospital, Grass Valley, CA, p. A64
CANALE, Joseph, Business Manager, Trenton Psychiatric Hospital, Trenton, NJ, p. A411
CANALEJO, Donald, Director Human Resources, Lower Keys Medical Center, Key West, FL, p. A127
CANARD, R. Shannon, Chief Executive Officer, Select Specialty Hospital–Jackson, Jackson, MS, p. A348
CANARIOS, Mike, Vice President and Chief Financial Officer, St. Jude Children's Research Hospital, Memphis, TN, p. A572
CANAVAN, Patrick J., PsyD, Chief Executive Officer, St. Elizabeths Hospital, Washington, DC, p. A117
CANCILLA, Deborah, Chief Information Officer, Grady Memorial Hospital, Atlanta, GA, p. A145
CANDIA, Gary R., FACHE Chief Executive Officer, Abington Health Lansdale Hospital, Lansdale, PA, p. A527
CANDILL, James W., M.D. President Medical Staff, Eye and Ear Clinic of Charleston, Charleston, WV, p. A671
CANDIO, Christine, Chief Executive Officer, Inova Alexandria Hospital, Alexandria, VA, p. A645
CANDULLO, Carl, Chief Information Officer, Munroe Regional Medical Center, Ocala, FL, p. A133
CANEDO, Jim, Chief Financial Officer, Pacific Hospital of Long Beach, Long Beach, CA, p. A68
CANFIELD, Brian, Commander, Womack Army Medical Center, Fort Bragg, NC, p. A453
CANIZARO, Tom, Vice President and Chief Financial Officer, South Central Regional Medical Center, Laurel, MS, p. A348
CANN–TAYLOR, Julie, R.N. Chief Operating Officer, Senior Vice President Patient Care Services and Chief Nursing Officer, Wyoming Medical Center, Casper, WY, p. A695
CANNIDA, Ieesha, Director Human Resources, Reliant Rehabilitation Hospital Dallas, Dallas, TX, p. A592
CANNING, John, Chief Financial Officer, Blythedale Children's Hospital, Valhalla, NY, p. A445
CANNON, C. Ron, M.D. Medical Director, River Oaks Hospital, Flowood, MS, p. A345
CANNON, Gayle, Director Human Resources, Childress Regional Medical Center, Childress, TX, p. A587
CANNON, Linda, Chief Medical Records Services, San Diego County Psychiatric Hospital, San Diego, CA, p. A85
CANOVA, Jr., Frank, Chief Financial Officer, CHRISTUS Health Shreveport–Bossier, Shreveport, LA, p. A277
CANOVACA, Frank, Director Management Information Systems, Metropolitan Hospital of Miami, Miami, FL, p. A131
CANTER, Danny, Manager Information Systems, Doctors Hospital Nelsonville, Nelsonville, OH, p. A486
CANTEY, Larry D., M.D. Chief Medical Officer, Fairfield Memorial Hospital, Winnsboro, SC, p. A554
CANTLEY, J. Scott, President and Chief Executive Officer, Marietta Memorial Hospital, Marietta, OH, p. A483
CANTON, David, D.O. Vice President Medical Affairs, Emanuel Medical Center, Turlock, CA, p. A93
CANTRELL, Dedra
Chief Information Officer, Emory University Hospital, Atlanta, GA, p. A145
Chief Information Officer, Emory University Hospital Midtown, Atlanta, GA, p. A145
Chief Information Officer, Wesley Woods Geriatric Hospital of Emory University, Atlanta, GA, p. A146
CANTRELL, Gary, President and Chief Executive Officer, St. Lucie Medical Center, Port St. Lucie, FL, p. A137
CANTU, Ray, D.O. Chief of Staff, Rice Medical Center, Eagle Lake, TX, p. A595
CANTU–LOPEZ, Lydia, Human Resources Representative, Solara Hospital Harlingen, Harlingen, TX, p. A602
CANVER, Charles, M.D. Chief Medical Officer, Provena United Samaritans Medical Center, Danville, IL, p. A179
CAPECE Jr., Vincent G., President and Chief Executive Officer, Middlesex Hospital, Middletown, CT, p. A110
CAPITELLI, Robert, M.D. Senior Vice President and Chief Medical Officer, St. Tammany Parish Hospital, Covington, LA, p. A265
CAPIZZI, Jennifer, Director Human Resources, H. B. Magruder Memorial Hospital, Port Clinton, OH, p. A487
CAPLAN, Marcie S., Vice President, UPMC Passavant, Pittsburgh, PA, p. A535
CAPLES, Greg, Chief Operating Officer, Summit Medical Center, Hermitage, TN, p. A566
CAPODIFERRO, Joseph, Chief Human and Learning Resources, Veterans Affairs New Jersey Health Care System, East Orange, NJ, p. A403
CAPPEL, Blaine, Director Information Systems, Memorial Health System, Abilene, KS, p. A230
CAPPELLO, Roger, M.D. Vice President Medical Affairs, Bon Secours Memorial Regional Medical Center, Mechanicsville, VA, p. A651
CAPPELLO, Thomas A., FACHE Director, Veterans Affairs Medical Center, Lake City, FL, p. A128
CAPPS, Kim, Chief Financial Officer, Hayes Green Beach Memorial Hospital, Charlotte, MI, p. A309
CAPPS, Rick, Chief Financial Officer, Cumberland County Hospital, Burkesville, KY, p. A248
CAPUANO, Terry Ann, R.N
Chief Operating Officer, Lehigh Valley Hospital, Allentown, PA, p. A517
Chief Operating Officer, Lehigh Valley Hospital–Muhlenberg, Bethlehem, PA, p. A518
CARACCIOLO, Kevin, Chief Human Resources Officer, Palm Beach Gardens Medical Center, Palm Beach Gardens, FL, p. A135
CARBALLO, Francisco R., M.D. Medical Director, Hospital HMA de Humacao, Humacao, PR, p. A701
CARBALLO, Jose E., Chief Executive Officer and Managing Director, Hospital San Pablo, Bayamon, PR, p. A700
CARBONE, Davide M., FACHE Chief Executive Officer, St. Mary's Medical Center, West Palm Beach, FL, p. A143
CARBONEL MASON, Wilma, Chief Nursing Officer, Fort Duncan Regional Medical Center, Eagle Pass, TX, p. A595
CARD, Dean, Chief Financial Officer, Kindred Hospital South Florida–Fort Lauderdale, Fort Lauderdale, FL, p. A123
CARDA, Greg, Chief Operating Officer, Poplar Bluff Regional Medical Center, Poplar Bluff, MO, p. A367
CARDALI, Paul, M.D. Chief of Staff, Lakeway Regional Hospital, Morristown, TN, p. A572
CARDAMONE, Stephen, D.O. Senior Vice President and Chief Medical Officer, Wheaton Franciscan Healthcare – The Wisconsin Heart Hospital, Wauwatosa, WI, p. A693
CARDEN, Lamar, M.D. Chief Medical Officer, Jack Hughston Memorial Hospital, Phenix City, AL, p. A25
CARDENAS, Mark, Director Plant Operations, Northern California Rehabilitation Hospital, Redding, CA, p. A82
CARDENAS, Michael E., M.D. Director Medical Services, Naval Hospital, Twentynine Palms, CA, p. A93
CARDENAS, Mitzi
Chief Information Officer, Truman Medical Center–Hospital Hill, Kansas City, MO, p. A363
Chief Information Officer, Truman Medical Center–Lakewood, Kansas City, MO, p. A363
CARDENAS, Noel J., FACHE Commander, San Antonio Military Medical Center, Fort Sam Houston, TX, p. A598
CARDILE, Eileen K., MS, President and Chief Executive Officer, Underwood–Memorial Hospital, Woodbury, NJ, p. A412
CARDIN, Deborah, MS, Chief Executive Officer, Jefferson County Health Center, Fairfield, IA, p. A219
CARDWELL, Marian, Chief Financial Officer, Potomac Valley Hospital, Keyser, WV, p. A673
CAREY, Ann, Vice President and Chief Information Officer, St. Vincent's Medical Center Riverside, Jacksonville, FL, p. A127
CAREY, Anne, Chief Nursing Officer, Heart of Florida Regional Medical Center, Davenport, FL, p. A121
CAREY, Bruce, Chief Executive Officer, Kindred Chicago–Central Hospital, Chicago, IL, p. A176
CAREY, Calvin, VP Finance and Support Services, Holy Rosary Healthcare, Miles City, MT, p. A377
CAREY, Debra D.
Chief Executive Officer, SUNY Downstate Medical Center University Hospital of Brooklyn,, NY, p. A437
Interim Chief Executive Officer, University Hospital of Brooklyn at Long Island College Hospital,, NY, p. A437
CAREY, Eric R., Vice President Information Systems and Chief Information Officer, Valley Hospital, Ridgewood, NJ, p. A409
CARGONARA, Douglas, Ph.D. Chief Information Officer, Pilgrim Psychiatric Center, Brentwood, NY, p. A422
CARIKER, Ann, Chief Operating Officer, Northeastern Nevada Regional Hospital, Elko, NV, p. A391
CARIKER, Kelly, Manager, Mid–Valley Hospital, Omak, WA, p. A663
CARISSIMI, Derek, Vice President Human Resources, Georgia Health Sciences Medical Center, Augusta, GA, p. A146
CARLE, Chris, Senior Vice President and Chief Operating Officer, St. Elizabeth Florence, Florence, KY, p. A250
CARLETON, David
Chief Information Officer, Heritage Valley Beaver, Beaver, PA, p. A518
Chief Information Officer, Sewickley Valley Hospital, (A Division of Valley Medical Facilities), Sewickley, PA, p. A538
CARLINO, James, Vice President Human Resources, Deborah Heart and Lung Center, Browns Mills, NJ, p. A402
CARLISLE, Charles, Director, East Mississippi State Hospital, Meridian, MS, p. A350
CARLISLE, Harald, Acting Chief Information Officer, Veterans Affairs Medical Center, Birmingham, AL, p. A17
CARLISLE, Mary Beth, Chief Executive Officer, Mildred Mitchell–Bateman Hospital, Huntington, WV, p. A672
CARLISLE, Sandy, Manager Human Resources, Holzer Medical Center – Jackson, Jackson, OH, p. A482
CARLOCK, Carey, Chief Executive Officer, Riveredge Hospital, Forest Park, IL, p. A182
CARLSON, Andrew, M.D. Vice President Medical Staff Services, Phoebe Sumter Medical Center, Americus, GA, p. A144
CARLSON, Bev, Chief Financial Officer, Delta County Memorial Hospital, Delta, CO, p. A99
CARLSON, Brian J., FACHE President and Chief Executive Officer, Lake View Memorial Hospital, Two Harbors, MN, p. A340
CARLSON, Carol, Director Marketing, Memorial Health Care Systems, Seward, NE, p. A389
CARLSON, Dan, Chief Financial Officer, Bay Area Medical Center, Marinette, WI, p. A685
CARLSON, Daniel, M.D
Senior Vice President and Chief Medical Officer, Leesburg Regional Medical Center, Leesburg, FL, p. A129
Senior Vice President Medical Affairs and Chief Medical Officer, The Villages Health System, The Villages, FL, p. A142
CARLSON, David J., D.O. Chief Medical Officer, Memorial Medical Center, Johnstown, PA, p. A526
CARLSON, Jamie N., Chief Human Resources Officer, Nebraska Heart Institute and Heart Hospital, Lincoln, NE, p. A385
CARLSON, Jeffrey, Chief Executive Officer, Mayo Clinic Health System in Waseca, Waseca, MN, p. A341
CARLSON, Kellie, Director Human Resources, Coastal Harbor Treatment Center, Savannah, GA, p. A159
CARLSON, Kim
Director Human Resources, Essentia Health Northern Pines, Aurora, MN, p. A328
Manager Human Resources, FirstLight Health System, Mora, MN, p. A336
CARLSON, Kurt, Chief Executive Officer, Otis R Bowen Center for Human Services, Warsaw, IN, p. A213

A778 Index of Health Care Professionals

Index of Health Care Professionals / Carter

Index of Health Care Professionals


CARLSON, Lisa, Chief Financial Officer, Sanford Medical Center Fargo, Fargo, ND, p. A465
CARLSON, Nancy
Chief Financial Officer, Crawford County Memorial Hospital, Denison, IA, p. A218
Chief Executive, Providence Little Company of Mary Medical Center San Pedro,, CA, p. A71
CARLSON, Pam, Senior Vice President and Chief Nursing Officer, Phoenix Children's Hospital, Phoenix, AZ, p. A36
CARLSON, Peter, Administrator, Aurora Psychiatric Hospital, Wauwatosa, WI, p. A693
CARLSON, Richard, Chief Financial Officer, Crawford Memorial Hospital, Robinson, IL, p. A192
CARLSON, Roland R., President and Chief Executive Officer, Pana Community Hospital, Pana, IL, p. A190
CARLSON, Stephen, M.D. President Medical Staff, St. Joseph's Hospital, Chippewa Falls, WI, p. A680
CARLSON, Stephen G., President and Chief Executive Officer, Community Medical Center, Missoula, MT, p. A377
CARLSON, Todd, M.D. Chief Medical Officer, Jefferson Healthcare, Port Townsend, WA, p. A664
CARLYLE, Dave, Director Human Resources, Wayne County Hospital, Corydon, IA, p. A217
CARMACK, Timothy W., Chief Financial Officer, Lucile Salter Packard Children's Hospital at Stanford, Palo Alto, CA, p. A79
CARMAIN, Jim, Vice President Financial and Information Services, Western Baptist Hospital, Paducah, KY, p. A257
CARMAN, Thomas H., President and Chief Executive Officer, Samaritan Medical Center, Watertown, NY, p. A446
CARMEN, Lee, Associate Vice President Health Care Information Systems, University of Iowa Hospitals and Clinics, Iowa City, IA, p. A221
CARMEN, Robert G., President, Adventist Health, Roseville, CA, p. B4
CARMICHAEL, Cindy, Interim Chief Executive Officer, Watonga Municipal Hospital, Watonga, OK, p. A507
CARMICHAEL, Craig, Vice President, Operations, St. Joseph Medical Center, Towson, MD, p. A294
CARMICHAEL, Lou Ann, Director Operations, South Lincoln Medical Center, Kemmerer, WY, p. A696
CARMIN, Ron, Vice President Fiscal Affairs, Mary Rutan Hospital, Bellefontaine, OH, p. A470
CARMODY, James, Vice President Human Resources, Wilkes–Barre General Hospital, Wilkes–Barre, PA, p. A542
CARMODY, Jane, R.N
Chief Nursing Officer, Alegent Health–Bergan Mercy Medical Center, Omaha, NE, p. A387
VP/Chief Nursing Executive, Alegent Health–Lakeside Hospital, Omaha, NE, p. A387
Chief Nursing Officer, Alegent Health–Mercy Hospital, Council Bluffs, IA, p. A217
CARMODY, Kerry, Chief Executive Officer, Providence Saint Joseph Medical Center, Burbank, CA, p. A56
CARNATHAN, Glenn, Vice President Human Resources, Baptist Hospital, Pensacola, FL, p. A136
CARNES, Ruth, Manager Human Resources, Jennings American Legion Hospital, Jennings, LA, p. A268
CARNEVALE, Raymond, Senior Vice President and Chief Operating Officer, Rome Memorial Hospital, Rome, NY, p. A442
CARNEY, Kevin, Senior Information Systems Analyst, Pine Creek Medical Center, Dallas, TX, p. A592
CARNEY, Michael J., Chief Executive Officer, Brentwood Behavioral HealthCare of Mississippi, Jackson, MS, p. A347
CARNEY, Stephen, M.D. Chief of Staff, Parkview Community Hospital Medical Center, Riverside, CA, p. A82
CARO, Vique, Chief Information Officer, Veterans Affairs Medical Center, Cincinnati, OH, p. A474
CAROL, Karin, Chief Operating Officer, Atlantic Shores Hospital, Fort Lauderdale, FL, p. A123
CAROLUS, Rhonda, Director of Nursing Operations, Northern Colorado Rehabilitation Hospital, Johnstown, CO, p. A102
CARON, Jacqueline, Chief Human Resources, Veterans Affairs Medical Center, Birmingham, AL, p. A17
CARON, Phillip A.
Chief Financial Officer, East Texas Medical Center Henderson, Henderson, TX, p. A603
Chief Financial Officer, East Texas Medical Center Jacksonville, Jacksonville, TX, p. A609
CARON Jr.,, William L., President, MaineHealth, Portland, ME, p. B83
CAROSELLI, Joseph P., Chief Executive Officer, Elks Rehab Hospital, Boise, ID, p. A166
CAROZZA, Sally, Director Human Resources, Western Pennsylvania Hospital, Pittsburgh, PA, p. A536
CARPEL, Emmett, M.D. Medical Director and Chief of Staff, Phillips Eye Institute, Minneapolis, MN, p. A335
CARPENTER, Curt, Manager Information Technology, Coquille Valley Hospital, Coquille, OR, p. A510
CARPENTER, Dan, Chief Financial Officer, Finley Hospital, Dubuque, IA, p. A219
CARPENTER, Dennis, Director Human Resources, Boscobel Area Health Care, Boscobel, WI, p. A679
CARPENTER, Elizabeth, Director Quality Assurance and Quality Improvement and Assistant Administrator, Promise Hospital of Miss Lou, Vidalia, LA, p. A279
CARPENTER, Jackie, Office Manager, Rock County Hospital, Bassett, NE, p. A381
CARPENTER, Kayla, Health Information Management Systems Officer, Northwest Mississippi Regional Medical Center, Clarksdale, MS, p. A344
CARPENTER, Leah A., Chief Executive Officer, Memorial Hospital Miramar, Miramar, FL, p. A132
CARPENTER, M. Troy, Chief Financial Officer, Kindred Hospital–Tucson, Tucson, AZ, p. A40
CARPENTER, Posie, MSN, Chief Administrative Officer, Santa Monica–UCLA Medical Center and Orthopaedic Hospital, Santa Monica, CA, p. A90
CARPENTER III,, William F., Chairman and Chief Executive Officer, LifePoint Hospitals, Inc., Brentwood, TN, p. B80
CARPER, Joleen, Director Quality and Risk, Tri–State Memorial Hospital, Clarkston, WA, p. A660
CARR, Charles E., Chief Executive Officer, Carilion Stonewall Jackson Hospital, Lexington, VA, p. A650
CARR, David, M.D. Physician Medical Director, The Rehabilitation Institute of St. Louis, Saint Louis, MO, p. A370
CARR, Deborah, Vice President Human Resources, Orange Regional Medical Center, Middletown, NY, p. A430
CARR, Diane
Chief Information Officer, Jacobi Medical Center,, NY, p. A433
Chief Information Officer, North Central Bronx Hospital,, NY, p. A436
CARR, Kevin, M.D. Chief of Staff, Southwest Health Center, Platteville, WI, p. A689
CARR, Randall, Director Human Resources, Parkwest Medical Center, Knoxville, TN, p. A568
CARR, Tim, Chief Financial Officer, Methodist Ambulatory Surgery Hospital, San Antonio, TX, p. A625
CARRANZA, Diana, Associate Director, Veterans Affairs Illiana Health Care System, Danville, IL, p. A179
CARRASCO, Anthony, Director Information Systems, Tri–City Regional Medical Center, Hawaiian Gardens, CA, p. A64
CARRASQUILLO, Carmen, M.D. Medical Director, Industrial Hospital, San Juan, PR, p. A703
CARREN, Donald M., Information Technology Leader, Anaheim Medical Center, Anaheim, CA, p. A53
CARRERA, Lavern H., Senior Vice President Human Resources, Northside Medical Center, Youngstown, OH, p. A492
CARRERO, Milton D., M.D. Medical Director, Dr. Ramon E. Betances Hospital–Mayaguez Medical Center Branch, Mayaguez, PR, p. A702
CARRIER, Lynn, Associate Director Administration and Support, Veterans Affairs Greater Los Angeles Healthcare System, Los Angeles, CA, p. A72
CARRIER, Patrick Brian, President and Chief Executive Officer, CHRISTUS Santa Rosa Health Care, San Antonio, TX, p. A624
CARRILLO, Irma, Director Human Resources, Ashford Presbyterian Community Hospital, San Juan, PR, p. A702
CARRILLO, Todd, Chief Information Officer, Yoakum County Hospital, Denver City, TX, p. A594
CARRILLO, Zulema, Chief Executive Officer, El Paso Psychiatric Center, El Paso, TX, p. A596
CARRINGER, Rick, Vice President Finance and Support Services, LeConte Medical Center, Sevierville, TN, p. A575
CARRISON, Dale, M.D. Chief of Staff, University Medical Center, Las Vegas, NV, p. A394
CARRITHERS, Mary Kay, Manager Health Information, Warren Memorial Hospital, Friend, NE, p. A383
CARROCINO, Joanne, FACHE President and Chief Executive Officer, Cape Regional Medical Center, Cape May Court House, NJ, p. A402
CARROLL, Allen P., Senior Vice President and Chief Executive Officer, Bon Secours St. Francis Hospital, Charleston, SC, p. A547
CARROLL, Dale, M.D. Senior Vice President Medical Affairs and Performance Improvement, Rockingham Memorial Hospital, Harrisonburg, VA, p. A649
CARROLL, David W., Chief Financial Officer, O'Connor Hospital, San Jose, CA, p. A88
CARROLL, Jack, Senior Director Human Resources, Spaulding Hospital for Continuing Medical Care Cambridge, Cambridge, MA, p. A299
CARROLL, Jack A., Ph.D. President and Chief Executive Officer, Magee Rehabilitation Hospital, Philadelphia, PA, p. A533
CARROLL, Jacqueline, Director Human Resources, Los Alamos Medical Center, Los Alamos, NM, p. A417
CARROLL, Jaime, Department Head, Walter Reed National Military Medical Center, Bethesda, MD, p. A290
CARROLL, James H., Chief Information Officer, St. John Medical Center, Westlake, OH, p. A491
CARROLL, Jason, Administrator and Chief Executive Officer, Leesville Rehabilitation Hospital, Leesville, LA, p. A272
CARROLL, Lawrence H., Director, Veterans Affairs Medical Center, San Francisco, CA, p. A87
CARROLL, Marsha, Director Financial Services, Screven County Hospital, Sylvania, GA, p. A160
CARROLL, Michael W., Administrator, Richland Parish Hospital, Delhi, LA, p. A265
CARROLL, Patricia, Senior Vice President and Chief Operating Officer, Saint Peter's University Hospital, New Brunswick, NJ, p. A407
CARROLL, Peggy, Chief Information Officer, Palos Community Hospital, Palos Heights, IL, p. A190
CARROLL, Richard, M.D
Chief Medical officer, Adventist Bolingbrook Hospital, Bolingbrook, IL, p. A174
Chief Medical Officer, Adventist GlenOaks Hospital, Glendale Heights, IL, p. A183
CARROLL, Sandy, Coordinator Human Resources, Norman Specialty Hospital, Norman, OK, p. A500
CARROLL, Susan, Chief Operating Officer, Inova Loudoun Hospital, Leesburg, VA, p. A650
CARROLL, Terri L., Vice President Financial Services, Hillsboro Area Hospital, Hillsboro, IL, p. A184
CARROLL, Tim, Chief Information Officer, Sunrise Canyon Hospital, Lubbock, TX, p. A614
CARROLL, Velma
Chief Information Officer, Augusta Health, Fishersville, VA, p. A648
Interim Chief Information Officer, Prince William Hospital, Manassas, VA, p. A651
CARRON, Patrick E., FACHE President and Chief Executive Officer, Perry County Memorial Hospital, Perryville, MO, p. A366
CARRUTH, Claude, Vice President and Chief Financial Officer, Henry Medical Center, Stockbridge, GA, p. A160
CARRUTH, Gregory, Head Information Management, Naval Hospital, Oak Harbor, WA, p. A663
CARRUTH, John M., Chief Executive Officer, Decatur County General Hospital, Parsons, TN, p. A574
CARRUTH, Keith, Chief Executive Officer, Regency Hospital of Covington, Covington, LA, p. A265
CARSON, Christine, Vice President Human Resources, St. Vincent Medical Center, Los Angeles, CA, p. A72
CARSON, Debbie, Director Human Resources, Promise Hospital of Vicksburg, Vicksburg, MS, p. A353
CARSON, Gregory W., Administrator, U. S. Air Force Clinic, Mountain Home AFB, ID, p. A169
CARSON, Jim, Director Human Resources, Henry County Health Center, Mount Pleasant, IA, p. A223
CARSON, Joe, Director Human Resources, Glen Oaks Hospital, Greenville, TX, p. A601
CARSON, Kara Jo, Chief Financial Officer, Pinckneyville Community Hospital, Pinckneyville, IL, p. A191
CARSON, Mitchell C., President and Chief Executive Officer, Longmont United Hospital, Longmont, CO, p. A104
CARSON, Terry M., Chief Executive Officer, Harrison Community Hospital, Cadiz, OH, p. A471
CARTER, Bruce C., President, United Hospital Center, Bridgeport, WV, p. A670
CARTER, Charla, Director Human Resources, Uvalde County Hospital Authority, Uvalde, TX, p. A632
CARTER, Cindy, Chief Nursing Officer, Northeast Regional Medical Center, Kirksville, MO, p. A363
CARTER, Dennis, M.D. Chief of Staff, Eastern Oklahoma Medical Center, Poteau, OK, p. A503
CARTER, Donna, MSN Chief Nursing Officer, Minden Medical Center, Minden, LA, p. A273
CARTER, Doug, Chief Financial Officer, Brookwood Medical Center, Birmingham, AL, p. A16
CARTER, Frank, Chief Financial Officer, Cornerstone Hospital of Huntington, Huntington, WV, p. A672
CARTER, Gary L., M.D. Medical Director of Quality, North Kansas City Hospital, North Kansas City, MO, p. A366
CARTER, Jason, Chief Executive Officer, Warm Springs Specialty Hospital, Luling, TX, p. A615
CARTER, Jessica Y., Chief Financial Officer, Crisp Regional Hospital, Cordele, GA, p. A150
CARTER, Lauren, Associate Administrator, Guadalupe Regional Medical Center, Seguin, TX, p. A627
CARTER, Len, Vice President Human Resources, FHN Memorial Hospital, Freeport, IL, p. A182
CARTER, Marcia, Director Human Resources, Bluegrass Community Hospital, Versailles, KY, p. A259
CARTER, Michael J., Chief Executive Officer, Memorial Hospital and Physician Group, Frederick, OK, p. A497
CARTER, Misty, Director Human Resources, Great Plains Regional Medical Center, Elk City, OK, p. A496

CARTER, Montez
Interim President and Chief Executive Officer, Good Samaritan Hospital, Greensboro, GA, p. A153
Vice President Operations, St. Mary's Health Care System, Athens, GA, p. A144
CARTER, Nebo, Chief Human Resources Officer, Singing River Health System, Pascagoula, MS, p. A351
CARTER, Priscilla, Chief Financial Officer, Mesa Hills Specialty Hospital, El Paso, TX, p. A596
CARTER, Rebecca W., MSN Vice President Patient Care and Chief Operating Officer, Transylvania Regional Hospital, Brevard, NC, p. A449
CARTER, Richard, District Chief Executive Officer, Hunt Memorial Hospital District, Greenville, TX, p. A602
CARTER, Richard, M.D. Chief Executive Officer, Physicians' Hospital in Anadarko, Anadarko, OK, p. A493
CARTER, Richard G., Chief Executive Officer, Valley View Medical Center, Fort Mohave, AZ, p. A32
CARTER, Scott, Chief Operating Officer, Center for Behavioral Medicine, Kansas City, MO, p. A361
CARTER, Teresa, Vice President and Chief Operating Officer, Medical Park Hospital, Winston–Salem, NC, p. A463
CARTER–ROBERTSON, Kira, Chief Executive Officer, Sparrow Specialty Hospital, Lansing, MI, p. A317
CARTHEW, Edward
Chief Human Resources Officer, Saint Joseph East, Lexington, KY, p. A253
Chief Human Resources Officer, Saint Joseph Hospital, Lexington, KY, p. A253
CARTWRIGHT, David, Director Management Information Systems, Danville Regional Medical Center, Danville, VA, p. A647
CARTWRIGHT, David A., Vice President Finance, Advocate Condell Medical Center, Libertyville, IL, p. A186
CARTWRIGHT, Kay B., R.N. Vice President and Chief Nursing Officer, Reid Hospital and Health Care Services, Richmond, IN, p. A211
CARTWRIGHT, Thomas, M.D. Chief of Staff, Witham Memorial Hospital, Lebanon, IN, p. A207
CARTY, Steven D., Chief Executive Officer, Mineral Community Hospital, Superior, MT, p. A379
CARUCCI, Dean, Chief Operating Officer, Overland Park Regional Medical Center, Overland Park, KS, p. A241
CARUGATI, Diane, Chief Operating Officer, Friends Hospital, Philadelphia, PA, p. A532
CARUSO, Charles, Chief Information Officer, Henrietta D. Goodall Hospital, Sanford, ME, p. A285
CARUSO, Diane M., MSN Chief Nursing Officer, HEALTHSOUTH Scottsdale Rehabilitation Hospital, Scottsdale, AZ, p. A38
CARUSO, Don, M.D. Chief Medical Officer, Cheshire Medical Center, Keene, NH, p. A398
CARUSO, Michael J., President and Chief Executive Officer, Ohio Valley Health Services and Education Corporation, Wheeling, WV, p. B98
CARUSO, Michael J., Chief Operating Officer, Ohio Valley Medical Center, Wheeling, WV, p. A676
CARVALHO, Robert M., M.D. Medical Director, Aurora Vista Del Mar Hospital, Ventura, CA, p. A94
CARVER, Christy, Administrator, Integrity Transitional Hospital, Denton, TX, p. A593
CARVER, Glenna, R.N. Chief Executive Officer, Texas Specialty Hospital at Dallas, Dallas, TX, p. A593
CARVER, Leota, Chief Financial Officer, Caribou Memorial Hospital and Living Center, Soda Springs, ID, p. A170
CASABONA, Nicholas, Chief Information Officer, Winthrop–University Hospital, Mineola, NY, p. A430
CASADY, W. Stephen, M.D. Chief of Staff, Putnam County Memorial Hospital, Unionville, MO, p. A372
CASAGRANDE, Judith, Chief Operating Officer, Saints Medical Center, Lowell, MA, p. A301
CASALOU, Robert F.
President and Chief Executive Officer, St. Joseph Mercy Hospital, Ypsilanti, MI, p. A326
President and Chief Executive Officer, St. Joseph Mercy Livingston Hospital, Howell, MI, p. A315
CASANOVA, Mark, Vice President and Chief Operating Officer, CHRISTUS Spohn Hospital Alice, Alice, TX, p. A577
CASANOVA, Robert Bernier, Chief Financial Officer, Industrial Hospital, San Juan, PR, p. A703
CASAREZ, Margaret, Chief Financial Officer, San Joaquin Valley Rehabilitation Hospital, Fresno, CA, p. A62
CASAS, Catherine, Executive Director, Woodland Hills Medical Center,, CA, p. A73
CASAZZA, Jerri, Manager Human Resources, Greystone Park Psychiatric Hospital, Morris Plains, NJ, p. A406
CASCIARI, Raymond, M.D. Chief Medical Officer, St. Joseph Hospital, Orange, CA, p. A78
CASE, Beth, Vice President Human Resources, St. Mary's Healthcare, Amsterdam, NY, p. A420

CASE, Cliff, Chief Financial Officer, Mineral Community Hospital, Superior, MT, p. A379
CASE, Cora, Chief Financial Officer, Renown South Meadows Medical Center, Reno, NV, p. A395
CASE, Ed, Executive Vice President and Chief Financial Officer, Rehabilitation Institute of Chicago, Chicago, IL, p. A177
CASE, Harvey
President, Vidant Beaufort Hospital, Washington, NC, p. A462
President, Vidant Pungo Hospital, Belhaven, NC, p. A448
CASE–WIRTH, Jill, Vice President and Chief Nursing Officer, Theda Clark Medical Center, Neenah, WI, p. A687
CASERTA, Kevin, M.D. Chief Medical Officer, Providence Centralia Hospital, Centralia, WA, p. A660
CASEY, Dina, Human Resources Officer, Lane County Hospital, Dighton, KS, p. A232
CASEY, John P., Administrator, Shodair Children's Hospital, Helena, MT, p. A376
CASEY, Joseph, Chief Financial Officer, Sturdy Memorial Hospital, Attleboro, MA, p. A295
CASEY, Karen J., MS, President and Chief Executive Officer, Columbia Center, Mequon, WI, p. A686
CASEY, Richard J., Assistant Vice President Operations, NorthShore University Health System Skokie Hospital, Skokie, IL, p. A194
CASEY, Timothy M., President and Chief Executive Officer, Montgomery Hospital Medical Center, Norristown, PA, p. A530
CASH, Jeff, Senior Vice President and Chief Information Officer, Mercy Medical Center, Cedar Rapids, IA, p. A215
CASHMAN, Gene, Chief Executive Officer, Select Specialty Hospital–Columbus, Columbus, OH, p. A477
CASHMAN, Tim, Chief Financial Officer, Gunnison Valley Hospital, Gunnison, CO, p. A102
CASHWELL, David
Chief Operating Officer, Montgomery Regional Hospital, Blacksburg, VA, p. A646
Chief Operating Officer, Osceola Regional Medical Center, Kissimmee, FL, p. A127
CASIANO, Manuel, M.D. Vice President Medical Affairs, Frederick Memorial Hospital, Frederick, MD, p. A291
CASILLAS, Rosalind, Director of Nursing, Lawrence Memorial Hospital, Walnut Ridge, AR, p. A52
CASIMIR, Kenneth, M.D. Medical Director, Mendota Mental Health Institute, Madison, WI, p. A684
CASKEY, Paul, M.D. Chief of Staff, Shriners Hospitals for Children, Spokane, WA, p. A667
CASNER, Trina, Chief Financial Officer and Chief Operating Officer, Pana Community Hospital, Pana, IL, p. A190
CASON, Diane, Supervisor Personnel and Payroll, Lake Butler Hospital Hand Surgery Center, Lake Butler, FL, p. A128
CASON, Randall R., FACHE President and Chief Executive Officer, Via Christi Hospital, Pittsburg, KS, p. A241
CASON, Steven, Chief Information Officer, Putnam General Hospital, Eatonton, GA, p. A152
CASON, Will, Vice President Human Resources, St. Rita's Medical Center, Lima, OH, p. A483
CASPERSON, Sean, Chief Resource Management, Martin Army Community Hospital, Fort Benning, GA, p. A153
CASPERSON, William, M.D. Vice President Medical Affairs, Memorial Hospital, Belleville, IL, p. A173
CASS, Paul, D.O. Chief Medical & Clinical Integration Officer, Wentworth–Douglass Hospital, Dover, NH, p. A397
CASSADY, Craig, Director of Nursing, Wiregrass Medical Center, Geneva, AL, p. A21
CASSADY, Richard L., Chief Financial Officer, Specialty Hospital at Kimball, Lakewood, NJ, p. A405
CASSAGNE, Nancy R., FACHE Chief Executive Officer, West Jefferson Medical Center, Marrero, LA, p. A272
CASSARA, Pamela, Chief Financial Officer, MetroSouth Medical Center, Blue Island, IL, p. A174
CASSEDY, Ryan, Chief Executive Officer, HEALTHSOUTH Rehabilitation Hospital of Fort Smith, Fort Smith, AR, p. A45
CASSEL, Kari, Senior Vice President and Chief Information Officer, Shands Jacksonville Medical Center, Jacksonville, FL, p. A126
CASSELS, William H., Administrator, DCH Regional Medical Center, Tuscaloosa, AL, p. A26
CASSENS, Ray, Vice President and Chief Financial Officer, Texas Health Presbyterian Hospital Plano, Plano, TX, p. A621
CASSIDAY, Cheryl, R.N. Director of Nursing, Chadron Community Hospital and Health Services, Chadron, NE, p. A382
CASSIDY, Doris B., Associate Director, Veterans Health Care System of the Ozarks, Fayetteville, AR, p. A44
CASSIDY, Erin
Chief Executive Officer, Nexus Specialty Hospital, Shenandoah, TX, p. A627
Chief Executive Officer, Nexus Specialty Hospital The Woodlands, Spring, TX, p. A628

CASSIDY, Hugh, Administrator, United Medical Healthwest–New Orleans, Gretna, LA, p. A267
CASSIDY, John W., M.D. President, Chief Executive Officer and Chief Medical Officer, Nexus Health Systems, Houston, TX, p. B94
CASSIDY, Joseph J., Vice President, Holy Redeemer Hospital and Medical Center, Meadowbrook, PA, p. A528
CASSIDY, Lori W., FACHE Assistant Vice President, Medical Center of Central Georgia, Macon, GA, p. A155
CASSIDY, Louise, Chief Executive Officer, Kindred Hospital Easton, Easton, PA, p. A522
CASSIDY, Patricia
President, Gottlieb Memorial Hospital, Melrose Park, IL, p. A187
Interim President and Chief Executive Officer, Loyola University Medical Center, Maywood, IL, p. A187
CASTANEDA, Edmundo, Chief Executive Officer, Sierra Medical Center, El Paso, TX, p. A596
CASTANEDA, Marissa, Chief Operating Officer and Director Marketing, Doctor's Hospital at Renaissance, Edinburg, TX, p. A595
CASTEEL, Karen, Director Human Resources, Palms of Pasadena Hospital, Saint Petersburg, FL, p. A138
CASTEEL, Lisa, Chief Financial Officer, Henry County Medical Center, Paris, TN, p. A574
CASTEEL, Rick
Vice President Management Information Systems and Chief Information Officer, Harford Memorial Hospital, Havre De Grace, MD, p. A292
Vice President Management Information Systems and Chief Information Officer, Upper Chesapeake Medical Center, Bel Air, MD, p. A289
CASTELLANOS, Miguel, M.D. Chief of Staff, Baptist Orange Hospital, Orange, TX, p. A619
CASTELLO, Frank V., M.D. Medical Director, Children's Specialized Hospital, New Brunswick, NJ, p. A406
CASTELLO, Fred, M.D. Chief Medical Officer, Augusta Health, Fishersville, VA, p. A648
CASTELLO, Lauren, Director Human Resources, Trinity Hospital Twin City, Dennison, OH, p. A479
CASTERLINE, Carolyn, Financial Director, Roosevelt Medical Center, Culbertson, MT, p. A374
CASTILLO, Edgar, Chief Financial Officer, Larkin Community Hospital, South Miami, FL, p. A139
CASTILLO, Paul, Chief Financial Officer, University of Michigan Hospitals and Health Centers, Ann Arbor, MI, p. A307
CASTILLO, Ralph, Chief Executive Officer, Morgan Memorial Hospital, Madison, GA, p. A156
CASTLE, Christopher M., Commander, Dwight David Eisenhower Army Medical Center, Fort Gordon, GA, p. A153
CASTLE, Dorothy, Director Human Resources, North Mississippi Medical Center–Eupora, Eupora, MS, p. A345
CASTLE, Eric, Director Information Services, Lawnwood Regional Medical Center, Fort Pierce, FL, p. A124
CASTLE, Kenneth, Chief Information Officer, Easton Hospital, Easton, PA, p. A522
CASTLE, Samantha, Director Human Resources and Performance Improvement, Ridge Behavioral Health System, Lexington, KY, p. A253
CASTLEBERRY, David L., Chief Executive Officer, Upson Regional Medical Center, Thomaston, GA, p. A160
CASTLEBERRY, Debi
Director Information System, St. David's Medical Center, Austin, TX, p. A581
Director Information System, St. David's Rehabilitation Center, Austin, TX, p. A581
CASTLEBERRY, Ginger, Chief Operating Officer, Valir Rehabilitation Hospital, Oklahoma City, OK, p. A502
CASTO, Sara, Executive Secretary, Pocahontas Memorial Hospital, Buckeye, WV, p. A670
CASTOR, Susan, Chief Nursing Officer, HEALTHSOUTH Rehabilitation Hospital of Toms River, Toms River, NJ, p. A411
CASTRIOTTA, Ralph, M.D. Medical Director, Carolina Center for Behavioral Health, Greer, SC, p. A551
CASTRO, Ana, Director Information Services and Clinical Information Services, Gerald Champion Regional Medical Center, Alamogordo, NM, p. A414
CASTRO, Craig
Chief Executive Officer, Clovis Community Medical Center, Clovis, CA, p. A57
Chief Information Officer, Community Regional Medical Center, Fresno, CA, p. A62
CASTRO, Pete, D.O. Chief of Staff, Heart of Texas Memorial Hospital, Brady, TX, p. A584
CASTRO, Ruben, Associate Administrator and Facility Information Security Officer, North Hills Hospital, North Richland Hills, TX, p. A618
CASTRO, Yamila, Director Human Resources, Hialeah Hospital, Hialeah, FL, p. A125

Index of Health Care Professionals / Chambless

Index of Health Care Professionals

CASTROMAN, Nellie, Chief Executive Officer, Select Specialty Hospital–Orlando, Orlando, FL, p. A134
CASTRONOVA, Paul, Chief Information Officer, North Canyon Medical Center, Gooding, ID, p. A168
CASWELL, Lori, Director Information Technology, Good Samaritan Medical Center, Brockton, MA, p. A298
CATALA, Lucy, Vice President Finance, Baylor Medical Center at Irving, Irving, TX, p. A609
CATALANO, Robert A., M.D. Chief Medical Officer, St. Luke's–Roosevelt Hospital Center, New York, NY, p. A437
CATALDO, Linda, Human Resources Secretary, Prevost Memorial Hospital, Donaldsonville, LA, p. A266
CATALIOTTI, Palmira, Vice President, Chief Financial Officer and Treasurer, Winthrop–University Hospital, Mineola, NY, p. A430
CATANIA, Joe, Chief Executive Officer, St. Anthony's Rehabilitation Hospital, Lauderdale Lakes, FL, p. A129
CATAUDELLA, Mary
Corporate Director Human Resources, LibertyHealth–Jersey City Medical Center, Jersey City, NJ, p. A405
Corporate Director Human Resources, Meadowlands Hospital Medical Center, Secaucus, NJ, p. A410
CATE, Maurine, Chief Executive Officer, McKenzie–Willamette Medical Center, Springfield, OR, p. A515
CATENA, Cornelio R., President and Chief Executive Officer, Wilkes–Barre General Hospital, Wilkes–Barre, PA, p. A542
CATES, Erin, Director Human Resources, Hill Country Memorial Hospital, Fredericksburg, TX, p. A600
CATES, Gary, President and Chief Executive Officer, ProMedica Defiance Regional Hospital, Defiance, OH, p. A479
CATES, Jessica, Fiscal Manager, Western State Hospital, Hopkinsville, KY, p. A252
CATES, Rodney
Senior Vice President Human Resources, Covenant Children's Hospital, Lubbock, TX, p. A613
Senior Vice President Human Resources, Covenant Medical Center, Lubbock, TX, p. A613
CATHEY Jr., James E., President and Chief Executive Officer, North Oaks Medical Center, Hammond, LA, p. A267
CATHEY Jr.,, James E., Chief Executive Officer, North Oaks Health System, Hammond, LA, p. B95
CATHEY, Michele, Administrator and Chief Executive Officer, Hamilton General Hospital, Hamilton, TX, p. A602
CATHEY, Walt, Administrator, Covenant Specialty Hospital, Lubbock, TX, p. A613
CATLETT, Joan, Director Human Resources, Valley General Hospital, Monroe, WA, p. A663
CATLIN, Rexford, Chief Executive Officer, Endless Mountain Health Systems, Montrose, PA, p. A529
CATT, Susan, Director Human Resources, North Valley Hospital, Whitefish, MT, p. A380
CATTALANI, Mark, M.D. Clinical Director, Richard H. Hutchings Psychiatric Center, Syracuse, NY, p. A444
CATTELL, JoAnne, Chief Nursing Officer, St. Petersburg General Hospital, Saint Petersburg, FL, p. A138
CATUCCI, Paul
Administrative Director Human Resources, Bon Secours St. Francis Medical Center, Midlothian, VA, p. A651
Director Human Resources, Bon Secours St. Mary's Hospital, Richmond, VA, p. A654
CAUBLE, David, Chief Financial Officer, St. Vincent's Blount, Oneonta, AL, p. A24
CAUDEL, Katie, Controller, Advanced Healthcare Medical Center, Ellington, MO, p. A359
CAUDEL–LOGSDON, Debbie, Director Information System, T. J. Samson Community Hospital, Glasgow, KY, p. A250
CAUDILL, Ralph, Director Information Systems, St. Mary's Hospital, Centralia, IL, p. A174
CAUGHELL, David, M.D. Chief of Staff, Jane Phillips Nowata Health Center, Nowata, OK, p. A500
CAUGHEY, Michelle, M.D. Physician In Chief, South San Francisco Medical Center, South San Francisco, CA, p. A91
CAULTON, Darryl, Chief Financial Officer, University of Miami Hospital, Miami, FL, p. A132
CAUSEY, Cynthia, Associate Administrator Human and Mission Services, McLeod Medical Center Dillon, Dillon, SC, p. A549
CAVA, Anthony V., Executive Director, Bayshore Community Hospital, Holmdel, NJ, p. A405
CAVAGNARO III, Charles E., M.D. President and Chief Executive Officer, Wing Memorial Hospital and Medical Centers, Palmer, MA, p. A303
CAVANAGH, Dru, R.N
Vice President Patient Care Services and Chief Nursing Officer, Chenango Memorial Hospital, Norwich, NY, p. A438
Interim Chief Executive Officer, Delaware Valley Hospital, Walton, NY, p. A446
Interim Chief Executive Officer, Delaware Valley Hospital, Walton, NY, p. A446
CAVANAGH, James, Chief Information Officer, St. Joseph's Regional Medical Center, Paterson, NJ, p. A408
CAVANAUGH, James, Chief Finance Officer, Wm. Jennings Bryan Dorn Veterans Affairs Medical Center, Columbia, SC, p. A549
CAVANAUGH, Paul, Director Human Resources, Friends Hospital, Philadelphia, PA, p. A532
CAVANESS, Patricia, Chief Clinical Officer, Kindred Hospital–San Diego, San Diego, CA, p. A85
CAVE, Rogelio, M.D. Medical Director, Roseland Community Hospital, Chicago, IL, p. A177
CAVENEY, Timothy, Chief Financial Officer, South Shore Hospital, Chicago, IL, p. A178
CAVERNO, John
Chief Human Resources Officer, Excela Frick Hospital, Mount Pleasant, PA, p. A530
Chief Human Resources Officer, Excela Health Westmoreland Hospital, Greensburg, PA, p. A524
CAVES, Donald, President, Wild Rose Community Memorial Hospital, Wild Rose, WI, p. A694
CAWLEY, Kevin J., Chief Executive Officer, Sheridan Community Hospital, Sheridan, MI, p. A323
CAWLEY, Patrick J., M.D. Medical Director, MUSC Medical Center of Medical University of South Carolina, Charleston, SC, p. A547
CAWTHON, David, Director Financial Services, Roosevelt Warm Springs Institute for Rehabilitation, Warm Springs, GA, p. A161
CAYER, Gerald, Executive Vice President and Chief Operating Officer, Franklin Memorial Hospital, Farmington, ME, p. A283
CAZAYOUX, John, Chief Financial Officer, Pointe Coupee General Hospital, New Roads, LA, p. A275
CEBALLOS, Gloria, MS, Interim President, Laurel Regional Hospital, Laurel, MD, p. A293
CEBRIK, Michael M., M.D. Director Medical Staff, Veterans Home and Hospital, Rocky Hill, CT, p. A111
CECCHETTINI, Diane E., R.N. President and Chief Executive Officer, MultiCare Health System, Tacoma, WA, p. B92
CECCHETTINI, Diane E., R.N. President and Chief Executive Officer, MultiCare Tacoma General Hospital, Tacoma, WA, p. A668
CECCONI, Thomas E., President and Chief Executive Officer, Mercy Medical Center, Canton, OH, p. A472
CECIL, Bruce, Chief Financial Officer, Fresno Surgical Hospital, Fresno, CA, p. A62
CECIL, Jason, Chief Information Officer, Capital Region Medical Center, Jefferson City, MO, p. A361
CECIL, Jeffrey, M.D. Chief of Staff, Platte County Memorial Hospital, Wheatland, WY, p. A698
CECIL, Jon C.
Chief Human Resource Officer, Cape Coral Hospital, Cape Coral, FL, p. A120
Chief Human Resource Officer, Gulf Coast Medical Center, Fort Myers, FL, p. A123
Chief Human Resource Officer, Lee Memorial Hospital, Fort Myers, FL, p. A124
CEDENO, Arturo, M.D. Medical Director, Hospital Buen Samaritano, Aguadilla, PR, p. A699
CEDOTAL, Kiley P., Chief Executive Officer, ICON Hospital, Humble, TX, p. A608
CEHELYK, Bohdan, M.D. Chief Medical Officer, East Mountain Hospital, Belle Mead, NJ, p. A401
CEKALLA, Bernie, Manager Human Resources, Albany Area Hospital and Medical Center, Albany, MN, p. A327
CELANO, Julie, Vice President Human Resources, Brigham and Women's Hospital, Boston, MA, p. A296
CELIA, Marc, FACHE Chief Executive Officer, Memorial Hermann Surgical Hospital Kingwood, Kingwood, TX, p. A611
CELLA, Ann S., R.N. Senior Vice President, Patient Care Services, St. Francis Hospital, Roslyn, NY, p. A442
CELLA, Robert, M.D
Vice President Medical Affairs, Berkshire Medical Center, Pittsfield, MA, p. A303
Vice President Medical Affairs, St. Peter's Hospital, Albany, NY, p. A420
CELLETTI, David, Chief Executive Officer, Northcoast Behavioral Healthcare System, Northfield, OH, p. A486
CELLUCCI, Jeff, Interim Chief Executive Officer, Kindred Hospital Northwest Indiana, Hammond, IN, p. A203
CELUCH, Paul, Vice President Human Resources and Support Services, Verdugo Hills Hospital, Glendale, CA, p. A63
CEMENO, Michael J., Chief Information Officer, Waterbury Hospital, Waterbury, CT, p. A112
CENTENO, Robert, M.D. Chief Medical Officer, Governor Juan F. Louis Hospital, Christiansted, VI, p. A704
CEPERO, Jesus, R.N. Vice President Nursing and Chief Nursing Officer, Meritus Medical Center, Hagerstown, MD, p. A292
CERCEO, Richard, Executive Vice President and Chief Operating Officer, Mercy Hospital and Medical Center, Chicago, IL, p. A176
CERONE, Shane, President, Beaumont Hospital – Royal Oak, Royal Oak, MI, p. A322
CERULLO, Timothy J., Chief Operating Officer, Largo Medical Center, Largo, FL, p. A128
CERVANTES, Mary Ann, District Director Management Information Systems, Matagorda Regional Medical Center, Bay City, TX, p. A582
CERVINO, Noel A., President and Chief Executive Officer, Civista Health, La Plata, MD, p. A292
CERVONI, Tom, M.D. Chief of Staff, Pattie A. Clay Regional Medical Center, Richmond, KY, p. A258
CESCA, Ken, Vice President Human Resources, MidState Medical Center, Meriden, CT, p. A110
CHA, Vicky, Assistant Chief Executive Officer, Lake Granbury Medical Center, Granbury, TX, p. A601
CHABALKO, John, M.D. Medical Director, Select Specialty Hospital–Wilmington, Wilmington, DE, p. A115
CHABALOWSKI, Edward, Chief Financial Officer, Temple University Hospital, Philadelphia, PA, p. A534
CHABNER, David, Director Information Services, Sky Lakes Medical Center, Klamath Falls, OR, p. A511
CHABOT, Judy, R.N. Chief Nursing Officer, Placentia–Linda Hospital, Placentia, CA, p. A80
CHADHA, Beenu, Chief Financial Officer, San Ramon Regional Medical Center, San Ramon, CA, p. A89
CHADWICK, Lionel K., Chief Executive Officer, Hi–Desert Medical Center, Joshua Tree, CA, p. A65
CHADWICK, Sharon M., Director Human Resources, Arrowhead Hospital, Glendale, AZ, p. A32
CHAFFEE, Jacob, M.D. Chief Medical Officer, Coulee Medical Center, Grand Coulee, WA, p. A662
CHAFFIN, Angela, Director Human Resources, Northeastern Nevada Regional Hospital, Elko, NV, p. A391
CHAFFIN, Linda, Director Medical Review, Baptist Memorial Hospital–Booneville, Booneville, MS, p. A344
CHAFFIN, Robert A., President and Chief Executive Officer, Ottawa Regional Hospital and Healthcare Center, Ottawa, IL, p. A190
CHAGRASULIS, Robert, M.D. Chief of Staff, Calais Regional Hospital, Calais, ME, p. A282
CHAHANOVICH, Jen, Chief Operating Officer, Pali Momi Medical Center, Aiea, HI, p. A163
CHAILDIN, Roberta, Manager Human Resources, Parrish Medical Center, Titusville, FL, p. A142
CHAISSON, Greg, M.D. Chief Medical Staff, Thibodaux Regional Medical Center, Thibodaux, LA, p. A278
CHAISSON, Rebecca, Interim Chief Financial Officer, Methodist McKinney Hospital, McKinney, TX, p. A616
CHALIAN, Christopher, M.D. Medical Director, Casa Colina Hospital for Rehabilitative Medicine, Pomona, CA, p. A80
CHALK, Jackie, Director Human Resources, HEALTHSOUTH Rehabilitation Hospital, Largo, FL, p. A128
CHALMERS, Bryan, Chief Financial Officer, Memorial Hospital, Craig, CO, p. A99
CHALONER, Robert S., President and Chief Executive Officer, Southampton Hospital, Southampton, NY, p. A443
CHAMBERLAIN, Denise, Chief Financial Officer, Paradise Valley Hospital, Phoenix, AZ, p. A36
CHAMBERLAIN, Joe, Interim Chief Executive Officer, MedCentral Health System, Mansfield, OH, p. B86
CHAMBERLIN, Kim, Vice President Patient Services and Chief Nursing Officer, Mercy Medical Center–North Iowa, Mason City, IA, p. A223
CHAMBERLIN, William, M.D. Chief Medical Officer, University of Illinois Hospital & Health Sciences System, Chicago, IL, p. A179
CHAMBERS, Barry M., CPA Chief Financial Officer, Ochsner Medical Center–Baton Rouge, Baton Rouge, LA, p. A262
CHAMBERS, Bradley, President, Medstar Union Memorial Hospital, Baltimore, MD, p. A288
CHAMBERS, Erin, M.D. Chief Medical Officer, Patients' Choice Medical Center of Erin, Erin, TN, p. A565
CHAMBERS, Jodi, M.D. Chief Medical Officer, St. Anthony Hospital, Lakewood, CO, p. A103
CHAMBERS, Pamela, Chief Executive Officer, Great Bend Regional Hospital, Great Bend, KS, p. A233
CHAMBERS, Regina, Assistant Vice President Human Resource, Rome Memorial Hospital, Rome, NY, p. A442
CHAMBERS, Susan, M.D. Administrator, Greil Memorial Psychiatric Hospital, Montgomery, AL, p. A23
CHAMBLEE, Jane, Manager Human Resources, North Mississippi Medical Center–Iuka, Iuka, MS, p. A347
CHAMBLESS, Kent, Chief Information Officer, Cornerstone Hospital of Houston – Bellaire, Houston, TX, p. A603
CHAMBLESS, Lesley
Vice President Human Resources, Carolinas Medical Center–Lincoln, Lincolnton, NC, p. A456
Assistant Vice President Workforce Relations, Carolinas Medical Center–NorthEast, Concord, NC, p. A451
CHAMBLESS, Marcy, Manager Business Office, Carl Vinson Veterans Affairs Medical Center, Dublin, GA, p. A152

Index of Health Care Professionals
Index of Health Care Professionals / Champagne

CHAMPAGNE, Charles, Chief Financial Officer, Northeast Rehabilitation Hospital, Salem, NH, p. A400
CHAMPAVANNARATH, Vilakon, Director Information Systems, Bartow Regional Medical Center, Bartow, FL, p. A118
CHAMPION, Joshua I., Director, Florida Hospital–Flagler, Palm Coast, FL, p. A135
CHAN, Bruce, Director Business Planning and Marketing, Sonora Regional Medical Center, Sonora, CA, p. A91
CHAN, Chiu Moon, Chairman, President and Chief Executive Officer, Dynacq Healthcare, Inc., Houston, TX, p. B49
CHAN, Fred, Chief Financial Officer, Intracare North Hospital, Houston, TX, p. A604
CHAN, Joyce, Chief Human Resources Officer, CentraCare Health System – Melrose, Melrose, MN, p. A334
CHAN, Marsha, PharmD Chief Quality Officer, St. Francis Medical Center, Lynwood, CA, p. A73
CHANAA, Ziad, M.D. Chief of Staff, Boone Memorial Hospital, Madison, WV, p. A673
CHANCE, Matt, Administrator, Baylor Medical Center at Uptown, Dallas, TX, p. A590
CHAND, Parveen, Chief Operating Officer, Creighton University Medical Center, Omaha, NE, p. A387
CHANDLER, Laurie, Financial Officer, Prairie Community Hospital, Terry, MT, p. A379
CHANDLER, Loren, Interim, Vice President and Chief Financial Officer, Holy Cross Hospital, Chicago, IL, p. A176
CHANDLER, Robert, M.D. Chief of Staff, Powell Valley Healthcare, Powell, WY, p. A697
CHANDLER, Ronald, Accountant II, Southwest Missouri Psychiatric Rehabilitation Center, El Dorado Springs, MO, p. A359
CHANDLER, Ryan, President and Chief Executive Officer, The Medical Center, Columbus, GA, p. A150
CHANDLER, Vincent, Director Information Services, Porterville Developmental Center, Porterville, CA, p. A81
CHANEZ, Adolfo, Vice President Finance and Chief Financial Officer, Saddleback Memorial Medical Center, Laguna Hills, CA, p. A66
CHANG, Alex
Chief Operating Officer, Englewood Community Hospital, Englewood, FL, p. A122
Vice President and Chief Operating Officer, Fawcett Memorial Hospital, Port Charlotte, FL, p. A136
CHANG, C. Joseph, President and Chief Executive Officer, East Valley Hospital Medical Center, Glendora, CA, p. A63
CHANG, Florence
Senior Vice President, Clinical Support Services and Chief Information Officer, MultiCare Good Samaritan Hospital, Puyallup, WA, p. A664
Senior Vice President, Clinical Support Services and Chief Information Officer, MultiCare Mary Bridge Children's Hospital and Health Center, Tacoma, WA, p. A668
Senior Vice President, Clinical Support Services and Chief Information Officer, MultiCare Tacoma General Hospital, Tacoma, WA, p. A668
CHANG, Sang–ick, M.D. Chief Medical Officer, Alameda County Medical Center, Oakland, CA, p. A77
CHANI, Swaranjik K., M.D. Chief of Staff, Caverna Memorial Hospital, Horse Cave, KY, p. A252
CHANNELL, Lesley
Assistant Vice President Human Resources, Dominion Hospital, Falls Church, VA, p. A647
Assistant Vice President Human Resources, Reston Hospital Center, Reston, VA, p. A654
CHANNING, Alan H.
President and Chief Executive Officer, Mount Sinai Hospital, Chicago, IL, p. A177
President and Chief Executive Officer, Schwab Rehabilitation Hospital, Chicago, IL, p. A178
CHANNING, Alan H., President and Chief Executive Officer, Sinai Health System, Chicago, IL, p. B118
CHANSKI, Jared, Administrator, Culberson Hospital, Van Horn, TX, p. A632
CHAPARRO, Natalia, Manager Human Resources, El Paso Children's Hospital, El Paso, TX, p. A596
CHAPIN, Andy, Director Information Technology, Elbert Memorial Hospital, Elberton, GA, p. A152
CHAPIN, Norman, M.D. Medical Director, Columbia Memorial Hospital, Hudson, NY, p. A427
CHAPIN, Ted G., Chief Executive Officer, Chilton Medical Center, Clanton, AL, p. A18
CHAPLIN, Steven, M.D. Medical Director, Kahi Mohala Behavioral Health, Ewa Beach, HI, p. A163
CHAPMAN, Alan, Director Information Systems, Louisiana Medical Center and Heart Hospital, Lacombe, LA, p. A269
CHAPMAN, Judy, Interim Director Information Systems, Lock Haven Hospital, Lock Haven, PA, p. A528
CHAPMAN, Marilyn, Director Human Resources, Sheehan Memorial Hospital, Buffalo, NY, p. A
CHAPMAN, Rick, Chief Information Officer, Kindred Hospital North Florida, Green Cove Springs, FL, p. A124
CHAPMAN, Roberta, Manager Human Resources, Appleton Medical Center, Appleton, WI, p. A678
CHAPMAN, Roland, Chief Information Officer, Northern Navajo Medical Center, Shiprock, NM, p. A418
CHAPMAN, Scott, Administrator, Manhattan Surgical Center,, KS, p. A238
CHAPMAN, Teresa, Vice President Human Resources, Marianjoy Rehabilitation Hospital, Wheaton, IL, p. A196
CHAPPELL, Brandee, Director of Nursing, LifeCare Hospitals of North Carolina, Rocky Mount, NC, p. A459
CHAPPELL, Robert, M.D. Vice President and Chief Medical Officer, Huntsville Hospital, Huntsville, AL, p. A22
CHAPPELL, Teresa, Chief Information Officer, Johnston Health, Smithfield, NC, p. A461
CHAPPLE, Scott, Chief Operating Officer, Oroville Hospital, Oroville, CA, p. A78
CHAPRNKA, Karen, Senior Vice President and Chief Operating Officer, Allegiance Health, Jackson, MI, p. A316
CHARBONNEAU, Elissa, D.O. Medical Director, New England Rehabilitation Hospital of Portland, Portland, ME, p. A285
CHARDAVOYNE, Alan, Controller, Elizabethtown Community Hospital, Elizabethtown, NY, p. A425
CHAREST, Richard
President, Landmark Medical Center, Woonsocket, RI, p. A545
Chief Executive Officer, Rehabilitation Hospital of Rhode Island, North Smithfield, RI, p. A544
CHARETTE, Deborah, Director of Nursing, East Mountain Hospital, Belle Mead, NJ, p. A401
CHARI, Ganesh, M.D. Chief of Staff, Oak Hill Hospital, Brooksville, FL, p. A120
CHARI, Ravi, M.D
Chief Medical Officer, Tristar Ashland City Medical Center, Ashland City, TN, p. A562
Chief Medical Officer, Tristar Centennial Medical Center, Nashville, TN, p. A573
CHARLES, Sally, Coordinator Human Resources, Grace Medical Center, Lubbock, TX, p. A614
CHARLES, Timothy L., President and Chief Executive Officer, Mercy Medical Center, Cedar Rapids, IA, p. A215
CHARLTON, Jr., Francis, M.D. Chief Medical Staff, St. Mary's Medical Center, San Francisco, CA, p. A87
CHARMEL, Patrick, President and Chief Executive Officer, Griffin Hospital, Derby, CT, p. A108
CHARTIER, Dianne, R.N. Chief Executive Officer, Vibra Hospital of Denver, Thornton, CO, p. A106
CHARTRAND, Gregg, Chief Financial Officer, Mercy Hospital, Moose Lake, MN, p. A336
CHASE, Brenda, Chief Operating Officer, Mercy Hospital Hot Springs, Hot Springs National Park, AR, p. A46
CHASE, Jean
Regional Manager Information Services, Aurora Lakeland Medical Center, Elkhorn, WI, p. A681
Regional Manager Information Services, Aurora Medical Center, Kenosha, WI, p. A683
Regional Manager Information Services, Aurora Memorial Hospital of Burlington, Burlington, WI, p. A679
CHASE, Kyle, Chief Financial Officer, Glacial Ridge Health System, Glenwood, MN, p. A332
CHASE, Layla, Chief Financial Officer, Springhill Medical Center, Springhill, LA, p. A278
CHASE, Pansy, Director Human Resources, Vidant Duplin Hospital, Kenansville, NC, p. A456
CHASE, Steven, Chief Information Officer, Craig General Hospital, Vinita, OK, p. A507
CHASE, Susan, Vice President, Carolinas Rehabilitation, Charlotte, NC, p. A450
CHASSE, Floyd, Vice President Human Resources, Mercy Regional Health Center,, KS, p. A238
CHASTAIN, James G., FACHE Director, Mississippi State Hospital, Whitfield, MS, p. A354
CHASTAIN, Stephen L., M.D. Medical Director, HEALTHSOUTH Rehabilitation Hospital, Dothan, AL, p. A19
CHASTANG, Mark J., FACHE Chief Operating Officer, Grady Memorial Hospital, Atlanta, GA, p. A145
CHASTANT, Lee, M.D. Chief Executive Officer, West Feliciana Parish Hospital, Saint Francisville, LA, p. A276
CHASTELAIN, Vincent, Director Business Development, River Oaks Hospital, New Orleans, LA, p. A275
CHATMAN, Jim, Chief Financial Officer, Maria Parham Medical Center, Henderson, NC, p. A454
CHATMAN, Mark, Director Human Resources, Fremont Hospital, Fremont, CA, p. A61
CHATMAN, Rosie, R.N. Associate Director Patient and Nursing Services, Veterans Affairs Medical Center, Northport, NY, p. A438
CHATTERJEE, Kanan, M.D. Chief of Staff, Veterans Affairs Medical Center, Lebanon, PA, p. A527
CHATTO, Paulette, Finance Officer, Northern Navajo Medical Center, Shiprock, NM, p. A418
CHAUDHRY, Deepak
Vice President Information Technology, Nexus Specialty Hospital, Shenandoah, TX, p. A627
Vice President Information Technology, Nexus Specialty Hospital The Woodlands, Spring, TX, p. A628
CHAUSSARD, David, Chief Executive Officer, Hillcrest Hospital Claremore, Claremore, OK, p. A495
CHAVA, N. Rao, M.D. Director, Central Alabama Veterans Health Care System, Montgomery, AL, p. A23
CHAVEZ, Delilah, Human Resources Assistant, Conejos County Hospital, La Jara, CO, p. A103
CHAVEZ, Irene, Senior Vice President and Area Manager, San Jose Medical Center, San Jose, CA, p. A88
CHAVEZ, Kevin, Administrator, Kindred Hospital of South Bay, Gardena, CA, p. A63
CHAVEZ, Margaret, Manager Human Resources, Hammond–Henry Hospital, Geneseo, IL, p. A182
CHAVEZ, Robert, Chief Financial Officer, Horsham Clinic, Ambler, PA, p. A518
CHAVEZ, Steve, Chief Financial Officer, St. John's Lutheran Hospital, Libby, MT, p. A377
CHAVEZ, Virgil, Chief Information Officer, Fort Defiance Indian Health Service Hospital, Fort Defiance, AZ, p. A32
CHAVIS, Anthony D., M.D. Vice President Medical Affairs and Patient Safety Officer, Community Hospital of the Monterey Peninsula, Monterey, CA, p. A75
CHAWLA, Nikki, M.D. Medical Director, Integris Seminole Medical Center, Seminole, OK, p. A504
CHAYER, Olivia, Lead Human Resources, York Hospital, York, ME, p. A286
CHAYKIN, Lee B., Chief Executive Officer, Westside Regional Medical Center, Plantation, FL, p. A136
CHEANEY, Theresa, Interim Chief Executive Officer, Chambers County Public Hospital District 1, Anahuac, TX, p. A578
CHEATWOOD, Elizabeth, Human Resource Director and Administrative Assistant, Jackson Parish Hospital, Jonesboro, LA, p. A268
CHEEK, Teddy, Chief Executive Officer, Medical Park Hospital, Hope, AR, p. A46
CHEEMA, Linde, Vice President Human Resources, Sequoia Hospital, Redwood City, CA, p. A82
CHEESEMAN, Karen, Director Human Resources, Mackinac Straits Health System, Saint Ignace, MI, p. A322
CHEEVER, Liz, Associate Administrator, Miracle Mile Medical Center, Los Angeles, CA, p. A70
CHELOFF, Alec, Chief Information Officer, Massachusetts Eye and Ear Infirmary, Boston, MA, p. A297
CHENEY, David, Chief Executive Officer, Banner Boswell Medical Center, Sun City, AZ, p. A39
CHENG, Becky, Chief Financial Officer, Corona Regional Medical Center, Corona, CA, p. A58
CHENSVOLD, Debrah, FACHE President and Chief Executive Officer, Palmer Lutheran Health Center, West Union, IA, p. A228
CHEPAK, Lois, R.N. Chief Clinical Officer, Eagleville Hospital, Eagleville, PA, p. A522
CHERNICH, Dale
Chief Information Officer, MedWest – Harris, Sylva, NC, p. A461
Chief Information Officer, MedWest – Swain, Bryson City, NC, p. A449
CHERNOW, David S., President and Chief Administrative Officer, Select Medical Corporation, Mechanicsburg, PA, p. B114
CHERONE, Nancy, Interim Chief Executive Officer, Nazareth Hospital, Philadelphia, PA, p. A533
CHERRY, Gay Nell, Director Human Resources, Rolling Plains Memorial Hospital, Sweetwater, TX, p. A630
CHERRY, Jean
Executive Vice President, Commonwealth Regional Specialty Hospital, Bowling Green, KY, p. A247
Executive Vice President and Chief Information Officer, Medical Center at Bowling Green, Bowling Green, KY, p. A248
Executive Vice President, Medical Center at Franklin, Franklin, KY, p. A250
Chief Information Officer, Medical Center at Scottsville, Scottsville, KY, p. A259
CHERRY, John I., M.D. Chief of Staff, Rock County Hospital, Bassett, NE, p. A381
CHERRY, Michael, Chief Financial Officer, Carolina Pines Regional Medical Center, Hartsville, SC, p. A551
CHERRY, Robert, M.D. Chief Medical Officer, Loyola University Medical Center, Maywood, IL, p. A187
CHERRY Jr., Vincent T., Chief Executive Officer, Davis Regional Medical Center, Statesville, NC, p. A461

A782 Index of Health Care Professionals

Index of Health Care Professionals / Christian

Index of Health Care Professionals

CHESLEY, Jeanine
Controller, HEALTHSOUTH Rehabilitation Hospital, Concord, NH, p. A397
Chief Executive Officer, New England Rehabilitation Hospital of Portland, Portland, ME, p. A285
CHESNE, Robert, M.D. Chief Medical Officer, Hollywood Presbyterian Medical Center, Los Angeles, CA, p. A69
CHESNOS, Richard C., Senior Vice President Finance and Chief Financial Officer, St. Clair Memorial Hospital, Pittsburgh, PA, p. A535
CHESSARE, John B., FACHE President and Chief Executive Officer, Greater Baltimore Medical Center, Baltimore, MD, p. A287
CHESSHIRE, Sandra, Chief Financial Officer, Shenandoah Medical Center, Shenandoah, IA, p. A226
CHESSIN, Neil A., Vice President, Jameson Hospital, New Castle, PA, p. A530
CHESSUM, George
Senior Vice President Information Systems and Chief Information Officer, Holy Family Medical Center, Des Plaines, IL, p. A180
Senior Vice President and Chief Information Officer, Our Lady of the Resurrection Medical Center, Chicago, IL, p. A177
Senior Vice President Information Systems and Chief Information Officer, Resurrection Medical Center, Chicago, IL, p. A177
Vice President Information Systems, Saint Francis Hospital, Evanston, IL, p. A181
Senior Vice President Information Systems and Chief Information Officer, Saint Joseph Hospital, Chicago, IL, p. A178
Chief Information Officer, West Suburban Medical Center, Oak Park, IL, p. A190
Chief Information Officer, Westlake Hospital, Melrose Park, IL, p. A187
CHESTEEN, Jimmy, Director Information Technology, Montfort Jones Memorial Hospital, Kosciusko, MS, p. A348
CHESTER, Julie, Director Human Resources, University Hospitals Case Medical Center, Cleveland, OH, p. A476
CHESTER, Kate, Senior Coordinator Public Relations, Providence St. Vincent Medical Center, Portland, OR, p. A514
CHESTER, Linnes L., USAF Administrator, Mike O'Callaghan Federal Hospital, Nellis AFB, NV, p. A394
CHESTER, William, Manager Human Resources, Veterans Affairs Medical Center, Grand Junction, CO, p. A102
CHESTNUT–RAULS, Monica, Vice President Human Resources, Peconic Bay Medical Center, Riverhead, NY, p. A441
CHEUNG, Alan, M.D. Vice President Medical Affairs, Castle Medical Center, Kailua, HI, p. A164
CHEUNG, Anna, President, St. Mary's Medical Center, San Francisco, CA, p. A87
CHEUNG, Marilou, Assistant Administrator Finance, Woodland Hills Medical Center,, CA, p. A73
CHEVERE, Carlos, M.D. Medical Director, I. Gonzalez Martinez Oncologic Hospital,, PR, p. A703
CHEVERTON, Dan, Director Information Systems, LewisGale Hospital at Pulaski, Pulaski, VA, p. A654
CHEW, Roy G., Ph.D. President, Kettering Medical Center, Kettering, OH, p. A482
CHEWNING III, Larry H., President and Chief Executive Officer, Nash Health Care Systems, Rocky Mount, NC, p. A460
CHEYNET, Sandee, Vice President Administrative Services, Bluefield Regional Medical Center, Bluefield, WV, p. A670
CHHABRA, Ankit
Director Finance, Fairview Hospital, Cleveland, OH, p. A475
Director Finance, Lakewood Hospital, Lakewood, OH, p. A482
CHIACCHIARO, Peter, Vice President Human Resources, St. Joseph Hospital, Bethpage, NY, p. A421
CHIANG, Jim, M.D. Chief of Staff, Boulder City Hospital, Boulder City, NV, p. A391
CHIANTELLA, Christopher, M.D. Chief of Staff, Inova Loudoun Hospital, Leesburg, VA, p. A650
CHIANTELLO, Charmaine, Chief Financial Officer, Aspirus Grand View Hospital, Ironwood, MI, p. A316
CHIARAMONTE, Michael J., Chief Executive Officer, Southern Maryland Hospital Center, Clinton, MD, p. A290
CHIARCHIARO, Martha, Vice President Human Resources, Clinton Hospital, Clinton, MA, p. A299
CHIAVETTA, Robert, Vice President Finance, United Memorial Medical Center, Batavia, NY, p. A421
CHICK, Melanie, Chief Executive Officer, Baylor Medical Center at Trophy Club, Trophy Club, TX, p. A631
CHICKEN, Kurt, Director Support Services, Palmer Lutheran Health Center, West Union, IA, p. A228
CHIEFFO, Ron, Chief Information Officer, Colorado River Medical Center, Needles, CA, p. A76
CHILCOTT, Stephen, Associate Director Human Resources, University of California, Davis Medical Center, Sacramento, CA, p. A84
CHILDERS, Bethany, Manager People Resources, Ogallala Community Hospital, Ogallala, NE, p. A387
CHILDERS, James R., Chief Financial Officer, Cobre Valley Regional Medical Center, Globe, AZ, p. A33
CHILDERS, Linda, Director Human Resources, Wallowa Memorial Hospital, Enterprise, OR, p. A510
CHILDRE Jr., Jimmy, Interim Chief Executive Officer, Washington County Regional Medical Center, Sandersville, GA, p. A158
CHILDS, Deborah, Chief Human Resources Officer, University of Michigan Hospitals and Health Centers, Ann Arbor, MI, p. A307
CHILDS, Joe, M.D. Vice President Medical Services, East Tennessee Children's Hospital, Knoxville, TN, p. A568
CHILDS, Michelle B., Executive Administrative Director Human Resources, Salinas Valley Memorial Healthcare System, Salinas, CA, p. A84
CHILDS, Steve, Chief Business Programs and Operations, Veterans Affairs Medical Center, Martinsburg, WV, p. A673
CHILES, John, M.D. Medical Director, Western State Hospital, Tacoma, WA, p. A668
CHILESKI, Andy, Chief Information Officer and Vice President Facilities, Berger Health System, Circleville, OH, p. A474
CHILL, Martha O'Regan, Executive Vice President Operations, Wellmont Holston Valley Medical Center, Kingsport, TN, p. A568
CHILTON, Alvin, Chief Financial Officer, Southeast Arizona Medical Center, Douglas, AZ, p. A31
CHIN, Ellyn, Vice President Finance, Gottlieb Memorial Hospital, Melrose Park, IL, p. A187
CHINBURG, Paul, M.D. Medical Director, Lane County Hospital, Dighton, KS, p. A232
CHINETTI, Peter J., Chief Financial Officer, Massachusetts Eye and Ear Infirmary, Boston, MA, p. A297
CHIOCO, Ernesto, M.D. Chief of Staff, Humboldt General Hospital, Humboldt, TN, p. A566
CHIODO, Deborah
Director Human Resources, Freeman Hospital West, Joplin, MO, p. A361
Director Human Resources, Freeman Neosho Hospital, Neosho, MO, p. A366
CHIOLO, Denise, Chief Human Resources Officer, Phoenixville Hospital, Phoenixville, PA, p. A534
CHIPMAN, Kim, Chief Clinical Officer, Kindred Hospital–White Rock, Dallas, TX, p. A591
CHIRCOP, Marc, Senior Vice President, Spectrum Health Butterworth Hospital, Grand Rapids, MI, p. A314
CHIRICHELLA, Joseph P., President and Chief Executive Officer, Deborah Heart and Lung Center, Browns Mills, NJ, p. A402
CHIRICO, Cathy, Director Human Resources, Edward John Noble Hospital of Gouverneur, Gouverneur, NY, p. A427
CHISENSKI, Walter, Director Information Technology, Casa Grande Regional Medical Center, Casa Grande, AZ, p. A31
CHISHOLM, Ken, Director Human Resources, Martha's Vineyard Hospital, Oak Bluffs, MA, p. A303
CHISHOLM, Lisa P., Troop Commander, Tripler Army Medical Center, Honolulu, HI, p. A164
CHISHOLM, Moody L.
President & Chief Executive Officer, St. Vincent's Medical Center Riverside, Jacksonville, FL, p. A127
President and Chief Executive Officer, St. Vincent's Medical Center Southside, Jacksonville, FL, p. A127
CHISHOLM, Sharon, Director Human Resources, Texas Health Presbyterian Hospital Allen, Allen, TX, p. A577
CHISLEY, Gyasi, Site Administrator and Chief Operating Officer, Mercy Hospital Anderson, Cincinnati, OH, p. A473
CHISSELL, Herbert G., M.D. Chief Medical Officer, Torrance State Hospital, Torrance, PA, p. A539
CHITAYAT, Ron, M.D. Chief Medical Staff, West Hills Hospital and Medical Center,, CA, p. A72
CHITTENDEN, Michael D., President, St. Vincent Carmel Hospital, Carmel, IN, p. A199
CHITTOM, Tommy, Vice President Information Services, East Alabama Medical Center, Opelika, AL, p. A24
CHIVERS, John, Chief Financial Officer, Lower Umpqua Hospital District, Reedsport, OR, p. A515
CHMIEL, Katherine Ann, MS, Chief Executive Officer, Massachusetts Hospital School, Canton, MA, p. A299
CHMIELEWSKI, Linda, R.N. Vice President Operations, St. Cloud Hospital, Saint Cloud, MN, p. A338
CHMURA, David, Manager Management Information Systems, Copper Queen Community Hospital, Bisbee, AZ, p. A31
CHOATE, Charlotte, Director Information Systems, Trinity Hospital of Augusta, Augusta, GA, p. A147
CHOATE, Michael, Interim Chief Financial Officer, St. Vincent General Hospital District, Leadville, CO, p. A103
CHODKOWSKI, Paul J., Chief Executive Officer, St. Anthony Summit Medical Center, Frisco, CO, p. A101
CHOINKA, Keith A., Vice President Information Systems and Chief Information Officer, St. Joseph Hospital, Nashua, NH, p. A399
CHOKSHI, Rajiv, M.D. Chief of Staff, Broward Health Medical Center, Fort Lauderdale, FL, p. A123
CHOLGER, Dave, Chief Financial Officer, Woodlawn Hospital, Rochester, IN, p. A211
CHONG, Johnnette, Chief Financial Officer, Los Angeles Community Hospital, Los Angeles, CA, p. A70
CHONGULIA, Terry, M.D. Chief of Staff, Walton Regional Medical Center, Monroe, GA, p. A156
CHOO, Michael C., M.D. Chief Executive Officer, Clinton Memorial Hospital, Wilmington, OH, p. A491
CHOO, Michael O.
Interim Chief Executive Officer, Anaheim General Hospital, Anaheim, CA, p. A53
President and Chief Executive Officer, Bellflower Medical Center, Bellflower, CA, p. A55
CHOPRA, Praveen, Chief Information and Supply Chain Officer, Children's Healthcare of Atlanta, Atlanta, GA, p. A145
CHORD, Ginger, Coordinator Human Resources, Sturgis Regional Hospital, Sturgis, SD, p. A560
CHOREY, Raymond M., President and Chief Executive Officer, Southeastern Ohio Regional Medical Center, Cambridge, OH, p. A471
CHOU, Rebecca, Director Information Systems, Palestine Regional Medical Center–East, Palestine, TX, p. A619
CHOW, Karen, Director Human Resources, Chinese Hospital, San Francisco, CA, p. A86
CHOWDHARY, Vijay K., M.D. Medical Director, Hampshire Memorial Hospital, Romney, WV, p. A675
CHOY, Ann N., Manager Human Resources and Payroll, Kuakini Medical Center, Honolulu, HI, p. A163
CHOY, Rose, Chief Financial Officer, Kahi Mohala Behavioral Health, Ewa Beach, HI, p. A163
CHRENCIK, Robert A., President and Chief Executive Officer, University of Maryland Medical System, Baltimore, MD, p. B138
CHRICEOL, Scooter, Chief Executive Officer, Monroe Surgical Hospital, Monroe, LA, p. A273
CHRISTENSEN, Cinthia S., JD Executive Vice President and Chief Operating Officer, Children's Hospital of Wisconsin, Milwaukee, WI, p. A686
CHRISTENSEN, David, M.D. Vice President Medical Affairs and Chief Medical Officer, Children's Hospital Central California, Madera, CA, p. A73
CHRISTENSEN, Earlene, Director Human Resources, Fayette County Memorial Hospital, Washington Court House, OH, p. A490
CHRISTENSEN, Elizabeth B., Director, Human Resources, Mercy Hospital of Portland, Portland, ME, p. A284
CHRISTENSEN, G. N., M.D. Chief Medical Officer, William Bee Ririe Hospital, Ely, NV, p. A391
CHRISTENSEN, Jay, FACHE Administrator, Mahaska Health Partnership, Oskaloosa, IA, p. A225
CHRISTENSEN, Jeffrey, Chief Executive Officer, HEALTHSOUTH Rehabilitation Institute of Tucson, Tucson, AZ, p. A40
CHRISTENSEN, Jim, Chief Executive Officer, Crittenden County Hospital, Marion, KY, p. A256
CHRISTENSEN, Marilyn, Director Information Technology, Milford Hospital, Milford, CT, p. A110
CHRISTENSEN, Mark, Assistant Administrator Finance and Chief Financial Officer, Cassia Regional Medical Center, Burley, ID, p. A167
CHRISTENSEN, Marti, Director of Psychiatric Nursing, Douglas County Community Mental Health Center, Omaha, NE, p. A388
CHRISTENSEN, Patricia, MSN Chief Operating Officer, Southern Maryland Hospital Center, Clinton, MD, p. A290
CHRISTENSEN, Sandra
Chief Financial Officer, Dallas County Hospital, Perry, IA, p. A225
Chief Executive Officer, Sheridan Memorial Hospital, Plentywood, MT, p. A378
CHRISTENSEN, W. R., M.D. Chief of Staff, East Texas Medical Center Pittsburg, Pittsburg, TX, p. A620
CHRISTENSEN–MORES, Donna, Director Human Resources, Myrtue Medical Center, Harlan, IA, p. A220
CHRISTENSON, Cindy, Chief Clinical Officer, Barrett Hospital & HealthCare, Dillon, MT, p. A375
CHRISTENSON, Lee, Administrator, Vista Health, Fayetteville, AR, p. A44
CHRISTENSON, Paul, Chief Financial Officer, Pampa Regional Medical Center, Pampa, TX, p. A620
CHRISTENSON, Ron, Chief Financial Officer, Morris County Hospital, Council Grove, KS, p. A232
CHRISTIAN, Bruce C., Chief Executive Officer, Adventist GlenOaks Hospital, Glendale Heights, IL, p. A183
CHRISTIAN, Charles, Chief Information Officer and Director Information Systems, Good Samaritan Hospital, Vincennes, IN, p. A212
CHRISTIAN, Glenn, Administrator, Mayo Clinic Health System in Cannon Falls, Cannon Falls, MN, p. A329

Index of Health Care Professionals
Index of Health Care Professionals / Christian

CHRISTIAN, Greg, Executive Director, Fontana Medical Center, Fontana, CA, p. A61
CHRISTIAN, Karolyne, Director Human Resources, Byrd Regional Hospital, Leesville, LA, p. A271
CHRISTIAN, Patricia L., R.N. Chief Executive Officer, John Umstead Hospital, Butner, NC, p. A450
CHRISTIANSEN, Anne, Chief Financial Officer, Pioneer Memorial Hospital and Health Services, Viborg, SD, p. A560
CHRISTIANSEN, Hilary, Chief Financial Officer, George C Grape Community Hospital, Hamburg, IA, p. A220
CHRISTIANSEN, Judy A., R.N. Chief Operating Officer, Ottawa Regional Hospital and Healthcare Center, Ottawa, IL, p. A190
CHRISTIANSEN, Kevin, Director Information Technology, University of Arizona Medical Center – University Campus, Tucson, AZ, p. A40
CHRISTIANSEN, Lance, Chief Information Officer, West Valley Medical Center, Caldwell, ID, p. A167
CHRISTIANSEN, Sara, Interim Director Human Resources, Sibley Medical Center, Arlington, MN, p. A327
CHRISTIANSON, Clark P., President and Chief Executive Officer, Providence Hospital, Mobile, AL, p. A23
CHRISTIANSON, Clinton J., FACHE President and Chief Executive Officer, Mercy Medical Center–Centerville, Centerville, IA, p. A216
CHRISTIANSON, Delano, Administrator, St. Michael's Hospital and Nursing Home, Sauk Centre, MN, p. A340
CHRISTIE, Andy, Chief Information Technology, Adair County Memorial Hospital, Greenfield, IA, p. A220
CHRISTIE, Janet L., Senior Vice President Human Resources, Shands at the University of Florida, Gainesville, FL, p. A124
CHRISTINE, Gerald, Chief Financial Officer, Lakewood Ranch Medical Center, Bradenton, FL, p. A119
CHRISTINE, Jerry, Chief Executive Officer, Putnam Community Medical Center, Palatka, FL, p. A135
CHRISTION, Lydia, Director Human Resources, HEALTHSOUTH Rehabilitation Hospital, Dothan, AL, p. A19
CHRISTISON, George, M.D. Medical Director, Patton State Hospital, Patton, CA, p. A80
CHRISTMAN, Lawrence, Chief Financial Officer and Chief Operating Officer, Riverview Hospital, Noblesville, IN, p. A210
CHRISTMAN, Lyndon J., President and Chief Executive Officer, Fayette County Memorial Hospital, Washington Court House, OH, p. A490
CHRISTMAN, Thomas C., Director Plant Operations, Kindred Hospital–St. Louis, Saint Louis, MO, p. A368
CHRISTOPHEL, Randal, Executive Vice President and Chief Financial Officer, Indiana University Health Goshen Hospital, Goshen, IN, p. A202
CHROBAK, Jeffrey, Vice President Finance and Chief Financial Officer, Sharon Regional Health System, Sharon, PA, p. A538
CHU, Edward, Chief Financial Officer, Leahi Hospital, Honolulu, HI, p. A163
CHUA, Jesus, M.D. Chief of Staff, Franklin Foundation Hospital, Franklin, LA, p. A266
CHUBB, John M., Chief Executive Officer, Community Regional Medical Center, Fresno, CA, p. A62
CHUGHTAI, Omar, Vice President and Chief Operating Officer, West Hills Hospital and Medical Center,, CA, p. A72
CHULACK, Peggy, Chief Administrative Officer and Chief Information Officer, Presbyterian Intercommunity Hospital, Whittier, CA, p. A96
CHUMBLEY, Bud, M.D. Chief Medical Officer, Scott & White Hospital at Round Rock, Round Rock, TX, p. A623
CHUN, Mirhee, Chief Financial Officer, Havenwyck Hospital, Auburn Hills, MI, p. A307
CHUNG, Maria, CPA Director Fiscal Services, Shriners Hospitals for Children–Boston, Boston, MA, p. A297
CHUNG, Raymond, M.D. Chief of Staff, Phoenix Veterans Affairs Health Care System, Phoenix, AZ, p. A36
CHUNN, Debbie, Director Medical Records, Bastrop Rehabilitation Hospital, Bastrop, LA, p. A262
CHURCH, Kim
  Manager Human Resources, G. Werber Bryan Psychiatric Hospital, Columbia, SC, p. A548
  Manager Human Resources, William S. Hall Psychiatric Institute, Columbia, SC, p. A548
CHURCHILL, Julie, Director Financial Services, The Hospital at Westlake Medical Center, Austin, TX, p. A582
CHURCHILL, Timothy A., President, Stephens Memorial Hospital, Norway, ME, p. A284
CHURCHWELL, Kevin B., M.D. Chief Executive Officer, Alfred I. duPont Hospital for Children, Wilmington, DE, p. A114
CHUSTZ, Mark, Administrator, Greene County Hospital, Eutaw, AL, p. A19
CIANCIOTTO CROYLE, Allison, Vice President of Human Resources, Mercy Medical Center, Rockville Centre, NY, p. A442
CIANFRANI, Michelle, Director Information Technology, Gilbert Hospital, Gilbert, AZ, p. A32
CIAREFELLA, Donna, Director Human Resources, Kindred Hospital Park View, Springfield, MA, p. A304
CICCARELLI, John, Chief Information Officer, Parkview Community Hospital Medical Center, Riverside, CA, p. A82
CICCARELLI, Thomas, Chief Information Officer, East Orange General Hospital, East Orange, NJ, p. A403
CICERO, James David, President and Chief Executive Officer, Ouachita County Medical Center, Camden, AR, p. A43
CICHA, Rhonda, Director Human Resources, Creedmoor Psychiatric Center,, NY, p. A432
CICHOCKI, David, Chief Fiscal Officer, Veterans Affairs Medical Center, Leeds, MA, p. A301
CICHOCKI, Gerald, M.D. Chief of Staff, Mt. San Rafael Hospital, Trinidad, CO, p. A106
CICIRETTI, Mary Louise, Director Human Resources, Riddle Hospital, Media, PA, p. A529
CIENCEWICKI, Michael, M.D. Vice President Medical Affairs, Raritan Bay Medical Center, Perth Amboy, NJ, p. A408
CIHA, Clayton, President and Chief Executive Officer, Alexian Brothers Behavioral Health Hospital, Hoffman Estates, IL, p. A184
CIHAK, Scott A., Chief Executive Officer, Kendall Regional Medical Center, Miami, FL, p. A131
CILLO, Laura A., Chief Operating Officer, West Boca Medical Center, Boca Raton, FL, p. A119
CIMINO, Anthony J., President and Chief Executive Officer, Robert Wood Johnson University Hospital at Hamilton, Hamilton, NJ, p. A404
CIMINO, Jr., Michael A., Chief Financial Officer, Banner Behavioral Health Hospital – Scottsdale, Scottsdale, AZ, p. A38
CINELLI, Kim, Administrator and Chief Executive Officer, Harper Hospital District Five, Harper, KS, p. A234
CINICOLA, John, M.D. Chief Medical Officer, Heritage Valley Beaver, Beaver, PA, p. A518
CIOFFI, Jack, M.D
  Senior Vice President and Chief Medical Officer, Legacy Mount Hood Medical Center, Gresham, OR, p. A511
  Senior Vice President and Chief Medical Officer, Legacy Salmon Creek Medical Center, Vancouver, WA, p. A668
CIOTA, Mark, M.D. Chief Executive Officer, Mayo Clinic Health System in Albert Lea, Albert Lea, MN, p. A327
CIRALDO, Lou, Information Services Representative, University Hospitals Geauga Medical Center, Chardon, OH, p. A472
CITA, Bob, Director Information Services, SEARHC MT. Edgecumbe Hospital, Sitka, AK, p. A30
CITAK, Michael, M.D. Chief Medical Officer, Lake Cumberland Regional Hospital, Somerset, KY, p. A259
CIVAN, Dino, Chief Information Officer, Kings County Hospital Center,, NY, p. A433
CIVIC, Dave, M.D. Associate Director Clinical Services, U. S. Public Health Service Phoenix Indian Medical Center, Phoenix, AZ, p. A37
CIVITELLO, Dean, Vice President Human Resources, Public Relations and Development, St. Joseph's Medical Center, Yonkers, NY, p. A447
CLACK, Lee, R.N. Chief Nursing Officer, Lake Wales Medical Center, Lake Wales, FL, p. A128
CLADOUHOS, Joseph, Chief Executive Officer, Syringa Hospital and Clinics, Grangeville, ID, p. A168
CLAIBORNE, Ronnie, M.D. Chief Medical Officer, Good Samaritan Hospital, Bakersfield, CA, p. A54
CLAIRMONT, Thomas
  President, Franklin Regional Hospital, Franklin, NH, p. A398
  President, Lakes Region General Hospital, Laconia, NH, p. A398
CLAIRMONT, Thomas, President, LRGHealthcare, Laconia, NH, p. B83
CLANCY, Joseph T., Chief Executive Officer, Peace River Regional Medical Center, Port Charlotte, FL, p. A137
CLANCY, Karen, Manager Information Systems Operations, Veterans Affairs Medical Center, Bath, NY, p. A421
CLANCY, Mikki
  Vice President and Chief Information Officer, Good Samaritan Hospital, Dayton, OH, p. A478
  Vice President and Chief Information Officer, Miami Valley Hospital, Dayton, OH, p. A478
CLAPP, Ann R., Director Human Resources, HEALTHSOUTH Rehabilitation Hospital of Texarkana, Texarkana, TX, p. A631
CLAPP, Mary, Controller, Henry County Hospital, Napoleon, OH, p. A485
CLAPP, Nicole, FACHE President and Chief Executive Officer, Grant Regional Health Center, Lancaster, WI, p. A684
CLAPSADDLE, Jason, Vice President Operations, McDowell Hospital, Marion, NC, p. A457
CLARK, Allan W., M.D. Medical Director, Southwood Psychiatric Hospital, Pittsburgh, PA, p. A535
CLARK, Amy, Vice President Human Resources, Medina Hospital, Medina, OH, p. A484
CLARK, Ben, Vice President and Chief Information Officer, Centra Lynchburg General Hospital, Lynchburg, VA, p. A650
CLARK, III, Bernard J., M.D. Medical Director, Alfred I. duPont Hospital for Children, Wilmington, DE, p. A114
CLARK, Chris, Chief Technology Officer, Elkview General Hospital, Hobart, OK, p. A497
CLARK, Cindy, Human Resource Consultant, Saint Joseph Mount Sterling, Mount Sterling, KY, p. A257
CLARK, Dale, Assistant Administrator and Director Human Resources, Wythe County Community Hospital, Wytheville, VA, p. A658
CLARK, David, Vice President Human Resources, Monongahela Valley Hospital, Monongahela, PA, p. A529
CLARK, Ed, M.D. Medical Director, Primary Children's Medical Center, Salt Lake City, UT, p. A640
CLARK, Ed, Vice President Finance, Specialty Hospital of Washington, Washington, DC, p. A117
CLARK, Estella, Chief Nursing Officer, Pikeville Medical Center, Pikeville, KY, p. A258
CLARK, Frank, Chief Information Officer, MUSC Medical Center of Medical University of South Carolina, Charleston, SC, p. A547
CLARK, Heather, Chief Executive Officer, Caldwell Memorial Hospital, Columbia, LA, p. A264
CLARK, Holly, Chief Operating Officer, Muskogee Regional Medical Center, Muskogee, OK, p. A499
CLARK, James A., M.P.H. Director, Veterans Affairs Medical Center, Decatur, GA, p. A151
CLARK, Jeff
  Director Information Systems, Graham Regional Medical Center, Graham, TX, p. A601
  Vice President Human Resources, Kadlec Medical Center, Richland, WA, p. A665
CLARK, Jeremy, Chief Executive Officer, Saint Francis Hospital–Bartlett, Bartlett, TN, p. A562
CLARK, John, Chief Financial Officer, Childrens Care Hospital and School, Sioux Falls, SD, p. A559
CLARK, Karen, MS Vice President Operations, Advocate South Suburban Hospital, Hazel Crest, IL, p. A184
CLARK, Karen, Director Administrative Services, Sonoma Developmental Center, Eldridge, CA, p. A60
CLARK, Karen S., Chief Financial Officer, St. Mary's Hospital, Streator, IL, p. A195
CLARK, Kathleen, President and Chief Executive Officer, Wilcox Memorial Hospital, Lihue, HI, p. A165
CLARK, Kaye, Assistant Director Human Resources Management, E. A. Conway Medical Center, Monroe, LA, p. A273
CLARK, Kent, M.D. Chief Medical Affairs and Quality, Waldo County General Hospital, Belfast, ME, p. A281
CLARK, Krystle, Director Medical Records, Mountrail County Medical Center, Stanley, ND, p. A468
CLARK, Lisa, Human Resources Officer, Holy Cross Hospital, Taos, NM, p. A418
CLARK, M. Victoria, Chief Executive Officer, La Paz Regional Hospital, Parker, AZ, p. A34
CLARK, Mark, Human Resources Liaison, U. S. Air Force Regional Hospital, Elmendorf AFB, AK, p. A28
CLARK, Mark A., Vice President Operations, St. Mary's Hospital, Centralia, IL, p. A174
CLARK, Michael
  Director Operations, Clay County Memorial Hospital, Henrietta, TX, p. A603
  Vice President Finance, FHN Memorial Hospital, Freeport, IL, p. A182
CLARK, Michael A., Administrator and Chief Executive Officer, Logan Regional Hospital, Logan, UT, p. A638
CLARK, N. Travis, President, Page Memorial Hospital, Luray, VA, p. A650
CLARK, Nancy, Vice President Human Resources, Regional Medical Center of San Jose, San Jose, CA, p. A88
CLARK, Patrick
  Senior Vice President Finance and Support Services, Avera Queen of Peace Hospital, Mitchell, SD, p. A558
  Manager Information Technology, Sunnyview Rehabilitation Hospital, Schenectady, NY, p. A443
CLARK, Paul, Senior Vice President and Chief Operating Officer, Munroe Regional Medical Center, Ocala, FL, p. A133
CLARK Jr., Ralph H., FACHE Chief Executive Officer, Medical Center Barbour, Eufaula, AL, p. A19
CLARK, Randal, Vice President Finance, Sebasticook Valley Health, Pittsfield, ME, p. A284
CLARK, Rebecca, Chief Nursing Officer, Two Rivers Behavioral Health System, Kansas City, MO, p. A363
CLARK, Richard, M.D. President, Medical Staff, Memorial Hospital of Sweetwater County, Rock Springs, WY, p. A697
CLARK, Richard, Chief Executive Officer, Poplar Springs Hospital, Petersburg, VA, p. A653
CLARK, Robert J., President and Chief Executive Officer, Bristol Bay Area Health Corporation, Dillingham, AK, p. A28

A784 Index of Health Care Professionals 

Index of Health Care Professionals / Cobb

Index of Health Care Professionals


CLARK, Robert L., M.D. Medical Director, Regional Hospital for Respiratory and Complex Care, Seattle, WA, p. A665
CLARK, Robin, Chief Nursing Officer, Select Specialty Hospital–Greensboro, Greensboro, NC, p. A454
CLARK, Ron, M.D. Vice President Clinical Activities and Chief Medical Officer, VCU Health System, Richmond, VA, p. A655
CLARK, Shannon, Chief Financial Officer, Drew Memorial Hospital, Monticello, AR, p. A49
CLARK, Sharon, Director Human Resources, Hillsboro Area Hospital, Hillsboro, IL, p. A184
CLARK, Shawn, Director Information Systems, The Physicians Centre Hospital, Bryan, TX, p. A586
CLARK, Steve, Chief Information Officer, Albemarle Health, Elizabeth City, NC, p. A452
CLARK, Teresa, Director of Nursing, Wichita County Health Center, Leoti, KS, p. A238
CLARK, Theo, Director Financial Services, Promise Hospital of Phoenix, Mesa, AZ, p. A34
CLARK, Thomas A., President and Chief Executive Officer, Avera Queen of Peace Hospital, Mitchell, SD, p. A558
CLARK, Tim
Director Human Resources, Moberly Regional Medical Center, Moberly, MO, p. A365
Chief Operating Officer, Promise Hospital of San Diego, San Diego, CA, p. A85
CLARK, Troy, Vice President Finance and Operations, Wellmont Bristol Regional Medical Center, Bristol, TN, p. A562
CLARK, William, M.D. Chief Clinical Affairs, Caro Center, Caro, MI, p. A308
CLARKE, James, M.D. Vice President Medical Affairs and Clinical Effectiveness, Ocean Medical Center, Brick Township, NJ, p. A402
CLARKE, Lisa, Interim Chief Financial Officer, Southwestern Medical Center, Lawton, OK, p. A498
CLARKSTON, Wendell, M.D. President Medical Staff, Saint Luke's South Hospital, Overland Park, KS, p. A241
CLAROS, Elizabeth, Administrator Personnel Services, Guam Memorial Hospital Authority, Tamuning, GU, p. A699
CLARRY, Patrick M., Vice President Human Resources, Providence Holy Family Hospital, Spokane, WA, p. A667
CLARY, Patrick, Vice President Human Resources, Providence Sacred Heart Medical Center & Children's Hospital, Spokane, WA, p. A667
CLATANOFF, Kris, Director Human Resources, St. Joseph Medical Center, Houston, TX, p. A606
CLAUDSON, Jackie, Administrator, South Big Horn County Hospital, Basin, WY, p. A695
CLAUDY, Frank, M.D. Vice President Medical Staff Affairs, Genesis Medical Center–Davenport, Davenport, IA, p. A217
CLAUNCH, Don, Senior Vice President, Chief Financial Officer and Chief Information Officer, Wyoming Medical Center, Casper, WY, p. A695
CLAUSEN, Patricia J., R.N. Chief Nurse Executive, Kaiser Permanente Downey Medical Center, Downey,, p. A59
CLAUSSEN, Tammy, Human Resources Executive, Tri Valley Health System, Cambridge, NE, p. A382
CLAVELL, Luis, M.D. Medical Director, San Jorge Children's Hospital, San Juan, PR, p. A703
CLAWSON, Tonya, Manager Human Resources, Mercy Medical Center–Centerville, Centerville, IA, p. A216
CLAXTON, Anthony, M.D. Clinical Director, Terrell State Hospital, Terrell, TX, p. A630
CLAXTON, Edmund, M.D. President, Medical Staff, Central Maine Medical Center, Lewiston, ME, p. A283
CLAXTON, Tracey, Controller, HEALTHSOUTH Rehabilitation Hospital of York, York, PA, p. A542
CLAY, David, Chief Operating Officer, Central Carolina Hospital, Sanford, NC, p. A460
CLAYMORE, Krystal, Chief Financial Officer, Great Plains Regional Medical Center, North Platte, NE, p. A386
CLAYPOOL, Blain
Chief Executive Officer, Renown Rehabilitation Hospital, Reno, NV, p. A395
Chief Executive Officer, Renown South Meadows Medical Center, Reno, NV, p. A395
CLAYTON, Edward, Chief Financial Officer, Phelps County Regional Medical Center, Rolla, MO, p. A367
CLAYTON, Kathy, Chief Financial Officer, Perry County Memorial Hospital, Tell City, IN, p. A212
CLAYTON, Kent G., President and Chief Executive Officer, Placentia–Linda Hospital, Placentia, CA, p. A80
CLAYTON, Philip A., President and Chief Executive Officer, Conway Medical Center, Conway, SC, p. A549
CLEARY, John J., Chief Executive Officer, West Suburban Medical Center, Oak Park, IL, p. A190
CLEARY, Steven R.
Vice President Finance, St. Joseph Medical Center, Kansas City, MO, p. A362
Vice President Finance, St. Mary's Medical Center, Blue Springs, MO, p. A355
CLECKLER, Jason, Chief Clinical Officer, Delta County Memorial Hospital, Delta, CO, p. A99
CLELAND, Dub, Chief Financial Officer, Oklahoma Surgical Hospital, Tulsa, OK, p. A506
CLELAND, William H., M.D. Chief Medical Officer, University Hospitals and Health System, University of Mississippi Medical Center, Jackson, MS, p. A348
CLEM, Sandra, Manager Information Management, Carl Vinson Veterans Affairs Medical Center, Dublin, GA, p. A152
CLEMEN, Linda, R.N. Vice President and Chief Nursing Officer, Katherine Shaw Bethea Hospital, Dixon, IL, p. A180
CLEMENS, Brian L.
President and Chief Executive Officer, Community Hospital, Oklahoma City, OK, p. A500
Chief Executive Officer, Northwest Surgical Hospital, Oklahoma City, OK, p. A501
CLEMENT, Bernie, Chief Information Officer, East Jefferson General Hospital, Metairie, LA, p. A273
CLEMENT, Kevin J., Chief Executive Officer, Siloam Springs Memorial Hospital, Siloam Springs, AR, p. A51
CLEMENT, Mark C., President and Chief Executive Officer, Rochester General Health System, Rochester, NY, p. B110
CLEMENTS, Christopher, Administrator, Kindred Hospital South Florida–Hollywood,, FL, p. A125
CLEMENTS, James, Chief Executive Officer, South Fulton Medical Center, Atlanta, GA, p. A146
CLEMENTS, Jill, Vice President Human Resources, Excela Latrobe Area Hospital, Latrobe, PA, p. A527
CLEMENTS, John R., Vice President and Chief Financial Officer, McCullough–Hyde Memorial Hospital, Oxford, OH, p. A487
CLEMENTS, Karen, R.N. Vice President, Chief Nursing Officer, The Acadia Hospital, Bangor, ME, p. A281
CLEMENTS, Larry E., Administrator, Wildwood Lifestyle Center and Hospital, Wildwood, GA, p. A162
CLEMENTS, Lynn
Director Human Resources, Shriners Hospitals for Children, Galveston Burns Hospital, Galveston, TX, p. A600
Director Human Resources, Shriners Hospitals for Children, Houston, Houston, TX, p. A606
CLEMMENSEN, J. Scott
Vice President Human Resources and Leadership Enhancement, Capital Health Medical Center–Hopewell, Pennington, NJ, p. A408
Vice President Human Resources and Leadership Enhancement, Capital Health Regional Medical Center, Trenton, NJ, p. A411
CLEMMER, Deb, Vice President Human Resources, Bothwell Regional Health Center, Sedalia, MO, p. A370
CLEMMONS, Mark, Director Information Systems, Community Memorial Healthcenter, South Hill, VA, p. A656
CLEMONS, Deneace, Chief Operating Officer, Twin Lakes Regional Medical Center, Leitchfield, KY, p. A252
CLEVELAND, Austin B., Chief Executive Officer, Select Specialty Hospital–Quad Cities, Davenport, IA, p. A217
CLEVELAND, Cynthia, Ph.D. Acting Associate Director, Veterans Affairs Medical Center, Birmingham, AL, p. A17
CLEVELAND, David, M.D. Chief Medical Officer, Shelby Baptist Medical Center, Alabaster, AL, p. A15
CLEVENGER, Jerry, Vice President Human Resources, Rowan Regional Medical Center, Salisbury, NC, p. A460
CLEVERSY, Stephanie
Manager Health Information Services, University Hospitals Conneaut Medical Center, Conneaut, OH, p. A478
Manager Health Information Systems, University Hospitals Geneva Medical Center, Geneva, OH, p. A481
CLICK, Glenn, Chief Financial Officer, Sequoyah Memorial Hospital, Sallisaw, OK, p. A504
CLICK, Mike, Administrator, Brownfield Regional Medical Center, Brownfield, TX, p. A585
CLIFF, Barbara J., FACHE President and Chief Executive Officer, Windber Medical Center, Windber, PA, p. A542
CLIFF, Tammy, R.N. Director Nursing Services, McKenzie Health System, Sandusky, MI, p. A322
CLIFFE, Peggy, Chief Executive Officer, Select Specialty Hospital–Wichita, Wichita, KS, p. A245
CLIFFORD, Michael J., Director Finance, Wayne Memorial Hospital, Honesdale, PA, p. A525
CLIFFORD, Ryan, M.D. Chief of Staff, Washakie Medical Center, Worland, WY, p. A698
CLIFTON, Gary, Chief Financial Officer, I–70 Community Hospital, Sweet Springs, MO, p. A371
CLIFTON–LEMAY, Sherri L., Director Human Resources, Natchez Regional Medical Center, Natchez, MS, p. A351
CLINE, Claire P., M.P.H. Senior Vice President Patient Care Services/CNO, Watauga Medical Center, Boone, NC, p. A449
CLINE, Vickie, Director Human Resources, Northwest Medical Center, Albany, MO, p. A355
CLINGENPEEL, Jeremy, Administrator and Chief Executive Officer, Hamilton County Hospital, Syracuse, KS, p. A243
CLINGER, Dallas, Administrator, Power County Hospital District, American Falls, ID, p. A166
CLINITE, Ed, D.O. Chief of Staff, Sonora Regional Medical Center, Sonora, CA, p. A91
CLINTON, David, M.D. Medical Director, Soldiers' Home in Holyoke, Holyoke, MA, p. A301
CLINTON, Lee, FACHE Vice President Operations, Perry County Memorial Hospital, Perryville, MO, p. A366
CLINTON, Lori, Chief Nursing Officer, Sparta Community Hospital, Sparta, IL, p. A194
CLIPP, Jerry, Manager Human Resources, Washakie Medical Center, Worland, WY, p. A698
CLISTER, Martha L., Director Human Resources, Canonsburg General Hospital, Canonsburg, PA, p. A520
CLONCH, Leslie, Vice President and Chief Information Officer, University Health Care System, Augusta, GA, p. A147
CLONTS, Jolene, Director Human Resources, Logan Regional Hospital, Logan, UT, p. A638
CLOSE, Debra, Chief Executive Officer, Dukes Memorial Hospital, Peru, IN, p. A210
CLOSNER, Shawn, Vice President Finance, St. Mary's Community Hospital, Nebraska City, NE, p. A386
CLOTHIER, Mark A., M.D. President Medical Staff, Mother Frances Hospital – Winnsboro, Winnsboro, TX, p. A635
CLOUD, Avery, Vice President and Chief Information Officer, New Hanover Regional Medical Center, Wilmington, NC, p. A462
CLOUD, Sylvia, Director Human Resources, Silver Lake Medical Center, Los Angeles, CA, p. A72
CLOUGH, James, Chief Executive Officer, Cleveland Area Hospital, Cleveland, OK, p. A495
CLOUGH, Jeanette G., President and Chief Executive Officer, Mount Auburn Hospital, Cambridge, MA, p. A299
CLOUGH, Richard, Chief Operating Officer, Robinson Memorial Hospital, Ravenna, OH, p. A487
CLOUGH, Sheila
President, Eagle River Memorial Hospital, Eagle River, WI, p. A680
President, Eagle River Memorial Hospital, Eagle River, WI, p. A680
President, Howard Young Medical Center, Woodruff, WI, p. A694
CLOUSE DAY, Sherry, Vice President Finance, Mercy Hospital Berryville, Berryville, AR, p. A42
CLOUTIER, Mary, Director Human Resources, Adventist Behavioral Health Rockville, Rockville, MD, p. A293
CLOUTIER, Michael, Director Information Services, Kennewick General Hospital, Kennewick, WA, p. A662
CLOVER, Robert, Assistant Superintendent, Logansport State Hospital, Logansport, IN, p. A207
CLUCK, Robert N., M.D. Vice President and Medical Director, Texas Health Arlington Memorial Hospital, Arlington, TX, p. A579
CLUTE, Gerald B., President and Chief Executive Officer, California Hospital Medical Center, Los Angeles, CA, p. A68
CLUTTS, Kathaleen, Director Human Resources, St. Alexius Hospital – Forest Park Campus, Saint Louis, MO, p. A369
CLYNE, Eileen, Director Human Resources, Christ Hospital, Jersey City, NJ, p. A405
CLYNE, Mary Ellen, Ph.D. President and Chief Executive Officer, Clara Maass Medical Center, Belleville, NJ, p. A401
CMIEL, Peggy, R.N. Chief Nursing Officer, Chinese Hospital, San Francisco, CA, p. A86
COAD, Christina D., Ph.D. Chief Administrative Officer, Jefferson Memorial Hospital, Ranson, WV, p. A675
COATES, Janet, President and Chief Executive Officer, Mother Frances Hospital – Winnsboro, Winnsboro, TX, p. A635
COATES, Jennifer, Coordinator Information Technology, Purcell Municipal Hospital, Purcell, OK, p. A503
COATS, Aaron, Information Technology Director, Mason District Hospital, Havana, IL, p. A183
COATS, Brenda, Director Human Resources, River Crest Hospital, San Angelo, TX, p. A624
COATS, John, M.D. Chief Medical Staff, Morehouse General Hospital, Bastrop, LA, p. A262
COATS, Kevin, Chief Financial Officer, Baylor Medical Center at Frisco, Frisco, TX, p. A600
COATSWORTH, Jeannine, Vice President Human Resources, Barlow Respiratory Hospital, Los Angeles, CA, p. A68
COBARRUBIAS, Ronnie O., Director Information Systems, Beverly Hospital, Montebello, CA, p. A75
COBARRUBIAS, Samuel, M.D. Chief of Staff, Clinch Memorial Hospital, Homerville, GA, p. A154
COBB, Jason E., FACHE Chief Executive Officer, Lakeview Regional Medical Center, Covington, LA, p. A265
COBB, Jeff, Information Technologist, Guthrie County Hospital, Guthrie Center, IA, p. A220
COBB, Maura, R.N. Chief Nursing Officer, Northridge Medical Center, Commerce, GA, p. A150

Index of Health Care Professionals

Index of Health Care Professionals / Cobb


COBB, Tammy, Chief Financial Officer, Jacksonville Medical Center, Jacksonville, AL, p. A22
COBBLE, Emlyn, Vice President and Chief Support Officer, Parkwest Medical Center, Knoxville, TN, p. A568
COBBS, Wendy
  Director Human Resources, Promise Hospital Baton Rouge, Baton Rouge, LA, p. A263
  Director of Human Resources, Promise Hospital of Baton Rouge, Baton Rouge, LA, p. A263
COBURN, Nate, Chief Financial Officer, Weiser Memorial Hospital, Weiser, ID, p. A171
COCCHI, Dean
  Chief Financial Officer, Kindred Hospital North Florida, Green Cove Springs, FL, p. A124
  Chief Financial Officer, Kindred Hospital Ocala, Ocala, FL, p. A133
COCHENNET, Bradley, Chief Executive Officer, Pagosa Springs Medical Center, Pagosa Springs, CO, p. A104
COCHRAN, Barry S., FACHE Administrator, Fayette Medical Center, Fayette, AL, p. A20
COCHRAN, Dan, Chief Operating Officer, Bingham Memorial Hospital, Blackfoot, ID, p. A166
COCHRAN, Daniel, Vice President and Chief Financial Officer, Shady Grove Adventist Hospital, Rockville, MD, p. A294
COCHRAN, Kay P., Vice President Human Resources, Twin County Regional Hospital, Galax, VA, p. A649
COCHRAN, Kenneth, FACHE President and Chief Executive Officer, East Liverpool City Hospital, East Liverpool, OH, p. A479
COCHRAN, Jr., Willie, M.D. Chief of Staff, Southern Regional Medical Center, Riverdale, GA, p. A158
COCHRANE, Andrew S.
  Chief Executive Officer, Maple Grove Hospital, Maple Grove, MN, p. A334
  President Hospital Operations, North Memorial Health Care, Robbinsdale, MN, p. A338
COCHRELL, Patricia, R.N. Executive Vice President and Chief Operating Officer, Harrison Medical Center, Bremerton, WA, p. A659
COCKER, Robert, Vice President Organizational Effectiveness, Grand Itasca Clinic and Hospital, Grand Rapids, MN, p. A332
COCKERHAM, Mary Ellen, Vice President Human Resources, Nazareth Hospital, Philadelphia, PA, p. A533
COCKING, Kathy, R.N. Vice President Operations, Barton Healthcare System, South Lake Tahoe, CA, p. A91
COCKRELL, Dennis, Director Human Resources, Gritman Medical Center, Moscow, ID, p. A169
COCKRELL, William, Administrator and Chief Executive Officer, Patient's Choice Medical Center of Claiborne County, Port Gibson, MS, p. A352
COCORULLO, Mark, Senior Vice President and Chief Financial Officer, Martin Health System, Stuart, FL, p. A139
CODER, Charles, Chief Financial Officer, Southside Regional Medical Center, Petersburg, VA, p. A653
CODY, Carolyn, M.D. Vice President Medical Affairs, BryanLGH Medical Center, Lincoln, NE, p. A385
CODY, Geraldine, Director Human Resources, Kingsboro Psychiatric Center,, NY, p. A433
CODY, James, Director, Veterans Affairs Medical Center, Syracuse, NY, p. A444
COE, Jason, M.D. Medical Director, Greenbrier Hospital, Covington, LA, p. A265
COE, Jason C., President and Chief Executive Officer, Hackettstown Regional Medical Center, Hackettstown, NJ, p. A404
COFFELL, Randy, Manager Human Resources, Mid-Valley Hospital, Omak, WA, p. A663
COFFEY, Bryan D., Chief Executive Officer, Sac-Osage Hospital, Osceola, MO, p. A366
COFFEY, C. Edward, M.D. Chief Executive Officer and Director Behavioral Health Services, Henry Ford Kingswood Hospital, Ferndale, MI, p. A312
COFFEY, Daniel B., President and Chief Executive Officer, The Acadia Hospital, Bangor, ME, p. A281
COFFEY, Dennis J., CPA Senior Vice President and Chief Financial Officer, J. Arthur Dosher Memorial Hospital, Southport, NC, p. A461
COFFEY, Joseph, Director Facility Administration, Rochester Psychiatric Center, Rochester, NY, p. A442
COFFEY, Judy
  Senior Vice President and Area Manager, San Rafael Medical Center, San Rafael, CA, p. A89
  Senior Vice President and Area Manager, Santa Rosa Medical Center, Santa Rosa, CA, p. A90
COFFEY, Kevin, Chief Financial Officer, Brookings Health System, Brookings, SD, p. A555
COFFEY, Timothy O., Senior Vice President Operations, Lake Charles Memorial Hospital, Lake Charles, LA, p. A271
COFFMAN, Douglas, Vice President and Chief Financial Officer, United Hospital Center, Bridgeport, WV, p. A670
COFFMAN, Joan, President and Chief Executive Officer, St. Joseph's Hospital, Chippewa Falls, WI, p. A680
COFFMAN BARNES, Julie, M.D. Chief Medical Officer, Redmond Regional Medical Center, Rome, GA, p. A158
COFIE, Daniel, M.D. Chief of Staff, Haywood Park Community Hospital, Brownsville, TN, p. A562
COFIELD, Robert, Dr.PH Chief Operating Officer and Associate Vice President, University of Virginia Medical Center, Charlottesville, VA, p. A646
COFINAS, Rebecca, Vice President and Chief Operating Executive Operations, Scripps Memorial Hospital-Encinitas, Encinitas, CA, p. A60
COFONE, Michael, Chief Financial Officer, Health Alliance Hospitals, Leominster, MA, p. A301
COGLEY, Richard, M.D. Senior Vice President Medical Affairs and Chief Medical Officer, Saint Vincent Health Center, Erie, PA, p. A523
COHEE, Jonathan, Chief Executive Officer, Vibra Hospital of Southeastern Michigan, Lincoln Park, MI, p. A318
COHEN, Aaron, Chief Financial Officer, Bellevue Hospital Center, New York, NY, p. A431
COHEN, Cindy, Director Human Resources, Stewart & Lynda Resnick Neuropsychiatric Hospital at UCLA, Los Angeles, CA, p. A72
COHEN, Gail C., Vice President Human Resources, Saint Clare's Health System, Denville, NJ, p. A403
COHEN, Ginger, Chief Nurse Executive, St. Luke's Rehabilitation Institute, Spokane, WA, p. A667
COHEN, Norman, M.D. Chief Medical Officer, Crossroads Community Hospital, Mount Vernon, IL, p. A188
COHEN, Philip A., Chief Executive Officer, Monterey Park Hospital, Monterey Park, CA, p. A75
COHEN, Robert, M.D. Chief Medical Officer, Sonoma Valley Hospital, Sonoma, CA, p. A91
COKER, Cindy, M.P.H. Vice President, Patient Care Services, Vidant Chowan Hospital, Edenton, NC, p. A452
COKER, John, Director Human Resource, Abington Health Lansdale Hospital, Lansdale, PA, p. A527
COKER, Raymond Kirk, M.D. Chief of Staff, Baptist Health Medical Center-Stuttgart, Stuttgart, AR, p. A51
COLAGUORI, Ronald J., Vice President Operations, St. Anthony's Hospital, Saint Petersburg, FL, p. A138
COLANDER, Charles, Vice President Information Systems and Chief Information Officer, Elmhurst Memorial Hospital,, IL, p. A181
COLANGELO, Nicholas, Chief Executive Officer, Clear Brook Lodge, Shickshinny, PA, p. A538
COLAS, Chuck, M.D. Medical Director, Surprise Valley Healthcare District, Cedarville, CA, p. A57
COLBERG, Gary R., FACHE President and Chief Executive Officer, Southeast Georgia Health System, Brunswick, GA, p. B120
COLBERG, Gary R., FACHE President and Chief Executive Officer, Southeast Georgia Health System Brunswick Campus, Brunswick, GA, p. A148
COLBERT, Carol, Director Human Resources, Trace Regional Hospital, Houston, MS, p. A347
COLBURN, Douglas, Chief Information Officer, Hughston Hospital, Columbus, GA, p. A149
COLBURN, Marj A., Facility Operating Officer, Risk Manager and Performance Improvement Coordinator, Hastings Regional Center, Hastings, NE, p. A384
COLBURN, Tim, President and Chief Executive Officer, Berger Health System, Circleville, OH, p. A474
COLCHER, Marian W., President and Chief Executive Officer, Valley Forge Medical Center and Hospital, Norristown, PA, p. A531
COLE, Annette E., R.N. Vice President and Chief Nursing Officer, Sky Lakes Medical Center, Klamath Falls, OR, p. A511
COLE, Beth, Director Information Services, Lewis-Gale Medical Center, Salem, VA, p. A655
COLE, Carlene, Manager Human Resources, Kittson Memorial Healthcare Center, Hallock, MN, p. A332
COLE, F. Sessions, M.D. Chief Medical Officer, St. Louis Children's Hospital, Saint Louis, MO, p. A370
COLE, Georgeanne, Chief Executive Officer, Rehabilitation Hospital of Southwest Virginia, Bristol, VA, p. A646
COLE Jr., Harry, Administrator, Georgiana Hospital, Georgiana, AL, p. A21
COLE, James B., Chief Executive Officer, Virginia Hospital Center – Arlington, Arlington, VA, p. A645
COLE, Jason
  Director Finance, Scott & White Hospital – Llano, Llano, TX, p. A613
  Senior Director Finance, Scott & White Hospital at Round Rock, Round Rock, TX, p. A623
COLE, Karen S., FACHE Chief Executive Officer, Shenandoah Medical Center, Shenandoah, IA, p. A226
COLE, Kelli, Chief Executive Officer, Kindred Hospital-San Francisco Bay Area, San Leandro, CA, p. A88
COLE, Lori, Director Information Management, Wayne Memorial Hospital, Goldsboro, NC, p. A453
COLE, Missy, Director Human Resources, HEALTHSOUTH Rehabilitation Hospital, Fayetteville, AR, p. A44
COLE, Robert, Chief Operating Officer, Connecticut Mental Health Center, New Haven, CT, p. A110
COLECCHI, Stephen, President and Chief Executive Officer, Robinson Memorial Hospital, Ravenna, OH, p. A487
COLEMAN, Alisa, Chief Executive Officer, Trigg County Hospital, Cadiz, KY, p. A248
COLEMAN, Andrea C., Chief Operating Officer, Penrose-St. Francis Health Services, Colorado Springs, CO, p. A98
COLEMAN, Curt, FACHE Chief Executive Officer, Jackson County Regional Health Center, Maquoketa, IA, p. A223
COLEMAN, Donna
  Director Professional Services, Jackson County Hospital District, Edna, TX, p. A595
  Director Human Resources, Texas Health Presbyterian Hospital Denton, Denton, TX, p. A594
COLEMAN, Doug, M.D. Chief of Staff, Jefferson Regional Medical Center, Pine Bluff, AR, p. A50
COLEMAN, James J., Ed.D. Director, Kalamazoo Psychiatric Hospital, Kalamazoo, MI, p. A316
COLEMAN, Jeff, Manager Information Systems, Navos, Seattle, WA, p. A665
COLEMAN, Jr., Jim L., Chief Operating Officer, Parkridge Medical Center, Chattanooga, TN, p. A563
COLEMAN, Keith T., Chief Financial Officer, Adena Health System, Chillicothe, OH, p. A472
COLEMAN, Lenon J., Interim Chief Human Resources Officer, Vanderbilt Hospital and Clinics, Nashville, TN, p. A574
COLEMAN, Melissa, Assistant Vice President Human Resources, Pikeville Medical Center, Pikeville, KY, p. A258
COLEMAN, Shane, Director Information Services, Delta Regional Medical Center, Greenville, MS, p. A346
COLERICK, Steven, Chief Executive Officer, Buena Vista Regional Medical Center, Storm Lake, IA, p. A227
COLETTA, Anthony V., M.D. Executive Vice President and Chief Medical Officer, Holy Redeemer Hospital and Medical Center, Meadowbrook, PA, p. A528
COLETTA, Sandra L., President and Chief Executive Officer, Kent County Memorial Hospital, Warwick, RI, p. A545
COLETTA, Tony, Vice President of Human Resources, Advocate Eureka Hospital, Eureka, IL, p. A181
COLEY, Brenda
  Executive Director, Metroplex Adventist Hospital, Killeen, TX, p. A610
  Executive Director, Rollins-Brook Community Hospital, Lampasas, TX, p. A611
COLGAN, Teresa, VP of Nursing, Great River Medical Center, West Burlington, IA, p. A228
COLKER, Rebecca, Chief Financial Officer, St. Mary's Hospital, Decatur, IL, p. A179
COLLAMORE, Beth, M.D. Chief of Staff, Cary Medical Center, Caribou, ME, p. A282
COLLAZO, Marian, Director Finance, Hospital San Cristobal, Coto Laurel, PR, p. A701
COLLIER, Gary, M.D. Vice President Medical Affairs and Chief Medical Officer, Miami Valley Hospital, Dayton, OH, p. A478
COLLIER, Jack, M.D. Chief of Staff, MountainView Hospital, Las Vegas, NV, p. A393
COLLIER, Lora, M.D. Chief Medical Staff, Integris Mayes County Medical Center, Pryor, OK, p. A503
COLLIER, Margaret P., Chief Executive Officer, SummitRidge Hospital, Lawrenceville, GA, p. A155
COLLIER, Russell J., FACHE President and Chief Executive Officer, Good Shepherd Medical Center-Marshall, Marshall, TX, p. A615
COLLIER, Scarlet, Chief Information Officer, Lane Regional Medical Center, Zachary, LA, p. A280
COLLIER, Shari, Chief Financial Officer, Overland Park Regional Medical Center, Overland Park, KS, p. A241
COLLIER, Tom, Manager Information Systems, Missouri Rehabilitation Center, Mount Vernon, MO, p. A365
COLLINS, Ava Jo, Vice President Operations, Ochsner Baptist Medical Center, New Orleans, LA, p. A274
COLLINS, Barry, D.O. Chief of Staff, Hillsdale Community Health Center, Hillsdale, MI, p. A315
COLLINS, Bobby, Director Human Resources, Mountain View Regional Medical Center, Norton, VA, p. A653
COLLINS, Chauncey, Director Operations, Austen Riggs Center, Stockbridge, MA, p. A305
COLLINS, David, Director for Administration, Naval Medical Center, Portsmouth, VA, p. A654
COLLINS, Dennis, Chief Financial Officer, The Brook Hospital – KMI, Louisville, KY, p. A255
COLLINS, Edmund, Chief Information Officer, Martin Health System, Stuart, FL, p. A139
COLLINS, Harold E., JD Chief Financial Officer, Franciscan Physicians Hospital, Munster, IN, p. A209


A786 Index of Health Care Professionals 

Index of Health Care Professionals / Connelly

COLLINS, Hugh, Interim Chief Executive Officer, Lakeside Memorial Hospital, Brockport, NY, p. A422
COLLINS, James M., President and Chief Executive Officer, St. Clair Memorial Hospital, Pittsburgh, PA, p. A535
COLLINS, Jeff, M.D
Chief Medical Officer, Providence Holy Family Hospital, Spokane, WA, p. A667
Chief Medical Officer, Providence Sacred Heart Medical Center & Children's Hospital, Spokane, WA, p. A667
COLLINS, Jeffrey A., Senior Vice President and Area Manager, Fresno Medical Center, Fresno, CA, p. A62
COLLINS, John F., President and Chief Executive Officer, Winthrop–University Hospital, Mineola, NY, p. A430
COLLINS, John R., Chief Financial Officer, Hemet Valley Medical Center, Hemet, CA, p. A64
COLLINS, Mark, Interim Chief Finance Officer, Rogue Valley Medical Center, Medford, OR, p. A512
COLLINS, Michael F., Chief Executive Officer, Merrimack Valley Hospital, Haverhill, MA, p. A300
COLLINS, Michael L., President and Chief Executive Officer, Jewish Hospital–Shelbyville, Shelbyville, KY, p. A259
COLLINS, Pam, Director Human Resources, Fairway Medical Center, Covington, LA, p. A265
COLLINS, Pamela, Vice President Chief Patient Services Officer, McCullough–Hyde Memorial Hospital, Oxford, OH, p. A487
COLLINS, Richard F., M.D. Executive Vice President and Chief Medical Officer, Jefferson Regional Medical Center, Jefferson Hills, PA, p. A525
COLLINS, Ricky M., M.D. Chief of Staff, Whitesburg ARH Hospital, Whitesburg, KY, p. A259
COLLINS, Rudy
Human Resources Business Partner, San Rafael Medical Center, San Rafael, CA, p. A89
Human Resources Business Partner, Santa Rosa Medical Center, Santa Rosa, CA, p. A90
COLLINS, Sandra, Chief Clinical Officer, Kindred Hospital–Philadelphia, Philadelphia, PA, p. A533
COLLINS, Sharon
Director Human Resources and Executive Administrative Assistant, Russell Regional Hospital, Russell, KS, p. A242
Chief Information Officer, Veterans Affairs Medical Center, Salem, VA, p. A656
COLLINS, Shaw, Director Information Technology, Methodist Hospitals, Gary, IN, p. A202
COLLINS, Terry, Chief Financial Officer, Aspen Valley Hospital District, Aspen, CO, p. A97
COLLINS, Thomas M., President, Chairman and Chief Executive Officer, Green Oaks Hospital, Dallas, TX, p. A591
COLLIPP, Dan, M.D. Chief of Staff, Wayne Memorial Hospital, Jesup, GA, p. A154
COLLISON, June, President, Community Hospital of San Bernardino, San Bernardino, CA, p. A84
COLLOTTA, Sharon
Director Human Resources, Mease Countryside Hospital, Safety Harbor, FL, p. A137
Director Human Resources, Mease Hospital Dunedin, Dunedin, FL, p. A122
Director Human Resources, Morton Plant Hospital, Clearwater, FL, p. A120
Director Team Resources, Morton Plant North Bay Hospital, New Port Richey, FL, p. A133
COLLURA, John
Executive Vice President Financial Services and Chief Financial Officer, Beth Israel Medical Center, New York, NY, p. A431
Executive Vice President and Chief Financial Officer, St. Luke's–Roosevelt Hospital Center, New York, NY, p. A437
COLMAN, Sandra, Director Human Resources, Cheyenne Regional Medical Center, Cheyenne, WY, p. A695
COLOMBO, Armando, Chief Executive Officer, Intermedical Hospital of South Carolina, Columbia, SC, p. A548
COLOMBO, Lisa, R.N. Vice President Patient Care Services and Chief Nursing Officer, Health Alliance Hospitals, Leominster, MA, p. A301
COLON, Daniel A., President and Chief Executive Officer, Saint Catherine Healthcare, LLC, Ashland, PA, p. B111
COLON, Daniel A.
President and Chief Executive Officer, Saint Catherine Medical Center Fountain Springs, Ashland, PA, p. A518
President and Chief Executive Officer, Saint Catherine Regional Hospital, Charlestown, IN, p. A199
COLON, Julio, Interim President and Chief Executive Officer, St. Luke's Episcopal Hospital, Ponce, PR, p. A702
COLON, Omar, M.D. Medical Director, HEALTHSOUTH Plano Rehabilitation Hospital, Plano, TX, p. A621
COLONES, Robert L., President and Chief Executive Officer, McLeod Regional Medical Center, Florence, SC, p. A550
COLORADO, Judy, R.N. Vice President, Patient Care Services, Kimball Medical Center, Lakewood, NJ, p. A405
COLOSIMO, Marie, Human Resources Officer, Veterans Affairs Pittsburgh Healthcare System, Pittsburgh, PA, p. A536
COLPO, Susan T., Chief Executive Officer, Life Line Hospital, Steubenville, OH, p. A488
COLSON, Curt, President and Chief Executive Officer, Clara Barton Hospital, Hoisington, KS, p. A234
COLSON, Wayne, Chief Financial Officer, College Station Medical Center, College Station, TX, p. A588
COLT, Darlene, R.N. Chief Nursing Officer, Spanish Peaks Regional Health Center, Walsenburg, CO, p. A106
COLTHARP, Missy, Director, Baptist Memorial Hospital–Union County, New Albany, MS, p. A351
COLTON, Jan, M.D. Acting Clinical Director, U. S. Public Health Service Indian Hospital, Pine Ridge, SD, p. A558
COLTRAIN, Penny, Director Human Resources, Vidant Beaufort Hospital, Washington, NC, p. A462
COLUCCI, Eugene, Vice President Finance, Greenwich Hospital, Greenwich, CT, p. A109
COLUCCIO, Medrice, R.N. Chief Executive Officer, Providence St. Peter Hospital, Olympia, WA, p. A663
COLUMBUS, Rebecca, Vice President Human Resources, River Region Medical Center, Vicksburg, MS, p. A353
COLVARD, Dusty, Manager Information Technology, Tehachapi Valley Healthcare District, Tehachapi, CA, p. A92
COLVIN, Garren
Senior Vice President and Chief Financial Officer, St. Elizabeth Edgewood, Edgewood, KY, p. A249
Senior Vice President Finance and Chief Financial Officer, St. Elizabeth Florence, Florence, KY, p. A250
Senior Vice President and Chief Financial Officer, St. Elizabeth Fort Thomas, Fort Thomas, KY, p. A250
COLVIN, Robert L., Administrator, Ouachita Community Hospital, West Monroe, LA, p. A279
COLVIN, William, Human Resources Officer, Homer Memorial Hospital, Homer, LA, p. A267
COLWELL, Darla, Director Human Resources and Marketing, Clay County Hospital, Flora, IL, p. A182
COLWELL, Dean, D.O. Vice President Medical Affairs, Doctors Hospital, Columbus, OH, p. A476
COLYER, Valeri J.
Director Human Resources, Dickenson Community Hospital, Clintwood, VA, p. A647
Director Human Resources, Norton Community Hospital, Norton, VA, p. A653
COMAIANNI, Sheri, Vice President Human Resources, Bakersfield Memorial Hospital, Bakersfield, CA, p. A54
COMBEST, Felton, M.D. Vice President Medical Affairs, Magnolia Regional Health Center, Corinth, MS, p. A345
COMBS, Barry, Chief Financial Officer, Cedar Crest Hospital, Belton, TX, p. A584
COMBS, Cindy, Supervisor Human Resources, Hampshire Memorial Hospital, Romney, WV, p. A675
COMBS, Jackie, Chief Operating and Nursing Officer, Hi–Desert Medical Center, Joshua Tree, CA, p. A65
COMBS, Mike, Manager Information Technology, Holdenville General Hospital, Holdenville, OK, p. A497
COMER, Fannessa, Chief Executive Officer, Northern Navajo Medical Center, Shiprock, NM, p. A418
COMER, Jennifer, M.D. Medical Director, Valle Vista Hospital, Greenwood, IN, p. A203
COMER, Randy, Chief Operating Officer, Athens–Limestone Hospital, Athens, AL, p. A16
COMER, Scott, Director Administrative Services, Marshall Medical Center, Placerville, CA, p. A80
COMERFORD, Jennifer, Manager Information Services, MidState Medical Center, Meriden, CT, p. A110
COMERFORD Jr., Thomas P., Superintendent, Clarks Summit State Hospital, Clarks Summit, PA, p. A520
COMFORT, Jeff, Vice President Administration, Northcoast Behavioral Healthcare System, Northfield, OH, p. A486
COMITTO, Judy, Vice President Information Services and Chief Information Officer, Trinitas Regional Medical Center, Elizabeth, NJ, p. A403
COMO, Cheryl A., R.N. Vice President Patient Services and Chief Nursing Officer, UPMC McKeesport, McKeesport, PA, p. A528
COMO, James, Director Human Resources, Chestnut Hill Hospital, Philadelphia, PA, p. A531
COMPTON, Brenda, Manager Information Technology, Plumas District Hospital, Quincy, CA, p. A81
COMPTON, Mark, Chief Financial Officer, Laughlin Memorial Hospital, Greeneville, TN, p. A566
COMPTON, Natasha, Chief Nursing Officer, Valley View Medical Center, Fort Mohave, AZ, p. A32
COMPTON, Ty, Chief Nursing Executive, Horton Community Hospital, Horton, KS, p. A235
COMPTON–OGLE, Carri, Administrative Officer, Heartland Behavioral Health Services, Nevada, MO, p. A366
COMSTOCK, John M., Chief Executive Officer, Cherokee Regional Medical Center, Cherokee, IA, p. A216
CONALLEN, Kathryn, Executive Director, Mercy Fitzgerald Hospital, Darby, PA, p. A521
CONANT, Cathy, Chief Human Resources and Personnel, Eastern Plumas Health Care District, Portola, CA, p. A81
CONANT, Sonya, Senior Director Human Resources, Alaska Native Medical Center, Anchorage, AK, p. A28
CONATY, Robert B., Executive Vice President Operations, Montefiore Medical Center,, NY, p. A434
CONAWAY, E. Edwin, M.D. Vice President Medical Affairs and Chief Medical Officer, Southeastern Ohio Regional Medical Center, Cambridge, OH, p. A471
CONCANNON, Margaret, Acting Administrator, Veterans Home and Hospital, Rocky Hill, CT, p. A111
CONCEPCION, Marco Reyes, Executive Director, Hospital Perea, Mayaguez, PR, p. A702
CONCEPCION, Walter, Chief Executive Officer, West Gables Rehabilitation Hospital, Miami, FL, p. A132
CONDE–STERLING, Tania, Executive Director, Hospital Del Maestro, San Juan, PR, p. A703
CONDINO, Deborah A., Site Administrator, St. John Macomb–Oakland Hospital, Oakland Center, Madison Heights, MI, p. A318
CONDIT, Edward, Executive Vice President and Chief Operating Officer, St. Mary's Hospital, Passaic, NJ, p. A408
CONDON, Joseph, Director Human Resources, Texas Health Harris Methodist Hospital Fort Worth, Fort Worth, TX, p. A599
CONDON, William, Deputy Administrative Officer, U. S. Public Health Service Indian Hospital, Fort Yates, ND, p. A466
CONDRY, Donna, Director Human Resources, Jones Regional Medical Center, Anamosa, IA, p. A214
CONE, Maryann, Chief Operating Officer, Sharp Grossmont Hospital, La Mesa, CA, p. A66
CONEJO, David, Chief Executive Officer, Red River Regional Hospital, Bonham, TX, p. A584
CONFALONE, Daniel, Chief Financial Officer, Good Shepherd Rehabilitation Hospital, Allentown, PA, p. A517
CONFORTI, James E., Chief Executive Officer, Memorial Medical Center, Modesto, CA, p. A75
CONGDON, James B., M.D. Medical Director, Horsham Clinic, Ambler, PA, p. A518
CONGER, Rex D., FACHE President and Chief Executive Officer, Perry Memorial Hospital, Princeton, IL, p. A192
CONGER, Sue, Chief Operating Officer, Eastside Psychiatric Hospital, Tallahassee, FL, p. A140
CONKLIN, Robin, R.N. Interim Chief Executive Officer, HEALTHSOUTH Rehabilitation Hospital of Southern Arizona, Tucson, AZ, p. A39
CONKLING, Victoria, Vice President Chief Nursing Officer, Delaware Valley Hospital, Walton, NY, p. A446
CONLEY, David, Chief Administrative Officer, SUNY Downstate Medical Center University Hospital of Brooklyn,, NY, p. A437
CONLEY, Joseph M., Chief Operating Officer, Concord Hospital, Concord, NH, p. A397
CONLEY, Kapua, Chief Executive Officer, Mesa View Regional Hospital, Mesquite, NV, p. A394
CONLEY, Kirkpatrick, Assistant Chief Executive Officer, Oro Valley Hospital, Oro Valley, AZ, p. A34
CONLEY, Melissa, Director Human Resources, Midwest Medical Center, Galena, IL, p. A182
CONLEY, Sue, Chief Executive Officer, Summit Medical Center, Van Buren, AR, p. A52
CONLEY, Teressa
Vice President and Chief Operating Officer, St. Rose Dominican Hospitals – Rose de Lima Campus, Henderson, NV, p. A392
Chief Operating Officer, St. Rose Dominican Hospitals – San Martin Campus, Las Vegas, NV, p. A394
Chief Operating Officer, St. Rose Dominican Hospitals – Siena Campus, Henderson, NV, p. A392
CONLEY, Thomas C., Senior Director Human Resources, Oconee Medical Center, Seneca, SC, p. A553
CONN, Kevin R.
Chief Executive Officer, HEALTHSOUTH Sunrise Rehabilitation Hospital, Fort Lauderdale, FL, p. A123
Interim Chief Executive Officer, HEALTHSOUTH Treasure Coast Rehabilitation Hospital, Vero Beach, FL, p. A142
CONNAUGHTON, Joanne, M.D. Chief Medical Officer, Kindred Hospital–Delaware County, Darby, PA, p. A521
CONNEL, Lorene, Chief Human Resources Management Service, Veterans Affairs Eastern Colorado Health Care System, Denver, CO, p. A100
CONNELL, Faith, Director of Nursing, Turning Point Hospital, Moultrie, GA, p. A157
CONNELL, Robert, PsyD, Superintendent, Larned State Hospital, Larned, KS, p. A237
CONNELLEY, Bertha, Director Human Resources, Austen Riggs Center, Stockbridge, MA, p. A305
CONNELLY, Jac, Chief Financial Officer, Rose Medical Center, Denver, CO, p. A100

Index of Health Care Professionals

Index of Health Care Professionals / Connelly

CONNELLY, Michael, President, Huggins Hospital, Wolfeboro, NH, p. A400
CONNELLY, Michael D., President and Chief Executive Officer, Catholic Health Partners, Cincinnati, OH, p. B28
CONNELLY, Steven, M.D. Chief Medical Officer, Park Nicollet Methodist Hospital, Saint Louis Park, MN, p. A339
CONNER, Chad, Interim Administrator, Green Clinic Surgical Hospital, Ruston, LA, p. A276
CONNER, Gary F., Chief Financial Officer, City of Hope's Helford Clinical Research Hospital, Duarte, CA, p. A59
CONNER, Gloria, Director Human Resources, WestEnd Hospital, Jennings, LA, p. A268
CONNER, Jeff, M.D. Chief Medical Staff, Loma Linda University Medical Center–Murrieta, Murrieta, CA, p. A76
CONNER, Laurie A., FACHE Vice President and Administrator, Mercy Medical Center – West Lakes, West Des Moines, IA, p. A228
CONNOLLY, Brian M., President and Chief Executive Officer, Oakwood Healthcare, Inc., Dearborn, MI, p. B96
CONNOLLY, James W., President and Chief Executive Officer, Ellis Hospital, Schenectady, NY, p. A443
CONNOLLY, Noreen B., MS Chief Nurse Executive, West Branch Regional Medical Center, West Branch, MI, p. A325
CONNOLLY, Teresa, MSN Chief Nursing Officer, Mayo Clinic Hospital, Phoenix, AZ, p. A36
CONNOR, Patrick, Chief Operating Officer, Columbia Hospital, West Palm Beach, FL, p. A142
CONNOR III, Paul J., President and Chief Executive Officer, Eastern Long Island Hospital, Greenport, NY, p. A427
CONNOR, William, Assistant Administrator and Director Human Resources, River Hospital, Alexandria Bay, NY, p. A420
CONNORS, Alfred, Senior Vice President Medical Affairs and Chief Medical Officer, MetroHealth Medical Center, Cleveland, OH, p. A475
CONNORS, Dennis, Executive Director, Glen Cove Hospital, Glen Cove, NY, p. A426
CONNORS, Lawrence J., Chief Operating Officer, St. Mary's Hospital Medical Center, Green Bay, WI, p. A682
CONNORS, Michael
  Senior Vice President and Chief Financial Officer, Cape Cod Hospital, Hyannis, MA, p. A301
  Senior Vice President and Chief Financial Officer, Falmouth Hospital, Falmouth, MA, p. A300
CONNY, Sophia, Deputy Administrative Officer, U. S. Public Health Service Indian Hospital, Pine Ridge, SD, p. A558
CONOCENTI, Paul, Chief Information Officer, City of Hope's Helford Clinical Research Hospital, Duarte, CA, p. A59
CONOLE, Charles P., FACHE Chief Executive Officer, Edward John Noble Hospital of Gouverneur, Gouverneur, NY, p. A427
CONOVER, Jevne, Administrator, LifeCare Hospitals of Wisconsin, Pewaukee, WI, p. A689
CONRAD, Elizabeth, Vice President Human Resources, Hospital of Saint Raphael, New Haven, CT, p. A110
CONRAD, Heidi, Vice President and Chief Financial Officer, Regions Hospital, Saint Paul, MN, p. A339
CONRAD, Terry, Interim CNO, Madison Memorial Hospital, Rexburg, ID, p. A170
CONRATH, Mark, Chief Financial Officer, Drumright Regional Hospital, Drumright, OK, p. A495
CONROW–VERVERIS, Stacy, Director Human Resources, Mineral Community Hospital, Superior, MT, p. A379
CONROY, Denis, Chief Financial Officer, Beverly Hospital, Beverly, MA, p. A295
CONROY, Joanne M., M.D. Executive Vice President and Chief Operating Officer, Morristown Medical Center, Morristown, NJ, p. A406
CONROY, Joseph, M.D. Vice President Medical Affairs, St. Mary Medical Center, Langhorne, PA, p. A526
CONROY, Mary Ann, Chief Executive Officer, Terre Haute Regional Hospital, Terre Haute, IN, p. A212
CONROY, Michael, Chief Financial Officer, Pine Creek Medical Center, Dallas, TX, p. A592
CONROY Jr., Robert B., Chief Executive Officer, St. Petersburg General Hospital, Saint Petersburg, FL, p. A138
CONROY, Tracy, Chief Executive Officer, Select Specialty Hospital–Evansville, Evansville, IN, p. A201
CONSIDINE, William H., President, Akron Children's Hospital, Akron, OH, p. A469
CONSIGLIO, Gayle
  Chief Information Officer, McLaren Flint, Flint, MI, p. A312
  Chief Information Officer, McLaren Lapeer Region, Lapeer, MI, p. A317
CONSIGNEY, Ginger, Vice President Human Resources, Lake Charles Memorial Hospital, Lake Charles, LA, p. A271
CONSOLVER, Roberta, Chief Clinical Officer, Kindred Hospital Sugar Land, Sugar Land, TX, p. A629
CONSTANTINO, Chris D., Executive Director, Elmhurst Hospital Center,, NY, p. A432
CONTE, John D., Director Facility Services, Wayne Memorial Hospital, Honesdale, PA, p. A525
CONTI, John, Director Finance, Shriners Hospitals for Children, Greenville, Greenville, SC, p. A550
CONTILLO, Nancy, Director Human Resources, Day Kimball Hospital, Putnam, CT, p. A111
CONTRERA, Yleana, Executive Director Human Resources, Hoboken University Medical Center, Hoboken, NJ, p. A404
CONWAY, Gerard, Chief Executive Officer, Aurora Las Encinas Hospital, Pasadena, CA, p. A79
CONWAY, Jimmy, M.D. President Medical Staff, Northwest Surgical Hospital, Oklahoma City, OK, p. A501
CONWAY, John Paul, Executive Vice President Human Resources, Oakwood Hospital & Medical Center–Dearborn, Dearborn, MI, p. A310
CONWELL, Heather, Chief Nursing Officer, Downey Regional Medical Center, Downey, CA, p. A59
CONWILL, Michael, Director Human Resources, Corpus Christi Medical Center, Corpus Christi, TX, p. A589
CONYERS, Lois
  Senior Vice President and Chief Financial Officer, Citrus Valley Medical Center–Inter–Community Campus, Covina, CA, p. A59
  Senior Vice President and Chief Financial Officer, Foothill Presbyterian Hospital, Glendora, CA, p. A63
COOK, Aaron, Director Information Services, Women and Children's Hospital, Lake Charles, LA, p. A271
COOK, Ann Fagan, Chief Information Officer, Parkview Hospital, Wheeler, TX, p. A634
COOK, Brandy, Chief Nursing Officer, Regional Rehabilitation Hospital, Phenix City, AL, p. A25
COOK, Brian, FACHE Chief Executive Officer, Capital Regional Medical Center, Tallahassee, FL, p. A140
COOK, David, Manager Information Systems, Advance Care Hospital, Hot Springs National Park, AR, p. A46
COOK, David, M.D. Chief Medical Officer, Presbyterian Hospital Huntersville, Huntersville, NC, p. A455
COOK, David, Vice President Human Resources, St. Louis Children's Hospital, Saint Louis, MO, p. A370
COOK, Diane, Chief Nursing Officer, Allegiance Specialty Hospital of Little Rock, Jacksonville, AR, p. A46
COOK, Elizabeth, Chief Information Officer, Mizell Memorial Hospital, Opp, AL, p. A24
COOK, Greg, Chief Financial Officer, Jackson Purchase Medical Center, Mayfield, KY, p. A256
COOK, Heidi, Chief Nursing Officer, Dr. John Warner Hospital, Clinton, IL, p. A179
COOK, Jaime, Director Human Resources, Riverside Tappahannock Hospital, Tappahannock, VA, p. A656
COOK, Jeff, Director Information Services, Medical Park Hospital, Hope, AR, p. A46
COOK, John
  Chief Financial Officer, Mercy Harvard Hospital, Harvard, IL, p. A183
  Vice President and Chief Financial Officer, Mercy Hospital and Trauma Center, Janesville, WI, p. A683
COOK, Katheryn, R.N. Nurse Executive, Veterans Affairs Medical Center, Cincinnati, OH, p. A474
COOK, Kevin S., President and Chief Executive Officer, Mercy St. Vincent Medical Center, Toledo, OH, p. A489
COOK, LaMont, Administrator, F. W. Huston Medical Center, Winchester, KS, p. A246
COOK, Linda, Vice President Human Resources, St. Joseph Hospital, Eureka, CA, p. A60
COOK, Lottie, Superintendent, Evansville Psychiatric Children Center, Evansville, IN, p. A201
COOK, Marcia, Director Information Technology, Bates County Memorial Hospital, Butler, MO, p. A356
COOK, Mark, Director Human Resources, Crossgates River Oaks Hospital, Brandon, MS, p. A344
COOK, Pamela W., Chief Financial Officer, Trace Regional Hospital, Houston, MS, p. A347
COOK, Patrick, Vice President Support Services, Morgan Memorial Hospital, Madison, GA, p. A156
COOK, Phillip, Administrator, Clinch Memorial Hospital, Homerville, GA, p. A154
COOK, Roger, Director Human Resources, Golden Valley Memorial Healthcare, Clinton, MO, p. A358
COOK, Ruth, Administrator, East Texas Medical Center Fairfield, Fairfield, TX, p. A597
COOK, Scott, Chief Financial Officer, Green Oaks Hospital, Dallas, TX, p. A591
COOK, Shelia, Director Information Systems, Presbyterian–Orthopaedic Hospital, Charlotte, NC, p. A451
COOK, Sheliah, Director Human Resources, Boone Memorial Hospital, Madison, WV, p. A673
COOK, Stacey, Director Human Resources, Civista Health, La Plata, MD, p. A292
COOK, Thomas J., Chief Executive Officer, UVA–HEALTHSOUTH Rehabilitation Hospital, Charlottesville, VA, p. A646
COOK, Thomas M., CPA Chief Financial Officer, St. Vincent Indianapolis Hospital, Indianapolis, IN, p. A205
COOK, Timothy W., President and Chief Executive Officer, Florida Hospital Heartland Medical Center, Sebring, FL, p. A139
COOK, Will L., President, UPMC Mercy, Pittsburgh, PA, p. A535
COOK, William, Associate Warden Business Service, California Mens Colony Hospital, San Luis Obispo, CA, p. A88
COOKE, Barbara
  Director Health Information Systems, Mount Vernon Hospital, Mount Vernon, NY, p. A430
  Director Health Information Systems, Sound Shore Medical Center of Westchester, New Rochelle, NY, p. A431
COOKE, David, Chief Nursing Officer, Sutter Surgical Hospital – North Valley, Yuba City, CA, p. A96
COOKE, Nancy, Chief Financial Officer, Weatherford Regional Medical Center, Weatherford, TX, p. A634
COOKSEY, Jill, Vice President Chief Nursing Officer, EMH Elyria Medical Center, Elyria, OH, p. A480
COOLEY, Lamar, R.N. Director of Nursing, Washington County Hospital and Nursing Home, Chatom, AL, p. A18
COOLEY, Stephen, M.D. Chairman Executive Committee Medical Staff, Naval Hospital, Oak Harbor, WA, p. A663
COOLEY, W. Carl, M.D. Chief Medical Officer, Crotched Mountain Rehabilitation Center, Greenfield, NH, p. A398
COOMBS, James, Chief Executive Officer, Grand River Hospital District, Rifle, CO, p. A105
COOMES, Larry, Chief Executive Officer, Palmdale Regional Medical Center, Palmdale, CA, p. A79
COONER, Suzanne, R.N. Vice President Operations, Grinnell Regional Medical Center, Grinnell, IA, p. A220
COONEY, Darlene, Director Nursing, Sumner Regional Medical Center, Wellington, KS, p. A245
COONEY, Lauri Ann, Director Nursing, Wheatland Memorial Healthcare, Harlowton, MT, p. A376
COOPER, Alisa, Manager Financial Resources, Michael E. DeBakey Veterans Affairs Medical Center, Houston, TX, p. A606
COOPER, Andrew, Manager, Information Services, McDowell Hospital, Marion, NC, p. A457
COOPER, Anthony J., FACHE President and Chief Executive Officer, Arnot Health, Elmira, NY, p. B11
COOPER, Casey, Chief Executive Officer, Cherokee Indian Hospital, Cherokee, NC, p. A451
COOPER, Chad D., President and Chief Executive Officer, St. Gabriel's Hospital, Little Falls, MN, p. A333
COOPER, Cliff, Chief Financial Officer, Wills Memorial Hospital, Washington, GA, p. A162
COOPER, Curtis, Manager Information Systems, Pioneers Medical Center, Meeker, CO, p. A104
COOPER, Dena, Chief Financial Officer, Campbellton Graceville Hospital, Graceville, FL, p. A124
COOPER, Dennis, Director Human Resources, Arkansas Methodist Medical Center, Paragould, AR, p. A50
COOPER, Donald, Director Information Systems, Harton Regional Medical Center, Tullahoma, TN, p. A576
COOPER, Donald C., Director, Veterans Affairs Central Iowa Health Care System, Des Moines, IA, p. A218
COOPER, Douglas, M.D. Chief Medical Officer, Grundy County Memorial Hospital, Grundy Center, IA, p. A220
COOPER Jr.,, Edwin H., MS, President and Chief Executive Officer, AcuityHealthcare, LP, Charlotte, NC, p. B4
COOPER, Hunt, M.D. Chief of Staff, Siloam Springs Memorial Hospital, Siloam Springs, AR, p. A51
COOPER, Ian, Chief Executive Officer, Kindred Hospital Cleveland–Gateway, Cleveland, OH, p. A475
COOPER, James C., Chief Operating Officer, Jefferson Regional Medical Center, Jefferson Hills, PA, p. A525
COOPER, Jeffrey M., President, Genesis Medical Center, DeWitt, De Witt, IA, p. A217
COOPER, Jerry, Manager Data Processing, Richland Hospital, Richland Center, WI, p. A690
COOPER, John C., Chief Executive Officer, Fremont Hospital, Fremont, CA, p. A61
COOPER, Joseph, M.D. Chief of Staff, Pender Memorial Hospital, Burgaw, NC, p. A449
COOPER, Kevin S., R.N. Administrator, LifeCare Hospitals of North Carolina, Rocky Mount, NC, p. A459
COOPER, MaryBeth, R.N. Chief Nursing Officer, Highland Community Hospital, Picayune, MS, p. A351
COOPER, Michael W., Chief Executive Officer, Breckinridge Memorial Hospital, Hardinsburg, KY, p. A251
COOPER, Pat, Comptroller, Conejos County Hospital, La Jara, CO, p. A103
COOPER, Scott, M.D. Chief Executive Officer, St. Barnabas Hospital,, NY, p. A436
COOPER, Sheri, Director Human Resources, Union General Hospital, Farmerville, LA, p. A266
COOPER, Tami, Acting Director of Nursing, Riverview Psychiatric Center, Augusta, ME, p. A281
COOPER, Tim, Chief Financial Officer, Prosser Memorial Hospital, Prosser, WA, p. A664

A788 Index of Health Care Professionals 

Index of Health Care Professionals / Cotterman


COOPER–LOHR, Willie, Chief Financial Officer, Barnesville Hospital, Barnesville, OH, p. A470
COOPERMAN, Todd, M.D. Medical Director, Rehabilitation Hospital of Tinton Falls, Tinton Falls, NJ, p. A410
COOPERSTEIN, Elizabeth, M.D. Chief Medical Officer, Wellmont Lonesome Pine Hospital, Big Stone Gap, VA, p. A645
COOPWOOD, Reginald W., M.D. President and Chief Executive Officer, Regional Medical Center at Memphis, Memphis, TN, p. A572
COORPENDER, William, Assistant Vice President Human Resources, North Florida Regional Medical Center, Gainesville, FL, p. A124
COOTS, Lawrence, M.D. Chief Medical Officer, Orange Park Medical Center, Orange Park, FL, p. A134
COPE, Brent A., Chief Executive Officer, Arizona Regional Medical Center, Mesa, AZ, p. A33
COPE, David
Chief Executive Officer, Marion Regional Hospital, Mullins, SC, p. A552
Chief Operating Officer, Mary Black Memorial Hospital, Spartanburg, SC, p. A553
COPE, Donald, Director Information Systems, Newman Regional Health, Emporia, KS, p. A232
COPELAND, Carolyn, Business Administrator, Madison State Hospital, Madison, IN, p. A208
COPELAND, Darlinda, Chief Operating Officer, Florida Hospital Memorial Medical Center, Daytona Beach, FL, p. A121
COPELAND, Dia, Administrator, Grimes St. Joseph Health Center, Navasota, TX, p. A618
COPELAND, Gail, Director Management Information Systems, CrossRidge Community Hospital, Wynne, AR, p. A52
COPELAND, John W., Chief Financial Officer, Crockett Hospital, Lawrenceburg, TN, p. A569
COPELAND Jr., Robert Y., FACHE Chief Executive Officer, Mercy McCune–Brooks Hospital, Carthage, MO, p. A357
COPELAND, Willie Mae, Chief Financial Officer, Harmon Memorial Hospital, Hollis, OK, p. A498
COPEN, Greg, Chief Information Officer, MedWest – Haywood, Clyde, NC, p. A451
COPENHAVER, Kathy, Director Human Resources, Haven Behavioral Health of Eastern Pennsylvania, Reading, PA, p. A536
COPES, Tammy, Director Information Systems, St. Mary's of Michigan Standish Hospital, Standish, MI, p. A323
COPPLE, Brad
President, Kishwaukee Community Hospital, DeKalb, IL, p. A180
President, Kishwaukee Community Hospital, DeKalb, IL, p. A180
President, Valley West Community Hospital, Sandwich, IL, p. A193
COPPOCK, R. Alan, FACHE President and Chief Executive Officer, Oak Tree Hospital, Corbin, KY, p. A249
CORBET, Mark, Interim Chief Financial Officer, LAC/University of Southern California Medical Center, Los Angeles, CA, p. A70
CORBI, Kelly, Chief Administrative Officer and Vice President Human Resources and Development, Meritus Medical Center, Hagerstown, MD, p. A292
CORBIN, Michelle, M.D. Chief of Staff, Powell County Medical Center, Deer Lodge, MT, p. A374
CORBIN, Phil, M.D. Chief Medical Officer, Parkview Noble Hospital, Kendallville, IN, p. A206
CORBIN, Scott, M.D. Chief of Staff, Northern Hospital of Surry County, Mount Airy, NC, p. A458
CORCORAN, Kevin, Chief Financial Officer, Westside Regional Medical Center, Plantation, FL, p. A136
CORCORAN, Linda, Chief Executive Officer, Aspire Behavioral Health of Conroe, Conroe, TX, p. A588
CORCORAN, Michael, Chief Financial Officer, Chesapeake Regional Medical Center, Chesapeake, VA, p. A646
CORCORAN, Nancy R., Senior Vice President Human Resources and Quality Service, Hackensack University Medical Center, Hackensack, NJ, p. A404
CORD, Jennifer, Vice President of Operations, Provena United Samaritans Medical Center, Danville, IL, p. A179
CORDEIRO, August B., FACHE President and Chief Executive Officer, Newport Hospital, Newport, RI, p. A544
CORDER, Earline, Chief Fiscal, Veterans Affairs Medical Center, Augusta, GA, p. A147
CORDER, Noralene, Chief Financial Officer, Seton Smithville Regional Hospital, Smithville, TX, p. A628
CORDER, Scott, Controller, HEALTHSOUTH Rehabilitation Hospital at Drake, Cincinnati, OH, p. A473
CORDIA, Jennifer, Vice President and Chief Nursing Executive, Christian Hospital, Saint Louis, MO, p. A368
CORDNER, Glenn D., Chief Executive Officer, Springfield Hospital, Springfield, VT, p. A644
CORDOLA, Craig, Chief Executive Officer, Memorial Hermann – Texas Medical Center, Houston, TX, p. A605
CORDOVA, Richard D., President and Chief Executive Officer, Children's Hospital Los Angeles, Los Angeles, CA, p. A69
CORDOVA, Sheila, Director Clinical Services and Chief Operating Officer, Aurora Charter Oak Hospital, Covina, CA, p. A58
CORDTS, Paul, Commander, Colonel Florence A. Blanchfield Army Community Hospital, Fort Campbell, KY, p. A250
COREA, Rohan, Director Healthcare Information Technology, Pacific Hospital of Long Beach, Long Beach, CA, p. A68
COREY, Mark, Chief Financial Officer, Behavioral Center of Michigan, Warren, MI, p. A324
CORFITS, Joe
Chief Financial Officer, Iowa Lutheran Hospital, Des Moines, IA, p. A218
Senior Vice President Finance, Iowa Methodist Medical Center, Des Moines, IA, p. A218
CORK, A. Scott, Chief Executive Officer, Hallmark Youthcare – Richmond, Richmond, VA, p. A655
CORK, Ronald J., President and Chief Executive Officer, Avera St. Anthony's Hospital, O'Neill, NE, p. A386
CORKERN, Kendall, Administrator, Serenity Springs Specialty Hospital, Farmerville, LA, p. A266
CORKERY, Thomas B., D.O. Chief Medical Officer, Canonsburg General Hospital, Canonsburg, PA, p. A520
CORLEY, Adam, M.D. Chief of Staff, Brazosport Regional Health System, Lake Jackson, TX, p. A611
CORLEY, Becky, Director Human Resources, Tyler Holmes Memorial Hospital, Winona, MS, p. A354
CORLEY, Craig, Chief Financial Officer, Thousand Oaks Surgical Hospital, Thousand Oaks, CA, p. A92
CORLEY, Janet, Accountant, Malvern Institute, Malvern, PA, p. A528
CORMIER, Laura, Director, Oconto Hospital & Medical Center, Oconto, WI, p. A688
CORN, Rick, Chief Information Officer, Huntsville Hospital, Huntsville, AL, p. A22
CORNAVA, Joanne, Director Human Resources, Marlton Rehabilitation Hospital, Marlton, NJ, p. A406
CORNEJO, C. Susan, Senior Vice President Finance and Chief Financial Officer, Providence Hospital, Mobile, AL, p. A23
CORNELIUS, Margaret E., Vice President Human Resources, Wyckoff Heights Medical Center,, NY, p. A438
CORNELIUS, Michelle
Director Human Resources for Northern Region, Eagle River Memorial Hospital, Eagle River, WI, p. A680
Director Human Resources, Howard Young Medical Center, Woodruff, WI, p. A694
Director Human Resources for the Northern Region, Sacred Heart–St. Mary's Hospitals, Rhinelander, WI, p. A690
CORNELIUS, Senta, Director Human Resources, West Valley Medical Center, Caldwell, ID, p. A167
CORNELL, John, Vice President Finance, Meadows Regional Medical Center, Vidalia, GA, p. A161
CORNETT, Sheila, Manager Human Resources, Hazard ARH Regional Medical Center, Hazard, KY, p. A251
CORNETT, Suzanne, Director Human Resources, Southern Kentucky Rehabilitation Hospital, Bowling Green, KY, p. A248
CORNICELLI, Kari, Chief Financial Officer, Sharp Grossmont Hospital, La Mesa, CA, p. A66
CORNING, Eileen M., Director Human Resources, Largo Medical Center, Largo, FL, p. A128
CORNWALL, Thomas, M.D. Medical Director, Holly Hill Hospital, Raleigh, NC, p. A459
CORNWELL, Cheryl, Chief Financial Officer, Great Falls Clinic Medical Center, Great Falls, MT, p. A376
CORONEL, Jorge, Chief Information Officer, Regional Hospital of Scranton, Scranton, PA, p. A538
CORPORA, Don, Senior Vice President Human Resources, Akron General Medical Center, Akron, OH, p. A469
CORRADINO, Richard L., Chief Financial Officer, Spanish Peaks Regional Health Center, Walsenburg, CO, p. A106
CORRADO, Theresa, Director Finance, St. Luke's Hospital – Quakertown Campus, Quakertown, PA, p. A536
CORREA, Elizabeth, Director Information Management, Big Spring State Hospital, Big Spring, TX, p. A584
CORREA, Maria de los Angeles, M.D. Medical Director, Hospital Metropolitan, San Juan, PR, p. A703
CORREA, Omar, Chief Operating Officer, Texas NeuroRehab Center, Austin, TX, p. A582
CORREA, Sharon, Associate Vice President, Glendale Adventist Medical Center, Glendale, CA, p. A63
CORREIA, Antonio, Chief Financial Officer, Holyoke Medical Center, Holyoke, MA, p. A300
CORREIA, Kathryn G., President and Chief Executive Officer, HealthEast Care System, Saint Paul, MN, p. B64
CORRIDON, Fran, Vice President Human Resources and Shared Services, Hackensack University Medical Center Mountainside, Montclair, NJ, p. A406
CORRIGAN, Paula, Vice President and Chief Financial Officer, OSF Saint James – John W. Albrecht Medical Center, Pontiac, IL, p. A192
CORRIGAN, Thomas L., Senior Vice President Finance, Managed Care and Chief Financial Officer, Christiana Care Health System, Newark, DE, p. A114
CORTI, Ronald, President and Chief Executive Officer, Community Hospital at Dobbs Ferry, Dobbs Ferry, NY, p. A425
CORTRIGHT, Michael, Chief Information Officer, Ralph H. Johnson Veterans Affairs Medical Center, Charleston, SC, p. A547
CORVINO, Frank A., President and Chief Executive Officer, Greenwich Hospital, Greenwich, CT, p. A109
CORWIN, Florence, Director for Administration, Pilgrim Psychiatric Center, Brentwood, NY, p. A422
CORWIN, R. William, M.D. Vice President and Chief Medical Officer, Miriam Hospital, Providence, RI, p. A544
CORWIN, Steven J., M.D. Chief Executive Officer, New York Presbyterian Healthcare System, New York, NY, p. B93
CORWIN, Steven J., M.D. Chief Executive Officer, New York–Presbyterian Hospital, New York, NY, p. A436
CORZINE, Judy, Administrative Director and Chief Information Officer, Stormont–Vail HealthCare, Topeka, KS, p. A244
COSBY, Bridget, Chief Executive Officer, Pauls Valley General Hospital, Pauls Valley, OK, p. A503
COSBY, Ernestine, Vice President Clinical Services and Chief Nursing Officer, Sheppard and Enoch Pratt Hospital, Baltimore, MD, p. A289
COSCO, John A., FACHE Administrator, Community Behavioral Health Hospital – Alexandria, Alexandria, MN, p. A327
COSGROVE, Delos, M.D. President and Chief Executive Officer, Cleveland Clinic Foundation, Cleveland, OH, p. A474
COSGROVE, Delos, M.D. President and Chief Executive Officer, Cleveland Clinic Health System, Cleveland, OH, p. B32
COSSAIRT, Vicki, Director Human Resources, Integris Grove General Hospital, Grove, OK, p. A497
COSSIO, Eduardo M., M.D. Chief of Staff, Morgan Memorial Hospital, Madison, GA, p. A156
COSTA, Christopher P., M.D. Chief of Staff, Gordon Memorial Hospital, Gordon, NE, p. A384
COSTA, Joe
Acting Chief Fiscal Officer, Brockton Veterans Affairs Medical Center, Brockton, MA, p. A298
Chief Financial Officer, Veterans Affairs Boston Healthcare System, Boston, MA, p. A297
COSTA, Mark E., Executive Director, Los Angeles Medical Center, Los Angeles, CA, p. A70
COSTA, Michael
Director Human Resources, Grimes St. Joseph Health Center, Navasota, TX, p. A618
Vice President Human Resources, St. Joseph Regional Health Center, Bryan, TX, p. A586
COSTANTINI, Polly, Director Human Resources, Hampton Behavioral Health Center, Westampton Township, NJ, p. A412
COSTANTINO, Mark J., M.D. Interim Chief Medical Officer, Athens Regional Medical Center, Athens, GA, p. A144
COSTANTINO, Vincent, Vice President Operations and Human Resources, Raritan Bay Medical Center, Perth Amboy, NJ, p. A408
COSTELLA, Jeane L., Vice President, Hudson Valley Hospital Center, Cortlandt Manor, NY, p. A424
COSTELLO, Benny, Chief Executive Officer, Promise Hospital of Miss Lou, Vidalia, LA, p. A279
COSTELLO, Jeff, Chief Financial Officer, Memorial Hospital of South Bend, South Bend, IN, p. A212
COSTIC, Andrew, Regional Chief Financial Officer, Abraham Lincoln Memorial Hospital, Lincoln, IL, p. A186
COSTIE, Glenn A., FACHE Director, Veterans Affairs Medical Center, Dayton, OH, p. A479
COTA, Scott, M.D. Director Medical Services, Naval Hospital, Lemoore, CA, p. A67
COTE, Mario, M.D. Chief of Staff and President Medical Staff, Illinois Valley Community Hospital, Peru, IL, p. A191
COTHRON, Robert, MSC, Administrator, U. S. Air Force Medical Center Keesler, Keesler AFB, MS, p. A348
COTSHOTT, Angelica, Chief Executive Officer, Kindred Hospital Melbourne, Melbourne, FL, p. A130
COTT, Gary, M.D. Executive Vice President Medical and Clinical Services, National Jewish Health, Denver, CO, p. A99
COTTER, Carole
Senior Vice President and Chief Information Officer, Emma Pendleton Bradley Hospital, East Providence, RI, p. A544
Vice President and Chief Information Officer, Miriam Hospital, Providence, RI, p. A544
Senior Vice President and Chief Information Officer, Rhode Island Hospital, Providence, RI, p. A544
COTTER, Richard W., Associate Director Operations, VA Butler Healthcare, Butler, PA, p. A519
COTTERMAN, Rob, Assistant Superintendent Program Services, Moccasin Bend Mental Health Institute, Chattanooga, TN, p. A563


 Index of Health Care Professionals A789

Index of Health Care Professionals

Index of Health Care Professionals

Index of Health Care Professionals / Cotti


COTTI, Matthew, Chief Financial Officer, Rehabilitation Hospital of Rhode Island, North Smithfield, RI, p. A544
COTTINGHAM, Jerod, Director Information Systems, Carlinville Area Hospital, Carlinville, IL, p. A174
COTTLE, Gil, Chief Financial Officer, St. Christopher's Hospital for Children, Philadelphia, PA, p. A533
COTTO, Hector L., M.D. Medical Director, Hospital San Francisco, San Juan, PR, p. A703
COTTON, Jerry, Interim COO, Baptist Medical Center Leake, Carthage, MS, p. A344
COTTON, Michael, Chief Financial Officer, Gadsden Regional Medical Center, Gadsden, AL, p. A20
COTTRELL, Christopher, M.D. Chief of Staff, Lake Pointe Medical Center, Rowlett, TX, p. A623
COTTRILL, Brian, Chief Information Officer, United Hospital Center, Bridgeport, WV, p. A670
COUCH, Beulah, Director Human Resources, Mary Breckinridge ARH Hospital, Hyden, KY, p. A252
COUCH, Bill, Chief Financial Officer, Ashley County Medical Center, Crossett, AR, p. A43
COUCH, George G., FACHE President and Chief Executive Officer, East Ohio Regional Hospital, Martins Ferry, OH, p. A484
COUCH, Lorie, Assistant Superintendent, Big Spring State Hospital, Big Spring, TX, p. A584
COUCH, Robert J., Chief Executive Officer, Medical Center of Manchester, Manchester, TN, p. A570
COUGHLIN, Ann, Director Human Resources, Boundary Community Hospital, Bonners Ferry, ID, p. A167
COUGHLIN, Cynthia, MS Chief Nursing Officer, Cheshire Medical Center, Keene, NH, p. A398
COUILLARD, John, Chief Financial Officer, Kindred Hospital Boston–North Shore, Peabody, MA, p. A303
COULLIETTE, Edwina, Manager Human Resources, St. Vincent's Medical Center Southside, Jacksonville, FL, p. A127
COULTAS, David, M.D. Vice President Clinical Affairs, University of Texas Health Science Center at Tyler, Tyler, TX, p. A632
COULTER, Barbara
Director Information Systems, Franciscan St. Francis Health – Indianapolis, Indianapolis, IN, p. A204
Director Information Systems, Franciscan St. Francis Health – Mooresville, Mooresville, IN, p. A209
COULTER, David C., Senior Vice President and Chief Executive Officer, WakeMed Cary Hospital, Cary, NC, p. A450
COULTER, Lisa, Director Human Resources, St. Christopher's Hospital for Children, Philadelphia, PA, p. A533
COUNTRYMAN, Cory, Interim Chief Executive Officer, Weatherford Regional Medical Center, Weatherford, TX, p. A634
COUNTY–TEEMER, Vickie, Coordinator Human Resources, Mitchell County Hospital, Camilla, GA, p. A148
COUNTZLER, John, Chief Executive Officer, Muhlenberg Community Hospital, Greenville, KY, p. A251
COURAGE, Kenneth F., Chief Executive Officer, Psychiatric Institute of Washington, Washington, DC, p. A117
COURIS, John D., President and Chief Executive Officer, Jupiter Medical Center, Jupiter, FL, p. A127
COURLISS, Richard, Chief Support Services, Cherry Hospital, Goldsboro, NC, p. A453
COURNYER, Tim, Chief Financial Officer, Morton General Hospital, Morton, WA, p. A663
COUROUNIS, Glenn, Vice President Human Resources, Lenox Hill Hospital, New York, NY, p. A433
COURREGE, Chad, Vice President Human Resources, Touro Infirmary, New Orleans, LA, p. A275
COURREGE, Gary, Chief Information Officer, Jennings American Legion Hospital, Jennings, LA, p. A268
COURTOIS, Harold, Administrator and Chief Executive Officer, Trego County–Lemke Memorial Hospital, Wakeeney, KS, p. A244
COURTOIS, Robert, Vice President Finance, Otsego Memorial Hospital, Gaylord, MI, p. A313
COURTWAY, Peter, Chief Information Officer, New Milford Hospital, New Milford, CT, p. A111
COUSAR, Myra, Director Human Resources, Baptist Memorial Hospital–Tipton, Covington, TN, p. A564
COUSENS, Tim, On–Site Administrator, Sage Memorial Hospital, Ganado, AZ, p. A32
COUSINEAU, Cathy, Director Human Resources, Woodland Hills Medical Center,, CA, p. A73
COUSINS, Kelly, Director Information Technology, Abbeville General Hospital, Abbeville, LA, p. A261
COUTURE, Elaine, R.N
Chief Executive Officer, Providence Holy Family Hospital, Spokane, WA, p. A667
Chief Executive Officer, Providence Sacred Heart Medical Center & Children's Hospital, Spokane, WA, p. A667
COVA, Charles J., President and Chief Executive Officer, Marian Medical Center, Santa Maria, CA, p. A90
COVA, Matthew, Chief Financial Officer, Northern Nevada Medical Center, Sparks, NV, p. A396
COVELL, Nancy, Director Human Resources, Cameron Memorial Community Hospital, Angola, IN, p. A197
COVERT, Charles O.
Chief Financial Officer, Saint Francis Hospital, Charleston, WV, p. A671
Vice President Finance, Thomas Memorial Hospital, South Charleston, WV, p. A676
COVERT, Michael H., FACHE Chief Executive Officer, Palomar Health, San Diego, CA, p. B99
COVERT, Rob, President and Chief Executive Officer, Oaklawn Hospital, Marshall, MI, p. A318
COVEY, Laird P., President, Central Maine Medical Center, Lewiston, ME, p. A283
COVEY, Staci, MS, President, Troy Community Hospital, Troy, PA, p. A539
COVIN, Charles
Chief Information Officer, Manchester Memorial Hospital, Manchester, CT, p. A109
Chief Information Officer, Rockville General Hospital, Vernon Rockville, CT, p. A112
COVINGTON, Casey, M.D. President Elect, Medical Staff, Jennie Stuart Medical Center, Hopkinsville, KY, p. A251
COVINGTON, Jerome, M.D. Chief Medical Officer, Lower Keys Medical Center, Key West, FL, p. A127
COWAN, Dale, M.D. Vice President Medical Affairs, Parma Community General Hospital, Parma, OH, p. A487
COWAN, Joshua, Chief Information Officer, St. Helena Hospital Clearlake, Clearlake, CA, p. A57
COWAN, Ronald M., Vice President Information Systems, Lewistown Hospital, Lewistown, PA, p. A527
COWDEN, Ella, Director Human Resources, Erlanger at Hutcheson, Fort Oglethorpe, GA, p. A153
COWGER, David, M.D. Senior Vice President Quality and Medical Affairs and Chief Medical Officer, Altoona Regional Health System, Altoona, PA, p. A517
COWIE, Cynthia, Chief Executive Officer, Southwest Regional Medical Center, Waynesburg, PA, p. A540
COWLES, Deborah, Vice President Human Resources, Flaget Memorial Hospital, Bardstown, KY, p. A247
COWLES, John, Chief Financial Officer, Silver Lake Medical Center, Los Angeles, CA, p. A72
COWLEY, Markie, Executive Vice President and Chief Operating Officer, Mission Hospital, Mission Viejo, CA, p. A74
COWLING, Michael, Chief Executive Officer, Palm Beach Gardens Medical Center, Palm Beach Gardens, FL, p. A135
COWLING, Phyllis A., CPA, President and Chief Executive Officer, United Regional Health Care System, Wichita Falls, TX, p. A635
COWPERTHWAIT, Cheri, Interim Chief Executive Officer, Lourdes Specialty Hospital of Southern New Jersey, Willingboro, NJ, p. A412
COX, Brenda, Director Human Resources, Scott & White Hospital at Round Rock, Round Rock, TX, p. A623
COX, Brian, Director Information Systems, Floyd Memorial Hospital and Health Services, New Albany, IN, p. A209
COX, Charles B., M.D. Chief of Staff, Woods Memorial Hospital, Etowah, TN, p. A565
COX, Courtney, Vice President Human Resources, UPMC Northwest, Seneca, PA, p. A538
COX, Danny, Chief Executive Officer, Atrium Medical Center, Stafford, TX, p. A628
COX, David W., Chief Financial Officer, Marin General Hospital, Greenbrae, CA, p. A64
COX, Debbie D., Administrative Director Human Resources, Central Texas Medical Center, San Marcos, TX, p. A627
COX, Dina, Director Human Resources, Kansas Rehabilitation Hospital, Topeka, KS, p. A244
COX, Dorothy, Manager Information Systems, Hackettstown Regional Medical Center, Hackettstown, NJ, p. A404
COX, F. Gregory, M.D. Chief of Staff, Parkway Regional Hospital, Fulton, KY, p. A250
COX, Gray, President, St. Francis Hospital and Health Services, Maryville, MO, p. A365
COX, Jack, M.D
Chief Quality Officer, Hoag Hospital Irvine, Irvine, CA, p. A65
Senior Vice President and Chief Quality Officer, Hoag Memorial Hospital Presbyterian, Newport Beach, CA, p. A76
COX, Jay, FACHE President and Chief Executive Officer, Tuomey Healthcare System, Sumter, SC, p. A554
COX, Keith, Administrator, LifeCare Hospitals of Shreveport, Shreveport, LA, p. A277
COX, Ken, Chief Financial Officer, St. Helena Parish Hospital, Greensburg, LA, p. A267
COX, Kenneth, M.D. Chief Medical Officer, Lucile Salter Packard Children's Hospital at Stanford, Palo Alto, CA, p. A79
COX, Kevin, Chief Financial Officer, Integris Grove General Hospital, Grove, OK, p. A497
COX, Leigh, Chief Information Officer, WellStar Windy Hill Hospital, Marietta, GA, p. A156
COX, Lynna B., Director Health Information Services, Anson General Hospital, Anson, TX, p. A579
COX, Matthew
Chief Financial Officer, Central Maine Medical Center, Lewiston, ME, p. A283
Senior Vice President and Chief Financial Officer, St. Vincent Infirmary Medical Center, Little Rock, AR, p. A48
COX, Randell, Director Data Processing, Bowie Memorial Hospital, Bowie, TX, p. A584
COX, Randy
Chief Information Officer, Lutheran Hospital of Indiana, Fort Wayne, IN, p. A201
Chief Information Officer, St. Joseph Hospital, Fort Wayne, IN, p. A202
COX, Raymond L., M.D. Chief Medical Officer, Providence Hospital, Washington, DC, p. A116
COX, Rosalie, Administrator, LifeCare Hospitals of Chester County, West Chester, PA, p. A541
COX, Sandra, Controller, Permian Regional Medical Center, Andrews, TX, p. A578
COX, Scott, Manager Information Systems, St. Vincent Salem Hospital, Salem, IN, p. A211
COX, Sheila, Director Human Resources, Cibola General Hospital, Grants, NM, p. A416
COX, Sherry, Chief Human Resources Officer, Ashe Memorial Hospital, Jefferson, NC, p. A455
COX, Steve, M.D. Chief Medical Officer, Fairfield Medical Center, Lancaster, OH, p. A482
COXE, Bob, M.D. Medical Director, Vanderbilt Stallworth Rehabilitation Hospital, Nashville, TN, p. A574
COY, Nelson, Director Human Resources, Tahoe Pacific Hospitals, Reno, NV, p. A395
COYE, Ed, Director Information Technology, Transylvania Regional Hospital, Brevard, NC, p. A449
COYLE, Joseph P., President and Chief Executive Officer, Southern Ocean Medical Center, Manahawkin, NJ, p. A406
COYLE, Michael F., Chief Executive Officer, West Holt Memorial Hospital, Atkinson, NE, p. A381
COYNE, Rose
Vice President and Chief Financial Officer, Cleveland Regional Medical Center, Shelby, NC, p. A460
Interim CFO, MedWest – Haywood, Clyde, NC, p. A451
COZART, Adrienne, Vice President Human Resources, University Medical Center, Lubbock, TX, p. A614
COZART, Phyllis, Director Human Resources, Haywood Park Community Hospital, Brownsville, TN, p. A562
CRABB, Ian, M.D. Medical Director, Nebraska Orthopaedic Hospital, Omaha, NE, p. A388
CRABB, Lindsay, Chief Executive Officer, Quartz Mountain Medical Center, Mangum, OK, p. A498
CRABBE, Amy
Vice President Human Resources, Charles A. Cannon Memorial Hospital, Linville, NC, p. A456
Senior Vice President Human Resources, Watauga Medical Center, Boone, NC, p. A449
CRABDREE, Nathan, Chief Financial Officer, Chesterfield General Hospital, Cheraw, SC, p. A547
CRABLE, W. Trent, Executive Vice President and Chief Operating Officer, Brooklyn Hospital Center,, NY, p. A431
CRABTREE, Douglas, Chief Executive Officer, Eastern Idaho Regional Medical Center, Idaho Falls, ID, p. A168
CRABTREE, Gordon, Chief Financial Officer, University of Utah Health Care – Hospital and Clinics, Salt Lake City, UT, p. A641
CRABTREE, Nathan, Chief Financial Officer, Springs Memorial Hospital, Lancaster, SC, p. A552
CRABTREE, Rick, Chief Operating Officer, Christus St. Vincent Regional Medical Center, Santa Fe, NM, p. A418
CRABTREE, Susan, Director Human Resources, Glendale Adventist Medical Center, Glendale, CA, p. A63
CRACOLICI, Frank J., President, St. Luke's–Roosevelt Hospital Center, New York, NY, p. A437
CRACROFT, Davis, M.D. Senior Director Medical Affairs, Scripps Mercy Hospital, San Diego, CA, p. A86
CRAFA, Regina, Vice President Human Resources, Bethesda Memorial Hospital, Boynton Beach, FL, p. A119
CRAFT, Christina, Director Information Systems, Washington County Hospital, Plymouth, NC, p. A458
CRAFT, Kirby, Chief Information Officer, Magee General Hospital, Magee, MS, p. A349
CRAFTS, Nicholas, Chief Operating Officer, St. Mary's Regional Medical Center, Enid, OK, p. A496
CRAIG, Celine, Director Human Resources, King's Daughters Medical Center, Brookhaven, MS, p. A344
CRAIG, Daniel, Warden, Iowa Medical and Classification Center, Oakdale, IA, p. A224
CRAIG, Donnette, Director Human Resources, CHRISTUS Coushatta Health Care Center, Coushatta, LA, p. A264


A790 Index of Health Care Professionals

Index of Health Care Professionals / Crouch

Index of Health Care Professionals


CRAIG, Emmett, Chief Human Resources Officer, Knapp Medical Center, Weslaco, TX, p. A634
CRAIG, Glenn L., Chief Operating Officer, University Medical Center, Lafayette, LA, p. A270
CRAIG, Jeff, Chief Human Resource Management, Veterans Affairs Maryland Health Care System–Baltimore Division, Baltimore, MD, p. A289
CRAIG, John D., Chief Financial Officer, St. Luke's Rehabilitation Institute, Spokane, WA, p. A667
CRAIG, Mary Anne, Chief Executive Officer, Kindred Hospital–Houston Northwest, Houston, TX, p. A605
CRAIG, Patrice, Manager Human Resources, Southern Arizona Veterans Affairs Health Care System, Tucson, AZ, p. A40
CRAIG, Paul A., R.N. Chief Human Resources and Risk Officer, UC San Diego Health System, San Diego, CA, p. A86
CRAIG, Rebecca W., Vice President and Chief Financial Officer, Wayne Memorial Hospital, Goldsboro, NC, p. A453
CRAIG, Scott, M.D. Medical Director, Van Matre HEALTHSOUTH Rehabilitation Hospital, Rockford, IL, p. A193
CRAIG, Tracy, Director Human Resources, Presbyterian Hospital Huntersville, Huntersville, NC, p. A455
CRAIG, William J., Chief Financial Officer, Howard Memorial Hospital, Nashville, AR, p. A49
CRAIGER, Lisa, Chief Nursing Officer, Jay County Hospital, Portland, IN, p. A210
CRAIGHTON, Michelle, Manager Finance, Franklin General Hospital, Hampton, IA, p. A220
CRAIGIE, Andrew, Chief Executive Officer, Garfield County Public Hospital District, Pomeroy, WA, p. A664
CRAIGIE, James N., M.D. Vice President Medical Affairs, McLeod Loris Healthcare, Loris, SC, p. A552
CRAIGIN, Jane, Chief Executive Officer, St. Vincent Williamsport Hospital, Williamsport, IN, p. A213
CRAIN, Allen, Director Human Resources, Rapides Regional Medical Center, Alexandria, LA, p. A261
CRAIN, Doris
  Vice President Information Services, Broward Health Medical Center, Fort Lauderdale, FL, p. A123
  Vice President and Chief Information Officer, Broward Health North, Deerfield Beach, FL, p. A122
CRAMBES, Terry, Manager Finance, Warren State Hospital, Warren, PA, p. A540
CRAMER, Brian J., Chief Executive Officer, Orthopaedic Hospital of Wisconsin – Glendale, Milwaukee, WI, p. A687
CRAMER, James R.
  Vice President and Chief Information Officer, Scottsdale Healthcare Shea Medical Center, Scottsdale, AZ, p. A38
  Chief Information Officer, Scottsdale Healthcare Thompson Peak Hospital, Scottsdale, AZ, p. A38
  Vice President and Chief Information Officer, Scottsdale Healthcare–Osborn Medical Center, Scottsdale, AZ, p. A38
CRANDALL, David, FACHE President and Chief Executive Officer, Hospital for Special Care, New Britain, CT, p. A110
CRANDALL, Jeff, M.D. Chief Medical Officer, Allen Memorial Hospital, Waterloo, IA, p. A227
CRANDELL, Kim O., Administrator, South Lyon Medical Center, Yerington, NV, p. A396
CRANE, Aaron
  Chief Financial Officer, Salem Hospital, Salem, OR, p. A515
  Chief Financial Officer, West Valley Hospital, Dallas, OR, p. A510
CRANE, Margaret W., Chief Executive Officer, Barlow Respiratory Hospital, Los Angeles, CA, p. A68
CRANFORD, Melvin, Chief Fiscal Services, Veterans Affairs Medical Center, Cheyenne, WY, p. A695
CRANMER, John, Chief Information Officer, Mayo Clinic Hospital, Phoenix, AZ, p. A36
CRANSTON, David C., M.D. Vice President Medical Staff Affairs, Grinnell Regional Medical Center, Grinnell, IA, p. A220
CRAPSER, Douglas, Executive Vice President, Harrington Memorial Hospital, Southbridge, MA, p. A304
CRATON, Deborah W., M.D. Chief Medical Officer, St. Vincent Dunn Hospital, Bedford, IN, p. A197
CRAVEN, Darcy, Interim President, Carolinas Hospital System, Florence, SC, p. A549
CRAWFORD, Angela, Director Human Resources, Cherry Hospital, Goldsboro, NC, p. A453
CRAWFORD, Arnita, Director Human Resources, The Woman's Hospital of Texas, Houston, TX, p. A607
CRAWFORD, Jim, Chief Financial Officer, Lawrence Medical Center, Moulton, AL, p. A24
CRAWFORD, John W., Chief Financial Officer, Okmulgee Memorial Hospital, Okmulgee, OK, p. A502
CRAWFORD, Lucinda, Vice President Financial Services, Vidant Duplin Hospital, Kenansville, NC, p. A456
CRAWFORD, Mark W., Chief Executive Officer, Northern Nevada Medical Center, Sparks, NV, p. A396
CRAWFORD, Robin, Vice President and Chief Financial Officer, Susan B. Allen Memorial Hospital, El Dorado, KS, p. A232
CRAWFORD, Susan, Manager Human Resources, Fayette County Hospital, Vandalia, IL, p. A195
CRAWFORD, Thomas
  Chicago Market Chief Information Officer, Louis A. Weiss Memorial Hospital, Chicago, IL, p. A176
  Administrator, St. Vincent Frankfort Hospital, Frankfort, IN, p. A202
CRAWFORD, Tom
  Vice President Human Resources, DeKalb Medical at Downtown Decatur, Decatur, GA, p. A151
  Vice President Human Resources, DeKalb Medical at Hillandale, Lithonia, GA, p. A155
CRAWFORD, Wendy, Director Human Resources, George L. Mee Memorial Hospital, King City, CA, p. A65
CRAYTON, Karen, Chief Executive Officer, AMG Specialty Hospital–Feliciana, Clinton, LA, p. A264
CREAL, Sharon, Vice President Financial Operations, Scripps Memorial Hospital–Encinitas, Encinitas, CA, p. A60
CREAMER, Ken, Chief Human Resource, Amarillo Veterans Affairs Health Care System, Amarillo, TX, p. A578
CREECH, Ginger, Chief Executive Officer, LTAC of Edmond, Edmond, OK, p. A496
CREECH, James, M.D. Chief of Staff, Avera Holy Family Hospital, Estherville, IA, p. A219
CREIGHTON, Brenda L., Director Human Resources, Hudson Hospital, Hudson, WI, p. A683
CREIGHTON, Janice, Human Resources Associate, Mental Health Institute, Mount Pleasant, IA, p. A224
CREIGHTON, Peggy F., R.N. Director of Nursing Services, Methodist Hospital Union County, Morganfield, KY, p. A256
CREPEAU, Diana, Director Human Resources, HEALTHSOUTH Rehabilitation Hospital of Colorado Springs, Colorado Springs, CO, p. A98
CREPS, Barbara, Director Human Resources and Accounting, Okeene Municipal Hospital, Okeene, OK, p. A500
CREQUE, J. C., Director Management Information Systems, Schneider Regional Medical Center, Saint Thomas, VI, p. A704
CRESPO, Rosaida M., Executive Director, Hospital San Carlos Borromeo, Moca, PR, p. A702
CRESPO, Waleska, Administrator, Hospital Hermanos Melendez, Bayamon, PR, p. A700
CRESSLEY, Pat, Vice President and Chief Financial Officer, Clearfield Hospital, Clearfield, PA, p. A520
CRESWELL, Linda, Director Human Resources, Texas Health Presbyterian Hospital–WNJ, Sherman, TX, p. A628
CREWS, Kimberly, Vice President Finance and Chief Financial Officer, High Point Regional Health System, High Point, NC, p. A455
CREWS, Michael E., Chief Financial Officer, Singing River Health System, Pascagoula, MS, p. A351
CRIBBS, Cyndie, Director of Nursing, Nor–Lea General Hospital, Lovington, NM, p. A417
CRIBBS, Susan, D.O. Chief of Staff, Tehachapi Valley Healthcare District, Tehachapi, CA, p. A92
CRIGER, Sara J., President, Mercy Hospital, Coon Rapids, MN, p. A330
CRILLY, Tom, Executive Vice President and Chief Financial Officer, Unity Hospital, Rochester, NY, p. A442
CRIM, Marcia, MSN, Chief Executive Officer, USMD Hospital at Arlington, Arlington, TX, p. A580
CRIPE, Kimberly C.
  President and Chief Executive Officer, Children's Hospital at Mission, Mission Viejo, CA, p. A74
  President and Chief Executive Officer, Children's Hospital of Orange County, Orange, CA, p. A78
CRIPPS, Hugh Don, M.D. Chief of Staff, DeKalb Community Hospital, Smithville, TN, p. A575
CRISANTI, John, M.D. Vice President Medical Affairs, Community Medical Center, Toms River, NJ, p. A411
CRISLER, Catherine, Executive Director Human Resources, Piedmont Fayette Hospital, Fayetteville, GA, p. A152
CRISLIP, David, Administrator, Methodist Healthcare–Fayette Hospital, Somerville, TN, p. A575
CRIST, Chris, Director Information Systems, Coffeyville Regional Medical Center, Coffeyville, KS, p. A231
CRISWELL, Jodie, Vice President Fiscal Services, Hammond–Henry Hospital, Geneseo, IL, p. A182
CRITTENDON, Cindy, M.D. Chief of Staff, Marlboro Park Hospital, Bennettsville, SC, p. A546
CRITTLE, Marsha, Director Human Resources, Huey P. Long Medical Center, Pineville, LA, p. A276
CRNKOVIC, A. Elaine, Chief Executive Officer, Cedar Springs Behavioral Health System, Colorado Springs, CO, p. A98
CROCKER, Daniel, M.D. Chief Medical Officer, LifeCare Hospitals of North Carolina, Rocky Mount, NC, p. A459
CROCKETT, Gary L., Administrator, Huey P. Long Medical Center, Pineville, LA, p. A276
CROCKETT, James Scott, M.D. Chief of Staff, Falls Community Hospital and Clinic, Marlin, TX, p. A615
CROCKETT, Kim, Director Management Information Systems, Shriners Hospitals for Children, Shreveport, Shreveport, LA, p. A277
CROCKETT, Mandy Lee, Director Human Resources, San Luis Valley Regional Medical Center, Alamosa, CO, p. A97
CROCKETT, Matt, Assistant Administrator and Chief Information Officer, Highline Medical Center, Burien, WA, p. A660
CROCKETT, Russ, Director Human Resources, Shriners Hospitals for Children–Intermountain, Salt Lake City, UT, p. A641
CROFFORD, Patricia, Vice President Human Resources, Flagstaff Medical Center, Flagstaff, AZ, p. A32
CROFT, Cheryl, Chairman Information Services, Mayo Clinic Jacksonville, Jacksonville, FL, p. A126
CROFT, Shauna, Chief Financial Officer, Power County Hospital District, American Falls, ID, p. A166
CROKER, James, Director Information Systems, St. Bernardine Medical Center, San Bernardino, CA, p. A85
CROMER, Tony, Chief Information Management, Martin Army Community Hospital, Fort Benning, GA, p. A153
CROMIKA, Mike, Director Information Services, Western Baptist Hospital, Paducah, KY, p. A257
CRONER, Robert, Executive Vice President and Chief Human Resources Officer, Children's Hospital of Philadelphia, Philadelphia, PA, p. A532
CRONIN, Annamarie, Director Human Resources, New England Rehabilitation Hospital, Woburn, MA, p. A306
CRONIN, David J., Regional Vice President Human Resources, Good Samaritan Medical Center, Brockton, MA, p. A298
CROOM, Jon–Paul, Chief Operating Officer, Walton Regional Medical Center, Monroe, GA, p. A156
CROOM Jr., Kennedy L., Administrator and Chief Executive Officer, Rhea Medical Center, Dayton, TN, p. A565
CROON, Dorwyn, M.D. President Medical Staff, Valdese General Hospital, Valdese, NC, p. A462
CROPLEY, Stacey, M.D. Chief Nursing Officer, Moore County Hospital District, Dumas, TX, p. A594
CROPPER, Douglas P., President and Chief Executive Officer, Genesis Health System, Davenport, IA, p. B54
CROPPER, Rosiland, M.D. Medical Director, Ascension Gonzales Rehabilitation Hospital, Gonzales, LA, p. A266
CROSBIE, John, Director Support Services, Indiana University Health Blackford Hospital, Hartford City, IN, p. A203
CROSBY, Dagmar, M.D. Chief of Staff, Klickitat Valley Health, Goldendale, WA, p. A661
CROSBY, Evalie M., CPA Vice President Finance and Chief Financial Officer, Alice Peck Day Memorial Hospital, Lebanon, NH, p. A398
CROSBY, Robert, Senior Vice President and Chief Financial Officer, Heywood Hospital, Gardner, MA, p. A300
CROSHAW, Diane, Vice President Human Resources, Bacharach Institute for Rehabilitation, Pomona, NJ, p. A409
CROSS, Carol, Chief Financial Officer, Texas Health Harris Methodist Hospital Stephenville, Stephenville, TX, p. A629
CROSS, Helene M., President and Chief Executive Officer, Fairbanks, Indianapolis, IN, p. A204
CROSS, Mark A., Chief Executive Officer, Marias Medical Center, Shelby, MT, p. A379
CROSSAN, Gary, Director Information Systems, Healdsburg District Hospital, Healdsburg, CA, p. A64
CROSSER, Roxanna, Vice President, Operations, OSF St. Mary Medical Center, Galesburg, IL, p. A182
CROSSEY, Robert, D.O. Chief Medical Officer, LifeCare Hospitals of Pittsburgh – Monroeville, Monroeville, PA, p. A529
CROSSIN, Robert J., Vice President Finance, Aria Health, Philadelphia, PA, p. A531
CROSSLEY, Beth, Director Information Systems, Chestnut Hill Hospital, Philadelphia, PA, p. A531
CROSSLEY, Kent, M.D. Acting Chief of Staff, Minneapolis Veterans Affairs Health Care System, Minneapolis, MN, p. A335
CROSTON, J. Kevin, M.D. Chief Medical Officer, North Memorial Health Care, Robbinsdale, MN, p. A338
CROTEAU, Christine, Acting Director, Edith Nourse Rogers Memorial Veterans Hospital, Bedford, MA, p. A295
CROTEAU, Gary, Assistant Vice President and Chief Information Officer, South County Hospital, Wakefield, RI, p. A545
CROTTY, Jr., Glenn, M.D. Executive Vice President and Chief Operating Officer, Charleston Area Medical Center, Charleston, WV, p. A671
CROTTY, Renee, Coordinator Marketing and Public Relations, Capital Medical Center, Olympia, WA, p. A663
CROUCH, Amy, Chief Financial Officer, DeKalb Health, Auburn, IN, p. A197
CROUCH, James, Vice President Technical Services, Northwest Medical Center, Albany, MO, p. A355
CROUCH, Matthew, Chief Executive Officer and Managing Director, Peachford Behavioral Health System, Atlanta, GA, p. A145

Index of Health Care Professionals

Index of Health Care Professionals / Croushore


CROUSHORE, Susan, President and Chief Executive Officer, Christ Hospital, Cincinnati, OH, p. A473
CROUT, Tom, MS Director Human Resources, Central Louisiana State Hospital, Pineville, LA, p. A276
CROW, Angie, Financial Director, The Center for Spinal Surgery, Nashville, TN, p. A573
CROW, Barbra, Chief Financial Officer, Little River Memorial Hospital, Ashdown, AR, p. A42
CROW, Beth, Associate Relations Representative, Grady Memorial Hospital, Delaware, OH, p. A479
CROW, Ralph, Director Information Technology and Systems, Sky Ridge Medical Center, Lone Tree, CO, p. A104
CROW, Ruth Ann, Administrator, Lake Whitney Medical Center, Whitney, TX, p. A635
CROWDER, Andy, Chief Information Officer, Florida Hospital, Orlando, FL, p. A134
CROWDER, Jerry W., President and Chief Executive Officer, Bradford Health Services, Birmingham, AL, p. B22
CROWDER, Lonna, Director of Nursing, Phillips County Hospital, Malta, MT, p. A377
CROWDER, Steve, Manager Information Technology, Natchitoches Regional Medical Center, Natchitoches, LA, p. A274
CROWE, Arthur, Director Information Systems, Peconic Bay Medical Center, Riverhead, NY, p. A441
CROWE, Danny, Chief Financial Officer, Parkway Medical Center, Decatur, AL, p. A18
CROWE, William R., President, Miners Medical Center, Hastings, PA, p. A524
CROWELL, Eric T.
President and Chief Executive Officer, Iowa Lutheran Hospital, Des Moines, IA, p. A218
President and Chief Executive Officer, Iowa Methodist Medical Center, Des Moines, IA, p. A218
CROWELL, Lynn, Chief Executive Officer, Arkansas Valley Regional Medical Center, La Junta, CO, p. A103
CROWL, Heather N., Chief Human Resources Officer, Kingman Regional Medical Center, Kingman, AZ, p. A33
CROWLEY, Amber, Vice President Human Resources, Avera Marshall Regional Medical Center, Marshall, MN, p. A334
CROWLEY, Cathleen, Chief Information Officer, Columbia Memorial Hospital, Hudson, NY, p. A427
CROWLEY, Daryl, Director Information Services, Memorial Medical Center of West Michigan, Ludington, MI, p. A318
CROWLEY, John, M.D. Medical Director, River Crest Hospital, San Angelo, TX, p. A624
CROWLEY, Sheryl, Chief Information Officer, Falmouth Hospital, Falmouth, MA, p. A300
CROWLEY, Thomas, President and Chief Executive Officer, Saint Elizabeth's Medical Center, Wabasha, MN, p. A341
CROWSON, Carol, Administrator, Beacon Children's Hospital, Luverne, AL, p. A22
CROWTHER, Bruce K., President and Chief Executive Officer, Northwest Community Hospital, Arlington Heights, IL, p. A172
CRUICKSHANK, James A., Chief Executive Officer, Trinity Hospital of Augusta, Augusta, GA, p. A147
CRUM, Dennis L., Vice President and Chief Financial Officer, Tift Regional Medical Center, Tifton, GA, p. A161
CRUMP, Michael C., Administrator, Villa Feliciana Medical Complex, Jackson, LA, p. A268
CRUMP, Rick, Chief Financial Officer, Lakeland Behavioral Health System, Springfield, MO, p. A371
CRUMPTON, Althea H., Administrator, Magee General Hospital, Magee, MS, p. A349
CRUMPTON, Elaine, Director Human Resources, Gunnison Valley Hospital, Gunnison, CO, p. A102
CRUNK, Frances H., Vice President and Chief Financial Officer, Florida Hospital Waterman, Tavares, FL, p. A141
CRUNKLETON, Kevin, Chief Financial Officer, Summit Surgical, LLC, Hutchinson, KS, p. A235
CRUSE, Adam, Chief Financial Officer, Three Rivers Medical Center, Louisa, KY, p. A254
CRUSE, Ray, Chief Executive Officer, Lakeland Community Hospital Watervliet, Watervliet, MI, p. A325
CRUTCHFIELD, David, Vice President and Chief Information Officer, Virginia Hospital Center – Arlington, Arlington, VA, p. A645
CRUTHIRDS, Leslie, Chief Human Resource Management Service, South Texas Veterans Health Care System, San Antonio, TX, p. A626
CRUTHIRDS, Richard, Director Information Systems, Peterson Regional Medical Center, Kerrville, TX, p. A610
CRUZ, Domingo, Senior Vice President Operations, San Jorge Children's Hospital, San Juan, PR, p. A703
CRUZ, Elyonel Ponton, Executive Director, Hospital Buen Samaritano, Aguadilla, PR, p. A699
CRUZ, Joseph V., Chief Information Officer, Ryder Memorial Hospital, Humacao, PR, p. A701
CRUZ, Julia, Chief Financial Officer, San Juan Capestrano Hospital, San Juan, PR, p. A703
CRUZ, Michael, Vice President Operations, Baptist St. Anthony Health System, Amarillo, TX, p. A578
CRUZ, Miguel, M.D. Medical Director, Bella Vista Hospital, Mayaguez, PR, p. A701
CUBB, Don, Chief Executive Officer, Regency Hospital of Odessa, Odessa, TX, p. A619
CUBELLIS, Guido J.
Chief Operating Officer, Nexus Specialty Hospital, Shenandoah, TX, p. A627
Chief Operating Officer, Nexus Specialty Hospital The Woodlands, Spring, TX, p. A628
CUBRE, Alan, M.D. Medical Director, Kindred Hospital–Sacramento, Folsom, CA, p. A60
CUELLAR, Eddie, Vice President Information Systems, Methodist Hospital, San Antonio, TX, p. A625
CUELLAR, Jacob, M.D. Chief Executive Officer, Peak Behavioral Health Services, Santa Teresa, NM, p. A418
CUERO, Liza, Coordinator Human Resources, Central Texas Rehabilitation Hospital, Austin, TX, p. A580
CUEVAS, Gilberto, Director Human Resources, Hospital De Damas, Ponce, PR, p. A702
CUEVAS, Jacki, Director Health Information Services, Regional Rehabilitation Hospital, Phenix City, AL, p. A25
CULBERSON, David K., Chief Executive Officer, San Joaquin General Hospital, French Camp, CA, p. A61
CULBERTSON, Laura, Director Human Resources, Rancho Springs Medical Center, Murrieta, CA, p. A76
CULLEN, John, M.D. Chief of Staff and Medical Director Long Term Care, Providence Valdez Medical Center, Valdez, AK, p. A30
CULLEN, John, Assistant Superintendent, Thomas B. Finan Center, Cumberland, MD, p. A291
CULLEN, Michael, Senior Vice President and Chief Financial Officer, South Shore Hospital, South Weymouth, MA, p. A304
CULLEN, Paul T., M.D. Vice President Medical Affairs, Washington Hospital, Washington, PA, p. A540
CULLITON, Gerald F., Director, Veterans Affairs Hudson Valley Health Care System–F.D. Roosevelt Hospital, Montrose, NY, p. A430
CULLIVER, Sandra, Director Human Resources, National Park Medical Center, Hot Springs, AR, p. A46
CULP, Christopher M., Commanding Officer, Naval Hospital Bremerton, Bremerton, WA, p. A659
CULP, Judy, Chief Financial Officer, Hill Regional Hospital, Hillsboro, TX, p. A603
CULUMBER, Janene, Vice President and Chief Financial Officer, H. Lee Moffitt Cancer Center and Research Institute, Tampa, FL, p. A140
CULVER, Shawna, Director Information Systems, Western Plains Medical Complex, Dodge City, KS, p. A232
CUMBEE, Lib, Director Information Systems, Providence Hospital, Columbia, SC, p. A548
CUMBIE, Dan L., Chief Nursing Officer, Flowers Hospital, Dothan, AL, p. A19
CUMMINGS, Brooke, Chief Financial Officer, LSU Bogalusa Medical Center, Bogalusa, LA, p. A263
CUMMINGS, Bruce D., President and Chief Executive Officer, Lawrence & Memorial Hospital, New London, CT, p. A111
CUMMINGS, Cindy, Chief Executive Officer, Putnam County Memorial Hospital, Unionville, MO, p. A372
CUMMINGS, Elmer, Vice President and Chief Financial Officer, Hardin Memorial Hospital, Elizabethtown, KY, p. A249
CUMMINGS, Greg, Chief Financial Officer, Texas Spine & Joint Hospital, Tyler, TX, p. A632
CUMMINGS, James, Vice President Human Resources, Lakeside Memorial Hospital, Brockport, NY, p. A422
CUMMINGS, Lisa, Director Outpatient Services, Copper Queen Community Hospital, Bisbee, AZ, p. A31
CUMMINGS, Steven, Chief Operating Officer and Chief Information Officer, Noble Hospital, Westfield, MA, p. A306
CUMMINS, Frank L.
Vice President Human Resources, John C. Lincoln Deer Valley Hospital, Phoenix, AZ, p. A35
Vice President Human Resources, John C. Lincoln North Mountain Hospital, Phoenix, AZ, p. A35
CUMMINS, Tom, M.D. Director Hospitalist Program, White River Medical Center, Batesville, AR, p. A42
CUNEO, Anthony J., Chief Operating Officer, Metropolitan St. Louis Psychiatric Center, Saint Louis, MO, p. A369
CUNLIFFE, Ronald, D.O. Chief of Staff, Highlands Medical Center, Sparta, TN, p. A576
CUNNINGHAM, Dale, M.D. Medical Director, HEALTHSOUTH Rehabilitation Hospital of Memphis, Memphis, TN, p. A571
CUNNINGHAM, Gail, Interim Chief Medical Officer, St. Joseph Medical Center, Towson, MD, p. A294
CUNNINGHAM, Henry, M.D. President Medical Staff, Kindred Hospital Tarrant County–Fort Worth Southwest, Fort Worth, TX, p. A599
CUNNINGHAM, James C., M.D. Chief Medical Officer, Cook Children's Medical Center, Fort Worth, TX, p. A598
CUNNINGHAM, James M., M.D. Vice President Medical Affairs, Medical Center of Central Georgia, Macon, GA, p. A155
CUNNINGHAM, Keith W., M.D. Medical Director, HEALTHSOUTH Scottsdale Rehabilitation Hospital, Scottsdale, AZ, p. A38
CUNNINGHAM, Kris, M.D. Chief of Staff, Wheatland Memorial Healthcare, Harlowton, MT, p. A376
CUNNINGHAM, Larmar, Chief Operating Officer, West Central Georgia Regional Hospital, Columbus, GA, p. A150
CUNNINGHAM, M. Edward, Chief Executive Officer, Crossroads Community Hospital, Mount Vernon, IL, p. A188
CUNNINGHAM, Michelle P., Chief Executive Officer, Highlands Hospital, Connellsville, PA, p. A521
CUNNINGHAM, Robert, Vice President Human Resources, Good Samaritan Hospital, Kearney, NE, p. A385
CUNNINGHAM, William, D.O. Chief Medical Officer, Metro Health Hospital, Wyoming, MI, p. A326
CUPP, Roy, Director Management Information Systems, Fayette Regional Health System, Connersville, IN, p. A199
CURBELO, Luis, Director Finance, Hospital Dr. Cayetano Coll Y Toste, Arecibo, PR, p. A700
CURCURUTO, James J., Senior Vice President Finance, St. Joseph's Medical Center, Yonkers, NY, p. A447
CURL, MaryAnn, M.D. Interim Chief of Staff, Charles George Veterans Affairs Medical Center, Asheville, NC, p. A448
CURLEE, Mindy, Coordinator Human Resources, Jackson County Hospital District, Edna, TX, p. A595
CURLING, Susan, M.D. Chief Medical Officer, Memorial Hermann Northeast, Humble, TX, p. A608
CURNEL, Robin, Chief Operating Officer and Chief Nursing Officer, Crittenden County Hospital, Marion, KY, p. A256
CURNOW, Annie, Coordinator Medical Staff and Public Relations, DeSoto Memorial Hospital, Arcadia, FL, p. A118
CURNUTT, Ann
Director Information Systems, Garfield Medical Center, Monterey Park, CA, p. A75
Director Information Systems, Monterey Park Hospital, Monterey Park, CA, p. A75
CURPHY, Rona, President and Chief Executive Officer, Casa Grande Regional Medical Center, Casa Grande, AZ, p. A31
CURRAN, Maria, Vice President Human Resources, VCU Health System, Richmond, VA, p. A655
CURRAN, Robert, Director Health Information Management, SSM St. Mary's Health Center, Saint Louis, MO, p. A369
CURRANS, Sheila, Chief Executive Officer, Harrison Memorial Hospital, Cynthiana, KY, p. A249
CURREN, Rob, Director Information Technology, Center for Behavioral Medicine, Kansas City, MO, p. A361
CURRIE, Patricia M., FACHE Chief Hospital Services, Scott and White Memorial Hospital, Temple, TX, p. A630
CURRIE, Scott D., Vice President and Chief Financial Officer, MidMichigan Medical Center–Midland, Midland, MI, p. A319
CURRIER, Donald L., Vice President Human Resources, Piedmont Medical Center, Rock Hill, SC, p. A553
CURRIGAN, Bernie, M.D. Chief Medical Officer, Providence Mount Carmel Hospital, Colville, WA, p. A660
CURRIN, Jr., John G., President, Alamance Regional Medical Center, Burlington, NC, p. A449
CURRIN, Sue, MS, Chief Executive Officer, San Francisco General Hospital Medical Center, San Francisco, CA, p. A87
CURRY, Cheryl, Vice President Finance, Avista Adventist Hospital, Louisville, CO, p. A104
CURRY, Jeffrey T.
Executive Vice President and Chief Financial Officer, Excela Frick Hospital, Mount Pleasant, PA, p. A530
Executive Vice President and Chief Financial Officer, Excela Health Westmoreland Hospital, Greensburg, PA, p. A524
Executive Vice President and Chief Financial Officer, Excela Latrobe Area Hospital, Latrobe, PA, p. A527
CURRY, Lori, Regional Chief Human Resources Officer, Providence Holy Cross Medical Center,, CA, p. A71
CURRY, Robert H., President and Chief Executive Officer, Citrus Valley Health Partners, Covina, CA, p. B32
CURRY, Robert H.
President and Chief Executive Officer, Citrus Valley Medical Center–Inter–Community Campus, Covina, CA, p. A59
President and Chief Executive Officer, Citrus Valley Medical Center–Queen of the Valley Campus, West Covina, CA, p. A95
CURRY, Stephen A., Director Information Services, Princeton Community Hospital, Princeton, WV, p. A675
CURTIN, Sean, Interim Chief Financial Officer, Massena Memorial Hospital, Massena, NY, p. A429
CURTIN, Thomas F., Vice President and Chief Financial Officer, Good Samaritan Hospital, Dayton, OH, p. A478
CURTIS, Edgar J., President and Chief Executive Officer, Memorial Health System, Springfield, IL, p. B87
CURTIS, Edgar J., President and Chief Executive Officer, Memorial Medical Center, Springfield, IL, p. A194
CURTIS, George, Director Information Technology Services, Upson Regional Medical Center, Thomaston, GA, p. A160


A792 Index of Health Care Professionals

Index of Health Care Professionals / Dane

CURTIS, Janis, Interim Director Information Technology, Duke Raleigh Hospital, Raleigh, NC, p. A459
CURTIS, Jeff, Chief Operating Officer, Greenwood Leflore Hospital, Greenwood, MS, p. A346
CURTIS, Lorna, Chief Financial Officer, Riverside Medical Center, Riverside, CA, p. A83
CURTIS, Lynda D., Senior Vice President and Executive Director, Bellevue Hospital Center, New York, NY, p. A431
CURTIS, Marilyn K., Vice President, Professional Services, Saint Francis Medical Center, Cape Girardeau, MO, p. A356
CURTIS, Michael, Administrator and Chief Executive Officer, Throckmorton County Memorial Hospital, Throckmorton, TX, p. A631
CURTIS, Scott A., Administrator and Chief Executive Officer, Kossuth Regional Health Center, Algona, IA, p. A214
CURVIN, Thomas J., M.D. Chief of Staff, Rankin Hospital District, Rankin, TX, p. A622
CUSANO, Susan, Director Human Resources, Four Winds Hospital, Katonah, NY, p. A428
CUSATIS, Michele A., Ph.D. Administrator, Waukesha County Mental Health Center, Waukesha, WI, p. A692
CUSENZ, Bruce J., M.D. Medical Director, Eastern Niagara Health System, Lockport, NY, p. A429
CUSHING, Heidi, Director Finance, Gordon Memorial Hospital, Gordon, NE, p. A384
CUSSINS, James, Chief Financial Officer, East Morgan County Hospital, Brush, CO, p. A98
CUSTER-MITCHELL, Marilyn J., President and Chief Executive Officer, Wabash County Hospital, Wabash, IN, p. A213
CUSUMANO, Margaret M., R.N. Chief Nursing Officer and Vice President Care Services, Vassar Brothers Medical Center, Poughkeepsie, NY, p. A441
CUTLER, Nancy, R.N. Vice President Patient Services/CNO, FHN Memorial Hospital, Freeport, IL, p. A182
CUTLER, Terry, Administrator and Chief Operating Officer, East Texas Medical Center Crockett, Crockett, TX, p. A589
CUTOLO, Jr., Edward, M.D. Chief of Staff, James A. Haley Veterans Hospital, Tampa, FL, p. A140
CUTRIGHT, Bruce E., MS Vice President Human Resources, Mary Lanning Healthcare, Hastings, NE, p. A384
CUTSFORTH, Shawn, Information Systems Officer, Pioneer Memorial Hospital, Heppner, OR, p. A511
CUTTER, Craig, Corporate Director Human Resources, Mountain Manor Treatment Center, Emmitsburg, MD, p. A291
CUTTS, W. Darrell, President and Chief Executive Officer, Piedmont Fayette Hospital, Fayetteville, GA, p. A152
CUZZOLA, Anthony, Vice President Rehabilitation Services, JFK Johnson Rehabilitation Institute, Edison, NJ, p. A403
CWYNAR, Jan, Vice President Operations, Regency Hospital of Minneapolis, Golden Valley, MN, p. A332
CYTLAK, David
Chief Financial Officer, Blanchard Valley Hospital, Findlay, OH, p. A480
Vice President Finance, Bluffton Hospital, Bluffton, OH, p. A471
CZAHOR, John, Chief Information Officer, Botsford Hospital, Farmington Hills, MI, p. A312
CZAJKA, Paul M., Chief Operating Officer, Fountain Valley Regional Hospital and Medical Center, Fountain Valley, CA, p. A61
CZEREW, Jane, Vice President Clinical Services, Quality Systems, Human Resources and Volunteer Services, Spectrum Health Zeeland Community Hospital, Zeeland, MI, p. A326
CZERMAK, Daniel, Chairman and President, AcuteCare Health System, Lakewood, NJ, p. B4
CZIPO, Kevin F., Executive Director and Chief Executive Officer, Stony Lodge Hospital, Ossining, NY, p. A440
CZUGALA, Matt, Manager Information Systems, Heartland Surgical Specialty Hospital, Overland Park, KS, p. A240
CZYZ, AnneMarie, R.N. Vice President for Clinical and Educational Services, St. Joseph's Hospital Health Center, Syracuse, NY, p. A444

## D

D'ACCURZIO, Albert, M.D. Medical Director, St. Elizabeth Medical Center, Utica, NY, p. A445
D'AGNES, Michael R., President and Chief Executive Officer, Raritan Bay Medical Center, Perth Amboy, NJ, p. A408
D'AGOSTINO, Becky, R.N. Director of Nursing, Baraga County Memorial Hospital, L'Anse, MI, p. A317
D'ALBERTO, Richard E., FACHE Chief Executive Officer, Laurens County Health Care System, Clinton, SC, p. A548
D'AMORE, Seanna, Director Human Resources, Elk Regional Health Center, Saint Marys, PA, p. A537
D'ANGELO, Elizabeth, M.D. Chief of Staff, Onslow Memorial Hospital, Jacksonville, NC, p. A455
D'ANGELO, Jennifer, Assistant Vice President Information Services, Christian Health Care Center, Wyckoff, NJ, p. A412
D'ANGELO, John, Chief Executive Officer, Banner Churchill Community Hospital, Fallon, NV, p. A391
D'ANGINA, Joseph, Area Finance Officer, Vallejo Medical Center, Vallejo, CA, p. A94
D'AQUILA, Richard, Executive Vice President and Chief Operating Officer, Yale–New Haven Hospital, New Haven, CT, p. A111
D'ASTOUS, Jacques, M.D. Chief of Staff, Shriners Hospitals for Children–Intermountain, Salt Lake City, UT, p. A641
D'ENBEAU, Richard, Chief Operating Officer, Mount Carmel New Albany Surgical Hospital, New Albany, OH, p. A486
D'ESMOND, C. Thomas, FACHE Administrator, Shriners Hospitals for Children–Boston, Boston, MA, p. A297
D'ETTORRE, Joseph A., Chief Executive Officer, Wyandot Memorial Hospital, Upper Sandusky, OH, p. A490
D'SOUZA, Carol, Director Human Resources, Casa Grande Regional Medical Center, Casa Grande, AZ, p. A31
DAANE, John, Information Systems Officer, Prairie du Chien Memorial Hospital, Prairie Du Chien, WI, p. A689
DABNEY, Ann, Manager Human Resources, Spring View Hospital, Lebanon, KY, p. A252
DACE, Linda, Vice President Finance, McDonough District Hospital, Macomb, IL, p. A186
DACOSTA, June
Acting Executive Director, Bronx Children's Psychiatric Center,, NY, p. A431
Acting Executive Director, Queens Children's Psychiatric Center,, NY, p. A436
DACUS, Mike
Vice President and Chief Financial Officer, Sheltering Arms Hospital South, Midlothian, VA, p. A651
Vice President Financial Services, Vidant Bertie Hospital, Windsor, NC, p. A463
DADLEZ, Christopher M., President and Chief Executive Officer, Mount Sinai Rehabilitation Hospital, Hartford, CT, p. A109
DADLEZ, Christopher M., President and Chief Executive Officer, Saint Francis Care, Inc., Hartford, CT, p. B111
DADLEZ, Christopher M., President and Chief Executive Officer, Saint Francis Hospital and Medical Center, Hartford, CT, p. A109
DADO, Joseph, Chief Information Officer, Memorial Medical Center, Johnstown, PA, p. A526
DAECH, Ed, Director Human Resources, Heartland Regional Medical Center, Marion, IL, p. A186
DAEGER, Brian, Vice President Financial Services, Margaret Mary Community Hospital, Batesville, IN, p. A197
DAGHER, Michel, D.O. Vice President and Chief Medical Officer, Banner Del E. Webb Medical Center, Sun City West, AZ, p. A39
DAGLIO, Michael, Chief Operating Officer, Danbury Hospital, Danbury, CT, p. A108
DAGUE, James O., President and Chief Executive Officer, Indiana University Health Goshen Hospital, Goshen, IN, p. A202
DAH, Cyrus E., Chief Financial Officer, Dameron Hospital, Stockton, CA, p. A91
DAHDUL, Adnan, M.D. Medical Director, HEALTHSOUTH Rehabilitation Hospital of Western Massachusetts, Ludlow, MA, p. A302
DAHL, James E., Chief Information Officer, Fort HealthCare, Fort Atkinson, WI, p. A681
DAHLBERG, Connie, Director Business and Employee, Sleepy Eye Medical Center, Sleepy Eye, MN, p. A340
DAHLEN, Gretchen M., FACHE Chief Executive Officer, Winneshiek Medical Center, Decorah, IA, p. A218
DAHLHAUSEN, Daniel J., M.D. Chief of Staff, Cannon Memorial Hospital, Pickens, SC, p. A553
DAHLING, James D., President and Chief Executive Officer, Children's Hospital of The King's Daughters, Norfolk, VA, p. A652
DAHLMAN, Kim, Administrator, Lost Rivers District Hospital, Arco, ID, p. A166
DAHLQUIST, Clay, M.D. Chief Medical Officer, Waverly Health Center, Waverly, IA, p. A228
DAHLSTRAND, David, Associate Chief of Staff Information Technology, Hunter Holmes McGuire Veterans Affairs Medical Center, Richmond, VA, p. A655
DAHLSTROM, Josiah, Administrator, Safe Haven Hospital of Pocatello, Pocatello, ID, p. A170
DAIGLE, Charles D.
Senior Vice President and Chief Operating Officer, Willis–Knighton Medical Center, Shreveport, LA, p. A277
Chief Operating Officer, WK Bossier Health Center, Bossier City, LA, p. A264
DAIGLE, Cheryl, R.N. Director of Nursing, Northern Maine Medical Center, Fort Kent, ME, p. A283
DAIGLE, Cindy, Chief Financial Officer, Houlton Regional Hospital, Houlton, ME, p. A283
DAIGLE, J. Barry, Manager Information Systems, University Medical Center, Lafayette, LA, p. A270
DAIKEN, Michael E., Chief Financial Officer, Highlands–Cashiers Hospital, Highlands, NC, p. A455
DAIKER, David, Chief Information Resource Management, Veterans Affairs Nebraska–Western Iowa Health Care System, Lincoln, NE, p. A386
DAILEY, Linda, Acting Chief Human Resources Officer, Veterans Affairs Medical Center, Augusta, GA, p. A147
DAILY, James L., President, Porter Medical Center, Middlebury, VT, p. A643
DAISLEY, Samuel, D.O. Vice President Medical Affairs, UPMC Horizon, Greenville, PA, p. A524
DAL COL, Richard, Vice President and Chief Medical Officer, Champlain Valley Physicians Hospital Medical Center, Plattsburgh, NY, p. A440
DALBY, William, Director Fiscal Services, Shriners Hospitals for Children, Northern California, Sacramento, CA, p. A84
DALE, Deborah, Chief Executive Officer, Select Specialty Hospital–Denver, Denver, CO, p. A100
DALE, Jae, Chief Executive Officer, Oro Valley Hospital, Oro Valley, AZ, p. A34
DALEBOUT, Kenneth, Chief Administrative Officer, Arroyo Grande Community Hospital, Arroyo Grande, CA, p. A54
DALEY, Chris, M.D. Chief of Staff, Estes Park Medical Center, Estes Park, CO, p. A101
DALEY, Robert, Vice President Fiscal and Information Technology Services, Black River Memorial Hospital, Black River Falls, WI, p. A679
DALL, Jamie, Director Finance and Support Operations, New Hampshire Hospital, Concord, NH, p. A397
DALLER, Sue, R.N. Assistant Administrator of Nursing, Hermann Area District Hospital, Hermann, MO, p. A360
DALLEY, Mark F., Administrator, Gunnison Valley Hospital, Gunnison, UT, p. A637
DALPIAZ, Joseph M., Director, Veterans Affairs Medical Center, Philadelphia, PA, p. A534
DALPOAS, Dolan, President and Chief Executive Officer, Abraham Lincoln Memorial Hospital, Lincoln, IL, p. A186
DALTON, Dayle, Vice President Human Resources, Los Robles Hospital and Medical Center, Thousand Oaks, CA, p. A92
DALTON, Eric
Chief Financial Officer, Memorial Medical Center, Modesto, CA, p. A75
Chief Financial Officer, Sutter Tracy Community Hospital, Tracy, CA, p. A93
DALTON, John, President and Chief Executive Officer, Inland Hospital, Waterville, ME, p. A285
DALTON, Ronald, M.D. Chief Medical Officer, NORTHSTAR Health System, Iron River, MI, p. A316
DALTON, Sandra L., R.N. Senior Vice President Patient Care Services and Chief Nursing Officer, Fletcher Allen Health Care, Burlington, VT, p. A643
DALTON, Wayne, Chief Financial Officer, Lakeview Hospital, Bountiful, UT, p. A637
DALTON, William S., M.D. President and Chief Executive Officer, H. Lee Moffitt Cancer Center and Research Institute, Tampa, FL, p. A140
DALY, Gail, Chief Operating Officer, St. Mary Medical Center, Long Beach, CA, p. A68
DALY, Sheila, President and Chief Executive Officer, Clinton Hospital, Clinton, MA, p. A299
DALY, Thomas M., Chief Financial Officer, University of Medicine and Dentistry of New Jersey–University Hospital, Newark, NJ, p. A407
DALY, Tim F., Chief Operating Officer, Antioch Medical Center, Antioch, CA, p. A53
DALY, William, Interim Chief Executive Officer, Pennsylvania Psychiatric Hospital, Harrisburg, PA, p. A524
DAMA, Sunil, M.D. Medical Director, Regency Hospital of Cincinnati, Cincinnati, OH, p. A474
DAMBOISE, Robin, Director Human Resources, Northern Maine Medical Center, Fort Kent, ME, p. A283
DAMM, Julie, Chief Financial Officer, Hancock County Memorial Hospital, Britt, IA, p. A215
DAMMEYER, Matt, Ph.D. Chief Operating Officer, Central Peninsula General Hospital, Soldotna, AK, p. A30
DAMODARAN, A. N., M.D. President Medical Staff, Indiana University Health Starke Hospital, Knox, IN, p. A206
DAMON, Chad, Chief Information Officer, St. Vincent Dunn Hospital, Bedford, IN, p. A197
DANCH, Stephen M., Chief Financial Officer, UPMC Hamot, Erie, PA, p. A523
DANDRIDGE, Thomas C., FACHE President and Chief Executive Officer, Regional Medical Center, Orangeburg, SC, p. A553
DANE, Jeff, Executive Vice President and Chief Financial Officer, University Medical Center, Lubbock, TX, p. A614

© 2012 AHA Guide Index of Health Care Professionals **A793**

Index of Health Care Professionals

DANG, Cynthia, Vice President Human Resources, North Hills Hospital, North Richland Hills, TX, p. A618

DANG, Minh, Vice President Finance, Robert Packer Hospital, Sayre, PA, p. A537

DANGERFIELD, Wesley, Community Chief Executive Officer, Summers County ARH Hospital, Hinton, WV, p. A672

DANIEL, Christopher W., Chief Financial Officer, Louisiana Medical Center and Heart Hospital, Lacombe, LA, p. A269

DANIEL, Dena, Director Information Systems, Jackson County Memorial Hospital, Altus, OK, p. A493

DANIEL, Lisa, Interim Chief Executive Officer, Memphis Mental Health Institute, Memphis, TN, p. A571

DANIEL, Patricia, Chief Information Officer, Lake Whitney Medical Center, Whitney, TX, p. A635

DANIEL, Richard, Administrator, Wedowee Hospital, Wedowee, AL, p. A26

DANIEL, Robin, Director of Human Resources, Northridge Medical Center, Commerce, GA, p. A150

DANIEL, Ron, Manager Information Systems, Matheny Medical and Educational Center, Peapack, NJ, p. A408

DANIEL, Vera W., Chief Human Resources Officer, Saint Louis University Hospital, Saint Louis, MO, p. A369

DANIEL, W. D., D.O. Chief of Staff, Medical Center of Manchester, Manchester, TN, p. A570

DANIEL, William, M.D. Chief Medical Officer, Booneville Community Hospital, Booneville, AR, p. A42

DANIELS, Andy
Chief Operating Officer, Bucyrus Community Hospital, Bucyrus, OH, p. A471
Vice President Non–Clinical Operations and Information Systems, Galion Community Hospital, Galion, OH, p. A480

DANIELS, Betty, M.D. Chief of Staff, St. Bernardine Medical Center, San Bernardino, CA, p. A85

DANIELS, Jeff, Chief Financial Officer, Bingham Memorial Hospital, Blackfoot, ID, p. A166

DANIELS, John, M.D. Medical Director, LifeCare Hospitals of Wisconsin, Pewaukee, WI, p. A689

DANIELS, Judy, Vice President Human Resources, Our Lady of Bellefonte Hospital, Ashland, KY, p. A247

DANIELS, Karen, MSN Chief Nursing Officer, Halifax Regional Medical Center, Roanoke Rapids, NC, p. A459

DANIELS, Kristin, Manager Human Resources, Sutter Center for Psychiatry, Sacramento, CA, p. A84

DANIELS, Mark, M.D. Vice President Physician Enterprise, Delnor Hospital, Geneva, IL, p. A182

DANIELS, S. Janette, Director Human Resources, HEALTHSOUTH Rehabilitation Hospital of Fort Smith, Fort Smith, AR, p. A45

DANIELS, Val C., Chief Financial Officer, Adventist Rehabilitation Hospital of Maryland, Rockville, MD, p. A293

DANIELS, W. Peter, FACHE President and Chief Executive Officer, Elmhurst Memorial Hospital,, IL, p. A181

DANIELS, Yelandra, M.D. Chief of Staff, Evans Memorial Hospital, Claxton, GA, p. A149

DANIELSON, David S., Senior Vice President Operations, Evergreen Hospital Medical Center, Kirkland, WA, p. A662

DANITZ, Doug, Director Information Technology, West Branch Regional Medical Center, West Branch, MI, p. A325

DANKER, Doug, Administrator, Mercy Hospital El Reno, El Reno, OK, p. A496

DANKERT, Sheri, Vice President Finance, Mayo Clinic Health System in Austin, Austin, MN, p. A328

DANKO, Douglas, President and Chief Executive Officer, Jameson Hospital, New Castle, PA, p. A530

DANN, Doreen, R.N. Chief Operating Officer, Victor Valley Community Hospital, Victorville, CA, p. A95

DANTIS, Gerry, Assistant Vice President Finance, SUNY Downstate Medical Center University Hospital of Brooklyn,, NY, p. A437

DANUSER, James, Chief Information Officer, Veterans Affairs Central Iowa Health Care System, Des Moines, IA, p. A218

DANZA, Frank J., Executive Director, Lenox Hill Hospital, New York, NY, p. A433

DAOUD, Joudat, M.D. Chief of Staff, Community Health Center of Branch County, Coldwater, MI, p. A310

DAQUIOAG, Francis, Controller, Kahuku Medical Center, Kahuku, HI, p. A164

DARBONNE, Tina, Chief Financial Officer, Central Louisiana State Hospital, Pineville, LA, p. A276

DARBY, Doug, Director Information Systems, Pioneers Memorial Healthcare District, Brawley, CA, p. A56

DARCEY, Patricia, R.N. Vice President/Chief Nursing Officer, Southampton Hospital, Southampton, NY, p. A443

DARDANO, Anthony, M.D. Chief Medical Officer, Delray Medical Center, Delray Beach, FL, p. A122

DARDEAU, Sean T., Chief Operating Officer, Trinity Medical Center, Birmingham, AL, p. A17

DARDEN, David B., Chief Executive Officer, Clinch Valley Medical Center, Richlands, VA, p. A654

DAREY, Roland, M.D. Medical Director, Wamego City Hospital, Wamego, KS, p. A244

DARLING, Rudy, Chief Operating Officer, Baxter Regional Medical Center, Mountain Home, AR, p. A49

DARNELL, Don, Chief Information Officer, Hamilton Memorial Hospital District, McLeansboro, IL, p. A187

DARNELL, Linda, Director Management Information Systems, King's Daughters' Hospital and Health Services, Madison, IN, p. A208

DARNELL, Vicki A., President and Chief Executive Officer, Ephraim McDowell Regional Medical Center, Danville, KY, p. A249

DARVIN, Ken, M.D. Chief of Staff, Stroud Regional Medical Center, Stroud, OK, p. A505

DARVISH, Adam, M.P.H. Chief Executive Officer, Kindred Hospital–Westminster, Westminster, CA, p. A96

DASARO, Lynda
Director Human Resources, Sutter Auburn Faith Hospital, Auburn, CA, p. A54
Director Human Resources, Sutter Roseville Medical Center, Roseville, CA, p. A83

DASCHER Jr., Norman E.
Chief Executive Officer, Samaritan Hospital, Troy, NY, p. A445
Executive Vice President, St. Mary's Hospital, Troy, NY, p. A445

DASKALAKIS, Tom G., Chief Operating Officer, West Chester Hospital, West Chester, OH, p. A491

DASS, Karla, Director Human Resources, Tri–County Hospital – Williston, Williston, FL, p. A143

DASSENKO, Dennis, Chief Information Officer, Essentia Health Duluth, Duluth, MN, p. A330

DATER, Suzanne, M.D. President Medical Staff, Bridgton Hospital, Bridgton, ME, p. A282

DAUBY, Randall W., Chief Executive Officer, Hamilton Memorial Hospital District, McLeansboro, IL, p. A187

DAUGHDRILL, Diane, Director Human Resources, Jefferson Davis Community Hospital, Prentiss, MS, p. A352

DAUGHDRILL, Richard, R.N. Chief Executive Officer, AMG Specialty Hospital–Slidell, Slidell, LA, p. A278

DAUGHERTY, Don, Director Information Systems, Fleming County Hospital, Flemingsburg, KY, p. A249

DAUGHERTY, Robert Alan, Chief Executive Officer, Mercy Regional Medical Center, Ville Platte, LA, p. A279

DAUGHERTY, Sam, Ed.D. President, Spectrum Health Reed City Hospital, Reed City, MI, p. A321

DAUGHERTY, Stephen J., Chief Executive Officer, Northside Hospital and Heart Institute, Saint Petersburg, FL, p. A138

DAUGHERTY, Thomas E., Administrator, Mecosta County Medical Center, Big Rapids, MI, p. A308

DAUGHTRY, Kaci, Director Human Resources, Andalusia Regional Hospital, Andalusia, AL, p. A15

DAUTERIVE, F. Ralph, M.D. Vice President Medical Affairs, Ochsner Medical Center–Baton Rouge, Baton Rouge, LA, p. A262

DAVANT, III, Charles, M.D. Chief Medical Officer, Blowing Rock Hospital, Blowing Rock, NC, p. A449

DAVE, Bhasker J., M.D. Superintendent, Mental Health Institute, Independence, IA, p. A221

DAVENPORT, Douglas, System Chief Financial Officer, Benefis Hospitals, Great Falls, MT, p. A376

DAVENPORT, Ginger, Director Human Resources, Texas Specialty Hospital at Dallas, Dallas, TX, p. A593

DAVENPORT, Julie, Chief Executive Officer, I–70 Community Hospital, Sweet Springs, MO, p. A371

DAVENPORT, Polly J., R.N. Chief Executive Officer, Ochsner Medical Center – North Shore, Slidell, LA, p. A278

DAVENPORT, Sally, Vice President of Patient Care Services & CNO, Ephraim McDowell Regional Medical Center, Danville, KY, p. A249

DAVENPORT, Sheilah, R.N. Chief Executive Officer and Superintendent, Clifton T. Perkins Hospital Center, Jessup, MD, p. A292

DAVES, Ronnie, Chief Executive Officer, Marlboro Park Hospital, Bennettsville, SC, p. A546

DAVID, Biff
Administrator, Evangeline Extended Care Hospital–Mamou, Mamou, LA, p. A272
Administrator, St. Landry Extended Care Hospital, Opelousas, LA, p. A276

DAVID, Daphne, Chief Operating Officer, Garden Park Medical Center, Gulfport, MS, p. A346

DAVID, Jeffrey, D.O. Chief Medical Officer, St. Mary's Medical Center, West Palm Beach, FL, p. A143

DAVID, Lim, Vice President Finance and Chief Financial Officer, St. Joseph Medical Center, Reading, PA, p. A537

DAVID, Myers M., Chief Information Officer, Iredell Memorial Hospital, Statesville, NC, p. A461

DAVID, R. Neal, Administrator and Chief of Staff, Madigan Healthcare System, Tacoma, WA, p. A668

DAVID, Robert
President and Chief Executive Officer, University Hospitals Conneaut Medical Center, Conneaut, OH, p. A478
President and Chief Executive Officer, University Hospitals Geneva Medical Center, Geneva, OH, p. A481

DAVIDOFF, Ravin, M.D. Chief Medical Officer, Boston Medical Center, Boston, MA, p. A296

DAVIDOW, Bruce B., Senior Vice President and Chief Operating Officer, Phelps Memorial Hospital Center, Sleepy Hollow, NY, p. A443

DAVIDOW, Daniel N., M.D. Medical Director, Cumberland Hospital, New Kent, VA, p. A651

DAVIDSON, Camille, Director Human Resources, Stanton County Hospital, Johnson, KS, p. A235

DAVIDSON, Charles O., M.D. Vice President Medical Affairs, Methodist Hospitals, Gary, IN, p. A202

DAVIDSON, Craig Val
Chief Executive Officer and Administrator, Beaver Valley Hospital, Beaver, UT, p. A637
Chief Executive Officer, Milford Valley Memorial Hospital, Milford, UT, p. A638

DAVIDSON, Diane, Senior Vice President Human Resources, Essentia Health Duluth, Duluth, MN, p. A330

DAVIDSON, Gary
Vice President and Chief Information Officer, Hospital of Saint Raphael, New Haven, CT, p. A110
Senior Vice President and Chief Information Officer, Lancaster General Health, Lancaster, PA, p. A526

DAVIDSON, Gary, M.D. Medical Director, Select Specialty Hospital–Johnstown, Johnstown, PA, p. A526

DAVIDSON, Gregg A., FACHE Chief Executive Officer, Skagit Valley Hospital, Mount Vernon, WA, p. A663

DAVIDSON, John, Vice President Human Resources, Sharon Regional Health System, Sharon, PA, p. A538

DAVIDSON, Kathleen, Vice President, Patient Care Services and Chief Nursing Officer, Norwood Hospital, Norwood, MA, p. A303

DAVIDSON, Nancy, Senior Vice President and Chief Financial Officer, Jackson County Memorial Hospital, Altus, OK, p. A493

DAVIDSON, Paulette, Chief Executive Officer, Bellevue Medical Center, Bellevue, NE, p. A382

DAVIDSON, Peter, M.D. Chief Medical Officer, Blue Mountain Recovery Center, Pendleton, OR, p. A513

DAVIDSON, Randy, M.D. Chief of Staff, Medical Center of Arlington, Arlington, TX, p. A579

DAVIDSON, Rocky, Chief Financial Officer, Hollywood Pavilion,, FL, p. A125

DAVIDSON, Rowena, Manager Business Office, LTAC of Edmond, Edmond, OK, p. A496

DAVIDSON, Sheila C., Vice President Human Resources, Mobile Infirmary Medical Center, Mobile, AL, p. A22

DAVIDSON, Tim, M.D. Chief Executive Physician Services, Providence St. Mary Medical Center, Walla Walla, WA, p. A669

DAVIDSON, Verno, R.N. Chief Nursing Officer, Vaughan Regional Medical Center, Selma, AL, p. A25

DAVIES, Donald, M.D. Chief of Staff, Valley View Regional Hospital, Ada, OK, p. A493

DAVIES, Janie, Chief Financial Officer, New Mexico Rehabilitation Center, Roswell, NM, p. A417

DAVILA, Susan, Administrator and Chief Executive Officer, Desert View Hospital, Pahrump, NV, p. A395

DAVIN, Joni, Director Information and Business Management Service Line, Veterans Affairs Eastern Kansas Health Care System, Topeka, KS, p. A244

DAVIN, Paul Robert, Vice President, Human Resources, Southampton Hospital, Southampton, NY, p. A443

DAVINI, John, Vice President, St. Rose Hospital, Hayward, CA, p. A64

DAVIS, A. Jack
Director Human Resources, Allegheny Valley Hospital, Natrona Heights, PA, p. A530
Vice President Human Resources, Canton–Potsdam Hospital, Potsdam, NY, p. A441

DAVIS, Adam
Director Information Technology, Cornerstone Hospital of SouthEast Arizona, Tucson, AZ, p. A39
Chief Information Officer, Cornerstone Hospital–West Monroe, West Monroe, LA, p. A279
Chief Information Officer, Solara Hospital Harlingen, Harlingen, TX, p. A602
Chief Information Officer, Solara Hospital Harlingen–Brownsville Campus, Brownsville, TX, p. A585

DAVIS, Amelia, Director of Nursing, CrossRidge Community Hospital, Wynne, AR, p. A52

DAVIS, Andrea, Assistant Administrator, Southern Hills Hospital and Medical Center, Las Vegas, NV, p. A393

DAVIS, Andy, President, St. Vincent's Birmingham, Birmingham, AL, p. A17

DAY, Scott, Vice President Human Resources, Exempla Lutheran Medical Center, Wheat Ridge, CO, p. A107

DAY, Sherry Clouse, CP
VP Finance/ Regional Chief Financial Officer, Mercy Hospital Aurora, Aurora, MO, p. A355
Chief Financial Officer, Mercy Hospital Cassville, Cassville, MO, p. A357
Chief Financial Officer, Mercy St. Francis Hospital, Mountain View, MO, p. A365

DAY, Therese, Chief Financial Officer, UMass Memorial Medical Center, Worcester, MA, p. A306

DAY, Timothy, Chief Administrative Officer, St. Luke's–Roosevelt Hospital Center, New York, NY, p. A437

DAY, Zed, Associate Vice President Information Technology, UK HealthCare Good Samaritan Hospital, Lexington, KY, p. A253

DE FARIA, Ludmila, M.D. Chief Medical Officer, Eastside Psychiatric Hospital, Tallahassee, FL, p. A140

DE FUR, Kyle, FACHE President, St. Vincent Indianapolis Hospital, Indianapolis, IN, p. A205

DE GARCIA, Carmen Bech, Director Human Resources, Lehigh Regional Medical Center, Lehigh Acres, FL, p. A129

DE HART, Kristen, Chief Executive Officer, Mid–America Rehabilitation Hospital, Shawnee Mission, KS, p. A243

DE HOYOS, Linda, M.D. Clinical Director, Thomas B. Finan Center, Cumberland, MD, p. A291

DE JESUS, Alexander, M.D. Medical Director, HEALTHSOUTH Rehabilitation Hospital of Sarasota, Sarasota, FL, p. A139

DE JESUS, Edwin, Comptroller, Hospital Santa Rosa, Guayama, PR, p. A701

DE LA PAZ, Christine, Director Human Resources, Aurora Charter Oak Hospital, Covina, CA, p. A58

DE LA PAZ, Eva
Regional Controller, Kindred Hospital Lafayette, Lafayette, LA, p. A270
Chief Financial Officer, Kindred Hospital–Corpus Christi, Corpus Christi, TX, p. A589

DE LA PENA, Will, Chief Financial Officer, Saint Francis Hospital and Health Centers, Poughkeepsie, NY, p. A441

DE LA TORRE, Ralph, M.D. Chairman and Chief Executive Officer, Steward Health Care System, LLC, Boston, MA, p. B124

DE LEON, Aurea, Chief Human Resources Officer, Hospital Universitario Dr. Ramon Ruiz Arnau, Bayamon, PR, p. A700

DE LONGO, Concepcion Quinones, M.D. Medical Director, University Pediatric Hospital, PR, p. A704

DE LOS REYES, Jay, Chief Operating Officer, HEALTHSOUTH Sunrise Rehabilitation Hospital, Fort Lauderdale, FL, p. A123

DE LOURDES ALEGRIA, Maria, Comptroller, Cardiovascular Center of Puerto Rico and the Caribbean, San Juan, PR, p. A702

DE PASQUALE, Edward, Chief Financial Officer, Memorial Medical Center, Johnstown, PA, p. A526

DE PIANO, Linda, Ph.D. Chief Executive Officer, Jerome Golden Center for Behavioral Health, Inc., West Palm Beach, FL, p. A142

DE PREZ, Bernadette, Chief Operating Officer, Skyridge Medical Center, Cleveland, TN, p. A564

DE ROBERTIS, Nicholas, M.D. Medical Director, St. Joseph's Medical Center, Yonkers, NY, p. A447

DE ROSA, James, Vice President Finance, Somerset Medical Center, Somerville, NJ, p. A410

DE SANTIAGO, Elizabeth, Director, Hospital Psiquiatrico Metropolitano, Cabo Rojo, PR, p. A700

DE TORRES, Francisco, M.D. Medical Director, Ashford Presbyterian Community Hospital, San Juan, PR, p. A702

DE VACA, Alessandra, Chief Administrative Officer, Hebrew Rehabilitation Center, Boston, MA, p. A297

DE VILLIERS, Willem, M.D. Chief Administrative Officer, UK HealthCare Good Samaritan Hospital, Lexington, KY, p. A253

DE VOSS, Gerald, Acting Administrator, Duane L. Waters Hospital, Jackson, MI, p. A316

DEAK, Terry, Chief Financial Officer, Colusa Regional Medical Center, Colusa, CA, p. A58

DEAKYNE, John R., Chief Financial Officer, Saint Mary's Regional Medical Center, Reno, NV, p. A395

DEAL, E. Chandler, M.D. Vice President Medical Affairs and Chief Medical Officer, Valley Baptist Medical Center–Harlingen, Harlingen, TX, p. A602

DEAL, Lisa, Budget Analyst, U. S. Public Health Service Indian Hospital, Eagle Butte, SD, p. A556

DEAL, Matt, Director Maintenance, Copper Basin Medical Center, Copperhill, TN, p. A564

DEAN, Donna
Chief Financial Officer, Osawatomie State Hospital, Osawatomie, KS, p. A240
Chief Financial Officer, Rainbow Mental Health Facility, Kansas City, KS, p. A236

DEAN, Douglas B., Chief Human Resources Officer, The Children's Hospital of Alabama, Birmingham, AL, p. A17

DEAN Jr., Douglas F., President and Chief Executive Officer, Elliot Hospital, Manchester, NH, p. A399

DEAN, Harrison M., FACHE Senior Vice President and Administrator, Baptist Health Medical Center – North Little Rock, North Little Rock, AR, p. A50

DEAN, Joel, Director Information Services, Piedmont Medical Center, Rock Hill, SC, p. A553

DEAN, Laura, Director Human Resources, Wilson Medical Center, Neodesha, KS, p. A239

DEAN, Linda, Chief Executive Officer, Good Shepherd Penn Partners Specialty Hospital at Rittenhouse, Philadelphia, PA, p. A532

DEAN, Lloyd H., President and Chief Executive Officer, Dignity Health, San Francisco, CA, p. B46

DEAN, Michele, Human Resources Specialist, Mid–Valley Hospital, Peckville, PA, p. A531

DEAN, Morre
Interim Chief Executive Officer, Littleton Adventist Hospital, Littleton, CO, p. A103
Chief Executive Officer, Parker Adventist Hospital, Parker, CO, p. A105

DEAN, Russell, Chief Executive Officer, LifeCare Hospital of Dayton, Miamisburg, OH, p. A485

DEAN, Thomas, M.D. Chief of Staff, Avera Weskota Memorial Hospital, Wessington Springs, SD, p. A561

DEANGELIS, Gene, Chief Fiscal Service, Veterans Affairs Medical Center, Cleveland, OH, p. A476

DEANGELO, Barbara, Director Human Resources, New York Westchester Square Medical Center,, NY, p. A435

DEANOGLIS, Jean, Director Management Information Systems, CHRISTUS Spohn Hospital Alice, Alice, TX, p. A577

DEANS, Ken, Chief Information Officer, Chesapeake Regional Medical Center, Chesapeake, VA, p. A646

DEARDORFF, Chad
Chief Financial Officer, Cornerstone Hospital of Bossier City, Bossier City, LA, p. A263
Group Chief Financial Officer, Cornerstone Hospital of SouthEast Arizona, Tucson, AZ, p. A39

DEARDORFF, John A., Chief Executive Officer, Fort Walton Beach Medical Center, Fort Walton Beach, FL, p. A124

DEARING, Bryan, Chief Executive Officer, Northridge Medical Center, Commerce, GA, p. A150

DEARMENT, Carol, Director Human Resources, Nor–Lea General Hospital, Lovington, NM, p. A417

DEARTH, Ron, Superintendent, Morton General Hospital, Morton, WA, p. A663

DEARY, Shirley, Director Human Resources, Glenbeigh Hospital and Outpatient Centers, Rock Creek, OH, p. A487

DEASON, Russell, Chief Information Officer, Naval Hospital, Pensacola, FL, p. A136

DEATER, Gary A., Vice President Administration, Human Resources and Risk Management, Witham Memorial Hospital, Lebanon, IN, p. A207

DEATON, David, Administrator and Chief Executive Officer, Little River Memorial Hospital, Ashdown, AR, p. A42

DEATON, Eric, Chief Executive Officer, Danville Regional Medical Center, Danville, VA, p. A647

DEATON, Michael, Chief Financial Officer, Chestatee Regional Hospital, Dahlonega, GA, p. A150

DEATON, Susan Renodin, Chief Human Resources Officer, Cumberland River Hospital, Celina, TN, p. A563

DEATON, Timothy C., Administrator, Complex Care Hospital at Tenaya, Las Vegas, NV, p. A392

DEAVERS, Nancy, R.N. Vice President and Chief Operating Officer, Oswego Hospital, Oswego, NY, p. A440

DEBARBA Jr., Daniel J., President and Chief Executive Officer, Norwalk Hospital, Norwalk, CT, p. A111

DEBARROS, Paula, Director Human Resources, Southwest Connecticut Mental Health System, Bridgeport, CT, p. A108

DEBBAS, Elias, M.D. President Medical Staff, Fort Washington Medical Center, Fort Washington, MD, p. A291

DEBBINK, Connie, Director Finance, Aurora Sheboygan Memorial Medical Center, Sheboygan, WI, p. A690

DEBBS, Ted, Administrator, Rusk State Hospital, Rusk, TX, p. A623

DEBLASIS, John, Senior Administrator, Belmont Community Hospital, Bellaire, OH, p. A470

DEBLIEUX, Dawna, Chief Nurse Executive, Natchitoches Regional Medical Center, Natchitoches, LA, p. A274

DEBLOIS, Arthur J., Interim President and Chief Executive Officer, Memorial Hospital of Rhode Island, Pawtucket, RI, p. A544

DEBLOIS, Georgean, M.D. Chairman Medical Staff, CJW Medical Center, Richmond, VA, p. A654

DEBOER, Cynthia D., Chief Financial Officer, Cedar Springs Behavioral Health System, Colorado Springs, CO, p. A98

DEBOER, K. C., Vice President, Avera St. Luke's Hospital, Aberdeen, SD, p. A555

DEBOLT, Larry, Chief Financial Officer, Bluffton Regional Medical Center, Bluffton, IN, p. A198

DEBORD, Thomas
President, Summa Barberton Citizens Hospital, Barberton, OH, p. A470
President, Summa Wadsworth–Rittman Hospital, Wadsworth, OH, p. A490

DEBUHR, Rhonda, R.N. Chief Clinical and Nursing Officer, Waverly Health Center, Waverly, IA, p. A228

DECAMP, Kay, Chief Human Resources Officer, Jack C. Montgomery Veterans Affairs Medical Center, Muskogee, OK, p. A499

DECAMPS, Daniel, M.D. Chief of Staff, Lake City Community Hospital, Lake City, SC, p. A552

DECELL, Daniela, Chief Executive Officer, Las Colinas Medical Center, Irving, TX, p. A609

DECHABERT, Rebecca, Acting Director Personnel, New York State Psychiatric Institute, New York, NY, p. A435

DECKARD, Rick, Chief Fiscal Service, Veterans Affairs Medical Center, Chillicothe, OH, p. A472

DECKARD, Steven, Vice President Human Resources, Indiana University Health Bloomington Hospital, Bloomington, IN, p. A198

DECKER, Barbara, R.N. Chief Nursing Officer, Provena St. Mary's Hospital, Kankakee, IL, p. A185

DECKER, Janice, Manager Human Resources, Senator Garrett W. Hagedorn Psychiatric Hospital, Glen Gardner, NJ, p. A

DECKER, Jeanine, Manager Human Resources, Arizona State Hospital, Phoenix, AZ, p. A35

DECKER, Kevin, Assistant Chief Executive Officer, Medical Center of South Arkansas, El Dorado, AR, p. A44

DECKER, Lisa K., Director Public Relations and Marketing, Franciscan St. Elizabeth Health – Lafayette Central, Lafayette, IN, p. A206

DECKER, Michael, President and Chief Executive Officer, Divine Savior Healthcare, Portage, WI, p. A689

DECORTE, Raymond P., M.D. Chief Medical Officer, East Jefferson General Hospital, Metairie, LA, p. A273

DECREMER, Dean, Chief Information Officer, Dickinson County Healthcare System, Iron Mountain, MI, p. A315

DEDECKER, Troy, Chief Executive Officer, Bartow Regional Medical Center, Bartow, FL, p. A118

DEE, Thomas A., Chief Executive Officer, Southwestern Vermont Medical Center, Bennington, VT, p. A643

DEEM, Sara, Director Operations, UC Health Surgical Hospital, West Chester, OH, p. A491

DEEMER, Miriam, Chief Executive Officer, Select Specialty Hospital–Grosse Pointe, Grosse Pointe Farms, MI, p. A314

DEEP, Noel, M.D. Chief Medical Staff, Langlade Memorial Hospital, Antigo, WI, p. A678

DEERFIELD, Della, Vice President Finance, Marcum and Wallace Memorial Hospital, Irvine, KY, p. A252

DEERING, Linda, R.N. Executive Vice President and Chief Operating Officer, Sherman Hospital, Elgin, IL, p. A181

DEES, Edith, Vice President Information Services and Chief Information Officer, Holy Spirit Hospital, Camp Hill, PA, p. A519

DEESE, Kim, R.N. Vice President/CNO, St. Vincent Medical Center, Los Angeles, CA, p. A72

DEETS, Daniel J., Chief Financial Officer, Hunterdon Medical Center, Flemington, NJ, p. A404

DEETS, Norm, Vice President and Chief Operating Officer, CGH Medical Center, Sterling, IL, p. A194

DEFAUW, Thomas D., FACHE President and Chief Executive Officer, Blue Water Health Services Corporation, Port Huron, MI, p. B22

DEFAUW, Thomas D., FACHE President and Chief Executive Officer, Port Huron Hospital, Port Huron, MI, p. A321

DEFAYE, Yael, Director, Information Technology, Rio Grande Hospital, Del Norte, CO, p. A99

DEFAZIO, Joseph J., Director Human Resources, Eastern Niagara Health System, Lockport, NY, p. A429

DEFER, Tamara, Director Human Resources, Baylor Regional Medical Center at Plano, Plano, TX, p. A621

DEFOORE, Richard G., FACHE Chief Executive Officer, Stamford Memorial Hospital, Stamford, TX, p. A628

DEFORD, Drexel
Chief Information Officer, Scripps Mercy Hospital, San Diego, CA, p. A86
Vice President and Chief Information Officer, Seattle Children's Hospital, Seattle, WA, p. A666

DEFRAIN, Douglas, Director Human Resources, Blanchard Valley Hospital, Findlay, OH, p. A480

DEFRANCESCO, Anthony, Associate Director, Veterans Affairs Long Beach Healthcare System, Long Beach, CA, p. A68

DEFURIO, Anthony C., Vice President and Chief Financial Officer, University of Colorado Hospital, Aurora, CO, p. A97

DEFURIO, Ken, President and Chief Executive Officer, Butler Health System, Butler, PA, p. A519

DEGEAR, David O., M.D. Vice President Medical Affairs, Westfields Hospital, New Richmond, WI, p. A688

Index of Health Care Professionals / Derby


DEGGES, Carla, R.N. Chief Clinical Officer, East Texas Medical Center Henderson, Henderson, TX, p. A603
DEGI, John, Director Human Resources, Henderson County Community Hospital, Lexington, TN, p. A569
DEGINA, Anthony M., President and Chief Executive Officer, Largo Medical Center, Largo, FL, p. A128
DEGRAND, Robert
Chief Information Officer, Community Memorial Hospital, Menomonee Falls, WI, p. A685
Chief Information Officer, Froedtert Memorial Lutheran Hospital, Milwaukee, WI, p. A686
DEGRAVELLE, Eric, Director Human Resources, Thibodaux Regional Medical Center, Thibodaux, LA, p. A278
DEGROFF, James, Director Technology and Network Services, St. Mary's Healthcare, Amsterdam, NY, p. A420
DEGROOT, Daniel, Chief Executive Officer, Community Memorial Hospital, Oconto Falls, WI, p. A688
DEGROOT, Randy, President and Chief Executive Officer, Community Health Center of Branch County, Coldwater, MI, p. A310
DEHAAN, Michael, M.D. President Medical Staff, West Suburban Medical Center, Oak Park, IL, p. A190
DEHAVEN, Bryce, Chief Financial Officer, Orange Park Medical Center, Orange Park, FL, p. A134
DEHEY, Arthur, Senior Vice President and Chief Financial Officer, Clifton Springs Hospital and Clinic, Clifton Springs, NY, p. A424
DEHNING, Cielo, M.D. Medical Director, Mid–America Rehabilitation Hospital, Shawnee Mission, KS, p. A243
DEICH, Faye L., R.N. Chief Operating Officer, Sacred Heart Hospital, Eau Claire, WI, p. A681
DEIS, Terrence G., President and Chief Executive Officer, Parma Community General Hospital, Parma, OH, p. A487
DEITZEN, Denise
Director, Aleda E. Lutz Veterans Affairs Medical Center, Saginaw, MI, p. A322
Acting Director, Veterans Affairs Medical Center, Battle Creek, MI, p. A308
DEJACO, Lynn S., Chief Financial Officer, FirstHealth Moore Regional Hospital, Pinehurst, NC, p. A458
DEJESUS, David, Vice President Human Resources, Southcoast Hospitals Group, Fall River, MA, p. A300
DEJONG, Jodi, Director Marketing, Pioneer Valley Hospital, West Valley City, UT, p. A642
DEJULIA, Jerome, M.D. Chief Medical Officer, Tyrone Hospital, Tyrone, PA, p. A539
DEKASTLE, Reuben J., Chief Nursing Officer, Weiser Memorial Hospital, Weiser, ID, p. A171
DEKEYZER, Ron, Regional Management Information Officer, CHRISTUS St. Frances Cabrini Hospital, Alexandria, LA, p. A261
DEKOK, Joni, Chief Nursing Officer, Sanford Sheldon Medical Center, Sheldon, IA, p. A226
DEKREY, Dale, MS Associate Director Operations and Resources, Veterans Affairs Health Care System, Fargo, ND, p. A466
DEKREY, Daniel, M.D. Chief of Staff, Sanford Bemidji Medical Center, Bemidji, MN, p. A328
DEL CASTILLO, Daniel, Chief Executive Officer, HEALTHSOUTH Rehabilitation Hospital, San Juan, PR, p. A703
DEL CHIARO, Terri
Chief Financial Officer, Mercy Hospital Fort Scott, Fort Scott, KS, p. A233
Vice President and Chief Financial Officer, Mercy Hospital Independence, Independence, KS, p. A235
DEL LOS SANTOS, Edwin, Director Information Systems, Fountain Valley Regional Hospital and Medical Center, Fountain Valley, CA, p. A61
DEL RIO, R. Maxilimien, M.D. Facility Director, Northern Virginia Mental Health Institute, Falls Church, VA, p. A648
DEL RIO, Tomas, Vice President Finance, University Hospital of Brooklyn at Long Island College Hospital,, NY, p. A437
DELA TORRE, Victor, Command Legal Officer, Naval Hospital, Lemoore, CA, p. A67
DELAGARDELLE, Pamela K., Chief Executive Officer, Grundy County Memorial Hospital, Grundy Center, IA, p. A220
DELAHANTY, Michael J., D.O. Medical Director, Edwin Shaw Rehab, Cuyahoga Falls, OH, p. A478
DELANEY, Diane, Vice President Human Resources, Sharp Memorial Hospital, San Diego, CA, p. A86
DELANEY, Margaret, Chief Information Officer, Mercy Hospital and Medical Center, Chicago, IL, p. A176
DELANEY, Michael, Chief Financial Officer, Two Rivers Behavioral Health System, Kansas City, MO, p. A363
DELANO, John
Vice President Chief Information Officer, Integris Baptist Medical Center, Oklahoma City, OK, p. A501
Vice President and Chief Information Officer, Integris Southwest Medical Center, Oklahoma City, OK, p. A501
DELANO, Michael, Administrator, Spearfish Regional Surgery Center, Spearfish, SD, p. A560
DELARDONIS, Virginia, Director Information Systems, Woodland Heights Medical Center, Lufkin, TX, p. A614
DELATTE, Sandra, Director Human Resources, Villa Feliciana Medical Complex, Jackson, LA, p. A268
DELBOCCIO, Suzanne, Chief Nursing Officer and Vice President Patient Care Services, Indiana University Health North Hospital, Carmel, IN, p. A199
DELELLO, Cory
Chief Financial Officer, Aurora Charter Oak Hospital, Covina, CA, p. A58
Chief Financial Officer, Aurora Vista Del Mar Hospital, Ventura, CA, p. A94
DELEON, Leo, Vice President Finance, Sentara Virginia Beach General Hospital, Virginia Beach, VA, p. A657
DELEON, Sherilene, Controller, HEALTHSOUTH Rehabilitation Hospital–Las Vegas, Las Vegas, NV, p. A393
DELFORGE, Gary L., Administrator, Odessa Memorial Healthcare Center, Odessa, WA, p. A663
DELGADO, Laurie
President, University Hospitals Bedford Medical Center, Cleveland, OH, p. A475
President, University Hospitals Richmond Medical Center, Cleveland, OH, p. A476
DELGADO, Pete, Chief Executive Officer, LAC/University of Southern California Medical Center, Los Angeles, CA, p. A70
DELIDUKA, John, M.D. Chief Medical Officer, Cascade Medical Center, Leavenworth, WA, p. A662
DELIEN, Rudie, Director Human Resources, Devereux Georgia Treatment Network, Kennesaw, GA, p. A154
DELISI III, Frank G., Chief Executive Officer, United Medical Center, Washington, DC, p. A117
DELK, Ray, FACHE Vice President Operations, Good Shepherd Medical Center–Marshall, Marshall, TX, p. A615
DELLA LANA, David, M.D. Chief of Staff, Fairchild Medical Center, Yreka, CA, p. A96
DELLA TORRE, Linda, Senior Vice President and Chief Operating Officer, Athens Regional Medical Center, Athens, GA, p. A144
DELLEA, Eugene A., President, Fairview Hospital, Great Barrington, MA, p. A300
DELLOCONO, John, Senior Vice President and Chief Financial Officer, CentraState Healthcare System, Freehold, NJ, p. A404
DELOACH, Jerrald, Chief Operating Officer, Citrus Memorial Health System, Inverness, FL, p. A126
DELONE, Lori, Chief Technology Officer, Halifax Health Medical Center of Daytona Beach, Daytona Beach, FL, p. A122
DELORENZO, David, Senior Director Human Resources, Sisters of Charity Hospital of Buffalo, Buffalo, NY, p. A423
DELUCA, Mike, Vice President Information Systems, Sarah Bush Lincoln Health Center, Mattoon, IL, p. A187
DELVEAUX, Joe, Manager Information Services, St. Francis Regional Medical Center, Shakopee, MN, p. A340
DEMARCO, Victor, Chief Financial Officer, Bronx–Lebanon Hospital Center Health Care System,, NY, p. A431
DEMARTINO, Pat, Chief Information Officer, Children's Specialized Hospital, New Brunswick, NJ, p. A406
DEMASIE, Dennis, Vice President Information Systems and Chief Information Officer, Rush–Copley Medical Center, Aurora, IL, p. A173
DEMATTEO, Kathleen, Chief Information Officer, Danbury Hospital, Danbury, CT, p. A108
DEMAY, Paul, Chief Information Officer, Northwest Medical Center, Springdale, AR, p. A51
DEMERS, Vickie, Chief Executive Officer, HEALTHSOUTH MountainView Regional Rehabilitation Hospital, Morgantown, WV, p. A674
DEMING, Mark, Controller, Oakwood Heritage Hospital, Taylor, MI, p. A324
DEMING, Peggy, Executive Vice President and Chief Financial Officer, University Health System, San Antonio, TX, p. A626
DEMING, Terra, Director Human Resources, Otsego Memorial Hospital, Gaylord, MI, p. A313
DEMONTGORENCY, Tara, Director Business Development, HEALTHSOUTH Bakersfield Rehabilitation Hospital, Bakersfield, CA, p. A54
DEMORROW, Dawn P., Chief Human Resources Service, Veterans Affairs Medical Center, Wilkes–Barre, PA, p. A542
DEMOTTE, Laura, Vice President Human Resources, Memorial Hospital Jacksonville, Jacksonville, FL, p. A126
DEMOURELLE, Steve, Chief Information Officer, Walter Olin Moss Regional Medical Center, Lake Charles, LA, p. A271
DEMPSEY, Charles, M.D. Medical Director, HEALTHSOUTH Rehabilitation Hospital of Spring Hill, Brooksville, FL, p. A120
DEMPSEY, Jeffrey, Vice President Operations, Mercy St. Charles Hospital, Oregon, OH, p. A486
DEMPSEY, John F., Vice President and Chief Financial Officer, Springfield Regional Medical Center, Springfield, OH, p. A488
DEMPSEY, Virginia B., President, Saint Joseph – London, London, KY, p. A254
DEMPSTER, John, President and Chief Executive Officer, Jefferson Regional Medical Center, Jefferson Hills, PA, p. A525
DEMURO, Rob, M.D. President Medical Staff, Elizabethtown Community Hospital, Elizabethtown, NY, p. A425
DENARDO, John J., Chief Executive Officer, University of Illinois Hospital & Health Sciences System, Chicago, IL, p. A179
DENARVAEZ, Margaret, President and Chief Executive Officer, Wellmont Health System, Kingsport, TN, p. B144
DENBO, John, Chief Executive Officer, Phelps County Regional Medical Center, Rolla, MO, p. A367
DENEFF, Randall, Vice President Finance, Mary Free Bed Rehabilitation Hospital, Grand Rapids, MI, p. A313
DENEN, Bruce, Manager Data Processing, Fayette County Memorial Hospital, Washington Court House, OH, p. A490
DENHAM, Stephanie, Chief Financial Officer and Human Resources Officer, Phillips County Hospital, Malta, MT, p. A377
DENIO, Arthur E., Vice President and Chief Financial Officer, NorthBay Medical Center, Fairfield, CA, p. A60
DENISIENKO, Mary, Vice President Human Resources, Palos Community Hospital, Palos Heights, IL, p. A190
DENISON, Brenda, Chief Financial Officer, Hamilton General Hospital, Hamilton, TX, p. A602
DENISON, Rita, Manager Information Systems, Sturgis Hospital, Sturgis, MI, p. A323
DENKER, Jill, Executive Director Human Resources, Lexington Regional Health Center, Lexington, NE, p. A385
DENMARK, Donald, M.D. Chief Medical Officer, Carondelet St. Joseph's Hospital, Tucson, AZ, p. A39
DENNEY, David, M.D. President Medical Staff, Medical West, Bessemer, AL, p. A16
DENNIS, Bradley, M.D. Chief Medical Officer, Brookwood Medical Center, Birmingham, AL, p. A16
DENNIS, Michael, Director, William J. McCord Adolescent and Treatment Center, Orangeburg, SC, p. A553
DENNISON, Cindy, Senior Director Rural Division, Mercy Willard Hospital, Willard, OH, p. A491
DENNO, Charles, Chief Financial Officer, Westwood Lodge Hospital, Westwood, MA, p. A306
DENNSTEDT, Crystal
Information Officer, North Texas State Hospital, Vernon, TX, p. A633
Chief Information Officer, North Texas State Hospital, Wichita Falls Campus, Wichita Falls, TX, p. A635
DENO, Mark S., Chief Executive Officer, HEALTHSOUTH Rehabilitation Hospital of Arlington, Arlington, TX, p. A579
DENO, Mary, Vice President Human Resources, Community Medical Center, Toms River, NJ, p. A411
DENSTEDT, Ron, Acting Director, Walter P. Reuther Psychiatric Hospital, Westland, MI, p. A325
DENT, Bruce, Director Human Resources, Park City Medical Center, Park City, UT, p. A639
DENTON, Charles L., Chief Executive Officer, Grenada Lake Medical Center, Grenada, MS, p. A346
DENTON, Christopher, Chief Financial Officer, Henrico Doctors' Hospital, Richmond, VA, p. A655
DENTON, Genise, Manager Human Resources, John J. Pershing Veterans Affairs Medical Center, Poplar Bluff, MO, p. A367
DENTON, Joe
Chief Financial Officer, Infirmary West, Mobile, AL, p. A22
Executive Vice President and Chief Financial Officer, Mobile Infirmary Medical Center, Mobile, AL, p. A22
DENTON, Tony, JD Chief Operating Officer, University of Michigan Hospitals and Health Centers, Ann Arbor, MI, p. A307
DENUCCI, Alex, Chief Financial Officer, Franciscan Hospital for Children, Boston, MA, p. A296
DEPAULO, Theron, Manager Information Systems, Providence Mount Carmel Hospital, Colville, WA, p. A660
DEPINHO, Ronald A., M.D. President, University of Texas M.D. Anderson Cancer Center, Houston, TX, p. A608
DEPKO, Mike, Director Information Technology, Brown County Hospital, Ainsworth, NE, p. A381
DEPONTE, Kathleen, M.D. Chief of Staff, Mountain View Regional Medical Center, Norton, VA, p. A653
DEPOYSTER, Avis, Director Human Resources, Brownfield Regional Medical Center, Brownfield, TX, p. A585
DEPRIEST, Paul Duane, M.D
Chief Medical Officer, UK HealthCare Good Samaritan Hospital, Lexington, KY, p. A253
Chief Medical Officer, University of Kentucky Albert B. Chandler Hospital, Lexington, KY, p. A253
DEQUARDO, John R., M.D. Superintendent, Colorado Mental Health Institute at Pueblo, Pueblo, CO, p. A105
DERBY, Richard P., Vice President Finance, Barton Healthcare System, South Lake Tahoe, CA, p. A91


© 2012 AHA Guide Index of Health Care Professionals **A797**

Index of Health Care Professionals

Index of Health Care Professionals

Index of Health Care Professionals / Derdeyn

DERDEYN, Paul, Director Fiscal Services and Plant Operations, Connecticut Valley Hospital, Middletown, CT, p. A110
DERENZIS, Vicki, Chief Financial Officer, Highlands Regional Medical Center, Sebring, FL, p. A139
DERFLINGER, Terri, Administrator, Mercy Hospital of Franciscan Sisters, Oelwein, IA, p. A224
DERNER, Monica, Chief Executive Officer and Chief Financial Officer, Modoc Medical Center, Alturas, CA, p. A53
DERNIER, Marty, Chief Financial Officer and Administrator, Kansas Rehabilitation Hospital, Topeka, KS, p. A244
DEROUEN, Jason, Director Management Information Systems, Grace Medical Center, Lubbock, TX, p. A614
DERRICK, Brian, Chief Financial Officer, Einstein Medical Center Philadelphia, Philadelphia, PA, p. A532
DERRICK, Niki, R.N. Chief Clinical Officer, Kindred Hospital–Bay Area St. Petersburg, Saint Petersburg, FL, p. A138
DERRINGTON, Ken R., Chief Financial Officer, Northern Colorado Rehabilitation Hospital, Johnstown, CO, p. A102
DERTZ, Donna, Director Human Resources, St. Bernard Hospital and Health Care Center, Chicago, IL, p. A178
DERUS, Charles, M.D. Vice President Medical Management, Advocate Good Samaritan Hospital, Downers Grove, IL, p. A180
DERUYTER, David N., M.D. President Medical Staff, Kindred Hospital–Atlanta, Atlanta, GA, p. A145
DESAI, Nimesh, M.D. Medical Director, Massena Memorial Hospital, Massena, NY, p. A429
DESAI, Shailesh, M.D. Chief of Staff, Baum Harmon Mercy Hospital, Primghar, IA, p. A225
DESALVO, Susan, Manager Human Resources, Veterans Affairs Medical Center, Bath, NY, p. A421
DESANCTIS, Mario, FACHE Director, Veterans Affairs Medical Center, Tomah, WI, p. A692
DESANTIS, Chris, Manager Human Resources, Shriners Hospitals for Children, Erie, Erie, PA, p. A523
DESANTIS, John
Chief Financial Officer, Glenwood Regional Medical Center, West Monroe, LA, p. A279
Chief Financial Officer, Ouachita Community Hospital, West Monroe, LA, p. A279
DESANTIS, Vincent, Vice President Finance, Phelps Memorial Hospital Center, Sleepy Hollow, NY, p. A443
DESCHAINE, Terry, Chief Executive Officer, Fredonia Regional Hospital, Fredonia, KS, p. A233
DESCHAMBEAU, Wayne G., President and Chief Executive Officer, Wayne Hospital, Greenville, OH, p. A481
DESCHENE, Normand E., FACHE President and Chief Executive Officer, Lowell General Hospital, Lowell, MA, p. A301
DESCHRYVER, Joseph, Chief Operating Officer, Sierra Vista Regional Medical Center, San Luis Obispo, CA, p. A88
DESHAIES, Roger, Chief Financial Officer, Fletcher Allen Health Care, Burlington, VT, p. A643
DESHAZO, Sheri, Chief Operating Officer, Kings Mountain Hospital, Kings Mountain, NC, p. A456
DESHIELDS, Michael S., M.D. Director Medical Affairs, Camden County Health Services Center, Blackwood, NJ, p. A402
DESIMONE, Maureen, Chief Operating Officer, Blythedale Children's Hospital, Valhalla, NY, p. A445
DESIMONE, Silvana, Chief Information Officer, Coney Island Hospital,, NY, p. A432
DESJEUNES, Carol, Chief Operating Officer, Psychiatric Institute of Washington, Washington, DC, p. A117
DESKINS, Juanita, Chief Operating Officer, Pikeville Medical Center, Pikeville, KY, p. A258
DESMARTEAU, Lisa Jo, Chief Financial Officer, Miami Jewish Home and Hospital for Aged, Miami, FL, p. A131
DESMOND, Heather, Chief Financial Officer, Bibb Medical Center, Centreville, AL, p. A18
DESMOND, P. Craig, President, Methodist Texsan Hospital, San Antonio, TX, p. A625
DESORMEAU, Mary, Chief Nursing Officer, Grand River Hospital District, Rifle, CO, p. A105
DESOTELLE, Robert C., President and Chief Executive Officer, Asheville Specialty Hospital, Asheville, NC, p. A448
DESOTO, David, M.D. Chief of Staff, National Park Medical Center, Hot Springs, AR, p. A46
DESOTO, James, M.D
Vice President Medical Affairs, Mercy Medical Center Redding, Redding, CA, p. A81
Vice President Medical Affairs, St. Elizabeth Community Hospital, Red Bluff, CA, p. A81
DESOUZA, Jacqueline
Chief Executive Officer, Lee's Summit Medical Center, Lee's Summit, MO, p. A364
Chief Operating Officer, Research Medical Center, Kansas City, MO, p. A362
DESPRES, Paul J., Chief Executive Officer, Eleanor Slater Hospital, Cranston, RI, p. A544
DESROCHES, Jeff, Manager Information Systems, Anaheim Regional Medical Center, Anaheim, CA, p. A53
DETOR, Robert E., Chief Executive Officer, South Oaks Hospital, Amityville, NY, p. A420
DETTERMAN, B. Lynn, Chief Executive Officer, Mercy Willard Hospital, Willard, OH, p. A491
DETTERMAN, Paula J., FACHE Chief Executive Officer, Mercer County Joint Township Community Hospital, Coldwater, OH, p. A476
DETTMER, Robert E., Deputy Commander for Health Services, Irwin Army Community Hospital, Junction City, KS, p. A236
DETWILER, Courtney, R.N. Administrator, Hampton Roads Specialty Hospital, Newport News, VA, p. A652
DEUEL, Teresa L., Chief Executive Officer, Hodgeman County Health Center, Jetmore, KS, p. A235
DEURMIER, Carol, Chief Executive Officer, St. Michael's Hospital Avera, Tyndall, SD, p. A560
DEUSTERMAN, Abe, Manager Information Technology, Essentia Health Fosston, Fosston, MN, p. A331
DEUTCHMAN, Adam, M.D. Chief of Staff, Steele Memorial Medical Center, Salmon, ID, p. A170
DEVABHAKTUNI, Venkata S., M.D. Medical Director, Bradford Health Services at Huntsville, Madison, AL, p. A22
DEVANEY, Catherine, Chief Executive Officer, HEALTHSOUTH Rehabilitation Hospital, Concord, NH, p. A397
DEVANEY, Ed, Vice President and Chief Operating Officer, Hackensack University Medical Center Mountainside, Montclair, NJ, p. A406
DEVANSKY, Gary W., Director, Veterans Affairs Medical Center, Coatesville, PA, p. A521
DEVAUGHN, Michael D.
Senior Vice President and Chief Financial Officer, WakeMed Cary Hospital, Cary, NC, p. A450
Senior Vice President Finance and Chief Financial Officer, WakeMed Raleigh Campus, Raleigh, NC, p. A459
DEVAULT, Jennifer, Vice President Associate Services, F. F. Thompson Hospital, Canandaigua, NY, p. A423
DEVAULT, Roseann M., Chief Financial Officer, Jefferson Memorial Hospital, Jefferson City, TN, p. A567
DEVENPORT, Genia, Administrator, New Mexico Rehabilitation Center, Roswell, NM, p. A417
DEVENUTO, Joseph, Vice President and Chief Information Officer, Norton Suburban Hospital, Louisville, KY, p. A255
DEVET, Reezie, Ph.D. President and Chief Executive Officer, McLaren Northern Michigan, Petoskey, MI, p. A320
DEVILLE, Linda F., Chief Executive Officer, Bunkie General Hospital, Bunkie, LA, p. A264
DEVIN, Brian V., Chief Operating Officer, Massachusetts Hospital School, Canton, MA, p. A299
DEVIN, Joe, Chief Executive Officer, Ocean Beach Hospital, Ilwaco, WA, p. A662
DEVINE, Christina, Director Human Resources, The Rehabilitation Institute of St. Louis, Saint Louis, MO, p. A370
DEVINE, Sarah, M.D. Chief of Staff, Myrtue Medical Center, Harlan, IA, p. A220
DEVINNEY, Sharon, Interim Chief Operating Officer, Madison Center and Hospital, South Bend, IN, p. A211
DEVITO, Joseph M., Vice President Finance and Chief Operating Officer, Geisinger–Bloomsburg Hospital, Bloomsburg, PA, p. A519
DEVLIN, James, Director Information Systems, St. Cloud Regional Medical Center, Saint Cloud, FL, p. A137
DEVOCELLE, Frank H., President and Chief Executive Officer, Olathe Medical Center, Olathe, KS, p. A240
DEVOL, Marjorie, M.D. Chief of Staff, Doctors Hospital Nelsonville, Nelsonville, OH, p. A486
DEVONEY, William, Chief Financial Officer, University of Illinois Hospital & Health Sciences System, Chicago, IL, p. A179
DEVORE, Pam, Financial Manager, Hillcrest Memorial Hospital, Simpsonville, SC, p. A553
DEVORE, Paul A., M.D. Medical Director, Gladys Spellman Specialty Hospital and Nursing Center, Cheverly, MD, p. A290
DEVRIES, Russell, Chief Business Operations, Keller Army Community Hospital, West Point, NY, p. A446
DEW, Douglas, M.D. President Medical Staff, Flagler Hospital, Saint Augustine, FL, p. A137
DEWALSCHE, Diane, R.N. Chief Operating Officer, Community Hospital of Long Beach, Long Beach, CA, p. A68
DEWALT, Stephen, Warden, Federal Medical Center, Lexington, KY, p. A253
DEWAN, Vijay, M.D. Clinical Director, Lincoln Regional Center, Lincoln, NE, p. A385
DEWBERRY, Doug, Chief Executive Officer and Administrator, Lanier Health Services, Valley, AL, p. A26
DEWBERRY, Robbie, Chief Executive Officer, Mitchell County Hospital, Colorado City, TX, p. A588
DEWERFF, Mike, Chief Financial Officer, Trinity Regional Medical Center, Fort Dodge, IA, p. A219
DEWISPELARE, Cheryl M., Chief Human Resources Officer, Veterans Affairs Medical Center, Omaha, NE, p. A388
DEWITT, Jocelyn, Chief Information Officer, University of Michigan Hospitals and Health Centers, Ann Arbor, MI, p. A307
DEWITT, Sarah, Director, Ogden Regional Medical Center, Ogden, UT, p. A639
DEWITT, Warren, M.D. Chief Medical Officer, Barnes–Kasson County Hospital, Susquehanna, PA, p. A539
DEXTER, Stephen P., President and Chief Executive Officer, Saint Francis Hospital, Charleston, WV, p. A671
DEXTER, Stephen P., President and Chief Executive Officer, Thomas Health System, Inc., South Charleston, WV, p. B129
DEXTER, Stephen P., President and Chief Executive Officer, Thomas Memorial Hospital, South Charleston, WV, p. A676
DEXTER, Sue, Administrative Department Leader Human Resources, McDonough District Hospital, Macomb, iL, p. A186
DHAWAN, Kamlesh, M.D. Chief of Staff, East Los Angeles Doctors Hospital, Los Angeles, CA, p. A69
DHINGRA, Ashok, M.D. Executive Medical Director, HEALTHSOUTH Deaconess Rehabilitation Hospital, Evansville, IN, p. A201
DHULIPALA, Vasudeva, M.D. Medical Director, HEALTHSOUTH Rehabilitation Hospital of Alexandria, Alexandria, LA, p. A261
DHUPER, Arti
Regional Director Human Resources, Chino Valley Medical Center, Chino, CA, p. A57
Regional Director Human Resources, Desert Valley Hospital, Victorville, CA, p. A95
Director Human Resources, San Dimas Community Hospital, San Dimas, CA, p. A86
DI BACCO, David J., Chief Operating Officer, Eastern Niagara Health System, Lockport, NY, p. A429
DI BERNARDO, Deborah, Chief Information Officer, St. Joseph's Medical Center, Yonkers, NY, p. A447
DI LORENZO, Anthony, Vice President Operations, NorthShore University Health System Skokie Hospital, Skokie, IL, p. A194
DI MARIA, Anthony, M.D. Medical Director, Jamaica Hospital Medical Center,, NY, p. A433
DI RIENZO, Louis, Chief Information Officer, Lake Shore Health Care Center, Irving, NY, p. A427
DI STEFANO, Anthony, Director Finance, Soldiers' Home in Holyoke, Holyoke, MA, p. A301
DIAL, Jeffery
Chief Operating Officer, Vidant Bertie Hospital, Windsor, NC, p. A463
Chief Operating Officer, Vidant Chowan Hospital, Edenton, NC, p. A452
DIAL, Marcia R., Administrator and Chief Executive Officer, Scotland County Hospital, Memphis, MO, p. A365
DIALTO, Margaret, Vice President Human Resources, Staten Island University Hospital,, NY, p. A437
DIAMOND, Anne, JD Chief Operating Officer, University of Connecticut Health Center, John Dempsey Hospital, Farmington, CT, p. A109
DIAMOND, Chris, Chief Executive Officer, Heritage Oaks Hospital, Sacramento, CA, p. A83
DIAMOND, Lester K., President, St. Dominic–Jackson Memorial Hospital, Jackson, MS, p. A348
DIAMOND, Robert
Vice President and Chief Information Officer, Putnam Hospital Center, Carmel, NY, p. A423
Chief Information Officer, Vassar Brothers Medical Center, Poughkeepsie, NY, p. A441
DIAMOND, Timothy, Chief Information Officer, La Rabida Children's Hospital, Chicago, IL, p. A176
DIAMOND, Vickie L., MS, President and Chief Executive Officer, Wyoming Medical Center, Casper, WY, p. A695
DIANGELO, John A.
Senior Vice President Finance and Chief Financial Officer, South Jersey Healthcare – Elmer Hospital, Elmer, NJ, p. A404
Senior Vice President Finance and Chief Financial Officer, South Jersey Healthcare – Regional Medical Center, Vineland, NJ, p. A411
DIANO, Robert, Director Human Resources, Broward Health Coral Springs, Coral Springs, FL, p. A121
DIAS, Walter, Vice President and Chief Operating Officer, Butler Hospital, Providence, RI, p. A544
DIAZ, Constantino, M.D. Chief of Staff, Newport Medical Center, Newport, TN, p. A574
DIAZ, Cristina, Director, Rush Oak Park Hospital, Oak Park, IL, p. A190
DIAZ, Felipe, M.D. Chief of Staff, Veterans Affairs Medical Center, Bath, NY, p. A421
DIAZ, Georgina, Chief Operating Officer, Palmetto General Hospital, Hialeah, FL, p. A125
DIAZ, Gloria, Executive Director, Hospital Santa Rosa, Guayama, PR, p. A701
DIAZ, Jesse, Chief Information Officer, Phoebe Putney Memorial Hospital, Albany, GA, p. A144

A798 Index of Health Care Professionals

Index of Health Care Professionals / Dix

Index of Health Care Professionals


DIAZ, Jorge Rodriguez, Director Human Resources, Hospital De La Concepcion, San German, PR, p. A702
DIAZ, Jose, Director Information Systems, Emory Johns Creek Hospital, Johns Creek, GA, p. A154
DIAZ, Octavio, M.D. Chief Medical Officer, Saint Vincent Hospital, Worcester, MA, p. A306
DIAZ, Paul J., President and Chief Executive Officer, Kindred Healthcare, Louisville, KY, p. B75
DIAZ, Rachael, Systems Operator, Coalinga Regional Medical Center, Coalinga, CA, p. A58
DIAZ, Ricardo, Chief Executive Officer, Shands Live Oak, Live Oak, FL, p. A129
DIAZ, Steve, M.D. Chief Medical Officer, MaineGeneral Medical Center–Waterville Campus, Waterville, ME, p. A286
DIAZ–LOPEZ, Emily, Director Human Resources, CHRISTUS Spohn Hospital Alice, Alice, TX, p. A577
DIBLIK, Donna, Chief Financial Officer, Our Lady of the Resurrection Medical Center, Chicago, IL, p. A177
DICESARE, Gayle, President and Chief Executive Officer, RiverValley Behavioral Health Hospital, Owensboro, KY, p. A257
DICESARE, Jan, Vice President Financial Operations, St. Vincent's East, Birmingham, AL, p. A17
DICK, David, Chief Executive Officer, Mitchell County Hospital Health Systems, Beloit, KS, p. A231
DICK, Lynette, Director of Support Services, Ellsworth County Medical Center, Ellsworth, KS, p. A232
DICK, Mollie, Coordinator Human Resources, Wayne County Hospital, Monticello, KY, p. A256
DICK, Myra, Manager Business Office, LTAC of Wichita, Wichita, KS, p. A245
DICKENS, Robert, Interim Chief Executive Officer, Auburn Regional Medical Center, Auburn, WA, p. A659
DICKERSON, Gene, M.D. Vice President Medical Affairs, Tuomey Healthcare System, Sumter, SC, p. A554
DICKERSON, Kathy, Chief Financial Officer, HEALTHSOUTH Rehabilitation Hospital of Arlington, Arlington, TX, p. A579
DICKERSON, Tammy, Director Human Resources, Carolinas Hospital System, Florence, SC, p. A549
DICKERSON, Taylor
Chief Information Officer, Lake City Medical Center, Lake City, FL, p. A128
Director Information Services, Ocala Regional Medical Center, Ocala, FL, p. A133
DICKERSON, Toby, Chief Information Resources Management Services, Durham Veterans Affairs Medical Center, Durham, NC, p. A452
DICKEY, John M., Chief Administrative Officer, Mayo Clinic Health System in Eau Claire, Eau Claire, WI, p. A681
DICKEY, Mark, Director Business Development, Valir Rehabilitation Hospital, Oklahoma City, OK, p. A502
DICKEY, Sarah J., Manager Personnel, Marshall Browning Hospital, Du Quoin, IL, p. A180
DICKEY Jr., W. P., Chief Executive Officer, Franklin County Memorial Hospital, Meadville, MS, p. A350
DICKINSON, Brett M., M.D
Chief of Staff, Parkland Health Center, Farmington, MO, p. A359
Chief of Staff, Parkland Health Center–Bonne Terre, Bonne Terre, MO, p. A355
DICKINSON, Galen, Chief Financial Officer, Cary Medical Center, Caribou, ME, p. A282
DICKMAN, Kathy, Director Information Technology, McCullough–Hyde Memorial Hospital, Oxford, OH, p. A487
DICKSON, Douglas, Senior Vice President Finance, Sierra View District Hospital, Porterville, CA, p. A81
DICKSON, James J., Administrator and Chief Executive Officer, Copper Queen Community Hospital, Bisbee, AZ, p. A31
DICKSON, Karen, Director, Human Resources, Maine Coast Memorial Hospital, Ellsworth, ME, p. A283
DICKSON, Lynette, Director Clinical Operations and Director of Nursing, District One Hospital, Faribault, MN, p. A331
DICKSON, Thomas C., Chief Executive Officer, Banner Thunderbird Medical Center, Glendale, AZ, p. A33
DICKSTEIN, Steve, Director, Newton Medical Center, Covington, GA, p. A150
DICROCE, Theresa M., M.D. Chief Medical Staff, North Valley Hospital, Tonasket, WA, p. A668
DICUS, Scott, M.D. Chief of Staff, White County Medical Center, Searcy, AR, p. A51
DIDENKO, Dima
Vice President and Chief Financial Officer, Florida Hospital Heartland Medical Center, Sebring, FL, p. A139
Vice President and Chief Financial Officer, Florida Hospital Wauchula, Wauchula, FL, p. A142
DIDIER, Debra, Vice President and Chief Financial Officer, Katherine Shaw Bethea Hospital, Dixon, IL, p. A180
DIEBLING, Tara, Chief Financial Officer, The Rehabilitation Institute of St. Louis, Saint Louis, MO, p. A370
DIECKMANN, Holli, Director Health Information, Sabetha Community Hospital, Sabetha, KS, p. A242
DIEDE, Dale, M.D. Medical Provider, Dahl Memorial Healthcare Association, Ekalaka, MT, p. A375
DIEDE, Shelby, Chief Financial Officer, Banner Lassen Medical Center, Susanville, CA, p. A92
DIEDERICH, J. Joseph
Executive Vice President and Chief Operating Officer, Oakwood Annapolis Hospital, Wayne, MI, p. A325
Executive Vice President and Chief Operating Officer, Oakwood Southshore Medical Center, Trenton, MI, p. A324
DIEDERICH, John A., Senior Vice President Operations and Chief Operating Officer, Rush–Copley Medical Center, Aurora, IL, p. A173
DIEDERICH, Thomas, Senior Vice President Human Resources, Phoenix Children's Hospital, Phoenix, AZ, p. A36
DIEGEL, James A., President and Chief Executive Officer, St. Charles Health System, Inc., Bend, OR, p. B122
DIEHL, Kent, M.D. Chief of Staff, Jacobson Memorial Hospital Care Center, Elgin, ND, p. A465
DIEHL, Michael, M.D. President, Ogden Regional Medical Center, Ogden, UT, p. A639
DIER, Joy, R.N. Vice President Clinical Services and Chief Nursing Officer, Texas Institute for Surgery at Texas Health Presbyterian Dallas, Dallas, TX, p. A592
DIERKENS, Janelle, Chief Administration Officer, New York State Psychiatric Institute, New York, NY, p. A435
DIERKER, Anne, Vice President Hospital Services, Pekin Hospital, Pekin, IL, p. A191
DIERS, Suzanne, R.N. Director Patient Care Services, Shriners Hospitals for Children, Portland, Portland, OR, p. A514
DIESFELD, James, M.D. President Medical Staff, Thorek Memorial Hospital, Chicago, IL, p. A178
DIESTEL, Peter, Senior Vice President and Chief Operating Officer, Valley Hospital, Ridgewood, NJ, p. A409
DIETER, Brian, President and Chief Executive Officer, Mary Greeley Medical Center, Ames, IA, p. A214
DIETERICH, Kevin, Director Information Services, Inland Hospital, Waterville, ME, p. A285
DIETRICK, Brian, Director Information Systems, Wilson Medical Center, Wilson, NC, p. A463
DIETSCHE, Jim, Chief Financial Officer, Bellin Memorial Hospital, Green Bay, WI, p. A682
DIETZ, Brian E., FACHE Interim President and Chief Executive Officer, St. Mary's Hospital, Streator, IL, p. A195
DIETZ, Gary, Director Information Technology Services, Walla Walla General Hospital, Walla Walla, WA, p. A669
DIETZ, Mark, Chief Medical Officer, New River Medical Center, Monticello, MN, p. A335
DIETZ, Michael, Chief Hospital Administration, U. S. Air Force Hospital, Hampton, VA, p. A649
DIEWALD, Wayne A., President, Genesis Medical Center–Davenport, Davenport, IA, p. A217
DIFRANCO, Vincent B., Chief Executive Officer, Community Hospital, Torrington, WY, p. A698
DIGGINS, Dana, Chief Financial Officer, Landmark Medical Center, Woonsocket, RI, p. A545
DIGNUM, Kirk, Ph.D. Chief Executive Officer, Mercy Regional Medical Center, Durango, CO, p. A100
DIGREGORIO, Connie L., Assistant Administrator, Cascade Valley Hospital and Clinics, Arlington, WA, p. A659
DIIESO, Nicholas T., R.N. Chief Operating Officer, Mount Auburn Hospital, Cambridge, MA, p. A299
DIIORIO, Emil, M.D. Chief Executive Officer, Surgical Specialty Center at Coordinated Health, Allentown, PA, p. A517
DILALLO, Kevin, Chief Executive Officer, Manatee Memorial Hospital, Bradenton, FL, p. A119
DILLARD, Evan S., FACHE President and Chief Executive Officer, Forrest General Hospital, Hattiesburg, MS, p. A346
DILLARD, Leigh, M.D. Chief of Staff, De Soto Regional Health System, Mansfield, LA, p. A272
DILLEHUNT, David B., Chief Information Officer, FirstHealth Moore Regional Hospital, Pinehurst, NC, p. A458
DILLON, Jim, Chief Financial Officer, Rangely District Hospital, Rangely, CO, p. A105
DILLON, Lorie, Chief Executive Officer, Geisinger HEALTHSOUTH Rehabilitation Hospital, Danville, PA, p. A521
DILLON, Mary E., MS Vice President Patient Care Services, Sisters of Charity Hospital of Buffalo, Buffalo, NY, p. A423
DILORENZO, Randolph, M.D. Medical Director, Syosset Hospital, Syosset, NY, p. A444
DILORETO, David, M.D. Executive Vice President and Chief Medical Officer, Saint Francis Hospital, Evanston, IL, p. A181
DIMARE, John, M.D. Medical Director, Foothill Presbyterian Hospital, Glendora, CA, p. A63
DIMAURO, Cynthia, M.D. Medical Director, Hillside Rehabilitation Hospital, Warren, OH, p. A490
DIMICHELE, Maria, Administrative Assistant, Kensington Hospital, Philadelphia, PA, p. A533
DIMMIG, Thomas, M.D. Medical Director, North Carolina Specialty Hospital, Durham, NC, p. A452
DINAN, Edward M., President and Chief Executive Officer, Lawrence Hospital Center, Bronxville, NY, p. A422
DINAUER, Cathy, MSN VP of Patient Care, Carson Tahoe Regional Healthcare, Carson City, NV, p. A391
DINGELDEIN, G. Peter, M.D. Chief Medical Officer, Wadley Regional Medical Center, Texarkana, TX, p. A631
DINGES, Brenda, Director of Nursing, Ness County Hospital, Ness City, KS, p. A239
DINGILIAN, John, M.D. Chief Medical Staff, Simi Valley Hospital and Health Care Services, Simi Valley, CA, p. A91
DINGLE, Steve, M.D. Chief Medical Officer, Arizona State Hospital, Phoenix, AZ, p. A35
DINGLER, Chance, M.D. Chief Medical Officer, Nocona General Hospital, Nocona, TX, p. A618
DINGMAN, III, Vincent, Chief Financial Officer, Columbia Memorial Hospital, Hudson, NY, p. A427
DINGO, Lynn, Director Human Resources, Crestwood Medical Center, Huntsville, AL, p. A21
DINHAM, Vilma L., R.N. Chief Nursing Officer, Encino Hospital Medical Center,, CA, p. A69
DINKHA, Duncan, M.D. Chief of Staff, Morrison Community Hospital, Morrison, IL, p. A188
DINKINS, Joseph, M.D. Chief Medical Staff, Mountain View Hospital, Payson, UT, p. A639
DINKINS, Vicki, Director Human Resources, Louis Smith Memorial Hospital, Lakeland, GA, p. A155
DINON, Nancy, Vice President Human Resources, Orlando Regional Medical Center, Orlando, FL, p. A134
DINSLAGE, Dennis, Vice President Finance and Chief Financial Officer, St. Francis Memorial Hospital, West Point, NE, p. A390
DINSMOOR, William S., Chief Financial Officer, Nebraska Medical Center, Omaha, NE, p. A388
DIOKNO, Ananias C., M.D. Executive Vice President and Chief Medical Officer, Beaumont Hospital – Royal Oak, Royal Oak, MI, p. A322
DION, Jeff, Chief Financial Officer, UMass Memorial–Marlborough Hospital, Marlborough, MA, p. A302
DION, Jeffrey P., Vice President Finance, St. Elizabeth's Medical Center, Brighton, MA, p. A298
DION, Michael J., R.N. Vice President Patient Care Services, Windham Hospital, Willimantic, CT, p. A113
DIONNE, Michele, Chief Executive Officer, Houston Physicians Hospital, Webster, TX, p. A634
DIONNE, Philip G., Chief Executive Officer, Ottumwa Regional Health Center, Ottumwa, IA, p. A225
DIPALMA, Maureen, Director Finance, Tewksbury Hospital, Tewksbury, MA, p. A305
DIPILLA, Victor, Vice President and Chief Business Development Officer, Christ Hospital, Cincinnati, OH, p. A473
DIRKS STEVENS, Amy, Chief Operating Officer, Provena Saint Joseph Medical Center, Joliet, IL, p. A185
DISANTO, Larry
Executive Vice President and Chief Operating Officer, Capital Health Medical Center–Hopewell, Pennington, NJ, p. A408
Executive Vice President and Chief Operating Officer, Capital Health Regional Medical Center, Trenton, NJ, p. A411
DISANZO, Frank, Vice President and Chief Information Officer, Saint Peter's University Hospital, New Brunswick, NJ, p. A407
DISCH, Catherine D., Executive Vice President and Chief Operating Officer, Truman Medical Center–Hospital Hill, Kansas City, MO, p. A363
DISHMAN, Leonardo, M.D. Chief Medical Officer, Alice Hyde Medical Center, Malone, NY, p. A429
DISPOTO, Martha, R.N. Chief Nursing Officer, Anaheim Regional Medical Center, Anaheim, CA, p. A53
DISTASIO, Stephen R., Acting Director, Veterans Affairs Black Hills Health Care System, Fort Meade, SD, p. A556
DISTEFANO, Guy, Chief Financial Officer, Hampton Behavioral Health Center, Westampton Township, NJ, p. A412
DISTL, Ron, Chief Executive Officer, MedCentral – Shelby Hospital, Shelby, OH, p. A488
DITTMANN, Jerry, Vice President Human Resources, Mount Nittany Medical Center, State College, PA, p. A539
DITTO, Debbie, CPA Controller, Lincoln Trail Behavioral Health System, Radcliff, KY, p. A258
DITURO, Beth, Divisional Chief Information Officer, Lenox Hill Hospital, New York, NY, p. A433
DIVELLO, Douglas F., President and Chief Executive Officer, Alice Hyde Medical Center, Malone, NY, p. A429
DIVER, Joseph, Vice President Information Services and Chief Information Officer, Bassett Medical Center, Cooperstown, NY, p. A424
DIVITO, Frank, Manager Information Systems, Jameson Hospital, New Castle, PA, p. A530
DIX, Georeg, Chief Information Officer, Olathe Medical Center, Olathe, KS, p. A240



Index of Health Care Professionals A799

Index of Health Care Professionals

Index of Health Care Professionals / Dix

DIX, Roger J., Senior Vice President and Chief Financial Officer, Hannibal Regional Hospital, Hannibal, MO, p. A360
DIXON, Debbie, Director Human Resources, Pampa Regional Medical Center, Pampa, TX, p. A620
DIXON, Del, Chief Information Officer, South Shore Hospital, South Weymouth, MA, p. A304
DIXON, Florine, Vice President Clinical Services, Memorial Hospital, Carthage, IL, p. A174
DIXON, Gregg, CP
Chief Financial Officer, Asheville Specialty Hospital, Asheville, NC, p. A448
Chief Financial Officer, Interfaith Medical Center,, NY, p. A433
DIXON, Matt, Chief Operating Officer, St. Mark's Hospital, Salt Lake City, UT, p. A641
DIXON, Michael, Director Human Resources, Self Regional Healthcare, Greenwood, SC, p. A551
DIXON, Sally J., President and Chief Executive Officer, Memorial Hospital, York, PA, p. A542
DIXON, Shannon, Manager Business Office, Weisbrod Memorial County Hospital, Eads, CO, p. A100
DIXON, Todd, R.N. Chief Executive Officer, Barrow Regional Medical Center, Winder, GA, p. A162
DIXON, Jr., Wynn L., Chief Executive Officer, Chesapeake Regional Medical Center, Chesapeake, VA, p. A646
DIZNEY, Donald R., Chairman and Chief Executive Officer, United Medical Corporation, Windermere, FL, p. B133
DIZON, Louis, M.D. Chief of Staff, Russell County Medical Center, Lebanon, VA, p. A650
DJOGAN, Djogan, Chief Financial Officer, George Nigh Rehabilitation Institute, Okmulgee, OK, p. A502
DMELLO, Artie, Director Case Management, Kindred Hospital Sugar Land, Sugar Land, TX, p. A629
DOAK, Mark, President and Chief Executive Officer, Davis Health System, Elkins, WV, p. B40
DOAK, Mark, President and Chief Executive Officer, Davis Memorial Hospital, Elkins, WV, p. A671
DOAN, Angela, Chief Financial Officer, Scott Memorial Hospital, Scottsburg, IN, p. A211
DOAN, Richard L., FACHE Chief Executive Officer, Barnesville Hospital, Barnesville, OH, p. A470
DOBALIAN, Derek, M.D. Chief of Staff, Tri–City Regional Medical Center, Hawaiian Gardens, CA, p. A64
DOBBINS, Jim, Vice President Human Resources, Lenoir Memorial Hospital, Kinston, NC, p. A456
DOBIN, Jennifer, Vice President Human Resources, Bayonne Medical Center, Bayonne, NJ, p. A401
DOBIZL, Howard
Director Information Technology Services, Howard Young Medical Center, Woodruff, WI, p. A694
Director Information Services for the Northern Region, Sacred Heart–St. Mary's Hospitals, Rhinelander, WI, p. A690
DOBLE, H. Peter, M.D. Director Medical Staff Affairs, St. Luke's Jerome Family Medical Center, Jerome, ID, p. A168
DOBOSENSKI, Dave, Chief Executive Officer, St. Croix Regional Medical Center, St. Croix Falls, WI, p. A691
DOBOSH, Jr., Joseph J., Vice President and Chief Financial Officer, Children's Specialized Hospital, New Brunswick, NJ, p. A406
DOBRAWA, Stanley
Area Technology Director, San Rafael Medical Center, San Rafael, CA, p. A89
Area Technology Director, Santa Rosa Medical Center, Santa Rosa, CA, p. A90
DOBRINSKI, Sandra, Director of Nursing, Comanche County Hospital, Coldwater, KS, p. A231
DOBROVICH, Michael, M.D. Chief Medical Officer, St. John Medical Center, Westlake, OH, p. A491
DOBSON, Glenda, Vice President Clinical Services, Louisiana Medical Center and Heart Hospital, Lacombe, LA, p. A269
DOBSON, Glenn E., Chief Financial Officer, NORTHSTAR Health System, Iron River, MI, p. A316
DOCKENDORFF, Patti, Director Finance, Tri–County Memorial Hospital, Whitehall, WI, p. A694
DOCKTER, Robert A., Administrator, Eureka Community Health Services Avera, Eureka, SD, p. A556
DODD, Eric, Chief Information Officer, Thorek Memorial Hospital, Chicago, IL, p. A178
DODD, John, Vice President Human Resources, Central Peninsula General Hospital, Soldotna, AK, p. A30
DODDS, Cheryl, M.D. Medical Director, Three Rivers Behavioral Health, West Columbia, SC, p. A554
DODDS, Rick A., Vice President Human Resources, Sonora Regional Medical Center, Sonora, CA, p. A91
DODDS, Sheryl, Chief Clinical Officer, Florida Hospital, Orlando, FL, p. A134
DODSON, Nancy, Chief Operating Officer, Gulf Coast Medical Center, Panama City, FL, p. A135
DODSON, Thomas, Executive Director, Buffalo Psychiatric Center, Buffalo, NY, p. A422
DOEDEN, Lynn, Chief Executive Officer, Decatur County Hospital and Cedar Living Center, Oberlin, KS, p. A240
DOEHRING, Christopher, M.D. Vice President Medical Affairs, Franciscan St. Francis Health – Indianapolis, Indianapolis, IN, p. A204
DOELING, Mariann, R.N. Administrator, Carrington Health Center, Carrington, ND, p. A464
DOGGETT, Sherri L., Vice President Patient Services, Mercy Medical Center–Centerville, Centerville, IA, p. A216
DOHERTY, Allison, Chief Financial Officer, The NeuroMedical Center Surgical Hospital, Baton Rouge, LA, p. A263
DOHERTY, Donna, R.N. Vice President of Nursing and Chief Nursing Officer, Jordan Hospital, Plymouth, MA, p. A304
DOHERTY, Randy, Administrator, Braintree Rehabilitation Hospital, Braintree, MA, p. A298
DOHERTY, Stephen, Chief Financial Officer, Forrest City Medical Center, Forrest City, AR, p. A45
DOI, Kathy, Executive Director Human Resources, Anaheim Regional Medical Center, Anaheim, CA, p. A53
DOIDGE, John C., Vice President Finance, Glencoe Regional Health Services, Glencoe, MN, p. A332
DOKSUM, Kathryn, Director Finance, Samaritan North Lincoln Hospital, Lincoln City, OR, p. A512
DOLAN, John, Chief Financial Officer, Covenant Hospital–Levelland, Levelland, TX, p. A612
DOLAN, Margaret, Director People Services, St. Elizabeth's Hospital, Belleville, IL, p. A173
DOLAN, Patricia R., R.N. Vice President/ Chief Nursing Officer, Florida Hospital Waterman, Tavares, FL, p. A141
DOLAN, Paul, M.D. Chief Medical Affairs Officer, Benefis Hospitals, Great Falls, MT, p. A376
DOLBEE, Hilary, Vice President and Chief Financial Officer, Pratt Regional Medical Center, Pratt, KS, p. A242
DOLES, Patty, Chief Financial Officer, Muskogee Regional Medical Center, Muskogee, OK, p. A499
DOLL, Ana S., Manager Human Resources, Adventist Rehabilitation Hospital of Maryland, Rockville, MD, p. A293
DOLLINGER, Michael, Personnel Administrator, Deer's Head Hospital Center, Salisbury, MD, p. A294
DOLLINS, Gary, Director Management Information Systems, Poplar Bluff Regional Medical Center, Poplar Bluff, MO, p. A367
DOLLINS, Mandy, R.N. Chief Nursing Officer, Five Rivers Medical Center, Pocahontas, AR, p. A50
DOLOHANTY–JOHNSON, Bridget, R.N. Vice President Patient Care Services, Parkview Whitley Hospital, Columbia City, IN, p. A199
DOMANICO, Lee, Chief Executive Officer, Marin General Hospital, Greenbrae, CA, p. A64
DOMEIER, Sandy, Director Patient Care Services, Sibley Medical Center, Arlington, MN, p. A327
DOMINGO, Connie, M.D. Medical Director, Weisman Children's Rehabilitation Hospital, Marlton, NJ, p. A406
DOMINGO, Ramon, M.D. Chief of Staff, McCamey County Hospital District, McCamey, TX, p. A616
DOMINGUE, Buffy, Chief Executive Officer, Lafayette Surgical Specialty Hospital, Lafayette, LA, p. A270
DOMINGUE, Kevin, Director Human Resources and Medical Affairs, Our Lady of Lourdes Regional Medical Center, Lafayette, LA, p. A270
DOMINGUEZ, Brenda, Director Human Resources, Cypress Creek Hospital, Houston, TX, p. A604
DOMINGUEZ, Isabel, Director Human Resources and Payroll, Cornerstone Hospital of SouthEast Arizona, Tucson, AZ, p. A39
DOMINGUEZ, Jerry A., CPA Chief Financial Officer, East Texas Medical Center Trinity, Trinity, TX, p. A631
DOMINGUEZ, Marie, Commander, General Leonard Wood Army Community Hospital, Fort Leonard Wood, MO, p. A360
DOMINSKI, Michelle, Human Resources Officer, VA Butler Healthcare, Butler, PA, p. A519
DOMINSKI, Paul, Vice President Human Resources, Park Nicollet Methodist Hospital, Saint Louis Park, MN, p. A339
DOMRES, Mary Jane, Director Materials Management and Administrator Information Technology, Cavalier County Memorial Hospital, Langdon, ND, p. A467
DONAHEY, Dick, Senior Vice President Human Resources, Alamance Regional Medical Center, Burlington, NC, p. A449
DONAHEY, Kenneth C., Chief Operating Officer, Hendersonville Medical Center, Hendersonville, TN, p. A566
DONAHUE, Brian, Chief Financial Officer, Portage Health, Hancock, MI, p. A314
DONAHUE, Debra, Senior Vice President and Chief Operating Officer, Champlain Valley Physicians Hospital Medical Center, Plattsburgh, NY, p. A440
DONAHUE, Elisabeth, Associate Director Human Resources, Jeanes Hospital, Philadelphia, PA, p. A532
DONAHUE, Leslie A., President and Chief Executive Officer, Piedmont Hospital, Atlanta, GA, p. A146
DONAHUE, Moreen, R.N. Chief Nursing Executive, Danbury Hospital, Danbury, CT, p. A108
DONAHUE, Patrick, Administrator, Methodist Hospital Union County, Morganfield, KY, p. A256
DONALD, Steve, M.D. Chief of Staff, Washington County Hospital and Nursing Home, Chatom, AL, p. A18
DONALDSON, Brooke G., Assistant Administrator Human Resources, Jackson Hospital, Marianna, FL, p. A130
DONALDSON, David, Director Human Resources, Castleview Hospital, Price, UT, p. A639
DONALDSON, Les, M.D. Chief of Staff, Roosevelt General Hospital, Portales, NM, p. A417
DONALDSON, Lori, Chief Financial Officer, UC San Diego Health System, San Diego, CA, p. A86
DONALDSON, Michelle, M.D. President Medical Staff, Livingston Memorial Hospital, Livingston, MT, p. A377
DONALDSON, Sherry, Director Human Resources, Barnwell County Hospital, Barnwell, SC, p. A546
DONALDSON, Tammy, Director of Nursing, Highlands Hospital, Connellsville, PA, p. A521
DONATELLE, Lawrence, M.D. Vice President Medical Affairs, St. Elizabeth Hospital, Appleton, WI, p. A678
DONENWIRTH, Karl, Vice President Information Services, Northcoast Behavioral Healthcare System, Northfield, OH, p. A486
DONGILLI, Jr., Paul, Ph.D. Executive Vice President and Chief Operating Officer, Madonna Rehabilitation Hospital, Lincoln, NE, p. A385
DONLEY, Brian, M.D. President, Lutheran Hospital, Cleveland, OH, p. A475
DONLIN, Michael T., FACHE Administrator, Floyd Valley Hospital, Le Mars, IA, p. A222
DONNELL, Dan, M.D. Chief of Staff, Midwest Regional Medical Center, Midwest City, OK, p. A499
DONNELLY, Gloria, Director Human Resources, Euclid Hospital, Euclid, OH, p. A480
DONOVAN, James W.
President and Chief Executive Officer, Miles Memorial Hospital, Damariscotta, ME, p. A283
President and Chief Executive Officer, St. Andrews Hospital and Healthcare Center, Boothbay Harbor, ME, p. A282
DONOVAN, Jenny, Director Human Resources, Wright Memorial Hospital, Trenton, MO, p. A372
DONOVAN, Kevin, Chief Executive Officer, Mt. Ascutney Hospital and Health Center, Windsor, VT, p. A644
DONOVAN, Mary, Controller, HEALTHSOUTH Rehabilitation Institute of Tucson, Tucson, AZ, p. A40
DONOVAN, Mike, Chief Financial Officer, Lemuel Shattuck Hospital, Jamaica Plain, MA, p. A301
DONOVAN, Patrick, M.D. Director Medical Staff, HEALTHSOUTH Rehabilitation Hospital, Fort Worth, TX, p. A598
DONOVAN, Terri, Chief Executive Officer, Wheatland Memorial Healthcare, Harlowton, MT, p. A376
DONSON, Elliott, Chief Information Specialist, Lincoln Hospital, Davenport, WA, p. A660
DONZE, Richard D., D.O. Senior Vice President Medical Affairs, Chester County Hospital, West Chester, PA, p. A541
DOODY, Kris A., R.N. Chief Executive Officer, Cary Medical Center, Caribou, ME, p. A282
DOOLEY, Jerry C., Chief Executive Officer, Georgetown Community Hospital, Georgetown, KY, p. A250
DOOLEY, Lisa, Health Information Officer, Middlesboro ARH Hospital, Middlesboro, KY, p. A256
DOOLEY, Mark J., Chief Executive Officer, Andalusia Regional Hospital, Andalusia, AL, p. A15
DOOLITTLE, Jon D., President and Chief Executive Officer, Northwest Medical Center, Albany, MO, p. A355
DOPSON, James, Director Human Resources, Ennis Regional Medical Center, Ennis, TX, p. A597
DOPSON, James D., M.D. Chief Medical Staff, East Texas Medical Center–Quitman, Quitman, TX, p. A622
DORAK, John, Chief Information Officer, Nicholas H. Noyes Memorial Hospital, Dansville, NY, p. A425
DORAN, Dave, Chief Financial Officer, Pondera Medical Center, Conrad, MT, p. A374
DORAN, Dennis J., President, Cambridge Medical Center, Cambridge, MN, p. A329
DORAN, Judy, R.N. Vice President of Hospital Services and Chief Nurse Executive, Stanly Regional Medical Center, Albemarle, NC, p. A448
DORAN, Ken, Interim Chief Financial Officer, Westlake Regional Hospital, Columbia, KY, p. A248
DORF, Jeffrey, M.D. Medical Director, Kindred Hospital–Albuquerque, Albuquerque, NM, p. A414
DORIA, Eugene, Chief Information Officer, Veterans Affairs Medical Center, Coatesville, PA, p. A521
DORIS, Doug, Chief Executive Officer, Central Carolina Hospital, Sanford, NC, p. A460
DORMAN, Charles M., FACHE Director, Veterans Affairs Medical Center, Wilmington, DE, p. A115

A800 Index of Health Care Professionals 

Index of Health Care Professionals / Drummond

DORMAN III, Harry G., FACHE President and Chief Executive Officer, Alice Peck Day Memorial Hospital, Lebanon, NH, p. A398
DORNHEGGEN, David, Chief Operating Officer, Good Samaritan Hospital, Cincinnati, OH, p. A473
DORNOFF, Edward G., Associate Director, Veterans Affairs Medical Center, Battle Creek, MI, p. A308
DOROGY, Sharon, Director Health Information Management, The Children's Institute of Pittsburgh, Pittsburgh, PA, p. A535
DOROTHY, Jonnie, Senior Director Human Resources, Massena Memorial Hospital, Massena, NY, p. A429
DORR, Amy, Vice President Human Resources, McLaren Lapeer Region, Lapeer, MI, p. A317
DORRIS, Patricia, Executive Director, Medical Center of Southeastern Oklahoma, Durant, OK, p. A495
DORRIS, Ronald E., Chief Executive Officer, Carrus Hospitals, Sherman, TX, p. B26
DORRIS, Ronald E.
Chief Executive Officer, Carrus Rehabilitation Hospital, Sherman, TX, p. A627
Chief Executive Officer, Carrus Specialty Hospital, Sherman, TX, p. A627
DORSCH, Anthony, Chief Financial Officer, Providence Alaska Medical Center, Anchorage, AK, p. A28
DORSEY, Lawrence T., Administrator, University Medical Center, Lafayette, LA, p. A270
DORSEY, Michael A., FACHE Chief Executive Officer, St. Joseph Medical Center, Kansas City, MO, p. A362
DORST, Jake, Vice President and Chief Information Officer, Meritus Medical Center, Hagerstown, MD, p. A292
DORUNDO, Cynthia M., President, UPMC McKeesport, McKeesport, PA, p. A528
DOSKOCIL, Mark, Acting Director, Veterans Affairs North Texas Health Care System, Dallas, TX, p. A593
DOSS, Justin, Chief Operating Officer, Blake Medical Center, Bradenton, FL, p. A119
DOSS, Mounir F.
Executive Vice President and Chief Financial Officer, Brookdale Hospital Medical Center,, NY, p. A431
Executive Vice President and Chief Financial Officer, Flushing Hospital Medical Center,, NY, p. A432
Executive Vice President and Chief Financial Officer, Jamaica Hospital Medical Center,, NY, p. A433
DOSSEY, Emily, Director Human Resources, Hamilton General Hospital, Hamilton, TX, p. A602
DOUBLE, Ron
Chief Information Officer, Parkview Hospital, Fort Wayne, IN, p. A201
Chief Information Officer, Parkview Noble Hospital, Kendallville, IN, p. A206
DOUCETTE, Elmer, Vice President and Chief Financial Officer, Eastern Maine Medical Center, Bangor, ME, p. A281
DOUCETTE, Julia, Director Human Resources, Phoenix Baptist Hospital, Phoenix, AZ, p. A36
DOUD, Tony, Controller, St. Mary's of Michigan Standish Hospital, Standish, MI, p. A323
DOUGH, Robert, M.D. Chief of Staff, Randolph Hospital, Asheboro, NC, p. A448
DOUGHERTY, Christopher J., Chief Executive Officer, Covenant Children's Hospital, Lubbock, TX, p. A613
DOUGHERTY, David, Chief Information Management Officer, Irwin Army Community Hospital, Junction City, KS, p. A236
DOUGHERTY, James, Commander, U. S. Air Force Medical Center Keesler, Keesler AFB, MS, p. A348
DOUGHERTY, Terry, Director Human Resources, Bryn Mawr Hospital, Bryn Mawr, PA, p. A519
DOUGHTY, Cathy, Vice President Human Resources, Sheppard and Enoch Pratt Hospital, Baltimore, MD, p. A289
DOUGHTY, Stephanie
Chief Financial Officer, Medical Center of the Rockies, Loveland, CO, p. A104
Chief Financial Officer, Poudre Valley Hospital, Fort Collins, CO, p. A101
DOUGLAS, Andy, Manager Information Technology, Burnett Medical Center, Grantsburg, WI, p. A682
DOUGLAS, Bill, Senior Vice President and Chief Financial Officer, Riverside Medical Center, Kankakee, IL, p. A185
DOUGLAS, Dora, Chief Financial Officer, Summersville Regional Medical Center, Summersville, WV, p. A676
DOUGLAS, Doug, Vice President Human Resources, AnMed Health Medical Center, Anderson, SC, p. A546
DOUGLAS, Errol, Director Human Resources, University of Miami Hospital, Miami, FL, p. A132
DOUGLAS, Jason T., Chief Executive Officer, Mercy Hospital, Moose Lake, MN, p. A336
DOUGLAS, Lesia, R.N. Vice President Patient Care Services and Chief Nurse Executive, Bon Secours Baltimore Health System, Baltimore, MD, p. A287
DOUGLAS, Paul, Vice President Human Resources, Baton Rouge General Medical Center, Baton Rouge, LA, p. A262
DOUGLAS, Phillip B., Chairman and Chief Executive Officer, LifeCare Management Services, Plano, TX, p. B80
DOUGLASS, Claudia, Chief Operating Officer, Piedmont Medical Center, Rock Hill, SC, p. A553
DOUKAS, Michael, Chief of Staff, Veterans Affairs Tennessee Valley Healthcare System, Nashville, TN, p. A574
DOUVILLE, Arthur, M.D. Chief Medical Officer, Good Samaritan Hospital, San Jose, CA, p. A88
DOVEL, Melissa, Manager Human Resources, Atrium Medical Center of Corinth, Corinth, TX, p. A588
DOVER, James F., FACHE President and Chief Executive Officer, O'Connor Hospital, San Jose, CA, p. A88
DOVI, Sebastian, M.D. Interim Chief Medical Officer, Saint Michael's Medical Center, Newark, NJ, p. A407
DOW, Alan, Interim Chief Financial Officer, Southern Coos Hospital and Health Center, Bandon, OR, p. A509
DOW, Norman, Director Finance, Sheehan Memorial Hospital, Buffalo, NY, p. A
DOWDELL, Dennis, Vice President Human Resources, Memorial Sloan–Kettering Cancer Center, New York, NY, p. A434
DOWDELL, Thomas C., FACHE Senior Vice President and Chief Operating Officer, Western Maryland Regional Medical Center, Cumberland, MD, p. A291
DOWDLE, Paula, Chief Operating Officer, Jefferson Healthcare, Port Townsend, WA, p. A664
DOWELL, Wade, M.D. Chief of Staff, South Sunflower County Hospital, Indianola, MS, p. A347
DOWGUN, Richard, Chief Information Officer, St. Francis Medical Center, Trenton, NJ, p. A411
DOWLING, Deanna, R.N. Chief Nursing Officer, Texas Specialty Hospital at Wichita Falls, Wichita Falls, TX, p. A635
DOWLING, Lisa, Manager Finance, Mercy Hospital Tishomingo, Tishomingo, OK, p. A505
DOWLING, Michael J., President and Chief Executive Officer, North Shore–Long Island Jewish Health System, Great Neck, NY, p. B95
DOWN, Melanie Falls, Site Manager, Crow/Northern Cheyenne Hospital, Crow Agency, MT, p. A374
DOWN, Philip B., President and Chief Executive Officer, Doctors Community Hospital, Lanham, MD, p. A292
DOWNEY, Brandon, Chief Operating Officer, Crossgates River Oaks Hospital, Brandon, MS, p. A344
DOWNEY, Daniel, Chief Fiscal Service, Veterans Administration New York Harbor Healthcare System,, NY, p. A437
DOWNEY, Patti L., Vice President, Human Resources, Liberty Hospital, Liberty, MO, p. A364
DOWNEY, Robert, Chief Financial Officer, Marshalltown Medical & Surgical Center, Marshalltown, IA, p. A223
DOWNEY, Susan, Chief Executive Officer, Kindred Hospital–Boston, Brighton, MA, p. A298
DOWNEY, William B., Chief Operating Officer, Riverside Behavioral Health Center, Hampton, VA, p. A649
DOWNEY, William B., President and Chief Executive Officer, Riverside Health System, Newport News, VA, p. B110
DOWNEY, William B.
Chief Operating Officer, Riverside Regional Medical Center, Newport News, VA, p. A652
President and Chief Executive Officer, Riverside Rehabilitation Institute, Newport News, VA, p. A652
DOWNING, David, M.D. Chief Medical Officer, Fort Defiance Indian Health Service Hospital, Fort Defiance, AZ, p. A32
DOWNS, Bryan, Director Information Systems, Central Peninsula General Hospital, Soldotna, AK, p. A30
DOWNS, Connie, Chief Financial Officer, Pennock Hospital, Hastings, MI, p. A315
DOWNS, Nancy, M.D. Vice President Medical Affairs, Memorial Hospital at Gulfport, Gulfport, MS, p. A346
DOWNS, Patricia, Director Human Resources, Northern Nevada Medical Center, Sparks, NV, p. A396
DOWNS, Sue, MSN, President, Flaget Memorial Hospital, Bardstown, KY, p. A247
DOXTATOR, Rick, Chief Financial Officer, Christus St. Vincent Regional Medical Center, Santa Fe, NM, p. A418
DOYEL, Brenda K., Chief Financial Officer, Sayre Memorial Hospital, Sayre, OK, p. A504
DOYLE, Barbara J., MS, Senior Vice President and Chief Executive Officer, Inova Mount Vernon Hospital, Alexandria, VA, p. A645
DOYLE, Dennis, Commanding Officer, William Beaumont Army Medical Center, El Paso, TX, p. A597
DOYLE, James F., Senior Vice President Finance and Chief Financial Officer, Elmhurst Memorial Hospital,, IL, p. A181
DOYLE, Jay, Chief Financial Officer, St. James Healthcare, Butte, MT, p. A374
DOYLE, John
Vice President Finance, Paoli Hospital, Paoli, PA, p. A531
Chief Financial Officer, Wenatchee Valley Hospital, Wenatchee, WA, p. A669
Assistant Vice President and Chief Financial Officer, Woodridge Hospital, Johnson City, TN, p. A568
DOYLE, Mark
Chief Financial Officer, Broward Health Medical Center, Fort Lauderdale, FL, p. A123
Chief Financial Officer, St. Vincent's Medical Center Riverside, Jacksonville, FL, p. A127
Chief Financial Officer, St. Vincent's Medical Center Southside, Jacksonville, FL, p. A127
DOYLE, Michael, M.D. Deputy Commander Clinical Services, Keller Army Community Hospital, West Point, NY, p. A446
DOYLE, Patricia S., R.N. Chief Nursing Officer, Regional Medical Center, Manchester, IA, p. A222
DOZIER, Carol, Chief Executive Officer, Ivinson Memorial Hospital, Laramie, WY, p. A696
DRABANT, Leah, Director of Finance, Complex Care Hospital at Ridgelake, Sarasota, FL, p. A138
DRAEHN, Donald, M.D. Chief of Staff, Scott & White Hospital – Brenham, Brenham, TX, p. A585
DRAGO, Susan, R.N. Chief Clinical Officer, Kindred Hospital North Florida, Green Cove Springs, FL, p. A124
DRAGOLOVIC, Goran, Chief Executive Officer, Barix Clinics of Ohio, Groveport, OH, p. A481
DRAIME, D. Eric, Vice President and Chief Financial Officer, Galion Community Hospital, Galion, OH, p. A480
DRAKE, Dan, VP, Patient Care Services, Albemarle Health, Elizabeth City, NC, p. A452
DRAPAL, Cindy, Interim Chief Executive Officer, George E. Weems Memorial Hospital, Apalachicola, FL, p. A118
DRAPER, Andy, Director Information Systems, TIRR Memorial Hermann, Houston, TX, p. A607
DRAPER, Vivian, Chief Financial Officer, U. S. Public Health Service Indian Hospital–Sells, Sells, AZ, p. A38
DRAYTON, Renee, Chief Human Resources, Prattville Baptist Hospital, Prattville, AL, p. A25
DREGNEY, Jim, Chief Financial Officer, Lakewood Health System, Staples, MN, p. A340
DREHER, Ronald, Finance Officer, Robert J. Dole Veterans Affairs Medical Center, Wichita, KS, p. A245
DREUSSI, Rob, Interim Director Information Systems, Ponca City Medical Center, Ponca City, OK, p. A503
DREW, Jeff, Fiscal Officer, Aleda E. Lutz Veterans Affairs Medical Center, Saginaw, MI, p. A322
DREW, Jim, Chief Information Officer, Baptist Hospital, Nashville, TN, p. A573
DREWETTE, Frederick J., Chief Financial Officer, Anaheim Regional Medical Center, Anaheim, CA, p. A53
DREXLER, Diane, R.N
Chief Nursing Officer, Yavapai Regional Medical Center – East, Prescott Valley, AZ, p. A37
Chief Nursing Officer, Yavapai Regional Medical Center, Prescott, AZ, p. A37
DRIFTMIER, Tammie, Director Human Resources, Clarinda Regional Health Center, Clarinda, IA, p. A216
DRIGGERS, Steve, M.D. Chief Medical Officer, Holy Family Memorial Medical Center, Manitowoc, WI, p. A685
DRINKWATER, Kenneth, Director Human Resources, Texas Health Harris Methodist Hospital Southlake, Southlake, TX, p. A628
DRINKWATER, Linda, Chief Financial Officer, Waldo County General Hospital, Belfast, ME, p. A281
DRINKWITZ, Jeremy, Chief Operating Officer, Sparks Regional Medical Center, Fort Smith, AR, p. A45
DRISCOLL, Angie, Director Human Resources, Los Alamitos Medical Center, Los Alamitos, CA, p. A68
DRISCOLL, Ann–Marie E., Director Human Resources, Saints Medical Center, Lowell, MA, p. A301
DRISCOLL, Nancy, R.N. Chief Nursing Officer, Longmont United Hospital, Longmont, CO, p. A104
DROBIL, Frank, Director Human Resources, McCurtain Memorial Hospital, Idabel, OK, p. A498
DROBOT, Michael D., Chief Executive Officer, Pacific Hospital of Long Beach, Long Beach, CA, p. A68
DROEGE, Marie T., President, Robert Packer Hospital, Sayre, PA, p. A537
DRONE, Marilyn, R.N. Vice President, CNO, St. Mary Medical Center, Apple Valley, CA, p. A54
DROPPERS, Larry, Chief Financial Officer, Walter Knox Memorial Hospital, Emmett, ID, p. A168
DROTTS, Jennifer, Manager Human Resources, Bigfork Valley Hospital, Bigfork, MN, p. A328
DROUILLARD, Jeanne, R.N. Chief Nursing Officer, Palmetto General Hospital, Hialeah, FL, p. A125
DROZD, Carol, Chief Operating Officer, St. Mark's Medical Center, La Grange, TX, p. A611
DRUCKENMILLER, Carol, R.N. Assistant Administrator and Chief Nursing Officer, University of South Alabama Children's and Women's Hospital, Mobile, AL, p. A23
DRUCKER, Steven C., President and Chief Executive Officer, Loretto Hospital, Chicago, IL, p. A176
DRUMMOND, Armand, Manager Human Resources, South Lincoln Medical Center, Kemmerer, WY, p. A696



Index of Health Care Professionals

Index of Health Care Professionals / Drummond


DRUMMOND, Michael, Chief Financial Officer, Runnells Specialized Hospital of Union County, Berkeley Heights, NJ, p. A401
DRUMWRIGHT, Douglas, Chief Executive Officer, Parkview Community Hospital Medical Center, Riverside, CA, p. A82
DRUMWRIGHT, Mary, Director Human Resources, Person Memorial Hospital, Roxboro, NC, p. A460
DRVARIC, David M., M.D. Chief of Staff, Shriners Hospitals for Children, Springfield, Springfield, MA, p. A305
DRY, Laurence, Vice President, Support and Ambulatory Services, Provena Saint Joseph Hospital, Elgin, IL, p. A181
DRYBURGH, Louise, Chief Executive Officer, First Care Health Center, Park River, ND, p. A468
DRYER, Len, Chief Financial Officer, Children's Hospital Colorado, Aurora, CO, p. A97
DRYMON, Lisa, Manager, Fairfax Community Hospital, Fairfax, OK, p. A496
DRZEWIECKI–BURGER, Mary Jo, Administrative Manager, Caro Center, Caro, MI, p. A308
DU PONT, Karen, Director Human Resources, Casa Colina Hospital for Rehabilitative Medicine, Pomona, CA, p. A80
DU RALL, Marty, Executive Director Human Resources, St. Vincent Indianapolis Hospital, Indianapolis, IN, p. A205
DUANE, Paul K.
Executive Vice President and Chief Financial Officer, Palmetto Health Baptist, Columbia, SC, p. A548
Executive Vice President and Chief Financial Officer, Palmetto Health Richland, Columbia, SC, p. A548
DUBE, Cynthia, M.D. Medical Director, Mayo Clinic Health System in Austin, Austin, MN, p. A328
DUBE, Sheri, Chief Operating Officer, St. David's North Austin Medical Center, Austin, TX, p. A581
DUBEN, Julie, Chief Clinical Officer, Kindred Hospital Northland, Kansas City, MO, p. A362
DUBICKI, Robert, Executive Vice President and Chief Operating Officer, Kingsbrook Jewish Medical Center,, NY, p. A433
DUBIS, John S., FACH
President and Chief Executive Officer, St. Elizabeth Edgewood, Edgewood, KY, p. A249
President and Chief Executive Officer, St. Elizabeth Edgewood, Edgewood, KY, p. A249
DUBIS, John S., FACHE President and Chief Executive Officer, St. Elizabeth Healthcare, Edgewood, KY, p. B122
DUBOIS, Brady, Interim Chief Executive Officer, Northern Louisiana Medical Center, Ruston, LA, p. A276
DUBOIS, Randy, Chief Executive Officer, Cushing Regional Hospital, Cushing, OK, p. A495
DUBOIS, Robbye N., Chief Executive Officer, Ethicus Hospital – Grapevine, Grapevine, TX, p. A601
DUBOSE, Alta, Chief Financial Officer, Marion Regional Hospital, Mullins, SC, p. A552
DUBROCA, Darryl S.
Chief Executive Officer and Managing Director, Spring Mountain Sahara, Las Vegas, NV, p. A393
Chief Executive Officer and Managing Director, Spring Mountain Treatment Center, Las Vegas, NV, p. A393
DUBROW, Melissa, Interim Administrative Officer, Waynesboro Hospital, Waynesboro, PA, p. A540
DUBRUL, Bill, Director Information Technology, St. Anthony's Hospital, Houston, TX, p. A606
DUBRUYNE, Sharon, Director Human Resources, College Hospital Costa Mesa, Costa Mesa, CA, p. A58
DUCEY, Ann, Chief Information Officer, Boys Town National Research Hospital, Omaha, NE, p. A387
DUCHAK, Douglas A., President and Chief Executive Officer, Englewood Hospital and Medical Center, Englewood, NJ, p. A404
DUCHARME, Maria, R.N. Interim Chief Nursing Officer, Miriam Hospital, Providence, RI, p. A544
DUCHEMIN, MaDena
Chief Human Resources Officer, Adirondack Medical Center, Saranac Lake, NY, p. A442
Assistant Administrator Human Resources, John Randolph Medical Center, Hopewell, VA, p. A649
DUCHENE, Pam, R.N. Vice President Patient Care Services, St. Joseph Hospital, Nashua, NH, p. A399
DUCHESNEAU, Angy, Senior Director Human Resources, Lakeview Hospital, Stillwater, MN, p. A340
DUCKOR, Steven, M.D. Chief of Staff, Chapman Medical Center, Orange, CA, p. A78
DUCKWORTH, Allison, Chief Operating Officer and Chief Nursing Officer, FirstHealth Richmond Memorial Hospital, Rockingham, NC, p. A459
DUCKWORTH, Bob, Director Information Systems, Medical West, Bessemer, AL, p. A16
DUCRO, Tom, Chief Financial Officer, UC Health Surgical Hospital, West Chester, OH, p. A491
DUDA, David, Senior Vice President and Chief Operating Officer, Riverside Medical Center, Kankakee, IL, p. A185
DUDA, Faye, R.N. Chief Nursing Officer, Long Beach Medical Center, Long Beach, NY, p. A429
DUDA, Thomas J., Chief Financial Officer, Hi–Desert Medical Center, Joshua Tree, CA, p. A65
DUDEK, Gerald, M.D. Chief of Staff, Mercy Hospital Cadillac, Cadillac, MI, p. A308
DUDLEY, III, Edward L., Senior Vice President and Chief Financial Officer, Catholic Medical Center, Manchester, NH, p. A399
DUDLEY, Kayleen, Interim Chief Executive Officer, Gothenburg Memorial Hospital, Gothenburg, NE, p. A384
DUES, Craig, D.O. Chief Medical Officer, Mercer County Joint Township Community Hospital, Coldwater, OH, p. A476
DUET, Angela, Director Information Technology, St. Charles Parish Hospital, Luling, LA, p. A272
DUETSCH, Stephen, Vice President Operations and Support, Spencer Hospital, Spencer, IA, p. A227
DUFF, Isabel, MS, Director, Veterans Affairs Long Beach Healthcare System, Long Beach, CA, p. A68
DUFF, James, Chief Executive Officer, Brentwood Hospital, Shreveport, LA, p. A277
DUFF, Jim, Chief Financial Officer, Colorado Mental Health Institute at Pueblo, Pueblo, CO, p. A105
DUFF, Mary Claire, CPA Chief Financial Officer, Ridgeview Psychiatric Hospital and Center, Oak Ridge, TN, p. A574
DUFFEE, Patrick, Director Medical Information Systems, Delta Medical Center, Memphis, TN, p. A571
DUFFEY, Victoria, Director of Nursing, Citizens Medical Center, Colby, KS, p. A231
DUFFIELD, Douglas, President and Chief Executive Officer, Florida Hospital Zephyrhills, Zephyrhills, FL, p. A143
DUFFIN, Kelly L., Operations Officer, Intermountain Medical Center, Murray, UT, p. A638
DUFFORD, Shawn, M.D. Vice President Medical Affairs and Chief Medical Officer, Exempla Saint Joseph Hospital, Denver, CO, p. A99
DUFFY, Daniel, D.O. Chief Medical Director, HealthSource Saginaw, Saginaw, MI, p. A322
DUFFY, Karen, R.N. Director Patient Care Services, BayCare Alliant Hospital, Dunedin, FL, p. A122
DUFFY, Kenneth, M.D. Medical Director, Seiling Community Hospital, Seiling, OK, p. A504
DUFFY, Mary Elizabeth, Senior Vice President and Chief Financial Officer, St. Luke's Cornwall Hospital, Newburgh, NY, p. A438
DUFFY, Pamela
Vice President Patient Care Services and Chief Nursing Officer, Kishwaukee Community Hospital, DeKalb, IL, p. A180
Vice President Patient Services and CNO, Valley West Community Hospital, Sandwich, IL, p. A193
DUFOUR, Lonnie L., Chief Operating Officer, Chief Information Officer and Director Human Resources, Bunkie General Hospital, Bunkie, LA, p. A264
DUGAL, John Charles, M.D. Medical Director, Community Specialty Hospital, Lafayette, LA, p. A270
DUGAN, Gary, M.D. Vice President Medical Affairs, DuBois Regional Medical Center, Du Bois, PA, p. A522
DUGAN, Margaret R., Executive Director, Greater Binghamton Health Center, Binghamton, NY, p. A421
DUGGAN, David, M.D. Medical Director, Upstate University Hospital, Syracuse, NY, p. A444
DUGGAN, Eileen, M.D. Medical Director, Crittenton Children's Center, Kansas City, MO, p. A361
DUGGAN, James E., Director Human Resources, Western Massachusetts Hospital, Westfield, MA, p. A306
DUGGAN, Michael, Chief Executive Officer, Detroit Medical Center, Detroit, MI, p. B46
DUGGAN, Tonya, Director Human Resources, Northern Louisiana Medical Center, Ruston, LA, p. A276
DUGGER, Sandy, Director Human Resources, Community Hospital, Torrington, WY, p. A698
DUHAIME, Robert A., R.N. Vice President–Operations/Chief Nurse Executive, Catholic Medical Center, Manchester, NH, p. A399
DUHE, Louis, Senior Director Information Technology, George Washington University Hospital, Washington, DC, p. A116
DUHON, Neal J., M.D. Chief of Staff, American Legion Hospital, Crowley, LA, p. A265
DUHON, Susan, Director Medical Records, St. James Parish Hospital, Lutcher, LA, p. A272
DUHON, Thomas, Director Human Resources, Heart Hospital of Lafayette, Lafayette, LA, p. A270
DUJON–REYNOLDS, Frances, Director Human Resources, Winnebago Mental Health Institute, Winnebago, WI, p. A694
DUKE, Deirdre J., Associate Executive Director Human Resources, North Shore University Hospital, Manhasset, NY, p. A429
DUKE, Gail R., Director Human Resources, Clarendon Memorial Hospital, Manning, SC, p. A552
DUKE, II, Lee M., M.D. Senior Vice President and Chief Physician Executive, Lancaster General Health, Lancaster, PA, p. A526
DUKE, Scott A., Chief Executive Officer, Glendive Medical Center, Glendive, MT, p. A375
DUKOFF, Ruth, M.D. Medical Director, North Star Behavioral Health System, Anchorage, AK, p. A28
DULBERGER, Philip M., M.D. Chief Executive Officer, IU Health Saxony Hospital, Fishers, IN, p. A
DUMONSEAU, Kent, Chief Financial Officer, Riverwood Healthcare Center, Aitkin, MN, p. A327
DUMONT, Rene, CIO/ Vice President Strategic Growth, St. Mary's Regional Medical Center, Lewiston, ME, p. A284
DUMSHA, Eileen, Manager Employee Relations, Weisman Children's Rehabilitation Hospital, Marlton, NJ, p. A406
DUNAWAY, James, Director Information Management, Mississippi State Hospital, Whitfield, MS, p. A354
DUNCAN, Charles, M.D. Medical Director, Kindred Hospital–San Antonio, San Antonio, TX, p. A625
DUNCAN, Cindy
Chief Operating Officer, Memorial Hospital and Physician Group, Frederick, OK, p. A497
Director Human Resources, Roosevelt General Hospital, Portales, NM, p. A417
DUNCAN, Darryl L., President and Chief Executive Officer, Monongalia General Hospital, Morgantown, WV, p. A674
DUNCAN, J. D., Director Human Resources, Pondera Medical Center, Conrad, MT, p. A374
DUNCAN, Jeremy, Director Information Systems, Lawrence Medical Center, Moulton, AL, p. A24
DUNCAN, Jimmy, Chief Human Resource Officer, North Colorado Medical Center, Greeley, CO, p. A102
DUNCAN, Lawrence, Chief Executive Officer, El Paso Children's Hospital, El Paso, TX, p. A596
DUNCAN, Lucinda, Chief Human Resources, Bayne–Jones Army Community Hospital, Fort Polk, LA, p. A266
DUNCAN, Lyman, Chief Financial Officer, San Juan Hospital, Monticello, UT, p. A638
DUNCAN, Michael J., System Chief Executive Officer, Chester County Hospital, West Chester, PA, p. A541
DUNCAN, Neal, Chief Executive Officer, Carson Tahoe Continuing Care Hospital, Carson City, NV, p. A391
DUNFORD, Ben, Chief Financial Officer, Texas Regional Medical Center, Sunnyvale, TX, p. A629
DUNFORD, Bill, Manager, Northside Hospital – Cherokee, Canton, GA, p. A148
DUNGAN, Janice L., Sr Vice President Clinical Services, Lake Regional Health System, Osage Beach, MO, p. A366
DUNHAM, David S., President, Mercy Medical Center Merced, Merced, CA, p. A74
DUNHAM, Shelly, R.N. Chief Executive Officer, Okeene Municipal Hospital, Okeene, OK, p. A500
DUNKER, Karla, Director Finance, Sedgwick County Health Center, Julesburg, CO, p. A102
DUNKIEL, Barbara, Director Human Resources, HEALTHSOUTH Sunrise Rehabilitation Hospital, Fort Lauderdale, FL, p. A123
DUNKIN, Jackie J., Director Human Resources, Platte Valley Medical Center, Brighton, CO, p. A98
DUNLAP, Mary Lou, Correctional Health Services Administrator, California Medical Facility, Vacaville, CA, p. A94
DUNLAY, Robert, M.D. Chief Medical Officer, Creighton University Medical Center, Omaha, NE, p. A387
DUNLOP, Jr., James H., CP
Senior Vice President and Chief Financial Officer, Kenmore Mercy Hospital, Kenmore, NY, p. A428
Senior Vice President Finance and Chief Financial Officer, Mercy Hospital, Buffalo, NY, p. A423
Chief Financial Officer, Sisters of Charity Hospital of Buffalo, Buffalo, NY, p. A423
DUNMAN, Robyn, Coordinator Human Resources, Kindred Hospital–Nashville, Nashville, TN, p. A573
DUNN, Adele, Director Human Resources, Larned State Hospital, Larned, KS, p. A237
DUNN, Audrey L., Director Human Resources, Hancock Medical Center, Bay Saint Louis, MS, p. A343
DUNN, Christopher, M.D. Vice President Medical Affairs, Sequoia Hospital, Redwood City, CA, p. A82
DUNN, Connie, Director Human Resources, Livingston Memorial Hospital, Livingston, MT, p. A377
DUNN, Daniel N., Vice President Operations, Wentworth–Douglass Hospital, Dover, NH, p. A397
DUNN, E. D., Vice President Human Resources, Virtua Memorial, Mount Holly, NJ, p. A406
DUNN, George, M.D. Senior Vice President Medical Affairs, Glen Cove Hospital, Glen Cove, NY, p. A426
DUNN, Jeffrey, Chief Executive Officer, North Georgia Medical Center, Ellijay, GA, p. A152
DUNN, Kim, Attorney–at–Law, Cordova Community Medical Center, Cordova, AK, p. A28


A802 Index of Health Care Professionals 

Index of Health Care Professionals / Easton

Index of Health Care Professionals

DUNN, Leonard, M.D. Chief Medical Officer, BayCare Alliant Hospital, Dunedin, FL, p. A122
DUNN, Marcy
Vice President Information Services and Chief Information Officer, Good Samaritan Hospital Medical Center, West Islip, NY, p. A446
Vice President Information Services and Chief Information Officer, Mercy Medical Center, Rockville Centre, NY, p. A442
Vice President Information Services and Chief Information Officer, St. Francis Hospital, Roslyn, NY, p. A442
DUNN, Margie, Director Human Resources, Middle Tennessee Mental Health Institute, Nashville, TN, p. A573
DUNN, Patrick A., R.N. Chief Nursing Officer, Lea Regional Medical Center, Hobbs, NM, p. A416
DUNN, Shawn, M.D. Medical Director, The NeuroMedical Center Surgical Hospital, Baton Rouge, LA, p. A263
DUNN, Sheila, Assistant Administrator Human Resources, Dale Medical Center, Ozark, AL, p. A24
DUNN, Terry, Director Information Technology, Battle Mountain General Hospital, Battle Mountain, NV, p. A391
DUNNE, Elizabeth, Chief Executive Officer, Providence Little Company of Mary Medical Center, Torrance, CA, p. A92
DUNNE, Penny, R.N. Director Human Resources, Samaritan Pacific Communities Hospital, Newport, OR, p. A513
DUNNING, David, Commander, Bayne–Jones Army Community Hospital, Fort Polk, LA, p. A266
DUNNING, Shane, Administrator, Carnegie Tri–County Municipal Hospital, Carnegie, OK, p. A494
DUNWOODY, Robert, Chief Financial Officer, Lawnwood Regional Medical Center, Fort Pierce, FL, p. A124
DUPLESSIS, Andre, Chief Operating Officer, Tulane–Lakeside Hospital, Metairie, LA, p. A273
DUPPER, Harold, Chief Financial Officer, Platte Valley Medical Center, Brighton, CO, p. A98
DUPPER, Larry L., Chief Financial Officer, Valley View Hospital, Glenwood Springs, CO, p. A101
DUPRE', Charlotte W., Chief Executive Officer, Central Mississippi Medical Center, Jackson, MS, p. A347
DUPREE, Lucy G., Director Human Resources, District One Hospital, Faribault, MN, p. A331
DUPREY, Irma, Administrator Medical Records, Hospital Universitario Dr. Ramon Ruiz Arnau, Bayamon, PR, p. A700
DUPUIS, Pamela M., R.N. Senior Vice President and Patient Care Services, Sound Shore Medical Center of Westchester, New Rochelle, NY, p. A431
DUQUE, Cynthia, R.N. Chief Operating Officer, Promise Hospital of East Los Angeles, Suburban Medical Center Campus, Paramount, CA, p. A79
DUQUETTE, Bill, Chief Executive Officer, Baptist Health South Florida, Homestead Hospital, Homestead, FL, p. A125
DUQUETTE, Connie, Director Human Resources, Sharp Memorial Hospital, San Diego, CA, p. A86
DURAKIEWICZ, Marek, M.D. Chief of Staff, Hickman Community Hospital, Centerville, TN, p. A563
DURBAK, Ivan, Chief Information Officer, Bronx–Lebanon Hospital Center Health Care System,, NY, p. A431
DURDEN, Rhonda, Chief Financial Officer, Emanuel Medical Center, Swainsboro, GA, p. A160
DURHAM, Bill, M.D. Chief Medical Officer, Oak Tree Hospital, Corbin, KY, p. A249
DURHAM, Josh, D.O. Chief of Staff, Clara Barton Hospital, Hoisington, KS, p. A234
DURHAM, Leslie, Vice President Information Systems, Bethesda Memorial Hospital, Boynton Beach, FL, p. A119
DURHAM, Linda, Director Human Resources, McNairy Regional Hospital, Selmer, TN, p. A575
DURHAM, Randy, Director Personnel, Memphis Mental Health Institute, Memphis, TN, p. A571
DURKIN, Patrick, Vice President Professional Services, Westlake Hospital, Melrose Park, IL, p. A187
DURNEY, Gerry, Chief Operating Officer, Good Samaritan Hospital, Suffern, NY, p. A444
DUROVICH, Christopher J., President and Chief Executive Officer, Children's Medical Center of Dallas, Dallas, TX, p. A590
DURR, Durinda, Vice President and Chief Nursing Officer, Rome Memorial Hospital, Rome, NY, p. A442
DURR, Jana, Director Human Resources, North Star Behavioral Health System, Anchorage, AK, p. A28
DURR, Michele, M.D. Medical Director, Webster County Community Hospital, Red Cloud, NE, p. A389
DURRENCE, Elizabeth, Chief Operating Officer, Kendall Regional Medical Center, Miami, FL, p. A131
DURST, Geoff, Vice President Finance, Avera St. Luke's Hospital, Aberdeen, SD, p. A555
DURST, Jennifer, Director Information Services, Washington County Hospital and Clinics, Washington, IA, p. A227
DURST, Sue, R.N. Vice President Plant Operations, McLaren Macomb, Mount Clemens, MI, p. A319
DURSTELER, Courtney, Chief Human Resources Officer, Franklin County Medical Center, Preston, ID, p. A170
DUSENBERY, Jack, President and Chief Executive Officer, Covenant Medical Center, Waterloo, IA, p. A228
DUTCHER, Phillip C., Chief Operating Officer, NCH Downtown Naples Hospital, Naples, FL, p. A133
DUTHE, Robert J., Vice President Corporate Management Information Systems, Albany Memorial Hospital, Albany, NY, p. A420
DUTLA, Nimal, M.D. Chief Medical Staff, Holzer Medical Center – Jackson, Jackson, OH, p. A482
DUTMERS, David, Team Leader Information and Technology Management, Spectrum Health United Hospital, Greenville, MI, p. A314
DUTTON, Angela, Chief Human Resources Management Service, Veterans Affairs Medical Center–Louisville, Louisville, KY, p. A255
DUTTON, Rebecca, Director Human Resources, Larue D. Carter Memorial Hospital, Indianapolis, IN, p. A204
DUVAL, John, Chief Executive Officer, VCU Health System, Richmond, VA, p. A655
DUVAL, Rob, Chief Human Resources Officer, Emma Pendleton Bradley Hospital, East Providence, RI, p. A544
DUVALL, Gary, Chief Information Resource Management, Jack C. Montgomery Veterans Affairs Medical Center, Muskogee, OK, p. A499
DUVALL, Richard, Director Support Services and Chief Operating Officer, Carthage Area Hospital, Carthage, NY, p. A424
DUVALL, Wendy, Chief Financial Officer, Barton County Memorial Hospital, Lamar, MO, p. A363
DVORAK, Robert M., Interim Chief Financial Officer, Salinas Valley Memorial Healthcare System, Salinas, CA, p. A84
DWIGHT, Kara, Chief of Staff, Down East Community Hospital, Machias, ME, p. A284
DWORKIN, Darren, Senior Vice President and Chief Information Officer, Cedars–Sinai Medical Center, Los Angeles, CA, p. A69
DWORKIN, Jack H., M.D. Vice President Medical Affairs and Chief Medical Officer, CentraState Healthcare System, Freehold, NJ, p. A404
DWORKIN, Paul, M.D. Physician–in–Chief, Connecticut Children's Medical Center, Hartford, CT, p. A109
DWOZAN, C. Richard, Chief Executive Officer, Habersham Medical Center, Demorest, GA, p. A151
DWYER, Cathy, Senior Administrator Information Systems, Burke Rehabilitation Hospital, White Plains, NY, p. A447
DWYER, James P., D.O
Chief Medical Officer, Virtua Marlton, Marlton, NJ, p. A406
Executive Vice President and Chief Medical Officer, Virtua Memorial, Mount Holly, NJ, p. A406
Executive Vice President and Chief Medical Officer, Virtua Voorhees, Voorhees, NJ, p. A412
DWYER, Nancy, Vice President Human Resources, Eastside Medical Center, Snellville, GA, p. A159
DWYER, William, Vice President Human Resources, Children's Specialized Hospital, New Brunswick, NJ, p. A406
DYBVIG, Rob, M.D. Chief Medical Officer, Osceola Medical Center, Osceola, WI, p. A688
DYCHE, Ginny, Director Community Relations, Aspen Valley Hospital District, Aspen, CO, p. A97
DYCUS, Steve, Director Marketing and Public Relations, Williamson Medical Center, Franklin, TN, p. A565
DYE, Blake A., President, St. Vincent Heart Center of Indiana, Indianapolis, IN, p. A205
DYE, Chris, Director Information Systems, Saint Joseph – Martin, Martin, KY, p. A256
DYER, Dave, Vice President and Chief Information Officer, Somerset Medical Center, Somerville, NJ, p. A410
DYER, Herb, Chief Executive Officer and Chief Operating Officer, Seton Medical Center Hays, Kyle, TX, p. A611
DYER, Kathleen
Vice President and Chief Information Officer, Adventist Behavioral Health Rockville, Rockville, MD, p. A293
Vice President and Chief Information Officer, Shady Grove Adventist Hospital, Rockville, MD, p. A294
DYER, Rebecca T., Administrator, Union General Hospital, Blairsville, GA, p. A147
DYESS, Lance K., M.D. Chief Medical Officer, Elba General Hospital, Elba, AL, p. A19
DYKE, Donna, Human Resources Officer, Kearney County Health Services, Minden, NE, p. A386
DYKEHOUSE, Rodney
Vice President Information Services, Oconomowoc Memorial Hospital, Oconomowoc, WI, p. A688
Senior Vice President Information Services, Waukesha Memorial Hospital, Waukesha, WI, p. A692
DYKES, Bradford W., President and Chief Executive Officer, Indiana University Health Bedford Hospital, Bedford, IN, p. A197
DYKES, Jennifer, Director Human Resources, Russell County Hospital, Russell Springs, KY, p. A258
DYKES, Nichole, Chief Financial Officer and Controller, HEALTHSOUTH Rehabilitation Hospital Midland–Odessa, Midland, TX, p. A616
DYKSTERHOUSE, Trevor J., President, Forest Health Medical Center, Ypsilanti, MI, p. A326
DYKSTRA, Janet H., Chief Executive Officer, Osceola Community Hospital, Sibley, IA, p. A226
DYRKACZ, Anna, Chief Financial Officer, Kindred Hospital Park View, Springfield, MA, p. A304
DZAU, Victor J., M.D. President and Chief Executive Officer, Duke University Health System, Durham, NC, p. B48
DZIEDZICKI, Ron, R.N. Chief Support Services Officer, University Hospitals Case Medical Center, Cleveland, OH, p. A476
DZIESINSKI, Ray R., Senior Vice President and Chief Financial Officer, Children's Medical Center of Dallas, Dallas, TX, p. A590

# E

EADIE, Reginald J., M.D
Vice President Medical Affairs, Harper University Hospital/Hutzel Women's Hospital, Detroit, MI, p. A310
President, Sinai–Grace Hospital, Detroit, MI, p. A311
EADY, Bruce, Chief Executive Officer, Howard A. Rusk Rehabilitation Center, Columbia, MO, p. A358
EAGEN, Mary K., R.N. Executive Vice President, Chief Nursing Officer, Parkland Health & Hospital System, Dallas, TX, p. A592
EAGER, David, Senior Vice President, Chief Financial Officer, Legacy Meridian Park Hospital, Tualatin, OR, p. A516
EAGERTON, Gregory S., Ph.D. Associate Director for Patient Care Services/Nurse Executive, Veterans Affairs Medical Center, Birmingham, AL, p. A17
EAGLEHOUSE, Louis, Site Director and Chief Information Officer, The Good Samaritan Hospital, Lebanon, PA, p. A527
EAKLE, Phyllis, Chief Financial Officer, Epic Medical Center, Eufaula, OK, p. A496
EAKS, C. Alan, Chief Executive Officer, Aurora Chicago Lakeshore Hospital, Chicago, IL, p. A175
EARDLEY, John, Chief Financial Officer, Twin Valley Behavioral Healthcare, Columbus, OH, p. A477
EARL, Anna, M.D. Chief of Staff, Liberty Medical Center, Chester, MT, p. A374
EARL, Mindy, Health Information Manager, Power County Hospital District, American Falls, ID, p. A166
EARLE, Audra, Chief Executive Officer, Watsonville Community Hospital, Watsonville, CA, p. A95
EARLE, Cletis, Vice President and Chief Information Officer, Wyckoff Heights Medical Center,, NY, p. A438
EARLEY, Robert, President and Chief Executive Officer, JPS Health Network, Fort Worth, TX, p. A599
EARLS, Sandra, Chief Financial Officer, Coalinga Regional Medical Center, Coalinga, CA, p. A58
EARLY, Elfie, Manager Data Services, Georgia Regional Hospital at Atlanta, Decatur, GA, p. A151
EARLY, Tom, Chief Financial Officer, Woodward Regional Hospital, Woodward, OK, p. A508
EARNSHAW, Dallas, Chief Executive Officer, Utah State Hospital, Provo, UT, p. A640
EASLEY, Marsha A., Chief Operating Officer, Orange Park Medical Center, Orange Park, FL, p. A134
EASON, Laurence, M.D. Chief Medical Officer, Providence Little Company of Mary Medical Center, Torrance, CA, p. A92
EASON, William, M.D. Medical Director, HEALTHSOUTH Cane Creek Rehabilitation Hospital, Martin, TN, p. A570
EASON SMEDLEY, Jessie, Chief Executive Officer, South Texas Rehabilitation Hospital, Brownsville, TX, p. A585
EASTBURG, Mark C., Ph.D. President and Chief Executive Officer, Pine Rest Christian Mental Health Services, Grand Rapids, MI, p. A313
EASTER, Thomas, M.D. President Medical Staff, San Antonio Community Hospital, Upland, CA, p. A94
EASTERWOOD, Diane J., Human Resources Business Partner, San Francisco Medical Center, San Francisco, CA, p. A87
EASTMAN, Brent, M.D
Chief Medical Officer, Scripps Green Hospital, La Jolla, CA, p. A65
Chief Medical Officer, Scripps Memorial Hospital–La Jolla, La Jolla, CA, p. A66
EASTMAN, David, Site Director, Ukiah Valley Medical Center, Ukiah, CA, p. A93
EASTMAN, Joseph F., Director Human Resources, Central Carolina Hospital, Sanford, NC, p. A460
EASTON, Laura J., R.N. President and Chief Executive Officer, Caldwell Memorial Hospital, Lenoir, NC, p. A456

© 2012 AHA Guide Index of Health Care Professionals **A803**

EATHERLY, Theresa, Chief Financial Officer, Doctor's Hospital – Tidwell, Houston, TX, p. A604

EATON, Ellen, Director Human Resources, Tift Regional Medical Center, Tifton, GA, p. A161

EATON, Jim, Chief Financial Officer, Wise Regional Health System, Decatur, TX, p. A593

EATON, Philip, Chief Executive Officer, HEALTHSOUTH Rehabilitation Hospital of Utah, Sandy, UT, p. A641

EAVENSON, J. Steven, Interim Vice President and Chief Financial Officer, Mercy Medical Center–Sioux City, Sioux City, IA, p. A226

EAVES, Clinton, Administrator, H. C. Watkins Memorial Hospital, Quitman, MS, p. A352

EBAUGH, Matthew T., Area Information Officer, San Diego Medical Center, San Diego, CA, p. A85

EBBETT, Patricia, Chief Human Resources Officer, Catawba Hospital, Catawba, VA, p. A646

EBERLE, Michele, Assistant Administrator, Mayo Clinic Health System – Chippewa Valley in Bloomer, Bloomer, WI, p. A679

EBERSOLE, Nathan, Controller, Calhoun–Liberty Hospital, Blountstown, FL, p. A118

EBERST, Laurie, R.N
President and Chief Executive Officer, St. John's Pleasant Valley Hospital, Camarillo, CA, p. A56
President and Chief Executive Officer, St. John's Regional Medical Center, Oxnard, CA, p. A78

EBERT, Cynthia, R.N. Chief Nursing Officer, Summit Healthcare Regional Medical Center, Show Low, AZ, p. A38

EBERT, Jr., Larry W., Chief Financial Officer, Northridge Medical Center, Commerce, GA, p. A150

EBERT, Michael, M.D. Chief of Staff, Veterans Affairs Connecticut Healthcare System, West Haven, CT, p. A113

EBERTH, Denise A., Director Human Resources, Allegan General Hospital, Allegan, MI, p. A307

EBINGER, William, M.D. President and Chief of Staff, Aurora Medical Center Grafton, Grafton, WI, p. A682

EBLIN, Steve E., Chief Executive Officer, Randolph Hospital, Asheboro, NC, p. A448

EBNER, Carl, Vice President Finance, Robinson Memorial Hospital, Ravenna, OH, p. A487

EBNER, Joseph, M.D. Chief Medical Officer, Speare Memorial Hospital, Plymouth, NH, p. A400

EBRI, Patrick, Ph.D
Vice President, Human Resources, Southeast Georgia Health System Brunswick Campus, Brunswick, GA, p. A148
Vice President Human Resources, Southeast Georgia Health System Camden Campus, Saint Marys, GA, p. A158

EBRIGHT, Brian, Chief Financial Officer, Arizona Spine and Joint Hospital, Mesa, AZ, p. A33

EBSEN, Mona, Chief Financial Officer, Kit Carson County Memorial Hospital, Burlington, CO, p. A98

ECCHER, Robbi, Vice President Human Resources, Sauk Prairie Memorial Hospital & Clinics, Prairie Du Sac, WI, p. A689

ECHELBERGER, Scott, Vice President, Operations, Catawba Valley Medical Center, Hickory, NC, p. A455

ECHOLS, Jane, Chief Executive Officer, Wills Memorial Hospital, Washington, GA, p. A162

ECKBERG, Stephen, Vice President Human Resources, St. Mary Medical Center, Apple Valley, CA, p. A54

ECKELS, Dan, Chief Financial Officer, Washington Regional Medical Center, Fayetteville, AR, p. A44

ECKENFELS, Susan, Chief Financial Officer, Ste. Genevieve County Memorial Hospital, Ste. Genevieve, MO, p. A371

ECKERD, Gayle
Chief Executive Officer, River Point Behavioral Health, Jacksonville, FL, p. A126
Chief Executive Officer, Wekiva Springs Center for Women, Jacksonville, FL, p. A127

ECKERT, Leslie, Chief Financial Officer, St. Elizabeth's Hospital, Belleville, IL, p. A173

ECKERT, Mark, Vice President Finance, Ochsner Medical Center – Kenner, Kenner, LA, p. A269

ECKERT, Mary L., President and Chief Executive Officer, Millcreek Community Hospital, Erie, PA, p. A523

ECKERT, Susan, R.N. Senior Vice President and Chief Nursing Officer, Medstar Washington Hospital Center, Washington, DC, p. A116

ECKES, Chad, Chief Information Officer, Midwestern Regional Medical Center, Zion, IL, p. A196

ECKMANN, John, Director Information Systems, Shenandoah Medical Center, Shenandoah, IA, p. A226

ECKSTEIN, William, Chief Financial Officer, Columbus Specialty Hospital, Columbus, GA, p. A149

EDDEY, Gary E., M.D. Medical Director, Matheny Medical and Educational Center, Peapack, NJ, p. A408

EDDINGTON, Tonya, Coordinator Human Resources, Select Specialty Hospital–Springfield, Springfield, MO, p. A371

EDDINS, Angela, Controller, HEALTHSOUTH Emerald Coast Rehabilitation Hospital, Panama City, FL, p. A135

EDDLEMAN, Patricia, Fiscal Officer, Heartland Behavioral Healthcare, Massillon, OH, p. A484

EDDY, Craig, M.D. Chief Medical Officer, The HealthCenter, Kalispell, MT, p. A377

EDELEN, Donald B., M.D. Vice President Medical Services and Quality Initiatives, Franciscan St. Elizabeth Health – Lafayette Central, Lafayette, IN, p. A206

EDELMAN, Marc D., Vice President Operations, Bristol Hospital, Bristol, CT, p. A108

EDELSTEIN, Hank, M.D. Chief of Staff, Trinity Hospital, Weaverville, CA, p. A95

EDENFIELD, Janet, Director Financial Services, Georgia Regional Hospital at Savannah, Savannah, GA, p. A159

EDGAR, Joseph H., Senior Vice President Operations, Gettysburg Hospital, Gettysburg, PA, p. A524

EDGAR, Nancy, Vice President Human Resources, Methodist Hospital, San Antonio, TX, p. A625

EDIE, Skip, Chief Information Officer, Carthage Area Hospital, Carthage, NY, p. A424

EDIN, Scott D., Chief Financial Officer, Amery Regional Medical Center, Amery, WI, p. A678

EDLER, Susie, Chief Executive Officer, Forest Park Medical Center, Dallas, TX, p. A591

EDMISSON, Jete, Chief Operating Officer and Chief Financial Officer, Cullman Regional Medical Center, Cullman, AL, p. A18

EDMONDS, Kelly, Chief Financial Officer, Western Maryland Hospital Center, Hagerstown, MD, p. A292

EDMONDSON, Bobby, Controller, Regional Rehabilitation Hospital, Phenix City, AL, p. A25

EDMONDSON, James H., Chief Executive Officer, Jacksonville Medical Center, Jacksonville, AL, p. A22

EDMONDSON, Theresa, Director, Walter B. Jones Alcohol and Drug Abuse Treatment Center, Greenville, NC, p. A454

EDMONSON, Cole, R.N. Vice President and Chief Nursing Officer, Texas Health Presbyterian Hospital Dallas, Dallas, TX, p. A592

EDMUNDSON, Reed, Administrator, Madison St. Joseph Health Center, Madisonville, TX, p. A615

EDNEY, Daniel, M.D. Chief of Staff, Promise Hospital of Vicksburg, Vicksburg, MS, p. A353

EDWARD, Virginia, R.N. Administrator and Chief Nursing Officer, West Anaheim Medical Center, Anaheim, CA, p. A53

EDWARDS, A. Jane, MSN Vice President, Patient Care Services, Blue Ridge Regional Hospital, Spruce Pine, NC, p. A461

EDWARDS, Annette, Chief Financial Officer, Odessa Memorial Healthcare Center, Odessa, WA, p. A663

EDWARDS, Becky, Manager Human Resources, Irwin County Hospital, Ocilla, GA, p. A157

EDWARDS Jr., Bob S., FACHE Chief Executive Officer, Banner Lassen Medical Center, Susanville, CA, p. A92

EDWARDS, Bruce
Vice President Human Resources, Heritage Valley Beaver, Beaver, PA, p. A518
Vice President Human Resources, Sewickley Valley Hospital, (A Division of Valley Medical Facilities), Sewickley, PA, p. A538

EDWARDS, Cathy, Director Organization and Talent Effectiveness, Bronson Battle Creek, Battle Creek, MI, p. A308

EDWARDS, Dana, Chief Financial Officer, HEALTHSOUTH Sea Pines Rehabilitation Hospital, Melbourne, FL, p. A130

EDWARDS, Danny R., Administrator, Complex Care Hospital at Ridgelake, Sarasota, FL, p. A138

EDWARDS, David, M.D. Chief Medical Officer, Banner Gateway Medical Center, Gilbert, AZ, p. A32

EDWARDS, David, Chief Financial Officer, SEARHC MT. Edgecumbe Hospital, Sitka, AK, p. A30

EDWARDS, Elizabeth, R.N. Director, Nursing Services, Sheridan Community Hospital, Sheridan, MI, p. A323

EDWARDS, Frank, M.D. Medical Director, Jones Memorial Hospital, Wellsville, NY, p. A446

EDWARDS, Gordon, Chief Financial Officer, Gundersen Lutheran Medical Center, La Crosse, WI, p. A683

EDWARDS, Gregg
Chief People Officer, Rogue Valley Medical Center, Medford, OR, p. A512
Chief People Officer, Three Rivers Medical Center, Grants Pass, OR, p. A511

EDWARDS, James, President, Hazleton General Hospital, Hazleton, PA, p. A525

EDWARDS, Jeff, Manager Information Services, Mendocino Coast District Hospital, Fort Bragg, CA, p. A61

EDWARDS, Jeffrey, M.D
Chief Medical Staff, Aspirus Grand View Hospital, Ironwood, MI, p. A316
Chief of Staff, Texas Health Harris Methodist Hospital Stephenville, Stephenville, TX, p. A629

EDWARDS, Jim, Executive Director of Information Technology, Gibson Area Hospital and Health Services, Gibson City, IL, p. A183

EDWARDS, John R., Administrator and Chief Executive Officer, Pacific Alliance Medical Center, Los Angeles, CA, p. A71

EDWARDS, Jon, Executive Director Finance, Fresno Heart and Surgical Hospital, Fresno, CA, p. A62

EDWARDS, Kathleen, Manager Information Systems Operation, HEALTHSOUTH Rehabilitation Hospital of Altoona, Altoona, PA, p. A517

EDWARDS, Mark, M.D. Chief Medical Officer, Lillian M. Hudspeth Memorial Hospital, Sonora, TX, p. A628

EDWARDS, Mark A., Chief Executive Officer, Livingston Hospital and Healthcare Services, Salem, KY, p. A258

EDWARDS, Marti, MSN Vice President Patient Care Services, Holy Family Medical Center, Des Plaines, IL, p. A180

EDWARDS, Michael R., Chief Executive Officer, Scott Regional Hospital, Morton, MS, p. A350

EDWARDS, Michelle, Executive Vice President Information Technology, Palmetto Health Baptist, Columbia, SC, p. A548

EDWARDS, Ramona, Chief Financial Officer, Mountrail County Medical Center, Stanley, ND, p. A468

EDWARDS, Rick
Vice President Finance Services, Hancock Regional Hospital, Greenfield, IN, p. A203
Director Information Systems, Howard County General Hospital, Columbia, MD, p. A290

EDWARDS, Steven D., President and Chief Executive Officer, CoxHealth, Springfield, MO, p. B40

EDWARDS, Steven D., President and Chief Executive Officer, Lester E. Cox Medical Centers, Springfield, MO, p. A371

EDWARDS, Susan, Vice President Human Resources, Culpeper Regional Hospital, Culpeper, VA, p. A647

EDWARDS, Susan A., President and Chief Executive Officer, ProHealth Care, Inc., Waukesha, WI, p. B104

EDWARDS, Teresa L., Vice President and Administrator, Sentara Leigh Hospital, Norfolk, VA, p. A652

EDWARDS, Terry, Controller, Kings Mountain Hospital, Kings Mountain, NC, p. A456

EDWARDS, Todd, Director Information Management Systems, Brazosport Regional Health System, Lake Jackson, TX, p. A611

EDWARDS, William, Information Technology Generalist, Wernersville State Hospital, Wernersville, PA, p. A540

EESLEY, Michael S., Chief Executive Officer, Centegra Health System, Crystal Lake, IL, p. B30

EESLEY, Michael S.
Chief Executive Officer, Centegra Hospital – McHenry, McHenry, IL, p. A187
Chief Executive Officer, Centegra Hospital – Woodstock, Woodstock, IL, p. A196

EFFEREN, Linda, M.D. Senior Vice President and Chief Medical Officer, South Nassau Communities Hospital, Oceanside, NY, p. A439

EFFERSON, Douglas P., FACHE Chief Executive Officer, De Soto Regional Health System, Mansfield, LA, p. A272

EGAN, Narci, Vice President and Chief Financial Officer, Beverly Hospital, Montebello, CA, p. A75

EGAN, Timothy C., Director, Human Resources, MountainView Regional Medical Center, Las Cruces, NM, p. A416

EGE, Garry, Chief Financial Officer, Coastal Harbor Treatment Center, Savannah, GA, p. A159

EGERTON, W. Eugene, M.D. Chief Medical Officer, Maryland General Hospital, Baltimore, MD, p. A288

EGGERS, Judy, Manager Human Resources, Alliance HealthCare System, Holly Springs, MS, p. A347

EHASZ, James, Chief Financial Officer, La Paz Regional Hospital, Parker, AZ, p. A34

EHINGER, Sue, Ph.D. Executive Vice President and Chief Operating Officer, Parkview Hospital, Fort Wayne, IN, p. A201

EHLER, Phyllis, Director Human Resources, Avera St. Benedict Hospital, Parkston, SD, p. A558

EHLERS, Jeffrey, Chief Financial Officer, Memorial Hospital of Union County, Marysville, OH, p. A484

EHLERS, Karan, Chief Financial Officer, West River Regional Medical Center, Hettinger, ND, p. A466

EHLINGER, Forrest, Vice President and Chief Financial Officer, Harrison Medical Center, Bremerton, WA, p. A659

EHLKE, Ranae, Administrative Secretary and Coordinator Risk Management and Human Resources, Kenmare Community Hospital, Kenmare, ND, p. A467

EHRAT, Michael, Chief Operating Officer, Skyline Medical Center, Nashville, TN, p. A573

EHRENBERGER, David, M.D. Chief Medical Officer, Avista Adventist Hospital, Louisville, CO, p. A104

EHRET, Charlene S., FACHE Director, James H. Quillen Veterans Affairs Medical Center, Mountain Home, TN, p. A572

EHRICH, Laurie, Chief Communications Officer, Wayne County Hospital, Corydon, IA, p. A217

EHRLICH, Frank, M.D. Chief Medical Officer, Kingston Hospital, Kingston, NY, p. A428

EHRLICH, Jane, President and Chief Executive Officer, Columbia Memorial Hospital, Hudson, NY, p. A427

Index of Health Care Professionals / Elwell

Index of Health Care Professionals

EHRLICH, Susan, M.D. Chief Executive Officer, San Mateo Medical Center, San Mateo, CA, p. A89
EHTISHAM, Saad, FACHE Chief Executive Officer, University Medical Center, Lebanon, TN, p. A569
EICHENAUER, Donald T., Chief Executive Officer, Wyoming County Community Hospital, Warsaw, NY, p. A446
EICHENBERGER, Daniel J., M.D. Medical Director, Floyd Memorial Hospital and Health Services, New Albany, IN, p. A209
EICHER, Kim D., Chief Executive Officer, St. Francis Health Care Centre, Green Springs, OH, p. A481
EICHMAN, Cynthia, President, Our Lady of Victory Hospital, Stanley, WI, p. A691
EIDAM, JoEllen, Chief Operating Officer, Adams Memorial Hospital, Decatur, IN, p. A200
EIDE, Tom, Chief Financial Officer, Prairie St. John's, Fargo, ND, p. A465
EIDSON, Charles, Assistant Administrator Human Resources, South Georgia Medical Center, Valdosta, GA, p. A161
EIG, Blair, M.D. Senior Vice President Medical Affairs, Holy Cross Hospital, Silver Spring, MD, p. A294
EIKE, Gail, Chief Financial Officer, Sanford Jackson Medical Center, Jackson, MN, p. A333
EIMERS, Katy, Human Resources Officer, Syringa Hospital and Clinics, Grangeville, ID, p. A168
EINBOND, Jeffrey, Director Facility Administration, South Beach Psychiatric Center,, NY, p. A436
EINSWEILER, Desiree, Interim Chief Executive Officer, Mitchell County Regional Health Center, Osage, IA, p. A224
EIPE, Joseph, M.D. Chief Medical Officer, Pacifica Hospital of the Valley,, CA, p. A71
EIQEL, Steve, Chief Financial Officer, Carroll County Memorial Hospital, Carrollton, KY, p. A248
EISCHEID, Randy, Director Information Systems, St. Anthony Regional Hospital, Carroll, IA, p. A215
EISELE, Karla, M.D. Clinical Director, State Hospital North, Orofino, ID, p. A170
EISEMANN, Bradley, Administrator, Crenshaw Community Hospital, Luverne, AL, p. A22
EISEN, Brian, Director Human Resources, Camden County Health Services Center, Blackwood, NJ, p. A402
EISENHAUER, Glenn, Vice President, Evangelical Community Hospital, Lewisburg, PA, p. A527
EISENMAN, Edward, Chief Executive Officer, Sunnyview Rehabilitation Hospital, Schenectady, NY, p. A443
EISENMANN, Claudia Ann, Chief Executive Officer, Select Specialty Hospital–Central Pennsylvania, Camp Hill, PA, p. A520
EISENRING, Richard, Chief Financial Officer, Holy Cross Hospital, Taos, NM, p. A418
EISENTRAGER, Steve, Administrator, Ohio Valley Medical Center, Springfield, OH, p. A488
EISENZOPH, Pete, Director Information Technology, Bay Area Medical Center, Marinette, WI, p. A685
EISMAN, Michael, M.D. Medical Director, Schuyler Hospital, Montour Falls, NY, p. A430
EISNER, Nina W., Chief Executive Officer and Managing Director, Ridge Behavioral Health System, Lexington, KY, p. A253
EITEL, Jeffrey, Chief Financial Officer, Littleton Adventist Hospital, Littleton, CO, p. A103
EITZEN, Jamie, Chief Financial Officer, Fairview Regional Medical Center, Fairview, OK, p. A496
EIXENBERGER, Timothy D., R.N. Chief Nursing Officer, St. Charles Medical Center – Bend, Bend, OR, p. A509
EKENGREN, Francie H., M.D. Chief Medical Officer, Wesley Medical Center, Wichita, KS, p. A246
EKEREN, Douglas R., Vice President Planning and Development, Avera Sacred Heart Hospital, Yankton, SD, p. A561
EKPO, Felix, Interim Manager Information Systems, Arrowhead Regional Medical Center, Colton, CA, p. A58
EKREM, Chris, Chief Executive Officer, Yoakum County Hospital, Denver City, TX, p. A594
EL MASRY, Waguih, M.D. Chief of Staff, Manatee Memorial Hospital, Bradenton, FL, p. A119
ELA, Sue
Executive Vice President and Chief Operating Officer, Aurora Medical Center of Oshkosh, Oshkosh, WI, p. A688
Executive Vice President and Chief Operating Officer, Aurora St. Luke's Medical Center, Milwaukee, WI, p. A686
ELAM, Moses D., M.D. Physician–in–Chief, Manteca Medical Center, Manteca, CA, p. A74
ELANGOVAN, N., M.D. Medical Director, Essex County Hospital Center, Cedar Grove, NJ, p. A402
ELARBEE, Vernon, Director of Human Resources, Florida Hospital North Pinellas, Tarpon Springs, FL, p. A141
ELBERT, Darlene M., R.N. Assistant Administrator and Chief Nursing Officer, Kossuth Regional Health Center, Algona, IA, p. A214
ELDER, Becky, Vice President Clinical Services, Perry County Memorial Hospital, Tell City, IN, p. A212
ELDER, Penny, Manager Human Resources, UC Health Surgical Hospital, West Chester, OH, p. A491
ELDER, Ronald J., Chief Executive Officer, Glenwood Regional Medical Center, West Monroe, LA, p. A279
ELDIB, Candace, Administrator, Batesville Specialty Hospital, Batesville, MS, p. A343
ELDIDY, Rene, M.D. Chief of Staff, CentraCare Health System – Long Prairie, Long Prairie, MN, p. A333
ELDRIDGE, Janet, Director Human Resources and Personnel, Brooks County Hospital, Quitman, GA, p. A157
ELDRIDGE, Jim, Area Financial Officer, Sacramento Medical Center, Sacramento, CA, p. A83
ELDRIDGE, Laurie, Chief Financial Officer, Marshall Medical Center, Placerville, CA, p. A80
ELDRIDGE, Lisa, Human Resources Officer, Thomas H. Boyd Memorial Hospital, Carrollton, IL, p. A174
ELEGANT, Bruce M., President and Chief Executive Officer, Rush Oak Park Hospital, Oak Park, IL, p. A190
ELFERT, Mike, Director Information Services, Lourdes Medical Center of Burlington County, Willingboro, NJ, p. A412
ELFORD, Dorothy J., Chief Executive Officer, Atrium Medical Center of Corinth, Corinth, TX, p. A588
ELGARICO, David, Chief Operating Officer, Rio Grande Regional Hospital, McAllen, TX, p. A615
ELGER, William, Executive Vice President and Chief Business and Finance Officer, University of Texas Medical Branch Hospitals, Galveston, TX, p. A600
ELICH, Liz, Vice President Human Resources, Frye Regional Medical Center, Hickory, NC, p. A455
ELIE, Charlene, Vice President Patient Care Services, Clinton Hospital, Clinton, MA, p. A299
ELIZALDE, David A., Director, Veterans Affairs Puget Sound Health Care System, Seattle, WA, p. A666
ELIZONDO, Diane, Director Human Resources, Harlingen Medical Center, Harlingen, TX, p. A602
ELKINGTON, Bruce
Regional Chief Information Officer, St. Clare Hospital, Lakewood, WA, p. A662
Regional Chief Information Officer, St. Francis Hospital, Federal Way, WA, p. A661
Vice President Information Technology, St. Joseph Medical Center, Tacoma, WA, p. A668
ELKINGTON, Mark, M.D. Chief Medical Officer, Willow Crest Hospital, Miami, OK, p. A499
ELKINS, James N., FACHE Director, Texas Center for Infectious Disease, San Antonio, TX, p. A626
ELKINS, Wendy, Director Operations, Dundy County Hospital, Benkelman, NE, p. A382
ELLARD, Ellen, Director Human Resources, Putnam General Hospital, Eatonton, GA, p. A152
ELLER, Jeff, FACHE President and Chief Executive Officer, Sonora Regional Medical Center, Sonora, CA, p. A91
ELLERBE, F. Dana, Assistant Administrator, Sutter Medical Center of Santa Rosa, Chanate Campus, Santa Rosa, CA, p. A90
ELLERBE, Suellyn, R.N. Executive Vice President, Chief Nursing Officer and Chief Operating Officer, Saint Clare's Health System, Denville, NJ, p. A403
ELLERT, William, M.D. Chief Medical Officer, Phoenix Baptist Hospital, Phoenix, AZ, p. A36
ELLEY, Michael, Chief Information Officer, Skaggs Regional Medical Center, Branson, MO, p. A356
ELLINGTON, Christopher, Executive Vice President and Chief Financial Officer, University of North Carolina Hospitals, Chapel Hill, NC, p. A450
ELLINGTON, Linda B., R.N. Interim Vice President and Chief Nursing Officer, Chatham Hospital, Siler City, NC, p. A460
ELLIOT, Anna, Head Information Technology, Dundy County Hospital, Benkelman, NE, p. A382
ELLIOTT, Barb, Chief Financial Officer, Fairbanks, Indianapolis, IN, p. A204
ELLIOTT, C. Layton, M.D. Chief of Staff, Witham Memorial Hospital, Lebanon, IN, p. A207
ELLIOTT, Charles M., M.D. Chief of Staff, Tippah County Hospital, Ripley, MS, p. A352
ELLIOTT Jr., Charles W., Chief Executive Officer, Johnston Health, Smithfield, NC, p. A461
ELLIOTT, Jim
Director Human Resources, Bryce Hospital, Tuscaloosa, AL, p. A26
Director Human Resources, Mary S Harper Geriatric Psychiatry Center, Tuscaloosa, AL, p. A26
ELLIOTT, Laura, Director Marketing and Human Resources, Evanston Regional Hospital, Evanston, WY, p. A696
ELLIOTT, Lee, Vice President Human Resources and Fund Development, Saint Francis Medical Center, Grand Island, NE, p. A384
ELLIOTT, Michael, Controller, Indianhead Medical Center, Shell Lake, WI, p. A691
ELLIOTT, R. James, Vice President Human Resources, The Charlotte Hungerford Hospital, Torrington, CT, p. A112
ELLIOTT, Robin, Personnel Officer, Community Memorial Hospital, Sumner, IA, p. A227
ELLIOTT, Shane, Associate Director Administration, Jerry L. Pettis Memorial Veterans Medical Center, Loma Linda, CA, p. A67
ELLIOTT, William T., Associate Administrator Administrative and Support Services, Hawaii State Hospital, Kaneohe, HI, p. A164
ELLIOTT MSN, Randi, Chief Nursing Officer, Baylor Medical Center at Frisco, Frisco, TX, p. A600
ELLIS, Amanda, Chief Financial Officer, Knox County Hospital, Barbourville, KY, p. A247
ELLIS, Betts, Administrator Institutional Relations, MUSC Medical Center of Medical University of South Carolina, Charleston, SC, p. A547
ELLIS, Bob, Director of Nursing, D. W. McMillan Memorial Hospital, Brewton, AL, p. A17
ELLIS, Dan C., Chief Executive Officer, Coteau des Prairies Hospital, Sisseton, SD, p. A560
ELLIS, Elmer G., FACHE President and Chief Executive Officer, East Texas Medical Center Regional Healthcare System, Tyler, TX, p. B49
ELLIS, Kelly, D.O. Chief Medical Officer, Tilden Community Hospital, Tilden, NE, p. A390
ELLIS, Lynn, Chief Financial Officer, LakeWood Health Center, Baudette, MN, p. A328
ELLIS, Michael J., Chief Executive Officer, Big Bend Regional Medical Center, Alpine, TX, p. A577
ELLIS, Nora, Market Chief Information Officer, MacNeal Hospital, Berwyn, IL, p. A173
ELLIS, Rich, Chief Operating Officer, Frye Regional Medical Center, Hickory, NC, p. A455
ELLIS, Seth, Chief Operating Officer, Motion Picture and Television Fund Hospital and Residential Services,, CA, p. A70
ELLIS, Susan, R.N. Vice President of Human Resources, Highlands Regional Medical Center, Prestonsburg, KY, p. A258
ELLIS, Thomas J., Vice President Human Resources, Mt. Washington Pediatric Hospital, Baltimore, MD, p. A288
ELLIS, Wendel, D.O. Chief Medical Staff, Greeley County Health Services, Tribune, KS, p. A244
ELLISH, Patti M., President and Chief Executive Officer, St. Tammany Parish Hospital, Covington, LA, p. A265
ELLISON, Darcy, R.N. Senior Vice President, Chief Nursing Officer and Inpatient Flow, St. Mary's Medical Center of Evansville, Evansville, IN, p. A201
ELLISON, Mike, Information Systems Lead, Summersville Regional Medical Center, Summersville, WV, p. A676
ELLISON, Patricia, Chief Financial Officer, Perry Memorial Hospital, Princeton, IL, p. A192
ELLISON, Tracey, Vice President Human Resources, Carroll Hospital Center, Westminster, MD, p. A294
ELLZEY, Bob S., FACHE President, Texas Health Harris Methodist Hospital Azle, Azle, TX, p. A582
ELMER, Dan, Vice President Finance, Morehead Memorial Hospital, Eden, NC, p. A452
ELMORE, Buddy, Chief Financial Officer, Sacred Heart Hospital of Pensacola, Pensacola, FL, p. A136
ELMORE, Ellen, M.D. Director Medical Services, Maniilaq Health Center, Kotzebue, AK, p. A29
ELMORE, Kevin, Chief Information Officer, Covenant Hospital–Levelland, Levelland, TX, p. A612
ELMORE, Nadine, Chief Executive Officer, Dahl Memorial Healthcare Association, Ekalaka, MT, p. A375
ELMORE, Thomas, Director Information System, National Park Medical Center, Hot Springs, AR, p. A46
ELMORE, Trent, Director Human Resources, Springs Memorial Hospital, Lancaster, SC, p. A552
ELROD, James K., FACHE President and Chief Executive Officer, Willis–Knighton Health System, Shreveport, LA, p. B146
ELSE, Ryan, M.D. Interim Vice President Medical Affairs, Mercy Hospital, Coon Rapids, MN, p. A330
ELSESSER, William, Director Professional Relations, Kindred Hospital North Houston, Houston, TX, p. A604
ELSIK, Kristina, Director Human Resources, DeTar Healthcare System, Victoria, TX, p. A633
ELSWICK, Shannon, President, Orlando Regional Medical Center, Orlando, FL, p. A134
ELTON, James, Chief Executive Officer, Select Long Term Care Hospital – Colorado Springs, Colorado Springs, CO, p. A98
ELWELL, Richard, Senior Vice President and Chief Financial Officer, Elliot Hospital, Manchester, NH, p. A399
ELWELL, Russell, M.D. Medical Director, Westfield Memorial Hospital, Westfield, NY, p. A446

© 2012 AHA Guide Index of Health Care Professionals **A805**

Index of Health Care Professionals

Index of Health Care Professionals / Ely

ELY, Thomas L., D.O. Chief Medical Officer, Gateway Medical Center, Clarksville, TN, p. A564
EMANUEL, Kate, Director Human Resources, Clarke County Hospital, Osceola, IA, p. A225
EMBERS, Tom, Assistant Administrator and Chief Operating Officer, William Newton Hospital, Winfield, KS, p. A246
EMBREE, Steve, Chief Financial Officer, Carolinas Hospital System, Florence, SC, p. A549
EMBREY, Jeffrey, M.D. Vice President Medical Affairs, Baylor Medical Center at Irving, Irving, TX, p. A609
EMBRY, Debra, Associate Administrator Employee Services, Atlanta Memorial Hospital, Atlanta, TX, p. A580
EMBURY, Stuart, M.D. Chief Medical Officer, Phelps Memorial Health Center, Holdrege, NE, p. A384
EMDUR, Larry, M.D. Chief of Staff, Promise Hospital of San Diego, San Diego, CA, p. A85
EMERICK, Ron, M.D. Chief of Staff, Doctor's Memorial Hospital, Perry, FL, p. A136
EMERSON, Cindy, Director Information Services, Mission Hospital, Mission Viejo, CA, p. A74
EMERSON, Marsha, Chief Support Officer, Craig General Hospital, Vinita, OK, p. A507
EMERSON, Sherri, Chief Executive Officer, Texas Health Heart & Vascular Hospital Arlington, Arlington, TX, p. A580
EMERY, Jeff, Chief Financial Officer and Chief Operating Officer, Gateways Hospital and Mental Health Center, Los Angeles, CA, p. A69
EMGE, Joann, Chief Executive Officer, Sparta Community Hospital, Sparta, IL, p. A194
EMMERICH, Melissa, M.D. President Medical Staff, Sacred Heart Hospital, Eau Claire, WI, p. A681
EMMINGER, Dianne, Vice President Information Services, ACMH Hospital, Kittanning, PA, p. A526
EMORY, Mark L., System Director Human Resources, Transylvania Regional Hospital, Brevard, NC, p. A449
EMTER, Melanie, Director Finance, Livingston Memorial Hospital, Livingston, MT, p. A377
ENCAPERA, Kimberly, M.D. Medical Director, Rehabilitation Hospital of Southern New Mexico, Las Cruces, NM, p. A416
ENCE, Michael, Computer Specialist, Sanpete Valley Hospital, Mount Pleasant, UT, p. A638
ENCKE, Faye, Director Information Management, HEALTHSOUTH Rehabilitation Hospital of Virginia, Richmond, VA, p. A655
ENDEN, Jay, M.D. Medical Director, Southside Hospital, Bay Shore, NY, p. A421
ENDERS Jr., Robert A., President, Chatham Hospital, Siler City, NC, p. A460
ENDERSON, Dan, Chief Financial Officer, Huguley Memorial Medical Center, Fort Worth, TX, p. A598
ENDICOTT, Sarah, M.D. Chief of Staff, North Runnels Hospital, Winters, TX, p. A636
ENDOM, Beth W., R.N. Vice President and Chief Nursing Officer, South Central Regional Medical Center, Laurel, MS, p. A348
ENDRES, Jack R., Administrator, East Texas Medical Center Jacksonville, Jacksonville, TX, p. A609
ENDRICH, Joseph, M.D. President and Chief Executive Officer, Weirton Medical Center, Weirton, WV, p. A676
ENG, Bland, Chief Executive Officer, Brandon Regional Hospital, Brandon, FL, p. A119
ENG, Jeffrey, M.D. Medical Director, HEALTHSOUTH Rehabilitation Hospital of Montgomery, Montgomery, AL, p. A24
ENGEL, David, Chief Executive Officer, Phillips County Hospital, Phillipsburg, KS, p. A241
ENGEL, Terry, Manager Information Technology, Oakes Community Hospital, Oakes, ND, p. A467
ENGELHART, Michael A., President, Advocate South Suburban Hospital, Hazel Crest, IL, p. A184
ENGELKEN, Joseph T., Chief Executive Officer, Tuba City Regional Health Care Corporation, Tuba City, AZ, p. A39
ENGESSER, Edward, Chief Financial Officer and Chief Information Officer, Barlow Respiratory Hospital, Los Angeles, CA, p. A68
ENGLAND, Dave, Director Human Resources, Lakeland Behavioral Health System, Springfield, MO, p. A371
ENGLAND, Donna, Director Medical Records, HEALTHSOUTH Rehabilitation Hospital of Fort Smith, Fort Smith, AR, p. A45
ENGLE, Dan, Chief Information Officer, Thayer County Health Services, Hebron, NE, p. A384
ENGLE, Heidi, Manager Information Technology, Glacial Ridge Health System, Glenwood, MN, p. A332
ENGLE, Steve, Chief Operations Officer, Mad River Community Hospital, Arcata, CA, p. A54
ENGLEHART, Jay, M.D. Medical Director, Southeast Missouri Mental Health Center, Farmington, MO, p. A359
ENGLEKING, David, M.D. Vice President Medical Affairs, CHRISTUS St. Patrick Hospital of Lake Charles, Lake Charles, LA, p. A271
ENGLERTH, Ladonna, Administrator, East Carroll Parish Hospital, Lake Providence, LA, p. A271
ENGLISH, Anne L., Director Human Resources, Chenango Memorial Hospital, Norwich, NY, p. A438
ENGLISH, Dennis, M.D. Vice President Medical Affairs, Magee–Womens Hospital of UPMC, Pittsburgh, PA, p. A535
ENGLISH, Jeff, Vice President Human Resources, St. Mary's Health Care System, Athens, GA, p. A144
ENGLISH, Julene, Director Human Resources, Kentfield Rehabilitation and Specialty Hospital, Kentfield, CA, p. A65
ENGLISH, Kathy L., R.N. Executive Vice President and Chief Operating Officer, Children's Hospital and Medical Center, Omaha, NE, p. A387
ENGLISH, Mark E., M.D. Chief of Staff, McKenzie Health System, Sandusky, MI, p. A322
ENGLISH, Nancy M., Chief Human Resources Officer, Banner Ironwood Medical Center, San Tan Valley, AZ, p. A38
ENGLUND, Paul, Chief Information Officer, Saints Medical Center, Lowell, MA, p. A301
ENGSTROM, Chad P., Director Human Resources, Westfields Hospital, New Richmond, WI, p. A688
ENGSTROM, Frederick, M.D. Medical Director, Brattleboro Retreat, Brattleboro, VT, p. A643
ENICKS, Charles, Chief Information Officer, University Hospitals and Health System, University of Mississippi Medical Center, Jackson, MS, p. A348
ENJADY, Rainey, Administrative Officer, Mescalero Public Health Service Indian Hospital, Mescalero, NM, p. A417
ENNEN, Philip L.
Vice President and Chief Executive Officer, Community Hospitals and Wellness Centers, Bryan, OH, p. A471
President and Chief Executive Officer, Community Hospitals and Wellness Centers–Montpelier, Montpelier, OH, p. A485
ENNIS, Virgil, Chief Information Officer, Helen Hayes Hospital, West Haverstraw, NY, p. A446
ENNS, Merle, Director Information Services, Prairie View, Newton, KS, p. A239
ENOCHS, Darren, Director Human Resources, Specialty Hospital of Mid–America, Overland Park, KS, p. A241
ENOKA, Christina, Director Human Resources and Risk Management, Kahi Mohala Behavioral Health, Ewa Beach, HI, p. A163
ENSLEY, Gordon, Chief Executive Officer, Lake District Hospital, Lakeview, OR, p. A512
ENSLEY, Terrasina, Director Human Resources, Fannin Regional Hospital, Blue Ridge, GA, p. A148
ENSMINGER, Jennifer, Chief Operating Officer, Pacific Hospital of Long Beach, Long Beach, CA, p. A68
ENSMINGER, Randy, M.D. Chief Medical Officer, Ocean Beach Hospital, Ilwaco, WA, p. A662
ENSRUDE, Layne, Chief Financial Officer, First Care Health Center, Park River, ND, p. A468
ENTENMANN, Kim, Director People Services, St. Joseph's Hospital, Chippewa Falls, WI, p. A680
ENTLER, Paul, D.O. Medical Director, Sparrow Specialty Hospital, Lansing, MI, p. A317
ENTWISTLE, David, Chief Executive Officer, University of Utah Health Care – Hospital and Clinics, Salt Lake City, UT, p. A641
ENTZMINGER, Julie, Manager Human Resources, Oakes Community Hospital, Oakes, ND, p. A467
EOLOFF, Eric J., Chief Operating Officer, Mercy Hospital St. Louis, Saint Louis, MO, p. A369
EPPERSON, Edward L., Chief Executive Officer, Carson Tahoe Regional Healthcare, Carson City, NV, p. A391
EPPERSON, Elysia, Director Human Resources, East Texas Medical Center Jacksonville, Jacksonville, TX, p. A609
EPPERSON, Jeff, Chief Financial Officer, Millwood Hospital, Arlington, TX, p. A579
EPPERSON, Kim, Director Business Development, River Oaks Hospital, New Orleans, LA, p. A275
EPPLER, Todd, Chief Executive Officer, Springhill Medical Center, Springhill, LA, p. A278
EPPS, Donna, Vice President and Chief Human Resources Officer, Lawrence & Memorial Hospital, New London, CT, p. A111
EPPS, Michelle, R.N. Chief Nursing Officer, Wellington Regional Medical Center, West Palm Beach, FL, p. A143
EPRIGHT, Janine L., Vice President and Chief Financial Officer, Gaylord Hospital, Wallingford, CT, p. A112
EPSTEIN, Michael, M.D. Senior Vice President Medical Affairs, All Children's Hospital, Saint Petersburg, FL, p. A138
EPSTEIN, Norman B., FACHE President, Chambersburg Hospital, Chambersburg, PA, p. A520
EPSTEIN, Norman B., FACHE President and Chief Executive Officer, Summit Health, Chambersburg, PA, p. B124
ERB, Judy, Vice President Patient Care Services and Chief Nursing Officer, Aultman Orrville Hospital, Orrville, OH, p. A487
ERBE, Allan D., Administrator, Riverside Behavioral Health Center, Hampton, VA, p. A649
ERDMAN, Donja, Chief Financial Officer, Marcus Daly Memorial Hospital, Hamilton, MT, p. A376
ERDMANN, Dorothy, Chief Executive Officer, Shawano Medical Center, Shawano, WI, p. A690
ERDMANN, Michael, M.D. Chief of Staff, Clement J. Zablocki Veterans Affairs Medical Center, Milwaukee, WI, p. A686
ERDOS, Joseph, M.D. Chief Information Officer, Veterans Affairs Connecticut Healthcare System, West Haven, CT, p. A113
ERENBERGER, Carol, Site Administrator, Carondelet Heart & Vascular Institute, Tucson, AZ, p. A39
ERGLE, Jeanine, Chief Financial Officer, Veterans Affairs Medical Center, Bay Pines, FL, p. A118
ERICH, Kevin R., President and Chief Executive Officer, Feather River Hospital, Paradise, CA, p. A79
ERICKSON, Brent, Administrator, Wright Patterson Medical Center, Wright–Patterson AFB, OH, p. A492
ERICKSON, Cindy, Chief Financial Officer, Sabine County Hospital, Hemphill, TX, p. A603
ERICKSON, Doug, Chief Financial Officer, Prague Community Hospital, Prague, OK, p. A503
ERICKSON, Karyn, Director Human Resources, Delta Medical Center, Memphis, TN, p. A571
ERICKSON, Nancy, Administrator Information Systems, Kossuth Regional Health Center, Algona, IA, p. A214
ERICKSON, Robert J., Chief Executive Officer, St. Francis Health Center, Topeka, KS, p. A244
ERICKSON, Ty W., Chief Executive Officer, Regina Medical Center, Hastings, MN, p. A332
ERICKSON, William A., Vice President and Chief Operating Officer, Sacred Heart–St. Mary's Hospitals, Rhinelander, WI, p. A690
ERICSON, Allen, Senior Vice President and Chief Operating Officer, Catholic Medical Center, Manchester, NH, p. A399
ERICSON, Kim
Vice President Finance, Fairview Lakes Health Services, Wyoming, MN, p. A342
Vice President Finance, Fairview Northland Medical Center, Princeton, MN, p. A337
ERKEN, Carole L., Human Resources Leader, Panorama City Medical Center,, CA, p. A71
ERLANDSON, Lesley, Human Resources Generalist, Mercy Hospital, Valley City, ND, p. A468
ERLICH, Ian, President and Chief Executive Officer, Maniilaq Health Center, Kotzebue, AK, p. A29
ERMANN, Bill, Interim Chief Executive Officer, Southwest Medical Center, Liberal, KS, p. A238
ERNDT, Robert, Site Manager, St. Mary Medical Center, Long Beach, CA, p. A68
ERNEST, Pam, R.N. CNO/ VP Patient Care Services, Franklin Memorial Hospital, Farmington, ME, p. A283
ERNST, William E., Administrator, Winkler County Memorial Hospital, Kermit, TX, p. A610
ERRICHETTI, Ann, M.D. President, Advocate Condell Medical Center, Libertyville, IL, p. A186
ERUKHIMOU, Jeffrey, M.D. Medical Director, Kindred Hospital–Heritage Valley, Beaver, PA, p. A518
ERVIN, Brad, Chief Executive Officer, Regency Hospital of Fort Worth, Fort Worth, TX, p. A599
ERVIN, Fulton
Senior Vice President and Chief Financial Officer, McLeod Medical Center Dillon, Dillon, SC, p. A549
Chief Financial Officer, McLeod Regional Medical Center, Florence, SC, p. A550
ERVIN, Richard, Chief Financial Officer, San Angelo Community Medical Center, San Angelo, TX, p. A624
ERVING–MENGEL, Tammi, Vice President, Chief Nursing Officer, High Point Regional Health System, High Point, NC, p. A455
ERWAY, Robert, Director for Administration, Bronx Psychiatric Center,, NY, p. A431
ERWIN, Connie, Manager, Samaritan Lebanon Community Hospital, Lebanon, OR, p. A512
ERWIN, Duane L., President and Chief Executive Officer, Aspirus, Inc., Wausau, WI, p. B14
ERWIN, Jerry A., Chief Human Resources Management Service, Veterans Affairs Medical Center, Dayton, OH, p. A479
ERWIN, Kermit, M.D. Medical Director, ProMedica Defiance Regional Hospital, Defiance, OH, p. A479
ESCAMILLA, Andrew G., R.N. Chief Executive Officer, Kindred Hospital Detroit, Detroit, MI, p. A311
ESCARDA, Ron, Chief Executive Officer, Fairfax Hospital, Kirkland, WA, p. A662
ESCHENBRENNER, Wade, Chief Financial Officer, Lexington Regional Health Center, Lexington, NE, p. A385
ESFANDIARI, Seifolah, M.D. Chief of Staff, Western Medical Center–Santa Ana, Santa Ana, CA, p. A89
ESKANDER, Nader, Director, Franciscan St. Anthony Health – Crown Point, Crown Point, IN, p. A200
ESKENAZI, Alan, Chief Executive Officer, Holliswood Hospital,, NY, p. A432

A806 Index of Health Care Professionals

FACKRELL, Sherlyn, Finance Controller, Grover C. Dils Medical Center, Caliente, NV, p. A391

FACTEAU, Patrick M., Chief Financial Officer, Adirondack Medical Center, Saranac Lake, NY, p. A442

FACULAK, Roger, Chief Financial Officer, Memorial Hermann Northwest Hospital, Houston, TX, p. A605

FACURI, Mark, Director Information Systems, Tri–City Medical Center, Oceanside, CA, p. A77

FADLER, Jeannie, R.N. Vice President, Patient Care Services, Saint Francis Medical Center, Cape Girardeau, MO, p. A356

FADOOL, Albert, Director Information Systems, Garden City Hospital, Garden City, MI, p. A313

FAEHNLE, Steve, M.D. Vice President Medical Affairs, Hendrick Health System, Abilene, TX, p. A577

FAGAN, Erin, Manager Human Resources, George Washington University Hospital, Washington, DC, p. A116

FAGAN, Michael, Chief Financial Officer, Huntington Hospital, Huntington, NY, p. A427

FAGAN–COOK, Ann, Administrator and Chief Executive Officer, Parkview Hospital, Wheeler, TX, p. A634

FAGERBERG, Lesley, Vice President Fiscal Services, Heart of the Rockies Regional Medical Center, Salida, CO, p. A105

FAGERSTROM, Joel, Executive Vice President and Chief Operating Officer, St. Luke's Hospital – Miners Campus, Coaldale, PA, p. A520

FAGG, Cindy, Fiscal Officer, Battle Mountain General Hospital, Battle Mountain, NV, p. A391

FAGIN, Beth, Manager Information Systems, St. Vincent's Medical Center Southside, Jacksonville, FL, p. A127

FAGUNDO, Ramon, M.D. Chief of Staff, Sistersville General Hospital, Sistersville, WV, p. A675

FAHD II, Charles F., Chief Executive Officer, Massena Memorial Hospital, Massena, NY, p. A429

FAHEY, Linda L., MS Vice President and Chief Nurse Executive, Decatur Memorial Hospital, Decatur, IL, p. A179

FAHEY, Walter, Chief Information Officer, Maimonides Medical Center,, NY, p. A434

FAHRLANDER, Jason, FACHE Chief Executive Officer, Hillcrest Medical Center, Tulsa, OK, p. A506

FAHS, Melvin H., Chief Executive Officer, Community Memorial Hospital, Hicksville, OH, p. A481

FAILE, J. Gene, Chief Executive Officer, Wilkes Regional Medical Center, North Wilkesboro, NC, p. A458

FAILING, Richard J., Chief Executive Officer, Kittson Memorial Healthcare Center, Hallock, MN, p. A332

FAILLA, Richard, Chief Executive Officer, Research Psychiatric Center, Kansas City, MO, p. A362

FAIN, Douglas, Director Computer Services, The University of Tennessee Medical Center, Knoxville, TN, p. A569

FAIRCHILD, David, M.D. Chief Medical Officer, Tufts Medical Center, Boston, MA, p. A297

FAIRCHILDS, Constance, R.N. Vice President Patient Care Services, Emanuel Medical Center, Turlock, CA, p. A93

FAIRCLOTH, Doug, Interim Chief Financial Officer, Elbert Memorial Hospital, Elberton, GA, p. A152

FAIRCLOTH, Gerald, Chief Executive Officer, Wayne Medical Center, Waynesboro, TN, p. A576

FAIRCLOTH, Karen, Chief Financial Officer, Memorial Hospital and Manor, Bainbridge, GA, p. A147

FAIRFAX, Tom, Director Information Systems, Bothwell Regional Health Center, Sedalia, MO, p. A370

FAISON, C. Forrest, Commander, Naval Medical Center, San Diego, CA, p. A85

FAKHRY, Wael, Senior Vice President and Chief Financial Officer, Indian River Medical Center, Vero Beach, FL, p. A142

FALANCE, Becky, Director Human Resources, Lovelace Rehabilitation Hospital, Albuquerque, NM, p. A414

FALASCO, Pam, Vice President, Chief Nursing Officer, Parma Community General Hospital, Parma, OH, p. A487

FALATKO, Michael J., FACHE President and Chief Executive Officer, Hills & Dales General Hospital, Cass City, MI, p. A309

FALBO, Susan, Vice President Human Resources, Wheeling Hospital, Wheeling, WV, p. A677

FALCK, Dennis, Chief Executive Officer, Warm Springs Rehabilitation Hospital, San Antonio, TX, p. A626

FALCON, Hugo, M.D. Director Medical Services, Piedmont Geriatric Hospital, Burkeville, VA, p. A646

FALCON, Spencer P., M.D. Vice President Medical Affairs, Samaritan Medical Center, Watertown, NY, p. A446

FALCONE, Robert E., M.D. Chief of Staff, Veterans Affairs Medical Center, Cincinnati, OH, p. A474

FALE, Randall J., FACHE Interim Chief Executive Officer, Arkansas State Hospital, Little Rock, AR, p. A47

FALIVENA, Richard, D.O. Vice President Medical Affairs, Cape Regional Medical Center, Cape May Court House, NJ, p. A402

FALKENBERRY, Lee, Director Information Systems, Monroe County Hospital, Monroeville, AL, p. A23

FALL, J. Mark, Chief Executive Officer, CareLink of Jackson, Jackson, MI, p. A316

FALL, Jennifer, Chief Information Officer, Gillette Children's Specialty Healthcare, Saint Paul, MN, p. A339

FALSETTI, Domonic F., M.D. Chief of Staff and Medical Director, Mount St. Mary's Hospital and Health Center, Lewiston, NY, p. A428

FALTERMAN, Jr., James B., M.D. Medical Director, University Medical Center, Lafayette, LA, p. A270

FALTZ, Lawrence L., M.D. Senior Vice President Medical Affairs and Medical Director, Phelps Memorial Hospital Center, Sleepy Hollow, NY, p. A443

FAMAKINWA, Abiodun, M.D. Acting Clinical Director, West Central Georgia Regional Hospital, Columbus, GA, p. A150

FANALE, James E., M.D. Senior Vice President System Development, Jordan Hospital, Plymouth, MA, p. A304

FANALE, Linda, Chief Financial Officer, Windber Medical Center, Windber, PA, p. A542

FANNIN, Allyson, Director Human Resources, LaSalle General Hospital, Jena, LA, p. A268

FANNIN, Pam, Coordinator Human Resources, LifeCare Hospital of Dayton, Miamisburg, OH, p. A485

FANNING, Linda T., R.N. Chief Nursing Officer, Mercy Hospital Oklahoma City, Oklahoma City, OK, p. A501

FANNING, Melinda, Chief Financial Officer and Controller, HEALTHSOUTH Southern Hills Rehabilitation Hospital, Princeton, WV, p. A675

FANNON, Susan, Chief Nursing Officer, Indian Path Medical Center, Kingsport, TN, p. A568

FANSELAU, Michael G., District Director Human Resources, Kindred Hospital–Sacramento, Folsom, CA, p. A60

FANTANO, Gene, Controller, Kindred Hospital–San Diego, San Diego, CA, p. A85

FARAH, Tony, M.D. President Medical Staff, Allegheny General Hospital, Pittsburgh, PA, p. A534

FARBER, Bobbi, M.D. Chief Medical Officer, St. Francis Hospital, Columbus, GA, p. A149

FARBER, Nancy D., Chief Executive Officer, Washington Hospital Healthcare System, Fremont, CA, p. A61

FARGASON, Crayton A., M.D. Medical Director, The Children's Hospital of Alabama, Birmingham, AL, p. A17

FARGUSON, Jack, Director Information Technology, Red River Regional Hospital, Bonham, TX, p. A584

FARHANG, Farzin, M.D. Medical Director, HEALTHSOUTH Rehabilitation Hospital–Las Vegas, Las Vegas, NV, p. A393

FARIA, Mary, FACHE Administrator, Seton Southwest Healthcare Center, Austin, TX, p. A581

FARINA, Albert M.
Chief Financial Officer, Mount Vernon Hospital, Mount Vernon, NY, p. A430
Senior Vice President and Chief Financial Officer, Sound Shore Medical Center of Westchester, New Rochelle, NY, p. A431

FARINA, Jonathan, Chief Information Officer, Brattleboro Memorial Hospital, Brattleboro, VT, p. A643

FARIS, Shellie, M.D. President Medical Staff, St. Francis Hospital and Health Services, Maryville, MO, p. A365

FARISH, Audra, Vice President Human Resources, Saint Joseph's Hospital of Atlanta, Atlanta, GA, p. A146

FARKAS, David, M.D
President Medical Staff, Aurora Medical Center, Kenosha, WI, p. A683
President Medical Staff, Aurora Memorial Hospital of Burlington, Burlington, WI, p. A679

FARKAS, Laura, Director Human Resources, Fairview Hospital, Great Barrington, MA, p. A300

FARLEY, H. Fred, FACH
President and Chief Operating Officer, Arnot Ogden Medical Center, Elmira, NY, p. A425
President and Chief Operating Officer, St. Joseph's Hospital, Elmira, NY, p. A426

FARMER, Guy, M.D. President Medical Staff, Calhoun Health Services, Calhoun City, MS, p. A344

FARMER, Kathleen, Assistant Administrator Finance and Chief Financial Officer, El Centro Regional Medical Center, El Centro, CA, p. A60

FARMER, Pat, Coordinator Human Resources and Safety Officer, Institute for Orthopaedic Surgery, Lima, OH, p. A482

FARMER, William, M.D. Chief of Staff, Evergreen Medical Center, Evergreen, AL, p. A20

FARNHAM, Diane, Acting Director Human Resources, Lallie Kemp Medical Center, Independence, LA, p. A268

FARNHAM, Krista, Chief Executive, Providence Seaside Hospital, Seaside, OR, p. A515

FARNSWORTH, Edward F., FACHE President, Capital Region Medical Center, Jefferson City, MO, p. A361

FARO, Joan, M.D. Chief Medical Officer, John T. Mather Memorial Hospital, Port Jefferson, NY, p. A440

FARR, Lorraine, Manager Human Resources, Georgia Regional Hospital at Atlanta, Decatur, GA, p. A151

FARR, Ralph, Chief Information Officer, University of Texas Medical Branch Hospitals, Galveston, TX, p. A600

FARR, Ronald
Senior Vice President and Chief Financial Officer, Frazier Rehab Institute, Louisville, KY, p. A254
Chief Financial Officer, Jewish Hospital, Louisville, KY, p. A254

FARR, William L., M.D. Chief Medical Officer, University Health Care System, Augusta, GA, p. A147

FARRAGE, Jim, M.D. Medical Director, Southern Kentucky Rehabilitation Hospital, Bowling Green, KY, p. A248

FARRELL, America S., FACHE Interim Chief Executive Officer, San Angelo Community Medical Center, San Angelo, TX, p. A624

FARRELL, Brenda, Vice President Finance, Brookhaven Memorial Hospital Medical Center, Patchogue, NY, p. A440

FARRELL, Darin, Chief Executive Officer, Arbuckle Memorial Hospital, Sulphur, OK, p. A505

FARRELL, George, M.D. Chief of Staff, Wythe County Community Hospital, Wytheville, VA, p. A658

FARRELL, Katie, Chief Operating Officer, Abington Health Lansdale Hospital, Lansdale, PA, p. A527

FARRELL, Lentz, Information Services Specialist, Silverton Hospital, Silverton, OR, p. A515

FARRELL, Michael J., FACHE Chief Executive Officer, Somerset Hospital, Somerset, PA, p. A538

FARRELL, Patrick J., Chief Executive Officer, Henrico Doctors' Hospital, Richmond, VA, p. A655

FARRELL, Roy, M.D. Chief Medical Officer, Carondelet Holy Cross Hospital, Nogales, AZ, p. A34

FARRELL, Steven E., M.D. Chief Medical Officer, Forrest General Hospital, Hattiesburg, MS, p. A346

FARRELL, Terence, Administrator, Herrin Hospital, Herrin, IL, p. A184

FARRELL, Teresa, Director Human Resources, Nacogdoches Medical Center, Nacogdoches, TX, p. A618

FARRELLY, Irene, Vice President and Chief Information Officer, Brooklyn Hospital Center,, NY, p. A431

FARRIS, Bain J., President and Chief Executive Officer, Exempla Saint Joseph Hospital, Denver, CO, p. A99

FARRIS, James R., FACHE Chief Executive Officer, Union County Hospital, Anna, IL, p. A172

FARRIS, Naomi, Director Human Resources, Atoka County Medical Center, Atoka, OK, p. A493

FARROW, Diane, Manager Information Technology and Systems, Willamette Valley Medical Center, McMinnville, OR, p. A512

FARROW, Ed, M.D. Chief Medical Staff, Epic Medical Center, Eufaula, OK, p. A496

FARSHAO, Nosratian, M.D. Chief Medical Staff, Memorial Hospital of Gardena, Gardena, CA, p. A63

FASANO, Philip, Chief Information Officer, Sacramento Medical Center, Sacramento, CA, p. A83

FATCH, Casey, Chief Operating Officer, Tri–City Medical Center, Oceanside, CA, p. A77

FATTIG, Marty, Administrator and Chief Executive Officer, Nemaha County Hospital, Auburn, NE, p. A381

FATULA, Suzette, Chief Financial Officer, Allen Parish Hospital, Kinder, LA, p. A269

FAUCHEAUX, Carolyn, Director Human Resources, St. Charles Parish Hospital, Luling, LA, p. A272

FAUCHEUX, Lisa, Director Human Resources, St. James Parish Hospital, Lutcher, LA, p. A272

FAUGHT, Charles J., Chief Financial Officer, Burnett Medical Center, Grantsburg, WI, p. A682

FAUL, Jennifer, Chief Operating Officer, Prairie St. John's, Fargo, ND, p. A465

FAULIS, Karen, Chief Operating Officer, Palmdale Regional Medical Center, Palmdale, CA, p. A79

FAULK Jr., A. Donald, FACHE President, Medical Center of Central Georgia, Macon, GA, p. A155

FAULK, Gordon, Administrator, Elmore Community Hospital, Wetumpka, AL, p. A27

FAULKNER, Charles A., FACHE Chief Executive Officer, Wiregrass Medical Center, Geneva, AL, p. A21

FAULKNER, Cindy, Chief Nursing Officer, Maria Parham Medical Center, Henderson, NC, p. A454

FAULKNER, David M., Chief Executive Officer, Fleming County Hospital, Flemingsburg, KY, p. A249

FAULKNER, Gary, Chief Executive Officer, Florence Community Healthcare, Florence, AZ, p. A32

FAULKNER, Kristi, Director Human Resources, United Regional Health Care System, Wichita Falls, TX, p. A635

FAULKNER, Laura, Chief Human Resource Management Service, Veterans Affairs Medical Center–Lexington, Lexington, KY, p. A254

FAULKNER, Mark T., President, Baptist Health Care Corporation, Pensacola, FL, p. B18

FAUST, Bill D., Administrator, Floyd County Medical Center, Charles City, IA, p. A216

FAVALE, Maria, FACHE Associate Director, Veterans Affairs Medical Center, Northport, NY, p. A438

Index of Health Care Professionals / Ferrans


FAVATA, Valerie, R.N. Chief Nursing Officer, Oswego Hospital, Oswego, NY, p. A440
FAVRET, John M., Director, Eastern State Hospital, Williamsburg, VA, p. A657
FAWNS, Bill, Interim Manager Information Systems, Kern Medical Center, Bakersfield, CA, p. A55
FAY, Brian, Director Information Systems, Sidney Health Center, Sidney, MT, p. A379
FAYE, Darryl, Chief Financial Officer, Cameron Memorial Community Hospital, Angola, IN, p. A197
FAYEN, Edward J., Associate Administrator Operations and Support, Washington Hospital Healthcare System, Fremont, CA, p. A61
FAYRE, Gail, M.D. Medical Director, Anna Jaques Hospital, Newburyport, MA, p. A302
FEAK, Christina, Chief Information Officer, Onslow Memorial Hospital, Jacksonville, NC, p. A455
FEAR, Frank, Chief Information Officer, Memorial Healthcare, Owosso, MI, p. A320
FEASEL, Jeff, Chief Executive Officer, Halifax Health Medical Center of Daytona Beach, Daytona Beach, FL, p. A122
FEASEL, Julie, Chief Executive Officer, Kindred Hospital Bay Area–Tampa, Tampa, FL, p. A141
FEATHER, Leroy P., Vice President Finance, Community Hospitals and Wellness Centers, Bryan, OH, p. A471
FEBUS, Steven, Chief Financial Officer, Pullman Regional Hospital, Pullman, WA, p. A664
FEDELE, Jerry J., President and Chief Executive Officer, Boca Raton Regional Hospital, Boca Raton, FL, p. A118
FEDER, Diane, MSN Senior Vice President and Chief Operating Officer, Witham Memorial Hospital, Lebanon, IN, p. A207
FEDER, Eric, Exec. VP, Chief Operating Officer, Bayfront Medical Center, Saint Petersburg, FL, p. A138
FEDERICO, Skip, Director Information Systems, Fairway Medical Center, Covington, LA, p. A265
FEDERINKO, David, Chief Information Officer, Allegan General Hospital, Allegan, MI, p. A307
FEDERSPIEL, John C., President and Chief Executive Officer, Hudson Valley Hospital Center, Cortlandt Manor, NY, p. A424
FEDORA, Deborah, Director Human Resources, Paoli Hospital, Paoli, PA, p. A531
FEE, Jeff, Chief Executive Officer, St. Patrick Hospital, Missoula, MT, p. A378
FEEMAN, Kimberly, Vice President Human Resources, The Good Samaritan Hospital, Lebanon, PA, p. A527
FEENEY, John, President and Chief Executive Officer, Berlin Memorial Hospital, Berlin, WI, p. A679
FEESS, David, President and Chief Executive Officer, Liberty Hospital, Liberty, MO, p. A364
FEGAN, Claudia, M.D. Chief Medical Officer, John H. Stroger Jr. Hospital of Cook County, Chicago, IL, p. A176
FEGAN, Theresa, Chief Clinical Officer, Tahoe Pacific Hospitals, Reno, NV, p. A395
FEGHALI, Georges, M.D
Senior Vice President Quality and Chief Medical Officer, Bethesda North Hospital, Cincinnati, OH, p. A472
Senior Vice President Quality and Chief Medical Officer, Good Samaritan Hospital, Cincinnati, OH, p. A473
FEHR, Mike, Vice President Operations and Chief Information Officer, Jupiter Medical Center, Jupiter, FL, p. A127
FEHR, Tracy, Executive Assistant and Director Human Resources, Red River Hospital, Wichita Falls, TX, p. A635
FEHRING, Marcia, Chief Financial Officer, Horn Memorial Hospital, Ida Grove, IA, p. A221
FEIDT, Leslie, Chief Information Officer, Erie County Medical Center, Buffalo, NY, p. A422
FEIKE, Jeffrey, President and Chief Administrative Officer, Fort Loudoun Medical Center, Lenoir City, TN, p. A569
FEIL, Julie, Accountant, Cavalier County Memorial Hospital, Langdon, ND, p. A467
FEILER, Kenneth H., Chief Executive Officer, Rose Medical Center, Denver, CO, p. A100
FEILNER, Margaret, Director Information Services, SSM St. Joseph Health Center, Saint Charles, MO, p. A368
FEINBERG, Daniel, M.D. Chief Medical Officer, Pennsylvania Hospital, Philadelphia, PA, p. A533
FEINBERG, David, M.D. Chief Executive Officer, Ronald Reagan University of California Los Angeles Medical Center, Los Angeles, CA, p. A71
FEINBERG, Jason, M.D
Vice President Medical Affairs and Chief Medical Officer, Geneva General Hospital, Geneva, NY, p. A426
Vice President Medical Affairs and Chief Medical Officer, Soldiers and Sailors Memorial Hospital of Yates County, Penn Yan, NY, p. A440
FEINOUR, Terry, Senior Vice President Corporate Services, Bayhealth Medical Center, Dover, DE, p. A114
FEIRN, Greg, Senior Vice President and Chief Financial Officer, Children's Hospital, New Orleans, LA, p. A274
FEISAL, J. Philip
Senior Vice President Acute Care Hospitals, Spartanburg Regional Medical Center, Spartanburg, SC, p. A554
Chief Executive Officer, Village Hospital, Greer, SC, p. A551
FEIST, Patricia, Manager Human Resources, Crook County Medical Services District, Sundance, WY, p. A697
FEIT, Marcy L., President and Chief Executive Officer, ValleyCare Medical Center, Pleasanton, CA, p. A80
FELBINGER, Richard, Senior Vice President and Chief Financial Officer, Borgess Medical Center, Kalamazoo, MI, p. A316
FELDHOUSE, Doreen, M.D. Chief of Staff, Dyersburg Regional Medical Center, Dyersburg, TN, p. A565
FELDMAN, David L., Executive Vice President and Treasurer, Circles of Care, Melbourne, FL, p. A130
FELDMAN, Mitchell S., Chief Executive Officer, West Boca Medical Center, Boca Raton, FL, p. A119
FELDMAN, Tom, Chief Financial Officer, East Ohio Regional Hospital, Martins Ferry, OH, p. A484
FELDSTEIN, Charles S., M.D. Vice President Medical Affairs, St. Rose Hospital, Hayward, CA, p. A64
FELEGE, Lester, Controller, New England Rehabilitation Hospital, Woburn, MA, p. A306
FELGAR, Alvin D., President and Chief Executive Officer, Frisbie Memorial Hospital, Rochester, NH, p. A400
FELICETTI, Jacqueline, Director Human Resources, Chester County Hospital, West Chester, PA, p. A541
FELICI, Brian K., Chief Executive Officer, Wetzel County Hospital, New Martinsville, WV, p. A674
FELICIANO, Jose R., Chief Executive Officer, Ryder Memorial Hospital, Humacao, PR, p. A701
FELICIANO, Lorenzo Gonzalez, M.D. Secretary of Health, Puerto Rico Department of Health, San Juan, PR, p. B106
FELICIANO, Lourdes, M.D. Chairman, Doctors' Center Hospital San Juan, San Juan, PR, p. A703
FELIX, Larry A., FACHE Chief Executive Officer, Ransom Memorial Hospital, Ottawa, KS, p. A240
FELIZ, Miriam, M.D. Medical Director, St. Catherine's Rehabilitation Hospital, North Miami, FL, p. A133
FELKNER, Joseph G., Senior Vice President and Chief Financial Officer, Palm Bay Hospital, Melbourne, FL, p. A130
FELL, David, M.D. Chief Medical Officer, Tulsa Spine and Specialty Hospital, Tulsa, OK, p. A507
FELLER, Julie, Director Human Resources, Grays Harbor Community Hospital, Aberdeen, WA, p. A659
FELLOWES, S. Gale, M.D. Chief Medical Officer, Memorial Health Care System, Chattanooga, TN, p. A563
FELLOWS, Steven A.
Executive Vice President and Chief Operating Officer, Goleta Valley Cottage Hospital, Santa Barbara, CA, p. A89
Executive Vice President and Chief Operating Officer, Santa Barbara Cottage Hospital, Santa Barbara, CA, p. A89
Executive Vice President and Chief Operating Officer, Santa Ynez Valley Cottage Hospital, Solvang, CA, p. A91
FELMLEE, Charles, Assistant Director Fiscal Services, Central Virginia Training Center, Madison Heights, VA, p. A650
FELTMAN, Steven, CPA Interim Chief Financial Officer, Virginia Regional Medical Center, Virginia, MN, p. A341
FELTON, David
President and Chief Executive Officer, Community Memorial Hospital, Hamilton, NY, p. A427
Manager Information Systems, Waldo County General Hospital, Belfast, ME, p. A281
FELTON, Debby, Chief Financial Officer, Central Arkansas Veterans Healthcare System, Little Rock, AR, p. A48
FELTS, Dave, Chief Information Systems, Logan Regional Hospital, Logan, UT, p. A638
FENDT, Phil, Chief Financial Officer, Memorial Community Health, Aurora, NE, p. A381
FENELLO, Michael A., Chief Executive Officer, St. Luke's McCall, McCall, ID, p. A169
FENER, Michael
Executive Director, Plainview Hospital, Plainview, NY, p. A440
Executive Director, Syosset Hospital, Syosset, NY, p. A444
FENGEL, Anna, Personnel Assistant, Mental Health Institute, Clarinda, IA, p. A216
FENN, Mark, Director Human Resources, Pulaski Memorial Hospital, Winamac, IN, p. A213
FENNELL, Charles, Vice President Information Management, St. Joseph's Hospital Health Center, Syracuse, NY, p. A444
FENSKE, Candace, Chief Executive Officer, Madelia Community Hospital, Madelia, MN, p. A334
FENSTERER, Rob, Director Information Services, Devereux Hospital and Children's Center of Florida, Melbourne, FL, p. A130
FENTON, Joanne, FACHE Chief Executive Officer, Northern Colorado Long Term Acute Hospital, Johnstown, CO, p. A102
FENWICK, Sandra, Chief Operating Officer, Children's Hospital Boston, Boston, MA, p. A296
FERCH, Wayne, President and Chief Executive Officer, Central Valley General Hospital, Hanford, CA, p. A64
FERETTO, Linda, Director Human Resources, Jerold Phelps Community Hospital, Garberville, CA, p. A62
FERGIE, Joy, Chief Financial Officer, Greenbrier Valley Medical Center, Ronceverte, WV, p. A675
FERGUS, Janie
Director and Chief Information Officer, Saint Joseph East, Lexington, KY, p. A253
Director and Chief Information Officer, Saint Joseph Hospital, Lexington, KY, p. A253
FERGUS, Linda, Manager Information Technology, Allegheny Valley Hospital, Natrona Heights, PA, p. A530
FERGUSON, Allison, Director Human Resources, Avoyelles Hospital, Marksville, LA, p. A272
FERGUSON, Bruce, Chief Financial Officer, Northwest Hospital & Medical Center, Seattle, WA, p. A665
FERGUSON, Cheryl L., Associate Administrator, Sanford Medical Center Canby, Canby, MN, p. A329
FERGUSON, Clifford, Director Information Technology and Systems, Bayshore Medical Center, Pasadena, TX, p. A620
FERGUSON, Deborah, Human Resources Consultant, Sentara Obici Hospital, Suffolk, VA, p. A656
FERGUSON, G. Thomas, Senior Vice President and Chief Human Resources Officer, New York–Presbyterian Hospital, New York, NY, p. A436
FERGUSON, Gary W., Executive Vice President and Chief Operating Officer, Christiana Care Health System, Newark, DE, p. A114
FERGUSON, Gordon B., President and Chief Executive Officer, Middle Tennessee Medical Center, Murfreesboro, TN, p. A573
FERGUSON, James E., Chief Executive Officer, Stonewall Memorial Hospital, Aspermont, TX, p. A580
FERGUSON, Karen, Director Human Resources, Johnson County Healthcare Center, Buffalo, WY, p. A695
FERGUSON, Louis D., Chief Financial Officer, Palestine Regional Medical Center–East, Palestine, TX, p. A619
FERGUSON, Michael, Chief Financial Officer, Harbor Oaks Hospital, New Baltimore, MI, p. A320
FERGUSON, Nina L., Director Human Resources, Little Colorado Medical Center, Winslow, AZ, p. A41
FERGUSON, Paul, Director Information Systems, Brownwood Regional Medical Center, Brownwood, TX, p. A585
FERGUSON, Randy, Chief Information Officer, Ridgecrest Regional Hospital, Ridgecrest, CA, p. A82
FERGUSON, Rick, Chief Executive Officer, Oklahoma Surgical Hospital, Tulsa, OK, p. A506
FERGUSON, Susan, Chief Operating Officer, Kindred Hospital–Delaware County, Darby, PA, p. A521
FERGUSON, Tonya, Director Human Resources, HEALTHSOUTH Rehabilitation Hospital of Virginia, Richmond, VA, p. A655
FERGUSON, Zeta, Chief Human Resources, Veterans Affairs Medical Center, Decatur, GA, p. A151
FERIA, Jorge, M.D. President Medical Staff, Wilma N. Vazquez Medical Center, Vega Baja, PR, p. A704
FERIGGNO, Sandie, Director Human Resources, Good Shepherd Medical Center, Longview, TX, p. A613
FERMANO, Joseph, Vice President Finance and Chief Financial Officer, Crotched Mountain Rehabilitation Center, Greenfield, NH, p. A398
FERNANDEZ, Alex, Chief Financial Officer, North Shore Medical Center, Miami, FL, p. A131
FERNANDEZ, Benigno J., M.D. Executive Medical Director, Laurel Ridge Treatment Center, San Antonio, TX, p. A625
FERNANDEZ, Bernardo, M.D. Chief Executive Officer, Cleveland Clinic Florida, Weston, FL, p. A143
FERNANDEZ, Emiliano, Director Information Services, Jerome Golden Center for Behavioral Health, Inc., West Palm Beach, FL, p. A142
FERNANDEZ, Genaro, M.D. Chief of Staff, Paradise Valley Hospital, National City, CA, p. A76
FERNANDEZ, Jean, Chief Information Officer, Milton Hospital, Milton, MA, p. A302
FERNANDEZ, John R., President and Chief Executive Officer, Massachusetts Eye and Ear Infirmary, Boston, MA, p. A297
FERNANDEZ, Jose L. Pimentel, Medical Director, Lafayette Hospital, Arroyo, PR, p. A700
FERNANDEZ, Manuel, Vice President Nursing, Larkin Community Hospital, South Miami, FL, p. A139
FERNANDEZ, Robert, M.D. Chief Medical Staff, Southern Maine Medical Center, Biddeford, ME, p. A282
FERNANDEZ, Tracey, Chief Financial Officer, Riverside Community Hospital, Riverside, CA, p. A83
FERNANDEZ–BRAVO, Grisel, R.N. Chief Nursing Officer, Memorial Hospital West, Pembroke Pines, FL, p. A135
FERNIANY, William, Ph.D. Chief Executive Officer, UAB Health System, Birmingham, AL, p. B132
FERRACANE, Tony, Vice President Human Resources, St. Mary Medical Center, Hobart, IN, p. A203
FERRANS, Richard, M.D. Vice President and Medical Information Officer, Memorial Hospital at Gulfport, Gulfport, MS, p. A346



Index of Health Care Professionals **A809**
Index of Health Care Professionals

Index of Health Care Professionals

Index of Health Care Professionals / Ferrante

FERRANTE, Fritz, Manager Information Services, Providence Kodiak Island Medical Center, Kodiak, AK, p. A29
FERRARA, Angela, Administrator, Baypointe Behavioral Health, Mobile, AL, p. A22
FERRARO, Christopher, Chief Financial Officer, Day Kimball Hospital, Putnam, CT, p. A111
FERREBEE, Mike, M.D. Vice President Medical Affairs, Monongalia General Hospital, Morgantown, WV, p. A674
FERRELL, David A.
Chief Executive Officer, Shriners Hospitals for Children, Galveston Burns Hospital, Galveston, TX, p. A600
Chief Executive Officer, Shriners Hospitals for Children, Houston, Houston, TX, p. A606
FERRELL, Ronald, Chief Information Officer, Veterans Affairs Medical Center, Albuquerque, NM, p. A415
FERRELLI, John J., Chief Operating Officer, Avanti Hospitals, El Segundo, CA, p. B15
FERRELLI, John J., Chief Executive Officer, Coast Plaza Hospital, Norwalk, CA, p. A77
FERREN, Alison, Vice President Information Technology and Chief Information Officer, Abington Memorial Hospital, Abington, PA, p. A517
FERRERI, Anthony C., President and Chief Executive Officer, Staten Island University Hospital,, NY, p. A437
FERRERO, Marcia L., MS Chief Nursing Officer, Heritage Valley Beaver, Beaver, PA, p. A518
FERRIELL, Kathleen, Chief Nursing Officer, Spring View Hospital, Lebanon, KY, p. A252
FERRIS, David, Chief Nursing Officer and Vice President Patient Care Services, Claxton–Hepburn Medical Center, Ogdensburg, NY, p. A439
FERRIS, Mark, M.D. Medical Director, Kindred Hospital–White Rock, Dallas, TX, p. A591
FERRONI, Karen, M.D. Medical Director, Holyoke Medical Center, Holyoke, MA, p. A300
FERRY, Jane, M.D. Vice President Medical Affairs, Grand View Hospital, Sellersville, PA, p. A538
FERRY, Thomas, Business Administrator, Oakwood Correctional Facility, Lima, OH, p. A483
FESENMEIER, James, M.D. Chief of Staff, Indiana University Health West Hospital, Avon, IN, p. A197
FESKO, Donald P., Chief Executive Officer and Administrator, Community Hospital, Munster, IN, p. A209
FESTA, J. Keith, M.D. Vice President Medical Affairs, Saint Francis Hospital and Health Centers, Poughkeepsie, NY, p. A441
FETTER, Lee F., President and Senior Executive Officer, St. Louis Children's Hospital, Saint Louis, MO, p. A370
FETTER, Trevor, President and Chief Executive Officer, TENET Healthcare Corporation, Dallas, TX, p. B127
FETTERS, Valerie, Chief Financial Officer, Hillsdale Community Health Center, Hillsdale, MI, p. A315
FEUER, Tammy, Chief Executive Officer, HEALTHSOUTH Rehabilitation Hospital of Vineland, Vineland, NJ, p. A411
FEUNNING, Charles, M.D. President Medical Staff, Summa Western Reserve Hospital, Cuyahoga Falls, OH, p. A478
FEUQUAY, Judith K., Chief Executive Officer, Nevada Regional Medical Center, Nevada, MO, p. A366
FICCHI, Adrienne, Vice President Information Management, Veterans Affairs Medical Center, Philadelphia, PA, p. A534
FICHTER, Craig R., Chief Financial Officer, Martin General Hospital, Williamston, NC, p. A462
FICKES, Catherine, R.N. President and Chief Executive Officer, St. Vincent Medical Center, Los Angeles, CA, p. A72
FICKLIN, Camille, Director Information Services, Family Health West, Fruita, CO, p. A101
FIDELI, Barbara, COO of Nonclinical, MetroSouth Medical Center, Blue Island, IL, p. A174
FIDLER, Soniya, Senior Director Human Resources, Yampa Valley Medical Center, Steamboat Springs, CO, p. A106
FIDUCIA, Karen A., FACHE President, Hospital Division, USMD Inc., Irving, TX, p. B140
FIEKER, Dan, D.O. Chief Medical Officer and Chief Operating Officer, St. Francis Health Center, Topeka, KS, p. A244
FIELD, Clifford, M.D. Medical Director, Kau Hospital, Pahala, HI, p. A165
FIELD, Kori, Director of Nursing, Brodstone Memorial Hospital, Superior, NE, p. A390
FIELD, Laurie, Director Human Resources, Eaton Rapids Medical Center, Eaton Rapids, MI, p. A312
FIELDER, Jaf, Vice President and Administrator, Willis–Knighton Medical Center, Shreveport, LA, p. A277
FIELDING, Laura M., Administrative Director Organizational Development, Holy Family Memorial Medical Center, Manitowoc, WI, p. A685
FIELDS Jr., Clarence, FACHE President and Chief Executive Officer, Goodall–Witcher Healthcare, Clifton, TX, p. A587
FIELDS, Donald R., Senior Community Chief Executive Officer, Hazard ARH Regional Medical Center, Hazard, KY, p. A251
FIELDS, Duane, Chief Financial Officer, Rush County Memorial Hospital, La Crosse, KS, p. A237
FIELDS, Glenn, Vice President Human Resources, Saint John's Health System, Anderson, IN, p. A197
FIELDS, Lexi M., Chief Financial Officer, Wallowa Memorial Hospital, Enterprise, OR, p. A510
FIELDS, Maura G., R.N. Chief Clinical Officer, North Valley Hospital, Whitefish, MT, p. A380
FIELDS, Sarah G., R.N. Vice President Nursing, North Kansas City Hospital, North Kansas City, MO, p. A366
FIERRO, Barbara, Director, Human Resources, St. Francis Hospital, Roslyn, NY, p. A442
FIGLIOZZI, Charles, CPA Vice President and Chief Financial Officer, New York Eye and Ear Infirmary, New York, NY, p. A435
FIGUEIREDO, Steve, Director, Dr. J. Corrigan Mental Health Center, Fall River, MA, p. A299
FIGUEROA, Maria, Director Human Resources, Ryder Memorial Hospital, Humacao, PR, p. A701
FIGUEROA, Roseann, Director Human Resources, Doctors Hospital of Laredo, Laredo, TX, p. A612
FIKE, Ruthita J.
Chief Executive Officer, Loma Linda University Behavioral Medicine Center, Redlands, CA, p. A82
Chief Executive Officer, Loma Linda University Behavioral Medicine Center, Redlands, CA, p. A82
Chief Executive Officer, Loma Linda University Medical Center, Loma Linda, CA, p. A67
Chief Executive Officer, Loma Linda University Medical Center, Loma Linda, CA, p. A67
FIKSE, David J., Chief Executive Officer, Northside Medical Center, Youngstown, OH, p. A492
FILBURN, Mandi, Director Human Resources, Twin Lakes Regional Medical Center, Leitchfield, KY, p. A252
FILER, Christine, Director Human Resources, HEALTHSOUTH Rehabilitation Hospital of Altoona, Altoona, PA, p. A517
FILIAK, Thomas, Chief Operating Officer, Auburn Community Hospital, Auburn, NY, p. A421
FILIPINI, Alfred, Manager Human Resources, Ancora Psychiatric Hospital, Ancora, NJ, p. A401
FILIPOWICZ, Thomas, M.D. Medical Director, St. Luke's Hospital – Quakertown Campus, Quakertown, PA, p. A536
FILKINS, James, Chief Information Officer, Norwegian American Hospital, Chicago, IL, p. A177
FILLER, Scott, Chief Executive Officer, HEALTHSOUTH Rehabilitation Hospital of Altoona, Altoona, PA, p. A517
FILLINGIM, Jed, Acting Chief Operating Officer and Associate Director, G.V. Montgomery Veterans Affairs Medical Center, Jackson, MS, p. A347
FILOSA, Frank, Fiscal Manager, Veterans Affairs Medical Center, Washington, DC, p. A117
FILPI, Jeanette, Chief Executive Officer, Pioneer Community Hospital of Patrick County, Stuart, VA, p. A656
FILSON, Debbie, Chief Financial Officer, Ashland Health Center, Ashland, KS, p. A230
FINAN Jr.,, John J., FACHE President and Chief Executive Officer, Franciscan Missionaries of Our Lady Health System, Inc., Baton Rouge, LA, p. B53
FINAN, Timothy J., FACH
President and Chief Executive Officer, Bradford Regional Medical Center, Bradford, PA, p. A519
President and Chief Executive Officer, Olean General Hospital, Olean, NY, p. A439
FINAN, Timothy J., FACHE President and Chief Executive Officer, Upper Allegheny Health System, Olean, NY, p. B140
FINCH, Debra A., Chief Operating Officer and Chief Nursing Officer, Carondelet St. Joseph's Hospital, Tucson, AZ, p. A39
FINCH, Joe, PsyD, Superintendent, Terrell State Hospital, Terrell, TX, p. A630
FINCH, John
Vice President Corporate Development, Benedictine Hospital, Kingston, NY, p. A428
Vice President Information Services, Kingston Hospital, Kingston, NY, p. A428
FINCH, Kenneth A., President and Chief Executive Officer, Huguley Memorial Medical Center, Fort Worth, TX, p. A598
FINCH, Kim, Chief Nursing Officer, Kosciusko Community Hospital, Warsaw, IN, p. A213
FINCH, Teresa, Chief Financial Officer, Trident Medical Center, Charleston, SC, p. A547
FINDLAY, Denice C., Director Human Resources, Community Hospital of San Bernardino, San Bernardino, CA, p. A84
FINE, Allan, Senior Vice President and Chief Strategy and Operations Officer, New York Eye and Ear Infirmary, New York, NY, p. A435
FINE, David J., Chief Executive Officer, St. Luke's Episcopal Health System, Houston, TX, p. B123
FINE, James, M.D. Executive Director Clinical Computing, Harborview Medical Center, Seattle, WA, p. A665
FINE, Peter S., FACHE President and Chief Executive Officer, Banner Health, Phoenix, AZ, p. B16
FINE, Stuart H., Chief Executive Officer, Grand View Hospital, Sellersville, PA, p. A538
FINELLI, Peter, Chief Financial Officer, Payson Regional Medical Center, Payson, AZ, p. A35
FINESTEIN, Brian, Chief Executive Officer, Easton Hospital, Easton, PA, p. A522
FINIZIO, John, President, St. Joseph Health Center, Warren, OH, p. A490
FINK, Eileen, Health Information Officer, North Big Horn Hospital District, Lovell, WY, p. A697
FINK, Kelley, Coordinator Human Resources, Sitka Community Hospital, Sitka, AK, p. A30
FINK, Renee, CPA Chief Financial Officer, Chase County Community Hospital, Imperial, NE, p. A384
FINLAYSON, Susan D., R.N. Senior Vice President and Chief Nursing Officer, Mercy Medical Center, Baltimore, MD, p. A288
FINLEY, Alan, Chief Operating Officer, Conway Regional Medical Center, Conway, AR, p. A43
FINLEY, Delvecchio, Chief Executive Officer, LAC–Harbor–University of California at Los Angeles Medical Center, Torrance, CA, p. A92
FINLEY, E. Jane, Senior Vice President and Executive Director, Kaiser Permanente Downey Medical Center, Downey,, p. A59
FINLEY, Edward, Administrator, Wray Community District Hospital, Wray, CO, p. A107
FINLEY, Kevan, Chief Executive Officer, Cedar Ridge Hospital, Oklahoma City, OK, p. A500
FINLEY, Mike, M.D. Chief Medical Officer, CHRISTUS St. Michael Health System, Texarkana, TX, p. A630
FINLEY, Tommy, Chief Information Officer, Rutherford Regional Medical Center, Rutherfordton, NC, p. A460
FINLEY, Waynea
System Director Human Resources, Warm Springs Rehabilitation Hospital, San Antonio, TX, p. A626
Corporate Director Human Resources, Warm Springs Specialty Hospital of Victoria, Victoria, TX, p. A633
FINN, Barry C., President and Chief Executive Officer, Rush–Copley Medical Center, Aurora, IL, p. A173
FINN, Patti, Assistant Administrator, Fulton County Health Center, Wauseon, OH, p. A491
FINNEGAN, Jay, Chief Executive Officer, Valley Hospital Medical Center, Las Vegas, NV, p. A394
FINNEY, Michele, Chief Executive Officer, Los Alamitos Medical Center, Los Alamitos, CA, p. A68
FINSTAD, Gary A., M.D. Chief of Staff, Kern Valley Healthcare District, Lake Isabella, CA, p. A66
FIORELLO, Tony, R.N. Chief Operating and Chief Nursing Officer, San Rafael Medical Center, San Rafael, CA, p. A89
FIORENZO, V. James, Executive Vice President and Chief Operating Officer, UPMC Hamot, Erie, PA, p. A523
FIORET, Phil, M.D. Vice President Medical Affairs, King's Daughters Medical Center, Ashland, KY, p. A247
FIOREY, Ramona, M.P.H. Commander, Moncrief Army Community Hospital, Fort Jackson, SC, p. A550
FIRES, Wiley M., Administrator, Shamrock General Hospital, Shamrock, TX, p. A627
FISCHELS, Diane, Senior Vice President and Chief Operating Officer, Mercy Medical Center–North Iowa, Mason City, IA, p. A223
FISCHER, Angie, Chief Financial Officer, Loring Hospital, Sac City, IA, p. A226
FISCHER, Chuck, Director Information Technology Systems, Teton Valley Hospital and Surgicenter, Driggs, ID, p. A168
FISCHER, James, R.N. Vice President Patient Care Services/Chief Nursing Officer, Munson Medical Center, Traverse City, MI, p. A324
FISCHER, Linda, Director Information Services, Huntington Hospital, Huntington, NY, p. A427
FISCHER, Lisa, Director Human Resources, Brown County Hospital, Ainsworth, NE, p. A381
FISCHER, Sandra, Director Human Resources, Veterans Affairs Medical Center, Salisbury, NC, p. A460
FISCHER, Sheri, Manager Human Resources, Grant Regional Health Center, Lancaster, WI, p. A684
FISCHER, Steven P., Chief Financial Officer, Beth Israel Deaconess Medical Center, Boston, MA, p. A296
FISCHER, Tamara, Chief Nursing Officer, Okeene Municipal Hospital, Okeene, OK, p. A500
FISER, David, Vice President and Chief Information Officer, Akron General Medical Center, Akron, OH, p. A469
FISH, Carrie L., Senior Vice President and Chief Operating Officer, Florida Hospital Waterman, Tavares, FL, p. A141

A810 Index of Health Care Professionals

Index of Health Care Professionals / Flood

Index of Health Care Professionals

FISH, Elizabeth
Senior Director Site Executive and Information Technology, Chester River Health System, Chestertown, MD, p. A290
Chief Information Officer, Dorchester General Hospital, Cambridge, MD, p. A290
Chief Information Officer, Memorial Hospital at Easton Maryland, Easton, MD, p. A291
FISH, Patsy, Chief Human Resources Management, James H. Quillen Veterans Affairs Medical Center, Mountain Home, TN, p. A572
FISHBACH, Ronald, M.D. Chief of Staff, St. Vincent Medical Center, Los Angeles, CA, p. A72
FISHBAIN, Ken, Chief Operating Officer, Gottlieb Memorial Hospital, Melrose Park, IL, p. A187
FISHBANE, Steven, M.D. Chief Medical Officer, Winthrop–University Hospital, Mineola, NY, p. A430
FISHEL, Linda, Manager Information Services, Edward John Noble Hospital of Gouverneur, Gouverneur, NY, p. A427
FISHER, Alan, Chief Executive Officer, Advanced Specialty Hospital of Toledo, Toledo, OH, p. A489
FISHER, Carol, Director of Nursing, Old Vineyard Behavioral Health Services, Winston–Salem, NC, p. A463
FISHER, David, Director Information Systems, Heart of Lancaster Regional Medical Center, Lititz, PA, p. A528
FISHER, David, M.D. Senior Vice President and Medical Director, Seattle Children's Hospital, Seattle, WA, p. A666
FISHER, David, Vice President Human Resources, Signature Healthcare Brockton Hospital, Brockton, MA, p. A298
FISHER, Dennis, Director Human Resources, Baptist Memorial Hospital–North Mississippi, Oxford, MS, p. A351
FISHER, Diane, R.N. VP, Patient Care Services, Otsego Memorial Hospital, Gaylord, MI, p. A313
FISHER, Jan E., President and Chief Executive Officer, Soldiers and Sailors Memorial Hospital, Wellsboro, PA, p. A540
FISHER, Jason B., Chief Executive Officer, St. Anthony's Hospital, Houston, TX, p. A606
FISHER, Jennifer A., Manager Human Resources, Henry County Hospital, Napoleon, OH, p. A485
FISHER, Kayla, M.D. Medical Director, Memphis Mental Health Institute, Memphis, TN, p. A571
FISHER, Kenneth, Associate Vice President Finance and Chief Financial Officer, University of Iowa Hospitals and Clinics, Iowa City, IA, p. A221
FISHER, Lynn, M.D. Chief of Staff, Rooks County Health Center, Plainville, KS, p. A242
FISHER, Lynne, R.N. Vice President of Patient Care Services, Vidant Beaufort Hospital, Washington, NC, p. A462
FISHER, Margaret A., Executive Director Human Resources, Specialty Hospital of Washington, Washington, DC, p. A117
FISHER, Michael, President and Chief Executive Officer, Cincinnati Children's Hospital Medical Center, Cincinnati, OH, p. A473
FISHER, Ryan, Director Human Resources, Bluffton Hospital, Bluffton, OH, p. A471
FISHER, Shawn, R.N. Director Clinical Services, Lakeside Memorial Hospital, Brockport, NY, p. A422
FISHER, Steven, M.D. President Medical Staff, Orthopaedic Hospital of Lutheran Health, Fort Wayne, IN, p. A201
FISHER, Thomas, Senior Vice President and Chief Financial Officer, The University of Tennessee Medical Center, Knoxville, TN, p. A569
FISHER, Tommie Ann, R.N. Director of Nursing, Clay County Hospital, Ashland, AL, p. A15
FISHER, William A., M.D. Executive Director, Creedmoor Psychiatric Center,, NY, p. A432
FISHKIN, Edward, M.D. Medical Director, Woodhull Medical and Mental Health Center,, NY, p. A438
FISHMANN, Andrew, M.D. Chairman, Medical Staff, Good Samaritan Hospital, Los Angeles, CA, p. A69
FISK, Anita, Director Human Resources, Okanogan Douglas District Hospital, Brewster, WA, p. A660
FISK, Art, Chief Information Officer, North Kansas City Hospital, North Kansas City, MO, p. A366
FISK, Kellee J., Vice President People Resources, Billings Clinic, Billings, MT, p. A373
FISNE, Joseph, Chief Information Officer, Pocono Medical Center, East Stroudsburg, PA, p. A522
FISSORI, Michele, Chief Financial Officer, North Star Behavioral Health System, Anchorage, AK, p. A28
FITCH, Duane, CPA Chief Financial Officer, Norwegian American Hospital, Chicago, IL, p. A177
FITCH, James A., Director Human Resources, CHRISTUS St. Catherine Hospital, Katy, TX, p. A610
FITCH, John A., Vice President Human Resources, Campbell County Memorial Hospital, Gillette, WY, p. A696
FITTS, Barry, Chief Information Officer, Trumbull Memorial Hospital, Warren, OH, p. A490
FITZ, Bette, Chief Nursing Officer, Garden City Hospital, Garden City, MI, p. A313
FITZ, J. D., M.D. Vice President Medical Affairs, MultiCare Good Samaritan Hospital, Puyallup, WA, p. A664
FITZ Jr., Thomas E., FACHE Interim Chief Executive Officer, St. Vincent Morrilton, Morrilton, AR, p. A49
FITZGERALD, Andy, Executive Vice President, Campbell County Memorial Hospital, Gillette, WY, p. A696
FITZGERALD, George, Regional Director Information Systems, LifeCare Hospitals of Pittsburgh, Pittsburgh, PA, p. A534
FITZGERALD, John L., Chief Executive Officer, Inova Fair Oaks Hospital, Fairfax, VA, p. A647
FITZGERALD, Larry, Chief Financial Officer, University of Virginia Medical Center, Charlottesville, VA, p. A646
FITZGERALD, Mike
Chief Financial Officer, St. Clare Hospital, Lakewood, WA, p. A662
Chief Financial Officer, St. Francis Hospital, Federal Way, WA, p. A661
Chief Financial Officer, St. Joseph Medical Center, Tacoma, WA, p. A668
FITZGERALD, Nancy D., Chief Operating Officer, CareLink of Jackson, Jackson, MI, p. A316
FITZGERALD, Patty, Staff Services, Charlevoix Area Hospital, Charlevoix, MI, p. A309
FITZGERALD, Tom, Manager Information Technology Service Delivery, Texas Health Presbyterian Hospital–WNJ, Sherman, TX, p. A628
FITZMAURICE, Dennis, Vice President, Professional Services, Our Lady of the Resurrection Medical Center, Chicago, IL, p. A177
FITZPATRICK, Daniel, Director Human Resources, Whitesburg ARH Hospital, Whitesburg, KY, p. A259
FITZPATRICK, James, M.D. Vice President Medical Affairs, Kenmore Mercy Hospital, Kenmore, NY, p. A428
FITZPATRICK, Paul, Manager Information Technology, Deaconess Medical Center, Spokane, WA, p. A667
FITZSIMMONS, Shawn, Director Information Technology Services, Community Medical Center, Toms River, NJ, p. A411
FIX, Judith A., R.N. Senior Vice President and Chief Nursing Officer, Long Beach Memorial Medical Center, Long Beach, CA, p. A68
FLACH, Shannan, Chief Executive Officer, Wamego City Hospital, Wamego, KS, p. A244
FLADER, Steve, Chief Financial Officer, Northwest Medical Center, Springdale, AR, p. A51
FLAHERTY, John, Controller, Fairlawn Rehabilitation Hospital, Worcester, MA, p. A306
FLAHERTY, Linda, R.N. Senior Vice President, Patient Care Services, McLean Hospital, Belmont, MA, p. A295
FLAHERTY, Patrick, Director Management Information, Naval Hospital Bremerton, Bremerton, WA, p. A659
FLAHERTY, Tom, Assistant Administrator, Los Angeles County Central Jail Hospital, Los Angeles, CA, p. A70
FLAIZ, Richard, M.D. President Medical Staff, Good Shepherd Health Care System, Hermiston, OR, p. A511
FLAKE, Robert, Chief Financial Officer, Yampa Valley Medical Center, Steamboat Springs, CO, p. A106
FLAKS, Jeffrey A., President and Chief Executive Officer, Hartford Hospital, Hartford, CT, p. A109
FLAKSMAN, Richard, M.D. Vice President Medical Affairs, OhioHealth Marion General Hospital, Marion, OH, p. A484
FLAKUS, Karleen, Director Human Resources, Winner Regional Healthcare Center, Winner, SD, p. A561
FLAMM, Cindy, Manager Quality, Choate Mental Health Center, Anna, IL, p. A172
FLANAGAN, Carl, CPA Chief Financial Officer, Basin Healthcare Center, Odessa, TX, p. A619
FLANAGAN, John, Chief Executive Officer, BCA Permian Basin, Midland, TX, p. A616
FLANAGAN, Michael J., Senior Vice President and Chief Operating Officer, St. Clair Memorial Hospital, Pittsburgh, PA, p. A535
FLANAGAN, Susan, Chief Operating Officer, Lucile Salter Packard Children's Hospital at Stanford, Palo Alto, CA, p. A79
FLANAGAN, Thomas, M.D. Medical Director, Aurora Behavioral Health Care, San Diego, CA, p. A85
FLANAGAN, Tom, Chief Operating Officer, Memorial Hermann – Texas Medical Center, Houston, TX, p. A605
FLANARY, Tresha, R.N. Chief Clinical Services Officer, Wamego City Hospital, Wamego, KS, p. A244
FLANDERS, Dave, Director Information Technology Systems, Emanuel Medical Center, Swainsboro, GA, p. A160
FLANDRY, Robert, M.D. Vice President and Chief Medical Officer, Spartanburg Regional Medical Center, Spartanburg, SC, p. A554
FLANIGAN, Erin, Vice President Human Resources, Wentworth–Douglass Hospital, Dover, NH, p. A397
FLANNERY, Donna M., Chief Executive Officer, Mercy Rehabilitation Hospital, Chesterfield, MO, p. A357
FLANNERY, Michael, M.D. Interim Chief of Staff, Roundup Memorial Healthcare, Roundup, MT, p. A378
FLANZ, Bruce J.
President and Chief Executive Officer, Flushing Hospital Medical Center,, NY, p. A432
President and Chief Executive Officer, Jamaica Hospital Medical Center,, NY, p. A433
FLASCHENRIEM, Julie, Chief Information Officer, Park Nicollet Methodist Hospital, Saint Louis Park, MN, p. A339
FLATT, G. Wayne, D.O. Chief Medical Director, Pushmataha Hospital & Home Health, Antlers, OK, p. A493
FLAVIN, Jan, Director Human Resources, Texas Health Harris Methodist Hospital Azle, Azle, TX, p. A582
FLECKENSTEIN, Casey, Medical and Surgical Nurse Manager, Monroe County Hospital, Forsyth, GA, p. A153
FLEEGEL, Monica, Director Human Resources, Mayo Clinic Health System in Albert Lea, Albert Lea, MN, p. A327
FLEENER, Mary Jane, Director of Clinical Services, Monroe Hospital, Bloomington, IN, p. A198
FLEENOR, Dennis, R.N. Chief Executive Officer, llano Specialty Hospital of Lubbock, Lubbock, TX, p. A614
FLEENOR, Sheila, Controller, Wellmont Lonesome Pine Hospital, Big Stone Gap, VA, p. A645
FLEER, Robert, M.D. Chief of Staff, Summersville Regional Medical Center, Summersville, WV, p. A676
FLEISCHER, Julie, M.D. President Medical Staff, Carlinville Area Hospital, Carlinville, IL, p. A174
FLEISCHMANN, Tim, Chief Financial Officer, Tuality Healthcare, Hillsboro, OR, p. A511
FLEITES, Fernando, Vice President Human Resources, CHRISTUS Santa Rosa Health Care, San Antonio, TX, p. A624
FLEMING, Ann, Senior Vice President, Quillen Rehabilitation Hospital, Johnson City, TN, p. A567
FLEMING, Dean, Chief Financial Officer, Athol Memorial Hospital, Athol, MA, p. A295
FLEMING, Michael, Chief People Officer, Banner Good Samaritan Medical Center, Phoenix, AZ, p. A35
FLEMING, Michelle, Chief Nursing Officer, Virginia Regional Medical Center, Virginia, MN, p. A341
FLEMING, Shane, Chief Financial Officer, Capital Health Regional Medical Center, Trenton, NJ, p. A411
FLEMING, William P., Chief Operating Officer, Norwood Hospital, Norwood, MA, p. A303
FLEMMING, Libby, Controller and Chief Information Officer, Louis Smith Memorial Hospital, Lakeland, GA, p. A155
FLESCH, Timothy A., President and Chief Executive Officer, St. Mary's Medical Center of Evansville, Evansville, IN, p. A201
FLETCHALL, Terry L., Administrator, Santiam Memorial Hospital, Stayton, OR, p. A516
FLETCHER, John, Chief Executive Officer, Patrick B. Harris Psychiatric Hospital, Anderson, SC, p. A546
FLETCHER, John R., Vice President and Chief Operating Officer, Hazleton General Hospital, Hazleton, PA, p. A525
FLETCHER, Kevin, Director Information Systems, Medical Center of McKinney, McKinney, TX, p. A616
FLETCHER, Michael, M.D. President Medical Staff, Hancock Regional Hospital, Greenfield, IN, p. A203
FLETCHER, Richard, Chief Operating Officer, Manatee Memorial Hospital, Bradenton, FL, p. A119
FLETCHER, Stephanie, Interim Chief Executive Officer, Berrien County Hospital, Nashville, GA, p. A157
FLETCHER, Steven, M.D. Chief of Staff, Baptist Health South Florida, Homestead Hospital, Homestead, FL, p. A125
FLETCHER–BROZENA, Jackie
Senior Vice President and Chief Operating Officer, Allied Services Rehabilitation Hospital, Scranton, PA, p. A537
Senior Vice President and Chief Operating Officer, John Heinz Institute of Rehabilitation Medicine, Wilkes–Barre, PA, p. A541
FLICKEMA, James D., VP, Professional & Ancillary Services, Otsego Memorial Hospital, Gaylord, MI, p. A313
FLICKINGER, Kenneth E., System Chief Financial Officer, Chester County Hospital, West Chester, PA, p. A541
FLINN, Charles, Chief Operating Officer, Kingston Hospital, Kingston, NY, p. A428
FLINT, Jennifer, Chief Financial Officer, Laird Hospital, Union, MS, p. A353
FLINT, Jr., Loring S., M.D. Senior Vice President Medical Affairs, Baystate Medical Center, Springfield, MA, p. A304
FLIPPO, Taya, Director, Mercy Hospital Berryville, Berryville, AR, p. A42
FLIS, James D., Chief Financial Officer, Livengrin Foundation, Bensalem, PA, p. A518
FLODEN, Scott, Chief Executive Officer, Promise Hospital of Phoenix, Mesa, AZ, p. A34
FLOOD, James, Director Information Systems, Claxton–Hepburn Medical Center, Ogdensburg, NY, p. A439
FLOOD, Nathan A., Chief Executive Officer, Hereford Regional Medical Center, Hereford, TX, p. A603

© 2012 AHA Guide Index of Health Care Professionals **A811**

FLOOD, Rebecca L., R.N. Senior Vice President Nursing, New York Methodist Hospital,, NY, p. A435

FLORENTINE, Erich
Chief People Officer, South Jersey Healthcare – Elmer Hospital, Elmer, NJ, p. A404
Chief People Officer, South Jersey Healthcare – Regional Medical Center, Vineland, NJ, p. A411

FLORENTINO, Paul, M.D. Director Medical Services, Walter Reed National Military Medical Center, Bethesda, MD, p. A290

FLORES, Cathy, R.N. Administrator, Chowchilla District Memorial Hospital, Chowchilla, CA, p. A57

FLORES, Christopher, Chief Financial Officer, Havasu Regional Medical Center, Lake Havasu City, AZ, p. A33

FLORES, Debbie, Chief Executive Officer, Banner Del E. Webb Medical Center, Sun City West, AZ, p. A39

FLORES, Debra A., MS, President and Administrator, Sentara CarePlex Hospital, Hampton, VA, p. A649

FLORES Jr., Ernest, Administrator, Dimmit County Memorial Hospital, Carrizo Springs, TX, p. A586

FLORES, Gerardo, R.N. Chief Operating Officer and Chief Nursing Officer, South Texas Regional Medical Center, Jourdanton, TX, p. A609

FLORES, Jeanne, Senior Vice President Human Resources and Organizational Development, Cedars–Sinai Medical Center, Los Angeles, CA, p. A69

FLORES–RAMIREZ, Rosie, Director Fiscal Services, Lanterman Developmental Center, Pomona, CA, p. A80

FLORKOWSKI, Doug, Chief Executive Officer, Lawrence County Memorial Hospital, Lawrenceville, IL, p. A186

FLOURNOY, Barbara, Administrator, Christus Dubuis Hospital of Port Arthur, Port Arthur, TX, p. A621

FLOWE, Kenneth, M.D. Chief Medical Officer, Person Memorial Hospital, Roxboro, NC, p. A460

FLOWERS, Deborah, Director Human Resources, Monroe County Hospital, Forsyth, GA, p. A153

FLOWERS, LaChelle, Administrative Assistant Human Resources, Sparrow Specialty Hospital, Lansing, MI, p. A317

FLOWERS, Michael, Director Information Management, Calhoun–Liberty Hospital, Blountstown, FL, p. A118

FLOYD, Duane, Vice President Human Resources and Professional Services, Watertown Regional Medical Center, Watertown, WI, p. A692

FLOYD, Gary, M.D. Executive Vice President Medical Affairs and Chief Medical Officer, JPS Health Network, Fort Worth, TX, p. A599

FLOYD, Greg, Chief Executive Officer, Kindred Hospital Richmond, Richmond, VA, p. A655

FLOYD, Jacqueline, Chief Nursing Officer, HEALTHSOUTH Rehabilitation Hospital of Fort Smith, Fort Smith, AR, p. A45

FLOYD, Kay A., R.N. Chief Executive Officer, Monroe County Hospital, Forsyth, GA, p. A153

FLOYD, Kiley, Administrator, Osborne County Memorial Hospital, Osborne, KS, p. A240

FLOYD, Richard B., President and Chief Executive Officer, Sherman Hospital, Elgin, IL, p. A181

FLUEGGE, Carol, Chief Operating Officer, Mercy Suburban Hospital, Norristown, PA, p. A530

FLUTY, Lisa, Director Information Services, Central Baptist Hospital, Lexington, KY, p. A253

FLYNN, Brian, Chief Human Resources Officer, Veterans Affairs Northern Indiana Health Care System, Fort Wayne, IN, p. A202

FLYNN, Brian T., Chief Executive Officer, Palms of Pasadena Hospital, Saint Petersburg, FL, p. A138

FLYNN, James P., M.D. President Medical Staff, Southwestern Regional Medical Center, Tulsa, OK, p. A507

FLYNN, Kristin, Manager Human Resources, French Hospital Medical Center, San Luis Obispo, CA, p. A88

FLYNN, Loretta, Director Human Resources, Gulf Coast Medical Center, Wharton, TX, p. A634

FLYNN, Matthew J., Senior Vice President and Chief Financial Officer, Northwestern Lake Forest Hospital, Lake Forest, IL, p. A186

FLYNN, Timothy C., M.D. Chief of Staff, Shands at the University of Florida, Gainesville, FL, p. A124

FOARD, Mesa, Director Information technology, William S. Hall Psychiatric Institute, Columbia, SC, p. A548

FOELSCH, Paul, Vice President Information Services and Chief Information Officer, Mercy Iowa City, Iowa City, IA, p. A221

FOELSKE, Loren
Vice President Finance, Kishwaukee Community Hospital, DeKalb, IL, p. A180
Vice President Finance, Valley West Community Hospital, Sandwich, IL, p. A193

FOGG, Robert W., Director Finance, Lake Taylor Transitional Care Hospital, Norfolk, VA, p. A652

FOGLER, Richard, M.D. Chairman Surgery and Chief Medical Officer, Brookdale Hospital Medical Center,, NY, p. A431

FOJTASEK, Georgia R., President and Chief Executive Officer, Allegiance Health, Jackson, MI, p. A316

FOLAND, Mary Ann, Manager Human Resources, Clinton Memorial Hospital, Wilmington, OH, p. A491

FOLAND, Pamela, Director Human Resources, Cox Monett, Monett, MO, p. A365

FOLEY, Crystal, Director Human Resources, Little River Medical Center, Rockdale, TX, p. A623

FOLEY, Daniel, M.D. Vice President Medical Affairs, United Hospital, Saint Paul, MN, p. A339

FOLEY, James T., CPA Vice President and Chief Financial Officer, Shore Medical Center, Somers Point, NJ, p. A410

FOLEY, John, Chief Information Officer, Allegheny General Hospital, Pittsburgh, PA, p. A534

FOLEY, Leah, Director Human Resources, Huguley Memorial Medical Center, Fort Worth, TX, p. A598

FOLEY, Michael, M.D. Chief Medical Officer, North Okaloosa Medical Center, Crestview, FL, p. A121

FOLEY, Michael, Director Information Systems, Saint Francis Medical Center, Grand Island, NE, p. A384

FOLEY, Regina, R.N. Vice President Nursing and Operations, Ocean Medical Center, Brick Township, NJ, p. A402

FOLEY, Sean, M.D. Medical Director, St. Vincent Rehabilitation Hospital, Sherwood, AR, p. A51

FOLK, Jeffrey R., M.D. Vice President Medical Affairs and Chief Medical Officer, Piedmont Newnan Hospital, Newnan, GA, p. A157

FOLKS, David G., M.D. Chief Medical Officer, New Hampshire Hospital, Concord, NH, p. A397

FOLKWEIN, Charles
Vice President Ancillary Services, St. Elizabeth Boardman Health Center, Boardman, OH, p. A471
Senior Vice President Ancillary Services and Information Technology, St. Elizabeth Health Center, Youngstown, OH, p. A492
Vice President Ancillary Services, St. Joseph Health Center, Warren, OH, p. A490

FOLL, Gary R., Chief Financial Officer, Atchison Hospital, Atchison, KS, p. A230

FOLLARD, Cheyenne, Chief Financial Officer, Central Vermont Medical Center, Berlin, VT, p. A643

FOLSKE, Lance, Chief Operating Officer, Cumberland Hall Hospital, Hopkinsville, KY, p. A251

FOLSOM, Tom, Manager Information Systems, Millinocket Regional Hospital, Millinocket, ME, p. A284

FOLSON, Catherine, MSN Chief Nursing Officer, Select Specialty Hospital–Pontiac, Pontiac, MI, p. A321

FOLTZ, Jeffry E., R.N. Vice President for Nursing, St. Joseph's Medical Center, Yonkers, NY, p. A447

FOLTZ, JoAnn M., R.N. Chief Executive Officer, Sanford Wheaton Medical Center, Wheaton, MN, p. A341

FONDESSY, Terrence, M.D. Vice President Medical Affairs, ProMedica Fostoria Community Hospital, Fostoria, OH, p. A480

FONSECA, Jesus, M.D. Chief of Staff, Lea Regional Medical Center, Hobbs, NM, p. A416

FONSECA, Melinda, Associate Director Human Resources, Rancho Los Amigos National Rehabilitation Center, Downey, CA, p. A59

FONT, Stephen, Coordinator Information Systems, Rochester Psychiatric Center, Rochester, NY, p. A442

FONTAINE, Melissa, Chief Operating Officer, UAMS Medical Center, Little Rock, AR, p. A48

FONTENOT, Brandon, M.D. Chief of Staff, Mercy Regional Medical Center, Ville Platte, LA, p. A279

FONTENOT, Cathi E., M.D. Medical Director, Interim LSU Public Hospital, New Orleans, LA, p. A274

FONTENOT, H. Jerrel, M.D. Medical Director, Ouachita Community Hospital, West Monroe, LA, p. A279

FONTENOT, Michael, Interim Chief Financial Officer, Oakdale Community Hospital, Oakdale, LA, p. A275

FONTENOT, Teri G., FACHE President and Chief Executive Officer, Woman's Hospital, Baton Rouge, LA, p. A263

FONTENOT, Terry J., Chief Executive Officer, Texas Regional Medical Center, Sunnyvale, TX, p. A629

FONZE, Tony
Vice President Information Services and Chief Information Officer, Carondelet Heart & Vascular Institute, Tucson, AZ, p. A39
Chief Information Officer, Carondelet Holy Cross Hospital, Nogales, AZ, p. A34
Chief Information Officer, Carondelet Health Network, Carondelet St. Joseph's Hospital, Tucson, AZ, p. A39
Chief Information Officer, Carondelet St. Mary's Hospital, Tucson, AZ, p. A39

FONZIE, Juril, Director Human Resources, Helena Regional Medical Center, Helena, AR, p. A46

FOOTE, Donald E., Fiscal Officer, Veterans Affairs Medical Center, Wilkes-Barre, PA, p. A542

FOOTE, John, Chief Information Officer, Veterans Affairs Medical Center, Manchester, NH, p. A399

FOOTE, Mark, Chief Financial Officer, Madera Community Hospital, Madera, CA, p. A73

FORAND, Angela, Director, William S. Hall Psychiatric Institute, Columbia, SC, p. A548

FORBES, Brenda, Controller, HEALTHSOUTH Rehabilitation Hospital of Fort Smith, Fort Smith, AR, p. A45

FORBES, Ronald O., M.D. Medical Director, Central State Hospital, Petersburg, VA, p. A653

FORBES–DANIELS, Kim, Chief Financial Officer, North Vista Hospital, North Las Vegas, NV, p. A394

FORD, Cindy, R.N. Chief Nursing Officer, Harrisburg Medical Center, Harrisburg, IL, p. A183

FORD, Connie, Vice President Human Resources, Indiana University Health La Porte Hospital, La Porte, IN, p. A206

FORD, Cora, Assistant Vice President Human Resources, Our Lady of the Lake Regional Medical Center, Baton Rouge, LA, p. A262

FORD, Douglas, M.D. Chief of Staff, Broward Health North, Deerfield Beach, FL, p. A122

FORD, James, Director Human Resources, Summit Medical Center, Van Buren, AR, p. A52

FORD, LaDonna, M.D. Medical Director, E. A. Conway Medical Center, Monroe, LA, p. A273

FORD, LeeAnn, Director Human Resources and Imaging, The Physicians Centre Hospital, Bryan, TX, p. A586

FORD Jr., Lloyd F., FACHE Chief Executive Officer, Riverview Regional Medical Center, Gadsden, AL, p. A20

FORD, Mary, Vice President and Chief Information Officer, Lakeland Regional Medical Center, Lakeland, FL, p. A128

FORD, Mike, Vice President Human Resources, Floyd Memorial Hospital and Health Services, New Albany, IN, p. A209

FORD, Tammy, Executive Director Human Resources, Greene County Medical Center, Jefferson, IA, p. A222

FORD, Timothy R., Chief Executive Officer, Blowing Rock Hospital, Blowing Rock, NC, p. A449

FORDE, Steve, Chief Financial Officer, Nelson County Health System, McVille, ND, p. A467

FORDHAM, Karen, Vice President Chief Operating Officer, Huron Valley–Sinai Hospital, Commerce Township, MI, p. A310

FORDYCE, Carol, Director of Patient Care Services, Sullivan County Memorial Hospital, Milan, MO, p. A365

FORDYCE, Michael L., President and Chief Executive Officer, Craig Hospital, Englewood, CO, p. A100

FORE, Larry T., Controller, Great Bend Regional Hospital, Great Bend, KS, p. A233

FOREMAN, Chris, Director, Phoebe Worth Medical Center, Sylvester, GA, p. A160

FOREMAN, Lee Ann
Vice President Human Resources, Mississippi Baptist Medical Center, Jackson, MS, p. A348
Vice President Human Resources, Mississippi Hospital for Restorative Care, Jackson, MS, p. A348

FORESE, Laura, M.D. Senior Vice President and Chief Medical Officer, New York–Presbyterian Hospital, New York, NY, p. A436

FORET, Robert, Chief Financial Officer, Yoakum Community Hospital, Yoakum, TX, p. A636

FORGE, Brenda J., Vice President Human Resources, St. Joseph Regional Medical Center, Lewiston, ID, p. A169

FORGEY, Roger, President and Chief Executive Officer, Erlanger at Hutcheson, Fort Oglethorpe, GA, p. A153

FORGEY, Warren, Executive Vice President Fiscal Services and Business Development, Schneck Medical Center, Seymour, IN, p. A211

FORGUES, Dan, Chief Financial Officer, Henrietta D. Goodall Hospital, Sanford, ME, p. A285

FORKEL, Todd, President and Chief Executive Officer, Avera St. Luke's Hospital, Aberdeen, SD, p. A555

FORKNER, Christine, Executive Vice President and Chief Financial Officer, National Jewish Health, Denver, CO, p. A99

FORMAN, Stuart, M.D. Chief Professional Services, Connecticut Valley Hospital, Middletown, CT, p. A110

FORMBY, Mary Beth, Chief Financial Officer, Lakewood Regional Medical Center, Lakewood, CA, p. A67

FORNERIS, Lori, R.N. Chief Clinical Officer, Loring Hospital, Sac City, IA, p. A226

FORNIER–JOHNSON, Michelle, Group Vice President Human Resources, St. Anthony Hospital, Lakewood, CO, p. A103

FORNOFF, Gerald A., Interim Chief Executive Officer, River Parishes Hospital, La Place, LA, p. A269

FORREST, Brian
Director Human Resources, Arnot Ogden Medical Center, Elmira, NY, p. A425
Vice President Human Resources, St. Joseph's Hospital, Elmira, NY, p. A426

FORREST, Jr., James L., Chief Financial Officer, Southeast Colorado Hospital District, Springfield, CO, p. A105

FORREST, Mary Helen, R.N. Chief Nursing Officer, UAMS Medical Center, Little Rock, AR, p. A48

Index of Health Care Professionals

Index of Health Care Professionals / Franke

FRANKE, Paul, M.D
Vice President Medical Affairs, Covenant Medical Center, Waterloo, IA, p. A228
Vice President Medical Affairs, Sartori Memorial Hospital, Cedar Falls, IA, p. A215
FRANKEL, Michele, Associate Executive Director Finance, Glen Cove Hospital, Glen Cove, NY, p. A426
FRANKENSTEIN, Richard, M.D. Vice President and Chief Medical Officer, Henry Mayo Newhall Memorial Hospital, Valencia, CA, p. A94
FRANKLIN, Barry L., Executive Vice President and Chief Financial Officer, Parma Community General Hospital, Parma, OH, p. A487
FRANKLIN, Clay, Chief Executive Officer, Plaza Medical Center of Fort Worth, Fort Worth, TX, p. A599
FRANKLIN, Hope, Coordinator Human Resources, Select Specialty Hospital–North Knoxville, Knoxville, TN, p. A568
FRANKLIN, James P., Administrator, Calhoun Health Services, Calhoun City, MS, p. A344
FRANKLIN, Michael A., FACHE President and Chief Executive Officer, Atlantic General Hospital, Berlin, MD, p. A289
FRANKLIN, Vicki L., Senior Vice President and Chief Operating Officer, Lake Regional Health System, Osage Beach, MO, p. A366
FRANKO, Stephen
Vice President Finance and Chief Financial Officer, Regional Hospital of Scranton, Scranton, PA, p. A538
Chief Financial Officer, Special Care Hospital, Nanticoke, PA, p. A530
Chief Financial Officer, Tyler Memorial Hospital, Tunkhannock, PA, p. A539
FRANKS, Charles, Chief Human Resources, Veterans Affairs Medical Center, Cleveland, OH, p. A476
FRANKS, Dennis, Vice President Operations, Doctors' Hospital of Michigan, Pontiac, MI, p. A320
FRANKS, Dennis, FACHE Chief Executive Officer, Neosho Memorial Regional Medical Center, Chanute, KS, p. A231
FRANSON, John K., M.D. Chief Medical Staff, Caribou Memorial Hospital and Living Center, Soda Springs, ID, p. A170
FRANTZ, Vincent, M.D. Chief of Staff, Plumas District Hospital, Quincy, CA, p. A81
FRANZ, Jerome, M.D. Chief Medical Staff, St. Luke's Hospital, San Francisco, CA, p. A87
FRANZ, Thomas, M.D. Medical Director, HEALTHSOUTH Harmarville Rehabilitation Hospital, Pittsburgh, PA, p. A534
FRANZBLAU, David R., M.D. Chief Medical Officer, Mercy St. Vincent Medical Center, Toledo, OH, p. A489
FRANZELLA, Susan, Human Resource Business Partner, San Jose Medical Center, San Jose, CA, p. A88
FRARDO, Virgil, M.D. Medical Director, HEALTHSOUTH Rehabilitation Hospital–Wichita Falls, Wichita Falls, TX, p. A635
FRASCA, Edith, Controller and Chief Financial Officer, The Pavilion, Champaign, IL, p. A175
FRASCELLA, Louis J., President and Chief Executive Officer, Lake Shore Health Care Center, Irving, NY, p. A427
FRASER, James, Chief Financial Officer, Ferrell Hospital, Eldorado, IL, p. A180
FRASER, John M., President and Chief Executive Officer, Nebraska Methodist Health System, Inc., Omaha, NE, p. B92
FRATE, Amy, Director of Nursing, Red River Hospital, Wichita Falls, TX, p. A635
FRATER, Chris, Chief Financial Officer, Lighthouse Care Center of Conway, Conway, SC, p. A549
FRATZKE, Mark, R.N. Chief Nursing Officer and Chief Operating Officer, Mayo Clinic Health System in Saint James, Saint James, MN, p. A338
FRAUENHOFER, Chris, Vice President Finance, Alice Hyde Medical Center, Malone, NY, p. A429
FRAUENPREIS, Kurt, M.D. Chief Medical Staff, Bear Valley Community Hospital, Big Bear Lake, CA, p. A55
FRAZIER, Amy, Supervisor Management Information Systems, Wetzel County Hospital, New Martinsville, WV, p. A674
FRAZIER, Derrick A., Chief Executive Officer, Southwest Georgia Regional Medical Center, Cuthbert, GA, p. A150
FRAZIER III, James P., Chief Executive Officer, Teche Regional Medical Center, Morgan City, LA, p. A273
FRAZIER, Joel L., M.D. Medical Director, Orthopedic Hospital, Oklahoma City, OK, p. A502
FRAZIER, Lee, FACHE Chief Executive Officer, St. Vincent Rehabilitation Hospital, Sherwood, AR, p. A51
FREAS, Mary Ann, Vice President and Chief Financial Officer, Southwest General Health Center, Middleburg Heights, OH, p. A485
FREDERIC, Donald J., FACHE Chief Executive Officer, Saint Mary's Regional Medical Center, Russellville, AR, p. A51
FREDERICK, Brenda, Director Human Resources, Laurel Ridge Treatment Center, San Antonio, TX, p. A625
FREDERICK, Gretchen A., R.N. Director Patient Care Services, Buffalo Hospital, Buffalo, MN, p. A329
FREDERICK, Lynn
Administrator, Mayo Clinic – Methodist Hospital, Rochester, MN, p. A338
Administrator, Mayo Clinic – Saint Marys Hospital, Rochester, MN, p. A338
FREDERICKS, Jack, Vice President Human Resources, Little Falls Hospital, Little Falls, NY, p. A428
FREDERICKS, Raymond F., President and Chief Executive Officer, JFK Health System, Edison, NJ, p. B74
FREDERICKS, Raymond F., President and CEO, JFK Medical Center, Edison, NJ, p. A403
FREDERICKSON, Kathy, Information Systems Site Lead, Sutter Delta Medical Center, Antioch, CA, p. A53
FREDETTE, Beth, Chief Information Officer, Children's Medical Center, Dayton, OH, p. A478
FREDRICH, Nancy, R.N. Chief Clinical Officer, Cooper County Memorial Hospital, Boonville, MO, p. A356
FREDRICK, Rick, Director Information Technology, Cottage Hospital, Woodsville, NH, p. A400
FREDRICKSON, Dennis, Chief Financial Officer, Phillips County Hospital, Phillipsburg, KS, p. A241
FREDRICKSON, Kelley, Director Information Services, Plaza Medical Center of Fort Worth, Fort Worth, TX, p. A599
FREDRICKSON, Mark A., M.D. Medical Director, HEALTHSOUTH Rehabilitation Hospital Midland–Odessa, Midland, TX, p. A616
FREEBERG, Wayne, Chief Information Officer, Cooley Dickinson Hospital, Northampton, MA, p. A303
FREEBURG, Rick, Chief Executive Officer, Baptist Health South Florida, Mariners Hospital, Tavernier, FL, p. A142
FREEBURN, Mark, Chief Executive Officer, HEALTHSOUTH Rehabilitation Hospital of Mechanicsburg, Mechanicsburg, PA, p. A529
FREED, David H., President and Chief Executive Officer, Nyack Hospital, Nyack, NY, p. A438
FREED, Glenn, D.O. Medical Director, St. Luke's Hospital – Miners Campus, Coaldale, PA, p. A520
FREED, Nancy, Chief Financial Officer, Seiling Community Hospital, Seiling, OK, p. A504
FREED, Stuart, M.D. Medical Director, Wenatchee Valley Hospital, Wenatchee, WA, p. A669
FREED–SIGURDSSON, Anna, M.D. Medical Director, Reliant Rehabilitation Hospital Dallas, Dallas, TX, p. A592
FREEDMAN, Barry R., President and Chief Executive Officer, Albert Einstein Healthcare Network, Philadelphia, PA, p. B7
FREEDMAN, Barry R., President and Chief Executive Officer, Einstein Medical Center Philadelphia, Philadelphia, PA, p. A532
FREEDMAN, Kenneth, M.D. Chief Medical Officer, Lemuel Shattuck Hospital, Jamaica Plain, MA, p. A301
FREEHOF, Leonard, Chief Executive Officer and Managing Director, Spring Valley Hospital Medical Center, Las Vegas, NV, p. A394
FREEL, Christopher, Chief Information Technologist, Okanogan Douglas District Hospital, Brewster, WA, p. A660
FREELAND, R. Alan, M.D. Chief Clinical Officer, Twin Valley Behavioral Healthcare, Columbus, OH, p. A477
FREEMAN, Amy E., President and Chief Executive Officer, Providence Hospital, Washington, DC, p. A116
FREEMAN, Brian, Vice President of Operations, Stanly Regional Medical Center, Albemarle, NC, p. A448
FREEMAN, Deanna, Administrator and Chief Executive Officer, Rawlins County Health Center, Atwood, KS, p. A230
FREEMAN, Donald, President and Chief Executive Officer, Preferred Management Corporation, Shawnee, OK, p. B102
FREEMAN, Elizabeth Joyce, Director, Veterans Affairs Palo Alto Health Care System, Palo Alto, CA, p. A79
FREEMAN, Jerry, Chief, Human Resources Management Services, Durham Veterans Affairs Medical Center, Durham, NC, p. A452
FREEMAN, Kimberlee, R.N. Vice President Patient Care Services and Chief Nursing Officer, Wayne Hospital, Greenville, OH, p. A481
FREEMAN, Louella, Chief Nursing Officer, Salinas Valley Memorial Healthcare System, Salinas, CA, p. A84
FREEMAN, Marianne, Vice President Human Resources, Rockdale Medical Center, Conyers, GA, p. A150
FREEMAN, Michael, Director Human Resources, Huhukam Memorial Hospital, Sacaton, AZ, p. A37
FREEMAN, Robert, Director Human Resources, Sparks Regional Medical Center, Fort Smith, AR, p. A45
FREEMAN, Tim, Administrator, Dubuis Hospital of Beaumont, Beaumont, TX, p. A583
FREEMAN, Wade, Regional Site Director, Mountain View Regional Medical Center, Norton, VA, p. A653
FREER, Carol V., M.D. Chief Medical Officer, Penn State Milton S. Hershey Medical Center, Hershey, PA, p. A525
FREESE–DECKER, Christina, President, Spectrum Health United Hospital, Greenville, MI, p. A314
FREIER, Toby, President, New Ulm Medical Center, New Ulm, MN, p. A336
FREIMARK, Jeffrey P., Chief Executive Officer, Miami Jewish Home and Hospital for Aged, Miami, FL, p. A131
FREITAG, Donald, M.D. Chief Medical Officer, Lynn County Hospital District, Tahoka, TX, p. A630
FRELING, Eric, M.D. Director Medical Staff Affairs, Memorial Hospital West, Pembroke Pines, FL, p. A135
FRENCH, Dean O., M.D. Chief of Staff, Faith Regional Health Services, Norfolk, NE, p. A386
FRENCH III, George E., FACHE Chief Executive Officer, Minden Medical Center, Minden, LA, p. A273
FRENCH, Holly, Chief Financial Officer, Newman Regional Health, Emporia, KS, p. A232
FRENCH, Jennifer, Director Organizational Quality, St. Vincent Clay Hospital, Brazil, IN, p. A198
FRENCH, William Chad, Chief Executive Officer, Kentucky River Medical Center, Jackson, KY, p. A252
FRERICHS, Craig, Chief Information Technology Service, Veterans Affairs Medical Center, Grand Junction, CO, p. A102
FRESH, John, Vice President Human Resources, Miners Medical Center, Hastings, PA, p. A524
FRESQUEZ, Juan, Chief Operating Officer, Houston Northwest Medical Center, Houston, TX, p. A604
FREUDENBERGER, Joe, Chief Executive Officer, OakBend Medical Center, Richmond, TX, p. A622
FREUND, Donna S., MSN Chief Nursing Officer, DeKalb Health, Auburn, IN, p. A197
FREW, Anne, Chief Executive Officer, Select Specialty Hospital–Erie, Erie, PA, p. A523
FREY, Jack, Business Manager, Greystone Park Psychiatric Hospital, Morris Plains, NJ, p. A406
FREY, Jeff, Business Administrator, Andrew McFarland Mental Health Center, Springfield, IL, p. A194
FREY, Mark A., President and Chief Executive Officer, Alexian Brothers Health System, Arlington Heights, IL, p. B8
FREY, Paul, Director Information Technology Applications, Indiana Orthopaedic Hospital, Indianapolis, IN, p. A204
FREY, Rachel, Director Human Resources, Athens–Limestone Hospital, Athens, AL, p. A16
FREYER, Mary, Chief Operating Officer, Little Company of Mary Hospital and Health Care Centers, Evergreen Park, IL, p. A181
FREYHOFER, Cornelia Sue, M.D. Medical Director, Moses Ludington Hospital, Ticonderoga, NY, p. A444
FREYMULLER, Robert S., Chief Executive Officer, Summerlin Hospital Medical Center, Las Vegas, NV, p. A394
FREYSINGER, Edward E., Chief Executive Officer, Providence Hood River Memorial Hospital, Hood River, OR, p. A511
FREYTAG, Peter, Senior Vice President Finance and Chief Financial Officer, Bristol Hospital, Bristol, CT, p. A108
FRIBERG, Deborah G.
President, Columbia St. Mary's Ozaukee Hospital, Mequon, WI, p. A686
President, Sacred Heart Rehabilitation Institute, Milwaukee, WI, p. A687
FRICK, Mark P., Vice President Human Resources, UPMC McKeesport, McKeesport, PA, p. A528
FRICK, Mary Jo, Director Finance, St. Catherine's Rehabilitation Hospital, North Miami, FL, p. A133
FRICKS, Tom, Interim Senior Vice President of Information Technology, Sacred Heart Medical Center at RiverBend, Springfield, OR, p. A516
FRIDOVICH, Mark, Ph.D. Administrator, Hawaii State Hospital, Kaneohe, HI, p. A164
FRIED, Guy, M.D. Chief Medical Officer, Magee Rehabilitation Hospital, Philadelphia, PA, p. A533
FRIED, Jeffrey M., FACHE President and Chief Executive Officer, Beebe Medical Center, Lewes, DE, p. A114
FRIEDBERG, Robert, President, Delnor Hospital, Geneva, IL, p. A182
FRIEDELL, Benjamin, Vice President Medical Affairs, Aurelia Osborn Fox Memorial Hospital, Oneonta, NY, p. A439
FRIEDEN, Robert
Vice President Information Systems, Genesis Medical Center, Illini Campus, Silvis, IL, p. A193
Vice President Information Systems, Genesis Medical Center–Davenport, Davenport, IA, p. A217
FRIEDENBACH, Daryl, Director Fiscal Services, Floyd Valley Hospital, Le Mars, IA, p. A222
FRIEDMAN, Greg, Director Information Technology, Children's Hospital of Richmond, Richmond, VA, p. A654
FRIEDMAN, Jonathan, Public Affairs Officer, Captain James A. Lovell Federal Health Care Center, North Chicago, IL, p. A189
FRIEDMAN, Lloyd, M.D. Vice President Medical Affairs and Chief Operating Officer, Milford Hospital, Milford, CT, p. A110
FRIEDMAN, Michael A., M.D. President and Chief Executive Officer, City of Hope's Helford Clinical Research Hospital, Duarte, CA, p. A59
FRIEDMAN, Peter, President and Chief Executive Officer, Newport Specialty Hospital, Tustin, CA, p. A93

**A814** Index of Health Care Professionals

Index of Health Care Professionals / Futrell

Index of Health Care Professionals


FRIEDMAN, Steven G., M.D. Interim Chief Medical Officer and Chair, Department of Surgery, New York Downtown Hospital, New York, NY, p. A435
FRIEDMAN, Steven H., Ph.D. Executive Vice President, Methodist Hospital of Chicago, Chicago, IL, p. A176
FRIEDRICH III, Daniel J., Chief Executive Officer, Blake Medical Center, Bradenton, FL, p. A119
FRIEL, Donald F., Executive Vice President, Holy Redeemer Hospital and Medical Center, Meadowbrook, PA, p. A528
FRIEL, John P., Chief Executive Officer, Oak Valley Hospital District, Oakdale, CA, p. A77
FRIELING, Jeff
Vice President Information Systems, Camden General Hospital, Camden, TN, p. A562
Vice President and Chief Information Officer, Jackson–Madison County General Hospital, Jackson, TN, p. A567
Chief Information Officer, Pathways of Tennessee, Jackson, TN, p. A567
FRIELING, Morris J., Chief Financial Officer, University of California, Irvine Healthcare, Orange, CA, p. A78
FRIEND, Lori
Director Human Resources, Integris Marshall County Medical Center, Madill, OK, p. A498
Human Resources Director, Integris Seminole Medical Center, Seminole, OK, p. A504
FRIER, Nancy, Chief Financial Officer, Eastern Oklahoma Medical Center, Poteau, OK, p. A503
FRIES, Bob, Director Fiscal Services, Colorado Mental Health Institute at Fort Logan, Denver, CO, p. A99
FRIES, Linda, Director Personnel, Ed Fraser Memorial Hospital and Baker Community Health Center, MacClenny, FL, p. A129
FRIESEN, Carol, Chief Executive Officer, Crete Area Medical Center, Crete, NE, p. A383
FRIESEN, Dale L., Chief Financial Officer, CareLink of Jackson, Jackson, MI, p. A316
FRIESEN, Lynette, Manager Human Resources, Henderson Health Care Services, Henderson, NE, p. A384
FRIESEN, Nancy, Chief Financial Officer, New River Medical Center, Monticello, MN, p. A335
FRIESEN, Quinton J., Executive Vice President and Chief Operating Officer, Greenwich Hospital, Greenwich, CT, p. A109
FRIGEN, Karen, Director Human Resources, Shriners Hospitals for Children, Twin Cities, Minneapolis, MN, p. A335
FRIGON, Shelby, Chief Financial Officer, Saint Luke's South Hospital, Overland Park, KS, p. A241
FRIGY, Alan, M.D. President Medical Staff, Pana Community Hospital, Pana, IL, p. A190
FRISBEE, Kent, Director Human Resources, Highlands Medical Center, Sparta, TN, p. A576
FRISBIE, Dawn, Chief Executive Officer, Select Specialty Hospital–Saginaw, Saginaw, MI, p. A322
FRITSCH, Phyllis, Administrator, Upland Hills Health, Dodgeville, WI, p. A680
FRITSCH, William, M.D. Medical Director, Landmark Hospital, Cape Girardeau, MO, p. A356
FRITSCHE, Jeff, Chief Financial Officer, Silverton Hospital, Silverton, OR, p. A515
FRITTS, Doris, R.N. Executive Director, Same Day Surgery Center, Rapid City, SD, p. A559
FRITTS, Jack, Vice President Finance and Chief Financial Officer, Grinnell Regional Medical Center, Grinnell, IA, p. A220
FRITTS, Robert
Chief Financial Officer, Grace Hospital, Morganton, NC, p. A458
Sr. Vice President, Chief Financial Officer, Valdese General Hospital, Valdese, NC, p. A462
FRITZ, John, D.O. Vice President Medical Affairs, Avera St. Luke's Hospital, Aberdeen, SD, p. A555
FRITZ, Thomas M., Chief Executive Officer, St. Luke's Rehabilitation Institute, Spokane, WA, p. A667
FRIZZELL, Neil, Chief Financial Officer, Freeman Regional Health Services, Freeman, SD, p. A557
FROCHTZWAJG, Stanley, M.D. Chief Medical Officer, Community Memorial Health System, Ventura, CA, p. A94
FROEBE, Tim, Vice President Human Resources, Mary Rutan Hospital, Bellefontaine, OH, p. A470
FROEMKE, Janet, Human Resources Officer, Lisbon Area Health Services, Lisbon, ND, p. A467
FROH, Chris, Senior Coordinator Human Resources, Select Specialty Hospital–Milwaukee, Milwaukee, WI, p. A687
FROHNHOFER, Erin J., Director Human Resources, Southwood Psychiatric Hospital, Pittsburgh, PA, p. A535
FROIMSON, Mark, President, Euclid Hospital, Euclid, OH, p. A480
FROIO, Ann M., Interim Chief Executive Officer, Arizona State Hospital, Phoenix, AZ, p. A35
FROISLAND, Jeffrey R., Chief Financial Officer, Mayo Clinic Hospital, Phoenix, AZ, p. A36
FROM, Leland, M.D. Vice President Medical Affairs, Beloit Health System, Beloit, WI, p. A679
FROMHOLD, John A., Chief Executive Officer, Hackensack University Medical Center Mountainside, Montclair, NJ, p. A406
FROMM, Robert, M.D. Senior Vice President and Chief Medical Officer, Maricopa Integrated Health System, Phoenix, AZ, p. A36
FROMMELT, William, Director Operations and Finance, River Falls Area Hospital, River Falls, WI, p. A690
FROSCH, James E., Director Finance, Texas Health Harris Methodist Hospital Cleburne, Cleburne, TX, p. A587
FROSCH, Kevin, Chief Financial Officer, Medina Regional Hospital, Hondo, TX, p. A603
FROST, Eric, Associate Vice President Human Resources, Upstate University Hospital, Syracuse, NY, p. A444
FROST, Joan, R.N. Chief Operating Officer/Chief Nursing Officer, Mercy Hospital Washington, Washington, MO, p. A372
FROST, Sarah, Associate Hospital Administrator, University of Arizona Medical Center – University Campus, Tucson, AZ, p. A40
FROST–KUNNEN, Jackie, Senior Vice President Operations, Mercy Medical Center–Des Moines, Des Moines, IA, p. A218
FRUGE, Janie, Chief Operating Officer and Chief Nursing Officer, West Calcasieu Cameron Hospital, Sulphur, LA, p. A278
FRUM, Judy, R.N. Chief Nursing Officer, Memorial Hospital Pembroke, Pembroke Pines, FL, p. A135
FRUM, R. David
President, Bridgton Hospital, Bridgton, ME, p. A282
President, Rumford Hospital, Rumford, ME, p. A285
FRY, Kenneth, Chief Financial Officer, Saint Alphonsus Regional Medical Center, Boise, ID, p. A166
FRY, Patrick E., Chief Executive Officer, Sutter Health, Sacramento, CA, p. B125
FRYE, Charles, Director Human Resources, Memorial Hospital of Sweetwater County, Rock Springs, WY, p. A697
FRYE, Darren, Manager, McLaren Bay Special Care, Bay City, MI, p. A308
FRYE Jr., Edward R., Chief Executive Officer, Clarendon Memorial Hospital, Manning, SC, p. A552
FRYE Jr., John W., Chief Executive Officer, Madera Community Hospital, Madera, CA, p. A73
FRYE, Kelly D., Director Human Resources, Montgomery General Hospital, Montgomery, WV, p. A673
FRYE, Terri, Manager Information Systems, Weston County Health Services, Newcastle, WY, p. A697
FUCCI, Thomas, Chief Operating Officer, Saint Vincent Health Center, Erie, PA, p. A523
FUCHS, Brian P., Chief Fiscal Service, James H. Quillen Veterans Affairs Medical Center, Mountain Home, TN, p. A572
FUCHS, Jonathan, Chief Information Officer, DeWitt Hospital, De Witt, AR, p. A44
FUCILE, Joanne, R.N. Vice President Patient Care Services, Spaulding Hospital for Continuing Medical Care North Shore, Salem, MA, p. A304
FUEHRER, Susan, Director, Veterans Affairs Medical Center, Cleveland, OH, p. A476
FUENTES, Frances, Coordinator Human Resources, HEALTHSOUTH Rehabilitation Hospital, San Juan, PR, p. A703
FUENTES Jr., Miguel A., President and Chief Executive Officer, Bronx–Lebanon Hospital Center Health Care System,, NY, p. A431
FUERSTENBERG, Donna, Fiscal Chief, Veterans Affairs Medical Center, Sheridan, WY, p. A697
FUGATTE, Cheryl, Vice President and Chief Nursing Officer, Jewish Hospital, Louisville, KY, p. A254
FUGAZY, Christopher, Chief Operating Officer, Jacobi Medical Center,, NY, p. A433
FUGITT, Kathy, Chief Information Officer, Ozark Health Medical Center, Clinton, AR, p. A43
FUHRMAN, Bradley, M.D. Physician in Chief, El Paso Children's Hospital, El Paso, TX, p. A596
FUHRMAN, Dennis, Vice President Finance, Essentia Health Fargo, Fargo, ND, p. A465
FUHS, Veronica, Chief Executive Officer, Lucas County Health Center, Chariton, IA, p. A216
FUJINAKA, Jason, Manager Information System, Wahiawa General Hospital, Wahiawa, HI, p. A165
FULCHER, Cathe, Superintendent, Evansville State Hospital, Evansville, IN, p. A201
FULKERSON, Judy, Director Human Resources, Greenview Regional Hospital, Bowling Green, KY, p. A248
FULKERSON, Richard, Director Fiscal Services, Shriners Hospitals for Children, Springfield, Springfield, MA, p. A305
FULKS, Gerald N., President and Chief Executive Officer, West Georgia Health, La Grange, GA, p. A155
FULKS, Pam, R.N. Chief Nursing Officer, Gila Regional Medical Center, Silver City, NM, p. A418
FULL, James M., FACHE President and Chief Executive Officer, Memorial Healthcare, Owosso, MI, p. A320
FULLBRIGHT, Gary D., Comptroller, Citizens Memorial Hospital, Bolivar, MO, p. A355
FULLER, Cheryl, Director Information Resources, Kansas Neurological Institute, Topeka, KS, p. A244
FULLER, Dale, Vice President and Chief Information Officer, Altoona Regional Health System, Altoona, PA, p. A517
FULLER, David W., Chief Executive Officer, North Okaloosa Medical Center, Crestview, FL, p. A121
FULLER, Debbie, Director Health Information Systems and Chief Information Officer, Doctors Medical Center, Modesto, CA, p. A75
FULLER, Jane, Director Human Resources, AMG Specialty Hospital–Lafayette Regional Campus, Lafayette, LA, p. A270
FULLER, Jill, Ph.D. President and Chief Executive Officer, Prairie Lakes Healthcare System, Watertown, SD, p. A560
FULLER, Lexie, Controller, Specialty Hospital of Meridian, Meridian, MS, p. A350
FULLER, Robert, Executive Vice President and Chief Operating Officer, Downey Regional Medical Center, Downey, CA, p. A59
FULTON, Lorna, Director Human Resources, Vibra Hospital of Denver, Thornton, CO, p. A106
FULTON, Lynn, Chief Executive Officer, Kewanee Hospital, Kewanee, IL, p. A186
FUNDERBURG, Michelle, Director Human Resources, Stephens Memorial Hospital, Breckenridge, TX, p. A584
FUNDERBURK, Mark, Executive Vice President and Administrator, University Medical Center, Lubbock, TX, p. A614
FUNG, Adrian, Director Information Systems, University Medical Center, Lebanon, TN, p. A569
FUNK, Gordon, Chief Executive Officer, Summit Surgical, LLC, Hutchinson, KS, p. A235
FUNK, Luann, Administrative Assistant and Manager Human Resources, Pana Community Hospital, Pana, IL, p. A190
FUNKHOUSER, Krisy L., Manager Human Resources, Willapa Harbor Hospital, South Bend, WA, p. A667
FUNKHOUSER, Lana, Vice President Human Resources, Indiana University Health West Hospital, Avon, IN, p. A197
FUQUA, David, Director Human Resources Management, LSU Medical Center–University Hospital, Shreveport, LA, p. A277
FUQUA, David G., Chief Executive Officer, Massac Memorial Hospital, Metropolis, IL, p. A188
FUQUA, Leon, Assistant Administrator, Wise Regional Health System, Decatur, TX, p. A593
FUREY, Warren, M.D. Vice President Medical Affairs, Mercy Hospital and Medical Center, Chicago, IL, p. A176
FURGURSON, Carol, Chief Operating Officer, Saint Louise Regional Hospital, Gilroy, CA, p. A63
FURLAN, Matthew
Chief Operating Officer, Appleton Medical Center, Appleton, WI, p. A678
Chief Operating Officer, Theda Clark Medical Center, Neenah, WI, p. A687
FURLONG, Marian M., R.N. Chief Executive Officer, Hudson Hospital, Hudson, WI, p. A683
FURLOW, Pete, Director Information Technology Services, Northeast Alabama Regional Medical Center, Anniston, AL, p. A15
FURMAN, John, Director Human Resources, Val Verde Regional Medical Center, Del Rio, TX, p. A593
FURMAN, Keith A., Chief Executive Officer, Lakeland Behavioral Health System, Springfield, MO, p. A371
FURNAS, David, Chief Information Officer, Gila Regional Medical Center, Silver City, NM, p. A418
FURNISS, Scott, Senior Vice President and Chief Financial Officer, Saint Agnes Hospital, Baltimore, MD, p. A288
FURRER, Susan, PsyD Acting Chief Operating Officer and Executive Director Behavioral Research and Training Institute, University of Medicine and Dentistry of New Jersey, University Behavioral Healthcare, Piscataway, NJ, p. A408
FUSCHILLO, Ronald, Chief Information Officer, Englewood Hospital and Medical Center, Englewood, NJ, p. A404
FUSCO, Kevin, Chief Operating Officer, Broward Health North, Deerfield Beach, FL, p. A122
FUSELIER, Gerald, Chief Operating Officer, Savoy Medical Center, Mamou, LA, p. A272
FUSELIER, Michael, FACHE Chief Financial Officer, Central Louisiana Surgical Hospital, Alexandria, LA, p. A261
FUSSELL, Eugene, M.D
Chief Medical Officer, St. John's Pleasant Valley Hospital, Camarillo, CA, p. A56
Chief Medical Officer, St. John's Regional Medical Center, Oxnard, CA, p. A78
FUTCH, Margaret A., Chief Executive Officer, HEALTHSOUTH Rehabilitation Hospital, Dothan, AL, p. A19
FUTRAL, Cindy, Director Human Resources, Elmore Community Hospital, Wetumpka, AL, p. A27
FUTRELL, Bradley, Chief Operating Officer, Hamilton Memorial Hospital District, McLeansboro, IL, p. A187

Index of Health Care Professionals

Index of Health Care Professionals / Fybel

FYBEL, Gary G., Senior Vice President and Chief Executive, Scripps Memorial Hospital–La Jolla, La Jolla, CA, p. A66

# G

GAAL, James G., M.D. Chief of Medical Staff, Jackson General Hospital, Ripley, WV, p. A675
GAASCH, Andrew
Chief Financial Officer, Parker Adventist Hospital, Parker, CO, p. A105
Chief Financial Officer, Porter Adventist Hospital, Denver, CO, p. A100
GABALDON, Karen, Chief Management Information Systems, Veterans Affairs Medical Center, West Palm Beach, FL, p. A143
GABARRO, Ralph, Chief Executive Officer, Mayo Regional Hospital, Dover–Foxcroft, ME, p. A283
GABAVICS, Mark, Director Human Resources, Shawano Medical Center, Shawano, WI, p. A690
GABEL, Christopher, Chief Operating Officer, Hollywood Pavilion,, FL, p. A125
GABEL, Marcia, Chief Financial Officer, Lane County Hospital, Dighton, KS, p. A232
GABEL, Phyllis, Chief Human Resource Officer, St. Luke's Rehabilitation Institute, Spokane, WA, p. A667
GABLENZ, Gordon, Vice President Finance, Ridgeview Medical Center, Waconia, MN, p. A341
GABORIAULT, Randall, Chief Information Officer, Christiana Care Health System, Newark, DE, p. A114
GABOW, Patricia A., M.D. Chief Executive Officer, Denver Health Medical Center, Denver, CO, p. A99
GABRIEL, Brenda, Director Human Resources, Harrison County Community Hospital, Bethany, MO, p. A355
GABRIEL, Scott F., Senior Vice President and Chief Operating Officer, Parkview Whitley Hospital, Columbia City, IN, p. A199
GABRIEL, Shirley, Chief Information Officer, University of Arizona Medical Center – University Campus, Tucson, AZ, p. A40
GABRIELE, Joan, Deputy Executive Director, Queens Hospital Center,, NY, p. A436
GABRIELSON, Nancy, Administrator and Chief Executive Officer, Iowa Specialty Hospital–Belmond, Belmond, IA, p. A214
GABRYEL, Timothy, M.D. Vice President Medical Affairs and Medical Director, Mercy Hospital, Buffalo, NY, p. A423
GACH, Peter, M.D. Chief of Staff, Northwest Medical Center, Margate, FL, p. A129
GADALLAH, Yousri, M.D. Chief Medical Officer, Pershing General Hospital, Lovelock, NV, p. A394
GADDIS, Cathryn, Director Human Resources, RiverValley Behavioral Health Hospital, Owensboro, KY, p. A257
GADE, Swami P., M.D. Medical Director, Tioga Medical Center, Tioga, ND, p. A468
GADEN, Paul, Vice President and Chief Operating Officer, CHRISTUS Spohn Hospital Corpus Christi Memorial, Corpus Christi, TX, p. A589
GADOMSKI, Veronica, R.N. Chief Nursing Officer, HEALTHSOUTH Rehabilitation Hospital, Albuquerque, NM, p. A414
GAEDE, John, Director Information Systems, El Centro Regional Medical Center, El Centro, CA, p. A60
GAENZLE, Jack, Senior Vice President Finance and Administration, UPMC Mercy, Pittsburgh, PA, p. A535
GAFFNEY, Laura, President and Chief Executive Officer, Interfaith Medical Center,, NY, p. A433
GAFFORD, Deborah, Chief Financial Officer, Menorah Medical Center, Overland Park, KS, p. A241
GAGE, Eileen, R.N
Vice President Nursing, Geneva General Hospital, Geneva, NY, p. A426
Vice President Nursing, Soldiers and Sailors Memorial Hospital of Yates County, Penn Yan, NY, p. A440
GAGE, Kevin, Chief Financial Officer, Stamford Hospital, Stamford, CT, p. A112
GAGE, Mark, D.O. Medical Director, Brookhaven Hospital, Tulsa, OK, p. A505
GAGLE, Stephen P., Manager Human Resources, Parkview Whitley Hospital, Columbia City, IN, p. A199
GAGLIO, Tony, Chief Financial Officer, Henry Ford Kingswood Hospital, Ferndale, MI, p. A312
GAGNON, Andy, Director Information Systems, Mercy Regional Health Center,, KS, p. A238
GAINDH, Ramesh, M.D. President Medical Staff, Parkview Adventist Medical Center, Brunswick, ME, p. A282
GAINER, Rolf B., Chief Executive Officer and Administrator, Brookhaven Hospital, Tulsa, OK, p. A505
GAINES, Jorie, Manager Information, Garfield County Public Hospital District, Pomeroy, WA, p. A664
GAIRE, Susan, M.D. President Medical Staff, Frisbie Memorial Hospital, Rochester, NH, p. A400
GAITAN, Alberto, M.D. Medical Director, O'Connor Hospital, Delhi, NY, p. A425
GAITER, Thomas E., M.D. Chief Medical Officer, Howard University Hospital, Washington, DC, p. A116
GAJ, Steve, Facility Chief Information Officer, Veterans Affairs Medical Center, Cleveland, OH, p. A476
GAJARE, N., M.D. Chief Clinical Affairs, Kalamazoo Psychiatric Hospital, Kalamazoo, MI, p. A316
GAJEWSKI, Christie, Director Human Resources, Pinckneyville Community Hospital, Pinckneyville, IL, p. A191
GALANDA, Chris, Chief Information Officer, Wilkes–Barre General Hospital, Wilkes–Barre, PA, p. A542
GALANG, Michael, M.D
Chief Information Officer, Mercy Hospital, Buffalo, NY, p. A423
Chief Information Officer, Sisters of Charity Hospital of Buffalo, Buffalo, NY, p. A423
GALATI, John P., President and Chief Executive Officer, Clifton Springs Hospital and Clinic, Clifton Springs, NY, p. A424
GALATI, Vicki L., Chief Financial Officer, Texas Health Specialty Hospital, Fort Worth, TX, p. A599
GALDIERI, Lou, R.N
Chief Operating Officer and Administrator, Mease Countryside Hospital, Safety Harbor, FL, p. A137
Chief Operating Officer and Administrator, Mease Hospital Dunedin, Dunedin, FL, p. A122
GALE, Donald I., M.D. Vice President Medical Affairs, Winter Haven Hospital, Winter Haven, FL, p. A143
GALE, Gabrielle, Chief Financial Officer, Forest View Psychiatric Hospital, Grand Rapids, MI, p. A313
GALE, Michael, Chief Financial Officer, Bournewood Health Systems, Brookline, MA, p. A298
GALES, Larry V., Director Human Resources, Coffey County Hospital, Burlington, KS, p. A231
GALFANO, Victor J., FACHE Chief Executive Officer, Regency Hospital of Northwest Indiana, East Chicago, IN, p. A200
GALINDO, Virgie, Chief Nurse Executive, Sutter Auburn Faith Hospital, Auburn, CA, p. A54
GALIPEAU, Michelle, Director Human Resources, St. Vincent's Birmingham, Birmingham, AL, p. A17
GALKOWSKI, James, Associate Director for Operations, Veterans Affairs Medical Center, Fayetteville, NC, p. A453
GALLA, Bernie
Interim Director Management Information Systems, Howard University Hospital, Washington, DC, p. A116
Director Information Services, Pikeville Medical Center, Pikeville, KY, p. A258
GALLAGHER, J. P., President, NorthShore University Health System Evanston Hospital, Evanston, IL, p. A181
GALLAGHER, James P., Chief Executive Officer, Summit Oaks Hospital, Summit, NJ, p. A410
GALLAGHER, Jeannie, Human Resource Generalist, East Morgan County Hospital, Brush, CO, p. A98
GALLAGHER, John, M.D. Chief Medical Officer, St. Mary's Medical Center of Evansville, Evansville, IN, p. A201
GALLAGHER, John, Chief Executive Officer, Stringfellow Memorial Hospital, Anniston, AL, p. A15
GALLAGHER, Joseph, Chief Executive Officer, Wyoming Behavioral Institute, Casper, WY, p. A695
GALLAGHER, Karen, Vice President Human Resources and Learning, Brooks Rehabilitation Hospital, Jacksonville, FL, p. A126
GALLAGHER, Keith W., FACHE Commander, Tripler Army Medical Center, Honolulu, HI, p. A164
GALLAGHER, Peter
Vice President and Chief Financial Officer, Bon Secours Memorial Regional Medical Center, Mechanicsville, VA, p. A651
Chief Financial Officer, Bon Secours St. Francis Medical Center, Midlothian, VA, p. A651
Chief Financial Officer, Bon Secours St. Mary's Hospital, Richmond, VA, p. A654
Senior Vice President and Chief Financial Officer, Bon Secours–Richmond Community Hospital, Richmond, VA, p. A654
GALLAGHER, Sean B., Chief Financial Officer, Houston Northwest Medical Center, Houston, TX, p. A604
GALLARDO, Ysidro, Associate Administrator Human Resources, Hazel Hawkins Memorial Hospital, Hollister, CA, p. A64
GALLATI, Todd, FACHE President and Chief Executive Officer, Trident Medical Center, Charleston, SC, p. A547
GALLAY, Emily, Vice President and Chief Information Officer, Lakeland Regional Medical Center–St. Joseph, Saint Joseph, MI, p. A322
GALLEGOS, Colleen, Director Human Resources, Guadalupe County Hospital, Santa Rosa, NM, p. A418
GALLES, Dan, Chief Financial Officer, San Dimas Community Hospital, San Dimas, CA, p. A86
GALLI, Jodi, Chief Nursing Officer, Eastern Maine Medical Center, Bangor, ME, p. A281
GALLIARDT, Scott, Chief Executive Officer, Acuity Hospital of South Texas, San Antonio, TX, p. A624
GALLIART, Mark, Chief Executive Officer, McBride Clinic Orthopedic Hospital, Oklahoma City, OK, p. A501
GALLIN, John I., M.D. Director, National Institutes of Health Clinical Center, Bethesda, MD, p. A289
GALLO, Cathy M., Vice President and Chief Nursing Officer, Levindale Hebrew Geriatric Center and Hospital, Baltimore, MD, p. A288
GALLO, James, Chief Human Resources Officer, St. Elizabeths Hospital, Washington, DC, p. A117
GALLO, Ronald, Director Human Resources, Blythedale Children's Hospital, Valhalla, NY, p. A445
GALLO, Scott, Assistant Vice President Talent, Midwestern Regional Medical Center, Zion, IL, p. A196
GALLOWAY, Crystal, Human Resources Generalist, Texas Health Specialty Hospital, Fort Worth, TX, p. A599
GALLOWAY, Nikki, Director Personnel and Administrative Secretary, Healthmark Regional Medical Center, DeFuniak Springs, FL, p. A122
GALLOWAY, Robert
Senior Vice President Finance and Chief Financial Officer, Cape Canaveral Hospital, Cocoa Beach, FL, p. A120
Senior Vice President Finance and Chief Financial Officer, Holmes Regional Medical Center, Melbourne, FL, p. A130
GALLUCCI, Kathleen, Chief Human Resources, Highland Hospital of Rochester, Rochester, NY, p. A441
GALLUCCI, Vince
Senior Vice President Human Resources, Mercy Medical Center, Oshkosh, WI, p. A688
Senior Vice President Human Resources, St. Elizabeth Hospital, Appleton, WI, p. A678
GALONSKY, Ronald J., Chief Operating Officer, O'Connor Hospital, San Jose, CA, p. A88
GALT, Nick, Chief Financial Officer, Las Colinas Medical Center, Irving, TX, p. A609
GALUSHA, Fred, Chief Information Officer, St. Luke's Rehabilitation Institute, Spokane, WA, p. A667
GALVA, Jorge, Executive Director, Hospital Manati Medical Center, Manati, PR, p. A701
GALVIN, Gary, M.D. Chief of Staff, Columbus Community Hospital, Columbus, WI, p. A680
GALVIN, Peter A., M.D. Director Medical Affairs, Peninsula Hospital Center,, NY, p. A
GALYON, Darlene, Director Human Resources, Choctaw Memorial Hospital, Hugo, OK, p. A498
GAMACHE, Cynde, R.N. Vice President and Chief Clinical Officer, Leesburg Regional Medical Center, Leesburg, FL, p. A129
GAMACHE, Edward L., President and Chief Executive Officer, Harbor Beach Community Hospital, Harbor Beach, MI, p. A315
GAMBERG, Elliott, Vice President Finance, New York Westchester Square Medical Center,, NY, p. A435
GAMBILL, Bill, Chief Financial Officer, Veterans Affairs Black Hills Health Care System, Fort Meade, SD, p. A556
GAMBILL, Dennis, Director Information Technology, Lakeside Memorial Hospital, Brockport, NY, p. A422
GAMBINO, Angela, R.N. Chief Nursing Officer, Hancock Medical Center, Bay Saint Louis, MS, p. A343
GAMBLE, Allen J., Comptroller, Bullock County Hospital, Union Springs, AL, p. A26
GAMBLE, Judy, Chief Financial Officer, Williamsburg Regional Hospital, Kingstree, SC, p. A551
GAMBLE, Kathleen, Fiscal Officer, Patton State Hospital, Patton, CA, p. A80
GAMBRELL Jr., Edward C., Administrator, Stephens County Hospital, Toccoa, GA, p. A161
GAMEL, Richard B., Administrator, Alegent Health Plainview Hospital, Plainview, NE, p. A389
GAMET, Nicki, R.N
VP/Chief Nursing Officer, Mercy Hospital Aurora, Aurora, MO, p. A355
Chief Nursing Officer, Mercy Hospital Cassville, Cassville, MO, p. A357
GAMINO, Randall, Director Perot Site, St. Joseph's Medical Center, Stockton, CA, p. A92
GAMMIERE, Thomas A., Senior Vice President and Chief Executive, Scripps Mercy Hospital, San Diego, CA, p. A86
GAMMON, Diane, Director Information Systems, Saint Francis Medical Center, Cape Girardeau, MO, p. A356
GAMMON, Sally T., FACHE President and Chief Executive Officer, Good Shepherd Rehabilitation Hospital, Allentown, PA, p. A517
GAMMON, Sally T., FACHE President and Chief Executive Officer, Good Shepherd Rehabilitation Network, Allentown, PA, p. B55
GANCI, Alan A., Director Finance and Controller, Lodi Community Hospital, Lodi, OH, p. A483

A816 Index of Health Care Professionals

GANCI, Deborah, Vice President Human Resources, Bellevue Hospital, Bellevue, OH, p. A470

GANDY, Patrick W., Chief Operating Officer, Lafayette General Medical Center, Lafayette, LA, p. A270

GANGEMI, Richard, M.D
Senior Vice President Academic, Medical Affairs and Chief Medical Officer, Newark–Wayne Community Hospital, Newark, NY, p. A438
Senior Vice President Academic and Medical Affairs, Rochester General Hospital, Rochester, NY, p. A441

GANGEMI–SOSA, Jeannith
Associate Executive Director, Elmhurst Hospital Center,, NY, p. A432
Senior Associate Executive Director, Lincoln Medical and Mental Health Center,, NY, p. A434
Senior Associate Executive Director, Queens Hospital Center,, NY, p. A436

GANGULY, Indranil, Vice President and Chief Information Officer, CentraState Healthcare System, Freehold, NJ, p. A404

GANN, Michele, Vice President Patient Services, Mercy Hospital Berryville, Berryville, AR, p. A42

GANN, Sherry, Administrator, Conway Regional Rehab Hospital, Conway, AR, p. A43

GANNON, Ronnie, Director Information Services, Southern Hills Medical Center, Nashville, TN, p. A573

GANNOTTA, Richard, Chief Operating Officer, Duke Raleigh Hospital, Raleigh, NC, p. A459

GANONG, Richard, M.D. Chief of Staff, Tahoe Forest Hospital District, Truckee, CA, p. A93

GANS, Bruce M., M.D. Executive Vice President and Chief Medical Officer, Kessler Institute for Rehabilitation, West Orange, NJ, p. A412

GANTNER, John
Executive Vice President Finance and Partner Company Operations, Jersey Shore University Medical Center, Neptune, NJ, p. A406
Executive Vice President Finance, Ocean Medical Center, Brick Township, NJ, p. A402
Executive Vice President Finance, Riverview Medical Center, Red Bank, NJ, p. A409
Executive Vice President Finance and Partner Company Operations, Southern Ocean Medical Center, Manahawkin, NJ, p. A406

GANTT, Cynthia J., Executive Officer, Naval Hospital, Twentynine Palms, CA, p. A93

GANTT, Debe, Chief Information Resource Management, Veterans Affairs Medical Center, Martinsburg, WV, p. A673

GANTT, Marsha, Interim Chief Nursing Officer, Barnwell County Hospital, Barnwell, SC, p. A546

GAPSTUR, Roxanna L., Ph.D. Chief Nursing Officer, Park Nicollet Methodist Hospital, Saint Louis Park, MN, p. A339

GARAY, Kenneth, M.D
Chief Medical Officer, LibertyHealth–Jersey City Medical Center, Jersey City, NJ, p. A405
Chief Medical Officer, Meadowlands Hospital Medical Center, Secaucus, NJ, p. A410

GARBANZOS, Del, Director Human Resources, Delano Regional Medical Center, Delano, CA, p. A59

GARBER, Jennifer Elizabeth, Vice President Human Resources, Emory Johns Creek Hospital, Johns Creek, GA, p. A154

GARBER, Mark, Vice President, Human Resources, Angel Medical Center, Franklin, NC, p. A453

GARCHA, Seema, M.D. Chief of Staff, Davis Regional Medical Center, Statesville, NC, p. A461

GARCIA, Aymette, Manager Human Resources, Wilma N. Vazquez Medical Center, Vega Baja, PR, p. A704

GARCIA, Carlos R., Vice President Clinical Services, Larkin Community Hospital, South Miami, FL, p. A139

GARCIA, Danette, Director Human Resources, HEALTHSOUTH Valley of the Sun Rehabilitation Hospital, Glendale, AZ, p. A33

GARCIA, Donna, Vice President, Finance, Presbyterian Hospital, Albuquerque, NM, p. A414

GARCIA, Felix, Director Health Information Services, Highlands Regional Medical Center, Sebring, FL, p. A139

GARCIA, Fernando, M.D. Chief of Staff, Avoyelles Hospital, Marksville, LA, p. A272

GARCIA, Gary, M.D. Chief of Staff, Mad River Community Hospital, Arcata, CA, p. A54

GARCIA, Georgina R., Chief Operating Officer, Fontana Medical Center, Fontana, CA, p. A61

GARCIA, Gerard, Acting Vice President Human Resources, University of Medicine and Dentistry of New Jersey–University Hospital, Newark, NJ, p. A407

GARCIA, Hector Troche, Director Human Resources, Cardiovascular Center of Puerto Rico and the Caribbean, San Juan, PR, p. A702

GARCIA, Idalia, Chief Human Resources Officer, State Psychiatric Hospital, San Juan, PR, p. A704

GARCIA, Irma, Job Coordinator, Rio Grande State Center/South Texas Health Care System, Harlingen, TX, p. A602

GARCIA, Joanne, Chief Operating Officer, Kindred Chicago–Central Hospital, Chicago, IL, p. A176

GARCIA, Joannie, CPA Director Finance, Hospital Perea, Mayaguez, PR, p. A702

GARCIA, Jose, Chief Human Resources Officer, San Juan City Hospital, San Juan, PR, p. A703

GARCIA, Kathleen, Controller, St. John's Episcopal Hospital–South Shore,, NY, p. A437

GARCIA, Lisa, Director Human Resources, Sunnyside Community Hospital, Sunnyside, WA, p. A667

GARCIA, Jr., Luis Mario, Director Human Resources, Methodist Sugar Land Hospital, Sugar Land, TX, p. A629

GARCIA, Margaret, Manager Human Resources, Baylor Medical Center at Frisco, Frisco, TX, p. A600

GARCIA, Michael, M.D. Medical Director, Leonard J. Chabert Medical Center, Houma, LA, p. A268

GARCIA, Michael R., Vice President Human Resources, SSM St. Joseph Health Center, Saint Charles, MO, p. A368

GARCIA, Robert W., M.D. Chief Medical Officer, Iraan General Hospital, Iraan, TX, p. A608

GARCIA, Roland
Senior Vice President and Chief Information Officer, Baptist Medical Center, Jacksonville, FL, p. A126
Senior Vice President and Chief Information Officer, Baptist Medical Center Beaches, Jacksonville Beach, FL, p. A127

GARCIA, Sharon, Human Resources Representative, Medina Regional Hospital, Hondo, TX, p. A603

GARCIA, Shawn, Manager Human Resources, Memorial Hospital Los Banos, Los Banos, CA, p. A73

GARCIA, Sylvia, Chief Accounting Officer, South Texas Spine and Surgical Hospital, San Antonio, TX, p. A626

GARCIA, Vicki, Vice President Human Resources, Roswell Park Cancer Institute, Buffalo, NY, p. A423

GARDINER, Karen, Director Fiscal Services, University Medical Center, Lafayette, LA, p. A270

GARDINER, Lisa, Director Marketing and Public Relations, Physicians Regional Medical Center – Pine Ridge, Naples, FL, p. A133

GARDNER, David, Manager Human Resources, Utah State Hospital, Provo, UT, p. A640

GARDNER, Donald F., Vice President Finance/Chief Financial Officer, Caldwell Memorial Hospital, Lenoir, NC, p. A456

GARDNER, Elizabeth C., R.N. Chief Nursing Officer, Hemet Valley Medical Center, Hemet, CA, p. A64

GARDNER, Guy, M.D
Chief Medical Affairs, Baptist Health Medical Center – North Little Rock, North Little Rock, AR, p. A50
Chief Medical Officer, Baptist Health Medical Center–Arkadelphia, Arkadelphia, AR, p. A42

GARDNER, Jacque, Administrative Assistant, Clinic Manager, Co–Chief Financial Officer and Chief Human Resources, McCone County Health Center, Circle, MT, p. A374

GARDNER, James D., M.D. Vice President and Chief Medical Officer, Waukesha Memorial Hospital, Waukesha, WI, p. A692

GARDNER Jr., James E., Chief Executive Officer, St. Anthony's Medical Center, Saint Louis, MO, p. A370

GARDNER, John, Chief Executive Officer, Yuma District Hospital, Yuma, CO, p. A107

GARDNER, Jonathan H., Chief Executive Officer, Southern Arizona Veterans Affairs Health Care System, Tucson, AZ, p. A40

GARDNER, Keith, Executive Vice President, Shriners Hospitals for Children, Tampa, FL, p. B118

GARDNER, Norman, M.D. President Medical Staff, Presentation Medical Center, Rolla, ND, p. A468

GARDNER, Patrick, M.D. Vice President Medical Affairs, St. Joseph's Community Hospital of West Bend, West Bend, WI, p. A693

GARDNER, Paul A., CPA, Administrator, George County Hospital, Lucedale, MS, p. A349

GARDNER, Robb, Chief Executive Officer, Henry County Health Center, Mount Pleasant, IA, p. A223

GARDNER, Russell W., Chief Financial Officer, Mount Carmel, Columbus, OH, p. A476

GARDNER, Sharon, Manager Information Systems, SSM St. Joseph Hospital West, Lake Saint Louis, MO, p. A363

GARDNER, Sharon R., Vice President Human Resources, Yuma Regional Medical Center, Yuma, AZ, p. A41

GARDNER, Zoe, Manager Human Resources, Sharp Chula Vista Medical Center, Chula Vista, CA, p. A57

GARES, Donna, R.N. President and Chief Executive Officer, San Jacinto Methodist Hospital, Baytown, TX, p. A582

GARFIELD, Mark, M.D. Vice President and Chief Medical Officer, Kaweah Delta Medical Center, Visalia, CA, p. A95

GARFINKEL, Leon, Director Information Services, University of Medicine and Dentistry of New Jersey, University Behavioral Healthcare, Piscataway, NJ, p. A408

GARISON, Jerri, R.N. President, Baylor Regional Medical Center at Plano, Plano, TX, p. A621

GARKO, Michael
Chief Financial Officer, Menifee Valley Medical Center, Sun City, CA, p. A92
Chief Financial Officer, Moreno Valley Community Hospital, Moreno Valley, CA, p. A75
Chief Financial Officer, St. Vincent Medical Center, Los Angeles, CA, p. A72

GARLAND, Anna, Director Human Resources, Fort Walton Beach Medical Center, Fort Walton Beach, FL, p. A124

GARLETS, Mary, Director Human Resources, Mayo Clinic Health System in Cannon Falls, Cannon Falls, MN, p. A329

GARMAN, Mary E., R.N. Chief Nursing Officer and Vice President Operations, Good Samaritan Hospital, Dayton, OH, p. A478

GARMAN, Michael, Chief Financial Officer, Avera St. Anthony's Hospital, O'Neill, NE, p. A386

GARNAS, David, Chief Executive Officer, Sedgwick County Health Center, Julesburg, CO, p. A102

GARNER, Douglas, Vice President, Thomas Hospital, Fairhope, AL, p. A20

GARNER, Ethnee, Vice President Nursing Services, Memorial Hospital, North Conway, NH, p. A399

GARNER, James H., Chief Financial Officer, Coffey County Hospital, Burlington, KS, p. A231

GARNER, Mario J., FACHE Chief Operating Officer, AMG Specialty Hospital–Lafayette Regional Campus, Lafayette, LA, p. A270

GARNER, William, M.D. Chief Medical Officer, Saint Catherine Regional Hospital, Charlestown, IN, p. A199

GARNETT, Mark, M.D. Chief of Staff, Hansford Hospital, Spearman, TX, p. A628

GAROFOLA, Aaron, Director Human Resources, Terre Haute Regional Hospital, Terre Haute, IN, p. A212

GARON, Jack, M.D. Chief Medical Officer, Mount Sinai Hospital, Chicago, IL, p. A177

GARONE, Marlene, M.D. Vice President Medical Affairs and Medical Director, Woman's Christian Association Hospital, Jamestown, NY, p. A428

GARRAMONE, Kathy
Chief Financial Officer, Jacobi Medical Center,, NY, p. A433
Chief Financial Officer, North Central Bronx Hospital,, NY, p. A436

GARRARD, Eric, Chief Executive Officer, HEALTHSOUTH Cane Creek Rehabilitation Hospital, Martin, TN, p. A570

GARRED, Sr., John, M.D. Chief Medical Officer, Burgess Health Center, Onawa, IA, p. A224

GARRETT, Alan H., President and Chief Executive Officer, St. Mary Medical Center, Apple Valley, CA, p. A54

GARRETT, Darlene, Chief Operating Officer, Parkview Huntington Hospital, Huntington, IN, p. A203

GARRETT, David B.
Chief Information Officer, Forsyth Medical Center, Winston–Salem, NC, p. A463
Senior Vice President Information Technology, Presbyterian Hospital, Charlotte, NC, p. A451
Chief Information Officer, Presbyterian Hospital Matthews, Matthews, NC, p. A457

GARRETT, Ginger, Regional Director Human Resources, Good Shepherd Medical Center–Marshall, Marshall, TX, p. A615

GARRETT, Jarren, Chief Administrative Officer, Baptist Orange Hospital, Orange, TX, p. A619

GARRETT, John, Chief Financial Officer, Cooper Green Mercy Hospital, Birmingham, AL, p. A16

GARRETT, Kevin C., M.D. Chief Medical Officer, Christus St. Vincent Regional Medical Center, Santa Fe, NM, p. A418

GARRETT, Lisa, Director Human Resources, Arizona Spine and Joint Hospital, Mesa, AZ, p. A33

GARRETT, Mark, Chief Information Officer, Shriners Hospitals for Children, Los Angeles, Los Angeles, CA, p. A72

GARRETT, Mykl, Executive Vice President and Chief Operating Officer, Trinity Bettendorf, Bettendorf, IA, p. A214

GARRETT, Regina, Director Health Information Management, Crossroads Community Hospital, Mount Vernon, IL, p. A188

GARRETT, Robert C., President and Chief Executive Officer, Hackensack University Medical Center, Hackensack, NJ, p. A404

GARRETT, Walter J., Chief Executive Officer, Welch Community Hospital, Welch, WV, p. A676

GARRICK, Renee, M.D. Chief Medical Officer, Westchester Medical Center, Valhalla, NY, p. A445

GARRIN, Paul, Chief Information Officer, Monmouth Medical Center, Long Branch, NJ, p. A405

GARRISON, Kenneth, M.D. Chief of Staff, Cumberland Memorial Hospital, Cumberland, WI, p. A680

GARRISON, Mark, Chief of Staff, Glenn Medical Center, Willows, CA, p. A96

GARRISON, Robert E., Chief Executive Officer, Southeast Health Center of Ripley County, Doniphan, MO, p. A358

GARRISON, Tina, Vice President, Operations, SSM DePaul Health Center, Bridgeton, MO, p. A356

Index of Health Care Professionals

Index of Health Care Professionals / Garrity

GARRITY, Nerissa, Chief Financial Officer, Kula Hospital, Kula, HI, p. A165
GARROW, Dina, Chief Nursing Officer and Chief Operating Officer, Kindred Hospital–Baldwin Park, Baldwin Park, CA, p. A55
GARROW, George, M.D. Senior Vice President and Chief Medical Officer, Western Maryland Regional Medical Center, Cumberland, MD, p. A291
GARRY, William, Chief Financial Officer, Edgefield County Hospital, Edgefield, SC, p. A549
GARSA, Arebi, Chief Financial Officer, Ashland Community Hospital, Ashland, OR, p. A509
GARSKE, Tom, Director Information Systems, Wiregrass Medical Center, Geneva, AL, p. A21
GARSKI, Mary Jo, Director Human Resources, Wellington Regional Medical Center, West Palm Beach, FL, p. A143
GARVEN, Charles, M.D. Vice President Medical Operations, Lakewood Hospital, Lakewood, OH, p. A482
GARVEY, Heather, Chief Financial Officer, Raulerson Hospital, Okeechobee, FL, p. A134
GARVEY, Thomas J., Chief Financial Officer, Mercy Hospital and Medical Center, Chicago, IL, p. A176
GARVIN, Henry, Chief Executive Officer, Conejos County Hospital, La Jara, CO, p. A103
GARVIN, Jan, Vice President Human Resources, Franciscan St. Elizabeth Health – Lafayette Central, Lafayette, IN, p. A206
GARVIN, Sarah C., Chief Executive Officer, Cypress Pointe Hospital East, Slidell, LA, p. A278
GARWOOD, III, William D., Associate Administrator and Chief Financial Officer, Angleton Danbury Medical Center, Angleton, TX, p. A579
GARY, Al, COO, Simpson General Hospital, Mendenhall, MS, p. A350
GARY, Stacci, Director Human Resources, Parkview Community Hospital Medical Center, Riverside, CA, p. A82
GARY, Stephen M., Senior Vice President and Chief Financial officer, Akron General Medical Center, Akron, OH, p. A469
GARZA, Chris, Director Patient Financial Services, Cornerstone Regional Hospital, Edinburg, TX, p. A595
GARZA, Ismelda, Director Information Systems, Comanche County Medical Center, Comanche, TX, p. A588
GARZA, Jennifer, Chief Operating Officer, The Woman's Hospital of Texas, Houston, TX, p. A607
GARZA, Kim, Vice President Human Resources, Samaritan Healthcare, Moses Lake, WA, p. A663
GARZA, Laura, Director Human Resources, Texas Specialty Hospital at Houston, Houston, TX, p. A607
GARZA, Tom, Director Fiscal and Support, Rio Grande State Center/South Texas Health Care System, Harlingen, TX, p. A602
GASAWAY, Rob, Chief Financial Officer, Galesburg Cottage Hospital, Galesburg, IL, p. A182
GASBARRA, Gary, Regional Chief Financial Officer, Provena Saint Joseph Medical Center, Joliet, IL, p. A185
GASCHO, Dwight, President and Chief Executive Officer, Scheurer Hospital, Pigeon, MI, p. A320
GASCHO, Gale E., Chief Executive Officer, Greater El Monte Community Hospital, South El Monte, CA, p. A91
GASH, Deborah
  Vice President and Chief Information Officer, Crittenton Children's Center, Kansas City, MO, p. A361
  Chief Information Officer, Saint Luke's Hospital of Kansas City, Kansas City, MO, p. A362
  Chief Information Officer, Saint Luke's South Hospital, Overland Park, KS, p. A241
GASKINS, Michael W., Executive Vice President and Chief Financial Officer, Hanover Hospital, Hanover, PA, p. A524
GASPAR, Deborah L., R.N. Chief Nursing Officer, Memorial Hospital of Sweetwater County, Rock Springs, WY, p. A697
GASPARD, H. J., Chief Executive Officer, HEALTHSOUTH Rehabilitation Hospital of Beaumont, Beaumont, TX, p. A583
GASPARINI, Michael L., Vice President Clinical Services and Chief Operating Officer, Western Missouri Medical Center, Warrensburg, MO, p. A372
GASQUE, James, M.D. Chief Hospital Services, U. S. Air Force Medical Center Keesler, Keesler AFB, MS, p. A348
GAST, Edwin A., Chief Executive Officer, Marshall Browning Hospital, Du Quoin, IL, p. A180
GASTON, Jan, Administrator, Jasper Memorial Hospital, Monticello, GA, p. A156
GASTON, Tammy, Chief Information Officer, Smith County Memorial Hospital, Smith Center, KS, p. A243
GATES, John
  Vice President Finance and Chief Financial Officer, California Pacific Medical Center, San Francisco, CA, p. A86
  Chief Financial Officer, St. Luke's Hospital, San Francisco, CA, p. A87
GATES, Margaret, Chief Human Resources, Harris Hospital, Newport, AR, p. A49
GATES, Philip E., M.D. Chief of Staff, Shriners Hospitals for Children, Shreveport, Shreveport, LA, p. A277
GATES, Polly, Senior Vice President and Chief Nursing Officer, Genesys Regional Medical Center, Grand Blanc, MI, p. A313
GATES, Rose, Director Human Resources, Hayward Area Memorial Hospital and Nursing Home, Hayward, WI, p. A683
GATES, Tracy, Chief Financial Officer, Jones Memorial Hospital, Wellsville, NY, p. A446
GATHERS, Mary, Director Information Systems, McKay–Dee Hospital Center, Ogden, UT, p. A639
GATHMAN, Michael, Chief Financial Officer, Veterans Affairs Medical Center, Spokane, WA, p. A667
GATI, Ken, M.D. Chief of Staff, Medical Center of South Arkansas, El Dorado, AR, p. A44
GATIEN, Lionel J., D.O. Chief of Staff, Kindred Hospital North Florida, Green Cove Springs, FL, p. A124
GATLIFF, Peggy, Chief Financial Officer, Edward White Hospital, Saint Petersburg, FL, p. A138
GATLIN, B. Lance, FACHE Administrator, Parmer Medical Center, Friona, TX, p. A600
GATMAITAN, Alfonso W., Chief Executive Officer, Indiana University Health Arnett Hospital, Lafayette, IN, p. A206
GATTO, Tony, Director Management Information Systems, Flushing Hospital Medical Center,, NY, p. A432
GAU, Kimberley A., FACHE Chief Executive Officer, Guttenberg Municipal Hospital, Guttenberg, IA, p. A220
GAUBERT, Steve C., Chief Financial Officer, Thibodaux Regional Medical Center, Thibodaux, LA, p. A278
GAUDREAU, Leo, Manager Plant and Property, Northwestern Medical Center, Saint Albans, VT, p. A644
GAUER, Natalie, Administrator, Milbank Area Hospital Avera, Milbank, SD, p. A557
GAUGHAN, Patty, Human Resource Administrative Officer, Nevada Regional Medical Center, Nevada, MO, p. A366
GAUL, Michael, Manager Information Systems, Atchison Hospital, Atchison, KS, p. A230
GAUNTT, Brandon, Director Information Systems, Hopkins County Memorial Hospital, Sulphur Springs, TX, p. A629
GAUSE, Garry L., President and Chief Executive Officer, Brookwood Medical Center, Birmingham, AL, p. A16
GAUTHIER, Bonnie B., President and Chief Executive Officer, The Hospital at Hebrew Health Care, West Hartford, CT, p. A113
GAUTHIER, Paul, Chief Information Resources Management, Veterans Affairs Montana Health Care System, Fort Harrison, MT, p. A375
GAUTNEY, Steven, Chief Executive Officer, Crisp Regional Hospital, Cordele, GA, p. A150
GAVALCHIK, Stephen M., FACHE Community Chief Executive Officer, Morgan County ARH Hospital, West Liberty, KY, p. A259
GAVENS, Mark R., Senior Vice President Clinical Care Services and Chief Operating Officer, Cedars–Sinai Medical Center, Los Angeles, CA, p. A69
GAVIN, Donald, Chief Financial Officer, Hillside Hospital, Pulaski, TN, p. A574
GAVIN, James M., Chief Financial Officer, St. Peter's Hospital, Albany, NY, p. A420
GAVIN, Joan, R.N. Chief Nursing Officer/Vice President, Patient Services, Shore Medical Center, Somers Point, NJ, p. A410
GAVIN, Linda, Associate Executive Director Marketing and Physician Recruitment, South Central Regional Medical Center, Laurel, MS, p. A348
GAVIN, Martin J., President and Chief Executive Officer, Connecticut Children's Medical Center, Hartford, CT, p. A109
GAVIN, Patrick, President, Crozer–Chester Medical Center, Upland, PA, p. A540
GAVIN, Tammy, Assistant Administrator and Chief Operating Officer, White River Medical Center, Batesville, AR, p. A42
GAVIOLI, R. Louis, M.D. Vice President Medical Affairs, St. Francis Medical Center, Monroe, LA, p. A273
GAVIS, Patricia, Chief Financial Officer, Ellenville Regional Hospital, Ellenville, NY, p. A425
GAVORA, George, Director Program Evaluation, Kingsboro Psychiatric Center,, NY, p. A433
GAVULIC, Melany, President & Chief Executive Officer, Hurley Medical Center, Flint, MI, p. A312
GAW, Kris
  Chief Operating Officer, Renown Regional Medical Center, Reno, NV, p. A395
  Chief Operating Officer, Renown Rehabilitation Hospital, Reno, NV, p. A395
  Chief Operating Officer, Renown South Meadows Medical Center, Reno, NV, p. A395
GAWLER, William, Chief Information Officer, Veterans Affairs Medical Center, Chillicothe, OH, p. A472
GAWNE, Bernard B., M.D. Vice President and Chief Medical Officer, Christ Hospital, Cincinnati, OH, p. A473
GAWORSKI, Mark, Vice President Finance, CFO, Spencer Hospital, Spencer, IA, p. A227
GAY, Chanda, Manager Human Resources, Jay Hospital, Jay, FL, p. A127
GAY, Christophe, M.D. Chief of Staff, Bellville General Hospital, Bellville, TX, p. A583
GAY, Don, Director Human Resources, West Hills Hospital, Reno, NV, p. A395
GAY, Kristi
  Chief Financial Officer, Memorial Medical Center – Livingston, Livingston, TX, p. A612
  Chief Financial Officer, Memorial Medical Center – Lufkin, Lufkin, TX, p. A614
  Chief Financial Officer, Memorial Medical Center – San Augustine, San Augustine, TX, p. A626
  Chief Financial Officer, Memorial Specialty Hospital, Lufkin, TX, p. A614
GAY, Vickie, Chief Executive Officer, Montgomery General Hospital, Montgomery, WV, p. A673
GAYLER, Lisa, Director Human Resources, Select Long Term Care Hospital – Colorado Springs, Colorado Springs, CO, p. A98
GAYMAN, Rob, Director Information Systems, Riverside Shore Memorial Hospital, Nassawadox, VA, p. A651
GAYNOR, Sheila, Director Human Resources, Perry County Memorial Hospital, Tell City, IN, p. A212
GAYNOR, Stanley J., FACHE President and Chief Executive Officer, Black River Memorial Hospital, Black River Falls, WI, p. A679
GAZIT, Sharyn D., Director Human Resources, Shriners Hospitals for Children–Boston, Boston, MA, p. A297
GEARHART, Danielle, Chief Executive Officer, Buchanan County Health Center, Independence, IA, p. A221
GEARY, David S., Chief Financial Officer, Cache Valley Specialty Hospital, North Logan, UT, p. A639
GEBHARD, Scott, Executive Vice President and Chief Operating Officer, JFK Medical Center, Edison, NJ, p. A403
GEBHART, Cheryl, Director Human Resources Providence Health Plan and Providence Medical Group, Providence Newberg Medical Center, Newberg, OR, p. A513
GEBHART, Jim, FACHE Chief Operating Officer, Hillcrest Baptist Medical Center, Waco, TX, p. A633
GEBHART Jr., Jim, FACHE President, Mercy Hospital Oklahoma City, Oklahoma City, OK, p. A501
GEBHART, Ronald J., M.D. Chief of Staff, Veterans Affairs Salt Lake City Health Care System, Salt Lake City, UT, p. A641
GEDDINGS, Toni, Director Human Resources, Cullman Regional Medical Center, Cullman, AL, p. A18
GEE, Brian, M.D. Director Emergency Services, Lander Regional Hospital, Lander, WY, p. A696
GEE, Kyle
  Chief Financial Officer, Beartooth Billings Clinic, Red Lodge, MT, p. A378
  Chief Financial Officer, Pioneer Medical Center, Big Timber, MT, p. A373
GEE, Thomas H., Administrator, Henry County Medical Center, Paris, TN, p. A574
GEERTS, Jodi, Chief Nursing Officer, Henry County Health Center, Mount Pleasant, IA, p. A223
GEHANT, David P., President and Chief Executive Officer, Boulder Community Hospital, Boulder, CO, p. A97
GEHEB, Michael, M.D
  Division President, Oakwood Heritage Hospital, Taylor, MI, p. A324
  Division President, Oakwood Hospital & Medical Center–Dearborn, Dearborn, MI, p. A310
GEHLAUF, Dee Ann, Senior Vice President Business and Organization Development, Marietta Memorial Hospital, Marietta, OH, p. A483
GEHLHAUSEN, Dorothy, Manager Human Resources, St. Mary's Warrick Hospital, Boonville, IN, p. A198
GEHRIG, Ryan, President, Mercy Hospital Fort Smith, Fort Smith, AR, p. A45
GEHRING, Jay, Director Information Systems, Ninnescah Valley Health System, Kingman, KS, p. A236
GEHRING, Sherry, R.N. Vice President Nursing, Inpatient Care and Chief Nursing Officer, Hancock Regional Hospital, Greenfield, IN, p. A203
GEHRING, Terri, Vice President Operations, McPherson Hospital, McPherson, KS, p. A238
GEIDT, Steve, Chief Executive Officer, Saddleback Memorial Medical Center, Laguna Hills, CA, p. A66
GEIER, Debra, M.D. President Medical Staff, Jamestown Regional Medical Center, Jamestown, ND, p. A466
GEIER, Peter E., Chief Executive Officer, Ohio State University Health System, Columbus, OH, p. B98
GEIER, Peter E., Chief Executive Officer, Ohio State University Medical Center, Columbus, OH, p. A477

A818 Index of Health Care Professionals

Index of Health Care Professionals / Gibbons

Index of Health Care Professionals

GEIGER, Cathy
Director Information Systems, Henry Ford Macomb Hospitals, Clinton Township, MI, p. A309
Director Information Services, St. Joseph Mercy Port Huron, Port Huron, MI, p. A321
GEIGER, Charles L., D.O. Chief of Staff, Belmont Community Hospital, Bellaire, OH, p. A470
GEIGER, Ralph, M.D. Chief of Staff, Sebastian River Medical Center, Sebastian, FL, p. A139
GEIGLE, Joseph, Director Human Resources, Fort Hamilton Hospital, Hamilton, OH, p. A481
GEIL, Kristie A., VP, Chief Nursing Officer, CGH Medical Center, Sterling, IL, p. A194
GEISSLER, Curt, President, Lakeview Hospital, Stillwater, MN, p. A340
GEISSLER, Michael E., Chief Executive Officer, Optima Specialty Hospital, Lafayette, LA, p. A270
GEIST, Jim, Chief Executive Officer, Capital Medical Center, Olympia, WA, p. A663
GEIST, Tammy, Chief Financial Officer, Presbyterian–Orthopaedic Hospital, Charlotte, NC, p. A451
GEITZ, Cheri, Director Human Resources, Ellsworth Municipal Hospital, Iowa Falls, IA, p. A222
GEIVER, Betsy, Chief Human Resources Officer, Sioux Falls VA Health Care System, Sioux Falls, SD, p. A560
GELDHOF, Jay
Director Information Systems, Greater El Monte Community Hospital, South El Monte, CA, p. A91
Director Information Systems, Whittier Hospital Medical Center, Whittier, CA, p. A96
GELFAND, Andrew, M.D. Medical Director, Our Children's House at Baylor, Dallas, TX, p. A592
GELL, Michael, Director Human Resources, Boys Town National Research Hospital, Omaha, NE, p. A387
GELLENBECK, Mary Ann, Chief Operating Officer, Butler County Medical Center, Hamilton, OH, p. A481
GELLER, Guy, Administrator and Chief Executive Officer, Beacham Memorial Hospital, Magnolia, MS, p. A349
GELLER, Harold S., Administrator, Othello Community Hospital, Othello, WA, p. A664
GELLER, Robert D., M.D. Vice President Medical Affairs, FHN Memorial Hospital, Freeport, IL, p. A182
GELLER, Warren, Executive Vice President and Chief Operating Officer, Englewood Hospital and Medical Center, Englewood, NJ, p. A404
GELMAN, Lawrence, M.D. Chief Executive Officer, Doctor's Hospital at Renaissance, Edinburg, TX, p. A595
GELORMINI, Frank, Chief Operating Officer, Community Medical Center, Toms River, NJ, p. A411
GEMMEL, Donald, Controller, Kindred Hospital South Florida–Hollywood,, FL, p. A125
GENDER, Aloma, MSN, Administrator and Chief Nursing Officer, CHRISTUS St. Michael Rehabilitation Hospital, Texarkana, TX, p. A630
GENEVRO, Thomas A., Vice President Human Resources, Butler Health System, Butler, PA, p. A519
GENGLER, Laraine, Chief Financial Officer, Lindsborg Community Hospital, Lindsborg, KS, p. A238
GENNA, Nick, Administrator, Treasure Valley Hospital, Boise, ID, p. A167
GENNRICH, Yvonne, Controller, Cook County North Shore Hospital, Grand Marais, MN, p. A332
GENOVA, Peter, Chief Information Officer, Long Beach Medical Center, Long Beach, NY, p. A429
GENOVESE, Vincent P., M.D. President Medical Staff, Muhlenberg Community Hospital, Greenville, KY, p. A251
GENSERT, Kurt, R.N. Vice President Operations, Platte Valley Medical Center, Brighton, CO, p. A98
GENTILE, Barbara, Vice President Chief Nursing Officer, Catskill Regional Medical Center, Harris, NY, p. A427
GENTILE, John, M.D
Vice President Medical Affairs, Alta Bates Summit Medical Center, Berkeley, CA, p. A55
Vice President Medical Affairs, Alta Bates Summit Medical Center – Summit Campus, Oakland, CA, p. A77
GENTILE, Joyce, Human Resource Benefits Specialist, Marshall Medical Center, Lewisburg, TN, p. A569
GENTILE, Lawrence, President and Chief Executive Officer, Redgate Memorial Recovery Center, Long Beach, CA, p. A68
GENTNER, Rocky, Chief Financial Officer, Newport Bay Hospital, Newport Beach, CA, p. A77
GENTRY, Cheryl G., Chief Executive Officer, Select Specialty Hospital–Beech Grove, Beech Grove, IN, p. A198
GENTRY, Gregg, Senior Vice President Human Resources, Erlanger Medical Center, Chattanooga, TN, p. A563
GENTRY, Jeanine, Chief Executive Officer, Mountain View Hospital District, Madras, OR, p. A512
GENTRY, Lee, FACHE Vice President and Administrator, Baptist Health Rehabilitation Institute, Little Rock, AR, p. A48
GEORGE, Alan E., Chief Executive Officer, Palestine Regional Medical Center–East, Palestine, TX, p. A619
GEORGE, Amanda, Assistant Controller, St. Vincent Morrilton, Morrilton, AR, p. A49
GEORGE, Brad, Director Information Systems, Parkland Medical Center, Derry, NH, p. A397
GEORGE, Denise, R.N. President and Chief Executive Officer, Northern Dutchess Hospital, Rhinebeck, NY, p. A441
GEORGE, Doug, Chief Financial Officer, VA Butler Healthcare, Butler, PA, p. A519
GEORGE, Gary
Regional Vice President Human Resources, Mercy St. Anne Hospital, Toledo, OH, p. A489
Regional Vice President Human Resources, Mercy St. Charles Hospital, Oregon, OH, p. A486
Regional Vice President Human Resources, Mercy St. Vincent Medical Center, Toledo, OH, p. A489
GEORGE, Jane, Controller, Methodist Healthcare–Fayette Hospital, Somerville, TN, p. A575
GEORGE, P. A., M.D. Chief of Staff, Madison Medical Center, Fredericktown, MO, p. A360
GEORGE, Patricia, Chief Information Officer, North Shore Medical Center, Salem, MA, p. A304
GEORGE, Shayne, Chief Executive Officer, Regional Medical Center–Bayonet Point, Hudson, FL, p. A125
GEORGE, Teresa, Vice President and Chief Operating Officer, Dell Children's Medical Center of Central Texas, Austin, TX, p. A580
GEORGE, Tracy L., Chief Financial Officer, St. James Parish Hospital, Lutcher, LA, p. A272
GEORGE, William, M.D. Chief of Staff, Beartooth Billings Clinic, Red Lodge, MT, p. A378
GEORGES, Angelo, M.D. President Medical and Dental Staff, Wheeling Hospital, Wheeling, WV, p. A677
GERARD, Alice M., President and Chief Executive Officer, McLaren Bay Region, Bay City, MI, p. A308
GERARD, Greg D., President, Saint Joseph Berea, Berea, KY, p. A247
GERATHS, Nathan L., Director, Veterans Affairs Edward Hines, Jr. Hospital, Hines, IL, p. A184
GERBER, Greg, M.D. Chief Medical Officer, Aurora Lakeland Medical Center, Elkhorn, WI, p. A681
GERBIG, Ralph, M.D. Chief of Staff, Johnson Memorial Health Services, Dawson, MN, p. A330
GERDTS, Elizabeth, Chief Nursing Officer, North Central Bronx Hospital,, NY, p. A436
GERETY, Meghan, M.D. Chief of Staff, Veterans Affairs Medical Center, Albuquerque, NM, p. A415
GERHART, Bobbie, President and Chief Executive Officer, Miami Valley Hospital, Dayton, OH, p. A478
GERHART, Paul, Chief Financial Officer, Sanford Canton–Inwood Medical Center, Canton, SD, p. A555
GERICK, Robert P., Interim Chief Executive Officer, Vibra Hospital of Fort Wayne, Fort Wayne, IN, p. A202
GERIG, Stacey L., Chief Executive Officer, Odessa Regional Medical Center, Odessa, TX, p. A619
GERING, Jeffrey T., Medical Center Director, Veterans Affairs Medical Center, Chillicothe, OH, p. A472
GERKE, Deborah, Chief Financial Officer, Complex Care Hospital at Tenaya, Las Vegas, NV, p. A392
GERLACH, George, Chief Executive Officer, Granite Falls Municipal Hospital and Manor, Granite Falls, MN, p. A332
GERLACH, Matthew S., Vice President and Chief Operating Officer, Glendale Memorial Hospital and Health Center, Glendale, CA, p. A63
GERMAN, Mike
Chief Financial Officer, Cape Coral Hospital, Cape Coral, FL, p. A120
Chief Financial Officer, Gulf Coast Medical Center, Fort Myers, FL, p. A123
GERMANN, William, M.D. Acting Chief of Staff, Veterans Affairs Medical Center, Dayton, OH, p. A479
GERMANY, Alan, Chief Financial Officer, Phoenix Baptist Hospital, Phoenix, AZ, p. A36
GERMUSKA, Natalie, Chief Executive Officer, Kindred Hospital–San Diego, San Diego, CA, p. A85
GERNDT, Angie, Human Resources Generalist, Central Community Hospital, Elkader, IA, p. A219
GERNHART, Diana, Chief Financial Officer, OHSU Hospital, Portland, OR, p. A514
GERRIOR, Marilyn, R.N. Chief Nursing Executive, Saint Louise Regional Hospital, Gilroy, CA, p. A63
GERRITS, Brad, Director Information Systems, Lakeview Medical Center, Rice Lake, WI, p. A690
GERSCH, Aaron, M.D. Chief of Staff, Albany Area Hospital and Medical Center, Albany, MN, p. A327
GERSHONE, Fern, Vice President Human Resources, Mille Lacs Health System, Onamia, MN, p. A336
GERSON, Elaine, Chief Clinical Officer and General Counsel, Aspen Valley Hospital District, Aspen, CO, p. A97
GERSTNER, Nancy, Manager Human Resources, Robert J. Dole Veterans Affairs Medical Center, Wichita, KS, p. A245
GERTEN, Michael E., Chief Executive Officer, Solara Hospital of Shawnee, Shawnee, OK, p. A504
GERTENBACH, Jennifer, Director Human Resources, Inova Fair Oaks Hospital, Fairfax, VA, p. A647
GERVAIN, Edward, Chief Operating Officer, Adventist La Grange Memorial Hospital, La Grange, IL, p. A186
GERVELER, Patrick M., Vice President Finance and Chief Financial Officer, Blessing Hospital, Quincy, IL, p. A192
GESSNER, Christopher, President, Children's Hospital of Pittsburgh of UPMC, Pittsburgh, PA, p. A534
GETMAN, Sylvia, President and Chief Executive Officer, The Aroostook Medical Center, Presque Isle, ME, p. A285
GETTINGER, Thomas, Executive Vice President and Chief Operating Officer, WakeMed Raleigh Campus, Raleigh, NC, p. A459
GETTINGS, Scott, M.D
Vice President and Chief Medical Officer, Holmes Regional Medical Center, Melbourne, FL, p. A130
Vice President Medical Affairs, Palm Bay Hospital, Melbourne, FL, p. A130
GETTO, Carl J., M.D. Senior Vice President Medical Affairs and Associate Dean Hospital Affairs, University of Wisconsin Hospital and Clinics, Madison, WI, p. A684
GETTYS, III, Roddey E., Chief Executive Officer, Baptist Easley Hospital, Easley, SC, p. A549
GETTYS, Sky, Chief Financial Officer, Fairfield Medical Center, Lancaster, OH, p. A482
GETWOOD, Charles, Assistant Chief Executive Officer, Calcasieu Oaks Geriatric Psychiatric Hospital, Lake Charles, LA, p. A271
GETZENDANER, Gail, Interim Director of Nursing, Missouri Rehabilitation Center, Mount Vernon, MO, p. A365
GEURTS, Chuck, Manager Management Information Services, Aurora BayCare Medical Center, Green Bay, WI, p. A682
GEWECKE, Tyler, Information Technology Technician, Fillmore County Hospital, Geneva, NE, p. A383
GFELLER, Michael, Director Information Systems, Medical Center of Plano, Plano, TX, p. A621
GHAFFARI, Bahram, Executive Director and Chief Financial Officer, Delano Regional Medical Center, Delano, CA, p. A59
GHANI, Jamal, Chief Operating Officer, Metro Health Hospital, Wyoming, MI, p. A326
GHERINGHELLI, Thomas, Chief Financial Officer, New England Baptist Hospital, Boston, MA, p. A297
GHERKE, Sheila, Director Human Resources, Minnie Hamilton HealthCare Center, Grantsville, WV, p. A672
GHEZZI, Keith T., M.D. Interim President and Chief Executive Officer, West Penn Allegheny Health System, Pittsburgh, PA, p. B144
GHIDOTTI, Craig, Vice President Human Resources, Southwestern Vermont Medical Center, Bennington, VT, p. A643
GHOSH, Tarun, Chief Information Officer, Fremont–Rideout Health Group, Marysville, CA, p. A74
GIAMALIS, John, Senior Vice President and Chief Financial Officer, Saint Francis Hospital and Medical Center, Hartford, CT, p. A109
GIANCOLA, Louis R., President and Chief Executive Officer, South County Hospital, Wakefield, RI, p. A545
GIANELLI, Arthur A., President and Chief Executive Officer, Nassau University Medical Center, East Meadow, NY, p. A425
GIANFORTUNE, Theresa, Chief Human Resources Officer, Marin General Hospital, Greenbrae, CA, p. A64
GIANG, Daniel, M.D. Vice President for Medical Administration, Loma Linda University Medical Center, Loma Linda, CA, p. A67
GIANGARDELLA, Mike, Vice President Finance and Administration, Salem Community Hospital, Salem, OH, p. A488
GIANNUZZI, Donna, R.N. Chief Patient Care Officer, Gulf Coast Medical Center, Fort Myers, FL, p. A123
GIANSANTE, Joseph, Vice President Human Resources, Ellis Hospital, Schenectady, NY, p. A443
GIARDINA, Deborah, Director Human Resources and Medical Staff Services, Rehabilitation Hospital of Fort Wayne, Fort Wayne, IN, p. A202
GIBBARD, Laura, Vice President Human Resources, McLaren Oakland, Pontiac, MI, p. A321
GIBBENS, Lori, Controller, HEALTHSOUTH Rehabilitation Hospital of Erie, Erie, PA, p. A523
GIBBERMAN, Val, M.D. Acting Chief of Staff, Veterans Affairs Medical Center, Hampton, VA, p. A649
GIBBONS, David
Chief Information Officer, Glendale Memorial Hospital and Health Center, Glendale, CA, p. A63
President, UPMC Northwest, Seneca, PA, p. A538



Index of Health Care Professionals A819

Index of Health Care Professionals
Index of Health Care Professionals / Gibbons

GIBBONS, H. Ray, FACHE Chief Executive Officer, Saint Alphonsus Medical Center – Baker City, Baker City, OR, p. A509
GIBBONS, Jason, Chief Financial Officer, Minidoka Memorial Hospital, Rupert, ID, p. A170
GIBBS, Marc, Interim Chief Information Officer, Brookhaven Memorial Hospital Medical Center, Patchogue, NY, p. A440
GIBBS–MCELVY, Shelana, M.D. Medical Director, HEALTHSOUTH Rehabilitation Hospital, Sewickley, PA, p. A538
GIBLER, W. Brian, M.D. President and Chief Executive Officer, University Hospital, Cincinnati, OH, p. A474
GIBSON, Amy, Chief Executive Officer, Jackson Medical Center, Jackson, AL, p. A22
GIBSON, Armetria, Human Resources Generalist, Kindred Hospital–Atlanta, Atlanta, GA, p. A145
GIBSON, Connie, R.N. Director Human Resources, Upstate Carolina Medical Center, Gaffney, SC, p. A550
GIBSON, Debra R., Chief Executive Officer, Select Specialty Hospital–Panama City, Panama City, FL, p. A135
GIBSON, Dick, Senior Vice President and Chief Information Officer, Legacy Emanuel Hospital and Health Center, Portland, OR, p. A514
GIBSON, Donald, M.D. Chief Medical Officer, Memorial Hermann Memorial City Medical Center, Houston, TX, p. A605
GIBSON III, Earnest, Administrator, Riverside General Hospital, Houston, TX, p. A606
GIBSON, Gerald, Director Human Resources, Walter P. Reuther Psychiatric Hospital, Westland, MI, p. A325
GIBSON, Joel, Vice President Human Resources, Henry Ford Macomb Hospitals, Clinton Township, MI, p. A309
GIBSON, Lori, Chief Human Resources Officer, Spectrum Health Special Care Hospital, Grand Rapids, MI, p. A314
GIBSON, Mary Helen, Director Human Resources, Floyd Valley Hospital, Le Mars, IA, p. A222
GIBSON, Megan, Nurse Manager, River Bend Hospital, West Lafayette, IN, p. A213
GIBSON, Miles, M.D. Chief of Staff, Russell County Hospital, Russell Springs, KY, p. A258
GIBSON, Robert, Senior Director Operating Services, Ottawa Regional Hospital and Healthcare Center, Ottawa, IL, p. A190
GIBSON, Valerie, Chief Operating Officer, Harper University Hospital/Hutzel Women's Hospital, Detroit, MI, p. A310
GIBSON, William R.
Chief Executive Officer, Hastings Regional Center, Hastings, NE, p. A384
Chief Executive Officer, Lincoln Regional Center, Lincoln, NE, p. A385
Chief Executive Officer, Norfolk Regional Center, Norfolk, NE, p. A386
GICZI, Mary Beth, Director Human Resources, HEALTHSOUTH Scottsdale Rehabilitation Hospital, Scottsdale, AZ, p. A38
GIDDINGS, Claudia, R.N. Chief Nursing Officer, Our Community Hospital, Scotland Neck, NC, p. A460
GIDDINGS, Wayne, Manager Management Information Systems, East Valley Hospital Medical Center, Glendora, CA, p. A63
GIDEON, Dawn M., Interim Chief Executive Officer, Doctors Medical Center–San Pablo Campus, San Pablo, CA, p. A89
GIEGER, Julie
Chief Financial Officer, Pioneer Community Hospital of Aberdeen, Aberdeen, MS, p. A343
Chief Financial Officer, Pioneer Community Hospital of Newton, Newton, MS, p. A351
Chief Financial Officer, Pioneer Community Hospital of Patrick County, Stuart, VA, p. A656
Chief Financial Officer, S. E. Lackey Memorial Hospital, Forest, MS, p. A346
GIEKEN, Lisa, Director Human Resources, Gothenburg Memorial Hospital, Gothenburg, NE, p. A384
GIENGER, Del, Director Financial Services, Frances Mahon Deaconess Hospital, Glasgow, MT, p. A375
GIESE, Angela C., Director Human Resources, Midwest Regional Medical Center, Midwest City, OK, p. A499
GIESE, Jon, Vice President and Chief Financial Officer, Simi Valley Hospital and Health Care Services, Simi Valley, CA, p. A91
GIESECKE, Guy, Chief Operations Officer, Baptist Hospitals of Southeast Texas, Beaumont, TX, p. A582
GIESKI, Denise S., MS, Chief Executive Officer, Tyler Memorial Hospital, Tunkhannock, PA, p. A539
GIFFORD, Dean, M.D. Chief of Staff, Wabash County Hospital, Wabash, IN, p. A213
GIFFORD, Ellen, Director Human Resources, Deaconess Hospital, Oklahoma City, OK, p. A500
GIGLIOTTI, Vicki, Chief Clinical Officer, Moab Regional Hospital, Moab, UT, p. A638
GIGOT, Kelly, Assistant Administrator and Chief Financial Officer, St. Vincent Hospital, Green Bay, WI, p. A682
GIJANTO, Charles
President, Baystate Northern Region, Baystate Franklin Medical Center, Greenfield, MA, p. A300
President, Baystate Mary Lane Hospital, Ware, MA, p. A305
GIL, Julio, Manager Information Services, Hazel Hawkins Memorial Hospital, Hollister, CA, p. A64
GILB, Robert, Director Information Services, Shriners Hospitals for Children–Chicago, Chicago, IL, p. A178
GILBERG, Ronald, M.D. Chief of Staff, Regional Medical Center–Bayonet Point, Hudson, FL, p. A125
GILBERT, Andrea F., FACHE President, Bryn Mawr Hospital, Bryn Mawr, PA, p. A519
GILBERT, Cameron R., Ph.D. President and Chief Executive Officer, Physicians Hospital System, Mishawaka, IN, p. B101
GILBERT, Carla, Controller, Cedar County Memorial Hospital, El Dorado Springs, MO, p. A359
GILBERT, Jack, Vice President Finance and Support Services, Advocate Illinois Masonic Medical Center, Chicago, IL, p. A175
GILBERT, Jeri, Director Human Resources, Watsonville Community Hospital, Watsonville, CA, p. A95
GILBERT, Kevin, R.N. Director Surgical and Operations, Wenatchee Valley Hospital, Wenatchee, WA, p. A669
GILBERT, Jr., Ronald, Chief Financial Officer, Soldiers and Sailors Memorial Hospital, Wellsboro, PA, p. A540
GILBERT, Thomas, Director Information Technology Services, Lake Cumberland Regional Hospital, Somerset, KY, p. A259
GILBERT, Thomas D., Chief Executive Officer, Wadley Regional Medical Center, Texarkana, TX, p. A631
GILBERT, William L., Chief Executive Officer, Deaconess Medical Center, Spokane, WA, p. A667
GILBERTSON, Gerry, FACHE Administrator, CentraCare Health System – Melrose, Melrose, MN, p. A334
GILBERTSON, Lesley, M.D. Executive and Medical Director, UC Health Surgical Hospital, West Chester, OH, p. A491
GILBREATH, Roy E., M.D. Vice President Medical Affairs, Georgetown Memorial Hospital, Georgetown, SC, p. A550
GILCHRIST, Doug, Chief Operating Officer, Summit Healthcare Regional Medical Center, Show Low, AZ, p. A38
GILDEA, Stephen, Chief Executive Officer, Tyrone Hospital, Tyrone, PA, p. A539
GILDON, Lisa, Chief Financial Officer, North Central Surgical Center, Dallas, TX, p. A592
GILES, Jared, Chief Operating Officer, Rancho Springs Medical Center, Murrieta, CA, p. A76
GILES, Steve, Chief Information Officer, Hollywood Presbyterian Medical Center, Los Angeles, CA, p. A69
GILES, William, Chief Financial Officer, Davis County Hospital, Bloomfield, IA, p. A215
GILGEN, Steve, Chief Financial Officer, Murphy Medical Center, Murphy, NC, p. A458
GILKEY, Edward, M.D. Vice President Medical Affairs, St. Luke's Hospital – Warren Campus, Phillipsburg, NJ, p. A408
GILL, Alexander, Interim Chief Executive Officer, Kindred Hospital Northland, Kansas City, MO, p. A362
GILL, Brian, Chief Executive Officer, Sonora Behavioral Health Hospital, Tucson, AZ, p. A40
GILL, Jan, Director Health Information Management Systems, HEALTHSOUTH Cane Creek Rehabilitation Hospital, Martin, TN, p. A570
GILL, Margaret, Chief Executive Officer, Memorial Health, Savannah, GA, p. A159
GILL, Mark, Vice President Finance and Chief Financial Officer, Cape Regional Medical Center, Cape May Court House, NJ, p. A402
GILL, Robert D., Chief Financial Officer, Woodwinds Health Campus, Woodbury, MN, p. A342
GILLEN, Kristin, R.N. Vice President of Patient Care Services, Three Rivers Medical Center, Grants Pass, OR, p. A511
GILLEN, Mark T., Director Finance and Operations, Owatonna Hospital, Owatonna, MN, p. A336
GILLEN, Michael J., FACHE President, Mercy Hospital Lebanon, Lebanon, MO, p. A364
GILLES, Ken
Chief Information Officer, Essentia Health Fargo, Fargo, ND, p. A465
Associate Chief Information Officer, Essentia Health St. Mary's Hospital – Detroit Lakes, Detroit Lakes, MN, p. A330
GILLESPIE, Anne, R.N. Associate Director Patient Care and Nursing Services, Jerry L. Pettis Memorial Veterans Medical Center, Loma Linda, CA, p. A67
GILLESPIE, Christina, Chief Financial Officer, Harrison County Community Hospital, Bethany, MO, p. A355
GILLESPIE, Karen, Director Human Resources, Anderson County Hospital, Garnett, KS, p. A233
GILLESPIE, Lisa, M.D. Chief Medical Officer, Rockdale Medical Center, Conyers, GA, p. A150
GILLESPIE, Lynn J., Vice President Human Resources and Organizational Development, OSF Saint Francis Medical Center, Peoria, IL, p. A191
GILLESPIE, Michele, Vice President of Operations, Southwest Medical Center, Liberal, KS, p. A238
GILLESPIE, Tim, Manager Information Systems, Richland Memorial Hospital, Olney, IL, p. A190
GILLETTE, Daniel, M.D. Clinical Director, Mental Health Institute, Cherokee, IA, p. A216
GILLETTE, Kathryn, Chief Executive Officer, Osceola Regional Medical Center, Kissimmee, FL, p. A127
GILLETTE, Paula, MSN Vice President Patient Care Services and Chief Nursing Officer, Newport Hospital, Newport, RI, p. A544
GILLETTE, Robert, Chief Information Officer, St. Elizabeth Medical Center, Utica, NY, p. A445
GILLETTE, Tom, Vice President and Chief Information Officer, Mount Sinai Medical Center, Miami Beach, FL, p. A132
GILLIAM, Eric, Administrator, Saint Joseph East, Lexington, KY, p. A253
GILLIAM, Leslie, Director Health Information Management, Dominion Hospital, Falls Church, VA, p. A647
GILLIAN, Tom, Chief Operating Officer, River Bend Hospital, West Lafayette, IN, p. A213
GILLIGAN, Candace L., Chief Executive Officer, Middle Tennessee Mental Health Institute, Nashville, TN, p. A573
GILLIS, Anne, Chief Financial Officer, Holy Cross Hospital, Silver Spring, MD, p. A294
GILLIS, Wayne, Interim Chief Executive Officer, Phoenix Baptist Hospital, Phoenix, AZ, p. A36
GILLMAN, Jerry E., Chief Executive Officer, Tri–County Hospital – Williston, Williston, FL, p. A143
GILMAN, Howard, M.D. Medical Executive, Christian Health Care Center, Wyckoff, NJ, p. A412
GILMAN, Kim, Chief Administrative Officer, Phoebe Worth Medical Center, Sylvester, GA, p. A160
GILMORE, Beverly, President and Chief Executive Officer, West Hills Hospital and Medical Center,, CA, p. A72
GILMORE, Hugh V., M.D. Vice President Medical Affairs, Seton Medical Center Williamson, Round Rock, TX, p. A623
GILMORE, Linda, Chief Nursing Officer/Chief Administrative Officer, Littleton Regional Hospital, Littleton, NH, p. A399
GILMORE, Phillip K., FACHE Chief Executive Officer, Ashley County Medical Center, Crossett, AR, p. A43
GILMORE, Stephen, Chief Financial Officer, Saint Vincent Hospital, Worcester, MA, p. A306
GILPEN, Mike, Director Human Resources, East Cooper Medical Center, Mount Pleasant, SC, p. A552
GILPIN, Ann C., President and Chief Executive Officer, Oswego Hospital, Oswego, NY, p. A440
GILPIN, Michael W., Vice President Human Resources, Sampson Regional Medical Center, Clinton, NC, p. A451
GILTNER, Michelle, Director Professional and Support Staff Services, University Hospitals Bedford Medical Center, Cleveland, OH, p. A475
GIN, Nancy, M.D. Area Associate Medical Director, Anaheim Medical Center, Anaheim, CA, p. A53
GINGHER, Barbara, R.N. Assistant Administrator for Patient Care Services, Baptist Medical Center Nassau, Fernandina Beach, FL, p. A123
GINN, Bobby, Chief Operating Officer, Crestwood Medical Center, Huntsville, AL, p. A21
GINSBERG, Ronald L., M.D. Vice President Medical Affairs, Northwest Hospital, Randallstown, MD, p. A293
GINSBURG, J. Lawrence, M.D. Vice President Medical Affairs, Evangelical Community Hospital, Lewisburg, PA, p. A527
GINTY, Neil W., Administrator, Louis Smith Memorial Hospital, Lakeland, GA, p. A155
GIOIA, Anthony, Chief Financial Officer, Indiana Orthopaedic Hospital, Indianapolis, IN, p. A204
GIOIA, Gregory J., Chief Fiscal and Administrative Services, Veterans Home and Hospital, Rocky Hill, CT, p. A111
GIONFRIDDO, Paul, MS Vice President Human Resources, Moses Taylor Hospital, Scranton, PA, p. A538
GIORDANO, Paul, Vice President Human Resources, South Nassau Communities Hospital, Oceanside, NY, p. A439
GIORDANO, Roger, M.D. Medical Director, HEALTHSOUTH Rehabilitation Hospital of Virginia, Richmond, VA, p. A655
GIOVANETTI, Victor, President and Chief Executive Officer, Lewis–Gale Medical Center, Salem, VA, p. A655
GIPSON, David N., Senior Vice President and Chief Clinical Operations Officer, Union Hospital, Elkton, MD, p. A291
GIRARD, Thomas, Vice President Human Resources, Pen Bay Medical Center, Rockport, ME, p. A285
GIRARDIER, Cheryl, Director Information Technology, Millcreek Community Hospital, Erie, PA, p. A523
GIRTEN, David M.
Corporate Director Financial Services, St. Vincent Seton Specialty Hospital, Indianapolis, IN, p. A205
Corporate Director Financial Services, St. Vincent Seton Specialty Hospital, Lafayette, IN, p. A207

**A820** Index of Health Care Professionals

Index of Health Care Professionals / Goldberg

Index of Health Care Professionals

GIRTY, Tara, Director Human Resources, Kiowa District Hospital and Manor, Kiowa, KS, p. A236
GISH, Christine, R.N. Acute Care Director, Mountain View Hospital District, Madras, OR, p. A512
GISH, Kevin, Chief Executive Officer, Essentia Health–Holy Trinity Hospital, Graceville, MN, p. A332
GISH, Mary L., R.N. Vice President and Chief Nursing Officer, Sierra Nevada Memorial Hospital, Grass Valley, CA, p. A64
GISI, Richard, M.D. Chief Medical Officer, Citrus Valley Medical Center–Inter–Community Campus, Covina, CA, p. A59
GISLESON, Joni, Director Finance, Palmer Lutheran Health Center, West Union, IA, p. A228
GISSEL, Betty, Vice President Human Resources, The University of Tennessee Medical Center, Knoxville, TN, p. A569
GITTELMAN, Michael B., Administrator, Bascom Palmer Eye Institute–Anne Bates Leach Eye Hospital, Miami, FL, p. A131
GIUDICE, William A., Vice President and Chief Financial Officer, Tallahassee Memorial HealthCare, Tallahassee, FL, p. A140
GIUGLIANO, Frank, M.D. Chief of Staff, Berwick Hospital Center, Berwick, PA, p. A518
GIULIANELLI, Victor, FACHE President and Chief Executive Officer, St. Mary's Healthcare, Amsterdam, NY, p. A420
GIVENS, Michael K., FACHE Administrator, St. Bernards Medical Center, Jonesboro, AR, p. A47
GIVENS, Scott H., Director Human Resources, Flowers Hospital, Dothan, AL, p. A19
GIVENS, Stephen K., Chief Operating Officer, Johnston Memorial Hospital, Abingdon, VA, p. A645
GIZZI, Jason, Controller, HEALTHSOUTH MountainView Regional Rehabilitation Hospital, Morgantown, WV, p. A674
GIZZI, Sam, President and Chief Executive Officer, Doctors' Hospital of Michigan, Pontiac, MI, p. A320
GLAD, Cory, Director Human Resources, Community Memorial Hospital, Cloquet, MN, p. A329
GLADE, James, Director Human Resources, Mountain West Medical Center, Tooele, UT, p. A641
GLADFELTER, Sharon, Health Information Officer, Brook Lane Health Services, Hagerstown, MD, p. A292
GLADSTONE, Art, R.N. Chief Operating Officer, Straub Clinic & Hospital, Honolulu, HI, p. A164
GLANZER, Elgin, Chief Financial Officer, Memorial Health System, Abilene, KS, p. A230
GLASER, Ruth, President, Pender Memorial Hospital, Burgaw, NC, p. A449
GLASNER, Greg, M.D. Chief Executive Officer, Essentia Health Fargo, Fargo, ND, p. A465
GLASS, Deborah, R.N. Chief Executive Officer, Whitman Hospital and Medical Center, Colfax, WA, p. A660
GLASS, Gordon, Chief Financial Officer, Golden Valley Memorial Healthcare, Clinton, MO, p. A358
GLASS, Steven, Chief Financial Officer, Cleveland Clinic Foundation, Cleveland, OH, p. A474
GLASSBURN, David, Interim Chief Financial Officer, Palm Drive Hospital, Sebastopol, CA, p. A90
GLASSCOCK, Gary M., President and Chief Executive Officer, Noland Health Services, Inc., Birmingham, AL, p. B94
GLASSMAN, Randy, Chief Financial Officer, Little Colorado Medical Center, Winslow, AZ, p. A41
GLAVES, Ann, Vice President Human Resources, St. Francis Regional Medical Center, Shakopee, MN, p. A340
GLAVIS, Edward S., Senior Vice President and Area Manager, Roseville Medical Center, Roseville, CA, p. A83
GLAZIER, Alisha, Compliance Officer and Director Health Information Management, Watonga Municipal Hospital, Watonga, OK, p. A507
GLAZIER, Steve, Chief Executive Officer, Saint Simons by–the–Sea Hospital, Saint Simons Island, GA, p. A158
GLEASON, Amanda, Director Human Resources, Indiana Orthopaedic Hospital, Indianapolis, IN, p. A204
GLEASON, Mike, Vice President and Chief Financial Officer, Shands Jacksonville Medical Center, Jacksonville, FL, p. A126
GLEASON, Ronald M., Chief Executive Officer, Liberty Medical Center, Chester, MT, p. A374
GLECKLER, John, Chief Financial Officer, St. Vincent's Medical Center, Bridgeport, CT, p. A108
GLEDHILL, John E., Chief Operating Officer, Central Valley Medical Center, Nephi, UT, p. A639
GLEISNER, Roger, Interim Chief Executive Officer, Rehoboth McKinley Christian Health Care Services, Gallup, NM, p. A416
GLEN, Diane M., Assistant Administrator, Barnes–Jewish West County Hospital, Saint Louis, MO, p. A368
GLENN, Jeannette, Vice President Human Resources, Education and Training, McLeod Regional Medical Center, Florence, SC, p. A550
GLENN, Mike, Administrator and Chief Executive Officer, Jefferson Healthcare, Port Townsend, WA, p. A664
GLENN, Sue, Director Administrative Services, Kalamazoo Psychiatric Hospital, Kalamazoo, MI, p. A316
GLENN, Susan, Chief Executive Officer, HEALTHSOUTH Rehabilitation Hospital, Kingsport, TN, p. A568
GLENN, Wil A., Director Communications, Larry B. Zieverink, Sr. Alcoholism Treatment Center, Raleigh, NC, p. A459
GLENNIE, Stacy, Director Health Information Services, Pratt Regional Medical Center, Pratt, KS, p. A242
GLENNING, Robert, Executive Vice President Finance and Chief Financial Officer, Hackensack University Medical Center, Hackensack, NJ, p. A404
GLEZEN, Joseph W., Director Human Resources, Southeastern Regional Medical Center, Lumberton, NC, p. A457
GLICKMAN, Bobby, M.D. Chief of Staff, Sutter Delta Medical Center, Antioch, CA, p. A53
GLIDDEN, Nancy, Chief Financial Officer, Calais Regional Hospital, Calais, ME, p. A282
GLIDDEN, Weldon, M.D. Chief of Staff, Chillicothe Hospital District, Chillicothe, TX, p. A587
GLIDEWELL Jr., Calvin E., Chief Executive Officer, Broward Health Medical Center, Fort Lauderdale, FL, p. A123
GLIELMI, Vincent D., D.O. Senior Vice President Medical Affairs, Ephrata Community Hospital, Ephrata, PA, p. A523
GLINIECKI, Charlene, Vice President Human Resources, El Camino Hospital, Mountain View, CA, p. A76
GLOCKNER, Cheri, Director Development, Carson Tahoe Regional Healthcare, Carson City, NV, p. A391
GLODOWSKI, Brenda, Chief Financial Officer, North Central Health Care, Wausau, WI, p. A693
GLOFF, Vickie, Accountant, Goodall–Witcher Healthcare, Clifton, TX, p. A587
GLOGGNER, Peter, Vice President Human Resources, Union Hospital, Elkton, MD, p. A291
GLONER, James, Senior Vice President, North Philadelphia Health System, Philadelphia, PA, p. A533
GLORIOSO, John, M.D. Deputy Commander Clinical Services, Weed Army Community Hospital, Fort Irwin, CA, p. A61
GLOSEMEYER, Talitha, M.P.H. Administrator, Norman Specialty Hospital, Norman, OK, p. A500
GLOSS, John, FACHE Administrator, Shriners Hospitals for Children, St. Louis, Saint Louis, MO, p. A369
GLOTZBACH, Karen, Acting Associate Director, Veterans Affairs Eastern Kansas Health Care System, Topeka, KS, p. A244
GLOTZBACK, Lee, Director Human Resources, Citrus Memorial Health System, Inverness, FL, p. A126
GLOVER, Doug, Controller, William S. Hall Psychiatric Institute, Columbia, SC, p. A548
GLOVER, Kenneth E., President and Chief Executive Officer, Dimensions Healthcare System, Cheverly, MD, p. B47
GLOVER, Kimberly, Director Information Systems, Lake City Community Hospital, Lake City, SC, p. A552
GLOVER, Sharon, Director Human Resources, Somerset Hospital, Somerset, PA, p. A538
GLOWA, Meghan, Director Human Resources, Sunnyview Rehabilitation Hospital, Schenectady, NY, p. A443
GLUBKA, Theresa, Chief Executive Officer, Sutter Solano Medical Center, Vallejo, CA, p. A94
GLUCHOWSKI, Jeanne, Executive Director, Conifer Park, Glenville, NY, p. A426
GLUECKERT, John W., Administrator, Montana State Hospital, Warm Springs, MT, p. A379
GLYER, David, Vice President Finance, Community Memorial Health System, Ventura, CA, p. A94
GLYNN, Cindy, Director Human Resources, Regional Rehabilitation Hospital, Phenix City, AL, p. A25
GLYNN, John, Senior Vice President and Chief Information Officer, Unity Hospital, Rochester, NY, p. A442
GLYNN, Margaret, M.D. Chief Medical Officer, North Mississippi Medical Center–Iuka, Iuka, MS, p. A347
GLYNN, Shari, Vice President Finance and Chief Financial Officer, Eaton Rapids Medical Center, Eaton Rapids, MI, p. A312
GNAM, Gwen, R.N. Chief Nursing Officer, Henry Ford Hospital, Detroit, MI, p. A310
GNANADEV, Dev, M.D. Medical Director, Arrowhead Regional Medical Center, Colton, CA, p. A58
GOACHER, Brad, Director Finance, Alton Memorial Hospital, Alton, IL, p. A172
GOAD, Dody, Administrator, Latimer County General Hospital, Wilburton, OK, p. A508
GOAD, Pat, Director Human Resources, Hillcrest Hospital Claremore, Claremore, OK, p. A495
GOBEL, Bret, Chief Financial Officer, Sierra Vista Hospital, Truth or Consequences, NM, p. A418
GOBELL, James, Chief Financial Officer, St. Luke's Regional Medical Center, Sioux City, IA, p. A227
GOBLE, Jonathan R., FACHE President and Chief Executive Officer, Indiana University Health North Hospital, Carmel, IN, p. A199
GOBLE, Mandy C., President and Chief Executive Officer, Mary Rutan Hospital, Bellefontaine, OH, p. A470
GOCHENOUR, Julia, Manager Information Systems, West River Regional Medical Center, Hettinger, ND, p. A466
GOCHIS, Paul D., M.D. Chief of Staff, St. Luke Community Hospital, Ronan, MT, p. A378
GODDARD, Donald, M.D. Chief Medical Officer, Heatherhill Care Communities, Chardon, OH, p. A472
GODDARD, Mark, M.D. Medical Director, HEALTHSOUTH Rehabilitation Hospital at Drake, Cincinnati, OH, p. A473
GODESKY, Susan, Director Information Technology, Nanticoke Memorial Hospital, Seaford, DE, p. A114
GODFREY, Kristine, Director Human Resources, Skyridge Medical Center, Cleveland, TN, p. A564
GODLEY, Patrick, Chief Financial Officer, Contra Costa Regional Medical Center, Martinez, CA, p. A74
GODSEY, Carol, Administrator, St. Mary's Warrick Hospital, Boonville, IN, p. A198
GODWIN, Jr., Herman A., M.D. Senior Vice President and Medical Director, Watauga Medical Center, Boone, NC, p. A449
GOEBEL, Bret, Finance Officer, Guadalupe County Hospital, Santa Rosa, NM, p. A418
GOEBEL, Dennis, Chief Executive Officer, Southwest Healthcare Services, Bowman, ND, p. A464
GOEBEL, Michael, Chief Executive Officer, Adventist Hinsdale Hospital, Hinsdale, IL, p. A184
GOEL, Amitabh, M.D. Chief Medical Officer, University Hospitals Geneva Medical Center, Geneva, OH, p. A481
GOELOE–ALSTON, Hendrina, Assistant Vice President Personnel, SUNY Downstate Medical Center University Hospital of Brooklyn,, NY, p. A437
GOERKE, Karleen, R.N. Chief Nursing Officer, Swedish Medical Center, Englewood, CO, p. A100
GOESER, Stephen L., FACHE President and Chief Executive Officer, Nebraska Methodist Hospital, Omaha, NE, p. A388
GOETTSCH, Barry, Chief Executive Officer, Marengo Memorial Hospital, Marengo, IA, p. A223
GOETZINGER, Susan, Chief Financial Officer, Riverton Memorial Hospital, Riverton, WY, p. A697
GOFF, Gary E., M.D. Medical Director, Texas Specialty Hospital at Dallas, Dallas, TX, p. A593
GOFF, Mark, Owner and Administrator, Community Specialty Hospital, Lafayette, LA, p. A270
GOFFNETT, Carol, Chief Executive Officer, Aspirus Grand View Hospital, Ironwood, MI, p. A316
GOFORTH, Annette, Manager Administrative Services, Central Prison Hospital, Raleigh, NC, p. A458
GOGGIN, Daniel, Chief Financial Officer, Memorial Hermann Sugar Land Hospital, Sugar Land, TX, p. A629
GOGGIN, Kathy, Director Administrative Services, Devereux Georgia Treatment Network, Kennesaw, GA, p. A154
GOGIA, Harmohinder, M.D. Chief Medical Officer, Western Medical Center Anaheim, Anaheim, CA, p. A53
GOGLIETTINO, Deborah
Senior Vice President Human Resources, Manchester Memorial Hospital, Manchester, CT, p. A109
Senior Vice President Human Resources, Rockville General Hospital, Vernon Rockville, CT, p. A112
GOHNER, Cindy, Vice President Clinical Services, Jamestown Regional Medical Center, Jamestown, ND, p. A466
GOINGS, Harold, Chief Human Resources, Veterans Affairs Greater Los Angeles Healthcare System, Los Angeles, CA, p. A72
GOLAS, Catherine, Administrator, Isham Health Center, Andover, MA, p. A295
GOLD, Joseph, M.D. Chief Medical Officer, McLean Hospital, Belmont, MA, p. A295
GOLDAMMER, Kyle, Chief Financial Officer, Sioux Falls Surgical Center, Sioux Falls, SD, p. A559
GOLDBERG, Andrew S., Associate Executive Director, Syosset Hospital, Syosset, NY, p. A444
GOLDBERG, David, M.D. Vice President Medical Affairs, Community Memorial Hospital, Menomonee Falls, WI, p. A685
GOLDBERG, David S., President, Baptist Health System, San Antonio, TX, p. A624
GOLDBERG, Edward M., President and Chief Executive Officer, St. Alexius Medical Center, Hoffman Estates, IL, p. A185
GOLDBERG, Frederick, M.D. Vice President Medical Affairs and Chief Medical Officer, Nathan Littauer Hospital and Nursing Home, Gloversville, NY, p. A426
GOLDBERG, Jonathan, Chief Information Officer, St. Peter's Hospital, Albany, NY, p. A420
GOLDBERG, Larry, President and Chief Executive Officer, Loyola University Health System, Maywood, IL, p. B
GOLDBERG, Paul R., Chief Financial Officer, LibertyHealth–Jersey City Medical Center, Jersey City, NJ, p. A405
GOLDBERG, Richard L., M.D. President, Medstar Georgetown University Hospital, Washington, DC, p. A116
GOLDBERG, Stanley, M.D. Chief of Staff, St. Mary Medical Center, Long Beach, CA, p. A68

Index of Health Care Professionals

Index of Health Care Professionals / Goldberg

GOLDBERG, Stephanie J., MSN Senior Vice President and Chief Nursing Officer, Hospital for Special Surgery, New York, NY, p. A433
GOLDBERGER, Joseph, M.D
Chief Medical Officer, Yavapai Regional Medical Center – East, Prescott Valley, AZ, p. A37
Chief Medical Officer, Yavapai Regional Medical Center, Prescott, AZ, p. A37
GOLDBLOOM, Alan L., M.D
President and Chief Executive Officer, Children's Hospitals and Clinics of Minnesota, Minneapolis, MN, p. A335
President and Chief Executive Officer, Children's Hospitals and Clinics of Minnesota, Saint Paul, MN, p. A339
GOLDBLOOM, Alan L., M.D. President and Chief Executive Officer, Children's Hospitals and Clinics of Minnesota, Minneapolis, MN, p. B31
GOLDEN, Joy, Chief Operating Officer, Lakeside Behavioral Health System, Memphis, TN, p. A571
GOLDENBERG, Dianne, Chief Executive Officer, Northwest Medical Center, Margate, FL, p. A129
GOLDFARB, Timothy M., Chief Executive Officer, Shands at the University of Florida, Gainesville, FL, p. A124
GOLDFARB, Timothy M., Chief Executive Officer, Shands HealthCare, Gainesville, FL, p. B117
GOLDFISHER, Anne M., R.N. Chief Nursing Officer, Santa Clara Medical Center, Santa Clara, CA, p. A90
GOLDFRACH, Andrew, Assistant Chief Executive Officer, Chestnut Hill Hospital, Philadelphia, PA, p. A531
GOLDMAN, Bruce, Chief Operating Officer, The HSC Pediatric Center, Washington, DC, p. A117
GOLDMAN, David, M.D. Vice President Medical Affairs and Education, Prince George's Hospital Center, Cheverly, MD, p. A290
GOLDMAN, Eric, Chief Executive Officer, Palms West Hospital, Loxahatchee, FL, p. A129
GOLDMAN, John S., Associate Director, Veterans Affairs Medical Center, Augusta, GA, p. A147
GOLDSCHMID, David, M.D. President Medical Staff, Seton Medical Center, Daly City, CA, p. A59
GOLDSMITH, Cheri L.
Director Financial Services, Parkland Health Center, Farmington, MO, p. A359
Director Financial Services, Parkland Health Center–Bonne Terre, Bonne Terre, MO, p. A355
GOLDSMITH, Dana L., M.D. Vice President Medical Affairs, Pen Bay Medical Center, Rockport, ME, p. A285
GOLDSMITH, Debra, Chief Executive Officer, Alegent Health Mercy Hospital, Corning, IA, p. A216
GOLDSTEIN, Allan, M.D. Medical Director and Chief of Staff, Select Specialty Hospital–Birmingham, Birmingham, AL, p. A16
GOLDSTEIN, Brian, M.D. Executive Vice President and Chief Operating Officer, University of North Carolina Hospitals, Chapel Hill, NC, p. A450
GOLDSTEIN, Charles, M.D. President Medical Staff, Riverside Shore Memorial Hospital, Nassawadox, VA, p. A651
GOLDSTEIN, Gary W., M.D. President and Chief Executive Officer, Kennedy Krieger Institute, Baltimore, MD, p. A287
GOLDSTEIN, Lisa, Executive Vice President and Chief Operating Officer, Hospital for Special Surgery, New York, NY, p. A433
GOLDSTEIN, Mark L., Chief Financial Officer, Anna Jaques Hospital, Newburyport, MA, p. A302
GOLDSTEIN, III, Nathan, M.D. Chief Medical Officer, Northwest Texas Healthcare System, Amarillo, TX, p. A578
GOLDSTEIN, Paul, Vice President Finance and Chief Financial Officer, Orlando Regional Medical Center, Orlando, FL, p. A134
GOLDSTEIN, Stephen, Director Information Systems, Regional Medical Center–Bayonet Point, Hudson, FL, p. A125
GOLDSTEIN, Steven I.
President and Chief Executive Officer, Highland Hospital of Rochester, Rochester, NY, p. A441
President and Chief Executive Officer, Strong Memorial Hospital of the University of Rochester, Rochester, NY, p. A442
GOLDSTEIN, Steven I., General Director and Chief Executive Officer, University of Rochester Medical Center, Rochester, NY, p. B139
GOLDSTEIN, Stuart, D.O. Chief of Staff, LewisGale Hospital at Pulaski, Pulaski, VA, p. A654
GOLDSTEIN, Wendy Z., President and Chief Executive Officer, Lutheran Medical Center,, NY, p. A434
GOLDSWORTHY, Patty, Interim Chief Executive Officer and Administrator, Pershing General Hospital, Lovelock, NV, p. A394
GOLDSZER, Robert, M.D. Senior Vice President and Chief Medical Officer, Mount Sinai Medical Center, Miami Beach, FL, p. A132
GOLER, Michael, M.D. Chief Medical Officer, South Lake Hospital, Clermont, FL, p. A120
GOLIER, Francis C., M.D. Chief of Staff, Community Hospital at Dobbs Ferry, Dobbs Ferry, NY, p. A425
GOLIGHTLY, Beverly, Director Information Technology, St. Vincent's East, Birmingham, AL, p. A17
GOLLAHER, Jeffrey, Chief Executive Officer, Hendricks Community Hospital, Hendricks, MN, p. A332
GOLOMB, Harvey, M.D. Chief Medical Officer, University of Chicago Medical Center, Chicago, IL, p. A179
GOLOVAN, Ronald, M.D. Vice President Medical Operations, Lutheran Hospital, Cleveland, OH, p. A475
GOMAN, Valerie, M.D. President Medical Staff, Baylor Medical Center at Waxahachie, Waxahachie, TX, p. A633
GOMBAR, Greg A.
Chief Financial Officer, Carolinas Medical Center, Charlotte, NC, p. A450
Chief Financial Officer, Carolinas Medical Center–Mercy, Charlotte, NC, p. A450
Chief Financial Officer, Carolinas Medical Center–University, Charlotte, NC, p. A450
GOMES, Carol, Director Operations, Stony Brook University Medical Center, Stony Brook, NY, p. A444
GOMES, Robert
Chief Executive Officer, Pioneer Memorial Hospital, Prineville, OR, p. A514
Chief Executive Officer, St. Charles Medical Center – Redmond, Redmond, OR, p. A515
GOMEZ, Carmen, Director Human Resources, North Shore Medical Center, Miami, FL, p. A131
GOMEZ, Gloria, M.D. Medical Director, East Mississippi State Hospital, Meridian, MS, p. A350
GOMEZ, Lynn M., Executive Director Human Resources, San Gorgonio Memorial Hospital, Banning, CA, p. A55
GOMEZ, Mike, Site Manager Medical Information Systems, Our Lady of Bellefonte Hospital, Ashland, KY, p. A247
GOMEZ, Robin, Administrator, Alvarado Hospital, San Diego, CA, p. A85
GOMEZ, Teresa, Chief Nursing Officer, Peninsula Hospital, Louisville, TN, p. A570
GONDER, Christie, Chief Nursing Officer, Sierra Vista Regional Medical Center, San Luis Obispo, CA, p. A88
GONGAWARE, Robert, Senior Vice President Finance, Indiana Regional Medical Center, Indiana, PA, p. A525
GONYEA, Sonja, Director Human Resources, United Memorial Medical Center, Batavia, NY, p. A421
GONZALES, D. V., Head Information Technology Management, Naval Medical Center, San Diego, CA, p. A85
GONZALES, Ed
Vice President Human Resources, St. John's Pleasant Valley Hospital, Camarillo, CA, p. A56
Vice President Human Resources, St. John's Regional Medical Center, Oxnard, CA, p. A78
GONZALES, Jan, Director Human Resources, North Valley Hospital, Tonasket, WA, p. A668
GONZALES, Mary Ann, M.D. Medical Director, Central Texas Rehabilitation Hospital, Austin, TX, p. A580
GONZALES, Pamela, Chief Operating Officer, Anson General Hospital, Anson, TX, p. A579
GONZALES, Patricia, Chief Executive Officer, Eastern Louisiana Mental Health System, Jackson, LA, p. A268
GONZALES, Rachel, R.N. Chief Executive Officer, Madison Memorial Hospital, Rexburg, ID, p. A170
GONZALEZ, Arthur A., FACHE Chief Executive Officer, Hennepin County Medical Center, Minneapolis, MN, p. A335
GONZALEZ, Aurelio, Chief Financial Officer, University Hospital and Medical Center, Tamarac, FL, p. A140
GONZALEZ, Dinah, Chief Financial Officer, Doctors Hospital of Laredo, Laredo, TX, p. A612
GONZALEZ, Elizabeth, Chief Financial Officer, Hospital Metropolitano Dr. Tito Mattei, Yauco, PR, p. A704
GONZALEZ, Erin, Director Human Resources and Education, Maryvale Hospital Medical Center, Phoenix, AZ, p. A36
GONZALEZ, Gilberto, Chief Executive Officer, Hospital Metropolitan, San Juan, PR, p. A703
GONZALEZ, Hugo, M.D. Chief Medical Officer, Sister Emmanuel Hospital, Miami, FL, p. A132
GONZALEZ, Jaime, Administrator, St. Catherine's Rehabilitation Hospital, North Miami, FL, p. A133
GONZALEZ, James R., Acting President and Chief Executive Officer, University of Medicine and Dentistry of New Jersey–University Hospital, Newark, NJ, p. A407
GONZALEZ, Jorge F., M.D. Chief Medical Officer, Florida Hospital Heartland Medical Center, Sebring, FL, p. A139
GONZALEZ, Jorge Matta, Executive Director, University Hospital, San Juan, PR, p. A704
GONZALEZ, Pedro J., Executive Director, Ashford Presbyterian Community Hospital, San Juan, PR, p. A702
GONZALEZ, Rainier, Chairman and Chief Executive Officer, Pacer Health Corporation, Miami Lakes, FL, p. B99
GONZALEZ, Rebecca
Director Human Resources, Parkview LaGrange Hospital, LaGrange, IN, p. A207
Manager Human Resources, Parkview Noble Hospital, Kendallville, IN, p. A206
GONZALEZ, Robert, M.D. Director, Ventura County Medical Center, Ventura, CA, p. A94
GONZALEZ, Sonia I., R.N. Chief Operating Officer, Oak Hill Hospital, Brooksville, FL, p. A120
GONZALEZ–FAJARDO, Ana, Human Resources Director, Palmetto General Hospital, Hialeah, FL, p. A125
GOOCH, Chris, Information Technology Director, Hermann Area District Hospital, Hermann, MO, p. A360
GOOCH, Matthew, Chief Operating Officer, Jennersville Regional Hospital, West Grove, PA, p. A541
GOOCH, Patricia Pidge", Chief Nursing Officer, Doctors Hospital of Manteca, Manteca, CA, p. A73
GOOD, Scott, Manager Information Services, Kearny County Hospital, Lakin, KS, p. A237
GOOD, Vance A., M.D. Chief Medical Staff, Troy Community Hospital, Troy, PA, p. A539
GOODALL, David, M.D. Chief Medical Staff, Deer River HealthCare Center, Deer River, MN, p. A330
GOODBALIAN, Terry, Vice President Finance and Chief Financial Officer, Henry Ford Macomb Hospitals, Clinton Township, MI, p. A309
GOODE, Galen, Chief Executive Officer, Hamilton Center, Terre Haute, IN, p. A212
GOODE, Lori, Director Human Resources, Baptist Memorial Hospital–Union County, New Albany, MS, p. A351
GOODE, Richard P., Chief Financial Officer, Cook Children's Medical Center, Fort Worth, TX, p. A598
GOODE, Vicky, Director Human Resources, LifeCare Hospitals of North Carolina, Rocky Mount, NC, p. A459
GOODIN, Debbie, Vice President Human Resources, Mills–Peninsula Health Services, Burlingame, CA, p. A56
GOODLETT, Lisa, Chief Financial Officer, Baptist Medical Center South, Montgomery, AL, p. A23
GOODMAN, Brenda, Chief Nursing Officer, Peach Regional Medical Center, Fort Valley, GA, p. A153
GOODMAN, David M., Ph.D. Chief Information Officer, Veterans Affairs Boston Healthcare System, Boston, MA, p. A297
GOODMAN, Larry J., M.D. Chief Executive Officer, Rush University Medical Center, Chicago, IL, p. B111
GOODMAN, Louis, Vice President Human Resources, UPMC Presbyterian Shadyside, Pittsburgh, PA, p. A535
GOODMAN, Mary Jo, Chief Operating Officer, Park Plaza Hospital, Houston, TX, p. A606
GOODMAN, Steven, Chief Operating Officer, Willow Crest Hospital, Miami, OK, p. A499
GOODNO, Janell, Chief Financial Officer, Stafford County Hospital, Stafford, KS, p. A243
GOODNOW, John H., Chief Executive Officer, Benefis Health System, Great Falls, MT, p. B21
GOODNOW, John H., Chief Executive Officer, Benefis Hospitals, Great Falls, MT, p. A376
GOODRICH, Brenda, D.O. Chief of Staff, Tyler Memorial Hospital, Tunkhannock, PA, p. A539
GOODRICH, C. Harlan, Vice President and Chief Information Officer, MidMichigan Medical Center–Midland, Midland, MI, p. A319
GOODRICH, Zane, Vice President Finance, East Tennessee Children's Hospital, Knoxville, TN, p. A568
GOODSON, Bradley R., Chief Executive Officer, Ochsner Baptist Medical Center, New Orleans, LA, p. A274
GOODSON, David, Chief Executive Officer, Select Specialty Hospital–Pensacola, Pensacola, FL, p. A136
GOODSTEIN, Ruth, Controller, HEALTHSOUTH Sunrise Rehabilitation Hospital, Fort Lauderdale, FL, p. A123
GOODWIN, Ervin, Manager Information Services, North Country Hospital and Health Center, Newport, VT, p. A644
GOODWIN, Jeremy, M.D. President, Medical Staff, Monroe County Hospital, Forsyth, GA, p. A153
GOODWIN, Keith D., President and Chief Executive Officer, East Tennessee Children's Hospital, Knoxville, TN, p. A568
GOODWIN, W. Jarrad, M.D. Director, University of Miami Hospital and Clinics, Miami, FL, p. A132
GOOLSBY, Elizabeth, Director, Veterans Affairs Medical Center, Fayetteville, NC, p. A453
GOPALAM, Gopinath, Chief Financial Officer, St. James Behavioral Health Hospital, Gonzales, LA, p. A267
GORBACH, Debbie, Vice President and Treasurer, Edwin Shaw Rehab, Cuyahoga Falls, OH, p. A478
GORBY, David, M.D. Interim Senior Vice President & Chief Medical Officer/VP Patient Safety & Quality, Nash Health Care Systems, Rocky Mount, NC, p. A460
GORBY, Karen S., FACHE Administrator, Mercy Memorial Hospital, Urbana, OH, p. A490
GORDIAN, Michael, Chief Financial Officer, Capital Regional Medical Center, Tallahassee, FL, p. A140

A822 Index of Health Care Professionals

Index of Health Care Professionals / Granger


GORDON, Dan, Chief Financial Officer, Feather River Hospital, Paradise, CA, p. A79
GORDON, Kevin, M.D. Chief of Staff, Medical Center of Southeastern Oklahoma, Durant, OK, p. A495
GORDON, Leilani, Director Human Resources and Payroll, Nye Regional Medical Center, Tonopah, NV, p. A396
GORDON, Mark M., Executive Vice President, Bon Secours St. Francis Medical Center, Midlothian, VA, p. A651
GORDON, Nancy Gail, R.N. CNO and VP of Nursing, Baptist Health South Florida, Homestead Hospital, Homestead, FL, p. A125
GORDON, Robert, Manager Information Systems, Halifax Regional Medical Center, Roanoke Rapids, NC, p. A459
GORDON, Steve, Director Human Resources, Lake City Medical Center, Lake City, FL, p. A128
GORDON, Steven R., President and Chief Executive Officer, Brattleboro Memorial Hospital, Brattleboro, VT, p. A643
GORDY, Joseph S., President, Flagler Hospital, Saint Augustine, FL, p. A137
GORE, Gary R., Chief Executive Officer, Marshall Health System, Guntersville, AL, p. B84
GORE, Tim, Chief Financial Officer, Rivendell Behavioral Health, Bowling Green, KY, p. A248
GOREAU, Judy, R.N. Director of Nursing, Eastside Psychiatric Hospital, Tallahassee, FL, p. A140
GOREE, Hal, Chief Information Officer, Franklin Foundation Hospital, Franklin, LA, p. A266
GOREY, Peter, Administrative Coordinator, Rockland Children's Psychiatric Center, Orangeburg, NY, p. A439
GORHAM, Jennie, D.O. Co–Medical Director, Missouri Rehabilitation Center, Mount Vernon, MO, p. A365
GORLEWSKI, Todd, Senior Vice President and Chief Financial Officer, St. Barnabas Hospital,, NY, p. A436
GORMAN, A. Alexander, Director Operations, Curry General Hospital, Gold Beach, OR, p. A510
GORMAN, Brandon, Controller, Bradley County Medical Center, Warren, AR, p. A52
GORMAN, Martha C., R.N. Vice President of Patient Care Services and Chief Nursing Officer, Gerald Champion Regional Medical Center, Alamogordo, NM, p. A414
GORMAN, Patricia, Chief Nurse Executive, Chinle Comprehensive Health Care Facility, Chinle, AZ, p. A31
GORMLEY, Maureen E., R.N. Chief Operating Officer, National Institutes of Health Clinical Center, Bethesda, MD, p. A289
GORMSEN, David, D.O. Chief Medical Officer, Mercy Medical Center, Canton, OH, p. A472
GORN, Angela, Vice President, Norton Sound Regional Hospital, Nome, AK, p. A29
GORRELL, Mark, Vice President Information Services, Baystate Medical Center, Springfield, MA, p. A304
GORS, Ann, Chief Executive Officer, Kentfield Rehabilitation and Specialty Hospital, Kentfield, CA, p. A65
GORSKI, William R., M.D. President and Chief Executive Officer, SwedishAmerican Hospital, Rockford, IL, p. A193
GORY, James, Chief Financial Officer, Northwest Medical Center, Winfield, AL, p. A27
GOSAR, Grace, M.D. Chief of Staff, Johnson County Healthcare Center, Buffalo, WY, p. A695
GOSCH, Shawn, Chief Financial Officer, Burgess Health Center, Onawa, IA, p. A224
GOSEY, J., M.D. Medical Director, Southern Surgical Hospital, Slidell, LA, p. A278
GOSHE, Nick, Chief Executive Officer, Rangely District Hospital, Rangely, CO, p. A105
GOSHIA, Rob, Chief Financial Officer, Paulding County Hospital, Paulding, OH, p. A487
GOSLINE, Peter L., Chief Executive Officer, Monadnock Community Hospital, Peterborough, NH, p. A400
GOSNELL, Dewey, Manager, Rush Oak Park Hospital, Oak Park, IL, p. A190
GOSNEY, Brett, Chief Executive Officer, Animas Surgical Hospital, Durango, CO, p. A100
GOSPODAREK, Robert E., President and Chief Executive Officer, Mercy St. Charles Hospital, Oregon, OH, p. A486
GOSS, Norma, R.N. COO/CNO, Flaget Memorial Hospital, Bardstown, KY, p. A247
GOSS, Richard, M.D. Medical Director, Harborview Medical Center, Seattle, WA, p. A665
GOSS, Roger, Director, Information Services, North Sunflower Medical Center, Ruleville, MS, p. A352
GOSSENS, Kevin, Director Human Resources, Riverside Medical Center, Waupaca, WI, p. A692
GOTTI, Sreekant, Director Information Systems, Desert Valley Hospital, Victorville, CA, p. A95
GOTTLIEB, Gary L., M.D. President and Chief Executive Officer, Partners HealthCare System, Inc., Boston, MA, p. B100
GOTTLIEB, Harold, M.D. Medical Director, CHRISTUS St. John Hospital, Nassau Bay, TX, p. A618
GOTTLIEB, Jonathan, M.D. Senior Vice President and Chief Medical Officer, University of Maryland Medical Center, Baltimore, MD, p. A289
GOTTLIEB, Michael, M.D. Chief Medical Officer, MetroWest Medical Center, Framingham, MA, p. A300
GOTTSCHALK, Jack, Interim Vice President Human Resources, Children's National Medical Center, Washington, DC, p. A116
GOTTSCHALK, M. Therese, President, Marian Health System, Tulsa, OK, p. B84
GOUGEON, Michele L., Executive Vice President and Chief Operating Officer, McLean Hospital, Belmont, MA, p. A295
GOUGH, Galal S., M.D. Chief of Staff, Coast Plaza Hospital, Norwalk, CA, p. A77
GOULD, Bill, Chief People Resource Officer, Winona Health, Winona, MN, p. A342
GOULD, Linda, Director Human Resources, Navarro Regional Hospital, Corsicana, TX, p. A589
GOULD, Lou, Vice President Human Resources, Harris County Hospital District, Houston, TX, p. A604
GOULD, Nita, Director Information Services, Parkside Hospital, Tulsa, OK, p. A506
GOULD, Robert, Chief Executive Officer, Banner Desert Medical Center, Mesa, AZ, p. A34
GOULET, James P., Vice President Operations, Columbus Community Hospital, Columbus, NE, p. A382
GOURLEY, Paul, M.D. Chief Hospital Services, U. S. Air Force Hospital, Hampton, VA, p. A649
GOVE, Cynthia A., Chief Operating Officer, Hampstead Hospital, Hampstead, NH, p. A398
GOVINDAIAH, Rajesh G., M.D. Chief Medical Officer, Memorial Medical Center, Springfield, IL, p. A194
GOWDER, Mike, Assistant Administrator, Union General Hospital, Blairsville, GA, p. A147
GOYAL, Alok, M.D. Medical Director, Kindred Hospital–Milwaukee, Greenfield, WI, p. A683
GOYNES, Jack, Director Information Resources, East Cooper Medical Center, Mount Pleasant, SC, p. A552
GOZIAH, Vicky, Software Administrator, Wesley Woods Long Term Care Hospital, Atlanta, GA, p. A146
GRABER, Donald, M.D. Medical Director, Richmond State Hospital, Richmond, IN, p. A211
GRABER, Ellen, Director, Human Resources, Skiff Medical Center, Newton, IA, p. A224
GRABOWSKI, Michael, M.D. President Medical Staff, Parkview Hospital, Fort Wayne, IN, p. A201
GRABUS, Christina, R.N. Chief Nursing Officer, Thomasville Medical Center, Thomasville, NC, p. A462
GRACE, Jeffery, M.D. Clinical Director, Buffalo Psychiatric Center, Buffalo, NY, p. A422
GRACE, Walter, Chief Executive Officer and Administrator, Baptist Memorial Hospital–Union County, New Albany, MS, p. A351
GRACER, Erik, M.D. Chief of Staff, San Ramon Regional Medical Center, San Ramon, CA, p. A89
GRACIA, Judy, Vice President Human Resources, St. Tammany Parish Hospital, Covington, LA, p. A265
GRACIA, Sandra C., M.D. Chief of Staff, Veterans Affairs Medical Center, San Juan, PR, p. A704
GRACIE, Michael, Chief Information Officer, Veterans Health Care System of the Ozarks, Fayetteville, AR, p. A44
GRADDY, Steve W.
Chief Financial Officer, Freeman Hospital West, Joplin, MO, p. A361
Chief Financial Officer, Freeman Neosho Hospital, Neosho, MO, p. A366
GRADNEY, Angel, Chief Executive Officer, Kindred Hospital East Houston, Channelview, TX, p. A587
GRADY, John M., Associate Director, Veterans Affairs Hudson Valley Health Care System–F.D. Roosevelt Hospital, Montrose, NY, p. A430
GRADY, Phillip L., Administrator, Holmes County Hospital and Clinics, Lexington, MS, p. A349
GRAEBER, Lawrence, Chief Executive Officer, Neshoba County General Hospital, Philadelphia, MS, p. A351
GRAEBER, Tod, Controller, Garrison Memorial Hospital, Garrison, ND, p. A466
GRAEBNER, David, Chief Administrative Officer, Aurora Sheboygan Memorial Medical Center, Sheboygan, WI, p. A690
GRAEBNER, Nancy Kay, President and Chief Executive Officer, Chelsea Community Hospital, Chelsea, MI, p. A309
GRAF, John, Senior Vice President, Watertown Regional Medical Center, Watertown, WI, p. A692
GRAFFIS, Richard, M.D. Executive Vice President and Chief Medical Officer, Indiana University Health University Hospital, Indianapolis, IN, p. A204
GRAFTON, Tina, Director Information Technology, Pinckneyville Community Hospital, Pinckneyville, IL, p. A191
GRAGG, Connie, Director Human Resources, Saint Mary's Regional Medical Center, Russellville, AR, p. A51
GRAGG, Martha, MSN, Chief Executive Officer, Sullivan County Memorial Hospital, Milan, MO, p. A365
GRAGNOLATI, Brian A., FACHE President and Chief Executive Officer, Suburban Hospital, Bethesda, MD, p. A290
GRAH, John A., FACHE Chief Executive Officer, Des Peres Hospital, Saint Louis, MO, p. A368
GRAHAM, Barry A., M.D. Vice President Medical Affairs, Avera Sacred Heart Hospital, Yankton, SD, p. A561
GRAHAM, Brenda, Chief Nursing Officer, Knox County Hospital, Barbourville, KY, p. A247
GRAHAM, C. Scott, D.O. Chief of Staff, Lake District Hospital, Lakeview, OR, p. A512
GRAHAM, Connie, Public Information Officer, Mercy Health Love County, Marietta, OK, p. A499
GRAHAM, David B., M.D. Senior Vice President and Chief Information Officer, Memorial Medical Center, Springfield, IL, p. A194
GRAHAM, Gerry J., Director Human Resources, Cottage Hospital, Woodsville, NH, p. A400
GRAHAM, J. Scott, Chief Executive Officer, Coulee Medical Center, Grand Coulee, WA, p. A662
GRAHAM, Jay
Interim Chief Financial Officer, Berwick Hospital Center, Berwick, PA, p. A518
Interim Chief Financial Officer, Brandywine Hospital, Coatesville, PA, p. A520
GRAHAM, Jeff, Chief Operating Officer, Adena Greenfield Medical Center, Greenfield, OH, p. A481
GRAHAM, Joe B., Chief Operating Officer, Nebraska Medical Center, Omaha, NE, p. A388
GRAHAM, John, Chief Financial Officer, Phoebe Worth Medical Center, Sylvester, GA, p. A160
GRAHAM, John R., President and Chief Executive Officer, St. Mary's of Michigan, Saginaw, MI, p. A322
GRAHAM, John W., Executive Vice President and Chief Operating Officer, Underwood–Memorial Hospital, Woodbury, NJ, p. A412
GRAHAM, Jon, Chief Financial Officer, Vidant Roanoke–Chowan Hospital, Ahoskie, NC, p. A448
GRAHAM, Kathryn, Director Communications and Community Relations, Novato Community Hospital, Novato, CA, p. A77
GRAHAM, Kimberley, R.N. Chief Nursing Officer and Chief Operating Officer, Broward Health Coral Springs, Coral Springs, FL, p. A121
GRAHAM, Larry M., FACHE President and Chief Executive Officer, Lake Charles Memorial Hospital, Lake Charles, LA, p. A271
GRAHAM, Michael, Director Human Resources, Community Hospital, Munster, IN, p. A209
GRAHAM, Shauna, Director Human Resources, Howard County Medical Center, Saint Paul, NE, p. A389
GRAHAM, Sheri S.
Director Human Resources and Administrative Services, Parkland Health Center, Farmington, MO, p. A359
Director Human Resources and Administrative Services, Parkland Health Center–Bonne Terre, Bonne Terre, MO, p. A355
GRAHAM, Sonja, Chief Executive Officer, North Oak Regional Medical Center, Senatobia, MS, p. A352
GRAHAM, Yolanda, M.D. Medical Director, Devereux Georgia Treatment Network, Kennesaw, GA, p. A154
GRAHE, Raymond A., Senior Vice President Strategic Ventures and Chief Financial Officer, Meritus Medical Center, Hagerstown, MD, p. A292
GRAMBY, Tiffany, Director Health Information Management and Privacy Officer, Barnesville Hospital, Barnesville, OH, p. A470
GRAMER, Johanna, Director Human Resources, Mimbres Memorial Hospital, Deming, NM, p. A415
GRAN, Daniel, Chief Executive Officer, Freeman Regional Health Services, Freeman, SD, p. A557
GRANADO–VILLAR, Deise, M.D. Chief Medical Officer and Senior Vice President Medical Affairs, Miami Children's Hospital, Miami, FL, p. A131
GRANATO, Jerome, M.D
Chief Medical Officer, Excela Frick Hospital, Mount Pleasant, PA, p. A530
Chief Medical Officer, Excela Health Westmoreland Hospital, Greensburg, PA, p. A524
Chief Medical Officer, Excela Latrobe Area Hospital, Latrobe, PA, p. A527
GRAND, Lawrence N., Executive Vice President and Chief Operating Officer, Hunterdon Medical Center, Flemington, NJ, p. A404
GRANDIOSI, Joe, Director Information Technology, Southern Hills Hospital and Medical Center, Las Vegas, NV, p. A393
GRANGER, Chris, M.D. President Medical Staff, Beauregard Memorial Hospital, De Ridder, LA, p. A265
GRANGER, Keith, President and Chief Executive Officer, Trinity Medical Center, Birmingham, AL, p. A17


Index of Health Care Professionals

Index of Health Care Professionals

Index of Health Care Professionals / Granger

GRANGER, Laura, Director, Human Resources, New Braunfels Regional Rehabilitation Hospital, New Braunfels, TX, p. A618
GRANGER, Robert P., President and Chief Executive Officer, St. Francis Hospital, Columbus, GA, p. A149
GRANNEMAN, Joe
Regional Chief Information Officer, Adventist GlenOaks Hospital, Glendale Heights, IL, p. A183
Chief Information Officer, Adventist Hinsdale Hospital, Hinsdale, IL, p. A184
GRANT, Cathy, R.N. Associate Vice President, Patient Services, Huron Valley–Sinai Hospital, Commerce Township, MI, p. A310
GRANT, Dan, Manager Business Office, Blue Mountain Recovery Center, Pendleton, OR, p. A513
GRANT, Dianna, M.D. Vice President Medical Management, Advocate Trinity Hospital, Chicago, IL, p. A175
GRANT, Howard R., M.D. President and Chief Executive Officer, Lahey Clinic Hospital, Burlington, MA, p. A298
GRANT, Larry, M.D. Chief Medical Officer, Coliseum Medical Centers, Macon, GA, p. A155
GRANT, Mikki, Chief Information Officer, Fort Belknap U. S. Public Health Service Indian Hospital, Harlem, MT, p. A376
GRANT, Pauline, FACHE Chief Executive Officer, Broward Health North, Deerfield Beach, FL, p. A122
GRANT, Samuel, Interim Chief Executive Officer, White Mountain Regional Medical Center, Springerville, AZ, p. A38
GRANT, William, Vice President Fiscal and Support Services, Laurens County Health Care System, Clinton, SC, p. A548
GRANTHAM, Candace, Chief Executive Officer, Cook Children's Northeast Hospital, Hurst, TX, p. A608
GRANTHAM, Charlie, Manager Information Systems, Marion Regional Hospital, Mullins, SC, p. A552
GRANTHAM, James, Administrator, Baptist Memorial Hospital–Booneville, Booneville, MS, p. A344
GRANTHAM, Keith, Director Information Technology, Covenant Medical Center, Saginaw, MI, p. A322
GRANVILLE, Brian, Director Information Technology, Buena Vista Regional Medical Center, Storm Lake, IA, p. A227
GRANVILLE, Sabrina M., Vice President Human Resources, Elliot Hospital, Manchester, NH, p. A399
GRANZOW, Steven L., Chief Executive Officer, Sheridan County Health Complex, Hoxie, KS, p. A235
GRASER, David, Chief Information Officer, Marquette General Health System, Marquette, MI, p. A318
GRASMEDER, Martin, M.D. Administrator, SEARHC MT. Edgecumbe Hospital, Sitka, AK, p. A30
GRASS, Linda J., Executive Director and Chief Executive Officer, Jeanes Hospital, Philadelphia, PA, p. A532
GRASSER, Tierney, Senior Vice President Finance, Olathe Medical Center, Olathe, KS, p. A240
GRATZ, Silvia, D.O. Chief Medical Officer, Fairmount Behavioral Health System, Philadelphia, PA, p. A532
GRATZMILLER, Annette, Director Information Services, HEALTHSOUTH Rehabilitation Hospital, Sewickley, PA, p. A538
GRAUE, Michael L., Executive Vice President and Chief Operating Officer, WellStar Kennestone Hospital, Marietta, GA, p. A156
GRAUER, David, Administrator, Intermountain Medical Center, Murray, UT, p. A638
GRAUPENSPERGER, Robert, Executive Vice President, Ephrata Community Hospital, Ephrata, PA, p. A523
GRAVENDER, Dave, Vice President and Chief Information Officer, Kaweah Delta Medical Center, Visalia, CA, p. A95
GRAVES, Amanda, Chief Information Systems, Veterans Affairs Medical Center, Washington, DC, p. A117
GRAVES, Buddy, Chief Information Officer, Southern Surgical Hospital, Slidell, LA, p. A278
GRAVES, Deanna, Chief Executive Officer, Texas Specialty Hospital at Lubbock, Lubbock, TX, p. A614
GRAVES, Jimmy, Administrator, Walthall County General Hospital, Tylertown, MS, p. A353
GRAVES, Robert L., Vice President and Administrator, Sentara Williamsburg Regional Medical Center, Williamsburg, VA, p. A657
GRAVES, Terri, Chief Financial Officer, Heartland Behavioral Health Services, Nevada, MO, p. A366
GRAY, Albert, Chief Executive Officer, The Children's Center, Bethany, OK, p. A494
GRAY, Anthony, Chief Financial Officer, LAC–Olive View–UCLA Medical Center,, CA, p. A70
GRAY, Clarence, Chief Financial Officer, Horizon Medical Center, Dickson, TN, p. A565
GRAY, David L., FACHE President, Baptist Hospital East, Louisville, KY, p. A254
GRAY, Gary, D.O. Chief Medical Officer, Natividad Medical Center, Salinas, CA, p. A84
GRAY, Herb, M.D. Chief Medical Officer, Falmouth Hospital, Falmouth, MA, p. A300
GRAY, Herman B., M.D. President, Children's Hospital of Michigan, Detroit, MI, p. A310
GRAY, James, M.D. Chief Medical Service, Amarillo Veterans Affairs Health Care System, Amarillo, TX, p. A578
GRAY, Jason, M.D. Chief Medical Officer, Mercy Medical Center, Roseburg, OR, p. A515
GRAY, Jeremy, Chief Executive Officer, Haywood Park Community Hospital, Brownsville, TN, p. A562
GRAY, Joshua, Director Information Technology, Coon Memorial Hospital and Home, Dalhart, TX, p. A590
GRAY, Judy, Vice President Human Resources, St. Peter's Hospital, Albany, NY, p. A420
GRAY, Karen D., Director Human Resources, Vibra Hospital of Southeastern Michigan, Lincoln Park, MI, p. A318
GRAY, Larry, President and Chief Executive Officer, Baptist Regional Medical Center, Corbin, KY, p. A248
GRAY, Leigh Cher, M.D. Chief of Staff, King's Daughters Medical Center, Brookhaven, MS, p. A344
GRAY, Mark, Chief Information Officer, McLaren Northern Michigan, Petoskey, MI, p. A320
GRAY, Mary, R.N. Director Information Technology and Special Project, Elba General Hospital, Elba, AL, p. A19
GRAY, Michelle, Nurse Executive, Atrium Medical Center of Corinth, Corinth, TX, p. A588
GRAY, Mike
Corporate Vice President Human Resources, East Texas Medical Center Rehabilitation Center, Tyler, TX, p. A632
Corporate Vice President Human Resources, East Texas Medical Center Specialty Hospital, Tyler, TX, p. A632
Corporate Vice President Human Resources, East Texas Medical Center Tyler, Tyler, TX, p. A632
GRAY, Patricia, Director Health Information Management, Cumberland Hall Hospital, Hopkinsville, KY, p. A251
GRAY, Penny, Administrator and Chief Executive Officer, Limestone Medical Center, Groesbeck, TX, p. A602
GRAY, Robert, Assistant Administrator Financial Services, Huntsville Memorial Hospital, Huntsville, TX, p. A608
GRAY, Tami, Chief Financial Officer, Irwin County Hospital, Ocilla, GA, p. A157
GRAY, Terry, Vice President Human Resources, Emanuel Medical Center, Turlock, CA, p. A93
GRAY, Thomas, M.D. Medical Director, Montana State Hospital, Warm Springs, MT, p. A379
GRAY, Val S., Chief Executive Officer, Helen Hayes Hospital, West Haverstraw, NY, p. A446
GRAY, Warren L., M.D. Chief of Staff, Indiana University Health Morgan Hospital, Martinsville, IN, p. A208
GRAYBEAL, Phillip
Chief Financial Officer, Page Memorial Hospital, Luray, VA, p. A650
Chief Financial Officer, Warren Memorial Hospital, Front Royal, VA, p. A648
GRAYBILL, Matthew P., Chief Operating Officer, Children's Medical Center, Dayton, OH, p. A478
GRAYBILL, Scott R., President and Chief Executive Officer, Community Hospital of Bremen, Bremen, IN, p. A198
GREASOM, Linda, Vice President Human Resources, Milford Regional Medical Center, Milford, MA, p. A302
GREBOSKY, Jamie, M.D. Vice President of Medical Affairs, Rogue Valley Medical Center, Medford, OR, p. A512
GRECO, Andrew, Chief Financial Officer, Calvary Hospital,, NY, p. A432
GRECO, Margaret, Chief Human Resources, Keller Army Community Hospital, West Point, NY, p. A446
GREELEY, Donna, Director Human Resources, Spalding Rehabilitation Hospital, Aurora, CO, p. A97
GREEN, Aimee, Director Human Resources, Stonewall Jackson Memorial Hospital, Weston, WV, p. A676
GREEN, Arnold, Senior Vice President and Chief Operating Officer, McLeod Loris Healthcare, Loris, SC, p. A552
GREEN, Barbara, Director Human Resources, O'Connor Hospital, Delhi, NY, p. A425
GREEN, Calvin, Chief Executive Officer, Riverside Medical Center, Franklinton, LA, p. A266
GREEN, Charles B., M.D. Surgeon General, Department of the Air Force, Washington, DC, p. B41
GREEN, Christine, Administrative Director Human Resources, Sutter Delta Medical Center, Antioch, CA, p. A53
GREEN, Darrin, M.D. Medical Director, De Queen Medical Center, De Queen, AR, p. A43
GREEN, David, Chief Human Resources, Veterans Affairs Medical Center, West Palm Beach, FL, p. A143
GREEN, David F., M.D. Chief Medical Officer, Concord Hospital, Concord, NH, p. A397
GREEN, David R., Administrator and Chief Executive Officer, El Centro Regional Medical Center, El Centro, CA, p. A60
GREEN, Gail P., R.N
Chief Nursing Officer, Renown Rehabilitation Hospital, Reno, NV, p. A395
Chief Nursing Officer, Renown South Meadows Medical Center, Reno, NV, p. A395
GREEN, Garry Kim, FACHE Administrator, Shriners Hospitals for Children, Shreveport, Shreveport, LA, p. A277
GREEN, Haley, Chief Financial Officer, Doctors Memorial Hospital, Bonifay, FL, p. A119
GREEN, Jack W., Administrator, Antelope Memorial Hospital, Neligh, NE, p. A386
GREEN, John
Vice President Human Resources, Iredell Memorial Hospital, Statesville, NC, p. A461
Vice President Finance, St. Peter's Hospital, Helena, MT, p. A376
GREEN, Judy, Director Human Resources, Putnam County Memorial Hospital, Unionville, MO, p. A372
GREEN, Julie, Vice President Human Resources, Cheshire Medical Center, Keene, NH, p. A398
GREEN, Karen, Chief Information Officer, Brooks Rehabilitation Hospital, Jacksonville, FL, p. A126
GREEN, Michael B., President and Chief Executive Officer, Concord Hospital, Concord, NH, p. A397
GREEN, Patrick, Chief Operating Officer, St. Anthony Hospital, Lakewood, CO, p. A103
GREEN, Peggy, Chief Operating Officer and Chief Nursing Officer, Saint Joseph – London, London, KY, p. A254
GREEN, Rhonda G., Administrator, Leonard J. Chabert Medical Center, Houma, LA, p. A268
GREEN, Ronnie, Director Information Systems, McBride Clinic Orthopedic Hospital, Oklahoma City, OK, p. A501
GREEN, Rose Marie, Director Human Resources, Humboldt General Hospital, Winnemucca, NV, p. A396
GREEN, Scott, M.D. Chief of Staff, St. Francis Memorial Hospital, West Point, NE, p. A390
GREEN, Steve, Comptroller, Jasper General Hospital, Bay Springs, MS, p. A343
GREEN, Susan, Chief Financial Officer, Lowell General Hospital, Lowell, MA, p. A301
GREEN, Warren A., President and Chief Executive Officer, LifeBridge Health, Baltimore, MD, p. B80
GREENBERG, Brigid, Interim Chief Executive Officer, GLOBALREHAB Hospital – Fort Worth, Fort Worth, TX, p. A598
GREENBERG, Mark, M.D
Chief Medical Officer, Cape Coral Hospital, Cape Coral, FL, p. A120
Medical Director, Gulf Coast Medical Center, Fort Myers, FL, p. A123
GREENE, Arthur, M.D. Vice President Medical Affairs, Sentara CarePlex Hospital, Hampton, VA, p. A649
GREENE, Barbara M., President, Franciscan Physicians Hospital, Munster, IN, p. A209
GREENE, Beth, Chief Operating Officer, Cherokee Indian Hospital, Cherokee, NC, p. A451
GREENE, Bradley, Chief Financial Officer, WellStar Douglas Hospital, Douglasville, GA, p. A151
GREENE Jr., Charles H., Administrator, Cordell Memorial Hospital, Cordell, OK, p. A495
GREENE, Dustin, Chief Operating Officer, Eastside Medical Center, Snellville, GA, p. A159
GREENE, Jr., Edward C., Assistant Vice President and Administrator, Russell County Medical Center, Lebanon, VA, p. A650
GREENE, Hugh, President and Chief Executive Officer, Baptist Health, Jacksonville, FL, p. B17
GREENE, Michael, Chief Executive Officer, Medical Center of Newark, Newark, OH, p. A486
GREENE, Queen, Director Human Resources, Baylor University Medical Center, Dallas, TX, p. A590
GREENE, Russ, Chief Executive Officer, Physicians' Specialty Hospital, Fayetteville, AR, p. A44
GREENER, Angela, Chief Administrative Officer, West Jefferson Medical Center, Marrero, LA, p. A272
GREENFIELD, Bruce A., M.D. Chief of Staff, California Hospital Medical Center, Los Angeles, CA, p. A68
GREENLEE, Kathryn M., R.N
Vice President, Clinical Services/CNO, ProMedica Bixby Hospital, Adrian, MI, p. A307
Vice President, Clinical Services/CNO, ProMedica Herrick Hospital, Tecumseh, MI, p. A324
GREENLY, John, Chief Financial Officer, Meadow Wood Behavioral Health System, New Castle, DE, p. A114
GREENMAN, Jennifer, Exec. Director, CIO, Bayfront Medical Center, Saint Petersburg, FL, p. A138
GREENMAN, Sharon, Director Human Resources, Melissa Memorial Hospital, Holyoke, CO, p. A102
GREENSPAN, Carrie, M.D. Chief of Staff, Broward Health Coral Springs, Coral Springs, FL, p. A121

A824 Index of Health Care Professionals

Index of Health Care Professionals / Grogan

GREENSTON, Matthew, M.D. Interim Chief Medical Officer, Catholic Medical Center, Manchester, NH, p. A399
GREENSWEIG, Gary, D.O
Chief Medical Officer, Petaluma Valley Hospital, Petaluma, CA, p. A80
Chief Medical Officer, Santa Rosa Memorial Hospital, Santa Rosa, CA, p. A90
GREENWOOD, Cathy, Manager Human Resources, LifeCare Hospitals of Dallas, Dallas, TX, p. A591
GREER, Eugene, Chief Information Officer, The HSC Pediatric Center, Washington, DC, p. A117
GREER, Nancy, R.N. Chief Nursing Officer, Saint Alphonsus Medical Center – Ontario, Ontario, OR, p. A513
GREER, Roxane, Coordinator Human Resources, Blowing Rock Hospital, Blowing Rock, NC, p. A449
GREER, Troy, Chief Executive Officer, Lovelace Westside Hospital, Albuquerque, NM, p. A414
GREER, William, Chief Information Officer, Veterans Affairs Medical Center, Birmingham, AL, p. A17
GREEVER, Suzanne, Chief Executive Officer, North Central Surgical Center, Dallas, TX, p. A592
GREGERSEN, Glenn, Director Information Technology, District One Hospital, Faribault, MN, p. A331
GREGG, Hunt, Director Information Systems, Texas Scottish Rite Hospital for Children, Dallas, TX, p. A592
GREGG, Richard, M.D. Medical Director, LifeCare Hospital of Dayton, Miamisburg, OH, p. A485
GREGG, Thomas, Interim President and Chief Executive Officer, St. Peter's Hospital, Helena, MT, p. A376
GREGONIS, Michael, Comptroller, Naval Hospital, Jacksonville, FL, p. A126
GREGORIAN, Myra, Vice President Human Resources, Long Beach Memorial Medical Center, Long Beach, CA, p. A68
GREGORICH, Miki, Director Human Resources, Pioneer Medical Center, Big Timber, MT, p. A373
GREGORIO, Louis J., FACHE Vice President Human Resources, Chambersburg Hospital, Chambersburg, PA, p. A520
GREGORY, Adina, Chief Nursing Officer, Great Bend Regional Hospital, Great Bend, KS, p. A233
GREGORY, Audrey, R.N. Chief Operating Officer, Saint Francis Hospital, Memphis, TN, p. A572
GREGORY, Dick, Ph.D
Chief Executive Officer, Center for Behavioral Medicine, Kansas City, MO, p. A361
Chief Executive Officer, Northwest Missouri Psychiatric Rehabilitation Center, Saint Joseph, MO, p. A368
GREGORY, Jan, Chief of Human Resources, Crittenden County Hospital, Marion, KY, p. A256
GREGORY, Nancy A.
Acting Director, Veterans Affairs Medical Center, Omaha, NE, p. A388
Acting Director, Veterans Affairs Nebraska–Western Iowa Health Care System, Lincoln, NE, p. A386
GREGORY, Shawn, Chief Financial Officer, South Bay Hospital, Sun City Center, FL, p. A140
GREGORY, Trip
Senior Vice President Human Resources, Palmetto Health Baptist, Columbia, SC, p. A548
Senior Vice President Human Resources, Palmetto Health Richland, Columbia, SC, p. A548
GREGOS, Ruth, Director Finance, Shriners Hospitals for Children, Tampa, Tampa, FL, p. A141
GREIMAN, Alan W., Administrator, Royal Oaks Hospital, Windsor, MO, p. A372
GREINER, Walter, Chief Financial Officer, AtlantiCare Regional Medical Center, Atlantic City, NJ, p. A401
GREMILLION, Karen, R.N. Chief Nursing Officer, Opelousas General Health System, Opelousas, LA, p. A276
GRENALDO, Paul, Executive Vice President and Chief Operating Officer, Doctors Community Hospital, Lanham, MD, p. A292
GRENDON, M. Todd, M.D. President Medical Staff, Saint Joseph Hospital, Chicago, IL, p. A178
GRENIER, Raymond, Chief Financial Officer, Northwest Texas Healthcare System, Amarillo, TX, p. A578
GRENNAN, Jr., M. Joseph, M.D
Vice President Medical Affairs, Boca Raton Regional Hospital, Boca Raton, FL, p. A118
Senior Vice President and Chief Medical Officer, Reading Hospital and Medical Center, West Reading, PA, p. A541
GRESKO, Teresa A., Chief Financial Officer, Kindred Hospital South Philadelphia, Philadelphia, PA, p. A533
GRESKOVICH, William, Chief Information Officer, Saint Agnes Hospital, Baltimore, MD, p. A288
GRESS, Jr., Harold M., Manager Management Information Systems, Fulton County Medical Center, Mc Connellsburg, PA, p. A528
GREW, Kate, MSN Vice President/Chief Nurse Executive, Carolinas Medical Center–NorthEast, Concord, NC, p. A451
GREW, Terry, Chief Business Office, Veterans Affairs Medical Center, Hampton, VA, p. A649
GRIBBIN, John T., FACHE President and Chief Executive Officer, CentraState Healthcare System, Freehold, NJ, p. A404
GRIBBIN, Karen, M.D. Chief of Staff, Jack C. Montgomery Veterans Affairs Medical Center, Muskogee, OK, p. A499
GRICUS, Peggy, R.N. Vice President, Patient Care Services/CNO, Silver Cross Hospital, New Lenox, IL, p. A189
GRIEP, John, M.D. Chief Medical Director, St. Catherine Hospital, East Chicago, IN, p. A200
GRIESS, Dan, Chief Executive Officer, Box Butte General Hospital, Alliance, NE, p. A381
GRIEST, Mary, Vice President Finance and Chief Financial Officer, Samaritan Regional Health System, Ashland, OH, p. A469
GRIFFIN, Angela, Privacy Officer, Wayne County Hospital, Monticello, KY, p. A256
GRIFFIN, Brad, Chief Operating Officer, Ocala Regional Medical Center, Ocala, FL, p. A133
GRIFFIN, Brian, Director Information Services, Springhill Medical Center, Springhill, LA, p. A278
GRIFFIN, Christopher B., Chief Executive Officer, D. W. McMillan Memorial Hospital, Brewton, AL, p. A17
GRIFFIN, Cindy, Director Human Resources, Medical Center Barbour, Eufaula, AL, p. A19
GRIFFIN, Dean A., President and Chief Executive Officer, Decatur General Hospital, Decatur, AL, p. A18
GRIFFIN, Donald, CPA Chief Financial Officer, New London Hospital, New London, NH, p. A399
GRIFFIN, James, Manager Information Systems, Martin General Hospital, Williamston, NC, p. A462
GRIFFIN, Jeannine, M.D. Chief of Staff, Memorial Medical Center, Port Lavaca, TX, p. A622
GRIFFIN, Maggi, Vice President and Chief Nursing Officer, John C. Lincoln North Mountain Hospital, Phoenix, AZ, p. A35
GRIFFIN, Matthew, M.D. Vice President Medical Affairs, Sinai–Grace Hospital, Detroit, MI, p. A311
GRIFFIN, Michael L., Chief Financial Officer, Butler County Medical Center, Hamilton, OH, p. A481
GRIFFIN, Paulette
Vice President Human Resources, Detroit Receiving Hospital/University Health Center, Detroit, MI, p. A310
Director Human Resources, Sinai–Grace Hospital, Detroit, MI, p. A311
GRIFFIN, Shirley, Director Health Information, North Mississippi Medical Center–Eupora, Eupora, MS, p. A345
GRIFFIN, Todd, M.D. Chief Medical Officer, Stony Brook University Medical Center, Stony Brook, NY, p. A444
GRIFFIN–MAHON, Selena, Assistant Vice President Human Resources, Bronx–Lebanon Hospital Center Health Care System,, NY, p. A431
GRIFFIS, Daniel, M.D. Medical Director, Plains Memorial Hospital, Dimmitt, TX, p. A594
GRIFFIS, Lisa, Chief Financial Officer and Business Office Manager, Specialty Hospital of Midwest City, Midwest City, OK, p. A499
GRIFFITH, David, M.D. Medical Director, Texas Center for Infectious Disease, San Antonio, TX, p. A626
GRIFFITH, Dena, Manager Information Systems, Kern Valley Healthcare District, Lake Isabella, CA, p. A66
GRIFFITH, Duane Lee, M.D. Chief of Staff, Texas Spine & Joint Hospital, Tyler, TX, p. A632
GRIFFITH, Dusty, Director Information Systems, Bolivar Medical Center, Cleveland, MS, p. A345
GRIFFITH, James, M.D. Associate Medical Director and Professional Chief of Staff, Kaiser Permanente Medical Center, Honolulu, HI, p. A163
GRIFFITH, James, Chief Operating Officer, Salinas Valley Memorial Healthcare System, Salinas, CA, p. A84
GRIFFITH, Jeanne, Chief Nursing Officer, Coryell Memorial Hospital, Gatesville, TX, p. A601
GRIFFITH, Keitha, Chief Nursing Officer, Medical Center of South Arkansas, El Dorado, AR, p. A44
GRIFFITH, Pamela, Director Administrative Services, Devereux Hospital and Children's Center of Florida, Melbourne, FL, p. A130
GRIFFITH, Patti, R.N. Chief Nursing Officer, Methodist Hospital for Surgery, Addison, TX, p. A577
GRIFFITH, Susan M., Chief Operations Officer, Eastern State Hospital, Lexington, KY, p. A253
GRIFFITH, Wayne B., FACHE Chief Executive Officer, Princeton Community Hospital, Princeton, WV, p. A675
GRIFFITHS, David, Vice President and Chief Financial Officer, Regional West Medical Center, Scottsbluff, NE, p. A389
GRIFFITHS, Mark
Director Management Information Systems, Incline Village Community Hospital, Incline Village, NV, p. A392
Chief Systems Innovation Officer, Tahoe Forest Hospital District, Truckee, CA, p. A93
GRIGG, William E., Senior Vice President and Chief Financial Officer, Methodist Hospital of Southern California, Arcadia, CA, p. A54
GRIGSBY, Stephen J., Chief Financial Officer, Jupiter Medical Center, Jupiter, FL, p. A127
GRIGSON, John A., Senior Vice President and Chief Financial Officer, Covenant Medical Center, Lubbock, TX, p. A613
GRILL, Laura D., R.N. Executive Vice President and Administrator, East Alabama Medical Center, Opelika, AL, p. A24
GRILLO, Alan, M.D. Chief of Staff, Spectrum Health Reed City Hospital, Reed City, MI, p. A321
GRILLO, Jorge C., Chief Information Officer, Canton–Potsdam Hospital, Potsdam, NY, p. A441
GRIM, Charles, D.D.S. Chief Executive Officer, William W. Hastings Indian Hospital, Tahlequah, OK, p. A505
GRIM, Mary Kay
Senior Vice President Human Resources, Lehigh Valley Hospital, Allentown, PA, p. A517
Senior Vice President Human Resources, Lehigh Valley Hospital–Muhlenberg, Bethlehem, PA, p. A518
GRIMALDI, Richard, President Medical Staff, Highlands Hospital, Connellsville, PA, p. A521
GRIMER, Ginny, Director Human Resources, George E. Weems Memorial Hospital, Apalachicola, FL, p. A118
GRIMES, Michael, Manager Human Resources, Kindred Hospital Bay Area–Tampa, Tampa, FL, p. A141
GRIMES, Pam, Director Human Resources, LTAC of Edmond, Edmond, OK, p. A496
GRIMES, Teresa G., Chief Executive Officer, Troy Regional Medical Center, Troy, AL, p. A26
GRIMES, Walter, Director Information Technology, Good Shepherd Medical Center–Marshall, Marshall, TX, p. A615
GRIMLEY, Karen A., R.N. Chief Nursing Officer, University of California, Irvine Healthcare, Orange, CA, p. A78
GRIMSHAW, Matthew, Chief Executive Officer, Mercy Medical Center, Williston, ND, p. A468
GRINDE, Brett, Network Manager, Lucas County Health Center, Chariton, IA, p. A216
GRINNELL, Steven, President and Chief Executive Officer, Lourdes Hospital, Paducah, KY, p. A257
GRINNEY, Jay F., President and Chief Executive Officer, HEALTHSOUTH Corporation, Birmingham, AL, p. B64
GRIP, Mark, Executive Director Business Development, Sierra Vista Hospital, Sacramento, CA, p. A84
GRISDELA, Michael, Chief Financial Officer, Karmanos Cancer Center, Detroit, MI, p. A311
GRISH, John, Assistant Executive Director and Chief Financial Officer, Howard University Hospital, Washington, DC, p. A116
GRISIER, Douglas, D.O. Medical Director, HEALTHSOUTH Rehabilitation Hospital of Erie, Erie, PA, p. A523
GRISNAK, Karen, R.N. Chief Operating Officer and Assistant Administrator Quality Services, Vallejo Medical Center, Vallejo, CA, p. A94
GRISSINGER, Matthew, Site Manager Information Systems, Indian Path Medical Center, Kingsport, TN, p. A568
GRISSLER, Brian G., President and Chief Executive Officer, Stamford Hospital, Stamford, CT, p. A112
GRISWOLD, Barbara, Chief Nursing Officer, Washington County Hospital and Clinics, Washington, IA, p. A227
GRITTNER, Linda
Vice President Human Resources, Providence Mount Carmel Hospital, Colville, WA, p. A660
Director Human Resources, Providence St. Joseph's Hospital, Chewelah, WA, p. A660
GROCE, David, Associate Administrator and Chief Financial Officer, Lincoln County Health System, Fayetteville, TN, p. A565
GROCHALA, Eugene
Vice President Information Systems, Capital Health Medical Center–Hopewell, Pennington, NJ, p. A408
Vice President Information Systems, Capital Health Regional Medical Center, Trenton, NJ, p. A411
GROENEWEG, Jennifer, R.N
Chief Clinical Officer, Great Lakes Specialty Hospital–Oak Campus, Grand Rapids, MI, p. A313
Director Nursing, LifeCare Hospitals of Wisconsin, Pewaukee, WI, p. A689
GROENIG, Matt, Vice President Finance, St. Luke's McCall, McCall, ID, p. A169
GROEPER, William E., Vice President Finance, Beloit Health System, Beloit, WI, p. A679
GROEPPER, Ronald, Senior Vice President and Area Manager, Sacramento Medical Center, Sacramento, CA, p. A83
GROESBECK, John
Area Finance Officer, San Rafael Medical Center, San Rafael, CA, p. A89
Area Finance Officer, Santa Rosa Medical Center, Santa Rosa, CA, p. A90
GROFF, Gerald D., M.D. Vice President Medical Affairs, Bassett Medical Center, Cooperstown, NY, p. A424
GROGAN, Dennis, M.D. Chief of Staff, Shriners Hospitals for Children, Tampa, Tampa, FL, p. A141

© 2012 AHA Guide Index of Health Care Professionals **A825**

Index of Health Care Professionals

Index of Health Care Professionals / Grogan

GROGAN, Ed, Vice President Information Services and Chief Information Officer, Calvert Memorial Hospital, Prince Frederick, MD, p. A293
GROGAN, Richard, Chief Executive Officer, Memorial Hospital of Salem County, Salem, NJ, p. A410
GROH, Charles, Interim Chief Information Officer, North Adams Regional Hospital, North Adams, MA, p. A303
GRONBACH, Sue, Director Human Resources, Providence Hospital, Southfield, MI, p. A323
GRONDA, Mark E., Vice President and Chief Financial Officer, Covenant Medical Center, Saginaw, MI, p. A322
GRONEMEYER, Pamella S., M.D. President Medical Staff, Red Bud Regional Hospital, Red Bud, IL, p. A192
GRONSETH, Timothy L., Vice President and Chief Financial Officer, Northfield Hospital, Northfield, MN, p. A336
GROOMS, Jr., Richard W., Vice President Human Resources, Providence Hospital, Columbia, SC, p. A548
GROS, Albert, M.D. Chief Medical Officer, St. David's South Austin Medical Center, Austin, TX, p. A581
GROS, Mark, Director Human Resources, United Medical Rehabilitation Hospital, Hammond, LA, p. A267
GROSDIDIER, Jonathan L., M.D. Chief of Staff, Memorial Hospital of Converse County, Douglas, WY, p. A696
GROSE, Jana, Director Management Information Systems, Massena Memorial Hospital, Massena, NY, p. A429
GROSKREUTZ, Kevin, Director Information Systems, St. Joseph's Hospital, Chippewa Falls, WI, p. A680
GROSS, Arthur K., FACHE Executive Vice President and Chief Information Officer, Henry Ford Wyandotte Hospital, Wyandotte, MI, p. A325
GROSS, Barry L., M.D. Executive Vice President and Chief Medical Officer, Riverside Regional Medical Center, Newport News, VA, p. A652
GROSS, Cathy, Director Health Information Management Systems, Wrangell Medical Center, Wrangell, AK, p. A30
GROSS, Cheryl, Director Human Resources, Edwards County Hospital and Healthcare Center, Kinsley, KS, p. A236
GROSS, Daniel, Senior Vice President Finance and Chief Financial Officer, Newton–Wellesley Hospital, Newton Lower Falls, MA, p. A303
GROSS, Denton, Director Information Services, Larue D. Carter Memorial Hospital, Indianapolis, IN, p. A204
GROSS, Kristin, Director Information Technology Center, Avera McKennan Hospital and University Health Center, Sioux Falls, SD, p. A559
GROSS, Lawrence, Executive Director, Central Oklahoma Community Mental Health Center, Norman, OK, p. A500
GROSS, Len, Director Human Resources, Sheridan Memorial Hospital, Sheridan, WY, p. A697
GROSS, Mark, Senior Business Director Finance, Mercy Health Partners, Lakeshore Campus, Shelby, MI, p. A323
GROSS, Melissa, Interim Administrator, Chester Mental Health Center, Chester, IL, p. A175
GROSS, Michael
Senior Vice President, Finance/Business Development, Ozarks Medical Center, West Plains, MO, p. A372
Chief Information Officer, Veterans Affairs Medical Center–Lexington, Lexington, KY, p. A254
GROSS, Paul, Human Services and Finance Officer, Larry B. Zieverink, Sr. Alcoholism Treatment Center, Raleigh, NC, p. A459
GROSS, Peter A., M.D. Senior Vice President and Chief Medical Officer, Hackensack University Medical Center, Hackensack, NJ, p. A404
GROSS, Randy, Chief Executive Officer, Plantation General Hospital, Plantation, FL, p. A136
GROSS, Tina, Director of Clinical Services, Sparrow Specialty Hospital, Lansing, MI, p. A317
GROSSET, Jessica
Director Information Technology, Mayo Clinic – Methodist Hospital, Rochester, MN, p. A338
Director Information Technology, Mayo Clinic – Saint Marys Hospital, Rochester, MN, p. A338
GROSSMAN, Drew, Chief Executive Officer, Broward Health Coral Springs, Coral Springs, FL, p. A121
GROSSMAN, Joseph
Chief Financial Officer, McDowell ARH Hospital, McDowell, KY, p. A256
Vice President Fiscal Affairs, Whitesburg ARH Hospital, Whitesburg, KY, p. A259
GROSSMAN, Marty, Director Information Technology, Christ Hospital, Jersey City, NJ, p. A405
GROSSMAN, Ray G., Vice President Human Resources, Memorial Medical Center – Livingston, Livingston, TX, p. A612
GROSSMAN, Robert I., M.D. Chief Executive Officer, NYU Langone Medical Center, New York, NY, p. A436
GROSSO, Michael, M.D. Senior Vice President Medical Affairs, Huntington Hospital, Huntington, NY, p. A427
GROVE, Wanda, Chief Executive Officer, Surprise Valley Healthcare District, Cedarville, CA, p. A57
GROVER, Amy, Director, Appalachian Behavioral Healthcare, Athens, OH, p. A470
GROWNEY, Daniel, M.D. Chief of Staff, York General Hospital, York, NE, p. A390
GROWSE, Michael, M.D. Clinical Director, Federal Medical Center, Lexington, KY, p. A253
GRUBB, Lois, Vice President Human Resources, Elmhurst Memorial Hospital,, IL, p. A181
GRUBB, Michael, Chief Operating Officer and Chief Financial Officer, Kindred Hospital of South Bay, Gardena, CA, p. A63
GRUBB, Nora, Chief Financial Officer, Big Sandy Medical Center, Big Sandy, MT, p. A373
GRUBBS, Stephen, Chief Executive Officer, Regional Hospital of Jackson, Jackson, TN, p. A567
GRUBER, Kreg, President, Memorial Hospital of South Bend, South Bend, IN, p. A212
GRUBER, Norman F., President and Chief Executive Officer, Salem Health, Salem, OR, p. B112
GRUBER, Norman F., President and Chief Executive Officer, Salem Hospital, Salem, OR, p. A515
GRUBER, Scott, M.D. Chief of Staff, John D. Dingell Veterans Affairs Medical Center, Detroit, MI, p. A311
GRUEBER, Cynthia M., Chief Operating Officer, OHSU Hospital, Portland, OR, p. A514
GRUEN, Jeremy, Director Information Systems, Pike County Memorial Hospital, Louisiana, MO, p. A364
GRUHONJIC, Osman, Chief Financial Officer, Frankfort Regional Medical Center, Frankfort, KY, p. A250
GRUN, Joseph, Chief Information Officer, New York State Psychiatric Institute, New York, NY, p. A435
GRUNDSTROM, David A., Chief Administrative Officer, Flambeau Hospital, Park Falls, WI, p. A689
GRUNER, Dean, M.D. President and Chief Executive Officer, ThedaCare, Inc., Appleton, WI, p. B129
GRUVER, Laquita, Fiscal Officer, Veterans Affairs Medical Center, Grand Junction, CO, p. A102
GRUZENSKY, Denton, Director Human Resources, Feather River Hospital, Paradise, CA, p. A79
GRYWALSKI, Jr., John S., CPA Chief Financial Officer, Saint Michael's Medical Center, Newark, NJ, p. A407
GRYZBEK, Thomas J., President, Franciscan St. Margaret Health – Hammond, Hammond, IN, p. A203
GRZYBOWSKI, John, M.D. Medical Director, Mayo Clinic Health System in Albert Lea, Albert Lea, MN, p. A327
GUACCIO, Anthony, Senior Vice President & Chief Operating Officer, Swedish Covenant Hospital, Chicago, IL, p. A178
GUAJARDO, Manuel G., M.D. Medical Director, Brownsville Doctors Hospital, Brownsville, TX, p. A585
GUAJARDO, Michael, Director Finance, CHRISTUS Spohn Hospital Alice, Alice, TX, p. A577
GUANCI, Robert, Vice President Operations, Bon Secours Maryview Medical Center, Portsmouth, VA, p. A654
GUARDIPEE, Lisa, Director, U. S. Public Health Service Indian Hospital, Fort Yates, ND, p. A466
GUARINI, Lucia A., Administrator, Essex County Hospital Center, Cedar Grove, NJ, p. A402
GUARINO, Celia, R.N. Vice President and Chief Nursing Officer, Holy Cross Hospital, Silver Spring, MD, p. A294
GUARINO, Kathleen, R.N. Vice President Patient Care Services, Mercy Hospital, Buffalo, NY, p. A423
GUARINO, Rick, M.D. Vice President Medical Affairs, Wilson Medical Center, Wilson, NC, p. A463
GUARNESCHELLI, Philip, Senior Vice President and Chief Operating Officer, Pinnacle Health System, Harrisburg, PA, p. A524
GUARRACINO, Joseph, Senior Vice President and Chief Financial Officer, Brooklyn Hospital Center,, NY, p. A431
GUARRERA, Frank, Executive Vice President and Chief Financial Officer, Motion Picture and Television Fund Hospital and Residential Services,, CA, p. A70
GUBERMAN, Wayne, Director Finance, Matheny Medical and Educational Center, Peapack, NJ, p. A408
GUELKER, Rhonda, Senior Director Finance, Rolling Plains Memorial Hospital, Sweetwater, TX, p. A630
GUERCI, Alan D., M.D
Chief Executive Officer, Mercy Medical Center, Rockville Centre, NY, p. A442
Chief Executive Officer, St. Francis Hospital, Roslyn, NY, p. A442
GUERRA, Tony, Chief Financial Officer and Chief Operating Officer, Sharp Coronado Hospital and Healthcare Center, Coronado, CA, p. A58
GUERRERO, Levi, M.D. Chief of Staff, Deckerville Community Hospital, Deckerville, MI, p. A310
GUERRERO, Marisa, Director Human Resources, Laredo Specialty Hospital, Laredo, TX, p. A612
GUERRERO, Silvia, Chief Accountant, Cornerstone Regional Hospital, Edinburg, TX, p. A595
GUERRIERO, Marianne, Nurse Executive, Christian Health Care Center, Wyckoff, NJ, p. A412
GUEST, Leona, Chief Nursing Unit, Hawaii State Hospital, Kaneohe, HI, p. A164
GUEVARA, Al, Vice President Operations, Brazosport Regional Health System, Lake Jackson, TX, p. A611
GUEVARA, Jesse, Senior Vice President and Chief Financial Officer, St. Francis Medical Center, Lynwood, CA, p. A73
GUEZ, Roberta H., Chief Operating Officer, Taunton State Hospital, Taunton, MA, p. A305
GUFFEY, Dale, Chief Financial Officer, Lower Keys Medical Center, Key West, FL, p. A127
GUFFEY, Jay, Senior Vice President and Chief Operating Officer, Mercy Hospital Springfield, Springfield, MO, p. A371
GUFFEY, Kerra, Chief Information Officer, Meriter Hospital, Madison, WI, p. A684
GUGLIELMO, Elaine, Vice President Human Resources and Organizational Development, Stamford Hospital, Stamford, CT, p. A112
GUIDERA, Kenneth, M.D. Chief of Staff, Shriners Hospitals for Children, Twin Cities, Minneapolis, MN, p. A335
GUIDRY, Carolyn, Business Manager, Community Specialty Hospital, Lafayette, LA, p. A270
GUIDRY, Floyd, M.D. Medical Director, Women and Children's Hospital, Lake Charles, LA, p. A271
GUIGNIER, Liz, Vice President Human Resources, Eisenhower Medical Center, Rancho Mirage, CA, p. A81
GUILFOIL, Thomas, Director Human Resources, Wing Memorial Hospital and Medical Centers, Palmer, MA, p. A303
GUILLORY, Cayle P., Administrator, Eunice Extended Care Hospital, Eunice, LA, p. A266
GUILLORY, Nicholas D., MSN, Administrator, Oceans Behavioral Hospital of Lake Charles, Lake Charles, LA, p. A271
GUILLOT, Karen, R.N. Chief Operating Officer, St. Charles Parish Hospital, Luling, LA, p. A272
GUIMARAES, Valerie, Director Human Resources, Livingston Regional Hospital, Livingston, TN, p. A570
GUIMOND, Stephen J., President and Chief Executive Officer, Saints Medical Center, Lowell, MA, p. A301
GUIN Jr., Jamie W., Chief Executive Officer, Lincoln County Health System, Fayetteville, TN, p. A565
GUINANE, Gerard, Vice President Human Resources and Diversity Management, Lakeland Regional Medical Center–St. Joseph, Saint Joseph, MI, p. A322
GUINANE, Jerry, Vice President Human Resources, SwedishAmerican Hospital, Rockford, IL, p. A193
GUINLE, Mary Lou, FACHE Chief Executive Officer, Select Specialty Hospital–Lexington, Lexington, KY, p. A253
GUINN, Judy, Chief Human Resources Officer, Graham Regional Medical Center, Graham, TX, p. A601
GUIRL, Nadine T.
Senior Vice President Human Resources, Oconomowoc Memorial Hospital, Oconomowoc, WI, p. A688
Senior Vice President Human Resources, Waukesha Memorial Hospital, Waukesha, WI, p. A692
GUITTE, Chris, Director Information Technology, Baylor Medical Center at Uptown, Dallas, TX, p. A590
GULARTE, Steven, Chief Executive Officer, Colorado–Fayette Medical Center, Weimar, TX, p. A634
GULBENKIAN, Karen, R.N. Director Patient Care Services, John C. Fremont Healthcare District, Mariposa, CA, p. A74
GULBIS, Shannan, Director Human Resources, Methodist Richardson Medical Center, Richardson, TX, p. A622
GULDE, James E., M.D. Medical Director, Dubuis Hospital of Paris, Paris, TX, p. A620
GULIHUR, Judith, Director Human Resources and Chief Financial Officer, McCamey County Hospital District, McCamey, TX, p. A616
GULL, Joann, Chief Nursing Officer, Elmhurst Hospital Center,, NY, p. A432
GULLINGSRUD, Timothy M., Chief Executive Officer, Hayward Area Memorial Hospital and Nursing Home, Hayward, WI, p. A683
GUMBINER, Carl H., M.D. Senior Vice President Medical Affairs and Chief Medical Officer, Children's Hospital and Medical Center, Omaha, NE, p. A387
GUMBS, Milton A., M.D. Vice President and Medical Director, Bronx–Lebanon Hospital Center Health Care System,, NY, p. A431
GUMMADI, Subhaker, M.D. President Medical Staff, Promise Hospital of Baton Rouge, Baton Rouge, LA, p. A263
GUNABALAN, Ryan, Chief Executive Officer, Behavioral Center of Michigan, Warren, MI, p. A324
GUNASEKARAN, Suresh, Assistant Vice President Information Resources, University of Texas Southwestern Medical Center, Dallas, TX, p. A593
GUNDA, Sharad, M.D. Chief of Staff, Franklin Foundation Hospital, Franklin, LA, p. A266
GUNDERSEN, Robert A., Market Chief Executive Officer, Kindred Hospital Northeast–Stoughton, Stoughton, MA, p. A305

A826 Index of Health Care Professionals

Index of Health Care Professionals / Hagy

Index of Health Care Professionals


GUNN, B. Joe, FACHE Interim Chief Executive Officer, Craig General Hospital, Vinita, OK, p. A507

GUNN, Deborah, Chief Information Officer, Veterans Affairs Medical Center, Salisbury, NC, p. A460

GUNN, John R., Executive Vice President and Chief Operating Officer, Memorial Sloan–Kettering Cancer Center, New York, NY, p. A434

GUNN, Robert, Vice President Human Resources, St. Joseph Mercy Port Huron, Port Huron, MI, p. A321

GUNNELS, Wheeler, M.D. Medical Director, Mizell Memorial Hospital, Opp, AL, p. A24

GUNNERSEN, Nils, Administrator, Bertrand Chaffee Hospital, Springville, NY, p. A443

GUNUKULA, Srinivas, M.D. Chief of Staff, Dallas Regional Medical Center, Mesquite, TX, p. A616

GUPTA, Apurv, M.D. Chief Medical Officer, Quincy Medical Center, Quincy, MA, p. A304

GUPTA, Arun, M.D. Vice President Medical Affairs, South Pointe Hospital, Warrensville Heights, OH, p. A490

GUPTA, Ashok K., M.D. Chief of Staff, Eaton Rapids Medical Center, Eaton Rapids, MI, p. A312

GUPTA, Vijay D., M.D. President and Chief Executive Officer, Franciscan Physicians Hospital, Munster, IN, p. A209

GURR, Lory, Chief Human Resources Division, Evans U. S. Army Community Hospital, Fort Carson, CO, p. A101

GURTO, Barbara, Manager Human Resources, University Hospitals Conneaut Medical Center, Conneaut, OH, p. A478

GURUNG, Anju, M.D. Chief Medical Officer, Mahnomen Health Center, Mahnomen, MN, p. A334

GUSHEE, Dean, M.D. Medical Director, Mason General Hospital, Shelton, WA, p. A666

GUSHO, Michael, Chief Financial Officer, St. Joseph Mercy Oakland, Pontiac, MI, p. A321

GUSSERT, Jeff, Director Operations, Dickinson County Healthcare System, Iron Mountain, MI, p. A315

GUSTAFSON, Brian, Chief Financial Officer, Veterans Affairs Montana Health Care System, Fort Harrison, MT, p. A375

GUSTAFSON, Michael, M.D. Chief Operating Officer, Faulkner Hospital, Boston, MA, p. A296

GUSTILO, Maria, M.D
- Medical Director, Osawatomie State Hospital, Osawatomie, KS, p. A240
- Medical Director, Rainbow Mental Health Facility, Kansas City, KS, p. A236

GUTH, Ron, Chief Financial Officer, Providence Hood River Memorial Hospital, Hood River, OR, p. A511

GUTHMILLER, Martin W., Chief Executive Officer, Orange City Area Health System, Orange City, IA, p. A224

GUTHRIE, Deborah S., Chief Executive Officer, HEALTHSOUTH Southern Hills Rehabilitation Hospital, Princeton, WV, p. A675

GUTIERREZ, Albert, FACHE President and Chief Executive Officer, Saint Joseph Regional Medical Center, Mishawaka, IN, p. A208

GUTIERREZ, Doris, Director Human Resources, Holy Cross Hospital, Chicago, IL, p. A176

GUTIERREZ, Lori, Chief Financial Officer, Rochelle Community Hospital, Rochelle, IL, p. A192

GUTIERREZ, Michael, Executive Director, Turquoise Lodge Hospital, Albuquerque, NM, p. A415

GUTIERREZ, Victor A., M.D. Medical Director, Allegiance Behavioral Health Center of Plainview, Plainview, TX, p. A621

GUTJAHR, Susan, Reimbursement Specialist, Sparta Community Hospital, Sparta, IL, p. A194

GUTMAN, Luisa, Senior Vice President and Chief Operating Officer, Holy Cross Hospital, Fort Lauderdale, FL, p. A123

GUTNICK, Michael, Senior Vice President Finance, Memorial Sloan–Kettering Cancer Center, New York, NY, p. A434

GUTOW, Andrew, M.D. Medical Director, Menlo Park Surgical Hospital, Menlo Park, CA, p. A74

GUTSCH, Michael, Chief Financial Officer, Southwest Health Center, Platteville, WI, p. A689

GUTSCHENRITTER, John, Chief Financial Officer, Wilson Medical Center, Neodesha, KS, p. A239

GUTTENBERG, Ellen, Chief Operating Officer, Frances Mahon Deaconess Hospital, Glasgow, MT, p. A375

GUTTIN, Enrique, M.D. Chief of Staff, Veterans Affairs Medical Center, Wilmington, DE, p. A115

GUTTMACHER, Laurence, M.D. Clinical Director, Rochester Psychiatric Center, Rochester, NY, p. A442

GUTZEIT, Michael, M.D. Chief Medical Officer, Children's Hospital of Wisconsin, Milwaukee, WI, p. A686

GUY, Ronald J., Chief Financial Officer, Capital Health Medical Center–Hopewell, Pennington, NJ, p. A408

GUYETTE, William, M.D. President Medical Staff, Livingston Hospital and Healthcare Services, Salem, KY, p. A258

GUZAN, David J., Chief Executive Officer, Fairway Medical Center, Covington, LA, p. A265

GUZMAN, Elizabeth, Chief Financial Officer, Metropolitan Hospital Center, New York, NY, p. A434

GWATKIN, Betty Ann, Vice President Human Resources, Northeastern Vermont Regional Hospital, Saint Johnsbury, VT, p. A644

GWYN, Brian
- President and Chief Executive Officer, Cleveland Regional Medical Center, Shelby, NC, p. A460
- President and Chief Executive Officer, Crawley Memorial Hospital, Boiling Springs, NC, p. A449
- President and Chief Executive Officer, Crawley Memorial Hospital, Boiling Springs, NC, p. A449
- President, Kings Mountain Hospital, Kings Mountain, NC, p. A456

GWYNN, Sherry, Administrative Director Human Resources, Care Regional Medical Center, Aransas Pass, TX, p. A579


## H


HAACK, Wanda, MSN Chief Nursing Officer, Genesis Medical Center, DeWitt, De Witt, IA, p. A217

HAACKE, David E., M.D. Chief of Staff, Collingsworth General Hospital, Wellington, TX, p. A634

HAAGENSON, Deb, R.N. Vice President of Patient Care, St. Joseph's Area Health Services, Park Rapids, MN, p. A337

HAAK, Thelma, Manager Health Information, Avera Dells Area Hospital, Dell Rapids, SD, p. A556

HAAK–MUSE, Margaret, Chief Financial Officer and Assistant Administrator, East Texas Medical Center–Mount Vernon, Mount Vernon, TX, p. A617

HAAR, Clare A., Chief Executive Officer, Eastern Niagara Health System, Lockport, NY, p. A429

HAAS, Christine, Manager Information Technology, Jersey Shore Hospital, Jersey Shore, PA, p. A525

HAAS, Marvin, Chief Administration and Finance Officer, Three Rivers Medical Center, Grants Pass, OR, p. A511

HAAS, Richard, FACHE President, Grandview Medical Center, Dayton, OH, p. A478

HAAS, Scott A., M.D. Chief Medical Officer, Eastern State Hospital, Lexington, KY, p. A253

HAAS, Susan, Director Human Resources, Aurora Behavioral Health Care, San Diego, CA, p. A85

HAASE, Patricia, Director Information Technology and Communications, Marian Medical Center, Santa Maria, CA, p. A90

HAASE, Ron, Vice President Human Resources, St. Mary's of Michigan, Saginaw, MI, p. A322

HAASKEN, Timothy W., Chief Financial Officer, Montgomery Regional Hospital, Blacksburg, VA, p. A646

HAATVEDT, Cy, M.D. Chief of Staff, Huron Regional Medical Center, Huron, SD, p. A557

HABASHY, Hany Mounir, M.D. Chief Medical Director, Methodist Extended Care Hospital, Memphis, TN, p. A571

HABIB, Noel, M.D. Chief Medical Officer, Huhukam Memorial Hospital, Sacaton, AZ, p. A37

HABOWSKI, Michael J., President and Chief Executive Officer, Ashtabula County Medical Center, Ashtabula, OH, p. A469

HACHENBERG, Dennis A., FACHE Chief Executive Officer, Anderson County Hospital, Garnett, KS, p. A233

HACHTEN II,, Richard A., FACHE President and Chief Executive Officer, Alegent Health, Omaha, NE, p. B7

HACKBARTH, John, CPA Senior Vice President Finance and Chief Financial Officer, Owensboro Medical Health System, Owensboro, KY, p. A257

HACKER, Kenneth, M.D. Chief of Staff, Progress West HealthCare Center, Saint Charles, MO, p. A367

HACKER, Leanne, Chief Financial Officer, Eastern New Mexico Medical Center, Roswell, NM, p. A417

HACKER, Mary Dee, R.N. Vice President, Patient Care Services and Chief Nursing Officer, Children's Hospital Los Angeles, Los Angeles, CA, p. A69

HACKER, Phillip, Chief Financial Officer, Citizens Medical Center, Victoria, TX, p. A633

HACKETT, Sylvia D., Vice President Human Resources, Rex Healthcare, Raleigh, NC, p. A459

HACKMAN, James, Corporate Vice President Human Resources, Florida Hospital Tampa, Tampa, FL, p. A140

HACKMAN, Paul, Chief Executive Officer, Ridgeview Institute, Smyrna, GA, p. A159

HACKNEY, Hannah, Director Accounting and Human Resources, DeWitt Hospital, De Witt, AR, p. A44

HACKSTEDDE, Anita, M.D. Vice President Medical Affairs, Salem Community Hospital, Salem, OH, p. A488

HADDAD, Nicholas, M.D. Acting Chief Medical Service, Aleda E. Lutz Veterans Affairs Medical Center, Saginaw, MI, p. A322

HADDAD, Phillip A., M.D. Chief Medical Officer, Solara Hospital of Shawnee, Shawnee, OK, p. A504

HADDADIN, Maen, M.D. President Medical Staff, Alegent Health Mercy Hospital, Corning, IA, p. A216

HADDEN, Kim E., R.N. Chief Nurse Executive, Riverside Medical Center, Riverside, CA, p. A83

HADDICAN, James, Vice President Finance, Gillette Children's Specialty Healthcare, Saint Paul, MN, p. A339

HADDIX, D. Parker, Chief Operating Officer, Davis Memorial Hospital, Elkins, WV, p. A671

HADDIX, Parker, Chief Executive Officer, William R. Sharpe, Jr. Hospital, Weston, WV, p. A676

HADDIX–HILL, Katherine, R.N. Chief Nursing Officer/Chief Operating Officer, Pender Memorial Hospital, Burgaw, NC, p. A449

HADEN, James E., President and Chief Executive Officer, Martha Jefferson Hospital, Charlottesville, VA, p. A646

HADJUK, Clare, Director Human Resources, Veterans Affairs Edward Hines, Jr. Hospital, Hines, IL, p. A184

HADLEY, Mike
- Chief Information Officer, Saint Francis Hospital, Memphis, TN, p. A572
- Director Information Systems, Saint Francis Hospital–Bartlett, Bartlett, TN, p. A562

HADLEY, Steven N., Chief Financial Officer, Kansas Medical Center, Andover, KS, p. A230

HADLEY, Susan, R.N. Director of Nursing, Dickinson County Healthcare System, Iron Mountain, MI, p. A315

HADZEGA, Angela, Chief Financial Officer, Kane Community Hospital, Kane, PA, p. A526

HADZIE, Daniel, M.D. Chief of Staff, Stonewall Memorial Hospital, Aspermont, TX, p. A580

HAEGER, Eric, M.D. President Medical Staff, Okanogan Douglas District Hospital, Brewster, WA, p. A660

HAEHN, Debra, Chief Financial Officer, Clay County Memorial Hospital, Henrietta, TX, p. A603

HAENELT, Michael, Chief Information Management, Weed Army Community Hospital, Fort Irwin, CA, p. A61

HAESEMEYER, Allan, M.D. Chief of Staff, Indianhead Medical Center, Shell Lake, WI, p. A691

HAEUSER, Jamie, Senior Vice President Operations, Woman's Hospital, Baton Rouge, LA, p. A263

HAFEN, Heather, Manager Human Resources, Sanpete Valley Hospital, Mount Pleasant, UT, p. A638

HAFFNER, Randall L., Ph.D. Chief Executive Officer, Porter Adventist Hospital, Denver, CO, p. A100

HAFFORD, Juliet, Director Human Resources, Oakwood Southshore Medical Center, Trenton, MI, p. A324

HAGAN, David J., M.D. Chief Medical Officer, Gibson Area Hospital and Health Services, Gibson City, IL, p. A183

HAGAN, Donald E., Chief Financial Officer, DeTar Healthcare System, Victoria, TX, p. A633

HAGAN, Eric, R.N. Vice President, Medical Center at Scottsville, Scottsville, KY, p. A259

HAGAN, Mary, Director Human Resources, Summit Park Hospital and Nursing Care Center, Pomona, NY, p. A440

HAGAN, Patrick J., President and Chief Operating Officer, Seattle Children's Hospital, Seattle, WA, p. A666

HAGELTHORN, Diane, Human Resources Generalist, Modoc Medical Center, Alturas, CA, p. A53

HAGEMANN, Margarethe, M.D. Chief of Staff, Veterans Affairs Medical Center, Memphis, TN, p. A572

HAGEN, Bruce P.
- President, Dublin Methodist Hospital, Dublin, OH, p. A479
- President, Grady Memorial Hospital, Delaware, OH, p. A479

HAGEN, Michael, Chief Executive Officer, Riverwood Healthcare Center, Aitkin, MN, p. A327

HAGEN, Paulette, Director Human Resources, Paynesville Area Health Care System, Paynesville, MN, p. A337

HAGENS, Gary, Chief Operating Officer and Vice President Medical Affairs, Advocate BroMenn Medical Center, Normal, IL, p. A189

HAGENSICKER, Janice, Chief Financial Officer, Rollins–Brook Community Hospital, Lampasas, TX, p. A611

HAGER, Jeff, M.D. President Medical Staff, North Mississippi Medical Center–Hamilton, Hamilton, AL, p. A21

HAGGARD, Tommy, Chief Executive Officer, Bluegrass Community Hospital, Versailles, KY, p. A259

HAGGERTY, Arthur, Director Information Systems, Madera Community Hospital, Madera, CA, p. A73

HAGGERTY, Bridget, Chief Information Officer, OHSU Hospital, Portland, OR, p. A514

HAGHIGHAT, Dennis, M.D. Vice President Medical Affairs, Mission Hospital, Mission Viejo, CA, p. A74

HAGLER, Dan, M.D. Vice President and Chief Medical Officer, Carolinas Medical Center–Union, Monroe, NC, p. A457

HAGOOD, Teena, Chief Nursing Officer, Kimble Hospital, Junction, TX, p. A609

HAGUE, Samuel, M.D. Chief of Staff, Integris Blackwell Regional Hospital, Blackwell, OK, p. A494

HAGY, Kelly, Director Human Resources and Professional Affairs, Northwest Medical Center, Winfield, AL, p. A27

HAGY, Michael, Chief Financial Officer, Pikeville Medical Center, Pikeville, KY, p. A258




Index of Health Care Professionals **A827**

Index of Health Care Professionals / Hahey


HAHEY, Joanne A., Senior Vice President and Chief Financial Officer, Jefferson Regional Medical Center, Jefferson Hills, PA, p. A525
HAHN, Annette, Director Human Resources, Rehabilitation Hospital of Wisconsin, Waukesha, WI, p. A692
HAHN, Bashirat, Chief Information Officer, MetroSouth Medical Center, Blue Island, IL, p. A174
HAHN, James W., Administrator, North Mississippi Medical Center–West Point, West Point, MS, p. A353
HAHN, Joseph, M.D. Chief of Staff, Cleveland Clinic Foundation, Cleveland, OH, p. A474
HAHN, Kenneth, M.D. Chief of Staff, South Peninsula Hospital, Homer, AK, p. A29
HAHN, Victoria J., Administrator and Chief Executive Officer, Wichita County Health Center, Leoti, KS, p. A238
HAILE, Michael, Senior Vice President and Chief Financial Officer, Faxton–St. Luke's Healthcare, Utica, NY, p. A445
HAILSTONE, Sherlyn, FACHE President, SSM Cardinal Glennon Children's Medical Center, Saint Louis, MO, p. A369
HAIM, Kelvin, M.D. Chief of Staff, North Georgia Medical Center, Ellijay, GA, p. A152
HAINES, Beverly J., R.N. Interim President, Patewood Memorial Hospital, Greenville, SC, p. A550
HAIR, Laurie, Chief Financial Officer, Phoebe Sumter Medical Center, Americus, GA, p. A144
HAIR, Troy, Chief Financial Officer, Abbeville General Hospital, Abbeville, LA, p. A261
HAIRGROVE, Heath
Administrator, Rehabilitation Hospital of DeQuincy, DeQuincy, LA, p. A266
Administrator, Tri Parish Rehabilitation Hospital, Leesville, LA, p. A272
HAIZLIP, Jr., Thomas M., M.D. Chief of Staff, Charles A. Cannon Memorial Hospital, Linville, NC, p. A456
HAJEK, Julie, Director Human Resources, St. David's North Austin Medical Center, Austin, TX, p. A581
HAKMILLER, Karl, M.D. Chief Medical Officer, South Baldwin Regional Medical Center, Foley, AL, p. A20
HALAKAN, Catherine, Senior Vice President, Albany Medical Center, Albany, NY, p. A420
HALAMKA, John, M.D. Chief Information Officer, Beth Israel Deaconess Medical Center, Boston, MA, p. A296
HALDEMAN, Larry, M.D. Executive Vice President and Chief Medical Officer, WellStar Windy Hill Hospital, Marietta, GA, p. A156
HALE, Becky, Director Human Resources, Hill Regional Hospital, Hillsboro, TX, p. A603
HALE, Byron, Chief Financial Officer, East Texas Medical Center Tyler, Tyler, TX, p. A632
HALE, Dana R., R.N. Vice President Nursing, Lawrence Memorial Hospital, Lawrence, KS, p. A237
HALE, Elizabeth, R.N. Vice President Patient Services and Chief Nursing Officer, Lawrence General Hospital, Lawrence, MA, p. A301
HALE, Nathan, Director Information Management, Howard Memorial Hospital, Nashville, AR, p. A49
HALE, Pat, Chief Financial Officer, Indian Path Medical Center, Kingsport, TN, p. A568
HALE, Vicki, Chief Financial Officer, NCH Downtown Naples Hospital, Naples, FL, p. A133
HALE, William R., Administrator, Carson Valley Medical Center, Gardnerville, NV, p. A392
HALEN, Catherine, Vice President Human Resources, Beebe Medical Center, Lewes, DE, p. A114
HALES, Brent, Chief Financial Officer, Uintah Basin Medical Center, Roosevelt, UT, p. A640
HALES, Joe, Director Information Systems, Primary Children's Medical Center, Salt Lake City, UT, p. A640
HALES Jr., John C., FACHE Interim Chief Executive Officer, Bamberg County Memorial Hospital, Bamberg, SC, p. A
HALES, Tom, CPA Chief Financial Officer, Crittenden County Hospital, Marion, KY, p. A256
HALEY, Bob, Interim Chief Executive Officer, Rainy Lake Medical Center, International Falls, MN, p. A333
HALEY, James, M.D. Senior Vice President and Chief Medical Officer, Unity Hospital, Rochester, NY, p. A442
HALEY, Kevin, Chief Financial Officer, Penn State Milton S. Hershey Medical Center, Hershey, PA, p. A525
HALEY, Michael E., President and Chief Executive Officer, Indiana University Health Ball Memorial Hospital, Muncie, IN, p. A209
HALFEN, John, M.D. Medical Director, Lakewood Health System, Staples, MN, p. A340
HALFEN, John
Administrator, Chief Executive Officer and Chief Financial Officer, Northern Inyo Hospital, Bishop, CA, p. A56
Administrator, Chief Executive Officer and Chief Financial Officer, Northern Inyo Hospital, Bishop, CA, p. A56
HALFERTY, Michael, M.D. President Medical Staff, Samaritan North Lincoln Hospital, Lincoln City, OR, p. A512
HALFHIDE, Jon W., President, St. Elizabeth Community Hospital, Red Bluff, CA, p. A81
HALFHILL, Patrick, Chief Financial Officer, Madison County Memorial Hospital, Madison, FL, p. A129
HALL, Alan, Chief Nursing Officer, St. Joseph's Behavioral Health Center, Stockton, CA, p. A91
HALL, Brenda, R.N. Vice President Patient Care Services, Yuma Regional Medical Center, Yuma, AZ, p. A41
HALL, Butch, Chief Financial Officer, Hardeman County Memorial Hospital, Quanah, TX, p. A622
HALL, Catherine, Manager Human Resources, Jefferson Hospital, Louisville, GA, p. A155
HALL, Charlene, Vice President Human Resources and Guest Support Services, Indiana University Health Morgan Hospital, Martinsville, IN, p. A208
HALL, Cindy, Coordinator Human Resources, Selby General Hospital, Marietta, OH, p. A484
HALL, Clara Cordelia, Chief Human Resources Officer, Breckinridge Memorial Hospital, Hardinsburg, KY, p. A251
HALL, Dan, R.N. Director of Nursing, St. John Owasso, Owasso, OK, p. A503
HALL, Dana, Director of Nursing, Quitman County Hospital, Marks, MS, p. A349
HALL, Darr, Chief Financial Officer, Nanticoke Memorial Hospital, Seaford, DE, p. A114
HALL, David, Chief Information Officer, Pineville Community Hospital Association, Pineville, KY, p. A258
HALL, David, M.D. Senior Vice President and Chief Medical Officer, St. Vincent Medical Center–North, Sherwood, AR, p. A51
HALL, David, Senior Vice President and Chief Operating Officer, The University of Tennessee Medical Center, Knoxville, TN, p. A569
HALL, Doug, Director Information Systems, Tri Valley Health System, Cambridge, NE, p. A382
HALL, Gary, Vice President of Information Technology, Estes Park Medical Center, Estes Park, CO, p. A101
HALL, George, M.D
Vice President Medical Affairs, St. Elizabeth Florence, Florence, KY, p. A250
Vice President Medical Affairs, St. Elizabeth Fort Thomas, Fort Thomas, KY, p. A250
HALL, Gerald, Director Resource Management, Naval Hospital, Oak Harbor, WA, p. A663
HALL, Herbert L., Administrator, Reception and Medical Center, Lake Butler, FL, p. A128
HALL, Jeanne, Director Information Systems, Shriners Hospitals for Children, St. Louis, Saint Louis, MO, p. A369
HALL, Jeffrey, M.D. Chief of Staff, Great River Medical Center, Blytheville, AR, p. A42
HALL, Jeremy, Assistant Administrator and Chief Financial Officer, Middlesboro ARH Hospital, Middlesboro, KY, p. A256
HALL, Jim
Budget Officer, Caswell Center, Kinston, NC, p. A456
Acting Chief Information Officer, Central Arkansas Veterans Healthcare System, Little Rock, AR, p. A48
HALL, Les, M.D
Chief Medical Officer, University of Missouri Hospitals and Clinics, Columbia, MO, p. A358
Chief of Staff, Women's and Children's Hospital, Columbia, MO, p. A358
HALL, Leslie, R.N. Senior Vice President–Chief Nursing Officer, Nash Health Care Systems, Rocky Mount, NC, p. A460
HALL, Linda, Administrator, Chillicothe Hospital District, Chillicothe, TX, p. A587
HALL, Marcia K., Chief Executive Officer, Sharp Coronado Hospital and Healthcare Center, Coronado, CA, p. A58
HALL, Mark
Chief Financial Officer, Bath Community Hospital, Hot Springs, VA, p. A650
Chief Financial Officer, Rehoboth McKinley Christian Health Care Services, Gallup, NM, p. A416
HALL, Mary A., Chief Medical Staff, McDowell ARH Hospital, McDowell, KY, p. A256
HALL, Melissa, Human Resources, Munising Memorial Hospital, Munising, MI, p. A319
HALL, Michael L., Chief Executive Officer, Avera Holy Family Hospital, Estherville, IA, p. A219
HALL, Mike, Risk Manager, Sistersville General Hospital, Sistersville, WV, p. A675
HALL Jr., Paul P., Chief Executive Officer and Chief Clinical Officer, Vibra Specialty Hospital of Dallas, Desoto, TX, p. A594
HALL, Robert, Chief Information Officer, Northern Hospital of Surry County, Mount Airy, NC, p. A458
HALL, Roger L.
President, Sacred Heart Hospital on the Emerald Coast, Miramar Beach, FL, p. A132
President, Sacred Heart Hospital on the Gulf, Port St. Joe, FL, p. A137
HALL, Sally, Manager Human Resources, South Texas Spine and Surgical Hospital, San Antonio, TX, p. A626
HALL, Stephanie, M.D. Chief Medical Officer, LAC/University of Southern California Medical Center, Los Angeles, CA, p. A70
HALL, Steve, Chief Financial Officer, Pekin Hospital, Pekin, IL, p. A191
HALL, Veronica, R.N. Chief Operating Officer, Henry Ford Hospital, Detroit, MI, p. A310
HALLADAY, Mark, Director Information Services, F. F. Thompson Hospital, Canandaigua, NY, p. A423
HALLAL, Joseph, M.D. Chief Medical Officer, Inova Fairfax Hospital, Falls Church, VA, p. A647
HALLATT, Jennifer
Chief Operating Officer, Mercy Harvard Hospital, Harvard, IL, p. A183
Administrator, Mercy Walworth Hospital and Medical Center, Lake Geneva, WI, p. A684
HALLER, III, William, M.D. Chief of Staff, Gadsden Regional Medical Center, Gadsden, AL, p. A20
HALLEY, Lisa, Vice President Human Resources, Holzer Medical Center, Gallipolis, OH, p. A480
HALLFORD, Wayne, Chief Executive Officer, Central Louisiana State Hospital, Pineville, LA, p. A276
HALLGREN, Hugh R., Chief Executive Officer, Sitka Community Hospital, Sitka, AK, p. A30
HALLIDAY, Lisa, Director Accounting Services, Taylor Regional Hospital, Hawkinsville, GA, p. A154
HALLIGAN, Ron, Vice President Support Services, Great River Medical Center, West Burlington, IA, p. A228
HALLISEY, Thomas, Vice President Information Management, Cortland Regional Medical Center, Cortland, NY, p. A424
HALLMAN, Ronald, Vice President Development and Public Relations, Porter Medical Center, Middlebury, VT, p. A643
HALLMARK, Todd, Chief Operating Officer, Choctaw Nation Health Care Center, Talihina, OK, p. A505
HALLY, Christine, Director Human Resources, Rochester Psychiatric Center, Rochester, NY, p. A442
HALMI, Denis J., M.D. President Medical Staff, Sentara Northern Virginia Medical Center, Woodbridge, VA, p. A657
HALPERN, Kevin G., Chief Executive Officer, Camden County Health Services Center, Blackwood, NJ, p. A402
HALPIN, Kim, Director Human Resources, Arms Acres, Carmel, NY, p. A423
HALSAN, Carole, R.N. Chief Executive Officer, Willapa Harbor Hospital, South Bend, WA, p. A667
HALSELL, David, Chief Financial Officer, Bothwell Regional Health Center, Sedalia, MO, p. A370
HALSTEAD, Doug, Manager Information Systems, Bartlett Regional Hospital, Juneau, AK, p. A29
HALTER, Kevin, Chief Executive Officer, Our Lady of Bellefonte Hospital, Ashland, KY, p. A247
HALTER, Michael P., Chief Executive Officer, Hahnemann University Hospital, Philadelphia, PA, p. A532
HALTER, Susan, M.D. Chief Medical Officer, Winneshiek Medical Center, Decorah, IA, p. A218
HALVERSON, Glen, Chief Operating Officer, Mammoth Hospital, Mammoth Lakes, CA, p. A73
HALVORSON, George C., Chairman and Chief Executive Officer, Kaiser Foundation Hospitals, Oakland, CA, p. B74
HALVORSON, Linda, Director Human Resources, Mountrail County Medical Center, Stanley, ND, p. A468
HALVORSON, Marla, Director Human Resources, St. Luke's Hospital, Duluth, MN, p. A330
HAMAM, Hisham, M.D. Chief of Staff, Northern Cochise Community Hospital, Willcox, AZ, p. A41
HAMANN, Barbara, Manager People Services, St. Nicholas Hospital, Sheboygan, WI, p. A690
HAMB, Aaron, M.D. Chief Medical Officer, Provident Hospital of Cook County, Chicago, IL, p. A177
HAMBLEN, Jeffrey J., Chief Executive Officer, Little Colorado Medical Center, Winslow, AZ, p. A41
HAMBLIN, James, Chief Financial Officer, White Mountain Regional Medical Center, Springerville, AZ, p. A38
HAMEL, Cathleen, MS Vice President and Chief Nursing Officer, Baxter Regional Medical Center, Mountain Home, AR, p. A49
HAMEL, Loren, M.D. President and Chief Executive Officer, Lakeland Healthcare, Saint Joseph, MI, p. B78
HAMEL, Loren, M.D
President and Chief Executive Officer, Lakeland Regional Medical Center–St. Joseph, Saint Joseph, MI, p. A322
President and Chief Executive Officer, Lakeland Specialty Hospital–Berrien Center, Berrien Center, MI, p. A308
HAMEL, Susan, Chief Nursing Officer, St. Luke's Hospital, Duluth, MN, p. A330
HAMILL, Dave H., President and Chief Executive Officer, Hampton Regional Medical Center, Varnville, SC, p. A554
HAMILTON, Aggie, Chief Human Resources, Veterans Affairs Montana Health Care System, Fort Harrison, MT, p. A375


**A828** Index of Health Care Professionals

Index of Health Care Professionals / Hansen


HAMILTON, Bruce
Vice President Human Resources, Lutheran Hospital of Indiana, Fort Wayne, IN, p. A201
Director Human Resources, Orthopaedic Hospital of Lutheran Health, Fort Wayne, IN, p. A201
HAMILTON, Chanda, Chief Information Officer, Clifton T. Perkins Hospital Center, Jessup, MD, p. A292
HAMILTON, Crystal, R.N. Chief Executive Officer, Maryvale Hospital Medical Center, Phoenix, AZ, p. A36
HAMILTON, Dan, Director Inpatient Services, Nor–Lea General Hospital, Lovington, NM, p. A417
HAMILTON, James, M.D. Chief of Staff, Habersham Medical Center, Demorest, GA, p. A151
HAMILTON, John B., FACHE Interim President and Chief Executive Officer, Central Washington Hospital, Wenatchee, WA, p. A669
HAMILTON, Joyce, Director Human Resources, McKenzie Regional Hospital, McKenzie, TN, p. A570
HAMILTON, Kay A., MS, President and Chief Executive Officer, Lewistown Hospital, Lewistown, PA, p. A527
HAMILTON, Mark C., M.D. President Medical Staff, Springfield Hospital, Springfield, VT, p. A644
HAMILTON, Michael E., Director, Veterans Affairs Illiana Health Care System, Danville, IL, p. A179
HAMILTON, Neal C., Chief Human Resources, James A. Haley Veterans Hospital, Tampa, FL, p. A140
HAMILTON, Phil, R.N. Chief Executive Officer, General John J. Pershing Memorial Hospital, Brookfield, MO, p. A356
HAMILTON, Richard C., Administrator, Harrison County Community Hospital, Bethany, MO, p. A355
HAMILTON, Robert, Chief Operating Officer, Provident Hospital of Cook County, Chicago, IL, p. A177
HAMILTON, Scott, Vice President and Chief Financial Officer, Parkwest Medical Center, Knoxville, TN, p. A568
HAMILTON, Terry, President, St. John Macomb–Oakland Hospital, Macomb Center, Warren, MI, p. A325
HAMILTON, Theresa, Chief Executive Officer, Fremont–Rideout Health Group, Marysville, CA, p. A74
HAMILTON, Tom, M.D. Chief of Staff, Decatur County General Hospital, Parsons, TN, p. A574
HAMILTON, William L., M.D. Chief Medical Officer, LDS Hospital, Salt Lake City, UT, p. A640
HAMILTON–BEYER, Maggie, Chief Financial Officer, Knoxville Hospital & Clinics, Knoxville, IA, p. A222
HAMILTON–CRAWFORD, Janice, Administrator, Southern Crescent Hospital for Specialty Care, Riverdale, GA, p. A158
HAMLIN, DeWayne, Director, Veterans Affairs Medical Center–Lexington, Lexington, KY, p. A254
HAMLIN, Faye, Manager Human Resources, Julian F. Keith Alcohol and Drug Abuse Treatment Center, Black Mountain, NC, p. A448
HAMLIN, Jeff, Director Finance, Oak Tree Hospital, Corbin, KY, p. A249
HAMLIN, Scott J., Chief Financial Officer, Cincinnati Children's Hospital Medical Center, Cincinnati, OH, p. A473
HAMM, David, President and Chief Executive Officer, Exempla Good Samaritan Medical Center, Lafayette, CO, p. A103
HAMMACK, Kathy, Chief Financial Officer, Western Medical Center–Santa Ana, Santa Ana, CA, p. A89
HAMMACK, Stanley K., Chief Executive Officer, University of South Alabama Hospitals, Mobile, AL, p. B139
HAMMER, Michael, Chief Executive Officer, Sanford Worthington Medical Center, Worthington, MN, p. A342
HAMMER, Rebecca J., Chief Financial Officer, Davis Memorial Hospital, Elkins, WV, p. A671
HAMMERAN, Kevin R., Executive Vice President and Chief Operating Officer, Miami Children's Hospital, Miami, FL, p. A131
HAMMES, Chris, FACHE President, Integris Baptist Medical Center, Oklahoma City, OK, p. A501
HAMMES, Paul, Senior Vice President and Chief Operating Officer, Forsyth Medical Center, Winston–Salem, NC, p. A463
HAMMETT, George, Director Human Resources, Carolina Center for Behavioral Health, Greer, SC, p. A551
HAMMETT, Richard A.
Chief Operating Officer, St. David's Medical Center, Austin, TX, p. A581
Chief Operating Officer, St. David's Rehabilitation Center, Austin, TX, p. A581
HAMMETT, Troy, Vice President and Chief Financial Officer, Doctors Hospital, Columbus, OH, p. A476
HAMMOND, Flora, M.D. Chief Medical Affairs, Rehabilitation Hospital of Indiana, Indianapolis, IN, p. A205
HAMMOND, Geoffrey, M.D. Medical Director, Larned State Hospital, Larned, KS, p. A237
HAMMOND, H. Michael, Administrator, Providence Medical Center, Wayne, NE, p. A390
HAMMOND, Kathy, Director Information Services, AnMed Health Medical Center, Anderson, SC, p. A546
HAMMOND, Michael
Chief Financial Officer, Lourdes Medical Center of Burlington County, Willingboro, NJ, p. A412
Chief Financial Officer, Mercy Medical Center, Springfield, MA, p. A305
Chief Financial Officer, Our Lady of Lourdes Medical Center, Camden, NJ, p. A402
HAMMOND, Thomas H., Chief Information Officer, St. Francis Medical Center, Monroe, LA, p. A273
HAMMONDS, Janie, Human Resources Officer, Columbus Community Hospital, Columbus, TX, p. A588
HAMMONDS, Laura, Assistant Administrator, Jasper Memorial Hospital, Monticello, GA, p. A156
HAMMONS, Mary, Chief Executive Officer, Delta Medical Center, Memphis, TN, p. A571
HAMON, Eric, Chief Financial Officer, Driscoll Children's Hospital, Corpus Christi, TX, p. A589
HAMONS, Janet, Vice President Human Resources, Hutchinson Regional Medical Center, Hutchinson, KS, p. A235
HAMONS, Spencer, Chief Information Officer, Holy Cross Hospital, Taos, NM, p. A418
HAMP, Matthew, Chief Operating Officer, Sisters of Charity Hospital of Buffalo, Buffalo, NY, p. A423
HAMPLE, David L., Chief Executive Officer, Montrose Memorial Hospital, Montrose, CO, p. A104
HAMPTON, Angie, Director Human Resources, Porter–Valparaiso Hospital Campus, Valparaiso, IN, p. A212
HAMPTON, David, M.D. Chief Medical Staff, Pampa Regional Medical Center, Pampa, TX, p. A620
HAMPTON, Debra C., Ph.D. Vice President, Administration and Chief Nursing Officer, Drake Center, Cincinnati, OH, p. A473
HAMPTON, Jeff, Director Information Systems, Lehigh Regional Medical Center, Lehigh Acres, FL, p. A129
HAMPTON, Laurie, Director Human Resources, Prairie du Chien Memorial Hospital, Prairie Du Chien, WI, p. A689
HAMRICK, Jan, Chief Financial Officer, Dodge County Hospital, Eastman, GA, p. A152
HAN, Ba, M.D. Clinical Director, Big Spring State Hospital, Big Spring, TX, p. A584
HAN, Kevin, Vice President and Chief Financial Officer, Stormont–Vail HealthCare, Topeka, KS, p. A244
HANAN, Rhonda Jean, Vice President of Patient Care, Mercy Hospital Ardmore, Ardmore, OK, p. A493
HANCOCK, Denise, Chief Financial Officer, Arbuckle Memorial Hospital, Sulphur, OK, p. A505
HANCOCK, J. Brian, M.D. Chief of Staff, Veterans Affairs Health Care System, Fargo, ND, p. A466
HANCOCK, Lori, Chief Business Officer, Veterans Affairs Medical Center, West Palm Beach, FL, p. A143
HANCOCK, Melinda, Interim Chief Financial Officer, Good Samaritan Hospital, Suffern, NY, p. A444
HANCOCK, Sharon, Director Human Resources, Drake Center, Cincinnati, OH, p. A473
HAND, Ronald E., Administrator, Oceans Behavioral Hospital of De Ridder, Deridder, LA, p. A266
HANDE, Vishwanath, M.D. Chief Medical Officer, Minnie Hamilton HealthCare Center, Grantsville, WV, p. A672
HANDELSMAN, Larry, M.D. Vice President Medical Affairs, Chelsea Community Hospital, Chelsea, MI, p. A309
HANDLER, Michael, M.D. Vice President Medical Administration, SSM St. Joseph Hospital West, Lake Saint Louis, MO, p. A363
HANDLEY, Charles R., Chief Financial Officer, Plaza Specialty Hospital, Houston, TX, p. A606
HANDLEY, Peter, M.D. Chief of Staff, Otsego Memorial Hospital, Gaylord, MI, p. A313
HANDLEY, Rhonda, Chief Financial Officer, Columbia Basin Hospital, Ephrata, WA, p. A661
HANDOL, Nelson, M.D. Medical Director, Laurel Oaks Behavioral Health Center, Dothan, AL, p. A19
HANDRICK, Carolyn, Manager Public Relations, Corning Hospital, Corning, NY, p. A424
HANDY, Steven P., CPA Senior Vice President, Chief Financial Officer and Chief Information Officer, Uniontown Hospital, Uniontown, PA, p. A540
HANEBRINK, Brad, D.O. Chief of Staff, Sheridan Memorial Hospital, Sheridan, WY, p. A697
HANEN, David G., Vice President and Chief Financial Officer, Fremont Area Medical Center, Fremont, NE, p. A383
HANEN, Marti, Director Human Resources, Providence Seaside Hospital, Seaside, OR, p. A515
HANENBURG, Thomas S., Chief Executive, Providence Medford Medical Center, Medford, OR, p. A512
HANEY, Judy, Chief Nursing Officer, Harris Hospital, Newport, AR, p. A49
HANEY, Kathryn, Chief Financial Officer, HEALTHSOUTH Valley of the Sun Rehabilitation Hospital, Glendale, AZ, p. A33
HANEY, Mark, Senior Vice President and Administrator, WellStar Paulding Hospital, Dallas, GA, p. A150
HANGER, Kelvin, Chief Executive Officer, Evendale Medical Center, Cincinnati, OH, p. A473
HANIGAN, Hank, Chief Operating Officer, Whidbey General Hospital, Coupeville, WA, p. A660
HANISCH, Denise, M.D. Chief of Staff, St. Mary's Healthcare Center, Pierre, SD, p. A558
HANKERD, Nanci, Manager Human Resources, Trinity Hospital, Weaverville, CA, p. A95
HANKINS, J. William, FACHE Chief Executive Officer, West Calcasieu Cameron Hospital, Sulphur, LA, p. A278
HANKINSON, Scott, Chief Financial Officer, Western Plains Medical Complex, Dodge City, KS, p. A232
HANKS, Claire H., R.N. Vice President and Chief Nursing Officer, Glendale Memorial Hospital and Health Center, Glendale, CA, p. A63
HANKS, John, Director Information Systems, East Tennessee Children's Hospital, Knoxville, TN, p. A568
HANKS, Tammy, Director Human Resources, Minidoka Memorial Hospital, Rupert, ID, p. A170
HANLEY, Darlene S., R.N. President and Chief Executive Officer, St. Lawrence Rehabilitation Center, Lawrenceville, NJ, p. A405
HANLEY, Janet, Chief Nursing Officer, Sharp Grossmont Hospital, La Mesa, CA, p. A66
HANLEY, Kathleen S., Chief Financial Officer, ProMedica Flower Hospital, Sylvania, OH, p. A489
HANLEY, Patrick, D.O. Interim Vice President Medical Affairs, Palmerton Hospital, Palmerton, PA, p. A531
HANLEY, Richard, Chief Operating Officer, Spring Harbor Hospital, Westbrook, ME, p. A286
HANLY, Donna, R.N. Senior Vice President and Chief Nursing Officer, Grant Medical Center, Columbus, OH, p. A476
HANNA, Mitchell J., Chief Executive Officer, Sutter Auburn Faith Hospital, Auburn, CA, p. A54
HANNA, Philip S., Administrator, Battle Mountain General Hospital, Battle Mountain, NV, p. A391
HANNA, Robb, Executive Director Information Technology, Lexington Regional Health Center, Lexington, NE, p. A385
HANNAH, Jill, Director Human Resources, James Cancer Hospital and Solove Research Institute, Columbus, OH, p. A476
HANNAH, Steve, Chief Operating Officer, Gordon Hospital, Calhoun, GA, p. A148
HANNAN, Barbara E., Chief Executive Officer, Select Specialty Hospital–Northeast New Jersey, Rochelle Park, NJ, p. A409
HANNERS, Brandy, Chief Financial Officer, Memorial Hospital, Martinsville, VA, p. A651
HANNERS, Rodney, Senior Vice President and Chief Operating Officer, Children's Hospital Los Angeles, Los Angeles, CA, p. A69
HANNON, Barbara A., MSN VP Nursing, Mount Desert Island Hospital, Bar Harbor, ME, p. A281
HANNON, Jennifer, Director Human Resources, Madison County Health Care System, Winterset, IA, p. A228
HANNON, Kay, Director Information Systems, Des Peres Hospital, Saint Louis, MO, p. A368
HANNON, Trish, FACHE President and Chief Executive Officer, New England Baptist Hospital, Boston, MA, p. A297
HANOLD, Gary, Director Management Information Systems, Angel Medical Center, Franklin, NC, p. A453
HANOVER, Kenneth, President and Chief Executive Officer, Beverly Hospital, Beverly, MA, p. A295
HANSEL, Jimmie W., Chief Executive Officer, Garden County Health Services, Oshkosh, NE, p. A388
HANSEN, Becky, Chief Financial Officer, Southwest Healthcare Services, Bowman, ND, p. A464
HANSEN, Chris, Senior Vice President Ambulatory Services and Chief Information Officer, The University of Kansas Hospital, Kansas City, KS, p. A236
HANSEN, Dawn, Regional Director Information Services, Wheaton Franciscan Healthcare – St. Joseph's, Milwaukee, WI, p. A687
HANSEN, Dennis, President, Shady Grove Adventist Hospital, Rockville, MD, p. A294
HANSEN, Gayle B., R.N
Chief Operating Officer, Mayo Clinic Health System in Fairmont, Fairmont, MN, p. A331
Chief Integration Officer, Mayo Clinic Health System in Saint James, Saint James, MN, p. A338
HANSEN, Jay, Director Information Services, Oconee Medical Center, Seneca, SC, p. A553
HANSEN, Kyle, Corporate Director Information Systems, Riverside Medical Center, Kankakee, IL, p. A185
HANSEN, Laurie
Associate Administrator, Emory Johns Creek Hospital, Johns Creek, GA, p. A154
Director Administrative Services, Johnson County Healthcare Center, Buffalo, WY, p. A695
HANSEN, Maggie, R.N. Chief Nursing Officer, Memorial Regional Hospital,, FL, p. A125


Index of Health Care Professionals

Index of Health Care Professionals

Index of Health Care Professionals / Hansen

HANSEN, Marcia A., R.N. Vice President Patient Services and Chief Nursing Officer, Ephrata Community Hospital, Ephrata, PA, p. A523
HANSEN, Michael T., FACHE President and Chief Executive Officer, Columbus Community Hospital, Columbus, NE, p. A382
HANSEN, Thomas N., M.D. Chief Executive Officer, Seattle Children's Hospital, Seattle, WA, p. A666
HANSMAN, Matthew, M.D. Chief of Staff, Sutter Maternity and Surgery Center of Santa Cruz, Santa Cruz, CA, p. A90
HANSON, Angie, R.N. Chief Nursing Officer, Howard Memorial Hospital, Nashville, AR, p. A49
HANSON, Bonnie, Chief Operating Officer, Dupont Hospital, Fort Wayne, IN, p. A201
HANSON, Carl, Administrator, Minidoka Memorial Hospital, Rupert, ID, p. A170
HANSON, Denise, Information Technology Specialist, St. Cloud Veterans Affairs Health Care System, Saint Cloud, MN, p. A338
HANSON, Gregory S., M.D. Chief Executive Officer, Clark Fork Valley Hospital, Plains, MT, p. A378
HANSON, Jane E., R.N. Chief Nursing Officer, Providence Medford Medical Center, Medford, OR, p. A512
HANSON, Jesica, Vice President and Chief Financial Officer, Bakersfield Memorial Hospital, Bakersfield, CA, p. A54
HANSON, Kristy, Chief Financial Officer, Mayo Clinic Health System – Northland in Barron, Barron, WI, p. A678
HANSON, Margaret, R.N. Interim President, Carney Hospital, Boston, MA, p. A296
HANSON, Mark C., M.D. Chief of Staff, Newton Medical Center, Covington, GA, p. A150
HANSON, Mary Ann, Director Personnel, Mental Health Institute, Cherokee, IA, p. A216
HANSON, Paul A., Chief Executive Officer, Sanford Bemidji Medical Center, Bemidji, MN, p. A328
HANSON, Rhonda, Director Human Resources, Huron Regional Medical Center, Huron, SD, p. A557
HANSON, Rita, M.D. Vice President Medical Affairs, Wheaton Franciscan Healthcare – St. Joseph's, Milwaukee, WI, p. A687
HANTOOT, Mark, M.D. Medical Director, Gateways Hospital and Mental Health Center, Los Angeles, CA, p. A69
HANYAK, Diana C., Chief Executive Officer, HEALTHSOUTH Tustin Rehabilitation Hospital, Tustin, CA, p. A93
HAPNEY, Sherry, Chief Financial Officer, HEALTHSOUTH Rehabilitation Hospital, Fort Worth, TX, p. A598
HAPPEL, Terry J., M.D
  Vice President and Chief Medical Officer, Chandler Regional Medical Center, Chandler, AZ, p. A31
  Vice President and Chief Medical Officer, Mercy Gilbert Medical Center, Gilbert, AZ, p. A32
HARA, Karen, Personnel Management Specialist, Hawaii State Hospital, Kaneohe, HI, p. A164
HARALDSON, Richard, Chief Executive Officer, Sidney Health Center, Sidney, MT, p. A379
HARALSON, Greg, Chief Operating Officer, Plaza Medical Center of Fort Worth, Fort Worth, TX, p. A599
HARARI, Jack L., M.D. Chief Medical Officer, West Boca Medical Center, Boca Raton, FL, p. A119
HARB, Gregory A., FACH
  Executive Vice President and Chief Operating Officer, Baystate Mary Lane Hospital, Ware, MA, p. A305
  Executive Vice President and Chief Operating Officer, Baystate Medical Center, Springfield, MA, p. A304
HARBAUGH, Charles, Director Human Resources, Mountain Lakes Medical Center, Clayton, GA, p. A149
HARBAUGH, Ken, Vice President and Chief Financial Officer, OSF Saint Francis Medical Center, Peoria, IL, p. A191
HARBERTS, Jerry, Information Technologist, Madison Hospital, Madison, MN, p. A334
HARBOR, Mike, Chief Financial Officer, Hardin Medical Center, Savannah, TN, p. A575
HARCHENKO, Vern, M.D. Chief of Staff, Garrison Memorial Hospital, Garrison, ND, p. A466
HARCOURT, Jenifer, Chief Operating Officer, RiverWoods Behavioral Health System, Riverdale, GA, p. A157
HARCOURT, Roxane, Chief Executive Officer, Streamwood Behavioral Health Center, Streamwood, IL, p. A195
HARCUP, Craig, M.D. Hospital Medical Director, Complex Care Hospital at Ridgelake, Sarasota, FL, p. A138
HARDEMAN, Diane, Director Personnel, Stephens County Hospital, Toccoa, GA, p. A161
HARDEN, Jean, Executive Director Human Resources, Baptist Hospital Northeast, La Grange, KY, p. A252
HARDESTY, Cynthia, Vice President and Chief Nursing Executive, Charles Cole Memorial Hospital, Coudersport, PA, p. A521
HARDIN, Cecil, CPA Chief Financial Officer, Catawba Hospital, Catawba, VA, p. A646
HARDIN, James, Human Resources Officer, Veterans Affairs Medical Center, Sheridan, WY, p. A697
HARDIN, Leslie, Chief Executive Officer and Chief Financial Officer, Seymour Hospital, Seymour, TX, p. A627
HARDIN, Mark, M.D. Medical Director, Ed Fraser Memorial Hospital and Baker Community Health Center, MacClenny, FL, p. A129
HARDIN, Nicholas, Chief Executive Officer, HEALTHSOUTH Sugar Land Rehabilitation Hospital, Sugar Land, TX, p. A629
HARDING, Catherine, M.D. Medical Director, HEALTHSOUTH Rehabilitation of Gadsden, Gadsden, AL, p. A20
HARDING, Christina, Vice President Finance, Mount Desert Island Hospital, Bar Harbor, ME, p. A281
HARDING, Denise, Director Human Resources, Plumas District Hospital, Quincy, CA, p. A81
HARDING, Edward A., FACHE President and Chief Executive Officer, Bay Area Medical Center, Marinette, WI, p. A685
HARDING, John R., Chief Executive Officer, Florida Hospital Tampa, Tampa, FL, p. A140
HARDING, Thomas, M.D. Medical Director, Milwaukee County Behavioral Health Division, Milwaukee, WI, p. A687
HARDISON, Gerald, Director Finance, Vidant Pungo Hospital, Belhaven, NC, p. A448
HARDMAN, Danny, Senior Vice President and Chief Nursing Officer, McAlester Regional Health Center, McAlester, OK, p. A499
HARDMAN, Wanda, Director Human Resources, Habersham Medical Center, Demorest, GA, p. A151
HARDOBY, Greg, Director Personnel, Runnells Specialized Hospital of Union County, Berkeley Heights, NJ, p. A401
HARDWICK, Garry, R.N. Chief Operating Officer, Newport Bay Hospital, Newport Beach, CA, p. A77
HARDY, Bob, Chief Operating Officer, Opelousas General Health System, Opelousas, LA, p. A276
HARDY, Eric S., Chief Financial Officer, Mesa View Regional Hospital, Mesquite, NV, p. A394
HARDY, Gregory, M.D. President Medical Staff, Stephens Memorial Hospital, Norway, ME, p. A284
HARDY, Janice, Chief Human Resources Management, Veterans Affairs Medical Center, Tuscaloosa, AL, p. A26
HARDY, John, Vice President Human Resources, Doctors Medical Center–San Pablo Campus, San Pablo, CA, p. A89
HARDY, Kevin, Chief Financial Officer, HEALTHSOUTH Treasure Coast Rehabilitation Hospital, Vero Beach, FL, p. A142
HARDY, Tom, D.O. Vice President Medical Affairs, Grandview Medical Center, Dayton, OH, p. A478
HARFF, Christine K., Chief Executive Officer, Sanford Medical Center Thief River Falls, Thief River Falls, MN, p. A340
HARGETT, Stephen A., Senior Vice President and Chief Financial Officer, Marina Del Rey Hospital, Marina Del Rey, CA, p. A74
HARGIS, Bryan J., FACHE Chief Executive Officer, St. Luke's Sugar Land Hospital, Sugar Land, TX, p. A629
HARGIS, Chris
  Chief Financial Officer, Providence Mount Carmel Hospital, Colville, WA, p. A660
  Chief Financial Officer, Providence St. Joseph's Hospital, Chewelah, WA, p. A660
HARGRAVE–THOMAS, Anne, Chief Executive Officer, Oakleaf Surgical Hospital, Eau Claire, WI, p. A681
HARGREAVES, Diane
  Vice President Human Resources, Provena Mercy Medical Center, Aurora, IL, p. A172
  Vice President Human Resources, Provena Saint Joseph Hospital, Elgin, IL, p. A181
HARGRODER, Ty, M.D. Chief of Staff, Acadia–St. Landry Hospital, Church Point, LA, p. A264
HARGROVE, Tressa B., Director Human Resources, Jackson Purchase Medical Center, Mayfield, KY, p. A256
HARING, Don, Vice President Finance and Treasurer, SwedishAmerican Hospital, Rockford, IL, p. A193
HARKEY, Shirley S., R.N. Vice President, Patient Services, Wayne Memorial Hospital, Goldsboro, NC, p. A453
HARKINS, Shelly, M.D. Chief Medical Officer, St. Elizabeth's Hospital, Belleville, IL, p. A173
HARKNESS, Charles, D.O. Vice President Medical Affairs, Southeast Alabama Medical Center, Dothan, AL, p. A19
HARLAN, Kevin W., President, Joint Township District Memorial Hospital, Saint Marys, OH, p. A488
HARLAN, Thomas M., Chief Executive Officer, Harbor Hospital of Southeast Texas, Beaumont, TX, p. A583
HARLAN, Thomas P., Administrator, Noland Hospital Birmingham, Birmingham, AL, p. A16
HARLE, Connie, Chief Nursing Officer, Range Regional Health Services, Hibbing, MN, p. A333
HARLESS, Andrea, Director Information Services, Wythe County Community Hospital, Wytheville, VA, p. A658
HARLESS, Jane, Director Information Services, Saint Francis Hospital, Charleston, WV, p. A671
HARLIN, Timothy, Chief Operating Officer, Hennepin County Medical Center, Minneapolis, MN, p. A335
HARLOVIC, Michael, R.N. Senior Vice President and Chief Operating Officer, Allegheny Valley Hospital, Natrona Heights, PA, p. A530
HARLOW, Donald, Director of Information Services, MountainView Regional Medical Center, Las Cruces, NM, p. A416
HARLOW, Lori, Chief Operating Officer, Skagit Valley Hospital, Mount Vernon, WA, p. A663
HARLOWE, Michael, President and Chief Executive Officer, Indiana University Health Tipton Hospital, Tipton, IN, p. A212
HARMAN, David L., Chief Executive Officer, Wallowa Memorial Hospital, Enterprise, OR, p. A510
HARMAN, Kenneth, Chief Executive Officer, Pioneers Medical Center, Meeker, CO, p. A104
HARMAN, Kimberly, Regional Manager Human Resources, Western State Hospital, Staunton, VA, p. A656
HARMER, Jon–Paul, M.D. Chief Medical Staff, Weatherford Regional Medical Center, Weatherford, TX, p. A634
HARMON, Amy, Chief Financial Officer, Kingfisher Regional Hospital, Kingfisher, OK, p. A498
HARMON, Cheryl A., Chief Financial Officer, Porter–Valparaiso Hospital Campus, Valparaiso, IN, p. A212
HARMON, David, D.O. Vice President Medical Services, RiverValley Behavioral Health Hospital, Owensboro, KY, p. A257
HARMON, Martin, Director Public Relations, Roosevelt Warm Springs Institute for Rehabilitation, Warm Springs, GA, p. A161
HARMS, Arlene, Chief Executive Officer, Rio Grande Hospital, Del Norte, CO, p. A99
HARMS, C. David, Chief Financial Officer, Kirby Medical Center, Monticello, IL, p. A188
HARMS, George, Chief Financial Officer, Good Samaritan Hospital, Kearney, NE, p. A385
HARMSEN, Constance A., FACHE Chief Executive Officer, Surgical Specialty Hospital of Arizona, Phoenix, AZ, p. A37
HARNED, Barbara, R.N. Chief Nursing Officer, Monroe County Hospital, Monroeville, AL, p. A23
HARNESS, Lorraine L., Administrator, Pike County Memorial Hospital, Louisiana, MO, p. A364
HARNESS, Phil, Chief Executive Officer, Doctor's Hospital, Leawood, KS, p. A237
HARNEY, Geraldine, Chief Financial Officer, U. S. Public Health Service Phoenix Indian Medical Center, Phoenix, AZ, p. A37
HARNEY, John, Chief Operating Officer, University of Colorado Hospital, Aurora, CO, p. A97
HARNING, Richard, Vice President Finance and Chief Financial Officer, Allegan General Hospital, Allegan, MI, p. A307
HARPER, Carrin, M.D. Chief Executive Officer, Haven Behavioral War Heroes Hospital, Pueblo, CO, p. A105
HARPER, Cindy, Director Information Systems, Westfield Memorial Hospital, Westfield, NY, p. A446
HARPER, Corwin N., Senior Vice President and Area Manager, Manteca Medical Center, Manteca, CA, p. A74
HARPER, David, Director, Site Information Systems, Advocate Eureka Hospital, Eureka, IL, p. A181
HARPER, Eric, Chief Information Officer, Southeastern Regional Medical Center, Lumberton, NC, p. A457
HARPER, Heather L., Chief Operating Officer, Southern Tennessee Medical Center, Winchester, TN, p. A576
HARPER, James F., Vice President and Chief Human Resources Officer, Georgetown Memorial Hospital, Georgetown, SC, p. A550
HARPER, Paul
  Interim Administrator, Kula Hospital, Kula, HI, p. A165
  Interim Administrator, Lanai Community Hospital, Lanai City, HI, p. A165
HARPER, R. Andrew, M.D. Medical Director, University of Texas Harris County Psychiatric Center, Houston, TX, p. A607
HARPER, Robert E., Chief Financial Officer, King's Daughters Hospital, Yazoo City, MS, p. A354
HARPER, Wally G., Vice President Human Resources, Gaylord Hospital, Wallingford, CT, p. A112
HARPER, William F., M.D. Chief of Staff, Central Texas Veterans Healthcare System, Temple, TX, p. A630
HARR, Donald, Controller, Ray County Memorial Hospital, Richmond, MO, p. A367
HARRAL, Carla, Chief Financial Officer, Surgical Hospital of Jonesboro, Jonesboro, AR, p. A47
HARREL, Mark, Chief Executive Officer, Phelps Memorial Health Center, Holdrege, NE, p. A384
HARRELL, Mike, Chief Financial Officer, Walton Rehabilitation Hospital, Augusta, GA, p. A147
HARRELL, Rex, Information Technologist, Salina Surgical Hospital, Salina, KS, p. A243
HARRELL, Steven W., FACHE Interim Chief Executive Officer, Bert Fish Medical Center, New Smyrna Beach, FL, p. A133
HARRELL, Thomas, Commander, U. S. Air Force Regional Hospital, Elmendorf AFB, AK, p. A28

A830 Index of Health Care Professionals

Index of Health Care Professionals

Index of Health Care Professionals / Hartmann

HARRIER, Margie, Medical Center Chief Operations Officer, Anaheim Medical Center, Anaheim, CA, p. A53
HARRIGAN, Robert, Vice President and Chief Operating Officer, Summa Health System, Akron, OH, p. A469
HARRILSON, Annette, Chief Clinical Officer, Kindred Hospital–Atlanta, Atlanta, GA, p. A145
HARRIMAN, Robert, M.D. Administrator, Gulf Breeze Hospital, Gulf Breeze, FL, p. A124
HARRINGTON, Dan, Chief Operating Officer and Director Human Resources, Williamsburg Regional Hospital, Kingstree, SC, p. A551
HARRINGTON, Hal, Director Human Resources, Natchez Community Hospital, Natchez, MS, p. A350
HARRINGTON, Jason, President and Chief Executive Officer, Lakes Regional Healthcare, Spirit Lake, IA, p. A227
HARRINGTON, Joseph P., President and Chief Executive Officer, Lodi Memorial Hospital, Lodi, CA, p. A67
HARRINGTON, Kathleen, Vice President Human Resources, Milton Hospital, Milton, MA, p. A302
HARRINGTON, Lane, R.N. Vice President Patient Care Services, Scotland Health Care System, Laurinburg, NC, p. A456
HARRINGTON, Michael L., Chief Operating Officer, Sarasota Memorial Hospital, Sarasota, FL, p. A139
HARRINGTON, Ron, Vice President and Chief Financial Officer, Gibson General Hospital, Princeton, IN, p. A210
HARRINGTON Jr.,, Russell D., FACHE President and Chief Executive Officer, Baptist Health, Little Rock, AR, p. B17
HARRIS, Andrew E., President and Chief Executive Officer, Blue Mountain Health System, Lehighton, PA, p. B21
HARRIS, Andrew E.
Chief Executive Officer, Gnaden Huetten Memorial Hospital, Lehighton, PA, p. A527
Chief Executive Officer, Palmerton Hospital, Palmerton, PA, p. A531
HARRIS, Angela, Chief Executive Officer, Kindred Hospital–Fort Worth, Fort Worth, TX, p. A599
HARRIS, II, Barry–Lewis, M.D. Chief of Staff, Veterans Affairs Gulf Coast Veterans Health Care System, Biloxi, MS, p. A344
HARRIS, Betty J., Director Human Resources, Brotman Medical Center, Culver City, CA, p. A59
HARRIS, Burt, Chief Financial Officer, Canyon Ridge Hospital, Chino, CA, p. A57
HARRIS, C. Martin, M.D
Chief Information Officer, Cleveland Clinic Children's Hospital for Rehabilitation, Cleveland, OH, p. A474
Chief Information Officer, Cleveland Clinic Foundation, Cleveland, OH, p. A474
Chief Information Officer, Fairview Hospital, Cleveland, OH, p. A475
Chief Information Officer, Lakewood Hospital, Lakewood, OH, p. A482
Chief Information Officer, Lutheran Hospital, Cleveland, OH, p. A475
HARRIS, David, M.D. President Medical Affairs, Biloxi Regional Medical Center, Biloxi, MS, p. A343
HARRIS, Deatrice, Supervisor Human Resources and Employment, Phoebe Sumter Medical Center, Americus, GA, p. A144
HARRIS, Debra, Director Medical Records, I–70 Community Hospital, Sweet Springs, MO, p. A371
HARRIS, Denise H., R.N. Chief Nursing Officer, Baptist Health South Florida, West Kendall Baptist Hospital, Miami, FL, p. A131
HARRIS, Donna
Director Human Resources, Hawthorn Children Psychiatric Hospital, Saint Louis, MO, p. A368
Chief Executive Officer, HEALTHSOUTH Rehabilitation Hospital of Jonesboro, Jonesboro, AR, p. A46
Director Human Resources, Metropolitan St. Louis Psychiatric Center, Saint Louis, MO, p. A369
Director Human Resources, St. Louis Psychiatric Rehabilitation Center, Saint Louis, MO, p. A370
HARRIS, Dory, Manager Human Resource, Teton Valley Hospital and Surgicenter, Driggs, ID, p. A168
HARRIS, Duane, Director Human Resources, Shadow Mountain Behavioral Health System, Tulsa, OK, p. A506
HARRIS, Howard, Vice President Human Resources, Regional Medical Center, Orangeburg, SC, p. A553
HARRIS, James D., M.D. Chief of Staff, Sanford Worthington Medical Center, Worthington, MN, p. A342
HARRIS, Janet Y., MSN, Chief Executive Officer and Chief Nursing Officer, University Hospitals and Health System, University of Mississippi Medical Center, Jackson, MS, p. A348
HARRIS, Janice, Director Human Resources, East El Paso Physicians Medical Center, El Paso, TX, p. A596
HARRIS, Jen, Director Health Information Management, Chase County Community Hospital, Imperial, NE, p. A384
HARRIS, Joanne, Director Human Resources, Mount Desert Island Hospital, Bar Harbor, ME, p. A281
HARRIS, John, Chief Executive Officer, Providence Memorial Hospital, El Paso, TX, p. A596
HARRIS, Julie, Chief Financial Officer, Winnie Community Hospital, Winnie, TX, p. A635
HARRIS, Kathy, Vice President, Mercy Hospital and Trauma Center, Janesville, WI, p. A683
HARRIS, Keri, M.D. Chief of Staff, Wyandot Memorial Hospital, Upper Sandusky, OH, p. A490
HARRIS, Larry, Director Administrative Services, Porterville Developmental Center, Porterville, CA, p. A81
HARRIS, Lee, Assistant Administrator Support Services, Memorial Hospital and Manor, Bainbridge, GA, p. A147
HARRIS, Lisa E., M.D. Chief Executive Officer and Medical Director, Wishard Health Services, Indianapolis, IN, p. A205
HARRIS, Marianna, Administrator, Webster County Community Hospital, Red Cloud, NE, p. A389
HARRIS, Mark D., Deputy Commander Clinical Services, DeWitt Army Community Hospital, Fort Belvoir, VA, p. A648
HARRIS, Merilyn, Administrator, Kau Hospital, Pahala, HI, p. A165
HARRIS, Mike
Chief Operating Officer, Continuous Care Centers of Tulsa, Tulsa, OK, p. A505
Interim Administrator, Genoa Community Hospital, Genoa, NE, p. A384
HARRIS, Miriam, Director Finance, Oklahoma Forensic Center, Vinita, OK, p. A507
HARRIS, Paula, Chief Executive Officer, Advanced Healthcare Medical Center, Ellington, MO, p. A359
HARRIS, R. Brian, M.D. Chief of Staff, Reeves Memorial Medical Center, Bernice, LA, p. A263
HARRIS, Robert M., M.D. President Medical and Dental Staff, Bergen Regional Medical Center, Paramus, NJ, p. A408
HARRIS, Sandra L., R.N. Senior Vice President and Chief Operating Officer, Texas Health Arlington Memorial Hospital, Arlington, TX, p. A579
HARRIS, Shelley, MSN Chief Nursing Officer, St. Elizabeth's Hospital, Belleville, IL, p. A173
HARRIS, Shelly, Chief Executive Officer, U. S. Public Health Service Indian Hospital, Rosebud, SD, p. A559
HARRIS, Stuart, M.D. Chief of Staff, Trigg County Hospital, Cadiz, KY, p. A248
HARRIS, Vena, Director Human Resources, Minneola District Hospital, Minneola, KS, p. A239
HARRIS, Wendell R., Ph.D. Chief Executive Officer, Bates County Memorial Hospital, Butler, MO, p. A356
HARRIS, William, Chief Information Resources Management, Veterans Affairs Central California Health Care System, Fresno, CA, p. A62
HARRISON, Alicia, Data Management Officer, Excelsior Springs Hospital, Excelsior Springs, MO, p. A359
HARRISON, Allen, Chief Executive Officer, St. David's North Austin Medical Center, Austin, TX, p. A581
HARRISON, Charles, Chief Executive Officer, San Bernardino Mountains Community Hospital District, Lake Arrowhead, CA, p. A66
HARRISON, Cindy, Vice President Human Resources, Chelsea Community Hospital, Chelsea, MI, p. A309
HARRISON, Dean M., President and Chief Executive Officer, Northwestern Memorial Healthcare, Chicago, IL, p. B96
HARRISON, Dean M., President and Chief Executive Officer, Northwestern Memorial Hospital, Chicago, IL, p. A177
HARRISON, Debra, MS Chief Nursing Officer, Mayo Clinic Jacksonville, Jacksonville, FL, p. A126
HARRISON, Douglas
Vice President Human Resources, Bon Secours St. Francis Hospital, Charleston, SC, p. A547
Vice President Human Resources, Roper Hospital, Charleston, SC, p. A547
HARRISON, Douglass, Vice President Operations, UPMC St. Margaret, Pittsburgh, PA, p. A536
HARRISON, Dyan, Manager Health Information, Ochiltree General Hospital, Perryton, TX, p. A620
HARRISON, Jo L., Vice President of Patient Care Services, Southwest Medical Center, Liberal, KS, p. A238
HARRISON, Scott, Director Information Systems, Twin Cities Community Hospital, Templeton, CA, p. A92
HARRON, Rick, Chief Financial Officer, Dominican Hospital, Santa Cruz, CA, p. A90
HARRY, Bruce, M.D. Clinical Director, Fulton State Hospital, Fulton, MO, p. A360
HARSHAWAT, Roopam, Chief Executive Officer, Harsha Behavioral Center, Terre Haute, IN, p. A212
HARSHBARGER, Catherine S., R.N. Chief Nursing Officer, Banner Lassen Medical Center, Susanville, CA, p. A92
HARSY, Brice, Chief Financial Officer, Marshall Browning Hospital, Du Quoin, IL, p. A180
HART, Cara, Director Human Resources, Morton Hospital and Medical Center, Taunton, MA, p. A305
HART, Charles E., MS, President and Chief Executive Officer, Regional Health, Rapid City, SD, p. B109
HART, Chet, Vice President Operations, Sentara CarePlex Hospital, Hampton, VA, p. A649
HART, Deborah, Chief Financial Officer, North Suburban Medical Center, Thornton, CO, p. A106
HART, Denise, Director Human Resources, Sullivan County Community Hospital, Sullivan, IN, p. A212
HART, Donna, Chief Information Officer, Provident Hospital of Cook County, Chicago, IL, p. A177
HART, Gary, M.D. Chief Medical Officer, Claxton–Hepburn Medical Center, Ogdensburg, NY, p. A439
HART, James, Chief Financial Officer, Hebrew Rehabilitation Center, Boston, MA, p. A297
HART, Joel A., FACHE President, Integris Baptist Regional Health Center, Miami, OK, p. A499
HART, John S., Administrator, East Texas Medical Center Clarksville, Clarksville, TX, p. A587
HART, Joline, Vice President Human Resources, Franklin Memorial Hospital, Farmington, ME, p. A283
HART, Linda, Vice President Finance, Grady Memorial Hospital, Chickasha, OK, p. A494
HART, Lisa, Chief Financial Officer, Elkview General Hospital, Hobart, OK, p. A497
HART, Michael, M.D. Medical Director, Stamford Memorial Hospital, Stamford, TX, p. A628
HART, Monique, Chief Financial Officer, Baptist Memorial Hospital–Tipton, Covington, TN, p. A564
HART, Pat, Director Human Resources, Three Rivers Medical Center, Louisa, KY, p. A254
HART, Richard H., M.D. President and Chief Executive Officer, Loma Linda University Adventist Health Sciences Center, Loma Linda, CA, p. B82
HART, Rick, Chief Financial Officer, Memorial Medical Center, Port Lavaca, TX, p. A622
HART, Scott, Controller, HEALTHSOUTH Lakeview Rehabilitation Hospital, Elizabethtown, KY, p. A249
HART, Steve, Controller, Kindred Hospital North Florida, Green Cove Springs, FL, p. A124
HART–FLYNN, Wilma, Vice President Patient Care Services/CNO, Illinois Valley Community Hospital, Peru, IL, p. A191
HARTE, Brian J., M.D. President, South Pointe Hospital, Warrensville Heights, OH, p. A490
HARTER, Dan, Manager Information Systems, Prosser Memorial Hospital, Prosser, WA, p. A664
HARTERT, Jim, M.D. Senior Vice President and Medical Director, Range Regional Health Services, Hibbing, MN, p. A333
HARTFORD, David, Administrator, Anoka–Metropolitan Regional Treatment Center, Anoka, MN, p. A327
HARTGRAVES, Steve L., Administrator and Chief Executive Officer, Graham Regional Medical Center, Graham, TX, p. A601
HARTLEY, Diane L., R.N. Director of Patient Care Services, Oakwood Annapolis Hospital, Wayne, MI, p. A325
HARTLEY, Joe
Director Information Systems, Hunt Memorial Hospital District, Greenville, TX, p. A602
Director Information Systems, Hunt Regional Community Hospital, Commerce, TX, p. A588
HARTLEY, Melinda D., R.N. Vice President Patient Care Services, Perry Hospital, Perry, GA, p. A157
HARTLEY, Michael W., Director Human Resources, Laredo Medical Center, Laredo, TX, p. A612
HARTLEY, Norma, Director Human Resources, Power County Hospital District, American Falls, ID, p. A166
HARTLEY, Wannah, Controller, Winkler County Memorial Hospital, Kermit, TX, p. A610
HARTLING, Ross, M.D. President Medical Staff, Cascade Valley Hospital and Clinics, Arlington, WA, p. A659
HARTMAN, Daphne, Chief Financial Officer, North Big Horn Hospital District, Lovell, WY, p. A697
HARTMAN, David, M.D. Chief of Staff, Franklin Hospital District, Benton, IL, p. A173
HARTMAN, Dennis, Chief Financial Officer, Excelsior Springs Hospital, Excelsior Springs, MO, p. A359
HARTMAN, Gregory
President and Chief Executive Officer, Seton Medical Center Austin, Austin, TX, p. A581
President and Chief Executive Officer, University Medical Center at Brackenridge, Austin, TX, p. A582
HARTMAN, Robert, M.D. Vice President Medical Affairs, Valley Hospital and Medical Center, Spokane Valley, WA, p. A667
HARTMAN, Susan, Chief Executive Officer, HEALTHSOUTH Nittany Valley Rehabilitation Hospital, Pleasant Gap, PA, p. A536
HARTMANN, Doreen, Vice President and Chief Financial Officer, Mercy Medical Center Merced, Merced, CA, p. A74
HARTMANN, Margot, Ph.D. President and Chief Executive Officer, Nantucket Cottage Hospital, Nantucket, MA, p. A302

Index of Health Care Professionals

Index of Health Care Professionals / Hartmann

HARTMANN, Peter M., M.D. Vice President Medical Affairs, York Hospital, York, PA, p. A543
HARTSELL, Scott, Chief Operating Officer, Brooksville Regional Hospital, Brooksville, FL, p. A119
HARTWICK, Bryan, Vice President Human Resources, Christian Hospital, Saint Louis, MO, p. A368
HARTWIG, Michael, M.D. Chief of Staff, Perry Memorial Hospital, Perry, OK, p. A503
HARTZELL, Dee, Manager Human Resources, St. Luke's Jerome Family Medical Center, Jerome, ID, p. A168
HARVEL, Norilina, Chief Financial Officer, Bonner General Hospital, Sandpoint, ID, p. A170
HARVEY, Anne, MSN Chief Nursing Officer, El Paso Specialty Hospital, El Paso, TX, p. A596
HARVEY, John, M.D
President and Chief Executive Officer, Oklahoma Heart Hospital, Oklahoma City, OK, p. A501
President and Chief Executive Officer, Oklahoma Heart Hospital, Oklahoma City, OK, p. A501
President and Chief Executive Officer, Oklahoma Heart Hospital South Campus, Oklahoma City, OK, p. A501
HARVEY, Kevin, Chief Financial Officer, McKenzie Regional Hospital, McKenzie, TN, p. A570
HARVEY, Linda, Chief Financial Officer, West Feliciana Parish Hospital, Saint Francisville, LA, p. A276
HARVEY, Michael, Chief Executive Officer, Community Memorial Hospital, Syracuse, NE, p. A390
HARVEY, Sally, R.N. Regional Administrator, Memorial Community Hospital and Health System, Blair, NE, p. A382
HARVEY, Stansel, FACHE Chief Executive Officer, Delta Regional Medical Center, Greenville, MS, p. A346
HARVILL, Brian
Vice President Financial Services, Vidant Bertie Hospital, Windsor, NC, p. A463
Vice President Financial Services, Vidant Chowan Hospital, Edenton, NC, p. A452
HARYASZ, Sandy, R.N. Chief Executive Officer, Page Hospital, Page, AZ, p. A34
HASAN, Farhana, M.D. Chief of Staff, Veterans Affairs Medical Center, Marion, IL, p. A187
HASBROUCK, Merritt J., President, Jackson Park Hospital and Medical Center, Chicago, IL, p. A176
HASHMI, Mubashir, Chief Information Officer, Pacifica Hospital of the Valley,, CA, p. A71
HASHMI, Stephenie, Chief Clinical Officer, Kindred Hospital Kansas City, Kansas City, MO, p. A362
HASKELL, Jeffrey, M.D. Chief Medical Staff, Lost Rivers District Hospital, Arco, ID, p. A166
HASKINS, Don, Administrative Director Human Resources, Southwest Mississippi Regional Medical Center, McComb, MS, p. A349
HASKINS, Randy
Director Information Systems, Mercy Medical Center–New Hampton, New Hampton, IA, p. A224
Director Information Systems, Mercy Medical Center–North Iowa, Mason City, IA, p. A223
HASKINS, Sandy, Interim Chief Executive Officer, Adventist Medical Center–Reedley, Reedley, CA, p. A82
HASLING, Debra, Director Medical Records, Lakeview Regional Medical Center, Covington, LA, p. A265
HASNI, Kamran, M.D. Chief of Medical Staff, Knox County Hospital, Barbourville, KY, p. A247
HASSAN, Tariq, M.D. Associate Director of Patient Care, Captain James A. Lovell Federal Health Care Center, North Chicago, IL, p. A189
HASSELBARTH, William C., Chief Financial Officer, Albany Medical Center, Albany, NY, p. A420
HASSELBRACK, Jeni, Director Human Resources, Gordon Hospital, Calhoun, GA, p. A148
HASSEMER, Robert J., Division Director Human Resources, Sacred Heart Hospital, Eau Claire, WI, p. A681
HASSLER, Robert, M.D. Director Medical Affairs, Brunswick Novant Medical Center, Bolivia, NC, p. A449
HASSON, Marie, M.D. Medical Director, Carrier Clinic, Belle Mead, NJ, p. A401
HASTIN, Kathy, Administrative Assistant Human Resources, River Valley Medical Center, Dardanelle, AR, p. A43
HASTINGS, David, Director Information Technology, Baton Rouge General Medical Center, Baton Rouge, LA, p. A262
HASTINGS, Kirk, Chief Information Technology, VA Butler Healthcare, Butler, PA, p. A519
HASTINGS, Sarah M., Vice President Human Resources, Ridgeview Medical Center, Waconia, MN, p. A341
HASTINGS–SMITH, Julie, Chief Financial Officer, Maryvale Hospital Medical Center, Phoenix, AZ, p. A36
HATALA, Alexander J., President and Chief Executive Officer, Our Lady of Lourdes Medical Center, Camden, NJ, p. A402
HATCH, Mary, Chief Financial Officer, Dixie Regional Medical Center, Saint George, UT, p. A640
HATCHER, Julie, Vice President Human Resources, O'Connor Hospital, San Jose, CA, p. A88
HATCHER, Melanie, Region Director Human Resources, Broward Health Imperial Point, Fort Lauderdale, FL, p. A123
HATCHER, Robert, Chief Financial Officer, Tulane Medical Center, New Orleans, LA, p. A275
HATFIELD, Chad, Chief Executive Officer, Plateau Medical Center, Oak Hill, WV, p. A674
HATFIELD, Jonathan, Supervisor Information Technology, Klickitat Valley Health, Goldendale, WA, p. A661
HATFIELD, Timothy A., Community Chief Executive Officer, Williamson ARH Hospital, South Williamson, KY, p. A259
HATHAWAY, Woody, Chief Financial Officer, Mt. San Rafael Hospital, Trinidad, CO, p. A106
HATLESTAD, Jill, Vice President Human Resources and Organizational Support, Glencoe Regional Health Services, Glencoe, MN, p. A332
HATTER, Rochelle, Chief Human Resources Officer, Roundup Memorial Healthcare, Roundup, MT, p. A378
HATTON, Julia
Chief Financial Officer, Nexus Specialty Hospital, Shenandoah, TX, p. A627
Chief Financial Officer, Nexus Specialty Hospital The Woodlands, Spring, TX, p. A628
HATTON, Tad, Chief Operating Officer, St. David's Round Rock Medical Center, Round Rock, TX, p. A623
HAUG, William F., FACHE Administrator, Kaiser Permanente Medical Center, Honolulu, HI, p. A163
HAUGE, Meri, R.N. Associate Director of Patient Care Services and Nurse Executive, St. Cloud Veterans Affairs Health Care System, Saint Cloud, MN, p. A338
HAUGEN, O. G., Director Resources, Naval Medical Center, San Diego, CA, p. A85
HAUGH, William, Chief Executive Officer, Logan Memorial Hospital, Russellville, KY, p. A258
HAUGO, Glenn, Chief Executive Officer, RC Hospital and Clinics, Olivia, MN, p. A336
HAUN, Richard, Chief Financial Officer, Wuesthoff Medical Center – Rockledge, Rockledge, FL, p. A137
HAUPERT, John M., FACHE Chief Executive Officer, Grady Memorial Hospital, Atlanta, GA, p. A145
HAUSAUER, Patricia K., Director Finance, Baptist Medical Center Nassau, Fernandina Beach, FL, p. A123
HAUSE, Eileen, Chief Executive Officer, Kensington Hospital, Philadelphia, PA, p. A533
HAUSER, Mark J., M.D. Chief Medical Officer, Baptist Health South Florida, Baptist Hospital of Miami, Miami, FL, p. A130
HAUSER, Michael, M.D. Chief Medical Officer, The HSC Pediatric Center, Washington, DC, p. A117
HAUSHALTER, Brandon, Chief Executive Officer, Bluffton Regional Medical Center, Bluffton, IN, p. A198
HAUSHALTER, Richard L., Chief Operating Officer, Rockingham Memorial Hospital, Harrisonburg, VA, p. A649
HAUSMANN, Jena, Executive Vice President and Chief Operating Officer, Children's Hospital Colorado, Aurora, CO, p. A97
HAUSMANN, Sherry, President, Via Christi Hospitals Wichita, Wichita, KS, p. A245
HAUSWIRTH, Michael
Chief Operating Officer, Aspirus Keweenaw Hospital, Laurium, MI, p. A317
Chief Operating Officer, Aspirus Ontonagon Hospital, Ontonagon, MI, p. A320
HAUSWIRTH, Renay, Chief Financial Officer, Palo Alto County Health System, Emmetsburg, IA, p. A219
HAVEL, Carol, R.N. Vice President Patient Care Services, Morris Hospital & Healthcare Centers, Morris, IL, p. A188
HAVEN, Adrian C., Site Manager, Gallup Indian Medical Center, Gallup, NM, p. A416
HAVERKAMP, Kathleen, M.D. Chief Medical Officer, Ellsworth Municipal Hospital, Iowa Falls, IA, p. A222
HAVRILLA, David A., Chief Financial Officer, Medstar Montgomery Medical Center, Olney, MD, p. A293
HAWK, James, M.D. Chief of Staff, Washington County Memorial Hospital, Potosi, MO, p. A367
HAWKINS, Bill, Director, Hiram W. Davis Medical Center, Petersburg, VA, p. A653
HAWKINS, Brian A., Director Medical Center, Veterans Affairs Medical Center, Washington, DC, p. A117
HAWKINS, Bryan, Controller, FirstHealth Montgomery Memorial Hospital, Troy, NC, p. A462
HAWKINS, Ellis, Senior Vice President and Chief Operating Officer, Phelps County Regional Medical Center, Rolla, MO, p. A367
HAWKINS, Hillary, M.D. Medical Director, Sheltering Arms Rehabilitation Hospital, Mechanicsville, VA, p. A651
HAWKINS, Janine, R.N. Chief Nursing Officer, Dameron Hospital, Stockton, CA, p. A91
HAWKINS, Jason F., President and Chief Executive Officer, Fulton County Medical Center, Mc Connellsburg, PA, p. A528
HAWKINS, Kidada
Interim President and Chief Operating Officer, St. Vincent's Blount, Oneonta, AL, p. A24
VP/COO Rural Hospital Operations, St. Vincent's Blount, Oneonta, AL, p. A24
Interim President and Chief Operating Officer, St. Vincent's St. Clair, Pell City, AL, p. A25
Vice President and Chief Operating Officer, St. Vincent's St. Clair, Pell City, AL, p. A25
HAWKINS, Roy, Acting Associate Director, Veterans Affairs Salt Lake City Health Care System, Salt Lake City, UT, p. A641
HAWKINS, Thomas J., Administrator, Central Prison Hospital, Raleigh, NC, p. A458
HAWKINS, Tim F., Chief Executive Officer, The Villages Health System, The Villages, FL, p. A142
HAWKINSON, Curtis R., Chief Executive Officer, Community Memorial Healthcare, Marysville, KS, p. A238
HAWLEY, Claudia, Director Human Resources, Mason General Hospital, Shelton, WA, p. A666
HAWLEY, Jason, Manager Information Services, Yuma District Hospital, Yuma, CO, p. A107
HAWLEY, William, Chief Executive Officer, Bluefield Regional Medical Center, Bluefield, WV, p. A670
HAWMAN, DeeDee, Director Human Resources, Lee's Summit Medical Center, Lee's Summit, MO, p. A364
HAWS, Kevin W., USN, Commanding Officer, U. S. Naval Hospital, Agana, GU, p. A699
HAWTHORNE, Douglas D., FACHE Chief Executive Officer, Texas Health Resources, Arlington, TX, p. B129
HAWTHORNE III, Henry, President and Chief Executive Officer, Columbus Regional Healthcare System, Whiteville, NC, p. A462
HAWTHORNE, Kimberly, Administrator, Mayo Clinic Health System – Franciscan Healthcare in Sparta, Sparta, WI, p. A691
HAXTOM, Moni, Interim Chief Financial Officer, Mercy Medical Center–North Iowa, Mason City, IA, p. A223
HAY, Jody, Director Human Resources, HEALTHSOUTH Nittany Valley Rehabilitation Hospital, Pleasant Gap, PA, p. A536
HAY, Morgan, Chief Financial Officer, Gerald Champion Regional Medical Center, Alamogordo, NM, p. A414
HAYDEN, Crystal, R.N. Chief Nursing Officer, Onslow Memorial Hospital, Jacksonville, NC, p. A455
HAYDEN, John
Senior Vice President and Chief Human Resources Officer, Bronson LakeView Hospital, Paw Paw, MI, p. A320
Vice President and Chief Human Resources Officer, Bronson Methodist Hospital, Kalamazoo, MI, p. A316
HAYDEN, Karen, Director Health Information Services, Performance Improvement and Risk Management, Valle Vista Hospital, Greenwood, IN, p. A203
HAYDEN, Patrick, M.D. Chief of Staff, Logan Memorial Hospital, Russellville, KY, p. A258
HAYDEN, Sheryl, Chief Financial Officer, Sierra Surgery Hospital, Carson City, NV, p. A391
HAYES, Brian T., Commander, David Grant Medical Center, Travis AFB, CA, p. A93
HAYES, Chris, Interim Corporate Director of Finance, Saint Mary's Hospital, Waterbury, CT, p. A112
HAYES, Deborah Marie, R.N. Chief Hospital Officer and Chief Nursing Officer, Christ Hospital, Cincinnati, OH, p. A473
HAYES, Donna, Controller, Decatur County General Hospital, Parsons, TN, p. A574
HAYES, Elaine, Controller, Sts. Mary & Elizabeth Hospital, Louisville, KY, p. A255
HAYES, Elizabeth, R.N. Director of Patient Services, Blowing Rock Hospital, Blowing Rock, NC, p. A449
HAYES, George E., FACHE President and Chief Executive Officer, Medical Center of the Rockies, Loveland, CO, p. A104
HAYES, James L., Director Human Resources, Western State Hospital, Hopkinsville, KY, p. A252
HAYES, James M., Chief Executive Officer, Trinity Muscatine, Muscatine, IA, p. A224
HAYES, Jim A., Chief Fiscal Service, Veterans Affairs Tennessee Valley Healthcare System, Nashville, TN, p. A574
HAYES, Karen, Chief Financial Officer, Phoebe North, Albany, GA, p. A144
HAYES, Kathe, Executive Director, Western New York Children's Psychiatric Center, West Seneca, NY, p. A446
HAYES, Kelly, Chief Financial Officer, North Texas Medical Center, Gainesville, TX, p. A600
HAYES, Kevin, M.D. Chief of Staff, Pioneer Community Hospital of Aberdeen, Aberdeen, MS, p. A343
HAYES, Kim, Director Human Resources, Bibb Medical Center, Centreville, AL, p. A18
HAYES, Marianne, Director Human Resources, Kremmling Memorial Hospital, Kremmling, CO, p. A102
HAYES, Michael, Chief Information Resource Management, Veterans Affairs Health Care System, Fargo, ND, p. A466

A832 Index of Health Care Professionals

Index of Health Care Professionals
Index of Health Care Professionals / Heichert

HEICHERT, Susan
Chief Information Officer, Mercy Hospital, Coon Rapids, MN, p. A330
Chief Information Officer, Unity Hospital, Fridley, MN, p. A331
HEIDER, John R., Vice President Finance, Augusta Health, Fishersville, VA, p. A648
HEIDT, Robert, Director Information Systems, Pembina County Memorial Hospital and Wedgewood Manor, Cavalier, ND, p. A464
HEIKKINEN, Todd, Director Rehabilitation Services, Orthopaedic Hospital of Wisconsin – Glendale, Milwaukee, WI, p. A687
HEILSBERG, Jim, Chief Financial Officer and Chief Information Officer, Whitman Hospital and Medical Center, Colfax, WA, p. A660
HEIM, Tonya, R.N. Vice President Patient Services and Chief Nursing Officer, Memorial Hospital and Health Care Center, Jasper, IN, p. A205
HEIMAN, Thomas, Assistant Vice President Information Services, John T. Mather Memorial Hospital, Port Jefferson, NY, p. A440
HEINDEL, Michael, Chief Operating Officer, North Vista Hospital, North Las Vegas, NV, p. A394
HEINEMANN, Don, Administrator and Chief Executive Officer, Blount Memorial Hospital, Maryville, TN, p. A570
HEINISCH, Sheri, Compliance Officer, Lisbon Area Health Services, Lisbon, ND, p. A467
HEINRICH, Mark T., D.O. President Medical Staff, Oroville Hospital, Oroville, CA, p. A78
HEINRICH, Michael G., Executive Vice President and Chief Financial Officer, Mercy Iowa City, Iowa City, IA, p. A221
HEINRICH, Timothy, Senior Vice President and Chief Operating Officer, Memorial Medical Center of West Michigan, Ludington, MI, p. A318
HEINRICHS, Alice, CPA Chief Financial Officer, Van Diest Medical Center, Webster City, IA, p. A228
HEINS, Patrick, Vice President Patient Care Services, Vidant Edgecombe Hospital, Tarboro, NC, p. A461
HEINSOHN, Carmel, M.D. Medical Director, Bournewood Health Systems, Brookline, MA, p. A298
HEINTZELMAN, Gayle M., President and Chief Executive Officer, Mercy Hospital Clermont, Batavia, OH, p. A470
HEINZE, Kyle, Coordinator Information Technology, Riveredge Hospital, Forest Park, IL, p. A182
HEINZMAN, Jerry, Senior Vice President and Chief Financial Officer, Sampson Regional Medical Center, Clinton, NC, p. A451
HEISE, Lance, Director Human Resources, Cascade Medical Center, Leavenworth, WA, p. A662
HEISE, Rosemarie, Vice President Finance, Indiana University Health Starke Hospital, Knox, IN, p. A206
HEISE, Teresa, Coordinator Management Information Systems, Pender Community Hospital, Pender, NE, p. A389
HEISER, Eric, Chief Information Resource Management, Sioux Falls VA Health Care System, Sioux Falls, SD, p. A560
HEISSER, Randy, M.D. Medical Director, Kindred Hospital–Chattanooga, Chattanooga, TN, p. A563
HEITZENRATER, James F., FACHE Chief Executive Officer, Alleghany Memorial Hospital, Sparta, NC, p. A461
HEITZMAN, Cynthia, R.N. Chief Nursing Officer, Seven Rivers Regional Medical Center, Crystal River, FL, p. A121
HELBERG, Ted, Vice President, Human Resources, The Acadia Hospital, Bangor, ME, p. A281
HELD, Karen, Site Coordinator Information Technology, St. Nicholas Hospital, Sheboygan, WI, p. A690
HELDRETH, Karen, Director Data Processing, Mercy Hospital El Reno, El Reno, OK, p. A496
HELFER, Cassandra, Chief Financial Officer, Ralph H. Johnson Veterans Affairs Medical Center, Charleston, SC, p. A547
HELFER, David, President, Texas Institute for Surgery at Texas Health Presbyterian Dallas, Dallas, TX, p. A592
HELGESON, Heidi E., M.D. Chief Medical Officer, Rio Grande Hospital, Del Norte, CO, p. A99
HELGET, Peggy, R.N. Vice President Patient Services and Chief Nursing Officer, Jennie Edmundson Hospital, Council Bluffs, IA, p. A217
HELLA, Timothy, Chief Information Officer, Otsego Memorial Hospital, Gaylord, MI, p. A313
HELLE, Dan, Human Resources Officer, Iowa City Veterans Affairs Health Care System, Iowa City, IA, p. A221
HELLELAND, Brian, Executive Vice President and Chief Operating Officer, St. Jude Medical Center, Fullerton, CA, p. A62
HELLER, Corey
Corporate Vice President and Chief Human Resources Officer, Baptist Health South Florida, Baptist Hospital of Miami, Miami, FL, p. A130
Corporate Vice President and Chief Human Resources Officer, Baptist Health South Florida, Homestead Hospital, Homestead, FL, p. A125
HELLER, Lisa, Manager Human Resources, Mercy Medical Center–New Hampton, New Hampton, IA, p. A224
HELLER, Michael, Chief Financial Officer, Corry Memorial Hospital, Corry, PA, p. A521
HELLER, Tom, Vice President Human Resources, Camden–Clark Medical Center, Parkersburg, WV, p. A674
HELLYER, Nancy R., Interim Chief Executive Officer, CHRISTUS Coushatta Health Care Center, Coushatta, LA, p. A264
HELM, Carrie, Chief Executive Officer, Arkansas Surgical Hospital, North Little Rock, AR, p. A49
HELM, Pamela E., Executive Director, Devereux Texas Treatment Network, League City, TX, p. A612
HELMANDOLLAR, Billy, Director Information Services, Wallace Thomson Hospital, Union, SC, p. A554
HELMS, Candace, Director Information Services, Good Samaritan Medical Center, West Palm Beach, FL, p. A142
HELMS, Sheryl, Vice President Human Resources, Good Samaritan Regional Medical Center, Corvallis, OR, p. A510
HELPER, Mark A., Vice President, Chief Financial Officer, Munson Medical Center, Traverse City, MI, p. A324
HELSEL, David S., M.D. Chief Executive Officer, Spring Grove Hospital Center, Baltimore, MD, p. A289
HELTON, Deirdre, Director Human Resources, Lakeway Regional Hospital, Morristown, TN, p. A572
HELTON, Fay, Director Medical Records, Red River Hospital, Wichita Falls, TX, p. A635
HELTON, Michelle, Director Human Resources, Wallace Thomson Hospital, Union, SC, p. A554
HELTON, Stephanie, Chief Financial Officer, Weatherford Regional Hospital, Weatherford, OK, p. A507
HELVIE, Charlotte, M.D. Chief of Staff, Northern Inyo Hospital, Bishop, CA, p. A56
HELWIG, Kent, Chief Executive Officer, Southwest Memorial Hospital, Cortez, CO, p. A99
HEMBREE, Greg, Chief Financial Officer, South Georgia Medical Center, Valdosta, GA, p. A161
HEMETER, Donald, Administrator, Wayne General Hospital, Waynesboro, MS, p. A353
HEMINGWAY, Elizabeth, Director Health Information, Fairlawn Rehabilitation Hospital, Worcester, MA, p. A306
HEMKER, Robert
Chief Financial Officer, Palomar Medical Center, Escondido, CA, p. A60
Chief Financial Officer, Pomerado Hospital, Poway, CA, p. A81
HEMMERT, Brian, Chief Executive Officer, Mesilla Valley Hospital, Las Cruces, NM, p. A416
HEMMING, Stuart, Chief Operating Officer, Portsmouth Regional Hospital, Portsmouth, NH, p. A400
HEMMINGER, Linda, MSN Assistant Administrator Clinical Services, Cass County Memorial Hospital, Atlantic, IA, p. A214
HEMPEL, Stephen, M.D. President Medical Staff, Lakeland Regional Medical Center–St. Joseph, Saint Joseph, MI, p. A322
HEMPHILL, Ruth, R.N. Chief Nursing Officer, Florida Hospital Zephyrhills, Zephyrhills, FL, p. A143
HEMPLER, Shannan, Director Human Resources, Norton County Hospital, Norton, KS, p. A239
HEMPLING, Randall, Chief Executive Officer, Shasta Regional Medical Center, Redding, CA, p. A82
HEMSCHOOT, Ed, Director Information Systems, Montgomery Hospital Medical Center, Norristown, PA, p. A530
HENDEE, Daniel D., Director, Veterans Affairs Northern Indiana Health Care System, Fort Wayne, IN, p. A202
HENDEL, Dawna, R.N. Chief Nursing Officer and Vice President Patient Care Services, Saint John's Health Center, Santa Monica, CA, p. A90
HENDEL, Diana, PharmD,
Chief Executive Officer, Community Hospital of Long Beach, Long Beach, CA, p. A68
Chief Executive Officer, Long Beach Memorial Medical Center, Long Beach, CA, p. A68
Chief Executive Officer, Miller Children's Hospital, Long Beach, CA, p. A68
HENDERSON, Andre, Director Information Systems, Mission Community Hospital, Valencia, CA, p. A94
HENDERSON, Anita, Director Human Resources, Pennock Hospital, Hastings, MI, p. A315
HENDERSON, Carol
Senior Vice President and Chief Talent Officer, Scottsdale Healthcare Shea Medical Center, Scottsdale, AZ, p. A38
Vice President Human Resources, Scottsdale Healthcare Thompson Peak Hospital, Scottsdale, AZ, p. A38
Vice President Human Resources, Scottsdale Healthcare–Osborn Medical Center, Scottsdale, AZ, p. A38
HENDERSON, Chad, Interim Director Management Information Systems, Valley View Regional Hospital, Ada, OK, p. A493
HENDERSON, Claudia, Chief Human Resources, St. Elizabeth's Medical Center, Brighton, MA, p. A298
HENDERSON, Darilyn, Human Resources Officer, Rice Medical Center, Eagle Lake, TX, p. A595
HENDERSON, David K., M.D. Deputy Director Clinical Care, National Institutes of Health Clinical Center, Bethesda, MD, p. A289
HENDERSON, David M., Director Human Resources, Summersville Regional Medical Center, Summersville, WV, p. A676
HENDERSON, Donald G., FACHE Chief Executive Officer, Central Florida Health Alliance, Leesburg, FL, p. B30
HENDERSON, Donald G., FACHE President and Chief Executive Officer, Leesburg Regional Medical Center, Leesburg, FL, p. A129
HENDERSON, Gail, Manager Human Resources, Lauderdale Community Hospital, Ripley, TN, p. A575
HENDERSON, Gary, Chief Information Resources Management Services, Veterans Affairs Medical Center, Huntington, WV, p. A673
HENDERSON, John, Administrator, Childress Regional Medical Center, Childress, TX, p. A587
HENDERSON, Kate, Vice President and Chief Operating Officer, University Medical Center at Brackenridge, Austin, TX, p. A582
HENDERSON, Kathy, Director Human Resources, Media and Public Relations, Willow Crest Hospital, Miami, OK, p. A499
HENDERSON, Larry, M.D. Medical Director, Greene County Hospital, Leakesville, MS, p. A349
HENDERSON, Lisa, Administrative Assistant, Palacios Community Medical Center, Palacios, TX, p. A619
HENDERSON, Maryanne, D.O. Medical Director, The Children's Institute of Pittsburgh, Pittsburgh, PA, p. A535
HENDERSON, Melody, R.N. Chief Operating Officer and Chief Nursing Officer, Golden Plains Community Hospital, Borger, TX, p. A584
HENDERSON, Mike, Director Human Resources, Forest View Psychiatric Hospital, Grand Rapids, MI, p. A313
HENDERSON, Peggy, Director Health Information, Stringfellow Memorial Hospital, Anniston, AL, p. A15
HENDERSON, Sherry, Vice President Financial Services and Chief Financial Officer, Frye Regional Medical Center, Hickory, NC, p. A455
HENDERSON, Teto E., Director Human Resources, Geary Community Hospital, Junction City, KS, p. A235
HENDERSON, Travis, M.D. Chief of Staff, Mobridge Regional Hospital, Mobridge, SD, p. A558
HENDERSON, Volante, Manager Human Resources, Walton Rehabilitation Hospital, Augusta, GA, p. A147
HENDERSON, W. Perry, Administrator, East Texas Medical Center Pittsburg, Pittsburg, TX, p. A620
HENDLER, Robert, M.D. Regional Chief Medical Officer, Centennial Medical Center, Frisco, TX, p. A600
HENDREN, Karen, Vice President of Finance, Mercy Hospital Ardmore, Ardmore, OK, p. A493
HENDRICK, William, Senior Vice President and Chief Operating Officer, The Good Samaritan Hospital, Lebanon, PA, p. A527
HENDRICKS, Barbara A., Vice President, Human Resources and Support Services, Nanticoke Memorial Hospital, Seaford, DE, p. A114
HENDRICKS, Marcia, R.N. Chief Executive Officer, Madison County Health Care System, Winterset, IA, p. A228
HENDRICKS, Nicole Smith, Vice President Operations, Belton Regional Medical Center, Belton, MO, p. A355
HENDRICKS, Vickie, Director Human Resources, Barstow Community Hospital, Barstow, CA, p. A55
HENDRICKSEN, Sherry L., MSN, Chief Executive Officer, Kindred Hospital Springfield, Springfield, IL, p. A194
HENDRICKSON, Craig L., President and Chief Executive Officer, Overlake Hospital Medical Center, Bellevue, WA, p. A659
HENDRICKSON, Roman, M.D. Medical Director, Ruby Valley Hospital, Sheridan, MT, p. A379
HENDRIX, Michael, Chief Financial Officer, Maine Coast Memorial Hospital, Ellsworth, ME, p. A283
HENDRIXSON, Mark, M.D. Chief Medical Officer, Jamestown Regional Medical Center, Jamestown, TN, p. A567
HENEGAR, Edward R., D.O. Vice President, Medical Affairs, Ozarks Medical Center, West Plains, MO, p. A372
HENES, Jean M., R.N. Director of Nursing, Avera Creighton Hospital, Creighton, NE, p. A383
HENINGER, Bev, Director Nursing, Kenmare Community Hospital, Kenmare, ND, p. A467
HENKE, Mark
Chief Financial Officer, Medical Center of South Arkansas, El Dorado, AR, p. A44
President and Chief Executive Officer, Northfield Hospital, Northfield, MN, p. A336
HENKEL, Robert J., FACHE President and Chief Executive Officer, Ascension Health, Saint Louis, MO, p. B11
HENKENIUS, Jim, Chief Financial Officer, Stewart Memorial Community Hospital, Lake City, IA, p. A222

A834 Index of Health Care Professionals

Index of Health Care Professionals / Herwig

Index of Health Care Professionals


HENLEY, Donald, Vice President Human Resources and Social Services, Grove City Medical Center, Grove City, PA, p. A524
HENLEY, John, M.D. Interim Director, Veterans Health Care System of the Ozarks, Fayetteville, AR, p. A44
HENNENBERG, Shayla, Director Human Resources, Essentia Health Ada, Ada, MN, p. A327
HENNESSEE, Debbie, Chief Financial Officer, Grandview Medical Center, Jasper, TN, p. A567
HENNESSEY, Ruth, Executive Vice President and Chief Administrative Officer, St. Francis Hospital, Roslyn, NY, p. A442
HENNESSY, Thomas G., President and Chief Executive Officer, Saint Francis Memorial Hospital, San Francisco, CA, p. A87
HENNIGAN, Michael, M.D. Medical Director, HEALTHSOUTH Emerald Coast Rehabilitation Hospital, Panama City, FL, p. A135
HENNIKE, Michael, Chief Executive Officer, Central Regional Hospital, Butner, NC, p. A450
HENNING, Charles, Program Director Business, Veterans Affairs Medical Center, Kansas City, MO, p. A363
HENOCH, Malcolm S., M.D. Chief Medical Officer, Oakwood Hospital & Medical Center–Dearborn, Dearborn, MI, p. A310
HENRICH, Christy, Controller, Kindred Hospital of Northern Indiana, Mishawaka, IN, p. A208
HENRIKSON, Mary, Chief Executive Officer, Carondelet St. Joseph's Hospital, Tucson, AZ, p. A39
HENRY, Anna, Chief Information Officer, Kimble Hospital, Junction, TX, p. A609
HENRY, Chris, Associate Administrator and Chief Financial Officer, Washington Hospital Healthcare System, Fremont, CA, p. A61
HENRY, Christopher, Chief Information Management, Carl R. Darnall Army Medical Center, Fort Hood, TX, p. A598
HENRY, Dane, Executive Vice President and Chief Operating Officer, DeKalb Medical at North Decatur, Decatur, GA, p. A151
HENRY, David, President and Chief Executive Officer, Northern Montana Hospital, Havre, MT, p. A376
HENRY, Debbie, Vice President Financial Services, North Arkansas Regional Medical Center, Harrison, AR, p. A45
HENRY, Don, M.D. President Medical and Dental Staff, Community Hospital, Munster, IN, p. A209
HENRY, Ginger, Chief Executive Officer, Prattville Baptist Hospital, Prattville, AL, p. A25
HENRY, Heather, Manager Information Systems, Hammond–Henry Hospital, Geneseo, IL, p. A182
HENRY Jr.,, Jake, President and Chief Executive Officer, Saint Francis Health System, Tulsa, OK, p. B111
HENRY, Jay, Chief Executive Officer, St. Charles Medical Center – Bend, Bend, OR, p. A509
HENRY, Joy, R.N. Director Nurses, Faith Community Hospital, Jacksboro, TX, p. A609
HENRY, Mandy, Administrator, Beacon Behavioral Hospital – New Orleans, New Orleans, LA, p. A274
HENRY, Patricia, Chief Financial Officer, Coastal Communities Hospital, Santa Ana, CA, p. A89
HENRY, Tim
  Accountant, Chatuge Regional Hospital and Nursing Home, Hiawassee, GA, p. A154
  Chief Financial Officer, Union General Hospital, Blairsville, GA, p. A147
HENRY, William
  Director Human Resources, East Texas Medical Center Henderson, Henderson, TX, p. A603
  Director Human Resources, East Texas Medical Center–Gilmer, Gilmer, TX, p. A601
  Director Human Resources, East Texas Medical Center–Quitman, Quitman, TX, p. A622
HENSEL, David, Director Financial Operations, Grady Memorial Hospital, Delaware, OH, p. A479
HENSKE, Terry, Director Human Resources, Memorial Hermann Northwest Hospital, Houston, TX, p. A605
HENSLER, Paul J., Chief Executive Officer, Kern Medical Center, Bakersfield, CA, p. A55
HENSLEY, Dena, Administrator, Yancey Community Medical Center, Burnsville, NC, p. A450
HENSLEY, Lori, Chief Human Resources Officer, Ness County Hospital, Ness City, KS, p. A239
HENSON, Judith, Chief Nursing Officer, Adena Health System, Chillicothe, OH, p. A472
HENSON, Maureen, Vice President Human Resources, Mercy Memorial Hospital System, Monroe, MI, p. A319
HENSON, Pam, Executive Director, Pathways of Tennessee, Jackson, TN, p. A567
HENSON, Steve, Vice President Operations, Saline Memorial Hospital, Benton, AR, p. A42
HENTON, Thomas, Chief Executive Officer, Weisbrod Memorial County Hospital, Eads, CO, p. A100
HENTZEN PAGE, Ann, M.D. Medical Director, Summit Surgical, LLC, Hutchinson, KS, p. A235
HENZE, Michael E., Chief Executive Officer, Lake Regional Health System, Osage Beach, MO, p. A366
HEPBURN, Margaret, R.N. President and Chief Executive Officer, Sierra Vista Regional Health Center, Sierra Vista, AZ, p. A38
HEPNER, Tim, M.D. Medical Director, St. John Owasso, Owasso, OK, p. A503
HERBECK, Marilyn, Coordinator Human Resources, Community Memorial Hospital, Staunton, IL, p. A194
HERBEK, Gary J., Chief Operating Officer, Civista Health, La Plata, MD, p. A292
HERBER, Matt, M.D. Chief of Staff, Avera Dells Area Hospital, Dell Rapids, SD, p. A556
HERBERT, Daniel, M.D. Medical Administrative Officer, Millinocket Regional Hospital, Millinocket, ME, p. A284
HERBERT, Don, Interim Chief Executive Officer, Star Valley Medical Center, Afton, WY, p. A695
HERBERT, Ed, Vice President Marketing and Communications, Woodridge Hospital, Johnson City, TN, p. A568
HERBERT, Janet, R.N. Chief Operating Officer, McKenzie Health System, Sandusky, MI, p. A322
HERBERT, Kevin, Chief Financial Officer, Oconee Medical Center, Seneca, SC, p. A553
HERBERT, Laurie, Vice President Operations, Three Rivers Health, Three Rivers, MI, p. A324
HERBERT, Peter N., M.D. Senior Vice President Medical Affairs and Chief of Staff, Yale–New Haven Hospital, New Haven, CT, p. A111
HERBERT, Suzanne, Chief Financial Officer, Mimbres Memorial Hospital, Deming, NM, p. A415
HERBST, Gary, Senior Vice President and Chief Financial Officer, Kaweah Delta Medical Center, Visalia, CA, p. A95
HERD, Jacqueline, R.N. Chief Nursing Officer, Atlanta Medical Center, Atlanta, GA, p. A145
HERDENER, Tony, Vice President Systems and Finance, Northeast Georgia Medical Center, Gainesville, GA, p. A153
HERDER, Debbie, Controller, Texas Specialty Hospital at Wichita Falls, Wichita Falls, TX, p. A635
HEREFORD, Michelle, Administrator, Transitional Care Hospital, Charlottesville, VA, p. A646
HERFINDAHL, Lowell D., Interim Chief Executive Officer, Linton Hospital, Linton, ND, p. A467
HERING, Kristine, R.N. Chief Nursing Officer, Speare Memorial Hospital, Plymouth, NH, p. A400
HERINK, Phil, Chief Executive Officer, Boise Behavioral Health Hospital, Boise, ID, p. A166
HERM, Ann, Associate Director Patient Care Services, John D. Dingell Veterans Affairs Medical Center, Detroit, MI, p. A311
HERMAN, David C., M.D. Chief Executive Officer, Vidant Health, Greenville, NC, p. B142
HERMAN, John J., Chief Operating Officer, Mercy Hospital, Buffalo, NY, p. A423
HERMAN, John W., Chief Executive Officer, Fairview Northland Medical Center, Princeton, MN, p. A337
HERMAN, Theresa, M.D. Chief Medical Officer and Chief Quality Officer, Dupont Hospital, Fort Wayne, IN, p. A201
HERMANN, Terri, R.N. Chief Nursing Officer, Franklin Hospital District, Benton, IL, p. A173
HERMANS, Louis H.
  Vice President Information Systems, JFK Johnson Rehabilitation Institute, Edison, NJ, p. A403
  Vice President Information Systems, JFK Medical Center, Edison, NJ, p. A403
HERMANSON, Patrick M., Administrator, Great Falls Clinic Medical Center, Great Falls, MT, p. A376
HERMOSILLO, Gilbert, Manager Information Services, Mendota Community Hospital, Mendota, IL, p. A188
HERN, Warren, President and Chief Executive Officer, Unity Hospital, Rochester, NY, p. A442
HERNANDEZ, Bernadette, R.N. Chief Operating Officer, Laredo Specialty Hospital, Laredo, TX, p. A612
HERNANDEZ Jr., George B., President and Chief Executive Officer, University Health System, San Antonio, TX, p. A626
HERNANDEZ, Hank, Chief Executive Officer, Las Palmas Del Sol Healthcare, El Paso, TX, p. A596
HERNANDEZ, Hector
  Chief Administrative Officer, Community Hospital of Huntington Park, Huntington Park, CA, p. A65
  Chief Executive Officer, East Los Angeles Doctors Hospital, Los Angeles, CA, p. A69
HERNANDEZ, Kim, Director Human Resources, AMG Specialty Hospital–Slidell, Slidell, LA, p. A278
HERNANDEZ, Leonard, Chief Executive Officer, Morton County Health System, Elkhart, KS, p. A232
HERNANDEZ, Luz Maria, Director Human Resources, I. Gonzalez Martinez Oncologic Hospital,, PR, p. A703
HERNANDEZ, Reyna, Chief Financial Officer, HEALTHSOUTH Rehabilitation Hospital of Miami, Miami, FL, p. A131
HERNANDEZ, Sandi, Controller, Lafayette General Surgical Hospital, Lafayette, LA, p. A270
HERNANDEZ, Tony, Director Information Technology, Fort Duncan Regional Medical Center, Eagle Pass, TX, p. A595
HERNANDEZ DROZDOWICZ, Diana, M.D. Medical Director, Rogers City Rehabilitation Hospital, Rogers City, MI, p. A321
HERNANDEZ–KEEBLE, Sonia, Superintendent, Rio Grande State Center/South Texas Health Care System, Harlingen, TX, p. A602
HERNANDEZ–LICHTL, Javier, Chief Executive Officer, Baptist Health South Florida, West Kendall Baptist Hospital, Miami, FL, p. A131
HERNDON, David N., M.D. Chief of Staff, Shriners Hospitals for Children, Galveston Burns Hospital, Galveston, TX, p. A600
HERNDON, Lori, President and Chief Executive Officer, AtlantiCare Regional Medical Center, Atlantic City, NJ, p. A401
HERR, Michael, Chief Financial Officer, Parkview Regional Hospital, Mexia, TX, p. A616
HERRARA, Espie, Chief Financial Officer, Peak Behavioral Health Services, Santa Teresa, NM, p. A418
HERRERA, Esmeraldo, M.D. Chief of Staff, Wayne Medical Center, Waynesboro, TN, p. A576
HERRERA, Georgina, M.D. Medical Director, Mesilla Valley Hospital, Las Cruces, NM, p. A416
HERRERA, Jocelyn A., Director Human Resources, Anaheim Medical Center, Anaheim, CA, p. A53
HERRERA, Veronica, Director Human Resources, Aurora Las Encinas Hospital, Pasadena, CA, p. A79
HERRERO, Carmelo, M.D. Medical Director, Hospital Oriente, Humacao, PR, p. A701
HERRICK, Stephen M., Ph.D. Director, Piedmont Geriatric Hospital, Burkeville, VA, p. A646
HERRIN, Curtis
  Chief Financial Officer, Toppenish Community Hospital, Toppenish, WA, p. A668
  Chief Financial Officer, Yakima Regional Medical and Cardiac Center, Yakima, WA, p. A669
HERRING, Jim, Senior Vice President, Children's Medical Center of Dallas, Dallas, TX, p. A590
HERRING, Randy, M.D. Chief of Staff, Coon Memorial Hospital and Home, Dalhart, TX, p. A590
HERRINGTON, Bruce, M.D. Chief Medical Officer, Louis Smith Memorial Hospital, Lakeland, GA, p. A155
HERRIOTT, Sue A., Director Human Resources, OSF St. Joseph Medical Center, Bloomington, IL, p. A173
HERRMAN, Edward, M.D. Assistant Administrator Patient Care Services, Integris Bass Pavilion, Enid, OK, p. A496
HERRMANN, Anna L., JD Assistant Administrator, Mayo Clinic Health System in New Prague, New Prague, MN, p. A336
HERRMANN, Deborah, M.D. Chief of Staff, I–70 Community Hospital, Sweet Springs, MO, p. A371
HERRMANN, Lee, Chief Healthcare Technology Officer, Santa Clara Valley Medical Center, San Jose, CA, p. A88
HERRMANN, Marty, M.D. Medical Director, Mayo Clinic Health System in New Prague, New Prague, MN, p. A336
HERRMANN, Sarah, R.N. Chief Nursing Officer, Select Specialty Hospital–Topeka, Topeka, KS, p. A244
HERRON, Katherine, Director Human Resources, Richard H. Hutchings Psychiatric Center, Syracuse, NY, p. A444
HERRON, Mary Beth, Director of Human Resources, Illinois Valley Community Hospital, Peru, IL, p. A191
HERRON, Michael, Chief Financial Officer, Southern Hills Hospital and Medical Center, Las Vegas, NV, p. A393
HERRON, Thomas L., FACHE Chief Executive Officer, Tristar Centennial Medical Center, Nashville, TN, p. A573
HERSEY, Robert, Chief Financial Officer, Northeastern Vermont Regional Hospital, Saint Johnsbury, VT, p. A644
HERSHBERGER, Scott, Acting Chief Information Management Services, Veterans Affairs Medical Center, Battle Creek, MI, p. A308
HERSOM, Deborah, Director Human Resources, HEALTHSOUTH Chattanooga Rehabilitation Hospital, Chattanooga, TN, p. A563
HERT, Rebecca, Director Human Resources, SouthCrest Hospital, Tulsa, OK, p. A507
HERTEL, Cheryl, Coordinator Human Resources, Stamford Memorial Hospital, Stamford, TX, p. A628
HERTZ, Roger
  Vice President, Jennie Edmundson Hospital, Council Bluffs, IA, p. A217
  Vice President Information Technology, Nebraska Methodist Hospital, Omaha, NE, p. A388
HERTZLER, Barbara, Chief Operating Officer, St. Joseph Mercy Oakland, Pontiac, MI, p. A321
HERWALDT, Debra J., Chief Financial Officer, Los Robles Hospital and Medical Center, Thousand Oaks, CA, p. A92
HERWIG, Brian J., Chief Operating Officer, Providence Medford Medical Center, Medford, OR, p. A512
HERWIG, Karen, Vice President Human Resources, Ashland Community Hospital, Ashland, OR, p. A509




Index of Health Care Professionals A835

Index of Health Care Professionals

Index of Health Care Professionals / Herzberg

HERZBERG, Deborah L., FACHE Chief Executive Officer, Davis County Hospital, Bloomfield, IA, p. A215
HERZBERG, Jami J., Assistant Vice President, Carolinas Rehabilitation, Charlotte, NC, p. A450
HERZBERG, Joseph W., Assistant Vice President Human Resources, WellStar Cobb Hospital, Austell, GA, p. A147
HERZOG, David, Chief Information Officer, Ventura County Medical Center, Ventura, CA, p. A94
HERZOG, Dean, Chief Financial Officer, Kona Community Hospital, Kealakekua, HI, p. A165
HERZOG, Mark P., President and Chief Executive Officer, Holy Family Memorial Medical Center, Manitowoc, WI, p. A685
HERZOG, Paul F., Chief Executive Officer, Memorial Medical Center, Las Cruces, NM, p. A416
HESCH, Dennis, Executive Vice President Finance and Chief Financial Officer, Carle Foundation Hospital, Urbana, IL, p. A195
HESS, Bob, Chief Information Officer, Bonner General Hospital, Sandpoint, ID, p. A170
HESS, Brian, Chief Executive Officer, Highlands Regional Medical Center, Sebring, FL, p. A139
HESS, Carolyn K., R.N. Administrator, Smith County Memorial Hospital, Smith Center, KS, p. A243
HESS, David F., M.D. President Medical Staff, Reynolds Memorial Hospital, Glen Dale, WV, p. A672
HESS, Matthew, Director Human Resources, Raleigh General Hospital, Beckley, WV, p. A670
HESS, Pamela, Chief Financial Officer, St. Joseph Hospital, Fort Wayne, IN, p. A202
HESS, Phil, Chief Executive Officer, Philhaven, Mount Gretna, PA, p. A529
HESS, Rita, R.N. Chief Nursing Officer, North Shore Medical Center, Miami, FL, p. A131
HESS, Steve
Vice President & Chief Information Officer, Medical Center of the Rockies, Loveland, CO, p. A104
Vice President Information Services and Chief Information Officer, University of Colorado Hospital, Aurora, CO, p. A97
HESSE, Fred, M.D. Medical Director, Arms Acres, Carmel, NY, p. A423
HESSELRODE, Renee, Director Health Information Management, Landmark Hospital, Cape Girardeau, MO, p. A356
HESSHEIMER, Susan, Director Human Resources, Johnson County Hospital, Tecumseh, NE, p. A390
HESSING, Jeffrey, M.D. Medical Director, Treasure Valley Hospital, Boise, ID, p. A167
HESSMAN, Mary Pat, Chief Fiscal, Veterans Affairs Medical Center, Northport, NY, p. A438
HESTER, Julie A., President and Chief Executive Officer, St. Francis Hospital, Wilmington, DE, p. A115
HESTER, Kathy, Chief Nursing Officer, Orange Park Medical Center, Orange Park, FL, p. A134
HESTER, Sharon
Site Manager Information Technology, St. Rose Dominican Hospitals – Rose de Lima Campus, Henderson, NV, p. A392
Site Manager Information Technology, St. Rose Dominican Hospitals – San Martin Campus, Las Vegas, NV, p. A394
Site Manager Information Technology, St. Rose Dominican Hospitals – Siena Campus, Henderson, NV, p. A392
HESTER, Steven, M.D. Vice President Medical Affairs, Norton Suburban Hospital, Louisville, KY, p. A255
HETLAGE, C. Kennon, FACHE Chief Executive Officer and Administrator, Memorial Hospital West, Pembroke Pines, FL, p. A135
HETLETVED, Beth, Director of Nurses, Garrison Memorial Hospital, Garrison, ND, p. A466
HETRICK, Robert G., Chief Financial Officer, Northern Hospital of Surry County, Mount Airy, NC, p. A458
HETT, Sam, Manager Human Resources, Satanta District Hospital, Satanta, KS, p. A243
HETTICH, E. Paul, Chief Financial Officer, BryLin Hospitals, Buffalo, NY, p. A422
HETTINGER, MaryLou, Director Quality Management, Devereux Children's Behavioral Health Center, Malvern, PA, p. A528
HETU, Maureen, Chief Information Officer, Our Lady of Lourdes Medical Center, Camden, NJ, p. A402
HETZ, Mark
Chief Information Officer, Rogue Valley Medical Center, Medford, OR, p. A512
Chief Information Officer, Three Rivers Medical Center, Grants Pass, OR, p. A511
HEURING, Ron, Director Information Systems, Perry County Memorial Hospital, Perryville, MO, p. A366
HEUSER, Keith E., Administrator, Mercy Hospital, Valley City, ND, p. A468
HEVER, Susan C., Director Human Resources, Brookhaven Memorial Hospital Medical Center, Patchogue, NY, p. A440
HEWIT, Craig, Executive Partner Information Technology and Chief Information Officer, Sanford Medical Center Fargo, Fargo, ND, p. A465
HEXUM, Gregory, Chief Financial Officer, Steele Memorial Medical Center, Salmon, ID, p. A170
HEYBOER Jr., Lester, President and Chief Executive Officer, HealthSource Saginaw, Saginaw, MI, p. A322
HEYDON, Larry, President and Chief Executive Officer, Johnson Memorial Hospital, Franklin, IN, p. A202
HEYE, John E., Chief Financial Officer, Maine Medical Center, Portland, ME, p. A284
HEYN, Matt, Administrator, Pawnee Valley Community Hospital, Larned, KS, p. A237
HEYWOOD, Matthew, Chief Operating Officer, New Hanover Regional Medical Center, Wilmington, NC, p. A462
HIATT, M. K., Administrator, Allendale County Hospital, Fairfax, SC, p. A549
HIATT, Tim, Chief Information Officer, Brodstone Memorial Hospital, Superior, NE, p. A390
HIBBERT, Paul, D.O. President Medical Staff, Illini Community Hospital, Pittsfield, IL, p. A192
HIBBS, Cathryn A., FACHE Chief Executive Officer, Deaconess Hospital, Oklahoma City, OK, p. A500
HIBEN, Daniel, Chief Executive Officer, Oswego Community Hospital, Oswego, KS, p. A240
HICCOX, Janelle, Director Human Resources, Lincoln Hospital, Davenport, WA, p. A660
HICKETHIER, Julie, R.N. Senior Vice President, Benefis Hospitals, Great Falls, MT, p. A376
HICKEY, Christopher, Chief Financial Officer, North Adams Regional Hospital, North Adams, MA, p. A303
HICKEY, Mairead, Ph.D. Executive Vice President and Chief Operating Officer, Brigham and Women's Hospital, Boston, MA, p. A296
HICKEY, Thomas P., Chief Executive Officer and Managing Director, Pembroke Hospital, Pembroke, MA, p. A303
HICKEY–BOYNTON, Meg, Director Human Resources and Marketing, Community Hospital of Anaconda, Anaconda, MT, p. A373
HICKLING, Karen, Director Human Resources, Palmdale Regional Medical Center, Palmdale, CA, p. A79
HICKMAN, George, Executive Vice President and Chief Information Officer, Albany Medical Center, Albany, NY, p. A420
HICKMAN, Louise, R.N. Vice President of Patient Care Services, Jefferson Regional Medical Center, Pine Bluff, AR, p. A50
HICKS, Angela, Controller, Our Community Hospital, Scotland Neck, NC, p. A460
HICKS, Crystal, R.N. Chief Nursing Officer, Harrison County Community Hospital, Bethany, MO, p. A355
HICKS, Joan, Chief Information Officer, University of Alabama Hospital, Birmingham, AL, p. A17
HICKS, Joe, Executive Director, Saint Barnabas Behavioral Health Center, Toms River, NJ, p. A411
HICKS, John R., President and Chief Executive Officer, Platte Valley Medical Center, Brighton, CO, p. A98
HICKS, Kevin J., President and Chief Executive Officer, Research Medical Center, Kansas City, MO, p. A362
HICKS, Shawnee, Director Human Resources, Magnolia Regional Medical Center, Magnolia, AR, p. A48
HICKS, Susan, Chief Operating Officer, Sky Ridge Medical Center, Lone Tree, CO, p. A104
HICKS, Terri, Chief Operating Officer and Chief Financial Officer, P & S Surgical Hospital, Monroe, LA, p. A273
HICKSON, Stan, FACHE Executive Vice President and Chief Operating Officer, Palmetto Health Richland, Columbia, SC, p. A548
HIDALGO, Humberto, M.D. Chief of Staff, South Texas Health System, Edinburg, TX, p. A595
HIEB, Dorothy, Director Human Resources, Sanford Medical Center Chamberlain, Chamberlain, SD, p. A555
HIEBERT, Leslie, Chief Financial Officer, Klickitat Valley Health, Goldendale, WA, p. A661
HIERS, Mitch, Director Information Services, Colquitt Regional Medical Center, Moultrie, GA, p. A157
HIGA, Russel, JD Regional Director Human Resources, Leahi Hospital, Honolulu, HI, p. A163
HIGDON, Kevin J., Chief Financial Officer, Thorek Memorial Hospital, Chicago, IL, p. A178
HIGGINBOTHAM, G. Douglas, Executive Director, South Central Regional Medical Center, Laurel, MS, p. A348
HIGGINBOTHAM, Michael, Chief Executive Officer, Texas Specialty Hospital at Houston, Houston, TX, p. A607
HIGGINS, Alana, Regional Information Management Executive, CHRISTUS St. Michael Health System, Texarkana, TX, p. A630
HIGGINS, John, Vice President Finance, Exempla Good Samaritan Medical Center, Lafayette, CO, p. A103
HIGGINS, Kevin A., Chief Financial Officer, Olmsted Medical Center, Rochester, MN, p. A338
HIGGINS, Larry, Vice President Human Resources, King's Daughters Medical Center, Ashland, KY, p. A247
HIGGINS, Myron, Chief Operating Officer, Mercer County Hospital, Aledo, IL, p. A172
HIGGINS, Susie, Chief Financial Officer, Grafton City Hospital, Grafton, WV, p. A672
HIGGINS, William, M.D. Vice President Medical Affairs, Hudson Valley Hospital Center, Cortlandt Manor, NY, p. A424
HIGGINS–BOWERS, Shirley, Vice President Human Resources, JFK Medical Center, Edison, NJ, p. A403
HIGGINSON, David, Senior Vice President and Chief Information Officer, Phoenix Children's Hospital, Phoenix, AZ, p. A36
HIGH, Kim, Chief Financial Officer, Baptist Memorial Hospital–Union County, New Albany, MS, p. A351
HIGHBAUGH, Michael, M.D. Medical Director, Baylor Specialty Hospital, Dallas, TX, p. A590
HIGHSMITH, Cameron, Chief Executive Officer, Cape Fear Valley – Bladen County Hospital, Elizabethtown, NC, p. A453
HIGHSMITH, Danette, Director Human Resources, Burke Medical Center, Waynesboro, GA, p. A162
HIGHTOWER, Bernita, Chief Human Resources, Martin Army Community Hospital, Fort Benning, GA, p. A153
HIGHTOWER, Skip
Chief Financial Officer, Grady General Hospital, Cairo, GA, p. A148
Senior Vice President and Chief Financial Officer, John D. Archbold Memorial Hospital, Thomasville, GA, p. A160
Senior Vice President and Chief Financial Officer, Mitchell County Hospital, Camilla, GA, p. A148
Senior Vice President and Chief Financial Officer, Pioneer Community Hospital of Early, Blakely, GA, p. A147
HIGHTOWER, Thomas, Chief Operating Officer, Grays Harbor Community Hospital, Aberdeen, WA, p. A659
HILAL, Marwan, M.D. Chief Medical Officer, University Hospitals Bedford Medical Center, Cleveland, OH, p. A475
HILAMAN, Brad L., M.D. Chief of Staff, J. Arthur Dosher Memorial Hospital, Southport, NC, p. A461
HILBERT, Frank, Senior Vice President and Chief Information Officer, McAlester Regional Health Center, McAlester, OK, p. A499
HILBERT, Laura, Interim Chief Operating Officer, Palms West Hospital, Loxahatchee, FL, p. A129
HILBURN, Diana, Vice President Information Technology and Chief Information Officer, Via Christi Hospitals Wichita, Wichita, KS, p. A245
HILDEBRAND, Richard D., M.D. Vice President Medical Affairs and Chief Medical Officer, St. Luke's Regional Medical Center, Sioux City, IA, p. A227
HILDEBRANDT, James, D.O. President Medical Staff, Sarah Bush Lincoln Health Center, Mattoon, IL, p. A187
HILDRETH, Beth, Vice President Human Resources, MedCentral – Mansfield Hospital, Mansfield, OH, p. A483
HILDWEIN, Robin, Chief Information Officer, Boca Raton Regional Hospital, Boca Raton, FL, p. A118
HILL, Bart, M.D. Vice President Medical Affairs, St. Luke's Regional Medical Center, Boise, ID, p. A167
HILL, Bettie, Chief Financial Officer, Poplar Springs Hospital, Petersburg, VA, p. A653
HILL, C. David, President, Integris Seminole Medical Center, Seminole, OK, p. A504
HILL, Cheryl
Vice President Human Resources, Columbia St. Mary's Hospital Milwaukee, Milwaukee, WI, p. A686
Vice President Human Resources, Columbia St. Mary's Ozaukee Hospital, Mequon, WI, p. A686
Vice President Human Resources, Sacred Heart Rehabilitation Institute, Milwaukee, WI, p. A687
HILL, David L., Chief Executive Officer, John C. Fremont Healthcare District, Mariposa, CA, p. A74
HILL, Deborah A., FACHE Chief Executive Officer, Summersville Regional Medical Center, Summersville, WV, p. A676
HILL, Douglas, M.D. Medical Director, Cascade Medical Center, Cascade, ID, p. A167
HILL, Duane N., Chief Executive Officer, Beaumont Bone and Joint Institute, Beaumont, TX, p. A582
HILL, Dwight, Vice President Human Resources, Northside Hospital, Atlanta, GA, p. A145
HILL, Herbert, Director Human Resources, Adventist Medical Center, Portland, OR, p. A513
HILL, Jackie, Chief Financial Officer, Brighton Center for Recovery, Brighton, MI, p. A308
HILL, James P., Senior Vice President Human Resources, Medstar Washington Hospital Center, Washington, DC, p. A116
HILL, Janice, R.N. Administrator, Baptist Memorial Restorative Care Hospital, Memphis, TN, p. A571
HILL, Jason, M.D. Chief Medical Officer, Choctaw Nation Health Care Center, Talihina, OK, p. A505
HILL, Jeff, Chief Executive Officer, Steele Memorial Medical Center, Salmon, ID, p. A170

A836 Index of Health Care Professionals

Index of Health Care Professionals / Hocum

Index of Health Care Professionals


HILL, Jill, Director Information Technology, Utah State Hospital, Provo, UT, p. A640
HILL, Jr., Joe B., Vice President Human Resources, Trident Medical Center, Charleston, SC, p. A547
HILL, John, Chief Executive Officer, Sacred Heart Medical Center at RiverBend, Springfield, OR, p. A516
HILL, Karen
Director Human Resources, Baylor Institute for Rehabilitation, Dallas, TX, p. A590
Coordinator Human Resources, Baylor Specialty Hospital, Dallas, TX, p. A590
Coordinator Human Resources, Our Children's House at Baylor, Dallas, TX, p. A592
HILL, Karen S., R.N. Chief Operating Officer and Chief Nursing Officer, Central Baptist Hospital, Lexington, KY, p. A253
HILL, Kent D., Director, Veterans Affairs Medical Center, Kansas City, MO, p. A363
HILL, Mary Beth, Coordinator Human Resources, Vidant Bertie Hospital, Windsor, NC, p. A463
HILL, Michael, M.D. Chief of Staff, LaFollette Medical Center, La Follette, TN, p. A569
HILL, Pamela German
Chief Financial Officer, Vista Medical Center East, Waukegan, IL, p. A196
Chief Financial Officer, Vista Medical Center West, Waukegan, IL, p. A196
HILL, Phillip, Interim Chief Executive Officer, Calhoun–Liberty Hospital, Blountstown, FL, p. A118
HILL, Ryan
Interim Chief Executive Officer, Essentia Health Ada, Ada, MN, p. A327
Chief Financial Officer, Essentia Health St. Mary's Hospital – Detroit Lakes, Detroit Lakes, MN, p. A330
HILL, Scott, Chief Executive Officer, Montgomery Regional Hospital, Blacksburg, VA, p. A646
HILL, Steven, Vice President Finance, University of Minnesota Medical Center, Fairview, Minneapolis, MN, p. A335
HILL, Stuart, Vice President and Treasurer, White County Medical Center, Searcy, AR, p. A51
HILL, Sue, Director Finance, Taylorville Memorial Hospital, Taylorville, IL, p. A195
HILL, Susan, Director Human Resources, East Texas Medical Center Clarksville, Clarksville, TX, p. A587
HILL, Terri, Director Human Resources, Pleasant Valley Hospital, Point Pleasant, WV, p. A675
HILL, Terri L., Vice President and Administrator, Union Hospital Clinton, Clinton, IN, p. A199
HILL–DAVIS, Nancy L., Vice President Human Resources and Risk Management, Mercy Hospital and Medical Center, Chicago, IL, p. A176
HILLARD, Jeffrey, FACHE Deputy Commander for Administration, Bayne–Jones Army Community Hospital, Fort Polk, LA, p. A266
HILLEBRAND, Jeffrey H., Chief Operating Officer, NorthShore University Health System Evanston Hospital, Evanston, IL, p. A181
HILLEGASS, Bonnie Essex, Chief Executive Officer, Harmon Medical and Rehabilitation Hospital, Las Vegas, NV, p. A392
HILLIARD, David J., D.O. Chief of Staff, Barnesville Hospital, Barnesville, OH, p. A470
HILLIARD, Eva, Director Human Resources, Sutter Davis Hospital, Davis, CA, p. A59
HILLIS, David W., President and Chief Executive Officer, Adcare Hospital of Worcester, Worcester, MA, p. A306
HILLMAN, Annette, Director Human Resources, Doctor's Hospital of Deer Creek, Leesville, LA, p. A271
HILLS, Cindi, Director Human Resources, Riverwood Healthcare Center, Aitkin, MN, p. A327
HILLS, Edward, D.D.S. Interim Chief Operating Officer, MetroHealth Medical Center, Cleveland, OH, p. A475
HILLS, Linda, Director Information Technology, Littleton Adventist Hospital, Littleton, CO, p. A103
HILMOE, Eric C., Chief Executive Officer, Sanford Canton–Inwood Medical Center, Canton, SD, p. A555
HILT, Monica
President, Sacred Heart Hospital, Tomahawk, WI, p. A692
President and Chief Operating Officer, Sacred Heart–St. Mary's Hospitals, Rhinelander, WI, p. A690
HILTON, Craig, Chief Executive Officer, Hampton Behavioral Health Center, Westampton Township, NJ, p. A412
HILTON, David, M.D. Medical Director, Hamilton Center, Terre Haute, IN, p. A212
HILTON, John, Operations Officer, Northern Cochise Community Hospital, Willcox, AZ, p. A41
HILTON, Lois, Director Human Resources, DeSoto Memorial Hospital, Arcadia, FL, p. A118
HILTON, Richard G., Associate Administrator and Chief Financial Officer, OCH Regional Medical Center, Starkville, MS, p. A353
HILTON, Shane, Vice President and Chief Financial Officer, Johnson City Medical Center, Johnson City, TN, p. A567
HILTON–SIEBERT, Stephanie, President and Chief Executive Officer, Salem Township Hospital, Salem, IL, p. A193
HILTUNEN, Theresa, Entity Information Officer, Penn Presbyterian Medical Center, Philadelphia, PA, p. A533
HIME, Judy, Director Human Resources, Gibson General Hospital, Trenton, TN, p. A576
HINCHEY, Paul P.
President and Chief Executive Officer, Candler Hospital, Savannah, GA, p. A158
President and Chief Executive Officer, St. Joseph's Hospital, Savannah, GA, p. A159
HINCKLEY, Fran, Chief Information Officer, Hebrew Rehabilitation Center, Boston, MA, p. A297
HINDERAKER, David, Chief Financial Officer, Prairie Lakes Healthcare System, Watertown, SD, p. A560
HINDMAN, Robbie, Vice President Patient Care Services and Chief Nursing Officer, Walker Baptist Medical Center, Jasper, AL, p. A22
HINDS, Bob, Executive Director, Bradford Health Services at Huntsville, Madison, AL, p. A22
HINDS, Nigel, Chief Financial Officer, Florida Hospital DeLand, DeLand, FL, p. A122
HINEMAN, Elizabeth, M.D. Chief Medical Staff, Scott County Hospital, Scott City, KS, p. A243
HINER, Jill, Vice President and Chief Financial Officer, Summa Western Reserve Hospital, Cuyahoga Falls, OH, p. A478
HINER, Peggy, Executive Secretary and Manager Human Resources, Wheatland Memorial Healthcare, Harlowton, MT, p. A376
HINES, Frederick W., President, Clarity Child Guidance Center, San Antonio, TX, p. A624
HINES, James, Chief Financial Officer, East Texas Medical Center Clarksville, Clarksville, TX, p. A587
HINES, Linda
Vice President and Site Executive, Baltimore Washington Medical Center, Glen Burnie, MD, p. A292
Vice President Information Technology and Information Systems, Kernan Orthopaedics and Rehabilitation, Baltimore, MD, p. A287
HINES, Randall, Interim Administrator, Central State Hospital, Milledgeville, GA, p. A156
HINES, Ron, Director Information Technology, Valley View Hospital, Glenwood Springs, CO, p. A101
HINESLEY, Jay, Assistant Chief Executive Officer, DeKalb Regional Medical Center, Fort Payne, AL, p. A20
HINKLE, David, Senior Vice President and Chief Information Officer, Nash Health Care Systems, Rocky Mount, NC, p. A460
HINKLE, Stacey, Director Information Technology, Banner Desert Medical Center, Mesa, AZ, p. A34
HINNER, William J.
Vice President Fiscal Services and Chief Financial Officer, Ministry Saint Michael's Hospital, Stevens Point, WI, p. A691
Vice President Finance and Chief Financial Officer, Saint Clare's Hospital, Weston, WI, p. A693
HINO, Raymond T., Chief Executive Officer, Mendocino Coast District Hospital, Fort Bragg, CA, p. A61
HINRICHS, Becky, Vice President Human Resources, Riverside Medical Center, Kankakee, IL, p. A185
HINRICHS, Michelle, Chief Nursing Officer, St. Joseph's Hospital and Health Center, Dickinson, ND, p. A465
HINRICHS, Sandy, Director Human Resources, Burnett Medical Center, Grantsburg, WI, p. A682
HINTON, George, Administrator, Aurora Sinai Medical Center, Milwaukee, WI, p. A686
HINTON, James H., President and Chief Executive Officer, Presbyterian Healthcare Services, Albuquerque, NM, p. B102
HINTON, Sharon, Chief Nursing Officer, Natchaug Hospital, Mansfield Center, CT, p. A109
HINTZE, Paul, M.D. Vice President Medical Affairs, Mercy Hospital St. Louis, Saint Louis, MO, p. A369
HIRKALER, Kim, Director Human Resources, Bon Secours Community Hospital, Port Jervis, NY, p. A440
HIROSE, Mivic, Executive Administrator, Laguna Honda Hospital and Rehabilitation Center, San Francisco, CA, p. A87
HIRSCH, Leslie D., FACHE President and Chief Executive Officer, Saint Clare's Health System, Denville, NJ, p. A403
HIRSCH, Michel Y., M.D. Chief Medical Staff, Prevost Memorial Hospital, Donaldsonville, LA, p. A266
HIRSCH, Ted W., Senior Executive Director, Kalispell Regional Medical Center, Kalispell, MT, p. A377
HIRSCHMAN, Debra L., MSN, Director, Veterans Affairs Medical Center, Sheridan, WY, p. A697
HIRSHBERG, Mark I., Chief Operating Officer, Bothwell Regional Health Center, Sedalia, MO, p. A370
HIRST, Barb, Vice President Human Resources and Chief Nursing Officer, Salem Community Hospital, Salem, OH, p. A488
HISAW, Shana, Chief Operating Officer, Acadia Abilene Hospital, Abilene, TX, p. A577
HISERODT, James, Senior Vice President Operations, Geneva General Hospital, Geneva, NY, p. A426
HISEY, Commie, D.O. Chief of Staff, Memorial Hospital, Gonzales, TX, p. A601
HITE–DAVIS, Anissa, Vice President Human Resources, St. Joseph's Hospital of Buckhannon, Buckhannon, WV, p. A670
HITT, Patricia A., Associate Director, Veterans Affairs Medical Center, Grand Junction, CO, p. A102
HITZLER, Ronald R., Administrator, Shriners Hospitals for Children, Shriners Burns Hospital, Cincinnati, Cincinnati, OH, p. A474
HIXENBAUGH, Cynthia, Director Human Resources, Pershing General Hospital, Lovelock, NV, p. A394
HIXSON, Kim, Chief Financial Officer, Avera Creighton Hospital, Creighton, NE, p. A383
HJEMBO, Philip, Chief Financial Officer, St. Elizabeth Hospital, Enumclaw, WA, p. A661
HLAHOL, Jan, Manager Human Resources, Cleveland Clinic Children's Hospital for Rehabilitation, Cleveland, OH, p. A474
HLAVENKA, Richard, Director Management Information Systems, Jamaica Hospital Medical Center,, NY, p. A433
HLUCHY, Nicholas, Business Analyst, Support Services Manager, Baton Rouge Rehabilitation Hospital, Baton Rouge, LA, p. A262
HO, Sylvia, Director Information Services, Grady Memorial Hospital, Chickasha, OK, p. A494
HO–SHING, Viodelda, Deputy Director Administration, Creedmoor Psychiatric Center,, NY, p. A432
HOACH, Ken, Assistant Vice President and Chief Information Officer, Emanuel Medical Center, Turlock, CA, p. A93
HOAG, Linda, Director Human Resources, St. Mary's Regional Medical Center, Enid, OK, p. A496
HOAGBIN, Joseph, M.D. Chief Quality Officer, Alegent Health–Mercy Hospital, Council Bluffs, IA, p. A217
HOAR, Brad, Director Information and Technology, Cedar Park Regional Medical Center, Cedar Park, TX, p. A587
HOAR, Tanya, Chief Financial Officer, Schoolcraft Memorial Hospital, Manistique, MI, p. A318
HOARD, Kaylee S., Chief Financial Officer, Cook Hospital and Convalescent Nursing Care Unit, Cook, MN, p. A329
HOARTY, Ranee, Business Manager Human Resources, Fillmore County Hospital, Geneva, NE, p. A383
HOBACK, Kim, Supervisor Information Systems, Athens–Limestone Hospital, Athens, AL, p. A16
HOBAN, Donna, M.D. Senior Vice President and Physician–in–Chief, Beaumont Hospital Grosse Pointe, Grosse Pointe, MI, p. A314
HOBAN, Douglas M., Vice President and Chief Financial Officer, Mercy Hospital Lebanon, Lebanon, MO, p. A364
HOBART, Robert, Director Management Information Systems, Heartland Behavioral Healthcare, Massillon, OH, p. A484
HOBBS, Donna, Nurse Executive, U. S. Public Health Service Indian Hospital–Sells, Sells, AZ, p. A38
HOBBS, Ed, Director Information Services, DeKalb Health, Auburn, IN, p. A197
HOBBS, Jan, M.D. Chief Medical Officer, Eastern New Mexico Medical Center, Roswell, NM, p. A417
HOBBS, Tommy, Chief Executive Officer, Illinois Valley Community Hospital, Peru, IL, p. A191
HOBECK, Susan, Chief Financial Officer, Community Memorial Hospital, Hicksville, OH, p. A481
HOBGOOD, Marcus, Director Information Services, LSU Medical Center–University Hospital, Shreveport, LA, p. A277
HOBSON, James M., President and Chief Executive Officer, Memorial Health Care System, Chattanooga, TN, p. A563
HOCE, N. Kristopher, Chief Operating Officer, Morton Plant Hospital, Clearwater, FL, p. A120
HOCHENBERG, Paul S., Senior Vice President Human Resources, Westchester Medical Center, Valhalla, NY, p. A445
HOCK, Douglas G., Senior Vice President Operations, Children's Medical Center of Dallas, Dallas, TX, p. A590
HOCKENBERRY, Michael A., Vice President Operations, Hanover Hospital, Hanover, PA, p. A524
HOCKENBURY, Debbie, Assistant Administrator and Chief Financial Officer, William Newton Hospital, Winfield, KS, p. A246
HOCKERT, Steve, Chief Executive Officer, Solara Hospital Conroe, Conroe, TX, p. A588
HOCKING, Barbara, R.N. Chief Operating Officer, Maine Coast Memorial Hospital, Ellsworth, ME, p. A283
HOCKING, Dale E.
Chief Financial Officer, Leesburg Regional Medical Center, Leesburg, FL, p. A129
Senior Vice President and Chief Financial Officer, The Villages Health System, The Villages, FL, p. A142
HOCUM, Timothy, Chief Financial Officer, Providence Kodiak Island Medical Center, Kodiak, AK, p. A29




Index of Health Care Professionals **A837**

Index of Health Care Professionals

Index of Health Care Professionals / Hodge

HODGE, Pamela, R.N. Chief Nursing Officer and Coordinator Performance Improvement, Jellico Community Hospital, Jellico, TN, p. A567
HODGES, Alan, Chief Operating Officer, Ochsner Medical Center – North Shore, Slidell, LA, p. A278
HODGES, Jay, Chief Financial Officer, Red River Regional Hospital, Bonham, TX, p. A584
HODGES, Joe, President, St. Anthony Hospital, Oklahoma City, OK, p. A502
HODGES, Randall H., President and Chief Executive Officer, CAMC Teays Valley Hospital, Hurricane, WV, p. A673
HODGES, Steve, Vice President Human Resources, Regional West Medical Center, Scottsbluff, NE, p. A389
HODGES, Teresa, Assistant Administrator, De Queen Medical Center, De Queen, AR, p. A43
HODGIN, Robin, R.N. Chief Administrator of Patient Care Services, Northern Hospital of Surry County, Mount Airy, NC, p. A458
HODGKINSON, Kimberly, Senior Vice President and Chief Financial Officer, St. Mary's Medical Center of Evansville, Evansville, IN, p. A201
HODGSON, Laurel, M.D. President Medical Staff, Doctors Medical Center–San Pablo Campus, San Pablo, CA, p. A89
HODSON, Don, M.D. Chief Medical Officer, St. Luke Hospital and Living Center, Marion, KS, p. A238
HOE, Adele, Director Human Resources, Castle Medical Center, Kailua, HI, p. A164
HOEFER, R. William, FACHE President, SSM St. Clare Health Center, Fenton, MO, p. A359
HOEFLE, Brian
Chief Financial Officer, Yavapai Regional Medical Center – East, Prescott Valley, AZ, p. A37
Chief Financial Officer, Yavapai Regional Medical Center, Prescott, AZ, p. A37
HOEFT, Thomas M., Executive Vice President and Chief Operating Officer, Huntington Hospital, Huntington, NY, p. A427
HOELL, Paul, M.D. President Medical Staff, New London Family Medical Center, New London, WI, p. A688
HOELSCHER, Steven C., Chief Operating Officer, Valley Regional Medical Center, Brownsville, TX, p. A585
HOEPPNER, David, M.D. Chief of Staff, Blue Ridge Regional Hospital, Spruce Pine, NC, p. A461
HOERTZ, Joanne, Vice President of Nursing, Brooks Rehabilitation Hospital, Jacksonville, FL, p. A126
HOFELICH, Kurt T., Vice President and Administrator, Sentara Obici Hospital, Suffolk, VA, p. A656
HOFER, Renee, Senior Vice President Fiscal Services, St. Joseph's Hospital of Buckhannon, Buckhannon, WV, p. A670
HOFF, David L., Chief Executive Officer, Wayne Memorial Hospital, Honesdale, PA, p. A525
HOFF, Linda, Chief Financial Officer, Meriter Hospital, Madison, WI, p. A684
HOFF, Margaret, Account Manager, Brown County Community Treatment Center, Green Bay, WI, p. A682
HOFFELD, Thomas, M.D. Chief of Staff, Spanish Peaks Regional Health Center, Walsenburg, CO, p. A106
HOFFER, Nolan, Chief Executive Officer, Southwest Idaho Advanced Care Hospital, Boise, ID, p. A166
HOFFMAN, Barbara, M.D. Chief Medical Officer, St. Christopher's Hospital for Children, Philadelphia, PA, p. A533
HOFFMAN, Brad, Administrative Director Human Resources, Shawnee Mission Medical Center, Shawnee Mission, KS, p. A243
HOFFMAN, Brian, Director Human Resources, Lancaster Regional Medical Center, Lancaster, PA, p. A526
HOFFMAN, Brian, M.D. Chief Medical Services, Veterans Affairs Boston Healthcare System, Boston, MA, p. A297
HOFFMAN, Cara, M.D. Chief of Staff, Parkway Medical Center, Decatur, AL, p. A18
HOFFMAN, Carole, Vice President, Parkridge Medical Center, Chattanooga, TN, p. A563
HOFFMAN, Charles, Vice President Financial Services and Chief Financial Officer, St. Joseph Mercy Livingston Hospital, Howell, MI, p. A315
HOFFMAN, Chris, Chief Operating Officer, Highlands Regional Medical Center, Prestonsburg, KY, p. A258
HOFFMAN, Daniel, M.D. Administrative Medical Director, Good Samaritan Regional Health Center, Mount Vernon, IL, p. A188
HOFFMAN, David E., M.D. Chief of Staff, North Big Horn Hospital District, Lovell, WY, p. A697
HOFFMAN, Debra, Manager Human Resources, Kern Valley Healthcare District, Lake Isabella, CA, p. A66
HOFFMAN, Glenn G., MS, Chief Executive Officer, Allegiance Behavioral Health Center of Plainview, Plainview, TX, p. A621
HOFFMAN, Howard, M.D. Medical Director, Psychiatric Institute of Washington, Washington, DC, p. A117
HOFFMAN, Jerry, Chief Financial Officer, Platte Health Center Avera, Platte, SD, p. A558
HOFFMAN, III, Joseph E.
Senior Vice President and Chief Financial Officer, Harford Memorial Hospital, Havre De Grace, MD, p. A292
Senior Vice President and Chief Financial Officer, Upper Chesapeake Medical Center, Bel Air, MD, p. A289
HOFFMAN, Mark, Chief Financial Officer, Oro Valley Hospital, Oro Valley, AZ, p. A34
HOFFMAN, Mary, Chief Financial Officer, Mayo Clinic Jacksonville, Jacksonville, FL, p. A126
HOFFMAN, Pamela S., Director of Human Resources, Monroe Hospital, Bloomington, IN, p. A198
HOFFMAN, Robert P., Vice President and Director Patient Care Services, Wilkes–Barre General Hospital, Wilkes–Barre, PA, p. A542
HOFFMAN, Todd, M.D. Medical Director, St. John Broken Arrow, Broken Arrow, OK, p. A494
HOFFMAN, Tom, Manager Information Systems, Wayne Memorial Hospital, Honesdale, PA, p. A525
HOFFMAN, Trudy, Executive Director, Northwest Center for Behavioral Health, Fort Supply, OK, p. A497
HOFFMAN, Val, Chief Financial Officer, Granite Falls Municipal Hospital and Manor, Granite Falls, MN, p. A332
HOFFMANN, Nancy, Vice President Finance, Carney Hospital, Boston, MA, p. A296
HOFFMANN, Wanda, Director Human Resources, River Oaks Hospital, New Orleans, LA, p. A275
HOFHEINS, Todd, Chief Financial Officer, Providence Regional Medical Center Everett, Everett, WA, p. A661
HOFIUS, Chuck, Chief Executive Officer, Perham Health, Perham, MN, p. A337
HOFMANN, Bill, M.D. Chief Medical Staff, Grays Harbor Community Hospital, Aberdeen, WA, p. A659
HOFSTETTER, Peter A., Chief Executive Officer, Holy Cross Hospital, Taos, NM, p. A418
HOGAN, Brian, Interim Chief Executive Officer, Baptist Rehabilitation–Germantown, Germantown, TN, p. A566
HOGAN, Judith, Comptroller and Director Resources and Logistics, Naval Hospital Bremerton, Bremerton, WA, p. A659
HOGAN, Michael, Chief Resource Management, General Leonard Wood Army Community Hospital, Fort Leonard Wood, MO, p. A360
HOGAN, Michael F., Ph.D. Commissioner, New York State Office of Mental Health, Albany, NY, p. B93
HOGAN, Richard H., CP
Chief Financial Officer, Landmark Hospital, Cape Girardeau, MO, p. A356
Chief Financial Officer, Landmark Hospital of Joplin, Joplin, MO, p. A361
HOGAN, Ronald E., Senior Vice President and Chief Financial Officer, St. Francis Medical Center, Monroe, LA, p. A273
HOGAN, Sean, President, SSM DePaul Health Center, Bridgeton, MO, p. A356
HOGAN, Timothy J., FACHE President, Riverview Medical Center, Red Bank, NJ, p. A409
HOGG, Donna, Supervisor Medical Records, Monroe County Hospital, Forsyth, GA, p. A153
HOHENBERGER, Joseph W., Chief Financial Officer, Mecosta County Medical Center, Big Rapids, MI, p. A308
HOHMANN, Terry, Chief Financial Officer, Kindred Hospital North Houston, Houston, TX, p. A604
HOKANSON, Lindee, Administrator, Idaho Falls Recovery Center, Idaho Falls, ID, p. A168
HOLBERT, Trisha, Vice President Human Resources, Mercy Hospital Springfield, Springfield, MO, p. A371
HOLBROOK, Chip, M.D. Chief of Staff, Simpson General Hospital, Mendenhall, MS, p. A350
HOLBROOK–PRESTON, Susan, Chief Operating Officer and Chief Nursing Officer, Indiana Heart Hospital, Indianapolis, IN, p. A204
HOLCOMB, Daxton, Chief Executive Officer, Freeman Neosho Hospital, Neosho, MO, p. A366
HOLCOMB, Holly, Chief Operating Officer, Childress Regional Medical Center, Childress, TX, p. A587
HOLCOMB, Ralph, Chief Information Officer, Good Shepherd Medical Center, Longview, TX, p. A613
HOLCOMB, Steven, M.D. Chief of Staff, Aurora Medical Center of Washington County, Hartford, WI, p. A683
HOLCOMBE, Sheryl, Administrative Assistant, Brownfield Regional Medical Center, Brownfield, TX, p. A585
HOLDEMAN, Royce, Chief Financial Officer, Mercy Hospital, Moundridge, KS, p. A239
HOLDEN, Angie, Chief Executive Officer, Regency Hospital of Cincinnati, Cincinnati, OH, p. A474
HOLDEN, Jay T., Vice President, Human Resources, Beaumont Hospital Grosse Pointe, Grosse Pointe, MI, p. A314
HOLDEN, Peter J., President and Chief Executive Officer, Jordan Hospital, Plymouth, MA, p. A304
HOLDEN, Tami, Director Human Resources, HEALTHSOUTH Bakersfield Rehabilitation Hospital, Bakersfield, CA, p. A54
HOLDER, Hal
Director Finance, SSM DePaul Health Center, Bridgeton, MO, p. A356
Vice President Finance, SSM St. Joseph Health Center, Saint Charles, MO, p. A368
Director Finance, SSM St. Joseph Hospital West, Lake Saint Louis, MO, p. A363
HOLDER, Joanna, Director Human Resources, Franklin Regional Medical Center, Louisburg, NC, p. A457
HOLDER, John, Chief Financial Officer, Mission Community Hospital, Valencia, CA, p. A94
HOLDER, Whitt
Chief Financial Officer, Physicians Surgical Hospital – Panhandle Campus, Amarillo, TX, p. A578
Chief Financial Officer, Physicians Surgical Hospital – Quail Creek, Amarillo, TX, p. A578
HOLDERMAN, Clay, Interim Administrator, Presbyterian Hospital, Albuquerque, NM, p. A414
HOLDERMAN, Wanda, Chief Executive Officer, Fresno Heart and Surgical Hospital, Fresno, CA, p. A62
HOLEKAMP, Nicholas, M.D. Medical Director, Ranken Jordan – A Pediatric Specialty Hospital, Maryland Heights, MO, p. A364
HOLEMAN, John, M.D. Chief of Staff, Methodist Hospital Union County, Morganfield, KY, p. A256
HOLGUIN, Mindee, Manager Human Resources, Sierra Vista Hospital, Truth or Consequences, NM, p. A418
HOLIDAY, Pam, Director Management Information Systems, Greene Memorial Hospital, Xenia, OH, p. A492
HOLINER, Joel, M.D. Executive Medical Director, Green Oaks Hospital, Dallas, TX, p. A591
HOLLAND, David
Chief Information Officer, Herrin Hospital, Herrin, IL, p. A184
Vice President Information Services, St. Joseph Memorial Hospital, Murphysboro, IL, p. A188
HOLLAND, Gabrielle, Chief Financial Officer, Irving Coppell Surgical Hospital, Irving, TX, p. A609
HOLLAND, Jeffrey S., Chief Executive Officer, Bayshore Medical Center, Pasadena, TX, p. A620
HOLLAND, Kevin, Chief Operating Officer, Singing River Health System, Pascagoula, MS, p. A351
HOLLAND, Kwi, Vice President Information Services, Knox Community Hospital, Mount Vernon, OH, p. A485
HOLLAND, Linda, Controller, Weston County Health Services, Newcastle, WY, p. A697
HOLLAND, Michael, M.D. Chief Executive Officer, Rehabilitation Hospital of Jennings, Jennings, LA, p. A268
HOLLAND, Robert, M.D. President Professional Staff, Columbia Memorial Hospital, Astoria, OR, p. A509
HOLLAND, Shannon S., R.N. Vice President of Patient Care Service, St. James Healthcare, Butte, MT, p. A374
HOLLAND, Sharron, Chief Financial Officer, Baptist Memorial Hospital–Huntingdon, Huntingdon, TN, p. A566
HOLLAND, Steve, M.D. Chief Medical Officer, Saint Mary's Hospital, Waterbury, CT, p. A112
HOLLANDER, Charles, M.D. Vice President and Chief Operating Officer, Hospital of Saint Raphael, New Haven, CT, p. A110
HOLLEMAN, Ivan, Chief Financial Officer, Baxter Regional Medical Center, Mountain Home, AR, p. A49
HOLLEMAN, James, M.D. Chief of Staff, St. Luke's Hospital, Columbus, NC, p. A451
HOLLEMAN, Stephen B., Chief Financial Officer, Shepherd Center, Atlanta, GA, p. A146
HOLLEY, Shay, M.D. President Medical Staff, Davis Hospital and Medical Center, Layton, UT, p. A638
HOLLIDAY, Michael T., Vice President Fiscal and Administrative Services, Van Wert County Hospital, Van Wert, OH, p. A490
HOLLIMAN, Emily L., President, Norwood Hospital, Norwood, MA, p. A303
HOLLINGER, Brad, Chairman and Chief Executive Officer, Vibra Healthcare, Mechanicsburg, PA, p. B142
HOLLINGER, Lori, Manager Human Resources, Fulton State Hospital, Fulton, MO, p. A360
HOLLINGSWORTH, Carl, Chief Financial Officer, St. Luke's Wood River Medical Center, Ketchum, ID, p. A168
HOLLINGSWORTH, Christine, Chief Financial Officer, Phoenix Veterans Affairs Health Care System, Phoenix, AZ, p. A36
HOLLINGSWORTH, Nancy, MSN, President and Chief Executive Officer, Saint Agnes Medical Center, Fresno, CA, p. A62
HOLLINGSWORTH, Sherri, Chief Human Resources Officer, University of Utah Health Care – Hospital and Clinics, Salt Lake City, UT, p. A641
HOLLIS, Tom, Chief Financial Officer, Ellett Memorial Hospital, Appleton City, MO, p. A355
HOLLMANN, Mark, M.D. Chief of Staff, Florida Hospital DeLand, DeLand, FL, p. A122
HOLLON, Kim Norton, FACHE Chief Executive Officer, Signature Healthcare Brockton Hospital, Brockton, MA, p. A298
HOLLOWAY, David, M.D. Chief Medical Officer, West Valley Hospital, Dallas, OR, p. A510

**A838** Index of Health Care Professionals

Index of Health Care Professionals / Horner

Index of Health Care Professionals

HOLLOWAY, Kary, Director Human Resources, Ocean Beach Hospital, Ilwaco, WA, p. A662
HOLLOWAY, Mary Ann, Manager Human Resources, Girard Medical Center, Girard, KS, p. A233
HOLLOWAY, Myra, Director Human Resources Management, Central State Hospital, Milledgeville, GA, p. A156
HOLLOWAY, W. David, M.D. Chief Medical Officer, Salem Hospital, Salem, OR, p. A515
HOLLOWELL, Robert, Director Information Systems, Swedish Medical Center, Englewood, CO, p. A100
HOLM, Mary Ann, Office Clerk, Tioga Medical Center, Tioga, ND, p. A468
HOLM, Pamela, R.N. Administrator, Perkins County Health Services, Grant, NE, p. A384
HOLM, Stan V., FACHE Chief Executive Officer, Midwest Regional Medical Center, Midwest City, OK, p. A499
HOLMAN, Diane, Manager Human Resources, Alta View Hospital, Sandy, UT, p. A641
HOLMAN, Steve, President, The Jewish Hospital, Cincinnati, OH, p. A474
HOLMAN, William R., FACHE President and Chief Executive Officer, Baton Rouge General Medical Center, Baton Rouge, LA, p. A262
HOLMES Jr., James M., President and Chief Executive Officer, Rappahannock General Hospital, Kilmarnock, VA, p. A650
HOLMES, James R., President and Chief Executive Officer, Redlands Community Hospital, Redlands, CA, p. A82
HOLMES, Jeremy, D.O. Chief of Staff, Kalkaska Memorial Health Center, Kalkaska, MI, p. A317
HOLMES, John, Business Manager, Ancora Psychiatric Hospital, Ancora, NJ, p. A401
HOLMES, John A., Chief Financial Officer, Ephrata Community Hospital, Ephrata, PA, p. A523
HOLMES, Mardy, Director Information Technology, Arkansas Methodist Medical Center, Paragould, AR, p. A50
HOLMES, Terry R., M.D. Clinical Director, Moccasin Bend Mental Health Institute, Chattanooga, TN, p. A563
HOLMES, William E., Chief Executive Officer, Moses Ludington Hospital, Ticonderoga, NY, p. A444
HOLMLUND, Billie, Director Information Services, Montana State Hospital, Warm Springs, MT, p. A379
HOLOM, Randall G., Chief Executive Officer, Frances Mahon Deaconess Hospital, Glasgow, MT, p. A375
HOLSCHBACH, Dennis, Chief Financial Officer and Director Human Resources, Ruby Valley Hospital, Sheridan, MT, p. A379
HOLST, Ken, Chief Financial Officer, Borgess–Lee Memorial Hospital, Dowagiac, MI, p. A311
HOLSTEEN, Marcie, Human Resources Officer, Wamego City Hospital, Wamego, KS, p. A244
HOLSTEN, Jack W., Chief Financial Officer, Vidant Medical Center, Greenville, NC, p. A454
HOLSTIEN, Bruce, President and Chief Executive Officer, Spartanburg Regional Healthcare System, Spartanburg, SC, p. B121
HOLSTON, James, M.D. Vice President and Chief Quality Officer, South Central Regional Medical Center, Laurel, MS, p. A348
HOLT, Annie, FACHE Chief Executive Officer, Alaska Regional Hospital, Anchorage, AK, p. A28
HOLT, Brian, Chief Executive Officer, Warm Springs Specialty Hospital of Victoria, Victoria, TX, p. A633
HOLT, Kory
  Division Controller Network Operations, Avera Dells Area Hospital, Dell Rapids, SD, p. A556
  Division Controller Network Operations, Avera Flandreau Hospital, Flandreau, SD, p. A556
HOLT, Mari J., R.N. Director Patient Care Services, Cambridge Medical Center, Cambridge, MN, p. A329
HOLT, Thomas A., Chief Financial Officer, Conroe Regional Medical Center, Conroe, TX, p. A588
HOLTHAUS, Julie K., Director Human Resources, Sabetha Community Hospital, Sabetha, KS, p. A242
HOLTHAUS, Monica, Chief Financial Officer, Community Health Care System, Onaga, KS, p. A240
HOLTZ, George, Manager Human Resources, Sharp Coronado Hospital and Healthcare Center, Coronado, CA, p. A58
HOLTZ, Mark, Chief Operating Officer, Overlook Medical Center, Summit, NJ, p. A410
HOLTZ, Noel, M.D. Chief Medical Officer, WellStar Douglas Hospital, Douglasville, GA, p. A151
HOLTZMAN, Michael, M.D. Medical Director, Kindred Hospital–St. Louis, Saint Louis, MO, p. A368
HOLUB, Gloria, Manager Communications, Oaklawn Psychiatric Center, Goshen, IN, p. A202
HOLYFIELD, Linda S., MSN, President and Chief Executive Officer, P & S Surgical Hospital, Monroe, LA, p. A273
HOLYOAK, Mark, Chief Executive Officer, Castleview Hospital, Price, UT, p. A639
HOLZER, Traci, Director Human Resources, Doctors Hospital of Manteca, Manteca, CA, p. A73
HOLZHEI, Gregory, D.O. Chief of Staff, Sparrow Clinton Hospital, Saint Johns, MI, p. A322
HOMA, Jim, Chief Executive Officer, Heatherhill Care Communities, Chardon, OH, p. A472
HOMAN, Cheryl, Administrative Director, Lima Memorial Health System, Lima, OH, p. A482
HOMAS, Dallas, Commander, Madigan Healthcare System, Tacoma, WA, p. A668
HOMER, Kenneth, M.D. Chief Medical Officer, Holy Cross Hospital, Fort Lauderdale, FL, p. A123
HOMERSKI, James, Director Information Services, Miners Medical Center, Hastings, PA, p. A524
HOMYK, David, Vice President Human Resources, Beaufort Memorial Hospital, Beaufort, SC, p. A546
HOMYK, Linda, Chief Nursing Officer, Sewickley Valley Hospital, (A Division of Valley Medical Facilities), Sewickley, PA, p. A538
HONAHNIE, De Alva, Chief Executive Officer, Hopi Health Care Center, Keams Canyon, AZ, p. A33
HONAINY, Hassan, M.D. President Medical Staff, LewisGale Hospital Alleghany, Low Moor, VA, p. A650
HONAKER, Linda, Vice President Financial Operations, Scripps Memorial Hospital–La Jolla, La Jolla, CA, p. A66
HONAKER, Robert, Associate Administrator and Chief Human Resources Officer, Pioneers Memorial Healthcare District, Brawley, CA, p. A56
HONAN, Thomas, Interim Chief Financial Officer, Loyola University Medical Center, Maywood, IL, p. A187
HONDLEY, Charles, Chief Financial Officer, Providence Memorial Hospital, El Paso, TX, p. A596
HONEA, Bert, M.D. Medical Director, McKee Medical Center, Loveland, CO, p. A104
HONEA, Bruce, Director Information Services, CHRISTUS Coushatta Health Care Center, Coushatta, LA, p. A264
HONERBRINK, Daniel, Vice President Finance and Chief Financial Officer, Fairmont General Hospital, Fairmont, WV, p. A671
HONEYCUTT, Cynthia, Director Human Resources, Moccasin Bend Mental Health Institute, Chattanooga, TN, p. A563
HONEYCUTT, Tammy, R.N. Director of Nursing, Jasper Memorial Hospital, Monticello, GA, p. A156
HONEYWELL, Robert, Site Administrator, Mercy Hospital Joplin, Joplin, MO, p. A361
HONKE, Richard, M.D. Chief of Staff, Avera St. Benedict Hospital, Parkston, SD, p. A558
HONSINGER, Melissa, Chief Operating Officer, Elks Rehab Hospital, Boise, ID, p. A166
HONTS, Gary, Chief Executive Officer, Creighton University Medical Center, Omaha, NE, p. A387
HOO–YOU, Hilary, Regional Administrator, Southwestern State Hospital, Thomasville, GA, p. A160
HOOD, Fred B., FACHE Administrator, North Mississippi Medical Center–Pontotoc Hospital and Nursing Home, Pontotoc, MS, p. A352
HOOD, Kathy, Administrative Assistant, Union General Hospital, Blairsville, GA, p. A147
HOOD, M. Michelle, President and Chief Executive Officer, Eastern Maine Healthcare Systems, Brewer, ME, p. B49
HOOD, Tom, Administrator, Tippah County Hospital, Ripley, MS, p. A352
HOOFMAN, Kevin, Director Management Information, White County Medical Center, Searcy, AR, p. A51
HOOK, Diane, Chief Financial Officer, Wayne County Hospital, Corydon, IA, p. A217
HOOK, Jeanette L., R.N. Chief Nursing Officer, Union County Hospital, Anna, IL, p. A172
HOOK, Linda, Chief Executive Officer, Promise Specialty Hospital of Salt Lake, Salt Lake City, UT, p. A640
HOOKER, Melvin, Chief Human Resources, Veterans Affairs Medical Center, Albuquerque, NM, p. A415
HOOKER, Rita, Administrative Director Information Services, Bon Secours St. Francis Health System, Greenville, SC, p. A550
HOOKS, Al, Senior Vice President and Chief Financial Officer, Nash Health Care Systems, Rocky Mount, NC, p. A460
HOOKS, Jr., Dwayne, R.N
  Chief Clinical Officer, MedWest – Harris, Sylva, NC, p. A461
  Chief Nursing Officer, MedWest – Haywood, Clyde, NC, p. A451
HOOPER, Andy
  Director Human Resources, Skyline Madison Campus, Madison, TN, p. A570
  Director Human Resources, Skyline Medical Center, Nashville, TN, p. A573
HOOPER, Grady, Chief Executive Officer, Seton Smithville Regional Hospital, Smithville, TX, p. A628
HOOPER, Helen, Director Human Resources, Southwestern Medical Center, Lawton, OK, p. A498
HOOPER, Joseph, Vice President Operations, OhioHealth Marion General Hospital, Marion, OH, p. A484
HOOPES, John L., Chief Executive Officer, Caribou Memorial Hospital and Living Center, Soda Springs, ID, p. A170
HOORNAERT, Jennifer, Chief Financial Officer, Carrington Health Center, Carrington, ND, p. A464
HOOSE, Gregory R., Chief Executive Officer, Straith Hospital for Special Surgery, Southfield, MI, p. A323
HOOVER, Alvin, FACHE Chief Executive Officer, King's Daughters Medical Center, Brookhaven, MS, p. A344
HOOVER, Dana, Chief Financial Officer, Hedrick Medical Center, Chillicothe, MO, p. A357
HOOVER, Garrett W., FACHE President and Chief Executive Officer, Nason Hospital, Roaring Spring, PA, p. A537
HOOVER, Jeremy, Chief Information Officer, Kiowa County Memorial Hospital, Greensburg, KS, p. A234
HOOVER, Kara, Controller and Director Human Resources, Keefe Memorial Hospital, Cheyenne Wells, CO, p. A98
HOOVER, Leon, Director Information Systems, Hendry Regional Medical Center, Clewiston, FL, p. A120
HOPE, Joseph D., D.O. President Medical Staff, Riddle Hospital, Media, PA, p. A529
HOPE, Lisa R., Director Human Resources, Muhlenberg Community Hospital, Greenville, KY, p. A251
HOPE, Steve, Vice President Corporate Services, Methodist Rehabilitation Center, Jackson, MS, p. A348
HOPE, IV, William, M.D. Chief of Medical Staff, Vidant Chowan Hospital, Edenton, NC, p. A452
HOPF, Georg J., President and Chief Executive Officer, Pacific Health Corporation, Tustin, CA, p. B99
HOPKINS, Frances F., Chief Financial Officer, Sabine Medical Center, Many, LA, p. A272
HOPKINS, Jason, Director Human Resources, Murray Medical Center, Chatsworth, GA, p. A149
HOPKINS, Kelli, Director Human Resources, H.S.C. Medical Center, Malvern, AR, p. A48
HOPKINS, Ken, Vice President Finance and Chief Financial Officer, Norman Regional Health System, Norman, OK, p. A500
HOPKINS, Laura, Director of Nursing, Mayo Clinic Health System in New Prague, New Prague, MN, p. A336
HOPKINS, Maura, R.N. Chief Nursing Officer, R M L Specialty Hospital, Hinsdale, IL, p. A184
HOPKINS, Paul, Chief Financial Officer, Harry S. Truman Memorial Veterans Hospital, Columbia, MO, p. A358
HOPKINS, Wade, Administrator, Southern Virginia Mental Health Institute, Danville, VA, p. A647
HOPKINS, William, Director Finance, Carolinas Rehabilitation, Charlotte, NC, p. A450
HOPP, Eva, Chief Nurse Executive, Pinckneyville Community Hospital, Pinckneyville, IL, p. A191
HOPPS, Deborah, Chief Executive Officer, HEALTHSOUTH Rehabilitation Hospital–Cityview, Fort Worth, TX, p. A598
HOPSON, W. Briggs, M.D. Clinical Medical Director, River Region Medical Center, Vicksburg, MS, p. A353
HORAN, Chris, M.D. Chief of Staff, Saint Mary's Regional Medical Center, Russellville, AR, p. A51
HORAN, Gary S., FACHE President and Chief Executive Officer, Trinitas Regional Medical Center, Elizabeth, NJ, p. A403
HORAN, Patrick, M.D. Chief of Staff, Town and Country Hospital, Tampa, FL, p. A141
HORAN, Sandra A., Executive Director, Margaretville Hospital, Margaretville, NY, p. A429
HORATH, Kevin, Director Human Resources, Decatur Memorial Hospital, Decatur, IL, p. A179
HORLANDER, Fred J., Vice President, Clark Memorial Hospital, Jeffersonville, IN, p. A205
HORN, Bill, Director Human Resources, Wickenburg Community Hospital, Wickenburg, AZ, p. A41
HORN, Jeff, Coordinator Information Systems, Jay County Hospital, Portland, IN, p. A210
HORN, LeeAnn, Chief Nurse Executive, Providence Kodiak Island Medical Center, Kodiak, AK, p. A29
HORN, Mike, M.D. Vice President Medical Affairs, Saint Francis Medical Center, Grand Island, NE, p. A384
HORN, Syndi, Director Information Systems, Memorial Hospital, Carthage, IL, p. A174
HORNBURG, Tom, Director Information Systems, Mason General Hospital, Shelton, WA, p. A666
HORNE, Barbara, R.N. Vice President and Chief Human Resource Development Officer, Indian River Medical Center, Vero Beach, FL, p. A142
HORNE, Beth, System Administrator Information Technology, Preston Memorial Hospital, Kingwood, WV, p. A673
HORNE, Eilene, Manager Human Resources, Mountain View Hospital, Idaho Falls, ID, p. A168
HORNE, Wallace J., M.D. Vice President Medical Affairs, Betsy Johnson Regional Hospital, Dunn, NC, p. A452
HORNER, Bryan, President and Chief Executive Officer, Shannon Medical Center, San Angelo, TX, p. A624
HORNER, Cheryl, Supervisor Data Processing, Community Memorial Hospital, Staunton, IL, p. A194
HORNER, James, Chief Information Officer, Veterans Affairs Medical Center, Portland, OR, p. A514

Index of Health Care Professionals / Horner

HORNER, John, Manager Business Office, Veterans Affairs Medical Center, Omaha, NE, p. A388
HORNER, John M., President and Chief Executive Officer, Major Hospital, Shelbyville, IN, p. A211
HORNING, Phyllis, Chief Financial Officer, Hamilton County Hospital, Syracuse, KS, p. A243
HORNUNG, Dona, Director Information and Technology Services, Doctors Hospital, Augusta, GA, p. A146
HORNUNG, Kurt, Director, Medical Center of Trinity, Trinity, FL, p. A142
HORNUUG, Joel, M.D. Chief Medical Officer, Morris County Hospital, Council Grove, KS, p. A232
HOROWITZ, Ira, M.D. Chief Medical Officer, Emory University Hospital, Atlanta, GA, p. A145
HORRAR, James L., President and Chief Executive Officer, QHR, Brentwood, TN, p. B106
HORRAS, Susan, Chief Financial Officer, Mahaska Health Partnership, Oskaloosa, IA, p. A225
HORROCKS, Chad, M.D. Chief of Staff, Teton Valley Hospital and Surgicenter, Driggs, ID, p. A168
HORSMAN, Sarah
Vice President Human Resources, MultiCare Good Samaritan Hospital, Puyallup, WA, p. A664
Senior Vice President Human Potential, MultiCare Mary Bridge Children's Hospital and Health Center, Tacoma, WA, p. A668
Senior Vice President Human Potential, MultiCare Tacoma General Hospital, Tacoma, WA, p. A668
HORST, Brad, Director Human Resources, Clear Lake Regional Medical Center, Webster, TX, p. A634
HORTON, Cynthia, M.D. Chief Medical Officer, Skyline Hospital, White Salmon, WA, p. A669
HORTON, Eileen M., Vice President, Patient Services/Chief Nursing Officer, Capital Health Regional Medical Center, Trenton, NJ, p. A411
HORTON, Greg, Director Support Services, State Hospital South, Blackfoot, ID, p. A166
HORTON, Jim, Chief Executive Officer, Pecos County Memorial Hospital, Fort Stockton, TX, p. A598
HORTON, Kenny, Director Information Systems, Walker Baptist Medical Center, Jasper, AL, p. A22
HORTON, Lynn M., Executive Director Human Resources, Fresno Heart and Surgical Hospital, Fresno, CA, p. A62
HORTON, Marie, Director Associate Relations, Bartow Regional Medical Center, Bartow, FL, p. A118
HORTON, Warren, Information Technologist, Baptist Health Medical Center–Stuttgart, Stuttgart, AR, p. A51
HORVAT, Kami, Chief Financial Officer, Doctors Hospital of West Covina, West Covina, CA, p. A95
HORVATH, Alex, Vice President Human Resources, Advocate BroMenn Medical Center, Normal, IL, p. A189
HORVATH, Dolores A., Chief Executive Officer, Pikes Peak Regional Hospital, Woodland Park, CO, p. A107
HOSFELD, Anne L., Chief Administrative Officer, Novato Community Hospital, Novato, CA, p. A77
HOSKINS, Michael, Chief Operating Officer, Fairview Park Hospital, Dublin, GA, p. A152
HOSKINS, Pearly Graham, M.D. President Medical Staff, Cape Fear Valley – Bladen County Hospital, Elizabethtown, NC, p. A453
HOSKINS, Shirley, Chief Operating Officer, Meadows Regional Medical Center, Vidalia, GA, p. A161
HOSLER, Steve, Regional Vice President Human Resources, Mercy Medical Center Redding, Redding, CA, p. A81
HOSTEENEZ, Vivie, Chief Financial Officer, U. S. Public Health Service Indian Hospital, San Carlos, AZ, p. A37
HOSTETLER, Barbara, Chief Operating Officer and Chief Nursing Officer, Regional Hospital for Respiratory and Complex Care, Seattle, WA, p. A665
HOSTETTER, Lynne, Vice President Human Resources, The HSC Pediatric Center, Washington, DC, p. A117
HOTA, Bala, Interim Chief Information Officer, John H. Stroger Jr. Hospital of Cook County, Chicago, IL, p. A176
HOTALING, Andrew, Chief Executive Officer, Forest View Psychiatric Hospital, Grand Rapids, MI, p. A313
HOTCHKISS, Jason, Controller, Teton Valley Hospital and Surgicenter, Driggs, ID, p. A168
HOTES, Lawrence S., M.D. Chief Medical Officer, New England Sinai Hospital and Rehabilitation Center, Stoughton, MA, p. A305
HOTT, Judith, Chief Executive Officer, Thomas B. Finan Center, Cumberland, MD, p. A291
HOTTENDORF, Catherine, MS, Executive Director, Franklin Hospital, Valley Stream, NY, p. A445
HOUGHTON, Roxan, Director Human Resources, Promise Hospital of Miss Lou, Vidalia, LA, p. A279
HOULE, David, Executive Vice President and Chief Financial Officer, The Hospital at Hebrew Health Care, West Hartford, CT, p. A113
HOULIHAN, David, M.D. Chief of Staff, Veterans Affairs Medical Center, Tomah, WI, p. A692
HOUMANN, Lars D., President, Florida Hospital, Orlando, FL, p. A134
HOUSE, Alan, Chief Financial Officer, Margaret R. Pardee Memorial Hospital, Hendersonville, NC, p. A454
HOUSE, David
Vice President, Baptist Health Extended Care Hospital, Little Rock, AR, p. A47
Vice President and Chief Information Officer, Baptist Health Medical Center – North Little Rock, North Little Rock, AR, p. A50
Vice President and Chief Information Officer, Baptist Health Medical Center–Arkadelphia, Arkadelphia, AR, p. A42
Vice President and Chief Information Officer, Baptist Health Medical Center–Little Rock, Little Rock, AR, p. A47
Vice President and Chief Information Officer, Baptist Health Rehabilitation Institute, Little Rock, AR, p. A48
HOUSE, Judy White, Director Human Resources, Houston Northwest Medical Center, Houston, TX, p. A604
HOUSER, Kirk, Director Administration, Naval Hospital Bremerton, Bremerton, WA, p. A659
HOUSER, Kris, M.D. Medical Director, Peninsula Hospital, Louisville, TN, p. A570
HOUSER, Robert, FACHE Chief Executive Officer, Blue Mountain Hospital, John Day, OR, p. A511
HOUSER–HANFELDER, Sallie, FACHE Director, Harry S. Truman Memorial Veterans Hospital, Columbia, MO, p. A358
HOUSH, Steven C., President, Fairview Lakes Health Services, Wyoming, MN, p. A342
HOUSLEY, Kristin, Chief Management Information Systems, South Lincoln Medical Center, Kemmerer, WY, p. A696
HOUSMAN, Hunter, M.D. Chief Medical Officer, Bourbon Community Hospital, Paris, KY, p. A258
HOUSTON, Anthony, Executive Vice President, St. Marys Health Center, Jefferson City, MO, p. A361
HOUSTON, Jerry, Director Information Systems, Jennie Stuart Medical Center, Hopkinsville, KY, p. A251
HOUSTON, Sally, M.D. Senior Vice President and Chief Medical Officer, Tampa General Hospital, Tampa, FL, p. A141
HOUSTON, Sandra Davis
Vice President Human Resources, California Hospital Medical Center, Los Angeles, CA, p. A68
Vice President Human Resources and Organizational Development, Glendale Memorial Hospital and Health Center, Glendale, CA, p. A63
HOUSTON, William J., M.D. Medical Director, Indiana University Health La Porte Hospital, La Porte, IN, p. A206
HOVAN, Keith A., President and Chief Executive Officer, Southcoast Hospitals Group, Fall River, MA, p. A300
HOVE, Barton A., President, Wellmont Bristol Regional Medical Center, Bristol, TN, p. A562
HOVENS, Michael R., M.D. Chief Medical Officer, Tri–Lakes Medical Center, Batesville, MS, p. A343
HOVHANESIAN, Joan, Vice President and Chief Information Officer, Shands at the University of Florida, Gainesville, FL, p. A124
HOWALT, Lyra, Chief Financial Officer, Central Carolina Hospital, Sanford, NC, p. A460
HOWARD, Catherine, Director Human Resources, Halifax Regional Health System, South Boston, VA, p. A656
HOWARD, Charles, M.D. Chief of Staff, St. Vincent Morrilton, Morrilton, AR, p. A49
HOWARD, Cindy, Director Financial Services, Oneida County Hospital, Malad City, ID, p. A169
HOWARD, Craig
Director, Veterans Affairs Medical Center, Canandaigua, NY, p. A423
Interim Director, Veterans Affairs Western New York Healthcare System–Buffalo Division, Buffalo, NY, p. A423
HOWARD, Daniel, Chief Financial Officer, Veterans Affairs Medical Center, Togus, ME, p. A285
HOWARD, Darcy, Chief Executive Officer and Chief Financial Officer, Logan County Hospital, Oakley, KS, p. A240
HOWARD, Eddie L.
Vice President and Chief Operating Officer, East Texas Medical Center Rehabilitation Center, Tyler, TX, p. A632
Vice President, Chief Operating Officer and Administrator, East Texas Medical Center Specialty Hospital, Tyler, TX, p. A632
HOWARD, Gary L., Senior Vice President, Chief Financial Officer and Corporate Compliance Officer, Hamilton Medical Center, Dalton, GA, p. A151
HOWARD, Greg M., Director Human Resource, Kingston Hospital, Kingston, NY, p. A428
HOWARD, Jill, R.N. Chief Operating Officer, Skyline Madison Campus, Madison, TN, p. A570
HOWARD, Katherine, Director Human Resources, Baptist Medical Center Nassau, Fernandina Beach, FL, p. A123
HOWARD, Loy M., President and Chief Executive Officer, Tanner Health System, Carrollton, GA, p. B126
HOWARD, Loy M., President and Chief Executive Officer, Tanner Medical Center, Carrollton, GA, p. A148
HOWARD, Norma N., Chief Executive Officer, Lindsay Municipal Hospital, Lindsay, OK, p. A498
HOWARD, Opal R., Director Human Resources, Florida Hospital DeLand, DeLand, FL, p. A122
HOWARD, Pamela B., R.N. Administrator, Lake Butler Hospital Hand Surgery Center, Lake Butler, FL, p. A128
HOWARD, Randy, M.D. Chief of Staff, Hendersonville Medical Center, Hendersonville, TN, p. A566
HOWARD, Roger, M.D. Senior Vice President and Medical Director, Beaumont Hospital – Troy, Troy, MI, p. A324
HOWARD, Roger, President and Chief Executive Officer, Dearborn County Hospital, Lawrenceburg, IN, p. A207
HOWARD, Ron, Chief Financial Officer, Holly Hill Hospital, Raleigh, NC, p. A459
HOWARD, Sabra, Manager Human Resources, Harlan ARH Hospital, Harlan, KY, p. A251
HOWARD, Stacy M., R.N. Chief Executive Officer, Kindred Hospital–St. Louis, Saint Louis, MO, p. A368
HOWARD, Teresa, Manager Human Resources, Yoakum County Hospital, Denver City, TX, p. A594
HOWARD, Tim, Chief Human Resources Officer, Fountain Valley Regional Hospital and Medical Center, Fountain Valley, CA, p. A61
HOWARD, Tom, Chief Financial Officer, Texas Health Presbyterian Hospital Flower Mound, Flower Mound, TX, p. A597
HOWARD, Win, Chief Executive Officer, Three Rivers Medical Center, Grants Pass, OR, p. A511
HOWARD–CROW, Dallis
Chief Human Resources Officer, Emory University Hospital Midtown, Atlanta, GA, p. A145
Chief Human Resources Officer, Wesley Woods Geriatric Hospital of Emory University, Atlanta, GA, p. A146
HOWART, Peg, Coordinator Human Resources and Benefits, Harlan County Health System, Alma, NE, p. A381
HOWAT, Greg, Vice President Human Resources, Eastern Maine Medical Center, Bangor, ME, p. A281
HOWDEN, Tim, Interim Chief Financial Officer, Grays Harbor Community Hospital, Aberdeen, WA, p. A659
HOWE, Debbie, Chief Executive Officer, Weatherford Regional Hospital, Weatherford, OK, p. A507
HOWE, Huberta Mayfield, Director Human Resources, Cooper Green Mercy Hospital, Birmingham, AL, p. A16
HOWE, James L., Chief Employee Relations, Pinnacle Pointe Hospital, Little Rock, AR, p. A48
HOWE, Mary Lenzini, Vice President Human Resources, Geisinger–Bloomsburg Hospital, Bloomsburg, PA, p. A519
HOWE, Scott W., Chief Executive Officer, Weeks Medical Center, Lancaster, NH, p. A398
HOWE, Vicki, Chief Information Officer, Ness County Hospital, Ness City, KS, p. A239
HOWELL, A. Todd, Chief Operating Officer, Columbus Regional Healthcare System, Whiteville, NC, p. A462
HOWELL, Amy M., Director Human Resources, St. Luke's Behavioral Health Center, Phoenix, AZ, p. A36
HOWELL, Bradley, Chief Executive Officer, Roundup Memorial Healthcare, Roundup, MT, p. A378
HOWELL, Carrie, Chief Financial Officer, Barstow Community Hospital, Barstow, CA, p. A55
HOWELL, Diana, Director Human Resources, Conroe Regional Medical Center, Conroe, TX, p. A588
HOWELL, Douglas
Interim President and Chief Executive Officer, Frazier Rehab Institute, Louisville, KY, p. A254
Interim President and Chief Executive Officer, Jewish Hospital, Louisville, KY, p. A254
HOWELL, Everette, M.D. Chief Medical Officer, The Center for Spinal Surgery, Nashville, TN, p. A573
HOWELL, Kathy A., Vice President Human Resources, Lexington Medical Center, West Columbia, SC, p. A554
HOWELL, Kathy A., R.N. Chief Executive Officer, Saint Luke's South Hospital, Overland Park, KS, p. A241
HOWELL, Marlin, Director Information Systems, Samaritan Healthcare, Moses Lake, WA, p. A663
HOWELL, Nathan, Chief Operating Officer, St. Elizabeth's Medical Center, Brighton, MA, p. A298
HOWELL, Pat, Chief Nursing Officer, Community Memorial Hospital, Syracuse, NE, p. A390
HOWELL, Patricia, M.D. President Medical Staff, Swedish Medical Center, Englewood, CO, p. A100
HOWELL, R. Edward, Vice President and Chief Executive Officer, University of Virginia Medical Center, Charlottesville, VA, p. A646
HOWELL, R. Edward, Vice President and Chief Executive Officer, UVA Health System, Charlottesville, VA, p. B140

A840 Index of Health Care Professionals

Index of Health Care Professionals / Hull

HOWELL, Ronene, Director Health Information Management, Bryce Hospital, Tuscaloosa, AL, p. A26
HOWELLS, Stephen, Chief Financial Officer, Kane County Hospital, Kanab, UT, p. A638
HOWERTER, Mark, M.D. President Medical Staff, Columbus Community Hospital, Columbus, NE, p. A382
HOWERTON, Shawn, M.D. President Medical Staff, Sampson Regional Medical Center, Clinton, NC, p. A451
HOWES, Constance A., President and Chief Executive Officer, Women & Infants Hospital of Rhode Island, Providence, RI, p. A545
HOY, Jonathan B., Chief Financial Officer, Durham Regional Hospital, Durham, NC, p. A452
HOYER, Scott, M.D. Vice President Quality and Chief Medical Officer, United Regional Health Care System, Wichita Falls, TX, p. A635
HOYOS, Kent, Chief Information Officer, Pomona Valley Hospital Medical Center, Pomona, CA, p. A80
HOYT, Nancy, R.N. Vice President Operations/Clinical and Chief Nursing Officer, Mercy Regional Medical Center, Durango, CO, p. A100
HRON, Janine, Chief Executive Officer, Crittenton Children's Center, Kansas City, MO, p. A361
HRUBIAK, Dan, Associate Computer Program Analyst, Western New York Children's Psychiatric Center, West Seneca, NY, p. A446
HRUBY, Deidre, Director of Patient Care, Madelia Community Hospital, Madelia, MN, p. A334
HSING, Shirley, Senior Vice President and Chief Financial Officer, North Oaks Medical Center, Hammond, LA, p. A267
HUANG, Benson, M.D. Medical Director, Laredo Specialty Hospital, Laredo, TX, p. A612
HUBBARD, Bill, Vice President, Operations, Carolinas Medical Center–NorthEast, Concord, NC, p. A451
HUBBARD, Daniel, Chief Financial Officer, Sioux Falls VA Health Care System, Sioux Falls, SD, p. A560
HUBBARD, David, Chief Executive Officer, Daniels Memorial Healthcare Center, Scobey, MT, p. A379
HUBBARD, Kathy, Manager Human Resources, Oneida County Hospital, Malad City, ID, p. A169
HUBBARD, Mark, Vice President Risk Management, Loma Linda University Behavioral Medicine Center, Redlands, CA, p. A82
HUBBARD, Norm, Executive Vice President, Seattle Cancer Care Alliance, Seattle, WA, p. A666
HUBBELL, John, Chief Financial Officer, Livingston Hospital and Healthcare Services, Salem, KY, p. A258
HUBBS, David, M.D. Chief Medical Staff, Grove Hill Memorial Hospital, Grove Hill, AL, p. A21
HUBBS III, Olas A., FACHE President and Chief Executive Officer, Memorial Hospital of Union County, Marysville, OH, p. A484
HUBELE, Suzanna D., M.D. Chief of Staff, Weiser Memorial Hospital, Weiser, ID, p. A171
HUBER, Joel, M.D. Chief of Staff, Avera Hand County Memorial Hospital & Clinic, Miller, SD, p. A557
HUBER, Timothy, Manager Financial Support, Mercy Hospital of Franciscan Sisters, Oelwein, IA, p. A224
HUBERT, Barney, Superintendent, Kansas Neurological Institute, Topeka, KS, p. A244
HUBERT, Maureen, Manager Management Information Services, Shriners Hospitals for Children, Erie, Erie, PA, p. A523
HUBERT, Michael, Vice President Human Resources, J. C. Blair Memorial Hospital, Huntingdon, PA, p. A525
HUBLER, Todd C., Chief Executive Officer, Williamson Memorial Hospital, Williamson, WV, p. A677
HUBLEY, Grover, M.D. President Medical Staff, Madison St. Joseph Health Center, Madisonville, TX, p. A615
HUBSCHMAN, Gary
Administrative Director Finance, Sutter Auburn Faith Hospital, Auburn, CA, p. A54
Administrative Director Finance, Sutter Roseville Medical Center, Roseville, CA, p. A83
HUCK, Karma, Chief Operating Officer, Scott County Hospital, Scott City, KS, p. A243
HUCKABEE, Mike, Network Administrator, Coryell Memorial Hospital, Gatesville, TX, p. A601
HUCKABY, Don, Chief Information Management Service, Veterans Affairs Eastern Colorado Health Care System, Denver, CO, p. A100
HUCKABY, Lee, Chief Executive Officer, Promise Hospital of Vicksburg, Vicksburg, MS, p. A353
HUCKSHORN, Kevin Ann, MSN, Director, Delaware Psychiatric Center, New Castle, DE, p. A114
HUDA, Edith, Director Human Resources, Daniels Memorial Healthcare Center, Scobey, MT, p. A379
HUDAK, Corey, Director Human Resources, Memorial Hospital, York, PA, p. A542
HUDDLESTON, J. Andrew, D.O. President Medical Staff, Bellevue Hospital, Bellevue, OH, p. A470
HUDDLESTON, Tina, Chief Nursing Officer, Baylor Medical Center at Trophy Club, Trophy Club, TX, p. A631
HUDGENS, Roselyn, Director Human Resources, Ballinger Memorial Hospital, Ballinger, TX, p. A582
HUDGINS, Paul
Associate Vice President Human Resources, Bascom Palmer Eye Institute–Anne Bates Leach Eye Hospital, Miami, FL, p. A131
Associate Vice President Human Resources, University of Miami Hospital and Clinics, Miami, FL, p. A132
HUDGINS, Thomas J., FACHE Administrator and Chief Executive Officer, Pinckneyville Community Hospital, Pinckneyville, IL, p. A191
HUDNELL, Sharon, R.N. Chief Nursing Officer, WK Bossier Health Center, Bossier City, LA, p. A264
HUDSON, C. R., Senior Vice President and Chief Financial Officer, Henry Mayo Newhall Memorial Hospital, Valencia, CA, p. A94
HUDSON, Donald C., President, Mercy Hospital of Folsom, Folsom, CA, p. A60
HUDSON, Gary Mikeal, Administrator, East Texas Medical Center Carthage, Carthage, TX, p. A586
HUDSON, Hamilton, Interim Chief Executive Officer, Wallace Thomson Hospital, Union, SC, p. A554
HUDSON, James, Assistant Chief Information Resource Management, Veterans Affairs Medical Center, Lake City, FL, p. A128
HUDSON, Janell, M.D. Chief Clinical Officer, Sanford Medical Center Thief River Falls, Thief River Falls, MN, p. A340
HUDSON, Kenneth J., Chief Financial Officer, Veterans Affairs Puget Sound Health Care System, Seattle, WA, p. A666
HUDSON, Kent, Chief Financial Officer, Ninnescah Valley Health System, Kingman, KS, p. A236
HUDSON, Larry C.
Executive Vice President and Chief Financial Officer, CAMC Teays Valley Hospital, Hurricane, WV, p. A673
Executive Vice President and Chief Financial Officer, Charleston Area Medical Center, Charleston, WV, p. A671
HUDSON, Lowell K., Chief Financial Officer, Glen Oaks Hospital, Greenville, TX, p. A601
HUDSON, Maggie, Director Operations and Financial Services, Santiam Memorial Hospital, Stayton, OR, p. A516
HUDSON, Marta, R.N. VP Patient Care Services, Community Hospital, McCook, NE, p. A386
HUDSON, Pamela, M.D. Chief Executive Officer, Crestwood Medical Center, Huntsville, AL, p. A21
HUDSON, Richard E., FACHE President and Chief Executive Officer, Wilson Medical Center, Wilson, NC, p. A463
HUDSON, Robbi, Chief Financial Officer, HEALTHSOUTH Rehabilitation Hospital, Fayetteville, AR, p. A44
HUDSPETH, Harvey, Executive Director Human Resources, Medical Center Health System, Odessa, TX, p. A619
HUDSPETH, Todd R., President and Chief Executive Officer, Jamestown Regional Medical Center, Jamestown, ND, p. A466
HUDSPITH, Tammie, Director Human Resources, River's Edge Hospital and Clinic, Saint Peter, MN, p. A339
HUEBBERS, Rodney N., Campus Administrator, Inova Fairfax Hospital, Falls Church, VA, p. A647
HUEBNER, Thomas W., President, Rutland Regional Medical Center, Rutland, VT, p. A644
HUEBNER, Timothy K., M.D. President Medical Affairs, Riverview Hospital Association, Wisconsin Rapids, WI, p. A694
HUELSKAMP, Donald P., Vice President Finance and Chief Financial Officer, Southeastern Ohio Regional Medical Center, Cambridge, OH, p. A471
HUENERGARDT, Sam, President and Chief Executive Officer, Central Texas Medical Center, San Marcos, TX, p. A627
HUERTA, Guillermo, M.D. Chief Medical Officer, Select Specialty Hospital–Omaha, Omaha, NE, p. A388
HUERTER, Holly
Vice President Human Resources, Jennie Edmundson Hospital, Council Bluffs, IA, p. A217
Vice President Human Resources, Nebraska Methodist Hospital, Omaha, NE, p. A388
HUETTL, Patricia, Vice President Finance and Chief Financial Officer, Holy Family Memorial Medical Center, Manitowoc, WI, p. A685
HUFF, Don, Interim Chief Information Officer, Mercy Hospital of Portland, Portland, ME, p. A284
HUFF, Jeff, Assistant Administrator Finance, Fayette Medical Center, Fayette, AL, p. A20
HUFF, Michael H., Chief Executive Officer, Hamilton Hospital, Olney, TX, p. A619
HUFF, Sally, Controller, Harrison Community Hospital, Cadiz, OH, p. A471
HUFFMAN, Cy, M.D. Chief Medical Officer, Erlanger Medical Center, Chattanooga, TN, p. A563
HUFFMAN, D Darlene, Director Human Resources, Princeton Community Hospital, Princeton, WV, p. A675
HUFFMAN, James, Chief Executive Officer and Administrator, Baptist Memorial Hospital–Desoto, Southaven, MS, p. A352
HUFFMAN, Joseph, Director Human Resources, HEALTHSOUTH MountainView Regional Rehabilitation Hospital, Morgantown, WV, p. A674
HUFFMAN, Sherry, Administrator Human Resources, Oakwood Heritage Hospital, Taylor, MI, p. A324
HUFFMAN, Steve, Chief Information Officer, Memorial Hospital of South Bend, South Bend, IN, p. A212
HUFFNER, William, M.D
Vice President Medical Affairs, Arnot Ogden Medical Center, Elmira, NY, p. A425
Chief Medical Officer and Senior Vice President Medical Affairs, St. Joseph's Hospital, Elmira, NY, p. A426
HUFFORD, Dustin, Chief Information Officer, Memorial Hospital, Fremont, OH, p. A480
HUFNAGEL, Keith, Director Human Resources, Stillwater Medical Center, Stillwater, OK, p. A505
HUFNAGEL, O. E., Chief Executive Officer, Okanogan Douglas District Hospital, Brewster, WA, p. A660
HUGGINS, Lois, Chief Human Resources Officer and Senior Vice President Human Resources, Rehabilitation Institute of Chicago, Chicago, IL, p. A177
HUGGINS, Michael C., Administrator Network System, Eastern Oklahoma Medical Center, Poteau, OK, p. A503
HUGHES, April, Chief Financial Officer, Peachford Behavioral Health System, Atlanta, GA, p. A145
HUGHES, Beth, President and Chief Executive Officer, Provena Saint Joseph Medical Center, Joliet, IL, p. A185
HUGHES, Christopher, M.D. Medical Director, Kindred Hospital Detroit, Detroit, MI, p. A311
HUGHES, Constance, Director of Nursing, West Gables Rehabilitation Hospital, Miami, FL, p. A132
HUGHES, David T., FACHE Senior Vice President Operations and Chief Operating Officer, Good Shepherd Health Care System, Hermiston, OR, p. A511
HUGHES, Edith M., President, Oakwood Southshore Medical Center, Trenton, MI, p. A324
HUGHES, Faye, Chief Nursing Officer and Chief Operating Officer, Medical Park Hospital, Hope, AR, p. A46
HUGHES, James, Director Human Resources, Lake Cumberland Regional Hospital, Somerset, KY, p. A259
HUGHES, Lee, Chief Executive Officer, Memorial Hospital of Texas County, Guymon, OK, p. A497
HUGHES, Letha, Chief Executive Officer, Medical Arts Hospital, Lamesa, TX, p. A611
HUGHES, Lonnie, Comptroller, Essex County Hospital Center, Cedar Grove, NJ, p. A402
HUGHES, Lori, R.N. Chief Nursing Officer, Vice President Operations and Patient Care Services, Cottage Hospital, Woodsville, NH, p. A400
HUGHES, Michael, M.D. Medical Director, Family Health West, Fruita, CO, p. A101
HUGHES, Michelle, Director Health Information Management, Madison River Oaks Medical Center, Canton, MS, p. A344
HUGHES, Philip, Chief Executive Officer, Community Medical Center of Izard County, Calico Rock, AR, p. A42
HUGHES, Robert, Executive Director, Coler–Goldwater Specialty Hospital and Nursing Facility, New York, NY, p. A432
HUGHES, Sandra
Chief Financial Officer, Clinch Memorial Hospital, Homerville, GA, p. A154
Executive Director Human Resources, Scripps Memorial Hospital–La Jolla, La Jolla, CA, p. A66
HUGHES, Tena, R.N. Program Director and Director Nursing, Bastrop Rehabilitation Hospital, Bastrop, LA, p. A262
HUGHES, Terry, Manager Management Information Systems, Nantucket Cottage Hospital, Nantucket, MA, p. A302
HUGHEY, James, Chief Financial Officer, Rockdale Medical Center, Conyers, GA, p. A150
HUGHSON, John, Chief Executive Officer, Burleson St. Joseph Health Center, Caldwell, TX, p. A586
HUGUELEY, Sandra, Assistant Administrator and Chief Nursing Officer, Methodist Extended Care Hospital, Memphis, TN, p. A571
HUHNKE, Ann, Chief Financial Officer, Lander Regional Hospital, Lander, WY, p. A696
HUIE, Robert D.
Executive Vice President and Chief Financial Officer, Willis–Knighton Medical Center, Shreveport, LA, p. A277
Chief Financial Officer, WK Bossier Health Center, Bossier City, LA, p. A264
HUISENGA, Jason, D.O. Chief Medical Staff, Buena Vista Regional Medical Center, Storm Lake, IA, p. A227
HULEFELD, Michael, Chief Executive Officer, Ochsner Medical Center, New Orleans, LA, p. A275
HULL, Betty, R.N. Director Patient Services, Coalinga Regional Medical Center, Coalinga, CA, p. A58
HULL, Brad, Chief Financial Officer, Dale Medical Center, Ozark, AL, p. A24
HULL, Dan, Chief Financial Officer, Healdsburg District Hospital, Healdsburg, CA, p. A64


Index of Health Care Professionals A841
Index of Health Care Professionals

HULL, Debbie, Chief Financial Officer, Fisher County Hospital District, Rotan, TX, p. A623

HULL, Grace, Director Human Resources, Nantucket Cottage Hospital, Nantucket, MA, p. A302

HULL, John, Chief Executive Officer, Seven Hills Behavioral Institute, Henderson, NV, p. A392

HULL, Kathy, President and Chief Executive Officer, Illini Community Hospital, Pittsfield, IL, p. A192

HULL, Ken, Director Human Resources, Inova Fairfax Hospital, Falls Church, VA, p. A647

HULLETT, Sandral, M.D. Chief Executive Officer and Medical Director, Cooper Green Mercy Hospital, Birmingham, AL, p. A16

HULLINGER, Scott, Chief Executive Officer, Two Rivers Behavioral Health System, Kansas City, MO, p. A363

HULSCHER, Ronald, Chief Financial Officer, Mark Reed Health Care District, McCleary, WA, p. A662

HULSE, Mark, Vice President and Chief Information Officer, H. Lee Moffitt Cancer Center and Research Institute, Tampa, FL, p. A140

HUME, Craig P., Chief Executive Officer, Surgical Specialty Center of Baton Rouge, Baton Rouge, LA, p. A263

HUMES, Ronny, Chief Operating Officer, Magnolia Regional Health Center, Corinth, MS, p. A345

HUMMEL, E. Joseph, Chief Strategy Officer, Southern Ocean Medical Center, Manahawkin, NJ, p. A406

HUMMELKE, Arlita, Manager Human Resources, Mercy Hospital Tishomingo, Tishomingo, OK, p. A505

HUMPHREY, Del, Administrator and Chief Executive Officer, Stonewall Hospital, Stonewall, LA, p. A278

HUMPHREY, James, Director Human and Educational Resources, Penrose–St. Francis Health Services, Colorado Springs, CO, p. A98

HUMPHREY, Jerel T., Chief Executive Officer, Wellington Regional Medical Center, West Palm Beach, FL, p. A143

HUMPHREY, Randy, Chief Financial Officer, Wesley Medical Center, Hattiesburg, MS, p. A347

HUMPHREY, Richard, Vice President Finance, Texas Health Harris Methodist Hospital Fort Worth, Fort Worth, TX, p. A599

HUMPHREYS, David J., M.D. Medical Director, River Park Hospital, Huntington, WV, p. A672

HUMPHREYS, L. Ray, Chief Executive Officer, Anderson Regional Medical Center, Meridian, MS, p. A350

HUMPHREYS, Ray, Chief Executive Officer, Anderson Regional Medical Center–South Campus, Meridian, MS, p. A350

HUMPHRIES, Stefan, M.D. Medical Director, St. Luke's Rehabilitation Institute, Spokane, WA, p. A667

HUMPHRIES, Vickie, Director Human Resources, Bon Secours Maryview Medical Center, Portsmouth, VA, p. A654

HUNGER, Dennis, Chief Executive Officer, Washington County Hospital and Clinics, Washington, IA, p. A227

HUNGERFORD, Daniel, Controller, HEALTHSOUTH Western Hills Rehabilitation Hospital, Parkersburg, WV, p. A674

HUNKE, Sonja, Director Human Resources, Providence Medical Center, Wayne, NE, p. A390

HUNSBERGER, Glenn, Director Management Information Systems, Palisades Medical Center, North Bergen, NJ, p. A407

HUNSBERGER, Tom, Vice President Human Resources, Riverview Hospital Association, Wisconsin Rapids, WI, p. A694

HUNSICKER, Elizabeth, Chief Operating Officer, Rose Medical Center, Denver, CO, p. A100

HUNT, D. Deann, Director Human Resources, Gibson General Hospital, Princeton, IN, p. A210

HUNT, Deloris, Corporate Vice President Human Resources, Harper University Hospital/Hutzel Women's Hospital, Detroit, MI, p. A310

HUNT, Jacquelyn, Vice President Clinical Support and Information Services, Bellin Memorial Hospital, Green Bay, WI, p. A682

HUNT, Jeff, Chief Executive Officer, Sunbury Community Hospital, Sunbury, PA, p. A539

HUNT, Linda A., President, St. Joseph's Hospital and Medical Center, Phoenix, AZ, p. A36

HUNT, Reta, Director of Nursing, Scott & White Hospital – Llano, Llano, TX, p. A613

HUNT, Ronald, Chief Executive Officer, Extended Care of Southwest Louisiana, Lake Charles, LA, p. A271

HUNT, Sharon, Administrator, W. J. Mangold Memorial Hospital, Lockney, TX, p. A613

HUNT, Tad M., MS, Chief Executive Officer, Litzenberg Memorial County Hospital, Central City, NE, p. A382

HUNT, William Robert, Chief Financial Officer, Reynolds Memorial Hospital, Glen Dale, WV, p. A672

HUNTER, Bart, Manager Information Technology, Effingham Hospital, Springfield, GA, p. A159

HUNTER, Byron, Vice President Human Resources, Cape Regional Medical Center, Cape May Court House, NJ, p. A402

HUNTER, David C., Chief Operating Officer, Parkview Noble Hospital, Kendallville, IN, p. A206

HUNTER, Fred, Chief Executive Officer, Marina Del Rey Hospital, Marina Del Rey, CA, p. A74

HUNTER, Jay, M.D. Chief of Staff, St. Joseph Regional Medical Center, Lewiston, ID, p. A169

HUNTER, Ken, R.N. Chief Executive Officer, Kimball Health Services, Kimball, NE, p. A385

HUNTER, Rick, Chief Financial Officer, Veterans Affairs Medical Center, Miami, FL, p. A132

HUNTER, Shelly, Chief Financial Officer, Mercy Hospital Joplin, Joplin, MO, p. A361

HUNTLEY, Devin, Vice President Operations, Community Medical Center, Missoula, MT, p. A377

HUPF, Angela, Vice President Human Resources and Community Relations, Memorial Health Center, Medford, WI, p. A685

HURD, Jacque, Vice President Human Resources, St. Bernards Medical Center, Jonesboro, AR, p. A47

HURD, Ross, Chief Information Officer, Lake Chelan Community Hospital, Chelan, WA, p. A660

HURLBUT, Marty, M.D. Medical Director, HEALTHSOUTH Rehabilitation Hospital, Fayetteville, AR, p. A44

HURLEY, Jeff, Vice President Human Resources, Flagler Hospital, Saint Augustine, FL, p. A137

HURRAY, Joan, Regional Director Information Services, St. Joseph Mercy Hospital, Ypsilanti, MI, p. A326

HURSCH, Diana, M.D. Chief of Staff, Buchanan General Hospital, Grundy, VA, p. A649

HURSH, John, Vice President Human Resources, Lester E. Cox Medical Centers, Springfield, MO, p. A371

HURST, James, Chief Fiscal Service, Veterans Affairs Medical Center, Oklahoma City, OK, p. A502

HURST, Steve, Information Technology Specialist, Haskell County Community Hospital, Stigler, OK, p. A504

HURT, Christie, M.D. Chief of Staff and Medical Director, Mercy Hospital Aurora, Aurora, MO, p. A355

HURT, Kelly, VP Human Resources, Great Plains Regional Medical Center, North Platte, NE, p. A386

HURT-STEFFEN, Sally, R.N. Chief Executive Officer, Sierra Providence East Medical Center, El Paso, TX, p. A596

HURTADO, Denise, Chief Financial Officer, Benson Hospital, Benson, AZ, p. A31

HURTADO, Raul, Chief Information Officer, Coleman County Medical Center, Coleman, TX, p. A588

HURWITZ, Steven, Vice President Human Resources, Seattle Children's Hospital, Seattle, WA, p. A666

HURZELER, Rosemary Johnson, President and Chief Executive Officer, The Connecticut Hospice, Branford, CT, p. A108

HUSEBY, Custer, Chief Executive Officer, Kindred Hospital Fargo, Fargo, ND, p. A465

HUSHER, Phil, Chief Financial Officer, Winner Regional Healthcare Center, Winner, SD, p. A561

HUSKEY, Jeff, Chief Executive Officer and Administrator, Clay County Memorial Hospital, Henrietta, TX, p. A603

HUSS, Cathy, Chief Financial Officer, LifeCare Medical Center, Roseau, MN, p. A338

HUSSAIN, Iftikhar

Chief Financial Officer, Mills–Peninsula Health Services, Burlingame, CA, p. A56

Chief Financial Officer, Sutter Maternity and Surgery Center of Santa Cruz, Santa Cruz, CA, p. A90

HUSTEDT, Dale, Associate Administrator Administrative Services, Rice Memorial Hospital, Willmar, MN, p. A342

HUSTON, Gary, D.O. Chief Medical Officer, University Hospitals Conneaut Medical Center, Conneaut, OH, p. A478

HUTCHENRIDER, E. Kenneth, President, Methodist Richardson Medical Center, Richardson, TX, p. A622

HUTCHENS, Steve, Vice President General Services, Grady Memorial Hospital, Chickasha, OK, p. A494

HUTCHESON, Jane, Administrator, Group Health Cooperative Central Hospital, Seattle, WA, p. A665

HUTCHESON, Larry, Chief Financial Officer and Director Administrative Services, Humboldt General Hospital, Winnemucca, NV, p. A396

HUTCHESON, Lou Ellen, M.D. Chief of Staff, Bacon County Hospital and Health System, Alma, GA, p. A144

HUTCHINS, Michael T., Administrator, Jay Hospital, Jay, FL, p. A127

HUTCHINS, Roger D., Chief Financial Officer, Doctors Hospital at White Rock Lake, Dallas, TX, p. A591

HUTCHINS, Sheri, Director Health Information Management, Muenster Memorial Hospital, Muenster, TX, p. A617

HUTCHINSON, Donna, Chief Financial Officer, Beaver Dam Community Hospitals, Beaver Dam, WI, p. A679

HUTCHINSON, James, CPA Chief Financial Officer, Affinity Medical Center, Massillon, OH, p. A484

HUTCHINSON, Red, Chief Information Officer, Franklin Regional Hospital, Franklin, NH, p. A398

HUTCHISON, Barbra, Director Medical Records, Richland Parish Hospital, Delhi, LA, p. A265

HUTCHISON, Dee, Acting Chief Executive Officer, U. S. Public Health Service Indian Hospital, Parker, AZ, p. A35

HUTCHISON, Florence N., M.D. Chief of Staff, Ralph H. Johnson Veterans Affairs Medical Center, Charleston, SC, p. A547

HUTCHISON, Harry, Vice President Fiscal Services, St. Bernards Medical Center, Jonesboro, AR, p. A47

HUTCHISON, Tammy, R.N. Director of Nursing, Gove County Medical Center, Quinter, KS, p. A242

HUTH, Richard, Chief Executive Officer, Doctor's Memorial Hospital, Perry, FL, p. A136

HUTH, Thomas, M.D. Vice President Medical Affairs, Reid Hospital and Health Care Services, Richmond, IN, p. A211

HUTKA, Michael, Interim Chief Executive Officer, Cornerstone Hospital of Austin, Austin, TX, p. A580

HUTSELL, Dick, Vice President Information Technology Services, Saint Louise Regional Hospital, Gilroy, CA, p. A63

HUTSELL, Richard, Vice President and Chief Information Officer, O'Connor Hospital, San Jose, CA, p. A88

HUTSON, Donald, Administrator and Chief Executive Officer, Baptist Memorial Hospital–North Mississippi, Oxford, MS, p. A351

HUTSON, Mark S., Chief Information Officer, Greenwood Leflore Hospital, Greenwood, MS, p. A346

HUTSON, Marty, Chief Financial Officer, St. Mary's Health Care System, Athens, GA, p. A144

HUTSON, Wayne

Chief Financial Officer, Union Hospital, Terre Haute, IN, p. A212

Chief Financial Officer, Union Hospital Clinton, Clinton, IN, p. A199

HUTT, Si, Chief Executive Officer, Ashley Regional Medical Center, Vernal, UT, p. A642

HUVAL, Shadelle, Director Finance, St. Martin Hospital, Breaux Bridge, LA, p. A264

HUYCKE, Mark, M.D. Chief of Staff, Veterans Affairs Medical Center, Oklahoma City, OK, p. A502

HYATT, Charlotte, MSN Vice President Clinical Services, Gaylord Hospital, Wallingford, CT, p. A112

HYATT, Cori

Director Human Resources, Midland Memorial Hospital, Midland, TX, p. A617

Director Human Resources, Midland Memorial Hospital, Midland, TX, p. A617

HYATT, David W., Interim Chief Executive Officer, Indiana University Health Starke Hospital, Knox, IN, p. A206

HYATT, Robert, M.D. Senior Vice President Medical Affairs, Lake Regional Health System, Osage Beach, MO, p. A366

HYATT, Ronnie, Senior Vice President Finance and Chief Financial Officer, Bon Secours St. Francis Health System, Greenville, SC, p. A550

HYDE, Cynthia, Interim Chief Information Officer, St. Mary's Medical Center of Evansville, Evansville, IN, p. A201

HYDE, Devon, Chief Operating Officer, Wuesthoff Medical Center – Rockledge, Rockledge, FL, p. A137

HYDE, Glen, M.D. Chief of Staff, INTEGRIS Canadian Valley Hospital, Yukon, OK, p. A508

HYDE, Jane E., President, Gettysburg Hospital, Gettysburg, PA, p. A524

HYDE, Keith, Chief Executive Officer, Providence Milwaukie Hospital, Milwaukie, OR, p. A513

HYDE, Robert, Human Resources Business Partner, Santa Clara Medical Center, Santa Clara, CA, p. A90

HYDE, Stephanie, Chief Executive Officer, Tyler Continuecare Hospital at Mother Frances, Tyler, TX, p. A632

HYDE, Stephen O., FACHE Chief Executive Officer, Southwestern Medical Center, Lawton, OK, p. A498

HYDE, Van D., MS, Chief Executive Officer, Sturgis Regional Hospital, Sturgis, SD, p. A560

HYDER, Shiraz, M.D. Director Medical Affairs, St. Alexius Medical Center, Bismarck, ND, p. A464

HYDOR, LouAnn, Director Information Integrity Management, Cardinal Hill Rehabilitation Hospital, Lexington, KY, p. A252

HYLAND, Donna W., President and Chief Executive Officer, Children's Healthcare of Atlanta, Atlanta, GA, p. A145

HYLTON, Heather, Chief Financial Officer, Plateau Medical Center, Oak Hill, WV, p. A674

HYMAN, Craig, Vice President Human Resources, Conway Medical Center, Conway, SC, p. A549

HYMANS, Daniel J., President, Memorial Medical Center – Ashland, Ashland, WI, p. A678

HYMBAUGH, Mitzi, Chief Personnel, Ringgold County Hospital, Mount Ayr, IA, p. A223

HYTOFF, Ronald A., FACHE President and Chief Executive Officer, Tampa General Hospital, Tampa, FL, p. A141

HYTRY, Steven, Chief Operating Officer, Aurora Las Encinas Hospital, Pasadena, CA, p. A79

Index of Health Care Professionals / Jablonover

Index of Health Care Professionals

## I


IANNONI, Joseph, Vice President Finance, Jordan Hospital, Plymouth, MA, p. A304
IBANEZ, Bella R., Budget Officer, Weed Army Community Hospital, Fort Irwin, CA, p. A61
IBRAHIM, Tajudeen, Interim Business Administrator, Elgin Mental Health Center, Elgin, IL, p. A180
ICENHOWER, Jeremy, Administrator and Chief Executive Officer, De Queen Medical Center, De Queen, AR, p. A43
ICKOWSKI, Michael F., Vice President Finance and Chief Financial Officer, Mount St. Mary's Hospital and Health Center, Lewiston, NY, p. A428
IDBEIS, Badr, M.D. Chief Executive Officer, Kansas Medical Center, Andover, KS, p. A230
IERARDI, Joseph P., Chief Executive Officer, Wayne Memorial Hospital, Jesup, GA, p. A154
IERO, Tony, Director Management Information Systems, North Philadelphia Health System, Philadelphia, PA, p. A533
IFTINIUK, Alan, Chief Executive Officer, French Hospital Medical Center, San Luis Obispo, CA, p. A88
IGLESIAS, Julio, M.D. Chief of Staff, Winn Parish Medical Center, Winnfield, LA, p. A279
IGNACIO, Manny, Controller, Riverside General Hospital, Houston, TX, p. A606
IGNACZAK, Thomas, M.D. Interim Vice President Medical Affairs, Bronson Battle Creek, Battle Creek, MI, p. A308
IGNAS, Ann, R.N. Chief Nurse Executive, Fairfield Memorial Hospital, Fairfield, IL, p. A182
IGNELZI, James, Interim Chief Executive Officer, Heartland Behavioral Healthcare, Massillon, OH, p. A484
IKNER, Don, Chief Executive Officer, Great Plains Regional Medical Center, Elk City, OK, p. A496
ILTIS, Michael T., Vice President Professional Services, Emanuel Medical Center, Turlock, CA, p. A93
IMADA, Ross, Director Information Systems, Shriners Hospitals for Children, Honolulu, Honolulu, HI, p. A164
IMBIMBO, Richard, Chief Financial Officer, St. Joseph Medical Center, Towson, MD, p. A294
IMLAY, Ralph, M.D. Chief of Staff, Harper Hospital District Five, Harper, KS, p. A234
IMLER, James R., Director Human Resources, Kimball Health Services, Kimball, NE, p. A385
IMSEIS, Mikhail, M.D. Chief of Staff, Ness County Hospital, Ness City, KS, p. A239
INCARNATI, Philip A., President and Chief Executive Officer, McLaren Health Care Corporation, Flint, MI, p. B86
INGALLS, Dawn, Regional Manager Human Resources, Avera Dells Area Hospital, Dell Rapids, SD, p. A556
INGE, Ray, Vice President Human Resources, Pomona Valley Hospital Medical Center, Pomona, CA, p. A80
INGHAM, Raymond V., Ph.D. President and Chief Executive Officer, Witham Memorial Hospital, Lebanon, IN, p. A207
INGLE, Richard M., M.D. Chief of Staff, Humboldt General Hospital, Winnemucca, NV, p. A396
INGLES, Kimberly, Director Human Resources, Winn Parish Medical Center, Winnfield, LA, p. A279
INGRAM, David, Director Management Information Systems, Medina Hospital, Medina, OH, p. A484
INGRAM, Herman, Director, Riverside Medical Center, Franklinton, LA, p. A266
INGRAM, J. Kevin, M.D. Chief of Staff, Riverland Medical Center, Ferriday, LA, p. A266
INGRAM, Karen, Director Human Resources, Baptist Memorial Hospital for Women, Memphis, TN, p. A571
INGRAM, Kim, Chief Executive Officer, Mountain Lakes Medical Center, Clayton, GA, p. A149
INGRAM, Peter
  Vice President and Chief Information Officer, Mount Sinai Hospital, Chicago, IL, p. A177
  Vice President and Chief Information Officer, Schwab Rehabilitation Hospital, Chicago, IL, p. A178
INGRAM, Todd, M.D. Chief of Staff, Baraga County Memorial Hospital, L'Anse, MI, p. A317
INGRODI, Travis, Flight Commander Resource Management, U. S. Air Force Hospital, Hampton, VA, p. A649
INGWERSON, Connie, Chief Financial Officer, Nemaha Valley Community Hospital, Seneca, KS, p. A243
INHOFE, Kyle, Chief Human Resources Officer, Veterans Affairs Medical Center, Oklahoma City, OK, p. A502
INHULSEN, Christopher, M.D. Chief of Staff, Flint River Community Hospital, Montezuma, GA, p. A156
INIGO–AGOSTINI, Emigdio, M.D. Board President, Clinica Espanola, Mayaguez, PR, p. A702
INMAN, Debbie
  Chief Nursing Officer, Physicians Surgical Hospital – Panhandle Campus, Amarillo, TX, p. A578
  Chief Nursing Officer, Physicians Surgical Hospital – Quail Creek, Amarillo, TX, p. A578
INMAN, Julie, Regional Executive Officer, Southeast Missouri Mental Health Center, Farmington, MO, p. A359
INNOCENTI Sr., John, President and Chief Executive Officer, UPMC Presbyterian Shadyside, Pittsburgh, PA, p. A535
INO, Alan, Chief Financial Officer, Good Samaritan Hospital, Los Angeles, CA, p. A69
INOUYE, Valerie, Chief Financial Officer, San Francisco General Hospital Medical Center, San Francisco, CA, p. A87
INSCHO, Kimberly, Vice President Community Relations and Human Resources, Margaret Mary Community Hospital, Batesville, IN, p. A197
INZANA, Lugene A., Vice President and Chief Financial and Support Services Officer, Lawrence & Memorial Hospital, New London, CT, p. A111
IPPOLITO, Mark, Administrator, Federal Correctional Institute Hospital, Littleton, CO, p. A103
IPSAN, Charlotte, President, Norton Suburban Hospital, Louisville, KY, p. A255
IQBAL, Nayyar, M.D. Director Medical Staff, Western State Hospital, Hopkinsville, KY, p. A252
IRANI, Glenn, M.D. Chief Medical Officer, Providence Tarzana Medical Center,, CA, p. A71
IRISH, Kevin, Chief Information Officer, Lakes Region General Hospital, Laconia, NH, p. A398
IRISH–CLARDY, Katherine, M.D. Chief Medical Officer, Sparks Regional Medical Center, Fort Smith, AR, p. A45
IRIZARRI, David, Director Management Information Systems, Plantation General Hospital, Plantation, FL, p. A136
IRIZARRY, Aixa
  Executive Director, Hospital HMA de Humacao, Humacao, PR, p. A701
  Executive Director, Hospital San Pablo Del Este, Fajardo, PR, p. A701
IRIZARRY, Lourdes, M.D. Chief of Staff, Albany Stratton Veterans Affairs Medical Center, Albany, NY, p. A420
IRUEGAS, Javier, Chief Executive Officer, Mission Regional Medical Center, Mission, TX, p. A617
IRVIN, Coy, M.D. Vice President and Chief Medical Officer, Baptist Hospital, Pensacola, FL, p. A136
IRVIN, Debbie, Director Health Information Management, BHC Alhambra Hospital, Rosemead, CA, p. A83
IRVIN, Donna, Director Human Resources, Southwest Surgical Hospital, Hurst, TX, p. A608
IRVIN, Miriam, CNO, HEALTHSOUTH Rehabilitation Hospital, Fayetteville, AR, p. A44
IRVIN, Thomas M., Administrator Human Resources, Ranken Jordan – A Pediatric Specialty Hospital, Maryland Heights, MO, p. A364
IRVINE, Laura, President, Methodist Dallas Medical Center, Dallas, TX, p. A592
IRVINE, Marvina, Chief Financial Officer, Pocahontas Memorial Hospital, Buckeye, WV, p. A670
IRVING, Mark, Manager Management Information Systems, OSF St. Francis Hospital, Escanaba, MI, p. A312
IRWIN, Gene, Chief Financial Officer, Jefferson County Health Center, Fairfield, IA, p. A219
IRWIN, Robert G., Vice President Information Systems, Robert Wood Johnson University Hospital, New Brunswick, NJ, p. A407
IRWIN, Ruth, Associate Director Clinical Operations, Stewart & Lynda Resnick Neuropsychiatric Hospital at UCLA, Los Angeles, CA, p. A72
ISAACS, Cynthia, Chief Executive Officer, Cornerstone Hospital of Huntington, Huntington, WV, p. A672
ISAACS, Diane, Director of Nursing, Ouachita County Medical Center, Camden, AR, p. A43
ISAACS, Linda, Vice President Human Resources, St. Luke's Hospital, San Francisco, CA, p. A87
ISAACS, Michael, Director Human Resources, Streamwood Behavioral Health Center, Streamwood, IL, p. A195
ISAACS, Stephen, M.D. Chief of Staff, Hugh Chatham Memorial Hospital, Elkin, NC, p. A453
ISAACSON, Alan, Vice President and Chief Operating Officer, Seton Shoal Creek Hospital, Austin, TX, p. A581
ISADO, Jose, M.D. Medical Director, Auxilio Mutuo Hospital, San Juan, PR, p. A702
ISEKE, Richard, M.D. Vice President Medical Affairs, Winchester Hospital, Winchester, MA, p. A306
ISEMANN, William R., President and Chief Executive Officer, KidsPeace Children's Hospital, Orefield, PA, p. A531
ISHAM, George J., M.D. Chief Health Officer and Medical Director Health Plan, Regions Hospital, Saint Paul, MN, p. A339
ISHIZUKA, Paul, Chief Financial Officer, University of Washington Medical Center, Seattle, WA, p. A666
ISHKANIAN, Gary, M.D. Vice President Medical Affairs, Mount Vernon Hospital, Mount Vernon, NY, p. A430
ISLER, Dorie, Director Human Resources, New Mexico Rehabilitation Center, Roswell, NM, p. A417
ISLEY, L. Lee, Chief Executive Officer, Granville Health System, Oxford, NC, p. A458
ISMAIL, Asad, M.D. Medical Director, Wellstone Regional Hospital, Jeffersonville, IN, p. A205
ISOM, Candace, Chief Operating Officer, Indiana University Health Paoli Hospital, Paoli, IN, p. A210
ISOM, Julie, Director Human Resources, Lakeview Hospital, Bountiful, UT, p. A637
ISOM, Ruby, Associate Vice President Human Resources, Loretto Hospital, Chicago, IL, p. A176
ISON, Tamara
  Chief Financial Officer, Spalding Regional Medical Center, Griffin, GA, p. A153
  Chief Financial Officer, Sylvan Grove Hospital, Jackson, GA, p. A154
ISOZAKI, Dan, Director Information Management, Los Robles Hospital and Medical Center, Thousand Oaks, CA, p. A92
ISRAEL, Alison, Controller, Martin County Hospital District, Stanton, TX, p. A628
ISRAEL, Michael D., President and Chief Executive Officer, Westchester Medical Center, Valhalla, NY, p. A445
ISSAI, Alice H.
  Chief Operating Officer, Los Angeles Medical Center, Los Angeles, CA, p. A70
  Chief Operating Officer, University of California, Irvine Healthcare, Orange, CA, p. A78
  Business Strategy and Finance Leader, West Los Angeles Medical Center, Los Angeles, CA, p. A72
ISSAI, Robert, President and Chief Executive Officer, Daughters of Charity Health System, Los Altos Hills, CA, p. B40
ITO, Derek, Director Human Resources, Shriners Hospitals for Children, Honolulu, Honolulu, HI, p. A164
IVCIC, Rebecca, Chief Financial Officer, Heatherhill Care Communities, Chardon, OH, p. A472
IVERSON, Kenneth J., USN, Commanding Officer, Naval Hospital, Camp Pendleton, CA, p. A56
IVES, Karen, Administrator, Harper County Community Hospital, Buffalo, OK, p. A494
IVES, Matthew, Interim Chief Executive Officer and Chief Financial Officer, Keokuk County Health Center, Sigourney, IA, p. A226
IVESON, Jr., William D., Clinical Operations Officer and Director Human Resources, Barnes–Kasson County Hospital, Susquehanna, PA, p. A539
IVESTER, Roger, Manager Information Systems, Habersham Medical Center, Demorest, GA, p. A151
IVESTER, Steve, Director Human Resources, Springbrook Behavioral Health System, Travelers Rest, SC, p. A554
IVEY, Bobbie, Director Human Resources, Chicot Memorial Medical Center, Lake Village, AR, p. A47
IVEY, Mark J., M.D. Medical Director, Great Lakes Specialty Hospital–Oak Campus, Grand Rapids, MI, p. A313
IVIE, Brian K., President, Mercy San Juan Medical Center, Carmichael, CA, p. A56
IVIE, Jack, Chief Operating Officer, St. Bernardine Medical Center, San Bernardino, CA, p. A85
IVORY, Brenda, Vice President Clinical Services and Chief Operating Officer, Harlingen Medical Center, Harlingen, TX, p. A602
IVY, Jay, R.N. Chief Executive Officer, NeuroMedical Center Rehabilitation Hospital, Baton Rouge, LA, p. A262
IWEIMRIN, Salvatore, R.N. Chief Executive Officer, Select Specialty Hospital–Cincinnati, Cincinnati, OH, p. A474
IYER, Raju, Chief Financial Officer, Regional Medical Center of San Jose, San Jose, CA, p. A88
IZAKOVIC, Martin, M.D. Vice President Medical Staff Affairs and Chief Medical Officer, Mercy Iowa City, Iowa City, IA, p. A221
IZQUIERDO, Elizabeth L., CPA, Chief Executive Officer, HEALTHSOUTH Rehabilitation Hospital of Miami, Miami, FL, p. A131
IZZI, Denine, Site Manager Information Systems, Robert Wood Johnson University Hospital Rahway, Rahway, NJ, p. A409
IZZO, Carolyn, Senior Vice President and Chief Operating Officer, Ellwood City Hospital, Ellwood City, PA, p. A522


## J


JABBARPOUR, Yad, M.D. Chief of Staff, Catawba Hospital, Catawba, VA, p. A646
JABLONOVER, Michael, M.D. President and Chief Executive Officer, Kernan Orthopaedics and Rehabilitation, Baltimore, MD, p. A287


© 2012 AHA Guide Index of Health Care Professionals **A843**

JABLONOWSKI, Gerard J., President and Chief Executive Officer, St. Francis Medical Center, Trenton, NJ, p. A411

JABLONSKI, Mark, Senior Vice President Human Resources, St. Jude Medical Center, Fullerton, CA, p. A62

JABOUR, John, Chief Information Officer, Ephrata Community Hospital, Ephrata, PA, p. A523

JACK, Claudia L., Director Associate Relations, Brooksville Regional Hospital, Brooksville, FL, p. A119

JACK, Dennis D., President and Chief Executive Officer, Golden Plains Community Hospital, Borger, TX, p. A584

JACKES, Frederick D., Assistant Administrator and Director Human Resources, Valley Forge Medical Center and Hospital, Norristown, PA, p. A531

JACKS, Anthony, Director Human Resources, Howard University Hospital, Washington, DC, p. A116

JACKSON, Anthony W., Chief Executive Officer, HEALTHSOUTH Rehabilitation Hospital, Rock Hill, SC, p. A553

JACKSON, Bryan G., Vice President and Chief Financial Officer, Jefferson Regional Medical Center, Pine Bluff, AR, p. A50

JACKSON, C. Keith, Chief Executive Officer, Springbrook Behavioral Health System, Travelers Rest, SC, p. A554

JACKSON, Carolyn, Chief Executive Officer, St. Christopher's Hospital for Children, Philadelphia, PA, p. A533

JACKSON, Cindy, Director Human Resources, Phelps Memorial Health Center, Holdrege, NE, p. A384

JACKSON, Courtney, Director Human Resources, Logan Memorial Hospital, Russellville, KY, p. A258

JACKSON, Daniel W., Chief Operating Officer, Inova Alexandria Hospital, Alexandria, VA, p. A645

JACKSON, Darryl, D.O. Chief of Staff, Prague Community Hospital, Prague, OK, p. A503

JACKSON, David, Chief Financial Officer, Baptist Medical Center Leake, Carthage, MS, p. A344

JACKSON, Fred L., FACHE Chief Executive Officer, King's Daughters Medical Center, Ashland, KY, p. A247

JACKSON, J. D., Chief Information Officer, Highlands Regional Medical Center, Prestonsburg, KY, p. A258

JACKSON, James, M.D. Chief of Staff, Cornerstone Hospital of Bossier City, Bossier City, LA, p. A263

JACKSON, James, Chief Operating Officer, Saint Francis Memorial Hospital, San Francisco, CA, p. A87

JACKSON, James, M.D. Vice President Medical Affairs, St. Joseph's Hospital, Savannah, GA, p. A159

JACKSON Jr., James H., Executive Director, Greenwood Leflore Hospital, Greenwood, MS, p. A346

JACKSON, Janice, Director Human Resources, Shands Lake Shore, Lake City, FL, p. A128

JACKSON, Jeffrey, M.D. Medical Director, Methodist Sugar Land Hospital, Sugar Land, TX, p. A629

JACKSON, Joanne, Administrator Human Resources, Community Relations and Quality Improvement, Amery Regional Medical Center, Amery, WI, p. A678

JACKSON, John J., President, FirstHealth Richmond Memorial Hospital, Rockingham, NC, p. A459

JACKSON, Judy, Director Health Information Management and Privacy Officer, Shodair Children's Hospital, Helena, MT, p. A376

JACKSON, Les, Manager Information Systems, Lower Keys Medical Center, Key West, FL, p. A127

JACKSON, Linda, Director Management Information Systems, Arkansas State Hospital, Little Rock, AR, p. A47

JACKSON, Linda, M.D. Chief of Staff, Lincoln County Health System, Fayetteville, TN, p. A565

JACKSON, Lori L., Director Human Resources, Verde Valley Medical Center, Cottonwood, AZ, p. A31

JACKSON, Lynn, Administrator, Northside Hospital Forsyth, Cumming, GA, p. A150

JACKSON, Max, M.D. Chief Medical Officer, Renown South Meadows Medical Center, Reno, NV, p. A395

JACKSON, Meg, Director Biomedical and Management Information Systems, Beauregard Memorial Hospital, De Ridder, LA, p. A265

JACKSON, Melinda, Director Human Resources, Bates County Memorial Hospital, Butler, MO, p. A356

JACKSON, Michelle, Chief Financial Officer, BHC Alhambra Hospital, Rosemead, CA, p. A83

JACKSON, Mike, President and Chief Executive Officer, Ephraim McDowell Fort Logan Hospital, Stanford, KY, p. A259

JACKSON, Reese, President and Chief Executive Officer, Forbes Regional Hospital, Monroeville, PA, p. A529

JACKSON, Robert, Chief Financial Officer, Alliance Health Center, Meridian, MS, p. A350

JACKSON Jr., Robert, Chief Executive Officer, Grove City Medical Center, Grove City, PA, p. A524

JACKSON, Samatha, M.D. Chief of Staff, Elkview General Hospital, Hobart, OK, p. A497

JACKSON, Stephen, M.D. Chief of Staff, Skyridge Medical Center, Cleveland, TN, p. A564

JACKSON, Susan E., R.N. Senior Vice President, Health Central, Ocoee, FL, p. A134

JACKSON, Suzanne B., FACHE Chief Executive Officer, Dominion Hospital, Falls Church, VA, p. A647

JACKSON, Tamara, R.N. Senior Vice President and Chief Nursing Officer, Firelands Regional Health System, Sandusky, OH, p. A488

JACKSON, Teresa, Chief Executive Officer, Choctaw Nation Health Care Center, Talihina, OK, p. A505

JACKSON, Thomas W., Chief Executive Officer, College Station Medical Center, College Station, TX, p. A588

JACKSON, Tina
Director Human Resources, Barrow Regional Medical Center, Winder, GA, p. A162
Manager Human Resources, Williamson Memorial Hospital, Williamson, WV, p. A677

JACKSON, Tom, Chief Financial Officer, Eastside Medical Center, Snellville, GA, p. A159

JACKSON, Tommy, Chief Executive Officer, Landmark Hospital of Athens, Athens, GA, p. A144

JACKSON, Tony, Director Information Technology, Sutter Amador Hospital, Jackson, CA, p. A65

JACKSON, Vance, FACH
Administrator and Chief Executive Officer, Hancock County Memorial Hospital, Britt, IA, p. A215
Interim Administrator, Palo Alto County Health System, Emmetsburg, IA, p. A219
Interim Chief Executive Officer, Regional Health Services of Howard County, Cresco, IA, p. A217

JACKSON, Vaughn, M.D. Chief of Staff, Conejos County Hospital, La Jara, CO, p. A103

JACO, Carol, R.N. Chief Operating Officer and Chief Nursing Officer, St. Francis Hospital, Litchfield, IL, p. A186

JACO, Mary, R.N. Director Patient Care Services and Chief Operating Officer, Shriners Hospitals for Children, Galveston Burns Hospital, Galveston, TX, p. A600

JACOB, Abraham, M.D. President Medical Staff, South Shore Hospital, Chicago, IL, p. A178

JACOB, Cheryl, Chief Operating Officer, Saddleback Memorial Medical Center, Laguna Hills, CA, p. A66

JACOBI, Robert, Chief Financial Officer, Bob Wilson Memorial Grant County Hospital, Ulysses, KS, p. A244

JACOBS, Andrea, Chief Operating Officer, South Pointe Hospital, Warrensville Heights, OH, p. A490

JACOBS, Andrew, M.D. Chief Medical Officer, Virginia Mason Medical Center, Seattle, WA, p. A666

JACOBS, Barbara Stewart, MSN Suburban Hospital Nursing and Patient Care Administrator, Suburban Hospital, Bethesda, MD, p. A290

JACOBS, David, Director Information Systems, Ashtabula County Medical Center, Ashtabula, OH, p. A469

JACOBS, Donna K., FACHE Director, Northern Arizona VA Health Care System, Prescott, AZ, p. A37

JACOBS, Ian, Chief, Human Resource Management Service, Louis A. Johnson Veterans Affairs Medical Center, Clarksburg, WV, p. A671

JACOBS, Joey, Chairman and Chief Executive Officer, Acadia Healthcare Company, Inc., Franklin, TN, p. B4

JACOBS, Jolene, Director Human Resources, Sparrow Ionia Hospital, Ionia, MI, p. A315

JACOBS, Julie, Director Human Resources, Oklahoma Forensic Center, Vinita, OK, p. A507

JACOBS, Mark, Director Information Services, Pomerene Hospital, Millersburg, OH, p. A485

JACOBS, Michael
Vice President Human Resources, Gladys Spellman Specialty Hospital and Nursing Center, Cheverly, MD, p. A290
Vice President Human Resources, Laurel Regional Hospital, Laurel, MD, p. A293
Vice President Human Resources, Prince George's Hospital Center, Cheverly, MD, p. A290

JACOBS, Mike, Director Information Technology, Logan County Hospital, Oakley, KS, p. A240

JACOBS, Richard, Vice President Finance and Chief Financial Officer, Canton–Potsdam Hospital, Potsdam, NY, p. A441

JACOBS, Robert, Regional Director Information Management, CHRISTUS Hospital–St. Elizabeth, Beaumont, TX, p. A583

JACOBS, Steven R., Chief Financial Officer, Central Washington Hospital, Wenatchee, WA, p. A669

JACOBSEN, Barry, Chief Executive Officer, Myrtue Medical Center, Harlan, IA, p. A220

JACOBSEN, John, M.D. Chief of Staff, Fillmore County Hospital, Geneva, NE, p. A383

JACOBSEN, William D., Chief Executive Officer, Carilion Franklin Memorial Hospital, Rocky Mount, VA, p. A655

JACOBSMEYER, Barbara, Chief Executive Officer, The Rehabilitation Institute of St. Louis, Saint Louis, MO, p. A370

JACOBSON, Andrea, Human Resource Officer, Cavalier County Memorial Hospital, Langdon, ND, p. A467

JACOBSON, Becky, Vice President Finance, St. Vincent Heart Center of Indiana, Indianapolis, IN, p. A205

JACOBSON, Carlton, Vice President Finance, Frank R. Howard Memorial Hospital, Willits, CA, p. A96

JACOBSON, Catherine A., President and Chief Executive Officer, Froedtert Memorial Lutheran Hospital, Milwaukee, WI, p. A686

JACOBSON, Gary, M.D. Chief Medical Officer, Pembroke Hospital, Pembroke, MA, p. A303

JACOBSON, Janet, Director Human Resources, Lakewood Health System, Staples, MN, p. A340

JACOBSON, Jenny, Manager Human Resources, Hillsboro Medical Center, Hillsboro, ND, p. A466

JACOBSON, John, Chief Financial Officer, Gibson Area Hospital and Health Services, Gibson City, IL, p. A183

JACOBSON, John L., Chief Executive Officer, Atchison Hospital, Atchison, KS, p. A230

JACOBSON, Peter, President, Essentia Health St. Mary's Hospital – Detroit Lakes, Detroit Lakes, MN, p. A330

JACOBSON, Randolph
Chief Financial Officer, Carrier Clinic, Belle Mead, NJ, p. A401
Chief Financial Officer, East Mountain Hospital, Belle Mead, NJ, p. A401

JACOBSON, Rodney D., Administrator, Bear Lake Memorial Hospital, Montpelier, ID, p. A169

JACOBSON, Shirley
Chief Financial Officer, Community Behavioral Health Hospital – Alexandria, Alexandria, MN, p. A327
Chief Financial Officer, Community Behavioral Health Hospital – St. Peter, Saint Peter, MN, p. A339

JACOBY, Jamie R., Chief Financial Officer, Memorial Hospital of Texas County, Guymon, OK, p. A497

JACQUES, Shane, Chief Financial Officer, Aspirus Keweenaw Hospital, Laurium, MI, p. A317

JACQUES, Teresa, Interim Chief Financial Officer, Adventist Medical Center–Reedley, Reedley, CA, p. A82

JADCZAK, Audrey, R.N
Vice President/Chief Nursing Officer, Lourdes Medical Center of Burlington County, Willingboro, NJ, p. A412
Chief Nursing Officer, Our Lady of Lourdes Medical Center, Camden, NJ, p. A402

JAEGER, Lee, FACHE Chief Executive Officer, St. Vincent Salem Hospital, Salem, IN, p. A211

JAFFE, David E., Chief Administrative Officer, Swedish/Edmonds, Edmonds, WA, p. A661

JAFFE, Gabriel, M.D. Vice President Medical Affairs, Doctors Community Hospital, Lanham, MD, p. A292

JAGER, Linda, Director Finance, Avera Weskota Memorial Hospital, Wessington Springs, SD, p. A561

JAGGI, Michael, D.O. Vice President and Chief Medical Officer, Hurley Medical Center, Flint, MI, p. A312

JAGODITZ, Chris, Chief Financial Officer, Cumberland Hall Hospital, Hopkinsville, KY, p. A251

JAHAN, Mohammad S., M.D. Clinical Director, Middle Tennessee Mental Health Institute, Nashville, TN, p. A573

JAHN, Andrew, Vice President Finance, Sonora Regional Medical Center, Sonora, CA, p. A91

JAHN, Barbara A., Chief Operating Officer, Exempla Saint Joseph Hospital, Denver, CO, p. A99

JAHN, David B., President and Chief Executive Officer, War Memorial Hospital, Sault Sainte Marie, MI, p. A323

JAHN, Gregory L., R.N. Chief Executive Officer, St. Luke's Behavioral Health Center, Phoenix, AZ, p. A36

JAHN, Kim C., Director Support Services, Manning Regional Healthcare Center, Manning, IA, p. A223

JAHN, Timothy, M.D. Medical Director and Liaison, St. Mary's Hospital Medical Center, Green Bay, WI, p. A682

JAHNIG, Jay A., Chief Executive Officer, Faulkton Area Medical Center, Faulkton, SD, p. A556

JAHRE, Jeffrey, M.D. Vice President Medical and Academic Affairs, St. Luke's University Hospital – Bethlehem Campus, Bethlehem, PA, p. A518

JAIN, Ashok, M.D. Chief of Staff, Oakwood Annapolis Hospital, Wayne, MI, p. A325

JAIN, Rajiv, M.D. Chief of Staff, Veterans Affairs Pittsburgh Healthcare System, Pittsburgh, PA, p. A536

JAIN, Sunita, M.D. Chief Medical Officer, Baptist Rehabilitation–Germantown, Germantown, TN, p. A566

JAKACKI, Timothy
President, ProMedica Bixby Hospital, Adrian, MI, p. A307
President, ProMedica Herrick Hospital, Tecumseh, MI, p. A324

JAKOUBECK, Denise, Director Human Resources, Hancock County Memorial Hospital, Britt, IA, p. A215

JAMAL, S., M.D. Medical Director, Faith Community Hospital, Jacksboro, TX, p. A609

JAMERSON, Mosella, Director Human Resources, Dorothea Dix Hospital, Raleigh, NC, p. A459

JAMES, Bruce, Chief Executive Officer, Union Hospital, Dover, OH, p. A479

JAMES, Carmelo, Chief Nursing Officer, East Los Angeles Doctors Hospital, Los Angeles, CA, p. A69

Index of Health Care Professionals

Index of Health Care Professionals / Jennette

JENNETTE, Brian, Chief Financial Officer, Northside Hospital – Cherokee, Canton, GA, p. A148
JENNEY, Karol A., Director Business Operations, Southwest Regional Rehabilitation Center, Battle Creek, MI, p. A308
JENNINGS, D. Arlo, Ph.D. Chief Information Officer, Mission Hospital, Asheville, NC, p. A448
JENNINGS, Donna, Vice President Quality and Ancillary Services, Mountain View Regional Medical Center, Norton, VA, p. A653
JENNINGS, Jeff, Chief Executive Officer, Select Specialty Hospital–South Dallas, De Soto, TX, p. A593
JENNINGS, Marilyn, Director Human Resources, Austin Surgical Hospital, Austin, TX, p. A580
JENNINGS, Mark
Director Information Systems, Northeast Georgia Medical Center, Gainesville, GA, p. A153
Chief Information Officer, Saint Anthony Hospital, Chicago, IL, p. A178
JENNINGS, Peter G., President and Chief Executive Officer, OSF St. Francis Hospital, Escanaba, MI, p. A312
JENNINGS, Reynold J., President and Chief Executive Officer, WellStar Health System, Marietta, GA, p. B144
JENNINGS, William M., President and Chief Executive Officer, Bridgeport Hospital, Bridgeport, CT, p. A108
JENSEN, Alice J., Chief Operating Officer, Geary Community Hospital, Junction City, KS, p. A235
JENSEN, Amy, Director Human Resources, Community Health Center of Branch County, Coldwater, MI, p. A310
JENSEN, Christopher, Chief Financial Officer, Three Rivers Behavioral Health, West Columbia, SC, p. A554
JENSEN, Dave, Director Human Resources, Performance Improvement and Risk Management, Mountain View Hospital, Gadsden, AL, p. A20
JENSEN, David M A, Chief Financial Officer, Oakland Mercy Hospital, Oakland, NE, p. A387
JENSEN, Donna, Director Clinical Services, Blue Mountain Hospital, Blanding, UT, p. A637
JENSEN, Eric, Chief Executive Officer, Regional Hospital for Respiratory and Complex Care, Seattle, WA, p. A665
JENSEN, Gail, Chief Financial Officer, Trego County–Lemke Memorial Hospital, Wakeeney, KS, p. A244
JENSEN, Jan, R.N. Chief Executive Officer and Administrator, William Bee Ririe Hospital, Ely, NV, p. A391
JENSEN, Janette, Manager Human Resources, Avera Holy Family Hospital, Estherville, IA, p. A219
JENSEN, Ken, Chief Financial Officer, ValleyCare Medical Center, Pleasanton, CA, p. A80
JENSEN, Kimberly, Vice President Human Resources, Avera Sacred Heart Hospital, Yankton, SD, p. A561
JENSEN, Leanna, Vice President Finance and Chief Financial Officer, Cobleskill Regional Hospital, Cobleskill, NY, p. A424
JENSEN, Mary, Controller, Mountain View Hospital, Gadsden, AL, p. A20
JENSEN, Michael E., President and Chief Executive Officer, Davis Hospital and Medical Center, Layton, UT, p. A638
JENSEN, Mons, Information Systems Team Leader, St. Helena Hospital, Saint Helena, CA, p. A84
JENSEN, Neal, Chief Executive Officer, Cobre Valley Regional Medical Center, Globe, AZ, p. A33
JENSEN, Paul, M.D. Chief of Staff, Regional Health Services of Howard County, Cresco, IA, p. A217
JENSEN, Renee K., Chief Executive Officer, Mark Reed Health Care District, McCleary, WA, p. A662
JENSEN, Ronald, Manager Finance, The Orthopedic Specialty Hospital, Murray, UT, p. A638
JENSEN, Sherry, Chief Financial Officer, Halifax Regional Medical Center, Roanoke Rapids, NC, p. A459
JENSEN, Steen, M.D. Chief of Staff, Seneca Healthcare District, Chester, CA, p. A57
JENSEN, Tom, Chief Executive Officer, Grays Harbor Community Hospital, Aberdeen, WA, p. A659
JENSEN, Troy, Director Human Resources, HEALTHSOUTH Rehabilitation Hospital of Utah, Sandy, UT, p. A641
JENSEN, Twyla, Director Human Resources, Pioneers Medical Center, Meeker, CO, p. A104
JENSEN, Vicki, Chief Human Resources Officer, Spectrum Health United Hospital, Greenville, MI, p. A314
JENSON, Cathy, Human Resources Generalist, Memorial Community Hospital and Health System, Blair, NE, p. A382
JENTZ, Amy, M.D. Chief of Staff, Sparrow Ionia Hospital, Ionia, MI, p. A315
JEPPI, Jessi, Director Human Resources, Rockford Center, Newark, DE, p. A114
JEPSON, Brian, Chief Operating Officer, Riverside Methodist Hospital, Columbus, OH, p. A477
JEPSON, Gary L., Chief Executive Officer, Pekin Hospital, Pekin, IL, p. A191
JEPSON, Jeanne, Director Human Resources, Hackettstown Regional Medical Center, Hackettstown, NJ, p. A404
JEPSON, Mark, Vice President, Silver Cross Hospital, New Lenox, IL, p. A189
JERANT, Steve, Vice President Information Technology, Forest Health Medical Center, Ypsilanti, MI, p. A326
JERGER, Greg, Chief Financial Officer, Memorial Health Care Systems, Seward, NE, p. A389
JERNIGAN, Donald L., Ph.D. President and Chief Executive Officer, Adventist Health System Sunbelt Health Care Corporation, Altamonte Springs, FL, p. B5
JERNIGAN, Pam, Chief Financial Officer, United Regional Medical Center, Manchester, TN, p. A570
JERNIGAN Jr., Robert F., Chief Executive Officer, Select Specialty Hospital–Durham, Durham, NC, p. A452
JEROME, Marivee, Senior Human Resources Business Partner, HEALTHSOUTH Rehabilitation Hospital of Sarasota, Sarasota, FL, p. A139
JESCH, Doug, Director Human Resources, Indiana University Health Starke Hospital, Knox, IN, p. A206
JESIOLOWSKI, Craig A., FACHE President, Saint Anne's Hospital, Fall River, MA, p. A299
JESSOP, Daniel E., CPA, Chief Executive Officer, Memorial Hospital of Carbon County, Rawlins, WY, p. A697
JESSUP, Stephen, Chief Financial Officer, Southwest Regional Rehabilitation Center, Battle Creek, MI, p. A308
JESTILA–PELTOLA, Gail, Chief Financial Officer, Baraga County Memorial Hospital, L'Anse, MI, p. A317
JESUDASS, Samson, M.D. Vice President Medical Affairs, Seton Medical Center Austin, Austin, TX, p. A581
JETER, Cynthia, Director Human Resources, Sutter Surgical Hospital – North Valley, Yuba City, CA, p. A96
JETER, John, Chief Financial Officer, Smyth County Community Hospital, Marion, VA, p. A651
JETER, John H., M.D. President and Chief Executive Officer, Hays Medical Center, Hays, KS, p. A234
JETER, Larry R., Chief Executive Officer, Chestatee Regional Hospital, Dahlonega, GA, p. A150
JETT, Alisa
Director Clinical Services, Regency Hospital of Florence, Florence, SC, p. A550
Chief Executive Officer, Regency Hospital of South Atlanta, East Point, GA, p. A152
JETTERGREN, Tess, Director Clinical Informatics, Essentia Health St. Mary's Medical Center, Duluth, MN, p. A330
JETTON, Dana, Chief Information Officer, Continuous Care Centers of Tulsa, Tulsa, OK, p. A505
JEUNEHOMME, Patti, Director Human Resources, Hot Springs County Memorial Hospital, Thermopolis, WY, p. A698
JEWELL, D. Keith
Senior Vice President and Chief Operating Officer, Franciscan St. Francis Health – Indianapolis, Indianapolis, IN, p. A204
Senior Vice President and Chief Operating Officer, Franciscan St. Francis Health – Mooresville, Mooresville, IN, p. A209
JEWETT, Lorraine M., Vice President and Chief Operating Officer, Bristol Bay Area Health Corporation, Dillingham, AK, p. A28
JEWETT, Sherri R., Chief Executive Officer, Valle Vista Hospital, Greenwood, IN, p. A203
JHA, Gautam, M.D. Chief of Staff, Salem Township Hospital, Salem, IL, p. A193
JILEK, Lea, Director Finance, HealthEast Bethesda Hospital, Saint Paul, MN, p. A339
JIMBOY, Twylla, Supervisor Human Resources, Lawton Indian Hospital, Lawton, OK, p. A498
JIMENEZ, Betzaida, Director Human Resources, Hospital de la Universidad de Puerto Rico/Dr. Federico Trilla, Carolina, PR, p. A700
JIMENEZ, Gerson, M.D. Medical Director, Hospital Episcopal San Lucas Guayama, Guayama, PR, p. A701
JIMENEZ, Mauricio, M.D. Chief Medical Officer, Kindred Hospital El Paso, El Paso, TX, p. A596
JIMENEZ–HERNANDEZ, Iris, Senior Vice President and Executive Director, Lincoln Medical and Mental Health Center,, NY, p. A434
JIMESON, Jean–Marie, Coordinator Human Resources, Kansas Spine Hospital, Wichita, KS, p. A245
JIMMERSON, Kevin, Business Manager, Mental Health Institute, Independence, IA, p. A221
JINRIGHT, Nicki, Chief Financial Officer, Elba General Hospital, Elba, AL, p. A19
JIRON, Feliciano, Chief Executive Officer, Los Alamos Medical Center, Los Alamos, NM, p. A417
JIROVEC, David, Director Finance, Ministry Good Samaritan Health Center, Merrill, WI, p. A686
JITH, Gayathri S., M.P.H. Vice President Operations, Valley Presbyterian Hospital,, CA, p. A72
JIVIDEN, Roxanne, Chief Executive Officer, Ohio Hospital for Child and Adolescent Psychiatry, Columbus, OH, p. A477
JOBBITT, Patty, Vice President Operations, Rehabilitation Institute of Michigan, Detroit, MI, p. A311
JOBE, Kathy, R.N. Chief Nursing Officer and Vice President Patient Care Services, Summa Barberton Citizens Hospital, Barberton, OH, p. A470
JOBE, Randy, Chief Operating Officer, Integris Baptist Regional Health Center, Miami, OK, p. A499
JOCHIM, Steven, Administrator, Cape Cod & Island Community Mental Health Center, Pocasset, MA, p. A304
JODWAY, Timothy, Chief Financial Officer, Garden City Hospital, Garden City, MI, p. A313
JOHE, David, M.D. President Medical Staff, Elk Regional Health Center, Saint Marys, PA, p. A537
JOHLMAN, Ed, Chief Financial Officer, Sheridan Memorial Hospital, Sheridan, WY, p. A697
JOHN, Aleyamma, R.N. Director of Nursing, Kensington Hospital, Philadelphia, PA, p. A533
JOHN, Julian, Chief Financial Officer, Kings County Hospital Center,, NY, p. A433
JOHN, Roger S., President and Chief Executive Officer, Great Plains Health Alliance, Inc., Phillipsburg, KS, p. B55
JOHNS, Dale, Administrator, Town and Country Hospital, Tampa, FL, p. A141
JOHNS, Dawn, Director Human Resources, Colquitt Regional Medical Center, Moultrie, GA, p. A157
JOHNS, Robert, Senior Vice President Administration, Rochelle Community Hospital, Rochelle, IL, p. A192
JOHNS, Thomas Bradford, M.D. Medical Director, Ridgeview Institute, Smyrna, GA, p. A159
JOHNS, Timothy, M.D. Chief Medical Officer and Board President, Gilbert Hospital, Gilbert, AZ, p. A32
JOHNSEN, Timothy J., President and Chief Executive Officer, Mercy Hospital Hot Springs, Hot Springs National Park, AR, p. A46
JOHNSON, Alan, Chief Information Officer, Doctors Community Hospital, Lanham, MD, p. A292
JOHNSON, Allen
Chief Financial Officer, Truman Medical Center–Hospital Hill, Kansas City, MO, p. A363
Chief Financial Officer, Truman Medical Center–Lakewood, Kansas City, MO, p. A363
JOHNSON, Andrew, Information Technology and Purchasing Officer, Windsor–Laurelwood Center for Behavioral Medicine, Willoughby, OH, p. A491
JOHNSON, Arlan D., Chief Executive Officer, Howard County Medical Center, Saint Paul, NE, p. A389
JOHNSON, Ashley F., Chief Financial Officer, Memorial Hospital Jacksonville, Jacksonville, FL, p. A126
JOHNSON, Audrey, Director Human Resources, Parkwood Behavioral Health System, Olive Branch, MS, p. A351
JOHNSON, Barbara
Chief Financial Officer, Essentia Health Duluth, Duluth, MN, p. A330
Chief Financial Officer, Essentia Health Northern Pines, Aurora, MN, p. A328
JOHNSON, Barbara Jo, R.N. Senior Vice President Human Resources Development, Centegra Hospital – Woodstock, Woodstock, IL, p. A196
JOHNSON, Belinda, R.N. Chief Nursing Officer/Chief Clinical Officer, Russellville Hospital, Russellville, AL, p. A25
JOHNSON, Betty, Associate Administrator, LSU Medical Center–University Hospital, Shreveport, LA, p. A277
JOHNSON, Beverly, Vice President Human Resources, North Kansas City Hospital, North Kansas City, MO, p. A366
JOHNSON, Billy, Chief Executive Officer, Coal County General Hospital, Coalgate, OK, p. A495
JOHNSON, Bonnie, R.N. Vice President of Patient Services, Perham Health, Perham, MN, p. A337
JOHNSON, Brenda
Director Human Resources, Baptist Memorial Hospital–Collierville, Collierville, TN, p. A564
Director Human Resources, North Mississippi Medical Center–West Point, West Point, MS, p. A353
JOHNSON, Bret
Chief Financial Officer, Bon Secours St. Francis Hospital, Charleston, SC, p. A547
Chief Financial Officer, Roper Hospital, Charleston, SC, p. A547
JOHNSON, Bryan, Administrator, The Orthopedic Specialty Hospital, Murray, UT, p. A638
JOHNSON, III, C. Thomas, Vice President Organizational Development and Chief Financial Officer, Southeastern Regional Medical Center, Lumberton, NC, p. A457
JOHNSON, Calvin D., Administrator, Kilmichael Hospital, Kilmichael, MS, p. A348
JOHNSON, Casey R., Chief Financial Officer, Sanford Medical Center Thief River Falls, Thief River Falls, MN, p. A340
JOHNSON, Charles, M.D. Chief of Staff, Renown Regional Medical Center, Reno, NV, p. A395
JOHNSON, Charlie, Vice President Finance and Chief Financial Officer, St. Mary's Hospital, Madison, WI, p. A684
JOHNSON, Chris, Assistant Administrator and Chief Financial Officer, Essentia Health Sandstone, Sandstone, MN, p. A339
JOHNSON, Craig, D.O. Medical Director, St. Vincent Clay Hospital, Brazil, IN, p. A198

**A846** Index of Health Care Professionals

Index of Health Care Professionals
Index of Health Care Professionals / Johnson

JOHNSON, Yvonne, M.D. President Medical Staff, Baptist Health South Florida, South Miami Hospital, Miami, FL, p. A130
JOHNSON–HATCHER, Dawn, Chief Financial Officer, Women and Children's Hospital, Lake Charles, LA, p. A271
JOHNSON–PHILLIPPE, Sue E., President and Chief Executive Officer, St. Joseph's Hospital of Buckhannon, Buckhannon, WV, p. A670
JOHNSRUD, Carolyn, Manager Human Resources, Missouri River Medical Center, Fort Benton, MT, p. A375
JOHNSRUD, Jill, Director of Nursing, Essentia Health–Holy Trinity Hospital, Graceville, MN, p. A332
JOHNSTON, Don, Chief Information Officer, San Joaquin General Hospital, French Camp, CA, p. A61
JOHNSTON, Jeffrey A., President, Mercy Hospital St. Louis, Saint Louis, MO, p. A369
JOHNSTON, Joe, Chief Executive Officer, Jay County Hospital, Portland, IN, p. A210
JOHNSTON, Kevin, M.D. Chief Medical Staff, Harney District Hospital, Burns, OR, p. A509
JOHNSTON, Lauren, Deputy Executive Director, Lincoln Medical and Mental Health Center,, NY, p. A434
JOHNSTON, Lori, Chief Financial Officer and Chief Operating Officer, ProMedica St. Luke's Hospital, Maumee, OH, p. A484
JOHNSTON, Michael V., M.D. Chief Medical Officer and Senior Vice President Medical Programs, Kennedy Krieger Institute, Baltimore, MD, p. A287
JOHNSTON, Monte, Manager Human Resources, Coquille Valley Hospital, Coquille, OR, p. A510
JOHNSTON, Phyllis, Director, Catawba Valley Medical Center, Hickory, NC, p. A455
JOHNSTON, Samantha, Chief Organizational Excellence, Memorial Hospital, Craig, CO, p. A99
JOHNSTON, Susan, Director Human Resources, East Alabama Medical Center, Opelika, AL, p. A24
JOHNSTON, Wayne, Director Information Systems, Ripon Medical Center, Ripon, WI, p. A690
JOINER, Wayne, Vice President Human Resources, The Medical Center, Columbus, GA, p. A150
JOLLY, Gaye, Chief Executive Officer, Roane Medical Center, Harriman, TN, p. A566
JOLLY, Jay P., Chief Executive Officer, Goodland Regional Medical Center, Goodland, KS, p. A233
JONAS, Stanley W., Chief Executive Officer, Alliance Community Hospital, Alliance, OH, p. A469
JONES, Alesia, Interim Chief Human Resources Officer, University of Alabama Hospital, Birmingham, AL, p. A17
JONES, Allan, Controller, HEALTHSOUTH Rehabilitation Hospital of Jonesboro, Jonesboro, AR, p. A46
JONES, Amelia, Chief Operating Officer, Oakland Regional Hospital, Southfield, MI, p. A323
JONES, Beth, Chief Operating Officer, Reeves Memorial Medical Center, Bernice, LA, p. A263
JONES, Bill, Administrator, Jackson County Hospital District, Edna, TX, p. A595
JONES, Bracken, Director Information Technology, Southern Virginia Mental Health Institute, Danville, VA, p. A647
JONES, Carol, Controller and Manager Business Office, Coryell Memorial Hospital, Gatesville, TX, p. A601
JONES, Catherine, Chief Nursing Officer, Ancora Psychiatric Hospital, Ancora, NJ, p. A401
JONES, Cheryl L., Director Human Resources and Education, Baptist St. Anthony Health System, Amarillo, TX, p. A578
JONES, Chris, Chief Executive Officer, Northern California Rehabilitation Hospital, Redding, CA, p. A82
JONES, Christian, Chief Executive Officer, Moberly Regional Medical Center, Moberly, MO, p. A365
JONES, Dale, Administrator, Noland Hospital Tuscaloosa, Tuscaloosa, AL, p. A26
JONES, Dan, Director Human Resources, Pike County Memorial Hospital, Louisiana, MO, p. A364
JONES, Dana, R.N. Chief Nursing Officer, Springhill Medical Center, Springhill, LA, p. A278
JONES, Darrell, Chief Executive Officer, Regency Hospital of Florence, Florence, SC, p. A550
JONES, David, Chief Financial Officer, Alexian Brothers Behavioral Health Hospital, Hoffman Estates, IL, p. A184
JONES, David C., Administrator, North Caddo Medical Center, Vivian, LA, p. A279
JONES, David L., Chief Financial Officer, Red Bud Regional Hospital, Red Bud, IL, p. A192
JONES, David R., Interim Chief Financial Officer, Mountain View Regional Medical Center, Norton, VA, p. A653
JONES, Deborah, Controller, Houston Hospital for Specialized Surgery, Houston, TX, p. A604
JONES, Derrick A., Administrator, Community Behavioral Health Hospital – Fergus Falls, Fergus Falls, MN, p. A331
JONES, Donald J., FACHE Administrator, North Mississippi Medical Center–Hamilton, Hamilton, AL, p. A21
JONES, Douglas
Regional Chief Information Officer, Providence Holy Cross Medical Center,, CA, p. A71
Regional Chief Information Officer, Providence Little Company of Mary Medical Center, Torrance, CA, p. A92
Interim Chief Information Officer, Providence Saint Joseph Medical Center, Burbank, CA, p. A56
JONES, Douglas T., President and Chief Executive Officer, Down East Community Hospital, Machias, ME, p. A284
JONES, Elaine, M.D. President Medical Staff, Roger Williams Medical Center, Providence, RI, p. A545
JONES, Evelyn, Director Human Resources, Choctaw Nation Health Care Center, Talihina, OK, p. A505
JONES, G.R. Sonny, Vice President Finance and Chief Financial Officer, St. Claire Regional Medical Center, Morehead, KY, p. A256
JONES, Glen M., Administrator, Red Bay Hospital, Red Bay, AL, p. A25
JONES, Greg, Chief Financial Officer, Wayne Memorial Hospital, Jesup, GA, p. A154
JONES, Gregory, M.D. Chief of Staff, Vidant Pungo Hospital, Belhaven, NC, p. A448
JONES, H. Roger, Chief Financial Officer, Straith Hospital for Special Surgery, Southfield, MI, p. A323
JONES, Ian V., M.D. Vice President Clinical Performance, Sherman Hospital, Elgin, IL, p. A181
JONES, J. Stephen, M.D. Chief of Staff, Muenster Memorial Hospital, Muenster, TX, p. A617
JONES, J. Thomas, President and Chief Executive Officer, West Virginia United Health System, Fairmont, WV, p. B145
JONES, Jeffery, Administrator, U. S. Air Force Regional Hospital, Elmendorf AFB, AK, p. A28
JONES, Jennifer L., Chief Financial Officer, Edwards County Hospital and Healthcare Center, Kinsley, KS, p. A236
JONES, Jeremy A., Administrator, Mercy Hospital Healdton, Healdton, OK, p. A497
JONES, John, M.D. Chief Medical Staff, Sanford Medical Center Chamberlain, Chamberlain, SD, p. A555
JONES, John R., Administrator, North Mississippi Medical Center–Eupora, Eupora, MS, p. A345
JONES, Johnnie M., Acting Chief Human Resource Management and Workforce Development Service, Veterans Affairs Gulf Coast Veterans Health Care System, Biloxi, MS, p. A344
JONES, Joyce, Director Human Resources, HEALTHSOUTH Rehabilitation Hospital, Kingsport, TN, p. A568
JONES, Julie L., R.N. Chief Nursing Officer, Beatrice Community Hospital and Health Center, Beatrice, NE, p. A382
JONES, Karen, M.D. Chief of Staff, Harris Hospital, Newport, AR, p. A49
JONES, Karen, Administrative Director Human Resources, Marion General Hospital, Marion, IN, p. A208
JONES, Kathleen, Vice President Finance and Chief Financial Officer, San Diego Hospice & The Institute of Palliative Medicine, San Diego, CA, p. A85
JONES, Kathy, Director Human Resources, Jackson Medical Center, Jackson, AL, p. A22
JONES, Ken M., Interim Chief Operating Officer, UCSF Medical Center, San Francisco, CA, p. A87
JONES, Kevin, Director Finance, Aurora Sinai Medical Center, Milwaukee, WI, p. A686
JONES, Kyle, Controller, Marshall Medical Center, Lewisburg, TN, p. A569
JONES, L. Val, M.D. Medical Director, Blue Mountain Hospital, Blanding, UT, p. A637
JONES, Lance W., Chief Executive Officer, Turkey Creek Medical Center, Knoxville, TN, p. A569
JONES, Larry, M.D. Chief Medical Officer, St. Mary's Hospital, Streator, IL, p. A195
JONES, Linda, Director Medical Records, Millwood Hospital, Arlington, TX, p. A579
JONES, Lola, R.N. Administrator, Chase County Community Hospital, Imperial, NE, p. A384
JONES, Lorrie Rickman, Ph.D. Director, Division of Mental Health, Department of Human Services, Springfield, IL, p. B48
JONES, Louis, Director Management Information Systems, Heart of Florida Regional Medical Center, Davenport, FL, p. A121
JONES, Lynda, Financial Officer, Riverland Medical Center, Ferriday, LA, p. A266
JONES, M. Steven, President, University Hospitals Geauga Medical Center, Chardon, OH, p. A472
JONES, Mark, Chief Financial Officer, Hill Country Memorial Hospital, Fredericksburg, TX, p. A600
JONES, Mark L., Chief Executive Officer, Pondera Medical Center, Conrad, MT, p. A374
JONES, Mark T., President, University Medical Center of Princeton at Plainsboro, Plainsboro, NJ, p. A409
JONES, Marsha, R.N. Director Nursing, King's Daughters Hospital, Yazoo City, MS, p. A354
JONES, Marshall, Senior Vice President Human Resources, Maricopa Integrated Health System, Phoenix, AZ, p. A36
JONES, Mary Jane, R.N. Chief Nursing Officer, Providence Little Company of Mary Medical Center San Pedro,, CA, p. A71
JONES, Maud, Manager Medical Records, TOPS Surgical Specialty Hospital, Houston, TX, p. A607
JONES, Melinda, R.N. Chief Nursing Officer, Morehouse General Hospital, Bastrop, LA, p. A262
JONES, Meredith, Chief Financial Officer, McNairy Regional Hospital, Selmer, TN, p. A575
JONES, Michael, M.D. Chief of Staff, Atchison Hospital, Atchison, KS, p. A230
JONES, Michael, Vice President and Chief Information Officer, Children's Hospital of Wisconsin, Milwaukee, WI, p. A686
JONES, Michael L., Ph.D. Chief Information Officer, Shepherd Center, Atlanta, GA, p. A146
JONES, Mike, Director Information Services, Marshall Medical Center, Placerville, CA, p. A80
JONES, Pat, Director Information Systems, River Oaks Hospital, Flowood, MS, p. A345
JONES, Percy E., M.D. Chief of Staff, Kindred Hospital–Greensboro, Greensboro, NC, p. A454
JONES, Philip L., Chief Financial Officer, Kindred Hospital–Nashville, Nashville, TN, p. A573
JONES, Phyllis, Chief Human Resources, Wm. Jennings Bryan Dorn Veterans Affairs Medical Center, Columbia, SC, p. A549
JONES, Ray, Vice President, Columbia Memorial Hospital, Hudson, NY, p. A427
JONES, Reginald, Business Manager, Georgia Regional Hospital at Atlanta, Decatur, GA, p. A151
JONES, Richard
Vice President and Chief Financial Officer, Boca Raton Regional Hospital, Boca Raton, FL, p. A118
Chief Financial Officer, Bon Secours Baltimore Health System, Baltimore, MD, p. A287
JONES, Richard, M.D. Medical Director, Reliant Rehabilitation Hospital North Texas, Richardson, TX, p. A622
JONES, Richard W., Chief Financial Officer, Reading Hospital and Medical Center, West Reading, PA, p. A541
JONES, Rita A., Chief Executive Officer, Dundy County Hospital, Benkelman, NE, p. A382
JONES, Rob, Chief Nursing Officer, Physicians' Medical Center, New Albany, IN, p. A209
JONES, Robert
Chief Executive Officer, McCready Health Services Foundation, Crisfield, MD, p. A290
Director Management Information Systems, St. Joseph Mercy Oakland, Pontiac, MI, p. A321
JONES, III, Robert, M.D. President Medical Staff, Jefferson Memorial Hospital, Ranson, WV, p. A675
JONES, Rodney B.
Interim Administrator, Kindred Hospital Pittsburgh–North Shore, Pittsburgh, PA, p. A534
Administrator, Kindred Hospital–Heritage Valley, Beaver, PA, p. A518
JONES, Ron, Chief Financial Officer, Butler County Health Care Center, David City, NE, p. A383
JONES, Ruth, Chief Operating Officer, Regency Hospital of Northwest Arkansas, Fayetteville, AR, p. A44
JONES, Scott, Chief Operating Officer, Midwestern Regional Medical Center, Zion, IL, p. A196
JONES, Shannon
Chief Financial Officer, Garfield County Public Hospital District, Pomeroy, WA, p. A664
Chief Operating Officer, Los Angeles Metropolitan Medical Center, Los Angeles, CA, p. A70
JONES, Sharon, Chief Financial Officer, Evergreen Medical Center, Evergreen, AL, p. A20
JONES, Sonja, Chief Financial Officer, Peninsula Hospital, Louisville, TN, p. A570
JONES, Stephen K., President and Chief Executive Officer, Robert Wood Johnson Health System & Network, New Brunswick, NJ, p. B110
JONES, Stephen K., President and Chief Executive Officer, Robert Wood Johnson University Hospital, New Brunswick, NJ, p. A407
JONES, Stephen K., M.D
Vice President Medical Staff Affairs, St. Rose Dominican Hospitals – Rose de Lima Campus, Henderson, NV, p. A392
Chief Medical Officer, St. Rose Dominican Hospitals – San Martin Campus, Las Vegas, NV, p. A394
Vice President Medical Staff Affairs, St. Rose Dominican Hospitals – Siena Campus, Henderson, NV, p. A392
JONES Jr., Stephen K., FACHE Chief Executive Officer, Clear Lake Regional Medical Center, Webster, TX, p. A634
JONES, Steven K., M.D. Medical Director, Advocate Eureka Hospital, Eureka, IL, p. A181
JONES, Tamera, Director Human Resources, Whittier Hospital Medical Center, Whittier, CA, p. A96

A848 Index of Health Care Professionals

# K

Index of Health Care Professionals / Kale

Index of Health Care Professionals

KALE, Debra
Vice President Human Resources, Cleveland Regional Medical Center, Shelby, NC, p. A460
Vice President Human Resources, Crawley Memorial Hospital, Boiling Springs, NC, p. A449
Director Human Resources, Kings Mountain Hospital, Kings Mountain, NC, p. A456
KALEEL, Reza, Executive Vice President and Chief Operating Officer, St. Mary's Hospital and Medical Center, Grand Junction, CO, p. A102
KALETKOWSKI, Chester B., President and Chief Executive Officer, South Jersey Healthcare, Vineland, NJ, p. B120
KALETKOWSKI, Chester B.
President and Chief Executive Officer, South Jersey Healthcare – Elmer Hospital, Elmer, NJ, p. A404
President and Chief Executive Officer, South Jersey Healthcare – Regional Medical Center, Vineland, NJ, p. A411
KALINA, Andrea, Vice President Human Resources and Organizational Advancement, St. Clair Memorial Hospital, Pittsburgh, PA, p. A535
KALKOWSKI, Kelly, Chief Executive Officer, Niobrara Valley Hospital, Lynch, NE, p. A386
KALKUT, Gary, M.D. Senior Vice President and Chief Medical Officer, Montefiore Medical Center,, NY, p. A434
KALL, Greg, Chief Information Officer, Summa Health System, Akron, OH, p. A469
KALLAL, Catherine, M.D. Chief Medical Officer, Holy Cross Hospital, Chicago, IL, p. A176
KALLEN–ZURY, Karen, Chief Executive Officer, Hollywood Pavilion,, FL, p. A125
KALLENBERGER, Dianna, Chief Manpower Branch, Irwin Army Community Hospital, Junction City, KS, p. A236
KALLEVIG, Daryl, Chief Information Officer, Riverwood Healthcare Center, Aitkin, MN, p. A327
KALONICK, Roger, Business Manager, North Alabama Regional Hospital, Decatur, AL, p. A18
KALSMAN, Stephen L., Area Finance Officer, San Jose Medical Center, San Jose, CA, p. A88
KALTHOFF, Stella, Administrative Assistant, Manager Human Resources and Coordinator Quality Improvement, Swift County–Benson Hospital, Benson, MN, p. A328
KALUA, Patricia, Chief Nurse Executive, Kona Community Hospital, Kealakekua, HI, p. A165
KAMBEROS, Peter N., Chief Operating Officer, Thorek Memorial Hospital, Chicago, IL, p. A178
KAMBHAMPATI, Radha, M.D. Vice President Medical Affairs, Allegheny Valley Hospital, Natrona Heights, PA, p. A530
KAMBIC, Phillip M., Chief Executive Officer, Riverside Medical Center, Kankakee, IL, p. A185
KAMBOJ, Pradeep, M.D. Chief Medical Staff, Tulare Regional Medical Center, Tulare, CA, p. A93
KAMERZELL, Rick, Vice President Operations, St. Thomas More Hospital, Canon City, CO, p. A98
KAMIKAWA, Cynthia, R.N. Vice President Nursing Emergency Department and Trauma and Chief Nursing Officer, Queen's Medical Center, Honolulu, HI, p. A164
KAMINSKI, Gene, Vice President Human Resources, McLaren Northern Michigan, Petoskey, MI, p. A320
KAMINSKI, Tammy, Director Human Resources, Alaska Regional Hospital, Anchorage, AK, p. A28
KAMINSKI, Toni, Director Human Resources, Medical Center Enterprise, Enterprise, AL, p. A19
KAMMERER, James M., Vice President Support Services, Great River Medical Center, West Burlington, IA, p. A228
KAMMERUD, Shawn, Manager Information Services, Osceola Medical Center, Osceola, WI, p. A688
KAMMIRE, Gordon, M.D. Chief of Staff, Wake Forest Baptist Health–Lexington Medical Center, Lexington, NC, p. A456
KAMOWSKI, David, Senior Vice President and Chief Information Officer, Rochester General Hospital, Rochester, NY, p. A441
KAMPS, Mary Jane
Chief Information Officer, Southern Maine Medical Center, Biddeford, ME, p. A282
Chief Information Officer, Union Hospital, Elkton, MD, p. A291
KAMPWERTH, Dennis, Director Management Information Systems, Gateway Regional Medical Center, Granite City, IL, p. A183
KANANI, Bhargav, M.D. Chief of Staff, Ste. Genevieve County Memorial Hospital, Ste. Genevieve, MO, p. A371
KANE, Addy, Chief Financial Officer, Roger Williams Medical Center, Providence, RI, p. A545
KANE, Audrey, Interim Chief Financial Officer, Prowers Medical Center, Lamar, CO, p. A103
KANE, Robert E., Administrator and Chief Executive Officer, Divine Providence Hospital, Williamsport, PA, p. A542
KANE, Terri, Administrator, Dixie Regional Medical Center, Saint George, UT, p. A640
KANG, Balvinder, M.D. Medical Director, BryLin Hospitals, Buffalo, NY, p. A422
KANIA, Kathy, Chief Information Officer, Staten Island University Hospital,, NY, p. A437
KANKEL, LeAnne, Vice President Human Relations, Barton Healthcare System, South Lake Tahoe, CA, p. A91
KANNADAY, Colleen, FACH
President, Advocate BroMenn Medical Center, Normal, IL, p. A189
President, Advocate Eureka Hospital, Eureka, IL, p. A181
KANSGEN, Mike, Director Information Services, Community Hospital, Grand Junction, CO, p. A101
KANTHILAL, S. K., M.D. President Medical Staff, Sarah D. Culbertson Memorial Hospital, Rushville, IL, p. A193
KANTO, William, M.D. Acting Senior Vice President and Chief Medical Officer, Georgia Health Sciences Medical Center, Augusta, GA, p. A146
KANTOS, Craig A., Chief Executive Officer, Riverside Medical Center, Waupaca, WI, p. A692
KANUCH, James A.
Vice President, Allegheny General Hospital, Pittsburgh, PA, p. A534
Vice President Finance, Forbes Regional Hospital, Monroeville, PA, p. A529
Vice President Finance, Western Pennsylvania Hospital, Pittsburgh, PA, p. A536
KANWAL, Neeraj, M.D. Vice President Medical Affairs, ProMedica Toledo Hospital, Toledo, OH, p. A489
KAPASKA, David, D.O. Regional President, Avera McKennan Hospital and University Health Center, Sioux Falls, SD, p. A559
KAPHINGS, Mary, Director Human Resources, Fairview Ridges Hospital, Burnsville, MN, p. A329
KAPLAN, Gary, M.D. Chairman and Chief Executive Officer, Virginia Mason Medical Center, Seattle, WA, p. A666
KAPLAN, Margaret B., Director, Veterans Affairs Medical Center, Wilkes–Barre, PA, p. A542
KAPLAN, Ronald, Chief Financial Officer, North Philadelphia Health System, Philadelphia, PA, p. A533
KAPLAN, Tamra, Chief Operating Officer, Long Beach Memorial Medical Center, Long Beach, CA, p. A68
KAPP, Becky, Administrator, Alta View Hospital, Sandy, UT, p. A641
KAPP III,, William K., M.D. President and Chief Executive Officer, Landmark Hospitals, Cape Girardeau, MO, p. B78
KAPTAIN–DAHLEN, Mari, Chief Operating Officer, Mercy Medical Center–Sioux City, Sioux City, IA, p. A226
KARADJOFF, Peter, President and Chief Executive Officer, St. Joseph Mercy Port Huron, Port Huron, MI, p. A321
KARAM, Chris, President and Chief Executive Officer, CHRISTUS St. Michael Health System, Texarkana, TX, p. A630
KARAM, Judith Ann, President and Chief Executive Officer, Sisters of Charity Health System, Cleveland, OH, p. B119
KARANAS, Andrew, M.D. Vice President Medical Affairs, SSM DePaul Health Center, Bridgeton, MO, p. A356
KARANJAI, Rajohn, M.D. Chief Medical Officer, Sidney Health Center, Sidney, MT, p. A379
KARASICK, Steve, Interim Vice President Human Resources, Piedmont Hospital, Atlanta, GA, p. A146
KARBER, Steven, M.D. Medical Director, Greene County Medical Center, Jefferson, IA, p. A222
KARDOW, Vivian
Chief Human Resources Officer, Memorial Hermann – Texas Medical Center, Houston, TX, p. A605
Chief Human Resources Officer, TIRR Memorial Hermann, Houston, TX, p. A607
KAREL, Thomas, Vice President Organization and Talent Effectiveness, Saint Mary's Health Care, Grand Rapids, MI, p. A314
KARES, Timothy, Chief Financial Officer, University of Arizona Medical Center – University Campus, Tucson, AZ, p. A40
KARGBO, Mary, Chief Executive Officer, Sheehan Memorial Hospital, Buffalo, NY, p. A
KARKENNY, James, Chief Executive Officer, Terence Cardinal Cooke Health Care Center, New York, NY, p. A437
KARL, Don, Chief Operating Officer, Las Palmas Del Sol Healthcare, El Paso, TX, p. A596
KARL, Peter J., President and Chief Executive Officer, Eastern Connecticut Health Network, Manchester, CT, p. B49
KARL, Peter J.
President and Chief Executive Officer, Manchester Memorial Hospital, Manchester, CT, p. A109
President and Chief Executive Officer, Rockville General Hospital, Vernon Rockville, CT, p. A112
KARL, Thomas P.
President, Parkland Health Center, Farmington, MO, p. A359
President, Parkland Health Center–Bonne Terre, Bonne Terre, MO, p. A355
KARMACH, Izabela, R.N. Administrator, San Diego County Psychiatric Hospital, San Diego, CA, p. A85
KARN, Deborah, Chief Executive Officer, Kindred Hospital–Delaware County, Darby, PA, p. A521
KARNAP, Fred W., Vice President Finance, Iredell Memorial Hospital, Statesville, NC, p. A461
KARNER, Diana M., R.N. Chief Nursing Officer, St. Luke's Hospital, San Francisco, CA, p. A87
KARNS, Kris, Ph.D
Chief Executive Officer, Kindred Hospital Lima, Lima, OH, p. A482
Chief Executive Officer, Kindred Hospital of Central Ohio, Mansfield, OH, p. A483
KARPF, Michael, M.D. Executive Vice President Health Affairs, UK HealthCare, Lexington, KY, p. B133
KARPMAN, Robert, M.D. Vice President Medical Affairs, Cortland Regional Medical Center, Cortland, NY, p. A424
KARRA, Sri, Chief Information Officer, Cooper Green Mercy Hospital, Birmingham, AL, p. A16
KARREN, Dinah, Director Human Resources, Bingham Memorial Hospital, Blackfoot, ID, p. A166
KARSTEN, Paul H., Vice President Finance and Chief Financial Officer, Pine Rest Christian Mental Health Services, Grand Rapids, MI, p. A313
KARTHEISER, Keri, Manager Human Resources, Aspirus Grand View Hospital, Ironwood, MI, p. A316
KARUSCHAK Jr., Michael, Chief Executive Officer, Amery Regional Medical Center, Amery, WI, p. A678
KARZON, Mark, Chief Executive Officer, U.S. Public Health Service Indian Hospital, Redlake, MN, p. A337
KASABIAN, Carolyn, Chief Financial Officer, St. Mary's Regional Medical Center, Lewiston, ME, p. A284
KASAN, Nita, Chief Operating Officer and Chief Nursing Officer, Sun Coast Hospital, Largo, FL, p. A128
KASBERGER, John, Vice President and Chief Financial Officer, Mercy Medical Center, Roseburg, OR, p. A515
KASEY, Jay D., Chief Operating Officer, Ohio State University Medical Center, Columbus, OH, p. A477
KASKIE, James R., President and Chief Executive Officer, KALEIDA Health, Buffalo, NY, p. A422
KASKO, Andre, D.O. Chief Medical Staff, Hi–Desert Medical Center, Joshua Tree, CA, p. A65
KASMAN, Glenn, President and Chief Executive Officer, MultiCare Good Samaritan Hospital, Puyallup, WA, p. A664
KASPER, Keith, Chief Financial Officer, Hospital of the University of Pennsylvania, Philadelphia, PA, p. A532
KASPER–COPE, Shelly, M.D. Chief of Staff, Tri Valley Health System, Cambridge, NE, p. A382
KASPERBAUER, Dwight, Vice President Human Resources, The University of Kansas Hospital, Kansas City, KS, p. A236
KASS, Andrew J A, M.D. Assistant Superintendent, Riverview Hospital for Children and Youth, Middletown, CT, p. A110
KASS, Bonnie, Chief Nursing Officer and Vice President Patient Care and Support Services, Huntington Memorial Hospital, Pasadena, CA, p. A80
KASSAB, Jerry, President and Chief Executive Officer, Lakeside Behavioral Healthcare–Princeton Plaza, Orlando, FL, p. A134
KASSAHN, Kristine, Chief Executive Officer, Fresno Surgical Hospital, Fresno, CA, p. A62
KASSER, Michael, Chief Financial Officer, Herrin Hospital, Herrin, IL, p. A184
KASSIS, Frederick, M.D. Chief of Staff, Rolling Plains Memorial Hospital, Sweetwater, TX, p. A630
KAST, Kevin F., President and Chief Executive Officer, St. Mary's Hospital, Decatur, IL, p. A179
KASTANIS, John N., FACHE Interim Chief Executive Officer, Temple University Hospital, Philadelphia, PA, p. A534
KATELEY, Trace, Manager Information Systems, San Bernardino Mountains Community Hospital District, Lake Arrowhead, CA, p. A66
KATEN–BAHENSKY, Donna, President and Chief Executive Officer, University of Wisconsin Hospital and Clinics, Madison, WI, p. A684
KATES, Josh, Information Technology Analyst, Andrew McFarland Mental Health Center, Springfield, IL, p. A194
KATES, Kenneth P., Chief Executive Officer, University of Iowa Hospitals and Clinics, Iowa City, IA, p. A221
KATHRINS, Richard J., President and Chief Executive Officer, Bacharach Institute for Rehabilitation, Pomona, NJ, p. A409
KATNENI, Jitendra P., M.D. Medical Director, Select Specialty Hospital–Flint, Flint, MI, p. A312
KATO, Laura, Vice President Human Resources, St. Francis Medical Center, Lynwood, CA, p. A73
KATSCHKE, Jr., R. William, M.D. Medical Director, Grover C. Dils Medical Center, Caliente, NV, p. A391
KATSIANIS, John, Chief Financial Officer, Christian Hospital, Saint Louis, MO, p. A368
KATZ, Jeffrey, M.D. Chief Medical Officer, Memorial Hermann – Texas Medical Center, Houston, TX, p. A605
KATZ, Mike, Director Information Systems, Logan Memorial Hospital, Russellville, KY, p. A258
KATZ, Mitchell H., M.D. Director, Los Angeles County–Department of Health Services, Los Angeles, CA, p. B82

A850 Index of Health Care Professionals

Index of Health Care Professionals / Kelley

Index of Health Care Professionals


KATZ, Richard, M.D. Vice President Medical Affairs, Mt. Washington Pediatric Hospital, Baltimore, MD, p. A288
KATZ, Robert, M.D. Vice President Clinical Affairs, University of New Mexico Hospitals, Albuquerque, NM, p. A415
KATZ, Stephen A., M.D. Chief Medical Officer and Senior Vice President Medical Affairs, Vassar Brothers Medical Center, Poughkeepsie, NY, p. A441
KATZ, Steven E., M.D. Chief Medical Officer, Jersey Shore Hospital, Jersey Shore, PA, p. A525
KATZIN, David, M.D. Chief Medical Officer, Central Carolina Hospital, Sanford, NC, p. A460
KAUFMAN, Bob, Fiscal Officer, Hiram W. Davis Medical Center, Petersburg, VA, p. A653
KAUFMAN, Cheryl, Director Health Information Management, Pasco Regional Medical Center, Dade City, FL, p. A121
KAUFMAN, Dan, Director Information Services, Paulding County Hospital, Paulding, OH, p. A487
KAUFMAN, Irvin A., M.D. Senior Vice President Health Affairs and Chief Medical Officer, Rady Children's Hospital – San Diego, San Diego, CA, p. A85
KAUFMAN, Mark, Director Human Resources, Lanterman Developmental Center, Pomona, CA, p. A80
KAUFMAN, Ronald L., M.D. Chief Medical Officer, Lakewood Regional Medical Center, Lakewood, CA, p. A67
KAUFMAN, Samuel, Chief Executive Officer and Managing Director, Desert Springs Hospital Medical Center, Las Vegas, NV, p. A392
KAUL, Stephanie, Chief Financial Officer, Platte County Memorial Hospital, Wheatland, WY, p. A698
KAUPA, Michael, Executive Vice President and Chief Operating Officer, Park Nicollet Methodist Hospital, Saint Louis Park, MN, p. A339
KAUPAS, Bill, Interim Chief Executive Officer, Twin Creeks Rehabilitation Hospital, Allen, TX, p. A577
KAUPPILA, Glenn, D.O. Chief of Staff, Aspirus Keweenaw Hospital, Laurium, MI, p. A317
KAUTZ, Terri, Manager Human Resources, Weiser Memorial Hospital, Weiser, ID, p. A171
KAUTZER, Kenneth A., Senior Vice President Finance and Treasurer, Saints Mary & Elizabeth Medical Center, Chicago, IL, p. A178
KAUZLARICH, Sidney A., M.D. Medical Director, Douglas County Community Mental Health Center, Omaha, NE, p. A388
KAVANAUGH, Paul B., President and Chief Executive Officer, Community Care Hospital, New Orleans, LA, p. A274
KAVAWAHA, Sean, Supervisor Information Technology and Information Systems, Pondera Medical Center, Conrad, MT, p. A374
KAVTARADZE, David, M.D. Chief of Staff, Crisp Regional Hospital, Cordele, GA, p. A150
KAY, Brian
  Chief Financial Officer, McLaren Bay Region, Bay City, MI, p. A308
  Chief Financial Officer, McLaren Bay Special Care, Bay City, MI, p. A308
KAY, Kirk, Chief Financial Officer, Veterans Affairs Medical Center, Omaha, NE, p. A388
KAY, Robert W., Senior Vice President and Chief Financial Officer, Memorial Medical Center, Springfield, IL, p. A194
KAYE, Jessie, Chief Executive Officer, Prairie View, Newton, KS, p. A239
KAZMIERCZAK, Stanley, Controller, Saint Joseph Hospital, Chicago, IL, p. A178
KAZMOUZ, Safwan, M.D. Chief Medical Director, HEALTHSOUTH Rehabilitation Hospital, Concord, NH, p. A397
KEAHEY, Kent A., FACHE President and Chief Executive Officer, Providence Health Center, Waco, TX, p. A633
KEANE, Dennis M.
  Vice President Finance and Chief Financial Officer, Community Hospital at Dobbs Ferry, Dobbs Ferry, NY, p. A425
  Vice President Finance and Chief Financial Officer, St. John's Riverside Hospital, Yonkers, NY, p. A447
KEANE, Fran, Vice President Human Resources, CentraState Healthcare System, Freehold, NJ, p. A404
KEARNEY, Lynn, VP Patient Services & Chief Nursing Officer, Robert Wood Johnson University Hospital Rahway, Rahway, NJ, p. A409
KEARNEY, M. Clark, Vice President Human Resources, Saint Mary's Hospital, Waterbury, CT, p. A112
KEARNS, James, Chief Information Officer, Delnor Hospital, Geneva, IL, p. A182
KEATHLEY, Wayne, M.P.H. President and Chief Operating Officer, Mount Sinai Hospital, New York, NY, p. A435
KEATON, Tony, Director Information Systems, Roane General Hospital, Spencer, WV, p. A676
KEATON, William A., Chief Executive Officer, Baylor Medical Center at Frisco, Frisco, TX, p. A600
KECK, Paul, M.D. President and Chief Executive Officer, Lindner Center of HOPE, Mason, OH, p. A484
KECKAN, William D., Chief Operating Officer, Marymount Hospital, Garfield Heights, OH, p. A481
KEDALIS, Bob, Director Business Development, Michiana Behavioral Health Center, Plymouth, IN, p. A210
KEDDINGTON, Richard, Chief Executive Officer, Select Specialty Hospital–Milwaukee, Milwaukee, WI, p. A687
KEE, Agnes, Financial Manager, Gallup Indian Medical Center, Gallup, NM, p. A416
KEEF, Shaun, Chief Financial Officer, Central Peninsula General Hospital, Soldotna, AK, p. A30
KEEFE, Dennis D., President and Chief Executive Officer, Care New England Health System, Providence, RI, p. B25
KEEFE, Mary Jo, R.N. Vice President Patient Care Services and Chief Nursing Officer, Chester River Health System, Chestertown, MD, p. A290
KEEFER, Russ, Chief Human Resources Officer, Kennewick General Hospital, Kennewick, WA, p. A662
KEEFOVER, Robert, M.D. Chief Medical Officer, William R. Sharpe, Jr. Hospital, Weston, WV, p. A676
KEEGAN, Julie, Vice President Finance, Craig Hospital, Englewood, CO, p. A100
KEEGAN, Justin, Director Support Services, Avera Gregory Hospital, Gregory, SD, p. A557
KEEL, Deborah C., Chief Executive Officer, North Fulton Regional Hospital, Roswell, GA, p. A158
KEEL, Patricia
  Chief Financial Officer, Good Shepherd Medical Center, Longview, TX, p. A613
  Chief Financial Officer, Good Shepherd Medical Center–Marshall, Marshall, TX, p. A615
KEELAN, John E., Administrator and Chief Executive Officer, Brodstone Memorial Hospital, Superior, NE, p. A390
KEELE, Paula, Manager Information Systems, Provena United Samaritans Medical Center, Danville, IL, p. A179
KEELER, Dave, Chief Financial Officer, Pipestone County Medical Center Avera, Pipestone, MN, p. A337
KEELER, Karl, Chief Executive Officer, Saint Alphonsus Medical Center – Nampa, Nampa, ID, p. A169
KEELEY, Brian E., President and Chief Executive Officer, Baptist Health South Florida, Coral Gables, FL, p. B18
KEELEY, Katherine, M.D. Chief of Staff, Sunrise Hospital and Medical Center, Las Vegas, NV, p. A394
KEELING, Kevin, Chief Financial Officer, St. Lucie Medical Center, Port St. Lucie, FL, p. A137
KEEN, Michael, Senior Vice President and Chief Financial Officer, Grand View Hospital, Sellersville, PA, p. A538
KEEN, Robert C., FACHE President and Chief Executive Officer, Hancock Regional Hospital, Greenfield, IN, p. A203
KEEN, Scott R., Chief Executive Officer, HEALTHSOUTH Rehabilitation Hospital of Western Massachusetts, Ludlow, MA, p. A302
KEENAN, Annette M., Chief Executive Officer, Webster County Memorial Hospital, Webster Springs, WV, p. A676
KEENAN, Harold, M.D. Chief Medical Officer, Garden County Health Services, Oshkosh, NE, p. A388
KEENAN, Jimmie O., Commander, Evans U. S. Army Community Hospital, Fort Carson, CO, p. A101
KEENAN, Richard, Senior Vice President Finance and Chief Financial Officer, Valley Hospital, Ridgewood, NJ, p. A409
KEENE, Kaaron, Vice President Patient Care Services, Memorial Health Center, Medford, WI, p. A685
KEENE, Kim, Vice President Professional Services, Thibodaux Regional Medical Center, Thibodaux, LA, p. A278
KEENE, Richard, Chief Financial Officer, Queen's Medical Center, Honolulu, HI, p. A164
KEENE, Russell G., Chief Executive Officer, Androscoggin Valley Hospital, Berlin, NH, p. A397
KEENEY, Mary Ellen, Vice President Human Resources, Thomas Jefferson University Hospital, Philadelphia, PA, p. A534
KEEVER, Jerry, Administrator, Sharkey–Issaquena Community Hospital, Rolling Fork, MS, p. A352
KEGLEY, Carl J., System Director Information Technology, Fairbanks Memorial Hospital, Fairbanks, AK, p. A29
KEGLEY, Sue, Director Human Resources, Onslow Memorial Hospital, Jacksonville, NC, p. A455
KEHRBERG, Mark, M.D. Chief Medical Officer, Calumet Medical Center, Chilton, WI, p. A680
KEHRBERG, Mark W., M.D. Senior Vice President and Chief Medical Officer, Mercy Medical Center, Oshkosh, WI, p. A688
KEHUS, Frank, Associate Director for Operations, Veterans Affairs Medical Center, Marion, IL, p. A187
KEILER, Susan, Chief Operating Officer, St. Mary's Regional Medical Center, Lewiston, ME, p. A284
KEILERS, Lance W., Administrator, Ballinger Memorial Hospital, Ballinger, TX, p. A582
KEIM, Jane T., Vice President Operations, The Children's Institute of Pittsburgh, Pittsburgh, PA, p. A535
KEIM, Richard, M.D. Chief Medical Officer, Spearfish Regional Surgery Center, Spearfish, SD, p. A560
KEIM, Thomas, Chief Executive Officer, Ste. Genevieve County Memorial Hospital, Ste. Genevieve, MO, p. A371
KEISER, Trish, Comptroller, Avera Gregory Hospital, Gregory, SD, p. A557
KEITEL, Kal, Manager Personnel Services, St. Anthony's Memorial Hospital, Effingham, IL, p. A180
KEITH, Bridgette, Director Human Resources, HEALTHSOUTH Northern Kentucky Rehabilitation Hospital, Edgewood, KY, p. A249
KEITH, Darlene, Chief Information Systems, Alleghany Memorial Hospital, Sparta, NC, p. A461
KEITH, David N., FACHE President and Chief Executive Officer, McAlester Regional Health Center, McAlester, OK, p. A499
KEITH, Lorraine, FACHE Chief Nursing Officer, St. Vincent's Medical Center Southside, Jacksonville, FL, p. A127
KELBAUGH, Brian, Chief Financial Officer, Grafton City Hospital, Grafton, WV, p. A672
KELBLY, Kevin, Senior Vice President Finance and Corporate Fiscal Affairs, Carroll Hospital Center, Westminster, MD, p. A294
KELL, Douglas B., Interim Chief Financial Officer, Carondelet Heart & Vascular Institute, Tucson, AZ, p. A39
KELLAR, Randy, Director Human Resources, Psychiatric Institute of Washington, Washington, DC, p. A117
KELLAR, Richard A., Administrator, Aurora West Allis Medical Center, West Allis, WI, p. A693
KELLEHER, John G., Manager Human Resources, Athol Memorial Hospital, Athol, MA, p. A295
KELLEHER, LaCinda, Director of Nursing, Colorado West Psychiatric Hospital, Grand Junction, CO, p. A101
KELLEHER, Mary, Vice President Human Resources, Holyoke Medical Center, Holyoke, MA, p. A300
KELLEHER, Patrick, M.D. Chief Medical Staff, Saint Joseph Berea, Berea, KY, p. A247
KELLENBARGER, Lance, Site Director Information Systems, St. Catherine Hospital, Garden City, KS, p. A233
KELLER, Allen, Director Human Resources, Sumner Regional Medical Center, Wellington, KS, p. A245
KELLER, Ann, Manager Health Information Management, Walton Rehabilitation Hospital, Augusta, GA, p. A147
KELLER, Diane R., Chief Executive Officer, Memorial Community Health, Aurora, NE, p. A381
KELLER, Gary I., President and Chief Executive Officer, Opelousas General Health System, Opelousas, LA, p. A276
KELLER, J. Michael, Vice President Operations, Newton Medical Center, Newton, KS, p. A239
KELLER, Jack M., Administrator, Hickman Community Hospital, Centerville, TN, p. A563
KELLER, James, Director Human Resources, NEA Baptist Memorial Hospital, Jonesboro, AR, p. A47
KELLER, Jane, R.N. Chief Executive Officer, Indiana Orthopaedic Hospital, Indianapolis, IN, p. A204
KELLER, Jim
  Director Information Services, Bronson Battle Creek, Battle Creek, MI, p. A308
  Site Director Information Services, Saint Mary's Health Care, Grand Rapids, MI, p. A314
KELLER, Justin, Director Information Technology, Murray County Medical Center, Slayton, MN, p. A340
KELLER, Mark, M.D. President Medical Staff, Wake Forest Baptist Health–Davie Hospital, Mocksville, NC, p. A457
KELLER, Marsha, Director Human Resources, Kane Community Hospital, Kane, PA, p. A526
KELLER, Maryalice, Vice President Brand and Talent Management, Unity Hospital, Rochester, NY, p. A442
KELLER, Michael J., Vice President Financial Affairs and Chief Financial Officer, Spaulding Hospital for Continuing Medical Care Cambridge, Cambridge, MA, p. A299
KELLER, Ruey, Acting Chief Information Officer, Veterans Affairs San Diego Healthcare System, San Diego, CA, p. A86
KELLER, Thomas, Executive Vice President and Chief Operating Officer, St. Anthony Shawnee Hospital, Shawnee, OK, p. A504
KELLER, Wendy, Director Health Information Management, Atrium Medical Center of Corinth, Corinth, TX, p. A588
KELLERMAN, Scott, Chief Financial Officer, Ely–Bloomenson Community Hospital, Ely, MN, p. A331
KELLEY, Ann, Director Human Resources, Hardin Memorial Hospital, Elizabethtown, KY, p. A249
KELLEY, Brent, Director Information Technology, Nor–Lea General Hospital, Lovington, NM, p. A417
KELLEY, Jalinda, Director, Chickasaw Nation Medical Center, Ada, OK, p. A493
KELLEY, Janice, Chief Financial Officer, Marshall County Hospital, Benton, KY, p. A247
KELLEY, Jim, Vice President Finance and Support Services, Advocate Lutheran General Hospital, Park Ridge, IL, p. A191
KELLEY, Mark A., M.D. Executive Vice President and Chief Medical Officer, Henry Ford Hospital, Detroit, MI, p. A310
KELLEY, Mary, Director Human Resources, The Outer Banks Hospital, Nags Head, NC, p. A458


© 2012 AHA Guide Index of Health Care Professionals **A851**

Index of Health Care Professionals

Index of Health Care Professionals / Kelley


KELLEY, Neal, Administrator, Seton Edgar B. Davis Hospital, Luling, TX, p. A614
KELLEY, R. Lewis, Administrator, Chatuge Regional Hospital and Nursing Home, Hiawassee, GA, p. A154
KELLEY, Randall L., President and Chief Executive Officer, Gaston Memorial Hospital, Gastonia, NC, p. A453
KELLEY, Sarah Jo, Director Human Resources, Ste. Genevieve County Memorial Hospital, Ste. Genevieve, MO, p. A371
KELLEY, Steven L., President and Chief Executive Officer, Ellenville Regional Hospital, Ellenville, NY, p. A425
KELLEY, Sue, Chief Financial Officer, Cordell Memorial Hospital, Cordell, OK, p. A495
KELLEY, Suzanne, Director Human Resources, North Suburban Medical Center, Thornton, CO, p. A106
KELLEY, Warren, Chief Information Officer, Reynolds Memorial Hospital, Glen Dale, WV, p. A672
KELLEY–ROBINSON, Kathleen, Manager Human Resources, Nebraska Orthopaedic Hospital, Omaha, NE, p. A388
KELLIHER, Brandon, IT Operations Officer, Great Plains Regional Medical Center, North Platte, NE, p. A386
KELLIHER, Michael, Vice President Human Resources, Brattleboro Memorial Hospital, Brattleboro, VT, p. A643
KELLING, Jim, M.D. Chief of Staff, Transylvania Regional Hospital, Brevard, NC, p. A449
KELLIS, Dana, M.D. Senior Vice President Medical Affairs and Chief Medical Officer, Pinnacle Health System, Harrisburg, PA, p. A524
KELLOGG, Brewster, D.O. Chief Medical Staff, Citizens Medical Center, Colby, KS, p. A231
KELLOGG, Jason, M.D. Chief of Staff, Newport Bay Hospital, Newport Beach, CA, p. A77
KELLS, Anne, Interim Chief Financial Officer, Appleton Area Health Services, Appleton, MN, p. A327
KELLUM, Craig, Director Management Information Systems, Cape Fear Valley – Bladen County Hospital, Elizabethtown, NC, p. A453
KELLY, Allen, R.N. Vice President Procedural Services & CNO, Riverside Medical Center, Kankakee, IL, p. A185
KELLY, Arthur C., Administrator and Chief Executive Officer, OCH Regional Medical Center, Starkville, MS, p. A353
KELLY, Ashley, Manager Human Resources, Middlesboro ARH Hospital, Middlesboro, KY, p. A256
KELLY, Brian
  Vice President Finance, Advocate South Suburban Hospital, Hazel Crest, IL, p. A184
  Acting Chief Fiscal Service, Veterans Affairs Medical Center, San Francisco, CA, p. A87
KELLY, Brian E., M.D. President Medical Staff, Saint Elizabeth's Medical Center, Wabasha, MN, p. A341
KELLY, Bruce, Chief Information Officer, Mercy Memorial Hospital System, Monroe, MI, p. A319
KELLY, Charles, D.O. Vice President Medical Affairs and Chief Medical Officer, Henry Ford Macomb Hospitals, Clinton Township, MI, p. A309
KELLY, Colan, Chief Financial Officer, Pineville Community Hospital Association, Pineville, KY, p. A258
KELLY, Daniel J., President and Chief Executive Officer, St. Mary's Community Hospital, Nebraska City, NE, p. A386
KELLY, Daniel R., Chief Executive Officer, McKenzie County Healthcare System, Watford City, ND, p. A468
KELLY, Debbie, Chief Executive Officer, South Texas Spine and Surgical Hospital, San Antonio, TX, p. A626
KELLY, Diane, R.N. Chief Operating Officer, Berkshire Medical Center, Pittsfield, MA, p. A303
KELLY, Edward, President, Milford Regional Medical Center, Milford, MA, p. A302
KELLY, John J., M.D. Chief of Staff, Abington Memorial Hospital, Abington, PA, p. A517
KELLY, Kathleen, M.D. Chief Medical Officer and Chief Quality Officer, SwedishAmerican Hospital, Rockford, IL, p. A193
KELLY, Kerry, Superintendent, Blue Mountain Recovery Center, Pendleton, OR, p. A513
KELLY, Laurence E., President and Chief Executive Officer, Nathan Littauer Hospital and Nursing Home, Gloversville, NY, p. A426
KELLY, Lynn, Vice President Human Resources, San Antonio Community Hospital, Upland, CA, p. A94
KELLY, Marcia, Manager, IT, Mercer County Hospital, Aledo, IL, p. A172
KELLY, Mark, Vice President Finance, St. Francis Medical Center, Trenton, NJ, p. A411
KELLY, Mark A., Chief Executive Officer, Select Specialty Hospital–Memphis, Memphis, TN, p. A572
KELLY, Maura, Vice President Fiscal Services, Pen Bay Medical Center, Rockport, ME, p. A285
KELLY, Maureen, R.N. Chief Nursing Officer, Roswell Park Cancer Institute, Buffalo, NY, p. A423
KELLY, Melissa, Chief Operating Officer, Pender Community Hospital, Pender, NE, p. A389
KELLY, Michael
  Vice President, Christian Hospital, Saint Louis, MO, p. A368
  Information Systems Account Executive, Progress West HealthCare Center, Saint Charles, MO, p. A367
KELLY, Michael, M.D. President Medical Staff, Raleigh General Hospital, Beckley, WV, p. A670
KELLY, Patrick, Director, Sioux Falls VA Health Care System, Sioux Falls, SD, p. A560
KELLY, Peter A., President and Chief Executive Officer, Christ Hospital, Jersey City, NJ, p. A405
KELLY, Roy, Facility Director, Hawthorn Center, Northville, MI, p. A320
KELLY, Scott A., Chief Executive Officer, Rogue Valley Medical Center, Medford, OR, p. A512
KELLY, Shannon, Director Human Resources, Morton General Hospital, Morton, WA, p. A663
KELLY, Steven G., President and Chief Executive Officer, Newton Medical Center, Newton, KS, p. A239
KELLY, Sylvia K., Chief Executive Officer, HEALTHSOUTH Rehabilitation Hospital, Albuquerque, NM, p. A414
KELLY, Thomas, Interim Chief Financial Officer, Geisinger–Community Medical Center, Scranton, PA, p. A537
KELLY, Jr., Thomas, Chief Financial Officer, Moses Taylor Hospital, Scranton, PA, p. A538
KELLY, Thomas F., M.D. Medical Director, Deer's Head Hospital Center, Salisbury, MD, p. A294
KELLY, Thomas J., M.P.H. Vice President Medical Affairs, Union Hospital, Dover, OH, p. A479
KELLY, Timothy J., M.D. Medical Director, Fairbanks, Indianapolis, IN, p. A204
KELLY, Virginia, Chief Financial Officer, Eastside Psychiatric Hospital, Tallahassee, FL, p. A140
KELSEY, Janet, Director Business, Evansville State Hospital, Evansville, IN, p. A201
KEM, Mark
  Vice President Finance and Chief Financial Officer, Chandler Regional Medical Center, Chandler, AZ, p. A31
  Vice President Finance and Chief Financial Officer, Mercy Gilbert Medical Center, Gilbert, AZ, p. A32
KEMKER, S. E., M.D. President Medical Staff, St. Vincent Salem Hospital, Salem, IN, p. A211
KEMMERER, Jan, Director of Nursing, Mitchell County Hospital Health Systems, Beloit, KS, p. A231
KEMP, Jennifer, Director Marketing and Public Relations, St. Thomas More Hospital, Canon City, CO, p. A98
KEMP, Kenneth, Director Information Systems, Carlsbad Medical Center, Carlsbad, NM, p. A415
KEMP, Thomas, Chief Information Officer, New York Hospital Queens,, NY, p. A435
KEMPIAK, Matthew, Director Human Resources and Administrative Services, Memorial Hospital of Gardena, Gardena, CA, p. A63
KEMPINSKI, Paul D., Chief Operating Officer, Alfred I. duPont Hospital for Children, Wilmington, DE, p. A114
KEMPSON, Dave, Chief Information Officer, Maricopa Integrated Health System, Phoenix, AZ, p. A36
KEMPTON, Dana, Associate Director and Chief Financial Officer, Redington–Fairview General Hospital, Skowhegan, ME, p. A285
KENAGY, John Jay, Ph.D. Senior Vice President and Chief Information Officer, Legacy Meridian Park Hospital, Tualatin, OR, p. A516
KENDALL, Abigail, Chief Nursing Officer and Chief Operating Officer, Cushing Regional Hospital, Cushing, OK, p. A495
KENDALL, Anthony
  Vice President Human Resources, Baptist Health Extended Care Hospital, Little Rock, AR, p. A47
  Vice President Human Resources, Baptist Health Medical Center – North Little Rock, North Little Rock, AR, p. A50
  Vice President Human Resources, Baptist Health Medical Center–Arkadelphia, Arkadelphia, AR, p. A42
  Vice President Human Resources, Baptist Health Medical Center–Little Rock, Little Rock, AR, p. A47
  Vice President Human Resources, Baptist Health Rehabilitation Institute, Little Rock, AR, p. A48
KENDALL, Kim, Director Human Resources, Lawrence County Memorial Hospital, Lawrenceville, IL, p. A186
KENDLER, Lisa
  Chief Financial Officer, Memorial Hermann Katy Hospital, Katy, TX, p. A610
  Chief Financial Officer, Memorial Hermann Memorial City Medical Center, Houston, TX, p. A605
KENDRICK, Donovan, M.D. Chief of Staff, Baptist Medical Center South, Montgomery, AL, p. A23
KENDRICK, Jim R., Chief Executive Officer, Longview Regional Medical Center, Longview, TX, p. A613
KENDRICK, Justin, Chief Operating Officer, Texoma Medical Center, Denison, TX, p. A593
KENDRICK, Michael, Chief Operating Officer, Des Peres Hospital, Saint Louis, MO, p. A368
KENDRICK, Ray
  Chief Human Resources Officer, Memorial Hospital Miramar, Miramar, FL, p. A132
  Chief Human Resources Officer, Memorial Regional Hospital,, FL, p. A125
KENKELEN, Maryann, Vice President Human Resources and Tenant Services, Kindred Hospital South Philadelphia, Philadelphia, PA, p. A533
KENNALLY, Kevin, M.D. Chief of Medical Staff, Sabetha Community Hospital, Sabetha, KS, p. A242
KENNEDY, Brad, Chief Executive Officer, HEALTHSOUTH Rehabilitation Hospital, Memphis, TN, p. A571
KENNEDY, Bruce, M.D. Chief Medical Officer, San Jacinto Methodist Hospital, Baytown, TX, p. A582
KENNEDY, Christopher, President, Viera Hospital, Melbourne, FL, p. A130
KENNEDY, Connie, Director Human Resources, Marlette Regional Hospital, Marlette, MI, p. A318
KENNEDY, Daniel, M.D. Chief of Staff, Sutter Davis Hospital, Davis, CA, p. A59
KENNEDY, Darla, Chief Information Officer, Newport Specialty Hospital, Tustin, CA, p. A93
KENNEDY, Diana, Director Human Resources, Meadowview Regional Medical Center, Maysville, KY, p. A256
KENNEDY, Elizabeth M., Administrator, J. Paul Jones Hospital, Camden, AL, p. A18
KENNEDY, Greg, Manager Human Resources, Windsor–Laurelwood Center for Behavioral Medicine, Willoughby, OH, p. A491
KENNEDY, Jay, Chief Operating Officer, Maria Parham Medical Center, Henderson, NC, p. A454
KENNEDY, Jerry, Administrator, Jefferson County Hospital, Fayette, MS, p. A345
KENNEDY, John, M.D. Vice President Medical Affairs, Mercy Health – Fairfield Hospital, Fairfield, OH, p. A480
KENNEDY, Kimberly, Manager Human Resources, Mendota Community Hospital, Mendota, IL, p. A188
KENNEDY, Mary, Chief Nursing Officer, Medina Hospital, Medina, OH, p. A484
KENNEDY, Pam, Vice President Regional Human Resources and Organizational Department, CHRISTUS St. Michael Health System, Texarkana, TX, p. A630
KENNEDY, R. Scott, M.D. Assistant Administrator and Chief Medical Officer, Olympic Medical Center, Port Angeles, WA, p. A664
KENNEDY, ReChelle, Chief Financial Officer, Kearny County Hospital, Lakin, KS, p. A237
KENNEDY, Ryan, Chief Operating Officer, Kingman Regional Medical Center, Kingman, AZ, p. A33
KENNEDY, Susan, Manager Human Resources, Presbyterian Hospital Matthews, Matthews, NC, p. A457
KENNEDY, Todd S., Executive Vice President and Chief Operating Officer, Providence Hospital, Mobile, AL, p. A23
KENNETH, Ron, M.D. Chief Medical Officer, West Valley Hospital, Goodyear, AZ, p. A33
KENNETT, David, Chief Financial Officer, Jersey Community Hospital, Jerseyville, IL, p. A185
KENNETT, Jerry, M.D. Chief Medical Officer, Boone Hospital Center, Columbia, MO, p. A358
KENNEY, Catherine, Chief Nursing Officer, Pampa Regional Medical Center, Pampa, TX, p. A620
KENNEY, Evan, Manager Information Technology Systems, Lee's Summit Medical Center, Lee's Summit, MO, p. A364
KENNEY, Mary Ellen, Chief Human Services, Veterans Affairs Medical Center, Manchester, NH, p. A399
KENNIFF, Peter B., CPA Chief Financial Officer, Mercy Suburban Hospital, Norristown, PA, p. A530
KENNINGTON, Lynn, Chief Financial Officer, Desert Springs Hospital Medical Center, Las Vegas, NV, p. A392
KENNINGTON, Milas H., Vice President, Human Resources, Western Medical Center–Santa Ana, Santa Ana, CA, p. A89
KENNY, Carolyn, Executive Vice President Clinical Care, Children's Healthcare of Atlanta, Atlanta, GA, p. A145
KENNY, Richard, Vice President Human Resources, Hallmark Health System, Melrose, MA, p. A302
KENNY, Thomas, Chief Executive Officer, Meadows Psychiatric Center, Centre Hall, PA, p. A520
KENT, Alan, Chief Executive Officer, Meadows Regional Medical Center, Vidalia, GA, p. A161
KENT, Blair, Administrator, Riverton Hospital, Riverton, UT, p. A640
KENT, David, M.D. Chief Medical Officer, Boise Behavioral Health Hospital, Boise, ID, p. A166
KENT, David, Director Human Resources, Bolivar Medical Center, Cleveland, MS, p. A345
KENT, Gerald P., Chief Executive Officer, Norristown State Hospital, Norristown, PA, p. A530
KENT, Michael, Chief Executive Officer, Muenster Memorial Hospital, Muenster, TX, p. A617


A852 Index of Health Care Professionals

Index of Health Care Professionals
Index of Health Care Professionals / Kilroy

KILROY, John E., Vice President and Chief Information Officer, Cape Cod Hospital, Hyannis, MA, p. A301
KIM, Eric, Chief Information Officer, Aurora Las Encinas Hospital, Pasadena, CA, p. A79
KIM, Paul, M.D. Chief of Staff, North Hills Hospital, North Richland Hills, TX, p. A618
KIM, Soon K., M.D. President and Chief Executive Officer, Aurora Behavioral Health Care, Corona, CA, p. B14
KIMBALL, Kevin, Vice President Information Technology, Roswell Park Cancer Institute, Buffalo, NY, p. A423
KIMBALL, Mark E., Administrator, Mitchell County Hospital, Camilla, GA, p. A148
KIMBALL, Sharon M., R.N. Vice President and Chief Nursing Officer, Caldwell Memorial Hospital, Lenoir, NC, p. A456
KIMBLE, Gail, Chief Human Resource Officer, Penn Presbyterian Medical Center, Philadelphia, PA, p. A533
KIMBLE, Gay, Director Human Resources, Susan B. Allen Memorial Hospital, El Dorado, KS, p. A232
KIMBLER, Christine M., R.N. Chief Operating Officer, FirstLight Health System, Mora, MN, p. A336
KIMBREW, Missey, Director Human Resources, Grafton City Hospital, Grafton, WV, p. A672
KIMBROUGH, Pam, M.D. Vice President Medical Affairs, Mercy Hospital Ardmore, Ardmore, OK, p. A493
KIMES, Kent, Director Information Systems, North Arkansas Regional Medical Center, Harrison, AR, p. A45
KIMMEL, Edra, M.D. Chief of Staff, Woman's Hospital, Flowood, MS, p. A346
KIMMEL, Kyle, Chief Financial Officer, Bacon County Hospital and Health System, Alma, GA, p. A144
KIMMEL, Stephen, Senior Vice President and Chief Financial Officer, Hendrick Health System, Abilene, TX, p. A577
KIMMES, Robert P., Chief Executive Officer, Clifton–Fine Hospital, Star Lake, NY, p. A443
KIMPLE, Robin, Director Information Services, Gettysburg Hospital, Gettysburg, PA, p. A524
KIMSAL, Ken, Chief Financial Officer, Russell County Hospital, Russell Springs, KY, p. A258
KIMSEY, Kerri, Director Human Resources, Arkansas Valley Regional Medical Center, La Junta, CO, p. A103
KINCAID, Bryan, Director Information Systems, Scotland Health Care System, Laurinburg, NC, p. A456
KINCAID, Kevin, Chief Executive Officer, Knoxville Hospital & Clinics, Knoxville, IA, p. A222
KINDER, Barbara, R.N. Chief Nursing Officer, Lake City Medical Center, Lake City, FL, p. A128
KINDER, Frederick, M.D. Chief of Staff, Willis–Knighton Medical Center, Shreveport, LA, p. A277
KINDERED, Deanne, Vice President Finance, Baylor Regional Medical Center at Plano, Plano, TX, p. A621
KINDRED, Bill, Chief Executive Officer, T. J. Samson Community Hospital, Glasgow, KY, p. A250
KINDRED, Bryan N., FACHE President and Chief Executive Officer, DCH Health System, Tuscaloosa, AL, p. B40
KING, Abner, Chief Operating Officer, Steele Memorial Medical Center, Salmon, ID, p. A170
KING, Alan N., FACHE President and Chief Executive Officer, Covenant Hospital Plainview, Plainview, TX, p. A621
KING, Amber, Director Human Resources, Northcrest Medical Center, Springfield, TN, p. A576
KING, Ashley, Chief Executive Officer, North Valley Health Center, Warren, MN, p. A341
KING, Bruce, President and Chief Executive Officer, New London Hospital, New London, NH, p. A399
KING, Chayne, Contracted Manager Information Technology, Mark Reed Health Care District, McCleary, WA, p. A662
KING, Chris, Director Information Services, OhioHealth Marion General Hospital, Marion, OH, p. A484
KING, Christopher, Director Operations and Administrative Services, Matheny Medical and Educational Center, Peapack, NJ, p. A408
KING, Craig, Coordinator Human Resources, Kindred Hospital Sugar Land, Sugar Land, TX, p. A629
KING, Davlin, Team Leader Human Resources, Mother Frances Hospital – Jacksonville, Jacksonville, TX, p. A609
KING, Debbie, Chief Executive Officer, Swisher Memorial Hospital District, Tulia, TX, p. A632
KING, Dennis P., Chief Executive Officer, Spring Harbor Hospital, Westbrook, ME, p. A286
KING, Don, Chief Operating Officer, Saint Thomas Hospital, Nashville, TN, p. A573
KING, Donna J., R.N. Vice President Clinical Operations and Chief Nursing Executive, Advocate Illinois Masonic Medical Center, Chicago, IL, p. A175
KING, Doug, M.D
  Medical Director, Pathways of Tennessee, Jackson, TN, p. A567
  Director Clinical Services, Western Mental Health Institute, Bolivar, TN, p. A562
KING, Ed, Chief Financial Officer, Downey Regional Medical Center, Downey, CA, p. A59
KING, Glenn
  Vice President, Chief Nursing Officer, MidMichigan Medical Center–Clare, Clare, MI, p. A309
  Vice President and Chief Nursing Officer, MidMichigan Medical Center–Gladwin, Gladwin, MI, p. A313
KING, Gordon A., Interim Chief Financial Officer, Saint Clare's Health System, Denville, NJ, p. A403
KING, Grace, Regional Director Human Resources, Broward Health North, Deerfield Beach, FL, p. A122
KING, Heath, Controller, Polk Medical Center, Cedartown, GA, p. A149
KING, Jamelle, Director Human Resources, Claremore Indian Hospital, Claremore, OK, p. A494
KING, James E., Corporate Director Information Technology, Reliant Rehabilitation Hospital Dallas, Dallas, TX, p. A592
KING, Jay, Vice President Human Resources, Mercy Hospitals of Bakersfield, Bakersfield, CA, p. A55
KING, Jim, Executive Vice President and Chief Operating Officer, Jackson County Memorial Hospital, Altus, OK, p. A493
KING, Joanie, Chief Financial Officer, Carteret General Hospital, Morehead City, NC, p. A457
KING, John T., M.D. Vice President Medical Staff Affairs, Franciscan St. Anthony Health – Crown Point, Crown Point, IN, p. A200
KING, Kim, Director Human Resources and Public Relations, Baptist Memorial Hospital–Huntingdon, Huntingdon, TN, p. A566
KING, Kirk, FACHE President, Texas Health Arlington Memorial Hospital, Arlington, TX, p. A579
KING, Linda, Chief Human Resources Management Service, Central Alabama Veterans Health Care System, Montgomery, AL, p. A23
KING, Louie, Interim Administrator, Teton Medical Center, Choteau, MT, p. A374
KING, Michael, Chief Financial Officer, El Camino Hospital, Mountain View, CA, p. A76
KING, Michael A., FACHE President and Chief Executive Officer, Camden–Clark Medical Center, Parkersburg, WV, p. A674
KING, Mike, Chief Operating Officer, Doctors Medical Center, Modesto, CA, p. A75
KING, Paul, M.D. Medical Director, Parkwood Behavioral Health System, Olive Branch, MS, p. A351
KING, Ray, M.D. Senior Vice President and Chief Medical Officer, Allegiance Health, Jackson, MI, p. A316
KING, Rich, Vice President Information Technology, West Virginia University Hospitals, Morgantown, WV, p. A674
KING, Sam, Chief Financial Officer, Renown Regional Medical Center, Reno, NV, p. A395
KING, Tamara, R.N. Chief Nurse Executive, Shepherd Center, Atlanta, GA, p. A146
KING, Thom, Chief Executive Officer, HEALTHSOUTH Rehabilitation Hospital, Florence, SC, p. A549
KING, Victoria, M.D. Chief Medical Officer, St. Thomas More Hospital, Canon City, CO, p. A98
KING ROBINSON, Jan, VP, Operations, Albemarle Health, Elizabeth City, NC, p. A452
KING–SCHREIBER, Susan, Vice President Human Resources, Franciscan St. Anthony Health – Michigan City, Michigan City, IN, p. A208
KINGHAM, Darrell L., CPA Vice President Finance, Beauregard Memorial Hospital, De Ridder, LA, p. A265
KINGSBURY, James A., President and Chief Executive Officer, UC Health, Cincinnati, OH, p. B133
KINGSLEY, Christi, Director Human Resources, West Calcasieu Cameron Hospital, Sulphur, LA, p. A278
KINGSLEY, Susan, Accountant, Kau Hospital, Pahala, HI, p. A165
KINGSTON, Peggy, Chief Executive Officer, Select Specialty Hospital–Pontiac, Pontiac, MI, p. A321
KINI, M. Narendra, M.D. President and Chief Executive Officer, Miami Children's Hospital, Miami, FL, p. A131
KINKAID, Gina, Vice President Human Resources, Newport Medical Center, Newport, TN, p. A574
KINKAID, Steve
  Vice President Technology, Nix Health Care System, San Antonio, TX, p. A625
  Director Information Systems, Palmerton Hospital, Palmerton, PA, p. A531
KINMAN, Brett, Chief Executive Officer, Forrest City Medical Center, Forrest City, AR, p. A45
KINNEY, Charles S., President and Chief Executive Officer, Westerly Hospital, Westerly, RI, p. A545
KINNEY, Janet, Chief Operating Officer, Northwest Florida Community Hospital, Chipley, FL, p. A120
KINSAUL, David, President and Chief Executive Officer, Children's Medical Center, Dayton, OH, p. A478
KINSEL, Mike, Controller, Federal Medical Center, Lexington, KY, p. A253
KINSEY, Daniel, M.D. Medical Director, Oaklawn Psychiatric Center, Goshen, IN, p. A202
KINSLOW, Kathleen, Ed.D. President and Chief Executive Officer, Aria Health, Philadelphia, PA, p. A531
KINTZ, Ronald J.
  Vice President and Treasurer, Arnot Ogden Medical Center, Elmira, NY, p. A425
  Senior Vice President Finance and Chief Financial Officer, St. Joseph's Hospital, Elmira, NY, p. A426
KINYON, Craig C., President, Reid Hospital and Health Care Services, Richmond, IN, p. A211
KINYON, David, Vice President of Operations and Outpatient Services, Three Rivers Medical Center, Grants Pass, OR, p. A511
KINYOUN, Nancy, Director Health Information Management, Hastings Regional Center, Hastings, NE, p. A384
KIO, Kenneth, Manager Human Resources, Albany Stratton Veterans Affairs Medical Center, Albany, NY, p. A420
KIPE, Larry, M.D. Chief of Staff, Memorial Hospital, Craig, CO, p. A99
KIPFER, Debra, Chief Financial Officer, Community Hospital of Bremen, Bremen, IN, p. A198
KIPPER, Tedd, Chief Operating Officer, Virginia Gay Hospital, Vinton, IA, p. A227
KIPREOS, Nicholas, M.D. Chief Medical Staff, Pioneer Community Hospital of Patrick County, Stuart, VA, p. A656
KIRBY, Adrienne, Ph.D. Chief Operating Officer, Cooper Health System, Camden, NJ, p. A402
KIRBY, Dale A., Chief Executive Officer, Colusa Regional Medical Center, Colusa, CA, p. A58
KIRBY, Elizabeth A., Director Human Resources, Aurora BayCare Medical Center, Green Bay, WI, p. A682
KIRBY II, James M., Chief Executive Officer, Margaret R. Pardee Memorial Hospital, Hendersonville, NC, p. A454
KIRBY, Jennifer, R.N. Chief Nursing Officer, George Washington University Hospital, Washington, DC, p. A116
KIRBY, Juliana Kay, R.N. Chief Nursing Officer and Director of Nursing, Tehachapi Valley Healthcare District, Tehachapi, CA, p. A92
KIRBY, Richard S., Executive Vice President and Chief Financial Officer, Community Memorial Hospital, Hamilton, NY, p. A427
KIRBY, Ruby, Administrator, Bolivar General Hospital, Bolivar, TN, p. A562
KIRCH, Cyndi, Vice President Human Resources, Mercy General Hospital, Sacramento, CA, p. A83
KIRCHER, Mark, Associate Vice President Finance, Norton Suburban Hospital, Louisville, KY, p. A255
KIRCHNER, Doris, Chief Executive Officer, Vail Valley Medical Center, Vail, CO, p. A106
KIRCHNER, Kent, M.D. Chief of Staff, G.V. Montgomery Veterans Affairs Medical Center, Jackson, MS, p. A347
KIRITANI, Tracy, Vice President and Chief Financial Officer, Clovis Community Medical Center, Clovis, CA, p. A57
KIRK, Darlene, Manager Finance, U. S. Public Health Service Indian Hospital, Crownpoint, NM, p. A415
KIRK Jr., H. Lee, President and Chief Executive Officer, Culpeper Regional Hospital, Culpeper, VA, p. A647
KIRK, Jean, Chief Financial Officer, Bennett County Hospital and Nursing Home, Martin, SD, p. A557
KIRK, Joe L., Executive Vice President, Freeman Hospital West, Joplin, MO, p. A361
KIRK, Paul, Vice President, Woman's Hospital, Baton Rouge, LA, p. A263
KIRK, Peggy, Senior Vice President Clinical Operations, Rehabilitation Institute of Chicago, Chicago, IL, p. A177
KIRK, Roger L., President and Chief Executive Officer, Bethesda Memorial Hospital, Boynton Beach, FL, p. A119
KIRK, Vanessa, Director of Nursing, Kiowa County Memorial Hospital, Greensburg, KS, p. A234
KIRK, Warren J., Chief Executive Officer, Doctors Medical Center, Modesto, CA, p. A75
KIRKBRIDE, Jim
  Director of Support Services, Pioneer Memorial Hospital, Prineville, OR, p. A514
  Director of Support Services, St. Charles Medical Center – Redmond, Redmond, OR, p. A515
KIRKER, Donna, R.N. Vice President Patient Services and Chief Nursing Officer, Glens Falls Hospital, Glens Falls, NY, p. A426
KIRKER, Lynda I., Chief Financial Officer, Flagler Hospital, Saint Augustine, FL, p. A137
KIRKHAM, Brett, Administrator, East Texas Medical Center Trinity, Trinity, TX, p. A631
KIRKHAM, Jeff, Chief Financial Officer, Community Hospital North, Indianapolis, IN, p. A204
KIRKS, Linda, Chief Financial Officer, Baptist Health System, San Antonio, TX, p. A624
KIRN, Galen, Administrator, California Mens Colony Hospital, San Luis Obispo, CA, p. A88
KIRSHNER, Arthur N., Chief Information Management, Winn Army Community Hospital, Hinesville, GA, p. A154

A854 Index of Health Care Professionals

Index of Health Care Professionals / Knipp

Index of Health Care Professionals


KIRSHNER, David, Senior Vice President and Chief Financial Officer, Children's Hospital Boston, Boston, MA, p. A296
KIRSON, Joel, M.D. Medical Director, Anchor Hospital, Atlanta, GA, p. A145
KIRSTEIN, Susan N., R.N. Chief Nursing Officer, Broadlawns Medical Center, Des Moines, IA, p. A218
KISER, Greg, Chief Executive Officer, Three Rivers Medical Center, Louisa, KY, p. A254
KISER II, James R., Chief Executive Officer, St. Joseph Hospital, Polson, MT, p. A378
KISER, Phyllis, Director Human Resources, Russell County Medical Center, Lebanon, VA, p. A650
KISER, Terry L.
Vice President and Chief Financial Officer, Georgetown Memorial Hospital, Georgetown, SC, p. A550
Chief Financial Officer, Waccamaw Community Hospital, Murrells Inlet, SC, p. A552
KISHNER, Janice, Chief Operating Officer and Nurse Executive, East Jefferson General Hospital, Metairie, LA, p. A273
KISKADDON, Robert, M.D. Chief Medical Officer, Margaret R. Pardee Memorial Hospital, Hendersonville, NC, p. A454
KISNER, Angela, Director Human Resources and Coordinator Medical Staff, Landmark Hospital, Cape Girardeau, MO, p. A356
KISTLER, Beckie, Controller, Our Lady of Peace, Louisville, KY, p. A255
KISTLER, Mike, Chief Executive Officer, Shadow Mountain Behavioral Health System, Tulsa, OK, p. A506
KITCHEN, Randy J., Chief Executive Officer, Dayton Rehabilitation Institute, Dayton, OH, p. A478
KITOWSKI, Jerome, M.D. Chief of Staff, Black River Memorial Hospital, Black River Falls, WI, p. A679
KITTELL, Elisabeth, Chief Financial Officer, Veterans Affairs Medical Center, Syracuse, NY, p. A444
KITTNER, Bonnie, R.N. Chief Nursing Officer, Mendocino Coast District Hospital, Fort Bragg, CA, p. A61
KITTRELL, Albert, M.D. Medical Director, Arkansas State Hospital, Little Rock, AR, p. A47
KIWALL, Walter J.
Executive Vice President and Chief Operating Officer, Mary Washington Hospital, Fredericksburg, VA, p. A648
Executive Vice President and Chief Operating Officer, Stafford Hospital, Stafford, VA, p. A656
KLARKOWSKI, Debbie, Manager Human Resources, Brown County Community Treatment Center, Green Bay, WI, p. A682
KLARNER, Lea Ann, Chief Executive Officer, Select Specialty Hospital–Fort Wayne, Fort Wayne, IN, p. A202
KLASSEN, Karen, Controller, HEALTHSOUTH Chattanooga Rehabilitation Hospital, Chattanooga, TN, p. A563
KLASSEN, Susan K., Chief Executive Officer and Administrator, Mahnomen Health Center, Mahnomen, MN, p. A334
KLAUKA, Floyd, Chief Financial Officer, Brook Lane Health Services, Hagerstown, MD, p. A292
KLAUSTERMEIER, Lisa, R.N. Chief Nursing Officer, Anderson Hospital, Maryville, IL, p. A187
KLAWITER, Thomas, Senior Vice President and Chief Operating Officer, Nix Health Care System, San Antonio, TX, p. A625
KLAWITER, Trey, Chief Operating Officer, Southwest General Hospital, San Antonio, TX, p. A626
KLAWITTER, Kyle, Vice President Human Resources, Summa Health System, Akron, OH, p. A469
KLEAM, Douglas V., Vice President and Chief Operating Officer, St. Vincent Medical Center, Los Angeles, CA, p. A72
KLEAS, Tara, Director Human Resources, HEALTHSOUTH Rehabilitation Hospital, Fort Worth, TX, p. A598
KLEEMAN, Debbie, Manager Information Systems, Perry County Memorial Hospital, Tell City, IN, p. A212
KLEEN, Kathy, Chief Nursing Officer, Tri–County Hospital, Wadena, MN, p. A341
KLEEN, Yachiel, M.D. Medical Director, Rehabilitation Hospital of Wisconsin, Waukesha, WI, p. A692
KLEIN, Aron, Vice President of Finance, Advocate Eureka Hospital, Eureka, IL, p. A181
KLEIN, Barbara, R.N. Director of Nursing, Arms Acres, Carmel, NY, p. A423
KLEIN, Cindy, Chief Financial Officer, Lamb Healthcare Center, Littlefield, TX, p. A612
KLEIN, Cindy C., Vice President Human Resources, PeaceHealth St. Joseph Medical Center, Bellingham, WA, p. A659
KLEIN, David G., M.D. Chief Operating Officer, Baylor All Saints Medical Center at Fort Worth, Fort Worth, TX, p. A598
KLEIN, Diany, Vice President Human Resources, Community Memorial Health System, Ventura, CA, p. A94
KLEIN, Edward A., Chief Financial Officer, Johnston Health, Smithfield, NC, p. A461
KLEIN, Eileen, Ph.D. Deputy Director Operations, South Beach Psychiatric Center,, NY, p. A436
KLEIN, Gerard D., Chief Executive Officer, Memorial Hospital of Sweetwater County, Rock Springs, WY, p. A697
KLEIN, Greg, Senior Director Finance, Presbyterian Hospital Matthews, Matthews, NC, p. A457
KLEIN, Jacqueline, Vice President Finance, Lakeview Medical Center, Rice Lake, WI, p. A690
KLEIN, Jerry, Chief Financial Officer, Lawrence County Memorial Hospital, Lawrenceville, IL, p. A186
KLEIN, Joel, Chief Executive Officer and Managing Director, Glen Oaks Hospital, Greenville, TX, p. A601
KLEIN, Julie, Chief Executive Officer, Sterling Regional MedCenter, Sterling, CO, p. A106
KLEIN, Kenneth, CPA Senior Vice President Finance and Chief Financial Officer, Menninger Clinic, Houston, TX, p. A605
KLEIN, Lynn E., Administrator, Mendota Community Hospital, Mendota, IL, p. A188
KLEIN, Ronald, M.D. Vice President and Chief Medical Officer, Brookhaven Memorial Hospital Medical Center, Patchogue, NY, p. A440
KLEINE, Doug, IT Director, St. Mary Medical Center, Apple Valley, CA, p. A54
KLEINHANZL, Thomas A., President and Chief Executive Officer, Frederick Memorial Hospital, Frederick, MD, p. A291
KLEINMAN, Richard, R.N. Manager Medical Informatics, Catalina Island Medical Center, Avalon, CA, p. A54
KLENKE, Lisa R., R.N. Vice President Patient Care Services, Mercer County Joint Township Community Hospital, Coldwater, OH, p. A476
KLEPIN, Michael R.
Administrator, Hunt Memorial Hospital District, Greenville, TX, p. A602
Administrator, Hunt Regional Community Hospital, Commerce, TX, p. A588
KLESACK, Debbie, Interim Chief Executive Officer, Bennett County Hospital and Nursing Home, Martin, SD, p. A557
KLEVEN, Brian, Chief Financial Officer, Alvarado Hospital, San Diego, CA, p. A85
KLEYMANN, Tiffany, Manager Human Resources, Greeley County Health Services, Tribune, KS, p. A244
KLICKSTEIN, Judith S., Chief Information Officer, Cambridge Health Alliance, Cambridge, MA, p. A299
KLIMEK, David, Chief Human Resources Officer, Olathe Medical Center, Olathe, KS, p. A240
KLIMP, Mary J., Chief Administrative Officer, Mayo Clinic Health System in New Prague, New Prague, MN, p. A336
KLINE, Donald E.
Chief Financial Officer and Vice President Operations, Mercy Allen Hospital, Oberlin, OH, p. A486
Senior Vice President Finance, St. Elizabeth Boardman Health Center, Boardman, OH, p. A471
Senior Vice President Finance, St. Elizabeth Health Center, Youngstown, OH, p. A492
Senior Vice President Finance, St. Joseph Health Center, Warren, OH, p. A490
KLINE, Julie, Senior Vice President Patient Services, Sonora Regional Medical Center, Sonora, CA, p. A91
KLINE, Mark W., M.D. Physician in Chief, Texas Children's Hospital, Houston, TX, p. A607
KLINGA, Maria, Director Management Information Systems, Silver Hill Hospital, New Canaan, CT, p. A110
KLINGENBERG, Pat, Director Human Resources, Towner County Medical Center, Cando, ND, p. A464
KLINGLER, Michael, M.D. Chief of Staff, Clay County Hospital, Flora, IL, p. A182
KLINGSEIS, Rob, Manager Information Systems, Community Hospital of Long Beach, Long Beach, CA, p. A68
KLINIKOWSKI, Angela, Director of Nursing, Vista Health, Fayetteville, AR, p. A44
KLINKER, Suzanne M., Director, Veterans Affairs Medical Center, Bay Pines, FL, p. A118
KLINKNER, Donna M., Chief Financial Officer, Madelia Community Hospital, Madelia, MN, p. A334
KLOC, Larry, Chief Financial Officer, Hopedale Medical Complex, Hopedale, IL, p. A185
KLOCK, Kathy, R.N. Senior Vice President Clinical Operations and Human Resources, Gundersen Lutheran Medical Center, La Crosse, WI, p. A683
KLOCKENGA, Kevin
President and Chief Executive Officer, Petaluma Valley Hospital, Petaluma, CA, p. A80
President and Chief Executive Officer, Santa Rosa Memorial Hospital, Santa Rosa, CA, p. A90
KLOCKMAN, Dena, Chief Financial Officer, Ogallala Community Hospital, Ogallala, NE, p. A387
KLOCKO, Daniel, Vice President Human Resources, Kootenai Medical Center, Coeur D'Alene, ID, p. A167
KLOEWER, Ron, Chief Information Officer, Montgomery County Memorial Hospital, Red Oak, IA, p. A225
KLOPFER, Rudy, Associate Director, Durham Veterans Affairs Medical Center, Durham, NC, p. A452
KLOSTERMAN, Mark D., FACHE President and Chief Executive Officer, St. Joseph's Hospital, Breese, IL, p. A174
KLOTZ, Carol, Director Human Resources, LifeCare Medical Center, Roseau, MN, p. A338
KLOTZ, Ken, M.D. Chief of Staff, Richard L. Roudebush Veterans Affairs Medical Center, Indianapolis, IN, p. A205
KLUGE, Thomas S., Chief Operating Officer, Halifax Regional Health System, South Boston, VA, p. A656
KLUGHERZ, Greg, Vice President Corporate Services and Chief Financial Officer, St. Cloud Hospital, Saint Cloud, MN, p. A338
KLUNE, Peter, Chief Executive Officer, Palo Verde Hospital, Blythe, CA, p. A56
KLUNK, Tim, Executive Director, Children's Hospital of Wisconsin–Fox Valley, Neenah, WI, p. A687
KLYCZEK, Mark F., President and Chief Executive Officer, Newark–Wayne Community Hospital, Newark, NY, p. A438
KMETZ, Thomas D., President, Kosair Children's Hospital, Louisville, KY, p. A254
KNAK, Roger, Administrator, Fairview Regional Medical Center, Fairview, OK, p. A496
KNAPHEIDE, Debbie, MSN, Site Administrator, Chief Nursing Officer and Chief Operating Officer, Carondelet Holy Cross Hospital, Nogales, AZ, p. A34
KNAPP, Anne, Chief Financial Officer, Valle Vista Hospital, Greenwood, IN, p. A203
KNAPP, Brian A., Vice President Operations, Fairview Ridges Hospital, Burnsville, MN, p. A329
KNAPP, Merlyn E., Chief Financial Officer, Saint Catherine Medical Center Fountain Springs, Ashland, PA, p. A518
KNAPP, Rhonda, Director Human Resources, Dahl Memorial Healthcare Association, Ekalaka, MT, p. A375
KNECHT, Brian J., Chief Operating Officer, Regional Medical Center of San Jose, San Jose, CA, p. A88
KNEDLER, Marie E., R.N
Vice President and Chief Operating Officer, Alegent Health–Bergan Mercy Medical Center, Omaha, NE, p. A387
Vice President and Chief Operating Officer, Alegent Health–Bergan Mercy Medical Center, Omaha, NE, p. A387
Vice President and Chief Operating Officer, Alegent Health–Mercy Hospital, Council Bluffs, IA, p. A217
Vice President and Chief Operating Officer, Alegent Health–Mercy Hospital, Council Bluffs, IA, p. A217
KNELL, Daniel J., MSN, President, Quincy Medical Center, Quincy, MA, p. A304
KNIEVEL, Lon, Chief Executive Officer, Tilden Community Hospital, Tilden, NE, p. A390
KNIGHT, Beth, Chief Nursing Officer, Nacogdoches Memorial Hospital, Nacogdoches, TX, p. A618
KNIGHT, Bethany, M.D. Chief of Staff, Community Medical Center of Izard County, Calico Rock, AR, p. A42
KNIGHT, Calvin K., President and Chief Executive Officer, John Muir Health, Walnut Creek, CA, p. B74
KNIGHT, Charles, Chief Financial Officer, Tippah County Hospital, Ripley, MS, p. A352
KNIGHT, Christopher D.
Chief Financial Officer, City Hospital, Martinsburg, WV, p. A673
Vice President Finance, Jefferson Memorial Hospital, Ranson, WV, p. A675
KNIGHT, Clif, M.D. Vice President Medical and Academic Affairs, Community Hospital North, Indianapolis, IN, p. A204
KNIGHT, Deana, Chief Executive Officer, Select Specialty Hospital–Greensboro, Greensboro, NC, p. A454
KNIGHT, Jennifer, Manager Human Resources, Waynesboro Hospital, Waynesboro, PA, p. A540
KNIGHT, Ken, Chief Financial Officer, Moab Regional Hospital, Moab, UT, p. A638
KNIGHT, Kimber, Chief Financial Officer, Braxton County Memorial Hospital, Gassaway, WV, p. A671
KNIGHT, Mark T., Executive Vice President and Chief Financial Officer, Jackson Health System, Miami, FL, p. A131
KNIGHT, Mary Ann, Chief Operating Officer, Medical Center of Trinity, Trinity, FL, p. A142
KNIGHT, Patricia, Vice President Human Resources, Tristar Centennial Medical Center, Nashville, TN, p. A573
KNIGHT, Russell M.
President and Chief Executive Officer, Mercy Medical Center–Dubuque, Dubuque, IA, p. A219
President and Chief Executive Officer, Mercy Medical Center–Dyersville, Dyersville, IA, p. A219
KNIGHT, Sue, CPA Chief Operating Officer, St. Elizabeth Hospital, Gonzales, LA, p. A267
KNIGHT, Terry, Public Information Officer and Administrative Assistant, California Mens Colony Hospital, San Luis Obispo, CA, p. A88
KNIGHT, Tim, Director Information Technology, Hot Springs County Memorial Hospital, Thermopolis, WY, p. A698
KNIGHT, Wayne, Director Finance, St. Vincent Clay Hospital, Brazil, IN, p. A198
KNIPP, Cindi, Director Human Resources, Rooks County Health Center, Plainville, KS, p. A242

Index of Health Care Professionals
Index of Health Care Professionals / Knittel

KNITTEL, Monty E., President and Chief Executive Officer, Walla Walla General Hospital, Walla Walla, WA, p. A669
KNIZLEY, Andrew, Chief Executive Officer, Houston Orthopedic and Spine Hospital, Bellaire, TX, p. A583
KNOBLOCH, Stanley
Chief Financial Officer, Sanford Luverne Medical Center, Luverne, MN, p. A334
Chief Financial Officer, Sanford Medical Center Rock Rapids, Rock Rapids, IA, p. A225
KNOCKE, Michael, Chief Information Officer, Kansas Spine Hospital, Wichita, KS, p. A245
KNODE, Scott, Chief Financial Officer, Veterans Memorial Hospital, Waukon, IA, p. A228
KNOERL, Thomas, Chief Financial Officer, Spectrum Health Reed City Hospital, Reed City, MI, p. A321
KNOKE, Debra R., Chief Executive Officer, Sequoyah Memorial Hospital, Sallisaw, OK, p. A504
KNOLL, Rolf W., M.D. Senior Vice President and Chief Medical Officer, Saint Francis Hospital and Medical Center, Hartford, CT, p. A109
KNOLL, Thomas, Site Director Finance, Community Memorial Hospital, Menomonee Falls, WI, p. A685
KNOST, Steve, Manager Facilities, UC Health Surgical Hospital, West Chester, OH, p. A491
KNOTT, Amy
Chief Financial Officer, Alegent Health–Bergan Mercy Medical Center, Omaha, NE, p. A387
Chief Financial Officer, Alegent Health–Mercy Hospital, Council Bluffs, IA, p. A217
KNOUS, Gail, Chief Executive Officer and Chief Compliance Officer, Basin Healthcare Center, Odessa, TX, p. A619
KNOWLAND, Richard
Area Chief Executive Officer, Promise Hospital Baton Rouge, Baton Rouge, LA, p. A263
Area Chief Executive Officer, Promise Hospital of Baton Rouge, Baton Rouge, LA, p. A263
Area Chief Executive Officer, Promise Hospital of Baton Rouge, Baton Rouge, LA, p. A263
KNOWLES, B. K., D.O. Chief of Staff, General John J. Pershing Memorial Hospital, Brookfield, MO, p. A356
KNOWLES, Christy, Chief Human Resources Officer, Coosa Valley Medical Center, Sylacauga, AL, p. A25
KNOWLES, John, Director Human Resources, Clinch Valley Medical Center, Richlands, VA, p. A654
KNOWLES, Lori, Director Human Resources, Park Plaza Hospital, Houston, TX, p. A606
KNOWLES, Petra, Chief Information Officer, PeaceHealth Southwest Medical Center, Vancouver, WA, p. A668
KNOWLES–SMITH, Peter, M.D. Medical Director, Bennett County Hospital and Nursing Home, Martin, SD, p. A557
KNOWLTON, Robert
Vice President, Baylor Specialty Hospital, Dallas, TX, p. A590
Vice President Finance, Our Children's House at Baylor, Dallas, TX, p. A592
KNOX, Dennis M., Chief Executive Officer, Western Medical Center Anaheim, Anaheim, CA, p. A53
KNOX, Jody, Administrator, Kindred Hospital Rancho, Rancho Cucamonga, CA, p. A81
KNOX, III, John J., Senior Vice President and Chief Information Officer, Carolinas Medical Center–University, Charlotte, NC, p. A450
KNOX, Jud, President, York Hospital, York, ME, p. A286
KNOX, Lisa, Manager Facility Automation, Terrell State Hospital, Terrell, TX, p. A630
KNOX, Roland, Chief Executive Officer, Northern Cochise Community Hospital, Willcox, AZ, p. A41
KNOX, Stacey A., Administrator, Rock County Hospital, Bassett, NE, p. A381
KNUDSEN, Mark, Director Fiscal Services, Shriners Hospitals for Children, Portland, Portland, OR, p. A514
KNUDSON, Jenny, Controller, Hiawatha Community Hospital, Hiawatha, KS, p. A234
KNUDSON, Veronica, Chief Operating Officer, Northwest Medical Center, Tucson, AZ, p. A40
KNUEVEN, Karen, Chief Nursing Officer, Olympia Medical Center, Los Angeles, CA, p. A71
KNULL, Ralph, Vice President Human Resources, Parma Community General Hospital, Parma, OH, p. A487
KNUTSON, Holly, Manager Information Technology, Kittson Memorial Healthcare Center, Hallock, MN, p. A332
KNUTSON, John P., M.D. Chief Medical Staff, Delta County Memorial Hospital, Delta, CO, p. A99
KNUTSON, Larry, Director Finance, CentraCare Health System – Long Prairie, Long Prairie, MN, p. A333
KNUTSON, Tanya, Director Human Resources, Mercy Hospital, Devils Lake, ND, p. A465
KOBBES ADAMS, Kathleen D., R.N. Chief Clinical Officer, Kindred Hospital–Tucson, Tucson, AZ, p. A40
KOBER, Merri, Director Information Services, Weatherford Regional Medical Center, Weatherford, TX, p. A634
KOBIS, David A., Senior Vice President and Chief Operating Officer, Bradford Regional Medical Center, Bradford, PA, p. A519
KOCH, Amanda, Director Human Resources, Greene Memorial Hospital, Xenia, OH, p. A492
KOCH, Cody, Director Human Resources, Saint Elizabeth Regional Medical Center, Lincoln, NE, p. A385
KOCH, Erich, Chief Financial Officer, West Hills Hospital, Reno, NV, p. A395
KOCH, Holly, Chief Financial Officer, Girard Medical Center, Girard, KS, p. A233
KOCH, Joseph G., Chief Executive Officer, Bourbon Community Hospital, Paris, KY, p. A258
KOCH, Robert, M.D. Chief Medical Staff, Cooper County Memorial Hospital, Boonville, MO, p. A356
KOCHEVAR, Vanessa
Chief Financial Officer, St. Mary's Regional Medical Center, Enid, OK, p. A496
Chief Financial Officer, Summerlin Hospital Medical Center, Las Vegas, NV, p. A394
KOCHIE, Daniel A., CPA Chief Financial Officer, Samaritan Hospital, Troy, NY, p. A445
KOCOUREK, Cathie A., Chief Administrative Officer, Aurora Medical Center – Manitowoc County, Two Rivers, WI, p. A692
KOCSIS, Dana, R.N. Vice President Nursing and Operations, Lodi Community Hospital, Lodi, OH, p. A483
KOCSIS, Violet, Vice President Human Resources and Development, Hunterdon Medical Center, Flemington, NJ, p. A404
KOEBNICK, Dale, Director Management Information Systems and Patient Access, Metroplex Adventist Hospital, Killeen, TX, p. A610
KOEHLER, Amy, Director Human Resources, Shelby Memorial Hospital, Shelbyville, IL, p. A193
KOEHLER, Maggie, Senior Vice President and Chief Financial Officer, Wilkes–Barre General Hospital, Wilkes–Barre, PA, p. A542
KOEHLER, Sherry, Chief Financial Officer, Greenville Regional Hospital, Greenville, IL, p. A183
KOEHLER, Suzanne, Vice President and Chief Support Officer, Methodist Medical Center of Oak Ridge, Oak Ridge, TN, p. A574
KOEHNE, Robert, Controller, Rehabilitation Hospital of Wisconsin, Waukesha, WI, p. A692
KOELE, Craig, Chief Executive Officer, Solara Hospital of Muskogee, Muskogee, OK, p. A500
KOENIG, Jr., Donald E., Executive Vice President and Chief Operating Officer, St. Elizabeth Health Center, Youngstown, OH, p. A492
KOENIG, Harris F., President and Chief Executive Officer, San Antonio Community Hospital, Upland, CA, p. A94
KOENIG, Mary, Chief Financial Officer, Vernon Memorial Healthcare, Viroqua, WI, p. A692
KOENIG, Thomas L., Vice President and Chief Operating Officer, Bon Secours St. Mary's Hospital, Richmond, VA, p. A654
KOEPKE, Eldon, Chief Financial Officer, Mitchell County Hospital Health Systems, Beloit, KS, p. A231
KOEPPEL–OLSEN, Carol, R.N. Vice President Patient Care Services, Fairview Ridges Hospital, Burnsville, MN, p. A329
KOESSL, Brenda, R.N. Director of Nursing Services, Frances Mahon Deaconess Hospital, Glasgow, MT, p. A375
KOESTER, Jean, Manager Human Resources, Limestone Medical Center, Groesbeck, TX, p. A602
KOFL, Andrea, Vice President Patient Care and Chief Nursing Executive, Mercy Medical Center Redding, Redding, CA, p. A81
KOHL, Kristi, M.D. Chief Medical Officer, Perkins County Health Services, Grant, NE, p. A384
KOHLBRENNER, Janis, R.N. Vice President Clinical Services and Chief Nursing Officer, Oneida Healthcare, Oneida, NY, p. A439
KOHLRUSS, Chuck, Vice President Human Resources and Operations Support, Holland Hospital, Holland, MI, p. A315
KOHRT, Nancy, Chief Financial Officer, Marengo Memorial Hospital, Marengo, IA, p. A223
KOINZAN, Leigh Jean, Director Finance, Boys Town National Research Hospital, Omaha, NE, p. A387
KOKJOHN, Bradley J., Chief Financial Officer, Fort Madison Community Hospital, Fort Madison, IA, p. A220
KOLAR, Stephen J., M.D
Vice President Medical Affairs, HealthEast Bethesda Hospital, Saint Paul, MN, p. A339
Vice President Medical Affairs, St. Joseph's Hospital, Saint Paul, MN, p. A339
KOLB, Fred L., Chief Executive Officer, Madison County Hospital, London, OH, p. A483
KOLB, Pat, Manager Information Technology, Clarendon Memorial Hospital, Manning, SC, p. A552
KOLESK, Stephen, M.D. Vice President and Chief Operating Officer, Virtua Memorial, Mount Holly, NJ, p. A406
KOLHEDE, Deborah, Vice President and Chief Operating Officer, St. Mary's Medical Center, San Francisco, CA, p. A87
KOLLMEYER, Sherry, Vice President Human Resources, Youth Villages Inner Harbour Campus, Douglasville, GA, p. A152
KOLMAN, Bret, CPA, Chief Executive Officer, Lafayette Regional Health Center, Lexington, MO, p. A364
KOLODZIEJCYK, Wanda, Director Human Resources, Cuero Community Hospital, Cuero, TX, p. A590
KOLODZIEJCZYK, Clayton, Chief Financial Officer, Meadowview Regional Medical Center, Maysville, KY, p. A256
KOLOSKY, John A., Executive Vice President and Chief Operating Officer, H. Lee Moffitt Cancer Center and Research Institute, Tampa, FL, p. A140
KOLOZSVARY, John, Chief Executive Officer, Southeast Michigan Surgical Hospital, Warren, MI, p. A325
KOLSETH, Shelley V., Chief Financial Officer, Memorial Hospital of Tampa, Tampa, FL, p. A141
KOMAN, Stuart, Ph.D. President and Chief Executive Officer, Walden Psychiatric Care, Waltham, MA, p. A305
KOMANDURI, Ramanujam, M.D. Chief of Staff, Veterans Affairs Southern Nevada Healthcare System, North Las Vegas, NV, p. A394
KOMAR, Ellen M., R.N. Vice President Patient Care Services, Stamford Hospital, Stamford, CT, p. A112
KOME, Hunter, Vice President Operations, Oconee Medical Center, Seneca, SC, p. A553
KOMENDA, John, Chief Financial Officer, Hendricks Regional Health, Danville, IN, p. A200
KOMINS, Jeff, M.D. Chief Medical Officer, Mercy Fitzgerald Hospital, Darby, PA, p. A521
KOMORNIK, Jeffrey, Director Human Resources, Milford Hospital, Milford, CT, p. A110
KOMOROSKI, Patrice L., R.N. Chief Executive Officer, Select Specialty Hospital–Madison, Madison, WI, p. A684
KONARSKI, Debbie, Chief Financial Officer, Chestnut Hill Hospital, Philadelphia, PA, p. A531
KONECNE, Robin, Manager Human Resources, Kit Carson County Memorial Hospital, Burlington, CO, p. A98
KONIGSBERG, Geri, Director Public Information, University of Texas Harris County Psychiatric Center, Houston, TX, p. A607
KONSAVAGE, Christian, M.D. Chief of Staff, Cumberland County Hospital, Burkesville, KY, p. A248
KONWINSKI, Theresa, R.N. Vice President Patient Care, ProMedica St. Luke's Hospital, Maumee, OH, p. A484
KOOIMAN, Thomas, Chief Executive Officer, Prairie Ridge Hospital and Health Services, Elbow Lake, MN, p. A331
KOON, Rion, Chief Information Management Division, William Beaumont Army Medical Center, El Paso, TX, p. A597
KOONTZ, Andrea, R.N. Vice President of Nursing Services, Community Hospital of Bremen, Bremen, IN, p. A198
KOOP, Steven, M.D. Medical Director, Gillette Children's Specialty Healthcare, Saint Paul, MN, p. A339
KOOS, Shaun, Administrator, Wenatchee Valley Hospital, Wenatchee, WA, p. A669
KOOY, Donald C., President and Chief Executive Officer, McLaren Flint, Flint, MI, p. A312
KOPEL, Samuel, M.D. Medical Director, Maimonides Medical Center,, NY, p. A434
KOPF, Chris, Chief Fiscal Officer, Summit Park Hospital and Nursing Care Center, Pomona, NY, p. A440
KOPFLE, Sue
Chief Human Resources Officer, University of Missouri Hospitals and Clinics, Columbia, MO, p. A358
Chief Human Resources Officer, Women's and Children's Hospital, Columbia, MO, p. A358
KOPINSKI, Donna, Chief Financial Officer, Crittenton Hospital Medical Center, Rochester, MI, p. A321
KOPINSKY, Kristen, Chief Operating Officer, Highlands Regional Medical Center, Sebring, FL, p. A139
KOPITA, Jeffrey, M.D. Chief Medical Officer and Vice President Medical Affairs, Baylor Medical Center at Garland, Garland, TX, p. A600
KOPMAN, Alan, FACHE President and Chief Executive Officer, New York Westchester Square Medical Center,, NY, p. A435
KOPP, Daniel, M.D. Senior Vice President and Chief Medical Officer, Faxton–St. Luke's Healthcare, Utica, NY, p. A445
KOPP, Greg, Chief Financial Officer, Regina Medical Center, Hastings, MN, p. A332
KOPPELMAN, Benjamin, President and Chief Executive Officer, St. Joseph's Area Health Services, Park Rapids, MN, p. A337
KOPPENHAVER, Colleen, Chief Financial Officer, Oaklawn Hospital, Marshall, MI, p. A318
KOPPERUD, Gordon, Director Operations, Sanford Westbrook Medical Center, Westbrook, MN, p. A341
KORBEL, Tamara, Director Management Information Systems, Ridgeview Medical Center, Waconia, MN, p. A341
KORDUCKI, Stanley R., President, Wood County Hospital, Bowling Green, OH, p. A471

A856 Index of Health Care Professionals

Index of Health Care Professionals / Kremer


KORICH, Frank, Vice President and Site Administrator, Soldiers and Sailors Memorial Hospital of Yates County, Penn Yan, NY, p. A440
KORN, Larry, Manager Finance, Southern Arizona Veterans Affairs Health Care System, Tucson, AZ, p. A40
KORN, Roy, M.D. Medical Director, Cobleskill Regional Hospital, Cobleskill, NY, p. A424
KORNBLATT, Lynne R., Vice President Human Resources, Einstein Medical Center Philadelphia, Philadelphia, PA, p. A532
KORNER, Kevin, Director Human Resources, Central Mississippi Medical Center, Jackson, MS, p. A347
KORNFIELD, Lee, M.D. Medical Director, Elks Rehab Hospital, Boise, ID, p. A166
KOROGI, Robin, Director, Veterans Affairs Montana Health Care System, Fort Harrison, MT, p. A375
KOROLY, Marla, M.D. Chief Medical Officer and Senior Vice President Medical Affairs, Northern Westchester Hospital, Mount Kisco, NY, p. A430
KORPELA, Donita, R.N. Director of Patient Care Services, Mercy Hospital, Moose Lake, MN, p. A336
KORSMO, Jeffrey, President and Chief Executive Officer, Via Christi Health, Wichita, KS, p. B142
KORTE, Fred, Chief Financial Officer, McLaren Oakland, Pontiac, MI, p. A321
KORTEMEYER, Jay, Chief Executive Officer, Brynn Marr Hospital, Jacksonville, NC, p. A455
KORTH, Mark, Chief Executive Officer, Mercy Medical Center Redding, Redding, CA, p. A81
KORTH, Paul, Chief Financial Officer, Cookeville Regional Medical Center, Cookeville, TN, p. A564
KORTH–WHITE, Kirsten, Vice President Operations, Mercy Hospital Grayling, Grayling, MI, p. A314
KORTUM, Joseph M., President and Chief Mission Officer, PeaceHealth Southwest Medical Center, Vancouver, WA, p. A668
KORYNTA, Vicky, Senior Vice President and Chief Operating Officer, Range Regional Health Services, Hibbing, MN, p. A333
KOSANOVICH, John, M.D. Vice President Medical Affairs, Covenant Medical Center, Saginaw, MI, p. A322
KOSANOVICH, John P., President, Watertown Regional Medical Center, Watertown, WI, p. A692
KOSCHKA, Ed, Network Vice President Information Technology and Chief Information Officer, Indiana Heart Hospital, Indianapolis, IN, p. A204
KOSCHKA, Edward, Network Vice President Information Technology and Chief Information Officer, Community Hospital North, Indianapolis, IN, p. A204
KOSE, William H., M.D
Senior Vice President Medical Affairs, Blanchard Valley Hospital, Findlay, OH, p. A480
Vice President Quality and Medical Affairs, Bluffton Hospital, Bluffton, OH, p. A471
KOSEK, Kevin, Chief Financial Officer, Iowa City Veterans Affairs Health Care System, Iowa City, IA, p. A221
KOSINA, Thomas, M.D. Chief of Staff, Winner Regional Healthcare Center, Winner, SD, p. A561
KOSLOW, Howard B., President and Chief Executive Officer, Promise Healthcare, Boca Raton, FL, p. B104
KOSLOW, Howard B., President and Chief Executive Officer, Promise Hospital of Miss Lou, Vidalia, LA, p. A279
KOSNOSKY, David, M.D. Chief Medical Officer, University Hospitals Geauga Medical Center, Chardon, OH, p. A472
KOSSEFF, Christopher O., President and Chief Executive Officer, University of Medicine and Dentistry of New Jersey, University Behavioral Healthcare, Piscataway, NJ, p. A408
KOSTER, John F., M.D. President and Chief Executive Officer, Providence Health & Services, Renton, WA, p. B105
KOSTER, Tracy, Director Human Resources, Carlinville Area Hospital, Carlinville, IL, p. A174
KOSTERS, Gregory J., D.O. Chief Medical Officer, Osceola Community Hospital, Sibley, IA, p. A226
KOSTOK, Barbara, Manager Human Resources, Punxsutawney Area Hospital, Punxsutawney, PA, p. A536
KOSTROUN, Deborah, Chief Operating Officer, Manatee Glens Hospital and Addiction Center, Bradenton, FL, p. A119
KOSTURKO, MaryEllen, R.N. Senior Vice President Patient Care Operations and Chief Nursing Officer, Bridgeport Hospital, Bridgeport, CT, p. A108
KOSYLA, Gail, Chief Financial Officer and Vice President Finance, St. Mary Medical Center, Langhorne, PA, p. A526
KOSZTYO, Carol, R.N. Vice President, Patient Care Services, Carrier Clinic, Belle Mead, NJ, p. A401
KOTEWICZ, Lori, Supervisor Human Resources, Aultman Orrville Hospital, Orrville, OH, p. A487
KOTIN, Kathy, Chief Financial Officer, Banner Good Samaritan Medical Center, Phoenix, AZ, p. A35
KOTRBA, Mitchell, Chief Financial Officer, North Valley Health Center, Warren, MN, p. A341
KOTSONIS, Robert, Chief Operating Officer, Northeast Rehabilitation Hospital, Salem, NH, p. A400
KOTTENBROOK, Susan, Chief Executive Officer, Red River Behavioral Center, Bossier City, LA, p. A264
KOTZEN, Michael S., Vice President and Chief Operating Officer, Virtua Voorhees, Voorhees, NJ, p. A412
KOUKOS, Dean, M.D. Chief Medical Staff, Barnwell County Hospital, Barnwell, SC, p. A546
KOUNTZ, David, M.D. Senior Vice President Medical Affairs, Jersey Shore University Medical Center, Neptune, NJ, p. A406
KOUPAL, Bernadette, Supervisor Business Office, Coordinator Information Systems and Administrative Assistant, Wagner Community Memorial Hospital Avera, Wagner, SD, p. A560
KOUTNER–RAUSCH, Geri, Director Human Resources, St. Lawrence Psychiatric Center, Ogdensburg, NY, p. A439
KOUTOUZOS, Connie L., R.N. COO/Vice President of Patient Care Services, NORTHSTAR Health System, Iron River, MI, p. A316
KOVACH, Andrew L.
Vice President Human Resources and Chief Administrative Officer, Morristown Medical Center, Morristown, NJ, p. A406
Vice President Human Resources and Chief Administrative Officer, Newton Medical Center, Newton, NJ, p. A407
Vice President Human Resources and Chief Administrative Officer, Overlook Medical Center, Summit, NJ, p. A410
KOVACS, Amber R., Chief Human Resources Officer, Banner Gateway Medical Center, Gilbert, AZ, p. A32
KOVACS, Elizabeth, R.N. Director of Nursing, Harrison Community Hospital, Cadiz, OH, p. A471
KOVASZNAY, Beatrice, M.D. Clinical Director, Capital District Psychiatric Center, Albany, NY, p. A420
KOVICH, Lynn, Assistant Commissioner, Division of Mental Health and Addiction Services, Department of Human Services, State of New Jersey, Trenton, NJ, p. B47
KOWALOFF, Harvey, M.D. Vice President Medical Affairs, Saint Anne's Hospital, Fall River, MA, p. A299
KOWALSKI, Richard S., FACHE President and Chief Executive Officer, OSF St. Mary Medical Center, Galesburg, IL, p. A182
KOWITT, Jack, Senior Vice President and Chief Information Officer, Parkland Health & Hospital System, Dallas, TX, p. A592
KOWNACKI, Dawn, Director Human Resources, Brooke Glen Behavioral Hospital, Fort Washington, PA, p. A523
KOZAI, Gerald T., President, St. Francis Medical Center, Lynwood, CA, p. A73
KOZEL, Joseph, M.D. President Medical Staff, Hoboken University Medical Center, Hoboken, NJ, p. A404
KOZEL, Kenneth D., FACH
President and Chief Executive Officer, Dorchester General Hospital, Cambridge, MD, p. A290
President and Chief Executive Officer, Memorial Hospital at Easton Maryland, Easton, MD, p. A291
KOZEL, Kenneth D., FACHE President and Chief Executive Officer, Shore Health System, Easton, MD, p. B118
KOZEL, Mary Ann, Chief Fiscal, Veterans Affairs Medical Center, Wilmington, DE, p. A115
KOZIK, Rhonda, Administrator, Norwood Health Center, Marshfield, WI, p. A685
KOZLOWSKI, Leon, Vice President Finance and Chief Financial Officer, Wyckoff Heights Medical Center,, NY, p. A438
KRABBENHOFT, Kelby K., President and Chief Executive Officer, Sanford Health, Sioux Falls, SD, p. B112
KRABLIN, Brett, M.D. Chief of Staff, Kingfisher Regional Hospital, Kingfisher, OK, p. A498
KRAEGER, Paul, Vice President Finance and Chief Financial Officer, Samaritan Medical Center, Watertown, NY, p. A446
KRAHNERT, John F., M.D. Chief Medical Officer, FirstHealth Moore Regional Hospital, Pinehurst, NC, p. A458
KRAJEWSKI, David
Vice President Finance, Levindale Hebrew Geriatric Center and Hospital, Baltimore, MD, p. A288
Vice President Finance, Northwest Hospital, Randallstown, MD, p. A293
KRAMER, Blake, Chief Executive Officer, Franklin Medical Center, Winnsboro, LA, p. A279
KRAMER, Cheri, Chief Administrative Officer, Mayo Clinic Health System in Lake City, Lake City, MN, p. A333
KRAMER, Danette, Chief Financial Officer, Regional Medical Center, Manchester, IA, p. A222
KRAMER, Janie, Chief Operating Officer, Sharp Memorial Hospital, San Diego, CA, p. A86
KRAMER, Jared, M.D. Chief of Staff, Howard County Medical Center, Saint Paul, NE, p. A389
KRAMER, Jon, Controller and Assistant Administrator, Northport Medical Center, Northport, AL, p. A24
KRAMER, Kathryn, M.D. President Medical Staff, Pekin Hospital, Pekin, IL, p. A191
KRAMER, Richard, Interim Chief Executive Officer, Southeast Louisiana Hospital, Mandeville, LA, p. A272
KRAMER, Sheila A., Chief Executive Officer, HEALTHSOUTH Rehabilitation Hospital of Cypress, Houston, TX, p. A604
KRAMER, Susan, Director of Human Resources, Levi Hospital, Hot Springs National Park, AR, p. A46
KRAML, Louis D., FACH
Chief Executive Officer, Bingham Memorial Hospital, Blackfoot, ID, p. A166
Chief Executive Officer, Mountain River Birthing and Surgery Center, Blackfoot, ID, p. A166
KRAMPITS, Carrie, Director Human Resources, McKenzie Health System, Sandusky, MI, p. A322
KRANZ, Marlene, Controller, Holton Community Hospital, Holton, KS, p. A234
KRASON, Jane E., R.N. Chief Executive Officer, Appalachian Behavioral Healthcare, Athens, OH, p. A470
KRASOVEC, Rudy, Director Human Resources, St. Mary–Corwin Medical Center, Pueblo, CO, p. A105
KRASS, Todd, R.N. Chief Executive Officer, Belton Regional Medical Center, Belton, MO, p. A355
KRAUKLIS, Gene
Regional Vice President Human Resources, Aurora Lakeland Medical Center, Elkhorn, WI, p. A681
Regional Vice President Human Resources, Aurora Medical Center, Kenosha, WI, p. A683
Regional Vice President Human Resources, Aurora Memorial Hospital of Burlington, Burlington, WI, p. A679
KRAUS, John, M.D. Chief Medical Officer, Bryn Mawr Rehabilitation Hospital, Malvern, PA, p. A528
KRAUSE, Donna, Chief Information Officer, Harry S. Truman Memorial Veterans Hospital, Columbia, MO, p. A358
KRAUSE, Kim, Director Human Resources, Baylor Jack and Jane Hamilton Heart and Vascular Hospital, Dallas, TX, p. A590
KRAUSE, Mary, Vice President Finance, Valley View Regional Hospital, Ada, OK, p. A493
KRAUSE, Michele, Chief Information Management Officer, Bassett Army Community Hospital, Fort Wainwright, AK, p. A29
KRAUSE, Michelle, Manager Human Resources, Veterans Affairs Medical Center, Leeds, MA, p. A301
KRAUSE, Steven, Manager Information Technology, Franciscan Physicians Hospital, Munster, IN, p. A209
KRAUSS, James D., President and Chief Executive Officer, Rockingham Memorial Hospital, Harrisonburg, VA, p. A649
KRAVETZ, Michael, M.D. Medical Director, HEALTHSOUTH Valley of the Sun Rehabilitation Hospital, Glendale, AZ, p. A33
KRAYNAK, Joseph, M.D. Chief Medical Officer, Abington Health Lansdale Hospital, Lansdale, PA, p. A527
KREATSOULAS, Nicholas, M.D
Vice President Medical Affairs, St. Elizabeth Boardman Health Center, Boardman, OH, p. A471
Senior Vice President and Chief Medical Officer, St. Elizabeth Health Center, Youngstown, OH, p. A492
Vice President Medical Affairs, St. Joseph Health Center, Warren, OH, p. A490
KREBS, Anne, Chief Financial Officer, Butler Health System, Butler, PA, p. A519
KREBS, Cindy, District Director Human Resources, Matagorda Regional Medical Center, Bay City, TX, p. A582
KREBS, George, M.D. Chief Medical Officer, Broughton Hospital, Morganton, NC, p. A457
KREBS, Teresa, Director Human Resources, North Texas Medical Center, Gainesville, TX, p. A600
KREBSBACH, Mayla, Chief Executive Officer, Aurora Vista Del Mar Hospital, Ventura, CA, p. A94
KREHBIEL, Beth, President and Chief Executive Officer, Fairview Ridges Hospital, Burnsville, MN, p. A329
KREIDER, Cheryl, Chief Operating Officer, Phoenixville Hospital, Phoenixville, PA, p. A534
KREIDER, Robert Q., President and Chief Executive Officer, Devereux, Villanova, PA, p. B46
KREIDLER, Marlene, Executive Director Human Resources, San Joaquin Community Hospital, Bakersfield, CA, p. A55
KREITEL, Nicole, Chief Financial Officer, Memorial Community Hospital and Health System, Blair, NE, p. A382
KREITINGER, Tate J., Chief Executive Officer, The HealthCenter, Kalispell, MT, p. A377
KREITZ, Don, Chief Executive Officer, Chapman Medical Center, Orange, CA, p. A78
KREITZER, Teri, Director Human Resources, Saint Francis Medical Center, Cape Girardeau, MO, p. A356
KRELL, G. Christopher, M.D. Chief of Staff, South Lincoln Medical Center, Kemmerer, WY, p. A696
KRELSTEIN, Michael, M.D. Medical Director, San Diego County Psychiatric Hospital, San Diego, CA, p. A85
KREMER, John, M.D. Chief Medical Officer, Lake Chelan Community Hospital, Chelan, WA, p. A660
KREMER, Ruth, Director Information Services, New River Medical Center, Monticello, MN, p. A335


Index of Health Care Professionals

Index of Health Care Professionals / Kren


KREN, John, Acting Chief Executive Officer, St. John's Medical Center and Living Center, Jackson, WY, p. A696
KRENYTZKY, S. Marc, M.D. Vice President Medical Affairs, Prince William Hospital, Manassas, VA, p. A651
KRESCH, Richard A., M.D. President and Chief Executive Officer, Ascend Health Corporation, New York, NY, p. B11
KRESS, Irene, Director Human Resources, OSF Holy Family Medical Center, Monmouth, IL, p. A188
KRESSE, Gregory, M.D. Chairman Medical Staff, Eureka Springs Hospital, Eureka Springs, AR, p. A44
KRETZ, Blake, President, Texas Health Harris Methodist Hospital Cleburne, Cleburne, TX, p. A587
KRETZINGER, Curt, Chief Operating Officer, Heartland Regional Medical Center, Saint Joseph, MO, p. A368
KREUSER, Michael, Director Fiscal Services, Milwaukee County Behavioral Health Division, Milwaukee, WI, p. A687
KREUTNER, Ron, Chief Financial Officer, Lodi Memorial Hospital, Lodi, CA, p. A67
KREUTZ, Cynthia, Chief Executive Officer, Spalding Rehabilitation Hospital, Aurora, CO, p. A97
KREUZER, Jay E., FACHE Chief Executive Officer, Kona Community Hospital, Kealakekua, HI, p. A165
KRICKBAUM, Robert, Chief Executive Officer, Edwards County Hospital and Healthcare Center, Kinsley, KS, p. A236
KRIEGER, Mark, Vice President and Chief Financial Officer, Barnes–Jewish Hospital, Saint Louis, MO, p. A368
KRIEGER, Robert, Interim Chief Operating Officer, Good Samaritan Hospital, San Jose, CA, p. A88
KRIEGER, Tim
  Director Information Systems, Betsy Johnson Regional Hospital, Dunn, NC, p. A452
  Director Information Systems, Morristown–Hamblen Healthcare System, Morristown, TN, p. A572
KRIKAVA, Joan, M.D. Director Medical Affairs, New Ulm Medical Center, New Ulm, MN, p. A336
KRISHNA, Doddanna, M.D. Chief of Staff, Antelope Valley Hospital, Lancaster, CA, p. A67
KRISHNAN, Devika, M.D. Clinical Director and Chief of Staff, Spring Grove Hospital Center, Baltimore, MD, p. A289
KRISHNASWAMY, Jaikumar, Chief Operating Officer, Cypress Fairbanks Medical Center, Houston, TX, p. A604
KRISSMAN, Roger, Chief Financial Officer, Desert Valley Hospital, Victorville, CA, p. A95
KRISTEL, John, Chief Executive Officer, Carlisle Regional Medical Center, Carlisle, PA, p. A520
KRISTOFF, Tina, Manager Human Resources, Alton Memorial Hospital, Alton, IL, p. A172
KRITZ, Howard
  Director Human Resources, Bellevue Hospital Center, New York, NY, p. A431
  Director, Coler–Goldwater Specialty Hospital and Nursing Facility, New York, NY, p. A432
KRITZ, John D., Senior Vice President and Chief Financial Officer, Range Regional Health Services, Hibbing, MN, p. A333
KRITZER, Tammy, Vice President Clinic Operations, Mayo Clinic Health System in Austin, Austin, MN, p. A328
KRIVENKO, Chuck, M.D. Chief Medical Officer, Clinical and Quality Services, Lee Memorial Hospital, Fort Myers, FL, p. A124
KRMPOTIC, Debra J., R.N. Chief Executive Officer, Banner Estrella Medical Center, Phoenix, AZ, p. A35
KRODEL, Scott, Director Information Systems, Johnson Memorial Hospital, Franklin, IN, p. A202
KROELL Jr., H. Scott, Chief Executive Officer, Liberty Regional Medical Center, Hinesville, GA, p. A154
KROESE, Robert D., FACHE Chief Executive Officer, Pella Regional Health Center, Pella, IA, p. A225
KROGEN, David, Controller, HEALTHSOUTH Rehabilitation Hospital of Southern Arizona, Tucson, AZ, p. A39
KROK, Stan, Chief Information Officer, Ann & Robert H. Lurie Children's Hospital of Chicago, Chicago, IL, p. A175
KROLL, Ronald, Chief Financial Officer, Mercy General Hospital, Sacramento, CA, p. A83
KRONENBERG, Paul J., M.D. President and Chief Executive Officer, Crouse Hospital, Syracuse, NY, p. A444
KROPP, Richard P.
  Vice President Human Resources, Lourdes Medical Center of Burlington County, Willingboro, NJ, p. A412
  Vice President Human Resources, Our Lady of Lourdes Medical Center, Camden, NJ, p. A402
KROSER, Jonathan, M.D. Chief of Staff, Northcrest Medical Center, Springfield, TN, p. A576
KROSOFF, Mary June, Chief Human Resources Officer, Highlands Hospital, Connellsville, PA, p. A521
KROUSE, Michael
  Chief Information Officer, Doctors Hospital, Columbus, OH, p. A476
  Senior Vice President Chief Information Officer, Dublin Methodist Hospital, Dublin, OH, p. A479
  Chief Information Officer Information Services, Grady Memorial Hospital, Delaware, OH, p. A479
  Chief Information Officer, Grant Medical Center, Columbus, OH, p. A476
  Chief Information Officer, Riverside Methodist Hospital, Columbus, OH, p. A477
KRUCZEK, Richard, Chief Executive Officer, HEALTHSOUTH Reading Rehabilitation Hospital, Reading, PA, p. A537
KRUCZLNICKI, David G., President and Chief Executive Officer, Glens Falls Hospital, Glens Falls, NY, p. A426
KRUEGER, Albert, M.D. Chief of Staff, Pioneers Medical Center, Meeker, CO, p. A104
KRUEGER, Christine, M.D. Chief of Staff, Munising Memorial Hospital, Munising, MI, p. A319
KRUEGER, David, Associate Director, Veterans Affairs Medical Center, Bath, NY, p. A421
KRUEGER, Ellen, Director Human Resources, Chadron Community Hospital and Health Services, Chadron, NE, p. A382
KRUEGER, Eric, Vice President, Finance and Chief Financial Officer, Sherman Hospital, Elgin, IL, p. A181
KRUEGER Jr., Harold L., Chief Executive Officer, Chadron Community Hospital and Health Services, Chadron, NE, p. A382
KRUEGER, James G., Ph.D. Chief Executive Officer, Rockefeller University Hospital, New York, NY, p. A436
KRUEGER, Mary T., President, Saint Clare's Hospital, Weston, WI, p. A693
KRUEGER, Pete, Director Human Resources, Borgess–Lee Memorial Hospital, Dowagiac, MI, p. A311
KRUGEL, Gary M., Senior Vice President Operations and Chief Financial Officer, Swedish Covenant Hospital, Chicago, IL, p. A178
KRUGER, Dale K., Chief Executive Officer and Chief Financial Officer, Tyler Healthcare Center Avera, Tyler, MN, p. A341
KRUMBERGER, Joanne, Associate Director, Veterans Affairs Palo Alto Health Care System, Palo Alto, CA, p. A79
KRUMMEL, Dere, Director Information Systems, Ochsner Medical Center – Kenner, Kenner, LA, p. A269
KRUMREY, Arthur J., Chief Information Officer, Loyola University Medical Center, Maywood, IL, p. A187
KRUMWIED, Robert D., President and Chief Executive Officer, Regional Mental Health Center, Merrillville, IN, p. A208
KRUSE, Victoria, Manager Human Resources, Franklin General Hospital, Hampton, IA, p. A220
KRUSIE, Kathleen R., Chief Executive Officer, St. Joseph Regional Health Center, Bryan, TX, p. A586
KRUT, Joyce, Vice President Information Systems, UPMC McKeesport, McKeesport, PA, p. A528
KRUYER–COLLINS, Emyle
  Director Human Resources, Doctor's Hospital and Neuromuscular Center, Bremen, IN, p. A198
  Vice President Human Resources, Unity Medical & Surgical Hospital, Mishawaka, IN, p. A208
KRUZEL, Janet, Health Information Manager, CentraCare Health System – Melrose, Melrose, MN, p. A334
KRUZICK, Michael, Acting Chief Financial Officer, Norwalk Hospital, Norwalk, CT, p. A111
KRUZNER, Melinda, Chief Financial Officer, Lexington Medical Center, West Columbia, SC, p. A554
KRYSTOF, Linda, Chief Nursing Officer, Antioch Medical Center, Antioch, CA, p. A53
KRYSTOWIAK, Thomas P.
  Vice President Finance, Berlin Memorial Hospital, Berlin, WI, p. A679
  Vice President Finance, Wild Rose Community Memorial Hospital, Wild Rose, WI, p. A694
KRYZANIAK, Larry, Chief Financial Officer, Hennepin County Medical Center, Minneapolis, MN, p. A335
KRZASTEK, Sue, Vice President Human Resources, Augusta Health, Fishersville, VA, p. A648
KRZJCI, David, Director Information Systems, Baylor Regional Medical Center at Grapevine, Grapevine, TX, p. A601
KU, Evelyn, Chief Nursing Officer, Monterey Park Hospital, Monterey Park, CA, p. A75
KUANGPARICHAT, Manoch, M.D. President Medical Staff, Excelsior Springs Hospital, Excelsior Springs, MO, p. A359
KUBACAK, Stephanie, M.D. Chief of Staff, Covenant Hospital–Levelland, Levelland, TX, p. A612
KUBALA, Joseph, Chief Financial Officer, St. Vincent Mercy Hospital, Elwood, IN, p. A200
KUBALL, Lana, Director Administrative Services, Lucas County Health Center, Chariton, IA, p. A216
KUBE, Don, M.D. Chief of Staff, Dickinson County Healthcare System, Iron Mountain, MI, p. A315
KUBIAK, Phillip J., President, Hampstead Hospital, Hampstead, NH, p. A398
KUBIAK, Richard, M.D. Vice President Medical Affairs, Peconic Bay Medical Center, Riverhead, NY, p. A441
KUBIK, James A., Administrator, Pawnee County Memorial Hospital, Pawnee City, NE, p. A389
KUBOTA, Andrea, Director Patient Care Services, Shriners Hospitals for Children, Honolulu, Honolulu, HI, p. A164
KUBOUSHEK, David, Chief, Fiscal Service, Durham Veterans Affairs Medical Center, Durham, NC, p. A452
KUBOW, Philip L., Senior Vice President Human Resources, Carle Foundation Hospital, Urbana, IL, p. A195
KUCERA, Kim, Chief Operating Officer, Mille Lacs Health System, Onamia, MN, p. A336
KUCHARSKI, Kathy, Director Management Information Systems, Brooks Memorial Hospital, Dunkirk, NY, p. A425
KUCK, Kathleen E., R.N. President and Chief Executive Officer, Pocono Medical Center, East Stroudsburg, PA, p. A522
KUCKEWICH, Mike, Director Information Systems, Terre Haute Regional Hospital, Terre Haute, IN, p. A212
KUCZORA, Paul, Chief Executive Officer, Grant–Blackford Mental Health Center, Marion, IN, p. A208
KUDLA, Ken
  Chief Information Officer, Salem Hospital, Salem, OR, p. A515
  Chief Information Officer, West Valley Hospital, Dallas, OR, p. A510
KUDRONOWICZ, Sherry, Administrator, Memorial Hospital of Lafayette County, Darlington, WI, p. A680
KUEHLER, Judy, M.D. President Medical Staff, King's Daughters' Hospital and Health Services, Madison, IN, p. A208
KUEHLER, Stephan A., Administrator, Knox County Hospital, Knox City, TX, p. A611
KUEHNEMUND, Bonnie, Comptroller, Heart of America Medical Center, Rugby, ND, p. A468
KUENNEN, Connie, Director Human Resources and Community Relations, Regional Health Services of Howard County, Cresco, IA, p. A217
KUENSTLER, Kristi, M.D. Chief of Staff, Texas Health Harris Methodist Hospital Azle, Azle, TX, p. A582
KUESER, Brian, M.D. Chief Medical Officer, Neosho Memorial Regional Medical Center, Chanute, KS, p. A231
KUESTERSTEFFEN, Vicki, Chief Executive Officer, J. D. McCarty Center for Children With Developmental Disabilities, Norman, OK, p. A500
KUFFLER, Julian, M.D. President Medical Staff, Mount Desert Island Hospital, Bar Harbor, ME, p. A281
KUHAR, Peggy A., R.N. Chief Nursing Officer, University Hospitals Geauga Medical Center, Chardon, OH, p. A472
KUHL, Patricia, Vice President Human Resources, Chester River Health System, Chestertown, MD, p. A290
KUHLE, Terri, Director Human Resources, St. Mary's Hospital, Decatur, IL, p. A179
KUHLMANN, Chris, Chief Financial Officer, Lakeland Community Hospital Watervliet, Watervliet, MI, p. A325
KUHLMANN, George, M.D. Chief of Staff, Cuyuna Regional Medical Center, Crosby, MN, p. A330
KUHLMANN, Michelle, M.D. Director Medical Staff, Thayer County Health Services, Hebron, NE, p. A384
KUHN, Anita, Controller, Texas County Memorial Hospital, Houston, MO, p. A360
KUHN, Brenda, Ph.D. Vice President Patient Care Services, Kettering Medical Center, Kettering, OH, p. A482
KUHN, Shawn, Facility Director Human Resources, Connecticut Valley Hospital, Middletown, CT, p. A110
KUHN, Steve, Chief Financial Officer, River Park Hospital, Huntington, WV, p. A672
KUHNS, Jay, Vice President Human Resources, All Children's Hospital, Saint Petersburg, FL, p. A138
KUIDA, Elliot H., Vice President and Chief Operating Officer, Martha Jefferson Hospital, Charlottesville, VA, p. A646
KUIPER, Evert J., President and Chief Executive Officer, Saint Anthony's Health Center, Alton, IL, p. A172
KUKELHAN, Alison, Manager Human Resources, Adams Memorial Hospital, Decatur, IN, p. A200
KUKLA, Steven F., Senior Vice President and Chief Financial Officer, Mercy Medical Center–Des Moines, Des Moines, IA, p. A218
KULIK, Alec G., Administrator, Cleveland Clinic Children's Hospital for Rehabilitation, Cleveland, OH, p. A474
KULISZ, Michael, D.O
  Chief Medical Officer, Kishwaukee Community Hospital, DeKalb, IL, p. A180
  Chief Medical Officer, Valley West Community Hospital, Sandwich, IL, p. A193
KULP, Paul, Director Human Resources, North Adams Regional Hospital, North Adams, MA, p. A303
KUMAR, Nanda, M.D. Chief of Staff, Northern California Rehabilitation Hospital, Redding, CA, p. A82
KUMAR, Puskoor, M.D. Administrator, Sundance Hospital, Arlington, TX, p. A579


**A858** Index of Health Care Professionals 

Index of Health Care Professionals / Laird

Index of Health Care Professionals

KUMAR, Raji, Chief Executive Officer, Dallas Medical Center, Dallas, TX, p. A591
KUMM, Mandy, Vice President Fiscal Services, Boone County Health Center, Albion, NE, p. A381
KUMMER, Margaret, Vice President Human Resources, Citizens Medical Center, Colby, KS, p. A231
KUNFERMAN, Debora A., Administrator and Chief Executive Officer, Cumberland Memorial Hospital, Cumberland, WI, p. A680
KUNIK, Cherie, R.N. Interim Vice President Patient Care Services & CNO, DeKalb Medical at North Decatur, Decatur, GA, p. A151
KUNNAPPILLY, Chester, M.D. Chief Medical Officer and Chief Quality Officer, San Mateo Medical Center, San Mateo, CA, p. A89
KUNSTLING, Ted, M.D. Chief Medical Officer, Duke Raleigh Hospital, Raleigh, NC, p. A459
KUNZ, Donna, Manager Human Resources, Saint Luke's South Hospital, Overland Park, KS, p. A241
KUNZ, Lisa, R.N. Chief Nursing Officer, Central Texas Rehabilitation Hospital, Austin, TX, p. A580
KUNZE, Gloria A., R.N. Vice President Operations, St. Joseph's Regional Medical Center, Paterson, NJ, p. A408
KUPFERSTEIN, Ron, Chief Executive Officer, Monrovia Memorial Hospital, Monrovia, CA, p. A75
KUPLEN, Carol, R.N. Chief Operating Officer and Chief Nursing Officer, St. Luke's University Hospital – Bethlehem Campus, Bethlehem, PA, p. A518
KURESKA, Kirk, Chief Executive Officer, RiverWoods Behavioral Health System, Riverdale, GA, p. A157
KURIAN, Santha, M.D. Chief of Staff, James E. Van Zandt Veterans Affairs Medical Center, Altoona, PA, p. A517
KURIGER, Frederick H., FACHE Chief Executive Officer, Catskill Regional Medical Center, Harris, NY, p. A427
KURTIAK, Mary Jo, Interim Chief Executive Officer, Senator Garrett W. Hagedorn Psychiatric Hospital, Glen Gardner, NJ, p. A
KURTZ, Marvin A.
Senior Vice President Finance and Chief Financial Officer, Florida Hospital Tampa, Tampa, FL, p. A140
Chief Financial Officer, Florida Hospital–Carrollwood, Tampa, FL, p. A140
KURTZ, Jr., Thomas F., Chief Operating Officer, Georgia Regional Hospital at Savannah, Savannah, GA, p. A159
KURZ, Kenneth R., M.D. Chief of Staff, MidState Medical Center, Meriden, CT, p. A110
KURZ, Sharon H., Ph.D. Chief Executive Officer, St. Elias Specialty Hospital, Anchorage, AK, p. A28
KURZENBERGER, Richard, Chief Financial Officer, Kingwood Pines Hospital, Kingwood, TX, p. A611
KUSHNER, Glenn, M.D. President Medical Staff, Westlake Hospital, Melrose Park, IL, p. A187
KUSLER, Julie, Manager Information Services, Avera St. Luke's Hospital, Aberdeen, SD, p. A555
KUTA, Daniel, R.N. Director of Nursing, Power County Hospital District, American Falls, ID, p. A166
KUTCH, John M., President, Trinity Health, Minot, ND, p. A467
KUTCHER, Gregory, M.D. President and Chief Executive Officer, Mayo Clinic Health System in Mankato, Mankato, MN, p. A334
KUTILEK, Richard J., Chief Operating Officer, Calvary Hospital,, NY, p. A432
KUYKENDALL, Kari, Human Resources Specialist, Pauls Valley General Hospital, Pauls Valley, OK, p. A503
KUZAS, Betsy, Executive Vice President and Chief Operating Officer, Phoenix Children's Hospital, Phoenix, AZ, p. A36
KUZMA, Gregory
Vice President and Chief Financial Officer, Flagstaff Medical Center, Flagstaff, AZ, p. A32
Vice President and Chief Financial Officer, Verde Valley Medical Center, Cottonwood, AZ, p. A31
KVASNICKA, John, M.D. Medical Director, St. John's Hospital, Saint Paul, MN, p. A339
KWASS, George, M.D. Chief of Staff, Merrimack Valley Hospital, Haverhill, MA, p. A300
KWIATEK, Susan, Associate Executive Director Patient Care Services, Glen Cove Hospital, Glen Cove, NY, p. A426
KWIESIELEWICZ, Nancy
Human Resources Business Partner, Ministry Good Samaritan Health Center, Merrill, WI, p. A686
Human Resources Representative, Saint Clare's Hospital, Weston, WI, p. A693
KYGER, David, M.D. Chief Medical Officer, Solara Hospital of Muskogee, Muskogee, OK, p. A500
KYHNELL, Koreen H., Vice President Human Resources, Indiana University Health Arnett Hospital, Lafayette, IN, p. A206
KYLE, James, M.D. Vice President Medical Affairs, St. Mary Medical Center, Apple Valley, CA, p. A54
KYLER, Yvonne, Director Human Resources, Texas Health Arlington Memorial Hospital, Arlington, TX, p. A579
KYLLO, Tom, Executive Vice President, Vail Valley Medical Center, Vail, CO, p. A106
KYNARD, Carmen, R.N. Chief Nursing Officer, Research Psychiatric Center, Kansas City, MO, p. A362
KYRIACOU, George M., President and Chief Executive Officer, Gaylord Hospital, Wallingford, CT, p. A112
KYWI, Alberto
Chief Information Officer, Goleta Valley Cottage Hospital, Santa Barbara, CA, p. A89
Chief Information Officer, Santa Barbara Cottage Hospital, Santa Barbara, CA, p. A89
Chief Information Officer, Santa Ynez Valley Cottage Hospital, Solvang, CA, p. A91

## L

L'HEUREUX, Dennis P., Chief Information Officer, Rockford Memorial Hospital, Rockford, IL, p. A193
L'ITALIEN, Mark, Director Information Services, Salem Community Hospital, Salem, OH, p. A488
LA CROIX, Kent, IT Supervisor, Schoolcraft Memorial Hospital, Manistique, MI, p. A318
LA FAVE, Jenny, Director, Sandhills Regional Medical Center, Hamlet, NC, p. A454
LA FRANCE, Pam
Vice President Human Resources, Community Hospital at Dobbs Ferry, Dobbs Ferry, NY, p. A425
Vice President Human Resources, St. John's Riverside Hospital, Yonkers, NY, p. A447
LA PORTE, Todd
Senior Vice President and Chief Financial Officer, Scottsdale Healthcare Shea Medical Center, Scottsdale, AZ, p. A38
Chief Financial Officer, Scottsdale Healthcare Thompson Peak Hospital, Scottsdale, AZ, p. A38
Senior Vice President and Chief Financial Officer, Scottsdale Healthcare–Osborn Medical Center, Scottsdale, AZ, p. A38
LA SOTA, John, Assistant Finance Officer, Clement J. Zablocki Veterans Affairs Medical Center, Milwaukee, WI, p. A686
LABAGNARA, James, M.D. Vice President Medical Affairs, St. Joseph's Regional Medical Center, Paterson, NJ, p. A408
LABAND, Andrew, Chief Information Officer, McLean Hospital, Belmont, MA, p. A295
LABARCA, Laurie, Executive Vice President and Chief Operating Officer, Via Christi Hospitals Wichita, Wichita, KS, p. A245
LABARGE, Robert J., Chief Executive Officer, Sturgis Hospital, Sturgis, MI, p. A323
LABELLA, Leonard, President and Chief Executive Officer, Verdugo Hills Hospital, Glendale, CA, p. A63
LABER, Susan, R.N. Chief Nursing Officer, Brandon Regional Hospital, Brandon, FL, p. A119
LABIAGA, Kimberly, Human Resources Leader, Fontana Medical Center, Fontana, CA, p. A61
LABINE, Lance C., Administrator, Dr. Dan C. Trigg Memorial Hospital, Tucumcari, NM, p. A418
LABONTE, Robin, Leader Financial Care, York Hospital, York, ME, p. A286
LABORIE, Sheree
Director Human Resources, Lakewood Hospital, Lakewood, OH, p. A482
Director Human Resources, Lutheran Hospital, Cleveland, OH, p. A475
LABRUM, Chad, Chief Financial Officer, Ashley Regional Medical Center, Vernal, UT, p. A642
LABUS, Susan, Chief Operating Officer, Pocono Medical Center, East Stroudsburg, PA, p. A522
LACASSE, Paul E., D.O. President and Chief Executive Officer, Botsford Hospital, Farmington Hills, MI, p. A312
LACEFIELD, Gayla, Director Human Resources, Howard Memorial Hospital, Nashville, AR, p. A49
LACEY, Carmen, R.N. President, Charles A. Cannon Memorial Hospital, Linville, NC, p. A456
LACEY, III, John W., M.D. Senior Vice President and Chief Medical Officer, The University of Tennessee Medical Center, Knoxville, TN, p. A569
LACEY, Ronald, M.D. Medical Director, Southwest Missouri Psychiatric Rehabilitation Center, El Dorado Springs, MO, p. A359
LACHANCE, Eric, Assistant Chief Executive Officer, Lake Wales Medical Center, Lake Wales, FL, p. A128
LACHANCE, Jeanne, Executive Vice President, Westerly Hospital, Westerly, RI, p. A545
LACHANCE, Mary Kay, Director Information Systems, St. John Macomb–Oakland Hospital, Macomb Center, Warren, MI, p. A325
LACHINA, Michael, M.D. Chief Medical Officer, Saint Francis Hospital, Memphis, TN, p. A572
LACHOWSKY, John, M.D. Chief Medical Officer, Mercy Hospital Ozark, Ozark, AR, p. A50
LACKEY, Lori, Chief Financial Officer, Sabetha Community Hospital, Sabetha, KS, p. A242
LACKEY, Thomas O., Administrator, Hale County Hospital, Greensboro, AL, p. A21
LACKNEY, Christopher J., Director Human Resources, Gifford Medical Center, Randolph, VT, p. A644
LACOT, Ivette, Director Human Resources, Hospital Episcopal San Lucas Guayama, Guayama, PR, p. A701
LACY, Edward L., FACHE Vice President and Administrator, Baptist Health Medical Center–Heber Springs, Heber Springs, AR, p. A45
LACY, John S., Senior Vice President Human Resources, Methodist Charlton Medical Center, Dallas, TX, p. A591
LACY, Leslie, Administrator, Cheyenne County Hospital, Saint Francis, KS, p. A242
LACY, Tyson, Chief Financial Officer, Lincoln Hospital, Davenport, WA, p. A660
LADAROLA, Sandra, Chief Nursing Officer, Waterbury Hospital, Waterbury, CT, p. A112
LADELY, Edward, Senior Vice President and Chief Financial Officer, Montgomery Hospital Medical Center, Norristown, PA, p. A530
LADENBURGER, Robert W., President and Chief Executive Officer, Exempla Healthcare, Inc., Denver, CO, p. B51
LADIANA, Red, Manager Information Systems, College Hospital Costa Mesa, Costa Mesa, CA, p. A58
LADNER, Warren, Chief Financial Officer, Natchez Community Hospital, Natchez, MS, p. A350
LAEL, Marielle, R.N. Chief Nursing Officer, Select Specialty Hospital–Fort Wayne, Fort Wayne, IN, p. A202
LAFERNEY, Jimmy, M.D. Vice President Medical Staff Affairs, Baylor Medical Center at Frisco, Frisco, TX, p. A600
LAFFERTY, Aline S., Vice President Human Resources, Henry Ford Wyandotte Hospital, Wyandotte, MI, p. A325
LAFFERTY, Douglas L., Chief Executive Officer, Plumas District Hospital, Quincy, CA, p. A81
LAFFEY, Leah, R.N. Chief Executive Officer, HEALTHSOUTH Rehabilitation Hospital, Sewickley, PA, p. A538
LAFINE, Amy, MSN, President and Chief Executive Officer, Provena St. Mary's Hospital, Kankakee, IL, p. A185
LAFLEUR, Cindy, President, Via Christi Rehabilitation Center, Wichita, KS, p. A245
LAFLEUR, Robert R., Chief Executive Officer, Cornerstone Hospital of Southwest Louisiana, Sulphur, LA, p. A278
LAFONE, Ken, Director Human Resources, Caswell Center, Kinston, NC, p. A456
LAFRANCOIS, Gregory, Chief Executive Officer, Prairie St. John's, Fargo, ND, p. A465
LAFRANCOIS, Mary, Vice President Human Resources, CHRISTUS Spohn Hospital Corpus Christi Memorial, Corpus Christi, TX, p. A589
LAGAARD, Scott, M.D. Chief of Staff, FirstLight Health System, Mora, MN, p. A336
LAGANA, Gina, Director Human Resources, Merrimack Valley Hospital, Haverhill, MA, p. A300
LAGASSE, David A., Senior Vice President Fiscal Affairs, McLean Hospital, Belmont, MA, p. A295
LAGASSE, Roger, Chief Financial Officer, Northern Maine Medical Center, Fort Kent, ME, p. A283
LAGNESE, John, M.D. Vice President Medical Affairs, UPMC St. Margaret, Pittsburgh, PA, p. A536
LAGUNZAD, Anastacia, M.D. Chief of Staff, Perry County Memorial Hospital, Tell City, IN, p. A212
LAHASKY, Doug, Chief Financial Officer, Acadia Vermilion Hospital, Lafayette, LA, p. A269
LAHATTE, Lawrence, M.D. Chief of Staff, Trinity Hospital of Augusta, Augusta, GA, p. A147
LAHAYE, Daniel, Manager, Savoy Medical Center, Mamou, LA, p. A272
LAHIDJANI, Jack, Chief Executive Officer, Miracle Mile Medical Center, Los Angeles, CA, p. A70
LAHOUT, Brenda, Chief Nurse Executive, Danville State Hospital, Danville, PA, p. A521
LAHTI, Molly, Director Human Resources, Parkland Medical Center, Derry, NH, p. A397
LAI, Iris, Chief Executive Officer, Alhambra Hospital Medical Center, Alhambra, CA, p. A53
LAIBINIS, Walter, M.D. Chief Medical Officer, Soldiers and Sailors Memorial Hospital, Wellsboro, PA, p. A540
LAIBLE, Anna, Administrator, Advocate Eureka Hospital, Eureka, IL, p. A181
LAIGN, Michael B., President and Chief Executive Officer, Holy Redeemer Hospital and Medical Center, Meadowbrook, PA, p. A528
LAIRD, David, President and Chief Executive Officer, Jewish Hospital & St. Mary's HealthCare, Louisville, KY, p. B73
LAIRD, Jeff, Controller, Stephens County Hospital, Toccoa, GA, p. A161

LAIRD, Melinda, MS Vice President Clinical Services, Wilson Medical Center, Wilson, NC, p. A463

LAISTER, Judy K., Director, Human Resources, Methodist Mansfield Medical Center, Mansfield, TX, p. A615

LAKE, Jane, Director Materials Management, St. Luke's Cornwall Hospital, Newburgh, NY, p. A438

LAKE, Nathan, Vice President Human Resources, Prairie Lakes Healthcare System, Watertown, SD, p. A560

LAKE, Peter M., M.D. Chief Medical Officer, Rogers Memorial Hospital, Oconomowoc, WI, p. A688

LAKEY, David L., M.D. Commissioner, Texas Department of State Health Services, Austin, TX, p. B128

LAKINS, Tom, Director Information Systems, Physicians Regional Medical Center, Knoxville, TN, p. A568

LAKNER, Stephen, M.D. President Medical and Affiliate Staff, Shady Grove Adventist Hospital, Rockville, MD, p. A294

LAKSHMANAN, Rekha, M.D. Medical Director, Mercy Continuing Care Hospital, Chesterfield, MO, p. A357

LALIBERTE, John, Assistant Vice President, Our Lady of Lourdes Memorial Hospital, Binghamton, NY, p. A422

LALLY, James M., M.D. Chief Medical Officer, Chino Valley Medical Center, Chino, CA, p. A57

LALLY, Michael K., Chief Executive Officer, Calais Regional Hospital, Calais, ME, p. A282

LALLY, Jr., Robert P., Vice President Finance, Medstar Franklin Square Medical Center, Baltimore, MD, p. A288

LAMADELEINE, Joseph, Chief Financial Officer, Veterans Affairs Connecticut Healthcare System, West Haven, CT, p. A113

LAMANTIA, Joseph, Executive Vice President and Chief Operating Officer, South Nassau Communities Hospital, Oceanside, NY, p. A439

LAMARCHE, Heather, Manager Human Resources, AMG Specialty Hospital – Lafayette, Lafayette, LA, p. A269

LAMARCHE, Marie, Director Human Resources, Harrison Medical Center, Bremerton, WA, p. A659

LAMB, Andrew, M.D. Chief of Staff, Alamance Regional Medical Center, Burlington, NC, p. A449

LAMB, Cindy, Director Human Resources, Marias Medical Center, Shelby, MT, p. A379

LAMB, Collin, Director Management Information Systems, St. Joseph Regional Medical Center, Lewiston, ID, p. A169

LAMB, Deanna, Director of Human Resources, Community Hospital–Fairfax, Fairfax, MO, p. A359

LAMB, Hope, Manager Human Resources, Kimble Hospital, Junction, TX, p. A609

LAMB, Timothy E., Commander, Martin Army Community Hospital, Fort Benning, GA, p. A153

LAMBERT, Amand, Director Human Resources, Allen Parish Hospital, Kinder, LA, p. A269

LAMBERT, Barbara, Director Healthcare Compliance, Eastern State Hospital, Williamsburg, VA, p. A657

LAMBERT, James M., FACHE President and Chief Executive Officer, Conway Regional Medical Center, Conway, AR, p. A43

LAMBERT, Karen A., President, Advocate Good Shepherd Hospital, Barrington, IL, p. A173

LAMBERT, Lynn, Chief Financial Officer, Wilson Medical Center, Wilson, NC, p. A463

LAMBERT, Paul, M.D. Chief of Staff, Veterans Affairs Medical Center, Boise, ID, p. A167

LAMBERT, Terry R., FACHE President, Lawrence Memorial Hospital, Walnut Ridge, AR, p. A52

LAMBKE, Michael, M.D. Medical Director, Redington–Fairview General Hospital, Skowhegan, ME, p. A285

LAMBORN, Cherie, Interim Vice President Human Resources, Springfield Regional Medical Center, Springfield, OH, p. A488

LAMBORN, Cheryl, Vice President Human Resources, Allegiance Health, Jackson, MI, p. A316

LAMBRECHT, Craig, M.D
Chief Operating Officer, Ashley Medical Center, Ashley, ND, p. A464

President and Chief Executive Officer, Medcenter One, Bismarck, ND, p. A464

LAMBRECHT, Rebecca, Manager Business Office and Chief Financial Officer, Alegent Health Plainview Hospital, Plainview, NE, p. A389

LAMBRECHT, Sandra, Chief Financial Officer, Haxtun Hospital District, Haxtun, CO, p. A102

LAMEN, Drake M., M.D. President and Chief Executive Officer, Chenango Memorial Hospital, Norwich, NY, p. A438

LAMEY, Rebecca, Vice President Human Resources, MaineGeneral Medical Center–Waterville Campus, Waterville, ME, p. A286

LAMIS, Pano, M.D. Medical Director, Atlanta Medical Center, Atlanta, GA, p. A145

LAMITIE, Timothy J., Deputy Director Administration, St. Lawrence Psychiatric Center, Ogdensburg, NY, p. A439

LAMLE, Sandra, Chief Financial Officer, Okeene Municipal Hospital, Okeene, OK, p. A500

LAMMERS, Sandra, Coordinator Human Resources and Finance, Alegent Health Mercy Hospital, Corning, IA, p. A216

LAMORELLA, Vincent M., Chief Financial Officer, Clarion Hospital, Clarion, PA, p. A520

LAMOUREUX, Bruce, Vice President and Chief Executive Officer, Providence Alaska Medical Center, Anchorage, AK, p. A28

LAMPARTER, David
Senior Vice President and Chief Financial Officer, John C. Lincoln Deer Valley Hospital, Phoenix, AZ, p. A35

Senior Vice President and Chief Financial Officer, John C. Lincoln North Mountain Hospital, Phoenix, AZ, p. A35

LAMPE, Michael, M.D. Chief of Staff, Kossuth Regional Health Center, Algona, IA, p. A214

LAMPTON, Brett, M.D. Chief of Staff, Baptist Memorial Hospital–North Mississippi, Oxford, MS, p. A351

LAMPTON, Lucius, M.D. Medical Director, Beacham Memorial Hospital, Magnolia, MS, p. A349

LANCASTER, Carlton, M.D. Medical Consultant, Hamilton Medical Center, Dalton, GA, p. A151

LANCASTER, Johnny, Chief Financial Officer, Vista Health, Fayetteville, AR, p. A44

LANCASTER, Tim, FACHE President and Chief Executive Officer, Hendrick Health System, Abilene, TX, p. A577

LANCE, Richard, Vice President Human Resources, Nix Health Care System, San Antonio, TX, p. A625

LANCET, Mark S., Administrator, Community Behavioral Health Hospital – Rochester, Rochester, MN, p. A338

LANCIOTTI, Kevin, Chief Financial Officer, McLaren Greater Lansing, Lansing, MI, p. A317

LAND, Beverly, Commanding Officer, Keller Army Community Hospital, West Point, NY, p. A446

LAND, David, D.O. Chief Medical Staff, Fort Duncan Regional Medical Center, Eagle Pass, TX, p. A595

LAND, Laura, Chief Human Resources Officer, OU Medical Center, Oklahoma City, OK, p. A502

LANDAU, Ken, Chief Financial Officer, Lake District Hospital, Lakeview, OR, p. A512

LANDERS, Alice, Administrative Director Operations, Texas Health Harris Methodist Hospital Hurst–Euless–Bedford, Bedford, TX, p. A583

LANDGARTEN, Steven, M.D. Chief Medical Officer, Hillcrest Medical Center, Tulsa, OK, p. A506

LANDIS, Bradlee, Chief Information Officer, Faith Community Hospital, Jacksboro, TX, p. A609

LANDIS, Steve, Director Information Services, St. Christopher's Hospital for Children, Philadelphia, PA, p. A533

LANDMAN, Paul, Director Human Resources, Ellwood City Hospital, Ellwood City, PA, p. A522

LANDRENEAU, Derrick, Director of Nursing, Baton Rouge Rehabilitation Hospital, Baton Rouge, LA, p. A262

LANDRETH, Jonathan, Chief Executive Officer, Lafayette Physical Rehabilitation Hospital, Lafayette, LA, p. A270

LANDRETH, Sandy, Director Human Resources, Seiling Community Hospital, Seiling, OK, p. A504

LANDRETH, Shannan, Information Systems, Livingston Hospital and Healthcare Services, Salem, KY, p. A258

LANDRY, Adam, Coordinator Computer Systems, Northern Maine Medical Center, Fort Kent, ME, p. A283

LANDRY, Candy, Chief Human Resource Officer, Eastside Psychiatric Hospital, Tallahassee, FL, p. A140

LANDRY, Donna, Interim Administrator, Heart Hospital of Lafayette, Lafayette, LA, p. A270

LANDRY, Ray A., Chief Executive Officer, Abbeville General Hospital, Abbeville, LA, p. A261

LANDRY, Wayne, Administrator and Chief Executive Officer, St. Catherine Memorial Hospital, New Orleans, LA, p. A275

LANDSMAN, Joseph, President and Chief Executive Officer, The University of Tennessee Medical Center, Knoxville, TN, p. A569

LANDSTROM, John
Director Human Resources, R M L Specialty Hospital, Hinsdale, IL, p. A184

Vice President Human Resources and Operations, RML Specialty Hospital, Chicago, IL, p. A177

LANDWEHR, Katie, Acting Associate Director, Veterans Affairs Medical Center, Omaha, NE, p. A388

LANE, David A., Deputy Commander Clinical Services, Tripler Army Medical Center, Honolulu, HI, p. A164

LANE, Kathy, Leader–ICU, Home Care, MedSurg, York Hospital, York, ME, p. A286

LANE, Kevin, D.O. Chief of Staff, Hardeman County Memorial Hospital, Quanah, TX, p. A622

LANE, Kevin, Vice President Information Systems, Silver Cross Hospital, New Lenox, IL, p. A189

LANE, Kim, Chief Fiscal Service, Overton Brooks Veterans Affairs Medical Center, Shreveport, LA, p. A277

LANE, Richard, Chief Financial Officer, Mid–America Rehabilitation Hospital, Shawnee Mission, KS, p. A243

LANE, Stacey
Executive Assistant Human Resources, Chambers Memorial Hospital, Danville, AR, p. A43

Director Human Resources, Hunt Regional Community Hospital, Commerce, TX, p. A588

LANE, Tommy, Chief Financial Officer, Lanier Health Services, Valley, AL, p. A26

LANER, Jr., Richard, Manager Information Systems, Miners' Colfax Medical Center, Raton, NM, p. A417

LANEY, Samuel Mark, M.D. President and Chief Executive Officer, Heartland Regional Medical Center, Saint Joseph, MO, p. A368

LANFORD, Alice Reed, FACHE Administrator, Shriners Hospitals for Children, Tampa, Tampa, FL, p. A141

LANG, Anne, Vice President Human Resources and Compliance and Privacy Officer, Winchester Hospital, Winchester, MA, p. A306

LANG, Cyndi, Director Information Services, French Hospital Medical Center, San Luis Obispo, CA, p. A88

LANG, David, Vice President Human Resources, Regional Medical Center of Hopkins County, Madisonville, KY, p. A255

LANG, Jr., Frank, M.D. Chief of Medicine, Sierra Nevada Memorial Hospital, Grass Valley, CA, p. A64

LANG, Gordon, M.D. Chief of Staff, Trego County–Lemke Memorial Hospital, Wakeeney, KS, p. A244

LANG, Irby, Vice President Human Resources, Anderson Regional Medical Center, Meridian, MS, p. A350

LANG, Jeffrey M., Chief Executive Officer, United Hospital District, Blue Earth, MN, p. A328

LANG, John Christopher, Chief Executive Officer, Cass Regional Medical Center, Harrisonville, MO, p. A360

LANG, Nicholas P., M.D
Chief of Staff, Central Arkansas Veterans Healthcare System, Little Rock, AR, p. A48

Chief Medical Officer, UAMS Medical Center, Little Rock, AR, p. A48

LANG, Patricia, M.D. Medical Director, Hot Springs Rehabilitation Center, Hot Springs National Park, AR, p. A46

LANG, Paula, Chief Executive Officer, Patient's Choice Medical Center, Belzoni, MS, p. A343

LANG, Richard, Ed.D. Vice President and Chief Information Officer, Doylestown Hospital, Doylestown, PA, p. A522

LANG, Richard T., Chief Financial Officer, Lewis County General Hospital, Lowville, NY, p. A429

LANG, Tony, Chief Information Officer, Bullock County Hospital, Union Springs, AL, p. A26

LANGAGER, Tyrone, M.D. Chief Medical Officer, Mountrail County Medical Center, Stanley, ND, p. A468

LANGBEHN, Cody, Chief Executive Officer, St. Luke's Wood River Medical Center, Ketchum, ID, p. A168

LANGBEHN, Jennifer, Medical Director, Mayo Clinic Health System in Saint James, Saint James, MN, p. A338

LANGBERG, Michael L., M.D. Senior Vice President Medical Affairs and Chief Medical Officer, Cedars–Sinai Medical Center, Los Angeles, CA, p. A69

LANGDON, Ashlee, Controller, Yalobusha General Hospital, Water Valley, MS, p. A353

LANGENBERG, Shannon, Director Human Resources, Jackson County Regional Health Center, Maquoketa, IA, p. A223

LANGER, Menachem, M.D. Chief Executive Officer, Cookeville Regional Medical Center, Cookeville, TN, p. A564

LANGFELDER, Richard, Executive Vice President and Chief Financial Officer, Lutheran Medical Center,, NY, p. A434

LANGLEY, Carol, Director Human Resources, Lake Granbury Medical Center, Granbury, TX, p. A601

LANGLEY, W. John, M.D. Chairman, East Cooper Medical Center, Mount Pleasant, SC, p. A552

LANGLITZ, Sara, Controller, Kindred Hospital–Houston, Houston, TX, p. A605

LANGLOIS, John
Vice President Finance, Citizens Baptist Medical Center, Talladega, AL, p. A26

Chief Financial Officer, Walker Baptist Medical Center, Jasper, AL, p. A22

LANGLOTZ, Karla, Director Human Resources, Central Florida Regional Hospital, Sanford, FL, p. A138

LANGMEAD, Paula A., Chief Executive Officer, Springfield Hospital Center, Sykesville, MD, p. A294

LANGROCK, Doug, M.D. Chief of Staff, Whidbey General Hospital, Coupeville, WA, p. A660

LANGSTON, Kimberly K., R.N. Executive Associate Director and Administrator, Scott and White Continuing Care Hospital, Temple, TX, p. A630

LANIG, Indria S., M.D. Medical Director, Northern Colorado Rehabilitation Hospital, Johnstown, CO, p. A102

LANKFORD, Deanna, Business Office Manager, Plano Specialty Hospital, Plano, TX, p. A621

LANNOYE, Craig, Vice President Operations, Wilson Memorial Hospital, Sidney, OH, p. A488

Index of Health Care Professionals / Lawhorn


LAWHORN, Renee, Director Medical Records, East Texas Medical Center Carthage, Carthage, TX, p. A586
LAWHORNE, Thomas, Chief Financial Officer, Regional Medical Center–Bayonet Point, Hudson, FL, p. A125
LAWLER, Anne, Director Human Resources, North Mississippi Medical Center–Hamilton, Hamilton, AL, p. A21
LAWLER, Kay, Business Office Manager, North Mississippi Medical Center–West Point, West Point, MS, p. A353
LAWLER, Patrick, Chief Executive Officer, Youth Villages Inner Harbour Campus, Douglasville, GA, p. A152
LAWLER, Steven, President, Vidant Medical Center, Greenville, NC, p. A454
LAWLESS, JoBeth, Director of Nursing, Nursing Services and Director Emergency Management Services, Lucas County Health Center, Chariton, IA, p. A216
LAWLESS, Rosalie, Director Human Resources, Fairlawn Rehabilitation Hospital, Worcester, MA, p. A306
LAWLOR, Kevin F., President and Chief Executive Officer, Huntington Hospital, Huntington, NY, p. A427
LAWONN, Kenneth
Senior Vice President Strategy & Technology, Alegent Health–Bergan Mercy Medical Center, Omaha, NE, p. A387
Senior Vice President Strategy and Technology, Alegent Health–Immanuel Medical Center, Omaha, NE, p. A387
Senior Vice President and Chief Information Officer, Alegent Health–Lakeside Hospital, Omaha, NE, p. A387
Senior Vice President and Chief Information Officer, Alegent Health–Mercy Hospital, Council Bluffs, IA, p. A217
Senior Vice President and Chief Information Officer, Alegent Health–Midlands Hospital, Papillion, NE, p. A389
LAWRENCE, Bruce, President and Chief Executive Officer, INTEGRIS Health, Oklahoma City, OK, p. B71
LAWRENCE, Dana, Interim Chief Executive Officer, Parkway Regional Hospital, Fulton, KY, p. A250
LAWRENCE, Jeffrey T., Chief Operating Officer, Denton Regional Medical Center, Denton, TX, p. A593
LAWRENCE, Jonathan I., President and Chief Executive Officer, Brooks Memorial Hospital, Dunkirk, NY, p. A425
LAWRENCE, Michael A., Chief Financial Officer, MacNeal Hospital, Berwyn, IL, p. A173
LAWRENCE, Rita, Director of Nursing, Doctors Hospital of West Covina, West Covina, CA, p. A95
LAWRENCE, Sandra A J
Executive Vice President and Chief Financial Officer, Children's Mercy Hospitals and Clinics, Kansas City, MO, p. A361
Executive Vice President and Chief Financial Officer, Children's Mercy South, Overland Park, KS, p. A240
LAWRENCE, Stephanie, Chief Financial Officer, Kentfield Rehabilitation and Specialty Hospital, Kentfield, CA, p. A65
LAWRENCE, Ursula, MSN Chief Nursing Officer, Central Carolina Hospital, Sanford, NC, p. A460
LAWRENCE, William P., President and Chief Executive Officer, McLaren Central Michigan, Mount Pleasant, MI, p. A319
LAWRENSON, Victoria
Chief Operating Officer, Bullock County Hospital, Union Springs, AL, p. A26
Chief Operating Officer, Crenshaw Community Hospital, Luverne, AL, p. A22
LAWSON, Alvin R., FACHE Chief Executive Officer, HEALTHSOUTH Western Hills Rehabilitation Hospital, Parkersburg, WV, p. A674
LAWSON, Beth, Chief Financial Officer and Director Governmental Affairs, Sunrise Canyon Hospital, Lubbock, TX, p. A614
LAWSON, David
Senior Vice President Human Resources, St. Clare Hospital, Lakewood, WA, p. A662
Senior Vice President Human Resources, St. Francis Hospital, Federal Way, WA, p. A661
Senior Vice President Human Resources, St. Joseph Medical Center, Tacoma, WA, p. A668
LAWSON, Doug, President, Baylor Regional Medical Center at Grapevine, Grapevine, TX, p. A601
LAWSON, Eric, Chief Financial Officer, North Florida Regional Medical Center, Gainesville, FL, p. A124
LAWSON, Judy, Director Information Services, Norton Community Hospital, Norton, VA, p. A653
LAWSON, Michael, Senior Vice President Operations, Grant Medical Center, Columbus, OH, p. A476
LAWSON, Michael E.
Director, Brockton Veterans Affairs Medical Center, Brockton, MA, p. A298
Director, Veterans Affairs Boston Healthcare System, Boston, MA, p. A297
LAWSON, Pam, Director Clinical Services, Select Specialty Hospital–Wilmington, Wilmington, DE, p. A115
LAWSON, Ralph E., Executive Vice President and Chief Financial Officer, Baptist Health South Florida, Baptist Hospital of Miami, Miami, FL, p. A130
LAWSON, Sandra K., Interim Director Fiscal Services, Shriners Hospitals for Children, St. Louis, Saint Louis, MO, p. A369
LAWSON, West, M.D
Chief Medical Officer, WakeMed Cary Hospital, Cary, NC, p. A450
Chief Medical Officer, WakeMed Raleigh Campus, Raleigh, NC, p. A459
LAWTON, Geoff, Vice President Operations, Littleton Adventist Hospital, Littleton, CO, p. A103
LAY, Sr., A. K., M.D. Chief Medical Officer, Jasper General Hospital, Bay Springs, MS, p. A343
LAY, Barbara, Chief Executive Officer, Pocahontas Memorial Hospital, Buckeye, WV, p. A670
LAYDEN, Lisa, Director of Finance, Highland Hospital, Charleston, WV, p. A671
LAYFIELD, Michael G., Chief Executive Officer, Drew Memorial Hospital, Monticello, AR, p. A49
LAYNE, Kristine, R.N. Chief Nursing Officer, Riverwood Healthcare Center, Aitkin, MN, p. A327
LAYTON, Ann, M.D. Chief of Staff, North Metro Medical Center, Jacksonville, AR, p. A46
LAYUGAN, Melvin, Director Human Resources, Horizon Specialty Hospital, Las Vegas, NV, p. A393
LAZARUS, David, M.D. Medical Director Clinical Affairs, Newton Medical Center, Newton, NJ, p. A407
LAZATIN, Lou, President and Chief Executive Officer, Saint John's Health Center, Santa Monica, CA, p. A90
LAZO, Nelson, Chief Executive Officer, Baptist Health South Florida, Doctors Hospital, Coral Gables, FL, p. A121
LAZROFF, Gary
Vice President Human Resources, St. John Medical Center, Westlake, OH, p. A491
Vice President Human Resources, St. Vincent Charity Medical Center, Cleveland, OH, p. A475
LAZURE, Lee A., Director Civil Service Commission, Douglas County Community Mental Health Center, Omaha, NE, p. A388
LAZZARO, III, Frank A., Chief Human Resources Officer, Phelps County Regional Medical Center, Rolla, MO, p. A367
LEA, Hampton P S, Chief Operating Officer, Eastern Louisiana Mental Health System, Jackson, LA, p. A268
LEA, Rich, Vice President Operations, Euclid Hospital, Euclid, OH, p. A480
LEACH, Craig, President and Chief Executive Officer, Torrance Memorial Medical Center, Torrance, CA, p. A92
LEACH, Leslie, Administrator, Memorial Specialty Hospital, Lufkin, TX, p. A614
LEACH, Mary Ann, Vice President and Chief Information Officer, Children's Hospital Colorado, Aurora, CO, p. A97
LEACH, Steven, M.D. Chief Medical Officer, University of Texas Southwestern Medical Center, Dallas, TX, p. A593
LEADER, Skip, Chief Information Officer, Choctaw Nation Health Care Center, Talihina, OK, p. A505
LEAHY, Jesse, M.D. Chief Medical Officer, Tri–County Memorial Hospital, Whitehall, WI, p. A694
LEAHY, Kevin D., President and Chief Executive Officer, Franciscan Alliance, Mishawaka, IN, p. B52
LEAHY, Mary P., Vice President Human Resources, St. Joseph Hospital, Orange, CA, p. A78
LEAHY, Rosanne, Vice President Nursing Services, CarolinaEast Medical Center, New Bern, NC, p. A458
LEAKE, Neta F., Administrative Assistant Human Resources, West Feliciana Parish Hospital, Saint Francisville, LA, p. A276
LEAKE, Sandy, MSN Associate Director, Nursing and Patient Care Services, Veterans Affairs Medical Center, Decatur, GA, p. A151
LEAKEY, Kim, R.N. Chief Nursing Officer, Lafayette Regional Health Center, Lexington, MO, p. A364
LEAL, Carlos, Chief Information Officer, Rio Grande Regional Hospital, McAllen, TX, p. A615
LEAL, Jorge E., Administrator, East Texas Medical Center–Gilmer, Gilmer, TX, p. A601
LEAL, Jr., Joseph M., M.D. Medical Director, Prairie Community Hospital, Terry, MT, p. A379
LEAMAN–CASE, Sheri, Administrator and Chief Executive Officer, St. Mary's of Michigan Standish Hospital, Standish, MI, p. A323
LEAMING, Larry E., Ph.D. Chief Executive Officer, Roosevelt General Hospital, Portales, NM, p. A417
LEAMON, Jim, Chief Financial Officer, J. F. K. Medical Center, Atlantis, FL, p. A118
LEAR, Richard, Director Information Systems, St. David's South Austin Medical Center, Austin, TX, p. A581
LEARY, Edward B., Chief Executive Officer, New Bedford Rehabilitation Hospital, New Bedford, MA, p. A302
LEARY, Matt, Chief Financial Officer, Wesley Medical Center, Wichita, KS, p. A246
LEARY, Matthew, Chief Financial Officer, Lee's Summit Medical Center, Lee's Summit, MO, p. A364
LEASURE, Sandie, Senior Vice President Human Resources, O'Bleness Memorial Hospital, Athens, OH, p. A470
LEAVER, William B., President and Chief Executive Officer, Iowa Health System, Des Moines, IA, p. B72
LEAVITT, Cynthia, R.N
Senior Vice President, Hospital Operations, Miles Memorial Hospital, Damariscotta, ME, p. A283
Senior Vice President, Hospital Operations, St. Andrews Hospital and Healthcare Center, Boothbay Harbor, ME, p. A282
LEAZER, Ronald, Chief Financial Officer, Gateway Regional Medical Center, Granite City, IL, p. A183
LEBARON, Bradley D., FACHE President and Chief Executive Officer, Uintah Basin Medical Center, Roosevelt, UT, p. A640
LEBARRON, Tere, Vice President Planning and Integration, University of Arizona Medical Center – University Campus, Tucson, AZ, p. A40
LEBEAU, Michelle, Vice President Human Resources, Champlain Valley Physicians Hospital Medical Center, Plattsburgh, NY, p. A440
LEBLANC, Ed, M.D. Vice President Medical Affairs, Seton Northwest Hospital, Austin, TX, p. A581
LEBLANC, Garon, Chief Plant Operations, Sage Rehabilitation Hospital, Baton Rouge, LA, p. A263
LEBLANC, Karen, Director, Applications, Samaritan Hospital, Troy, NY, p. A445
LEBLANC, Stephen J., Chief Operating Officer, Dartmouth–Hitchcock Medical Center, Lebanon, NH, p. A398
LEBLANC, Terry, Chief Operating Officer, New London Hospital, New London, NH, p. A399
LEBOWITZ, Howard, M.D. Chief Medical Officer, Specialty Hospital at Kimball, Lakewood, NJ, p. A405
LEBRON, Sonia M., Human Resources Specialist, Industrial Hospital, San Juan, PR, p. A703
LEBRUN, James, Chief Executive Officer, Gordon Memorial Hospital, Gordon, NE, p. A384
LECHMAN, Brenda, Director Human Resources, Haxtun Hospital District, Haxtun, CO, p. A102
LECHOCO, Bing, Director Human Resources, Specialty Hospital of Washington–Hadley, Washington, DC, p. A117
LECKER, Marijo, Vice President, Martha Jefferson Hospital, Charlottesville, VA, p. A646
LECONTE, Chantal, Chief Executive Officer, Memorial Hospital Pembroke, Pembroke Pines, FL, p. A135
LEDBETTER, Joy, Director Human Resources, Methodist Medical Center of Illinois, Peoria, IL, p. A191
LEDDEN, Edwin L., Assistant Administrator, Henry County Medical Center, Paris, TN, p. A574
LEDER, Larry, Chief Financial Officer, Promise Hospital of Miss Lou, Vidalia, LA, p. A279
LEDERER, Jane, R.N. Vice President and Chief Nursing Officer, Kingsbrook Jewish Medical Center,, NY, p. A433
LEDERMAN, Joel, Director Information Systems, Community Health Center of Branch County, Coldwater, MI, p. A310
LEDERMAN, Mark, Chief Information Officer, Interfaith Medical Center,, NY, p. A433
LEDET, Cathi, Comptroller, University Behavioral Health of Denton, Denton, TX, p. A594
LEDFORD, Maribeth, Director Human Resources, Henry Medical Center, Stockbridge, GA, p. A160
LEDGERWOOD, Linda, Director Human Resources, Whitman Hospital and Medical Center, Colfax, WA, p. A660
LEDOUX, Roger C., Chief Executive Officer, Byrd Regional Hospital, Leesville, LA, p. A271
LEDYARD, Robin, M.P.H. President, Community Hospital East, Indianapolis, IN, p. A204
LEE, Bryan, Chief Operating Officer, Eliza Coffee Memorial Hospital, Florence, AL, p. A20
LEE, Bryan R., Chief Financial Officer, Kingwood Medical Center, Kingwood, TX, p. A611
LEE, Byong, Manager Information Technology and PACS Administrator, Limestone Medical Center, Groesbeck, TX, p. A602
LEE, Cheryl D., R.N. Vice President Patient Care Services, Chief Executive Nurse and Compliance Officer, Sheltering Arms Hospital South, Midlothian, VA, p. A651
LEE, Dana, M.D. Chief of Staff, North Hawaii Community Hospital, Kamuela, HI, p. A164
LEE, Deborah, Chief Nursing Officer, Community Westview Hospital, Indianapolis, IN, p. A204
LEE, Don, Chief Information Officer, Metropolitan Hospital Center, New York, NY, p. A434
LEE, Dwight A., M.D. Chief Medical Officer, Doctors Hospital at White Rock Lake, Dallas, TX, p. A591
LEE, Eric A., President and Chief Executive Officer, Jennie Stuart Medical Center, Hopkinsville, KY, p. A251
LEE, Gina, Chief Financial Officer, Fort Lauderdale Hospital, Fort Lauderdale, FL, p. A123
LEE, Helen, Manager Information Systems, Chinese Hospital, San Francisco, CA, p. A86


A862 Index of Health Care Professionals

Index of Health Care Professionals / Leonard

Index of Health Care Professionals


LEE, James Y., Executive Vice President and Chief Operating Officer, Lawrence Hospital Center, Bronxville, NY, p. A422
LEE, Jeannie, Director Human Resources, Marshall County Hospital, Benton, KY, p. A247
LEE, Jenny, Human Resources Generalist, Essentia Health–Holy Trinity Hospital, Graceville, MN, p. A332
LEE, John Paul, M.D. Chief of Staff, S. E. Lackey Memorial Hospital, Forest, MS, p. A346
LEE, John R., Chief Executive Officer, Mat–Su Regional Medical Center, Palmer, AK, p. A30
LEE, Joseph, M.D. President Medical Staff, Riverside Community Hospital, Riverside, CA, p. A83
LEE, Karen, MSN Chief Nursing Officer, Belton Regional Medical Center, Belton, MO, p. A355
LEE, Karen, Director Human Resources, Gallup Indian Medical Center, Gallup, NM, p. A416
LEE, Kayleen R., Chief Executive Officer, Sioux Center Community Hospital and Health Center Avera, Sioux Center, IA, p. A226
LEE, Larry, Chief Financial Officer, United Hospital District, Blue Earth, MN, p. A328
LEE, Mary Ann, Chief Nursing Officer, HEALTHSOUTH Rehabilitation Hospital of Austin, Austin, TX, p. A580
LEE, Mary C., Manager Human Resources, Jonathan M. Wainwright Memorial VA Medical Center, Walla Walla, WA, p. A669
LEE, Mihi, Chief Financial Officer, Coast Plaza Hospital, Norwalk, CA, p. A77
LEE, Nancy, R.N. Vice President Patient Care Services and Chief Nursing Officer, Stanford Hospital and Clinics, Palo Alto, CA, p. A79
LEE, Nathan W., Chief Executive Officer, Mary Breckinridge ARH Hospital, Hyden, KY, p. A252
LEE, Noel, Administrative Director and Chief Information Officer, Mercy Medical Center Merced, Merced, CA, p. A74
LEE, Patrick, Chief Executive Officer, Continuum Rehabilitation Hospital of North Texas, Flower Mound, TX, p. A597
LEE, Randall, Vice President and Chief Operating Officer, Baptist Health South Florida, Baptist Hospital of Miami, Miami, FL, p. A130
LEE, Robbin M., Chief Operating Officer, J. F. K. Medical Center, Atlantis, FL, p. A118
LEE, Robert H., President, Raulerson Hospital, Okeechobee, FL, p. A134
LEE, Stacey, Chief Financial Officer, Johnson Memorial Health Services, Dawson, MN, p. A330
LEE, Stephen, President, Baptist Medical Center Nassau, Fernandina Beach, FL, p. A123
LEE, T. Kim, CPA, Chief Executive Officer, Bowie Memorial Hospital, Bowie, TX, p. A584
LEE, Tami, MSN Chief Nursing Officer, Lancaster Regional Medical Center, Lancaster, PA, p. A526
LEE, Terry, M.D. Chief of Staff, Garfield Medical Center, Monterey Park, CA, p. A75
LEE, Thomas G., Chief Financial Officer, Medicine Lodge Memorial Hospital, Medicine Lodge, KS, p. A239
LEE, Victor N., FACHE President and Chief Executive Officer, Boone County Health Center, Albion, NE, p. A381
LEE, Vincent H. S., FACHE Regional Chief Executive Officer, Leahi Hospital, Honolulu, HI, p. A163
LEECH, James J., Commander, William Beaumont Army Medical Center, El Paso, TX, p. A597
LEEDOM, Hope, Director Human Resources, Beauregard Memorial Hospital, De Ridder, LA, p. A265
LEEGSTRA, Ruurd, Chief Financial Officer, Silver Hill Hospital, New Canaan, CT, p. A110
LEEKA, Andrew B., President and Chief Executive Officer, Good Samaritan Hospital, Los Angeles, CA, p. A69
LEEPER, Kevin, Chief Executive Officer, Scott & White Hospital – Llano, Llano, TX, p. A613
LEESER, Robert, M.D. Chief Medical Officer, Hayes Green Beach Memorial Hospital, Charlotte, MI, p. A309
LEET, Arabella, M.D. Chief of Staff, Shriners Hospitals for Children, Honolulu, Honolulu, HI, p. A164
LEFEVRE, Denise, Chief Information Officer, Oroville Hospital, Oroville, CA, p. A78
LEFEVRE, Steve, Administrator, Fisher County Hospital District, Rotan, TX, p. A623
LEFF, Marc, Vice President Human Resources, Maimonides Medical Center,, NY, p. A434
LEFFLER, Stephen, Chief Medical Officer, Fletcher Allen Health Care, Burlington, VT, p. A643
LEFKOW, Frances, Director Human Resources, La Rabida Children's Hospital, Chicago, IL, p. A176
LEFTWICH, Hal W., FACHE Chief Executive Officer, Fishermen's Hospital, Marathon, FL, p. A129
LEGASPI, Johnson, Director Information Systems, Alhambra Hospital Medical Center, Alhambra, CA, p. A53
LEGEL, Tom, Vice President Finance and Information, Kootenai Medical Center, Coeur D'Alene, ID, p. A167
LEGENDZIEWICZ, Henry, Senior Vice President and Chief Financial Officer, Nathan Littauer Hospital and Nursing Home, Gloversville, NY, p. A426
LEGER, Lynn, Director Information Systems, Ridgeview Institute, Smyrna, GA, p. A159
LEGERE, Tina Marie, Chief Executive Officer, Parkland Medical Center, Derry, NH, p. A397
LEGG, Alyce, Vice President Human Resources, Samaritan Regional Health System, Ashland, OH, p. A469
LEGGETT, G. Raymond, Chief Executive Officer, CarolinaEast Medical Center, New Bern, NC, p. A458
LEGRAND, Daniel, M.D. Chief Medical Officer, St. Vincent Indianapolis Hospital, Indianapolis, IN, p. A205
LEGRAND III,, Edwin C., Executive Director, Mississippi State Department of Mental Health, Jackson, MS, p. B91
LEHMANN, Robert J., Chief Executive Officer, Keystone Newport News, Newport News, VA, p. A652
LEHNER, Bill, Director Management Information Systems, Amery Regional Medical Center, Amery, WI, p. A678
LEHNER, Deborah, Administrator, Greeley County Health Services, Tribune, KS, p. A244
LEIBENHAUT, Mark, M.D. Chief of Staff, Sutter Medical Center, Sacramento, Sacramento, CA, p. A84
LEIBHAM, Geri, Manager Business Office, Salina Surgical Hospital, Salina, KS, p. A243
LEIBMAN, Maurice, M.D. Chief Medical Officer, Memorial Hermann Northwest Hospital, Houston, TX, p. A605
LEICHMAN, Ann Marie, R.N. Vice President Patient Care Services and Chief Nursing Officer, Valley Hospital, Ridgewood, NJ, p. A409
LEICHNER, Raymond, Director Finance, Abington Health Lansdale Hospital, Lansdale, PA, p. A527
LEIDY, R. Grant, Vice President Finance, Deborah Heart and Lung Center, Browns Mills, NJ, p. A402
LEIF, Sue, R.N. Director Human Resources, Annie Jeffrey Memorial County Health Center, Osceola, NE, p. A388
LEIGH, Cindy, Chief Operating Officer, Fairbanks, Indianapolis, IN, p. A204
LEIMGRUBER, Jeffrey A., President, Hillcrest Hospital, Cleveland, OH, p. A475
LEINEN, Rick, Chief Financial Officer, Montgomery County Memorial Hospital, Red Oak, IA, p. A225
LEIS, Jr., James L., Chief Financial Officer, Doctor's Memorial Hospital, Perry, FL, p. A136
LEISCHNER, Lindsay, R.N
Administrator and Chief Executive Officer, Avera Dells Area Hospital, Dell Rapids, SD, p. A556
Administrator and Chief Executive Officer, Avera Flandreau Hospital, Flandreau, SD, p. A556
LEISE, Karen, Coordinator Human Resources, Saunders Medical Center, Wahoo, NE, p. A390
LEISHER, George, Vice President Human Resources, Northridge Hospital Medical Center–Roscoe Boulevard Campus,, CA, p. A70
LEISHER, Kenneth W., Chief Executive Officer, Heart of the Rockies Regional Medical Center, Salida, CO, p. A105
LEIST, Vincent, President and Chief Executive Officer, North Arkansas Regional Medical Center, Harrison, AR, p. A45
LEITE, Dolores
Chief Human Resource Executive, Jacobi Medical Center,, NY, p. A433
Chief Human Resource Executive, North Central Bronx Hospital,, NY, p. A436
LEITENBERGER, Donna, Director Information Services, Edward White Hospital, Saint Petersburg, FL, p. A138
LEITNER, Mark, Chief Executive Officer, East Texas Medical Center Henderson, Henderson, TX, p. A603
LEJEUNE, Dolores N., R.N. President and Chief Executive Officer, St. Elizabeth Hospital, Gonzales, LA, p. A267
LEJSEK, Shari, Administrator, Patients' Hospital of Redding, Redding, CA, p. A82
LELAND, Joni, Director Human Resources, Memorial Hospital, Gonzales, TX, p. A601
LELEUX, Ross, Chief Information Officer, Iberia Medical Center, New Iberia, LA, p. A274
LEM, Alan
Vice President Finance, Fairview Ridges Hospital, Burnsville, MN, p. A329
Vice President Finance, Fairview Southdale Hospital, Edina, MN, p. A331
LEMAIRE, Joseph M., Executive Vice President and Chief Financial Officer, Holy Name Medical Center, Teaneck, NJ, p. A410
LEMAIRE, Suzanne, Manager Health Information Management Services and Corporate Compliance Officer, Scheurer Hospital, Pigeon, MI, p. A320
LEMAISTRE, Collin, Chief Operating Officer, Nacogdoches Medical Center, Nacogdoches, TX, p. A618
LEMANSKI, Dennis R., D.O. Senior Vice President Medical Affairs and Medical Education/CMO, Henry Ford Wyandotte Hospital, Wyandotte, MI, p. A325
LEMAR, Homer, M.D. Deputy Commander Clinical Services, William Beaumont Army Medical Center, El Paso, TX, p. A597
LEMASTERS, Deb, Director Human Resources, Woodlawn Hospital, Rochester, IN, p. A211
LEMIEUX, Harry, Chief Information and Innovation Officer, Morton Hospital and Medical Center, Taunton, MA, p. A305
LEMIEUX, Kandie, Administrative Assistant and Director Human Resources, Northern Rockies Medical Center, Cut Bank, MT, p. A374
LEMMER, Donn J., Vice President Finance, West Shore Medical Center, Manistee, MI, p. A318
LEMMONS, Tracy G., Director Human Resources, Mercy McCune–Brooks Hospital, Carthage, MO, p. A357
LEMON, Brian J., Chief Executive Officer, MacNeal Hospital, Berwyn, IL, p. A173
LEMON, Donna, Director Human Resources, Ward Memorial Hospital, Monahans, TX, p. A617
LEMON, Marc, Administrator, Kindred Hospital Ocala, Ocala, FL, p. A133
LEMON, Rita, Director Human Resources, Avera Queen of Peace Hospital, Mitchell, SD, p. A558
LEMON, Thomas R., Chief Executive Officer, Otsego Memorial Hospital, Gaylord, MI, p. A313
LEMONS, Elizabeth, Chief Operating Officer, Middle Tennessee Medical Center, Murfreesboro, TN, p. A573
LEMONS, Tania, Controller, East Texas Medical Center–Quitman, Quitman, TX, p. A622
LEMONTE, David, Chief Executive Officer, Memorial Medical Center – Livingston, Livingston, TX, p. A612
LENAHAN, Kevin
Director Corporate Accounting, Budgets, Grants and Reimbursements, Newton Medical Center, Newton, NJ, p. A407
Vice President Finance and Chief Financial Officer, Overlook Medical Center, Summit, NJ, p. A410
LENAMOND, Kevin, Information Management Service Line Executive, Michael E. DeBakey Veterans Affairs Medical Center, Houston, TX, p. A606
LENARD, Gary, Director Human Resources, Hendricks Regional Health, Danville, IN, p. A200
LENCIONI, Kathi, Chief Executive Officer, Sharp Mesa Vista Hospital, San Diego, CA, p. A86
LENEAVE, Mark, Administrator, Meadowbrook Rehabilitation Hospital, Gardner, KS, p. A233
LENKEVICH, Ellen R., Chief Nursing Officer, Florida Hospital–Flagler, Palm Coast, FL, p. A135
LENKOWSKI, Thomas, Chief Financial Officer, Martha's Vineyard Hospital, Oak Bluffs, MA, p. A303
LENNARTZ, Randal, Vice President Finance, Highland District Hospital, Hillsboro, OH, p. A482
LENNEN, Anthony B., President, Community Hospital South, Indianapolis, IN, p. A204
LENOIR, Frank, Executive Director Human Resources, Mercy Hospital Washington, Washington, MO, p. A372
LENTENBRINK, Laura, Vice President, Human Resources, Borgess Medical Center, Kalamazoo, MI, p. A316
LENTZ, Darrell, Chief Executive Officer, Sun Coast Hospital, Largo, FL, p. A128
LENZ, Jan, Chief Nursing Officer, Athens–Limestone Hospital, Athens, AL, p. A16
LENZ, Roger W., Interim Chief Executive Officer, Oakland Mercy Hospital, Oakland, NE, p. A387
LENZO, Julie, Director Business Office, Specialty Hospital of Albuquerque, Albuquerque, NM, p. A415
LEO, Elizabeth, Vice President Human Resources, Regional Hospital of Scranton, Scranton, PA, p. A538
LEON, Anne R., Administrator, Kindred Hospital–Bay Area, Pasadena, TX, p. A620
LEON, Daniel, Chief Financial Officer, Sherman Oaks Hospital,, CA, p. A71
LEON, Luis, Regional Chief Executive Officer, Paradise Valley Hospital, National City, CA, p. A76
LEONARD, Bradley M., M.D. Vice President Medical Affairs, Baylor Regional Medical Center at Plano, Plano, TX, p. A621
LEONARD, Donavan, Chief Financial Officer, Baptist Memorial Hospital–Booneville, Booneville, MS, p. A344
LEONARD, Edward F., Executive Vice President and Chief Operating Officer, White Plains Hospital Center, White Plains, NY, p. A447
LEONARD, James C., M.D. President and Chief Executive Officer, Carle Foundation Hospital, Urbana, IL, p. A195
LEONARD, Kathy, Manager Human Resources, Community Howard Specialty Hospital, Kokomo, IN, p. A206
LEONARD, Kevin, Vice President for Finance and Chief Financial Officer, New England Sinai Hospital and Rehabilitation Center, Stoughton, MA, p. A305


 Index of Health Care Professionals A863

LEONARD, Leland, M.D. Administrator, Fort Defiance Indian Health Service Hospital, Fort Defiance, AZ, p. A32

LEONARD, Mark, Vice President Finance, Beaumont Hospital – Troy, Troy, MI, p. A324

LEONARD, Mark T.
Chief Executive Officer, Dickenson Community Hospital, Clintwood, VA, p. A647
Chief Executive Officer, Norton Community Hospital, Norton, VA, p. A653

LEONARD, Robert, Director Information Services, Sierra Vista Regional Medical Center, San Luis Obispo, CA, p. A88

LEONARD, Roger, M.D. Vice President Medical Affairs, Medstar Montgomery Medical Center, Olney, MD, p. A293

LEONARD, William H., President, Carolinas Medical Center–University, Charlotte, NC, p. A450

LEONARD, William J., USN, Commanding Officer, Naval Hospital, Lemoore, CA, p. A67

LEONDAR, Kimberly, Director Human Resources, Texas Health Harris Methodist Hospital Stephenville, Stephenville, TX, p. A629

LEONE, Ellen, R.N. Chief Nursing Officer, University of Connecticut Health Center, John Dempsey Hospital, Farmington, CT, p. A109

LEONELIS, Lisa, Chief Information Officer, Veterans Affairs Salt Lake City Health Care System, Salt Lake City, UT, p. A641

LEONHARDT, Darrell, Senior Vice President Information Systems, Arkansas Children's Hospital, Little Rock, AR, p. A47

LEONHARDT, Gary, M.D. Clinical Director, Walter B. Jones Alcohol and Drug Abuse Treatment Center, Greenville, NC, p. A454

LEOPARD, Jimmy, FACHE Chief Executive Officer, Wagoner Community Hospital, Wagoner, OK, p. A507

LEPE, Patti, Chief Financial Officer, Parkview Community Hospital Medical Center, Riverside, CA, p. A82

LEPORE, Timothy J., FACS Medical Director, Nantucket Cottage Hospital, Nantucket, MA, p. A302

LEPP, Jerry, Acting Chief Executive Officer, Ashley Medical Center, Ashley, ND, p. A464

LEPPKE, Ben, Chief Information Officer, Satanta District Hospital, Satanta, KS, p. A243

LEQUEUX, Veronica, Vice President Human Resources, Blake Medical Center, Bradenton, FL, p. A119

LEQUIRE, Mark, M.D. Chief of Staff, Vaughan Regional Medical Center, Selma, AL, p. A25

LERCH, Gail, R.N
Vice President, Kapiolani Medical Center for Women & Children, Honolulu, HI, p. A163
Vice President Human Resources, Pali Momi Medical Center, Aiea, HI, p. A163
Executive Vice President Human Resources, Straub Clinic & Hospital, Honolulu, HI, p. A164

LERNER, Wayne M., DPH, President and Chief Executive Officer, Holy Cross Hospital, Chicago, IL, p. A176

LEROY, Joseph B., M.D. Clinical Director, Southwestern State Hospital, Thomasville, GA, p. A160

LEROY, Kurt, Manager Information Management, Lanier Health Services, Valley, AL, p. A26

LEROY, Michael
Senior Vice President and Chief Information Officer, Detroit Receiving Hospital/University Health Center, Detroit, MI, p. A310
Senior Vice President and Chief Information Officer, Harper University Hospital/Hutzel Women's Hospital, Detroit, MI, p. A310

LESCHKE, Gwenn, Vice President Human Resources, Advocate Condell Medical Center, Libertyville, IL, p. A186

LESINS, Ross, Chief Information Officer, Casa Colina Hospital for Rehabilitative Medicine, Pomona, CA, p. A80

LESLIE, Bruce, M.D. Chief of Staff, Grant Memorial Hospital, Petersburg, WV, p. A674

LESLIE, Desdemona, Finance Officer, U. S. Public Health Service Indian Hospital–Whiteriver, Whiteriver, AZ, p. A40

LESLIE, Donald P., M.D. Medical Director, Shepherd Center, Atlanta, GA, p. A146

LESLIE, Frank, Vice President Operations, Highlands–Cashiers Hospital, Highlands, NC, p. A455

LESLIE, Kelly, Chief Financial Officer, Ferry County Memorial Hospital, Republic, WA, p. A665

LESOING–LUCS, Jennifer, Vice President and Chief Financial Officer, BryanLGH Medical Center, Lincoln, NE, p. A385

LESTER, James, Director Fiscal Services, Shriners Hospitals for Children, Shriners Burns Hospital, Cincinnati, Cincinnati, OH, p. A474

LESTER, Mark, M.D. Vice President and Chief Quality Officer, Texas Health Presbyterian Hospital Dallas, Dallas, TX, p. A592

LESTER, Ron, Chief Human Resources, Veterans Affairs Medical Center, Cheyenne, WY, p. A695

LESTER, William, M.D. Vice President Medical Affairs, Cardinal Hill Rehabilitation Hospital, Lexington, KY, p. A252

LETELLIER, Jean–Pierre, M.D. Chief of Staff, Memorial Hospital, Seminole, TX, p. A627

LETH, Rence, Administrator, Riverside Center for Behavioral Medicine, Riverside, CA, p. A83

LETSON, Robert F., Chief Executive Officer, South Peninsula Hospital, Homer, AK, p. A29

LETT, Bryan W., Chief Executive Officer, Michiana Behavioral Health Center, Plymouth, IN, p. A210

LETT, Tammy, R.N. Chief Nursing Officer, Greenville Regional Hospital, Greenville, IL, p. A183

LEU, Christopher, Chief Executive Officer, Texas Health Harris Methodist Hospital Stephenville, Stephenville, TX, p. A629

LEUNG, Lawrence, M.D. Chief of Staff, Veterans Affairs Palo Alto Health Care System, Palo Alto, CA, p. A79

LEVELING, Jim, Director Information Technology, Kansas City Orthopaedic Institute, Leawood, KS, p. A237

LEVENSON, Adam, Manager Information Systems, Lakeside Medical Center, Belle Glade, FL, p. A118

LEVENSON, Marc, M.D. Director, Veterans Affairs Medical Center, Manchester, NH, p. A399

LEVER, Roger, M.D. President Medical Staff, The Outer Banks Hospital, Nags Head, NC, p. A458

LEVERETT, Carey O., Vice President Information Services, Meritus Medical Center, Hagerstown, MD, p. A292

LEVERICH, Karen, Chief Executive Officer, Specialty Hospital of Mid–America, Overland Park, KS, p. A241

LEVERING, Theresa, Director Human Resources, Doctors Hospital of Sarasota, Sarasota, FL, p. A138

LEVI, Allen, Director Information Services, Ephraim McDowell Regional Medical Center, Danville, KY, p. A249

LEVI, John, Director of Human Resources, St. Lawrence Rehabilitation Center, Lawrenceville, NJ, p. A405

LEVINE, Alexandra, M.D
Chief Medical Officer, City of Hope's Helford Clinical Research Hospital, Duarte, CA, p. A59
Medical Director, University of Southern California–Norris Cancer Hospital, Los Angeles, CA, p. A72

LEVINE, Larry L., President and Chief Executive Officer, Blythedale Children's Hospital, Valhalla, NY, p. A445

LEVINE, Marty, Vice President Human Resources, Windham Hospital, Willimantic, CT, p. A113

LEVINE, Michelle, Director Human Resources, Long Beach Medical Center, Long Beach, NY, p. A429

LEVINE, Peter H., M.D. Executive Medical Director Behavioral Health Services, Adventist Behavioral Health Rockville, Rockville, MD, p. A293

LEVINE, Robert V., Executive Vice President and Chief Operating Officer, Flushing Hospital Medical Center,, NY, p. A432

LEVISON, Julie, Director Human Resources, Providence Medford Medical Center, Medford, OR, p. A512

LEVITAN, Kenneth, Vice President Information Systems, Einstein Medical Center Philadelphia, Philadelphia, PA, p. A532

LEVITZ, Michele, Director Finance, St. Luke's Hospital – Miners Campus, Coaldale, PA, p. A520

LEVLEIT, Spencer, Director Information Technology, Unicoi County Memorial Hospital, Erwin, TN, p. A565

LEVY, Brian, M.D. Medical Director, LTAC of Edmond, Edmond, OK, p. A496

LEVY, Scott S., M.D. Vice President and Chief Medical Officer, Doylestown Hospital, Doylestown, PA, p. A522

LEVY, Susan M., M.D. Vice President Medical Affairs, Levindale Hebrew Geriatric Center and Hospital, Baltimore, MD, p. A288

LEWANDOWSKI, James, Vice President Corporate Human Resources, Alexian Brothers Behavioral Health Hospital, Hoffman Estates, IL, p. A184

LEWANDOWSKI, Terri, Director Financial Services, Our Lady of Victory Hospital, Stanley, WI, p. A691

LEWELLEN, Thomas, D.O. Chief of Staff, Delta Memorial Hospital, Dumas, AR, p. A44

LEWERKE, Jane, Manager Human Resources, Northern Arizona VA Health Care System, Prescott, AZ, p. A37

LEWGOOD, Tony, Administrator, Shriners Hospitals for Children–Lexington, Lexington, KY, p. A253

LEWIS, Angel, Executive Director Human Resources, Cookeville Regional Medical Center, Cookeville, TN, p. A564

LEWIS, Barbara, Chief Nursing Officer, Integris Seminole Medical Center, Seminole, OK, p. A504

LEWIS, Brinsley B., Chief Executive Officer, Florida Hospital–Carrollwood, Tampa, FL, p. A140

LEWIS, III, Carlisle, Senior Vice President Legal and Human Resources, Sharp Mesa Vista Hospital, San Diego, CA, p. A86

LEWIS, Chris, M.D. Vice President Medical Affairs, Mercy Hospital Independence, Independence, KS, p. A235

LEWIS, Colleen, Director Human Resources, Texas NeuroRehab Center, Austin, TX, p. A582

LEWIS, Curtis, M.D. Chief of Staff, Grady Memorial Hospital, Atlanta, GA, p. A145

LEWIS, Dana, Director Clinical Services, Southern Kentucky Rehabilitation Hospital, Bowling Green, KY, p. A248

LEWIS, Dave, Director Information Services, St. Francis Hospital and Health Services, Maryville, MO, p. A365

LEWIS, Jr., Donald C., Vice President and Chief Financial Officer, Coffee Regional Medical Center, Douglas, GA, p. A151

LEWIS, Doug, Chief Financial Officer, Elks Rehab Hospital, Boise, ID, p. A166

LEWIS, Eric, Chief Executive Officer, Olympic Medical Center, Port Angeles, WA, p. A664

LEWIS, Frank, Ph.D. Chief Executive Officer, Oklahoma NeuroSpecialty Center, Tulsa, OK, p. A506

LEWIS, George, Executive Director, Bayview Behavioral Health Campus, Chula Vista, CA, p. A57

LEWIS, George E., M.D. Medical Officer, Nebraska Penal and Correctional Hospital, Lincoln, NE, p. A385

LEWIS, Gerry
Chief Information Officer, Seton Edgar B. Davis Hospital, Luling, TX, p. A614
Chief Information Officer, Seton Highland Lakes, Burnet, TX, p. A586
Chief Information Officer, Seton Medical Center Austin, Austin, TX, p. A581
Chief Information Officer, Seton Medical Center Williamson, Round Rock, TX, p. A623
Chief Information Officer, Seton Northwest Hospital, Austin, TX, p. A581
Chief Information Officer, Seton Shoal Creek Hospital, Austin, TX, p. A581
Chief Information Officer, University Medical Center at Brackenridge, Austin, TX, p. A582

LEWIS, Gina, Director Human Resources, HEALTHSOUTH Rehabilitation Hospital–Las Vegas, Las Vegas, NV, p. A393

LEWIS, Gordon, Chief Executive Officer, Burnett Medical Center, Grantsburg, WI, p. A682

LEWIS, J. Steve, Director Finance, Youth Villages Inner Harbour Campus, Douglasville, GA, p. A152

LEWIS, Jackie, Director Human Resources, Bacon County Hospital and Health System, Alma, GA, p. A144

LEWIS, Jacob, Chief Financial Officer, Mark Twain St. Joseph's Hospital, San Andreas, CA, p. A84

LEWIS, Jo, Director Human Resources, Providence Tarzana Medical Center,, CA, p. A71

LEWIS, John I., President and Chief Executive Officer, ACMH Hospital, Kittanning, PA, p. A526

LEWIS, Kashion, Director Human Resources, Mayhill Hospital, Denton, TX, p. A594

LEWIS, Kenneth S., JD, President and Chief Executive Officer, Union Hospital, Elkton, MD, p. A291

LEWIS, Kent, Director Information Services, Southwestern Medical Center, Lawton, OK, p. A498

LEWIS, Libby, Chief Financial Officer, CHRISTUS Jasper Memorial Hospital, Jasper, TX, p. A609

LEWIS, Luther J., FACHE Chief Executive Officer, Five Rivers Medical Center, Pocahontas, AR, p. A50

LEWIS, Marie, Human Resources Liaison, Veterans Affairs Medical Center, Saint Louis, MO, p. A370

LEWIS, Mary Jo, FACHE President and Chief Executive Officer, Sumner Regional Medical Center, Gallatin, TN, p. A566

LEWIS, Michael, Chief Operating Officer, Mother Frances Hospital – Jacksonville, Jacksonville, TX, p. A609

LEWIS, Nan M., Administrator, East Central Regional Hospital, Augusta, GA, p. A146

LEWIS, Nicholas P., Chief Operating Officer, Lourdes Hospital, Paducah, KY, p. A257

LEWIS, Pam, Chief Compliance Officer, William R. Sharpe, Jr. Hospital, Weston, WV, p. A676

LEWIS, Paul, Chief Executive Officer, Holy Rosary Healthcare, Miles City, MT, p. A377

LEWIS, Rayburn, M.D. Executive, Swedish Medical Center–Cherry Hill Campus, Seattle, WA, p. A666

LEWIS, Rick, Chief Information Officer, Chester Regional Medical Center, Chester, SC, p. A547

LEWIS, Robin, Chief Financial Officer, Kiowa District Hospital and Manor, Kiowa, KS, p. A236

LEWIS, Ron, M.D. Medical Director, Dubuis Hospital of Lake Charles, Lake Charles, LA, p. A271

LEWIS, Rosalind, R.N. Chief Nursing Officer, Community Health Care System, Onaga, KS, p. A240

LEWIS, Sharon
Director Information Systems, Forbes Regional Hospital, Monroeville, PA, p. A529
Chief Nursing Officer, Glenwood Regional Medical Center, West Monroe, LA, p. A279

LEWIS, Sheila, Administrator, Harmon Memorial Hospital, Hollis, OK, p. A498

LEWIS, Shirley,Chinle Comprehensive Health Care Facility, Chinle, AZ, p. A31

Index of Health Care Professionals
Index of Health Care Professionals / Lipham

LIPHAM, Mary Sue, Controller, St. Luke's The Woodlands Hospital, The Woodlands, TX, p. A631
LIPINSKI, Gary, M.D
Regional Vice President and Chief Medical Officer, Adventist Hinsdale Hospital, Hinsdale, IL, p. A184
Regional Vice President and Chief Medical Officer, Adventist La Grange Memorial Hospital, La Grange, IL, p. A186
LIPINSKI, Jim
Regional Chief Financial Officer, Franciscan St. Anthony Health – Michigan City, Michigan City, IN, p. A208
Chief Financial Officer, Franciscan St. Margaret Health – Hammond, Hammond, IN, p. A203
LIPKIND, Ethan, President and Chief Executive Officer, Deckerville Community Hospital, Deckerville, MI, p. A310
LIPMAN, Brian, M.D. Vice President Medical Affairs, Oconomowoc Memorial Hospital, Oconomowoc, WI, p. A688
LIPMAN, Henry D.
Executive Vice President and Chief Financial Officer, Franklin Regional Hospital, Franklin, NH, p. A398
Sr. VP/Financial Strategy and External Relations, Lakes Region General Hospital, Laconia, NH, p. A398
LIPNER, Zach, Vice President Human Resources, Newark Beth Israel Medical Center, Newark, NJ, p. A407
LIPPERT, Brandt, Vice President Human Resources, Adena Greenfield Medical Center, Greenfield, OH, p. A481
LIPPINCOTT, Ken, M.D. Chief of Staff, North Mississippi State Hospital, Tupelo, MS, p. A353
LIPSCOMB, Tracy, Vice President Financial Services and Chief Financial Officer, Garrett County Memorial Hospital, Oakland, MD, p. A293
LIPSKY, Janice G., R.N. System Vice President Human Resources and Organizational Development, St. Vincent's Medical Center Riverside, Jacksonville, FL, p. A127
LIPSTEIN, Steven H., President and Chief Executive Officer, BJC HealthCare, Saint Louis, MO, p. B21
LIRA, Mayra, Human Resources Specialist, Peak Behavioral Health Services, Santa Teresa, NM, p. A418
LISA, Mark P., FACHE Chief Executive Officer, Doctors Hospital of Manteca, Manteca, CA, p. A73
LISAK, Lawrence D., Superintendent, Larue D. Carter Memorial Hospital, Indianapolis, IN, p. A204
LISCHALK, Beki, Director Human Resources, Jefferson Healthcare, Port Townsend, WA, p. A664
LISELL, Susan C., Vice President of Clinical Services, LifeCare Medical Center, Roseau, MN, p. A338
LISENBY, Michael, M.D. Vice President and Chief Medical Officer, East Alabama Medical Center, Opelika, AL, p. A24
LISH, David, Director Human Resources, Sierra Vista Hospital, Sacramento, CA, p. A84
LISKE, Thomas, M.D. Chief Medical Officer, Kindred Hospital–Sycamore, Sycamore, IL, p. A195
LISONBEE, Rodney
Chief Financial Officer, American Fork Hospital, American Fork, UT, p. A637
Chief Financial Officer, Orem Community Hospital, Orem, UT, p. A639
Chief Financial Officer, Utah Valley Regional Medical Center, Provo, UT, p. A640
LISTER, Jack, Director Human Resources, Takoma Regional Hospital, Greeneville, TN, p. A566
LISTON, Denise R., R.N. Vice President Clinical and Support Services, Garrett County Memorial Hospital, Oakland, MD, p. A293
LISTON, John, Chief Financial Officer, Port Huron Hospital, Port Huron, MI, p. A321
LISZEWSKI, Richard S., Chief Executive Officer, Memorial Hospital Los Banos, Los Banos, CA, p. A73
LITAKER, Thomas, Chief Financial Officer, Skagit Valley Hospital, Mount Vernon, WA, p. A663
LITE, Myron, Director Human Resources, Fitzgibbon Hospital, Marshall, MO, p. A364
LITE, Randy, Vice President, Molokai General Hospital, Kaunakakai, HI, p. A165
LITKE, Robert, Chief Information Officer, Mille Lacs Health System, Onamia, MN, p. A336
LITOVITZ, Gary, M.D. Medical Director, Dominion Hospital, Falls Church, VA, p. A647
LITTLE, Christopher M., Vice President and Chief Financial Officer, Ellwood City Hospital, Ellwood City, PA, p. A522
LITTLE, Gary, M.D. Medical Director, George Washington University Hospital, Washington, DC, p. A116
LITTLE, James E., Chief Financial Officer, Siloam Springs Memorial Hospital, Siloam Springs, AR, p. A51
LITTLE, James P., M.D. Medical Director, HEALTHSOUTH Rehabilitation Hospital, Kingsport, TN, p. A568
LITTLE, Lou, Senior Vice President and Administrator, WellStar Windy Hill Hospital, Marietta, GA, p. A156
LITTLE, Steven N., President and Chief Executive Officer, Agnesian HealthCare, Fond Du Lac, WI, p. A681
LITTLE, Suzanne, Human Resources Specialist, Columbia Basin Hospital, Ephrata, WA, p. A661
LITTLE, Vicky, Director Human Resources, Effingham Hospital, Springfield, GA, p. A159
LITTLE, William, Chief Executive Officer, Highlands Medical Center, Sparta, TN, p. A576
LITTLEFIELD, Karen, Manager Human Resources, Waldo County General Hospital, Belfast, ME, p. A281
LITTLESON, Steven G., FACHE President, Jersey Shore University Medical Center, Neptune, NJ, p. A406
LITTLETON, Robert, Administrator, Ray County Memorial Hospital, Richmond, MO, p. A367
LITTRELL, Jeremy, Director Human Resources, Brodstone Memorial Hospital, Superior, NE, p. A390
LITTRELL, Mark, Chief Executive Officer, Lincoln Prairie Behavioral Health Center, Springfield, IL, p. A194
LITZ, Thomas H., FACHE President an Chief Executive Officer, St. Luke's Hospital – Warren Campus, Phillipsburg, NJ, p. A408
LITZENBERG, Karen, Public Information Officer, Sonoma Developmental Center, Eldridge, CA, p. A60
LIUZZA, Jed, Vice President Human Resources, Mercy Hospital Hot Springs, Hot Springs National Park, AR, p. A46
LIVELY, Carol, Chief Executive Officer, Hardeman County Memorial Hospital, Quanah, TX, p. A622
LIVELY, Corey, Chief Executive Officer, Elkview General Hospital, Hobart, OK, p. A497
LIVENGOOD, Annette, Vice President Human Resources, Garrett County Memorial Hospital, Oakland, MD, p. A293
LIVESAY, Jr., William, D.O. Medical Director, HEALTHSOUTH Rehabilitation Hospital of Charleston, Charleston, SC, p. A547
LIVIN, Lee, Chief Financial Officer, Wishard Health Services, Indianapolis, IN, p. A205
LIVINGSTON, Adrienne, Director Human Resources, Kingwood Pines Hospital, Kingwood, TX, p. A611
LIVINGSTON, Carolyn, Director Human Resources, Salt Lake Regional Medical Center, Salt Lake City, UT, p. A641
LIVINGSTON, Charles
Administrator, Dakota Plains Surgical Center, Aberdeen, SD, p. A555
Chief Executive Officer, Midwest Surgical Hospital, Omaha, NE, p. A388
LIVINGSTON, Keith
Senior Vice President and Chief Information Officer, Appleton Medical Center, Appleton, WI, p. A678
Senior Vice President and Chief Information Officer, Theda Clark Medical Center, Neenah, WI, p. A687
LIVINGSTON, Rod, Manager Information Technology, Marlette Regional Hospital, Marlette, MI, p. A318
LIVINGSTON, Sam, Information Resource Consultant, G. Werber Bryan Psychiatric Hospital, Columbia, SC, p. A548
LIVSEY, Don, Vice President and Chief Information Officer, Children's Hospital and Research Center at Oakland, Oakland, CA, p. A77
LLANO, Manuel R.
Chief Executive Officer, Atlantic Shores Hospital, Fort Lauderdale, FL, p. A123
Chief Executive Officer, Focus Healthcare of Florida, Cooper City, FL, p. A121
Chief Executive Officer, Fort Lauderdale Hospital, Fort Lauderdale, FL, p. A123
LLEWELLYN, Michael R., Chief Operating Officer, Laguna Honda Hospital and Rehabilitation Center, San Francisco, CA, p. A87
LLOYD, Carey, M.D. Chief Medical Officer, Brigham City Community Hospital, Brigham City, UT, p. A637
LLOYD, John K., President and Chief Executive Officer, Meridian Health, Neptune, NJ, p. B89
LLOYD, Richard, D.O. Chief of Staff, Harbor Beach Community Hospital, Harbor Beach, MI, p. A315
LLOYD, Russell E., Associate Director Resources, Central Texas Veterans Healthcare System, Temple, TX, p. A630
LLOYD, Susan, Chief Health Information Management and Revenue Administration, Veterans Affairs Medical Center, Augusta, GA, p. A147
LO, Wesley, Regional Chief Executive Officer, Maui Memorial Medical Center, Wailuku, HI, p. A165
LOADER, Clifford, Chief Financial Officer, Banner Desert Medical Center, Mesa, AZ, p. A34
LOAFMAN, Mark, M.D. Vice President Medical Affairs, Norwegian American Hospital, Chicago, IL, p. A177
LOBBAN, Victoria, Interim Vice President Finance, Norwood Hospital, Norwood, MA, p. A303
LOBECK, Charles C., Administrator, Shriners Hospitals for Children, Twin Cities, Minneapolis, MN, p. A335
LOCHBRUNNER, Linda, Chief Financial Officer, E. A. Conway Medical Center, Monroe, LA, p. A273
LOCKARD, Dennis, Vice President Fiscal Services and Chief Financial Officer, Wayne Hospital, Greenville, OH, p. A481
LOCKCUFF, Todd, Chief Financial Officer, Inova Alexandria Hospital, Alexandria, VA, p. A645
LOCKE, Christopher, Chief Operating Officer, Spalding Regional Medical Center, Griffin, GA, p. A153
LOCKE, Marianne, R.N. Associate Director Patient Care Services, Northern Arizona VA Health Care System, Prescott, AZ, p. A37
LOCKE, Stuart, Interim Chief Executive Officer, Southern Kentucky Rehabilitation Hospital, Bowling Green, KY, p. A248
LOCKEE, W. Brad, M.D. Chief of Staff, Alegent Health Plainview Hospital, Plainview, NE, p. A389
LOCKERD, Marie Paul, M.D. Chief Medical Officer, Sanford Jackson Medical Center, Jackson, MN, p. A333
LOCKHART, Jimmy Wayne, M.D. Medical Director, HEALTHSOUTH Treasure Coast Rehabilitation Hospital, Vero Beach, FL, p. A142
LOCKLAIR, Deborah, FACHE Administrator, McLeod Medical Center Dillon, Dillon, SC, p. A549
LOCKLEAR, Ann, Vice President, Human Resources, Scotland Health Care System, Laurinburg, NC, p. A456
LOCKWOOD, Melissa, Chief Executive Officer, Preston Memorial Hospital, Kingwood, WV, p. A673
LODGE, James S., Chief Human Resources, Veterans Affairs Ann Arbor Healthcare System, Ann Arbor, MI, p. A307
LOE, Cindy, Director of Nursing, Essentia Health Northern Pines, Aurora, MN, p. A328
LOEB, Katherine, R.N. Interim Vice President, Patient Care Services, Holy Cross Hospital, Chicago, IL, p. A176
LOEBL, John, Chief Executive Officer, Kearny County Hospital, Lakin, KS, p. A237
LOEFFELHOLZ, Tim, Account Executive Information Technology, Finley Hospital, Dubuque, IA, p. A219
LOERA, Arnold, M.D. Vice President and Medical Director, Bristol Bay Area Health Corporation, Dillingham, AK, p. A28
LOERINC, Albert, M.D. Medical Director, New Bedford Rehabilitation Hospital, New Bedford, MA, p. A302
LOEWENSTEIN, Howard, Chief Information Resource Management Services, Jesse Brown Veterans Affairs Chicago Health Care System, Chicago, IL, p. A176
LOFFING, David, Chief Operating Officer, University of Illinois Hospital & Health Sciences System, Chicago, IL, p. A179
LOFGRAN, Reid, D.O. Chief of Staff, North Canyon Medical Center, Gooding, ID, p. A168
LOFGREN, Richard P., M.D. Vice President Health Care Operations, University of Kentucky Albert B. Chandler Hospital, Lexington, KY, p. A253
LOFTON, Kevin E., FACHE President and Chief Executive Officer, Catholic Health Initiatives, Englewood, CO, p. B27
LOFTUS, John, M.D. Chief of Staff, Oakland Medical Center, Oakland, CA, p. A77
LOFTUS, Philip, Ph.D
Vice President and Chief Information Officer, Aurora Medical Center of Oshkosh, Oshkosh, WI, p. A688
Vice President and Chief Information Officer, Aurora Psychiatric Hospital, Wauwatosa, WI, p. A693
Vice President and Chief Information Officer, Aurora St. Luke's Medical Center, Milwaukee, WI, p. A686
LOFTUS, Terry, M.D. Chief Medical Officer, Banner Boswell Medical Center, Sun City, AZ, p. A39
LOGAN, Brad, Chief Financial Officer, Sycamore Shoals Hospital, Elizabethton, TN, p. A565
LOGAN, Denise, Director Human Resources, Specialty Rehabilitation Hospital, Coushatta, LA, p. A264
LOGAN, Heather, Assistant Administrator Diagnostic and Support Services, Cascade Valley Hospital and Clinics, Arlington, WA, p. A659
LOGAN, Martha, Chief Executive Officer, United Regional Medical Center, Manchester, TN, p. A570
LOGAN, Mitch, Director Finance, Northside Hospital Forsyth, Cumming, GA, p. A150
LOGAN, Renee, Chief Financial Officer, Murray County Medical Center, Slayton, MN, p. A340
LOGAN, Sarah, Manager Human Resources, Morgan Memorial Hospital, Madison, GA, p. A156
LOGAR, Michael, Assistant Superintendent, Larue D. Carter Memorial Hospital, Indianapolis, IN, p. A204
LOGIE, Eric, Director Information Systems, Alvarado Hospital, San Diego, CA, p. A85
LOGIE, William, Vice President Human Resources, The University of Toledo Medical Center, Toledo, OH, p. A489
LOGSDON, Diane, Vice President Planning and Development, Hardin Memorial Hospital, Elizabethtown, KY, p. A249
LOGSDON, Terri, Chief Financial Officer, Hickory Trail Hospital, Desoto, TX, p. A594
LOHMAN, Eric, M.D. Chief of Staff, Meadowview Regional Medical Center, Maysville, KY, p. A256
LOHMEIER, Justin, M.D. Chief of Staff, Baptist Memorial Hospital–Union County, New Albany, MS, p. A351
LOHR, Daniel E., Senior Vice President and Chief Financial Officer, The William W. Backus Hospital, Norwich, CT, p. A111

A866 Index of Health Care Professionals 

Index of Health Care Professionals / Manzanero

Index of Health Care Professionals


MALAMED, Michael, M.D. Chief of Staff, Sherman Oaks Hospital,, CA, p. A71
MALANEY, Scott C., President and Chief Executive Officer, Blanchard Valley Health System, Findlay, OH, p. B21
MALANEY, Scott C., President and Chief Executive Officer, Blanchard Valley Hospital, Findlay, OH, p. A480
MALASTO, Thomas A., Chief Executive Officer, Indiana Heart Hospital, Indianapolis, IN, p. A204
MALATEK, Jennifer, Chief Executive Officer, New Braunfels Regional Rehabilitation Hospital, New Braunfels, TX, p. A618
MALAVE ROSARIO, Javier E., Executive Director, Cardiovascular Center of Puerto Rico and the Caribbean, San Juan, PR, p. A702
MALBROUGH, Christie, Director of Nursing, Pioneer Community Hospital of Newton, Newton, MS, p. A351
MALCOLM, Nathaniel, Chief Operating Officer, Lakewood Regional Medical Center, Lakewood, CA, p. A67
MALCOLMSON, James F., M.D. Chief of Staff, Sierra Vista Hospital, Truth or Consequences, NM, p. A418
MALCOM, Leesa, Director Human Resources, Baldwin Park Medical Center, Baldwin Park, CA, p. A55
MALDONADO, Diraida, Administrator, Hospital de la Universidad de Puerto Rico/Dr. Federico Trilla, Carolina, PR, p. A700
MALDONADO, Wanda, Director Human Resources, University Hospital, San Juan, PR, p. A704
MALEK, Frank, Chief Financial Officer, Northern Louisiana Medical Center, Ruston, LA, p. A276
MALEY, Shelley, Director Human Resources, St. Luke's Hospital – Quakertown Campus, Quakertown, PA, p. A536
MALIK, Amir, M.D. Cardiologist, Plaza Medical Center of Fort Worth, Fort Worth, TX, p. A599
MALIK, Azfar, M.D. Chief Executive Officer and Chief Medical Officer, CenterPointe Hospital, Saint Charles, MO, p. A367
MALIN, Seth, M.D. President Medical and Dental Staff, Delaware County Memorial Hospital, Drexel Hill, PA, p. A522
MALINA, Joanne J., M.D. Chief of Staff, Veterans Affairs Hudson Valley Health Care System–F.D. Roosevelt Hospital, Montrose, NY, p. A430
MALISH, Richard, M.D. Deputy Commander Clinical Services, Winn Army Community Hospital, Hinesville, GA, p. A154
MALLAH, Isaac
President and Chief Executive Officer, South Florida Baptist Hospital, Plant City, FL, p. A136
President and Chief Executive Officer, St. Joseph's Hospital, Tampa, FL, p. A141
MALLERY, Edwina, Vice President Information Systems, Lafayette General Medical Center, Lafayette, LA, p. A270
MALLETT, Teresa, Director Accounting and Health Information Management, Madison Community Hospital, Madison, SD, p. A557
MALLIK, Subodh, M.D. Chief of Staff, Pecos County Memorial Hospital, Fort Stockton, TX, p. A598
MALLON, Lisa, Interim President and Chief Executive Officer, J. C. Blair Memorial Hospital, Huntingdon, PA, p. A525
MALLORY, Cheryl, M.D. Chief Medical Officer, Syringa Hospital and Clinics, Grangeville, ID, p. A168
MALLOY, Peter, Chief Information Officer, Cheshire Medical Center, Keene, NH, p. A398
MALM, Brad, Director Human Resources and Education, Lindsborg Community Hospital, Lindsborg, KS, p. A238
MALMSTROM, Ron, Information Research Specialist, Parsons State Hospital and Training Center, Parsons, KS, p. A241
MALONE, Ginger L., MSN Chief Nursing Officer, North Memorial Health Care, Robbinsdale, MN, p. A338
MALONE, John T., President and Chief Executive Officer, UPMC Hamot, Erie, PA, p. A523
MALONE, Maureen A., Chief Operating Officer, Arrowhead Regional Medical Center, Colton, CA, p. A58
MALONE, Michael, Vice President and Chief Human Resources Officer, Virginia Hospital Center – Arlington, Arlington, VA, p. A645
MALONE, Sherry, Director Human Resources, Twin Rivers Regional Medical Center, Kennett, MO, p. A363
MALONE, Thomas, M.D. President, Harper University Hospital/Hutzel Women's Hospital, Detroit, MI, p. A310
MALONEY, Jay, M.D. Chief of Staff, St. John's Lutheran Hospital, Libby, MT, p. A377
MALONEY, Patrick, Interim Chief Executive Officer, Spring Hill Regional Hospital, Spring Hill, FL, p. A139
MALONEY, Paul V., Chief Financial Officer, Natchaug Hospital, Mansfield Center, CT, p. A109
MALONEY, Richard J., M.P.H. Commissioner, Summit Park Hospital and Nursing Care Center, Pomona, NY, p. A440
MALONEY, Tom, Chief Financial Officer, Atrium Medical Center, Middletown, OH, p. A485
MALOTT, Deanna, Director Human Resources, Henry County Hospital, New Castle, IN, p. A209
MALOTT, Gregg, Chief Financial Officer, Pulaski Memorial Hospital, Winamac, IN, p. A213
MALOTTE, Rebecca, Executive Director and Chief Nursing Officer, The Heart Hospital at Deaconess Gateway, Newburgh, IN, p. A210
MALTE, Robert H., Chief Executive Officer, Evergreen Hospital Medical Center, Kirkland, WA, p. A662
MALZEWSKI, Mike, Chief Financial Officer, St. Joseph's Community Hospital of West Bend, West Bend, WI, p. A693
MAMANGAKIS, John P., Senior Vice President, Sound Shore Medical Center of Westchester, New Rochelle, NY, p. A431
MAMARY, Glenn, Chief Information Officer, Hunterdon Medical Center, Flemington, NJ, p. A404
MAMBOURG, Rolland, M.D
Vice President Medical Affairs, Saint Mary's Health Care, Grand Rapids, MI, p. A314
Vice President Physician Services, St. Joseph Mercy Hospital, Ypsilanti, MI, p. A326
MANALO, Francisco, Director of Information Services, Florida Hospital North Pinellas, Tarpon Springs, FL, p. A141
MANAS, Julie, President and Chief Executive Officer, Sacred Heart Hospital, Eau Claire, WI, p. A681
MANCHESTER, George A., M.D
Executive Vice President and Chief Medical Officer, Muncy Valley Hospital, Muncy, PA, p. A530
Executive Vice President Medical Affairs, Williamsport Regional Medical Center, Williamsport, PA, p. A542
MANCHUR, Fred M., President and Chief Executive Officer, Kettering Health Network, Dayton, OH, p. B75
MANDANAS, Renato, M.D. Vice President Medical Affairs, Oswego Hospital, Oswego, NY, p. A440
MANDEL, David, M.D. Chief of Staff, East Texas Medical Center Trinity, Trinity, TX, p. A631
MANDELL, James, M.D. President and Chief Executive Officer, Children's Hospital Boston, Boston, MA, p. A296
MANDERINO, Michelle, Chief Human Resources, Malcom Randall Veterans Affairs Medical Center, Gainesville, FL, p. A124
MANDHAN, Narain, M.D. President Medical Staff, Kirby Medical Center, Monticello, IL, p. A188
MANDI, Deepak, M.D. Chief of Staff, Veterans Affairs Medical Center, West Palm Beach, FL, p. A143
MANDRACCHIA, Vincent, DPM Chief Medical Officer, Broadlawns Medical Center, Des Moines, IA, p. A218
MANEEN, Vincent S., Chief Financial Officer, Oneida Healthcare, Oneida, NY, p. A439
MANESS, Judith A., FACHE President and Chief Executive Officer, Mount St. Mary's Hospital and Health Center, Lewiston, NY, p. A428
MANESTRINA, Robert, Vice President Human Resources, Underwood–Memorial Hospital, Woodbury, NJ, p. A412
MANFULL, Debra, Interim Chief Executive Officer, State Hospital North, Orofino, ID, p. A170
MANGAL, Ajay, M.D. Chief Executive Officer, Butler County Medical Center, Hamilton, OH, p. A481
MANGANO, Richard, Administrator and Chief Executive Officer, Malvern Institute, Malvern, PA, p. A528
MANGIN, Paul, Vice President Finance, Mercy Medical Center–Clinton, Clinton, IA, p. A216
MANGIONE, Ellen, M.D. Chief of Staff, Veterans Affairs Eastern Colorado Health Care System, Denver, CO, p. A100
MANGONA, John, Chief Information Officer and Compliance Officer, Saratoga Hospital, Saratoga Springs, NY, p. A443
MANGUM, Rozanne, Administrative Assistant and Director Human Resources, Grover C. Dils Medical Center, Caliente, NV, p. A391
MANHEIMER, Dean, Senior Vice President Human Resources, Northwestern Memorial Hospital, Chicago, IL, p. A177
MANI, C. K., M.D. Chief of Staff, Memorial Medical Center – Livingston, Livingston, TX, p. A612
MANIGOLD, David O., M.D. President Medical Staff, Ottawa Regional Hospital and Healthcare Center, Ottawa, IL, p. A190
MANIS, G. Scott, Chief Executive Officer, Doctors Hospital at White Rock Lake, Dallas, TX, p. A591
MANKER, Marcia, Chief Executive Officer, Orange Coast Memorial Medical Center, Fountain Valley, CA, p. A61
MANKINS, Mark L., M.D. Chief of Staff, Hamilton Hospital, Olney, TX, p. A619
MANKOSKI, Susan, Vice President Human Resources, St. Marys Health Center, Jefferson City, MO, p. A361
MANLAGNIT, Maybelle, Senior Accounting Officer, Metropolitan State Hospital, Norwalk, CA, p. A77
MANLEY, John, Director Information Systems, Jackson General Hospital, Ripley, WV, p. A675
MANLEY, Warren, Administrator, Dorminy Medical Center, Fitzgerald, GA, p. A152
MANN, Brian, Chief Executive Officer, Select Specialty Hospital–Danville, Danville, PA, p. A521
MANN, Joel, Administrator Information Systems, J. D. McCarty Center for Children With Developmental Disabilities, Norman, OK, p. A500
MANN, Lindsay K., Chief Executive Officer, Kaweah Delta Medical Center, Visalia, CA, p. A95
MANN, Scott, M.D. Medical Director, Dorothea Dix Hospital, Raleigh, NC, p. A459
MANN, Thomas, M.D. Chief of Staff, Dorminy Medical Center, Fitzgerald, GA, p. A152
MANN, Todd, President and Chief Executive Officer, Harlingen Medical Center, Harlingen, TX, p. A602
MANNICH, H. Andrew, Chief Operating Officer, St. Louis Psychiatric Rehabilitation Center, Saint Louis, MO, p. A370
MANNING, Andra, Manager Business Office, Baylor Medical Center at Uptown, Dallas, TX, p. A590
MANNING, Angela, Director Health Information Services, HEALTHSOUTH Sunrise Rehabilitation Hospital, Fort Lauderdale, FL, p. A123
MANNING, Bain, Director Human Resources, Leonard J. Chabert Medical Center, Houma, LA, p. A268
MANNING, Donald, M.D. Clinical Director, Georgia Regional Hospital at Savannah, Savannah, GA, p. A159
MANNING, Jay, M.D. Chief of Staff, Vidant Beaufort Hospital, Washington, NC, p. A462
MANNING, JoAnn, Chief Financial Officer, Emory Johns Creek Hospital, Johns Creek, GA, p. A154
MANNING, Kimberly, Chief Nursing Officer, Washington County Hospital, Plymouth, NC, p. A458
MANNING, Laura, Administrative Director, Corning Hospital, Corning, NY, p. A424
MANNING, Lori, Administrator Human Resources, Western State Hospital, Tacoma, WA, p. A668
MANNING, Thomas, M.D. Medical Director, Mountain View Hospital District, Madras, OR, p. A512
MANNION, Stephen, Assistant Vice President Information Systems Customer Service, Medstar Franklin Square Medical Center, Baltimore, MD, p. A288
MANNIX, Mary N., FACHE President and Chief Executive Officer, Augusta Health, Fishersville, VA, p. A648
MANNS, Bill, Chief Operating Officer, Alameda County Medical Center, Oakland, CA, p. A77
MANOCHA, Lovelesh, M.D. Chief Medical Officer, Acuity Hospital of South Texas, San Antonio, TX, p. A624
MANOHARA, Anand, Associate Administrator, Good Samaritan Hospital, Bakersfield, CA, p. A54
MANOR, Lisa, Chief Clinical Officer, Kindred Hospital–Nashville, Nashville, TN, p. A573
MANSFIELD, Al, Chief Financial Officer, Saint Vincent Health Center, Erie, PA, p. A523
MANSFIELD, David, M.D. Chief of Staff, El Paso Specialty Hospital, El Paso, TX, p. A596
MANSFIELD, Deena, Director Human Resources, Ashley Regional Medical Center, Vernal, UT, p. A642
MANSFIELD, Jean, Director Human Resources, McLean Hospital, Belmont, MA, p. A295
MANSFIELD, Jodi J., Interim President and Chief Executive Officer, University of Arizona Medical Center – University Campus, Tucson, AZ, p. A40
MANSFIELD, Kevin, Director Human Resources, Davis Hospital and Medical Center, Layton, UT, p. A638
MANSFIELD, Robert, Chief Executive Officer, Red River Hospital, Wichita Falls, TX, p. A635
MANSFIELD, Stephen L., FACHE President and Chief Executive Officer, Methodist Health System, Dallas, TX, p. B89
MANSIUS, Marian Rose, Assistant General Minister, Sisters of Saint Francis, Syracuse, NY, p. B119
MANSKE, Lou Ann, Director Human Resources, Madonna Rehabilitation Hospital, Lincoln, NE, p. A385
MANSON, David, Manager Human Resources, Santa Clara Valley Medical Center, San Jose, CA, p. A88
MANSON, III, William T., President, AnMed Health Medical Center, Anderson, SC, p. A546
MANSOOR, Ureej, M.D. Chief of Staff, Southeast Health Center of Ripley County, Doniphan, MO, p. A358
MANSUE, Amy B., President and Chief Executive Officer, Children's Specialized Hospital, New Brunswick, NJ, p. A406
MANSURE, John F., FACHE President, Greer Memorial Hospital, Greer, SC, p. A551
MANTE, Laurie, Administrator and Vice President, Eddy Cohoes Rehabilitation Center, Cohoes, NY, p. A424
MANTELL, Amy, Vice President Human Resources, Mercy Hospital of Folsom, Folsom, CA, p. A60
MANTERNACH, Paul, M.D. Senior Vice President Physician Integration, Mercy Medical Center–North Iowa, Mason City, IA, p. A223
MANTOOTH, Chuck, President, Watauga Medical Center, Boone, NC, p. A449
MANUEL, Shasta, Executive Director Finance, St. Anthony Hospital, Oklahoma City, OK, p. A502
MANUS, Kim, Chief Financial Officer, Newport Hospital and Health Services, Newport, WA, p. A663
MANZ, Louis, Director Information and Communication Services, Chatham Hospital, Siler City, NC, p. A460
MANZANERO, Bienvenido, M.D. Medical Director, Hampstead Hospital, Hampstead, NH, p. A398

Index of Health Care Professionals

Index of Health Care Professionals / Manzella


MANZELLA, Arlene, Administrator, Norfolk Psychiatric Center, Norfolk, VA, p. A652
MANZER, Andrew R., President and Chief Executive Officer, Schuyler Hospital, Montour Falls, NY, p. A430
MANZO, Arnie, Vice President Human Resources, Saint Barnabas Medical Center, Livingston, NJ, p. A405
MANZOOR, Amir, M.D. Medical Director, Select Specialty Hospital–Panama City, Panama City, FL, p. A135
MAO, Chi C., M.D. Medical Director, Select Specialty Hospital–Houston, Houston, TX, p. A606
MAPES, Kevin
Regional Information Technology Director, Providence Medical Center, Kansas City, KS, p. A236
Regional Information Technology Director, Saint John Hospital, Leavenworth, KS, p. A237
Director Kansas Division System and Technology Service Center, St. Francis Health Center, Topeka, KS, p. A244
MAPLES, Rickie, Interim Chief Financial Officer, Southeast Health Center of Ripley County, Doniphan, MO, p. A358
MAPPIN, F Gregory, M.D. Vice President Medical Affairs, Self Regional Healthcare, Greenwood, SC, p. A551
MARANO, Angeline M., Chief Operating Officer, Memorial Regional Hospital,, FL, p. A125
MARAS, Greg, Vice President Human Resources, Meadville Medical Center, Meadville, PA, p. A528
MARCANO, Norma, Chief Operating Officer, San Juan City Hospital, San Juan, PR, p. A703
MARCANTANO, Mark, Executive Vice President and Chief Operating Officer, Women & Infants Hospital of Rhode Island, Providence, RI, p. A545
MARCANTEL, Bill, Chief Information Systems, Allen Parish Hospital, Kinder, LA, p. A269
MARCELLAIS, Duane, Information Technology Specialist, Public Health Service Indian Hospital – Quentin N. Burdick Memorial Health Facility, Belcourt, ND, p. A464
MARCELLINO, David, Executive Vice President and Chief Financial Officer, Botsford Hospital, Farmington Hills, MI, p. A312
MARCH, Riley, Manager Information Technology, Southeast Health Center of Ripley County, Doniphan, MO, p. A358
MARCHAND, Gary G., President and Chief Executive Officer, Memorial Hospital at Gulfport, Gulfport, MS, p. A346
MARCHANT, Joseph, Administrator, Bibb Medical Center, Centreville, AL, p. A18
MARCHETTI, Mark E., President and Chief Executive Officer, Ashland Community Hospital, Ashland, OR, p. A509
MARCHLEWSKI, Anthony, M.D. President Medical and Psychological Staff, Bellin Psychiatric Center, Green Bay, WI, p. A682
MARCOGLIESE, John, Vice President Financial Operations, Rye Hospital Center, Rye, NY, p. A442
MARCOVICI, Mia, M.D. Chief Medical Officer, Norristown State Hospital, Norristown, PA, p. A530
MARCRUM, Jennifer, Chief Financial Officer, Sumner County Hospital District One, Caldwell, KS, p. A231
MARCUM, Derrick, Director Information Systems, Missouri Baptist Medical Center, Saint Louis, MO, p. A369
MARCUS, Donald H., M.D. Medical Director, Los Angeles Medical Center, Los Angeles, CA, p. A70
MARCUS, Stuart, M.D. Senior Vice President and Chief Medical Officer, St. Vincent's Medical Center, Bridgeport, CT, p. A108
MARCZAK, Stanley, Chief Financial Officer, Mayo Clinic Health System in Mankato, Mankato, MN, p. A334
MARCZEWSKI, Les, M.D. Chief Medical Officer, Loring Hospital, Sac City, IA, p. A226
MARDEN–RESNIK, Hilary, Vice President Human Resources, Hennepin County Medical Center, Minneapolis, MN, p. A335
MARDINI, George, M.D. Chief of Staff, Battle Mountain General Hospital, Battle Mountain, NV, p. A391
MAREK, Kyle, Manager Information Services, Carteret General Hospital, Morehead City, NC, p. A457
MAREK, Rick, Vice President Medical Information Systems, Warm Springs Rehabilitation Hospital, San Antonio, TX, p. A626
MARGENAU, Randall, Chief Information Officer, William S. Middleton Memorial Veterans Hospital, Madison, WI, p. A684
MARGETTS, Marty, Senior Vice President Human Resources, Physicians Regional Medical Center, Knoxville, TN, p. A568
MARGO, John G., Vice President Human Resources, Oneida Healthcare, Oneida, NY, p. A439
MARGOLIS, Marilyn, Chief Nursing Officer, Emory Johns Creek Hospital, Johns Creek, GA, p. A154
MARGOLIS, Ron, Chief Information Officer, University of New Mexico Hospitals, Albuquerque, NM, p. A415
MARGOLSKEE, Howard, M.D. Chief of Staff, Sebasticook Valley Health, Pittsfield, ME, p. A284
MARGOT, Skip, Vice President Patient Care Services and Chief Nurse Executive, Shady Grove Adventist Hospital, Rockville, MD, p. A294
MARGUGLIO, Paul, M.D. Chief of Staff, Healdsburg District Hospital, Healdsburg, CA, p. A64
MARGULIS, Richard T., Executive Vice President and Chief Operating Officer, Brookhaven Memorial Hospital Medical Center, Patchogue, NY, p. A440
MARIETTA, John, M.D
Chief Medical Officer, St. David's Medical Center, Austin, TX, p. A581
Chief Medical Officer, St. David's Rehabilitation Center, Austin, TX, p. A581
MARIETTA, Megan, Chief Operating Officer, Kingwood Medical Center, Kingwood, TX, p. A611
MARIETTA, Richard, M.D. Medical Director, Clear Lake Regional Medical Center, Webster, TX, p. A634
MARINELLI, Samuel, Vice President Finance and Chief Financial Officer, Chester River Health System, Chestertown, MD, p. A290
MARINELLI, Steve, Chief Financial Officer, Northwest Mississippi Regional Medical Center, Clarksdale, MS, p. A344
MARINELLO, Anthony, Chief Executive Officer, Mountain Vista Medical Center, Mesa, AZ, p. A34
MARINI, Frank, Vice President and Chief Information Officer, TMC Healthcare, Tucson, AZ, p. A40
MARINO, A. Michael, M.D. Senior Vice President Medical Administration, Greenwich Hospital, Greenwich, CT, p. A109
MARINO, Marchita H., Vice President Human Resources, Wuesthoff Medical Center – Rockledge, Rockledge, FL, p. A137
MARINOFF, Peter, Director Operations, Paul Oliver Memorial Hospital, Frankfort, MI, p. A312
MARION, Ben, Chief Executive Officer and Managing Director, Turning Point Hospital, Moultrie, GA, p. A157
MARION, Sue, Manager Business Office, Knox County Hospital, Knox City, TX, p. A611
MARIOTTI, Denise, Chief Human Resources Officer, Pennsylvania Hospital, Philadelphia, PA, p. A533
MARK, Curtis, M.D. Chief Medical Officer, Pioneer Memorial Hospital and Health Services, Viborg, SD, p. A560
MARK, Joseph M.
Chief Executive Officer, Redwood Memorial Hospital, Fortuna, CA, p. A61
President and Chief Executive Officer, St. Joseph Hospital, Eureka, CA, p. A60
MARKANT, David, Director Information Systems, Clifton Springs Hospital and Clinic, Clifton Springs, NY, p. A424
MARKEL, Michael J., MSN Executive Director of Operations, St. Joseph Mercy Livingston Hospital, Howell, MI, p. A315
MARKER, Sheri L., Vice President Human Resources, Rush University Medical Center, Chicago, IL, p. A178
MARKETTI, Dean M., Chief Information Officer, Morris Hospital & Healthcare Centers, Morris, IL, p. A188
MARKGRAF, Janelle, Director Human Resources, Langlade Memorial Hospital, Antigo, WI, p. A678
MARKHAM, Barbara, Chief Financial Officer, Glendive Medical Center, Glendive, MT, p. A375
MARKHAM, Marlin, Chief Financial Officer, Wilkes Regional Medical Center, North Wilkesboro, NC, p. A458
MARKHAM, Patricia A., Administrator and Chief Executive Officer, Cass County Memorial Hospital, Atlantic, IA, p. A214
MARKOS, Dennis R., Chief Executive Officer, Ed Fraser Memorial Hospital and Baker Community Health Center, MacClenny, FL, p. A129
MARKOVICH, Stephen, M.D. President, Riverside Methodist Hospital, Columbus, OH, p. A477
MARKOWITZ, Bruce J., President and Chief Executive Officer, Palisades Medical Center, North Bergen, NJ, p. A407
MARKOWITZ, Stuart, M.D. Chief Medical Officer, Hartford Hospital, Hartford, CT, p. A109
MARKOWSKI, Stan, Chief Financial Officer, Palmetto Lowcountry Behavioral Health, Charleston, SC, p. A547
MARKS, Craig J., FACHE President, Mark Twain St. Joseph's Hospital, San Andreas, CA, p. A84
MARKS, Jerry, Chief Financial Officer, St. Vincent Frankfort Hospital, Frankfort, IN, p. A202
MARKS, Michael, M.D. Chief of Staff, Norwalk Hospital, Norwalk, CT, p. A111
MARKS, Stanley, M.D
Chief Medical Officer, Memorial Hospital Miramar, Miramar, FL, p. A132
Chief Medical Officer, Memorial Hospital Pembroke, Pembroke Pines, FL, p. A135
Chief Medical Officer, Memorial Regional Hospital,, FL, p. A125
MARKSTROM, Susan, M.D. Chief of Staff, St. Cloud Veterans Affairs Health Care System, Saint Cloud, MN, p. A338
MARKWITH, Candace L., Chief Executive Officer, Sierra Vista Regional Medical Center, San Luis Obispo, CA, p. A88
MARLER, Ruth, Chief Operating Officer/Chief Nursing Officer, Johnston Health, Smithfield, NC, p. A461
MARLEY, Charles, D.O. Vice President Medical Affairs, Gettysburg Hospital, Gettysburg, PA, p. A524
MARLEY, Kim, M.D. Chief Medical Officer, Windber Medical Center, Windber, PA, p. A542
MARLEY, Lee
VP/Information Services Chief Application Officer, Presbyterian Hospital, Albuquerque, NM, p. A414
VP/Information Services Chief Application Officer, Presbyterian Kaseman Hospital, Albuquerque, NM, p. A414
MARLEY, Mark E., FACHE Chief Executive Officer, Natchitoches Regional Medical Center, Natchitoches, LA, p. A274
MARLEY, Michael, Chief Information Officer, Veterans Affairs Medical Center, Leeds, MA, p. A301
MARLGE, Charles G., M.D. Chief of Staff, Marias Medical Center, Shelby, MT, p. A379
MARLOW, Billy, Administrator/CEO, North Sunflower Medical Center, Ruleville, MS, p. A352
MARLOW, Gary, M.D. President Medical Staff, Texas Health Presbyterian Hospital–WNJ, Sherman, TX, p. A628
MARMANDE, Susanne, Administrator, Infirmary Long Term Acute Care Hospital, Mobile, AL, p. A22
MARNELL, George, Director, Veterans Affairs Medical Center, Albuquerque, NM, p. A415
MARNEY, Terri A., R.N. Director of Nursing, Plains Regional Medical Center, Clovis, NM, p. A415
MAROC, Genice, FACHE Administrator and Chief Executive Officer, Cox Monett, Monett, MO, p. A365
MARON, Michael, President and Chief Executive Officer, Holy Name Medical Center, Teaneck, NJ, p. A410
MAROSTICA, L. Anthony, Director Human Resources, Spanish Peaks Regional Health Center, Walsenburg, CO, p. A106
MAROTTA, Diane, Vice President Human Resources, John T. Mather Memorial Hospital, Port Jefferson, NY, p. A440
MAROUN, Christiane, M.D. Chief of Staff, Childrens Care Hospital and School, Sioux Falls, SD, p. A559
MARPLE, Anthony, Vice President of Strategy, Mercy Hospital of Portland, Portland, ME, p. A284
MARQUARDT, Robert C., FACHE President and Chief Executive Officer, Fairmont General Hospital, Fairmont, WV, p. A671
MARQUES, John, Vice President Human Resources, University of Arizona Medical Center – University Campus, Tucson, AZ, p. A40
MARQUES, Tony, Director Information Systems, Grace Cottage Hospital, Townshend, VT, p. A644
MARR, Debbie, Administrative Assistant and Director Human Resources, Fredonia Regional Hospital, Fredonia, KS, p. A233
MARRA, Mary Anne, R.N. Vice President/Chief Nursing Officer, East Orange General Hospital, East Orange, NJ, p. A403
MARREEL, Richard, Chief Information Officer, BryanLGH Medical Center, Lincoln, NE, p. A385
MARRERO, Jose, Director Finance, San Jorge Children's Hospital, San Juan, PR, p. A703
MARRERO, Norma, Executive Administrator, Doctors' Center Hospital San Juan, San Juan, PR, p. A703
MARRONI, Denise, Chief Financial Officer, Providence Centralia Hospital, Centralia, WA, p. A660
MARS, Martha, R.N. Director of Nursing, St. John Broken Arrow, Broken Arrow, OK, p. A494
MARSALIS, Joyce, Manager Human Resources, Roane Medical Center, Harriman, TN, p. A566
MARSCH, Jean, Director Human Resources, St. Vincent Hospital, Green Bay, WI, p. A682
MARSEE, DeWayne, Director Information Systems, Joint Township District Memorial Hospital, Saint Marys, OH, p. A488
MARSH, Amy, Chief Financial Officer, Integris Baptist Regional Health Center, Miami, OK, p. A499
MARSH, Daniel L., Director, West Texas VA Health Care System, Big Spring, TX, p. A584
MARSH, Leslie, Chief Executive Officer, Lexington Regional Health Center, Lexington, NE, p. A385
MARSH, Linda, Vice President Financial Services and Chief Financial Officer, Alhambra Hospital Medical Center, Alhambra, CA, p. A53
MARSH, Mark A., Chief Executive Officer, Greenview Regional Hospital, Bowling Green, KY, p. A248
MARSH, Jr., Murray S., Chief Financial Officer, Warren General Hospital, Warren, PA, p. A540
MARSH, Paul, Director Information Systems, Parkridge Medical Center, Chattanooga, TN, p. A563
MARSHALL, Deborah K., Vice President Public Relations, Good Samaritan Hospital, Suffern, NY, p. A444
MARSHALL, Debra, Director Human Resources, Bradley County Medical Center, Warren, AR, p. A52
MARSHALL, Glen, Chief Executive Officer, Kennewick General Hospital, Kennewick, WA, p. A662
MARSHALL, James L., Chief Executive Officer, Mercy Hospital, Devils Lake, ND, p. A465
MARSHALL, Jerry, Director Information Systems, United Regional Health Care System, Wichita Falls, TX, p. A635


A872 Index of Health Care Professionals 

Index of Health Care Professionals / Martucci


MARSHALL, John A., Chief Executive Officer, Horizon Medical Center, Dickson, TN, p. A565
MARSHALL, Ken, M.D. Chief Medical Officer, Indiana University Health Bloomington Hospital, Bloomington, IN, p. A198
MARSHALL, Kenneth P., Senior Vice President and Chief Operating Officer, University of Louisville Hospital, Louisville, KY, p. A255
MARSHALL, Michael, Vice President Finance and Chief Financial Officer, Anderson Hospital, Maryville, IL, p. A187
MARSHALL, Michael D., Administrator and Chief Executive Officer, Bryan W. Whitfield Memorial Hospital, Demopolis, AL, p. A19
MARSHALL, Robert, Vice President and Chief Operating Officer, University of Texas Health Science Center at Tyler, Tyler, TX, p. A632
MARSHALL, Robert E., Chief Executive Officer, Montevista Hospital, Las Vegas, NV, p. A393
MARSHALL, Sherrie, Health Information Management Services Director, The Rehabilitation Institute of St. Louis, Saint Louis, MO, p. A370
MARSILIO, Lisa, Vice President and Administrator, Good Shepherd Specialty Hospital, Bethlehem, PA, p. A518
MARSO, Paul, Vice President Human Resources, St. Mary's Healthcare Center, Pierre, SD, p. A558
MARSTELLER, Brent A., President and Chief Executive Officer, Cabell Huntington Hospital, Huntington, WV, p. A672
MARTANIUK, Jean, Director Personnel, Mt. Ascutney Hospital and Health Center, Windsor, VT, p. A644
MARTEL, Ron, Director for Administration, Naval Hospital, Pensacola, FL, p. A136
MARTENS, Angela, Controller, Cumberland Memorial Hospital, Cumberland, WI, p. A680
MARTENS, Troy, Chief Operating Officer, Trinity Regional Medical Center, Fort Dodge, IA, p. A219
MARTI, Maria L., Director Fiscal Services, Auxilio Mutuo Hospital, San Juan, PR, p. A702
MARTIN, Amy, Director Human Resources, Mary Black Memorial Hospital, Spartanburg, SC, p. A553
MARTIN, Antonio D., Senior Vice President and Executive Director, Kings County Hospital Center,, NY, p. A433
MARTIN, Barbara J., R.N
  President and Chief Executive Officer, Vista Medical Center East, Waukegan, IL, p. A196
  President and Chief Executive Officer, Vista Medical Center West, Waukegan, IL, p. A196
MARTIN, Billy, Human Resource Analyst, Blue Mountain Recovery Center, Pendleton, OR, p. A513
MARTIN, Brent, Chief Executive Officer, LifeCare Specialty Hospital of North Louisiana, Ruston, LA, p. A276
MARTIN, Bruce A., Vice President Human Resources, CarolinaEast Medical Center, New Bern, NC, p. A458
MARTIN, C. Gregory, M.D. Chief Medical Officer, Emerson Hospital, Concord, MA, p. A299
MARTIN, Carl, President and Chief Executive Officer, Morehead Memorial Hospital, Eden, NC, p. A452
MARTIN, Carmen, Associate Administrator, Auxilio Mutuo Hospital, San Juan, PR, p. A702
MARTIN, Cary, Chief Executive Officer, Houston Healthcare System, Warner Robins, GA, p. B69
MARTIN, Cary, Chief Executive Officer, Houston Medical Center, Warner Robins, GA, p. A161
MARTIN, Cathy, Administrator, Sterlington Rehabilitation Hospital, Sterlington, LA, p. A278
MARTIN Jr.,, Charles N., Chairman and Chief Executive Officer, Vanguard Health System, Nashville, TN, p. B141
MARTIN, Cherie, FACHE Chief Executive Officer, Banner Behavioral Health Hospital – Scottsdale, Scottsdale, AZ, p. A38
MARTIN, Cheryl
  Manager Human Resources, Columbia Memorial Hospital, Astoria, OR, p. A509
  Chief Information Officer, Tuomey Healthcare System, Sumter, SC, p. A554
MARTIN, Christine M.
  Chief Financial Officer, Crawley Memorial Hospital, Boiling Springs, NC, p. A449
  Chief Financial Officer, St. Luke's Hospital, Columbus, NC, p. A451
MARTIN, Clifford G., M.D. President Medical Staff, St. Nicholas Hospital, Sheboygan, WI, p. A690
MARTIN, Connie
  Administrator, Physicians Medical Center, Houma, LA, p. A268
  Director Human Resources, Trinity Hospital of Augusta, Augusta, GA, p. A147
MARTIN, Corey, M.D. Director Medical Affairs, Buffalo Hospital, Buffalo, MN, p. A329
MARTIN, David, Supervisor Human Resources, Sequoyah Memorial Hospital, Sallisaw, OK, p. A504
MARTIN, David, M.D. Vice President Medical Staff Affairs, St. David's Round Rock Medical Center, Round Rock, TX, p. A623
MARTIN, David, Chief Operating Officer, Valley Hospital and Medical Center, Spokane Valley, WA, p. A667
MARTIN, David T., President, UPMC Passavant, Pittsburgh, PA, p. A535
MARTIN, Dean, M.D. Medical Director, Shadow Mountain Behavioral Health System, Tulsa, OK, p. A506
MARTIN, Deanna, MSN, Chief Executive Officer, HEALTHSOUTH Desert Canyon Rehabilitation Hospital, Las Vegas, NV, p. A392
MARTIN, Deborah, Assistant Administrator, Skagit Valley Hospital, Mount Vernon, WA, p. A663
MARTIN, Debra, Director of Nursing, Hamilton General Hospital, Hamilton, TX, p. A602
MARTIN, Donna, R.N. Chief Nursing Officer, Ochsner Baptist Medical Center, New Orleans, LA, p. A274
MARTIN, Elizabeth J., Vice President and Administrator, Riverside Tappahannock Hospital, Tappahannock, VA, p. A656
MARTIN, Emily Howard, Administrator, Commonwealth Regional Specialty Hospital, Bowling Green, KY, p. A247
MARTIN, Eva, M.D. Chief of Staff, Carl Vinson Veterans Affairs Medical Center, Dublin, GA, p. A152
MARTIN, Garry, Chief Fiscal, Veterans Affairs North Texas Health Care System, Dallas, TX, p. A593
MARTIN, Greg, President, Integris Grove General Hospital, Grove, OK, p. A497
MARTIN, Gregg
  Manager Management Information Systems, Arnot Ogden Medical Center, Elmira, NY, p. A425
  Chief Information Officer, St. Joseph's Hospital, Elmira, NY, p. A426
  Senior Vice President and Chief Operating Officer, Tuomey Healthcare System, Sumter, SC, p. A554
MARTIN, Harvey C., M.D. Medical Director, Red River Hospital, Wichita Falls, TX, p. A635
MARTIN, Holly, Human Resources Leader, Iowa Specialty Hospital–Clarion, Clarion, IA, p. A216
MARTIN, Jack, Director Human Resources, Texas Institute for Surgery at Texas Health Presbyterian Dallas, Dallas, TX, p. A592
MARTIN, James C., M.D
  Vice President and Chief Medical Officer, CHRISTUS Santa Rosa Health Care, San Antonio, TX, p. A624
  Vice President and Chief Medical Officer, CHRISTUS Santa Rosa Hospital – New Braunfels, New Braunfels, TX, p. A618
MARTIN, James D.
  Chief Financial Officer, Hawthorn Children Psychiatric Hospital, Saint Louis, MO, p. A368
  Chief Financial Officer, Metropolitan St. Louis Psychiatric Center, Saint Louis, MO, p. A369
  Chief Financial Officer, St. Louis Psychiatric Rehabilitation Center, Saint Louis, MO, p. A370
MARTIN, James W., D.D.S. Chief of Staff, Baptist Memorial Hospital–Tipton, Covington, TN, p. A564
MARTIN, Jeanene R., M.P.H
  Senior Vice President Human Resources, WakeMed Cary Hospital, Cary, NC, p. A450
  Senior Vice President Human Resources, WakeMed Raleigh Campus, Raleigh, NC, p. A459
MARTIN, Jeffrey H., M.D. Chief of Staff, Murphy Medical Center, Murphy, NC, p. A458
MARTIN, Jeffrey L., President, Ministry Saint Michael's Hospital, Stevens Point, WI, p. A691
MARTIN, Kelly, Chief Financial Officer, Fairchild Medical Center, Yreka, CA, p. A96
MARTIN, Kenneth A., M.D. Chief of Staff, Arkansas Surgical Hospital, North Little Rock, AR, p. A49
MARTIN, Kevin, M.P.H. Administrator, Shriners Hospitals for Children–Intermountain, Salt Lake City, UT, p. A641
MARTIN, Leslie, Associate Administrator, McKee Medical Center, Loveland, CO, p. A104
MARTIN, Macky, Director Human Resources, Fairview Regional Medical Center, Fairview, OK, p. A496
MARTIN, Patrick, Director Information Systems, Calvary Hospital,, NY, p. A432
MARTIN, Patrick, M.D. Medical Director, Wilmington Treatment Center, Wilmington, NC, p. A462
MARTIN, Patrick J., President and Chief Executive Officer, Fisher–Titus Medical Center, Norwalk, OH, p. A486
MARTIN, Paul J., Director Human Resources, Los Angeles Medical Center, Los Angeles, CA, p. A70
MARTIN, Ric, Information Specialist, Madison State Hospital, Madison, IN, p. A208
MARTIN, Richard A., MS
  Chief Nursing Officer, Hoag Hospital Irvine, Irvine, CA, p. A65
  Senior Vice President and Chief Nursing Officer, Hoag Memorial Hospital Presbyterian, Newport Beach, CA, p. A76
MARTIN, Rick, Vice President of Ancillary and Support Services, St. Charles Medical Center – Bend, Bend, OR, p. A509
MARTIN, Rozanne, Assistant Administrator Human Resources, Highline Medical Center, Burien, WA, p. A660
MARTIN, Sharon E., M.D. President Medical Staff, Fulton County Medical Center, Mc Connellsburg, PA, p. A528
MARTIN, Steve
  Chief Information Officer, CHRISTUS Santa Rosa Health Care, San Antonio, TX, p. A624
  Chief Information Officer, CHRISTUS Santa Rosa Hospital – New Braunfels, New Braunfels, TX, p. A618
MARTIN, Susan, Vice President Finance, Middlesex Hospital, Middletown, CT, p. A110
MARTIN, Thomas J., Chief Executive Officer, Lincoln Hospital, Davenport, WA, p. A660
MARTIN, Tom, Vice President and Chief Information Officer, Evergreen Hospital Medical Center, Kirkland, WA, p. A662
MARTIN, Val, Director Financial Management Services Center, Veterans Affairs Salt Lake City Health Care System, Salt Lake City, UT, p. A641
MARTIN, Valene J., Administrative Director Human Resources, Community Hospital of Long Beach, Long Beach, CA, p. A68
MARTIN–FORMAN, Marty Ann, Chief Operating Officer, Fulton State Hospital, Fulton, MO, p. A360
MARTIN–PRATT, Diane, Director Information Systems, Niagara Falls Memorial Medical Center, Niagara Falls, NY, p. A438
MARTINCHICK, Jim, M.D. Chief of Staff, Ivinson Memorial Hospital, Laramie, WY, p. A696
MARTINEZ, Albino
  Director Budget and Finance, Miners' Colfax Medical Center, Raton, NM, p. A417
  Director Finance and Budget, New Mexico Behavioral Health Institute at Las Vegas, Las Vegas, NM, p. A417
MARTINEZ, Beverly, Director of Nursing, Rio Grande Hospital, Del Norte, CO, p. A99
MARTINEZ, Carlos J., Director Resource Management, Naval Medical Center, Portsmouth, VA, p. A654
MARTINEZ, Edward, Chief Information Officer, Miami Children's Hospital, Miami, FL, p. A131
MARTINEZ, Fernando, Vice President and Chief Information Officer, Jackson Health System, Miami, FL, p. A131
MARTINEZ, Frank, Vice President Human Resources, West Jefferson Medical Center, Marrero, LA, p. A272
MARTINEZ Jr., Fred, Chief Executive Officer, St. Charles Parish Hospital, Luling, LA, p. A272
MARTINEZ, Jose, M.D. Chief of Staff, Trinity Hospital Twin City, Dennison, OH, p. A479
MARTINEZ, Josue, Coordinator Information Systems, University Hospital, San Juan, PR, p. A704
MARTINEZ, Kristen, Coordinator Human Resources, Kindred Hospital–La Mirada, La Mirada, CA, p. A66
MARTINEZ, Marcos, Chief Business Operations, Winn Army Community Hospital, Hinesville, GA, p. A154
MARTINEZ, Michelle, Interim Chief Executive Officer, U. S. Public Health Service Indian Hospital–Whiteriver, Whiteriver, AZ, p. A40
MARTINEZ, Regina M., Director Human Resources, La Paz Regional Hospital, Parker, AZ, p. A34
MARTINEZ, Steve, Executive Director and Administrator, New Mexico Behavioral Health Institute at Las Vegas, Las Vegas, NM, p. A417
MARTINEZ, Virginia, Manager Human Resources, Copper Queen Community Hospital, Bisbee, AZ, p. A31
MARTING, Bill, Senior Vice President and Chief Financial Officer, The University of Kansas Hospital, Kansas City, KS, p. A236
MARTINO, Anthony
  Chief Executive Officer, Select Specialty Hospital–Laurel Highlands, Latrobe, PA, p. A527
  Interim Chief Executive Officer, Select Specialty Hospital–Pittsburgh/UPMC, Pittsburgh, PA, p. A535
MARTINO, Michael, M.D. Chief of Staff, Arkansas Valley Regional Medical Center, La Junta, CO, p. A103
MARTINSON, Erling, M.D. Medical Director, Nelson County Health System, McVille, ND, p. A467
MARTINSON, Tiffany, Director Human Resources, Norton Sound Regional Hospital, Nome, AK, p. A29
MARTIRANO, Michael, M.D. President Medical Staff, Elmhurst Memorial Hospital,, IL, p. A181
MARTOCCIO, Debi, R.N. Chief Operating Officer, Florida Hospital at Connerton Long Term Acute Care, Land O'Lakes, FL, p. A128
MARTS, Teresa, M.D. Chief Medical Staff, Community Memorial Hospital, Burke, SD, p. A555
MARTUCCI, Kathleen, Director Human Resources, Helen Hayes Hospital, West Haverstraw, NY, p. A446


Index of Health Care Professionals

Index of Health Care Professionals

Index of Health Care Professionals / Marver


MARVER, Stacy, Director Information Technology, Saint Clare's Hospital, Weston, WI, p. A693
MARX, Edward, Vice President and Chief Information Officer, Texas Health Harris Methodist Hospital Azle, Azle, TX, p. A582
MARX, Tomasine
Chief Financial Officer, St. John Hospital and Medical Center, Detroit, MI, p. A311
Chief Financial Officer, St. John Macomb–Oakland Hospital, Macomb Center, Warren, MI, p. A325
Chief Financial Officer, St. John Macomb–Oakland Hospital, Oakland Center, Madison Heights, MI, p. A318
Chief Financial Officer, St. John River District Hospital, East China, MI, p. A311
MARX, Troy, Director Human Resources, Upland Hills Health, Dodgeville, WI, p. A680
MARX, William, M.D. Chief of Staff, Veterans Affairs Medical Center, Syracuse, NY, p. A444
MARXEN, Leah, Administrator and Chief Executive Officer, Stewart Memorial Community Hospital, Lake City, IA, p. A222
MARZINZIK, John A., Vice President Finance, Frisbie Memorial Hospital, Rochester, NH, p. A400
MASCHER, Troy, Director Information Systems, Via Christi Hospital, Pittsburg, KS, p. A241
MASCIARELLI, Filippo, M.D. Chief of Staff, Denton Regional Medical Center, Denton, TX, p. A593
MASH, Bob, Chief Executive Officer, Red Rock Behavioral Hospital, Las Vegas, NV, p. A393
MASHAK–EKERN, Jane, Fiscal Officer, Veterans Affairs Medical Center, Tomah, WI, p. A692
MASHINSKI, John
Senior Vice President Human Resources, Bon Secours–DePaul Medical Center, Norfolk, VA, p. A652
Vice President Human Resources, Mary Immaculate Hospital, Newport News, VA, p. A652
MASI, George V., Chief Operating Officer, Harris County Hospital District, Houston, TX, p. A604
MASKELL, Denise, Chief Information Officer, Springfield Hospital Center, Sykesville, MD, p. A294
MASKUS, Jane, Vice President and Chief Information Officer, Lawrence Memorial Hospital, Lawrence, KS, p. A237
MASLYN, Jay T., Chief Financial Officer, Nicholas H. Noyes Memorial Hospital, Dansville, NY, p. A425
MASON, Bill A., Chief Executive Officer, Meadow Wood Behavioral Health System, New Castle, DE, p. A114
MASON, Cheryl S., Chief Financial Officer, Regional Medical Center, Orangeburg, SC, p. A553
MASON, Jane G., Chief Clinical Officer, Kindred Hospital of Northern Indiana, Mishawaka, IN, p. A208
MASON, Kathy, Chief Operating Officer, Atrium Medical Center of Corinth, Corinth, TX, p. A588
MASON, Keith, Chief Executive Officer, Bailey Medical Center, Owasso, OK, p. A502
MASON, Ray, Interim Chief Executive Officer, Liberty Dayton Regional Medical Center, Liberty, TX, p. A612
MASON, Reginald, M.D. President Medical Staff, Riverside Tappahannock Hospital, Tappahannock, VA, p. A656
MASON, Sally, Director Human Resources, Golden Plains Community Hospital, Borger, TX, p. A584
MASON, Sam, Director Management Information Systems, Northwest Texas Healthcare System, Amarillo, TX, p. A578
MASON, Sandra, Director Nursing Services and Senior Nurse Executive, Naval Hospital, Twentynine Palms, CA, p. A93
MASON, Steve, Assistant Superintendent and Chief Operating Officer, Clifton T. Perkins Hospital Center, Jessup, MD, p. A292
MASON, William R., Chief Operating Officer, Brooke Glen Behavioral Hospital, Fort Washington, PA, p. A523
MASONER, Carolyn, Director Information Services, Saint Luke's North Hospital – Barry Road, Kansas City, MO, p. A362
MASOOD, Shahid, M.D. Clinical Director, Mildred Mitchell–Bateman Hospital, Huntington, WV, p. A672
MASSE, Roger A., FACHE Chief Executive Officer, Ellsworth County Medical Center, Ellsworth, KS, p. A232
MASSENGALE, David, Chief Financial Officer, Taylor Regional Hospital, Campbellsville, KY, p. A248
MASSENGILL, Leigh, Chief Executive Officer, Medical Center of Trinity, Trinity, FL, p. A142
MASSEY, Gina, Vice President Human Resources, Clarity Child Guidance Center, San Antonio, TX, p. A624
MASSEY, Kimberly, Controller, Cobb Memorial Hospital, Royston, GA, p. A158
MASSEY, Rocco K., Community Chief Executive Officer, Beckley ARH Hospital, Beckley, WV, p. A670
MASSEY, Steven, President and Chief Executive Officer, Westfields Hospital, New Richmond, WI, p. A688
MASSIE, Jamie, Chief Financial Officer, Coal County General Hospital, Coalgate, OK, p. A495
MASSIELLO, Martin, Senior Vice President and Chief Operating Officer, Eisenhower Medical Center, Rancho Mirage, CA, p. A81
MASSIET, Jill, R.N. Vice President Patient Care, Baptist Health Medical Center–Little Rock, Little Rock, AR, p. A47
MASSIMILLA, John P., FACHE Vice President Administration, Chambersburg Hospital, Chambersburg, PA, p. A520
MASSMAN, Patty, Director of Nursing, Granite Falls Municipal Hospital and Manor, Granite Falls, MN, p. A332
MASSMANN, Jerry
Chief Financial Officer, Children's Hospitals and Clinics of Minnesota, Minneapolis, MN, p. A335
Chief Financial Officer, Children's Hospitals and Clinics of Minnesota, Saint Paul, MN, p. A339
MAST, Dave
Chief Financial Officer, Providence Holy Cross Medical Center,, CA, p. A71
Chief Financial Officer, Providence Saint Joseph Medical Center, Burbank, CA, p. A56
MAST, Duane, M.D. Medical Director, Hocking Valley Community Hospital, Logan, OH, p. A483
MAST, Joelle, Ph.D. Chief Medical Officer, Blythedale Children's Hospital, Valhalla, NY, p. A445
MASTERS, Ken, Director Information Systems, Mercy McCune–Brooks Hospital, Carthage, MO, p. A357
MASTERS, Kim, M.D. Medical Director, Saint Simons by–the–Sea Hospital, Saint Simons Island, GA, p. A158
MASTERS, Regina, R.N. Director of Nursing, Continuing Care Hospital, Lexington, KY, p. A253
MASTERSON, David J., Chief Executive Officer, Sampson Regional Medical Center, Clinton, NC, p. A451
MASTERSON, Paul, Chief Financial Officer, Genesis HealthCare System, Zanesville, OH, p. A492
MASTERSON, Sammie, Chief Human Resources Officer, Harney District Hospital, Burns, OR, p. A509
MASTERTON, William J., Chief Executive Officer, Coastal Carolina Hospital, Hardeeville, SC, p. A551
MASTRO, Mary Lou, President, Linden Oaks Hospital at Edward, Naperville, IL, p. A189
MASTROIANNI, Tom, Vice President Human Resources, Lawrence Hospital Center, Bronxville, NY, p. A422
MASTROPIETRO, N. A., M.D. Medical Director, Lancaster Regional Medical Center, Lancaster, PA, p. A526
MATA, Maribel, Director Information Services, Doctors Hospital of Laredo, Laredo, TX, p. A612
MATA–GUERRERO, Rita, Nurse Director, Weslaco Rehabilitation Hospital, Weslaco, TX, p. A634
MATAI, Divya, Chief Operating Officer and Chief Financial Officer, Jack Hughston Memorial Hospital, Phenix City, AL, p. A25
MATEJKA, Cheryl
Chief Financial Officer, Mercy Hospital St. Louis, Saint Louis, MO, p. A369
Chief Financial Officer, Mercy Hospital Washington, Washington, MO, p. A372
MATENS, Brett, Chief Operating Officer, St. David's South Austin Medical Center, Austin, TX, p. A581
MATHAI, Matt, M.D. Medical Director, Select Specialty Hospital–Milwaukee, Milwaukee, WI, p. A687
MATHEIS, Tracey, Chief Financial Officer, Moberly Regional Medical Center, Moberly, MO, p. A365
MATHER, Kelly, Chief Executive Officer, Sonoma Valley Hospital, Sonoma, CA, p. A91
MATHERS, Martha, COO/VP, Our Lady of Peace, Louisville, KY, p. A255
MATHES, Lisa L., Director of Human Resources, Southwest Medical Center, Liberal, KS, p. A238
MATHEW, Bob, Director Finance, Griffin Memorial Hospital, Norman, OK, p. A500
MATHEW, Finny, Chief Operating Officer, Kosciusko Community Hospital, Warsaw, IN, p. A213
MATHEW, Jefy, M.D. Chief of Staff, St. Luke's The Woodlands Hospital, The Woodlands, TX, p. A631
MATHEW, Mammen, M.D. Chief Rehabilitation Medicine, Woodrow Wilson Rehabilitation Center, Fishersville, VA, p. A648
MATHEWS, Hilary G., R.N. Administrator, Mayo Clinic Jacksonville, Jacksonville, FL, p. A126
MATHEWS, Patrick J., Chief Executive Officer and Chief Financial Officer, St. Joseph Medical Center, Houston, TX, p. A606
MATHEWS, Paul G., CPA, Administrator, Hardtner Medical Center, Olla, LA, p. A275
MATHEWSON, Patricia, Chief Nursing Officer, Tulare Regional Medical Center, Tulare, CA, p. A93
MATHIAS, Debra
Chief Operating Officer, Children's Hospital at Mission, Mission Viejo, CA, p. A74
Chief Operating Officer, Children's Hospital of Orange County, Orange, CA, p. A78
MATHIEU, Jan, Director Human Resources, Heartland Surgical Specialty Hospital, Overland Park, KS, p. A240
MATHIEU, Karen, Director Human Resources, Bear Valley Community Hospital, Big Bear Lake, CA, p. A55
MATHIS, Linda, Director Human Resources, Muskogee Regional Medical Center, Muskogee, OK, p. A499
MATHIS, Rebecca, Vice President and Chief Financial Officer, Adventist Hinsdale Hospital, Hinsdale, IL, p. A184
MATHIS, Susan, Chief Operating Officer, CenterPointe Hospital, Saint Charles, MO, p. A367
MATHURIN, Jr., Emile, M.D. Medical Director, HEALTHSOUTH Rehabilitation Hospital, Humble, TX, p. A608
MATHURIN, Venra, Vice President Human Resources, Interfaith Medical Center,, NY, p. A433
MATICH, Philip, M.D. Vice President Medical Affairs, St. Joseph Mercy Port Huron, Port Huron, MI, p. A321
MATLACK, Ross A., FACHE Chief Executive Officer, RiverView Health, Crookston, MN, p. A330
MATLOCK, Mike, M.D. Chief Medical Officer, Providence St. Peter Hospital, Olympia, WA, p. A663
MATNEY, James L., President and Chief Executive Officer, Colquitt Regional Medical Center, Moultrie, GA, p. A157
MATNEY, Tim, Chief Financial Officer, Logan Regional Medical Center, Logan, WV, p. A673
MATRELLA, Sandra, Manager Finance, Buffalo Hospital, Buffalo, MN, p. A329
MATSIL, Robyn, Human Resources Director, Vista Medical Center West, Waukegan, IL, p. A196
MATSINGER, John, M.D. Medical Director, Virtua Berlin, Berlin, NJ, p. A402
MATTA, Lalita, M.D. Chief Medical Officer and Vice President Medical Affairs, UMass Memorial–Marlborough Hospital, Marlborough, MA, p. A302
MATTERN, Dean
President and Chief Executive Officer, Community Memorial Hospital, Turtle Lake, ND, p. A468
President and Chief Executive Officer, Garrison Memorial Hospital, Garrison, ND, p. A466
MATTES, Bryan, Associate Administrator, CrossRidge Community Hospital, Wynne, AR, p. A52
MATTES, Daniel
Chief Executive Officer, Midwest Orthopedic Specialty Hospital, Franklin, WI, p. A681
President, Wheaton Franciscan Healthcare – Franklin, Franklin, WI, p. A682
President, Wheaton Franciscan Healthcare – St. Francis, Milwaukee, WI, p. A687
MATTES, James A., President and Chief Executive Officer, Grande Ronde Hospital, La Grande, OR, p. A512
MATTES, Mark D., R.N. Assistant Administrator/Patient Care Services, Golden Valley Memorial Healthcare, Clinton, MO, p. A358
MATTEUCCI, Dolly, Interim Executive Director, Napa State Hospital, Napa, CA, p. A76
MATTHEWS, Adora, M.D. Medical Director, HEALTHSOUTH Rehabilitation Hospital, Florence, SC, p. A549
MATTHEWS, Bertt, Director Human Resources, Cushing Memorial Hospital, Leavenworth, KS, p. A237
MATTHEWS, Bryan C., Acting Director, Jack C. Montgomery Veterans Affairs Medical Center, Muskogee, OK, p. A499
MATTHEWS, Carol, Director Human Resources, Saline Memorial Hospital, Benton, AR, p. A42
MATTHEWS, Carole, Vice President Patient Care, Wood County Hospital, Bowling Green, OH, p. A471
MATTHEWS, Clinton, President and Chief Executive Officer, Reading Hospital and Medical Center, West Reading, PA, p. A541
MATTHEWS, Deborah, Administrator, Tanner Medical Center–Villa Rica, Villa Rica, GA, p. A161
MATTHEWS, Edward, Interim Chief Executive Officer, Victor Valley Community Hospital, Victorville, CA, p. A95
MATTHEWS, Gwen, MSN, Chief Executive Officer, Ukiah Valley Medical Center, Ukiah, CA, p. A93
MATTHEWS, Kenneth, Manager Information Technology, Guadalupe County Hospital, Santa Rosa, NM, p. A418
MATTHEWS, Ted, Chief Executive Officer, Eastland Memorial Hospital, Eastland, TX, p. A595
MATTHEY, Michael, Facility Chief Information Officer, Louis A. Johnson Veterans Affairs Medical Center, Clarksburg, WV, p. A671
MATTHIAS, Mark, M.D. Vice President of Medical Affairs, St. Cloud Hospital, Saint Cloud, MN, p. A338
MATTICE, Thomas, Director, Richard L. Roudebush Veterans Affairs Medical Center, Indianapolis, IN, p. A205
MATTINGLY, Marty, Vice President Human Resources, Methodist Hospital, Henderson, KY, p. A251
MATTIS, Nancy, Chief Patient Care Services, Catalina Island Medical Center, Avalon, CA, p. A54
MATTIS, Paul, Vice President Finance, Titusville Area Hospital, Titusville, PA, p. A539
MATTISON, Kenneth R., President and Chief Executive Officer, Florida Hospital Waterman, Tavares, FL, p. A141


A874 Index of Health Care Professionals

Index of Health Care Professionals / McCallister

Index of Health Care Professionals


MATTKE, Roger, Chief Financial Officer, Lafayette General Medical Center, Lafayette, LA, p. A270
MATTLY, Sheila, Chief Nursing Officer, Wayne County Hospital, Corydon, IA, p. A217
MATTON, Jeffrey A., President and Chief Executive Officer, Medstar Good Samaritan Hospital, Baltimore, MD, p. A288
MATTSON, Jodi, Director of Nursing, Cedar Springs Behavioral Health System, Colorado Springs, CO, p. A98
MATTSON, Wayne, Management Information Systems Specialist, Rogers Memorial Hospital, Oconomowoc, WI, p. A688
MATUK, Liz, Executive Director, Administrative and Clinical Services, Cleveland Clinic Florida, Weston, FL, p. A143
MATZEK, Eileen, Director Information Technology, Advocate Condell Medical Center, Libertyville, IL, p. A186
MATZENBACHER, Elaine, Chief Financial Officer, Washington County Hospital, Nashville, IL, p. A189
MATZIGKEIT, Linda, Senior Vice President Human Resources, Children's Healthcare of Atlanta, Atlanta, GA, p. A145
MAULDIN, Rick, Director Information Services, Atlanta Memorial Hospital, Atlanta, TX, p. A580
MAURER, Gregory L., Administrator, Elmore Medical Center, Mountain Home, ID, p. A169
MAURER, Jackie, Fiscal Officer, Julian F. Keith Alcohol and Drug Abuse Treatment Center, Black Mountain, NC, p. A448
MAURER, Marjorie A., MSN Vice President Operations and Chief Nursing Executive, Advocate Good Samaritan Hospital, Downers Grove, IL, p. A180
MAURER, Marsha L., R.N. Interim Chief Operating Officer, Beth Israel Deaconess Medical Center, Boston, MA, p. A296
MAURICE, Timothy, Chief Financial Officer, University of California, Davis Medical Center, Sacramento, CA, p. A84
MAURICIO, Roberto, M.D. Chief of Staff, Cumberland River Hospital, Celina, TN, p. A563
MAURIELLO, Renee, R.N. Vice President, Patient Care Services, Mercy Medical Center, Rockville Centre, NY, p. A442
MAURIN, Michael J., Chief Financial Officer, Southern Surgical Hospital, Slidell, LA, p. A278
MAUST, Richard, Chief Information Officer, Jacksonville Medical Center, Jacksonville, AL, p. A22
MAVROMATIS, Lou, Vice President Data Processing, Southern Maryland Hospital Center, Clinton, MD, p. A290
MAWYER, David, Chief Financial Officer, Western State Hospital, Staunton, VA, p. A656
MAXIE, Bryan K., Administrator, Marion General Hospital, Columbia, MS, p. A345
MAXWELL, Dale, Senior VP Chief Financial Officer, Presbyterian Kaseman Hospital, Albuquerque, NM, p. A414
MAXWELL, David, Vice President Operations, Saint John's Health System, Anderson, IN, p. A197
MAXWELL, Jody, Manager Business Office, Smith County Memorial Hospital, Smith Center, KS, p. A243
MAXWELL, John, M.D. Chief of Staff, Glenwood Regional Medical Center, West Monroe, LA, p. A279
MAXWELL, Kevin, M.D. Chief of Staff, Glendive Medical Center, Glendive, MT, p. A375
MAXWELL, Ronnie, Director Information Systems, Glenwood Regional Medical Center, West Monroe, LA, p. A279
MAY, Brandon, Chief Financial Officer, Bartow Regional Medical Center, Bartow, FL, p. A118
MAY, Carol, Chief Financial Officer, Vice President Finance and Operations, Sauk Prairie Memorial Hospital & Clinics, Prairie Du Sac, WI, p. A689
MAY, Frank, Chief Executive Officer, Yampa Valley Medical Center, Steamboat Springs, CO, p. A106
MAY, John, Chief Financial Officer, Wetzel County Hospital, New Martinsville, WV, p. A674
MAY, Kevin B.
  Chief Financial Officer, Blowing Rock Hospital, Blowing Rock, NC, p. A449
  System Director Finance, Charles A. Cannon Memorial Hospital, Linville, NC, p. A456
  Chief Financial Officer, Watauga Medical Center, Boone, NC, p. A449
MAY, Randy
  Executive Director, Griffin Memorial Hospital, Norman, OK, p. A500
  Interim Executive Director, Jim Taliaferro Community Mental Health, Lawton, OK, p. A498
MAY, Ronald B., M.D. Vice President Medical Affairs, CarolinaEast Medical Center, New Bern, NC, p. A458
MAY, Scott, Area Director Technology, Santa Clara Medical Center, Santa Clara, CA, p. A90
MAY, Sonja, Director Human Resources, Morton County Health System, Elkhart, KS, p. A232
MAY, Troy, Chief Information Officer, University of Louisville Hospital, Louisville, KY, p. A255
MAY, Walter E., President and Chief Executive Officer, Pikeville Medical Center, Pikeville, KY, p. A258
MAYER, Karen, VP Patient Care Services, Rush Oak Park Hospital, Oak Park, IL, p. A190
MAYER, Monica, M.D. Clinical Director, Public Health Service Indian Hospital – Quentin N. Burdick Memorial Health Facility, Belcourt, ND, p. A464
MAYES, James C., Manager Information Technology and Chief Security Officer, Palo Verde Hospital, Blythe, CA, p. A56
MAYES, Shelley, Director of Medical Information Services, Southwest Medical Center, Liberal, KS, p. A238
MAYEUX, Michael, Chief Financial Officer, Teche Regional Medical Center, Morgan City, LA, p. A273
MAYEWSKI, Raymond, M.D
  Chief Medical Officer, Highland Hospital of Rochester, Rochester, NY, p. A441
  Chief Medical Officer, Strong Memorial Hospital of the University of Rochester, Rochester, NY, p. A442
MAYFIELD, Dianne, Director, Texas Health Harris Methodist Hospital Cleburne, Cleburne, TX, p. A587
MAYFIELD, Michael Bradley, M.D. Chief of Staff, Chicot Memorial Medical Center, Lake Village, AR, p. A47
MAYHEW, Nicholas, Vice President and Chief Financial Officer, Rome Memorial Hospital, Rome, NY, p. A442
MAYHLE, Douglas, M.D. Medical Director, Nicholas H. Noyes Memorial Hospital, Dansville, NY, p. A425
MAYLE, Connie, Vice President Administrative Services, UPMC Horizon, Greenville, PA, p. A524
MAYNARD, Amy, Acting Chief Finance Service, Central Texas Veterans Healthcare System, Temple, TX, p. A630
MAYNARD, John, Director Information Systems, Ottawa Regional Hospital and Healthcare Center, Ottawa, IL, p. A190
MAYNARD, Rhonda, Chief Financial Officer, Physicians Regional Medical Center, Knoxville, TN, p. A568
MAYO, Andrew, Chief Executive Officer and Managing Director, North Star Behavioral Health System, Anchorage, AK, p. A28
MAYO, Cindy, Chief Executive, Providence Centralia Hospital, Centralia, WA, p. A660
MAYO, Hal, Chief Financial Officer, Liberty Dayton Regional Medical Center, Liberty, TX, p. A612
MAYO, Michael A., FACHE President, Baptist Medical Center, Jacksonville, FL, p. A126
MAYO, Randy, Director Information Technology, William Newton Hospital, Winfield, KS, p. A246
MAYO, Sarah, Vice President Financial and Information Services, Lenoir Memorial Hospital, Kinston, NC, p. A456
MAYORAL, Jorge, M.D. Medical Director, Rehabilitation Hospital of Rhode Island, North Smithfield, RI, p. A544
MAYS, Christine, R.N
  Chief Operating Officer and Chief Nurse Executive, Saint Joseph East, Lexington, KY, p. A253
  Chief Operating Officer and Chief Nurse Executive, Saint Joseph Hospital, Lexington, KY, p. A253
MAYSILLES, Nancy, R.N. Chief Nursing Officer, Medical Center of Trinity, Trinity, FL, p. A142
MAYSON, Mark J., M.D. Medical Director, Palmetto Health Baptist, Columbia, SC, p. A548
MAZO, Scott, Vice President Human Resources, Northwest Medical Center, Margate, FL, p. A129
MAZOUR, Linda, M.D. President, Franklin County Memorial Hospital, Franklin, NE, p. A383
MAZUR, Geoff, Director Information Technology, Charles Cole Memorial Hospital, Coudersport, PA, p. A521
MAZUR, Robert, Vice President Human Resources, Capital Region Medical Center, Jefferson City, MO, p. A361
MAZZA, Mary, Director Human Resources, HEALTHSOUTH Rehabilitation Hospital of Western Massachusetts, Ludlow, MA, p. A302
MAZZEO, Paul, M.D. Chief of Staff, Beaufort Memorial Hospital, Beaufort, SC, p. A546
MAZZOLA, Joe, D.O
  Sr. Vice President Medical Affairs/Chief Quality Officer, Grace Hospital, Morganton, NC, p. A458
  Sr. Vice President Medical Affairs/Chief Quality Officer, Valdese General Hospital, Valdese, NC, p. A462
MAZZORANO, Tony, Chief Executive Officer, Palm Springs General Hospital, Hialeah, FL, p. A125
MAZZUCA, Darryl, Director Management Information Systems, Little Company of Mary Hospital and Health Care Centers, Evergreen Park, IL, p. A181
MBENGA, Saul, Manager Information Technology, Alliance HealthCare System, Holly Springs, MS, p. A347
MCADAMS, David, Chief Financial Officer, Lindner Center of HOPE, Mason, OH, p. A484
MCAFEE, Thomas J., President, Northwestern Lake Forest Hospital, Lake Forest, IL, p. A186
MCALISTER, Michael, Chief Executive Officer, Select Specialty Hospital–Nashville, Nashville, TN, p. A573
MCALLISTER, Guy, Assistant Vice President and Chief Information Officer, Tift Regional Medical Center, Tifton, GA, p. A161
MCALOON, Richard, Vice President Human Resources, Hartford Hospital, Hartford, CT, p. A109
MCANALLY, Eileen, Senior Vice President Human Resources, Lankenau Medical Center, Wynnewood, PA, p. A542
MCANDREW, Michael, Chief Executive Officer, Hopkins County Memorial Hospital, Sulphur Springs, TX, p. A629
MCARTHUR, Ronald L., Chief Executive Officer, Summit Healthcare Regional Medical Center, Show Low, AZ, p. A38
MCARTOR, Dana, R.N. Director of Nursing, Perkins County Health Services, Grant, NE, p. A384
MCAULIFFE, Gregory, M.D. Chief Medical Officer, San Luis Valley Regional Medical Center, Alamosa, CO, p. A97
MCAULIFFE, John, M.D. Medical Director, Sauk Prairie Memorial Hospital & Clinics, Prairie Du Sac, WI, p. A689
MCBEE, Gala, Administrator, George Nigh Rehabilitation Institute, Okmulgee, OK, p. A502
MCBEE Jr.,, Harold A., President, Mid Atlantic Health Management, Inc., Stevensville, MD, p. B89
MCBEE, Marie, Chief Executive Officer, Warwick Manor Behavioral Health, East New Market, MD, p. A291
MCBRATNEY, Kathleen, M.D. President, Cushing Memorial Hospital, Leavenworth, KS, p. A237
MCBREARTY, Michael, M.D. Vice President Medical Affairs, Thomas Hospital, Fairhope, AL, p. A20
MCBRIDE, Anne, Chief Financial Officer, Regional Hospital for Respiratory and Complex Care, Seattle, WA, p. A665
MCBRIDE, Brandon, Chief Operating Officer, Logan Regional Hospital, Logan, UT, p. A638
MCBRIDE, Dan, M.D. Chief of Staff, Spring Valley Hospital Medical Center, Las Vegas, NV, p. A394
MCBRIDE, Grace, Vice President Acute Care Services, St. Marys Health Center, Jefferson City, MO, p. A361
MCBRIDE, Kate, Chief Operating Officer, Poplar Springs Hospital, Petersburg, VA, p. A653
MCBRIDE, Michael J., FACHE President and Chief Executive Officer, St. Mary's Hospital and Medical Center, Grand Junction, CO, p. A102
MCBRIDE, Norman L., FACHE Vice President and Chief Operating Officer, CHRISTUS Spohn Hospital Kleberg, Kingsville, TX, p. A610
MCBRIDE, III, Thomas Y., Executive Vice President and Chief Financial Officer, Gwinnett Hospital System, Lawrenceville, GA, p. A155
MCBROOM, Mike, FACHE Vice President Human Resources, Hendrick Health System, Abilene, TX, p. A577
MCBROOM, Robert, M.D. Medical Director, Texas Specialty Hospital at Wichita Falls, Wichita Falls, TX, p. A635
MCBRYDE, Richard, Senior Vice President and Chief Operating Officer, North Arkansas Regional Medical Center, Harrison, AR, p. A45
MCCABE, Jack H., FACHE Administrator, CHRISTUS St. Catherine Hospital, Katy, TX, p. A610
MCCABE, Jim, Chief Financial Officer, Promise Hospital of San Diego, San Diego, CA, p. A85
MCCABE, John B., M.D. Chief Executive Officer, Upstate University Hospital, Syracuse, NY, p. A444
MCCABE, Mary, Chief Financial Officer, North Colorado Medical Center, Greeley, CO, p. A102
MCCABE, Patrick, Senior Vice President Finance and Chief Financial Officer, Bridgeport Hospital, Bridgeport, CT, p. A108
MCCABE Jr., Patrick G., FACHE President and Chief Executive Officer, Levi Hospital, Hot Springs National Park, AR, p. A46
MCCABE, Steve, Chief Executive Officer, Hill Crest Behavioral Health Services, Birmingham, AL, p. A16
MCCAFFERTY, Michael, Chief Executive Officer, Sheridan Memorial Hospital, Sheridan, WY, p. A697
MCCAHILL, Mary, Chief Nursing Officer, Thorek Memorial Hospital, Chicago, IL, p. A178
MCCAIN, Rebecca, Chief Financial Officer and Assistant Administrator, Electra Memorial Hospital, Electra, TX, p. A597
MCCALEB, Marg, Chief Human Resources Management, Veterans Affairs Black Hills Health Care System, Fort Meade, SD, p. A556
MCCALL, Brad
  President and Chief Executive Officer, Physicians Surgical Hospital – Panhandle Campus, Amarillo, TX, p. A578
  President and Chief Executive Officer, Physicians Surgical Hospital – Quail Creek, Amarillo, TX, p. A578
MCCALL, Cynde, R.N. Chief Nursing Officer, Select Specialty Hospital–Omaha, Omaha, NE, p. A388
MCCALL, Harlo, Chief Nursing Officer, Summit Medical Center, Van Buren, AR, p. A52
MCCALL, Lee, Administrator, Winston Medical Center, Louisville, MS, p. A349
MCCALLISTER, Bob, Director Human Resources, Baptist Memorial Hospital–Golden Triangle, Columbus, MS, p. A345
MCCALLISTER, Darla, Chief Financial Officer, Lakeside Women's Hospital, Oklahoma City, OK, p. A501
MCCALLISTER, Diane, M.D. Chief Medical Officer, Porter Adventist Hospital, Denver, CO, p. A100

Index of Health Care Professionals

Index of Health Care Professionals / McCallister

MCCALLISTER, Sean, Administrator, Providence Valdez Medical Center, Valdez, AK, p. A30
MCCAMPBELL, Kellie, Coordinator Human Resources, Kindred Hospital–Chattanooga, Chattanooga, TN, p. A563
MCCAMPBELL, Marcia, M.D. Chief Medical Officer, Shasta Regional Medical Center, Redding, CA, p. A82
MCCANCE, Chad, M.D. Chief of Staff, Cass County Memorial Hospital, Atlantic, IA, p. A214
MCCANDLESS, Barbara
Vice President Human Resources, Organization Development, Albany Memorial Hospital, Albany, NY, p. A420
Corporate Vice President Human Resources, Samaritan Hospital, Troy, NY, p. A445
MCCANN, Barbara, Director Human Resources, Sunrise Canyon Hospital, Lubbock, TX, p. A614
MCCANN, Joseph, Chief Information Officer, Saint Francis Hospital and Health Centers, Poughkeepsie, NY, p. A441
MCCANN, Kyle, Chief Operating Officer, SouthCrest Hospital, Tulsa, OK, p. A507
MCCANN, Lew, Director Management Information Systems, OSF Holy Family Medical Center, Monmouth, IL, p. A188
MCCANNA, Peter J., Executive Vice President Administration and Chief Financial Officer, Northwestern Memorial Hospital, Chicago, IL, p. A177
MCCARLEY, Bobby, Director Information Management, Searcy Hospital, Mount Vernon, AL, p. A24
MCCARTAN, Mary E., Manager Human Resources, Veterans Affairs Long Beach Healthcare System, Long Beach, CA, p. A68
MCCARTER, Scott, Chief Information Officer, Karmanos Cancer Center, Detroit, MI, p. A311
MCCARTER, Jr., Thomas G., M.D. Chief Medical Officer, Lankenau Medical Center, Wynnewood, PA, p. A542
MCCARTHY, Brian, Director Information Systems, Memorial Hospital of Salem County, Salem, NJ, p. A410
MCCARTHY, Linda M., R.N. VP/ Chief Nursing Officer, Citrus Memorial Health System, Inverness, FL, p. A126
MCCARTHY, Maureen, M.D. Chief of Staff, Veterans Affairs Medical Center, Salem, VA, p. A656
MCCARTHY, Robert R., Vice President Finance and Chief Financial Officer, Chenango Memorial Hospital, Norwich, NY, p. A438
MCCARTHY, Steve, Assistant Administrator Business Operations, Upland Hills Health, Dodgeville, WI, p. A680
MCCARTHY, Sue, Chief Financial Officer, Grady Memorial Hospital, Atlanta, GA, p. A145
MCCARTHY, Teresa, Interim Director Human Resources, McDowell Hospital, Marion, NC, p. A457
MCCARTHY, Tim, President Puerto Rico Division, First Hospital Panamericano, Cidra, PR, p. A700
MCCARTY, Bernie, Director Facilities, Hoopeston Regional Health Center, Hoopeston, IL, p. A185
MCCARTY, Daniel P., Chief Operating Officer, Orange City Area Health System, Orange City, IA, p. A224
MCCARTY, Maryland, Director Information Systems, Atlanta Medical Center, Atlanta, GA, p. A145
MCCARTY, Pat, Director Human Resources, Pushmataha Hospital & Home Health, Antlers, OK, p. A493
MCCARTY, Wendy, Director Human Resources, Hillsboro Community Hospital, Hillsboro, KS, p. A234
MCCASKILL, Linda A. W.
Market Chief Executive Officer, Kindred Hospital–Aurora, Aurora, CO, p. A97
Chief Executive Officer, Kindred Hospital–Denver, Denver, CO, p. A99
MCCASLIN, Anna, Chief Financial Officer, Nebraska Orthopaedic Hospital, Omaha, NE, p. A388
MCCAUGHEY, James, Chief Strategy Officer, Lucile Salter Packard Children's Hospital at Stanford, Palo Alto, CA, p. A79
MCCAULEY, Bryan, Associate Executive Director, Riverview Regional Medical Center, Gadsden, AL, p. A20
MCCAULEY, Cynthia, Chief Financial Officer, Good Samaritan Medical Center, West Palm Beach, FL, p. A142
MCCAULEY, Dudley, Controller, Lincoln County Medical Center, Ruidoso, NM, p. A417
MCCAULEY, Sue E., Director Finance, Baum Harmon Mercy Hospital, Primghar, IA, p. A225
MCCAULEY, W. Roger, Senior Vice President Administration and Chief Financial Officer, UPMC Northwest, Seneca, PA, p. A538
MCCAWLEY, Thomas J., Manager Human Resources, CGH Medical Center, Sterling, IL, p. A194
MCCLAID, Michael, M.D. President Medical Staff, Community Hospital of Bremen, Bremen, IN, p. A198
MCCLAIN, David, Executive Vice President Operations, Tahlequah City Hospital, Tahlequah, OK, p. A505
MCCLAIN, Richard, M.D. Chief Medical Officer, Chickasaw Nation Medical Center, Ada, OK, p. A493
MCCLALLEN, Gerald, President Medical Staff, St. Joseph Memorial Hospital, Murphysboro, IL, p. A188
MCCLANAHAN, Gary, Chief Information Officer, Sequoyah Memorial Hospital, Sallisaw, OK, p. A504
MCCLANAHAN, Sher, Chief Operating Officer, Bethesda North Hospital, Cincinnati, OH, p. A472
MCCLANAHAN, William, M.D. Chief of Staff, St. Vincent's St. Clair, Pell City, AL, p. A25
MCCLARIGAN, Linda, R.N. Vice President, Patient Care Services, Alice Hyde Medical Center, Malone, NY, p. A429
MCCLASKEY, Cynthia, Ph.D. Director, Southwestern Virginia Mental Health Institute, Marion, VA, p. A651
MCCLEESE, Randy, Vice President Information Services and Chief Information Officer, St. Claire Regional Medical Center, Morehead, KY, p. A256
MCCLELLAN, Ashley, Chief Executive Officer, Medical Center of Lewisville, Lewisville, TX, p. A612
MCCLENDON, Pat, MSN Chief Nursing Officer, Palmdale Regional Medical Center, Palmdale, CA, p. A79
MCCLINTICK, Cliff, Chief Information Officer, Lindner Center of HOPE, Mason, OH, p. A484
MCCLOSKEY, Louis, Chief Human Resources, Veterans Affairs Medical Center, Wilmington, DE, p. A115
MCCLUNG, Brett, President, Texas Health Harris Methodist Hospital Southwest Fort Worth, Fort Worth, TX, p. A599
MCCLUNG, Eric, Chief Information Management Division, Reynolds Army Community Hospital, Fort Sill, OK, p. A497
MCCLUNG, James W., Assistant Chief Executive Officer, Northern Louisiana Medical Center, Ruston, LA, p. A276
MCCLUNG, Lyle, M.D. Chief of Staff, Carilion Stonewall Jackson Hospital, Lexington, VA, p. A650
MCCLURE, Dan, Chief Information Officer, Hi–Desert Medical Center, Joshua Tree, CA, p. A65
MCCLURE, Gwenda, USAF Chief Nursing Officer, Mimbres Memorial Hospital, Deming, NM, p. A415
MCCLURE, Jan, Chief Executive Officer, Hill Regional Hospital, Hillsboro, TX, p. A603
MCCLURE, Joseph, Chief Executive Officer, Advanced Care Hospital of Montana, Billings, MT, p. A373
MCCLURE, Joy, Chief Financial Officer, Ashe Memorial Hospital, Jefferson, NC, p. A455
MCCLURG, Cathy, Director Human Resources, William Newton Hospital, Winfield, KS, p. A246
MCCLURG, Chris, Chief Financial Officer, Pattie A. Clay Regional Medical Center, Richmond, KY, p. A258
MCCLURKAN, Mac
Chief Information Officer, HealthEast Bethesda Hospital, Saint Paul, MN, p. A339
Chief Information Officer, St. John's Hospital, Saint Paul, MN, p. A339
Chief Information Officer, Woodwinds Health Campus, Woodbury, MN, p. A342
MCCLUSKEY, Tabb, M.D. Chief Medical Officer, Hendricks Community Hospital, Hendricks, MN, p. A332
MCCLUSKEY, Zachary, Chief Operating Officer, StoneCrest Medical Center, Smyrna, TN, p. A575
MCCLUSKY, Derek, M.D. Chief of Staff, Northern Louisiana Medical Center, Ruston, LA, p. A276
MCCLYMONDS, Bruce, President and Chief Executive Officer, West Virginia University Hospitals, Morgantown, WV, p. A674
MCCOBB, David
Chief Information Officer, Citrus Valley Medical Center–Inter–Community Campus, Covina, CA, p. A59
Chief Information Officer, Foothill Presbyterian Hospital, Glendora, CA, p. A63
MCCOIC, Kristie, Director Human Resources, St. Joseph's Health Services, Hillsboro, WI, p. A683
MCCOLE–WICHER, Sharon, R.N. Chief Nursing Officer, San Francisco General Hospital Medical Center, San Francisco, CA, p. A87
MCCOLLOUGH, Kristy, Assistant Administrator and Chief Financial Officer, Integris Mayes County Medical Center, Pryor, OK, p. A503
MCCOLLUM, Ken, Vice President, Human Resources, NorthBay Medical Center, Fairfield, CA, p. A60
MCCOLLUM, Rodger, Chief Executive Officer, Snoqualmie Valley Hospital, Snoqualmie, WA, p. A667
MCCOLM, Denni, Chief Information Officer, Citizens Memorial Hospital, Bolivar, MO, p. A355
MCCOMAS, James, Vice President Operations, Hutchinson Regional Medical Center, Hutchinson, KS, p. A235
MCCOMAS, Marc, Executive Director, Haven Behavioral Senior Care of North Denver, Thornton, CO, p. A106
MCCOMBS, III, William, Ph.D. Chief Information Officer, Scott and White Memorial Hospital, Temple, TX, p. A630
MCCONAHY, Richard L., Interim Chief Executive Officer, Pampa Regional Medical Center, Pampa, TX, p. A620
MCCONAUGHY, Chris, Chief Nursing Officer, Paradise Valley Hospital, Phoenix, AZ, p. A36
MCCONNELL, George, Director, Earle E. Morris Alcohol and Drug Treatment Center, Columbia, SC, p. A548
MCCONNELL, John D., M.D. Chief Executive Officer, Wake Forest Baptist Health, Winston–Salem, NC, p. B143
MCCONNELL, Patrick G., Chief Financial Officer, West Park Hospital, Cody, WY, p. A696
MCCONNELL, Ron, Chief Operating Officer, Altoona Regional Health System, Altoona, PA, p. A517
MCCORKLE Jr., Philip H., President and Chief Executive Officer, Saint Mary's Health Care, Grand Rapids, MI, p. A314
MCCORMACK, Cynthia, MS, Director, Veterans Affairs Medical Center, Cheyenne, WY, p. A695
MCCORMACK, J. David, President and Chief Executive Officer, Northeast Alabama Regional Medical Center, Anniston, AL, p. A15
MCCORMACK, Jane, R.N. Vice President, Chief Nursing Officer and Nursing and Patient Care Services, Unity Hospital, Rochester, NY, p. A442
MCCORMACK, Julie M., R.N. Administrator, Integris Blackwell Regional Hospital, Blackwell, OK, p. A494
MCCORMICK, Dee Dawn, Director Personnel and Human Resources, Coon Memorial Hospital and Home, Dalhart, TX, p. A590
MCCORMICK, Jason, Vice President Finance and Chief Financial Officer, Family Health West, Fruita, CO, p. A101
MCCORMICK, Jayne
Chief Medical Officer CDS, Presbyterian Hospital, Albuquerque, NM, p. A414
Chief Medical Officer CDS, Presbyterian Kaseman Hospital, Albuquerque, NM, p. A414
MCCORMICK, John, Chief Financial Officer, Oak Valley Hospital District, Oakdale, CA, p. A77
MCCORMICK, Karen, Director Client Services, St. John Macomb–Oakland Hospital, Oakland Center, Madison Heights, MI, p. A318
MCCORMICK, Pam, Director Human Resources, Permian Regional Medical Center, Andrews, TX, p. A578
MCCOWN, Fran, Administrator, Haskell Memorial Hospital, Haskell, TX, p. A603
MCCOY, Andrea C., M.D. Chief Medical Officer, Jeanes Hospital, Philadelphia, PA, p. A532
MCCOY, Craig, Chief Executive Officer, Emory Johns Creek Hospital, Johns Creek, GA, p. A154
MCCOY, Elizabeth, Chief Human Resources Management, Stony Brook University Medical Center, Stony Brook, NY, p. A444
MCCOY, Jessica, Director Human Resources, Cedar Springs Behavioral Health System, Colorado Springs, CO, p. A98
MCCOY, Mike, Chief Operating Officer, Saint Mary's Regional Medical Center, Russellville, AR, p. A51
MCCOY, Paul, Director Human Resources, Mayers Memorial Hospital District, Fall River Mills, CA, p. A60
MCCOY, Shawn W., Chief Administrative Officer, Deaconess Hospital, Evansville, IN, p. A201
MCCOY, Stephanie, President and Chief Executive Officer, Jackson General Hospital, Ripley, WV, p. A675
MCCRACKEN, Ann B., M.D
President Medical Staff, Solara Hospital Harlingen, Harlingen, TX, p. A602
Chief Medical Director, Solara Hospital Harlingen–Brownsville Campus, Brownsville, TX, p. A585
MCCRANIE, Robbie, Director Human Resources, Plano Specialty Hospital, Plano, TX, p. A621
MCCRAW, Elizabeth, Vice President, Human Resources, Gaston Memorial Hospital, Gastonia, NC, p. A453
MCCRAW, Nicki, Assistant Vice President Human Resources, Harborview Medical Center, Seattle, WA, p. A665
MCCREA, Kim, Chief Human Resources Officer, Ortonville Area Health Services, Ortonville, MN, p. A336
MCCREA, Mary Anne, Chief Nursing Officer, Creighton University Medical Center, Omaha, NE, p. A387
MCCREA, Yvette, Chief Human Resources, Winn Army Community Hospital, Hinesville, GA, p. A154
MCCREARY, Michael, Chief of Services, Mercy Hospital Washington, Washington, MO, p. A372
MCCRIMMON, Scott, Manager Information Technology, Northern Arizona VA Health Care System, Prescott, AZ, p. A37
MCCUE, Cathy, Director Human Resources, St. Anthony's Hospital, Houston, TX, p. A606
MCCUE, Jack D., M.D. Senior Vice President and Interim Chief Medical Officer, Regional Medical Center at Memphis, Memphis, TN, p. A572
MCCUE, Robert N., Vice President Finance, Mid Coast Hospital, Brunswick, ME, p. A282
MCCUE, Steven
Chief Financial Officer, Clinton Hospital, Clinton, MA, p. A299
Chief Financial Officer, UMass Memorial–Marlborough Hospital, Marlborough, MA, p. A302
MCCULLEY, Larry W., President and Chief Executive Officer, Touchette Regional Hospitals, Centreville, IL, p. A175
MCCULLOCH, Liz, Chief Information Resource Management Systems, Veterans Affairs Medical Center, Cheyenne, WY, p. A695

A876 Index of Health Care Professionals

Index of Health Care Professionals / McGee

Index of Health Care Professionals


MCCULLOUGH, Barbara A., Vice President Human Resources, Washington Hospital, Washington, PA, p. A540
MCCULLOUGH, Bobby, Chief Operating Officer, Central Florida Regional Hospital, Sanford, FL, p. A138
MCCULLOUGH, Michael
Chief Financial Officer, Lutheran Hospital of Indiana, Fort Wayne, IN, p. A201
Chief Financial Officer, Orthopaedic Hospital of Lutheran Health, Fort Wayne, IN, p. A201
Chief Financial Officer, Rehabilitation Hospital of Fort Wayne, Fort Wayne, IN, p. A202
MCCULLOUGH, Paula, VP Patient Care Services, St. Vincent's Blount, Oneonta, AL, p. A24
MCCULLOUGH, Sharon, Director Human Resources, Indiana Heart Hospital, Indianapolis, IN, p. A204
MCCULLOUGH, Wadra, Chief Nursing Officer, Spalding Regional Medical Center, Griffin, GA, p. A153
MCCUMBER, Tracy, Manager Information Systems, Chenango Memorial Hospital, Norwich, NY, p. A438
MCCUMMINGS, James, Executive Director, Kingsboro Psychiatric Center,, NY, p. A433
MCCUNE, Becky, Director Human Resources, Community Relations and Education, Coffeyville Regional Medical Center, Coffeyville, KS, p. A231
MCCUNE, Connie, Vice President Human Resources, Via Christi Hospital, Pittsburg, KS, p. A241
MCCUNE, William, President, Delaware County Memorial Hospital, Drexel Hill, PA, p. A522
MCCURDY, Brent, Director Management Information, St. Croix Regional Medical Center, St. Croix Falls, WI, p. A691
MCCURDY, Carol, Chief Information Officer, Chickasaw Nation Medical Center, Ada, OK, p. A493
MCCURRY, Mark, M.D. Chief of Staff, Haskell County Community Hospital, Stigler, OK, p. A504
MCCUTCHAN, Matt, Chief Financial Officer, Greater Regional Medical Center, Creston, IA, p. A217
MCCUTCHEON, Edna I., Chief Executive Officer, Torrance State Hospital, Torrance, PA, p. A539
MCCUTCHEON, Henry, Chief Executive Officer, Lake City Community Hospital, Lake City, SC, p. A552
MCCUTCHEON, Norma J., R.N
Senior Vice President Operations, Wheaton Franciscan Healthcare – St. Joseph's, Milwaukee, WI, p. A687
Senior Vice President Operations, Wheaton Franciscan Healthcare – The Wisconsin Heart Hospital, Wauwatosa, WI, p. A693
MCDADE, Jo Ann, Assistant Administrator Finance, Arkansas State Hospital, Little Rock, AR, p. A47
MCDANALD, Matt, M.D. Chief Medical Officer, Baptist Hospital Northeast, La Grange, KY, p. A252
MCDANEL, Joyce
Vice President Human Resources and Education, Iowa Lutheran Hospital, Des Moines, IA, p. A218
Vice President Human Resources, Iowa Methodist Medical Center, Des Moines, IA, p. A218
MCDANIEL, Amy, Chief Financial Officer, Iowa Specialty Hospital–Clarion, Clarion, IA, p. A216
MCDANIEL, Burton, M.D. Medical Director, Roosevelt Warm Springs Institute for Rehabilitation, Warm Springs, GA, p. A161
MCDANIEL, Graciela, Chief Financial Officer, Veterans Affairs Medical Center, Philadelphia, PA, p. A534
MCDANIEL, Kim, Director Human Resources, HEALTHSOUTH Rehabilitation Hospital of Montgomery, Montgomery, AL, p. A24
MCDANIEL, LaDonna, Financial Manager, Prattville Baptist Hospital, Prattville, AL, p. A25
MCDANIEL, Lisa, Assistant Administrator Human Resources, Kittitas Valley Community Hospital, Ellensburg, WA, p. A661
MCDANIEL, Ruth A., Chief Executive Officer, Spring View Hospital, Lebanon, KY, p. A252
MCDANIEL, Suzie Q., Director Human Resources, Bay Area Hospital, Coos Bay, OR, p. A510
MCDANIEL, Jr., W. Burton, M.D. Physician Executive, Roosevelt Warm Springs LTAC Hospital, Warm Springs, GA, p. A161
MCDAVID, Clarence, Vice President Human Resources, Rose Medical Center, Denver, CO, p. A100
MCDERMOTT, James, M.D. Chief of Staff, Sedan City Hospital, Sedan, KS, p. A243
MCDERMOTT, Margaret, Chief Executive Officer, Saints Mary & Elizabeth Medical Center, Chicago, IL, p. A178
MCDERMOTT, Thomas, Vice President Finance, Fayette County Memorial Hospital, Washington Court House, OH, p. A490
MCDERMOTT, Vincent, Executive Director Finance, Faulkner Hospital, Boston, MA, p. A296
MCDEVITT, Chuck, Chief Information Officer, Self Regional Healthcare, Greenwood, SC, p. A551
MCDEVITT, Mike, Chief Information Officer, The Children's Hospital of Alabama, Birmingham, AL, p. A17
MCDIVITT, Robert P., FACHE Director, Veterans Affairs Ann Arbor Healthcare System, Ann Arbor, MI, p. A307
MCDONALD, Bruce M., M.D. Senior Vice President Medical Affairs, Bridgeport Hospital, Bridgeport, CT, p. A108
MCDONALD, Buck, Chief Financial Officer, St. Helena Hospital Clearlake, Clearlake, CA, p. A57
MCDONALD, Edward A.
Senior Vice President and Chief Financial Officer, St. Helena Hospital, Saint Helena, CA, p. A84
Chief Financial Officer, St. Helena Hospital–Center for Behavioral Health, Vallejo, CA, p. A94
MCDONALD, Elizabeth, Director Human Resources, Wayne Memorial Hospital, Honesdale, PA, p. A525
MCDONALD, Frank, D.O. Chief of Staff, Southeast Colorado Hospital District, Springfield, CO, p. A105
MCDONALD, Gary
Assistant Administrator Human Resources, Stone County Medical Center, Mountain View, AR, p. A49
Assistant Administrator Human Resources, White River Medical Center, Batesville, AR, p. A42
MCDONALD, Gregory, Vice President Finance and Chief Financial Officer, Roswell Park Cancer Institute, Buffalo, NY, p. A423
MCDONALD, Jeff, Chief Executive Officer, Canyon Ridge Hospital, Chino, CA, p. A57
MCDONALD, John, D.O. President and Chief of Medical Staff, Good Shepherd Medical Center–Marshall, Marshall, TX, p. A615
MCDONALD, Joseph D., President and Chief Executive Officer, Catholic Health System, Buffalo, NY, p. B29
MCDONALD, Kathy, Director Personnel, Covenant Hospital–Levelland, Levelland, TX, p. A612
MCDONALD, Larry, Director Human Resources, Miami Jewish Home and Hospital for Aged, Miami, FL, p. A131
MCDONALD, Lauren, M.D. Medical Director and Medical Staff President, Vibra Specialty Hospital of Dallas, Desoto, TX, p. A594
MCDONALD, Mark, M.D. President, Institute for Orthopaedic Surgery, Lima, OH, p. A482
MCDONALD, Michael, Chief Executive Officer, The Vines, Ocala, FL, p. A134
MCDONALD, Rick, Chief Financial Officer, Anson General Hospital, Anson, TX, p. A579
MCDONALD, Rosalind S., MSN Vice President Nursing Services, Lenoir Memorial Hospital, Kinston, NC, p. A456
MCDONALD, Steve, Director Information Systems, Northside Hospital and Heart Institute, Saint Petersburg, FL, p. A138
MCDONALD, Stuart, M.D. President Medical Staff, Kindred Hospital–Fort Worth, Fort Worth, TX, p. A599
MCDONALD, Susan, M.D. Vice President, St. Joseph's Medical Center, Stockton, CA, p. A92
MCDONALD, William A., President and Chief Executive Officer, St. Joseph's Regional Medical Center, Paterson, NJ, p. A408
MCDONALD–UPTON, Ann, Chief Nursing Officer, St. Joseph Mercy Oakland, Pontiac, MI, p. A321
MCDONNELL, Michael J.
Vice President and Chief Operations Officer, Sheltering Arms Hospital South, Midlothian, VA, p. A651
Vice President and Chief Operating Officer, Sheltering Arms Rehabilitation Hospital, Mechanicsville, VA, p. A651
MCDONNELL, Nancy, Manager Information Systems, Illinois Valley Community Hospital, Peru, IL, p. A191
MCDONNELL, Stephen C., Senior Vice President, Chief Financial Officer and Chief Operating Officer, Sibley Memorial Hospital, Washington, DC, p. A117
MCDONOUGH, Jeffrey, Assistant Vice President Human Resources, Vassar Brothers Medical Center, Poughkeepsie, NY, p. A441
MCDONOUGH, JoAnn, Director Operations and Chief Nursing Officer, Crittenton Children's Center, Kansas City, MO, p. A361
MCDONOUGH, Sharon, Chief Executive Officer, First Street Hospital, Bellaire, TX, p. A583
MCDOUGAL, Pedro, M.D. Medical Director, Weslaco Rehabilitation Hospital, Weslaco, TX, p. A634
MCDOUGAL Jr., Tom R., President and Chief Executive Officer, Medical West, Bessemer, AL, p. A16
MCDOUGLE, Mark, Executive Vice President and Chief Operating Officer, Maimonides Medical Center,, NY, p. A434
MCDOWELL, III, Arthur V., M.D. Vice President Clinical Affairs, Middlesex Hospital, Middletown, CT, p. A110
MCDOWELL, Charles
Chief Human Resources Officer, ProMedica Flower Hospital, Sylvania, OH, p. A489
Corporate Vice President Human Resources, ProMedica Fostoria Community Hospital, Fostoria, OH, p. A480
MCDOWELL, Jane, FACHE Administrator, Jefferson County Hospital, Waurika, OK, p. A507
MCDOWELL, Jean, Chief Financial Officer, Kindred Hospital–Dallas, Dallas, TX, p. A591
MCDOWELL, Jon, FACHE Chief Operating Officer, The Rehabilitation Institute of St. Louis, Saint Louis, MO, p. A370
MCDOWELL, Jon C., Vice President Human Resources, Bayhealth Medical Center, Dover, DE, p. A114
MCDOWELL, Paul L., Vice President Finance and Chief Financial Officer, King's Daughters Medical Center, Ashland, KY, p. A247
MCDOWELL, Richard, Chief Financial Officer, Ridge Behavioral Health System, Lexington, KY, p. A253
MCDRURY, Martha M., R.N. Chief Operating Officer and Chief Nursing Officer, Holy Family Hospital and Medical Center, Methuen, MA, p. A302
MCDUFF, Raoul, Director Human Resources, Palm Drive Hospital, Sebastopol, CA, p. A90
MCEACHERN, John, Controller, Sebastian River Medical Center, Sebastian, FL, p. A139
MCELDOWNEY, Erin, Manager Human Resources, Haven Senior Horizons, Phoenix, AZ, p. A35
MCELFRESH, Jim, Manager Human Resources, Norfolk Regional Center, Norfolk, NE, p. A386
MCELLIGOTT, Daniel P., FACHE President and Chief Executive Officer, Saint Francis Medical Center, Grand Island, NE, p. A384
MCELRATH, Matthew, Chief Human Resources Officer, Keck Hospital of USC, Los Angeles, CA, p. A70
MCELROY, Maria Elena, Vice President Human Resources, HEALTHSOUTH Rehabilitation Hospital of Southern Arizona, Tucson, AZ, p. A39
MCELROY, Sherry, Director Health Information Management, Osceola Community Hospital, Sibley, IA, p. A226
MCELROY, Wayne, Administrator, Pickens County Medical Center, Carrollton, AL, p. A18
MCENROY, Karolyn, Business Office Manager, Oakland Mercy Hospital, Oakland, NE, p. A387
MCENTEE, Chris, Network Specialist, Van Buren County Hospital, Keosauqua, IA, p. A222
MCEUEN, Jacqueline, Coordinator Human Resources, Bellville General Hospital, Bellville, TX, p. A583
MCEVILLY, Kerrie, Director Finance and Information Systems, Stevens Community Medical Center, Morris, MN, p. A336
MCEVOY, Lawrence R., M.D. Chief Executive Officer, Memorial Health System, Colorado Springs, CO, p. A98
MCEWEN, David S., Vice President Operations, Port Huron Hospital, Port Huron, MI, p. A321
MCEWEN, Mary Louise, Superintendent, Riverview Psychiatric Center, Augusta, ME, p. A281
MCEWEN, Michelle, President and Chief Executive Officer, Speare Memorial Hospital, Plymouth, NH, p. A400
MCFADDEN, Ian, President and Chief Executive Officer, Methodist Hospitals, Gary, IN, p. A202
MCFALL, Cathy, Human Resources Manager, Kiowa County Memorial Hospital, Greensburg, KS, p. A234
MCFALL, Vicky, Chief Executive Officer, Monroe County Medical Center, Tompkinsville, KY, p. A259
MCFARLAND, Kenneth, President and Chief Executive Officer, Mission Hospital, Mission Viejo, CA, p. A74
MCFARLAND, Nita, Director of Nursing, Ninnescah Valley Health System, Kingman, KS, p. A236
MCFARLAND, Rhonda, Director Human Resources, Carolinas Medical Center–Union, Monroe, NC, p. A457
MCFARLAND, Rodney, M.D. Medical Director, Freeman Neosho Hospital, Neosho, MO, p. A366
MCFARLAND, Tracee, Chief Financial Officer, Claiborne County Hospital, Tazewell, TN, p. A576
MCFARLIN, Andrew, Director Information Services, Johnson Memorial Hospital, Stafford Springs, CT, p. A112
MCFAUL, Joan, Vice President Information Technology and Chief Information Officer, Glens Falls Hospital, Glens Falls, NY, p. A426
MCFERRAN, Virginia
Chief Information Officer, Ronald Reagan University of California Los Angeles Medical Center, Los Angeles, CA, p. A71
Chief Information Officer, Santa Monica–UCLA Medical Center and Orthopaedic Hospital, Santa Monica, CA, p. A90
MCGAHEY, Nikki, Information Officer, Jefferson County Hospital, Waurika, OK, p. A507
MCGARIGLE, Kristine, President, Ministry Good Samaritan Health Center, Merrill, WI, p. A686
MCGARVEY, Missy, Director Computer Information Systems, Twin Valley Behavioral Healthcare, Columbus, OH, p. A477
MCGAUGH, Jamie, Controller, Atoka County Medical Center, Atoka, OK, p. A493
MCGEACHEY, Edward J., President and Chief Executive Officer, Southern Maine Medical Center, Biddeford, ME, p. A282
MCGEE, Jessica
Chief Financial Officer, AMG Specialty Hospital – Lafayette, Lafayette, LA, p. A269
Chief Financial Officer, AMG Specialty Hospital–Slidell, Slidell, LA, p. A278


 Index of Health Care Professionals **A877**

MCGEE, Ken W.
Vice President Operations, Cornerstone Hospital of Houston – Bellaire, Houston, TX, p. A603
Vice President Hospital Development, Solara Hospital Harlingen–Brownsville Campus, Brownsville, TX, p. A585

MCGEE, Mark F., M.D. Chief Clinical Officer, Appalachian Behavioral Healthcare, Athens, OH, p. A470

MCGEE, Terry, Chief Operations Officer, Central State Hospital, Milledgeville, GA, p. A156

MCGILL, Cindy, Senior Vice President Human Resources, Presbyterian Kaseman Hospital, Albuquerque, NM, p. A414

MCGILL, Steve, Chief Financial Officer, Wabash General Hospital, Mount Carmel, IL, p. A188

MCGILL, Timothy W., Chief Executive Officer, River Park Hospital, Mc Minnville, TN, p. A570

MCGILVRAY, Greg, Chief Financial Officer, Medical Center Enterprise, Enterprise, AL, p. A19

MCGIMSEY, Erika, Controller, Jewish Hospital–Shelbyville, Shelbyville, KY, p. A259

MCGINLEY, Clement, M.D. Vice President Medical Affairs, Gnaden Huetten Memorial Hospital, Lehighton, PA, p. A527

MCGINNIS, Ronald, M.D. Medical Director, The University of Toledo Medical Center, Toledo, OH, p. A489

MCGINTY, Daniel B., Administrator, Essentia Health St. Mary's Medical Center, Duluth, MN, p. A330

MCGLADE, James, Director Human Resources, United Hospital, Saint Paul, MN, p. A339

MCGLEW, Timothy, Chief Executive Officer, Kern Valley Healthcare District, Lake Isabella, CA, p. A66

MCGLONE, Robert, Vice President Human Resources, Rapid City Regional Hospital, Rapid City, SD, p. A559

MCGLORY, Joyce, Vice President Human Resources, Methodist Hospitals, Gary, IN, p. A202

MCGLOTHLIN, Wylie, M.D. Chief Medical Officer, Henry County Hospital, New Castle, IN, p. A209

MCGOLDRICK, Margaret M., Executive Vice President and Administrator, Abington Memorial Hospital, Abington, PA, p. A517

MCGONNELL, James, Chief Financial Officer, Memorial Medical Center, Las Cruces, NM, p. A416

MCGOVERN, Julia, Vice President Human Resources, Chilton Hospital, Pompton Plains, NJ, p. A409

MCGOVERN, Pam, Director Technology, Huggins Hospital, Wolfeboro, NH, p. A400

MCGOWAN, Donna, Administrator, Lane County Hospital, Dighton, KS, p. A232

MCGOWAN, Gloria, Chief Financial Officer, Wiregrass Medical Center, Geneva, AL, p. A21

MCGOWAN, Marion A., Executive Vice President and Chief Operating Officer, Lancaster General Health, Lancaster, PA, p. A526

MCGOWEN, Bernard A., M.D. Medical Director, Kindred Hospital Tarrant County–Arlington, Arlington, TX, p. A579

MCGOWIN, III, Norman F., M.D. Chief of Staff, L. V. Stabler Memorial Hospital, Greenville, AL, p. A21

MCGRAIL, Robert, Chief Financial Officer, West Branch Regional Medical Center, West Branch, MI, p. A325

MCGRATH, Denise B., Chief Executive Officer, HEALTHSOUTH Sea Pines Rehabilitation Hospital, Melbourne, FL, p. A130

MCGRATH, Lynn, M.D. Vice President Medical Affairs, Deborah Heart and Lung Center, Browns Mills, NJ, p. A402

MCGRAW, Karin, Director, Veterans Affairs Medical Center, Beckley, WV, p. A670

MCGRAW, Scott, M.D. Medical Director, Irving Coppell Surgical Hospital, Irving, TX, p. A609

MCGREAHAM, David S., M.D. Vice President Medical Affairs, Munson Medical Center, Traverse City, MI, p. A324

MCGREGOR, Julie
Vice President and Chief People Officer, Jewish Hospital, Louisville, KY, p. A254
Director Human Resources, Sts. Mary & Elizabeth Hospital, Louisville, KY, p. A255

MCGREGOR, Randy, M.D. Medical Director, Fairbanks Memorial Hospital, Fairbanks, AK, p. A29

MCGREW, David S., Chief Financial Officer, Santa Clara Valley Medical Center, San Jose, CA, p. A88

MCGUE, Lisa, Controller, HEALTHSOUTH Northern Kentucky Rehabilitation Hospital, Edgewood, KY, p. A249

MCGUFFIN, Patty, R.N. Chief Nursing Officer, Allen County Hospital, Iola, KS, p. A235

MCGUIGAN, Kevin, M.D. Medical Director, St. Lawrence Rehabilitation Center, Lawrenceville, NJ, p. A405

MCGUIGAN, Timothy, Chief Human Resources, Veterans Affairs Medical Center, Salem, VA, p. A656

MCGUINNESS, Patrick, Chief Information Management, Keller Army Community Hospital, West Point, NY, p. A446

MCGUIRE, Ann M., Vice President Human Resources, Indiana University Health Ball Memorial Hospital, Muncie, IN, p. A209

MCGUIRE, Cynthia, Chief Operating Officer, Adirondack Medical Center, Saranac Lake, NY, p. A442

MCGUIRE, Glenn, Chief Financial Officer, LaFollette Medical Center, La Follette, TN, p. A569

MCGUIRE, H. Aryon, Administrator, E. A. Conway Medical Center, Monroe, LA, p. A273

MCGUIRE, Jay, Director Information Systems, Southeast Hospital, Cape Girardeau, MO, p. A357

MCGUIRE, Karen, Chief Financial Officer, Audubon County Memorial Hospital, Audubon, IA, p. A214

MCGUIRL, Mary, Director Information Systems, Oneida Healthcare, Oneida, NY, p. A439

MCGURK, Kevin, Controller, Bellin Psychiatric Center, Green Bay, WI, p. A682

MCHALE, John, Vice President Management Information Systems, Lower Bucks Hospital, Bristol, PA, p. A519

MCHUGH, Frank, Chief Financial Officer, Provena St. Mary's Hospital, Kankakee, IL, p. A185

MCHUGH, Michael J., M.D. Medical Director, Cleveland Clinic Children's Hospital for Rehabilitation, Cleveland, OH, p. A474

MCHUGH, William, M.D. Chief Medical Officer, Trinitas Regional Medical Center, Elizabeth, NJ, p. A403

MCILROY, Gail, Director Medical Records, Texas Specialty Hospital at Wichita Falls, Wichita Falls, TX, p. A635

MCILWAIN, Lisa
Vice President Human Resources, Miles Memorial Hospital, Damariscotta, ME, p. A283
Vice President Human Resources, St. Andrews Hospital and Healthcare Center, Boothbay Harbor, ME, p. A282

MCINTIRE, Jo, Chief Nursing Officer, Adams Memorial Hospital, Decatur, IN, p. A200

MCINTOSH, Charles, Senior Director Human Resources, University of Minnesota Medical Center, Fairview, Minneapolis, MN, p. A335

MCINTOSH, Joe, Director Management Information Systems, Logansport State Hospital, Logansport, IN, p. A207

MCINTOSH, Tyler, Chief Financial Officer, Creek Nation Community Hospital, Okemah, OK, p. A500

MCINTYRE, Cindy, R.N. Administrative Director Clinical Services, Magee General Hospital, Magee, MS, p. A349

MCINTYRE, Daniel J., President and Chief Executive Officer, The Charlotte Hungerford Hospital, Torrington, CT, p. A112

MCINTYRE, Kathleen, Province Leader, American Province of Little Company of Mary Sisters, Evergreen Park, IL, p. B9

MCINTYRE, Scott, FACHE Chief Executive Officer, Haskell County Community Hospital, Stigler, OK, p. A504

MCIWAIN, John, Director Human Resources, Wayne Memorial Hospital, Jesup, GA, p. A154

MCKARRY, Victor, M.D. President Medical Staff, Resurrection Medical Center, Chicago, IL, p. A177

MCKAY, Daniel E., Chief Executive Officer, Northwest Medical Center, Springdale, AR, p. A51

MCKAY, Danny H., Administrator, Noxubee General Hospital, Macon, MS, p. A349

MCKAY, Michael, Manager Information Systems, Wickenburg Community Hospital, Wickenburg, AZ, p. A41

MCKAY, Ronda, MSN Vice President Patient Care Services, Chief Nursing Officer, Community Hospital, Munster, IN, p. A209

MCKEE, Jed, M.D. Medical Director, Select Specialty Hospital–Topeka, Topeka, KS, p. A244

MCKEE, Robert J.
Vice President and Chief Human Resources Officer, Clearfield Hospital, Clearfield, PA, p. A520
Vice President Human Resources, DuBois Regional Medical Center, Du Bois, PA, p. A522

MCKEE, Scott, Chief Operating Officer, Wheeling Hospital, Wheeling, WV, p. A677

MCKEE, Jr., Willis P., M.D. Chief Medical Officer, Frankfort Regional Medical Center, Frankfort, KY, p. A250

MCKEEBY, Jon W., Chief Information Officer, National Institutes of Health Clinical Center, Bethesda, MD, p. A289

MCKEEN, Marcia, Director Human Resources, Twin Valley Behavioral Healthcare, Columbus, OH, p. A477

MCKELDIN, Pat, Human Resource Business Partner, Manteca Medical Center, Manteca, CA, p. A74

MCKELVEY, Robert
Director Information System, Mergers and Integrations, Indiana University Health Ball Memorial Hospital, Muncie, IN, p. A209
Chief Information Officer, Indiana University Health Blackford Hospital, Hartford City, IN, p. A203

MCKENNA, Bertine C., Ph.D. Executive Vice President and Chief Operating Officer, Bassett Medical Center, Cooperstown, NY, p. A424

MCKENNA, Chris, Director Human Resources, Manatee Glens Hospital and Addiction Center, Bradenton, FL, p. A119

MCKENNA, Dennis, M.D. Interim Vice President Medical Affairs, Albany Medical Center, Albany, NY, p. A420

MCKENNA, Donald, President and Chief Executive Officer, St. Mary's Health Care System, Athens, GA, p. A144

MCKENNA, John F., Chief Executive Officer and Managing Director, Rockford Center, Newark, DE, p. A114

MCKENNA, Kathleen, Public Affairs Leader, South Sacramento Medical Center, Sacramento, CA, p. A84

MCKENNA, Michael, M.D. Vice President Medical Management, Advocate Lutheran General Hospital, Park Ridge, IL, p. A191

MCKENNA, Quinn, Chief Operating Officer, University of Utah Health Care – Hospital and Clinics, Salt Lake City, UT, p. A641

MCKENZIE, Christine, Director Human Resources, Lake Norman Regional Medical Center, Mooresville, NC, p. A457

MCKENZIE, Jackie, Director Administrative Services, Beacham Memorial Hospital, Magnolia, MS, p. A349

MCKENZIE, Ryan, R.N. Director of Nursing, Aurora Behavioral Health System–Glendale, Glendale, AZ, p. A32

MCKENZIE, Susan Beth, Vice President Human Resources, St. Mary's Medical Center, Huntington, WV, p. A673

MCKENZIE, William G., Interim Administrator, Evergreen Medical Center, Evergreen, AL, p. A20

MCKENZIE, William G., President, Chief Executive Officer and Chairman, Gilliard Health Services, Montgomery, AL, p. B54

MCKEON, John, Vice President Human Resources, Kingsbrook Jewish Medical Center,, NY, p. A433

MCKEON, Vanessa, Interim Chief Financial Officer, University of Texas Harris County Psychiatric Center, Houston, TX, p. A607

MCKEOWN, Colleen, Senior Vice President and Area Manager, Hayward Medical Center, Hayward, CA, p. A64

MCKERNAN, Stephen W., Chief Executive Officer, University of New Mexico Hospitals, Albuquerque, NM, p. A415

MCKIDDY, Paul, Director Information Technology, Monroe County Medical Center, Tompkinsville, KY, p. A259

MCKIE, Kathy, Director Human Resources, Montrose Memorial Hospital, Montrose, CO, p. A104

MCKIMMY, Doyle L., FACH
Chief Executive Officer, Jewell County Hospital, Mankato, KS, p. A238
Chief Executive Officer, Washington County Hospital, Washington, KS, p. A245

MCKINLEY, Bryan, Chief Financial Officer, St. Mark's Hospital, Salt Lake City, UT, p. A641

MCKINLEY, Ernie, Chief Information Officer, University Medical Center, Las Vegas, NV, p. A394

MCKINLEY, Ivy, Director Human Resources, Our Lady of the Resurrection Medical Center, Chicago, IL, p. A177

MCKINLEY, Katie, Assistant Administrator/Nursing, Southwest Mississippi Regional Medical Center, McComb, MS, p. A349

MCKINLEY, Mike, Information Security Officer, West Texas VA Health Care System, Big Spring, TX, p. A584

MCKINLEY, Ronald, Ph.D. Vice President Human Resources and Employee Services, University of Texas Medical Branch Hospitals, Galveston, TX, p. A600

MCKINLEY, Jr., Rudolph, Vice President Operations and Chief Operating Officer, East Tennessee Children's Hospital, Knoxville, TN, p. A568

MCKINNEY, Carol, Director Information Services, Western Missouri Medical Center, Warrensburg, MO, p. A372

MCKINNEY, Dan, Administrator, Hermann Area District Hospital, Hermann, MO, p. A360

MCKINNEY, Diane, R.N. Vice President Patient Care Service, Decatur County Memorial Hospital, Greensburg, IN, p. A203

MCKINNEY, Jenny, Director Information Systems, Grant Memorial Hospital, Petersburg, WV, p. A674

MCKINNEY, Paul, Administrator, Martin County Hospital District, Stanton, TX, p. A628

MCKINNEY, Sally, Director Human Resources, Woodland Heights Medical Center, Lufkin, TX, p. A614

MCKINNEY, Sheila A., President, Texas Health Presbyterian Hospital Allen, Allen, TX, p. A577

MCKINNEY, Tressy, Director Information Services, Research Medical Center, Kansas City, MO, p. A362

MCKINNON, Ronald A., Chief Executive Officer, Benson Hospital, Benson, AZ, p. A31

MCKINNON, Scott, President and Chief Executive Officer, Memorial Hospital, North Conway, NH, p. A399

MCKINSTRY, Scott, M.D. Chief of Staff, Corpus Christi Medical Center, Corpus Christi, TX, p. A589

MCKNELLY, Lorenzo, D.O. Chief of Staff, Capital Region Medical Center, Jefferson City, MO, p. A361

MCKNIGHT, Craig L., Senior Vice President and Chief Financial Officer, Phoenix Children's Hospital, Phoenix, AZ, p. A36

MCKNIGHT, Richard B., Senior Vice President and Chief Information Officer, Presbyterian Hospital Huntersville, Huntersville, NC, p. A455

MCKOY, Lori, Business Partner, Pender Memorial Hospital, Burgaw, NC, p. A449

MCKULA, Tim, Vice President Information Systems and Chief Information Officer, Rehabilitation Institute of Chicago, Chicago, IL, p. A177

Index of Health Care Professionals / McQuiston

Index of Health Care Professionals

MCLAIN, Allen, M.D. Chief of Staff, Grisell Memorial Hospital District One, Ransom, KS, p. A242
MCLAIN, Cindy, Chief Executive Officer, Select Specialty Hospital–Fort Smith, Fort Smith, AR, p. A45
MCLAIN, Jerry, M.D. Chief of Staff, Chadron Community Hospital and Health Services, Chadron, NE, p. A382
MCLAIN, Kathy, Chief Financial Officer, Childress Regional Medical Center, Childress, TX, p. A587
MCLAIN, Terri L., FACHE President, Mercy Hospital Washington, Washington, MO, p. A372
MCLARTY, Walter L., Chief Human Resources Officer, Good Samaritan Hospital, Cincinnati, OH, p. A473
MCLAUGHLIN, Christine, Chief Financial Officer, Millinocket Regional Hospital, Millinocket, ME, p. A284
MCLAUGHLIN, Colleen, Director Employee Relations, Auburn Community Hospital, Auburn, NY, p. A421
MCLAUGHLIN, Gary, Vice President Finance and Chief Financial Officer, Overlake Hospital Medical Center, Bellevue, WA, p. A659
MCLAUGHLIN, Jason, Chief Financial Officer, McKenzie–Willamette Medical Center, Springfield, OR, p. A515
MCLAUGHLIN, Kathryn, Vice President and Chief Nursing Officer, Pacific Hospital of Long Beach, Long Beach, CA, p. A68
MCLAUGHLIN, Kevin, Director Information Systems, Saint Catherine Regional Hospital, Charlestown, IN, p. A199
MCLAUGHLIN, Maribeth, R.N. Vice President Patient Care Services, Magee–Womens Hospital of UPMC, Pittsburgh, PA, p. A535
MCLAUGHLIN, Neil R., R.N
Interim President, Hampshire Memorial Hospital, Romney, WV, p. A675
President, War Memorial Hospital, Berkeley Springs, WV, p. A670
MCLAUGHLIN, Pamela, Chief Financial Officer, HEALTHSOUTH Rehabilitation Hospital of Austin, Austin, TX, p. A580
MCLAUGHLIN, Sherry, Director Human Resources, Forrest City Medical Center, Forrest City, AR, p. A45
MCLAUGHLIN, Suzanne G., R.N. Chief Nursing Officer and Vice President Patient Care, St. Elizabeth's Medical Center, Brighton, MA, p. A298
MCLAUGHLIN, William J., Administrator, Thomas Hospital, Fairhope, AL, p. A20
MCLAURIN, Monty E., President and Chief Executive Officer, Indian Path Medical Center, Kingsport, TN, p. A568
MCLAURIN, Rod, Director Information Systems, Marlboro Park Hospital, Bennettsville, SC, p. A546
MCLEAN, Anthony, President, St. Francis Hospital, Federal Way, WA, p. A661
MCLEAN, Beatrice J., Director, Searcy Hospital, Mount Vernon, AL, p. A24
MCLEAN, Bill, Senior Vice President Human Resources, Avera McKennan Hospital and University Health Center, Sioux Falls, SD, p. A559
MCLEAN, Chris J., Chief Financial Officer, Methodist Healthcare Memphis Hospitals, Memphis, TN, p. A572
MCLEAN, Georgia, Director Human Resources, Mount Sinai Medical Center, Miami Beach, FL, p. A132
MCLEAN, Michael A., Chief Executive Officer, Regency Hospital of Northwest Arkansas, Fayetteville, AR, p. A44
MCLEAN, Nicole, Chief Nursing Officer, Select Specialty Hospital–Flint, Flint, MI, p. A312
MCLELLAN, Ava, Coordinator Human Resources, HEALTHSOUTH Rehabilitation Hospital of Spring Hill, Brooksville, FL, p. A120
MCLENDON, Carla
Director Human Resources, Appling Healthcare System, Baxley, GA, p. A147
Director Information Resource Management Services, Charles George Veterans Affairs Medical Center, Asheville, NC, p. A448
MCLENDON, Connie, Director Human Resources, Piedmont Mountainside Hospital, Jasper, GA, p. A154
MCLENDON, John, Senior Vice President and Chief Information Officer, Adventist Bolingbrook Hospital, Bolingbrook, IL, p. A174
MCLENNAN, Marlene, Controller, Monroe County Hospital, Forsyth, GA, p. A153
MCLEOD, Sheldon, Chief Operating Officer, North Central Bronx Hospital,, NY, p. A436
MCLIN, Robert D., President and Chief Executive Officer, Good Samaritan Hospital, Vincennes, IN, p. A212
MCLISTER, Charles, Chief Executive Officer, Fairmount Behavioral Health System, Philadelphia, PA, p. A532
MCLOONE, Paul, M.D
Chief Medical Officer, Trinity Bettendorf, Bettendorf, IA, p. A214
Chief Medical Officer, Trinity Rock Island, Rock Island, IL, p. A192
MCMAHON, Chris, Chief Operating Officer, The Medical Center of Southeast Texas, Port Arthur, TX, p. A622
MCMAHON, Elaine, Administrator, Kwajalein Hospital, Kwajalein Island, MH, p. A699
MCMAHON, Eugene J., M.D. President and Chief Executive Officer, Provena Saint Joseph Hospital, Elgin, IL, p. A181
MCMAHON, Nancy, Vice President Human Resources, Miriam Hospital, Providence, RI, p. A544
MCMANUS, Kathleen A., Executive Vice President/Chief Operating Officer, Munson Medical Center, Traverse City, MI, p. A324
MCMANUS, Lawrence E., President and Chief Executive Officer, Catholic Health Services of Long Island, Rockville Centre, NY, p. B29
MCMANUS, Michael T., Chief Operating Officer, Memorial Hospital, Belleville, IL, p. A173
MCMANUS, Ronald, Senior Vice President Clinical Services and Business Entities, Peconic Bay Medical Center, Riverhead, NY, p. A441
MCMANUS, Tim
Interim Chief Executive Officer, CJW Medical Center, Richmond, VA, p. A654
President and Chief Executive Officer, Reston Hospital Center, Reston, VA, p. A654
MCMASTER, Sandra
Regional Chief Information Officer, Kauai Veterans Memorial Hospital, Waimea, HI, p. A165
Regional Chief Information Officer, Samuel Mahelona Memorial Hospital, Kapaa, HI, p. A164
MCMATH, Mark W., Chief Information Officer, Indiana University Health Bloomington Hospital, Bloomington, IN, p. A198
MCMENAMIN, Anneliese, Vice President Human Resources, Kennedy Memorial Hospitals–University Medical Center, Cherry Hill, NJ, p. A403
MCMICHEN, Diane, Director Human Resources, DeKalb Regional Medical Center, Fort Payne, AL, p. A20
MCMILLAN, Deborah, Director Human Resources, Glenn Medical Center, Willows, CA, p. A96
MCMILLAN, Don, Chief Information Officer, Sacred Heart Medical Center, Eugene, OR, p. A510
MCMILLAN, Douglas A., Administrator and Chief Executive Officer, West Park Hospital, Cody, WY, p. A696
MCMILLAN, Irene, Chief Financial Officer, Sierra Vista Hospital, Sacramento, CA, p. A84
MCMILLAN, James, Vice President Finance, Capital Region Medical Center, Jefferson City, MO, p. A361
MCMILLAN, Jon R., Chief Financial Officer, Beatrice Community Hospital and Health Center, Beatrice, NE, p. A382
MCMILLAN, Linda, Human Resources Specialist, Choctaw Health Center, Philadelphia, MS, p. A351
MCMILLAN, Sheila, Chief Financial Officer, Park Nicollet Methodist Hospital, Saint Louis Park, MN, p. A339
MCMILLAN, William, M.D. Vice President Medical Affairs, Norman Regional Health System, Norman, OK, p. A500
MCMILLAN, William I., FACHE Chief Executive Officer, Curry General Hospital, Gold Beach, OR, p. A510
MCMILLEN, Eric, Interim Chief Executive Officer, Ochsner Medical Center–Baton Rouge, Baton Rouge, LA, p. A262
MCMINN, Melvin, Director Human Resources, Wernersville State Hospital, Wernersville, PA, p. A540
MCMORROUGH, Jerry L., Vice President Human Resources, Medical Center of Arlington, Arlington, TX, p. A579
MCMULLEN, Ronald B., President, Christian Hospital, Saint Louis, MO, p. A368
MCMULLEN, Thomas A.
Chief Financial Officer, Kindred Hospital–Delaware County, Darby, PA, p. A521
Chief Financial Officer, Kindred Hospital–Philadelphia, Philadelphia, PA, p. A533
MCMURRAY, Jean Ann, R.N. Chief Nursing Officer, Jacksonville Medical Center, Jacksonville, AL, p. A22
MCMURRAY, Sean S., FACHE Vice President and Chief Executive Officer, Johnston Memorial Hospital, Abingdon, VA, p. A645
MCMURREN, MaryAnne, R.N. Administrator and Chief Executive Officer, Cottage Grove Community Hospital, Cottage Grove, OR, p. A510
MCMURRY, Timothy, Associate Director Operations, Iowa City Veterans Affairs Health Care System, Iowa City, IA, p. A221
MCNABB, Teresita, R.N. Vice President Nursing Services, Terrebonne General Medical Center, Houma, LA, p. A268
MCNAIR, Lisa, CP
Senior Vice President and Chief Financial Officer, Burleson St. Joseph Health Center, Caldwell, TX, p. A586
Senior Vice President and Chief Financial Officer, Grimes St. Joseph Health Center, Navasota, TX, p. A618
Senior Vice President and Chief Financial Officer, St. Joseph Regional Health Center, Bryan, TX, p. A586
MCNAIR, Michael H., Chief Executive Officer, Sandhills Regional Medical Center, Hamlet, NC, p. A454
MCNALLY, Joseph, M.D. Medical Director, Streamwood Behavioral Health Center, Streamwood, IL, p. A195
MCNALLY, Kathy, Chief Nursing Officer, HEALTHSOUTH Rehabilitation Hospital at Drake, Cincinnati, OH, p. A473
MCNALLY, Lou-Ann, Director Human Resources, Claxton–Hepburn Medical Center, Ogdensburg, NY, p. A439
MCNAMARA, Marilyn, M.D. Vice President Medical Affairs, Southwest General Health Center, Middleburg Heights, OH, p. A485
MCNAMARA, Mike, Chief Information Officer, George L. Mee Memorial Hospital, King City, CA, p. A65
MCNAMARA, Steve, Chief Financial Officer, Orange Coast Memorial Medical Center, Fountain Valley, CA, p. A61
MCNAMARA, Thomas, D.O. Vice President Medical Management, WellStar Cobb Hospital, Austell, GA, p. A147
MCNAMARA, Timothy M.
Senior Vice President Human Resources, Bradford Regional Medical Center, Bradford, PA, p. A519
Senior Vice President Human Resources, Olean General Hospital, Olean, NY, p. A439
MCNAMARA, Tom, Director Information Technology, Community Hospital of the Monterey Peninsula, Monterey, CA, p. A75
MCNAUGHTON, Richard, Chief Information Management Service, Veterans Affairs Medical Center, Togus, ME, p. A285
MCNEA, Melvin, Chief Operating Officer, Great Plains Regional Medical Center, North Platte, NE, p. A386
MCNEECE, Steve, Chief Executive Officer, Community Hospital of Anaconda, Anaconda, MT, p. A373
MCNEEL, Wakelin, M.D. Medical Director, BHC Alhambra Hospital, Rosemead, CA, p. A83
MCNEICE, Keith, Vice President and Chief Information Officer, Carolinas Medical Center–NorthEast, Concord, NC, p. A451
MCNEIL, Greg R., Chief Executive Officer, Lincoln County Hospital, Lincoln, KS, p. A238
MCNEIL, John, President and Chief Executive Officer, Eastern Regional Medical Center, Philadelphia, PA, p. A532
MCNEIL, Karen
Chief Nursing Officer, University Hospitals Conneaut Medical Center, Conneaut, OH, p. A478
Chief Nursing Officer, University Hospitals Geneva Medical Center, Geneva, OH, p. A481
MCNEILL, Michael, Chief Financial Management, Veterans Affairs Medical Center, Albuquerque, NM, p. A415
MCNETT, Dale, M.D. Medical Director, Warren General Hospital, Warren, PA, p. A540
MCNEY, Jim, Vice President Finance and Chief Financial Officer, North Kansas City Hospital, North Kansas City, MO, p. A366
MCNULTY III,, Joseph S., President and Chief Executive Officer, Pioneer Health Services, Magee, MS, p. B102
MCNULTY, Stephanie, Chief Operating Officer, St. Petersburg General Hospital, Saint Petersburg, FL, p. A138
MCNULTY, Tim, Vice President Human Resources, Grace Cottage Hospital, Townshend, VT, p. A644
MCNUTT, Pamela
Vice President Information Systems, Methodist Charlton Medical Center, Dallas, TX, p. A591
Senior Vice President and Chief Information Officer, Methodist Dallas Medical Center, Dallas, TX, p. A592
Senior Vice President and Chief Information Officer, Methodist Mansfield Medical Center, Mansfield, TX, p. A615
MCOLVIN, Tom, Executive Director, Sagamore Children's Psychiatric Center, Dix Hills, NY, p. A425
MCPHERSON, Archie, M.D. Vice President and Chief Medical Officer, Virginia Hospital Center – Arlington, Arlington, VA, p. A645
MCPHERSON, Lon, M.D. Senior Vice President Medical Affairs and Chief Quality Officer, Munroe Regional Medical Center, Ocala, FL, p. A133
MCPHERSON, Rhonda, Vice President Human Resources, Fayette Regional Health System, Connersville, IN, p. A199
MCPHETRES, Joyce, Vice President Human Resources, Bridgton Hospital, Bridgton, ME, p. A282
MCQUADE, Linda, Director Information Management, Kindred Hospital South Florida–Hollywood,, FL, p. A125
MCQUAID, Bill, Assistant Vice President and Chief Information Officer, Parkview Adventist Medical Center, Brunswick, ME, p. A282
MCQUAID, David P., FACHE President and Chief Operating Officer, Thomas Jefferson University Hospital, Philadelphia, PA, p. A534
MCQUAIDE, Teresa A., Chief Executive Officer, Trenton Psychiatric Hospital, Trenton, NJ, p. A411
MCQUEEN, Elbert T., President and Chief Executive Officer, Central Georgia Rehabilitation Hospital, Macon, GA, p. A155
MCQUILLAN, Kent, Chief Information Officer, Summit Healthcare Regional Medical Center, Show Low, AZ, p. A38
MCQUILLEN, D. Paul, D.O. Chief of Staff, Mercy Medical Center–New Hampton, New Hampton, IA, p. A224
MCQUISTAN, Bob, Vice President Finance, York General Hospital, York, NE, p. A390
MCQUISTON, Mike, Director Human Resources, Wise Regional Health System, Decatur, TX, p. A593

 Index of Health Care Professionals A879

Index of Health Care Professionals
Index of Health Care Professionals / McRae

MCRAE, Paul, M.D. Chief of Staff, Bayfront Medical Center, Saint Petersburg, FL, p. A138
MCROBERTS, Susan, R.N. Vice President and Chief Nursing Officer, Franciscan St. Francis Health – Indianapolis, Indianapolis, IN, p. A204
MCRORIE, Sherri, Director Human Resources, Anson Community Hospital, Wadesboro, NC, p. A462
MCRORY, Diana, Director Human Resources, Doctor's Memorial Hospital, Perry, FL, p. A136
MCSHAY, Kristi, Chief Executive Officer, Arizona Spine and Joint Hospital, Mesa, AZ, p. A33
MCSWAIN, Marilyn, MSN, Administrator, Lake Charles Memorial Hospital for Women, Lake Charles, LA, p. A271
MCSWEENEY, Greg, M.D. Vice President Medical Affairs, Carney Hospital, Boston, MA, p. A296
MCTAGGART, Jac, Chief Executive Officer, Hillsboro Medical Center, Hillsboro, ND, p. A466
MCTAGUE, Jerome, JD, Administrator and Chief Executive Officer, Physician's Choice Hospital – Fremont, Fremont, OH, p. A480
MCTIGRIT, Chris, Manager Information Technology, Delta Memorial Hospital, Dumas, AR, p. A44
MCTIGUE, Michael
Chief Information Officer, Clara Maass Medical Center, Belleville, NJ, p. A401
Chief Information Officer, Saint Barnabas Medical Center, Livingston, NJ, p. A405
MCVAY, Randall, Chief Executive Officer, Ocala Regional Medical Center, Ocala, FL, p. A133
MCVEIGH, Kevin
Interim Chief Human Resources Officer, Banner Behavioral Health Hospital – Scottsdale, Scottsdale, AZ, p. A38
Chief Human Resources Officer, Banner Desert Medical Center, Mesa, AZ, p. A34
MCVEY, Eric A., M.D. Vice President and Chief Medical Officer, Mississippi Baptist Medical Center, Jackson, MS, p. A348
MCVEY, Lynn, President and Chief Executive Officer, Meadowlands Hospital Medical Center, Secaucus, NJ, p. A410
MCVEY, Marty, Chief Executive Officer, Spring Branch Medical Center, Houston, TX, p. A606
MCVEY, Timothy J., Chief Financial Officer, Mission Regional Medical Center, Mission, TX, p. A617
MCVICKER, Sandra I., MSN, Chief Executive Officer, University Hospital McDuffie, Thomson, GA, p. A160
MCWATTERS III, David M., President and Chief Executive Officer, Highland Hospital, Charleston, WV, p. A671
MCWAY, Jacob, Senior Vice President and Chief Financial Officer, Lester E. Cox Medical Centers, Springfield, MO, p. A371
MCWHIRT, Robert, Vice President Patient Care Services and Chief Nursing Executive, Calvert Memorial Hospital, Prince Frederick, MD, p. A293
MCWHORTER III, John B., President, Baylor University Medical Center, Dallas, TX, p. A590
MCWHORTER, Sharon, Director Information Systems, Ephraim McDowell Fort Logan Hospital, Stanford, KY, p. A259
MCWILLIAMS, Terrence R., M.D. Vice President Medical Affairs, Newport Hospital, Newport, RI, p. A544
MEACHAM, Sherry, Coordinator Human Resources, Select Specialty Hospital–Winston–Salem, Winston–Salem, NC, p. A463
MEACHAM, Steve, Vice President Finance, King's Daughters' Hospital and Health Services, Madison, IN, p. A208
MEACHAM, Verna, Chief Executive Officer, Fort Washington Medical Center, Fort Washington, MD, p. A291
MEACHEM, Michelle, Director Human Resources, Elizabethtown Community Hospital, Elizabethtown, NY, p. A425
MEAD, Barbara, Executive Director, Lourdes Counseling Center, Richland, WA, p. A665
MEAD, Linda, Director Human Resources, Margaretville Hospital, Margaretville, NY, p. A429
MEAD, Richard, Senior Director Human Resources, Saint Francis Memorial Hospital, San Francisco, CA, p. A87
MEAD, Rick, Human Resources Leader, Oakland Medical Center, Oakland, CA, p. A77
MEADE, Jeff, M.D. Chief Medical Officer, Watertown Regional Medical Center, Watertown, WI, p. A692
MEADE, Robert C., Chief Executive Officer, Doctors Hospital of Sarasota, Sarasota, FL, p. A138
MEADOR, Debra, Assistant Administrator, Stonewall Memorial Hospital, Aspermont, TX, p. A580
MEADOWS, Barbara, Chief Financial Manager, Captain James A. Lovell Federal Health Care Center, North Chicago, IL, p. A189
MEADOWS, Danny, M.D. Medical Director, Logansport State Hospital, Logansport, IN, p. A207
MEADOWS, Hal, M.D. Chief Medical Officer, Banner Lassen Medical Center, Susanville, CA, p. A92
MEADOWS, Julia, Chief Financial Officer, Virginia Gay Hospital, Vinton, IA, p. A227
MEADOWS, Michael J., Chief Executive Officer, Livingston Regional Hospital, Livingston, TN, p. A570
MEADOWS, Nancy, Chief Financial Officer, Methodist Hospital, San Antonio, TX, p. A625
MEADOWS, Peri, Director Human Resources, Rhea Medical Center, Dayton, TN, p. A565
MEANS, Dennis, M.D. Vice President Medical Affairs, Carilion New River Valley Medical Center, Christiansburg, VA, p. A646
MEANS, Jr., William H., Administrator, Bastrop Rehabilitation Hospital, Bastrop, LA, p. A262
MEARNS, Stephanie, Vice President Patient Care Services and Chief Nurse Executive, Seton Medical Center, Daly City, CA, p. A59
MEARS, Terry, Director Information Systems, Durham Regional Hospital, Durham, NC, p. A452
MECHLING, Glenn C., FACH
Senior Vice President Human Resources, Muncy Valley Hospital, Muncy, PA, p. A530
Senior Vice President Human Resources, Williamsport Regional Medical Center, Williamsport, PA, p. A542
MEDAGLIA, Guy A., President and Chief Executive Officer, Saint Anthony Hospital, Chicago, IL, p. A178
MEDCIROS, Ron, Director Applied Information Technology, Worcester State Hospital, Worcester, MA, p. A306
MEDEIROS, Barbara, R.N. Chief Nurse Executive, Memorial Hospital Los Banos, Los Banos, CA, p. A73
MEDEIROS, Katherine, President and Chief Executive Officer, Sierra Nevada Memorial Hospital, Grass Valley, CA, p. A64
MEDEROS, Ana J., Chief Executive Officer, Palmetto General Hospital, Hialeah, FL, p. A125
MEDINA, Alberto, Information Technology Senior Consultant, Hospital Manati Medical Center, Manati, PR, p. A701
MEDINA, Alma, R.N. Chief Executive Officer, Cornerstone Regional Hospital, Edinburg, TX, p. A595
MEDINA, Betsmari, Director Human Resources, Dr. Ramon E. Betances Hospital–Mayaguez Medical Center Branch, Mayaguez, PR, p. A702
MEDINA, Ed, M.D. Medical Director, Phillips County Hospital, Malta, MT, p. A377
MEDINA, Eleanor, M.D. Chief Medical Officer, Behavioral Center of Michigan, Warren, MI, p. A324
MEDINA, Luz D., Controller, Hospital Hermanos Melendez, Bayamon, PR, p. A700
MEDINA, Marco, Chief Information Officer, Stanton County Hospital, Johnson, KS, p. A235
MEDINA, Shelbie, Chief People Officer, Buchanan County Health Center, Independence, IA, p. A221
MEDIRATTA, Ravinder P., M.D. Chief of Staff, Bronson LakeView Hospital, Paw Paw, MI, p. A320
MEDLEY, Adron, M.D. Chief Medical Staff, Northern Rockies Medical Center, Cut Bank, MT, p. A374
MEDLEY, Barry, Director Information Systems, Cook Medical Center–A Campus of Tift Regional Medical Center, Adel, GA, p. A144
MEDLEY, Dennis, Administrator, Physicians' Medical Center, New Albany, IN, p. A209
MEDLEY, Wathen, M.D. Chief Medical Officer, Owensboro Medical Health System, Owensboro, KY, p. A257
MEDLIN, John, Chief Nursing Officer, North Carolina Specialty Hospital, Durham, NC, p. A452
MEDLOCK, Beth, Manager Information Technology, Jackson Hospital, Marianna, FL, p. A130
MEDLOCK, Darci, Manager Human Resources, St. Vincent Dunn Hospital, Bedford, IN, p. A197
MEDOVICH, Lisa
Senior Vice President and Chief Financial Officer, Hillside Rehabilitation Hospital, Warren, OH, p. A490
Senior Vice President and Chief Financial Officer, Northside Medical Center, Youngstown, OH, p. A492
Senior Vice President and Chief Financial Officer, Trumbull Memorial Hospital, Warren, OH, p. A490
MEDRANO, Ruben, M.D. President Medical Staff, OSF Holy Family Medical Center, Monmouth, IL, p. A188
MEDRANO, Samuel, M.D. Chief of Staff, Colusa Regional Medical Center, Colusa, CA, p. A58
MEDUNA, Leo L., M.D. Chief Medical Officer, Saunders Medical Center, Wahoo, NE, p. A390
MEE, Thomas, R.N. Vice President Operations, McLaren Lapeer Region, Lapeer, MI, p. A317
MEEHAN, Neil S., D.O. Chief Medical Officer and Chief Medical Information Officer, Lawrence General Hospital, Lawrence, MA, p. A301
MEEK, Julie, Vice President Finance, Kadlec Medical Center, Richland, WA, p. A665
MEEKER, Brian, D.O. President Medical Staff, Virginia Gay Hospital, Vinton, IA, p. A227
MEEKER, Mark, D.O. Medical Staff President, OSF St. Mary Medical Center, Galesburg, IL, p. A182
MEEKINS, Lance, Administrator, Nocona General Hospital, Nocona, TX, p. A618
MEEKINS, Michelle, Manager Human Resources, Sentara Virginia Beach General Hospital, Virginia Beach, VA, p. A657
MEEKS, Julia M., Chief Operating Officer, Specialty Hospital of Lorain, Amherst, OH, p. A469
MEENK, Susan
Vice President Service Area, Providence Centralia Hospital, Centralia, WA, p. A660
Vice President Service Area, Providence St. Peter Hospital, Olympia, WA, p. A663
MEERT, Tiffany, Chief Operating Officer, Northern Nevada Medical Center, Sparks, NV, p. A396
MEESE, Larry, Chief Executive Officer, Jackson Hospital, Marianna, FL, p. A130
MEESIG, Deborah, M.D. Chief of Staff, Veterans Affairs Medical Center, Chillicothe, OH, p. A472
MEGEHEE, Mark, Vice President and Chief Information Officer, Decatur General Hospital, Decatur, AL, p. A18
MEGGS, Christi, Director Human Resources, Marlboro Park Hospital, Bennettsville, SC, p. A546
MEGLI, Cami, Controller, Morrison Community Hospital, Morrison, IL, p. A188
MEGOW, Kimberly, M.D. Chief Medical Officer, South Georgia Medical Center, Valdosta, GA, p. A161
MEGUIAR, Ramon V., M.D. Senior Vice President and Chief Medical Officer, Memorial Health, Savannah, GA, p. A159
MEHAFFEY, M. Beth, Vice President Human Resources, Baptist Medical Center, Jacksonville, FL, p. A126
MEHARG, John, Director Health Information Technology, Norman Regional Health System, Norman, OK, p. A500
MEHINDRU, Vinay, M.D
Vice President/Chief Medical Officer, Florida Hospital Waterman, Tavares, FL, p. A141
Medical Director, Wuesthoff Medical Center – Rockledge, Rockledge, FL, p. A137
MEHLER, Philip, M.D. Chief Medical Officer, Denver Health Medical Center, Denver, CO, p. A99
MEHRINGER, Todd, Director Information Systems, Memorial Hospital and Health Care Center, Jasper, IN, p. A205
MEHTA, Kalpana, Chief Fiscal Services, Jesse Brown Veterans Affairs Chicago Health Care System, Chicago, IL, p. A176
MEHTA, Raj, Chief Financial Officer, Medina Memorial Hospital, Medina, NY, p. A429
MEHUS, James, M.D. Chief of Staff, Sanford Medical Center Mayville, Mayville, ND, p. A467
MEIAR, Cindy, Human Resources and Payroll Coordinator, Trego County–Lemke Memorial Hospital, Wakeeney, KS, p. A244
MEIDINGER, Duane, Vice President Finance, Walla Walla General Hospital, Walla Walla, WA, p. A669
MEIDINGER, Sue, Manager Business Office, Linton Hospital, Linton, ND, p. A467
MEIER, Suzanne S., System Director, Compensation and Human Resources Technology, Memorial Hermann Memorial City Medical Center, Houston, TX, p. A605
MEIER, Timothy
Chief Financial Officer, Alegent Health–Lakeside Hospital, Omaha, NE, p. A387
Chief Financial Officer, Alegent Health–Midlands Hospital, Papillion, NE, p. A389
MEIERGERD, Jean, Chief Information Officer, St. Francis Memorial Hospital, West Point, NE, p. A390
MEIERS, Dawn, Coordinator Medical Staff and Personnel Services, Southeast Michigan Surgical Hospital, Warren, MI, p. A325
MEIGS, Jeffrey L., Chief Financial Officer, Louis A. Weiss Memorial Hospital, Chicago, IL, p. A176
MEIGS, Jr., John, M.D. Chief of Staff, Bibb Medical Center, Centreville, AL, p. A18
MEINDEL, Nympha, R.N. Chief Information Officer, North Shore University Hospital, Manhasset, NY, p. A429
MEINHART, Richard, Manager Information Systems, Daviess Community Hospital, Washington, IN, p. A213
MEINKOTH, Jennifer, Chief Information Officer, Memorial Hospital, Belleville, IL, p. A173
MEIS, Fred J., Chief Executive Officer, Kearney County Health Services, Minden, NE, p. A386
MEISNER, Anne, MSN, President and Chief Executive Officer, Midwestern Regional Medical Center, Zion, IL, p. A196
MEISSNER, Shari, Chief Financial Officer, Liberty Medical Center, Chester, MT, p. A374
MEISTER, Steven, M.D. Chief of Staff, Avera Marshall Regional Medical Center, Marshall, MN, p. A334
MEITZ, Mary, Vice President Finance, Bronson Methodist Hospital, Kalamazoo, MI, p. A316
MEKALA, Bhavani P., M.D. President Medical Staff, Christ Hospital, Jersey City, NJ, p. A405
MEKHJIAN, Hagop, M.D. Medical Director, Ohio State University Medical Center, Columbus, OH, p. A477
MELAHN, Will L., M.D. Vice President Medical Affairs and Chief Medical Officer, St. Claire Regional Medical Center, Morehead, KY, p. A256

A880 Index of Health Care Professionals

Index of Health Care Professionals / Meyer

MELANCON, Derek, Director Human Resources and Marketing, Springhill Medical Center, Springhill, LA, p. A278
MELANCON, Mary, Chief Financial Officer, Abrom Kaplan Memorial Hospital, Kaplan, LA, p. A269
MELAND, Jeff, M.D. Vice President, Chief Medical Officer, Northfield Hospital, Northfield, MN, p. A336
MELARAGNO, Robert, Vice President Finance, O'Bleness Memorial Hospital, Athens, OH, p. A470
MELARAGNO, Tony, M.D. Chief Administrative Officer, Legacy Good Samaritan Hospital and Medical Center, Portland, OR, p. A514
MELBOURNE, John, M.D. Medical Director, Conifer Park, Glenville, NY, p. A426
MELBY, Gina, Chief Executive Officer, J. F. K. Medical Center, Atlantis, FL, p. A118
MELBY, Larry, Chief Executive Officer, Select Specialty Hospital–Palm Beach, Lake Worth, FL, p. A128
MELCHIODE, J. D., Chief Operating Officer, MountainView Hospital, Las Vegas, NV, p. A393
MELCHIOR, Eric L., Executive Vice President and Chief Financial Officer, Greater Baltimore Medical Center, Baltimore, MD, p. A287
MELENDEZ, Alma, Controller, Dimmit County Memorial Hospital, Carrizo Springs, TX, p. A586
MELENDEZ, Eddie, Director Human Resources, Brownsville Doctors Hospital, Brownsville, TX, p. A585
MELENDEZ, Pedro
Administrator, Centro De Salud Conductual Menonita–CIMA, Aibonito, PR, p. A699
Administrator, Hospital Menonita De Cayey, Cayey, PR, p. A700
Administrator, Mennonite General Hospital, Aibonito, PR, p. A699
MELGAR, Sergio L., Vice President Health Affairs and Chief Financial Officer, UK HealthCare Good Samaritan Hospital, Lexington, KY, p. A253
MELIN, Craig N., President and Chief Executive Officer, Cooley Dickinson Hospital, Northampton, MA, p. A303
MELL, Kevin, Vice President Operations, Medstar Montgomery Medical Center, Olney, MD, p. A293
MELL, Vicki, Vice President Human Resources, Ohio Valley General Hospital, McKees Rocks, PA, p. A528
MELLETT, David, Chief Financial Officer, Boone County Hospital, Boone, IA, p. A215
MELLO, Brett, Chief Information Officer, Rehoboth McKinley Christian Health Care Services, Gallup, NM, p. A416
MELLO, Paul, Manager Data Processing, Metropolitan State Hospital, Norwalk, CA, p. A77
MELLON, Monte, M.D. Chief of Staff, Catalina Island Medical Center, Avalon, CA, p. A54
MELSON, Benjamin B., CPA Executive Vice President and Chief Financial Officer, Texas Children's Hospital, Houston, TX, p. A607
MELTON, Georgia, Associate Vice President Human Resources, University of Texas Health Science Center at Tyler, Tyler, TX, p. A632
MELTON, Linda Dickey, Vice President Human Resources, North Arkansas Regional Medical Center, Harrison, AR, p. A45
MELTVEDT, Jr., Robert, M.D. Vice President Medical Affairs, Warren Memorial Hospital, Front Royal, VA, p. A648
MELTZER, David B., Chief Financial Officer, Texas Health Presbyterian Hospital Denton, Denton, TX, p. A594
MELTZER, Neil M., President and Chief Operating Officer, Sinai Hospital of Baltimore, Baltimore, MD, p. A289
MELVILLE, Carol, Director Human Resources, West Houston Medical Center, Houston, TX, p. A608
MELVIN, Susan, D.O. Chief Medical Officer, Long Beach Memorial Medical Center, Long Beach, CA, p. A68
MELZER, Douglas L., Chief Executive Officer, Long Beach Medical Center, Long Beach, NY, p. A429
MENCHINI, August F., Director Human Resources, Eastern Long Island Hospital, Greenport, NY, p. A427
MENDELOWITZ, Susan, Executive Vice President and Chief Operating Officer, Bergen Regional Medical Center, Paramus, NJ, p. A408
MENDENHALL, David, Chief Information Officer, Hutchinson Regional Medical Center, Hutchinson, KS, p. A235
MENDEZ, Aaron, Director Management Information Systems, Hospital De La Concepcion, San German, PR, p. A702
MENDEZ, Alex A., Senior Vice President and Chief Financial Officer, Mount Sinai Medical Center, Miami Beach, FL, p. A132
MENDEZ, Kim K., Ed.D. Vice President and Chief Nursing Officer, Brookhaven Memorial Hospital Medical Center, Patchogue, NY, p. A440
MENDEZ, Lincoln S., Chief Executive Officer, Baptist Health South Florida, South Miami Hospital, Miami, FL, p. A130
MENDIOLA, Rosie L., Director Information Systems, South Texas Health System, Edinburg, TX, p. A595
MENDOZA, Dana, Chief Information Officer, Maui Memorial Medical Center, Wailuku, HI, p. A165
MENDOZA, Glenda, Acting Chief Executive Officer, The Hospital at Craig Ranch, McKinney, TX, p. A616
MENDOZA, Yolanda, Director Human Resources, Rehabilitation Hospital of Southern New Mexico, Las Cruces, NM, p. A416
MENENDEZ, Deborah, VP Human Resources, Bayfront Medical Center, Saint Petersburg, FL, p. A138
MENGEL, Nancy, Director Information Technology, Inova Loudoun Hospital, Leesburg, VA, p. A650
MENGLE, Scott, Vice President Human Resources, St. Joseph Medical Center, Reading, PA, p. A537
MENKES, Jeffrey, President and Chief Executive Officer, New York Downtown Hospital, New York, NY, p. A435
MENNONNA, Guy, Senior Vice President Human Resources, Bergen Regional Medical Center, Paramus, NJ, p. A408
MENON, Rema, M.D. Clinical Director, Parsons State Hospital and Training Center, Parsons, KS, p. A241
MENOR, Peter, Vice President Operations, Chandler Regional Medical Center, Chandler, AZ, p. A31
MENSCH, Alan, M.D. Senior Vice President Medical Affairs, Plainview Hospital, Plainview, NY, p. A440
MENSEN, Amy, Chief Administrative Officer, Regional Medical Center, Manchester, IA, p. A222
MENTON, Timothy P., Interim Chief Executive Officer, Westlake Regional Hospital, Columbia, KY, p. A248
MERCADO, Leda Marta R, Chief Operating Officer, Hospital Menonita De Cayey, Cayey, PR, p. A700
MERCADO, Sylvia, Executive Director, University Pediatric Hospital,, PR, p. A704
MERCENE, Maro, Chief Information Officer, Los Angeles Metropolitan Medical Center, Los Angeles, CA, p. A70
MERCER, David, Coordinator Information Systems, Baptist Memorial Hospital–Union City, Union City, TN, p. A576
MERCER, Shawna, Director Human Resources, Kansas Neurological Institute, Topeka, KS, p. A244
MERCER, William, M.D. Director, Peterson Rehabilitation Hospital, Wheeling, WV, p. A676
MERCHANT, Ron, M.D. Medical Director, Schick Shadel Hospital, Seattle, WA, p. A666
MERCIECA, Rita, R.N. Executive Director, Forest Hills Hospital,, NY, p. A432
MERCIER, Linda, MSN, Chief Executive Officer, Houston Northwest Medical Center, Houston, TX, p. A604
MERCIER, Rita, Manager Finance, James A. Haley Veterans Hospital, Tampa, FL, p. A140
MERCURI, Ralph, Vice President and Chief Financial Officer, Major Hospital, Shelbyville, IN, p. A211
MERCURIO, Paul, M.D. Medical Director, Summit Park Hospital and Nursing Care Center, Pomona, NY, p. A440
MEREDITH, Linda, MSN Chief Operating Officer, Scott & White Hospital – Llano, Llano, TX, p. A613
MEREDITH, Stephen L., Chief Executive Officer, Twin Lakes Regional Medical Center, Leitchfield, KY, p. A252
MEREK, Gloria, Director of Nursing, Springfield Hospital Center, Sykesville, MD, p. A294
MERILLO, Myra, Supervisor Health Information Management, HEALTHSOUTH Rehabilitation Hospital of Spring Hill, Brooksville, FL, p. A120
MERIWETHER, Wayne, Chief Operating Officer, Methodist Hospital, Henderson, KY, p. A251
MERK, Richard, Executive Vice President, Allegiance Behavioral Health Center of Plainview, Plainview, TX, p. A621
MERK, Richard T., Chief Executive Officer, Bienville Medical Center, Arcadia, LA, p. A261
MERKEL, Earl, M.D. Chief of Staff, Russell Regional Hospital, Russell, KS, p. A242
MERKLE, Greg, Director Information Systems, Sheppard and Enoch Pratt Hospital, Baltimore, MD, p. A289
MERKLE, Richard E., Chief Human Resources Officer, Geisinger Medical Center, Danville, PA, p. A521
MERKLEY, Jason R., Chief Executive Officer, Brookings Health System, Brookings, SD, p. A555
MERLI, Geno, M.D. Chief Medical Officer, Thomas Jefferson University Hospital, Philadelphia, PA, p. A534
MERLIS, Laurence M., President and Chief Executive Officer, Abington Memorial Hospital, Abington, PA, p. A517
MERRED, Mehdi, Chief Executive Officer, Quincy Valley Medical Center, Quincy, WA, p. A664
MERRELL, Bruce, FACHE President, St. Mary's Hospital, Centralia, IL, p. A174
MERRIGAN, Mary C., Manager Public Relations, Sanford Vermillion Medical Center, Vermillion, SD, p. A560
MERRILL, Chuck, M.D. Vice President Medical Affairs, Marian Medical Center, Santa Maria, CA, p. A90
MERRILL, Mark H., President, Valley Health System, Winchester, VA, p. B141
MERRILL, Michael, M.D. Interim Vice President Medical Affairs, United Memorial Medical Center, Batavia, NY, p. A421
MERRILL, Rick W., President and Chief Executive Officer, Cook Children's Medical Center, Fort Worth, TX, p. A598
MERRITT, Bradley, M.D. Medical Director, Trinity Mother Frances Rehabilitation Hospital, Tyler, TX, p. A632
MERRITT, Janet, Chief Financial Officer, St. Vincent Williamsport Hospital, Williamsport, IN, p. A213
MERRY, Duane, Chief Information Officer, Little Falls Hospital, Little Falls, NY, p. A428
MERRYMAN, Scott
Chief Financial Officer, CHRISTUS Coushatta Health Care Center, Coushatta, LA, p. A264
Chief Financial Officer, CHRISTUS Spohn Hospital Corpus Christi Memorial, Corpus Christi, TX, p. A589
MERRYWELL, Paul, Chief Information Officer, Sycamore Shoals Hospital, Elizabethton, TN, p. A565
MERSON, Wendy, Chief Executive Officer, Windmoor Healthcare of Clearwater, Clearwater, FL, p. A120
MERTZ, John, Chief Information Officer, South Nassau Communities Hospital, Oceanside, NY, p. A439
MERVAK, Gary, Chief Financial Officer, Northwest Medical Center, Margate, FL, p. A129
MERVES, Ed, M.D. Medical Director, Coastal Harbor Treatment Center, Savannah, GA, p. A159
MERWIN, Robert W., Chief Executive Officer, Mills–Peninsula Health Services, Burlingame, CA, p. A56
MESA, Diana, Director Human Resources, Pecos County Memorial Hospital, Fort Stockton, TX, p. A598
MESA, Gustavo, Chief Information Officer, San Juan City Hospital, San Juan, PR, p. A703
MESAROS, Dennis, Chief Operating Officer, Providence Centralia Hospital, Centralia, WA, p. A660
MESIC, John, M.D. Chief Medical Officer, Sutter Auburn Faith Hospital, Auburn, CA, p. A54
MESSELT, Mary Jo, Director Human Resources, Mercy Hospital Logan County, Guthrie, OK, p. A497
MESSER, Bristol, Chief Executive Officer, McCurtain Memorial Hospital, Idabel, OK, p. A498
MESSERSMITH, Darrell, Director Information Systems, Platte Valley Medical Center, Brighton, CO, p. A98
MESSERSMITH, Scott E., Director Human Resources, Columbus Community Hospital, Columbus, NE, p. A382
MESSINA, Daniel J., Ph.D. Senior Vice President and Chief Operating Officer, CentraState Healthcare System, Freehold, NJ, p. A404
MESSMER, Joseph, Interim Chief Executive Officer, St. Mary's Healthcare Center, Pierre, SD, p. A558
MESTAN, Robert E., M.D. Chief of Staff, Perry Memorial Hospital, Princeton, IL, p. A192
MESTEMACHER, Christine, M.D. President Medical Staff, Baptist Memorial Hospital for Women, Memphis, TN, p. A571
METCALF, Mike, Chief Administrative Officer, Essentia Health Duluth, Duluth, MN, p. A330
METCALF, Peter, M.D. President Medical Staff, Genesis Medical Center, Illini Campus, Silvis, IL, p. A193
METCALFE, Kevan, Chief Executive Officer, Corona Regional Medical Center, Corona, CA, p. A58
METHE, Joan, Chief Information Officer, Mercy Medical Center, Springfield, MA, p. A305
METHVEN, George, M.D. Chief Medical Staff, Cedar County Memorial Hospital, El Dorado Springs, MO, p. A359
METHVEN, Jeffrey M., Vice President Ambulatory Services and Chief Human Resources Officer, Saratoga Hospital, Saratoga Springs, NY, p. A443
METHVIN, Jeff, Manager Information Technology, St. Luke Hospital and Living Center, Marion, KS, p. A238
METIKO, Olushola, M.D. Medical Director, Central Prison Hospital, Raleigh, NC, p. A458
METIVIER, Roberta, Vice President Human Resources and Administrator, Western Main Nursing Home, Stephens Memorial Hospital, Norway, ME, p. A284
METOYER, Derek, M.D. Chief of Staff, Opelousas General Health System, Opelousas, LA, p. A276
METTS, Michael, Chief Financial Officer, Odessa Regional Medical Center, Odessa, TX, p. A619
METZ, Bruce, Ph.D. Chief Information Officer, Lahey Clinic Hospital, Burlington, MA, p. A298
METZ, Carl, Vice President Human Resources, Ephraim McDowell Regional Medical Center, Danville, KY, p. A249
METZ, Karen, Chief Executive Officer, Physicians Regional Medical Center, Knoxville, TN, p. A568
METZGER, John, Controller, NorthKey Community Care, Covington, KY, p. A249
MEURER, Bryan, Director Information Systems, Mat–Su Regional Medical Center, Palmer, AK, p. A30
MEWHIRTER, Michael, Chief Financial Officer, Florida Hospital North Pinellas, Tarpon Springs, FL, p. A141
MEYER, Anthony, M.D. Medical Director, Aurora Psychiatric Hospital, Wauwatosa, WI, p. A693
MEYER, Cheryl, Director Human Resources, Palmer Lutheran Health Center, West Union, IA, p. A228

Index of Health Care Professionals

Index of Health Care Professionals

Index of Health Care Professionals / Meyer

MEYER, Daniel T., Chief Administrative Officer, Aurora BayCare Medical Center, Green Bay, WI, p. A682
MEYER, Eugene W., President and Chief Executive Officer, Lawrence Memorial Hospital, Lawrence, KS, p. A237
MEYER, Francis, Vice President Information Systems Technology, KALEIDA Health, Buffalo, NY, p. A422
MEYER, Gary, M.D. Chief of Staff, Grand River Hospital District, Rifle, CO, p. A105
MEYER, Gary A., President and Chief Executive Officer, Schneck Medical Center, Seymour, IN, p. A211
MEYER, Gordon, Director Human Resources, Oakland Regional Hospital, Southfield, MI, p. A323
MEYER, James E., President and Chief Executive Officer, MedCentral – Mansfield Hospital, Mansfield, OH, p. A483
MEYER, Jeffrey K., Chief Executive Officer, Osceola Medical Center, Osceola, WI, p. A688
MEYER, Joe S., Chief Financial Officer, Scott County Hospital, Scott City, KS, p. A243
MEYER, John, M.D. Chief of Staff, Medina Regional Hospital, Hondo, TX, p. A603
MEYER, Karen, Vice President Finance and Chief Financial Officer, Rush Memorial Hospital, Rushville, IN, p. A211
MEYER, Kris, R.N. Director of Nursing, Pawnee County Memorial Hospital, Pawnee City, NE, p. A389
MEYER, Kurt A., Vice President Human Resources, Elkhart General Healthcare System, Elkhart, IN, p. A200
MEYER, Lori, Interim Chief Financial Officer, South Peninsula Hospital, Homer, AK, p. A29
MEYER, Mark, Vice President and Chief Financial Officer, Texas Health Presbyterian Hospital Dallas, Dallas, TX, p. A592
MEYER, Nate, Director Finance, Douglas County Hospital, Alexandria, MN, p. A327
MEYER, Philip A., Director Finance, Dearborn County Hospital, Lawrenceburg, IN, p. A207
MEYER, Richard A., Chief Financial Officer, Mary Black Memorial Hospital, Spartanburg, SC, p. A553
MEYER, Robert L., President and Chief Executive Officer, Phoenix Children's Hospital, Phoenix, AZ, p. A36
MEYER, Robin, Vice President Support Services, Decatur County Memorial Hospital, Greensburg, IN, p. A203
MEYER, Roger, M.D. Chief of Staff, Warren Memorial Hospital, Friend, NE, p. A383
MEYER, Thomas, Vice President Finance, Morris Hospital & Healthcare Centers, Morris, IL, p. A188
MEYER, Timothy, M.D. Chief of Staff, Memorial Medical Center – Neillsville, Neillsville, WI, p. A688
MEYER, Wessel, M.D. Chief of Staff, Veterans Affairs Central California Health Care System, Fresno, CA, p. A62
MEYER–UYEHARA, Cathy, Administrator, Hale Ho'ola Hamakua, Honokaa, HI, p. A163
MEYERHOFER, Cheri, Vice President Human Resources, PeaceHealth Southwest Medical Center, Vancouver, WA, p. A668
MEYERS, Ann M., Chief Executive Officer, Mayo Clinic Hospital, Phoenix, AZ, p. A36
MEYERS, Audrey, President and Chief Executive Officer, Valley Hospital, Ridgewood, NJ, p. A409
MEYERS, Betty, Chief Financial Officer, Crook County Medical Services District, Sundance, WY, p. A697
MEYERS, Brent, Administrator, Beaver County Memorial Hospital, Beaver, OK, p. A494
MEYERS, Dennis, R.N. President and Chief Executive Officer, Manchester Memorial Hospital, Manchester, KY, p. A256
MEYERS, Larry, Chief Information Officer, Wilson Memorial Hospital, Sidney, OH, p. A488
MEYERS, Mark A., President, Glendale Memorial Hospital and Health Center, Glendale, CA, p. A63
MEYERS, Russell
  President and Chief Executive Officer, Midland Memorial Hospital, Midland, TX, p. A617
  President and Chief Executive Officer, Midland Memorial Hospital, Midland, TX, p. A617
MEYERS, Steve, Director Human Resources, New York Community Hospital,, NY, p. A435
MEYERS, William, Chief Information Officer, St. Luke's Hospital, Chesterfield, MO, p. A357
MEZA, Casey
  Chief Executive Officer, Clearwater Valley Hospital and Clinics, Orofino, ID, p. A169
  Chief Executive Officer, St. Mary's Hospital, Cottonwood, ID, p. A168
MEZA, Eduardo, M.D. Medical Director, Prairie St. John's, Fargo, ND, p. A465
MEZA, Lourdes, Coordinator Human Resources, Doctors Hospital of West Covina, West Covina, CA, p. A95
MEZZA, Nicholas, Chief Executive Officer, LifeCare Hospitals of Mechanicsburg, Mechanicsburg, PA, p. A529
MEZZAROBA, Albert, Chief Executive Officer, Lower Bucks Hospital, Bristol, PA, p. A519
MIANO, Christena, Human Resources Director, Medical Center of Trinity, Trinity, FL, p. A142
MICHAEL, Amy J., Chief Operating Officer, Sullivan County Memorial Hospital, Milan, MO, p. A365
MICHAEL, Don, Chief Financial Officer, Jay County Hospital, Portland, IN, p. A210
MICHAEL, Liz, Vice President Patient Care Services and Chief Nursing Officer, Stillwater Medical Center, Stillwater, OK, p. A505
MICHAEL, Lois, Vice President Human Resources, Torrance Memorial Medical Center, Torrance, CA, p. A92
MICHAELS, Hilary, Executive Director, Specialty Hospital at Kimball, Lakewood, NJ, p. A405
MICHAELSON, Linda, Director Human Resources, Lake District Hospital, Lakeview, OR, p. A512
MICHALEK, Debra, Chief Financial Officer, Kindred Hospital–Louisville, Louisville, KY, p. A254
MICHALSKI, Barb, Manager Human Resources, Flambeau Hospital, Park Falls, WI, p. A689
MICHALSKI, Gene, President and Chief Executive Officer, Beaumont Health System, Royal Oak, MI, p. B20
MICHALSKI, Gene, Executive Vice President and Chief Operating Officer, Beaumont Hospital – Royal Oak, Royal Oak, MI, p. A322
MICHEL, Diane, Vice President Nursing, Children's Hospital, New Orleans, LA, p. A274
MICHEL, George J., Chief Operating Officer, Larkin Community Hospital, South Miami, FL, p. A139
MICHEL, Linda, Administrator, North Valley Hospital, Tonasket, WA, p. A668
MICHEL–OGBORN, Deborah, Chief Information Resource Management, Malcom Randall Veterans Affairs Medical Center, Gainesville, FL, p. A124
MICHELETTI, Denise D., R.N. Director, Central Virginia Training Center, Madison Heights, VA, p. A650
MICHELETTI, Susan C., Chief Operating Officer, San Ramon Regional Medical Center, San Ramon, CA, p. A89
MICHELL, Pamela W., R.N. Vice President and Chief Nursing Officer, Munroe Regional Medical Center, Ocala, FL, p. A133
MICIOTTO, Joseph M., Administrator, LSU Medical Center–University Hospital, Shreveport, LA, p. A277
MICKELSON, Ryan, Chief Executive Officer, Mountrail County Medical Center, Stanley, ND, p. A468
MICKENS, Walt, President and Chief Executive Officer, Queen of the Valley Medical Center, Napa, CA, p. A76
MICKIEWICZ, Nanette, M.D. President and Chief Medical Officer, Dominican Hospital, Santa Cruz, CA, p. A90
MIDDENDORF, Bruce, M.D. Chief Medical Officer, St. Mary's Health Care System, Athens, GA, p. A144
MIDDLETON, Jackie, Vice President Human Resources, Methodist Dallas Medical Center, Dallas, TX, p. A592
MIDGETT, Ronnie, Chief Financial Officer, Colleton Medical Center, Walterboro, SC, p. A554
MIEDLER, Michael, M.D. Chief Medical Officer, Continuing Care Hospital, Lexington, KY, p. A253
MIER, David, Chief Financial Officer, El Paso Children's Hospital, El Paso, TX, p. A596
MIESNER, Gail, Chief Financial Officer, Memorial Hospital, Chester, IL, p. A175
MIGAUD, Christy, Controller, Ochsner Baptist Medical Center, New Orleans, LA, p. A274
MIGNOSNA, Gary, Vice President Human Resources, UPMC Passavant, Pittsburgh, PA, p. A535
MIGOYA, Carlos A., President and Chief Executive Officer, Jackson Health System, Miami, FL, p. A131
MIKELA, Mary, Vice President Mission Stewardship, Saint Anthony's Health Center, Alton, IL, p. A172
MIKELL, Jeffrey, M.D. Chief Medical Officer, Wesley Woods Long Term Care Hospital, Atlanta, GA, p. A146
MIKES, James, Administrator, Heartland Long Term Acute Care Hospital, Saint Joseph, MO, p. A368
MIKHAIL, Ashraf, M.D. Medical Director, Brynn Marr Hospital, Jacksonville, NC, p. A455
MIKI, Nobuyuki, M.D. Vice President Medical Affairs, Kuakini Medical Center, Honolulu, HI, p. A163
MIKITARIAN Jr., George, Chief Executive Officer, Parrish Medical Center, Titusville, FL, p. A142
MIKITKA, Joseph, Vice President Human Resources, Sacred Heart Hospital, Allentown, PA, p. A517
MIKKELSON, Tom, M.D. Interim Chief Operating Officer, Touchette Regional Hospitals, Centreville, IL, p. A175
MIKLAVIC, Kirk, Director, Human Resources, Central Maine Medical Center, Lewiston, ME, p. A283
MIKLOS, Maggie, Director Human Resources, Northside Hospital and Heart Institute, Saint Petersburg, FL, p. A138
MIKULIC, Jeannie, Director Human Resources, Providence Portland Medical Center, Portland, OR, p. A514
MIKUTOWSKI, Melody, Chief Human Resources Management, Veterans Affairs Medical Center, Portland, OR, p. A514
MILAND, Shelly, Vice President Finance and Chief Financial Officer, Texas Health Harris Methodist Hospital Hurst–Euless–Bedford, Bedford, TX, p. A583
MILANES, Carlos, Chief Executive Officer and Managing Director, Aiken Regional Medical Centers, Aiken, SC, p. A546
MILANO, Arthur D., Vice President Human Resources, Berkshire Medical Center, Pittsfield, MA, p. A303
MILATOVICH, Natasha, Association Vice President Human Resources, White Memorial Medical Center, Los Angeles, CA, p. A73
MILAZZO, John, Chief Financial Officer, River Region Medical Center, Vicksburg, MS, p. A353
MILBRANDT, David, M.D. Vice President Medical Affairs, Fairview Lakes Health Services, Wyoming, MN, p. A342
MILBURN, Sandra, Director Human Resources, HEALTHSOUTH Rehabilitation Hospital of Memphis, Memphis, TN, p. A571
MILES, Brenda, Chief Executive Officer, Hill Country Specialty Hospital, New Braunfels, TX, p. A618
MILES, David K., President and Chief Executive Officer, The Children's Institute of Pittsburgh, Pittsburgh, PA, p. A535
MILES, John, Chief Financial Officer, Piedmont Fayette Hospital, Fayetteville, GA, p. A152
MILES, Kerry
  Site Director, Providence Centralia Hospital, Centralia, WA, p. A660
  Chief Information Officer, Providence St. Peter Hospital, Olympia, WA, p. A663
MILES, Laverne, Chief Operating Officer, Fort Defiance Indian Health Service Hospital, Fort Defiance, AZ, p. A32
MILES, Paul V.
  Chief Operating Officer, Morgan County ARH Hospital, West Liberty, KY, p. A259
  Vice President Administration, Whitesburg ARH Hospital, Whitesburg, KY, p. A259
MILES, Senta, Director Human Resources, Medical Center of McKinney, McKinney, TX, p. A616
MILIAN, Tony, Chief Financial Officer, Palm Springs General Hospital, Hialeah, FL, p. A125
MILICEVIC, Heather, Director Human Resources, Summa Western Reserve Hospital, Cuyahoga Falls, OH, p. A478
MILLARD, James M., President and Chief Executive Officer, Kenmore Mercy Hospital, Kenmore, NY, p. A428
MILLER, Alan B., President and Chief Executive Officer, Universal Health Services, Inc., King of Prussia, PA, p. B134
MILLER, Alicia, Director Human Resources, Aspen Valley Hospital District, Aspen, CO, p. A97
MILLER, Amy A., Human Resources Assistant, Hawarden Community Hospital, Hawarden, IA, p. A221
MILLER, Annette, M.D. Medical Staff Chairman, Brown County Hospital, Ainsworth, NE, p. A381
MILLER, Aubrey, M.D. Chief of Staff, Lexington Medical Center, West Columbia, SC, p. A554
MILLER, Barb, Director Human Resources, St. Gabriel's Hospital, Little Falls, MN, p. A333
MILLER, Barbara, Manager Business Office, Tri–County Hospital – Williston, Williston, FL, p. A143
MILLER, Barbara H., M.D. Chief Medical Officer, Newman Memorial Hospital, Shattuck, OK, p. A504
MILLER, Berry, M.D. Chief Medical Officer, Cameron Memorial Community Hospital, Angola, IN, p. A197
MILLER, Beth, Controller, HEALTHSOUTH Harmarville Rehabilitation Hospital, Pittsburgh, PA, p. A534
MILLER, Blaine K., Administrator, Republic County Hospital, Belleville, KS, p. A230
MILLER, Brian, Administrator and Chief Executive Officer, Dallas County Medical Center, Fordyce, AR, p. A45
MILLER, Bryan, Chief Operating Officer, Plantation General Hospital, Plantation, FL, p. A136
MILLER, Chad, Chief Financial Officer, Bolivar Medical Center, Cleveland, MS, p. A345
MILLER, Charles, D.O. Chief of Staff, Unicoi County Memorial Hospital, Erwin, TN, p. A565
MILLER, Charles F., President and Chief Executive Officer, Piedmont Medical Center, Rock Hill, SC, p. A553
MILLER, Christi, Manager Human Resources, West River Regional Medical Center, Hettinger, ND, p. A466
MILLER, Christine
  Vice President Human Resources, Hanover Hospital, Hanover, PA, p. A524
  Chief Human Resources Management Services, Veterans Affairs Medical Center, Togus, ME, p. A285
MILLER, Connie, Vice President Human Resources, Overland Park Regional Medical Center, Overland Park, KS, p. A241
MILLER, Dan, Vice President Finance, Forest Health Medical Center, Ypsilanti, MI, p. A326
MILLER, Daniel
  Vice President Human Resources, EMH Elyria Medical Center, Elyria, OH, p. A480
  Chief Operating Officer, Swedish Medical Center, Englewood, CO, p. A100

A882 Index of Health Care Professionals

Index of Health Care Professionals / Mills

Index of Health Care Professionals


MILLER, David, Chief Financial Officer, Sturgis Hospital, Sturgis, MI, p. A323
MILLER, David L., Chief Information Officer, UAMS Medical Center, Little Rock, AR, p. A48
MILLER, David R., President, River Falls Area Hospital, River Falls, WI, p. A690
MILLER, David T., Vice President and Chief Financial Officer, Children's Medical Center, Dayton, OH, p. A478
MILLER, Debra
Administrator, Crosbyton Clinic Hospital, Crosbyton, TX, p. A590
Senior Vice President Human Resources, Petaluma Valley Hospital, Petaluma, CA, p. A80
Vice President Human Resources, Santa Rosa Memorial Hospital, Santa Rosa, CA, p. A90
MILLER, Dennis E., FACHE Chief Executive Officer, Williamson Medical Center, Franklin, TN, p. A565
MILLER, Derek, Senior Vice President and Chief Financial Officer, Southeast Alabama Medical Center, Dothan, AL, p. A19
MILLER, Dianne, Director Health Information Management, Van Matre HEALTHSOUTH Rehabilitation Hospital, Rockford, IL, p. A193
MILLER, Dionne, Chief Operating Officer, Sutter Roseville Medical Center, Roseville, CA, p. A83
MILLER, Donald, Vice President and Chief Financial Officer, Queen of the Valley Medical Center, Napa, CA, p. A76
MILLER, Donald, M.D. Chief of Staff, Washington County Hospital and Clinics, Washington, IA, p. A227
MILLER, Duane, Senior Vice President Finance, Carson City Hospital, Carson City, MI, p. A309
MILLER, Eileen, Director Human Resources, Northern Dutchess Hospital, Rhinebeck, NY, p. A441
MILLER, Elaine G., Director of Nursing, Oaklawn Psychiatric Center, Goshen, IN, p. A202
MILLER, Elizabeth, CPA Chief Financial Officer, Stamford Memorial Hospital, Stamford, TX, p. A628
MILLER, Eric, M.D. Chief of Staff, Beaver Dam Community Hospitals, Beaver Dam, WI, p. A679
MILLER, Gary, Chief Executive Officer, Peak View Behavioral Health, Colorado Springs, CO, p. A98
MILLER, Gary E., M.D. Medical Director, Kingwood Pines Hospital, Kingwood, TX, p. A611
MILLER, Gary L.
Regional Director Information Systems, Saint Joseph Regional Medical Center, Mishawaka, IN, p. A208
Regional Director Information Systems, Saint Joseph Regional Medical Center–Plymouth Campus, Plymouth, IN, p. A210
MILLER, Gary P., President and Chief Executive Officer, St. Alexius Medical Center, Bismarck, ND, p. A464
MILLER, Gene, Chief Executive Officer, Northeastern Nevada Regional Hospital, Elko, NV, p. A391
MILLER Jr., George N., Chief Executive Officer, Okmulgee Memorial Hospital, Okmulgee, OK, p. A502
MILLER, Greg, Senior Vice President Operations, Shands Jacksonville Medical Center, Jacksonville, FL, p. A126
MILLER, Gwyn, Director Human Resources, Klickitat Valley Health, Goldendale, WA, p. A661
MILLER, Harvey, Director, G. Werber Bryan Psychiatric Hospital, Columbia, SC, p. A548
MILLER, Heidi, Chief Executive Officer, Kindred Hospital–Tucson, Tucson, AZ, p. A40
MILLER, Helen M., Director Human Resources, War Memorial Hospital, Berkeley Springs, WV, p. A670
MILLER, J. D., M.D
Chief Medical Officer, Hazard ARH Regional Medical Center, Hazard, KY, p. A251
Vice President Medical Affairs, Morgan County ARH Hospital, West Liberty, KY, p. A259
Vice President Medical Affairs, Williamson ARH Hospital, South Williamson, KY, p. A259
MILLER, J. Todd, Vice President and Chief Operating Officer, Alice Peck Day Memorial Hospital, Lebanon, NH, p. A398
MILLER, Jackie, D.O. Chief of Staff, Northwest Medical Center, Albany, MO, p. A355
MILLER, James, CPA Chief Financial Officer, AMG Specialty Hospital–Lafayette Regional Campus, Lafayette, LA, p. A270
MILLER, James, Director Human Resources, Lakeside Behavioral Health System, Memphis, TN, p. A571
MILLER, James D., M.D. Chief Medical Officer, Memorial Hospital of Carbondale, Carbondale, IL, p. A174
MILLER, James I., President and Chief Executive Officer, Renown Health, Reno, NV, p. B110
MILLER, James J., Vice President and Chief Financial Officer, Henry Ford Wyandotte Hospital, Wyandotte, MI, p. A325
MILLER, Jason, Chief Operating Officer, The BridgeWay, North Little Rock, AR, p. A50
MILLER, Jeff, Chief Operating Officer, Citizens Memorial Hospital, Bolivar, MO, p. A355
MILLER, Jeffrey S., President and Chief Executive Officer, High Point Regional Health System, High Point, NC, p. A455
MILLER, John
Vice President Information Services, Medcenter One, Bismarck, ND, p. A464
Chief Financial Officer, St. Mary's Hospital Medical Center, Green Bay, WI, p. A682
MILLER Jr., John A., FACHE Chief Executive Officer, AnMed Health Medical Center, Anderson, SC, p. A546
MILLER Jr.,, John A., FACHE Chief Executive Officer, AnMed Health, Anderson, SC, p. B10
MILLER, Jon, Team Leader Accounting and Information Services, Hancock Regional Hospital, Greenfield, IN, p. A203
MILLER, Judy, Director Human Resources, Town and Country Hospital, Tampa, FL, p. A141
MILLER, Julie, Chief Operating Officer, Williamson Medical Center, Franklin, TN, p. A565
MILLER, Kay J., MS Chief Nursing Officer, Medical Center of the Rockies, Loveland, CO, p. A104
MILLER, Kelli, Vice President Human Resources, Mary Free Bed Rehabilitation Hospital, Grand Rapids, MI, p. A313
MILLER, Ken, Chief Financial Officer, Paris Regional Medical Center, Paris, TX, p. A620
MILLER, Kevin J., FACHE President and Chief Executive Officer, Hutchinson Regional Medical Center, Hutchinson, KS, p. A235
MILLER, Kim, Chief Information Officer, Bowdle Hospital, Bowdle, SD, p. A555
MILLER, Kimberly J., FACHE Chief Executive Officer, Beaver Dam Community Hospitals, Beaver Dam, WI, p. A679
MILLER, Kris, Director Human Resources, Spectrum Health Reed City Hospital, Reed City, MI, p. A321
MILLER, Leanne R., Director Human Resources, Community Hospital, McCook, NE, p. A386
MILLER, Leighton, Chief Information Officer, Meade District Hospital, Meade, KS, p. A239
MILLER, Linda, R.N. Senior Vice President Operations and Chief Nursing Officer, Our Lady of Lourdes Memorial Hospital, Binghamton, NY, p. A422
MILLER, Lisa, Director Human Resources, Hendry Regional Medical Center, Clewiston, FL, p. A120
MILLER, Lisa, R.N. Director of Nursing, North Sunflower Medical Center, Ruleville, MS, p. A352
MILLER, Lisa, Administrator, Specialty Rehabilitation Hospital of Luling, Luling, LA, p. A272
MILLER, Lynn J., Vice President Financial Services, Oaklawn Psychiatric Center, Goshen, IN, p. A202
MILLER, Mark A., FACHE Chief Executive Officer, Memorial Health System, Abilene, KS, p. A230
MILLER, Marty, Vice President and Chief Information Officer, Children's Hospital Los Angeles, Los Angeles, CA, p. A69
MILLER, Mary, Vice President Finance and Business Development, Mt. Washington Pediatric Hospital, Baltimore, MD, p. A288
MILLER, Matthew, M.D. Vice President Medical Affairs, Danbury Hospital, Danbury, CT, p. A108
MILLER, Michele, Chief Financial Officer, Community Memorial Hospital, Oconto Falls, WI, p. A688
MILLER, Nancy, R.N. Chief Nursing Officer, Van Matre HEALTHSOUTH Rehabilitation Hospital, Rockford, IL, p. A193
MILLER, Nate, Chief Executive Officer, Surgical Hospital of Jonesboro, Jonesboro, AR, p. A47
MILLER, Nicole, Director Human Resources, Riverside Shore Memorial Hospital, Nassawadox, VA, p. A651
MILLER, Peter, FACHE Chief Executive Officer, Specialty Hospital of Washington–Hadley, Washington, DC, p. A117
MILLER, Phil, Chief Financial Officer, Shelby Memorial Hospital, Shelbyville, IL, p. A193
MILLER, Redonda, M.D. Vice President Medical Affairs, Johns Hopkins Hospital, Baltimore, MD, p. A287
MILLER, Richard
Administrator Finance, Banner Thunderbird Medical Center, Glendale, AZ, p. A33
Administrator and Chief Executive Officer, Norton County Hospital, Norton, KS, p. A239
Vice President Finance, University of Chicago Medical Center, Chicago, IL, p. A179
MILLER, Richard P., Chief Executive Officer, Virtua Health, Marlton, NJ, p. B143
MILLER, Rick
Chief Financial Officer, District One Hospital, Faribault, MN, p. A331
President and Chief Operating Officer, Nationwide Children's Hospital, Columbus, OH, p. A477
MILLER, Rip, Chief Executive Officer, The Hospital at Westlake Medical Center, Austin, TX, p. A582
MILLER, Robert, Chief Executive Officer, Coshocton County Memorial Hospital, Coshocton, OH, p. A478
MILLER, Rod, Chief Information Technology, Community Hospital, Torrington, WY, p. A698
MILLER, Sam, Chief Operating Officer, North Sunflower Medical Center, Ruleville, MS, p. A352
MILLER, Scott
Director Information Services, Forrest City Medical Center, Forrest City, AR, p. A45
Chief Financial Officer, Schick Shadel Hospital, Seattle, WA, p. A666
MILLER, Sharon, Chief Information Officer, Community Howard Regional Hospital, Kokomo, IN, p. A206
MILLER, Shelly, R.N. Chief Executive Officer, Orthopaedic Hospital of Lutheran Health, Fort Wayne, IN, p. A201
MILLER, Sherry L., Director Human Resources, Springfield Hospital Center, Sykesville, MD, p. A294
MILLER, Stan, Executive Director Human Resources, St. Thomas More Hospital, Canon City, CO, p. A98
MILLER, Stephen R., Chief Executive Officer, Kosciusko Community Hospital, Warsaw, IN, p. A213
MILLER, Steve, Chief Information Officer, Oklahoma Heart Hospital, Oklahoma City, OK, p. A501
MILLER, Steven, Chief Financial Officer, Seven Rivers Regional Medical Center, Crystal River, FL, p. A121
MILLER, Stuart P., M.D. Medical Director, HEALTHSOUTH Sea Pines Rehabilitation Hospital, Melbourne, FL, p. A130
MILLER, Susan, Financial Administrator, Faulkton Area Medical Center, Faulkton, SD, p. A556
MILLER, Tamara, Administrator, Madison Community Hospital, Madison, SD, p. A557
MILLER, Tammie, Director Marketing and Public Relations, Plateau Medical Center, Oak Hill, WV, p. A674
MILLER, Ted, Chief Financial Officer, Floyd Memorial Hospital and Health Services, New Albany, IN, p. A209
MILLER, Thomas, M.D. Medical Director, University of Utah Health Care – Hospital and Clinics, Salt Lake City, UT, p. A641
MILLER, Tim C., M.D. Vice President, Chief Medical Officer and Director Academy Affairs, OSF Saint Francis Medical Center, Peoria, IL, p. A191
MILLER, Tish, Chief Financial Officer, John C. Fremont Healthcare District, Mariposa, CA, p. A74
MILLER, Todd, Chief Executive Officer and Chief Restructuring Officer, Peninsula Hospital Center,, NY, p. A
MILLER, Wanda, R.N. Director of Clinical Services, Asheville Specialty Hospital, Asheville, NC, p. A448
MILLER, Wayne, D.O. Associate Chief Medical Officer, Mercy Suburban Hospital, Norristown, PA, p. A530
MILLER, Jr., Wentz J., Managing Director and Chief Financial Officer, Integris Baptist Medical Center, Oklahoma City, OK, p. A501
MILLER, William, Coordinator Management Information Systems, Livengrin Foundation, Bensalem, PA, p. A518
MILLER, William P., President and Chief Executive Officer, Caro Community Hospital, Caro, MI, p. A309
MILLER–BALFOUR, Pam, Director Human Resources, Socorro General Hospital, Socorro, NM, p. A418
MILLER–COLLETTE, Melody M., Director Human Resources, North Okaloosa Medical Center, Crestview, FL, p. A121
MILLER–PHIPPS, Julie K., Senior Vice President and Executive Director, Anaheim Medical Center, Anaheim, CA, p. A53
MILLHORN, Melanie, Director Human Resources, SEARHC MT. Edgecumbe Hospital, Sitka, AK, p. A30
MILLIGAN, Corbi, M.D. Chief of Staff, StoneCrest Medical Center, Smyrna, TN, p. A575
MILLION, Brenda, R.N. Vice President and Chief Nursing Officer, St. Bernards Medical Center, Jonesboro, AR, p. A47
MILLIRONS, Dennis C., FACHE President, Sanford Medical Center Fargo, Fargo, ND, p. A465
MILLIS, Priscilla, Chief Executive Officer, Lakeway Regional Hospital, Morristown, TN, p. A572
MILLNER, Jane, Director Community Relations and Development, St. Lawrence Rehabilitation Center, Lawrenceville, NJ, p. A405
MILLS, Bryan A., President and Chief Executive Officer, Community Health Network, Indianapolis, IN, p. B33
MILLS, Chip, Director Information Technology, Sentara Obici Hospital, Suffolk, VA, p. A656
MILLS, Craig, Senior Financial Advisor, Park City Medical Center, Park City, UT, p. A639
MILLS, Craig J.
Vice President Human Resources, Sacred Heart Medical Center, Eugene, OR, p. A510
Regional Vice President of Culture and People, Sacred Heart Medical Center at RiverBend, Springfield, OR, p. A516
MILLS, Dennis, Director Human Resources, San Ramon Regional Medical Center, San Ramon, CA, p. A89
MILLS, John C., Senior Vice President Operations, Fairview Hospital, Cleveland, OH, p. A475
MILLS, Marianne, R.N. Chairperson, Stanton County Hospital, Johnson, KS, p. A235
MILLS, Nikki, Director Human Resources and Operations, Buffalo Hospital, Buffalo, MN, p. A329



Index of Health Care Professionals **A883**

Index of Health Care Professionals

Index of Health Care Professionals / Mills

MILLS, Randy, Vice President Operations and Business Development, Northcrest Medical Center, Springfield, TN, p. A576
MILLS, Scott, M.D. Vice President Medical Staff Administration and Chief Medical Officer, Mid Coast Hospital, Brunswick, ME, p. A282
MILLS, Stephanie, Vice President Information and Materials Systems, Our Lady of the Lake Regional Medical Center, Baton Rouge, LA, p. A262
MILLS, Stephen, Chief Executive Officer, Dubuis Health System, Houston, TX, p. B48
MILLS, Stephen S., President and Chief Executive Officer, New York Hospital Queens,, NY, p. A435
MILLS, Vicki L., Chief Financial Officer, Anderson County Hospital, Garnett, KS, p. A233
MILLS, William, M.D
Senior Vice President Quality and Professional Affairs, Bradford Regional Medical Center, Bradford, PA, p. A519
Senior Vice President Quality and Professional Affairs, Olean General Hospital, Olean, NY, p. A439
MILLS, William H., Associate Director, Veterans Affairs Medical Center, Lebanon, PA, p. A527
MILLS–MATHEWS, Marcy, Director Human Resources, Palms West Hospital, Loxahatchee, FL, p. A129
MILLSAPS, Janet
Chief Human Resources Officer, MedWest – Harris, Sylva, NC, p. A461
Vice President Human Resources, MedWest – Haywood, Clyde, NC, p. A451
MILLSTEAD, Bart, Administrator, Memorial Hospital of Carbondale, Carbondale, IL, p. A174
MILNE, C. Dean, D.O. Medical Director, Complex Care Hospital at Tenaya, Las Vegas, NV, p. A392
MILNES, Lynn, Chief Executive Officer, Decatur County Hospital, Leon, IA, p. A222
MILONE, Sheri, Chief Executive Officer and Administrator, Lovelace Women's Hospital, Albuquerque, NM, p. A414
MILOVICH, David, Vice President Human Resources, Saint Mary's Regional Medical Center, Reno, NV, p. A395
MILTENBERGER, Cynthia, Director Organizational Effectiveness, Cass Regional Medical Center, Harrisonville, MO, p. A360
MILTON, Paul A., Executive Vice President and Chief Operating Officer, Ellis Hospital, Schenectady, NY, p. A443
MILTON, Rhonda, Director Human Resources, Summit Behavioral Healthcare, Cincinnati, OH, p. A474
MILVET, Jr., Robert W., Chief Financial Officer, Preston Memorial Hospital, Kingwood, WV, p. A673
MIMOSO, Michael, FACHE President and Chief Executive Officer, Kimball Medical Center, Lakewood, NJ, p. A405
MIMS, Staci, Chief Nursing Officer, Dorminy Medical Center, Fitzgerald, GA, p. A152
MIMS, Wanda, Director, Veterans Affairs Medical Center, San Juan, PR, p. A704
MINCY, Lowney, Director Information Services, Southside Hospital, Bay Shore, NY, p. A421
MINDEN, Philip, Chief Executive Officer, Pasco Regional Medical Center, Dade City, FL, p. A121
MINDER, George, Chief Executive Officer, Big Horn County Memorial Hospital, Hardin, MT, p. A376
MINDINGAL, Talford, Chief Resource Management Division, San Antonio Military Medical Center, Fort Sam Houston, TX, p. A598
MINEAR, Michael N., Chief Information Officer, University of California, Davis Medical Center, Sacramento, CA, p. A84
MINER, Greg, Administrator, Siouxland Surgery Center, Dakota Dunes, SD, p. A556
MINER, John
Chief Financial Officer, Kindred Hospital–Bay Area St. Petersburg, Saint Petersburg, FL, p. A138
Chief Financial Officer, Kindred Hospital–Central Tampa, Tampa, FL, p. A141
MINES, Kathryn, Director Human Resources, St. Joseph's Hospital, Breese, IL, p. A174
MINGLE, Regina, Senior Vice President and Chief Leadership Officer, Lancaster General Health, Lancaster, PA, p. A526
MINGS, William, M.D. Medical Director, Carl Albert Community Mental Health Center, McAlester, OK, p. A499
MINGUS, Linda, Director Human Resources, Aurora Medical Center of Oshkosh, Oshkosh, WI, p. A688
MINICK, Mark J., President and Chief Executive Officer, Van Wert County Hospital, Van Wert, OH, p. A490
MINIER, Mary, Vice President Operations, Indiana University Health White Memorial Hospital, Monticello, IN, p. A208
MINISSALE, Joseph, Interim President, Methodist McKinney Hospital, McKinney, TX, p. A616
MINK, Linda, R.N. Vice President Clinical Service Line Development, Ivinson Memorial Hospital, Laramie, WY, p. A696
MINKEN, Stanley, M.D. Chief Medical Officer, Chester River Health System, Chestertown, MD, p. A290
MINKOWITZ, Sam, Chief Financial Officer, Woodland Heights Medical Center, Lufkin, TX, p. A614
MINNICK, Paul E., R.N. Vice President Patient Services, Beebe Medical Center, Lewes, DE, p. A114
MINNICK, Peggy, R.N. Chief Executive Officer, BHC Alhambra Hospital, Rosemead, CA, p. A83
MINNIS, Rosanne, Business Officer, Rochester Psychiatric Center, Rochester, NY, p. A442
MINON, Maria, M.D
Vice President Medical Affairs and Chief Medical Officer, Children's Hospital at Mission, Mission Viejo, CA, p. A74
Vice President Medical Affairs and Chief Medical Officer, Children's Hospital of Orange County, Orange, CA, p. A78
MINOR, Beverly, Chief Human Resources, Schleicher County Medical Center, Eldorado, TX, p. A597
MINOR, Denise, R.N. Chief Nursing Officer, Lutheran Hospital, Cleveland, OH, p. A475
MINTONYE, Traci, Chief Financial Officer, River Hospital, Alexandria Bay, NY, p. A420
MIR, Sidney, M.D. Vice President Medical Affairs and Chief Medical Officer, Bon Secours Baltimore Health System, Baltimore, MD, p. A287
MIRABELLA, Ilene, Director Human Resources, New Bedford Rehabilitation Hospital, New Bedford, MA, p. A302
MIRANDA, A. Greg, D.O. President Medical Staff, St. Joseph's Hospital, Highland, IL, p. A184
MIRANDA, Ada S., M.D
Medical Director, Hospital Dr. Cayetano Coll Y Toste, Arecibo, PR, p. A700
Medical Director, Hospital Metropolitano Dr. Susoni, Arecibo, PR, p. A700
MIRANDA, Jay S., Chief Executive Officer, Coral Gables Hospital, Coral Gables, FL, p. A121
MIRANDA, Juliet, Chief Nursing Officer, Tri–City Regional Medical Center, Hawaiian Gardens, CA, p. A64
MIRANDA, Vicki, Vice President Human Resources, Dominican Hospital, Santa Cruz, CA, p. A90
MIRANDA, Victor Hernandez, M.D. Chief of Staff, Mennonite General Hospital, Aibonito, PR, p. A699
MIRDITA, Anthony, Chief Financial Officer, Putnam Hospital Center, Carmel, NY, p. A423
MIRE, Nona, Director Information Systems, Our Lady of Lourdes Regional Medical Center, Lafayette, LA, p. A270
MIRISOLA, Virginia, Fiscal Director, Spaulding Hospital for Continuing Medical Care North Shore, Salem, MA, p. A304
MIRONTI, Denise, Senior Vice President Patient Care Services, Cortland Regional Medical Center, Cortland, NY, p. A424
MIRZA, Irfan, Chief Financial Officer, Plantation General Hospital, Plantation, FL, p. A136
MIRZABEGIAN, Edward, Chief Executive Officer, Antelope Valley Hospital, Lancaster, CA, p. A67
MISCHLER, Kathy, Director Human Resources, HEALTHSOUTH Rehabilitation Hospital, Sewickley, PA, p. A538
MISHRA, Sanjeeb, M.D. Chief of Staff, Civista Health, La Plata, MD, p. A292
MISIASZEK, Yvonne, Service Unit Director, Crow/Northern Cheyenne Hospital, Crow Agency, MT, p. A374
MISITANO, Anthony F., President and Chief Executive Officer, Post Acute Medical, LLC, Camp Hill, PA, p. B102
MISKIMEN, Theresa, M.D. Vice President Medical Services, University of Medicine and Dentistry of New Jersey, University Behavioral Healthcare, Piscataway, NJ, p. A408
MISKO, Michael, M.D. Vice President Medical Staff Services and Chief Medical Officer, Western Missouri Medical Center, Warrensburg, MO, p. A372
MISLAN, Tim, MS Vice President Patient Care Services, Missouri Baptist Medical Center, Saint Louis, MO, p. A369
MISTRETTA, Mike, Vice President Information Systems and Chief Information Officer, MedCentral – Mansfield Hospital, Mansfield, OH, p. A483
MISTROT, Cindi, Associate Administrator, South Texas Health System, Edinburg, TX, p. A595
MITCHAM, Debbie, Chief Financial Officer, Northside Hospital, Atlanta, GA, p. A145
MITCHAM, Jerry, Interim President and Chief Executive Officer, Booneville Community Hospital, Booneville, AR, p. A42
MITCHEL, David M., Chief Executive Officer, Avoyelles Hospital, Marksville, LA, p. A272
MITCHELL, Adonna, Director Fiscal Services, North Mississippi Medical Center–Eupora, Eupora, MS, p. A345
MITCHELL, Andrew J., President and Chief Executive Officer, Peconic Bay Medical Center, Riverhead, NY, p. A441
MITCHELL, Barbara, Senior Vice President Marketing and Human Resources, Valley Medical Center, Renton, WA, p. A664
MITCHELL, Brenda, Director Human Resources, Roseland Community Hospital, Chicago, IL, p. A177
MITCHELL, Bryan, Director Information Systems, Fairfield Memorial Hospital, Fairfield, IL, p. A182
MITCHELL, Chris, Director Information Systems, Manatee Glens Hospital and Addiction Center, Bradenton, FL, p. A119
MITCHELL, Clifton, Manager Human Resources, Southwestern State Hospital, Thomasville, GA, p. A160
MITCHELL, Connie, Ph.D. Chief Information Officer, Creedmoor Psychiatric Center,, NY, p. A432
MITCHELL, Dan, Chief Operating Officer, Radius Specialty Hospital Boston, Boston, MA, p. A297
MITCHELL, Debbie, Director Human Resources, Woodrow Wilson Rehabilitation Center, Fishersville, VA, p. A648
MITCHELL, Elizabeth C., Vice President and Administrator, Specialty Hospital of Meridian, Meridian, MS, p. A350
MITCHELL, Errol, Vice President, Integris Southwest Medical Center, Oklahoma City, OK, p. A501
MITCHELL, Gary W., FACHE Chief Executive Officer, Newman Memorial Hospital, Shattuck, OK, p. A504
MITCHELL Jr., Harold E., CPA, Administrator and Chief Executive Officer, Bradley County Medical Center, Warren, AR, p. A52
MITCHELL, Jack C., FACHE Chief Executive Officer, HEALTHSOUTH Rehabilitation Hospital, Fayetteville, AR, p. A44
MITCHELL, Jodie, Facility Financial Director, Sturgis Regional Hospital, Sturgis, SD, p. A560
MITCHELL, John W., Administrator, Delta County Memorial Hospital, Delta, CO, p. A99
MITCHELL, Joseph J., President, Trinity Hospital Twin City, Dennison, OH, p. A479
MITCHELL, Judi, Vice President Human Resources, Navos, Seattle, WA, p. A665
MITCHELL, Kathy
Director Human Resources, Lakeview Medical Center, Rice Lake, WI, p. A690
Chief Nursing Officer, Muhlenberg Community Hospital, Greenville, KY, p. A251
MITCHELL, Kenneth W., M.D. Medical Director, St. David's North Austin Medical Center, Austin, TX, p. A581
MITCHELL, Kent, Chief Financial Officer, Hamilton Memorial Hospital District, McLeansboro, IL, p. A187
MITCHELL, Larry, M.D. Chief of Staff, Clinch Valley Medical Center, Richlands, VA, p. A654
MITCHELL, Lee, Chief Financial Officer, Red River Hospital, Wichita Falls, TX, p. A635
MITCHELL, Lori J., Chief Financial Officer, Harborview Medical Center, Seattle, WA, p. A665
MITCHELL, Marsha, Director Human Resources, Fleming County Hospital, Flemingsburg, KY, p. A249
MITCHELL, Mary S., Chief Resource Management Services, Veterans Affairs Medical Center, Birmingham, AL, p. A17
MITCHELL, Morris, Director Human Resources, Poplar Springs Hospital, Petersburg, VA, p. A653
MITCHELL, Naomi, Director Human Resources, Kentucky River Medical Center, Jackson, KY, p. A252
MITCHELL, Perry, M.D. Chief of Staff, Little Colorado Medical Center, Winslow, AZ, p. A41
MITCHELL, Rebekah, Chief Financial Officer, Madison County Health Care System, Winterset, IA, p. A228
MITCHELL, Richard R., Director Information Technology, Eagleville Hospital, Eagleville, PA, p. A522
MITCHELL, Sarah
Director Finance, Mary S Harper Geriatric Psychiatry Center, Tuscaloosa, AL, p. A26
Chief Financial Officer, Tilden Community Hospital, Tilden, NE, p. A390
MITCHELL, Sheena, Director Human Resources, Lafayette General Medical Center, Lafayette, LA, p. A270
MITCHELL, Steve, Chief Operating Officer, Memorial Medical Center, Modesto, CA, p. A75
MITCHELL, Stuart, Executive Vice President and Chief Operating Officer, Palm Bay Hospital, Melbourne, FL, p. A130
MITCHELL, Timothy, R.N. Chief Nursing Officer, Complex Care Hospital at Ridgelake, Sarasota, FL, p. A138
MITCHELL III, Walton F., Director, Catawba Hospital, Catawba, VA, p. A646
MITCHELL, William J., M.D. Chief Medical Officer, Lovelace Westside Hospital, Albuquerque, NM, p. A414
MITHUN, Robert, M.D. Physician in Chief, San Francisco Medical Center, San Francisco, CA, p. A87
MITRICK, Joseph M., FACHE President, Baptist Medical Center Beaches, Jacksonville Beach, FL, p. A127
MITRY, Norman F., President and Chief Executive Officer, Heritage Valley Beaver, Beaver, PA, p. A518
MITRY, Norman F., President and Chief Executive Officer, Heritage Valley Health System, Beaver, PA, p. B68
MITRY, Norman F., President and Chief Executive Officer, Sewickley Valley Hospital, (A Division of Valley Medical Facilities), Sewickley, PA, p. A538
MITTEER, Brian R., Chief Executive Officer, Cortland Regional Medical Center, Cortland, NY, p. A424

A884 Index of Health Care Professionals

Index of Health Care Professionals / Montante

Index of Health Care Professionals

MITTELSTAEDT, Doug, Vice President Human Resources, Children's Hospital, New Orleans, LA, p. A274
MITZNER, Jennifer C.
Chief Financial Officer, Hoag Hospital Irvine, Irvine, CA, p. A65
Senior Vice President Finance and Chief Financial Officer, Hoag Memorial Hospital Presbyterian, Newport Beach, CA, p. A76
MIYAMOTO, Faye, Vice President Human Resources, Rehabilitation Hospital of the Pacific, Honolulu, HI, p. A164
MIYASAWA, Patricia, CPA Director Fiscal Service, Shriners Hospitals for Children, Honolulu, Honolulu, HI, p. A164
MIYAUCHI, Kimberly, R.N. Chief Nursing Officer, Kingman Regional Medical Center, Kingman, AZ, p. A33
MIZE, William D., Interim Chief Executive Officer, Trousdale Medical Center, Hartsville, TN, p. A566
MIZELL, Patricia A., Chief Financial Officer, Riverside Medical Center, Franklinton, LA, p. A266
MIZELL, Philip L., M.D. Medical Director, The BridgeWay, North Little Rock, AR, p. A50
MIZELLE, Shelley, Chief Resource Management Division, Reynolds Army Community Hospital, Fort Sill, OK, p. A497
MIZER, Alison, Chief Financial Officer, St. Anthony North Hospital, Westminster, CO, p. A106
MIZEUR, Tracy, M.D. President Medical Staff, Abraham Lincoln Memorial Hospital, Lincoln, IL, p. A186
MIZIA, Robert, Director Information Systems and Chief Information Officer, Underwood–Memorial Hospital, Woodbury, NJ, p. A412
MIZONO, Gary, M.D. Physician–in–Chief, San Rafael Medical Center, San Rafael, CA, p. A89
MIZRACH, Kenneth H., Director, Veterans Affairs New Jersey Health Care System, East Orange, NJ, p. A403
MLADY, Celine M., Chief Executive Officer, Osmond General Hospital, Osmond, NE, p. A388
MO, Lin H., President and Chief Executive Officer, New York Community Hospital,, NY, p. A435
MOAD, Harold, Chief Operating Officer, Elkview General Hospital, Hobart, OK, p. A497
MOAK, Jennifer, Business Office Manager, Lawrence County Hospital, Monticello, MS, p. A350
MOAK, Mike, Chief Information Officer, Southwest Mississippi Regional Medical Center, McComb, MS, p. A349
MOAKLER, Thomas J., Chief Executive Officer, Houlton Regional Hospital, Houlton, ME, p. A283
MOALLEMIAN, Patrick, Chief Executive Officer and Managing Director, Arbour H. R. I. Hospital, Brookline, MA, p. A298
MOATS, Susan, R.N. Vice President of Patient Care Services and Chief Nursing Officer, The Heart Hospital Baylor Plano, Plano, TX, p. A621
MOBERG, Kirk, M.D. Executive Vice President and Chief Medical Officer, Carle Foundation Hospital, Urbana, IL, p. A195
MOBLEY, Barbara, Chief Executive Officer, Methodist Rehabilitation Hospital, Dallas, TX, p. A592
MOBLEY, Dana, Chief Information Officer, Our Community Hospital, Scotland Neck, NC, p. A460
MOBLEY, Paul, D.O. Clinical Director, Claremore Indian Hospital, Claremore, OK, p. A494
MOBLEY, Robert L., M.D. Executive Vice President Medical Affairs and Quality, St. Dominic–Jackson Memorial Hospital, Jackson, MS, p. A348
MOCK, Presley, M.D. Chief of Staff, Texas Institute for Surgery at Texas Health Presbyterian Dallas, Dallas, TX, p. A592
MOCK, Sara, Director Administrative Services, Kansas Neurological Institute, Topeka, KS, p. A244
MOCKLIN, Kevin, M.D. Director Medical Staff, Lake Charles Memorial Hospital, Lake Charles, LA, p. A271
MODLIN, Stacy, Chief Operating Officer, Northwest Medical Center, Margate, FL, p. A129
MOE, Aldean J., Chief Operating Officer, Alpena Regional Medical Center, Alpena, MI, p. A307
MOE, Terrance D., M.D. President Medical Staff, Eagle River Memorial Hospital, Eagle River, WI, p. A680
MOEBIUS, Geoffrey D., Chief Executive Officer, Physicians Regional Medical Center – Pine Ridge, Naples, FL, p. A133
MOEEN, Farida, M.D. Chief Operating Officer, Doctor's Hospital – Tidwell, Houston, TX, p. A604
MOELLER, Jerry G., FACHE President and Chief Executive Officer, Stillwater Medical Center, Stillwater, OK, p. A505
MOEN, Daniel J., Chief Executive Officer, LHP Hospital Group, Plano, TX, p. B79
MOEN, Daniel P., President and Chief Executive Officer, Mercy Medical Center, Springfield, MA, p. A305
MOEN, Kelly, Interim Chief Executive Officer, Memorial Medical Center – Neillsville, Neillsville, WI, p. A688
MOEN, Nellie, Coordinator Human Resources, Kindred Hospital–Bay Area, Pasadena, TX, p. A620
MOFFAT, Dodi, Supervisor Human Resources, Garden County Health Services, Oshkosh, NE, p. A388
MOFFATT, Dan, Chief Information Officer, Sanford Bemidji Medical Center, Bemidji, MN, p. A328
MOFFATT, Tracey, Chief Operating Officer, Wellmont Hancock County Hospital, Sneedville, TN, p. A575
MOFFET, Chris, Director Information Services, Bob Wilson Memorial Grant County Hospital, Ulysses, KS, p. A244
MOFFITT, Mark, Chief Information Officer, Adena Health System, Chillicothe, OH, p. A472
MOFFITT, Scott, Director Information Systems, Sanford Sheldon Medical Center, Sheldon, IA, p. A226
MOGHISSI, Etie, M.D. Chief Medical Staff, Centinela Hospital Medical Center, Inglewood, CA, p. A65
MOGLER, Rick A., Director Human Resources, Passavant Area Hospital, Jacksonville, IL, p. A185
MOHAMMADBHOY, Kayum, M.D. Chief of Staff, DeSoto Memorial Hospital, Arcadia, FL, p. A118
MOHAMMED, Ehtaisham, M.D. Chief Medical Officer, Sibley Medical Center, Arlington, MN, p. A327
MOHAMMED, Larry, Director Information Systems, Town and Country Hospital, Tampa, FL, p. A141
MOHAN, Amite, Executive Director, Shore Rehabilitation Hospital, Brick, NJ, p. A402
MOHAN, Prabha, M.D. President Medical Staff, Texas Health Presbyterian Hospital Kaufman, Kaufman, TX, p. A610
MOHANTY, Prasanna, Assistant Administrator Finance, Los Angeles Medical Center, Los Angeles, CA, p. A70
MOHESKY, Deb, Chief Financial Officer, Carondelet St. Mary's Hospital, Tucson, AZ, p. A39
MOHLER, Brittany, Director Human Resources, Deer River HealthCare Center, Deer River, MN, p. A330
MOHNKERN, Pearl, Vice President Human Resources, Advance Care Hospital, Hot Springs National Park, AR, p. A46
MOHR, Angela, R.N. Vice President of Nursing, St. Anthony Shawnee Hospital, Shawnee, OK, p. A504
MOHR, Steve
Senior Vice President Finance and Chief Financial Officer, Loma Linda University Behavioral Medicine Center, Redlands, CA, p. A82
Senior Vice President Finance and Chief Financial Officer, Loma Linda University Medical Center, Loma Linda, CA, p. A67
MOK, Michelle, Chief Financial Officer, Saint John's Health Center, Santa Monica, CA, p. A90
MOKFI, Shaya, M.D. Medical Director and President Medical Staff, Kindred Hospital of Northern Indiana, Mishawaka, IN, p. A208
MOKIAO, Lei, Coordinator Human Resources, Molokai General Hospital, Kaunakakai, HI, p. A165
MOLACEK, Shane, Chief Information Officer, Valley County Health System, Ord, NE, p. A388
MOLAI, Ashton, M.D. Chief Medical Officer, Wilkes Regional Medical Center, North Wilkesboro, NC, p. A458
MOLINA, Isabel, M.D. Chief Medical Officer, Lamb Healthcare Center, Littlefield, TX, p. A612
MOLINA, John, Chief Executive Officer, U. S. Public Health Service Phoenix Indian Medical Center, Phoenix, AZ, p. A37
MOLINA, Luis
Vice President Finance and Chief Financial Officer, Community Hospital, Munster, IN, p. A209
Chief Financial Officer, St. Catherine Hospital, East Chicago, IN, p. A200
MOLINARI, Michael, M.D. Chief of Staff, Corona Regional Medical Center, Corona, CA, p. A58
MOLINARO, Frank L., Chief Executive Officer, Arrowhead Hospital, Glendale, AZ, p. A32
MOLINO, C. Gene, Associate Director, Veterans Affairs Medical Center, Wilkes–Barre, PA, p. A542
MOLITOR, Margie, R.N. Chief Executive Officer, Washakie Medical Center, Worland, WY, p. A698
MOLL, Ben, Assistant Chief Financial Officer, Nashoba Valley Medical Center, Ayer, MA, p. A295
MOLL, Gudrun, R.N. Chief Nursing Officer, St. John's Regional Medical Center, Oxnard, CA, p. A78
MOLLER, Lynn, Chief Financial Officer, Community Memorial Hospital, Redfield, SD, p. A559
MOLLESTON, Julie, Executive Director Human Resources and Customer Services, University of California, Irvine Healthcare, Orange, CA, p. A78
MOLLOHAN, Joan, Vice President Human Resources, Ochsner Medical Center, New Orleans, LA, p. A275
MOLLOY, Kevin, Senior Vice President and Chief Operating Officer, Beth Israel Medical Center, New York, NY, p. A431
MOLLOY, Reuben D., Chief Information Officer, Governor Juan F. Louis Hospital, Christiansted, VI, p. A704
MOLMEN, David R., Chief Executive Officer, Altru Health System, Grand Forks, ND, p. A466
MOLTHEN, Barbara, Director Human Resources, Aurora Psychiatric Hospital, Wauwatosa, WI, p. A693
MOLYNEUX, Phyllis, Associate Administrator Human Resources and Education, Williamson Medical Center, Franklin, TN, p. A565
MOMEYER, Polly, Manager Human Resources, Millcreek Community Hospital, Erie, PA, p. A523
MON, Kathy, Vice President Operations, The Hospital at Hebrew Health Care, West Hartford, CT, p. A113
MONAGHAN, Aimee, Administrator, Compass Behavioral Center of Crowley, Crowley, LA, p. A265
MONAHAN, Jane, Director Human Resources, Monroe Clinic, Monroe, WI, p. A687
MONARCH, Beth, Executive Vice President and Chief Operating Officer, Cardinal Hill Rehabilitation Hospital, Lexington, KY, p. A252
MONASTERIO, Eugene A., M.D. Medical Director, Children's Hospital of Richmond, Richmond, VA, p. A654
MONCHER, Daniel J., Vice President and Chief Financial Officer, Firelands Regional Health System, Sandusky, OH, p. A488
MONCRIEF, Bill, ORH IT Client Executive, Oakland Regional Hospital, Southfield, MI, p. A323
MONCZEWSKI, Patricia, Chief Operating Officer, Mercy General Hospital, Sacramento, CA, p. A83
MONDRAGON, Donald, M.D. Deputy Commander Clinical Services, Reynolds Army Community Hospital, Fort Sill, OK, p. A497
MONETTE, Steven, Chief Financial Officer, Valley Regional Hospital, Claremont, NH, p. A397
MONEY, Rory, Manager Human Resources, Methodist McKinney Hospital, McKinney, TX, p. A616
MONG, Mary, R.N. Chief Operating Officer, Coney Island Hospital,, NY, p. A432
MONGE, A. John, Vice President Operations, Castle Medical Center, Kailua, HI, p. A164
MONGE, Catherine, Senior Vice President Operations, Medstar Washington Hospital Center, Washington, DC, p. A116
MONGE, Peter W., President, Medstar Montgomery Medical Center, Olney, MD, p. A293
MONGELL, Mitchell P., FACHE Chief Executive Officer, Colleton Medical Center, Walterboro, SC, p. A554
MONGER, Kenneth, Chief Financial Officer, Shawano Medical Center, Shawano, WI, p. A690
MONGER, Lloyd, Chief Executive Officer, Jackson Parish Hospital, Jonesboro, LA, p. A268
MONGER, Shelton, Director Information Technology, Wayne Hospital, Greenville, OH, p. A481
MONGOVEN, Pat, Director Information Systems, Winter Haven Hospital, Winter Haven, FL, p. A143
MONIACI, Cathy, Chief Operating Officer, Shriners Hospitals for Children, Houston, Houston, TX, p. A606
MONICAL, Robert, President and Chief Executive Officer, McPherson Hospital, McPherson, KS, p. A238
MONJE, Mary Anne
Chief Financial Officer, Greater El Monte Community Hospital, South El Monte, CA, p. A91
Chief Financial Officer and Chief Operating Officer, Whittier Hospital Medical Center, Whittier, CA, p. A96
MONKRES, Paula, Administrative Assistant and Director Human Resources, Nocona General Hospital, Nocona, TX, p. A618
MONROE, Ginny, Chief Operating Officer, Newport Hospital and Health Services, Newport, WA, p. A663
MONROE, Janet J., R.N. Chief Executive Officer, Greystone Park Psychiatric Hospital, Morris Plains, NJ, p. A406
MONROE, Mary, Chief Information Officer, Veterans Affairs Medical Center, Tomah, WI, p. A692
MONROIG, Domingo, Administrator, Castaner General Hospital, Castaner, PR, p. A700
MONSANTO, Monte, Chief Information Systems, Russell County Hospital, Russell Springs, KY, p. A258
MONSON, Kerry, Vice President Finance and Chief Financial Officer, Mercy Medical Center, Williston, ND, p. A468
MONSON, Mark, Chief Operating Officer, Beaver Dam Community Hospitals, Beaver Dam, WI, p. A679
MONSOUR, Mitchell D., Interim Chief Executive Officer, Williamsburg Regional Hospital, Kingstree, SC, p. A551
MONSRUD, Michele, Director Human Resources, Walton Regional Medical Center, Monroe, GA, p. A156
MONTAG, Kathy, Administrator Health Care, State Correctional Institution at Camp Hill, Camp Hill, PA, p. A520
MONTAGNESE, Robert A., President and Chief Executive Officer, Licking Memorial Hospital, Newark, OH, p. A486
MONTALBO, Tripp, Chief Operating Officer, Huntsville Memorial Hospital, Huntsville, TX, p. A608
MONTALVO, Eladio, Chief Operating Officer, Doctors Hospital of Laredo, Laredo, TX, p. A612
MONTALVO, Jose, M.D. Medical Director, Hospital Del Maestro, San Juan, PR, p. A703
MONTALVO, Juan F., M.D. Chief of Staff, Doctors Hospital of Laredo, Laredo, TX, p. A612
MONTANO, Mayra, Director Information Systems, Hospital Metropolitano Dr. Susoni, Arecibo, PR, p. A700
MONTANTE, Carl, Director Information Systems and Information Technology, Shriners Hospitals for Children, Portland, Portland, OR, p. A514


Index of Health Care Professionals A885

Index of Health Care Professionals / Montanye

MONTANYE, Cherelle, Chief Executive Officer, Ellsworth Municipal Hospital, Iowa Falls, IA, p. A222
MONTECALVO, Anthony, M.D. Chief Medical Executive, Danville State Hospital, Danville, PA, p. A521
MONTELLA, Alan J., Assistant Administrator Finance, Sullivan County Community Hospital, Sullivan, IN, p. A212
MONTENEGRO, Diana, Director Human Resources, Baptist Health South Florida, South Miami Hospital, Miami, FL, p. A130
MONTENEGRO, Robert, M.D. Chief of Staff, Glacial Ridge Health System, Glenwood, MN, p. A332
MONTERA, Julie, Director Information Technology, Sutter Medical Center, Sacramento, Sacramento, CA, p. A84
MONTES, Ernesto, Director Finance, Castaner General Hospital, Castaner, PR, p. A700
MONTES, Lisa K., Chief Executive Officer, Del Amo Hospital, Torrance, CA, p. A92
MONTEYNE, Peter J., M.D. Chief Medical Staff, Promise Hospital Baton Rouge, Baton Rouge, LA, p. A263
MONTEZ, Beverly, Manager Business Office, Otto Kaiser Memorial Hospital, Kenedy, TX, p. A610
MONTGOMERY, Angie, Director Human Resources, Peninsula Hospital, Louisville, TN, p. A570
MONTGOMERY, Bennie, R.N. Chief Nursing Officer and Chief Operations Officer, Kindred Hospital of Riverside, Perris, CA, p. A80
MONTGOMERY, Charles, M.D. Medical Director, Logansport Memorial Hospital, Logansport, IN, p. A207
MONTGOMERY, Dewery, Chief Operating Officer, Holmes County Hospital and Clinics, Lexington, MS, p. A349
MONTGOMERY, George H., Chief Executive Officer, Schoolcraft Memorial Hospital, Manistique, MI, p. A318
MONTGOMERY, Jackie, Director Human Resources, MetroSouth Medical Center, Blue Island, IL, p. A174
MONTGOMERY, James T., FACHE President, Touro Infirmary, New Orleans, LA, p. A275
MONTGOMERY, Jennifer
Vice President, Nursing, Port Huron Hospital, Port Huron, MI, p. A321
Chief Nursing Officer, Rochelle Community Hospital, Rochelle, IL, p. A192
Chief Financial Officer, Washakie Medical Center, Worland, WY, p. A698
MONTGOMERY, Lisa P., Administrator Finance and Support Services, MUSC Medical Center of Medical University of South Carolina, Charleston, SC, p. A547
MONTGOMERY, Mark, M.D. Vice President Quality and Medical Affairs, St. Joseph Regional Health Center, Bryan, TX, p. A586
MONTGOMERY, Mary Jim, R.N. Chief Operating Officer, Crisp Regional Hospital, Cordele, GA, p. A150
MONTGOMERY, Michael J., President and Chief Executive Officer, Cleo Wallace Centers Hospital, Westminster, CO, p. A106
MONTGOMERY II, Raymond W., FACHE President and Chief Executive Officer, White County Medical Center, Searcy, AR, p. A51
MONTGOMERY, Robert, Chief Financial Officer, Shriners Hospitals for Children–Lexington, Lexington, KY, p. A253
MONTGOMERY, Tina, Chief Financial Officer, Sidney Health Center, Sidney, MT, p. A379
MONTGOMERY, Traci, Manager Human Resources, Patients' Hospital of Redding, Redding, CA, p. A82
MONTOUR, Vina, Director Information Technology, U. S. Public Health Service Phoenix Indian Medical Center, Phoenix, AZ, p. A37
MONTROSS, Susan D.
Vice President Human Resources, Allied Services Rehabilitation Hospital, Scranton, PA, p. A537
Vice President Human Resources, John Heinz Institute of Rehabilitation Medicine, Wilkes–Barre, PA, p. A541
MONVESKY, Kimberly, Chief Financial Officer, Pikes Peak Regional Hospital, Woodland Park, CO, p. A107
MONZINGO, Ashley, Human Resources, Accounts Payable and Payroll, TOPS Surgical Specialty Hospital, Houston, TX, p. A607
MOODY, David, Vice President Human Resources, Salina Regional Health Center, Salina, KS, p. A242
MOODY, Heather, Chief Human Resource Management, Hunter Holmes McGuire Veterans Affairs Medical Center, Richmond, VA, p. A655
MOODY, James, Chief Financial Officer, Donalsonville Hospital, Donalsonville, GA, p. A151
MOODY, Michael
Senior Vice President and Chief Financial Officer, John Muir Behavioral Health Center, Concord, CA, p. A58
Chief Financial Officer, John Muir Medical Center, Concord, Concord, CA, p. A58
Senior Vice President and Chief Financial Officer, John Muir Medical Center, Walnut Creek, Walnut Creek, CA, p. A95
MOODY, Michael L., Market Chief Executive Officer, Kindred Hospital–Louisville, Louisville, KY, p. A254
MOODY, Vicky, Director Human Resources, Houlton Regional Hospital, Houlton, ME, p. A283
MOON, Diane
Chief Financial Officer, Inland Valley Medical Center, Wildomar, CA, p. A96
Chief Financial Officer, Rancho Springs Medical Center, Murrieta, CA, p. A76
MOON, Gina, Vice President Finance, New London Family Medical Center, New London, WI, p. A688
MOON, John, Associate Director, Veterans Affairs Eastern Kansas Health Care System, Topeka, KS, p. A244
MOON, Lori, R.N. Vice President Clinical Operations/ Business Development, McDonough District Hospital, Macomb, IL, p. A186
MOON, Lynn, Director Human Resources, Lock Haven Hospital, Lock Haven, PA, p. A528
MOON, Robert, Senior Vice President Northern Region and Chief Financial Officer, Mercy St. Charles Hospital, Oregon, OH, p. A486
MOONEY, Beth, R.N. Chief Nursing Officer, HEALTHSOUTH Valley of the Sun Rehabilitation Hospital, Glendale, AZ, p. A33
MOONEY, Jamie, Vice President and Chief Information Officer, Hospital for Special Surgery, New York, NY, p. A433
MOONEY, Jimmy, Chief Executive Officer, Willingway Hospital, Statesboro, GA, p. A160
MOONEY, Katharine, R.N. Chief Nursing Officer, Upstate University Hospital, Syracuse, NY, p. A444
MOONEY, Robert W., M.D. Medical Director, Willingway Hospital, Statesboro, GA, p. A160
MOONEY, Susan E., M.D. Vice President and Chief Medical Officer, Alice Peck Day Memorial Hospital, Lebanon, NH, p. A398
MOONEY, Thomas, M.D. President Executive Committee Medical Staff, Naval Medical Center, Portsmouth, VA, p. A654
MOORE III, Ben, President and Chief Executive Officer, River Hospital, Alexandria Bay, NY, p. A420
MOORE, Betty, Business Manager, North Mississippi Medical Center–Iuka, Iuka, MS, p. A347
MOORE, Bill, Chief Human Resources, El Centro Regional Medical Center, El Centro, CA, p. A60
MOORE, Bob, FACHE Chief Executive Officer, Lancaster Regional Medical Center, Lancaster, PA, p. A526
MOORE, Brandon, Administrator and Chief Executive Officer, Park Place Surgical Hospital, Lafayette, LA, p. A270
MOORE, Brett, CPA Assistant Administrator Finance, Sutter Amador Hospital, Jackson, CA, p. A65
MOORE, C. Thomas, Chief Financial Officer, Regional Medical Center of Hopkins County, Madisonville, KY, p. A255
MOORE, Carrie, Director Human Resources, Meadowbrook Rehabilitation Hospital, Gardner, KS, p. A233
MOORE, Christie, Director Human Resources, Reliant Rehabilitation Hospital Mid–Cities, Bedford, TX, p. A583
MOORE, Courtney, CPA Chief Financial Officer, Morgan Memorial Hospital, Madison, GA, p. A156
MOORE, Dana
Senior Vice President Information Services, St. Anthony Hospital, Lakewood, CO, p. A103
Senior Vice President Information Services, St. Anthony North Hospital, Westminster, CO, p. A106
MOORE, Darrell W., Chief Executive Officer, Parkridge Medical Center, Chattanooga, TN, p. A563
MOORE, Debra, Chief Executive Officer, Parkside Hospital, Tulsa, OK, p. A506
MOORE, Debra L., Senior Vice President, Memorial Health Care System, Chattanooga, TN, p. A563
MOORE, Diane C., Chief Financial Officer, Copper Queen Community Hospital, Bisbee, AZ, p. A31
MOORE, Donald F., Director, Jerry L. Pettis Memorial Veterans Medical Center, Loma Linda, CA, p. A67
MOORE, Donna, Director Human Resources, Belmont Community Hospital, Bellaire, OH, p. A470
MOORE, Dylan, Controller, Rogers City Rehabilitation Hospital, Rogers City, MI, p. A321
MOORE, Edward H., President and Chief Executive Officer, Harrington Memorial Hospital, Southbridge, MA, p. A304
MOORE, Elizabeth, Chief Operating Officer, Silver Hill Hospital, New Canaan, CT, p. A110
MOORE, Emily, Director Human Resources and Information Technology, Haskell Memorial Hospital, Haskell, TX, p. A603
MOORE, Emmett E., JD, Chief Executive Officer, Reliant Healthcare Partners, Addison, TX, p. B109
MOORE, Gary, Chief Executive Officer, Shoshone Medical Center, Kellogg, ID, p. A168
MOORE, Greg, CPA, Interim Chief Executive Officer, Pioneers Memorial Healthcare District, Brawley, CA, p. A56
MOORE, James D., FACHE Chief Executive Officer, Integris Southwest Medical Center, Oklahoma City, OK, p. A501
MOORE, Jane, Director, Fiscal Services, Quitman County Hospital, Marks, MS, p. A349
MOORE, Jason H., Vice President and Chief Operating Officer, Tallahassee Memorial HealthCare, Tallahassee, FL, p. A140
MOORE, Jay, M.D. Vice President, Medical Affairs, SSM DePaul Health Center, Bridgeton, MO, p. A356
MOORE, Jeannie, Director Human Resources, Northern Hospital of Surry County, Mount Airy, NC, p. A458
MOORE, John, M.D. Medical Director, Granite County Medical Center, Philipsburg, MT, p. A378
MOORE, John
Administrator, Hiawatha Community Hospital, Hiawatha, KS, p. A234
Chief Executive Officer, South Lake Hospital, Clermont, FL, p. A120
MOORE, John G.
Chief Financial Officer, Anson Community Hospital, Wadesboro, NC, p. A462
Vice President and Chief Financial Officer, Carolinas Medical Center–Union, Monroe, NC, p. A457
MOORE, Kadie, Director Human Resources, Vidant Edgecombe Hospital, Tarboro, NC, p. A461
MOORE, Kandi, Administrator, Specialists Hospital – Shreveport, Shreveport, LA, p. A277
MOORE, Karen, Vice President Information Technology and Chief Information Officer, Southern Regional Medical Center, Riverdale, GA, p. A158
MOORE, Karen O., R.N. President and Chief Executive Officer, UMass Memorial–Marlborough Hospital, Marlborough, MA, p. A302
MOORE, Kathy D., Chief Operating Officer, St. Luke's Regional Medical Center, Boise, ID, p. A167
MOORE, Kermit, R.N. Chief Operating Officer and Chief Nursing Officer, Nemaha County Hospital, Auburn, NE, p. A381
MOORE, Kerry, M.D. Chief of Staff, Carilion Tazewell Community Hospital, Tazewell, VA, p. A656
MOORE, Kim, Director Operations, Woodridge Hospital, Johnson City, TN, p. A568
MOORE, Kim S., President and Chief Executive Officer, Saint Elizabeth Regional Medical Center, Lincoln, NE, p. A385
MOORE, Larry E., Chief Financial Officer, Cumberland Medical Center, Crossville, TN, p. A564
MOORE, Lauralinda, Manager Finance, CHRISTUS Spohn Hospital Kleberg, Kingsville, TX, p. A610
MOORE, Leigh, Administrative Assistant Human Resources, H. C. Watkins Memorial Hospital, Quitman, MS, p. A352
MOORE, Linda, Manager Human Resources, Seymour Hospital, Seymour, TX, p. A627
MOORE, Lois Jean, FACHE Administrator, University of Texas Harris County Psychiatric Center, Houston, TX, p. A607
MOORE, Marcia, Vice President, Tomball Regional Medical Center, Tomball, TX, p. A631
MOORE, Margaret, Manager Business Office, Sabine County Hospital, Hemphill, TX, p. A603
MOORE, Mark E., President and Chief Executive Officer, Indiana University Health Bloomington Hospital, Bloomington, IN, p. A198
MOORE, Matthew, Senior Vice President and Chief Financial Officer, St. Francis Hospital, Columbus, GA, p. A149
MOORE, Megan K., Vice President and Administrator, Riverside Walter Reed Hospital, Gloucester, VA, p. A649
MOORE, Melinda, Chief Human Resources Officer, Banner Lassen Medical Center, Susanville, CA, p. A92
MOORE, Michael L., Chief Executive Officer, Regency Hospital of Jackson, Jackson, MS, p. A348
MOORE, Mike, Chief Financial Officer, Jane Phillips Medical Center, Bartlesville, OK, p. A494
MOORE, Mindy S., Chief Executive Officer, Cornerstone Hospital of SouthEast Arizona, Tucson, AZ, p. A39
MOORE, Monty, Director Information Services, Summit Surgical, LLC, Hutchinson, KS, p. A235
MOORE, Neil J.
Chief Financial Officer, Laurel Regional Hospital, Laurel, MD, p. A293
Chief Financial Officer, Prince George's Hospital Center, Cheverly, MD, p. A290
MOORE, Nelda, Director Data Processing, Memorial Hospital and Manor, Bainbridge, GA, p. A147
MOORE, Paul, Chief Information Officer, Connecticut Mental Health Center, New Haven, CT, p. A110
MOORE, Paula, R.N. Chief Nursing Officer, Twin Cities Community Hospital, Templeton, CA, p. A92
MOORE, Phyllis, Director Information Systems and Data Center, Doctors Medical Center–San Pablo Campus, San Pablo, CA, p. A89

A886 Index of Health Care Professionals

Index of Health Care Professionals / Morquecho

Index of Health Care Professionals

MOORE, Richard
Director Information Technology, Hawthorn Children Psychiatric Hospital, Saint Louis, MO, p. A368
Director Information Technology, Metropolitan St. Louis Psychiatric Center, Saint Louis, MO, p. A369
Director Information Technology, St. Louis Psychiatric Rehabilitation Center, Saint Louis, MO, p. A370
MOORE, Rick
Chief Information Officer, Bethesda North Hospital, Cincinnati, OH, p. A472
Chief Information Officer, Good Samaritan Hospital, Cincinnati, OH, p. A473
MOORE, Rita, Director Finance, Boscobel Area Health Care, Boscobel, WI, p. A679
MOORE, Robin A., Vice President Human Resources, Concord Hospital, Concord, NH, p. A397
MOORE, Rodney, M.D. Vice President Medical Affairs, Cape Canaveral Hospital, Cocoa Beach, FL, p. A120
MOORE, Sandee, Chief Operating Officer, Eastern Idaho Regional Medical Center, Idaho Falls, ID, p. A168
MOORE, Sandra, Director Human Resources, Mayo Clinic Health System – Chippewa Valley in Bloomer, Bloomer, WI, p. A679
MOORE, Sandy, Interim CFO, Mercer County Hospital, Aledo, IL, p. A172
MOORE, Sheriann, Service Unit Director, U. S. Public Health Service Indian Hospital, Winnebago, NE, p. A390
MOORE, Steve, Chief Financial Officer, Southern Tennessee Medical Center, Winchester, TN, p. A576
MOORE, Susan B., Interim Chief Financial Officer, UCSF Medical Center, San Francisco, CA, p. A87
MOORE, Susan L., R.N. Director Nursing, Thayer County Health Services, Hebron, NE, p. A384
MOORE, Tim, Chief Accounting Officer and Vice President Ancillary Services, Blessing Hospital, Quincy, IL, p. A192
MOORE, Tim, M.D. Chief of Staff, Brownwood Regional Medical Center, Brownwood, TX, p. A585
MOORE, Tim, R.N
Chief Information Officer, Hoag Hospital Irvine, Irvine, CA, p. A65
Senior Vice President and Chief Information Officer, Hoag Memorial Hospital Presbyterian, Newport Beach, CA, p. A76
MOORE, Vernon, Chief Business and Finance, University of Texas Health Science Center at Tyler, Tyler, TX, p. A632
MOORE, Warren E., Executive Vice President and Chief Operating Officer, Children's Specialized Hospital, New Brunswick, NJ, p. A406
MOORE, William, Chief Information Officer, Parrish Medical Center, Titusville, FL, p. A142
MOORE, William T., Chief Executive Officer, Atlanta Medical Center, Atlanta, GA, p. A145
MOORE–HARDY, Cynthia, President and Chief Executive Officer, Lake Health, Concord Township, OH, p. A477
MOOREHOUSE, Brett, FACHE Vice President and Chief Operating Officer, Ranken Jordan – A Pediatric Specialty Hospital, Maryland Heights, MO, p. A364
MOORER, Thad, Chief Information Officer, Eastside Psychiatric Hospital, Tallahassee, FL, p. A140
MOORHEAD, David, M.D. Chief Medical Officer, Florida Hospital, Orlando, FL, p. A134
MOORMAN, Gary L., D.O. Vice President Medical Affairs, Fisher–Titus Medical Center, Norwalk, OH, p. A486
MOORMAN, Kristi, Supervisor Human Resources, Share Medical Center, Alva, OK, p. A493
MOOTS, Eric, Vice President and Chief Financial Officer, Adventist GlenOaks Hospital, Glendale Heights, IL, p. A183
MORA, Fernando, Vice President Management Information Systems, Hospital Interamericano De Medicina Avanzada, Caguas, PR, p. A700
MORACA, Lynn, Director Human Resources, Lodi Community Hospital, Lodi, OH, p. A483
MORAHAN, John R., FACHE President and Chief Executive Officer, St. Joseph Medical Center, Reading, PA, p. A537
MORALES, Carlos, Manager Data Processing, Valley Baptist Medical Center–Brownsville, Brownsville, TX, p. A585
MORALES, Carmela, M.D. Chief of Staff, University Medical Center of El Paso, El Paso, TX, p. A597
MORALES, Daniza
Chief Information Officer, Hospital Menonita De Cayey, Cayey, PR, p. A700
Manager Information System, Mennonite General Hospital, Aibonito, PR, p. A699
MORALES, Elsie, Chief Financial Officer, Hospital Universitario Dr. Ramon Ruiz Arnau, Bayamon, PR, p. A700
MORALES, Joel, Chief Financial Officer, Fort Duncan Regional Medical Center, Eagle Pass, TX, p. A595
MORALES, John R., Chief Financial Officer, John H. Stroger Jr. Hospital of Cook County, Chicago, IL, p. A176
MORALES, Juan A., MSN, Health System Director, Veterans Affairs Tennessee Valley Healthcare System, Nashville, TN, p. A574
MORALES, Marilyn, Assistant Administrator and Chief Operating Officer, Ashford Presbyterian Community Hospital, San Juan, PR, p. A702
MORALES, Steve, Director Human Resources, Sutter Medical Center of Santa Rosa, Chanate Campus, Santa Rosa, CA, p. A90
MORALES, Trish, Director Human Resources, Lakewood Ranch Medical Center, Bradenton, FL, p. A119
MORAN, Colleen M., Director Human Resources, Spaulding Hospital for Continuing Medical Care North Shore, Salem, MA, p. A304
MORAN, Debbie, Executive Director, Carl Albert Community Mental Health Center, McAlester, OK, p. A499
MORAN, Janet, Vice President Human Resources, Lourdes Medical Center of Burlington County, Willingboro, NJ, p. A412
MORAN, Marian, Chief Information Officer, St. Mary Medical Center, Langhorne, PA, p. A526
MORAN, Mark J., President and Chief Executive Officer, MetroHealth Medical Center, Cleveland, OH, p. A475
MORAN, Tim, Interim Chief Executive Officer, Mountain West Medical Center, Tooele, UT, p. A641
MORANDEIRA, Ana, Director Marketing, San Juan Capestrano Hospital, San Juan, PR, p. A703
MORASKO, Jerome, President and Chief Executive Officer, Avita Health System, Galion, OH, p. B16
MORASKO, Jerome
Chief Executive Officer, Bucyrus Community Hospital, Bucyrus, OH, p. A471
President and Chief Executive Officer, Galion Community Hospital, Galion, OH, p. A480
MORASKO, Robert A., Chief Executive Officer, Campbell County Memorial Hospital, Gillette, WY, p. A696
MORDECAI, Steve, Director Human Resources, Griffin Hospital, Derby, CT, p. A108
MOREAU, Brian, Director Data Processing, Marcus Daly Memorial Hospital, Hamilton, MT, p. A376
MOREAU, Kim, Assistant Vice President Information Systems, Carroll Hospital Center, Westminster, MD, p. A294
MOREAU, Steven C., Chief Executive Officer, St. Joseph Hospital, Orange, CA, p. A78
MOREFIELD, Terri, Deputy Chief Human Resources Division, Bassett Army Community Hospital, Fort Wainwright, AK, p. A29
MOREH, Swenda, Chief Executive Officer, Kindred Hospital–Baldwin Park, Baldwin Park, CA, p. A55
MOREIN, Sandy, Chief Operating Officer, Mercy Regional Medical Center, Ville Platte, LA, p. A279
MORELAND, John, M.D. Chief Medical Officer, Marcus Daly Memorial Hospital, Hamilton, MT, p. A376
MORELAND, Tresha, Vice President Human Resources, Fremont–Rideout Health Group, Marysville, CA, p. A74
MORELLI, Gerald, Director Human Resources, Veterans Affairs Medical Center, Philadelphia, PA, p. A534
MORELLO, Salvatore, Vice President Finance, The Mount Sinai Hospital of Queens,, NY, p. A437
MORENO, Raymond, M.D. Vice President Medical Affairs, Tift Regional Medical Center, Tifton, GA, p. A161
MORESI, Randy, Chief Executive Officer, North Hills Hospital, North Richland Hills, TX, p. A618
MORETTE, Joseph M., Executive Vice President, Methodist Rehabilitation Center, Jackson, MS, p. A348
MORETZ, Sandy, R.N. Chief Operating Officer and Vice President Patient Care Services, Twin County Regional Hospital, Galax, VA, p. A649
MOREY, Scott, Chief Nursing Officer, Maryvale Hospital Medical Center, Phoenix, AZ, p. A36
MORGAN, Craig, Chief Executive Officer, Knox County Hospital, Barbourville, KY, p. A247
MORGAN, Daniel R., Chief Operating Officer, Bay Medical Center, Panama City, FL, p. A135
MORGAN, David, Interim Chief Executive Officer, Johnson Memorial Hospital, Stafford Springs, CT, p. A112
MORGAN, Derek, Director Human Resources, Avista Adventist Hospital, Louisville, CO, p. A104
MORGAN, Dwight, Vice President Human Resources, Aurora St. Luke's Medical Center, Milwaukee, WI, p. A686
MORGAN, Janet, Manager Human Resources, Lander Regional Hospital, Lander, WY, p. A696
MORGAN, Jeff, Director Information Systems, Northeastern Nevada Regional Hospital, Elko, NV, p. A391
MORGAN, Jeffrey, Associate Executive Director and Chief Financial Officer, Carlisle Regional Medical Center, Carlisle, PA, p. A520
MORGAN, Jennifer, Chief Executive Officer and Managing Director, Anchor Hospital, Atlanta, GA, p. A145
MORGAN, Kelly C., President and Chief Executive Officer, Mercy Medical Center, Roseburg, OR, p. A515
MORGAN, Larry, Controller, T. J. Samson Community Hospital, Glasgow, KY, p. A250
MORGAN, Lori, M.D. Chief Administrative Officer, Legacy Emanuel Hospital and Health Center, Portland, OR, p. A514
MORGAN, Mace, Director Information Systems, Minden Medical Center, Minden, LA, p. A273
MORGAN, Margaret, Director Human Resources, Centinela Hospital Medical Center, Inglewood, CA, p. A65
MORGAN, Matthew, Manager Human Resources, Lakeside Medical Center, Belle Glade, FL, p. A118
MORGAN, Michelle C., Chief Human Resource Manager, Saint Anthony Hospital, Chicago, IL, p. A178
MORGAN, Norma J., Chief Executive Officer, Effingham Hospital, Springfield, GA, p. A159
MORGAN, Nyle, Chief Information Officer, Sheridan Memorial Hospital, Sheridan, WY, p. A697
MORGAN, Rebecca
Senior Director Human Resources, Pioneer Memorial Hospital, Prineville, OR, p. A514
Senior Director Human Resources, St. Charles Medical Center – Bend, Bend, OR, p. A509
Senior Director Human Resources, St. Charles Medical Center – Redmond, Redmond, OR, p. A515
MORGAN, Richard P., M.D. Chief of Staff, Sanford Luverne Medical Center, Luverne, MN, p. A334
MORGAN, Samuel, Senior Vice President Financial Operations, Culpeper Regional Hospital, Culpeper, VA, p. A647
MORGAN, Susan, Chief Financial Officer, Mercy Regional Health Center,, KS, p. A238
MORGAN, Teresa
Chief Financial Officer, McGehee–Desha County Hospital, McGehee, AR, p. A48
Assistant Vice President Human Resources, Shannon Medical Center, San Angelo, TX, p. A624
MORGAN, Timothy J., Chief Financial Officer, Maryville Scott Nolan Center, Des Plaines, IL, p. A180
MORGAN, Vicky, Director Information Services, Centinela Hospital Medical Center, Inglewood, CA, p. A65
MORGAN, Victor, Chief Financial Officer, MidMichigan Medical Center–Gratiot, Alma, MI, p. A307
MORGAN, W. Hugh, M.D. Chief Medical Staff, Edgefield County Hospital, Edgefield, SC, p. A549
MORGENROTH, Betsy, Director Human Resources, Hoopeston Regional Health Center, Hoopeston, IL, p. A185
MORGESE, Vincent, M.D. Vice President Medical Affairs, Queen of the Valley Medical Center, Napa, CA, p. A76
MORIARTY, Bill, M.D. Chief Medical Officer, Bay Area Hospital, Coos Bay, OR, p. A510
MORILLO, Jose F., Chief Executive Officer, Charlotte Regional Medical Center, Punta Gorda, FL, p. A137
MORIN, Linda, Director of Nursing, Copper Queen Community Hospital, Bisbee, AZ, p. A31
MORISSETTE, Daniel, Senior Vice President Finance and Administration, The University of Toledo Medical Center, Toledo, OH, p. A489
MORISSETTE, Philip, Chief Financial Officer, Bridgton Hospital, Bridgton, ME, p. A282
MORITZ, Mary, Administrator Human Resources, Humboldt County Memorial Hospital, Humboldt, IA, p. A221
MORK Jr., David L., FACHE Chief Executive Officer, Select Specialty Hospital–Augusta, Augusta, GA, p. A147
MORKEL, Derek, Chief Executive Officer, HealthTech Management Services, Franklin, TN, p. B67
MORLEY, Jr., Andrew P., M.D. Senior Vice President and Chief Medical Officer, The Medical Center, Columbus, GA, p. A150
MORLEY, Denise M., Director Human Resources, Wyoming County Community Hospital, Warsaw, NY, p. A446
MORLOCK, Paul, Vice President Human Resources, Stanly Regional Medical Center, Albemarle, NC, p. A448
MORNELLI, Ronald, Senior Vice President Operations and Chief Operating Officer, Olean General Hospital, Olean, NY, p. A439
MORNINGSTAR, Tim, Blue Star, Unity Medical & Surgical Hospital, Mishawaka, IN, p. A208
MORON, David, M.D. Clinical Director, Rio Grande State Center/South Texas Health Care System, Harlingen, TX, p. A602
MORONY, David, Chief Financial Officer, Casa Colina Hospital for Rehabilitative Medicine, Pomona, CA, p. A80
MOROSES, Mark, Vice President and Chief Information Officer, St. Luke's–Roosevelt Hospital Center, New York, NY, p. A437
MORQUECHO, Adam
Director Information Systems, Garden Grove Hospital and Medical Center, Garden Grove, CA, p. A63
Director Information Technology, Huntington Beach Hospital, Huntington Beach, CA, p. A65
Director Information Technology, La Palma Intercommunity Hospital, La Palma, CA, p. A66
Director Information Technology, West Anaheim Medical Center, Anaheim, CA, p. A53

MORREALE, Daniel, Vice President and Chief Information Officer, Kingsbrook Jewish Medical Center,, NY, p. A433

MORREALE, Gene, President and Chief Executive Officer, Oneida Healthcare, Oneida, NY, p. A439

MORRELL, Dan, Manager Information Systems, Sierra Vista Hospital, Truth or Consequences, NM, p. A418

MORRICAL, Michael G., Chief Operating Officer, University Medical Center, Lebanon, TN, p. A569

MORRIS, Alexander, Corporate Director Human Resources, Fort Washington Medical Center, Fort Washington, MD, p. A291

MORRIS, Beverly
Vice President Human Resources, Kettering Medical Center, Kettering, OH, p. A482
Vice President Human Resources, Sycamore Medical Center, Miamisburg, OH, p. A485

MORRIS, Christopher
Director Human Resources, Wheaton Franciscan Healthcare – Elmbrook Memorial, Brookfield, WI, p. A679
Director Human Resources, Wheaton Franciscan Healthcare – St. Joseph's, Milwaukee, WI, p. A687
Director Human Resources, Wheaton Franciscan Healthcare – The Wisconsin Heart Hospital, Wauwatosa, WI, p. A693

MORRIS, Darrel, Chief Executive Officer, Drumright Regional Hospital, Drumright, OK, p. A495

MORRIS, David W., Chief Executive Officer, Highlands Behavioral Health System, Littleton, CO, p. A103

MORRIS, Debbie M., Director Human Resources, Marcus Daly Memorial Hospital, Hamilton, MT, p. A376

MORRIS, Dennis, Area Finance Officer, Oakland Medical Center, Oakland, CA, p. A77

MORRIS, Don, Vice President Human Resources, Wesley Medical Center, Wichita, KS, p. A246

MORRIS, Douglas
Chief Financial Officer, St. Francis Health Care Centre, Green Springs, OH, p. A481
Chief Financial Officer, Vibra Hospital of Southeastern Michigan, Lincoln Park, MI, p. A318

MORRIS, Dwain, Vice President and Chief Financial Officer, University of Texas M.D. Anderson Cancer Center, Houston, TX, p. A608

MORRIS, Elaine F., Administrator, Methodist Ambulatory Surgery Hospital, San Antonio, TX, p. A625

MORRIS, George, Vice President Information Technology and Chief Information Officer, Northwest Community Hospital, Arlington Heights, IL, p. A172

MORRIS, Gerry, Administrator, Magnolia Behavioral Healthcare, Lacombe, LA, p. A269

MORRIS, Janet, Director Human Resources, HEALTHSOUTH Lakeview Rehabilitation Hospital, Elizabethtown, KY, p. A249

MORRIS, Janice, Accountant, CrossRidge Community Hospital, Wynne, AR, p. A52

MORRIS, Jarrett, Vice President Finance, Carolinas Medical Center–Lincoln, Lincolnton, NC, p. A456

MORRIS, Jeffrey, M.D
Medical Director, Summa Barberton Citizens Hospital, Barberton, OH, p. A470
Vice President Medical Affairs, Summa Wadsworth–Rittman Hospital, Wadsworth, OH, p. A490

MORRIS, Jim, Vice President Finance, Baptist Hospital East, Louisville, KY, p. A254

MORRIS, Jimmy L., Chief Executive Officer and Administrator, Lynn County Hospital District, Tahoka, TX, p. A630

MORRIS, Jody, President and Chief Executive Officer, Franklin Regional Medical Center, Louisburg, NC, p. A457

MORRIS, John, M.D. Chief of Staff, Cullman Regional Medical Center, Cullman, AL, p. A18

MORRIS, Lisa, Vice President Human Resources, Swedish Medical Center, Englewood, CO, p. A100

MORRIS, Marsha, Manager Information Services, Fairview Park Hospital, Dublin, GA, p. A152

MORRIS, Michael, Administrator, Bellville General Hospital, Bellville, TX, p. A583

MORRIS, Paul G., Chief Financial Officer, Alaska Regional Hospital, Anchorage, AK, p. A28

MORRIS, R. Randall, Administrator, West Carroll Memorial Hospital, Oak Grove, LA, p. A275

MORRIS, Rosanna D., R.N. CNO & Senior VP Patient Care Services, Nebraska Medical Center, Omaha, NE, p. A388

MORRIS, Shawna, Senior Vice President Operations and Chief Operating Officer, Menninger Clinic, Houston, TX, p. A605

MORRIS, Terri, Manager Information Systems, Methodist Richardson Medical Center, Richardson, TX, p. A622

MORRIS, Toni, Chief Executive Officer, Sutter Surgical Hospital – North Valley, Yuba City, CA, p. A96

MORRIS, Tony, Business Manager, Mental Health Institute, Cherokee, IA, p. A216

MORRIS, Wayne, Chief Financial Officer, Veterans Affairs Medical Center, Marion, IL, p. A187

MORRIS, Will, Director Information Technology, Tri–Lakes Medical Center, Batesville, MS, p. A343

MORRISON, Christopher, Deputy Chief Executive Officer, Trenton Psychiatric Hospital, Trenton, NJ, p. A411

MORRISON, Deane, Chief Information Officer, Concord Hospital, Concord, NH, p. A397

MORRISON, Dianne, Director Human Resources, Mizell Memorial Hospital, Opp, AL, p. A24

MORRISON, Gary, Chief Operating Officer, Karmanos Cancer Center, Detroit, MI, p. A311

MORRISON, Greg, M.D. Vice President Medical Affairs, Grant Medical Center, Columbus, OH, p. A476

MORRISON, Kathy E., Executive Director Human Resources, St. Catherine Hospital, Garden City, KS, p. A233

MORRISON, Leon M., M.D. Vice President Medical Staff Services, Carteret General Hospital, Morehead City, NC, p. A457

MORRISON, Mark, Director Support Services, Shriners Hospitals for Children, Philadelphia, Philadelphia, PA, p. A533

MORRISON, Maureen, Vice President Financial Services, Advocate Trinity Hospital, Chicago, IL, p. A175

MORRISON, Michael, Chief Financial Officer, Hendersonville Medical Center, Hendersonville, TN, p. A566

MORRISON, Sarah, Vice President Clinical Services, Shepherd Center, Atlanta, GA, p. A146

MORRISSETT, Barbara, Vice President Human Resources, St. Mary's Medical Center, San Francisco, CA, p. A87

MORRISSETTE, Daniel, Chief Financial Officer, Stanford Hospital and Clinics, Palo Alto, CA, p. A79

MORRISSEY, Joseph V., President, Milton Hospital, Milton, MA, p. A302

MORRISSEY, Moira, Chief Operating Officer and General Counsel, Four Winds Hospital, Katonah, NY, p. A428

MORRISSEY, Una E., R.N. Senior Vice President, Chief Nursing Officer and Chief Operating Officer, New York Community Hospital,, NY, p. A435

MORROW, Jennifer, Director Human Resources, San Joaquin Valley Rehabilitation Hospital, Fresno, CA, p. A62

MORROW, Pat, Director Human Resources, Walker Baptist Medical Center, Jasper, AL, p. A22

MORROW, Randy, Vice President and Chief Operating Officer, Boone Hospital Center, Columbia, MO, p. A358

MORROW, Renee, Business Manager, Meadowbrook Rehabilitation Hospital, Gardner, KS, p. A233

MORROW, Robert, M.D. Chief of Staff, McDowell Hospital, Marion, NC, p. A457

MORROW, W. Robert, M.D. Senior Vice President and Medical Director, Arkansas Children's Hospital, Little Rock, AR, p. A47

MORSE, Cayce, Administrative Assistant, Frio Regional Hospital, Pearsall, TX, p. A620

MORSE, Larry, Chief Executive Officer and Administrator, Johnson Regional Medical Center, Clarksville, AR, p. A43

MORSE, Patrick, M.D. President Medical Staff, West Branch Regional Medical Center, West Branch, MI, p. A325

MORSE, Rebecca, Chief Human Resources Officer, Palo Verde Hospital, Blythe, CA, p. A56

MORSTAD, Joan, Director Information Systems, Coliseum Medical Centers, Macon, GA, p. A155

MORTENSEN, Shane, Chief Financial Officer, San Luis Valley Regional Medical Center, Alamosa, CO, p. A97

MORTENSSON, Marcie, Chief Human Resources Officer, Tahoe Forest Hospital District, Truckee, CA, p. A93

MORTH, Paul, Vice President Finance, Medcenter One, Bismarck, ND, p. A464

MORTINSEN, Roy, M.D. Chief of Staff, Sanford Vermillion Medical Center, Vermillion, SD, p. A560

MORTON, David, M.D. Chief Medical Officer, St. Anthony's Medical Center, Saint Louis, MO, p. A370

MORTON, Denise, Chief Financial Officer, Veterans Affairs Medical Center – Alexandria, Pineville, LA, p. A276

MORTON, Robert, M.D. Medical Director, Rolling Hills Hospital, Ada, OK, p. A493

MORTON, Stan C., FACHE President, Texas Health Presbyterian Hospital Denton, Denton, TX, p. A594

MORTON, Stephanie, Chief Information Officer, Providence Alaska Medical Center, Anchorage, AK, p. A28

MORTOZA, Angela, Administrator, Adair County Memorial Hospital, Greenfield, IA, p. A220

MOSCATO, Mary K., Chief Operating Officer–Hebrew Rehabilitation Center and Hebrew Senior Life Health Care Services, Hebrew Rehabilitation Center, Boston, MA, p. A297

MOSCHITTA, Philip C., Director, Veterans Affairs Medical Center, Northport, NY, p. A438

MOSCHKAU, Don, Director Human Resources, Fairview Lakes Health Services, Wyoming, MN, p. A342

MOSCOSO, Ricardo, M.D. Medical Director, University Hospital, San Juan, PR, p. A704

MOSELEY, Thomas, M.D. President Medical Staff, North Country Hospital and Health Center, Newport, VT, p. A644

MOSELY, Chisty, Director Information Management, Saint Simons by–the–Sea Hospital, Saint Simons Island, GA, p. A158

MOSER, Brenda, Vice President Finance, Regional Health Services of Howard County, Cresco, IA, p. A217

MOSER, Joseph, M.D. Vice President Medical Staff Affairs, Anne Arundel Medical Center, Annapolis, MD, p. A287

MOSER, Neal, M.D. Medical Director, HEALTHSOUTH Northern Kentucky Rehabilitation Hospital, Edgewood, KY, p. A249

MOSER, Stan, President and Chief Executive Officer, Bozeman Deaconess Hospital, Bozeman, MT, p. A373

MOSER, Thomas B., Chief Operating Officer, Forbes Regional Hospital, Monroeville, PA, p. A529

MOSER, Tracy, Director Human Resources, Upper Valley Medical Center, Troy, OH, p. A490

MOSES, Deana, Manager Human Resources, Lincoln County Medical Center, Ruidoso, NM, p. A417

MOSES, Gregory, M.D. President Medical Staff, Camden–Clark Medical Center, Parkersburg, WV, p. A674

MOSESIAN, Robert, Controller, HEALTHSOUTH Bakersfield Rehabilitation Hospital, Bakersfield, CA, p. A54

MOSHIER, John, Director Human Resources, Clara Barton Hospital, Hoisington, KS, p. A234

MOSHIRPUR, Jasmin, M.D
Dean and Medical Director, Elmhurst Hospital Center,, NY, p. A432
Chief Medical Officer, Queens Hospital Center,, NY, p. A436

MOSHOFSKY, Bill, M.D. Chief of Staff, Sacred Heart Medical Center, Eugene, OR, p. A510

MOSIER, Dawn, Director Human Resources, HEALTHSOUTH Rehabilitation Institute of Tucson, Tucson, AZ, p. A40

MOSIER, John, D.O. Chief of Staff, Herington Municipal Hospital, Herington, KS, p. A234

MOSKOWITZ, Samuel E., President, Medstar Franklin Square Medical Center, Baltimore, MD, p. A288

MOSLEY, Brian, Coordinator Human Resources and Payroll Benefits, Kindred Hospital–San Antonio, San Antonio, TX, p. A625

MOSLEY, Tonja, Chief Financial Officer, Heart of Florida Regional Medical Center, Davenport, FL, p. A121

MOSS, Austin, Vice President Human Resources, Jennie Stuart Medical Center, Hopkinsville, KY, p. A251

MOSS, C. Renee, M.D. Chief Medical Officer, Riverside Rehabilitation Institute, Newport News, VA, p. A652

MOSS, Misty, Director Business Administration, Logansport State Hospital, Logansport, IN, p. A207

MOSS, Ray, Vice President and Chief Information Officer, Valley Presbyterian Hospital,, CA, p. A72

MOSS, Stuart, Chief Financial Officer, Marlton Rehabilitation Hospital, Marlton, NJ, p. A406

MOSSOFF, Alan, Chief Financial Officer, Northern Dutchess Hospital, Rhinebeck, NY, p. A441

MOSSOP, Karen, Director Human Resources, Montgomery County Emergency Service, Norristown, PA, p. A530

MOST, Kevin, D.O. Vice President Medical Affairs, Central DuPage Hospital, Winfield, IL, p. A196

MOTONAGA, Gregg, M.D. Chief of Staff, Central Peninsula General Hospital, Soldotna, AK, p. A30

MOTTE, Michael J.
Chief Executive Officer, St. Alexius Hospital – Broadway Campus, Saint Louis, MO, p. A369
Chief Executive Officer, St. Alexius Hospital – Forest Park Campus, Saint Louis, MO, p. A369

MOUGHON, Edward, Superintendent, Big Spring State Hospital, Big Spring, TX, p. A584

MOUISSET, Rena B., Director Human Resources and Contract Compliance, St. Martin Hospital, Breaux Bridge, LA, p. A264

MOULTHROP, David L., Ph.D. President and Chief Executive Officer, Rogers Memorial Hospital, Oconomowoc, WI, p. A688

MOUNIE, Mike, Director Finance, Sentara Obici Hospital, Suffolk, VA, p. A656

MOUNT, Mary H., Administrative Officer, Fort Belknap U. S. Public Health Service Indian Hospital, Harlem, MT, p. A376

MOUNTAIN, J. Michael, Chief Financial Officer, RiverValley Behavioral Health Hospital, Owensboro, KY, p. A257

MOUREY, Jerry, Vice President Information Technology and Chief Information Officer, Aspirus Wausau Hospital, Wausau, WI, p. A693

MOUSA, Ayman, Ph.D. Chief Executive Officer, Pacifica Hospital of the Valley,, CA, p. A71

MOUSTAKAKIS, John, Senior Vice President Information Systems and Chief Information Officer, Westchester Medical Center, Valhalla, NY, p. A445

MOVER, Michael, Chief Information Officer, Riverview Hospital, Noblesville, IN, p. A210

MOWDER, Kristan, Director Administration and Patient Care Services, Eastern State Hospital, Lexington, KY, p. A253

MOYA, Linda, Director Human Resources, Mesilla Valley Hospital, Las Cruces, NM, p. A416

MOYER, Dale, Vice President Information Systems, Evangelical Community Hospital, Lewisburg, PA, p. A527

MOYER, Douglas J., Chief Executive Officer, Mary Black Memorial Hospital, Spartanburg, SC, p. A553

Index of Health Care Professionals / Murphy

MOYER, Ed, Chief Operating Officer, Emory–Adventist Hospital, Smyrna, GA, p. A159
MOYER, Mark, Vice President and Chief Financial Officer, Presbyterian Hospital, Charlotte, NC, p. A451
MOYER, Patricia M., Chief Financial Officer, Herington Municipal Hospital, Herington, KS, p. A234
MOYER, William E., President, St. Luke's Hospital – Miners Campus, Coaldale, PA, p. A520
MOYNIER, Ryan, Chief Financial Officer, Castleview Hospital, Price, UT, p. A639
MRAMOR, Joann, Director Human Resources, Seven Rivers Regional Medical Center, Crystal River, FL, p. A121
MRUK, Donald, M.D. President Medical Staff, Athol Memorial Hospital, Athol, MA, p. A295
MUCCILLI, Pamela M., Vice President and Chief Information Officer, The William W. Backus Hospital, Norwich, CT, p. A111
MUCKENFUSS, Penny, Chief Nursing Officer, Lighthouse Care Center of Conway, Conway, SC, p. A549
MUDD, Karen, Director Marketing and Public Affairs, Sutter Tracy Community Hospital, Tracy, CA, p. A93
MUDRY, Janel, Chief Operating Officer, Southwest Regional Medical Center, Waynesburg, PA, p. A540
MUELLER, Arthur, Director Management Information Systems, Cuero Community Hospital, Cuero, TX, p. A590
MUELLER, Charles, M.D. Chief of Staff, Texas County Memorial Hospital, Houston, MO, p. A360
MUELLER, Jeff T., M.D. Medical Director, Mayo Clinic Hospital, Phoenix, AZ, p. A36
MUELLER, Michael E., Chief Financial Officer, Health Central, Ocoee, FL, p. A134
MUELLER, Paul A., Chief Operating Officer, Rogers Memorial Hospital, Oconomowoc, WI, p. A688
MUELLER, Robert, M.D. Chief of Staff, Madison County Hospital, London, OH, p. A483
MUELLER, Robert
  Director Human Resources, West Suburban Medical Center, Oak Park, IL, p. A190
  Director Human Resources, Westlake Hospital, Melrose Park, IL, p. A187
MUHS, David, Chief Financial Officer, Henry County Health Center, Mount Pleasant, IA, p. A223
MULDER, Dale R., President and Chief Executive Officer, Kindred Rehabilitation Hospital Clear Lake, Webster, TX, p. A634
MULDER, Sherri, Director Information Technology, Clay County Hospital, Ashland, AL, p. A15
MULDER, Steven, M.D. President and Chief Executive Officer, Hutchinson Area Health Care, Hutchinson, MN, p. A333
MULDERIG, Marsha L., R.N. Chief Nursing Officer, Crisp Regional Hospital, Cordele, GA, p. A150
MULDOON, Patrick L., FACHE President and Chief Executive Officer, Health Alliance Hospitals, Leominster, MA, p. A301
MULDOON, Sean R., M.D. Senior Vice President & Chief Medical Officer–Kindred Healthcare, Hospital Division, Kindred Hospital Northland, Kansas City, MO, p. A362
MULKEY, Peter, Chief Operating Officer, Clinch Valley Medical Center, Richlands, VA, p. A654
MULLAHEY, Mike, Operations Manager, Albany Stratton Veterans Affairs Medical Center, Albany, NY, p. A420
MULLANEY, Ruth, Personnel Officer, Dorothea Dix Psychiatric Center, Bangor, ME, p. A281
MULLANEY, Susan, Administrator, Sunnyside Medical Center, Clackamas, OR, p. A509
MULLEN, Ellen, M.D. Chief of Staff, Iberia Medical Center, New Iberia, LA, p. A274
MULLEN, Gary, Chief Information Officer, Madison County Health Care System, Winterset, IA, p. A228
MULLEN, Ron, Superintendent, Mental Health Institute, Mount Pleasant, IA, p. A224
MULLEN, Thomas R., President and Chief Executive Officer, Mercy Medical Center, Baltimore, MD, p. A288
MULLENAX, Paul, Business Manager, Wyoming State Hospital, Evanston, WY, p. A696
MULLENS, Allen, M.D. Chief Medical Staff, Norton Community Hospital, Norton, VA, p. A653
MULLER, A. Gary, FACHE President and Chief Executive Officer, Marquette General Health System, Marquette, MI, p. A318
MULLER, Dorothy A., Director Human Resources, Holliswood Hospital,, NY, p. A432
MULLER, Lynn, Chief Financial Officer, North Metro Medical Center, Jacksonville, AR, p. A46
MULLER, Oz, Director Human Resources, Porter Adventist Hospital, Denver, CO, p. A100
MULLER, Ralph W., President and Chief Executive Officer, University of Pennsylvania Health System, Philadelphia, PA, p. B139
MULLER, William, M.D. Vice President Medical Affairs, Milford Regional Medical Center, Milford, MA, p. A302
MULLIGAN, Marie, R.N. Vice President Nursing, John T. Mather Memorial Hospital, Port Jefferson, NY, p. A440
MULLIGAN, Michael, M.D. President Medical Staff, Anderson Hospital, Maryville, IL, p. A187
MULLIGAN, Regina, Vice President Nursing, Nathan Littauer Hospital and Nursing Home, Gloversville, NY, p. A426
MULLINGS, Donna, Director of Nursing, Assumption Community Hospital, Napoleonville, LA, p. A274
MULLINGS, Paul, Chief Operating Officer, Howard University Hospital, Washington, DC, p. A116
MULLINS, Cindy, Director Information Technology, Saint Mary's Regional Medical Center, Reno, NV, p. A395
MULLINS, Debbie, Director, Saint Joseph – London, London, KY, p. A254
MULLINS, Erin, D.O. Chief Medical Staff, Dickenson Community Hospital, Clintwood, VA, p. A647
MULLINS Jr., John David, Administrator, Clinton County Hospital, Albany, KY, p. A247
MULLINS, Kem, FACHE Senior Vice President and Hospital President, WellStar Cobb Hospital, Austell, GA, p. A147
MULLINS, Larry, Chief Information Officer, W. J. Mangold Memorial Hospital, Lockney, TX, p. A613
MULLINS, Larry A., FACHE President and Chief Executive Officer, Samaritan Health Services, Corvallis, OR, p. B112
MULLINS, Tommy H., Administrator, Boone Memorial Hospital, Madison, WV, p. A673
MULLNER, Darla, Director Human Resources, Rush–Copley Medical Center, Aurora, IL, p. A173
MULLOTH, Rajan, M.D. President Medical Staff, Mid–Valley Hospital, Peckville, PA, p. A531
MULVEHILL, Mitch, Senior Vice President and Chief Financial Officer, Texas Health Presbyterian Hospital–WNJ, Sherman, TX, p. A628
MULVIHILL, Jody, Vice President Finance, The Children's Institute of Pittsburgh, Pittsburgh, PA, p. A535
MUMMA, Barbara, Vice President Human Resources, Ephrata Community Hospital, Ephrata, PA, p. A523
MUNCH, David, M.D. Vice President and Chief Clinical and Quality Officer, Exempla Lutheran Medical Center, Wheat Ridge, CO, p. A107
MUNDAY, Kathy, Chief Financial Officer, Veterans Affairs Sierra Nevada Health Care System, Reno, NV, p. A395
MUNDY, Mark J., President and Chief Executive Officer, New York Methodist Hospital,, NY, p. A435
MUNDY, Stephens M., President and Chief Executive Officer, Champlain Valley Physicians Hospital Medical Center, Plattsburgh, NY, p. A440
MUNFORD, Thedosia, Senior Vice President and Chief Nursing Officer, Providence Hospital, Washington, DC, p. A116
MUNGER, Jonas, M.D. Chief Medical Staff, Moab Regional Hospital, Moab, UT, p. A638
MUNGER, Richard, Administrator, Mount Grant General Hospital, Hawthorne, NV, p. A392
MUNGER, Victor, Vice President Human Resources, Quincy Medical Center, Quincy, MA, p. A304
MUNGOVAN, Sandy, Chief Information Officer, LAC–Harbor–University of California at Los Angeles Medical Center, Torrance, CA, p. A92
MUNHOLLAND, Cleta
  Administrator, Louisiana Extended Care Hospital West Monroe, West Monroe, LA, p. A279
  Administrator, Specialty Extended Care of Monroe, Monroe, LA, p. A273
MUNIAK, Daniel, M.D. Chief Medical Officer, Garfield County Health Center, Jordan, MT, p. A376
MUNIR, Amjad, M.D. Medical Director, HEALTHSOUTH Chattanooga Rehabilitation Hospital, Chattanooga, TN, p. A563
MUNOZ, Astro, Chief Executive Officer, Hospital Pavia–Hato Rey, San Juan, PR, p. A703
MUNOZ, Beverly, Chief Executive Officer, Rehabilitation Hospital of Southern New Mexico, Las Cruces, NM, p. A416
MUNOZ, Natalie
  Director of Clinical Services, Nexus Specialty Hospital, Shenandoah, TX, p. A627
  Director of Clinical Services, Nexus Specialty Hospital The Woodlands, Spring, TX, p. A628
MUNOZ, Sylvia, Director Human Resources, Promise Hospital of East Los Angeles, Suburban Medical Center Campus, Paramount, CA, p. A79
MUNOZ, Thalia H., Administrator, Starr County Memorial Hospital, Rio Grande City, TX, p. A622
MUNRO, Stuart J., M.D. Clinical Director, Center for Behavioral Medicine, Kansas City, MO, p. A361
MUNSEY, Brenda, Senior Human Resources Business Partner, Saint Alphonsus Medical Center – Ontario, Ontario, OR, p. A513
MUNSON, Bill, Vice President and Chief Financial Officer, Boulder Community Hospital, Boulder, CO, p. A97
MUNSON, Jennifer, Chief Financial Officer, Okanogan Douglas District Hospital, Brewster, WA, p. A660
MUNSON, Joan, Manager Information Systems, Fairchild Medical Center, Yreka, CA, p. A96
MUNSON, John, Vice President and Chief Financial Officer, St. Anthony Regional Hospital, Carroll, IA, p. A215
MUNSON, Kris, Director Human Resources, Arbour H. R. I. Hospital, Brookline, MA, p. A298
MUNTZ, Tim, President and Chief Executive Officer, St. Margaret's Hospital, Spring Valley, IL, p. A194
MUNYAN, Lori, Director, Human Resources, HEALTHSOUTH Rehabilitation Hospital of Toms River, Toms River, NJ, p. A411
MUR, Ahmad, M.D. Acting Medical Director, Senator Garrett W. Hagedorn Psychiatric Hospital, Glen Gardner, NJ, p. A
MURANSKY, Ed, Owner, Surgical Hospital at Southwoods, Youngstown, OH, p. A492
MURCHISON, Sandra, Director Medical Records, Coosa Valley Medical Center, Sylacauga, AL, p. A25
MURDOCH, William, M.D. Medical Director, Loma Linda University Behavioral Medicine Center, Redlands, CA, p. A82
MURDOCK, Guy
  Vice President Human Resources, Healthbridge Children's Hospital of Houston, Houston, TX, p. A604
  Vice President Human Resources, Nexus Specialty Hospital, Shenandoah, TX, p. A627
  Vice President Human Resources, Nexus Specialty Hospital The Woodlands, Spring, TX, p. A628
MURDOCK–LANGAN, Patricia, Medical Director, Alegent Health–Lakeside Hospital, Omaha, NE, p. A387
MURDY, James B., Chief Financial Officer, Belmont Community Hospital, Bellaire, OH, p. A470
MURFORD, Tracy, Director Human Resources, Cardinal Hill Rehabilitation Hospital, Lexington, KY, p. A252
MURPHY, Brian, M.D
  Chief of Staff, Monroe Hospital, Bloomington, IN, p. A198
  Chief of Staff, Valley View Hospital, Glenwood Springs, CO, p. A101
MURPHY, Bruce, M.D. President and Chief Executive Officer, Arkansas Heart Hospital, Little Rock, AR, p. A47
MURPHY, Charles J., Associate Vice President Human Resources, Strong Memorial Hospital of the University of Rochester, Rochester, NY, p. A442
MURPHY, Christy, Director Health Information Systems, Crossgates River Oaks Hospital, Brandon, MS, p. A344
MURPHY, Dale, M.D. Vice President Medical Affairs, Summa Health System, Akron, OH, p. A469
MURPHY, Dennis M., Executive Vice President and Chief Operating Officer, Northwestern Memorial Hospital, Chicago, IL, p. A177
MURPHY, Elizabeth A., R.N. Vice President for Patient Care Services, Saint Mary's Health Care, Grand Rapids, MI, p. A314
MURPHY, J. Patrick, Chief Financial Officer, North Baldwin Infirmary, Bay Minette, AL, p. A16
MURPHY, James, Chief Executive Officer, South Texas Surgical Hospital, Corpus Christi, TX, p. A589
MURPHY, Janice, President, Fairview Hospital, Cleveland, OH, p. A475
MURPHY, Jeffrey J., Executive Vice President and Chief Executive Officer, Saint Francis Hospital, Evanston, IL, p. A181
MURPHY, Jim, Interim Administrator, Keefe Memorial Hospital, Cheyenne Wells, CO, p. A98
MURPHY, John, Chief Financial Officer, Renaissance Hospital, Groves, TX, p. A602
MURPHY, John B., M.D. Vice President Medical Affairs and Chief Medical Officer, Rhode Island Hospital, Providence, RI, p. A544
MURPHY, John M., M.D
  President and Chief Executive Officer, Danbury Hospital, Danbury, CT, p. A108
  Executive Director and Senior Vice President, New Milford Hospital, New Milford, CT, p. A111
MURPHY, John M., M.D. President, Western Connecticut Healthcare, Inc., Danbury, CT, p. B145
MURPHY, Joseph, Chief Executive Officer, Arbour Hospital, Boston, MA, p. A295
MURPHY, Judy, Director Human Resources, Southwest General Health Center, Middleburg Heights, OH, p. A485
MURPHY, Julia, Chief Nursing Officer, Logan Memorial Hospital, Russellville, KY, p. A258
MURPHY, Julie, Chief Financial Officer, Saint Luke's North Hospital – Barry Road, Kansas City, MO, p. A362
MURPHY, Kathy, Site Manager, Mescalero Public Health Service Indian Hospital, Mescalero, NM, p. A417
MURPHY, Kelly, Director Human Resources, Family Health West, Fruita, CO, p. A101


Index of Health Care Professionals **A889**

Index of Health Care Professionals
Index of Health Care Professionals / Murphy

MURPHY, Kevin G.
Senior Vice President Finance and Chief Financial Officer, Manchester Memorial Hospital, Manchester, CT, p. A109
Senior Vice President Finance and Chief Financial Officer, Rockville General Hospital, Vernon Rockville, CT, p. A112
MURPHY, Linda, Chief Financial Officer, Osborne County Memorial Hospital, Osborne, KS, p. A240
MURPHY, Lionel, Chief Executive Officer, Southeast Regional Medical Center, Kentwood, LA, p. A269
MURPHY, Lynda J., Vice President Human Resources, Logansport Memorial Hospital, Logansport, IN, p. A207
MURPHY, Martha, Vice President Human Resources, St. Joseph Mercy Oakland, Pontiac, MI, p. A321
MURPHY, Michael, M.D. Chief Medical Officer, Sharp Grossmont Hospital, La Mesa, CA, p. A66
MURPHY, Michael, CPA, President and Chief Executive Officer, Sharp HealthCare, San Diego, CA, p. B117
MURPHY, Michael D., Chief Executive Officer, Abilene Regional Medical Center, Abilene, TX, p. A577
MURPHY, Michael J., Director, Veterans Affairs Health Care System, Fargo, ND, p. A466
MURPHY, Neil W., R.N
Senior Vice President and Chief Nursing Officer, Centegra Hospital – McHenry, McHenry, IL, p. A187
Senior Vice President, Chief Nursing Officer, Centegra Hospital – Woodstock, Woodstock, IL, p. A196
MURPHY, Patrick, Vice President Finance, Thomas Hospital, Fairhope, AL, p. A20
MURPHY, Patrick J., M.D. Chief of Staff, Three Rivers Hospital, Waverly, TN, p. A576
MURPHY, Richard J., President and Chief Executive Officer, Richmond University Medical Center,, NY, p. A436
MURPHY, Rita, Director Human Resources, Cobre Valley Regional Medical Center, Globe, AZ, p. A33
MURPHY, Steve, Director Networks, Good Samaritan Regional Health Center, Mount Vernon, IL, p. A188
MURPHY, Steven, Executive Director, Devereux Hospital and Children's Center of Florida, Melbourne, FL, p. A130
MURPHY, Susan G., Chief Operating Officer, Santa Clara Medical Center, Santa Clara, CA, p. A90
MURPHY, Terry
President and Chief Executive Officer, Bayhealth Medical Center, Dover, DE, p. A114
Director Information Services, Phoenixville Hospital, Phoenixville, PA, p. A534
MURPHY, Therese, Chief Nursing Officer, Florida Hospital at Connerton Long Term Acute Care, Land O'Lakes, FL, p. A128
MURPHY, Thomas, M.D. Vice President Medical Affairs, Children's Medical Center, Dayton, OH, p. A478
MURPHY, Tim, Vice President, Human Resources, Mercy Hospital Fort Smith, Fort Smith, AR, p. A45
MURPHY, Tom, Chief Executive Officer, Weiser Memorial Hospital, Weiser, ID, p. A171
MURPHY–FROBISH, Erin, Vice President Human Resources, Morris Hospital & Healthcare Centers, Morris, IL, p. A188
MURRAY, Brian, M.D. Medical Director, Erie County Medical Center, Buffalo, NY, p. A422
MURRAY, Brian, Chief Financial Officer, Gunnison Valley Hospital, Gunnison, UT, p. A637
MURRAY, Cindy, R.N. Chief Nursing Officer and Chief Operating Officer, Baylor Medical Center at Waxahachie, Waxahachie, TX, p. A633
MURRAY, Diana, Director Information Systems, Grand River Hospital District, Rifle, CO, p. A105
MURRAY, Eric, Manager Public Relations, Kremmling Memorial Hospital, Kremmling, CO, p. A102
MURRAY, Geno, President and Chief Executive Officer, Charles A. Dean Memorial Hospital, Greenville, ME, p. A283
MURRAY, Gerald, President and Chief Executive Officer, Altoona Regional Health System, Altoona, PA, p. A517
MURRAY, James Patrick, FACHE Chief Executive Officer, Peterson Regional Medical Center, Kerrville, TX, p. A610
MURRAY, Jana, Manager Medical Records, Mercy St. Francis Hospital, Mountain View, MO, p. A365
MURRAY, Kent, M.D. Chief of Staff, Robert J. Dole Veterans Affairs Medical Center, Wichita, KS, p. A245
MURRAY, Kevin J., Senior Vice President, John T. Mather Memorial Hospital, Port Jefferson, NY, p. A440
MURRAY, Michael, Chief Executive Officer, San Gabriel Valley Medical Center, San Gabriel, CA, p. A87
MURRAY, Patricia M., Information Officer, Southern Inyo Healthcare District, Lone Pine, CA, p. A67
MURRAY, Sherri, Chief Financial Officer, Montgomery General Hospital, Montgomery, WV, p. A673
MURRAY, Susan, Director Information Services, Trident Medical Center, Charleston, SC, p. A547
MURRAY, Wesley E., Chief Executive Officer, Texas County Memorial Hospital, Houston, MO, p. A360
MURRELL, Joseph, Chief Executive Officer, Wayne County Hospital, Monticello, KY, p. A256
MURREY, Mady, R.N. Vice President and Administrator, MultiCare Mary Bridge Children's Hospital and Health Center, Tacoma, WA, p. A668
MURRILL, Mike, Vice President and Chief Financial Officer, Adventist Bolingbrook Hospital, Bolingbrook, IL, p. A174
MURROW, Carol, Vice President Business Development, Skaggs Regional Medical Center, Branson, MO, p. A356
MURRY, Jim, Chief Information Officer, University of California, Irvine Healthcare, Orange, CA, p. A78
MURTHA, Patrick J., Chief Executive Officer, Regency Hospital of Toledo, Sylvania, OH, p. A489
MURTHY, Bangalore, M.D. Director Medical Staff, Jackson Park Hospital and Medical Center, Chicago, IL, p. A176
MURTOS, Kristen, FACHE President, NorthShore University Health System Skokie Hospital, Skokie, IL, p. A194
MURZYN, Derek, Chief Executive Officer, Kindred Hospital–Greensboro, Greensboro, NC, p. A454
MUSACK, Scott, Chief Information Officer, Silver Lake Medical Center, Los Angeles, CA, p. A72
MUSSELMAN, Bud, Chief Operating Officer and Chief Financial Officer, Highline Medical Center, Burien, WA, p. A660
MUSSELWHITE, Ronald P., Vice President Human Resources, Peninsula Hospital Center,, NY, p. A
MUSSMAN, Rebekah, Chief Financial Officer, Kearney County Health Services, Minden, NE, p. A386
MUSSO, Lewis C., Vice President Human Resources, Trinity Health System, Steubenville, OH, p. A489
MUSTAFA, Mahmoud, Director Information Systems, Sheehan Memorial Hospital, Buffalo, NY, p. A
MUSTIAN, J. Perry, President, Archbold Medical Center, Thomasville, GA, p. B10
MUSTIAN, J. Perry, President and Chief Executive Officer, John D. Archbold Memorial Hospital, Thomasville, GA, p. A160
MUSUMECI, Maryann, Director, Veterans Affairs Medical Center,, NY, p. A437
MUTARELLI, Richard, Chief Financial Officer, Munroe Regional Medical Center, Ocala, FL, p. A133
MUTCHLER, Roger, Manager Information Technology, Aultman Orrville Hospital, Orrville, OH, p. A487
MUTZIGER, John, M.D. Chief Medical Officer, Laird Hospital, Union, MS, p. A353
MWANIKI, Mary
Chief Financial Officer, Reliant Rehabilitation Hospital Dallas, Dallas, TX, p. A592
Chief Financial Officer, Reliant Rehabilitation Hospital Mid–Cities, Bedford, TX, p. A583
Chief Financial Officer, Reliant Rehabilitation Hospital North Texas, Richardson, TX, p. A622
MWEBE, David, M.D. Chief of Staff, Osmond General Hospital, Osmond, NE, p. A388
MYATT, Kevin A., Senior Vice President Human Resources, Yale–New Haven Hospital, New Haven, CT, p. A111
MYBURGH, Ronell, Administrator, Healthbridge Childrens Rehabilitation Hospital, Orange, CA, p. A78
MYCROFT, Tina, Vice President and Chief Financial Officer, St. Joseph Hospital, Orange, CA, p. A78
MYDLER, Todd, M.D. Chief Medical Officer, Parker Adventist Hospital, Parker, CO, p. A105
MYER, Amber, Director Medical Records, Throckmorton County Memorial Hospital, Throckmorton, TX, p. A631
MYERS, Adam L., M.D. Chief Medical Officer, Methodist Mansfield Medical Center, Mansfield, TX, p. A615
MYERS, April, Administrator, Kindred Hospital–La Mirada, La Mirada, CA, p. A66
MYERS, Becky, Human Resources Specialist, Illini Community Hospital, Pittsfield, IL, p. A192
MYERS, Carl, M.D. Vice President Medical Affairs and Chief Medical Officer, Yuma Regional Medical Center, Yuma, AZ, p. A41
MYERS, Chuck, M.D. Chief of Staff, Palo Pinto General Hospital, Mineral Wells, TX, p. A617
MYERS, Craig G., Chief Executive Officer, Coastal Communities Hospital, Santa Ana, CA, p. A89
MYERS, Dan, Controller, Kossuth Regional Health Center, Algona, IA, p. A214
MYERS, Doug, Senior Vice President and Chief Financial Officer, Children's Hospital and Research Center at Oakland, Oakland, CA, p. A77
MYERS, Douglas, Executive Vice President, Chief Financial Officer and Interim Chief Operating Officer, Children's National Medical Center, Washington, DC, p. A116
MYERS, Edward W., Chief Executive Officer, St. Luke's Medical Center, Phoenix, AZ, p. A36
MYERS, Frederick, M.D. Chief Medical Officer, Takoma Regional Hospital, Greeneville, TN, p. A566
MYERS, Jeffrey D., President and Chief Executive Officer, Hamilton Health Care System, Inc., Dalton, GA, p. B56
MYERS, Jeffrey D., President and Chief Executive Officer, Hamilton Medical Center, Dalton, GA, p. A151
MYERS, Jerry, M.D. Chief Executive Officer, Kell West Regional Hospital, Wichita Falls, TX, p. A635
MYERS, Jim, Chief Financial Officer, Indiana University Health Bloomington Hospital, Bloomington, IN, p. A198
MYERS, Karen, Vice President Financial Services, Stoughton Hospital Association, Stoughton, WI, p. A691
MYERS, Katie, Chief Financial Officer, Alleghany Memorial Hospital, Sparta, NC, p. A461
MYERS, Keith G., Chairman and Chief Executive Officer, LHC Group, Lafayette, LA, p. B79
MYERS, Kevin, Director Information Systems, Lake Granbury Medical Center, Granbury, TX, p. A601
MYERS, Kimberly, Director Human Resources, Guthrie County Hospital, Guthrie Center, IA, p. A220
MYERS, Lisa, Director Human Resources, Heritage Oaks Hospital, Sacramento, CA, p. A83
MYERS, Lynne L., Executive Vice President and Chief Operating Officer, Meriter Hospital, Madison, WI, p. A684
MYERS, Mark, M.D. Chief Medical Officer, Continuous Care Centers of Tulsa, Tulsa, OK, p. A505
MYERS, Michael D., Chief Executive Officer, Veterans Memorial Hospital, Waukon, IA, p. A228
MYERS, Michelle F., Manager Human Resources, Florida Hospital Wauchula, Wauchula, FL, p. A142
MYERS, Paul, M.D. Neonatologist and Chief Medical Officer, Children's Hospital of Wisconsin–Fox Valley, Neenah, WI, p. A687
MYERS, Philip, M.D. Vice President Medical Affairs, Samaritan Regional Health System, Ashland, OH, p. A469
MYERS, Robert T., Chief Operating Officer, Parkview LaGrange Hospital, LaGrange, IN, p. A207
MYERS, Russ, Senior Vice President and Chief Operating Officer, Yakima Valley Memorial Hospital, Yakima, WA, p. A669
MYERS, Shane P., Chief Operating Officer, Iberia Medical Center, New Iberia, LA, p. A274
MYERS, Sheri, Vice President Patient Care Services, McLaren Central Michigan, Mount Pleasant, MI, p. A319
MYERS, Steve, Assistant Administrator, Advanced Healthcare Medical Center, Ellington, MO, p. A359
MYERS, Tara, Director Human Resources, AnMed Health Rehabilitation Hospital, Anderson, SC, p. A546
MYERS, William, Chief Operating Officer, Montgomery County Emergency Service, Norristown, PA, p. A530
MYHRE, Jane, MS Director Health Information, Chippewa County–Montevideo Hospital, Montevideo, MN, p. A335
MYLA, Sara, M.D. Chief of Staff, Fountain Valley Regional Hospital and Medical Center, Fountain Valley, CA, p. A61
MYLES, Lee T., Chief Executive Officer, St. Mary's Regional Medical Center, Lewiston, ME, p. A284
MYNARK, Richard H., Chief Executive Officer, Pulaski Memorial Hospital, Winamac, IN, p. A213
MYSTER, Jennifer, President, Buffalo Hospital, Buffalo, MN, p. A329

# N

NABEL, Elizabeth, M.D
President, Brigham and Women's Hospital, Boston, MA, p. A296
President, Faulkner Hospital, Boston, MA, p. A296
NABER, Mary, Senior Vice President Worklife Services, St. John Hospital and Medical Center, Detroit, MI, p. A311
NACHIMUTHU, Anbu, Chief Financial Officer, Atrium Medical Center of Corinth, Corinth, TX, p. A588
NACHTIGAL, Amy, Chief Financial Officer, Saint Luke's Hospital of Kansas City, Kansas City, MO, p. A362
NACHTRIEB, Han, Vice President Human Resources, Seattle Cancer Care Alliance, Seattle, WA, p. A666
NACION, Glenn, Vice President Human Resources, Trinitas Regional Medical Center, Elizabeth, NJ, p. A403
NADEAU, Barbara, Chief Human Resources, Veterans Affairs Medical Center, White River Junction, VT, p. A644
NADEAU, Steve, Senior Vice President Human Resources, Gwinnett Hospital System, Lawrenceville, GA, p. A155
NADER, Keoni, Director Human Resources, Louis A. Weiss Memorial Hospital, Chicago, IL, p. A176
NADER, Mary, Director Applications, Spectrum Health Special Care Hospital, Grand Rapids, MI, p. A314
NADKARNI, Manasi, M.D. Vice President Medical Affairs, Trinity Muscatine, Muscatine, IA, p. A224
NADOLNY, Stephanie, Vice President Clinical Services, Spaulding Rehabilitation Hospital Cape Cod, East Sandwich, MA, p. A299
NADONE, John, Chief Financial Officer, Southwest Memorial Hospital, Cortez, CO, p. A99

A890 Index of Health Care Professionals

Index of Health Care Professionals
Index of Health Care Professionals / Neely

NAEVE, Clayton, Vice President and Chief Information Officer, St. Jude Children's Research Hospital, Memphis, TN, p. A572
NAFZIGER, Laurie N., President and Chief Executive Officer, Oaklawn Psychiatric Center, Goshen, IN, p. A202
NAFZIGER, Steve, M.D. Vice President Medical Affairs, Parkview Medical Center, Pueblo, CO, p. A105
NAGALA, Vani, M.D. Chief Medical Officer, Oakes Community Hospital, Oakes, ND, p. A467
NAGEL, Donna, Director Human Resources, Continuous Care Centers of Tulsa, Tulsa, OK, p. A505
NAGLE, Jolene, Director Medical Records, Peterson Rehabilitation Hospital, Wheeling, WV, p. A676
NAGLE, Mike, Director Financial Services, Jerold Phelps Community Hospital, Garberville, CA, p. A62
NAGLER, Harris M., M.D. President, Beth Israel Medical Center, New York, NY, p. A431
NAGLER, Richard, M.D. Chief of Staff, Mayo Clinic Health System – Northland in Barron, Barron, WI, p. A678
NAGLOSKY, Paul, Administrator, Indianhead Medical Center, Shell Lake, WI, p. A691
NAGOWSKI, Michael, President and Chief Executive Officer, Cape Fear Valley Health System, Fayetteville, NC, p. B24
NAGOWSKI, Michael
  President and Chief Executive Officer, Cape Fear Valley Medical Center, Fayetteville, NC, p. A453
  President and Chief Executive Officer, Highsmith–Rainey Specialty Hospital, Fayetteville, NC, p. A453
NAGY, Jeff, Chief Financial Officer, River Bend Hospital, West Lafayette, IN, p. A213
NAGY, Kimberly, R.N. Vice President Operations and Chief Nurse Executive, Northwestern Lake Forest Hospital, Lake Forest, IL, p. A186
NAIBERK, Donald T., Administrator, Butler County Health Care Center, David City, NE, p. A383
NAILLON, Marcia, Chief Operating Officer and Administrative Registered Nurse, North Valley Hospital, Tonasket, WA, p. A668
NAIR, Chand, M.D. Medical Director, Brooke Glen Behavioral Hospital, Fort Washington, PA, p. A523
NAIR, Vijayachandran, M.D. Chief of Staff, John J. Pershing Veterans Affairs Medical Center, Poplar Bluff, MO, p. A367
NAJJAR, Maher, M.D. Medical Director, Kindred Hospital Chicago–Northlake, Northlake, IL, p. A189
NAKAGAWA, Marc
  Vice President and Chief Financial Officer, Transylvania Regional Hospital, Brevard, NC, p. A449
  Chief Financial Officer, Trinity Hospital of Augusta, Augusta, GA, p. A147
NAKAMOTO, Kenneth, M.D. Vice President Medical Affairs, Pomona Valley Hospital Medical Center, Pomona, CA, p. A80
NAKASUJI, Jody, Chief Financial Officer, LAC–Harbor–University of California at Los Angeles Medical Center, Torrance, CA, p. A92
NALDI, Robert, Chief Financial Officer, Maimonides Medical Center,, NY, p. A434
NALEPPA, Peggy, President and Chief Executive Officer, Peninsula Regional Health System, Salisbury, MD, p. A294
NALL, Brian, Chief Executive Officer, Benewah Community Hospital, Saint Maries, ID, p. A170
NALL, Wes, Administrator, Grove Hill Memorial Hospital, Grove Hill, AL, p. A21
NALLE, Tambara, Chief Financial Officer, Eastern State Hospital, Lexington, KY, p. A253
NALLI, Jonathan, Chief Executive Officer, Porter–Valparaiso Hospital Campus, Valparaiso, IN, p. A212
NALLS, Jacqueline, Chief Financial Officer, Phoenixville Hospital, Phoenixville, PA, p. A534
NANCE, Sally S., Chief Executive Officer, Excelsior Springs Hospital, Excelsior Springs, MO, p. A359
NANDIN, Dalia, Manager Human Resources, Kindred Rehabilitation Hospital Clear Lake, Webster, TX, p. A634
NANIA, James A., System Vice President and Chief Financial Officer, Hallmark Health System, Melrose, MA, p. A302
NANTZ, Mark S., FACHE Chief Executive Officer, Bon Secours St. Francis Health System, Greenville, SC, p. A550
NAPIER, Lisa, Chief Financial Officer, Atlanta Medical Center, Atlanta, GA, p. A145
NAPIER, Randy L.
  Administrator, Frazier Rehab Institute, Louisville, KY, p. A254
  President and Chief Executive Officer, Southern Indiana Rehabilitation Hospital, New Albany, IN, p. A209
NAPIER, Troy
  Chief Information Officer, Baptist Hospitals of Southeast Texas, Beaumont, TX, p. A582
  Director, Baptist Orange Hospital, Orange, TX, p. A619
NAPIERALA, Edward A., Chief Executive Officer, West Branch Regional Medical Center, West Branch, MI, p. A325
NAPOLI, Mark, M.D. Chief of Staff, P & S Surgical Hospital, Monroe, LA, p. A273
NAPOLITANO, Mary Pat
  Director Human Resources, Specialty Hospital at Kimball, Lakewood, NJ, p. A405
  Director Human Resources, Specialty Hospital at Monmouth, Long Branch, NJ, p. A405
NAPP, Marc L., M.D. Vice President Medical Affairs, Lenox Hill Hospital, New York, NY, p. A433
NAPPER, Rick D., President and Chief Executive Officer, Magnolia Regional Health Center, Corinth, MS, p. A345
NAQVI, Shahid, M.D. President Medical Staff, Floyd Valley Hospital, Le Mars, IA, p. A222
NARAMORE, G. Harold, M.D. Chief Medical Officer and In house Legal Counsel, Blount Memorial Hospital, Maryville, TN, p. A570
NARAYAN, Satish, M.D. Medical Director, Glen Oaks Hospital, Greenville, TX, p. A601
NARBUTAS, Virgis
  Chief Executive Officer, Garden Grove Hospital and Medical Center, Garden Grove, CA, p. A63
  Chief Executive Officer, Huntington Beach Hospital, Huntington Beach, CA, p. A65
  Chief Executive Officer, La Palma Intercommunity Hospital, La Palma, CA, p. A66
  Chief Executive Officer, West Anaheim Medical Center, Anaheim, CA, p. A53
NARDO, Jeff, Director Human Resources, Brynn Marr Hospital, Jacksonville, NC, p. A455
NARROW, Ann, Director of Nursing, River Hospital, Alexandria Bay, NY, p. A420
NARY, Ed, Director Information Technology and Chief Compliance Officer, Wilbarger General Hospital, Vernon, TX, p. A633
NASEM, Charles D., FACHE President and Chief Executive Officer, Louisiana Medical Center and Heart Hospital, Lacombe, LA, p. A269
NASET–PAYNE, Janet, R.N. Chief Operating Officer, Van Diest Medical Center, Webster City, IA, p. A228
NASH, Gayle, R.N. Chief Nursing Officer, MountainView Regional Medical Center, Las Cruces, NM, p. A416
NASH, Ira, M.D. Chief Medical Officer, Mount Sinai Hospital, New York, NY, p. A435
NASH, Jeff, Director Information Technology and Services, Mary Black Memorial Hospital, Spartanburg, SC, p. A553
NASH, Jerry A., Chief Executive Officer, Conroe Regional Medical Center, Conroe, TX, p. A588
NASH, John D., President and Chief Executive Officer, Franciscan Hospital for Children, Boston, MA, p. A296
NASH, Robert, M.D. Chief of Staff, Richland Memorial Hospital, Olney, IL, p. A190
NASH, Tim, M.D. Chief of Staff, Marshall Medical Center, Lewisburg, TN, p. A569
NASIR, Iqbal, M.D. Chief of Staff, Oakwood Southshore Medical Center, Trenton, MI, p. A324
NASK, Frank P., President and Chief Executive Officer, Broward Health, Fort Lauderdale, FL, p. B23
NASR, Anthony, M.D. Chief Medical Staff, Feather River Hospital, Paradise, CA, p. A79
NASRALLA, Anthony J., FACHE President and Chief Executive Officer, Titusville Area Hospital, Titusville, PA, p. A539
NASS, Mike
  Vice President and Chief Financial Officer, St. John's Hospital, Saint Paul, MN, p. A339
  Vice President and Chief Financial Officer, St. Joseph's Hospital, Saint Paul, MN, p. A339
NASSIEF, Raymond, Senior Vice President Operations and Clinical Transformation, John Muir Medical Center, Walnut Creek, Walnut Creek, CA, p. A95
NASSIF, Jason, Chief Operating Officer, LTAC Hospital of Greenwood, Greenwood, MS, p. A346
NATALONI, Tom, Senior Director Information Technology, Hahnemann University Hospital, Philadelphia, PA, p. A532
NATEMAN, Barry A., Director Human Resources, Community Memorial Healthcenter, South Hill, VA, p. A656
NATHAN, James R.
  President, Cape Coral Hospital, Cape Coral, FL, p. A120
  President and Chief Executive Officer, Gulf Coast Medical Center, Fort Myers, FL, p. A123
NATHAN, James R., President and Chief Executive Officer, Lee Memorial Health System, Fort Myers, FL, p. B79
NATHAN, James R., President, Lee Memorial Hospital, Fort Myers, FL, p. A124
NATHAN, Matthew L., Surgeon General, Bureau of Medicine and Surgery, Department of the Navy, Washington, DC, p. B23
NATHANSON, Andrea, Director Finance, Baystate Franklin Medical Center, Greenfield, MA, p. A300
NATIONS, Mary Kay, Chief Financial Officer, Kindred Hospital–New Orleans, New Orleans, LA, p. A274
NATRAJAN, Sunil, M.D. Medical Director, Kindred Hospital–Tucson, Tucson, AZ, p. A40
NATZKE, Kenneth J., President and Chief Executive Officer, OSF St. Joseph Medical Center, Bloomington, IL, p. A173
NAU, James, Manager Computer and Applications Support, Delaware Psychiatric Center, New Castle, DE, p. A114
NAUGLE, Gary, Senior Vice President Human Resources, Altoona Regional Health System, Altoona, PA, p. A517
NAUMAN, Michael B., Senior Vice President and Chief Information Officer, OSF Saint Francis Medical Center, Peoria, IL, p. A191
NAVARRO, Danielle, R.N. Chief Nursing Officer, Guthrie County Hospital, Guthrie Center, IA, p. A220
NAVARRO, Tess, Chief Financial Officer, Laguna Honda Hospital and Rehabilitation Center, San Francisco, CA, p. A87
NAVAS, Manuel, M.D. Medical Director, Hospital San Pablo Del Este, Fajardo, PR, p. A701
NAWROCKI, Bernie
  Administrative Director Finance, ProMedica Bixby Hospital, Adrian, MI, p. A307
  Administrative Director Finance, ProMedica Herrick Hospital, Tecumseh, MI, p. A324
NAWROCKI, Edward
  President, St. Luke's Hospital – Anderson Campus, Easton, PA, p. A522
  President, St. Luke's Hospital – Quakertown Campus, Quakertown, PA, p. A536
NAY, Clifford D., Executive Director, Scott Memorial Hospital, Scottsburg, IN, p. A211
NAYAK, Raghu, Chief Executive Officer, Hind General Hospital, Hobart, IN, p. A203
NAZ, Haroon, Chief Executive Officer, Pinnacle Hospital, Crown Point, IN, p. A200
NAZE, Jesse, Chief Financial Officer, Fall River Hospital, Hot Springs, SD, p. A557
NDOW, Emmanuel, Chief Information Officer, Marion General Hospital, Marion, IN, p. A208
NEAL, Birgitta, Data Entry and Information Technologist, Stamford Memorial Hospital, Stamford, TX, p. A628
NEAL, Bob, Director Information Technology, Sparrow Ionia Hospital, Ionia, MI, p. A315
NEAL, Gerald D., Chief Executive Officer and Administrator, Guthrie County Hospital, Guthrie Center, IA, p. A220
NEAL, Greg
  Chief Operating Officer, Wellmont Bristol Regional Medical Center, Bristol, TN, p. A562
  President and Chief Executive Officer, Wellmont Hawkins County Memorial Hospital, Rogersville, TN, p. A575
NEAL, John C., Chief Executive Officer, Hood Memorial Hospital, Amite, LA, p. A261
NEAL, Roger, Vice President and Chief Information Officer, Duncan Regional Hospital, Duncan, OK, p. A495
NEALE, Debra, R.N. Chief Nursing Officer, O'Connor Hospital, Delhi, NY, p. A425
NEALON, James, M.D. President Medical Staff, Silverton Hospital, Silverton, OR, p. A515
NEALON, Patricia, Director, VA Butler Healthcare, Butler, PA, p. A519
NEAMAN, Mark R., President and Chief Executive Officer, NorthShore University HealthSystem, Evanston, IL, p. B95
NEAPOLITAN, David, Chief Financial Officer, Emanuel Medical Center, Turlock, CA, p. A93
NEAT, Gary, Director Information Management Systems, Taylor Regional Hospital, Campbellsville, KY, p. A248
NECAS, Kevin
  Chief Financial Officer, University of Missouri Hospitals and Clinics, Columbia, MO, p. A358
  Chief Financial Officer, Women's and Children's Hospital, Columbia, MO, p. A358
NECCI, Mindy, Director Human Resources, Aurora West Allis Medical Center, West Allis, WI, p. A693
NECHANICKY, Jeff, Assistant Director, Richard L. Roudebush Veterans Affairs Medical Center, Indianapolis, IN, p. A205
NEECE, Patrick, Chief Information Officer, Jefferson Regional Medical Center, Pine Bluff, AR, p. A50
NEEDHAM, Kim
  Assistant Chief Executive Officer, Vista Medical Center East, Waukegan, IL, p. A196
  Assistant Chief Executive Officer, Vista Medical Center West, Waukegan, IL, p. A196
NEEDHAM, Tracy, Director of Nursing, Sutter Davis Hospital, Davis, CA, p. A59
NEEDMAN, Herbert G., President and Chief Executive Officer, Temple Community Hospital, Los Angeles, CA, p. A72
NEELAGARU, Narasimhulu, M.D. Chief of Staff, Northridge Medical Center, Commerce, GA, p. A150
NEELEY, Scott, M.D. Chief Medical Officer, St. Alexius Medical Center, Hoffman Estates, IL, p. A185
NEELY, Cindy, Administrator, Mercy Hospital Columbus, Columbus, KS, p. A232
NEELY, Dale, Chief Operating Officer, Capital Regional Medical Center, Tallahassee, FL, p. A140


Index of Health Care Professionals A891

NEELY, Joseph H., FACHE Chief Executive Officer, SouthCrest Hospital, Tulsa, OK, p. A507

NEELY, Randall, Chief Executive Officer, Simpson General Hospital, Mendenhall, MS, p. A350

NEERGHEEN, Chabilal, M.D. Medical Director, Western Massachusetts Hospital, Westfield, MA, p. A306

NEESEN, Cindy, Director of Information Technology, Butler County Health Care Center, David City, NE, p. A383

NEET, Bradley D., FACHE President and Chief Executive Officer, Mary Lanning Healthcare, Hastings, NE, p. A384

NEFF, Mark J., FACHE President and Chief Executive Officer, St. Claire Regional Medical Center, Morehead, KY, p. A256

NEFF, Mary L., R.N. Chief Operating Officer and Chief Nursing Officer, Mercy Hospital Cadillac, Cadillac, MI, p. A308

NEFF, Mary Beth, Director Human Resources, Sistersville General Hospital, Sistersville, WV, p. A675

NEFF, William, M.D
Chief Medical Officer, Medical Center of the Rockies, Loveland, CO, p. A104
Chief Medical Officer, Poudre Valley Hospital, Fort Collins, CO, p. A101

NEGOSHIAN, Carol, MSN Chief Nursing Officer, Putnam Community Medical Center, Palatka, FL, p. A135

NEGRO, Frank, Interim Chief Information Officer, New York Downtown Hospital, New York, NY, p. A435

NEGRON, Manuel, Chief Information Technology Service, Veterans Affairs Medical Center, San Juan, PR, p. A704

NEIKIRK, Richard, Chief Executive Officer, Cumberland County Hospital, Burkesville, KY, p. A248

NEILSON, Bill, M.D. Vice President Medical Affairs, Baptist St. Anthony Health System, Amarillo, TX, p. A578

NEILSON–BEALE, Carol, Chief Financial Officer, Cypress Creek Hospital, Houston, TX, p. A604

NEIMAN, Carla, Chief Financial Officer, Clark Fork Valley Hospital, Plains, MT, p. A378

NEITZEL, Monte, Chief Executive Officer, Greater Regional Medical Center, Creston, IA, p. A217

NELL, Rocio, M.D. Chief Executive Officer, Montgomery County Emergency Service, Norristown, PA, p. A530

NELL, Sergio, Director Information Systems, Watsonville Community Hospital, Watsonville, CA, p. A95

NELSON, Allison
Chief Financial Officer, Sanford Deuel County Medical Center, Clear Lake, SD, p. A556
Chief Financial Officer, Sanford Medical Center Canby, Canby, MN, p. A329

NELSON, Barbara J., Ph.D. Chief Nursing Executive, Sutter Roseville Medical Center, Roseville, CA, p. A83

NELSON, Betty, Director of Marketing and Development, Lindsborg Community Hospital, Lindsborg, KS, p. A238

NELSON, Bill, Chief Executive Officer, Mille Lacs Health System, Onamia, MN, p. A336

NELSON, Brian, M.D. Chief Medical Officer, Cache Valley Specialty Hospital, North Logan, UT, p. A639

NELSON, Brock D., President and Chief Executive Officer, Regions Hospital, Saint Paul, MN, p. A339

NELSON, Carol, Director Human Resources, Montevista Hospital, Las Vegas, NV, p. A393

NELSON, Charles, Chief Executive Officer, Aspirus Keweenaw Hospital, Laurium, MI, p. A317

NELSON, David, M.D. Medical Director, Barlow Respiratory Hospital, Los Angeles, CA, p. A68

NELSON, David A., President and Chief Executive Officer, St. Francis Healthcare Campus, Breckenridge, MN, p. A329

NELSON, Dawn, Director Human Resources, St. Vincent General Hospital District, Leadville, CO, p. A103

NELSON, Deana, R.N. Executive Vice President and Chief Operating Officer, Tampa General Hospital, Tampa, FL, p. A141

NELSON, Evan, M.D. Medical Director, New Mexico Rehabilitation Center, Roswell, NM, p. A417

NELSON, Fritz, Administrator, Ochsner Extended Care Hospital of Kenner, Kenner, LA, p. A269

NELSON, Jack, Senior Vice President and Chief Information Officer, Mount Sinai Hospital, New York, NY, p. A435

NELSON, Jackie, Director Human Resources, Hansford Hospital, Spearman, TX, p. A628

NELSON, James, M.D. Chief Medical Staff, Lake Wales Medical Center, Lake Wales, FL, p. A128

NELSON, James J., Senior Vice President Finance and Strategic Planning, Fort HealthCare, Fort Atkinson, WI, p. A681

NELSON, Jeffrey, M.D. Chief of Staff, Nor–Lea General Hospital, Lovington, NM, p. A417

NELSON, Jeri, Chief Financial Officer, Eastern Plumas Health Care District, Portola, CA, p. A81

NELSON, Joseph, M.D. President Medical Staff, Lewis–Gale Medical Center, Salem, VA, p. A655

NELSON, Katey, Director Human Resources, Sevier Valley Medical Center, Richfield, UT, p. A640

NELSON, Kathleen, R.N. Chief Nursing Officer, Eastern Idaho Regional Medical Center, Idaho Falls, ID, p. A168

NELSON, Kathy
Chief Financial Officer, Marshall Medical Center North, Guntersville, AL, p. A21
Chief Financial Officer, Marshall Medical Center South, Boaz, AL, p. A17
Director Marketing and Strategic Planning, Valley General Hospital, Monroe, WA, p. A663

NELSON, Kenneth W., Superintendent, Bridgewater State Hospital, Bridgewater, MA, p. A298

NELSON, Kerri, Chief Financial Officer, Memorial Medical Center of West Michigan, Ludington, MI, p. A318

NELSON, Linda M., R.N. Director of Nursing Services, Chippewa County–Montevideo Hospital, Montevideo, MN, p. A335

NELSON, Lisa M., MS, Chief Executive Officer, Reliant Rehabilitation Hospital Abilene, Abilene, TX, p. A577

NELSON, Lucy, Director Finance, Maniilaq Health Center, Kotzebue, AK, p. A29

NELSON, Lynn M., R.N. Chief Operating Officer, St. John's Riverside Hospital, Yonkers, NY, p. A447

NELSON, Marlin Pete, Vice President Fiscal Services, Divine Savior Healthcare, Portage, WI, p. A689

NELSON, Martha
Chief Financial Officer, Antelope Memorial Hospital, Neligh, NE, p. A386
Chief Financial Officer, Niobrara Valley Hospital, Lynch, NE, p. A386

NELSON, Meredith, Chief Financial Officer, Valley View Medical Center, Fort Mohave, AZ, p. A32

NELSON, Michael
Chief Financial Officer, Kindred Hospital–Greensboro, Greensboro, NC, p. A454
Executive Vice President and Chief Financial Officer, Pomona Valley Hospital Medical Center, Pomona, CA, p. A80

NELSON, Michael E., Chief Financial Officer, Riveredge Hospital, Forest Park, IL, p. A182

NELSON, Mike, Chief Financial Officer, Saint Anthony's Health Center, Alton, IL, p. A172

NELSON, Nan
Chief Financial Officer, Oconomowoc Memorial Hospital, Oconomowoc, WI, p. A688
Vice President Finance, Waukesha Memorial Hospital, Waukesha, WI, p. A692

NELSON, Nick, Director Support Services, Adams Memorial Hospital, Decatur, IN, p. A200

NELSON, Nicole
Director Human Resources, Cloud County Health Center, Concordia, KS, p. A232
Human Resources Coordinator, Select Specialty Hospital–Omaha, Omaha, NE, p. A388

NELSON, Raymond, Acting Chief Information Resource Management, Veterans Affairs Health Care System, Fargo, ND, p. A466

NELSON, Rhonda, Chief Nursing Officer, Forrest City Medical Center, Forrest City, AR, p. A45

NELSON, RimaAnn O., Director, Veterans Affairs Medical Center, Saint Louis, MO, p. A370

NELSON, Rodney M., Chief Executive Officer, Mackinac Straits Health System, Saint Ignace, MI, p. A322

NELSON, Sally I., Chief Executive Officer, Huntsville Memorial Hospital, Huntsville, TX, p. A608

NELSON, Sean, Deputy Director, Veterans Affairs Medical Center, Cleveland, OH, p. A476

NELSON, Selena, Chief Financial Officer, Fallon Medical Complex, Baker, MT, p. A373

NELSON, Shelby, Chief Executive Officer, Platte County Memorial Hospital, Wheatland, WY, p. A698

NELSON, Siri, Chief Administrative Officer, Sutter Lakeside Hospital, Lakeport, CA, p. A66

NELSON, Stewart R., Chief Financial Officer, Halifax Regional Health System, South Boston, VA, p. A656

NELSON, Tammy, Manager Human Resources, Southwest Health Center, Platteville, WI, p. A689

NELSON, Thomas, M.D. Director Emergency Room, Gibson General Hospital, Trenton, TN, p. A576

NELSON, Tom, Director Human Resources, Mitchell County Regional Health Center, Osage, IA, p. A224

NELSON, Tricia, Chief Financial Officer, RiverWoods Behavioral Health System, Riverdale, GA, p. A157

NELSON, William, M.D. Medical Director, Riverview Psychiatric Center, Augusta, ME, p. A281

NELSON–JONES, Susan, Director Human Resources, Tehachapi Valley Healthcare District, Tehachapi, CA, p. A92

NEMI, Neil, Administrator Facility Information Center, Richard H. Hutchings Psychiatric Center, Syracuse, NY, p. A444

NEONAKIS, Stephanie W., Manager, University Hospitals Richmond Medical Center, Cleveland, OH, p. A476

NESBIT, Steven, D.O. Chief Medical Officer, Via Christi Hospitals Wichita, Wichita, KS, p. A245

NESBIT, Tom, Director Human Resources, Kendall Regional Medical Center, Miami, FL, p. A131

NESMITH, Nikki, Chief Nursing Officer, Evans Memorial Hospital, Claxton, GA, p. A149

NESPOLI, John L., Chief Executive Officer, Sacred Heart Hospital, Allentown, PA, p. A517

NESS, David L., Vice President Operations, Grinnell Regional Medical Center, Grinnell, IA, p. A220

NESS, Edwin, President and Chief Executive Officer, Munson Healthcare, Traverse City, MI, p. B92

NESS, Edwin, President and Chief Executive Officer, Munson Medical Center, Traverse City, MI, p. A324

NESS, Jon, Chief Executive Officer, Kootenai Medical Center, Coeur D'Alene, ID, p. A167

NESSEL, Mark
Executive Vice President and Chief Operating Officer, Lourdes Medical Center of Burlington County, Willingboro, NJ, p. A412
Chief Operating Officer, Our Lady of Lourdes Medical Center, Camden, NJ, p. A402

NESSELBUSH, Robert, President, Rochester General Hospital, Rochester, NY, p. A441

NESTER, Darlene
Market Chief Human Resources Officer, Coastal Carolina Hospital, Hardeeville, SC, p. A551
Chief Human Resources Officer, Hilton Head Hospital, Hilton Head Island, SC, p. A551

NESTER WOLFE, Cheryl R., R.N. Senior Vice President Operations and Chief Nursing Officer, Salem Hospital, Salem, OR, p. A515

NESTO, Richard W., M.D. Executive Vice President and Chief Medical Officer, Lahey Clinic Hospital, Burlington, MA, p. A298

NETH, Marvin, Administrator, Callaway District Hospital, Callaway, NE, p. A382

NETTERVILLE, Chad, Administrator, Field Memorial Community Hospital, Centreville, MS, p. A344

NETTLES, Alexander, M.D. Chief of Staff, Monroe County Hospital, Monroeville, AL, p. A23

NETTLES, Angela F., Director Human Resources, KershawHealth, Camden, SC, p. A546

NETTLES, Robert, Director Human Resources, MountainView Hospital, Las Vegas, NV, p. A393

NEUENDORF, David A., FACHE President and Chief Executive Officer, Audrain Medical Center, Mexico, MO, p. A365

NEUENDORF, Deborah, Vice President Administration, Hudson Valley Hospital Center, Cortlandt Manor, NY, p. A424

NEUENDORF, Michael, Chief Executive Officer, Wesley Medical Center, Hattiesburg, MS, p. A347

NEUMAN, Keith A.
Chief Information Officer, Dupont Hospital, Fort Wayne, IN, p. A201
Chief Information Officer, Rehabilitation Hospital of Fort Wayne, Fort Wayne, IN, p. A202

NEUMAN, Michael J., Vice President Finance, Kennedy Krieger Institute, Baltimore, MD, p. A287

NEUMAN, Richard, Assistant Administrator and Chief Human Resources Officer, Olympic Medical Center, Port Angeles, WA, p. A664

NEUMANN, Charles W., President and Chief Executive Officer, St. Joseph Medical Center, Towson, MD, p. A294

NEUMANN, Jamie, Director Human Resources, Iroquois Memorial Hospital and Resident Home, Watseka, IL, p. A195

NEUVIRTH, Stephanie, Chief Human Resource and Diversity Officer, City of Hope's Helford Clinical Research Hospital, Duarte, CA, p. A59

NEVAREZ, Domingo, Chief Executive Officer, Hospital de la Universidad de Puerto Rico/Dr. Federico Trilla, Carolina, PR, p. A700

NEVAREZ, Michele, Chief Human Resources Officer, Platte County Memorial Hospital, Wheatland, WY, p. A698

NEVILL, David S., Chief Executive Officer, Lovelace Medical Center, Albuquerque, NM, p. A414

NEVILLE, Bette, R.N. Interim CNO and Director of Nursing, Mercy Hospital of Portland, Portland, ME, p. A284

NEVILLE, Joyce, Chief Nursing Officer, River Parishes Hospital, La Place, LA, p. A269

NEVIN, Janice E., M.D. Chief Medical Officer, Christiana Care Health System, Newark, DE, p. A114

NEVINSKI, Lois, Manager Information Services, Buffalo Hospital, Buffalo, MN, p. A329

NEW, Cathy, Vice President Clinical Services, St. Francis Hospital and Health Services, Maryville, MO, p. A365

NEWBERRY–FERGUSON, Linda, Chief Executive Officer, Kindred Hospital–Milwaukee, Greenfield, WI, p. A683

NEWBY, Doug, Chief Information Officer, Highlands Medical Center, Scottsboro, AL, p. A25

NEWBY, Nancy M., FACHE President and Chief Executive Officer, Washington County Hospital, Nashville, IL, p. A189

Index of Health Care Professionals / Nieves

Index of Health Care Professionals

NEWCOMB, James, M.D. Vice President Medical, Ochsner Medical Center – North Shore, Slidell, LA, p. A278
NEWCOMB, Mike, D.O
Senior Vice President and Chief Operating Officer, Legacy Meridian Park Hospital, Tualatin, OR, p. A516
Senior Vice President and Chief Operating Officer, Legacy Mount Hood Medical Center, Gresham, OR, p. A511
NEWCOMB, Nancy, Director Human Resources, Jennersville Regional Hospital, West Grove, PA, p. A541
NEWELL, Dan, Chief Financial Officer, Highlands Medical Center, Scottsboro, AL, p. A25
NEWELL, Janice
Chief Information Officer, Swedish Medical Center–Cherry Hill Campus, Seattle, WA, p. A666
Chief Information Officer, Swedish Medical Center–First Hill, Seattle, WA, p. A666
NEWELL, Ryan, M.D. Chief of Staff, Plateau Medical Center, Oak Hill, WV, p. A674
NEWEY, Mark, D.O. Chief of Staff, Mercy Hospital Healdton, Healdton, OK, p. A497
NEWHOUSE, Paul R., Chief Executive Officer, Kindred Hospital West–Jefferson, Marrero, LA, p. A272
NEWLAND, Judy, R.N. Director, Incline Village Community Hospital, Incline Village, NV, p. A392
NEWLAND, Kathie, Controller, Wheatland Memorial Healthcare, Harlowton, MT, p. A376
NEWLAND, Tammy, Coordinator Human Resources, Scotland County Hospital, Memphis, MO, p. A365
NEWMAN, Billy, Department Head, Naval Hospital, Lemoore, CA, p. A67
NEWMAN, Cynthia, Manager Human Resources, Petersburg Medical Center, Petersburg, AK, p. A30
NEWMAN, Diane, Administrator, Johnson County Hospital, Tecumseh, NE, p. A390
NEWMAN, Douglas A., Chief Executive Officer, LaSalle General Hospital, Jena, LA, p. A268
NEWMAN, Edith, Interim Administrator, John J. Madden Mental Health Center, Hines, IL, p. A184
NEWMAN, Greg, M.D. Chief of Staff, Parkview Regional Hospital, Mexia, TX, p. A616
NEWMAN, James, M.D. President Medical Staff, Kennewick General Hospital, Kennewick, WA, p. A662
NEWMAN, Julie, Vice President Finance, Tahlequah City Hospital, Tahlequah, OK, p. A505
NEWMAN, Kari, Director Human Resources, Dayton General Hospital, Dayton, WA, p. A661
NEWMAN, Kurt, M.D. President and Chief Executive Officer, Children's National Medical Center, Washington, DC, p. A116
NEWMAN, Martin, M.D. Chief Medical Officer, Aurora Behavioral Health System–Glendale, Glendale, AZ, p. A32
NEWMAN, Thomas M., Vice President Finance, UPMC St. Margaret, Pittsburgh, PA, p. A536
NEWMILLER, Vicki, Chief Operating Officer, Great Falls Clinic Medical Center, Great Falls, MT, p. A376
NEWMYER, Terry
President and Chief Executive Officer, St. Helena Hospital, Saint Helena, CA, p. A84
President and Chief Executive Officer, St. Helena Hospital Clearlake, Clearlake, CA, p. A57
President and Chief Executive Officer, St. Helena Hospital–Center for Behavioral Health, Vallejo, CA, p. A94
NEWPOWER, Nicole, Coordinator Human Resources, Kindred Hospital–Fort Worth, Fort Worth, TX, p. A599
NEWQUIST, Dennis, Director Information Systems, Abilene Regional Medical Center, Abilene, TX, p. A577
NEWSOM, Jamie, Director Information Systems, Williamsburg Regional Hospital, Kingstree, SC, p. A551
NEWSOM, Paul, Chief Operating Officer, Kentuckiana Medical Center, Clarksville, IN, p. A199
NEWSOME, Gary D., President and Chief Executive Officer, Health Management Associates, Naples, FL, p. B62
NEWSOME, Samuel C., M.D. President Medical Staff, Pioneer Community Hospital of Stokes, Danbury, NC, p. A451
NEWTON, Carmen, Manager Human Resources, Corpus Christi Specialty Hospital, Corpus Christi, TX, p. A589
NEWTON, Gail, R.N. Vice President Patient Care Services, St. Luke's Hospital – Warren Campus, Phillipsburg, NJ, p. A408
NEWTON, John, Vice President Financial and Support Services and Chief Financial Officer, Memorial Hospital, North Conway, NH, p. A399
NEWTON, Keith, Chief Executive Officer, South Baldwin Regional Medical Center, Foley, AL, p. A20
NEWTON, Mark, President and Chief Executive Officer, Swedish Covenant Hospital, Chicago, IL, p. A178
NEWTON, Milissa, Supervisor Human Resources, Good Samaritan Hospital, Bakersfield, CA, p. A54
NEWTON, Steven R., President, Baylor All Saints Medical Center at Fort Worth, Fort Worth, TX, p. A598
NEWTON, Susan, Chief Financial Officer, Broward Health Imperial Point, Fort Lauderdale, FL, p. A123
NEWTON, Terri, Chief Nursing Officer, Lakewood Regional Medical Center, Lakewood, CA, p. A67
NEWTON, Wilma, Executive Vice President and Chief Financial Officer, St. Vincent's Birmingham, Birmingham, AL, p. A17
NG, Anthony, M.D. Vice President and Chief Medical Officer, The Acadia Hospital, Bangor, ME, p. A281
NG, Thomas T., Chief Information Officer, Collingsworth General Hospital, Wellington, TX, p. A634
NG, Vincent, Director, Veterans Affairs Medical Center, Providence, RI, p. A545
NGUYEN, Dat, M.D. Chief of Staff, ValleyCare Medical Center, Pleasanton, CA, p. A80
NGUYEN, Eileen, Administrator, Renaissance Hospital, Groves, TX, p. A602
NGUYEN, Hao, M.D. Medical Director, Lanterman Developmental Center, Pomona, CA, p. A80
NGUYEN, Nicholas, M.D. Interim Medical Director, Metropolitan St. Louis Psychiatric Center, Saint Louis, MO, p. A369
NGUYEN, Vicki, Chief Financial Officer, Good Samaritan Hospital, Bakersfield, CA, p. A54
NIAZI, A., M.D. Chief of Staff, Anson Community Hospital, Wadesboro, NC, p. A462
NIAZI, Sultan, Chief Financial Officer, Arms Acres, Carmel, NY, p. A423
NIBLOCK, Christine, Chief Financial Officer, Sheridan County Health Complex, Hoxie, KS, p. A235
NICASTRO, Pam, Director Human Resources, Kenmore Mercy Hospital, Kenmore, NY, p. A428
NICELY, David E., Chief Executive Officer, Johnson City Medical Center, Johnson City, TN, p. A567
NICELY, Dennis, Chief Executive Officer, Landmark Hospital of Joplin, Joplin, MO, p. A361
NICHELSON, Kathleen, Director Human Resources, Horsham Clinic, Ambler, PA, p. A518
NICHOLAS, Connie, Interim Chief Executive Officer, L. V. Stabler Memorial Hospital, Greenville, AL, p. A21
NICHOLS, Arthur W., President and Chief Executive Officer, Cheshire Medical Center, Keene, NH, p. A398
NICHOLS, Barbara, R.N. President and Chief Executive Officer, Corry Memorial Hospital, Corry, PA, p. A521
NICHOLS, Bryan, Chief Financial Officer, The Heart Hospital Baylor Plano, Plano, TX, p. A621
NICHOLS, Dia, Chief Executive Officer, John Randolph Medical Center, Hopewell, VA, p. A649
NICHOLS, Dwight J., M.D. Chief of Staff, Stephens Memorial Hospital, Breckenridge, TX, p. A584
NICHOLS, Gretchen, R.N. Chief Administrative Officer, Legacy Mount Hood Medical Center, Gresham, OR, p. A511
NICHOLS, James, Chief Information Officer, Veterans Affairs Medical Center, Syracuse, NY, p. A444
NICHOLS, Laura L., Team Leader Human Resources, Hancock Regional Hospital, Greenfield, IN, p. A203
NICHOLS, Lorraine, Director Information Services, Alice Peck Day Memorial Hospital, Lebanon, NH, p. A398
NICHOLS, Mark, FACHE Chief Executive Officer, LewisGale Hospital at Pulaski, Pulaski, VA, p. A654
NICHOLS, Mark, R.N. Director of Nurses, Liberty Dayton Regional Medical Center, Liberty, TX, p. A612
NICHOLS, Michael, Corporate Vice President Information Technology, Touchette Regional Hospitals, Centreville, IL, p. A175
NICHOLS, Owen, PsyD, President and Chief Executive Officer, NorthKey Community Care, Covington, KY, p. A249
NICHOLS, Richard, Administrator, Sutter Maternity and Surgery Center of Santa Cruz, Santa Cruz, CA, p. A90
NICHOLS, Robert R., M.D. Vice President Medical Affairs, Mercy Hospital Fort Scott, Fort Scott, KS, p. A233
NICHOLS, Robin
Chief Financial Officer, Betsy Johnson Regional Hospital, Dunn, NC, p. A452
Chief Financial Officer, Coshocton County Memorial Hospital, Coshocton, OH, p. A478
NICHOLS, Sharon, D.O. Chief of Staff, Clark Fork Valley Hospital, Plains, MT, p. A378
NICHOLS, Stephen, Chief Executive Officer, Quitman County Hospital, Marks, MS, p. A349
NICHOLS, Suzanne, Director Human Resources, Muleshoe Area Medical Center, Muleshoe, TX, p. A618
NICHOLS, Terry, Interim Chief Executive Officer, Horton Community Hospital, Horton, KS, p. A235
NICHOLS, Theodore, M.D. Senior Vice President Medical Affairs, Lake Health, Concord Township, OH, p. A477
NICHOLSON, Britain, M.D. Chief Medical Officer, Massachusetts General Hospital, Boston, MA, p. A297
NICHOLSON, Cindy, Director Human Resources, Shelby Baptist Medical Center, Alabaster, AL, p. A15
NICHOLSON, Donna, Chief Nursing Officer, Gadsden Regional Medical Center, Gadsden, AL, p. A20
NICHOLSON, Kevin, Chief Executive Officer, Trillium Specialty Hospital–East Valley, Mesa, AZ, p. A34
NICHOLSON, Kristin, Coordinator Human Resources, Genesis Medical Center, DeWitt, De Witt, IA, p. A217
NICHOLSON, Molly, R.N. Vice President of Patient Care/Chief Nurse Executive, Provena United Samaritans Medical Center, Danville, IL, p. A179
NICHOLSON, Tim, Chief Executive Officer, Encore Healthcare, Columbia, MD, p. B50
NICKEL, Craig, M.D. Chief of Staff, Lindsborg Community Hospital, Lindsborg, KS, p. A238
NICKEL, Kathleen, Director Communications, Mercy Medical Center, Roseburg, OR, p. A515
NICKELL, Janice, Administrative Assistant, Glen Rose Medical Center, Glen Rose, TX, p. A601
NICKELL, Jerry, Vice President Human Resource and Mission, Saint Alphonsus Medical Center – Baker City, Baker City, OR, p. A509
NICKELL, Sarah, Vice President Human Resources, Mercy Regional Medical Center, Lorain, OH, p. A483
NICKELS, John, M.D. President Medical Staff, Grace Hospital, Cleveland, OH, p. A475
NICKRAND, Tami, Director Information Technology, Harbor Beach Community Hospital, Harbor Beach, MI, p. A315
NICODEMUS, Lowell, Director Information Systems, Hendricks Regional Health, Danville, IN, p. A200
NICOLAY, Donald, M.D. Chief Medical Officer, Community Hospital, Grand Junction, CO, p. A101
NICOLETTA, Nicholas
Corporate Vice President and Chief Financial Officer, Bassett Medical Center, Cooperstown, NY, p. A424
Vice President and Chief Financial Officer, O'Connor Hospital, Delhi, NY, p. A425
NICOLL, C. Diana, M.D. Chief of Staff, Veterans Affairs Medical Center, San Francisco, CA, p. A87
NICOLSON, Lynne T., M.D. Medical Director, Sunnyview Rehabilitation Hospital, Schenectady, NY, p. A443
NICOSIA, Chris, Chief Financial Officer, Corpus Christi Medical Center, Corpus Christi, TX, p. A589
NIECE, Pam, Director Human Resources, Orem Community Hospital, Orem, UT, p. A639
NIELAN, Nicole, Director Information Technology, Kimball Health Services, Kimball, NE, p. A385
NIELSEN, Colleen, Director Operations, St. Joseph Hospital, Polson, MT, p. A378
NIELSEN, Gregory A., President, Great Plains Regional Medical Center, North Platte, NE, p. A386
NIELSEN, Gwen, Manager Human Resources, Indianhead Medical Center, Shell Lake, WI, p. A691
NIELSEN, Jeri, Compliance Officer, Mental Health Institute, Clarinda, IA, p. A216
NIELSEN, Kristine, Interim Chief Human Resources Officer, Creighton University Medical Center, Omaha, NE, p. A387
NIELSEN, LuAnn, R.N. Chief Nursing Officer, Franklin County Medical Center, Preston, ID, p. A170
NIELSEN, Sandy J., Director, Veterans Affairs Medical Center, Spokane, WA, p. A667
NIELSEN, Wayne, Director Human Resources, Ocala Regional Medical Center, Ocala, FL, p. A133
NIELSON, Curtis, Director Finance, South Lincoln Medical Center, Kemmerer, WY, p. A696
NIELSON, Lars, M.D. Chief Medical Officer, Weeks Medical Center, Lancaster, NH, p. A398
NIELSON, P. Douglas, M.D. Chief of Staff, Kahuku Medical Center, Kahuku, HI, p. A164
NIEMANN, Lynne, Director Nurses and Patient Care, Community Memorial Hospital, Sumner, IA, p. A227
NIEMER, Peggy, Vice President Human Resources, Children's Hospital of Wisconsin, Milwaukee, WI, p. A686
NIEMEYER, Bruce, Director Human Resources, Yadkin Valley Community Hospital, Yadkinville, NC, p. A463
NIEMEYER, Romaine, President and Chief Executive Officer, Holy Spirit Hospital, Camp Hill, PA, p. A519
NIENHUESER, Roberta, Chief Financial Officer, Fitzgibbon Hospital, Marshall, MO, p. A364
NIERMAN, David M., M.D. Vice President and Chief Medical Officer, The Mount Sinai Hospital of Queens,, NY, p. A437
NIERMAN, Peter, M.D. Chief Medical Officer, Aurora Chicago Lakeshore Hospital, Chicago, IL, p. A175
NIERMAN, Stephen, Chief Operating Officer, South Florida Baptist Hospital, Plant City, FL, p. A136
NIES, Lynn, Human Resources Officer, Veterans Affairs Medical Center, Erie, PA, p. A523
NIESE, Mel, Chief Fiscal Service, Veterans Affairs Palo Alto Health Care System, Palo Alto, CA, p. A79
NIESSINK, Henry
Regional Director Information Technology Services, Mercy Medical Center Redding, Redding, CA, p. A81
Senior Manager Information Technology Systems, St. Elizabeth Community Hospital, Red Bluff, CA, p. A81
NIEVES, Caridad, Chief Nursing Officer and Chief Operating Officer, Coral Gables Hospital, Coral Gables, FL, p. A121

Index of Health Care Professionals

Index of Health Care Professionals / Nieves

NIEVES, Deborah, Director Management Information Systems, Hospital San Francisco, San Juan, PR, p. A703
NIEVES, Erick, M.D. Medical Director, Hospital San Carlos Borromeo, Moca, PR, p. A702
NIEVES, Jesus, Chief Executive Officer, Bella Vista Hospital, Mayaguez, PR, p. A701
NIEVES, Jose, Director Information Systems, Hospital San Carlos Borromeo, Moca, PR, p. A702
NIEVES, Patria, Director, Hospital Metropolitano Dr. Susoni, Arecibo, PR, p. A700
NIGHMAN, Mike, Facility Coordinator Information Systems, Shelby Baptist Medical Center, Alabaster, AL, p. A15
NIGHTENGALE, Randy, Chief Financial Officer, North Valley Hospital, Whitefish, MT, p. A380
NIGHTINGALE, Mark, Senior Administrator, Merrimack Valley Hospital, Haverhill, MA, p. A300
NIGRIN, Daniel, M.D. Vice President Information Services and Chief Information Officer, Children's Hospital Boston, Boston, MA, p. A296
NIHALANI, Sunil, M.D. Chief Medical Staff, Lake Wales Medical Center, Lake Wales, FL, p. A128
NIKOLIC, Srbo, Chief Financial Officer, Hartgrove Hospital, Chicago, IL, p. A175
NILES, Heather, Director Human Resources Operations, Mercy Harvard Hospital, Harvard, IL, p. A183
NILES, Richard, M.D. Chief of Staff, Seymour Hospital, Seymour, TX, p. A627
NILL, Michael, M.D. President Medical Staff, Marietta Memorial Hospital, Marietta, OH, p. A483
NILSSON, Keith, Chief Financial Officer, Cleveland Clinic Florida, Weston, FL, p. A143
NINNEMAN, David, Associate Director, Veterans Affairs Medical Center, Cincinnati, OH, p. A474
NINU, Christine, Chief Operating Officer, Kindred Hospital–Milwaukee, Greenfield, WI, p. A683
NIPPER, Nathan, Vice President and Chief Operating Officer, Piedmont Newnan Hospital, Newnan, GA, p. A157
NISSENBAUM, Mark, M.D. Chief of Staff, Veterans Affairs Medical Center, Tuscaloosa, AL, p. A26
NIX, Bo, Chief Information Officer, Madison Valley Medical Center, Ennis, MT, p. A375
NIX, D. Mark, President and Chief Executive Officer, Infirmary Health System, Mobile, AL, p. B71
NIX, Monica, Administrator, Bethesda Rehabilitation Hospital, Baton Rouge, LA, p. A262
NIXDORF, David L., Director Support Services, Frances Mahon Deaconess Hospital, Glasgow, MT, p. A375
NIXON, Margaret, Director Human Resources, St. Vincent Medical Center–North, Sherwood, AR, p. A51
NIXON, Myra, Director Human Resources, HEALTHSOUTH Rehabilitation Hospital, Concord, NH, p. A397
NOAK, Amy, Director Human Resources, St. David's Round Rock Medical Center, Round Rock, TX, p. A623
NOAKES, Timothy J., Chief Financial Officer, Memorial Hospital Los Banos, Los Banos, CA, p. A73
NOBBE, Donna, Director Information Systems, Margaret Mary Community Hospital, Batesville, IN, p. A197
NOBLE, James S., Senior Vice President Finance and Chief Financial Officer, Huntington Memorial Hospital, Pasadena, CA, p. A80
NOBLE, Kerry L., Administrator, Pemiscot Memorial Health System, Hayti, MO, p. A360
NOBLE, Mallie S., Administrator, Mary Breckinridge ARH Hospital, Hyden, KY, p. A252
NOBLE, Paula, Chief Financial Officer and Treasurer, Ann & Robert H. Lurie Children's Hospital of Chicago, Chicago, IL, p. A175
NOBLE, Stacy, Administrator, Southeast Rehabilitation Hospital, Lake Village, AR, p. A47
NOBLIN, Jeff, FACHE Chief Executive Officer, Crockett Hospital, Lawrenceburg, TN, p. A569
NOCITA, Shawn, Chief Information Resource Management, James E. Van Zandt Veterans Affairs Medical Center, Altoona, PA, p. A517
NOCKERTS, Steven R., Chief Executive Officer, Richland Hospital, Richland Center, WI, p. A690
NOCKET, Patricia, Assistant Vice President Clinical Nursing Services, Saint Francis Hospital and Health Centers, Poughkeepsie, NY, p. A441
NOE, J. Thomas, Director Human Resources, Charles Cole Memorial Hospital, Coudersport, PA, p. A521
NOEL, Angie, Administrative Director Human Resources, Texas Health Presbyterian Hospital Plano, Plano, TX, p. A621
NOEL, III, Philip J., Assistant Administrator and Chief Operating Officer, Baptist Health System, San Antonio, TX, p. A624
NOEL, Vicki, Vice President Human Resources, Southern Ohio Medical Center, Portsmouth, OH, p. A487
NOFFSINGER, Sandy, Executive Assistant, Risk Manager and Director Marketing, Dundy County Hospital, Benkelman, NE, p. A382
NOGA, James W., Chief Information Officer, Massachusetts General Hospital, Boston, MA, p. A297
NOGLER, Wendy, Director Human Resources, Lincoln County Health System, Fayetteville, TN, p. A565
NOGUERAS, Juan, M.D. Chief of Staff, Cleveland Clinic Florida, Weston, FL, p. A143
NOHELTY, Pete, Chief Information Officer, Sacred Heart Hospital, Eau Claire, WI, p. A681
NOHOS, Janet G., Executive Vice President, St. Bernard Hospital and Health Care Center, Chicago, IL, p. A178
NOKELS, Kevin J., FACHE Vice President and Chief Operating Officer, Alegent Health–Midlands Hospital, Papillion, NE, p. A389
NOKES, Gregory B., Vice President Human Resources, Middlesex Hospital, Middletown, CT, p. A110
NOLAN, Barbara, Manager Human Resources, Warm Springs Medical Center, Warm Springs, GA, p. A161
NOLAN, Heather, Director Information Services, Northern Louisiana Medical Center, Ruston, LA, p. A276
NOLAN, Jennifer, President and Chief Executive Officer, Our Lady of Peace, Louisville, KY, p. A255
NOLAN, Matthew, Director Facilities and Operations, Elizabethtown Community Hospital, Elizabethtown, NY, p. A425
NOLAN, Michael J.
- Area Chief Operating Officer and Safety, Promise Hospital of Baton Rouge, Baton Rouge, LA, p. A263
- Area Safety Director, Promise Hospital of Baton Rouge, Baton Rouge, LA, p. A263

NOLAN, Patrick B., President and Chief Executive Officer, Warren Memorial Hospital, Front Royal, VA, p. A648
NOLAN, Rosemary, R.N
- Chief Operating Officer and Chief Nursing Officer, Heritage Valley Beaver, Beaver, PA, p. A518
- Chief Operating Officer and Chief Nursing Officer, Sewickley Valley Hospital, (A Division of Valley Medical Facilities), Sewickley, PA, p. A538

NOLEN, Benny, President, Saint Joseph Mount Sterling, Mount Sterling, KY, p. A257
NOLL, Gerald A., Chief Financial Officer, Rogers Memorial Hospital, Oconomowoc, WI, p. A688
NOLL, Keith, President, York Hospital, York, PA, p. A543
NOLL, Linda
- Executive Director Human Resources, Mercy Hospital Fort Scott, Fort Scott, KS, p. A233
- Executive Director Human Resources, Mercy Hospital Independence, Independence, KS, p. A235

NOLLETTE, Karen, Chief Financial Officer, West Holt Memorial Hospital, Atkinson, NE, p. A381
NOLT, Lori, Director Information Technology, Philhaven, Mount Gretna, PA, p. A529
NOLTING, Evelyn, Chief Executive Officer and Managing Director, River Oaks Hospital, New Orleans, LA, p. A275
NOONAN, Cindy, Chief Operating Officer, ValleyCare Medical Center, Pleasanton, CA, p. A80
NOONAN, Kathryn, Director Information Management, Lemuel Shattuck Hospital, Jamaica Plain, MA, p. A301
NORBURY, Denise, Regional Executive Officer, Southwest Missouri Psychiatric Rehabilitation Center, El Dorado Springs, MO, p. A359
NORBY, Kim, Chief Information Officer, Burgess Health Center, Onawa, IA, p. A224
NORBY, Michael, Interim Chief Financial Officer, Harris County Hospital District, Houston, TX, p. A604
NORD, Gay, Chief Executive Officer, Methodist Hospital, San Antonio, TX, p. A625
NORD, Stanley K., Chief Financial Officer, West Houston Medical Center, Houston, TX, p. A608
NORDAHL, Richard E., Chief Executive Officer, Sanford Sheldon Medical Center, Sheldon, IA, p. A226
NORDING, Rodney, Vice President Organizational Support, Mayo Clinic Health System in Austin, Austin, MN, p. A328
NORDSTROM, Katie, Director Human Resources, Beartooth Billings Clinic, Red Lodge, MT, p. A378
NORDSTROM, Tawnya, Director Human Resources, Centennial Peaks Hospital, Louisville, CO, p. A104
NORDWICK, Thomas Joseph, Executive Director, Adams Memorial Hospital, Decatur, IN, p. A200
NOREEN, James, M.D. Chief Medical Officer, Regina Medical Center, Hastings, MN, p. A332
NOREEN, Ron, Director Information Services, Comanche County Memorial Hospital, Lawton, OK, p. A498
NOREM, Ashley, Chief Information Systems, Indiana University Health Starke Hospital, Knox, IN, p. A206
NOREN, Mary Kay, Chief Executive Officer, Eastern Shore Hospital Center, Cambridge, MD, p. A290
NOREN, Tom, M.D. Chief Medical Officer, Marquette General Health System, Marquette, MI, p. A318
NORGAARD, Margaret B.
- Chief Executive Officer, Poplar Community Hospital, Poplar, MT, p. A378
- Chief Executive Officer, Trinity Hospital, Wolf Point, MT, p. A380

NORICK, Laurence, M.D. Clinical Director, U. S. Public Health Service Indian Hospital, Parker, AZ, p. A35
NORIEGA, Donna, Chief Operating Officer, Arizona State Hospital, Phoenix, AZ, p. A35
NORMAN, Debbie, Director Human Resources, Central Louisiana Surgical Hospital, Alexandria, LA, p. A261
NORMAN, Jimmy, Chief Financial Officer, Mountain Lakes Medical Center, Clayton, GA, p. A149
NORMAN, Julie, Chief Financial Officer, Yadkin Valley Community Hospital, Yadkinville, NC, p. A463
NORMAN, Lori, Chief Financial Officer, HEALTHSOUTH Rehabilitation of Gadsden, Gadsden, AL, p. A20
NORMAN, Mark, Administrator, Pioneer Community Hospital of Newton, Newton, MS, p. A351
NORMAN, Mary, R.N. Chief Nursing Officer, Bear Valley Community Hospital, Big Bear Lake, CA, p. A55
NORMAN, Michael L., Executive Vice President and Chief Operating Officer, Landmark Hospital, Cape Girardeau, MO, p. A356
NORMAN, Robin, Senior Vice President and Chief Financial Officer, Virginia Hospital Center – Arlington, Arlington, VA, p. A645
NORMAN, Rolf, Chief Financial Officer, Sunnyside Medical Center, Clackamas, OR, p. A509
NORMINGTON–SLAY, Jeremy, FACHE Chief Executive Officer, Moundview Memorial Hospital & Clinics, Friendship, WI, p. A682
NORO, Sharon, Chief Executive Officer, Select Specialty Hospital–Youngstown, Youngstown, OH, p. A492
NORONHA, Augusto A., Vice President Finance and Chief Financial Officer, Missouri Baptist Medical Center, Saint Louis, MO, p. A369
NORQUEST, Cathy, Director Human Resources, York General Hospital, York, NE, p. A390
NORR–MCPHILLIPS, Karina, Associate Executive Director Human Resources, Franklin Hospital, Valley Stream, NY, p. A445
NORRIS, Charles, Chief Executive Officer, Memorial Hospital, Gonzales, TX, p. A601
NORRIS, Doug, Administrator and Chief Operating Officer, Western Medical Center–Santa Ana, Santa Ana, CA, p. A89
NORRIS, John, M.D. Chief Medical Officer, Johnson Memorial Hospital, Franklin, IN, p. A202
NORRIS, Marsha, Director Information Systems, Ste. Genevieve County Memorial Hospital, Ste. Genevieve, MO, p. A371
NORRIS, Phil, Chief Financial Officer, Great River Medical Center, Blytheville, AR, p. A42
NORRIS, Timothy, Chief Financial Officer, Greene County General Hospital, Linton, IN, p. A207
NORTH, Scott L., FACH
- Chief Executive Officer, St. John's Hospital, Saint Paul, MN, p. A339
- Chief Executive Officer, St. Joseph's Hospital, Saint Paul, MN, p. A339
- Chief Executive Officer, Woodwinds Health Campus, Woodbury, MN, p. A342

NORTHERN, Gail M., Director Human Resources, Blue Mountain Hospital, Blanding, UT, p. A637
NORTHROP, Dale, Vice President Finance, Castle Medical Center, Kailua, HI, p. A164
NORTHROP, James, Director, Southern Nevada Adult Mental Health Services, Las Vegas, NV, p. A393
NORTHUP, Jeffrey, D.O. Chief Medical Officer, Summit Healthcare Regional Medical Center, Show Low, AZ, p. A38
NORTON, Andrew J., M.D. Senior Vice President Medical Affairs, Froedtert Memorial Lutheran Hospital, Milwaukee, WI, p. A686
NORTON, Bruce J., Senior Vice President and Chief Financial Officer, Sierra Vista Regional Health Center, Sierra Vista, AZ, p. A38
NORTON, Debbie, Chief Financial Officer, Medical Center Barbour, Eufaula, AL, p. A19
NORTON, Julie, Chief Financial Officer, Avera McKennan Hospital and University Health Center, Sioux Falls, SD, p. A559
NORTON, Lizette, Associate Vice President Human Resources Management, Loma Linda University Medical Center, Loma Linda, CA, p. A67
NORTON, Meg, Senior Vice President and Chief Operating Officer, Rady Children's Hospital – San Diego, San Diego, CA, p. A85
NORTON, Robert G., President and Chief Executive Officer, North Shore Medical Center, Salem, MA, p. A304
NORWOOD, Jay, Acting Superintendent, Kerrville State Hospital, Kerrville, TX, p. A610
NORWOOD, Lyle, M.D. Chief of Staff, Hughston Hospital, Columbus, GA, p. A149

A894 Index of Health Care Professionals

Index of Health Care Professionals / O'Hare

Index of Health Care Professionals

NOSACKA, Mark, Chief Executive Officer, Good Samaritan Medical Center, West Palm Beach, FL, p. A142
NOSBISCH, Don, Director Human Resources, Floyd County Medical Center, Charles City, IA, p. A216
NOSEWORTHY, Ed, President and Chief Executive Officer, Florida Hospital Fish Memorial, Orange City, FL, p. A134
NOSEWORTHY, John, M.D. President and Chief Executive Officer, Mayo Clinic Health System, Rochester, MN, p. B85
NOTARIANNI, Bob, Administrator, Noland Hospital Anniston, Anniston, AL, p. A15
NOTEMAN, Laurali, Director Human Resources, Kane County Hospital, Kanab, UT, p. A638
NOTTIDGE, Andrew, Director Human Resources, Physicians Regional Medical Center – Pine Ridge, Naples, FL, p. A133
NOTTINGHAM, Cheryl, Chief Financial Officer, Atlantic General Hospital, Berlin, MD, p. A289
NOUNA, Nabil, M.D. Chief of Staff, Allegan General Hospital, Allegan, MI, p. A307
NOVAK, Adam, Chief Executive Officer, Kindred Hospital Peoria, Peoria, IL, p. A191
NOVAK, Christopher, Chief Operating Officer, Alexian Brothers Behavioral Health Hospital, Hoffman Estates, IL, p. A184
NOVAK, Edward, President and Chief Executive Officer, Sacred Heart Hospital, Chicago, IL, p. A178
NOVAK, Georgene, Director Human Resources, Littleton Regional Hospital, Littleton, NH, p. A399
NOVAK, James, Vice President, Human Resources, St. Francis Medical Center, Monroe, LA, p. A273
NOVAK, Kristen, Manager Human Resources, River Falls Area Hospital, River Falls, WI, p. A690
NOVAK, Michael, Vice President Operations, Saint Mary's Hospital, Waterbury, CT, p. A112
NOVAK, Sharon, CPA Vice President Finance, Pike Community Hospital, Waverly, OH, p. A491
NOVOA, Jose E., M.D. Medical Director, Cardiovascular Center of Puerto Rico and the Caribbean, San Juan, PR, p. A702
NOVOTNY, Mark, M.D. Chief Medical Officer, Southwestern Vermont Medical Center, Bennington, VT, p. A643
NOWACHEK, Debra S., Director Human Resources, Grinnell Regional Medical Center, Grinnell, IA, p. A220
NOWAK, Shelley A., Chief Executive Officer, Lakeside Behavioral Health System, Memphis, TN, p. A571
NOWELL, Laura
  Chief Financial Officer, Cornerstone Hospital–West Monroe, West Monroe, LA, p. A279
  Vice President Accounting and Finance, Solara Hospital Harlingen, Harlingen, TX, p. A602
NOWICKI, Becky, Director Human Resources, Michiana Behavioral Health Center, Plymouth, IN, p. A210
NOWICKI, Zigmund, Director Human Resources, Catskill Regional Medical Center, Harris, NY, p. A427
NOWLAND, Bob, M.D. Chief of Staff, Texas Health Harris Methodist Hospital Hurst–Euless–Bedford, Bedford, TX, p. A583
NOWLIN, Jeffrey D., Executive Vice President and Chief Operating Officer, Gwinnett Hospital System, Lawrenceville, GA, p. A155
NOWLIN, Patricia, Director of Accounting, Cooper County Memorial Hospital, Boonville, MO, p. A356
NOWLING, Tara, Director Human Resources, Monroe County Hospital, Monroeville, AL, p. A23
NOYES, Debra, Chief Financial Officer, Putnam Community Medical Center, Palatka, FL, p. A135
NUCKLES, Craig, Chief Executive Officer, Managing and Regional Vice President, Timberlawn Mental Health System, Dallas, TX, p. A593
NUDD, Brandon M., Director, Organizational Development, Park Ridge Health, Hendersonville, NC, p. A454
NUDENCE, Robert, M.D. Chief of Staff, Highlands Regional Medical Center, Sebring, FL, p. A139
NUGENT, Carlene, Chief Clinical Officer, Kindred Hospital South Florida–Hollywood,, FL, p. A125
NUNAMAKER, Michael, FACHE Chief Executive Officer, Grady Memorial Hospital, Chickasha, OK, p. A494
NUNELLEY, Preston, M.D. Chief Medical Officer, Central Baptist Hospital, Lexington, KY, p. A253
NUNEZ, Carlos, Director Management Information Systems, First Hospital Panamericano, Cidra, PR, p. A700
NUNEZ, Milton, Chief Financial Officer, Woodhull Medical and Mental Health Center,, NY, p. A438
NUNLEY, Julie, R.N. Chief Executive Officer, Banner Ironwood Medical Center, San Tan Valley, AZ, p. A38
NUNLEY, Penny, Vice President Human Resources, Hannibal Regional Hospital, Hannibal, MO, p. A360
NUNN, Chalmers, M.D. Chief Medical Officer and Senior Vice President, Centra Lynchburg General Hospital, Lynchburg, VA, p. A650
NUNNELLEY, Greg, Director Human Resources, Pineville Community Hospital Association, Pineville, KY, p. A258
NUNNERY, Reece, Chief Financial Officer, Southwest Mississippi Regional Medical Center, McComb, MS, p. A349
NUNNES, Maria, Director Information Systems, Gnaden Huetten Memorial Hospital, Lehighton, PA, p. A527
NURICK, Paul E., Chief Executive Officer, Kittitas Valley Community Hospital, Ellensburg, WA, p. A661
NUSBAUM, Neil, M.D. Chief of Staff, Veterans Affairs Medical Center, Leeds, MA, p. A301
NUSS, Michelle, M.D. Chief Medical Officer, West Virginia University Hospitals, Morgantown, WV, p. A674
NUTTER, Robert, COO, Vice President of Human Resources and Support Services, Mercy Hospital of Portland, Portland, ME, p. A284
NWANGBURUKA, Okechukwu, M.D. Medical Director, Sierra Vista Hospital, Sacramento, CA, p. A84
NYBERG, Amy, Chief Strategy Officer, Beaver Dam Community Hospitals, Beaver Dam, WI, p. A679
NYBERG, Becky T., Chief Financial Officer, Bloomington Meadows Hospital, Bloomington, IN, p. A198
NYHUS, Corey, M.D. President Medical Staff, Perham Health, Perham, MN, p. A337
NYIKES, Debra, Director Finance and Chief Financial Officer, Cleveland Clinic Children's Hospital for Rehabilitation, Cleveland, OH, p. A474
NYKAMP, Robert, Vice President and Chief Operating Officer, Pine Rest Christian Mental Health Services, Grand Rapids, MI, p. A313
NYLUND, Barbara, M.D. Chief of Staff, Novato Community Hospital, Novato, CA, p. A77
NYP, Randall G., FACH
  President and Chief Executive Officer, Providence Medical Center, Kansas City, KS, p. A236
  President and Chief Executive Officer, Saint John Hospital, Leavenworth, KS, p. A237
NYSTROM, Janet, Manager Human Resources, Progress West HealthCare Center, Saint Charles, MO, p. A367

## O

O'BRIEN, Charles, M.D. President, Sanford University of South Dakota Medical Center, Sioux Falls, SD, p. A559
O'BRIEN, Dan, D.O. Medical Director, Indiana University Health Paoli Hospital, Paoli, IN, p. A210
O'BRIEN, Darcey, Chief Executive Officer, Integris Clinton Regional Hospital, Clinton, OK, p. A495
O'BRIEN, David, M.D. Senior Vice President, COO, St. Mary Medical Center, Apple Valley, CA, p. A54
O'BRIEN, Elizabeth, Chief Financial Officer, Northern Nevada Adult Mental Health Services, Sparks, NV, p. A395
O'BRIEN, Gracie, Chief Information Officer, Sequoia Hospital, Redwood City, CA, p. A82
O'BRIEN, Jane E., M.D. Medical Director, Franciscan Hospital for Children, Boston, MA, p. A296
O'BRIEN, John, Chief Executive Officer, Manning Regional Healthcare Center, Manning, IA, p. A223
O'BRIEN, John, M.D. Chief of Staff, Natchez Regional Medical Center, Natchez, MS, p. A351
O'BRIEN, John A., FACH
  Chief Operating Officer, Laurel Regional Hospital, Laurel, MD, p. A293
  President, Prince George's Hospital Center, Cheverly, MD, p. A290
O'BRIEN, John G., President and Chief Executive Officer, UMass Memorial Health Care, Inc., Worcester, MA, p. B133
O'BRIEN, John G., President and Chief Executive Officer, UMass Memorial Medical Center, Worcester, MA, p. A306
O'BRIEN, Karen, Director Human Resources, Gerald Champion Regional Medical Center, Alamogordo, NM, p. A414
O'BRIEN, Kelly, Vice President Operations, Riverview Medical Center, Red Bank, NJ, p. A409
O'BRIEN, Kevin, Chief Operating Officer, Newman Memorial Hospital, Shattuck, OK, p. A504
O'BRIEN, Laureen
  Chief Information Officer, Providence Newberg Medical Center, Newberg, OR, p. A513
  Chief Information Officer, Providence Portland Medical Center, Portland, OR, p. A514
O'BRIEN, Mary
  Administrator, Aurora St. Luke's Medical Center, Milwaukee, WI, p. A686
  Director Information Systems and Telecommunications, New York Westchester Square Medical Center,, NY, p. A435
O'BRIEN, Maureen, Chief Operating Officer, Redwood City Medical Center, Redwood City, CA, p. A82
O'BRIEN, Renee, Director Human Resources, Greater Binghamton Health Center, Binghamton, NY, p. A421
O'BRIEN, Timothy, M.D. Chief of Staff, Ashtabula County Medical Center, Ashtabula, OH, p. A469
O'BRIEN, Yvonne M., MS Chief of Nursing, Pella Regional Health Center, Pella, IA, p. A225
O'BRYANT, G. Mark, President and Chief Executive Officer, Tallahassee Memorial HealthCare, Tallahassee, FL, p. A140
O'CONNELL, Cynthia, M.D. Chief of Staff, Carl R. Darnall Army Medical Center, Fort Hood, TX, p. A598
O'CONNOR, Annalise, Director Human Resources, Sierra Nevada Memorial Hospital, Grass Valley, CA, p. A64
O'CONNOR, Christopher M., President and Chief Executive Officer, Hospital of Saint Raphael, New Haven, CT, p. A110
O'CONNOR, Daniel
  Vice President Human Resources, Munroe Regional Medical Center, Ocala, FL, p. A133
  Chief Information Officer, United Memorial Medical Center, Batavia, NY, p. A421
O'CONNOR, David, Executive Vice President and Chief Financial Officer, Gaston Memorial Hospital, Gastonia, NC, p. A453
O'CONNOR, Delia, Chief Executive Officer, Anna Jaques Hospital, Newburyport, MA, p. A302
O'CONNOR, Dennis, M.D. Medical Director, Ira Davenport Memorial Hospital, Bath, NY, p. A421
O'CONNOR, Ellen, Chief Nursing Officer, Jacobi Medical Center,, NY, p. A433
O'CONNOR, J. T., M.D. Medical Director, Mercy Health Love County, Marietta, OK, p. A499
O'CONNOR, James, Executive Vice President, St. Charles Hospital, Port Jefferson, NY, p. A440
O'CONNOR, Kathy, Vice President, Finance and Chief Financial Officer, St. Joseph Mercy Hospital, Ypsilanti, MI, p. A326
O'CONNOR, Marcia, Chief Executive Officer, Choctaw Memorial Hospital, Hugo, OK, p. A498
O'CONNOR, Michael, M.D. Chief Medical Officer, Banner Ironwood Medical Center, San Tan Valley, AZ, p. A38
O'CONNOR, Michael F., Senior Vice President Finance, York Hospital, York, PA, p. A543
O'CONNOR, Nicholas, Vice President and Chief Information Officer, Plainview Hospital, Plainview, NY, p. A440
O'CONNOR, Patrick, Chief Operating Officer, Morris Hospital & Healthcare Centers, Morris, IL, p. A188
O'CONNOR, Steve, Manager Human Resources, Kern Medical Center, Bakersfield, CA, p. A55
O'CONNOR, Thomas, President, United Hospital, Saint Paul, MN, p. A339
O'CONNOR, Timothy, Executive Vice President and Chief Financial Officer, Lahey Clinic Hospital, Burlington, MA, p. A298
O'DAY, Ken, Supervisor Information Systems, Corry Memorial Hospital, Corry, PA, p. A521
O'DELL, Darrell, Director Information Services, Good Samaritan Hospital, San Jose, CA, p. A88
O'DELL, Janet, Administrative Director, Eastern Louisiana Mental Health System, Jackson, LA, p. A268
O'DONNELL, Chris, Director for Administration, Naval Hospital, Pensacola, FL, p. A136
O'DONNELL, Michael, Chief Financial Officer, Peconic Bay Medical Center, Riverhead, NY, p. A441
O'DONNELL, Patrick W., CP
  Senior Vice President and Chief Operating Officer, Chambersburg Hospital, Chambersburg, PA, p. A520
  Vice President Finance, Waynesboro Hospital, Waynesboro, PA, p. A540
O'DONNELL, Randall L., Ph.D
  President and Chief Executive Officer, Children's Mercy Hospitals and Clinics, Kansas City, MO, p. A361
  President and Chief Executive Officer, Children's Mercy South, Overland Park, KS, p. A240
O'DONOGHUE, Brian, M.D. Chief Medical Officer, Breckinridge Memorial Hospital, Hardinsburg, KY, p. A251
O'FLANAGAN, Jayne, Director Human Resources, Incline Village Community Hospital, Incline Village, NV, p. A392
O'GORMAN, Jr., Thomas
  Assistant Administrator and Chief Financial Officer, East Texas Medical Center Pittsburg, Pittsburg, TX, p. A620
  Chief Financial Officer, East Texas Medical Center–Gilmer, Gilmer, TX, p. A601
O'HALLA, Mark S., President and Chief Executive Officer, McLaren Macomb, Mount Clemens, MI, p. A319
O'HARA, Denise, Vice President Human Resources, Wilson Medical Center, Wilson, NC, p. A463
O'HARA, Kathleen, Vice President Human Resources, Erie County Medical Center, Buffalo, NY, p. A422
O'HARA, Michael
  Senior Executive Director Human Resources, Houston Medical Center, Warner Robins, GA, p. A161
  Senior Executive Director, Perry Hospital, Perry, GA, p. A157
O'HARE, Rose Ann, R.N. Vice President Patient Services, Lawrence Hospital Center, Bronxville, NY, p. A422


Index of Health Care Professionals **A895**

O'KEEFE, Charles, Director Health Information Services, HEALTHSOUTH Rehabilitation Hospital of Tallahassee, Tallahassee, FL, p. A140

O'KEEFE, James M., President and Chief Executive Officer, Mile Bluff Medical Center, Mauston, WI, p. A685

O'KEEFE, John, Chief Executive Officer, Select Specialty Hospital–Gulf Coast, Gulfport, MS, p. A346

O'KEEFE, Kathy, Director Operations, Pilgrim Psychiatric Center, Brentwood, NY, p. A422

O'KEEFE, Michael N., President and Chief Executive Officer, Evangelical Community Hospital, Lewisburg, PA, p. A527

O'KEEFFE, Maureen, Vice President Human Resources, St. Luke's Regional Medical Center, Boise, ID, p. A167

O'LASKEY, Bonnie, Vice President Human Resources, Edward White Hospital, Saint Petersburg, FL, p. A138

O'LEARY, Daniel H., M.D. Chief Medical Officer, Health Alliance Hospitals, Leominster, MA, p. A301

O'LEARY, Kevin J., Senior Vice President and Chief Financial Officer, Exeter Hospital, Exeter, NH, p. A398

O'LEARY, Megan A., Vice President Human Resources and Rehabilitation Services, McKenzie–Willamette Medical Center, Springfield, OR, p. A515

O'LEARY, Rand, Senior Vice President and Chief Operating Officer, Henry Ford Wyandotte Hospital, Wyandotte, MI, p. A325

O'LOUGHLIN, James F., President and Chief Executive Officer, Memorial Hospital Jacksonville, Jacksonville, FL, p. A126

O'MALLEY, Erin, M.D. Chief Clinical Officer, Kindred Hospital North Houston, Houston, TX, p. A604

O'MALLEY, John, FACHE Chief Executive Officer, Select Specialty Hospital–Ann Arbor, Ypsilanti, MI, p. A326

O'MALLEY, Jon P., Chief Executive Officer, Select Specialty Hospital–Macomb County, Mount Clemens, MI, p. A319

O'MALLEY, Mary Jo, R.N. Vice President Diagnostics and Support Services, Oconomowoc Memorial Hospital, Oconomowoc, WI, p. A688

O'MALLEY, Terry, Vice President Human Resources, Frederick Memorial Hospital, Frederick, MD, p. A291

O'MALLEY, Trevor, Site Manager, Provena Saint Joseph Hospital, Elgin, IL, p. A181

O'NEAL, Michael, Administrator and Chief Executive Officer, George C Grape Community Hospital, Hamburg, IA, p. A220

O'NEAL, Nancy L., Interim Administrator, Lakeside Medical Center, Belle Glade, FL, p. A118

O'NEIL, Jeremy, Manager Finance, Providence Valdez Medical Center, Valdez, AK, p. A30

O'NEIL, Linda B., R.N. Chief Executive Officer, Hospital for Extended Recovery, Norfolk, VA, p. A652

O'NEIL Jr., Mark T., President and Chief Executive Officer, Hilton Head Hospital, Hilton Head Island, SC, p. A551

O'NEILL, Bonnie, Vice President Employee Services, Northern Montana Hospital, Havre, MT, p. A376

O'NEILL, Jeannine, Director Information Systems, South Baldwin Regional Medical Center, Foley, AL, p. A20

O'NEILL, Joseph J., M.D. Vice President Medical Affairs, South County Hospital, Wakefield, RI, p. A545

O'NEILL, Michael, M.D. Chief Medical Officer, Eastside Medical Center, Snellville, GA, p. A159

O'NEILL, Michelle, M.D. President Medical Staff, Fairfield Memorial Hospital, Fairfield, IL, p. A182

O'NEILL, Stephan, Vice President Information Services, Hartford Hospital, Hartford, CT, p. A109

O'NEILL, Stephen, Clinical Director, Norfolk Regional Center, Norfolk, NE, p. A386

O'REAR, Caleb F., Chief Executive Officer, Denton Regional Medical Center, Denton, TX, p. A593

O'REAR, Christie, Human Resources Officer, Collingsworth General Hospital, Wellington, TX, p. A634

O'ROURKE, Kenneth, Administrator, Beck Behavioral Hospital, Baton Rouge, LA, p. A262

O'SHAUGHNESSY, Bryan, Chief Information Officer, Ellwood City Hospital, Ellwood City, PA, p. A522

O'SHAUGHNESSY, Jon C., Chief Executive Officer, Millwood Hospital, Arlington, TX, p. A579

O'SHEA, James E.
Administrator, Springbrook Hospital, Brooksville, FL, p. A120
Administrator, Willough Healthcare System, Naples, FL, p. A133

O'SHIELDS, Hugh, M.D. President Medical Staff, Trinity Medical Center, Birmingham, AL, p. A17

O'SULLIVAN, Barbara, M.D. Medical Director, Rockefeller University Hospital, New York, NY, p. A436

O'SULLIVAN, Colin
Administrator, Complex Care Hospital of Idaho, Meridian, ID, p. A169
Administrator, Tahoe Pacific Hospitals, Reno, NV, p. A395

OAKES, Julie P., R.N. Manager Risk and Quality, Ocean Beach Hospital, Ilwaco, WA, p. A662

OAKES, Patti
Director Human Resources, Medical Center of the Rockies, Loveland, CO, p. A104
Interim Vice President Human Resources, Poudre Valley Hospital, Fort Collins, CO, p. A101

OAKS, Dana, Chief Executive Officer, Columbia Hospital, West Palm Beach, FL, p. A142

OATES, John
Director Information Systems, Geneva General Hospital, Geneva, NY, p. A426
Director Information Systems, Soldiers and Sailors Memorial Hospital of Yates County, Penn Yan, NY, p. A440

OATES, Susie, Assistant Superintendent for Administration, Southwestern State Hospital, Thomasville, GA, p. A160

OBENLAND, Kathleen, Director Public Affairs, Providence St. Mary Medical Center, Walla Walla, WA, p. A669

OBER, Kathleen, M.D. Chief Medical Officer, Blue Hill Memorial Hospital, Blue Hill, ME, p. A282

OBER, Tammy L., Chief Executive Officer, Lancaster Rehabilitation Hospital, Lancaster, PA, p. A526

OBERG, Roger B., Chief Executive Officer, St. Vincent General Hospital District, Leadville, CO, p. A103

OBERHEU, Todd, Chief Executive Officer, Spanish Peaks Regional Health Center, Walsenburg, CO, p. A106

OBERHOLTZER, Curt, Assistant Administrator Human Resources and Organizational Development, Bay Area Medical Center, Marinette, WI, p. A685

OBERMAN, Shannon, Coordinator Human Resources, Select Specialty Hospital–Wilmington, Wilmington, DE, p. A115

OBERMIER, Jenny, VP, Director of Nursing, York General Hospital, York, NE, p. A390

OBERRIEDER, Marsha, Vice President Operations, Northwestern Lake Forest Hospital, Lake Forest, IL, p. A186

OBERST, Larry, Vice President Finance, Spectrum Health Special Care Hospital, Grand Rapids, MI, p. A314

OBRYCKI, Travis, Director Information Systems, Memorial Medical Center – Neillsville, Neillsville, WI, p. A688

OCASIO, J. Manuel, Vice President Human Resources, Holy Cross Hospital, Silver Spring, MD, p. A294

OCCHIOGROSSO, Kathleen, Vice President Human Resources, St. Mary's Hospital, Troy, NY, p. A445

OCHOA, Nikki
Interim Chief Financial Officer, St. Joseph's Behavioral Health Center, Stockton, CA, p. A91
Interim Chief Financial Officer, St. Joseph's Medical Center, Stockton, CA, p. A92

OCHOA, Ricardo, Chief Fiscal Officer, Veterans Affairs Medical Center, San Juan, PR, p. A704

OCHOA, Yolanda, Director Human Resources, Acuity Hospital of South Texas, San Antonio, TX, p. A624

OCHS, David T., President and Chief Executive Officer, OSF Saint James – John W. Albrecht Medical Center, Pontiac, IL, p. A192

OCHS, Kristine, R.N. Administrator, Grisell Memorial Hospital District One, Ransom, KS, p. A242

OCHSENDORF, Derrick, Manager Information Technology and Systems, Johnson Memorial Health Services, Dawson, MN, p. A330

OCKERS, Thomas, President and Chief Executive Officer, Brookhaven Memorial Hospital Medical Center, Patchogue, NY, p. A440

OCON, Paul, R.N. Chief Nursing Officer, El Paso Children's Hospital, El Paso, TX, p. A596

OCTAVIANI, Raul, M.D. Chief Medical Officer, Radius Specialty Hospital Boston, Boston, MA, p. A297

ODATO, David, Chief Administrative and Chief Human Resources Officer, UCSF Medical Center, San Francisco, CA, p. A87

ODDIS, Joseph M., Chief Executive Officer, Bon Secours Maryview Medical Center, Portsmouth, VA, p. A654

ODEGAARD, Daniel D., Chief Executive Officer, Bigfork Valley Hospital, Bigfork, MN, p. A328

ODELL, Cheryl, Chief Nursing Officer, Sharp Mesa Vista Hospital, San Diego, CA, p. A86

ODEN, Greg, M.D. Medical Director and Chief of Staff, Select Specialty Hospital–Jackson, Jackson, MS, p. A348

ODOM, Keli, Chief Operating Officer, North Central Surgical Center, Dallas, TX, p. A592

ODOM, Mary, Accountant, Larned State Hospital, Larned, KS, p. A237

ODOM, Robbin, R.N. Chief Nursing Officer, Women and Children's Hospital, Lake Charles, LA, p. A271

ODUBELA, Abayomi, M.D. Chief Medical Officer, Inland Valley Medical Center, Wildomar, CA, p. A96

OEHLERS, Randi, Site Director Management Information Systems, Mercy Hospital Cadillac, Cadillac, MI, p. A308

OEHLKE, Tammy, Director Human Resources, St. Mark's Medical Center, La Grange, TX, p. A611

OEHM, Janice, Manager Business Office, Johnson County Hospital, Tecumseh, NE, p. A390

OEHRING, David J., Chief Financial Officer, Spectrum Health United Hospital, Greenville, MI, p. A314

OELMAN, Mary B., R.N. Chief Operating Officer and Chief Clinical Officer, Barlow Respiratory Hospital, Los Angeles, CA, p. A68

OESTREICH, Alyssa, Chief Operating Officer, Odessa Memorial Healthcare Center, Odessa, WA, p. A663

OESTREICH, Pearl, Director Human Resources, Scott & White Hospital – Llano, Llano, TX, p. A613

OETTING, Phyllis, Director Human Resources, Mitchell County Hospital Health Systems, Beloit, KS, p. A231

OETZEL, Gerald P., Chief Financial Officer, Jeanes Hospital, Philadelphia, PA, p. A532

OFFUTT, Dan, Manager Finance, Knox County Hospital, Knox City, TX, p. A611

OFNER, Lori, Vice President Human Resources, Easton Hospital, Easton, PA, p. A522

OGATA, Edward S., M.D. Chief Medical Officer, Ann & Robert H. Lurie Children's Hospital of Chicago, Chicago, IL, p. A175

OGAWA, Quin, Vice President and Chief Financial Officer, Kuakini Medical Center, Honolulu, HI, p. A163

OGBURN, Wayne, FACHE Administrator, Rankin Hospital District, Rankin, TX, p. A622

OGDEN, Judy, Director Information Technology, Franklin Medical Center, Winnsboro, LA, p. A279

OGDEN, Michael L., President and Chief Executive Officer, Little Falls Hospital, Little Falls, NY, p. A428

OGEDA, Fidel, M.D. Chief of Staff, Medical Arts Hospital, Lamesa, TX, p. A611

OGG, Tom, Vice President Information Services and Chief Information Officer, Akron Children's Hospital, Akron, OH, p. A469

OGILVIE, Patrick, M.D. Chief Medical Officer, Mark Reed Health Care District, McCleary, WA, p. A662

OGILVIE, Richard, Chief Information Officer, Southwestern Vermont Medical Center, Bennington, VT, p. A643

OGLESBY, Darrell M., Administrator, Putnam General Hospital, Eatonton, GA, p. A152

OGLESBY, Michele, Manager Human Resources, Eastern Oklahoma Medical Center, Poteau, OK, p. A503

OGORZALEK, Ed, Chief Financial Officer, Rutland Regional Medical Center, Rutland, VT, p. A644

OHE, Darin, Chief Financial Officer, Richard P. Stadter Psychiatric Center, Grand Forks, ND, p. A466

OHE, Gregory P., President and Chief Executive Officer, Health Central, Ocoee, FL, p. A134

OHL, Connie, Acting Chief Human Resources, Veterans Affairs Illiana Health Care System, Danville, IL, p. A179

OHLE, Rick L., Chief Operating Officer, St. Mary's of Michigan, Saginaw, MI, p. A322

OHMART, Dean, Assistant Administrator and Chief Financial Officer, Ransom Memorial Hospital, Ottawa, KS, p. A240

OHNOUTKA, Debra, Chief Nursing Officer, St. Joseph Medical Center, Kansas City, MO, p. A362

OHRT, James M., M.D. Director Medical Staff, Henderson Health Care Services, Henderson, NE, p. A384

OISHI, Gregg, Senior Vice President and Chief Operating Officer, Kuakini Medical Center, Honolulu, HI, p. A163

OJEDA, Filiberto J., Director Quality Improvement, Risk Management and Information System, Greenwood County Hospital, Eureka, KS, p. A233

OKABE, David
Senior Vice President, Chief Financial Officer and Treasurer, Kapiolani Medical Center for Women & Children, Honolulu, HI, p. A163
Executive Vice President, Chief Financial Officer and Treasurer, Pali Momi Medical Center, Aiea, HI, p. A163
Executive Vice President, Chief Financial Officer and Treasurer, Straub Clinic & Hospital, Honolulu, HI, p. A164
Executive Vice President, Chief Financial Officer and Treasurer, Wilcox Memorial Hospital, Lihue, HI, p. A165

OKAMOTO, Gary, M.D. Senior Vice President and Chief Medical Executive, Rehabilitation Hospital of the Pacific, Honolulu, HI, p. A164

OKASHIMA, Mark, Area Finance Officer, South San Francisco Medical Center, South San Francisco, CA, p. A91

OKECHUKWU, Vitalis C., M.D. President Medical Staff, Kindred Hospital Lafayette, Lafayette, LA, p. A270

OKERSON, Alan, Director Information Technology, Kenmare Community Hospital, Kenmare, ND, p. A467

OKESON, Keith, President and Chief Executive Officer, LifeCare Medical Center, Roseau, MN, p. A338

OKSENDAHL, Elaine, Administrator, Schick Shadel Hospital, Seattle, WA, p. A666

OKUHARA, Mary, Director Human Resources, Lakewood Regional Medical Center, Lakewood, CA, p. A67

OLANDER, Scott, Vice President and Chief Financial Officer, Yakima Valley Memorial Hospital, Yakima, WA, p. A669

Index of Health Care Professionals / Orsini

Index of Health Care Professionals

OLAZAGASTI, Rafael, M.D. Vice President Medical Affairs and Network Development, Benedictine Hospital, Kingston, NY, p. A428
OLDEN, R. Don, Chief Executive Officer, Wahiawa General Hospital, Wahiawa, HI, p. A165
OLDER, Michael, M.D. President Medical Staff, Nashoba Valley Medical Center, Ayer, MA, p. A295
OLDHAM, Benjamin, M.D. Chief of Staff, East Georgia Regional Medical Center, Statesboro, GA, p. A160
OLDHAM, John M., M.D. Senior Vice President and Chief of Staff, Menninger Clinic, Houston, TX, p. A605
OLDHAM, Lawrence, Chief Financial Officer, Austin Surgical Hospital, Austin, TX, p. A580
OLDS, Susan, Chief Financial Officer, St. Anthony's Hospital, Saint Petersburg, FL, p. A138
OLEJNIK, Marilyn A., Vice President Finance, Porter Medical Center, Middlebury, VT, p. A643
OLESON, Chuck, Chief Information Officer, Butler Health System, Butler, PA, p. A519
OLEY, Edwin M., President and Chief Executive Officer, Mercy Regional Medical Center, Lorain, OH, p. A483
OLINDE, Chad E., Administrator and Chief Executive Officer, Pointe Coupee General Hospital, New Roads, LA, p. A275
OLINGER, Richard P., Chief Financial Officer, Millcreek Community Hospital, Erie, PA, p. A523
OLINGER, Terry, System Chief Human Resources Officer, Benefis Hospitals, Great Falls, MT, p. A376
OLIPHANT, Gerald P., Executive Vice President and Chief Operating Officer, Good Samaritan Hospital, Cincinnati, OH, p. A473
OLIVA, Anthony F., D.O. Sr. Vice President & Chief Medical Officer, Borgess Medical Center, Kalamazoo, MI, p. A316
OLIVA, Damaso, M.D. Chief Medical Officer, Southwest General Hospital, San Antonio, TX, p. A626
OLIVA, George, Associate Information Systems Analyst, Lanterman Developmental Center, Pomona, CA, p. A80
OLIVARES, Rafael, Controller, Starr County Memorial Hospital, Rio Grande City, TX, p. A622
OLIVAS, Ray, Chief Fiscal Service, West Texas VA Health Care System, Big Spring, TX, p. A584
OLIVE, Alan C., Chief Executive Officer, Providence Newberg Medical Center, Newberg, OR, p. A513
OLIVEIRA, Edgar, M.D
Chief Medical Staff, Linton Hospital, Linton, ND, p. A467
Chief of Staff, Wishek Community Hospital and Clinics, Wishek, ND, p. A468
OLIVENCIA, Humberto, M.D. Medical Director, Hospital Perea, Mayaguez, PR, p. A702
OLIVER, Athan, Administrator and Chief Executive Officer, Iberia Rehabilitation Hospital, New Iberia, LA, p. A274
OLIVER, David, Director Information Systems, King's Daughters Medical Center, Ashland, KY, p. A247
OLIVER, Julie, Chief Human Resources Officer, Mayo Clinic Health System in Mankato, Mankato, MN, p. A334
OLIVER, Karen, Vice President Human Resources, West Florida Hospital, Pensacola, FL, p. A136
OLIVER, Vincent, Administrator, Island Hospital, Anacortes, WA, p. A659
OLIVERA, Sue, Vice President, Aultman Hospital, Canton, OH, p. A472
OLIVERIO, John D., President and Chief Executive Officer, Wheaton Franciscan Healthcare, Wheaton, IL, p. B145
OLIVIER, Edward, Chief Financial Officer, Charles A. Dean Memorial Hospital, Greenville, ME, p. A283
OLIVIERI, Michael, Chief Financial Officer, Lower Bucks Hospital, Bristol, PA, p. A519
OLLER, Darrell, Director Information Systems, Abraham Lincoln Memorial Hospital, Lincoln, IL, p. A186
OLLI, Cindy, R.N. Chief Nursing Officer, Schoolcraft Memorial Hospital, Manistique, MI, p. A318
OLLIE, Edwin J., Executive Vice President and Chief Financial Officer, New Hanover Regional Medical Center, Wilmington, NC, p. A462
OLLIS, Linda Neu, FACHE Chief Operating Officer, Monongalia General Hospital, Morgantown, WV, p. A674
OLLSON, Joanne, Vice President Human Resources, Noble Hospital, Westfield, MA, p. A306
OLM, Brad, Director Human Resources, Edgerton Hospital and Health Services, Edgerton, WI, p. A681
OLMO, Blanca, Director Finance, University Pediatric Hospital,, PR, p. A704
OLMSTEAD, David, Associate Administrator and Director Human Resources, Lake Pointe Medical Center, Rowlett, TX, p. A623
OLMSTEAD, Linda, Director Human Resources, Northwest Hospital & Medical Center, Seattle, WA, p. A665
OLS, Timothy A., FACHE President and Chief Executive Officer, Sarah Bush Lincoln Health Center, Mattoon, IL, p. A187
OLSCAMP, Karen E., Chief Executive Officer, Baltimore Washington Medical Center, Glen Burnie, MD, p. A292
OLSEN, Ryan, Vice President of Operations, St. Jude Medical Center, Fullerton, CA, p. A62
OLSEN, Sabrina, Chief Financial Officer, Duke University Hospital, Durham, NC, p. A452
OLSON, Carol, Administrator, Community Behavioral Health Hospital – St. Peter, Saint Peter, MN, p. A339
OLSON, Cheryl, Chief Human Resources Officer, Othello Community Hospital, Othello, WA, p. A664
OLSON, Christine K., MSN, Chief Administrative Officer and Chief Nursing Executive, Aurora Medical Center, Kenosha, WI, p. A683
OLSON, David, Interim President, St. Joseph's Community Hospital of West Bend, West Bend, WI, p. A693
OLSON, Diana
Chief Human Resources Officer, Mercy Tiffin Hospital, Tiffin, OH, p. A489
Chief Human Resources Officer, Mercy Willard Hospital, Willard, OH, p. A491
OLSON, Eric, Chief Financial Officer, Providence Portland Medical Center, Portland, OR, p. A514
OLSON, Forrest, M.D. Chief Medical Officer, Enloe Medical Center, Chico, CA, p. A57
OLSON, Gary R., President and Chief Executive Officer, St. Luke's Hospital, Chesterfield, MO, p. A357
OLSON, Gregory A., President and Chief Executive Officer, Memorial Health Center, Medford, WI, p. A685
OLSON, John L., M.D. Medical Director, Lakeview Medical Center, Rice Lake, WI, p. A690
OLSON, John N., Chief Executive Officer, Walter Knox Memorial Hospital, Emmett, ID, p. A168
OLSON, Kent, Administrator and Chief Executive Officer, Philip Health Services, Philip, SD, p. A558
OLSON, Kevin, Director Information Systems, St. Anthony Hospital, Oklahoma City, OK, p. A502
OLSON, Lynn R., Director Human Resources, Hendricks Community Hospital, Hendricks, MN, p. A332
OLSON, Lynn W., President and Chief Executive Officer, Hannibal Regional Hospital, Hannibal, MO, p. A360
OLSON, Marcia, Business Office Manager, Webster County Community Hospital, Red Cloud, NE, p. A389
OLSON, MariBeth, R.N. Vice President Patient Care Services, Mercy Hospital, Coon Rapids, MN, p. A330
OLSON, Michael R., Administrator, American Fork Hospital, American Fork, UT, p. A637
OLSON, Randall M., Chief Executive Officer, Lane Regional Medical Center, Zachary, LA, p. A280
OLSON, Rick, M.D. Chief of Staff, Sunnyside Medical Center, Clackamas, OR, p. A509
OLSON, Tim
Senior Vice President Finance, Appleton Medical Center, Appleton, WI, p. A678
Senior Vice President Finance, Theda Clark Medical Center, Neenah, WI, p. A687
OLSON, William, Director Finance, Providence St. Vincent Medical Center, Portland, OR, p. A514
OLSSON, Clifford Lee, Chief Financial Officer, Tuba City Regional Health Care Corporation, Tuba City, AZ, p. A39
OLSSON, Dave, Director of Marketing, Aspirus Keweenaw Hospital, Laurium, MI, p. A317
OLSZEWSKI, Joseph, Director Information Services, Aria Health, Philadelphia, PA, p. A531
OMAN, Michelle, D.O. Chief Medical Officer, Essentia Health Northern Pines, Aurora, MN, p. A328
OMAR, Sharif, Chief Executive Officer, Pottstown Memorial Medical Center, Pottstown, PA, p. A536
OMEL, John, Interim Vice President Human Resources, Good Samaritan Hospital, San Jose, CA, p. A88
OMER, Robert W., FACHE Chief Executive Officer and Administrator, Southeast Colorado Hospital District, Springfield, CO, p. A105
OMMEN, Ronald A., Interim Chief Executive Officer, Paynesville Area Health Care System, Paynesville, MN, p. A337
OMOLARA, Khar, M.D. Chief Medical Staff, Jefferson County Hospital, Fayette, MS, p. A345
OMOTUNDE, Olukayode S., M.D. Chief Medical Staff, First Care Health Center, Park River, ND, p. A468
OMRAN, Yasser, M.D. President Medical Staff, Pomerene Hospital, Millersburg, OH, p. A485
OMTA, Stephen R., Chief Operating Officer, PeaceHealth St. Joseph Medical Center, Bellingham, WA, p. A659
ONG, Jesus M., President, South Shore Hospital, Chicago, IL, p. A178
ONG, Richard B., Chief Information Officer, Saint Vincent Health Center, Erie, PA, p. A523
ONIFATHER, Jeff, Chief Financial Officer, Cornerstone of Medical Arts Center Hospital, Fresh Meadows, NY, p. A426
ONTIVEROS Jr., Alfredo, Chief Executive Officer, East El Paso Physicians Medical Center, El Paso, TX, p. A596
OOSTRA, Randall D., FACHE President and Chief Executive Officer, ProMedica Health System, Toledo, OH, p. B104
OPDAHL, Jim
Administrator, Jacobson Memorial Hospital Care Center, Elgin, ND, p. A465
Interim Chief Executive Officer, Wishek Community Hospital and Clinics, Wishek, ND, p. A468
OPHEIKENS, Robyn, Assistant Administrator Human Resources, St. Mark's Hospital, Salt Lake City, UT, p. A641
OPIE, Timothy, M.D. President Professional Staff, Providence Seaside Hospital, Seaside, OR, p. A515
OPPENHEIM, Steven, M.D. Vice President Medical Affairs, San Diego Hospice & The Institute of Palliative Medicine, San Diego, CA, p. A85
OPPITO, Glenn, Vice President Human Resources, Monmouth Medical Center, Long Branch, NJ, p. A405
OQUENDO, Tanja, Vice President Human Resources, Spectrum Health Butterworth Hospital, Grand Rapids, MI, p. A314
ORAM–SMITH, Jeffrey C., M.D. Chief Medical Officer, Penrose–St. Francis Health Services, Colorado Springs, CO, p. A98
ORCUTT, David, Chief Executive Officer, Lake Granbury Medical Center, Granbury, TX, p. A601
ORDYNA, Daniel, Chief Executive Officer, Willamette Valley Medical Center, McMinnville, OR, p. A512
ORE, Ruta, Director Human Resources, Pottstown Memorial Medical Center, Pottstown, PA, p. A536
OREAR, Kathy, Director Human Resources, Newman Regional Health, Emporia, KS, p. A232
OREB, Denny, Interim Chief Executive Officer, Orthopedic Hospital, Oklahoma City, OK, p. A502
OREGEL, Omar, Controller, Kindred Hospital–Ontario, Ontario, CA, p. A78
OREY, Lon, Vice President Human Resources, Presbyterian Intercommunity Hospital, Whittier, CA, p. A96
ORFANOS, John G., M.D. Chief of Staff, Cornerstone Regional Hospital, Edinburg, TX, p. A595
ORIOL, Albert, Vice President Information Management and Chief Information Officer, Rady Children's Hospital – San Diego, San Diego, CA, p. A85
ORIOLI, Sherri, Director Personnel Systems, University of Texas Harris County Psychiatric Center, Houston, TX, p. A607
ORLANDI, Mary, Manager Human Resources, Carney Hospital, Boston, MA, p. A296
ORLANDO, Anthony T., Senior Vice President Finance, Englewood Hospital and Medical Center, Englewood, NJ, p. A404
ORLANDO, Charles, Senior Vice President and Chief Financial Officer, Sinai Hospital of Baltimore, Baltimore, MD, p. A289
ORLANDO, Joseph S., President, Bergen Regional Medical Center, Paramus, NJ, p. A408
ORLANDO, Lorraine, Vice President Human Resources, New York Hospital Queens,, NY, p. A435
ORLOWSKI, Janis M., M.D. Senior Vice President Medical Affairs and Chief Medical Officer, Medstar Washington Hospital Center, Washington, DC, p. A116
ORMAN Jr., Bernard A., Administrator, Samaritan Memorial Hospital, Macon, MO, p. A364
ORME, Dave, Chief Information Officer, Rehabilitation Hospital of the Pacific, Honolulu, HI, p. A164
ORMOND, Evalyn, Chief Executive Officer, Union General Hospital, Farmerville, LA, p. A266
ORMOND, Jack, Chief Financial Officer, Cuba Memorial Hospital, Cuba, NY, p. A424
ORMS, J. Michael, M.D. Chief of Staff, East Texas Medical Center Fairfield, Fairfield, TX, p. A597
ORMSBY, Joan, Vice President, West Suburban Medical Center, Oak Park, IL, p. A190
ORNELAS, Henry, Chief Operating Officer, LAC/University of Southern California Medical Center, Los Angeles, CA, p. A70
ORONA, Rene, M.D. Chief of Staff, Marshall Medical Center, Placerville, CA, p. A80
OROZCO, Jorge, Chief Executive Officer, Rancho Los Amigos National Rehabilitation Center, Downey, CA, p. A59
ORR, Lindell W., Interim Chief Executive Officer, St. Cloud Regional Medical Center, Saint Cloud, FL, p. A137
ORR, Shirley, R.N. Chief Nursing Officer, Holdenville General Hospital, Holdenville, OK, p. A497
ORR, Stephanie, R.N. Chief Nursing Officer, Steele Memorial Medical Center, Salmon, ID, p. A170
ORRELL, Carolyn, Chief Information Officer, Saint Mary's Hospital, Waterbury, CT, p. A112
ORRELL, Linda, Interim Chief Nursing Officer, Drew Memorial Hospital, Monticello, AR, p. A49
ORRICK, Charles H., Administrator, Donalsonville Hospital, Donalsonville, GA, p. A151
ORRISON, Pat, Director Information Services, Marianjoy Rehabilitation Hospital, Wheaton, IL, p. A196
ORSAG, Melanie, Director Health Information Services, Cedar Crest Hospital, Belton, TX, p. A584
ORSINI, Bob, Chief Operating Officer, Walton Rehabilitation Hospital, Augusta, GA, p. A147


Index of Health Care Professionals A897

ORSINI, John
  Executive Vice President and Chief Financial Officer, Holy Family Medical Center, Des Plaines, IL, p. A180
  Executive Vice President Finance and Chief Financial Officer, Resurrection Medical Center, Chicago, IL, p. A177
  Chief Financial Officer, Saint Francis Hospital, Evanston, IL, p. A181
  Chief Financial Officer, West Suburban Medical Center, Oak Park, IL, p. A190
  Chief Financial Officer, Westlake Hospital, Melrose Park, IL, p. A187
ORSINI, Thomas J., President and Chief Executive Officer, Lake Taylor Transitional Care Hospital, Norfolk, VA, p. A652
ORSKEY, David, Administrator, Physicians Care Surgical Hospital, Royersford, PA, p. A537
ORT, Linda, Chief Financial Officer, Piggott Community Hospital, Piggott, AR, p. A50
ORTEGA, Cesar, M.D. Chief of Staff, Doctor's Hospital – Tidwell, Houston, TX, p. A604
ORTEGA, Debbie, Chief Human Resource Officer and Vice President Administrative Services, Huntington Memorial Hospital, Pasadena, CA, p. A80
ORTEGA, Jose, Administrator and Chief Operating Officer, Greater El Monte Community Hospital, South El Monte, CA, p. A91
ORTEGA, Juan Carlos, M.D. Chief of Staff, Colorado–Fayette Medical Center, Weimar, TX, p. A634
ORTHAUS, Denis, Director Human Resources, Philhaven, Mount Gretna, PA, p. A529
ORTIZ, Bienvenido, Coordinator Information Systems, Hospital De Damas, Ponce, PR, p. A702
ORTIZ, Jr., Blas, Assistant Superintendent and Public Information Officer, Rio Grande State Center/South Texas Health Care System, Harlingen, TX, p. A602
ORTIZ, Carlos, M.D. Senior Vice President Medical Services, F. F. Thompson Hospital, Canandaigua, NY, p. A423
ORTIZ, Edson, Chief Information Officer, Hospital Metropolitano Dr. Tito Mattei, Yauco, PR, p. A704
ORTIZ, Evelyn Padilla
  Director Human Resources, Hospital Menonita De Cayey, Cayey, PR, p. A700
  Director Human Resources, Mennonite General Hospital, Aibonito, PR, p. A699
ORTIZ, Felix, Administrator, I. Gonzalez Martinez Oncologic Hospital,, PR, p. A703
ORTIZ, Jorge Garcia, Executive Director, Industrial Hospital, San Juan, PR, p. A703
ORTIZ, Jose O., Chief Financial Officer, Ryder Memorial Hospital, Humacao, PR, p. A701
ORTIZ, Migdalia, Director Human Resources, Hospital San Carlos Borromeo, Moca, PR, p. A702
ORTIZ, Milagros, CPA Chief Financial Officer, Ashford Presbyterian Community Hospital, San Juan, PR, p. A702
ORTIZ, Norma, M.D. Medical Director, Hospital Hermanos Melendez, Bayamon, PR, p. A700
ORTIZ, Vicent, Chief Information Officer, Hospital Dr. Cayetano Coll Y Toste, Arecibo, PR, p. A700
ORTIZ VARGAS, Ruth M., Administrator, Lafayette Hospital, Arroyo, PR, p. A700
ORTIZ–BITNER, Olivia, Acting Chief Financial Officer, Veterans Affairs Greater Los Angeles Healthcare System, Los Angeles, CA, p. A72
ORTOLANI, Philip A., Vice President Operations, Mid Coast Hospital, Brunswick, ME, p. A282
ORTON, Sharon, Director Information Services and Technology, Corpus Christi Medical Center, Corpus Christi, TX, p. A589
OSANTOSKI, Tina, Director Human Resources, Harbor Beach Community Hospital, Harbor Beach, MI, p. A315
OSBAHR, Leah, Administrator, Washington County Memorial Hospital, Potosi, MO, p. A367
OSBERG, Art, M.D. Vice President and Chief Medical Officer, Ocala Regional Medical Center, Ocala, FL, p. A133
OSBERG III, James, Ph.D. Director, Dorothea Dix Hospital, Raleigh, NC, p. A459
OSBORN, Matt, M.D. Chief of Staff, Integris Baptist Regional Health Center, Miami, OK, p. A499
OSBORN, Tom, D.O. Chief Medical Staff, Holdenville General Hospital, Holdenville, OK, p. A497
OSBORNE, Anna, Chief Human Resources Management Service, West Texas VA Health Care System, Big Spring, TX, p. A584
OSBORNE, Jay, M.D. Senior Vice President Medical Affairs, Northside Medical Center, Youngstown, OH, p. A492
OSBORNE, Kimberly, Vice President and Chief Financial Officer, Eisenhower Medical Center, Rancho Mirage, CA, p. A81
OSBORNE, Matt, Flight Chief Medical Information Systems, Wright Patterson Medical Center, Wright–Patterson AFB, OH, p. A492
OSBORNE, Phil, Director Information Technology, Bourbon Community Hospital, Paris, KY, p. A258

OSBORNE, Sandra, Director Information Systems, Monongahela Valley Hospital, Monongahela, PA, p. A529
OSBORNE, Terry W., CPA, Chief Executive Officer, American Legion Hospital, Crowley, LA, p. A265
OSBURN, Jerry, Administrator, Covenant Hospital–Levelland, Levelland, TX, p. A612
OSCADAL, Martin
  Vice President Human Resources, St. Elizabeth Edgewood, Edgewood, KY, p. A249
  Senior Vice President Human Resources, St. Elizabeth Florence, Florence, KY, p. A250
  Senior Vice President Human Resources, St. Elizabeth Fort Thomas, Fort Thomas, KY, p. A250
OSEGARD, Jeff, Chief Information Officer, Lakewood Health System, Staples, MN, p. A340
OSER, William F., M.D. Senior Vice President and Chief Medical Officer, JFK Medical Center, Edison, NJ, p. A403
OSINSKI, Kathleen, Chief Human Resources Service, John D. Dingell Veterans Affairs Medical Center, Detroit, MI, p. A311
OSKIN, Jeffrey, Vice President Ancillary and Support Services, Florida Hospital Tampa, Tampa, FL, p. A140
OSLIN, Dave, M.D. Chief of Staff, Veterans Affairs Medical Center, Philadelphia, PA, p. A534
OSMUS, Richard D., Chief Executive Officer, Abbeville Area Medical Center, Abbeville, SC, p. A546
OSSE, John M., Interim Chief Executive Officer, Winner Regional Healthcare Center, Winner, SD, p. A561
OSSELLO, Susan, Chief Financial Officer, Granite County Medical Center, Philipsburg, MT, p. A378
OSTASZEWSKI, Patricia, MS, Chief Executive Officer, HEALTHSOUTH Rehabilitation Hospital of Toms River, Toms River, NJ, p. A411
OSTBERG, Melissa, Chief Financial Officer, Marias Medical Center, Shelby, MT, p. A379
OSTBLOOM, Jan, Human Resources Consultant, Our Lady of Peace, Louisville, KY, p. A255
OSTEEN, Tom J., Director Area Technology, Manteca Medical Center, Manteca, CA, p. A74
OSTER, Rebecca, Director Human Resources, HealthSource Saginaw, Saginaw, MI, p. A322
OSTERBERG, Valerie, Chief Financial Officer, Sanford Vermillion Medical Center, Vermillion, SD, p. A560
OSTERHOLM, Tim, Administrator and Chief Executive Officer, St. Vincent Medical Center–North, Sherwood, AR, p. A51
OSTERHOUT, David, Assistant Superintendent and Chief Financial Officer, El Paso Psychiatric Center, El Paso, TX, p. A596
OSTERLAND, Linda, Director Information Services, St. John River District Hospital, East China, MI, p. A311
OSTERLY, Eric, Chief Financial Officer, Florida Hospital Fish Memorial, Orange City, FL, p. A134
OSTRANDER, Maria DC, R.N. Chief Nurse Executive, San Antonio State Hospital, San Antonio, TX, p. A626
OSTRANDER, Mark, Vice President Financial Services, Community Medical Center, Toms River, NJ, p. A411
OSTRANDER, Thomas, Vice President Human Resources, Sparrow Hospital, Lansing, MI, p. A317
OSTROWSKI, Lawrence, M.D. Chief Clinical Officer, Summit Behavioral Healthcare, Cincinnati, OH, p. A474
OSTROWSKY, Barry, President and Chief Executive Officer, Barnabas Health, West Orange, NJ, p. B19
OSWALD, Kathy, Senior Vice President and Chief Human Resources Officer, Henry Ford Hospital, Detroit, MI, p. A310
OSWALD, Michelle, Director of Information Systems, Community Hospital–Fairfax, Fairfax, MO, p. A359
OSWALD, Traci L., Vice President Human Resources, Galion Community Hospital, Galion, OH, p. A480
OSWALD, Wesley W., Interim Chief Executive Officer, Memorial Hospital, Fremont, OH, p. A480
OSWALT, Charles, Vice President and Chief Financial Officer, Levi Hospital, Hot Springs National Park, AR, p. A46
OTERO, Victoria, Director Human Resources, HEALTHSOUTH Rehabilitation Hospital, Albuquerque, NM, p. A414
OTHMAN, Sami, Regional Site Director Information Process Services, Mercy Allen Hospital, Oberlin, OH, p. A486
OTHOLE, Jean, Chief Executive Officer, U. S. Public Health Service Indian Hospital, Zuni, NM, p. A419
OTIS, Deb, Director Information Systems, Spring Hill Regional Hospital, Spring Hill, FL, p. A139
OTT, Christopher, M.D. Interim Chief Medical Officer, St. Anthony Hospital, Lakewood, CO, p. A103
OTT, Darin, D.O. Chief of Staff, Kane County Hospital, Kanab, UT, p. A638
OTT, Kathryn Lynne, MSN Vice President Patient Care Services/Chief Nursing Officer, Fitzgibbon Hospital, Marshall, MO, p. A364
OTT, Ronald H.
  President, Excela Frick Hospital, Mount Pleasant, PA, p. A530
  President, Excela Health Westmoreland Hospital, Greensburg, PA, p. A524

OTT, Ryan, Chief Executive Officer, Integra Specialty Hospital, Muncie, IN, p. A209
OTTATI, David, President and Chief Executive Officer, Florida Hospital–Flagler, Palm Coast, FL, p. A135
OTTE, Elaine, Chief Operating Officer, Clarinda Regional Health Center, Clarinda, IA, p. A216
OTTMAR, Kellie, Manager Information Services, East Adams Rural Hospital, Ritzville, WA, p. A665
OTTO, Sara, Director Human Resources, North Canyon Medical Center, Gooding, ID, p. A168
OTTO, Steve
  Chief Executive Officer, Skyline Madison Campus, Madison, TN, p. A570
  Chief Executive Officer, Skyline Medical Center, Nashville, TN, p. A573
OTTONE, Robert, Administrator, Maniilaq Health Center, Kotzebue, AK, p. A29
OTWELL, Robert, Chief Executive Officer, Maury Regional Hospital, Columbia, TN, p. A564
OUBRE, Chris, Director Information Systems, Singing River Health System, Pascagoula, MS, p. A351
OUBRE Jr., Nathaniel L., Senior Vice President and Area Manager, Oakland Medical Center, Oakland, CA, p. A77
OUELETTE, Lisa, Director Human Resources, Beaumont Hospital – Troy, Troy, MI, p. A324
OUELLETTE, Demetra, Chief Operating Officer, Rehabilitation Hospital of Rhode Island, North Smithfield, RI, p. A544
OUSEY, Tracy, Director Human Resources, Washington County Hospital and Clinics, Washington, IA, p. A227
OVANDO, Benjamin, Chief Operations Officer, Rancho Los Amigos National Rehabilitation Center, Downey, CA, p. A59
OVERBEY, Bill
  Chief Financial Officer and Chief Information Officer, Hays Medical Center, Hays, KS, p. A234
  Chief Financial Officer, Pawnee Valley Community Hospital, Larned, KS, p. A237
OVERBY, Roger, Executive Director Information Systems, Greene County Medical Center, Jefferson, IA, p. A222
OVEREEM, Mark, Chief Financial Officer, Centinela Hospital Medical Center, Inglewood, CA, p. A65
OVERMAN, David S.
  Chief Operating Officer, Children's Hospitals and Clinics of Minnesota, Minneapolis, MN, p. A335
  Chief Operating Officer, Children's Hospitals and Clinics of Minnesota, Saint Paul, MN, p. A339
OVERSTREET, Alyson, Chief Financial Officer, Washington County Hospital and Nursing Home, Chatom, AL, p. A18
OVERSTREET, Amy, Director Human Resources, Trousdale Medical Center, Hartsville, TN, p. A566
OVERSTREET, Kristie, Administrator, Greenbrier Hospital, Covington, LA, p. A265
OWCZARZAK, Margaret, Facility Chief Information Officer, Veterans Affairs Western New York Healthcare System–Buffalo Division, Buffalo, NY, p. A423
OWEN, Laura, Senior Vice President and Chief Executive Officer, Mother Frances Hospital – Tyler, Tyler, TX, p. A632
OWEN, Ronald S., FACHE Chief Executive Officer, Southeast Alabama Medical Center, Dothan, AL, p. A19
OWEN, Sabrina, Human Resources Officer, Veterans Affairs Central Iowa Health Care System, Des Moines, IA, p. A218
OWEN, Sandra, Director Fiscal and Accounting, Harper Hospital District Five, Harper, KS, p. A234
OWEN–PLIETZ, Carrie, Chief Executive Officer, Sutter Medical Center, Sacramento, Sacramento, CA, p. A84
OWENS, Betina, Chief Information Officer, LSU Bogalusa Medical Center, Bogalusa, LA, p. A263
OWENS, Beverly, Controller, Central Georgia Rehabilitation Hospital, Macon, GA, p. A155
OWENS, Brian, Chief Operating Officer, Lindner Center of HOPE, Mason, OH, p. A484
OWENS, Craig A., Senior Vice President and Administrator, WellStar Douglas Hospital, Douglasville, GA, p. A151
OWENS, Diane, Administrator, St. David's Rehabilitation Center, Austin, TX, p. A581
OWENS, Jonathan, Chief Executive Officer, Rush County Memorial Hospital, La Crosse, KS, p. A237
OWENS, Leon, Director, Caswell Center, Kinston, NC, p. A456
OWENS, Loma, Data Manager, Southwestern State Hospital, Thomasville, GA, p. A160
OWENS, Mark, M.D. Vice President Medical Affairs, Mercy San Juan Medical Center, Carmichael, CA, p. A56
OWENS, Pamela, Director Health Information Management, Hanover Hospital, Hanover, PA, p. A524
OWENS, Richard, Chief Financial Officer, D. W. McMillan Memorial Hospital, Brewton, AL, p. A17
OWENS, Shawn, Chief Operating Officer, Laurel Ridge Treatment Center, San Antonio, TX, p. A625
OWENS, Stephanie, Manager Human Resources, McDowell ARH Hospital, McDowell, KY, p. A256

# P

PANZA Jr., Louis J., President and Chief Executive Officer, Monongahela Valley Hospital, Monongahela, PA, p. A529

PANZARINO, Peter J., M.D. Chief Medical Officer, Catskill Regional Medical Center, Harris, NY, p. A427

PANZETTA, Frank, Director Human Resources, St. Joseph's Hospital Health Center, Syracuse, NY, p. A444

PAOLUCCI, Benjamin, D.O. Chief of Staff, Southeast Michigan Surgical Hospital, Warren, MI, p. A325

PAPA, Alan, President, Akron General Medical Center, Akron, OH, p. A469

PAPACOSTAS, Arthur C., M.D
Vice President and Chief Information Officer, Jeanes Hospital, Philadelphia, PA, p. A532
Vice President and Chief Information Officer, Temple University Hospital, Philadelphia, PA, p. A534

PAPADAKOS, James, Chief Financial Officer, Signature Healthcare Brockton Hospital, Brockton, MA, p. A298

PAPALIA, Fern, Vice President, Patient Care Services, Community Medical Center, Toms River, NJ, p. A411

PAPALIA, John P., FACHE Chief Executive Officer, Warren General Hospital, Warren, PA, p. A540

PAPANIA, Barry A., Administrator, Nicholas County Hospital, Carlisle, KY, p. A248

PAPE, Becky A., R.N. Chief Executive Officer, Samaritan Lebanon Community Hospital, Lebanon, OR, p. A512

PAPE, Carolyn, Director Human Resources, Whidbey General Hospital, Coupeville, WA, p. A660

PAPPAN, Clayton, Director Human Resources and Marketing, South Central Kansas Medical Center, Arkansas City, KS, p. A230

PAPPAS, Charles, M.D. Chief Operating Officer, Bascom Palmer Eye Institute–Anne Bates Leach Eye Hospital, Miami, FL, p. A131

PAPPAS, Kirk, M.D. Physician–in–Chief, Santa Rosa Medical Center, Santa Rosa, CA, p. A90

PAPPAS, Nanette, Manager Business Office, Colorado Acute Long Term Hospital, Denver, CO, p. A99

PAPPAS, Nick, Chief Information Officer, Downey Regional Medical Center, Downey, CA, p. A59

PAPPAS, Sharon H., R.N. Chief Nursing Officer, Porter Adventist Hospital, Denver, CO, p. A100

PAPPAS, Sheryl L., Chief Financial Officer, Sanford Medical Center Webster, Webster, SD, p. A561

PAPPONE, Lisa, Chief Executive Officer, Arbour–Fuller Hospital, Attleboro, MA, p. A295

PARADIS, Brian, Chief Operating Officer, Florida Hospital, Orlando, FL, p. A134

PARADIS, James, Vice President Administration, Riddle Hospital, Media, PA, p. A529

PARADIS, Jeanne, Director Information Services, The Acadia Hospital, Bangor, ME, p. A281

PARASIDA, Tammy, Manager Business Office, Peterson Rehabilitation Hospital, Wheeling, WV, p. A676

PARAUDA, Martina A., Director, Veterans Administration New York Harbor Healthcare System,, NY, p. A437

PARAVISINI, Nilda, Director Human Resources, Hospital Manati Medical Center, Manati, PR, p. A701

PARCELLS, Patrick, Senior Vice President and Administrator, Riverside Regional Medical Center, Newport News, VA, p. A652

PARDE, Erin, Vice President, Finance and Operations, Liberty Hospital, Liberty, MO, p. A364

PARDUE, Cherie, Interim Chief Information Officer, Children's National Medical Center, Washington, DC, p. A116

PARDUE, Michelle, M.D. Chief Medical Staff, Springhill Medical Center, Springhill, LA, p. A278

PAREEK, Yogesh, M.D. Clinical Director, Brown County Community Treatment Center, Green Bay, WI, p. A682

PARENT, Paula A., R.N. Director Human Resources and Nursing Administration, Cary Medical Center, Caribou, ME, p. A282

PARENTEAU, Michael, Vice President and Chief Financial Officer, Providence St. Mary Medical Center, Walla Walla, WA, p. A669

PARIS, David, Chief Executive Officer, Perry County General Hospital, Richton, MS, p. A352

PARIS, Gregory A., FACHE Chief Executive Officer, Monroe County Hospital, Albia, IA, p. A214

PARIS, John, M.D. Chief Medical Officer, Riverview Hospital, Noblesville, IN, p. A210

PARIS, Richard, M.D. Chief Medical Officer, Somerset Medical Center, Somerville, NJ, p. A410

PARIS, Trevor, M.D. Medical Director, Brooks Rehabilitation Hospital, Jacksonville, FL, p. A126

PARISH, Karen, Director Information Systems, Orange Park Medical Center, Orange Park, FL, p. A134

PARISH, Thomas, Chief Financial Officer, Howard County Medical Center, Saint Paul, NE, p. A389

PARK, Bockhi, Chief Operating Officer, Sherman Oaks Hospital,, CA, p. A71

PARK, Denten, Chief Executive Officer, MountainView Regional Medical Center, Las Cruces, NM, p. A416

PARK, Eddie, Acting Director Human Resources, Metropolitan State Hospital, Norwalk, CA, p. A77

PARK, Gary L., President, University of North Carolina Hospitals, Chapel Hill, NC, p. A450

PARK, Ron, Chief Financial Officer, Somerset Hospital, Somerset, PA, p. A538

PARK, Theron, Chief Executive Officer, Providence Portland Medical Center, Portland, OR, p. A514

PARKER, Alyson, Director, Florida Hospital–Flagler, Palm Coast, FL, p. A135

PARKER, Audrey, Budget Analyst, U. S. Public Health Service Indian Hospital, Winnebago, NE, p. A390

PARKER, Christopher J., R.N. Chief Nursing Officer, Memorial Hospital at Easton Maryland, Easton, MD, p. A291

PARKER, Cythia, Fiscal Director, Washington County Regional Medical Center, Sandersville, GA, p. A158

PARKER, Janie, Chief Financial Officer, Hardin County General Hospital, Rosiclare, IL, p. A193

PARKER, Jim, M.D. President Medical Staff, Southeastern Regional Medical Center, Lumberton, NC, p. A457

PARKER, Judy Goforth, Ph.D. Administrator, Chickasaw Nation Medical Center, Ada, OK, p. A493

PARKER, Marty, Chief Information Officer, Carolinas Hospital System, Florence, SC, p. A549

PARKER, Michael, M.D. Chief of Staff, Sharon Hospital, Sharon, CT, p. A111

PARKER, Paula, Chief Financial Officer, Wyoming County Community Hospital, Warsaw, NY, p. A446

PARKER, Robert, Chief Executive Officer, Meadowview Regional Medical Center, Maysville, KY, p. A256

PARKER, Rodney, Senior Associate Executive Director, Coney Island Hospital,, NY, p. A432

PARKER, Scott, M.D. Medical Director, Baptist Easley Hospital, Easley, SC, p. A549

PARKER, Teresa, Vice President and Chief Nursing Officer, Baptist Medical Center South, Montgomery, AL, p. A23

PARKER, Thomas, Chief Executive Officer, Upper Valley Medical Center, Troy, OH, p. A490

PARKER, Tina, Director Human Resources, HEALTHSOUTH Rehabilitation Hospital Midland–Odessa, Midland, TX, p. A616

PARKER, Valerie, M.D. Clinical Director, U. S. Public Health Service Indian Hospital, Rosebud, SD, p. A559

PARKES, Brian, M.D. Chief Medical Officer, Scotland Health Care System, Laurinburg, NC, p. A456

PARKEY, Kasey, Coordinator Payroll and Benefits, Kindred Hospital–Corpus Christi, Corpus Christi, TX, p. A589

PARKHILL, Cherie, Chief Financial Officer, Crosbyton Clinic Hospital, Crosbyton, TX, p. A590

PARKHURST, James E., President and Chief Executive Officer, Newport Bay Hospital, Newport Beach, CA, p. A77

PARKINSON, Michelle A., Director Human Resources, Prairie St. John's, Fargo, ND, p. A465

PARKS, Audrey, Senior Administrative Director Information Technology, Salinas Valley Memorial Healthcare System, Salinas, CA, p. A84

PARKS, Cary, Chief Information Resource Management, Veterans Affairs Medical Center, Hampton, VA, p. A649

PARKS, Dave, Chief Information Officer, Three Rivers Health, Three Rivers, MI, p. A324

PARKS, Ginger, Director Human Resources, Cape Fear Valley – Bladen County Hospital, Elizabethtown, NC, p. A453

PARKS, Jim, Chief Operating Officer, Box Butte General Hospital, Alliance, NE, p. A381

PARKS, Michelle, Administrator, RiverValley Behavioral Health Hospital, Owensboro, KY, p. A257

PARKS, Richard H., FACHE President and Chief Executive Officer, Covenant Health System, Lubbock, TX, p. B39

PARKS, Richard H., FACHE President and Chief Executive Officer, Covenant Medical Center, Lubbock, TX, p. A613

PARKS, Sherry, R.N. Chief Nursing Officer, Saint Alphonsus Regional Medical Center, Boise, ID, p. A166

PARKS, Shirley, Manager Human Resources, Weston County Health Services, Newcastle, WY, p. A697

PARKS, Vicki, Vice President, Murray–Calloway County Hospital, Murray, KY, p. A257

PARMER, David N., President and Chief Executive Officer, Baptist Hospitals of Southeast Texas, Beaumont, TX, p. A582

PARMER, Dennis, M.D. Chief Medical Staff, Community Hospital of Long Beach, Long Beach, CA, p. A68

PARNEL, George, Chief Financial Officer, Clifton T. Perkins Hospital Center, Jessup, MD, p. A292

PARNELL, Dennis, Senior Vice President Human Resources, Suburban Hospital, Bethesda, MD, p. A290

PAROBEK, James, President, Sts. Mary & Elizabeth Hospital, Louisville, KY, p. A255

PAROBY, Carmen, Chief Executive Officer, West Florida Community Care Center, Milton, FL, p. A132

PAROD, Daniel A., Senior Vice President Hospital and Administrative Affairs, Rockford Memorial Hospital, Rockford, IL, p. A193

PAROSKI, Margaret, M.D. Executive Vice President and Chief Medical Officer, KALEIDA Health, Buffalo, NY, p. A422

PARR, Lynnette, Chief Financial Officer, Down East Community Hospital, Machias, ME, p. A284

PARRA, Michelle, Director Human Resources, Kindred Hospital of South Bay, Gardena, CA, p. A63

PARRILLA, Ramon, M.D. Chief Medical Officer, First Hospital Panamericano, Cidra, PR, p. A700

PARRINELLO, Kathleen M., Ph.D. Chief Operating Officer, Strong Memorial Hospital of the University of Rochester, Rochester, NY, p. A442

PARRINO, Thomas, M.D. Chief of Staff, Veterans Affairs Medical Center, White River Junction, VT, p. A644

PARRIS, Jill, Network Vice President Human Resources, Community Hospital North, Indianapolis, IN, p. A204

PARRIS, Pat, Chief Financial Officer, University Hospital McDuffie, Thomson, GA, p. A160

PARRIS, Timothy, President and Chief Executive Officer, Cirrus Health, Dallas, TX, p. B32

PARRISH, Becky, Director Human Resources, Southern Virginia Regional Medical Center, Emporia, VA, p. A647

PARRISH, E. Al, Director Human Resources, Southampton Memorial Hospital, Franklin, VA, p. A648

PARRISH, James G., FACHE Chief Executive Officer, Humboldt General Hospital, Winnemucca, NV, p. A396

PARRISH, Jerry A., Vice President, AnMed Health Medical Center, Anderson, SC, p. A546

PARRISH, Pamela, Director Information Systems, Brunswick Novant Medical Center, Bolivia, NC, p. A449

PARRISH, Priscilla, Chief Financial Officer, Blake Medical Center, Bradenton, FL, p. A119

PARRISH, Suann, Chief Financial Officer, Yoakum County Hospital, Denver City, TX, p. A594

PARROTT, Keith, FACHE President, Princeton Baptist Medical Center, Birmingham, AL, p. A16

PARRY, Timothy, R.N. Vice President Nursing, Highland District Hospital, Hillsboro, OH, p. A482

PARSEGHIAN, Donald, Chief Financial Officer, Meadowlands Hospital Medical Center, Secaucus, NJ, p. A410

PARSON, Taft, M.D. Medical Director, Henry Ford Kingswood Hospital, Ferndale, MI, p. A312

PARSONS, Brad, Administrator and Chief Executive Officer, NEA Baptist Memorial Hospital, Jonesboro, AR, p. A47

PARSONS, Elizabeth, Human Resources Business Partner, Baptist Easley Hospital, Easley, SC, p. A549

PARSONS, Jamie, Vice President Human Resources, Johnson City Medical Center, Johnson City, TN, p. A567

PARSONS, Jeff Jeffery, Administrator, Westbury Community Hospital, Houston, TX, p. A608

PARSONS, Lauren, M.D. Clinical Director, North Texas State Hospital, Wichita Falls Campus, Wichita Falls, TX, p. A635

PARSONS, Roger, Senior Vice President Finance, San Antonio Community Hospital, Upland, CA, p. A94

PARSONS, Suzanne, Vice President Human Resources, UMass Memorial–Marlborough Hospital, Marlborough, MA, p. A302

PARSONS, Terri L., Administrator, Advanced Care Hospital of White County, Searcy, AR, p. A51

PARSONS, Vicki L.
Regional Vice President Human Resources, Covenant Medical Center, Waterloo, IA, p. A228
Regional Vice President Human Resources, Mercy Hospital of Franciscan Sisters, Oelwein, IA, p. A224
Regional Vice President Human Resources, Sartori Memorial Hospital, Cedar Falls, IA, p. A215

PARTAMIAN, Gregory A., Chief Operating Officer, Crittenton Hospital Medical Center, Rochester, MI, p. A321

PARTEE, Paris I., Associate Administrator and Director Human Resources, John H. Stroger Jr. Hospital of Cook County, Chicago, IL, p. A176

PARTENZA, John, Vice President and Treasurer, Northern Westchester Hospital, Mount Kisco, NY, p. A430

PARTHEMORE, Warrenette, Director Human Resources, Memorial Hospital, Fremont, OH, p. A480

PARTIN, Gary, M.D. President Medical Staff, Westlake Regional Hospital, Columbia, KY, p. A248

PARUCH, Randy J., Director, Information Systems, Holland Hospital, Holland, MI, p. A315

PARUNGAO, AMy, Director of Nursing, Rehabilitation Hospital of the Pacific, Honolulu, HI, p. A164

PARVEZ, Syed, M.D. Administrator, Community General Hospital, Dilley, TX, p. A594

PASANEN, Wayne, M.D. Vice President Medical Affairs, Lowell General Hospital, Lowell, MA, p. A301

PASCASIO, Robert A., FACHE Chief Executive Officer, Hancock Medical Center, Bay Saint Louis, MS, p. A343

PASCOE, John, M.D. Executive Medical Director, Timberlawn Mental Health System, Dallas, TX, p. A593

Index of Health Care Professionals

Index of Health Care Professionals / Pawlowski

PAWLOWSKI, Phil
Vice President Finance and Chief Financial Officer, Ashtabula County Medical Center, Ashtabula, OH, p. A469
Chief Financial Officer, Glenbeigh Hospital and Outpatient Centers, Rock Creek, OH, p. A487
PAWOLA, Ken
Chief Operating Officer, R M L Specialty Hospital, Hinsdale, IL, p. A184
Chief Operating Officer, RML Specialty Hospital, Chicago, IL, p. A177
PAXSON, Gary, Chief Information Officer, White River Medical Center, Batesville, AR, p. A42
PAYAWAL, Roy, Executive Vice President Finance, Sacred Heart Hospital, Chicago, IL, p. A178
PAYLOR, Tarry, Director Human Resources, Children's Hospital of Michigan, Detroit, MI, p. A310
PAYNE, Cary J., Interim Chief Executive Officer, Lawrence Medical Center, Moulton, AL, p. A24
PAYNE, Gary, President and Chief Executive Officer, Cardinal Hill Healthcare System, Lexington, KY, p. B25
PAYNE, Gary, Chief Executive Officer, Cardinal Hill Rehabilitation Hospital, Lexington, KY, p. A252
PAYNE, James, Director Information Systems, Southern Tennessee Medical Center, Winchester, TN, p. A576
PAYNE, Janet S.
Vice President Human Resources, Provena Covenant Medical Center, Urbana, IL, p. A195
Vice President Human Resources, Provena United Samaritans Medical Center, Danville, IL, p. A179
PAYNE, Jason, Administrator, John C. Stennis Memorial Hospital, De Kalb, MS, p. A345
PAYNE, Jeffery L., Vice President Human Resources, Lakeland Regional Medical Center, Lakeland, FL, p. A128
PAYNE, Judy, R.N. Chief Operating Officer, Turning Point Hospital, Moultrie, GA, p. A157
PAYNE, Kenneth G., Chief Financial Officer, Holzer Medical Center, Gallipolis, OH, p. A480
PAYNE, Michael, M.D. Chief of Staff, Dallas County Medical Center, Fordyce, AR, p. A45
PAYNE, Michael E., Administrator, Girard Medical Center, Girard, KS, p. A233
PAYNE, Rick, Director Information Systems, Santa Rosa Medical Center, Milton, FL, p. A132
PAYNE, Steven, Chief Financial Officer, Salt Lake Regional Medical Center, Salt Lake City, UT, p. A641
PAYTON, Becky J., Vice President Human Resources, Mercy Hospital Oklahoma City, Oklahoma City, OK, p. A501
PAYTON, J. Ronald, Director Human Resources, Gateway Regional Medical Center, Granite City, IL, p. A183
PAZ, Harold L., M.D. Chief Executive Officer, Penn State Milton S. Hershey Medical Center, Hershey, PA, p. A525
PAZDERNIK, Mary, Chief Financial Officer, Mahnomen Health Center, Mahnomen, MN, p. A334
PEA, Gary, Chief Financial Officer, Glenn Medical Center, Willows, CA, p. A96
PEA, Richard, Director Human Resources, Memorial Hospital and Health Care Center, Jasper, IN, p. A205
PEABODY, Joyce L., M.D. Vice President and Chief Medical Officer, Saratoga Hospital, Saratoga Springs, NY, p. A443
PEABODY, Kim, Chief Operating Officer, The Brook Hospital – KMI, Louisville, KY, p. A255
PEABODY, Paul, Chief Information Officer, Palomar Medical Center, Escondido, CA, p. A60
PEACE, James, M.D. Chief of Staff, Olympia Medical Center, Los Angeles, CA, p. A71
PEACE III, Lother E., President and Chief Executive Officer, Russell Medical Center, Alexander City, AL, p. A15
PEACH, Larry, Assistant Administrator and Chief Financial Officer, Mendota Community Hospital, Mendota, IL, p. A188
PEACOCK, Gary G., Senior Vice President and Chief Financial Officer, Decatur Memorial Hospital, Decatur, IL, p. A179
PEACOCK, Steve, Assistant Vice President, Plaza Specialty Hospital, Houston, TX, p. A606
PEAK, Daniel, M.D. Chief Medical Staff, Southampton Memorial Hospital, Franklin, VA, p. A648
PEAL, Chip, Chief Executive Officer, Frankfort Regional Medical Center, Frankfort, KY, p. A250
PEARCE, Charles T.
Chief Financial and Information Officer, Kalispell Regional Medical Center, Kalispell, MT, p. A377
CFIO, The HealthCenter, Kalispell, MT, p. A377
PEARCE, Edward, M.D. Chief of Staff, Caldwell Memorial Hospital, Lenoir, NC, p. A456
PEARCE, Kelly, Vice President of Operations, SSM St. Clare Health Center, Fenton, MO, p. A359
PEARCH, William, Chief Information Officer, Yukon–Kuskokwim Delta Regional Hospital, Bethel, AK, p. A28
PEARCY, Joetta J., Human Resources Director, Glendive Medical Center, Glendive, MT, p. A375
PEARLMAN, Helen, Nurse Executive, Minneapolis Veterans Affairs Health Care System, Minneapolis, MN, p. A335
PEARSALL, Craig K., Director Human Resources, Lourdes Counseling Center, Richland, WA, p. A665
PEARSALL, Cynthia, Chief Nursing Officer, Fairfield Medical Center, Lancaster, OH, p. A482
PEARSALL, Tracy, Director Human Resources, Arkansas State Hospital, Little Rock, AR, p. A47
PEARSON, Bruce, FACH
Executive Vice President and Chief Executive Officer, John C. Lincoln Deer Valley Hospital, Phoenix, AZ, p. A35
Executive Vice President and Chief Executive Officer, John C. Lincoln North Mountain Hospital, Phoenix, AZ, p. A35
PEARSON, David, Chief Information Officer, St. Luke's Hospital, Columbus, NC, p. A451
PEARSON, Dawn, Director Human Resources, HEALTHSOUTH Rehabilitation Hospital of Vineland, Vineland, NJ, p. A411
PEARSON, George, Director Human Resources Management Service, Veterans Affairs Medical Center, Coatesville, PA, p. A521
PEARSON, Gregory, Associate Executive Director Finance, Riverview Regional Medical Center, Gadsden, AL, p. A20
PEARSON, Kellie, Director Human Resources, Lower Bucks Hospital, Bristol, PA, p. A519
PEARSON, Linnie, Coordinator Human Resources and Benefits, Montfort Jones Memorial Hospital, Kosciusko, MS, p. A348
PEARSON, Madelyn, R.N. Sr. Vice President Patient Care Services, Englewood Hospital and Medical Center, Englewood, NJ, p. A404
PEARSON, Marshall, Director Management Information Systems, St. David's North Austin Medical Center, Austin, TX, p. A581
PEARSON, Matthew Paul, Chief Executive Officer, Select Specialty Hospital–Western Missouri, Kansas City, MO, p. A362
PEARSON, Sandra, Manager Human Resources, St. Vincent Rehabilitation Hospital, Sherwood, AR, p. A51
PEART, Carol, Chief Financial Officer, Aurora Chicago Lakeshore Hospital, Chicago, IL, p. A175
PEASNALL, Arlene F., Senior Vice President Human Resources, Kaiser Permanente Medical Center, Honolulu, HI, p. A163
PEBURN, Eric, Chief Financial Officer, Halifax Health Medical Center of Daytona Beach, Daytona Beach, FL, p. A122
PECHACEK, Judith, R.N. Vice President Patient Care, Fairview Southdale Hospital, Edina, MN, p. A331
PECHOUS, Bryan, M.D. Vice President Medical Affairs, Finley Hospital, Dubuque, IA, p. A219
PECK, Bob, Interim Chief Executive Officer, Wesley Rehabilitation Hospital, Wichita, KS, p. A246
PECK, Darin, M.D. Chief of Staff, Charles A. Dean Memorial Hospital, Greenville, ME, p. A283
PECK, Gary V.
Interim Chief Executive Officer, East Adams Rural Hospital, Ritzville, WA, p. A665
Chief Operating Officer, Providence Mount Carmel Hospital, Colville, WA, p. A660
PECK, Kathey, Manager Health Information, Caribou Memorial Hospital and Living Center, Soda Springs, ID, p. A170
PECK, Kay E., Ph.D
Chief Executive Officer, Kindred Hospital–Amarillo, Amarillo, TX, p. A578
Chief Executive Officer, Kindred Rehabilitation Hospital, Amarillo, TX, p. A578
PECK, Lori, Vice President Finance, Memorial Health Center, Medford, WI, p. A685
PECK, Michael D., Assistant Administrator, Caribou Memorial Hospital and Living Center, Soda Springs, ID, p. A170
PECK, Thomas R., Chief Executive Officer, Franciscan St. Elizabeth Health – Crawfordsville, Crawfordsville, IN, p. A199
PEDERSEN, Alan, Vice President Human Resources, Cayuga Medical Center at Ithaca, Ithaca, NY, p. A428
PEDERSEN, Darren, Coordinator Information Technology, Weisman Children's Rehabilitation Hospital, Marlton, NJ, p. A406
PEDERSEN, Paul E., M.D. Vice President and Chief Medical Officer, OSF St. Joseph Medical Center, Bloomington, IL, p. A173
PEDERSON, Karn, Manager Health Information Management, McKenzie County Healthcare System, Watford City, ND, p. A468
PEDERSON, Randall K., Chief Executive Officer, Tioga Medical Center, Tioga, ND, p. A468
PEDLEY, Joe, CPA Vice President and Chief Financial Officer, Lawrence Memorial Hospital, Lawrence, KS, p. A237
PEDLOW, Bernadette R., Senior Vice President Business and Chief Operating Officer, Albany Medical Center, Albany, NY, p. A420
PEDROZA, Fernando
Director Information Systems, Medical Center of the Rockies, Loveland, CO, p. A104
Chief Information Officer, Poudre Valley Hospital, Fort Collins, CO, p. A101
PEEBLES, Robert J., President and Chief Executive Officer, Mercy Medical Center–Sioux City, Sioux City, IA, p. A226
PEED, Nancy, Administrator and Chief Executive Officer, Peach Regional Medical Center, Fort Valley, GA, p. A153
PEEK, Michael Scott, Chief Executive Officer, Chambers Memorial Hospital, Danville, AR, p. A43
PEELGREN, Jim, Chief Information Officer, Tulare Regional Medical Center, Tulare, CA, p. A93
PEER, Julie, Vice President Finance, Brookville Hospital, Brookville, PA, p. A519
PEERY, Lori, Chief Human Resource Management Services, Veterans Affairs Palo Alto Health Care System, Palo Alto, CA, p. A79
PEET, Carole, MSN, President and Chief Executive Officer, St. Anthony North Hospital, Westminster, CO, p. A106
PEET, Melodie J., Superintendent, Riverview Hospital for Children and Youth, Middletown, CT, p. A110
PEETERS, Marie, Director Human Resources, Mercy Iowa City, Iowa City, IA, p. A221
PEGE, Diane, M.D. Vice President Medical Affairs, Sutter Lakeside Hospital, Lakeport, CA, p. A66
PEHRSON, Timothy T., Chief Executive Officer, McKay–Dee Hospital Center, Ogden, UT, p. A639
PEIFFER, Paul V.
Executive Vice President and Chief Operating Officer, River Oaks Hospital, Flowood, MS, p. A345
Chief Operating Officer, Woman's Hospital, Flowood, MS, p. A346
PEKOFSKE, Robert, Vice President Finance, Advocate Christ Medical Center, Oak Lawn, IL, p. A189
PELACCIA, Joseph, President and Chief Executive Officer, Milford Hospital, Milford, CT, p. A110
PELLE, Fred L., FACH
Chief Executive Officer, Jackson Purchase Medical Center, Mayfield, KY, p. A256
President and Chief Executive Officer, Wellmont Hancock County Hospital, Sneedville, TN, p. A575
PELLECCHIA, Joseph, M.D. Chief of Staff, Veterans Affairs Medical Center–Lexington, Lexington, KY, p. A254
PELLEGRINO, Cynthia Miller, Chief Executive Officer, Western Maryland Hospital Center, Hagerstown, MD, p. A292
PELLETIER, Stephen, Leader Guest Services, York Hospital, York, ME, p. A286
PELLICONE, John T., M.D. Medical Director, Helen Hayes Hospital, West Haverstraw, NY, p. A446
PELSMAN, Mara, Chief Executive Officer, Gateways Hospital and Mental Health Center, Los Angeles, CA, p. A69
PELTIER, Robert, M.D. Senior Vice President and Chief Medical Officer, North Oaks Medical Center, Hammond, LA, p. A267
PELTOLA, Gene, President and Chief Executive Officer, Yukon–Kuskokwim Delta Regional Hospital, Bethel, AK, p. A28
PELTON, Deborah, R.N. Chief Nursing Officer, Texas Spine & Joint Hospital, Tyler, TX, p. A632
PELZ, Thomas, M.D. Chief of Staff, Boscobel Area Health Care, Boscobel, WI, p. A679
PEMBERTON, John S., Director Human Resources, Tuba City Regional Health Care Corporation, Tuba City, AZ, p. A39
PENA, Julie, Director Finance, Community Howard Specialty Hospital, Kokomo, IN, p. A206
PENCE, Julie, Associate Director Human Resources, Highland District Hospital, Hillsboro, OH, p. A482
PENDER, John, M.D. Medical Director, Texas Health Specialty Hospital, Fort Worth, TX, p. A599
PENDERGAST, Debra, Senior Vice President Patient Care Services and Chief Nursing Officer, John Muir Medical Center, Walnut Creek, Walnut Creek, CA, p. A95
PENDERGAST, Jim, Administrator Human Resources, University of New Mexico Hospitals, Albuquerque, NM, p. A415
PENDERGRAFT, Tina, Chief Nursing Officer, Satanta District Hospital, Satanta, KS, p. A243
PENDLETON, Debbie, Human Resources Specialist, Weslaco Rehabilitation Hospital, Weslaco, TX, p. A634
PENDLETON, Gretchen, Chief Human Resources Officer, Mercy Suburban Hospital, Norristown, PA, p. A530
PENDLETON, Kevin, Chief Information Technology, Lakeside Behavioral Health System, Memphis, TN, p. A571
PENDLETON, Timothy, M.D. President Medical Staff, Brookville Hospital, Brookville, PA, p. A519
PENICK, Lisa, R.N. Chief Nursing Officer, Carroll County Memorial Hospital, Carrollton, KY, p. A248
PENKA, Steven, President and Chief Executive Officer, Athol Memorial Hospital, Athol, MA, p. A295

A902 Index of Health Care Professionals 

Index of Health Care Professionals

Index of Health Care Professionals / Pert

PERT, Robert M., Vice President Finance and Chief Financial Officer, United Regional Health Care System, Wichita Falls, TX, p. A635
PERUSSE, Margo, Administrator and Chief Nursing Officer, La Palma Intercommunity Hospital, La Palma, CA, p. A66
PESKIN, Ted, M.D. Acute Care Medical Director, Hilo Medical Center, Hilo, HI, p. A163
PESSAGNO, Paul, Chief Financial Officer, Richard L. Roudebush Veterans Affairs Medical Center, Indianapolis, IN, p. A205
PETER, David, M.D
Senior Vice President Medical Affairs and Chief Medical Director, Akron General Medical Center, Akron, OH, p. A469
Senior Vice President Medical Affairs and Chief Medical Officer, Lodi Community Hospital, Lodi, OH, p. A483
PETER, Douglas G., M.D. Chief Medical Officer, Gallup Indian Medical Center, Gallup, NM, p. A416
PETER, Edith S., Chief Financial Officer and Vice President Finance, Cooley Dickinson Hospital, Northampton, MA, p. A303
PETER, Jan D., Vice President Fiscal Services and Chief Financial Officer, Good Shepherd Health Care System, Hermiston, OR, p. A511
PETERMAN, Tammy, R.N. Executive Vice President, Chief Operating Officer and Chief Nursing Officer, The University of Kansas Hospital, Kansas City, KS, p. A236
PETERMEIER, Jill, Senior Executive Human Resources, Marshalltown Medical & Surgical Center, Marshalltown, IA, p. A223
PETERS, Allen, President and Chief Executive Officer, Raleigh General Hospital, Beckley, WV, p. A670
PETERS, Bill, Acting Director of Psychiatry, Brainerd Regional Human Services Center, Brainerd, MN, p. A328
PETERS, Brian, Chief Information Officer, St. Vincent Indianapolis Hospital, Indianapolis, IN, p. A205
PETERS, Bruce, Vice President and Chief Operating Officer, Bakersfield Memorial Hospital, Bakersfield, CA, p. A54
PETERS, Cindy, Chief Information Officer, Oak Hill Hospital, Brooksville, FL, p. A120
PETERS, Connie, R.N. Operations Leader and Regional Health Administrator, Alegent Health–Memorial Hospital, Schuyler, NE, p. A389
PETERS, Dave, Chief Human Resources Officer, Veterans Affairs Nebraska–Western Iowa Health Care System, Lincoln, NE, p. A386
PETERS, Gerald, Vice President Information Technologies and Chief Information Officer, Lake Health, Concord Township, OH, p. A477
PETERS, Jan, Vice President Human Resources, Saint Vincent Hospital, Worcester, MA, p. A306
PETERS, John, Chief Financial Officer, St. Joseph's Hospital and Medical Center, Phoenix, AZ, p. A36
PETERS, Ken
Director Human Resources Management, Bellin Memorial Hospital, Green Bay, WI, p. A682
Director Human Resources, Bellin Psychiatric Center, Green Bay, WI, p. A682
PETERS, Mark J., M.D. President and Chief Executive Officer, East Jefferson General Hospital, Metairie, LA, p. A273
PETERS, Patrick, Chief Executive Officer, Mt. Graham Regional Medical Center, Safford, AZ, p. A37
PETERS, Regina, Chief Executive Officer, Stroud Regional Medical Center, Stroud, OK, p. A505
PETERS, Stephen D., Administrator, Dubuis Hospital of Alexandria, Alexandria, LA, p. A261
PETERS, Sue, Vice President Human Resources, Munson Medical Center, Traverse City, MI, p. A324
PETERS, Violeta, R.N. Chief Executive Officer, Specialty Hospital at Monmouth, Long Branch, NJ, p. A405
PETERSEN, Brenda, Director Human Resources, Sanford Wheaton Medical Center, Wheaton, MN, p. A341
PETERSEN, Debbie, Chief Operating Officer and Chief Nursing Officer, Spalding Rehabilitation Hospital, Aurora, CO, p. A97
PETERSEN, Gary, Chief Operating Officer, Sunnyside Medical Center, Clackamas, OR, p. A509
PETERSEN, Julie, Chief Executive Officer, Prosser Memorial Hospital, Prosser, WA, p. A664
PETERSEN, Keith J., Chief Executive Officer, Phoebe Sumter Medical Center, Americus, GA, p. A144
PETERSEN, Richard W., President and Chief Executive Officer, Maine Medical Center, Portland, ME, p. A284
PETERSON, Anne, Vice President Human Resources and Support Services, Licking Memorial Hospital, Newark, OH, p. A486
PETERSON, Bill
Director Human Resources, John F. Kennedy Memorial Hospital, Indio, CA, p. A65
Chief Human Resources Director, Sierra Vista Regional Medical Center, San Luis Obispo, CA, p. A88
PETERSON, Bonnie, Chief Operating Officer and Vice President Clinical Services, Richard P. Stadter Psychiatric Center, Grand Forks, ND, p. A466
PETERSON, Brent A., Administrator, Cherry County Hospital, Valentine, NE, p. A390
PETERSON, Bruce, Chief Information Officer, Rome Memorial Hospital, Rome, NY, p. A442
PETERSON, Chad, Chief Information Officer, Sanford Northwood Deaconess Health Center, Northwood, ND, p. A467
PETERSON, Cheryl, Business Office Manager, Surgical Institute of Reading, Wyomissing, PA, p. A542
PETERSON, Cindy, Vice President and Chief Information Officer, Henry Mayo Newhall Memorial Hospital, Valencia, CA, p. A94
PETERSON, Dane C., Chief Operating Officer, Emory University Hospital Midtown, Atlanta, GA, p. A145
PETERSON, Daniel, Chief Human Resource Management Service, Central Arkansas Veterans Healthcare System, Little Rock, AR, p. A48
PETERSON, David
Manager Human Resources, Gunnison Valley Hospital, Gunnison, UT, p. A637
Regional Chief Information Officer, Memorial Health Care System, Chattanooga, TN, p. A563
Regional Chief Information Officer, St. Vincent Infirmary Medical Center, Little Rock, AR, p. A48
PETERSON, Dennis, Chief Information Officer, George E. Weems Memorial Hospital, Apalachicola, FL, p. A118
PETERSON, Douglas R., President and Chief Executive Officer, Chippewa Valley Hospital and Oakview Care Center, Durand, WI, p. A680
PETERSON, Dustin, Chief Financial Officer, Providence Medical Center, Wayne, NE, p. A390
PETERSON, Erica, Chief Financial Officer, Sanford Medical Center Chamberlain, Chamberlain, SD, p. A555
PETERSON, Gary, M.D. Vice President Medical Affairs and Medical Director, St. Luke's Hospital, Duluth, MN, p. A330
PETERSON, James, Senior Vice President Finance, Habersham Medical Center, Demorest, GA, p. A151
PETERSON, Jeff, M.D. Chief of Staff, Essentia Health Ada, Ada, MN, p. A327
PETERSON, Jeffrey, M.D. Medical Director, Cooperstown Medical Center, Cooperstown, ND, p. A465
PETERSON, John, Vice President Information Systems, Longmont United Hospital, Longmont, CO, p. A104
PETERSON, Josilyn, Chief Financial Officer, Ballinger Memorial Hospital, Ballinger, TX, p. A582
PETERSON, Julie, Chief Financial Officer, Sutter Delta Medical Center, Antioch, CA, p. A53
PETERSON, Kathy, Director Information Services, OSF Saint Anthony Medical Center, Rockford, IL, p. A192
PETERSON, Katie, R.N. Director of Nursing, Pender Community Hospital, Pender, NE, p. A389
PETERSON, Larry, Chief Financial Officer, Allen County Hospital, Iola, KS, p. A235
PETERSON, Margaret R., R.N. Chief Executive Officer, Desert Valley Hospital, Victorville, CA, p. A95
PETERSON, Mercy, Interim Chief Executive Officer, Nye Regional Medical Center, Tonopah, NV, p. A396
PETERSON, Michael, Vice President Ancillary and Support Services and Chief Information Officer, Sebasticook Valley Health, Pittsfield, ME, p. A284
PETERSON, Philip, Executive Vice President and Chief Financial Officer, Mercy Medical Center, Cedar Rapids, IA, p. A215
PETERSON, Randall, President and Chief Executive Officer, Stormont–Vail HealthCare, Topeka, KS, p. A244
PETERSON, Robert
Chief Financial Officer, Hackettstown Regional Medical Center, Hackettstown, NJ, p. A404
Chief Operating Officer, West Florida Hospital, Pensacola, FL, p. A136
PETERSON, Ron, FACHE President and Chief Executive Officer, Baxter Regional Medical Center, Mountain Home, AR, p. A49
PETERSON, Ron, Chief Information Officer, Pottstown Memorial Medical Center, Pottstown, PA, p. A536
PETERSON, Ronald R., President, Johns Hopkins Health System, Baltimore, MD, p. B74
PETERSON, Ronald R., President, Johns Hopkins Hospital, Baltimore, MD, p. A287
PETERSON, Scott, Vice President of People and Organizational Development, Peninsula Regional Health System, Salisbury, MD, p. A294
PETERSON, Seth, Director Information Services, Coshocton County Memorial Hospital, Coshocton, OH, p. A478
PETERSON, Shelley, Vice President Patient Services and Chief Nursing Officer, St. Mary's Hospital and Medical Center, Grand Junction, CO, p. A102
PETERSON, Stephen, Director Information Systems, Garrett County Memorial Hospital, Oakland, MD, p. A293
PETERSON, Steven G., Chief Executive Officer, Signature Hospital Corporation, Houston, TX, p. B118
PETERSON, Thomas, M.D. Chief Executive Officer, Richard P. Stadter Psychiatric Center, Grand Forks, ND, p. A466
PETERSON, Tim, M.D. Chief of Staff, Meeker Memorial Hospital, Litchfield, MN, p. A333
PETERSON, Tracie, R.N. Chief Nursing Officer, Great Lakes Specialty Hospital–Oak Campus, Grand Rapids, MI, p. A313
PETIK, Jason, Chief Executive Officer, Sidney Regional Medical Center, Sidney, NE, p. A389
PETRE, Patrick A., Chief Executive Officer, Arrowhead Regional Medical Center, Colton, CA, p. A58
PETRECCIA, David, M.D. Physician Advisor, Placentia–Linda Hospital, Placentia, CA, p. A80
PETRICK, Teresa G., President, UPMC St. Margaret, Pittsburgh, PA, p. A536
PETRIE, Lori, Chief Financial Officer, Mercy Regional Medical Center, Ville Platte, LA, p. A279
PETRILLO, Nancy, Director Human Resources, Matheny Medical and Educational Center, Peapack, NJ, p. A408
PETRINA, Robert
Chief Financial Officer, Alta Bates Summit Medical Center, Berkeley, CA, p. A55
Chief Financial Officer, Alta Bates Summit Medical Center – Summit Campus, Oakland, CA, p. A77
PETRINO, Robert, M.D. Chief of Staff, Northwest Medical Center, Springdale, AR, p. A51
PETRITZ, Jennifer J., Director Human Resources, University of Washington Medical Center, Seattle, WA, p. A666
PETRO, Lisa, Director Human Resources, Southwest Regional Medical Center, Waynesburg, PA, p. A540
PETROFF, Thomas, D.O. Vice President Medical Affairs, McLaren Greater Lansing, Lansing, MI, p. A317
PETROV, John R., Vice President Human Resources, Fairmont General Hospital, Fairmont, WV, p. A671
PETROVICH, Lawrence, M.D. Chief Medical Officer, York Hospital, York, ME, p. A286
PETRUCCI, Peter E., M.D. Vice President Patient Safety, Quality and Medical Affairs, Sibley Memorial Hospital, Washington, DC, p. A117
PETTEY, Robbie, Chief Financial Officer, National Park Medical Center, Hot Springs, AR, p. A46
PETTIJOHN, Trent, M.D. Chief Medical Officer, The Heart Hospital Baylor Plano, Plano, TX, p. A621
PETTINATO, Paul J., M.D. Chief Information Officer, Signature Healthcare Brockton Hospital, Brockton, MA, p. A298
PETTIT, Donny, Chief Financial Officer, Coon Memorial Hospital and Home, Dalhart, TX, p. A590
PETTIT, Harlan, M.D. Chief of Staff, Fishermen's Hospital, Marathon, FL, p. A129
PETTITE, Shirley F., Chief, Human Resources, Veterans Affairs Tennessee Valley Healthcare System, Nashville, TN, p. A574
PETTUS, Lisa, Manager Information Systems, Cherry Hospital, Goldsboro, NC, p. A453
PETTY, Jane, Director Human Resources, Hillside Hospital, Pulaski, TN, p. A574
PETTY, Kent
Chief Information Officer, Wellmont Hancock County Hospital, Sneedville, TN, p. A575
Chief Information Officer, Wellmont Holston Valley Medical Center, Kingsport, TN, p. A568
PETTY, Russ, M.D. Chief of Staff, Towner County Medical Center, Cando, ND, p. A464
PETTY, Vicki, Manager Human Resources, Wayne Medical Center, Waynesboro, TN, p. A576
PETZEL, Robert A., M.D. Under Secretary for Health, Department of Veterans Affairs, Washington, DC, p. B42
PEYERL, John, Chief Financial Officer, Redwood Area Hospital, Redwood Falls, MN, p. A337
PEYOK, David M., Chief Executive Officer, Cimarron Memorial Hospital, Boise City, OK, p. A494
PEZZIA, Marlene, Director, Tomball Regional Medical Center, Tomball, TX, p. A631
PFAFF, Joni, Chief Nursing Officer, Grisell Memorial Hospital District One, Ransom, KS, p. A242
PFAFF, Karen, Director Human Resources, Carroll County Memorial Hospital, Carrollton, MO, p. A357
PFAFF, Wanda, Vice President Human Resources, St. Alexius Medical Center, Bismarck, ND, p. A464
PFAU, Beth, M.D. Chief Medical Officer, Larue D. Carter Memorial Hospital, Indianapolis, IN, p. A204
PFEFFER, Wayne L., FACHE Director, Veterans Affairs Medical Center–Louisville, Louisville, KY, p. A255
PFEIFER, Mark P., M.D. Senior Vice President and Chief Medical Officer, University of Louisville Hospital, Louisville, KY, p. A255
PFEIFER, Michael, Chief Executive Officer, Presentation Medical Center, Rolla, ND, p. A468
PFEIFFER, James A., FACHE President and Chief Executive Officer, Self Regional Healthcare, Greenwood, SC, p. A551
PFEIFFER, Margaret, R.N. Vice President Patient Care Services, Good Samaritan Hospital, Los Angeles, CA, p. A69

Index of Health Care Professionals / Pinkosky

Index of Health Care Professionals

PFISTER, Joann M.
Director Human Resources, Providence Milwaukie Hospital, Milwaukie, OR, p. A513
Director Human Resources, Providence Willamette Falls Medical Center, Oregon City, OR, p. A513
PFISTER, Pam, Associate Administrator, Morrison Community Hospital, Morrison, IL, p. A188
PFISTER, Scott, Chief Financial Officer, Gateway Medical Center, Clarksville, TN, p. A564
PFITZER, Anthony D., FACHE Chief Executive Officer, Grimes St. Joseph Health Center, Navasota, TX, p. A618
PFRANK, Kym
Senior Vice President and Chief Information Officer, Union Hospital, Terre Haute, IN, p. A212
Vice President Information Systems, Union Hospital Clinton, Clinton, IN, p. A199
PHAIRE, Jean C., Executive Vice President Patient Care Services and Chief Nursing Executive, United Medical Center, Washington, DC, p. A117
PHAM, K., M.D. Chief of Staff, Winkler County Memorial Hospital, Kermit, TX, p. A610
PHARR, Ryan, M.D. Chief Medical Staff, Salem Memorial District Hospital, Salem, MO, p. A370
PHELAN, Cynthia, Vice President Human Resources, Lawrence General Hospital, Lawrence, MA, p. A301
PHELPS, Britton, Chief Executive Officer, Southern Virginia Regional Medical Center, Emporia, VA, p. A647
PHELPS, Craig, M.D. Chief of Staff, Great Plains Regional Medical Center, Elk City, OK, p. A496
PHELPS, David E., President and Chief Executive Officer, Berkshire Health Systems, Inc., Pittsfield, MA, p. B21
PHELPS, Joel, Chief Operating Officer, Salina Regional Health Center, Salina, KS, p. A242
PHELPS, Kathleen, Director Human Resources, Treasure Valley Hospital, Boise, ID, p. A167
PHELPS, M. Randell, Chief Executive Officer, Gunnison Valley Hospital, Gunnison, CO, p. A102
PHELPS, Mark H., M.D. Chief of Staff and Medical Director, Jerold Phelps Community Hospital, Garberville, CA, p. A62
PHILBRICK, Teri, Chief Executive Officer, Oklahoma Center for Orthopedic and Multi–Specialty Surgery, Oklahoma City, OK, p. A501
PHILIPP, Joseph, M.D. Chief Medical Officer, Mercy Regional Health Center,, KS, p. A238
PHILIPS III, Grady W., Chief Executive Officer, Memorial Hospital, Martinsville, VA, p. A651
PHILIPS, J. Michael, Chief Strategy Officer, San Juan Regional Medical Center, Farmington, NM, p. A416
PHILLIPE, James R., President, Holzer Medical Center, Gallipolis, OH, p. A480
PHILLIPPE II, James R., President, Holzer Medical Center – Jackson, Jackson, OH, p. A482
PHILLIPS, Alan, M.D. Interim Administrator, Hot Springs Rehabilitation Center, Hot Springs National Park, AR, p. A46
PHILLIPS, Alan M., Controller, HEALTHSOUTH Rehabilitation Hospital of Virginia, Richmond, VA, p. A655
PHILLIPS, Annette S., President and Chief Executive Officer, Mercy Memorial Hospital System, Monroe, MI, p. A319
PHILLIPS, Barry
Executive Director Human Resources, Camden General Hospital, Camden, TN, p. A562
Director Human Resources, Pathways of Tennessee, Jackson, TN, p. A567
PHILLIPS, Bill, Vice President Information Services, University Health System, San Antonio, TX, p. A626
PHILLIPS, Chance, Chief Financial Officer, Oak Hill Hospital, Brooksville, FL, p. A120
PHILLIPS, Charles, Chief Executive Officer, Jefferson Davis Community Hospital, Prentiss, MS, p. A352
PHILLIPS, Courtney, Chief Financial Officer, Delta Regional Medical Center, Greenville, MS, p. A346
PHILLIPS, David, Chief Operating Officer, Barnesville Hospital, Barnesville, OH, p. A470
PHILLIPS, David L.
Chief Executive Officer, St. John Broken Arrow, Broken Arrow, OK, p. A494
President and Chief Executive Officer, St. John Owasso, Owasso, OK, p. A503
PHILLIPS, Donna, President, Bryn Mawr Rehabilitation Hospital, Malvern, PA, p. A528
PHILLIPS, Donna Z., M.D. Chief Executive Officer, HEALTHSOUTH Rehabilitation Hospital of Fredericksburg, Fredericksburg, VA, p. A648
PHILLIPS, Glenn, Director Information Systems, Gadsden Regional Medical Center, Gadsden, AL, p. A20
PHILLIPS, Heath, Chief Executive Officer, HEALTHSOUTH Rehabilitation Hospital of Tallahassee, Tallahassee, FL, p. A140
PHILLIPS, J. Randall, FACHE Chief Executive Officer, North Alabama Regional Hospital, Decatur, AL, p. A18
PHILLIPS, John
Vice President Information Systems, Burleson St. Joseph Health Center, Caldwell, TX, p. A586
Vice President Information System, Grimes St. Joseph Health Center, Navasota, TX, p. A618
Vice President Information Services, St. Joseph Regional Health Center, Bryan, TX, p. A586
PHILLIPS, John E., FACHE President and Chief Executive Officer, Methodist Mansfield Medical Center, Mansfield, TX, p. A615
PHILLIPS, Joseph, Director Information Systems, Aurelia Osborn Fox Memorial Hospital, Oneonta, NY, p. A439
PHILLIPS, Kimberly A., Chief Financial Officer, The Children's Home of Pittsburgh, Pittsburgh, PA, p. A535
PHILLIPS, Lionel J., Vice President Financial Services, Fauquier Hospital, Warrenton, VA, p. A657
PHILLIPS, Lori, Vice President and Chief Nursing Officer, Gibson General Hospital, Princeton, IN, p. A210
PHILLIPS, Margaret, Director Human Resources, Memorial Hospital, North Conway, NH, p. A399
PHILLIPS, Michael, Chief Executive Officer, Elkhorn Valley Rehabilitation Hospital, Casper, WY, p. A695
PHILLIPS, Michael T., FACHE Chief Executive Officer, Vibra Hospital of San Diego, San Diego, CA, p. A86
PHILLIPS, Pam, Chief Human Resource Officer, Wiregrass Medical Center, Geneva, AL, p. A21
PHILLIPS, Richard, Chief Financial Officer, Desert Regional Medical Center, Palm Springs, CA, p. A78
PHILLIPS, Robert, Administrator, Walker Baptist Medical Center, Jasper, AL, p. A22
PHILLIPS, Steve, Information Officer, Greene County General Hospital, Linton, IN, p. A207
PHILLIPS, Tammy, Director Information Services, Medical Center of Arlington, Arlington, TX, p. A579
PHILLIPS, Terry, Director Information Technology, Maury Regional Hospital, Columbia, TN, p. A564
PHILLIPS, Todd, M.D. Interim Vice President, Medical Affairs, Kimball Medical Center, Lakewood, NJ, p. A405
PHIPPS, Bonnie, President and Chief Executive Officer, Saint Agnes Hospital, Baltimore, MD, p. A288
PHIPPS, Jackie G., Director Human Resources, Johnston Memorial Hospital, Abingdon, VA, p. A645
PHIPPS–ADAMS, Holly, Vice President Human Resources, Medstar Union Memorial Hospital, Baltimore, MD, p. A288
PIARULLI, Sue, Administrative Director Operations, Paradise Valley Hospital, Phoenix, AZ, p. A36
PIATKOWSKI, John S., M.D
President and Chief Executive Officer, Carilion New River Valley Medical Center, Christiansburg, VA, p. A646
Chief Executive Officer, Carilion Tazewell Community Hospital, Tazewell, VA, p. A656
PIATKOWSKI, Shannon
Director Information Technology, Blake Medical Center, Bradenton, FL, p. A119
Chief Information Officer, Brandon Regional Hospital, Brandon, FL, p. A119
PIAZZA, Tony, Director Human Resources, Titus Regional Medical Center, Mount Pleasant, TX, p. A617
PICCIONE, Jennifer, Chief Nursing and Clinical Services Officer, Madison County Hospital, London, OH, p. A483
PICCONE, Robert, President, Clear Brook Manor, Wilkes–Barre, PA, p. A541
PICKEL, Joseph, Director Resource Management, Walter Reed National Military Medical Center, Bethesda, MD, p. A290
PICKENS, Troy, Chief Financial Officer, Barnwell County Hospital, Barnwell, SC, p. A546
PICKETT, Beverly, R.N. Chief Nursing Officer, Oklahoma Surgical Hospital, Tulsa, OK, p. A506
PICKETT, Lisa C., M.D. Chief Medical Officer, Durham Regional Hospital, Durham, NC, p. A452
PICKOFF, Robert M., M.D. Vice President Medical Affairs, Glens Falls Hospital, Glens Falls, NY, p. A426
PICOU, Timothy, Manager Information Technology, Lower Umpqua Hospital District, Reedsport, OR, p. A515
PIEKARCZYK, Wally, Chief Financial Officer, Iberia Medical Center, New Iberia, LA, p. A274
PIEMONT, Joseph G., Executive Vice President and Chief Operating Officer, Carolinas Medical Center–Mercy, Charlotte, NC, p. A450
PIEPER, Blaine, Chief Executive Officer, Ohio County Hospital, Hartford, KY, p. A251
PIERCE, Eddie, M.D. Chief Medical Staff, Kearney County Health Services, Minden, NE, p. A386
PIERCE, Eva, Chief Information Officer, Corcoran District Hospital, Corcoran, CA, p. A58
PIERCE, Jennifer, Administrative Director of Finance, St. Anthony Shawnee Hospital, Shawnee, OK, p. A504
PIERCE, Kenneth, Chief Financial Officer, Brookhaven Hospital, Tulsa, OK, p. A505
PIERCE, Laura, Chief Administrative Officer Human Resources, Memorial Medical Center, Las Cruces, NM, p. A416
PIERCE, Margaret H., Executive Director, Baldwin Park Medical Center, Baldwin Park, CA, p. A55
PIERCE, Michael L., Chief Executive Officer, HEALTHSOUTH Rehabilitation Hospital of Memphis, Memphis, TN, p. A571
PIERCE, Pat, Director Information Systems, Lakewood Regional Medical Center, Lakewood, CA, p. A67
PIERCE, Trent, R.N. Chief Executive Officer, HEALTHSOUTH Rehabilitation Hospital, Fort Worth, TX, p. A598
PIERDON, Steven, M.D. Executive Vice President and Chief Medical Officer, Geisinger Wyoming Valley Medical Center, Wilkes Barre, PA, p. A541
PIERESCHI, Giovanni, Vice President Management Information Systems, Hospital HMA de Humacao, Humacao, PR, p. A701
PIERRE, Letonia, Coordinator Human Resources, Assumption Community Hospital, Napoleonville, LA, p. A274
PIERSON, Kari, Manager, Howard County Medical Center, Saint Paul, NE, p. A389
PIERSON, Marc, M.D. Vice President Clinical Information and Quality, PeaceHealth St. Joseph Medical Center, Bellingham, WA, p. A659
PIERSON, Richard, Executive Director, UAMS Medical Center, Little Rock, AR, p. A48
PIETRANGELO, Steve, Director Information Services, War Memorial Hospital, Sault Sainte Marie, MI, p. A323
PIETRO, Daniel, M.D. Medical Director, Sturdy Memorial Hospital, Attleboro, MA, p. A295
PIETSCH, Al, CPA Senior Vice President and Chief Financial Officer, Baltimore Washington Medical Center, Glen Burnie, MD, p. A292
PIFER, Eric, M.D. Chief Medical Officer, El Camino Hospital, Mountain View, CA, p. A76
PIFKO, Duane, Interim Director Financial Services, Drake Center, Cincinnati, OH, p. A473
PIGG, Charles, Chief Information Officer, St. Bernards Medical Center, Jonesboro, AR, p. A47
PIGG, Russell, Chief Executive Officer, Eliza Coffee Memorial Hospital, Florence, AL, p. A20
PIGOTT, John, M.D. Chief Medical Officer, Tulane Medical Center, New Orleans, LA, p. A275
PIGOTT, Randall, Chief Financial Officer, Marion General Hospital, Columbia, MS, p. A345
PIKE, David, Interim Chief Financial Officer, Fleming County Hospital, Flemingsburg, KY, p. A249
PIKE, David R., Chief Financial Officer, Lower Oconee Community Hospital, Glenwood, GA, p. A153
PIKE, Irving, M.D. Chief Medical Officer, John Muir Medical Center, Walnut Creek, Walnut Creek, CA, p. A95
PIKE, Pauline, Chief Operating Officer, Beverly Hospital, Beverly, MA, p. A295
PIKE, Randi, Director of Nursing, Pioneer Medical Center, Big Timber, MT, p. A373
PIKE, Ronald F., M.D. Medical Director, Adcare Hospital of Worcester, Worcester, MA, p. A306
PIKE, Tim, M.D. Chief Medical Officer, Portsmouth Regional Hospital, Portsmouth, NH, p. A400
PIKER, John F., M.D. Medical Director, Villa Feliciana Medical Complex, Jackson, LA, p. A268
PIL, Pieter, M.D. Chief Medical Staff, Martha's Vineyard Hospital, Oak Bluffs, MA, p. A303
PILARCZYK, Penny, Vice President Human Resources, Advocate Lutheran General Hospital, Park Ridge, IL, p. A191
PILE, Larry, Director Human Resources, Deaconess Hospital, Evansville, IN, p. A201
PILLION, Scott, Chief Executive Officer, Helen Newberry Joy Hospital, Newberry, MI, p. A320
PILONG, Alfred E., President and Chief Executive Officer, Winchester Medical Center, Winchester, VA, p. A657
PILOT, Dave, Chief Financial Officer, Mayo Clinic Health System in Albert Lea, Albert Lea, MN, p. A327
PINA, Ignacio, Director Administrative Services, Lanterman Developmental Center, Pomona, CA, p. A80
PINAC, Gil, Chief Executive Officer, Crowley Rehabilitation Hospital, Crowley, LA, p. A265
PINCUS, Emil R., M.D. Medical Director, Stony Lodge Hospital, Ossining, NY, p. A440
PINE, Richard M., President and Chief Executive Officer, Livengrin Foundation, Bensalem, PA, p. A518
PINEIRO, Carlos M.
President, Hospital HMA de Humacao, Humacao, PR, p. A701
President, Hospital Interamericano De Medicina Avanzada, Caguas, PR, p. A700
PING, Patricia, Director Information Services, Gibson General Hospital, Princeton, IN, p. A210
PINKELMAN, Janet, Director Human Resources, Faith Regional Health Services, Norfolk, NE, p. A386
PINKERTON, Patricia, Vice President and Chief Financial Officer, Sheppard and Enoch Pratt Hospital, Baltimore, MD, p. A289
PINKOSKY, Frank, Senior Vice President, Robert Packer Hospital, Sayre, PA, p. A537

Index of Health Care Professionals / Pourier

Index of Health Care Professionals


POLLINGTON, Karen, VP Patient Care, Northern Montana Hospital, Havre, MT, p. A376
POLLOCK, Jeffrey, Chief Information Officer, Wentworth–Douglass Hospital, Dover, NH, p. A397
POLLOCK, Maureen King, Chief Executive Officer, Eagleville Hospital, Eagleville, PA, p. A522
POLLOCK, Tina, R.N. Chief Nursing Officer, Dallas Regional Medical Center, Mesquite, TX, p. A616
POLO, Fabian, Chief Operating Officer, Our Children's House at Baylor, Dallas, TX, p. A592
POLONSKY, Dana, Vice President of Clinical Services, Craig Hospital, Englewood, CO, p. A100
POLONSKY, Kenneth, M.D. Chief Executive Officer, University of Chicago Medical Center, Chicago, IL, p. A179
POLOVICH, Joyce, Manager Information Systems, Western Pennsylvania Hospital, Pittsburgh, PA, p. A536
POLSELLI, Donna, Chief Operating Officer, Franciscan Hospital for Children, Boston, MA, p. A296
POLSTER, Peggy, Manager Personnel and Administrative Assistant, Falls Community Hospital and Clinic, Marlin, TX, p. A615
POLTRACK, Andrew, M.D. Chief of Staff, Margaret Mary Community Hospital, Batesville, IN, p. A197
POLZIN, Greg, Chief Financial Officer, Iowa Specialty Hospital–Belmond, Belmond, IA, p. A214
POMA, Frank W.
Interim President, St. John Hospital and Medical Center, Detroit, MI, p. A311
President, St. John River District Hospital, East China, MI, p. A311
PONCE, Agustin, Supervisor Maintenance, Castaner General Hospital, Castaner, PR, p. A700
PONCE, Joseph A., Chief Information Management, Dwight David Eisenhower Army Medical Center, Fort Gordon, GA, p. A153
PONCE, Martha, Director Information Technologies and Telecommunications, Saint John's Health Center, Santa Monica, CA, p. A90
POND, Dwight, TIS Boise, Saint Alphonsus Regional Medical Center, Boise, ID, p. A166
POND–BELL, Michele, R.N. Administrator Nursing, Cassia Regional Medical Center, Burley, ID, p. A167
PONDER, David, Information Technology Officer, Claremore Indian Hospital, Claremore, OK, p. A494
PONETA, Jan, Director Information Services, Jefferson Regional Medical Center, Crystal City, MO, p. A358
PONT, Allan, M.D. Vice President Medical Affairs, California Pacific Medical Center, San Francisco, CA, p. A86
PONTASCH, Erich, M.D. Chief of Staff, Mercy St. Anne Hospital, Toledo, OH, p. A489
PONTI, Mary–Anne D., R.N. Chief Operating Officer and Chief Nurse Executive, McLaren Northern Michigan, Petoskey, MI, p. A320
PONTICELLO, Nat, Vice President Human Resources, Nebraska Medical Center, Omaha, NE, p. A388
PONTIOUS, Becky, Human Resources/Accounting, Loring Hospital, Sac City, IA, p. A226
PONTREMOLI, Del, Director Human Resources, Spaulding Rehabilitation Hospital Cape Cod, East Sandwich, MA, p. A299
POOCH, Fred, Supervisor Information Technology, Johnson County Hospital, Tecumseh, NE, p. A390
POOK, Lots, Chief Information Officer, National Jewish Health, Denver, CO, p. A99
POOL, Roxana J., M.P.H. Chief Executive Officer, Hillside Hospital, Pulaski, TN, p. A574
POOLAW, Bryce, M.D. Clinical Director, Lawton Indian Hospital, Lawton, OK, p. A498
POOLE, Andrew J., Chief Financial Officer, Riverside Hospital, South Bend, IN, p. A212
POOLE, Karen, Chief Operating Officer, Boca Raton Regional Hospital, Boca Raton, FL, p. A118
POOLE, Ken, Coordinator Information Systems, Stone County Medical Center, Mountain View, AR, p. A49
POOLE, Rob, Director, Jane Phillips Medical Center, Bartlesville, OK, p. A494
POOLE–ADAMS, Veronica, R.N
Vice President, Chief Operating Officer and Chief Nursing Executive, Cleveland Regional Medical Center, Shelby, NC, p. A460
Vice President and Chief Nursing Officer, Crawley Memorial Hospital, Boiling Springs, NC, p. A449
POORE, J. Michael
Chief Executive Officer, MedWest – Harris, Sylva, NC, p. A461
Chief Executive Officer, MedWest – Swain, Bryson City, NC, p. A449
POORE, Justin, D.O. Chief Medical Staff, Cloud County Health Center, Concordia, KS, p. A232
POORE, Timothy T., Chief Executive Officer, HEALTHSOUTH East Valley Rehabilitation Hospital, Mesa, AZ, p. A34
POORTEN, Kevin P., President and Chief Executive Officer, Kish Health System, De Kalb, IL, p. B78
POPE, Alan R., M.D
Vice President, Medical Affairs, Lourdes Medical Center of Burlington County, Willingboro, NJ, p. A412
Vice President Medical Affairs, Our Lady of Lourdes Medical Center, Camden, NJ, p. A402
POPE, Brad, Vice President Human Resources, Memorial Health Care System, Chattanooga, TN, p. A563
POPE, Eddie
Director Information Systems, Pioneer Community Hospital of Patrick County, Stuart, VA, p. A656
Chief Information Officer, S. E. Lackey Memorial Hospital, Forest, MS, p. A346
POPE, J. Larry, Vice President Finance, Baptist Easley Hospital, Easley, SC, p. A549
POPE, James W., FACHE President and Chief Executive Officer, Sylvania Franciscan Health, Toledo, OH, p. B126
POPE, Lona
Director Financial Services, Shriners Hospitals for Children, Galveston Burns Hospital, Galveston, TX, p. A600
Director Fiscal Services, Shriners Hospitals for Children, Houston, Houston, TX, p. A606
POPE, Richard, Vice President Human Resources, Jackson County Memorial Hospital, Altus, OK, p. A493
POPE, Robert, Information Technology Director and Ministry Liaison, Saint John's Health System, Anderson, IN, p. A197
POPKIN, Barbara, R.N. Associate Executive Director Patient Care Services, Franklin Hospital, Valley Stream, NY, p. A445
POPKIN, Steve, Chief Executive Officer, Silver Lake Medical Center, Los Angeles, CA, p. A72
POPKO, George A., Senior Vice President and Chief Financial Officer, Christ Hospital, Jersey City, NJ, p. A405
POPLAWSKI, Steven, M.D. Medical Director, Forest Health Medical Center, Ypsilanti, MI, p. A326
POPOVICH, Cal, Vice President Information Technology, All Children's Hospital, Saint Petersburg, FL, p. A138
POPOVICH, John, M.D. President and Chief Executive Officer, Henry Ford Hospital, Detroit, MI, p. A310
POPP, Adam, Director Information Systems, Avera St. Benedict Hospital, Parkston, SD, p. A558
POPP, Jason, Chief of Medical Staff, Rochelle Community Hospital, Rochelle, IL, p. A192
POPP, Susan, Controller, Kindred Hospital–Fort Worth, Fort Worth, TX, p. A599
POQUETTE, Gary R., FACHE Chief Executive Officer, Niobrara Health and Life Center, Lusk, WY, p. A697
PORRATA, Carlos, CPA Chief Financial Officer, Hospital Episcopal San Lucas Guayama, Guayama, PR, p. A701
PORTCHY, Mindy, Manager Human Resources, Mark Reed Health Care District, McCleary, WA, p. A662
PORTELA, Joyce, President, Washington Adventist Hospital, Takoma Park, MD, p. A294
PORTEN, Hank J., FACHE President and Chief Executive Officer, Holyoke Medical Center, Holyoke, MA, p. A300
PORTER, Billy, Chief Executive Officer, Paris Regional Medical Center, Paris, TX, p. A620
PORTER, Cedric, M.D. President Medical Staff, Emanuel Medical Center, Swainsboro, GA, p. A160
PORTER, Dan, Vice President and Chief Financial Officer, Ottumwa Regional Health Center, Ottumwa, IA, p. A225
PORTER, Dorothy L., Director of Compliance/Risk/Quality, Asheville Specialty Hospital, Asheville, NC, p. A448
PORTER, Glen, Vice President Human Resources, Essentia Health St. Mary's Medical Center, Duluth, MN, p. A330
PORTER, Greg, Chief Financial Officer, Rio Grande Hospital, Del Norte, CO, p. A99
PORTER, James, M.D. Vice President Medical Affairs, Deaconess Hospital, Evansville, IN, p. A201
PORTER, Janet E., Ph.D. Executive Vice President and Chief Operating Officer, Dana–Farber Cancer Institute, Boston, MA, p. A296
PORTER, Jody, R.N. Senior Vice President Patient Care Services and Chief Nursing Officer, Greater Baltimore Medical Center, Baltimore, MD, p. A287
PORTER Jr., John M., President and Chief Executive Officer, Ephrata Community Hospital, Ephrata, PA, p. A523
PORTER, John T., President and Chief Executive Officer, Avera Health, Sioux Falls, SD, p. B15
PORTER, Joyce, Chief Human Resources Officer, Adams County Regional Medical Center, Seaman, OH, p. A488
PORTER, Lance, Assistant Chief Executive Officer, Galesburg Cottage Hospital, Galesburg, IL, p. A182
PORTER, Lisa, Director Human Resources, Leadership and Education, Veterans Affairs Salt Lake City Health Care System, Salt Lake City, UT, p. A641
PORTER, Patricia, Chief Financial Officer, South Oaks Hospital, Amityville, NY, p. A420
PORTER, Sharon, Chief Financial Officer, Massachusetts Hospital School, Canton, MA, p. A299
PORTER, Stephen D., President, Sentara Princess Anne Hospital, Virginia Beach, VA, p. A657
PORTER, T. J., Director Human Resources, Bennett County Hospital and Nursing Home, Martin, SD, p. A557
PORTNER, Barry, M.D. Chief of Staff, Prowers Medical Center, Lamar, CO, p. A103
PORTNER, Michael, M.D. Chief Medical Staff, Bolivar Medical Center, Cleveland, MS, p. A345
PORTWOOD, David A., Chief Operating Officer, Coliseum Medical Centers, Macon, GA, p. A155
PORTWOOD, Lee, Chief Information Officer, Mother Frances Hospital – Jacksonville, Jacksonville, TX, p. A609
PORWOLL, Amy, Vice President of Information Systems, St. Cloud Hospital, Saint Cloud, MN, p. A338
POSAR, Steven, M.D. Chief of Medicine, Doctor's Hospital and Neuromuscular Center, Bremen, IN, p. A198
POSCH, David R., Chief Executive Officer, Vanderbilt Hospital and Clinics, Nashville, TN, p. A574
POSCH, Tim B., Business Manager and Director Personnel, Parsons State Hospital and Training Center, Parsons, KS, p. A241
POSECAI, Scott J., Executive Vice President and Chief Financial Officer, Ochsner Medical Center, New Orleans, LA, p. A275
POSEY, Dawn, Chief Operating Officer, Promise Hospital of Vicksburg, Vicksburg, MS, p. A353
POSEY, M. Kenneth, FACHE Administrator, Jasper General Hospital, Bay Springs, MS, p. A343
POSMOGA, Paul, Chief Financial Officer, Twin Cities Community Hospital, Templeton, CA, p. A92
POST, Kevin, D.O. Chief Medical Officer, Hegg Memorial Health Center Avera, Rock Valley, IA, p. A226
POST, Kimberly, R.N. Vice President and Administrator, Scottsdale Healthcare Thompson Peak Hospital, Scottsdale, AZ, p. A38
POSTERNACK, Charles, M.D. Chief Medical Officer, J. F. K. Medical Center, Atlantis, FL, p. A118
POSTLER–SLATTERY, Diane, Ph.D. President and Chief Operating Officer, Aspirus Wausau Hospital, Wausau, WI, p. A693
POSTLETHWAIT, Betsy, Chief Operating Officer, Princeton Baptist Medical Center, Birmingham, AL, p. A16
POSTON, Ann, Director Financial Services, Roosevelt Warm Springs LTAC Hospital, Warm Springs, GA, p. A161
POSTON, Anne, Human Resources Officer, Lake City Community Hospital, Lake City, SC, p. A552
POSTULKA, Carol, Administrative Coordinator, Avera Gregory Hospital, Gregory, SD, p. A557
POTEETE, Robin
Manager Human Resources, Wellmont Hancock County Hospital, Sneedville, TN, p. A575
Manager Human Resources, Wellmont Hawkins County Memorial Hospital, Rogersville, TN, p. A575
POTHAST, Joyce, Vice President Human and Environmental Services, Van Wert County Hospital, Van Wert, OH, p. A490
POTTENGER, Jay, Administrator, Missouri River Medical Center, Fort Benton, MT, p. A375
POTTER, Carolyn, Director Human Resources, McLaren Central Michigan, Mount Pleasant, MI, p. A319
POTTER, Joe, M.D. Chief of Staff, Integris Marshall County Medical Center, Madill, OK, p. A498
POTTER, Rhonda, Director Human Resources, De Soto Regional Health System, Mansfield, LA, p. A272
POTTER, Sterling, M.D. Chief of Staff, Castleview Hospital, Price, UT, p. A639
POTTER, Steve, Manager Business and Information Systems, Clifton–Fine Hospital, Star Lake, NY, p. A443
POTTER, Val, Director Human Resources, St. Vincent Salem Hospital, Salem, IN, p. A211
POTTI, Esther, M.D. Chief Medical Staff, Sanford Bagley Medical Center, Bagley, MN, p. A328
POTTORFF, Jimmy, Interim Administrator, Walter Olin Moss Regional Medical Center, Lake Charles, LA, p. A271
POTTS, Mary Ann, Director Personnel, Community Hospitals and Wellness Centers, Bryan, OH, p. A471
POUGNAUD, Teresa, Vice President Human Resources, McLeod Loris Healthcare, Loris, SC, p. A552
POULLARD, James, Chief Executive Officer, Kindred Hospital Midtown, Houston, TX, p. A604
POULTON, Connie, Vice President Colleague Relations, Alliance Community Hospital, Alliance, OH, p. A469
POUND, Robert, Administrator, Oceans Behavioral Hospital of Kentwood, Kentwood, LA, p. A269
POUND, Steven, Vice President Human Resources, Hamilton Medical Center, Dalton, GA, p. A151
POUND, Terry, Chief Financial Officer, Rice County District Hospital, Lyons, KS, p. A238
POURIER, William, Service Unit Director, U. S. Public Health Service Indian Hospital, Pine Ridge, SD, p. A558

Index of Health Care Professionals / Povich



POVICH, Mark, D.O. Medical Director, OSF St. Francis Hospital, Escanaba, MI, p. A312
POWE, Lee, Director Management Information Systems, Hugh Chatham Memorial Hospital, Elkin, NC, p. A453
POWEL, Linda J., M.D. Medical Director, Odessa Memorial Healthcare Center, Odessa, WA, p. A663
POWELL, Candy, Administrator, Collingsworth General Hospital, Wellington, TX, p. A634
POWELL, Charles, Chief Financial Officer, Arkansas Surgical Hospital, North Little Rock, AR, p. A49
POWELL, Claudia, R.N. Director of Nursing, Melissa Memorial Hospital, Holyoke, CO, p. A102
POWELL, D. Jerome, M.D
Chief Information Officer, Highland Hospital of Rochester, Rochester, NY, p. A441
Chief Information Officer, Strong Memorial Hospital of the University of Rochester, Rochester, NY, p. A442
POWELL, Darla, Administrative Assistant, Mayhill Hospital, Denton, TX, p. A594
POWELL, Dian, Chief Executive Officer, Roseland Community Hospital, Chicago, IL, p. A177
POWELL, Frank R., Chief Financial Officer, Houston Medical Center, Warner Robins, GA, p. A161
POWELL, Holly
Interim Administrator, Dubuis Hospital of Shreveport, Shreveport, LA, p. A277
Administrator, Dubuis Hospital of Texarkana, Texarkana, TX, p. A631
POWELL, Jackie, Director Human Resources, Pemiscot Memorial Health System, Hayti, MO, p. A360
POWELL, Jimmy, Manager Human Resources, Harry S. Truman Memorial Veterans Hospital, Columbia, MO, p. A358
POWELL, Kay, Director Human Resources, CHRISTUS Jasper Memorial Hospital, Jasper, TX, p. A609
POWELL, Lorie, Chief Executive Officer, Select Specialty Hospital–Flint, Flint, MI, p. A312
POWELL, Mary Lou, MSN Chief Nursing Officer, Rex Healthcare, Raleigh, NC, p. A459
POWELL, Michele, Chief Executive Officer, Select Rehabilitation Hospital of Denton, Denton, TX, p. A594
POWELL, Parker, Administrator, Prairie Community Hospital, Terry, MT, p. A379
POWELL, Robyn L., Chief Financial Officer, Marion General Hospital, Marion, IN, p. A208
POWELL, Sharon, Director Human Resources, Walter Olin Moss Regional Medical Center, Lake Charles, LA, p. A271
POWELL, Steven, M.D. Chief Medical Officer, New London Hospital, New London, NH, p. A399
POWELL, Traci, Director Human Resources, HEALTHSOUTH Emerald Coast Rehabilitation Hospital, Panama City, FL, p. A135
POWELL, Troy, Chief Executive Officer, HEALTHSOUTH Rehabilitation Hospital of Charleston, Charleston, SC, p. A547
POWELL, Virginia, Director Finance, Wilmington Treatment Center, Wilmington, NC, p. A462
POWELL–STAFFORD, Valerie L., Chief Operating Officer, Doctors Hospital of Sarasota, Sarasota, FL, p. A138
POWELSON, Jeffrey A., Chief Executive Officer, Broaddus Hospital, Philippi, WV, p. A674
POWER, Bob
Vice President Information Services, Good Samaritan Regional Medical Center, Corvallis, OR, p. A510
Vice President Information Services, Samaritan Lebanon Community Hospital, Lebanon, OR, p. A512
POWER, Robert, Associate Executive Director Finance, Southside Hospital, Bay Shore, NY, p. A421
POWERS, Anthony, Vice President Patient Care Services, Baptist Regional Medical Center, Corbin, KY, p. A248
POWERS, Charles, M.D. Administrative Medical Director, WK Bossier Health Center, Bossier City, LA, p. A264
POWERS, Donald, Chairman, President and Chief Executive Officer, Community Healthcare System, Hammond, IN, p. B37
POWERS, Jack, Director Human Resources, Central Washington Hospital, Wenatchee, WA, p. A669
POWERS, Jamekia, Assistant Director Human Resources, Georgia Regional Hospital at Savannah, Savannah, GA, p. A159
POWERS, Kelli, Chief Executive Officer, Athens–Limestone Hospital, Athens, AL, p. A16
POWERS, Marcia, Vice President Human Resources, Norwegian American Hospital, Chicago, IL, p. A177
POWERS, Melinda, D.O. Chief of Staff, Jackson County Memorial Hospital, Altus, OK, p. A493
POWERS, Michael K., FACHE Chief Executive Officer, Fairbanks Memorial Hospital, Fairbanks, AK, p. A29
POWERS, Paul A., Vice President and Chief Financial Officer, Lakeland Regional Medical Center, Lakeland, FL, p. A128
POWERS, Richard, M.D. Chief of Staff, Palm Drive Hospital, Sebastopol, CA, p. A90
POWERS, Ryan, Chief Financial Officer, Spectrum Health Zeeland Community Hospital, Zeeland, MI, p. A326
POWRIE, Raymond, M.D. Senior Vice President Quality and Clinical Effectiveness, Women & Infants Hospital of Rhode Island, Providence, RI, p. A545
POYNTER, Carmen, Director Human Resources, Rockcastle Regional Hospital and Respiratory Care Center, Mount Vernon, KY, p. A257
POZNIAK, Richard A., Director Marketing and Communications, Hallmark Health System, Melrose, MA, p. A302
PRABHU, Asha, M.D. Chief Medical Officer, Warren State Hospital, Warren, PA, p. A540
PRACHEIL, Michael, Chief Financial Officer, Thayer County Health Services, Hebron, NE, p. A384
PRACHT, Matthew, Vice President Finance, Scotland Health Care System, Laurinburg, NC, p. A456
PRADA, Janina
Director Information Technology, El Paso Children's Hospital, El Paso, TX, p. A596
Director Information Services, University Medical Center of El Paso, El Paso, TX, p. A597
PRAGER, Jay E., Chief Executive Officer, Reynolds Memorial Hospital, Glen Dale, WV, p. A672
PRAKASH, Amitabh, M.D. Chief Medical Officer, Anaheim Regional Medical Center, Anaheim, CA, p. A53
PRATER, Jeff, Chief Executive Officer, Granite County Medical Center, Philipsburg, MT, p. A378
PRATER, Marsha A., Ph.D. Senior Vice President and Chief Nursing Officer, Memorial Medical Center, Springfield, IL, p. A194
PRATER, Robin, Director Human Resources, Howard A. Rusk Rehabilitation Center, Columbia, MO, p. A358
PRATHER, Bobbie L., Chief Financial Officer, Central Baptist Hospital, Lexington, KY, p. A253
PRATI, Richard, Chief Operating Officer, Fort Duncan Regional Medical Center, Eagle Pass, TX, p. A595
PRATT, Bonnie, R.N. Chief Nursing Officer, Lakeview Regional Medical Center, Covington, LA, p. A265
PRATT, Debbie, Chief Financial Officer, Washington County Memorial Hospital, Potosi, MO, p. A367
PRATT, Elizabeth, Director Health Information Management, University Behavioral Health of Denton, Denton, TX, p. A594
PRATT, Lisa, Vice President Human Resources, Memorial Hospital of Rhode Island, Pawtucket, RI, p. A544
PRATT, Mary Ellen, FACHE Chief Executive Officer, St. James Parish Hospital, Lutcher, LA, p. A272
PRATT, Timothy J., M.D. Vice President of Medical Affairs/Chief Medical Officer, SSM St. Clare Health Center, Fenton, MO, p. A359
PRAY, Jan, Coordinator Payroll and Benefits, Kindred Hospital Boston–North Shore, Peabody, MA, p. A303
PRAYWELL, Hunter, Vice President Information Technology and Chief Information Officer, Queen's Medical Center, Honolulu, HI, p. A164
PRAZNIK, Gary, Chief Information Officer, Waccamaw Community Hospital, Murrells Inlet, SC, p. A552
PREAU, William, M.D. Medical Director, Fairway Medical Center, Covington, LA, p. A265
PRECHT, James, Chief Financial Officer, Goodland Regional Medical Center, Goodland, KS, p. A233
PRENGLER, Irving, M.D. Vice President Medical Staff Affairs, Baylor University Medical Center, Dallas, TX, p. A590
PRENTISS, Kristin, Chief Financial Officer, Specialty Hospital at Monmouth, Long Branch, NJ, p. A405
PREPIERI, Tim, Director Human Resources, Watonga Municipal Hospital, Watonga, OK, p. A507
PRESS, Christopher E., FACHE President, Blanchard Valley Regional Health Center, Blanchard Valley Hospital, Findlay, OH, p. A480
PRESS, Robert, M.D. Chief Medical Officer, NYU Langone Medical Center, New York, NY, p. A436
PRESSER, Jonathan, Vice President Finance and Operations, Norton Audubon Hospital, Louisville, KY, p. A254
PRESSMAN, Eric, D.O. Chair Department of Medicine, Englewood Community Hospital, Englewood, FL, p. A122
PREST, Craig, Director Operation Services, Humboldt General Hospital, Winnemucca, NV, p. A396
PRESTON, Troy, Director Human Resources, Schuyler Hospital, Montour Falls, NY, p. A430
PRESTRIDGE, Tim, Chief Financial Officer, LewisGale Hospital Alleghany, Low Moor, VA, p. A650
PRETE, Mark, M.D. Vice President Medical Affairs, The Charlotte Hungerford Hospital, Torrington, CT, p. A112
PRETTYMAN, Edgar E., PsyD, Chief Executive Officer, Texas NeuroRehab Center, Austin, TX, p. A582
PREUSS, Heather, M.D. Medical Director, Fall River Hospital, Hot Springs, SD, p. A557
PREWITT, Connie F., Chief Financial Officer, Billings Clinic, Billings, MT, p. A373
PREWITT, Ron, President, Lee Regional Medical Center, Pennington Gap, VA, p. A653
PRIBYL, Stephen J., FACHE Chief Executive Officer, District One Hospital, Faribault, MN, p. A331
PRICE, Alysia, Director Human Resources, Colleton Medical Center, Walterboro, SC, p. A554
PRICE, Brad H., Vice President Finance and Operations, Wellmont Holston Valley Medical Center, Kingsport, TN, p. A568
PRICE, Cecil, M.D. Director, Wake Forest University Health Service, Winston–Salem, NC, p. A463
PRICE, Eric, Financial Specialist, Senior, State Hospital South, Blackfoot, ID, p. A166
PRICE, Fred, R.N. Chief Executive Officer, Monroe Hospital, Bloomington, IN, p. A198
PRICE, Harrison, Interim President and Chief Executive Officer, Cornerstone Healthcare Group, Dallas, TX, p. B38
PRICE, Jeffrey, Director Information Technology, Nevada Regional Medical Center, Nevada, MO, p. A366
PRICE, John D., Chief Financial Officer, FirstHealth Richmond Memorial Hospital, Rockingham, NC, p. A459
PRICE, Julie
Chief Financial Officer, Rooks County Health Center, Plainville, KS, p. A242
Chief Financial Officer, Union County General Hospital, Clayton, NM, p. A415
PRICE, Kevin A., Vice President and Chief Operating Officer, Sparrow Clinton Hospital, Saint Johns, MI, p. A322
PRICE, Kim, Chief Executive Officer, Franklin General Hospital, Hampton, IA, p. A220
PRICE, Larry, Assistant Administrator, Limestone Medical Center, Groesbeck, TX, p. A602
PRICE, Lori, President, Saint Joseph Regional Medical Center–Plymouth Campus, Plymouth, IN, p. A210
PRICE, Lorraine B., Associate Director, Veterans Affairs Medical Center, Hampton, VA, p. A649
PRICE, Manuel, Director Information Systems, Brookwood Medical Center, Birmingham, AL, p. A16
PRICE, Norma Jean, Manager Personnel, Riverland Medical Center, Ferriday, LA, p. A266
PRICE, Norman M., FACHE Chief Executive Officer and Administrator, Southwest Health Systems, Mccomb, MS, p. B121
PRICE, Norman M., FACHE Chief Executive Officer, Southwest Mississippi Regional Medical Center, McComb, MS, p. A349
PRICE, Peggy Cain, Vice President and Chief Operating Officer, Exempla Lutheran Medical Center, Wheat Ridge, CO, p. A107
PRICE, Sam, Executive Vice President Finance/Chief Financial Officer, East Alabama Medical Center, Opelika, AL, p. A24
PRICE, Shari, Director Information Services, Baptist Hospital East, Louisville, KY, p. A254
PRICE, Sheila C., R.N. Chief Nursing Officer/Vice President of Nursing, Angel Medical Center, Franklin, NC, p. A453
PRICE, Shelby, Chief Executive Officer, Louisiana State Hospitals, Baton Rouge, LA, p. B83
PRICE, Toni, Director Human Resources, Lincoln County Medical Center, Troy, MO, p. A372
PRICE, Wendy, Manager Human Resources, Nicholas County Hospital, Carlisle, KY, p. A248
PRICHARD, Barbara, Assistant Administrator, South Sunflower County Hospital, Indianola, MS, p. A347
PRIDDY, III, Ernest C., Chief Financial Officer, Old Vineyard Behavioral Health Services, Winston–Salem, NC, p. A463
PRIDDY, Steven L., M.D. Vice President Physician Affairs and Chief Medical Officer, St. Vincent Carmel Hospital, Carmel, IN, p. A199
PRIDEAUX, Heather, Director Finance, Rawlins County Health Center, Atwood, KS, p. A230
PRIEBE, Cedric T., M.D
Vice President and Chief Information Officer, Butler Hospital, Providence, RI, p. A544
Senior Vice President and Chief Information Officer, Kent County Memorial Hospital, Warwick, RI, p. A545
Senior Vice President and Chief Information Officer, Women & Infants Hospital of Rhode Island, Providence, RI, p. A545
PRIEBE, Debbie, Administrator, Physicians Behavioral Hospital, Shreveport, LA, p. A277
PRIEST, Claude, Chief Financial Officer, Prairie Ridge Hospital and Health Services, Elbow Lake, MN, p. A331
PRIEST, David, Director Information Systems, Charlevoix Area Hospital, Charlevoix, MI, p. A309
PRIEST, Geoff, M.D. Chief Medical Officer, Meriter Hospital, Madison, WI, p. A684
PRIEST, Mike, M.D. Chief of Staff, Pawhuska Hospital, Pawhuska, OK, p. A503
PRIESTLEY, Betty, Manager Business Office, Texas Specialty Hospital at Houston, Houston, TX, p. A607
PRIESTLEY, Carlos W., Chief Operating Officer, Providence Little Company of Mary Medical Center San Pedro,, CA, p. A71

A908 Index of Health Care Professionals 

Index of Health Care Professionals / Pyrah

Index of Health Care Professionals

PRIMEAUX, Pam, Chief Financial Officer, Jennings American Legion Hospital, Jennings, LA, p. A268
PRINCE, Clay C., Chief Medical Officer, Madison Memorial Hospital, Rexburg, ID, p. A170
PRINCE, Gayle, Director Human Resources, Washington County Regional Medical Center, Sandersville, GA, p. A158
PRINCE, Sue, Director Information Systems, Northern Westchester Hospital, Mount Kisco, NY, p. A430
PRINCE, Thomas A., Vice President Operations and Human Resources, Northeast Rehabilitation Hospital, Salem, NH, p. A400
PRINCIPE, Hector Cintron, M.D. Director, Hospital Universitario Dr. Ramon Ruiz Arnau, Bayamon, PR, p. A700
PRINGLE–MILLER, Letitia, Administrative Director, Tuomey Healthcare System, Sumter, SC, p. A554
PRINTY, Wayne
Chief Financial Officer and Senior Vice President Finance, Miles Memorial Hospital, Damariscotta, ME, p. A283
Chief Financial Officer and Senior Vice President Finance, St. Andrews Hospital and Healthcare Center, Boothbay Harbor, ME, p. A282
PRINTZ, David, Vice President and Chief Information Officer, Central DuPage Hospital, Winfield, IL, p. A196
PRIOLA, Pat, Chief Financial Officer, Jerome Golden Center for Behavioral Health, Inc., West Palm Beach, FL, p. A142
PRIORE, Jacqueline, Chief Nursing Officer, Samaritan Hospital, Troy, NY, p. A445
PRISELAC, Thomas M., President and Chief Executive Officer, Cedars–Sinai Medical Center, Los Angeles, CA, p. A69
PRISTER, James R.
President and Chief Executive Officer, R M L Specialty Hospital, Hinsdale, IL, p. A184
President and Chief Executive Officer, RML Specialty Hospital, Chicago, IL, p. A177
PRITCHARD, Joann, Chief Financial Officer, Veterans Affairs Medical Center, Erie, PA, p. A523
PRITCHARD, Teresa, Vice President, Yakima Valley Memorial Hospital, Yakima, WA, p. A669
PRITCHETT, Greg, Controller, Cuero Community Hospital, Cuero, TX, p. A590
PRITHVIRAJ, Panju, M.D. President Medical Staff, H. B. Magruder Memorial Hospital, Port Clinton, OH, p. A487
PRIVETT, David, Deputy Director, Western New York Children's Psychiatric Center, West Seneca, NY, p. A446
PROBASCO, Brent, Chief Financial Officer, Cass Regional Medical Center, Harrisonville, MO, p. A360
PROBSTFIELD, Dan, Senior Vice President and Chief Financial Officer, Lake Regional Health System, Osage Beach, MO, p. A366
PROBUS, Kimberly, Chief Executive Officer, Kindred Hospital–Bay Area St. Petersburg, Saint Petersburg, FL, p. A138
PROCHILO, John F., Chief Executive Officer and Administrator, Northeast Rehabilitation Hospital, Salem, NH, p. A400
PROCHNOW, Bryan, Chief Financial Officer, Matagorda Regional Medical Center, Bay City, TX, p. A582
PROCTOR, Deborah A., President and Chief Executive Officer, St. Joseph Health, Orange, CA, p. B122
PROCTOR, III, Folsom, M.D. Vice President and Chief Medical Officer, Piedmont Mountainside Hospital, Jasper, GA, p. A154
PROCTOR, George M., Senior Vice President and Executive Director, Woodhull Medical and Mental Health Center,, NY, p. A438
PROCTOR, Ken, Director Human Resources, Mayo Regional Hospital, Dover–Foxcroft, ME, p. A283
PROCTOR, Sandra, R.N. Chief Nurse Executive, Memorial Medical Center, Modesto, CA, p. A75
PROCTOR, Stephen, Director of Human Resources/Risk, Russellville Hospital, Russellville, AL, p. A25
PROCTOR, Steven M., President, Matheny Medical and Educational Center, Peapack, NJ, p. A408
PROEHL, Sheila R., Chief Financial Officer, Hudson Hospital, Hudson, WI, p. A683
PROKOSCH, Brian, M.D. Vice President Medical Affairs, St. Francis Regional Medical Center, Shakopee, MN, p. A340
PRONI, John, CPA Manager Finance, BayCare Alliant Hospital, Dunedin, FL, p. A122
PROSKE, Donna, MS Executive Vice President, Chief Operating Officer and Chief Nursing Executive, Staten Island University Hospital,, NY, p. A437
PROTHERO, Marie, MSN, Chief Executive Officer, Utah Valley Specialty Hospital, Provo, UT, p. A640
PROTO, Robert, Director Information Systems, Torrance Memorial Medical Center, Torrance, CA, p. A92
PROTOS, George, Director Human Resources, Healdsburg District Hospital, Healdsburg, CA, p. A64
PROUD, James, Vice President Human Resources and Marketing, Uniontown Hospital, Uniontown, PA, p. A540
PROULX, David R., Assistant Vice President Operations, Valley West Community Hospital, Sandwich, IL, p. A193
PROVENZANO, Jeff, Chief Financial Officer, Mayo Regional Hospital, Dover–Foxcroft, ME, p. A283
PRUIETT, Bobby, Chief Financial Officer, Texoma Medical Center, Denison, TX, p. A593
PRUIETT, Linda, Vice President Human Resources, Sky Ridge Medical Center, Lone Tree, CO, p. A104
PRUITT, Angela L., Director Health Information Management and Quality Improvement, Timberlawn Mental Health System, Dallas, TX, p. A593
PRUITT, Michael W., Interim Administrator, Coleman County Medical Center, Coleman, TX, p. A588
PRUNCHUNAS, Edward M., Senior Vice President and Chief Financial Officer, Cedars–Sinai Medical Center, Los Angeles, CA, p. A69
PRUNOSKE, Mark, Chief Financial Officer and Senior Vice President Finance, F. F. Thompson Hospital, Canandaigua, NY, p. A423
PRUSATIS, Michael, Vice President Finance, Sinai–Grace Hospital, Detroit, MI, p. A311
PRYBYLO, Mary, President and Chief Executive Officer, St. Joseph Hospital, Bangor, ME, p. A281
PRYOR, David, Chief Operating Officer, Chilton Medical Center, Clanton, AL, p. A18
PRYOR, Dennis P., Administrator, Salem Memorial District Hospital, Salem, MO, p. A370
PRYOR, Robert W., M.D. President and Chief Executive Officer, Scott & White Healthcare, Temple, TX, p. B113
PRYOR, Shanna, R.N. Chief Nursing Officer, Helena Regional Medical Center, Helena, AR, p. A46
PRYOR, Vincent, Senior Vice President Finance and Chief Financial Officer, Edward Hospital, Naperville, IL, p. A189
PRYOR, William B., Senior Vice President Human Resources, Cape Fear Valley Medical Center, Fayetteville, NC, p. A453
PRZYBYLSKI, David, Interim Controller, Sparrow Specialty Hospital, Lansing, MI, p. A317
PSAILA, Justin P., M.D. Vice President Medical Affairs, St. Luke's Hospital – Anderson Campus, Easton, PA, p. A522
PSHEA, Pam, R.N. Chief Nursing Officer, San Ramon Regional Medical Center, San Ramon, CA, p. A89
PUCKETT, Doug, President and Chief Executive Officer, Indiana University Health Morgan Hospital, Martinsville, IN, p. A208
PUCKETT, Kimberly, Manager Human Resources, Carroll County Memorial Hospital, Carrollton, KY, p. A248
PUCKETT, Kristi, Director Human Resources, Grande Ronde Hospital, La Grande, OR, p. A512
PUENTES, Francisco, Human Resource Officer, San Diego County Psychiatric Hospital, San Diego, CA, p. A85
PUETZER, Mary, MS Chief Operating Officer, Select Specialty Hospital–Milwaukee, Milwaukee, WI, p. A687
PUFFENBERGER, James, Vice President and Chief Financial Officer, Reid Hospital and Health Care Services, Richmond, IN, p. A211
PUGH, Janelle, Vice President Finance and Operations, Saint Joseph Mount Sterling, Mount Sterling, KY, p. A257
PUGH, William H., Senior Vice President Corporate Finance and Chief Financial Officer, Pinnacle Health System, Harrisburg, PA, p. A524
PUGSLEY, Tim, Manager Information Technology, Nebraska Orthopaedic Hospital, Omaha, NE, p. A388
PUHY, Dorothy E., Executive Vice President and Chief Financial Officer, Dana–Farber Cancer Institute, Boston, MA, p. A296
PUJOLS–MCKEE, Ana, M.D. Chief Medical Officer and Associate Executive Director, Penn Presbyterian Medical Center, Philadelphia, PA, p. A533
PUKALA, Shirley, R.N. Assistant Administrator of Operations, St. Lawrence Rehabilitation Center, Lawrenceville, NJ, p. A405
PULASKI, Jason, Controller, HEALTHSOUTH Reading Rehabilitation Hospital, Reading, PA, p. A537
PULCO, Dominic J., Executive Vice President Finance and Chief Financial Officer, VCU Health System, Richmond, VA, p. A655
PULEO, Mark, Vice President and Chief Human Resources Officer, Henry Mayo Newhall Memorial Hospital, Valencia, CA, p. A94
PULIDO, Michael, Process Leader Human Resources, Heartland Regional Medical Center, Saint Joseph, MO, p. A368
PULLARKAT, Sajit, Chief Executive Officer and Managing Director, Centennial Hills Hospital Medical Center, Las Vegas, NV, p. A392
PULLEY, Bob, Interim Chief Financial Officer, Lehigh Regional Medical Center, Lehigh Acres, FL, p. A129
PULLIN, Dennis W., Chief Executive Officer, Medstar Harbor Hospital, Baltimore, MD, p. A288
PULLMAN, Debbie, Director Finance, Avera Hand County Memorial Hospital & Clinic, Miller, SD, p. A557
PULLMAN, Jayson, Chief Executive Officer, Hawarden Community Hospital, Hawarden, IA, p. A221
PULSIPHER, Gary W., President and Chief Executive Officer, Mercy Hospital Joplin, Joplin, MO, p. A361
PUNJABI, Rishab, Chief Financial Officer, Kindred Hospital–New Jersey Morris County, Dover, NJ, p. A403
PUNZIRUDU, Debbie, Controller, HEALTHSOUTH Rehabilitation Hospital of Spring Hill, Brooksville, FL, p. A120
PURANIK, Prakash, M.D. Chief of Staff, Beckley ARH Hospital, Beckley, WV, p. A670
PURCELL, Sandra, Administrative Director Business and Financial Services, Illini Community Hospital, Pittsfield, IL, p. A192
PURCELL, Terry
Vice President Support Services and Ambulatory Care, Gnaden Huetten Memorial Hospital, Lehighton, PA, p. A527
Director Information Services, Lea Regional Medical Center, Hobbs, NM, p. A416
Vice President Ambulatory Care and Support Services, Palmerton Hospital, Palmerton, PA, p. A531
PURDY, Bruce, M.D. Chief of Staff, Muleshoe Area Medical Center, Muleshoe, TX, p. A618
PURGETT, Thomas, M.D. Chief Medical Staff, Baylor Regional Medical Center at Grapevine, Grapevine, TX, p. A601
PURINGTON, Denise, Vice President and Chief Information Officer, Elliot Hospital, Manchester, NH, p. A399
PURINTON, Sandy, Chief Nursing Officer, Trego County–Lemke Memorial Hospital, Wakeeney, KS, p. A244
PUROHIT, Amish, Chief Executive Officer, Huhukam Memorial Hospital, Sacaton, AZ, p. A37
PUROHIT, Kumar, Chief Financial Officer, Rockford Center, Newark, DE, p. A114
PURRINGTON, Janice, Coordinator Medical Records, Avera Hand County Memorial Hospital & Clinic, Miller, SD, p. A557
PURSLEY, Roger, Chief Executive Officer, Western Mental Health Institute, Bolivar, TN, p. A562
PURTELL, Greg, Vice President Human Resources, McLaren Bay Special Care, Bay City, MI, p. A308
PURTLE, Mark, M.D
Vice President Medical Affairs, Iowa Lutheran Hospital, Des Moines, IA, p. A218
Vice President Medical Affairs, Iowa Methodist Medical Center, Des Moines, IA, p. A218
PURUSHOTHAM, Sanjay, Executive Director Information Systems, Bon Secours Baltimore Health System, Baltimore, MD, p. A287
PURVANCE, Clint, M.D. Chief Medical Officer, Barton Healthcare System, South Lake Tahoe, CA, p. A91
PURVES, Stephen A., FACHE President and Chief Executive Officer, Munroe Regional Medical Center, Ocala, FL, p. A133
PURVIS, Jay, Administrator, Wabash General Hospital, Mount Carmel, IL, p. A188
PURVIS, Michael L., Chief Executive Officer, Cook Medical Center–A Campus of Tift Regional Medical Center, Adel, GA, p. A144
PURVIS, Mike, Chief Administrative Officer, Sutter Medical Center of Santa Rosa, Chanate Campus, Santa Rosa, CA, p. A90
PUSTINA, Karl, Assistant Administrator Finance, Upland Hills Health, Dodgeville, WI, p. A680
PUSZKARSKA, Lucyna M., M.D. Medical Director, Riveredge Hospital, Forest Park, IL, p. A182
PUTHOFF, Timothy, Chief Executive Officer, Gateway Medical Center, Clarksville, TN, p. A564
PUTNAM, Mark, M.D. Medical Director, Haven Behavioral Health of Eastern Pennsylvania, Reading, PA, p. A536
PUTNAM, Stewart C., Executive Vice President and Chief Operating Officer, Unity Hospital, Rochester, NY, p. A442
PUTNAM, Timothy L., FACHE President and Chief Executive Officer, Margaret Mary Community Hospital, Batesville, IN, p. A197
PUU, Linda, Chief Nursing Officer, Kaiser Permanente Medical Center, Honolulu, HI, p. A163
PUVOGEL, LuAnn, R.N. Administrator, Salina Surgical Hospital, Salina, KS, p. A243
PUZO, Thomas C., President and Chief Operating Officer, Cornerstone of Medical Arts Center Hospital, Fresh Meadows, NY, p. A426
PUZZUTO, David, M.D. Vice President Medical Affairs and Chief Medical Officer, Waterbury Hospital, Waterbury, CT, p. A112
PYE, Irma L., Senior Vice President and Chief Human Resource Officer, Valley Baptist Medical Center–Harlingen, Harlingen, TX, p. A602
PYLE, David, M.D. Vice President Medical Affairs, St. Bernards Medical Center, Jonesboro, AR, p. A47
PYLE, Diana, Director Human Resources, Cedar County Memorial Hospital, El Dorado Springs, MO, p. A359
PYLE, Julia, R.N. Chief Nursing Officer, Newman Regional Health, Emporia, KS, p. A232
PYLE, Rick, Director Information Systems, Harrisburg Medical Center, Harrisburg, IL, p. A183
PYPER, Thomas, Chief Executive Officer, Trinity Hospital, Weaverville, CA, p. A95
PYRAH, Scott, Director Information Systems, Elks Rehab Hospital, Boise, ID, p. A166

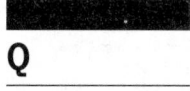

PYTLEWSKI, David, M.D. Clinical Director, Eastern Shore Hospital Center, Cambridge, MD, p. A290

PYTLINSKI, Doug, Vice President Administration, Alton Memorial Hospital, Alton, IL, p. A172

# Q

QUACH, Steve, M.D. Chief Medical Officer, University of Texas Medical Branch Hospitals, Galveston, TX, p. A600

QUACKENBUSH, Kirk, M.D. Chief of Staff, Platte Valley Medical Center, Brighton, CO, p. A98

QUADRI, Rob, Director Management Information Systems, Barton Healthcare System, South Lake Tahoe, CA, p. A91

QUAGLIATA, Joseph A., President and Chief Executive Officer, South Nassau Communities Hospital, Oceanside, NY, p. A439

QUALLS, Brenda, Chief Financial Officer, Oconee Regional Medical Center, Milledgeville, GA, p. A156

QUALLS, Judi, Director Human Resources, Elba General Hospital, Elba, AL, p. A19

QUALLS Jr., Paul E.
Chief Executive Officer, Solara Hospital Harlingen, Harlingen, TX, p. A602
Chief Executive Officer, Solara Hospital Harlingen–Brownsville Campus, Brownsville, TX, p. A585

QUAM, David, M.D. Area Medical Director, Fontana Medical Center, Fontana, CA, p. A61

QUANSTROM, Julie, Director Information Systems and Reimbursement Specialist, Wilson Medical Center, Neodesha, KS, p. A239

QUARANTE, Dino, Chief Financial Officer, Aurora Behavioral Health System–Glendale, Glendale, AZ, p. A32

QUARLES, Christopher, M.D. Director Medical Services, Naval Hospital, Jacksonville, FL, p. A126

QUARTIER, Michael J., Vice President Administration and Human Resources, Huntington Hospital, Huntington, NY, p. A427

QUATTROCCHI, Robert, President and Chief Executive Officer, Northside Healthcare System, Atlanta, GA, p. B96

QUATTROCCHI, Robert, President and Chief Executive Officer, Northside Hospital, Atlanta, GA, p. A145

QUEBEDEAUX, Jay, Chief Executive Officer, North Metro Medical Center, Jacksonville, AR, p. A46

QUEEN, J. R., USN, Commanding Officer, Naval Hospital Beaufort, Beaufort, SC, p. A546

QUENAN, James, M.D. Chief Medical Officer, Amery Regional Medical Center, Amery, WI, p. A678

QUICHOCHO, Vince, Manager Information Systems, Guam Memorial Hospital Authority, Tamuning, GU, p. A699

QUIGLEY, Michelle Ann, MS Vice President and Chief Nursing Officer, Valley Presbyterian Hospital,, CA, p. A72

QUIGLEY, Scott, Director Information Services, Grays Harbor Community Hospital, Aberdeen, WA, p. A659

QUIGLEY, Stephen J., Chief Executive Officer, Southwood Psychiatric Hospital, Pittsburgh, PA, p. A535

QUILLEN, Suzanne, R.N. Chief Executive Officer, Advanced Care Hospital of Southern New Mexico, Las Cruces, NM, p. A416

QUILLIN, Gayla, Administrator, Promise Specialty Hospital of Southeast Texas, Nederland, TX, p. A618

QUINLAN, Christine, MS Chief Nursing Officer, Alexian Brothers Behavioral Health Hospital, Hoffman Estates, IL, p. A184

QUINLAN, Michael, M.D. Chief of Staff, Audrain Medical Center, Mexico, MO, p. A365

QUINLAN, Patrick J., M.D. Chief Executive Officer, Ochsner Health System, New Orleans, LA, p. B97

QUINLAN, Patrick J., M.D. Chief Executive Officer, Ochsner Medical Center, New Orleans, LA, p. A275

QUINLIVAN, John, Chief Executive Officer, Redmond Regional Medical Center, Rome, GA, p. A158

QUINLIVAN, Kathy, Director Management Information Systems, Avera Sacred Heart Hospital, Yankton, SD, p. A561

QUINN, Clifton, Chief Executive Officer, Regency Hospital of Meridian, Meridian, MS, p. A350

QUINN, Donna, Vice President Operations and Quality, Driscoll Children's Hospital, Corpus Christi, TX, p. A589

QUINN, Jennifer, Quality and Safety Coordinator, Shawano Medical Center, Shawano, WI, p. A690

QUINN, John A., Chief Executive Officer, Spalding Regional Medical Center, Griffin, GA, p. A153

QUINN, Mary Anna, Vice President, St. Jude Children's Research Hospital, Memphis, TN, p. A572

QUINONES, Arnaldo, Chief Information Officer, Ashford Presbyterian Community Hospital, San Juan, PR, p. A702

QUINONES, Yolanda, Director Finance, I. Gonzalez Martinez Oncologic Hospital,, PR, p. A703

QUINONEZ, Yolanda, Chief Financial Officer, Hospital de la Universidad de Puerto Rico/Dr. Federico Trilla, Carolina, PR, p. A700

QUINT–BOUZID, Marjorie, Chief Nursing Officer and Vice President Patient Care Services, Fort Washington Medical Center, Fort Washington, MD, p. A291

QUINTANA, Jacob, Administrator, Care Regional Medical Center, Aransas Pass, TX, p. A579

QUINTANA, Jay, Vice President Operations, Cornerstone Hospital–West Monroe, West Monroe, LA, p. A279

QUINTANA, Sonya, R.N. Chief Nursing Officer, Osceola Regional Medical Center, Kissimmee, FL, p. A127

QUINTANA–HAMMON, Selene, Chief Executive Officer, University Behavioral Health of El Paso, El Paso, TX, p. A597

QUINTANAR, Humberto, Chief Information Officer, Antelope Valley Hospital, Lancaster, CA, p. A67

QUINTO, Mike
Chief Information Officer, Blowing Rock Hospital, Blowing Rock, NC, p. A449
Chief Information Officer, Charles A. Cannon Memorial Hospital, Linville, NC, p. A456
Chief Information Officer, Watauga Medical Center, Boone, NC, p. A449

QUINTON, Ben, Chief Executive Officer, Lander Regional Hospital, Lander, WY, p. A696

QUINTON, Byron, Chief Executive Officer, Clarion Hospital, Clarion, PA, p. A520

QUIRIN, Julie L., FACH
Chief Executive Officer, Saint Luke's Cancer Institute, Kansas City, MO, p. A362
Chief Executive Officer, Saint Luke's Hospital of Kansas City, Kansas City, MO, p. A362

QUIRING, Robert, Vice President Human Resources, Integris Baptist Medical Center, Oklahoma City, OK, p. A501

QUIRK, Pamela, Director of Nursing, Soldiers' Home in Holyoke, Holyoke, MA, p. A301

QUIRKE, David, Vice President Information Services, Frederick Memorial Hospital, Frederick, MD, p. A291

QUIROGA, Pam, Vice President Human Resources, South Oaks Hospital, Amityville, NY, p. A420

QUIST, Ryan, Administrative Assistant, Biggs–Gridley Memorial Hospital, Gridley, CA, p. A64

QUITO, Arturo L., M.D. Chief of Staff, Erlanger Bledsoe Hospital, Pikeville, TN, p. A574

# R

RAAB, Daniel J., President and Chief Executive Officer, Taylorville Memorial Hospital, Taylorville, IL, p. A195

RAB, Shafiq, Chief Information Officer, Orange Regional Medical Center, Middletown, NY, p. A430

RABAGO, Janie, Chief Accountant, San Antonio State Hospital, San Antonio, TX, p. A626

RABALAIS, David, M.D. Chief Medical Staff, Lane Regional Medical Center, Zachary, LA, p. A280

RABALAIS, Michael, Chief Executive Officer, Oceans Specialty Hospital of Gretna, Gretna, LA, p. A267

RABELO, Wilfredo, Chief Operating Officer, Hospital Episcopal San Lucas Guayama, Guayama, PR, p. A701

RABER, Conrad, Chief Information Resources Management Service, Durham Veterans Affairs Medical Center, Durham, NC, p. A452

RABIDEAU, Ray, M.D. Medical Director, Memorial Hospital, North Conway, NH, p. A399

RABIN, Barry, M.D. Medical Director, Linden Oaks Hospital at Edward, Naperville, IL, p. A189

RABINOWITZ, Abraham, Assistant Finance Officer, William S. Middleton Memorial Veterans Hospital, Madison, WI, p. A684

RABINOWITZ, Stephen, Executive Director, Manhattan Psychiatric Center–Ward's Island, New York, NY, p. A434

RABORN, Janelle, Chief Operating Officer, Lovelace Women's Hospital, Albuquerque, NM, p. A414

RABUKA, Mickey, Administrator, Florala Memorial Hospital, Florala, AL, p. A20

RACHAL, I. M., Chief Fiscal Service, South Texas Veterans Health Care System, San Antonio, TX, p. A626

RACHESKY, Ingrid, M.D. President Medical Staff, Bay Medical Center, Panama City, FL, p. A135

RACHUIG, Sue, Director Information Services, Tulane Medical Center, New Orleans, LA, p. A275

RACKLIFFE, David, Assistant Vice President Information Services, Bristol Hospital, Bristol, CT, p. A108

RACKOVAN, Patricia G., Senior Vice President & Chief Nurse Executive, JFK Medical Center, Edison, NJ, p. A403

RACZEK, James, M.D. Sr. Vice President of Operations and Chief Medical Officer, Eastern Maine Medical Center, Bangor, ME, p. A281

RADANDT, Jeremiah, Chief Financial Officer, Primary Children's Medical Center, Salt Lake City, UT, p. A640

RADCLIFF, Joey, Chief Financial Officer, Five Rivers Medical Center, Pocahontas, AR, p. A50

RADCLIFFE, Eric, M.D. Medical Director, United Hospital Center, Bridgeport, WV, p. A670

RADEMACHER, Frank, Director, Information Systems, St. Joseph Mercy Livingston Hospital, Howell, MI, p. A315

RADEMAKER, John, M.D. Medical Director, Physicians' Medical Center, New Albany, IN, p. A209

RADENHEIMER, Tony, Network Administrator, River Park Hospital, Huntington, WV, p. A672

RADER, Herbert, M.D. Vice President and Medical Director, New York Community Hospital,, NY, p. A435

RADER, Mark, FACHE Chief Executive Officer, University Hospital and Medical Center, Tamarac, FL, p. A140

RADER, Michael E., M.D. Vice President and Medical Director, Nyack Hospital, Nyack, NY, p. A438

RADFORD, Joanna, Chief Human Resources Officer, Shoshone Medical Center, Kellogg, ID, p. A168

RADFORD, Juanita, Coordinator Team Resource, South Florida Baptist Hospital, Plant City, FL, p. A136

RADKE, Sam, Vice President of Finance, Estes Park Medical Center, Estes Park, CO, p. A101

RADLOFF, Diane M., President and Chief Executive Officer, St. John Macomb–Oakland Hospital, Oakland Center, Madison Heights, MI, p. A318

RADOTICH, Maureen, Director Human Resources, Providence Valdez Medical Center, Valdez, AK, p. A30

RADUNSKY, Daniel, M.D. Medical Staff President, Union County General Hospital, Clayton, NM, p. A415

RADZEVICH, Jason, Vice President Finance, Milton Hospital, Milton, MA, p. A302

RAETHEL, Kathryn A., M.P.H. President and Chief Executive Officer, Castle Medical Center, Kailua, HI, p. A164

RAFALA, Paula, Director, Human Resources, Memorial Medical Center, Modesto, CA, p. A75

RAFALSKI, Mark, CPA Chief Financial Officer, Indiana University Health La Porte Hospital, La Porte, IN, p. A206

RAFFERTY, Diane
Chief Operating Officer, Brotman Medical Center, Culver City, CA, p. A59
Chief Executive Officer, University of Arizona Medical Center – University Campus, Tucson, AZ, p. A40

RAFFERTY, Joseph, Chief Executive Officer, Healthbridge Children's Hospital of Houston, Houston, TX, p. A604

RAFFERTY, Joyce, Vice President Finance, Champlain Valley Physicians Hospital Medical Center, Plattsburgh, NY, p. A440

RAFFERTY, Patrick W.
Executive Vice President and Chief Operating Officer, Community Behavioral Health Center, Fresno, CA, p. A62
Executive Vice President and Chief Operating Officer, Community Regional Medical Center, Fresno, CA, p. A62

RAFFETY, Leannette, Administrative Generalist, Stroud Regional Medical Center, Stroud, OK, p. A505

RAFFOUL, John, Senior Vice President Finance, White Memorial Medical Center, Los Angeles, CA, p. A73

RAFUS, Matthew, Chief Information Officer, Veterans Affairs Medical Center, White River Junction, VT, p. A644

RAGEL, Larry, Chief Financial Officer, St. John's Hospital, Springfield, IL, p. A194

RAGGIO, James J., Chief Executive Officer, Lompoc Valley Medical Center, Lompoc, CA, p. A67

RAGLE, Bertha, Director Personnel, CrossRidge Community Hospital, Wynne, AR, p. A52

RAGON, Rebecca, Coordinator Public Relations and Marketing, Pomerene Hospital, Millersburg, OH, p. A485

RAGONA, Robert A., Vice President Finance, Eastern Long Island Hospital, Greenport, NY, p. A427

RAGONE, Dale, Interim Chief Information Officer, Bayshore Community Hospital, Holmdel, NJ, p. A405

RAGOTHAMAN, Krishna, M.D. Chief of Staff, Mercy St. Charles Hospital, Oregon, OH, p. A486

RAGSDALE, Mary, Director Human Resources, Broughton Hospital, Morganton, NC, p. A457

RAGSDALE, Sara, D.O. Chief Medical Staff, Newport Hospital and Health Services, Newport, WA, p. A663

RAGSDALE, Sarah, R.N. Chief Nursing Officer, Smith County Memorial Hospital, Smith Center, KS, p. A243

RAGU, Alliri, M.D. Chief of Staff, Stewart–Webster Hospital, Richland, GA, p. A157

RAHAMAN, Suara, M.D. Chief Medical Staff, Bolivar General Hospital, Bolivar, TN, p. A562

RAHDERT, Richard, M.D. Medical Director, River Bend Hospital, West Lafayette, IN, p. A213

RAHMAN, Randy
Chief Information Officer, Yavapai Regional Medical Center – East, Prescott Valley, AZ, p. A37
Chief Information Officer, Yavapai Regional Medical Center, Prescott, AZ, p. A37

RAHMAN, Syed, M.D. Chief of Staff, Horizon Specialty Hospital, Las Vegas, NV, p. A393

Index of Health Care Professionals / Rasina


RAHN, Douglas L., Senior Vice President and Chief Operating Officer, Memorial Medical Center, Springfield, IL, p. A194
RAICA, Dagmar Ann, R.N. Chief Nursing Officer, Marquette General Health System, Marquette, MI, p. A318
RAINA, Suresh, M.D. Vice President Medical Staff and Chief Medical Officer, Palisades Medical Center, North Bergen, NJ, p. A407
RAINBOLT, Mike, Chief Financial Officer, Rivendell Behavioral Health Services of Arkansas, Benton, AR, p. A42
RAINDL, Donna, Manager Business Office, Lynn County Hospital District, Tahoka, TX, p. A630
RAINER, George P., Senior Vice President Human Resources, Winthrop–University Hospital, Mineola, NY, p. A430
RAINES, Chris, Chief Fiscal Services, Veterans Affairs Medical Center, Beckley, WV, p. A670
RAINES, Diane, R.N. Senior Vice President & CNO, Baptist Medical Center Beaches, Jacksonville Beach, FL, p. A127
RAINES, Joy, Coordinator Human Resources, Kindred Hospital Tarrant County–Fort Worth Southwest, Fort Worth, TX, p. A599
RAINEY, Jackie, Assistant Administrator and Controller, Atlanta Memorial Hospital, Atlanta, TX, p. A580
RAINS, Celeste, D.O. Chief of Staff, Logan County Hospital, Oakley, KS, p. A240
RAINS, Debbie, Coordinator Health Information Management, Erlanger Bledsoe Hospital, Pikeville, TN, p. A574
RAINS, Gail, R.N. Director Patient Care Services, Shriners Hospitals for Children, Shreveport, Shreveport, LA, p. A277
RAINS, Jeff G., Chief Executive Officer, DeKalb Regional Medical Center, Fort Payne, AL, p. A20
RAINS, Paul, MSN, President, St. Joseph's Behavioral Health Center, Stockton, CA, p. A91
RAINS, Steve, Director Information Services, McKee Medical Center, Loveland, CO, p. A104
RAINSTEIN, Miguel, M.D. Acting Chief of Staff, Veterans Affairs Western New York Healthcare System–Buffalo Division, Buffalo, NY, p. A423
RAISNER, Gary, Chief Operating Officer, Norristown State Hospital, Norristown, PA, p. A530
RAJATATNAM, Richard, M.D. Area Medical Director, Riverside Medical Center, Riverside, CA, p. A83
RAJPARA, Suresh, M.D. Chief Medical Officer, Jerome Golden Center for Behavioral Health, Inc., West Palm Beach, FL, p. A142
RAJSKI, Dianna, President and Chief Executive Officer, Childrens Care Hospital and School, Sioux Falls, SD, p. A559
RAJU, Ramanathan, M.D. Chief Executive Officer, Cook County Bureau of Health Services, Chicago, IL, p. B38
RAK, Roger, Director Human Resources, South Shore Hospital, Chicago, IL, p. A178
RAK, Ronald C., JD, Chief Executive Officer, Saint Peter's University Hospital, New Brunswick, NJ, p. A407
RAKES–STEPHENS, Kim, M.D. Chief Medical Staff, Colleton Medical Center, Walterboro, SC, p. A554
RAKOV, Robert, M.D. Chief Medical Officer, Cogdell Memorial Hospital, Snyder, TX, p. A628
RALPH, Chandler M., President and Chief Executive Officer, Adirondack Medical Center, Saranac Lake, NY, p. A442
RALPH, Stephen A., President and Chief Executive Officer, Huntington Memorial Hospital, Pasadena, CA, p. A80
RALSTIN, Char, Director of Nursing, Haven Senior Horizons, Phoenix, AZ, p. A35
RALSTON, Mary Beth, Manager Human Resources, North Georgia Medical Center, Ellijay, GA, p. A152
RAMAEKERS, Gina, Director Human Resources, St. Anthony Regional Hospital, Carroll, IA, p. A215
RAMAGE, Gary, M.D. Chief Medical Officer, McKenzie County Healthcare System, Watford City, ND, p. A468
RAMAN, Jayashree, Vice President and Chief Information Officer, Reading Hospital and Medical Center, West Reading, PA, p. A541
RAMAZANI, Regina, Chief Financial Officer, Garden Park Medical Center, Gulfport, MS, p. A346
RAMBHATLA, Kamalakar, M.D. Chief of Staff, Greater El Monte Community Hospital, South El Monte, CA, p. A91
RAMER, Gary, Manager Information Management, Jonathan M. Wainwright Memorial VA Medical Center, Walla Walla, WA, p. A669
RAMEY, Charles W., Vice President, Sentara Northern Virginia Medical Center, Woodbridge, VA, p. A657
RAMEY, Jan, MSN Chief Nursing Officer, Person Memorial Hospital, Roxboro, NC, p. A460
RAMEY, Michael, Director Human Resources, The Heart Hospital Baylor Plano, Plano, TX, p. A621
RAMEY, Rita, Director Information Systems, Buchanan General Hospital, Grundy, VA, p. A649
RAMEY, Steve, Chief Financial Officer, Southampton Memorial Hospital, Franklin, VA, p. A648
RAMIREZ, Conrad, Director Information Services, St. Mary's Regional Medical Center, Enid, OK, p. A496
RAMIREZ, Corazon, M.D. Chief Executive Officer, Physician Synergy Group, Irving, TX, p. B101
RAMIREZ, Corazon, M.D. Chief Executive Officer, Pine Creek Medical Center, Dallas, TX, p. A592
RAMIREZ, Eddy, Vice President Operations, Ochsner Medical Center – Kenner, Kenner, LA, p. A269
RAMIREZ, Eleanor, R.N. Executive Vice President and Chief Operating Officer, Saint John's Health Center, Santa Monica, CA, p. A90
RAMIREZ, Jaime, Chief Executive Officer, McCamey County Hospital District, McCamey, TX, p. A616
RAMIREZ, Marcos, Manager Human Resources, Baylor Medical Center at Waxahachie, Waxahachie, TX, p. A633
RAMIREZ, Willie, Manager Labor Relations, Laguna Honda Hospital and Rehabilitation Center, San Francisco, CA, p. A87
RAMLO, Ricki, Vice President Human Resources, Jamestown Regional Medical Center, Jamestown, ND, p. A466
RAMMLER, Linda, R.N. Chief Nursing Officer, Bonner General Hospital, Sandpoint, ID, p. A170
RAMOS, Cecilia, M.D. Chief of Staff, Lompoc Valley Medical Center, Lompoc, CA, p. A67
RAMOS, Eduardo, M.D. Medical Director, HEALTHSOUTH Rehabilitation Hospital, San Juan, PR, p. A703
RAMOS, Eric, M.D. Chief Medical Officer, Doctors Medical Center, Modesto, CA, p. A75
RAMOS, Holly, R.N. Chief Clinical Officer, Kindred Hospital–Ontario, Ontario, CA, p. A78
RAMOS, Jet, Head Staff Administration, Naval Hospital, Camp Pendleton, CA, p. A56
RAMOS, Norma, Chief Financial Officer, Baylor Medical Center at Carrollton, Carrollton, TX, p. A586
RAMOS, Raymond, Vice President and Chief Operating Officer, CHRISTUS Spohn Hospital Beeville, Beeville, TX, p. A583
RAMPAGE, Bruce E., Chief Executive Officer, NORTHSTAR Health System, Iron River, MI, p. A316
RAMPP, Randal D., M.D. Chief Medical Officer, River Park Hospital, Mc Minnville, TN, p. A570
RAMSAY, Kathy, R.N. Director Communications and Development, Rooks County Health Center, Plainville, KS, p. A242
RAMSEY, Beryl O., FACHE Chief Executive Officer, Methodist Willowbrook Hospital, Houston, TX, p. A605
RAMSEY, Bill, Director Human Resources, Ochsner Baptist Medical Center, New Orleans, LA, p. A274
RAMSEY, David L., President and Chief Executive Officer, Charleston Area Medical Center, Charleston, WV, p. A671
RAMSEY, David L., President and Chief Executive Officer, Charleston Area Medical Center Health System, Inc., Charleston, WV, p. B30
RAMSEY, Gina B., Vice President Financial Services and Chief Financial Officer, Wake Forest Baptist Medical Center, Winston–Salem, NC, p. A463
RAMSEY, James, Vice President Finance, Carolinas Medical Center–NorthEast, Concord, NC, p. A451
RAMSEY, Lisa, Chief Financial Officer, Greenwood County Hospital, Eureka, KS, p. A233
RAMSEY, Paul G., Chief Executive Officer, UW Medicine, Seattle, WA, p. B140
RAMSEY, Roy M., Executive Director, Bradford Health Services at Warrior Lodge, Warrior, AL, p. A26
RAMSEY, Steve, Chief Financial Officer, Powell Valley Healthcare, Powell, WY, p. A697
RAMSEY, Tara, M.D. President Medical Staff, Passavant Area Hospital, Jacksonville, IL, p. A185
RAMSEY, Thomas, Chief Financial Officer, River Parishes Hospital, La Place, LA, p. A269
RAMTHUN, Jane, Chief Financial Officer, Story County Medical Center, Nevada, IA, p. A224
RANA, Irfan, M.D. Chief of Staff, Cozby–Germany Hospital, Grand Saline, TX, p. A601
RAND, David, M.D. Chief of Staff, Torrance Memorial Medical Center, Torrance, CA, p. A92
RAND, Kevin, M.D. Clinical Director, Chinle Comprehensive Health Care Facility, Chinle, AZ, p. A31
RAND, Richard, Director Human Resources, Ely–Bloomenson Community Hospital, Ely, MN, p. A331
RANDALL, Bryan J.
Vice President Finance and Chief Financial Officer, Heritage Valley Beaver, Beaver, PA, p. A518
Vice President Finance and Chief Financial Officer, Sewickley Valley Hospital, (A Division of Valley Medical Facilities), Sewickley, PA, p. A538
RANDALL, Cherry, Business Officer, Greater Binghamton Health Center, Binghamton, NY, p. A421
RANDALL, JoEllen, Administrative Director Human Resources, Ottumwa Regional Health Center, Ottumwa, IA, p. A225
RANDALL, Kenneth W., Chief Executive Officer, Artesia General Hospital, Artesia, NM, p. A415
RANDALL, Ralph X., FACHE Chief Executive Officer, Jefferson Hospital, Louisville, GA, p. A155
RANDLE, Emily, Vice President Operations, Orange Coast Memorial Medical Center, Fountain Valley, CA, p. A61
RANDLE, Michael, Chief Financial Officer, Homer Memorial Hospital, Homer, LA, p. A267
RANDOLPH, Arianne, Director Human Resources, Pikes Peak Regional Hospital, Woodland Park, CO, p. A107
RANDOLPH, Bruce, Chief Information Technology, Arizona State Hospital, Phoenix, AZ, p. A35
RANDOLPH, Geoffrey, M.D. Chief Medical Officer, Lutheran Hospital of Indiana, Fort Wayne, IN, p. A201
RANDOLPH, Karsten, Vice President Finance/Chief Financial Officer, Park Ridge Health, Hendersonville, NC, p. A454
RANDOLPH, Jr., Leonard M., M.D
Senior Vice President and Chief Medical Officer, Mercy Hospital Anderson, Cincinnati, OH, p. A473
Senior Vice President and Divisional Chief Medical Officer, Mercy Hospital Mount Airy, Cincinnati, OH, p. A473
RANDOLPH, Linda, Director Personnel Services, Washington County Hospital and Nursing Home, Chatom, AL, p. A18
RANERI, Samuel
Senior Vice President Operations and Business Development, Excela Frick Hospital, Mount Pleasant, PA, p. A530
Senior Vice President Operations and Business Development, Excela Health Westmoreland Hospital, Greensburg, PA, p. A524
Senior Vice President Operations and Business Development, Excela Latrobe Area Hospital, Latrobe, PA, p. A527
RANGAVIZ, Rassoul, Chief Financial Officer, Copley Hospital, Morrisville, VT, p. A643
RANGHELLI, Gloria, Deputy Chief Financial Officer, Coler–Goldwater Specialty Hospital and Nursing Facility, New York, NY, p. A432
RANKIN, Beverley A., R.N. Vice President & Chief Nursing Officer, Alice Peck Day Memorial Hospital, Lebanon, NH, p. A398
RANKIN III, Fred M.
President and Chief Executive Officer, Mary Washington Hospital, Fredericksburg, VA, p. A648
President and Chief Executive Officer, Stafford Hospital, Stafford, VA, p. A656
RANKIN III,, Fred M., President and Chief Executive Officer, Mary Washington Healthcare, Fredericksburg, VA, p. B84
RANNEY, Timothy, M.D. Vice President Medical Affairs and Chief Medical Officer, Missouri Baptist Medical Center, Saint Louis, MO, p. A369
RANNIGER, Kathy, Director Finance, Hawarden Community Hospital, Hawarden, IA, p. A221
RANSOM, Jim, Chief Executive Officer, Reliant Rehabilitation Hospital North Texas, Richardson, TX, p. A622
RANSOM, Natalie, Chief Nursing Officer, Southern Hills Hospital and Medical Center, Las Vegas, NV, p. A393
RANTZ III,, August J., Founder and Chief Executive Officer, AMG Integrated Healthcare Management, Lafayette, LA, p. B9
RAO, Gutti, M.D. Medical Director, LTAC Hospital of Greenwood, Greenwood, MS, p. A346
RAO, Kalapala, M.D. Medical Director, HEALTHSOUTH Western Hills Rehabilitation Hospital, Parkersburg, WV, p. A674
RAO, Noel, M.D. Medical Director, Marianjoy Rehabilitation Hospital, Wheaton, IL, p. A196
RAO, Raghu, M.D. Chief of Staff, Helen Newberry Joy Hospital, Newberry, MI, p. A320
RAPAPORT, Gary D., Chief Executive Officer, Sutter Delta Medical Center, Antioch, CA, p. A53
RAPENSKE, Jennifer, Manager Financial Services, Mercy Medical Center–New Hampton, New Hampton, IA, p. A224
RAPP, David, Chief Information Officer, Wheeling Hospital, Wheeling, WV, p. A677
RAPP, Larry, M.D. Chief Medical Officer, Prairie Ridge Hospital and Health Services, Elbow Lake, MN, p. A331
RAPP, Peter F., Vice President and Executive Director, OHSU Hospital, Portland, OR, p. A514
RAPP, Robin, R.N. Chief Executive Officer, Kindred Hospital–Ontario, Ontario, CA, p. A78
RAPP, Ron, Controller, Charles Cole Memorial Hospital, Coudersport, PA, p. A521
RAREY, Kanute, Chief Executive Officer, Carroll County Memorial Hospital, Carrollton, KY, p. A248
RARICK, Karen
Director Information Technology, Schuylkill Medical Center – East Norwegian Street, Pottsville, PA, p. A536
Director Information Systems, Schuylkill Medical Center – South Jackson Street, Pottsville, PA, p. A536
RASCHKE, Judy, Director Human Resources, Pipestone County Medical Center Avera, Pipestone, MN, p. A337
RASH, Doug, Director Information Technology, Ferrell Hospital, Eldorado, IL, p. A180
RASH, Martin S., Chairman and Chief Executive Officer, RegionalCare Hospital Partners, Brentwood, TN, p. B109
RASINA, Stacia, Director Human Resources, Promise Hospital of San Diego, San Diego, CA, p. A85


Index of Health Care Professionals

© 2012 AHA Guide Index of Health Care Professionals A911

Index of Health Care Professionals

Index of Health Care Professionals / Rask


RASK, Brenda, Vice President Operations, Carrington Health Center, Carrington, ND, p. A464
RASKE, Jamie, Information Technology Lead, St. Mary's Healthcare Center, Pierre, SD, p. A558
RASMUSSEN, David D., Chief Executive Officer, Russell County Hospital, Russell Springs, KY, p. A258
RASMUSSEN, Diane, Director Human Resources, Cambridge Medical Center, Cambridge, MN, p. A329
RASMUSSEN, Kyle, Chief Executive Officer, Meeker Memorial Hospital, Litchfield, MN, p. A333
RASMUSSEN, Renee, Senior Vice President and Chief Financial Officer, Allen Memorial Hospital, Waterloo, IA, p. A227
RASMUSSEN, Roger, Chief Administrative Officer, Newport Hospital and Health Services, Newport, WA, p. A663
RASMUSSEN, Scott, Director Human Resources, Lincoln Regional Center, Lincoln, NE, p. A385
RASMUSSEN, Steven, M.D. Medical Director, Butler Hospital, Providence, RI, p. A544
RASMUSSON, Duane, Vice President Human Resources, St. Cloud Hospital, Saint Cloud, MN, p. A338
RASOOL, Chaudri, D.O. Chief of Staff, Palmer Lutheran Health Center, West Union, IA, p. A228
RASOR, Linda, R.N. Chief Executive Officer, Plains Memorial Hospital, Dimmitt, TX, p. A594
RASPER, Deborah Y., FACHE Administrator, St. Vincent Mercy Hospital, Elwood, IN, p. A200
RASTER, Robert, M.D. Medical Director, Michiana Behavioral Health Center, Plymouth, IN, p. A210
RATCLIFF, David, M.D. Chief Medical Affairs, Washington Regional Medical Center, Fayetteville, AR, p. A44
RATCLIFF, Paul, Director Information Services, Baylor Medical Center at Carrollton, Carrollton, TX, p. A586
RATCLIFFE, Alma, M.D. Executive Vice President Medical Staff and Business Development, Saint Clare's Health System, Denville, NJ, p. A403
RATCLIFFE, Denise, Executive Vice President and Chief Operating Officer, Christian Health Care Center, Wyckoff, NJ, p. A412
RATH, Marilyn, Co–Director Management Information Systems and Chief Information Officer, Day Kimball Hospital, Putnam, CT, p. A111
RATHBUN, Lori, Vice President Operations, Mercy Medical Center–Centerville, Centerville, IA, p. A216
RATLIFF, Ada, Chief Information Officer, Patient's Choice Medical Center of Claiborne County, Port Gibson, MS, p. A352
RATLIFF, Kim, Director Health Information Management, Southwestern Virginia Mental Health Institute, Marion, VA, p. A651
RATLIFF, Maggie, Chief Information Officer, St. Joseph Medical Center, Kansas City, MO, p. A362
RATLIFF, Steve, Director Information, Guadalupe Regional Medical Center, Seguin, TX, p. A627
RATLIFF, Thomas W., M.D. President Medical Staff, Saint Francis Hospital–Bartlett, Bartlett, TN, p. A562
RATLIFFE, Kathy, Director Human Resources, Tuality Healthcare, Hillsboro, OR, p. A511
RATNAKAR, Nitesh, M.D. Chief Medical Officer, Davis Memorial Hospital, Elkins, WV, p. A671
RATNER, Jeffrey, M.D. Senior Vice President Medical Affairs, Mount Nittany Medical Center, State College, PA, p. A539
RATTRAY, Cindy Stewart, Director Human Resources, Jewish Hospital–Shelbyville, Shelbyville, KY, p. A259
RATTRAY, Scott, Vice President and Chief Information Officer, Saint Joseph's Hospital of Atlanta, Atlanta, GA, p. A146
RAU, John, President and Chief Executive Officer, Stevens Community Medical Center, Morris, MN, p. A336
RAU, Robin, Chief Executive Officer, Miller County Hospital, Colquitt, GA, p. A149
RAUCH, Deena R., R.N. Chief Nursing Officer, Gritman Medical Center, Moscow, ID, p. A169
RAUCH, Scott C., Vice President Human Resources, Reid Hospital and Health Care Services, Richmond, IN, p. A211
RAUCH, Scott L., M.D. President, McLean Hospital, Belmont, MA, p. A295
RAUCHER, Beth, M.D. Senior Vice President and Chief Medical Officer, Lutheran Medical Center,, NY, p. A434
RAUH, Cindy, R.N. Vice President and Chief Nursing Officer, Duncan Regional Hospital, Duncan, OK, p. A495
RAUPERS, Debra, MSN Chief Nursing Officer, Corning Hospital, Corning, NY, p. A424
RAUSCH, Steve, Manager Information Technology, Hillsdale Community Health Center, Hillsdale, MI, p. A315
RAUSCHER, Andrew, M.D. Medical Director, Little Falls Hospital, Little Falls, NY, p. A428
RAVELING, Lynn, Chief Financial Officer, Pocahontas Community Hospital, Pocahontas, IA, p. A225
RAVI, Nathan, M.D. Chief of Staff, Veterans Affairs Medical Center, Saint Louis, MO, p. A370
RAVLIN, Suzanne M., Director Human Resources, Katherine Shaw Bethea Hospital, Dixon, IL, p. A180
RAWLINGS, Linda, Director Human Resources and Personnel, Three Rivers Hospital, Waverly, TN, p. A576
RAWSON, Richard L.
  President and Chief Executive Officer, Hanford Community Medical Center, Hanford, CA, p. A64
  Chief Executive Officer, Loma Linda University Medical Center–Murrieta, Murrieta, CA, p. A76
RAWSTHORNE, Larry, M.D. Senior Vice President Medical Affairs, Sparrow Hospital, Lansing, MI, p. A317
RAY, Beverly, Director Human Resources, Dyersburg Regional Medical Center, Dyersburg, TN, p. A565
RAY, Denise, Senior Vice President and Chief Operating Officer, Piedmont Hospital, Atlanta, GA, p. A146
RAY, Donald, Vice President of Operations, Maryland General Hospital, Baltimore, MD, p. A288
RAY, Dwayne, Chief Financial Officer, Medical Center of McKinney, McKinney, TX, p. A616
RAY, Elaine, Administrator, Choate Mental Health Center, Anna, IL, p. A172
RAY, Holly, Director Human Resources, Mid–America Rehabilitation Hospital, Shawnee Mission, KS, p. A243
RAY, Jerilyn, Manager Human Resources, St. Elizabeth Hospital, Enumclaw, WA, p. A661
RAY, Kirk M., Chief Executive Officer, DeKalb Health, Auburn, IN, p. A197
RAY, Lisa, R.N. Vice President, Patient Care Services, Murray–Calloway County Hospital, Murray, KY, p. A257
RAY, Rachel, Chief Financial Officer, Unity Medical Center, Grafton, ND, p. A466
RAY, Roger A., M.D. Executive Vice President and Chief Medical Officer, Carolinas Medical Center, Charlotte, NC, p. A450
RAY, Todd A., Director Human Resources, Greenville Regional Hospital, Greenville, IL, p. A183
RAYL, Cheryl, Chief Executive Officer, Allegiance Specialty Hospital Permian Basin, Midland, TX, p. A616
RAYMER, Chris, R.N
  Chief Operating Officer and Chief Nursing Officer, Great River Medical Center, Blytheville, AR, p. A42
  Interim Chief Operating Officer, South Mississippi County Regional Medical Center, Osceola, AR, p. A50
RAYMOND, Jane, Vice President and Chief Operating Officer, Reston Hospital Center, Reston, VA, p. A654
RAYMOND, Michael, M.D. Chief Medical Officer, NorthShore University Health System Skokie Hospital, Skokie, IL, p. A194
RAYMOND, Mindy, Vice President Human Resources, Boca Raton Regional Hospital, Boca Raton, FL, p. A118
RAYMOND, Scott, Director Information Systems, Orange Coast Memorial Medical Center, Fountain Valley, CA, p. A61
RAYNAUD, Eugene
  Administrator, Shriners Hospitals for Children, Spokane, WA, p. A667
  Interim Chief Executive Officer and Administrator, Shriners Hospitals for Children, Los Angeles, Los Angeles, CA, p. A72
RAYNER, Evan J., Chief Executive Officer, Healdsburg District Hospital, Healdsburg, CA, p. A64
RAYNER, Susan, M.D. Executive Vice President, Schwab Rehabilitation Hospital, Chicago, IL, p. A178
RAYNES, Anthony, M.D. Psychiatrist in Chief, Arbour H. R. I. Hospital, Brookline, MA, p. A298
RAYNES, Scott, President and Chief Executive Officer, Northcrest Medical Center, Springfield, TN, p. A576
RAYUDU, Subbu, M.D. Chief of Staff, Alliance HealthCare System, Holly Springs, MS, p. A347
RAZAGHI, Ahmad, Chief Executive Officer, Sage Memorial Hospital, Ganado, AZ, p. A32
RAZAK, Mohamed, M.D. Chief of Staff, Heart of Florida Regional Medical Center, Davenport, FL, p. A121
RAZMIC, Tammy, Associate Administrator Finance and Chief Financial Officer, Inova Mount Vernon Hospital, Alexandria, VA, p. A645
RAZO, Virginia, Chief Operating Officer, Incline Village Community Hospital, Incline Village, NV, p. A392
RAZVI, Mohammed, M.D. Chief of Staff, Iroquois Memorial Hospital and Resident Home, Watseka, IL, p. A195
REA, Jerry A., Ph.D. Superintendent, Parsons State Hospital and Training Center, Parsons, KS, p. A241
REA, Noel, Chief Executive Officer, Wrangell Medical Center, Wrangell, AK, p. A30
READ, Richard
  Chief Financial Officer, Haywood Park Community Hospital, Brownsville, TN, p. A562
  Chief Financial Officer, Regional Hospital of Jackson, Jackson, TN, p. A567
READ, Susan, Director Information Technology Support, Great Bend Regional Hospital, Great Bend, KS, p. A233
READING, Matt, Director Human Resources, Indiana Regional Medical Center, Indiana, PA, p. A525
READY, Janet L., President and Chief Operating Officer, Vassar Brothers Medical Center, Poughkeepsie, NY, p. A441
REAGAN, David, M.D. Chief of Staff, James H. Quillen Veterans Affairs Medical Center, Mountain Home, TN, p. A572
REAGAN Jr., James H., Ph.D. Chief Executive Officer, Morris County Hospital, Council Grove, KS, p. A232
REAL, Lawrence A., M.D. Medical Director, Belmont Center for Comprehensive Treatment, Philadelphia, PA, p. A531
REALE, Kelli, Vice President Human Resources, Magee–Womens Hospital of UPMC, Pittsburgh, PA, p. A535
REAM, Tom, Regional Chief Information Officer, Sutter Auburn Faith Hospital, Auburn, CA, p. A54
REAMER, Roger J., Chief Executive Officer, Memorial Health Care Systems, Seward, NE, p. A389
REANDEAU, Michael
  Chief Information Officer, Mills–Peninsula Health Services, Burlingame, CA, p. A56
  Regional Chief Information Officer, Sutter Maternity and Surgery Center of Santa Cruz, Santa Cruz, CA, p. A90
REANO, Paul, Chief Executive Officer, Atoka County Medical Center, Atoka, OK, p. A493
REARDON, Jerry, Director Information Systems, Catawba Valley Medical Center, Hickory, NC, p. A455
REBLOCK, Kimberly, M.D. Chief Operating Officer, The Children's Home of Pittsburgh, Pittsburgh, PA, p. A535
RECA, Sr., Thomas, Senior Vice President Finance and Chief Financial Officer, Staten Island University Hospital,, NY, p. A437
RECHSTEINER, Hans, M.D. Chief of Staff, Burnett Medical Center, Grantsburg, WI, p. A682
RECKDENWALD, Jeanine, Assistant Vice President Human Resources, Bristol Hospital, Bristol, CT, p. A108
RECKERT, Sandy, Director Communications and Public Affairs, Johns Hopkins Bayview Medical Center, Baltimore, MD, p. A287
RECUPERO, David, Chief Financial Officer, San Gorgonio Memorial Hospital, Banning, CA, p. A55
RECUPERO, Patricia R., JD, President and Chief Executive Officer, Butler Hospital, Providence, RI, p. A544
RED THUNDER, Charlene, Chief Executive Officer, U. S. Public Health Service Indian Hospital, Eagle Butte, SD, p. A556
REDD, Dakota, R.N
  Chief Clinical Officer, Kindred Hospital–St. Louis, Saint Louis, MO, p. A368
  Chief Nursing Officer, The Rehabilitation Institute of St. Louis, Saint Louis, MO, p. A370
REDD, James, M.D. Chief Medical Officer, San Juan Hospital, Monticello, UT, p. A638
REDDEN, Robert, Site Director Information Technology, Community Hospital of San Bernardino, San Bernardino, CA, p. A84
REDDICK, Lisa, Director Organizational Resources, Tri–County Hospital, Wadena, MN, p. A341
REDDICK, Michelle, Director Human Resources, Turning Point Hospital, Moultrie, GA, p. A157
REDDICK, Shawn, Director Information Management, Flint River Community Hospital, Montezuma, GA, p. A156
REDDING, Lisa, Manager Human Resources, Morgan County ARH Hospital, West Liberty, KY, p. A259
REDDY, Dipak, Director Information Technology, Miracle Mile Medical Center, Los Angeles, CA, p. A70
REDDY, Krishna K., M.D. President Medical Staff, Lanier Health Services, Valley, AL, p. A26
REDDY, Lex, Chief Executive Officer, Chino Valley Medical Center, Chino, CA, p. A57
REDDY, Prem, M.D. Interim President and Chief Executive Officer, Prime Healthcare Services, Ontario, CA, p. B103
REDHORSE–CHARLEY, Gloria, Director Human Resources, Northern Navajo Medical Center, Shiprock, NM, p. A418
REDING, Janeen K., Director Human Resources, St. Anthony Hospital, Pendleton, OR, p. A513
REDINGTON, James, M.D. Chief of Staff, Bath Community Hospital, Hot Springs, VA, p. A650
REDMON, Gary, Chief Financial Officer, South Texas Regional Medical Center, Jourdanton, TX, p. A609
REDMOND, Michael, Senior Vice President and Chief Operating Officer, Crotched Mountain Rehabilitation Center, Greenfield, NH, p. A398
REDMOND, Paula, Controller, HEALTHSOUTH Tustin Rehabilitation Hospital, Tustin, CA, p. A93
REDUTO, Lawrence A., M.D. President and Chief Medical Officer, St. Joseph Hospital, Bethpage, NY, p. A421
REECE, Courtney, Chief Financial Officer, Piedmont Newnan Hospital, Newnan, GA, p. A157
REECE, Jeff, Chief Executive Officer, Chesterfield General Hospital, Cheraw, SC, p. A547
REECE, Morris A.
  EVP/COO, Laird Hospital, Union, MS, p. A353
  Executive Vice President and Chief Operating Officer, Rush Foundation Hospital, Meridian, MS, p. A350
REECER, Jeff, Chief Operating Officer, Texas Health Presbyterian Hospital Denton, Denton, TX, p. A594


**A912** Index of Health Care Professionals

Index of Health Care Professionals / Reites

Index of Health Care Professionals


REED, Cindy, Director Community Relations, Austin State Hospital, Austin, TX, p. A580
REED, Dianne, Director Information Systems, Higgins General Hospital, Bremen, GA, p. A148
REED, Fred, M.D. Chief of Staff, Lincoln Hospital, Davenport, WA, p. A660
REED, Gregory C., FACHE Chief Executive Officer, United General Hospital, Sedro Woolley, WA, p. A666
REED, Hollis, M.D. Chief of Staff, Veterans Affairs Medical Center – Alexandria, Pineville, LA, p. A276
REED, Jan A., CPA, Administrator and Chief Executive Officer, Electra Memorial Hospital, Electra, TX, p. A597
REED, Jason, President and Chief Executive Officer, Oceans Healthcare, Lake Charles, LA, p. B97
REED, John E., M.D. Medical Director, Baptist Memorial Hospital–Golden Triangle, Columbus, MS, p. A345
REED, Karen
Chief Nursing Officer, Pioneer Memorial Hospital, Prineville, OR, p. A514
Interim Chief Nursing Officer, St. Charles Medical Center – Redmond, Redmond, OR, p. A515
REED, Kathleen, Manager Human Resources, Missouri Baptist Sullivan Hospital, Sullivan, MO, p. A371
REED, Kirby, Director Information Systems, Jasper County Hospital, Rensselaer, IN, p. A211
REED, Leslie, Chief Financial Officer, Wright Memorial Hospital, Trenton, MO, p. A372
REED, Lester, M.D
Vice President Medical Affairs and Acute Care, MultiCare Mary Bridge Children's Hospital and Health Center, Tacoma, WA, p. A668
Vice President Medical Affairs and Acute Care, MultiCare Tacoma General Hospital, Tacoma, WA, p. A668
REED, Linda
Vice President and Chief Information Officer, Morristown Medical Center, Morristown, NJ, p. A406
Vice President Information Systems and Chief Information Officer, Newton Medical Center, Newton, NJ, p. A407
Vice President and Chief Information Officer, Overlook Medical Center, Summit, NJ, p. A410
REED, Marie, Director Human Resources, Antelope Valley Hospital, Lancaster, CA, p. A67
REED, Rick, Interim Chief Executive Officer, Palm Drive Hospital, Sebastopol, CA, p. A90
REED, Ronald R., President and Chief Executive Officer, Mercy Iowa City, Iowa City, IA, p. A221
REED, Victoria L., FACHE Chief Executive Officer, James B. Haggin Memorial Hospital, Harrodsburg, KY, p. A251
REEDER, Robert, FACHE Chief Executive Officer, Columbia Basin Hospital, Ephrata, WA, p. A661
REEDER, Wendy, R.N. Chief Nursing Officer, Harrison Memorial Hospital, Cynthiana, KY, p. A249
REEF, Marion, Chief Executive Officer, Select Specialty Hospital–Winston–Salem, Winston–Salem, NC, p. A463
REEFER, John C., M.D. Director, Butler Health System, Butler, PA, p. A519
REEG, Kari, Manager Human Resources, Genoa Community Hospital, Genoa, NE, p. A384
REEL, Stephanie L., Vice President Information Services, Johns Hopkins Hospital, Baltimore, MD, p. A287
REES, Adam, Executive Vice President and Chief Administrative Officer, Mayo Clinic Health System in Austin, Austin, MN, p. A328
REES, Brenda, Chief Financial Officer, Memorial Hospital of Carbon County, Rawlins, WY, p. A697
REES, Elizabeth, Chief Clinical Officer, Specialty Hospital of Albuquerque, Albuquerque, NM, p. A415
REES, Jeff, Director Information Systems, Bacharach Institute for Rehabilitation, Pomona, NJ, p. A409
REES, Matthew, Chief Executive Officer, Mayers Memorial Hospital District, Fall River Mills, CA, p. A60
REESE, Bert
Chief Information Officer, Sentara Leigh Hospital, Norfolk, VA, p. A652
Chief Information Officer, Sentara Norfolk General Hospital, Norfolk, VA, p. A653
Chief Information Officer, Sentara Princess Anne Hospital, Virginia Beach, VA, p. A657
REESE, Kathie, Administrator, Dubuis Hospital of Paris, Paris, TX, p. A620
REESE, Linda, Administrator, Telecare Heritage Psychiatric Health Center, Oakland, CA, p. A77
REESE, Maryann, FACHE President and Chief Executive Officer, St. Elizabeth's Hospital, Belleville, IL, p. A173
REESE, Pamela A., FACHE Chief Clinical Officer, Citizens Memorial Hospital, Bolivar, MO, p. A355
REESE, Sandra, Administrator, Lower Umpqua Hospital District, Reedsport, OR, p. A515
REESE, Willis L., Administrator, Falls Community Hospital and Clinic, Marlin, TX, p. A615
REETZ, Brenda, R.N. Chief Operating Officer, Greene County General Hospital, Linton, IN, p. A207
REETZ, Renee, Director Human Resources, St. Mary's of Michigan Standish Hospital, Standish, MI, p. A323
REEVE, Jay A., President and Chief Executive Officer, Eastside Psychiatric Hospital, Tallahassee, FL, p. A140
REEVES, Amy D., Director Human Resources, Cedar Park Regional Medical Center, Cedar Park, TX, p. A587
REEVES, Carol, Interim Area Finance Officer, Santa Clara Medical Center, Santa Clara, CA, p. A90
REEVES, Cory, Chief Financial Officer, Gordon Hospital, Calhoun, GA, p. A148
REEVES, Jennifer, Chief Nursing Officer, Texas Specialty Hospital at Lubbock, Lubbock, TX, p. A614
REEVES, Katy, Vice President Human Resources, Fauquier Hospital, Warrenton, VA, p. A657
REEVES, Kaylene, Director, Tahoe Pacific Hospitals, Reno, NV, p. A395
REEVES, Mike
Vice President, St. John Medical Center, Tulsa, OK, p. A507
Chief Information Officer, St. John Owasso, Owasso, OK, p. A503
REEVES, Pamela, M.D. Director, John D. Dingell Veterans Affairs Medical Center, Detroit, MI, p. A311
REEVES, Rachel, Manager Human Resources, Kindred Hospital Victoria, Victoria, TX, p. A633
REEVES, Steve, M.D. Chief Medical Officer, Greater Regional Medical Center, Creston, IA, p. A217
REEVES, William C., D.O. Chief of Staff, Mercy Hospital of Defiance, Defiance, OH, p. A479
REGAN, Christine, Vice President Human Resources, Massachusetts Eye and Ear Infirmary, Boston, MA, p. A297
REGEHR, Stan, President and Chief Executive Officer, Nemaha Valley Community Hospital, Seneca, KS, p. A243
REGIER, Donald, M.D. Chief Medical Officer, Sedgwick County Health Center, Julesburg, CO, p. A102
REGIER, Marion, Chief Executive Officer, Hillsboro Community Hospital, Hillsboro, KS, p. A234
REGLING, Anne, Interim Chief Financial Officer, Bronson Battle Creek, Battle Creek, MI, p. A308
REGULA, John
Chief Information Officer, Allied Services Rehabilitation Hospital, Scranton, PA, p. A537
Chief Information Officer, John Heinz Institute of Rehabilitation Medicine, Wilkes–Barre, PA, p. A541
REHM, Janice, Manager Human Resources, University of South Alabama Children's and Women's Hospital, Mobile, AL, p. A23
REHMER, Patricia, Commissioner, Connecticut Department of Mental Health and Addiction Services, Hartford, CT, p. B38
REICH, Joel R., M.D
Senior Vice President Medical Affairs, Manchester Memorial Hospital, Manchester, CT, p. A109
Senior Vice President Medical Affairs, Rockville General Hospital, Vernon Rockville, CT, p. A112
REICHARD, Steve, Manager Information Systems, Brigham City Community Hospital, Brigham City, UT, p. A637
REICHFIELD, Michael L., President, Doctors Hospital, Columbus, OH, p. A476
REICHMAN, Joseph, M.D. Vice President Medical Affairs and Clinical Effectiveness, Riverview Medical Center, Red Bank, NJ, p. A409
REID, Barbara S., Chief Financial Officer, Willingway Hospital, Statesboro, GA, p. A160
REID, Bev, Chief Financial Officer, St. Luke Hospital and Living Center, Marion, KS, p. A238
REID, Jim
Vice President and Chief Information Officer, Covenant Children's Hospital, Lubbock, TX, p. A613
Vice President and Chief Information Officer, Covenant Medical Center, Lubbock, TX, p. A613
REID, Karl, Chief Information Officer, Minneapolis Veterans Affairs Health Care System, Minneapolis, MN, p. A335
REID, Kenneth G., President and Chief Executive Officer, Carlinville Area Hospital, Carlinville, IL, p. A174
REID, Parlane, M.D. Chief Medical Officer, Sarasota Memorial Hospital, Sarasota, FL, p. A139
REID, Richard, Chief Financial Officer, Sonoma Valley Hospital, Sonoma, CA, p. A91
REID, Stephanie, R.N. Vice President of Quality and Chief Nursing Officer, Carroll Hospital Center, Westminster, MD, p. A294
REID, Timothy, M.D. Chief Medical Staff, Carroll County Memorial Hospital, Carrollton, MO, p. A357
REIDER, Rodney D., Chief Operating Officer, Saint Alphonsus Regional Medical Center, Boise, ID, p. A166
REIDY, Margaret, M.D. Vice President Medical Affairs, UPMC Presbyterian Shadyside, Pittsburgh, PA, p. A535
REIF, Richard A., President and Chief Executive Officer, Doylestown Hospital, Doylestown, PA, p. A522
REIFF, Troy T.
Corporate Director Operations, St. Vincent Seton Specialty Hospital, Indianapolis, IN, p. A205
Corporate Director Operations, St. Vincent Seton Specialty Hospital, Lafayette, IN, p. A207
REIFFENBERGER, Daniel, M.D. Chief Medical Staff, Prairie Lakes Healthcare System, Watertown, SD, p. A560
REIFSNYDER, Daniel, M.D. President Medical and Dental Staff, Lewistown Hospital, Lewistown, PA, p. A527
REILEY, Peggy J., R.N. Senior Vice President and Chief Clinical Officer, Scottsdale Healthcare Shea Medical Center, Scottsdale, AZ, p. A38
REILLY, Brian, Chief Financial Officer, Hahnemann University Hospital, Philadelphia, PA, p. A532
REILLY, Dennis A., President and Chief Executive Officer, Little Company of Mary Hospital and Health Care Centers, Evergreen Park, IL, p. A181
REILLY, Jeff
Senior Vice President Operations, Bon Secours Community Hospital, Port Jervis, NY, p. A440
Senior Vice President Operations, St. Anthony Community Hospital, Warwick, NY, p. A446
REILLY, John, M.D. Vice President Medical Affairs and Chief Medical Officer, Mercy Medical Center, Rockville Centre, NY, p. A442
REILLY, Richard, Deputy Executive Director, Syosset Hospital, Syosset, NY, p. A444
REILLY, Robert, Vice President and Chief Financial Officer, Anne Arundel Medical Center, Annapolis, MD, p. A287
REILLY, Tiffany, Director Human Resources, Childrens Care Hospital and School, Sioux Falls, SD, p. A559
REIMER, Arlo, M.D. Chief of Staff, Kearny County Hospital, Lakin, KS, p. A237
REIMER, Charm, Chief Financial Officer, Western State Hospital, Tacoma, WA, p. A668
REIMER, Lanny, M.D. Chief Medical Staff, Weston County Health Services, Newcastle, WY, p. A697
REIMER, Randy, Chief Financial Officer, Adventist Behavioral Health Rockville, Rockville, MD, p. A293
REIMER, Ronda, R.N. Chief Nursing Officer, Davis County Hospital, Bloomfield, IA, p. A215
REIN, Mitchell S., M.D. Chief Medical Officer, North Shore Medical Center, Salem, MA, p. A304
REINART, Greg, Chief Financial Officer, Hereford Regional Medical Center, Hereford, TX, p. A603
REINEKE, Marilyn, Director Human Resources, Mercy Hospital of Defiance, Defiance, OH, p. A479
REINER, Rosemary, MSN Vice President and Chief Clinical Officer, The Villages Health System, The Villages, FL, p. A142
REINERT, Chad, Director Information Technology, Hamilton General Hospital, Hamilton, TX, p. A602
REINHARD, Diane, R.N. Vice President of Patient Care Services, Craig Hospital, Englewood, CO, p. A100
REINHARD, James S., M.D. Commissioner, Virginia Department of Mental Health, Richmond, VA, p. B143
REINHARD, Russ, Chief Executive, Providence Willamette Falls Medical Center, Oregon City, OR, p. A513
REINHART, Jeffery, M.D. Chief of Staff, Drew Memorial Hospital, Monticello, AR, p. A49
REINKE, Bradley, M.D. Chief of Staff, Dameron Hospital, Stockton, CA, p. A91
REINKE, N. Sue, Vice President Human Resources, Lewistown Hospital, Lewistown, PA, p. A527
REISELT, Doug
Vice President and Chief Information Officer, Baptist Memorial Hospital – Memphis, Memphis, TN, p. A571
Vice President and Chief Information Officer, Baptist Memorial Hospital–Collierville, Collierville, TN, p. A564
REISLER, Harold, Controller, Methodist Hospital of Chicago, Chicago, IL, p. A176
REISMAN, Ernestine O., Vice President Human Resources, Down East Community Hospital, Machias, ME, p. A284
REISMAN, Ronald, M.D
Chief Medical Director, St. Vincent Seton Specialty Hospital, Indianapolis, IN, p. A205
rireisma@stvincent.org, St. Vincent Seton Specialty Hospital, Lafayette, IN, p. A207
REISNER, Monica, Director Human Resources Operations, Wilcox Memorial Hospital, Lihue, HI, p. A165
REISSENER, Nancy
Acting Director, James A. Haley Veterans Hospital, Tampa, FL, p. A140
Acting Director, Malcom Randall Veterans Affairs Medical Center, Gainesville, FL, p. A124
REISZ, Carol, Chief Financial Officer, North Caddo Medical Center, Vivian, LA, p. A279
REITER, Scott, D.O. Chief of Staff, Scheurer Hospital, Pigeon, MI, p. A320
REITES, Tammy, Vice President Patient Financial Services, Children's Hospital, New Orleans, LA, p. A274

REITINGER, Thomas A., Interim Chief Executive Officer, Sacred Heart Medical Center, Eugene, OR, p. A510

REITZ, Brent, Vice President and Administrator, Adventist Rehabilitation Hospital of Maryland, Rockville, MD, p. A293

REITZ, Judy A., Sc.D. Executive Vice President and Chief Operating Officer, Johns Hopkins Hospital, Baltimore, MD, p. A287

REITZ, Robert, Ph.D. Regional Executive Officer, Fulton State Hospital, Fulton, MO, p. A360

RELPH, Daren, Chief Executive Officer, Wayne County Hospital, Corydon, IA, p. A217

REMALEY, Anne, Vice President Human Resources, ACMH Hospital, Kittanning, PA, p. A526

REMARK, Christopher, Chief Operating Officer, Aultman Hospital, Canton, OH, p. A472

REMBECKI, Roger, M.D. Chief of Staff, Missouri Baptist Sullivan Hospital, Sullivan, MO, p. A371

REMBIS, Michael A., FACHE Chief Executive Officer, Hollywood Presbyterian Medical Center, Los Angeles, CA, p. A69

REMIGIO, Odalys, Assistant Vice President, Finance, Baptist Health South Florida, West Kendall Baptist Hospital, Miami, FL, p. A131

REMILLARD, Jean D., M.D. Chief Medical Officer/Chief Quality Officer, Lovelace Medical Center, Albuquerque, NM, p. A414

REMILLARD, John R., President, Aurelia Osborn Fox Memorial Hospital, Oneonta, NY, p. A439

REMINGTON, Amanda
Director Human Resources, Spalding Regional Medical Center, Griffin, GA, p. A153
Director Human Resources, Sylvan Grove Hospital, Jackson, GA, p. A154

REMSPECHER, Mark, Director Human Resources, Southeast Missouri Mental Health Center, Farmington, MO, p. A359

REMSTEIN, Robert, D.O
Vice President Medical Affairs, Capital Health Medical Center–Hopewell, Pennington, NJ, p. A408
Vice President Medical Affairs, Capital Health Regional Medical Center, Trenton, NJ, p. A411

RENDON, Eloise, Director Human Resources, Twin Cities Community Hospital, Templeton, CA, p. A92

RENEDO, David, M.D. Chief of Staff, St. Joseph Hospital, Bangor, ME, p. A281

RENEY, Michael, Chief Financial Officer, Brigham and Women's Hospital, Boston, MA, p. A296

RENFREE, Mark, Chief Financial Officer, La Rabida Children's Hospital, Chicago, IL, p. A176

RENIER, Hugh, M.D
Vice President Medical Affairs, Essentia Health Duluth, Duluth, MN, p. A330
Vice President Medical Affairs, Essentia Health St. Mary's Medical Center, Duluth, MN, p. A330

RENNALLS–ATKINSON, Angela, R.N. Interim Chief Executive Officer, Schneider Regional Medical Center, Saint Thomas, VI, p. A704

RENNEKER, Dave, Chief Financial Officer, HEALTHSOUTH Rehabilitation Hospital, Humble, TX, p. A608

RENNEKER, James M., MSN Chief Operating Officer and Chief Nursing Officer, Louis A. Weiss Memorial Hospital, Chicago, IL, p. A176

RENNER, Dianne, Director Human Resources, Logansport State Hospital, Logansport, IN, p. A207

RENO, III, William, M.D. President Medical Staff, Wesley Medical Center, Hattiesburg, MS, p. A347

RENSHAW, Dee, Chief Executive Officer, Henryetta Medical Center, Henryetta, OK, p. A497

RENSHAW, Preston, M.D. Chief Medical Officer, Avera St. Anthony's Hospital, O'Neill, NE, p. A386

RENTFRO, Donald, Chief Executive Officer, Natchez Community Hospital, Natchez, MS, p. A350

RENTSCH, Richard E., President, Stroud Regional Medical Center, Stroud, OK, p. A505

RENTZ, Norman G., President and Chief Executive Officer, Cannon Memorial Hospital, Pickens, SC, p. A553

REOHR, Sara, Regional Controller, West Gables Rehabilitation Hospital, Miami, FL, p. A132

REPAC, Kimberly S., Senior Vice President and Chief Financial Officer, Western Maryland Regional Medical Center, Cumberland, MD, p. A291

REPASS, Lois, Quality Assurance Specialist and Coordinator Performance Improvement, Northern Nevada Adult Mental Health Services, Sparks, NV, p. A395

REPINO, Thomas, Executive Director Ancillary Services, Connally Medical Center, Floresville, TX, p. A597

REPLOGLE, Raymond L., President and Chief Executive Officer, Continuous Care Centers of Tulsa, Tulsa, OK, p. A505

REQUIERME, Glenn P., Director Information Technology, Kindred Hospital–Baldwin Park, Baldwin Park, CA, p. A55

RERYCH, Stephen, M.D. President Medical Staff, Pleasant Valley Hospital, Point Pleasant, WV, p. A675

RESCH–SILVESTRI, Jennifer, Director Public Affairs, Fontana Medical Center, Fontana, CA, p. A61

RESENDEZ, James R., Chief Executive Officer, South Texas Regional Medical Center, Jourdanton, TX, p. A609

RESENDEZ, Linda, R.N. Chief Executive Officer, South Texas Health System, Edinburg, TX, p. A595

RESETAR, Gayle L.
Vice President and Chief Operating Officer, Georgetown Memorial Hospital, Georgetown, SC, p. A550
Chief Operating Officer, Waccamaw Community Hospital, Murrells Inlet, SC, p. A552

RESNEDER, Norma, Senior Vice President Human Resources and Organizational Development, Valley Presbyterian Hospital, , CA, p. A72

RESSLER, David R., Chief Executive Officer, Aspen Valley Hospital District, Aspen, CO, p. A97

RESSLER, Dennis, Chief Financial Officer, St. Joseph Hospital and Health Center, Kokomo, IN, p. A206

RESTREPO, Macarena, Manager Business Office, Sister Emmanuel Hospital, Miami, FL, p. A132

RESTREPO, Nicolas, M.D. Vice President Medical Affairs, Winchester Medical Center, Winchester, VA, p. A657

RESTUCCIA, Michael, Chief Information Officer, Hospital of the University of Pennsylvania, Philadelphia, PA, p. A532

RESTUM, William H., Ph.D. President, Rehabilitation Institute of Michigan, Detroit, MI, p. A311

RETALIC, Tammy B., R.N. Vice President Nursing and Patient and Family Centered Care, Hebrew Rehabilitation Center, Boston, MA, p. A297

RETTGER, Linda, M.D. President Medical Staff, Kane Community Hospital, Kane, PA, p. A526

RETTIG, Linda, Director Financial Services, Washington County Hospital, Washington, KS, p. A245

RETZLAFF, Nancy, Director Human Resources, OakBend Medical Center, Richmond, TX, p. A622

REULAND, Charlie, Sc.D. Executive Vice President and Chief Operating Officer, Johns Hopkins Bayview Medical Center, Baltimore, MD, p. A287

REUTER, Mark, M.D. Medical Director and Chief of Staff, Memorial Health Center, Medford, WI, p. A685

REVELS, Beverly, Director Human Resources, Sutter Amador Hospital, Jackson, CA, p. A65

REVERMAN, Larry, Director Information Systems, Clark Memorial Hospital, Jeffersonville, IN, p. A205

REVIEL, Jackie, R.N. Vice President Patient Care Services, Beauregard Memorial Hospital, De Ridder, LA, p. A265

REWERTS, Karen
Vice President Finance, SSM Cardinal Glennon Children's Medical Center, Saint Louis, MO, p. A369
Vice President Finance and Chief Financial Officer, SSM St. Clare Health Center, Fenton, MO, p. A359

REX–WALLER, John G., Chief Executive Officer, National Surgical Hospitals, Chicago, IL, p. B92

REXFORD, Linda, Director Human Resources, Weeks Medical Center, Lancaster, NH, p. A398

REXROAD, Ann, Director Information Technology, Grafton City Hospital, Grafton, WV, p. A672

REXWINKLE, Lori, Chief Nursing Officer, Coffeyville Regional Medical Center, Coffeyville, KS, p. A231

REYES, Arnold, Administrator, U. S. Penitentiary Infirmary, Lewisburg, PA, p. A527

REYES, Raul, M.D. Medical Director, San Juan City Hospital, San Juan, PR, p. A703

REYMAN, Reed, President and Chief Executive Officer, St. Joseph's Hospital and Health Center, Dickinson, ND, p. A465

REYNEN, Mark, D.O. President Medical Staff, Avera Queen of Peace Hospital, Mitchell, SD, p. A558

REYNOLDS, Angela D., Chief Financial Officer, Lewis–Gale Medical Center, Salem, VA, p. A655

REYNOLDS, Benjamin, Director Information Systems, Brookville Hospital, Brookville, PA, p. A519

REYNOLDS, Denise, Chief Nursing Officer, Memorial Hospital Miramar, Miramar, FL, p. A132

REYNOLDS, George, M.D. Vice President, Chief Information Officer and Chief Medical Information Officer, Children's Hospital and Medical Center, Omaha, NE, p. A387

REYNOLDS, Hope, Executive Director Human Resources and Support Services, Margaret R. Pardee Memorial Hospital, Hendersonville, NC, p. A454

REYNOLDS, James B., M.D. Medical Director, Northwest Missouri Psychiatric Rehabilitation Center, Saint Joseph, MO, p. A368

REYNOLDS, Jay, M.D. Chief Operating Officer and Chief Medical Officer, The Aroostook Medical Center, Presque Isle, ME, p. A285

REYNOLDS, Mark, Controller, Central State Hospital, Louisville, KY, p. A254

REYNOLDS, Phyllis, R.N. VP, Nursing, Beaumont Hospital Grosse Pointe, Grosse Pointe, MI, p. A314

REYNOLDS, Randee, Interim President, Parkview Adventist Medical Center, Brunswick, ME, p. A282

REYNOLDS, Ray, Chief Executive Officer, Glen Rose Medical Center, Glen Rose, TX, p. A601

REYNOLDS, Richard M., President and Chief Executive Officer, MidMichigan Health, Midland, MI, p. B90

REYNOLDS, Robert, Director Information Systems, Mary Rutan Hospital, Bellefontaine, OH, p. A470

REYNOLDS, Ronald J., President, Muncy Valley Hospital, Muncy, PA, p. A530

REYNOLDS, Rosalyne, Administrator, Northern Nevada Adult Mental Health Services, Sparks, NV, p. A395

REYNOLDS, Stephen Curtis, President and Chief Executive Officer, Baptist Memorial Health Care Corporation, Memphis, TN, p. B19

REYNOLDS, Teresa, Chief Operating Officer, MedWest – Haywood, Clyde, NC, p. A451

REYNOLDS, Terry, M.D. Chief of Staff, Southeast Georgia Health System Brunswick Campus, Brunswick, GA, p. A148

REYNOLDS, Todd, Chief Information Officer, Memorial Medical Center – Ashland, Ashland, WI, p. A678

REYNOLDS, Vance V., CPA, Chief Executive Officer, Texas Health Presbyterian Hospital–WNJ, Sherman, TX, p. A628

REYNOLDS–GOSSETTE, Youdie, Controller, Wilma N. Vazquez Medical Center, Vega Baja, PR, p. A704

REZAC, Pamela J., Regional President, Avera Sacred Heart Hospital, Yankton, SD, p. A561

RHEE, Carolyn F., Chief Executive Officer, LAC–Olive View–UCLA Medical Center, , CA, p. A70

RHEINHEIMER, Rick, Chief Clinical Officer, Kindred Hospital–Chattanooga, Chattanooga, TN, p. A563

RHINE, Kathleen, Vice President Administrative Services and Chief Operating Officer, St. Joseph Mercy Hospital, Ypsilanti, MI, p. A326

RHINEHART, Jennie R., Administrator and Chief Executive Officer, Community Hospital, Tallassee, AL, p. A26

RHOADES, Charles E., M.D. Chief Executive Officer, Kansas City Orthopaedic Institute, Leawood, KS, p. A237

RHOADES, Cory, Chief Financial Officer, Willamette Valley Medical Center, McMinnville, OR, p. A512

RHOADES, Mark, Vice President and Chief Human Resources Officer, Duncan Regional Hospital, Duncan, OK, p. A495

RHOADES, Shelly, Chief Financial Officer, Clarion Psychiatric Center, Clarion, PA, p. A520

RHOADS, Pam, Chief Financial Officer, Fairfax Hospital, Kirkland, WA, p. A662

RHODEN, Patty, Chief Financial Officer, Banner Estrella Medical Center, Phoenix, AZ, p. A35

RHODES, Eric, Assistant Vice President of Operations, Provena Covenant Medical Center, Urbana, IL, p. A195

RHODES, Helen, R.N. Associate Director Operations, Veterans Affairs Northern Indiana Health Care System, Fort Wayne, IN, p. A202

RHODES, J. Gary, FACHE Chief Executive Officer, Kane Community Hospital, Kane, PA, p. A526

RHODES, Kay, R.N. Chief Nursing Officer, Redmond Regional Medical Center, Rome, GA, p. A158

RHODES, Lee, Chief Executive Officer, Central Montana Medical Center, Lewistown, MT, p. A377

RHODES, Liz, Director Information Services, Specialty Hospital Jacksonville, Jacksonville, FL, p. A126

RHODES, Robert
Chief Information Officer, Houston Medical Center, Warner Robins, GA, p. A161
Director Information Systems, Perry Hospital, Perry, GA, p. A157

RHODES, Roger, Chief Executive Officer, Baylor Surgical Hospital at Fort Worth, Fort Worth, TX, p. A598

RHODES, Sally, MSN, Administrative Director, Institute for Orthopaedic Surgery, Lima, OH, p. A482

RHUDY, Kenneth D., Chief Executive Officer, Brooks County Hospital, Quitman, GA, p. A157

RIAL, Joanne, Chief Financial Officer, Cumberland Hospital, New Kent, VA, p. A651

RIALS, Joe, Director Fiscal Services, North Mississippi State Hospital, Tupelo, MS, p. A353

RIALS, Loren, Chief Financial Officer, Heartland Regional Medical Center, Marion, IL, p. A186

RIANO, Omaira D., Chief Nursing Officer, HEALTHSOUTH Sunrise Rehabilitation Hospital, Fort Lauderdale, FL, p. A123

RIAZ, Mohammad, M.D. Chief of Staff, Raulerson Hospital, Okeechobee, FL, p. A134

RICARD, Joan M., R.N. Chief Operating Officer, Southern Arizona Veterans Affairs Health Care System, Tucson, AZ, p. A40

RICARTTI, Rebecca R., Interim Director Human Resources, Garfield Medical Center, Monterey Park, CA, p. A75

RICCI, David A., President and Chief Executive Officer, Saint Michael's Medical Center, Newark, NJ, p. A407

RICCIO, John A., M.D. Chief Medical Officer, Auburn Community Hospital, Auburn, NY, p. A421

Index of Health Care Professionals / Rigdon

Index of Health Care Professionals

RICCIONI, Mich
Chief Financial Officer, Petaluma Valley Hospital, Petaluma, CA, p. A80
Chief Financial Officer, Santa Rosa Memorial Hospital, Santa Rosa, CA, p. A90
RICCITELLI, Anthony, Chief Operating Officer, Worcester State Hospital, Worcester, MA, p. A306
RICCITELLI, Vincent, Vice President and Chief Financial Officer, Hoboken University Medical Center, Hoboken, NJ, p. A404
RICE, Amy, Chief Financial Officer, Helena Regional Medical Center, Helena, AR, p. A46
RICE, Ann Madden, Chief Executive Officer, University of California, Davis Medical Center, Sacramento, CA, p. A84
RICE, Craig, Director Information, Schneck Medical Center, Seymour, IN, p. A211
RICE, David, M.D. Vice President Medical Affairs, Northport Medical Center, Northport, AL, p. A24
RICE, James W., Director, Veterans Affairs Medical Center, Iron Mountain, MI, p. A315
RICE, Mark, CPA Controller, Jersey Shore Hospital, Jersey Shore, PA, p. A525
RICE, Peter, M.D. Medical Director, PeaceHealth Ketchikan Medical Center, Ketchikan, AK, p. A29
RICE, R. Timothy, President and Chief Executive Officer, Cone Health, Greensboro, NC, p. A454
RICE, Thomas J., FACH
President and Chief Executive Officer, Englewood Community Hospital, Englewood, FL, p. A122
President and Chief Executive Officer, Fawcett Memorial Hospital, Port Charlotte, FL, p. A136
RICE, Thomas R., FACHE President and Chief Operating Officer, Southern Plains Medical Group, Oklahoma City, OK, p. B120
RICE, Tim, President and Chief Executive Officer, Lakewood Health System, Staples, MN, p. A340
RICH, Dan, Director Finance, Texas Health Presbyterian Hospital Allen, Allen, TX, p. A577
RICH, Jeri
Assistant Administrator and Chief Financial Officer, Hunt Memorial Hospital District, Greenville, TX, p. A602
Assistant Administrator and Chief Financial Officer, Hunt Regional Community Hospital, Commerce, TX, p. A588
RICH, John, System Director Information Technology, Indiana University Health Arnett Hospital, Lafayette, IN, p. A206
RICH, Judy F., President and Chief Executive Officer, TMC Healthcare, Tucson, AZ, p. A40
RICH, Kori, Chief Executive Officer, The Physicians Centre Hospital, Bryan, TX, p. A586
RICH, Mark, Director Information Services, Ashley Regional Medical Center, Vernal, UT, p. A642
RICH, Philip, M.D. Chief Medical Officer, West Hills Hospital, Reno, NV, p. A395
RICH, Travis, Chief Executive Officer, GLOBALREHAB Hospital – San Antonio, San Antonio, TX, p. A624
RICH–MCLERRAN, Andrea, Chief Executive Officer, Cumberland River Hospital, Celina, TN, p. A563
RICHARD, Brent, Administrative Director Information Systems, Southern Ohio Medical Center, Portsmouth, OH, p. A487
RICHARD, Brian, Director Information Technology, Gaylord Hospital, Wallingford, CT, p. A112
RICHARD, Charlene, Director Human Resources, Harrington Memorial Hospital, Southbridge, MA, p. A304
RICHARD, Christina, Administrator, Kindred Hospital Tarrant County–Arlington, Arlington, TX, p. A579
RICHARD, Larry, M.D. Chief Medical Staff, Decatur County Hospital, Leon, IA, p. A222
RICHARD, Marilyn, Director Human Resources, Daviess Community Hospital, Washington, IN, p. A213
RICHARD, Scott, Vice President Finance and Chief Financial Officer, St. Elizabeth Hospital, Gonzales, LA, p. A267
RICHARD, Tim, IT Coordinator, Crawford Memorial Hospital, Robinson, IL, p. A192
RICHARDS, Amy, Accounting, Franklin County Memorial Hospital, Franklin, NE, p. A383
RICHARDS, Frank
Chief Information Officer, Geisinger Medical Center, Danville, PA, p. A521
Chief Information Officer, Geisinger Wyoming Valley Medical Center, Wilkes Barre, PA, p. A541
RICHARDS, Jaena, Chief Financial Officer, Powell County Medical Center, Deer Lodge, MT, p. A374
RICHARDS, Joan K., President and Chief Executive Officer, Crozer–Keystone Health System, Springfield, PA, p. B40
RICHARDS, Jon, Chief Financial Officer, Newport Medical Center, Newport, TN, p. A574
RICHARDS, Jonathan, Chief Financial Officer, David Grant Medical Center, Travis AFB, CA, p. A93
RICHARDS, Kyle, Chief Executive Officer, Waverly Health Center, Waverly, IA, p. A228
RICHARDS, Nate, Director Information Technology, Mitchell County Hospital Health Systems, Beloit, KS, p. A231
RICHARDS, Richard M., Chief Executive Officer, Northern Idaho Advanced Care Hospital, Post Falls, ID, p. A170
RICHARDS, Robert J., Vice President Finance and Chief Financial Officer, The Good Samaritan Hospital, Lebanon, PA, p. A527
RICHARDS, Sheila K., Director Human Resources, Baylor Medical Center at Carrollton, Carrollton, TX, p. A586
RICHARDS, Steve, M.D. Chief Medical Officer, Texas Scottish Rite Hospital for Children, Dallas, TX, p. A592
RICHARDS, Thom, Director Information Technology, Knoxville Hospital & Clinics, Knoxville, IA, p. A222
RICHARDS, Tim, Executive Vice President and Chief Financial Officer, KidsPeace Children's Hospital, Orefield, PA, p. A531
RICHARDS, Timothy, Chief Financial Officer, Roxborough Memorial Hospital, Philadelphia, PA, p. A533
RICHARDS, Tricia, Director Human Resources, Valley County Health System, Ord, NE, p. A388
RICHARDSON, April, M.D. Medical Director, Springbrook Behavioral Health System, Travelers Rest, SC, p. A554
RICHARDSON, David, M.D. Chief of Staff, Delta Medical Center, Memphis, TN, p. A571
RICHARDSON, Denise, R.N. Senior Vice President and Chief Nursing Officer, St. Barnabas Hospital,, NY, p. A436
RICHARDSON, Greg, Director Human Resources, Newton Medical Center, Covington, GA, p. A150
RICHARDSON, Irene, Chief Financial Officer, Memorial Hospital of Sweetwater County, Rock Springs, WY, p. A697
RICHARDSON, Jana
Interim Chief Financial Officer, Stone County Medical Center, Mountain View, AR, p. A49
Chief Financial Officer, White River Medical Center, Batesville, AR, p. A42
RICHARDSON, Jane, Vice President Human Resources, St. Vincent Heart Center of Indiana, Indianapolis, IN, p. A205
RICHARDSON, Janice, Chief Executive Officer and Managing Director, Rivendell Behavioral Health, Bowling Green, KY, p. A248
RICHARDSON, Judy, M.D. President Medical Staff, Mid–Columbia Medical Center, The Dalles, OR, p. A516
RICHARDSON, Karen K., Senior Vice President and Chief Financial Officer, Providence Health Center, Waco, TX, p. A633
RICHARDSON, Keith, Chief Financial Officer, Adventist La Grange Memorial Hospital, La Grange, IL, p. A186
RICHARDSON, Kevin, M.D. Chief of Staff, Southwest Mississippi Regional Medical Center, McComb, MS, p. A349
RICHARDSON, Mark D., FACHE President and Chief Executive Officer, Great River Medical Center, West Burlington, IA, p. A228
RICHARDSON, Matthew, Director Human Resources, HEALTHSOUTH Rehabilitation Hospital, Memphis, TN, p. A571
RICHARDSON, Michael, Director Information Services, Alaska Regional Hospital, Anchorage, AK, p. A28
RICHARDSON Jr., Nathaniel, Interim President, Parkway Medical Center, Decatur, AL, p. A18
RICHARDSON, Shazetta, Director of Nursing, Cypress Creek Hospital, Houston, TX, p. A604
RICHARDSON, Terika, M.P.H. Associate Administrator, Spotsylvania Regional Medical Center, Fredericksburg, VA, p. A648
RICHARDSON, Terrie, Coordinator Human Resources, Select Specialty Hospital–Augusta, Augusta, GA, p. A147
RICHARDSON, Timothy J., M.D. Chief of Staff, Veterans Affairs Medical Center, Togus, ME, p. A285
RICHARDSON, Todd, Regional Vice President Information Services, Mercy Hospital of Franciscan Sisters, Oelwein, IA, p. A224
RICHARDSON, William T., President and Chief Executive Officer, Tift Regional Medical Center, Tifton, GA, p. A161
RICHARDT, Claudia, Director Human Resources and Organization Development, St. Mary's Medical Center of Evansville, Evansville, IN, p. A201
RICHARDVILLE, Craig
Senior Vice President and Chief Information Officer, Carolinas Medical Center, Charlotte, NC, p. A450
Senior Vice President, Carolinas Medical Center–Mercy, Charlotte, NC, p. A450
Chief Information Officer, Carolinas Rehabilitation, Charlotte, NC, p. A450
Chief Information Officer, Cleveland Regional Medical Center, Shelby, NC, p. A460
RICHASON, Amie, Chief Human Resources Officer, Mercy Allen Hospital, Oberlin, OH, p. A486
RICHENS, Ken, Chief Information Officer, Central Valley Medical Center, Nephi, UT, p. A639
RICHER, R. David, Chief Executive Officer, Fairlawn Rehabilitation Hospital, Worcester, MA, p. A306
RICHERT, Ed, M.D. Chief of Staff, Modoc Medical Center, Alturas, CA, p. A53
RICHETTI, Michael, Chief Financial Officer, Chilton Hospital, Pompton Plains, NJ, p. A409
RICHEY, Cheryl, Director of Finance, St. Mary's Warrick Hospital, Boonville, IN, p. A198
RICHHART, David, Vice President Fiscal Services, Community Medical Center, Missoula, MT, p. A377
RICHIE, Kevin P., Senior Human Resources Business Partner, Saint Joseph – London, London, KY, p. A254
RICHMAN, Jonathan, M.D. Chief of Staff, Chase County Community Hospital, Imperial, NE, p. A384
RICHMAN, Timothy, President, Calumet Medical Center, Chilton, WI, p. A680
RICHMOND, Andy, Director Information Technology, Choctaw Memorial Hospital, Hugo, OK, p. A498
RICHOUX, Jacquelyn, Chief Financial Officer, Field Memorial Community Hospital, Centreville, MS, p. A344
RICHTER, Daniel, M.D. Chief of Staff, Alegent Health–Community Memorial Hospital, Missouri Valley, IA, p. A223
RICK, Bob, Vice President Information Technology, USMD Hospital at Arlington, Arlington, TX, p. A580
RICKARD, Debra, R.N. Chief Nursing Officer, Galesburg Cottage Hospital, Galesburg, IL, p. A182
RICKARD, Patricia, Vice President Human Resources, Central Vermont Medical Center, Berlin, VT, p. A643
RICKARD, Sheryl, Chief Executive Officer, Bonner General Hospital, Sandpoint, ID, p. A170
RICKER, Roger, Director Marketing and Public Relations, Peninsula Hospital, Louisville, TN, p. A570
RICKS, Cecil, Interim Chief Financial Officer, Madison Memorial Hospital, Rexburg, ID, p. A170
RICKS, Edward, Vice President and Chief Information Officer, Beaufort Memorial Hospital, Beaufort, SC, p. A546
RICKS, Michael, Chief Operating Officer, St. Joseph's Medical Center, Stockton, CA, p. A92
RICO, Richard, Vice President and Chief Financial Officer, Sky Lakes Medical Center, Klamath Falls, OR, p. A511
RIDALL, Jackie, Director Human Resources, Berwick Hospital Center, Berwick, PA, p. A518
RIDDELL, Barbara, Vice President Information Services, Atlantic General Hospital, Berlin, MD, p. A289
RIDDER, Terri, Director Human Resources, St. Francis Memorial Hospital, West Point, NE, p. A390
RIDDLE, Alecia, Manager Human Resources, Desert View Hospital, Pahrump, NV, p. A395
RIDDLE Sr., Brian L., FACHE Chief Executive Officer, Emanuel Medical Center, Swainsboro, GA, p. A160
RIDDLE, Kent, Interim President, Mary Free Bed Rehabilitation Hospital, Grand Rapids, MI, p. A313
RIDGE, Burt, Director of Information Technology, Mountain View Hospital District, Madras, OR, p. A512
RIDGWAY, Leah, M.D. President Medical Staff, Shawnee Mission Medical Center, Shawnee Mission, KS, p. A243
RIDINGS, Patty, Director of Nursing, Girard Medical Center, Girard, KS, p. A233
RIDLEY, Pam, Director Information Systems, Henry County Medical Center, Paris, TN, p. A574
RIDOUT, Les, Human Resources Officer, Ohio State University Medical Center, Columbus, OH, p. A477
RIEBER, Jim, Director Information Systems, Perham Health, Perham, MN, p. A337
RIECHERS, Thomas, M.D. Chief Medical Staff, Mercy Hospital Washington, Washington, MO, p. A372
RIEDEL, Jennifer, Chief Operating Officer, Fairmount Behavioral Health System, Philadelphia, PA, p. A532
RIEDLINGER, Joann, Vice President Nursing and Manager Information Systems, Bucyrus Community Hospital, Bucyrus, OH, p. A471
RIEG, Kevin, M.D. President Medical Staff, Via Christi Rehabilitation Center, Wichita, KS, p. A245
RIEGE, Michael J., Chief Executive Officer, Virginia Gay Hospital, Vinton, IA, p. A227
RIEGER, Bill, Chief Information Officer, Flagler Hospital, Saint Augustine, FL, p. A137
RIEGER, Michael S., Vice President and Chief Financial Officer, Mercy Medical Center, Canton, OH, p. A472
RIEGERT, Patricia, Director Fiscal Services, Danville State Hospital, Danville, PA, p. A521
RIEMER–MATUZAK, Stephanie J., Chief Executive Officer, Mercy Hospital Grayling, Grayling, MI, p. A314
RIESEBERG, Eric F., President, Specialty Hospitals of America, LLC, Portsmouth, NH, p. B121
RIESER, Michael, M.D. Medical Director, Ridge Behavioral Health System, Lexington, KY, p. A253
RIETSEMA, Wouter, M.D. Chief Quality and Information Officer, Champlain Valley Physicians Hospital Medical Center, Plattsburgh, NY, p. A440
RIGAS, Warren Alston, Executive Vice President and Chief Operating Officer, Floyd Medical Center, Rome, GA, p. A158
RIGBY, Holly, Senior Vice President and Chief Operating Officer, Windber Medical Center, Windber, PA, p. A542
RIGDON, Edward, M.D. Chief Medical Officer, Crossgates River Oaks Hospital, Brandon, MS, p. A344

RIGDON, Pam, Director Nursing, Laird Hospital, Union, MS, p. A353

RIGGALL, Ian, Manager Data Processing, Barstow Community Hospital, Barstow, CA, p. A55

RIGGLE, Linda, R.N. Vice President Patient Care Services and Chief Nursing Executive, French Hospital Medical Center, San Luis Obispo, CA, p. A88

RIGGS, Chris, Chief Financial Officer, Pender Memorial Hospital, Burgaw, NC, p. A449

RIGGS, Debra, Chief Financial Officer, Caverna Memorial Hospital, Horse Cave, KY, p. A252

RIGHTMYER, Gerald, M.D. Chief of Staff, Methodist Hospital, Henderson, KY, p. A251

RIGNEY, Alice, Chief Human Resources Officer, Abbeville Area Medical Center, Abbeville, SC, p. A546

RIGSBEE, Cristina, Chief Operating Officer, Granville Health System, Oxford, NC, p. A458

RIGSBY, Brent, Chief Financial Officer, Southwest Georgia Regional Medical Center, Cuthbert, GA, p. A150

RIGSBY, Diane, Chief Information Officer, Capital Hospice, Arlington, VA, p. A645

RIGSBY, Jimmy, Chief Executive Officer, Campbellton Graceville Hospital, Graceville, FL, p. A124

RIKER, Sharon, Manager Data Processing, Okmulgee Memorial Hospital, Okmulgee, OK, p. A502

RILEY, Betty, Chief Financial Officer, Ellsworth Municipal Hospital, Iowa Falls, IA, p. A222

RILEY, Colleen, M.D. Medical Director, Laguna Honda Hospital and Rehabilitation Center, San Francisco, CA, p. A87

RILEY, Daniel J., Chief Financial Officer, UAMS Medical Center, Little Rock, AR, p. A48

RILEY, Diane, Controller, HEALTHSOUTH Deaconess Rehabilitation Hospital, Evansville, IN, p. A201

RILEY, Doug, Director Information Services, Skagit Valley Hospital, Mount Vernon, WA, p. A663

RILEY, Edward E., Chief Executive Officer, Greenwood County Hospital, Eureka, KS, p. A233

RILEY, Joe B., President and Chief Executive Officer, Jackson Hospital and Clinic, Montgomery, AL, p. A24

RILEY, John, Chief Financial Officer, Harrisburg Medical Center, Harrisburg, IL, p. A183

RILEY, Kenneth, Director Information Systems, Wing Memorial Hospital and Medical Centers, Palmer, MA, p. A303

RILEY, Mike, Senior Vice President and Chief Operating Officer, Presbyterian–Orthopaedic Hospital, Charlotte, NC, p. A451

RILEY, Randy
Chief Financial Officer, Center for Behavioral Medicine, Kansas City, MO, p. A361
Fiscal and Administrative Manager, Northwest Missouri Psychiatric Rehabilitation Center, Saint Joseph, MO, p. A368

RILEY, Robert, Chief Financial Officer, Prince William Hospital, Manassas, VA, p. A651

RILEY, Susan, Director Human Resources, HEALTHSOUTH Rehabilitation Hospital of Miami, Miami, FL, p. A131

RILEY, Tim, Vice President, Hendrick Center for Extended Care, Abilene, TX, p. A577

RILEY, Jr., William, M.D. Chief of Staff, Memorial Hermann Sugar Land Hospital, Sugar Land, TX, p. A629

RIMA, Pat, Health Care Manager, State Penitentiary Hospital, Walla Walla, WA, p. A669

RIMAR, Stephen, M.D. Senior Vice President Medical Affairs, New York Hospital Queens,, NY, p. A435

RIMEL, Jeff, Chief Financial Officer, Cibola General Hospital, Grants, NM, p. A416

RINALDI, Anthony, Executive Vice President, Fairview Hospital, Great Barrington, MA, p. A300

RINALDI, Daniel, Chief Financial Officer, Ellis Hospital, Schenectady, NY, p. A443

RINAUDO, Helen, Vice President Human Resources, Saint Francis Hospital and Health Centers, Poughkeepsie, NY, p. A441

RINDFLEISCH, Jody, Manager Human Resources, Redwood Area Hospital, Redwood Falls, MN, p. A337

RINDLER, Kyle, Director Information Systems, Mercer County Joint Township Community Hospital, Coldwater, OH, p. A476

RINDLISBACHER, Diane
Manager Information Systems, American Fork Hospital, American Fork, UT, p. A637
Manager Information Systems, Orem Community Hospital, Orem, UT, p. A639
Director Information Systems, Utah Valley Regional Medical Center, Provo, UT, p. A640

RINEHART, Dallas, Director Operations and Information Services, Wellmont Bristol Regional Medical Center, Bristol, TN, p. A562

RINEHART, Rick, Chief Information Officer, Carle Foundation Hospital, Urbana, IL, p. A195

RINEY, Steven, Vice President Information Technology and Chief Information Officer, Methodist Medical Center of Illinois, Peoria, IL, p. A191

RING, Brian K., Chief Operating Officer, Henry County Hospital, New Castle, IN, p. A209

RING, Cynthia, Vice President Human Resources, Health Alliance Hospitals, Leominster, MA, p. A301

RING, Melissa, Ph.D. Chief Operating Officer, Southeast Missouri Mental Health Center, Farmington, MO, p. A359

RINGE, Kathy, Director Human Resources, Sage Rehabilitation Hospital, Baton Rouge, LA, p. A263

RINGER, Dave, M.D. Chief of Staff, Good Samaritan Hospital, Greensboro, GA, p. A153

RINGER, Joann, Chief Operating Officer, Miami Valley Hospital, Dayton, OH, p. A478

RINGLER, Judith A., Chief Information Resources Management, Veterans Affairs Medical Center, San Francisco, CA, p. A87

RINKS, Kevin, Chief Financial Officer, Walton Regional Medical Center, Monroe, GA, p. A156

RINTOUL, Alexander M., Chief Executive Officer, The Medical Center at Elizabeth Place, Dayton, OH, p. A478

RION, Trey, Chief Information Officer, West Calcasieu Cameron Hospital, Sulphur, LA, p. A278

RIORDAN, Michael C., President and Chief Executive Officer, Greenville Hospital System, Greenville, SC, p. B56

RIOS, Cindy, Chief Financial Officer, Medical Center of Southeastern Oklahoma, Durant, OK, p. A495

RIPPE, Diana, Financial Services Executive, Tri Valley Health System, Cambridge, NE, p. A382

RIPPERGER, Ted, Administrative Director Human Resources, Atrium Medical Center, Middletown, OH, p. A485

RIPPEY, Wesley E., M.D. Chief Medical Officer, Adventist Medical Center, Portland, OR, p. A513

RISBY, Emile, M.D. Clinical Director, Georgia Regional Hospital at Atlanta, Decatur, GA, p. A151

RISER, Donna, Administrator, S. E. Lackey Memorial Hospital, Forest, MS, p. A346

RISH, Matthew, Vice President Finance, St. Vincent Charity Medical Center, Cleveland, OH, p. A475

RISHA, Holly, Administrative Director Human Resources, College Hospital, Cerritos, CA, p. A57

RISINGER, Jennifer, M.D. Chief of Staff, Palmetto Health Richland, Columbia, SC, p. A548

RISK II, Carl W., Administrator, St. Vincent Jennings Hospital, North Vernon, IN, p. A210

RISLOW, Deb, Chief Information Officer, Gundersen Lutheran Medical Center, La Crosse, WI, p. A683

RISPOLI, Anthony C.
Vice President Finance, Anderson Regional Medical Center, Meridian, MS, p. A350
Vice President Finance, Anderson Regional Medical Center–South Campus, Meridian, MS, p. A350

RISSE, Thomas
Chief Financial Officer and Vice President Business Services, Kaiser Permanente Medical Center, Honolulu, HI, p. A163
Chief Financial Officer, Providence St. Peter Hospital, Olympia, WA, p. A663

RISSI, Daniel, M.D. Vice President, Chief Medical and Clinical Operations Officer, Lawrence & Memorial Hospital, New London, CT, p. A111

RITCHIE, Ann, Director Human Resources, Ochsner St. Anne General Hospital, Raceland, LA, p. A276

RITCHIE, Bruce, Vice President of Finance and Chief Financial Officer, Peninsula Regional Health System, Salisbury, MD, p. A294

RITCHIE, Jim, Director Management Information Systems, South Shore Hospital, Chicago, IL, p. A178

RITCHIE, Shannan, Chief Operating Officer, Lakewood Hospital, Lakewood, OH, p. A482

RITON, John, Director Information Services, Memorial Hospital of Tampa, Tampa, FL, p. A141

RITTENOUR, Melanie, Director Human Resources, Paulding County Hospital, Paulding, OH, p. A487

RITTER, J. Trees, D.O. Chief of Staff, French Hospital Medical Center, San Luis Obispo, CA, p. A88

RITTER, Randall, Associate Director, Veterans Affairs Ann Arbor Healthcare System, Ann Arbor, MI, p. A307

RITTER, Robert G., Associate Director, Harry S. Truman Memorial Veterans Hospital, Columbia, MO, p. A358

RITTMAN, Todd, Director of Nursing, Larue D. Carter Memorial Hospital, Indianapolis, IN, p. A204

RITZ, Robert P., Chief Executive Officer, St. John's Hospital, Springfield, IL, p. A194

RIVARD, Betty, Vice President Human Resources, Gillette Children's Specialty Healthcare, Saint Paul, MN, p. A339

RIVAS, Ramon Rodriguez, M.D. Medical Director, Hospital San Cristobal, Coto Laurel, PR, p. A701

RIVAS, Ray, Chief Financial Officer, Chapman Medical Center, Orange, CA, p. A78

RIVERA, Anthony, Director Human Resources, Hartgrove Hospital, Chicago, IL, p. A175

RIVERA, Catherine, Nurse Manager, Kindred Hospital–San Diego, San Diego, CA, p. A85

RIVERA, Christina, Director Human Resources, Southwest General Hospital, San Antonio, TX, p. A626

RIVERA, Cristina, Chief Executive Officer, Allen County Hospital, Iola, KS, p. A235

RIVERA, Enrique, Chief Financial Officer, Bella Vista Hospital, Mayaguez, PR, p. A701

RIVERA, Gabriel, Controller, First Hospital Panamericano, Cidra, PR, p. A700

RIVERA, Ivonne, Director Finance, Hospital Oriente, Humacao, PR, p. A701

RIVERA, Joe, Chief Information Technology Officer, Laredo Medical Center, Laredo, TX, p. A612

RIVERA, Jose Garcia, Director Human Resources, Hospital Buen Samaritano, Aguadilla, PR, p. A699

RIVERA, Luis, Director Human Resources, San Juan Capestrano Hospital, San Juan, PR, p. A703

RIVERA, Maria, Director Human Resources, Westside Regional Medical Center, Plantation, FL, p. A136

RIVERA, Marta, Executive Director, First Hospital Panamericano, Cidra, PR, p. A700

RIVERA, Philip, Chief Operating Officer, Memorial Medical Center, Las Cruces, NM, p. A416

RIVERA-JIMENEZ, Carmen E., Director Information Management, Hospital Buen Samaritano, Aguadilla, PR, p. A699

RIVERA-POL, Noriselle, Vice President Finance, Hospital Manati Medical Center, Manati, PR, p. A701

RIVERS, Guy, Chief Financial Officer, Columbia Memorial Hospital, Astoria, OR, p. A509

RIVERS, Kenneth I.
Chief Executive Officer, Inland Valley Medical Center, Wildomar, CA, p. A96
Chief Executive Officer, Rancho Springs Medical Center, Murrieta, CA, p. A76

RIVERS, Rose, R.N. Chief Nursing Officer, St. Vincent's Medical Center Riverside, Jacksonville, FL, p. A127

RIVES, Patricia, R.N. Chief Nursing Officer, Western Medical Center–Santa Ana, Santa Ana, CA, p. A89

RIVEST, Jeffrey A., FACHE President and Chief Executive Officer, University of Maryland Medical Center, Baltimore, MD, p. A289

RIZK, Magdy, M.D. Chief of Staff, West Houston Medical Center, Houston, TX, p. A608

RIZK, Norman, M.D. Interim Chief Medical Officer, Stanford Hospital and Clinics, Palo Alto, CA, p. A79

RIZK, Rob, Information Technology Director, Good Shepherd Health Care System, Hermiston, OR, p. A511

ROACH, David, Vice President Information Systems, Kadlec Medical Center, Richland, WA, p. A665

ROACH, Dee A., M.D. Chief of Staff, Mitchell County Hospital, Colorado City, TX, p. A588

ROACH, Donna, Chief Information Officer, Borgess Medical Center, Kalamazoo, MI, p. A316

ROACH, Geoff, Director Human Resources, Forks Community Hospital, Forks, WA, p. A661

ROACH, Maureen
Chief Financial Officer, Kindred Hospital Kansas City, Kansas City, MO, p. A362
Senior Chief Financial Officer, Kindred Hospital–St. Louis, Saint Louis, MO, p. A368

ROACH, Steven P., Chief Executive Officer, Nashoba Valley Medical Center, Ayer, MA, p. A295

ROADCAP, Carla, MSN, Chief Executive Officer, Good Shepherd Medical Center–Linden, Linden, TX, p. A612

ROADER, Charles, Vice President Finance, Edgerton Hospital and Health Services, Edgerton, WI, p. A681

ROARK, Chris, Chief Information Officer, Stillwater Medical Center, Stillwater, OK, p. A505

ROARK, Robert, Director Human Resources, Laughlin Memorial Hospital, Greeneville, TN, p. A566

ROARTY, Maureen, Vice President Human Resources, Nassau University Medical Center, East Meadow, NY, p. A425

ROAT, David, D.O. Acting Medical Director, Ancora Psychiatric Hospital, Ancora, NJ, p. A401

ROATH, Lee, System Chief Information Officer, Benefis Hospitals, Great Falls, MT, p. A376

ROATH, Shawna, Director Human Resources, Crittenton Children's Center, Kansas City, MO, p. A361

ROB, Lee, Director Human Resources, Pioneer Community Hospital of Aberdeen, Aberdeen, MS, p. A343

ROBB, Joy, Vice President Human Resources, Prairie View, Newton, KS, p. A239

ROBB, Lee, Director Human Resources, Covington County Hospital, Collins, MS, p. A345

ROBBINS, Dan, Information Technology and Account Executive, St. Vincent Medical Center, Los Angeles, CA, p. A72

Index of Health Care Professionals / Rock

Index of Health Care Professionals

ROBBINS, Danielle A., Vice President Human Resources, St. Catherine of Siena Medical Center, Smithtown, NY, p. A443
ROBBINS, Howard M., M.D. Senior Vice President and Chief Medical Officer, Martin Health System, Stuart, FL, p. A139
ROBBINS, James, M.D. Director, Phoenix Veterans Affairs Health Care System, Phoenix, AZ, p. A36
ROBBINS, Juanita D., Chief Operating and Development Officer, Kernan Orthopaedics and Rehabilitation, Baltimore, MD, p. A287
ROBBINS, Kenneth, M.D. Chief Medical Officer, Straub Clinic & Hospital, Honolulu, HI, p. A164
ROBBIO, Joan M., Senior Vice President and Chief Human Resources Officer, Lahey Clinic Hospital, Burlington, MA, p. A298
ROBEANO, Karen, MS Chief Nursing Officer, Riverside Methodist Hospital, Columbus, OH, p. A477
ROBERGE, Jeremy
Director Reimbursement, Androscoggin Valley Hospital, Berlin, NH, p. A397
Chief Financial Officer, Huggins Hospital, Wolfeboro, NH, p. A400
ROBERSON, Imelda, Director Finance, St. Vincent's St. Clair, Pell City, AL, p. A25
ROBERSON, Lynda, Senior Program Director, Rusk State Hospital, Rusk, TX, p. A623
ROBERSON, Madeleine, Chief Executive Officer, Presbyterian–St. Luke's Medical Center, Denver, CO, p. A100
ROBERTS, Alden, M.D. Chief Medical Officer, PeaceHealth Southwest Medical Center, Vancouver, WA, p. A668
ROBERTS, Allyson, CPA Chief Financial Officer, Nor–Lea General Hospital, Lovington, NM, p. A417
ROBERTS, Barbara, Chief Financial Officer, Veterans Affairs Medical Center–Louisville, Louisville, KY, p. A255
ROBERTS, Brad, Network Administrator, Swisher Memorial Hospital District, Tulia, TX, p. A632
ROBERTS, Cathy, Director Human Resources, Mercy Regional Medical Center, Durango, CO, p. A100
ROBERTS, Charles, M.D. Medical Director, Children's Mercy South, Overland Park, KS, p. A240
ROBERTS, Curt L., Chief Executive Officer, Select Specialty Hospital–Dallas, Carrollton, TX, p. A586
ROBERTS, Cyndi, Director Human Resources, Plaza Medical Center of Fort Worth, Fort Worth, TX, p. A599
ROBERTS, Floyd, M.D. Chief Medical Officer, Baton Rouge General Medical Center, Baton Rouge, LA, p. A262
ROBERTS, Glen, Chief Financial Officer, Delta Medical Center, Memphis, TN, p. A571
ROBERTS, Greg, Superintendent, Oregon State Hospital, Salem, OR, p. A515
ROBERTS, Jack, Director Information Systems, Twin County Regional Hospital, Galax, VA, p. A649
ROBERTS, John, Director Information Systems, Mena Regional Health System, Mena, AR, p. A49
ROBERTS, Jonelle A., Chief Financial Officer, Cleo Wallace Centers Hospital, Westminster, CO, p. A106
ROBERTS, Kenneth D., President, John T. Mather Memorial Hospital, Port Jefferson, NY, p. A440
ROBERTS, Kevin A., FACHE President and Chief Executive Officer, Glendale Adventist Medical Center, Glendale, CA, p. A63
ROBERTS, Lisa, Chief Operating Officer, Purcell Municipal Hospital, Purcell, OK, p. A503
ROBERTS, Mark, President, Muskogee Community Hospital, Muskogee, OK, p. A499
ROBERTS, Matthew S., Chief Executive Officer, The Medical Center of Southeast Texas, Port Arthur, TX, p. A622
ROBERTS, Michele, Hospital Recruiter, Kindred Hospital–Greensboro, Greensboro, NC, p. A454
ROBERTS, Mickey, Director Information Systems, Huey P. Long Medical Center, Pineville, LA, p. A276
ROBERTS, Pamela W., Chief Executive Officer, McNairy Regional Hospital, Selmer, TN, p. A575
ROBERTS, Paul, Chief of Staff and Deputy Commander for Administration, Reynolds Army Community Hospital, Fort Sill, OK, p. A497
ROBERTS, Phillip, Vice President Finance and Chief Financial Officer, Columbus Community Hospital, Columbus, WI, p. A680
ROBERTS, Robert C.
Vice President, Baptist Health Extended Care Hospital, Little Rock, AR, p. A47
Senior Vice President Financial Services, Baptist Health Medical Center – North Little Rock, North Little Rock, AR, p. A50
Vice President and Chief Financial Officer, Baptist Health Medical Center–Arkadelphia, Arkadelphia, AR, p. A42
Senior Vice President Financial Services, Baptist Health Medical Center–Little Rock, Little Rock, AR, p. A47
Senior Vice President, Baptist Health Rehabilitation Institute, Little Rock, AR, p. A48
ROBERTS, Roslyn, Manager, Northside Hospital – Cherokee, Canton, GA, p. A148
ROBERTS, Shane H., Chief Executive Officer, St. Luke Community Hospital, Ronan, MT, p. A378
ROBERTS, Teresa, Chief Financial Officer, Ringgold County Hospital, Mount Ayr, IA, p. A223
ROBERTSON, Bradley, Chief Financial Officer, Saint Francis Hospital, Memphis, TN, p. A572
ROBERTSON, Carla, Interim Chief Executive Officer, Saline Memorial Hospital, Benton, AR, p. A42
ROBERTSON, Casey, Chief Executive Officer, Woodland Heights Medical Center, Lufkin, TX, p. A614
ROBERTSON, Darcy, Financial Officer, Northern Cochise Community Hospital, Willcox, AZ, p. A41
ROBERTSON, Gary W., Chief Executive Officer, Ferry County Memorial Hospital, Republic, WA, p. A665
ROBERTSON, James, Chief Executive Officer, Mt. San Rafael Hospital, Trinidad, CO, p. A106
ROBERTSON, Jean, M.D. Chief Information Officer, Fairfield Medical Center, Lancaster, OH, p. A482
ROBERTSON, Jimmy, Chief Financial Officer, Baptist Memorial Hospital–Golden Triangle, Columbus, MS, p. A345
ROBERTSON, John L., Administrator, West Central Georgia Regional Hospital, Columbus, GA, p. A150
ROBERTSON, Larry, Chief Executive Officer, Texas Health Center for Diagnostic & Surgery, Plano, TX, p. A621
ROBERTSON, Laura, R.N
Chief Executive Officer, Banner Baywood Medical Center, Mesa, AZ, p. A34
Chief Executive Officer, Banner Heart Hospital, Mesa, AZ, p. A34
ROBERTSON, Michelle, R.N
President and Chief Executive Officer, Seton Highland Lakes, Burnet, TX, p. A586
President and Chief Executive Officer, Seton Medical Center Williamson, Round Rock, TX, p. A623
President and Chief Executive Officer, Seton Northwest Hospital, Austin, TX, p. A581
ROBERTSON, Mike, President and Chief Executive Officer, Piedmont Mountainside Hospital, Jasper, GA, p. A154
ROBERTSON, Patricia L., Executive Vice President, Mary Immaculate Hospital, Newport News, VA, p. A652
ROBERTSON, Steve
Vice President, Kapiolani Medical Center for Women & Children, Honolulu, HI, p. A163
Senior Vice President, Pali Momi Medical Center, Aiea, HI, p. A163
Executive Vice President and Chief Information Officer, Straub Clinic & Hospital, Honolulu, HI, p. A164
Executive Vice President Revenue Cycle Management and Chief Information Officer, Wilcox Memorial Hospital, Lihue, HI, p. A165
ROBERTSON, Tana, Chief Operating Officer, McCamey County Hospital District, McCamey, TX, p. A616
ROBERTSON, William G., President and Chief Executive Officer, Adventist HealthCare, Rockville, MD, p. B6
ROBERTSON–KECK, Karen, Vice President Human Resources, Medstar Franklin Square Medical Center, Baltimore, MD, p. A288
ROBERTSTAD, John R., FACH
President, Oconomowoc Memorial Hospital, Oconomowoc, WI, p. A688
President, Waukesha Memorial Hospital, Waukesha, WI, p. A692
ROBESON, Ricky
Administrator, AMG Specialty Hospital–Denham Springs, Denham Springs, LA, p. A265
Chief Executive Officer, AMG Specialty Hospital–Houma, Houma, LA, p. A267
ROBICHEAUX, Warren, Administrator, East Texas Medical Center–Quitman, Quitman, TX, p. A622
ROBINS, Scott, M.D
Chief Medical Officer, Covenant Children's Hospital, Lubbock, TX, p. A613
Chief Medical Officer, Covenant Medical Center, Lubbock, TX, p. A613
ROBINSON, Alan, Chief Financial Officer, Logan Regional Hospital, Logan, UT, p. A638
ROBINSON, Bradley, Chief Financial Officer, Evans U. S. Army Community Hospital, Fort Carson, CO, p. A101
ROBINSON, Chris, M.D. Chief of Staff, Lincoln County Medical Center, Ruidoso, NM, p. A417
ROBINSON, Dan, Vice President Operations, Poudre Valley Hospital, Fort Collins, CO, p. A101
ROBINSON, David, D.O. Medical Director, St. Joseph's Behavioral Health Center, Stockton, CA, p. A91
ROBINSON, Girard, M.D. Chief Medical Officer, Spring Harbor Hospital, Westbrook, ME, p. A286
ROBINSON, Glenn A., Chief Executive Officer, Hillcrest Baptist Medical Center, Waco, TX, p. A633
ROBINSON, Helen, Chief Clinical Officer, Ellenville Regional Hospital, Ellenville, NY, p. A425
ROBINSON, Jack, Chief Financial Officer, St. Joseph's Regional Medical Center, Paterson, NJ, p. A408
ROBINSON, James, Chief Financial Officer, George E. Weems Memorial Hospital, Apalachicola, FL, p. A118
ROBINSON III, James L., PsyD, Director, Veterans Affairs Medical Center, Memphis, TN, p. A572
ROBINSON, John, M.D. Clinical Director, U.S. Public Health Service Indian Hospital, Redlake, MN, p. A337
ROBINSON, Lance, Associate Director, Amarillo Veterans Affairs Health Care System, Amarillo, TX, p. A578
ROBINSON, Mark, Associate Administrator and Chief Financial Officer, Hazel Hawkins Memorial Hospital, Hollister, CA, p. A64
ROBINSON, Mark, FACHE Chief Executive Officer, Lake City Medical Center, Lake City, FL, p. A128
ROBINSON, Michael
Chief Executive Officer, Bon Secours Memorial Regional Medical Center, Mechanicsville, VA, p. A651
Executive Vice President and Administrator, Bon Secours–Richmond Community Hospital, Richmond, VA, p. A654
ROBINSON, Nellie C., R.N. Executive Vice President, Patient Services & Chief Nursing Officer, Children's National Medical Center, Washington, DC, p. A116
ROBINSON, Pat, Manager Accounting, St. Vincent Rehabilitation Hospital, Sherwood, AR, p. A51
ROBINSON, Patricia C., Chief Executive Officer, Edgefield County Hospital, Edgefield, SC, p. A549
ROBINSON, Paul H., M.D. Medical Director, American Fork Hospital, American Fork, UT, p. A637
ROBINSON, Phillip D., Chief Executive Officer, Lankenau Medical Center, Wynnewood, PA, p. A542
ROBINSON, Richard H., Chief Executive Officer, Yakima Regional Medical and Cardiac Center, Yakima, WA, p. A669
ROBINSON, Stephen, Chief Operating Officer, Lakeview Regional Medical Center, Covington, LA, p. A265
ROBINSON, Thaddeus, Chief Information Officer, Welch Community Hospital, Welch, WV, p. A676
ROBINSON, Tim, Executive Vice President, Chief Financial and Administrative Officer and Treasurer, Nationwide Children's Hospital, Columbus, OH, p. A477
ROBINSON, Vance, Chief Information Officer, Homer Memorial Hospital, Homer, LA, p. A267
ROBINSON, William, Director Human Resources, HEALTHSOUTH Rehabilitation Hospital of Erie, Erie, PA, p. A523
ROBINSON, William J., Senior Vice President and Treasurer, Shands at the University of Florida, Gainesville, FL, p. A124
ROBINSON–WHITE, Chakilla, Chief Operating Officer, Doctors Hospital at White Rock Lake, Dallas, TX, p. A591
ROBISCH, Christine, Senior Vice President and Area Manager, San Francisco Medical Center, San Francisco, CA, p. A87
ROBISON, Bruce, Vice President and Chief Information Officer, Lester E. Cox Medical Centers, Springfield, MO, p. A371
ROBISON, Deborah, R.N. Interim Chief Executive Officer, Atlanta Memorial Hospital, Atlanta, TX, p. A580
ROBISON, Keith, Chief Information Officer, Woman's Christian Association Hospital, Jamestown, NY, p. A428
ROBISON, Neely, Director Human Resources, The BridgeWay, North Little Rock, AR, p. A50
ROBISON, Wendell, M.D. Chief of Staff, Veterans Affairs Medical Center, Sheridan, WY, p. A697
ROBITAILLE, Mark E., President and Chief Executive Officer, Martin Health System, Stuart, FL, p. A139
ROBSON, Alan M., M.D. Senior Vice President and Medical Director, Children's Hospital, New Orleans, LA, p. A274
ROBSON, Marcia, R.N. Chief Nursing Officer, Ozarks Medical Center, West Plains, MO, p. A372
ROBSON, Melissa, President, Prince William Hospital, Manassas, VA, p. A651
ROBY, William J., Executive Vice President, Mountain Manor Treatment Center, Emmitsburg, MD, p. A291
ROCA, Robert, M.D. Vice President Medical Affairs, Sheppard and Enoch Pratt Hospital, Baltimore, MD, p. A289
ROCHE, Alana, Director Human Resources, Louisiana Medical Center and Heart Hospital, Lacombe, LA, p. A269
ROCHE, Kathleen M., R.N. Executive Vice President and Chief Operating Officer, Saint Francis Hospital and Medical Center, Hartford, CT, p. A109
ROCHE, Lori, Chief Operating Officer, Wyoming County Community Hospital, Warsaw, NY, p. A446
ROCHE, Richard J., Vice President Human Resources and Support Services, Memorial Health, Savannah, GA, p. A159
ROCHMAN, F. Daniel, M.D. President Medical Staff, Memorial Medical Center – Ashland, Ashland, WI, p. A678
ROCK, Brian, Director Information Systems, Culpeper Regional Hospital, Culpeper, VA, p. A647

Index of Health Care Professionals

Index of Health Care Professionals / Rock

ROCK, Michael, M.D
Chief Medical Officer, Mayo Clinic – Methodist Hospital, Rochester, MN, p. A338
Chief Medical Officer, Mayo Clinic – Saint Marys Hospital, Rochester, MN, p. A338
ROCK, Ron, Chief Executive Officer, Northwest Specialty Hospital, Post Falls, ID, p. A170
ROCKSMITH, Eugenio, M.D. Medical Director, HEALTHSOUTH Rehabilitation Hospital of Vineland, Vineland, NJ, p. A411
ROCKWELL, Jane, Director Support Services, North Metro Medical Center, Jacksonville, AR, p. A46
ROCKWOOD, John D., President, Medstar National Rehabilitation Network, Washington, DC, p. A116
RODDEN, Celeste, Chief Information Officer, Hillcrest Hospital Claremore, Claremore, OK, p. A495
RODDY, Thomas, Assistant Administrator, Sandhills Regional Medical Center, Hamlet, NC, p. A454
RODDY, Tim, M.D. Vice President Medical Affairs, Swedish/Edmonds, Edmonds, WA, p. A661
RODDY, Walt, Director Information Management Systems, Natchez Regional Medical Center, Natchez, MS, p. A351
RODEN, George
Vice President Human Resources, Mercy Hospital Aurora, Aurora, MO, p. A355
Vice President Human Resources, Mercy Hospital Cassville, Cassville, MO, p. A357
RODENBAUGH, Cathy, Director Human Resources, Holy Rosary Healthcare, Miles City, MT, p. A377
RODGE, Mark, Director Information Systems, Eaton Rapids Medical Center, Eaton Rapids, MI, p. A312
RODGERS, April, Vice President, Human Resources, Holy Name Medical Center, Teaneck, NJ, p. A410
RODGERS, Jamie, Chief Executive Officer, Covington County Hospital, Collins, MS, p. A345
RODGERS, Larry, Chief Executive Officer, Scenic Mountain Medical Center, Big Spring, TX, p. A584
RODGERS, Susan K., MSN Chief Operating Officer, Lovelace Medical Center, Albuquerque, NM, p. A414
RODGES, Teresa, Executive Director Marketing and Public Relations, McLaren Oakland, Pontiac, MI, p. A321
RODIER, James Barton, M.D. Chief Quality Officer, Health Central, Ocoee, FL, p. A134
RODOWICZ, Darlene, Chief Financial Officer, Berkshire Medical Center, Pittsfield, MA, p. A303
RODRIGUES, Pablo, M.D. Medical Director, Kindred Hospital–Amarillo, Amarillo, TX, p. A578
RODRIGUEZ, Alex
Vice President and Chief Information Officer, St. Elizabeth Edgewood, Edgewood, KY, p. A249
Vice President and Chief Information Officer, St. Elizabeth Florence, Florence, KY, p. A250
Vice President and Chief Information Officer, St. Elizabeth Fort Thomas, Fort Thomas, KY, p. A250
RODRIGUEZ, Alfred, M.D. President Medical Staff, Texas Health Presbyterian Hospital Plano, Plano, TX, p. A621
RODRIGUEZ, Ben A., Chief Executive Officer, Florida Medical Center, Fort Lauderdale, FL, p. A123
RODRIGUEZ, Candie, Director Human Resources, Hospital San Cristobal, Coto Laurel, PR, p. A701
RODRIGUEZ, Catherine, Chief Financial Officer, Ventura County Medical Center, Ventura, CA, p. A94
RODRIGUEZ, Edgardo, Director Management Information Systems, Auxilio Mutuo Hospital, San Juan, PR, p. A702
RODRIGUEZ, Enrique, M.D. Medical Director, llano Specialty Hospital of Lubbock, Lubbock, TX, p. A614
RODRIGUEZ, Jaime, Chief Financial Officer, San Juan City Hospital, San Juan, PR, p. A703
RODRIGUEZ, Jose Luis, Chief Executive Officer, Hospital Pavia–Santurce, San Juan, PR, p. A703
RODRIGUEZ, Jose O., M.D. Medical Director, Castaner General Hospital, Castaner, PR, p. A700
RODRIGUEZ, Joseph, Chief Executive Officer, Acadia Vermilion Hospital, Lafayette, LA, p. A269
RODRIGUEZ, Laura, Director Medical Records, Hospital Del Maestro, San Juan, PR, p. A703
RODRIGUEZ, Leticia, Controller, Ward Memorial Hospital, Monahans, TX, p. A617
RODRIGUEZ, Lizzette, Director Finance, Hospital San Francisco, San Juan, PR, p. A703
RODRIGUEZ, Luis, M.D. Chief of Staff, Vidant Roanoke–Chowan Hospital, Ahoskie, NC, p. A448
RODRIGUEZ, Marco, Chief Financial Officer, Navarro Regional Hospital, Corsicana, TX, p. A589
RODRIGUEZ, Mario, Chief Executive Officer, Laredo Specialty Hospital, Laredo, TX, p. A612
RODRIGUEZ, Maritza
Chief Financial Officer, Hospital Dr. Cayetano Coll Y Toste, Arecibo, PR, p. A700
Chief Financial Officer, Hospital Metropolitan, San Juan, PR, p. A703
RODRIGUEZ, Martha, Chief Financial Officer, Sunnyside Community Hospital, Sunnyside, WA, p. A667
RODRIGUEZ, Patricia, Senior Vice President and Area Manager, South Sacramento Medical Center, Sacramento, CA, p. A84
RODRIGUEZ, Ramon J., President and Chief Executive Officer, Wyckoff Heights Medical Center,, NY, p. A438
RODRIGUEZ, Roy, Chief Executive Officer, Promise Hospital of San Diego, San Diego, CA, p. A85
RODRIGUEZ, Rufus, M.D. Medical Director, Mayo Clinic Health System in Fairmont, Fairmont, MN, p. A331
RODRIGUEZ, Tony, Director Human Resources, South Texas Rehabilitation Hospital, Brownsville, TX, p. A585
RODRIGUEZ, Vilma, Director Human Resources, Hospital San Pablo Del Este, Fajardo, PR, p. A701
RODRIGUEZ, Wilfredo, M.D. Chief of Staff, Veterans Affairs Medical Center, Battle Creek, MI, p. A308
RODRIQUEZ, Daisy, Director Human Resources, Fort Duncan Regional Medical Center, Eagle Pass, TX, p. A595
ROE, Barbara, Vice President and Director Human Resources, Christus St. Vincent Regional Medical Center, Santa Fe, NM, p. A418
ROE, Paula, Assistant Vice President Operations, St. Elizabeth Grant, Williamstown, KY, p. A260
ROE, Timothy
Chief Information Officer, Hillside Rehabilitation Hospital, Warren, OH, p. A490
Chief Information Officer, Northside Medical Center, Youngstown, OH, p. A492
ROE, Timothy J., President and Chief Executive Officer, Rehabilitation Hospital of the Pacific, Honolulu, HI, p. A164
ROEBKEN, Curtis, M.D. Chief Medical Staff, Kentfield Rehabilitation and Specialty Hospital, Kentfield, CA, p. A65
ROEDER, Donna, Chief Financial Officer, Jackson County Regional Health Center, Maquoketa, IA, p. A223
ROEDER, Werner, M.D. Vice President Medical Affairs, Lawrence Hospital Center, Bronxville, NY, p. A422
ROEDERER, Chris, Vice President Human Resources, Tampa General Hospital, Tampa, FL, p. A141
ROEHRICH, Jeff, Chief Financial Officer, Spearfish Regional Surgery Center, Spearfish, SD, p. A560
ROEHRLE, Andreas, Director Finance, Sentara Williamsburg Regional Medical Center, Williamsburg, VA, p. A657
ROEL, Jennifer, Chief Executive Officer, Mountain Valley Regional Rehabilitation Hospital, Prescott Valley, AZ, p. A37
ROEMER, Dennis, Senior Vice President and Chief Financial Officer, Georgia Health Sciences Medical Center, Augusta, GA, p. A146
ROESER, William, President and Chief Executive Officer, Sparrow Ionia Hospital, Ionia, MI, p. A315
ROESLER, Bruce E., FACHE President and Chief Executive Officer, Mercy Medical Center–New Hampton, New Hampton, IA, p. A224
ROETMAN, James D., President and Chief Executive Officer, Pocahontas Community Hospital, Pocahontas, IA, p. A225
ROFF, Lynette A., Director, Veterans Affairs Eastern Colorado Health Care System, Denver, CO, p. A100
ROGALSKI, Robert, Chief Executive Officer, Excela Health, Greensburg, PA, p. B51
ROGALSKI, Ted, Chief Executive Officer, Mercer County Hospital, Aledo, IL, p. A172
ROGAN, Edie, Manager Human Resources, Eastern State Hospital, Williamsburg, VA, p. A657
ROGENESS, Graham, M.D. Medical Director, Clarity Child Guidance Center, San Antonio, TX, p. A624
ROGERS, Aaron, Chief Executive Officer, Mountainview Medical Center, White Sulphur Springs, MT, p. A379
ROGERS, Bard, M.D. Chief of Staff, Golden Plains Community Hospital, Borger, TX, p. A584
ROGERS, David, Chief Executive Officer, Sanford Medical Center Webster, Webster, SD, p. A561
ROGERS, Doris, Vice President Human Resources, Saint Luke's Hospital of Kansas City, Kansas City, MO, p. A362
ROGERS, Emily, Manager Human Resources, Community Westview Hospital, Indianapolis, IN, p. A204
ROGERS, Gregory H., President, MidMichigan Medical Center–Midland, Midland, MI, p. A319
ROGERS, James E., Executive Director, Sonoma Developmental Center, Eldridge, CA, p. A60
ROGERS, James H., FACHE Regional Vice President, HEALTHSOUTH Rehabilitation Hospital, Columbia, SC, p. A548
ROGERS, Jared, M.D. Chief Medical Officer, Provena Covenant Medical Center, Urbana, IL, p. A195
ROGERS, Joan, R.N. Chief Nursing Officer, St. Helena Hospital Clearlake, Clearlake, CA, p. A57
ROGERS, Joel, Chief Operating Officer, Minidoka Memorial Hospital, Rupert, ID, p. A170
ROGERS, Joseph J., Vice President and Chief Operating Officer, Redwood Memorial Hospital, Fortuna, CA, p. A61
ROGERS, Judith, R.N. Senior Vice President Operations, Holy Cross Hospital, Silver Spring, MD, p. A294
ROGERS, Kathy, Vice President Marketing, Conejos County Hospital, La Jara, CO, p. A103
ROGERS, Keith
Administrator, Advance Care Hospital, Hot Springs National Park, AR, p. A46
Interim Administrator, Advance Care Hospital of Fort Smith, Fort Smith, AR, p. A45
ROGERS, LaDonna, Director Human Resources, T. J. Samson Community Hospital, Glasgow, KY, p. A250
ROGERS, Lucy, Chief Information Resource Management Systems, Veterans Affairs North Texas Health Care System, Dallas, TX, p. A593
ROGERS, Mark E., Chief Executive Officer and Administrator, Pushmataha Hospital & Home Health, Antlers, OK, p. A493
ROGERS, Mark G.
Interim Vice President Finance and Chief Financial Officer, Genesis Medical Center, Illini Campus, Silvis, IL, p. A193
Interim Vice President Finance and Chief Financial Officer, Genesis Medical Center–Davenport, Davenport, IA, p. A217
ROGERS, Matt, Chief Financial Officer, Philhaven, Mount Gretna, PA, p. A529
ROGERS, Michael, Vice President Fiscal Services, Brattleboro Memorial Hospital, Brattleboro, VT, p. A643
ROGERS, Paul
Chief Financial Officer, Crittenden Regional Hospital, West Memphis, AR, p. A52
Chief Financial Officer, Mena Regional Health System, Mena, AR, p. A49
Chief Financial Officer, Mineral Area Regional Medical Center, Farmington, MO, p. A359
ROGERS, Randy, Chief Financial Officer, Vaughan Regional Medical Center, Selma, AL, p. A25
ROGERS, Rhonda, Chief Financial Officer, Nacogdoches Medical Center, Nacogdoches, TX, p. A618
ROGERS, Rich
Senior Vice President Support Services and Chief Information Officer, Cape Canaveral Hospital, Cocoa Beach, FL, p. A120
Senior Vice President Support Services and Chief Information Officer, Holmes Regional Medical Center, Melbourne, FL, p. A130
ROGERS, Richard, Administrator, Boscobel Area Health Care, Boscobel, WI, p. A679
ROGERS, Richard K., FACHE Vice President Human Resources, Wayne Memorial Hospital, Goldsboro, NC, p. A453
ROGERS, II, Robert T., M.D. Medical Director, Canton–Potsdam Hospital, Potsdam, NY, p. A441
ROGERS, Scott, Chief Operating Officer, Bear Valley Community Hospital, Big Bear Lake, CA, p. A55
ROGERS, Sherry L., MS Chief Nursing Officer, Redington–Fairview General Hospital, Skowhegan, ME, p. A285
ROGERS, Valerie J., Director of Nursing, William W. Hastings Indian Hospital, Tahlequah, OK, p. A505
ROGERS, W. Kent, Chief Executive Officer, Valley View Regional Hospital, Ada, OK, p. A493
ROGERS, William, Chief Medical Officer, Gilmore Memorial Regional Medical Center, Amory, MS, p. A343
ROGNESS, Robin, Vice President and Chief Financial Officer, Mercy Hospital of Folsom, Folsom, CA, p. A60
ROGOZ, Brian, Vice President Finance and Treasurer, The Hospital of Central Connecticut, New Britain, CT, p. A110
ROHAN, Colleen, Director Human Resources, Little Company of Mary Hospital and Health Care Centers, Evergreen Park, IL, p. A181
ROHAN, Heather J., Chief Executive Officer, Aventura Hospital and Medical Center, Aventura, FL, p. A118
ROHLAND, John, Director Information Technology, Tri–County Memorial Hospital, Whitehall, WI, p. A694
ROHRBACH, Dan D., President and Chief Executive Officer, Southwest Health Center, Platteville, WI, p. A689
ROHRBACH, William K., Vice President Fiscal Affairs, Memorial Hospital, Towanda, PA, p. A539
ROHRER, Harry
Chief Financial Officer, Bascom Palmer Eye Institute–Anne Bates Leach Eye Hospital, Miami, FL, p. A131
Chief Financial Officer, University of Miami Hospital and Clinics, Miami, FL, p. A132
ROHRER, Mark, M.D. Chief Medical Officer, Kindred Hospital–Boston, Brighton, MA, p. A298
ROHRICH, George A., Chief Executive Officer, Memorial Hospital, Craig, CO, p. A99
ROIG, Emilio, M.D. Network Medical Director, Devereux Hospital and Children's Center of Florida, Melbourne, FL, p. A130
ROIZ, JoAnn, Director Human Resources, HEALTHSOUTH Tustin Rehabilitation Hospital, Tustin, CA, p. A93
ROJAS, Anna, Chief Executive Officer, Kindred Hospital Tarrant County–Fort Worth Southwest, Fort Worth, TX, p. A599

A918 Index of Health Care Professionals

Index of Health Care Professionals

Index of Health Care Professionals / Rosno


ROSNO, Shawn, Deputy Director Operations, Elmira Psychiatric Center, Elmira, NY, p. A426
ROSS, Aletha, Vice President Human Resources, Ingalls Memorial Hospital, Harvey, IL, p. A183
ROSS, Candace, Coordinator Human Resources, HEALTHSOUTH Western Hills Rehabilitation Hospital, Parkersburg, WV, p. A674
ROSS, Carmella, Manager Human Resources, The Hospital at Hebrew Health Care, West Hartford, CT, p. A113
ROSS, Charles, M.D. Vice President Medical Affairs, Chilton Hospital, Pompton Plains, NJ, p. A409
ROSS, Craig A., M.D. Chief of Staff, College Hospital Costa Mesa, Costa Mesa, CA, p. A58
ROSS, David, President and Chief Executive Officer, St. Joseph Hospital, Nashua, NH, p. A399
ROSS, Hoyt, Chief Executive Officer, Kindred Hospital North Florida, Green Cove Springs, FL, p. A124
ROSS, Jacqueline, Chief Human Resources Officer, Veterans Affairs Medical Center, Spokane, WA, p. A667
ROSS, James E., Chief Operating Officer, Camden General Hospital, Camden, TN, p. A562
ROSS, James E., FACHE President and Chief Executive Officer, Chester River Health System, Chestertown, MD, p. A290
ROSS, James E., Vice President and Chief Operating Officer, Jackson–Madison County General Hospital, Jackson, TN, p. A567
ROSS, James H., Chief Executive Officer, University of Missouri Health Care, Columbia, MO, p. B139
ROSS, James H., Chief Executive Officer, University of Missouri Hospitals and Clinics, Columbia, MO, p. A358
ROSS, Jay, Chief Financial Officer, St. Joseph's Area Health Services, Park Rapids, MN, p. A337
ROSS, Jeffrey, M.D. Medical Director, Specialty Hospital of Albuquerque, Albuquerque, NM, p. A415
ROSS, John, Vice President, Franciscan St. Francis Health – Mooresville, Mooresville, IN, p. A209
ROSS, John M., Vice President Finance and Chief Financial Officer, Rochelle Community Hospital, Rochelle, IL, p. A192
ROSS, Joseph, Chief Financial Officer, Livingston Regional Hospital, Livingston, TN, p. A570
ROSS, Joseph P., President and Chief Executive Officer, Meritus Medical Center, Hagerstown, MD, p. A292
ROSS, Kathy
  Chief Information Officer, Providence Hospital, Mobile, AL, p. A23
  Chief Information Officer, Sacred Heart Hospital of Pensacola, Pensacola, FL, p. A136
ROSS, Kelly, M.D. Chief of Staff, Mitchell County Regional Health Center, Osage, IA, p. A224
ROSS, Lisa, Human Resources Officer, Greater Regional Medical Center, Creston, IA, p. A217
ROSS, Phil, Chief Executive Officer, Surgical Hospital of Oklahoma, Oklahoma City, OK, p. A502
ROSS, Robert, M.D. Chief of Staff, Ortonville Area Health Services, Ortonville, MN, p. A336
ROSS, Robert, Executive Vice President and Chief Operating Officer, St. Luke's Cornwall Hospital, Newburgh, NY, p. A438
ROSS, Samuel Lee, MS, Chief Executive Officer, Bon Secours Baltimore Health System, Baltimore, MD, p. A287
ROSS Jr., Semmes, Administrator, Lawrence County Hospital, Monticello, MS, p. A350
ROSS, Shana, Director Human Resources, Adventist Bolingbrook Hospital, Bolingbrook, IL, p. A174
ROSS, Zeff, FACHE Senior Vice President and Chief Executive Officer, Memorial Regional Hospital,, FL, p. A125
ROSS–COLE, Melissa, Director Human Resources, Regency Hospital of Northwest Arkansas, Fayetteville, AR, p. A44
ROSS–SPANG, Carol, Senior Vice President, Methodist Healthcare Memphis Hospitals, Memphis, TN, p. A572
ROSSDALE, Robert, Deputy Executive Director, Queens Hospital Center,, NY, p. A436
ROSSETTI, Stephen J., Ph.D. President and Chief Executive Officer, Saint Luke Institute, Silver Spring, MD, p. A294
ROSSFELD, John
  Interim Chief Executive Officer, Daviess Community Hospital, Washington, IN, p. A213
  Interim Chief Executive Officer, Newman Regional Health, Emporia, KS, p. A232
ROSSI, Alfred N., M.D. Chief Executive Officer, Hopedale Medical Complex, Hopedale, IL, p. A185
ROSSI, Coleen, Director Quality Services, HEALTHSOUTH Rehabilitation Hospital of Toms River, Toms River, NJ, p. A411
ROSSI, Frank J., Senior Vice President Human Resources, Cook Children's Medical Center, Fort Worth, TX, p. A598
ROSSI, Lawrence, M.D. Clinical Director, Trenton Psychiatric Hospital, Trenton, NJ, p. A411
ROSSI, Mark F., Chief Operating Officer and General Counsel, Hopedale Medical Complex, Hopedale, IL, p. A185
ROSSITTO, Erica, R.N. Chief Nursing Officer, North Suburban Medical Center, Thornton, CO, p. A106
ROSSMAN, Greg, Chief Human Resource Officer, Denver Health Medical Center, Denver, CO, p. A99
ROSSMANN, Barbara, President and Chief Executive Officer, Henry Ford Macomb Hospitals, Clinton Township, MI, p. A309
ROSSMANN, Samuel H., Chief Executive Officer, TOPS Surgical Specialty Hospital, Houston, TX, p. A607
ROSSYION, Stephanie, Chief Clinical Officer, Kindred Hospital Lafayette, Lafayette, LA, p. A270
ROSVOLD, Robert, Director Finance, Virtua Voorhees, Voorhees, NJ, p. A412
ROTELLA, William, Vice President Human Resources, University of North Carolina Hospitals, Chapel Hill, NC, p. A450
ROTENBERRY–BAGGETT, Katie, Administrative Assistant and Human Resources, Yalobusha General Hospital, Water Valley, MS, p. A353
ROTERT, Jeffrey J., Chief Operating Officer, Sanford Worthington Medical Center, Worthington, MN, p. A342
ROTH, Anna M., Chief Executive Officer, Contra Costa Regional Medical Center, Martinez, CA, p. A74
ROTH, Chris, Chief Executive Officer, St. Luke's Regional Medical Center, Boise, ID, p. A167
ROTH III, Edward J., President and Chief Executive Officer, Aultman Hospital, Canton, OH, p. A472
ROTH III,, Edward J., President and Chief Executive Officer, Aultman Health Foundation, Canton, OH, p. B14
ROTH, Eugene, Vice President Information Services, Mercy Hospital St. Louis, Saint Louis, MO, p. A369
ROTH, Norman G., Executive Vice President and Chief Operating Officer, Bridgeport Hospital, Bridgeport, CT, p. A108
ROTH, Steven, Vice President Informatics and Chief Information Officer, Pinnacle Health System, Harrisburg, PA, p. A524
ROTHE, Brian, Site Director Information Systems, Castle Medical Center, Kailua, HI, p. A164
ROTHERY, Daniel J., President, Boone Hospital Center, Columbia, MO, p. A358
ROTHMAN, Marc, M.D. Medical Director, Friends Hospital, Philadelphia, PA, p. A532
ROTHSCHILD, Marylee, M.D. Chief of Staff, Veterans Affairs Medical Center–Louisville, Louisville, KY, p. A255
ROTHSTEIN, Fred C., M.D. President, University Hospitals Case Medical Center, Cleveland, OH, p. A476
ROTHSTEIN, Robert, M.D. Vice President Medical Affairs, Suburban Hospital, Bethesda, MD, p. A290
ROTKER, Jonathan, M.D. Chief of Staff, Southern Hills Medical Center, Nashville, TN, p. A573
ROTSTED, Scott, Chief Executive Officer, HEALTHSOUTH Rehabilitation Hospital of Petersburg, Petersburg, VA, p. A653
ROTY, Chris, President, Baptist Hospital Northeast, La Grange, KY, p. A252
ROUBIDEAUX, Yvette, M.P.H. Director, U. S. Indian Health Service, Rockville, MD, p. B132
ROUND, Valerie, Chief Executive Officer, St. John Sapulpa, Sapulpa, OK, p. A504
ROUNDS, George, M.D. Chief of Staff, Bigfork Valley Hospital, Bigfork, MN, p. A328
ROUNDY, Ann, Vice President Employee Services, Columbus Community Hospital, Columbus, WI, p. A680
ROUNSLEY, Karen, Controller, HEALTHSOUTH Chesapeake Rehabilitation Hospital, Salisbury, MD, p. A294
ROUSH, Barbara, Chief Operating Officer, Sierra Vista Hospital, Sacramento, CA, p. A84
ROUSH, D. Channing, President, Carolinas Medical Center–Mercy, Charlotte, NC, p. A450
ROUSH, Sharon L., Chief Executive Officer, South Bay Hospital, Sun City Center, FL, p. A140
ROUSSEAU, Mickie, Director Human Resources, Terrebonne General Medical Center, Houma, LA, p. A268
ROUSSEL, Steve, Vice President Finance, Baylor Medical Center at Waxahachie, Waxahachie, TX, p. A633
ROUX, Roger, Senior Vice President Financial Affairs and Chief Financial Officer, Rady Children's Hospital – San Diego, San Diego, CA, p. A85
ROUZER, Cindy, Director Human Resources, Spooner Health System, Spooner, WI, p. A691
ROVITO, Kevin, Interim Chief Financial Officer, Jackson Hospital, Marianna, FL, p. A130
ROWAN, Dan, M.D. President Medical Staff, Little Company of Mary Hospital and Health Care Centers, Evergreen Park, IL, p. A181
ROWAN, R. C., Director Human Resources, Neosho Memorial Regional Medical Center, Chanute, KS, p. A231
ROWAND, Sean, Chief Information Officer, Veterans Affairs Medical Center, Erie, PA, p. A523
ROWE, Bart, Director Information Technology, St. Joseph Medical Center, Reading, PA, p. A537
ROWE, Brenda, Chief Executive Officer, Kindred Hospital–Dallas, Dallas, TX, p. A591
ROWE, Chad D., Director Human Resources, Aspirus Keweenaw Hospital, Laurium, MI, p. A317
ROWE, Jeanne M., M.D. Chief Medical Officer, Shore Medical Center, Somers Point, NJ, p. A410
ROWE, Linda, R.N. Chief Nursing Officer, Carson Valley Medical Center, Gardnerville, NV, p. A392
ROWE, Paul W., Director Information Technology, St. Francis Hospital, Wilmington, DE, p. A115
ROWE, Scott, Chief Executive Officer, HEALTHSOUTH Chattanooga Rehabilitation Hospital, Chattanooga, TN, p. A563
ROWELL, Jim H., Vice President Human Resources, Rutherford Regional Medical Center, Rutherfordton, NC, p. A460
ROWEN, Jennifer, Director Human Resources, Allegiance Specialty Hospital of Little Rock, Jacksonville, AR, p. A46
ROWLAND, Claire, Director Human Resources, Acadia Vermilion Hospital, Lafayette, LA, p. A269
ROWLAND, Martha Tolbert, Vice President Finance, Middle Tennessee Medical Center, Murfreesboro, TN, p. A573
ROWLAND, Michael, M.D. Vice President Medical Affairs, Franklin Memorial Hospital, Farmington, ME, p. A283
ROWLAND, Robert, M.D. Medical Director, HEALTHSOUTH Rehabilitation Hospital of Tallahassee, Tallahassee, FL, p. A140
ROWLANDS, Dewey R., Vice President Finance and Chief Financial Officer, Oneida Healthcare, Oneida, NY, p. A439
ROWLEY, Michael, Chief Executive Officer, Salt Lake Behavioral Health, Salt Lake City, UT, p. A641
ROWLEY, Tim, Chief Operating Officer, Perkins County Health Services, Grant, NE, p. A384
ROWSHAN, Omid, M.D. President Medical Staff, Lower Bucks Hospital, Bristol, PA, p. A519
ROY, Joel, Manager Information Systems, The Brook Hospital – KMI, Louisville, KY, p. A255
ROY, Rock, Professional Services Director, Power County Hospital District, American Falls, ID, p. A166
ROY, Schindelheim, M.D. Chief of Staff, George L. Mee Memorial Hospital, King City, CA, p. A65
ROYAL, Jennifer A., Administrator, Burke Medical Center, Waynesboro, GA, p. A162
ROYAL, Keli, Director Human Resources, Shenandoah Medical Center, Shenandoah, IA, p. A226
ROYAL, Ty, Executive Director of Support Services and Human Resources, Gibson Area Hospital and Health Services, Gibson City, IL, p. A183
ROYER, Jerry, M.D. Chief Medical Officer, San Joaquin General Hospital, French Camp, CA, p. A61
ROYER, Thomas C., M.D. Interim Chief Executive Officer, Parkland Health & Hospital System, Dallas, TX, p. A592
ROYSTER, Randy, Vice President Human Resources, Lovelace Medical Center, Albuquerque, NM, p. A414
ROZARIO, Nirmala, M.D. Chief of Staff, Veterans Affairs Medical Center, Spokane, WA, p. A667
ROZELL, Becky, Chief Human Resources Officer, Madison County Hospital, London, OH, p. A483
ROZENFELD, Jon, Executive Vice President and Chief Operating Officer, St. Mary's Hospital, Madison, WI, p. A684
ROZMUS, Mike, Director Information Systems, Rockingham Memorial Hospital, Harrisonburg, VA, p. A649
ROZNOVSKY, Karen, Director Human Resources, Yoakum Community Hospital, Yoakum, TX, p. A636
RUBAR, Jackie, Administrative Assistant and Director Human Resources, Leesville Rehabilitation Hospital, Leesville, LA, p. A272
RUBE, David M., M.D. Clinical Director, Queens Children's Psychiatric Center,, NY, p. A436
RUBENS, Deborah, Director Human Resources, Shriners Hospitals for Children, Northern California, Sacramento, CA, p. A84
RUBERDALL, Stephen, M.D. Chief Medical Officer, Grady General Hospital, Cairo, GA, p. A148
RUBERTE, Henry, Administrator, Hospital San Gerardo, San Juan, PR, p. A703
RUBERTI, Charlene, Director Information Technology Development, Ancora Psychiatric Hospital, Ancora, NJ, p. A401
RUBIN, Amir Dan, President and Chief Executive Officer, Stanford Health Care, Palo Alto, CA, p. B123
RUBIN, Amir Dan, President and Chief Executive Officer, Stanford Hospital and Clinics, Palo Alto, CA, p. A79
RUBIN, Linda, Chief Operating Officer, Spectrum Health Reed City Hospital, Reed City, MI, p. A321
RUBIN, Richard, M.D. Chief Medical Officer, St. Mary's Hospital, Troy, NY, p. A445
RUBIN, Vincent, Chief Financial Officer, Brotman Medical Center, Culver City, CA, p. A59
RUBINATE, Donna, R.N. Chief Operating Officer, Good Samaritan Medical Center, Brockton, MA, p. A298
RUBINSTEIN, Mitchell, M.D. Vice President Medical Affairs, Valley Hospital, Ridgewood, NJ, p. A409


**A920** Index of Health Care Professionals

Index of Health Care Professionals / Ryan

Index of Health Care Professionals

RUBIO, Felipe, M.D. Medical Director, Kindred Hospital–Dayton, Dayton, OH, p. A478
RUBLE, Charalene, Chief Nursing Officer, llano Specialty Hospital of Lubbock, Lubbock, TX, p. A614
RUCHTI, Kevin, Coordinator Information Systems, Grant Regional Health Center, Lancaster, WI, p. A684
RUCHTI, Robert D., R.N. Interim Chief Executive Officer, Buchanan General Hospital, Grundy, VA, p. A649
RUCKEL, Michael R., Vice President Finance, Decatur County Memorial Hospital, Greensburg, IN, p. A203
RUCKER, Craig
Senior Vice President and Chief Financial Officer, Bethesda North Hospital, Cincinnati, OH, p. A472
Senior Vice President and Chief Financial Officer, Good Samaritan Hospital, Cincinnati, OH, p. A473
RUCKER, Sheryl, Chief Information Officer, Edgerton Hospital and Health Services, Edgerton, WI, p. A681
RUDD, Barry, Chief Information Officer, Mayo Clinic Health System in Waycross, Waycross, GA, p. A162
RUDD, John, Chief Financial Officer, Cayuga Medical Center at Ithaca, Ithaca, NY, p. A428
RUDDEN, Elizabeth, Vice President Human Resources, Connecticut Children's Medical Center, Hartford, CT, p. A109
RUDEK, Charles M., Chief Information Officer, UPMC St. Margaret, Pittsburgh, PA, p. A536
RUDIN, Joel, Chief Executive Officer, New England Rehabilitation Hospital, Woburn, MA, p. A306
RUDIS, Lorrie, Director Human Resources, Crotched Mountain Rehabilitation Center, Greenfield, NH, p. A398
RUDISILL, Lynne
Controller, Select Specialty Hospital–Knoxville, Knoxville, TN, p. A568
Controller, Select Specialty Hospital–North Knoxville, Knoxville, TN, p. A568
RUDITZ, Bettiann S., Chief Nursing Officer, Broward Health North, Deerfield Beach, FL, p. A122
RUDOLF, Steven, Vice President Human Resources, Baptist Hospital East, Louisville, KY, p. A254
RUDOLPH, Dawn, Chief Executive Officer, Saint Thomas Hospital, Nashville, TN, p. A573
RUDZIK, Donna, Director Human Resources, Hopkins County Memorial Hospital, Sulphur Springs, TX, p. A629
RUE, Robert, Controller, Ellenville Regional Hospital, Ellenville, NY, p. A425
RUECKERT, Sebastian, M.D. Chief Medical Officer, Christian Hospital, Saint Louis, MO, p. A368
RUEDISUELI, Amy, Chief Financial Officer, McKenzie Health System, Sandusky, MI, p. A322
RUELLO, Rocky, Vice President Human Resources, Mercy Hospital St. Louis, Saint Louis, MO, p. A369
RUFAT, Berta, Controller, Baptist Health South Florida, South Miami Hospital, Miami, FL, p. A130
RUFF, Michael, Chief Financial Officer, Scenic Mountain Medical Center, Big Spring, TX, p. A584
RUFF, Victoria, M.D. Medical Director, Select Specialty Hospital–Columbus, Columbus, OH, p. A477
RUFFING, Jr., John J., M.D. Chief of Staff, Box Butte General Hospital, Alliance, NE, p. A381
RUFFOLO, Joseph A., President and Chief Executive Officer, Niagara Falls Memorial Medical Center, Niagara Falls, NY, p. A438
RUGE, Randy, Chief Operating Officer, Paulding County Hospital, Paulding, OH, p. A487
RUGGERO, Robert, Senior Vice President Operations, Lourdes Medical Center of Burlington County, Willingboro, NJ, p. A412
RUHLEN, Michael, M.D. Chief Medical Officer, Carolinas Medical Center–Mercy, Charlotte, NC, p. A450
RUIZ, Ismael, Chief Information Officer, Doctors' Center Hospital San Juan, San Juan, PR, p. A703
RUIZ, Javier, M.D. Medical Director, Intracare North Hospital, Houston, TX, p. A604
RUIZ, Jesse, Chief Executive Officer, Select Specialty Hospital–Houston, Houston, TX, p. A606
RUIZ, Mary, Chief Executive Officer, Manatee Glens Hospital and Addiction Center, Bradenton, FL, p. A119
RUIZ, Ralph, Director Information Technology and Services, Kendall Regional Medical Center, Miami, FL, p. A131
RUIZ, Tony, Chief Operating Officer, Medical Center Health System, Odessa, TX, p. A619
RUKAVINA, Mark, M.D. Chief Medical Staff, Marcum and Wallace Memorial Hospital, Irvine, KY, p. A252
RUKSTAD, Julie, Chief Financial Officer, Olympic Medical Center, Port Angeles, WA, p. A664
RUMANS, Mark C., M.D. Physician in Chief, Billings Clinic, Billings, MT, p. A373
RUMBAUGH, Bruce, M.D. Director Patient Care, Atoka County Medical Center, Atoka, OK, p. A493
RUMFORD, Darren K., Chief Financial Officer, Geary Community Hospital, Junction City, KS, p. A235
RUMMEL, Jennifer
Director Human Resources, East Texas Medical Center Athens, Athens, TX, p. A580
Director Human Resources, East Texas Medical Center Fairfield, Fairfield, TX, p. A597
RUNKE, David, Chief Financial Officer, Riverside County Regional Medical Center, Moreno Valley, CA, p. A76
RUNT, David, Chief Information Officer, Banner Del E. Webb Medical Center, Sun City West, AZ, p. A39
RUNYAN, Duane, Chief Executive Officer and Managing Director, Rivendell Behavioral Health Services of Arkansas, Benton, AR, p. A42
RUNYAN, Mark, Director Information Services, Salt Lake Regional Medical Center, Salt Lake City, UT, p. A641
RUOTOLO, Frank, Chief Information Officer, Gateway Medical Center, Clarksville, TN, p. A564
RUPERT, Duke, President and Chief Executive Officer, Western Pennsylvania Hospital, Pittsburgh, PA, p. A536
RUPERT, James M., Chief Fiscal Services, Veterans Affairs Medical Center, Battle Creek, MI, p. A308
RUPERT, Michael J., Chief Financial Officer, Veterans Affairs Long Beach Healthcare System, Long Beach, CA, p. A68
RUPP, Robert, Chief Executive Officer, Harris Hospital, Newport, AR, p. A49
RUPPEL, Rick, Chief Financial Officer, Memorial Hospital, Fremont, OH, p. A480
RUPPERT SCHILLER, Kerri
Senior Vice President and Chief Financial Officer, Children's Hospital at Mission, Mission Viejo, CA, p. A74
Senior Vice President and Chief Financial Officer, Children's Hospital of Orange County, Orange, CA, p. A78
RUSCITTO, Kathryn H., President, St. Joseph's Hospital Health Center, Syracuse, NY, p. A444
RUSH, Ann Marie, Chief Financial Officer, Penobscot Valley Hospital, Lincoln, ME, p. A284
RUSH, Christopher, Vice President and Administrator, Rush Foundation Hospital, Meridian, MS, p. A350
RUSH, Cindy, Director Human Resources, Clay County Medical Center, Clay Center, KS, p. A231
RUSH, Domenica, Chief Executive Officer, Sierra Vista Hospital, Truth or Consequences, NM, p. A418
RUSH, Donald J., Chief Executive Officer, Providence Kodiak Island Medical Center, Kodiak, AK, p. A29
RUSH, Ed, President and Chief Executive Officer, Iredell Memorial Hospital, Statesville, NC, p. A461
RUSH, Jeff W.
Interim Vice President Finance, Angel Medical Center, Franklin, NC, p. A453
Chief Financial Officer, Wallace Thomson Hospital, Union, SC, p. A554
RUSH, Matthew, President and Chief Executive Officer, Hayes Green Beach Memorial Hospital, Charlotte, MI, p. A309
RUSHIN, Denise, Director Human Resources, Poplar Bluff Regional Medical Center, Poplar Bluff, MO, p. A367
RUSHING, R. Lynn, Chief Executive Officer, Brook Lane Health Services, Hagerstown, MD, p. A292
RUSHING, Robyn, Administrator, Lakeview Specialty Hospital and Rehabilitation Center, Waterford, WI, p. A692
RUSHING, Tracy, Executive Assistant Human Resources and Payroll, Pioneer Community Hospital of Newton, Newton, MS, p. A351
RUSHNELL, Christi C., Vice President Information Technology, Palm Bay Hospital, Melbourne, FL, p. A130
RUSK, Scott, M.D. Vice President Medical Administration, Mercy Hospital of Portland, Portland, ME, p. A284
RUSKAN II, Jeff, Chief Executive Officer, HEALTHSOUTH Rehabilitation Hospital of Virginia, Richmond, VA, p. A655
RUSKOWSKI, David, President, Franciscan St. Anthony Health – Crown Point, Crown Point, IN, p. A200
RUSSAKOFF, David, M.D. Chief Medical Officer, Princeton Baptist Medical Center, Birmingham, AL, p. A16
RUSSEL, Kimberly A., President and Chief Executive Officer, BryanLGH Health System, Lincoln, NE, p. B23
RUSSELL, Dardanella, Chief Human Resources Management Service, Veterans Affairs Hudson Valley Health Care System–F.D. Roosevelt Hospital, Montrose, NY, p. A430
RUSSELL, Dee B., M.D. Vice President & Chief of Medical Affairs, Floyd Medical Center, Rome, GA, p. A158
RUSSELL, Donald
Vice President, Adventist GlenOaks Hospital, Glendale Heights, IL, p. A183
Regional Vice President Human Resources, Adventist Hinsdale Hospital, Hinsdale, IL, p. A184
RUSSELL, Erin, Controller, Kindred Hospital–San Antonio, San Antonio, TX, p. A625
RUSSELL, Eunice, Manager Human Resources, Arrowhead Behavioral Health Hospital, Maumee, OH, p. A484
RUSSELL, Freda, Interim Chief Executive Officer, Three Rivers Hospital, Waverly, TN, p. A576
RUSSELL, Georgette, Vice President of Talent & Organizational Effectiveness, Carson City Hospital, Carson City, MI, p. A309
RUSSELL, John D., President and Chief Executive Officer, Columbus Community Hospital, Columbus, WI, p. A680
RUSSELL, Jon
Vice President Information Systems, Kettering Medical Center, Kettering, OH, p. A482
Chief Information Officer, Sycamore Medical Center, Miamisburg, OH, p. A485
RUSSELL, Karen, Director Human Resources, Perry Memorial Hospital, Princeton, IL, p. A192
RUSSELL, Kathy, R.N. Chief Nursing Officer, Bluegrass Community Hospital, Versailles, KY, p. A259
RUSSELL, Kim, M.D. Chief of Staff, Scott & White Hospital – Llano, Llano, TX, p. A613
RUSSELL, Linda, Director Human Resources, Kindred Hospital–Indianapolis, Indianapolis, IN, p. A204
RUSSELL, Linda B., Chief Executive Officer, The Woman's Hospital of Texas, Houston, TX, p. A607
RUSSELL, Marvin
Corporate Senior Vice President Human Resources, Beth Israel Medical Center, New York, NY, p. A431
Senior Vice President Human Resources, St. Luke's–Roosevelt Hospital Center, New York, NY, p. A437
RUSSELL, Michelle L., Administrator, Community Howard Specialty Hospital, Kokomo, IN, p. A206
RUSSELL, Nancy, Chief Financial Officer, Clifton–Fine Hospital, Star Lake, NY, p. A443
RUSSELL, Robert, Chief Operating Officer, Atlanta Medical Center, Atlanta, GA, p. A145
RUSSELL, Robert J., Associate Executive Director Operations, Penn Presbyterian Medical Center, Philadelphia, PA, p. A533
RUSSELL, Shelia, Director Human Resources, Jamestown Regional Medical Center, Jamestown, TN, p. A567
RUSSELL, Sherrie
Vice President and Chief Information Officer, Alexian Brothers Behavioral Health Hospital, Hoffman Estates, IL, p. A184
Chief Information Officer, St. Alexius Medical Center, Hoffman Estates, IL, p. A185
RUSSELL, Thomas, Chief Executive Officer, Adventist Medical Center, Portland, OR, p. A513
RUSSELL, Tim, Administrator, Stillwater Community Hospital, Columbus, MT, p. A374
RUSSELL, William B., Chief Executive Officer, Three Rivers Health, Three Rivers, MI, p. A324
RUSSELL-COOK, Donna, President, St. Elizabeth Hospital, Enumclaw, WA, p. A661
RUSSO, Arthur, M.D. Director Medical Affairs, Harrington Memorial Hospital, Southbridge, MA, p. A304
RUSSO, Kimberly, Chief Operating Officer, George Washington University Hospital, Washington, DC, p. A116
RUSSO, Michael, Chief Administrative Officer, Saint Anthony's Health Center, Alton, IL, p. A172
RUSSO, Paul, Director, Veterans Affairs Medical Center, Miami, FL, p. A132
RUTH, Joseph, Executive Vice President and Chief Operating Officer, Sparrow Hospital, Lansing, MI, p. A317
RUTHER, Randy, Vice President Finance and Chief Financial Officer, Little Company of Mary Hospital and Health Care Centers, Evergreen Park, IL, p. A181
RUTHERFORD, Cynthia, Manager Business Office, Hood Memorial Hospital, Amite, LA, p. A261
RUTHERFORD, Dennis E., Chief Financial Officer, Palo Verde Hospital, Blythe, CA, p. A56
RUTHERFORD, George W., Vice President and Chief Operating Officer, Sparrow Ionia Hospital, Ionia, MI, p. A315
RUTHERFORD, Michael, Chief Financial Officer, Ohio State University Medical Center, Columbus, OH, p. A477
RUTHERFORD, Theresa, R.N. Chief Operating Officer, St. Mary's Hospital, Decatur, IL, p. A179
RUTKOWSKI, James C., Chief Financial Officer, Southwest Regional Medical Center, Waynesburg, PA, p. A540
RUTLEDGE, Geri, Director Business, East Mississippi State Hospital, Meridian, MS, p. A350
RUTLEDGE, Virginia, Assistant Administrator, Barton County Memorial Hospital, Lamar, MO, p. A363
RUTTER, James, M.D. Chief of Staff, Integris Grove General Hospital, Grove, OK, p. A497
RUWOLDT, Steven T., Chief Executive Officer, Salem Community Hospital, Salem, OH, p. A488
RUYTER, Mary J., Chief Executive Officer, Sanford Jackson Medical Center, Jackson, MN, p. A333
RYALS, Billie, Human Resources Director, Sullivan County Memorial Hospital, Milan, MO, p. A365
RYAN, Chris, Chief Information Officer, Auburn Community Hospital, Auburn, NY, p. A421
RYAN, Christina M., R.N. Chief Executive Officer, The Women's Hospital, Newburgh, IN, p. A210

RYAN, Colleen
Director Management Information Systems, Landmark Medical Center, Woonsocket, RI, p. A545
Chief Information Officer and Vice President Professional Services, Rehabilitation Hospital of Rhode Island, North Smithfield, RI, p. A544

RYAN, Cory, M.D. Chief of Staff, Wayne County Hospital, Monticello, KY, p. A256

RYAN, David, Vice President Human Resources, Falmouth Hospital, Falmouth, MA, p. A300

RYAN, Debora, R.N. Vice President Patient Care, St. Francis Regional Medical Center, Shakopee, MN, p. A340

RYAN, Dennis, Senior Vice President and Chief Financial Officer, Children's Hospital of The King's Daughters, Norfolk, VA, p. A652

RYAN, Frank, Chief Financial Officer, Veterans Affairs Medical Center, Manchester, NH, p. A399

RYAN, J. Thomas, M.D
Executive Vice President and Chief Medical Officer, Mary Washington Hospital, Fredericksburg, VA, p. A648
Executive Vice President and Chief Medical Officer, Stafford Hospital, Stafford, VA, p. A656

RYAN, Jacqueline, Director Human Resources, Mayo Clinic Health System in Lake City, Lake City, MN, p. A333

RYAN, Kimberly, Chief Executive Officer, Eastside Medical Center, Snellville, GA, p. A159

RYAN, Lisa M., Coordinator Human Resources, Hampstead Hospital, Hampstead, NH, p. A398

RYAN, Maria, Ph.D. Chief Executive Officer, Cottage Hospital, Woodsville, NH, p. A400

RYAN, Michael
Administrator, Mayo Clinic Health System – Oakridge in Osseo, Osseo, WI, p. A689
Senior Vice President Finance, Memorial Hospital of Rhode Island, Pawtucket, RI, p. A544

RYAN, Michael J., Chief Executive Officer, Herington Municipal Hospital, Herington, KS, p. A234

RYAN, Patrice
Vice President Human Resources, Goleta Valley Cottage Hospital, Santa Barbara, CA, p. A89
Vice President Human Resources, Santa Barbara Cottage Hospital, Santa Barbara, CA, p. A89
Vice President Human Resources, Santa Ynez Valley Cottage Hospital, Solvang, CA, p. A91

RYAN, Raymond, M.D. Chief of Staff, Fayette County Hospital, Vandalia, IL, p. A195

RYAN, Rebecca, Interim Director Human Resources and Employee Health, Ukiah Valley Medical Center, Ukiah, CA, p. A93

RYAN, Stacy, Corporate Director Human Resources, Warren General Hospital, Warren, PA, p. A540

RYAN, Tim, Director Finance, Centennial Peaks Hospital, Louisville, CO, p. A104

RYAN, Jr., Timothy J., Director Human Resources, Lewis County General Hospital, Lowville, NY, p. A429

RYBA, Janice L., JD, Chief Executive Officer, St. Mary Medical Center, Hobart, IN, p. A203

RYBA, Thomas L., Chief Executive Officer, Lighthouse Care Center of Conway, Conway, SC, p. A549

RYBA, Tomi S., President and Chief Executive Officer, El Camino Hospital, Mountain View, CA, p. A76

RYBOLT, Andrew
Vice President and Chief Financial Officer, Redwood Memorial Hospital, Fortuna, CA, p. A61
Chief Financial Officer, St. Joseph Hospital, Eureka, CA, p. A60

RYCHENER, Michelle, Chief Operating Officer, Henry County Hospital, Napoleon, OH, p. A485

RYDER, Doug, Vice President Clinical Operations and Service Lines, Advocate Good Shepherd Hospital, Barrington, IL, p. A173

RYDER, Jeff, Director Information Systems, Saint Joseph Mount Sterling, Mount Sterling, KY, p. A257

RYDER, Jennifer, Director of Nursing, Mercy Continuing Care Hospital, Chesterfield, MO, p. A357

RYDER, John, Administrator and Chief Executive Officer, Borgess–Pipp Hospital, Plainwell, MI, p. A320

RYDER, Rebecca L., R.N. President and Chief Executive Officer, Franklin Memorial Hospital, Farmington, ME, p. A283

RYDER, Robert
Chief Executive Officer, St. Mary–Corwin Medical Center, Pueblo, CO, p. A105
Chief Executive Officer, St. Thomas More Hospital, Canon City, CO, p. A98

RYDER, Ronald, D.O. President of the Medical Staff, Robert Wood Johnson University Hospital at Hamilton, Hamilton, NJ, p. A404

RYERSON, Nancy, Director Information Systems, Central Florida Regional Hospital, Sanford, FL, p. A138

RYKERT, Lauren P., Senior Vice President, The Methodist Hospital, Houston, TX, p. A607

RYLAND, Jennifer M., R.N. Chief Administrative Officer, Jackson Medical Center, Jackson, AL, p. A22

RYLE, Barry, Chief Information Officer, Oswego Hospital, Oswego, NY, p. A440

RYLE, Deborah L., Administrator and Chief Executive Officer, St. David's Round Rock Medical Center, Round Rock, TX, p. A623

## S

SAAL, A. Kim, M.D. President Medical Staff, Mount Auburn Hospital, Cambridge, MA, p. A299

SAALFELD, Thomas, Senior Vice President and Chief Operating Officer, St. Elizabeth Fort Thomas, Fort Thomas, KY, p. A250

SAAVEDRA, JayLynn, Chief Information Officer, U. S. Public Health Service Indian Hospital, Parker, AZ, p. A35

SAAVEDRA, John, Service Area Director Human Resources, Providence Saint Joseph Medical Center, Burbank, CA, p. A56

SABA, Fadi, M.D. Chief of Staff, Edward White Hospital, Saint Petersburg, FL, p. A138

SABA, Francis M., Chief Executive Officer, Milford Regional Medical Center, Milford, MA, p. A302

SABAHI, Mojtaba, M.D. Chief of Staff, Promise Hospital of East Los Angeles, Suburban Medical Center Campus, Paramount, CA, p. A79

SABANDIT, Elizabeth, Director Human Resources, Alhambra Hospital Medical Center, Alhambra, CA, p. A53

SABELLA, Deborah, R.N. Chief Executive Officer, Landmark Hospital of Columbia, Columbia, MO, p. A358

SABHARRWAL, Parajeet, Administrator, Minimally Invasive Surgery Center, Lenexa, KS, p. A237

SABIA, John, M.D. Medical Director, Northern Dutchess Hospital, Rhinebeck, NY, p. A441

SABIN, Bridget, Director Human Resources, Madison Hospital, Madison, MN, p. A334

SABIN, Margaret D., President and Chief Executive Officer, Penrose–St. Francis Health Services, Colorado Springs, CO, p. A98

SABITTI, Jesse, M.D. Chief Medical Officer, Kenmare Community Hospital, Kenmare, ND, p. A467

SABOTTA, John, Director Information Systems, St. Margaret's Hospital, Spring Valley, IL, p. A194

SABUS, Matthew, Director Information Systems, Boone County Hospital, Boone, IA, p. A215

SACCO, Frank V., FACHE President and Chief Executive Officer, Memorial Healthcare System,, FL, p. B87

SACHDEV, Aruna, M.D. Medical Director, Massachusetts Hospital School, Canton, MA, p. A299

SACHS, III, Henry T., M.D. Medical Director, Emma Pendleton Bradley Hospital, East Providence, RI, p. A544

SACHTLEBEN, Michael, Chief Operating Officer, Medstar Georgetown University Hospital, Washington, DC, p. A116

SACK, Michael V., President and Chief Executive Officer, Hallmark Health System, Melrose, MA, p. A302

SACKETT, John, Chief Executive Officer, Avista Adventist Hospital, Louisville, CO, p. A104

SACKMANN, Charles, M.D. Chief of Staff, East Adams Rural Hospital, Ritzville, WA, p. A665

SACKRISON, Jeffrey N., FACH
President, Vidant Bertie Hospital, Windsor, NC, p. A463
President, Vidant Chowan Hospital, Edenton, NC, p. A452

SADA, Judy, Chief Financial Officer, Memorial Hospital Miramar, Miramar, FL, p. A132

SADAU, Ernie W., President and Chief Executive Officer, CHRISTUS Health, Irving, TX, p. B31

SADLER, Joy, Director Human Resources, Bear River Valley Hospital, Tremonton, UT, p. A642

SADR, Farrokh, M.D. Chief Medical Officer, Sacred Heart Hospital, Allentown, PA, p. A517

SADVARY, Thomas J., FACHE President and Chief Executive Officer, Scottsdale Healthcare, Scottsdale, AZ, p. B114

SAENZ, Luis J Rodriquez, M.D. Medical Director, Hospital Menonita De Cayey, Cayey, PR, p. A700

SAFDIE, Ezra R., Associate Director, Veterans Affairs Medical Center, San Francisco, CA, p. A87

SAFF, Eric, Senior Vice President and Chief Information Officer, John Muir Behavioral Health Center, Concord, CA, p. A58

SAFFORD, Ronald, Administrator, Palestine Regional Rehabilitation Center, Palestine, TX, p. A619

SAFIAN, Keith F., President and Chief Executive Officer, Phelps Memorial Hospital Center, Sleepy Hollow, NY, p. A443

SAFLEY, Thomas, Chief Financial Officer, St. Joseph Regional Medical Center, Lewiston, ID, p. A169

SAFYER, Steven M., M.D. President and Chief Executive Officer, Montefiore Medical Center,, NY, p. A434

SAGAN, John, Vice President Finance, St. Mary's Healthcare, Amsterdam, NY, p. A420

SAGAR, Karen S., Vice President Human Resources, Franciscan St. Francis Health – Indianapolis, Indianapolis, IN, p. A204

SAGEMAN, Scott, M.D. Vice President and Chief Medical Officer, St. Joseph Hospital, Eureka, CA, p. A60

SAGMIT, Rodney, Chief Information Management, Veterans Affairs Long Beach Healthcare System, Long Beach, CA, p. A68

SAHA, Sanjay K., Executive Vice President, Operations, Wake Forest Baptist Medical Center, Winston–Salem, NC, p. A463

SAHLSTROM, Christopher, M.D. Chief of Staff, Mat–Su Regional Medical Center, Palmer, AK, p. A30

SAHMAUNT, Sarabeth, Supervisory Accountant, Lawton Indian Hospital, Lawton, OK, p. A498

SAIA, Carrie L., R.N. Interim Chief Executive Officer, Holton Community Hospital, Holton, KS, p. A234

SAINTZ, Jeffrey, Vice President Human Resources, Titusville Area Hospital, Titusville, PA, p. A539

SAIYED, Ashfaq, M.D. Medical Director, Irwin County Hospital, Ocilla, GA, p. A157

SAJID, Muhammad W., M.D. Medical Director, Lincoln Trail Behavioral Health System, Radcliff, KY, p. A258

SALANGER, Matthew J., President and Chief Executive Officer, United Health Services, Binghamton, NY, p. B133

SALANGER, Matthew J., President and Chief Executive Officer, United Health Services Hospitals–Binghamton, Binghamton, NY, p. A422

SALAS, Victor, M.D. President Medical Staff, Jones Regional Medical Center, Anamosa, IA, p. A214

SALAZAR, Juan, Director Human Resources, St. Luke's Episcopal Hospital, Ponce, PR, p. A702

SALAZAR, Kathy, Manager Human Resources, Michael E. DeBakey Veterans Affairs Medical Center, Houston, TX, p. A606

SALAZAR, Linda C., Information Technology Leader, Baldwin Park Medical Center, Baldwin Park, CA, p. A55

SALAZAR, Margie, Director Human Resources, Valley Regional Medical Center, Brownsville, TX, p. A585

SALAZAR, Pamela, M.D. Chief of Staff, Walton Rehabilitation Hospital, Augusta, GA, p. A147

SALCEDO, Nydimar, Chief Human Resources Officer, Castaner General Hospital, Castaner, PR, p. A700

SALDIVAR, Duke, Chief Executive Officer, HEALTHSOUTH Rehabilitation Hospital of Austin, Austin, TX, p. A580

SALEM, Gary, M.D. Vice President Medical Affairs, McLaren Lapeer Region, Lapeer, MI, p. A317

SALEM, Michael, M.D. President and Chief Executive Officer, National Jewish Health, Denver, CO, p. A99

SALERNO, Thomas A., President, St. Mary Medical Center, Long Beach, CA, p. A68

SALGADO, Joe, M.D. Chief of Staff, Artesia General Hospital, Artesia, NM, p. A415

SALGUERO, Otto
Chief Information Officer, Excela Frick Hospital, Mount Pleasant, PA, p. A530
Chief Information Officer, Excela Health Westmoreland Hospital, Greensburg, PA, p. A524
Chief Information Officer, Excela Latrobe Area Hospital, Latrobe, PA, p. A527

SALINAS, Daniel, M.D. Senior Vice President and Chief Medical Officer, Children's Healthcare of Atlanta, Atlanta, GA, p. A145

SALISBURY, Dennis, M.D. Vice President for Medical Affairs, St. James Healthcare, Butte, MT, p. A374

SALISBURY, Margaret A., Director Marketing, Runnells Specialized Hospital of Union County, Berkeley Heights, NJ, p. A401

SALISBURY, Renee A., Director Human Resources, Kewanee Hospital, Kewanee, iL, p. A186

SALISBURY, Rick, M.D. President Medical Staff, Samaritan Lebanon Community Hospital, Lebanon, OR, p. A512

SALISBURY, Tracy
Director Human Resources, Central State Hospital, Petersburg, VA, p. A653
Director Human Resources, Hiram W. Davis Medical Center, Petersburg, VA, p. A653

SALLER, William
Chief Financial Officer, North Hills Hospital, North Richland Hills, TX, p. A618
Chief Financial Officer, Rio Grande Regional Hospital, McAllen, TX, p. A615

SALLEY, Wanda, Administrative Director Human Resources, Gulf Coast Medical Center, Panama City, FL, p. A135

SALLIS, Tom, Director Information Systems, Sparks Regional Medical Center, Fort Smith, AR, p. A45

SALLOUM, Fadi, M.D. Medical Director, Select Specialty Hospital–Pontiac, Pontiac, MI, p. A321

SALMAN, Wael, M.D. Vice President Medical Affairs, Memorial Healthcare, Owosso, MI, p. A320

Index of Health Care Professionals / Santos

Index of Health Care Professionals

SALMON, Chuck, Chief Executive, Swedish/Issaquah, Issaquah, WA, p. A662
SALMON, Gretchen, M.D. Medical Director, Hale Ho'ola Hamakua, Honokaa, HI, p. A163
SALMON, Robert J.
Chief Executive Officer, Sanford Deuel County Medical Center, Clear Lake, SD, p. A556
Chief Executive Officer, Sanford Medical Center Canby, Canby, MN, p. A329
SALNAS, Todd, Chief Operating Officer, Santa Rosa Memorial Hospital, Santa Rosa, CA, p. A90
SALO, Saliba, Chief Operating Officer, Northridge Hospital Medical Center–Roscoe Boulevard Campus,, CA, p. A70
SALOME, Jenny, Chief Financial Officer and Assistant Administrator, Northwest Hills Surgical Hospital, Austin, TX, p. A581
SALOMON, Kathryn, Director Human Resources, Kona Community Hospital, Kealakekua, HI, p. A165
SALOUM, Herbert A., M.D. Medical Director, St. Michael's Hospital Avera, Tyndall, SD, p. A560
SALSBERRY, David, Chief Financial Officer, JPS Health Network, Fort Worth, TX, p. A599
SALTAFORMAGGIO, Cheri, Chief Executive Officer, St. Charles Surgical Hospital, New Orleans, LA, p. A275
SALTZMAN, Ronald, M.D. Chief of Staff, Saddleback Memorial Medical Center, Laguna Hills, CA, p. A66
SALVADOR, Ed, Chief Financial Officer, St. Jude Medical Center, Fullerton, CA, p. A62
SALVATI, Mario, Director Fiscal Services, Shriners Hospitals for Children, Philadelphia, Philadelphia, PA, p. A533
SALVINO, Sonia, Vice President Finance, University Hospitals Case Medical Center, Cleveland, OH, p. A476
SALVITTI, Alfred, Chief Financial Officer, Eagleville Hospital, Eagleville, PA, p. A522
SALVITTI, Alfred P., Chief Financial Officer, Friends Hospital, Philadelphia, PA, p. A532
SALVO, Stephen, Vice President Human Resources, Anna Jaques Hospital, Newburyport, MA, p. A302
SALVO, Thomas, Associate Executive Director Human Resources, Glen Cove Hospital, Glen Cove, NY, p. A426
SALYER, Steven, Chief Executive Officer, Sebastian River Medical Center, Sebastian, FL, p. A139
SALZBERG, Ron, Executive Director Human Resources, Saddleback Memorial Medical Center, Laguna Hills, CA, p. A66
SAM, Charlene, Manager Health Information, Choctaw Health Center, Philadelphia, MS, p. A351
SAMET, Kenneth A., President and Chief Executive Officer, MedStar Health, Columbia, MD, p. B86
SAMILO, Nick, Vice President Fiscal Services and Chief Financial Officer, Stanly Regional Medical Center, Albemarle, NC, p. A448
SAMMARCO, Michael, M.D. Chief Financial Officer, Erie County Medical Center, Buffalo, NY, p. A422
SAMMER, Edwin, M.D. Vice President and Chief Medical Officer, Lakeland Regional Medical Center, Lakeland, FL, p. A128
SAMMONS, Craig, Chief Financial Officer, Sky Ridge Medical Center, Lone Tree, CO, p. A104
SAMMONS, James, M.D. Vice President Medical Affairs, Sentara Williamsburg Regional Medical Center, Williamsburg, VA, p. A657
SAMPLES, Beth A.
Vice President Human Resources, CAMC Teays Valley Hospital, Hurricane, WV, p. A673
Vice President Human Resources, Charleston Area Medical Center, Charleston, WV, p. A671
SAMPLES, Patience M., R.N. Chief Nursing Officer, East Morgan County Hospital, Brush, CO, p. A98
SAMPSON, Arthur J., FACHE Executive Director, Miriam Hospital, Providence, RI, p. A544
SAMPSON, Bob
Vice President Human Resources, Providence Regional Medical Center Everett, Everett, WA, p. A661
Vice President Human Resources, Redwood Memorial Hospital, Fortuna, CA, p. A61
SAMPSON, Cherie L., Director Human Resources, San Diego Medical Center, San Diego, CA, p. A85
SAMPSON, Jill, Director Human Resources, Lemuel Shattuck Hospital, Jamaica Plain, MA, p. A301
SAMS, Tricia, M.D. Medical Director, Memorial Health Care Systems, Seward, NE, p. A389
SAMSON, Ley, Director Management Information Systems, Clear Lake Regional Medical Center, Webster, TX, p. A634
SAMUDRALA, Siresha, M.D. Medical Director, Mercy Rehabilitation Hospital, Chesterfield, MO, p. A357
SAMUEL, Guy, Director Human Resources, St. Petersburg General Hospital, Saint Petersburg, FL, p. A138
SAMUELS, Steven, M.D. Medical Director, Kindred Hospital Indianapolis South, Greenwood, IN, p. A203
SAMUELS, Tammy, Director Human Resources, Union County Hospital, Anna, IL, p. A172
SAMYN, Mike, Vice President, Finance and Chief Financial Officer, St. Mary Mercy Hospital, Livonia, MI, p. A318
SAMZ, Jeff, Chief Operating Officer, Huntsville Hospital, Huntsville, AL, p. A22
SAN FILIPPO, Bruce, M.D. Chief Medical Officer, Memorial Medical Center, Las Cruces, NM, p. A416
SANBORN, Michael, FACHE President, Baylor Medical Center at Carrollton, Carrollton, TX, p. A586
SANBORN, Randall, Director Information Technology, HealthSource Saginaw, Saginaw, MI, p. A322
SANCHEZ, Carmen, Director Human Resources, Hospital Dr. Cayetano Coll Y Toste, Arecibo, PR, p. A700
SANCHEZ, Freddie T., Director Information Systems, Placentia–Linda Hospital, Placentia, CA, p. A80
SANCHEZ, Jacqueline, Director Human Resources, Los Angeles Metropolitan Medical Center, Los Angeles, CA, p. A70
SANCHEZ, John, Vice President Human Resources, White Plains Hospital Center, White Plains, NY, p. A447
SANCHEZ, Jon, M.D. Chief of Staff, Bluegrass Community Hospital, Versailles, KY, p. A259
SANCHEZ, Jose R., President and Chief Executive Officer, Norwegian American Hospital, Chicago, IL, p. A177
SANCHEZ, Nancy, Senior Vice President and Vice Dean Human Resources, NYU Langone Medical Center, New York, NY, p. A436
SANCHEZ, Patty, Site Manager Human Resources, Adventist La Grange Memorial Hospital, La Grange, IL, p. A186
SANCHEZ, Rachel, Director Information Systems, Providence Little Company of Mary Medical Center San Pedro,, CA, p. A71
SANCHEZ, Rebecca, R.N. Director of Nursing, Texas Center for Infectious Disease, San Antonio, TX, p. A626
SANCHEZ–BICKLEY, Michelle
Vice President Human Resources, Renown Regional Medical Center, Reno, NV, p. A395
Vice President Human Resources, Renown Rehabilitation Hospital, Reno, NV, p. A395
Vice President Human Resources, Renown South Meadows Medical Center, Reno, NV, p. A395
SANCHEZ–JIMENEZ, Aida, M.D. Chief Medical Officer, Osceola Regional Medical Center, Kissimmee, FL, p. A127
SANDBERG, Todd, Chief Executive Officer, Sibley Medical Center, Arlington, MN, p. A327
SANDENE, Jeff, Chief Finance, Sanford University of South Dakota Medical Center, Sioux Falls, SD, p. A559
SANDER, Cindy, Coordinator Human Resources, Kindred Hospital–St. Louis, Saint Louis, MO, p. A368
SANDER, Wendy, Director Human Resources, Riverside Medical Center, Riverside, CA, p. A83
SANDERS, Amy, Chief Human Resources, Captain James A. Lovell Federal Health Care Center, North Chicago, IL, p. A189
SANDERS, David, Chief Financial Officer, Jackson Parish Hospital, Jonesboro, LA, p. A268
SANDERS, David S., Chief Executive Officer, Fannin Regional Hospital, Blue Ridge, GA, p. A148
SANDERS, Gale H., Director, Gadsden Regional Medical Center, Gadsden, AL, p. A20
SANDERS, Harv, Chief Financial Officer, Rhea Medical Center, Dayton, TN, p. A565
SANDERS, Jeff, Chief Operating Officer, Maine Medical Center, Portland, ME, p. A284
SANDERS, Jeffrey, M.D. Chief of Staff, Carson Tahoe Regional Healthcare, Carson City, NV, p. A391
SANDERS, John W., President, OhioHealth Marion General Hospital, Marion, OH, p. A484
SANDERS, Kelly, Vice President Human Resources, Good Shepherd Health Care System, Hermiston, OR, p. A511
SANDERS, Kris, Chief Financial Officer, Methodist Extended Care Hospital, Memphis, TN, p. A571
SANDERS, Lee Anne, Director Human Resources, Cozby–Germany Hospital, Grand Saline, TX, p. A601
SANDERS, Michael B., President and Chief Executive Officer, Monroe Clinic, Monroe, WI, p. A687
SANDERS, Robert, M.D. Chief Medical Officer, Texoma Medical Center, Denison, TX, p. A593
SANDERS, Ryan, Director Information Services, Doctors Hospital of Columbus, Columbus, GA, p. A149
SANDERS, Steve, Chief Financial Officer, Washington County Hospital and Clinics, Washington, IA, p. A227
SANDERS, Susie Sherrod, Budget Officer, Cherry Hospital, Goldsboro, NC, p. A453
SANDERS, Thomas J., FACHE Director, Robert J. Dole Veterans Affairs Medical Center, Wichita, KS, p. A245
SANDERS, Todd, Manager Finance, Alta View Hospital, Sandy, UT, p. A641
SANDERSON, Kevin, Director Information Systems, Goodland Regional Medical Center, Goodland, KS, p. A233
SANDIFER, Ron, Chief Information Officer, Community Memorial Health System, Ventura, CA, p. A94
SANDIFER, Tawny, R.N. Vice President Patient Care, Capital Region Medical Center, Jefferson City, MO, p. A361
SANDIN, James H., M.D. Assistant Administrator Medical Affairs, Hunt Memorial Hospital District, Greenville, TX, p. A602
SANDLER, Vivian, Director Human Resources, Memorial Regional Hospital South,, FL, p. A125
SANDLIN, Keith, Chief Executive Officer, Cartersville Medical Center, Cartersville, GA, p. A148
SANDLIN, Michael, M.D. Chief of Staff, Okmulgee Memorial Hospital, Okmulgee, OK, p. A502
SANDORA, George, Vice President Finance, Allegheny Valley Hospital, Natrona Heights, PA, p. A530
SANDOVAL, Yvonne, Director of Nursing Operations, Rehabilitation Hospital of Southern New Mexico, Las Cruces, NM, p. A416
SANDS, Tiffany, Manager Health Information, Arbuckle Memorial Hospital, Sulphur, OK, p. A505
SANDSTROM, C. Bruce, Vice President and Chief Financial Officer, The Aroostook Medical Center, Presque Isle, ME, p. A285
SANFORD, Lisa, VP Patient Care/CNO, Holy Rosary Healthcare, Miles City, MT, p. A377
SANFORD, Sharon K., Director Human Resources, Jersey Community Hospital, Jerseyville, IL, p. A185
SANGER, David, M.D. Chief Medical Officer, Pawnee Valley Community Hospital, Larned, KS, p. A237
SANGHI, Harishankar, M.D. Clinical Director, St. Lawrence Psychiatric Center, Ogdensburg, NY, p. A439
SANKARAN, Jaya, M.D. Chief of Staff, St. Mary's of Michigan Standish Hospital, Standish, MI, p. A323
SANKOORIKAL, Joseph, M.D. Chief Medical Staff, Kansas Rehabilitation Hospital, Topeka, KS, p. A244
SANKOVICH, Mary Lou, MSN, Chief Executive Officer and Chief Nursing Officer, Vibra Hospital of Mahoning Valley, Boardman, OH, p. A471
SANKOVITZ, Patrick, M.D. Chief Medical Officer, St. Anthony North Hospital, Westminster, CO, p. A106
SANS, Heather, Human Resource Generalist, Edwin Shaw Rehab, Cuyahoga Falls, OH, p. A478
SANTAMARIA, Mark A., President, MidMichigan Medical Center–Gratiot, Alma, MI, p. A307
SANTANA, Leticia, Administrator Medical Records, Hospital Hermanos Melendez, Bayamon, PR, p. A700
SANTANGELO, Charles J., CP
Executive Vice President and Chief Financial Officer, Muncy Valley Hospital, Muncy, PA, p. A530
Executive Vice President and Chief Financial Officer, Williamsport Regional Medical Center, Williamsport, PA, p. A542
SANTANGELO, John, Director Information Technology, Cleveland Clinic Florida, Weston, FL, p. A143
SANTANGELO, Linda, Ph.D. Director, Desert Willow Treatment Center, Las Vegas, NV, p. A392
SANTIAGO, Alejandro, Director Finance, Doctors' Center Hospital San Juan, San Juan, PR, p. A703
SANTIAGO, Carlos T., Director Human Resources, Hospital Oncologico Andres Grillasca, Ponce, PR, p. A702
SANTIAGO, Eddie, M.D. Medical Director, Specialty Hospital at Monmouth, Long Branch, NJ, p. A405
SANTIAGO, Manuel, Chief Information Officer, Hospital Metropolitan, San Juan, PR, p. A703
SANTIAGO, Orlando, Human Resources Officer, Hospital Del Maestro, San Juan, PR, p. A703
SANTIAGO, Sugehi, Director, Hospital San Francisco, San Juan, PR, p. A703
SANTISTEVAN, Vivian, Chief Human Resources, Fort Defiance Indian Health Service Hospital, Fort Defiance, AZ, p. A32
SANTMAN, Kim D., Vice President Finance, St. Margaret's Hospital, Spring Valley, IL, p. A194
SANTORE, Richard, M.D. Chief Medical Officer, Sharp Memorial Hospital, San Diego, CA, p. A86
SANTOS, Alfred, Administrator, Lincoln County Medical Center, Ruidoso, NM, p. A417
SANTOS, David, Chief Operating Officer (VP Operations), St. Helena Hospital Clearlake, Clearlake, CA, p. A57
SANTOS, George, M.D. Executive Medical Director, West Oaks Hospital, Houston, TX, p. A608
SANTOS, Hugo, Vice President Human Resources, Children's Hospital Los Angeles, Los Angeles, CA, p. A69
SANTOS, Ismael, Director Human Resources, Valle Vista Hospital, Greenwood, IN, p. A203
SANTOS, Joseph C., M.P.H. Deputy Secretary for Hospital Administration, Commonwealth Health Center, Saipan, MP, p. A699
SANTOS, Lori, Vice President Finance, Albany Memorial Hospital, Albany, NY, p. A420

Index of Health Care Professionals
Index of Health Care Professionals / Santos

SANTOS, Thomas, R.N. Chief Nursing Officer and Director Quality Services, Parkview Community Hospital Medical Center, Riverside, CA, p. A82
SANTULLI, Patricia, Director Human Resources, Elmira Psychiatric Center, Elmira, NY, p. A426
SANVILLE, David, Vice President Finance, Gifford Medical Center, Randolph, VT, p. A644
SANZ, Lawrence A., Senior Vice President Finance and Chief Financial Officer, Midland Memorial Hospital, Midland, TX, p. A617
SANZ, Sean M., Chief Operating Officer, Rowan Regional Medical Center, Salisbury, NC, p. A460
SAPOLIS, Richard, Director Clinical Operations, First Hospital Wyoming Valley, Wilkes–Barre, PA, p. A541
SAPPINGTON–CRITTENDEN, Shana, Chief Operating Officer, Westside Regional Medical Center, Plantation, FL, p. A136
SAQUATON, Antonio, M.D. Chief Medical Officer, Select Specialty Hospital–Omaha, Omaha, NE, p. A388
SARBACHER, James, Chief Information Officer, State Hospital North, Orofino, ID, p. A170
SARDANA, Sadhana, M.D. Clinical Director, Rockland Children's Psychiatric Center, Orangeburg, NY, p. A439
SARDONE, Frank J., President and Chief Executive Officer, Bronson Healthcare Group, Inc., Kalamazoo, MI, p. B22
SARDONE, Frank J.
President and Chief Executive Officer, Bronson LakeView Hospital, Paw Paw, MI, p. A320
President and Chief Executive Officer, Bronson Methodist Hospital, Kalamazoo, MI, p. A316
SARGEANT, Marty
Chief Operating Officer, City of Hope's Helford Clinical Research Hospital, Duarte, CA, p. A59
Chief Operating Officer, Cleveland Clinic Florida, Weston, FL, p. A143
SARGENT, J. Dale, M.D
Chief Medical Officer, Wellmont Hancock County Hospital, Sneedville, TN, p. A575
Chief Medical Officer, Wellmont Holston Valley Medical Center, Kingsport, TN, p. A568
SARGENT, Kimberly, Vice President Patient Services, St. Luke's Hospital – Miners Campus, Coaldale, PA, p. A520
SARGENT, Patrick D., Commander, Carl R. Darnall Army Medical Center, Fort Hood, TX, p. A598
SARGENT, Reed
Assistant Administrator Finance, Garfield Memorial Hospital and Clinics, Panguitch, UT, p. A639
Assistant Administrator Finance, Valley View Medical Center, Cedar City, UT, p. A637
SARIAN, Michael, Chief Executive Officer, Hollywood Community Hospital, Los Angeles, CA, p. A69
SARLE, C. Richard, FACHE President and Chief Executive Officer, Carrier Clinic, Belle Mead, NJ, p. A401
SARMENTO, Joann, Manager Human Resources, Fairchild Medical Center, Yreka, CA, p. A96
SARNECKI, Robert (Bob), Chief Information Officer, Kingman Regional Medical Center, Kingman, AZ, p. A33
SARRICO, Christine, Chief Financial Officer, Saint Agnes Medical Center, Fresno, CA, p. A62
SARWAR, Mohammed, M.D. Medical Director, Walter Olin Moss Regional Medical Center, Lake Charles, LA, p. A271
SASS, Judy A., Chief Human Resources Officer, McGehee–Desha County Hospital, McGehee, AR, p. A48
SASS, Kevin, FACHE Senior Executive Officer, Doctors Hospital of Columbus, Columbus, GA, p. A149
SASSER, Kelley, Director Information Systems, Florida Hospital Zephyrhills, Zephyrhills, FL, p. A143
SATEY, Phil, Vice President Human Resources, Valdese General Hospital, Valdese, NC, p. A462
SATKOSKI, Linda L., R.N. Chief Operating Officer, Indiana University Health La Porte Hospital, La Porte, IN, p. A206
SATO, James T., FACHE Chief Executive Officer, Helena Regional Medical Center, Helena, AR, p. A46
SATROM, William, Chief Financial Officer, Jackson County Hospital District, Edna, TX, p. A595
SATTAR, Parhez, Senior Director Information Technology, Grande Ronde Hospital, La Grande, OR, p. A512
SATTLER, Alan, President, ProMedica Flower Hospital, Sylvania, OH, p. A489
SATTLER, Sharon, Human Resources Officer, Ferry County Memorial Hospital, Republic, WA, p. A665
SAUCEDO, Jesse, Chief Financial Officer, Heartland Surgical Specialty Hospital, Overland Park, KS, p. A240
SAUER, Bernie, Director Information Technology, San Gabriel Valley Medical Center, San Gabriel, CA, p. A87
SAUER, Mary R., R.N. Chief Nursing Officer, Lakewood Hospital, Lakewood, OH, p. A482
SAUERS, Preston, Chief Financial Officer, Ellsworth County Medical Center, Ellsworth, KS, p. A232
SAUK, Michael, Chief Information Officer, University of Wisconsin Hospital and Clinics, Madison, WI, p. A684
SAUL, Thomas, Interim Chief Operating Officer, Culpeper Regional Hospital, Culpeper, VA, p. A647
SAULLO, Nancy, Director Human Resources, Warren State Hospital, Warren, PA, p. A540
SAULNIER, Robert, R.N. Chief Nurse Executive, Columbus Specialty Hospital, Columbus, GA, p. A149
SAULS, Randy, Chief Executive Officer and Administrator, South Georgia Medical Center, Valdosta, GA, p. A161
SAUM, Anita, Director Human Resources, Rehabilitation Hospital of Tinton Falls, Tinton Falls, NJ, p. A410
SAUNAITIS, Tammy, Chief Human Resources Officer, Meriter Hospital, Madison, WI, p. A684
SAUNDERS, Candice, Senior Vice President and Administrator, WellStar Kennestone Hospital, Marietta, GA, p. A156
SAUNDERS, John R., M.D. Senior Vice President Medical Affairs and Chief Medical Officer, Greater Baltimore Medical Center, Baltimore, MD, p. A287
SAUNDERS, Jonathan, Chief Financial Officer, Baylor Medical Center at Trophy Club, Trophy Club, TX, p. A631
SAUNDERS, Kristi K., Director and Compliance Officer, Calais Regional Hospital, Calais, ME, p. A282
SAUNDERS, M. Patricia, R.N. Vice President Nursing, Hanover Hospital, Hanover, PA, p. A524
SAUNDERS, Rosanne C., Senior Vice President and Chief Human Resources Officer, Jefferson Regional Medical Center, Jefferson Hills, PA, p. A525
SAUNDERS, Theodore, Assistant Controller, Wesley Woods Long Term Care Hospital, Atlanta, GA, p. A146
SAVAGE, Josh, Chief Financial Officer, Brownfield Regional Medical Center, Brownfield, TX, p. A585
SAVAGE, Kim, Interim Controller, Charlton Memorial Hospital, Folkston, GA, p. A152
SAVAGE, Robert L., President and Chief Executive Officer, Saint Francis Hospital and Health Centers, Poughkeepsie, NY, p. A441
SAVAGE, Steve, Chief Operating Officer, BCA Stonecrest Hospital, Detroit, MI, p. A310
SAVAGE–TRACY, Elizabeth, Vice President and Human Resources Officer, Winchester Medical Center, Winchester, VA, p. A657
SAVERESE, Joseph, Director Information Systems, New York Methodist Hospital,, NY, p. A435
SAVINO, Linda A., MS, Chief Executive Officer, Rehabilitation Hospital of Tinton Falls, Tinton Falls, NJ, p. A410
SAVITCH, Lane A., President, Kadlec Medical Center, Richland, WA, p. A665
SAVOY III, F. Peter, Chief Executive Officer, Acadia–St. Landry Hospital, Church Point, LA, p. A264
SAVOY, Greg, M.D. Chief Medical Officer, Savoy Medical Center, Mamou, LA, p. A272
SAVOY, Remi, Administrator, Oceans Behavioral Hospital of Opelousas, Opelousas, LA, p. A275
SAVSTROM, Curt, Chief Financial Officer and Chief Information Officer, River's Edge Hospital and Clinic, Saint Peter, MN, p. A339
SAWA, Kendall, R.N. Vice President Patient Care Services, PeaceHealth Ketchikan Medical Center, Ketchikan, AK, p. A29
SAWDEY, Don, M.D. Medical Director, Daniels Memorial Healthcare Center, Scobey, MT, p. A379
SAWYER, Anne, Chief Financial Officer, Wayne County Hospital, Monticello, KY, p. A256
SAWYER, Colleen A., MSN,
Executive Director, Mohawk Valley Psychiatric Center, Utica, NY, p. A445
Executive Director, Richard H. Hutchings Psychiatric Center, Syracuse, NY, p. A444
SAWYER, Dorothy, Chief Executive Officer, Carondelet St. Mary's Hospital, Tucson, AZ, p. A39
SAWYER, Gregory D., M.D. Vice President Physician Practices, Yakima Valley Memorial Hospital, Yakima, WA, p. A669
SAWYER, John, Executive Director, Porterville Developmental Center, Porterville, CA, p. A81
SAWYER, Robert, Senior Project Specialist, Spaulding Hospital for Continuing Medical Care North Shore, Salem, MA, p. A304
SAWYER, Scott, Chief Financial Officer, Community Medical Center, Falls City, NE, p. A383
SAWYER, Stephen
Chief Financial Officer, Dickenson Community Hospital, Clintwood, VA, p. A647
Chief Financial Officer, Norton Community Hospital, Norton, VA, p. A653
SAXTON, Beth, R.N. Vice President Patient Care Services, Yuma District Hospital, Yuma, CO, p. A107
SAYDACK, Roger, Interim Chief Operating Officer, Sacred Heart Medical Center at RiverBend, Springfield, OR, p. A516
SAYLER, Beth, Director Human Resources, Regency Hospital of Covington, Covington, LA, p. A265
SAYLER, Elizabeth, M.D. Chief of Staff, Lead–Deadwood Regional Hospital, Deadwood, SD, p. A556
SAYLER, Mark, Chief Financial Officer, Curry General Hospital, Gold Beach, OR, p. A510
SAYLER, Roger, Finance Officer, Veterans Affairs Health Care System, Fargo, ND, p. A466
SAYLER, Timothy, President and Chief Executive Officer, St. Joseph Regional Medical Center, Lewiston, ID, p. A169
SAYLOR, Craig M., Vice President and Chief Operating Officer, Somerset Hospital, Somerset, PA, p. A538
SAYLOR, Richard F., M.D. Chief Medical Officer, Pottstown Memorial Medical Center, Pottstown, PA, p. A536
SAYLORS, Julie, Controller, AnMed Health Rehabilitation Hospital, Anderson, SC, p. A546
SAYRE, Amy, Director Human Resources, General John J. Pershing Memorial Hospital, Brookfield, MO, p. A356
SAYRE, Michelle, R.N. Chief Nursing Officer, Arrowhead Regional Medical Center, Colton, CA, p. A58
SCAFIDI, Frank, Vice President and Chief Information Officer, Georgetown Memorial Hospital, Georgetown, SC, p. A550
SCALISE, Paul, M.D. Chief Pulmonary Medicine and Internal Medicine, Hospital for Special Care, New Britain, CT, p. A110
SCALLEN, Jr., Joseph, Chief Financial Officer, Children's Hospital of Michigan, Detroit, MI, p. A310
SCALLON, Jean, Chief Executive Officer, Bloomington Meadows Hospital, Bloomington, IN, p. A198
SCANLON, Dennis P., Vice President Finance, Doctors Community Hospital, Lanham, MD, p. A292
SCANLON, Donald, Chief Financial Officer, Mount Sinai Hospital, New York, NY, p. A435
SCANLON, Jill, Director Human Resources, Northern Colorado Rehabilitation Hospital, Johnstown, CO, p. A102
SCANLON, John, DPM Chief Medical Officer, Chestnut Hill Hospital, Philadelphia, PA, p. A531
SCANLON, Shaun J., Senior Vice President Finance and Chief Financial Officer, Vail Valley Medical Center, Vail, CO, p. A106
SCANNELL, Stephen J., Chief Financial Officer, McLaren Northern Michigan, Petoskey, MI, p. A320
SCARANO, Jenaro, M.D. Medical Director, St. Luke's Episcopal Hospital, Ponce, PR, p. A702
SCARBORO, Parrish, Chief Operating Officer, John F. Kennedy Memorial Hospital, Indio, CA, p. A65
SCARBOROUGH, Scott, CPA, Interim Executive Director, The University of Toledo Medical Center, Toledo, OH, p. A489
SCARPINO, David
Senior Vice President and Chief Financial Officer, Benedictine Hospital, Kingston, NY, p. A428
Senior Vice President Finance and Chief Financial Officer, Kingston Hospital, Kingston, NY, p. A428
Chief Financial Officer, Margaretville Hospital, Margaretville, NY, p. A429
SCARROW, Lloyd, Chief Executive Officer, Physicians Medical Center of Santa Fe Hospital, Santa Fe, NM, p. A418
SCENNA, Maria, Chief Operating Officer, St. Christopher's Hospital for Children, Philadelphia, PA, p. A533
SCEPANSKI, Theresa, Vice President People and Organizational Development, University Health System, San Antonio, TX, p. A626
SCERCY, Charles, Chief Executive Officer, Snowden at Fredericksburg, Fredericksburg, VA, p. A648
SCHAAB, Ben, VP Fiscal Services/ Chief Financial Officer, CGH Medical Center, Sterling, IL, p. A194
SCHAACK, Gregory J., CP
Vice President and Chief Financial Officer, Candler Hospital, Savannah, GA, p. A158
Vice President and Chief Financial Officer, St. Joseph's Hospital, Savannah, GA, p. A159
SCHAAF, Jerry, M.D. Chief Medical Officer, Shenandoah Medical Center, Shenandoah, IA, p. A226
SCHAAF, Kay, Chief Nursing Officer, Prairie Community Hospital, Terry, MT, p. A379
SCHABERG, Dennis, M.D. Chief Medicine, Veterans Affairs Greater Los Angeles Healthcare System, Los Angeles, CA, p. A72
SCHADE, Sue, Chief Information Officer, Brigham and Women's Hospital, Boston, MA, p. A296
SCHAEFBAUER, Brian, Director Information Technology, Mobridge Regional Hospital, Mobridge, SD, p. A558
SCHAEFER, Becky, Chief Financial Officer, University of Utah Neuropsychiatric Institute, Salt Lake City, UT, p. A641
SCHAEFER, Carol, Human Resources, Hermann Area District Hospital, Hermann, MO, p. A360
SCHAEFER, Daniel, Vice President Information Services, Mayo Clinic Health System – Franciscan Healthcare in La Crosse, La Crosse, WI, p. A684
SCHAEFER, Jamie
Vice President Finance, Avera Sacred Heart Hospital, Yankton, SD, p. A561
Vice President Finance, Milbank Area Hospital Avera, Milbank, SD, p. A557

A924 Index of Health Care Professionals

Index of Health Care Professionals

Index of Health Care Professionals / Schmieg

SCHMIEG, Greg
Executive Director, Roosevelt Warm Springs Institute for Rehabilitation, Warm Springs, GA, p. A161
Executive Director, Roosevelt Warm Springs LTAC Hospital, Warm Springs, GA, p. A161
SCHMIEGE, Ardis, Chief Financial Officer, Cascade Valley Hospital and Clinics, Arlington, WA, p. A659
SCHMIER, Joe, Director Human Resources, Payroll & Employee Health, Community Medical Center, Missoula, MT, p. A377
SCHMIT–CLINE, Annette, M.D. Medical Director, Mayo Clinic Health System in Springfield, Springfield, MN, p. A340
SCHMITGEN, Jamie, Chair Human Resources, Mayo Clinic Hospital, Phoenix, AZ, p. A36
SCHMITT, John, Senior Vice President and Chief Financial Officer, Kingsbrook Jewish Medical Center,, NY, p. A433
SCHMITT, Joseph, Chief Information Officer, St. Elizabeth's Medical Center, Brighton, MA, p. A298
SCHMITT, III, Joseph, Senior Vice President Finance and Chief Financial Officer, Henry Ford Hospital, Detroit, MI, p. A310
SCHMITT, Karl, M.D. Chief of Staff, St. Elizabeth Edgewood, Edgewood, KY, p. A249
SCHMITT, Michael, Chief Executive Officer, Kindred Hospital–Atlanta, Atlanta, GA, p. A145
SCHMITT, Jr., Milton G., M.D. Chief Medical Officer, Rockford Memorial Hospital, Rockford, IL, p. A193
SCHMITT, Peggy, President and Chief Executive Officer, North Kansas City Hospital, North Kansas City, MO, p. A366
SCHMITT II, Robert C., Chief Executive Officer, Gibson Area Hospital and Health Services, Gibson City, IL, p. A183
SCHMITT, Thomas M., Chief Executive Officer, Kansas Spine Hospital, Wichita, KS, p. A245
SCHMITTER, Angela, Director Health Information Management, Scotland County Hospital, Memphis, MO, p. A365
SCHMITZ, Bonnie, Chief Financial Officer, Waupun Memorial Hospital, Waupun, WI, p. A693
SCHMITZ, Brenda, Manager Finance, Central Alabama Veterans Health Care System, Montgomery, AL, p. A23
SCHMITZ, Christopher, Director Human Resources, Stoughton Hospital Association, Stoughton, WI, p. A691
SCHMITZ, Joseph, Chief Financial Officer, St. Cloud Veterans Affairs Health Care System, Saint Cloud, MN, p. A338
SCHMITZ, Vince
Senior Vice President and Chief Financial Officer, MultiCare Mary Bridge Children's Hospital and Health Center, Tacoma, WA, p. A668
Senior Vice President and Chief Financial Officer, MultiCare Tacoma General Hospital, Tacoma, WA, p. A668
SCHNACK, Tim H.
Chief Financial Officer, Alegent Health–Immanuel Medical Center, Omaha, NE, p. A387
Chief Financial Officer, Alegent Health–Memorial Hospital, Schuyler, NE, p. A389
SCHNEDLER, Lisa W., FACHE Chief Executive Officer and Administrator, Van Buren County Hospital, Keosauqua, IA, p. A222
SCHNEE, Lee, M.D. Chief Medical Staff, Holton Community Hospital, Holton, KS, p. A234
SCHNEEBERGER, Marie, Director of Health, Madelia Community Hospital, Madelia, MN, p. A334
SCHNEIDER, Barbara, R.N. Chief Executive Officer, Brotman Medical Center, Culver City, CA, p. A59
SCHNEIDER, Barry S., Chief Executive Officer, Western Arizona Regional Medical Center, Bullhead City, AZ, p. A31
SCHNEIDER, Brenda, Chief Financial Officer, Skyline Hospital, White Salmon, WA, p. A669
SCHNEIDER, Brian, Chief Financial Officer, Dupont Hospital, Fort Wayne, IN, p. A201
SCHNEIDER, C. W., President and Chief Executive Officer, Northwest Hospital & Medical Center, Seattle, WA, p. A665
SCHNEIDER, Carol L., Chief Operating Officer, John H. Stroger Jr. Hospital of Cook County, Chicago, IL, p. A176
SCHNEIDER, Catherine, M.D. Chief Medical Officer, Mt. Ascutney Hospital and Health Center, Windsor, VT, p. A644
SCHNEIDER, David R., Executive Director, Langlade Memorial Hospital, Antigo, WI, p. A678
SCHNEIDER, Doug, Director Information Systems, Raulerson Hospital, Okeechobee, FL, p. A134
SCHNEIDER, Greg, Director Information Technology, Winnebago Mental Health Institute, Winnebago, WI, p. A694
SCHNEIDER, H. Frank, Chief Executive Officer, Select Specialty Hospital–Wilmington, Wilmington, DE, p. A115
SCHNEIDER, Jessie, Director Human Resources, Community Memorial Healthcare, Marysville, KS, p. A238
SCHNEIDER, John, Human Resources Director, Putnam Community Medical Center, Palatka, FL, p. A135
SCHNEIDER, Ken
Chair Human Resources, Mayo Clinic – Methodist Hospital, Rochester, MN, p. A338
Chair Human Resources, Mayo Clinic – Saint Marys Hospital, Rochester, MN, p. A338
SCHNEIDER, Maureen, MSN Senior Vice President Clinical Program Development and Chief Operating Officer, Somerset Medical Center, Somerville, NJ, p. A410
SCHNEIDER, Palmer, Administrator, Van Diest Medical Center, Webster City, IA, p. A228
SCHNEIDER, Shanon, Chief Information Officer, Greeley County Health Services, Tribune, KS, p. A244
SCHNEIDER, Stacie A., Manager Human Resources, Aurora Medical Center – Manitowoc County, Two Rivers, WI, p. A692
SCHNEIDER, Stephen, Manager Information Services, Alaska Psychiatric Institute, Anchorage, AK, p. A28
SCHNEIDER, Valerie, Director Human Resources, Gove County Medical Center, Quinter, KS, p. A242
SCHNEIDER, William, Chief Financial Officer, St. Joseph's Hospital and Health Center, Dickinson, ND, p. A465
SCHNEIDERMAN, Henry, M.D. Vice President Medical Services and Physician in Chief, The Hospital at Hebrew Health Care, West Hartford, CT, p. A113
SCHNELL, Dawn, Chief Nursing Officer, Sanford Jackson Medical Center, Jackson, MN, p. A333
SCHNELL, Mary, R.N. Chief Nursing Officer, Howard A. Rusk Rehabilitation Center, Columbia, MO, p. A358
SCHNIEDERS, Michael H., President and Chief Executive Officer, Good Samaritan Hospital, Kearney, NE, p. A385
SCHNIER, Martin, D.O. Chief of Staff, West Texas VA Health Care System, Big Spring, TX, p. A584
SCHNOOR, Jeff, Director Information Technology and Systems, North Suburban Medical Center, Thornton, CO, p. A106
SCHOCK, Carl, Superintendent, Austin State Hospital, Austin, TX, p. A580
SCHOCK, Marilyn, Chief Executive Officer, McKee Medical Center, Loveland, CO, p. A104
SCHODDE, Joseph, Vice President Financial Services, Charlevoix Area Hospital, Charlevoix, MI, p. A309
SCHOELL, Mark C., Chief Executive Officer, United Memorial Medical Center, Batavia, NY, p. A421
SCHOELLER, Betsy V., Director Human Resources and Education, Mary Greeley Medical Center, Ames, IA, p. A214
SCHOEN, Greg, M.D. Regional Medical Director, Fairview Northland Medical Center, Princeton, MN, p. A337
SCHOEN, Lynn, Chief Executive Officer, Kindred Hospital–Dayton, Dayton, OH, p. A478
SCHOENDIENST, Gerald A., Chief Executive Officer, Jeff Davis Hospital, Hazlehurst, GA, p. A154
SCHOENECKER, Perry L., M.D. Chief of Staff, Shriners Hospitals for Children, St. Louis, Saint Louis, MO, p. A369
SCHOENHOLTZ, Jack C., M.D. President, Chief Executive Officer, Administrator and Medical Director, Rye Hospital Center, Rye, NY, p. A442
SCHOENIG, Tom
System Director Information Services, Desert Springs Hospital Medical Center, Las Vegas, NV, p. A392
Regional Director Information Services, Valley Hospital Medical Center, Las Vegas, NV, p. A394
SCHOEPLEIN, Kevin D., President, OSF Healthcare System, Peoria, IL, p. B99
SCHOETTLE, Steve, M.D. Chief Medical Staff, Ozark Health Medical Center, Clinton, AR, p. A43
SCHOFIELD, John, Chief Information Officer, Flagstaff Medical Center, Flagstaff, AZ, p. A32
SCHOFIELD, Sherry, Director Human Resources, Memorial Hospital, Martinsville, VA, p. A651
SCHOLEFIELD, Robert, Chief Operating Officer, St. Elizabeth Medical Center, Utica, NY, p. A445
SCHOLER, Duane, Chief Executive Officer, Arizona Orthopedic Surgical Hospital, Chandler, AZ, p. A31
SCHOLTEN, Ted, Chief Operating Officer, Rehabilitation Hospital of Fort Wayne, Fort Wayne, IN, p. A202
SCHOLZ, Suzanne, Director Medical Records, Horsham Clinic, Ambler, PA, p. A518
SCHON, John, Administrator and Chief Executive Officer, Dickinson County Healthcare System, Iron Mountain, MI, p. A315
SCHONEBERY, Jeremy, Director Information Technology, Heart of America Medical Center, Rugby, ND, p. A468
SCHONLAU, Dan, Chief Financial Officer, Nebraska Heart Institute and Heart Hospital, Lincoln, NE, p. A385
SCHOOLER, Richard D., M.D. Chief Medical Officer, Freeman Hospital West, Joplin, MO, p. A361
SCHOOLER, Rick
Vice President and Chief Information Officer, Orlando Regional Medical Center, Orlando, FL, p. A134
Vice President Information Services, Orlando Regional South Seminole Hospital, Longwood, FL, p. A129
SCHOOMAKER, Eric B., Surgeon General, Department of the Army, Office of the Surgeon General, Falls Church, VA, p. B41
SCHOONMAKER, John T., Senior Vice President and Chief Financial Officer, Texas Scottish Rite Hospital for Children, Dallas, TX, p. A592
SCHOPER, Marian, Manager Human Resources, Mayo Clinic Health System in Springfield, Springfield, MN, p. A340
SCHOR, Mark, Chief Executive Officer, First Hospital Wyoming Valley, Wilkes–Barre, PA, p. A541
SCHORI, Melissa, M.D. Medical Director, Lincoln Medical and Mental Health Center,, NY, p. A434
SCHOTT, Connie, Administrative Assistant, Florida Hospital Memorial Medical Center, Daytona Beach, FL, p. A121
SCHOU, Howard, Chief Financial Officer, Franklin Hospital District, Benton, IL, p. A173
SCHOULTIES, Daniel L., M.D. Vice President Medical Affairs, Good Samaritan Hospital, Dayton, OH, p. A478
SCHOWENGERDT, Daniel, M.D. Chief of Staff, Comanche County Hospital, Coldwater, KS, p. A231
SCHRADER, Guillermo, M.D. Acting Medical Director, Eastern State Hospital, Williamsburg, VA, p. A657
SCHRAEDER, David, Director Information Systems, Russell Regional Hospital, Russell, KS, p. A242
SCHRAMM, Michael, Chief Executive Officer, Rice Memorial Hospital, Willmar, MN, p. A342
SCHRAMM, Steven R., Chief Financial Officer, Mountain View Hospital, Payson, UT, p. A639
SCHRECK, Rhonda, Director Human Resources, Keokuk Area Hospital, Keokuk, IA, p. A222
SCHREEG, Timothy M., President and Chief Executive Officer, Jasper County Hospital, Rensselaer, IN, p. A211
SCHREIBER, Anne, Manager Human Resources, Fairfax Hospital, Kirkland, WA, p. A662
SCHREIBER, Mary Jo, R.N. Vice President Patient Services, Winter Haven Hospital, Winter Haven, FL, p. A143
SCHREIBER, Matthew, M.D. Chief Medical Officer, Piedmont Hospital, Atlanta, GA, p. A146
SCHREIBER, Rob, M.D. Chief Medical Officer, Hebrew Rehabilitation Center, Boston, MA, p. A297
SCHREIER, Scott, Chief Information Officer, Mt. Ascutney Hospital and Health Center, Windsor, VT, p. A644
SCHREIER, Susan, R.N. Chief Nursing Executive, Rockford Memorial Hospital, Rockford, IL, p. A193
SCHREINER, David L., FACHE President and Chief Executive Officer, Katherine Shaw Bethea Hospital, Dixon, IL, p. A180
SCHREITMUELLER, Julie, Chief Operating Officer, Story County Medical Center, Nevada, IA, p. A224
SCHREIVOGEL, Herman, Chief Executive Officer, Lincoln Community Hospital and Nursing Home, Hugo, CO, p. A102
SCHRODER, Loren D., Chief Financial Officer, Phelps Memorial Health Center, Holdrege, NE, p. A384
SCHROEDER, Christine, R.N. Chief Nursing Officer, Carrington Health Center, Carrington, ND, p. A464
SCHROEDER, Cygnet, D.O. Medical Director, HEALTHSOUTH Rehabilitation Hospital of Fort Smith, Fort Smith, AR, p. A45
SCHROEDER, Gary, Chief Financial Officer, Dayton General Hospital, Dayton, WA, p. A661
SCHROEDER, Larry, Chief Executive Officer, Sauk Prairie Memorial Hospital & Clinics, Prairie Du Sac, WI, p. A689
SCHROEDER, Rick, Chief Executive Officer, North Big Horn Hospital District, Lovell, WY, p. A697
SCHROEDL, Greg, M.D. Vice President Medical and Chief Quality Officer, Northwest Hospital & Medical Center, Seattle, WA, p. A665
SCHROER, Patricia A., President and Chief Executive Officer, Mercy Hospital Anderson, Cincinnati, OH, p. A473
SCHROFFEL, Bruce, President and Chief Executive Officer, University of Colorado Hospital, Aurora, CO, p. A97
SCHROYER, Mike, Chief Operating Officer, St. Vincent Heart Center of Indiana, Indianapolis, IN, p. A205
SCHROYER, Renee, Chief Financial Officer, Sutter Surgical Hospital – North Valley, Yuba City, CA, p. A96
SCHRUM, Andrew, Director Information Systems, Washington County Memorial Hospital, Potosi, MO, p. A367
SCHRUMPF, Jason, President, Missouri Delta Medical Center, Sikeston, MO, p. A371
SCHUBERT, Bob, Director Human Resources, Scott & White Hospital – Brenham, Brenham, TX, p. A585
SCHUCKMAN, Tim, Chief Financial Officer, Jennie M. Melham Memorial Medical Center, Broken Bow, NE, p. A382
SCHUE, Janine
Senior Vice President People Resources, Newark–Wayne Community Hospital, Newark, NY, p. A438
Senior Vice President Human Resources, Rochester General Hospital, Rochester, NY, p. A441
SCHUELER, Joe, Chief Financial Officer, Morrow County Hospital, Mount Gilead, OH, p. A485
SCHUESSLER, Donald, M.D. Medical Director, Edward John Noble Hospital of Gouverneur, Gouverneur, NY, p. A427
SCHUESSLER, Dwight, Chief Information Officer, Iowa City Veterans Affairs Health Care System, Iowa City, IA, p. A221
SCHUESSLER, Joel, Interim Vice President Human Resources, DeKalb Medical at North Decatur, Decatur, GA, p. A151
SCHUETT, Susan M., Chief Information Officer, Olmsted Medical Center, Rochester, MN, p. A338

A926 Index of Health Care Professionals

Index of Health Care Professionals / Scott


SCHUETZ, Charles D., Chief Executive Officer, University General Hospital, Houston, TX, p. A607
SCHUETZ, Jill, Manager Human Resources, LifeCare Hospitals of Wisconsin, Pewaukee, WI, p. A689
SCHUITEMAN, Jackson, Chief Financial Officer, Sioux Center Community Hospital and Health Center Avera, Sioux Center, IA, p. A226
SCHUKNECHT, Amy, Manager Human Resources, Lynn County Hospital District, Tahoka, TX, p. A630
SCHULER, Allison, R.N. Chief Nursing Officer, Montfort Jones Memorial Hospital, Kosciusko, MS, p. A348
SCHULER, G. Wayne, Chief Executive Officer, Cleveland Regional Medical Center, Cleveland, TX, p. A587
SCHULER, Kathy, R.N. Vice President of Patient Care Services, Winchester Hospital, Winchester, MA, p. A306
SCHULER, William, M.D. President Medical Staff, Mendota Community Hospital, Mendota, IL, p. A188
SCHULHOF, Alicia, Chief Operating Officer, Brandon Regional Hospital, Brandon, FL, p. A119
SCHULTE, James E., Chief Executive Officer, Redwood Area Hospital, Redwood Falls, MN, p. A337
SCHULTE, Joyce, Chief Executive Officer, Ellinwood District Hospital, Ellinwood, KS, p. A232
SCHULTE, Mark, Chief Executive Officer, Avera Creighton Hospital, Creighton, NE, p. A383
SCHULTEIS, Chris, Vice President/Chief Financial Officer, Southampton Hospital, Southampton, NY, p. A443
SCHULTHEIS, David, Chief Financial Officer, Devereux Children's Behavioral Health Center, Malvern, PA, p. A528
SCHULTHEIS, Hal, Director Information Systems, Hendersonville Medical Center, Hendersonville, TN, p. A566
SCHULTZ, Bradley
Chief Financial Officer, Skyline Madison Campus, Madison, TN, p. A570
Chief Financial Officer, Skyline Medical Center, Nashville, TN, p. A573
SCHULTZ, David W., FACHE Executive Vice President and Chief Operating Officer, Overlake Hospital Medical Center, Bellevue, WA, p. A659
SCHULTZ, Diana, Chief Executive Officer, Kindred Hospital–Corpus Christi, Corpus Christi, TX, p. A589
SCHULTZ, Jacky, R.N. Executive Vice President and Chief Operating Officer, Suburban Hospital, Bethesda, MD, p. A290
SCHULTZ, Karl W., M.D. Chief of Staff, Elkhart General Healthcare System, Elkhart, IN, p. A200
SCHULTZ, Kim, Manager Information, Connally Medical Center, Floresville, TX, p. A597
SCHULTZ, Mary Kay, Director Human Resources, Sturgis Hospital, Sturgis, MI, p. A323
SCHULTZ, Rachelle H., President and Chief Executive Officer, Winona Health, Winona, MN, p. A342
SCHULZ, Charles K., Chief Executive Officer, York General Hospital, York, NE, p. A390
SCHULZ, Larry A., Chief Executive Officer, Lake Region Healthcare Corporation, Fergus Falls, MN, p. A331
SCHULZ, Marcie, Director Patient Care, Sakakawea Medical Center, Hazen, ND, p. A466
SCHULZ, Richard, Chief Executive Officer, HEALTHSOUTH Scottsdale Rehabilitation Hospital, Scottsdale, AZ, p. A38
SCHUMACHER, Ann, R.N. Vice President and Chief Operating Officer, Alegent Health–Immanuel Medical Center, Omaha, NE, p. A387
SCHUMACHER, Debbie
Chief Human Resources, Clearwater Valley Hospital and Clinics, Orofino, ID, p. A169
Manager Human Resource, St. Mary's Hospital, Cottonwood, ID, p. A168
SCHUMACHER, Kevin, Director of Information Services, LifeCare Medical Center, Roseau, MN, p. A338
SCHUMACHER, Linda, Chief Operating Officer, Chinese Hospital, San Francisco, CA, p. A86
SCHUMACHER, Rod, Chief Executive Officer, Roswell Regional Hospital, Roswell, NM, p. A417
SCHUMM, Herbert, M.D. Vice President Medical Affairs, St. Rita's Medical Center, Lima, OH, p. A483
SCHUPP, Frank, Chief Executive Officer, Flint River Community Hospital, Montezuma, GA, p. A156
SCHURKAMP, Christine, Human Resources Director, Spectrum Health Gerber Memorial, Fremont, MI, p. A312
SCHUSTER, Catherine, Chief Information Officer, Northern Dutchess Hospital, Rhinebeck, NY, p. A441
SCHUSTER, Christine C., President and Chief Executive Officer, Emerson Hospital, Concord, MA, p. A299
SCHUSTER, Emmett C., President and Chief Executive Officer, Gibson General Hospital, Princeton, IN, p. A210
SCHUSTER, Jolene, Director Information Technology, Trego County–Lemke Memorial Hospital, Wakeeney, KS, p. A244
SCHUSTER, Lexie, Vice President Human Resources, Good Samaritan Hospital, Los Angeles, CA, p. A69
SCHUTTER, Mark E., Ph.D. Superintendent and Chief Executive Officer, Logansport State Hospital, Logansport, IN, p. A207
SCHWAB, Bob, M.D. Chief Quality Officer, Texas Health Presbyterian Hospital Denton, Denton, TX, p. A594
SCHWAB, Caryn A., Executive Director, The Mount Sinai Hospital of Queens,, NY, p. A437
SCHWABENBAUER, Mary Ann, Director Information Technology, Elk Regional Health Center, Saint Marys, PA, p. A537
SCHWAGER, Mary A., Director Human Resources, Antelope Memorial Hospital, Neligh, NE, p. A386
SCHWALL, Garry, Chief Operating Officer, Winthrop–University Hospital, Mineola, NY, p. A430
SCHWAN, Joni, Director Human Resources, Excelsior Springs Hospital, Excelsior Springs, MO, p. A359
SCHWANER, III, Charles, Chief Financial Officer, Doctors Hospital of Sarasota, Sarasota, FL, p. A138
SCHWANKE, Daniel, President, ProMedica Fostoria Community Hospital, Fostoria, OH, p. A480
SCHWARM, Tony, President, Missouri Baptist Sullivan Hospital, Sullivan, MO, p. A371
SCHWARTZ, Ave, Chief Information Officer, Austen Riggs Center, Stockbridge, MA, p. A305
SCHWARTZ, Jonathon, M.D. Medical Director and Chief Medical Officer, Spaulding Hospital for Continuing Medical Care Cambridge, Cambridge, MA, p. A299
SCHWARTZ, Judy, M.D. Chief Medical Officer, Knox Community Hospital, Mount Vernon, OH, p. A485
SCHWARTZ, Kenneth V., M.D. Medical Director, Griffin Hospital, Derby, CT, p. A108
SCHWARTZ, Kim K., Director Human Resources and Physician Clinics, Boone County Hospital, Boone, IA, p. A215
SCHWARTZ, Michael J., Interim President, Morton Hospital and Medical Center, Taunton, MA, p. A305
SCHWARTZ, Peggy, Vice President Human Resources, Wayne Hospital, Greenville, OH, p. A481
SCHWARTZ, Peter
Manager Information Services, Carrier Clinic, Belle Mead, NJ, p. A401
Director Information Systems, East Mountain Hospital, Belle Mead, NJ, p. A401
SCHWARTZ, Roberta, Executive Vice President, The Methodist Hospital, Houston, TX, p. A607
SCHWARTZ, Ronald, M.D. Medical Director, Masonicare Health Center, Wallingford, CT, p. A112
SCHWARTZ, Sharon, Director Medical Records, Scott & White Hospital – Brenham, Brenham, TX, p. A585
SCHWARZBACH, Jerry, M.D. Medical Director, East Texas Medical Center Rehabilitation Center, Tyler, TX, p. A632
SCHWARZKOPF, Ruth, R.N. Chief Nursing Officer, West Boca Medical Center, Boca Raton, FL, p. A119
SCHWEAGEL, Glen
Vice President Finance, Barnes–Jewish St. Peters Hospital, Saint Peters, MO, p. A370
Chief Financial Officer, Progress West HealthCare Center, Saint Charles, MO, p. A367
SCHWEERS, Michele, Vice President Human Resources, Kimball Medical Center, Lakewood, NJ, p. A405
SCHWEICKHARDT, Mary Jo, Vice President Human Resources, Medstar Georgetown University Hospital, Washington, DC, p. A116
SCHWEIGERT, Matthew B., Administrator, Mercy Continuing Care Hospital, Chesterfield, MO, p. A357
SCHWEIGERT, Nicole, Director Human Resources, Texas Health Presbyterian Hospital Flower Mound, Flower Mound, TX, p. A597
SCHWEIGHART, Karen, MS, Administrator, Andrew McFarland Mental Health Center, Springfield, IL, p. A194
SCHWEIKART, Jay
Chief Financial Officer, Kindred Hospital Chicago–Northlake, Northlake, IL, p. A189
Chief Financial Officer, Kindred Hospital–Sycamore, Sycamore, IL, p. A195
SCHWEISS, Sue, Director of Nursing, Sleepy Eye Medical Center, Sleepy Eye, MN, p. A340
SCHWEITZER, Alex, Superintendent and Chief Executive Officer, North Dakota State Hospital, Jamestown, ND, p. A467
SCHWEITZER, Michael, M.D. Chief Medical Officer, St. Vincent Healthcare, Billings, MT, p. A373
SCHWEITZER, Tammy, Chief Financial Officer, Grisell Memorial Hospital District One, Ransom, KS, p. A242
SCHWEIZER, Brenda, Coordinator Human Resources, Kindred Hospital of Northern Indiana, Mishawaka, IN, p. A208
SCHWENZFEIER, Jeni, Chief Financial Officer, Kittson Memorial Healthcare Center, Hallock, MN, p. A332
SCHWERZLER, Ron, M.D. Director Medical Services, Serenity Lane, Eugene, OR, p. A510
SCHWIND, David, Chief Financial Officer, Capital Hospice, Arlington, VA, p. A645
SCHWIND, Mary, R.N. Chief Clinical Officer, Kindred Hospital–San Francisco Bay Area, San Leandro, CA, p. A88
SCHWINGLER, Joyce, Chief Financial Officer, Eureka Community Health Services Avera, Eureka, SD, p. A556
SCHWOEBLE, Walter, Vice President Human Resources, Akron Children's Hospital, Akron, OH, p. A469
SCIALDONE, Michael A., Chief Financial Officer, Memorial Health System, Colorado Springs, CO, p. A98
SCIARRO, Jason
President and Chief Operating Officer, Centegra Hospital – McHenry, McHenry, IL, p. A187
Chief Operating Officer, Centegra Hospital – Woodstock, Woodstock, IL, p. A196
SCIBELLI, Tony, Vice President Human Resources and Operations, Faxton–St. Luke's Healthcare, Utica, NY, p. A445
SCIESZINSKI, Robert C., Vice President Finance, Ministry Door County Medical Center, Sturgeon Bay, WI, p. A691
SCIONTI, Jeff, Chief Operating Officer, Parkland Medical Center, Derry, NH, p. A397
SCIORTINO, John E., Senior Vice President and Chief Operating Officer, New York Hospital Queens,, NY, p. A435
SCIOSCIA, Angela, M.D. Chief Medical Officer, UC San Diego Health System, San Diego, CA, p. A86
SCIOTTI, Joanne, Director Information Technology, Jennersville Regional Hospital, West Grove, PA, p. A541
SCIULLO, Armando, D.O. Chief of Staff, Grove City Medical Center, Grove City, PA, p. A524
SCIURBA, John, Vice President and Chief Financial Officer, White Plains Hospital Center, White Plains, NY, p. A447
SCLAIR, Max
Vice President Human Resources, Brookdale Hospital Medical Center,, NY, p. A431
Vice President Human Resources, Flushing Hospital Medical Center,, NY, p. A432
Vice President Human Resources, Jamaica Hospital Medical Center,, NY, p. A433
SCLAMA, Tony, M.D. Vice President Medical Affairs, Medstar Franklin Square Medical Center, Baltimore, MD, p. A288
SCOBIE, Robbin, Vice President Nursing, Aurelia Osborn Fox Memorial Hospital, Oneonta, NY, p. A439
SCOCCIA, Vincent, D.O. Chief Medical Staff, Nye Regional Medical Center, Tonopah, NV, p. A396
SCOGGINS, Kim, Administrator, Polk Medical Center, Cedartown, GA, p. A149
SCOPAC, Paul A., Vice President of Operations and Chief Operating Officer, Oneida Healthcare, Oneida, NY, p. A439
SCOPELLITI, Joseph A., M.D. President and Chief Executive Officer, Guthrie Healthcare System, Sayre, PA, p. B56
SCORZELLI, Gerard, Chief Financial Officer, Albany Stratton Veterans Affairs Medical Center, Albany, NY, p. A420
SCOTT, Arthur B., Vice President Operations, North Adams Regional Hospital, North Adams, MA, p. A303
SCOTT, Camille, Administrator, Forks Community Hospital, Forks, WA, p. A661
SCOTT, Charles F., President and Chief Executive Officer, Henry Medical Center, Stockbridge, GA, p. A160
SCOTT, Colleen M., Vice President Finance, Waterbury Hospital, Waterbury, CT, p. A112
SCOTT, Craig, Interim Director Management Information Systems, University of Miami Hospital, Miami, FL, p. A132
SCOTT, David W., President and Chief Executive Officer, Ohio Valley General Hospital, McKees Rocks, PA, p. A528
SCOTT, Debbie, Chief Operating Officer, Davis County Hospital, Bloomfield, IA, p. A215
SCOTT, Doug, Director Human Resources, Jacksonville Medical Center, Jacksonville, AL, p. A22
SCOTT, Ernie, Director Human Resources, Natchitoches Regional Medical Center, Natchitoches, LA, p. A274
SCOTT, Ginger, Vice President Human Resources, Columbus Regional Healthcare System, Whiteville, NC, p. A462
SCOTT, Heath, M.D. Chief of Staff, King's Daughters Hospital, Yazoo City, MS, p. A354
SCOTT, James, M.D. Vice President Medical Affairs, Candler Hospital, Savannah, GA, p. A158
SCOTT, Jeffrey, Chief Information Officer, St. Joseph Hospital and Health Center, Kokomo, IN, p. A206
SCOTT, Jerry, Chief Operating Officer, Navos, Seattle, WA, p. A665
SCOTT, Jon W., Chief Executive Officer, Select Specialty Hospital–Topeka, Topeka, KS, p. A244
SCOTT, Joseph F., FACHE President and Chief Executive Officer, LibertyHealth–Jersey City Medical Center, Jersey City, NJ, p. A405
SCOTT, Kimberley, Director Health Care Services, Kansas Neurological Institute, Topeka, KS, p. A244
SCOTT, Kurt M., FACHE Administrator, LSU Bogalusa Medical Center, Bogalusa, LA, p. A263
SCOTT, M Daryl, Assistant Vice President, Jefferson Regional Medical Center, Pine Bluff, AR, p. A50
SCOTT, Robert F., Vice President Human Resources, Advocate Good Shepherd Hospital, Barrington, IL, p. A173


Index of Health Care Professionals

Index of Health Care Professionals

Index of Health Care Professionals / Scott


SCOTT, Ron, Vice President Human Resources, Queen of the Valley Medical Center, Napa, CA, p. A76
SCOTT, Seth, M.D. Chief of Staff, George County Hospital, Lucedale, MS, p. A349
SCOTT, Stacy, Director of Nursing, Sabetha Community Hospital, Sabetha, KS, p. A242
SCOTT, Steve, Chief Operating Officer, Sheridan Community Hospital, Sheridan, MI, p. A323
SCOTT, Susan, Director Medical Records, Beartooth Billings Clinic, Red Lodge, MT, p. A378
SCOTT, Thomas, Chief Operating Officer, Chilton Hospital, Pompton Plains, NJ, p. A409
SCOTT, Vanda
Chief Executive Officer, Select Specialty Hospital–Knoxville, Knoxville, TN, p. A568
Chief Executive Officer, Select Specialty Hospital–Knoxville, Knoxville, TN, p. A568
Chief Executive Officer, Select Specialty Hospital–North Knoxville, Knoxville, TN, p. A568
SCOTT, Vigil, Resource Management Flight Commander, Wright Patterson Medical Center, Wright–Patterson AFB, OH, p. A492
SCOTT, William, M.D. Vice President Medical Affairs, Regional Medical Center of San Jose, San Jose, CA, p. A88
SCOTT, William, Chief Financial Officer, Specialty Hospital of Mid–America, Overland Park, KS, p. A241
SCOTT, William P., M.D. Chief of Staff, River Valley Medical Center, Dardanelle, AR, p. A43
SCOTTEN, Dianne, Chief Clinical Officer, Central Montana Medical Center, Lewistown, MT, p. A377
SCOTTO, Dan, Director Data Processing, Eastern Long Island Hospital, Greenport, NY, p. A427
SCOWN, Kent, Director Operations and Information Services, Jerold Phelps Community Hospital, Garberville, CA, p. A62
SCRASE, David R., M.D. Executive Senior Vice President and Chief Operating Officer, Presbyterian Kaseman Hospital, Albuquerque, NM, p. A414
SCREMIN, Karen, Vice President Finance, Exempla Lutheran Medical Center, Wheat Ridge, CO, p. A107
SCRIBER, Rachel, Director of Marketing & Public Relations, Medical Center of South Arkansas, El Dorado, AR, p. A44
SCRIVO, Jr., Joseph A., Director Human Resources, Mercy Hospital, Buffalo, NY, p. A423
SCRUGGS, Kisha, Chief Financial Officer, Brentwood Hospital, Shreveport, LA, p. A277
SCRUGGS, Sherry
Administrator, Gibson General Hospital, Trenton, TN, p. A576
Administrator, Humboldt General Hospital, Humboldt, TN, p. A566
Administrator, Milan General Hospital, Milan, TN, p. A572
SCULCO, Thomas P., M.D. Surgeon–in–Chief and Medical Director, Hospital for Special Surgery, New York, NY, p. A433
SCULLY, Charles
Chief Information Officer, Renown Regional Medical Center, Reno, NV, p. A395
Chief Information Officer, Renown Rehabilitation Hospital, Reno, NV, p. A395
Chief Information Officer, Renown South Meadows Medical Center, Reno, NV, p. A395
SCULLY, Trish
Manager Employment Services, Massachusetts Hospital School, Canton, MA, p. A299
Director Human Resources, Taunton State Hospital, Taunton, MA, p. A305
SCURLOCK, Scott, Chief Information Officer, Doctors Memorial Hospital, Bonifay, FL, p. A119
SCZYGELSKI, Sidney C., Senior Vice President Finance and Chief Financial Officer, Aspirus Wausau Hospital, Wausau, WI, p. A693
SEABORN, Scott, Administrator, St. Joseph Memorial Hospital, Murphysboro, IL, p. A188
SEAFORD, Jeff, Director Human Resources, Hugh Chatham Memorial Hospital, Elkin, NC, p. A453
SEAGO, Terri, Chief Financial Officer, Baptist Memorial Hospital–Collierville, Collierville, TN, p. A564
SEAGRAVES, David H., Chief Executive Officer, Cobb Memorial Hospital, Royston, GA, p. A158
SEAGROVES, Matthew, Chief Financial Officer, Brooksville Regional Hospital, Brooksville, FL, p. A119
SEAHORN, Martha, R.N. Chief Nurse Office, Shelby Baptist Medical Center, Alabaster, AL, p. A15
SEAL, John, Director Human Resources, Riverside Medical Center, Franklinton, LA, p. A266
SEAL, Ronald T., Chief Executive Officer, Texoma Medical Center, Denison, TX, p. A593
SEALE, Corey A., Administrator, Moreno Valley Community Hospital, Moreno Valley, CA, p. A75
SEALE, Edward, Chief Information Officer, New Horizons Health Systems, Owenton, KY, p. A257
SEALE, Paul E., FACHE Chief Operating Officer, Upstate University Hospital, Syracuse, NY, p. A444
SEALS, Carol, Chief Financial Officer, Indiana University Health Ball Memorial Hospital, Muncie, IN, p. A209
SEALS, Frank, Chief Financial Officer, Reeves County Hospital, Pecos, TX, p. A620
SEALS, Molly
Senior Vice President Human Resources and Learning, St. Elizabeth Boardman Health Center, Boardman, OH, p. A471
Senior Vice President Human Resources and Learning, St. Elizabeth Health Center, Youngstown, OH, p. A492
Senior Vice President Human Resources and Learning, St. Joseph Health Center, Warren, OH, p. A490
SEALS, Robert, D.O. Medical Director, Carson City Hospital, Carson City, MI, p. A309
SEARBY, Tonya L., Chief Human Resources, Veterans Affairs Medical Center, Marion, IL, p. A187
SEARLE, Anne, Chief Information Officer, University Medical Center of Princeton at Plainsboro, Plainsboro, NJ, p. A409
SEARLE, Reynolds, Director Information Systems, Fairfield Memorial Hospital, Winnsboro, SC, p. A554
SEARS, Frank, Vice President Information Services, Memorial Hospital of Carbondale, Carbondale, IL, p. A174
SEARS, Marilyn, President and Chief Executive Officer, Shelby Memorial Hospital, Shelbyville, IL, p. A193
SEARS, Michael A., Chief Financial Officer, Wayne Medical Center, Waynesboro, TN, p. A576
SEARS, Michelle, Director Information Systems, Helen Newberry Joy Hospital, Newberry, MI, p. A320
SEASE, Peggy, Vice President Human Resources, Southeast Alabama Medical Center, Dothan, AL, p. A19
SEAVER, Roger E., President and Chief Executive Officer, Henry Mayo Newhall Memorial Hospital, Valencia, CA, p. A94
SEAY, Lisa, Director Human Resources, Baylor Medical Center at Irving, Irving, TX, p. A609
SEBASTIAN, Peggy A., R.N. President and Chief Executive Officer, St. Joseph's Hospital, Highland, IL, p. A184
SEBASTIANELLI, Joseph T., President and Chief Executive Officer, Jefferson Health System, Radnor, PA, p. B73
SEBEK, Brenda Jean, R.N. Chief Nursing Officer, St. Mary's Community Hospital, Nebraska City, NE, p. A386
SECHI, Patricia, Chief Operating Officer, North Shore Medical Center, Miami, FL, p. A131
SECKINGER, Jenn, Chief Financial Officer, Community Memorial Hospital, Syracuse, NE, p. A390
SECKINGER, Mark R., Administrator and Chief Executive Officer, Hardin Memorial Hospital, Kenton, OH, p. A482
SECOR, Diane K., Director Human Resources, Lawrence Medical Center, Moulton, AL, p. A24
SECOR, Jr., Richard, M.D. Chief of Staff, Mineral Area Regional Medical Center, Farmington, MO, p. A359
SECORA, Charles, M.D. Interim Chief Executive Officer, Miners' Colfax Medical Center, Raton, NM, p. A417
SEDGWICK, Sally, Manager Public Relations and Marketing, Bigfork Valley Hospital, Bigfork, MN, p. A328
SEDIGHI, Hooman, M.D. President and Chief Executive Officer, GLOBALREHAB, Dallas, TX, p. B54
SEEDER, Rachael, Controller, Santiam Memorial Hospital, Stayton, OR, p. A516
SEEHAFER, Kevin
Chief Financial Officer, Kenmare Community Hospital, Kenmare, ND, p. A467
Chief Financial Officer, Trinity Health, Minot, ND, p. A467
SEEKINS, DeAnne
Director, Durham Veterans Affairs Medical Center, Durham, NC, p. A452
Director, Veterans Affairs Medical Center, Hampton, VA, p. A649
SEELEY, Kevin, Chief Information Officer, Mike O'Callaghan Federal Hospital, Nellis AFB, NV, p. A394
SEELMAN, Michael, Chief Operating Officer, Northside Medical Center, Youngstown, OH, p. A492
SEELY, Paula, Manager Human Resources, Kossuth Regional Health Center, Algona, IA, p. A214
SEEMS, Steven, Director of Information Technology, Phillips County Hospital, Phillipsburg, KS, p. A241
SEEVER, Jennifer, Regional Chief Financial Officer, Sedan City Hospital, Sedan, KS, p. A243
SEGAL, Jonathan, Chief Financial Officer, New York State Psychiatric Institute, New York, NY, p. A435
SEGELEON, Kurt, Director Health Information Management, Kindred Hospital–Pittsburgh, Oakdale, PA, p. A531
SEGIN, Robert
Chief Financial Officer, Virtua Berlin, Berlin, NJ, p. A402
Executive Vice President & Chief Financial Officer, Virtua Marlton, Marlton, NJ, p. A406
Chief Financial Officer, Virtua Memorial, Mount Holly, NJ, p. A406
SEGLER, Randall K., FACHE Chief Executive Officer, Comanche County Memorial Hospital, Lawton, OK, p. A498
SEGRAVES, Steven, M.D. Medical Director, Research Psychiatric Center, Kansas City, MO, p. A362
SEHRT, Lori, Chief Financial Officer, McKee Medical Center, Loveland, CO, p. A104
SEIBERT, Nancy, Director Human Resources, Franklin Hospital District, Benton, IL, p. A173
SEID, Lynette, Area Chief Financial Officer, San Diego Medical Center, San Diego, CA, p. A85
SEIDE, Rob, Manager Marketing and Communications, St. Luke's Hospital, San Francisco, CA, p. A87
SEIDEN, Michael V., President and Chief Executive Officer, Fox Chase Cancer Center–American Oncologic Hospital, Philadelphia, PA, p. A532
SEIDL, Doris A., Vice President Human Resources, Port Huron Hospital, Port Huron, MI, p. A321
SEIDLER, Richard A., FACH
President and Chief Executive Officer, Trinity Bettendorf, Bettendorf, IA, p. A214
President and Chief Executive Officer, Trinity Rock Island, Rock Island, IL, p. A192
SEIFER, Jill, Vice President Human Resources, Oaklawn Psychiatric Center, Goshen, IN, p. A202
SEIGLER, Leslie G., Executive Assistant and Coordinator Human Resources, Edgefield County Hospital, Edgefield, SC, p. A549
SEILER, Edward H., Director, Veterans Affairs Medical Center, Huntington, WV, p. A673
SEILER, Gregory A., Chief Executive Officer, Rio Grande Regional Hospital, McAllen, TX, p. A615
SEITZ, Stewart R., Chief Executive Officer, Gladys Spellman Specialty Hospital and Nursing Center, Cheverly, MD, p. A290
SEKULIC, Milan, M.D. Chief of Staff, Titus Regional Medical Center, Mount Pleasant, TX, p. A617
SELBOVITZ, Leslie, M.D. Senior Vice President Medical Affairs, Newton–Wellesley Hospital, Newton Lower Falls, MA, p. A303
SELBY, Eric, R.N. Chief Nursing Officer, Chicot Memorial Medical Center, Lake Village, AR, p. A47
SELDEN, Thomas A., FACHE President and Chief Executive Officer, Southwest General Health Center, Middleburg Heights, OH, p. A485
SELENKE, Darcy, M.D. Chief of Staff, Mercy Hospital Columbus, Columbus, KS, p. A232
SELEY, Jim, Chief Information Officer, Clay County Medical Center, Clay Center, KS, p. A231
SELF, Debbie, Chief Financial Officer, North Georgia Medical Center, Ellijay, GA, p. A152
SELF, Douglas, Chief Operating Officer, Carson Tahoe Regional Healthcare, Carson City, NV, p. A391
SELF, Joshua, Chief Operating Officer, Barrow Regional Medical Center, Winder, GA, p. A162
SELFRIDGE, Tara, Manager Human Resources, Purcell Municipal Hospital, Purcell, OK, p. A503
SELHORST, Sonya, Administrator, Mercy Hospital of Defiance, Defiance, OH, p. A479
SELIGMAN, Joel, President and Chief Executive Officer, Northern Westchester Hospital, Mount Kisco, NY, p. A430
SELIGMAN, Morris H., M.D. Chief Medical Officer and Chief Medical Information Officer, Sycamore Shoals Hospital, Elizabethton, TN, p. A565
SELL, Paula, Director Human Resources, Allen County Hospital, Iola, KS, p. A235
SELLA, John, Chief Financial Officer, Spectrum Health Gerber Memorial, Fremont, MI, p. A312
SELLARDS, Michael G., Chief Executive Officer, Pallottine Health Services, Huntington, WV, p. B99
SELLARDS, Michael G., President and Chief Executive Officer, St. Mary's Medical Center, Huntington, WV, p. A673
SELLERS, Larry W., M.D. Chief Medical Officer, Mercy Medical Center–Sioux City, Sioux City, IA, p. A226
SELLERS, Laura, Director Information Systems, Youth Villages Inner Harbour Campus, Douglasville, GA, p. A152
SELLERS, Liz, R.N. Chief Nursing Officer, Southwest Memorial Hospital, Cortez, CO, p. A99
SELLERS, Regena, Chief Nursing Officer, Three Rivers Behavioral Health, West Columbia, SC, p. A554
SELLERS, Robert R., President, Clay County Hospital, Flora, IL, p. A182
SELLHEIM, Kevin, Chief Executive Officer, Sleepy Eye Medical Center, Sleepy Eye, MN, p. A340
SELLICK, Kathleen Ann, President and Chief Executive Officer, Rady Children's Hospital – San Diego, San Diego, CA, p. A85
SELLS, Angie Phelps, Manager Human Resources, Harrison County Hospital, Corydon, IN, p. A199
SELLS, Matt, CPA Chief Financial Officer, Brown County Hospital, Ainsworth, NE, p. A381


A928 Index of Health Care Professionals 

Index of Health Care Professionals / Shapiro

Index of Health Care Professionals


SELMAN, David G.
Corporate Vice President Information Resources, ProMedica Bay Park Hospital, Oregon, OH, p. A486
Vice President Information, ProMedica Flower Hospital, Sylvania, OH, p. A489
Corporate Vice President Information Resources, ProMedica Fostoria Community Hospital, Fostoria, OH, p. A480
Chief Information Officer, ProMedica Toledo Hospital, Toledo, OH, p. A489
SELMAN, J. Peter, Administrator and Chief Executive Officer, Baptist Medical Center East, Montgomery, AL, p. A23
SELMON, Patricia, Director Public Relations and Chief Human Resources, Jefferson County Hospital, Fayette, MS, p. A345
SELPH, Wendy, Director Human Resources, Dodge County Hospital, Eastman, GA, p. A152
SELTMAN, Pam, Director Human Resources, Rush County Memorial Hospital, La Crosse, KS, p. A237
SELTZER, Paul, M.D. Chief of Staff, Columbia Hospital, West Palm Beach, FL, p. A142
SELVAGGI, Richard, M.D. Chief of Staff, Hunt Regional Community Hospital, Commerce, TX, p. A588
SELVAM, A. Panneer, M.D. Chief of Staff, Northern Arizona VA Health Care System, Prescott, AZ, p. A37
SELVIDGE, Sandra, Chief Fiscal Service, Veterans Affairs Medical Center, Cincinnati, OH, p. A474
SELZ, Timothy P., Vice President, Orange Regional Medical Center, Middletown, NY, p. A430
SEMAR, Dale, Controller, Medina Regional Hospital, Hondo, TX, p. A603
SEMELSBERGER, Kimberly, Vice President Financial Operations, Miners Medical Center, Hastings, PA, p. A524
SEMERDJIAN, Gregory, M.D. Senior Vice President Medical Affairs, St. Joseph Medical Center, Tacoma, WA, p. A668
SEMINGSON, John H., Chief Executive Officer, Ruby Valley Hospital, Sheridan, MT, p. A379
SEMRAD, Marianne, Associate Director Administrative Services, Captain James A. Lovell Federal Health Care Center, North Chicago, IL, p. A189
SENDAYDIEGO, Fe, Director Information Systems, Sonoma Valley Hospital, Sonoma, CA, p. A91
SENELICK, Richard, M.D. Medical Director, HEALTHSOUTH Rehabilitation Institute of San Antonio, San Antonio, TX, p. A625
SENESAC, Marc, Vice President Human Resources, Advocate Illinois Masonic Medical Center, Chicago, IL, p. A175
SENGER, Richard, Chief Financial Officer, Portsmouth Regional Hospital, Portsmouth, NH, p. A400
SENGER, Tricia, Chief Financial Officer, Elmore Medical Center, Mountain Home, ID, p. A169
SENKER, Thomas J., FACHE President and Chief Executive Officer, Newton Medical Center, Newton, NJ, p. A407
SENKO, Mark, Chief Executive Officer, Vibra Hospital of Northwestern Indiana, Crown Point, IN, p. A200
SENNEFF, Robert G., FACHE President and Chief Executive Officer, Graham Hospital, Canton, IL, p. A174
SENNETT, Nancy, R.N. Vice President Nursing Services, Franciscan St. Elizabeth Health – Crawfordsville, Crawfordsville, IN, p. A199
SENNISH, James, Vice President Human Resources, Firelands Regional Health System, Sandusky, OH, p. A488
SEO, Harlan, Accountant, Hale Ho'ola Hamakua, Honokaa, HI, p. A163
SEPCOSKI, John, Director Information Technology, Barnes–Kasson County Hospital, Susquehanna, PA, p. A539
SEPICH, Charles E., FACHE Director, Hunter Holmes McGuire Veterans Affairs Medical Center, Richmond, VA, p. A655
SEPP Jr., Howard W., FACHE Vice President and Administrator, Southeast Georgia Health System Camden Campus, Saint Marys, GA, p. A158
SEPPANEN, Carol, Director Human Resources, Baraga County Memorial Hospital, L'Anse, MI, p. A317
SERAFIN, Deborah J., Vice President Human Resources, Mount St. Mary's Hospital and Health Center, Lewiston, NY, p. A428
SERAPHINE, Jeffrey G., FACHE Division President, Duke LifePoint Healthcare, Brentwood, TN, p. B48
SERENO, Joe, Interim Chief Financial Officer, Southwest General Hospital, San Antonio, TX, p. A626
SERENO, Joseph, Chief Financial Officer, Lovelace Women's Hospital, Albuquerque, NM, p. A414
SERFLING, G. Aubrey, President and Chief Executive Officer, Eisenhower Medical Center, Rancho Mirage, CA, p. A81
SERGEANT, James R., Chief Executive Officer, Sierra Surgery Hospital, Carson City, NV, p. A391
SERKETICH, Steve, Manager Information Services, Aurora Sheboygan Memorial Medical Center, Sheboygan, WI, p. A690
SERLE, John, President and Chief Executive Officer, Lourdes Medical Center, Pasco, WA, p. A664
SERNULKA, John M., President and Chief Executive Officer, Carroll Hospital Center, Westminster, MD, p. A294
SERNYAK, Michael, M.D. Director, Connecticut Mental Health Center, New Haven, CT, p. A110
SERRANO, Jorge L. Matta, Administrator, Auxilio Mutuo Hospital, San Juan, PR, p. A702
SERRATT, Jim, Chief Executive Officer, Willow Springs Center, Reno, NV, p. A395
SERRILL, G. B., Chief Operating Officer, Wesley Medical Center, Wichita, KS, p. A246
SESSA, Bonnie, Vice President and Chief Information Officer, Beth Israel Medical Center, New York, NY, p. A431
SESSIONS, Tracey, Administrator, State Hospital South, Blackfoot, ID, p. A166
SESSLER, Connie, Director Human Resources, ProMedica St. Luke's Hospital, Maumee, OH, p. A484
SETCHEL, David P., Vice President Operations, Bon Secours–DePaul Medical Center, Norfolk, VA, p. A652
SETILI, Rick, Manager Information Systems, Warren General Hospital, Warren, PA, p. A540
SETTELMEYER, Camille, Assistant Administrator Clinical Services, Mercy Hospital, Valley City, ND, p. A468
SETTLE, Andrea, Director Human Resources, Taylor Regional Hospital, Campbellsville, KY, p. A248
SETTLES, Laura, Director Human Resources, Baylor Medical Center at Garland, Garland, TX, p. A600
SETZKORN–MEYER, Marsha, Director Public Relations and Marketing, Hillsboro Community Hospital, Hillsboro, KS, p. A234
SEUFERER, Stanley, D.O. Chief of Staff, Memorial Medical Center of West Michigan, Ludington, MI, p. A318
SEVENICH, Mark, Director Human Resources, Owatonna Hospital, Owatonna, MN, p. A336
SEVERANCE, Matthew J., FACHE Chief Executive Officer, Roper Hospital, Charleston, SC, p. A547
SEVILLIAN, Clarence, President and Chief Executive Officer, McLaren Oakland, Pontiac, MI, p. A321
SEWELL, Lance, Chief Financial Officer, South Lake Hospital, Clermont, FL, p. A120
SEXTON, Cheryl, Director Nursing Operations, South Texas Rehabilitation Hospital, Brownsville, TX, p. A585
SEXTON, Cindy
Chief Financial Officer, St. David's North Austin Medical Center, Austin, TX, p. A581
Chief Financial Officer, St. David's Round Rock Medical Center, Round Rock, TX, p. A623
SEXTON, James J., FACHE President and Chief Executive Officer, Henry Ford Wyandotte Hospital, Wyandotte, MI, p. A325
SEXTON, Kevin
Director Information Systems, Greenbrier Valley Medical Center, Ronceverte, WV, p. A675
Director Information Systems, Raleigh General Hospital, Beckley, WV, p. A670
SEXTON, Kevin J., President and Chief Executive Officer, Holy Cross Hospital, Silver Spring, MD, p. A294
SEXTON, William J., Administrator, Wyoming State Hospital, Evanston, WY, p. A696
SEXTON, William P., Chief Executive Officer, Prairie du Chien Memorial Hospital, Prairie Du Chien, WI, p. A689
SEY, Mark, Vice President and Chief Administrative Officer, Lodi Memorial Hospital, Lodi, CA, p. A67
SEYBOLD, Henry, Senior Vice President and Chief Financial Officer, Rockford Memorial Hospital, Rockford, IL, p. A193
SEYMOUR, Anthea, Chief Operating Officer, St. Elizabeths Hospital, Washington, DC, p. A117
SEYMOUR, Galen, M.D. Chief of Staff, Horton Community Hospital, Horton, KS, p. A235
SEYMOUR, Jose, Chief Information Resource Management, James A. Haley Veterans Hospital, Tampa, FL, p. A140
SEYMOUR, Kathy, Acting Chief Human Resources Management Service, Aleda E. Lutz Veterans Affairs Medical Center, Saginaw, MI, p. A322
SGANGA, Fred S., Interim Chief Executive Officer, Stony Brook University Medical Center, Stony Brook, NY, p. A444
SHACKELFORD, Gerald, Staff Support Specialist, Texas Center for Infectious Disease, San Antonio, TX, p. A626
SHADLE, Jacque, Chief Executive Officer, Baton Rouge Rehabilitation Hospital, Baton Rouge, LA, p. A262
SHADOWEN, Michael, M.D. Chief of Staff, T. J. Samson Community Hospital, Glasgow, KY, p. A250
SHADWICK, Shirley A., Administrator Human Resources, Desert Springs Hospital Medical Center, Las Vegas, NV, p. A392
SHAFER, Duane, Chief Financial Officer, Titus Regional Medical Center, Mount Pleasant, TX, p. A617
SHAFER, Robert
Vice President Finance, Mercy Medical Center–Dubuque, Dubuque, IA, p. A219
Vice President Finance, Mercy Medical Center–Dyersville, Dyersville, IA, p. A219
SHAFER, Timothy, M.D. Medical Director, Grace Cottage Hospital, Townshend, VT, p. A644
SHAFFER, Linda, Director Human Resources, ProMedica Defiance Regional Hospital, Defiance, OH, p. A479
SHAFFER, Michael, Vice President Fiscal Services, St. Joseph's Hospital Health Center, Syracuse, NY, p. A444
SHAFFER, Sarah Dale, Director Human Resources, Northwest Mississippi Regional Medical Center, Clarksdale, MS, p. A344
SHAFICI, Khaled, M.D. President Medical Staff, Cornerstone Hospital–West Monroe, West Monroe, LA, p. A279
SHAH, Aman Ali, M.D. Chief Medical Staff, Lake Whitney Medical Center, Whitney, TX, p. A635
SHAH, Avani D., M.D. Chief of Medical Staff, Medstar St. Mary's Hospital, Leonardtown, MD, p. A293
SHAH, Chetan, M.D. Chief of Staff, Rhea Medical Center, Dayton, TN, p. A565
SHAH, Girishkumar, M.D. Clinical Director, Southeast Louisiana Hospital, Mandeville, LA, p. A272
SHAH, Gita, M.D. Vice President Medical Affairs, Laurel Regional Hospital, Laurel, MD, p. A293
SHAH, Jayendra H., M.D. Chief Medical Officer, Southern Arizona Veterans Affairs Health Care System, Tucson, AZ, p. A40
SHAH, Paresh, Director Information Systems, Reston Hospital Center, Reston, VA, p. A654
SHAH, Rizwan, M.D. Medical Director, HEALTHSOUTH Rehabilitation Hospital of Arlington, Arlington, TX, p. A579
SHAH, Shalin
Chief Financial Officer, Northside Hospital and Heart Institute, Saint Petersburg, FL, p. A138
Chief Operating Officer, Regional Medical Center–Bayonet Point, Hudson, FL, p. A125
SHAH, Vital, M.D. Director, Central State Hospital, Louisville, KY, p. A254
SHAHAN, Mary Jo, Vice President and Chief Financial Officer, West Virginia University Hospitals, Morgantown, WV, p. A674
SHAHAN, Matthew, Director Information Systems, Glendive Medical Center, Glendive, MT, p. A375
SHAHEEN, Jim, President, Strategic Behavioral Health, LLC, Memphis, TN, p. B124
SHAHRYAR, Syed, M.D. Medical Director, Promise Hospital of Phoenix, Mesa, AZ, p. A34
SHAHSAVARI, Mehan, M.D. Chief of Staff, Norman Specialty Hospital, Norman, OK, p. A500
SHAHZADA, Kamran, M.D. Chief Medical Staff, South Central Kansas Medical Center, Arkansas City, KS, p. A230
SHALLASH, Anthony J., M.D. Interim Medical Director, Franklin Hospital, Valley Stream, NY, p. A445
SHALLOCK, James R., Chief Financial Officer, OakBend Medical Center, Richmond, TX, p. A622
SHAMBLES, Terry W., Interim Chief Executive Officer, Perry Memorial Hospital, Perry, OK, p. A503
SHANAHAN, Thomas, Chief Financial Officer and Senior Vice President, Raritan Bay Medical Center, Perth Amboy, NJ, p. A408
SHANKLES, Ellen, Chief Executive Officer, GLOBALREHAB Hospital – Dallas, Dallas, TX, p. A591
SHANLEY, Diane, Deputy Service Unit Director, U. S. Public Health Service Indian Hospital–Sells, Sells, AZ, p. A38
SHANLEY, Kevin, Vice President Finance and Chief Financial Officer, Morristown Medical Center, Morristown, NJ, p. A406
SHANLEY, Linda, Vice President and Chief Information Officer, Saint Francis Hospital and Medical Center, Hartford, CT, p. A109
SHANNON, David A., Chief Executive Officer, Penobscot Valley Hospital, Lincoln, ME, p. A284
SHANNON, Greg, Director Human Resources, Ozarks Medical Center, West Plains, MO, p. A372
SHANNON, John Jay, M.D. Chief Medical Officer, Parkland Health & Hospital System, Dallas, TX, p. A592
SHANNON, Richard, M.D. Chief of Staff, Montrose Memorial Hospital, Montrose, CO, p. A104
SHANNON, Ruth, Director Human Resources, Sharp Grossmont Hospital, La Mesa, CA, p. A66
SHAPIRO, David, M.D
Vice President Medical Affairs and Chief Medical Officer, Columbia St. Mary's Hospital Milwaukee, Milwaukee, WI, p. A686
Vice President Medical Affairs and Chief Medical Officer, Columbia St. Mary's Ozaukee Hospital, Mequon, WI, p. A686
Vice President Medical Affairs and Chief Medical Officer, Sacred Heart Rehabilitation Institute, Milwaukee, WI, p. A687
SHAPIRO, Edward R., M.D. Medical Director and Chief Executive Officer, Austen Riggs Center, Stockbridge, MA, p. A305
SHAPIRO, Ira, M.D. Chief Medical Officer, St. Mary's Regional Medical Center, Lewiston, ME, p. A284
SHAPIRO, Louis A., President and Chief Executive Officer, Hospital for Special Surgery, New York, NY, p. A433
SHAPIRO, Marc, M.D. Chief Medical Officer, St. Helena Hospital Clearlake, Clearlake, CA, p. A57

SHAPIRO, Robert S., Senior Vice President and Chief Financial Officer, Forest Hills Hospital,, NY, p. A432

SHAPIRO, Steven D., M.D
Chief Medical Officer, Bon Secours St. Francis Hospital, Charleston, SC, p. A547
Vice President Medical Affairs, Roper Hospital, Charleston, SC, p. A547

SHARANGPANI, Rojesh, M.D. Chief of Staff, Capital Medical Center, Olympia, WA, p. A663

SHARFSTEIN, Steven S., M.D. President and Chief Executive Officer, Sheppard and Enoch Pratt Hospital, Baltimore, MD, p. A289

SHARMA, Aika, M.D. President Medical Staff, Alameda Hospital, Alameda, CA, p. A53

SHARMA, Chandra, M.D. Chief of Staff, Welch Community Hospital, Welch, WV, p. A676

SHARMA, Roger, Chief Financial Officer, Citrus Valley Medical Center–Queen of the Valley Campus, West Covina, CA, p. A95

SHARP, Barry
Director, Iowa City Veterans Affairs Health Care System, Iowa City, IA, p. A221
Acting Director, Minneapolis Veterans Affairs Health Care System, Minneapolis, MN, p. A335

SHARP, Charles S., Chief Executive Officer, Wilmington Treatment Center, Wilmington, NC, p. A462

SHARP, Cindy, M.D. Chief Medical Officer, Madison Valley Medical Center, Ennis, MT, p. A375

SHARP, Gina, Executive Director, Linden Oaks Hospital at Edward, Naperville, IL, p. A189

SHARP, Julie
Supervisor Human Resources, Chase County Community Hospital, Imperial, NE, p. A384
Chief Operations Officer, Falls Community Hospital and Clinic, Marlin, TX, p. A615

SHARP, Raymond, Vice President and Chief Information Officer, CGH Medical Center, Sterling, IL, p. A194

SHARP, Richard, M.D. Medical Director, CHRISTUS St. Michael Rehabilitation Hospital, Texarkana, TX, p. A630

SHARPNACK, Linton, R.N. Director Nursing, Heatherhill Care Communities, Chardon, OH, p. A472

SHARRER, Steven, Vice President Human Resources, Saint John's Health Center, Santa Monica, CA, p. A90

SHARTLE, William, Senior Vice President Human Resources, Holy Spirit Hospital, Camp Hill, PA, p. A519

SHARUM, Melinda
Director of Human Resources, Mercy Hospital Ardmore, Ardmore, OK, p. A493
Director Human Resources, Mercy Hospital Healdton, Healdton, OK, p. A497

SHARY, Dave, Administrator Human Resources, Ridgecrest Regional Hospital, Ridgecrest, CA, p. A82

SHATAVA, Angie, Director Human Resources, Adair County Memorial Hospital, Greenfield, IA, p. A220

SHATILLA, Maggie, M.D. Chief of Staff, Bamberg County Memorial Hospital, Bamberg, SC, p. A

SHATRAW, Thomas, Director Human Resources, Samaritan Medical Center, Watertown, NY, p. A446

SHAUB, Diane, Director Human Resources, Dublin Methodist Hospital, Dublin, OH, p. A479

SHAUGHNESSY, Mary
Vice President Finance, Spaulding Rehabilitation Hospital, Boston, MA, p. A297
Vice President Finance, Spaulding Rehabilitation Hospital Cape Cod, East Sandwich, MA, p. A299

SHAULL, Ty, Chief Operating Officer, Wyandot Memorial Hospital, Upper Sandusky, OH, p. A490

SHAVER, John, Chief Financial Officer, Noble Hospital, Westfield, MA, p. A306

SHAVER, Robert D., M.D. Vice President Medical Affairs, The Good Samaritan Hospital, Lebanon, PA, p. A527

SHAW, Barbara, Nursing Manager/ Chief Nursing Officer, Brighton Center for Recovery, Brighton, MI, p. A308

SHAW, Brigitte W., Chief Operating Officer, Pepin Heart Hospital, Florida Hospital Tampa, Tampa, FL, p. A140

SHAW, David
Vice President and Chief Operating Officer, Susan B. Allen Memorial Hospital, El Dorado, KS, p. A232
Vice President Information Systems, Wishard Health Services, Indianapolis, IN, p. A205

SHAW, David B., Chief Executive Officer and Administrator, Nor–Lea General Hospital, Lovington, NM, p. A417

SHAW, Douglas A., Chief Executive Officer, Mad River Community Hospital, Arcata, CA, p. A54

SHAW, Gary, Administrator, Alaska Native Medical Center, Anchorage, AK, p. A28

SHAW, Gene, Chief Information Officer, Yuma Regional Medical Center, Yuma, AZ, p. A41

SHAW, Greg, Vice President and Chief Financial Officer, Audrain Medical Center, Mexico, MO, p. A365

SHAW, J. Michael, Chief Executive Officer, Rusk County Memorial Hospital and Nursing Home, Ladysmith, WI, p. A684

SHAW, Jan, Director Personnel, River Bend Hospital, West Lafayette, IN, p. A213

SHAW, John C., M.D. Medical Director, Southern Indiana Rehabilitation Hospital, New Albany, IN, p. A209

SHAW, Karen, Chief Nursing Officer and Director of Clinical Services, St. Vincent Jennings Hospital, North Vernon, IN, p. A210

SHAW, Kathy, Chief Executive Officer, Haven Senior Horizons, Phoenix, AZ, p. A35

SHAW, Kendra, Manager Information Services, Mayo Clinic Health System in Red Wing, Red Wing, MN, p. A337

SHAW, Mandy, M.D. Chief of Staff, Sidney Regional Medical Center, Sidney, NE, p. A389

SHAW, Mary, Chief Operating Officer, Essentia Health St. Mary's Hospital of Superior, Superior, WI, p. A692

SHAW, Michael R., Chief Executive Officer, Kindred Hospital–Albuquerque, Albuquerque, NM, p. A414

SHAW, Patrick, Chief Executive Officer, Grafton City Hospital, Grafton, WV, p. A672

SHAW, Robert C., President and Chief Executive Officer, Thousand Oaks Surgical Hospital, Thousand Oaks, CA, p. A92

SHAW, Ted, Interim Chief Financial Officer, East Jefferson General Hospital, Metairie, LA, p. A273

SHAW, Violet, R.N. Director of Nursing, Grafton City Hospital, Grafton, WV, p. A672

SHAWGO, Darla, Director Human Resources, Sparta Community Hospital, Sparta, IL, p. A194

SHEA, Drew, Assistant Chief Financial Officer, Coastal Carolina Hospital, Hardeeville, SC, p. A551

SHEA, Peter H., M.D. Senior Vice President and Chief Medical Officer, The William W. Backus Hospital, Norwich, CT, p. A111

SHEAGREN, Craig, Vice President Finance, Sarah Bush Lincoln Health Center, Mattoon, IL, p. A187

SHEALY, Keith, M.D. Chief of Staff, Springs Memorial Hospital, Lancaster, SC, p. A552

SHEAR, Larry, Administrative Assistant, Norwood Health Center, Marshfield, WI, p. A685

SHEARER, Christopher, M.D. Chief Medical Officer, John C. Lincoln North Mountain Hospital, Phoenix, AZ, p. A35

SHEARER, Ron, M.D. Regional Medical Director, Peace Harbor Hospital, Florence, OR, p. A510

SHEEHAN, John, Chief Executive Officer, Douglas County Community Mental Health Center, Omaha, NE, p. A388

SHEEHAN, John C., FACHE Executive Vice President and Chief Operating Officer, St. Luke's Hospital, Cedar Rapids, IA, p. A215

SHEEHAN, Karen, Director Information Systems, Swedish Covenant Hospital, Chicago, IL, p. A178

SHEEHAN, Terrence P., M.D. Medical Director, Adventist Rehabilitation Hospital of Maryland, Rockville, MD, p. A293

SHEEHY, Earl N., Chief Executive Officer, Dr. John Warner Hospital, Clinton, IL, p. A179

SHEEHY, Joseph, Chief Executive Officer and Managing Director, The Pavilion, Champaign, IL, p. A175

SHEERIN, Rick, Vice President Fiscal Services, Floyd Medical Center, Rome, GA, p. A158

SHEETS, Cindy, Chief Information Officer, Mount Carmel, Columbus, OH, p. A476

SHEETS, Jennifer, R.N. Chief Executive Officer, Kindred Hospital–Charleston, Charleston, SC, p. A547

SHEETS, Jim, Administrator, LDS Hospital, Salt Lake City, UT, p. A640

SHEFFIELD, J D, D.O. President Medical Staff, Coryell Memorial Hospital, Gatesville, TX, p. A601

SHEFFO, Gregory, M.D. Chief Medical Officer, Clearfield Hospital, Clearfield, PA, p. A520

SHEHAN, Mary, R.N. Senior Vice President and Chief Nursing Officer, Swedish Covenant Hospital, Chicago, IL, p. A178

SHEHATA, Adel R., M.D. Medical Director, Desert Springs Hospital Medical Center, Las Vegas, NV, p. A392

SHEHATA, Nady, M.D. Vice President Medical Affairs, Sisters of Charity Hospital of Buffalo, Buffalo, NY, p. A423

SHEHI, G. Michael, M.D. Interim Chief Executive Officer, Mountain View Hospital, Gadsden, AL, p. A20

SHELBURNE, John D., M.D. Chief of Staff, Durham Veterans Affairs Medical Center, Durham, NC, p. A452

SHELBY, Dennis R., Chief Executive Officer, Wilson Medical Center, Neodesha, KS, p. A239

SHELBY, Joyce, Manager Human Resources, Hardin County General Hospital, Rosiclare, IL, p. A193

SHELDON, Diana, CNO, Stone County Medical Center, Mountain View, AR, p. A49

SHELDON, Donald S., M.D. President and Chief Executive Officer, EMH Elyria Medical Center, Elyria, OH, p. A480

SHELDON, Lyle Ernest, FACHE President and Chief Executive Officer, Harford Memorial Hospital, Havre De Grace, MD, p. A292

SHELDON, Lyle Ernest, FACHE President and Chief Executive Officer, Upper Chesapeake Health System, Bel Air, MD, p. B140

SHELDON, Lyle Ernest, FACHE President and Chief Executive Officer, Upper Chesapeake Medical Center, Bel Air, MD, p. A289

SHELDON, Mo S., Chief Operating Officer, Glen Rose Medical Center, Glen Rose, TX, p. A601

SHELDON, Richard, M.D. Vice President Medical Affairs, San Gorgonio Memorial Hospital, Banning, CA, p. A55

SHELFORD, Dave, Assistant Superintendent, Richmond State Hospital, Richmond, IN, p. A211

SHELL, Steve, Chief Executive Officer, West Hills Hospital, Reno, NV, p. A395

SHELLEY, Jim, Manager Operations, Madison Center and Hospital, South Bend, IN, p. A211

SHELOR, Bonnie, Vice President Human Resources, Bon Secours Memorial Regional Medical Center, Mechanicsville, VA, p. A651

SHELT, Elizabeth, Civilian Personnel Officer, Dwight David Eisenhower Army Medical Center, Fort Gordon, GA, p. A153

SHELTON, Carl, M.D. Medical Director, HEALTHSOUTH Southern Hills Rehabilitation Hospital, Princeton, WV, p. A675

SHELTON, Carol, Director Human Resources, Lovelace Women's Hospital, Albuquerque, NM, p. A414

SHELTON, Darlene, Coordinator Team Resources, BayCare Alliant Hospital, Dunedin, FL, p. A122

SHELTON, Jeffrey D., Chief Executive Officer, Harlan County Health System, Alma, NE, p. A381

SHELTON, John
President and Chief Executive Officer, DeKalb Medical at Downtown Decatur, Decatur, GA, p. A151
Executive Vice President and Chief Operating Officer, DeKalb Medical at Downtown Decatur, Decatur, GA, p. A151
President and Chief Executive Officer, DeKalb Medical at Hillandale, Lithonia, GA, p. A155
Chief Operating Officer, DeKalb Medical at Hillandale, Lithonia, GA, p. A155
President and Chief Executive Officer, DeKalb Medical at North Decatur, Decatur, GA, p. A151

SHELTON, John, President and Chief Executive Officer, DeKalb Regional Health System, Decatur, GA, p. B41

SHELTON, Kathy
Director Human Resources, East Texas Medical Center Pittsburg, Pittsburg, TX, p. A620
Director Human Resources, East Texas Medical Center–Mount Vernon, Mount Vernon, TX, p. A617

SHELTON, Scott, Executive Vice President and Chief Financial Officer, Miami Valley Hospital, Dayton, OH, p. A478

SHELVOCK, Kathy, R.N. Assistant Administrator Patient Care Services, Fairchild Medical Center, Yreka, CA, p. A96

SHENKER, Charles, M.D. Chief of Staff, Aventura Hospital and Medical Center, Aventura, FL, p. A118

SHEPARD, Charles, M.D. Medical Director, Winona Health, Winona, MN, p. A342

SHEPARD, Karen
Senior Vice President and Chief Financial Officer, Pioneer Memorial Hospital, Prineville, OR, p. A514
Senior Vice President Finance and Chief Financial Officer, St. Charles Medical Center – Bend, Bend, OR, p. A509
Senior Vice President Finance and Chief Financial Officer, St. Charles Medical Center – Redmond, Redmond, OR, p. A515

SHEPHARD, Russ, Senior Systems Analyst, Dyersburg Regional Medical Center, Dyersburg, TN, p. A565

SHEPHERD, Stephen C., Chief Executive Officer, Candler County Hospital, Metter, GA, p. A156

SHEPLER, Mary, R.N. Vice President and Chief Nursing Officer, Exempla Saint Joseph Hospital, Denver, CO, p. A99

SHEPPARD, Sharon, Manager Human Resources, Sycamore Shoals Hospital, Elizabethton, TN, p. A565

SHEPPARD, Varinya, R.N. Chief Nursing Officer, St. Elizabeth Medical Center, Utica, NY, p. A445

SHERBELL, Stanley, M.D. Executive Vice President Medical Affairs, New York Methodist Hospital,, NY, p. A435

SHERBONDY, Lori, Director Human Resources, Battle Mountain General Hospital, Battle Mountain, NV, p. A391

SHERBUN, Michael, Ph.D. Chief Executive Officer, Cedar Hills Hospital, Portland, OR, p. A513

SHERER, Susan, Chief Information Resource Management, Veterans Affairs Medical Center, Dayton, OH, p. A479

SHERIDAN, Bridget, Chief Human Resources Officer, Beaver Dam Community Hospitals, Beaver Dam, WI, p. A679

SHERIDAN, Cheryl, R.N
Senior Vice President and Chief Nursing Officer, Newark–Wayne Community Hospital, Newark, NY, p. A438
Senior Vice President Patient Care Services, Rochester General Hospital, Rochester, NY, p. A441

SHERIDAN, Elizabeth, Chief Operating Officer, South Jersey Healthcare – Regional Medical Center, Vineland, NJ, p. A411

Index of Health Care Professionals / Shumway

Index of Health Care Professionals


SHERIDAN Jr., John P., President and Chief Executive Officer, Cooper Health System, Camden, NJ, p. A402
SHERLIN, Anthony, Director Information Systems, DeKalb Regional Medical Center, Fort Payne, AL, p. A20
SHERMAN, Frederick C., M.D. Chief Medical Officer, The Children's Home of Pittsburgh, Pittsburgh, PA, p. A535
SHERMAN, James, Executive Director Hospital Operations, Tri–City Regional Medical Center, Hawaiian Gardens, CA, p. A64
SHERMAN, Shelly, Director Human Resources, Mercy Hospital Clermont, Batavia, OH, p. A470
SHERMAN, Stephanie, Chief Human Resources Officer, West Boca Medical Center, Boca Raton, FL, p. A119
SHERON, William E., Chief Executive Officer, Wooster Community Hospital, Wooster, OH, p. A491
SHERRARD, Mark, D.O. Chief Medical Officer and Senior Vice President Medical Affairs, Mercy Memorial Hospital System, Monroe, MI, p. A319
SHERRETT, John, Chief Financial Officer and Chief Operating Officer, Forks Community Hospital, Forks, WA, p. A661
SHERRILL, Angela
Chief Information Officer, Laird Hospital, Union, MS, p. A353
Corporate Director Information System, Rush Foundation Hospital, Meridian, MS, p. A350
Corporate Director Information System, Specialty Hospital of Meridian, Meridian, MS, p. A350
SHERROD, Mike, Chief Executive Officer, Coliseum Northside Hospital, Macon, GA, p. A155
SHERROD, Rhonda Kay, MSN, Administrator, Shands Lake Shore, Lake City, FL, p. A128
SHERRY, Bernard, President and Chief Executive Officer, Baptist Hospital, Nashville, TN, p. A573
SHERWOOD, Charlotte, Chief Financial Officer, North Sunflower Medical Center, Ruleville, MS, p. A352
SHERWOOD, Rose, Information Technology Specialist, Kingfisher Regional Hospital, Kingfisher, OK, p. A498
SHETH, Shishir, M.D. President Medical Staff, Sacred Heart–St. Mary's Hospitals, Rhinelander, WI, p. A690
SHETLER, Charles L., CPA Chief Financial Officer, Indiana University Health Bedford Hospital, Bedford, IN, p. A197
SHETTLESWORTH, Amanda, Director Human Resources, Bloomington Meadows Hospital, Bloomington, IN, p. A198
SHEW, Angel
Director Area Technology, Redwood City Medical Center, Redwood City, CA, p. A82
Director Area Technology, South San Francisco Medical Center, South San Francisco, CA, p. A91
SHEWBRIDGE, Rick, M.D. Vice President Medical Operations, Medina Hospital, Medina, OH, p. A484
SHICKOLOVICH, William, Chief Information Officer, Tufts Medical Center, Boston, MA, p. A297
SHIELDS, Anna, Executive Director Information Systems, Santa Rosa Memorial Hospital, Santa Rosa, CA, p. A90
SHIELDS, Charlie, Chief Operating Officer, Truman Medical Center–Lakewood, Kansas City, MO, p. A363
SHIELDS, Diane, Chief Human Resources Officer, Alpena Regional Medical Center, Alpena, MI, p. A307
SHIELDS, Leanne, Chief Financial Officer, Spring Valley Hospital Medical Center, Las Vegas, NV, p. A394
SHIEPE, Clifford, President and Chief Executive Officer, Tri–City Regional Medical Center, Hawaiian Gardens, CA, p. A64
SHIFF, Mary Treacy, Chief Financial Officer, Kindred Chicago–Central Hospital, Chicago, IL, p. A176
SHIFFER, W. Frank, Interim Chief Financial Officer, Johnson Memorial Hospital, Stafford Springs, CT, p. A112
SHIFFERMILLER, William, M.D. Vice President Medical Affairs, Nebraska Methodist Hospital, Omaha, NE, p. A388
SHIHADY, Sharon, Director Human Resources, HEALTHSOUTH Cane Creek Rehabilitation Hospital, Martin, TN, p. A570
SHILKAITIS, Mary, Vice President Patient Care and Chief Nursing Officer, Rush–Copley Medical Center, Aurora, IL, p. A173
SHIMAMOTO, Kevin, Director Information Technology, Sierra View District Hospital, Porterville, CA, p. A81
SHINAMAN, Keith C McLean, Senior Vice President Finance, Baystate Medical Center, Springfield, MA, p. A304
SHINE, Kenneth, M.D. Executive Vice Chancellor, University of Texas System, Austin, TX, p. B139
SHINICK, Mary K., Vice President Human Resources, Nyack Hospital, Nyack, NY, p. A438
SHININGER, Kimberly R., Director Human Resources, Wabash County Hospital, Wabash, IN, p. A213
SHIPIERSKI, Sally, Controller, Geisinger HEALTHSOUTH Rehabilitation Hospital, Danville, PA, p. A521
SHIPLEY, Kurt
Chief Financial Officer, Jordan Valley Medical Center, West Jordan, UT, p. A642
Chief Financial Officer, Pioneer Valley Hospital, West Valley City, UT, p. A642
SHIPP, Geraldine H., Director of Risk Management, Sampson Regional Medical Center, Clinton, NC, p. A451
SHIPP, Rhonda, Chief Financial Officer, Ozark Health Medical Center, Clinton, AR, p. A43
SHIPPY, Angela, M.D. Vice President Medical Affairs, St. Luke's Episcopal Hospital, Houston, TX, p. A606
SHIRAH, Anita, Director Human Resources, University of South Alabama Medical Center, Mobile, AL, p. A23
SHIRLEN, David
Vice President Human Resources, Grace Hospital, Morganton, NC, p. A458
Vice President Human Resources, Valdese General Hospital, Valdese, NC, p. A462
SHIRLEY, Christian, Director Human Resources, Geisinger HEALTHSOUTH Rehabilitation Hospital, Danville, PA, p. A521
SHIRLEY, Douglas E., Senior Executive Vice President and Chief Financial Officer, Cooper Health System, Camden, NJ, p. A402
SHIRLEY, Phil, Director Information Resource Management, Broughton Hospital, Morganton, NC, p. A457
SHIRLEY, Steve, Chief Information Officer, Parkview Medical Center, Pueblo, CO, p. A105
SHISLER, Pearl, Director Human Resources, HEALTHSOUTH Treasure Coast Rehabilitation Hospital, Vero Beach, FL, p. A142
SHIVERY, Toni
Vice President Human Resources, Harford Memorial Hospital, Havre De Grace, MD, p. A292
Vice President Human Resources, Upper Chesapeake Medical Center, Bel Air, MD, p. A289
SHMERLING, James E., President and Chief Executive Officer, Children's Hospital Colorado, Aurora, CO, p. A97
SHOBE, Franklin, Administrator and Chief Executive Officer, Black Hills Surgery Center, Rapid City, SD, p. A558
SHOBE, Susan, Director Administration and Support Services, Alton Mental Health Center, Alton, IL, p. A172
SHOCKEY, Kathryn L., Director Human Resources, Lead–Deadwood Regional Hospital, Deadwood, SD, p. A556
SHOCKLEY, Mary, Director Human Resources, Russell Medical Center, Alexander City, AL, p. A15
SHOCKNEY, Brian T., FACHE Chief Operating Officer, Indiana University Health Arnett Hospital, Lafayette, IN, p. A206
SHOEMAKER, Larry D., M.D. Chief Medical Officer, Singing River Health System, Pascagoula, MS, p. A351
SHOEMAKER, Robert, M.D. Chief of Staff Community Heart and Vascular, Indiana Heart Hospital, Indianapolis, IN, p. A204
SHOEN, Jay, Controller, LifeCare Hospitals of Mechanicsburg, Mechanicsburg, PA, p. A529
SHOEN, Timothy, M.D. Vice President Medical Staff Services, St. Mary's Healthcare, Amsterdam, NY, p. A420
SHOENER, Carl, Chief Information Officer, Hazleton General Hospital, Hazleton, PA, p. A525
SHOMAKER, Susan, Director Information Management Systems, J. Arthur Dosher Memorial Hospital, Southport, NC, p. A461
SHONNARD, John, M.D. Medical Director, UPMC Northwest, Seneca, PA, p. A538
SHONTZ, Maggie, VP, Human Resources, MacNeal Hospital, Berwyn, IL, p. A173
SHOOK, Rod, Chief Financial Officer, Wagoner Community Hospital, Wagoner, OK, p. A507
SHOOKS, Charles, M.D. Chief of Staff, Windham Hospital, Willimantic, CT, p. A113
SHOPLAND, George, Chief Executive Officer, Manatee Palms Youth Services, Bradenton, FL, p. A119
SHOR, Joel, M.D. Chief of Staff, Bluefield Regional Medical Center, Bluefield, WV, p. A670
SHORB, Gary S., President and Chief Executive Officer, Methodist Le Bonheur Healthcare, Memphis, TN, p. B89
SHORES, David G., D.O. President Medical Staff, Fairview Park Hospital, Dublin, GA, p. A152
SHORES, Larry, M.D. Executive Medical Director, Cedar Springs Behavioral Health System, Colorado Springs, CO, p. A98
SHORK, Michael, M.D. Director Information Systems Services, Mercy St. Charles Hospital, Oregon, OH, p. A486
SHORT, Kathy, D.O. Family Practice, Carroll County Memorial Hospital, Carrollton, KY, p. A248
SHORT, M. Andrew, Vice President Information Services, Samaritan Medical Center, Watertown, NY, p. A446
SHORT, Margaret W., Coordinator Information Technology, Webster County Memorial Hospital, Webster Springs, WV, p. A676
SHORT, Peter H., M.D. Senior Vice President Medical Affairs, Beverly Hospital, Beverly, MA, p. A295
SHORT, Steve, Executive Vice President Finance and Administration, Tampa General Hospital, Tampa, FL, p. A141
SHORT, Ted, Chief Financial Officer, Fairview Park Hospital, Dublin, GA, p. A152
SHORT, W. L., M.D. Chief Medical Officer, Memorial Health System, Abilene, KS, p. A230
SHOUKAIR, Sami, M.D. Chief Medical Officer, La Palma Intercommunity Hospital, La Palma, CA, p. A66
SHOUP, Chris, President, Methodist Hospital for Surgery, Addison, TX, p. A577
SHOUSE, Shellie, Chief Financial Officer, Bluegrass Community Hospital, Versailles, KY, p. A259
SHOWERS, Russell H., Vice President Human Resources, Valley Hospital, Ridgewood, NJ, p. A409
SHOWS, Carla
Payroll Clerk, George County Hospital, Lucedale, MS, p. A349
Payroll Clerk, Greene County Hospital, Leakesville, MS, p. A349
SHRADER, David, M.D. Chief of Staff, Star Valley Medical Center, Afton, WY, p. A695
SHREEVE, Susan
Chief Financial Officer, Belton Regional Medical Center, Belton, MO, p. A355
Chief Financial Officer, Research Medical Center, Kansas City, MO, p. A362
Chief Financial Officer, Research Psychiatric Center, Kansas City, MO, p. A362
SHREVE, Susan, Executive Director Information Technology, Boone Memorial Hospital, Madison, WV, p. A673
SHREVES, Melissa, Director Human Resources, Monongalia General Hospital, Morgantown, WV, p. A674
SHREWSBURY, Kim, Vice President and Chief Financial Officer, Decatur General Hospital, Decatur, AL, p. A18
SHRIVER, Debra, R.N. Chief Nurse Executive, Trinity Regional Medical Center, Fort Dodge, IA, p. A219
SHROADES, David W., Vice President Technology Services, Alliance Community Hospital, Alliance, OH, p. A469
SHRODER, Robert W.
President and Chief Executive Officer, St. Elizabeth Health Center, Youngstown, OH, p. A492
President and Chief Executive Officer, St. Joseph Health Center, Warren, OH, p. A490
SHROFF, Rajendra, M.D. Administrative Medical Director, St. Mary's Hospital, Centralia, IL, p. A174
SHROYER, Linda K., Administrator, Potomac Valley Hospital, Keyser, WV, p. A673
SHUBIN, Allan, Chief Financial Officer, Pacific Alliance Medical Center, Los Angeles, CA, p. A71
SHUEY, Keith, M.D. Chief Medical Staff, Johnson County Hospital, Tecumseh, NE, p. A390
SHUFFIELD, Sean, Regional Chief Information Officer, St. Joseph Medical Center, Towson, MD, p. A294
SHUFFIELD, Shawn, Executive Director Information Services, Saline Memorial Hospital, Benton, AR, p. A42
SHUFFLEBARGER, Tom, Chief Operating Officer, The Children's Hospital of Alabama, Birmingham, AL, p. A17
SHUFORD, Little, Manager Medical Information, Kindred Hospital–Greensboro, Greensboro, NC, p. A454
SHUGARMAN, Mark D., President and Chief Executive Officer, Floyd Memorial Hospital and Health Services, New Albany, IN, p. A209
SHUGHART, Deborah A., Vice President and Chief Financial Officer, Fulton County Medical Center, Mc Connellsburg, PA, p. A528
SHUGRUE, Dianne, MSN Senior Vice President Operations and Chief Operating Officer, Glens Falls Hospital, Glens Falls, NY, p. A426
SHULER, Conrad K., M.D. Chief Medical Officer, Oconee Medical Center, Seneca, SC, p. A553
SHULER, Trish, Chief Clinical Officer, Landmark Hospital of Joplin, Joplin, MO, p. A361
SHULIK, David, Vice President and Chief Financial Officer, UPMC Horizon, Greenville, PA, p. A524
SHULKIN, David J., M.D. President and Chief Executive Officer, Morristown Medical Center, Morristown, NJ, p. A406
SHULL, Jennifer, R.N. Chief Nursing Officer, Florida Hospital Fish Memorial, Orange City, FL, p. A134
SHULL, Kenneth A., FACHE Chief Executive Officer, St. Luke's Hospital, Columbus, NC, p. A451
SHULMAN, Lawrence N., M.D. Senior Vice President Medical Affairs and Chief Medical Officer, Dana–Farber Cancer Institute, Boston, MA, p. A296
SHULTS, Randi L., Chief Executive Officer, North Carolina Specialty Hospital, Durham, NC, p. A452
SHULTZ, P. Stephen, M.D. Vice President Medical Affairs, Mayo Clinic Health System – Franciscan Healthcare in La Crosse, La Crosse, WI, p. A684
SHUMAN, Betty, Director Human Resources, Wesley Rehabilitation Hospital, Wichita, KS, p. A246
SHUMAN, Daniel, D.O. Chief Medical Officer, Ashland Health Center, Ashland, KS, p. A230
SHUMATE, Karen J., R.N. Chief Operating Officer, Lawrence Memorial Hospital, Lawrence, KS, p. A237
SHUMWAY, Barbara, Director Human Resources, North Big Horn Hospital District, Lovell, WY, p. A697
SHUMWAY, Donald L., Chief Executive Officer, Crotched Mountain Rehabilitation Center, Greenfield, NH, p. A398

Index of Health Care Professionals / Shupp


SHUPP, Susie, Director Human Resources, Nemaha County Hospital, Auburn, NE, p. A381
SHUSTER, Jamie, Director Associate Relations, Anderson Regional Medical Center–South Campus, Meridian, MS, p. A350
SHUTE, Keith M., M.D. Senior Vice President Medical Affairs and Clinical Services, Androscoggin Valley Hospital, Berlin, NH, p. A397
SHUTE, Leonard J.
Chief Financial Officer, Highland Hospital of Rochester, Rochester, NY, p. A441
Chief Financial Officer, Strong Memorial Hospital of the University of Rochester, Rochester, NY, p. A442
SHUTER, Mark H., President and Chief Executive Officer, Adena Health System, Chillicothe, OH, p. A472
SHUTTA, Rudolph, Chief Financial Officer, Bear Valley Community Hospital, Big Bear Lake, CA, p. A55
SHUTTLESWORTH, Mitzi, Director Human Resources, East Texas Medical Center Carthage, Carthage, TX, p. A586
SHYAVITZ, Linda, President and Chief Executive Officer, Sturdy Memorial Hospital, Attleboro, MA, p. A295
SIAL, Jay, Chief Financial Officer, University of Kentucky Albert B. Chandler Hospital, Lexington, KY, p. A253
SIBLEY, Jeri, Director Revenue Cycle, Riverside Tappahannock Hospital, Tappahannock, VA, p. A656
SICA, Vincent A., President and Chief Executive Officer, DeSoto Memorial Hospital, Arcadia, FL, p. A118
SICILIA, Bruce, M.D. Medical Director, HEALTHSOUTH Rehabilitation Hospital of York, York, PA, p. A542
SIDDIQI, Ather, M.D
Medical Director, Nexus Specialty Hospital, Shenandoah, TX, p. A627
Medical Director, Nexus Specialty Hospital The Woodlands, Spring, TX, p. A628
SIDDIQUI, Hugh, Senior Applications Analyst, Linden Oaks Hospital at Edward, Naperville, IL, p. A189
SIDES, Tim
Chief Financial Officer, Aurora Behavioral Health Care, San Diego, CA, p. A85
Chief Financial Officer, Aurora Las Encinas Hospital, Pasadena, CA, p. A79
SIEBE, Sonya, Manager Human Resources, San Mateo Medical Center, San Mateo, CA, p. A89
SIEBENALER, Christopher, Administrator and Chief Executive Officer, Methodist Sugar Land Hospital, Sugar Land, TX, p. A629
SIEBERT, Kristy, Manager Finance, John J. Pershing Veterans Affairs Medical Center, Poplar Bluff, MO, p. A367
SIEBERT, Matt, Assistant Administrator of Ancillary Services, Hermann Area District Hospital, Hermann, MO, p. A360
SIEBRECHT, Kaylee, Director Human Resources, Story County Medical Center, Nevada, IA, p. A224
SIEFKIN, Allan, M.D. Chief Medical Officer, University of California, Davis Medical Center, Sacramento, CA, p. A84
SIEGEL, Fredric, M.D. Chief of Staff, Desert View Hospital, Pahrump, NV, p. A395
SIEGEL, Lesley, M.D. Medical Director, Riverview Hospital for Children and Youth, Middletown, CT, p. A110
SIEGELMAN, Gary M., M.D. Senior Vice President and Chief Medical Officer, Bayhealth Medical Center, Dover, DE, p. A114
SIEGFRIED, Bryan, M.D. President Medical Staff, Community Memorial Hospital, Staunton, IL, p. A194
SIEGLEN, Linda, M.D. Vice President Medical Affairs, University Medical Center of Princeton at Plainsboro, Plainsboro, NJ, p. A409
SIEK, Terry, MSN Chief Nursing Officer, Hays Medical Center, Hays, KS, p. A234
SIELEMAN, Sharron, R.N. VP, Nursing, Central Maine Medical Center, Lewiston, ME, p. A283
SIEMER, Brenda, Director of Information Technology, Harrison County Community Hospital, Bethany, MO, p. A355
SIEWERT, Charles
Director Human Resources, Buffalo Psychiatric Center, Buffalo, NY, p. A422
Director Human Resources, Western New York Children's Psychiatric Center, West Seneca, NY, p. A446
SIFERS, Carl, Director Information Technology and System Services, Centerpoint Medical Center, Independence, MO, p. A360
SIFFRING, Connie K., Chief Executive Officer, Select Specialty Hospital–Midland, Midland, TX, p. A617
SIGEL, Jay, M.D. Chief Medical Staff, Crane Memorial Hospital, Crane, TX, p. A589
SIGLER, Wes, Chief Executive Officer, Tri–Lakes Medical Center, Batesville, MS, p. A343
SIGLIN, Martin, M.D. Vice President Medical Affairs, Louis A. Weiss Memorial Hospital, Chicago, IL, p. A176
SIGNOR, Kristin, Director Finance, Sunnyview Rehabilitation Hospital, Schenectady, NY, p. A443
SIGSBURY, John R., President and Chief Executive Officer, Emanuel Medical Center, Turlock, CA, p. A93
SILARD, Kathleen A., R.N. Executive Vice President Operations and Chief Operating Officer, Stamford Hospital, Stamford, CT, p. A112
SILKWORTH, Jim, Chief Human Resources Officer, Our Lady of Lourdes Memorial Hospital, Binghamton, NY, p. A422
SILL–LEAHY, Janet, Manager Human Resources, Schick Shadel Hospital, Seattle, WA, p. A666
SILLIMAN, Walter, Chief Information Officer, Ouachita County Medical Center, Camden, AR, p. A43
SILLS, Doug, Chief Executive Officer, River Region Medical Center, Vicksburg, MS, p. A353
SILLS, John M., Chief Information Officer, Health Central, Ocoee, FL, p. A134
SILSBEE, Dave, Chief Information Officer, Cary Medical Center, Caribou, ME, p. A282
SILSBY, Harry, M.D. Medical Director, Intermountain Hospital, Boise, ID, p. A166
SILVA, Carmen, R.N. Chief Operating Officer, Doctors Hospital of Manteca, Manteca, CA, p. A73
SILVA, Lori, Director Human Resources, Mt. San Rafael Hospital, Trinidad, CO, p. A106
SILVA, Margaret, Executive Assistant and Coordinator Human Resources, Promise Hospital of San Antonio, San Antonio, TX, p. A625
SILVA, Raul, M.D. Executive Director, Rockland Children's Psychiatric Center, Orangeburg, NY, p. A439
SILVER, Michael R., M.D. Vice President Medical Affairs, Rush Oak Park Hospital, Oak Park, IL, p. A190
SILVER, Timothy, M.D. Medical Director, Sheltering Arms Hospital South, Midlothian, VA, p. A651
SILVERHATBAND, Darlene J., Supervisory Human Resource Specialist, Chinle Comprehensive Health Care Facility, Chinle, AZ, p. A31
SILVERMAN, Daniel C., M.D
Senior Vice President Medical Affairs, Albany Memorial Hospital, Albany, NY, p. A420
Chief Medical Officer, Acute Care Troy, Samaritan Hospital, Troy, NY, p. A445
Vice President and Chief Medical Officer, Sinai Hospital of Baltimore, Baltimore, MD, p. A289
SILVERMAN, Glen, Chief Executive Officer, Madison River Oaks Medical Center, Canton, MS, p. A344
SILVERSTEIN, Joel, M.D. Chief Medical Officer, Copley Hospital, Morrisville, VT, p. A643
SILVERTHORNE, Samuel, Chief Information Officer, U. S. Air Force Medical Center Keesler, Keesler AFB, MS, p. A348
SILVEUS, Patrick, M.D. Medical Director, Kosciusko Community Hospital, Warsaw, IN, p. A213
SILVIA, Charles B., M.D. Chief Medical Officer and Vice President Medical Affairs, Peninsula Regional Health System, Salisbury, MD, p. A294
SILVIA, Clarence J., President and Chief Executive Officer, The Hospital of Central Connecticut, New Britain, CT, p. A110
SIMCHUK, Cathy J., Chief Operating Officer, Providence Holy Family Hospital, Spokane, WA, p. A667
SIMIA, Greg
Chief Financial Officer, Bon Secours Maryview Medical Center, Portsmouth, VA, p. A654
Interim Chief Financial Officer, Bon Secours–DePaul Medical Center, Norfolk, VA, p. A652
Chief Financial Officer, Mary Immaculate Hospital, Newport News, VA, p. A652
SIMKINS, Palma, Chief Human Resources Management Services, Veterans Affairs Medical Center, Battle Creek, MI, p. A308
SIMMONS, Angela L., Chief Executive Officer, HEALTHSOUTH Rehabilitation Hospital, Humble, TX, p. A608
SIMMONS, Brad, Chief Operating Officer, Saint Luke's Hospital of Kansas City, Kansas City, MO, p. A362
SIMMONS, Daniel F., Senior Vice President and Treasurer, Monongahela Valley Hospital, Monongahela, PA, p. A529
SIMMONS, David, M.D. Chief of Staff, Grenada Lake Medical Center, Grenada, MS, p. A346
SIMMONS, Donald, M.D. Chief Medical Staff, Good Shepherd Medical Center–Linden, Linden, TX, p. A612
SIMMONS, Dorlynn, Chief Executive Officer, Mescalero Public Health Service Indian Hospital, Mescalero, NM, p. A417
SIMMONS, Eileen, Chief Financial Officer, Magee–Womens Hospital of UPMC, Pittsburgh, PA, p. A535
SIMMONS, Kermit, Administrator, Louisiana Extended Care Hospital of Natchitoches, Natchitoches, LA, p. A274
SIMMONS, Leslie, Executive Vice President and Chief Operating Officer, Carroll Hospital Center, Westminster, MD, p. A294
SIMMONS, Linda V., President and Chief Executive Officer, Decatur County Memorial Hospital, Greensburg, IN, p. A203
SIMMONS, Nancy B., Executive Vice President and Chief Administrative Officer, Good Samaritan Hospital Medical Center, West Islip, NY, p. A446
SIMMONS, Preston M., Chief Operating Officer, Providence Regional Medical Center Everett, Everett, WA, p. A661
SIMMONS, Randy, President and Chief Executive Officer, Paris Community Hospital, Paris, IL, p. A190
SIMMONS, Roger
Chief Financial Officer, Coliseum Medical Centers, Macon, GA, p. A155
Chief Financial Officer, Coliseum Northside Hospital, Macon, GA, p. A155
SIMMONS, Steven, Chief Human Resources Officer, Hahnemann University Hospital, Philadelphia, PA, p. A532
SIMMONS, Terry E., Chief Nursing Officer, Madison County Health Care System, Winterset, IA, p. A228
SIMMONS, Tim C., Chief Executive Officer, West Oaks Hospital, Houston, TX, p. A608
SIMMONS, William, President and Chief Executive Officer, St. Luke's Patients Medical Center, Pasadena, TX, p. A620
SIMMS, Jennifer, Director Human Resources, University Medical Center, Lafayette, LA, p. A270
SIMMS, John L., President and Chief Executive Officer, Scott & White Hospital – Brenham, Brenham, TX, p. A585
SIMMS, Sr., Michael S., Vice President Human Resources, Northeast Alabama Regional Medical Center, Anniston, AL, p. A15
SIMODEJKA, John E., President and Chief Executive Officer, Schuylkill Health System, Pottsville, PA, p. B113
SIMODEJKA, John E.
President and Chief Executive Officer, Schuylkill Medical Center – East Norwegian Street, Pottsville, PA, p. A536
President and Chief Executive Officer, Schuylkill Medical Center – South Jackson Street, Pottsville, PA, p. A536
SIMON, Anha, Director Human Resources, Winnie Community Hospital, Winnie, TX, p. A635
SIMON, Ashley, Chief Financial Officer, Kansas Surgery and Recovery Center, Wichita, KS, p. A245
SIMON, Deborah R., R.N. President and Chief Executive Officer, Methodist Medical Center of Illinois, Peoria, IL, p. A191
SIMON, Keri, Executive Director, Women's and Children's Hospital, Columbia, MO, p. A358
SIMON, Lloyd, M.D. Medical Director, Eastern Long Island Hospital, Greenport, NY, p. A427
SIMON, Patricia, Manager Information Systems, Veterans Affairs Medical Center, Canandaigua, NY, p. A423
SIMON, Paul, M.D. Medical Director, Cornerstone Hospital of SouthEast Arizona, Tucson, AZ, p. A39
SIMON, Richard, M.D. Chief of Staff, University of Connecticut Health Center, John Dempsey Hospital, Farmington, CT, p. A109
SIMON, Stuart, M.D. Medical Director, North Central Surgical Center, Dallas, TX, p. A592
SIMON, Teresa, Director Information Systems, Nacogdoches Medical Center, Nacogdoches, TX, p. A618
SIMON, Thresa, M.D. Medical Director, Poplar Springs Hospital, Petersburg, VA, p. A653
SIMONDS, Brock, Interim Chief Financial Officer, Chatham Hospital, Siler City, NC, p. A460
SIMONE, James M., Vice President and Chief Financial Officer, EMH Elyria Medical Center, Elyria, OH, p. A480
SIMONIN, Steven J., Chief Executive Officer, Iowa Specialty Hospital–Clarion, Clarion, IA, p. A216
SIMONS, Chris, Director Health Information Management and Utilization Review, Spring Harbor Hospital, Westbrook, ME, p. A286
SIMONS, Janice, FACHE Chief Executive Officer, Medina Regional Hospital, Hondo, TX, p. A603
SIMONSON, John F., M.D. President Medical Staff, Memorial Community Hospital and Health System, Blair, NE, p. A382
SIMONSON, Paul, Vice President, Trinity Health, Minot, ND, p. A467
SIMPATICO, Thomas, M.D. Facility Director and Network System Manager, Chicago–Read Mental Health Center, Chicago, IL, p. A175
SIMPSON, Bob, Vice President Finance, Methodist Richardson Medical Center, Richardson, TX, p. A622
SIMPSON, Chris, Chief Executive Officer, Cornerstone Hospital–West Monroe, West Monroe, LA, p. A279
SIMPSON, Dana, Manager Human Resources, Riverview Regional Medical Center, Gadsden, AL, p. A20
SIMPSON, Katrina, Director Human Resources, Valley View Regional Hospital, Ada, OK, p. A493
SIMPSON, Keith J., Chief Operating Officer, Jennings American Legion Hospital, Jennings, LA, p. A268
SIMPSON, Jr., Lee A., Chief Executive Officer, Kindred Hospital Tulsa, Tulsa, OK, p. A506
SIMPSON, Linda, Vice President Human Resources, Grant Medical Center, Columbus, OH, p. A476
SIMPSON, Pamela, Director Human Resources, Select Specialty Hospital–Houston, Houston, TX, p. A606
SIMPSON, Richard, M.D. Chief of Staff, Fairmont General Hospital, Fairmont, WV, p. A671


A932 Index of Health Care Professionals

Index of Health Care Professionals / Slavin

SIMPSON Jr., Robert E., M.P.H. President and Chief Executive Officer, Brattleboro Retreat, Brattleboro, VT, p. A643
SIMPSON–TUGGLE, Delois, Vice President Human Resources and Organizational Development and Chief Human Resources Officer, Greater Baltimore Medical Center, Baltimore, MD, p. A287
SIMS, Abraham
Interim Chief Executive Officer, Reliant Rehabilitation Hospital Central Texas, Round Rock, TX, p. A623
Chief Executive Officer, Reliant Rehabilitation Hospital North Houston, Shenandoah, TX, p. A627
SIMS, B. Wayne, President and Chief Executive Officer, KVC Psychiatric Hospital, Kansas City, KS, p. A236
SIMS, Brian, Director Administrative Services, Knoxville Hospital & Clinics, Knoxville, IA, p. A222
SIMS, Jason, M.D. Chief Medical Officer, Cleveland Area Hospital, Cleveland, OK, p. A495
SIMS, Kathleen
Vice President Operations, Manchester Memorial Hospital, Manchester, CT, p. A109
Vice President Operations, Rockville General Hospital, Vernon Rockville, CT, p. A112
SIMS, Mark E., Chief Executive Officer, StoneCrest Medical Center, Smyrna, TN, p. A575
SIMS, Tina, Director Human Resources, Methodist Extended Care Hospital, Memphis, TN, p. A571
SIMS, W. Larry, Chief Financial Officer and Vice President Financial Services, Colquitt Regional Medical Center, Moultrie, GA, p. A157
SIMS, Wanda
Chief Information Officer, Baptist Medical Center East, Montgomery, AL, p. A23
Chief Information Officer, Baptist Medical Center South, Montgomery, AL, p. A23
SINCICH, Robert, Vice President Human Resources, Ashtabula County Medical Center, Ashtabula, OH, p. A469
SINCLAIR, Brad, Chief Financial Officer, Crossgates River Oaks Hospital, Brandon, MS, p. A344
SINCLAIR, Deb Arend, Vice President Human Resources, DeKalb Health, Auburn, IN, p. A197
SINCLAIR, Jan, Director Personnel, Oaklawn Hospital, Marshall, MI, p. A318
SINCLAIR, Jennifer, Vice President Finance, St. Dominic–Jackson Memorial Hospital, Jackson, MS, p. A348
SINCLAIR, Kathy, Vice President Human Resources, Spartanburg Regional Medical Center, Spartanburg, SC, p. A554
SINCLAIR, Laura, Director Human Resources, Kansas City Orthopaedic Institute, Leawood, KS, p. A237
SINCLAIR, Michael, Chief Executive Officer, Rooks County Health Center, Plainville, KS, p. A242
SINCOCK, Gregory M., Information Technology Leader, West Los Angeles Medical Center, Los Angeles, CA, p. A72
SINEK, James J., President and Chief Executive Officer, Faith Regional Health Services, Norfolk, NE, p. A386
SINEK, James J., President and Chief Executive Officer, Faith Regional Health Services, Norfolk, NE, p. B52
SINGAL, Manisha, M.D. Medical Director, Specialty Hospital of Washington, Washington, DC, p. A117
SINGER, Donna, Chief Executive Officer, Blue Mountain Hospital, Blanding, UT, p. A637
SINGER, Susan, Director Human Resources, New York Eye and Ear Infirmary, New York, NY, p. A435
SINGH, Inderjit, M.D. Clinical Director, Pilgrim Psychiatric Center, Brentwood, NY, p. A422
SINGH, Prableen, Chief Information Officer, Newton Medical Center, Newton, KS, p. A239
SINGH–SANDHU, Mohinder S., M.D. President Medical Staff, Henry Ford Wyandotte Hospital, Wyandotte, MI, p. A325
SINGLE, John L., Chief Executive Officer, Huron Regional Medical Center, Huron, SD, p. A557
SINGLES, James L., Chief Financial Officer, Marlette Regional Hospital, Marlette, MI, p. A318
SINGLETARY, Robert G., President and Chief Executive Officer, Maria Parham Medical Center, Henderson, NC, p. A454
SINGLETON, Al, M.D. Chief Psychiatry and Chief Medical Staff, Colorado Mental Health Institute at Pueblo, Pueblo, CO, p. A105
SINGLETON, J. Knox, President and Chief Executive Officer, Inova Health System, Falls Church, VA, p. B71
SINGLETON, Larry, Chief Financial Officer, Lakeside Medical Center, Belle Glade, FL, p. A118
SINGLETON, Roy, Director Computer Information Systems, Palmdale Regional Medical Center, Palmdale, CA, p. A79
SINICROPE, Jr., Frank J., Vice President Financial Services, Princeton Community Hospital, Princeton, WV, p. A675
SINISI, Albert, Director Information Systems, Doctors' Hospital of Michigan, Pontiac, MI, p. A320
SINISI, Linda, Intity Information Officer, Pennsylvania Hospital, Philadelphia, PA, p. A533
SINNER, James E., President and Chief Executive Officer, Medina Memorial Hospital, Medina, NY, p. A429
SINNER, Laurie K., Director Human Resources, Community Hospital, Grand Junction, CO, p. A101
SINNOTT, James, M.D. Chief Medical Staff, Coquille Valley Hospital, Coquille, OR, p. A510
SINOTTE, Brian, Chief Operating Officer, Porter–Valparaiso Hospital Campus, Valparaiso, IN, p. A212
SIOSON, Stephanie
Director Human Resources, Garden Grove Hospital and Medical Center, Garden Grove, CA, p. A63
Director Human Resources, Huntington Beach Hospital, Huntington Beach, CA, p. A65
Director Human Resources, La Palma Intercommunity Hospital, La Palma, CA, p. A66
Director Human Resources, West Anaheim Medical Center, Anaheim, CA, p. A53
SIPEK, John, Supervisor Client Services, Aurora Medical Center of Washington County, Hartford, WI, p. A683
SIREK, David, Chief Information Officer, Myrtue Medical Center, Harlan, IA, p. A220
SIRK, David R., Chief Executive Officer, Vaughan Regional Medical Center, Selma, AL, p. A25
SIRK, Donald, Director Information Systems, Medstar St. Mary's Hospital, Leonardtown, MD, p. A293
SIROIS, Peter, Interim Chief Executive Officer, Northern Maine Medical Center, Fort Kent, ME, p. A283
SIROTTA, Ted D., Chief Financial Officer, Northwestern Medical Center, Saint Albans, VT, p. A644
SISARCICK, Barbara, Administrator, Peterson Rehabilitation Hospital, Wheeling, WV, p. A676
SISK, Glenn C., President, Coosa Valley Medical Center, Sylacauga, AL, p. A25
SISK, Jack, Chief Financial Officer, Punxsutawney Area Hospital, Punxsutawney, PA, p. A536
SISK, Katie, Director Human Resources, Hiawatha Community Hospital, Hiawatha, KS, p. A234
SISK, Lori, R.N. Chief Nursing Officer, Sanford Medical Center Canby, Canby, MN, p. A329
SISK, Rodney, Chief Financial Officer, Fannin Regional Hospital, Blue Ridge, GA, p. A148
SISLER, Debbie, Director Human Resources, Vidant Roanoke–Chowan Hospital, Ahoskie, NC, p. A448
SISLER, Rebecca, Director Human Resources, Box Butte General Hospital, Alliance, NE, p. A381
SISON, Joseph, M.D. Medical Director, Heritage Oaks Hospital, Sacramento, CA, p. A83
SISSON, Travis, Chief Operating Officer, Wesley Medical Center, Hattiesburg, MS, p. A347
SISSON, William G., President, Central Baptist Hospital, Lexington, KY, p. A253
SISTO, Steven A., Senior Vice President and Chief Operating Officer, Methodist Hospital of Southern California, Arcadia, CA, p. A54
SITARIK, Sherrie, President and Chief Executive Officer, Orlando Health, Orlando, FL, p. B98
SITTA, Nasser, M.D. President Medical Staff, Fauquier Hospital, Warrenton, VA, p. A657
SITTIG, Kevin, M.D. Senior Associate Dean and Chief Medical Officer, LSU Medical Center–University Hospital, Shreveport, LA, p. A277
SITTLOW, Jo, Senior Director of Patient Care and Chief Nursing Officer, Lakeview Hospital, Stillwater, MN, p. A340
SIVESS, Chuck, Vice President Human Resources, Providence Health Center, Waco, TX, p. A633
SIVLEY, Susanna S., Chief Personnel Officer, Highlands Medical Center, Scottsboro, AL, p. A25
SIX, Deborah, Coordinator Data Processing, Wayne Memorial Hospital, Jesup, GA, p. A154
SIZEMORE, Darin, Controller, Bell Hospital, Ishpeming, MI, p. A316
SKAARE, Dolores, R.N. Chief Nursing Officer, Plantation General Hospital, Plantation, FL, p. A136
SKABELUND, Hoyt, Administrator, Plains Regional Medical Center, Clovis, NM, p. A415
SKADEN, John, Chief Financial Officer, Saint Joseph's Hospital, Marshfield, WI, p. A685
SKAGGS, Lynda, Chief Nursing Officer, Fleming County Hospital, Flemingsburg, KY, p. A249
SKALA, Pat
Chief Information Officer, Laguna Honda Hospital and Rehabilitation Center, San Francisco, CA, p. A87
Chief Information Officer, San Francisco General Hospital Medical Center, San Francisco, CA, p. A87
SKARULIS, Patricia, Vice President Information Systems, Memorial Sloan–Kettering Cancer Center, New York, NY, p. A434
SKARZYNSKI, Joseph, M.D
Medical Director, Jacobi Medical Center,, NY, p. A433
Medical Director, North Central Bronx Hospital,, NY, p. A436
SKEANS, John, Chief Financial Officer, St. Anthony's Medical Center, Saint Louis, MO, p. A370
SKELDON, Timothy K., Senior Vice President and Chief Financial Officer, Parrish Medical Center, Titusville, FL, p. A142
SKELLEY, Dennis B., President and Chief Executive Officer, Walton Rehabilitation Hospital, Augusta, GA, p. A147
SKELTON, Jeff, Chief Financial Officer, Carolina Center for Behavioral Health, Greer, SC, p. A551
SKELTON, John, Director Finance, Temple Community Hospital, Los Angeles, CA, p. A72
SKIDMORE, Jocelyn, Director Finance, St. Francis Hospital and Health Services, Maryville, MO, p. A365
SKIEM, Paul
Senior Vice President Human Resources, Holy Family Medical Center, Des Plaines, IL, p. A180
Senior Vice President Human Resources, Resurrection Medical Center, Chicago, IL, p. A177
Senior Vice President Human Resources, Saint Francis Hospital, Evanston, IL, p. A181
SKILLINGS, Charles E., President and Chief Executive Officer, St. Anthony Shawnee Hospital, Shawnee, OK, p. A504
SKILLINGS, Lois N., MSN, President and Chief Executive Officer, Mid Coast Hospital, Brunswick, ME, p. A282
SKILLMAN, Sally, Director Human Resources, Shriners Hospitals for Children, Shriners Burns Hospital, Cincinnati, Cincinnati, OH, p. A474
SKINNER, Eileen F., FACHE President and Chief Executive Officer, Mercy Hospital of Portland, Portland, ME, p. A284
SKINNER, Gwendolyn, Executive Director, Devereux Georgia Treatment Network, Kennesaw, GA, p. A154
SKINNER, Jeannette, FACHE Chief Executive Officer, Wuesthoff Medical Center – Melbourne, Melbourne, FL, p. A130
SKINNER, Jon C., Chief Executive Officer, Baylor Institute for Rehabilitation, Dallas, TX, p. A590
SKINNER, Marjorie, Director Finance, Pershing General Hospital, Lovelock, NV, p. A394
SKINNER, Ross, Director Information Systems, Payson Regional Medical Center, Payson, AZ, p. A35
SKLAMBERG, Todd, President, Sunrise Hospital and Medical Center, Las Vegas, NV, p. A394
SKLAR, Joel, M.D. Chief Medical Officer, Marin General Hospital, Greenbrae, CA, p. A64
SKOGSBERGH, Jim H., President and Chief Executive Officer, Advocate Health Care, Oak Brook, IL, p. B6
SKORICH, Brenda, Manager Business and Medical Records, Virginia Regional Medical Center, Virginia, MN, p. A341
SKORNIAK, Stan, MS Associate Medical Center Director, John J. Pershing Veterans Affairs Medical Center, Poplar Bluff, MO, p. A367
SKOV, Randy, Vice President, Mid–Columbia Medical Center, The Dalles, OR, p. A516
SKRINDE, Tracie, Director Human Resources, United General Hospital, Sedro Woolley, WA, p. A666
SKRIPPS, Michele M., R.N. Administrator, AnMed Health Rehabilitation Hospital, Anderson, SC, p. A546
SKULA, Erika, Chief Financial Officer, Manchester Memorial Hospital, Manchester, KY, p. A256
SKVARENINA, Michael, Assistant Vice President Information Systems, Holy Name Medical Center, Teaneck, NJ, p. A410
SKYLES, Jill, R.N. Chief Nursing Officer, Barnes–Jewish St. Peters Hospital, Saint Peters, MO, p. A370
SLABA, Bryan, Chief Executive Officer, Wagner Community Memorial Hospital Avera, Wagner, SD, p. A560
SLACK, Martin R., Chief Executive Officer, Gulf Coast Medical Center, Wharton, TX, p. A634
SLADKY, Todd J., Chief Financial Officer, Great River Medical Center, West Burlington, IA, p. A228
SLAGLE, Amy, M.D. President Medical Staff, Menominee Tribal Clinic, Shawano Medical Center, Shawano, WI, p. A690
SLANE, Eric, M.D. Chief of Staff, Grant Regional Health Center, Lancaster, WI, p. A684
SLATE, Clyde, Assistant Superintendent Administrative Services, Memphis Mental Health Institute, Memphis, TN, p. A571
SLATE, Sonny, Chief Operating Officer, Georgia Regional Hospital at Atlanta, Decatur, GA, p. A151
SLATER, Craig M., M.D. Chief Medical Officer, Columbus Regional Healthcare System, Whiteville, NC, p. A462
SLATER, Jan, Chief Executive Officer, Oklahoma State University Medical Center, Tulsa, OK, p. A506
SLATTERY, Greg, Vice President Information, Community Hospitals and Wellness Centers, Bryan, OH, p. A471
SLATTERY, Sue, Director Human Resources, St. Luke's Hospital, Cedar Rapids, IA, p. A215
SLATTMAN, Robin, Chief Nursing Officer, Memorial Hospital of Union County, Marysville, OH, p. A484
SLAVIN, Kevin J., FACHE President and Chief Executive Officer, East Orange General Hospital, East Orange, NJ, p. A403
SLAVIN, Peter L., M.D. President, Massachusetts General Hospital, Boston, MA, p. A297

Index of Health Care Professionals

SLAWITSKY, Bruce, Vice President Human Resources, Hospital for Special Surgery, New York, NY, p. A433

SLAWKOWSKI, Ken, Interim Director Information Systems, Holy Cross Hospital, Chicago, IL, p. A176

SLAYDON, Cindy, Chief Nursing Executive, Sparks Regional Medical Center, Fort Smith, AR, p. A45

SLAYTON, Lisa C., Senior Vice President Human Resources, Bon Secours St. Francis Health System, Greenville, SC, p. A550

SLAYTON, Val, M.D. Vice President Medical Affairs, Sts. Mary & Elizabeth Hospital, Louisville, KY, p. A255

SLEDGE, Cynthia Moore, M.D. Medical Director, Bryce Hospital, Tuscaloosa, AL, p. A26

SLEPIN, Robert, Vice President and Chief Information Officer, John C. Lincoln North Mountain Hospital, Phoenix, AZ, p. A35

SLETTE, Katie, Director Human Resources and Marketing, Windom Area Hospital, Windom, MN, p. A342

SLICK, Lois, Director Human Resources, LakeWood Health Center, Baudette, MN, p. A328

SLIETER Jr., Richard G., Administrator, Community Behavioral Health Hospital – Baxter, Baxter, MN, p. A328

SLIGER, Susan, Director Human Resources, War Memorial Hospital, Sault Sainte Marie, MI, p. A323

SLINGERLAND, Micki J.
Chief Operating Officer, Tristar Ashland City Medical Center, Ashland City, TN, p. A562
Chief Operating Officer, Tristar Centennial Medical Center, Nashville, TN, p. A573

SLIPKOVICH, Daniel S., Chief Executive Officer, Capella Healthcare, Franklin, TN, p. B24

SLITER, Elizabeth, M.D. Chairman Medical Staff, Decatur County Hospital and Cedar Living Center, Oberlin, KS, p. A240

SLIWA, James, M.D. Chief Medical Officer, Rehabilitation Institute of Chicago, Chicago, IL, p. A177

SLIWINSKI, Jeff, Chief Financial Officer, Clear Lake Regional Medical Center, Webster, TX, p. A634

SLIWINSKI, Ron, Chief Operations Officer, University of Wisconsin Hospital and Clinics, Madison, WI, p. A684

SLOAN, Gary, Chief Executive Officer, San Ramon Regional Medical Center, San Ramon, CA, p. A89

SLOAN, Ronald A., FACHE President, The Outer Banks Hospital, Nags Head, NC, p. A458

SLOAN, Steve, Chief Financial Officer, Lake Cumberland Regional Hospital, Somerset, KY, p. A259

SLOCUM, Brandon H., Senior Vice President and Chief Financial Officer, Medical West, Bessemer, AL, p. A16

SLOCUM, Gregg Y., Chief Financial Officer, Valley Forge Medical Center and Hospital, Norristown, PA, p. A531

SLONAKER, Jody, Chief Fiscal Section, Veterans Affairs Medical Center, Martinsburg, WV, p. A673

SLONIM, Sheryl A., Executive Vice President and Chief Nursing Officer, Holy Name Medical Center, Teaneck, NJ, p. A410

SLONINA, Marrianne, Director Human Resources, Georgetown Community Hospital, Georgetown, KY, p. A250

SLUBOWSKI, Michael A., Chief Executive Officer, Sisters of Charity of Leavenworth Health System, Denver, CO, p. B119

SLUSHER, Michael, Community Chief Executive Officer, Middlesboro ARH Hospital, Middlesboro, KY, p. A256

SLY-SMITH, Michelle, Chief Executive Officer, Sullivan County Community Hospital, Sullivan, IN, p. A212

SLYTER, Mark F., FACHE President and Chief Executive Officer, Mississippi Baptist Health System, Jackson, MS, p. B90

SMALE, Cindy, Director Human Resources, Indiana University Health Bedford Hospital, Bedford, IN, p. A197

SMALL, Annette, R.N. Chief Executive Officer, St. Mary's Medical Center, Blue Springs, MO, p. A355

SMALL, Deborah C., R.N. Chief Nursing Officer, Fairview Hospital, Cleveland, OH, p. A475

SMALL, Jonathan, Chief Operations Information and Technology, John D. Dingell Veterans Affairs Medical Center, Detroit, MI, p. A311

SMALL, Terry L., Assistant Chief Executive Officer, William R. Sharpe, Jr. Hospital, Weston, WV, p. A676

SMALLWOOD, Vicki, Chief Information Officer, Veterans Affairs Medical Center, Tuscaloosa, AL, p. A26

SMALTZ, Herb, Chief Information Officer, Ohio State University Medical Center, Columbus, OH, p. A477

SMANIK, Robert E., FACHE President and Chief Executive Officer, Day Kimball Hospital, Putnam, CT, p. A111

SMARR, Susan, M.D. Physician–in–Chief, Santa Clara Medical Center, Santa Clara, CA, p. A90

SMART, Dan, Chief Information Management Officer, Permian Regional Medical Center, Andrews, TX, p. A578

SMART, George J.
VP Finance & IT, Alpena Regional Medical Center, Alpena, MI, p. A307
Vice President Finance and System Services, Spectrum Health Zeeland Community Hospital, Zeeland, MI, p. A326

SMART, Paul, CPA Chief Financial Officer, Franklin County Medical Center, Preston, ID, p. A170

SMART, Robert M., Chief Executive Officer, Reliant Rehabilitation Hospital Mid–Cities, Bedford, TX, p. A583

SMEEKS, Frank C., M.D. Chief Medical Officer, Frye Regional Medical Center, Hickory, NC, p. A455

SMESNEY, Michael, Chief Executive Officer, Renaissance Healthcare Systems, Houston, TX, p. B109

SMESNY, Michael
Chief Financial Officer, Kindred Hospital El Paso, El Paso, TX, p. A596
Region Chief Financial Officer, Kindred Hospital–Amarillo, Amarillo, TX, p. A578

SMESTAD, Craig, M.D. Chief Medical Officer, Brandon Regional Hospital, Brandon, FL, p. A119

SMILEY, Christy, Director Human Resources, Audrain Medical Center, Mexico, MO, p. A365

SMIRZ, Lynda Ann, M.D. Chief Medical Officer, Indiana University Health North Hospital, Carmel, IN, p. A199

SMITH, Alan H.
Chief Financial Officer, Garden Grove Hospital and Medical Center, Garden Grove, CA, p. A63
Chief Financial Officer, Huntington Beach Hospital, Huntington Beach, CA, p. A65
Chief Financial Officer, La Palma Intercommunity Hospital, La Palma, CA, p. A66
Chief Financial Officer, West Anaheim Medical Center, Anaheim, CA, p. A53

SMITH, Andrew, M.D. Chief Medical Staff, Guttenberg Municipal Hospital, Guttenberg, IA, p. A220

SMITH, Andrew
Chief Information Management, Madigan Healthcare System, Tacoma, WA, p. A668
CFO, St. Petersburg General Hospital, Saint Petersburg, FL, p. A138

SMITH, Barbara H., Senior Vice President & Chief Operating Officer, Robert Wood Johnson University Hospital at Hamilton, Hamilton, NJ, p. A404

SMITH, Becky, Manager Human Resources, McKenzie County Healthcare System, Watford City, ND, p. A468

SMITH, Bennie, Director Human Resources and Risk Management, Lady of the Sea General Hospital, Cut Off, LA, p. A265

SMITH, Bernie, Chief Financial Officer, Troy Community Hospital, Troy, PA, p. A539

SMITH, Beth, Controller, Mercy Hospital, Valley City, ND, p. A468

SMITH, Bethany, Controller, HEALTHSOUTH Cane Creek Rehabilitation Hospital, Martin, TN, p. A570

SMITH, Bobby, Vice President Physician Services and Quality, Illinois Valley Community Hospital, Peru, IL, p. A191

SMITH, Bradley, President and Chief Executive Officer, Rush Memorial Hospital, Rushville, IN, p. A211

SMITH, Brenda, Director Financial Services, Alliance Health Center, Meridian, MS, p. A350

SMITH, Brent, M.D. Chief Medical Officer and Vice President Clinical Integration, Edward Hospital, Naperville, IL, p. A189

SMITH, Brent, Chief Financial Officer, Jennersville Regional Hospital, West Grove, PA, p. A541

SMITH, Brian
Executive Vice President and Chief Operating Officer, St. Rita's Medical Center, Lima, OH, p. A483
Chief Operating Officer, Wamego City Hospital, Wamego, KS, p. A244

SMITH, Carl, Director Information Systems, King's Daughters Medical Center, Brookhaven, MS, p. A344

SMITH, Chris, Vice President Information Technology, North Oaks Medical Center, Hammond, LA, p. A267

SMITH, Cindy, Chief Executive Officer, Kindred Hospital–Sycamore, Sycamore, IL, p. A195

SMITH, Coke R., M.D. Medical Director, Sunnyside Community Hospital, Sunnyside, WA, p. A667

SMITH, Connie, President and Chief Executive Officer, Commonwealth Health Corporation, Bowling Green, KY, p. B33

SMITH, Connie
Chief Executive Officer, Medical Center at Bowling Green, Bowling Green, KY, p. A248
Chief Executive Officer and Chief Operating Officer, Medical Center at Scottsville, Scottsville, KY, p. A259

SMITH, Dale, Director Human Resources, Texas Health Harris Methodist Hospital Hurst–Euless–Bedford, Bedford, TX, p. A583

SMITH, Dan, Director Human Resources, Memorial Hospital, Carthage, IL, p. A174

SMITH, Daniel
Interim Chief Executive Officer, Sugar Land Surgical Hospital, Sugar Land, TX, p. A629
Chief Financial Officer, TOPS Surgical Specialty Hospital, Houston, TX, p. A607

SMITH, Daniel B.
Vice President Finance, Good Samaritan Regional Medical Center, Corvallis, OR, p. A510
Vice President Finance, Samaritan Albany General Hospital, Albany, OR, p. A509
Vice President Finance, Samaritan Lebanon Community Hospital, Lebanon, OR, p. A512

SMITH, Daniel W., Chief Financial Officer, Pioneers Memorial Healthcare District, Brawley, CA, p. A56

SMITH, Danny
Director Human Resources, Bryan W. Whitfield Memorial Hospital, Demopolis, AL, p. A19
Chief Financial Officer, Redmond Regional Medical Center, Rome, GA, p. A158

SMITH, Darline, R.N. Vice President Patient Care Services and Chief Nursing Officer, St. Francis Medical Center, Monroe, LA, p. A273

SMITH, Darrin, Vice President Human Resources, Parkview Medical Center, Pueblo, CO, p. A105

SMITH, Darwin K., Vice President Human Resources, Union Hospital, Dover, OH, p. A479

SMITH, David
Vice President Rehabilitation Services, Baylor Institute for Rehabilitation, Dallas, TX, p. A590
Manager Data Center, Huguley Memorial Medical Center, Fort Worth, TX, p. A598
Senior Director Human Resources, Marquette General Health System, Marquette, MI, p. A318
Chief Financial Officer, Memorial Regional Hospital,, FL, p. A125

SMITH, David A., Vice President and Chief Operating Officer, Avista Adventist Hospital, Louisville, CO, p. A104

SMITH, David B., Assistant Vice President Information Services, Medstar Harbor Hospital, Baltimore, MD, p. A288

SMITH, David N., M.D. Vice President Medical Affairs, Rowan Regional Medical Center, Salisbury, NC, p. A460

SMITH, Debra, Chief Executive Officer, St. Joseph's Health Services, Hillsboro, WI, p. A683

SMITH, Denise
Director Financial Services, Florida State Hospital, Chattahoochee, FL, p. A120
Director Health Information, HEALTHSOUTH Chattanooga Rehabilitation Hospital, Chattanooga, TN, p. A563

SMITH, Dennis H., Director, Veterans Affairs Maryland Health Care System–Baltimore Division, Baltimore, MD, p. A289

SMITH, Dennis J., Chief Operating Officer, James Cancer Hospital and Solove Research Institute, Columbus, OH, p. A476

SMITH, Denny R., Administrator, Camden General Hospital, Camden, TN, p. A562

SMITH, Diana B., Chief Financial Officer, Texas Specialty Hospital at Dallas, Dallas, TX, p. A593

SMITH, Diane, Chief Nursing Officer, Baptist Health Extended Care Hospital, Little Rock, AR, p. A47

SMITH, Dick, Director Human Resources, West Park Hospital, Cody, WY, p. A696

SMITH, Donna P., R.N. Vice President Patient Care Services and Chief Nursing Officer, Clifton Springs Hospital and Clinic, Clifton Springs, NY, p. A424

SMITH, Donnie
Chief Human Resources Officer, Laird Hospital, Union, MS, p. A353
Director Human Resources, Rush Foundation Hospital, Meridian, MS, p. A350

SMITH, Doug, Chief Financial Officer, McKay–Dee Hospital Center, Ogden, UT, p. A639

SMITH, Douglas, Chief Financial Officer, Mesilla Valley Hospital, Las Cruces, NM, p. A416

SMITH Jr., Edward H., Interim Chief Executive Officer, St. Anthony Regional Hospital, Carroll, IA, p. A215

SMITH, Eric, Chief Financial Officer, East Georgia Regional Medical Center, Statesboro, GA, p. A160

SMITH, Ericka, Chief Operating Officer, Monterey Park Hospital, Monterey Park, CA, p. A75

SMITH, Eugene, Chief Information Officer, Maniilaq Health Center, Kotzebue, AK, p. A29

SMITH, Gary, Manager Information Technology, Paynesville Area Health Care System, Paynesville, MN, p. A337

SMITH, Gene, Senior Vice President Operations, AMG Specialty Hospital–Slidell, Slidell, LA, p. A278

SMITH, Gregory
Chief Information Officer, Covenant Medical Center, Waterloo, IA, p. A228
Senior Vice President and Chief Information Officer, Wheaton Franciscan Healthcare – St. Francis, Milwaukee, WI, p. A687
Senior Vice President and Chief Information Officer, Wheaton Franciscan Healthcare – The Wisconsin Heart Hospital, Wauwatosa, WI, p. A693

Index of Health Care Professionals / Smith

Index of Health Care Professionals


SMITH, Gretchen, Vice President Nursing and Compliance and Risk, Rush Memorial Hospital, Rushville, IN, p. A211
SMITH, Harley, President, Washington County Hospital, Plymouth, NC, p. A458
SMITH, Heather
Director Information Services, Holy Cross Hospital, Silver Spring, MD, p. A294
Director Finance, Meyersdale Medical Center, Meyersdale, PA, p. A529
SMITH, Jack, Acting Chief Information Resources Management Service, Veterans Affairs Sierra Nevada Health Care System, Reno, NV, p. A395
SMITH, James E.
Superintendent, North Texas State Hospital, Vernon, TX, p. A633
Superintendent, North Texas State Hospital, Wichita Falls Campus, Wichita Falls, TX, p. A635
SMITH, James L., Chief Financial Officer, Greeley County Health Services, Tribune, KS, p. A244
SMITH, James M., M.D. Medical Director, Bastrop Rehabilitation Hospital, Bastrop, LA, p. A262
SMITH, Janet, Chief Financial Officer, Troy Regional Medical Center, Troy, AL, p. A26
SMITH, Jeanna, Administrative Assistant and Human Resources Officer, Polk Medical Center, Cedartown, GA, p. A149
SMITH, Jeff, Chief Information Officer, Holy Cross Hospital, Fort Lauderdale, FL, p. A123
SMITH, Jeffrey
Chief Executive Officer, Kindred Rehabilitation Hospital Northeast Houston, Humble, TX, p. A608
Senior Vice President and Chief Operating Officer, Mercy Medical Center, Canton, OH, p. A472
SMITH, Jill, Administrative Coordinator, J. Paul Jones Hospital, Camden, AL, p. A18
SMITH, Jim, Director Information Systems, Mineral Area Regional Medical Center, Farmington, MO, p. A359
SMITH, Jimmy, Coordinator Clinical Information Technology, Chilton Medical Center, Clanton, AL, p. A18
SMITH, Jo Beth
Director Support Services and Human Resources, Decatur County Hospital, Leon, IA, p. A222
Director Human Resources, Medical Arts Hospital, Lamesa, TX, p. A611
SMITH, Joanne C., M.D. President and Chief Executive Officer, Rehabilitation Institute of Chicago, Chicago, IL, p. A177
SMITH, Jodi, Administrative Assistant Human Resources, Eureka Springs Hospital, Eureka Springs, AR, p. A44
SMITH, John, Chief Executive Officer, Coffeyville Regional Medical Center, Coffeyville, KS, p. A231
SMITH, Jonathan, Chief Financial Officer, Blue Ridge Regional Hospital, Spruce Pine, NC, p. A461
SMITH, Joseph B., Vice President Finance, Medstar Union Memorial Hospital, Baltimore, MD, p. A288
SMITH, Joseph S., Chief Executive Officer, Boone County Hospital, Boone, IA, p. A215
SMITH, Josh, Vice President Human Resources, Palmetto Lowcountry Behavioral Health, Charleston, SC, p. A547
SMITH, Judy, M.D. Medical Director, Roswell Park Cancer Institute, Buffalo, NY, p. A423
SMITH, Julia
Chief Financial Officer, Kindred Hospital–Charleston, Charleston, SC, p. A547
Chief Financial Officer, Kindred Hospital–Chattanooga, Chattanooga, TN, p. A563
SMITH, Julie, R.N. Director of Nursing, Jersey Community Hospital, Jerseyville, IL, p. A185
SMITH, Justin
Interim Chief Executive Officer, Kindred Hospital Dallas Central, Dallas, TX, p. A591
Administrator, Kindred Hospital–White Rock, Dallas, TX, p. A591
SMITH, Karen, Interim Chief Executive Officer, Coffey County Hospital, Burlington, KS, p. A231
SMITH, Karen S., Director Information Services, Chilton Hospital, Pompton Plains, NJ, p. A409
SMITH, Karyl, Director Human Resources, LAC–Harbor–University of California at Los Angeles Medical Center, Torrance, CA, p. A92
SMITH, Kathleen, Interim Vice President Human Resources, Glens Falls Hospital, Glens Falls, NY, p. A426
SMITH, Kelli, M.D. Chief of Staff, Magee General Hospital, Magee, MS, p. A349
SMITH, Kelly C., Chief Operating Officer, Oakwood Heritage Hospital, Taylor, MI, p. A324
SMITH, Ken, Chief Financial Officer, Cooperstown Medical Center, Cooperstown, ND, p. A465
SMITH, Kenneth, M.D. Chief of Staff, John C. Fremont Healthcare District, Mariposa, CA, p. A74
SMITH, Kevin, Vice President Finance and Support Services, Rehabilitation Institute of Michigan, Detroit, MI, p. A311
SMITH, Kevin E., Chief Operating Officer, Scott & White Hospital – Taylor, Taylor, TX, p. A630
SMITH, Kevin F., President and Chief Executive Officer, Winchester Hospital, Winchester, MA, p. A306
SMITH, Kevin M., Director Human Resources, Indian Path Medical Center, Kingsport, TN, p. A568
SMITH, Lana, Director Human Resources, Davis Regional Medical Center, Statesville, NC, p. A461
SMITH, Larry, Senior Vice President and Chief Financial Officer, Valley Medical Center, Renton, WA, p. A664
SMITH, Lawrence, M.D. Senior Vice President and Chief Medical Officer, Forest Hills Hospital,, NY, p. A432
SMITH, Leighton B., M.D. Vice President Medical Affairs, Northwest Community Hospital, Arlington Heights, IL, p. A172
SMITH, Leora, Information System and Health Information Management Team Leader, Phelps Memorial Health Center, Holdrege, NE, p. A384
SMITH, Lex, Chief Executive Officer, George L. Mee Memorial Hospital, King City, CA, p. A65
SMITH, Linda, FACHE Chief Executive Officer, Santa Clara Valley Medical Center, San Jose, CA, p. A88
SMITH, Linda C., M.D. Medical Director, HEALTHSOUTH Rehabilitation Hospital of Beaumont, Beaumont, TX, p. A583
SMITH, Linda D., Director, Veterans Affairs Medical Center, Cincinnati, OH, p. A474
SMITH, Linda T., Director Human Resources, Clay County Hospital, Ashland, AL, p. A15
SMITH, Linda V., Director Human Resources, Englewood Community Hospital, Englewood, FL, p. A122
SMITH, Lori, Chief Financial Officer, Meade District Hospital, Meade, KS, p. A239
SMITH, Lorie, Director Human Resources, Nason Hospital, Roaring Spring, PA, p. A537
SMITH, Jr., Louis G., Chief Executive Officer, Memorial Hermann Northeast, Humble, TX, p. A608
SMITH, Marisa, Director Information Services, East Georgia Regional Medical Center, Statesboro, GA, p. A160
SMITH, Mark H., M.D. Chief of Staff, Iowa City Veterans Affairs Health Care System, Iowa City, IA, p. A221
SMITH, Mark T., CPA, President, Sycamore Medical Center, Miamisburg, OH, p. A485
SMITH, Marshall E., FACHE Chief Executive Officer, New River Medical Center, Monticello, MN, p. A335
SMITH, Martha, Chief Operating Officer, Kapiolani Medical Center for Women & Children, Honolulu, HI, p. A163
SMITH, Mary Clare, M.D. Medical Director, Western State Hospital, Staunton, VA, p. A656
SMITH, Marybeth
Director Human Resources, Saint Francis Hospital, Charleston, WV, p. A671
Director Human Resources, Thomas Memorial Hospital, South Charleston, WV, p. A676
SMITH, Matthew, Operations Director Finance and Support Services, Alegent Health–Community Memorial Hospital, Missouri Valley, IA, p. A223
SMITH, Melinda, Chief Information Systems, H. C. Watkins Memorial Hospital, Quitman, MS, p. A352
SMITH, Melissa
Controller, Select Specialty Hospital–Jackson, Jackson, MS, p. A348
Vice President and Controller, Select Specialty Hospital–Wilmington, Wilmington, DE, p. A115
SMITH, Michael, Director Support Services and Information Technology, Medina Regional Hospital, Hondo, TX, p. A603
SMITH, Michael K., D.O. Vice President Medical Affairs, McLaren Macomb, Mount Clemens, MI, p. A319
SMITH, Michael K., Regional Administrator, Mercy Hospital Ozark, Ozark, AR, p. A50
SMITH, Michelle, Coordinator Human Resources, Baton Rouge Rehabilitation Hospital, Baton Rouge, LA, p. A262
SMITH, Michelle T., R.N. Chief Nursing Officer, Greenville Memorial Hospital, Greenville, SC, p. A550
SMITH, Mickey, Chief Executive Officer, Oak Hill Hospital, Brooksville, FL, p. A120
SMITH, Mike
Chief Information Officer, Cape Coral Hospital, Cape Coral, FL, p. A120
Chief Information Officer, Gulf Coast Medical Center, Fort Myers, FL, p. A123
Chief Information Officer, Lee Memorial Hospital, Fort Myers, FL, p. A124
SMITH, Nadine, Director Human Resources, Reeves County Hospital, Pecos, TX, p. A620
SMITH, Neil, M.D. Chief Medical Officer, Fairview Hospital, Cleveland, OH, p. A475
SMITH, Nekisha, Director Medical Records, Riverland Medical Center, Ferriday, LA, p. A266
SMITH, Norine, Chief Executive Officer, U. S. Public Health Service Indian Hospital, Cass Lake, MN, p. A329
SMITH, Ollie, Vice President Human Resources, Paris Community Hospital, Paris, IL, p. A190
SMITH, Pam, Director Human Resources, East Liverpool City Hospital, East Liverpool, OH, p. A479
SMITH, Patrick, M.D. Chief Medical Officer, Arrowhead Hospital, Glendale, AZ, p. A32
SMITH, Paul, Chief Financial Officer, Kindred Hospital of Riverside, Perris, CA, p. A80
SMITH, Paula
Senior Vice President Chief Information Officer, Oakwood Annapolis Hospital, Wayne, MI, p. A325
Chief Information Officer, Oakwood Heritage Hospital, Taylor, MI, p. A324
Leader Information Services and Chief Information Officer, Oakwood Hospital & Medical Center–Dearborn, Dearborn, MI, p. A310
Vice President Information Services and Chief Information Officer, Oakwood Southshore Medical Center, Trenton, MI, p. A324
SMITH, Peg, Vice President and Chief Nursing Officer, Chandler Regional Medical Center, Chandler, AZ, p. A31
SMITH, Peyton A., Chief Executive Officer, Lower Oconee Community Hospital, Glenwood, GA, p. A153
SMITH, Phyllis
Vice President Human Resources, Tahlequah City Hospital, Tahlequah, OK, p. A505
Associate Director, Veterans Affairs Medical Center, Birmingham, AL, p. A17
SMITH, Randall, Executive Vice President, Jackson Park Hospital and Medical Center, Chicago, IL, p. A176
SMITH, Rebecca, Vice President and Chief Operating Officer, Caldwell Memorial Hospital, Lenoir, NC, p. A456
SMITH, Rhonda, Director Human Resources, Shriners Hospitals for Children, Portland, Portland, OR, p. A514
SMITH, Rhonda E., R.N
Vice President Patient Care Services and Chief Nursing Officer, Union Hospital, Terre Haute, IN, p. A212
Chief Nursing Officer, Union Hospital Clinton, Clinton, IN, p. A199
SMITH, Rich, Vice President Human Resources, Sunnyside Medical Center, Clackamas, OR, p. A509
SMITH, Richard C., Senior Vice President and Chief Financial Officer, JFK Medical Center, Edison, NJ, p. A403
SMITH, Rick, Director Information Systems, Jamestown Regional Medical Center, Jamestown, TN, p. A567
SMITH, Robert, Chief Information Officer, Fulton State Hospital, Fulton, MO, p. A360
SMITH, Robert M., M.D. Acting Director, Veterans Affairs San Diego Healthcare System, San Diego, CA, p. A86
SMITH, Robin S., Chief Nursing Officer, Indiana University Health White Memorial Hospital, Monticello, IN, p. A208
SMITH, Rodney, VP Support Services, Harrisburg Medical Center, Harrisburg, IL, p. A183
SMITH, Rodney R., Chief Executive Officer, Lawnwood Regional Medical Center, Fort Pierce, FL, p. A124
SMITH, Ron, Chief Financial Officer, Wickenburg Community Hospital, Wickenburg, AZ, p. A41
SMITH, Roy, Chief Financial Officer, Onslow Memorial Hospital, Jacksonville, NC, p. A455
SMITH, Ryan J., Administrator, Mayo Clinic Health System in Saint James, Saint James, MN, p. A338
SMITH, Ryan K., Chief Executive Officer, Memorial Hospital of Converse County, Douglas, WY, p. A696
SMITH, Sandra K., Chief Executive Officer, Deer's Head Hospital Center, Salisbury, MD, p. A294
SMITH, Sandra L., Administrator, Adena Greenfield Medical Center, Greenfield, OH, p. A481
SMITH, Scott, M.D. Chief of Staff, Adams Memorial Hospital, Decatur, IN, p. A200
SMITH, Scott D., Chief Financial Officer, Adams County Regional Medical Center, Seaman, OH, p. A488
SMITH, Scott M.
Chief Executive Officer, Bolivar Medical Center, Cleveland, MS, p. A345
Chief Executive Officer, Lake Wales Medical Center, Lake Wales, FL, p. A128
SMITH, Seneca, Chief Operating Officer, Creek Nation Community Hospital, Okemah, OK, p. A500
SMITH, Shane, M.D. Physician, Sanford Sheldon Medical Center, Sheldon, IA, p. A226
SMITH, Sherry, Manager Human Resources, Dallas County Hospital, Perry, IA, p. A225
SMITH, Sherry Bea, R.N. Chief Executive Officer and Chief Financial Officer, Lead–Deadwood Regional Hospital, Deadwood, SD, p. A556
SMITH, Shirley M., Chief Financial Officer, Andalusia Regional Hospital, Andalusia, AL, p. A15
SMITH, Sid, Director Information Resources, Larned State Hospital, Larned, KS, p. A237

Index of Health Care Professionals

Index of Health Care Professionals / Smith

SMITH, Stephen, Administrator, Selby General Hospital, Marietta, OH, p. A484
SMITH, Stephen B., M.D. Chief Medical Officer, Nebraska Medical Center, Omaha, NE, p. A388
SMITH, Steve
Chief Financial Officer, Albany Area Hospital and Medical Center, Albany, MN, p. A327
Chief Financial Officer, Kansas Heart Hospital, Wichita, KS, p. A245
SMITH, Steven
Chief Financial Officer, Kindred Hospital Detroit, Detroit, MI, p. A311
Chief Financial Officer, Lea Regional Medical Center, Hobbs, NM, p. A416
Chief Information Officer, Saints Mary & Elizabeth Medical Center, Chicago, IL, p. A178
SMITH, Steven L., Chief Executive Officer, Matagorda Regional Medical Center, Bay City, TX, p. A582
SMITH, Tammy, Director Human Resources, St. Vincent Morrilton, Morrilton, AR, p. A49
SMITH, Ted, Chief Executive Officer, Savoy Medical Center, Mamou, LA, p. A272
SMITH, Teresa, Chief Financial Officer, Memorial Hospital, Carthage, IL, p. A174
SMITH, Terrance, M.D. Chairman Medical Staff, Sanford Deuel County Medical Center, Clear Lake, SD, p. A556
SMITH, Thomas, Chief Information Officer, NorthShore University Health System Evanston Hospital, Evanston, IL, p. A181
SMITH III, Thomas C., FACHE Director, Central Texas Veterans Healthcare System, Temple, TX, p. A630
SMITH, Thomas G., Administrator and Chief Executive Officer, Audubon County Memorial Hospital, Audubon, IA, p. A214
SMITH, Tiffany, Director Human Resources, Wellstone Regional Hospital, Jeffersonville, IN, p. A205
SMITH, Tim
Director Information Systems, Iroquois Memorial Hospital and Resident Home, Watseka, IL, p. A195
Chief Executive Officer, Sharp Memorial Hospital, San Diego, CA, p. A86
SMITH, Todd A., Chief Executive Officer, Aurora Charter Oak Hospital, Covina, CA, p. A58
SMITH, Tommy J., President and Chief Executive Officer, Baptist Healthcare System, Louisville, KY, p. B18
SMITH, Tracy, Director Human Resources, Mercy St. Francis Hospital, Mountain View, MO, p. A365
SMITH, Trevor, Chief Management Information Services, Gunnison Valley Hospital, Gunnison, CO, p. A102
SMITH, Trueman, M.D. Chief Medical Officer, Livingston Regional Hospital, Livingston, TN, p. A570
SMITH, Tyson, M.D
Chief Medical Officer, MedWest – Haywood, Clyde, NC, p. A451
Vice President Medical Affairs, St. Mary's Medical Center, Huntington, WV, p. A673
SMITH, Vincent
Chief Information Officer, Elmhurst Hospital Center,, NY, p. A432
Chief Information Officer, Queens Hospital Center,, NY, p. A436
SMITH, W. Stuart, Executive Director and Vice President Clinical Operations, MUSC Medical Center of Medical University of South Carolina, Charleston, SC, p. A547
SMITH, Wayne, Interim President and Chief Executive Officer, Southeast Hospital, Cape Girardeau, MO, p. A357
SMITH, Wayne, President and Chief Executive Officer, SoutheastHEALTH, Cape Girardeau, MO, p. B120
SMITH, Wayne T., Chairman, President and Chief Executive Officer, Community Health Systems, Inc., Franklin, TN, p. B33
SMITH, Wendell, Chief Operating Officer, St. James Behavioral Health Hospital, Gonzales, LA, p. A267
SMITH, William R., Chief Executive Officer and Director Human Resources, Virginia Regional Medical Center, Virginia, MN, p. A341
SMITH, Windell, Chief Operating Officer, Mayo Clinic Health System in Waycross, Waycross, GA, p. A162
SMITH CALLIHAN, Nanette, Vice President Human Resources, New England Sinai Hospital and Rehabilitation Center, Stoughton, MA, p. A305
SMITH–HILL, Janet
Senior Vice President Human Resources, Forsyth Medical Center, Winston–Salem, NC, p. A463
Senior Vice President Human Resources, Presbyterian Hospital, Charlotte, NC, p. A451
SMITH–NEVINS, Sharon, Executive Director, Metropolitan State Hospital, Norwalk, CA, p. A77
SMITHERS, John, Network Specialist, River Hospital, Alexandria Bay, NY, p. A420
SMITHHART, Paula, Director Human Resources, Coryell Memorial Hospital, Gatesville, TX, p. A601
SMITHMIER, Kenneth L., President and Chief Executive Officer, Decatur Memorial Hospital, Decatur, IL, p. A179
SMOCK, Tait, Manager Information Systems, Pella Regional Health Center, Pella, IA, p. A225
SMOCYNSKI, Nancy, Director Payroll, Personnel and Human Resources, Kindred Hospital–Pittsburgh, Oakdale, PA, p. A531
SMOKER, Bret, M.D. Clinical Director, PHS Santa Fe Indian Hospital, Santa Fe, NM, p. A418
SMOLEN, John F., FACHE President and Chief Executive Officer, Western Missouri Medical Center, Warrensburg, MO, p. A372
SMOLIK, Anton, M.D. Chief of Medical Staff, Harlan County Health System, Alma, NE, p. A381
SMOLIK, James Christian, Chief Executive Officer, Riverton Memorial Hospital, Riverton, WY, p. A697
SMOOT, Brannon, M.D. Medical Director, Austin Surgical Hospital, Austin, TX, p. A580
SMOOT, Steve, Administrator, Utah Valley Regional Medical Center, Provo, UT, p. A640
SMOOT, Todd, Chief Information Officer, Jefferson Memorial Hospital, Ranson, WV, p. A675
SMOTHERS, Carol, M.D. Chief of Staff, Pointe Coupee General Hospital, New Roads, LA, p. A275
SMOTHERS, Kevin, M.D. Senior Vice President Medical Affairs and Chief Medical and Quality Officer, Carroll Hospital Center, Westminster, MD, p. A294
SMOTHERS, Margaret Shawn, Administrator, Kenmare Community Hospital, Kenmare, ND, p. A467
SMOTHERS, Mark, M.D. Chief Medical Staff, Holmes County Hospital and Clinics, Lexington, MS, p. A349
SNAPP, III, William R.
Vice President and Chief Financial Officer, Ephraim McDowell Fort Logan Hospital, Stanford, KY, p. A259
Vice President Finance and Chief Financial Officer, Ephraim McDowell Regional Medical Center, Danville, KY, p. A249
SNAVELY, Gretchen, Director Human Resources, Holton Community Hospital, Holton, KS, p. A234
SNEDEGAR, Michael, Chief Financial Officer, Bourbon Community Hospital, Paris, KY, p. A258
SNEDIGAR, Rudy C., Administrator and Chief Executive Officer, Barton County Memorial Hospital, Lamar, MO, p. A363
SNEED, Jim, Chief Financial Officer, Lauderdale Community Hospital, Ripley, TN, p. A575
SNELGROVE, Steven C., Chief Executive Officer, Wake Forest Baptist Health–Lexington Medical Center, Lexington, NC, p. A456
SNELL, Donald F., Executive Vice President and Chief Operating Officer, Lahey Clinic Hospital, Burlington, MA, p. A298
SNELL, Peggy, Chief Finance Officer, Cherry County Hospital, Valentine, NE, p. A390
SNELL, Steve, M.D. Chief of Staff, Southwestern Medical Center, Lawton, OK, p. A498
SNENK, Don, Chief Financial Officer, Mercy Fitzgerald Hospital, Darby, PA, p. A521
SNIDER, Charles, Vice President Human Resources, Oak Hill Hospital, Brooksville, FL, p. A120
SNIDER, George A., Vice President Human Resources, BryanLGH Medical Center, Lincoln, NE, p. A385
SNIDER, Glenn R., M.D. Chief of Staff, Louis A. Johnson Veterans Affairs Medical Center, Clarksburg, WV, p. A671
SNIDER, Tim, Senior Vice President and Chief Financial Officer, Upper Valley Medical Center, Troy, OH, p. A490
SNIDER, Timothy, Manager Information Systems, Fannin Regional Hospital, Blue Ridge, GA, p. A148
SNIDERMAN, Howard, Chief Operating Officer, Fairfield Medical Center, Lancaster, OH, p. A482
SNIFFEN, Michael J., FACHE President and Chief Executive Officer, St. Mary's Hospital, Passaic, NJ, p. A408
SNODGRASS, Liz, Chief Financial Officer, Trigg County Hospital, Cadiz, KY, p. A248
SNOOK, Joel, Chief Financial Officer, Arrowhead Hospital, Glendale, AZ, p. A32
SNOW, Brian, Manager Information Systems, Appling Healthcare System, Baxley, GA, p. A147
SNOW, Charlyn, Director Human Resources, Northwest Texas Healthcare System, Amarillo, TX, p. A578
SNOW, David, Area Information Officer, Woodland Hills Medical Center,, CA, p. A73
SNOW, Dorothy, M.D. Chief of Staff, Veterans Affairs Maryland Health Care System–Baltimore Division, Baltimore, MD, p. A289
SNOW, Meldon L., Chief Executive Officer, Murray County Medical Center, Slayton, MN, p. A340
SNOWDEN, Raymond W., President and Chief Executive Officer, Memorial Hospital and Health Care Center, Jasper, IN, p. A205
SNYDER, Alice, Vice President, Chief Nursing Officer, OSF St. Mary Medical Center, Galesburg, IL, p. A182
SNYDER, Dallas, Chief Financial Officer, Springfield Hospital Center, Sykesville, MD, p. A294
SNYDER, Daniel J., Chief Executive Officer, University of Miami Hospital, Miami, FL, p. A132
SNYDER, David, M.D. Chief of Staff, DeKalb Medical at Downtown Decatur, Decatur, GA, p. A151
SNYDER, David, Chief Information Officer and Vice President Information Technology, Ellis Hospital, Schenectady, NY, p. A443
SNYDER, Jeffrey, Chief Executive Officer, Mercy Suburban Hospital, Norristown, PA, p. A530
SNYDER, John, Executive Vice President and Chief Operating Officer, Carle Foundation Hospital, Urbana, IL, p. A195
SNYDER, Kristy, Director Human Resources, Fulton County Health Center, Wauseon, OH, p. A491
SNYDER, Marilyn, Chief Information Officer, Liberty Medical Center, Chester, MT, p. A374
SNYDER, Marjorie, M.D. Clinical Director, Dorothea Dix Psychiatric Center, Bangor, ME, p. A281
SNYDER, Mary E., Chief Operations Officer, Montrose Memorial Hospital, Montrose, CO, p. A104
SNYDER, Norman, M.D. Medical Director, Vista Health, Fayetteville, AR, p. A44
SNYDER, R. Brad, Chief Operating Officer, Torrance State Hospital, Torrance, PA, p. A539
SNYDER, Renae, Chief Financial Officer, Sakakawea Medical Center, Hazen, ND, p. A466
SNYDER Jr., Robert E., President, Orlando Regional South Seminole Hospital, Longwood, FL, p. A129
SNYDER, Ron, Chief Financial Officer, Hardin Memorial Hospital, Kenton, OH, p. A482
SNYDER, Steven, Vice President Human Resources, Franciscan Hospital for Children, Boston, MA, p. A296
SNYDER, Tony, Administrator and Chief Executive Officer, Pomerene Hospital, Millersburg, OH, p. A485
SNYDER, Vicky, Chief Operating Officer and Chief Financial Officer, Medina Hospital, Medina, OH, p. A484
SNYDER, Wendy
Director Finance, University Hospitals Conneaut Medical Center, Conneaut, OH, p. A478
Director Finance, University Hospitals Geneva Medical Center, Geneva, OH, p. A481
SOARES, Denise C., R.N. Executive Director, Harlem Hospital Center, New York, NY, p. A432
SOARES, Jair C., M.D. Executive Director, University of Texas Harris County Psychiatric Center, Houston, TX, p. A607
SOBECK, Brenda, Director of Human Resources, Jones Memorial Hospital, Wellsville, NY, p. A446
SOBIECK, Bridget, Director of Nursing, Cook County North Shore Hospital, Grand Marais, MN, p. A332
SOCHA, Jake, Chief Executive Officer, Kindred Hospital Park View, Springfield, MA, p. A304
SODERHOLM, Jon, President, Avera Heart Hospital of South Dakota, Sioux Falls, SD, p. A559
SOEKORO, Julie, Chief Financial Officer, Trinity Medical Center, Birmingham, AL, p. A17
SOHN, Steven, M.D. President Medical Staff, Dallas County Hospital, Perry, IA, p. A225
SOILEAU, D. Kirk, Chief Executive Officer, Oakdale Community Hospital, Oakdale, LA, p. A275
SOK, James E., FACH
President and Chief Executive Officer, Sheltering Arms Hospital South, Midlothian, VA, p. A651
President and Chief Executive Officer, Sheltering Arms Rehabilitation Hospital, Mechanicsville, VA, p. A651
SOKOLA, Thomas P., Chief Administrative Officer, Geisinger Medical Center, Danville, PA, p. A521
SOKOLOW, Norman J., Chairman and Chief Executive Officer, Cornerstone of Medical Arts Center Hospital, Fresh Meadows, NY, p. A426
SOKOLOWSKI, Magdalena, R.N. Director of Nursing, St. Lawrence Rehabilitation Center, Lawrenceville, NJ, p. A405
SOKUNBI, Dolamu, M.D. Chief of Staff, Nacogdoches Medical Center, Nacogdoches, TX, p. A618
SOLAIMAN, Shereen, Vice President Human Resources, Riverside Methodist Hospital, Columbus, OH, p. A477
SOLAZZO, Mark J.
Senior Vice President and Chief Operating Officer, Forest Hills Hospital,, NY, p. A432
Executive Vice President and Chief Operating Officer, Franklin Hospital, Valley Stream, NY, p. A445
Regional Chief Operating Officer, Syosset Hospital, Syosset, NY, p. A444
SOLBERG, Bradley, FACHE Chief Executive Officer, Hammond–Henry Hospital, Geneseo, IL, p. A182
SOLDATIS, Jeffrey J., M.D. Chairman Medical Executive Committee, Indiana Orthopaedic Hospital, Indianapolis, IN, p. A204
SOLDO, Stephen, M.D. Chief Medical Officer, Saint Agnes Medical Center, Fresno, CA, p. A62
SOLEM, Terry S., System Vice President Human Resources, Provena Saint Joseph Medical Center, Joliet, IL, p. A185

A936 Index of Health Care Professionals

Index of Health Care Professionals / Spears


SOLER, Eddie, Chief Financial Officer, Florida Hospital, Orlando, FL, p. A134
SOLHEIM, John H., Chief Executive Officer, Cuyuna Regional Medical Center, Crosby, MN, p. A330
SOLIE, Carol M., M.D. Chief Medical Officer, Wyoming Medical Center, Casper, WY, p. A695
SOLIMAN, Russell
System Manager Client Services and Management Information Services, Provena Saint Joseph Medical Center, Joliet, IL, p. A185
Director Information Services, Provena St. Mary's Hospital, Kankakee, IL, p. A185
SOLIMON, Russ, Chief Information Officer, Adventist La Grange Memorial Hospital, La Grange, IL, p. A186
SOLIN, Andrea, Chief Financial Officer, Lovelace Rehabilitation Hospital, Albuquerque, NM, p. A414
SOLINSKI, Ruth, Vice President Organizational Development, Bell Hospital, Ishpeming, MI, p. A316
SOLIS, Gloria, R.N. Chief Operating Officer and Chief Nursing Officer, Saint Luke's East Hospital, Lee's Summit, MO, p. A364
SOLIVAN, Jose E.
Chief Financial Officer, Hospital Menonita De Cayey, Cayey, PR, p. A700
Chief Financial Officer, Mennonite General Hospital, Aibonito, PR, p. A699
SOLIVAN, Miguel A., Administrator, Hospital Oriente, Humacao, PR, p. A701
SOLLE, Craig E., President and Chief Executive Officer, Pike Community Hospital, Waverly, OH, p. A491
SOLLENBERGER, Donna K., Executive Vice President and Chief Executive Officer, University of Texas Medical Branch Hospitals, Galveston, TX, p. A600
SOLOMON, Elizabeth, R.N. Regional Quality/Risk Director and Interim Chief Nursing Officer, HEALTHSOUTH Rehabilitation Hospital–Las Vegas, Las Vegas, NV, p. A393
SOLOMON, John, M.D. Director, South Carolina Department of Corrections Hospital, Columbia, SC, p. A548
SOLOMON, Steven, Vice President Human Resources, Garden City Hospital, Garden City, MI, p. A313
SOLORZANO, Rosa, Interim Director Human Resources, Toppenish Community Hospital, Toppenish, WA, p. A668
SOLOW, Jodie, Director Human Resources, Chatham Hospital, Siler City, NC, p. A460
SOLVERSON, Paul, Interim Chief Information Officer, Centegra Hospital – Woodstock, Woodstock, IL, p. A196
SOMBAR, Jr., Michael J., Chief Financial Officer, Jefferson Hospital, Louisville, GA, p. A155
SOMERVILLE, Jacqueline G., R.N. Senior Vice President for Patient Care Services and Chief Nursing Officer, Brigham and Women's Hospital, Boston, MA, p. A296
SOMERVILLE, Susan, R.N. Executive Director, North Shore University Hospital, Manhasset, NY, p. A429
SOMISETTY, Sreedhar, M.D. Chief Medical Officer, Mahaska Health Partnership, Oskaloosa, IA, p. A225
SOMMERS, Belinda, Chief Information Officer, Lake Charles Memorial Hospital, Lake Charles, LA, p. A271
SOMMERS, Thomas W., FACHE President and Chief Executive Officer, Beatrice Community Hospital and Health Center, Beatrice, NE, p. A382
SONDERMAN, Betty, Manager Human Resources, Ridgeview Institute, Smyrna, GA, p. A159
SONDERMAN, Thomas, M.D. Vice President and Chief Medical Officer, Columbus Regional Hospital, Columbus, IN, p. A199
SONENREICH, Steven D., President and Chief Executive Officer, Mount Sinai Medical Center, Miami Beach, FL, p. A132
SONG, Daniel, Chief Financial Officer, Monterey Park Hospital, Monterey Park, CA, p. A75
SONGER, Lucille, Acting Chief Operating Officer, Athol Memorial Hospital, Athol, MA, p. A295
SONNENBERG, Martha, M.D. Chief of Staff, Brotman Medical Center, Culver City, CA, p. A59
SONNENBERG, Stephanie, Director Information Management Systems, ProMedica Defiance Regional Hospital, Defiance, OH, p. A479
SONNENBERG, William, M.D. President Medical Staff, Titusville Area Hospital, Titusville, PA, p. A539
SONNENSCHEIN, Silvia, M.D. Chief of Staff, Kohala Hospital, Kohala, HI, p. A165
SONS, Regina K., Administrative Director Human Resources and Volunteer Services Associate Ethics and Compliance Officer, Mineral Area Regional Medical Center, Farmington, MO, p. A359
SONTHEIMER, Dan, M.D. Vice President Medical Affairs, Lester E. Cox Medical Centers, Springfield, MO, p. A371
SOOD, Harish, M.D. Medical Director, Long Beach Medical Center, Long Beach, NY, p. A429
SOOHOO, Richard
Chief Financial Officer, Sutter Davis Hospital, Davis, CA, p. A59
Chief Financial Officer, Sutter Medical Center, Sacramento, Sacramento, CA, p. A84
SOPER, Brent, Chief Financial Officer, San Joaquin Community Hospital, Bakersfield, CA, p. A55
SOPER, Thomas, D.O. Medical Director, Sterling Regional MedCenter, Sterling, CO, p. A106
SOPKO, Jeffrey
West Region Director of HR, Kindred Hospital Northland, Kansas City, MO, p. A362
District Director Human Resources, Kindred Hospital–San Diego, San Diego, CA, p. A85
SOPT, Michael, M.D. Chief of Staff, Brooks County Hospital, Quitman, GA, p. A157
SORAN, Andrei, Chief Executive Officer, MetroWest Medical Center, Framingham, MA, p. A300
SORBELLO, Bud, Director Management Information Systems, Hudson Valley Hospital Center, Cortlandt Manor, NY, p. A424
SORENSEN, Todd, M.D. Chief Executive Officer, Regional West Medical Center, Scottsbluff, NE, p. A389
SORENSON Jr.,, Charles W., M.D. Chief Executive Officer, Intermountain Healthcare, Inc, Salt Lake City, UT, p. B72
SORENSON, Dennis, Supervisor Information Technology, South Haven Health System, South Haven, MI, p. A323
SORENSON, Ed, Vice President Finance and Chief Financial Officer, Community Hospital of San Bernardino, San Bernardino, CA, p. A84
SORENSON, Euretta, R.N. Chief Nursing Officer, New River Medical Center, Monticello, MN, p. A335
SORENSON, Shannon, Chief Executive Officer, Brown County Hospital, Ainsworth, NE, p. A381
SOREY, Sharon, R.N. Regional Administrator, Mercy Hospital Paris, Paris, AR, p. A50
SORIANO, Luis, M.D. Chief of Staff, Pocahontas Memorial Hospital, Buckeye, WV, p. A670
SORIANO, Miriam, M.D. Chief Medical Staff, Ashland Community Hospital, Ashland, OR, p. A509
SORRELL, Sr., Ralph W., Chief Financial Officer, Adena Greenfield Medical Center, Greenfield, OH, p. A481
SOSA–GUERRERO, Sandra, Chief Executive Officer, Larkin Community Hospital, South Miami, FL, p. A139
SOSENKO, Alexander, M.D. Chief of Staff, Silver Cross Hospital, New Lenox, IL, p. A189
SOSTMAN, Dirk, M.D. Executive Vice President, Chief Medical Officer and Chief Academic Officer, The Methodist Hospital, Houston, TX, p. A607
SOSTROM, Cynthia, Chief Information Officer, Veterans Affairs Medical Center, Sheridan, WY, p. A697
SOTERAKIS, Jack, M.D. Executive Vice President Medical Affairs, St. Francis Hospital, Roslyn, NY, p. A442
SOTO, Manuel Ramirez, M.D. Medical Director, Hospital Metropolitano Dr. Tito Mattei, Yauco, PR, p. A704
SOTOMAYOR, Eduardo, Director, Caribbean Medical Center, Fajardo, PR, p. A701
SOTOS, Steven, M.D. President Medical Staff, LifeCare Hospitals of Pittsburgh, Pittsburgh, PA, p. A534
SOTTILE, Frank, M.D. Interim Chief Executive Officer, Crittenton Hospital Medical Center, Rochester, MI, p. A321
SOUDERS, Stuart, Coordinator Human Resources, William S. Middleton Memorial Veterans Hospital, Madison, WI, p. A684
SOUKUP, Paul, Chief Financial Officer, St. Luke Community Hospital, Ronan, MT, p. A378
SOULE, Frederick L., Interim Chief Executive Officer, Yadkin Valley Community Hospital, Yadkinville, NC, p. A463
SOURBEER, Jay C., Commanding Officer, Naval Hospital, Twentynine Palms, CA, p. A93
SOUSA, Francine, Director Management Information Service, New England Sinai Hospital and Rehabilitation Center, Stoughton, MA, p. A305
SOUSLEY, Dennis, Vice President of Clinical Services, Fitzgibbon Hospital, Marshall, MO, p. A364
SOUTHARD, Suzanne, Director Finance, Community Hospital–Fairfax, Fairfax, MO, p. A359
SOUTHERS, Nancy J., Vice President and Chief Financial Officer, The HSC Pediatric Center, Washington, DC, p. A117
SOUTHWORTH, Barbara, R.N. Associate Director for Patient Care Services, Veterans Affairs Medical Center, Marion, IL, p. A187
SOUTHWORTH, Scott, M.D. Medical Director, South Davis Community Hospital, Bountiful, UT, p. A637
SOUZA, Al, Chief Executive Officer, Los Angeles Community Hospital, Los Angeles, CA, p. A70
SOUZA, Darlene, Vice President, St. Joseph Health Services of Rhode Island, North Providence, RI, p. A544
SOUZA, Greg, Vice President Human Resources, Lucile Salter Packard Children's Hospital at Stanford, Palo Alto, CA, p. A79
SOVETSKHY, Ed, Director Information Services, Portsmouth Regional Hospital, Portsmouth, NH, p. A400
SOWA, Phillip E., Chief Executive Officer, Saint Louis University Hospital, Saint Louis, MO, p. A369
SOWDER, Sam, Director Information Systems, Southwest General Hospital, San Antonio, TX, p. A626
SOWDERS, Dale, President and Chief Executive Officer, Holland Hospital, Holland, MI, p. A315
SOWELL, Ronald G.
Executive Vice President, Commonwealth Regional Specialty Hospital, Bowling Green, KY, p. A247
Executive Vice President, Medical Center at Bowling Green, Bowling Green, KY, p. A248
Executive Vice President, Medical Center at Franklin, Franklin, KY, p. A250
Chief Financial Officer, Medical Center at Scottsville, Scottsville, KY, p. A259
SOWERS, Kevin W., MSN, Chief Executive Officer, Duke University Hospital, Durham, NC, p. A452
SOWLE, Karolee M., FACHE Chief Executive Officer, Desert Regional Medical Center, Palm Springs, CA, p. A78
SPACKMAN, Jared, Chief Financial Officer, Davis Hospital and Medical Center, Layton, UT, p. A638
SPACONE, Alan, M.D. Chief Medical Officer, Tuba City Regional Health Care Corporation, Tuba City, AZ, p. A39
SPACONE, Celia, M.D. Director Operations, Buffalo Psychiatric Center, Buffalo, NY, p. A422
SPALDING, Marsha, M.D. Medical Director, Sunrise Canyon Hospital, Lubbock, TX, p. A614
SPANGLER, Elizabeth L., M.D
Vice President Medical Affairs and Chief Medical Officer, CAMC Teays Valley Hospital, Hurricane, WV, p. A673
Vice President Medical Affairs, Charleston Area Medical Center, Charleston, WV, p. A671
SPANGLER, Wendell J., M.D. Chief of Staff, Paulding County Hospital, Paulding, OH, p. A487
SPANN, Chuck, Chief Executive Officer, Northwest Medical Center, Winfield, AL, p. A27
SPANN, Debbie, Director Human Resources, Morehouse General Hospital, Bastrop, LA, p. A262
SPANN, Lori, Director Human Resources, Iberia Medical Center, New Iberia, LA, p. A274
SPANO, Dennis, M.D. Medical Director, Mayo Clinic Health System in Lake City, Lake City, MN, p. A333
SPANO, Jason, Manager Information Technology, Prowers Medical Center, Lamar, CO, p. A103
SPARACINO, Michael, M.D. Chief Medical Staff, River's Edge Hospital and Clinic, Saint Peter, MN, p. A339
SPARE, John, Accountant, Parsons State Hospital and Training Center, Parsons, KS, p. A241
SPARKMAN, Dena C., FACHE Community Chief Executive Officer, Whitesburg ARH Hospital, Whitesburg, KY, p. A259
SPARKMAN, Jill, Director Human Resources, Odessa Regional Medical Center, Odessa, TX, p. A619
SPARKS, Gary R., Administrator, CrossRidge Community Hospital, Wynne, AR, p. A52
SPARKS, Jason, Director, Human Resources, HEALTHSOUTH Rehabilitation Hospital at Drake, Cincinnati, OH, p. A473
SPARKS, Jennifer, Human Resources Generalist, Complex Care Hospital at Ridgelake, Sarasota, FL, p. A138
SPARKS, Richard G., President and Chief Executive Officer, Appalachian Regional Healthcare System, Boone, NC, p. B10
SPARLING, Nicki, Manager Human Resources, Major Hospital, Shelbyville, IN, p. A211
SPARPANA, Eileen, Director Finance, Dickinson County Healthcare System, Iron Mountain, MI, p. A315
SPARROW, Francis D., M.D. Medical Director, Philhaven, Mount Gretna, PA, p. A529
SPARTZ, Dale A., Vice President Human Resources, Stanford Hospital and Clinics, Palo Alto, CA, p. A79
SPARZO, John, M.D. Vice President Medical Affairs, Hendricks Regional Health, Danville, IN, p. A200
SPATH, Deborah, R.N. Associate Director Patient and Nurses Services, Albany Stratton Veterans Affairs Medical Center, Albany, NY, p. A420
SPAUDE, Paul A., FACHE President and Chief Executive Officer, Borgess Medical Center, Kalamazoo, MI, p. A316
SPEAR, James, Executive Vice President and Chief Financial Officer, Central DuPage Hospital, Winfield, IL, p. A196
SPEARE, Mark
Senior Associate Director Human Resources, Ronald Reagan University of California Los Angeles Medical Center, Los Angeles, CA, p. A71
Senior Associate Director Patient Relations and Human Resources, Santa Monica–UCLA Medical Center and Orthopaedic Hospital, Santa Monica, CA, p. A90
SPEARS, David, D.O. Chief of Staff, Selby General Hospital, Marietta, OH, p. A484
SPEARS, James, Chief Financial Officer, Harrison Memorial Hospital, Cynthiana, KY, p. A249
SPEARS, LaLana, Supervisor Accounting, Claremore Indian Hospital, Claremore, OK, p. A494


Index of Health Care Professionals

Index of Health Care Professionals

Index of Health Care Professionals / Spears

SPEARS, Michael, Vice President of Human Resources, St. Anthony Shawnee Hospital, Shawnee, OK, p. A504
SPEARS, Tim, D.O. Chief of Staff, Allen County Hospital, Iola, KS, p. A235
SPEASE, Dorothy, Manager Business Office, Douglas County Memorial Hospital, Armour, SD, p. A555
SPECK, Michelle A., Vice President Human Resources, UPMC Bedford Memorial, Everett, PA, p. A523
SPECKS, Gracie, MS, Director, Veterans Affairs Medical Center – Alexandria, Pineville, LA, p. A276
SPEECH, Thomas, M.D. Director, Winnebago Mental Health Institute, Winnebago, WI, p. A694
SPEES, Jonathan, Chief Financial Officer, Keck Hospital of USC, Los Angeles, CA, p. A70
SPEES, M. Shane, President and Chief Executive Officer, Baptist Health System, Birmingham, AL, p. B18
SPEIDEL, Francis X., M.D. Chief Executive Officer, St. Luke's Hospital at the Vintage, Houston, TX, p. A607
SPEIGHT, Becky, Chief Financial Officer, Bailey Medical Center, Owasso, OK, p. A502
SPEIGHT, Marianne, Vice President Information System and Chief Information Officer, Cincinnati Children's Hospital Medical Center, Cincinnati, OH, p. A473
SPEIGHTS, Rosetta, R.N. Chief Nursing Officer, Vista Medical Center West, Waukegan, IL, p. A196
SPEKTOR, Mark, M.D. President and Chief Executive Officer, Bayonne Medical Center, Bayonne, NJ, p. A401
SPELL, Dale, Chief Executive Officer, Appling Healthcare System, Baxley, GA, p. A147
SPELL, Kenneth R., Vice President Operations, Baptist Health South Florida, Homestead Hospital, Homestead, FL, p. A125
SPELLACY, Tara, Director Human Resources, Braintree Rehabilitation Hospital, Braintree, MA, p. A298
SPENCE, Monte, Chief Operating Officer, Rehabilitation Hospital of Indiana, Indianapolis, IN, p. A205
SPENCE, Terri
Chief Information Officer, Bon Secours Maryview Medical Center, Portsmouth, VA, p. A654
Vice President Information Services, Mary Immaculate Hospital, Newport News, VA, p. A652
SPENCE, William, Director, Roseland Community Hospital, Chicago, IL, p. A177
SPENCER, C. Dale, Chief Financial Officer, Community Hospital, Torrington, WY, p. A698
SPENCER, James, Chief Financial Officer, Mildred Mitchell–Bateman Hospital, Huntington, WV, p. A672
SPENCER, John, Director Human Resources, Alleghany Memorial Hospital, Sparta, NC, p. A461
SPENCER, Marianne, R.N. Vice President Operations and Chief Operating Officer, Edward Hospital, Naperville, IL, p. A189
SPENCER, Marie, Chief Nursing Officer and Senior Administrator, Burke Rehabilitation Hospital, White Plains, NY, p. A447
SPENCER, Mike, Chief Information Officer, Henry County Hospital, New Castle, IN, p. A209
SPENCER, Misti, Director Inpatient Services, Selby General Hospital, Marietta, OH, p. A484
SPENCER, Rachelle, Administrator, Kindred Hospital Arizona–Phoenix, Phoenix, AZ, p. A35
SPENCER, Richard, M.D. Clinical Director, Utah State Hospital, Provo, UT, p. A640
SPENCER, Susan, Chief Financial Officer, Samaritan Memorial Hospital, Macon, MO, p. A364
SPENCER, Todd, M.D. Chief Medical Staff, Adventist Medical Center–Reedley, Reedley, CA, p. A82
SPENCER, Tom, Chief Financial Officer, Kindred Hospital Tarrant County–Fort Worth Southwest, Fort Worth, TX, p. A599
SPENST, Brett, Vice President Finance and Operations, Kettering Medical Center, Kettering, OH, p. A482
SPERLING, Louis, Vice President Human Resources, Rhode Island Hospital, Providence, RI, p. A544
SPEZIA, Anthony, President and Chief Executive Officer, Covenant Health, Knoxville, TN, p. B39
SPICER, Ceina, R.N. Chief Operating Officer, Elba General Hospital, Elba, AL, p. A19
SPICER, John R., President and Chief Executive Officer, Mount Vernon Hospital, Mount Vernon, NY, p. A430
SPICER, John R., President and Chief Executive Officer, Sound Shore Health System, New Rochelle, NY, p. B120
SPICER, John R., President and Chief Executive Officer, Sound Shore Medical Center of Westchester, New Rochelle, NY, p. A431
SPICER, Michael J., President and Chief Executive Officer, St. Joseph's Medical Center, Yonkers, NY, p. A447
SPICER, Sam, M.D. Vice President Medical Affairs, New Hanover Regional Medical Center, Wilmington, NC, p. A462
SPIDLE, Tara, Controller, Decatur County Hospital, Leon, IA, p. A222
SPIEGEL, Kevin M., FACHE Chief Executive Officer, Methodist Healthcare Memphis Hospitals, Memphis, TN, p. A572
SPIER, Deborah, Administrator, Oceans Behavioral Hospital of Greater New Orleans, Kenner, LA, p. A269
SPIER, Scott A., M.D. Senior Vice President Medical Affairs, Mercy Medical Center, Baltimore, MD, p. A288
SPIGEL, Michael, Executive Vice President & Chief Operating Officer, Brooks Rehabilitation Hospital, Jacksonville, FL, p. A126
SPIKE, Colleen A., Chief Executive Officer, River's Edge Hospital and Clinic, Saint Peter, MN, p. A339
SPILLERS, David S., Chief Executive Officer, Huntsville Hospital, Huntsville, AL, p. A22
SPILLERS, David S., Chief Executive Officer, Huntsville Hospital Health System, Huntsville, AL, p. B69
SPINA, Lori, Vice President Human Resources, Good Samaritan Hospital Medical Center, West Islip, NY, p. A446
SPINHARNEY, Sarah, Senior Vice President, Baptist Health System, San Antonio, TX, p. A624
SPINOLO, Jorge, M.D. Chief of Staff, Henry Medical Center, Stockbridge, GA, p. A160
SPITULNIK, Aric, President and Chief Operating Officer, Levindale Hebrew Geriatric Center and Hospital, Baltimore, MD, p. A288
SPIVAK, Natalie, Director Information Services, Oaklawn Hospital, Marshall, MI, p. A318
SPIVEY, David A., President and Chief Executive Officer, St. Mary Mercy Hospital, Livonia, MI, p. A318
SPIVEY, Sue, Administrator, Irwin County Hospital, Ocilla, GA, p. A157
SPOELMAN, Roger
President and Chief Executive Officer, Mercy Health Partners, Hackley Campus, Muskegon, MI, p. A319
President and Chief Executive Officer, Mercy Health Partners, Mercy Campus, Muskegon, MI, p. A319
SPONG, Bernadette, Chief Financial Officer, Rex Healthcare, Raleigh, NC, p. A459
SPONSLER, Betsy A., Chief Financial Officer, Valley Hospital Medical Center, Las Vegas, NV, p. A394
SPOON, Barry, M.D. Chief of Staff, Mercy St. Francis Hospital, Mountain View, MO, p. A365
SPOONER, Allan M., Interim President and Chief Executive Officer, St. Rose Dominican Hospitals – Rose de Lima Campus, Henderson, NV, p. A392
SPOONER, Christopher, M.D. Chief of Staff, Southeast Arizona Medical Center, Douglas, AZ, p. A31
SPOONER, Jennifer, Controller, HEALTHSOUTH Rehabilitation Hospital of Tallahassee, Tallahassee, FL, p. A140
SPOONER, William T.
Senior Vice President and Chief Information Officer, Sharp Grossmont Hospital, La Mesa, CA, p. A66
Senior Vice President and Chief Information Officer, Sharp Memorial Hospital, San Diego, CA, p. A86
Senior Vice President Information Systems, Sharp Mesa Vista Hospital, San Diego, CA, p. A86
SPRADLIN, John, Information Systems Director, Franklin Foundation Hospital, Franklin, LA, p. A266
SPRAGG, Cherie, R.N. Senior Vice President Nursing Services, Fisher–Titus Medical Center, Norwalk, OH, p. A486
SPRAGGINS, Tommy, Director Information Services, Russell Medical Center, Alexander City, AL, p. A15
SPRAGUE, F. Remington, M.D
Chief Medical Officer, Mercy Health Partners, Hackley Campus, Muskegon, MI, p. A319
Chief Medical Officer, Mercy Health Partners, Mercy Campus, Muskegon, MI, p. A319
SPRAGUE, Sharon, Director Therapeutic Services, Dorothea Dix Psychiatric Center, Bangor, ME, p. A281
SPRATLING, Larry, M.D. Chief Medical Officer, Banner Baywood Medical Center, Mesa, AZ, p. A34
SPRAY, William R., Chief Executive Officer, Harton Regional Medical Center, Tullahoma, TN, p. A576
SPRIGGS, Larry, Controller, HEALTHSOUTH Rehabilitation Institute of San Antonio, San Antonio, TX, p. A625
SPRING, Jason A., FACHE Chief Executive Officer, North Valley Hospital, Whitefish, MT, p. A380
SPRINGATE, Brian, Chief Nursing Officer, Bourbon Community Hospital, Paris, KY, p. A258
SPRINGER, David, M.D. President Medical Staff, Sanford Medical Center Rock Rapids, Rock Rapids, IA, p. A225
SPRINGER, Madge, Director Human Resources, Florida Hospital Waterman, Tavares, FL, p. A141
SPRINGER, Theresa, Chief Financial Officer, OSF Holy Family Medical Center, Monmouth, IL, p. A188
SPRINGMANN, Tressa, Chief Information Officer, Greater Baltimore Medical Center, Baltimore, MD, p. A287
SPRINKLE, Joseph, Chief Information Officer, Doctor's Memorial Hospital, Perry, FL, p. A136
SPROUT, Merry, R.N. Chief Nursing Officer, Antelope Memorial Hospital, Neligh, NE, p. A386
SPROWL, Chris, M.D. Vice President, PeaceHealth St. Joseph Medical Center, Bellingham, WA, p. A659
SPRUIT, Jr., Jacob, Chief Financial Officer, South Fulton Medical Center, Atlanta, GA, p. A146
SPRUYT, James, Chief Executive Officer, Cumberland Hall Hospital, Hopkinsville, KY, p. A251
SPUHLER, Richard, Chief Executive Officer, Brigham City Community Hospital, Brigham City, UT, p. A637
SPURGEON, Karen, Chief Financial Officer, Lake Chelan Community Hospital, Chelan, WA, p. A660
SPURGEON, Sharon A., Chief Executive Officer, Coalinga Regional Medical Center, Coalinga, CA, p. A58
SPURLOCK, Shirley, Director Human Resources, Millwood Hospital, Arlington, TX, p. A579
SPYROW, Florence, President, Genesis Medical Center, Illini Campus, Silvis, IL, p. A193
SQUIRES, Danny, Vice President and Chief Financial Officer, Wake Forest Baptist Health–Lexington Medical Center, Lexington, NC, p. A456
SQUIRES, David, Senior Vice President, Cheyenne Regional Medical Center, Cheyenne, WY, p. A695
SQUIRES, Paula C., Senior Vice President Human Resources, Baystate Medical Center, Springfield, MA, p. A304
SREBINSKI, Ron, Chief Financial Officer, Caro Community Hospital, Caro, MI, p. A309
SREERAMA, Ravi K., M.D. Chief of Staff, East Texas Medical Center Clarksville, Clarksville, TX, p. A587
SRIBNICK, Wayne, M.D. Senior Vice President and Chief Medical Officer, Providence Hospital, Columbia, SC, p. A548
SRINIVASAN, Rajachandran, M.D. Medical Director, Porterville Developmental Center, Porterville, CA, p. A81
SRIPADA, Subra
Senior Vice President and Chief Information Officer, Beaumont Hospital – Royal Oak, Royal Oak, MI, p. A322
Senior Vice President and Chief Information Officer, Beaumont Hospital – Troy, Troy, MI, p. A324
Senior Vice President and Chief Information Officer, Beaumont Hospital Grosse Pointe, Grosse Pointe, MI, p. A314
SRIVASTAVA, Mohit, M.D. Chief of Staff, Bunkie General Hospital, Bunkie, LA, p. A264
SROCK, Timothy G., Vice President Human Resources, McLaren Flint, Flint, MI, p. A312
ST CLAIR, Jeffery M., President and Chief Executive Officer, Springhill Memorial Hospital, Mobile, AL, p. A23
ST GEORGE, Scott, Senior Vice President and Chief Financial Officer, St. Mary's Hospital, Troy, NY, p. A445
ST MARTIN, Lee Anne, Director Operations, Soldiers' Home in Holyoke, Holyoke, MA, p. A301
ST. AMANT, Tracy, Director Human Resources, Phoebe North, Albany, GA, p. A144
ST. CLAIR, Jeffery M., President and Chief Executive Officer, Springhill Memorial Hospital, Mobile, AL, p. A23
ST. GEORGE, George H., FACHE Chief Executive Officer, Screven County Hospital, Sylvania, GA, p. A160
ST. JOHN, Ryan, Assistant Administrator, Summers County ARH Hospital, Hinton, WV, p. A672
ST. JULIEN, Linda M., R.N. CNO/COO of Clinical, MetroSouth Medical Center, Blue Island, IL, p. A174
ST. LEGER, John, Chief Executive Officer, Select Specialty Hospital–McKeesport, McKeesport, PA, p. A528
ST. MARTIN, Andrew, M.D. Chief of Staff, River Parishes Hospital, La Place, LA, p. A269
STAAB, Mary, Director Finance, Cordova Community Medical Center, Cordova, AK, p. A28
STABILE, Barry, Chief Operating Officer, Springfield Hospital Center, Sykesville, MD, p. A294
STACEY, Brian
Chief Financial Officer, Elmhurst Hospital Center,, NY, p. A432
Chief Financial Officer, Queens Hospital Center,, NY, p. A436
STACEY, Rulon F., FACHE President and Chief Executive Officer, Poudre Valley Health System, Fort Collins, CO, p. B102
STACIE, Beverly, Director Human Resources, Clifton T. Perkins Hospital Center, Jessup, MD, p. A292
STACK, R. Timothy, FACHE President and Chief Executive Officer, Piedmont Healthcare, Atlanta, GA, p. B101
STACKHOUSE, Jenni, Chief Financial Officer, River Point Behavioral Health, Jacksonville, FL, p. A126
STACKHOUSE, Rebecca J., Associate Director, Wm. Jennings Bryan Dorn Veterans Affairs Medical Center, Columbia, SC, p. A549
STACKHOUSE, Sharon, Assistant Administrator and Director Risk Management, Peachford Behavioral Health System, Atlanta, GA, p. A145
STACY, James, Director Human Resources, Southwest Missouri Psychiatric Rehabilitation Center, El Dorado Springs, MO, p. A359
STADLER, James J., M.D. Associate Administrator Medical Services, Guam Memorial Hospital Authority, Tamuning, GU, p. A699

A938 Index of Health Care Professionals

Index of Health Care Professionals / Steele

Index of Health Care Professionals

STADLER, Thomas, M.D. Vice President Medical Affairs and Chief Medical Officer, Madonna Rehabilitation Hospital, Lincoln, NE, p. A385
STADNYK, Sheldon, M.D. Chief Medical Officer, North Colorado Medical Center, Greeley, CO, p. A102
STAFFORD, Cindy, Chief Executive Officer, Allegiance Specialty Hospital of Little Rock, Jacksonville, AR, p. A46
STAFFORD, Walt, Director Information Technology, Chatuge Regional Hospital and Nursing Home, Hiawassee, GA, p. A154
STAGG, Kevin, Executive Vice President Finance and Chief Financial Officer, Christian Health Care Center, Wyckoff, NJ, p. A412
STAGGS, Nathan, President and Chief Executive Officer, St. Mark's Medical Center, La Grange, TX, p. A611
STAGNER, Barbara, Director Human Resources, Palo Pinto General Hospital, Mineral Wells, TX, p. A617
STAHL, Anthony, Director Human Resources, Florida Hospital Heartland Medical Center, Sebring, FL, p. A139
STAHL, Daniel, M.D. Medical Director, Mayo Clinic Health System in Waseca, Waseca, MN, p. A341
STAHL, Daniel, D.O. Chief of Staff, Rush Memorial Hospital, Rushville, IN, p. A211
STAHL, Ronald, M.D. Chief Medical Officer, Crouse Hospital, Syracuse, NY, p. A444
STAHL, William D., Chief Operating Officer, Rooks County Health Center, Plainville, KS, p. A242
STAHLKUPPE, Robert F., M.D. Chief of Staff, Chatuge Regional Hospital and Nursing Home, Hiawassee, GA, p. A154
STAIGER, Tom, M.D. Medical Director, University of Washington Medical Center, Seattle, WA, p. A666
STALCUP, Connie, Manager Information Systems, Murphy Medical Center, Murphy, NC, p. A458
STALCUP, Linda, Chief Executive Officer, Stevens County Hospital, Hugoton, KS, p. A235
STALEY, John H., Ph.D. Senior Associate Director and Interim Chief Operating Officer, University of Iowa Hospitals and Clinics, Iowa City, IA, p. A221
STALKER, Neil, M.D. Chief of Staff, Dukes Memorial Hospital, Peru, IN, p. A210
STALL, Kristi, Chief Human Resources Officer, Mahnomen Health Center, Mahnomen, MN, p. A334
STALLINGS, Elizabeth, Chief Operating Officer, John Muir Behavioral Health Center, Concord, CA, p. A58
STALLWORTH, Monica, M.D. Chief of Staff, Western Maryland Hospital Center, Hagerstown, MD, p. A292
STALLWORTH, Terresa, M.D. Clinical Director, San Antonio State Hospital, San Antonio, TX, p. A626
STALNAKER, Avah, Chief Executive Officer, Stonewall Jackson Memorial Hospital, Weston, WV, p. A676
STAMAS, Peter, M.D. Vice President Medical Affairs, Saint Joseph's Hospital, Marshfield, WI, p. A685
STAMATERIS, Connie, M.D. Director Medical Services, Naval Hospital, Pensacola, FL, p. A136
STAMBAUGH, Lynn E., R.N. Chief Executive Officer, Sarah D. Culbertson Memorial Hospital, Rushville, IL, p. A193
STAMPER, Lana, Chief Executive Officer, Riverland Medical Center, Ferriday, LA, p. A266
STAMPOHAR, Jeffry, Chief Executive Officer, Deer River HealthCare Center, Deer River, MN, p. A330
STANCILL, Linda, Vice President and Chief Financial Officer, St. Joseph Health System, Tawas City, MI, p. A324
STANDEFFER, Luke, Administrator, Northport Medical Center, Northport, AL, p. A24
STANDER, Paul, M.D. Chief Medical Officer, Banner Good Samaritan Medical Center, Phoenix, AZ, p. A35
STANDISH, James F., Chief Financial Officer, Masonicare Health Center, Wallingford, CT, p. A112
STANDRIDGE, Debra K.
President, Wheaton Franciscan Healthcare – Elmbrook Memorial, Brookfield, WI, p. A679
President, Wheaton Franciscan Healthcare – St. Joseph's, Milwaukee, WI, p. A687
President, Wheaton Franciscan Healthcare – The Wisconsin Heart Hospital, Wauwatosa, WI, p. A693
STANEK, Janet, Executive Vice President, Stormont–Vail HealthCare, Topeka, KS, p. A244
STANFIELD, Alma, Director Human Resources, WellStar Cobb Hospital, Austell, GA, p. A147
STANFILL, Timothy, Chief Financial Officer, Summit Medical Center, Hermitage, TN, p. A566
STANFORD, Brian, Director Human Resources, Biloxi Regional Medical Center, Biloxi, MS, p. A343
STANGE KOLO, Tracey, Vice President Human Resources, UPMC St. Margaret, Pittsburgh, PA, p. A536
STANGL, Abbey, Chief Financial Officer, Manning Regional Healthcare Center, Manning, IA, p. A223
STANGL, William, Chief Executive Officer, Mountain View Regional Hospital, Casper, WY, p. A695
STANIC, Steve M.
Vice President and Chief Information Officer, Mississippi Baptist Medical Center, Jackson, MS, p. A348
Vice President and Chief Information Officer, Mississippi Hospital for Restorative Care, Jackson, MS, p. A348
STANLEY, Cassandra, Director Personnel, Eastern Shore Hospital Center, Cambridge, MD, p. A290
STANLEY, Ed
Director Information Systems, Barrow Regional Medical Center, Winder, GA, p. A162
Director Information Systems, Walton Regional Medical Center, Monroe, GA, p. A156
STANLEY, Jennifer, M.D. President Medical Staff, St. Vincent Jennings Hospital, North Vernon, IN, p. A210
STANLEY, John T.
Vice President Planning and Information Systems, Riverside Regional Medical Center, Newport News, VA, p. A652
Vice President Planning and Information Systems, Riverside Rehabilitation Institute, Newport News, VA, p. A652
STANLEY, Lynda, Senior Vice President and Chief Operating Officer, J. Arthur Dosher Memorial Hospital, Southport, NC, p. A461
STANLEY, Mark, Director Fiscal Services, Middle Tennessee Mental Health Institute, Nashville, TN, p. A573
STANLEY, Robert
Chief Financial Officer, llano Specialty Hospital of Lubbock, Lubbock, TX, p. A614
Chief Financial Officer, Texas Specialty Hospital at Lubbock, Lubbock, TX, p. A614
STANNARD, Mark, M.D. Chief of Staff, Hudson Hospital, Hudson, WI, p. A683
STANSEL, Robert, Vice President of Human Resources, Estes Park Medical Center, Estes Park, CO, p. A101
STANSKI, Vickie, Financial Analyst, Parkview LaGrange Hospital, LaGrange, IN, p. A207
STANTON, Lowell, Chief Financial Officer, Methodist Sugar Land Hospital, Sugar Land, TX, p. A629
STANTON, Melanie, R.N. Chief Nursing Officer, Sycamore Shoals Hospital, Elizabethton, TN, p. A565
STANTON, Mike, D.O. Medical Director, Baylor Medical Center at Trophy Club, Trophy Club, TX, p. A631
STANUSH, Chris, Director Information Management, San Antonio State Hospital, San Antonio, TX, p. A626
STAPLES, Deborah L., Chief Operating Officer, Pennsylvania Hospital, Philadelphia, PA, p. A533
STAPLES, Janet, Vice President Human Resources, South Central Regional Medical Center, Laurel, MS, p. A348
STAPLETON, Carla J., Director Human Resources, Paul B. Hall Regional Medical Center, Paintsville, KY, p. A257
STAPLETON, Michael, MS, President and Chief Executive Officer, F. F. Thompson Hospital, Canandaigua, NY, p. A423
STAPLETON, Robert, Director Administration, Richard H. Hutchings Psychiatric Center, Syracuse, NY, p. A444
STARA, Jeanne, R.N. Chief Nursing Officer, Ponca City Medical Center, Ponca City, OK, p. A503
STARBIRD, William, M.D. Chief of Staff, Marlette Regional Hospital, Marlette, MI, p. A318
STAREN, Edgar, M.D. Senior Vice President Medical Affairs, Midwestern Regional Medical Center, Zion, IL, p. A196
STARESINIC, Barbara, Director Human Resources, Hi–Desert Medical Center, Joshua Tree, CA, p. A65
STARK, Charles A., FACHE Chief Executive Officer, Columbus Regional Healthcare System, Columbus, GA, p. B32
STARK, David, Chief Financial Officer, Lancaster Rehabilitation Hospital, Lancaster, PA, p. A526
STARK, Donna, Director Human Resources, Baylor Regional Medical Center at Grapevine, Grapevine, TX, p. A601
STARK, Jared, Executive Director, Franciscan St. Francis Health – Mooresville, Mooresville, IN, p. A209
STARK, Patricia Ann, R.N. CNO, Florida Hospital DeLand, DeLand, FL, p. A122
STARK, Randy, Vice President Human Resources and Support Services, Cobleskill Regional Hospital, Cobleskill, NY, p. A424
STARK, Steve, Chief Information Officer, Cass County Memorial Hospital, Atlantic, IA, p. A214
STARKEBAUM, Gordon, M.D. Chief of Staff, Veterans Affairs Puget Sound Health Care System, Seattle, WA, p. A666
STARKES, Henry, M.D. Medical Director, Biggs–Gridley Memorial Hospital, Gridley, CA, p. A64
STARKEY, Shelly, Personnel Coordinator, Cook County North Shore Hospital, Grand Marais, MN, p. A332
STARLING, James F., M.D. Chief Medical Officer, Danville Regional Medical Center, Danville, VA, p. A647
STARLING, Mark, M.D. Chief Medical Officer, Banner Heart Hospital, Mesa, AZ, p. A34
STARLING, Susan, President and Chief Executive Officer, Marcum and Wallace Memorial Hospital, Irvine, KY, p. A252
STARMANN–HARRISON, Mary, FACHE President and Chief Executive Officer, Hospital Sisters Health System, Springfield, IL, p. B69
STARNES, Gregory D., Chief Executive Officer, Fayette County Hospital, Vandalia, IL, p. A195
STARNS, Mark, Administrator, Pinnacle Specialty Hospital, Tulsa, OK, p. A506
STARON, Willard, Chief Financial Officer, Crittenton Children's Center, Kansas City, MO, p. A361
STARR, Kay, Manager Human Resources, Vernon Memorial Healthcare, Viroqua, WI, p. A692
STARR, Linda, Director of Nursing, Horsham Clinic, Ambler, PA, p. A518
STASIK, Randall, President and Chief Executive Officer, Spectrum Health Gerber Memorial, Fremont, MI, p. A312
STASIKELIS, Peter J., M.D. Chief of Staff, Shriners Hospitals for Children, Greenville, Greenville, SC, p. A550
STASKIN, David
Director Human Resources, HEALTHSOUTH Rehabilitation Hospital of Mechanicsburg, Mechanicsburg, PA, p. A529
Director Human Resources, LifeCare Hospitals of Mechanicsburg, Mechanicsburg, PA, p. A529
STASTNY, Eric, Vice President Human Resources, Emerson Hospital, Concord, MA, p. A299
STASTNY, Mark
Vice President Information Technology, Laureate Psychiatric Clinic and Hospital, Tulsa, OK, p. A506
Vice President Information Technology, Saint Francis Hospital, Tulsa, OK, p. A506
STATA, Stephen C., Interim Chief Technology Officer, Northwestern Medical Center, Saint Albans, VT, p. A644
STATEN, Gary L., Chief Executive Officer, Trace Regional Hospital, Houston, MS, p. A347
STATEN, James, Senior Vice President Finance, Yale–New Haven Hospital, New Haven, CT, p. A111
STATES, Chuck, Director Information Systems, Punxsutawney Area Hospital, Punxsutawney, PA, p. A536
STATON, Donna, Chief Information Officer, Fauquier Hospital, Warrenton, VA, p. A657
STATON, Paul
Chief Financial Officer, Ronald Reagan University of California Los Angeles Medical Center, Los Angeles, CA, p. A71
Chief Financial Officer, Santa Monica–UCLA Medical Center and Orthopaedic Hospital, Santa Monica, CA, p. A90
STATUTO, Richard, President and Chief Executive Officer, Bon Secours Health System, Inc., Marriottsville, MD, p. B22
STATZ, Lila, M.D. Chief of Staff, Haxtun Hospital District, Haxtun, CO, p. A102
STAUFFER, Keith, Regional Chief Information Officer, Carrington Health Center, Carrington, ND, p. A464
STAUSS, Laura, Director of Human Resources, Huggins Hospital, Wolfeboro, NH, p. A400
STAZINSKI, Larry, Vice President Finance, Franciscan St. Anthony Health – Crown Point, Crown Point, IN, p. A200
STEAD, William, Associate Vice Chancellor for Health Affairs, Director Informatics Center and Chief Strategy and Information Officer, Vanderbilt Hospital and Clinics, Nashville, TN, p. A574
STEADHAM, Emily, Administrative Assistant Human Resources and Public Relations, Grove Hill Memorial Hospital, Grove Hill, AL, p. A21
STEADHAM, Mark B., President and Chief Executive Officer, Morris Hospital & Healthcare Centers, Morris, IL, p. A188
STEBBINS, Deborah E., FACHE Chief Executive Officer, Alameda Hospital, Alameda, CA, p. A53
STEBBINS, Michael, Director Organization and Talent Effectiveness, Mercy Hospital Cadillac, Cadillac, MI, p. A308
STEBBINS, Trish, Director Management Information Systems, Florida Hospital Fish Memorial, Orange City, FL, p. A134
STECKEL, Cindy, Vice President Chief Nurse and Operations Executive, Scripps Memorial Hospital–La Jolla, La Jolla, CA, p. A66
STECKER, Tim, Chief Financial Officer, Kindred Hospital–Denver, Denver, CO, p. A99
STECKLER, Michael J., President and Chief Executive Officer, Jennie M. Melham Memorial Medical Center, Broken Bow, NE, p. A382
STED, Charles A., Chief Executive Officer, Hawaii Pacific Health, Honolulu, HI, p. B57
STEED, Robert A., Director Information Systems, Capital Regional Medical Center, Tallahassee, FL, p. A140
STEELE, Chrys, Director Information Systems, Springs Memorial Hospital, Lancaster, SC, p. A552
STEELE, David, Vice President and Chief Information Officer, St. Francis Hospital, Columbus, GA, p. A149
STEELE Jr.,, Glenn, Ph.D. President and Chief Executive Officer, Geisinger Health System, Danville, PA, p. B54
STEELE, Mark, M.D
Chief Medical Officer, Truman Medical Center–Hospital Hill, Kansas City, MO, p. A363
Chief Medical Officer, Truman Medical Center–Lakewood, Kansas City, MO, p. A363

Index of Health Care Professionals

Index of Health Care Professionals / Steele

STEELE, Michael, M.D. Chief of Staff, Perry County Memorial Hospital, Perryville, MO, p. A366
STEELE, Terry L., Vice President Finance and Chief Financial Officer, Holland Hospital, Holland, MI, p. A315
STEELE, Tina, Chief Executive Officer and Chief Financial Officer, Fairfax Community Hospital, Fairfax, OK, p. A496
STEELMAN, Jeffrey, Director Information Systems, LewisGale Hospital Alleghany, Low Moor, VA, p. A650
STEENPORT, John, Director Information Technology, Portage Health, Hancock, MI, p. A314
STEEVENS, Alan, Director Information Management, St. Clare Hospital and Health Services, Baraboo, WI, p. A678
STEFANEK, Allen, Chief Financial Officer, Hollywood Presbyterian Medical Center, Los Angeles, CA, p. A69
STEFANOWICZ, Alex
Vice President Human Resources, USMD Hospital at Arlington, Arlington, TX, p. A580
Vice President Human Resources, USMD Hospital at Fort Worth, Fort Worth, TX, p. A599
STEFFEN, Elly, Chief Executive Officer and Administrator, Continuing Care Hospital at St. Luke's, Cedar Rapids, IA, p. A215
STEFFEN, Keith E., President and Chief Executive Officer, OSF Saint Francis Medical Center, Peoria, IL, p. A191
STEFFENS, Aaron, Chief Operating Officer, Mercy Hospital Oklahoma City, Oklahoma City, OK, p. A501
STEFKA, Darryl, Administrator, Cuero Community Hospital, Cuero, TX, p. A590
STEFL, William, Director Information Systems, Mercy Health Partners, Hackley Campus, Muskegon, MI, p. A319
STEFO, Andrew, Senior Vice President Finance and Chief Financial Officer, Ingalls Memorial Hospital, Harvey, IL, p. A183
STEFOVIC, John W., M.D. President Medical Staff, Saint Catherine Medical Center Fountain Springs, Ashland, PA, p. A518
STEGALL, Christopher A.
Regional Chief Financial Officer and Chief Operating Officer, Promise Hospital Baton Rouge, Baton Rouge, LA, p. A263
Regional Chief Financial Officer and Chief Operating Officer, Promise Hospital of Vicksburg, Vicksburg, MS, p. A353
STEGALL, Paula, R.N. Chief Nurse Executive, Anson Community Hospital, Wadesboro, NC, p. A462
STEGGE, Sherri, Director Human Resources, Vallejo Medical Center, Vallejo, CA, p. A94
STEICHEN, Barry L.
Executive Vice President, Chief Administrative Officer and Chief Financial Officer, Laureate Psychiatric Clinic and Hospital, Tulsa, OK, p. A506
Executive Vice President and Chief Financial Officer, Saint Francis Hospital, Tulsa, OK, p. A506
STEICHEN, Elizabeth, Human Resources, Lewis and Clark Specialty Hospital, Yankton, SD, p. A561
STEIDLE, Ernie, Chief Operating Officer, Woodrow Wilson Rehabilitation Center, Fishersville, VA, p. A648
STEIG, Nancy, Director Fiscal Services, Mayo Clinic Health System – Oakridge in Osseo, Osseo, WI, p. A689
STEIGER, Nancy, R.N. Chief Executive Officer and Chief Mission Officer, PeaceHealth St. Joseph Medical Center, Bellingham, WA, p. A659
STEIGMAN, Don S., Chief Operating Officer, Jackson Health System, Miami, FL, p. A131
STEIGMEYER, Robert P., President and Chief Executive Officer, Geisinger–Community Medical Center, Scranton, PA, p. A537
STEIMEL, Ronald, Vice President Administration and Chief Operating Officer, Mercy Medical Center, Rockville Centre, NY, p. A442
STEIN, Eric H., FACHE President and Chief Executive Officer, Cobleskill Regional Hospital, Cobleskill, NY, p. A424
STEIN, Keith L., M.D
Senior Vice President Medical Affairs and Chief Medical Officer, Baptist Medical Center, Jacksonville, FL, p. A126
Chief Medical Officer, Baptist Medical Center Beaches, Jacksonville Beach, FL, p. A127
STEIN, Patrick, M.D. Clinical Director, Western New York Children's Psychiatric Center, West Seneca, NY, p. A446
STEIN, Richard, M.D. Chief of Staff, Bay Area Medical Center, Marinette, WI, p. A685
STEIN, Robert, M.D. Vice President Medical Management, Advocate Christ Medical Center, Oak Lawn, IL, p. A189
STEIN, Robert, Chief Executive Officer, Kindred Hospital–Houston, Houston, TX, p. A605
STEIN, Sandra, Chief Human Resources Management, Veterans Affairs Central California Health Care System, Fresno, CA, p. A62
STEIN, Sheldon J., President and Chief Executive Officer, Mt. Washington Pediatric Hospital, Baltimore, MD, p. A288
STEINBERG, Dina, Chief People Resources Officer, Banner Estrella Medical Center, Phoenix, AZ, p. A35
STEINBERG, James P., M.D. Chief Medical Officer, Emory University Hospital Midtown, Atlanta, GA, p. A145
STEINBERG, Jeffrey, M.D. Chief Executive Officer, Louis A. Weiss Memorial Hospital, Chicago, IL, p. A176
STEINBERG, Marc E., Vice President Community Relations and Physician Recruitment, Passavant Area Hospital, Jacksonville, IL, p. A185
STEINBLOCK, Matthew, Systems Administrator, Community Memorial Hospital, Syracuse, NE, p. A390
STEINER, Dana, R.N. Executive Director of Nursing Services, Lexington Regional Health Center, Lexington, NE, p. A385
STEINER, Garith W., Chief Executive Officer and Administrator, Vernon Memorial Healthcare, Viroqua, WI, p. A692
STEINER, J. Scott, Chief Operating Officer, MacNeal Hospital, Berwyn, IL, p. A173
STEINER, Jeffrey T., Vice President Finance, Memorial Hospital at Gulfport, Gulfport, MS, p. A346
STEINER, Julie, Manager Marketing and Public Relations, Vernon Memorial Healthcare, Viroqua, WI, p. A692
STEINER, Thomas, Chief Operating Officer, Beebe Medical Center, Lewes, DE, p. A114
STEINES, Jeanne, D.O. Medical Director, Connecticut Mental Health Center, New Haven, CT, p. A110
STEINGALL, Patricia, R.N. Vice President, Patient Care Services, Hunterdon Medical Center, Flemington, NJ, p. A404
STEINHART, Curt, M.D. Chief Medical Officer, OU Medical Center, Oklahoma City, OK, p. A502
STEINKIRCHNER, Jim, Regional Controller, HEALTHSOUTH Rehabilitation Hospital, Sewickley, PA, p. A538
STEINKRUGER, Roger W., Chief Executive Officer, Tri Valley Health System, Cambridge, NE, p. A382
STEINKUHLER, Diane, Administrative Assistant Human Resources, I–70 Community Hospital, Sweet Springs, MO, p. A371
STEINLE, Carrie, Chief Human Resources, South Texas Regional Medical Center, Jourdanton, TX, p. A609
STEINMANN, David
VP/COO, Mercy Hospital Aurora, Aurora, MO, p. A355
Chief Operating Officer, Mercy Hospital Cassville, Cassville, MO, p. A357
STEINMANN, Robin, Administrative Director Human Resources, Anderson Hospital, Maryville, IL, p. A187
STEITZ, David P., Interim Chief Executive Officer, Mineral Area Regional Medical Center, Farmington, MO, p. A359
STELIGA, Kymm, Human Resources Specialist, Belmont Center for Comprehensive Treatment, Philadelphia, PA, p. A531
STELL, G. Max, M.D. Medical Director, Minden Medical Center, Minden, LA, p. A273
STELLING, Jonathan, M.D. Chief Medical Officer, St. Mary's Community Hospital, Nebraska City, NE, p. A386
STELLY, Donna, Human Resources Coordinator, Kindred Hospital Lafayette, Lafayette, LA, p. A270
STELTENPOHL, Robert, Controller, Southern Indiana Rehabilitation Hospital, New Albany, IN, p. A209
STELTER, Carolyn, M.D. Chief of Staff, Minnesota Valley Health Center, Le Sueur, MN, p. A333
STELZER, Jason, Director Human Resources, St. Clare Hospital and Health Services, Baraboo, WI, p. A678
STEMMERMAN, Jill, R.N. Vice President Nursing, Saint Anthony Hospital, Chicago, IL, p. A178
STENBERG Jr., Arnold T., Executive Vice President and Chief Administrative Officer, All Children's Hospital, Saint Petersburg, FL, p. A138
STENDEL–FREELS, Robin, Coordinator Human Resources, Specialty Hospital of Albuquerque, Albuquerque, NM, p. A415
STENERSON, David, Vice President Fiscal Services and Chief Financial Officer, OSF Saint Anthony Medical Center, Rockford, IL, p. A192
STENGER, Michael J., Interim President and Chief Executive Officer, Iroquois Memorial Hospital and Resident Home, Watseka, IL, p. A195
STENGER, Sandra, Acting Chief Human Resources, Veterans Affairs Medical Center, Cincinnati, OH, p. A474
STENSON, Richard, President and Chief Executive Officer, Tuality Healthcare, Hillsboro, OR, p. A511
STENSRUD, Kirk A., Chief Executive Officer, Glacial Ridge Health System, Glenwood, MN, p. A332
STEPANSKY, David, M.D. Chief Medical Officer, Phoenixville Hospital, Phoenixville, PA, p. A534
STEPHANY, Mark, Executive Director, Elmira Psychiatric Center, Elmira, NY, p. A426
STEPHENS, Bernard B., Chief Financial Officer, Bradford Health Services at Huntsville, Madison, AL, p. A22
STEPHENS, Billy E., Vice President Information Technology, Infirmary West, Mobile, AL, p. A22
STEPHENS, Carrie, Coordinator Information Systems, Saunders Medical Center, Wahoo, NE, p. A390
STEPHENS, Dana, Director Information Technology, St. Elizabeth's Hospital, Belleville, IL, p. A173
STEPHENS, Donita, Director Financial Services, Choctaw Health Center, Philadelphia, MS, p. A351
STEPHENS, Eddy, Vice President Information Technology, Mobile Infirmary Medical Center, Mobile, AL, p. A22
STEPHENS, Ellen, Vice President Information Services, Mercy Hospital Oklahoma City, Oklahoma City, OK, p. A501
STEPHENS, Larry
Chief Financial Officer, Collingsworth General Hospital, Wellington, TX, p. A634
Chief Financial Officer, Kimble Hospital, Junction, TX, p. A609
Chief Financial Officer, Schleicher County Medical Center, Eldorado, TX, p. A597
STEPHENS, Michael R.
President and Market Leader, Mercy Hospital Mount Airy, Cincinnati, OH, p. A473
President and Market Leader, Mercy Hospital Western Hills, Cincinnati, OH, p. A473
STEPHENS, Norman F., President and Chief Executive Officer, Portneuf Medical Center, Pocatello, ID, p. A170
STEPHENS, Peggy, M.D. Superintendent and Medical Director, Madison State Hospital, Madison, IN, p. A208
STEPHENS, Terry A., Chief Executive Officer, River Park Hospital, Huntington, WV, p. A672
STEPHENSON, Ben, M.D. Chief of Staff, Phillips County Hospital, Phillipsburg, KS, p. A241
STEPHENSON, Darlene, Vice President Operations, Mary Immaculate Hospital, Newport News, VA, p. A652
STEPHENSON, John, M.D. Chief of Staff, Mackinac Straits Health System, Saint Ignace, MI, p. A322
STEPHENSON, Melinda, Chief Executive Officer, Kingwood Medical Center, Kingwood, TX, p. A611
STEPHENSON, Penny, Chief Financial Officer, Ellinwood District Hospital, Ellinwood, KS, p. A232
STEPHENSON, Steve R., M.D. Executive Vice President and Chief Operating Officer, Iowa Methodist Medical Center, Des Moines, IA, p. A218
STEPP, Dana, Human Resources Officer, Marcum and Wallace Memorial Hospital, Irvine, KY, p. A252
STERBACH, Maureen, Vice President Human Resources, St. Joseph's Hospital and Medical Center, Phoenix, AZ, p. A36
STERLING, Jacci, R.N. Chief Nursing Executive, Sutter Maternity and Surgery Center of Santa Cruz, Santa Cruz, CA, p. A90
STERLING, Julie, Manager Information System, South Sunflower County Hospital, Indianola, MS, p. A347
STERLING, Michelle, R.N. Acting Chief Nursing Officer, Rancho Los Amigos National Rehabilitation Center, Downey, CA, p. A59
STERLING, Terrie, R.N. Chief Operating Officer, Our Lady of the Lake Regional Medical Center, Baton Rouge, LA, p. A262
STERMER, Susan, Director Finance, LifeCare Hospitals of Wisconsin, Pewaukee, WI, p. A689
STERN, Barry, Chief Financial Officer, Long Beach Medical Center, Long Beach, NY, p. A429
STERN, James, M.D. Senior Vice President Medical Staff, Kindred Hospital South Florida–Hollywood,, FL, p. A125
STERNBERG, Janet, President and Chief Executive Officer, Huron Medical Center, Bad Axe, MI, p. A307
STERNBERG, Paul, M.D. Professor and Chairman, Vanderbilt Hospital and Clinics, Nashville, TN, p. A574
STESNEY–RIDENOUR, Chris, Vice President Operations, Beaumont Hospital Grosse Pointe, Grosse Pointe, MI, p. A314
STETTHEIMER, Timothy
Vice President and Chief Information Officer, St. Vincent's Birmingham, Birmingham, AL, p. A17
Regional Chief Information Officer, St. Vincent's Blount, Oneonta, AL, p. A24
STEUSSY, William, Chief Financial Officer, Greene County Medical Center, Jefferson, IA, p. A222
STEUTER, Krista, Director Human Resources, Catalina Island Medical Center, Avalon, CA, p. A54
STEVEN, Eva, Chief Financial Officer, Roosevelt General Hospital, Portales, NM, p. A417
STEVENS, Ann Marie, Chief Executive Officer, Mid–Valley Hospital, Peckville, PA, p. A531
STEVENS, Berton, Director Information Systems, Memorial Medical Center, Las Cruces, NM, p. A416
STEVENS, Bryan N., Chief Financial Officer, Highland Community Hospital, Picayune, MS, p. A351
STEVENS, Chris E., Chief Information Officer, Billings Clinic, Billings, MT, p. A373
STEVENS, Diane L., MS Director Human Resources and Compliance Officer, Huntsville Memorial Hospital, Huntsville, TX, p. A608
STEVENS, Dori, Chief Nursing Officer, Sutter Delta Medical Center, Antioch, CA, p. A53
STEVENS, Emily, Chief Nursing Officer, Mat–Su Regional Medical Center, Palmer, AK, p. A30
STEVENS, George, Chief Financial Officer, University Medical Center, Las Vegas, NV, p. A394

A940 Index of Health Care Professionals

Index of Health Care Professionals / Stone

STEVENS, Janis, Director Human Resources, Raulerson Hospital, Okeechobee, FL, p. A134
STEVENS, Kelly, Manager Human Resources, St. Joseph Memorial Hospital, Murphysboro, IL, p. A188
STEVENS, Lianne, Vice President Information Technology, Nebraska Medical Center, Omaha, NE, p. A388
STEVENS, Lisa, Chief Clinical Officer and Chief Operating Officer, Northern California Rehabilitation Hospital, Redding, CA, p. A82
STEVENS, Rick, Chief Administrative Officer, St. Luke's Hospital, San Francisco, CA, p. A87
STEVENS, Robert, President and Chief Executive Officer, Ridgeview Medical Center, Waconia, MN, p. A341
STEVENS, Saundra J., Chief Executive Officer, Adams County Regional Medical Center, Seaman, OH, p. A488
STEVENS, Shelbourn, President, Brunswick Novant Medical Center, Bolivia, NC, p. A449
STEVENS, Susan, Director Human Resources, The HealthCenter, Kalispell, MT, p. A377
STEVENS, Tammy, Chief Operating Officer, Madison County Memorial Hospital, Madison, FL, p. A129
STEVENS, Tom, Director Personnel, Morehead Memorial Hospital, Eden, NC, p. A452
STEVENS, Velinda, President, Kalispell Regional Medical Center, Kalispell, MT, p. A377
STEVENSON, Angelia, Manager Finance, Veterans Affairs Medical Center, Tuscaloosa, AL, p. A26
STEVENSON, John, M.D. Senior Vice President and Chief Medical Officer, South Shore Hospital, South Weymouth, MA, p. A304
STEVENSON, Michael, Administrator, Murphy Medical Center, Murphy, NC, p. A458
STEVENSON, William, M.D. Chief of Staff, Fayette County Memorial Hospital, Washington Court House, OH, p. A490
STEVERSON, Denise, Director Human Resources, Dorminy Medical Center, Fitzgerald, GA, p. A152
STEVES, Sonja
Senior Vice President Human Resources and Marketing, Legacy Emanuel Hospital and Health Center, Portland, OR, p. A514
Vice President Marketing, Legacy Good Samaritan Hospital and Medical Center, Portland, OR, p. A514
Vice President Human Resources and Marketing, Legacy Meridian Park Hospital, Tualatin, OR, p. A516
Senior Vice President Human Resources, Legacy Mount Hood Medical Center, Gresham, OR, p. A511
Vice President Human Resources, Legacy Salmon Creek Medical Center, Vancouver, WA, p. A668
STEWARD, Rachel, Manager Human Resources, Bailey Medical Center, Owasso, OK, p. A502
STEWARD, Todd E., Chief Executive Officer, St. David's South Austin Medical Center, Austin, TX, p. A581
STEWART, Charles L., Chief Executive Officer, Poplar Bluff Regional Medical Center, Poplar Bluff, MO, p. A367
STEWART, Charles R., Vice President Business, Finance and Corporate Compliance, Southern Maryland Hospital Center, Clinton, MD, p. A290
STEWART, Christine R., FACHE Chief Executive Officer, Russellville Hospital, Russellville, AL, p. A25
STEWART, Clint, Vice President Finance/Business Operations, McDowell Hospital, Marion, NC, p. A457
STEWART, Craig, Chief Financial Officer, Gila Regional Medical Center, Silver City, NM, p. A418
STEWART, Daphne, Director Human Resources, Southeast Louisiana Hospital, Mandeville, LA, p. A272
STEWART, David K., Senior Vice President and Chief Financial Officer, Providence Hospital, Columbia, SC, p. A548
STEWART, Debbie, Human Resources Officer, Herington Municipal Hospital, Herington, KS, p. A234
STEWART, Dianne, Controller, Burke Medical Center, Waynesboro, GA, p. A162
STEWART, Evelyn G., Chief Executive Officer, El Paso LTAC Hospital, El Paso, TX, p. A596
STEWART, Hedda, Director Human Resources, Neshoba County General Hospital, Philadelphia, MS, p. A351
STEWART, Inez, Vice President, Children's Hospital Boston, Boston, MA, p. A296
STEWART, Jane, Director Information Services, J. F. K. Medical Center, Atlantis, FL, p. A118
STEWART, John, Director Finance, Burke Rehabilitation Hospital, White Plains, NY, p. A447
STEWART, Joseph A., President and Chief Executive Officer, Sierra View District Hospital, Porterville, CA, p. A81
STEWART, Kendall, M.D. Medical Director, Southern Ohio Medical Center, Portsmouth, OH, p. A487
STEWART, Marc, M.D. Vice President and Medical Director, Seattle Cancer Care Alliance, Seattle, WA, p. A666
STEWART, Marian, M.D. Chief of Staff, Jay Hospital, Jay, FL, p. A127
STEWART, Nova
Chief Information Officer, Chapman Medical Center, Orange, CA, p. A78
Chief Information Officer, Western Medical Center Anaheim, Anaheim, CA, p. A53
Chief Information Officer, Western Medical Center–Santa Ana, Santa Ana, CA, p. A89
STEWART, Patty, Chief Financial Officer, Memorial Hospital, Gonzales, TX, p. A601
STEWART, Paul, M.D. Medical Director, Kindred Hospital Las Vegas–Sahara, Las Vegas, NV, p. A393
STEWART, Paul R., President and Chief Executive Officer, Sky Lakes Medical Center, Klamath Falls, OR, p. A511
STEWART, Paula, M.D. Medical Director, HEALTHSOUTH Lakeshore Rehabilitation Hospital, Birmingham, AL, p. A16
STEWART, Ronnelle, Chief Human Resources Officer, Brookwood Medical Center, Birmingham, AL, p. A16
STEWART, Russell L., M.D. Chief Medical Officer, Braxton County Memorial Hospital, Gassaway, WV, p. A671
STEWART, Scott, M.D. Vice President Medical Management, Good Samaritan Medical Center, Brockton, MA, p. A298
STEWART, Scott, Manager Information Services, Rochelle Community Hospital, Rochelle, IL, p. A192
STEWART, Stephanie C., Executive Director, Human Resources, Saint Thomas Hospital, Nashville, TN, p. A573
STEWART, Steve, Director Information Technology, Henry County Health Center, Mount Pleasant, IA, p. A223
STEWART, Terry, Director Information Systems, Dauterive Hospital, New Iberia, LA, p. A274
STEWART, Tim, Chief Information Officer, Abbeville Area Medical Center, Abbeville, SC, p. A546
STICKLE, Edwin, M.D. Chief Medical Officer, United General Hospital, Sedro Woolley, WA, p. A666
STICKLER, Debra, Chief Information Officer, Veterans Affairs Medical Center, Lebanon, PA, p. A527
STIEB, Pamela, Chief Financial Officer, Sterling Regional MedCenter, Sterling, CO, p. A106
STIEGMANN, Greg, M.D. Vice President Clinical Affairs, University of Colorado Hospital, Aurora, CO, p. A97
STIEKES, Robert, Chief Financial Officer, Peace River Regional Medical Center, Port Charlotte, FL, p. A137
STIFF, Patrick, Coordinator Information Technology, Madison County Memorial Hospital, Madison, FL, p. A129
STIGLEMAN, Randy, President and Chief Executive Officer, Stewart–Webster Hospital, Richland, GA, p. A157
STIGLER, Barker, M.D. Chief of Staff, Burleson St. Joseph Health Center, Caldwell, TX, p. A586
STIGLER, Harold, Chief Executive Officer, Southwest Surgical Hospital, Hurst, TX, p. A608
STIGLIANESE, Amber, Manager Human Resources, Coalinga Regional Medical Center, Coalinga, CA, p. A58
STIKELEATHER, Janie, Director Marketing and Community Relations, Davis Regional Medical Center, Statesville, NC, p. A461
STILES, Suzanne, Chief Human Resources Officer & Sr. Vice President/Administrative and Support Services, Lakes Region General Hospital, Laconia, NH, p. A398
STILLER, Brian, Director, Veterans Affairs Medical Center, Togus, ME, p. A285
STILLMAN, Dennis, Interim Chief Financial Officer, Bartlett Regional Hospital, Juneau, AK, p. A29
STILLMAN, Elizabeth M., Acting Director, Colorado Mental Health Institute at Fort Logan, Denver, CO, p. A99
STILLMAN, Michelle, Director of Care Management, Asheville Specialty Hospital, Asheville, NC, p. A448
STILLO, Joseph, M.D. Medical Director, HEALTHSOUTH Rehabilitation Hospital of Toms River, Toms River, NJ, p. A411
STILLWORD, Joseph, Chief of Staff, Putnam Community Medical Center, Palatka, FL, p. A135
STILTNER, Wanda, Director Human Resources, Buchanan General Hospital, Grundy, VA, p. A649
STIMPSON, Jared, Chief Financial Officer, Evanston Regional Hospital, Evanston, WY, p. A696
STIMSON–RUSIN, Judi, Chief Financial Officer, Palm Beach Gardens Medical Center, Palm Beach Gardens, FL, p. A135
STINNETT, Ron, Chief Executive Officer, Los Angeles Metropolitan Medical Center, Los Angeles, CA, p. A70
STINSON, Katy, Director Information Services, Medical Center of Southeastern Oklahoma, Durant, OK, p. A495
STINSON, Martha, Director, Columbia Hospital, West Palm Beach, FL, p. A142
STIPE, Christopher R., FACHE Chief Executive Officer, Clarinda Regional Health Center, Clarinda, IA, p. A216
STIRE, David R., President and Chief Executive Officer, Jane Phillips Medical Center, Bartlesville, OK, p. A494
STIRLE, Roger, Business Manager, Mental Health Institute, Clarinda, IA, p. A216
STITZER, Philip, D.O. Chief Medical Officer, Moberly Regional Medical Center, Moberly, MO, p. A365
STOB, David, Chief Financial Officer, Kindred Hospital Seattle–Northgate, Seattle, WA, p. A665
STOBO, John D., M.D. Senior Vice President Health Sciences and Services, University of California–Systemwide Administration, Oakland, CA, p. B138
STOCK, Constance, M.D. Chief of Staff, Sturgis Regional Hospital, Sturgis, SD, p. A560
STOCK, Greg K., Chief Executive Officer, Thibodaux Regional Medical Center, Thibodaux, LA, p. A278
STOCK, Neil, Director Technology and Facilities, Mercy Regional Medical Center, Durango, CO, p. A100
STOCKHAUSEN, Christopher, Chief Financial Officer, UPMC McKeesport, McKeesport, PA, p. A528
STOCKLEY, Selena, Chief Operating Officer, Shadow Mountain Behavioral Health System, Tulsa, OK, p. A506
STOCKS, Alton, Commander, Walter Reed National Military Medical Center, Bethesda, MD, p. A290
STOCKSTILL, Mark, R.N. Administrator, Highland Community Hospital, Picayune, MS, p. A351
STOCKTON, Kevin, Chief Executive Officer, Northwest Medical Center, Tucson, AZ, p. A40
STOCKTON, Linda, Chief Financial Officer, Pasco Regional Medical Center, Dade City, FL, p. A121
STOCKTON, Rick
Chief Executive Officer, Promise Hospital of Bossier City, Bossier City, LA, p. A264
Chief Executive Officer, Promise Hospital of Louisiana – Shreveport Campus, Shreveport, LA, p. A277
STOCKWELL, David, Interim Director, Veterans Affairs Medical Center, Boise, ID, p. A167
STODDARD, Mark R., President, Central Valley Medical Center, Nephi, UT, p. A639
STODDARD, Mark R., President and Chairman, Rural Health Group, Nephi, UT, p. B110
STOECKELER, Joel, M.D. Chief of Staff, Baldwin Area Medical Center, Baldwin, WI, p. A678
STOECKMAN, Bill, Chief Information Officer, Spearfish Regional Surgery Center, Spearfish, SD, p. A560
STOEKE, Jason, Director Management Information Systems, Community Memorial Hospital, Cloquet, MN, p. A329
STOFFERSON, Laura, Director of Nursing, Ellsworth County Medical Center, Ellsworth, KS, p. A232
STOJAKOVICH, Edward R.
Chief Financial Officer, Dominion Hospital, Falls Church, VA, p. A647
Chief Financial Officer, Reston Hospital Center, Reston, VA, p. A654
STOKER, Rick, Director Management Information Systems, Horizon Medical Center, Dickson, TN, p. A565
STOKES, Elia, Chief Financial Officer, Plaza Medical Center of Fort Worth, Fort Worth, TX, p. A599
STOKES, Gary L., Chief Executive Officer, Nacogdoches Medical Center, Nacogdoches, TX, p. A618
STOKES, Priscilla, MS Vice President Patient Care and Chief Nursing Officer, St. Luke's Regional Medical Center, Sioux City, IA, p. A227
STOKES, Randell G., Administrator, LifeCare Hospitals of San Antonio, San Antonio, TX, p. A625
STOKES, Richard, CPA Chief Financial Officer, Clarendon Memorial Hospital, Manning, SC, p. A552
STOKES, Tina, Manager Human Resources, Regency Hospital of Florence, Florence, SC, p. A550
STOLBA, Robert J., Chief Financial Officer, Mason District Hospital, Havana, IL, p. A183
STOLDT, Garrick J., Vice President and Chief Financial Officer, Saint Peter's University Hospital, New Brunswick, NJ, p. A407
STOLLER, Theo, Director Human Resources, Jacobson Memorial Hospital Care Center, Elgin, ND, p. A465
STOLTZ, Kyla, Vice President Human Resources, Centerpoint Medical Center, Independence, MO, p. A360
STOLTZ, Lori, Chief Financial Officer, Benewah Community Hospital, Saint Maries, ID, p. A170
STOLTZFUS, William F., Interim Chief Financial Officer, Hendry Regional Medical Center, Clewiston, FL, p. A120
STOLYAR, Edward B., D.O. Director Management Information Systems, New York Community Hospital,, NY, p. A435
STOLZE, Jeffery
Vice President Human Resources, Trinity Bettendorf, Bettendorf, IA, p. A214
Vice President Human Resources, Trinity Rock Island, Rock Island, IL, p. A192
STOMBERG, LeAnn, Chief Financial Officer, Minneapolis Veterans Affairs Health Care System, Minneapolis, MN, p. A335
STOMP, Gregory, Chief Executive Officer, Cooperstown Medical Center, Cooperstown, ND, p. A465
STONE, Bud, Director Information Systems, Eastern State Hospital, Lexington, KY, p. A253
STONE, Dan, Community Chief Executive Officer, Harlan ARH Hospital, Harlan, KY, p. A251

Index of Health Care Professionals

Index of Health Care Professionals / Stone

STONE, Darlene, Senior Vice President Human Resources, The Villages Health System, The Villages, FL, p. A142
STONE, David, Director Information Systems, Titus Regional Medical Center, Mount Pleasant, TX, p. A617
STONE, Duncan, D.D.S. Chief Medical Staff, Mississippi State Hospital, Whitfield, MS, p. A354
STONE, Eric, Commander, U. S. Air Force Hospital, Hampton, VA, p. A649
STONE, Janice, Vice President Clinical Integration, Spectrum Health Gerber Memorial, Fremont, MI, p. A312
STONE, Jeanette, Vice President Operations, Baptist Health South Florida, South Miami Hospital, Miami, FL, p. A130
STONE, Jeff, Director Human Resources, Marshall Medical Center North, Guntersville, AL, p. A21
STONE, Joanna, Chief Nursing Officer, Livingston Hospital and Healthcare Services, Salem, KY, p. A258
STONE, John, Director Information Services and Chief Information Officer, Fairmont General Hospital, Fairmont, WV, p. A671
STONE, Michelle, D.O. Chief Medical Staff, Community Memorial Healthcare, Marysville, KS, p. A238
STONE, Richard, M.D. Medical Director, Metropolitan Hospital Center, New York, NY, p. A434
STONE, Ronald W., Regional Chief Human Resource Officer, Long Island Jewish Medical Center,, NY, p. A434
STONE, Susan, Director Human Resources, Claiborne County Hospital, Tazewell, TN, p. A576
STONE, Susan, R.N. Chief Nursing Officer and VP of Patient Care Services, Sharp Memorial Hospital, San Diego, CA, p. A86
STONE, Terry, Chief Financial Officer and Chief Information Officer, Willapa Harbor Hospital, South Bend, WA, p. A667
STONE, Thomas J., FACHE Chief Executive Officer, Monroe County Hospital, Monroeville, AL, p. A23
STONE, Timothy D., Executive Vice President and Chief Operating Officer, Decatur Memorial Hospital, Decatur, IL, p. A179
STONEBURG, John, Chief Information Officer, Tuality Healthcare, Hillsboro, OR, p. A511
STONEHOCKER, Lori, D.O. Chief Medical Staff, Dundy County Hospital, Benkelman, NE, p. A382
STONER, Courtney E., Director Marketing Operations, HEALTHSOUTH Rehabilitation Hospital of York, York, PA, p. A542
STONER, Donald, M.D. Chief Medical Officer, Halifax Health Medical Center of Daytona Beach, Daytona Beach, FL, p. A122
STONER, James, Chief Financial Officer, Lake Norman Regional Medical Center, Mooresville, NC, p. A457
STONER, Steve, Chief Information Officer, Richard L. Roudebush Veterans Affairs Medical Center, Indianapolis, IN, p. A205
STOOPS, Stephens, M.D
Chief Medical Officer, St. Joseph Medical Center, Kansas City, MO, p. A362
Chief Medical Officer, St. Mary's Medical Center, Blue Springs, MO, p. A355
STOPPER, Jim, Interim Chief Financial Officer, Evangelical Community Hospital, Lewisburg, PA, p. A527
STORCK, William H., Chief Financial Officer, Community Memorial Healthcare, Marysville, KS, p. A238
STORER, William, M.D. Medical Director, St. Vincent Heart Center of Indiana, Indianapolis, IN, p. A205
STOREY, Kam, Director Human Resources, Sebastian River Medical Center, Sebastian, FL, p. A139
STOREY, Kevin, Chief Executive Officer, Comanche County Medical Center, Comanche, TX, p. A588
STOREY, Paul, Chief Executive Officer, Greenbrier Valley Medical Center, Ronceverte, WV, p. A675
STORIALE, Paul D., Senior Vice President Finance and Chief Financial Officer, Robert Wood Johnson University Hospital, New Brunswick, NJ, p. A407
STORM, Dave, Director Business Support, St. Anthony's Memorial Hospital, Effingham, IL, p. A180
STORMANNS, Thomas, Chief Executive Officer, Wellstone Regional Hospital, Jeffersonville, IN, p. A205
STORMS, Bruce, M.D. Chief of Staff, Grady Memorial Hospital, Chickasha, OK, p. A494
STORR, Katie, Director Personnel, Mississippi State Hospital, Whitfield, MS, p. A354
STORTO, David E., President, Spaulding Rehabilitation Hospital, Boston, MA, p. A297
STORTZUM, Christopher, M.D. President Medical Staff, McDonough District Hospital, Macomb, IL, p. A186
STORY, Lawrence, Chief Executive Officer, Behavioral Hospital of Bellaire, Houston, TX, p. A603
STOTTLEMYRE, Georgan L., Director Human Resources, Northern Inyo Hospital, Bishop, CA, p. A56
STOUGH, Joe, Chief Operating Officer, Infirmary West, Mobile, AL, p. A22
STOUGH, Robin
Chief Financial Officer, Belmont Pines Hospital, Youngstown, OH, p. A492
Chief Financial Officer, Windsor–Laurelwood Center for Behavioral Medicine, Willoughby, OH, p. A491
STOUT, Bess, Director Human Resources, LaFollette Medical Center, La Follette, TN, p. A569
STOUT, Deana, Vice President Financial Services, Medstar Good Samaritan Hospital, Baltimore, MD, p. A288
STOUT, Don, Administrator, Fond Du Lac County Mental Health Center, Fond Du Lac, WI, p. A681
STOUT, Patsy, Director Personnel, Richland Parish Hospital, Delhi, LA, p. A265
STOUT, Sandy, Director Human Resources, Vista Health, Fayetteville, AR, p. A44
STOUT–TORRES, Sherri, Chief Nursing Officer, Watsonville Community Hospital, Watsonville, CA, p. A95
STOVALL, Richard G., Senior Vice President Fiscal Services and Chief Financial Officer, Southern Regional Medical Center, Riverdale, GA, p. A158
STOVALL, Susan M., Chief Executive Officer, Kindred Hospital Rome, Rome, GA, p. A158
STOVER, Angie, Administrative Assistant, Surgical Hospital of Jonesboro, Jonesboro, AR, p. A47
STOVER, Benny, Vice President Finance, Mercy Hospital Rogers, Rogers, AR, p. A50
STOVER, Christina, Chief Executive Officer, HEALTHSOUTH Rehabilitation Hospital of Northern Virginia, Aldie, VA, p. A645
STOVER, George M., Chief Executive Officer, Rice County District Hospital, Lyons, KS, p. A238
STOVER, Raymond
President, MidMichigan Medical Center–Clare, Clare, MI, p. A309
President and Chief Executive Officer, MidMichigan Medical Center–Gladwin, Gladwin, MI, p. A313
STOVER, Ryan, Chief Financial Officer, Norton County Hospital, Norton, KS, p. A239
STOVER, Thomas L., M.D. President and Chief Executive Officer, Akron General Health System, Akron, OH, p. B7
STOVERINK, Mike, Chief Financial Officer, Richland Memorial Hospital, Olney, IL, p. A190
STOWELL, Dana A., Chief Information Officer, McCurtain Memorial Hospital, Idabel, OK, p. A498
STOWMAN, Amber, Controller, Lisbon Area Health Services, Lisbon, ND, p. A467
STOY, Gale, Manager Information Systems, Mid Coast Hospital, Brunswick, ME, p. A282
STOY, Thomas, M.D. Chief of Staff, St. Gabriel's Hospital, Little Falls, MN, p. A333
STOYANOFF, Pamela, Executive Vice President and Chief Operating Officer, Methodist Dallas Medical Center, Dallas, TX, p. A592
STRABEL, Elizabeth, M.D. Chief Medical Staff, Divine Savior Healthcare, Portage, WI, p. A689
STRACHAN, Eileen, Coordinator Human Resources, Kindred Hospital–Sycamore, Sycamore, IL, p. A195
STRACHAN, Ronald
Chief Information Officer, WellStar Douglas Hospital, Douglasville, GA, p. A151
Senior Vice President and Chief Information Officer, WellStar Kennestone Hospital, Marietta, GA, p. A156
STRACK, Kirk, Vice President and Chief Financial Officer, Clark Memorial Hospital, Jeffersonville, IN, p. A205
STRADER, Lynn, Chief Financial Officer, CJW Medical Center, Richmond, VA, p. A654
STRAHAN, Greg, Chief Operating Officer, Owensboro Medical Health System, Owensboro, KY, p. A257
STRAIN, Donna, Director Human Resources, Ray County Memorial Hospital, Richmond, MO, p. A367
STRAND, Edward A., CPA Chief Financial Officer, Lake Region Healthcare Corporation, Fergus Falls, MN, p. A331
STRANGE, John, President and Chief Executive Officer, St. Luke's Hospital, Duluth, MN, p. A330
STRANGE, Roger, Chief Information Officer, St. Vincent Heart Center of Indiana, Indianapolis, IN, p. A205
STRASH, Shawn G., Chief Executive Officer, Paradise Valley Hospital, Phoenix, AZ, p. A36
STRASSNER III, Lawrence F., R.N. Vice President, Patient Care Services and Chief Nursing Officer, Medstar Franklin Square Medical Center, Baltimore, MD, p. A288
STRATTON, Doug, Chief Resource Management Division, Bassett Army Community Hospital, Fort Wainwright, AK, p. A29
STRATTON, Jim, Vice President Finance, Graham Hospital, Canton, IL, p. A174
STRATTON, Joe, Chief Executive Officer, Kit Carson County Memorial Hospital, Burlington, CO, p. A98
STRATTON, Mary, Director Human Resources, River Park Hospital, Huntington, WV, p. A672
STRAUGHAN, John, Director Information Technology, Wallowa Memorial Hospital, Enterprise, OR, p. A510
STRAUMANIS, John P., M.D. Vice President Medical Affairs and Chief Medical Officer, Kernan Orthopaedics and Rehabilitation, Baltimore, MD, p. A287
STRAUSBAUGH, Andy, Vice President Finance and Operations, Norton Brownsboro Hospital, Louisville, KY, p. A255
STRAUSS, Alan
Chief Financial Officer, Carondelet Holy Cross Hospital, Nogales, AZ, p. A34
Chief Financial Officer, Carondelet St. Joseph's Hospital, Tucson, AZ, p. A39
STRAUSS, Andrejs, M.D. Interim Vice President Medical Affairs, Beebe Medical Center, Lewes, DE, p. A114
STRAUSS, Thomas J., President and Chief Executive Officer, Summa Health System, Akron, OH, p. A469
STRAUSS, Thomas J., President and Chief Executive Officer, Summa Health System, Akron, OH, p. B124
STRAWN, Keith A., Vice President Human Resources, New Hanover Regional Medical Center, Wilmington, NC, p. A462
STRAWSER, Debbie A., Director Human Resources, Lindner Center of HOPE, Mason, OH, p. A484
STRAYER, Lorna, Senior Vice President Administration and Business Development, Fisher–Titus Medical Center, Norwalk, OH, p. A486
STRAYHAM, Joan, R.N. Interim Chief Executive Officer, Northwest Mississippi Regional Medical Center, Clarksdale, MS, p. A344
STRECK, William F., M.D. President and Chief Executive Officer, Bassett Healthcare Network, Cooperstown, NY, p. B19
STRECK, William F., M.D. President and Chief Executive Officer, Bassett Medical Center, Cooperstown, NY, p. A424
STRECKER, Dede, Chief Nursing Officer, White River Medical Center, Batesville, AR, p. A42
STRECKER, Kevin, President, Via Christi Hospital, Wichita, KS, p. A245
STREET, Rex, Senior Vice President and Chief Financial Officer, Alamance Regional Medical Center, Burlington, NC, p. A449
STREET, Scott, President and Chief Executive Officer, Mercy Hospital Rogers, Rogers, AR, p. A50
STREETER, Alan W., Chief Financial Officer, Mitchell County Regional Health Center, Osage, IA, p. A224
STREETER, Robert, M.D. Vice President Medical Affairs, Mercy Medical Center Merced, Merced, CA, p. A74
STREETT, David, M.D. Medical Director, Pinnacle Pointe Hospital, Little Rock, AR, p. A48
STREICH, Rebecca, Manager Human Resources and Education Manager, Hutchinson Area Health Care, Hutchinson, MN, p. A333
STRENGTH, Perry, Director Information Services, San Antonio Community Hospital, Upland, CA, p. A94
STREVY, Sonia R., Chief Nursing Officer, Wabash County Hospital, Wabash, IN, p. A213
STREYLE, Edward, MS Senior Vice President and Chief Nursing Officer, Maryland General Hospital, Baltimore, MD, p. A288
STRIBLEN, Becky, Director Human Resources, Moab Regional Hospital, Moab, UT, p. A638
STRICKER, Sean, Chief Executive Officer, Select Specialty Hospital–San Antonio, San Antonio, TX, p. A626
STRICKER, Steven, M.D. Physician in Chief, Vallejo Medical Center, Vallejo, CA, p. A94
STRICKLAND, Barrie, Chief Financial Officer, TIRR Memorial Hermann, Houston, TX, p. A607
STRICKLAND, Connie, Chief Executive Officer, Select Specialty Hospital–Oklahoma City, Oklahoma City, OK, p. A502
STRICKLAND, Gina, Administrative Assistant and Director Human Resources, Little River Memorial Hospital, Ashdown, AR, p. A42
STRICKLAND, Lee, Regional Director Information Technology, Park Ridge Health, Hendersonville, NC, p. A454
STRICKLAND, Morris S., Chief Financial Officer, Helen Keller Hospital, Sheffield, AL, p. A25
STRICKLAND, Samuel A., Chief Financial Officer, Red Bay Hospital, Red Bay, AL, p. A25
STRICKLAND, Wallace, President and Chief Executive Officer, Rush Health Systems, Meridian, MS, p. B110
STRICKLING, Keith, Chief Accountant, Jay Hospital, Jay, FL, p. A127
STRIEBY, John F., Chief Executive Officer, Nix Health Care System, San Antonio, TX, p. A625
STRING, Sherrie, Vice President Human Resources, Via Christi Hospitals Wichita, Wichita, KS, p. A245
STRITTMATTER, Brenda M., Patient Services Officer, Berger Health System, Circleville, OH, p. A474
STRITTMATTER, Julie, Director Human Resources, Baylor All Saints Medical Center at Fort Worth, Fort Worth, TX, p. A598
STROBEL, Jane, Interim Chief Financial Officer, Mercy Regional Medical Center, Durango, CO, p. A100
STROBEL, Rand, Vice President Information Technology, Valley Medical Center, Renton, WA, p. A664

A942 Index of Health Care Professionals

Index of Health Care Professionals / Sullivan

Index of Health Care Professionals

STRODE, Marc, Chief Executive Officer, Val Verde Regional Medical Center, Del Rio, TX, p. A593
STROEMEL, Douglas M.
President, Mercy Hospital Aurora, Aurora, MO, p. A355
President, Mercy Hospital Cassville, Cassville, MO, p. A357
STROHE, Tommy, Interim Chief Executive Officer, LTAC Hospital of Greenwood, Greenwood, MS, p. A346
STROHMYER, Jeffrey, M.D. Chief Medical Officer, Alegent Health–Midlands Hospital, Papillion, NE, p. A389
STROMBERG, Audrey, Administrator, Roosevelt Medical Center, Culbertson, MT, p. A374
STROMSTAD, Darlene, FACHE President and Chief Executive Officer, Waterbury Hospital, Waterbury, CT, p. A112
STRONG, David
Chief Financial Officer/Vice President Finance, Skaggs Regional Medical Center, Branson, MO, p. A356
Vice President and Chief Financial Officer, Southeast Hospital, Cape Girardeau, MO, p. A357
STRONG, David W., President, Rex Healthcare, Raleigh, NC, p. A459
STRONG, Douglas, Chief Executive Officer, University of Michigan Hospitals and Health Centers, Ann Arbor, MI, p. A307
STRONG, Tricia, Chief Financial Officer, Cumberland River Hospital, Celina, TN, p. A563
STROP, Judith, Director Finance, Rusk County Memorial Hospital and Nursing Home, Ladysmith, WI, p. A684
STROPLE, Kenneth, President and Chief Executive Officer, Downey Regional Medical Center, Downey, CA, p. A59
STROSNIDER, Preston, M.D. Vice President Medical Affairs, Conway Medical Center, Conway, SC, p. A549
STROSS, Daniel, Chief Information Officer, Genesys Regional Medical Center, Grand Blanc, MI, p. A313
STROUD, Teresa, Chief Financial Officer, Salem Township Hospital, Salem, IL, p. A193
STROUGH, Joe, Administrator, Mobile Infirmary Medical Center, Mobile, AL, p. A22
STROUSE, Thomas, M.D. Medical Director, Stewart & Lynda Resnick Neuropsychiatric Hospital at UCLA, Los Angeles, CA, p. A72
STRUBEL, Kim, Vice President, Edwin Shaw Rehab, Cuyahoga Falls, OH, p. A478
STRUCHTEMEYER, Glen E., Director, Central Alabama Veterans Health Care System, Montgomery, AL, p. A23
STRUCK, Tony, Chief Financial Officer, Yuma Regional Medical Center, Yuma, AZ, p. A41
STRUGATZ, Joshua, Associate Executive Director Operations, Glen Cove Hospital, Glen Cove, NY, p. A426
STRUMWASSER, Todd, M.D. Chief Executive, Swedish Medical Center–First Hill, Seattle, WA, p. A666
STRUYK, Douglas A., President and Chief Executive Officer, Christian Health Care Center, Wyckoff, NJ, p. A412
STRZEMPKO, Stanley, M.D. Vice President Medical Affairs and Chief Medical Officer, Noble Hospital, Westfield, MA, p. A306
STUART, Donald W., Associate Director, Albany Stratton Veterans Affairs Medical Center, Albany, NY, p. A420
STUART, Jimmy D.
Administrator, Riverview Regional Medical Center North, Carthage, TN, p. A562
Administrator, Riverview Regional Medical Center South, Carthage, TN, p. A563
STUART, Philip J., Administrator and Chief Executive Officer, Tomah Memorial Hospital, Tomah, WI, p. A692
STUART, Robin, Interim Administrator, Morrill County Community Hospital, Bridgeport, NE, p. A382
STUART, Sharon, R.N. Chief Executive Officer, Cornerstone Hospital of South Houston, Houston, TX, p. A603
STUBBLEFIELD, Greg
Vice President and Administrator, Baptist Health Medical Center–Arkadelphia, Arkadelphia, AR, p. A42
Vice President and Administrator, Baptist Health Medical Center–Little Rock, Little Rock, AR, p. A47
STUBBS, Don
Vice President Human Resources, Candler Hospital, Savannah, GA, p. A158
Vice President Human Resources, St. Joseph's Hospital, Savannah, GA, p. A159
STUBBS, Karen, Chief Nursing Officer, Northwest Medical Center, Tucson, AZ, p. A40
STUBBS, Richard, M.D. Vice President Medical Affairs, Casa Grande Regional Medical Center, Casa Grande, AZ, p. A31
STUBER, Joseph A., President and Chief Executive Officer, Perry County Memorial Hospital, Tell City, IN, p. A212
STUCK, Julie, R.N. Vice President Patient Services, Hocking Valley Community Hospital, Logan, OH, p. A483
STUCKY, Nancy, Director Human Resources and Public Relations, Ninnescah Valley Health System, Kingman, KS, p. A236
STUCZYNSKI, Joseph, Assistant Administrator Finance and Support, Memorial Hospital Pembroke, Pembroke Pines, FL, p. A135
STUDEBAKER, Shelly, Director Management Information Systems, Clinch Memorial Hospital, Homerville, GA, p. A154
STUDLEY, Brett, M.D. Chief of Staff, Beatrice Community Hospital and Health Center, Beatrice, NE, p. A382
STUENKEL, Kurt, FACHE President and Chief Executive Officer, Floyd Medical Center, Rome, GA, p. A158
STUERSEL, Marie, Director Human Resources, Seneca Healthcare District, Chester, CA, p. A57
STUEVE, Jo W., Co–Chief Operating Officer, Children's Mercy Hospitals and Clinics, Kansas City, MO, p. A361
STULL, Regenia, R.N. Chief Nurse Executive, Phelps County Regional Medical Center, Rolla, MO, p. A367
STULTS, Kim, Director Education, Bellevue Hospital, Bellevue, OH, p. A470
STULTZ, James R.
Senior Vice President Human Resources, East Ohio Regional Hospital, Martins Ferry, OH, p. A484
Senior Vice President Human Resources, Ohio Valley Medical Center, Wheeling, WV, p. A676
STUMBAUGH, Terri, R.N. Director Patient Care Services, Johnson Regional Medical Center, Clarksville, AR, p. A43
STUMBO, Kathy, President, Saint Joseph – Martin, Martin, KY, p. A256
STUMP, Jerry, Chief Financial Officer, Good Samaritan Hospital, Vincennes, IN, p. A212
STUMPF, Robert, M.D. President Medical Staff, Columbia Center, Mequon, WI, p. A686
STUMPO, Barbara J., R.N. Vice President Patient Care Services, Griffin Hospital, Derby, CT, p. A108
STURANS, Joanne, Vice President Human Resources, Phelps Memorial Hospital Center, Sleepy Hollow, NY, p. A443
STURGEON, Jim, Area Director Human Resources, Kindred Hospital Las Vegas–Sahara, Las Vegas, NV, p. A393
STURGIS, Daniel, Ph.D. Director Psychology, Norfolk Regional Center, Norfolk, NE, p. A386
STURGIS, Gayle, Vice President Nursing, Glencoe Regional Health Services, Glencoe, MN, p. A332
STURGIS, James D., Director Human Resources, Texas Scottish Rite Hospital for Children, Dallas, TX, p. A592
STURGIS, Jonathan, Chief Financial Officer, San Jacinto Methodist Hospital, Baytown, TX, p. A582
STURGIS, Paul, Vice President Human Resources, Rehabilitation Institute of Michigan, Detroit, MI, p. A311
STURM, Brenda L., MSN Vice President of Nursing, Daviess Community Hospital, Washington, IN, p. A213
STURSA, Robin, Chief Information Officer, St. Vincent Charity Medical Center, Cleveland, OH, p. A475
STYER, Brent, Director Information Technology, Whitesburg ARH Hospital, Whitesburg, KY, p. A259
STYLES, Kelly R., Vice President and Chief Information Officer, Connecticut Children's Medical Center, Hartford, CT, p. A109
SUAREZ, Jose David, M.D. Chief of Staff, Larkin Community Hospital, South Miami, FL, p. A139
SUAREZ, Lauren, Chief Executive Officer, Kindred Hospital Seattle–Northgate, Seattle, WA, p. A665
SUAREZ, Orlando, Manager Information Technology, Larkin Community Hospital, South Miami, FL, p. A139
SUBER, Mandy, Controller, Calhoun Health Services, Calhoun City, MS, p. A344
SUBLETTE, Elizabeth
Chief Financial Officer, Providence Milwaukie Hospital, Milwaukie, OR, p. A513
Chief Finance Officer, Providence Willamette Falls Medical Center, Oregon City, OR, p. A513
SUCH, William
Chief Executive Officer, Wesley Woods Geriatric Hospital of Emory University, Atlanta, GA, p. A146
Chief Executive Officer, Wesley Woods Long Term Care Hospital, Atlanta, GA, p. A146
SUCHER, Randy, Executive Vice President, Springhill Memorial Hospital, Mobile, AL, p. A23
SUCHER, Therese O., Senior Vice President Operations, Southern Regional Medical Center, Riverdale, GA, p. A158
SUDA, Shirley, M.D. Area Medical Director, Woodland Hills Medical Center,, CA, p. A73
SUDDARTH, Jonathan, D.O. Chief of Staff, Madison County Health Care System, Winterset, IA, p. A228
SUDDUTH, Anthony G., CPA Chief Financial Officer, T. J. Samson Community Hospital, Glasgow, KY, p. A250
SUDDUTH, Debbie, Director Information Services, Heritage Medical Center, Shelbyville, TN, p. A575
SUDICKY, Mary, Chief Financial Officer, St. Mary Medical Center, Hobart, IN, p. A203
SUDOLCAN, Joseph, M.D. Medical Director, Reagan Memorial Hospital, Big Lake, TX, p. A584
SUDOMIR, Joey, Chief Information Officer, Texas Health Harris Methodist Hospital Southlake, Southlake, TX, p. A628
SUEHS, JoAnne, Manager Human Resources, Chapman Medical Center, Orange, CA, p. A78
SUEIRO, Edwin, Administrator, Hospital De Damas, Ponce, PR, p. A702
SUFFIS, Joanne
Vice President Human Resources, Swedish Medical Center–Cherry Hill Campus, Seattle, WA, p. A666
Vice President Human Resources, Swedish Medical Center–First Hill, Seattle, WA, p. A666
SUGAR, Bev, Associate Administrator and Director Human Resources, Inova Mount Vernon Hospital, Alexandria, VA, p. A645
SUGG, Amy, Director Human Resources, Scott Regional Hospital, Morton, MS, p. A350
SUGHRUE, Timothy H., Chief Executive Officer, Rapid City Regional Hospital, Rapid City, SD, p. A559
SUGIYAMA, Deborah, President, NorthBay Medical Center, Fairfield, CA, p. A60
SUHR, Nancy, Manager Human Resources, Pender Community Hospital, Pender, NE, p. A389
SUIRE, Bridget, Acting Administrator, MMO Rehabilitation and Wellness Center, Plaquemine, LA, p. A276
SUITTER, Marie, Chief Financial Officer, The Acadia Hospital, Bangor, ME, p. A281
SUKIN, Debra F.
Chief Executive Officer, St. Luke's Lakeside Hospital, The Woodlands, TX, p. A631
Chief Executive Officer, St. Luke's The Woodlands Hospital, The Woodlands, TX, p. A631
SUKSI, Eugene, Chief Executive Officer, Sutter Coast Hospital, Crescent City, CA, p. A59
SULIK, Sandra, M.D. Vice President Medical Affairs, St. Joseph's Hospital Health Center, Syracuse, NY, p. A444
SULIT, Maria Teresa, Director Human Resources, Holly Hill Hospital, Raleigh, NC, p. A459
SULLIVAN, Christopher, M.D. Chief Medical Officer, Centerpoint Medical Center, Independence, MO, p. A360
SULLIVAN, Craig, Chief Financial Officer, Hickman Community Hospital, Centerville, TN, p. A563
SULLIVAN, Danita S., R.N. Chief Nursing Officer, Tulane Medical Center, New Orleans, LA, p. A275
SULLIVAN, David, Director Human Resources, Doctors Hospital, Columbus, OH, p. A476
SULLIVAN, Donald, M.D. Medical Director, HEALTHSOUTH Rehabilitation Hospital, Memphis, TN, p. A571
SULLIVAN, George, Director Management Information Systems, Mary Lanning Healthcare, Hastings, NE, p. A384
SULLIVAN, Jamie, Chief Operating Officer, Cooper Green Mercy Hospital, Birmingham, AL, p. A16
SULLIVAN, Jennie, Director Finance, Wray Community District Hospital, Wray, CO, p. A107
SULLIVAN, Jennifer, Senior Vice President Finance and Chief Financial Officer, St. James Mercy Health System, Hornell, NY, p. A427
SULLIVAN, John
Vice President Human Resources, Health Central, Ocoee, FL, p. A134
President, Medstar Washington Hospital Center, Washington, DC, p. A116
Chief Executive Officer, Mount Pleasant Hospital, Mount Pleasant, SC, p. A552
SULLIVAN, Jude, Chief Clinical Officer, Kindred Hospital–La Mirada, La Mirada, CA, p. A66
SULLIVAN, Keith, Associate Director, Veterans Affairs Medical Center, Chillicothe, OH, p. A472
SULLIVAN, Marie, R.N. Chief Nursing Officer and Administrator, Northeast Rehabilitation Hospital, Salem, NH, p. A400
SULLIVAN, Mark J., Vice President Human Resources, Western Maryland Regional Medical Center, Cumberland, MD, p. A291
SULLIVAN, Martha, Chief Information Officer, Harrison Memorial Hospital, Cynthiana, KY, p. A249
SULLIVAN, Mary Patricia, R.N. Chief Nursing Officer, Overlook Medical Center, Summit, NJ, p. A410
SULLIVAN, Maurita, Administrator, Mayo Clinic Health System – Northland in Barron, Barron, WI, p. A678
SULLIVAN, Michael, M.D. Chief Medical Officer, Northern Maine Medical Center, Fort Kent, ME, p. A283
SULLIVAN, Michael Dean, M.D. Chief of Staff, Mercy Hospital El Reno, El Reno, OK, p. A496
SULLIVAN, Patrick L., FACHE Director, Captain James A. Lovell Federal Health Care Center, North Chicago, IL, p. A189
SULLIVAN, Patrick L., Chief Operating Officer, St. John's Episcopal Hospital–South Shore,, NY, p. A437
SULLIVAN, Theresa, Chief Operating Officer, Cuyuna Regional Medical Center, Crosby, MN, p. A330
SULLIVAN, Thomas, Vice President Fiscal Services, Harrington Memorial Hospital, Southbridge, MA, p. A304
SULLIVAN, Wardell, Director Human Resources, Touchette Regional Hospitals, Centreville, IL, p. A175

Index of Health Care Professionals

Index of Health Care Professionals / Sullivan

SULLIVAN, William, Chief Financial Officer, Mount Auburn Hospital, Cambridge, MA, p. A299
SULOG, Amy, Comptroller, Naval Hospital, Twentynine Palms, CA, p. A93
SULSER, Jamey, Director Human Resources, South Davis Community Hospital, Bountiful, UT, p. A637
SULU, Dorothy, Chief Financial Officer, Hopi Health Care Center, Keams Canyon, AZ, p. A33
SUMMERER, Mike H., M.D. Chief Executive Officer, University of Connecticut Health Center, John Dempsey Hospital, Farmington, CT, p. A109
SUMMERS, Andrew, Vice President Business Operations, Texas Institute for Surgery at Texas Health Presbyterian Dallas, Dallas, TX, p. A592
SUMMERS, Barbara, President, Community Hospital North, Indianapolis, IN, p. A204
SUMMERS, Curtis, Chief Executive Officer, Summit Medical Center, Edmond, OK, p. A496
SUMMERS, David A.
Chief Financial Officer, Tristar Ashland City Medical Center, Ashland City, TN, p. A562
Chief Financial Officer, Tristar Centennial Medical Center, Nashville, TN, p. A573
SUMMERS, Heather, Director, Chickasaw Nation Medical Center, Ada, OK, p. A493
SUMMERS, Jeff, M.D. Medical Director, Select Specialty Hospital–North Knoxville, Knoxville, TN, p. A568
SUMMERS, Paul, Chief Financial Officer, Delaware Valley Hospital, Walton, NY, p. A446
SUMMERS, Sharon K., R.N. Executive Vice President and Chief Operating Officer, FHN Memorial Hospital, Freeport, IL, p. A182
SUMMERS, Stephen M., FACHE Chief Executive Officer, Wise Regional Health System, Decatur, TX, p. A593
SUMMERSETT III, James A., FACHE President and Chief Executive Officer, Knapp Medical Center, Weslaco, TX, p. A634
SUMMERVILLE, Wendell, Chief Financial Officer, Bryce Hospital, Tuscaloosa, AL, p. A26
SUMNER, Clara M., Senior Vice President and Chief Executive Officer, Medical Center at Franklin, Franklin, KY, p. A250
SUMNER, J. Andrew, M.D. Vice President Medical Affairs, Southern Maryland Hospital Center, Clinton, MD, p. A290
SUMNER, Jack R., Assistant Administrator Finance, Providence Newberg Medical Center, Newberg, OR, p. A513
SUMRA, K. S., M.D. Chief of Staff, Pembina County Memorial Hospital and Wedgewood Manor, Cavalier, ND, p. A464
SUMRALL, Mary Ellen, Chief Nursing Officer, Baptist Memorial Hospital–Golden Triangle, Columbus, MS, p. A345
SUMTER, Rob, Executive Vice President and Chief Operating Officer, Regional Medical Center at Memphis, Memphis, TN, p. A572
SUND, Lynn A., R.N. Senior Vice President, Administrator and Chief Nursing Executive, Laureate Psychiatric Clinic and Hospital, Tulsa, OK, p. A506
SUND, Lynn A., MS, Senior Vice President, Administrator and Chief Nursing Executive, Saint Francis Hospital, Tulsa, OK, p. A506
SUND, Lynn A., R.N. Senior Vice President, Administrator and Chief Nursing Executive, Saint Francis Hospital, Tulsa, OK, p. A506
SUNDBERG, Nita, Director Human Resources, Three Rivers Behavioral Health, West Columbia, SC, p. A554
SUNDBY, Stephen, Interim Chief Executive Officer, Cordova Community Medical Center, Cordova, AK, p. A28
SUNDIN, Jon, M.D. Medical Director, The Orthopedic Specialty Hospital, Murray, UT, p. A638
SUNDQUIST, Philip, M.D. Chief Medical Staff, Lucas County Health Center, Chariton, IA, p. A216
SUNDRUD, Diane
Director Human Resources, Essentia Health Fosston, Fosston, MN, p. A331
Human Resource Service Partner, Essentia Health St. Mary's Hospital – Detroit Lakes, Detroit Lakes, MN, p. A330
SUNGA, Marcos N., M.D. Chief of Staff, Hardin County General Hospital, Rosiclare, IL, p. A193
SUNKAVALLE, Krishna, M.D. Chief Medical Officer, Hamlin Memorial Hospital, Hamlin, TX, p. A602
SUNQUIST, Joanne, Chief Information Officer, Hennepin County Medical Center, Minneapolis, MN, p. A335
SUNTRAPAK, Todd, Interim Chief Executive Officer, Children's Hospital Central California, Madera, CA, p. A73
SUPPAN, Marchelle, DPM, President and Chief Executive Officer, Aultman Orrville Hospital, Orrville, OH, p. A487
SUPPLEE, Linda, Chief Executive Officer, Select Specialty Hospital–Zanesville, Zanesville, OH, p. A492
SURANI, Salim, M.D. Medical Director, Kindred Hospital–Corpus Christi, Corpus Christi, TX, p. A589
SURBER, Randy, Chief Operating Officer, Florida Hospital DeLand, DeLand, FL, p. A122
SURESH, Srinivasan, M.D. Chief Medical Information Officer, Children's Hospital of Michigan, Detroit, MI, p. A310
SURKALA, Karen, Vice President, Westfield Memorial Hospital, Westfield, NY, p. A446
SURL, Deepak, Chief Information Officer, Eastern New Mexico Medical Center, Roswell, NM, p. A417
SURO, Marta R Mercado, Chief Operating Officer, Mennonite General Hospital, Aibonito, PR, p. A699
SUROWITZ, Dale, Chief Executive, Providence Tarzana Medical Center,, CA, p. A71
SURRATT, Shawn, M.D. Chief of Staff, Memorial Hospital and Manor, Bainbridge, GA, p. A147
SURROCK, Lester, Chief Financial Officer, Nix Health Care System, San Antonio, TX, p. A625
SUSI, Jeffrey L., President and Chief Executive Officer, Indian River Medical Center, Vero Beach, FL, p. A142
SUSICK, Nancy, MSN, President, Beaumont Hospital – Troy, Troy, MI, p. A324
SUSSMAN, Andrew, M.D. Chief Operating Officer, UMass Memorial Medical Center, Worcester, MA, p. A306
SUSTERICH, Tim, Chief Financial Officer, Metro Health Hospital, Wyoming, MI, p. A326
SUTER, Brian, Chief Financial Officer, Mayo Clinic Health System in Fairmont, Fairmont, MN, p. A331
SUTER, Mia, Senior Vice President Organizational Development, Owensboro Medical Health System, Owensboro, KY, p. A257
SUTHERLAND, Jenna, Manager Human Resources, Denton Regional Medical Center, Denton, TX, p. A593
SUTHERLAND, Shea, Chief Financial Officer, Midwest Regional Medical Center, Midwest City, OK, p. A499
SUTHERLIN, Shara, R.N. Director Patient Care Services, South Peninsula Hospital, Homer, AK, p. A29
SUTIKA, John, President, DuBois Regional Medical Center, Du Bois, PA, p. A522
SUTTLES, Robert W.
Vice President Human Resources, Cape Canaveral Hospital, Cocoa Beach, FL, p. A120
Vice President Human Resources, Holmes Regional Medical Center, Melbourne, FL, p. A130
Vice President Human Resources, Palm Bay Hospital, Melbourne, FL, p. A130
SUTTON, DeAnn, Chief Executive Officer, Heritage Park Surgical Hospital, Sherman, TX, p. A627
SUTTON, Elaine, Chief Information Officer, General John J. Pershing Memorial Hospital, Brookfield, MO, p. A356
SUTTON, Fred, M.D. Chief Medical Officer, Harris County Hospital District, Houston, TX, p. A604
SUTTON, Janet, M.D. Medical Director, McLaren Bay Special Care, Bay City, MI, p. A308
SUTTON, Julie, Director Performance Improvement, State Hospital South, Blackfoot, ID, p. A166
SUTTON, Michele K., Executive Vice President and Chief Operating Officer, North Oaks Medical Center, Hammond, LA, p. A267
SUTTON, Pat, Director Human Resources, Dearborn County Hospital, Lawrenceburg, IN, p. A207
SUTTON, Rhonda, Director Human Resources, Richland Hospital, Richland Center, WI, p. A690
SUTTON, Richard O., Chief Executive Officer, North Colorado Medical Center, Greeley, CO, p. A102
SUTTON, Thomas, Associate Director, Malcom Randall Veterans Affairs Medical Center, Gainesville, FL, p. A124
SUVER, James A., FACHE Chief Executive Officer, Ridgecrest Regional Hospital, Ridgecrest, CA, p. A82
SUYENAGA, Lee, Chief Executive Officer, Whittier Hospital Medical Center, Whittier, CA, p. A96
SUZUKI, Daniel, M.D. Medical Director, Aurora Las Encinas Hospital, Pasadena, CA, p. A79
SVENDSEN, Mark Deyo, M.D. Medical Director, Mayo Clinic Health System – Red Cedar in Menomonie, Menomonie, WI, p. A685
SVENSSON, Travis, M.D. Medical Director, Fremont Hospital, Fremont, CA, p. A61
SVETLIK, Joe, Vice President Finance, Reedsburg Area Medical Center, Reedsburg, WI, p. A690
SVIHOVEC, Angelia K., Chief Executive Officer, Mobridge Regional Hospital, Mobridge, SD, p. A558
SWAB, Joseph, Chief Financial Officer, Muhlenberg Community Hospital, Greenville, KY, p. A251
SWAB, Joseph A., Chief Financial Officer, Iroquois Memorial Hospital and Resident Home, Watseka, IL, p. A195
SWAGERTY, Jill, Director Human Resources, Union County General Hospital, Clayton, NM, p. A415
SWAIN, Art, Vice President Support Services, Joint Township District Memorial Hospital, Saint Marys, OH, p. A488
SWAINE, Richard P., President, Beaumont Hospital Grosse Pointe, Grosse Pointe, MI, p. A314
SWALLER, Pat, R.N. Chief Operating Officer, Placentia–Linda Hospital, Placentia, CA, p. A80
SWAN, Dennis A., President and Chief Executive Officer, Sparrow Health System, Lansing, MI, p. B121
SWAN, Dennis A., President and Chief Executive Officer, Sparrow Hospital, Lansing, MI, p. A317
SWANGER, Cae, Chief Information Officer, Riverside Community Hospital, Riverside, CA, p. A83
SWANGER, Carol, Chief Nursing Officer, Kansas Rehabilitation Hospital, Topeka, KS, p. A244
SWANK, Georgia, Chief Nursing Officer, Ridge Behavioral Health System, Lexington, KY, p. A253
SWANSON, Darlene, Business Manager, Hillsboro Medical Center, Hillsboro, ND, p. A466
SWANSON, Peter, Assistant Administrator Fiscal Services, Island Hospital, Anacortes, WA, p. A659
SWARTOUT, Judi, Chief Financial Officer, Sutter Coast Hospital, Crescent City, CA, p. A59
SWARTOUT, Paula, HR Manager, Dickinson County Healthcare System, Iron Mountain, MI, p. A315
SWARTWOOD, Philip, Director Information Systems, Grove City Medical Center, Grove City, PA, p. A524
SWARTZ, Edward, Chief Financial Officer, Spring Grove Hospital Center, Baltimore, MD, p. A289
SWARTZ, Michael J., Medical Center Director, Veterans Affairs Medical Center, Bath, NY, p. A421
SWASAND, Berri, M.D. Chief of Staff, Shoshone Medical Center, Kellogg, ID, p. A168
SWAUNCY, Felicia, Chief Financial Officer, Lakeside Behavioral Health System, Memphis, TN, p. A571
SWEDIEN, Scott, Director Information Services, Baldwin Area Medical Center, Baldwin, WI, p. A678
SWEDISH, Joseph R., President and Chief Executive Officer, Trinity Health, Novi, MI, p. B130
SWEENEY, Mary, Vice President Colleague Services and Development, St. Mary Medical Center, Langhorne, PA, p. A526
SWEENEY, Michael, Chief Information Officer, Fox Chase Cancer Center–American Oncologic Hospital, Philadelphia, PA, p. A532
SWEENEY, Rick, Director Information Services, Creighton University Medical Center, Omaha, NE, p. A387
SWEENEY, Tracey, Director Business and Support Services, Montana State Hospital, Warm Springs, MT, p. A379
SWEET, Constance, M.D. President Medical Staff, Memorial Hospital, Towanda, PA, p. A539
SWEET, Mary, Administrator, Kiowa County Memorial Hospital, Greensburg, KS, p. A234
SWEET, Renae, Chief Financial Officer, Surprise Valley Healthcare District, Cedarville, CA, p. A57
SWEETNICH, Ed, Director Human Resources, Mercer County Joint Township Community Hospital, Coldwater, OH, p. A476
SWEEZEY, Trish, R.N. Chief Nursing Officer, New London Hospital, New London, NH, p. A399
SWEGER, Pamela K., Director Human Resources, Atchison Hospital, Atchison, KS, p. A230
SWENSON, Cathy, Chief Executive Officer, Nelson County Health System, McVille, ND, p. A467
SWENSON, Daniel J., Chief Executive Officer, CentraCare Health System – Long Prairie, Long Prairie, MN, p. A333
SWENSON, Diane, Director of Staff Services and Chief Nursing Officer, Carrus Specialty Hospital, Sherman, TX, p. A627
SWENSON, Jeff, M.D. Chief of Staff, Minidoka Memorial Hospital, Rupert, ID, p. A170
SWENSON, Jennifer, President, Fort Hamilton Hospital, Hamilton, OH, p. A481
SWENSON, Kirstin D., Director Human Resources, Regina Medical Center, Hastings, MN, p. A332
SWENSON, Nena, Financial Manager, Tahoe Pacific Hospitals, Reno, NV, p. A395
SWENSON, Nina, Director Business Services, Newport Bay Hospital, Newport Beach, CA, p. A77
SWENSON, Paula C., R.N. Vice President and Chief Nursing Officer, St. Catherine Hospital, East Chicago, IN, p. A200
SWENSON, Roberta, R.N. Vice President of Patient Services, Estes Park Medical Center, Estes Park, CO, p. A101
SWENSON, Wade, M.D. Chief of Staff, Lake Region Healthcare Corporation, Fergus Falls, MN, p. A331
SWENSON, Warren, Chief Financial Officer, United Medical Rehabilitation Hospital, Hammond, LA, p. A267
SWICEGOOD, Debbie, Director Human Resources, Vidant Chowan Hospital, Edenton, NC, p. A452
SWICK, Michael D., President and Chief Executive Officer, Lima Memorial Health System, Lima, OH, p. A482
SWIDERSKI, Tom, Chief Financial Officer, Orthopaedic Hospital of Wisconsin – Glendale, Milwaukee, WI, p. A687
SWIFT, Brian M., Senior Administrator Plant Operations, Burke Rehabilitation Hospital, White Plains, NY, p. A447

A944 Index of Health Care Professionals 

Index of Health Care Professionals / Tarlow

Index of Health Care Professionals


SWIFT, David
Vice President Human Resources, Volunteer and Community Services, Kernan Orthopaedics and Rehabilitation, Baltimore, MD, p. A287
Vice President Human Resources, Maryland General Hospital, Baltimore, MD, p. A288
SWIFT, Kyle, Chief Executive Officer, Medical Center of South Arkansas, El Dorado, AR, p. A44
SWIFT, Mark, D.O. President Medical Staff, East Liverpool City Hospital, East Liverpool, OH, p. A479
SWIFT, Nick, Chief Financial Officer, Maury Regional Hospital, Columbia, TN, p. A564
SWILLEY Jr., Bryanie W.
Chief Executive Officer, Jordan Valley Medical Center, West Jordan, UT, p. A642
Chief Executive Officer, Pioneer Valley Hospital, West Valley City, UT, p. A642
SWIM, Murray, Chief Human Resources Officer, Montgomery Hospital Medical Center, Norristown, PA, p. A530
SWINDELL, Terry
Controller, Bolivar General Hospital, Bolivar, TN, p. A562
Chief Financial Officer, Camden General Hospital, Camden, TN, p. A562
Controller, Gibson General Hospital, Trenton, TN, p. A576
Chief Financial Officer, Humboldt General Hospital, Humboldt, TN, p. A566
SWINFARD, Ronald W., M.D. President and Chief Executive Officer, Lehigh Valley Health Network, Allentown, PA, p. B79
SWINFARD, Ronald W., M.D
President and Chief Executive Officer, Lehigh Valley Hospital, Allentown, PA, p. A517
President and Chief Executive Officer, Lehigh Valley Hospital–Muhlenberg, Bethlehem, PA, p. A518
SWINGLE, Dale, Vice President Information Services, Robert Packer Hospital, Sayre, PA, p. A537
SWINT, Ken, Vice President Finance and Chief Financial Officer, ProMedica Fostoria Community Hospital, Fostoria, OH, p. A480
SWINT, Patricia, Director Information Technology, ProMedica St. Luke's Hospital, Maumee, OH, p. A484
SWISHER, Gena, Vice President Nursing, Hampshire Memorial Hospital, Romney, WV, p. A675
SWISHER, Kay, Vice President and Chief Operating Officer, Laurens County Health Care System, Clinton, SC, p. A548
SWISHER, Reagan, Director Human Resources, Iowa Specialty Hospital–Belmond, Belmond, IA, p. A214
SWISSHELM, Patricia, Acting Chief Fiscal Service, Veterans Affairs Medical Center–Lexington, Lexington, KY, p. A254
SWITZEN, Seth, M.D. Chief of Staff, St. Mary's Regional Medical Center, Enid, OK, p. A496
SWOBODA, Mary, R.N. Chief Nursing Officer, Skiff Medical Center, Newton, IA, p. A224
SWOFFORD, Lisa, Director Administrative Services, Ozark Health Medical Center, Clinton, AR, p. A43
SWOOPES, Patrick R., Administrator, Diamond Grove Center for Children and Adolescents, Louisville, MS, p. A349
SWOPE, Jon D., President and Chief Executive Officer, Mercy Hospital Springfield, Springfield, MO, p. A371
SWORD, Russ D., FACHE Interim Chief Executive Officer, Chicot Memorial Medical Center, Lake Village, AR, p. A47
SYED, Mamoon, Vice President Human Resources, Rady Children's Hospital – San Diego, San Diego, CA, p. A85
SYKES, Angel, Director Human Resources, Memorial Hospital and Manor, Bainbridge, GA, p. A147
SYKES, Christina, Director Human Resources, Labette Health, Parsons, KS, p. A241
SYKES, Lisa
IS/Communications Director, Anson Community Hospital, Wadesboro, NC, p. A462
Director Information Services, Carolinas Medical Center–Union, Monroe, NC, p. A457
SYLVESTER, Sandy, Chief Operating Officer, Okanogan Douglas District Hospital, Brewster, WA, p. A660
SYLVIA–HUTCHINSON, Doreen M., Vice President Operations and Chief Nurse Executive, Fairview Hospital, Great Barrington, MA, p. A300
SYNDER, Judy, Director Human Resources, Olympia Medical Center, Los Angeles, CA, p. A71
SYPIEN, Troy, Director Information Technology and Systems, Medical City Dallas Hospital, Dallas, TX, p. A591
SZABO, Cathy, Director Human Resources, Caverna Memorial Hospital, Horse Cave, KY, p. A252
SZABO, Charleen R., FACHE Director, Veterans Affairs Medical Center, West Palm Beach, FL, p. A143
SZABO, Sandor, M.D. Chief of Staff, Veterans Affairs Long Beach Healthcare System, Long Beach, CA, p. A68
SZALADOS, James E., M.D. Vice President Medical Affairs, Lakeside Memorial Hospital, Brockport, NY, p. A422
SZCZEPANSKI, Bernadette S.
Vice President, Human Resources Development, Centegra Hospital – McHenry, McHenry, IL, p. A187
Vice President Human Resources Development, Centegra Hospital – Woodstock, Woodstock, IL, p. A196
SZCZUROWSKI, Richard, Director Human Resources, Norristown State Hospital, Norristown, PA, p. A530
SZEKELY, Lauraine, R.N. Senior Vice President, Patient Care, Northern Westchester Hospital, Mount Kisco, NY, p. A430
SZENCZY, Catherine
Senior Vice President and Chief Information Officer, Medstar Georgetown University Hospital, Washington, DC, p. A116
Senior Vice President and Chief Information Officer, Medstar Union Memorial Hospital, Baltimore, MD, p. A288
SZYMANSKI, Candra, Chief Operating Officer, UMass Memorial–Marlborough Hospital, Marlborough, MA, p. A302


# T


TAAFFE, Janette, Administrator Human Resources, St. Luke's Hospital, Chesterfield, MO, p. A357
TABB, Kevin, M.D. President and Chief Executive Officer, Beth Israel Deaconess Medical Center, Boston, MA, p. A296
TABBAH, Isam, M.D. Chief of Staff, Harrison Community Hospital, Cadiz, OH, p. A471
TABIBI, Wasae S., M.D. President Medical Staff, Plaza Specialty Hospital, Houston, TX, p. A606
TABOADO, Ketty, Chief Financial Officer, Gladys Spellman Specialty Hospital and Nursing Center, Cheverly, MD, p. A290
TABOR, Britt, Senior Vice President and Chief Financial Officer, Erlanger Medical Center, Chattanooga, TN, p. A563
TABOR, Jeffrey, Director Human Resources, Jackson General Hospital, Ripley, WV, p. A675
TABOR, Randy, Chief Financial Officer, Lady of the Sea General Hospital, Cut Off, LA, p. A265
TABUENCA, Arnold, M.D. Medical Director, Riverside County Regional Medical Center, Moreno Valley, CA, p. A76
TACHOVSKY, Barbara J., President, Paoli Hospital, Paoli, PA, p. A531
TADROS, Magdy, M.D. Medical Director, Meadowbrook Rehabilitation Hospital, Gardner, KS, p. A233
TADURAN, Virgilio, M.D. Chief Medical Officer, Satanta District Hospital, Satanta, KS, p. A243
TADYCH, Michael C., Associate Director, Veterans Affairs Sierra Nevada Health Care System, Reno, NV, p. A395
TAFFE, Patrick, Vice President Information Services, North Memorial Health Care, Robbinsdale, MN, p. A338
TAFOYA, Debbie, Vice President and Chief Information Officer, Huntington Memorial Hospital, Pasadena, CA, p. A80
TAFOYA, Debra, Director Human Resources, Complex Care Hospital at Tenaya, Las Vegas, NV, p. A392
TAFT, Kenneth L., Executive Vice President and Chief Operating Officer, Bronson Methodist Hospital, Kalamazoo, MI, p. A316
TAFUR, Mario, M.D. Chief of Staff, St. Luke's Behavioral Health Center, Phoenix, AZ, p. A36
TAGAI, Lee, Director Human Resources, Lafayette Regional Health Center, Lexington, MO, p. A364
TAGGART, Travis, Director Information Technology, RiverValley Behavioral Health Hospital, Owensboro, KY, p. A257
TAHBO, Robin, Financial Management Officer, U. S. Public Health Service Indian Hospital, Parker, AZ, p. A35
TAINPEAH, Cynthia, Administrator, Creek Nation Community Hospital, Okemah, OK, p. A500
TAIT, Darlene, Director Human Resources, Charlton Memorial Hospital, Folkston, GA, p. A152
TAKES, Kay, R.N. Vice President Patient Care Services and Chief Nursing Officer, Mercy Medical Center–Dubuque, Dubuque, IA, p. A219
TALALAI, James, Senior Vice President and Chief Information Officer, Baylor Institute for Rehabilitation, Dallas, TX, p. A590
TALBOT, Angela, Manager Human Resources, Hamilton County Hospital, Syracuse, KS, p. A243
TALBOT, Lisa, Director Human Resources, St. David's South Austin Medical Center, Austin, TX, p. A581
TALBOT, Robert, Director Human Resources, Baylor Medical Center at Uptown, Dallas, TX, p. A590
TALBOT, Tom, Chief Executive Officer, Community Mental Health Center, Lawrenceburg, IN, p. A207
TALBOTT, Drew, Vice President Operations, Via Christi Hospital, Pittsburg, KS, p. A241
TALENTO, Rick, Senior Vice President and Chief Financial Officer, Providence Hospital, Washington, DC, p. A116
TALLANT–BALL, Mary Jo, Director Health Information Systems, Dallas Medical Center, Dallas, TX, p. A591
TALLARICO, Dominica, Chief Operating Officer, Advocate Christ Medical Center, Oak Lawn, IL, p. A189
TALLERY, Jeremy, D.O. Chief of Staff, Hermann Area District Hospital, Hermann, MO, p. A360
TALLEY, Amanda, Human Resources Director, Highlands–Cashiers Hospital, Highlands, NC, p. A455
TALLEY, Cyndi, Director Information Systems, Greenview Regional Hospital, Bowling Green, KY, p. A248
TALLEY, Stephanie S.
Director Human Resources, Centennial Medical Center, Frisco, TX, p. A600
Associate Administrator and Director Human Resources, Dallas Medical Center, Dallas, TX, p. A591
TALLMAN, Derrick, Chief Executive Officer, Western Massachusetts Hospital, Westfield, MA, p. A306
TALLON, Joe, Vice President Finance, Salina Regional Health Center, Salina, KS, p. A242
TALLON, Richard, Chief Financial Officer, Jefferson County Hospital, Waurika, OK, p. A507
TALLURI, Jay, M.D. Chief Medical Officer, East Morgan County Hospital, Brush, CO, p. A98
TALMO, Michael S., Chief Executive Officer, Vista Health Texarkana, Texarkana, AR, p. A51
TAM, David A., FACHE Chief Administrative Officer, Pomerado Hospital, Poway, CA, p. A81
TAMAR, Earl J., Chief Executive Officer, Galesburg Cottage Hospital, Galesburg, IL, p. A182
TAMBURELLO, Leonardo, Divisional Chief Financial Officer, New York Community Hospital,, NY, p. A435
TAMMINEN, John, M.D. President Medical Staff, Carilion Giles Community Hospital, Pearisburg, VA, p. A653
TANAKA, Steven, Chief Information Officer, Pomerado Hospital, Poway, CA, p. A81
TANDY, Gary R., Chief Financial Officer, General John J. Pershing Memorial Hospital, Brookfield, MO, p. A356
TANG, Shirley, R.N. Chief Nursing Officer, Garfield Medical Center, Monterey Park, CA, p. A75
TANGEMAN, Todd, Director Human Resources, Newton Medical Center, Newton, KS, p. A239
TANGUAY, Denis, Chief Information Officer, Central Maine Medical Center, Lewiston, ME, p. A283
TANIS, Earl P., Senior Vice President Financial Operations, Bayhealth Medical Center, Dover, DE, p. A114
TANKEL, Nancy, R.N. Chief Nurse Executive, Woodland Hills Medical Center,, CA, p. A73
TANNA, Manish, M.D. President Medical Staff, Holy Family Medical Center, Des Plaines, IL, p. A180
TANNENBAUM, Scott, M.D. Medical Director, HEALTHSOUTH Sunrise Rehabilitation Hospital, Fort Lauderdale, FL, p. A123
TANNER, Arlan, Chief Information Officer, Kit Carson County Memorial Hospital, Burlington, CO, p. A98
TANNER, Douglas, Chief Executive Officer, Washington County Hospital and Nursing Home, Chatom, AL, p. A18
TANNER, James, M.D. Vice President and Chief Medical Officer, St. Vincent Infirmary Medical Center, Little Rock, AR, p. A48
TANNER, Kaylee, Human Resources Business Partner, Abraham Lincoln Memorial Hospital, Lincoln, IL, p. A186
TANNER, Laureen K., FACHE President and Chief Executive Officer, Ranken Jordan – A Pediatric Specialty Hospital, Maryland Heights, MO, p. A364
TANNER, Sharon M., President, Albemarle Health, Elizabeth City, NC, p. A452
TANTHOREY, Geoff, Director Information Systems, Granville Health System, Oxford, NC, p. A458
TAPIA, Francis, M.D. President Medical Staff, Terre Haute Regional Hospital, Terre Haute, IN, p. A212
TAPIA, Leonard, Chief Financial Officer, Alta Vista Regional Hospital, Las Vegas, NM, p. A417
TAPLETT, Dean, Controller, Quincy Valley Medical Center, Quincy, WA, p. A664
TAPPAN, Hugh C., President and Chief Executive Officer, Wesley Medical Center, Wichita, KS, p. A246
TAPPER, Shane, Director Management Information Systems, Fort Madison Community Hospital, Fort Madison, IA, p. A220
TARANTINO, Kathryn, Vice President Administration, Robert Wood Johnson University Hospital Rahway, Rahway, NJ, p. A409
TARAR, Ahmad, M.D. Medical Director, Heartland Behavioral Health Services, Nevada, MO, p. A366
TARASOVICH, James
Chief Financial Officer, Mayo Clinic Health System in Saint James, Saint James, MN, p. A338
Chief Financial Officer, Mayo Clinic Health System in Springfield, Springfield, MN, p. A340
TARBELL, Tim, Assistant Administrator Support Services, Scott & White Hospital – Taylor, Taylor, TX, p. A630
TARBET, Joyce, M.D. Chief Medical Officer, Murray County Medical Center, Slayton, MN, p. A340
TARBET, Michele T., R.N. Chief Executive Officer, Sharp Grossmont Hospital, La Mesa, CA, p. A66
TARLOW, Eli, Chief Information Officer, Bellevue Hospital Center, New York, NY, p. A431

Index of Health Care Professionals

Index of Health Care Professionals / Tarnowski


TARNOWSKI, Tim, Chief Information Officer, University of Kentucky Albert B. Chandler Hospital, Lexington, KY, p. A253
TARR, John S., M.D. Chief Medical Officer, Gunnison Valley Hospital, Gunnison, CO, p. A102
TARRANT, Jeffrey S., FACH
President, Integris Bass Baptist Health Center, Enid, OK, p. A496
President, Integris Bass Pavilion, Enid, OK, p. A496
TARRANT, Maureen, Chief Executive Officer, Sky Ridge Medical Center, Lone Tree, CO, p. A104
TARTAGLIA, Judith C., President and Chief Executive Officer, Central Vermont Medical Center, Berlin, VT, p. A643
TARULLI, Pamela, Senior Vice President Human Resources, Good Samaritan Hospital, Suffern, NY, p. A444
TARWATER, Michael C., Chief Executive Officer, Carolinas HealthCare System, Charlotte, NC, p. B25
TASSEY, Karen, MS Chief Operating Officer, Albany Memorial Hospital, Albany, NY, p. A420
TASSO, Tina, Manager Human Resources, The Orthopedic Specialty Hospital, Murray, UT, p. A638
TATE, Charlene, M.D. Chief Medical Staff and Clinical Services, Eleanor Slater Hospital, Cranston, RI, p. A544
TATE, Charles, Director Information Technology, Lallie Kemp Medical Center, Independence, LA, p. A268
TATE, James, M.D. Chief of Staff, Patients' Hospital of Redding, Redding, CA, p. A82
TATE, Jean, Manager Human Resources, RiverView Health, Crookston, MN, p. A330
TATE, Jodie, Director Human Resources, Westerly Hospital, Westerly, RI, p. A545
TATE, Kimberly J., Director Human Resources, Meadows Psychiatric Center, Centre Hall, PA, p. A520
TATELBAUM, Ronald, M.D. Interim Vice President Medical Affairs, Putnam Hospital Center, Carmel, NY, p. A423
TATNALL, Andrew, Chief Executive Officer, Select Specialty Hospital–Atlanta, Atlanta, GA, p. A146
TATRO, Chad, Supervisor Information Systems, Northeast Regional Medical Center, Kirksville, MO, p. A363
TATUM, Martha F., Chief Executive Officer, Evans Memorial Hospital, Claxton, GA, p. A149
TATUM, Robert, M.D. Chief of Staff, Madison River Oaks Medical Center, Canton, MS, p. A344
TATUM, Stanley D., FACHE Chief Executive Officer, St. Mary's Regional Medical Center, Enid, OK, p. A496
TAUNER, Gary, Chief Operating Officer, St. John's Medical Center and Living Center, Jackson, WY, p. A696
TAUNTON, David, M.D. Chief of Staff, Texas Health Harris Methodist Hospital Southlake, Southlake, TX, p. A628
TAVAKOLI, Kenda, Vice President Information Technology and Chief Information Officer, Sibley Memorial Hospital, Washington, DC, p. A117
TAVARY, James, Chief Executive Officer, Wickenburg Community Hospital, Wickenburg, AZ, p. A41
TAVASOLI, Reza, Information Officer, Orthopedic Hospital, Oklahoma City, OK, p. A502
TAVENNER, Matt, Assistant Administrator, Jackson Purchase Medical Center, Mayfield, KY, p. A256
TAWNEY, Michael W., D.O. Vice President Medical Affairs, Port Huron Hospital, Port Huron, MI, p. A321
TAYLOR, Adam, Manager Information Technology, Northern Inyo Hospital, Bishop, CA, p. A56
TAYLOR, Alfred P., Chief Executive Officer, Stanly Regional Medical Center, Albemarle, NC, p. A448
TAYLOR, Alice, MSN, Chief Executive Officer, Broward Health Imperial Point, Fort Lauderdale, FL, p. A123
TAYLOR, Alvin, Chief Human Resources, Five Rivers Medical Center, Pocahontas, AR, p. A50
TAYLOR, Anthony, Manager Information Technology, Cherokee Indian Hospital, Cherokee, NC, p. A451
TAYLOR, Beth, Director Human Resources, Newton–Wellesley Hospital, Newton Lower Falls, MA, p. A303
TAYLOR, Cecilia, Chief Financial Officer, Midwestern Regional Medical Center, Zion, IL, p. A196
TAYLOR, Cherie, Chief Executive Officer, Northern Rockies Medical Center, Cut Bank, MT, p. A374
TAYLOR, Cheryl, R.N. Director of Nursing, Henry Ford Kingswood Hospital, Ferndale, MI, p. A312
TAYLOR, Christina, Director Human Resources, The Brook Hospital – KMI, Louisville, KY, p. A255
TAYLOR, Clay, Chief Financial Officer, Covenant Hospital Plainview, Plainview, TX, p. A621
TAYLOR, Dana Shantel, Director of Organizational Development, Fairfield Memorial Hospital, Fairfield, IL, p. A182
TAYLOR, David, Vice President Information Systems and Chief Information Officer, Stamford Hospital, Stamford, CT, p. A112
TAYLOR, Diana, Administrator, Sabine County Hospital, Hemphill, TX, p. A603
TAYLOR, Dwayne, Chief Executive Officer, Sycamore Shoals Hospital, Elizabethton, TN, p. A565
TAYLOR, Gary, Manager Information Services, Paris Community Hospital, Paris, IL, p. A190
TAYLOR, Gene, Chief Financial Officer, Princeton Baptist Medical Center, Birmingham, AL, p. A16
TAYLOR, Gregory, Chief Financial Officer, Cornerstone Hospital of Austin, Austin, TX, p. A580
TAYLOR, Gregory W., M.D. Vice President and Chief Operating Officer, High Point Regional Health System, High Point, NC, p. A455
TAYLOR, Iris, R.N. President, Detroit Receiving Hospital/University Health Center, Detroit, MI, p. A310
TAYLOR, James H., FACHE President and Chief Executive Officer, University of Louisville Hospital, Louisville, KY, p. A255
TAYLOR, Janet, CPA Chief Financial Officer, Ozarks Community Hospital, Springfield, MO, p. A371
TAYLOR, Janey, Chief Information and Technology, Overton Brooks Veterans Affairs Medical Center, Shreveport, LA, p. A277
TAYLOR, Jeff
Senior Vice President Finance, Magnolia Regional Health Center, Corinth, MS, p. A345
Vice President Finance, St. Luke's Regional Medical Center, Boise, ID, p. A167
TAYLOR, Jim, Chief Business Office, Malcom Randall Veterans Affairs Medical Center, Gainesville, FL, p. A124
TAYLOR, Joel, Administrator, Citizens Baptist Medical Center, Talladega, AL, p. A26
TAYLOR, Judd, Chief Financial Officer, Ogden Regional Medical Center, Ogden, UT, p. A639
TAYLOR, Julia, Area Director Human Resources, Kindred Hospital–Charleston, Charleston, SC, p. A547
TAYLOR, Julie, Chief Executive Officer, West Valley Medical Center, Caldwell, ID, p. A167
TAYLOR, Kendra, Director Inpatient Nursing, Salem Township Hospital, Salem, IL, p. A193
TAYLOR, Kent, Director Human Resources, Riverside Walter Reed Hospital, Gloucester, VA, p. A649
TAYLOR, Kevin C.
Chief Operating Officer, John D. Archbold Memorial Hospital, Thomasville, GA, p. A160
Chief Operating Officer, Mitchell County Hospital, Camilla, GA, p. A148
TAYLOR, Kimberly, Chief Operating Officer, Upstate Carolina Medical Center, Gaffney, SC, p. A550
TAYLOR, Konnie, Chief Financial Officer, Carl Albert Community Mental Health Center, McAlester, OK, p. A499
TAYLOR, Lee, M.D. Vice President and Chief Medical Officer, Southeast Hospital, Cape Girardeau, MO, p. A357
TAYLOR, Loren L., Chief Executive Officer, North Memorial Health Care, Robbinsdale, MN, p. A338
TAYLOR, Mark R., FACHE President and Chief Executive Officer, Columbia St. Mary's Hospital Milwaukee, Milwaukee, WI, p. A686
TAYLOR, Meredith, Comptroller, South Sunflower County Hospital, Indianola, MS, p. A347
TAYLOR, Merle, Vice President Operations, UPMC McKeesport, McKeesport, PA, p. A528
TAYLOR, Michael
Chief Information Officer, Bon Secours St. Francis Hospital, Charleston, SC, p. A547
Chief Information Officer, Roper Hospital, Charleston, SC, p. A547
Vice President Financial Services and Chief Financial Officer, St. Rose Hospital, Hayward, CA, p. A64
TAYLOR, Michael V.
Senior Vice President Human Resources, Sentara Leigh Hospital, Norfolk, VA, p. A652
Vice President Human Resources, Sentara Princess Anne Hospital, Virginia Beach, VA, p. A657
TAYLOR, Mimi
Corporate Vice President Information Technology, Baptist Health South Florida, Baptist Hospital of Miami, Miami, FL, p. A130
Corporate Vice President Information Technology, Baptist Health South Florida, Homestead Hospital, Homestead, FL, p. A125
Vice President Information Technology, Baptist Health South Florida, Mariners Hospital, Tavernier, FL, p. A142
Vice President Information Technology, Baptist Health South Florida, South Miami Hospital, Miami, FL, p. A130
TAYLOR, Patricia, Director, Patient Care Services, Vidant Bertie Hospital, Windsor, NC, p. A463
TAYLOR, Patrick, M.D. President and Chief Executive Officer, Holy Cross Hospital, Fort Lauderdale, FL, p. A123
TAYLOR, Paul
Administrator, Ozarks Community Hospital, Gravette, AR, p. A45
Administrator, Ozarks Community Hospital, Springfield, MO, p. A371
TAYLOR, Renie, Administrator, Stone County Medical Center, Mountain View, AR, p. A49
TAYLOR, Richard, Chief Financial Officer, Western Mental Health Institute, Bolivar, TN, p. A562
TAYLOR, Richard S., M.D. Chief Medical Officer, Cape Fear Valley Medical Center, Fayetteville, NC, p. A453
TAYLOR, Rob, Corporate Director Human Resources, East Los Angeles Doctors Hospital, Los Angeles, CA, p. A69
TAYLOR, Robbie, Director Human Resources, North Sunflower Medical Center, Ruleville, MS, p. A352
TAYLOR, III, Robert, M.D. Vice President Medical Affairs, Our Lady of Lourdes Memorial Hospital, Binghamton, NY, p. A422
TAYLOR, Ross, M.D. Clinical Director, Austin State Hospital, Austin, TX, p. A580
TAYLOR, Scott J., President and Chief Executive Officer, St. Catherine Hospital, Garden City, KS, p. A233
TAYLOR, Shawnia, Chief Financial Officer, Richardson Medical Center, Rayville, LA, p. A276
TAYLOR, Shelia, Director, Taylor Hardin Secure Medical Facility, Tuscaloosa, AL, p. A26
TAYLOR, Stacy, Chief Financial Officer, Nemaha County Hospital, Auburn, NE, p. A381
TAYLOR, Steven L., Chief Executive Officer, Harrison County Hospital, Corydon, IN, p. A199
TAYLOR, Susan L., Chief Executive Officer, College Hospital Costa Mesa, Costa Mesa, CA, p. A58
TAYLOR, Terry, Associate Director, Veterans Affairs Medical Center, Dayton, OH, p. A479
TAYLOR, Tim, Chief Operating Officer, Warren State Hospital, Warren, PA, p. A540
TAYLOR, Todd, Chief Executive Officer, Stafford County Hospital, Stafford, KS, p. A243
TAYLOR, Tony, Vice President Operations, Colleton Medical Center, Walterboro, SC, p. A554
TAYLOR, Tyrone, Chief Financial Officer, Veterans Affairs New Jersey Health Care System, East Orange, NJ, p. A403
TAYLOR, Venus, Director Human Resources, BHC Alhambra Hospital, Rosemead, CA, p. A83
TCHELEBI, Mounzer, M.D. Medical Director, Wyckoff Heights Medical Center,, NY, p. A438
TEAFORD, Carrie, Vice President Finance, Baptist Hospital, Nashville, TN, p. A573
TEAGUE, Anna B., M.D. Chief of Staff, Veterans Affairs Medical Center, Fayetteville, NC, p. A453
TEAGUE, Dean, Chief Operating Officer, Calvert Memorial Hospital, Prince Frederick, MD, p. A293
TEAL, Dianne P., MSN Vice President Clinical Operations, CHRISTUS St. Patrick Hospital of Lake Charles, Lake Charles, LA, p. A271
TEAS, Gregory, M.D. Chief Medical Officer, Alexian Brothers Behavioral Health Hospital, Hoffman Estates, IL, p. A184
TEASDALE, Peggy, Director Human Resources, Southeast Health Center of Ripley County, Doniphan, MO, p. A358
TEBA, Luis, M.D. Vice President and Chief Medical Officer, Gaylord Hospital, Wallingford, CT, p. A112
TEBBE, James, M.D. Vice President Medical Affairs, Ochsner Medical Center – Kenner, Kenner, LA, p. A269
TEDDER, Cookie, Human Resources Manager, Texas Health Center for Diagnostic & Surgery, Plano, TX, p. A621
TEDESCHI, Anthony, M.D. Chief Operating Officer, Norwegian American Hospital, Chicago, IL, p. A177
TEEL, Kenneth R., President, Presbyterian Hospital of Rockwall, Rockwall, TX, p. A623
TEETER, Richard, Chief Financial Officer, Muenster Memorial Hospital, Muenster, TX, p. A617
TEEUWEN, Pat, Director Team Resources, St. Joseph's Hospital, Tampa, FL, p. A141
TEFERA, Tad, Vice President Finance, Ohio Valley General Hospital, McKees Rocks, PA, p. A528
TEFFETELLER, Scott L.
President and Chief Executive Officer, Union Hospital, Terre Haute, IN, p. A212
President and Chief Executive Officer, Union Hospital Clinton, Clinton, IN, p. A199
TEISSONNIERE, Maria T., Director Public Relations, Hospital Oncologico Andres Grillasca, Ponce, PR, p. A702
TEITELBAUM, Karen
Executive Vice President and Chief Operating Officer, Mount Sinai Hospital, Chicago, IL, p. A177
Executive Vice President and Chief Operating Officer, Schwab Rehabilitation Hospital, Chicago, IL, p. A178
TEJADA, Vanessa, Manager Human Resources, HEALTHSOUTH Rehabilitation Institute of San Antonio, San Antonio, TX, p. A625
TEJEDA, Nicholas, Chief Operating Officer, Twin Cities Community Hospital, Templeton, CA, p. A92
TELITZ, Rita, Director Human Resources, Rusk County Memorial Hospital and Nursing Home, Ladysmith, WI, p. A684
TELL, Marjorie, Vice President Information Technology, Riverview Hospital Association, Wisconsin Rapids, WI, p. A694


A946 Index of Health Care Professionals

Index of Health Care Professionals / Thomas

Index of Health Care Professionals

TELLER, Michele, Director Human Resources, Fishermen's Hospital, Marathon, FL, p. A129
TELLO, Anthoney M., M.D. Medical Director, Medcenter One, Bismarck, ND, p. A464
TELLOR, Tammy, Acting Director Human Resources, Choate Mental Health Center, Anna, IL, p. A172
TELTHORSTER, Marcia M., Vice President Human Resources, University Medical Center of Princeton at Plainsboro, Plainsboro, NJ, p. A409
TEMECK, Barbara, M.D. Chief of Staff, Veterans Affairs Edward Hines, Jr. Hospital, Hines, IL, p. A184
TEMPELMEYER, Zak, M.D. Chief Medical Staff, Community Memorial Hospital, Syracuse, NE, p. A390
TEMPEST, Wendy, Director Human Resources, Northern California Rehabilitation Hospital, Redding, CA, p. A82
TEMPLE, John, Director Information Systems, York General Hospital, York, NE, p. A390
TEMPLETON, Carrie E., FACHE Chief Executive Officer, Lafayette General Surgical Hospital, Lafayette, LA, p. A270
TEMPLETON, Gary, M.D. Medical Director, Regency Hospital of Northwest Arkansas, Fayetteville, AR, p. A44
TEMPLETON, Parker, FACHE Chief Executive Officer, Franklin Foundation Hospital, Franklin, LA, p. A266
TEMPLETON, Sheryl, Chief Financial Officer, Scotland County Hospital, Memphis, MO, p. A365
TEMPLETON, III, William, M.D. Medical Director, Clark Memorial Hospital, Jeffersonville, IN, p. A205
TEMPLIN, Nancy, Vice President Finance and Chief Financial Officer, All Children's Hospital, Saint Petersburg, FL, p. A138
TENENBAUM, Jordan, Chief Executive Officer, Select Specialty Hospital–St. Louis, Saint Charles, MO, p. A367
TENHOUSE, Steven, Chief Executive Officer, Kirby Medical Center, Monticello, IL, p. A188
TENNANT, Gail, Director, H. Douglas Singer Mental Health and Developmental Center, Rockford, IL, p. A192
TENNISON, Gary, D.O. Chief of Staff, Crawford Memorial Hospital, Robinson, IL, p. A192
TENNYSON, Guy, Director Information Systems and Telecommunications, San Ramon Regional Medical Center, San Ramon, CA, p. A89
TENNYSON, Ruby, Director Administration, Naval Hospital, Jacksonville, FL, p. A126
TENREIRO, Edgardo, Chief Operating Officer, Baton Rouge General Medical Center, Baton Rouge, LA, p. A262
TEODO, Paul M., Chief Operating Officer, Holy Cross Hospital, Chicago, IL, p. A176
TEPEDINO, Michael, M.D. Chief of Staff, Harton Regional Medical Center, Tullahoma, TN, p. A576
TEPEDINO, Miguel, M.D. Chief Medicine, Lake City Medical Center, Lake City, FL, p. A128
TEPPER, Gil, M.D. Chief of Staff, Miracle Mile Medical Center, Los Angeles, CA, p. A70
TERAN, Maria, Personnel Officer, Ventura County Medical Center, Ventura, CA, p. A94
TERBUSH, Jennifer, Director of Nursing, Hills & Dales General Hospital, Cass City, MI, p. A309
TERHORST, Tom, Director Human Resources, Aurora Medical Center of Washington County, Hartford, WI, p. A683
TERPSTRA, Dale, D.O. Medical Director, Spectrum Health Zeeland Community Hospital, Zeeland, MI, p. A326
TERRELL, Freddie, M.D. Chief of Staff, Clark Regional Medical Center, Winchester, KY, p. A260
TERRELL, Greg, Senior Vice President and Chief Operating Officer, Norman Regional Health System, Norman, OK, p. A500
TERRELL, Jay, Manager Management Information Systems, Riverview Regional Medical Center, Gadsden, AL, p. A20
TERRELL, Michael T., Chief Financial Officer, Brandon Regional Hospital, Brandon, FL, p. A119
TERRINONI, Gary G., Chief Financial Officer and Senior Vice President, Kennedy Memorial Hospitals–University Medical Center, Cherry Hill, NJ, p. A403
TERRIO, James, M.D. Chief Medical Officer, Evans U. S. Army Community Hospital, Fort Carson, CO, p. A101
TERRY, Sr., Darrell K., Senior Vice President Operations, Newark Beth Israel Medical Center, Newark, NJ, p. A407
TERRY, Micheal, President and Chief Executive Officer, Salina Regional Health Center, Salina, KS, p. A242
TERRY, Richard, Vice President & Chief Information Officer, Carson City Hospital, Carson City, MI, p. A309
TERRYBERRY, Daniel S., M.D. Chief Medical Officer, Albemarle Health, Elizabeth City, NC, p. A452
TERTEL, Jenifer K., Director Human Resources, Medical City Dallas Hospital, Dallas, TX, p. A591
TERWILLIGER, James, Vice President Operations, UPMC Presbyterian Shadyside, Pittsburgh, PA, p. A535
TESKE, Mark, Chief Financial Officer, Hill Crest Behavioral Health Services, Birmingham, AL, p. A16
TESSARZIK, Connie, Business Manager, Riverview Hospital for Children and Youth, Middletown, CT, p. A110
TESSNEER, Michael, Chief Executive Officer, Minnesota Department of Human Services, Saint Paul, MN, p. B90
TEST, Russell A., Chief Executive Officer, Select Specialty Hospital–Gainesville, Gainesville, FL, p. A124
TETER, Heather, Chief Financial Officer, Los Alamos Medical Center, Los Alamos, NM, p. A417
TETZ, Warren, Senior Vice President and Chief Operating Officer, Glendale Adventist Medical Center, Glendale, CA, p. A63
TETZLAFF, Sue, Vice President of Nursing, War Memorial Hospital, Sault Sainte Marie, MI, p. A323
TEUBNER, Sandra, Chief Financial Officer, St. Aloisius Medical Center, Harvey, ND, p. A466
TEUFEL, George, Vice President Finance, Advocate Good Shepherd Hospital, Barrington, IL, p. A173
TEUMER, Chris, Vice President and Chief Information Officer, Newark–Wayne Community Hospital, Newark, NY, p. A438
TEW, Brian, Vice President and Chief Information Officer, Catholic Medical Center, Manchester, NH, p. A399
TEWKSBURY, Randy E., Vice President Finance, Lewistown Hospital, Lewistown, PA, p. A527
THACKER, Bruce, Controller, Madison St. Joseph Health Center, Madisonville, TX, p. A615
THACKER, Roland, Chief Financial Officer, Hughston Hospital, Columbus, GA, p. A149
THALL, Barry, M.D. Medical Director, Los Robles Hospital and Medical Center, Thousand Oaks, CA, p. A92
THAMES, Thomas B., M.D
Vice President Medical Affairs, Sentara Princess Anne Hospital, Virginia Beach, VA, p. A657
Interim President, Sentara Virginia Beach General Hospital, Virginia Beach, VA, p. A657
Vice President Medical Affairs, Sentara Virginia Beach General Hospital, Virginia Beach, VA, p. A657
THARASRI, Luke, Administrator, Kindred Hospital–Los Angeles, Los Angeles, CA, p. A70
THARP, Stephen, M.D. Medical Director, St. Vincent Frankfort Hospital, Frankfort, IN, p. A202
THATE, Mark
Vice President Human Resources, Kishwaukee Community Hospital, DeKalb, IL, p. A180
Vice President Human Resources, Valley West Community Hospital, Sandwich, IL, p. A193
THAW, James G., President and Chief Executive Officer, Athens Regional Medical Center, Athens, GA, p. A144
THAXTON, James D., Chief Operating Officer, Baylor University Medical Center, Dallas, TX, p. A590
THAYER, Gilbert M., M.D. Chief Medical Staff, Hardin Medical Center, Savannah, TN, p. A575
THEBARGE, Steven, Chief Operating Officer and Chief Financial Officer, Dorothea Dix Psychiatric Center, Bangor, ME, p. A281
THEILER, Brian, President and Chief Executive Officer, Tri–County Memorial Hospital, Whitehall, WI, p. A694
THEIRING, James, Interim Chief Executive Officer, Mission Community Hospital, Valencia, CA, p. A94
THEISEN, Janet
Chief Information Officer, Sanford Tracy Medical Center, Tracy, MN, p. A340
Chief Information Officer, Sanford Westbrook Medical Center, Westbrook, MN, p. A341
THELEN, Brent, Associate Director, John D. Dingell Veterans Affairs Medical Center, Detroit, MI, p. A311
THEMELIS, Carol, Vice President Human Resources, Frisbie Memorial Hospital, Rochester, NH, p. A400
THERIOT, Lyle, Director Human Resources, Lakeview Regional Medical Center, Covington, LA, p. A265
THERIOT, Paul, Chief Operating Officer, Gadsden Regional Medical Center, Gadsden, AL, p. A20
THEROULT, Thomas N., Chief Executive Officer, Select Specialty Hospital–Omaha, Omaha, NE, p. A388
THERRIEN, Charles D., Chief Executive Officer, Maine Coast Memorial Hospital, Ellsworth, ME, p. A283
THEUS, Thomas L., M.D. Chief of Medicine, Doctors Hospital of Columbus, Columbus, GA, p. A149
THEUS, Will, M.D. Chief of Staff, Gordon Hospital, Calhoun, GA, p. A148
THIBODEAU, Jan, Director Human Resources, HEALTHSOUTH Southern Hills Rehabilitation Hospital, Princeton, WV, p. A675
THIBODEAUX, Annette, Director Human Resources, Savoy Medical Center, Mamou, LA, p. A272
THIBODEAUX, Douglas, M.D. Chief Medical Officer, OakBend Medical Center, Richmond, TX, p. A622
THIEL, Scott, M.D. Chief of Staff, Boone County Hospital, Boone, IA, p. A215
THIELE, Rosemary, Chief Executive Officer, Progressive Hospital, Las Vegas, NV, p. A393
THIELEN, Kurt, Manager Business Office, Minneapolis Veterans Affairs Health Care System, Minneapolis, MN, p. A335
THIELKE, Jayne, Chief Financial Officer, Swift County–Benson Hospital, Benson, MN, p. A328
THIELST, Christina B., Chief Operating Officer, Ventura County Medical Center, Ventura, CA, p. A94
THIEMAN, Richard, Chief Financial Officer, Wilbarger General Hospital, Vernon, TX, p. A633
THIESFELD, Rebecca A., Executive Director Human Resources, Cuyuna Regional Medical Center, Crosby, MN, p. A330
THIESSEN, David, Associate Director Support Services, Missouri Rehabilitation Center, Mount Vernon, MO, p. A365
THIGPEN, Kevin, Vice President Human Resources, Athens Regional Medical Center, Athens, GA, p. A144
THILGES, Michael, Chief Financial Officer, Clarke County Hospital, Osceola, IA, p. A225
THIMIS, Nicholas, Chief Information Officer, West Jefferson Medical Center, Marrero, LA, p. A272
THOENDEL, Victor, M.D. Chief Medical Officer, Butler County Health Care Center, David City, NE, p. A383
THOMAS, Adeeb, M.D. Vice President Medical Affairs, St. Vincent's East, Birmingham, AL, p. A17
THOMAS, Amy, Vice President Finance, Memorial Hospital, Belleville, IL, p. A173
THOMAS, Brian E., Administrator, Alton Mental Health Center, Alton, IL, p. A172
THOMAS, Brian N., Senior Vice President and Chief Operating Officer, Jefferson Regional Medical Center, Pine Bluff, AR, p. A50
THOMAS, Brook, Chief Financial Officer, West Boca Medical Center, Boca Raton, FL, p. A119
THOMAS, IV, Calvin, Chief Operating Officer, St. Lucie Medical Center, Port St. Lucie, FL, p. A137
THOMAS, Chris, FACHE President and Chief Executive Officer, Community Hospital, Grand Junction, CO, p. A101
THOMAS, Cristina, Vice President and Chief Information Officer, Mercy Medical Center–Des Moines, Des Moines, IA, p. A218
THOMAS, Curt, Administrator, Ness County Hospital, Ness City, KS, p. A239
THOMAS, Dan, Chief Executive Officer, Laurel Ridge Treatment Center, San Antonio, TX, p. A625
THOMAS, Debbie, Chief Operating Officer, Dorminy Medical Center, Fitzgerald, GA, p. A152
THOMAS, Debora, Chief Financial Officer, Florida Hospital Memorial Medical Center, Daytona Beach, FL, p. A121
THOMAS, Denise, Chief Financial Officer, Spring View Hospital, Lebanon, KY, p. A252
THOMAS, Drake, Chief Information Officer, CarePartners Health Services, Asheville, NC, p. A448
THOMAS, Geogy, M.D. Chief of Staff, Jellico Community Hospital, Jellico, TN, p. A567
THOMAS, James, Chief Financial Officer, Montfort Jones Memorial Hospital, Kosciusko, MS, p. A348
THOMAS, Jennifer, Director Public Relations, Lake Butler Hospital Hand Surgery Center, Lake Butler, FL, p. A128
THOMAS, Joan, Chief Financial Officer, Brunswick Novant Medical Center, Bolivia, NC, p. A449
THOMAS, Jody, Director Human Resources, Texas Health Harris Methodist Hospital Southwest Fort Worth, Fort Worth, TX, p. A599
THOMAS, John, Chief Operating Officer, San Mateo Medical Center, San Mateo, CA, p. A89
THOMAS, John A., M.D. Chief Medical Staff, Culberson Hospital, Van Horn, TX, p. A632
THOMAS, John H., M.D. Chief of Staff, Healthmark Regional Medical Center, DeFuniak Springs, FL, p. A122
THOMAS, Karen A., R.N
Vice President and Chief Information Officer, Bryn Mawr Hospital, Bryn Mawr, PA, p. A519
Chief Information Officer, Bryn Mawr Rehabilitation Hospital, Malvern, PA, p. A528
Acting Vice President and Chief Information Officer, Lankenau Medical Center, Wynnewood, PA, p. A542
Vice President and Chief Information Officer, Paoli Hospital, Paoli, PA, p. A531
THOMAS, Keith, M.D. Chief of Staff, Blue Mountain Hospital, John Day, OR, p. A511
THOMAS, Kimberly A., R.N. Chief Executive Officer, Select Specialty Hospital–Akron, Akron, OH, p. A469
THOMAS, Kirk E., Vice President Operations, Lewistown Hospital, Lewistown, PA, p. A527
THOMAS, Lizbeth, M.D. Vice President Medical Affairs, Fairview Ridges Hospital, Burnsville, MN, p. A329
THOMAS, Maggie, Vice President Human Resources and Practice Management, South County Hospital, Wakefield, RI, p. A545
THOMAS, Michael, Associate Administrator, Wayne County Hospital, Corydon, IA, p. A217
THOMAS, Michael P., Administrator, Meade District Hospital, Meade, KS, p. A239
THOMAS, Michael S., President and Chief Administrative Officer, John Muir Medical Center, Concord, Concord, CA, p. A58

© 2012 AHA Guide Index of Health Care Professionals **A947**

Index of Health Care Professionals
Index of Health Care Professionals / Thomas

THOMAS, Mitchell T., Chief Financial Officer, Presbyterian Intercommunity Hospital, Whittier, CA, p. A96
THOMAS, Nathan, M.D. President Medical Staff, Meyersdale Medical Center, Meyersdale, PA, p. A529
THOMAS, Nicky, Director Human Resources, Baptist Memorial Hospital–Union City, Union City, TN, p. A576
THOMAS, Paula, R.N. Vice President Patient Services, UPMC Bedford Memorial, Everett, PA, p. A523
THOMAS, Renae, Chief Financial Officer, Mother Frances Hospital – Winnsboro, Winnsboro, TX, p. A635
THOMAS, Robert, Administrator, Columbus Community Hospital, Columbus, TX, p. A588
THOMAS, Ronald J., Coordinator Information Systems, North Alabama Regional Hospital, Decatur, AL, p. A18
THOMAS, Ruth, Chief Operating Officer, Mercy Fitzgerald Hospital, Darby, PA, p. A521
THOMAS, Scott C., Administrative Director Human Resources/Communication, Granville Health System, Oxford, NC, p. A458
THOMAS, Shawn M., Director Human Resources, Payson Regional Medical Center, Payson, AZ, p. A35
THOMAS, Spencer, Chief Executive Officer, Newport Medical Center, Newport, TN, p. A574
THOMAS, Stephanie, Chief Operating Officer, Denver Health Medical Center, Denver, CO, p. A99
THOMAS, Sue
Manager Human Resources, Beckley ARH Hospital, Beckley, WV, p. A670
Director Human Resources, Mercy Regional Medical Center, Ville Platte, LA, p. A279
THOMAS, Thomas S., Chief Financial Officer, Peninsula Hospital Center,, NY, p. A
THOMAS, Tracy, Director Human Resources, Cumberland Hall Hospital, Hopkinsville, KY, p. A251
THOMAS, Wanda W., Director Health Information, Neosho Memorial Regional Medical Center, Chanute, KS, p. A231
THOMAS, Warner L., FACHE System President and Chief Operating Officer, Ochsner Medical Center, New Orleans, LA, p. A275
THOMAS, Jr., William, M.D. Medical Director Clinical and Internal Affairs, Molokai General Hospital, Kaunakakai, HI, p. A165
THOMAS–FOLDS, Lana, System Director Human Resources, Jack Hughston Memorial Hospital, Phenix City, AL, p. A25
THOMASKUTTY, Christopher G., Vice President Corporate Affairs, Mercy Medical Center, Baltimore, MD, p. A288
THOMASON, Joe D., Chief Executive Officer, Centennial Medical Center, Frisco, TX, p. A600
THOMASON, Richard, FACHE Chief Executive Officer, Pender Community Hospital, Pender, NE, p. A389
THOMASON, Rose, Interim Vice President Human Resources, JPS Health Network, Fort Worth, TX, p. A599
THOMASSON, Mark, Vice President Human Resources, Providence Memorial Hospital, El Paso, TX, p. A596
THOMPSON, Alan, M.D. President Medical Staff, Warm Springs Medical Center, Warm Springs, GA, p. A161
THOMPSON, Albert, M.D. Chief of Staff, Charlton Memorial Hospital, Folkston, GA, p. A152
THOMPSON, Angela S., Vice President Human Resources and Support Services, Indiana University Health North Hospital, Carmel, IN, p. A199
THOMPSON, Becki, Controller, Oakes Community Hospital, Oakes, ND, p. A467
THOMPSON, Belinda, Coordinator Human Resources, HEALTHSOUTH Chesapeake Rehabilitation Hospital, Salisbury, MD, p. A294
THOMPSON, Betsy, Director Human Resources, Northern Virginia Mental Health Institute, Falls Church, VA, p. A648
THOMPSON, Bobby, Director Information Technology, Stephens Memorial Hospital, Breckenridge, TX, p. A584
THOMPSON, C. Lynn, M.D. Vice President Medical Affairs, Lima Memorial Health System, Lima, OH, p. A482
THOMPSON, Chad, Chief Financial Officer, Lallie Kemp Medical Center, Independence, LA, p. A268
THOMPSON, Charolette, Chief Financial Officer, Reeves Memorial Medical Center, Bernice, LA, p. A263
THOMPSON, Cheryl, Chief Nursing Officer, Garden Park Medical Center, Gulfport, MS, p. A346
THOMPSON, Chris
Chief Financial Officer, Delta Community Medical Center, Delta, UT, p. A637
Chief Financial Officer, Fillmore Community Medical Center, Fillmore, UT, p. A637
Chief Financial Officer, Sanpete Valley Hospital, Mount Pleasant, UT, p. A638
Chief Financial Officer, Sevier Valley Medical Center, Richfield, UT, p. A640
THOMPSON, Cindy, Chief Financial Officer, Northwest Surgical Hospital, Oklahoma City, OK, p. A501
THOMPSON, Craig B., M.D. President and Chief Executive Officer, Memorial Sloan–Kettering Cancer Center, New York, NY, p. A434
THOMPSON, Dale, Chief Operating Officer, Western State Hospital, Tacoma, WA, p. A668
THOMPSON, David, M.D. Chief of Staff, Richardson Medical Center, Rayville, LA, p. A276
THOMPSON, David
Chief Financial Officer, St. Anthony Hospital, Lakewood, CO, p. A103
Chief Financial Officer, St. Anthony Summit Medical Center, Frisco, CO, p. A101
THOMPSON, David M., Chief Executive Officer, Sutter Tracy Community Hospital, Tracy, CA, p. A93
THOMPSON, Deborah A., Director, William S. Middleton Memorial Veterans Hospital, Madison, WI, p. A684
THOMPSON, Donna K., Chief Executive Officer, Allegiance Health Center of Ruston, Ruston, LA, p. A276
THOMPSON, Douglas, Director Information Systems, Brookdale Hospital Medical Center,, NY, p. A431
THOMPSON, Dwight, Chief Financial Officer, Altru Health System, Grand Forks, ND, p. A466
THOMPSON, Elaine C., Ph.D. President and Chief Executive Officer, Lakeland Regional Medical Center, Lakeland, FL, p. A128
THOMPSON, Frederick G., Ph.D. President, Anson Community Hospital, Wadesboro, NC, p. A462
THOMPSON, Helen, Interim Director, Indian Health Service Hospital, Rapid City, SD, p. A558
THOMPSON, James H., FACHE Owner and Chief Executive Officer, Healthmark Regional Medical Center, DeFuniak Springs, FL, p. A122
THOMPSON, Jane, Administrator and Chief Operating Officer, York General Hospital, York, NE, p. A390
THOMPSON, Jeff, M.D. Chief of Staff, DeKalb Regional Medical Center, Fort Payne, AL, p. A20
THOMPSON, Jeffrey E., M.D. Chief Executive Officer, Gundersen Lutheran Medical Center, La Crosse, WI, p. A683
THOMPSON, Jerry
Chief Financial Officer, Sanford Tracy Medical Center, Tracy, MN, p. A340
Chief Financial Officer, Sanford Westbrook Medical Center, Westbrook, MN, p. A341
THOMPSON, John W., M.D. Chief of Staff, Eastern Louisiana Mental Health System, Jackson, LA, p. A268
THOMPSON, Kevin
Chief Financial Officer, Sharp Memorial Hospital, San Diego, CA, p. A86
Chief Financial Officer, Sharp Mesa Vista Hospital, San Diego, CA, p. A86
THOMPSON, Kim, Chief Executive Officer, Fulton County Hospital, Salem, AR, p. A51
THOMPSON, Linda
Chief Operating Officer, Fairfax Community Hospital, Fairfax, OK, p. A496
Vice President Human Resources, New England Baptist Hospital, Boston, MA, p. A297
THOMPSON, Lisa, MSN Director of Nursing, Hiawatha Community Hospital, Hiawatha, KS, p. A234
THOMPSON, Mark, Vice President Finance and Chief Financial Officer, Lourdes Hospital, Paducah, KY, p. A257
THOMPSON, Mark, M.D. Chief Medical Officer, Monroe Clinic, Monroe, WI, p. A687
THOMPSON, Mark, Vice President Financial Services, Rapid City Regional Hospital, Rapid City, SD, p. A559
THOMPSON, Matthew J., Chief Executive Officer, Carson City Hospital, Carson City, MI, p. A309
THOMPSON, Melissa, M.D. Chief Medical Officer, Adair County Memorial Hospital, Greenfield, IA, p. A220
THOMPSON, Michael S., Chief Executive Officer, Frio Regional Hospital, Pearsall, TX, p. A620
THOMPSON, Michael W., Chief Executive Officer, HEALTHSOUTH Rehabilitation of Gadsden, Gadsden, AL, p. A20
THOMPSON, Michele T., Deputy Chief Operating Officer, Provident Hospital of Cook County, Chicago, IL, p. A177
THOMPSON, Ormand P., Administrator, North Baldwin Infirmary, Bay Minette, AL, p. A16
THOMPSON, Pamela, Chief Operations Officer, Huhukam Memorial Hospital, Sacaton, AZ, p. A37
THOMPSON, Patricia
Treasurer and Chief Financial Officer, Geneva General Hospital, Geneva, NY, p. A426
Treasurer and Chief Financial Officer, Soldiers and Sailors Memorial Hospital of Yates County, Penn Yan, NY, p. A440
THOMPSON, Ranae M., MSN Director Patient Care Services, Shriners Hospitals for Children, Greenville, Greenville, SC, p. A550
THOMPSON, Robert, M.D. Chief of Staff, Mission Community Hospital, Valencia, CA, p. A94
THOMPSON, Sarah, Vice President Operations, Tift Regional Medical Center, Tifton, GA, p. A161
THOMPSON, Shari, M.D. President Medical Staff, Fitzgibbon Hospital, Marshall, MO, p. A364
THOMPSON, Sherene, Director Human Resources, Methodist Willowbrook Hospital, Houston, TX, p. A605
THOMPSON, Sheri, Director Information Technology, Crete Area Medical Center, Crete, NE, p. A383
THOMPSON, Sonja, Deputy Commander Clinical Services, Martin Army Community Hospital, Fort Benning, GA, p. A153
THOMPSON, Stuart, Director Human Resources, Cleveland Clinic Florida, Weston, FL, p. A143
THOMPSON, Susan K., President and Chief Executive Officer, Trinity Regional Medical Center, Fort Dodge, IA, p. A219
THOMPSON, Susie, Executive Director Fiscal Services, Hamilton Center, Terre Haute, IN, p. A212
THOMPSON, Terry, Director Information Services, North Star Behavioral Health System, Anchorage, AK, p. A28
THOMPSON, Sr., Timothy L., Senior Vice President and Chief Information Officer, The Methodist Hospital, Houston, TX, p. A607
THOMPSON, Tina H., Coordinator Human Resources, FirstHealth Montgomery Memorial Hospital, Troy, NC, p. A462
THOMPSON, Tom, Vice President and Chief Financial Officer, Raleigh General Hospital, Beckley, WV, p. A670
THOMPSON, Trinise, Director Human Resources, St. Luke's Medical Center, Phoenix, AZ, p. A36
THOMPSON, William, M.D. Chief Medical Officer, Baptist Hospital, Nashville, TN, p. A573
THOMPSON, William P., President and Chief Executive Officer, SSM Health Care, Saint Louis, MO, p. B122
THOMSEN, Greg, FACHE Chief Executive Officer, Columbus Specialty Hospital, Columbus, GA, p. A149
THOMSEN, Jan, Director Human Resources, Tyler County Hospital, Woodville, TX, p. A636
THOMSEN, Sue, Chief Financial Officer, South Texas Rehabilitation Hospital, Brownsville, TX, p. A585
THOMSEN, Vicki, Director Human Resources, Aurora Behavioral Health System–Glendale, Glendale, AZ, p. A32
THOMSON, Doug, M.D. Chief Medical Officer, Commonwealth Regional Specialty Hospital, Bowling Green, KY, p. A247
THOMSON, Ken, M.D. Medical Director, Sugar Land Surgical Hospital, Sugar Land, TX, p. A629
THOMSON, Nicole, Chief Financial Officer, Saint Louise Regional Hospital, Gilroy, CA, p. A63
THOMSON, Sean, CPA Chief Financial Officer, Spotsylvania Regional Medical Center, Fredericksburg, VA, p. A648
THOMSON, Steven, M.D. Medical Director, Heartland Behavioral Healthcare, Massillon, OH, p. A484
THORDARSON, G. Thor, President and Chief Executive Officer, Indiana University Health La Porte Hospital, La Porte, IN, p. A206
THORE, Joe, Chief Operating Officer, Ashe Memorial Hospital, Jefferson, NC, p. A455
THOREEN, Peter W., FACHE President and Chief Executive Officer, St. Luke's Regional Medical Center, Sioux City, IA, p. A227
THORESON, Scott D., FACHE Administrator, Mayo Clinic Health System in Springfield, Springfield, MN, p. A340
THORGUSON, Kimberly, M.D. Chief of Staff, Teche Regional Medical Center, Morgan City, LA, p. A273
THORN, III, Eugene A., Vice President Finance and Chief Financial Officer, Union Hospital, Dover, OH, p. A479
THORNE, Dana, Administrator Human Resources, Valley Hospital Medical Center, Las Vegas, NV, p. A394
THORNE, Paul, M.D. Chief Medical Director, St. Cloud Regional Medical Center, Saint Cloud, FL, p. A137
THORNE Jr., William, Chief Executive Officer, Acoma–Canoncito–Laguna Hospital, Acoma, NM, p. A414
THORNELL, Timothy, FACHE Chief Executive Officer, Lea Regional Medical Center, Hobbs, NM, p. A416
THORNQUIST, Betsy, Chief Information Officer, St. Vincent's Medical Center, Bridgeport, CT, p. A108
THORNSBERRY, Michael, M.D. Chief of Staff, Veterans Affairs Medical Center, Birmingham, AL, p. A17
THORNTON, Bob, Exec. VP, Chief Financial Officer, Bayfront Medical Center, Saint Petersburg, FL, p. A138
THORNTON, Cayetano, Chief Information Officer, Walter Reed National Military Medical Center, Bethesda, MD, p. A290
THORNTON, Dale E., M.P.H. President and Chief Executive Officer, Mercy Tiffin Hospital, Tiffin, OH, p. A489
THORNTON, Daryl W., Chief Operating Officer, Kansas Medical Center, Andover, KS, p. A230
THORNTON, Jillisa, Director of Nursing, Coastal Harbor Treatment Center, Savannah, GA, p. A159
THORNTON Jr.,, Robert M., Chief Executive Officer, Sunlink Health Systems, Atlanta, GA, p. B125
THORNTON, Timothy J., Chief Financial Officer, Russell Medical Center, Alexander City, AL, p. A15

**A948** Index of Health Care Professionals

Index of Health Care Professionals / Tomlin

Index of Health Care Professionals


THORPE, Linda, Chief Executive Officer, East Morgan County Hospital, Brush, CO, p. A98
THORPE, Paul, M.D. Chief of Staff, Wilson Memorial Hospital, Sidney, OH, p. A488
THORPE, Wendy, Area Director Information Systems, St. Joseph Hospital, Eureka, CA, p. A60
THORSEN, Erik, Chief Executive Officer, Columbia Memorial Hospital, Astoria, OR, p. A509
THORWALD, Robert, Chief Information Officer, Washington Hospital Healthcare System, Fremont, CA, p. A61
THOTA, Suresh, M.D. Chief of Staff, Volunteer Community Hospital, Martin, TN, p. A570
THOTAKURA, Raj, M.D. Medical Director, Old Vineyard Behavioral Health Services, Winston–Salem, NC, p. A463
THRASHER, Barton, M.D. Chief of Staff, Methodist Healthcare–Fayette Hospital, Somerville, TN, p. A575
THRASHER, Charlotte, Vice President and Chief Operating Officer, Seton Medical Center Austin, Austin, TX, p. A581
THREEWITS, Sheree, Director Human Resources, Manatee Memorial Hospital, Bradenton, FL, p. A119
THRUSH, Warren, Coordinator Human Resources, Brookville Hospital, Brookville, PA, p. A519
THULI, Karen, Coordinator Information Systems, Upland Hills Health, Dodgeville, WI, p. A680
THUN, Todd, Director Human Resources, Montana State Hospital, Warm Springs, MT, p. A379
THUNELL, Adam, Chief Operating Officer and Vice President Operations, Community Memorial Health System, Ventura, CA, p. A94
THURMER, DeAnn, Chief Operating Officer, Waupun Memorial Hospital, Waupun, WI, p. A693
THURMOND, David, Chief Information Resource Management Service, Veterans Affairs Medical Center – Alexandria, Pineville, LA, p. A276
THURMOND, Jeff, Vice President Information Systems, Baptist Regional Medical Center, Corbin, KY, p. A248
THURSTON, Leigh, Vice President Information Systems, Community Medical Center, Missoula, MT, p. A377
THURSTON, Richard, M.D. Chief of Staff, Benewah Community Hospital, Saint Maries, ID, p. A170
THURSTON, Thomas, M.D. Medical Director, J. D. McCarty Center for Children With Developmental Disabilities, Norman, OK, p. A500
THYGESON, Cindy, M.D. Director Medical Affairs, Sutter Center for Psychiatry, Sacramento, CA, p. A84
TIBBETT, Cheryl, Chief Financial Officer, Charlotte Regional Medical Center, Punta Gorda, FL, p. A137
TIBBITS, Richard M., Vice President and Chief Operating Officer, Loma Linda University Medical Center–Murrieta, Murrieta, CA, p. A76
TIBBITTS, Thomas, Interim Chief Executive Officer, Allen Memorial Hospital, Waterloo, IA, p. A227
TIBBS, E. W., President and Chief Executive Officer, Centra Southside Community Hospital, Farmville, VA, p. A648
TICE, Darlette, Chief Nursing Officer, Manatee Memorial Hospital, Bradenton, FL, p. A119
TICE, Heidi, Chief Financial Officer, Cheyenne County Hospital, Saint Francis, KS, p. A242
TICE, Kirk C., President and Chief Executive Officer, Robert Wood Johnson University Hospital Rahway, Rahway, NJ, p. A409
TICE, Linda, Director Information Systems, Riverton Memorial Hospital, Riverton, WY, p. A697
TICHENOR, John, Chief Financial Officer, Ohio County Hospital, Hartford, KY, p. A251
TIEDT, Jerry, Director Information Systems, Waverly Health Center, Waverly, IA, p. A228
TIEFENTHALER BSN, MSN, MHA, Brenda Marie, R.N. Vice President Patient Care and Informatics, Spencer Hospital, Spencer, IA, p. A227
TIEMENS, Linda, Chief Executive Officer, Select Specialty Hospital–Tulsa Midtown, Tulsa, OK, p. A506
TIEMEYER, Nancy, Director Health Information Management, George C Grape Community Hospital, Hamburg, IA, p. A220
TIERNAN, Kelley, Chief Financial Officer, Claxton–Hepburn Medical Center, Ogdensburg, NY, p. A439
TIERNEY, Mark A., Chief Financial Officer, Manatee Memorial Hospital, Bradenton, FL, p. A119
TIETJEN, George, M.D. Chief of Staff, Wayne Memorial Hospital, Honesdale, PA, p. A525
TIGGELAAR, Tom, Vice President Finance, Mayo Clinic Health System – Franciscan Healthcare in La Crosse, La Crosse, WI, p. A684
TILLER, Gary L., Chief Executive Officer, Ninnescah Valley Health System, Kingman, KS, p. A236
TILLETT, Grant, Director Information Technologies, Prairie Lakes Healthcare System, Watertown, SD, p. A560
TILLIRSON, Mike, D.O. Executive Vice President and Chief Medical Officer, AnMed Health Medical Center, Anderson, SC, p. A546
TILLMAN, Barry, M.D. Chief Medical Staff, Promise Hospital of Miss Lou, Vidalia, LA, p. A279
TILLMAN, Jill, Assistant Chief Executive Officer, Brandywine Hospital, Coatesville, PA, p. A520
TILLMAN, Kanner, Chief Financial Officer, Encino Hospital Medical Center,, CA, p. A69
TILLMAN, Michael, Vice President Patient Services and Chief Operating Officer, United Hospital Center, Bridgeport, WV, p. A670
TILSON, Natalie, Controller, HEALTHSOUTH Rehabilitation Hospital, Kingsport, TN, p. A568
TILTON, David P., President and Chief Executive Officer, AtlantiCare, Egg Harbor Township, NJ, p. B14
TILUS, Sheryl, R.N. Vice President Clinical Services/Chief Nursing Officer, Skaggs Regional Medical Center, Branson, MO, p. A356
TIMANUS, Anthony, Chief Executive Officer, Avera Gregory Hospital, Gregory, SD, p. A557
TIMBERS, Christopher T., Vice President and Chief Information Officer, Suburban Hospital, Bethesda, MD, p. A290
TIMLIN, Marie, R.N. Chief Nursing Officer, Yampa Valley Medical Center, Steamboat Springs, CO, p. A106
TIMM, Mark
Director Human Resources, Yavapai Regional Medical Center – East, Prescott Valley, AZ, p. A37
Director Human Resources, Yavapai Regional Medical Center, Prescott, AZ, p. A37
TIMM, Matt, M.D. Medical Director, Pender Community Hospital, Pender, NE, p. A389
TIMMER, Kari, Chief Financial Officer, Hegg Memorial Health Center Avera, Rock Valley, IA, p. A226
TIMMERMAN, Candace, Director Human Resources, Avera Creighton Hospital, Creighton, NE, p. A383
TIMMERMAN, Jo, Manager Accounting, Norwood Health Center, Marshfield, WI, p. A685
TIMMONS, Bret, D.O. Chief Medical Staff, Power County Hospital District, American Falls, ID, p. A166
TIMMONS, William, Chief Executive Officer, Los Ninos Hospital, Phoenix, AZ, p. A36
TIMPE, Ronald, Associate Administrator, Buchanan County Health Center, Independence, IA, p. A221
TINCH, Paula, Interim Chief Financial Officer, Newark–Wayne Community Hospital, Newark, NY, p. A438
TINCHER, Pat, Director Finance, Langlade Memorial Hospital, Antigo, WI, p. A678
TINDALL, Patricia, Chief Executive Officer, Lyndon B. Johnson Tropical Medical Center, Pago Pago, AS, p. A699
TINDLE, Jeff A., Chief Executive Officer, Carroll County Memorial Hospital, Carrollton, MO, p. A357
TINDLE, Tim, Chief Information Officer, Harris County Hospital District, Houston, TX, p. A604
TINGLE, Billy, Director Information Systems and Respiratory Therapy, Avoyelles Hospital, Marksville, LA, p. A272
TINGSTAD, Jonathan, Vice President and Chief Financial Officer, Seattle Cancer Care Alliance, Seattle, WA, p. A666
TINKER, Peter, Chief Human Resources Officer, Veterans Affairs Medical Center,, NY, p. A437
TINNEY, Sean, FACHE President and Chief Operating Officer, St. Vincent's East, Birmingham, AL, p. A17
TINSA, Udom, M.D. Medical Director, Ashley Medical Center, Ashley, ND, p. A464
TINSLEY, Austin, M.D. Chief Medical Officer, Poplar Bluff Regional Medical Center, Poplar Bluff, MO, p. A367
TINSLEY III, Edward D., Chief Executive Officer, McLeod Loris Healthcare, Loris, SC, p. A552
TINSLEY, Kay
Vice President Fiscal Services, Good Samaritan Regional Health Center, Mount Vernon, IL, p. A188
Vice President Finance, St. Mary's Hospital, Centralia, IL, p. A174
TINTLE, Keith D., Chief Executive Officer, Timpanogos Regional Hospital, Orem, UT, p. A639
TIPPIN, Philip, M.D. Chief of Staff, Chambers Memorial Hospital, Danville, AR, p. A43
TIPPIN, Russell, Chief Executive Officer, Permian Regional Medical Center, Andrews, TX, p. A578
TIPPS, Linda, Director Human Resources, Southern Tennessee Medical Center, Winchester, TN, p. A576
TIPTON, Peggy, Chief Operating Officer and Chief Nursing Officer, Oklahoma Heart Hospital, Oklahoma City, OK, p. A501
TIPTON, Silvia A., Chief Financial Officer and Director Human Resources, Throckmorton County Memorial Hospital, Throckmorton, TX, p. A631
TIRA, Cheryl, Director Information Systems, Columbus Community Hospital, Columbus, NE, p. A382
TIRMAN, Kerry R., FACHE President, Mississippi Baptist Medical Center, Jackson, MS, p. A348
TISCHLER, James F., M.D. Chief of Staff, Veterans Affairs Medical Center, Coatesville, PA, p. A521
TISDALE, Willis E., Director Human Resources, Shriners Hospitals for Children, Greenville, Greenville, SC, p. A550
TISDALL, Renae, Chief Financial Officer, Mobridge Regional Hospital, Mobridge, SD, p. A558
TISSIER, Becky, Chief Fiscal Service, Veterans Affairs Illiana Health Care System, Danville, IL, p. A179
TITSWORTH, Sue, Director Human Resources, Coleman County Medical Center, Coleman, TX, p. A588
TITTLE, JoDee, Human Resources Director, Mountain View Hospital District, Madras, OR, p. A512
TITUS, Marilyn, Vice President and Chief Operating Officer, Hillside Rehabilitation Hospital, Warren, OH, p. A490
TOADVINE, Stephen, M.D. Chief Medical Officer, Hardin Memorial Hospital, Elizabethtown, KY, p. A249
TOBEY, Shelley R., R.N. Chief Operating Officer and Chief Nursing Officer, Texas Health Presbyterian Hospital Flower Mound, Flower Mound, TX, p. A597
TOBIN, Hugh, Chief Financial Officer, DeKalb Regional Medical Center, Fort Payne, AL, p. A20
TOBIN, Timothy, M.D. Chief of Staff, Longview Regional Medical Center, Longview, TX, p. A613
TOBIN, Timothy C., FACHE President and Chief Executive Officer, Spotsylvania Regional Medical Center, Fredericksburg, VA, p. A648
TOBLER, Randy, M.D. Chief Medical Officer, Scotland County Hospital, Memphis, MO, p. A365
TOBON–STEVENS, Paula, Associate Administrator, Angleton Danbury Medical Center, Angleton, TX, p. A579
TODD, Bob, Director Information Systems, Mount Auburn Hospital, Cambridge, MA, p. A299
TODD, David, M.D. President Medical Staff, Memorial Specialty Hospital, Lufkin, TX, p. A614
TODD, Dianna, Director Human Resources, Boulder City Hospital, Boulder City, NV, p. A391
TODD, Fred O., Senior Vice President Finance, McLeod Loris Healthcare, Loris, SC, p. A552
TODD, James, Chief Financial Officer, River Oaks Hospital, New Orleans, LA, p. A275
TODD, Jansen, D.O. Chief of Staff, Woodland Heights Medical Center, Lufkin, TX, p. A614
TODD, Robbie, Director Information Technology, Horn Memorial Hospital, Ida Grove, IA, p. A221
TODD, Steve J., Chief Operating Officer, St. Luke Community Hospital, Ronan, MT, p. A378
TODOROW, Thomas, Chief Financial Officer, Children's Hospital of Philadelphia, Philadelphia, PA, p. A532
TOEBBE, Nelson, Chief Executive Officer, St. John's Episcopal Hospital–South Shore,, NY, p. A437
TOEDT, Michael E., M.D. Director Clinical Services, Cherokee Indian Hospital, Cherokee, NC, p. A451
TOERING, Marla, Chief Operating Officer, Sioux Center Community Hospital and Health Center Avera, Sioux Center, IA, p. A226
TOFANI, Gerald, Chief Financial Officer, Monmouth Medical Center, Long Branch, NJ, p. A405
TOL, Daryl, Chief Executive Officer, Florida Hospital Memorial Medical Center, Daytona Beach, FL, p. A121
TOLBERT, Sue, Chief Financial Officer, Earl K. Long Medical Center, Baton Rouge, LA, p. A262
TOLEFREE, Paulette, Chief Nursing Officer, Bradley County Medical Center, Warren, AR, p. A52
TOLLEFSON, Sue, Coordinator Payroll Personnel, Granite Falls Municipal Hospital and Manor, Granite Falls, MN, p. A332
TOLLESON, Kerry, Chief Financial Officer, Creighton University Medical Center, Omaha, NE, p. A387
TOLLEY, Cherie, Chief Executive Officer, Palmetto Lowcountry Behavioral Health, Charleston, SC, p. A547
TOLOSKY, Mark R., FACHE President and Chief Executive Officer, Baystate Health, Inc., Springfield, MA, p. B20
TOLOSKY, Mark R., FACHE President and Chief Executive Officer, Baystate Medical Center, Springfield, MA, p. A304
TOLOZA, Eileen, M.D. Chief of Staff, Peterson Regional Medical Center, Kerrville, TX, p. A610
TOLSON, Rick, Chief Administrative Officer and Chief Human Resources Officer, Christ Hospital, Cincinnati, OH, p. A473
TOM, Adrian, Supervisor Management Information Systems, Hopi Health Care Center, Keams Canyon, AZ, p. A33
TOMAS, George, Director Information Services, Griffin Hospital, Derby, CT, p. A108
TOMASINO, Tom, Administrator and Chief Executive Officer, Whidbey General Hospital, Coupeville, WA, p. A660
TOMASSETTI, Dennis, Chief Financial Officer, UPMC Passavant, Pittsburgh, PA, p. A535
TOMBERLIN, Terri, Manager Human Resources, Curry General Hospital, Gold Beach, OR, p. A510
TOMIMOTO, Ty, Acting Vice President Financial Affairs, Rehabilitation Hospital of the Pacific, Honolulu, HI, p. A164
TOMLIN, Kerry W., Associate Administrator, Clay County Hospital, Ashland, AL, p. A15

Index of Health Care Professionals

Index of Health Care Professionals / Tomlinson

TOMLINSON, Charles M., M.D. Vice President and Chief Medical Officer, Crawley Memorial Hospital, Boiling Springs, NC, p. A449
TOMLINSON, Daniel, Chair Human Resources, Mayo Clinic Jacksonville, Jacksonville, FL, p. A126
TOMLINSON, David
Senior Vice President, Chief Information Officer, Centegra Hospital – McHenry, McHenry, IL, p. A187
Senior Vice President, Chief Information Officer, Centegra Hospital – Woodstock, Woodstock, IL, p. A196
TOMLINSON, Sallie, Manager Human Resources, Arbuckle Memorial Hospital, Sulphur, OK, p. A505
TOMO, Ronald A., Vice President and Chief Information Officer, Nassau University Medical Center, East Meadow, NY, p. A425
TOMORY, Gerald, M.D
Regional Medical Director, Kauai Veterans Memorial Hospital, Waimea, HI, p. A165
Regional Medical Director, Samuel Mahelona Memorial Hospital, Kapaa, HI, p. A164
TOMPKINS, Charles, M.D. Chief of Staff, Crenshaw Community Hospital, Luverne, AL, p. A22
TOMPKINS, John, Administrator, Pioneer Community Hospital of Aberdeen, Aberdeen, MS, p. A343
TOMPKINS, Kim, Director Information Services, DeTar Healthcare System, Victoria, TX, p. A633
TOMPKINS, Ronald G., M.D. Chief of Staff and Director Research, Shriners Hospitals for Children–Boston, Boston, MA, p. A297
TONA, Vinod, M.D. President Medical Staff, Regency Hospital of Florence, Florence, SC, p. A550
TONEY, Mark, President and Chief Executive Officer, Brookdale Hospital Medical Center,, NY, p. A431
TONEY, Scott, R.N. Chief Nursing Officer, HEALTHSOUTH Northern Kentucky Rehabilitation Hospital, Edgewood, KY, p. A249
TONG, Cheryl, Chief Financial Officer, Antelope Valley Hospital, Lancaster, CA, p. A67
TONGATE, Scott, Chief Executive Officer, Lauderdale Community Hospital, Ripley, TN, p. A575
TONJES, Ken, Chief Financial Officer, PeaceHealth Ketchikan Medical Center, Ketchikan, AK, p. A29
TONNU, Lannie, Senior Vice President and Chief Financial Officer, Children's Hospital Los Angeles, Los Angeles, CA, p. A69
TOOKE, Landon, Chief Executive Officer, Reeves Memorial Medical Center, Bernice, LA, p. A263
TOOKE, Michael, M.D
Vice President Medical Affairs, Dorchester General Hospital, Cambridge, MD, p. A290
Chief Medical Officer, Memorial Hospital at Easton Maryland, Easton, MD, p. A291
TOOKE, Ryan, Interim Chief Executive Officer, Rosebud Health Care Center, Forsyth, MT, p. A375
TOOKER, Deby, Director Human Resources, Surgical Specialty Hospital of Arizona, Phoenix, AZ, p. A37
TOOLE, LaDon
Administrator, Brooks County Hospital, Quitman, GA, p. A157
Chief Operating Officer and Administrator, Grady General Hospital, Cairo, GA, p. A148
Chief Operating Officer and Administrator, Grady General Hospital, Cairo, GA, p. A148
TOOLE, Patricia, Vice President Human Resources, East Mountain Hospital, Belle Mead, NJ, p. A401
TOOLE, Trish, Vice President Administrative Services, Carrier Clinic, Belle Mead, NJ, p. A401
TOOLEY, Stan, President and Chief Executive Officer, Southwest Regional Rehabilitation Center, Battle Creek, MI, p. A308
TOOMEY, Richard Kirk, FACHE President and Chief Executive Officer, Beaufort Memorial Hospital, Beaufort, SC, p. A546
TOON, William, Director Information Technology, Wesley Medical Center, Hattiesburg, MS, p. A347
TOPALSKY, George V., M.D. Vice President Medical Operations, Marymount Hospital, Garfield Heights, OH, p. A481
TOPMILLER, Darrell, Director Finance, Fulton County Health Center, Wauseon, OH, p. A491
TOPP III, Walter W., Administrator, Houston Hospital for Specialized Surgery, Houston, TX, p. A604
TOPPER, David, Chief Executive Officer, Alta Healthcare System, Los Angeles, CA, p. B9
TOPPER, John E., Senior Vice President and Chief Financial Officer, Mercy Medical Center, Baltimore, MD, p. A288
TORCHIA, Joseph, M.D. Senior Vice President Medical Affairs and Chief Medical Officer, Holy Spirit Hospital, Camp Hill, PA, p. A519
TORCHIA, Jude, Chief Executive Officer, OrthoColorado Hospital, Lakewood, CO, p. A103
TORDESILLAS, Victor, Director Human Resources, Arrowhead Regional Medical Center, Colton, CA, p. A58
TORMANEN, John, Director Mission and Human Resources, St. Joseph's Area Health Services, Park Rapids, MN, p. A337
TORN, Michael, Chief Executive Officer, Edgewood Surgical Hospital, Transfer, PA, p. A539
TOROSSIAN, Lynn M., President, Huron Valley–Sinai Hospital, Commerce Township, MI, p. A310
TORRES, Harvey, Vice President Finance and Chief Financial Officer, Harlingen Medical Center, Harlingen, TX, p. A602
TORRES AYALA, Eugenio, Director Information Systems, Cardiovascular Center of Puerto Rico and the Caribbean, San Juan, PR, p. A702
TORTELLA, Anthony, Chief Financial Officer, Fairmount Behavioral Health System, Philadelphia, PA, p. A532
TOSADO, Damaris, Manager Human Resources, Veterans Affairs Medical Center, San Juan, PR, p. A704
TOSI, Stephen, M.D. Chief Medical Officer, UMass Memorial Medical Center, Worcester, MA, p. A306
TOSTENSON, Brad, Chief Information Officer, Essentia Health–Holy Trinity Hospital, Graceville, MN, p. A332
TOSTI, Debra, Interim Chief Executive Officer, Tewksbury Hospital, Tewksbury, MA, p. A305
TOTH, Jackie, Administrator, Acute Care Specialty Hospital of Aultman, Canton, OH, p. A472
TOUPS, Sharon A., Senior Vice President and Chief Operating Officer, St. Tammany Parish Hospital, Covington, LA, p. A265
TOURIGNY, Barry, Vice President Human Resources and Organizational Development, Cabell Huntington Hospital, Huntington, WV, p. A672
TOUROS, Krista, Assistant Administrator Finance, Sutter Lakeside Hospital, Lakeport, CA, p. A66
TOUSIGNANT, Grace, R.N. Chief Nursing Officer, Aspirus Keweenaw Hospital, Laurium, MI, p. A317
TOUVELLE, Cynthia, R.N. Senior Director Care Management and Chief Nursing Officer, Barnesville Hospital, Barnesville, OH, p. A470
TOWERS, Darleen, Director Human Resources, Lake Whitney Medical Center, Whitney, TX, p. A635
TOWLE, Michael, Vice President Finance, Alice Hyde Medical Center, Malone, NY, p. A429
TOWLE, Sonya, Director Human Resources, Mercy Hospital, Moose Lake, MN, p. A336
TOWN, Alex, Chief Financial Officer, Tri–State Memorial Hospital, Clarkston, WA, p. A660
TOWNER, Chad, Chief Executive Officer, Dupont Hospital, Fort Wayne, IN, p. A201
TOWNES, Tim, Director Information Systems, Trinity Medical Center, Birmingham, AL, p. A17
TOWNLEY, Nancy, R.N. Senior Vice President Operations, United Regional Health Care System, Wichita Falls, TX, p. A635
TOWNSDIN–WOODRUFF, Patricia J., President and Chief Executive Officer, Minnesota Valley Health Center, Le Sueur, MN, p. A333
TOWNSEND, Cathy, Chief Nursing Officer, Banner Ironwood Medical Center, San Tan Valley, AZ, p. A38
TOWNSEND, Dona E., Chief Nursing Officer, Northeastern Nevada Regional Hospital, Elko, NV, p. A391
TOWNSEND, Gary, Chief Information Officer, Hurley Medical Center, Flint, MI, p. A312
TOWNSEND, Roxane A., M.D
Chief Executive Officer, Earl K. Long Medical Center, Baton Rouge, LA, p. A262
Chief Executive Officer, Interim LSU Public Hospital, New Orleans, LA, p. A274
TOWNSEND, Roxane A., M.D. Chief Executive Officer, LSU Health Care Services Division, Baton Rouge, LA, p. B83
TOWNSEND, Tanya
Chief Information Officer, St. Mary's Hospital Medical Center, Green Bay, WI, p. A682
Chief Information Officer, St. Vincent Hospital, Green Bay, WI, p. A682
TOWNSEND, Theodore E., FACHE President and Chief Executive Officer, St. Luke's Hospital, Cedar Rapids, IA, p. A215
TOWNSLEY, Malcolm, M.D. Chief of Staff, St. Anthony Hospital, Pendleton, OR, p. A513
TOY, Linda, Director Information Systems, Havasu Regional Medical Center, Lake Havasu City, AZ, p. A33
TOYE, Lawrence J., Chief Financial Officer, Kindred Hospital–Boston, Brighton, MA, p. A298
TOZER, Charles, Chief Executive Officer, Spectrum Health Special Care Hospital, Grand Rapids, MI, p. A314
TOZIER, Kenneth, M.D. Chief of Surgery, Milan General Hospital, Milan, TN, p. A572
TRACEY, Karen, Chief Human Resources, Select Specialty Hospital–Greensboro, Greensboro, NC, p. A454
TRACHTA, Michael D., FACHE Executive Vice President and Chief Operating Officer, Mercy Medical Center, Cedar Rapids, IA, p. A215
TRACKWELL, Anita M., R.N. Chief Nursing Officer, Johnson Memorial Hospital, Franklin, IN, p. A202
TRACY, Allen R., Senior Vice President and Chief Financial Officer, St. John Medical Center, Westlake, OH, p. A491
TRACY, Larry, FACHE Chief Operating Officer, Barnes–Jewish West County Hospital, Saint Louis, MO, p. A368
TRACY, Timothy J., Chief Executive Officer, Sanford Vermillion Medical Center, Vermillion, SD, p. A560
TRAHAN, Lyman, Chief Executive Officer, Abrom Kaplan Memorial Hospital, Kaplan, LA, p. A269
TRAHERN, Sheri
Chief Financial Officer, St. Mary–Corwin Medical Center, Pueblo, CO, p. A105
Chief Administrative Officer and Chief Financial Officer, St. Thomas More Hospital, Canon City, CO, p. A98
TRAIL, Alan, Director Information Systems, Muhlenberg Community Hospital, Greenville, KY, p. A251
TRAINER, Michael, Chief Financial Officer, Akron Children's Hospital, Akron, OH, p. A469
TRAINOR, Karyn, Director Human Resources, St. Patrick Hospital, Missoula, MT, p. A378
TRAINOR, Sara, Chief Financial Officer, Community Memorial Hospital, Sumner, IA, p. A227
TRAISTER, Lynne, Controller, Rehabilitation Hospital of Tinton Falls, Tinton Falls, NJ, p. A410
TRAMMELL, Angela, Controller, Trinity Hospital Twin City, Dennison, OH, p. A479
TRAMMELL, Patrick, Chief Executive Officer, Cherokee Medical Center, Centre, AL, p. A18
TRAMP, Francis G., President, Burgess Health Center, Onawa, IA, p. A224
TRAN, Khiem, M.D. Acting Chief of Staff, Veterans Affairs Illiana Health Care System, Danville, IL, p. A179
TRAN, Lac, Senior Vice President Information Services, Rush University Medical Center, Chicago, IL, p. A178
TRAN, Liz, Director Human Resources, Bellflower Medical Center, Bellflower, CA, p. A55
TRANQUILLO, Stephen, Chief Information Officer, Thomas Jefferson University Hospital, Philadelphia, PA, p. A534
TRANTALIS, Cary, R.N. Vice President Operations, Windham Hospital, Willimantic, CT, p. A113
TRANTHAM, Susan, Director Human Resources, HEALTHSOUTH Rehabilitation Hospital, Florence, SC, p. A549
TRAUB, Bruce, Chief Financial Officer, University Medical Center of Princeton at Plainsboro, Plainsboro, NJ, p. A409
TRAUTMAN, Robert J., Chief Executive Officer, Regency Hospital of Hattiesburg, Hattiesburg, MS, p. A347
TRAVIS, David A.
Chief Financial Officer, East Texas Medical Center Athens, Athens, TX, p. A580
Chief Financial Officer, East Texas Medical Center Fairfield, Fairfield, TX, p. A597
TRAVIS, Dee Dee, Director Community Relations, Calais Regional Hospital, Calais, ME, p. A282
TRAVIS, Stephen, M.D. Chief of Staff, Mercy Hospital Logan County, Guthrie, OK, p. A497
TRAYLOR, Jerri Sue, Manager Human Resources, The Women's Hospital, Newburgh, IN, p. A210
TRAYLOR, Robert, Flight Commander Medical Information Systems, U. S. Air Force Regional Hospital, Elmendorf AFB, AK, p. A28
TRAYNOR, Karen, Chief Financial Officer, Richland Hospital, Richland Center, WI, p. A690
TRCZINSKI, Judi, Vice President and Chief Human Resources Officer, Hospital for Special Care, New Britain, CT, p. A110
TREACY, Nancy, Director Finance, Cambridge Medical Center, Cambridge, MN, p. A329
TREACY–SHIFF, Mary, Vice President Finance, Advocate Good Samaritan Hospital, Downers Grove, IL, p. A180
TREADWAY, Michael G., Controller, Trinity Mother Frances Rehabilitation Hospital, Tyler, TX, p. A632
TREADWELL, Karen, Director Human Resources, Lake Martin Community Hospital, Dadeville, AL, p. A18
TREASE, Kevin, Chief Information Officer, Antelope Memorial Hospital, Neligh, NE, p. A386
TREASURE, Jeffrey S., Senior Vice President Finance and Chief Financial Officer, Glens Falls Hospital, Glens Falls, NY, p. A426
TREASURE, Martin
Director Human Resources, Schuylkill Medical Center – East Norwegian Street, Pottsville, PA, p. A536
Director Human Resources, Schuylkill Medical Center – South Jackson Street, Pottsville, PA, p. A536
TREFNEY, Frank, M.D. Chief Medical Staff, Williamsburg Regional Hospital, Kingstree, SC, p. A551
TREGLOWN, Brad, Director Information Systems, Redmond Regional Medical Center, Rome, GA, p. A158
TREHAN, Rajeev, M.D. Chief of Staff, Veterans Affairs Eastern Kansas Health Care System, Topeka, KS, p. A244
TREMAINE, Richard, Associate Director, Veterans Affairs Medical Center, Leeds, MA, p. A301
TREMBLAY, Marilyn, Director Information, Regional Medical Center, Orangeburg, SC, p. A553

A950 Index of Health Care Professionals 

Index of Health Care Professionals / Turgeon

Index of Health Care Professionals


TREMBLE, John, Chief Financial Officer, St. Croix Regional Medical Center, St. Croix Falls, WI, p. A691
TREMBULAK, Frank J., Executive Vice President and Chief Operating Officer, Geisinger Medical Center, Danville, PA, p. A521
TREMONTI, Carl
Chief Financial Officer, Mease Countryside Hospital, Safety Harbor, FL, p. A137
Chief Financial Officer, Mease Hospital Dunedin, Dunedin, FL, p. A122
Chief Financial Officer, Morton Plant Hospital, Clearwater, FL, p. A120
Chief Financial Officer, Morton Plant North Bay Hospital, New Port Richey, FL, p. A133
TREMONTI, Yvette, Vice President Human Resources, H. Lee Moffitt Cancer Center and Research Institute, Tampa, FL, p. A140
TRENARY, Thomas J., President, Baylor Medical Center at Garland, Garland, TX, p. A600
TRENDE, Gary D., FACH
Associate Director, Veterans Affairs Medical Center, Tuscaloosa, AL, p. A26
Chief Operating Officer, Veterans Affairs Tennessee Valley Healthcare System, Nashville, TN, p. A574
TRENKLE, Kevan, Chief Executive Officer, Citizens Medical Center, Colby, KS, p. A231
TRENT, Cindy, Manager Personnel, Fall River Hospital, Hot Springs, SD, p. A557
TREPAGNIER, Katherine, Director Human Resources, River Parishes Hospital, La Place, LA, p. A269
TRESSA, John, MSN, Chief Executive Officer, Park Plaza Hospital, Houston, TX, p. A606
TRETINA, Mike, Vice President and Chief Financial Officer, Mary Greeley Medical Center, Ames, IA, p. A214
TRETTER, Stan, M.D. President Medical Staff, Memorial Hospital and Health Care Center, Jasper, IN, p. A205
TREUTLEIN, Scott, M.D. Medical Director, Wyoming County Community Hospital, Warsaw, NY, p. A446
TREVATHAN, Dave, Director Information Systems, Rose Medical Center, Denver, CO, p. A100
TREVINO, Carlos, Chief Operating Officer, Mission Regional Medical Center, Mission, TX, p. A617
TREVINO, Guillermo, M.D. President Medical Staff, Wayne Hospital, Greenville, OH, p. A481
TREVINO, Paul, Administrator, CHRISTUS Hospital–St. Elizabeth, Beaumont, TX, p. A583
TREVISANI, Michael F., M.D
Vice President Medical Affairs and Chief Medical Officer, Chenango Memorial Hospital, Norwich, NY, p. A438
Executive Vice President and Chief Medical Officer, Delaware Valley Hospital, Walton, NY, p. A446
TREXLER, Don, Chief Executive Officer, Cypress Pointe Surgical Hospital, Hammond, LA, p. A267
TRIBBLE, Terry, Chief Financial Officer, East Central Regional Hospital, Augusta, GA, p. A146
TRICE, Richard
Director Operations, University Hospitals Conneaut Medical Center, Conneaut, OH, p. A478
Director Operations, University Hospitals Geneva Medical Center, Geneva, OH, p. A481
TRIEBES, David G., Chief Executive Officer, Samaritan Albany General Hospital, Albany, OR, p. A509
TRIGG, Pat, Coordinator Personnel and Credentialing, El Campo Memorial Hospital, El Campo, TX, p. A595
TRIGG, Terry, Director Human Resources, Wesley Medical Center, Hattiesburg, MS, p. A347
TRIGIANI, Charles, D.O. Medical Director, Hampton Behavioral Health Center, Westampton Township, NJ, p. A412
TRILIVAS, Judy, Vice President and Chief Operating Officer, The Mount Sinai Hospital of Queens,, NY, p. A437
TRIMBLE, Charley O., Chief Executive Officer, Grace Medical Center, Lubbock, TX, p. A614
TRIMBLE, Deborah, R.N. Chief Executive Officer, Paul B. Hall Regional Medical Center, Paintsville, KY, p. A257
TRIMBLE, Donald, CPA Chief Financial Officer, Vibra Specialty Hospital of Dallas, Desoto, TX, p. A594
TRIMBLE, Kevin T., FACHE President and Chief Executive Officer, Saint Luke's North Hospital – Barry Road, Kansas City, MO, p. A362
TRIMBLE, Melody, Chief Executive Officer, Sparks Regional Medical Center, Fort Smith, AR, p. A45
TRIMM, Robert M., Chief Administrative Officer, Mayo Clinic Health System in Waycross, Waycross, GA, p. A162
TRIMMER, Mary R., Interim Chief Operating Officer, Mount Carmel, Columbus, OH, p. A476
TRIMMER, Matt, Director Information Services, Mercy Medical Center–Dubuque, Dubuque, IA, p. A219
TRINIDAD, Terry, Director Management Information Systems, Clearfield Hospital, Clearfield, PA, p. A520
TRIPLETT, John, D.O. President Medical Staff, Saint Joseph – Martin, Martin, KY, p. A256
TRITTIN, Kim, Manager Human Resources, Mayo Clinic Health System in Red Wing, Red Wing, MN, p. A337
TROCINO, Mark
Chief Information Officer, DeKalb Medical at Hillandale, Lithonia, GA, p. A155
Chief Information Officer, DeKalb Medical at North Decatur, Decatur, GA, p. A151
TROGMAN, Richard, FACHE Chief Operating Officer, Woodland Hills Medical Center,, CA, p. A73
TROLLOPE, Grant, Chief Financial Officer, Northeastern Nevada Regional Hospital, Elko, NV, p. A391
TROMBLEY, Barb, Director Financial Services, Munising Memorial Hospital, Munising, MI, p. A319
TROMPETER, Dawn, Vice President Finance, Ottawa Regional Hospital and Healthcare Center, Ottawa, IL, p. A190
TRONCONE, Michael T., Chief Human Resources Officer, Calvary Hospital,, NY, p. A432
TROSCLAIR, Andree, Vice President Human Resources, Arkansas Children's Hospital, Little Rock, AR, p. A47
TROSIN, Jill A., R.N. Chief Nursing Officer, Memorial Hospital, Fremont, OH, p. A480
TROTTER, Wally, Director Human Resources, Mountain View Hospital, Payson, UT, p. A639
TROUSDALE, Cindy, Chief Financial Officer, Verdugo Hills Hospital, Glendale, CA, p. A63
TROUT, Gene, Chief Financial Officer, Canonsburg General Hospital, Canonsburg, PA, p. A520
TROUTMAN, Gary, CP
Chief Financial Officer, Baptist Hospitals of Southeast Texas, Beaumont, TX, p. A582
Chief Financial Officer, Baptist Orange Hospital, Orange, TX, p. A619
TROWER, Brad, Chief Executive Officer, Jenkins County Hospital, Millen, GA, p. A156
TROWERS, Boswell, Director, Marion–Citrus Mental Health Centers, Ocala, FL, p. A133
TROXELL, Larry, Chief Executive Officer, Seiling Community Hospital, Seiling, OK, p. A504
TROY, Peggy N., President and Chief Executive Officer, Children's Hospital and Health System, Milwaukee, WI, p. B31
TROY, Peggy N.
President and Chief Executive Officer, Children's Hospital of Wisconsin, Milwaukee, WI, p. A686
President and Chief Executive Officer, Children's Hospital of Wisconsin–Fox Valley, Neenah, WI, p. A687
TROYER, David, Chief Information Officer, Veterans Affairs Northern Indiana Health Care System, Fort Wayne, IN, p. A202
TROYER, Devin, M.D. Medical Director, HEALTHSOUTH Rehabilitation Hospital, Columbia, SC, p. A548
TROYO, Glynda, Chief Executive Officer, St. Theresa Specialty Hospital, Metairie, LA, p. A273
TRUAX, Bradley, M.D. Senior Vice President Medical Affairs and Chief Medical Officer, St. James Mercy Health System, Hornell, NY, p. A427
TRUAX, Christopher, Chief Executive Officer, Morrow County Hospital, Mount Gilead, OH, p. A485
TRUE, Janet E., M.D. Clinical Director, Kerrville State Hospital, Kerrville, TX, p. A610
TRUEBLOOD, Susan, Chief Executive Officer, Georgia Regional Hospital at Atlanta, Decatur, GA, p. A151
TRUESDALE, Jr., Fred A., Administrator, North Mississippi Medical Center–Iuka, Iuka, MS, p. A347
TRUITT, Louise, Vice President Human Resources, Capital Regional Medical Center, Tallahassee, FL, p. A140
TRUITT, Ron, Director Information Services, Palms of Pasadena Hospital, Saint Petersburg, FL, p. A138
TRUJILLO, Jesse, Chief Information Officer, St. Mark's Hospital, Salt Lake City, UT, p. A641
TRUKENMILLER, Denise, Director Human Resources, Burgess Health Center, Onawa, IA, p. A224
TRUMAN, Mark, Vice President of Operations, Floyd Memorial Hospital and Health Services, New Albany, IN, p. A209
TRUMP, Donald L., M.D. President and Chief Executive Officer, Roswell Park Cancer Institute, Buffalo, NY, p. A423
TRUNFIO, Joseph A., Ph.D. President and Chief Executive Officer, Atlantic Health, Morristown, NJ, p. B14
TRUSSELL, Robert, Administrator, Foundation Surgical Hospital of San Antonio, San Antonio, TX, p. A624
TRUWIT, Jonathon D., M.D. Chief Medical Officer, University of Virginia Medical Center, Charlottesville, VA, p. A646
TRZNADEL, Marc, Chief Nursing Officer, Loretto Hospital, Chicago, IL, p. A176
TSALATE, Cynthia, Human Resource Specialist, U. S. Public Health Service Indian Hospital, Zuni, NM, p. A419
TSAMBIRAS, Petros, M.D. Chief of Staff, Pasco Regional Medical Center, Dade City, FL, p. A121
TSENG, Allen, Administrative Director, Texas Health Harris Methodist Hospital Southwest Fort Worth, Fort Worth, TX, p. A599
TSO, Ronald, Chief Executive Officer, Chinle Comprehensive Health Care Facility, Chinle, AZ, p. A31
TSUI–WU, Jane, Interim Chief Information Officer, Stony Brook University Medical Center, Stony Brook, NY, p. A444
TUBBS, John, M.D. Chief of Staff, West Holt Memorial Hospital, Atkinson, NE, p. A381
TUBBS, Mary Beth, Chief Executive Officer, Acuity Specialty Hospital of New Jersey, Atlantic City, NJ, p. A401
TUCK, April E., Senior Director Human Resources, Copley Hospital, Morrisville, VT, p. A643
TUCKER, Carol, Worklife Services Consultant, Brighton Center for Recovery, Brighton, MI, p. A308
TUCKER, Carolyn, Director Human Resources, Island Hospital, Anacortes, WA, p. A659
TUCKER, Cathy, Director Human Resources, Iraan General Hospital, Iraan, TX, p. A608
TUCKER, Jr., G. Edward, Vice President Corporate Services, Forrest General Hospital, Hattiesburg, MS, p. A346
TUCKER, Gary, Senior Vice President Operations and Chief Operating Officer, Mount St. Mary's Hospital and Health Center, Lewiston, NY, p. A428
TUCKER, H. Jaquita, Executive Director Human Resources, Providence Hospital, Mobile, AL, p. A23
TUCKER, John A., Chief Executive Officer, Iberia Medical Center, New Iberia, LA, p. A274
TUCKER, John R., FACHE Administrator, Atmore Community Hospital, Atmore, AL, p. A16
TUCKER, Joseph B., Senior Vice President and Chief Financial Officer, Fort Washington Medical Center, Fort Washington, MD, p. A291
TUCKER, Joshua, Chief Executive Officer, Mercy Hospital Logan County, Guthrie, OK, p. A497
TUCKER, Lisa, Chief Information Officer, University Hospital McDuffie, Thomson, GA, p. A160
TUCKER, Rebecca
Chief Financial Officer, Integris Bass Baptist Health Center, Enid, OK, p. A496
Chief Financial Officer, Integris Bass Pavilion, Enid, OK, p. A496
TUCKER, Robert, M.D. Chief Medical Officer, Murray–Calloway County Hospital, Murray, KY, p. A257
TUCKER, Ron, Business Office Manager, Kiowa County Memorial Hospital, Greensburg, KS, p. A234
TUCKER, Sidney, Chief Executive Officer, North Runnels Hospital, Winters, TX, p. A636
TUCKER, Steven E., President and Chief Operating Officer, Memorial Medical Center, Johnstown, PA, p. A526
TUDOR, Nathan, Administrator and Chief Executive Officer, Otto Kaiser Memorial Hospital, Kenedy, TX, p. A610
TUELL, William J., MSN, Facility Director, Commonwealth Center for Children and Adolescents, Staunton, VA, p. A656
TUFTS, Patrick, M.D. Medical Director, Mineral Community Hospital, Superior, MT, p. A379
TULISIAK, Thomas, M.D. President, Medina Hospital, Medina, OH, p. A484
TULLMAN, Stephen M., Chief Executive Officer, Phoenixville Hospital, Phoenixville, PA, p. A534
TUMA, Bonnie, Human Resources Team Lead, National Institutes of Health Clinical Center, Bethesda, MD, p. A289
TUMLIN, Richard, Chief Operating Officer, Southern Hills Medical Center, Nashville, TN, p. A573
TUMMURU, Ramireddy K., M.D. Chief Medical Officer, Porter–Valparaiso Hospital Campus, Valparaiso, IN, p. A212
TUNGATE, Rex A.
Administrator, Casey County Hospital, Liberty, KY, p. A254
Administrator, Jane Todd Crawford Hospital, Greensburg, KY, p. A251
TUNNELL, Richard, Director Information Systems Technology and Health Management Information Systems, University of Medicine and Dentistry of New Jersey–University Hospital, Newark, NJ, p. A407
TUNNEY, Niona, Director Human Resources, Cochran Memorial Hospital, Morton, TX, p. A617
TUNSON, Lynn, Manager Medical Records, Complex Care Hospital at Tenaya, Las Vegas, NV, p. A392
TUPPER, Dave, Chief Executive Officer and Administrator, Horizon Specialty Hospital, Las Vegas, NV, p. A393
TUPPER, Kevin, Director Information Technology, Windham Hospital, Willimantic, CT, p. A113
TUPPONCE, David, M.D. Chief Medical Officer, Paradise Valley Hospital, Phoenix, AZ, p. A36
TURCO, Joseph, Director Human Resources, Columbus Regional Hospital, Columbus, IN, p. A199
TUREK, Beth, Site Manager Information Systems, Advocate South Suburban Hospital, Hazel Crest, IL, p. A184
TURGEON, Jim, Vice President Finance, Allegiance Behavioral Health Center of Plainview, Plainview, TX, p. A621


© 2012 AHA Guide Index of Health Care Professionals **A951**

Index of Health Care Professionals

Index of Health Care Professionals / Turk


TURK, Edward, Vice President Finance, Scripps Mercy Hospital, San Diego, CA, p. A86
TURKAL, Nick, M.D. President and Chief Executive Officer, Aurora Health Care, Milwaukee, WI, p. B15
TURKAL–BARRETT, Kari, Flight Commander Resource Management Officer, Mike O'Callaghan Federal Hospital, Nellis AFB, NV, p. A394
TURKEL, Brooks, Chief Executive Officer, Regional Hospital of Scranton, Scranton, PA, p. A538
TURLEY, Mary Ann, D.O. Medical Director, John C. Lincoln Deer Valley Hospital, Phoenix, AZ, p. A35
TURLEY, Susan S., Chief Financial Officer, Doctor's Hospital at Renaissance, Edinburg, TX, p. A595
TURMAN, Anna, Chief Information Officer, Chadron Community Hospital and Health Services, Chadron, NE, p. A382
TURNA, Tarlochan, M.D. Medical Director, Mayo Clinic Health System in Cannon Falls, Cannon Falls, MN, p. A329
TURNBULL, James, Vice President and Chief Information Officer, University of Utah Health Care – Hospital and Clinics, Salt Lake City, UT, p. A641
TURNER, Amy, Director Human Resources, Butler County Medical Center, Hamilton, OH, p. A481
TURNER, Bill, Vice President Human Resources, Valir Rehabilitation Hospital, Oklahoma City, OK, p. A502
TURNER, Brenda C.
Chief Human Resources Officer, Palomar Medical Center, Escondido, CA, p. A60
Chief Human Resources Officer, Pomerado Hospital, Poway, CA, p. A81
TURNER, Carol, President and Chief Executive Officer, Atrium Medical Center, Middletown, OH, p. A485
TURNER, Cindy R., Chief Executive Officer, Bacon County Hospital and Health System, Alma, GA, p. A144
TURNER, Dale, Vice President Human Resources, Reedsburg Area Medical Center, Reedsburg, WI, p. A690
TURNER, Dane J., Director Human Resources, West Branch Regional Medical Center, West Branch, MI, p. A325
TURNER, Deborah, Vice President Human Resources, St. Luke's Cornwall Hospital, Newburgh, NY, p. A438
TURNER, Farell, Chief Financial Officer, Appling Healthcare System, Baxley, GA, p. A147
TURNER, Farrell, Interim Administrator, Charlton Memorial Hospital, Folkston, GA, p. A152
TURNER, Glenda, Director Personnel, Oakwood Correctional Facility, Lima, OH, p. A483
TURNER, Jeff, FACHE Chief Executive Officer, Moore County Hospital District, Dumas, TX, p. A594
TURNER, John E., President and Chief Executive Officer, Behavioral Centers of America, Nashville, TN, p. B20
TURNER, Kathy, Director Human Resources, East Texas Medical Center Trinity, Trinity, TX, p. A631
TURNER, Kelly, Senior Vice President Finance and Chief Financial Officer, Glendale Adventist Medical Center, Glendale, CA, p. A63
TURNER, Linda, Manager Health Information Management, Brown County Community Treatment Center, Green Bay, WI, p. A682
TURNER, Marc, Chief Operating Officer, Palmetto Lowcountry Behavioral Health, Charleston, SC, p. A547
TURNER, Mark J., President and Chief Executive Officer, Memorial Hospital, Belleville, IL, p. A173
TURNER, Mark S., Chief Executive Officer, San Gorgonio Memorial Hospital, Banning, CA, p. A55
TURNER, Melissa, Senior Vice President Human Resources, Bridgeport Hospital, Bridgeport, CT, p. A108
TURNER, Michael, M.D. Chief of Staff, Abbeville Area Medical Center, Abbeville, SC, p. A546
TURNER, Nancy, Director Communications, Sutter Roseville Medical Center, Roseville, CA, p. A83
TURNER, Pamela, Executive Director, Bronx Psychiatric Center,, NY, p. A431
TURNER, Patricia, R.N. Director of Nursing, Sac–Osage Hospital, Osceola, MO, p. A366
TURNER, Randy, Chief Human Resource Management Services, Veterans Affairs Medical Center, Boise, ID, p. A167
TURNER, Robert A., Chief Executive Officer, Select Specialty Hospital–Longview, Longview, TX, p. A613
TURNER, Robert L., Ph.D. Chief Executive Officer, Holly Hill Hospital, Raleigh, NC, p. A459
TURNER, Saundra G., Director Human Resources, Jefferson Regional Medical Center, Crystal City, MO, p. A358
TURNER, Shelly, Chief Clinical Services Officer, Medical Center of Manchester, Manchester, TN, p. A570
TURNER, Sherrilyn, Director Human Resources, Southeast Colorado Hospital District, Springfield, CO, p. A105
TURNER, Spencer, Chief Executive Officer, Texas Health Presbyterian Hospital Flower Mound, Flower Mound, TX, p. A597
TURNER, Steve, Director Information Technology, Salem Township Hospital, Salem, IL, p. A193
TURNER, Wade, M.D. Chief of Staff, William Newton Hospital, Winfield, KS, p. A246
TURNEY, Brian, Chief Executive Officer, Kingman Regional Medical Center, Kingman, AZ, p. A33
TURNEY, Larry, Administrator, Cochran Memorial Hospital, Morton, TX, p. A617
TURNEY, Vern
Director Information Services, Lourdes Counseling Center, Richland, WA, p. A665
Director Information Technology, Lourdes Medical Center, Pasco, WA, p. A664
TURNQUIST, Carrie, Director Human Resources, Buena Vista Regional Medical Center, Storm Lake, IA, p. A227
TURPEN, Joann, Director Human Resources, Chilton Medical Center, Clanton, AL, p. A18
TURSKY, Martin, President and Chief Executive Officer, Firelands Regional Health System, Sandusky, OH, p. A488
TURSO, Janet, Controller, HEALTHSOUTH Rehabilitation Hospital of Toms River, Toms River, NJ, p. A411
TUSA, Edward A., Chief Financial Officer, Mayo Clinic Health System in Cannon Falls, Cannon Falls, MN, p. A329
TUSCANY, Joanne E.
Director Worklife Services, St. John Macomb–Oakland Hospital, Macomb Center, Warren, MI, p. A325
Director Work life Services, St. John Macomb–Oakland Hospital, Oakland Center, Madison Heights, MI, p. A318
TUSTEN, Jay, Chief Executive Officer, Stanton County Hospital, Johnson, KS, p. A235
TUTTLE, Jamie, Coordinator Human Resources, Warren Memorial Hospital, Friend, NE, p. A383
TUTTLE, William A., Interim Chief Executive Officer, Baptist Memorial Hospital–Tipton, Covington, TN, p. A564
TVEIT, Charles, Chief Operating Officer, Lake District Hospital, Lakeview, OR, p. A512
TWARDY, Cindi, Manager Human Resources, Meeker Memorial Hospital, Litchfield, MN, p. A333
TWIDALE, Margaret, Manager Information Systems, Kane Community Hospital, Kane, PA, p. A526
TWIDWELL, Lisa, Administrator, Madison Medical Center, Fredericktown, MO, p. A360
TWILLIGEAR, Cindy, Manager Human Resources, Veterans Affairs Medical Center – Alexandria, Pineville, LA, p. A276
TWO BEARS, Eric, Chief Information Officer, Pioneer Community Hospital of Newton, Newton, MS, p. A351
TYE, Angie, Director Human Resources, Waverly Health Center, Waverly, IA, p. A228
TYLER, Alan J., FACHE Director, Veterans Affairs Medical Center, Tuscaloosa, AL, p. A26
TYLER, Holley, R.N. Chief Nursing Officer, Valley Regional Medical Center, Brownsville, TX, p. A585
TYLER, James E., Vice President and Administrator, Carilion Giles Community Hospital, Pearisburg, VA, p. A653
TYLER, Philene, Chief Finance Officer, Chinle Comprehensive Health Care Facility, Chinle, AZ, p. A31
TYLER, Richard, Corporate Director Human Resources, Conway Regional Medical Center, Conway, AR, p. A43
TYLER, Rick, M.D. Vice President Medical Affairs, CHRISTUS Hospital–St. Elizabeth, Beaumont, TX, p. A583
TYLER, Rosamond M., Administrator, Tyler Holmes Memorial Hospital, Winona, MS, p. A354
TYLER, Tanya
Vice President Human Resources, Memorial Medical Center – Lufkin, Lufkin, TX, p. A614
Vice President Human Resources, Memorial Specialty Hospital, Lufkin, TX, p. A614
TYLKOWSKI, Chester, M.D. Chief of Staff, Shriners Hospitals for Children–Lexington, Lexington, KY, p. A253
TYNER, W. Russell, President and Chief Executive Officer, Baptist Health, Montgomery, AL, p. B17
TYNES, Jr., L. Lee, M.D. Medical Director, Central Louisiana State Hospital, Pineville, LA, p. A276
TYRA, Diana, Director Health Information, Kentucky River Medical Center, Jackson, KY, p. A252
TYRA, J. Allen, Chief Executive Officer, Crossgates River Oaks Hospital, Brandon, MS, p. A344
TYRRELL, Lawrence, Chief Financial Officer, Pacifica Hospital of the Valley,, CA, p. A71
TYRRELL, Shawn O., R.N. VP/Chief Nursing Officer, Adventist Hinsdale Hospital, Hinsdale, IL, p. A184
TYSON, Bill, Chief Information Officer, Veterans Affairs Medical Center, Miami, FL, p. A132
TYSON, Charlotte C., Chief Operating Officer, Lewis–Gale Medical Center, Salem, VA, p. A655
TYSON, Peggy, Director Human Resources, Research Psychiatric Center, Kansas City, MO, p. A362


## U


UBBING, Mina H., President and Chief Executive Officer, Fairfield Medical Center, Lancaster, OH, p. A482
UBER, Charlotte M., Chief Executive Officer, Warren State Hospital, Warren, PA, p. A540
UDALL, Ben, M.D. Chief of Staff, Kimble Hospital, Junction, TX, p. A609
UDALL, Jared, Chief Financial Officer, Rehabilitation Hospital of Southern New Mexico, Las Cruces, NM, p. A416
UFFER, Mark H., Chief Executive Officer, Colorado River Medical Center, Needles, CA, p. A76
UGHOUWA, Ejiro, M.D. Chief of Staff, Allen Parish Hospital, Kinder, LA, p. A269
UHLENKOTT, Muriel R., Human Resources Officer, Tri–State Memorial Hospital, Clarkston, WA, p. A660
UHLER, Denis, Manager Information Systems, Auburn Regional Medical Center, Auburn, WA, p. A659
UHLIK, Allen, M.D. Chief of Staff, Copper Basin Medical Center, Copperhill, TN, p. A564
UHLIR, Tricia, Chief Executive Officer, Fall River Hospital, Hot Springs, SD, p. A557
ULAND, Jonas S., Executive Director, Greene County General Hospital, Linton, IN, p. A207
ULBRICHT, John E., Chief Operating Officer, Laredo Medical Center, Laredo, TX, p. A612
ULBRICHT, William G., President, St. Anthony's Hospital, Saint Petersburg, FL, p. A138
ULDRICH, Patricia, R.N. Chief Nursing Officer, St. James Mercy Health System, Hornell, NY, p. A427
ULICNY, Gary R., Ph.D. President and Chief Executive Officer, Shepherd Center, Atlanta, GA, p. A146
ULLRICH, Nathan, M.D. Chief Medical Officer, Whitman Hospital and Medical Center, Colfax, WA, p. A660
ULMER, Carlton
Chief Executive Officer, Gulf Coast Medical Center, Panama City, FL, p. A135
Chief Operating Officer, Redmond Regional Medical Center, Rome, GA, p. A158
ULMER, Carol, Chief Executive Officer, Select Specialty Hospital–Sioux Falls, Sioux Falls, SD, p. A559
ULMER, Dean, Manager Information Services, Hot Springs Rehabilitation Center, Hot Springs National Park, AR, p. A46
ULREY, Chris, Director Management Information Systems, St. Luke's Behavioral Health Center, Phoenix, AZ, p. A36
ULRICH Jr., James P., President and Chief Executive Officer, Community Hospital, McCook, NE, p. A386
ULRICH, Tanya, Director Human Resources, Forbes Regional Hospital, Monroeville, PA, p. A529
ULSETH, Randy, Chief Executive Officer, FirstLight Health System, Mora, MN, p. A336
UMBEL, Gigi, Director Finance, University Hospitals Bedford Medical Center, Cleveland, OH, p. A475
UMPHREY, Thomas, Senior Vice President Human Resources, The Aroostook Medical Center, Presque Isle, ME, p. A285
UNDERWOOD, Debbie, Manager Human Resources, Plains Memorial Hospital, Dimmitt, TX, p. A594
UNDERWOOD, Ken, Chief Executive Officer, Hazel Hawkins Memorial Hospital, Hollister, CA, p. A64
UNDERWOOD, Mal, Interim Sr. VP and Chief Financial Officer, DeKalb Medical at North Decatur, Decatur, GA, p. A151
UNDERWOOD, Martha, Chief Human Resources Officer, Baptist Hospital, Nashville, TN, p. A573
UNDERWOOD, Patricia A., Chief Financial Officer, Magee Rehabilitation Hospital, Philadelphia, PA, p. A533
UNDERWOOD, Vickie, Director Human Resources, Wyandot Memorial Hospital, Upper Sandusky, OH, p. A490
UNELL, Deonna, Chief Executive Officer, Irving Coppell Surgical Hospital, Irving, TX, p. A609
UNG, Oon Soo, Chief Financial Officer, Columbia Hospital, West Palm Beach, FL, p. A142
UNGER, Kevin L., FACHE President and Chief Executive Officer, Poudre Valley Hospital, Fort Collins, CO, p. A101
UNRATH, Amy, Administrator Human Resources, St. Mary's Hospital Medical Center, Green Bay, WI, p. A682
UNRUH, Greg, Chief Executive Officer, Community Health Care System, Onaga, KS, p. A240
UNTCH, Matt, Controller, Research Psychiatric Center, Kansas City, MO, p. A362
UNZEN, John, Chief Financial Officer, Mille Lacs Health System, Onamia, MN, p. A336
UPADHYAY, Yogendra, M.D. Senior Vice President Medical Affairs, South Oaks Hospital, Amityville, NY, p. A420
UPCHURCH, Jim, M.D. Chief Medical Officer, Crow/Northern Cheyenne Hospital, Crow Agency, MT, p. A374
UPDIKE, Wanda, M.D. Chief of Staff, Salt Lake Regional Medical Center, Salt Lake City, UT, p. A641


**A952** Index of Health Care Professionals

UPFIELD, Jaclyn, Chief Operating Officer, G. Werber Bryan Psychiatric Hospital, Columbia, SC, p. A548

UPHAM, Kevin, Chief Human Resources Officer, Minneapolis Veterans Affairs Health Care System, Minneapolis, MN, p. A335

UPTON, Daniel, Vice President and Chief Financial Officer, Doylestown Hospital, Doylestown, PA, p. A522

UPTON, Scott, Administrator, Jane Phillips Nowata Health Center, Nowata, OK, p. A500

URADNIK, Michael, Chief Operating Officer, Fairfax Hospital, Kirkland, WA, p. A662

URBACH, Marlene, Chief Human Resources Officer, Doctors Hospital at White Rock Lake, Dallas, TX, p. A591

URBAN, Dan, Vice President of Finance, Monroe Hospital, Bloomington, IN, p. A198

URBAN, Frank
Chief Financial Officer, River Crest Hospital, San Angelo, TX, p. A624
Chief Financial Officer, Southwood Psychiatric Hospital, Pittsburgh, PA, p. A535

URBAN, Louise, R.N. Senior Vice President Patient Care Services and Chief Nursing Officer, Jefferson Regional Medical Center, Jefferson Hills, PA, p. A525

URBAN, Thomas S., Market Leader and President, Mercy Health – Fairfield Hospital, Fairfield, OH, p. A480

URBAN, Tom, Director Human Resources, Wills Memorial Hospital, Washington, GA, p. A162

URBANCSIK, Don
Director Finance, Euclid Hospital, Euclid, OH, p. A480
Director Finance, Lutheran Hospital, Cleveland, OH, p. A475

URBANSKI, Joanne, President and Chief Executive Officer, South Haven Health System, South Haven, MI, p. A323

URBANSKI, Pamela A., R.N. Chief Nursing Officer, Senior Vice President, Patient Care Services, Mercy Memorial Hospital System, Monroe, MI, p. A319

URBISTONDO, Lisa, Chief Financial Officer, Peach Regional Medical Center, Fort Valley, GA, p. A153

URDANETA, Alfonso, M.D. President Medical Staff, Washington County Hospital, Nashville, IL, p. A189

URLAUB, Charles J., President and Chief Executive Officer, Mercy Hospital, Buffalo, NY, p. A423

UROFSKY, Michele L., Executive Vice President and Chief Administrative Officer, Holy Redeemer Hospital and Medical Center, Meadowbrook, PA, p. A528

URVAND, Leslie O., Administrator, St. Luke's Hospital, Crosby, ND, p. A465

URZAK, Staci, Director Patient Care Services, Regional Health Services of Howard County, Cresco, IA, p. A217

USELMAN, Krista, Chief Executive Officer, HEALTHSOUTH Rehabilitation Hospital of North Houston, Conroe, TX, p. A588

USHAK, Don, Director Information Systems, New York Eye and Ear Infirmary, New York, NY, p. A435

USHER, David, Chief Financial Officer, Kimball Health Services, Kimball, NE, p. A385

USHER, Paul L., President and Chief Executive Officer, Marion General Hospital, Marion, IN, p. A208

USHIJIMA, Arthur A., President and Chief Executive Officer, Queen's Health Systems, Honolulu, HI, p. B108

USHIJIMA, Arthur A., President, Queen's Medical Center, Honolulu, HI, p. A164

UTECHT, Dawan, Chief Executive Officer, Community Behavioral Health Center, Fresno, CA, p. A62

UTECHT, Thomas, M.D. Chief Quality Officer, Community Regional Medical Center, Fresno, CA, p. A62

UTEMARK, Paul, Chief Executive Officer, Fillmore County Hospital, Geneva, NE, p. A383

UTLEY, Donna, Vice President Human Resources, Mercy San Juan Medical Center, Carmichael, CA, p. A56

UTLEY, Kelly, Chief Financial Officer, Sidney Regional Medical Center, Sidney, NE, p. A389

UTTARO, Thomas, Executive Director, South Beach Psychiatric Center,, NY, p. A436

UTTENDORFSKY, Rob, Director Information Management, Lewis County General Hospital, Lowville, NY, p. A429

UTTERBACK, Julie, Vice President and Chief Financial Officer, Methodist Medical Center of Oak Ridge, Oak Ridge, TN, p. A574

UY, Rogelio, M.D. Chief of Staff, Middlesboro ARH Hospital, Middlesboro, KY, p. A256

UYEMURA, Monte, M.D. Chief of Staff, Wray Community District Hospital, Wray, CO, p. A107

UZZELL, Justina M.
Chief Human Resources Officer, Banner Baywood Medical Center, Mesa, AZ, p. A34
Chief People Resources Officer, Banner Heart Hospital, Mesa, AZ, p. A34

# V

VAAGENES, Carl P., Chief Executive Officer, Douglas County Hospital, Alexandria, MN, p. A327

VAALER, Mark, M.D
Chief Medical Officer, South Florida Baptist Hospital, Plant City, FL, p. A136
Vice President Medical Staff Affairs, St. Joseph's Hospital, Tampa, FL, p. A141

VACHEK, Paul, Vice President of Finance/Operations, Saint Alphonsus Medical Center – Ontario, Ontario, OR, p. A513

VACHON, Scott, Director Information Technology, Littleton Regional Hospital, Littleton, NH, p. A399

VADEN, Jim, Director Information Systems, Lauderdale Community Hospital, Ripley, TN, p. A575

VAGANEK, Joseph B., Chief Financial Officer, Edward John Noble Hospital of Gouverneur, Gouverneur, NY, p. A427

VAGUE, Jeff, Regional Manager Information Systems, Mercy Hospitals of Bakersfield, Bakersfield, CA, p. A55

VAHLBERG, Susan, Director Employee and Community Relations, Walter Knox Memorial Hospital, Emmett, ID, p. A168

VAIL, B. J., Director Information Systems, Morehouse General Hospital, Bastrop, LA, p. A262

VAIL, Bryan, Chief Information Officer, Clement J. Zablocki Veterans Affairs Medical Center, Milwaukee, WI, p. A686

VAIL, Lisa M., R.N. Vice President, Patient Care, Liberty Hospital, Liberty, MO, p. A364

VAIL, Lucy M., Director Human Resources & Partner Relations, Sparrow Clinton Hospital, Saint Johns, MI, p. A322

VAIL, Ronald, M.D. Chief of Staff, Lower Umpqua Hospital District, Reedsport, OR, p. A515

VAIL, Terrence, Acting Chief Human Resources Management Services, Veterans Affairs Medical Center, San Francisco, CA, p. A87

VAILLANCOURT, Alex, Chief Information Officer, Christ Hospital, Cincinnati, OH, p. A473

VAILLANCOURT, Stacy, Vice President Marketing, Communications, Advocacy and Human Resources, Saint Agnes Medical Center, Fresno, CA, p. A62

VAIOLETI, Stephany, Administrator, Kahuku Medical Center, Kahuku, HI, p. A164

VAKHARIA, Mahaveer, M.D. Medical Director, RiverWoods Behavioral Health System, Riverdale, GA, p. A157

VALBUENA, Richard, M.D. Medical Director, Latimer County General Hospital, Wilburton, OK, p. A508

VALDERA, Trummell, Senior Vice President and Chief Human Resources Officer, Jackson Health System, Miami, FL, p. A131

VALDERAZ, Leonard, Administrator, Sunrise Canyon Hospital, Lubbock, TX, p. A614

VALDESPINO, Gustavo A., President and Chief Executive Officer, Valley Presbyterian Hospital,, CA, p. A72

VALDEZ, Alex, JD, Chief Executive Officer, Christus St. Vincent Regional Medical Center, Santa Fe, NM, p. A418

VALDEZ, Mary, Chief Operating Officer, South Texas Rehabilitation Hospital, Brownsville, TX, p. A585

VALENTE, Anthony, M.D. Vice President Medical Affairs, Hazleton General Hospital, Hazleton, PA, p. A525

VALENTI, James N., FACHE President and Chief Executive Officer, University Medical Center of El Paso, El Paso, TX, p. A597

VALENTIN, Taira, Interim Director Finance, Hospital Buen Samaritano, Aguadilla, PR, p. A699

VALENTINE, Gregory
Superintendent, Osawatomie State Hospital, Osawatomie, KS, p. A240
Superintendent, Rainbow Mental Health Facility, Kansas City, KS, p. A236

VALENTINE, Lisa R., Chief Operating Officer, Henrico Doctors' Hospital, Richmond, VA, p. A655

VALENTINE, Mark, President and Chief Executive Officer, The Heart Hospital Baylor Plano, Plano, TX, p. A621

VALENTINE, Robert A., Regional Administrator, Alegent Health–Community Memorial Hospital, Missouri Valley, IA, p. A223

VALENTO, Jessica, Director Information Systems, Range Regional Health Services, Hibbing, MN, p. A333

VALK, Keith, Vice President Human Resources, Aurelia Osborn Fox Memorial Hospital, Oneonta, NY, p. A439

VALLADOLID, Sara, M.D. Medical Director, Sage Memorial Hospital, Ganado, AZ, p. A32

VALLES, John, Senior Vice President and Chief Financial Officer, Loretto Hospital, Chicago, IL, p. A176

VALLEY, Curt, Customer Site Manager, McLaren Bay Region, Bay City, MI, p. A308

VALLIANT, Mary T., MS, Chief Executive Officer, Barnwell County Hospital, Barnwell, SC, p. A546

VALLIDO, Gabe, Chief Information Officer, Naval Hospital, Camp Pendleton, CA, p. A56

VALLIERE, George, Chief Executive Officer, Claremore Indian Hospital, Claremore, OK, p. A494

VALLIERE, Mark, M.D. Senior Vice President Medical Affairs and Chief Medical Officer, Mercy Medical Center, Cedar Rapids, IA, p. A215

VALLIERRE, Walter, Chief Administrative Officer, St. Elizabeths Hospital, Washington, DC, p. A117

VAMPRINE, Laurene, Senior Vice President Information Systems, Erlanger Medical Center, Chattanooga, TN, p. A563

VAN ARKEL, Terence, Vice President and Chief Financial Officer, Doctors Hospital, Augusta, GA, p. A146

VAN ARSDAL, Al, Director Human Resources, Covenant Medical Center, Saginaw, MI, p. A322

VAN BOENING, Jon, President and Chief Executive Officer, Bakersfield Memorial Hospital, Bakersfield, CA, p. A54

VAN BREE, Margaret M., Dr.PH, Chief Executive Officer, St. Luke's Episcopal Hospital, Houston, TX, p. A606

VAN BUREN, Shelly, Director Human Resources, Frances Mahon Deaconess Hospital, Glasgow, MT, p. A375

VAN BUSKIRK, George F., M.D. Chief of Staff, Veterans Affairs Medical Center, Bay Pines, FL, p. A118

VAN CAMP, Keith, Vice President Information Services, St. Dominic-Jackson Memorial Hospital, Jackson, MS, p. A348

VAN CLEAVE, Bruce L., M.D
Senior Vice President and Chief Medical Officer, Aurora Medical Center of Oshkosh, Oshkosh, WI, p. A688
Senior Vice President and Chief Medical Officer, Aurora St. Luke's Medical Center, Milwaukee, WI, p. A686

VAN CLEAVE, Vanetta, Chief Financial Officer, Yukon–Kuskokwim Delta Regional Hospital, Bethel, AK, p. A28

VAN DE KREEKE, Jeffrey, Senior Vice President Finance, Froedtert Memorial Lutheran Hospital, Milwaukee, WI, p. A686

VAN DECAR, Tama, M.D. Chief Medical Officer, Fort Walton Beach Medical Center, Fort Walton Beach, FL, p. A124

VAN DEE, Keith, Director Human Resources, Drew Memorial Hospital, Monticello, AR, p. A49

VAN DER HORST, Hendrik, Chief Information Officer, Ira Davenport Memorial Hospital, Bath, NY, p. A421

VAN DONSELAAR, Lois J., R.N. Vice President & Chief Nursing Officer, Borgess Medical Center, Kalamazoo, MI, p. A316

VAN DRIEL, Allen, FACHE Chief Operating Officer, Chadron Community Hospital and Health Services, Chadron, NE, p. A382

VAN ELSLANDER, Ken, Director, Brighton Center for Recovery, Brighton, MI, p. A308

VAN GHELUWE, Betty, Chief Operating Officer, Elmore Medical Center, Mountain Home, ID, p. A169

VAN GORDER, Chris D., FACHE President and Chief Executive Officer, Scripps Health, San Diego, CA, p. B114

VAN GRINSVEN, Gerard, President and Chief Executive Officer, Henry Ford West Bloomfield Hospital, West Bloomfield, MI, p. A325

VAN GUNDY, Milt, M.D. President Medical Staff, Marshalltown Medical & Surgical Center, Marshalltown, IA, p. A223

VAN HEININGEN, Robert, Vice President Human Resources, Johnson Memorial Hospital, Stafford Springs, CT, p. A112

VAN HEUSEN, Melanie, Director Human Resources, Gateways Hospital and Mental Health Center, Los Angeles, CA, p. A69

VAN HOFF, Cynthia, Chief Financial Officer, Sutter Solano Medical Center, Vallejo, CA, p. A94

VAN HORN, Allan, M.D. President Medical Staff, Methodist Charlton Medical Center, Dallas, TX, p. A591

VAN HORN, William, M.D. Medical Director, Lighthouse Care Center of Conway, Conway, SC, p. A549

VAN HYNING, Jill, Director Human Resources, Richland Memorial Hospital, Olney, IL, p. A190

VAN KAMPEN, Cindy, Chief Nursing Officer, North Ottawa Community Hospital, Grand Haven, MI, p. A313

VAN LOON, Glen, M.D. Chief of Staff, Marshall County Hospital, Benton, KY, p. A247

VAN LOOY, James, M.D. Chief Medical Executive, Altru Health System, Grand Forks, ND, p. A466

VAN LUVEN, Audrey C., Senior Vice President and Chief Human Resources Officer, Christiana Care Health System, Newark, DE, p. A114

VAN MATRE, Jennifer, Director Finance and Information Technology, Trinity Hospital, Weaverville, CA, p. A95

VAN MEETEREN, Robert, President and Chief Executive Officer, Reedsburg Area Medical Center, Reedsburg, WI, p. A690

Index of Health Care Professionals

Index of Health Care Professionals / Van Meter

VAN METER, Rex, President, INTEGRIS Canadian Valley Hospital, Yukon, OK, p. A508
VAN NORMAN, Steven, M.D. Medical Director, Dixie Regional Medical Center, Saint George, UT, p. A640
VAN NOY, William J., Chief Financial Officer, Tehachapi Valley Healthcare District, Tehachapi, CA, p. A92
VAN RYBROEK, Greg, Chief Executive Officer, Mendota Mental Health Institute, Madison, WI, p. A684
VAN SCOYK, Mitch, Manager Information Systems, Delta County Memorial Hospital, Delta, CO, p. A99
VAN STRATEN, Elizabeth, President and Chief Executive Officer, St. Bernard Hospital and Health Care Center, Chicago, IL, p. A178
VAN STRATTON, Kate, Manager Human Resources, University Hospitals Geneva Medical Center, Geneva, OH, p. A481
VAN VICKLE, Robin, Chief Financial Officer, Bristow Medical Center, Bristow, OK, p. A494
VAN VRANKEN, Arthur, M.D. Chief Medical Officer, Essentia Health–Holy Trinity Hospital, Graceville, MN, p. A332
VAN VRANKEN, Matthew, President, Spectrum Health Hospital Group, Spectrum Health Butterworth Hospital, Grand Rapids, MI, p. A314
VAN VRANKEN, Ross, Chief Executive Officer, University of Utah Neuropsychiatric Institute, Salt Lake City, UT, p. A641
VAN WHY, Susan, Director Human Resources, St. Luke's Hospital – Miners Campus, Coaldale, PA, p. A520
VAN WINKLE, Melanie, Chief Financial Officer, Mammoth Hospital, Mammoth Lakes, CA, p. A73
VAN ZANTEN, Niko, M.D. Chief of Staff, Sac–Osage Hospital, Osceola, MO, p. A366
VANASKIE, William F., Executive Vice President and Chief Operating Officer, Maricopa Integrated Health System, Phoenix, AZ, p. A36
VANBEEK, Jan, Chief Executive Officer, Crook County Medical Services District, Sundance, WY, p. A697
VANBOEKEL, Tony, Director Information Systems, Shasta Regional Medical Center, Redding, CA, p. A82
VANCE, Amy
  Executive Vice President and Chief Operating Officer, Presbyterian Hospital, Charlotte, NC, p. A451
  Executive Vice President and Chief Operating Officer, Presbyterian Hospital Matthews, Matthews, NC, p. A457
VANCE, Ellen B.
  Vice President Human Resources, Sheltering Arms Hospital South, Midlothian, VA, p. A651
  Vice President and Chief Human Resource Officer, Sheltering Arms Rehabilitation Hospital, Mechanicsville, VA, p. A651
VANCE, Mark, M.D. Chief Medical Officer, Quincy Valley Medical Center, Quincy, WA, p. A664
VANCE, Stacie, Vice President Clinical Services, Indiana Orthopaedic Hospital, Indianapolis, IN, p. A204
VANCONIA, R. Brent, President, St. Marys Health Center, Jefferson City, MO, p. A361
VANCOURT, Bernie, Chief Operating Officer, Bay Area Medical Center, Marinette, WI, p. A685
VANDENBARK, Heather, Human Resources Specialist, State Hospital North, Orofino, ID, p. A170
VANDENBERG, Andra, Director Human Resources, Butler County Health Care Center, David City, NE, p. A383
VANDENBOSCH, Darryl, Vice President and Chief Financial Officer, St. Bernardine Medical Center, San Bernardino, CA, p. A85
VANDENHOVEN, Tom, Chief Financial Officer, Takoma Regional Hospital, Greeneville, TN, p. A566
VANDER EYCK, Theresa, Administrator, Community Behavioral Health Hospital – Bemidji, Bemidji, MN, p. A328
VANDERHOOFT, J. Eric, M.D. President Medical Staff, St. Mark's Hospital, Salt Lake City, UT, p. A641
VANDERMARK, Jay H., Chief Financial Officer, Veterans Affairs Northern Indiana Health Care System, Fort Wayne, IN, p. A202
VANDERPOOL, Lee, Vice President, Dominican Hospital, Santa Cruz, CA, p. A90
VANDERSLICE, Doug, Vice President and Chief Financial Officer, St. Louis Children's Hospital, Saint Louis, MO, p. A370
VANDERSTEK, Eliott R., Chief Fiscal Service, Veterans Affairs Eastern Colorado Health Care System, Denver, CO, p. A100
VANDERSTOUW, Karl, Director Management Information Systems, Lenoir Memorial Hospital, Kinston, NC, p. A456
VANDERVLIET, William, M.D. Vice President Medical Affairs, Holland Hospital, Holland, MI, p. A315
VANDERWEGE, Larry, Administrator and Chief Executive Officer, Lindsborg Community Hospital, Lindsborg, KS, p. A238
VANDERWERF, Quinten, M.D. Chief Medical Officer, Eisenhower Medical Center, Rancho Mirage, CA, p. A81
VANDETTE, Joan, Vice President Human Resources, Brooks Memorial Hospital, Dunkirk, NY, p. A425
VANDEVEER Jr., Alden M., FACHE Chief Executive Officer, Kiowa District Hospital and Manor, Kiowa, KS, p. A236
VANDEWATER, David T., President and Chief Executive Officer, Ardent Health Services, Nashville, TN, p. B10
VANDEWEGE, Dana, Director Human Resources, Capital Medical Center, Olympia, WA, p. A663
VANDORT, Patti J., MSN Vice President Nursing/Chief Nursing Officer, Holland Hospital, Holland, MI, p. A315
VANDRUFF, John, M.D. Chief of Staff, Payson Regional Medical Center, Payson, AZ, p. A35
VANEK, James, Chief Executive Officer, Lavaca Medical Center, Hallettsville, TX, p. A602
VANES, Wendell, Chief Financial Officer, Saint Mary's Regional Medical Center, Russellville, AR, p. A51
VANGARI, Veena, R.N. Director of Nursing, Trinity Hospital, Weaverville, CA, p. A95
VANHAREN, James, M.D. Medical Director, Forest View Psychiatric Hospital, Grand Rapids, MI, p. A313
VANHOUWELING, Mason, Chief Operating Officer, Spring Valley Hospital Medical Center, Las Vegas, NV, p. A394
VANMARCKE, Thibaut, Chief Operating Officer, Medical Center of Trinity, Trinity, FL, p. A142
VANMEETREN, Victoria J., President, St. Rose Dominican Hospitals – San Martin Campus, Las Vegas, NV, p. A394
VANNESS II, William C., M.D. President, Community Hospital of Anderson and Madison County, Anderson, IN, p. A197
VANNETT, Vince, Director Human Resources, Jellico Community Hospital, Jellico, TN, p. A567
VANNOY, Patricia, Controller, Oakwood Southshore Medical Center, Trenton, MI, p. A324
VANOSDOL, Thomas J., President, Saint John's Health System, Anderson, IN, p. A197
VANSANT, Pam, Vice President and Chief Operating Officer, The Jewish Hospital, Cincinnati, OH, p. A474
VANSANT, Scott, M.D. Chief Medical Officer, Central State Hospital, Milledgeville, GA, p. A156
VANVEEN, Thomas, M.D. Chief Medical Officer, Santiam Memorial Hospital, Stayton, OR, p. A516
VANWICHEN, Ward C., Chief Executive Officer, Phillips County Hospital, Malta, MT, p. A377
VANWYHE, Brenda, Senior Vice President Finance and Chief Financial Officer, Rush–Copley Medical Center, Aurora, IL, p. A173
VARA, John, M.D. Chief of Staff, Veterans Affairs Medical Center, Miami, FL, p. A132
VARA, Raymond
  Chief Executive Officer, Kapiolani Medical Center for Women & Children, Honolulu, HI, p. A163
  Chief Executive Officer, Pali Momi Medical Center, Aiea, HI, p. A163
  Chief Executive Officer, Straub Clinic & Hospital, Honolulu, HI, p. A164
VARELA, Nancy, Director Human Resources, Patton State Hospital, Patton, CA, p. A80
VARGA, Patrick, Chief Operating Officer, Mercy Medical Center Redding, Redding, CA, p. A81
VARGAS, Jose L., M.D. Medical Director, West Gables Rehabilitation Hospital, Miami, FL, p. A132
VARGAS, Laura, Chief Executive Officer and Managing Director, San Juan Capestrano Hospital, San Juan, PR, p. A703
VARGAS, Margie, Director Human Resources, Memorial Hospital Pembroke, Pembroke Pines, FL, p. A135
VARGAS, Marisol, Director Finance, Hospital Del Maestro, San Juan, PR, p. A703
VARGAS, Nancy
  Director Human Resources, Mark Twain St. Joseph's Hospital, San Andreas, CA, p. A84
  Chief Human Resources, St. Joseph's Behavioral Health Center, Stockton, CA, p. A91
  Vice President Human Resources, St. Joseph's Medical Center, Stockton, CA, p. A92
VARGHESE, Roy, M.D. Chief of Staff, Mary Breckinridge ARH Hospital, Hyden, KY, p. A252
VARGHESE, Shibu, Vice President Human Resources, University of Texas M.D. Anderson Cancer Center, Houston, TX, p. A608
VARIAN, Grant, M.D. Medical Director, Mary Rutan Hospital, Bellefontaine, OH, p. A470
VARK, Lawrence, M.D. Chief Medical Officer, Creek Nation Community Hospital, Okemah, OK, p. A500
VARLAND, Drew, Chief Nursing Officer and Chief Operating Officer, Pioneers Medical Center, Meeker, CO, p. A104
VARLEY, Kevin
  Chief Financial Officer, Kindred Hospital–Heritage Valley, Beaver, PA, p. A518
  Chief Financial Officer, Kindred Hospital–Pittsburgh, Oakdale, PA, p. A531
VARNADO, Anjanette, M.D. Chief Medical Officer, St. Helena Parish Hospital, Greensburg, LA, p. A267
VARNADO, Darryl, Vice President Human Resources, University of Colorado Hospital, Aurora, CO, p. A97
VARNADO, Krystyna, Director Human Resources, Garden Park Medical Center, Gulfport, MS, p. A346
VARNADOE, Milo, Director Information Systems, Warm Springs Medical Center, Warm Springs, GA, p. A161
VARNER, Terry, Administrator, Yalobusha General Hospital, Water Valley, MS, p. A353
VARTELAS, Helene M., Acting Chief Executive Officer, Connecticut Valley Hospital, Middletown, CT, p. A110
VASHISHTA, Ashok, M.D
  Vice President Medical Affairs, McLaren Bay Region, Bay City, MI, p. A308
  Vice President Medical Affairs, McLaren Central Michigan, Mount Pleasant, MI, p. A319
VASKELIS, Glenna L., CPA, President and Administrator, Sequoia Hospital, Redwood City, CA, p. A82
VASQUEZ, Alberto, Administrator, Garfield Memorial Hospital and Clinics, Panguitch, UT, p. A639
VASQUEZ, Chris, Executive Vice President and Chief Operating Officer, University Health System, San Antonio, TX, p. A626
VASQUEZ, George
  Chief Technology Officer, Clovis Community Medical Center, Clovis, CA, p. A57
  Vice President Information Services, Community Behavioral Health Center, Fresno, CA, p. A62
VASQUEZ, Miguel, Chief Financial Officer, Sister Emmanuel Hospital, Miami, FL, p. A132
VASQUEZ, Nelson, Vice President Finance, Jackson Park Hospital and Medical Center, Chicago, IL, p. A176
VASQUEZ, Patty, Administrator, Cozby–Germany Hospital, Grand Saline, TX, p. A601
VASS, Kathy, Head Human Resources, Naval Hospital, Oak Harbor, WA, p. A663
VASSALL, John, M.D
  Chief Medical Officer, Swedish Medical Center–Cherry Hill Campus, Seattle, WA, p. A666
  Chief Medical Officer, Swedish Medical Center–First Hill, Seattle, WA, p. A666
VASSAR, Debra, Chief Nursing Officer, Arkansas Methodist Medical Center, Paragould, AR, p. A50
VASUNAGA, Amy, Chief Nurse Executive, Leahi Hospital, Honolulu, HI, p. A163
VATH, Richard, M.D. Vice President Medical Affairs, Our Lady of the Lake Regional Medical Center, Baton Rouge, LA, p. A262
VATSAVAI, Sundararama R., M.D. Medical Director, Baton Rouge Rehabilitation Hospital, Baton Rouge, LA, p. A262
VAUGHAN, Amanda, Chief Financial Officer, St. Catherine Hospital, Garden City, KS, p. A233
VAUGHAN, Brandon, Chief Financial Officer, Jacobson Memorial Hospital Care Center, Elgin, ND, p. A465
VAUGHAN, Brian, Chief Financial Officer, Lovelace Medical Center, Albuquerque, NM, p. A414
VAUGHAN, Page H., Chief Executive Officer, Chester Regional Medical Center, Chester, SC, p. A547
VAUGHAN, Peggy, M.D
  Senior Vice President Medical Affairs, Harford Memorial Hospital, Havre De Grace, MD, p. A292
  Senior Vice President Medical Affairs, Upper Chesapeake Medical Center, Bel Air, MD, p. A289
VAUGHAN, Rob, Chief Financial Officer, Carilion New River Valley Medical Center, Christiansburg, VA, p. A646
VAUGHN, Anita, Administrator and Chief Executive Officer, Baptist Memorial Hospital for Women, Memphis, TN, p. A571
VAUGHN, Barbara, Interim Chief Nursing Officer and Chief Operating Officer, Baylor Medical Center at Garland, Garland, TX, p. A600
VAUGHN, Dennise
  Vice President Corporate Resources, Edward Hospital, Naperville, IL, p. A189
  Vice President Corporate Resources, Linden Oaks Hospital at Edward, Naperville, IL, p. A189
VAUGHN, Kerry, Chief Information Officer, St. Mary's Health Care System, Athens, GA, p. A144
VAUGHN, Kevin P., Chief Financial Officer, Kansas Spine Hospital, Wichita, KS, p. A245
VAUGHN, Lindsey, M.D. President Medical Staff, Sentara Obici Hospital, Suffolk, VA, p. A656
VAUGHN, Michael, Chief Financial Officer, Monroe County Hospital, Monroeville, AL, p. A23
VAUGHN, Sandy, Director Information Services, Baylor All Saints Medical Center at Fort Worth, Fort Worth, TX, p. A598
VAUGHN, Ted W., Director Human Resources, Trinity Regional Medical Center, Fort Dodge, IA, p. A219
VAUGHT, Richard H., Administrator, William Newton Hospital, Winfield, KS, p. A246
VAZIRI, H. Kevin, President, Woodland Healthcare, Woodland, CA, p. A96
VAZQUEZ, Brunilda, Medical Director, State Psychiatric Hospital, San Juan, PR, p. A704
VAZQUEZ, Emilio, M.D. Chief Medical Officer, DeKalb Health, Auburn, IN, p. A197

**A954** Index of Health Care Professionals

VAZQUEZ, Francisco, Associate Director, Michael E. DeBakey Veterans Affairs Medical Center, Houston, TX, p. A606

VAZQUEZ, Manuel J., Executive Administrator, Hospital Oncologico Andres Grillasca, Ponce, PR, p. A702

VEENSTRA, Henry A., President, Spectrum Health Zeeland Community Hospital, Zeeland, MI, p. A326

VEGA, James, Director Information Systems, Palm Beach Gardens Medical Center, Palm Beach Gardens, FL, p. A135

VEGA, Maria, Director Human Resources, Auxilio Mutuo Hospital, San Juan, PR, p. A702

VEILLETTE, David, President and Chief Executive Officer, Western Regional Medical Center, Goodyear, AZ, p. A33

VEILLEUX, Jeffrey
Senior Vice President and Chief Financial Officer, Swedish Medical Center–Cherry Hill Campus, Seattle, WA, p. A666
Executive Vice President and Chief Financial Officer, Swedish Medical Center–First Hill, Seattle, WA, p. A666

VEILLON, Paul, CP
Chief Financial Officer, Advance Care Hospital, Hot Springs National Park, AR, p. A46
Chief Financial Officer, Advance Care Hospital of Fort Smith, Fort Smith, AR, p. A45
Chief Financial Officer, Mercy Continuing Care Hospital, Chesterfield, MO, p. A357

VEIT, Kathy, Director Health Information Services, Loring Hospital, Sac City, IA, p. A226

VEITH, Terry, Director Management Information Systems, Franciscan St. Anthony Health – Michigan City, Michigan City, IN, p. A208

VEITZ, Larry W., Chief Executive Officer, Spearfish Regional Hospital, Spearfish, SD, p. A560

VELA, Manuel, President and Chief Executive Officer, Valley Baptist Health System, Harlingen, TX, p. B141

VELASQUEZ, Alfred T., Area Information Officer, Riverside Medical Center, Riverside, CA, p. A83

VELASQUEZ, Carolina, Chief Information Officer, Uvalde County Hospital Authority, Uvalde, TX, p. A632

VELASQUEZ, Lin, Vice President Human Resources, Saint Louise Regional Hospital, Gilroy, CA, p. A63

VELASQUEZ, Roberto, M.D. Medical Director, Hospital Oncologico Andres Grillasca, Ponce, PR, p. A702

VELEZ, Pablo, Chief Executive Officer, Sharp Chula Vista Medical Center, Chula Vista, CA, p. A57

VELLINGA, David H., FACHE President and Chief Executive Officer, Mercy Medical Center–Des Moines, Des Moines, IA, p. A218

VELOSO, Kwang, Director Information Systems, Curry General Hospital, Gold Beach, OR, p. A510

VELTRI, Frank, M.D. President Medical Staff, Palo Alto County Health System, Emmetsburg, IA, p. A219

VELTRI, Gregory M., Chief Information Officer, Denver Health Medical Center, Denver, CO, p. A99

VELUSWAMY, Ragupathy, M.D. Vice President Medical Affairs, Wilkes–Barre General Hospital, Wilkes–Barre, PA, p. A542

VENABLE, Mark, Interim Director Human Resources, Shriners Hospitals for Children, St. Louis, Saint Louis, MO, p. A369

VENABLE, Robert, M.D. Chief Medical Staff, Washington County Hospital, Plymouth, NC, p. A458

VENANZI, William, M.D. Chief Medical Officer, Wright Patterson Medical Center, Wright–Patterson AFB, OH, p. A492

VENDETTI, Marilouise, M.D. Chief Medical Officer, AtlantiCare Regional Medical Center, Atlantic City, NJ, p. A401

VENEREO, Miguel, M.D. Director Medical Staff, Memorial Hospital West, Pembroke Pines, FL, p. A135

VENGCO, Joel L., MS Vice President and Chief Information Officer, Baystate Health, Baystate Mary Lane Hospital, Ware, MA, p. A305

VENHUIZEN, Pamela, Chief Human Resources Officer, Cooperstown Medical Center, Cooperstown, ND, p. A465

VENNES, Lorrie, Chief Financial Officer, Broadwater Health Center, Townsend, MT, p. A379

VENTAMEGLIA, Tom, Director Information Systems, Crittenton Hospital Medical Center, Rochester, MI, p. A321

VENTRESS, William L., Chief Executive Officer, Moccasin Bend Mental Health Institute, Chattanooga, TN, p. A563

VENTURELLA, James, Chief Information Officer, UPMC Presbyterian Shadyside, Pittsburgh, PA, p. A535

VENUTO, Cindy, Public Information Officer, Bear Valley Community Hospital, Big Bear Lake, CA, p. A55

VENUTO, Frank, Vice President Human Resources, Baltimore Washington Medical Center, Glen Burnie, MD, p. A292

VENUTO, Kenneth, Chief Financial Officer, St. Joseph's Hospital, Chippewa Falls, WI, p. A680

VENZANT, Shamada, Manager Health Information, Specialty Hospital of Winnfield, Winnfield, LA, p. A279

VERA, Luis F., M.D. Medical Director, Kensington Hospital, Philadelphia, PA, p. A533

VERBEKE, Lori, Chief Financial Officer, Timberlawn Mental Health System, Dallas, TX, p. A593

VERBUS, John R., Senior Vice President and Chief Operating Officer, Frederick Memorial Hospital, Frederick, MD, p. A291

VERCRUYSSE, Craig, Chief Information Officer, California Pacific Medical Center, San Francisco, CA, p. A86

VERDEJA, Juan–Carlos, M.D. President of Medical Staff, Baptist Health South Florida, West Kendall Baptist Hospital, Miami, FL, p. A131

VERDON, Chris, Director Finance, Phillips Eye Institute, Minneapolis, MN, p. A335

VERGNE, Roger T., Chief Fiscal Service, Hunter Holmes McGuire Veterans Affairs Medical Center, Richmond, VA, p. A655

VERGOS, Katherine, Chief Operating Officer, Ripon Medical Center, Ripon, WI, p. A690

VERMILLION, Kerry
Senior Vice President Finance and Chief Financial Officer, Baptist Hospital, Pensacola, FL, p. A136
Senior Vice President Finance and Chief Financial Officer, Gulf Breeze Hospital, Gulf Breeze, FL, p. A124

VERNERE, Mike, Executive Officer, Naval Hospital, Jacksonville, FL, p. A126

VERNON, Janice, Supervisory Information Technology Specialist, John J. Pershing Veterans Affairs Medical Center, Poplar Bluff, MO, p. A367

VERNON, Justin, Chief Operating Officer, Crittenden Regional Hospital, West Memphis, AR, p. A52

VERNON–YOUNG, Karen, Vice President Human Resources and Communications, CarePartners Health Services, Asheville, NC, p. A448

VERRET, Dean, Vice President Financial Services, Terrebonne General Medical Center, Houma, LA, p. A268

VERRETTE, Paula, M.D. Vice President Quality and Performance Improvement and Chief Medical Officer, Huntington Memorial Hospital, Pasadena, CA, p. A80

VERSECKES, Mike, Financial Officer, Terrell State Hospital, Terrell, TX, p. A630

VERZI, Dennis, Executive Director, St. Catherine of Siena Medical Center, Smithtown, NY, p. A443

VESTER, Nancy
Vice President Information Technology, Leesburg Regional Medical Center, Leesburg, FL, p. A129
Vice President and Chief Information Officer, The Villages Health System, The Villages, FL, p. A142

VETTER, Rich, M.D. Associate Chief, Essentia Health St. Mary's Hospital – Detroit Lakes, Detroit Lakes, MN, p. A330

VIALL, John, M.D. Vice President Medical Affairs, Holzer Medical Center, Gallipolis, OH, p. A480

VICCELLIO, Cathrine, Chief Nursing Officer, Select Long Term Care Hospital – Colorado Springs, Colorado Springs, CO, p. A98

VICENTE, Oscar, Chief Financial Officer, Palmetto General Hospital, Hialeah, FL, p. A125

VICENTI, Darren, M.D. Clinical Director, Hopi Health Care Center, Keams Canyon, AZ, p. A33

VICK, Dan J., M.D. Vice President of Medical Affairs and Chief Medical Officer, Oneida Healthcare, Oneida, NY, p. A439

VICK, David, Chief Information Officer, Elkhart General Healthcare System, Elkhart, IN, p. A200

VICKERS, Cynthia, R.N. Assistant Administrator for Nursing Services, Memorial Hospital and Manor, Bainbridge, GA, p. A147

VICKERS, Dave, Chief Financial Officer, Los Alamitos Medical Center, Los Alamitos, CA, p. A68

VICKERY, Ian, Director Information Technology, D. W. McMillan Memorial Hospital, Brewton, AL, p. A17

VICKNAIR, Joseph, Chief Information Officer, P & S Surgical Hospital, Monroe, LA, p. A273

VICKROY, Joseph, M.D. Medical Director, HEALTHSOUTH Rehabilitation Hospital of Utah, Sandy, UT, p. A641

VIDAURRE, Victor, Assistant Vice President Human Resources, St. Elizabeth Hospital, Gonzales, LA, p. A267

VIDRINE, Charmaine, CPA Chief Financial Officer, American Legion Hospital, Crowley, LA, p. A265

VIEIRA, Terri, Vice President Operations, Sebasticook Valley Health, Pittsfield, ME, p. A284

VIELKIND, James, Chief Financial Officer, Little Falls Hospital, Little Falls, NY, p. A428

VIENNEAU, Marie E., R.N. Chief Executive Officer, Millinocket Regional Hospital, Millinocket, ME, p. A284

VIERKANT, Matthew, M.D. President Medical Staff, Mother Frances Hospital – Jacksonville, Jacksonville, TX, p. A609

VIGGERS, Andreas, Director Human Resources, Providence Little Company of Mary Medical Center San Pedro,, CA, p. A71

VIGIL, Kevin, Director Information Systems, Los Alamos Medical Center, Los Alamos, NM, p. A417

VIGUS, Ronald J., Chief Executive Officer, Newberry County Memorial Hospital, Newberry, SC, p. A553

VILAR, Ramon J., Administrator, Wilma N. Vazquez Medical Center, Vega Baja, PR, p. A704

VILHAUER, Beverly, Chief Operating Officer and Chief Financial Officer, Linton Hospital, Linton, ND, p. A467

VILLA, Alex, Chief Executive Officer, Fallbrook Hospital, Fallbrook, CA, p. A60

VILLAFANI, J. Mario, M.D. Chief of Staff, Kingwood Medical Center, Kingwood, TX, p. A611

VILLAFLOR, Osias, M.D. Chief Medical Staff, Nicholas County Hospital, Carlisle, KY, p. A248

VILLALOBOS, Max
Senior Vice President, Vacaville Medical Center, Vacaville, CA, p. A94
Senior Vice President and Area Manager, Vallejo Medical Center, Vallejo, CA, p. A94

VILLANO, Jeremi, M.D. Chief of Staff, Crook County Medical Services District, Sundance, WY, p. A697

VILLANUEVA, Alice A.
Senior Vice President Human Resources, John Muir Behavioral Health Center, Concord, CA, p. A58
Vice President Human Resources, John Muir Medical Center, Concord, Concord, CA, p. A58
Senior Vice President Human Resources, John Muir Medical Center, Walnut Creek, Walnut Creek, CA, p. A95

VILLANUEVA, Jeffrey D., Vice President and Administrator, Rollins–Brook Community Hospital, Lampasas, TX, p. A611

VILLANUEVA, Yvette, Senior Associate Executive Director, Woodhull Medical and Mental Health Center,, NY, p. A438

VILLARAZA, II, Christopher, M.D. Chief Medical Staff, Grafton City Hospital, Grafton, WV, p. A672

VILLARREAL, Troy, Chief Executive Officer, Medical Center of Plano, Plano, TX, p. A621

VILLARREAL, Xavier, Chief Executive Officer, Navarro Regional Hospital, Corsicana, TX, p. A589

VILLEGAS, Lorraine, Manager Human Resources, Paradise Valley Hospital, National City, CA, p. A76

VILLEGAS, William, Chief Financial Officer, Jellico Community Hospital, Jellico, TN, p. A567

VILUMS, Karl, Chief Financial Officer, Ivinson Memorial Hospital, Laramie, WY, p. A696

VINAS, Elmo, Director Human Resources, Franklin Foundation Hospital, Franklin, LA, p. A266

VINCENT, Ben, FACHE Chief Executive Officer, Braxton County Memorial Hospital, Gassaway, WV, p. A671

VINCENT, Cynthia, Vice President Finance, St. Francis Regional Medical Center, Shakopee, MN, p. A340

VINCENT, David, Director Information Systems, Canonsburg General Hospital, Canonsburg, PA, p. A520

VINCENT, Larry, Director Human Resources, Delta County Memorial Hospital, Delta, CO, p. A99

VINCENT, Mitch, Vice President Organizational Support, Range Regional Health Services, Hibbing, MN, p. A333

VINCENT, Sherril, Vice President Finance/CFO, Alexian Brothers Acute Care Ministries, St. Alexius Medical Center, Hoffman Estates, IL, p. A185

VINNAKOTA, Radha, M.D. President Medical Staff, Robert Wood Johnson University Hospital Rahway, Rahway, NJ, p. A409

VINSEL, Douglas B., FACHE Chief Executive Officer, Duke Raleigh Hospital, Raleigh, NC, p. A459

VINSON, Roy C., Chief Executive Officer, Lubbock Heart Hospital, Lubbock, TX, p. A614

VINYARD, Roy G., FACHE President and Chief Executive Officer, Asante Health System, Medford, OR, p. B11

VIOLETTE, Brenda, M.D. Director Medical Staff, Firelands Regional Health System, Sandusky, OH, p. A488

VIOLI, Ronald L., Chief Executive Officer, Wheeling Hospital, Wheeling, WV, p. A677

VIPOND, Kathleen, Assistant Administrator and Director, Abraham Lincoln Memorial Hospital, Lincoln, IL, p. A186

VIPPERMAN, Mark, President and Chief Executive Officer, Memorial Medical Center of West Michigan, Ludington, MI, p. A318

VIRGEN, Tomas, R.N. Chief Operating Officer, El Centro Regional Medical Center, El Centro, CA, p. A60

VISAGGIO, Stella, Chief Operating Officer, Hackettstown Regional Medical Center, Hackettstown, NJ, p. A404

VISCARDO, William, M.D. Chief Medical Officer, Adirondack Medical Center, Saranac Lake, NY, p. A442

VISGER, John, M.D. Chief Medical Staff, Gritman Medical Center, Moscow, ID, p. A169

VISH, Nancy, Ph.D. President, Baylor Jack and Jane Hamilton Heart and Vascular Hospital, Dallas, TX, p. A590

VITALE, Lisa, Director Human Resources, Van Matre HEALTHSOUTH Rehabilitation Hospital, Rockford, IL, p. A193

VITALE, Nickolas A.
Executive Vice President and Chief Financial Officer, Beaumont Hospital – Royal Oak, Royal Oak, MI, p. A322
Senior Vice President and Chief Financial Officer, Beaumont Hospital Grosse Pointe, Grosse Pointe, MI, p. A314

VITALI, Vincent, Vice President and Chief Information Officer, Advocate BroMenn Medical Center, Normal, IL, p. A189

VITALIS, Lee Ann, Executive Director Human Resources, St. Croix Regional Medical Center, St. Croix Falls, WI, p. A691

VITIELLO, Jon, Chief Financial Officer, Mercy Hospital Oklahoma City, Oklahoma City, OK, p. A501

VITO, Christopher A., President and Chief Executive Officer, Rehabilitation Institutes of Nevada, Las Vegas, NV, p. A393

VITRANO, Craig, M.D. Medical Director, St. Elizabeth Hospital, Gonzales, LA, p. A267

VIVIANO, Paul S., Chief Executive Officer, UC San Diego Health System, San Diego, CA, p. A86

VIVIT, Romeo, Chief Surgeon, U. S. Public Health Service Indian Hospital, Rosebud, SD, p. A559

VIVODA, Michael, Chief Executive Officer, Cadence Health, Winfield, IL, p. B23

VIVODA, Michael, President, Central DuPage Hospital, Winfield, IL, p. A196

VLARS, Scott, Chief Information Technology Services, Veterans Affairs Medical Center, Wilmington, DE, p. A115

VLODARCHYK, Coreen, R.N. Vice President, Patient Care Services and Chief Nursing Officer, Barnes–Jewish Hospital, Saint Louis, MO, p. A368

VOECKS, Barbara, Chief Information Officer, Ortonville Area Health Services, Ortonville, MN, p. A336

VOELKEL, Jonathon, Administrator, Wilbarger General Hospital, Vernon, TX, p. A633

VOELKER, Dolph, Director Information Services, Indiana University Health Goshen Hospital, Goshen, IN, p. A202

VOELKER, Justin, Chief Financial Officer, Valley Hospital and Medical Center, Spokane Valley, WA, p. A667

VOGEL, Corey, M.D. Chief of Staff, Aurora BayCare Medical Center, Green Bay, WI, p. A682

VOGEL, Lynn H., Vice President and Chief Information Officer, University of Texas M.D. Anderson Cancer Center, Houston, TX, p. A608

VOGELSANG, Mark, Director Information Services, Providence Holy Family Hospital, Spokane, WA, p. A667

VOGENTIZ, William, M.D. Medical Director, AnMed Health Rehabilitation Hospital, Anderson, SC, p. A546

VOGT, Allen J., Chief Executive Officer, Cook Hospital and Convalescent Nursing Care Unit, Cook, MN, p. A329

VOGT, Dennis, Director Information Technology, Madison County Hospital, London, OH, p. A483

VOHS, Lester, Chief Information Management, Osawatomie State Hospital, Osawatomie, KS, p. A240

VOISARD, Victor, Director Human Resources, San Gabriel Valley Medical Center, San Gabriel, CA, p. A87

VOISELLE, Dana, Director Human Resources, Baptist Medical Center Beaches, Jacksonville Beach, FL, p. A127

VOLANTO, John, Vice President and Chief Information Officer, Nyack Hospital, Nyack, NY, p. A438

VOLENTINE, Robert, Director Information Services, Cibola General Hospital, Grants, NM, p. A416

VOLINSKI, Douglas R., Vice President and Chief Financial Officer, Duncan Regional Hospital, Duncan, OK, p. A495

VOLK, Marita, M.D. Director Medical Services and Chief of Staff, Euclid Hospital, Euclid, OH, p. A480

VOLKERDING, Elizabeth, Director Workforce Excellence, San Juan Regional Medical Center, Farmington, NM, p. A416

VOLKMAR, Larry E., Chief Executive Officer, Banner Good Samaritan Medical Center, Phoenix, AZ, p. A35

VOLOCH, Bill, Interim Chief Executive Officer, Medical Center of Aurora, Aurora, CO, p. A97

VOLPE, Buddy, Director Human Resources, Peterson Regional Medical Center, Kerrville, TX, p. A610

VOLPE, Michele M., Executive Director and Chief Executive Officer, Penn Presbyterian Medical Center, Philadelphia, PA, p. A533

VOLTAIRE, Adler, Chief Administrative Officer, Interim LSU Public Hospital, New Orleans, LA, p. A274

VON BEHREN, Rachel, Director Financial Services, Jones Regional Medical Center, Anamosa, IA, p. A214

VON ZYCHLIN, Claus
President and Chief Executive Officer, Mount Carmel, Columbus, OH, p. A476
Executive Vice President and Chief Operating Officer, Mount Carmel St. Ann's, Westerville, OH, p. A491

VONDERAU, Mary, Vice President Strategy and Operations, Provena Mercy Medical Center, Aurora, IL, p. A172

VONDERFECHT, Dennis, President and Chief Executive Officer, Mountain States Health Alliance, Johnson City, TN, p. B91

VONK, Gail, Director Human Resources and Marketing, Sioux Center Community Hospital and Health Center Avera, Sioux Center, IA, p. A226

VOORDE, Christine T., Chief Executive Officer, Kindred Hospital of Northern Indiana, Mishawaka, IN, p. A208

VOORHEES, Michael, MS, Executive Director, East Mountain Hospital, Belle Mead, NJ, p. A401

VOSBURGH, Margaret, Chief Operating Officer, Stanford Hospital and Clinics, Palo Alto, CA, p. A79

VOSBURGH, Mary M., R.N
Vice President Nursing and Chief Nursing Officer, Arnot Ogden Medical Center, Elmira, NY, p. A425
Vice President Nursing and Chief Nursing Officer, St. Joseph's Hospital, Elmira, NY, p. A426

VOSS, Kathy, Director Human Resources, New River Medical Center, Monticello, MN, p. A335

VOSS, Robert
Chief Financial Officer, Laredo Specialty Hospital, Laredo, TX, p. A612
Chief Financial Officer, New Braunfels Regional Rehabilitation Hospital, New Braunfels, TX, p. A618

VOSS, Wayne M., Chief Executive Officer, Methodist West Houston Hospital, Houston, TX, p. A605

VOSSBERG, Brad, M.D. Chief Rehabilitation, Community Howard Specialty Hospital, Kokomo, IN, p. A206

VOSSLER, Jeffrey W., Vice President Financial Services, Joint Township District Memorial Hospital, Saint Marys, OH, p. A488

VOTAW, Anthony, Chief Information Officer, Cayuga Medical Center at Ithaca, Ithaca, NY, p. A428

VOWELL, John H., Interim Chief Executive Officer, Bartlett Regional Hospital, Juneau, AK, p. A29

VOZOS, Frank J., FACS, Executive Director, Monmouth Medical Center, Long Branch, NJ, p. A405

VRAZEL, Desiree, Director of Nurses, El Campo Memorial Hospital, El Campo, TX, p. A595

VRBA, Frank, Chief Information Officer, Annie Jeffrey Memorial County Health Center, Osceola, NE, p. A388

VUCHAK, Jerry
Vice President Information Systems, Barnes–Jewish Hospital, Saint Louis, MO, p. A368
Vice President Information Systems, Barnes–Jewish West County Hospital, Saint Louis, MO, p. A368

VUGRINEC, Barbara P., Vice President Information Systems, Beebe Medical Center, Lewes, DE, p. A114

VUKICH, David, M.D. Senior Vice President, Chief Medical Officer and Chief Quality Officer, Shands Jacksonville Medical Center, Jacksonville, FL, p. A126

VUKOVICH, Pamela S.
Senior Vice President, Chief Financial Officer and Treasurer, Legacy Emanuel Hospital and Health Center, Portland, OR, p. A514
Senior Vice President, Chief Financial Officer and Treasurer, Legacy Good Samaritan Hospital and Medical Center, Portland, OR, p. A514
Senior Vice President and Chief Financial Officer, Legacy Salmon Creek Medical Center, Vancouver, WA, p. A668

VUKSTA, Jeanne, Chief Financial Officer, Bacharach Institute for Rehabilitation, Pomona, NJ, p. A409

VUOCOLO, Philip, M.D. Chief Medical Officer, Monadnock Community Hospital, Peterborough, NH, p. A400

# W

WAARALA, Kirsten, D.O. Vice President Medical Services, Garden City Hospital, Garden City, MI, p. A313

WABLE, Chad W., President and Chief Executive Officer, Saint Mary's Hospital, Waterbury, CT, p. A112

WACHTEL, R. Andrew, FACHE Chief Executive Officer, Ponca City Medical Center, Ponca City, OK, p. A503

WACHTER, Hal, Director Information Systems, University Hospital of Brooklyn at Long Island College Hospital,, NY, p. A437

WACK, Mark, Chief Financial Officer, Biloxi Regional Medical Center, Biloxi, MS, p. A343

WADDELL, Lesa, Director Human Resources, Marengo Memorial Hospital, Marengo, IA, p. A223

WADE, Donna, Senior Director Human Resources, Comanche County Memorial Hospital, Lawton, OK, p. A498

WADE, Glenn, Director Information Systems, Highlands Medical Center, Sparta, TN, p. A576

WADE, Hong, Chief Financial Officer, Sweeny Community Hospital, Sweeny, TX, p. A629

WADE, Jonathan O., President and Chief Executive Officer, Mercy St. Francis Hospital, Mountain View, MO, p. A365

WADE, Karen, Chief Information Officer, U. S. Public Health Service Indian Hospital-Sells, Sells, AZ, p. A38

WADE, Linda, Chief Executive Officer, HEALTHSOUTH Rehabilitation Hospital of Montgomery, Montgomery, AL, p. A24

WADE, Nancy, M.D. Chief of Staff, Hills & Dales General Hospital, Cass City, MI, p. A309

WADEWITZ, Martin, Interim Chief Executive Officer, Angel Medical Center, Franklin, NC, p. A453

WAFFORD, Marty, Chief Financial Officer, Chickasaw Nation Medical Center, Ada, OK, p. A493

WAGERS, Rick, Senior Executive Vice President and Chief Financial Officer, Regional Medical Center at Memphis, Memphis, TN, p. A572

WAGES, N. Gary, FACHE Interim Chief Executive Officer, Cushing Memorial Hospital, Leavenworth, KS, p. A237

WAGGENER, Yvonne, Chief Financial Officer, San Bernardino Mountains Community Hospital District, Lake Arrowhead, CA, p. A66

WAGGONER, Craig, Chief Operating Officer, Clovis Community Medical Center, Clovis, CA, p. A57

WAGGONER, Jeff, M.D. Chief of Staff, Weisbrod Memorial County Hospital, Eads, CO, p. A100

WAGGONER, Michelle, Vice President Human Resources and Physician Services, Community Memorial Hospital, Hicksville, OH, p. A481

WAGNER, Alan, Chief Operating Officer, Coulee Medical Center, Grand Coulee, WA, p. A662

WAGNER, Arthur, Senior Vice President and Executive Director, Coney Island Hospital,, NY, p. A432

WAGNER, Barry, D.O. President and Chief Executive Officer, Cumberland Medical Center, Crossville, TN, p. A564

WAGNER, Dale
Chief Financial Officer, Kindred Hospital–Los Angeles, Los Angeles, CA, p. A70
Chief Financial Officer, Kindred Hospital–Westminster, Westminster, CA, p. A96

WAGNER, David D., Chief Information Management Service, Veterans Affairs Gulf Coast Veterans Health Care System, Biloxi, MS, p. A344

WAGNER, Elaine, M.D. Commander, Naval Medical Center, Portsmouth, VA, p. A654

WAGNER, Jack W., Executive Vice President and Chief Financial Officer, Shawnee Mission Medical Center, Shawnee Mission, KS, p. A243

WAGNER, Janet, R.N. Chief Executive Officer, Sutter Davis Hospital, Davis, CA, p. A59

WAGNER, Karen L., CPA Director Fiscal Services, Shriners Hospitals for Children, Erie, Erie, PA, p. A523

WAGNER, Linda, Chief Financial Officer, Sanford Worthington Medical Center, Worthington, MN, p. A342

WAGNER, Linda S., MSN, Interim Chief Executive Officer, Seneca Healthcare District, Chester, CA, p. A57

WAGNER, Randall J., Chief Operating Officer, Saint Mary's Health Care, Grand Rapids, MI, p. A314

WAGNER, Russell R., Senior Vice President and Chief Financial Officer, Holy Redeemer Hospital and Medical Center, Meadowbrook, PA, p. A528

WAGNER, Sherry, Director Human Resources, Oklahoma Center for Orthopedic and Multi–Specialty Surgery, Oklahoma City, OK, p. A501

WAGNER, Suzie, Director Human Resources, HEALTHSOUTH Rehabilitation Hospital of Alexandria, Alexandria, LA, p. A261

WAGNER, Terry, Chief Information Officer, Upstate University Hospital, Syracuse, NY, p. A444

WAGNER, Timothy, M.D. Chief Medical Staff, Yoakum Community Hospital, Yoakum, TX, p. A636

WAGNER, Vanessa, Chief Financial Officer, Lawrence Memorial Hospital, Walnut Ridge, AR, p. A52

WAGNON, LaNell, Director Medical Records, Comanche County Hospital, Coldwater, KS, p. A231

WAGNON, William, Chief Executive Officer, MountainView Hospital, Las Vegas, NV, p. A393

WAGONER, Dean, Director Human Resources, Good Samaritan Hospital, Vincennes, IN, p. A212

WAHL, Gene O., Chief Financial Officer, North Dakota State Hospital, Jamestown, ND, p. A467

WAHL, Josephine Sclafani, R.N. VP, Patient Care Services & CNO, Henry Ford Wyandotte Hospital, Wyandotte, MI, p. A325

WAHL, Tony, Chief Executive Officer, Texas Spine & Joint Hospital, Tyler, TX, p. A632

WAHLMEIER, James E., President and Chief Executive Officer, Cloud County Health Center, Concordia, KS, p. A232

WAHLUND, Keith, Vice President Human Resources, Essentia Health Fargo, Fargo, ND, p. A465

WAIBEL, David, M.D. Medical Director, Clarks Summit State Hospital, Clarks Summit, PA, p. A520

WAIND, Mark, Administrative Director Information Services, Altru Health System, Grand Forks, ND, p. A466

WAITE, Douglas, M.D. Vice President Medical Affairs, Day Kimball Hospital, Putnam, CT, p. A111

Index of Health Care Professionals / Wallenhaupt

Index of Health Care Professionals


WAITE, Douglas D.
Chief Financial Officer, Seton Edgar B. Davis Hospital, Luling, TX, p. A614
Senior Vice President and Chief Financial Officer, Seton Highland Lakes, Burnet, TX, p. A586
Chief Financial Officer, Seton Medical Center Austin, Austin, TX, p. A581
Senior Vice President and Chief Financial Officer, Seton Medical Center Williamson, Round Rock, TX, p. A623
Chief Financial Officer, Seton Northwest Hospital, Austin, TX, p. A581
Chief Financial Officer, Seton Shoal Creek Hospital, Austin, TX, p. A581
Chief Financial Officer, University Medical Center at Brackenridge, Austin, TX, p. A582
WAITES, Cherri, Chief Financial Officer, Palacios Community Medical Center, Palacios, TX, p. A619
WAJDA, David, Chief Financial Officer, Nazareth Hospital, Philadelphia, PA, p. A533
WAKEFIELD, Brett
Vice President Human Resources, Gottlieb Memorial Hospital, Melrose Park, IL, p. A187
Director Human Resources, Thorek Memorial Hospital, Chicago, IL, p. A178
WAKEFIELD, Mamie
Vice President Finance and Chief Financial Officer, Emma Pendleton Bradley Hospital, East Providence, RI, p. A544
Chief Financial Officer, Miriam Hospital, Providence, RI, p. A544
Senior Vice President and Chief Financial Officer, Rhode Island Hospital, Providence, RI, p. A544
WAKEMAN, Daniel L., President, ProMedica St. Luke's Hospital, Maumee, OH, p. A484
WAKIM, Tina, Vice President Information, Northside Hospital, Atlanta, GA, p. A145
WAKSMONSKI, Teresa, Chief Fiscal Service, James E. Van Zandt Veterans Affairs Medical Center, Altoona, PA, p. A517
WAKULCHIK, Grace, R.N. Chief Operating Officer, Akron Children's Hospital, Akron, OH, p. A469
WALAS, Steven, Chief Executive Officer, HEALTHSOUTH Chesapeake Rehabilitation Hospital, Salisbury, MD, p. A294
WALCEK, Peter, Vice President Finance, Wentworth–Douglass Hospital, Dover, NH, p. A397
WALCZAK, Charles, FACH
Administrator, Shriners Hospitals for Children, Erie, Erie, PA, p. A523
Administrator, Shriners Hospitals for Children, Springfield, Springfield, MA, p. A305
WALDBART, Andy, Department Manager, Heart of the Rockies Regional Medical Center, Salida, CO, p. A105
WALDBILLIG, Karla, Director Human Resources, Finley Hospital, Dubuque, IA, p. A219
WALDEN, Anita, Vice President and Chief Nursing Officer, Decatur General Hospital, Decatur, AL, p. A18
WALDEN, Kristy, R.N. Interim Administrator, Kindred Hospital–Indianapolis, Indianapolis, IN, p. A204
WALDO, Allen J., CPA, Chief Executive Officer, Cooper County Memorial Hospital, Boonville, MO, p. A356
WALDO, Bruce, Chief Executive Officer, Aurora Behavioral Health System–Glendale, Glendale, AZ, p. A32
WALDO, Gail, Director Information Technology, Rockdale Medical Center, Conyers, GA, p. A150
WALDOW, Dee, Chief Financial Officer, Palo Pinto General Hospital, Mineral Wells, TX, p. A617
WALDRON, Michele, Vice President and Chief Financial Officer, Children's Hospital Central California, Madera, CA, p. A73
WALDRON, Ray, Director Information Technology, Gordon Memorial Hospital, Gordon, NE, p. A384
WALDROP, Cathy, Director, Hospital Nursing Services, North Mississippi Medical Center–Pontotoc Hospital and Nursing Home, Pontotoc, MS, p. A352
WALDROUP, Gerald E., Senior Vice President, Good Samaritan Hospital, Vincennes, IN, p. A212
WALDRUM, Michael, M.D. Chief Executive Officer, University of Alabama Hospital, Birmingham, AL, p. A17
WALDY, Byron, Director Human Resources, St. Francis Health Center, Topeka, KS, p. A244
WALENTA, Jason, M.D. Medical Director, Willow Springs Center, Reno, NV, p. A395
WALERSTEIN, Steven, M.D. Executive Vice President and Medical Director, Nassau University Medical Center, East Meadow, NY, p. A425
WALI, Jyotika, M.D. Chief of Staff, Kindred Hospital–Brea, Brea, CA, p. A56
WALIGURA, R. Curtis, D.O. Vice President Medical Affairs, Chief Medical Officer, UPMC McKeesport, McKeesport, PA, p. A528
WALKER, Alene, Director Human Resources, Quincy Valley Medical Center, Quincy, WA, p. A664
WALKER, Andrew, Chief Financial Officer, Johnson Memorial Hospital, Franklin, IN, p. A202
WALKER, Angela, M.D. Medical Director, HEALTHSOUTH Rehabilitation Hospital, Albuquerque, NM, p. A414
WALKER, Austin, Accounting Manager, Kindred Hospital Northland, Kansas City, MO, p. A362
WALKER, Beth, R.N. President, FirstHealth Montgomery Memorial Hospital, Troy, NC, p. A462
WALKER, Bruce, R.N. Chief Executive Officer, Ascension Gonzales Rehabilitation Hospital, Gonzales, LA, p. A266
WALKER, C. O., M.D. Chief of Staff, Donalsonville Hospital, Donalsonville, GA, p. A151
WALKER, Carol, Chief Financial Officer, Oklahoma Heart Hospital, Oklahoma City, OK, p. A501
WALKER, Chad A., Director Human Resources, Caldwell Medical Center, Princeton, KY, p. A258
WALKER, Cheri, R.N. Chief Nursing Officer, King's Daughters Medical Center, Brookhaven, MS, p. A344
WALKER, Codie, Chief Financial Officer, Veterans Affairs Medical Center, Salem, VA, p. A656
WALKER, Donna, Chief Nurse Executive, Weeks Medical Center, Lancaster, NH, p. A398
WALKER, Gale N., President and Chief Executive Officer, Avera St. Benedict Hospital, Parkston, SD, p. A558
WALKER, Gary, Commander, U. S. Air Force Regional Hospital, Eglin AFB, FL, p. A122
WALKER, Gregory J., Chief Executive Officer, Wentworth–Douglass Hospital, Dover, NH, p. A397
WALKER, Jan
Director Human Resources, Centra Lynchburg General Hospital, Lynchburg, VA, p. A650
Director Human Resources, Glenwood Regional Medical Center, West Monroe, LA, p. A279
WALKER, Jerry
Interim Regional Chief Executive Officer, Kauai Veterans Memorial Hospital, Waimea, HI, p. A165
Interim Regional Chief Executive Officer, Samuel Mahelona Memorial Hospital, Kapaa, HI, p. A164
WALKER, John E., FACHE Chief Executive Officer, Logan Regional Medical Center, Logan, WV, p. A673
WALKER, Jon, M.D. Chief of Staff, Wise Regional Health System, Decatur, TX, p. A593
WALKER, Kevin, Vice President Operations, Research Psychiatric Center, Kansas City, MO, p. A362
WALKER, Kristie, Director Human Resources, Montgomery Regional Hospital, Blacksburg, VA, p. A646
WALKER, Larry D., Chief Operating Officer, Glenwood Regional Medical Center, West Monroe, LA, p. A279
WALKER, Larry Joe, Administrator and Chief Executive Officer, Hardy Wilson Memorial Hospital, Hazlehurst, MS, p. A347
WALKER, Lawrence, M.D. Chief of Staff, San Bernardino Mountains Community Hospital District, Lake Arrowhead, CA, p. A66
WALKER, LeRoy
Vice President Human Resources, St. Rose Dominican Hospitals – San Martin Campus, Las Vegas, NV, p. A394
Vice President Human Resources, St. Rose Dominican Hospitals – Siena Campus, Henderson, NV, p. A392
WALKER, Lynette, R.N. Executive Director Human Resources, Central Baptist Hospital, Lexington, KY, p. A253
WALKER, Mary, Manager Information Technology, HEALTHSOUTH Rehabilitation Hospital–Wichita Falls, Wichita Falls, TX, p. A635
WALKER, Melissa, Senior Vice President and Chief Financial Officer, McAlester Regional Health Center, McAlester, OK, p. A499
WALKER, Michael, D.O. Chief of Staff, East Texas Medical Center–Mount Vernon, Mount Vernon, TX, p. A617
WALKER, Paul A., Senior Vice President and Chief Operating Officer, Kennedy Memorial Hospitals–University Medical Center, Cherry Hill, NJ, p. A403
WALKER, Pia, Director Human Resources, Carolinas Medical Center–Mercy, Charlotte, NC, p. A450
WALKER, Randy
Vice President, Methodist Dallas Medical Center, Dallas, TX, p. A592
Director Nursing Services, State Hospital South, Blackfoot, ID, p. A166
WALKER, Renee, Director Human Resources, Bastrop Rehabilitation Hospital, Bastrop, LA, p. A262
WALKER, Robert L., President and Chief Executive Officer, Texas Scottish Rite Hospital for Children, Dallas, TX, p. A592
WALKER, Ronald P., Interim Chief Financial Officer, United Medical Center, Washington, DC, p. A117
WALKER, Steven, Chief Executive Officer, South Hampton Community Hospital, Dallas, TX, p. A592
WALKER, Suzi, Manager Business Office, Cozby–Germany Hospital, Grand Saline, TX, p. A601
WALKER, Tim, Manager Information Services, PeaceHealth Ketchikan Medical Center, Ketchikan, AK, p. A29
WALKER, Troy, Director Finance, St. Clare Hospital and Health Services, Baraboo, WI, p. A678
WALKER, Tyree, Chief Human Resources Officer, Vidant Medical Center, Greenville, NC, p. A454
WALKER Jr., William J., Chief Executive Officer, Memorial Hospital and Manor, Bainbridge, GA, p. A147
WALKLEY, Peter, M.D
Chief of Staff, Franklin Regional Hospital, Franklin, NH, p. A398
Chief Medical Officer, Lakes Region General Hospital, Laconia, NH, p. A398
WALL, Daniel J., President and Chief Executive Officer, Emma Pendleton Bradley Hospital, East Providence, RI, p. A544
WALL, J. C., M.D. Chief of Staff, Stones River Hospital, Woodbury, TN, p. A576
WALL, Kathryn S.
Executive Vice President Human Resources and Organizational Development, Mary Washington Hospital, Fredericksburg, VA, p. A648
Executive Vice President Human Resources and Organizational Development, Stafford Hospital, Stafford, VA, p. A656
WALL, Michael L., President, Northridge Hospital Medical Center–Roscoe Boulevard Campus,, CA, p. A70
WALLACE, Arthur, Chief Financial Officer, Broward Health Coral Springs, Coral Springs, FL, p. A121
WALLACE, Bernadine L., MSN Chief Nursing Officer and Chief Operating Officer, Marion General Hospital, Marion, IN, p. A208
WALLACE, Brenda, R.N. Chief Nursing Officer, Ouachita Community Hospital, West Monroe, LA, p. A279
WALLACE, Carolyn, Director Human Resources, Connecticut Mental Health Center, New Haven, CT, p. A110
WALLACE, David T., Chief Executive Officer, Woodward Regional Hospital, Woodward, OK, p. A508
WALLACE, Debbye, Chief Operating Officer, Hill Country Memorial Hospital, Fredericksburg, TX, p. A600
WALLACE, Dianne, County Information Manager, Douglas County Community Mental Health Center, Omaha, NE, p. A388
WALLACE, Donna Geiken, Chief Operating Officer and Chief Financial Officer, Hopkins County Memorial Hospital, Sulphur Springs, TX, p. A629
WALLACE, Glenn, Chief Operating Officer, Medical Center of Plano, Plano, TX, p. A621
WALLACE, Jo Lynn, Vice President of Nursing, Rogue Valley Medical Center, Medford, OR, p. A512
WALLACE, Kelly, Senior Vice President and Chief Financial Officer, Seattle Children's Hospital, Seattle, WA, p. A666
WALLACE, Linda, Director Human Resources, Sierra Medical Center, El Paso, TX, p. A596
WALLACE, Mark A., President and Chief Executive Officer, Texas Children's Hospital, Houston, TX, p. A607
WALLACE, Mark T., Director Human Resources, Lodi Memorial Hospital, Lodi, CA, p. A67
WALLACE, Melanie, Manager Human Resources, Sutter Tracy Community Hospital, Tracy, CA, p. A93
WALLACE, Michael S., President and Chief Executive Officer, Fort HealthCare, Fort Atkinson, WI, p. A681
WALLACE, Nancy
Vice President Human Resources, Alegent Health–Bergan Mercy Medical Center, Omaha, NE, p. A387
Vice President Human Resources, Alegent Health–Immanuel Medical Center, Omaha, NE, p. A387
Vice President Human Resources, Alegent Health–Lakeside Hospital, Omaha, NE, p. A387
Vice President Human Resources, Alegent Health–Memorial Hospital, Schuyler, NE, p. A389
Senior Vice President Human Resources, Alegent Health–Mercy Hospital, Council Bluffs, IA, p. A217
Interim Senior Vice President Human Resources, Alegent Health–Midlands Hospital, Papillion, NE, p. A389
WALLACE, Patrick L., Administrator, East Texas Medical Center Athens, Athens, TX, p. A580
WALLACE, Penny, Chief Financial Officer, Guadalupe Regional Medical Center, Seguin, TX, p. A627
WALLACE, Richard, Assistant Administrator, Chief Financial Officer and Controller, Tyler County Hospital, Woodville, TX, p. A636
WALLACE, Rick D., FACHE President and Chief Executive Officer, San Juan Regional Medical Center, Farmington, NM, p. A416
WALLACE, Sandra, Chief Financial Officer, Parkwood Behavioral Health System, Olive Branch, MS, p. A351
WALLACE, Tabatha, Director Human Resources, Pasco Regional Medical Center, Dade City, FL, p. A121
WALLACE-MOORE, Patrice, Chief Executive Officer and Executive Director, Arms Acres, Carmel, NY, p. A423
WALLEN, Carla, Manager Human Resources, Cass Regional Medical Center, Harrisonville, MO, p. A360
WALLENHAUPT, Stephen, M.D. Executive Vice President Medical Affairs, Presbyterian Hospital, Charlotte, NC, p. A451

Index of Health Care Professionals

Index of Health Care Professionals / Waller

WALLER, Kenneth, Fiscal Administrator, Deer's Head Hospital Center, Salisbury, MD, p. A294
WALLER, Patricia A., R.N. Assistant Administrator Patient Care Services, Newton Medical Center, Covington, GA, p. A150
WALLER, Tracy, Interim Chief Information Officer, Cook Children's Medical Center, Fort Worth, TX, p. A598
WALLING, John R., President, River Bend Hospital, West Lafayette, IN, p. A213
WALLIS, Carla, Director Human Resources, North Ottawa Community Hospital, Grand Haven, MI, p. A313
WALLIS, Eric, R.N. Vice President Patient Care and Chief Nursing Officer, OhioHealth Marion General Hospital, Marion, OH, p. A484
WALLMAN, Gerald H., Administrator, Doctors Hospital of West Covina, West Covina, CA, p. A95
WALLS, Randy, Manager Information Services, Fairbanks, Indianapolis, IN, p. A204
WALLSCHLAEGER, Erich, Chief Financial Officer, Cedar Park Regional Medical Center, Cedar Park, TX, p. A587
WALMSLEY III, George J., CPA, President and Chief Executive Officer, North Philadelphia Health System, Philadelphia, PA, p. A533
WALMUS, Adam C., Director, Michael E. DeBakey Veterans Affairs Medical Center, Houston, TX, p. A606
WALSER, Bill, Coordinator Technology, Cameron Regional Medical Center, Cameron, MO, p. A356
WALSH, Barbara, Chief Executive Officer, Specialty Hospital Jacksonville, Jacksonville, FL, p. A126
WALSH, Bob, R.N. Chief Operating Officer, Grady Memorial Hospital, Delaware, OH, p. A479
WALSH, Debbie, MSN, Chief Executive Officer, Fountain Valley Regional Hospital and Medical Center, Fountain Valley, CA, p. A61
WALSH, Gerard M.
Senior Vice President and Chief Operating Officer, Dorchester General Hospital, Cambridge, MD, p. A290
Senior Vice President and Chief Operating Officer, Memorial Hospital at Easton Maryland, Easton, MD, p. A291
WALSH, John, M.D. Chief Medical Officer, Florida Hospital–Flagler, Palm Coast, FL, p. A135
WALSH, John, Chief Fiscal Services, Veterans Affairs Hudson Valley Health Care System–F.D. Roosevelt Hospital, Montrose, NY, p. A430
WALSH, Kate, President and Chief Executive Officer, Boston Medical Center, Boston, MA, p. A296
WALSH, Ken, Chief Financial Officer, St. Luke's Medical Center, Phoenix, AZ, p. A36
WALSH, Kevin, Administrator, Wake Forest Baptist Health–Davie Hospital, Mocksville, NC, p. A457
WALSH, Kim, Chief Nursing Officer, Signature Healthcare Brockton Hospital, Brockton, MA, p. A298
WALSH, Len, Executive Vice President and Chief Operating Officer, St. Barnabas Hospital,, NY, p. A436
WALSH, Leon, Chief Financial Officer, Petersburg Medical Center, Petersburg, AK, p. A30
WALSH, Marcia S., M.P.H. Chief Operating Officer, Community Health Care System, Onaga, KS, p. A240
WALSH, Marilyn J., Vice President Human Resources, Kent County Memorial Hospital, Warwick, RI, p. A545
WALSH, Marlene, Vice President and Administrator, Girard Medical Center, Philadelphia, PA, p. A532
WALSH, Mary Beth, M.D. Chief Executive Officer, Burke Rehabilitation Hospital, White Plains, NY, p. A447
WALSH, Michael, Senior Vice President Finance and Chief Financial Officer, Abington Memorial Hospital, Abington, PA, p. A517
WALSH, Richard, Executive Vice President and Chief Operating Officer, SwedishAmerican Hospital, Rockford, IL, p. A193
WALSH, Richard J., Ph.D. Chief Human Resources Officer, Durham Regional Hospital, Durham, NC, p. A452
WALSH, Shawn, Chief Operating Officer, Rockford Center, Newark, DE, p. A114
WALSH, Timothy J., Chief Executive Officer, Martha's Vineyard Hospital, Oak Bluffs, MA, p. A303
WALSH, William P.
Senior Vice President and Executive Director, Jacobi Medical Center,, NY, p. A433
Executive Director, North Central Bronx Hospital,, NY, p. A436
WALSTATLER, Bennett, M.D. President, Spectrum Health United Hospital, Greenville, MI, p. A314
WALSTON, John, Chief Information Officer, Southern Arizona Veterans Affairs Health Care System, Tucson, AZ, p. A40
WALTER, Gayle, Director of Nursing, Thomas B. Finan Center, Cumberland, MD, p. A291
WALTER, Melissa, Chief Financial Officer, Clarinda Regional Health Center, Clarinda, IA, p. A216
WALTER, Stephen
Senior Vice President and Chief Financial Officer, Community Behavioral Health Center, Fresno, CA, p. A62
Senior Vice President and Chief Financial Officer, Community Regional Medical Center, Fresno, CA, p. A62
WALTERS, Anthony, Chief Executive Officer, Springwoods Behavioral Health Hospital, Fayetteville, AR, p. A44
WALTERS, David, D.O. Vice President and Chief Medical Officer, Botsford Hospital, Farmington Hills, MI, p. A312
WALTERS, Joan, MSN, Administrator, Prague Community Hospital, Prague, OK, p. A503
WALTERS, Julie, Chief Nursing Officer, Hillsdale Community Health Center, Hillsdale, MI, p. A315
WALTERS, Kevin
Chief Financial Officer, St. Rose Dominican Hospitals – Rose de Lima Campus, Henderson, NV, p. A392
Chief Financial Officer, St. Rose Dominican Hospitals – San Martin Campus, Las Vegas, NV, p. A394
Chief Financial Officer, St. Rose Dominican Hospitals – Siena Campus, Henderson, NV, p. A392
WALTERS, Mary, Chief Nursing Officer, Central Community Hospital, Elkader, IA, p. A219
WALTERS, Patrick, Interim Chief Executive Officer, Inova Loudoun Hospital, Leesburg, VA, p. A650
WALTERS, Wayne, Chief Executive Officer, Baptist Medical Center Leake, Carthage, MS, p. A344
WALTHALL, Wayne, Interim Chief Financial Officer, Oklahoma State University Medical Center, Tulsa, OK, p. A506
WALTHER, Robert H., Chief Financial Officer, Peterson Regional Medical Center, Kerrville, TX, p. A610
WALTMAN, DeeDee, Information Officer, Garden County Health Services, Oshkosh, NE, p. A388
WALTON, Brian, Vice President and Chief Financial Officer, Baptist St. Anthony Health System, Amarillo, TX, p. A578
WALTON, Carlyle L. E., Chief Executive Officer, Metroplex Adventist Hospital, Killeen, TX, p. A610
WALTON, Charles, Corporate Director Human Resources, Shenandoah Memorial Hospital, Woodstock, VA, p. A657
WALTON, Gary, M.D. Chief Medical Officer, Hill Hospital of Sumter County, York, AL, p. A27
WALTON, Georgian, Director Human Resources, Elbert Memorial Hospital, Elberton, GA, p. A152
WALTON, Greg, Chief Information Officer, El Camino Hospital, Mountain View, CA, p. A76
WALTON, Harold, M.D. Chief of Staff, Bayshore Medical Center, Pasadena, TX, p. A620
WALTON, Robert M., Director, Veterans Affairs Medical Center, White River Junction, VT, p. A644
WALTZ, Brenda M., FACHE Chief Executive Officer, Garden Park Medical Center, Gulfport, MS, p. A346
WALZ, Pat, President and Chief Executive Officer, Yuma Regional Medical Center, Yuma, AZ, p. A41
WAMSLEY, Marie, Chief Financial Officer, Memorial Hospital of Lafayette County, Darlington, WI, p. A680
WANG, Alan, M.D. Chief Medical Officer, Emory Johns Creek Hospital, Johns Creek, GA, p. A154
WANGER, David S.
Chief Executive Officer, Florence Hospital at Anthem, Florence, AZ, p. A32
Chief Executive Officer, Gilbert Hospital, Gilbert, AZ, p. A32
WANGLER, Patricia, Chief Executive Officer, Essentia Health Fosston, Fosston, MN, p. A331
WANGSMO, Gary L., Chief Financial Officer, George L. Mee Memorial Hospital, King City, CA, p. A65
WANGSNESS, Erik, Chief Executive Officer, Jellico Community Hospital, Jellico, TN, p. A567
WANNER, David, Chief Information Officer, St. Mary's of Michigan, Saginaw, MI, p. A322
WANTLAND, Margaret, Chief Financial Officer, Kindred Hospital–Albuquerque, Albuquerque, NM, p. A414
WANTZ, Steve, Senior Vice President Human Resources and Administration, Indiana University Health University Hospital, Indianapolis, IN, p. A204
WAPPELHORST, Andrea, Chief Nursing Officer, TOPS Surgical Specialty Hospital, Houston, TX, p. A607
WARD, Brook, Executive Vice President, Washington Hospital, Washington, PA, p. A540
WARD, Cary, M.D. Chief Medical Officer, Saint Elizabeth Regional Medical Center, Lincoln, NE, p. A385
WARD, David M., Senior Vice President and Chief Financial Officer, Cabell Huntington Hospital, Huntington, WV, p. A672
WARD, Greg
Chief Financial Officer and Vice President Operations, Carlinville Area Hospital, Carlinville, IL, p. A174
Senior Director Clinical Services, Copley Hospital, Morrisville, VT, p. A643
WARD, Henry J., Vice President and Chief Financial Officer, Westfield Memorial Hospital, Westfield, NY, p. A446
WARD, James, M.D
Chief Medical Officer, Sacred Heart Hospital of Pensacola, Pensacola, FL, p. A136
President Medical Staff, USMD Hospital at Arlington, Arlington, TX, p. A580
WARD, Jeanne L., R.N. President and Chief Executive Officer, Oconee Medical Center, Seneca, SC, p. A553
WARD, Kenneth
Director Information Services, Shriners Hospitals for Children, Springfield, Springfield, MA, p. A305
Regional Director Information Services, Shriners Hospitals for Children–Boston, Boston, MA, p. A297
WARD, Kevin J., Vice President and Chief Financial Officer, New York Hospital Queens,, NY, p. A435
WARD, Kristen, Coordinator Human Resources, Kindred Hospital–Boston, Brighton, MA, p. A298
WARD, Lesli, Vice President Human Resources, Shands Jacksonville Medical Center, Jacksonville, FL, p. A126
WARD, Lisa, Director Management Information Systems, Columbus Regional Healthcare System, Whiteville, NC, p. A462
WARD, Louise, Vice President Financial and Support Services, Roane General Hospital, Spencer, WV, p. A676
WARD, Michael, Director Information Services, Anderson Hospital, Maryville, IL, p. A187
WARD, Robert, Chief Executive Officer, Highlands Regional Rehabilitation Hospital, El Paso, TX, p. A596
WARD, Sandy, Administrator, Johnson County Healthcare Center, Buffalo, WY, p. A695
WARD, Silva, Director Human Resources, Center for Behavioral Medicine, Kansas City, MO, p. A361
WARD, Stormy, Chief Nurse Executive, Big Spring State Hospital, Big Spring, TX, p. A584
WARD, Virginia, Human Resources Officer, Naval Hospital, Twentynine Palms, CA, p. A93
WARD, Wendy, Director Human Resources, Mercy Hospital El Reno, El Reno, OK, p. A496
WARD–PRESSON, Kathryn M., R.N. Associate Director for Patient Care Services, Durham Veterans Affairs Medical Center, Durham, NC, p. A452
WARDA, Paul, Chief Financial Officer, Medstar Georgetown University Hospital, Washington, DC, p. A116
WARDELL, Kevin S., President, Norton Hospital, Louisville, KY, p. A255
WARDELL, Patrick R., Chief Executive Officer, Cambridge Health Alliance, Cambridge, MA, p. A299
WARDEN, Michael S.
Senior Vice President Information Technology, Banner Good Samaritan Medical Center, Phoenix, AZ, p. A35
Senior Vice President and Chief Information Officer, Banner Heart Hospital, Mesa, AZ, p. A34
Senior Vice President and Chief Information Officer, East Morgan County Hospital, Brush, CO, p. A98
WARDWELL, Robert D.
Chief Financial Officer, St. John's Pleasant Valley Hospital, Camarillo, CA, p. A56
Chief Financial Officer, St. John's Regional Medical Center, Oxnard, CA, p. A78
WARE, Bobbie K., R.N. Vice President/Patient Care/Chief Nursing Officer, Mississippi Baptist Medical Center, Jackson, MS, p. A348
WARE, Bobbie K., FACHE Chief Executive Officer and Chief Nursing Officer, Mississippi Hospital for Restorative Care, Jackson, MS, p. A348
WARE, Judy, Director Human Resources, Johnson Memorial Hospital, Franklin, IN, p. A202
WARE, Karen, Director Human Resources, Integris Blackwell Regional Hospital, Blackwell, OK, p. A494
WARE, Scott T., Chief Operating Officer, Western Baptist Hospital, Paducah, KY, p. A257
WARE, Shannon, President and Chief Executive Officer, Eastern State Hospital, Lexington, KY, p. A253
WAREING, Colleen, Vice President Patient Care Services, Atlantic General Hospital, Berlin, MD, p. A289
WARFIELD, William, Chief Human Resources Management, Veterans Affairs Boston Healthcare System, Boston, MA, p. A297
WARLITNER, Todd, Vice President Business Operations, The Outer Banks Hospital, Nags Head, NC, p. A458
WARM, Ira, Senior Vice President Human Resources, Brooklyn Hospital Center,, NY, p. A431
WARMAN, Debbie, Vice President Human Resources, MetroHealth Medical Center, Cleveland, OH, p. A475
WARMAN Jr., Harold C., FACHE President and Chief Executive Officer, Highlands Regional Medical Center, Prestonsburg, KY, p. A258
WARMBOLD, Steve, Director Information Management Service Line, Veterans Affairs Medical Center, Saint Louis, MO, p. A370

A958 Index of Health Care Professionals

Index of Health Care Professionals / Weaver

Index of Health Care Professionals


WARMERDAM, David, Chief Financial Officer, Brynn Marr Hospital, Jacksonville, NC, p. A455
WARNER, John, M.D. Chief Executive Officer, University of Texas Southwestern Medical Center, Dallas, TX, p. A593
WARNER, Norma, Area Director Health Information Management, Kindred Hospital–Fort Worth, Fort Worth, TX, p. A599
WARNER–PACHECO, Paula, Chief Human Resources, Rio Grande Hospital, Del Norte, CO, p. A99
WARNOCK, Dawn, Director Medical Records, Taylor Regional Hospital, Hawkinsville, GA, p. A154
WARREN, Beka, R.N. Interim Chief Clinical Officer, Memorial Hospital, Craig, CO, p. A99
WARREN, Bradley J., Senior Vice President and Chief People Officer, Memorial Medical Center, Springfield, IL, p. A194
WARREN, Danny, Chief Financial Officer, Lake Wales Medical Center, Lake Wales, FL, p. A128
WARREN, Gorman, Chief Financial Officer, Texas Health Harris Methodist Hospital Southlake, Southlake, TX, p. A628
WARREN, Jennifer, Chief Financial Officer, Purcell Municipal Hospital, Purcell, OK, p. A503
WARREN, Karen, Fiscal Officer, Porterville Developmental Center, Porterville, CA, p. A81
WARREN, Larry, Chief Executive Officer, Howard University Hospital, Washington, DC, p. A116
WARREN, Linda, Director Human Resources, Cogdell Memorial Hospital, Snyder, TX, p. A628
WARREN, Merritt, M.D. Medical Director and Chief of Staff, Brookings Health System, Brookings, SD, p. A555
WARREN, Michael D., President, Good Samaritan Regional Health Center, Mount Vernon, IL, p. A188
WARREN, Richard
Vice President Health Information Systems, Allegiance Health, Jackson, MI, p. A316
Chief Information Officer, Hillcrest Baptist Medical Center, Waco, TX, p. A633
WARREN, Roger D., M.D. Administrator, Hanover Hospital, Hanover, KS, p. A234
WARREN, Ron, Director Information Systems, Loretto Hospital, Chicago, IL, p. A176
WARREN, Sarah, Coordinator Human Resources, Hickory Trail Hospital, Desoto, TX, p. A594
WARREN, Seth C. R., President, Franciscan St. James Hospital and Health Centers, Olympia Fields, IL, p. A190
WARREN, Shanna, Director Human Resources, Medical Center of Plano, Plano, TX, p. A621
WARREN, Terri, Chief Financial Officer, Dyersburg Regional Medical Center, Dyersburg, TN, p. A565
WARREN Jr., Wm. Michael, Chief Executive Officer, The Children's Hospital of Alabama, Birmingham, AL, p. A17
WARRINER, Ken, Chief Financial Officer, Madison River Oaks Medical Center, Canton, MS, p. A344
WARRINGTON, Sr., James E., M.D. Chief of Staff, Quitman County Hospital, Marks, MS, p. A349
WARSING, Tracy, M.D. Site Leader Chief of Staff, Mayo Clinic Health System – Franciscan Healthcare in Sparta, Sparta, WI, p. A691
WARTCHOW, Leann, Assistant Chief Executive Officer and Certified Risk Manager, Lost Rivers District Hospital, Arco, ID, p. A166
WAS, Gregory J., CPA Chief Financial Officer, Melissa Memorial Hospital, Holyoke, CO, p. A102
WASDEN, Mitchell L., Ed.D. Chief Operating Officer, Women's and Children's Hospital, Columbia, MO, p. A358
WASDEN, Ricky, Manager Information Technology, Jefferson Hospital, Louisville, GA, p. A155
WASEMILLER–SMITH, Lisa, M.D. Chief Medical Officer, Lakeside Women's Hospital, Oklahoma City, OK, p. A501
WASHAM, Jim M., Director Human Resources, Silverton Hospital, Silverton, OR, p. A515
WASHAM, Mark, Chief Information Officer, Shriners Hospitals for Children, Shriners Burns Hospital, Cincinnati, Cincinnati, OH, p. A474
WASHBURN, Tonya, M.D. Medical Director, Valir Rehabilitation Hospital, Oklahoma City, OK, p. A502
WASHECKA, James, Chief Financial Officer, Easton Hospital, Easton, PA, p. A522
WASHINGTON, Carolyn, Director of Human Resources, Doctor's Hospital – Tidwell, Houston, TX, p. A604
WASHINGTON, Glen A., Senior Vice President and Chief Operating Officer, Cabell Huntington Hospital, Huntington, WV, p. A672
WASHINGTON, Lorraine, Vice President Human Resources, St. Dominic–Jackson Memorial Hospital, Jackson, MS, p. A348
WASHINGTON, Lydia, Controller, Acuity Hospital of South Texas, San Antonio, TX, p. A624
WASHINGTON, Reginald, M.D. Chief Medical Officer, Presbyterian–St. Luke's Medical Center, Denver, CO, p. A100
WASHINGTON, Stephanie, Director Community Relations and Human Resources, King's Daughters Hospital, Yazoo City, MS, p. A354
WASIUK, Pauline, Director Human Resources, Southern Virginia Mental Health Institute, Danville, VA, p. A647
WASSALL, Dianne, Director Human Resources, St. Joseph Medical Center, Towson, MD, p. A294
WASSILAK, Leighton, Manager, Information Systems/ Telecommunications, SSM St. Clare Health Center, Fenton, MO, p. A359
WASSON, Phil, Chief Information Officer, SwedishAmerican Hospital, Rockford, IL, p. A193
WATERBURY, Brad, Director Human Resources, Bonner General Hospital, Sandpoint, ID, p. A170
WATERCUTTER, William, Director Management Information System, Upper Valley Medical Center, Troy, OH, p. A490
WATERS, Danny, Director Information Technology and Systems, South Bay Hospital, Sun City Center, FL, p. A140
WATERS, Eric, Vice President Operations, Pen Bay Medical Center, Rockport, ME, p. A285
WATERS, Gina, Director Human Resources, Evans Memorial Hospital, Claxton, GA, p. A149
WATERS, Glenn D., FACH
President, Mease Countryside Hospital, Safety Harbor, FL, p. A137
President and Chief Executive Officer, Mease Hospital Dunedin, Dunedin, FL, p. A122
President, Morton Plant Hospital, Clearwater, FL, p. A120
WATERS, Glenn D., FACHE President, Morton Plant Mease Health Care, Clearwater, FL, p. B91
WATERS, Glenn D., FACHE President, Morton Plant North Bay Hospital, New Port Richey, FL, p. A133
WATERS, Karen, Chief Nursing Officer, St. Mary's Warrick Hospital, Boonville, IN, p. A198
WATERS, Mickey, Director Information Technology, Conway Medical Center, Conway, SC, p. A549
WATERS, Patrick, Director Information Technology, Marshall County Hospital, Benton, KY, p. A247
WATERS, Stephen F., M.D. Medical Director, Atlantic General Hospital, Berlin, MD, p. A289
WATERS, Victor, M.D. Chief of Staff, Sioux Falls VA Health Care System, Sioux Falls, SD, p. A560
WATERSTON, Judith C., MS, President and Chief Executive Officer, New England Sinai Hospital and Rehabilitation Center, Stoughton, MA, p. A305
WATHEN, Cheryl, Interim Chief Financial Officer, Deaconess Hospital, Evansville, IN, p. A201
WATHEN, James A., Chief Executive Officer, Southern Coos Hospital and Health Center, Bandon, OR, p. A509
WATKINS, Anne Marie, R.N. Chief Nursing Officer, Rancho Springs Medical Center, Murrieta, CA, p. A76
WATKINS, Chris, Director of Information Technology, Craig Hospital, Englewood, CO, p. A100
WATKINS, Pamela, Chief Financial Officer, Veterans Affairs Medical Center, Decatur, GA, p. A151
WATKINS, Scott, Director, Employment/Employee Relations, Catholic Medical Center, Manchester, NH, p. A399
WATKINS, William D., Chief Administrative Officer, Bluffton Hospital, Bluffton, OH, p. A471
WATLAND, Judy A., R.N. Chief Nursing Officer, O'Connor Hospital, San Jose, CA, p. A88
WATRY, Margaret, Director of Patient Care Services and Nurse Executive, Phillips Eye Institute, Minneapolis, MN, p. A335
WATSON, Betty A., Chief Financial Officer, Syringa Hospital and Clinics, Grangeville, ID, p. A168
WATSON, Brent, M.D. Chief Medical Staff, Roane General Hospital, Spencer, WV, p. A676
WATSON, Christopher, M.D. Chief Medical Officer, Bellin Memorial Hospital, Green Bay, WI, p. A682
WATSON, Dean, M.D. Chief Medical Officer, Tallahassee Memorial HealthCare, Tallahassee, FL, p. A140
WATSON, Deborah, Senior Vice President and Chief Operating Officer, Bayhealth Medical Center, Dover, DE, p. A114
WATSON, Dolores, Director Health Information Management, Arms Acres, Carmel, NY, p. A423
WATSON, Heath
Controller, HEALTHSOUTH Rehabilitation Hospital, Dothan, AL, p. A19
Controller, HEALTHSOUTH Rehabilitation Hospital of Montgomery, Montgomery, AL, p. A24
WATSON, James B., Chief Executive Officer, Ira Davenport Memorial Hospital, Bath, NY, p. A421
WATSON, Jim, Chief Financial Officer, OU Medical Center, Oklahoma City, OK, p. A502
WATSON, Kathy, R.N. Administrator and Chief Nursing Officer, The Center for Spinal Surgery, Nashville, TN, p. A573
WATSON, Kerry, President, Durham Regional Hospital, Durham, NC, p. A452
WATSON, Linda, Director, G.V. Montgomery Veterans Affairs Medical Center, Jackson, MS, p. A347
WATSON, Luke, M.D. Chief of Staff, Pacific Hospital of Long Beach, Long Beach, CA, p. A68
WATSON, Mary Lou, MS Vice President Nursing, Medstar St. Mary's Hospital, Leonardtown, MD, p. A293
WATSON, Michelle, Chief Operating Officer and Chief Nursing Officer, Livingston Regional Hospital, Livingston, TN, p. A570
WATSON, Nancy, Director Human Resources, Mercy Hospital, Coon Rapids, MN, p. A330
WATSON, Scott, JD Vice President Human Resources and Support Services, Mercy Hospital Joplin, Joplin, MO, p. A361
WATSON, Shane, Chief Executive Officer, Red Bud Regional Hospital, Red Bud, IL, p. A192
WATSON, Teresa C., Vice President Administration, Carolinas Medical Center–Lincoln, Lincolnton, NC, p. A456
WATSON, Thelma Ruth, M.D. Medical Director, Schneider Regional Medical Center, Saint Thomas, VI, p. A704
WATSON, Trey, Network Administrator, Sumner County Hospital District One, Caldwell, KS, p. A231
WATSON, Vicki, Manager Human Resources, Select Specialty Hospital–Jackson, Jackson, MS, p. A348
WATSON, Virgil, Administrator, Sumner County Hospital District One, Caldwell, KS, p. A231
WATT, Andrew, M.D. Vice President, Chief Information Officer and Chief Medical Information Officer, Southern New Hampshire Medical Center, Nashua, NH, p. A399
WATT, Ella, Chief Financial Officer, University of New Mexico Hospitals, Albuquerque, NM, p. A415
WATT, Tracy, Director Information Systems, Jackson Purchase Medical Center, Mayfield, KY, p. A256
WATTERS, Greg, Chief Financial Officer, El Paso Specialty Hospital, El Paso, TX, p. A596
WATTOO, Dost, M.D. Chief of Staff, Valley Hospital Medical Center, Las Vegas, NV, p. A394
WATTS, Gary, M.D. Chief Medical Officer, Mayhill Hospital, Denton, TX, p. A594
WATTS, Hugh, M.D. Chief of Staff, Shriners Hospitals for Children, Los Angeles, Los Angeles, CA, p. A72
WATTS, Larry, Chief Medical Officer, Hays Medical Center, Hays, KS, p. A234
WATTS–JOHNSON, Christine M., Assistant Vice President, Madera Community Hospital, Madera, CA, p. A73
WAUN, Cynthia, Chief Operating Officer and Risk Manager, Brynn Marr Hospital, Jacksonville, NC, p. A455
WAUTERS, Ron, Chief Financial Officer, Pella Regional Health Center, Pella, IA, p. A225
WAY, Harold, Chief Financial Officer and Chief Operating Officer, San Gabriel Valley Medical Center, San Gabriel, CA, p. A87
WAYNE, Jim, Chief Financial Officer, OSF St. Francis Hospital, Escanaba, MI, p. A312
WAYNE, Kenneth, M.D. Chief Medical Officer, Ottumwa Regional Health Center, Ottumwa, IA, p. A225
WAYRAUCH, Karen, Interim Director Information Systems, East Ohio Regional Hospital, Martins Ferry, OH, p. A484
WEADICK, James F., Administrator and Chief Executive Officer, Newton Medical Center, Covington, GA, p. A150
WEAR, Sondra, Director Financial Services, Eureka Springs Hospital, Eureka Springs, AR, p. A44
WEATHERFORD, Dennis, Chief Executive Officer, Putnam County Hospital, Greencastle, IN, p. A202
WEATHERFORD, Ted, Chief Financial Officer, Howard A. Rusk Rehabilitation Center, Columbia, MO, p. A358
WEATHERWAX, Marlene, Vice President and Chief Financial Officer, Columbus Regional Hospital, Columbus, IN, p. A199
WEAVER, Angie L., Director Human Resources, Gilmore Memorial Regional Medical Center, Amory, MS, p. A343
WEAVER, Daryl W., Chief Executive Officer, King's Daughters Hospital, Yazoo City, MS, p. A354
WEAVER, Douglas K., FACHE President, Integris Mayes County Medical Center, Pryor, OK, p. A503
WEAVER, Jason
Director Information Systems, Crockett Hospital, Lawrenceburg, TN, p. A569
Finance Manager, Maple Grove Hospital, Maple Grove, MN, p. A334
WEAVER, Jeff, Chief Financial Officer, Morton County Health System, Elkhart, KS, p. A232
WEAVER, Joe, Chief Operating Officer and Vice President Operations, Northeast Alabama Regional Medical Center, Anniston, AL, p. A15
WEAVER, Judy, MS, Chief Executive Officer, Acuity Specialty Hospital – Ohio Valley, Steubenville, OH, p. A488
WEAVER, Kim, CPA Chief Financial Officer, Sumner Regional Medical Center, Wellington, KS, p. A245
WEAVER, Kimberli, Chief Nursing Officer, L. V. Stabler Memorial Hospital, Greenville, AL, p. A21
WEAVER, Nancy, Vice President of Nursing, Chief Nursing Officer, Carson City Hospital, Carson City, MI, p. A309
WEAVER, William, Chief Executive Officer, Dover Behavioral Health System, Dover, DE, p. A114


 Index of Health Care Professionals **A959**

Index of Health Care Professionals
Index of Health Care Professionals / Webb

WEBB Jr., Charles L., Administrator, Lincoln Trail Behavioral Health System, Radcliff, KY, p. A258
WEBB, Craig R., M.D. Deputy Commander for Clinical Services, Irwin Army Community Hospital, Junction City, KS, p. A236
WEBB, David, Chief Financial Officer, NEA Baptist Memorial Hospital, Jonesboro, AR, p. A47
WEBB, Dee, Vice President Human Resources, St. Bernardine Medical Center, San Bernardino, CA, p. A85
WEBB, Denise, Administrator, Virginia Beach Psychiatric Center, Virginia Beach, VA, p. A657
WEBB, Donald, Chief Financial Officer, Williamson Medical Center, Franklin, TN, p. A565
WEBB, Gary, Director Human Resources, Corry Memorial Hospital, Corry, PA, p. A521
WEBB, Herbert, M.D. Chief Medical Officer, Providence Little Company of Mary Medical Center San Pedro,, CA, p. A71
WEBB, Jeffrey D., CPA Chief Financial Officer, Jasper County Hospital, Rensselaer, IN, p. A211
WEBB, Joseph, Chief Operating Officer, Northwest Mississippi Regional Medical Center, Clarksdale, MS, p. A344
WEBB, Karen, M.D
Chief Medical Officer, Des Peres Hospital, Saint Louis, MO, p. A368
Chief Medical Officer, Saint Louis University Hospital, Saint Louis, MO, p. A369
WEBB, Kevin C., Ph.D. President, ProMedica Toledo Hospital, Toledo, OH, p. A489
WEBB, Kimberly, Chief Financial Officer, Cheyenne Regional Medical Center, Cheyenne, WY, p. A695
WEBB, Linda, R.N. Chief Nursing Executive, Pulaski Memorial Hospital, Winamac, IN, p. A213
WEBB, Lisa, Vice President Finance and Chief Financial Officer, Saint Francis Medical Center, Grand Island, NE, p. A384
WEBB, Patricia G., Senior Vice President Human Resources, UMass Memorial Medical Center, Worcester, MA, p. A306
WEBB, Paula, Chief Financial Officer, Lake Butler Hospital Hand Surgery Center, Lake Butler, FL, p. A128
WEBB, Renick, M.D. Chief Medical Director, Central Louisiana Surgical Hospital, Alexandria, LA, p. A261
WEBB, Robin, Director Human Resources, Perry Memorial Hospital, Perry, OK, p. A503
WEBB, Steven B., FACHE Administrator, Baptist Health Medical Center–Stuttgart, Stuttgart, AR, p. A51
WEBB, W. Larry, Senior Vice President and Chief Financial Officer, Athens Regional Medical Center, Athens, GA, p. A144
WEBBER, Cathy, Chief Information Officer, Franklin County Memorial Hospital, Franklin, NE, p. A383
WEBBER, Chelsea, Director Human Resources, LifeCare Hospitals of Pittsburgh – Monroeville, Monroeville, PA, p. A529
WEBBER, Deborah G., Chief Operating Officer, Anaheim Regional Medical Center, Anaheim, CA, p. A53
WEBBER, Joyce, Chief Financial Officer, Spalding Rehabilitation Hospital, Aurora, CO, p. A97
WEBDALE, Ralph, Vice President Finance, Brooks Memorial Hospital, Dunkirk, NY, p. A425
WEBER, Ayanna, Director Human Resources, Huron Valley–Sinai Hospital, Commerce Township, MI, p. A310
WEBER, Barbara, Chief Operating Officer, Advocate Lutheran General Hospital, Park Ridge, IL, p. A191
WEBER, Jr., Ernest P., Interim Chief Information Officer, SUNY Downstate Medical Center University Hospital of Brooklyn,, NY, p. A437
WEBER, Frank, Chief Executive Officer, Select Specialty Hospital–Charleston, Charleston, WV, p. A671
WEBER, Gordon, Chief Operating Officer, Clarks Summit State Hospital, Clarks Summit, PA, p. A520
WEBER, James, D.O. Chief of Staff, Washington County Memorial Hospital, Potosi, MO, p. A367
WEBER, Michael T., President and Chief Executive Officer, Health Quest Systems, Inc., Lagrangeville, NY, p. B64
WEBER, Pete M., President and Chief Executive Officer, Gordon Hospital, Calhoun, GA, p. A148
WEBER, Rebecca
Senior Vice President and Chief Information Officer, Jersey Shore University Medical Center, Neptune, NJ, p. A406
Senior Vice President and Chief Information Officer, Ocean Medical Center, Brick Township, NJ, p. A402
Senior Vice President Information Technology, Riverview Medical Center, Red Bank, NJ, p. A409
Senior Vice President and Chief Information Officer, Southern Ocean Medical Center, Manahawkin, NJ, p. A406
WEBER, Robert, M.D. Chief Medical Staff, Watsonville Community Hospital, Watsonville, CA, p. A95
WEBER, Tiffany, Chief Financial Officer, Perkins County Health Services, Grant, NE, p. A384
WEBSTER, Cindy, Vice President Financial Services, Licking Memorial Hospital, Newark, OH, p. A486
WEBSTER, Janice, Director Human Resources, West Oaks Hospital, Houston, TX, p. A608
WEBSTER, Joanne, Director Human Resources, Community Hospital of the Monterey Peninsula, Monterey, CA, p. A75
WEBSTER, Kathleen, R.N. Vice President Patient Services, Hudson Valley Hospital Center, Cortlandt Manor, NY, p. A424
WEBSTER, Kim, Manager Information Systems, Franklin Regional Medical Center, Louisburg, NC, p. A457
WEBSTER, Mark
President and Chief Executive Officer, Claxton–Hepburn Medical Center, Ogdensburg, NY, p. A439
Vice President Finance, Hudson Valley Hospital Center, Cortlandt Manor, NY, p. A424
WEBSTER, Odetta, Director Human Resources, Shriners Hospitals for Children, Spokane, WA, p. A667
WEBSTER, William W., FACHE Chief Executive Officer, Medical Center Health System, Odessa, TX, p. A619
WECKENBORG, Janet, FACHE VP Operations, Capital Region Medical Center, Jefferson City, MO, p. A361
WEDEL, Sandy, Director Human Resources, Ellsworth County Medical Center, Ellsworth, KS, p. A232
WEDGEWORTH, Joyce, Financial Clerk, Hill Hospital of Sumter County, York, AL, p. A27
WEE, Donald, Chief Executive Officer, Tri–State Memorial Hospital, Clarkston, WA, p. A660
WEED, III, John, M.D. Medical Director, Little River Medical Center, Rockdale, TX, p. A623
WEED, Warren
Director Human Resources, River Oaks Hospital, Flowood, MS, p. A345
Director Associate Relations, Woman's Hospital, Flowood, MS, p. A346
WEEKLEY, Steve, Director Information Technology, Cooper County Memorial Hospital, Boonville, MO, p. A356
WEEKS, Donnie J., FACHE President and Chief Executive Officer, KershawHealth, Camden, SC, p. A546
WEEKS, James, Chief Information Officer, Greenwich Hospital, Greenwich, CT, p. A109
WEEKS, Margaret, Manager Personnel, Tippah County Hospital, Ripley, MS, p. A352
WEEKS, Steven Douglas, FACHE Senior Vice President and Administrator, Baptist Health Medical Center–Little Rock, Little Rock, AR, p. A47
WEELDREYER, Jim, Manager Information Technology, Pershing General Hospital, Lovelock, NV, p. A394
WEEMS, Reva, Director Human Resources, Crossroads Community Hospital, Mount Vernon, IL, p. A188
WEERTS, Michael, Director Human Resources, Grand River Hospital District, Rifle, CO, p. A105
WEG, Jennifer, R.N. Chief Nursing Officer, Sanford Worthington Medical Center, Worthington, MN, p. A342
WEGG, Daniel, M.D. Medical Director, St. Vincent Randolph Hospital, Winchester, IN, p. A213
WEGHORST, George, M.D. Chief Medical Officer, Providence Newberg Medical Center, Newberg, OR, p. A513
WEGLARZ, Ron, Chief Operating Officer, Streamwood Behavioral Health Center, Streamwood, IL, p. A195
WEGNER, Mike, Chief Financial Officer, Via Christi Hospitals Wichita, Wichita, KS, p. A245
WEHLING, Robert D., Interim Chief Financial Officer, Saint Alphonsus Medical Center – Baker City, Baker City, OR, p. A509
WEHNER, Jill, Vice President Financial Services, Harbor Beach Community Hospital, Harbor Beach, MI, p. A315
WEHR, Julie, Director Human Resources, Odessa Memorial Healthcare Center, Odessa, WA, p. A663
WEHRMEISTER, Erica, Chief Operating Officer, Lutheran Hospital of Indiana, Fort Wayne, IN, p. A201
WEIDAUER, Shannon, Director Human Resources, Inland Valley Medical Center, Wildomar, CA, p. A96
WEIDEMANN, Donald, Administrator, Union County General Hospital, Clayton, NM, p. A415
WEIDER, Will
Chief Information Officer, Calumet Medical Center, Chilton, WI, p. A680
Chief Information Officer, Eagle River Memorial Hospital, Eagle River, WI, p. A680
Chief Information Officer, Mercy Medical Center, Oshkosh, WI, p. A688
Chief Information Officer, Ministry Saint Michael's Hospital, Stevens Point, WI, p. A691
Chief Information Officer, Saint Joseph's Hospital, Marshfield, WI, p. A685
Chief Information Officer, St. Elizabeth Hospital, Appleton, WI, p. A678
WEIDMAN, Samuel G., Executive Vice President and Chief Financial Officer, Children's Hospital of Richmond, Richmond, VA, p. A654
WEIDNER, Deborah, M.D. Chief Medical Officer, Natchaug Hospital, Mansfield Center, CT, p. A109
WEIDNER, James, President, Cullman Regional Medical Center, Cullman, AL, p. A18
WEIDNER, Peter
Director Management Information Systems, Community Hospital at Dobbs Ferry, Dobbs Ferry, NY, p. A425
Director Management Information Systems, St. John's Riverside Hospital, Yonkers, NY, p. A447
WEIGEL, Cherry, Director Health Information Management, RC Hospital and Clinics, Olivia, MN, p. A336
WEIGEL, Christine H., R.N. Clinical Operating Officer, McBride Clinic Orthopedic Hospital, Oklahoma City, OK, p. A501
WEIL, David S., Senior Vice President and Administrator, Saint Francis Hospital South, Tulsa, OK, p. A506
WEIL, Robert, M.D. President, Lakewood Hospital, Lakewood, OH, p. A482
WEILAND, David, M.D. VP Medical Affairs, Bayfront Medical Center, Saint Petersburg, FL, p. A138
WEILENMAN, Shelly L., R.N. Chief Nursing Officer, Coastal Carolina Hospital, Hardeeville, SC, p. A551
WEINBAUM, Frederic, M.D. Executive Vice President Operations and Chief Medical Officer, Southampton Hospital, Southampton, NY, p. A443
WEINBERG, Assa, M.D. Chief of Staff, Temple Community Hospital, Los Angeles, CA, p. A72
WEINBERG, Meryl, Executive Director, Metropolitan Hospital Center, New York, NY, p. A434
WEINBERG, Mitch, M.D. Chief of Staff, Evergreen Hospital Medical Center, Kirkland, WA, p. A662
WEINER, Gary
Vice President Information Technology, Chief Information Officer, Community Hospital, Munster, IN, p. A209
Chief Information Officer, St. Catherine Hospital, East Chicago, IN, p. A200
Vice President Information Technology and Chief Information Officer, St. Mary Medical Center, Hobart, IN, p. A203
WEINER, Jack, President and Chief Executive Officer, St. Joseph Mercy Oakland, Pontiac, MI, p. A321
WEINER, Jerome, M.D. Senior Vice President Medical Affairs, Good Samaritan Hospital Medical Center, West Islip, NY, p. A446
WEINER, Martin E., M.D. Chief of Staff, Seton Edgar B. Davis Hospital, Luling, TX, p. A614
WEINGARTNER, Ronald, Chief Operating Officer, St. Charles Hospital, Port Jefferson, NY, p. A440
WEINHOLD, Chantal, Executive Director, Long Island Jewish Medical Center,, NY, p. A434
WEINHOLD, Robert, Chief Executive Officer, Foundations Behavioral Health, Doylestown, PA, p. A522
WEINKRANTZ, Alan, Chief Financial Officer, University of Medicine and Dentistry of New Jersey, University Behavioral Healthcare, Piscataway, NJ, p. A408
WEINMANN, Shannon, Director Human Resources, Community Medical Center, Falls City, NE, p. A383
WEINMEISTER, Kurt, Executive Vice President and Chief Operating Officer, Pomona Valley Hospital Medical Center, Pomona, CA, p. A80
WEINMEISTER III, Oscar K., Chief Executive Officer, Blue Ridge Regional Hospital, Spruce Pine, NC, p. A461
WEINREIS, Brian, Vice President Operations and Finance, Abbott Northwestern Hospital, Minneapolis, MN, p. A334
WEINSTEIN, Barry S., Chief Financial Officer, Four Winds Hospital, Katonah, NY, p. A428
WEINSTEIN, Brian, M.D. Chief of Staff, Westside Regional Medical Center, Plantation, FL, p. A136
WEINSTEIN, Gary B., President and Chief Executive Officer, Washington Hospital, Washington, PA, p. A540
WEINSTEIN, James, M.D. President and Chief Executive Officer, Dartmouth–Hitchcock Medical Center, Lebanon, NH, p. A398
WEINSTEIN, Jay S., Chief Operating Officer, St. Anthony Hospital, Lakewood, CO, p. A103
WEINSTEIN, Roslyn, Chief Operating Officer, Kings County Hospital Center,, NY, p. A433
WEINSTOCK, Dean R., R.N. Executive Director, Pilgrim Psychiatric Center, Brentwood, NY, p. A422
WEINTZ, Charles, D.O. Chief of Staff, Stanton County Hospital, Johnson, KS, p. A235
WEIS, Charles
Chief Financial Officer, Mount Sinai Hospital, Chicago, IL, p. A177
Chief Financial Officer, Schwab Rehabilitation Hospital, Chicago, IL, p. A178
WEIS, Harry, Chief Executive Officer, Natividad Medical Center, Salinas, CA, p. A84
WEIS, Maurine, Vice President Patient Care Service and Chief Nursing Officer, ProMedica Bay Park Hospital, Oregon, OH, p. A486
WEIS, Shirley
Chief Administrative Officer, Mayo Clinic – Methodist Hospital, Rochester, MN, p. A338
Chief Administrative Officer, Mayo Clinic – Saint Marys Hospital, Rochester, MN, p. A338

A960 Index of Health Care Professionals 

Index of Health Care Professionals / Westerheide

WEIS, Wade, Senior Director Finance, Grande Ronde Hospital, La Grande, OR, p. A512
WEISE, Charles, M.D. Medical Director, Highland Hospital, Charleston, WV, p. A671
WEISENFREUND, Jochanan, M.D. Senior Vice President Academic and Medical Affairs, Interfaith Medical Center,, NY, p. A433
WEISFIELD, Phyllis, Chief Executive Officer and Managing Director, Horsham Clinic, Ambler, PA, p. A518
WEISHAPL, Natasha, Manager Business Office and Human Resources, Decatur County Hospital and Cedar Living Center, Oberlin, KS, p. A240
WEISNER, Brad, Executive Vice President and Chief Operating Officer, Nash Health Care Systems, Rocky Mount, NC, p. A460
WEISS, Allen S., M.D. President and Chief Executive Officer, NCH Downtown Naples Hospital, Naples, FL, p. A133
WEISS, Barry J., Chairman of the Board, College Health Enterprises, Santa Fe Springs, CA, p. B32
WEISS, Clay, Administrator, Northwest Texas Surgery Center, Amarillo, TX, p. A578
WEISS, David, Vice President Information System, Alton Memorial Hospital, Alton, IL, p. A172
WEISS, Gary, Chief Financial Officer, NorthShore University Health System Evanston Hospital, Evanston, IL, p. A181
WEISS, Linda W., FACHE Director, Albany Stratton Veterans Affairs Medical Center, Albany, NY, p. A420
WEISS, Phyllis, Director Human Resources, Alameda Hospital, Alameda, CA, p. A53
WEISS, Terri, Chief Financial Officer, Reliant Rehabilitation Hospital North Houston, Shenandoah, TX, p. A627
WEISSENBERGER, Ralf, Director Information Systems, White Memorial Medical Center, Los Angeles, CA, p. A73
WEISSER, Lisa, Supervisor Finance, Wagner Community Memorial Hospital Avera, Wagner, SD, p. A560
WEISUL, Jonathan, M.D
 Vice President Medical Affairs and Chief Medical Officer, CHRISTUS Coushatta Health Care Center, Coushatta, LA, p. A264
 Chief Medical Officer and Vice President Innovation, Community Medical Center, Missoula, MT, p. A377
WELCH, Abbey, Director Human Resources, Harmon Memorial Hospital, Hollis, OK, p. A498
WELCH, Andrew, Director, Amarillo Veterans Affairs Health Care System, Amarillo, TX, p. A578
WELCH, Bonnie, Chief Information Officer, St. James Mercy Health System, Hornell, NY, p. A427
WELCH, Bryant, Chief Human Resources, Washington Hospital Healthcare System, Fremont, CA, p. A61
WELCH, Charolotte, Chief Nursing Officer, Haskell Memorial Hospital, Haskell, TX, p. A603
WELCH, David, M.D. Medical Director, Clifton–Fine Hospital, Star Lake, NY, p. A443
WELCH, David, Director Information Technology, Simpson General Hospital, Mendenhall, MS, p. A350
WELCH, Donald E., Chief Operating Officer, Florida Hospital Zephyrhills, Zephyrhills, FL, p. A143
WELCH, Douglas, Chief Executive Officer, Doctors Hospital, Augusta, GA, p. A146
WELCH, Jeffery L., Chief Operating Officer, Delray Medical Center, Delray Beach, FL, p. A122
WELCH, Kenneth, M.D. Chief Medical Officer, Banner Estrella Medical Center, Phoenix, AZ, p. A35
WELCH, Melissa, Director Health Information Management, Oakdale Community Hospital, Oakdale, LA, p. A275
WELCH, Rosemary C., R.N. Vice President and Chief Nursing Officer, Medstar National Rehabilitation Network, Washington, DC, p. A116
WELCH, Shelly, R.N. Senior Vice President and Chief Nursing Officer, North Oaks Medical Center, Hammond, LA, p. A267
WELCH, Tony
 VP Human Resources, Englewood Community Hospital, Englewood, FL, p. A122
 Vice President Human Resources, Fawcett Memorial Hospital, Port Charlotte, FL, p. A136
WELCH, William L., FACHE Chief Executive Officer, Jefferson Community Health Center, Fairbury, NE, p. A383
WELDAY, Douglas D., Executive Vice President and Chief Financial Officer, Oakwood Hospital & Medical Center–Dearborn, Dearborn, MI, p. A310
WELDER, Linda R., M.D. Chief of Staff, Highland District Hospital, Hillsboro, OH, p. A482
WELDING, Theodore L., Administrator, Kindred Hospital South Florida–Fort Lauderdale, Fort Lauderdale, FL, p. A123
WELDON, Jim, Chief Information Officer, St. Anthony's Medical Center, Saint Louis, MO, p. A370
WELDON, Marie L., FACHE Director, South Texas Veterans Health Care System, San Antonio, TX, p. A626
WELDON, William W., Ph.D. Interim Chief Executive Officer, Cogdell Memorial Hospital, Snyder, TX, p. A628
WELDY, Alan, Vice President Human Resources, Compliance and Legal Services, Indiana University Health Goshen Hospital, Goshen, IN, p. A202
WELKER, Suzanne, Chief Human Resources Officer and Vice President Marketing Strategy, Berger Health System, Circleville, OH, p. A474
WELKIE, Katy, R.N. Administrator and Chief Executive Officer, Primary Children's Medical Center, Salt Lake City, UT, p. A640
WELL, Molly, Chief Nursing Officer, Martin General Hospital, Williamston, NC, p. A462
WELLENDORF, Sharon A., Chief Nursing Officer, Horn Memorial Hospital, Ida Grove, IA, p. A221
WELLENDORF, Tracey, M.D. Chief of Staff, St. Anthony Regional Hospital, Carroll, IA, p. A215
WELLING, Lynn, Commander, Naval Hospital, Jacksonville, FL, p. A126
WELLING, Richard, M.D. Chief of Staff, Bartlett Regional Hospital, Juneau, AK, p. A29
WELLMANN, Jane, Chief Financial Officer, Scott & White Hospital – Brenham, Brenham, TX, p. A585
WELLS, A. Shane
 Chief Financial Officer, Cornerstone Hospital of Houston – Bellaire, Houston, TX, p. A603
 Chief Financial Officer, Solara Hospital Harlingen–Brownsville Campus, Brownsville, TX, p. A585
WELLS, Alphe, Vice President Human Resources and Support Services, Delta Regional Medical Center, Greenville, MS, p. A346
WELLS, Carol, R.N. Chief Nursing Officer, Central Louisiana Surgical Hospital, Alexandria, LA, p. A261
WELLS, Dale, Senior Vice President Finance and Operations, Alliance Community Hospital, Alliance, OH, p. A469
WELLS, Jason, Chief Human Resources Management Service, Veterans Affairs Health Care System, Fargo, ND, p. A466
WELLS, Jonathan, Supervisor Information Technology, Kansas Surgery and Recovery Center, Wichita, KS, p. A245
WELLS, Mary S., R.N. Chief Executive Officer, Community Memorial Hospital, Sumner, IA, p. A227
WELLS, Scott E., MSN Chief Nursing Officer, St. Francis Health Center, Topeka, KS, p. A244
WELLS, Valerie
 Manager Human Resources, HEALTHSOUTH Rehabilitation Hospital, Humble, TX, p. A608
 Manager Human Resources, HEALTHSOUTH Rehabilitation Hospital of North Houston, Conroe, TX, p. A588
WELSH, Cari, Interim Chief Financial Officer, Fountain Valley Regional Hospital and Medical Center, Fountain Valley, CA, p. A61
WELSH, Luckey, Interim Director, Cherry Hospital, Goldsboro, NC, p. A453
WENGER, Cheryl, Manager Health Information and Quality Assurance, Hiawatha Community Hospital, Hiawatha, KS, p. A234
WENGER, Jill, Vice President Human Resources, McPherson Hospital, McPherson, KS, p. A238
WENGER–KELLER, David, M.D. Chief of Staff, Fort Madison Community Hospital, Fort Madison, IA, p. A220
WENGERD, Gary, Vice President Finance and Chief Financial Officer, Mercy Regional Medical Center, Lorain, OH, p. A483
WENTZ, Robert J., President and Chief Executive Officer, Oroville Hospital, Oroville, CA, p. A78
WENTZEL, Chris, M.D. Interim Medical Director, Corning Hospital, Corning, NY, p. A424
WENZEL, Matthew J., Chief Executive Officer, Hedrick Medical Center, Chillicothe, MO, p. A357
WERFT, Ronald C., President and Chief Executive Officer, Cottage Health System, Santa Barbara, CA, p. B39
WERFT, Ronald C.
 President and Chief Executive Officer, Goleta Valley Cottage Hospital, Santa Barbara, CA, p. A89
 President and Chief Executive Officer, Santa Barbara Cottage Hospital, Santa Barbara, CA, p. A89
 President and Chief Executive Officer, Santa Ynez Valley Cottage Hospital, Solvang, CA, p. A91
WERKOWSKI, Richard F., Chief Financial Officer, Speare Memorial Hospital, Plymouth, NH, p. A400
WERNECKE, Jennie, Human Resources Manager, Dr. John Warner Hospital, Clinton, IL, p. A179
WERNER, Don, Chief Executive Officer, Lady of the Sea General Hospital, Cut Off, LA, p. A265
WERNER, Edward, Director Human Resources, HEALTHSOUTH Reading Rehabilitation Hospital, Reading, PA, p. A537
WERNER, Julie, Chief Operating Officer, Community Memorial Hospital, Syracuse, NE, p. A390
WERNER, Kurt, M.D. Chief of Staff, Veterans Affairs Montana Health Care System, Fort Harrison, MT, p. A375
WERNER, Mark D., M.D. Executive Vice President and Chief Medical Officer, Carilion Medical Center, Roanoke, VA, p. A655
WERNER, Sandy, Director Human Resources, Simi Valley Hospital and Health Care Services, Simi Valley, CA, p. A91
WERNER, Todd S., Chief Executive Officer, Banner Gateway Medical Center, Gilbert, AZ, p. A32
WERNICK, Joel, President and Chief Executive Officer, Phoebe Putney Health System, Albany, GA, p. B101
WERNICK, Joel, President and Chief Executive Officer, Phoebe Putney Memorial Hospital, Albany, GA, p. A144
WERNKE, Chris, Chief Operating Officer, Dominican Hospital, Santa Cruz, CA, p. A90
WERRBACH, John P., Chief Executive Officer, Alexian Brothers Medical Center, Elk Grove Village, IL, p. A181
WERTH–SWEENEY, Stacey, Facility Operating Officer, Lincoln Regional Center, Lincoln, NE, p. A385
WERTHMAN, Ronald J., Vice President Finance, Chief Financial Officer and Treasurer, Johns Hopkins Hospital, Baltimore, MD, p. A287
WERTZ, Barbara
 Vice President Patient Care Services, Providence Medical Center, Kansas City, KS, p. A236
 Vice President Patient Care Services, Saint John Hospital, Leavenworth, KS, p. A237
WERTZ, Jackie, Director Human Resources, George C Grape Community Hospital, Hamburg, IA, p. A220
WERTZ, Randy S., Chief Executive Officer, Golden Valley Memorial Healthcare, Clinton, MO, p. A358
WESCOTT, Lisle, President, SSM St. Joseph Hospital West, Lake Saint Louis, MO, p. A363
WESENER DIECK, Jill, Director Human Resources, Tri–County Memorial Hospital, Whitehall, WI, p. A694
WESLEY, Deb, MSN Chief Nursing Officer, The Children's Hospital of Alabama, Birmingham, AL, p. A17
WESLEY, Jim
 Interim Senior Vice President and Chief Information Officer, John Muir Medical Center, Concord, Concord, CA, p. A58
 Interim Chief Information Officer, John Muir Medical Center, Walnut Creek, Walnut Creek, CA, p. A95
WESLEY, Lois Sprengeler, Director Quality Management, U. S. Public Health Service Indian Hospital, San Carlos, AZ, p. A37
WESSELS, Jana, Associate Vice President Human Resources, University of Iowa Hospitals and Clinics, Iowa City, IA, p. A221
WESSON, Jim D., Vice President and Administrator, CHRISTUS Santa Rosa Hospital – New Braunfels, New Braunfels, TX, p. A618
WEST, Arthur, Chief Financial Officer, Hialeah Hospital, Hialeah, FL, p. A125
WEST, Dan, Director Information Technology Systems, Middle Tennessee Medical Center, Murfreesboro, TN, p. A573
WEST, David, Chief Operating Officer, Deckerville Community Hospital, Deckerville, MI, p. A310
WEST, Heather, Director Human Resources, Lakeland Community Hospital Watervliet, Watervliet, MI, p. A325
WEST, James R., President and Chief Executive Officer, Presbyterian Intercommunity Hospital, Whittier, CA, p. A96
WEST, Joanell, Human Resources Generalist, Methodist Healthcare–Fayette Hospital, Somerville, TN, p. A575
WEST, Judy, Vice President Human Resources, Maine Medical Center, Portland, ME, p. A284
WEST, Karen M., Administrator Support Services, Wild Rose Community Memorial Hospital, Wild Rose, WI, p. A694
WEST, Margaret M., MS, Chief Executive Officer, Magnolia Regional Medical Center, Magnolia, AR, p. A48
WEST, Michael A., Chief Executive Officer, Rothman Specialty Hospital, Bensalem, PA, p. A518
WEST, Michael C., M.D. Chief of Staff, McCurtain Memorial Hospital, Idabel, OK, p. A498
WEST, Michele, Director Human Resources, Doctors Medical Center, Modesto, CA, p. A75
WEST, Steve, M.D. Chief Medical Officer, Capital Regional Medical Center, Tallahassee, FL, p. A140
WEST, Steven J., Chief Executive Officer, Indiana University Health Blackford Hospital, Hartford City, IN, p. A203
WEST, Tamara, R.N. Vice President Patient Care, Nicholas H. Noyes Memorial Hospital, Dansville, NY, p. A425
WEST, Warren K., FACHE Chief Executive Officer, Littleton Regional Hospital, Littleton, NH, p. A399
WEST, William, M.D. Chief of Staff, Edgerton Hospital and Health Services, Edgerton, WI, p. A681
WESTBROOK, Kenneth K., President and Chief Executive Officer, Integrated Healthcare, Santa Ana, CA, p. B71
WESTENFELDER, Grant, M.D. Chief Medical Officer, Midwest Medical Center, Galena, IL, p. A182
WESTENHOFER, Steve, Chief Executive Officer, Mimbres Memorial Hospital, Deming, NM, p. A415
WESTER, K. Scott, FACHE President and Chief Executive Officer, Our Lady of the Lake Regional Medical Center, Baton Rouge, LA, p. A262
WESTERHEIDE, Karen, Chief Financial Officer, Veterans Affairs Medical Center, Saint Louis, MO, p. A370

Index of Health Care Professionals

Index of Health Care Professionals

Index of Health Care Professionals / Westfall

WESTFALL, Gay, Senior Vice President Human Resources, Sacramento Medical Center, Sacramento, CA, p. A83
WESTFIELD, Brian W., MSN, Director, Jonathan M. Wainwright Memorial VA Medical Center, Walla Walla, WA, p. A669
WESTGARD, David E., M.D. Chief Medical Officer, Olmsted Medical Center, Rochester, MN, p. A338
WESTMAN, Ken, Chief Executive Officer, Barrett Hospital & HealthCare, Dillon, MT, p. A375
WESTMORELAND, Penny
Chief Financial Officer, Lakeland Community Hospital, Haleyville, AL, p. A21
Chief Financial Officer, Russellville Hospital, Russellville, AL, p. A25
WESTON, Betty, Chief Human Resources Officer, U. S. Public Health Service Phoenix Indian Medical Center, Phoenix, AZ, p. A37
WESTON, Nancy R., R.N. Vice President Nursing Services, Memorial Hospital, Belleville, IL, p. A173
WESTON, Terry, M.D. Vice President Physician Services, MedCentral – Mansfield Hospital, Mansfield, OH, p. A483
WESTON–HALL, Patricia, Chief Executive Officer, Glenbeigh Hospital and Outpatient Centers, Rock Creek, OH, p. A487
WESTOVER, Gerald, M.D. Medical Director, Upper Connecticut Valley Hospital, Colebrook, NH, p. A397
WESTPHAL, James, M.D. Medical Director, Hawaii State Hospital, Kaneohe, HI, p. A164
WESTRICH, Vern, President and Chief Executive Officer, Haven Behavioral Healthcare, Nashville, TN, p. B56
WETHERS, Darren E., M.D. President Medical Staff, SSM St. Mary's Health Center, Saint Louis, MO, p. A369
WETHINGTON, Bud, Chief Executive Officer, Tomball Regional Medical Center, Tomball, TX, p. A631
WETHINGTON, Patti, R.N. Chief Nursing Officer, Spectrum Health Gerber Memorial, Fremont, MI, p. A312
WEVER, Kurt, M.D. Chief of Staff, Pikes Peak Regional Hospital, Woodland Park, CO, p. A107
WEXLER, Erik G., President and Chief Executive Officer, Saint Vincent Hospital, Worcester, MA, p. A306
WEYHMULLER, Gary J., Chief Operating Officer, Fox Chase Cancer Center–American Oncologic Hospital, Philadelphia, PA, p. A532
WEYMOUTH, Deborah K., Executive Director and Senior Vice President, New Milford Hospital, New Milford, CT, p. A111
WEYMOUTH, Linda, Chief Financial Officer, Manatee Palms Youth Services, Bradenton, FL, p. A119
WHALEN, David, Chief Executive Officer, Twin Cities Hospital, Niceville, FL, p. A133
WHALEN, Eileen, R.N. Executive Director, Harborview Medical Center, Seattle, WA, p. A665
WHALEN, Patti, Manager Human Resources, Wichita County Health Center, Leoti, KS, p. A238
WHALEN, Scott, FACHE President and Chief Executive Officer, Saint Vincent Health Center, Erie, PA, p. A523
WHALEN, Scott, FACHE President and Chief Executive Officer, Saint Vincent Health System, Erie, PA, p. B112
WHALEN, Scott, FACHE President and Chief Executive Officer, Westfield Memorial Hospital, Westfield, NY, p. A446
WHALEN, Thomas
Chief Financial Officer, Braintree Rehabilitation Hospital, Braintree, MA, p. A298
Vice President Finance, Good Samaritan Medical Center, Brockton, MA, p. A298
WHALEN, Thomas, M.D. Chief Medical Officer, Lehigh Valley Hospital–Muhlenberg, Bethlehem, PA, p. A518
WHALEY, Alan R., Administrator, Infirmary West, Mobile, AL, p. A22
WHALEY, Joseph, Chief, Human Resources Management Service, Veterans Affairs Medical Center, Fayetteville, NC, p. A453
WHARTON, Joe H., M.D. Chief of Staff, Bradley County Medical Center, Warren, AR, p. A52
WHEAT, Ken, Chief Operating Officer, Desert Regional Medical Center, Palm Springs, CA, p. A78
WHEAT, Melissa, Manager Human Resources, Infirmary West, Mobile, AL, p. A22
WHEAT, Terry, R.N. Acting Administrator, Shriners Hospitals for Children–Chicago, Chicago, IL, p. A178
WHEATLEY, Jane, Chief Executive Officer, Taylor Regional Hospital, Campbellsville, KY, p. A248
WHEATLEY, Jason
Manager Information Systems, Provena Covenant Medical Center, Urbana, IL, p. A195
Manager Information Systems, Provena United Samaritans Medical Center, Danville, IL, p. A179
WHEATLEY, Richard, Chief Information Officer, Cape Regional Medical Center, Cape May Court House, NJ, p. A402
WHEATON, David, Director Human Resources, Blue Hill Memorial Hospital, Blue Hill, ME, p. A282
WHEELAN, Kevin, M.D. Medical Director, Baylor Jack and Jane Hamilton Heart and Vascular Hospital, Dallas, TX, p. A590
WHEELER, Barb, Business Manager, Mental Health Institute, Mount Pleasant, IA, p. A224
WHEELER, Brent, Vice President Ancillary and Support Services, McLaren Flint, Flint, MI, p. A312
WHEELER, Butch, FACHE Chief Executive Officer, Hughston Hospital, Columbus, GA, p. A149
WHEELER, Dana
Director Human Resources, South Bay Hospital, Sun City Center, FL, p. A140
Director Human Resources, Venice Regional Medical Center, Venice, FL, p. A142
WHEELER, Dane, Chief Financial Officer, Adams Memorial Hospital, Decatur, IN, p. A200
WHEELER, Dawne, Chief Executive Officer, Select Specialty Hospital–Canton, Canton, OH, p. A472
WHEELER, Deborah, Director Human Resources, North Carolina Specialty Hospital, Durham, NC, p. A452
WHEELER, James A., Vice President Human Relations and Community Development, Androscoggin Valley Hospital, Berlin, NH, p. A397
WHEELER, Jim, Executive Vice President and Chief Financial Officer, South Haven Health System, South Haven, MI, p. A323
WHEELER, Joan, R.N. Administrator, Runnells Specialized Hospital of Union County, Berkeley Heights, NJ, p. A401
WHEELER, Katrina, Chief Financial Officer, Mayo Clinic Health System in Waycross, Waycross, GA, p. A162
WHEELER, Kevin, Information Technology Leader, Walnut Creek Medical Center, Walnut Creek, CA, p. A95
WHEELER, Lois, Manager Human Resources, F. W. Huston Medical Center, Winchester, KS, p. A246
WHEELER, Lynette, MSN Chief Nursing Officer, Truman Medical Center–Lakewood, Kansas City, MO, p. A363
WHEELER, Pam, Manager Human Resources, Scott County Hospital, Scott City, KS, p. A243
WHEELER, Rebecca, Director Finance, Baldwin Park Medical Center, Baldwin Park, CA, p. A55
WHEELER, Robert
Controller, HEALTHSOUTH Rehabilitation Hospital, Florence, SC, p. A549
Vice President Human Resources, South Shore Hospital, South Weymouth, MA, p. A304
WHEELER, Terry J., Chief Executive Officer, Cypress Fairbanks Medical Center, Houston, TX, p. A604
WHEELER, Zach, Senior Vice President Human Resources, John D. Archbold Memorial Hospital, Thomasville, GA, p. A160
WHEELESS, Jane, Director Human Resources, Crosbyton Clinic Hospital, Crosbyton, TX, p. A590
WHELAN, Doris, Chief Information Officer, Moberly Regional Medical Center, Moberly, MO, p. A365
WHELAN, Laurie A., Senior Vice President Finance and Chief Financial Officer, Hospital for Special Care, New Britain, CT, p. A110
WHELAN, Melissa, Director Health Information, Brighton Center for Recovery, Brighton, MI, p. A308
WHELAN, Thomas, President, Lodi Community Hospital, Lodi, OH, p. A483
WHELAN, Wendy, Director Talent, Southwestern Regional Medical Center, Tulsa, OK, p. A507
WHERRY, Richard, M.D. Chief of Staff, Chestatee Regional Hospital, Dahlonega, GA, p. A150
WHERRY, Robin, Risk Manager and Director Quality Assurance and Health Information Management, HEALTHSOUTH MountainView Regional Rehabilitation Hospital, Morgantown, WV, p. A674
WHETSTINE, Tyler, Director of Information Systems, Citrus Memorial Health System, Inverness, FL, p. A126
WHETTON, Matthew, Chief Business Administration, Veterans Affairs Central California Health Care System, Fresno, CA, p. A62
WHICHARD, Forrest, Chief Financial Officer, Ochsner Medical Center – North Shore, Slidell, LA, p. A278
WHIDDON, William, Chief Financial Officer, The Medical Center of Southeast Texas, Port Arthur, TX, p. A622
WHILDEN, Sean
Chief Financial Officer, Houston Medical Center, Warner Robins, GA, p. A161
Chief Financial Officer, Perry Hospital, Perry, GA, p. A157
WHILES, David
Director Health Information Systems, Midland Memorial Hospital, Midland, TX, p. A617
Director Health Information Systems, Midland Memorial Hospital, Midland, TX, p. A617
WHILLOCK, Mary C., R.N. Associate Nursing Officer and Chief Operating Officer, Florida Hospital–Carrollwood, Tampa, FL, p. A140
WHIPKEY, Jared, Chief Financial Officer, Barrow Regional Medical Center, Winder, GA, p. A162
WHIPPLE, Glenn, Chief Information Officer, Dameron Hospital, Stockton, CA, p. A91
WHIPPLE, James, Administrator and Chief Executive Officer, Marshall Medical Center, Placerville, CA, p. A80
WHITAKER, Charles, Director Information Technology, Madison Parish Hospital, Tallulah, LA, p. A278
WHITAKER, David D., FACHE President and Chief Executive Officer, Norman Regional Health System, Norman, OK, p. A500
WHITAKER, Doris, Vice President Human Resources, Booneville Community Hospital, Booneville, AR, p. A42
WHITAKER, E. Berton, FACHE Chief Executive Officer, Regional Medical Center of Hopkins County, Madisonville, KY, p. A255
WHITAKER, James B., President, Circles of Care, Melbourne, FL, p. A130
WHITAKER, Jimmy, Director Information Systems, Central Carolina Hospital, Sanford, NC, p. A460
WHITAKER, Neil, M.D
Chief Medical Director, Orem Community Hospital, Orem, UT, p. A639
Medical Director, Utah Valley Regional Medical Center, Provo, UT, p. A640
WHITE, A. Randle, M.D. Chief Medical Staff, Greenwood Leflore Hospital, Greenwood, MS, p. A346
WHITE, Al, CPA Senior Vice President Business Services, Broadlawns Medical Center, Des Moines, IA, p. A218
WHITE, Andrea, Chief Executive Officer, Select Specialty Hospital–Birmingham, Birmingham, AL, p. A16
WHITE, Beverly, MS, Facility Director, Mary S Harper Geriatric Psychiatry Center, Tuscaloosa, AL, p. A26
WHITE, Brian M., President and Chief Operating Officer, Northwest Hospital, Randallstown, MD, p. A293
WHITE, Bruce D., Chief Executive Officer, Knox Community Hospital, Mount Vernon, OH, p. A485
WHITE, Charles, Chief Administrative Officer, Upper Connecticut Valley Hospital, Colebrook, NH, p. A397
WHITE, Chris L., Administrator, Catskill Regional Medical Center, Callicoon, NY, p. A423
WHITE, Cindy, CPA Assistant Vice President and Chief Financial Officer, INTEGRIS Canadian Valley Hospital, Yukon, OK, p. A508
WHITE, Cole, Director Finance, Kremmling Memorial Hospital, Kremmling, CO, p. A102
WHITE, Darrell, R.N. Administrator, Tristar Ashland City Medical Center, Ashland City, TN, p. A562
WHITE, Debbie
Chief Financial Officer, CHRISTUS St. Frances Cabrini Hospital, Alexandria, LA, p. A261
Chief Financial Officer, CHRISTUS St. Patrick Hospital of Lake Charles, Lake Charles, LA, p. A271
WHITE, Deborah, Director Human Resources, Maniilaq Health Center, Kotzebue, AK, p. A29
WHITE, Debra, Chief Nursing Officer, Saint Luke's Hospital of Kansas City, Kansas City, MO, p. A362
WHITE, Diane B., Director Human Resources, Jerome Golden Center for Behavioral Health, Inc., West Palm Beach, FL, p. A142
WHITE, Donna, Director Human Resources, HEALTHSOUTH Rehabilitation Hospital of Charleston, Charleston, SC, p. A547
WHITE, Doug, Chief Executive Officer, Grand Strand Regional Medical Center, Myrtle Beach, SC, p. A552
WHITE, Dudley R., Administrator and Chief Executive Officer, Concho County Hospital, Eden, TX, p. A595
WHITE, Gary B., M.D. Chief Medical Staff, Uintah Basin Medical Center, Roosevelt, UT, p. A640
WHITE, Harold, Vice Chancellor, LSU Medical Center–University Hospital, Shreveport, LA, p. A277
WHITE, J. B., Director Information Systems, River Region Medical Center, Vicksburg, MS, p. A353
WHITE, James, M.D. Chief of Staff, Riverton Memorial Hospital, Riverton, WY, p. A697
WHITE, James P., M.D. Chief Medical Officer, Integris Baptist Medical Center, Oklahoma City, OK, p. A501
WHITE Jr., James R., Chief Executive Officer, Pioneer Community Hospital of Stokes, Danbury, NC, p. A451
WHITE, Jean, Vice President Finance, Avera Heart Hospital of South Dakota, Sioux Falls, SD, p. A559
WHITE, Jeffrey L., Senior Vice President and Chief Financial Officer, Beaufort Memorial Hospital, Beaufort, SC, p. A546
WHITE, Jim
Chief Information Officer, Lompoc Valley Medical Center, Lompoc, CA, p. A67
Chief Financial Officer, Parkside Hospital, Tulsa, OK, p. A506
WHITE, Joanne, Chief Information Officer, Wood County Hospital, Bowling Green, OH, p. A471
WHITE, Jody, Executive Vice President and Chief Operating Officer, Lowell General Hospital, Lowell, MA, p. A301
WHITE, Joe
Chief Financial Officer, Central Texas Hospital, Cameron, TX, p. A586
Chief Financial Officer, Lake Whitney Medical Center, Whitney, TX, p. A635

A962 Index of Health Care Professionals 

Index of Health Care Professionals / Wiggins

Index of Health Care Professionals


WHITE, John, M.D. Medical Director, Parkside Hospital, Tulsa, OK, p. A506
WHITE, John D., Chief Financial Officer, Wythe County Community Hospital, Wytheville, VA, p. A658
WHITE, John R., Chief Executive Officer, Klickitat Valley Health, Goldendale, WA, p. A661
WHITE, Kathy, Interim Chief Operating Officer, Doctors Medical Center–San Pablo Campus, San Pablo, CA, p. A89
WHITE, Kay, Director Human Resources and Diversity, Marion Regional Hospital, Mullins, SC, p. A552
WHITE, Kelli, Manager Human Resources, CenterPointe Hospital, Saint Charles, MO, p. A367
WHITE, Kevin A., Administrator, Medicine Lodge Memorial Hospital, Medicine Lodge, KS, p. A239
WHITE, Linda, Director Fiscal Services, Memphis Mental Health Institute, Memphis, TN, p. A571
WHITE, Linda E., President and Chief Executive Officer, Deaconess Health System, Evansville, IN, p. B40
WHITE, Lindy P., President and Chief Executive Officer, Smyth County Community Hospital, Marion, VA, p. A651
WHITE, Louise, R.N
Vice President Patient Care Services and Chief Nursing Officer, Children's Hospital at Mission, Mission Viejo, CA, p. A74
Vice President Patient Care Services and Chief Nursing Officer, Children's Hospital of Orange County, Orange, CA, p. A78
WHITE, Lynwood R., Vice President Finance, Randolph Hospital, Asheboro, NC, p. A448
WHITE, Mark, Director Information Services, Mount Desert Island Hospital, Bar Harbor, ME, p. A281
WHITE, Mary M., Chief Executive Officer, Swedish Medical Center, Englewood, CO, p. A100
WHITE, Mary–Louise, M.D. Chief Executive Officer, Dr. Solomon Carter Fuller Mental Health Center, Boston, MA, p. A296
WHITE, Nathan, Director Information Systems, Caldwell Memorial Hospital, Lenoir, NC, p. A456
WHITE, Olinda, Chief Financial Officer, Wrangell Medical Center, Wrangell, AK, p. A30
WHITE, Padraic, Interim Administrator, Ward Memorial Hospital, Monahans, TX, p. A617
WHITE, Patricia, Vice President Human Resources, Seton Medical Center, Daly City, CA, p. A59
WHITE, Randall, Chief Executive Officer, Fayette Regional Health System, Connersville, IN, p. A199
WHITE, Randy, Chief Nursing Officer, Baptist Memorial Hospital–Union County, New Albany, MS, p. A351
WHITE, Robert, Director Information Technology, Helena Regional Medical Center, Helena, AR, p. A46
WHITE, Robin, Assistant Vice President Human Resources, Parkview Adventist Medical Center, Brunswick, ME, p. A282
WHITE, Sabrina, Coordinator Human Resources, Select Specialty Hospital–Charleston, Charleston, WV, p. A671
WHITE, Shelia, Director Human Resources, Bon Secours–Richmond Community Hospital, Richmond, VA, p. A654
WHITE, Shirley, Director Human Resources, Ashley County Medical Center, Crossett, AR, p. A43
WHITE, Steve, M.D. Chief Medical Officer, Guadalupe Regional Medical Center, Seguin, TX, p. A627
WHITE, Terri, Commissioner, Oklahoma Department of Mental Health and Substance Abuse Services, Oklahoma City, OK, p. B98
WHITE, Thomas, Director Human Resources, Blue Ridge Regional Hospital, Spruce Pine, NC, p. A461
WHITE, Wayne, Director Computer Services, Sage Memorial Hospital, Ganado, AZ, p. A32
WHITE, Wendy
Vice President Human Resources, CHRISTUS Health Shreveport–Bossier, Shreveport, LA, p. A277
Regional Vice President Human Resources, CHRISTUS St. Frances Cabrini Hospital, Alexandria, LA, p. A261
Assistant Administrator Human Resources, CHRISTUS St. Patrick Hospital of Lake Charles, Lake Charles, LA, p. A271
WHITE, Wesley D., Chief Financial Officer, Community Hospital, Grand Junction, CO, p. A101
WHITE, Willie, M.D. Director Medical Staff, J. Paul Jones Hospital, Camden, AL, p. A18
WHITE, Woody, Chief Financial Officer, Wellington Regional Medical Center, West Palm Beach, FL, p. A143
WHITE HOUSE, Judy, Vice President Human Resources, St. Mary's Hospital and Medical Center, Grand Junction, CO, p. A102
WHITE–JACOBS, Mary Beth, R.N. Vice President Patient Care Services, Black River Memorial Hospital, Black River Falls, WI, p. A679
WHITEAKER, Les, Vice President and Chief Financial Officer, Memorial Medical Center – Ashland, Ashland, WI, p. A678
WHITED, Brian, M.D. Medical Director, Mayo Clinic Health System in Mankato, Mankato, MN, p. A334
WHITED, Steve, Chief Executive Officer, Minnie Hamilton HealthCare Center, Grantsville, WV, p. A672
WHITEHEAD, Alva W., M.D. Vice President Medical Services, McLeod Regional Medical Center, Florence, SC, p. A550
WHITEHEAD, David, President and Chief Executive Officer, The William W. Backus Hospital, Norwich, CT, p. A111
WHITEHORN, Jeffrey T., Chief Executive Officer, Summit Medical Center, Hermitage, TN, p. A566
WHITEHOUSE, Edward J., Chief Executive Officer, Sylvan Grove Hospital, Jackson, GA, p. A154
WHITEHURST, Carolyn, Director Human Resources, Texas Health Presbyterian Hospital Kaufman, Kaufman, TX, p. A610
WHITEHURST, Rob, Chief, Office of Information and Technology, Veterans Affairs Ann Arbor Healthcare System, Ann Arbor, MI, p. A307
WHITELEY, Earl S., Administrator, Calhoun Memorial Hospital, Arlington, GA, p. A144
WHITELOCK, Kim, Chief Executive Officer, Valley Hospital Phoenix, Phoenix, AZ, p. A37
WHITENACK, Barbara, Manager Human Resources, St. Vincent Mercy Hospital, Elwood, IN, p. A200
WHITENACK, John, Chief Operating Officer, Greystone Park Psychiatric Hospital, Morris Plains, NJ, p. A406
WHITESIDE, Patrick, Director Information Systems, Spectrum Health Gerber Memorial, Fremont, MI, p. A312
WHITESIDE, Timothy, M.D. Chief of Staff, Wahiawa General Hospital, Wahiawa, HI, p. A165
WHITETHORNE, Priscilla, Chief Executive Officer, U. S. Public Health Service Indian Hospital–Sells, Sells, AZ, p. A38
WHITFIELD, Bruce, Vice President and Chief Financial Officer, St. Patrick Hospital, Missoula, MT, p. A378
WHITFIELD Jr., Charles H., President and Chief Executive Officer, Laughlin Memorial Hospital, Greeneville, TN, p. A566
WHITFIELD, Jay, Chief Financial Officer, Baylor University Medical Center, Dallas, TX, p. A590
WHITFIELD, Teresa L., MS Director Quality and Outcomes, Eastern Plumas Health Care District, Portola, CA, p. A81
WHITING, Barbara, Director Health Information Management, Promise Hospital of Vicksburg, Vicksburg, MS, p. A353
WHITLEY, Kathleen, M.D. Director Clinical and Professional Service, Worcester State Hospital, Worcester, MA, p. A306
WHITLEY, Pam, R.N. Chief Operating Officer and Chief Nursing Officer, Green Oaks Hospital, Dallas, TX, p. A591
WHITLOCK, Jr., James A., M.D. Medical Director, Northeast Rehabilitation Hospital, Salem, NH, p. A400
WHITLOCK, Nancy, Manager Human Resources, Summers County ARH Hospital, Hinton, WV, p. A672
WHITMAN, Bill, Chief Operating Officer, JPS Health Network, Fort Worth, TX, p. A599
WHITMER, Carl, President and Chief Executive Officer, IASIS Healthcare, Franklin, TN, p. B70
WHITMORE, Ray B., Chief Financial Officer, McCurtain Memorial Hospital, Idabel, OK, p. A498
WHITMORE, W. Patrick, Chief Financial Officer, Medical Center of Plano, Plano, TX, p. A621
WHITNEY, Donald, Director Human Resources, Kindred Hospital–Albuquerque, Albuquerque, NM, p. A414
WHITNEY, Nancy, Chief Financial Officer, St. Francis Healthcare Campus, Breckenridge, MN, p. A329
WHITNUM, Rhonda, Director Health Improvement Management, Prague Community Hospital, Prague, OK, p. A503
WHITSON, Charles P., CPA Senior Vice President Finance, Lake Charles Memorial Hospital, Lake Charles, LA, p. A271
WHITT, Charles Christopher, Chief Nursing Officer, River Park Hospital, Huntington, WV, p. A672
WHITTAKER, Shawn, Chief Nursing Officer, Miller County Hospital, Colquitt, GA, p. A149
WHITTAKER, Sheena, M.D. President Medical Staff, Maine Coast Memorial Hospital, Ellsworth, ME, p. A283
WHITTEMORE, Marjorie, Director Human Resources, Rio Grande Regional Hospital, McAllen, TX, p. A615
WHITTEN, Cynthia, R.N. Chief Executive Officer, Select Specialty Hospital–Springfield, Springfield, MO, p. A371
WHITTENBURG, Pat, Director Human Resources and Corporate Compliance Officer, Cumberland Medical Center, Crossville, TN, p. A564
WHITTIER, John J., Vice President Finance, Hampstead Hospital, Hampstead, NH, p. A398
WHITTINGTON, Bruce
Vice President Human Resources, Hays Medical Center, Hays, KS, p. A234
Vice President Human Resources, Pawnee Valley Community Hospital, Larned, KS, p. A237
WHITTINGTON, Carol, Chief Human Resources Officer, Sacred Heart Hospital of Pensacola, Pensacola, FL, p. A136
WHITTINGTON, Hilary, Chief Financial Officer, Jefferson Healthcare, Port Townsend, WA, p. A664
WHITTINGTON, Laurie A., Chief Operating Officer, Memorial Hospital of Union County, Marysville, OH, p. A484
WHITTINGTON, Shane, Chief Financial Officer, Caldwell Medical Center, Princeton, KY, p. A258
WHITTLE, Ingrid, Chief Executive Officer, Cedar Crest Hospital, Belton, TX, p. A584
WHITTLE, Timothy E., M.D. Chief Medical Staff, North Mississippi Medical Center–West Point, West Point, MS, p. A353
WHOLLEY, Diane, Director Fiscal Services, Bridgewater State Hospital, Bridgewater, MA, p. A298
WHYTE, Alec, M.D. Clinical Director, Elmira Psychiatric Center, Elmira, NY, p. A426
WIBBENMEYER, Christopher, Director Human Resources, Perry County Memorial Hospital, Perryville, MO, p. A366
WIBBENS, Cheryl, M.D. Vice President Medical Staff Affairs, Memorial Hospital of South Bend, South Bend, IN, p. A212
WIBORG, Shelley, MS Chief Nursing Officer, Mercer County Hospital, Aledo, IL, p. A172
WICKE, III, Julius, Vice President Finance and Hospital Financial Officer, Baylor Jack and Jane Hamilton Heart and Vascular Hospital, Dallas, TX, p. A590
WICKE, Regina, Chief Financial Officer, Columbus Community Hospital, Columbus, TX, p. A588
WICKENS, Jeanne, Chief Financial Officer, Allegiance Health, Jackson, MI, p. A316
WICKER, Kenneth R., Chief Executive Officer, Brooksville Regional Hospital, Brooksville, FL, p. A119
WICKIZER, Jr., Boyd, M.D. Chief Medical Officer, Southside Regional Medical Center, Petersburg, VA, p. A653
WICKLINE, Melissa, Director Marketing, Greenbrier Valley Medical Center, Ronceverte, WV, p. A675
WICKLUND, Grant, President and Chief Executive Officer, Exempla Lutheran Medical Center, Wheat Ridge, CO, p. A107
WIDEMAN, Jeff, Director Information Systems, Gilmore Memorial Regional Medical Center, Amory, MS, p. A343
WIDENER, Michael, Chief Financial Officer, J. C. Blair Memorial Hospital, Huntingdon, PA, p. A525
WIDENER, William, Administrator and Chief Executive Officer, Kremmling Memorial Hospital, Kremmling, CO, p. A102
WIDHELM, Timothy, M.D. Chief of Staff, Memorial Community Health, Aurora, NE, p. A381
WIDNER, Eric W., President, Oakwood Annapolis Hospital, Wayne, MI, p. A325
WIDRA, Linda S., FACHE Chief Operating Officer, Lakewood Ranch Medical Center, Bradenton, FL, p. A119
WIEBE, Robert, M.D. Chief Medical Officer, Mercy General Hospital, Sacramento, CA, p. A83
WIEBOLT, Jani M., President and Chief Executive Officer, Essentia Health St. Joseph's Medical Center, Brainerd, MN, p. A328
WIECK, Jennifer, Business Manager, Genoa Community Hospital, Genoa, NE, p. A384
WIECZOREK, Pawel, Director Information Technology, BryLin Hospitals, Buffalo, NY, p. A422
WIEGAND, Deborah, R.N. Administrator, CHRISTUS Jasper Memorial Hospital, Jasper, TX, p. A609
WIEMANN, Michael, M.D. President, Providence Hospital, Southfield, MI, p. A323
WIENAND, Michael, Manager Human Resources, Clarion Hospital, Clarion, PA, p. A520
WIENER, Mark S., President, Springfield Regional Medical Center, Springfield, OH, p. A488
WIENS, Ron, Chief Financial Officer, Shodair Children's Hospital, Helena, MT, p. A376
WIENTJES, Keri, Director Human Resources, Mobridge Regional Hospital, Mobridge, SD, p. A558
WIEPKING, Deb, MSN Chief Clinical Officer, Valley View Hospital, Glenwood Springs, CO, p. A101
WIERMAN, James L., M.D. Chief of Staff, Borgess–Lee Memorial Hospital, Dowagiac, MI, p. A311
WIERZBICKI, Barb, Manager Human Resources, Select Specialty Hospital–Downriver, Taylor, MI, p. A324
WIESNER, Gerald, Administrator, Miami County Medical Center, Paola, KS, p. A241
WIEWIORA, Nancy, Chief Operating Officer, Vibra Hospital of San Diego, San Diego, CA, p. A86
WIEWORA, Ron, M.D. Chief Medical Officer, Lakeside Medical Center, Belle Glade, FL, p. A118
WIGGINS, Carla, Director Human Resources, Livingston Hospital and Healthcare Services, Salem, KY, p. A258
WIGGINS, John, Chief Financial Officer, Evans Memorial Hospital, Claxton, GA, p. A149
WIGGINS, Josh
Vice President Controller, MidMichigan Medical Center–Clare, Clare, MI, p. A309
Vice President and Controller, MidMichigan Medical Center–Gladwin, Gladwin, MI, p. A313
WIGGINS, Mike, M.D. Chief of Staff, Laurens County Health Care System, Clinton, SC, p. A548


© 2012 AHA Guide Index of Health Care Professionals **A963**

WIGGINS, Stephen P., Director, Western State Hospital, Hopkinsville, KY, p. A252

WIGGINTON, Gwynn, Controller, El Campo Memorial Hospital, El Campo, TX, p. A595

WIGHTMAN, Lori, FACHE President, Unity Hospital, Fridley, MN, p. A331

WIGINGTON, James, M.D. Chief of Staff, Heart of the Rockies Regional Medical Center, Salida, CO, p. A105

WIGNALL, Terry A.
Director Human Resources, St. Vincent Seton Specialty Hospital, Indianapolis, IN, p. A205
Director Human Resources, St. Vincent Seton Specialty Hospital, Lafayette, IN, p. A207

WIIK, Jennifer, Chief Nursing Officer, Ortonville Area Health Services, Ortonville, MN, p. A336

WIJEWARDANE, Chamath, Director Information Technology, OCH Regional Medical Center, Starkville, MS, p. A353

WILBANKS, John F., FACH
Chief Operating Officer, Baptist Medical Center, Jacksonville, FL, p. A126
Chief Operating Officer, Baptist Medical Center Beaches, Jacksonville Beach, FL, p. A127

WILBERDING, Deborah, Controller, Rush Oak Park Hospital, Oak Park, IL, p. A190

WILBUR, Jennifer, Interim Chief Financial Officer, East Adams Rural Hospital, Ritzville, WA, p. A665

WILBUR, Thomas W., Chief Executive Officer and Superintendent, Newport Hospital and Health Services, Newport, WA, p. A663

WILBURN, Sue, Vice President Human Resources and Organizational Development, East Tennessee Children's Hospital, Knoxville, TN, p. A568

WILCHER, Greta
Senior Vice President and Chief Financial Officer, Mercy Hospital Fort Smith, Fort Smith, AR, p. A45
Senior Vice President and Chief Financial Officer, Mercy Hospital Waldron, Waldron, AR, p. A52

WILCOX, Billy, Chief Financial Officer, Specialty Hospital Jacksonville, Jacksonville, FL, p. A126

WILCOX, Jack, Chief Financial Officer, Ennis Regional Medical Center, Ennis, TX, p. A597

WILCOX, James, Chief Executive Officer, El Paso Specialty Hospital, El Paso, TX, p. A596

WILCOX, William H., President and Chief Executive Officer, United Surgical Partners International, Addison, TX, p. B134

WILCZEK, Joseph, Chief Executive Officer, St. Elizabeth Hospital, Enumclaw, WA, p. A661

WILD, James, M.D. Medical Director, Lake Shore Health Care Center, Irving, NY, p. A427

WILD, Jane, Director Information Technology, St. Mary's Hospital and Medical Center, Grand Junction, CO, p. A102

WILD, Mary Lou, Vice President Patient Care Services, Sarah Bush Lincoln Health Center, Mattoon, IL, p. A187

WILD, William, Chief Executive Officer, LTAC of Wichita, Wichita, KS, p. A245

WILDE, Gary, President and Chief Executive Officer, Community Memorial Health System, Ventura, CA, p. A94

WILDEBRANDT, David, Administrator, Baptist Hospital, Pensacola, FL, p. A136

WILDER, Janet, Coordinator Human Resources, Knox County Hospital, Barbourville, KY, p. A247

WILDER, Jeanine, Director Human Resources, Nicholas H. Noyes Memorial Hospital, Dansville, NY, p. A425

WILDER, John, Director Information Systems, Spaulding Hospital for Continuing Medical Care Cambridge, Cambridge, MA, p. A299

WILDER, Kathy, R.N. Chief Clinical Officer, Medical Center Barbour, Eufaula, AL, p. A19

WILDER, Norman, M.D. Vice President Medical Affairs, Alaska Regional Hospital, Anchorage, AK, p. A28

WILDER, Norman, Director Information Systems, Alta Vista Regional Hospital, Las Vegas, NM, p. A417

WILES, Michelle, Vice President Human Resources, Bon Secours Baltimore Health System, Baltimore, MD, p. A287

WILEY, Chuck, Manager Information Systems, Harrison County Hospital, Corydon, IN, p. A199

WILEY, Donald J., President and Chief Executive Officer, St. Joseph's Medical Center, Stockton, CA, p. A92

WILEY, Mark, Manager Information Systems Development, UPMC Bedford Memorial, Everett, PA, p. A523

WILEY, Rebecca J., R.N. Director, Wm. Jennings Bryan Dorn Veterans Affairs Medical Center, Columbia, SC, p. A549

WILFONG, Mario, Vice President Finance and Administration, UPMC Bedford Memorial, Everett, PA, p. A523

WILFORD, Linda, CPA Senior Vice President and Chief Financial Officer, Holy Cross Hospital, Fort Lauderdale, FL, p. A123

WILHELM, Bruce W., Vice President Human Resources, Bassett Medical Center, Cooperstown, NY, p. A424

WILHELM, Christine, Vice President Operations, Charlevoix Area Hospital, Charlevoix, MI, p. A309

WILHELM, Connie, Chief Financial Officer, Swisher Memorial Hospital District, Tulia, TX, p. A632

WILHELM, Jr., John O., Senior Vice President and Chief Financial Officer, Emerson Hospital, Concord, MA, p. A299

WILHELM, Paul, M.D. Chief of Staff, Kiowa District Hospital and Manor, Kiowa, KS, p. A236

WILHELMSEN Jr., Thomas E., President and Chief Executive Officer, Southern New Hampshire Medical Center, Nashua, NH, p. A399

WILHITE, Jade, Manager Human Resource, Memorial Hospital, Craig, CO, p. A99

WILHITE, James, Director Systems Information, North Mississippi State Hospital, Tupelo, MS, p. A353

WILHITE, Jerald, Administrator Human Resources, Heartland Behavioral Healthcare, Massillon, OH, p. A484

WILHITE, Milton, Chief Financial Officer, Plains Memorial Hospital, Dimmitt, TX, p. A594

WILHOIT, Ellen, President and Chief Administrative Officer, LeConte Medical Center, Sevierville, TN, p. A575

WILHOITE, David, CP
Senior Vice President Finance and Chief Financial Officer, Sumner Regional Medical Center, Gallatin, TN, p. A566
Senior Vice President Finance and Chief Financial Officer, Trousdale Medical Center, Hartsville, TN, p. A566

WILK, Leonard E., Vice President and Chief Administrative Officer, Aurora Medical Center Grafton, Grafton, WI, p. A682

WILK, Michael, Vice President Financial Services and Chief Financial Officer, Pocono Medical Center, East Stroudsburg, PA, p. A522

WILK, Terry, Chief Information Officer, Henry Medical Center, Stockbridge, GA, p. A160

WILKE, Julie, Vice President and Chief Financial Officer, Monroe Clinic, Monroe, WI, p. A687

WILKE, Kris, Manager Health Information, Granite Falls Municipal Hospital and Manor, Granite Falls, MN, p. A332

WILKEN, Thomas
Vice President Human Resources, Seton Medical Center Williamson, Round Rock, TX, p. A623
Vice President Human Resources, Seton Shoal Creek Hospital, Austin, TX, p. A581

WILKENS, Carie, Director of Human Resources, Carson Tahoe Regional Healthcare, Carson City, NV, p. A391

WILKERSON, Donald H., Chief Executive Officer, St. David's Medical Center, Austin, TX, p. A581

WILKERSON, Jacquelyn, R.N. Chief Nursing Officer, Conway Regional Medical Center, Conway, AR, p. A43

WILKERSON, Michelle, Director Human Resources, Paradise Valley Hospital, Phoenix, AZ, p. A36

WILKERSON, Scott, Interim Senior Vice President and Chief Financial Officer, Sparrow Hospital, Lansing, MI, p. A317

WILKES, Chris, MS Director Human Resources, Blount Memorial Hospital, Maryville, TN, p. A570

WILKES, Wendell, Chief Financial Officer, Byrd Regional Hospital, Leesville, LA, p. A271

WILKIE, Paula, Chief Financial Officer, Presentation Medical Center, Rolla, ND, p. A468

WILKINSON, David, M.D. Chief of Staff, Columbus Community Hospital, Columbus, TX, p. A588

WILKINSON, Paul G., Chief Operating Officer, Providence St. Peter Hospital, Olympia, WA, p. A663

WILKINSON, Robyn, Senior Vice President Human Resources, Mercy Medical Center–Des Moines, Des Moines, IA, p. A218

WILKINSON, Steven D., President and Chief Executive Officer, Menorah Medical Center, Overland Park, KS, p. A241

WILL, DeDe, Director Finance, Douglas County Community Mental Health Center, Omaha, NE, p. A388

WILL–MOWERY, Nicki L., Ph.D. Chief Executive Officer, Lower Keys Medical Center, Key West, FL, p. A127

WILLAMS, Kyle, Chief Information Officer, Kirby Medical Center, Monticello, IL, p. A188

WILLAMS, Mike, Chief Information Officer, FHN Memorial Hospital, Freeport, IL, p. A182

WILLARD, Craig, Director Information Technology and Systems, Frankfort Regional Medical Center, Frankfort, KY, p. A250

WILLARS, Susan, Vice President Human Resources, Mission Regional Medical Center, Mission, TX, p. A617

WILLE, Lesley A., Administrator and Executive Director, South Bay Medical Center,, CA, p. A72

WILLE, Matt, Chief Executive Officer, Dallas County Hospital, Perry, IA, p. A225

WILLEKE, Louis R., Administrator, Refugio County Memorial Hospital, Refugio, TX, p. A622

WILLEMSEN, Jane, Chief Administrative Officer, John Muir Medical Center, Walnut Creek, Walnut Creek, CA, p. A95

WILLERT, Todd, Administrator, Story County Medical Center, Nevada, IA, p. A224

WILLET, Terry, Chief Executive Officer, Allen Parish Hospital, Kinder, LA, p. A269

WILLETT, Richard, Chief Executive Officer, Redington–Fairview General Hospital, Skowhegan, ME, p. A285

WILLETT, Simon, Director Administrative Operations, South Texas Veterans Health Care System, San Antonio, TX, p. A626

WILLETT, Terry, Chief Financial Officer, Bunkie General Hospital, Bunkie, LA, p. A264

WILLETT, Vita M., Administrator and Executive Director, Riverside Medical Center, Riverside, CA, p. A83

WILLEY, Randy
Business Manager, Lincoln Regional Center, Lincoln, NE, p. A385
Business Manager, Norfolk Regional Center, Norfolk, NE, p. A386

WILLHITE, Jean, Director Human Resources, Sutter Solano Medical Center, Vallejo, CA, p. A94

WILLIAMS, Alec, Chief Information Officer, Samaritan Regional Health System, Ashland, OH, p. A469

WILLIAMS, Althea, Senior Vice President Human Resources, Grady Memorial Hospital, Atlanta, GA, p. A145

WILLIAMS, Antoinette, Chief Nursing Officer, John H. Stroger Jr. Hospital of Cook County, Chicago, IL, p. A176

WILLIAMS, Arthur, M.D. Medical Director, Braintree Rehabilitation Hospital, Braintree, MA, p. A298

WILLIAMS, Ashley, Manager Human Resources, Southern Inyo Healthcare District, Lone Pine, CA, p. A67

WILLIAMS, Avilla, MS, President, INTEGRIS Health Edmond, Edmond, OK, p. A495

WILLIAMS, Beverly, R.N. Chief Nursing Officer, Washington County Memorial Hospital, Potosi, MO, p. A367

WILLIAMS, Bob, President and Chief Executive Officer, Baptist St. Anthony Health System, Amarillo, TX, p. A578

WILLIAMS, Brian, Director Information Systems, St. Joseph's Hospital of Buckhannon, Buckhannon, WV, p. A670

WILLIAMS, Brit, M.D. President Medical Staff, Dr. John Warner Hospital, Clinton, IL, p. A179

WILLIAMS, Cara, Director Human Resources, Scripps Memorial Hospital–Encinitas, Encinitas, CA, p. A60

WILLIAMS, Carrie, R.N. Chief Nursing Officer, Henry County Hospital, New Castle, IN, p. A209

WILLIAMS, Catherine, M.D. Medical Director, Lewis County General Hospital, Lowville, NY, p. A429

WILLIAMS, Cecille, Assistant Administrator, Shamrock General Hospital, Shamrock, TX, p. A627

WILLIAMS, Cheryl, Director Human Resources, Seton Edgar B. Davis Hospital, Luling, TX, p. A614

WILLIAMS, Christopher, M.D. Chief of Staff, Keefe Memorial Hospital, Cheyenne Wells, CO, p. A98

WILLIAMS, Claudia, R.N. CNO, Washington Regional Medical Center, Fayetteville, AR, p. A44

WILLIAMS, Dana, Assistant Administrator and Chief Financial Officer, Baptist Memorial Hospital–North Mississippi, Oxford, MS, p. A351

WILLIAMS, Dana D., Chief Executive Officer, Jennings American Legion Hospital, Jennings, LA, p. A268

WILLIAMS, Daniel J., Senior Director Finance, Truman Medical Center–Lakewood, Kansas City, MO, p. A363

WILLIAMS, Darek, Director Human Resources, Elgin Mental Health Center, Elgin, IL, p. A180

WILLIAMS, Darlene, R.N. Administrator, Memorial Medical Center – San Augustine, San Augustine, TX, p. A626

WILLIAMS, David, Director Information Technology, Franklin Hospital District, Benton, IL, p. A173

WILLIAMS, David L., M.D. Chief Medical Officer, St. Joseph Hospital and Health Center, Kokomo, IN, p. A206

WILLIAMS, David R., President and Chief Executive Officer, Rapides Regional Medical Center, Alexandria, LA, p. A261

WILLIAMS, Deanna, R.N. Director of Nursing, Bacon County Hospital and Health System, Alma, GA, p. A144

WILLIAMS, Debra, Senior Vice President Human Resources, Parkview Hospital, Fort Wayne, IN, p. A201

WILLIAMS, Dionne, Director Human Resources, Vaughan Regional Medical Center, Selma, AL, p. A25

WILLIAMS, Gary, Chief Financial Officer, Gulf Coast Medical Center, Wharton, TX, p. A634

WILLIAMS, Ginger, M.D. Chief Medical Officer, Oaklawn Hospital, Marshall, MI, p. A318

WILLIAMS, Homer, Chief Civilian Personnel Branch, Reynolds Army Community Hospital, Fort Sill, OK, p. A497

WILLIAMS, Jackie, Director Human Resources, Madison River Oaks Medical Center, Canton, MS, p. A344

WILLIAMS, James, M.D
Chief Medical Staff, Granville Health System, Oxford, NC, p. A458
Chief of Staff, Riverside Medical Center, Waupaca, WI, p. A692

WILLIAMS, James, Chief Nursing Officer, University Hospitals Bedford Medical Center, Cleveland, OH, p. A475

WILLIAMS, James M., D.O. Vice President Medical Affairs, Community Westview Hospital, Indianapolis, IN, p. A204

WILLIAMS, Jay, Director Information Services, Presbyterian–St. Luke's Medical Center, Denver, CO, p. A100

Index of Health Care Professionals / Wilson

Index of Health Care Professionals

WILLIAMS, Jeremy, Chief Financial Officer, Banner Boswell Medical Center, Sun City, AZ, p. A39
WILLIAMS, Jim, Chief Financial Officer, Minden Medical Center, Minden, LA, p. A273
WILLIAMS, Joan, Administrative Assistant, Lamb Healthcare Center, Littlefield, TX, p. A612
WILLIAMS, John
Chief Financial Officer, Upson Regional Medical Center, Thomaston, GA, p. A160
Chief Information Officer, Veterans Affairs Medical Center, Bay Pines, FL, p. A118
WILLIAMS, John G., President and Chief Executive Officer, Barton Healthcare System, South Lake Tahoe, CA, p. A91
WILLIAMS, Judith L., Director Human Resources, Davis Memorial Hospital, Elkins, WV, p. A671
WILLIAMS, Julie, Chief Financial Officer, Smith County Memorial Hospital, Smith Center, KS, p. A243
WILLIAMS, Karen
Director Human Resources, CHRISTUS St. Michael Rehabilitation Hospital, Texarkana, TX, p. A630
Chief Financial Officer, Streamwood Behavioral Health Center, Streamwood, IL, p. A195
WILLIAMS, Kenneth, Chief Information Officer, Veterans Affairs Medical Center, Fayetteville, NC, p. A453
WILLIAMS, L. Dale, M.D. Vice President and Chief Medical Director, High Point Regional Health System, High Point, NC, p. A455
WILLIAMS, Lauren, R.N. Vice President of Professional Services and Chief Nursing Officer, Lawrence & Memorial Hospital, New London, CT, p. A111
WILLIAMS, Linda, Director of Nursing, Villa Feliciana Medical Complex, Jackson, LA, p. A268
WILLIAMS, Lynn
Vice President, Commonwealth Regional Specialty Hospital, Bowling Green, KY, p. A247
Vice President Human Resources, Medical Center at Bowling Green, Bowling Green, KY, p. A248
Vice President Human Resources, Medical Center at Scottsville, Scottsville, KY, p. A259
WILLIAMS, Margaret, Chief Financial Officer, Baptist Memorial Hospital for Women, Memphis, TN, p. A571
WILLIAMS, Margo L., R.N. Chief Nursing Officer, Anderson County Hospital, Garnett, KS, p. A233
WILLIAMS, Mark, M.D. Chief Medical Officer, Atrium Medical Center, Middletown, OH, p. A485
WILLIAMS, Mark, Chief Financial Officer, Citrus Memorial Health System, Inverness, FL, p. A126
WILLIAMS, Mary, Director Human Resources, Medina Memorial Hospital, Medina, NY, p. A429
WILLIAMS, Michael, FACHE Administrator, Fairfield Memorial Hospital, Winnsboro, SC, p. A554
WILLIAMS, Michael D., President and Chief Executive Officer, Community Hospital Corporation, Plano, TX, p. B37
WILLIAMS, Michael L., FACHE Vice President Human Resources, Community Howard Regional Hospital, Kokomo, IN, p. A206
WILLIAMS, Michael R., M.D. Chief Executive Officer, Hill Country Memorial Hospital, Fredericksburg, TX, p. A600
WILLIAMS, Michelle, Administrator, Sedan City Hospital, Sedan, KS, p. A243
WILLIAMS, Mickey, Manager Information Technology, Moccasin Bend Mental Health Institute, Chattanooga, TN, p. A563
WILLIAMS, Mike, Accountant, Limestone Medical Center, Groesbeck, TX, p. A602
WILLIAMS, Pamela G., Director Human Resources, White County Medical Center, Searcy, AR, p. A51
WILLIAMS, Pamela S., Vice President Human Resources, Medstar Harbor Hospital, Baltimore, MD, p. A288
WILLIAMS, Paul, Director Human Resources, Mission Community Hospital, Valencia, CA, p. A94
WILLIAMS Sr., Perry E., Administrator and Chief Executive Officer, Alliance HealthCare System, Holly Springs, MS, p. A347
WILLIAMS, R. Martin, Director Financial Services, Cox Monett, Monett, MO, p. A365
WILLIAMS, R. D., Administrator and Chief Executive Officer, Ashe Memorial Hospital, Jefferson, NC, p. A455
WILLIAMS, Randy, Director Management Information Systems, Maria Parham Medical Center, Henderson, NC, p. A454
WILLIAMS, Rhonda Y., Chief Executive Officer, Trillium Specialty Hospital–West Valley, Sun City, AZ, p. A39
WILLIAMS, Rich, Director Human Resources, Upson Regional Medical Center, Thomaston, GA, p. A160
WILLIAMS, Richard, Chief Operating Officer, Southwest Mississippi Regional Medical Center, McComb, MS, p. A349
WILLIAMS, Robert, Director Information Systems, Lake Pointe Medical Center, Rowlett, TX, p. A623
WILLIAMS, Robert D., Chief Executive Officer, Special Care Hospital, Nanticoke, PA, p. A530
WILLIAMS, Roby D., Administrator, Hardin County General Hospital, Rosiclare, IL, p. A193
WILLIAMS, Rod, Manager Information Systems, Citizens Medical Center, Colby, KS, p. A231
WILLIAMS, Rodney W., M.D. Vice President Medical Affairs, Good Samaritan Hospital, Suffern, NY, p. A444
WILLIAMS, Roger, Chief Financial Officer, New Horizons Health Systems, Owenton, KY, p. A257
WILLIAMS, Ronald, M.D. Medical Director, Landmark Hospital of Joplin, Joplin, MO, p. A361
WILLIAMS, Sandi, Manager Business Officer, Garfield County Health Center, Jordan, MT, p. A376
WILLIAMS, Sandra
Chief Financial Officer, Cape Fear Valley – Bladen County Hospital, Elizabethtown, NC, p. A453
Chief Financial Officer, Cape Fear Valley Medical Center, Fayetteville, NC, p. A453
WILLIAMS, Scott, Chief Operating Officer, Shelby Baptist Medical Center, Alabaster, AL, p. A15
WILLIAMS, Sean J., President and Chief Financial Officer, Mercy Medical Center–Clinton, Clinton, IA, p. A216
WILLIAMS, Shane, Director Information Systems, Davis Hospital and Medical Center, Layton, UT, p. A638
WILLIAMS, Sharon, Vice President Finance and Information Technology, Avera Marshall Regional Medical Center, Marshall, MN, p. A334
WILLIAMS, Sheila, Chief Executive Officer, H.S.C. Medical Center, Malvern, AR, p. A48
WILLIAMS, Stephanie, R.N. Chief Nursing Officer, Washington Hospital Healthcare System, Fremont, CA, p. A61
WILLIAMS, Stephen, President, Norton Healthcare, Louisville, KY, p. B96
WILLIAMS, Thomas, D.O. Chief of Staff, Sullivan County Memorial Hospital, Milan, MO, p. A365
WILLIAMS, Tina, Chief Financial Officer, Alaska Psychiatric Institute, Anchorage, AK, p. A28
WILLIAMS, Todd, M.D. President Medical Staff, Eastern Idaho Regional Medical Center, Idaho Falls, ID, p. A168
WILLIAMS, Tom, Director Human Resources, Lake Regional Health System, Osage Beach, MO, p. A366
WILLIAMS, Tonja, R.N. President and Chief Executive Officer, Continuing Care Hospital, Lexington, KY, p. A253
WILLIAMS, Warren, CPA Director Fiscal Services, Mississippi State Hospital, Whitfield, MS, p. A354
WILLIAMS, Jr., Wendell H., M.D. Medical Director, Specialty Hospital Jacksonville, Jacksonville, FL, p. A126
WILLIAMS, Winifred
Vice President Human Resources, Providence Medical Center, Kansas City, KS, p. A236
Vice President Human Resources, Saint John Hospital, Leavenworth, KS, p. A237
WILLIAMS–WHITE, Reba, M.D. Chief of Staff, Renaissance Hospital Terrell, Terrell, TX, p. A630
WILLIAMSON, John, Human Resources Site Manager, Baptist Health South Florida, Mariners Hospital, Tavernier, FL, p. A142
WILLIAMSON, Johnny, M.D. Chief Medical Officer, Hartgrove Hospital, Chicago, IL, p. A175
WILLIAMSON, Marilyn
Director Human Resources, Osawatomie State Hospital, Osawatomie, KS, p. A240
Chief Human Resources Officer, Rainbow Mental Health Facility, Kansas City, KS, p. A236
WILLIAMSON, Sharon, Chief Information Technology, Robert J. Dole Veterans Affairs Medical Center, Wichita, KS, p. A245
WILLIAMSON, William P., M.D. Medical Director, Frazier Rehab Institute, Louisville, KY, p. A254
WILLIE, David, Chief Financial Officer, PeaceHealth Southwest Medical Center, Vancouver, WA, p. A668
WILLINGHAM, Alex, M.D. Medical Director, Warm Springs Rehabilitation Hospital, San Antonio, TX, p. A626
WILLINGHAM, Debbie, Administrative Assistant, Field Memorial Community Hospital, Centreville, MS, p. A344
WILLINGHAM, John, Chief Executive Officer and Managing Director, Carolina Center for Behavioral Health, Greer, SC, p. A551
WILLIS, Bill, Director Information Technology, River Point Behavioral Health, Jacksonville, FL, p. A126
WILLIS, Joy, Acting Chief Fiscal Service, G.V. Montgomery Veterans Affairs Medical Center, Jackson, MS, p. A347
WILLIS, Kathy, M.D. Medical Director, Lallie Kemp Medical Center, Independence, LA, p. A268
WILLIS, Mona M.
Director Human Resources, Landmark Medical Center, Woonsocket, RI, p. A545
Director Human Resources, Rehabilitation Hospital of Rhode Island, North Smithfield, RI, p. A544
WILLIS, Rebecca, Chief Nursing Officer, Sampson Regional Medical Center, Clinton, NC, p. A451
WILLIS, Sandra, Manager Human Resources, Citizens Baptist Medical Center, Talladega, AL, p. A26
WILLIS, Sherita, M.D. Chief of Staff, South Mississippi County Regional Medical Center, Osceola, AR, p. A50
WILLIS, Toni, M.D. Medical Director, Reliant Rehabilitation Hospital Mid–Cities, Bedford, TX, p. A583
WILLIS, Traci, Chief Executive Officer, Lovelace Rehabilitation Hospital, Albuquerque, NM, p. A414
WILLIS, Walt, M.D. Medical Director, Neshoba County General Hospital, Philadelphia, MS, p. A351
WILLIS, Wendy L., Assistant Vice President Human Resources, Ochsner Medical Center – Kenner, Kenner, LA, p. A269
WILLIS, William L., Administrator, Dubuis Hospital of Lake Charles, Lake Charles, LA, p. A271
WILLMANN, Adam, Administrator, Pioneer Community Hospital of Early, Blakely, GA, p. A147
WILLMON, Brian, M.D. Medical Director, Plains Regional Medical Center, Clovis, NM, p. A415
WILLMORE, Lois, Supervisor Health Information Management, Cedar County Memorial Hospital, El Dorado Springs, MO, p. A359
WILLMS, Frederick, M.D. Vice President Medical Affairs, Piedmont Fayette Hospital, Fayetteville, GA, p. A152
WILLS, Kim, Chief Operating Officer, Cook Medical Center–A Campus of Tift Regional Medical Center, Adel, GA, p. A144
WILLS, Laura S., Administrator, Noland Hospital Shelby, Alabaster, AL, p. A15
WILLS, Lawrence E., Vice President Operations, OSF St. Joseph Medical Center, Bloomington, IL, p. A173
WILLS, Michele, Registered Health Information Administrator, Caro Center, Caro, MI, p. A308
WILLS, Shannon, Director Human Resources, Delray Medical Center, Delray Beach, FL, p. A122
WILLSIE, Brett, Manager Human Resources, Sentara Williamsburg Regional Medical Center, Williamsburg, VA, p. A657
WILLWERTH, Deborah J., R.N. Chief Operating Officer, Lancaster Regional Medical Center, Lancaster, PA, p. A526
WILMOT, Joan, Chief Fiscal Officer, Veterans Affairs Medical Center, White River Junction, VT, p. A644
WILSON, Alice, FACHE Vice President Administration, St. Luke's Hospital – Warren Campus, Phillipsburg, NJ, p. A408
WILSON, Amy, M.D. Medical Director, Baylor Institute for Rehabilitation, Dallas, TX, p. A590
WILSON, Andrew, M.D. Interim Chief Medical Officer, Salinas Valley Memorial Healthcare System, Salinas, CA, p. A84
WILSON, Ann, Acting Director Human Resources, Hopedale Medical Complex, Hopedale, IL, p. A185
WILSON, Becky, Manager Human Resources, Allegiance Specialty Hospital of Kilgore, Kilgore, TX, p. A610
WILSON, Bill, Chief Financial Officer, North Carolina Specialty Hospital, Durham, NC, p. A452
WILSON, Bobbie, Director Human Resources, Crete Area Medical Center, Crete, NE, p. A383
WILSON, Brian, D.O. Medical Staff President, Spencer Hospital, Spencer, IA, p. A227
WILSON, Carolyn, President, University of Minnesota Medical Center, Fairview, Minneapolis, MN, p. A335
WILSON, Charlene J., Vice President Human Resources, St. Francis Hospital, Wilmington, DE, p. A115
WILSON, Charles
Chief Human Resources Officer, Penn State Milton S. Hershey Medical Center, Hershey, PA, p. A525
Director Information Systems, St. Mary's Medical Center, Huntington, WV, p. A673
WILSON, Cheryl A., Chief Operating Officer, Rapides Regional Medical Center, Alexandria, LA, p. A261
WILSON, Christopher, M.D. Inpatient Medical Director, South Texas Rehabilitation Hospital, Brownsville, TX, p. A585
WILSON, Cynthia, M.D. Chief of Staff, Mercy Hospital Rogers, Rogers, AR, p. A50
WILSON, David C., President and Chief Executive Officer, Shelby Baptist Medical Center, Alabaster, AL, p. A15
WILSON, David R., M.D. Chief of Staff, St. Vincent's Blount, Oneonta, AL, p. A24
WILSON, Deanna, VP Patient Care Services/Site Manager, Aspirus Ontonagon Hospital, Ontonagon, MI, p. A320
WILSON, Deb, Director Human Resources, Kalispell Regional Medical Center, Kalispell, MT, p. A377
WILSON, Deborah J., Senior Vice President and Chief Financial Officer, Lawrence General Hospital, Lawrence, MA, p. A301
WILSON, Dottie, Director Human Resources, Pickens County Medical Center, Carrollton, AL, p. A18
WILSON, Eleanor, R.N. Vice President and Chief Operating Officer, Doylestown Hospital, Doylestown, PA, p. A522
WILSON, Elizabeth M., Coordinator Human Resources, Regency Hospital of Cincinnati, Cincinnati, OH, p. A474
WILSON, Jr., Floyd, Executive Vice President Human Resources, Metro Health Hospital, Wyoming, MI, p. A326
WILSON, Greg, Chief Operating Officer and Chief Financial Officer, Paynesville Area Health Care System, Paynesville, MN, p. A337

© 2012 AHA Guide Index of Health Care Professionals A965

Index of Health Care Professionals

Index of Health Care Professionals / Wilson

WILSON, Hamlin J.
Senior Vice President Human Resources, Wellmont Bristol Regional Medical Center, Bristol, TN, p. A562
Senior Vice President Human Resources, Wellmont Holston Valley Medical Center, Kingsport, TN, p. A568
WILSON, Harold E., Chief Executive Officer, Eastern State Hospital, Medical Lake, WA, p. A662
WILSON, Hugh D., Interim Chief Executive Officer, Phoebe North, Albany, GA, p. A144
WILSON, James D., Chief Executive Officer, Lakewood Ranch Medical Center, Bradenton, FL, p. A119
WILSON, Jason, Administrator, Valley View Medical Center, Cedar City, UT, p. A637
WILSON, Jim
Vice President Information Technology, Promise Hospital of East Los Angeles, Suburban Medical Center Campus, Paramount, CA, p. A79
Vice President Information Technology, Promise Hospital of San Diego, San Diego, CA, p. A85
WILSON, Jodi, Site Administrator, Diley Ridge Medical Center, Canal Winchester, OH, p. A472
WILSON, John P., Chief Financial Officer, Heartland Regional Medical Center, Saint Joseph, MO, p. A368
WILSON, John R., Vice President, Human Resources, Murray–Calloway County Hospital, Murray, KY, p. A257
WILSON, John W., Chief Executive Officer, Warren Memorial Hospital, Friend, NE, p. A383
WILSON, Kim, Interim Director of Nursing, Benewah Community Hospital, Saint Maries, ID, p. A170
WILSON, Kim, M.D. Chief of Staff, Tri–State Memorial Hospital, Clarkston, WA, p. A660
WILSON, Kim A., R.N
Chief Operating Officer, St. John's Pleasant Valley Hospital, Camarillo, CA, p. A56
Chief Operating Officer, St. John's Regional Medical Center, Oxnard, CA, p. A78
WILSON, Kimberly P.
Associate Vice President, UK HealthCare Good Samaritan Hospital, Lexington, KY, p. A253
Director Human Resources, University of Kentucky Albert B. Chandler Hospital, Lexington, KY, p. A253
WILSON, Lerae, R.N. Vice President Patient Services and Chief Nursing Officer, St. Claire Regional Medical Center, Morehead, KY, p. A256
WILSON, Linde Finsrud, Chief Executive Officer, Sharon Regional Health System, Sharon, PA, p. A538
WILSON, Lois, Controller, Roger Mills Memorial Hospital, Cheyenne, OK, p. A494
WILSON, Mark, M.D. Chief of Staff, Cooper Green Mercy Hospital, Birmingham, AL, p. A16
WILSON, Mary L., M.D. Area Medical Director, Panorama City Medical Center,, CA, p. A71
WILSON, Nancy, Chief Nurse Executive, Wilcox Memorial Hospital, Lihue, HI, p. A165
WILSON, Nancy V., Chief Financial Officer, Kindred Hospital–La Mirada, La Mirada, CA, p. A66
WILSON, Patricia, Vice President Human Resources, Englewood Hospital and Medical Center, Englewood, NJ, p. A404
WILSON, Preshie
Vice President Finance, Baylor All Saints Medical Center at Fort Worth, Fort Worth, TX, p. A598
Vice President Finance Services, Baylor Regional Medical Center at Grapevine, Grapevine, TX, p. A601
WILSON, Rhonda, Director Human Resources, Mayo Clinic Health System – Oakridge in Osseo, Osseo, WI, p. A689
WILSON, Robert, D.O. Director Medical Services, Eagleville Hospital, Eagleville, PA, p. A522
WILSON, Robert, M.D. Chief of Staff, Southeast Georgia Health System Camden Campus, Saint Marys, GA, p. A158
WILSON, Robert E.
Vice President and Chief Information Officer, Crozer–Chester Medical Center, Upland, PA, p. A540
Vice President and Chief Information Officer, Delaware County Memorial Hospital, Drexel Hill, PA, p. A522
WILSON, Roger D., M.D. Medical Director, St. John Sapulpa, Sapulpa, OK, p. A504
WILSON, Roy, M.D. Medical Director, St. Louis Psychiatric Rehabilitation Center, Saint Louis, MO, p. A370
WILSON, Sherry, R.N. Chief Nursing Officer Long Term Care, Mayers Memorial Hospital District, Fall River Mills, CA, p. A60
WILSON, Stephan A., Chief Financial Officer, Montrose Memorial Hospital, Montrose, CO, p. A104
WILSON, Terrance E.
President and Chief Executive Officer, Franciscan St. Elizabeth Health – Lafayette Central, Lafayette, IN, p. A206
President and Chief Executive Officer, St. Elizabeth East, Lafayette, IN, p. A207
WILSON, Terry, Director Human Resources and Compliance, Doctors Hospital Nelsonville, Nelsonville, OH, p. A486
WILSON, Vicki, Chief Human Resources Officer, Dixie Regional Medical Center, Saint George, UT, p. A640
WILSON, William, Interim Chief Financial Officer, Valley Presbyterian Hospital,, CA, p. A72
WILSON, William G., President and Chief Executive Officer, Jackson County Memorial Hospital, Altus, OK, p. A493
WILSON, Yolande, Chief Executive Officer, Kindred Hospital Boston–North Shore, Peabody, MA, p. A303
WILSON–NEIL, Carla, Chief Operating Officer, Pennock Hospital, Hastings, MI, p. A315
WILTERMOOD, Michael C., President and Chief Executive Officer, Enloe Medical Center, Chico, CA, p. A57
WILTROUT, Terry, Chief Executive Officer, Canonsburg General Hospital, Canonsburg, PA, p. A520
WIMMER, Donna, Director Human Resources, Franciscan St. Anthony Health – Crown Point, Crown Point, IN, p. A200
WIMMER, Keri, R.N. Patient Care Director, CentraCare Health System – Melrose, Melrose, MN, p. A334
WIMSATT, Michael, Director Human Resources, Piedmont Geriatric Hospital, Burkeville, VA, p. A646
WIN, Aye Mya, M.D. Chief Medical Staff, Western Plains Medical Complex, Dodge City, KS, p. A232
WINBERY, Ben, Chief Financial Officer, Montevista Hospital, Las Vegas, NV, p. A393
WINCH, James, Vice President Finance, Essentia Health St. Joseph's Medical Center, Brainerd, MN, p. A328
WINCHESTER, David, Interim Vice President and Chief Financial Officer, Memorial Health Care System, Chattanooga, TN, p. A563
WINDER, Todd V., Administrator and Chief Executive Officer, Oneida County Hospital, Malad City, ID, p. A169
WINDHAM, Hailey, Chief Information Management, San Antonio Military Medical Center, Fort Sam Houston, TX, p. A598
WINDHAM, Joel R.
Director Human Resources, Regional Hospital of Jackson, Jackson, TN, p. A567
Director Human Resources, Trinity Medical Center, Birmingham, AL, p. A17
WINDHAM, Michael, Chief Nursing Officer, Doctor's Memorial Hospital, Perry, FL, p. A136
WINDHAM, Vann, Chief Financial Officer, L. V. Stabler Memorial Hospital, Greenville, AL, p. A21
WINDLE, Jane, R.N. Director of Nurses, North Mississippi Medical Center–West Point, West Point, MS, p. A353
WINEGARNER, Rodney, Chief Financial Officer, Mercy Hospitals of Bakersfield, Bakersfield, CA, p. A55
WINEGEART, Steve, Chief Financial Officer, Wadley Regional Medical Center, Texarkana, TX, p. A631
WINEINGER, Stephanie, Director of Nursing, Greeley County Health Services, Tribune, KS, p. A244
WINFIELD, Gary, M.D. Medical Director, Memorial Hospital Jacksonville, Jacksonville, FL, p. A126
WINFREE, Kersey, M.D. Chief Medical Officer, St. Anthony Hospital, Oklahoma City, OK, p. A502
WINFREY, John W., Vice President Finance and Chief Financial Officer, DCH Regional Medical Center, Tuscaloosa, AL, p. A26
WING, Mitch, Network Administrator, Cloud County Health Center, Concordia, KS, p. A232
WING, Susan M., R.N. Chief Operating Officer, Falmouth Hospital, Falmouth, MA, p. A300
WING, Yakesun, Business Strategy and Finance Leader, Walnut Creek Medical Center, Walnut Creek, CA, p. A95
WINGATE, Phyllis A., Division President, Carolinas Medical Center–NorthEast, Concord, NC, p. A451
WINGET, Mary, Director Human Resources, Minden Medical Center, Minden, LA, p. A273
WINGFIELD, Gena, Senior Vice President and Chief Financial Officer, Arkansas Children's Hospital, Little Rock, AR, p. A47
WINIARSKI, Michael H., FACHE Vice President and Chief Financial Officer, Tuomey Healthcare System, Sumter, SC, p. A554
WINKELHAKE, Doug, President, Norton Brownsboro Hospital, Louisville, KY, p. A255
WINKELMEYER, Edwin, Director Human Resources, Abilene Regional Medical Center, Abilene, TX, p. A577
WINKLE, Derek, Director Human Resources, Morristown–Hamblen Healthcare System, Morristown, TN, p. A572
WINKLER, Gordon W., Administrator and Chief Executive Officer, Ringgold County Hospital, Mount Ayr, IA, p. A223
WINKLER, Walter, Chief Executive Officer, Keokuk Area Hospital, Keokuk, IA, p. A222
WINN, Bill, Chief Information Officer, Ivinson Memorial Hospital, Laramie, WY, p. A696
WINN, Eleyce, Assistant Administrator, Clarendon Memorial Hospital, Manning, SC, p. A552
WINN, George, Chief Executive Officer, Evanston Regional Hospital, Evanston, WY, p. A696
WINN, Holly, Vice President Human Resources and Ancillary Services, Black River Memorial Hospital, Black River Falls, WI, p. A679
WINN, Karla, Chief Information Officer, Greater Regional Medical Center, Creston, IA, p. A217
WINN, Michael R., Director, Central Arkansas Veterans Healthcare System, Little Rock, AR, p. A48
WINN, Roger P., President, UPMC Bedford Memorial, Everett, PA, p. A523
WINNENBERG, William
Chief Information Officer, Pioneer Memorial Hospital, Prineville, OR, p. A514
Chief Information Officer, St. Charles Medical Center – Bend, Bend, OR, p. A509
Chief Information Officer, St. Charles Medical Center – Redmond, Redmond, OR, p. A515
WINNER, Douglas, Chief Financial Officer, Providence Hospital, Southfield, MI, p. A323
WINRIGHT, Donna, Director Human Resources and Senior Services, Kearny County Hospital, Lakin, KS, p. A237
WINSELL, Susan, Vice President Human Resources, Marian Medical Center, Santa Maria, CA, p. A90
WINSETT, Gracia, Chief Financial Officer, Wellstone Regional Hospital, Jeffersonville, IN, p. A205
WINSLOW, Grover C., M.D. Chief of Staff, Sabine County Hospital, Hemphill, TX, p. A603
WINSTON, Bob, M.D. Medical Director, Acadia Vermilion Hospital, Lafayette, LA, p. A269
WINTER, Jan, Chief Executive Officer, Bristow Medical Center, Bristow, OK, p. A494
WINTER, Jon R., D.O. Chief of Staff, Camden General Hospital, Camden, TN, p. A562
WINTER, Mike, Vice President and Chief Financial Officer, Baylor Medical Center at Garland, Garland, TX, p. A600
WINTERS, Gene, Chief Financial Officer, Dallas Regional Medical Center, Mesquite, TX, p. A616
WINTERS, Janice, Controller, Pickens County Medical Center, Carrollton, AL, p. A18
WINTERS, Joyce, MSN, Administrator, Kindred Hospital–Brea, Brea, CA, p. A56
WINTERS, Mary Ellen, Director Human Resources, Mena Regional Health System, Mena, AR, p. A49
WINTHROP, Michael, President, Bellevue Hospital, Bellevue, OH, p. A470
WIRKKULA, James, M.D. Chief Medical Officer, Ellett Memorial Hospital, Appleton City, MO, p. A355
WIRTHGEN, Doug
Facility Chief Information Officer, Jerry L. Pettis Memorial Veterans Medical Center, Loma Linda, CA, p. A67
Chief Information Officer, Veterans Affairs Palo Alto Health Care System, Palo Alto, CA, p. A79
WIRTZ, Carman, Vice President Human Resources, Memorial Hospital of Union County, Marysville, OH, p. A484
WISCHKAEMPER, Jo Nell, Administrator, Lamb Healthcare Center, Littlefield, TX, p. A612
WISDOM, Karen J., Executive Vice President and Chief Operating Officer, Hamilton Medical Center, Dalton, GA, p. A151
WISE, Gregory, M.D
Vice President Medical Affairs, Kettering Medical Center, Kettering, OH, p. A482
Vice President Medical Affairs, Sycamore Medical Center, Miamisburg, OH, p. A485
WISE, Jennifer, Chief Nursing Officer, Franklin Foundation Hospital, Franklin, LA, p. A266
WISE, Jerry, Controller, Mercy Rehabilitation Hospital, Chesterfield, MO, p. A357
WISE, Jerry R., Administrator and Vice President, Hart County Hospital, Hartwell, GA, p. A153
WISE, Robert P., FACHE President and Chief Executive Officer, Hunterdon Medical Center, Flemington, NJ, p. A404
WISEMAN, Roger D., Chief Financial Officer, MetroWest Medical Center, Framingham, MA, p. A300
WISNER, Donna, Chief Financial Officer, Dr. John Warner Hospital, Clinton, IL, p. A179
WISNIESKI, Thomas, Director, Veterans Affairs Gulf Coast Veterans Health Care System, Biloxi, MS, p. A344
WISNIEWSKI, Cass, Interim Chief Financial Officer, Hurley Medical Center, Flint, MI, p. A312
WISNIEWSKI, Richard, Senior Vice President Finance and Chief Financial Officer, Mount Nittany Medical Center, State College, PA, p. A539
WISNOSKI, Joseph, Vice President Finance and Chief Financial Officer, John T. Mather Memorial Hospital, Port Jefferson, NY, p. A440
WISS, Albert, Chief Financial Officer, Share Medical Center, Alva, OK, p. A493

**A966** Index of Health Care Professionals 

Index of Health Care Professionals / Woodbeck

Index of Health Care Professionals


WISSEL, Andrew
Director Human Resources, Mount Sinai Hospital, Chicago, IL, p. A177
Director Human Resources, Schwab Rehabilitation Hospital, Chicago, IL, p. A178
WISSLER, James, President and Chief Executive Officer, Hanover Hospital, Hanover, PA, p. A524
WISWELL, Ashleigh, Director Human Resources, Moore County Hospital District, Dumas, TX, p. A594
WITENSKE, James, Chief Information Officer, Jefferson Regional Medical Center, Jefferson Hills, PA, p. A525
WITHERSPOON, Lynn, Vice President and Chief Information Officer, Ochsner Medical Center, New Orleans, LA, p. A275
WITHIAM, Cathy, Director Human Resources, McBride Clinic Orthopedic Hospital, Oklahoma City, OK, p. A501
WITHROW, Pat, M.D. Vice President Medical Affairs, Western Baptist Hospital, Paducah, KY, p. A257
WITKO, James F., M.D. Chief Medical Officer, Halifax Regional Health System, South Boston, VA, p. A656
WITKOWICZ, Victor J., Senior Vice President and Chief Financial Officer, Madonna Rehabilitation Hospital, Lincoln, NE, p. A385
WITKOWSKI, Richard J., Director Management Information Systems, Mount St. Mary's Hospital and Health Center, Lewiston, NY, p. A428
WITMER, Bruce, M.D. Medical Director, Fresno Surgical Hospital, Fresno, CA, p. A62
WITMER, Craig, Chief Information Officer, Providence Tarzana Medical Center,, CA, p. A71
WITT, David, Chief Financial Officer, CHRISTUS St. John Hospital, Nassau Bay, TX, p. A618
WITT, James, Chief Operations Officer, Memorial Hermann Memorial City Medical Center, Houston, TX, p. A605
WITT, Jana, Chief Executive Officer, Cedar County Memorial Hospital, El Dorado Springs, MO, p. A359
WITT, Laura, Administrator Human Resources, Banner Thunderbird Medical Center, Glendale, AZ, p. A33
WITT, Michael, Director of Information Technology, Two Rivers Behavioral Health System, Kansas City, MO, p. A363
WITT, Michael A., M.D. Chief of Staff, Murray Medical Center, Chatsworth, GA, p. A149
WITT, Sarah, Director Human Resources, Richmond State Hospital, Richmond, IN, p. A211
WITT, Stephen, President and Chief Executive Officer, College Hospital, Cerritos, CA, p. A57
WITT, Thomas J., M.D
President and Chief Executive Officer, Mayo Clinic Health System in Cannon Falls, Cannon Falls, MN, p. A329
President and Chief Executive Officer, Mayo Clinic Health System in Lake City, Lake City, MN, p. A333
President and Chief Executive Officer, Mayo Clinic Health System in Red Wing, Red Wing, MN, p. A337
WITTE, Kari, Director of Patient Care, Windom Area Hospital, Windom, MN, p. A342
WITTERSTAETER, Ellen, Chief Operating Officer, Fort Walton Beach Medical Center, Fort Walton Beach, FL, p. A124
WITTES, Robert E., M.D. Physician in Chief, Memorial Sloan–Kettering Cancer Center, New York, NY, p. A434
WITTHAUS, Denise, Assistant Administrator Finance, Hermann Area District Hospital, Hermann, MO, p. A360
WITTHAUS, Patricia, Director Information Services, Valley Regional Hospital, Claremont, NH, p. A397
WITTMAN, Thomas, Chief Information Officer, Jewish Hospital, Louisville, KY, p. A254
WITTON, David, Manager Information Systems, St. John's Medical Center and Living Center, Jackson, WY, p. A696
WITTROCK, Edward A., Vice President Regional System, Mayo Clinic Health System – Chippewa Valley in Bloomer, Bloomer, WI, p. A679
WIZDA, Jerome, Commander, U. S. Air Force Hospital, Hampton, VA, p. A649
WODICKA, Mary Jo, Director Human Resources, Wheaton Franciscan Healthcare – All Saints, Racine, WI, p. A689
WOELTJEN, Bill, Chief Financial Officer, Sarasota Memorial Hospital, Sarasota, FL, p. A139
WOEN, Linda, Director Human Resources, Yuma Rehabilitation Hospital, Yuma, AZ, p. A41
WOERNER, Steve, Chief Executive Officer, Driscoll Children's Hospital, Corpus Christi, TX, p. A589
WOFFORD, Stephanie, Controller, Salem Memorial District Hospital, Salem, MO, p. A370
WOHLFARDT, Diana, Director Human Resources, Nashville General Hospital, Nashville, TN, p. A573
WOHLFORD, Steve, Chief Operating Officer–Hospital Services, Johnson Memorial Hospital, Franklin, IN, p. A202
WOIRHAYE, Ted, R.N. Director of Nursing, Ruby Valley Hospital, Sheridan, MT, p. A379
WOJNO, Kathy, R.N. Chief Nursing Officer, Hollywood Presbyterian Medical Center, Los Angeles, CA, p. A69
WOJTALA, Barbara, Chief Executive Officer, Regency Hospital Cleveland East, Cleveland, OH, p. A475
WOJTALEWICZ, Jeanette, Vice President Finance, Saint Elizabeth Regional Medical Center, Lincoln, NE, p. A385
WOJTOWICZ, Linda, R.N. Senior Vice President and Chief Operations Officer, TMC Healthcare, Tucson, AZ, p. A40
WOLAK, Robert, Chief Information Resource Management Service, G.V. Montgomery Veterans Affairs Medical Center, Jackson, MS, p. A347
WOLBERS, Chad, Chief Operating Officer, Finley Hospital, Dubuque, IA, p. A219
WOLCOTT, Daniel, President, Takoma Regional Hospital, Greeneville, TN, p. A566
WOLD, Lynn, Chief Operation Officer, St. Luke's Regional Medical Center, Sioux City, IA, p. A227
WOLF, Brenda J., President and Chief Executive Officer, La Rabida Children's Hospital, Chicago, IL, p. A176
WOLF, Bryan, M.D. Senior Vice President and Chief Information Officer, Children's Hospital of Philadelphia, Philadelphia, PA, p. A532
WOLF, Edward H., President and Chief Executive Officer, Lakeview Medical Center, Rice Lake, WI, p. A690
WOLF, Jack, Vice President Information Systems, Montefiore Medical Center,, NY, p. A434
WOLF, John, Chief Human Resources Officer, Jupiter Medical Center, Jupiter, FL, p. A127
WOLF, Laura J., President, Franciscan Sisters of Christian Charity Sponsored Ministries, Inc., Manitowoc, WI, p. B53
WOLF, Marc, Director Human Resources, St. Barnabas Hospital,, NY, p. A436
WOLF, R. Chris, Chief Executive Officer, Payson Regional Medical Center, Payson, AZ, p. A35
WOLF, Randall, Vice President Finance, Perry County Memorial Hospital, Perryville, MO, p. A366
WOLF, Stephanne, Chief Nursing Officer, Morris County Hospital, Council Grove, KS, p. A232
WOLF, Terry Gerigk, Director, Veterans Affairs Pittsburgh Healthcare System, Pittsburgh, PA, p. A536
WOLF–ROSENBLUM, Stephanie, M.D. Chief Medical Officer, Southern New Hampshire Medical Center, Nashua, NH, p. A399
WOLFE, John, Chief Financial Officer, Saint Elizabeth's Medical Center, Wabasha, MN, p. A341
WOLFE, Judy, Chief Executive Officer, Corpus Christi Specialty Hospital, Corpus Christi, TX, p. A589
WOLFE, Kari, M.D. Medical Director, Seton Shoal Creek Hospital, Austin, TX, p. A581
WOLFE, Lois, Director Human Resources, Geisinger–Community Medical Center, Scranton, PA, p. A537
WOLFE, Mitchell, M.D. Chief of Staff, Clay County Memorial Hospital, Henrietta, TX, p. A603
WOLFE, Philip R., President and Chief Executive Officer, Gwinnett Hospital System, Lawrenceville, GA, p. A155
WOLFE, Stephen A., President and Chief Executive Officer, Indiana Regional Medical Center, Indiana, PA, p. A525
WOLFE, Teresa E., Manager Human Resources, Kansas Heart Hospital, Wichita, KS, p. A245
WOLFENBARGER, Carol C., R.N. Chief Operating Officer and Chief Nursing Executive, Jefferson Memorial Hospital, Jefferson City, TN, p. A567
WOLFF, Cathy, Vice President Financial Services and Chief Financial Officer, Yuma District Hospital, Yuma, CO, p. A107
WOLFF, David, Director Information Technology, Newberry County Memorial Hospital, Newberry, SC, p. A553
WOLFF, Ellen, R.N. Chief Nursing Officer/Senior VP/Patient Care Services, Lakes Region General Hospital, Laconia, NH, p. A398
WOLFF, Patrice P., Director Information Services, Westfields Hospital, New Richmond, WI, p. A688
WOLFF, Susan, Chief Information Officer, NCH Downtown Naples Hospital, Naples, FL, p. A133
WOLFF, Whitney, M.D. Medical Director, Taunton State Hospital, Taunton, MA, p. A305
WOLFGANG, Tony, Chief Financial Officer, Veterans Affairs Medical Center, Coatesville, PA, p. A521
WOLFMAN, Barry A., Chief Executive Officer and Managing Director, George Washington University Hospital, Washington, DC, p. A116
WOLFORD, Dennis A., FACHE Chief Executive Officer, Macon County General Hospital, Lafayette, TN, p. A569
WOLIN, Harry, Administrator and Chief Executive Officer, Mason District Hospital, Havana, IL, p. A183
WOLLEBEN, Robert G., Chief Executive Officer, Trumbull Memorial Hospital, Warren, OH, p. A490
WOLOSZYN, Daniel B., Chief Executive Officer, Rehabilitation Hospital of Indiana, Indianapolis, IN, p. A205
WOLTEMATH, Kelli, D.O. Chief Medical Staff, George C Grape Community Hospital, Hamburg, IA, p. A220
WOLTER, Nicholas, M.D. President and Chief Executive Officer, Billings Clinic, Billings, MT, p. A373
WOLTERMAN, Daniel J., President and Chief Executive Officer, Memorial Hermann Healthcare System, Houston, TX, p. B87
WOLTHER, Eunice, Public Information Officer, Colorado Mental Health Institute at Pueblo, Pueblo, CO, p. A105
WOLTHUIZEN, Dianne, Director Human Resources, Sanford Sheldon Medical Center, Sheldon, IA, p. A226
WOLZ, John, M.D. Chief Medical Staff, Yuma District Hospital, Yuma, CO, p. A107
WOMEODU, Robin, M.D. Chief Medical Officer, Methodist Healthcare Memphis Hospitals, Memphis, TN, p. A572
WONES, Robert, M.D. Vice President and Associate Chief of Staff, University Hospital, Cincinnati, OH, p. A474
WONG, Art, Chief Financial Officer, Heritage Oaks Hospital, Sacramento, CA, p. A83
WONG, Davies, M.D. Medical Director, Kindred Hospital–San Diego, San Diego, CA, p. A85
WONG, Dionne, Vice President and Chief Human Resources Officer, Broward Health Medical Center, Fort Lauderdale, FL, p. A123
WOOD, Bill, Director Human Resources, South Haven Health System, South Haven, MI, p. A323
WOOD, Cathy, Director Human Resources, Memorial Hospital at Gulfport, Gulfport, MS, p. A346
WOOD, Cheryl L., Chief Engineering and Technology, Veterans Affairs Medical Center, Spokane, WA, p. A667
WOOD, Clyde, Chief Executive Officer, Volunteer Community Hospital, Martin, TN, p. A570
WOOD, David, Director Acute Care Services, Lewis County General Hospital, Lowville, NY, p. A429
WOOD, David P., FACHE Medical Center Director, Veterans Affairs Medical Center, Oklahoma City, OK, p. A502
WOOD, Deb, Vice President Human Resources, Kaweah Delta Medical Center, Visalia, CA, p. A95
WOOD, Fred, M.D. Medical Director, Cassia Regional Medical Center, Burley, ID, p. A167
WOOD, Gerry, Information Technologist, Kalamazoo Psychiatric Hospital, Kalamazoo, MI, p. A316
WOOD, Gregory C., Chief Executive Officer, Scotland Health Care System, Laurinburg, NC, p. A456
WOOD, James, Director Human Resources, Memorial Medical Center of West Michigan, Ludington, MI, p. A318
WOOD, James B., Chief Human Resources Officer, Halifax Regional Medical Center, Roanoke Rapids, NC, p. A459
WOOD, Joseph T., Vice President and Chief Information Officer, The Medical Center, Columbus, GA, p. A150
WOOD, Ken, President and Chief Executive Officer, North Hawaii Community Hospital, Kamuela, HI, p. A164
WOOD, Kenneth W.
President and Chief Executive Officer, Grace Hospital, Morganton, NC, p. A458
President and Chief Executive Officer, Valdese General Hospital, Valdese, NC, p. A462
WOOD, Lawrence, M.D. Chief Medical Officer, Littleton Adventist Hospital, Littleton, CO, p. A103
WOOD, Lisa Mae, Chief Financial Officer, Gritman Medical Center, Moscow, ID, p. A169
WOOD, Michael K., M.D. Chief Medical Officer, Mills–Peninsula Health Services, Burlingame, CA, p. A56
WOOD, Richard, Chief Financial Officer, Seton Medical Center, Daly City, CA, p. A59
WOOD, Robert, Chief Fiscal Services, Jack C. Montgomery Veterans Affairs Medical Center, Muskogee, OK, p. A499
WOOD, Robin, Director Information Systems, Platte County Memorial Hospital, Wheatland, WY, p. A698
WOOD, Sandy
Director Patient Care Services, Doctors Hospital Nelsonville, Nelsonville, OH, p. A486
Vice President Patient Services, Pleasant Valley Hospital, Point Pleasant, WV, p. A675
WOOD, Tina, Vice President Finance, Harper University Hospital/Hutzel Women's Hospital, Detroit, MI, p. A310
WOOD, Troy, Chief Operating Officer, Lakeview Hospital, Bountiful, UT, p. A637
WOOD, William E., M.D. Chief of Staff, Sequoyah Memorial Hospital, Sallisaw, OK, p. A504
WOODALL, Jay, Chief Executive Officer, Corpus Christi Medical Center, Corpus Christi, TX, p. A589
WOODALL, Lois, Director Human Resources, Lighthouse Care Center of Conway, Conway, SC, p. A549
WOODALL, Matt, Director Information Management, SSM DePaul Health Center, Bridgeton, MO, p. A356
WOODARD, Victor, Manager Information Technology, Dodge County Hospital, Eastman, GA, p. A152
WOODARD–THOMPSON, Charlesetta, President and Chief Executive Officer, Erlanger Health System, Chattanooga, TN, p. B50
WOODARD–THOMPSON, Charlesetta, President and Chief Executive Officer, Erlanger Medical Center, Chattanooga, TN, p. A563
WOODBECK, Terry L., Administrator, Tulsa Spine and Specialty Hospital, Tulsa, OK, p. A507

Index of Health Care Professionals

Index of Health Care Professionals / Woodford

WOODFORD, Margo, Assistant Administrator, Mayo Clinic Health System in Springfield, Springfield, MN, p. A340
WOODFORD, Steve, Chief Financial Officer, East Cooper Medical Center, Mount Pleasant, SC, p. A552
WOODFORD, Wayne, Executive Vice President and Chief Financial Officer, St. Joseph Hospital, Bangor, ME, p. A281
WOODIN, Joseph L., President and Chief Executive Officer, Gifford Medical Center, Randolph, VT, p. A644
WOODLAND, John, M.D. Medical Director, Vail Valley Medical Center, Vail, CO, p. A106
WOODLIFF, Brian K., President and Chief Executive Officer, Tahlequah City Hospital, Tahlequah, OK, p. A505
WOODLOCK, David J., Administrator, Four Winds Hospital, Saratoga Springs, NY, p. A442
WOODRICH, John T., President and Chief Operating Officer, BryanLGH Medical Center, Lincoln, NE, p. A385
WOODRUFF, Kathy, R.N. Chief Nursing Officer, Marshall Medical Center North, Guntersville, AL, p. A21
WOODRUFF, Stephen, M.D. Chief Medical Officer, NEA Baptist Memorial Hospital, Jonesboro, AR, p. A47
WOODS, Bob, Chief Information Officer, ValleyCare Medical Center, Pleasanton, CA, p. A80
WOODS, Brian, Director Human Resources, Stones River Hospital, Woodbury, TN, p. A576
WOODS, Cheryl, Chief Nursing Officer, Ochsner Medical Center – North Shore, Slidell, LA, p. A278
WOODS, Daniel J., President and Chief Executive Officer, St. Anthony's Memorial Hospital, Effingham, IL, p. A180
WOODS, Jr., Duane L., Chief Financial Officer, Fisher–Titus Medical Center, Norwalk, OH, p. A486
WOODS, Fred, Chief Financial Officer, The BridgeWay, North Little Rock, AR, p. A50
WOODS, Jennifer, R.N. Chief Nursing Officer, McLaren Northern Michigan, Petoskey, MI, p. A320
WOODS, Josh, Director Information Systems, Camden–Clark Medical Center, Parkersburg, WV, p. A674
WOODS, Julia, MSN Vice President and Chief Nursing Officer, Saint Luke's South Hospital, Overland Park, KS, p. A241
WOODS, Matthew, Executive Vice President Finance and Chief Financial Officer, Winchester Hospital, Winchester, MA, p. A306
WOODS, Rashawn, Director Human Resources, Shriners Hospitals for Children, Los Angeles, Los Angeles, CA, p. A72
WOODS, Suzanne, President and Chief Executive Officer, Flowers Hospital, Dothan, AL, p. A19
WOODS, Suzanne, R.N. Vice President Nursing and Chief Nursing Officer, Palm Bay Hospital, Melbourne, FL, p. A130
WOODS–NYCE, Karen, Chief Executive Officer, Twin Valley Behavioral Healthcare, Columbus, OH, p. A477
WOODWARD, Andy, Chief Financial Officer, Forrest General Hospital, Hattiesburg, MS, p. A346
WOODWARD, Ashley, Interim Chief Executive Officer, Valley County Health System, Ord, NE, p. A388
WOODWARD, David E., Executive Director, Devereux Children's Behavioral Health Center, Malvern, PA, p. A528
WOODWARD, James L., President and Chief Executive Officer, Meriter Hospital, Madison, WI, p. A684
WOODWARD, Kevin, Chief Financial Officer, Biggs–Gridley Memorial Hospital, Gridley, CA, p. A64
WOODWARD, Martin D., Director Acute Care Services, Larry B. Zieverink, Sr. Alcoholism Treatment Center, Raleigh, NC, p. A459
WOODWARD, Russell, M.D. Chief Medical Officer, Methodist Hospital, San Antonio, TX, p. A625
WOODWARD, Teresa, Director Human Resources, Landmark Hospital of Joplin, Joplin, MO, p. A361
WOODWARD, Will, Director Finance, Mercy Hospital Clermont, Batavia, OH, p. A470
WOODYARD, Elizabeth, MSN, Chief Executive Officer, Petersburg Medical Center, Petersburg, AK, p. A30
WOODYARD, Nancy, Chief Financial Officer, Neosho Memorial Regional Medical Center, Chanute, KS, p. A231
WOOL, Julius, Executive Director, Queens Hospital Center,, NY, p. A436
WOOLF, Louis J., President, Hebrew Rehabilitation Center, Boston, MA, p. A297
WOOLLEN, Susan, R.N. Director of Nursing, Lafayette General Surgical Hospital, Lafayette, LA, p. A270
WOOLLEY, Diane, Vice President Human Resources, Waterbury Hospital, Waterbury, CT, p. A112
WOOLLEY, Jacqueline, Vice President Human Resources, St. Joseph Hospital, Nashua, NH, p. A399
WOOLLEY, Sheila, R.N. Vice President, Patient Care Services, Wentworth–Douglass Hospital, Dover, NH, p. A397
WOOLSTENHULME, Daren, Chief Financial Officer, HEALTHSOUTH Rehabilitation Hospital of Utah, Sandy, UT, p. A641
WOOTEN, Mark D., M.D. Chief of Staff, Veterans Affairs Northern Indiana Health Care System, Fort Wayne, IN, p. A202
WORDEN, Jerry L., Chief Financial Officer, Marquette General Health System, Marquette, MI, p. A318
WORDEN, Kieth Anne, Director Human Resources, Mildred Mitchell–Bateman Hospital, Huntington, WV, p. A672
WORKMAN, Jennifer, Director Human Resources, Jane Phillips Medical Center, Bartlesville, OK, p. A494
WORKMAN, John R.
  Chief Executive Officer, Athens Regional Medical Center, Athens, TN, p. A562
  Chief Executive Officer, Woods Memorial Hospital, Etowah, TN, p. A565
WORKMAN, Mark, M.D. Chief Medical Officer, West Jefferson Medical Center, Marrero, LA, p. A272
WORLEY Jr., John C., Chief Executive Officer, Cache Valley Specialty Hospital, North Logan, UT, p. A639
WORLEY, Kathy, Director Human Resources, Brigham City Community Hospital, Brigham City, UT, p. A637
WORLEY, Steve, President and Chief Executive Officer, Children's Hospital, New Orleans, LA, p. A274
WORRELL, James W., Chief Financial Officer, Pioneers Medical Center, Meeker, CO, p. A104
WORRICK, Gerald M., President and Chief Executive Officer, Ministry Door County Medical Center, Sturgeon Bay, WI, p. A691
WORSOWICZ, Gregory, M.D. Medical Director, Howard A. Rusk Rehabilitation Center, Columbia, MO, p. A358
WORTHAM, Christopher, Chief Executive Officer, HEALTHSOUTH Rehabilitation Hospital Midland–Odessa, Midland, TX, p. A616
WORTHAM, Stephanie, Director Financial Services, Norman Specialty Hospital, Norman, OK, p. A500
WORTHAM, Turner, Chief Financial Officer, Grand Strand Regional Medical Center, Myrtle Beach, SC, p. A552
WORTHINGTON, Diane, Director Human Resources, Placentia–Linda Hospital, Placentia, CA, p. A80
WORTMAN, Rand J., Chief Executive Officer, Kadlec Medical Center, Richland, WA, p. A665
WOZNIAK, Gregory T., President and Chief Executive Officer, St. Mary Medical Center, Langhorne, PA, p. A526
WOZNIAK, Ilona, Vice President and Chief Operating Officer, WellStar Cobb Hospital, Austell, GA, p. A147
WOZNIAK, Peter, R.N. Chief Executive Officer, Venice Regional Medical Center, Venice, FL, p. A142
WOZNIAK, Susan C., R.N. Senior Vice President and Chief Operating Officer, OSF Saint Francis Medical Center, Peoria, IL, p. A191
WRAALSTAD, Kimber L., FACHE Administrator and Chief Executive Officer, Cook County North Shore Hospital, Grand Marais, MN, p. A332
WRAGGE, Jean, Director of Nurses, Limestone Medical Center, Groesbeck, TX, p. A602
WRATTEN, Carol, M.D. Interim Chief Medical Officer, Baptist Health System, San Antonio, TX, p. A624
WRAY, Char, Vice President Chief Clinical Operations and Chief Information Officer, EMH Elyria Medical Center, Elyria, OH, p. A480
WRAY, Christine R., President, Medstar St. Mary's Hospital, Leonardtown, MD, p. A293
WRAY, Dean, Vice President Finance, Southern Ohio Medical Center, Portsmouth, OH, p. A487
WRAY, Robert, D.O. Chief Medical Staff, Edwards County Hospital and Healthcare Center, Kinsley, KS, p. A236
WRAY, Thomas, Director Information, Geisinger–Bloomsburg Hospital, Bloomsburg, PA, p. A519
WREN, Mark A., M.D. Medical Director, HEALTHSOUTH Rehabilitation Hospital of Texarkana, Texarkana, TX, p. A631
WREN, Patricia J., Chief Human Resources Officer, Hospital of the University of Pennsylvania, Philadelphia, PA, p. A532
WREN, Timothy, Chief Financial Officer, Abbeville Area Medical Center, Abbeville, SC, p. A546
WRIGHT, Ann L., R.N. Assistant Central Delivery System CNO, Presbyterian Hospital, Albuquerque, NM, p. A414
WRIGHT, Betsy T., President and Chief Executive Officer, Woman's Christian Association Hospital, Jamestown, NY, p. A428
WRIGHT, Brady, Information Technology Network Administrator, Washington County Hospital and Nursing Home, Chatom, AL, p. A18
WRIGHT, Charles T., President and Chief Executive Officer, St. James Healthcare, Butte, MT, p. A374
WRIGHT, Christopher Kemp
  Chief Executive Officer, Riverside Hospital of Louisiana, Alexandria, LA, p. A261
  Chief Executive Officer, Specialty Hospital of Winnfield, Winnfield, LA, p. A279
WRIGHT, Claudia, Director Health Information Management, Weatherford Regional Hospital, Weatherford, OK, p. A507
WRIGHT, Connie, Director Human Resources, Texas Health Presbyterian Hospital Dallas, Dallas, TX, p. A592
WRIGHT, Dan
  Vice President Human Resources, Children's Mercy Hospitals and Clinics, Kansas City, MO, p. A361
  Vice President Human Resources, Children's Mercy South, Overland Park, KS, p. A240
WRIGHT, Daniel, Director Information Technology, Saint Alphonsus Medical Center – Nampa, Nampa, ID, p. A169
WRIGHT, Dawn, Director Human Resources, Artesia General Hospital, Artesia, NM, p. A415
WRIGHT, Debra J., R.N. Chief Executive Officer, Howard Memorial Hospital, Nashville, AR, p. A49
WRIGHT, Ivan, M.D. Vice President Medical Affairs, Trinity Health System, Steubenville, OH, p. A489
WRIGHT, James, M.D. Chief Financial Officer, Cypress Fairbanks Medical Center, Houston, TX, p. A604
WRIGHT, Janet, R.N. Vice President Patient Care Executive, Lourdes Medical Center, Pasco, WA, p. A664
WRIGHT, Jean, M.D. Chief Medical Officer, Carolinas Medical Center–NorthEast, Concord, NC, p. A451
WRIGHT, Joe, Chief Financial Officer, Mitchell County Hospital, Colorado City, TX, p. A588
WRIGHT, Julie M., Director Human Resources, Ridgeview Psychiatric Hospital and Center, Oak Ridge, TN, p. A574
WRIGHT, Krista, Director Human Resources, St. Vincent Frankfort Hospital, Frankfort, IN, p. A202
WRIGHT, Linda, Director Information, Ottawa County Health Center, Minneapolis, KS, p. A239
WRIGHT, Lucius, M.D. Chief of Staff, Jackson–Madison County General Hospital, Jackson, TN, p. A567
WRIGHT, Margaret, President, Palos Community Hospital, Palos Heights, IL, p. A190
WRIGHT, Mark, Vice President, Aultman Hospital, Canton, OH, p. A472
WRIGHT, Mark J., Vice President Finance, Aurelia Osborn Fox Memorial Hospital, Oneonta, NY, p. A439
WRIGHT, Mary Lynne, R.N. President, Madison Hospital, Madison, AL, p. A22
WRIGHT, Patricia, Personal Analyst, San Joaquin General Hospital, French Camp, CA, p. A61
WRIGHT, Peter J., Chief Operating Officer, Littleton Regional Hospital, Littleton, NH, p. A399
WRIGHT II, Phil A., Chief Executive Officer, Southampton Memorial Hospital, Franklin, VA, p. A648
WRIGHT, Phillip L., FACHE Chief Executive Officer, Santa Rosa Medical Center, Milton, FL, p. A132
WRIGHT, Randall P., Executive Vice President and Chief Operating Officer, Texas Children's Hospital, Houston, TX, p. A607
WRIGHT, Rick, President and Chief Executive Officer, McLaren Greater Lansing, Lansing, MI, p. A317
WRIGHT, Robert, M.D. Chief of Staff, Washington County Regional Medical Center, Sandersville, GA, p. A158
WRIGHT, Roger, Director Human Resources, Porterville Developmental Center, Porterville, CA, p. A81
WRIGHT, Rory, M.D. President Medical Staff, Orthopaedic Hospital of Wisconsin – Glendale, Milwaukee, WI, p. A687
WRIGHT, Roy, FACH
  President and Chief Executive Officer, Cape Canaveral Hospital, Cocoa Beach, FL, p. A120
  President, Palm Bay Hospital, Melbourne, FL, p. A130
WRIGHT, Ruth, Director Information Services, Erlanger at Hutcheson, Fort Oglethorpe, GA, p. A153
WRIGHT, Sandra, Acting Chief Information Technology Services, Central Texas Veterans Healthcare System, Temple, TX, p. A630
WRIGHT, Sandra Gayle, Ed.D. Chief Executive Officer, Tyler County Hospital, Woodville, TX, p. A636
WRIGHT, Stephanie, Director Human Resources Management, Veterans Affairs San Diego Healthcare System, San Diego, CA, p. A86
WRIGHT, Stephen C., M.D. Chief Medical Officer, Faulkner Hospital, Boston, MA, p. A296
WRIGHT, Stephen F.
  President and Chief Executive Officer, CHRISTUS Health Shreveport–Bossier, Shreveport, LA, p. A277
  President and Chief Executive Officer, CHRISTUS St. Frances Cabrini Hospital, Alexandria, LA, p. A261
  President and Chief Executive Officer, CHRISTUS St. Patrick Hospital of Lake Charles, Lake Charles, LA, p. A271
WRIGHT, Stuart M., CPA Chief Financial Officer, Upstate University Hospital, Syracuse, NY, p. A444
WRIGHT, Tony, Chief Financial Officer, Mercy McCune–Brooks Hospital, Carthage, MO, p. A357
WRINN, Denise, Vice President Financial Services and Chief Financial Officer, Cortland Regional Medical Center, Cortland, NY, p. A424

Index of Health Care Professionals / Young

WROBLEWSKI, Edmund, M.D
  Vice President Medical Affairs and Chief Medical Officer, Goleta Valley Cottage Hospital, Santa Barbara, CA, p. A89
  Vice President Medical Affairs and Chief Medical Officer, Santa Barbara Cottage Hospital, Santa Barbara, CA, p. A89
  Vice President Medical Affairs and Chief Medical Officer, Santa Ynez Valley Cottage Hospital, Solvang, CA, p. A91
WROGG, Frank, Director Information Technology, Mayo Clinic Health System – Red Cedar in Menomonie, Menomonie, WI, p. A685
WU, Jonathan, M.D. President and Chairman, AHMC & Healthcare, Inc., Alhambra, CA, p. B7
WU, Kenneth, M.D. Medical Director, Marlton Rehabilitation Hospital, Marlton, NJ, p. A406
WUEBBELS, Carman, R.N. Chief Nursing Officer, Mason District Hospital, Havana, IL, p. A183
WUESTE, David, Director Information Services, University of Southern California–Norris Cancer Hospital, Los Angeles, CA, p. A72
WUKITSCH, Michael, Chief Human Resources Officer, Children's Hospital Colorado, Aurora, CO, p. A97
WURGLER, Brad D., Chief Financial Officer, Perham Health, Perham, MN, p. A337
WURTH, Jackie, Director of Nursing, Cumberland Hall Hospital, Hopkinsville, KY, p. A251
WURTH, Marie, Vice President Human Resources and Public Relations Officer, Sierra Vista Regional Health Center, Sierra Vista, AZ, p. A38
WURTZEL, Leann, Director Human Resources, Mayo Clinic Health System – Red Cedar in Menomonie, Menomonie, WI, p. A685
WYANT, Sandy, Director Human Resources, St. Mary's Medical Center, West Palm Beach, FL, p. A143
WYATT, Basil, Chief Financial Officer, Continuous Care Centers of Tulsa, Tulsa, OK, p. A505
WYATT, Charles, M.D. Medical Director, AMG Specialty Hospital–Lafayette Regional Campus, Lafayette, LA, p. A270
WYATT, Jana, Chief Executive Officer, Mizell Memorial Hospital, Opp, AL, p. A24
WYATT, Leslie G., Senior Vice President Children's Services and Executive Director, Children's Hospital of Richmond, Richmond, VA, p. A654
WYATT, Vincent N., Chief Financial Officer, Fort Walton Beach Medical Center, Fort Walton Beach, FL, p. A124
WYDICK, Sue, Director Human Resources, Ohio County Hospital, Hartford, KY, p. A251
WYDRA, Lana, Vice President Human Resources, Nathan Littauer Hospital and Nursing Home, Gloversville, NY, p. A426
WYERS, Michael, Chief Financial Officer, Englewood Community Hospital, Englewood, FL, p. A122
WYLES, Rick, Chief Financial Officer, McLaren Flint, Flint, MI, p. A312
WYLIE, Eugene, Chief Human Resources Officer, Jerry L. Pettis Memorial Veterans Medical Center, Loma Linda, CA, p. A67
WYLIE, Patrick, Director Information Systems, Petaluma Valley Hospital, Petaluma, CA, p. A80
WYMAN, Alan, Chief Information Officer, Providence Hospital, Washington, DC, p. A116
WYMAN, Jill, Interim Director Human Resources, Baystate Franklin Medical Center, Greenfield, MA, p. A300
WYNES, Jim Bob, Director Human Resources, Southwest Memorial Hospital, Cortez, CO, p. A99
WYNN, Chester A., President and Chief Executive Officer, Passavant Area Hospital, Jacksonville, IL, p. A185
WYNN, Katherine, Director Human Resource, Oklahoma Heart Hospital, Oklahoma City, OK, p. A501
WYNN, Paige, Chief Financial Officer, Dorminy Medical Center, Fitzgerald, GA, p. A152
WYRSCH, Steven J., R.N. Senior Vice President, Operations and Chief Operating Officer, Memorial Hospital, North Conway, NH, p. A399
WYSE, Gene, D.O. Medical Director, Hastings Regional Center, Hastings, NE, p. A384
WYSE, LaMar L., Chief Operating Officer, Doctors Hospital Nelsonville, Nelsonville, OH, p. A486
WYSONG–HARDER, Alyson, Chief Executive Officer, Heartland Behavioral Health Services, Nevada, MO, p. A366

## X

XAOCHAY, Billy, Manager Information Technology, Blue Mountain Hospital, Blanding, UT, p. A637
XINIS, James J., President and Chief Executive Officer, Calvert Memorial Hospital, Prince Frederick, MD, p. A293
XIPPOLITOS, Lee Anne, R.N. Chief Nursing Officer, Stony Brook University Medical Center, Stony Brook, NY, p. A444

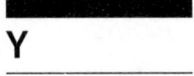

## Y

YABLONKA, Eric, Vice President and Chief Information Officer, University of Chicago Medical Center, Chicago, IL, p. A179
YAEGER, Eric, M.D. Medical Director, Kindred Hospital–Denver, Denver, CO, p. A99
YAHNER, Michael, Chief Financial Officer, Torrance State Hospital, Torrance, PA, p. A539
YAHYA, Zuhair, M.D. Chief Medical Officer, San Dimas Community Hospital, San Dimas, CA, p. A86
YAJKO, Gene, Director Human Resources, Soldiers and Sailors Memorial Hospital, Wellsboro, PA, p. A540
YAKLIC, Jerome, M.D. Chief of Staff, Huron Medical Center, Bad Axe, MI, p. A307
YAKLIN, Shelleye, President and Chief Executive Officer, North Ottawa Community Hospital, Grand Haven, MI, p. A313
YAMADA, Chrissy, CPA Senior Vice President Finance, Evergreen Hospital Medical Center, Kirkland, WA, p. A662
YAMADA, Jeff, Assistant Vice President, Yakima Valley Memorial Hospital, Yakima, WA, p. A669
YAMAKAWA, Mark, Chief Operating Officer, Queen's Medical Center, Honolulu, HI, p. A164
YAN, James, M.D. Chief of Staff, Chinese Hospital, San Francisco, CA, p. A86
YANAI, Christopher, Warden and Chief Executive Officer, Oakwood Correctional Facility, Lima, OH, p. A483
YANCY, Daniel, Administrator and Chief Executive Officer, Winnie Community Hospital, Winnie, TX, p. A635
YANEZ, Maria J., Chief Financial Officer, Baptist Health South Florida, Doctors Hospital, Coral Gables, FL, p. A121
YANKOWSKI, Edward, Chief Human Resources Management Service, Veterans Affairs Medical Center, Northport, NY, p. A438
YANNI, Anthony, M.D. Vice President Medical Affairs, Regional Hospital of Scranton, Scranton, PA, p. A538
YANNI, Jason, Senior Financial Analyst, Presbyterian Hospital Huntersville, Huntersville, NC, p. A455
YARBOROUGH, Dianne, Director Information Systems, Doctors Hospital at White Rock Lake, Dallas, TX, p. A591
YARBOROUGH, James, FACHE Interim Chief Executive Officer, Elbert Memorial Hospital, Elberton, GA, p. A152
YARDLEY, Jean, Budget Officer, Dorothea Dix Hospital, Raleigh, NC, p. A459
YARN, Jayce, Director Information Technology, Marias Medical Center, Shelby, MT, p. A379
YAROCH, Julie, D.O
  Vice President Medical Affairs, ProMedica Bixby Hospital, Adrian, MI, p. A307
  Vice President Medical Affairs, ProMedica Herrick Hospital, Tecumseh, MI, p. A324
YARRAMSETTI, Sri, Director Information Systems, Mission Regional Medical Center, Mission, TX, p. A617
YASKO, Joyce M., Ph.D. Chief Operating Officer, Roswell Park Cancer Institute, Buffalo, NY, p. A423
YATES, Ann C., R.N. Director Patient Care and Clinical Services, St. Vincent Mercy Hospital, Elwood, IN, p. A200
YATES, Gary R., M.D
  Senior Vice President and Chief Medical Officer, Sentara Leigh Hospital, Norfolk, VA, p. A652
  Chief Medical Officer, Sentara Norfolk General Hospital, Norfolk, VA, p. A653
YATES, James R., M.D. Chief of Staff, Jacksonville Medical Center, Jacksonville, AL, p. A22
YATES, Rob, Chief Executive Officer, Intracare North Hospital, Houston, TX, p. A604
YATES, Vinson, President, Grant Medical Center, Columbus, OH, p. A476
YATSATTIE, Clyde, Administrative Officer, U. S. Public Health Service Indian Hospital, Zuni, NM, p. A419
YAWN, Roy A., M.D. President and Chief Executive Officer, Olmsted Medical Center, Rochester, MN, p. A338
YAWORSKY, Jason
  Chief Information Officer, Bradford Regional Medical Center, Bradford, PA, p. A519
  Senior Vice President Information Systems and Chief Information Officer, Olean General Hospital, Olean, NY, p. A439
YAZAWA, Albert, M.D. Regional Medical Director, Leahi Hospital, Honolulu, HI, p. A163
YAZZIE, Bennie C., Interim Chief Executive Officer, Gallup Indian Medical Center, Gallup, NM, p. A416
YEAGER, Dianne, Chief Executive Officer, Crane Memorial Hospital, Crane, TX, p. A589
YEAGER, Kevin, Vice President Fiscal Services, Holzer Medical Center – Jackson, Jackson, OH, p. A482
YEAST, John, M.D. Director Medical Affairs, Saint Luke's Hospital of Kansas City, Kansas City, MO, p. A362
YEASTED, G. Alan, M.D. Senior Vice President and Chief Medical Officer, St. Clair Memorial Hospital, Pittsburgh, PA, p. A535
YEATES, Alan H., Vice President Fiscal Services, Wyandot Memorial Hospital, Upper Sandusky, OH, p. A490
YEATES, Diane, Chief Operating Officer, Terrebonne General Medical Center, Houma, LA, p. A268
YECHOOR, Siva, M.D. Medical Director, Arrowhead Behavioral Health Hospital, Maumee, OH, p. A484
YECNY, Rick, Chief Executive Officer, Peace Harbor Hospital, Florence, OR, p. A510
YEDVAB, Lauren, Senior Vice President, New York Methodist Hospital,, NY, p. A435
YEE, Brenda, MSN, Chief Executive Officer, Chinese Hospital, San Francisco, CA, p. A86
YEH, Ada, R.N. Chief Operating Officer and Chief Nursing Officer, Chapman Medical Center, Orange, CA, p. A78
YESITIS, Dawn, Director Human Resources, John C. Fremont Healthcare District, Mariposa, CA, p. A74
YETMAN, Robert, M.D. Medical Director, Healthbridge Children's Hospital of Houston, Houston, TX, p. A604
YEUNG, Christopher A., M.D. Chief of Staff, Surgical Specialty Hospital of Arizona, Phoenix, AZ, p. A37
YI, Brenda, Director Medical Resource Management and Chief Financial Officer, U. S. Air Force Medical Center Keesler, Keesler AFB, MS, p. A348
YI, Sok, M.D. President Medical Staff, Culpeper Regional Hospital, Culpeper, VA, p. A647
YILMAZ, Mehmet, M.D. Medical Director, Southwest Regional Rehabilitation Center, Battle Creek, MI, p. A308
YIM, Janet, Director Information Services, St. Mary Mercy Hospital, Livonia, MI, p. A318
YINGLING, Barbara, R.N. Vice President and Chief Nursing Officer, Mercy Medical Center, Canton, OH, p. A472
YITTA, Prasad, M.D. Medical Director, River Hospital, Alexandria Bay, NY, p. A420
YOAKUM, Jerrie, Director Human Resources, Ilano Specialty Hospital of Lubbock, Lubbock, TX, p. A614
YOCHELSON, Michael R., M.D. Vice President and Medical Director, Medstar National Rehabilitation Network, Washington, DC, p. A116
YOCHUM, Richard E., President and Chief Executive Officer, Pomona Valley Hospital Medical Center, Pomona, CA, p. A80
YODER, Cathy
  Chief Financial Officer, South Florida Baptist Hospital, Plant City, FL, p. A136
  Chief Financial Officer, St. Joseph's Hospital, Tampa, FL, p. A141
YOKLEY, Dorothy, Assistant Administrator, Hickman Community Hospital, Centerville, TN, p. A563
YON, Robin, Site Finance Director, Mercy Health – Fairfield Hospital, Fairfield, OH, p. A480
YOO, George, M.D. Chief Medical Officer, Karmanos Cancer Center, Detroit, MI, p. A311
YOON, Chris, M.D. Medical Director, HEALTHSOUTH Bakersfield Rehabilitation Hospital, Bakersfield, CA, p. A54
YORDY, Alan R., President and Chief Mission Officer, PeaceHealth, Bellevue, WA, p. B100
YORK, Chris, FACHE Chief Operating Officer, Baylor Regional Medical Center at Grapevine, Grapevine, TX, p. A601
YORK, Don, Vice President Human Resources, Sky Lakes Medical Center, Klamath Falls, OR, p. A511
YORK, Jack, Director Information Systems, Bingham Memorial Hospital, Blackfoot, ID, p. A166
YORK, Linda, Manager Human Resources, Memorial Hospital of Converse County, Douglas, WY, p. A696
YORK, Mary, Vice President Human Resources, Memorial Medical Center, Johnstown, PA, p. A526
YORK, Russell W.
  Chief Financial Officer, Mississippi Baptist Medical Center, Jackson, MS, p. A348
  Vice President and Chief Financial Officer, Mississippi Hospital for Restorative Care, Jackson, MS, p. A348
YOSHII, Brian, Vice President Information Technology, Kaiser Permanente Medical Center, Honolulu, HI, p. A163
YOSKO, Kathleen C., President and Chief Executive Officer, Marianjoy Rehabilitation Hospital, Wheaton, IL, p. A196
YOST, Carla J., R.N. Chief Operating Officer, Mercy Regional Health Center,, KS, p. A238
YOST, David, M.D. Clinical Director, U. S. Public Health Service Indian Hospital–Whiteriver, Whiteriver, AZ, p. A40
YOST, James, Director Management Information Systems, Meadowlands Hospital Medical Center, Secaucus, NJ, p. A410
YOUNES, Steven, Vice President, Chief Human Resources Officer and Employment Counsel, St. Vincent's Medical Center, Bridgeport, CT, p. A108
YOUNG, Angela, Human Resources Officer, Veterans Affairs Medical Center, Chillicothe, OH, p. A472
YOUNG, Ann, Vice President Community and Staff Relations, Mercy Medical Center–Centerville, Centerville, IA, p. A216



Index of Health Care Professionals

YOUNG, Barry, Director Human Resources, Western Mental Health Institute, Bolivar, TN, p. A562

YOUNG, Bev, Director Human Resources, Frankfort Regional Medical Center, Frankfort, KY, p. A250

YOUNG, Beverly, Director Human Resources, Memorial Hospital of Carbon County, Rawlins, WY, p. A697

YOUNG, Bryce A.
Chief Operating Officer, Hays Medical Center, Hays, KS, p. A234
Chief Operating Officer, Pawnee Valley Community Hospital, Larned, KS, p. A237

YOUNG, Chris, Vice President and Chief Information Officer, Saint Thomas Hospital, Nashville, TN, p. A573

YOUNG, David
Vice President External Operations, Sumner Regional Medical Center, Gallatin, TN, p. A566
Senior Vice President Planning and Technology, Trousdale Medical Center, Hartsville, TN, p. A566

YOUNG, Eric, M.D. Chief of Staff, Veterans Affairs Ann Arbor Healthcare System, Ann Arbor, MI, p. A307

YOUNG, Eric L.
Vice President Finance and Chief Financial Officer, Marietta Memorial Hospital, Marietta, OH, p. A483
Chief Financial Officer, Selby General Hospital, Marietta, OH, p. A484

YOUNG, J. Phillip, FACHE Chief Executive Officer, Southern Tennessee Medical Center, Winchester, TN, p. A576

YOUNG, James, Senior Vice President Finance and Chief Financial Officer, Howard County General Hospital, Columbia, MD, p. A290

YOUNG, James, M.D. Chief of Staff, McGehee–Desha County Hospital, McGehee, AR, p. A48

YOUNG, Jeffrey D.
Chief Information Officer, Children's Hospitals and Clinics of Minnesota, Minneapolis, MN, p. A335
Chief Information Officer, Children's Hospitals and Clinics of Minnesota, Saint Paul, MN, p. A339

YOUNG, Jeremie, M.D. Chief of Staff, Tri–County Hospital – Williston, Williston, FL, p. A143

YOUNG, Jimmy, Chief Financial Officer, Gilmore Memorial Regional Medical Center, Amory, MS, p. A343

YOUNG, John, Interim CEO, MedWest – Haywood, Clyde, NC, p. A451

YOUNG, Joyce, R.N. VP, Patient Services & Chief Nursing Officer, St. Joseph Mercy Livingston Hospital, Howell, MI, p. A315

YOUNG, Judy, Chief Financial Officer, Acadia–St. Landry Hospital, Church Point, LA, p. A264

YOUNG, Kathlene A., FACHE President and Chief Executive Officer, St. Joseph Hospital and Health Center, Kokomo, IN, p. A206

YOUNG, Kevin, FACHE President and Chief Executive Officer, Adventist Behavioral Health Rockville, Rockville, MD, p. A293

YOUNG, Kimberly, Chief Financial Officer, Baptist Memorial Hospital–Desoto, Southaven, MS, p. A352

YOUNG, Lori, Manager Health Information Management, Sumner Regional Medical Center, Wellington, KS, p. A245

YOUNG, Martha, Director Human Resources, Cumberland County Hospital, Burkesville, KY, p. A248

YOUNG, Mary, Director Human Resources, Colorado Mental Health Institute at Pueblo, Pueblo, CO, p. A105

YOUNG, Mathew, Manager Information Systems, Boscobel Area Health Care, Boscobel, WI, p. A679

YOUNG, Michael, Chief Financial Officer, Mad River Community Hospital, Arcata, CA, p. A54

YOUNG, Michael A., FACHE President and Chief Executive Officer, Pinnacle Health System, Harrisburg, PA, p. A524

YOUNG, Nancy, Director Human Resources,, Lake Chelan Community Hospital, Chelan, WA, p. A660

YOUNG, Pam, Human Resources Leader, Davis County Hospital, Bloomfield, IA, p. A215

YOUNG, Patty, R.N. Hospital Director of Nursing, Ashland Health Center, Ashland, KS, p. A230

YOUNG, Russ, Network Administrator, Wheatland Memorial Healthcare, Harlowton, MT, p. A376

YOUNG, Russell T., Chief Financial Officer, Central Florida Regional Hospital, Sanford, FL, p. A138

YOUNG, Rusty, Chief Financial Officer, Brownsville Doctors Hospital, Brownsville, TX, p. A585

YOUNG, Sandra G., Vice President Human Resources, Missouri Baptist Medical Center, Saint Louis, MO, p. A369

YOUNG, Stephanie, Chief Information Technology, Aleda E. Lutz Veterans Affairs Medical Center, Saginaw, MI, p. A322

YOUNG, Steve, Director Information Systems, Baylor Medical Center at Frisco, Frisco, TX, p. A600

YOUNG, Steven W., Director, Veterans Affairs Salt Lake City Health Care System, Salt Lake City, UT, p. A641

YOUNG, Susan M.
Chief Executive Officer, Mayhill Hospital, Denton, TX, p. A594
Chief Executive Officer, University Behavioral Health of Denton, Denton, TX, p. A594

YOUNG, Tammy, Controller, HEALTHSOUTH Lakeshore Rehabilitation Hospital, Birmingham, AL, p. A16

YOUNG, Terri, Vice President Human Resources, Alfred I. duPont Hospital for Children, Wilmington, DE, p. A114

YOUNG, Tyce, Patient Services Officer, Clay County Medical Center, Clay Center, KS, p. A231

YOUNG Jr., William A., President and Chief Executive Officer, St. John Medical Center, Westlake, OH, p. A491

YOUNG–HISE, Teri R., Director of Nursing, Waldo County General Hospital, Belfast, ME, p. A281

YOUNGBLOOD, Elizabeth
President, Baylor Specialty Hospital, Dallas, TX, p. A590
President, Our Children's House at Baylor, Dallas, TX, p. A592

YOUNGBLOOD, Erin R., Chief Human Resources Officer, Behavioral Center of Michigan, Warren, MI, p. A324

YOUNGER, Lonnie D., Chief Financial Officer, Huntsville Hospital, Huntsville, AL, p. A22

YOUNGS, Patsy, President, Texas Health Presbyterian Hospital Kaufman, Kaufman, TX, p. A610

YOUNKIN, Ken, Comptroller, J. D. McCarty Center for Children With Developmental Disabilities, Norman, OK, p. A500

YOUREE, Ben, Interim Chief Executive Officer, Dyersburg Regional Medical Center, Dyersburg, TN, p. A565

YOURZEK, Tari, Chief Nursing Officer, Boundary Community Hospital, Bonners Ferry, ID, p. A167

YOUSAITIS, Zoe, Director Human.Resources, Eagleville Hospital, Eagleville, PA, p. A522

YOUSO, Michael, Chief Executive Officer, Grand Itasca Clinic and Hospital, Grand Rapids, MN, p. A332

YOX, John, Senior Vice President and Chief Operating Officer, St. Catherine Hospital, Garden City, KS, p. A233

YU, Alex, Chief Financial Officer, Tri–City Medical Center, Oceanside, CA, p. A77

YU, Derrick, Administrator, Toppenish Community Hospital, Toppenish, WA, p. A668

YUCHA, Scott, Director Information Technology, Sunbury Community Hospital, Sunbury, PA, p. A539

YUEN, Kit, R.N. Interim Chief Nursing Officer, New York Downtown Hospital, New York, NY, p. A435

YUHAS, John, D.O. Medical Director, St. Francis Health Care Centre, Green Springs, OH, p. A481

YULICH, Michael, Director Information Services, Mercy Suburban Hospital, Norristown, PA, p. A530

YUNGMANN, Michael, Chief Executive Officer, Southside Regional Medical Center, Petersburg, VA, p. A653

YUNIS, Norm, M.D. Medical Director, Regency Hospital of Minneapolis, Golden Valley, MN, p. A332

YUNUSOV, Ed, Coordinator Facility Information Center, Queens Children's Psychiatric Center,, NY, p. A436

YURKIEWICZ, Sharon, Chief Executive Officer, Kindred Hospital–Wyoming Valley, Wilkes Barre, PA, p. A541

YUST, Randall C., Chief Operating Officer and Chief Financial Officer, Indiana University Health North Hospital, Carmel, IN, p. A199

# Z

ZABAWSKI, Denise, Vice President Information Services and Chief Information Officer, Nationwide Children's Hospital, Columbus, OH, p. A477

ZABIELSKI, Gerald C., M.D. Chief Medical Staff, Wright Memorial Hospital, Trenton, MO, p. A372

ZABINSKY, Hadley, Chief Information Officer, Harrington Memorial Hospital, Southbridge, MA, p. A304

ZACHARIASEN, Keith, Chief Financial Officer, Wamego City Hospital, Wamego, KS, p. A244

ZACHARY, Beth D., President and Chief Executive Officer, White Memorial Medical Center, Los Angeles, CA, p. A73

ZACHARY, Kevin, Chief Executive Officer, Parkview Regional Hospital, Mexia, TX, p. A616

ZACHRICH, Jane, Chief Nursing Officer, Community Memorial Hospital, Hicksville, OH, p. A481

ZADYLAK, Robert, M.D. Vice President Medical Management, Advocate Illinois Masonic Medical Center, Chicago, IL, p. A175

ZAFONTE, Ross, D.O. Chief, Physical Medicine and Rehabilitation and Vice President Medical Affairs, Research and Education, Spaulding Rehabilitation Hospital, Boston, MA, p. A297

ZAGER, Joseph P., Vice President and Administrator, Riverside Shore Memorial Hospital, Nassawadox, VA, p. A651

ZAGERMAN, Robert, Chief Financial Officer, Brooke Glen Behavioral Hospital, Fort Washington, PA, p. A523

ZAGLAMA, Chris, Director Information Services, Southwest Regional Medical Center, Waynesburg, PA, p. A540

ZAGLUL, Jose, M.D. Chief Medical Officer, Manatee Glens Hospital and Addiction Center, Bradenton, FL, p. A119

ZAHN, Chip, Chief Operating Officer, Las Colinas Medical Center, Irving, TX, p. A609

ZAIDBERG, Edward A., Senior Vice President Finance, New York Methodist Hospital,, NY, p. A435

ZAIDI, Syed A., M.D. Chief of Staff, Lauderdale Community Hospital, Ripley, TN, p. A575

ZAJAC, Walter
Senior Vice President and Chief Financial Officer, Dorchester General Hospital, Cambridge, MD, p. A290
Senior Vice President and Chief Financial Officer, Memorial Hospital at Easton Maryland, Easton, MD, p. A291

ZAJEC, Doris A.
Human Resources Business Partner, Marymount Hospital, Garfield Heights, OH, p. A481
Director Human Resources, South Pointe Hospital, Warrensville Heights, OH, p. A490

ZAJIC, Holly, Vice President Human Resources and Physician Services, Ivinson Memorial Hospital, Laramie, WY, p. A696

ZAKAI, Aminadav, M.D. Medical Director, Arbour–Fuller Hospital, Attleboro, MA, p. A295

ZALDIVAR, Rogelio, M.D. Medical Director, Westchester General Hospital, Miami, FL, p. A132

ZALMAN, Tisha, Chief Executive Officer, El Campo Memorial Hospital, El Campo, TX, p. A595

ZALOUDEK, Lisa, Chief Human Resources Officer, Ponca City Medical Center, Ponca City, OK, p. A503

ZALUD, Nicolette, Customer Site Manager, McLaren Central Michigan, Mount Pleasant, MI, p. A319

ZALUSKI, Heather, M.D. President Medical Staff, Shodair Children's Hospital, Helena, MT, p. A376

ZAMBITO, Paolo, Chief Executive Officer, Ochsner Medical Center – Kenner, Kenner, LA, p. A269

ZAMBRANA, David, R.N. Chief Operating Officer and Chief Nursing Officer, University of Miami Hospital, Miami, FL, p. A132

ZAMBRINI, Christine, Chief Operating Officer and Chief Nursing Officer, Henry Ford West Bloomfield Hospital, West Bloomfield, MI, p. A325

ZAMORA, Don, Director Human Resources, Parkway Medical Center, Decatur, AL, p. A18

ZAMORA DE AGUERO, Hilde, Human Resources Site Director, Baptist Health South Florida, West Kendall Baptist Hospital, Miami, FL, p. A131

ZANE, Kristi, Chief Human Resources Officer, Crawford Memorial Hospital, Robinson, IL, p. A192

ZANI, Carl, Director Information Systems, Memorial Hospital of Union County, Marysville, OH, p. A484

ZANKMAN, Lisa, Senior Vice President Human Resources, Beth Israel Deaconess Medical Center, Boston, MA, p. A296

ZAPPALA, Phyllis
Vice President Human Resources, Danbury Hospital, Danbury, CT, p. A108
Senior Vice President Human Resources, New Milford Hospital, New Milford, CT, p. A111

ZAPPALA, Phyllis F.
Senior Vice President, Danbury Hospital, Danbury, CT, p. A108
Senior Vice President Human Resources, New Milford Hospital, New Milford, CT, p. A111

ZARA, George A., President and Chief Executive Officer, Providence Hospital, Columbia, SC, p. A548

ZARAK, Tamie, Director Human Resources, Memorial Medical Center – Neillsville, Neillsville, WI, p. A688

ZAREN, Douglas, FACHE Administrator, Memorial Regional Hospital South,, FL, p. A125

ZARITSKY, Arno, M.D. Senior Vice President Clinical Services, Children's Hospital of The King's Daughters, Norfolk, VA, p. A652

ZARRILLA, Peter, Vice President and Chief Human Resources Officer, Lowell General Hospital, Lowell, MA, p. A301

ZASTOCKI, Deborah, FACHE President and Chief Executive Officer, Chilton Hospital, Pompton Plains, NJ, p. A409

ZASTOUPIL, Rockford, President and Chief Executive Officer, St. Aloisius Medical Center, Harvey, ND, p. A466

ZAUNER, Mike, Chief Executive Officer, Sierra Vista Hospital, Sacramento, CA, p. A84

ZAVATCHEN, Nancy, Director Information Technology, Cullman Regional Medical Center, Cullman, AL, p. A18

ZAVODNICK, Jacquelyn, M.D. Medical Director, Devereux Children's Behavioral Health Center, Malvern, PA, p. A528

ZAWACKI, Brenda, Manager Human Resources, Providence Kodiak Island Medical Center, Kodiak, AK, p. A29

ZAWISZA, Walter, Chief Financial Officer, Veterans Affairs Ann Arbor Healthcare System, Ann Arbor, MI, p. A307

# AHA Membership Categories

*The American Hospital Association is primarily an organization of hospitals and related institutions. Its object, according to its bylaws, is "to promote high–quality health care and health services for all the people through leadership in the development of public policy, leadership in the representation and advocacy of hospital and health care organization interests, and leadership in the provision of services to assist hospitals and health care organizations in meeting the health care needs of their communities."*

## Institutional Members

**Hospitals or health services organizations or systems which provide a continuum of integrated, community health resources and which include at least one licensed hospital that is owned, leased, managed or religiously sponsored.**

Institutional members include hospitals, health care systems, integrated delivery systems, and physician hospital organizations (PHOs) and health maintenance organizations (HMOs) wholly or partially owned by or owning a member hospital or system. An Institutional member hospital, health care system or integrated delivery system may, at its discretion and upon approval of a membership application by the Association chief executive officer, extend membership to the health care provider organizations, other than a hospital that it owns, leases, or fully controls.

### Freestanding Health Care Provider Organizations

These are health provider organizations, other than registered hospitals, that provide patient care services, including, but not limited to, ambulatory, preventive, rehabilitative, specialty, post–acute and continuing care, as well as physician groups, health insurance services, and staff and group model health maintenance organizations without a hospital component. Freestanding Health Care Provider Organizations members are not owned or controlled by an Institutional member hospital, health care system or integrated delivery system member. They may, however, be part of an organization eligible for, but not holding, Institutional membership.

### Other Organizations

This category includes organizations interested in the objectives of the American Hospital Association, but not eligible for Institutional or Freestanding Health Care Provider Organization Membership. Organizations eligible for Other membership shall include, but not be limited to, associations, societies, foundations, corporations, educational and academic institutions, companies, government agencies, international health providers, and organizations having an interest in and a desire to support the objectives of the Association.

### Provisional Members

Hospitals that are in the planning or construction stage and that, on completion, will be eligible for institutional membership. Provisional membership may also be granted to applicant institutions that cannot, at present, meet the requirements of Institutional or Freestanding Health Care Provider Organization membership.

### Government Institution Group Members

Groups of government hospitals operated by the same unit of government may obtain institutional membership under a group plan. Membership dues are based on a special schedule set forth in the bylaws of the AHA.

*U.S. hospitals and hospitals in areas associated with the U.S. that are Institutional members of the American Hospital Association are included in the list of hospitals in section A. Canadian Institutional members of the American Hospital Association are listed below.*

## Canada

**ALBERTA**

**Lamont:** LAMONT HEALTH CARE CENTRE, P.O. Bag 10, Zip T0B 2R0; tel. 780/895–2211; Harold James, Executive Director

**MANITOBA**

**Winnipeg:** RIVERVIEW HEALTH CENTRE, 1 Morley Avenue East, Zip R3L 2P4; tel. 204/452–3411; Norman R. Kasian, President and Chief Executive Officer

**ONTARIO**

**London:** ST. JOSEPH'S HEALTH CENTRE, P.O. Box 5777, Zip N6A 4V2; tel. 519/646–6000; Gillian Kernaghan, M.D., President and Chief Executive Officer

**Renfrew:** RENFREW VICTORIA HOSPITAL, 499 Raglan Street North, Zip K7V 1P6; tel. 613/432–4851; Randy V. Penney, Executive Director

**Thornhill:** SHOULDICE HOSPITAL, 7750 Bayview Avenue, Zip L3T 4A3; tel. 905/889–1125; John Hughes, Chief Administrative Officer

**Toronto:** MOUNT SINAI HOSPITAL, 600 University Avenue, Zip M5G 1X5; tel. 416/586–4800; Joseph Mapa, FACHE, President and Chief Executive Officer

**QUEBEC**

**Montreal:** MOUNT SINAI HOSPITAL CENTER, 5690 Cavendish Cote St-Luc', Zip H4W 1S7; tel. 514/369–2222; Michel Amar, Executive Director

▮▮▮▮▮▮

# Associated University Programs in Health Administration

### CALIFORNIA

**San Diego:** CALIFORNIA COLLEGE SAN DIEGO, 2820 Camino Del Rio South, Suite 300, Zip 92108–3821; tel. 619/295–5784; Barbara Thomas, Chief Operations Officer

**San Francisco:** GOLDEN GATE UNIVERSITY, 536 Mission Street, Univ Library, Zip 94105–2968; tel. 415/442–7242; Steven Dunlap, Head Technical Services

### IOWA

**Iowa City:** DEPARTMENT OF HEALTH MANAGEMENT AND POLICY, UNIVERSITY OF IOWA, 105 River Street, N232A CPHB, Zip 52246; tel. 319/384–3830; Keith Mueller, Ph.D., Professor and Head

### MARYLAND

**Bethesda:** NAVAL SCHOOL OF HEALTH SCIENCES, Naval Medical Command, National Region, Zip 20889–5611; tel. 301/295–1251

### MISSOURI

**Columbia:** UNIVERSITY OF MISSOURI, HEALTH MANAGEMENT AND INFORMATICS, CE707 Clinical Support and Education Building, DC 00600, One Hospital Drive, Zip 65212; tel. 573/882–6179; Lanis Hicks, Ph.D., Professor and Associate Chair

### PENNSYLVANIA

**University Park:** PENNSYLVANIA STATE UNIVERSITY, 604 Ford Building, Zip 16802; tel. 814/863–2859; Dennis Shea, Department Head

### TEXAS

**Brooks AFB:** U. S. AIR FORCE SCHOOL OF AEROSPACE MEDICINE, USAFSAM–CCE, Zip 78235–5301; tel. 210/536–4251; Colonel Richard E. Bachmann, Jr., Commander

**San Antonio:** ARMY–BAYLOR UNIVERSITY PROGRAM IN HEALTH CARE ADMINISTRATION, 3151 Scott Road, Building 2841, Zip 78234–6135; tel. 210/221–6443; Lieutenant Colonel M. Nicholas Coppola, Program Director
TRINITY UNIVERSITY, One Trinity Place, #58, Zip 78212–7200; tel. 210/736–8107; Mary E. Stefl, Ph.D., Chairman

**Sheppard AFB:** U. S. AIR FORCE SCHOOL OF HEALTH CARE SCIENCES, Building 1900, MST/114, Academic Library, Zip 76311; tel. 817/851–2511

### PUERTO RICO

**San Juan:** SCHOOL OF PUBLIC HEALTH, P.O. Box 5067, Zip 00936; tel. 809/767–9626; Orlando Nieves, Dean

# Hospital Schools of Nursing

**NEW YORK**

**Elmira:** ARNOT–OGDEN MEMORIAL HOSPITAL School of Nursing

**PENNSYLVANIA**

**New Castle:** JAMESON HOSPITAL School of Nursing

# Nonhospital Preacute and Postacute Care Facilities

## ALABAMA

**Fort Rucker:** LYSTER ARMY HEALTH CLINIC, Andrews Lane, Building 301, Zip 36362–5000; tel. 334/255–7359; Colonel Patrick N. Denman, Commander

**Maxwell Afb:** MAXWELL CLINIC, 300 Twining Street, Zip 36112–6027; tel. 334/953–7801; Colonel Bart O. Iddins, Commander

## ALASKA

**Anchorage:** ALASKA VETERANS AFFAIRS HEALTHCARE SYSTEM, 2925 Debarr Road, Zip 99508–2989; tel. 907/257–6930; Alex Spector, Director

## ARIZONA

**Davis–Monthan AFB:** U. S. AIR FORCE CLINIC, 4175 South Alamo Avenue, Zip 85707–4405; tel. 520/228–2930

**Fort Huachuca:** RAYMOND W. BLISS ARMY HEALTH CENTER, 45001 Winrow Avenue, Zip 85613–7040; tel. 520/533–2350; Colonel Thomas W. Smith, M.D., MSC, Commander

**Glendale:** U. S. AIR FORCE HOSPITAL LUKE, Luke AFB, 7219 North Litchfield Road, Zip 85309–1525; tel. 623/856–7502; Colonel Schuyler K. Geller, Commander

## ARKANSAS

**Jacksonville:** U. S. AIR FORCE CLINIC LITTLE ROCK, Little Rock AFB, Zip 72099–5057; tel. 501/987–7411; Colonel Rebecca A. Russell, USAF, Commander

## CALIFORNIA

**Beale AFB:** U. S. AIR FORCE HOSPITAL, 15301 Warren Shingle Road, Zip 95903–1907; tel. 530/634–4838; Lieutenant Colonel Robert G. Quinn, MSC, USAF, FACHE, Administrator

**Edwards AFB:** U. S. AIR FORCE CLINIC, 10 Hospital Road, Building 5500, Zip 93524–1730; tel. 661/277–2010; Colonel Sally Petty, Commander

**Los Angeles:** DEPARTMENT OF VETERANS AFFAIRS, OUTPATIENT CLINIC, 351 East Temple Street, Zip 90012; tel. 213/253–5000; Jules Morevac, Ph.D., Director

**Martinez:** VETERANS AFFAIRS NORTHERN CALIFORNIA HEALTH SYSTEM, 150 Muir Road, Zip 94553; tel. 925/372–2000; Lawrence S. Sandler, Director

**Moss Beach:** SETON MEDICAL CENTER COASTSIDE, 600 Marine Boulevard, Zip 94038–9641; tel. 650/563–7100; Lorraine P. Auerbach, President and Chief Executive Officer

**Port Hueneme:** NAVAL AMBULATORY CARE CENTER, Zip 93043; tel. 805/982–6301; Major Frederick White, Officer–in–Charge

**San Francisco:** VETERANS AFFAIRS OUTPATIENT CLINIC, 4150 Clement Street, Zip 94121; tel. 415/221–4810; Lawrence C. Stewart, Director

**Sepulveda:** VETERANS AFFAIRS MEDICAL CENTER, 16111 Plummer Street, Zip 91343; tel. 818/891–7711; Charles M. Doorman, Acting Director

**Vandenberg AFB:** U. S. AIR FORCE HOSPITAL, 338 South Dakota Street, Zip 93437–6307; tel. 805/606–1110; Commander Janice Wallace, Commander

**Winterhaven:** U. S. PUBLIC HEALTH SERVICE INDIAN HOSPITAL, P.O. Box 1368, Zip 85366–1368; tel. 760/572–0217; Kent Smalley, M.D., Acting Chief Executive Officer and Clinical Director

## COLORADO

**Las Animas:** SOUTHERN COLORADO HEALTHCARE SYSTEM, P.O. Box 390, Zip 81054–0390; tel. 719/456–1260; Stuart C. Collyer, Director

**USAF Academy:** U. S. AIR FORCE ACADEMY CLINIC, 4102 Pinion Drive, Zip 80840–4000; tel. 719/333–5102; Colonel Alan B. Berg, Commander

## CONNECTICUT

**Groton:** NAVAL HOSPITAL, 1 Wahoo Drive, Box 600, Zip 06349–5600; tel. 860/694–3261

**Newington:** VETERANS AFFAIRS MEDICAL CENTER–NEWINGTON CAMPUS, 555 Willard Avenue, Zip 06111–2600; tel. 860/666–6951; Roger L. Johnson, Director

## DELAWARE

**Dover:** U. S. AIR FORCE HOSPITAL DOVER, 300 Tuskegee Boulevard, Zip 19902–7307; tel. 302/677–2525; Colonel Genanne Hansen–Bayless, Administrator

**New Castle:** CHRISTIANA CARE VISITING NURSE ASSOCIATION, One Reads Way, Zip 19720; tel. 302/327–8200; Lynn C. Jones, President

PHYSICAL THERAPY PLUS, 1 Reads Way, Suite 300, Zip 19720; tel. 302/326–8755; Stephen Rombach, Director

**Newark:** CHRISTIANA CARE IMAGING CENTER, 4751 Ogletown–Stanton Road, Zip 19713; tel. 302/731–9800; Charles Baxter, Director

CHRISTIANA SURGICENTER, 4755 Ogletown–Stanton Road, Zip 19718; tel. 302/733–6900; Margaret Wojcik, Coordinator

HEALTH CARE CENTER AT CHRISTIANA, 200 Hygeia Drive, Zip 19714

**Wilmington:** EUGENE DUPONT PREVENTIVE MEDICINE AND REHABILITATION INSTITUTE, 3506 Kennett Pike, Zip 19807; tel. 302/655–4041

## FLORIDA

**Jacksonville:** BAPTIST HOME HEALTH CARE, 3563 Philips Highway, Suite 202, Zip 32207; tel. 904/202–4300; Diane Jones, Director

BAPTIST OCCUPATIONAL HEALTH, 1325 San Marco Boulevard, Suite 301, Zip 32207; tel. 904/202–2395; Donna Snider, Director

BAPTIST PRIMARY CARE, 3563 Philips Highway, Suite 101, Zip 32207; tel. 904/376–3744; Berl O'Malley, Administrator

PAVILION INFUSION THERAPY, 3563 Philips Highway, Suite 202, Zip 32207; tel. 904/202–5730; Diane Jones, Director

PSYCHIATRIC AND PSYCHOLOGICAL CARE, 4160 University Boulevard South, Zip 32216; tel. 904/376–3800; Mark A. Masters, Ph.D., Director

**Key West:** NAVAL REGIONAL MEDICAL CLINIC, 1500 Douglas Circle, Zip 33040; tel. 305/293–4613; Commander Stephen Lanier, Officer–in–Charge

**MacDill AFB:** U. S. AIR FORCE HOSPITAL, 8415 Bayshore Boulevard, Zip 33621–1607; tel. 813/827–9521

**Patrick AFB:** U. S. AIR FORCE CLINIC, 1381 South Patrick Drive, Zip 32925–3606; tel. 407/494–8102; Colonel William Swindling, Commanding Officer

**Tyndall AFB:** U. S. AIR FORCE CLINIC, 340 Magnolia Avenue, Zip 32403–5612; tel. 850/283–7515; Colonel Michael J. Murphy, Commander

## GEORGIA

**Calhoun:** ALLIANT HEALTH PLANS, INC., 401 South Wall Street, Suite 201, Zip 30701; tel. 706/629–8848; Judy Pair, Chief Executive Officer

GEORGIA HEALTH PLUS, 401 South Wall Street, Suite 201, Zip 30701; tel. 706/629–1833

**Columbus:** AZALEA TRACE, 910 Talbotton Road, Zip 31901; tel. 706/323–9513; Todd West, Administrator

HAMILTON HOUSE NURSING CENTER/ADULT LIVING CENTER, 1911 Hamilton Road, Zip 31901; tel. 706/571–1850; John Sims, Administrator

**Moody AFB:** U. S. AIR FORCE HOSPITAL MOODY, 3278 Mitchell Boulevard, Zip 31699–1500; tel. 229/257–3772

**Robins AFB:** U. S. AIR FORCE CLINIC, 655 Seventh Street, Zip 31098–2227; tel. 912/327–7996; Colonel John A. Lee, USAF, MSC, Commander

**Rome:** CENTREX, 420 East Second Avenue, Zip 30161; tel. 706/235–1006; Dee B. Russell, M.D., Chief Executive Officer

COMMUNITY HOSPICECARE, P.O. Box 233, Zip 30162–0233; tel. 706/232–0807; Kurt Stuenkel, FACHE, President and Chief Executive Officer

FLOYD HOME HEALTH AGENCY, P.O. Box 6248, Zip 30162–6248; tel. 706/802–4600; Kurt Stuenkel, FACHE, President and Chief Executive Officer

FLOYD MEDICAL OUTPATIENT SURGERY, P.O. Box 233, Zip 30162–0233; tel. 706/802–2070; Kurt Stuenkel, FACHE, President and Chief Executive Officer

FLOYD REHABILITATION CENTER, P.O. Box 233, Zip 30162–0233; tel. 706/802–2091; Kurt Stuenkel, FACHE, President and Chief Executive Officer

## HAWAII

**Honolulu:** KAISER MOANALUA, 3288 Moanalua Road, Zip 96819–1469; tel. 808/432–0000; Melodee J. Deutsch, MS, M.P.H., Director Quality

MALUHIA HOSPITAL, 1027 Hala Drive, Zip 96817; tel. 808/832–5874; Sally T. Ishikawa, Administrator

VA PACIFIC ISLANDS HEALTHCARE SYSTEM, 459 Patterson Road, Zip 96819; tel. 808/541–1582; James E. Hastings, M.D., Director

**Pearl Harbor:** NAVAL REGIONAL MEDICAL CLINIC, Box 121, Building 1750, Zip 96860–5080; tel. 808/471–3025; Captain Joseph Moore, Commanding Officer

## ILLINOIS

**Great Lakes:** NAVAL HEALTH CLINIC GREAT LAKES, 3001A Sixth Street, Zip 60088–5230; tel. 847/688–4560; Captain Thomas E. McGue, Commanding Officer

**Oak Forest:** OAK FOREST HEALTH CENTER OF COOK COUNTY, 15900 South Cicero Avenue, Zip 60452–4006; tel. 708/687–7200; Sylvia Edwards, Chief Operating Officer

**Peoria Heights:** SAINT CLARE HOME, 5533 North Galena Road, Zip 61614–4499; tel. 309/682–5428; Candy Conover, Administrator

**Scott AFB:** SCOTT MEDICAL CENTER, 310 West Losey Street, Zip 62225–5252; tel. 618/256–7456; Colonel Bret D. Burton, Commander

## KANSAS

**Fort Leavenworth:** MUNSON ARMY HEALTH CENTER, 550 Pope Avenue, Zip 66027–2332; tel. 913/684–6420; Colonel David Bitterman, Commander

**Great Bend:** ST. ROSE AMBULATORY & SURGERY CENTER, 3515 Broadway Street, Zip 67530–3633; tel. 620/792–2511; Leanne M. Irsik, R.N., Senior Vice President and Administrator

**Wichita:** U. S. AIR FORCE HOSPITAL, 59570 Leavenworth Street, Suite 6E4, Zip 67221–5300; tel. 316/759–5421

## LOUISIANA

**Barksdale AFB:** U. S. AIR FORCE CLINIC, 243 Curtiss Road, Suite 100, Zip 71110–5300; tel. 318/456–6004; Colonel James M. Benge, Commander

**New Orleans:** NAVAL MEDICAL CLINIC, 1 Sanctuary Drive, Zip 70142–5300; tel. 504/678–2400

VETERANS AFFAIRS MEDICAL CENTER, 1601 Perdido Street, Zip 70112–1262; tel. 504/568–0811; Julie A. Catellier, Director

## MAINE

**Damariscotta:** COVE'S EDGE, 26 Schooner Street, Zip 04543; tel. 207/563–4645; Judy McGuire, Administrator

MILES MEDICAL GROUP, INC., 35 Miles Street, Zip 04543; tel. 207/563–1234; Stacey Miller–Friant, Director

**Kennebunk:** SOUTHERN MAINE HEALTH AND HOME SERVICES, P.O. Box 739, Zip 04043; tel. 207/985–4767; Elaine Brady, R.N., Executive Director

## MARYLAND

**Andrews AFB:** MALCOLM GROW MEDICAL CLINIC, 1050 West Perimeter, Suite B5–10, Zip 20762–6600; tel. 240/857–3001; Colonel Rudolph Cachuela, Commanding Officer

**Annapolis:** NAVAL MEDICAL CLINIC, 50 Rodgers Road, Zip 21402; tel. 410/293–1330; Captain Francis R. MacMahon, MC, USN, Commanding Officer

**Baltimore:** ST. AGNES HEALTH SERVICES, 900 Caton Avenue, Zip 21229; tel. 410/368–2945; Peter Clay, Senior Vice President Managed Care

ST. AGNES HOME CARE AND HOSPICE, 3421 Benson Avenue, Suite G100, Zip 21227; tel. 410/368–2825; Robin Dowell, Director

**Ellicott City:** ST. AGNES NURSING AND REHABILITATION CENTER, 3000 North Ridge Road, Zip 21043; tel. 410/461–7577; Barbara A. Gustke, R.N., Administrator Extended Care Facility

**Fort George G Meade:** KIMBROUGH ARMY HEALTH CENTER, 2480 Llewellyn Avenue, Zip 20755; tel. 301/677–4171; Colonel Billie J. Mielcarek, Commanding Officer

**Fort Howard:** VETERANS AFFAIRS MARYLAND HEALTH CARE SYSTEM–FORT HOWARD DIVISION, 9600 North Point Road, Zip 21052–9989; tel. 410/477–1800; Patricia Vicari, Director

**Patuxent River:** NAVAL MEDICAL CLINIC, 47149 Buse Road, Zip 20670–5370; tel. 301/342–1418; Captain R. J. McCormick–Boyle, Commanding Officer

## MASSACHUSETTS

**Boston:** JOSLIN DIABETES CENTER, One Joslin Place, Zip 02215; tel. 617/732–2400; Kenneth E. Quickel, M.D., President and Chief Executive Officer

**Springfield:** BAY STATE VISITING NURSE ASSOCIATION AND HOSPICE, 50 Maple Street, Zip 01105; tel. 413/781–5070; Ruth Odgren, President

**Turners Falls:** FARREN CARE CENTER, 340 Montague City Road, Zip 01376–9983; tel. 413/774–3111; James Clifford, Administrator

## MICHIGAN

**Big Rapids:** MECOSTA HEALTH SERVICES, 650 Linden Street, Zip 49307; tel. 231/796–3200; Gail Bullard, Director

**Detroit:** ST. JOHN DETROIT RIVERVIEW CENTER, 7733 East Jefferson Avenue, Zip 48214–2598; tel. 313/499–4000; Joseph M. Tasse, FACHE, President and Chief Executive Officer

ST. JOHN NORTHEAST COMMUNITY HOSPITAL, 4777 East Outer Drive, Zip 48234–0401; tel. 313/369–9100

**Port Huron:** MARWOOD MANOR NURSING HOME, 1300 Beard Street, Zip 48060; tel. 818/982–2594; Brian Oberly, Administrator

TRI–HOSPITAL E.M.S., 309 Grand River Street, Zip 48060; tel. 313/985–7115; Ken Cummings, Chief Executive Officer

WILLOW ENTERPRISES, INC., 1221 Pine Grove Avenue, Zip 48060; tel. 313/989–3737

**Saline:** ST. JOSEPH MERCY SALINE HOSPITAL, 400 West Russell Street, Zip 48176–1183; tel. 734/429–1500; Robert F. Casalou, President and Chief Executive Officer

**Sault Sainte Marie:** SAULT SAINTE MARIE TRIBAL HEALTH AND HUMAN SERVICES CENTER, 2864 Ashmun Street, Zip 49783; tel. 906/495–5651; Russell Vizina, Division Director Health

**Warren:** HENRY FORD MACOMB HOSPITAL–WARREN CAMPUS, 13355 East Ten Mile Road, Zip 48089–2048; tel. 586/759–7300; Barbara Rossmann, President and Chief Executive Officer

## MINNESOTA

**Saint Paul:** HEALTHEAST CARE, INC., 1690 University Avenue W, Suite 370, Zip 55104–3729; tel. 651/232–5070

HEALTHEAST HOME CARE, INC., 1700 University Avenue, Zip 55104; tel. 651/232–2800; Catherine Barr, Vice President Home Health

HEALTHEAST MEDICAL RESEARCH INSTITUTE, 559 Capitol Boulevard, Zip 55103; tel. 651/232–2300

## MISSISSIPPI

**Columbus:** U. S. AIR FORCE CLINIC, 201 Independence, Suite 101, Zip 39701–5300; tel. 662/434–2297; Colonel Dave Armstrong, Commander

## MISSOURI

**Independence:** SURGI–CARE CENTER OF INDEPENDENCE, 2311 Redwood Avenue, Zip 64057; tel. 816/373–7995

**Whiteman AFB:** U. S. AIR FORCE CLINIC WHITEMAN, 331 Sijan Avenue, Zip 65305–5001; tel. 660/687–1194; Lieutenant Colonel David Wilmot, USAF, MSC, Administrator

## MONTANA

**Malmstrom AFB:** U. S. AIR FORCE CLINIC, Zip 59402–5300; tel. 406/731–3863; Colonel David L. Doty, Administrator

**Miles City:** VETERANS AFFAIRS MEDICAL CENTER, 210 South Winchester Avenue, Zip 59301–4742; tel. 406/232–3060

## NEBRASKA

**Grand Island:** GRAND ISLAND DIVISION, 2211 North Broadwell Avenue, Zip 68803–2196; tel. 308/382–3660; Gary N. Nugent, Chief Executive Officer

**North Platte:** GREAT PLAINS PHO, INC., P.O. Box 1167, Zip 69103; tel. 308/535–7496; Todd Hlavaty, M.D., Chairman

**Offutt AFB:** EHRLING BERGQUIST HOSPITAL, 2501 Capehart Road, Zip 68113–2160; tel. 402/294–7312; Colonel Howard Googins, Deputy Commander

## NEW HAMPSHIRE

**Portsmouth:** NAVAL MEDICAL CLINIC, Building H–1, Zip 03801; tel. 207/439–1000; Captain F. M. Richardson, Commanding Officer

## NEW JERSEY

**Atlantic City:** ATLANTICARE SURGERY CENTER, 1925 Pacific Avenue, Zip 08401; tel. 609/407–2200; William Aarons, M.D., President

**Egg Harbor City:** ATLANTICARE BEHAVIORAL HEALTH, 2511 Fire Road, Suite B10, Zip 08234; tel. 609/272–6392; Julia Drew, President and Chief Executive Officer

ATLANTICARE HEALTH SERVICES, 2500 English Creek Avenue, Building C., Zip 08234; tel. 609/272–6392; Donald Parker, President and Chief Executive Officer

**Fort Monmouth:** PATTERSON ARMY HEALTH CLINIC, Stephenson Avenue, Building 1075, Zip 07703–5504; tel. 908/532–1266; Colonel Don Speers, Commander

**Jersey City:** ST. FRANCIS HOSPITAL, 25 McWilliams Place, Zip 07302–1698; tel. 201/418–1000

**Millburn:** ATLANTIC HOME CARE AND HOSPICE, 33 Bleeker Street, Zip 07041; tel. 973/379–8400; Susan Quinn, Administrator

**Morristown:** ALLIANCE IMAGING CENTER, 65 Maple Street, Zip 07960; tel. 973/267–5700; Barbara Picorale, Administrator

**Succasunna:** DIALYSIS CENTER OF NORTHWEST NEW JERSEY, 170 Righter Road, Zip 07876; tel. 973/584–1117; Carol Cahill, Administrator

## NEW MEXICO

**Albuquerque:** ALBUQUERQUE IHS HEALTH CENTER, 801 Vassar Drive N.E., Zip 87106–2799; tel. 505/248–4000; Maria Rickert, Chief Executive Officer

**Cannon AFB:** U. S. AIR FORCE CLINIC, 208 West Casablanca Avenue, Zip 88103–5300; tel. 505/784–6318; Lieutenant Colonel Michelle Pufall, Administrator

**Holloman AFB:** U. S. AIR FORCE CLINIC, 280 First Street, Zip 88330–8273; tel. 505/572–5587

**Kirtland AFB:** U. S. AIR FORCE CLINIC–KIRTLAND, 2050 A Second Street S.E., Zip 87117–5559; tel. 505/846–3547; Colonel Regina Aune, Commander

## NEW YORK

**Bronx:** MORRISANIA DIAGNOSTIC AND TREATMENT CENTER, 1225 Gerard Avenue, Zip 10452; tel. 718/960–2777; Victor Hernandez, Administrator

SEGUNDO RUIZ BELVIS DIAGNOSTIC AND TREATMENT CENTER, 545 East 142nd Street, Zip 10454; tel. 718/579–4000; Victor Hernandez, Administrator

**Brooklyn:** CUMBERLAND DIAGNOSTIC AND TREATMENT CENTER, 100 North Portland Avenue, Zip 11205; tel. 718/260–7500; Candis Best, Administrator

DR. SUSAN SMITH NURSING REHABILITATION CENTER, 594 Albany Avenue, Zip 11203; tel. 718/245–7000; Peola Small, Chief Operating Officer

EAST NEW YORK DIAGNOSTIC AND TREATMENT CENTER, 2094 Pitkin Avenue, Zip 11207; tel. 718/240–0400; Yvette Isaac, Administrator

**Buffalo:** MERCY NURSING FACILITY, 565 Abbott Road, Zip 14220; tel. 716/828–2301; Christine Kluckhohn, President, Continuing Care

NAZARETH HOME, 291 West North Street, Zip 14201; tel. 716/881–2323; Christine Kluckhohn, President, Continuing Care

ST. CATHERINE LABOURE, 2157 Main Street, Zip 14214; tel. 716/862–1451; Christine Kluckhohn, President, Continuing Care

ST. FRANCIS OF BUFFALO, 34 Benwood Avenue, Zip 14214; tel. 716/862–2500; Christine Kluckhohn, President, Continuing Care

**Cheektowaga:** MCAULEY SETON HOME CARE, 2875 Union Road, Suite 14, Zip 14227; tel. 716/685–4870; Mark A. Sullivan, President and Senior Administrative Officer

MERCY HOME CARE, 2875 Union Road, Suite 14, Zip 14227; tel. 716/685–4870; Mark A. Sullivan, President and Senior Administrative Officer

**Dunkirk:** ST. VINCENT'S HOME, 319 Washington Avenue, Zip 14048; tel. 716/366–2066; J. Thomas Briody, Senior Vice President Long Term Care and Ambulatory Services

**Fort Drum:** U. S. ARMY MEDICAL DEPARTMENT ACTIVITY, 11050 Mount Belvedere Boulevard, Zip 13602–5004; tel. 315/772–4024; Colonel Mark W. Thompson, MC, Commander

**Kenmore:** MCAULEY RESIDENCE, 1503 Military Road, Zip 14217; tel. 716/447–6600; Christine Kluckhohn, President, Continuing Care

**Lancaster:** ST. ELIZABETH'S HOME, 5539 Broadway, Zip 14086; tel. 716/683–5150; Christine Kluckhohn, President, Continuing Care

**New York:** GOUVERNEUR HOSPITAL, 227 Madison Street, Zip 10002; tel. 212/238–7000; Gregory M. Kaladjian, Executive Director

RENAISSANCE DIAGNOSTIC AND TREATMENT CENTER, 215 West 125 Street, Zip 10027; tel. 212/932–6500; Rose Garcia, Administrator

**Olean:** ST. JOSEPH MANOR, 2211 West State Street, Zip 14760; tel. 716/372–7810; Christine Kluckhohn, President, Continuing Care

**Orchard Park:** FATHER BAKER MANOR, 6400 Powers Road, Zip 14127; tel. 716/667–0001; Christine Kluckhohn, President, Continuing Care

**Staten Island:** SEA VIEW HOSPITAL REHABILITATION CENTER AND HOME, 460 Brielle Avenue, Zip 10314; tel. 212/390–8181; Jane M. Lyons, Executive Director

**Tuckahoe:** HOME NURSING ASSOCIATION OF WESTCHESTER, 69 Main Street, Zip 10707; tel. 919/961–2818; Mary Wehrberger, Director

**Williamsville:** ST. FRANCIS OF WILLIAMSVILLE, 147 Reist Street, Zip 14221; tel. 716/633–5400; Christine Kluckhohn, President, Continuing Care

## NORTH CAROLINA

**Cherry Point:** NAVAL HOSPITAL, PSC Box 8023, Zip 28533–0023; tel. 252/466–0266; Captain John Burgess, Commanding Officer

**Jefferson:** AMH SEGRAVES CARE CENTER, 200 Hospital Avenue, Zip 28640; tel. 336/246–7101; R. D. Williams, Administrator and Chief Executive Officer

**Seymour Johnson AFB:** U. S. AIR FORCE HOSPITAL SEYMOUR JOHNSON, 1050 Curtis Avenue, Zip 27531–5300; tel. 919/722–1812; Colonel Donna M. Lake, Commanding Officer

**Southern Pines:** ST. JOSEPH OF THE PINES HOSPITAL, 590 Central Drive, Zip 28387; tel. 910/246–1000; Ken Cormier, President and Chief Executive Officer

**Wilson:** WILMED NURSING CARE CENTER, 1705 Tarboro Street S.W., Zip 27893–3428; tel. 252/399–8998; Gene Fulcher, Administrator

## NORTH DAKOTA

**Grand Forks AFB:** U. S. AIR FORCE HOSPITAL, 220 G Street, Zip 58205–6332; tel. 701/747–5391

**Minot:** U. S. AIR FORCE REGIONAL HOSPITAL, 10 Missile Avenue, Zip 58705–5024; tel. 701/723–5103; Colonel Lawrence Riddles, Commander

## OHIO

**Cleveland:** KAISER PERMANENTE, 1001 Lakeside, Zip 44114; tel. 216/362–2000; Patricia Kennedy–Scott, President

METROHEALTH CENTER FOR SKILLED NURSING CARE, 4229 Pearl Road, Zip 44109; tel. 216/957–3675; Yvette Bozman, Administrator

**Columbus:** OHIOHEALTH GROUP, 445 Hutchinson Avenue, Suite 300, Zip 43235–5677; tel. 614/566–0123; John Burns, Chief Executive Officer

VETERANS AFFAIRS OUTPATIENT CLINIC, 420 North James Road, Zip 43219–1834; tel. 614/257–5200; Lillian Thone, Chief Executive Officer

**Worthington:** HOMEREACH, 404 East Wilson Bridge Road, Suite H., Zip 43085; tel. 614/566–0888; Fran Baby, Vice President Home and Hospice Services

## OKLAHOMA

**Altus:** U. S. AIR FORCE CLINIC ALTUS, 301 North First Street, Zip 73523–5005; tel. 580/481–5204; Colonel Charles W. Cotta, USAF, Commander

**Clinton:** U. S. PUBLIC HEALTH SERVICE INDIAN HOSPITAL, Route 1, Box 3060, Zip 73601–9303; tel. 580/323–2884; Terri Schmidt, Director

**Enid:** U. S. AIR FORCE CLINIC, Vance AFB, Building 810, Zip 73705–5000; tel. 405/249–7494; Lieutenant Colonel Andrew F. Love, MSC, USAF, Commander Medical Group

**Eufaula:** EUFALA INDIAN HEALTH CENTER, 800 Forest Avenue, Zip 74432; tel. 918/689–2547; Shelly Crow, Health System Administrator

**Okmulgee:** OKMULGEE INDIAN HEALTH SYSTEM, 1313 East 20th, Zip 74447; tel. 918/758–1926; Steve Landsberry, Administrator

**Sapulpa:** SAPULPA INDIAN HEALTH CENTER, 1125 East Clevelend, Zip 74066; tel. 918/224–9310; Judy Aaron, Health System Administrator

**Tinker AFB:** U. S. AIR FORCE HOSPITAL TINKER, 5700 Arnold Street, Zip 73145; tel. 405/736–2084; Colonel Lloyd A. Reinke, Commander

**Tulsa:** WARREN CLINIC, 6600 South Yale Avenue, Zip 74136; tel. 918/502–7300; James Kaltenbachner, Senior Vice President

## OREGON

**White City:** VETERANS AFFAIRS DOMICILIARY, Zip 97503; tel. 503/826–2111; Frank Drake, Director

## PENNSYLVANIA

**Chester:** COMMUNITY HOSPITAL, DIVISION OF THE CROZER–CHESTER MEDICAL CENTER, Ninth and Wilson Streets, Zip 19013–2098; tel. 610/494–0700; Kevin Caputo, M.D., Vice President Operations

**Dallastown:** WELLSPAN MEDICAL GROUP, 757 South Pleasant Avenue, Zip 17313; tel. 717/851–6515

**Warminster:** ABINGTON MEMORIAL HEALTH CENTER – WARMINSTER CAMPUS, 225 Newtown Road, Zip 18974–5221; tel. 215/441–6600; Katie Farrell, Chief Executive Officer

**York:** SOUTH CENTRAL PREFERRED, 45 Monument Road, Suite 200, Zip 17403; tel. 717/741–9511; Charles H. Chodroff, M.D., Executive Director

WELLSPAN HEALTH CARE SERVICES, 1001 South George Street, Zip 17405; tel. 717/851–2121; Bruce M. Bartels, President

## RHODE ISLAND

**Newport:** NAVAL HOSPITAL, 1 Riggs Road, Zip 02841–1002; tel. 401/841–3771; Captain Andre Greedan, Deputy Commander

## SOUTH CAROLINA

**Shaw AFB:** U. S. AIR FORCE HOSPITAL SHAW, 431 Meadowlark Street, Zip 29152–5019; tel. 803/895–6324; Colonel Troy Molnar, Commander

## SOUTH DAKOTA

**Ellsworth AFB:** U. S. AIR FORCE CLINIC, 2900 Doolittle Drive, Zip 57706–4821; tel. 605/385–3201; Colonel Chris Gray, Commanding Officer

## TEXAS

**Abilene:** U. S. AIR FORCE CLINIC, 697 Hospital Road, Zip 79607–1367; tel. 915/696–5429; Major John G. Wiseman, Administrator

**Corpus Christi:** CORPUS CHRISTI MEDICAL CENTER – NORTHWEST, 13725 Northwest Boulevard, Zip 78410–5199; tel. 361/767–4400; Jay Woodall, Chief Executive Officer

NAVAL HOSPITAL, 10651 E Street, Zip 78419–5131; tel. 361/961–2688; Captain James P. Rice, Commanding Officer

**Dallas:** SURGICARE OF TRAVIS CENTER, INC., 13355 Noel Road, Suite 650, Zip 75240–6694; tel. 713/520–1782

**El Paso:** VETERANS AFFAIRS HEALTHCARE CENTER, 5001 North Piedras Street, Zip 79930–4211; tel. 915/564–6100; Edward Valenzuela, Director

**Houston:** GRAMERCY OUTPATIENT SURGERY CENTER. LTD., 2727 Gramercy, Zip 77025; tel. 713/660–6900; Hamel Patel, Administrator

WEST HOUSTON SURGICARE, 970 Campbell Road, Zip 77024; tel. 713/461–3547

**Laughlin AFB:** U. S. AIR FORCE HOSPITAL, 590 Mitchell Boulevard, Zip 78843–5200; tel. 210/298–6311

**San Antonio:** U. S. AIR FORCE CLINIC BROOKS, Building 615, Zip 78235–5300; tel. 210/536–2087; Lieutenant Colonel Donald Sampson, Commanding Officer

WILFORD HALL AMBULATORY SURGICAL CENTER, 2200 Bergquist Drive, Suite 1, Zip 78236–9908; tel. 210/292–7412; Brigadier General Thomas Travis, Commanding Officer

**Sheppard AFB:** U. S. AIR FORCE REGIONAL HOSPITAL–SHEPPARD, 149 Hart Street, Suite 1, Zip 76311–3478; tel. 940/676–5874; Lieutenant Colonel Lance Rogers, Administrator

**Universal City:** U. S. AIR FORCE CLINIC RANDOLPH, 221 3rd Street West, Zip 78150–4801; tel. 210/652–5701; Lieutenant Colonel Dennis E. Franks, Administrator

**Webster:** BAY AREA SURGICARE CENTER, 502 Medical Center Boulevard, Zip 77598; tel. 281/332–2433; Carol Simons, Administrator

## VIRGINIA

**Fort Eustis:** MCDONALD ARMY HEALTH CENTER, Jefferson Avenue, Zip 23604–5548; tel. 757/314–7501; Colonel Cass Scott, Administrator

**Fort Lee:** KENNER ARMY HEALTH CENTER, 700 24th Street, Zip 23801–1716; tel. 804/734–9256; Colonel Vivian T. Hutson, Commander

**Quantico:** NAVAL REGIONAL MEDICAL CLINIC, 3259 Catlin Avenue, Zip 22134; tel. 703/784–1699; Captain Mary E. Neill, USN, Commanding Officer

## WASHINGTON

**Fairchild AFB:** U. S. AIR FORCE CLINIC, 701 Hospital Loop, Suite 102, Zip 99011–8701; tel. 509/247–5217; Colonel Barbara Jefts, Commanding Officer

## WISCONSIN

**Green Bay:** UNITY HOSPICE, P.O. Box 28345, Zip 54324–8345; tel. 920/494–0225; Donald Seibel, Executive Director

## WYOMING

**Cheyenne:** U. S. AIR FORCE HOSPITAL, 6900 Alden Drive, Zip 82005–3913; tel. 307/773–2045; Major Brenda Bullard, Administrator

# Provisional Hospitals

*This listing includes organizations that, as of June 1, 2011, were in the planning or construction stage and that, on completion, will be eligible for Institutional membership. Some hospitals are granted provisional membership for reasons related to other Association requirements. Hospitals classified as provisional members for reasons other than being under construction are indicated by a bullet ( ● ).*

## ALABAMA

**Butler:** CHOCTAW GENERAL HOSPITAL, 401 Vanity Fair Avenue, Zip 36904; tel. 205/459–9100; J. W. Cowan, Administrator

## CALIFORNIA

**Ontario:** ONTARIO MEDICAL CENTER, 2295 South Vineyard Avenue, Zip 91761–7925; tel. 909/724–5000; Yvonne Roddy–Sturm, R.N., Chief Nurse Executive

## NEW MEXICO

**Rio Rancho:** PRESBYTERIAN RUST MEDICAL CENTER, 2400 Unser Boulevard S.E., Zip 87124–3392; tel. 505/253–7878; Jeff McBee, Administrator

## SOUTH DAKOTA

**Aberdeen:** SANFORD MEDICAL CENTER ABERDEEN, 3015 3rd Avenue S.E., Zip 57401–5418; tel. 605/725–1700; Gordon Larson, Chief Executive Officer

## TEXAS

**College Station:** SCOTT & WHITE HOSPITAL – COLLEGE STATION, 700 Scott & White Drive, Zip 77845; tel. 800/299–1212; Jason Jennings, Chief Executive Officer

## WISCONSIN

**Janesville:** ST. MARY'S JANESVILLE HOSPITAL, 3400 East Racine Steeet, Zip 53546; tel. 608/373–8000; Kerry Swanson, President

# Associate Members

## Ambulatory Centers and Home Care Agencies

### United States

#### FLORIDA

NEMOURS CHILDREN'S CLINIC, 807 Children's Way, Jacksonville, Zip 32207; tel. 904/390–3600; William A. Cover, Administrator

#### NEW HAMPSHIRE

DARTMOUTH COLLEGE HEALTH SERVICE, 7 Rope Ferry Road, Hanover, Zip 03755–1421; tel. 603/650–1400; John H. Turco, M.D., Director

#### PENNSYLVANIA

WILLS EYE HOSPITAL, 840 Walnut Street, Philadelphia, Zip 19107–5109; tel. 215/928–3000; Joseph P. Bilson, Executive Director

## Blue Cross Plans

### United States

#### ARIZONA

BLUE CROSS AND BLUE SHIELD OF ARIZONA, Box 13466, Phoenix, Zip 85002–3466; tel. 602/864–4541; Vishu Jhaveri, M.D., Senior Vice President and Chief Medical Officer

#### PENNSYLVANIA

HIGHMARK BLUE CROSS BLUE SHIELD, 120 Fifth Avenue Place, Suite 3014, Pittsburgh, Zip 15222; tel. 412/544–7646; Sandra R. Tomlinson, Senior Vice President, Provider Services

*The members listed in **bold** are Associate Advantage members.* © 2012 AHA Guide

# Other Members

## UNITED STATES

### Alliance:

PREMIER, INC., 13034 Ballantyne Corporate Place, Charlotte, North Carolina Zip 28277–1498; tel. 704/816–5353; Susan DeVore, President and Chief Executive Officer; www.premierinc.com

THE NEW JERSEY COUNCIL OF TEACHING HOSPITALS, 154 West State Street, Trenton, New Jersey Zip 08608; tel. 609/656–9600; J. Richard Goldstein, MD, President; www.njcth.org

UNIVERSITY HEALTHSYSTEM CONSORTIUM, INC., 155 North Wacker Drive, Chicago, Illinois Zip 60606–1787; tel. 630/954–1700; Irene M. Thompson, President and Chief Executive Officer; www.uhc.edu

VHA, INC., PO Box 140909, Irving, Texas Zip 75014–0909; tel. 972/830–0253; Curtis W. Nonomaque, President and Chief Executive Officer; www.vha.com

### Architecture:

BURT HILL, 400 Morgan Center, 101 East Diamond Street, Butler, Pennsylvania Zip 16001–5977; tel. 724/285–4761; John E. Brock, Vice President; www.burthill.com

DEVENNEY GROUP ARCHITECTS, 201 West Indian School Road, Phoenix, Arizona Zip 85013–3203; tel. 602/943–8950; Julie Barkenbush, Chief Executive Officer; www.devenneygroup.com

EARL SWENSSON ASSOCIATES, INC., 2100 West End Avenue, Suite 1200, Nashville, Tennessee Zip 37203; tel. 615/329–9445; Richard L. Miller, President; www.esarch.com

HDR ARCHITECTURE, INC., 8404 Indian Hills Drive, Omaha, Nebraska Zip 68114; tel. 402/399–1000; Doug Wignall, Executive Vice President; www.hdrinc.com

MATTHEI AND COLIN ASSOCIATES, 332 South Michigan Avenue, Suite 614, Chicago, Illinois Zip 60604; tel. 312/939–4002; Ronald G. Kobold, Managing Partner

MESSER CONSTRUCTION COMPANY, 5158 Fishwick Drive, Cincinnati, Ohio Zip 45216; tel. 513/242–1541; Tiffany Witham, Director Marketing; www.messer.com

MMC CONTRACTORS, 4717 F. Street, Omaha, Nebraska Zip 68117–1404; tel. 402/861–0681; Patrick Ryan, Senior Project Manager; www.mmcontractors.com

PERKINS & WILL, INC., 617 West Seventh Street, Suite 1200, Los Angeles, California Zip 90017–3830; tel. 312/755–0770; Timothy Pettigrew, Associate, Healthcare Knowledge Coordinator; www.perkinswill.com

RLF, 4750 New Broad Street, Orlando, Florida Zip 32814–6422; tel. 407/647–1039; Vincent Della Donna, Senior Healthcare Architect; www.rlfae.com

SMITHGROUP, INC., 301 Battery Street, San Francisco, California Zip 94104–4250; tel. 415/227–0100; James T. Hannon, Senior Vice President; www.sf.smithgroup.com

### Bank:

**BANK OF AMERICA, 101 South Tryon Street, Charlotte, North Carolina Zip 28255–0001; tel. 704/388–2255; Gayle Higaki, Senior Vice President; www.bankofamerica.com**

WELLS FARGO SECURITIES, 230 West Monroe Street, Chicago, Illinois Zip 60606–4703; tel. 312/845–9779; Philip J. Kaplan, Vice President; www.wellsfargo.com

### Communication Systems Org:

**AT & T, 1010 Wilshire Boulevard, Room 1240, Los Angeles, California Zip 90017; tel. 805/648–2463; Deborah Sunday, Director Product Marketing Management**

---

AVAILITY, LLC, 740 East Campbell Road, Suite 1000, Richardson, Texas Zip 75081–1886; tel. 904/470–4984; Andrea Overman, Director, Marketing; www.availity.com

BECKER'S HOSPITAL REVIEW, 315 Vernon Avenue, Glencoe, Illinois Zip 60022–2136; tel. 800/417–2035; Scott Becker, Publisher; www.beckersasc.com

**COOPER SIGNAGE & GRAPHICS, INC., 2405 Lance Court, Loganville, Georgia Zip 30052–4613; tel. 800/297–2324; Randy R. Cooper, President; www.sinsystems.org**

### Construction Firm:

KBR BUILDING GROUP, 10 Cadillac Drive, Suite 460, Brentwood, Tennessee Zip 37027–5096; tel. 615/742–6610; Michael Pierle, Executive Vice President

### Consulting Firm:

**ACUSTAF SOFTWARE, 7601 France Avenue, Suite 575, Edina, Minnesota Zip 55435–5968; tel. 952/831–4122; Terry Suby, President; www.acustafsoftware.com**

ARAMARK, 1101 Market Street, Philadelphia, Pennsylvania Zip 19107–2988; tel. 215/238–4054; Anthony C. Stanowski, Vice President Industrial Relations; www.aramark.com

ATHENA HEALTH, 1500 Urban Center Drive, Suite 500, Birmingham, Alabama Zip 35242–2566; tel. 205/970–3330; Jerry C. Smith, Vice President Finance; www.athenahealth.com

**BMGI, 1200 17th Street, Suite 180, Denver, Colorado Zip 80202–5815; tel. 303/827–0010; Scott McAllister, Senior Performance Excellence Consultant; www.bmgi.com/default.aspx**

**BOXWOOD TECHNOLOGY, INC, 11350 McCormick Road, Suite 101, Hunt Valley, Maryland Zip 21031; tel. 888/491–8833; John Bell, Chairman; www.boxwoodtech.com**

**BURWOOD GROUP, INC., 125 South Wacker Drive, Suite 2950, Chicago, Illinois Zip 60602; tel. 312/327–4600; Mark Theoharous, President; www.burwood.com**

**CARE TECH SOLUTIONS, 901 Wilshire Drive, Suite 100, Troy, Michigan Zip 48084; tel. 248/823–9000; Colleen Hanley, Vice President, Marketing, Communications and Government Affairs; www.caretech.com**

CAREMEDIC, 800 Carillon Parkway, Suite 250, Saint Petersburg, Florida Zip 33716; tel. 727/329–7838; Richard Nelli, Vice President Product and Solution Management; www.caremedic.com

CATALYST LEARNING COMPANY, 310 West Liberty Street, Suite 403, Louisville, Kentucky Zip 40202–3015; tel. 502/584–7337; M. Lynn Fischer, Founder and Chief Executive Officer; www.catalystlearning.com

COMPASS GROUP, INC., 2181 Victory Parkway, Cincinnati, Ohio Zip 45206; tel. 513/241–0142; Cary Gutbezahl, President; www.compassgroupinc.com

COMPASS LEXECON, 332 South Michigan Avenue, Suite 1300, Chicago, Illinois Zip 60604; tel. 312/322–0200; Ben Brighoff, Senior Analyst; www.lexecon.com

CONIFER HEALTH SOLUTIONS, 2401 Internet Boulevard, Suite 201, Frisco, Texas Zip 75034–5977; tel. 972/335–6120; Vanessa Harris, Senior Market Research Specialist; www.coniferhealth.com

**COPYRIGHT CLEARANCE CENTER, 222 Rosewood Drive, Danvers, Massachusetts Zip 01923–4520; tel. 978/646–2633; Stephanie Fox, Alliances Director; www.copyright.com**

**DEVELOPMENT DIMENSIONS INTERNATIONAL, 1225 Washington Pike, Bridgeville, Pennsylvania Zip 15017–2838; tel. 412/257–3623; Colby Fazio, Marketing Consultant; www.ddiworld.com**

**DIXON HUGHES GOODMAN, 102 First Street, Suite 201, Hudson, Ohio Zip 44236–5386; tel. 330/650–1752; Jim Yanci, Principal; www.dhgllp.com**

---

DRAEGER, 3135 Quarry Road, Telford, Pennsylvania Zip 18969–1042; tel. 215/660–2310; Susan Thornton, Senior Marketing Manager, Information Technology Solutions; www.draeger.com

ECLIPSYS, 76 Batterson Park Road, Farmington, Connecticut Zip 06032; tel. 860/246–3000; Marvin S. Goldwasser, Vice President Product Marketing, Patient Flow and Performance Management; www.eclipsys.com

ELSEVIER, INC., 3251 Riverport Lane, Maryland Heights, Missouri Zip 63043–4816; tel. 314/447–8000; Christian Rockwell, Director; www.clinicaldecisionsupport.com

EMDAT, 6180 Verona Road, Suite 200, Fitchburg, Wisconsin Zip 53719–1945; tel. 608/270–6400; Laura Lowe, Director Field Marketing; www.emdat.com

ERDMAN, P.O. Box 44975, Madison, Wisconsin Zip 53744–4975; tel. 608/410–8000; Molly Hamm, Research Librarian; www.erdman.com

ERNST & YOUNG, 41 South High Street, Columbus, Ohio Zip 43215–6101; tel. 949/437–0220; Jonathan G. Weaver, Partner

**ERNST & YOUNG, 5 Times Square, 14th Floor, New York, New York Zip 10036–6530; tel. 212/773–3000; Frank Bresz, Senior Manager; www.ey.com/global/content.nsf/us/home**

**EXECUTIVE HEALTH RESOURCES, INC., 15 Campus Boulevard, Suite 200, Newtown Square, Pennsylvania Zip 19073; tel. 610/446–6100; Robert Corrato, President and Chief Executive Officer; www.ehrdocs.com**

FIDELITY INVESTMENTS, 100 Magellan Way, Mail Zone KW23, Covington, Kentucky Zip 41015–1987; tel. 859/386–3117; John Campbell, Manager; www.fmr.com

GENERAL PHYSICS CORPORATION, 300 East Big Beaver Road, Suite 300, Troy, Michigan Zip 48083–1265; tel. 248/526–5500; Sue Martin, Vice President Marketing; www.wwwgpworldwide.com

**GETWELLNETWORK, INC., 7920 Norfolk Avenue, 11th Floor, Bethesda, Maryland Zip 20814–2500; tel. 240/482–3200; Michael B. O'Neil, Jr., President and Chief Executive Officer; www.getwellnetwork.com**

**GLOBAL HEALTHCARE EXCHANGE, LLC, 1315 West Century Drive, Louisville, Colorado Zip 80027–9560; tel. 720/887–7000; Karen Conway, Director Industry Programs; www.ghx.com**

GOLDMAN, SACHS AND COMPANY, 200 West Street, New York, New York Zip 10282–2198; Calla Frett, Director

GREAT AMERICAN INSURANCE GROUP, 301 East 4th Street, 21st Floor North, Cincinnati, Ohio Zip 45202–4201; tel. 513/763–6165; Merita Sohn, Marketing Manager; www.greatamericaninsurance.com

**H. R. S. INTERNATIONAL, 25 East Washington, 6th Floor, Chicago, Illinois Zip 60602; tel. 312/236–7770; Carrie Parks, Marketing Specialist; www.hrsolutions.com**

HEALTHPORT, 925 North Point Parkway, Alpharetta, Georgia Zip 30005–5210; tel. 770/360–1700; Catherine Valyi, Director Marketing; www.healthport.com

INTEGRATED HEALTHCARE STRATEGIES, tel. 612/339–0919; Julie McCauley, Senior Vice President, Corporate; www.ihstrategies.com

**INTERWOVEN, 160 East Tasman Drive, San Jose, California Zip 95134; tel. 408/774–2000; Joe Cowan, Chief Executive Officer and Director; www.interwoven.com**

IPROTEAN, LLC, 12255 El Camino Real, Suite 300, San Diego, California Zip 92130–4087; tel. 800/771–9490; Gordon R. Clark, President and Chief Executive Officer; www.iprotean.com

J. A. THOMAS & ASSOCIATES, 3715 Northside Parkway, 100 Northcreek, Suite 200, Atlanta, Georgia Zip 30327; tel. 770/438–8537; Melissa Dickinson, Coordinator Marketing; www.jathomas.com

---

**KAUFMAN HALL, 5202 Old Orchard Road, Suite N700, Skokie, Illinois Zip 60077; tel. 847/441–8780; Jason H. Sussman, Partner; www.kaufmanhall.com**

**KROLL ONTRACK, INC., 18350 Mount Langley Street, Suite 110, Fountain Valley, California Zip 92708; tel. 800/872–2599; Stacey May, Manager; www.krollontrack.com**

KURT SALMON ASSOCIATES, 1355 Peachtree Street N.E., Suite 900, Atlanta, Georgia Zip 30309–0900; tel. 404/892–0321; Wendi B. Farris, Administrative Assistant; www.kurtsalmon.com

KYRUUS, INC., 121 High Street, 4th Floor, Boston, Massachusetts Zip 02210; tel. 617/419–2060; David Hood, Marketing Director; www.kyruus.com

LATHAM AND WATKINS, LLP, 633 West 5th Street, Suite 4000, Los Angeles, California Zip 90071; tel. 213/485–1234; Daniel K. Settelmayer, Partner; www.lw.com

**LEXISNEXIS, 1000 Alderman Drive, Alpharetta, Georgia Zip 30005; tel. 404/577–1779; Sarah J. Stansberry, Senior Director, Marketing; www.lexisnexis.com**

**LIVEPROCESS, 271 Grove Avenue, Building D., Verona, New Jersey Zip 07044; tel. 973/571–2500; Nathaniel Weiss, Chief Executive Officer; www.liveprocess.com**

**MARITZ, INC., 1375 North Highway Drive, Fenton, Missouri Zip 63099; tel. 636/827–4000; Amy Kramer, Healthcare Section Strategist; www.maritz.com**

MCDONALD HOPKINS, LLC, 600 Superior Avenue East, Suite 2100, Cleveland, Ohio Zip 44114–2690; tel. 216/348–5400; Richard S. Cooper, Member; www.mcdonaldhopkins.com

MCKESSON PROVIDER TECHNOLOGIES, 5995 Windward Parkway, Alpharetta, Georgia Zip 30005; tel. 404/338–3519; Jocelyn B. Green, Legal Assistant

NES ASSOCIATES, LLC, 6363 Walker Lane, Suite 130, Alexandria, Virginia Zip 22310–3261; tel. 703/224–2607; Mark Rose, Director Healthcare Programs; www.nesassociates.com

**NVOQ, 1715 38th Street, Boulder, Colorado Zip 80301–2603; tel. 720/562–4500; Charles Corfield, Chief Executive Officer; www.mvoq.com**

O.C. TANNER COMPANY, 1930 South State Street, Salt Lake City, Utah Zip 84115–2311; tel. 801/493–3310; Cordell Clinger, Manager Exhibits; www.octanner.com

**OBJECTIVE HEALTH, A MCKINSEY SOLUTION FOR HEALTHCARE PROVIDERS, 404 Wyman Street, Suite 300, Waltham, Massachusetts Zip 02451–1241; tel. 781/522–3264; Kimberly Peters, Coordinator Marketing; www.objectivehealth.com**

**PACKETMOTION, INC., 260 Santa Ana Court, Sunnyvale, California Zip 94085–4512; tel. 408/449–4300; Ravi Khatod, Senior Vice President, Sales and Business Development; www.packetmotion.com**

**PEER CONSULTING, 2856 80Th Avenue S.E., Suite 200, Mercer Island, Washington Zip 98040–2984; tel. 206/236–1300; Linus Diedling, Executive Advisory Services Leader; www.peerconsulting.net**

PHYSICIAN WELLNESS SERVICES, 5000 West 36th Street, Suite 360, Minneapolis, Minnesota Zip 55416; tel. 877/731–3949; Lori Brostrom, Director, Marketing; www.physicianwellnessservices.com

PIVOTHEALTH, LLC, 5200 Maryland Way, Suite 300, Brentwood, Tennessee Zip 37027; tel. 615/983–4000; Howard D. Jewell, Executive Vice President; www.pivothealth.com

**POLICY TECHNOLOGIES INTERNATIONAL, INC., 346 Grand Loop, Rexburg, Idaho Zip 83440; tel. 208/359–8123; Josh Perry, Director Marketing; www.policytech.com**

**PREMIERE GLOBAL SERVICES, 3280 Peachtree Road N.W., Suite 1000, Atlanta, Georgia Zip 30305–2422; tel. 404/543–9449; Mark H. Horne, Vice President Marketing, Notifications and Reminders; www.premiereglobal.com**

**PRESS GANEY ASSOCIATES, INC., 404 Columbia Place, South Bend, Indiana Zip 46601–2315; tel. 800/232–8032; Gwendalyn Hadley, Marketing Manager; www.pressganey.com**

PROFESSIONAL RESEARCH CONSULTANTS, INC., 11326 P. Street, Omaha, Nebraska Zip 68137–2316; tel. 800/428–7455; Janna Binder, Director Marketing and Public Relations; www.prconline.com

QUAMMEN HEALTH CARE CONSULTANTS, 522B Brandies Circle, Suite 4, Murfreesboro, Tennessee Zip 37128–4873; tel. 407/539–2015; Robecca Quammen, President; www.quammengroup.com

**QUEST SOFTWARE, 6500 Emerald Parkway, Suite 400, Dublin, Ohio Zip 43016–6234; tel. 949/754–8000; Connie West, Director Marketing; www.quest.com**

RYCAN, P.O. Box 306, Marshall, Minnesota Zip 56258–0306; tel. 800/201–3324; Marg Louwagie, Administrative Assistant; www.rycan.com

**SAMUELI INSTITUTE, 1737 King Street, Suite 600, Alexandria, Virginia Zip 22314–2764; tel. 703/299–4800; Bonnie R. Sakallaris, Vice President Optimal Healing Environments; www.siib.org**

SCHNEIDER ELECTRIC, 1415 South Roselle Road, Palatine, Illinois Zip 60067-7337; Mailing Address 903 East 130th Drive, Thornton, Colorado Zip 80241–1104; tel. 303/475–6632; Hugh K. Denning, National Account Manager–Healthcare; www.schneider–electric.com

SHERIDAN HEALTHCARE, INC., 1613 North Harrison Parkway, Suite 200, Sunrise, Florida Zip 33323–2853; tel. 954/838–2749; Terri Burgess, Director Operations, Business Development; www.sheridanhealthcare.com

**SIEMENS HEALTHCARE, 51 Valley Stream Parkway, Malvern, Pennsylvania Zip 19355; tel. 610/448–4500; Barbara Sivek, Senior Director Industry Relations; www.medical.siemens.com**

SIPS CONSULTS, 550 North Main Street, Suite 207, Duncanville, Texas Zip 75116–3660; tel. 972/572–1988; Donnie Payne, Business Manager; www.sipsconsults.com

SODEXO HEALTH CARE, 86 Hopmeadow Street, Simsbury, Connecticut Zip 06089; tel. 860/325–1220; Shirley Palmieri, Director Creative Services; www.sodexo.com

SOYRING CONSULTING, 880 21st Avenue North, Saint Petersburg, Florida Zip 33704; tel. 727/822–8774; Adam Higman, Consultant; www.soyringconsulting.com

SPECIALTYCARE, 3100 West End Avenue, Suite 800, Nashville, Tennessee Zip 37203; tel. 615/345–5400; Nancy R. Becker, Director Corporate Services and Product Development; www.specialtycare.net

**STOCKAMP AND ASSOCIATES, INC., 6000 S.W. Meadows Road, Suite 300, Lake Oswego, Oregon Zip 97035; tel. 503/303–1200; Karen Andrews, Senior Marketing Manager; www.stockamp.com**

STRATFORD FIDELITY, 901 Marquette Avenue, Suite 2200, Minneapolis, Minnesota Zip 55402–3721; tel. 877/815–6366; Gary D. Aden, Senior Vice President; www.stratfordfidelity.com

STROUDWATER ASSOCIATES, 50 Sewall Street, Suite 102, Portland, Maine Zip 04102–2646; tel. 207/221–8255; Marc Voyvodich, Chief Executive Officer

SULLIVAN, COTTER AND ASSOCIATES, INC., 3011 West Grand Boulevard, Suite 2800, Detroit, Michigan Zip 48202–3096; tel. 313/872–1760; Michael Stewart, Managing Director; www.sullivancotter.com

SURGICAL CARE AFFILIATES, P.O. Box 382491, Birmingham, Alabama Zip 35238–2491; tel. 205/545–2759; Joe T. Clark, Executive Vice President; www.scasurgery.com

**SURGICAL INFORMATION SYSTEMS, 11605 Haynes Bridge Road, Alpharetta, Georgia Zip 30004; tel. 678/507–1706; Kelly R. Pinkerton, Manager Marketing; www.sisfirst.com**

**SYSCOM SERVICES, INC, 1010 Wayne Avenue, Suite 320, Silver Spring, Maryland Zip 20910; tel. 301/768–0118; Lee Weinstein, President; www.syscomservices.com**

**TESTSOURCE, 4344 Plainfield Avenue N.E., Grand Rapids, Michigan Zip 49525; tel. 800/691–3737; Mark Wiersma, President; www.testsource.com**

THE HSM GROUP, LTD, 8777 East Via de Ventura #188, Scottsdale, Arizona Zip 85258; tel. 480/947–8078; Sheryl Bronkesh, President; www.hsmgroup.com

THE JACKSON GROUP, INC., 219 1st Avenue S.W., Hickory, North Carolina Zip 28602–2922; tel. 828/328–8968; Alan Jackson, President; www.thejacksongroup.com

TIAA CREF, 8500 Andrew Carnegie Boulevard, B208, Charlotte, North Carolina Zip 28262–8500; tel. 704/988–8064; Kevin S. Nazworth, Vice President Healthcare Market; www.tiaa–cref.org

TRUVEN HEALTH ANALYTICS, 6200 South Syracuse Way, Suite 300, Greenwood Village, Colorado Zip 80111; tel. 303/486–6400; Julie Weigel, Vice President; www.thomsonreuters.com

**VECNA, 6404 Ivy Lane, Suite 500, Greenbelt, Maryland Zip 20770; tel. 240/965–4500; Daniel Theobold, President**

VENDOR CREDENTIALING SERVICE, INC., 616 Cypress Creek Parkway, Suite 800, Houston, Texas Zip 77090–3029; tel. 281/863–9500; Troy Kyle, President and Chief Executive Officer; www.vcsdatabase.com

**VERITY, INC, 5758 West Las Positas Boulevard, Suite 100, Pleasanton, California Zip 94588; tel. 925/598–3003; Michael Pliner, President; www.verity.com**

**WASTE MANAGEMENT, 1001 Fannin St. Suite 4000, Houston, Texas Zip 77002–6711; tel. 713/265–1352; Bill Turpin, Director Strategic Development**

WESTERN HEALTHCARE ALLIANCE, tel. 970/683–5223; Carolyn S. Bruce, Chief Executive Officer; www.wha1.org

XANITOS, 3809 West Chester Pike, Suite 210, Newtown Square, Pennsylvania Zip 19073–2304; tel. 484/654–2300; Graeme A. Crothall, Chairman and Chief Executive Officer; www.xanitos.com

ZIX CORPORATION, 2711 North Haskell Avenue, Suite 2200, Dallas, Texas Zip 75204–2961; tel. 214/370–2241; Geoffrey R. Bibby, Vice President, Corporate Marketing; www.zixcorp.com

### Educational Services:

NATIONAL RURAL HEALTH RESOURCE CENTER, 600 East Superior Street, Suite 404, Duluth, Minnesota Zip 55802; tel. 218/727–9390; Terry J. Hill, Executive Director; www.ruralcenter.org

THE APPRENTICE CORPORATION, PO BOX 693, Buffalo, New York Zip 14207–0693; tel. 716/877–1000; Anton Scheepers, Consultant; www.theapprenticedoctor.com

### Food Service Management:

PRINCE FOOD SYSTEMS, INC., 11001 South Wilcrest Drive, Suite 200, Houston, Texas Zip 77099–4329; tel. 281/568–3131; Steve Caudle, Chief Operating Officer; www.princefoodsystems.com

### Fund Raising:

**IMAGINE NATION BOOKS, 282 Century Place, Suite 2000, Louisville, Colorado Zip 80027–1677; tel. 303/527–5461; Jim Burnett, Vice President, Corporate Division; www.booksarefun.com**

### Health Promotion Facility:

**HEALTHWAYS, 701 Cool Springs Boulevard, Franklin, Tennessee Zip 37067–2697; tel. 615/614–4571; Suzanne Shepard, Director, Government Strategy**

### Hospice:

HOSPICE OF THE VALLEY, 1510 East Flower Street, Phoenix, Arizona Zip 85014–5698; tel. 602/530–6900; Susan Levine, Executive Director; www.hov.org

### Information Systems:

**ALLSCRIPTS, 3 Ravinia Drive, Suite 1100, Atlanta, Georgia Zip 30346–2134; tel. 800/654–0889; Shari A. Cox, Director, Strategic Programs**

CERNER CORPORATION, 2800 Rockcreek Parkway, Kansas City, Missouri Zip 64117; tel. 816/221–1024; Brandon Most, Manager; www.cerner.com

DESIGN CLINICALS, 5200 Southcenter Boulevard, Suite 250, Seattle, Washington Zip 98188–7911; tel. 888/633–7320; Dewey Howell, Chief Executive Officer; www.designclinicals.com

**IMPRIVATA, INC., 10 Maguire Road Building 4, Lexington, Massachusetts Zip 02421–3110; tel. 781/674–2700; Ed Gaudel, Chief Marketing Officer; www.imprivata.com**

KPMG LLP, 303 East Wacker Drive, 19th Floor, Chicago, Illinois Zip 60601; tel. 312/665–2073; Edward J. Giniat, National Line of Business Leader, Healthcare and Pharmaceuticals Practice

SCC SOFT COMPUTER, 5400 Tech Data Drive, Clearwater, Florida Zip 33760–3116; tel. 727/789–0100; Gilbert Hakim, Chief Executive Officer; www.softcomputer.com

### Insurance Broker:

**AMERICAN FIDELITY ASSURANCE COMPANY, 2000 North Classen Boulevard, Oklahoma City, Oklahoma Zip 73106; tel. 877/967–5748; Brian Mauck, National Sales Director; www.af–group.com**

*The members listed in* **bold** *are Associate Advantage members.* © 2012 AHA Guide

BOSTON MUTUAL LIFE INSURANCE COMPANY, 120 Royall Street, Canton, Massachusetts Zip 02021; tel. 781/828–7000; Peter Tillson, Vice President; www.bostonmutual.com

CHUBB INSURANCE, P.O. Box 2002, Simsbury, Connecticut Zip 06070; tel. 860/408–2017; Kimberly Holmes, Assistant Vice President Healthcare; www.chubb.com

DYE & ESKIN, 1324 Vincent Place, Mc Lean, Virginia Zip 22101; tel. 703/556–0744; Rick Eskin, President

G. E. FINANCIAL, GE Appliance Park Building, Suite 100, Louisville, Kentucky Zip 40225; tel. 502/254–1756; Greg Miller, Director Business Development; www.ge.com

ING EMPLOYEE BENEFITS, 20 Washington Avenue South, Minneapolis, Minnesota Zip 55401; tel. 612/372–1122; Steve Pitzer, Vice President

LOYAL INSURANCE, 423 Westport Road, Suite 201, Kansas City, Missouri Zip 64111; tel. 816/841–3597; Michael Reidy, Vice President

LTC FINANCIAL PARTNERS, 5110 Carillon Point, Kirkland, Washington Zip 98033–7388; tel. 866/471–4072; Dan Cahn, Senior Vice President Business Development; www.ltcfp.com

MEDICAL PROTECTIVE, 5814 Reed Road, Fort Wayne, Indiana Zip 46835; tel. 260/486–0814; Bruce Whitmore, Hospital and Facilities Sales Leader; www.medpro.com

NEBCO, 1264 Knollwood Drive West, West Chester, Pennsylvania Zip 19380; tel. 877/739–3330; James M. Mattison, Vice President; www.nebenefit.com

THE ALLEN J. FLOOD COMPANIES, INC., 2 Madison Avenue, Larchmont, New York Zip 10538; tel. 914/834–9326; Allen J. Flood, President; www.ajfusa.com

UNITED CONCORDIA COMPANY, INC., 4401 Deer Path Road, Harrisburg, Pennsylvania Zip 17110; tel. 717/260–6800; Brett Altland, Product Development Analyst; www.ucci.com

VALIC, 2929 Allen Parkway (L6–40), Houston, Texas Zip 77019–2111; tel. 713/831–6128; Nicole Mott, Associate Director Marketing; www.valic.com

### Managed Care/Utilization:

CENTENE CORPORATION, 111 East Capitol Street, Suite 500, Jackson, Mississippi Zip 39201; tel. 601/863–0835; K. Michael Bailey, Vice President; www.centene.com

### Manufacturer/Supplier:

AMERISOURCE BERGEN, 1300 Morris Drive, Chesterbrook, Pennsylvania Zip 19087–5559; tel. 610/727–2441; Claire Biermaas, Manager Market Development; www.amerisourcebergen.com

AMGEN, INC., 1 Amgen Center Drive, Thousand Oaks, California Zip 91320; tel. 805/447–2106; Debra Litwak, President and Chief Executive Officer; www.amgen.com

BAXTER HEALTHCARE CORPORATION, Route 120 and Wilson Road, Round Lake, Illinois Zip 60073; tel. 847/270–5440; Tom Progar, Vice President Marketing Strategy and Operations; www.baxter.com

BIOMEDIX, 178 East Ninth Street, Saint Paul, Minnesota Zip 55101; tel. 651/762–4010; Lyndsay Toensing, Director of Marketing Communications and Events; www.biomedix.com

BOSTON SCIENTIFIC, 100 Boston Scientific Way, Marlborough, Massachusetts Zip 01752–1234; tel. 508/683–4000; David Wilson, Senior Manager Health Economics and Reimbursement; www.bostonscientific.com

CANON USA, One Canon Plaza, Lake Success, New York, Zip 11042–1110; tel. 516/328–5000; Mary Kay Galvin, Consultant; www.canon.com

CAREFUSION CORPORATION, 3750 Torrey View Court, San Diego, California Zip 92130–2622; tel. 858/617–2000; Jocelyn Ochinang, Senior Associate, Market Research; www.carefusion.com

DA COTT ENERGY SERVICES, LTD., 4545 Bissonnet, Suite 125, Bellaire, Texas Zip 77401; tel. 713/664–8600; Steven D. Guy, Managing Partner; www.decott.com

EXTENSION, INC, 6435 West Jefferson Boulevard, Suite 201, Fort Wayne, Indiana Zip 46804–6203; tel. 877/207–3753; Whitney St. Pierre, Director Marketing; www.opentheredbox.com

GE HEALTHCARE, 3000 North Grandview Boulevard, Waukesha, Wisconsin Zip 53188; tel. 262/312–7915; Patrick Connolly, Information Management and Strategy Manager; www.gehealthcare.com

HILL–ROM, 1069 State Route 46 East, Batesville, Indiana Zip 47006–9167; tel. 812/934–7958; Thomas J. Jeffers, Director Government Relations; www.hill-rom.com

JOHNSON & JOHNSON, 829 Williamsburg Boulevard, Downingtown, Pennsylvania Zip 19335–4124; tel. 610/518–7295; Larry Westfall, Director Healthcare Quality Alliances

KWALU LLC, 1835 Savoy Drive, Suite 200, Atlanta, Georgia Zip 30341–1073; tel. 678/690–5600; Chad Langville, Director, Business Development; www.kwalu.com

LESLIE CONTROLS, INC., 12501 Telecom Drive, Temple Terrace, Florida Zip 33637–0906; tel. 813/978–1000; Tina Ware, Marketing Manager; www.lesliecontrols.com

LILLY USA, LLC, Lilly Corporate Center–DC 5021, Indianapolis, Indiana Zip 46285–4113; tel. 317/277–8173; John H. Poulin, Advisor Professional Relations; www.lilly.com

MAXXVAULT, LLC, 6820 Taylorsville Road, Finchville, Kentucky Zip 40022–6785; tel. 516/880–6800; John Jones, Director Healthcare Solutions; www.maxxvault.com

MEDTRONIC, INC, 8200 Coral Sea Street NE, Mounds View, MN Zip 55112–4391; tel. 763/526–2947; Stephanie Waite, Administrative Assistant; www.medtronic.com

MISSION LINEN SUPPLY, P O Box 1299, Santa Barbara, California Zip 93102–1299; tel. 805/730–3715; Kimberly Garden, Director Marketing; www.missionlinen.com

OTSUKA AMERICA PHARMACEUTICAL, INC., 2440 Research Boulevard, Rockville, Maryland Zip 20850; tel. 301/990–0030; Jennifer Greaney, Director; www.otsuka.com

PFIZER, INC., 500 Arcola Road, F6221, Collegeville, Pennsylvania Zip 19426–3982; tel. 484/865–3291; Jon Stelzmiller, Vice President Institutional Sales

RICOH/IKON, 101 North Wacker Drive, Suite 1850, Chicago, Illinois Zip 60606–1751; tel. 312/252–4498; Patricia Brown, Manager; www.ikon.com

UMF CORPORATION, 4709 Golf Road, Suite 300A, Skokie, Illinois Zip 60076–1231; tel. 847/920–0370; Red Degala, Director Finance; www.perfectclean.com

WAKO DIAGNOSTICS, 1025 Terra Bella Avenue, Suite A., Mountain View, California Zip 94043–1829; tel. 650/210–9153; Audrey Long, Director, Marketing

### Metro Hospital Assn:

HOSPITAL ASSOCIATION OF SOUTHERN CALIFORNIA, 515 South Figueroa Street, Suite 1300, Los Angeles, California Zip 90071–3300; tel. 213/538–0700; James D. Barber, President; www.hasc.org

### National Health Care Prof Assn:

AMERICAN DENTAL ASSOCIATION, 211 East Chicago Avenue, Chicago, Illinois Zip 60611–2678; tel. 312/440–2500; Sheila A. Strock, Senior Manager, Interprofessional Relations; www.ada.org

NATIONAL ASSOCIATION FOR HEALTHCARE QUALITY, 4700 West Lake Avenue, Glenview, Illinois Zip 60025–1468; tel. 847/375–4867; Stacy Sochacki, Executive Director

### Network:

CENTURA HEALTH, 188 Inverness Drive West, Suite 500, Englewood, Colorado Zip 80112–5204; tel. 303/290–6500; Gary Campbell, Chief Executive Officer; www.centura.org

### Nursing Facility/Unit:

ST. MARY'S HOSPITAL FOR CHILDREN, 29–01 216th Street, Bayside, New York Zip 11360; tel. 718/281–8500; Eileen Chisari, Executive Vice President and Administrator

### Other:

3N, 505 North Brand Boulevard, Suite 700, Glendale, California Zip 91203; tel. 818/230–9728; Steve Kirchmeier, Vice President Healthcare; www.3nonline.com

ACCRETIVE HEALTH, 401 North Michigan Avenue, Suite 2700, Chicago, Illinois Zip 60611–4255; tel. 312/324–5477; Jennifer Johnson, Manager Physician Advisory Program; www.accretivehealth.com

ACS, A XEROX COMPANY, 2828 North Haskell Avenue, Dallas, Texas Zip 75204–2909; tel. 214/584–5408; Holly Hartman, Manager Marketing Healthcare Provice Solutions; www.acs-hcs.com

AD ASTRA, INC., P O Box 3534, Silver Spring, Maryland Zip 20918–3534; tel. 301/408–4242; Lena Toolsie, President; www.ad-astrainc.com

AEROSCOUT, 1300 Island Drive, Suite 202, Redwood City, California Zip 94065; tel. 650/596–2994; Gabi Daniely, Vice President Marketing and Product Strategy; www.aeroscout.com

AG MEDICAL SYSTEMS, INC., 13 Prosper Court, Lake In The Hills, Illinois Zip 60156–9603; tel. 800/262–2344; Denise Hammer, Manager, Marketing Business Development

AGILITY RECOVERY SOLUTIONS, 11030 Circle Point Road, Suite 450, Westminster, Colorado Zip 80020–2791; tel. 877/495–9615; Jenny Boyd, Director Marketing Account; www.agilityrecovery.com

AMERICA'S BLOOD CENTERS, 725 15th Street N.W., Suite 700, Washington, District of Columbia Zip 20005; tel. 202/393–5725; Jim MacPherson, Executive Director

AMERICAN ACADEMY OF PHYSICIAN ASSISTANTS, 2318 Mill Road, Suite 1300, Alexandria, Virginia Zip 22314–6833; tel. 703/836–2272; James G. Potter, Interim Chief Executive Officer; www.aapa.org

AMERICAN ASSOCIATION FOR WOUND CARE MANAGEMENT, 4109 Glenrose Street, Kensington, Maryland Zip 20895–3718; tel. 301/933–2200; Jule Crider, Executive Director; www.aawcm.org

AMERICAN ASSOCIATION OF NURSE ANESTHETISTS, 222 South Prospect Avenue, Park Ridge, Illinois Zip 60068–4001; tel. 847/655–1100; John F. Garde, Interim Executive Director; www.aana.com

AMERICAN BOARD OF INTERNAL MEDICINE, 510 Walnut Street, Suite 1700, Philadelphia, Pennsylvania Zip 19106; tel. 215/446–3500; Kevin P. Caviston, Strategic Relations Liaison; www.abim.org

AMERICAN BOARD OF MEDICAL SPECIALTIES, 222 North La Salle Street, Suite 1500, Chicago, Illinois Zip 60601–1003; tel. 847/491–9091; Kevin B. Weiss, President and Chief Executive Officer; www.abms.org

AMERICAN COLLEGE OF HEALTHCARE EXECUTIVES, One North Franklin, Suite 1700, Chicago, Illinois Zip 60606–4425; tel. 312/424–2800; Thomas C. Dolan, President and Chief Executive Officer; www.ache.org

AMERICAN DENTAL EDUCATION ASSOCIATION, 1400 K Street N.W., Suite 1100, Washington, District of Columbia Zip 20005; tel. 202/289–7201; Richard Valachovic, Executive Director; www.adea.org

AMERICAN HEALTH INFORMATION MANAGEMENT ASSOCIATION, 233 North Michigan Avenue, Suite 2150, Chicago, Illinois Zip 60601–5806; tel. 312/233–1100; David A. Sweet, Director Library Services

AMERINET, INC., 500 Commonwealth Drive, Warrendale, Pennsylvania Zip 15086–7516; tel. 877/711–5700; Randall Walter, Vice President Marketing; www.amerinet-gpo.com

AMN HEALTHCARE, INC., 12400 High Bluff Drive, Suite 100, San Diego, California Zip 92130–3581; tel. 866/871–8519; Steve Wehn, Senior Vice President of Corporate Development

ANTHELIO HEALTHCARE SOLUTIONS INC, tel. 214/257–7000; Mary Gael Senko, Brand Manager; www.antheliohealth.com

APOGEE PHYSICIANS, 2525 East Camelback Road, Suite 1100, Phoenix, Arizona Zip 85016–4282; tel. 602/778–3600; Michael Gregory, MD, Chairman; www.apogeephysicians.com

ARC GROUP ASSOCIATES, 330 South Warminster Road, Suite 345, Hatboro, Pennsylvania Zip 19040; tel. 215/881–9500; Eric Malakoff, Vice President Sales and Marketing; www.arcgroup.net

ARMED FORCES INSTITUTE OF PATHOLOGY, 6825 16th Street N.W., Building 54, Washington, District of Columbia Zip 20306–6000; tel. 202/782–2100; Colonel Renata Greenspan, Director; www.afip.osd.mil

ASSOCIATION OF PERIOPERATIVE REGISTERED NURSES, 2170 South Parker Road, Suite 400, Denver, Colorado Zip 80231; tel. 303/755–6304; Linda Groah, Executive Director and Chief Executive Officer; www.aorn.org

**BERNARD HODES GROUP, 220 East 42nd Street, 14th Floor, New York, New York Zip 10017; tel. 888/438–9911; Karen Hart, Senior Vice President Healthcare Division; www.hodes.com**

**BEST UPON REQUEST, 8170 Corporate Park Drive, Suite 300, Cincinnati, Ohio Zip 45242; tel. 513/605–7800; Kirsten Lecky, Vice President Business Development; bestuponrequest.com**

BKD, LLP, P.O. Box 1190, Springfield, Missouri Zip 65801–1900; tel. 417/831–7283; www.bkd.com

BLUE CROSS AND BLUE SHIELD ASSOCIATION, 225 North Michigan Avenue, Chicago, Illinois Zip 60601–7680; tel. 312/297–6000; Scott P. Serota, President and Chief Executive Officer; www.bcbs.com

CANON BUSINESS SOLUTIONS, 300 Commerce Square Boulevard, Burlington, New Jersey Zip 08016–1270; tel. 847/706–3411; Paul T. Murphy, Director Strategic Contract Support; www.solutions.canon.com

**CAP SITE INC., 85 South Prospect Street, Burlington, Vermont Zip 05401–3444; tel. 802/383–0675; Gino Johnson, Senior Vice President; www.capsite.com**

**CARETECH SOLUTIONS, INC., tel. 248/823–0800; Paula Gwyn, Senior Manager Business Development; www.caretechsolutions.com**

**CCM ADVISORS, LLC, 190 South La Salle Street, Suite 2800, Chicago, Illinois Zip 60603; tel. 312/444–6200; Michael Randall, Director Sales and Marketing; www.ahafunds.org**

**CERTIPHI SCREENING, INC., 1105 Industrial Highway, Southampton, Pennsylvania Zip 18966; tel. 888/260–1370; Tony D'Orazio, President; www.certiphi.com**

CHAN HEALTHCARE AUDITORS, 231 South Bemiston Avenue, Suite 300, Saint Louis, Missouri Zip 63105; tel. 314/802–2008; Dan Clayton, Director, Knowledge Management; www.chanllc.com

**CISCO SYSTEMS, 165 Needletree Lane, Glastonbury, Connecticut Zip 06033; tel. 860/657–8127; Michael Haymaker, Director Healthcare Industry Marketing; www.cisco.com**

**CLAREDI CORPORATION, 2525 Lake Park Boulevard, Salt Lake City, Utah Zip 84120; tel. 801/982–3001; www.claredi.com**

**COMPUTER ASSOCIATES, One Computer Associates Plaza, Islandia, New York Zip 11749; tel. 800/225–5224; Michael McDermand, Vice President Healthcare; www.ca.com**

**CONCUITY, INCORPORATED, 200 North Fairway Drive Suite 182, Vernon Hills, Illinois Zip 60061–1861; tel. 847/465–6003; James Farrar, Vice President Sales; www.concuity.com**

COVENANT HOSPICE, 5041 North 12th Avenue, Pensacola, Florida Zip 32504; tel. 850/433–2155; Dale O. Knee, President and Chief Executive Officer; www.covenanthospice.org

CRANEWARE, INC., 3340 Peachtree Road N.E. Suite 850, Atlanta, Georgia Zip 30326–1072; tel. 404/364–2037; Ann Marie Brown, Executive Vice President Marketing; www.craneware.com

CRIMSHIELD INC., 4121 East Valley Auto Drive, Suite 116, Mesa, Arizona Zip 85206–4632; tel. 888/422–2547; Denny Dobbins, Legal Counsel

**CYRACOM, 5780 North Swan Road, Tucson, Arizona Zip 85718–4527; tel. 800/713–4950; Jeremy Woan, President and Chief Executive Officer; www.cyracom.com**

CUSHMAN & WAKEFIELD, 107 Elm Street, 4 Stamford Plaza, 8th Floor, Stamford, Connecticut Zip 06902–3834; tel. 203/326–5829; Alina Schoepfer, Market Analysis Specialist; www.cushwake.com

DEPARTMENT OF AIR FORCE MEDICAL SERVICE, HQ USAF/SG, Bolling AFB, District of Columbia Zip 20332–6188; tel. 202/545–6700

DEPARTMENT OF THE ARMY, OFFICE OF THE SURGEON GENERAL, 5109 Leesburg Pike, Falls Church, Virginia Zip 22041–3258; tel. 202/690–6467

DEPARTMENT OF THE NAVY, BUREAU OF MEDICINE AND SURGERY, 2300 East Street N.W., Washington, District of Columbia Zip 20372–5300; tel. 202/762–3701; Rear Admiral Adam M. Robinson, Surgeon General

DEPARTMENT OF VETERANS AFFAIRS, 810 Vermont Avenue NW, Washington, District of Columbia Zip 20420–0001; tel. 202/273–5400; Michael J Kussman, MD, Acting Undersecretary of Health; www.va.gov/health/default.asp

DEPARTMENT OF VETERANS AFFAIRS, 201 Walnut Avenue, Suite 201, Vallejo, California Zip 94592–1107; Linda Pierce, Director, Sierra Pacific Network

DHHS, PUBLIC HEALTH SERVICE, INDIAN HEALTH SERVICE, DIVISION OF BUSINESS OFFICE ENHANCEMENT, 12300 Twinbrook Parkway, Suite 360–57, Rockville, Maryland Zip 20852; tel. 301/443–0227; Frank Martin, Management Analyst; www.ihs.gov

**DILIGENT, A DIVISION OF ARJO, 2349 West Lake Street, Suite 250, Addison, Illinois Zip 60101–6183; tel. 800/323–1245; Andy Hepburn, Vice President; www.arjousa.com**

**DIVERSIFIED INVESTMENT ADVISORS, 4 Manhattanville Road, Purchase, New York Zip 10577; tel. 914/697–8952; Eric Henon, Vice President; www.divinvest.com**

DNV HEALTHCARE, INC., 400 Techne Center Drive, Suite 350, Milford, Ohio Zip 45150–2792; tel. 513/388–4863; Beverly J. Eller, Manager Business Operations; www.dnvhealthcareinc.com

**EKTRON, INC., 542 Amherst Street, Nashua, New Hampshire Zip 03063–1016; tel. 603/594–0249; Richard Brown, Director Channel, Alliances and Healthcare; www.ektron.com**

EMERGENCY CONSULTANTS, INC., 4075 Copper Ridge Drive, Traverse City, Michigan Zip 49684–4796; tel. 800/253–1795; James Johnson, President; www.eci–med.com

FTI HEALTHCARE, 5310 Maryland Way, Suite 250, Brentwood, Tennessee Zip 37027–5370; tel. 615/324–8500; Iain Briggs, Senior Managing Director; www.ftihealthcare.com

FUOCO GROUP, 200 Parkway Drive South, Suite 302, Hauppauge, New York Zip 11788–2024; tel. 631/360–1700; Lou J. Fuoco, Managing Director; www.fuoco.com

HEALTHCARE BUSINESS ASSOCIATES, P.O. Box 1188, Rancho Mirage, California Zip 92270–1188; tel. 888/292–6929; Jack C. Nixon, President

HEALTH PARK HOSPITALITY, 181 South Northwest Highway, Barrington, Illinois Zip 60010–4607; tel. 847/842–8366; Dominic Chiovari, President and Chief Executive Officer

**HIPAA ACADEMY, 14225 University Avenue, Suite 240, Waukee, Iowa Zip 50263; tel. 515/453–8247; Lorna L. Waggoner, Director Business Development**

HIRERIGHT, 5151 California Avenue, Irvine, California Zip 92617–3059; tel. 800/400–2761; Bob Sparanese, Manager Product Marketing; www.hireright.com

**HMS, 355 Quartermaster Court, Jeffersonville, Indiana Zip 47130–3670; tel. 812/704–5747; Rich Flaherty, Vice President Sales and Marketing; www.hms.com**

HOOPER, LUNDY & BOOKMAN, INC., 1875 Century Park East, Suite 1600, Los Angeles, California Zip 90067; tel. 310/551–8111; Lloyd Bookman, Partner; www.health–law.com

HQ ACC/SGMS, 162 Dodd, Suite 100, Langley AFB, Virginia Zip 23665–1995

HQ AETC/SGAL, 63 Main Circle, Suite 3, Randolph AFB, Texas Zip 78150–4549

HQ AFMC/SGAR, 4225 Logistics Avenue, N–209, Dayton, Ohio Zip 45433–5761; tel. 937/656–3655; Alice Rohrbach

HQ AFSPC/SGAL, 150 Vandenberg Street, Suite 1105, Petterson AFB, Colorado Zip 80914–4550

HQ AMC/SGSL, 203 West Losey Street, Room 1180, Scott AFB, Illinois Zip 62225–5219

HQ PACAF/SGAL, 25 East Street, Suite D1, Hickam AFB, Hawaii Zip 96853–5418

HQ USAFA/SGAL, Pinion Drive, Building 4102, Suite 3, USAF Academy, Colorado Zip 80840

**HR SOLUTIONS, INC., 25 East Washington Street, Suite 600, Chicago, Illinois Zip 60602; tel. 312/236–7170; Kevin Sheridan, Senior Vice President – HR Optimization; www.hrsolutionsinc.com**

**HYLAND SOFTWARE, INC., 28500 Clemens Road, Westlake, Ohio Zip 44145; tel. 440/788–5814; Michael Kortan, Director Health Care Solutions; www.onbase.com**

**I.D. EXPERTS, 10300 S.W. Greenburg Road, Suite 570, Portland, Oregon Zip 97223–5410; tel. 866/726–4271; Sally Gray, Manager Sales Support; www.idexpertcorp.com**

**IDENTITY FORCE, 1257 Worcester Road, Suite 308, Framingham, Massachusetts Zip 01701; tel. 508/788–6660; Mike Lawson, Vice President; www.identityforce.com**

INTERNATIONAL ASSOCIATION FOR HEALTHCARE SECURITY AND SAFETY, P.O. Box 5038, Glendale Heights, Illinois Zip 60139; tel. 630/529–3913; Nancy Felesena, Executive Assistant; www.iahss.org

IPC THE HOSPITALIST COMPANY, INC., 4605 Lankershim Boulevard, Hollywood, CA Zip 91602–1818; tel. 818/766–3502; Todd J. Kislak, Vice President Marketing and Development; www.hospitalist.com

**IRONPORT, 950 Elm Avenue, San Bruno, California Zip 94066; tel. 650/989–6500; Jeff Williams, Vice President Sales; www.ironport.com**

JACKSON HEALTHCARE, 2655 North Winds Parkway, Alpharetta, Georgia Zip 30009; tel. 770/643–5500; Robert S. Schlotman, Chief Marketing Officer; www.jacksonhealthcare.com

JANI–KING, 16885 Dallas Parkway, Addison, Texas Zip 75001; tel. 972/991–0900; Bob Carabajal, Director Healthcare Services; www.janiking.com

KFORCE HEALTHCARE, 1001 East Palm Avenue, Tampa, Florida Zip 33605–3551; tel. 800/397–9814; LeAnn Dinehart, Project Manager; https://www.kforce.com

LIFE LINE SCREENING, 6150 Oak Tree Boulevard, Suite 200, Independence, Ohio Zip 44131–2569; tel. 800/897–9177; Kellie D. Privette, Senior Vice President; www.lifelinescreening.com

LODGENET INTERACTIVE CORPORATION, 3900 West Innovation Street, Sioux Falls, South Dakota Zip 57107; tel. 605/988–1418; Stacy Forsch, Administrative Assistant II; www.lodgenet.com

**MAGELLAN HEALTH SERVICES, 6950 Columbia Gateway Drive, Columbia, Maryland Zip 21046; tel. 314/387–4000; Rick Lee, President Employer Solutions; www.magellanhealth.com**

MEDCOR, INC., P.O. Box 550, McHenry, Illinois Zip 60051–0550; tel. 815/363–9500; Jerry Jaskowiak, Vice President Sales; www.medcor.com

MEDIMPACT HEALTHCARE SYSTEMS, INC, 10680 Treena Street, San Diego, California Zip 92128; tel. 858/566–2727; Dana Felthouse, Vice President Marketing; www.medimpact.com

MEDQUIST TRANSCRIPTIONS LTD, 9009 Carothers Parkway, Suite C–2, Franklin, Tennessee Zip 37067–1704; tel. 615/798–6000; Michael Zinn, Manager Sales and Marketing Support Center; www.medquist.com

METLIFE RESOURCES, 400 Atrium Drive, Somerset, New Jersey Zip 08873–4162; tel. 732/652–1268; Ty Minnich, Vice President; www.metlife.com

MODERN HEALTHCARE, 360 North Michigan Avenue, Chicago, Illinois Zip 60601–3806; tel. 312/649–5491; Fawn Lopez, Publisher; www.modernhealthcare.com

MRI INTERNATIONAL, INC./CLAIMS SERVICING OF AMERICA, 5330 South Durango Drive, Las Vegas, Nevada Zip 89113–1835; tel. 702/396–8822; Linda Martinez

NAVAL REGIONAL MEDICAL CENTER, PSC 1005, Box 36, FPO, Armed Forces Africa, Canada, E Zip 09593–0136

**NOBLIS, 3150 Fairview Park South, Falls Church, Virginia Zip 22042; tel. 703/610–2255; Alan Dowling, Executive Director; www.mitretek.org**

PERKINELMER GENETICS, INC., P.O. Box 219, Bridgeville, Pennsylvania Zip 15017; tel. 412/220–2300; Joseph M. Quashnock, Laboratory Director; www.perkinelmergenetics.com

**PILAT, 460 U.S. Highway 22 West Suite 408, Whitehouse Station, New Jersey Zip 08889–3447; tel. 908/823–9417; Travis Lupo, Director Business Development; www.pilat–nai.com**

PRICEWATERHOUSE COOPERS, 300 Madison Avenue, New York, New York Zip 10017–6232; tel. 813/348–7457; Betty Croft, Senior Manager Business Information Services; www.pwc.com

QUADRAMED CORPORATION, 12110 Sunset Hills Road, Suite 600, Reston, Virginia Zip 20190; tel. 800/393–0278; Laura Adams, Director Manager; www.quadramed.com

RF TECHNOLOGIES, 3125 North 126th Street, Brookfield, Wisconsin Zip 53005; tel. 800/669–9946; Glenn Jonas, President and Chief Executive Officer; www.rft.com

ROSARIO INCORPORATED, 501 Burwood Drive, Winston Salem, North Carolina Zip 27127; tel. 866/279–8485; Sandra R. Rosario, Director/Owner; www.rosarioinc.com

SIMPLEX GRINNELL, 50 Technology Drive, Westminster, Massachusetts Zip 01441; tel. 978/731–8486; Suzanne Rahall, Marketing Manager, Healthcare Communications; www.simplexgrinnell.com

SMITHS MEDICAL CRITICAL CARE, 160 Weymouth Street, Rockland, Massachusetts Zip 02370–1136; tel. 781/792–2555; Eugene Stavtsev, Senior Global Market Research Analyst; www.smiths–medical.com

ST. LOUIS EYE SURGERY, 12990 Manchester Road, Suite 103, Saint Louis, Missouri Zip 63131–1860; tel. 314/686–4220; Melanie Kofron, Administrator

*The members listed in **bold** are Associate Advantage members.*

© 2012 AHA Guide

SUBWAY, 325 Bic Drive, Milford, Connecticut Zip 06461; tel. 800/888–4848; Joanne Kilgore, Global Account Manager; www.subway.com

**TANDBERG, 29 Norfolk Avenue, Peabody, Massachusetts Zip 01960; tel. 978/531–1516; Luke Leininger, Senior Product Manager, Healthcare TelePresence; www.tandberg.com**

**TEAMHEALTH, 265 Brookview Town Center Way, Suite 400, Knoxville, Tennessee Zip 37919; tel. 865/293–5486; Tracy Young, Vice President Communication; www.teamhealth.com**

THE ADVISORY BOARD COMPANY, 2445 M Street N.W., Washington, District of Columbia Zip 20037–2403; tel. 202/266–5600; Britton Perry, Associate Director, Information Resource Center; www.advisory.com

THE AMERICAN COLLEGE OF OBSTETRICIANS AND GYNECOLOGISTS, 409 12th Street, S.W., Washington, District of Columbia Zip 20024–2188; tel. 202/638–5577; Hal Lawrence, Executive Vice President; www.acog.org

THE GOVERNANCE INSTITUTE, 9685 Via Excelencia, Suite 100, San Diego, California Zip 92126–7500; tel. 858/909–0811; Jona Raasch, President and Chief Executive Officer; www.governanceinstitute.com

THE JEWISH GUILD FOR THE BLIND, 15 West 65th Street, New York, New York Zip 10023; tel. 212/769–6200; Alan R. Morse, President and Chief Executive Officer; www.jgb.org

THE RISK MANAGEMENT AND PATIENT SAFETY INSTITUTE, 6215 West St. Joseph Highway, Lansing, Michigan Zip 48917; tel. 517/886–8352; Patricia A. Dextrom, Merchandising Manager

**THE WALKER COMPANY, 4848 Hastings Drive, Lake Oswego, Oregon Zip 97035; tel. 503/534–9461; Larry W. Walker, Principal; www.walkercompany.com**

THEREX, INC., 341 Cool Springs Boulevard, Franklin, Tennessee Zip 37067; tel. 615/236–2550; Michael G. Skiera, President and Chief Executive Officer; www.therex.us

**THERMO USCS, 120 Bishop's Way, Brookfield, Wisconsin Zip 53008; tel. 262/784–5600; Christine Miller, Executive Vice President Healthcare Group; www.thermo.com**

**TRANSUNION, LLC, 445 Hutchinson Avenue, Suite 800, Columbus, Ohio Zip 43235; tel. 614/785–6411; Martin Callahan, Vice President Business Development; www.transunion.com**

TRAVELERS INSURANCE COMPANY, One Tower Square, Hartford, Connecticut Zip 06183–1134; tel. 860/277–9830; Wayne Tryon, Director Business Development; www.travelers.com

U. S. ARMY MEDICAL COMMAND, 2050 Worth Road, Suite 10, San Antonio, Texas Zip 78234–6010; tel. 210/221–2212; Ann Russell Potter

UNIFORM DATA SYSTEM FOR MEDICAL REHABILITATION, 270 Northpointe Parkway, Suite 300, Amherst, New York Zip 14228; tel. 716/817–7800; Beth Demakos, Associate Product Manager; www.udsmr.org

**VERGE SOLUTIONS, LLC, 710 Johnnie Dodds Boulevard, Suite 202, Mount Pleasant, South Carolina Zip 29464–3045; tel. 843/628–4168; Katie Layman, Marketing Manager; www.verge–solutions.com**

**VERISYS CORPORATION, 1001 North Fairfax Avenue, Suite 640, Alexandria, Virginia Zip 22314–1798; tel. 703/535–1471; John Benson, Chief Operating Officer; www.verisys.com/**

**VERSUS TECHNOLOGY, INC., 2600 Miller Creek Road, Traverse City, Michigan Zip 49684; tel. 231/946–5868; Stephanie Bertschy, Director Marketing; www.versustech.com**

**VERTICAL CLAIMS MANAGEMENT, L.L.C., Three Gateway Center, 15 North, Pittsburgh, Pennsylvania Zip 15222; tel. 800/501–6248; Clare Bello, President; www.vcm–llc.com**

VETERANS AFFAIRS EASTERN REGION OFFICE, 9600 North Point Road, Fort Howard, Maryland Zip 21052

**VOCERA COMMUNICATIONS, 525 Race Street, Suite 150, San Jose, California Zip 95126–3495; tel. 408/882–5100; Diana Cropley, Marketing Program Specialist; www.vocera.com**

VISN 1 OFFICE, 200 Spring Road, Building 61, Bedford, Massachusetts Zip 01730

VISN 2 OFFICE, P O Box 8980, Albany, New York Zip 12208–0980; tel. 518/626–5000

VISN 3 OFFICE, 130 West Kingsbridge Road, Building 16, Bronx, New York Zip 10468; tel. 718/584–9000; Michael A Sabo, Director

VISN 4 OFFICE, Delafield Road, Pittsburgh, Pennsylvania Zip 15240

VISN 5 OFFICE, 849 International Drive, Suite 275, Linthicum Heights, Maryland Zip 21090

VISN 6 OFFICE, 300 West Morgan Street, Suite 1402, Durham, North Carolina Zip 27701

VISN 7 OFFICE, 3700 Crestwood Parkway NE, Suite 260, Duluth, Georgia Zip 30096–5585

VISN 8 OFFICE, P O Box 406, Bay Pines, Florida Zip 33744

VISN 9 OFFICE, 1310 24th Avenue South, Nashville, Tennessee Zip 37212–2637

VISN 10 OFFICE, 11500 Northlake Drive, Suite 200, Cincinnati, Ohio Zip 45259–1655

VISN 11 OFFICE, P O Box 134002, Ann Arbor, Michigan Zip 48113–4002; Linda Belton, Network Director

VISN 12 OFFICE, P O Box 5000, Building 18, Hines, Illinois Zip 60141–5000; tel. 708/202–8400; Renee Oshinski, Acting Network Director

VISN 15 OFFICE, 4801 Linwood Boulevard, Kansas City, Missouri Zip 64128; James R Floyd, Director

VISN 16 OFFICE, 1600 East Woodrow Wilson Drive, Suite A, 3rd Floor, Jackson, Mississippi Zip 39216; tel. 601/364–7901; Rica Lewis Payton, Deputy Network Director

VISN 17 OFFICE, 2301 East Lamar Boulevard, Suite 650, Arlington, Texas Zip 76006–7435

VISN 18 OFFICE, 6950 E Williams Field Road, Mesa, Arizona Zip 85212–6033; tel. 602/222–2681; Patricia A McKlem, Director; www.va.gov/VISN18

VISN 19 OFFICE, 4100 East Mississippi Avenue, Suite 510, Glendale, Colorado Zip 80222

VISN 20 OFFICE, 1601 4th Plain Boulevard, Building 17, Suite 402, Vancouver, Washington Zip 95661; tel. 360/619–5925

VISN 21 OFFICE, 201 Walnut Avenue, Mare Island, California Zip 94592

VISN 22 OFFICE, 5901 East Seventh Street, Long Beach, California Zip 90822; tel. 562/826–8000; Kenneth J. Clark, FACHE, Director

VISN 23 OFFICE, 5445 Minnehaha Avenue South, 2nd Floor, Minneapolis, Minnesota Zip 55417; tel. 612/727–5967; Robert A. Petzel, MD, Network Director; www.visn23.med.va.gov

WIGGIN AND DANA, LLP, P.O. Box 1832, New Haven, Connecticut Zip 06508–1832; tel. 203/498–4400; Maureen Weaver, Partner

WITT/KIEFFER, 2015 Spring Road, Suite 510, Oak Brook, Illinois Zip 60523; tel. 630/990–1370; James W. Gauss, Senior Advisor to Chief Executive Officer and Senior Vice President

### Other Health Related:

SOMNIA ANESTHESIA, 10 Commerce Drive, New Rochelle, New York Zip 10801–5214; tel. 877/795–5788; Marc E. Koch, MD, MBA, Chief Executive Officer and President; www.somniainc.com

### Recruitment Services:

**B. E. SMITH, 9777 Ridge Drive, Suite 300, Lenexa, Kansas Zip 66219–9746; tel. 913/752–4533; Allison Murphy, Marketing Manager; www.besmith.com**

DOCCAFE.COM, R5435 Star Dust Lane, Ringle, Wisconsin Zip 54471–9743; 3045; tel. 715/302–8881; Laura Fitzsimmons, Managing Member; www.doccafe.com

UNITED ANESTHESIA, P.O. Box 1847, Kernsville North Carolina, Zip 27285–1847; tel. 800/334–8320; Tracy Strother–Mayer, Chief Operating Officer; www.unitedanesthesia.com

### Regional Health Care Assn:

TEXAS ORGANIZATION OF RURAL & COMMUNITY HOSPITALS, P.O. Box 14547, Austin, Texas Zip 78761; tel. 512/873–0045; David Pearson, President and Chief Executive Officer; www.torchnet.org

# CANADA

### Consulting Firm:

IMPARK, 601 West Cordova Street, Suite 300, Vancouver, BC Zip V6B 1G1; tel. 604/331–7216; Jeffrey Powell, Coordinator Marketing; www.impark.com

**RADICALOGIC TECHNOLOGIES, INC., 77 Peter Street, Suite 300, Toronto, Ontario Zip M5V 2G4; tel. 416/410–8456; Colin Hung, Vice President Marketing and Alliances; www.rl–solutions.com**

### National Hospital Assn:

CANADIAN HEALTHCARE ASSOCIATION, 17 York Street, Suite 100, Ottawa, Ontario, Canada Zip K1N 9J6; tel. 613/241–8005; Pamela Fralick, President and Chief Executive Officer

### Other:

**HALOGEN SOFTWARE CORPORATION, 495 March Road, Suite 500, Ottawa, Ontario Zip K2K 3G1; tel. 613/270–1011; Lorna Daly, Channel Manager Healthcare; www.halogensoftware.com**

INTERNATIONAL MEDICAL INTERPRETERS ASSOCIATION, 80 Corporatate Drive, Suite 305, Toronto, Zip M1H 3G5; tel. 416/296–0842; Izabel Arocha, Executive Director; www.imiaweb.org

### Provincial Hospital Assn:

ONTARIO HOSPITAL ASSOCIATION, 200 Front Street West, Suite 2800, Toronto, Ontario Zip M5V 3L1; tel. 416/205–1300; Warren Di Clemente, Vice President Educational Services and Operations; www.oha.com

# FOREIGN

# ALBANIA

### Other:

AMERICAN HOSPITAL, Rruga Lord Bayron – Laprake, Tirane, Zip 10026; tel. 003/235–7535; Klodian Allaybeu, Chief Executive Officer; www.spitaliamerican.com

# BAHAMAS

### Other:

PRINCESS MARGARET HOSPITAL, P.O. Box N–8200, Nassau, tel. 242/322–2861; Coralie Adderley, Chief Hospital Administrator; www.phabahamas.org

# BAHRAIN

### Other:

INTERNATIONAL HOSPITAL OF BAHRAIN, P.O. Box 1084, Manama, F. S. Zeerah, President

# BANGLADESH

### Consulting Firm:

U. S. BANGLADESH FOUNDATION, House 32, Road 10, Block D., Banani, Dhaka, Zip 1213; tel. 880/881–3070; Mohammad Zahurul Haque, Chief Executive Officer; www.banglasoy.com/usbdf.htm

# BERMUDA

### Other:

KING EDWARD VII MEMORIAL HOSPITAL, P.O. Box HM1023, Hamilton, L. Keitha Bassett, Health Sciences Librarian

# BRAZIL

### Consulting Firm:

CONSORCIO PAULISTA DE SAUDE, Rua Gironda 37, Sao Paulo, Zip 01435–040; tel. 551/885–7472; Marcos Gurger do Amaral, Director; www.consorciopaulistadesaude.com.br

TRIUNFO PARTICIPACOES E INVESTIMENTOS, S.A., Rua Olimpiadas 205 Conjunto 142/143, Sao Paulo, Zip 04551000; tel. 551/169–3999; Dorival Pagani, Director; www.tpisa.com.br/

**Manufacturer/Supplier:**

GOCIL SERVICOS DE VIGILANCIA E SEGURANCA LIDA,
Avenida Conselheiro Rodrigues Alves, 352, Sao Paulo,
Zip Sao Paulo; Marcos Gurger do Amaral, Consultant;
www.gocil.com.br

**Other:**

HOSPITAL SAMARITANO, Rua Conselheiro Brotero, 1486,
Sao Paulo, Zip 01232–010; Jose Antonio de Lima,
General Superintendent; www.samaritano.com.br

## COLOMBIA

**Other:**

ASOCIACION COLOMBIANA DE HOSPITALES Y CLINICAS,
Carrera 4, No 73–15, Bogota, Juan Carlos Giraldo
Valencia, Director General; www.achc.org.co

## ECUADOR

**Other:**

JUNTA DE BENEFICENCIA DE GUAYAQUIL, P.O. Box
09–01–789, Guayaquil, Lautaro Aspiazu Wright,
Director; www.jbg.org.ec

## GEORGIA

**Other:**

MEDI CLUB GEORGIA, 22A, Tashkenti Street, Tbilisi,
Zip 0160; tel. 995/225–1991; Dimitri Makhatadze,
General Director; www.mediclubgeorgia.ge

## GERMANY

**Other:**

HQ USAFE/SGPXL, Unit 3050, Box 130, Ramstein AB,
Armed Forces Africa, Canada, E Zip 09094–5001

## GREECE

**Other:**

DIAGNOSTIC AND THERAPEUTIC CENTRE OF ATHENS
HYGEIA, S A, 4 Erythrou Stavrou & Kifissiap, Athens,
Andreas Kartapanis, General Manager

## HONG KONG

**Consulting Firm:**

QUALITY HEALTHCARE MEDICAL SERVICES LIMITED, 303
Des Voeux Road Central, 4th Floor, Sheung Wan,
Zip 00000; Philip Choy, Director; www.qhms.com

## ISRAEL

**Other:**

HADASSAH MEDICAL ORGANIZATION, Box 12000,
Jerusalem, Zip 91120; Ehud Kokia, Director General;
www.hadassah.org.il

## JAPAN

**Other:**

KAMEDA MEDICAL CENTER AND CLINICS, 929 Higashi–Cho,
Kamogawa City, Zip 296–8602; John C. Wocher,
Executive Vice President; www.kameda.com
NAVAL REGIONAL MEDICAL CENTER, U.S. Naval Base, FPO,
Armed Forces Pacific Zip 96362
ST. LUKE'S INTERNATIONAL HOSPITAL, 10–1 Akashi–Cho,
Chuo–Ku, Tokyo 104, Shigeaki Hinohara, Honorary
President

## JORDAN

**Other:**

SPECIALTY HOSPITAL, P.O. Box 930186, Amman,
Zip 11193; Fawzi Al–Hammouri, General Manager;
www.specialty–hospital.com

## LEBANON

**Other:**

AMERICAN UNIVERSITY OF BEIRUT MEDICAL CENTER, 3 Dag
Hammarskjold Plaza, 8th Floor, New York, New York
Zip 10017–2303; Munthir Kuzayli, Medical Center
Director
SAINT GEORGE HOSPITAL, P.O. Box 166378, Beirut,
Zip 1100–2807; Ziad Kamel, Administrative Director;
www.stgeorgehospital.org

## MEXICO

**Consulting Firm:**

ASOCIACION NACIONAL DE HOSPITALES PRIVADOS, Av
Ejercito Nacional Mexicano No 613 Col Granada,
Mexico City, Roberto Simon Sauma, President

**Other:**

CONSORCIO MEXICANO DE HOSPITALES, A.C., Galeana
#600–12, San Pedro Garza Garcia, Zip 66230;
tel. 528/040–5901; Humberto Javier Potes Gonzalez,
Chief Executive Officer
SHRINERS HOSPITAL FOR CHILDREN, Av Del Iman 257, Col
Pedregal de Santa Ursula, Delegacion Coyoacan,
Mexico City, Zip 04600; Araceli Nagore, Administrator

## MYANMAR

**Other:**

ASIA ROYAL GENERAL HOSPITAL, 14 Baho Street,
Sanchaung Township, Yangon, Zip 11162;
tel. 951/153–8055; Myat Thu, Managing Director;
www.asiaroyalmedical.com

## NETHERLANDS ANTILLES

**Other:**

SINT MAARTEN MEDICAL CENTER FOUNDATION, Welgelegen
Road 30 Ut 1 Cay Hill, Sint Maarten,
tel. 599/543–1111; George Scot, General Director

## PANAMA

**Other:**

CLINICA HOSPITAL SAN FERNANDO, S. A., Dept PTY 1663,
P.O. Box 25207, Miami, Florida Zip 33102–5207;
tel. 507/229–1699; Edgardo Fernandez, Medical
Director; www.hospitalsanfernando.com

## PERU

**Other:**

BRITISH AMERICAN HOSPITAL, Avenue Alfredo Salazar 3 Era,
Lima 27, tel. 511/712–3000; Gonzalo Garrido–Lecca,
Director; www.angloamericana.com.pe

## PHILIPPINES

**Ambulatory Care Center:**

DEPARTMENT OF VETERANS AFFAIRS, OUTPATIENT CLINIC,
Pasay City, APO, Zip 96440; tel. 632/833–4566;
Artemio Arugay, Commander; www.va.gov

**Other:**

ST. LUKE'S MEDICAL CENTER, 279 East Rodriguez Sr
Boulevard, Quezon City, Jose F. G. Ledesma, Chief
Executive Officer

## SAUDI ARABIA

**Other:**

ABDUL RAHMAN AL MISHARI GENERAL HOSPITAL, Olaya,
Riyadh 11564, Abdul Rahman Al Mishari, President
AL HAMMADI HOSPITAL, P.O. Box 55004, Riyadh,
Zip 11534; Mohammed Al Hammadi, Executive Director
MUHAMMAD SALEH BASHARAHIL HOSPITAL, P.O. Box
10505, Madinah Road, Omora Gadida, Makkah,
tel. 009/520–4444; Turki M. Basharahil, General
Manager

## TURKEY

**Other:**

ANADOLU MEDICAL CENTER, Cumhuriyet Mahallesi 2255
Sokak Gebze, Kocaeli, Zip 41400; Robert Gerard Kiely,
President and Chief Executive Officer;
www.anadolusaglik.org
ISTANBUL MEMORIAL HOSPITAL, Piyale Pasa Bulvari,
Okmeydani, Istanbul, Zip 80270; Sevin Suekinci,
Assistant Medical Director and Coordinator Quality
MEDICANA INTERNATIONAL ANKARA HOSPITAL, Sogutozu
Caddesi 2165 Sokak No. 6, Ankara, Zip 06520;
tel. 905/749–0384; Oguz Engiz, Chief Executive
Officer; www.medicana.com

## UNITED ARAB EMIRATES

**Other:**

AMERICAN HOSPITAL–DUBAI, P.O. Box 59, Dubai, Saeed M.
Almulla, Chairman

*The members listed in* **bold** *are Associate Advantage members.* © 2012 AHA Guide

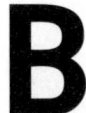

# B

**Health Care Systems,
Networks
and Alliances**

Section B

# Introduction

This section includes listings for networks, health care systems and alliances.

## Health Care Systems

To reflect the diversity that exists among health care organizations, this publication uses the term health care system to identify both multihospital and diversified single hospital systems.

### Multihospital Systems

A multihospital health care system is two or more hospitals owned, leased, sponsored, or contract managed by a central organization.

### Single Hospital Systems

Single, freestanding member hospitals may be categorized as health care systems by bringing into membership three or more, and at least 25 percent, of their owned or leased non–hospital preacute and postacute health care organizations. (For purposes of definition, health care delivery is the availability of professional healthcare staff during all hours of the organization's operations). Organizations provide, or provide and finance, diagnostic, therapeutic, and/or consultative patient or client services that normally precede or follow acute, inpatient, hospitalization; or that serve to prevent or substitute for such hospitalization. These services are provided in either a freestanding facility not eligible for licensure as a hospital under state statue or through one that is a subsidiary of a hospital.

The first part of this section is an alphabetical list of multihospital health care systems. Each system listed contains two or more hospitals, which are listed under the system by state. Data for this section were compiled from the 2010 *Annual Survey* and the membership information base as published in section A of the *AHA Guide*.

One of the following codes appears after the name of each system listed to indicate the type of organizational control reported by that system:

| | |
|---|---|
| **CC** | Catholic (Roman) church–related system, not–for–profit |
| **CO** | Other church–related system, not–for–profit |
| **NP** | Other not–for–profit system, including nonfederal, governmental systems |
| **IO** | Investor–owned, for profit system |
| **FG** | Federal Government |

One of the following codes appears after the name of each hospital to indicate how that hospital is related to the system:

| | |
|---|---|
| **O** | Owned |
| **L** | Leased |
| **S** | Sponsored |
| **CM** | Contract–managed |

## Health System Classification System

An identification system for Health Systems was developed jointly by the American Hospital Association's Health Research and Education Trust and Health Forum, and the University of California-Berkeley.[1] A health system is assigned to one of five categories based on how much they differentiate and centralize their hospital services, physician arrangements, and provider-based insurance products. Differentiation refers to the number of different products or services that the organization offers. Centralization refers to whether decision-making and service delivery emanate from the system level more so than individual hospitals.

### Categories:

*Centralized Health System:* A delivery system in which the system centrally organizes individual hospital service delivery, physician arrangements, and insurance product development. The number of different products/services that are offered across the system is moderate.

*Centralized Physician/Insurance Health System:* A delivery system with highly centralized physician arrangements and insurance product development. Within this group, hospital services are relatively decentralized with individual hospitals having discretion over the array of services they offer. The number of different products/services that are offered across the system is moderate.

*Moderately Centralized Health System:* A delivery system that is distinguished by the presence of both centralized and decentralized activity for hospital services, physician arrangements, and insurance product development. For example, a system within this group may have centralized care of expensive, high technology services, such as open heart surgery, but allows individual hospitals to provide an array of other health services based on local needs. The number of different products/services that are offered across the system is moderate.

*Decentralized Health System:* A delivery system with a high degree of decentralized of hospital services, physician arrangements, and insurance product development. Within this group, systems may lack an overarching structure for coordination. Service and product differentiation is high, which may explain why centralization is hard to achieve. In this group, the system may simply service a role in sharing information and providing administrative support to highly developed local delivery systems centered around hospitals.

*Independent Hospital System:* A delivery system with limited differentiation in hospital services, physician arrangements, and insurance product development. These systems are largely horizontal affiliations of autonomous hospitals.

*No Assignment:* For some systems sufficient data from the Annual Survey were not available to determine a cluster assignment.

The second part of this section lists health care systems indexed geographically by state and city. Every effort has been made to be as inclusive and accurate as possible. However, as in all efforts of this type, there may be omissions. For further information, write to the Section for Health Care Systems, American Hospital Association, 155 N. Wacker Drive, Chicago, IL 60606.

## Networks

The *AHA Guide* shows listings of networks. A network is defined as a group of hospitals, physicians, other providers, insurers and/or community agencies that work together to coordinate and deliver a broad spectrum of services to their community. Organizations listed represent the lead or hub of the network activity. Networks are listed by state, then alphabetically by name including participating partners.

The network identification process has purposely been designed to capture networks of varying organization type. Sources include but are not limited to the following: *AHA Annual Survey,* national, state and metropolitan associations, national news and periodical searches, and the networks and their health care providers themselves. Therefore, networks are included regardless of whether a hospital or healthcare system is the network lead. When an individual hospital does appear in the listing, it is indicative of the role the hospital plays as the network lead. In addition, the network listing is **not** mutually exclusive of the hospital, health care system or alliance listings within this publication.

Networks are very fluid in their composition as goals evolve and partners change. Therefore, some of the networks included in this listing may have dissolved, reformed, or simply been renamed as this section was being produced for publication.

The network identification process is an ongoing and responsive initiative. As more information is collected and validated, it will be made available in other venues, in addition to the *AHA Guide.* For more information concerning the network identification process, please contact The American Hospital Association Resource Center at 312/422–2050.

## Alliances

An alliance is a formal organization, usually owned by shareholders/members, that works on behalf of its individual members in the provision of services and products and in the promotion of activities and ventures. The organization functions under a set of bylaws or other written rules to which each member agrees to abide.

Alliances are listed alphabetically by name. Its members are listed alphabetically by state, city, and then by member name.

[1] Bazzoli, CJ; Shortell, SM; Dubbs, N; Chan, C; and Kralovec, P; ''A Taxonomy of Health networks and Systems: Bringing Order Out of Chaos'' *Health Services Research*, February; 1999

# Statistics for Multihospital Health Care Systems and their Hospitals

The following tables describing multihospital health care systems refers to information in section B of the 2013 *AHA Guide*.

Table 1 shows the number of multihospital health care systems by type of control. Table 2 provides a breakdown of the number of systems that own, lease, sponsor or contract manage hospitals within each control category. Table 3 gives the number of hospitals and beds in each control category as well as total hospitals and beds. Finally, Table 4 shows the percentage of hospitals and beds in each control category.

For more information on multihospital health care systems, please write to the Section for Health Care Systems, 155 N. Wacker Drive, Chicago, Illinois 60606 or call 312/422–3000.

### Table 1. Multihospital Health Care Systems, by Type of Organizaton Control

| Type of Control | Code | Number of Systems |
|---|---|---|
| Catholic (Roman) church–related | CC | 37 |
| Other church–related | CO | 12 |
| Subtotal, church–related | | 49 |
| Other not–for–profit | NP | 284 |
| Subtotal, not–for–profit | | 333 |
| Investor Owned | IO | 80 |
| Federal Government | FG | 5 |
| Total | | 418 |

### Table 2. Multihospital Health Care Systems, by Type of Ownership and Control

| Type of Ownership | Catholic Church–Related (CC) | Other Church–Related (CO) | Total Church–Related (CC + CO) | Other Not–for–Profit (NP) | Total Not–for–Profit (CC, CO, + NP) | Investor–Owned (IO) | Federal Govern–ment (FG) | All Systems |
|---|---|---|---|---|---|---|---|---|
| Systems that only own, lease or sponsor | 31 | 8 | 39 | 255 | 294 | 74 | 5 | 373 |
| Systems that only contract–manage | 0 | 0 | 0 | 1 | 1 | 2 | 0 | 3 |
| Systems that manage, own, lease, or sponsor | 6 | 4 | 10 | 28 | 38 | 4 | 0 | 42 |
| Total | 37 | 12 | 49 | 284 | 333 | 80 | 5 | 418 |

### Table 3. Hospitals and Beds in Multihospital Health Care Systems, by Type of Ownership and Control

| Type of Ownership | Catholic Church–Related (CC) H | B | Other Church–Related (CO) H | B | Total Church–Related (CC + CO) H | B | Other Not–for–Profit (NP) H | B | Total Not–for–Profit (CC, CO, + NP) H | B | Investor–Owned (IO) H | B | Federal Govern–ment (FG) H | B | All Systems H | B |
|---|---|---|---|---|---|---|---|---|---|---|---|---|---|---|---|---|
| Owned, leased or sponsored | 544 | 102,364 | 105 | 21,996 | 649 | 124,360 | 1,398 | 300,819 | 2,047 | 425,179 | 1,288 | 150,842 | 213 | 38,217 | 3,548 | 614,238 |
| Contract–managed | 39 | 1,470 | 6 | 546 | 45 | 2,016 | 84 | 5,687 | 129 | 7,703 | 129 | 8,681 | 0 | 0 | 258 | 16,384 |
| Total | 583 | 103,834 | 111 | 22,542 | 694 | 126,376 | 1,482 | 306,506 | 2,176 | 432,882 | 1,417 | 159,523 | 213 | 38,217 | 3,806 | 630,622 |

**H** = hospitals; **B** = beds.

### Table 4. Hospitals and Beds in Multihospital Health Care Systems, by Type of Ownership and Control as a Percentage of All Systems

| Type of Ownership | Catholic Church–Related (CC) H | B | Other Church–Related (CO) H | B | Total Church–Related (CC + CO) H | B | Other Not–for–Profit (NP) H | B | Total Not–for–Profit (CC, CO, + NP) H | B | Investor–Owned (IO) H | B | Federal Govern–ment (FG) H | B | All Systems H | B |
|---|---|---|---|---|---|---|---|---|---|---|---|---|---|---|---|---|
| Owned, leased or sponsored | 15.3 | 16.7 | 3.0 | 3.6 | 18.3 | 20.2 | 39.4 | 49.0 | 57.7 | 69.2 | 36.3 | 24.6 | 6.0 | 6.2 | 100.0 | 100.0 |
| Contract–managed | 15.1 | 9.0 | 2.3 | 3.3 | 17.4 | 12.3 | 32.6 | 34.7 | 50.0 | 47.0 | 50.0 | 53.0 | 0.0 | 0.0 | 100.0 | 100.0 |
| Total | 15.3 | 16.5 | 2.9 | 3.6 | 18.2 | 20.0 | 38.9 | 48.6 | 57.2 | 68.6 | 37.2 | 25.3 | 5.6 | 6.1 | 100.0 | 100.0 |

**H** = hospitals; **B** = beds.
*Please note that figures may not always equal the provided subtotal or total percentages due to rounding.

**0091: ACADIA HEALTHCARE COMPANY, INC.** (IO)
830 Crescent Centre Drive, Suite 610, Franklin, TN
Zip 37067–7323; tel. 615/861–6000; Joey Jacobs, Chairman and
Chief Executive Officer
**(Independent Hospital System)**

**ARIZONA:** SONORA BEHAVIORAL HEALTH HOSPITAL (O, 56 beds) 6050 North
Corona Road, Tucson, AZ Zip 85704–1096; tel. 520/469–8700; Brian
Gill, Chief Executive Officer

**DELAWARE:** MEADOW WOOD BEHAVIORAL HEALTH SYSTEM (O, 53 beds)
575 South Dupont Highway, New Castle, DE Zip 19720–4600;
tel. 302/328–3330; Bill A. Mason, Chief Executive Officer
**Web address:** www.meadowwoodhospital.com

**LOUISIANA:** ACADIA VERMILION HOSPITAL (O, 54 beds) 2520 North
University Avenue, Lafayette, LA Zip 70507–5306; tel. 337/234–5614;
Joseph Rodriguez, Chief Executive Officer
**Web address:** www.vermilionhospital.com

**MICHIGAN:** HARBOR OAKS HOSPITAL (O, 45 beds) 35031 23 Mile Road,
New Baltimore, MI Zip 48047–3649; tel. 586/725–5777; Sari
Abromovich, Chief Executive Officer
**Web address:** www.harboroaks.com

**MISSOURI:** LAKELAND BEHAVIORAL HEALTH SYSTEM (O, 66 beds) 440
South Market Street, Springfield, MO Zip 65806–2026;
tel. 417/865–5581; Keith A. Furman, Chief Executive Officer
**Web address:** www.lakeland–hospital.com

**NEVADA:** SEVEN HILLS BEHAVIORAL INSTITUTE (O, 58 beds) 3021 West
Horizon Ridge Parkway, Henderson, NV Zip 89052–3990;
tel. 702/646–5000; John Hull, Chief Executive Officer

**OKLAHOMA:** ROLLING HILLS HOSPITAL (O, 44 beds) 1000 Rolling Hills Lane,
Ada, OK Zip 74820–9415; tel. 580/436–3600; John Baker, Chief
Executive Officer
**Web address:** www.rollinghillshospital.com

**PENNSYLVANIA:** SOUTHWOOD PSYCHIATRIC HOSPITAL (O, 112 beds) 2575
Boyce Plaza Road, Pittsburgh, PA Zip 15241–3925; tel. 412/257–2290;
Stephen J. Quigley, Chief Executive Officer
**Web address:** www.southwoodhospital.com

**TEXAS:** ACADIA ABILENE HOSPITAL (O, 58 beds) 4225 Woods Place, Abilene,
TX Zip 79602–7991, Mailing Address: P.O. Box 5559, Zip 79608;
tel. 325/698–6600; Shana Hisaw, Chief Operating Officer
**Web address:** www.acadiaabilene.com

RED RIVER HOSPITAL (O, 66 beds) 1505 Eighth Street, Wichita Falls, TX
Zip 76301–3106; tel. 940/322–3171; Robert Mansfield, Chief Executive
Officer
**Web address:** www.redriverhospital.com

**VIRGINIA:** MOUNT REGIS CENTER (O, 25 beds) 405 Kimball Avenue, Salem,
VA Zip 24153–6299; tel. 540/389–4761; Gail S. Basham, Chief
Executive Officer

| | | |
|---|---|---|
| **Owned, leased, sponsored:** | 11 hospitals | 637 beds |
| **Contract–managed:** | 0 hospitals | 0 beds |
| **Totals:** | 11 hospitals | 637 beds |

**0640: ACUITYHEALTHCARE, LP** (IO)
10200 Mallard Creek Road, Suite 300, Charlotte, NC
Zip 28262–9705; tel. 877/228–4893; Edwin H. Cooper, Jr., MS,
President and Chief Executive Officer
**(Independent Hospital System)**

**ARIZONA:** TRILLIUM SPECIALTY HOSPITAL–EAST VALLEY (O, 60 beds) 215
South Power Road, Mesa, AZ Zip 85206–5235; tel. 480/985–6992;
Kevin Nicholson, Chief Executive Officer
**Web address:** www.trilliumhospital.net

TRILLIUM SPECIALTY HOSPITAL–WEST VALLEY (O, 120 beds) 13818 North
Thunderbird Boulevard, Sun City, AZ Zip 85351–2574; tel. 623/977–1325;
Rhonda Y. Williams, Chief Executive Officer
**Web address:** www.trilliumhospital.net

**NEW JERSEY:** ACUITY SPECIALTY HOSPITAL OF NEW JERSEY (O, 30 beds)
1925 Pacific Avenue, Atlantic City, NJ Zip 08401–6713;
tel. 609/441–8160; Mary Beth Tubbs, Chief Executive Officer
**Web address:** www.acuityhealthcare.net

**NORTH CAROLINA:** CAROLINAS SPECIALTY HOSPITAL (O, 38 beds) 2001
Vail Avenue, 7th Floor, Charlotte, NC Zip 28207; tel. 704/379–6450;
Susan R. Davis, Chief Executive Officer
**Web address:** www.cshnc.org

**OHIO:** ACUITY SPECIALTY HOSPITAL – OHIO VALLEY (O, 40 beds) 380
Summit Avenue, 3rd Floor, Steubenville, OH Zip 43952;
tel. 740/283–7600; Judy Weaver, MS, Chief Executive Officer
**Web address:** www.acuityhealthcare.net

**TEXAS:** ACUITY HOSPITAL OF SOUTH TEXAS (O, 30 beds) 718 Lexington
Avenue, San Antonio, TX Zip 78212–4768; tel. 210/572–4600; Scott
Galliardt, Chief Executive Officer
**Web address:** www.acuityhealthcare.net

ICON HOSPITAL (O, 42 beds) 19211 Mckay Boulevard, Humble, TX
Zip 77338–5502; tel. 281/883–5500; Kiley P. Cedotal, Chief Executive
Officer
**Web address:** www.acuityhealthcare.net

| | | |
|---|---|---|
| **Owned, leased, sponsored:** | 7 hospitals | 360 beds |
| **Contract–managed:** | 0 hospitals | 0 beds |
| **Totals:** | 7 hospitals | 360 beds |

**0414: ACUTECARE HEALTH SYSTEM** (IO)
500 River Avenue, Suite 150, Lakewood, NJ Zip 08701–4743;
tel. 732/364–0800; Daniel Czermak, Chairman and President

**NEW JERSEY:** SPECIALTY HOSPITAL AT KIMBALL (O, 25 beds) 600 River
Avenue, 4 West, Lakewood, NJ Zip 08701; tel. 732/942–3588; Hilary
Michaels, Executive Director
**Web address:** www.acutecarehs.com

SPECIALTY HOSPITAL AT MONMOUTH (O, 25 beds) 300 Second Avenue,
Long Branch, NJ Zip 07740; tel. 732/923–5037; Violeta Peters, R.N., Chief
Executive Officer
**Web address:** www.acutecarehs.com

| | | |
|---|---|---|
| **Owned, leased, sponsored:** | 2 hospitals | 50 beds |
| **Contract–managed:** | 0 hospitals | 0 beds |
| **Totals:** | 2 hospitals | 50 beds |

**★0235: ADVENTIST HEALTH** (CO)
2100 Douglas Boulevard, Roseville, CA Zip 95661–3898, Mailing
Address: P.O. Box 619002, Zip 95661–9002; tel. 916/781–2000;
Robert G. Carmen, President
**(Moderately Centralized Health System)**

**CALIFORNIA:** ADVENTIST MEDICAL CENTER–REEDLEY (L, 44 beds) 372
West Cypress Avenue, Reedley, CA Zip 93654–2199; tel. 559/638–8155;
Sandy Haskins, Interim Chief Executive Officer
**Web address:** www.skdh.org

CENTRAL VALLEY GENERAL HOSPITAL (O, 30 beds) 1025 North Douty
Street, Hanford, CA Zip 93230–3722, Mailing Address: P.O. Box 480,
Zip 93232–0480; tel. 559/583–2100; Wayne Ferch, President and Chief
Executive Officer
**Web address:** www.hanfordhealth.com

FEATHER RIVER HOSPITAL (O, 54 beds) 5974 Pentz Road, Paradise, CA
Zip 95969–5509; tel. 530/877–9361; Kevin R. Erich, President and Chief
Executive Officer
**Web address:** www.frhosp.org

---

For explanation of codes following names, see page B2.
★ Indicates Type III membership in the American Hospital Association.

FRANK R. HOWARD MEMORIAL HOSPITAL (L, 25 beds) One Madrone Street, Willits, CA Zip 95490–4225; tel. 707/459–6801; Rick Bockmann, Chief Executive Officer
**Web address:** www.howardhospital.com

GLENDALE ADVENTIST MEDICAL CENTER (O, 414 beds) 1509 Wilson Terrace, Glendale, CA Zip 91206–4098; tel. 818/409–8000; Kevin A. Roberts, FACHE, President and Chief Executive Officer
**Web address:** www.glendaleadventist.com

HANFORD COMMUNITY MEDICAL CENTER (O, 94 beds) 450 Greenfield Avenue, Hanford, CA Zip 93230–3513; tel. 559/582–9000; Richard L. Rawson, President and Chief Executive Officer

SAN JOAQUIN COMMUNITY HOSPITAL (O, 255 beds) 2615 Chester Avenue, Bakersfield, CA Zip 93301–2006, Mailing Address: P.O. Box 2615, Zip 93303–2615; tel. 661/395–3000; Robert J. Beehler, President and Chief Executive Officer
**Web address:** www.sanjoaquinhospital.org

SIMI VALLEY HOSPITAL AND HEALTH CARE SERVICES (O, 97 beds) 2975 North Sycamore Drive, Simi Valley, CA Zip 93065–1201; tel. 805/955–6000; Caroline Esparza, Interim Chief Executive Officer
**Web address:** www.simivalleyhospital.com

SONORA REGIONAL MEDICAL CENTER (O, 152 beds) 1000 Greenley Road, Sonora, CA Zip 95370–4819; tel. 209/536–5000; Jeff Eller, FACHE, President and Chief Executive Officer
**Web address:** www.sonorahospital.org

ST. HELENA HOSPITAL (O, 116 beds) 10 Woodland Road, Saint Helena, CA Zip 94574; tel. 707/963–3611; Terry Newmyer, President and Chief Executive Officer
**Web address:** www.sthelenahospital.org

ST. HELENA HOSPITAL CLEARLAKE (O, 25 beds) 15630 18th Avenue, Clearlake, CA Zip 95422–9339, Mailing Address: P.O. Box 6720, Zip 95422–6720; tel. 707/994–6486; Terry Newmyer, President and Chief Executive Officer
**Web address:** www.adventisthealth.org

ST. HELENA HOSPITAL–CENTER FOR BEHAVIORAL HEALTH (O, 30 beds) 525 Oregon Street, Vallejo, CA Zip 94590–3201; tel. 707/648–2200; Terry Newmyer, President and Chief Executive Officer
**Web address:** www.sthelenahospital.org/Behavioral/

UKIAH VALLEY MEDICAL CENTER (O, 62 beds) 275 Hospital Drive, Ukiah, CA Zip 95482–4531; tel. 707/462–3111; Gwen Matthews, R.N., MSN, Chief Executive Officer
**Web address:** www.adventisthealth.org

WHITE MEMORIAL MEDICAL CENTER (O, 280 beds) 1720 Cesar E Chavez Avenue, Los Angeles, CA Zip 90033–2481; tel. 323/268–5000; Beth D. Zachary, President and Chief Executive Officer
**Web address:** www.whitememorial.com

**HAWAII:** CASTLE MEDICAL CENTER (O, 160 beds) 640 Ulukahiki Street, Kailua, HI Zip 96734–4498; tel. 808/263–5500; Kathryn A. Raethel, R.N., M.P.H., President and Chief Executive Officer
**Web address:** www.castlemed.com

**OREGON:** ADVENTIST MEDICAL CENTER (O, 252 beds) 10123 S.E. Market Street, Portland, OR Zip 97216–2599; tel. 503/257–2500; Thomas Russell, Chief Executive Officer
**Web address:** www.adventisthealthnw.com

TILLAMOOK COUNTY GENERAL HOSPITAL (L, 25 beds) 1000 Third Street, Tillamook, OR Zip 97141–3430; tel. 503/842–4444; Larry Davy, President and Chief Executive Officer
**Web address:** www.tcgh.com

**WASHINGTON:** WALLA WALLA GENERAL HOSPITAL (O, 37 beds) 1025 South Second Avenue, Walla Walla, WA Zip 99362–1398, Mailing Address: P.O. Box 1398, Zip 99362–0309; tel. 509/525–0480; Monty E. Knittel, President and Chief Executive Officer
**Web address:** www.wwgh.com

| | | |
|---|---|---|
| **Owned, leased, sponsored:** | 18 hospitals | 2152 beds |
| **Contract-managed:** | 0 hospitals | 0 beds |
| **Totals:** | 18 hospitals | 2152 beds |

★4165: **ADVENTIST HEALTH SYSTEM SUNBELT HEALTH CARE CORPORATION** (CO)
900 Hope Way, Altamonte Springs, FL Zip 32714–1502; tel. 407/357–1000; Donald L. Jernigan, Ph.D., President and Chief Executive Officer
**(Decentralized Health System)**

**COLORADO:** AVISTA ADVENTIST HOSPITAL (O, 114 beds) 100 Health Park Drive, Louisville, CO Zip 80027–9583; tel. 303/673–1000; John Sackett, Chief Executive Officer
**Web address:** www.avistahospital.org

LITTLETON ADVENTIST HOSPITAL (O, 202 beds) 7700 South Broadway Street, Littleton, CO Zip 80122–2628; tel. 303/730–8900; Morre Dean, Interim Chief Executive Officer
**Web address:** www.centura.org

PARKER ADVENTIST HOSPITAL (O, 142 beds) 9395 Crown Crest Boulevard, Parker, CO Zip 80138; tel. 303/269–4000; Morre Dean, Chief Executive Officer
**Web address:** www.parkerhospital.org

PORTER ADVENTIST HOSPITAL (O, 239 beds) 2525 South Downing Street, Denver, CO Zip 80210–5876; tel. 303/778–1955; Randall L. Haffner, Ph.D., Chief Executive Officer
**Web address:** www.centura.org

**FLORIDA:** FLORIDA HOSPITAL (O, 2170 beds) 601 East Rollins Street, Orlando, FL Zip 32803–1489; tel. 407/303–6611; Lars D. Houmann, President
**Web address:** www.flhosp.org

FLORIDA HOSPITAL AT CONNERTON LONG TERM ACUTE CARE (O, 8 beds) 9441 Health Center Drive, Land O'Lakes, FL Zip 34637–5837; tel. 813/903–3701; Debi Martoccio, R.N., Chief Operating Officer
**Web address:** www.elevatinghealthcare.org

FLORIDA HOSPITAL DELAND (O, 156 beds) 701 West Plymouth Avenue, DeLand, FL Zip 32720; tel. 386/943–4522; Mark LaRose, President and Chief Executive Officer
**Web address:** www.fhdeland.org

FLORIDA HOSPITAL FISH MEMORIAL (O, 175 beds) 1055 Saxon Boulevard, Orange City, FL Zip 32763–8468; tel. 386/917–5000; Ed Noseworthy, President and Chief Executive Officer
**Web address:** www.fhfishmemorial.org

FLORIDA HOSPITAL HEARTLAND MEDICAL CENTER (O, 222 beds) 4200 Sun'n Lake Boulevard, Sebring, FL Zip 33872–1986, Mailing Address: P.O. Box 9400, Zip 33871–9400; tel. 863/314–4466; Timothy W. Cook, President and Chief Executive Officer
**Web address:** www.fhheartland.org/

FLORIDA HOSPITAL MEMORIAL MEDICAL CENTER (O, 396 beds) 301 Memorial Medical Parkway, Daytona Beach, FL Zip 32117–5167; tel. 386/676–6000; Daryl Tol, Chief Executive Officer
**Web address:** www.floridahospitalmemorial.org

FLORIDA HOSPITAL NORTH PINELLAS (L, 150 beds) 1395 South Pinellas Avenue, Tarpon Springs, FL Zip 34689–3721; tel. 727/942–5000; Bruce Bergherm, Chief Executive Officer
**Web address:** www.hemh.com

FLORIDA HOSPITAL TAMPA (O, 320 beds) 3100 East Fletcher Avenue, Tampa, FL Zip 33613–4688; tel. 813/971–6000; John R. Harding, Chief Executive Officer
**Web address:** www.uch.org

FLORIDA HOSPITAL WATERMAN (O, 204 beds) 1000 Waterman Way, Tavares, FL Zip 32778–5266; tel. 352/253–3333; Kenneth R. Mattison, President and Chief Executive Officer
**Web address:** www.fhwat.org

FLORIDA HOSPITAL WAUCHULA (O, 25 beds) 533 West Carlton Street, Wauchula, FL Zip 33873; tel. 863/773–3101; Linda Adler, Administrator
**Web address:** www.fhheartland.org

FLORIDA HOSPITAL ZEPHYRHILLS (O, 154 beds) 7050 Gall Boulevard, Zephyrhills, FL Zip 33541–1399; tel. 813/788–0411; Douglas Duffield, President and Chief Executive Officer
**Web address:** www.fhzeph.org

FLORIDA HOSPITAL–CARROLLWOOD (O, 59 beds) 7171 North Dale Mabry Highway, Tampa, FL Zip 33614–2699; tel. 813/932–2222; Brinsley B. Lewis, Chief Executive Officer
**Web address:** www.uch.org

Section B

For explanation of codes following names, see page B2.
★ Indicates Type III membership in the American Hospital Association.

FLORIDA HOSPITAL–FLAGLER (O, 99 beds) 60 Memorial Medical Parkway, Palm Coast, FL Zip 32164; tel. 386/586–2000; David Ottati, President and Chief Executive Officer
**Web address:** www.fhms.com

**GEORGIA:** EMORY–ADVENTIST HOSPITAL (O, 52 beds) 3949 South Cobb Drive S.E., Smyrna, GA Zip 30080–6300; tel. 770/434–0710; Dennis Kiley, President
**Web address:** www.emoryadventist.org

GORDON HOSPITAL (O, 80 beds) 1035 Red Bud Road, Calhoun, GA Zip 30701–2082, Mailing Address: P.O. Box 12938, Zip 30703–7013; tel. 706/629–2895; Pete M. Weber, President and Chief Executive Officer
**Web address:** www.gordonhospital.com

**ILLINOIS:** ADVENTIST BOLINGBROOK HOSPITAL (O, 148 beds) 500 Remington Boulevard, Bolingbrook, IL Zip 60440; tel. 630/312–5000; Rick Mace, Chief Executive Officer
**Web address:** www.keepingyouwell.com/abh/

ADVENTIST GLENOAKS HOSPITAL (O, 141 beds) 701 Winthrop Avenue, Glendale Heights, IL Zip 60139–1403; tel. 630/545–8000; Bruce C. Christian, Chief Executive Officer
**Web address:** www.keepingyouwell.com

ADVENTIST HINSDALE HOSPITAL (O, 271 beds) 120 North Oak Street, Hinsdale, IL Zip 60521–3890; tel. 630/856–9000; Michael Goebel, Chief Executive Officer
**Web address:** www.keepingyouwell.com

ADVENTIST LA GRANGE MEMORIAL HOSPITAL (O, 179 beds) 5101 South Willow Spring Road, La Grange, IL Zip 60525–2680; tel. 708/245–9000; Lary Davis, President and Chief Executive Officer
**Web address:** www.keepingyouwell.com

**KANSAS:** SHAWNEE MISSION MEDICAL CENTER (O, 374 beds) 9100 West 74th Street, Shawnee Mission, KS Zip 66204–4004, Mailing Address: Box 2923, Zip 66201–1323; tel. 913/676–2000; Ken J. Bacon, President and Chief Executive Officer
**Web address:** www.shawneemission.org

**KENTUCKY:** MANCHESTER MEMORIAL HOSPITAL (O, 63 beds) 210 Marie Langdon Drive, Manchester, KY Zip 40962–9156; tel. 606/598–5104; Dennis Meyers, R.N., President and Chief Executive Officer
**Web address:** www.manchestermemorial.org

**NORTH CAROLINA:** PARK RIDGE HEALTH (O, 98 beds) 100 Hospital Drive, Hendersonville, NC Zip 28792–5272; tel. 828/684–8501; Jimm Bunch, President and Chief Executive Officer
**Web address:** www.parkridgehealth.org

**TENNESSEE:** JELLICO COMMUNITY HOSPITAL (L, 31 beds) 188 Hospital Lane, Jellico, TN Zip 37762–4400; tel. 423/784–7252; Erik Wangsness, Chief Executive Officer
**Web address:** www.jellicohospital.com

TAKOMA REGIONAL HOSPITAL (C, 100 beds) 401 Takoma Avenue, Greeneville, TN Zip 37743–4647; tel. 423/639–3151; Daniel Wolcott, President
**Web address:** www.takoma.org

**TEXAS:** CENTRAL TEXAS MEDICAL CENTER (O, 178 beds) 1301 Wonder World Drive, San Marcos, TX Zip 78666–7544; tel. 512/353–8979; Sam Huenergardt, President and Chief Executive Officer
**Web address:** www.ctmc.org

HUGULEY MEMORIAL MEDICAL CENTER (O, 188 beds) 11801 South Freeway, Fort Worth, TX Zip 76134, Mailing Address: P.O. Box 6337, Zip 76115–0337; tel. 817/293–9110; Kenneth A. Finch, President and Chief Executive Officer
**Web address:** www.huguley.org

METROPLEX ADVENTIST HOSPITAL (O, 177 beds) 2201 South Clear Creek Road, Killeen, TX Zip 76549–4110; tel. 254/526–7523; Carlyle L. E. Walton, Chief Executive Officer
**Web address:** www.mplex.org

ROLLINS–BROOK COMMUNITY HOSPITAL (O, 35 beds) 608 North Key Avenue, Lampasas, TX Zip 76550, Mailing Address: P.O. Box 589, Zip 76550; tel. 512/556–3682; Jeffrey D. Villanueva, Vice President and Administrator
**Web address:** www.mplex.org

**WISCONSIN:** CHIPPEWA VALLEY HOSPITAL AND OAKVIEW CARE CENTER (O, 75 beds) 1220 Third Avenue West, Durand, WI Zip 54736–1600, Mailing Address: P.O. Box 224, Zip 54736–0224; tel. 715/672–4211; Douglas R. Peterson, President and Chief Executive Officer
**Web address:** www.keepingyouwell.com

| Owned, leased, sponsored: | 32 hospitals | 6925 beds |
|---|---|---|
| Contract–managed: | 1 hospital | 100 beds |
| **Totals:** | 33 hospitals | 7025 beds |

---

**★0214:  ADVENTIST HEALTHCARE** (NP)
1801 Research Boulevard, Suite 400, Rockville, MD Zip 20850; tel. 301/315–3030; William G. Robertson, President and Chief Executive Officer
**(Centralized Health System)**

**MARYLAND:** ADVENTIST BEHAVIORAL HEALTH ROCKVILLE (O, 283 beds) 14901 Broschart Road, Rockville, MD Zip 20850–3395; tel. 301/251–4500; Kevin Young, FACHE, President and Chief Executive Officer
**Web address:** www.adventistbehavioralhealth.com

ADVENTIST REHABILITATION HOSPITAL OF MARYLAND (O, 77 beds) 9909 Medical Center Drive, Rockville, MD Zip 20850; tel. 240/864–6000; Brent Reitz, Vice President and Administrator
**Web address:** www.adventistrehab.com

SHADY GROVE ADVENTIST HOSPITAL (O, 327 beds) 9901 Medical Center Drive, Rockville, MD Zip 20850–3395; tel. 240/826–6000; Dennis Hansen, President
**Web address:** www.adventisthealthcare.com

WASHINGTON ADVENTIST HOSPITAL (O, 204 beds) 7600 Carroll Avenue, Takoma Park, MD Zip 20912–6392; tel. 301/891–7600; Joyce Newmyer, President
**Web address:** www.adventisthealthcare.com

**NEW JERSEY:** HACKETTSTOWN REGIONAL MEDICAL CENTER (O, 111 beds) 651 Willow Grove Street, Hackettstown, NJ Zip 07840–1792; tel. 908/852–5100; Jason C. Coe, President and Chief Executive Officer
**Web address:** www.hrmcnj.org

| Owned, leased, sponsored: | 5 hospitals | 1002 beds |
|---|---|---|
| Contract–managed: | 0 hospitals | 0 beds |
| **Totals:** | 5 hospitals | 1002 beds |

---

**★0064:  ADVOCATE HEALTH CARE** (NP)
2025 Windsor Drive, Oak Brook, IL Zip 60523; tel. 630/990–5018; Jim H. Skogsbergh, President and Chief Executive Officer
**(Moderately Centralized Health System)**

**ILLINOIS:** ADVOCATE BROMENN MEDICAL CENTER (O, 200 beds) 1304 Franklin Avenue, Normal, IL Zip 61761, Mailing Address: P.O. Box 2850, Bloomington, Zip 61702–2850; tel. 309/454–1400; Colleen Kannaday, FACHE, President
**Web address:** www.bromenn.org

ADVOCATE CHRIST MEDICAL CENTER (O, 672 beds) 4440 West 95th Street, Oak Lawn, IL Zip 60453–2699; tel. 708/684–8000; Kenneth W. Lukhard, President
**Web address:** www.advocatehealth.com/christ

ADVOCATE CONDELL MEDICAL CENTER (O, 269 beds) 801 South Milwaukee Avenue, Libertyville, IL Zip 60048–3199; tel. 847/362–2900; Dominica Tallerico, M.D., President
**Web address:** www.advocatehealth.com/condell/

ADVOCATE EUREKA HOSPITAL (O, 18 beds) 101 South Major Street, Eureka, IL Zip 61530; tel. 309/467–2371; Colleen Kannaday, FACHE, President
**Web address:** www.advocatehealth.com/bromenn

ADVOCATE GOOD SAMARITAN HOSPITAL (O, 326 beds) 3815 Highland Avenue, Downers Grove, IL Zip 60515–1590; tel. 630/275–5900; David S. Fox, President
**Web address:** www.advocatehealth.com/gsam

ADVOCATE GOOD SHEPHERD HOSPITAL (O, 169 beds) 450 West Highway 22, Barrington, IL Zip 60010–1901; tel. 847/381–0123; Karen A. Lambert, President
**Web address:** www.advocatehealth.com

*For explanation of codes following names, see page B2.*
★ *Indicates Type III membership in the American Hospital Association.*

Section B

ADVOCATE ILLINOIS MASONIC MEDICAL CENTER (O, 335 beds) 836 West Wellington Avenue, Chicago, IL Zip 60657–5193; tel. 773/975–1600; Susan Nordstrom Lopez, President
**Web address:** www.advocatehealth.com/masonic

ADVOCATE LUTHERAN GENERAL HOSPITAL (O, 624 beds) 1775 Dempster Street, Park Ridge, IL Zip 60068–1174; tel. 847/723–2210; Anthony A. Armada, President
**Web address:** www.advocatehealth.com

ADVOCATE SOUTH SUBURBAN HOSPITAL (O, 225 beds) 17800 South Kedzie Avenue, Hazel Crest, IL Zip 60429–0989; tel. 708/799–8000; Michael A. Engelhart, President
**Web address:** www.advocatehealth.com/ssub/

ADVOCATE TRINITY HOSPITAL (O, 188 beds) 2320 East 93rd Street, Chicago, IL Zip 60617–9984; tel. 773/967–2000; Jonathan R. Bruss, President
**Web address:** www.advocatehealth.com/trinity

| | | |
|---|---|---|
| Owned, leased, sponsored: | 10 hospitals | 3026 beds |
| Contract–managed: | 0 hospitals | 0 beds |
| Totals: | 10 hospitals | 3026 beds |

**0312: AHMC & HEALTHCARE, INC.** (IO)
55 South Raymond Avenue, Suite 105, Alhambra, CA Zip 91801–7100; tel. 626/457–9600; Jonathan Wu, M.D., President and Chairman
**(Independent Hospital System)**

**CALIFORNIA:** ALHAMBRA HOSPITAL MEDICAL CENTER (O, 144 beds) 100 South Raymond Avenue, Alhambra, CA Zip 91801–3199, Mailing Address: P.O. Box 510, Zip 91802–0510; tel. 626/570–1606; Iris Lai, Chief Executive Officer
**Web address:** www.alhambrahospital.com

ANAHEIM REGIONAL MEDICAL CENTER (O, 223 beds) 1111 West La Palma Avenue, Anaheim, CA Zip 92801–2881; tel. 714/774–1450; Donald A. Lorack, Jr., Chief Executive Officer
**Web address:** www.anaheimregionalmc.com

GARFIELD MEDICAL CENTER (O, 210 beds) 525 North Garfield Avenue, Monterey Park, CA Zip 91754–1205; tel. 626/573–2222; David J. Batista, Chief Executive Officer
**Web address:** www.garfieldmedicalcenter.com

GREATER EL MONTE COMMUNITY HOSPITAL (O, 46 beds) 1701 Santa Anita Avenue, South El Monte, CA Zip 91733–3411; tel. 626/579–7777; Gale E. Gascho, Chief Executive Officer
**Web address:** www.greaterelmonte.com

MONTEREY PARK HOSPITAL (O, 101 beds) 900 South Atlantic Boulevard, Monterey Park, CA Zip 91754–4780; tel. 626/570–9000; Philip A. Cohen, Chief Executive Officer
**Web address:** www.montereyparkhosp.com

SAN GABRIEL VALLEY MEDICAL CENTER (O, 231 beds) 438 West Las Tunas Drive, San Gabriel, CA Zip 91776–1216, Mailing Address: P.O. Box 1507, Zip 91778–1507; tel. 626/289–5454; Michael Murray, Chief Executive Officer
**Web address:** www.sgvmc.org

WHITTIER HOSPITAL MEDICAL CENTER (O, 81 beds) 9080 Colima Road, Whittier, CA Zip 90605–1600; tel. 562/945–3561; Lee Suyenaga, Chief Executive Officer
**Web address:** www.whittierhospital.com

| | | |
|---|---|---|
| Owned, leased, sponsored: | 7 hospitals | 1036 beds |
| Contract–managed: | 0 hospitals | 0 beds |
| Totals: | 7 hospitals | 1036 beds |

**★0247: AKRON GENERAL HEALTH SYSTEM** (NP)
400 Wabash Avenue, Akron, OH Zip 44307–2433; tel. 330/344–6000; Thomas L. Stover, M.D., President and Chief Executive Officer
**(Moderately Centralized Health System)**

**OHIO:** AKRON GENERAL MEDICAL CENTER (O, 474 beds) 400 Wabash Avenue, Akron, OH Zip 44307–2433; tel. 330/344–6000; Alan Papa, President
**Web address:** www.akrongeneral.org

EDWIN SHAW REHAB (O, 38 beds) 330 Broadway Street East, Cuyahoga Falls, OH Zip 44221–3342; tel. 330/436–0910; Kim Strubel, Vice President
**Web address:** www.edwinshaw.com

LODI COMMUNITY HOSPITAL (O, 25 beds) 225 Elyria Street, Lodi, OH Zip 44254–1096; tel. 330/948–1222; Thomas Whelan, President
**Web address:** www.lodihospital.org

| | | |
|---|---|---|
| Owned, leased, sponsored: | 3 hospitals | 537 beds |
| Contract–managed: | 0 hospitals | 0 beds |
| Totals: | 3 hospitals | 537 beds |

**1685: ALBERT EINSTEIN HEALTHCARE NETWORK** (NP)
5501 Old York Road, Philadelphia, PA Zip 19141–3098; tel. 215/456–7890; Barry R. Freedman, President and Chief Executive Officer
**(Independent Hospital System)**

**PENNSYLVANIA:** BELMONT CENTER FOR COMPREHENSIVE TREATMENT (O, 147 beds) 4200 Monument Road, Philadelphia, PA Zip 19131–1625; tel. 215/877–2000; Sharon A. Bergen, Chief Operating Officer
**Web address:** www.einstein.edu

EINSTEIN MEDICAL CENTER PHILADELPHIA (O, 652 beds) 5501 Old York Road, Philadelphia, PA Zip 19141–3098; tel. 215/456–7890; Barry R. Freedman, President and Chief Executive Officer
**Web address:** www.einstein.edu

MONTGOMERY HOSPITAL MEDICAL CENTER (O, 177 beds) 1301 Powell Street, Norristown, PA Zip 19401–3377, Mailing Address: P.O. Box 992, Zip 19404–0992; tel. 610/270–2000; Timothy M. Casey, President and Chief Executive Officer
**Web address:** www.montgomeryhospital.org

| | | |
|---|---|---|
| Owned, leased, sponsored: | 3 hospitals | 976 beds |
| Contract–managed: | 0 hospitals | 0 beds |
| Totals: | 3 hospitals | 976 beds |

**0278: ALEGENT HEALTH** (CO)
12809 West Dodge Road, Omaha, NE Zip 68154; tel. 402/343–4000; Richard A. Hachten, II, FACHE, President and Chief Executive Officer
**(Moderately Centralized Health System)**

**IOWA:** ALEGENT HEALTH MERCY HOSPITAL (O, 22 beds) 603 Rosary Drive, Corning, IA Zip 50841–1685; tel. 641/322–3121; Debra Goldsmith, Chief Executive Officer
**Web address:** www.alegent.com

ALEGENT HEALTH–COMMUNITY MEMORIAL HOSPITAL (O, 16 beds) 631 North Eighth Street, Missouri Valley, IA Zip 51555–1199; tel. 712/642–2784; Robert A. Valentine, Regional Administrator
**Web address:** www.alegent.org

ALEGENT HEALTH–MERCY HOSPITAL (O, 163 beds) 800 Mercy Drive, Council Bluffs, IA Zip 51503–3128, Mailing Address: P.O. Box 1C, Zip 51502–3001; tel. 712/328–5000; Marie E. Knedler, R.N., Vice President and Chief Operating Officer
**Web address:** www.alegent.com/mercy

**NEBRASKA:** ALEGENT HEALTH MERCY CARE CENTER (O, 250 beds) 1870 South 75th Street, Omaha, NE Zip 68124; tel. 402/398–6800; Joyce Gibbs, Vice President

ALEGENT HEALTH PLAINVIEW HOSPITAL (O, 16 beds) 704 North Third Street, Plainview, NE Zip 68769, Mailing Address: P.O. Box 489, Zip 68769–0489; tel. 402/582–4245; Richard B. Gamel, Administrator
**Web address:** www.plainviewhealth.org

ALEGENT HEALTH–BERGAN MERCY MEDICAL CENTER (O, 320 beds) 7500 Mercy Road, Omaha, NE Zip 68124–2319; tel. 402/398–6060; Marie E. Knedler, R.N., Vice President and Chief Operating Officer
**Web address:** www.alegent.com/bergan

ALEGENT HEALTH–IMMANUEL MEDICAL CENTER (O, 285 beds) 6901 North 72nd Street, Omaha, NE Zip 68122–1799; tel. 402/572–2121; Ann Schumacher, MSN, R.N., Vice President and Chief Operating Officer
**Web address:** www.alegent.com/immanuel

For explanation of codes following names, see page B2.
★ Indicates Type III membership in the American Hospital Association.

ALEGENT HEALTH–LAKESIDE HOSPITAL (O, 160 beds) 16901 Lakeside Hills Court, Omaha, NE Zip 68130–2318; tel. 402/717–8000; Cindy Alloway, Vice President and Chief Operating Officer
**Web address:** www.alegent.org

ALEGENT HEALTH–MEMORIAL HOSPITAL (O, 25 beds) 104 West 17th Street, Schuyler, NE Zip 68661–1396; tel. 402/352–2441; Connie Peters, R.N., Operations Leader and Regional Health Administrator
**Web address:** www.alegent.org

ALEGENT HEALTH–MIDLANDS HOSPITAL (O, 54 beds) 11111 South 84th Street, Papillion, NE Zip 68046–4122; tel. 402/593–3000; Kevin J. Nokels, FACHE, Vice President and Chief Operating Officer
**Web address:** www.alegent.org/midlands

MEMORIAL COMMUNITY HOSPITAL AND HEALTH SYSTEM (O, 25 beds) 810 North 22nd Street, Blair, NE Zip 68008–1199, Mailing Address: P.O. Box 250, Zip 68008–0250; tel. 402/426–2182; Sally Harvey, R.N., Regional Administrator
**Web address:** www.mchhs.org

| | | |
|---|---|---|
| Owned, leased, sponsored: | 11 hospitals | 1336 beds |
| Contract–managed: | 0 hospitals | 0 beds |
| Totals: | 11 hospitals | 1336 beds |

---

**0065: ALEXIAN BROTHERS HEALTH SYSTEM** (CC)
3040 Salt Creek Lane, Arlington Heights, IL Zip 60005; tel. 847/463–8910; Mark A. Frey, President and Chief Executive Officer
**(Centralized Health System)**

| | | |
|---|---|---|
| Owned, leased, sponsored: | 0 hospitals | 0 beds |
| Contract–managed: | 0 hospitals | 0 beds |
| Totals: | 0 hospitals | 0 beds |

---

**0413: ALLEGIANCE HEALTH MANAGEMENT** (IO)
504 Texas Street, Suite 200, Shreveport, LA Zip 71101; tel. 318/226–8202; Rock Bordelon, President and Chief Executive Officer
**(Independent Hospital System)**

**ARKANSAS:** ALLEGIANCE SPECIALTY HOSPITAL OF LITTLE ROCK (O, 40 beds) 1400 Braden Street, Jacksonville, AR Zip 72076–3721; tel. 501/985–7026; Cindy Stafford, Chief Executive Officer
**Web address:** www.allegiancespecialtyhospitaloflr.com

RIVER VALLEY MEDICAL CENTER (O, 35 beds) 200 North Third Street, Dardanelle, AR Zip 72834–3802, Mailing Address: P.O. Box 578, Zip 72834–0578; tel. 479/229–4677; Jodi Love, R.N., Chief Executive Officer

**TEXAS:** ALLEGIANCE BEHAVIORAL HEALTH CENTER OF PLAINVIEW (O, 20 beds) 2601 Dimmit Road, 4th Floor, Plainview, TX Zip 79072; tel. 806/296–9191; Glenn G. Hoffman, MS, Chief Executive Officer
**Web address:** www.ahmgt.com

ALLEGIANCE SPECIALTY HOSPITAL OF KILGORE (O, 60 beds) 1612 South Henderson Boulevard, Kilgore, TX Zip 75662–3594; tel. 903/984–3505; Sherry Bustin, Chief Executive Officer
**Web address:** www.ahmgt.com

ALLEGIANCE SPECIALTY HOSPITAL PERMIAN BASIN (O, 48 beds) 207 Tradewinds Boulevard, Midland, TX Zip 79706–2807; tel. 432/699–3215; Cheryl Rayl, Chief Executive Officer
**Web address:** www.ahmgt.com

| | | |
|---|---|---|
| Owned, leased, sponsored: | 5 hospitals | 203 beds |
| Contract–managed: | 0 hospitals | 0 beds |
| Totals: | 5 hospitals | 203 beds |

---

**0317: ALLIANT MANAGEMENT SERVICES** (IO)
2650 Eastpoint Parkway, Suite 300, Louisville, KY Zip 40223–5135; tel. 502/992–3525; Timothy L. Jarm, President and Chief Executive Officer
**(Moderately Centralized Health System)**

**ILLINOIS:** FAIRFIELD MEMORIAL HOSPITAL (C, 55 beds) 303 N.W. 11th Street, Fairfield, IL Zip 62837–1203; tel. 618/842–2611; Katherine Bunting, Chief Executive Officer
**Web address:** www.fairfieldmemorial.org

FAYETTE COUNTY HOSPITAL (O, 110 beds) 650 West Taylor Street, Vandalia, IL Zip 62471–1296; tel. 618/283–1231; Gregory D. Starnes, Chief Executive Officer
**Web address:** www.fayettecountyhospital.org

FERRELL HOSPITAL (C, 25 beds) 1201 Pine Street, Eldorado, IL Zip 62930–1634; tel. 618/273–3361; Tom Barry, President and Chief Executive Officer
**Web address:** www.ferrellhosp.org

FRANKLIN HOSPITAL DISTRICT (C, 25 beds) 201 Bailey Lane, Benton, IL Zip 62812–1969; tel. 618/439–3161; Hervey E. Davis, Chief Executive Officer
**Web address:** www.franklinhospital.net

PARIS COMMUNITY HOSPITAL (C, 25 beds) 721 East Court Street, Paris, IL Zip 61944; tel. 217/465–4141; Randy Simmons, President and Chief Executive Officer
**Web address:** www.pariscommunityhospital.com

WABASH GENERAL HOSPITAL (C, 25 beds) 1418 College Drive, Mount Carmel, IL Zip 62863–2638; tel. 618/262–8621; Jay Purvis, Administrator
**Web address:** www.wabashgeneral.com

**INDIANA:** GIBSON GENERAL HOSPITAL (C, 70 beds) 1808 Sherman Drive, Princeton, IN Zip 47670–1043; tel. 812/385–3401; Emmett C. Schuster, President and Chief Executive Officer
**Web address:** www.gibsongeneral.com

PERRY COUNTY MEMORIAL HOSPITAL (C, 25 beds) 1 Hospital Road, Tell City, IN Zip 47586–0362; tel. 812/547–7011; Joseph A. Stuber, President and Chief Executive Officer
**Web address:** www.pchospital.org

WABASH COUNTY HOSPITAL (C, 50 beds) 710 North East Street, Wabash, IN Zip 46992–1924, Mailing Address: P.O. Box 548, Zip 46992–0548; tel. 260/563–3131; Marilyn J. Custer–Mitchell, President and Chief Executive Officer
**Web address:** www.wchospital.com

**KENTUCKY:** BRECKINRIDGE MEMORIAL HOSPITAL (C, 43 beds) 1011 Old Highway 60, Hardinsburg, KY Zip 40143–2597; tel. 270/756–7000; Michael W. Cooper, Chief Executive Officer
**Web address:** www.breckhealth.org

CARROLL COUNTY MEMORIAL HOSPITAL (C, 25 beds) 309 11th Street, Carrollton, KY Zip 41008–1400; tel. 502/732–4321; Kanute Rarey, Chief Executive Officer
**Web address:** www.ccmhosp.com

CAVERNA MEMORIAL HOSPITAL (C, 25 beds) 1501 South Dixie Street, Horse Cave, KY Zip 42749–1477; tel. 270/786–2191; Alan B. Alexander, Chief Executive Officer
**Web address:** www.cavernahospital.com

JAMES B. HAGGIN MEMORIAL HOSPITAL (C, 25 beds) 464 Linden Avenue, Harrodsburg, KY Zip 40330–1862; tel. 859/734–5441; Victoria L. Reed, R.N., FACHE, Chief Executive Officer
**Web address:** www.hagginhosp.org

LIVINGSTON HOSPITAL AND HEALTHCARE SERVICES (C, 25 beds) 131 Hospital Drive, Salem, KY Zip 42078–8043; tel. 270/988–2299; Mark A. Edwards, Chief Executive Officer
**Web address:** www.lhhs.org

MUHLENBERG COMMUNITY HOSPITAL (C, 105 beds) 440 Hopkinsville Street, Greenville, KY Zip 42345–1172, Mailing Address: P.O. Box 387, Zip 42345–0387; tel. 270/338–8000; John Countzler, Chief Executive Officer
**Web address:** www.mchky.org

RUSSELL COUNTY HOSPITAL (C, 25 beds) 153 Dowell Road, Russell Springs, KY Zip 42642–4236, Mailing Address: P.O. Box 1610, Zip 42642–1610; tel. 270/866–4141; David D. Rasmussen, Chief Executive Officer
**Web address:** www.russellcohospital.org

TWIN LAKES REGIONAL MEDICAL CENTER (C, 75 beds) 910 Wallace Avenue, Leitchfield, KY Zip 42754–1499; tel. 270/259–9400; Stephen L. Meredith, Chief Executive Officer
**Web address:** www.tlrmc.com

---

For explanation of codes following names, see page B2.
★ Indicates Type III membership in the American Hospital Association.

© 2012 AHA Guide

**NORTH CAROLINA:** HUGH CHATHAM MEMORIAL HOSPITAL (C, 208 beds) 180 Parkwood Drive, Elkin, NC Zip 28621–0560, Mailing Address: P.O. Box 560, Zip 28621–0560; tel. 336/527–7000; David Loving, Chief Executive Officer
**Web address:** www.hughchatham.org

**TENNESSEE:** PATIENTS' CHOICE MEDICAL CENTER OF ERIN (C, 25 beds) 5001 East Main Street, Erin, TN Zip 37061–0489, Mailing Address: P.O. Box 489, Zip 37061–0489; tel. 931/289–4211; Gladys Anderson, Interim CEO
**Web address:** www.pcmc–erintn.com/

| | | |
|---|---|---|
| Owned, leased, sponsored: | 1 hospital | 110 beds |
| Contract–managed: | 18 hospitals | 881 beds |
| Totals: | 19 hospitals | 991 beds |

---

**★0041: ALLINA HEALTH** (NP)
2925 Chicago Avenue, Minneapolis, MN Zip 55407, Mailing Address: P.O. Box 43, Zip 55440; tel. 612/262–5000; Ken Paulus, President and Chief Executive Officer
**(Moderately Centralized Health System)**

**MINNESOTA:** ABBOTT NORTHWESTERN HOSPITAL (O, 649 beds) 800 East 28th Street, Minneapolis, MN Zip 55407–3799; tel. 612/863–4000; Ben Bache-Wiig, M.D., President
**Web address:** www.abbottnorthwestern.com

BUFFALO HOSPITAL (O, 44 beds) 303 Catlin Street, Buffalo, MN Zip 55313–1947; tel. 763/682–1212; Jennifer Myster, President
**Web address:** www.buffalohospital.org

CAMBRIDGE MEDICAL CENTER (O, 78 beds) 701 South Dellwood Street, Cambridge, MN Zip 55008–1920; tel. 763/689–7700; Dennis J. Doran, President
**Web address:** www.allina.com/ahs/cambridge.nsf

HUTCHINSON AREA HEALTH CARE (C, 177 beds) 1095 Highway 15 South, Hutchinson, MN Zip 55350–3182; tel. 320/234–5000; Steven Mulder, M.D., President and Chief Executive Officer
**Web address:** www.hahc–hmc.com

MERCY HOSPITAL (O, 251 beds) 4050 Coon Rapids Boulevard, Coon Rapids, MN Zip 55433–2586; tel. 763/236–6000; Sara J. Criger, President
**Web address:** www.allinamercy.org

NEW ULM MEDICAL CENTER (O, 45 beds) 1324 Fifth Street North, New Ulm, MN Zip 56073–1553; tel. 507/217–5000; Toby Freier, President
**Web address:** www.newulmmedicalcenter.com

OWATONNA HOSPITAL (O, 43 beds) 2250 N.W. 26th Street, Owatonna, MN Zip 55060–5503; tel. 507/451–3850; David L. Albrecht, President
**Web address:** www.owatonnahospital.com

PHILLIPS EYE INSTITUTE (O, 8 beds) 2215 Park Avenue, Minneapolis, MN Zip 55404–3756; tel. 612/775–8800; Joan M. Arbach, Interim President
**Web address:** www.allina.com

ST. FRANCIS REGIONAL MEDICAL CENTER (C, 86 beds) 1455 St. Francis Avenue, Shakopee, MN Zip 55379–3380; tel. 952/428–3000; Michael A. Baumgartner, President
**Web address:** www.stfrancis–shakopee.com

UNITED HOSPITAL (O, 398 beds) 333 North Smith Avenue, Saint Paul, MN Zip 55102–2389; tel. 651/241–8000; Thomas O'Connor, President
**Web address:** www.allina.com

UNITY HOSPITAL (O, 220 beds) 550 Osborne Road N.E., Fridley, MN Zip 55432–2799; tel. 763/236–5000; Lori Wightman, R.N., MSN, FACHE, President
**Web address:** www.allina.com

**WISCONSIN:** RIVER FALLS AREA HOSPITAL (O, 25 beds) 1629 East Division Street, River Falls, WI Zip 54022–1571; tel. 715/425–6155; David R. Miller, President
**Web address:** www.allina.com

| | | |
|---|---|---|
| Owned, leased, sponsored: | 10 hospitals | 1761 beds |
| Contract–managed: | 2 hospitals | 263 beds |
| Totals: | 12 hospitals | 2024 beds |

**0187: ALTA HEALTHCARE SYSTEM** (IO)
10780 Santa Monica Boulevard, Suite 400, Los Angeles, CA Zip 90025–7616; tel. 310/943–4500; David Topper, Chief Executive Officer

**CALIFORNIA:** HOLLYWOOD COMMUNITY HOSPITAL (O, 45 beds) 6245 De Longpre Avenue, Los Angeles, CA Zip 90028–9001; tel. 323/462–2271; Michael Sarian, Chief Executive Officer
**Web address:** www.hollywoodcommunityhospital.com

LOS ANGELES COMMUNITY HOSPITAL (O, 180 beds) 4081 East Olympic Boulevard, Los Angeles, CA Zip 90023–3330; tel. 323/267–0477; Al Souza, Chief Executive Officer

| | | |
|---|---|---|
| Owned, leased, sponsored: | 2 hospitals | 225 beds |
| Contract–managed: | 0 hospitals | 0 beds |
| Totals: | 2 hospitals | 225 beds |

---

**2295: AMERICAN PROVINCE OF LITTLE COMPANY OF MARY SISTERS** (CC)
9350 South California Avenue, Evergreen Park, IL Zip 60805–2595; tel. 708/229–5491; Sister Kathleen McIntyre, Province Leader
**(Moderately Centralized Health System)**

**ILLINOIS:** LITTLE COMPANY OF MARY HOSPITAL AND HEALTH CARE CENTERS (O, 298 beds) 2800 West 95th Street, Evergreen Park, IL Zip 60805–2795; tel. 708/422–6200; Dennis A. Reilly, President and Chief Executive Officer
**Web address:** www.lcmh.org

**INDIANA:** MEMORIAL HOSPITAL AND HEALTH CARE CENTER (O, 135 beds) 800 West Ninth Street, Jasper, IN Zip 47546–2516; tel. 812/996–2345; Raymond W. Snowden, President and Chief Executive Officer
**Web address:** www.mhhcc.org

| | | |
|---|---|---|
| Owned, leased, sponsored: | 2 hospitals | 433 beds |
| Contract–managed: | 0 hospitals | 0 beds |
| Totals: | 2 hospitals | 433 beds |

---

**0644: AMG INTEGRATED HEALTHCARE MANAGEMENT** (IO)
101 La Rue France, Suite 500, Lafayette, LA Zip 70508–3144; tel. 337/269–9828; August J. Rantz, III, Founder and Chief Executive Officer
**(Independent Hospital System)**

**KANSAS:** LTAC OF WICHITA (O, 26 beds) 8080 East Pawnee Street, Wichita, KS Zip 67207–5475; tel. 316/682–0004; William Wild, Chief Executive Officer

**LOUISIANA:** AMG SPECIALTY HOSPITAL – LAFAYETTE (O, 58 beds) 310 Youngsville Highway, Lafayette, LA Zip 70508; tel. 337/839–9880; Jason Branson, Chief Executive Officer
**Web address:** www.amglafayette.com

AMG SPECIALTY HOSPITAL–DENHAM SPRINGS (O, 117 beds) 8375 Florida Boulevard, Denham Springs, LA Zip 70726; tel. 225/665–2664; Ricky Robeson, Administrator
**Web address:** www.amgihm.com/ltac_of_denham_springs

AMG SPECIALTY HOSPITAL–FELICIANA (O, 16 beds) 9725 Grace Lane, Clinton, LA Zip 70722; tel. 225/683–1600; Karen Crayton, Chief Executive Officer
**Web address:** www.amgihm.com/ltac_of_feliciana

AMG SPECIALTY HOSPITAL–HOUMA (O, 40 beds) 629 Dunn Street, Houma, LA Zip 70360–4707; tel. 985/274–0001; Ricky Robeson, Chief Executive Officer

AMG SPECIALTY HOSPITAL–SLIDELL (O, 40 beds) 1400 Lindberg Drive, Slidell, LA Zip 70458–8056; tel. 985/326–0440; Richard Daughdrill, R.N., Chief Executive Officer
**Web address:** www.acadianamanagementgroup.com

LAFAYETTE PHYSICAL REHABILITATION HOSPITAL (O, 32 beds) 307 Polly Lane, Lafayette, LA Zip 70508–4960; tel. 337/314–1111; Jonathan Landreth, Chief Executive Officer

NEUROMEDICAL CENTER REHABILITATION HOSPITAL (O, 23 beds) 10101 Park Rowe Avenue, Suite 500, Baton Rouge, LA Zip 70810; tel. 225/906–2999; Jay Ivy, R.N., Chief Executive Officer
**Web address:** www.theneuromedicalcenter.com

For explanation of codes following names, see page B2.
★ Indicates Type III membership in the American Hospital Association.

**MISSISSIPPI:** LTAC HOSPITAL OF GREENWOOD (O, 40 beds) 1401 River Road Floor 2, Greenwood, MS Zip 38930–4030; tel. 662/459–2681; Tommy Strohe, Interim Chief Executive Officer
**Web address:** www.amgihm.com/ltac_of_greenwood

**OKLAHOMA:** LTAC OF EDMOND (O, 37 beds) 1100 East Ninth Street, Edmond, OK Zip 73034–5755; tel. 405/341–8150; Ginger Creech, Chief Executive Officer
**Web address:** www.amgihm.com

| | | |
|---|---|---|
| Owned, leased, sponsored: | 10 hospitals | 429 beds |
| Contract–managed: | 0 hospitals | 0 beds |
| Totals: | 10 hospitals | 429 beds |

---

● **0389: ANMED HEALTH** (NP)
800 North Fant Street, Anderson, SC Zip 29621–5793; tel. 864/512–1000; John A. Miller, Jr., FACHE, Chief Executive Officer
**(Moderately Centralized Health System)**

**SOUTH CAROLINA:** ANMED HEALTH MEDICAL CENTER (O, 382 beds) 800 North Fant Street, Anderson, SC Zip 29621–5793; tel. 864/512–1000; John A. Miller, Jr., FACHE, Chief Executive Officer
**Web address:** www.anmedhealth.org

| | | |
|---|---|---|
| Owned, leased, sponsored: | 1 hospital | 382 beds |
| Contract–managed: | 0 hospitals | 0 beds |
| Totals: | 1 hospital | 382 beds |

---

★ **0866: APPALACHIAN REGIONAL HEALTHCARE SYSTEM** (NP)
336 Deerfield Road, Boone, NC Zip 28607–5008, Mailing Address: P.O. Box 2600, Zip 28607–2600; tel. 828/262–4100; Richard G. Sparks, President and Chief Executive Officer

**NORTH CAROLINA:** BLOWING ROCK HOSPITAL (C, 97 beds) 418 Chestnut Street, Blowing Rock, NC Zip 28605–0148, Mailing Address: P.O. Box 148, Zip 28605–0148; tel. 828/295–3136; Timothy R. Ford, Chief Executive Officer
**Web address:** www.apprhs.org

CHARLES A. CANNON MEMORIAL HOSPITAL (C, 35 beds) 434 Hospital Drive, Linville, NC Zip 28646, Mailing Address: P.O. Box 767, Zip 28646; tel. 828/737–7000; Carmen Lacey, MSN, R.N., President
**Web address:** www.apprhs.org

WATAUGA MEDICAL CENTER (C, 99 beds) 336 Deerfield Road, Boone, NC Zip 28607–5008, Mailing Address: P.O. Box 2600, Zip 28607–2600; tel. 828/262–4100; Chuck Mantooth, President
**Web address:** www.apprhs.org

| | | |
|---|---|---|
| Owned, leased, sponsored: | 0 hospitals | 0 beds |
| Contract–managed: | 3 hospitals | 231 beds |
| Totals: | 3 hospitals | 231 beds |

---

**0145: APPALACHIAN REGIONAL HEALTHCARE, INC.** (NP)
2285 Executive Drive, Suite 400, Lexington, KY Zip 40505–4810, Mailing Address: P.O. Box 8086, Zip 40533–8086; tel. 859/226–2440; Jerry Haynes, President and Chief Executive Officer
**(Decentralized Health System)**

**KENTUCKY:** HARLAN ARH HOSPITAL (O, 137 beds) 81 Ball Park Road, Harlan, KY Zip 40831–1792; tel. 606/573–8100; Dan Stone, Community Chief Executive Officer
**Web address:** www.arh.org

HAZARD ARH REGIONAL MEDICAL CENTER (O, 308 beds) 100 Medical Center Drive, Hazard, KY Zip 41701–1000; tel. 606/439–6600; Donald R. Fields, Senior Community Chief Executive Officer
**Web address:** www.arh.org

MARY BRECKINRIDGE ARH HOSPITAL (O, 25 beds) 130 Kate Ireland Drive, Hyden, KY Zip 41749–0000, Mailing Address: P.O. Box 447–A, Zip 41749–0000; tel. 606/672–2901; Mallie S. Noble, Administrator
**Web address:** www.frontiernursing.org

MCDOWELL ARH HOSPITAL (O, 25 beds) Route 122, McDowell, KY Zip 41647, Mailing Address: P.O. Box 247, Zip 41647–0247; tel. 606/377–3400; Russell Barker, Community Chief Executive Officer
**Web address:** www.arh.org

MIDDLESBORO ARH HOSPITAL (O, 96 beds) 3600 West Cumberland Avenue, Middlesboro, KY Zip 40965–2614, Mailing Address: P.O. Box 340, Zip 40965–0340; tel. 606/242–1100; Michael Slusher, Community Chief Executive Officer
**Web address:** www.arh.org/middlesboro

MORGAN COUNTY ARH HOSPITAL (L, 25 beds) 476 Liberty Road, West Liberty, KY Zip 41472–2049, Mailing Address: P.O. Box 579, Zip 41472–0579; tel. 606/743–3186; Stephen M. Gavalchik, FACHE, Community Chief Executive Officer
**Web address:** www.arh.org

WHITESBURG ARH HOSPITAL (O, 82 beds) 240 Hospital Road, Whitesburg, KY Zip 41858–1254; tel. 606/633–3600; Dena C. Sparkman, FACHE, Community Chief Executive Officer
**Web address:** www.arh.org/whitesburg

WILLIAMSON ARH HOSPITAL (O, 123 beds) 260 Hospital Drive, South Williamson, KY Zip 41503–4072; tel. 606/237–1710; Timothy A. Hatfield, Community Chief Executive Officer
**Web address:** www.arh.org

**WEST VIRGINIA:** BECKLEY ARH HOSPITAL (O, 167 beds) 306 Stanaford Road, Beckley, WV Zip 25801–3142; tel. 304/255–3000; Rocco K. Massey, Community Chief Executive Officer
**Web address:** www.arh.org

SUMMERS COUNTY ARH HOSPITAL (L, 61 beds) Terrace Street, Hinton, WV Zip 25951–2407, Mailing Address: Drawer 940, Zip 25951–0940; tel. 304/466–1000; Wesley Dangerfield, Community Chief Executive Officer
**Web address:** www.arh.org

| | | |
|---|---|---|
| Owned, leased, sponsored: | 10 hospitals | 1049 beds |
| Contract–managed: | 0 hospitals | 0 beds |
| Totals: | 10 hospitals | 1049 beds |

---

★ **0104: ARCHBOLD MEDICAL CENTER** (NP)
910 South Broad Street, Thomasville, GA Zip 31792–6113; tel. 229/228–2739; J. Perry Mustian, President
**(Moderately Centralized Health System)**

**GEORGIA:** BROOKS COUNTY HOSPITAL (L, 25 beds) 903 North Court Street, Quitman, GA Zip 31643–1315, Mailing Address: P.O. Box 5000, Zip 31643–5000; tel. 229/263–4171; Kenneth D. Rhudy, Chief Executive Officer
**Web address:** www.archbold.org

GRADY GENERAL HOSPITAL (L, 48 beds) 1155 Fifth Street S.E., Cairo, GA Zip 39828–0360, Mailing Address: P.O. Box 360, Zip 39828–0360; tel. 229/377–1150; LaDon Toole, Chief Operating Officer and Administrator
**Web address:** www.archbold.org

JOHN D. ARCHBOLD MEMORIAL HOSPITAL (O, 328 beds) 915 Gordon Avenue, Thomasville, GA Zip 31792–6614, Mailing Address: P.O. Box 1018, Zip 31799–1018; tel. 229/228–2000; J. Perry Mustian, President and Chief Executive Officer
**Web address:** www.archbold.org

MITCHELL COUNTY HOSPITAL (L, 181 beds) 90 East Stephens Street, Camilla, GA Zip 31730–1836, Mailing Address: P.O. Box 639, Zip 31730–0639; tel. 229/336–5284; Mark E. Kimball, Administrator
**Web address:** www.archbold.org

| | | |
|---|---|---|
| Owned, leased, sponsored: | 4 hospitals | 582 beds |
| Contract–managed: | 0 hospitals | 0 beds |
| Totals: | 4 hospitals | 582 beds |

---

★ **0069: ARDENT HEALTH SERVICES** (IO)
1 Burton Hills Boulevard, Suite 250, Nashville, TN Zip 37215; tel. 615/296–3000; David T. Vandewater, President and Chief Executive Officer
**(Moderately Centralized Health System)**

---

For explanation of codes following names, see page B2.
★ Indicates Type III membership in the American Hospital Association.
● Single hospital health care system

**NEW MEXICO:** LOVELACE MEDICAL CENTER (O, 263 beds) 601 Martin Luther King Avenue N.E., Albuquerque, NM Zip 87102–3670; tel. 505/727–8000; David S. Nevill, Chief Executive Officer
**Web address:** www.lovelace.com

LOVELACE REHABILITATION HOSPITAL (O, 80 beds) 505 Elm Street N.E., Albuquerque, NM Zip 87102–2500; tel. 505/727–4700; Traci Willis, Chief Executive Officer
**Web address:** www.lovelace.com

LOVELACE WESTSIDE HOSPITAL (O, 80 beds) 10501 Golf Course Road N.W., Albuquerque, NM Zip 87114–5000, Mailing Address: P.O. Box 25555, Zip 87125–0555; tel. 505/727–2000; Troy Greer, Chief Executive Officer
**Web address:** www.lovelacesandia.com

LOVELACE WOMEN'S HOSPITAL (O, 120 beds) 4701 Montgomery Boulevard N.E., Albuquerque, NM Zip 87109–1251, Mailing Address: P.O. Box 25555, Zip 87125–0555; tel. 505/727–7800; Sheri Milone, Chief Executive Officer and Administrator
**Web address:** www.lovelace.com

ROSWELL REGIONAL HOSPITAL (O, 26 beds) 117 East 19th Street, Roswell, NM Zip 88201; tel. 575/627–7000; Rod Schumacher, Chief Executive Officer
**Web address:** www.roswellregional.com

**OKLAHOMA:** BAILEY MEDICAL CENTER (O, 37 beds) 10502 North 110th East Avenue, Owasso, OK Zip 74055; tel. 918/376–8000; Keith Mason, Chief Executive Officer
**Web address:** www.baileymedicalcenter.com

CUSHING REGIONAL HOSPITAL (O, 95 beds) 1027 East Cherry Street, Cushing, OK Zip 74023–4101, Mailing Address: P.O. Box 1409, Zip 74023–1409; tel. 918/225–2915; Randy DuBois, Chief Executive Officer
**Web address:** www.hillcrest.com

HENRYETTA MEDICAL CENTER (O, 41 beds) Dewey Bartlett & Main Streets, Henryetta, OK Zip 74437–6820, Mailing Address: P.O. Box 1269, Zip 74437–1269; tel. 918/650–1100; Dee Renshaw, Chief Executive Officer
**Web address:** www.henryettamedicalcenter.com

HILLCREST HOSPITAL CLAREMORE (O, 89 beds) 1202 North Muskogee Place, Claremore, OK Zip 74017–3036; tel. 918/341–2556; David Chaussard, Chief Executive Officer
**Web address:** www.hillcrestclaremore.com

HILLCREST MEDICAL CENTER (O, 537 beds) 1120 South Utica, Tulsa, OK Zip 74104–4090; tel. 918/579–1000; Jason Fahrlander, FACHE, Chief Executive Officer
**Web address:** www.hillcrest.com

SOUTHCREST HOSPITAL (O, 160 beds) 8801 South 101st East Avenue, Tulsa, OK Zip 74133–5716; tel. 918/294–4000; Joseph H. Neely, FACHE, Chief Executive Officer
**Web address:** www.southcresthospital.com

| | | |
|---|---|---|
| Owned, leased, sponsored: | 11 hospitals | 1528 beds |
| Contract–managed: | 0 hospitals | 0 beds |
| Totals: | 11 hospitals | 1528 beds |

---

**★0809:  ARNOT HEALTH** (NP)
600 Roe Avenue, Elmira, NY Zip 14905–1629; tel. 607/737–4100; Anthony J. Cooper, FACHE, President and Chief Executive Officer
**(Independent Hospital System)**

**NEW YORK:** ARNOT OGDEN MEDICAL CENTER (O, 244 beds) 600 Roe Avenue, Elmira, NY Zip 14905–1629; tel. 607/737–4100; H. Fred Farley, R.N., Ph.D., FACHE, President and Chief Operating Officer
**Web address:** www.aomc.org

IRA DAVENPORT MEMORIAL HOSPITAL (O, 156 beds) 7571 State Route 54, Bath, NY Zip 14810–9590; tel. 607/776–8500; James B. Watson, Chief Executive Officer
**Web address:** www.davenportandtaylor.org

ST. JOSEPH'S HOSPITAL (O, 212 beds) 555 St. Joseph's Boulevard, Elmira, NY Zip 14901–3223; tel. 607/733–6541; H. Fred Farley, R.N., Ph.D., FACHE, President and Chief Operating Officer
**Web address:** www.stjosephs.org

| | | |
|---|---|---|
| Owned, leased, sponsored: | 3 hospitals | 612 beds |
| Contract–managed: | 0 hospitals | 0 beds |
| Totals: | 3 hospitals | 612 beds |

---

**★0094:  ASANTE HEALTH SYSTEM** (NP)
2650 Siskiyou Boulevard, Suite 200, Medford, OR Zip 97504–8170; tel. 541/789–4100; Roy G. Vinyard, FACHE, President and Chief Executive Officer
**(Moderately Centralized Health System)**

**OREGON:** ROGUE VALLEY MEDICAL CENTER (O, 307 beds) 2825 East Barnett Road, Medford, OR Zip 97504–8332; tel. 541/789–7000; Scott A. Kelly, Chief Executive Officer
**Web address:** www.asante.org

THREE RIVERS MEDICAL CENTER (O, 107 beds) 500 S.W. Ramsey Avenue, Grants Pass, OR Zip 97527; tel. 541/472–7000; Win Howard, Chief Executive Officer
**Web address:** www.asante.org

| | | |
|---|---|---|
| Owned, leased, sponsored: | 2 hospitals | 414 beds |
| Contract–managed: | 0 hospitals | 0 beds |
| Totals: | 2 hospitals | 414 beds |

---

**0638:  ASCEND HEALTH CORPORATION** (IO)
32 East 57th Street, 17th Floor, New York, NY Zip 10022–2513; Richard A. Kresch, M.D., President and Chief Executive Officer
**(Independent Hospital System)**

**ARIZONA:** VALLEY HOSPITAL PHOENIX (O, 122 beds) 3550 East Pinchot Avenue, Phoenix, AZ Zip 85018–7434; tel. 602/957–4000; Kim Whitelock, Chief Executive Officer
**Web address:** www.valleyhospital–phoenix.com

**OREGON:** CEDAR HILLS HOSPITAL (O, 78 beds) 10300 S.W. Eastridge Street, Portland, OR Zip 97225–5004; tel. 503/944–5000; Michael Sherbun, Ph.D., Chief Executive Officer
**Web address:** www.cedarhillshospital.com

**TEXAS:** BEHAVIORAL HOSPITAL OF BELLAIRE (O, 70 beds) 5314 Dashwood Drive, Houston, TX Zip 77081–4603; tel. 713/600–9500; Lawrence Story, Chief Executive Officer
**Web address:** www.bhbhospital.com

MAYHILL HOSPITAL (O, 59 beds) 2809 South Mayhill Road, Denton, TX Zip 76208–5910; tel. 940/239–3000; Susan M. Young, Chief Executive Officer
**Web address:** www.mayhillhospital.com

UNIVERSITY BEHAVIORAL HEALTH OF DENTON (O, 104 beds) 2026 West University Drive, Denton, TX Zip 76201–0644; tel. 940/320–8100; Susan M. Young, Chief Executive Officer
**Web address:** www.ubhdenton.net

UNIVERSITY BEHAVIORAL HEALTH OF EL PASO (O, 163 beds) 1900 Denver Avenue, El Paso, TX Zip 79902–3008; tel. 915/544–4000; Selene Quintana–Hammon, Chief Executive Officer
**Web address:** www.ubhelpaso.com/

**UTAH:** SALT LAKE BEHAVIORAL HEALTH (O, 118 beds) 3802 South 700 East, Salt Lake City, UT Zip 84106–1182; tel. 801/264–6000; Michael Rowley, Chief Executive Officer
**Web address:** www.saltlakebehavioralhealth.com

| | | |
|---|---|---|
| Owned, leased, sponsored: | 7 hospitals | 714 beds |
| Contract–managed: | 0 hospitals | 0 beds |
| Totals: | 7 hospitals | 714 beds |

---

**★0198:  ASCENSION HEALTH** (CC)
4600 Edmundson Road, Saint Louis, MO Zip 63134–3806; tel. 314/733–8000; Robert J. Henkel, FACHE, President and Chief Executive Officer
**(Decentralized Health System)**

**ALABAMA:** PROVIDENCE HOSPITAL (S, 349 beds) 6801 Airport Boulevard, Mobile, AL Zip 36608–3785, Mailing Address: P.O. Box 850429, Zip 36685–0429; tel. 251/633–1000; Clark P. Christianson, President and Chief Executive Officer
**Web address:** www.providencehospital.org

ST. VINCENT'S BIRMINGHAM (S, 439 beds) 810 St. Vincent's Drive, Birmingham, AL Zip 35205–1695, Mailing Address: P.O. Box 12407, Zip 35202–2407; tel. 205/939–7000; Andy Davis, President
**Web address:** www.stvhs.com

Section B

ST. VINCENT'S BLOUNT (S, 40 beds) 150 Gilbreath, Oneonta, AL Zip 35121–2534, Mailing Address: P.O. Box 1000, Zip 35121–1000; tel. 205/274–3000; Kidada Hawkins, Interim President and Chief Operating Officer
**Web address:** www.stvhs.com

ST. VINCENT'S EAST (S, 336 beds) 50 Medical Park East Drive, Birmingham, AL Zip 35235–9987; tel. 205/838–3000; Sean Tinney, FACHE, President and Chief Operating Officer
**Web address:** www.stvhs.com

ST. VINCENT'S ST. CLAIR (S, 36 beds) 2805 Doctor John Haynes Drive, Pell City, AL Zip 35125–1499; tel. 205/338–3301; Kidada Hawkins, Interim President and Chief Operating Officer
**Web address:** www.stvhs.com

**ARIZONA:** CARONDELET HEART & VASCULAR INSTITUTE (S, 58 beds) 4888 North Stone Avenue, Tucson, AZ Zip 85704; tel. 520/696–2365; Carol Erenberger, Site Administrator
**Web address:** www.carondelet.org

CARONDELET HOLY CROSS HOSPITAL (S, 56 beds) 1171 West Target Range Road, Nogales, AZ Zip 85621–2496; tel. 520/285–3000; Debbie Knapheide, MSN, Site Administrator, Chief Nursing Officer and Chief Operating Officer
**Web address:** www.carondelet.org

CARONDELET ST. JOSEPH'S HOSPITAL (S, 449 beds) 350 North Wilmot Road, Tucson, AZ Zip 85711–2678; tel. 520/296–3211; Mary Henrikson, Chief Executive Officer
**Web address:** www.carondelet.org

CARONDELET ST. MARY'S HOSPITAL (S, 429 beds) 1601 West St. Mary's Road, Tucson, AZ Zip 85745–2682; tel. 520/872–3000; Dorothy Sawyer, Chief Executive Officer
**Web address:** www.carondelet.org

**CONNECTICUT:** ST. VINCENT'S MEDICAL CENTER (S, 396 beds) 2800 Main Street, Bridgeport, CT Zip 06606–4292; tel. 203/576–5454; Susan L. Davis, R.N., Ed.D., FACHE, President and Chief Executive Officer
**Web address:** www.stvincents.org

**DISTRICT OF COLUMBIA:** PROVIDENCE HOSPITAL (S, 506 beds) 1150 Varnum Street N.E., Washington, DC Zip 20017–2104; tel. 202/269–7000; Amy E. Freeman, President and Chief Executive Officer
**Web address:** www.provhosp.org

**FLORIDA:** SACRED HEART HOSPITAL OF PENSACOLA (S, 458 beds) 5151 North Ninth Avenue, Pensacola, FL Zip 32504–8795, Mailing Address: P.O. Box 2700, Zip 32513–2700; tel. 850/416–7000; Susan L. Davis, R.N., Ed.D., FACHE, President and Chief Executive Officer
**Web address:** www.sacred–heart.org

SACRED HEART HOSPITAL ON THE EMERALD COAST (S, 58 beds) 7800 Highway 98 West, Miramar Beach, FL Zip 32550; tel. 850/278–3000; Roger L. Hall, President
**Web address:** www.sacredheartemerald.org

SACRED HEART HOSPITAL ON THE GULF (S, 25 beds) 3801 East Highway 98, Port St. Joe, FL Zip 32456–5318; tel. 850/229–5600; Roger L. Hall, President
**Web address:** www.sacred–heart.org/gulf/

ST. VINCENT'S MEDICAL CENTER RIVERSIDE (S, 501 beds) 1 Shircliff Way, Jacksonville, FL Zip 32204–2982, Mailing Address: P.O. Box 2982, Zip 32203–2982; tel. 904/308–7300; Moody L. Chisholm, President & Chief Executive Officer
**Web address:** www.jaxhealth.com

ST. VINCENT'S MEDICAL CENTER SOUTHSIDE (S, 221 beds) 4201 Belfort Road, Jacksonville, FL Zip 32216; tel. 904/296–3700; Moody L. Chisholm, President and Chief Executive Officer
**Web address:** www.jaxhealth.com

**IDAHO:** ST. JOSEPH REGIONAL MEDICAL CENTER (S, 136 beds) 415 Sixth Street, Lewiston, ID Zip 83501–0816; tel. 208/743–2511; Timothy Sayler, President and Chief Executive Officer
**Web address:** www.sjrmc.org

**ILLINOIS:** ALEXIAN BROTHERS BEHAVIORAL HEALTH HOSPITAL (O, 141 beds) 1650 Moon Lake Boulevard, Hoffman Estates, IL Zip 60194–5000; tel. 847/882–1600; Clayton Ciha, President and Chief Executive Officer
**Web address:** www.abbhh.org

ALEXIAN BROTHERS MEDICAL CENTER (O, 370 beds) 800 Biesterfield Road, Elk Grove Village, IL Zip 60007–3397; tel. 847/437–5500; John P. Werrbach, Chief Executive Officer
**Web address:** www.alexian.org

ST. ALEXIUS MEDICAL CENTER (O, 305 beds) 1555 Barrington Road, Hoffman Estates, IL Zip 60169–1019; tel. 847/843–2000; Edward M. Goldberg, President and Chief Executive Officer
**Web address:** www.stalexius.org

**INDIANA:** SAINT JOHN'S HEALTH SYSTEM (S, 185 beds) 2015 Jackson Street, Anderson, IN Zip 46016–4339; tel. 765/649–2511; Thomas J. VanOsdol, President
**Web address:** www.saintjohns.stvincent.org

ST. JOSEPH HOSPITAL AND HEALTH CENTER (S, 137 beds) 1907 West Sycamore Street, Kokomo, IN Zip 46901–4197, Mailing Address: P.O. Box 9010, Zip 46904–9010; tel. 765/452–5611; Kathlene A. Young, MS, FACHE, President and Chief Executive Officer
**Web address:** www.stjoseph.stvincent.org

ST. MARY'S WARRICK HOSPITAL (S, 35 beds) 1116 Millis Avenue, Boonville, IN Zip 47601–0629; tel. 812/897–4800; Carol Godsey, Administrator
**Web address:** www.stmarys.org/warrick

ST. MARY'S MEDICAL CENTER OF EVANSVILLE (S, 430 beds) 3700 Washington Avenue, Evansville, IN Zip 47750–0002; tel. 812/485–4000; Timothy A. Flesch, President and Chief Executive Officer
**Web address:** www.stmarys.org

ST. VINCENT CARMEL HOSPITAL (S, 104 beds) 13500 North Meridian Street, Carmel, IN Zip 46032; tel. 317/582–7000; Michael D. Chittenden, President
**Web address:** www.stvincent.org

ST. VINCENT CLAY HOSPITAL (S, 25 beds) 1206 East National Avenue, Brazil, IN Zip 47834–2797, Mailing Address: P.O. Box 489, Zip 47834–0489; tel. 812/442–2500; Jerry Laue, Administrator
**Web address:** www.stvincent.org

ST. VINCENT DUNN HOSPITAL (S, 25 beds) 1600 23rd Street, Bedford, IN Zip 47421–4704; tel. 812/275–3331; Deborah Bruner, Chief Executive Officer
**Web address:** www.stvincent.org/st–vincent–dunn

ST. VINCENT FRANKFORT HOSPITAL (S, 25 beds) 1300 South Jackson Street, Frankfort, IN Zip 46041–3394, Mailing Address: P.O. Box 669, Zip 46041–0669; tel. 765/656–3000; Thomas Crawford, Administrator
**Web address:** www.stvincent.org

ST. VINCENT HEART CENTER OF INDIANA (S, 107 beds) 10580 North Meridian Street, Indianapolis, IN Zip 46290; tel. 317/583–5000; Blake A. Dye, President
**Web address:** www.theheartcenter.com

ST. VINCENT INDIANAPOLIS HOSPITAL (S, 873 beds) 2001 West 86th Street, Indianapolis, IN Zip 46260–1991, Mailing Address: P.O. Box 40970, Zip 46240–0970; tel. 317/338–2345; Kyle De Fur, FACHE, President
**Web address:** www.stvincent.org

ST. VINCENT JENNINGS HOSPITAL (S, 25 beds) 301 Henry Street, North Vernon, IN Zip 47265–1097; tel. 812/352–4200; Carl W. Risk, II, Administrator
**Web address:** www.stvincent.org

ST. VINCENT MERCY HOSPITAL (S, 25 beds) 1331 South A Street, Elwood, IN Zip 46036–1942; tel. 765/552–4600; Deborah Y. Rasper, FACHE, Administrator
**Web address:** www.stvincent.org

ST. VINCENT RANDOLPH HOSPITAL (S, 25 beds) 473 Greenville Avenue, Winchester, IN Zip 47394–2235, Mailing Address: P.O. Box 407, Zip 47394–0407; tel. 765/584–0004; Francis G. Albarano, Administrator
**Web address:** www.stvincent.org

ST. VINCENT SALEM HOSPITAL (S, 25 beds) 911 North Shelby Street, Salem, IN Zip 47167–1694; tel. 812/883–5881; Lee Jaeger, FACHE, Chief Executive Officer
**Web address:** www.wcmhospital.org

ST. VINCENT SETON SPECIALTY HOSPITAL (S, 30 beds) 1501 Hartford Street, Lafayette, IN Zip 47904; tel. 765/236–8900; Peter H. Alexander, Administrator
**Web address:** www.stvincent.org

ST. VINCENT SETON SPECIALTY HOSPITAL (S, 74 beds) 8050 Township Line Road, Indianapolis, IN Zip 46260; tel. 317/415–8353; Peter H. Alexander, Administrator
**Web address:** www.stvincent.org/

For explanation of codes following names, see page B2.
★ Indicates Type III membership in the American Hospital Association.

ST. VINCENT WILLIAMSPORT HOSPITAL (S, 16 beds) 412 North Monroe Street, Williamsport, IN Zip 47993–0215; tel. 765/762–4000; Jane Craigin, Chief Executive Officer
**Web address:** www.stvincent.org

**MARYLAND:** SAINT AGNES HOSPITAL (S, 372 beds) 900 Caton Avenue, Baltimore, MD Zip 21229–5299; tel. 410/368–6000; Bonnie Phipps, President and Chief Executive Officer
**Web address:** www.stagnes.org

**MICHIGAN:** BORGESS MEDICAL CENTER (S, 387 beds) 1521 Gull Road, Kalamazoo, MI Zip 49048–1640; tel. 269/226–7000; Paul A. Spaude, FACHE, President and Chief Executive Officer
**Web address:** www.borgess.com

BORGESS–LEE MEMORIAL HOSPITAL (S, 25 beds) 420 West High Street, Dowagiac, MI Zip 49047–1943; tel. 269/782–8681; John Ryder, Interim Chief Executive Officer
**Web address:** www.borgess.com

BORGESS–PIPP HOSPITAL (S, 43 beds) 411 Naomi Street, Plainwell, MI Zip 49080–1222; tel. 269/685–6811; John Ryder, Administrator and Chief Executive Officer
**Web address:** www.borgess.com

BRIGHTON CENTER FOR RECOVERY (S, 99 beds) 12851 Grand River Road, Brighton, MI Zip 48116–8506; tel. 810/227–1211; Ken Van Elslander, Director
**Web address:** www.brightonhospital.org

GENESYS REGIONAL MEDICAL CENTER (S, 410 beds) One Genesys Parkway, Grand Blanc, MI Zip 48439–8066; tel. 810/606–5000; Elizabeth Aderholdt, President
**Web address:** www.genesys.org

PROVIDENCE HOSPITAL (S, 430 beds) 16001 West Nine Mile Road, Southfield, MI Zip 48075–4818, Mailing Address: P.O. Box 2043, Zip 48037–2043; tel. 248/424–3000; Michael Wiemann, M.D., President
**Web address:** www.providence–stjohnhealth.org

ST. JOHN HOSPITAL AND MEDICAL CENTER (S, 680 beds) 22101 Moross Road, Detroit, MI Zip 48236–2172; tel. 313/343–4000; Frank W. Poma, Interim President
**Web address:** www.stjohn.org

ST. JOHN MACOMB–OAKLAND HOSPITAL, MACOMB CENTER (S, 336 beds) 11800 East Twelve Mile Road, Warren, MI Zip 48093–3494; tel. 586/573–5000; Terry Hamilton, President
**Web address:** www.stjohnprovidence.org/macomb

ST. JOHN MACOMB–OAKLAND HOSPITAL, OAKLAND CENTER (S, 157 beds) 27351 Dequindre, Madison Heights, MI Zip 48071–3499; tel. 248/967–7000; Diane M. Radloff, President and Chief Executive Officer
**Web address:** www.stjohnprovidence.org/oakland

ST. JOHN RIVER DISTRICT HOSPITAL (S, 68 beds) 4100 River Road, East China, MI Zip 48054–2909; tel. 810/329–7111; Frank W. Poma, President
**Web address:** www.stjohn.org

ST. JOSEPH HEALTH SYSTEM (S, 20 beds) 200 Hemlock Street, Tawas City, MI Zip 48763–9237, Mailing Address: P.O. Box 659, Zip 48764–0659; tel. 989/362–3411; Ann M. Balfour, R.N., Administrator
**Web address:** www.sjhsys.org

ST. MARY'S OF MICHIGAN (S, 228 beds) 800 South Washington Avenue, Saginaw, MI Zip 48601–2551; tel. 989/907–8000; John R. Graham, President and Chief Executive Officer
**Web address:** www.stmarysofmichigan.org

ST. MARY'S OF MICHIGAN STANDISH HOSPITAL (S, 68 beds) 805 West Cedar Street, Standish, MI Zip 48658–9526; tel. 989/846–4521; Sheri Leaman–Case, Administrator and Chief Executive Officer
**Web address:** www.stmarysofmichigan.org/standish

**MISSOURI:** ST. JOSEPH MEDICAL CENTER (S, 239 beds) 1000 Carondelet Drive, Kansas City, MO Zip 64114–4673; tel. 816/942–4400; Michael A. Dorsey, FACHE, Chief Executive Officer
**Web address:** www.carondelethealth.org

ST. MARY'S MEDICAL CENTER (S, 131 beds) 201 West R. D. Mize Road, Blue Springs, MO Zip 64014–2518; tel. 816/228–5900; Annette Small, R.N., Chief Executive Officer
**Web address:** www.carondelethealth.org

**NEW YORK:** MOUNT ST. MARY'S HOSPITAL AND HEALTH CENTER (S, 425 beds) 5300 Military Road, Lewiston, NY Zip 14092–1903; tel. 716/297–4800; Judith A. Maness, FACHE, President and Chief Executive Officer
**Web address:** www.msmh.org

OUR LADY OF LOURDES MEMORIAL HOSPITAL (S, 154 beds) 169 Riverside Drive, Binghamton, NY Zip 13905–4246; tel. 607/798–5111; David Patak, President and Chief Executive Officer
**Web address:** www.lourdes.com

ST. MARY'S HEALTHCARE (S, 310 beds) 427 Guy Park Avenue, Amsterdam, NY Zip 12010–1095; tel. 518/842–1900; Victor Giulianelli, FACHE, President and Chief Executive Officer
**Web address:** www.smha.org

**TENNESSEE:** BAPTIST HOSPITAL (S, 425 beds) 2000 Church Street, Nashville, TN Zip 37236–0002; tel. 615/284–5555; Bernard Sherry, President and Chief Executive Officer
**Web address:** www.baptisthospital.com

HICKMAN COMMUNITY HOSPITAL (S, 65 beds) 135 East Swan Street, Centerville, TN Zip 37033–1446; tel. 931/729–4271; Jack M. Keller, Administrator
**Web address:** www.hickmanhospital.com

MIDDLE TENNESSEE MEDICAL CENTER (S, 286 beds) 1700 Medical Center Parkway, Murfreesboro, TN Zip 37129–2245; tel. 615/396–4100; Gordon B. Ferguson, President and Chief Executive Officer
**Web address:** www.mtmc.org

SAINT THOMAS HOSPITAL (S, 395 beds) 4220 Harding Road, Nashville, TN Zip 37205–2095, Mailing Address: P.O. Box 380, Zip 37202–0380; tel. 615/222–2111; Dawn Rudolph, Chief Executive Officer
**Web address:** www.stthomas.org

**TEXAS:** DELL CHILDREN'S MEDICAL CENTER OF CENTRAL TEXAS (S, 176 beds) 4900 Mueller Boulevard, Austin, TX Zip 78723–3079; tel. 512/324–0000; Robert I. Bonar, Jr., President and Chief Executive Officer
**Web address:** www.dellchildrens.net

PROVIDENCE HEALTH CENTER (S, 647 beds) 6901 Medical Parkway, Waco, TX Zip 76712–7998, Mailing Address: P.O. Box 2589, Zip 76702–2589; tel. 254/751–4000; Kent A. Keahey, FACHE, President and Chief Executive Officer
**Web address:** www.providence.net

SETON EDGAR B. DAVIS HOSPITAL (S, 25 beds) 130 Hays Street, Luling, TX Zip 78648–3207; tel. 830/875–7000; Neal Kelley, Administrator
**Web address:** www.seton.net

SETON HIGHLAND LAKES (S, 25 beds) 3201 South Water Street, Burnet, TX Zip 78611–7219, Mailing Address: P.O. Box 1219, Zip 78611–7219; tel. 512/715–3000; Michelle Robertson, R.N., President and Chief Executive Officer
**Web address:** www.seton.net

SETON MEDICAL CENTER AUSTIN (S, 425 beds) 1201 West 38th Street, Austin, TX Zip 78705–1006; tel. 512/324–1000; Gregory Hartman, President and Chief Executive Officer
**Web address:** www.seton.net

SETON MEDICAL CENTER HAYS (O, 84 beds) 6001 Kyle Parkway, Kyle, TX Zip 78640–6112, Mailing Address: 6001 Kyle Prkway, Zip 78640–6112; tel. 512/504–5000; Herb Dyer, Chief Executive Officer and Chief Operating Officer
**Web address:** www.seton.net

SETON MEDICAL CENTER WILLIAMSON (S, 135 beds) 201 Seton Parkway, Round Rock, TX Zip 78665; tel. 512/324–4000; Michelle Robertson, R.N., President and Chief Executive Officer
**Web address:** www.seton.net/williamson

SETON NORTHWEST HOSPITAL (S, 121 beds) 11113 Research Boulevard, Austin, TX Zip 78759–5236; tel. 512/324–6000; Michelle Robertson, R.N., President and Chief Executive Officer
**Web address:** www.seton.net

SETON SHOAL CREEK HOSPITAL (S, 84 beds) 3501 Mills Avenue, Austin, TX Zip 78731–6391; tel. 512/324–2000; Alan Isaacson, Vice President and Chief Operating Officer
**Web address:** www.seton.net

SETON SMITHVILLE REGIONAL HOSPITAL (O, 12 beds) 800 East Highway 71, Smithville, TX Zip 78957; tel. 512/237–3214; Grady Hooper, Chief Executive Officer
**Web address:** www.srhnet.org

For explanation of codes following names, see page B2.
★ Indicates Type III membership in the American Hospital Association.

SETON SOUTHWEST HEALTHCARE CENTER (S, 17 beds) 7900 F. M. 1826, Austin, TX Zip 78737; tel. 512/324–9000; Mary Faria, FACHE, Administrator
**Web address:** www.seton.net

UNIVERSITY MEDICAL CENTER AT BRACKENRIDGE (S, 241 beds) 601 East 15th Street, Austin, TX Zip 78701–1996; tel. 512/324–7000; Gregory Hartman, President and Chief Executive Officer
**Web address:** www.seton.net

**WASHINGTON:** LOURDES COUNSELING CENTER (S, 20 beds) 1175 Carondelet Drive, Richland, WA Zip 99354–3300; tel. 509/943–9104; Barbara Mead, Executive Director
**Web address:** www.lourdeshealth.net

LOURDES MEDICAL CENTER (S, 35 beds) 520 North Fourth Avenue, Pasco, WA Zip 99301–2568, Mailing Address: P.O. Box 2568, Zip 99302–2568; tel. 509/547–7704; John Serle, President and Chief Executive Officer
**Web address:** www.lourdeshealth.net

**WISCONSIN:** COLUMBIA ST. MARY'S HOSPITAL MILWAUKEE (S, 306 beds) 2301 North Lake Drive, Milwaukee, WI Zip 53211–4508; tel. 414/291–1000; Mark R. Taylor, FACHE, President and Chief Executive Officer
**Web address:** www.columbia–stmarys.org

COLUMBIA ST. MARY'S OZAUKEE HOSPITAL (S, 152 beds) 13111 North Port Washington Road, Mequon, WI Zip 53097–2416; tel. 262/243–7300; Deborah G. Friberg, President
**Web address:** www.columbia–stmarys.org

SACRED HEART REHABILITATION INSTITUTE (S, 20 beds) 2025 East Newport Avenue, Milwaukee, WI Zip 53211–2906; tel. 414/298–6700; Deborah G. Friberg, President
**Web address:** www.columbia–stmarys.com

| | | |
|---|---|---|
| Owned, leased, sponsored: | 77 hospitals | 15753 beds |
| Contract–managed: | 0 hospitals | 0 beds |
| Totals: | 77 hospitals | 15753 beds |

**0519:  ASPIRUS, INC.** (NP)
425 Pine Ridge Boulevard, Wausau, WI Zip 54401–4123; tel. 715/847–2118; Duane L. Erwin, President and Chief Executive Officer
**(Moderately Centralized Health System)**

**MICHIGAN:** ASPIRUS KEWEENAW HOSPITAL (O, 25 beds) 205 Osceola Street, Laurium, MI Zip 49913–2134; tel. 906/337–6500; Charles Nelson, Chief Executive Officer
**Web address:** www.aspiruskeweenaw.org

ASPIRUS ONTONAGON HOSPITAL (O, 18 beds) 601 South Seventh Street, Ontonagon, MI Zip 49953–1448; tel. 906/884–8000; Michael Hauswirth, Chief Operating Officer
**Web address:** www.aspirus–ontonagon.org

**WISCONSIN:** ASPIRUS WAUSAU HOSPITAL (O, 262 beds) 333 Pine Ridge Boulevard, Wausau, WI Zip 54401–4187; tel. 715/847–2121; Diane Postler–Slattery, Ph.D., President and Chief Operating Officer
**Web address:** www.aspirus.org

MEMORIAL HEALTH CENTER (O, 124 beds) 135 South Gibson Street, Medford, WI Zip 54451–1696; tel. 715/748–8100; Gregory A. Olson, President and Chief Executive Officer
**Web address:** www.memhc.com

| | | |
|---|---|---|
| Owned, leased, sponsored: | 4 hospitals | 429 beds |
| Contract–managed: | 0 hospitals | 0 beds |
| Totals: | 4 hospitals | 429 beds |

**★0865:  ATLANTIC HEALTH** (NP)
475 South Street, Morristown, NJ Zip 07962, Mailing Address: P.O. Box 1905, Zip 07962–1905; tel. 973/660–3270; Joseph A. Trunfio, Ph.D., President and Chief Executive Officer
**(Moderately Centralized Health System)**

**NEW JERSEY:** MORRISTOWN MEDICAL CENTER (O, 649 beds) 100 Madison Avenue, Morristown, NJ Zip 07962–1956; tel. 973/971–5000; David J. Shulkin, M.D., President and Chief Executive Officer
**Web address:** www.atlantichealth.org/Morristown/

NEWTON MEDICAL CENTER (O, 140 beds) 175 High Street, Newton, NJ Zip 07860–1004; tel. 973/383–2121; Thomas J. Senker, FACHE, President and Chief Executive Officer
**Web address:** www.atlantichealth.org

OVERLOOK MEDICAL CENTER (O, 299 beds) 99 Beauvoir Avenue, Summit, NJ Zip 07902–0220; tel. 908/522–2000; Alan R. Lieber, President
**Web address:** www.atlantichealth.org/Overlook

| | | |
|---|---|---|
| Owned, leased, sponsored: | 3 hospitals | 1088 beds |
| Contract–managed: | 0 hospitals | 0 beds |
| Totals: | 3 hospitals | 1088 beds |

**● ★0293:  ATLANTICARE** (NP)
2500 English Creek Avenue, Building 500, Suite 501, Egg Harbor Township, NJ Zip 08234; tel. 609/407–2309; David P. Tilton, President and Chief Executive Officer
**(Centralized Health System)**

ATLANTICARE REGIONAL MEDICAL CENTER (O, 538 beds) 1925 Pacific Avenue, Atlantic City, NJ Zip 08401–6713; tel. 609/441–8994; Lori Herndon, President and Chief Executive Officer
**Web address:** www.atlanticare.org

| | | |
|---|---|---|
| Owned, leased, sponsored: | 1 hospital | 538 beds |
| Contract–managed: | 0 hospitals | 0 beds |
| Totals: | 1 hospital | 538 beds |

**0859:  AULTMAN HEALTH FOUNDATION** (NP)
2600 Sixth Street S.W., Canton, OH Zip 44710–1702; Edward J. Roth, III, President and Chief Executive Officer

**OHIO:** AULTMAN HOSPITAL (O, 612 beds) 2600 Sixth Street S.W., Canton, OH Zip 44710–1702; tel. 330/452–9911; Edward J. Roth, III, President and Chief Executive Officer
**Web address:** www.aultman.com

AULTMAN ORRVILLE HOSPITAL (O, 25 beds) 832 South Main Street, Orrville, OH Zip 44667–2208; tel. 330/682–3010; Marchelle Suppan, DPM, President and Chief Executive Officer
**Web address:** www.aultmanorrville.org

| | | |
|---|---|---|
| Owned, leased, sponsored: | 2 hospitals | 637 beds |
| Contract–managed: | 0 hospitals | 0 beds |
| Totals: | 2 hospitals | 637 beds |

**0360:  AURORA BEHAVIORAL HEALTH CARE** (IO)
4238 Green River Road, Corona, CA Zip 92882; tel. 951/549–8032; Soon K. Kim, M.D., President and Chief Executive Officer
**(Independent Hospital System)**

**ARIZONA:** AURORA BEHAVIORAL HEALTH SYSTEM–GLENDALE (O, 80 beds) 6015 West Peoria Avenue, Glendale, AZ Zip 85302–1201; tel. 623/344–4400; Bruce Waldo, Chief Executive Officer
**Web address:** www.aurorabehavioral.com

**CALIFORNIA:** AURORA BEHAVIORAL HEALTH CARE (O, 80 beds) 11878 Avenue of Industry, San Diego, CA Zip 92128–3423; tel. 858/487–3200; James S. Plummer, Chief Executive Officer
**Web address:** www.aurorasandiego.com

AURORA CHARTER OAK HOSPITAL (O, 95 beds) 1161 East Covina Boulevard, Covina, CA Zip 91724–1599; tel. 626/966–1632; Todd A. Smith, Chief Executive Officer
**Web address:** www.aurorabehavioral.com

AURORA LAS ENCINAS HOSPITAL (O, 138 beds) 2900 East Del Mar Boulevard, Pasadena, CA Zip 91107–4399; tel. 626/795–9901; Gerard Conway, Chief Executive Officer
**Web address:** www.lasencinashospital.com

AURORA VISTA DEL MAR HOSPITAL (O, 87 beds) 801 Seneca Street, Ventura, CA Zip 93001–1411; tel. 805/653–6434; Mayla Krebsbach, Chief Executive Officer
**Web address:** www.vistadelmarhospital.com

For explanation of codes following names, see page B2.
★ Indicates Type III membership in the American Hospital Association.
● Single hospital health care system

**ILLINOIS:** AURORA CHICAGO LAKESHORE HOSPITAL (O, 108 beds) 4840 North Marine Drive, Chicago, IL Zip 60640–4296; tel. 773/878–9700; C. Alan Eaks, Chief Executive Officer
**Web address:** www.chicagolakeshorehospital.com

| Owned, leased, sponsored: | 6 hospitals | 588 beds |
|---|---|---|
| Contract–managed: | 0 hospitals | 0 beds |
| Totals: | 6 hospitals | 588 beds |

---

**★2215: AURORA HEALTH CARE** (NP)
3000 West Montana, Milwaukee, WI Zip 53215–3268, Mailing Address: P.O. Box 341880, Zip 53234–1880; tel. 414/647–3000; Nick Turkal, M.D., President and Chief Executive Officer
**(Centralized Health System)**

**WISCONSIN:** AURORA BAYCARE MEDICAL CENTER (O, 159 beds) 2845 Greenbrier Road, Green Bay, WI Zip 54311, Mailing Address: P.O. Box 8900, Zip 54308; tel. 920/288–8000; Daniel T. Meyer, Chief Administrative Officer
**Web address:** www.aurorabaycare.com

AURORA LAKELAND MEDICAL CENTER (O, 75 beds) W3985 County Road NN, Elkhorn, WI Zip 53121–4389; tel. 262/741–2000; Vicki Lewis, R.N., MS, FACHE, Vice President and Chief Administrative Officer
**Web address:** www.aurorahealthcare.org

AURORA MEDICAL CENTER (O, 73 beds) 10400 South 75th Street, Kenosha, WI Zip 53142; tel. 262/948–5600; Christine K. Olson, R.N., MSN, Chief Administrative Officer and Chief Nursing Executive
**Web address:** www.aurorahealthcare.org

AURORA MEDICAL CENTER – MANITOWOC COUNTY (O, 66 beds) 5000 Memorial Drive, Two Rivers, WI Zip 54241–2399; tel. 920/794–5000; Cathie A. Kocourek, Chief Administrative Officer
**Web address:** www.aurorahealthcare.org

AURORA MEDICAL CENTER GRAFTON (O, 81 beds) 975 Port Washington Road, Grafton, WI Zip 53024–9201; tel. 262/329–1000; Leonard E. Wilk, Vice President and Chief Administrative Officer
**Web address:** www.aurorahealthcare.org

AURORA MEDICAL CENTER OF OSHKOSH (O, 61 beds) 855 North Westhaven Drive, Oshkosh, WI Zip 54904; tel. 920/456–6000; Jeffrey Bard, Vice President Operations
**Web address:** www.aurorahealthcare.com

AURORA MEDICAL CENTER OF WASHINGTON COUNTY (O, 45 beds) 1032 East Sumner Street, Hartford, WI Zip 53027–1698; tel. 262/673–2300; Lisa Just, Vice President and Chief Administrative Officer
**Web address:** www.aurorahealthcare.org

AURORA MEDICAL CENTER SUMMIT (O, 71 beds) 36500 Aurora Drive, Summit, WI Zip 53066–4899; tel. 262/434–1000; Daniel J. Bonk, Chief Executive Officer
**Web address:** www.aurorahealthcare.org

AURORA MEMORIAL HOSPITAL OF BURLINGTON (O, 65 beds) 252 McHenry Street, Burlington, WI Zip 53105–1828; tel. 262/767–6000; Vicki Lewis, R.N., MS, FACHE, Vice President and Chief Administrative Officer
**Web address:** www.aurorahealthcare.org

AURORA PSYCHIATRIC HOSPITAL (O, 65 beds) 1220 Dewey Avenue, Wauwatosa, WI Zip 53213–2598; tel. 414/454–6600; Peter Carlson, Administrator
**Web address:** www.aurorahealthcare.org

AURORA SHEBOYGAN MEMORIAL MEDICAL CENTER (O, 130 beds) 2629 North Seventh Street, Sheboygan, WI Zip 53083–4998; tel. 920/451–5000; David Graebner, Chief Administrative Officer
**Web address:** www.aurorahealthcare.org

AURORA SINAI MEDICAL CENTER (O, 188 beds) 945 North 12th Street, Milwaukee, WI Zip 53233–1337, Mailing Address: P.O. Box 342, Zip 53201–0342; tel. 414/219–2000; George Hinton, Administrator
**Web address:** www.aurorahealthcare.org

AURORA ST. LUKE'S MEDICAL CENTER (O, 710 beds) 2900 West Oklahoma Avenue, Milwaukee, WI Zip 53215–4330, Mailing Address: P.O. Box 2901, Zip 53201–2901; tel. 414/649–6000; Mary O'Brien, Administrator
**Web address:** www.aurorahealthcare.org

AURORA WEST ALLIS MEDICAL CENTER (O, 220 beds) 8901 West Lincoln Avenue, West Allis, WI Zip 53227–2409, Mailing Address: P.O. Box 27901, Zip 53227–0901; tel. 414/328–6000; Richard A. Kellar, Administrator
**Web address:** www.aurorahealthcare.org

| Owned, leased, sponsored: | 14 hospitals | 2009 beds |
|---|---|---|
| Contract–managed: | 0 hospitals | 0 beds |
| Totals: | 14 hospitals | 2009 beds |

---

**0869: AVANTI HOSPITALS** (IO)
222 North Sepulveda Boulevard, Suite 950, El Segundo, CA Zip 90245–5614; tel. 310/356–0550; John J. Ferrelli, Chief Operating Officer

**CALIFORNIA:** COAST PLAZA HOSPITAL (O, 123 beds) 13100 Studebaker Road, Norwalk, CA Zip 90650–2531; tel. 562/868–3751; John J. Ferrelli, Chief Executive Officer
**Web address:** www.coastplaza.com

COMMUNITY HOSPITAL OF HUNTINGTON PARK (O, 157 beds) 2623 East Slauson Avenue, Huntington Park, CA Zip 90255–2900; tel. 323/583–1931; Hector Hernandez, Chief Administrative Officer
**Web address:** www.chhp.org

EAST LOS ANGELES DOCTORS HOSPITAL (O, 127 beds) 4060 East Whittier Boulevard, Los Angeles, CA Zip 90023–2526; tel. 323/268–5514; Hector Hernandez, Chief Executive Officer
**Web address:** www.elalax.com

MEMORIAL HOSPITAL OF GARDENA (O, 172 beds) 1145 West Redondo Beach Boulevard, Gardena, CA Zip 90247–3528; tel. 310/532–4200; Araceli Lonergan, Chief Executive Officer
**Web address:** www.mhglax.com/

| Owned, leased, sponsored: | 4 hospitals | 579 beds |
|---|---|---|
| Contract–managed: | 0 hospitals | 0 beds |
| Totals: | 4 hospitals | 579 beds |

---

**★5255: AVERA HEALTH** (CC)
3900 West Avera Drive, Suite 301, Sioux Falls, SD Zip 57108; tel. 605/322–4700; John T. Porter, President and Chief Executive Officer
**(Decentralized Health System)**

**IOWA:** AVERA HOLY FAMILY HOSPITAL (O, 25 beds) 826 North Eighth Street, Estherville, IA Zip 51334–1598; tel. 712/362–2631; Michael L. Hall, Chief Executive Officer
**Web address:** www.avera–holyfamily.org

FLOYD VALLEY HOSPITAL (C, 25 beds) 714 Lincoln Street N.E., Le Mars, IA Zip 51031–3314; tel. 712/546–7871; Michael T. Donlin, FACHE, Administrator
**Web address:** www.floydvalleyhospital.org

HEGG MEMORIAL HEALTH CENTER AVERA (C, 85 beds) 1202 21st Avenue, Rock Valley, IA Zip 51247–1497; tel. 712/476–8000; Glenn Zevenbergen, Chief Executive Officer
**Web address:** www.hegghc.org

OSCEOLA COMMUNITY HOSPITAL (C, 25 beds) Ninth Avenue North, Sibley, IA Zip 51249–0258, Mailing Address: P.O. Box 258, Zip 51249–0258; tel. 712/754–2574; Janet H. Dykstra, Chief Executive Officer
**Web address:** www.osceolacommunityhospital.org

SIOUX CENTER COMMUNITY HOSPITAL AND HEALTH CENTER AVERA (C, 90 beds) 605 South Main Avenue, Sioux Center, IA Zip 51250–1398; tel. 712/722–1271; Kayleen R. Lee, Chief Executive Officer
**Web address:** www.schospital.org

**MINNESOTA:** AVERA MARSHALL REGIONAL MEDICAL CENTER (O, 25 beds) 300 South Bruce Street, Marshall, MN Zip 56258–3900; tel. 507/532–9661; Mary B. Maertens, FACHE, President and Chief Executive Officer
**Web address:** www.averamarshall.org

PIPESTONE COUNTY MEDICAL CENTER AVERA (C, 25 beds) 916 4th Avenue S.W., Pipestone, MN Zip 56164–0370; tel. 507/825–5811; Bradley D. Burris, Chief Executive Officer
**Web address:** www.pcmchealth.org

TYLER HEALTHCARE CENTER AVERA (C, 56 beds) 240 Willow Street, Tyler, MN Zip 56178–0280, Mailing Address: P.O. Box 280, Zip 56178–0280; tel. 507/247–5521; Dale K. Kruger, Chief Executive Officer and Chief Financial Officer
**Web address:** www.averamckennan.org/amck/regionalfacilities/tyler/

Section B

For explanation of codes following names, see page B2.
★ Indicates Type III membership in the American Hospital Association.

**NEBRASKA:** AVERA CREIGHTON HOSPITAL (O, 54 beds) 1503 Main Street, Creighton, NE Zip 68729–0186, Mailing Address: P.O. Box 186, Zip 68729–0186; tel. 402/358–5700; Mark Schulte, Chief Executive Officer
**Web address:** www.avera.org/creighton/

AVERA ST. ANTHONY'S HOSPITAL (O, 25 beds) 302 North Second Street, O'Neill, NE Zip 68763–1514, Mailing Address: P.O. Box 270, Oneill, Zip 68763–0270; tel. 402/336–2611; Ronald J. Cork, President and Chief Executive Officer
**Web address:** www.avera.org/st-anthonys

**SOUTH DAKOTA:** AVERA DE SMET MEMORIAL HOSPITAL (L, 14 beds) 306 Prairie Avenue S.W., De Smet, SD Zip 57231, Mailing Address: P.O. Box 160, Zip 57231; tel. 605/854–3329; Janice Schardin, R.N., MS, Administrator and Chief Executive Officer
**Web address:** www.desmetmemorial.org

AVERA DELLS AREA HOSPITAL (L, 23 beds) 909 North Iowa Avenue, Dell Rapids, SD Zip 57022–1231; tel. 605/428–5431; Lindsay Leischner, R.N., Administrator and Chief Executive Officer
**Web address:** www.avera.org

AVERA FLANDREAU HOSPITAL (L, 18 beds) 214 North Prairie Street, Flandreau, SD Zip 57028–1243; tel. 605/997–2433; Lindsay Leischner, R.N., Administrator and Chief Executive Officer
**Web address:** www.flandreaumedical.org

AVERA GREGORY HOSPITAL (O, 63 beds) 400 Park Avenue, Gregory, SD Zip 57533–0400, Mailing Address: P.O. Box 408, Zip 57533–0408; tel. 605/835–8394; Anthony Timanus, Chief Executive Officer
**Web address:** www.gregoryhealthcare.org

AVERA HAND COUNTY MEMORIAL HOSPITAL & CLINIC (L, 19 beds) 300 West Fifth Street, Miller, SD Zip 57362–1238; tel. 605/853–2421; Bryan Breitling, Administrator
**Web address:** www.avera.org

AVERA MCKENNAN HOSPITAL AND UNIVERSITY HEALTH CENTER (O, 400 beds) 800 East 21st Street, Sioux Falls, SD Zip 57105–1096, Mailing Address: P.O. Box 5045, Zip 57117–5045; tel. 605/322–8000; David Kapaska, D.O., Regional President
**Web address:** www.averamckennan.org

AVERA QUEEN OF PEACE HOSPITAL (O, 196 beds) 525 North Foster, Mitchell, SD Zip 57301–2999; tel. 605/995–2000; Thomas A. Clark, President and Chief Executive Officer
**Web address:** www.averaqueenofpeace.org

AVERA SACRED HEART HOSPITAL (O, 293 beds) 501 Summit Avenue, Yankton, SD Zip 57078–3899; tel. 605/668–8000; Pamela J. Rezac, Regional President
**Web address:** www.averasacredheart.com

AVERA ST. BENEDICT HOSPITAL (O, 100 beds) 401 West Glynn Drive, Parkston, SD Zip 57366–2031; tel. 605/928–3311; Gale N. Walker, President and Chief Executive Officer
**Web address:** www.averastbenedict.org

AVERA ST. LUKE'S HOSPITAL (O, 270 beds) 305 South State Street, Aberdeen, SD Zip 57402–4450; tel. 605/622–5000; Todd Forkel, President and Chief Executive Officer
**Web address:** www.averastlukes.org

AVERA WESKOTA MEMORIAL HOSPITAL (L, 23 beds) 604 First Street N.E., Wessington Springs, SD Zip 57382; tel. 605/539–1201; Gaea Blue, Administrator and Chief Executive Officer
**Web address:** www.averaweskota.org

EUREKA COMMUNITY HEALTH SERVICES AVERA (C, 6 beds) 410 Ninth Street, Eureka, SD Zip 57437–0517, Mailing Address: P.O. Box 517, Zip 57437–0517; tel. 605/284–2661; Robert A. Dockter, Administrator
**Web address:** www.avera.org

LANDMANN–JUNGMAN MEMORIAL HOSPITAL AVERA (C, 19 beds) 600 Billars Street, Scotland, SD Zip 57059–2026; tel. 605/583–2226; Lee Baldwin, Administrator and Chief Executive Officer
**Web address:** www.ljmh.org

MARSHALL COUNTY HEALTHCARE CENTER AVERA (C, 18 beds) 413 Ninth Street, Britton, SD Zip 57430; tel. 605/448–2253; Nick Fosness, Chief Executive Officer
**Web address:** www.avera.org

MILBANK AREA HOSPITAL AVERA (L, 25 beds) 901 East Virgil Avenue, Milbank, SD Zip 57252; tel. 605/432–4538; Natalie Gauer, Administrator
**Web address:** www.averamilbank.org

PLATTE HEALTH CENTER AVERA (C, 65 beds) 601 East Seventh, Platte, SD Zip 57369–2123, Mailing Address: P.O. Box 200, Zip 57369–0200; tel. 605/337–3364; Mark Burket, Chief Executive Officer
**Web address:** www.phcavera.org

ST. MICHAEL'S HOSPITAL AVERA (C, 25 beds) 410 West 16th Avenue, Tyndall, SD Zip 57066, Mailing Address: P.O. Box 27, Zip 57066–0027; tel. 605/589–3341; Carol Deurmier, Chief Executive Officer
**Web address:** www.avera.org/

WAGNER COMMUNITY MEMORIAL HOSPITAL AVERA (C, 20 beds) 513 Third Street S.W., Wagner, SD Zip 57380, Mailing Address: P.O. Box 280, Zip 57380–0280; tel. 605/384–3611; Bryan Slaba, Chief Executive Officer
**Web address:** www.avera.org

| | | |
|---|---|---|
| **Owned, leased, sponsored:** | 16 hospitals | 1573 beds |
| **Contract–managed:** | 12 hospitals | 459 beds |
| **Totals:** | 28 hospitals | 2032 beds |

---

**★0633: AVITA HEALTH SYSTEM** (NP)
269 Portland Way South, Galion, OH Zip 44833–2399; tel. 419/468–4841; Jerome Morasko, President and Chief Executive Officer
**(Independent Hospital System)**

**OHIO:** BUCYRUS COMMUNITY HOSPITAL (O, 25 beds) 629 North Sandusky Avenue, Bucyrus, OH Zip 44820–1821; tel. 419/562–4677; Jerome Morasko, Chief Executive Officer
**Web address:** www.bchonline.org

GALION COMMUNITY HOSPITAL (O, 35 beds) 269 Portland Way South, Galion, OH Zip 44833–2399; tel. 419/468–4841; Jerome Morasko, President and Chief Executive Officer
**Web address:** www.galionhospital.org

| | | |
|---|---|---|
| **Owned, leased, sponsored:** | 2 hospitals | 60 beds |
| **Contract–managed:** | 0 hospitals | 0 beds |
| **Totals:** | 2 hospitals | 60 beds |

---

**★0194: BANNER HEALTH** (NP)
1441 North 12th Street, Phoenix, AZ Zip 85006–2837, Mailing Address: P.O. Box 25489, Zip 85002–5489; tel. 602/747–4000; Peter S. Fine, FACHE, President and Chief Executive Officer
**(Decentralized Health System)**

**ALASKA:** FAIRBANKS MEMORIAL HOSPITAL (L, 217 beds) 1650 Cowles Street, Fairbanks, AK Zip 99701–5998; tel. 907/452–8181; Michael K. Powers, FACHE, Chief Executive Officer
**Web address:** www.bannerhealth.com

**ARIZONA:** BANNER BAYWOOD MEDICAL CENTER (O, 340 beds) 6644 East Baywood Avenue, Mesa, AZ Zip 85206–1797; tel. 480/321–2000; Laura Robertson, R.N., Chief Executive Officer
**Web address:** www.bannerhealth.com

BANNER BEHAVIORAL HEALTH HOSPITAL – SCOTTSDALE (O, 95 beds) 7575 East Earll Drive, Scottsdale, AZ Zip 85251–6915; tel. 480/941–7500; Cherie Martin, R.N., MSN, FACHE, Chief Executive Officer
**Web address:** www.bannerhealth.com

BANNER BOSWELL MEDICAL CENTER (O, 489 beds) 10401 West Thunderbird Boulevard, Sun City, AZ Zip 85351–3004, Mailing Address: P.O. Box 1690, Zip 85372–1690; tel. 623/832–4000; David Cheney, Chief Executive Officer
**Web address:** www.sunhealth.org

BANNER DEL E. WEBB MEDICAL CENTER (O, 373 beds) 14502 West Meeker Boulevard, Sun City West, AZ Zip 85375–5299, Mailing Address: P.O. Box 5169, Zip 85376–5169; tel. 623/214–4000; Debbie Flores, Chief Executive Officer
**Web address:** www.sunhealth.org

BANNER DESERT MEDICAL CENTER (O, 583 beds) 1400 South Dobson Road, Mesa, AZ Zip 85202–9879; tel. 480/412–3000; Robert Gould, Chief Executive Officer
**Web address:** www.bannerhealth.com

BANNER ESTRELLA MEDICAL CENTER (O, 214 beds) 9201 West Thomas Road, Phoenix, AZ Zip 85037–3332; tel. 623/327–4000; Debra J. Krmpotic, R.N., Chief Executive Officer
**Web address:** www.bannerhealth.com

For explanation of codes following names, see page B2.
★ Indicates Type III membership in the American Hospital Association.

BANNER GATEWAY MEDICAL CENTER (O, 177 beds) 1900 North Higley Road, Gilbert, AZ Zip 85234; tel. 480/543–2000; Todd S. Werner, Chief Executive Officer
**Web address:** www.bannerhealth.com

BANNER GOOD SAMARITAN MEDICAL CENTER (O, 640 beds) 1111 East McDowell Road, Phoenix, AZ Zip 85006–2666, Mailing Address: P.O. Box 2989, Zip 85062–2989; tel. 602/239–2000; Larry E. Volkmar, Chief Executive Officer
**Web address:** www.bannerhealth.com

BANNER HEART HOSPITAL (O, 111 beds) 6750 East Baywood Avenue, Mesa, AZ Zip 85206; tel. 480/854–5000; Laura Robertson, R.N., Chief Executive Officer
**Web address:** www.bannerhealth.com

BANNER IRONWOOD MEDICAL CENTER (O, 36 beds) 37000 North Gantzel Road, San Tan Valley, AZ Zip 85140–7303; tel. 480/394–4000; Julie Nunley, R.N., Chief Executive Officer
**Web address:** www.bannerhealth.com

BANNER THUNDERBIRD MEDICAL CENTER (O, 480 beds) 5555 West Thunderbird Road, Glendale, AZ Zip 85306–4696; tel. 602/865–5555; Thomas C. Dickson, Chief Executive Officer
**Web address:** www.bannerhealth.com

PAGE HOSPITAL (C, 25 beds) 501 North Navajo Drive, Page, AZ Zip 86040, Mailing Address: P.O. Box 1447, Zip 86040–1447; tel. 928/645–2424; Sandy Haryasz, R.N., Chief Executive Officer
**Web address:** www.bannerhealth.com

**CALIFORNIA:** BANNER LASSEN MEDICAL CENTER (O, 25 beds) 1800 Spring Ridge Drive, Susanville, CA Zip 96130–4809; tel. 530/252–2000; Bob S. Edwards, Jr., FACHE, Chief Executive Officer
**Web address:** www.bannerhealth.com

**COLORADO:** EAST MORGAN COUNTY HOSPITAL (L, 19 beds) 2400 West Edison Street, Brush, CO Zip 80723–1640; tel. 970/842–6200; Linda Thorpe, Chief Executive Officer
**Web address:** www.emchbrush.com

MCKEE MEDICAL CENTER (O, 121 beds) 2000 Boise Avenue, Loveland, CO Zip 80538–4281; tel. 970/669–4640; Marilyn Schock, Chief Executive Officer
**Web address:** www.mckeeloveland.com

NORTH COLORADO MEDICAL CENTER (L, 258 beds) 1801 16th Street, Greeley, CO Zip 80634; tel. 970/352–4121; Richard O. Sutton, Chief Executive Officer
**Web address:** www.ncmcgreeley.com

STERLING REGIONAL MEDCENTER (O, 25 beds) 615 Fairhurst Street, Sterling, CO Zip 80751–0500; tel. 970/522–0122; Julie Klein, Chief Executive Officer
**Web address:** www.bannerhealth.com

**NEBRASKA:** OGALLALA COMMUNITY HOSPITAL (L, 18 beds) 2601 North Spruce Street, Ogallala, NE Zip 69153–2465; tel. 308/284–4011; Sharon Lind, MSN, Chief Executive Officer
**Web address:** www.bannerhealth.com

**NEVADA:** BANNER CHURCHILL COMMUNITY HOSPITAL (O, 40 beds) 801 East Williams Avenue, Fallon, NV Zip 89406–3052; tel. 775/867–7000; John D'Angelo, Chief Executive Officer
**Web address:** www.bannerhealth.com

**WYOMING:** COMMUNITY HOSPITAL (O, 25 beds) 2000 Campbell Drive, Torrington, WY Zip 82240–1597; tel. 307/532–4181; Vincent B. DiFranco, Chief Executive Officer
**Web address:** www.bannerhealth.com

PLATTE COUNTY MEMORIAL HOSPITAL (L, 25 beds) 201 14th Street, Wheatland, WY Zip 82201–3201, Mailing Address: P.O. Box 848, Zip 82201–0848; tel. 307/322–3636; Shelby Nelson, Chief Executive Officer
**Web address:** www.bannerhealth.com

WASHAKIE MEDICAL CENTER (L, 25 beds) 400 South 15th Street, Worland, WY Zip 82401–3531, Mailing Address: P.O. Box 700, Zip 82401–0700; tel. 307/347–3221; Margie Molitor, R.N., Chief Executive Officer
**Web address:** www.washakiemedicalcenter.com

| | | |
|---|---|---|
| Owned, leased, sponsored: | 22 hospitals | 4336 beds |
| Contract–managed: | 1 hospital | 25 beds |
| **Totals:** | 23 hospitals | 4361 beds |

★**0005: BAPTIST HEALTH** (CO)
800 Prudential Drive, Jacksonville, FL Zip 32207; tel. 904/202–4011; Hugh Greene, President and Chief Executive Officer
**(Independent Hospital System)**

**FLORIDA:** BAPTIST MEDICAL CENTER (O, 844 beds) 800 Prudential Drive, Jacksonville, FL Zip 32207–8203; tel. 904/202–2000; Michael A. Mayo, FACHE, President
**Web address:** www.e–baptisthealth.com

BAPTIST MEDICAL CENTER BEACHES (O, 136 beds) 1350 13th Avenue South, Jacksonville Beach, FL Zip 32250–3205; tel. 904/627–2900; Joseph M. Mitrick, FACHE, President
**Web address:** www.e–baptisthealth.com

BAPTIST MEDICAL CENTER NASSAU (O, 52 beds) 1250 South 18th Street, Fernandina Beach, FL Zip 32034–3098; tel. 904/321–3500; Stephen Lee, President
**Web address:** www.e–baptisthealth.com

| | | |
|---|---|---|
| Owned, leased, sponsored: | 3 hospitals | 1032 beds |
| Contract–managed: | 0 hospitals | 0 beds |
| **Totals:** | 3 hospitals | 1032 beds |

★**0150: BAPTIST HEALTH** (NP)
301 Brown Springs Road, Montgomery, AL Zip 36117; tel. 334/273–4400; W. Russell Tyner, President and Chief Executive Officer
**(Centralized Health System)**

**ALABAMA:** BAPTIST MEDICAL CENTER EAST (O, 182 beds) 400 Taylor Road, Montgomery, AL Zip 36117–3512, Mailing Address: P.O. Box 241267, Zip 36124–1267; tel. 334/277–8330; J. Peter Selman, Administrator and Chief Executive Officer
**Web address:** www.baptistfirst.org

BAPTIST MEDICAL CENTER SOUTH (O, 386 beds) 2105 East South Boulevard, Montgomery, AL Zip 36116–2498, Mailing Address: Box 11010, Zip 36111–0010; tel. 334/288–2100; Robin Barca, Chief Executive Officer
**Web address:** www.baptistfirst.org

PRATTVILLE BAPTIST HOSPITAL (O, 56 beds) 124 South Memorial Drive, Prattville, AL Zip 36067–3619, Mailing Address: P.O. Box 681630, Zip 36067–1638; tel. 334/365–0651; Ginger Henry, Chief Executive Officer
**Web address:** www.baptistfirst.org

| | | |
|---|---|---|
| Owned, leased, sponsored: | 3 hospitals | 624 beds |
| Contract–managed: | 0 hospitals | 0 beds |
| **Totals:** | 3 hospitals | 624 beds |

★**0355: BAPTIST HEALTH** (NP)
9601 Interstate 630, Exit 7, Little Rock, AR Zip 72205–7299; tel. 501/202–2000; Russell D. Harrington, Jr., FACHE, President and Chief Executive Officer
**(Centralized Physician/Insurance Health System)**

**ARKANSAS:** BAPTIST HEALTH EXTENDED CARE HOSPITAL (O, 37 beds) 9601 Interstate 630, Exit 7, 10th Floor, Little Rock, AR Zip 72205–7202; tel. 501/202–1070; Mike Perkins, Administrator
**Web address:** www.baptist–health.com

BAPTIST HEALTH MEDICAL CENTER – NORTH LITTLE ROCK (O, 220 beds) 3333 Springhill Drive, North Little Rock, AR Zip 72117–2922; tel. 501/202–3000; Harrison M. Dean, FACHE, Senior Vice President and Administrator
**Web address:** www.baptist–health.org

BAPTIST HEALTH MEDICAL CENTER–ARKADELPHIA (L, 25 beds) 3050 Twin Rivers Drive, Arkadelphia, AR Zip 71923–4299; tel. 870/245–2622; Greg Stubblefield, Vice President and Administrator
**Web address:** www.baptist–health.org

BAPTIST HEALTH MEDICAL CENTER–HEBER SPRINGS (O, 25 beds) 1800 Bypass Road, Heber Springs, AR Zip 72543–9135; tel. 501/887–3000; Edward L. Lacy, FACHE, Vice President and Administrator
**Web address:** www.baptist–health.com

For explanation of codes following names, see page B2.
★ Indicates Type III membership in the American Hospital Association.

BAPTIST HEALTH MEDICAL CENTER–LITTLE ROCK (O, 703 beds) 9601 Interstate 630, Exit 7, Little Rock, AR Zip 72205–7299; tel. 501/202–2000; Steven Douglas Weeks, FACHE, Senior Vice President and Administrator **Web address:** www.baptist–health.org

BAPTIST HEALTH MEDICAL CENTER–STUTTGART (L, 49 beds) North Buerkle Road, Stuttgart, AR Zip 72160–3420, Mailing Address: P.O. Box 1905, Zip 72160–1905; tel. 870/673–3511; Steven B. Webb, FACHE, Administrator **Web address:** www.baptist–health.org

BAPTIST HEALTH REHABILITATION INSTITUTE (O, 100 beds) 9601 Interstate 630, Exit 7, Little Rock, AR Zip 72205–7249; tel. 501/202–7000; Lee Gentry, FACHE, Vice President and Administrator **Web address:** www.baptist–health.com

| | | |
|---|---|---|
| Owned, leased, sponsored: | 7 hospitals | 1159 beds |
| Contract–managed: | 0 hospitals | 0 beds |
| Totals: | 7 hospitals | 1159 beds |

---

**★0185: BAPTIST HEALTH CARE CORPORATION** (NP)
1717 North E Street, Suite 320, Pensacola, FL Zip 32501, Mailing Address: P.O. Box 17500, Zip 32522–7500; tel. 850/434–4011; Mark T. Faulkner, President
**(Moderately Centralized Health System)**

**ALABAMA:** ATMORE COMMUNITY HOSPITAL (L, 49 beds) 401 Medical Park Drive, Atmore, AL Zip 36502–3091; tel. 251/368–2500; John R. Tucker, FACHE, Administrator **Web address:** www.ebaptisthealthcare.org

**FLORIDA:** BAPTIST HOSPITAL (O, 339 beds) 1000 West Moreno, Pensacola, FL Zip 32501–2393, Mailing Address: P.O. Box 17500, Zip 32522–7500; tel. 850/434–4011; David Wildebrandt, Administrator **Web address:** www.ebaptisthealthcare.org

GULF BREEZE HOSPITAL (O, 77 beds) 1110 Gulf Breeze Parkway, Gulf Breeze, FL Zip 32561; tel. 850/934–2000; Robert Harriman, M.D., Administrator **Web address:** www.ebaptisthealthcare.org

JAY HOSPITAL (L, 55 beds) 14114 South Alabama Street, Jay, FL Zip 32565–1070; tel. 850/675–8000; Michael T. Hutchins, Administrator **Web address:** www.bhcpns.org/jayhospital/

| | | |
|---|---|---|
| Owned, leased, sponsored: | 4 hospitals | 520 beds |
| Contract–managed: | 0 hospitals | 0 beds |
| Totals: | 4 hospitals | 520 beds |

---

**★0122: BAPTIST HEALTH SOUTH FLORIDA** (NP)
6855 Red Road, Suite 600, Coral Gables, FL Zip 33143–3632; tel. 786/662–7111; Brian E. Keeley, President and Chief Executive Officer
**(Centralized Physician/Insurance Health System)**

BAPTIST HEALTH SOUTH FLORIDA, BAPTIST HOSPITAL OF MIAMI (O, 672 beds) 8900 North Kendall Drive, Miami, FL Zip 33176–2197; tel. 786/596–1960; Bo Boulenger, Chief Executive Officer **Web address:** www.baptisthealth.net

BAPTIST HEALTH SOUTH FLORIDA, DOCTORS HOSPITAL (O, 146 beds) 5000 University Drive, Coral Gables, FL Zip 33146–2094; tel. 786/308–3000; Nelson Lazo, Chief Executive Officer **Web address:** www.baptisthealth.net

BAPTIST HEALTH SOUTH FLORIDA, HOMESTEAD HOSPITAL (O, 142 beds) 975 Baptist Way, Homestead, FL Zip 33033–7600; tel. 786/243–8000; Bill Duquette, Chief Executive Officer **Web address:** www.baptisthealth.net

BAPTIST HEALTH SOUTH FLORIDA, MARINERS HOSPITAL (O, 25 beds) 91500 Overseas Highway, Tavernier, FL Zip 33070–2547; tel. 305/434–3000; Rick Freeburg, Chief Executive Officer **Web address:** www.baptisthealth.net

BAPTIST HEALTH SOUTH FLORIDA, SOUTH MIAMI HOSPITAL (O, 357 beds) 6200 S.W. 73rd Street, Miami, FL Zip 33143–9990; tel. 786/662–4000; Lincoln S. Mendez, Chief Executive Officer **Web address:** www.baptisthealth.net

BAPTIST HEALTH SOUTH FLORIDA, WEST KENDALL BAPTIST HOSPITAL (O, 133 beds) 9555 S.W. 162nd Avenue, Miami, FL Zip 33196; tel. 786/467–2000; Javier Hernandez–Lichtl, Chief Executive Officer **Web address:** www.westkendallbaptist.com

| | | |
|---|---|---|
| Owned, leased, sponsored: | 6 hospitals | 1475 beds |
| Contract–managed: | 0 hospitals | 0 beds |
| Totals: | 6 hospitals | 1475 beds |

---

**0265: BAPTIST HEALTH SYSTEM** (IO)
215 East Quincy, Suite 200, San Antonio, TX Zip 78216; tel. 210/297–1040

| | | |
|---|---|---|
| Owned, leased, sponsored: | 0 hospitals | 0 beds |
| Contract–managed: | 0 hospitals | 0 beds |
| Totals: | 0 hospitals | 0 beds |

---

**0345: BAPTIST HEALTH SYSTEM** (CO)
3201 4th Avenue South, Birmingham, AL Zip 35222–1723, Mailing Address: P.O. Box 830605, Zip 35283–0605; tel. 205/715–5319; M. Shane Spees, President and Chief Executive Officer
**(Centralized Physician/Insurance Health System)**

**ALABAMA:** CITIZENS BAPTIST MEDICAL CENTER (O, 116 beds) 604 Stone Avenue, Talladega, AL Zip 35160–2217, Mailing Address: P.O. Box 978, Zip 35160–0978; tel. 256/362–8111; Joel Taylor, Administrator **Web address:** www.bhsala.com

PRINCETON BAPTIST MEDICAL CENTER (O, 337 beds) 701 Princeton Avenue S.W., Birmingham, AL Zip 35211–1305; tel. 205/783–3000; Keith Parrott, FACHE, President **Web address:** www.bhsala.com

SHELBY BAPTIST MEDICAL CENTER (O, 266 beds) 1000 First Street North, Alabaster, AL Zip 35007–0488; tel. 205/620–8100; David C. Wilson, President and Chief Executive Officer **Web address:** www.bhsala.com

WALKER BAPTIST MEDICAL CENTER (O, 236 beds) 3400 Highway 78 East, Jasper, AL Zip 35501–8956, Mailing Address: P.O. Box 3547, Zip 35502–3547; tel. 205/387–4000; Robert Phillips, Administrator **Web address:** www.bhsala.com

| | | |
|---|---|---|
| Owned, leased, sponsored: | 4 hospitals | 955 beds |
| Contract–managed: | 0 hospitals | 0 beds |
| Totals: | 4 hospitals | 955 beds |

---

**★0315: BAPTIST HEALTHCARE SYSTEM** (CO)
4007 Kresge Way, Louisville, KY Zip 40207–4677; tel. 502/896–5000; Tommy J. Smith, President and Chief Executive Officer
**(Moderately Centralized Health System)**

**KENTUCKY:** BAPTIST HOSPITAL EAST (O, 519 beds) 4000 Kresge Way, Louisville, KY Zip 40207–4676; tel. 502/897–8100; David L. Gray, FACHE, President **Web address:** www.baptisteast.com

BAPTIST HOSPITAL NORTHEAST (O, 108 beds) 1025 New Moody Lane, La Grange, KY Zip 40031–0559; tel. 502/222–5388; Chris Roty, President **Web address:** www.baptistnortheast.com

BAPTIST REGIONAL MEDICAL CENTER (O, 273 beds) 1 Trillium Way, Corbin, KY Zip 40701–8420; tel. 606/528–1212; Larry Gray, President and Chief Executive Officer **Web address:** www.baptistregional.com

CENTRAL BAPTIST HOSPITAL (O, 344 beds) 1740 Nicholasville Road, Lexington, KY Zip 40503–1499; tel. 859/260–6100; William G. Sisson, President **Web address:** www.centralbap.com

HARDIN MEMORIAL HOSPITAL (C, 268 beds) 913 North Dixie Avenue, Elizabethtown, KY Zip 42701; tel. 270/737–1212; Dennis B. Johnson, Chief Executive Officer **Web address:** www.hmh.net

---

For explanation of codes following names, see page B2.
★ Indicates Type III membership in the American Hospital Association.

PATTIE A. CLAY REGIONAL MEDICAL CENTER (C, 66 beds) 801 Eastern Bypass, Richmond, KY Zip 40475–2405, Mailing Address: P.O. Box 1600, Zip 40476–2603; tel. 859/623–3131; Todd Jones, President and Chief Executive Officer
**Web address:** www.pattieaclay.org

WESTERN BAPTIST HOSPITAL (O, 320 beds) 2501 Kentucky Avenue, Paducah, KY Zip 42003–3200; tel. 270/575–2100; Larry O. Barton, FACHE, President
**Web address:** www.westernbaptist.com

| | | |
|---|---|---|
| Owned, leased, sponsored: | 5 hospitals | 1564 beds |
| Contract–managed: | 2 hospitals | 334 beds |
| Totals: | 7 hospitals | 1898 beds |

---

**★1625: BAPTIST MEMORIAL HEALTH CARE CORPORATION** (NP)
350 North Humphreys Boulevard, Memphis, TN Zip 38120–2177; tel. 901/227–5117; Stephen Curtis Reynolds, President and Chief Executive Officer
**(Decentralized Health System)**

**ARKANSAS:** NEA BAPTIST MEMORIAL HOSPITAL (O, 100 beds) 3024 Stadium Boulevard, Jonesboro, AR Zip 72401–7493; tel. 870/972–7000; Brad Parsons, Administrator and Chief Executive Officer
**Web address:** www.neabaptist.com

**MISSISSIPPI:** BAPTIST MEMORIAL HOSPITAL–BOONEVILLE (L, 114 beds) 100 Hospital Street, Booneville, MS Zip 38829–3359; tel. 662/720–5000; James Grantham, Administrator
**Web address:** www.bmhcc.org

BAPTIST MEMORIAL HOSPITAL–DESOTO (O, 249 beds) 7601 Southcrest Parkway, Southaven, MS Zip 38671–4742; tel. 662/772–4000; James Huffman, Chief Executive Officer and Administrator
**Web address:** www.bmhcc.org

BAPTIST MEMORIAL HOSPITAL–GOLDEN TRIANGLE (O, 249 beds) 2520 Fifth Street North, Columbus, MS Zip 39705–2095, Mailing Address: P.O. Box 1307, Zip 39703–1307; tel. 662/244–1000; Paul Cade, Administrator and Chief Executive Officer
**Web address:** www.bmhcc.org

BAPTIST MEMORIAL HOSPITAL–NORTH MISSISSIPPI (O, 217 beds) 2301 South Lamar Boulevard, Oxford, MS Zip 38655–5373, Mailing Address: P.O. Box 946, Zip 38655–6002; tel. 662/232–8100; Donald Hutson, Administrator and Chief Executive Officer
**Web address:** www.bmhcc.org

BAPTIST MEMORIAL HOSPITAL–UNION COUNTY (L, 153 beds) 200 State Highway 30 West, New Albany, MS Zip 38652–3112; tel. 662/538–7631; Walter Grace, Chief Executive Officer and Administrator
**Web address:** www.bmhcc.org

**TENNESSEE:** BAPTIST MEMORIAL HOSPITAL – MEMPHIS (O, 642 beds) 6019 Walnut Grove Road, Memphis, TN Zip 38120–2173; tel. 901/226–5000; Derick Ziegler, Administrator and Chief Executive Officer
**Web address:** www.baptistonline.org

BAPTIST MEMORIAL HOSPITAL FOR WOMEN (O, 140 beds) 6225 Humphreys Boulevard, Memphis, TN Zip 38120–2373; tel. 901/227–9000; Anita Vaughn, Administrator and Chief Executive Officer
**Web address:** www.bmhcc.org

BAPTIST MEMORIAL HOSPITAL–COLLIERVILLE (O, 81 beds) 1500 West Poplar Avenue, Collierville, TN Zip 38017–0601; tel. 901/861–9400; Kyle Armstrong, Administrator
**Web address:** www.bmhcc.org

BAPTIST MEMORIAL HOSPITAL–HUNTINGDON (O, 33 beds) 631 R.B. Wilson Drive, Huntingdon, TN Zip 38344–1727; tel. 731/986–4461; Susan M. Breeden, Administrator and Chief Executive Officer
**Web address:** www.bmhcc.org

BAPTIST MEMORIAL HOSPITAL–TIPTON (O, 50 beds) 1995 Highway 51 South, Covington, TN Zip 38019–3635; tel. 901/476–2621; William A. Tuttle, Interim Chief Executive Officer
**Web address:** www.bmhcc.org

BAPTIST MEMORIAL HOSPITAL–UNION CITY (O, 88 beds) 1201 Bishop Street, Union City, TN Zip 38261–5403, Mailing Address: P.O. Box 310, Zip 38281–0310; tel. 731/885–2410; Barry Bondurant, Administrator and Chief Executive Officer
**Web address:** www.bmhcc.org

BAPTIST MEMORIAL RESTORATIVE CARE HOSPITAL (O, 30 beds) 6019 Walnut Grove Road, Memphis, TN Zip 38120–2113; tel. 901/226–1400; Janice Hill, R.N., Administrator
**Web address:** www.baptistonline.org/facilities/restorativecare

BAPTIST REHABILITATION–GERMANTOWN (O, 58 beds) 2100 Exeter Road, Germantown, TN Zip 38138–3978; tel. 901/757–1350; Brian Hogan, Interim Chief Executive Officer
**Web address:** www.bmhcc.org

| | | |
|---|---|---|
| Owned, leased, sponsored: | 14 hospitals | 2204 beds |
| Contract–managed: | 0 hospitals | 0 beds |
| Totals: | 14 hospitals | 2204 beds |

---

**★0118: BARNABAS HEALTH** (NP)
95 Old Short Hills Road, West Orange, NJ Zip 07052; tel. 973/322–4000; Barry Ostrowsky, President and Chief Executive Officer
**(Moderately Centralized Health System)**

**NEW JERSEY:** CLARA MAASS MEDICAL CENTER (O, 429 beds) One Clara Maass Drive, Belleville, NJ Zip 07109–3557; tel. 973/450–2000; Mary Ellen Clyne, Ph.D., President and Chief Executive Officer
**Web address:** www.sbhcs.com

COMMUNITY MEDICAL CENTER (O, 489 beds) 99 Route 37 West, Toms River, NJ Zip 08755–6423; tel. 732/557–8051; Stephanie L. Bloom, FACHE, President and Chief Executive Officer
**Web address:** www.barnabashealth.org

KIMBALL MEDICAL CENTER (O, 240 beds) 600 River Avenue, Lakewood, NJ Zip 08701–4281; tel. 732/363–1900; Michael Mimoso, FACHE, President and Chief Executive Officer
**Web address:** www.barnabashealth.org

MONMOUTH MEDICAL CENTER (O, 337 beds) 300 Second Avenue, Long Branch, NJ Zip 07740–6303; tel. 732/222–5200; Frank J. Vozos, M.D., FACS, Executive Director
**Web address:** www.sbhcs.com

NEWARK BETH ISRAEL MEDICAL CENTER (O, 402 beds) 201 Lyons Avenue, Newark, NJ Zip 07112–2027; tel. 973/926–7000; John A. Brennan, M.D., M.P.H., President and Chief Executive Officer
**Web address:** www.sbhcs.com

SAINT BARNABAS BEHAVIORAL HEALTH CENTER (O, 40 beds) 1691 Highway 9, Toms River, NJ Zip 08755–1245; tel. 732/914–1688; Joe Hicks, Executive Director
**Web address:** www.barnabashealth.org/

SAINT BARNABAS MEDICAL CENTER (O, 597 beds) 94 Old Short Hills Road, Livingston, NJ Zip 07039–5672; tel. 973/322–5000; John F. Bonamo, M.D., MS, Executive Director
**Web address:** www.sbhcs.com

| | | |
|---|---|---|
| Owned, leased, sponsored: | 7 hospitals | 2534 beds |
| Contract–managed: | 0 hospitals | 0 beds |
| Totals: | 7 hospitals | 2534 beds |

---

**★0528: BASSETT HEALTHCARE NETWORK** (NP)
1 Atwell Road, Cooperstown, NY Zip 13326–1301; tel. 607/547–3456; William F. Streck, M.D., President and Chief Executive Officer
**(Independent Hospital System)**

**NEW YORK:** AURELIA OSBORN FOX MEMORIAL HOSPITAL (O, 220 beds) 1 Norton Avenue, Oneonta, NY Zip 13820–2629; tel. 607/432–2000; John R. Remillard, President
**Web address:** www.aofoxhospital.com

BASSETT MEDICAL CENTER (O, 164 beds) One Atwell Road, Cooperstown, NY Zip 13326–1394; tel. 607/547–3100; William F. Streck, M.D., President and Chief Executive Officer
**Web address:** www.bassett.org

COBLESKILL REGIONAL HOSPITAL (O, 40 beds) 178 Grandview Drive, Cobleskill, NY Zip 12043–5144; tel. 518/254–3456; Eric H. Stein, FACHE, President and Chief Executive Officer
**Web address:** www.cobleskillhospital.org

For explanation of codes following names, see page B2.
★ Indicates Type III membership in the American Hospital Association.

**Section B**

LITTLE FALLS HOSPITAL (O, 59 beds) 140 Burwell Street, Little Falls, NY Zip 13365–1725; tel. 315/823–1000; Michael L. Ogden, President and Chief Executive Officer
**Web address:** www.lfhny.org

O'CONNOR HOSPITAL (O, 16 beds) 460 Andes Road, State Route 28, Delhi, NY Zip 13753; tel. 607/746–0300; Daniel M. Ayres, Chief Executive Officer
**Web address:** www.oconnorhosp.org

| Owned, leased, sponsored: | 5 hospitals | 499 beds |
| Contract–managed: | 0 hospitals | 0 beds |
| Totals: | 5 hospitals | 499 beds |

---

★**0095:  BAYLOR HEALTH CARE SYSTEM** (CO)
3500 Gaston Avenue, Dallas, TX Zip 75246; tel. 214/820–0111; Joel T. Allison, President and Chief Executive Officer
**(Centralized Health System)**

**TEXAS:** BAYLOR ALL SAINTS MEDICAL CENTER AT FORT WORTH (O, 606 beds) 1400 Eighth Avenue, Fort Worth, TX Zip 76104–4192; tel. 817/926–2544; Steven R. Newton, President
**Web address:** www.baylorhealth.com

BAYLOR INSTITUTE FOR REHABILITATION (O, 87 beds) 909 North Washington Avenue, Dallas, TX Zip 75246–1520; tel. 214/820–9300; Jon C. Skinner, Chief Executive Officer
**Web address:** www.bhcs.com

BAYLOR MEDICAL CENTER AT GARLAND (O, 240 beds) 2300 Marie Curie Drive, Garland, TX Zip 75042–5706; tel. 972/487–5000; Thomas J. Trenary, President
**Web address:** www.baylorhealth.com

BAYLOR MEDICAL CENTER AT IRVING (L, 222 beds) 1901 North MacArthur Boulevard, Irving, TX Zip 75061; tel. 972/579–8100; Cindy K. Schamp, President
**Web address:** www.baylorhealth.com

BAYLOR MEDICAL CENTER AT WAXAHACHIE (O, 54 beds) 1405 West Jefferson Street, Waxahachie, TX Zip 75165–2275; tel. 972/923–7000; Jay Fox, President
**Web address:** www.bhcs.com

BAYLOR ORTHOPEDIC AND SPINE HOSPITAL AT ARLINGTON (O, 24 beds) 707 Highlander Boulevard, Arlington, TX Zip 76015–4319; tel. 817/583–7100; Allan Beck, Chief Executive Officer
**Web address:** www.baylorarlington.com

BAYLOR REGIONAL MEDICAL CENTER AT GRAPEVINE (O, 274 beds) 1650 West College Street, Grapevine, TX Zip 76051–1650; tel. 817/481–1588; Doug Lawson, President
**Web address:** www.bhcs.com

BAYLOR REGIONAL MEDICAL CENTER AT PLANO (O, 112 beds) 4700 Alliance Boulevard, Plano, TX Zip 75093; tel. 469/814–2000; Jerri Garison, R.N., President
**Web address:** www.baylorhealth.com

BAYLOR SPECIALTY HOSPITAL (O, 61 beds) 3504 Swiss Avenue, Dallas, TX Zip 75204–6224; tel. 214/820–9700; Elizabeth Youngblood, President
**Web address:** www.bhcs.com

BAYLOR UNIVERSITY MEDICAL CENTER (O, 933 beds) 3500 Gaston Avenue, Dallas, TX Zip 75246–2088; tel. 214/820–0111; John B. McWhorter, III, President
**Web address:** www.baylorhealth.com

OUR CHILDREN'S HOUSE AT BAYLOR (O, 54 beds) 3504 Swiss Avenue, Dallas, TX Zip 75204–6224; tel. 214/820–9838; Elizabeth Youngblood, President
**Web address:** www.bhcs.com

| Owned, leased, sponsored: | 11 hospitals | 2667 beds |
| Contract–managed: | 0 hospitals | 0 beds |
| Totals: | 11 hospitals | 2667 beds |

---

★**1095:  BAYSTATE HEALTH, INC.** (NP)
759 Chestnut Street, Springfield, MA Zip 01199–0001; tel. 413/794–0000; Mark R. Tolosky, JD, FACHE, President and Chief Executive Officer
**(Centralized Physician/Insurance Health System)**

**MASSACHUSETTS:** BAYSTATE FRANKLIN MEDICAL CENTER (O, 90 beds) 164 High Street, Greenfield, MA Zip 01301–2613; tel. 413/773–0211; Charles Gijanto, President, Baystate Northern Region
**Web address:** www.baystatehealth.com

BAYSTATE MARY LANE HOSPITAL (O, 31 beds) 85 South Street, Ware, MA Zip 01082–1697; tel. 413/967–6211; Charles Gijanto, President
**Web address:** www.baystatehealth.com

BAYSTATE MEDICAL CENTER (O, 659 beds) 759 Chestnut Street, Springfield, MA Zip 01199–0001; tel. 413/794–0000; Mark R. Tolosky, JD, FACHE, President and Chief Executive Officer
**Web address:** www.baystatehealth.org

| Owned, leased, sponsored: | 3 hospitals | 780 beds |
| Contract–managed: | 0 hospitals | 0 beds |
| Totals: | 3 hospitals | 780 beds |

---

★**9575:  BEAUMONT HEALTH SYSTEM** (NP)
3711 West 13 Mile Road, Royal Oak, MI Zip 48073–6767; tel. 248/898–5000; Gene Michalski, President and Chief Executive Officer
**(Centralized Health System)**

**MICHIGAN:** BEAUMONT HOSPITAL – ROYAL OAK (O, 1070 beds) 3601 West Thirteen Mile Road, Royal Oak, MI Zip 48073–6712; tel. 248/898–5000; Shane Cerone, President
**Web address:** www.beaumonthospitals.com

BEAUMONT HOSPITAL – TROY (O, 394 beds) 44201 Dequindre Road, Troy, MI Zip 48085–1117; tel. 248/964–5000; Nancy Susick, MSN, President
**Web address:** www.beaumonthospitals.com

BEAUMONT HOSPITAL GROSSE POINTE (O, 250 beds) 468 Cadieux Road, Grosse Pointe, MI Zip 48230–1507; tel. 313/473–1000; Richard P. Swaine, President
**Web address:** www.beaumont.edu

| Owned, leased, sponsored: | 3 hospitals | 1714 beds |
| Contract–managed: | 0 hospitals | 0 beds |
| Totals: | 3 hospitals | 1714 beds |

---

**0362:  BEHAVIORAL CENTERS OF AMERICA** (IO)
3100 West End Avenue, Suite 1000, Nashville, TN Zip 37203; tel. 615/463–3200; John E. Turner, President and Chief Executive Officer
**(Independent Hospital System)**

BCA STONECREST HOSPITAL (O, 90 beds) 15000 Gratiot Avenue, Detroit, MI Zip 48205–1973; tel. 313/245–0600; Steve Savage, Chief Operating Officer
**Web address:** www.bcastonecrestcenter.com

**OHIO:** OHIO HOSPITAL FOR CHILD AND ADOLESCENT PSYCHIATRY (O, 68 beds) 880 Greenlawn Avenue, Columbus, OH Zip 43223–2616; tel. 614/449–9664; Roxanne Jividen, Chief Executive Officer
**Web address:** www.bca-corp.com

TEN LAKES CENTER (O, 16 beds) 819 North First Street, 3rd Floor, Dennison, OH Zip 44621; tel. 740/922–7499; Laura Blackburn, Administrator
**Web address:** www.tenlakescenter.com/

**TEXAS:** BCA PERMIAN BASIN (O, 64 beds) 3300 South FM 1788, Midland, TX Zip 79706–2601; tel. 432/561–5915; John Flanagan, Chief Executive Officer
**Web address:** www.bcapermianbasin.com/

CEDAR CREST HOSPITAL (O, 50 beds) 3500 I–35 South, Belton, TX Zip 76513; tel. 254/939–2100; Ingrid Whittle, Chief Executive Officer
**Web address:** www.cedarcresthospital.com

| Owned, leased, sponsored: | 5 hospitals | 288 beds |
| Contract–managed: | 0 hospitals | 0 beds |
| Totals: | 5 hospitals | 288 beds |

---

**0545:  BENEDICTINE SISTERS OF THE ANNUNCIATION** (CC)
7520 University Drive, Bismarck, ND Zip 58504–9653; tel. 701/255–1520; Sister Susan Berger, Prioress
**(Moderately Centralized Health System)**

For explanation of codes following names, see page B2.
★ Indicates Type III membership in the American Hospital Association.

**NORTH DAKOTA:** GARRISON MEMORIAL HOSPITAL (S, 22 beds) 407 Third Avenue S.E., Garrison, ND Zip 58540–7235; tel. 701/463–2275; Dean Mattern, President and Chief Executive Officer
**Web address:** www.garrisonmh.com

ST. ALEXIUS MEDICAL CENTER (S, 281 beds) 900 East Broadway, Bismarck, ND Zip 58501–4586, Mailing Address: P.O. Box 5510, Zip 58506–5510; tel. 701/530–7000; Gary P. Miller, President and Chief Executive Officer
**Web address:** www.st.alexius.org

| | | |
|---|---|---|
| Owned, leased, sponsored: | 2 hospitals | 303 beds |
| Contract–managed: | 0 hospitals | 0 beds |
| Totals: | 2 hospitals | 303 beds |

**0538:  BENEFIS HEALTH SYSTEM** (NP)
1101 26th Street South, Great Falls, MT Zip 59405; tel. 406/455–5000; John H. Goodnow, Chief Executive Officer
**(Moderately Centralized Health System)**

**MONTANA:** BENEFIS HOSPITALS (O, 438 beds) 1101 26th Street South, Great Falls, MT Zip 59405–5104; tel. 406/455–5000; John H. Goodnow, Chief Executive Officer
**Web address:** www.benefis.org

MISSOURI RIVER MEDICAL CENTER (C, 52 beds) 1501 St. Charles Street, Fort Benton, MT Zip 59442–0249, Mailing Address: P.O. Box 249, Zip 59442–0249; tel. 406/622–3331; Jay Pottenger, Administrator
**Web address:** www.mrmcfb.org

| | | |
|---|---|---|
| Owned, leased, sponsored: | 1 hospital | 438 beds |
| Contract–managed: | 1 hospital | 52 beds |
| Totals: | 2 hospitals | 490 beds |

**★2435:  BERKSHIRE HEALTH SYSTEMS, INC.** (NP)
725 North Street, Pittsfield, MA Zip 01201–4124; tel. 413/447–2743; David E. Phelps, President and Chief Executive Officer
**(Independent Hospital System)**

**MASSACHUSETTS:** BERKSHIRE MEDICAL CENTER (O, 278 beds) 725 North Street, Pittsfield, MA Zip 01201–4124; tel. 413/447–2000; Diane Kelly, R.N., Chief Operating Officer
**Web address:** www.berkshirehealthsystems.com

FAIRVIEW HOSPITAL (O, 24 beds) 29 Lewis Avenue, Great Barrington, MA Zip 01230–1713; tel. 413/528–0790; Eugene A. Dellea, President
**Web address:** www.berkshirehealthsystems.com

| | | |
|---|---|---|
| Owned, leased, sponsored: | 2 hospitals | 302 beds |
| Contract–managed: | 0 hospitals | 0 beds |
| Totals: | 2 hospitals | 302 beds |

**★0051:  BJC HEALTHCARE** (NP)
4901 Forest Park Avenue, Suite 1200, Saint Louis, MO Zip 63108–1401; tel. 314/747–9322; Steven H. Lipstein, President and Chief Executive Officer
**(Centralized Health System)**

**ILLINOIS:** ALTON MEMORIAL HOSPITAL (O, 253 beds) One Memorial Drive, Alton, IL Zip 62002–6722; tel. 618/463–7311; David A. Braasch, President
**Web address:** www.altonmemorialhospital.org

CLAY COUNTY HOSPITAL (C, 18 beds) 911 Stacy Burk Drive, Flora, IL Zip 62839–1823, Mailing Address: P.O. Box 280, Zip 62839–0280; tel. 618/662–2131; Robert R. Sellers, President
**Web address:** www.claycountyhospital.org

**MISSOURI:** BARNES–JEWISH HOSPITAL (O, 1305 beds) 1 Barnes–Jewish Hospital Plaza, Saint Louis, MO Zip 63110–1003; tel. 314/747–3000; Richard J. Liekweg, President
**Web address:** www.barnesjewish.org

BARNES–JEWISH ST. PETERS HOSPITAL (O, 113 beds) 10 Hospital Drive, Saint Peters, MO Zip 63376–1659; tel. 636/916–9000; John Antes, President
**Web address:** www.bjsph.org/

BARNES–JEWISH WEST COUNTY HOSPITAL (O, 77 beds) 12634 Olive Boulevard, Saint Louis, MO Zip 63141–6337; tel. 314/996–8000; Larry Tracy, FACHE, Chief Operating Officer
**Web address:** www.barnesjewishwestcounty.org

BOONE HOSPITAL CENTER (L, 360 beds) 1600 East Broadway, Columbia, MO Zip 65201–5844; tel. 573/815–8000; Daniel J. Rothery, President
**Web address:** www.boone.org

CHRISTIAN HOSPITAL (O, 262 beds) 11133 Dunn Road, Saint Louis, MO Zip 63136–6119; tel. 314/653–5000; Ronald B. McMullen, President
**Web address:** www.bjc.org

MISSOURI BAPTIST MEDICAL CENTER (O, 448 beds) 3015 North Ballas Road, Saint Louis, MO Zip 63131–2329; tel. 314/996–5000; Joan Magruder, President
**Web address:** www.missouribaptistmedicalcenter.org

MISSOURI BAPTIST SULLIVAN HOSPITAL (O, 56 beds) 751 Sappington Bridge Road, Sullivan, MO Zip 63080–2354; tel. 573/468–4186; Tony Schwarm, President
**Web address:** www.missouribaptistsullivan.org

PARKLAND HEALTH CENTER (O, 98 beds) 1101 West Liberty Street, Farmington, MO Zip 63640–1921; tel. 573/756–6451; Thomas P. Karl, President
**Web address:** www.parklandhealthcenter.org

PARKLAND HEALTH CENTER–BONNE TERRE (O, 6 beds) 7245 Raider Road, Bonne Terre, MO Zip 63628–3767; tel. 573/358–1400; Thomas P. Karl, President
**Web address:** www.parklandhealthcenter.org

PROGRESS WEST HEALTHCARE CENTER (O, 42 beds) Two Progress Point, Saint Charles, MO Zip 63368–2208; tel. 636/344–2273; John Antes, President
**Web address:** www.progresswesthealthcare.org

ST. LOUIS CHILDREN'S HOSPITAL (O, 250 beds) One Children's Place, Saint Louis, MO Zip 63110–1002; tel. 314/454–6000; Lee F. Fetter, President and Senior Executive Officer
**Web address:** www.stlouischildrens.org

| | | |
|---|---|---|
| Owned, leased, sponsored: | 12 hospitals | 3270 beds |
| Contract–managed: | 1 hospital | 18 beds |
| Totals: | 13 hospitals | 3288 beds |

**★0852:  BLANCHARD VALLEY HEALTH SYSTEM** (NP)
1900 South Main Street, Findlay, OH Zip 45840–1214; tel. 419/423–4500; Scott C. Malaney, President and Chief Executive Officer

**OHIO:** BLANCHARD VALLEY HOSPITAL (O, 181 beds) 1900 South Main Street, Findlay, OH Zip 45840; tel. 419/423–4500; Scott C. Malaney, President and Chief Executive Officer
**Web address:** www.bvhealthsystem.org

BLUFFTON HOSPITAL (O, 25 beds) 139 Garau Street, Bluffton, OH Zip 45817–0048; tel. 419/358–9010; William D. Watkins, Chief Administrative Officer
**Web address:** www.bvhealthsystem.org

| | | |
|---|---|---|
| Owned, leased, sponsored: | 2 hospitals | 206 beds |
| Contract–managed: | 0 hospitals | 0 beds |
| Totals: | 2 hospitals | 206 beds |

**0300:  BLUE MOUNTAIN HEALTH SYSTEM** (NP)
211 North 12th Street, Lehighton, PA Zip 18235–1138; tel. 610/377–1300; Andrew E. Harris, President and Chief Executive Officer
**(Independent Hospital System)**

**PENNSYLVANIA:** GNADEN HUETTEN MEMORIAL HOSPITAL (O, 186 beds) 211 North 12th Street, Lehighton, PA Zip 18235–1138; tel. 610/377–1300; Andrew E. Harris, Chief Executive Officer
**Web address:** www.bluemountainhealthsystem.org

For explanation of codes following names, see page B2.
★ Indicates Type III membership in the American Hospital Association.

Section B

PALMERTON HOSPITAL (O, 60 beds) 135 Lafayette Avenue, Palmerton, PA Zip 18071–1596; tel. 610/826–3141; Andrew E. Harris, Chief Executive Officer
**Web address:** www.bmhs.com

| Owned, leased, sponsored: | 2 hospitals | 246 beds |
|---|---|---|
| Contract–managed: | 0 hospitals | 0 beds |
| Totals: | 2 hospitals | 246 beds |

---

★**0053: BLUE WATER HEALTH SERVICES CORPORATION** (NP)
1221 Pine Grove Avenue, Port Huron, MI Zip 48061–5011; tel. 810/989–3717; Thomas D. DeFauw, FACHE, President and Chief Executive Officer
**(Independent Hospital System)**

**MICHIGAN:** MARWOOD MANOR NURSING HOME (O, 106 beds) 1300 Beard Street, Port Huron, MI Zip 48060; tel. 818/982–2594; Brian Oberly, Administrator

PORT HURON HOSPITAL (O, 186 beds) 1221 Pine Grove Avenue, Port Huron, MI Zip 48060–3511; tel. 810/987–5000; Thomas D. DeFauw, FACHE, President and Chief Executive Officer
**Web address:** www.porthuronhospital.org

| Owned, leased, sponsored: | 2 hospitals | 292 beds |
|---|---|---|
| Contract–managed: | 0 hospitals | 0 beds |
| Totals: | 2 hospitals | 292 beds |

---

★**5085: BON SECOURS HEALTH SYSTEM, INC.** (CC)
1505 Marriottsville Road, Marriottsville, MD Zip 21104–1399; tel. 410/442–5511; Richard Statuto, President and Chief Executive Officer
**(Moderately Centralized Health System)**

**KENTUCKY:** OUR LADY OF BELLEFONTE HOSPITAL (O, 151 beds) St. Christopher Drive, Ashland, KY Zip 41101, Mailing Address: P.O. Box 789, Zip 41105–0789; tel. 606/833–3333; Kevin Halter, Chief Executive Officer
**Web address:** www.olbh.com

**MARYLAND:** BON SECOURS BALTIMORE HEALTH SYSTEM (O, 89 beds) 2000 West Baltimore Street, Baltimore, MD Zip 21223–1597; tel. 410/362–3000; Samuel Lee Ross, M.D., MS, Chief Executive Officer
**Web address:** www.bonsecoursbaltimore.com

**NEW YORK:** BON SECOURS COMMUNITY HOSPITAL (O, 187 beds) 160 East Main Street, Port Jervis, NY Zip 12771–2245, Mailing Address: P.O. Box 1014, Zip 12771–1014; tel. 845/858–7000; Jeff Reilly, Senior Vice President Operations
**Web address:** www.bonsecourscommunityhosp.org

GOOD SAMARITAN HOSPITAL (O, 308 beds) 255 Lafayette Avenue, Suffern, NY Zip 10901–4869; tel. 845/368–5000; Philip A. Patterson, Chief Executive Officer
**Web address:** www.goodsamhosp.org

ST. ANTHONY COMMUNITY HOSPITAL (O, 73 beds) 15 Maple Avenue, Warwick, NY Zip 10990–1028; tel. 845/986–2276; Jeff Reilly, Senior Vice President Operations
**Web address:** www.stanthonycommunityhosp.org

**SOUTH CAROLINA:** BON SECOURS ST. FRANCIS HEALTH SYSTEM (O, 331 beds) One St. Francis Drive, Greenville, SC Zip 29601–3207; tel. 864/255–1000; Mark S. Nantz, FACHE, Chief Executive Officer
**Web address:** www.stfrancishealth.org

**VIRGINIA:** BON SECOURS MARYVIEW MEDICAL CENTER (O, 466 beds) 3636 High Street, Portsmouth, VA Zip 23707–3270; tel. 757/398–2200; Joseph M. Oddis, Chief Executive Officer
**Web address:** www.bonsecourshamptonroads.com

BON SECOURS MEMORIAL REGIONAL MEDICAL CENTER (O, 225 beds) 8260 Atlee Road, Mechanicsville, VA Zip 23116–1844; tel. 804/764–6000; Michael Robinson, Chief Executive Officer
**Web address:** www.bonsecours.com

BON SECOURS ST. FRANCIS MEDICAL CENTER (O, 130 beds) 13710 St. Francis Boulevard, Midlothian, VA Zip 23114–3267; tel. 804/594–7300; Mark M. Gordon, Executive Vice President
**Web address:** www.bonsecours.com/sfmc/default.asp

BON SECOURS ST. MARY'S HOSPITAL (O, 391 beds) 5801 Bremo Road, Richmond, VA Zip 23226–1907; tel. 804/285–2011; Toni R. Ardabell, R.N., Chief Executive Officer
**Web address:** www.bonsecours.com

BON SECOURS–DEPAUL MEDICAL CENTER (O, 238 beds) 150 Kingsley Lane, Norfolk, VA Zip 23505–4650; tel. 757/889–5000; John E. Barrett, III, Chief Executive Officer
**Web address:** www.bonsecourshamptonroads.com

BON SECOURS–RICHMOND COMMUNITY HOSPITAL (O, 101 beds) 1500 North 28th Street, Richmond, VA Zip 23223–5396, Mailing Address: P.O. Box 27184, Zip 23261–7184; tel. 804/225–1700; Michael Robinson, Executive Vice President and Administrator
**Web address:** www.bonsecours.com

MARY IMMACULATE HOSPITAL (O, 232 beds) 2 Bernardine Drive, Newport News, VA Zip 23602–4499; tel. 757/886–6000; Patricia L. Robertson, Executive Vice President
**Web address:** www.bonsecourshamptonroads.com

| Owned, leased, sponsored: | 13 hospitals | 2922 beds |
|---|---|---|
| Contract–managed: | 0 hospitals | 0 beds |
| Totals: | 13 hospitals | 2922 beds |

---

**2455: BRADFORD HEALTH SERVICES** (IO)
2101 Magnolia Avenue South, Suite 518, Birmingham, AL Zip 35205; tel. 205/251–7753; Jerry W. Crowder, President and Chief Executive Officer

**ALABAMA:** BRADFORD HEALTH SERVICES AT HUNTSVILLE (O, 84 beds) 1600 Browns Ferry Road, Madison, AL Zip 35758–9769, Mailing Address: P.O. Box 176, Zip 35758–0176; tel. 256/461–7272; Bob Hinds, Executive Director
**Web address:** www.bradfordhealth.com

BRADFORD HEALTH SERVICES AT WARRIOR LODGE (O, 100 beds) 1189 Allbritt Road, Warrior, AL Zip 35180, Mailing Address: P.O. Box 129, Zip 35180–0129; tel. 205/647–1945; Roy M. Ramsey, Executive Director
**Web address:** www.bradfordhealth.com

| Owned, leased, sponsored: | 2 hospitals | 184 beds |
|---|---|---|
| Contract–managed: | 0 hospitals | 0 beds |
| Totals: | 2 hospitals | 184 beds |

---

★**0595: BRONSON HEALTHCARE GROUP, INC.** (NP)
301 John Street, Kalamazoo, MI Zip 49007–5345; tel. 269/341–6000; Frank J. Sardone, President and Chief Executive Officer
**(Independent Hospital System)**

**MICHIGAN:** BRONSON BATTLE CREEK (O, 218 beds) 300 North Avenue, Battle Creek, MI Zip 49017–3307; tel. 269/966–8000; Denise Brooks–Williams, President and Chief Executive Officer
**Web address:** www.bchealth.com

BRONSON LAKEVIEW HOSPITAL (O, 35 beds) 408 Hazen Street, Paw Paw, MI Zip 49079–1019, Mailing Address: P.O. Box 209, Zip 49079–0209; tel. 269/657–3141; Frank J. Sardone, President and Chief Executive Officer
**Web address:** www.bronsonhealth.com/lakeview

BRONSON METHODIST HOSPITAL (O, 368 beds) 601 John Street, Kalamazoo, MI Zip 49007–5346; tel. 269/341–6000; Frank J. Sardone, President and Chief Executive Officer
**Web address:** www.bronsonhealth.com

| Owned, leased, sponsored: | 3 hospitals | 621 beds |
|---|---|---|
| Contract–managed: | 0 hospitals | 0 beds |
| Totals: | 3 hospitals | 621 beds |

---

For explanation of codes following names, see page B2.
★ Indicates Type III membership in the American Hospital Association.

Section B

★**3115: BROWARD HEALTH** (NP)
303 S.E. 17th Street, Fort Lauderdale, FL Zip 33316–2510;
tel. 954/355–5100; Frank P. Nask, President and Chief Executive
Officer

**FLORIDA:** BROWARD HEALTH CORAL SPRINGS (O, 182 beds) 3000 Coral
Hills Drive, Coral Springs, FL Zip 33065; tel. 954/344–3000; Drew
Grossman, Chief Executive Officer
**Web address:** www.browardhealth.org

BROWARD HEALTH IMPERIAL POINT (O, 180 beds) 6401 North Federal
Highway, Fort Lauderdale, FL Zip 33308–1495; tel. 954/776–8500; Alice
Taylor, R.N., MSN, Chief Executive Officer
**Web address:** www.browardhealth.org

BROWARD HEALTH MEDICAL CENTER (O, 656 beds) 1600 South Andrews
Avenue, Fort Lauderdale, FL Zip 33316–2510; tel. 954/355–4400; Calvin E.
Glidewell, Jr., Chief Executive Officer
**Web address:** www.browardhealth.org

BROWARD HEALTH NORTH (O, 360 beds) 201 East Sample Road, Deerfield
Beach, FL Zip 33064–3502; tel. 954/941–8300; Pauline Grant, FACHE, Chief
Executive Officer
**Web address:** www.browardhealth.org

| Owned, leased, sponsored: | 4 hospitals | 1378 beds |
|---|---|---|
| Contract–managed: | 0 hospitals | 0 beds |
| Totals: | 4 hospitals | 1378 beds |

★**0400: BRYANLGH HEALTH SYSTEM** (NP)
1600 South 48th Street, Lincoln, NE Zip 68506;
tel. 402/489–0200; Kimberly A. Russel, President and Chief
Executive Officer
**(Centralized Physician/Insurance Health System)**

**NEBRASKA:** BRYANLGH MEDICAL CENTER (O, 346 beds) 1600 South 48th
Street, Lincoln, NE Zip 68506–1283; tel. 402/489–0200; John T.
Woodrich, President and Chief Operating Officer
**Web address:** www.bryanlgh.org

CRETE AREA MEDICAL CENTER (O, 24 beds) 2910 Betten Drive, Crete, NE
Zip 68333–0220, Mailing Address: P.O. Box 220, Zip 68333–0220;
tel. 402/826–2102; Carol Friesen, Chief Executive Officer
**Web address:** www.creteareamedicalcenter.com

| Owned, leased, sponsored: | 2 hospitals | 370 beds |
|---|---|---|
| Contract–managed: | 0 hospitals | 0 beds |
| Totals: | 2 hospitals | 370 beds |

**9655: BUREAU OF MEDICINE AND SURGERY, DEPARTMENT
OF THE NAVY** (FG)
2300 East Street N.W., Washington, DC Zip 20372–5300;
tel. 202/762–3701; Rear Admiral Matthew L. Nathan, Surgeon
General
**(Independent Hospital System)**

**CALIFORNIA:** NAVAL HOSPITAL (O, 16 beds) 937 Franklin Avenue, Lemoore,
CA Zip 93246–5004; tel. 559/998–4421; Captain William J. Leonard,
USN, Commanding Officer
**Web address:** www.lemoore.med.navy.mil

NAVAL HOSPITAL (O, 72 beds) Santa Margarita Road, Building H100, Camp
Pendleton, CA Zip 92055–5191, Mailing Address: P.O. Box 555191,
Zip 92055–5191; tel. 760/725–1304; Captain Kenneth J. Iverson, MC, USN,
Commanding Officer
**Web address:** www.cpen.med.navy.mil

NAVAL HOSPITAL (O, 39 beds) Twentynine Palms, CA Zip 92278;
tel. 760/830–2190; Captain Jay C. Sourbeer, Commanding Officer
**Web address:** www.nhtp.med.navy.mil/nhtp

NAVAL MEDICAL CENTER (O, 285 beds) 34800 Bob Wilson Drive, San Diego,
CA Zip 92134–5000; tel. 619/532–6400; Rear Admiral C. Forrest Faison,
Commander
**Web address:** www.nmcsd.med.navy.mil

**FLORIDA:** NAVAL HOSPITAL (O, 64 beds) 2080 Child Street, Jacksonville, FL
Zip 32214–5000; tel. 904/542–7300; Captain Lynn Welling, Commander
**Web address:** www.navalhospitaljax.com

NAVAL HOSPITAL (O, 32 beds) 6000 West Highway 98, Pensacola, FL
Zip 32512–0003; tel. 850/505–6413; Maureen Padden, Commander
**Web address:** www.psaweb.pcola.med.navy.mil

**GUAM:** U. S. NAVAL HOSPITAL (O, 55 beds) Agana, GU Zip 96910; FPO,
APtel. 671/344–9340; Captain Kevin W. Haws, USN, Commanding Officer
**Web address:** www.med.navy.mil/sites/nmw/commands

**MARYLAND:** WALTER REED NATIONAL MILITARY MEDICAL CENTER (O, 240
beds) 8901 Wisconsin Avenue, Bethesda, MD Zip 20889–5600;
tel. 301/295–4611; Rear Admiral Alton Stocks, Commander
**Web address:** www.bethesda.med.navy.mil

**NORTH CAROLINA:** NAVAL HOSPITAL (O, 117 beds) Camp Lejeune, NC
Zip 28547–0100; tel. 910/450–4300; Captain Daniel J. Zinder,
Commanding Officer
**Web address:** www.med.navy.mil/sites/nhcl

**SOUTH CAROLINA:** NAVAL HOSPITAL BEAUFORT (O, 20 beds) 1 Pinckney
Boulevard, Beaufort, SC Zip 29902–6148; tel. 843/228–5301; Captain J.
R. Queen, MSC, USN, Commanding Officer
**Web address:** www.beaufortnavalhospital.com/

**VIRGINIA:** NAVAL MEDICAL CENTER (O, 274 beds) 620 John Paul Jones
Circle, Portsmouth, VA Zip 23708–2197; tel. 757/953–5000; Rear
Admiral Elaine Wagner, M.D., Commander
**Web address:** www.nmcp.med.navy.mil

**WASHINGTON:** NAVAL HOSPITAL (O, 29 beds) 3475 North Saratoga Street,
Oak Harbor, WA Zip 98278–8800; tel. 360/257–9500; Captain Susan
Lickenstein, Commander
**Web address:** www.med.navy.mil/sites/nhoh/Pages/default.aspx

NAVAL HOSPITAL BREMERTON (O, 40 beds) One Boone Road, Bremerton,
WA Zip 98312–1898; tel. 360/475–4000; Captain Christopher M. Culp,
Commanding Officer
**Web address:** www.med.navy.mil/sites/nhbrem

| Owned, leased, sponsored: | 13 hospitals | 1283 beds |
|---|---|---|
| Contract–managed: | 0 hospitals | 0 beds |
| Totals: | 13 hospitals | 1283 beds |

★**0813: CADENCE HEALTH** (NP)
25 North Winfield Road, Winfield, IL Zip 60190; tel. 630/933–1600;
Michael Vivoda, Chief Executive Officer

**ILLINOIS:** CENTRAL DUPAGE HOSPITAL (O, 344 beds) 25 North Winfield
Road, Winfield, IL Zip 60190; tel. 630/933–1600; Michael Vivoda,
President
**Web address:** www.cdh.org

DELNOR HOSPITAL (O, 159 beds) 300 Randall Road, Geneva, IL
Zip 60134–4200; tel. 630/208–3000; Robert Friedberg, President
**Web address:** www.delnor.com

| Owned, leased, sponsored: | 2 hospitals | 503 beds |
|---|---|---|
| Contract–managed: | 0 hospitals | 0 beds |
| Totals: | 2 hospitals | 503 beds |

**0113: CANCER TREATMENT CENTERS OF AMERICA** (IO)
1336 Basswood Road, Schaumburg, IL Zip 60173;
tel. 847/342–7400; Stephen B. Bonner, President and Chief
Executive Officer

**ARIZONA:** WESTERN REGIONAL MEDICAL CENTER (O, 24 beds) 14200 West
Fillmore Street, Goodyear, AZ Zip 85338–3005; tel. 623/207–3000;
David Veillette, President and Chief Executive Officer
**Web address:** www.cancercenter.com/western–hospital.cfm

**ILLINOIS:** MIDWESTERN REGIONAL MEDICAL CENTER (O, 73 beds) 2520
Elisha Avenue, Zion, IL Zip 60099–2587; tel. 847/872–4561; Anne
Meisner, MSN, President and Chief Executive Officer
**Web address:** www.cancercenter.com

**OKLAHOMA:** SOUTHWESTERN REGIONAL MEDICAL CENTER (O, 43 beds)
10109 East 79th Street, Tulsa, OK Zip 74133–4564;
tel. 918/286–5000; Steve Mackin, President and Chief Executive Officer
**Web address:** www.cancercenter.com

Section B

For explanation of codes following names, see page B2.
★ Indicates Type III membership in the American Hospital Association.

**PENNSYLVANIA:** EASTERN REGIONAL MEDICAL CENTER (O, 22 beds) 1331 East Wyoming Avenue, Philadelphia, PA Zip 19124; tel. 800/294–8333; John McNeil, President and Chief Executive Officer
**Web address:** www.cancercenter.com

| Owned, leased, sponsored: | 4 hospitals | 162 beds |
|---|---|---|
| Contract–managed: | 0 hospitals | 0 beds |
| Totals: | 4 hospitals | 162 beds |

★**0124:  CAPE COD HEALTHCARE, INC.** (NP)
88 Lewis Bay Road, Hyannis, MA Zip 02601–5210; tel. 508/862–5121; Michael K. Lauf, President and Chief Executive Officer
**(Centralized Health System)**

**MASSACHUSETTS:** CAPE COD HOSPITAL (O, 259 beds) 27 Park Street, Hyannis, MA Zip 02601–5230; tel. 508/771–1800; Jason M. Adams, Chief Operating Officer
**Web address:** www.capecodhealth.org

FALMOUTH HOSPITAL (O, 95 beds) 100 Ter Heun Drive, Falmouth, MA Zip 02540–2599; tel. 508/548–5300; Susan M. Wing, R.N., Chief Operating Officer
**Web address:** www.capecodhealth.org

| Owned, leased, sponsored: | 2 hospitals | 354 beds |
|---|---|---|
| Contract–managed: | 0 hospitals | 0 beds |
| Totals: | 2 hospitals | 354 beds |

**0835:  CAPE FEAR VALLEY HEALTH SYSTEM** (NP)
1638 Owen Drive, Fayetteville, NC Zip 28304, Mailing Address: P.O. Box 2000, Zip 28302–2000; tel. 910/615–4000; Michael Nagowski, President and Chief Executive Officer
**(Moderately Centralized Health System)**

**NORTH CAROLINA:** CAPE FEAR VALLEY – BLADEN COUNTY HOSPITAL (O, 26 beds) 501 South Poplar Street, Elizabethtown, NC Zip 28337–0398, Mailing Address: P.O. Box 398, Zip 28337–0398; tel. 910/862–5100; Cameron Highsmith, Chief Executive Officer
**Web address:** www.bchn.org

CAPE FEAR VALLEY MEDICAL CENTER (O, 666 beds) 1638 Owen Drive, Fayetteville, NC Zip 28304–3431, Mailing Address: P.O. Box 2000, Zip 28302–2000; tel. 910/615–4000; Michael Nagowski, President and Chief Executive Officer
**Web address:** www.capefearvalley.com

HIGHSMITH–RAINEY SPECIALTY HOSPITAL (O, 133 beds) 150 Robeson Street, Fayetteville, NC Zip 28301–5570; tel. 910/615–1000; Michael Nagowski, President and Chief Executive Officer
**Web address:** www.capefearvalley.com

| Owned, leased, sponsored: | 3 hospitals | 825 beds |
|---|---|---|
| Contract–managed: | 0 hospitals | 0 beds |
| Totals: | 3 hospitals | 825 beds |

**0337:  CAPELLA HEALTHCARE** (IO)
501 Corporate Centre Drive, Suite 200, Franklin, TN Zip 37067; tel. 615/764–3000; Daniel S. Slipkovich, Chief Executive Officer
**(Moderately Centralized Health System)**

**ALABAMA:** JACKSONVILLE MEDICAL CENTER (O, 69 beds) 1701 Pelham Road South, Jacksonville, AL Zip 36265–3399, Mailing Address: P.O. Box 999, Zip 36265–0999; tel. 256/435–4970; James H. Edmondson, Chief Executive Officer
**Web address:** www.jmchealth.com

PARKWAY MEDICAL CENTER (O, 120 beds) 1874 Beltline Road S.W., Decatur, AL Zip 35601–5509, Mailing Address: P.O. Box 2211, Zip 35609–2211; tel. 256/350–2211; Nathaniel Richardson, Jr., Interim President
**Web address:** www.parkwaymedicalcenter.com

**ARKANSAS:** NATIONAL PARK MEDICAL CENTER (O, 181 beds) 1910 Malvern Avenue, Hot Springs, AR Zip 71901–7799; tel. 501/321–1000; Jerry D. Mabry, FACHE, Chief Executive Officer
**Web address:** www.nationalparkmedical.com

SAINT MARY'S REGIONAL MEDICAL CENTER (O, 137 beds) 1808 West Main Street, Russellville, AR Zip 72801–2724; tel. 479/968–2841; Donald J. Frederic, FACHE, Chief Executive Officer
**Web address:** www.saintmarysregional.com

**MISSOURI:** MINERAL AREA REGIONAL MEDICAL CENTER (O, 98 beds) 1212 Weber Road, Farmington, MO Zip 63640–3325; tel. 573/756–4581; David P. Steitz, Interim Chief Executive Officer
**Web address:** www.marmc.net

**OKLAHOMA:** MUSKOGEE COMMUNITY HOSPITAL (L, 45 beds) 2900 North Main Street, Muskogee, OK Zip 74401–4078; tel. 918/687–7777; Mark Roberts, President
**Web address:** www.mch–ok.com

MUSKOGEE REGIONAL MEDICAL CENTER (L, 194 beds) 300 Rockefeller Drive, Muskogee, OK Zip 74401–5081; tel. 918/682–5501; Kevin N. Fowler, Chief Executive Officer
**Web address:** www.muskogeehealth.com

SOUTHWESTERN MEDICAL CENTER (O, 178 beds) 5602 S.W. Lee Boulevard, Lawton, OK Zip 73505–9635; tel. 580/531–4700; Stephen O. Hyde, FACHE, Chief Executive Officer
**Web address:** www.swmconline.com

**OREGON:** WILLAMETTE VALLEY MEDICAL CENTER (O, 88 beds) 2700 S.E. Stratus Avenue, McMinnville, OR Zip 97128–6498; tel. 503/472–6131; Daniel Ordyna, Chief Executive Officer
**Web address:** www.wvmcweb.com

**TENNESSEE:** DEKALB COMMUNITY HOSPITAL (O, 52 beds) 520 West Main Street, Smithville, TN Zip 37166–0640, Mailing Address: P.O. Box 640, Zip 37166–0640; tel. 615/215–5000; Robert M. Luther, Interim Executive Officer
**Web address:** www.dekalbcommunityhospital.com

GRANDVIEW MEDICAL CENTER (O, 68 beds) 1000 Highway 28, Jasper, TN Zip 37347–3638; tel. 423/837–9500; Bruce A. Baldwin, Chief Executive Officer
**Web address:** www.grandviewhospital.com

HIGHLANDS MEDICAL CENTER (O, 44 beds) 401 Sewell Road, Sparta, TN Zip 38583–1299; tel. 931/738–9211; William Little, Chief Executive Officer
**Web address:** www.whitecountyhospital.com

RIVER PARK HOSPITAL (O, 125 beds) 1559 Sparta Street, Mc Minnville, TN Zip 37110–1316; tel. 931/815–4000; Timothy W. McGill, Chief Executive Officer
**Web address:** www.riverparkhospital.com

STONES RIVER HOSPITAL (O, 60 beds) 324 Doolittle Road, Woodbury, TN Zip 37190–1140; tel. 615/563–4001; Robert M. Luther, Interim Chief Executive Officer
**Web address:** www.stonesriverhospital.com

**WASHINGTON:** CAPITAL MEDICAL CENTER (O, 110 beds) 3900 Capital Mall Drive S.W., Olympia, WA Zip 98502–5026, Mailing Address: P.O. Box 19002, Zip 98507–9002; tel. 360/754–5858; Jim Geist, Chief Executive Officer
**Web address:** www.capitalmedical.com

| Owned, leased, sponsored: | 15 hospitals | 1569 beds |
|---|---|---|
| Contract–managed: | 0 hospitals | 0 beds |
| Totals: | 15 hospitals | 1569 beds |

★**0297:  CAPITAL HEALTH** (NP)
750 Brunswick Avenue, Trenton, NJ Zip 08638–4174; tel. 609/394–6000; Al Maghazehe, Ph.D., FACHE, Chief Executive Officer
**(Independent Hospital System)**

**NEW JERSEY:** CAPITAL HEALTH MEDICAL CENTER–HOPEWELL (O, 223 beds) 1 Capital Way, Pennington, NJ Zip 08534; tel. 609/303–4000; Al Maghazehe, Ph.D., FACHE, Chief Executive Officer
**Web address:** www.capitalhealth.org

CAPITAL HEALTH REGIONAL MEDICAL CENTER (O, 226 beds) 750 Brunswick Avenue, Trenton, NJ Zip 08638–4174; tel. 609/394–6000; Al Maghazehe, Ph.D., FACHE, Chief Executive Officer
**Web address:** www.capitalhealth.org

---

For explanation of codes following names, see page B2.
★ Indicates Type III membership in the American Hospital Association.

| | | |
|---|---|---|
| Owned, leased, sponsored: | 2 hospitals | 449 beds |
| Contract–managed: | 0 hospitals | 0 beds |
| Totals: | 2 hospitals | 449 beds |

**0301: CARDINAL HILL HEALTHCARE SYSTEM** (NP)
2050 Versailes Road, Lexington, KY Zip 40504; tel. 859/254–5701;
Gary Payne, President and Chief Executive Officer
**(Independent Hospital System)**

**KENTUCKY:** CARDINAL HILL REHABILITATION HOSPITAL (O, 108 beds) 2050
Versailles Road, Lexington, KY Zip 40504–1405; tel. 859/254–5701;
Gary Payne, Chief Executive Officer
**Web address:** www.cardinalhill.org

CARDINAL HILL SPECIALTY HOSPITAL (O, 32 beds) 85 North Grand Avenue,
Fort Thomas, KY Zip 41075; tel. 859/572–3880; Janice Bauer, Administrator

| | | |
|---|---|---|
| Owned, leased, sponsored: | 2 hospitals | 140 beds |
| Contract–managed: | 0 hospitals | 0 beds |
| Totals: | 2 hospitals | 140 beds |

**★0099: CARE NEW ENGLAND HEALTH SYSTEM** (NP)
45 Willard Avenue, Providence, RI Zip 02905–3218;
tel. 401/453–7900; Dennis D. Keefe, President and Chief Executive
Officer
**(Centralized Health System)**

**RHODE ISLAND:** BUTLER HOSPITAL (O, 117 beds) 345 Blackstone
Boulevard, Providence, RI Zip 02906–4829; tel. 401/455–6200; Patricia
R. Recupero, M.D., JD, President and Chief Executive Officer
**Web address:** www.butler.org

KENT COUNTY MEMORIAL HOSPITAL (O, 306 beds) 455 Tollgate Road,
Warwick, RI Zip 02886–2770; tel. 401/737–7000; Sandra L. Coletta,
President and Chief Executive Officer
**Web address:** www.kentri.org

WOMEN & INFANTS HOSPITAL OF RHODE ISLAND (O, 247 beds) 101 Dudley
Street, Providence, RI Zip 02905–2499; tel. 401/274–1100; Constance A.
Howes, President and Chief Executive Officer
**Web address:** www.womenandinfants.org

| | | |
|---|---|---|
| Owned, leased, sponsored: | 3 hospitals | 670 beds |
| Contract–managed: | 0 hospitals | 0 beds |
| Totals: | 3 hospitals | 670 beds |

**★0070: CARILION CLINIC** (NP)
Belleview at Jefferson Street, Roanoke, VA Zip 24014, Mailing
Address: P.O. Box 13727, Zip 24036–3727; tel. 540/981–7000;
Nancy Howell Agee, President and Chief Executive Officer
**(Moderately Centralized Health System)**

**VIRGINIA:** BEDFORD MEMORIAL HOSPITAL (O, 124 beds) 1613 Oakwood
Street, Bedford, VA Zip 24523–0688, Mailing Address: P.O. Box 688,
Zip 24523–0688; tel. 540/586–2441; Patti Jurkus, President and Chief
Executive Officer
**Web address:** www.bmhva.com

CARILION FRANKLIN MEMORIAL HOSPITAL (O, 32 beds) 180 Floyd Avenue,
Rocky Mount, VA Zip 24151–1389; tel. 540/483–5277; William D. Jacobsen,
Chief Executive Officer
**Web address:** www.carilion.com

CARILION GILES COMMUNITY HOSPITAL (O, 25 beds) 159 Hartley Way,
Pearisburg, VA Zip 24134–2471; tel. 540/921–6000; James E. Tyler, Vice
President and Administrator
**Web address:** www.carilion.com

CARILION MEDICAL CENTER (O, 624 beds) Belleview at Jefferson Street,
Roanoke, VA Zip 24014, Mailing Address: P.O. Box 13367, Zip 24033–3367;
tel. 540/981–7000; Nancy Howell Agee, President and Chief Executive
Officer
**Web address:** www.carilionclinic.org

CARILION NEW RIVER VALLEY MEDICAL CENTER (O, 146 beds) 2900 Lamb
Circle, Christiansburg, VA Zip 24073–5041, Mailing Address: P.O. Box 5,
Radford, Zip 24143–0005; tel. 540/731–2000; John S. Piatkowski, M.D.,
President and Chief Executive Officer
**Web address:** www.carilionclinic.org

CARILION STONEWALL JACKSON HOSPITAL (O, 25 beds) 1 Health Circle,
Lexington, VA Zip 24450–2492; tel. 540/458–3300; Charles E. Carr, Chief
Executive Officer
**Web address:** www.carilionclinic.com

CARILION TAZEWELL COMMUNITY HOSPITAL (O, 7 beds) 141 Ben Bolt
Avenue, Tazewell, VA Zip 24651–9700; tel. 276/988–8700; John S.
Piatkowski, M.D., Chief Executive Officer
**Web address:** www.carilionclinic.org

| | | |
|---|---|---|
| Owned, leased, sponsored: | 7 hospitals | 983 beds |
| Contract–managed: | 0 hospitals | 0 beds |
| Totals: | 7 hospitals | 983 beds |

**★0705: CAROLINAS HEALTHCARE SYSTEM** (NP)
1000 Blythe Boulevard, Charlotte, NC Zip 28203–5871, Mailing
Address: P.O. Box 32861, Zip 28232–2861; tel. 704/355–2000;
Michael C. Tarwater, Chief Executive Officer
**(Moderately Centralized Health System)**

**NORTH CAROLINA:** ANSON COMMUNITY HOSPITAL (O, 125 beds) 500
Morven Road, Wadesboro, NC Zip 28170–2745; tel. 704/694–5131;
Frederick G. Thompson, Ph.D., President
**Web address:** www.carolinasmedicalcenter.org

CAROLINAS MEDICAL CENTER (O, 874 beds) 1000 Blythe Boulevard,
Charlotte, NC Zip 28203–5871, Mailing Address: P.O. Box 32861,
Zip 28232–2861; tel. 704/355–2000; Spencer Lilly, Interim President
**Web address:** www.carolinasmedicalcenter.org

CAROLINAS MEDICAL CENTER–LINCOLN (O, 90 beds) 433 McAlister Road,
Lincolnton, NC Zip 28092; tel. 980/212–2000; Peter W. Acker, President
**Web address:** www.cmc–lincoln.org

CAROLINAS MEDICAL CENTER–MERCY (O, 303 beds) 2001 Vail Avenue,
Charlotte, NC Zip 28207–1289; tel. 704/304–5000; D. Channing Roush,
President
**Web address:** www.carolinashealthcare.org

CAROLINAS MEDICAL CENTER–NORTHEAST (O, 450 beds) 920 Church Street
North, Concord, NC Zip 28025–2983; tel. 704/403–3000; Phyllis A.
Wingate, Division President
**Web address:** www.carolinashealthcare.org

CAROLINAS MEDICAL CENTER–UNION (L, 239 beds) 600 Hospital Drive,
Monroe, NC Zip 28112–6000, Mailing Address: P.O. Box 5003,
Zip 28111–5003; tel. 704/283–3100; Michael Lutes, President
**Web address:** www.cmc–union.org

CAROLINAS MEDICAL CENTER–UNIVERSITY (O, 130 beds) 8800 North Tryon
Street, Charlotte, NC Zip 28262–8415, Mailing Address: P.O. Box 560727,
Zip 28256–0727; tel. 704/863–6000; William H. Leonard, President
**Web address:** www.carolinashealthcare.org

CAROLINAS REHABILITATION (O, 169 beds) 1100 Blythe Boulevard, Charlotte,
NC Zip 28203–5864; tel. 704/355–4300; Robert G. Larrison, Jr., President
**Web address:** www.carolinasrehabilitation.org

CLEVELAND REGIONAL MEDICAL CENTER (L, 364 beds) 201 East Grover
Street, Shelby, NC Zip 28150; tel. 704/487–3000; Brian Gwyn, President
and Chief Executive Officer
**Web address:** www.clevelandregional.org

COLUMBUS REGIONAL HEALTHCARE SYSTEM (C, 107 beds) 500 Jefferson
Street, Whiteville, NC Zip 28472–9987; tel. 910/642–8011; Henry
Hawthorne, III, President and Chief Executive Officer
**Web address:** www.crhealthcare.org

CRAWLEY MEMORIAL HOSPITAL (L, 51 beds) 315 West College Avenue,
Boiling Springs, NC Zip 28017, Mailing Address: P.O. Box 996,
Zip 28017–0996; tel. 704/434–9466; Brian Gwyn, President and Chief
Executive Officer
**Web address:** www.carolinas.org

GRACE HOSPITAL (C, 117 beds) 2201 South Sterling Street, Morganton, NC
Zip 28655–4058; tel. 828/580–5000; Kenneth W. Wood, President and
Chief Executive Officer
**Web address:** www.gracehcs.org

For explanation of codes following names, see page B2.
★ Indicates Type III membership in the American Hospital Association.

KINGS MOUNTAIN HOSPITAL (L, 72 beds) 706 West King Street, Kings Mountain, NC Zip 28086–2708; tel. 980/487–5000; Brian Gwyn, President
**Web address:** www.carolinas.org

MURPHY MEDICAL CENTER (C, 191 beds) 3990 U.S. Highway 64 East Alt, Murphy, NC Zip 28906–7917; tel. 828/837–8161; Michael Stevenson, Administrator
**Web address:** www.murphymedical.org

SCOTLAND HEALTH CARE SYSTEM (C, 152 beds) 500 Lauchwood Drive, Laurinburg, NC Zip 28352–5599; tel. 910/291–7000; Gregory C. Wood, Chief Executive Officer
**Web address:** www.scotlandhealth.org

ST. LUKE'S HOSPITAL (C, 35 beds) 101 Hospital Drive, Columbus, NC Zip 28722–9473; tel. 828/894–3311; Kenneth A. Shull, FACHE, Chief Executive Officer
**Web address:** www.saintlukeshospital.com

STANLY REGIONAL MEDICAL CENTER (C, 102 beds) 301 Yadkin Street, Albemarle, NC Zip 28001–3448, Mailing Address: P.O. Box 1489, Zip 28002–1489; tel. 704/984–4000; Alfred P. Taylor, Chief Executive Officer
**Web address:** www.stanly.org

VALDESE GENERAL HOSPITAL (O, 155 beds) 720 Malcolm Boulevard, Valdese, NC Zip 28690, Mailing Address: P.O. Box 700, Zip 28690–0700; tel. 828/874–2251; Kenneth W. Wood, President and Chief Executive Officer
**Web address:** www.blueridgehealth.org

WILKES REGIONAL MEDICAL CENTER (C, 98 beds) 1370 West D Street, North Wilkesboro, NC Zip 28659–3506, Mailing Address: P.O. Box 609, Zip 28659–0609; tel. 336/651–8100; J. Gene Faile, Chief Executive Officer
**Web address:** www.wilkesregional.org

**SOUTH CAROLINA:** BON SECOURS ST. FRANCIS HOSPITAL (C, 179 beds) 2095 Henry Tecklenburg Drive, Charleston, SC Zip 29414–0001; tel. 843/402–1000; Allen P. Carroll, Senior Vice President and Chief Executive Officer
**Web address:** www.ropersaintfrancis.com

CANNON MEMORIAL HOSPITAL (C, 42 beds) 123 West G. Acker Drive, Pickens, SC Zip 29671–2739, Mailing Address: P.O. Box 188, Zip 29671–0188; tel. 864/878–4791; Norman G. Rentz, President and Chief Executive Officer
**Web address:** www.cannonhospital.org

MOUNT PLEASANT HOSPITAL (C, 50 beds) 3500 North Highway 17, Mount Pleasant, SC Zip 29466–9123; tel. 843/606–7000; John Sullivan, Chief Executive Officer
**Web address:** www.mymountpleasanthospital.com

ROPER HOSPITAL (C, 342 beds) 316 Calhoun Street, Charleston, SC Zip 29401–1125; tel. 843/724–2000; Matthew J. Severance, FACHE, Chief Executive Officer
**Web address:** www.ropersaintfrancis.com

| | | |
|---|---|---|
| Owned, leased, sponsored: | 12 hospitals | 3022 beds |
| Contract–managed: | 11 hospitals | 1415 beds |
| **Totals:** | 23 hospitals | 4437 beds |

---

**0656: CARRUS HOSPITALS** (IO)
1810 West U.S. Highway 82, Sherman, TX Zip 75092–7069; tel. 903/870–2600; Ronald E. Dorris, Chief Executive Officer
**(Independent Hospital System)**

**TEXAS:** CARRUS REHABILITATION HOSPITAL (O, 24 beds) 1810 West U.S. Highway 82, Suite 100, Sherman, TX Zip 75092–7069; tel. 903/870–2600; Ronald E. Dorris, Chief Executive Officer
**Web address:** www.carrushospital.com

CARRUS SPECIALTY HOSPITAL (O, 16 beds) 1810 West U.S. Highway 82, Sherman, TX Zip 75092–7069; tel. 903/870–2600; Ronald E. Dorris, Chief Executive Officer
**Web address:** www.carrushospital.com

| | | |
|---|---|---|
| Owned, leased, sponsored: | 2 hospitals | 40 beds |
| Contract–managed: | 0 hospitals | 0 beds |
| **Totals:** | 2 hospitals | 40 beds |

---

**★0136: CATHOLIC HEALTH EAST** (CC)
3805 West Chester Pike, Suite 100, Newtown Square, PA Zip 19073; tel. 610/355–2000; Judith M. Persichilli, Chief Executive Officer
**(Decentralized Health System)**

**DELAWARE:** ST. FRANCIS HOSPITAL (O, 214 beds) Seventh and Clayton Streets, Wilmington, DE Zip 19805–0500, Mailing Address: P.O. Box 2500, Zip 19805–0500; tel. 302/421–4100; Julie A. Hester, President and Chief Executive Officer
**Web address:** www.stfrancishealthcare.org

**FLORIDA:** HOLY CROSS HOSPITAL (O, 571 beds) 4725 North Federal Highway, Fort Lauderdale, FL Zip 33308–4668, Mailing Address: P.O. Box 23460, Zip 33307–3460; tel. 954/771–8000; Patrick Taylor, M.D., President and Chief Executive Officer
**Web address:** www.holy–cross.com

SOUTH FLORIDA BAPTIST HOSPITAL (S, 147 beds) 301 North Alexander Street, Plant City, FL Zip 33563–9058, Mailing Address: Drawer H, Zip 33564–9058; tel. 813/757–1200; Isaac Mallah, President and Chief Executive Officer
**Web address:** www.sjbhealth.org

ST. ANTHONY'S HOSPITAL (S, 395 beds) 1200 Seventh Avenue North, Saint Petersburg, FL Zip 33705–1388, Mailing Address: P.O. Box 12588, Zip 33733–2588; tel. 727/825–1100; William G. Ulbricht, President
**Web address:** www.stanthonys.com/

ST. JOSEPH'S HOSPITAL (S, 883 beds) 3001 West Martin Luther King Boulevard, Tampa, FL Zip 33607–6387, Mailing Address: P.O. Box 4227, Zip 33677–4227; tel. 813/870–4000; Isaac Mallah, President and Chief Executive Officer
**Web address:** www.sjbhealth.org

**GEORGIA:** GOOD SAMARITAN HOSPITAL (O, 25 beds) 1201 Siloam Highway, Greensboro, GA Zip 30642–2811; tel. 706/453–7331; Montez Carter, Interim President and Chief Executive Officer
**Web address:** www.stmarysgoodsam.org

SAINT JOSEPH'S HOSPITAL OF ATLANTA (O, 258 beds) 5665 Peachtree Dunwoody Road N.E., Atlanta, GA Zip 30342–1764; tel. 678/843–7001; Scott Schmidly, Chief Executive Officer
**Web address:** www.stjosephsatlanta.org

ST. MARY'S HEALTH CARE SYSTEM (O, 165 beds) 1230 Baxter Street, Athens, GA Zip 30606–3791; tel. 706/389–3000; Donald McKenna, President and Chief Executive Officer
**Web address:** www.stmarysathens.com

**MAINE:** MERCY HOSPITAL OF PORTLAND (O, 168 beds) 144 State Street, Portland, ME Zip 04101–3795; tel. 207/879–3000; Eileen F. Skinner, FACHE, President and Chief Executive Officer
**Web address:** www.mercyhospital.com

**MASSACHUSETTS:** FARREN CARE CENTER (O, 72 beds) 340 Montague City Road, Turners Falls, MA Zip 01376–9983; tel. 413/774–3111; James Clifford, Administrator

MERCY MEDICAL CENTER (O, 221 beds) 271 Carew Street, Springfield, MA Zip 01104–2398, Mailing Address: P.O. Box 9012, Zip 01102–9012; tel. 413/748–9000; Daniel P. Moen, President and Chief Executive Officer
**Web address:** www.mercycares.com

**NEW JERSEY:** LOURDES MEDICAL CENTER OF BURLINGTON COUNTY (O, 221 beds) 218–A Sunset Road, Willingboro, NJ Zip 08046–1162; tel. 609/835–2900; Mark Nessel, Executive Vice President and Chief Operating Officer
**Web address:** www.lourdesnet.org

OUR LADY OF LOURDES MEDICAL CENTER (O, 391 beds) 1600 Haddon Avenue, Camden, NJ Zip 08103–3117; tel. 856/757–3500; Alexander J. Hatala, President and Chief Executive Officer
**Web address:** www.lourdesnet.org

SAINT MICHAEL'S MEDICAL CENTER (O, 207 beds) 111 Central Avenue, Newark, NJ Zip 07102–2094; tel. 973/877–5549; David A. Ricci, President and Chief Executive Officer
**Web address:** www.smmcnj.org

ST. FRANCIS MEDICAL CENTER (O, 163 beds) 601 Hamilton Avenue, Trenton, NJ Zip 08629–1986; tel. 609/599–5000; Gerard J. Jablonowski, President and Chief Executive Officer
**Web address:** www.stfrancismedical.com

---

For explanation of codes following names, see page B2.
★ Indicates Type III membership in the American Hospital Association.

**NEW YORK:** ALBANY MEMORIAL HOSPITAL (O, 165 beds) 600 Northern Boulevard, Albany, NY Zip 12204–1083; tel. 518/471–3221; Steven P. Boyle, Executive Vice President
**Web address:** www.nehealth.com

SAMARITAN HOSPITAL (O, 134 beds) 2215 Burdett Avenue, Troy, NY Zip 12180–2475; tel. 518/271–3300; Norman E. Dascher, Jr., Chief Executive Officer
**Web address:** www.nehealth.com

ST. JAMES MERCY HEALTH SYSTEM (O, 222 beds) 411 Canisteo Street, Hornell, NY Zip 14843–2197; tel. 607/324–8000; Mary E. LaRowe, FACHE, President and Chief Executive Officer
**Web address:** www.stjamesmercy.org

ST. MARY'S HOSPITAL (O, 293 beds) 1300 Massachusetts Avenue, Troy, NY Zip 12180–1695; tel. 518/268–5000; Norman E. Dascher, Jr., Executive Vice President
**Web address:** www.setonhealth.org

ST. PETER'S HOSPITAL (O, 487 beds) 315 South Manning Boulevard, Albany, NY Zip 12208–1789; tel. 518/525–1550; Steven P. Boyle, Executive Vice President
**Web address:** www.sphcs.org

SUNNYVIEW REHABILITATION HOSPITAL (O, 115 beds) 1270 Belmont Avenue, Schenectady, NY Zip 12308–2104; tel. 518/382–4500; Edward Eisenman, Chief Executive Officer
**Web address:** www.sunnyview.org

**NORTH CAROLINA:** ST. JOSEPH OF THE PINES HOSPITAL (O, 204 beds) 590 Central Drive, Southern Pines, NC Zip 28387; tel. 910/246–1000; Ken Cormier, President and Chief Executive Officer

**PENNSYLVANIA:** MERCY FITZGERALD HOSPITAL (O, 391 beds) 1500 South Lansdowe Avenue, Darby, PA Zip 19023; tel. 610/237–4000; Kathryn Conallen, Executive Director
**Web address:** www.mercyhealth.org

MERCY SUBURBAN HOSPITAL (O, 126 beds) 2701 DeKalb Pike, Norristown, PA Zip 19401–1820; tel. 610/278–2000; Jeffrey Snyder, Chief Executive Officer
**Web address:** www.mercyhealth.org

NAZARETH HOSPITAL (O, 233 beds) 2601 Holme Avenue, Philadelphia, PA Zip 19152–2096; tel. 215/335–6000; Nancy Cherone, Interim Chief Executive Officer
**Web address:** www.nazarethhospital.org

ST. MARY MEDICAL CENTER (O, 315 beds) 1201 Langhorne–Newtown Road, Langhorne, PA Zip 19047–1234; tel. 215/710–2000; Gregory T. Wozniak, President and Chief Executive Officer
**Web address:** www.stmaryhealthcare.org

| | | |
|---|---|---|
| Owned, leased, sponsored: | 26 hospitals | 6786 beds |
| Contract–managed: | 0 hospitals | 0 beds |
| Totals: | 26 hospitals | 6786 beds |

★**0092:   CATHOLIC HEALTH INITIATIVES** (CC)
198 Inverness Drive West, Suite 800, Englewood, CO Zip 80112–5202; tel. 303/298–9100; Kevin E. Lofton, FACHE, President and Chief Executive Officer
**(Decentralized Health System)**

**ARKANSAS:** ST. VINCENT INFIRMARY MEDICAL CENTER (S, 409 beds) Two St. Vincent Circle, Little Rock, AR Zip 72205–5499; tel. 501/552–3000; Peter D. Banko, FACHE, President and Chief Executive Officer
**Web address:** www.stvincenthealth.com

ST. VINCENT MEDICAL CENTER–NORTH (S, 58 beds) 2215 Wildwood Avenue, Sherwood, AR Zip 72120; tel. 501/552–7100; Tim Osterholm, Administrator and Chief Executive Officer
**Web address:** www.stvincenthealth.com

ST. VINCENT MORRILTON (S, 25 beds) 4 Hospital Drive, Morrilton, AR Zip 72110–4510; tel. 501/977–2300; Thomas E. Fitz, Jr., FACHE, Interim Chief Executive Officer
**Web address:** www.stanthonysmorrilton.com/

**COLORADO:** MERCY REGIONAL MEDICAL CENTER (S, 82 beds) 1010 Three Springs Boulevard, Durango, CO Zip 81301–5089; tel. 970/247–4311; Kirk Dignum, Ph.D., Chief Executive Officer
**Web address:** www.mercydurango.org

PENROSE–ST. FRANCIS HEALTH SERVICES (S, 405 beds) 2222 North Nevada Avenue, Colorado Springs, CO Zip 80907–6799, Mailing Address: P.O. Box 7021, Zip 80933–7021; tel. 719/776–5000; Margaret D. Sabin, President and Chief Executive Officer
**Web address:** www.penrosestfrancis.org

ST. ANTHONY HOSPITAL (S, 222 beds) 11600 West Second Place, Lakewood, CO Zip 80228–1527; tel. 720/321–0000; Jeffrey Brickman, FACHE, President and Chief Executive Officer
**Web address:** www.stanthonyhosp.org

ST. ANTHONY NORTH HOSPITAL (S, 138 beds) 2551 West 84th Avenue, Westminster, CO Zip 80031; tel. 303/426–2151; Carole Peet, R.N., MSN, President and Chief Executive Officer
**Web address:** www.stanthonynorth.org

ST. ANTHONY SUMMIT MEDICAL CENTER (S, 34 beds) 340 Peak One Drive, Frisco, CO Zip 80443, Mailing Address: P.O. Box 738, Zip 80443–0738; tel. 970/668–3300; Paul J. Chodkowski, Chief Executive Officer
**Web address:** www.summitmedicalcenter.org

ST. MARY–CORWIN MEDICAL CENTER (S, 202 beds) 1008 Minnequa Avenue, Pueblo, CO Zip 81004–3798; tel. 719/557–4000; Robert Ryder, Chief Executive Officer
**Web address:** www.centura.org

ST. THOMAS MORE HOSPITAL (S, 55 beds) 1338 Phay Avenue, Canon City, CO Zip 81212–2221; tel. 719/285–2000; Robert Ryder, Chief Executive Officer
**Web address:** www.stmhospital.org

**IOWA:** MERCY MEDICAL CENTER – WEST LAKES (O, 82 beds) 1755 59th Place, West Des Moines, IA Zip 50266–7736; tel. 515/358–8000; Laurie A. Conner, FACHE, Vice President and Administrator
**Web address:** www.mercywestlakes.org/

MERCY MEDICAL CENTER–CENTERVILLE (S, 45 beds) 1 St. Joseph's Drive, Centerville, IA Zip 52544–8055; tel. 641/437–4111; Clinton J. Christianson, FACHE, President and Chief Executive Officer
**Web address:** www.mercycenterville.org

MERCY MEDICAL CENTER–DES MOINES (S, 567 beds) 1111 6th Avenue, Des Moines, IA Zip 50314–2611; tel. 515/247–3121; David H. Vellinga, FACHE, President and Chief Executive Officer
**Web address:** www.mercydesmoines.org

**KANSAS:** ST. CATHERINE HOSPITAL (S, 110 beds) 401 East Spuce Street, Garden City, KS Zip 67846–5679; tel. 620/272–2561; Scott J. Taylor, President and Chief Executive Officer
**Web address:** www.stcath-hosp.org

ST. ROSE AMBULATORY & SURGERY CENTER (S, 0 beds) 3515 Broadway Street, Great Bend, KS Zip 67530–3633; tel. 620/792–2511; Leanne M. Irsik, R.N., Senior Vice President and Administrator

**KENTUCKY:** CONTINUING CARE HOSPITAL (S, 45 beds) 150 North Eagle Creek Drive, 5th Floor, Lexington, KY Zip 40509; tel. 859/967–5744; Tonja Williams, MSN, R.N., President and Chief Executive Officer

FLAGET MEMORIAL HOSPITAL (S, 40 beds) 4305 New Shepherdsville Road, Bardstown, KY Zip 40004; tel. 502/350–5000; Sue Downs, R.N., MSN, President
**Web address:** www.flaget.com

SAINT JOSEPH – LONDON (S, 89 beds) 310 East Ninth Street, London, KY Zip 40741–1299; tel. 606/330–6000; Virginia B. Dempsey, President
**Web address:** www.saintjosephhealthsystem.org

SAINT JOSEPH – MARTIN (S, 25 beds) 11203 Main Street, Martin, KY Zip 41649–0910; tel. 606/285–6400; Kathy Stumbo, President
**Web address:** www.saintjosephmartin.org

SAINT JOSEPH BEREA (S, 25 beds) 305 Estill Street, Berea, KY Zip 40403–1909; tel. 859/986–3151; Greg D. Gerard, President
**Web address:** www.saintjosephberea.org

SAINT JOSEPH EAST (S, 144 beds) 150 North Eagle Creek Drive, Lexington, KY Zip 40509–1807; tel. 859/967–5000; Eric Gilliam, Administrator
**Web address:** www.sjhlex.org

SAINT JOSEPH HOSPITAL (S, 366 beds) One St. Joseph Drive, Lexington, KY Zip 40504–3754; tel. 859/278–3436; Ken D. Haynes, President
**Web address:** www.sjhlex.org

SAINT JOSEPH MOUNT STERLING (S, 56 beds) 50 Sterling Avenue, Mount Sterling, KY Zip 40353–1158, Mailing Address: P.O. Box 7, Zip 40353–0007; tel. 859/497–6000; Benny Nolen, President
**Web address:** www.sjhlex.org

Section B

For explanation of codes following names, see page B2.
★ Indicates Type III membership in the American Hospital Association.

**MARYLAND:** ST. JOSEPH MEDICAL CENTER (S, 320 beds) 7601 Osler Drive, Towson, MD Zip 21204–7582; tel. 410/337–1000; Charles W. Neumann, President and Chief Executive Officer
**Web address:** www.sjmcmd.org

**MINNESOTA:** ALBANY AREA HOSPITAL AND MEDICAL CENTER (S, 17 beds) 300 Third Avenue, Albany, MN Zip 56307–9363; tel. 320/845–2121; Sandra Day, Administrator, Chief Nursing Officer
**Web address:** www.albanyareahospital.com

LAKEWOOD HEALTH CENTER (S, 59 beds) 600 Main Avenue South, Baudette, MN Zip 56623–2855; tel. 218/634–2120; Jason Breuer, Administrator
**Web address:** www.lakewoodhealthcenter.org

ST. FRANCIS HEALTHCARE CAMPUS (S, 145 beds) 2400 St. Francis Drive, Breckenridge, MN Zip 56520–1298; tel. 218/643–3000; David A. Nelson, President and Chief Executive Officer
**Web address:** www.sfcare.org

ST. GABRIEL'S HOSPITAL (S, 25 beds) 815 Second Street S.E., Little Falls, MN Zip 56345–3596; tel. 320/632–5441; Chad D. Cooper, President and Chief Executive Officer
**Web address:** www.stgabriels.com

ST. JOSEPH'S AREA HEALTH SERVICES (S, 25 beds) 600 Pleasant Avenue, Park Rapids, MN Zip 56470–1432; tel. 218/732–3311; Benjamin Koppelman, President and Chief Executive Officer
**Web address:** www.sjahs.org

**NEBRASKA:** GOOD SAMARITAN HOSPITAL (S, 229 beds) 10 East 31st Street, Kearney, NE Zip 68847–2926, Mailing Address: P.O. Box 1990, Zip 68848–1990; tel. 308/865–7100; Michael H. Schnieders, President and Chief Executive Officer
**Web address:** www.gshs.org

NEBRASKA HEART INSTITUTE AND HEART HOSPITAL (S, 52 beds) 7500 South 91st Street, Lincoln, NE Zip 68526; tel. 402/327–2700; Thomas Burnell, Chief Executive Officer
**Web address:** www.neheart.com

SAINT ELIZABETH REGIONAL MEDICAL CENTER (S, 260 beds) 555 South 70th Street, Lincoln, NE Zip 68510–2462; tel. 402/219–8000; Kim S. Moore, President and Chief Executive Officer
**Web address:** www.saintelizabethonline.com

SAINT FRANCIS MEDICAL CENTER (S, 200 beds) 2620 West Faidley Avenue, Grand Island, NE Zip 68803–4297, Mailing Address: P.O. Box 9804, Zip 68802–9804; tel. 308/384–4600; Daniel P. McElligott, FACHE, President and Chief Executive Officer
**Web address:** www.saintfrancisgi.org

ST. MARY'S COMMUNITY HOSPITAL (S, 18 beds) 1314 Third Avenue, Nebraska City, NE Zip 68410–1930; tel. 402/873–3321; Daniel J. Kelly, President and Chief Executive Officer
**Web address:** www.stmaryshospitalnecity.org

**NEW JERSEY:** SAINT CLARE'S HEALTH SYSTEM (S, 426 beds) 25 Pocono Road, Denville, NJ Zip 07834–2954; tel. 973/625–6000; Leslie D. Hirsch, FACHE, President and Chief Executive Officer
**Web address:** www.saintclares.org

**NORTH DAKOTA:** CARRINGTON HEALTH CENTER (S, 49 beds) 800 North Fourth Street, Carrington, ND Zip 58421–1217, Mailing Address: P.O. Box 461, Zip 58421–0461; tel. 701/652–3141; Mariann Doeling, R.N., Administrator
**Web address:** www.carringtonhealthcenter.org

LISBON AREA HEALTH SERVICES (S, 25 beds) 905 Main Street, Lisbon, ND Zip 58054–0353, Mailing Address: P.O. Box 353, Zip 58054–0353; tel. 701/683–5241; Peggy Larson, Administrator
**Web address:** www.lisbonhospital.com

MERCY HOSPITAL (S, 25 beds) 1031 Seventh Street N.E., Devils Lake, ND Zip 58301–2798; tel. 701/662–2131; James L. Marshall, Chief Executive Officer
**Web address:** www.mercyhospitaldl.com

MERCY HOSPITAL (S, 19 beds) 570 Chautauqua Boulevard, Valley City, ND Zip 58072–3199; tel. 701/845–6400; Keith E. Heuser, Administrator
**Web address:** www.mercyhospitalvalleycity.org

MERCY MEDICAL CENTER (S, 25 beds) 1301 15th Avenue West, Williston, ND Zip 58801–3896; tel. 701/774–7400; Matthew Grimshaw, Chief Executive Officer
**Web address:** www.mercy–williston.org

OAKES COMMUNITY HOSPITAL (S, 20 beds) 1200 North Seventh Street, Oakes, ND Zip 58474–2502; tel. 701/742–3291; Lee Boyles, Chief Executive Officer
**Web address:** www.oakeshospital.com

ST. JOSEPH'S HOSPITAL AND HEALTH CENTER (S, 25 beds) 30 Seventh Street West, Dickinson, ND Zip 58601–4399; tel. 701/456–4000; Reed Reyman, President and Chief Executive Officer
**Web address:** www.stjoeshospital.org

**OHIO:** GOOD SAMARITAN HOSPITAL (S, 520 beds) 375 Dixmyth Avenue, Cincinnati, OH Zip 45220–2489; tel. 513/862–1400; David Dornheggen, Chief Operating Officer
**Web address:** www.trihealth.com

GOOD SAMARITAN HOSPITAL (S, 400 beds) 2222 Philadelphia Drive, Dayton, OH Zip 45406–1813; tel. 937/734–2612; Eloise Broner, President and Chief Executive Officer
**Web address:** www.goodsamdayton.com

**OREGON:** MERCY MEDICAL CENTER (S, 141 beds) 2700 Stewart Parkway, Roseburg, OR Zip 97471–1297; tel. 541/673–0611; Kelly C. Morgan, President and Chief Executive Officer
**Web address:** www.mercyrose.org

ST. ANTHONY HOSPITAL (S, 25 beds) 1601 S.E. Court Avenue, Pendleton, OR Zip 97801–3297; tel. 541/276–5121; Jim Schlenker, Interim President and Chief Executive Officer
**Web address:** www.sahpendleton.org

**PENNSYLVANIA:** ST. JOSEPH MEDICAL CENTER (S, 180 beds) 2500 Bernville Road, Reading, PA Zip 19605, Mailing Address: P.O. Box 316, Zip 19603–0316; tel. 610/378–2000; John R. Morahan, FACHE, President and Chief Executive Officer
**Web address:** www.thefutureofhealthcare.org

**SOUTH DAKOTA:** GETTYSBURG MEMORIAL HOSPITAL (S, 60 beds) 606 East Garfield Avenue, Gettysburg, SD Zip 57442–1398; tel. 605/765–2480; Mark Schmidt, President and Chief Executive Officer
**Web address:** www.st–marys.com

ST. MARY'S HEALTHCARE CENTER (S, 164 beds) 800 East Dakota Avenue, Pierre, SD Zip 57501–3313; tel. 605/224–3100; Joseph Messmer, Interim Chief Executive Officer
**Web address:** www.st–marys.com

**TENNESSEE:** MEMORIAL HEALTH CARE SYSTEM (S, 336 beds) 2525 De Sales Avenue, Chattanooga, TN Zip 37404–1161; tel. 423/495–2525; James M. Hobson, President and Chief Executive Officer
**Web address:** www.memorial.org

**WASHINGTON:** ST. ANTHONY HOSPITAL (O, 80 beds) 11567 Canterwood Boulevard N.W., Gig Harbor, WA Zip 98332–5812; tel. 253/530–2000; Kurt Schley, President
**Web address:** www.fhshealth.org/

ST. CLARE HOSPITAL (S, 98 beds) 11315 Bridgeport Way S.W., Lakewood, WA Zip 98499–3004; tel. 253/588–1711; Kathy Bressler, President
**Web address:** www.fhshealth.org

ST. ELIZABETH HOSPITAL (S, 25 beds) 1450 Battersby Avenue, Enumclaw, WA Zip 98022–0218, Mailing Address: P.O. Box 218, Zip 98022–0218; tel. 360/825–2505; Donna Russell–Cook, President
**Web address:** www.fhshealth.org

ST. FRANCIS HOSPITAL (S, 110 beds) 34515 Ninth Avenue South, Federal Way, WA Zip 98003–6799; tel. 253/944–8100; Anthony McLean, President
**Web address:** www.fhshealth.org

ST. JOSEPH MEDICAL CENTER (S, 299 beds) 1717 South J Street, Tacoma, WA Zip 98405–3004, Mailing Address: P.O. Box 2197, Zip 98401–2197; tel. 253/426–4101; Syd Bersante, President
**Web address:** www.fhshealth.org

| | | |
|---|---|---|
| Owned, leased, sponsored: | 55 hospitals | 7626 beds |
| Contract–managed: | 0 hospitals | 0 beds |
| Totals: | 55 hospitals | 7626 beds |

**★5155: CATHOLIC HEALTH PARTNERS** (CC)
615 Elsinore Place, Cincinnati, OH Zip 45202; tel. 513/639–2800; Michael D. Connelly, President and Chief Executive Officer
**(Moderately Centralized Health System)**

For explanation of codes following names, see page B2.
★ Indicates Type III membership in the American Hospital Association.

**KENTUCKY:** LOURDES HOSPITAL (O, 277 beds) 1530 Lone Oak Road, Paducah, KY Zip 42003–7900, Mailing Address: P.O. Box 7100, Zip 42002–7100; tel. 270/444–2444; Steven Grinnell, President and Chief Executive Officer
**Web address:** www.lourdes–pad.org

MARCUM AND WALLACE MEMORIAL HOSPITAL (O, 25 beds) 60 Mercy Court, Irvine, KY Zip 40336–1331; tel. 606/723–2115; Susan Starling, President and Chief Executive Officer
**Web address:** www.marcumandwallace.org

**OHIO:** INSTITUTE FOR ORTHOPAEDIC SURGERY (O, 8 beds) 801 Medical Drive, Suite B., Lima, OH Zip 45804; tel. 419/224–7586; Sally Rhodes, R.N., MSN, Administrative Director
**Web address:** www.ioshospital.com

MERCY ALLEN HOSPITAL (O, 25 beds) 200 West Lorain Street, Oberlin, OH Zip 44074–1077; tel. 440/775–1211; Susan Bowers, R.N., President and Chief Nursing Officer
**Web address:** www.mercyonline.org/mercy_allen_hospital.aspx

MERCY HEALTH – FAIRFIELD HOSPITAL (O, 228 beds) 3000 Mack Road, Fairfield, OH Zip 45014; tel. 513/870–7000; Thomas S. Urban, Market Leader and President
**Web address:** www.e–mercy.com

MERCY HOSPITAL ANDERSON (O, 188 beds) 7500 State Road, Cincinnati, OH Zip 45255–2492; tel. 513/624–4500; Patricia A. Schroer, President and Chief Executive Officer
**Web address:** www.e–mercy.com

MERCY HOSPITAL CLERMONT (O, 119 beds) 3000 Hospital Drive, Batavia, OH Zip 45103–1921; tel. 513/732–8200; Gayle M. Heintzelman, President and Chief Executive Officer
**Web address:** www.e–mercy.com

MERCY HOSPITAL MOUNT AIRY (O, 170 beds) 2446 Kipling Avenue, Cincinnati, OH Zip 45239–6650; tel. 513/853–5000; Michael R. Stephens, President and Market Leader
**Web address:** www.e–mercy.com

MERCY HOSPITAL OF DEFIANCE (O, 23 beds) 1404 East Second Street, Defiance, OH Zip 43512; tel. 419/782–8444; Sonya Selhorst, Administrator
**Web address:** www.ehealthconnection.com/regions/toledo/

MERCY HOSPITAL WESTERN HILLS (O, 156 beds) 3131 Queen City Avenue, Cincinnati, OH Zip 45238–2396; tel. 513/389–5000; Michael R. Stephens, President and Market Leader
**Web address:** www.e–mercy.com

MERCY MEMORIAL HOSPITAL (O, 25 beds) 904 Scioto Street, Urbana, OH Zip 43078–2200; tel. 937/653–5231; Karen S. Gorby, R.N., MSN, FACHE, Administrator
**Web address:** www.health–partners.org

MERCY REGIONAL MEDICAL CENTER (O, 259 beds) 3700 Kolbe Road, Lorain, OH Zip 44053–1697; tel. 440/960–4000; Edwin M. Oley, President and Chief Executive Officer
**Web address:** www.community–health–partners.com

MERCY ST. ANNE HOSPITAL (O, 96 beds) 3404 West Sylvania Avenue, Toledo, OH Zip 43623; tel. 419/407–2663; Bradley J. Bertke, President and Chief Executive Officer
**Web address:** www.mercyweb.org

MERCY ST. CHARLES HOSPITAL (O, 271 beds) 2600 Navarre Avenue, Oregon, OH Zip 43616–3297; tel. 419/696–7200; Robert E. Gospodarek, President and Chief Executive Officer
**Web address:** www.mercyweb.org

MERCY ST. VINCENT MEDICAL CENTER (O, 431 beds) 2213 Cherry Street, Toledo, OH Zip 43608–2691; tel. 419/251–3232; Kevin S. Cook, President and Chief Executive Officer
**Web address:** www.mercyweb.org

MERCY TIFFIN HOSPITAL (O, 51 beds) 45 St. Lawrence Drive, Tiffin, OH Zip 44883–0727; tel. 419/455–7000; Dale E. Thornton, M.P.H., President and Chief Executive Officer
**Web address:** www.mercyweb.org

MERCY WILLARD HOSPITAL (O, 25 beds) 1100 Neal Zick Road, Willard, OH Zip 44890–9287; tel. 419/964–5000; B. Lynn Detterman, Chief Executive Officer
**Web address:** www.mercyweb.org

SPRINGFIELD REGIONAL MEDICAL CENTER (O, 254 beds) 100 Medical Center Drive, Springfield, OH Zip 45504–2687; tel. 937/325–0531; Mark S. Wiener, President
**Web address:** www.communityhospital.com

ST. ELIZABETH BOARDMAN HEALTH CENTER (O, 128 beds) 8401 Market Street, Boardman, OH Zip 44512–6777; tel. 330/729–2929; Eugenia Aubel, President
**Web address:** www.ehealthconnection.com/regions/youngstown/content/show_facility.asp?facility_id=190

ST. ELIZABETH HEALTH CENTER (O, 429 beds) 1044 Belmont Avenue, Youngstown, OH Zip 44504–1096, Mailing Address: P.O. Box 1790, Zip 44501–1790; tel. 330/746–7211; Robert W. Shroder, President and Chief Executive Officer
**Web address:** www.hmpartners.org

ST. JOSEPH HEALTH CENTER (O, 138 beds) 667 Eastland Avenue S.E., Warren, OH Zip 44484–4531; tel. 330/841–4000; John Finizio, President
**Web address:** www.hmpartners.org

ST. RITA'S MEDICAL CENTER (O, 415 beds) 730 West Market Street, Lima, OH Zip 45801–4670; tel. 419/227–3361; Robert O. Baxter, President
**Web address:** www.stritas.org

THE JEWISH HOSPITAL (O, 209 beds) 4777 East Galbraith Road, Cincinnati, OH Zip 45236–2725; tel. 513/686–3000; Steve Holman, President
**Web address:** www.jewishhospitalcincinnati.com/

| | | |
|---|---|---|
| Owned, leased, sponsored: | 23 hospitals | 3950 beds |
| Contract–managed: | 0 hospitals | 0 beds |
| **Totals:** | 23 hospitals | 3950 beds |

**0233: CATHOLIC HEALTH SERVICES OF LONG ISLAND** (CC)
992 North Village Avenue, 1st Floor, Rockville Centre, NY Zip 11570; tel. 516/705–3700; Lawrence E. McManus, President and Chief Executive Officer
**(Centralized Physician/Insurance Health System)**

**NEW YORK:** GOOD SAMARITAN HOSPITAL MEDICAL CENTER (O, 531 beds) 1000 Montauk Highway, West Islip, NY Zip 11795–4927; tel. 631/376–3000; Nancy B. Simmons, Executive Vice President and Chief Administrative Officer
**Web address:** www.good–samaritan–hospital.org

MERCY MEDICAL CENTER (O, 196 beds) 1000 North Village Avenue, Rockville Centre, NY Zip 11570–1000; tel. 516/705–2525; Alan D. Guerci, M.D., Chief Executive Officer
**Web address:** www.mercymedicalcenter.chsli.org

ST. CATHERINE OF SIENA MEDICAL CENTER (O, 503 beds) 50 Route 25–A, Smithtown, NY Zip 11787–1348; tel. 631/862–3000; Dennis Verzi, Executive Director
**Web address:** www.stcatherinemedicalcenter.org

ST. CHARLES HOSPITAL (O, 289 beds) 200 Belle Terre Road, Port Jefferson, NY Zip 11777–1928; tel. 631/474–6000; James O'Connor, Executive Vice President
**Web address:** www.stcharleshospital.chsli.org

ST. FRANCIS HOSPITAL (O, 312 beds) 100 Port Washington Boulevard, Roslyn, NY Zip 11576–1353; tel. 516/562–6000; Alan D. Guerci, M.D., Chief Executive Officer
**Web address:** www.stfrancisheartcenter.chsli.org

| | | |
|---|---|---|
| Owned, leased, sponsored: | 5 hospitals | 1831 beds |
| Contract–managed: | 0 hospitals | 0 beds |
| **Totals:** | 5 hospitals | 1831 beds |

**★0234: CATHOLIC HEALTH SYSTEM** (CC)
2121 Main Street, Suite 300, Buffalo, NY Zip 14214; tel. 716/862–2410; Joseph D. McDonald, President and Chief Executive Officer
**(Independent Hospital System)**

FATHER BAKER MANOR (O, 160 beds) 6400 Powers Road, Orchard Park, NY Zip 14127; tel. 716/667–0001; Christine Kluckhohn, President, Continuing Care

KENMORE MERCY HOSPITAL (O, 315 beds) 2950 Elmwood Avenue, Kenmore, NY Zip 14217–1390; tel. 716/447–6100; James M. Millard, President and Chief Executive Officer
**Web address:** www.chsbuffalo.org

MCAULEY RESIDENCE (O, 160 beds) 1503 Military Road, Kenmore, NY Zip 14217; tel. 716/447–6600; Christine Kluckhohn, President, Continuing Care

For explanation of codes following names, see page B2.
★ Indicates Type III membership in the American Hospital Association.

MERCY HOSPITAL (O, 436 beds) 565 Abbott Road, Buffalo, NY
Zip 14220–2095; tel. 716/826–7000; Charles J. Urlaub, President and Chief
Executive Officer
**Web address:** www.chsbuffalo.org

MERCY NURSING FACILITY (O, 74 beds) 565 Abbott Road, Buffalo, NY
Zip 14220; tel. 716/828–2301; Christine Kluckhohn, President, Continuing
Care

NAZARETH HOME (O, 125 beds) 291 West North Street, Buffalo, NY
Zip 14201; tel. 716/881–2323; Christine Kluckhohn, President, Continuing
Care

SISTERS OF CHARITY HOSPITAL OF BUFFALO (O, 467 beds) 2157 Main
Street, Buffalo, NY Zip 14214–2692; tel. 716/862–1000; Peter U.
Bergmann, President and Chief Executive Officer
**Web address:** www.chsbuffalo.org

ST. CATHERINE LABOURE (O, 80 beds) 2157 Main Street, Buffalo, NY
Zip 14214; tel. 716/862–1451; Christine Kluckhohn, President, Continuing
Care

ST. ELIZABETH'S HOME (O, 117 beds) 5539 Broadway, Lancaster, NY
Zip 14086; tel. 716/683–5150; Christine Kluckhohn, President, Continuing
Care

ST. FRANCIS OF BUFFALO (O, 120 beds) 34 Benwood Avenue, Buffalo, NY
Zip 14214; tel. 716/862–2500; Christine Kluckhohn, President, Continuing
Care

ST. FRANCIS OF WILLIAMSVILLE (O, 142 beds) 147 Reist Street, Williamsville,
NY Zip 14221; tel. 716/633–5400; Christine Kluckhohn, President,
Continuing Care

ST. JOSEPH MANOR (O, 22 beds) 2211 West State Street, Olean, NY
Zip 14760; tel. 716/372–7810; Christine Kluckhohn, President, Continuing
Care

| | | |
|---|---|---|
| Owned, leased, sponsored: | 12 hospitals | 2218 beds |
| Contract–managed: | 0 hospitals | 0 beds |
| Totals: | 12 hospitals | 2218 beds |

---

★**0298: CENTEGRA HEALTH SYSTEM** (NP)
385 Millennium Drive, Crystal Lake, IL Zip 60012;
tel. 815/788–5800; Michael S. Eesley, Chief Executive Officer
**(Centralized Health System)**

ILLINOIS: CENTEGRA HOSPITAL – MCHENRY (O, 173 beds) 4201 Medical
Center Drive, McHenry, IL Zip 60050–9506; tel. 815/344–5000; Michael
S. Eesley, Chief Executive Officer
**Web address:** www.centegra.org

CENTEGRA HOSPITAL – WOODSTOCK (O, 135 beds) 3701 Doty Road,
Woodstock, IL Zip 60098–7509, Mailing Address: P.O. Box 1990,
Zip 60098–1990; tel. 815/338–2500; Michael S. Eesley, Chief Executive
Officer
**Web address:** www.centegra.org

| | | |
|---|---|---|
| Owned, leased, sponsored: | 2 hospitals | 308 beds |
| Contract–managed: | 0 hospitals | 0 beds |
| Totals: | 2 hospitals | 308 beds |

---

●**0634: CENTERRE HEALTHCARE** (IO)
5250 Virginia Way, Suite 240, Brentwood, TN Zip 37027–7576;
tel. 615/846–9508; Patrick A. Foster, President and Chief Executive
Officer

PENNSYLVANIA: LANCASTER REHABILITATION HOSPITAL (O, 10 beds) 675
Good Drive, Lancaster, PA Zip 17601–2426; tel. 717/406–3000; Tammy
L. Ober, Chief Executive Officer
**Web address:** www.lancastergeneral.org

| | | |
|---|---|---|
| Owned, leased, sponsored: | 1 hospital | 10 beds |
| Contract–managed: | 0 hospitals | 0 beds |
| Totals: | 1 hospital | 10 beds |

---

**2265: CENTRA HEALTH, INC.** (NP)
1920 Atherholt Road, Lynchburg, VA Zip 24501–1104;
tel. 434/200–3000; W. Michael Bryant, President and Chief
Executive Officer
**(Moderately Centralized Health System)**

VIRGINIA: CENTRA LYNCHBURG GENERAL HOSPITAL (O, 1081 beds) 1920
Atherholt Road, Lynchburg, VA Zip 24501–1104; tel. 434/200–4700; W.
Michael Bryant, President and Chief Executive Officer
**Web address:** www.centrahealth.com

CENTRA SOUTHSIDE COMMUNITY HOSPITAL (O, 86 beds) 800 Oak Street,
Farmville, VA Zip 23901–1199; tel. 434/392–8811; E. W. Tibbs, President
and Chief Executive Officer
**Web address:** www.centrasouthside.com

| | | |
|---|---|---|
| Owned, leased, sponsored: | 2 hospitals | 1167 beds |
| Contract–managed: | 0 hospitals | 0 beds |
| Totals: | 2 hospitals | 1167 beds |

---

★**0184: CENTRACARE HEALTH SYSTEM** (NP)
1406 Sixth Avenue North, Saint Cloud, MN Zip 56303;
tel. 320/251–2700; Terence Pladson, M.D., President and Chief
Executive Officer
**(Moderately Centralized Health System)**

MINNESOTA: CENTRACARE HEALTH SYSTEM – LONG PRAIRIE (O, 20 beds)
20 Ninth Street S.E., Long Prairie, MN Zip 56347–1404;
tel. 320/732–2141; Daniel J. Swenson, Chief Executive Officer
**Web address:** www.centracare.com

CENTRACARE HEALTH SYSTEM – MELROSE (O, 93 beds) 525 Main Street
West, Melrose, MN Zip 56352–1098; tel. 320/256–4231; Gerry Gilbertson,
FACHE, Administrator
**Web address:** www.centracare.com

ST. CLOUD HOSPITAL (O, 467 beds) 1406 Sixth Avenue North, Saint Cloud,
MN Zip 56303–1901; tel. 320/251–2700; Craig J. Broman, FACHE,
President, St. Cloud Hospital
**Web address:** www.centracare.com

| | | |
|---|---|---|
| Owned, leased, sponsored: | 3 hospitals | 580 beds |
| Contract–managed: | 0 hospitals | 0 beds |
| Totals: | 3 hospitals | 580 beds |

---

**0856: CENTRAL FLORIDA HEALTH ALLIANCE** (NP)
600 East Dixie Avenue, Leesburg, FL Zip 34748–5925;
tel. 352/323–5762; Donald G. Henderson, FACHE, Chief Executive
Officer

FLORIDA: LEESBURG REGIONAL MEDICAL CENTER (O, 316 beds) 600 East
Dixie Avenue, Leesburg, FL Zip 34748–5999; tel. 352/323–5762; Donald
G. Henderson, FACHE, President and Chief Executive Officer
**Web address:** www.cfhalliance.org

THE VILLAGES HEALTH SYSTEM (O, 198 beds) 1451 El Camino Real, The
Villages, FL Zip 32159; tel. 352/751–8000; Tim F. Hawkins, Chief Executive
Officer
**Web address:** www.cfhalliance.org

| | | |
|---|---|---|
| Owned, leased, sponsored: | 2 hospitals | 514 beds |
| Contract–managed: | 0 hospitals | 0 beds |
| Totals: | 2 hospitals | 514 beds |

---

★**0955: CHARLESTON AREA MEDICAL CENTER HEALTH
SYSTEM, INC.** (NP)
501 Morris Street, Charleston, WV Zip 25301–1300, Mailing
Address: P.O. Box 1547, Zip 25326–1547; tel. 304/388–5432;
David L. Ramsey, President and Chief Executive Officer
**(Independent Hospital System)**

WEST VIRGINIA: CAMC TEAYS VALLEY HOSPITAL (O, 70 beds) 1400 Hospital
Drive, Hurricane, WV Zip 25526–9202; tel. 304/757–1700; Randall H.
Hodges, President and Chief Executive Officer
**Web address:** www.camc.org

---

For explanation of codes following names, see page B2.
★ Indicates Type III membership in the American Hospital Association.
● Single hospital health care system

© 2012 AHA Guide

CHARLESTON AREA MEDICAL CENTER (O, 795 beds) 501 Morris Street, Charleston, WV Zip 25301–1300, Mailing Address: P.O. Box 1547, Zip 25326–1547; tel. 304/388–5432; David L. Ramsey, President and Chief Executive Officer
**Web address:** www.camc.org

| Owned, leased, sponsored: | 2 hospitals | 865 beds |
|---|---|---|
| Contract–managed: | 0 hospitals | 0 beds |
| **Totals:** | 2 hospitals | 865 beds |

**0407:  CHILDREN'S HOSPITAL AND HEALTH SYSTEM** (NP)
9000 West Wisconsin Avenue, Milwaukee, WI Zip 53226–4810, Mailing Address: P.O. Box 1997, Zip 53201–1997; tel. 414/226–2000; Peggy N. Troy, President and Chief Executive Officer
**(Independent Hospital System)**

**WISCONSIN:** CHILDREN'S HOSPITAL OF WISCONSIN (O, 296 beds) 9000 West Wisconsin Avenue, Milwaukee, WI Zip 53226–4810, Mailing Address: P.O. Box 1997, Zip 53201–1997; tel. 414/266–2000; Peggy N. Troy, President and Chief Executive Officer
**Web address:** www.chw.org

CHILDREN'S HOSPITAL OF WISCONSIN KENOSHA CLINIC (O, 19 beds) 8500 75th Street, Suite 101, Kenosha, WI Zip 53142; tel. 262/653–2260; Peggy N. Troy, President and Chief Executive Officer

CHILDREN'S HOSPITAL OF WISCONSIN–FOX VALLEY (O, 42 beds) 130 Second Avenue, 3rd Floor South, Neenah, WI Zip 54956; tel. 920/969–7900; Peggy N. Troy, President and Chief Executive Officer
**Web address:** www.chw.org

| Owned, leased, sponsored: | 3 hospitals | 357 beds |
|---|---|---|
| Contract–managed: | 0 hospitals | 0 beds |
| **Totals:** | 3 hospitals | 357 beds |

**0331:  CHILDREN'S HOSPITALS AND CLINICS OF MINNESOTA** (NP)
2525 Chicago Avenue South, Minneapolis, MN Zip 55404; tel. 612/813–6100; Alan L. Goldbloom, M.D., President and Chief Executive Officer
**(Moderately Centralized Health System)**

**MINNESOTA:** CHILDREN'S HOSPITALS AND CLINICS OF MINNESOTA (O, 347 beds) 2525 Chicago Avenue South, Minneapolis, MN Zip 55404–9976; tel. 612/813–6100; Alan L. Goldbloom, M.D., President and Chief Executive Officer
**Web address:** www.childrensmn.org

CHILDREN'S HOSPITALS AND CLINICS OF MINNESOTA (O, 133 beds) 345 North Smith Avenue, Saint Paul, MN Zip 55102–2392; tel. 651/220–6000; Alan L. Goldbloom, M.D., President and Chief Executive Officer
**Web address:** www.childrensmn.org

| Owned, leased, sponsored: | 2 hospitals | 480 beds |
|---|---|---|
| Contract–managed: | 0 hospitals | 0 beds |
| **Totals:** | 2 hospitals | 480 beds |

● ★**0131:  CHRISTIANA CARE HEALTH SYSTEM** (NP)
501 West 14th Street, Wilmington, DE Zip 19801–1013, Mailing Address: P.O. Box 1668, Zip 19899; tel. 302/733–1000; Robert J. Laskowski, M.D., President and Chief Executive Officer
**(Moderately Centralized Health System)**

**DELAWARE:** CHRISTIANA CARE HEALTH SYSTEM (O, 988 beds) 4755 Ogletown–Stanton Road, Newark, DE Zip 19718–0002, Mailing Address: P.O. Box 6001, Zip 19726–6001; tel. 302/733–1000; Robert J. Laskowski, M.D., President and Chief Executive Officer
**Web address:** www.christianacare.org

| Owned, leased, sponsored: | 1 hospital | 988 beds |
|---|---|---|
| Contract–managed: | 0 hospitals | 0 beds |
| **Totals:** | 1 hospital | 988 beds |

★**0192:  CHRISTUS HEALTH** (CC)
6363 North Highway 161, Suite 450, Irving, TX Zip 75038; tel. 214/492–8500; Ernie W. Sadau, President and Chief Executive Officer
**(Moderately Centralized Health System)**

**ARKANSAS:** MAGNOLIA REGIONAL MEDICAL CENTER (C, 49 beds) 101 Hospital Drive, Magnolia, AR Zip 71753–2416, Mailing Address: P.O. Box 629, Zip 71754–0629; tel. 870/235–3000; Margaret M. West, MS, Chief Executive Officer
**Web address:** www.magnoliahospital.org

**LOUISIANA:** CHRISTUS COUSHATTA HEALTH CARE CENTER (O, 25 beds) 1635 Marvel Street, Coushatta, LA Zip 71019–9022, Mailing Address: P.O. Box 589, Zip 71019–0589; tel. 318/932–2000; Nancy R. Hellyer, Interim Chief Executive Officer
**Web address:** www.christuscoushatta.org

CHRISTUS HEALTH SHREVEPORT–BOSSIER (O, 302 beds) One St. Mary Place, Shreveport, LA Zip 71101–4399; tel. 318/681–4500; Stephen F. Wright, President and Chief Executive Officer
**Web address:** www.christusschumpert.org

CHRISTUS ST. FRANCES CABRINI HOSPITAL (O, 281 beds) 3330 Masonic Drive, Alexandria, LA Zip 71301–3899; tel. 318/487–1122; Stephen F. Wright, President and Chief Executive Officer
**Web address:** www.christushealth.org/sfcabrini

CHRISTUS ST. PATRICK HOSPITAL OF LAKE CHARLES (O, 228 beds) 524 Dr. Michael Debakey Drive, Lake Charles, LA Zip 70601–5799, Mailing Address: P.O. Box 3401, Zip 70602–3401; tel. 337/436–2511; Stephen F. Wright, President and Chief Executive Officer
**Web address:** www.stpatrickhospital.org

NATCHITOCHES REGIONAL MEDICAL CENTER (C, 78 beds) 501 Keyser Avenue, Natchitoches, LA Zip 71457–6036, Mailing Address: P.O. Box 2009, Zip 71457–2009; tel. 318/214–4200; Mark E. Marley, FACHE, Chief Executive Officer
**Web address:** www.natchitocheshospital.org

**NEW MEXICO:** CHRISTUS ST. VINCENT REGIONAL MEDICAL CENTER (O, 195 beds) 455 St. Michael's Drive, Santa Fe, NM Zip 87505–7663, Mailing Address: P.O. Box 2107, Zip 87504–2107; tel. 505/983–3361; Alex Valdez, JD, Chief Executive Officer
**Web address:** www.stvin.org

**TEXAS:** CHRISTUS HOSPITAL–ST. ELIZABETH (O, 456 beds) 2830 Calder Avenue, Beaumont, TX Zip 77702–1809, Mailing Address: P.O. Box 5405, Zip 77726–5405; tel. 409/892–7171; Paul Trevino, Administrator
**Web address:** www.christushospital.org

CHRISTUS JASPER MEMORIAL HOSPITAL (L, 50 beds) 1275 Marvin Hancock Drive, Jasper, TX Zip 75951–4995; tel. 409/384–5461; Deborah Wiegand, R.N., Administrator
**Web address:** www.christusjasper.org

CHRISTUS SANTA ROSA HEALTH CARE (O, 778 beds) 333 North Santa Rosa Street, San Antonio, TX Zip 78207–3108; tel. 210/704–4184; Patrick Brian Carrier, President and Chief Executive Officer
**Web address:** www.christussantarosa.org

CHRISTUS SANTA ROSA HOSPITAL – NEW BRAUNFELS (O, 112 beds) 600 North Union Avenue, New Braunfels, TX Zip 78130–4191; tel. 830/606–9111; Jim D. Wesson, Vice President and Administrator
**Web address:** www.christussantarosa.org

CHRISTUS SPOHN HOSPITAL ALICE (O, 114 beds) 2500 East Main Street, Alice, TX Zip 78332–4169; tel. 361/661–8000; Mark Casanova, Vice President and Chief Operating Officer
**Web address:** www.christusspohn.org/locations_alice.htm

CHRISTUS SPOHN HOSPITAL BEEVILLE (L, 49 beds) 1500 East Houston Street, Beeville, TX Zip 78102–5312; tel. 361/354–2000; Raymond Ramos, Vice President and Chief Operating Officer
**Web address:** www.christusspohn.org

CHRISTUS SPOHN HOSPITAL CORPUS CHRISTI MEMORIAL (O, 800 beds) 2606 Hospital Boulevard, Corpus Christi, TX Zip 78405–1818, Mailing Address: P.O. Box 5280, Zip 78465–5280; tel. 361/902–4000; Paul Gaden, Vice President and Chief Operating Officer
**Web address:** www.christusspohn.org

CHRISTUS SPOHN HOSPITAL KLEBERG (O, 77 beds) 1311 General Cavazos Boulevard, Kingsville, TX Zip 78363–1197; tel. 361/595–1661; Norman L. McBride, FACHE, Vice President and Chief Operating Officer
**Web address:** www.christusspohn.org

For explanation of codes following names, see page B2.
★ Indicates Type III membership in the American Hospital Association.
● Single hospital health care system

Section B

CHRISTUS ST. CATHERINE HOSPITAL (O, 102 beds) 701 Fry Road, Katy, TX Zip 77450; tel. 281/599–5700; Jack H. McCabe, FACHE, Administrator **Web address:** www.christusstcatherine.org

CHRISTUS ST. JOHN HOSPITAL (O, 121 beds) 18300 St. John Drive, Nassau Bay, TX Zip 77058–6302; tel. 281/333–5503; Thomas Permetti, Regional Chief Operating Officer and Administrator **Web address:** www.christusstjohn.org

CHRISTUS ST. MICHAEL HEALTH SYSTEM (O, 312 beds) 2600 St. Michael Drive, Texarkana, TX Zip 75503–2372; tel. 903/614–1000; Chris Karam, President and Chief Executive Officer **Web address:** www.christusstmichael.org

CHRISTUS ST. MICHAEL REHABILITATION HOSPITAL (O, 50 beds) 2400 St. Michael Drive, Texarkana, TX Zip 75503; tel. 903/614–4000; Aloma Gender, R.N., MSN, Administrator and Chief Nursing Officer **Web address:** www.christusstmichael.org

RICE MEDICAL CENTER (C, 15 beds) 600 South Austin Road, Eagle Lake, TX Zip 77434–3298, Mailing Address: P.O. Box 277, Zip 77434–0277; tel. 979/234–5571; James D. Janek, Chief Executive Officer **Web address:** www.ricemedicalcenter.org

| | | |
|---|---|---|
| Owned, leased, sponsored: | 17 hospitals | 4052 beds |
| Contract–managed: | 3 hospitals | 142 beds |
| Totals: | 20 hospitals | 4194 beds |

**0350: CIRRUS HEALTH** (IO)
9301 North Central Expressway, Suite 360, Dallas, TX Zip 75231; tel. 214/217–0100; Timothy Parris, President and Chief Executive Officer
**(Independent Hospital System)**

BAYLOR MEDICAL CENTER AT TROPHY CLUB (O, 20 beds) 2850 East State Highway 114, Trophy Club, TX Zip 76262; tel. 817/837–4600; Melanie Chick, Chief Executive Officer **Web address:** www.tc–mc.com

NORTH TEXAS HOSPITAL (O, 16 beds) 2801 South Mayhill Road, Denton, TX Zip 76208–5910; tel. 940/220–0600; Judith Schiros, Chief Executive Officer and Administrator **Web address:** www.northtexashospital.com

| | | |
|---|---|---|
| Owned, leased, sponsored: | 2 hospitals | 36 beds |
| Contract–managed: | 0 hospitals | 0 beds |
| Totals: | 2 hospitals | 36 beds |

**0101: CITRUS VALLEY HEALTH PARTNERS** (NP)
210 West San Bernardino Road, Covina, CA Zip 91723; tel. 626/331–7331; Robert H. Curry, President and Chief Executive Officer

**CALIFORNIA:** CITRUS VALLEY MEDICAL CENTER–INTER–COMMUNITY CAMPUS (O, 252 beds) 210 West San Bernardino Road, Covina, CA Zip 91723–1901, Mailing Address: P.O. Box 6108, Zip 91722–5108; tel. 626/331–7331; Robert H. Curry, President and Chief Executive Officer **Web address:** www.cvhp.org

CITRUS VALLEY MEDICAL CENTER–QUEEN OF THE VALLEY CAMPUS (O, 263 beds) 1115 South Sunset Avenue, West Covina, CA Zip 91790–3940, Mailing Address: P.O. Box 1980, Zip 91793–1980; tel. 626/962–4011; Robert H. Curry, President and Chief Executive Officer **Web address:** www.cvhp.org

FOOTHILL PRESBYTERIAN HOSPITAL (O, 105 beds) 250 South Grand Avenue, Glendora, CA Zip 91741–4218; tel. 626/963–8411; Diana Lugo–Zenner, R.N., Administrator **Web address:** www.cvhp.org

| | | |
|---|---|---|
| Owned, leased, sponsored: | 3 hospitals | 620 beds |
| Contract–managed: | 0 hospitals | 0 beds |
| Totals: | 3 hospitals | 620 beds |

**★0212: CLEVELAND CLINIC HEALTH SYSTEM** (NP)
9500 Euclid, Cleveland, OH Zip 44195–5108; tel. 216/444–2200; Delos Cosgrove, M.D., President and Chief Executive Officer
**(Centralized Health System)**

**FLORIDA:** CLEVELAND CLINIC FLORIDA (O, 155 beds) 3100 Weston Road, Weston, FL Zip 33331–3602; tel. 954/659–6001; Bernardo Fernandez, M.D., Chief Executive Officer **Web address:** www.clevelandclinic.org/florida

**OHIO:** CLEVELAND CLINIC CHILDREN'S HOSPITAL FOR REHABILITATION (O, 25 beds) 2801 Martin Luther King Jr. Drive, Cleveland, OH Zip 44104–3865; tel. 216/448–6400; Michael J. McHugh, M.D., Medical Director **Web address:** www.clevelandclinic.org/childrenshospital

CLEVELAND CLINIC FOUNDATION (O, 1267 beds) 9500 Euclid Avenue, Cleveland, OH Zip 44195–5108; tel. 216/444–2200; Delos Cosgrove, M.D., President and Chief Executive Officer **Web address:** www.clevelandclinic.org

EUCLID HOSPITAL (O, 231 beds) 18901 Lake Shore Boulevard, Euclid, OH Zip 44119–1090; tel. 216/531–9000; Mark Froimson, President **Web address:** www.euclidhospital.org

FAIRVIEW HOSPITAL (O, 375 beds) 18101 Lorain Avenue, Cleveland, OH Zip 44111–5656; tel. 216/476–7000; Janice Murphy, President **Web address:** www.fairviewhospital.org

HILLCREST HOSPITAL (O, 406 beds) 6780 Mayfield Road, Cleveland, OH Zip 44124–2202; tel. 440/312–4500; Jeffrey A. Leimgruber, President **Web address:** www.hillcresthospital.org

LAKEWOOD HOSPITAL (O, 250 beds) 14519 Detroit Avenue, Lakewood, OH Zip 44107–4383; tel. 216/521–4200; Robert Weil, M.D., President **Web address:** www.lakewoodhospital.org

LUTHERAN HOSPITAL (O, 182 beds) 1730 West 25th Street, Cleveland, OH Zip 44113–3170; tel. 216/696–4300; Brian Donley, M.D., President **Web address:** www.lutheranhospital.org

MARYMOUNT HOSPITAL (O, 232 beds) 12300 McCracken Road, Garfield Heights, OH Zip 44125–2975; tel. 216/581–0500; Joanne Zeroske, President and Chief Executive Officer **Web address:** www.marymount.org

MEDINA HOSPITAL (O, 110 beds) 1000 East Washington Street, Medina, OH Zip 44256–2170; tel. 330/725–1000; Thomas Tulisiak, M.D., President **Web address:** www.medinahospital.org

SOUTH POINTE HOSPITAL (O, 172 beds) 20000 Harvard Road, Warrensville Heights, OH Zip 44122–7099; tel. 216/491–6000; Brian J. Harte, M.D., President **Web address:** www.southpointehospital.org

| | | |
|---|---|---|
| Owned, leased, sponsored: | 11 hospitals | 3405 beds |
| Contract–managed: | 0 hospitals | 0 beds |
| Totals: | 11 hospitals | 3405 beds |

**0076: COLLEGE HEALTH ENTERPRISES** (IO)
11627 Telegraph Road, Suite 200, Santa Fe Springs, CA Zip 90670; tel. 562/923–9449; Barry J. Weiss, Chairman of the Board

**CALIFORNIA:** COLLEGE HOSPITAL (O, 157 beds) 10802 College Place, Cerritos, CA Zip 90703–1579; tel. 562/924–9581; Stephen Witt, President and Chief Executive Officer **Web address:** www.collegehospitals.com

COLLEGE HOSPITAL COSTA MESA (O, 122 beds) 301 Victoria Street, Costa Mesa, CA Zip 92627–7131; tel. 949/642–2734; Susan L. Taylor, Chief Executive Officer **Web address:** www.collegehospitalcm.com

| | | |
|---|---|---|
| Owned, leased, sponsored: | 2 hospitals | 279 beds |
| Contract–managed: | 0 hospitals | 0 beds |
| Totals: | 2 hospitals | 279 beds |

**★0161: COLUMBUS REGIONAL HEALTHCARE SYSTEM** (NP)
707 Center Street, Suite 400, Columbus, GA Zip 31901; tel. 706/660–6100; Charles A. Stark, FACHE, Chief Executive Officer
**(Centralized Health System)**

**GEORGIA:** AZALEA TRACE (O, 110 beds) 910 Talbotton Road, Columbus, GA Zip 31901; tel. 706/323–9513; Todd West, Administrator

For explanation of codes following names, see page B2.
★ Indicates Type III membership in the American Hospital Association.

© 2012 AHA Guide

Section B

DOCTORS HOSPITAL OF COLUMBUS (O, 171 beds) 616 19th Street, Columbus, GA Zip 31901–1528, Mailing Address: P.O. Box 2188, Zip 31902–2188; tel. 706/494–4262; Kevin Sass, FACHE, Senior Executive Officer
**Web address:** www.doctorshospital.net

HAMILTON HOUSE NURSING CENTER/ADULT LIVING CENTER (O, 128 beds) 1911 Hamilton Road, Columbus, GA Zip 31901; tel. 706/571–1850; John Sims, Administrator

HUGHSTON HOSPITAL (O, 100 beds) 100 Frist Court, Columbus, GA Zip 31908–7188, Mailing Address: P.O. Box 7188, Zip 31908–7188; tel. 706/576–2100; Butch Wheeler, FACHE, Chief Executive Officer
**Web address:** www.hughstonhospital.com

MARION MEMORIAL NURSING HOME (O, 70 beds) Highway 41, Buena Vista, GA Zip 31803, Mailing Address: P.O. Box 197, Zip 31803; tel. 229/649–7100; Barbara Mitchell, Administrator

THE MEDICAL CENTER (O, 497 beds) 710 Center Street, Columbus, GA Zip 31901–1527, Mailing Address: P.O. Box 951, Zip 31902–0951; tel. 706/571–1000; Ryan Chandler, President and Chief Executive Officer
**Web address:** www.columbusregional.com

| | | |
|---|---|---|
| **Owned, leased, sponsored:** | 6 hospitals | 1076 beds |
| **Contract–managed:** | 0 hospitals | 0 beds |
| **Totals:** | 6 hospitals | 1076 beds |

---

**0520:  COMMONWEALTH HEALTH CORPORATION** (NP)
800 Park Street, Bowling Green, KY Zip 42101–2356; tel. 270/745–1500; Connie Smith, President and Chief Executive Officer
**(Moderately Centralized Health System)**

**KENTUCKY:** COMMONWEALTH REGIONAL SPECIALTY HOSPITAL (O, 28 beds) 250 Park Drive, 6th Floor, Bowling Green, KY Zip 42101, Mailing Address: P.O. Box 90010, Zip 42101; tel. 270/796–6200; Emily Howard Martin, Administrator
**Web address:** www.commonwealthregionalspecialtyhospital.org

MEDICAL CENTER AT BOWLING GREEN (O, 337 beds) 250 Park Street, Bowling Green, KY Zip 42101–1795, Mailing Address: P.O. Box 90010, Zip 42102–9010; tel. 270/745–1000; Connie Smith, Chief Executive Officer
**Web address:** www.themedicalcenter.org

MEDICAL CENTER AT FRANKLIN (O, 25 beds) 1100 Brookhaven Road, Franklin, KY Zip 42134–2746; tel. 270/598–4800; Clara M. Sumner, Senior Vice President and Chief Executive Officer
**Web address:** www.themedicalcenterfranklin.org

MEDICAL CENTER AT SCOTTSVILLE (O, 135 beds) 456 Burnley Road, Scottsville, KY Zip 42164–6355; tel. 270/622–2800; Eric Hagan, R.N., Vice President
**Web address:** www.mcbg.org/scottsville

| | | |
|---|---|---|
| **Owned, leased, sponsored:** | 4 hospitals | 525 beds |
| **Contract–managed:** | 0 hospitals | 0 beds |
| **Totals:** | 4 hospitals | 525 beds |

---

**0401:  COMMUNITY HEALTH NETWORK** (NP)
7330 Shadeland Station, Indianapolis, IN Zip 46256–3957; tel. 317/355–1411; Bryan A. Mills, President and Chief Executive Officer

**INDIANA:** COMMUNITY HOSPITAL EAST (O, 233 beds) 1500 North Ritter Avenue, Indianapolis, IN Zip 46219–3095; tel. 317/355–1411; Robin Ledyard, M.D., M.P.H., President
**Web address:** www.ecommunity.org

COMMUNITY HOSPITAL NORTH (O, 389 beds) 7150 Clearvista Drive, Indianapolis, IN Zip 46256; tel. 317/621–6262; Barbara Summers, President
**Web address:** www.ecommunity.com

COMMUNITY HOSPITAL OF ANDERSON AND MADISON COUNTY (O, 173 beds) 1515 North Madison Avenue, Anderson, IN Zip 46011–3453; tel. 765/298–4242; William C. Vanness, II, M.D., President
**Web address:** www.communityanderson.com

COMMUNITY HOSPITAL SOUTH (O, 108 beds) 1402 East County Line Road South, Indianapolis, IN Zip 46227; tel. 317/887–7000; Anthony B. Lennen, President
**Web address:** www.ecommunity.com

COMMUNITY HOWARD REGIONAL HOSPITAL (O, 152 beds) 3500 South Lafountain Street, Kokomo, IN Zip 46904–9011, Mailing Address: P.O. Box 9011, Zip 46904–9011; tel. 765/453–0702; James P. Alender, President and Chief Executive Officer
**Web address:** www.howardregional.org

COMMUNITY HOWARD SPECIALTY HOSPITAL (O, 30 beds) 829 North Dixon Road, Kokomo, IN Zip 46901–7709; tel. 765/452–6700; Michelle L. Russell, Administrator
**Web address:** www.howardregional.org

COMMUNITY WESTVIEW HOSPITAL (O, 68 beds) 3630 Guion Road, Indianapolis, IN Zip 46222–1699; tel. 317/924–6661; Jon P. Anderson, CPA, Chief Executive Officer
**Web address:** www.westviewhospital.org

INDIANA HEART HOSPITAL (O, 56 beds) 8075 North Shadeland Avenue, Indianapolis, IN Zip 46250; tel. 317/621–8000; Thomas A. Malasto, Chief Executive Officer
**Web address:** www.hearthospital.com

| | | |
|---|---|---|
| **Owned, leased, sponsored:** | 8 hospitals | 1209 beds |
| **Contract–managed:** | 0 hospitals | 0 beds |
| **Totals:** | 8 hospitals | 1209 beds |

---

**★0080:  COMMUNITY HEALTH SYSTEMS, INC.** (IO)
4000 Meridian Boulevard, Franklin, TN Zip 37067–6325, Mailing Address: P.O. Box 689020, Zip 37068–9020; tel. 615/465–7000; Wayne T. Smith, Chairman, President and Chief Executive Officer
**(Decentralized Health System)**

**ALABAMA:** CHEROKEE MEDICAL CENTER (O, 45 beds) 400 Northwood Drive, Centre, AL Zip 35960–1023; tel. 256/927–5531; Patrick Trammell, Chief Executive Officer
**Web address:** www.cherokeemedicalcenter.com

CRESTWOOD MEDICAL CENTER (O, 150 beds) One Hospital Drive, Huntsville, AL Zip 35801–3403; tel. 256/429–4000; Pamela Hudson, M.D., Chief Executive Officer
**Web address:** www.crestwoodmedcenter.com

DEKALB REGIONAL MEDICAL CENTER (O, 115 beds) 200 Medical Center Drive, Fort Payne, AL Zip 35968–3415, Mailing Address: P.O. Box 680778, Zip 35968–1608; tel. 256/845–3150; Jeff G. Rains, Chief Executive Officer
**Web address:** www.dekalbregional.com

FLOWERS HOSPITAL (O, 235 beds) 4370 West Main Street, Dothan, AL Zip 36305–4000, Mailing Address: P.O. Box 6907, Zip 36302–6907; tel. 334/793–5000; Suzanne Woods, President and Chief Executive Officer
**Web address:** www.flowershospital.com

GADSDEN REGIONAL MEDICAL CENTER (O, 299 beds) 1007 Goodyear Avenue, Gadsden, AL Zip 35903–1195; tel. 256/494–4000; Stephen G. Pennington, Chief Executive Officer
**Web address:** www.gadsdenregional.com

L. V. STABLER MEMORIAL HOSPITAL (O, 61 beds) 29 L. V. Stabler Drive, Greenville, AL Zip 36037–3800; tel. 334/382–2671; Connie Nicholas, Interim Chief Executive Officer
**Web address:** www.lvstabler.com

MEDICAL CENTER ENTERPRISE (O, 117 beds) 400 North Edwards Street, Enterprise, AL Zip 36330; tel. 334/347–0584; Jeffrey M. Brannon, Chief Executive Officer
**Web address:** www.mcehospital.com

SOUTH BALDWIN REGIONAL MEDICAL CENTER (L, 110 beds) 1613 North McKenzie Street, Foley, AL Zip 36535–2299; tel. 251/949–3400; Keith Newton, Chief Executive Officer
**Web address:** www.southbaldwinrmc.com

TRINITY MEDICAL CENTER (O, 379 beds) 800 Montclair Road, Birmingham, AL Zip 35213–1984; tel. 205/592–1000; Keith Granger, President and Chief Executive Officer
**Web address:** www.bhsala.com

**ALASKA:** MAT–SU REGIONAL MEDICAL CENTER (O, 74 beds) 2500 South Woodworth Loop, Palmer, AK Zip 99645, Mailing Address: P.O. Box 1687, Zip 99645–1687; tel. 907/861–6000; John R. Lee, Chief Executive Officer
**Web address:** www.matsuregional.com

---

For explanation of codes following names, see page B2.
★ Indicates Type III membership in the American Hospital Association.

**ARIZONA:** NORTHWEST MEDICAL CENTER (O, 270 beds) 6200 North La Cholla Boulevard, Tucson, AZ Zip 85741–3599; tel. 520/742–9000; Kevin Stockton, Chief Executive Officer
**Web address:** www.northwestmedicalcenter.com

ORO VALLEY HOSPITAL (O, 144 beds) 1551 East Tangerine Road, Oro Valley, AZ Zip 85737; tel. 520/901–3500; Jae Dale, Chief Executive Officer
**Web address:** www.nmcorovalley.com

PAYSON REGIONAL MEDICAL CENTER (L, 44 beds) 807 South Ponderosa Street, Payson, AZ Zip 85541–5599; tel. 928/474–3222; R. Chris Wolf, Chief Executive Officer
**Web address:** www.paysonhospital.com

WESTERN ARIZONA REGIONAL MEDICAL CENTER (O, 139 beds) 2735 Silver Creek Road, Bullhead City, AZ Zip 86442–8303; tel. 928/763–2273; Barry S. Schneider, Chief Executive Officer
**Web address:** www.warmc.com

**ARKANSAS:** FORREST CITY MEDICAL CENTER (L, 70 beds) 1601 Newcastle Road, Forrest City, AR Zip 72335; tel. 870/261–0000; Brett Kinman, Chief Executive Officer
**Web address:** www.forrestcitymedicalcenter.com

HARRIS HOSPITAL (O, 104 beds) 1205 McLain Street, Newport, AR Zip 72112–3533; tel. 870/523–8911; Robert Rupp, Chief Executive Officer
**Web address:** www.harrishospital.com

HELENA REGIONAL MEDICAL CENTER (L, 100 beds) 1801 Martin Luther King Drive, Helena, AR Zip 72342, Mailing Address: P.O. Box 788, Zip 72342–0788; tel. 870/338–5800; James T. Sato, FACHE, Chief Executive Officer
**Web address:** www.helenarmc.com

MEDICAL CENTER OF SOUTH ARKANSAS (L, 120 beds) 700 West Grove Street, El Dorado, AR Zip 71730–4416, Mailing Address: P.O. Box 1998, Zip 71731–1998; tel. 870/863–2000; Kyle Swift, Chief Executive Officer
**Web address:** www.themedcenter.net

SILOAM SPRINGS MEMORIAL HOSPITAL (O, 43 beds) 205 East Jefferson Street, Siloam Springs, AR Zip 72761–3697; tel. 479/524–4141; Kevin J. Clement, Chief Executive Officer
**Web address:** www.ssmh.us

**CALIFORNIA:** BARSTOW COMMUNITY HOSPITAL (L, 23 beds) 555 South Seventh Avenue, Barstow, CA Zip 92311–3043; tel. 760/256–1761; S. Sean Fowler, Chief Executive Officer
**Web address:** www.barstowhospital.com

FALLBROOK HOSPITAL (L, 86 beds) 624 East Elder Street, Fallbrook, CA Zip 92028–3099; tel. 760/728–1191; Alex Villa, Chief Executive Officer
**Web address:** www.fallbrookhospital.com

WATSONVILLE COMMUNITY HOSPITAL (O, 106 beds) 75 Nielson Street, Watsonville, CA Zip 95076–2468; tel. 831/724–4741; Audra Earle, Chief Executive Officer
**Web address:** www.watsonvillehospital.com

**FLORIDA:** LAKE WALES MEDICAL CENTER (O, 131 beds) 410 South 11th Street, Lake Wales, FL Zip 33853–4256; tel. 863/676–1433; Scott M. Smith, Chief Executive Officer
**Web address:** www.lakewalesmedicalcenter.com

NORTH OKALOOSA MEDICAL CENTER (O, 110 beds) 151 Redstone Avenue S.E., Crestview, FL Zip 32539–6026; tel. 850/689–8100; David W. Fuller, Chief Executive Officer
**Web address:** www.northokaloosa.com

**GEORGIA:** FANNIN REGIONAL HOSPITAL (O, 50 beds) 2855 Old Highway 5, Blue Ridge, GA Zip 30513–6248; tel. 706/632–3711; David S. Sanders, Chief Executive Officer
**Web address:** www.fanninregionalhospital.com

TRINITY HOSPITAL OF AUGUSTA (O, 105 beds) 2260 Wrightsboro Road, Augusta, GA Zip 30904–4726; tel. 706/481–7000; James A. Cruickshank, Chief Executive Officer
**Web address:** www.trinityofaugusta.com

**ILLINOIS:** CROSSROADS COMMUNITY HOSPITAL (O, 41 beds) 8 Doctors Park Road, Mount Vernon, IL Zip 62864–6224; tel. 618/244–5500; M. Edward Cunningham, Chief Executive Officer
**Web address:** www.crossroadscommunityhospital.com

GALESBURG COTTAGE HOSPITAL (O, 119 beds) 695 North Kellogg Street, Galesburg, IL Zip 61401–2885; tel. 309/343–8131; Earl J. Tamar, Chief Executive Officer
**Web address:** www.cottagehospital.com

GATEWAY REGIONAL MEDICAL CENTER (O, 337 beds) 2100 Madison Avenue, Granite City, IL Zip 62040–4799; tel. 618/798–3000; Mark Bethell, Chief Executive Officer
**Web address:** www.gatewayregional.net

HEARTLAND REGIONAL MEDICAL CENTER (O, 92 beds) 3333 West DeYoung, Marion, IL Zip 62959; tel. 618/998–7000; Stephen Lunn, Chief Executive Officer
**Web address:** www.heartlandregional.com

METROSOUTH MEDICAL CENTER (O, 180 beds) 12935 South Gregory Street, Blue Island, IL Zip 60406–2470; tel. 708/597–2000; Enrique Beckmann, M.D., Ph.D., President and Chief Executive Officer
**Web address:** www.metrosouthmedicalcenter.com

RED BUD REGIONAL HOSPITAL (O, 140 beds) 325 Spring Street, Red Bud, IL Zip 62278–1194; tel. 618/282–3831; Shane Watson, Chief Executive Officer
**Web address:** www.redbudhospital.com

UNION COUNTY HOSPITAL (L, 47 beds) 517 North Main Street, Anna, IL Zip 62906–1696; tel. 618/833–4511; James R. Farris, FACHE, Chief Executive Officer
**Web address:** www.unioncountyhospital.com

VISTA MEDICAL CENTER EAST (O, 192 beds) 1324 North Sheridan Road, Waukegan, IL Zip 60085–2181; tel. 847/360–3000; Barbara J. Martin, R.N., President and Chief Executive Officer
**Web address:** www.vistahealth.com

VISTA MEDICAL CENTER WEST (O, 67 beds) 2615 Washington Street, Waukegan, IL Zip 60085–4988; tel. 847/249–3900; Barbara J. Martin, R.N., President and Chief Executive Officer
**Web address:** www.vistahealth.com

**INDIANA:** BLUFFTON REGIONAL MEDICAL CENTER (O, 79 beds) 303 South Main Street, Bluffton, IN Zip 46714–2529; tel. 260/824–3210; Brandon Haushalter, Chief Executive Officer
**Web address:** www.blufftonregional.com

DUKES MEMORIAL HOSPITAL (O, 25 beds) 275 West 12th Street, Peru, IN Zip 46970–1698; tel. 765/472–8000; Debra Close, Chief Executive Officer
**Web address:** www.dukesmemorialhosp.com

DUPONT HOSPITAL (O, 131 beds) 2520 East Dupont Road, Fort Wayne, IN Zip 46825; tel. 260/416–3000; Chad Towner, Chief Executive Officer
**Web address:** www.thedupontdifference.com

KOSCIUSKO COMMUNITY HOSPITAL (O, 72 beds) 2101 East Dubois Drive, Warsaw, IN Zip 46580–3288; tel. 574/267–3200; Stephen R. Miller, Chief Executive Officer
**Web address:** www.kch.com

LUTHERAN HOSPITAL OF INDIANA (O, 396 beds) 7950 West Jefferson Boulevard, Fort Wayne, IN Zip 46804–1677; tel. 260/435–7001; Brian Bauer, Chief Executive Officer
**Web address:** www.lutheranhospital.com

ORTHOPAEDIC HOSPITAL OF LUTHERAN HEALTH (O, 44 beds) 7952 West Jefferson Boulevard, Fort Wayne, IN Zip 46804–4140; tel. 260/435–2999; Shelly Miller, R.N., Chief Executive Officer
**Web address:** www.theorthohospital.com

PORTER–VALPARAISO HOSPITAL CAMPUS (O, 276 beds) 814 La Porte Avenue, Valparaiso, IN Zip 46383–5898; tel. 219/263–4600; Jonathan Nalli, Chief Executive Officer
**Web address:** www.porterhealth.org

REHABILITATION HOSPITAL OF FORT WAYNE (O, 36 beds) 7970 West Jefferson Boulevard, Fort Wayne, IN Zip 46804–4140; tel. 260/435–6100; Ted Scholten, Chief Operating Officer
**Web address:** www.rehabhospital.com

ST. JOSEPH HOSPITAL (O, 191 beds) 700 Broadway, Fort Wayne, IN Zip 46802–1493; tel. 260/425–3000; Eric N. Looper, Chief Executive Officer
**Web address:** www.stjoehospital.com

**KENTUCKY:** KENTUCKY RIVER MEDICAL CENTER (L, 54 beds) 540 Jett Drive, Jackson, KY Zip 41339–9620; tel. 606/666–6000; William Chad French, Chief Executive Officer
**Web address:** www.kentuckyrivermc.com

PARKWAY REGIONAL HOSPITAL (O, 70 beds) 2000 Holiday Lane, Fulton, KY Zip 42041–8468; tel. 270/472–2522; Dana Lawrence, Interim Chief Executive Officer
**Web address:** www.parkwayregionalhospital.com

For explanation of codes following names, see page B2.
★ Indicates Type III membership in the American Hospital Association.

THREE RIVERS MEDICAL CENTER (O, 80 beds) Highway 644, Louisa, KY Zip 41230–9632, Mailing Address: P.O. Box 769, Zip 41230–0769; tel. 606/638–9451; Greg Kiser, Chief Executive Officer
**Web address:** www.threeriversmedicalcenter.com

**LOUISIANA:** BYRD REGIONAL HOSPITAL (O, 60 beds) 1020 West Fertitta Boulevard, Leesville, LA Zip 71446–4645; tel. 337/239–9041; Roger C. LeDoux, Chief Executive Officer
**Web address:** www.byrdregional.com

NORTHERN LOUISIANA MEDICAL CENTER (O, 91 beds) 401 East Vaughn Avenue, Ruston, LA Zip 71270–5950; tel. 318/254–2100; Brady Dubois, Interim Chief Executive Officer
**Web address:** www.northernlouisianamedicalcenter.com

WOMEN AND CHILDREN'S HOSPITAL (O, 88 beds) 4200 Nelson Road, Lake Charles, LA Zip 70605–4118; tel. 337/474–6370; Bryan S. Bateman, Chief Executive Officer
**Web address:** www.women–childrens.com

**MISSISSIPPI:** RIVER REGION MEDICAL CENTER (O, 297 beds) 2100 Highway 61 North, Vicksburg, MS Zip 39183, Mailing Address: P.O. Box 590, Zip 39181–0590; tel. 601/883–5000; Doug Sills, Chief Executive Officer
**Web address:** www.riverregion.com

WESLEY MEDICAL CENTER (O, 211 beds) 5001 Hardy Street, Hattiesburg, MS Zip 39402–1366, Mailing Address: P.O. Box 16509, Zip 39404–6509; tel. 601/268–8000; Michael Neuendorf, Chief Executive Officer
**Web address:** www.wesley.com

**MISSOURI:** MOBERLY REGIONAL MEDICAL CENTER (O, 94 beds) 1515 Union Avenue, Moberly, MO Zip 65270–9449; tel. 660/263–8400; Christian Jones, Chief Executive Officer
**Web address:** www.moberlyhospital.com

NORTHEAST REGIONAL MEDICAL CENTER (L, 115 beds) 315 South Osteopathy, Kirksville, MO Zip 63501–8599, Mailing Address: P.O. Box C8502, Zip 63501–8599; tel. 660/785–1000; Eric A. Barber, Chief Executive Officer
**Web address:** www.nermc.com

**NEVADA:** MESA VIEW REGIONAL HOSPITAL (O, 25 beds) 1299 Bertha Howe Avenue, Mesquite, NV Zip 89027; tel. 702/346–8040; Kapua Conley, Chief Executive Officer
**Web address:** www.mesaviewhospital.com

**NEW JERSEY:** MEMORIAL HOSPITAL OF SALEM COUNTY (O, 110 beds) 310 Woodstown Road, Salem, NJ Zip 08079–2080; tel. 856/935–1000; Richard Grogan, Chief Executive Officer
**Web address:** www.salemhospitalnj.org

**NEW MEXICO:** ALTA VISTA REGIONAL HOSPITAL (O, 52 beds) 104 Legion Drive, Las Vegas, NM Zip 87701; tel. 505/426–3500; Maridel Acosta, Chief Executive Officer
**Web address:** www.altavistaregionalhospital.com

CARLSBAD MEDICAL CENTER (O, 127 beds) 2430 West Pierce Street, Carlsbad, NM Zip 88220–3597; tel. 575/887–4105; Chad Campbell, Chief Executive Officer
**Web address:** www.carlsbadmedicalcenter.com

EASTERN NEW MEXICO MEDICAL CENTER (O, 149 beds) 405 West Country Club Road, Roswell, NM Zip 88201–5209; tel. 505/622–8170; ,
**Web address:** www.enmmc.com

LEA REGIONAL MEDICAL CENTER (O, 214 beds) 5419 North Lovington Highway, Hobbs, NM Zip 88240–9125, Mailing Address: P.O. Box 3000, Zip 88241–9501; tel. 575/492–5000; Timothy Thornell, FACHE, Chief Executive Officer
**Web address:** www.learegionalmedical.com

MIMBRES MEMORIAL HOSPITAL (O, 99 beds) 900 West Ash Street, Deming, NM Zip 88030–4098, Mailing Address: P.O. Box 710, Zip 88031–0710; tel. 575/546–2761; Steve Westenhofer, Chief Executive Officer
**Web address:** www.mimbresmemorial.com

MOUNTAINVIEW REGIONAL MEDICAL CENTER (O, 142 beds) 4311 East Lohman Avenue, Las Cruces, NM Zip 88011–8255; tel. 575/556–7600; Denten Park, Chief Executive Officer
**Web address:** www.mountainviewregional.com

**NORTH CAROLINA:** MARTIN GENERAL HOSPITAL (L, 49 beds) 310 South McCaskey Road, Williamston, NC Zip 27892–2150, Mailing Address: P.O. Box 1128, Zip 27892–1128; tel. 252/809–6179; Jodi Beauregard, Chief Executive Officer
**Web address:** www.martingeneral.com

**OHIO:** AFFINITY MEDICAL CENTER (O, 112 beds) 875 Eighth Street N.E., Massillon, OH Zip 44646–8503, Mailing Address: P.O. Box 805, Zip 44648–8503; tel. 330/832–8761; Ronald L. Bierman, Chief Executive Officer
**Web address:** www.affinitymedicalcenter.com

HILLSIDE REHABILITATION HOSPITAL (O, 65 beds) 8747 Squires Lane N.E., Warren, OH Zip 44484–1649; tel. 330/841–3700; Marilyn Titus, Vice President and Chief Operating Officer
**Web address:** www.valleycarehealth.net

NORTHSIDE MEDICAL CENTER (O, 373 beds) 500 Gypsy Lane, Youngstown, OH Zip 44501–0240; tel. 330/884–1000; David J. Fikse, Chief Executive Officer
**Web address:** www.valleycarehealth.net

TRUMBULL MEMORIAL HOSPITAL (O, 292 beds) 1350 East Market Street, Warren, OH Zip 44482–6628; tel. 330/841–9011; Robert G. Wolleben, Chief Executive Officer
**Web address:** www.valleycarehealth.net

**OKLAHOMA:** DEACONESS HOSPITAL (O, 273 beds) 5501 North Portland Avenue, Oklahoma City, OK Zip 73112–2099; tel. 405/604–6000; Cathryn A. Hibbs, FACHE, Chief Executive Officer
**Web address:** www.deaconessokc.com

PONCA CITY MEDICAL CENTER (O, 72 beds) 1900 North 14th Street, Ponca City, OK Zip 74601–2099; tel. 580/765–3321; R. Andrew Wachtel, FACHE, Chief Executive Officer
**Web address:** www.poncamedcenter.com

WOODWARD REGIONAL HOSPITAL (L, 44 beds) 900 17th Street, Woodward, OK Zip 73801–2448; tel. 580/256–5511; David T. Wallace, Chief Executive Officer
**Web address:** www.woodwardhospital.com

**OREGON:** MCKENZIE–WILLAMETTE MEDICAL CENTER (O, 113 beds) 1460 G Street, Springfield, OR Zip 97477–4197; tel. 541/726–4400; Maurine Cate, Chief Executive Officer
**Web address:** www.mckweb.com

**PENNSYLVANIA:** BERWICK HOSPITAL CENTER (O, 341 beds) 701 East 16th Street, Berwick, PA Zip 18603–2397; tel. 570/759–5000; Ronald R. Beer, Chief Executive Officer
**Web address:** www.berwick–hospital.com

BRANDYWINE HOSPITAL (O, 164 beds) 201 Reeceville Road, Coatesville, PA Zip 19320–1536; tel. 610/383–8000; Bryan Burklow, Chief Executive Officer
**Web address:** www.brandywinehospital.com

CHESTNUT HILL HOSPITAL (O, 135 beds) 8835 Germantown Avenue, Philadelphia, PA Zip 19118–2718; tel. 215/248–8200; John D. Cacciamani, Chief Executive Officer
**Web address:** www.chhealthsystem.com

EASTON HOSPITAL (O, 231 beds) 250 South 21st Street, Easton, PA Zip 18042–3892; tel. 610/250–4000; Brian Finestein, Chief Executive Officer
**Web address:** www.easton–hospital.com

FIRST HOSPITAL WYOMING VALLEY (O, 107 beds) 562 Wyoming Avenue, Wilkes–Barre, PA Zip 18704–3721; tel. 570/552–3900; Mark Schor, Chief Executive Officer
**Web address:** www.firsthospital.net/Pages/home.aspx

JENNERSVILLE REGIONAL HOSPITAL (O, 59 beds) 1015 West Baltimore Pike, West Grove, PA Zip 19390–9459; tel. 610/869–1000; Charles A. Davis, Chief Executive Officer
**Web address:** www.jennersville.com

LOCK HAVEN HOSPITAL (O, 59 beds) 24 Cree Drive, Lock Haven, PA Zip 17745–2699; tel. 570/893–5000; John A. Zidansek, Chief Executive Officer
**Web address:** www.lockhavenhospital.com

MEMORIAL HOSPITAL (O, 100 beds) 325 South Belmont Street, York, PA Zip 17403–2609, Mailing Address: P.O. Box 15118, Zip 17405–7118; tel. 717/843–8623; Sally J. Dixon, President and Chief Executive Officer
**Web address:** www.mhyork.org

MID–VALLEY HOSPITAL (O, 25 beds) 1400 Main Street, Peckville, PA Zip 18452–2009; tel. 570/383–5500; Ann Marie Stevens, Chief Executive Officer
**Web address:** www.mth.org

MOSES TAYLOR HOSPITAL (O, 217 beds) 700 Quincy Avenue, Scranton, PA Zip 18510–1724; tel. 570/340–2100; Justin Davis, Chief Executive Officer
**Web address:** www.mth.org

For explanation of codes following names, see page B2.
★ Indicates Type III membership in the American Hospital Association.

PHOENIXVILLE HOSPITAL (O, 118 beds) 140 Nutt Road, Phoenixville, PA Zip 19460–3900, Mailing Address: P.O. Box 3001, Zip 19460–0916; tel. 610/983–1000; Stephen M. Tullman, Chief Executive Officer
**Web address:** www.phoenixvillehospital.com

POTTSTOWN MEMORIAL MEDICAL CENTER (O, 234 beds) 1600 East High Street, Pottstown, PA Zip 19464–5093; tel. 610/327–7000; Sharif Omar, Chief Executive Officer
**Web address:** www.pottstownmemorial.com

REGIONAL HOSPITAL OF SCRANTON (O, 224 beds) 746 Jefferson Avenue, Scranton, PA Zip 18510–1624; tel. 570/348–7100; Brooks Turkel, Chief Executive Officer
**Web address:** www.regionalhospitalofscranton.net

SPECIAL CARE HOSPITAL (O, 64 beds) 128 West Washington Street, Nanticoke, PA Zip 18634–3113; tel. 570/735–5000; Robert D. Williams, Chief Executive Officer
**Web address:** www.specialcarehospital.net

SUNBURY COMMUNITY HOSPITAL (O, 76 beds) 350 North Eleventh Street, Sunbury, PA Zip 17801–1611; tel. 570/286–3333; Jeff Hunt, Chief Executive Officer
**Web address:** www.sunburyhospital.com

TYLER MEMORIAL HOSPITAL (O, 58 beds) 880 State Road 6 West, Tunkhannock, PA Zip 18657–6149; tel. 570/836–2161; Denise S. Gieski, MS, Chief Executive Officer
**Web address:** www.tylermemorialhospital.net

WILKES–BARRE GENERAL HOSPITAL (O, 372 beds) 575 North River Street, Wilkes–Barre, PA Zip 18764–0001; tel. 570/829–8111; Cornelio R. Catena, President and Chief Executive Officer
**Web address:** www.wvhc.org

**SOUTH CAROLINA:** CAROLINAS HOSPITAL SYSTEM (O, 436 beds) 805 Pamplico Highway, Florence, SC Zip 29505–6050, Mailing Address: P.O. Box 100550, Zip 29502–0550; tel. 843/674–5000; Darcy Craven, Interim President
**Web address:** www.carolinashospital.com

CHESTERFIELD GENERAL HOSPITAL (L, 59 beds) 711 Chesterfield Highway, Cheraw, SC Zip 29520; tel. 843/537–7881; Jeff Reece, Chief Executive Officer
**Web address:** www.chesterfieldgeneral.com

MARION REGIONAL HOSPITAL (O, 124 beds) 2829 East Highway 76, Mullins, SC Zip 29574–6035, Mailing Address: P.O. Drawer 1150, Marion, Zip 29571–1150; tel. 843/431–2000; David Cope, Chief Executive Officer
**Web address:** www.carolinashospitalmarion.com/Pages/Home.aspx

MARLBORO PARK HOSPITAL (L, 102 beds) 1138 Cheraw Highway, Bennettsville, SC Zip 29512–0738; tel. 843/479–2881; Ronnie Daves, Chief Executive Officer
**Web address:** www.marlboroparkhospital.com

MARY BLACK MEMORIAL HOSPITAL (O, 181 beds) 1700 Skylyn Drive, Spartanburg, SC Zip 29307–1061, Mailing Address: P.O. Box 3217, Zip 29304–3217; tel. 864/573–3000; Douglas J. Moyer, Chief Executive Officer
**Web address:** www.maryblack.org

SPRINGS MEMORIAL HOSPITAL (O, 186 beds) 800 West Meeting Street, Lancaster, SC Zip 29720–2298; tel. 803/286–1214; Douglas T. Arbour, Chief Executive Officer
**Web address:** www.springsmemorial.com

**TENNESSEE:** DYERSBURG REGIONAL MEDICAL CENTER (O, 110 beds) 400 East Tickle Street, Dyersburg, TN Zip 38024–3120; tel. 731/285–2410; Ben Youree, Interim Chief Executive Officer
**Web address:** www.dyersburgregionalmc.com

GATEWAY MEDICAL CENTER (O, 247 beds) 651 Dunlop Lane, Clarksville, TN Zip 37040–5015, Mailing Address: P.O. Box 31629, Zip 37040–0028; tel. 931/502–1000; Timothy Puthoff, Chief Executive Officer
**Web address:** www.ghsystem.com

HAYWOOD PARK COMMUNITY HOSPITAL (O, 36 beds) 2545 North Washington Avenue, Brownsville, TN Zip 38012–1610; tel. 731/772–4110; Jeremy Gray, Chief Executive Officer
**Web address:** www.haywoodparkcommunity.com

HENDERSON COUNTY COMMUNITY HOSPITAL (O, 36 beds) 200 West Church Street, Lexington, TN Zip 38351–2014; tel. 731/968–3646; Jack S. Buck, Chief Executive Officer
**Web address:** www.hendersoncchospital.com

HERITAGE MEDICAL CENTER (O, 70 beds) 2835 Highway 231 North, Shelbyville, TN Zip 37160–7327; tel. 931/685–5433; Daniel Buckner, Interim Chief Executive Officer
**Web address:** www.heritagemedicalcenter.com

LAKEWAY REGIONAL HOSPITAL (O, 135 beds) 726 McFarland Street, Morristown, TN Zip 37814–3990; tel. 423/586–2302; Priscilla Millis, Chief Executive Officer
**Web address:** www.lakewayregionalhospital.com

MCKENZIE REGIONAL HOSPITAL (O, 34 beds) 161 Hospital Drive, McKenzie, TN Zip 38201–1636; tel. 731/352–5344; Darrell Blaylock, Chief Executive Officer
**Web address:** www.mckenzieregionalhospital.com

MCNAIRY REGIONAL HOSPITAL (O, 45 beds) 705 East Poplar Avenue, Selmer, TN Zip 38375–1828; tel. 731/645–3221; Pamela W. Roberts, Chief Executive Officer
**Web address:** www.mcnairyregionalhospital.com

REGIONAL HOSPITAL OF JACKSON (O, 120 beds) 367 Hospital Boulevard, Jackson, TN Zip 38305–2080; tel. 731/661–2000; Stephen Grubbs, Chief Executive Officer
**Web address:** www.regionalhospitaljackson.com/Pages/Home.aspx

SKYRIDGE MEDICAL CENTER (O, 208 beds) 2305 Chambliss Avenue N.W., Cleveland, TN Zip 37311–3847, Mailing Address: P.O. Box 3060, Zip 37320–3060; tel. 423/559–6000; R. Coleman Foss, Chief Executive Officer
**Web address:** www.skyridgemedicalcenter.net

VOLUNTEER COMMUNITY HOSPITAL (O, 65 beds) 161 Mount Pelia Road, Martin, TN Zip 38237–3811; tel. 731/587–4261; Clyde Wood, Chief Executive Officer
**Web address:** www.volunteercommunityhospital.com

**TEXAS:** ABILENE REGIONAL MEDICAL CENTER (O, 205 beds) 6250 U.S. Highway 83, Abilene, TX Zip 79606–5299; tel. 325/428–1000; Michael D. Murphy, Chief Executive Officer
**Web address:** www.abileneregional.com

BIG BEND REGIONAL MEDICAL CENTER (O, 25 beds) 2600 Highway 118 North, Alpine, TX Zip 79830–2002; tel. 432/837–3447; Michael J. Ellis, Chief Executive Officer
**Web address:** www.bigbendhealthcare.com

BROWNWOOD REGIONAL MEDICAL CENTER (O, 168 beds) 1501 Burnet Drive, Brownwood, TX Zip 76801–5933, Mailing Address: P.O. Box 760, Zip 76804–0760; tel. 325/646–8541; Claude E. Camp, III, Chief Executive Officer
**Web address:** www.brmc–cares.com

CEDAR PARK REGIONAL MEDICAL CENTER (O, 77 beds) 1401 Medical Parkway, Cedar Park, TX Zip 78613–7763; tel. 512/528–7000; Tim P. Adams, FACHE, Chief Executive Officer
**Web address:** www.cedarparkregional.com

COLLEGE STATION MEDICAL CENTER (O, 166 beds) 1604 Rock Prairie Road, College Station, TX Zip 77845–8345, Mailing Address: P.O. Box 10000, Zip 77842–3500; tel. 979/764–5100; Thomas W. Jackson, Chief Executive Officer
**Web address:** www.csmedcenter.com

DETAR HEALTHCARE SYSTEM (O, 222 beds) 506 East San Antonio Street, Victoria, TX Zip 77901–6060, Mailing Address: P.O. Box 2089, Zip 77902–2089; tel. 361/575–7441; William R. Blanchard, Chief Executive Officer
**Web address:** www.detar.com

HILL REGIONAL HOSPITAL (O, 66 beds) 101 Circle Drive, Hillsboro, TX Zip 76645–2670; tel. 254/580–8500; Jan McClure, Chief Executive Officer
**Web address:** www.chs.net

LAKE GRANBURY MEDICAL CENTER (L, 83 beds) 1310 Paluxy Road, Granbury, TX Zip 76048–5655; tel. 817/573–2273; David Orcutt, Chief Executive Officer
**Web address:** www.lakegranburymedicalcenter.com

LAREDO MEDICAL CENTER (O, 326 beds) 1700 East Saunders Avenue, Laredo, TX Zip 78041–5401, Mailing Address: Drawer 2068, Zip 78044–2068; tel. 956/796–5000; Timothy E. Schmidt, Chief Executive Officer
**Web address:** www.laredomedical.com

For explanation of codes following names, see page B2.
★ Indicates Type III membership in the American Hospital Association.

LONGVIEW REGIONAL MEDICAL CENTER (O, 127 beds) 2901 North Fourth Street, Longview, TX Zip 75605–5191, Mailing Address: P.O. Box 14000, Zip 75607–4000; tel. 903/758–1818; Jim R. Kendrick, Chief Executive Officer
**Web address:** www.longviewregional.com

NAVARRO REGIONAL HOSPITAL (O, 148 beds) 3201 West State Highway 22, Corsicana, TX Zip 75110–2469; tel. 903/654–6800; Xavier Villarreal, Chief Executive Officer
**Web address:** www.navarrohospital.com

SAN ANGELO COMMUNITY MEDICAL CENTER (O, 131 beds) 3501 Knickerbocker Road, San Angelo, TX Zip 76904–7698; tel. 325/949–9511; America S. Farrell, FACHE, Interim Chief Executive Officer
**Web address:** www.sacmc.com

SCENIC MOUNTAIN MEDICAL CENTER (O, 75 beds) 1601 West 11th Place, Big Spring, TX Zip 79720–4198; tel. 432/263–1211; Larry Rodgers, Chief Executive Officer
**Web address:** www.smmccares.com

SOUTH TEXAS REGIONAL MEDICAL CENTER (O, 67 beds) 1905 Highway 97 East, Jourdanton, TX Zip 78026–1504; tel. 830/769–3515; James R. Resendez, Chief Executive Officer
**Web address:** www.strmc.com

TOMBALL REGIONAL MEDICAL CENTER (O, 289 beds) 605 Holderrieth Street, Tomball, TX Zip 77375–0889, Mailing Address: P.O. Box 889, Zip 77377–0889; tel. 281/401–7500; Bud Wethington, Chief Executive Officer
**Web address:** www.tomballregionalmedicalcenter.com

WEATHERFORD REGIONAL MEDICAL CENTER (O, 82 beds) 713 East Anderson Street, Weatherford, TX Zip 76086–9971; tel. 817/596–8751; Cory Countryman, Interim Chief Executive Officer
**Web address:** www.weatherfordregional.com

WOODLAND HEIGHTS MEDICAL CENTER (O, 115 beds) 505 South John Redditt Drive, Lufkin, TX Zip 75904–3157, Mailing Address: P.O. Box 150610, Zip 75915–0610; tel. 936/634–8311; Casey Robertson, Chief Executive Officer
**Web address:** www.woodlandheights.net

**UTAH:** MOUNTAIN WEST MEDICAL CENTER (O, 31 beds) 2055 North Main, Tooele, UT Zip 84074–2794; tel. 435/843–3600; Tim Moran, Interim Chief Executive Officer
**Web address:** www.mountainwestmc.com

**VIRGINIA:** SOUTHAMPTON MEMORIAL HOSPITAL (O, 72 beds) 100 Fairview Drive, Franklin, VA Zip 23851–1206, Mailing Address: P.O. Box 817, Zip 23851–0817; tel. 757/569–6100; Phil A. Wright, II, Chief Executive Officer
**Web address:** www.smhfranklin.com

SOUTHERN VIRGINIA REGIONAL MEDICAL CENTER (O, 80 beds) 727 North Main Street, Emporia, VA Zip 23847–1274; tel. 434/348–4400; Britton Phelps, Chief Executive Officer
**Web address:** www.svrmc.com

SOUTHSIDE REGIONAL MEDICAL CENTER (O, 300 beds) 200 Medical Park Boulevard, Petersburg, VA Zip 23805; tel. 804/765–5000; Michael Yungmann, Chief Executive Officer
**Web address:** www.srmconline.com

**WASHINGTON:** DEACONESS MEDICAL CENTER (O, 388 beds) 800 West Fifth Avenue, Spokane, WA Zip 99204–2803, Mailing Address: P.O. Box 248, Zip 99210–0248; tel. 509/458–5800; William L. Gilbert, Chief Executive Officer
**Web address:** www.deaconess–spokane.org

VALLEY HOSPITAL AND MEDICAL CENTER (O, 123 beds) 12606 East Mission Avenue, Spokane Valley, WA Zip 99216–1090; tel. 509/924–6650; Dennis Barts, Chief Executive Officer
**Web address:** www.valleyhospital.org

**WEST VIRGINIA:** BLUEFIELD REGIONAL MEDICAL CENTER (O, 240 beds) 500 Cherry Street, Bluefield, WV Zip 24701–3390; tel. 304/327–1100; William Hawley, Chief Executive Officer
**Web address:** www.bluefield.org

GREENBRIER VALLEY MEDICAL CENTER (O, 113 beds) 202 Maplewood Avenue, Ronceverte, WV Zip 24970–0497, Mailing Address: P.O. Box 497, Zip 24970–0497; tel. 304/647–4411; Paul Storey, Chief Executive Officer
**Web address:** www.gvmc.com

PLATEAU MEDICAL CENTER (O, 25 beds) 430 Main Street, Oak Hill, WV Zip 25901–3455; tel. 304/469–8600; Chad Hatfield, Chief Executive Officer
**Web address:** www.plateaumedicalcenter.com

**WYOMING:** EVANSTON REGIONAL HOSPITAL (O, 42 beds) 190 Arrowhead Drive, Evanston, WY Zip 82930–9266; tel. 307/789–3636; George Winn, Chief Executive Officer
**Web address:** www.evanstonregionalhospital.com

| | | |
|---|---|---|
| Owned, leased, sponsored: | 132 hospitals | 17730 beds |
| Contract–managed: | 0 hospitals | 0 beds |
| Totals: | 132 hospitals | 17730 beds |

**0249: COMMUNITY HEALTHCARE SYSTEM** (NP)
901 MacArthur Boulevard, Hammond, IN Zip 46321–2959; tel. 219/836–1600; Donald Powers, Chairman, President and Chief Executive Officer
**(Independent Hospital System)**

**INDIANA:** COMMUNITY HOSPITAL (O, 449 beds) 901 MacArthur Boulevard, Munster, IN Zip 46321–2959; tel. 219/836–1600; Donald P. Fesko, Chief Executive Officer and Administrator
**Web address:** www.comhs.org

ST. CATHERINE HOSPITAL (O, 189 beds) 4321 Fir Street, East Chicago, IN Zip 46312–3097; tel. 219/392–1700; JoAnn Birdzell, Chief Executive Officer and Administrator
**Web address:** www.stcatherinehospital.org

ST. MARY MEDICAL CENTER (O, 190 beds) 1500 South Lake Park Avenue, Hobart, IN Zip 46342–6699; tel. 219/942–0551; Janice L. Ryba, JD, Chief Executive Officer
**Web address:** www.comhs.org

| | | |
|---|---|---|
| Owned, leased, sponsored: | 3 hospitals | 828 beds |
| Contract–managed: | 0 hospitals | 0 beds |
| Totals: | 3 hospitals | 828 beds |

**★0384: COMMUNITY HOSPITAL CORPORATION** (NP)
5801 Tennyson Parkway, Suite 550, Plano, TX Zip 75024; tel. 972/943–6400; Michael D. Williams, President and Chief Executive Officer
**(Independent Hospital System)**

**NEW MEXICO:** ARTESIA GENERAL HOSPITAL (L, 43 beds) 702 North 13th Street, Artesia, NM Zip 88210–1199; tel. 575/748–3333; Kenneth W. Randall, Chief Executive Officer
**Web address:** www.artesiageneral.com

**TEXAS:** BAPTIST HOSPITALS OF SOUTHEAST TEXAS (O, 394 beds) 3080 College Street, Beaumont, TX Zip 77701–4689, Mailing Address: P.O. Box 1591, Zip 77704–1591; tel. 409/212–5000; David N. Parmer, President and Chief Executive Officer
**Web address:** www.mhbh.org

BAPTIST ORANGE HOSPITAL (O, 40 beds) 608 Strickland Drive, Orange, TX Zip 77630–4717; tel. 409/883–9361; Jarren Garrett, Chief Administrative Officer
**Web address:** www.baptistorangehospital.org

ST. MARK'S MEDICAL CENTER (O, 48 beds) One St. Mark's Place, La Grange, TX Zip 78945; tel. 979/242–2200; Nathan Staggs, President and Chief Executive Officer
**Web address:** www.smmctx.org

YOAKUM COMMUNITY HOSPITAL (L, 25 beds) 1200 Carl Ramert Drive, Yoakum, TX Zip 77995–4198, Mailing Address: P.O. Box 753, Zip 77995–0753; tel. 361/293–2321; Karen Barber, Chief Executive Officer
**Web address:** www.yoakumhospital.com

| | | |
|---|---|---|
| Owned, leased, sponsored: | 5 hospitals | 550 beds |
| Contract–managed: | 0 hospitals | 0 beds |
| Totals: | 5 hospitals | 550 beds |

**1085: COMMUNITY MEDICAL CENTERS** (NP)
Fresno and Maddy Drive, Fresno, CA Zip 93721, Mailing Address: P.O. Box 1232, Zip 93715–1232; tel. 559/459–6000; Tim A. Joslin, President and Chief Executive Officer
**(Moderately Centralized Health System)**

For explanation of codes following names, see page B2.
★ Indicates Type III membership in the American Hospital Association.

**CALIFORNIA:** CLOVIS COMMUNITY MEDICAL CENTER (O, 109 beds) 2755 Herndon Avenue, Clovis, CA Zip 93611–6800; tel. 559/324–4000; Craig Castro, Chief Executive Officer
**Web address:** www.communitymedical.org

COMMUNITY BEHAVIORAL HEALTH CENTER (O, 60 beds) 7171 North Cedar Avenue, Fresno, CA Zip 93720–3311; tel. 559/449–8000; Dawan Utecht, Chief Executive Officer
**Web address:** www.communitymedical.org

COMMUNITY REGIONAL MEDICAL CENTER (O, 677 beds) 2823 Fresno Street, Fresno, CA Zip 93721–1324; tel. 559/459–6000; John M. Chubb, Chief Executive Officer
**Web address:** www.communitymedical.org

| Owned, leased, sponsored: | 3 hospitals | 846 beds |
|---|---|---|
| Contract–managed: | 0 hospitals | 0 beds |
| Totals: | 3 hospitals | 846 beds |

**0339: CONEMAUGH HEALTH SYSTEM** (NP)
1086 Franklin Street, Johnstown, PA Zip 15905–4398; tel. 814/534–9000; Scott A. Becker, President and Chief Executive Officer
**(Centralized Physician/Insurance Health System)**

**PENNSYLVANIA:** MEMORIAL MEDICAL CENTER (O, 525 beds) 1086 Franklin Street, Johnstown, PA Zip 15905–4398; tel. 814/534–9000; Steven E. Tucker, President and Chief Operating Officer
**Web address:** www.conemaugh.org

MEYERSDALE MEDICAL CENTER (O, 20 beds) 200 Hospital Drive, Meyersdale, PA Zip 15552–1249; tel. 814/634–5911; Mary L. Libengood, President
**Web address:** www.conemaugh.org

MINERS MEDICAL CENTER (O, 30 beds) 290 Haida Avenue, Hastings, PA Zip 16646, Mailing Address: P.O. Box 689, Zip 16646–0689; tel. 814/247–3100; William R. Crowe, President
**Web address:** www.minersmedicalcenter.org

| Owned, leased, sponsored: | 3 hospitals | 575 beds |
|---|---|---|
| Contract–managed: | 0 hospitals | 0 beds |
| Totals: | 3 hospitals | 575 beds |

**0014: CONNECTICUT DEPARTMENT OF MENTAL HEALTH AND ADDICTION SERVICES** (NP)
410 Capitol Avenue, Hartford, CT Zip 06106, Mailing Address: P.O. Box 341431, Zip 06134–1431; tel. 860/418–7000; Patricia Rehmer, Commissioner
**(Independent Hospital System)**

**CONNECTICUT:** CONNECTICUT MENTAL HEALTH CENTER (O, 39 beds) 34 Park Street, New Haven, CT Zip 06508–1842, Mailing Address: P.O. Box 1842, Zip 06508–1842; tel. 203/974–7144; Michael Sernyak, M.D., Director
**Web address:** www.dmhas.state.ct.us/lmha.htm

CONNECTICUT VALLEY HOSPITAL (O, 537 beds) Eastern Drive, Middletown, CT Zip 06457–3947, Mailing Address: PO BOX 351, Zip 06457–7023; tel. 860/262–5000; Helene M. Vartelas, Acting Chief Executive Officer

SOUTHWEST CONNECTICUT MENTAL HEALTH SYSTEM (O, 62 beds) 97 Middle Street, Bridgeport, CT Zip 06604; tel. 203/551–7400; James M. Pisciotta, Chief Executive Officer
**Web address:** www.ct.gov/dmhas/cwp/view.asp?a=2946&q=378936

| Owned, leased, sponsored: | 3 hospitals | 638 beds |
|---|---|---|
| Contract–managed: | 0 hospitals | 0 beds |
| Totals: | 3 hospitals | 638 beds |

**★0127: CONTINUUM HEALTH PARTNERS** (NP)
555 West 57th Street, New York, NY Zip 10019; tel. 212/523–8130; Stanley Brezenoff, President and Chief Executive Officer
**(Moderately Centralized Health System)**

**NEW YORK:** BETH ISRAEL MEDICAL CENTER (O, 840 beds) First Avenue and 16th Street, New York, NY Zip 10003–3803; tel. 212/420–2000; Harris M. Nagler, M.D., President
**Web address:** www.bethisraelny.org

NEW YORK EYE AND EAR INFIRMARY (O, 32 beds) 310 East 14th Street, New York, NY Zip 10003–4201; tel. 212/979–4000; D. McWilliams Kessler, President and Chief Executive Officer
**Web address:** www.nyee.edu

ST. LUKE'S–ROOSEVELT HOSPITAL CENTER (O, 711 beds) 1111 Amsterdam Avenue, New York, NY Zip 10025–1716; tel. 212/523–4000; Frank J. Cracolici, President
**Web address:** www.slrhc.org

| Owned, leased, sponsored: | 3 hospitals | 1583 beds |
|---|---|---|
| Contract–managed: | 0 hospitals | 0 beds |
| Totals: | 3 hospitals | 1583 beds |

**0016: COOK COUNTY BUREAU OF HEALTH SERVICES** (NP)
1900 West Polk Street, Suite 200, Chicago, IL Zip 60612; tel. 312/864–6820; Ramanathan Raju, M.D., Chief Executive Officer
**(Independent Hospital System)**

**ILLINOIS:** JOHN H. STROGER JR. HOSPITAL OF COOK COUNTY (O, 460 beds) 1901 West Harrison Street, Chicago, IL Zip 60612–3785; tel. 312/864–6000; Carol L. Schneider, Chief Operating Officer
**Web address:** www.cookcountyhealth.net

OAK FOREST HEALTH CENTER OF COOK COUNTY (O, 95 beds) 15900 South Cicero Avenue, Oak Forest, IL Zip 60452–4006; tel. 708/687–7200; Sylvia Edwards, Chief Operating Officer

PROVIDENT HOSPITAL OF COOK COUNTY (O, 25 beds) 500 East 51st Street, Chicago, IL Zip 60615–2494; tel. 312/572–2000; Robert Hamilton, Chief Operating Officer
**Web address:** www.ccbhs.org/pages/ProvidentHospitalofCookCounty.htm

| Owned, leased, sponsored: | 3 hospitals | 580 beds |
|---|---|---|
| Contract–managed: | 0 hospitals | 0 beds |
| Totals: | 3 hospitals | 580 beds |

**0905: CORNERSTONE HEALTHCARE GROUP** (IO)
2200 Ross Avenue, suite 3060, Dallas, TX Zip 75201–2708; tel. 469/621–6700; Harrison Price, Interim President and Chief Executive Officer
**(Independent Hospital System)**

**ARIZONA:** CORNERSTONE HOSPITAL OF SOUTHEAST ARIZONA (O, 54 beds) 7220 East Rosewood Drive, Tucson, AZ Zip 85710; tel. 520/546–4595; Mindy S. Moore, Chief Executive Officer
**Web address:** www.chghospitals.com

**LOUISIANA:** CORNERSTONE HOSPITAL OF BOSSIER CITY (O, 54 beds) 4900 Medical Drive, Bossier City, LA Zip 71112–4596; tel. 318/747–9500; Sheri Burnette, R.N., Chief Executive Officer and Administrator
**Web address:** www.chghospitals.com/

CORNERSTONE HOSPITAL OF SOUTHWEST LOUISIANA (O, 30 beds) 703 Cypress Street, Sulphur, LA Zip 70663; tel. 337/527–1102; Robert R. Lafleur, Chief Executive Officer
**Web address:** www.cornerstonehealthcaregroup.com

CORNERSTONE HOSPITAL–WEST MONROE (O, 40 beds) 6198 Cypress Street, West Monroe, LA Zip 71291–9010; tel. 318/396–5600; Chris Simpson, Chief Executive Officer
**Web address:** www.cornerstonehealthcaregroup.com

**TEXAS:** CORNERSTONE HOSPITAL OF AUSTIN (O, 128 beds) 4207 Burnet Road, Austin, TX Zip 78756–3396; tel. 512/706–1900; Michael Hutka, Interim Chief Executive Officer
**Web address:** www.chghospitals.com/cha.html

CORNERSTONE HOSPITAL OF HOUSTON – BELLAIRE (O, 130 beds) 5314 Dashwood, Houston, TX Zip 77081; tel. 713/295–5300; James Camp, R.N., Chief Executive Officer
**Web address:** www.chghospitals.com

CORNERSTONE HOSPITAL OF SOUTH HOUSTON (O, 30 beds) 1919 Labranch 7GWS Street, Houston, TX Zip 77002; tel. 713/756–8660; Sharon Stuart, R.N., Chief Executive Officer
**Web address:** www.chghospitals.com

For explanation of codes following names, see page B2.
★ Indicates Type III membership in the American Hospital Association.

Section B

SOLARA HOSPITAL HARLINGEN–BROWNSVILLE CAMPUS (O, 41 beds) 333 Lorenaly Drive, Brownsville, TX Zip 78526; tel. 956/546–0808; Paul E. Qualls, Jr., Chief Executive Officer
**Web address:** www.solarahc.com/shcbr.html

**WEST VIRGINIA:** CORNERSTONE HOSPITAL OF HUNTINGTON (O, 28 beds) 2900 First Avenue, Two East, Huntington, WV Zip 25702; tel. 304/399–2600; Cynthia Isaacs, Chief Executive Officer
**Web address:** www.chghospitals.com

| | | |
|---|---|---|
| **Owned, leased, sponsored:** | 9 hospitals | 535 beds |
| **Contract–managed:** | 0 hospitals | 0 beds |
| **Totals:** | 9 hospitals | 535 beds |

---

**★0103: COTTAGE HEALTH SYSTEM** (NP)
Pueblo at Bath Streets, Santa Barbara, CA Zip 93105, Mailing Address: P.O. Box 689, Zip 93102–0689; tel. 805/569–7290; Ronald C. Werft, President and Chief Executive Officer
**(Independent Hospital System)**

**CALIFORNIA:** GOLETA VALLEY COTTAGE HOSPITAL (O, 78 beds) 351 South Patterson Avenue, Santa Barbara, CA Zip 93111–2496, Mailing Address: Box 6306, Zip 93160–6306; tel. 805/967–3411; Ronald C. Werft, President and Chief Executive Officer
**Web address:** www.sbch.org

SANTA BARBARA COTTAGE HOSPITAL (O, 345 beds) 400 West Pueblo Street, Santa Barbara, CA Zip 93105–4390, Mailing Address: P.O. Box 689, Zip 93102–0689; tel. 805/682–7111; Ronald C. Werft, President and Chief Executive Officer
**Web address:** www.cottagehealthsystem.org

SANTA YNEZ VALLEY COTTAGE HOSPITAL (O, 10 beds) 2050 Viborg Road, Solvang, CA Zip 93463–2295; tel. 805/688–6431; Ronald C. Werft, President and Chief Executive Officer
**Web address:** www.cottagehealthsystem.org

| | | |
|---|---|---|
| **Owned, leased, sponsored:** | 3 hospitals | 433 beds |
| **Contract–managed:** | 0 hospitals | 0 beds |
| **Totals:** | 3 hospitals | 433 beds |

---

**★0123: COVENANT HEALTH** (NP)
100 Fort Sanders West Boulevard, Knoxville, TN Zip 37922; tel. 865/531–5555; Anthony Spezia, President and Chief Executive Officer
**(Centralized Health System)**

**TENNESSEE:** FORT LOUDOUN MEDICAL CENTER (L, 40 beds) 550 Fort Loudoun Medical Center Drive, Lenoir City, TN Zip 37772–5673; tel. 865/271–6000; Jeffrey Feike, President and Chief Administrative Officer
**Web address:** www.covenanthealth.com

FORT SANDERS REGIONAL MEDICAL CENTER (O, 402 beds) 1901 West Clinch Avenue, Knoxville, TN Zip 37916–2307; tel. 865/541–1111; Keith Altshuler, President and Chief Administrative Officer
**Web address:** www.covenanthealth.com

LECONTE MEDICAL CENTER (O, 123 beds) 742 Middle Creek Road, Sevierville, TN Zip 37862–5019, Mailing Address: P.O. Box 8005, Zip 37864–8005; tel. 865/446–7000; Ellen Wilhoit, President and Chief Administrative Officer
**Web address:** www.lecontemedicalcenter.com

METHODIST MEDICAL CENTER OF OAK RIDGE (O, 255 beds) 990 Oak Ridge Turnpike, Oak Ridge, TN Zip 37830–6976, Mailing Address: P.O. Box 2529, Zip 37831–2529; tel. 865/835–1000; Michael Belbeck, President and Chief Administrative Officer
**Web address:** www.mmcoakridge.com

MORRISTOWN–HAMBLEN HEALTHCARE SYSTEM (O, 143 beds) 908 West Fourth Street North, Morristown, TN Zip 37814–3894, Mailing Address: P.O. Box 1178, Zip 37816–1178; tel. 423/586–4231; Gordon Lintz, Chief Administrative Officer
**Web address:** www.mhhs1.org

PARKWEST MEDICAL CENTER (O, 297 beds) 9352 Park West Boulevard, Knoxville, TN Zip 37923–4325, Mailing Address: P.O. Box 22993, Zip 37933–0993; tel. 865/373–1000; Rick Lassiter, President and Chief Administrative Officer
**Web address:** www.yesparkwest.com

ROANE MEDICAL CENTER (O, 36 beds) 412 Devonia Street, Harriman, TN Zip 37748–0489, Mailing Address: P.O. Box 489, Zip 37748–0489; tel. 865/882–1323; Gaye Jolly, Chief Executive Officer
**Web address:** www.roanemedical.com

| | | |
|---|---|---|
| **Owned, leased, sponsored:** | 7 hospitals | 1296 beds |
| **Contract–managed:** | 0 hospitals | 0 beds |
| **Totals:** | 7 hospitals | 1296 beds |

---

**★0036: COVENANT HEALTH SYSTEM** (NP)
3615 19th Street, Lubbock, TX Zip 79410–1201; tel. 806/725–0447; Richard H. Parks, FACHE, President and Chief Executive Officer
**(Centralized Health System)**

**TEXAS:** COVENANT CHILDREN'S HOSPITAL (O, 73 beds) 4000 24th Street, Lubbock, TX Zip 79410–1218; tel. 806/725–1011; Christopher J. Dougherty, Chief Executive Officer
**Web address:** www.covenanthealth.org

COVENANT HOSPITAL PLAINVIEW (L, 68 beds) 2601 Dimmitt Road, Plainview, TX Zip 79072–1833; tel. 806/296–5531; Alan N. King, FACHE, President and Chief Executive Officer
**Web address:** www.covenantplainview.org

COVENANT HOSPITAL–LEVELLAND (L, 22 beds) 1900 South College Avenue, Levelland, TX Zip 79336–6508; tel. 806/894–4963; Jerry Osburn, Administrator
**Web address:** www.covenanthealth.org

COVENANT MEDICAL CENTER (O, 607 beds) 3615 19th Street, Lubbock, TX Zip 79410–1201, Mailing Address: P.O. Box 1201, Zip 79408–1201; tel. 806/725–0000; Richard H. Parks, FACHE, President and Chief Executive Officer
**Web address:** www.covenanthealth.org

COVENANT SPECIALTY HOSPITAL (O, 56 beds) 3815 20th Street, Lubbock, TX Zip 79410; tel. 806/725–9200; Walt Cathey, Administrator
**Web address:** www.covenanthealth.org/view/Facilities/Specialty_Hospital

| | | |
|---|---|---|
| **Owned, leased, sponsored:** | 5 hospitals | 826 beds |
| **Contract–managed:** | 0 hospitals | 0 beds |
| **Totals:** | 5 hospitals | 826 beds |

---

**★5885: COVENANT HEALTH SYSTEMS, INC.** (CC)
100 Ames Pond Drive, Suite 102, Tewksbury, MA Zip 01876–1293; tel. 978/654–6363; David R. Lincoln, President and Chief Executive Officer
**(Moderately Centralized Health System)**

**MAINE:** ST. JOSEPH HOSPITAL (O, 84 beds) 360 Broadway, Bangor, ME Zip 04401–3897, Mailing Address: P.O. Box 403, Zip 04402–0403; tel. 207/262–1000; Mary Prybylo, President and Chief Executive Officer
**Web address:** www.sjhhealth.com

ST. MARY'S REGIONAL MEDICAL CENTER (O, 171 beds) 330 Sabattus Street, Lewiston, ME Zip 04240, Mailing Address: P.O. Box 291, Zip 04243–0291; tel. 207/777–8100; Lee T. Myles, Chief Executive Officer
**Web address:** www.stmarysmaine.com

**NEW HAMPSHIRE:** ST. JOSEPH HOSPITAL (O, 144 beds) 172 Kinsley Street, Nashua, NH Zip 03061–2013; tel. 603/882–3000; David Ross, President and Chief Executive Officer
**Web address:** www.stjosephhospital.com

| | | |
|---|---|---|
| **Owned, leased, sponsored:** | 3 hospitals | 399 beds |
| **Contract–managed:** | 0 hospitals | 0 beds |
| **Totals:** | 3 hospitals | 399 beds |

---

For explanation of codes following names, see page B2.
★ Indicates Type III membership in the American Hospital Association.

**0179: COXHEALTH** (NP)
1423 North Jefferson Avenue, Springfield, MO Zip 65802–1988;
tel. 417/269–3108; Steven D. Edwards, President and Chief
Executive Officer
**(Centralized Physician/Insurance Health System)**

**MISSOURI:** COX MONETT (O, 25 beds) 801 North Lincoln Avenue, Monett,
MO Zip 65708–1641; tel. 417/235–3144; Genice Maroc, FACHE,
Administrator and Chief Executive Officer
**Web address:** www.coxhealth.com

LESTER E. COX MEDICAL CENTERS (O, 646 beds) 1423 North Jefferson
Street, Springfield, MO Zip 65802–1988; tel. 417/269–3000; Steven D.
Edwards, President and Chief Executive Officer
**Web address:** www.coxhealth.com

| | | |
|---|---|---|
| Owned, leased, sponsored: | 2 hospitals | 671 beds |
| Contract–managed: | 0 hospitals | 0 beds |
| Totals: | 2 hospitals | 671 beds |

★**0008: CROZER–KEYSTONE HEALTH SYSTEM** (NP)
100 West Sproul Road, Springfield, PA Zip 19064;
tel. 610/338–8205; Joan K. Richards, President and Chief Executive
Officer
**(Moderately Centralized Health System)**

**PENNSYLVANIA:** CROZER–CHESTER MEDICAL CENTER (O, 507 beds) One
Medical Center Boulevard, Upland, PA Zip 19013–3995;
tel. 610/447–2000; Patrick Gavin, President
**Web address:** www.crozer.org

DELAWARE COUNTY MEMORIAL HOSPITAL (O, 213 beds) 501 North
Lansdowne Avenue, Drexel Hill, PA Zip 19026–1114; tel. 610/284–8100;
William McCune, President
**Web address:** www.crozer.org

| | | |
|---|---|---|
| Owned, leased, sponsored: | 2 hospitals | 720 beds |
| Contract–managed: | 0 hospitals | 0 beds |
| Totals: | 2 hospitals | 720 beds |

●**0334: CYPRESS HEALTH SYSTEMS** (IO)
106 Preston Day Circle, Benton, LA Zip 71006; tel. 318/965–9914;
Kim B. Bird, President and Chief Executive Officer
**(Independent Hospital System)**

**MONTANA:** POWELL COUNTY MEDICAL CENTER (C, 16 beds) 1101 Texas
Avenue, Deer Lodge, MT Zip 59722–1828; tel. 406/846–2212; Alan Bird,
Chief Executive Officer
**Web address:** www.pcmh.org

| | | |
|---|---|---|
| Owned, leased, sponsored: | 0 hospitals | 0 beds |
| Contract–managed: | 1 hospital | 16 beds |
| Totals: | 1 hospital | 16 beds |

★**1075: DAUGHTERS OF CHARITY HEALTH SYSTEM** (CC)
26000 Altamont Road, Los Altos Hills, CA Zip 94022;
tel. 650/917–4500; Robert Issai, President and Chief Executive
Officer
**(Moderately Centralized Health System)**

**CALIFORNIA:** O'CONNOR HOSPITAL (O, 202 beds) 2105 Forest Avenue, San
Jose, CA Zip 95128–1471; tel. 408/947–2500; James F. Dover, FACHE,
President and Chief Executive Officer
**Web address:** www.oconnorhospital.org

SAINT LOUISE REGIONAL HOSPITAL (O, 93 beds) 9400 No Name Uno, Gilroy,
CA Zip 95020–3528; tel. 408/848–2000; Joanne E. Allen, President and
Chief Executive Officer
**Web address:** www.dochs.org

SETON MEDICAL CENTER (O, 429 beds) 1900 Sullivan Avenue, Daly City, CA
Zip 94015–2229; tel. 650/992–4000; Lorraine P. Auerbach, President and
Chief Executive Officer
**Web address:** www.setonmedicalcenter.org

SETON MEDICAL CENTER COASTSIDE (O, 116 beds) 600 Marine Boulevard,
Moss Beach, CA Zip 94038–9641; tel. 650/563–7100; Lorraine P.
Auerbach, President and Chief Executive Officer

ST. FRANCIS MEDICAL CENTER (O, 323 beds) 3630 East Imperial Highway,
Lynwood, CA Zip 90262–2636; tel. 310/900–8900; Gerald T. Kozai,
President
**Web address:** www.dochs.org

ST. VINCENT MEDICAL CENTER (O, 271 beds) 2131 West Third Street, Los
Angeles, CA Zip 90057–7992, Mailing Address: P.O. Box 57992,
Zip 90057–7992; tel. 213/484–7111; Catherine Fickes, R.N., President and
Chief Executive Officer
**Web address:** www.stvincentmedicalcenter.com

| | | |
|---|---|---|
| Owned, leased, sponsored: | 6 hospitals | 1434 beds |
| Contract–managed: | 0 hospitals | 0 beds |
| Totals: | 6 hospitals | 1434 beds |

★**0864: DAVIS HEALTH SYSTEM** (NP)
Reed Street and Gorman Avenue, Elkins, WV Zip 26241, Mailing
Address: P.O. Box 1697, Zip 26241–1697; tel. 304/636–3300;
Mark Doak, President and Chief Executive Officer

**WEST VIRGINIA:** BROADDUS HOSPITAL (O, 72 beds) 1 Healthcare Drive,
Philippi, WV Zip 26416–1051, Mailing Address: P.O. Box 930,
Zip 26416–1051; tel. 304/457–1760; Jeffrey A. Powelson, Chief
Executive Officer
**Web address:** www.davishealthsystem.org/

DAVIS MEMORIAL HOSPITAL (O, 90 beds) Gorman Avenue and Reed Street,
Elkins, WV Zip 26241, Mailing Address: P.O. Box 1484, Zip 26241–1484;
tel. 304/636–3300; Mark Doak, President and Chief Executive Officer
**Web address:** www.davishealthsystem.com

| | | |
|---|---|---|
| Owned, leased, sponsored: | 2 hospitals | 162 beds |
| Contract–managed: | 0 hospitals | 0 beds |
| Totals: | 2 hospitals | 162 beds |

**1825: DCH HEALTH SYSTEM** (NP)
809 University Boulevard East, Tuscaloosa, AL Zip 35401;
tel. 205/759–7111; Bryan N. Kindred, FACHE, President and Chief
Executive Officer
**(Moderately Centralized Health System)**

**ALABAMA:** DCH REGIONAL MEDICAL CENTER (O, 405 beds) 809 University
Boulevard East, Tuscaloosa, AL Zip 35401–9961; tel. 205/759–7111;
William H. Cassels, Administrator
**Web address:** www.dchsystem.com

FAYETTE MEDICAL CENTER (L, 167 beds) 1653 Temple Avenue North,
Fayette, AL Zip 35555–1314, Mailing Address: P.O. Drawer 710,
Zip 35555–0710; tel. 205/932–5966; Barry S. Cochran, FACHE,
Administrator
**Web address:** www.dchsystem.com

NORTHPORT MEDICAL CENTER (O, 196 beds) 2700 Hospital Drive,
Northport, AL Zip 35476; tel. 205/333–4500; Luke Standeffer, Administrator
**Web address:** www.dchsystem.com

| | | |
|---|---|---|
| Owned, leased, sponsored: | 3 hospitals | 768 beds |
| Contract–managed: | 0 hospitals | 0 beds |
| Totals: | 3 hospitals | 768 beds |

★**0313: DEACONESS HEALTH SYSTEM** (NP)
600 Mary Street, Evansville, IN Zip 47747; tel. 812/450–5000;
Linda E. White, President and Chief Executive Officer
**(Centralized Health System)**

**INDIANA:** DEACONESS HOSPITAL (O, 541 beds) 600 Mary Street, Evansville,
IN Zip 47747–0001; tel. 812/450–5000; Shawn W. McCoy, Chief
Administrative Officer
**Web address:** www.deaconess.com

THE WOMEN'S HOSPITAL (O, 74 beds) 4199 Gateway Boulevard, Newburgh,
IN Zip 47630; tel. 812/842–4200; Christina M. Ryan, R.N., Chief Executive
Officer
**Web address:** www.deaconess.com

For explanation of codes following names, see page B2.
★ Indicates Type III membership in the American Hospital Association.
● Single hospital health care system

**B40** Health Care Systems, Networks and Alliances

© 2012 AHA Guide

| Owned, leased, sponsored: | 2 hospitals | 615 beds |
|---|---|---|
| Contract–managed: | 0 hospitals | 0 beds |
| Totals: | 2 hospitals | 615 beds |

| Owned, leased, sponsored: | 9 hospitals | 478 beds |
|---|---|---|
| Contract–managed: | 0 hospitals | 0 beds |
| Totals: | 9 hospitals | 478 beds |

**0330: DEKALB REGIONAL HEALTH SYSTEM** (NP)
2701 North Decatur Road, Decatur, GA Zip 30033;
tel. 404/501–1000; John Shelton, President and Chief Executive Officer
**(Independent Hospital System)**

**GEORGIA:** DEKALB MEDICAL AT DOWNTOWN DECATUR (O, 44 beds) 450 North Candler Street, Decatur, GA Zip 30030–2671; tel. 404/501–6700; John Shelton, President and Chief Executive Officer
**Web address:** www.dekalbmedicalcenter.org

DEKALB MEDICAL AT HILLANDALE (O, 100 beds) 2801 DeKalb Medical Parkway, Lithonia, GA Zip 30058; tel. 404/501–8700; John Shelton, President and Chief Executive Officer
**Web address:** www.dekalbmedical.org

DEKALB MEDICAL AT NORTH DECATUR (O, 436 beds) 2701 North Decatur Road, Decatur, GA Zip 30033–5995; tel. 404/501–1000; John Shelton, President and Chief Executive Officer
**Web address:** www.dekalbmedical.org

| Owned, leased, sponsored: | 3 hospitals | 580 beds |
|---|---|---|
| Contract–managed: | 0 hospitals | 0 beds |
| Totals: | 3 hospitals | 580 beds |

**9495: DEPARTMENT OF THE AIR FORCE** (FG)
1420 Pentagon, Room 4E1084, Washington, DC Zip 20330–1420;
tel. 202/767–4765; Lieutenant General Charles B. Green, M.D., Surgeon General
**(Independent Hospital System)**

**ALASKA:** U. S. AIR FORCE REGIONAL HOSPITAL (O, 64 beds) 5955 Zeamer Avenue, Elmendorf AFB, AK Zip 99506–3700; tel. 907/580–3006; Colonel Thomas Harrell, Commander
**Web address:** www.elmendorf.af.mil/

**CALIFORNIA:** DAVID GRANT MEDICAL CENTER (O, 110 beds) 101 Bodin Circle, Travis AFB, CA Zip 94535–1800; tel. 707/423–7300; Colonel Brian T. Hayes, Commander
**Web address:** www.travis.af.mil/units/dgmc/index.asp

**FLORIDA:** U. S. AIR FORCE REGIONAL HOSPITAL (O, 57 beds) 307 Boatner Road, Suite 114, Eglin AFB, FL Zip 32542–1282; tel. 850/883–8221; Colonel Gary Walker, Commander
**Web address:** www.eglin.af.mil

**IDAHO:** U. S. AIR FORCE CLINIC (O, 10 beds) 90 Hope Drive, Building 600, Mountain Home AFB, ID Zip 83648–5300; tel. 208/828–7610; Lieutenant Colonel Gregory W. Carson, Administrator

**ILLINOIS:** SCOTT MEDICAL CENTER (O, 18 beds) 310 West Losey Street, Scott AFB, IL Zip 62225–5252; tel. 618/256–7456; Colonel Bret D. Burton, Commander

**MISSISSIPPI:** U. S. AIR FORCE MEDICAL CENTER KEESLER (O, 56 beds) 301 Fisher Street, Room 1A132, Keesler AFB, MS Zip 39534–2519; tel. 228/376–2550; Colonel Robert Cothron, USAF, MSC, Administrator
**Web address:** www.keesler.af.mil

**NEVADA:** MIKE O'CALLAGHAN FEDERAL HOSPITAL (O, 46 beds) 4700 Las Vegas Boulevard North, Suite 2419, Nellis AFB, NV Zip 89191–6601; tel. 702/653–2000; Colonel Christian Benjamin, USAF, MC, Commander
**Web address:** www.lasvegas.va.gov/

**OHIO:** WRIGHT PATTERSON MEDICAL CENTER (O, 52 beds) 4881 Sugar Maple Drive, Wright–Patterson AFB, OH Zip 45433–5529; tel. 937/257–9144; Brent Erickson, Administrator
**Web address:** www.wpafb.af.mil/units/wpmc/

**VIRGINIA:** U. S. AIR FORCE HOSPITAL (O, 65 beds) 77 Nealy Avenue, Hampton, VA Zip 23665–2080; tel. 757/764–6969; Colonel Eric Stone, Commander
**Web address:** www.jble.af.mil

**9395: DEPARTMENT OF THE ARMY, OFFICE OF THE SURGEON GENERAL** (FG)
5109 Leesburg Pike, Falls Church, VA Zip 22041;
tel. 703/681–3000; Lieutenant General Eric B. Schoomaker, Surgeon General
**(Moderately Centralized Health System)**

**ALASKA:** BASSETT ARMY COMMUNITY HOSPITAL (O, 24 beds) 1060 Gaffney Road, Box 7400, Fort Wainwright, AK Zip 99703–7400, Mailing Address: 1060 Gaffney Road, Box 7440, Zip 99703–7440; tel. 907/361–5172; Colonel George Appenzeller, Commander
**Web address:** www.alaska.amedd.army.mil

**CALIFORNIA:** WEED ARMY COMMUNITY HOSPITAL (O, 27 beds) Inner Loop Road and 4th Street, Building 166, Fort Irwin, CA Zip 92310–5065, Mailing Address: P.O. Box 105109, Zip 92310–5109; tel. 760/380–3108; Colonel Michael L. Kiefer, Commander
**Web address:** www.irwin.amedd.army.mil

**COLORADO:** EVANS U. S. ARMY COMMUNITY HOSPITAL (O, 57 beds) 1650 Cochrane Circle, Building 7500, Fort Carson, CO Zip 80913–5101; tel. 719/526–7200; Colonel Jimmie O. Keenan, Commander
**Web address:** www.evans.amedd.army.mil

**GEORGIA:** DWIGHT DAVID EISENHOWER ARMY MEDICAL CENTER (O, 125 beds) Hospital Drive, Fort Gordon, GA Zip 30905–5650; tel. 706/787–5811; Commander Christopher M. Castle, Commander
**Web address:** www.ddeamc.amedd.army.mil

MARTIN ARMY COMMUNITY HOSPITAL (O, 57 beds) 7950 Martin Loop, Fort Benning, GA Zip 31905–5648, Mailing Address: 7950 Martin Loop, B9200, Room 010, Zip 31905–5648; tel. 706/544–2516; Colonel Timothy E. Lamb, Commander
**Web address:** www.martin.amedd.army.mil

WINN ARMY COMMUNITY HOSPITAL (O, 79 beds) 1061 Harmon Avenue, Hinesville, GA Zip 31314–5674, Mailing Address: 1061 Harmon Avenue, Suite 2311B, Zip 31314–5674; tel. 912/435–6965; Colonel Ronald Place, M.D., Commander
**Web address:** www.winn.amedd.army.mil/

**HAWAII:** TRIPLER ARMY MEDICAL CENTER (O, 198 beds) 1 Jarret White Road, Honolulu, HI Zip 96859–5000; tel. 808/433–6661; Brigadier General Keith W. Gallagher, FACHE, Commander
**Web address:** www.tamc.amedd.army.mil

**KANSAS:** IRWIN ARMY COMMUNITY HOSPITAL (O, 44 beds) 600 Caisson Hill Road, Junction City, KS Zip 66442–5037; tel. 785/239–7000; Colonel Barry R. Pockrandt, Commander
**Web address:** www.iach.amedd.army.mil/

**KENTUCKY:** COLONEL FLORENCE A. BLANCHFIELD ARMY COMMUNITY HOSPITAL (O, 66 beds) 650 Joel Drive, Fort Campbell, KY Zip 42223; tel. 270/798–8040; Colonel Paul Cordts, Commander
**Web address:** www.campbell.amedd.army.mil/

IRELAND ARMY COMMUNITY HOSPITAL (O, 33 beds) 289 Ireland Avenue, Fort Knox, KY Zip 40121–5111; tel. 502/624–9333; Colonel Cornelius C. Maher, Commander
**Web address:** www.iach.knox.amedd.army.mil/

**LOUISIANA:** BAYNE–JONES ARMY COMMUNITY HOSPITAL (O, 22 beds) 1585 3rd Street, Fort Polk, LA Zip 71459–5102; tel. 337/531–3928; Colonel David Dunning, Commander
**Web address:** www.polk.amedd.army.mil

**MARSHALL ISLANDS:** KWAJALEIN HOSPITAL (O, 14 beds) U.S. Army Kwajalein Atoll, Kwajalein Island, MH Zip 96960, Mailing Address: Box 1702, APO, APZip 96555–5000; tel. 805/355–2225; Elaine McMahon, Administrator

**MISSOURI:** GENERAL LEONARD WOOD ARMY COMMUNITY HOSPITAL (O, 54 beds) 126 Missouri Avenue, Fort Leonard Wood, MO Zip 65473–8952; tel. 573/596–0414; Colonel Marie Dominguez, Commander
**Web address:** www.amedd.army.mil

For explanation of codes following names, see page B2.
★ Indicates Type III membership in the American Hospital Association.

Section B

**NEW YORK:** KELLER ARMY COMMUNITY HOSPITAL (O, 31 beds) 900 Washington Road, West Point, NY Zip 10996–1197, Mailing Address: U.S. Military Academy, Building 900, Zip 10996–1197; tel. 845/938–5169; Colonel Beverly Land, Commanding Officer
**Web address:** www.kach.amedd.army.mil/

**NORTH CAROLINA:** WOMACK ARMY MEDICAL CENTER (O, 156 beds) Normandy Drive, Fort Bragg, NC Zip 28307–5000; tel. 910/907–6000; Colonel Brian Canfield, Commander
**Web address:** www.wamc.amedd.army.mil/

**OKLAHOMA:** REYNOLDS ARMY COMMUNITY HOSPITAL (O, 43 beds) 4301 Mow Way Road, Fort Sill, OK Zip 73503–6300; tel. 580/458–3000; Colonel Jennifer L. Bedick, Commander
**Web address:** www.rach.sill.amedd.army.mil

**SOUTH CAROLINA:** MONCRIEF ARMY COMMUNITY HOSPITAL (O, 60 beds) 4500 Stuart Street, Fort Jackson, SC Zip 29207–5720; tel. 803/751–2160; Colonel Ramona Fiorey, MSN, M.P.H., Commander
**Web address:** www.moncrief.amedd.army.mil

**TEXAS:** CARL R. DARNALL ARMY MEDICAL CENTER (O, 109 beds) 36000 Darnall Loop, Fort Hood, TX Zip 76544–5095; tel. 254/288–8000; Colonel Patrick D. Sargent, Commander
**Web address:** www.crdamc.amedd.army.mil

SAN ANTONIO MILITARY MEDICAL CENTER (O, 226 beds) 3851 Roger Brookes Drive, Fort Sam Houston, TX Zip 78234–6200; tel. 210/916–4141; Colonel Noel J. Cardenas, FACHE, Commander
**Web address:** www.bamc.amedd.army.mil

WILLIAM BEAUMONT ARMY MEDICAL CENTER (O, 209 beds) 5005 North Piedras Street, El Paso, TX Zip 79920–5001; tel. 915/742–2121; Colonel Dennis Doyle, Commanding Officer
**Web address:** www.wbamc.amedd.army.mil

**VIRGINIA:** DEWITT ARMY COMMUNITY HOSPITAL (O, 46 beds) 9501 Farrell Road, Fort Belvoir, VA Zip 22060–5901, Mailing Address: 9501 Farrell Road, Suite GC11, Zip 22060–5901; tel. 703/805–0510; Colonel Susan Annicelli, Commander
**Web address:** www.dewitt.wramc.amedd.army.mil

**WASHINGTON:** MADIGAN HEALTHCARE SYSTEM (O, 235 beds) Fitzsimmons Drive, Building 9040, Tacoma, WA Zip 98431–1100; tel. 253/968–1110; Colonel Dallas Homas, Commander
**Web address:** www.mamc.amedd.army.mil

| | | |
|---|---|---|
| Owned, leased, sponsored: | 22 hospitals | 1915 beds |
| Contract-managed: | 0 hospitals | 0 beds |
| Totals: | 22 hospitals | 1915 beds |

**9295: DEPARTMENT OF VETERANS AFFAIRS** (FG)
810 Vermont Avenue N.W., Washington, DC Zip 20420; tel. 202/273–5781; Robert A. Petzel, M.D., Under Secretary for Health
**(Decentralized Health System)**

**ALABAMA:** CENTRAL ALABAMA VETERANS HEALTH CARE SYSTEM (O, 321 beds) 215 Perry Hill Road, Montgomery, AL Zip 36109–3798; tel. 334/272–4670; Glen E. Struchtemeyer, Director
**Web address:** www.centralalabama.va.gov/

VETERANS AFFAIRS MEDICAL CENTER (O, 151 beds) 700 South 19th Street, Birmingham, AL Zip 35233–1927; tel. 205/933–8101; Rica Lewis–Payton, Director
**Web address:** www.va.gov/sta/guide/home.asp

VETERANS AFFAIRS MEDICAL CENTER (O, 381 beds) 3701 Loop Road, Tuscaloosa, AL Zip 35404–5015; tel. 205/554–2000; Alan J. Tyler, MS, FACHE, Director
**Web address:** www.tuscaloosa.va.gov

**ARIZONA:** NORTHERN ARIZONA VA HEALTH CARE SYSTEM (O, 137 beds) 500 Highway 89 North, Prescott, AZ Zip 86313–5000; tel. 928/445–4860; Donna K. Jacobs, FACHE, Director
**Web address:** www.va.gov/sta/guide/home.asp

PHOENIX VETERANS AFFAIRS HEALTH CARE SYSTEM (O, 197 beds) 650 East Indian School Road, Phoenix, AZ Zip 85012–1892; tel. 602/277–5551; James Robbins, M.D., Director
**Web address:** www.phoenix.med.va.gov

SOUTHERN ARIZONA VETERANS AFFAIRS HEALTH CARE SYSTEM (O, 285 beds) 3601 South 6th Avenue, Tucson, AZ Zip 85723–0002; tel. 520/792–1450; Jonathan H. Gardner, Chief Executive Officer
**Web address:** www.tucson.va.gov

**ARKANSAS:** CENTRAL ARKANSAS VETERANS HEALTHCARE SYSTEM (O, 551 beds) 4300 West Seventh Street, Little Rock, AR Zip 72205–5484; tel. 501/257–1000; Michael R. Winn, Director
**Web address:** www.va.gov/sta/guide/home.asp

VETERANS HEALTH CARE SYSTEM OF THE OZARKS (O, 72 beds) 1100 North College Avenue, Fayetteville, AR Zip 72703–6995; tel. 479/443–4301; John Henley, M.D., Interim Director
**Web address:** www.va.gov/sta/guide/home.asp

**CALIFORNIA:** JERRY L. PETTIS MEMORIAL VETERANS MEDICAL CENTER (O, 97 beds) 11201 Benton Street, Loma Linda, CA Zip 92357; tel. 909/825–7084; Donald F. Moore, Director
**Web address:** www.lomalinda.va.gov

VETERANS AFFAIRS CENTRAL CALIFORNIA HEALTH CARE SYSTEM (O, 54 beds) 2615 East Clinton Avenue, Fresno, CA Zip 93703–2223; tel. 559/225–6100; Alan S. Perry, Director
**Web address:** www.va.gov/sta/guide/home.asp

VETERANS AFFAIRS GREATER LOS ANGELES HEALTHCARE SYSTEM (O, 1087 beds) 11301 Wilshire Boulevard, Los Angeles, CA Zip 90073–1003; tel. 310/478–3711; Donna M. Beiter, R.N., MSN, Director
**Web address:** www.va.gov/sta/guide/home.asp

VETERANS AFFAIRS LONG BEACH HEALTHCARE SYSTEM (O, 234 beds) 5901 East 7th Street, Long Beach, CA Zip 90822–5201; tel. 562/826–8000; Isabel Duff, MS, Director
**Web address:** www.va.gov/sta/guide/home.asp

VETERANS AFFAIRS MEDICAL CENTER (O, 244 beds) 4150 Clement Street, San Francisco, CA Zip 94121–1598; tel. 415/221–4810; Lawrence H. Carroll, Director
**Web address:** www.va.gov/sta/guide/home.asp

VETERANS AFFAIRS PALO ALTO HEALTH CARE SYSTEM (O, 808 beds) 3801 Miranda Avenue, Palo Alto, CA Zip 94304–1207; tel. 650/493–5000; Elizabeth Joyce Freeman, Director
**Web address:** www.va.gov/sta/guide/home.asp

VETERANS AFFAIRS SAN DIEGO HEALTHCARE SYSTEM (O, 232 beds) 3350 LaJolla Village Drive, San Diego, CA Zip 92161–0002; tel. 858/552–8585; Robert M. Smith, M.D., Acting Director
**Web address:** www.sandiego.va.gov

**COLORADO:** SOUTHERN COLORADO HEALTHCARE SYSTEM (O, 299 beds) Las Animas, CO Zip 81054–0390; tel. 719/456–1260; Stuart C. Collyer, Director

VETERANS AFFAIRS EASTERN COLORADO HEALTH CARE SYSTEM (O, 252 beds) 1055 Clermont Street, Denver, CO Zip 80220–3877; tel. 303/399–8020; Lynette A. Roff, Director
**Web address:** www.va.gov/sta/guide/home.asp

VETERANS AFFAIRS MEDICAL CENTER (O, 23 beds) 2121 North Avenue, Grand Junction, CO Zip 81501–6499; tel. 970/242–0731; William R. Berryman, M.D., Acting Director
**Web address:** www.va.gov/sta/guide/home.asp

**CONNECTICUT:** VETERANS AFFAIRS CONNECTICUT HEALTHCARE SYSTEM (O, 160 beds) 950 Campbell Avenue, West Haven, CT Zip 06516–2770; tel. 203/932–5711; John Callahan, Acting Director
**Web address:** www.va.gov/sta/guide/home.asp

**DELAWARE:** VETERANS AFFAIRS MEDICAL CENTER (O, 120 beds) 1601 Kirkwood Highway, Wilmington, DE Zip 19805–4989; tel. 302/994–2511; Charles M. Dorman, FACHE, Director
**Web address:** www.va.gov/wilmington

**DISTRICT OF COLUMBIA:** VETERANS AFFAIRS MEDICAL CENTER (O, 291 beds) 50 Irving Street N.W., Washington, DC Zip 20422–0002; tel. 202/745–8100; Brian A. Hawkins, Director Medical Center
**Web address:** www.washingtondc.va.gov/

**FLORIDA:** JAMES A. HALEY VETERANS HOSPITAL (O, 93 beds) 13000 Bruce B. Downs Boulevard, Tampa, FL Zip 33612–4798; tel. 813/972–2000; Nancy Reissener, Acting Director
**Web address:** www.va.gov/visn8/tampa

MALCOM RANDALL VETERANS AFFAIRS MEDICAL CENTER (O, 222 beds) 1601 S.W. Archer Road, Gainesville, FL Zip 32608–1197; tel. 352/376–1611; Nancy Reissener, Acting Director
**Web address:** www.northflorida.va.gov/

For explanation of codes following names, see page B2.
★ Indicates Type III membership in the American Hospital Association.

VETERANS AFFAIRS MEDICAL CENTER (O, 291 beds) 10000 Bay Pines Boulevard, Bay Pines, FL Zip 33744, Mailing Address: P.O. Box 5005, Zip 33744–5005; tel. 727/398–6661; Suzanne M. Klinker, Director
**Web address:** www.baypines.va.gov/

VETERANS AFFAIRS MEDICAL CENTER (O, 133 beds) 7305 North Military Trail, West Palm Beach, FL Zip 33410–6400; tel. 561/422–8262; Charleen R. Szabo, FACHE, Director
**Web address:** www.va.gov/sta/guide/home.asp

VETERANS AFFAIRS MEDICAL CENTER (O, 281 beds) 1201 N.W. 16th Street, Miami, FL Zip 33125–1624; tel. 305/575–7000; Paul Russo, Director
**Web address:** www.va.gov/miami

VETERANS AFFAIRS MEDICAL CENTER (O, 180 beds) 619 South Marion Avenue, Lake City, FL Zip 32025–5898; tel. 386/755–3016; Thomas A. Cappello, M.P.H., FACHE, Director
**Web address:** www.va.gov/sta/guide/home.asp

**GEORGIA:** CARL VINSON VETERANS AFFAIRS MEDICAL CENTER (O, 178 beds) 1826 Veterans Boulevard, Dublin, GA Zip 31021–3620; tel. 478/272–1210; J. Mark Anderson, Acting Director
**Web address:** www.va.gov/sta/guide/home.asp

VETERANS AFFAIRS MEDICAL CENTER (O, 239 beds) 1670 Clairmont Road, Decatur, GA Zip 30033–4004; tel. 404/321–6111; James A. Clark, M.P.H., Director
**Web address:** www.atlanta.va.gov/

VETERANS AFFAIRS MEDICAL CENTER (O, 338 beds) 1 Freedom Way, Augusta, GA Zip 30904–6285; tel. 706/733–0188; Patricia O. Pittman, Acting Director
**Web address:** www.augusta.va.gov/

**IDAHO:** VETERANS AFFAIRS MEDICAL CENTER (O, 79 beds) 500 West Fort Street, Boise, ID Zip 83702–4598; tel. 208/422–1000; David Stockwell, Interim Director
**Web address:** www.va.gov/directory/guide/home.asp

**ILLINOIS:** CAPTAIN JAMES A. LOVELL FEDERAL HEALTH CARE CENTER (O, 103 beds) 3001 Green Bay Road, North Chicago, IL Zip 60064–3049; tel. 847/688–1900; Patrick L. Sullivan, FACHE, Director
**Web address:** www.lovell.fhcc.va.gov

JESSE BROWN VETERANS AFFAIRS CHICAGO HEALTH CARE SYSTEM (O, 240 beds) 820 South Damen, Chicago, IL Zip 60612–3776; tel. 312/569–8387; Michael A. Anaya, Sr., FACHE, Medical Center Director
**Web address:** www.va.gov/sta/guide/home.asp

VETERANS AFFAIRS EDWARD HINES, JR. HOSPITAL (O, 385 beds) Fifth Avenue & Roosevelt Road, Hines, IL Zip 60141–5000, Mailing Address: P.O. Box 5000, Zip 60141–5000; tel. 708/202–8387; Nathan L. Geraths, Director
**Web address:** www.va.gov/sta/guide/home.asp

VETERANS AFFAIRS ILLIANA HEALTH CARE SYSTEM (O, 245 beds) 1900 East Main Street, Danville, IL Zip 61832–5198; tel. 217/554–3000; Michael E. Hamilton, Director
**Web address:** www.va.gov/sta/guide/home.asp

VETERANS AFFAIRS MEDICAL CENTER (O, 55 beds) 2401 West Main Street, Marion, IL Zip 62959–1194; tel. 618/997–5311; Paul Bockelman, Director
**Web address:** www.marion.va.gov

**INDIANA:** RICHARD L. ROUDEBUSH VETERANS AFFAIRS MEDICAL CENTER (O, 209 beds) 1481 West Tenth Street, Indianapolis, IN Zip 46202–2884; tel. 317/554–0000; Thomas Mattice, Director
**Web address:** www.indianapolis.va.gov

VETERANS AFFAIRS NORTHERN INDIANA HEALTH CARE SYSTEM (O, 105 beds) 2121 Lake Avenue, Fort Wayne, IN Zip 46805–5347; tel. 260/460–1310; Daniel D. Hendee, Director
**Web address:** www.va.gov/sta/guide/home.asp

**IOWA:** IOWA CITY VETERANS AFFAIRS HEALTH CARE SYSTEM (O, 83 beds) 601 Highway 6 West, Iowa City, IA Zip 52246–2208; tel. 319/339–7100; Barry Sharp, Director
**Web address:** www.iowacity.va.gov/

VETERANS AFFAIRS CENTRAL IOWA HEALTH CARE SYSTEM (O, 255 beds) 3600 30th Street, Des Moines, IA Zip 50310–5774; tel. 515/699–5999; Donald C. Cooper, Director
**Web address:** www.va.centra/iowa.va.gov

**KANSAS:** ROBERT J. DOLE VETERANS AFFAIRS MEDICAL CENTER (O, 41 beds) 5500 East Kellogg, Wichita, KS Zip 67218; tel. 316/685–2221; Thomas J. Sanders, FACHE, Director
**Web address:** www.va.gov/sta/guide/home.asp

VETERANS AFFAIRS EASTERN KANSAS HEALTH CARE SYSTEM (O, 213 beds) 2200 Gage Boulevard, Topeka, KS Zip 66622–0002; tel. 785/350–3111; John Moon, Associate Director
**Web address:** www.va.gov/sta/guide/home.asp

**KENTUCKY:** VETERANS AFFAIRS MEDICAL CENTER–LEXINGTON (O, 138 beds) 1101 Veterans Drive, Lexington, KY Zip 40502; tel. 859/233–4511; DeWayne Hamlin, Director
**Web address:** www.va.gov/sta/guide/home.asp

VETERANS AFFAIRS MEDICAL CENTER–LOUISVILLE (O, 116 beds) 800 Zorn Avenue, Louisville, KY Zip 40206–1499; tel. 502/287–5500; Wayne L. Pfeffer, FACHE, Director
**Web address:** www.louisville.va.gov

**LOUISIANA:** OVERTON BROOKS VETERANS AFFAIRS MEDICAL CENTER (O, 119 beds) 510 East Stoner Avenue, Shreveport, LA Zip 71101–4295; tel. 318/221–8411; Shirley Bealer, Director
**Web address:** www.va.gov/sta/guide/home.asp

VETERANS AFFAIRS MEDICAL CENTER – ALEXANDRIA (O, 143 beds) 2495 Shreveport Highway, 71 N., Pineville, LA Zip 71360, Mailing Address: P.O. Box 69004, Alexandria, Zip 71306–9004; tel. 318/466–2205; Gracie Specks, MS, Director
**Web address:** www.va.gov/sta/guide/home.asp

**MAINE:** VETERANS AFFAIRS MEDICAL CENTER (O, 167 beds) 1 VA Center, Togus, ME Zip 04330; tel. 207/623–8411; Brian Stiller, Director
**Web address:** www.visn1.med.va.gov/togus/

**MARYLAND:** VETERANS AFFAIRS MARYLAND HEALTH CARE SYSTEM–BALTIMORE DIVISION (O, 452 beds) 10 North Greene Street, Baltimore, MD Zip 21201–1524; tel. 410/605–7001; Dennis H. Smith, Director
**Web address:** www.va.gov/sta/guide/home.asp

**MASSACHUSETTS:** BROCKTON VETERANS AFFAIRS MEDICAL CENTER (O, 375 beds) 940 Belmont Street, Brockton, MA Zip 02401–5596; tel. 508/583–4500; Michael E. Lawson, Director
**Web address:** www.va.gov/sta/guide/home.asp

EDITH NOURSE ROGERS MEMORIAL VETERANS HOSPITAL (O, 147 beds) 200 Springs Road, Bedford, MA Zip 01730–1198; tel. 781/687–2000; Christine Croteau, Acting Director
**Web address:** www.va.gov/sta/guide/home.asp

VETERANS AFFAIRS BOSTON HEALTHCARE SYSTEM (O, 361 beds) 1400 VFW Parkway, Boston, MA Zip 02132; tel. 617/232–9500; Michael E. Lawson, Director
**Web address:** www.va.gov/sta/guide/home.asp

VETERANS AFFAIRS MEDICAL CENTER (O, 167 beds) 421 North Main Street, Leeds, MA Zip 01053–9764; tel. 413/582–3000; Roger L. Johnson, Director
**Web address:** www.va.gov/sta/guide/home.asp

**MICHIGAN:** ALEDA E. LUTZ VETERANS AFFAIRS MEDICAL CENTER (O, 100 beds) 1500 Weiss Street, Saginaw, MI Zip 48602–5298; tel. 989/497–2500; Denise Deitzen, Director
**Web address:** www.saginaw.va.gov/

JOHN D. DINGELL VETERANS AFFAIRS MEDICAL CENTER (O, 188 beds) 4646 John R Street, Detroit, MI Zip 48201–1932; tel. 313/576–1000; Pamela Reeves, M.D., Director
**Web address:** www.va.gov/sta/guide/home.asp

VETERANS AFFAIRS ANN ARBOR HEALTHCARE SYSTEM (O, 105 beds) 2215 Fuller Road, Ann Arbor, MI Zip 48105–2399; tel. 734/769–7100; Robert P. McDivitt, FACHE, Director
**Web address:** www.annarbor.va.gov

VETERANS AFFAIRS MEDICAL CENTER (O, 313 beds) 5500 Armstrong Road, Battle Creek, MI Zip 49037; tel. 269/966–5600; Denise Deitzen, Acting Director
**Web address:** www.battlecreek.va.gov/

VETERANS AFFAIRS MEDICAL CENTER (O, 17 beds) 325 East H Street, Iron Mountain, MI Zip 49801–4792; tel. 906/774–3300; James W. Rice, Director
**Web address:** www.va.gov/sta/guide/home.asp

**MINNESOTA:** MINNEAPOLIS VETERANS AFFAIRS HEALTH CARE SYSTEM (O, 305 beds) One Veterans Drive, Minneapolis, MN Zip 55417–2399; tel. 612/725–2000; Barry Sharp, Acting Director
**Web address:** www.minneapolis.va.gov

ST. CLOUD VETERANS AFFAIRS HEALTH CARE SYSTEM (O, 388 beds) 4801 Veterans Drive, Saint Cloud, MN Zip 56303–2099; tel. 320/252–1670; Barry I. Bahl, Director
**Web address:** www.stcloud.va.gov

For explanation of codes following names, see page B2.
★ Indicates Type III membership in the American Hospital Association.

**MISSISSIPPI:** G.V. MONTGOMERY VETERANS AFFAIRS MEDICAL CENTER (O, 323 beds) 1500 East Woodrow Wilson Drive, Jackson, MS Zip 39216–5199; tel. 601/364–1201; Linda Watson, Director
**Web address:** www.va.gov

VETERANS AFFAIRS GULF COAST VETERANS HEALTH CARE SYSTEM (O, 392 beds) 400 Veterans Avenue, Biloxi, MS Zip 39531–2410; tel. 228/523–5000; Thomas Wisnieski, Director
**Web address:** www.va.gov/biloxi

**MISSOURI:** HARRY S. TRUMAN MEMORIAL VETERANS HOSPITAL (O, 126 beds) 800 Hospital Drive, Columbia, MO Zip 65201–5275; tel. 573/814–6000; Sallie Houser-Hanfelder, FACHE, Director
**Web address:** www.columbiamo.va.gov

JOHN J. PERSHING VETERANS AFFAIRS MEDICAL CENTER (O, 58 beds) 1500 North Westwood Boulevard, Poplar Bluff, MO Zip 63901–3318; tel. 573/686–4151; Marjorie Hedstrom, Director
**Web address:** www.poplarbluff.va.gov

VETERANS AFFAIRS MEDICAL CENTER (O, 356 beds) 915 North Grand, Saint Louis, MO Zip 63106–1621; tel. 314/652–4100; RimaAnn O. Nelson, Director
**Web address:** www.va.gov/sta/guide/home.asp

VETERANS AFFAIRS MEDICAL CENTER (O, 157 beds) 4801 East Linwood Boulevard, Kansas City, MO Zip 64128–2226; tel. 816/861–4700; Kent D. Hill, Director
**Web address:** www.va.gov/sta/guide/home.asp

**MONTANA:** VETERANS AFFAIRS MONTANA HEALTH CARE SYSTEM (O, 65 beds) 1892 Williams Street, Fort Harrison, MT Zip 59636, Mailing Address: P.O. Box 1500, Zip 59636–1500; tel. 406/442–6410; Robin Korogi, Director
**Web address:** www.va.gov/sta/guide/home.asp

**NEBRASKA:** VETERANS AFFAIRS MEDICAL CENTER (O, 100 beds) 4101 Woolworth Avenue, Omaha, NE Zip 68105–1873; tel. 402/346–8800; Nancy A. Gregory, Acting Director
**Web address:** www.va.gov/sta/guide/home.asp

VETERANS AFFAIRS NEBRASKA–WESTERN IOWA HEALTH CARE SYSTEM (O, 186 beds) 600 South 70th Street, Lincoln, NE Zip 68510–2493; tel. 402/489–3802; Nancy A. Gregory, Acting Director
**Web address:** www.nebraska.va.gov/visitors/lincoln.asp

**NEVADA:** VETERANS AFFAIRS SIERRA NEVADA HEALTH CARE SYSTEM (O, 64 beds) 1000 Locust Street, Reno, NV Zip 89502–2597; tel. 775/786–7200; Kurt W. Schlegelmilch, M.D., FACHE, Director
**Web address:** www.reno.va.gov

VETERANS AFFAIRS SOUTHERN NEVADA HEALTHCARE SYSTEM (O, 57 beds) North Las Vegas, NV Zip 89036; tel. 702/636–3000; John Bright, Director
**Web address:** www.va.gov/sta/guide/home.asp

**NEW HAMPSHIRE:** VETERANS AFFAIRS MEDICAL CENTER (O, 90 beds) 718 Smyth Road, Manchester, NH Zip 03104–4098; tel. 603/624–4366; Marc Levenson, M.D., Director
**Web address:** www.va.gov/sta/guide/home.asp

**NEW JERSEY:** VETERANS AFFAIRS NEW JERSEY HEALTH CARE SYSTEM (O, 414 beds) 385 Tremont Avenue, East Orange, NJ Zip 07018–1095; tel. 973/676–1000; Kenneth H. Mizrach, Director
**Web address:** www.va.gov/sta/guide/home.asp

**NEW MEXICO:** VETERANS AFFAIRS MEDICAL CENTER (O, 281 beds) 1501 San Pedro S.E., Albuquerque, NM Zip 87108–5138; tel. 505/265–1711; George Marnell, Director
**Web address:** www.southwest.va.gov/albuquerque/

**NEW YORK:** ALBANY STRATTON VETERANS AFFAIRS MEDICAL CENTER (O, 148 beds) 113 Holland Avenue, Albany, NY Zip 12208–3473; tel. 518/626–5000; Linda W. Weiss, MS, FACHE, Director
**Web address:** www.va.gov/sta/guide/home.asp

ST. ALBANS PRIMARY AND EXTENDED CARE CENTER (O, 100 beds) 179Th Street And Linden Boulevard, Jamaica, NY Zip 11425–0001;

VETERANS ADMINISTRATION NEW YORK HARBOR HEALTHCARE SYSTEM (O, 517 beds) 800 Poly Place, Brooklyn, NY Zip 11209–7104; tel. 718/630–3500; Martina A. Parauda, Director
**Web address:** www.nyharbor.va.gov

VETERANS AFFAIRS HUDSON VALLEY HEALTH CARE SYSTEM–F.D. ROOSEVELT HOSPITAL (O, 356 beds) Montrose, NY Zip 10548; tel. 914/737–4400; Gerald F. Culliton, Director

VETERANS AFFAIRS MEDICAL CENTER (O, 359 beds) 76 Veterans Avenue, Bath, NY Zip 14810–0842; tel. 607/664–4000; Michael J. Swartz, Medical Center Director
**Web address:** www.bath.va.gov

VETERANS AFFAIRS MEDICAL CENTER (O, 196 beds) 400 Fort Hill Avenue, Canandaigua, NY Zip 14424–1159; tel. 585/394–2000; Craig Howard, Director
**Web address:** www.va.gov/sta/guide/home.asp

VETERANS AFFAIRS MEDICAL CENTER (O, 325 beds) 130 West Kingsbridge Road, Bronx, NY Zip 10468–3992; tel. 718/584–9000; Maryann Musumeci, Director
**Web address:** www.va.gov/sta/guide/home.asp

VETERANS AFFAIRS MEDICAL CENTER (O, 502 beds) 79 Middleville Road, Northport, NY Zip 11768–2293; tel. 631/261–4400; Philip C. Moschitta, Director
**Web address:** www.va.gov/sta/guide/home.asp

VETERANS AFFAIRS MEDICAL CENTER (O, 154 beds) 800 Irving Avenue, Syracuse, NY Zip 13210–2716; tel. 315/425–4400; James Cody, Director
**Web address:** www.syracuse.va.gov

VETERANS AFFAIRS WESTERN NEW YORK HEALTHCARE SYSTEM–BATAVIA DIVISION (O, 128 beds) 222 Richmond Avenue, Batavia, NY Zip 14020–1288; tel. 585/297–1000; Royce Calhoun, Assistant Director
**Web address:** www.buffalo.va.gov/batavia.asp

VETERANS AFFAIRS WESTERN NEW YORK HEALTHCARE SYSTEM–BUFFALO DIVISION (O, 113 beds) 3495 Bailey Avenue, Buffalo, NY Zip 14215–1129; tel. 716/834–9200; Craig Howard, Interim Director
**Web address:** www.va.gov/visns/visn02

**NORTH CAROLINA:** CHARLES GEORGE VETERANS AFFAIRS MEDICAL CENTER (O, 116 beds) 1100 Tunnel Road, Asheville, NC Zip 28805–2087; tel. 828/298–7911; Cynthia Breyfogle, Director
**Web address:** www.asheville.va.gov/

DURHAM VETERANS AFFAIRS MEDICAL CENTER (O, 265 beds) 508 Fulton Street, Durham, NC Zip 27705–3897; tel. 919/286–0411; DeAnne Seekins, Director
**Web address:** www.va.gov

VETERANS AFFAIRS MEDICAL CENTER (O, 56 beds) 2300 Ramsey Street, Fayetteville, NC Zip 28301–3899; tel. 910/488–2120; Elizabeth Goolsby, Director
**Web address:** www.fayettevillenc.va.gov

VETERANS AFFAIRS MEDICAL CENTER (O, 171 beds) 1601 Brenner Avenue, Salisbury, NC Zip 28144–2559; tel. 704/638–9000; Anthony L. Dawson, FACHE, Interim Director
**Web address:** www.salisbury.va.gov

**NORTH DAKOTA:** VETERANS AFFAIRS HEALTH CARE SYSTEM (O, 77 beds) 2101 Elm Street North, Fargo, ND Zip 58102–2498; tel. 701/232–3241; Michael J. Murphy, Director
**Web address:** www.va.gov/sta/guide/home.asp

**OHIO:** VETERANS AFFAIRS MEDICAL CENTER (O, 592 beds) 10701 East Boulevard, Cleveland, OH Zip 44106–1702; tel. 216/791–3800; Susan Fuehrer, Director
**Web address:** www.va.gov/sta/guide/home.asp

VETERANS AFFAIRS MEDICAL CENTER (O, 297 beds) 17273 State Route 104, Chillicothe, OH Zip 45601–8608; tel. 740/773–1141; Jeffrey T. Gering, Medical Center Director
**Web address:** www.va.gov/sta/guide/home.asp

VETERANS AFFAIRS MEDICAL CENTER (O, 269 beds) 3200 Vine Street, Cincinnati, OH Zip 45220–2288; tel. 513/475–6300; Linda D. Smith, Director
**Web address:** www.cincinnati.va.gov/

VETERANS AFFAIRS MEDICAL CENTER (O, 370 beds) 4100 West Third Street, Dayton, OH Zip 45428–1002; tel. 937/268–6511; Glenn A. Costie, FACHE, Director
**Web address:** www.va.gov/sta/guide/home.asp

**OKLAHOMA:** JACK C. MONTGOMERY VETERANS AFFAIRS MEDICAL CENTER (O, 111 beds) 1011 Honor Heights Drive, Muskogee, OK Zip 74401–1318; tel. 918/683–3261; Bryan C. Matthews, Acting Director
**Web address:** www.muskogee.va.gov

For explanation of codes following names, see page B2.
★ Indicates Type III membership in the American Hospital Association.

Section B

VETERANS AFFAIRS MEDICAL CENTER (O, 192 beds) 921 N.E. 13th Street, Oklahoma City, OK Zip 73104–5028; tel. 405/456–1000; David P. Wood, FACHE, Medical Center Director
**Web address:** www.oklahoma.va.gov

**OREGON:** VETERANS AFFAIRS DOMICILIARY (O, 1075 beds) White City, OR Zip 97503; tel. 503/826–2111; Frank Drake, Director

VETERANS AFFAIRS MEDICAL CENTER (O, 149 beds) 3710 S.W. U.S. Veterans Hospital Road, Portland, OR Zip 97239, Mailing Address: P.O. Box 1034, Zip 97207–1034; tel. 503/220–8262; John E. Patrick, Director
**Web address:** www.va.gov/sta/guide/home.asp

VETERANS AFFAIRS ROSEBURG HEALTHCARE SYSTEM (O, 88 beds) 913 N.W. Garden Valley Boulevard, Roseburg, OR Zip 97470–6513; tel. 541/440–1000; Carol Bogedain, FACHE, Director
**Web address:** www.va.gov/sta/guide/home.asp

**PENNSYLVANIA:** JAMES E. VAN ZANDT VETERANS AFFAIRS MEDICAL CENTER (O, 68 beds) 2907 Pleasant Valley Boulevard, Altoona, PA Zip 16602–4305; tel. 814/943–8164; Charles T. Becker, Acting Director
**Web address:** www.altoona.va.gov

VA BUTLER HEALTHCARE (O, 66 beds) 325 New Castle Road, Butler, PA Zip 16001–2480; tel. 724/287–4781; Patricia Nealon, Director
**Web address:** www.butler.va.gov

VETERANS AFFAIRS MEDICAL CENTER (O, 306 beds) 1400 Black Horse Hill Road, Coatesville, PA Zip 19320–2040; tel. 610/384–7711; Gary W. Devansky, Director
**Web address:** www.va.gov/sta/guide/home.asp

VETERANS AFFAIRS MEDICAL CENTER (O, 26 beds) 135 East 38th Street, Erie, PA Zip 16504–1559; tel. 814/860–2576; Michael Adelman, M.D., Director
**Web address:** www.va.gov/sta/guide/home.asp

VETERANS AFFAIRS MEDICAL CENTER (O, 213 beds) 1700 South Lincoln Avenue, Lebanon, PA Zip 17042–7529; tel. 717/272–6621; Robert W. Callahan, Jr., Director
**Web address:** www.lebanon.va.gov

VETERANS AFFAIRS MEDICAL CENTER (O, 134 beds) 3900 Woodland Avenue, Philadelphia, PA Zip 19104–4594; tel. 215/823–5800; Joseph M. Dalpiaz, Director

VETERANS AFFAIRS MEDICAL CENTER (O, 173 beds) 1111 East End Boulevard, Wilkes–Barre, PA Zip 18711–0030; tel. 570/824–3521; Margaret B. Kaplan, Director
**Web address:** www.va.gov/vamcwb

VETERANS AFFAIRS PITTSBURGH HEALTHCARE SYSTEM (O, 447 beds) University Drive, Pittsburgh, PA Zip 15240–1001; tel. 412/688–6000; Terry Gerigk Wolf, Director
**Web address:** www.pittsburgh.va.gov/

**PUERTO RICO:** VETERANS AFFAIRS MEDICAL CENTER (O, 330 beds) 10 Casia Street, San Juan, PR Zip 00921–3201; tel. 787/641–7582; Wanda Mims, Director
**Web address:** www.va.gov/visn8/sanjuan

**RHODE ISLAND:** VETERANS AFFAIRS MEDICAL CENTER (O, 73 beds) 830 Chalkstone Avenue, Providence, RI Zip 02908–4799; tel. 401/273–7100; Vincent Ng, Director
**Web address:** www.providence.va.gov/

**SOUTH CAROLINA:** RALPH H. JOHNSON VETERANS AFFAIRS MEDICAL CENTER (O, 98 beds) 109 Bee Street, Charleston, SC Zip 29401–5799; tel. 843/577–5011; Carolyn L. Adams, Director
**Web address:** www.va.gov/sta/guide/home.asp

WM. JENNINGS BRYAN DORN VETERANS AFFAIRS MEDICAL CENTER (O, 109 beds) 6439 Garners Ferry Road, Columbia, SC Zip 29209–1639; tel. 803/776–4000; Rebecca J. Wiley, R.N., Director
**Web address:** www.columbiasc.va.gov/

**SOUTH DAKOTA:** SIOUX FALLS VA HEALTH CARE SYSTEM (O, 98 beds) 2501 West 22nd Street, Sioux Falls, SD Zip 57105–9920, Mailing Address: P.O. Box 5046, Zip 57117–5046; tel. 605/336–3230; Patrick Kelly, Director
**Web address:** www.siouxfalls.va.gov

VETERANS AFFAIRS BLACK HILLS HEALTH CARE SYSTEM (O, 308 beds) 113 Comanche Road, Fort Meade, SD Zip 57741–1099; tel. 605/720–7170; Stephen R. DiStasio, Acting Director
**Web address:** www.va.gov/sta/guide/home.asp

**TENNESSEE:** JAMES H. QUILLEN VETERANS AFFAIRS MEDICAL CENTER (O, 483 beds) Mountain Home, TN Zip 37684–5002; tel. 423/926–1171; Charlene S. Ehret, FACHE, Director
**Web address:** www.va.gov

VETERANS AFFAIRS MEDICAL CENTER (O, 280 beds) 1030 Jefferson Avenue, Memphis, TN Zip 38104–2193; tel. 901/523–8990; James L. Robinson, III, PsyD, Director
**Web address:** www.memphis.va.gov

VETERANS AFFAIRS TENNESSEE VALLEY HEALTHCARE SYSTEM (O, 260 beds) 1310 24th Avenue South, Nashville, TN Zip 37212–2637; tel. 615/327–4751; Juan A. Morales, R.N., MSN, Health System Director
**Web address:** www.tennesseevalley.va.gov

**TEXAS:** AMARILLO VETERANS AFFAIRS HEALTH CARE SYSTEM (O, 69 beds) 6010 West Amarillo Boulevard, Amarillo, TX Zip 79106–1992; tel. 806/355–9703; Andrew Welch, Director
**Web address:** www.va.gov/sta/guide/home.asp

CENTRAL TEXAS VETERANS HEALTHCARE SYSTEM (O, 1532 beds) 1901 Veterans Memorial Drive, Temple, TX Zip 76504–7493; tel. 254/778–4811; Thomas C. Smith, III, FACHE, Director
**Web address:** www.central–texas.med.va.gov

MICHAEL E. DEBAKEY VETERANS AFFAIRS MEDICAL CENTER (O, 739 beds) 2002 Holcombe Boulevard, Houston, TX Zip 77030–4298; tel. 713/791–1414; Adam C. Walmus, Director
**Web address:** www.houston.va.gov

SOUTH TEXAS VETERANS HEALTH CARE SYSTEM (O, 838 beds) 7400 Merton Minter Boulevard, San Antonio, TX Zip 78284–5799; tel. 210/617–5140; Marie L. Weldon, FACHE, Director
**Web address:** www.vasthcs.med.va.gov

VETERANS AFFAIRS NORTH TEXAS HEALTH CARE SYSTEM (O, 875 beds) 4500 South Lancaster Road, Dallas, TX Zip 75216–7167; tel. 214/742–8387; Mark Doskocil, Acting Director
**Web address:** www.va.gov/sta/guide/home.asp

WEST TEXAS VA HEALTH CARE SYSTEM (O, 149 beds) 300 Veterans Boulevard, Big Spring, TX Zip 79720–5500; Big Springs, tel. 432/263–7361; Daniel L. Marsh, Director
**Web address:** www.bigspring.va.gov/about/

**UTAH:** VETERANS AFFAIRS SALT LAKE CITY HEALTH CARE SYSTEM (O, 121 beds) 500 Foothill Drive, Salt Lake City, UT Zip 84148–0002; tel. 801/582–1565; Steven W. Young, Director
**Web address:** www.saltlakecity.va.gov/

**VERMONT:** VETERANS AFFAIRS MEDICAL CENTER (O, 60 beds) 215 North Main Street, White River Junction, VT Zip 05009–0001; tel. 802/291–6206; Robert M. Walton, Director
**Web address:** www.va.gov/sta/guide/home.asp

**VIRGINIA:** HUNTER HOLMES MCGUIRE VETERANS AFFAIRS MEDICAL CENTER (O, 317 beds) 1201 Broad Rock Boulevard, Richmond, VA Zip 23249–0002; tel. 804/675–5000; Charles E. Sepich, FACHE, Director
**Web address:** www.va.gov/sta/guide/home.asp

VETERANS AFFAIRS MEDICAL CENTER (O, 395 beds) 100 Emancipation Drive, Hampton, VA Zip 23667–0001; tel. 757/722–9961; DeAnne Seekins, Director
**Web address:** www.va.gov/sta/guide/home.asp

VETERANS AFFAIRS MEDICAL CENTER (O, 298 beds) 1970 Roanoke Boulevard, Salem, VA Zip 24153–6478; tel. 540/982–2463; Miguel H. LaPuz, M.D., Director
**Web address:** www.salem.va.gov

**WASHINGTON:** JONATHAN M. WAINWRIGHT MEMORIAL VA MEDICAL CENTER (O, 14 beds) 77 Wainwright Drive, Walla Walla, WA Zip 99362–3994; tel. 509/525–5200; Brian W. Westfield, MSN, Director
**Web address:** www.va.gov/sta/guide/home.asp

VETERANS AFFAIRS MEDICAL CENTER (O, 70 beds) 4815 North Assembly Street, Spokane, WA Zip 99205–6197; tel. 509/434–7200; Sandy J. Nielsen, Director
**Web address:** www.va.gov/sta/guide/home.asp

VETERANS AFFAIRS PUGET SOUND HEALTH CARE SYSTEM (O, 358 beds) 1660 South Columbian Way, Seattle, WA Zip 98108–1597; tel. 206/762–1010; David A. Elizalde, Director
**Web address:** www.va.gov/sta/guide/home.asp

Section B

For explanation of codes following names, see page B2.
★ Indicates Type III membership in the American Hospital Association.

**WEST VIRGINIA:** LOUIS A. JOHNSON VETERANS AFFAIRS MEDICAL CENTER (O, 71 beds) 1 Medical Center Drive, Clarksburg, WV Zip 26301–4199; tel. 304/623–3461; Beth Brown, Director
**Web address:** www.clarksburg.va.gov

VETERANS AFFAIRS MEDICAL CENTER (O, 40 beds) 200 Veterans Avenue, Beckley, WV Zip 25801–6499; tel. 304/255–2121; Karin McGraw, Director
**Web address:** www.va.gov/sta/guide/home.asp

VETERANS AFFAIRS MEDICAL CENTER (O, 80 beds) 1540 Spring Valley Drive, Huntington, WV Zip 25704–9300; tel. 304/429–6741; Edward H. Seiler, Director
**Web address:** www.huntington.va.gov/

VETERANS AFFAIRS MEDICAL CENTER (O, 246 beds) 510 Butler Avenue, Martinsburg, WV Zip 25401–0205; tel. 304/263–0811; Ann Brown, Director
**Web address:** www.va.gov/sta/guide/home.asp

**WISCONSIN:** CLEMENT J. ZABLOCKI VETERANS AFFAIRS MEDICAL CENTER (O, 370 beds) 5000 West National Avenue, Milwaukee, WI Zip 53295; tel. 414/384–2000; Robert H. Beller, FACHE, Director
**Web address:** www.va.gov/sta/guide/home.asp

VETERANS AFFAIRS MEDICAL CENTER (O, 71 beds) 500 East Veterans Street, Tomah, WI Zip 54660; tel. 608/372–3971; Mario DeSanctis, FACHE, Director
**Web address:** www.tomah.va.gov

WILLIAM S. MIDDLETON MEMORIAL VETERANS HOSPITAL (O, 86 beds) 2500 Overlook Terrace, Madison, WI Zip 53705–2286; tel. 608/256–1901; Deborah A. Thompson, Director
**Web address:** www.madison.va.gov

**WYOMING:** VETERANS AFFAIRS MEDICAL CENTER (O, 21 beds) 2360 East Pershing Boulevard, Cheyenne, WY Zip 82001–5392; tel. 307/778–7550; Cynthia McCormack, MS, Director
**Web address:** www.cheyenne.va.gov/

VETERANS AFFAIRS MEDICAL CENTER (O, 185 beds) 1898 Fort Road, Sheridan, WY Zip 82801–8320; tel. 307/672–3473; Debra L. Hirschman, R.N., MSN, Director
**Web address:** www.va.gov/sta/guide/home.asp

| | | |
|---|---|---|
| Owned, leased, sponsored: | 138 hospitals | 33437 beds |
| Contract–managed: | 0 hospitals | 0 beds |
| Totals: | 138 hospitals | 33437 beds |

---

**★2145:   DETROIT MEDICAL CENTER** (NP)
3990 John R., Detroit, MI Zip 48201; tel. 313/745–1250; Michael Duggan, Chief Executive Officer

| | | |
|---|---|---|
| Owned, leased, sponsored: | 0 hospitals | 0 beds |
| Contract–managed: | 0 hospitals | 0 beds |
| Totals: | 0 hospitals | 0 beds |

---

**0845:   DEVEREUX** (NP)
444 Devereux Drive, Villanova, PA Zip 19085, Mailing Address: P.O. Box 638, Zip 19085–0638; tel. 610/520–3000; Robert Q. Kreider, President and Chief Executive Officer
**(Independent Hospital System)**

**FLORIDA:** DEVEREUX HOSPITAL AND CHILDREN'S CENTER OF FLORIDA (O, 100 beds) 8000 Devereux Drive, Melbourne, FL Zip 32940–7907; tel. 321/242–9100; Steven Murphy, Executive Director
**Web address:** www.devereux.org

**GEORGIA:** DEVEREUX GEORGIA TREATMENT NETWORK (O, 187 beds) 1291 Stanley Road N.W., Kennesaw, GA Zip 30152–4359; tel. 770/427–0147; Gwendolyn Skinner, Executive Director
**Web address:** www.devereuxga.org

**PENNSYLVANIA:** DEVEREUX CHILDREN'S BEHAVIORAL HEALTH CENTER (O, 33 beds) 655 Sugartown Road, Malvern, PA Zip 19355–0275, Mailing Address: P.O. Box 275, Zip 19355–0275; tel. 610/296–6820; David E. Woodward, Executive Director
**Web address:** www.devereux.org

**TEXAS:** DEVEREUX TEXAS TREATMENT NETWORK (O, 57 beds) 1150 Devereux Drive, League City, TX Zip 77573–2043; tel. 281/335–1000; Pamela E. Helm, Executive Director
**Web address:** www.devereux.org

| | | |
|---|---|---|
| Owned, leased, sponsored: | 4 hospitals | 377 beds |
| Contract–managed: | 0 hospitals | 0 beds |
| Totals: | 4 hospitals | 377 beds |

---

**★5205:   DIGNITY HEALTH** (CC)
185 Berry Street, Suite 300, San Francisco, CA Zip 94107–1773; tel. 415/438–5500; Lloyd H. Dean, President and Chief Executive Officer
**(Decentralized Health System)**

**ARIZONA:** CHANDLER REGIONAL MEDICAL CENTER (O, 224 beds) 1955 West Frye Road, Chandler, AZ Zip 85224–4230; tel. 480/728–3000; Tim Bricker, President and Chief Executive Officer
**Web address:** www.chandlerregional.com

MERCY GILBERT MEDICAL CENTER (S, 212 beds) 3555 South Val Vista Road, Gilbert, AZ Zip 85297; tel. 480/728–8000; Tim Bricker, President and Chief Executive Officer
**Web address:** www.mercygilbert.org

ST. JOSEPH'S HOSPITAL AND MEDICAL CENTER (S, 697 beds) 350 West Thomas Road, Phoenix, AZ Zip 85013–4496, Mailing Address: P.O. Box 2071, Zip 85001–2071; tel. 602/406–3000; Linda A. Hunt, President
**Web address:** www.stjosephs–phx.org

**CALIFORNIA:** ARROYO GRANDE COMMUNITY HOSPITAL (O, 67 beds) 345 South Halcyon Road, Arroyo Grande, CA Zip 93420–3899; tel. 805/489–4261; Kenneth Dalebout, Chief Administrative Officer
**Web address:** www.arroyograndehospital.org

BAKERSFIELD MEMORIAL HOSPITAL (O, 255 beds) 420 34th Street, Bakersfield, CA Zip 93301–2237; tel. 661/327–1792; Jon Van Boening, President and Chief Executive Officer
**Web address:** www.bakersfieldmemorial.org

CALIFORNIA HOSPITAL MEDICAL CENTER (O, 318 beds) 1401 South Grand Avenue, Los Angeles, CA Zip 90015–3010; tel. 213/748–2411; Gerald B. Clute, President and Chief Executive Officer
**Web address:** www.chmcla.org

COMMUNITY HOSPITAL OF SAN BERNARDINO (O, 321 beds) 1805 Medical Center Drive, San Bernardino, CA Zip 92411–1214; tel. 909/887–6333; June Collison, President
**Web address:** www.chsb.org

DOMINICAN HOSPITAL (S, 276 beds) 1555 Soquel Drive, Santa Cruz, CA Zip 95065–1794; tel. 831/462–7700; Nanette Mickiewicz, M.D., President and Chief Medical Officer
**Web address:** www.dominicanhospital.org

FRENCH HOSPITAL MEDICAL CENTER (O, 112 beds) 1911 Johnson Avenue, San Luis Obispo, CA Zip 93401–4131; tel. 805/543–5353; Alan Iftiniuk, Chief Executive Officer
**Web address:** www.frenchmedicalcenter.org

GLENDALE MEMORIAL HOSPITAL AND HEALTH CENTER (O, 334 beds) 1420 South Central Avenue, Glendale, CA Zip 91204–2508; tel. 818/502–1900; Mark A. Meyers, President
**Web address:** www.glendalememorial.com

MARIAN MEDICAL CENTER (S, 256 beds) 1400 East Church Street, Santa Maria, CA Zip 93454–5906; tel. 805/739–3000; Charles J. Cova, President and Chief Executive Officer
**Web address:** www.marianmedicalcenter.org

MARK TWAIN ST. JOSEPH'S HOSPITAL (O, 30 beds) 768 Mountain Ranch Road, San Andreas, CA Zip 95249–9707; tel. 209/754–3521; Craig J. Marks, FACHE, President
**Web address:** www.marktwainhospital.com

MERCY GENERAL HOSPITAL (S, 286 beds) 4001 J Street, Sacramento, CA Zip 95819–3600; tel. 916/453–4545; Phyllis Baltz, Interim President
**Web address:** www.mercygeneral.org

MERCY HOSPITAL OF FOLSOM (S, 106 beds) 1650 Creekside Drive, Folsom, CA Zip 95630–3405; tel. 916/983–7400; Donald C. Hudson, President
**Web address:** www.mercyfolsom.org

MERCY HOSPITALS OF BAKERSFIELD (S, 269 beds) 2215 Truxtun Avenue, Bakersfield, CA Zip 93301–3698, Mailing Address: P.O. Box 119, Zip 93302–0119; tel. 661/632–5000; Russell V. Judd, President
**Web address:** www.mercybakersfield.org

---

For explanation of codes following names, see page B2.
★ Indicates Type III membership in the American Hospital Association.

Section B

MERCY MEDICAL CENTER MERCED (S, 186 beds) 333 Mercy Avenue, Merced, CA Zip 95340–8319; tel. 209/564–5000; David S. Dunham, President
**Web address:** www.mercymercedcares.org

MERCY MEDICAL CENTER MOUNT SHASTA (S, 33 beds) 914 Pine Street, Mount Shasta, CA Zip 96067–2143; tel. 530/926–6111; Kenneth E. S. Platou, President
**Web address:** www.mercymtshasta.org

MERCY MEDICAL CENTER REDDING (S, 261 beds) 2175 Rosaline Avenue, Redding, CA Zip 96001–2509, Mailing Address: P.O. Box 496009, Zip 96049–6009; tel. 530/225–6000; Mark Korth, Chief Executive Officer
**Web address:** www.mercy.org

MERCY SAN JUAN MEDICAL CENTER (S, 359 beds) 6501 Coyle Avenue, Carmichael, CA Zip 95608–0306, Mailing Address: P.O. Box 479, Zip 95609–0479; tel. 916/537–5000; Brian K. Ivie, President
**Web address:** www.mercysanjuan.org

METHODIST HOSPITAL OF SACRAMENTO (O, 325 beds) 7500 Hospital Drive, Sacramento, CA Zip 95823–5477; tel. 916/423–3000; Eugene Bassett, Interim President and Chief Executive Officer
**Web address:** www.methodistsacramento.org

NORTHRIDGE HOSPITAL MEDICAL CENTER–ROSCOE BOULEVARD CAMPUS (O, 371 beds) 18300 Roscoe Boulevard, Northridge, CA Zip 91328–4167; tel. 818/885–8500; Michael L. Wall, President
**Web address:** www.northridgehospital.org

OAK VALLEY HOSPITAL DISTRICT (O, 150 beds) 350 South Oak Street, Oakdale, CA Zip 95361–3519; tel. 209/847–3011; John P. Friel, Chief Executive Officer
**Web address:** www.oakvalleycares.org

SAINT FRANCIS MEMORIAL HOSPITAL (O, 239 beds) 900 Hyde Street, San Francisco, CA Zip 94109–4899, Mailing Address: P.O. Box 7726, Zip 94120–7726; tel. 415/353–6000; Thomas G. Hennessy, President and Chief Executive Officer
**Web address:** www.saintfrancismemorial.org

SEQUOIA HOSPITAL (O, 153 beds) 170 Alameda De Las Pulgas, Redwood City, CA Zip 94062–2799; tel. 650/369–5811; Glenna L. Vaskelis, CPA, President and Administrator
**Web address:** www.sequoiahospital.org

SIERRA NEVADA MEMORIAL HOSPITAL (O, 121 beds) 155 Glasson Way, Grass Valley, CA Zip 95945–5723, Mailing Address: P.O. Box 1029, Zip 95945–1029; tel. 530/274–6000; Katherine Medeiros, President and Chief Executive Officer
**Web address:** www.snmh.org

ST. BERNARDINE MEDICAL CENTER (S, 250 beds) 2101 North Waterman Avenue, San Bernardino, CA Zip 92404–4836; tel. 909/883–8711; Steven R. Barron, President
**Web address:** www.stbernardinemedicalcenter.com

ST. ELIZABETH COMMUNITY HOSPITAL (S, 65 beds) 2550 Sister Mary Columba Drive, Red Bluff, CA Zip 96080–4397; tel. 530/529–8000; Jon W. Halfhide, President
**Web address:** www.mercy.org

ST. JOHN'S PLEASANT VALLEY HOSPITAL (S, 127 beds) 2309 Antonio Avenue, Camarillo, CA Zip 93010–1414; tel. 805/389–5800; Laurie Eberst, R.N., President and Chief Executive Officer
**Web address:** www.stjohnshealth.org

ST. JOHN'S REGIONAL MEDICAL CENTER (S, 266 beds) 1600 North Rose Avenue, Oxnard, CA Zip 93030–3723; tel. 805/988–2500; Laurie Eberst, R.N., President and Chief Executive Officer
**Web address:** www.stjohnshealth.org

ST. JOSEPH'S BEHAVIORAL HEALTH CENTER (S, 35 beds) 2510 North California Street, Stockton, CA Zip 95204–5502; tel. 209/461–2000; Paul Rains, R.N., MSN, President
**Web address:** www.stjosephscanhelp.org

ST. JOSEPH'S MEDICAL CENTER (S, 273 beds) 1800 North California Street, Stockton, CA Zip 95204–6019, Mailing Address: P.O. Box 213008, Zip 95213–3008; tel. 209/943–2000; Donald J. Wiley, President and Chief Executive Officer
**Web address:** www.stjosephsCARES.org

ST. MARY MEDICAL CENTER (S, 165 beds) 1050 Linden Avenue, Long Beach, CA Zip 90813, Mailing Address: P.O. Box 887, Zip 90801–0887; tel. 562/491–9000; Thomas A. Salerno, President
**Web address:** www.stmarymedicalcenter.org

ST. MARY'S MEDICAL CENTER (S, 232 beds) 450 Stanyan Street, San Francisco, CA Zip 94117–1079; tel. 415/668–1000; Anna Cheung, President
**Web address:** www.stmarysmedicalcenter.com

WOODLAND HEALTHCARE (O, 111 beds) 1325 Cottonwood Street, Woodland, CA Zip 95695–5199; tel. 530/662–3961; H. Kevin Vaziri, President
**Web address:** www.woodlandhealthcare.org

**NEVADA:** ST. ROSE DOMINICAN HOSPITALS – ROSE DE LIMA CAMPUS (S, 129 beds) 102 East Lake Mead Parkway, Henderson, NV Zip 89015–5524; tel. 702/616–5000; Allan M. Spooner, Interim President and Chief Executive Officer
**Web address:** www.strosecares.com

ST. ROSE DOMINICAN HOSPITALS – SAN MARTIN CAMPUS (O, 147 beds) 8280 West Warm Springs Road, Las Vegas, NV Zip 89113; tel. 702/492–8000; Victoria J. VanMeetren, President
**Web address:** www.strosehospitals.org

ST. ROSE DOMINICAN HOSPITALS – SIENA CAMPUS (S, 219 beds) 3001 St. Rose Parkway, Henderson, NV Zip 89052; tel. 702/616–5000; Rod A. Davis, FACHE, President and Chief Executive Officer
**Web address:** www.strosehospitals.com

| Owned, leased, sponsored: | 37 hospitals | 7980 beds |
|---|---|---|
| Contract–managed: | 0 hospitals | 0 beds |
| **Totals:** | 37 hospitals | 7980 beds |

---

**0029:  DIMENSIONS HEALTHCARE SYSTEM** (NP)
3001 Hospital Drive, 3rd Floor, Cheverly, MD Zip 20785; tel. 301/583–4000; Kenneth E. Glover, President and Chief Executive Officer
**(Moderately Centralized Health System)**

**MARYLAND:** LAUREL REGIONAL HOSPITAL (O, 124 beds) 7300 Van Dusen Road, Laurel, MD Zip 20707–9266; tel. 301/725–4300; Gloria Ceballos, R.N., MS, Interim President
**Web address:** www.laurelregionalhospital.org

PRINCE GEORGE'S HOSPITAL CENTER (O, 411 beds) 3001 Hospital Drive, Cheverly, MD Zip 20785–1189; tel. 301/618–2000; John A. O'Brien, FACHE, President
**Web address:** www.princegeorgeshospital.org

| Owned, leased, sponsored: | 2 hospitals | 535 beds |
|---|---|---|
| Contract–managed: | 0 hospitals | 0 beds |
| **Totals:** | 2 hospitals | 535 beds |

---

**0010:  DIVISION OF MENTAL HEALTH AND ADDICTION SERVICES, DEPARTMENT OF HUMAN SERVICES, STATE OF NEW JERSEY** (NP)
Capital Center, P.O. Box 727, Trenton, NJ Zip 08625–0727; tel. 609/777–0702; Lynn Kovich, Assistant Commissioner
**(Independent Hospital System)**

**NEW JERSEY:** ANCORA PSYCHIATRIC HOSPITAL (O, 500 beds) 301 Spring Garden Road, Ancora, NJ Zip 08037–9699; tel. 609/561–1700; Allan Boyer, Chief Executive Officer
**Web address:** www.peoplefirstnurses.nj.gov/ancora.htm

ARTHUR BRISBANE CHILDREN TREATMENT CENTER (O, 92 beds) County Road 524, Farmingdale, NJ Zip 07727, Mailing Address: P.O. Box 625, Zip 07727; Vincent Giampeitro, Chief Executive Officer

GREYSTONE PARK PSYCHIATRIC HOSPITAL (O, 557 beds) 59 Koch Avenue, Morris Plains, NJ Zip 07950–1005; tel. 973/538–1800; Janet J. Monroe, R.N., Chief Executive Officer
**Web address:** www.state.nj.us/humanservices/pfnurse/greystone.htm

SENATOR GARRETT W. HAGEDORN PSYCHIATRIC HOSPITAL (O, 288 beds) 200 Sanatorium Road, Glen Gardner, NJ Zip 08826–3291; tel. 908/537–2141; Mary Jo Kurtiak, Interim Chief Executive Officer
**Web address:** www.state.nj.us

For explanation of codes following names, see page B2.
★ Indicates Type III membership in the American Hospital Association.

TRENTON PSYCHIATRIC HOSPITAL (O, 392 beds) Route 29 and Sullivan Way, Trenton, NJ Zip 08628–3425, Mailing Address: P.O. Box 7500, West Trenton, Zip 08628–7500; tel. 609/633–1500; Teresa A. McQuaide, Chief Executive Officer
**Web address:** www.nj.gov/

| Owned, leased, sponsored: | 5 hospitals | 1829 beds |
|---|---|---|
| Contract–managed: | 0 hospitals | 0 beds |
| Totals: | 5 hospitals | 1829 beds |

---

**0536: DIVISION OF MENTAL HEALTH, DEPARTMENT OF HUMAN SERVICES** (NP)
319 East Madison Street, S–3B, Springfield, IL Zip 62701; tel. 217/785–6023; Lorrie Rickman Jones, Ph.D., Director
**(Independent Hospital System)**

**ILLINOIS:** ALTON MENTAL HEALTH CENTER (O, 165 beds) 4500 College Avenue, Alton, IL Zip 62002–5099; tel. 618/474–3800; Brian E. Thomas, Administrator

CHESTER MENTAL HEALTH CENTER (O, 245 beds) Chester Road, Chester, IL Zip 62233–0031, Mailing Address: Box 31, Zip 62233–0031; tel. 618/826–4571; Melissa Gross, Interim Administrator

CHICAGO–READ MENTAL HEALTH CENTER (O, 200 beds) 4200 North Oak Park Avenue, Chicago, IL Zip 60634–1457; tel. 773/794–4000; Thomas Simpatico, M.D., Facility Director and Network System Manager

CHOATE MENTAL HEALTH CENTER (O, 79 beds) 1000 North Main Street, Anna, IL Zip 62906–1699; tel. 618/833–5161; Elaine Ray, Administrator

ELGIN MENTAL HEALTH CENTER (O, 500 beds) 750 South State Street, Elgin, IL Zip 60123–7692; tel. 847/742–1040; Amparo Lopez, Region Executive Director
**Web address:** www.dhs.state.il.us

H. DOUGLAS SINGER MENTAL HEALTH AND DEVELOPMENTAL CENTER (O, 162 beds) 4402 North Main Street, Rockford, IL Zip 61103–1278; tel. 815/987–7096; Gail Tennant, Director

JOHN J. MADDEN MENTAL HEALTH CENTER (O, 150 beds) 1200 South First Avenue, Hines, IL Zip 60141; tel. 708/338–7202; Edith Newman, Interim Administrator

| Owned, leased, sponsored: | 7 hospitals | 1501 beds |
|---|---|---|
| Contract–managed: | 0 hospitals | 0 beds |
| Totals: | 7 hospitals | 1501 beds |

---

**★0226: DUBUIS HEALTH SYSTEM** (CC)
1700 West Loop South, Suite 1100A, Houston, TX Zip 77027–3007; tel. 713/277–2300; Stephen Mills, Chief Executive Officer
**(Independent Hospital System)**

**ARKANSAS:** ADVANCE CARE HOSPITAL (C, 26 beds) 300 Werner Street, 3rd Floor East, Hot Springs National Park, AR Zip 71913; tel. 501/609–4300; Keith Rogers, Administrator
**Web address:** www.dubuis.org

ADVANCE CARE HOSPITAL OF FORT SMITH (C, 25 beds) 7301 Rogers Avenue, 4th Floor, Fort Smith, AR Zip 72917; tel. 479/314–4900; Keith Rogers, Interim Administrator
**Web address:** www.dubuis.org

**GEORGIA:** SOUTHERN CRESCENT HOSPITAL FOR SPECIALTY CARE (C, 30 beds) 11 Upper Riverdale Road S.W., 6th Floor, Riverdale, GA Zip 30274; tel. 770/897–7603; Janice Hamilton–Crawford, Administrator

**IOWA:** CONTINUING CARE HOSPITAL AT ST. LUKE'S (C, 17 beds) 1026 A Avenue N.E., 6th Floor, Cedar Rapids, IA Zip 52402; tel. 319/369–8142; Elly Steffen, Chief Executive Officer and Administrator
**Web address:** www.stlukescr.org

**LOUISIANA:** DUBUIS HOSPITAL OF ALEXANDRIA (O, 33 beds) 3330 Masonic Drive, 4th Floor, Alexandria, LA Zip 71301; tel. 318/448–6505; Stephen D. Peters, Administrator
**Web address:** www.dubuis.org

DUBUIS HOSPITAL OF LAKE CHARLES (O, 23 beds) 524 Dr. Michael DeBakey Drive, 5th Floor, Lake Charles, LA Zip 70601–5725; tel. 337/491–7752; William L. Willis, Administrator
**Web address:** www.dubuis.com

DUBUIS HOSPITAL OF SHREVEPORT (O, 36 beds) One St. Mary Place, 6th Floor, Shreveport, LA Zip 71101; tel. 318/221–3802; Holly Powell, Interim Administrator
**Web address:** www.dubuis.org

**MISSOURI:** MERCY CONTINUING CARE HOSPITAL (O, 54 beds) 13190 South Outer Forty Road, Chesterfield, MO Zip 63017–5917; tel. 314/392–6380; Matthew B. Schweigert, Administrator
**Web address:** www.dubuis.org

**TEXAS:** CHRISTUS DUBUIS HOSPITAL OF BRYAN (O, 30 beds) 1600 Joseph Drive, 2nd Floor, Bryan, TX Zip 77802; tel. 979/821–5000; Randy E. Johnson, Administrator
**Web address:** www.dubuis.org

CHRISTUS DUBUIS HOSPITAL OF PORT ARTHUR (O, 15 beds) 3600 Gates Boulevard, Port Arthur, TX Zip 77642; tel. 409/989–5300; Barbara Flournoy, Administrator
**Web address:** www.dubuis.org

DUBUIS HOSPITAL OF BEAUMONT (O, 51 beds) 2830 Calder Avenue, 4th Floor, Beaumont, TX Zip 77702; tel. 409/899–8154; Tim Freeman, Administrator
**Web address:** www.dubuis.org

DUBUIS HOSPITAL OF CORPUS CHRISTI (O, 22 beds) 600 Elizabeth Street, 3rd Floor, Corpus Christi, TX Zip 78404; tel. 361/881–3223; Diane Kaiser, Administrator
**Web address:** www.dubuis.org

DUBUIS HOSPITAL OF PARIS (O, 25 beds) 865 Deshong Drive, 5th Floor, Paris, TX Zip 75462; tel. 903/782–2960; Kathie Reese, Administrator
**Web address:** www.dubuis.org

DUBUIS HOSPITAL OF TEXARKANA (O, 49 beds) 2400 St. Michael Drive, 2nd Floor, Texarkana, TX Zip 75503–2372; tel. 903/614–7600; Holly Powell, Administrator
**Web address:** www.dubuis.org

| Owned, leased, sponsored: | 10 hospitals | 338 beds |
|---|---|---|
| Contract–managed: | 4 hospitals | 98 beds |
| Totals: | 14 hospitals | 436 beds |

---

**0861: DUKE LIFEPOINT HEALTHCARE** (IO)
103 Powell Court, Brentwood, TN Zip 37027–5079; Jeffrey G. Seraphine, FACHE, Division President

**NORTH CAROLINA:** MARIA PARHAM MEDICAL CENTER (O, 102 beds) 566 Ruin Creek Road, Henderson, NC Zip 27536–2957; tel. 252/438–4143; Robert G. Singletary, President and Chief Executive Officer
**Web address:** www.mariaparham.com

PERSON MEMORIAL HOSPITAL (O, 110 beds) 615 Ridge Road, Roxboro, NC Zip 27573–4630; tel. 336/599–2121; Chad Brown, M.P.H., Chief Executive Officer
**Web address:** www.personhospital.com

**VIRGINIA:** TWIN COUNTY REGIONAL HOSPITAL (O, 86 beds) 200 Hospital Drive, Galax, VA Zip 24333–2283; tel. 276/236–8181; Jon D. Applebaum, President and Chief Executive Officer
**Web address:** www.tcrh.org

| Owned, leased, sponsored: | 3 hospitals | 298 beds |
|---|---|---|
| Contract–managed: | 0 hospitals | 0 beds |
| Totals: | 3 hospitals | 298 beds |

---

**★0190: DUKE UNIVERSITY HEALTH SYSTEM** (NP)
201 Trent Drive, Durham, NC Zip 27710, Mailing Address: P.O. Box 3701, Zip 27710–3701; tel. 919/684–2255; Victor J. Dzau, M.D., President and Chief Executive Officer
**(Centralized Health System)**

**NORTH CAROLINA:** DUKE RALEIGH HOSPITAL (O, 148 beds) 3400 Wake Forest Road, Raleigh, NC Zip 27609–7373, Mailing Address: P.O. Box 28280, Zip 27611–8280; tel. 919/954–3000; Douglas B. Vinsel, FACHE, Chief Executive Officer
**Web address:** www.dukehealthraleigh.org

DUKE UNIVERSITY HOSPITAL (O, 813 beds) 2301 Erwin Road, Durham, NC Zip 27710–0001, Mailing Address: P.O. Box 3708, Zip 27710–3708; tel. 919/684–8111; Kevin W. Sowers, R.N., MSN, Chief Executive Officer
**Web address:** www.dukehealth.org

For explanation of codes following names, see page B2.
★ Indicates Type III membership in the American Hospital Association.

DURHAM REGIONAL HOSPITAL (L, 202 beds) 3643 North Roxboro Road, Durham, NC Zip 27704–2763; tel. 919/470–4000; Kerry Watson, President
**Web address:** www.durhamregional.org

| | | |
|---|---|---|
| **Owned, leased, sponsored:** | 3 hospitals | 1163 beds |
| **Contract–managed:** | 0 hospitals | 0 beds |
| **Totals:** | 3 hospitals | 1163 beds |

● **0286:  DYNACQ HEALTHCARE, INC.** (IO)
10304 Interstate 10 East, Suite 369, Houston, TX Zip 77029; tel. 713/367–2000; Chiu Moon Chan, Chairman, President and Chief Executive Officer
**(Independent Hospital System)**

**TEXAS:** SURGERY SPECIALTY HOSPITALS OF AMERICA (O, 37 beds) 4301B Vista, Pasadena, TX Zip 77504; tel. 713/378–3000; Celia Barrera, Administrator

| | | |
|---|---|---|
| **Owned, leased, sponsored:** | 1 hospital | 37 beds |
| **Contract–managed:** | 0 hospitals | 0 beds |
| **Totals:** | 1 hospital | 37 beds |

★ **1895:  EAST TEXAS MEDICAL CENTER REGIONAL HEALTHCARE SYSTEM** (NP)
1000 South Beckham Street, Tyler, TX Zip 75701–1996, Mailing Address: P.O. Box 6400, Zip 75711–6400; tel. 903/535–6211; Elmer G. Ellis, FACHE, President and Chief Executive Officer
**(Centralized Physician/Insurance Health System)**

EAST TEXAS MEDICAL CENTER ATHENS (L, 117 beds) 2000 South Palestine Street, Athens, TX Zip 75751–5610; tel. 903/676–1000; Patrick L. Wallace, Administrator

EAST TEXAS MEDICAL CENTER CARTHAGE (L, 37 beds) 409 Cottage Road, Carthage, TX Zip 75633–1466, Mailing Address: P.O. Box 549, Zip 75633–0549; tel. 903/693–3841; Gary Mikeal Hudson, Administrator
**Web address:** www.etmc.org

EAST TEXAS MEDICAL CENTER CLARKSVILLE (L, 36 beds) 3000 West Main Street, Clarksville, TX Zip 75426, Mailing Address: P.O. Box 1270, Zip 75426–1270; tel. 903/427–6400; John S. Hart, Administrator
**Web address:** www.etmc.org

EAST TEXAS MEDICAL CENTER CROCKETT (L, 49 beds) 1100 Loop 304 East, Crockett, TX Zip 75835–1810; tel. 936/546–3862; Terry Cutler, Administrator and Chief Operating Officer
**Web address:** www.etmc.org

EAST TEXAS MEDICAL CENTER FAIRFIELD (L, 20 beds) 125 Newman Street, Fairfield, TX Zip 75840–1499; tel. 903/389–2121; Ruth Cook, Administrator
**Web address:** www.etmc.org

EAST TEXAS MEDICAL CENTER HENDERSON (O, 47 beds) 300 Wilson Street, Henderson, TX Zip 75652–5956; tel. 903/657–7541; Mark Leitner, Chief Executive Officer
**Web address:** www.etmc.org/etmchenderson

EAST TEXAS MEDICAL CENTER JACKSONVILLE (O, 38 beds) 501 South Ragsdale Street, Jacksonville, TX Zip 75766–2413; tel. 903/541–5000; Jack R. Endres, Administrator
**Web address:** www.etmc.org

EAST TEXAS MEDICAL CENTER PITTSBURG (L, 25 beds) 2701 Highway 271 North, Pittsburg, TX Zip 75686–1032; tel. 903/946–5000; W. Perry Henderson, Administrator
**Web address:** www.etmc.org

EAST TEXAS MEDICAL CENTER REHABILITATION CENTER (O, 49 beds) 701 Olympic Plaza Circle, Tyler, TX Zip 75701–1996; tel. 903/596–3000; Eddie L. Howard, Vice President and Chief Operating Officer
**Web address:** www.etmc.org

EAST TEXAS MEDICAL CENTER SPECIALTY HOSPITAL (O, 36 beds) 1000 South Beckham, 5th Floor, Tyler, TX Zip 75701; tel. 903/596–3600; Eddie L. Howard, Vice President, Chief Operating Officer and Administrator
**Web address:** www.etmc.org

EAST TEXAS MEDICAL CENTER TRINITY (L, 22 beds) 317 Prospect Drive, Trinity, TX Zip 75862, Mailing Address: P.O. Box 3169, Zip 75862; tel. 936/744–1100; Brett Kirkham, Administrator
**Web address:** www.etmc.org

EAST TEXAS MEDICAL CENTER TYLER (O, 450 beds) 1000 South Beckham Street, Tyler, TX Zip 75701–1996, Mailing Address: Box 6400, Zip 75711–6400; tel. 903/597–0351; Robert B. Evans, Administrator and Chief Executive Officer
**Web address:** www.etmc.org

EAST TEXAS MEDICAL CENTER–GILMER (O, 35 beds) 712 North Wood Street, Gilmer, TX Zip 75644–1751; tel. 903/841–7100; Jorge E. Leal, Administrator
**Web address:** www.etmc.org

EAST TEXAS MEDICAL CENTER–MOUNT VERNON (L, 30 beds) 500 Highway 37 South, Mount Vernon, TX Zip 75457–3602, Mailing Address: P.O. Box 477, Zip 75457–0477; tel. 903/537–8000; David Bailey, Administrator
**Web address:** www.etmc.org

EAST TEXAS MEDICAL CENTER–QUITMAN (L, 25 beds) 117 Winnsboro Street, Quitman, TX Zip 75783–2144, Mailing Address: P.O. Box 1000, Zip 75783–1000; tel. 903/763–6300; Warren Robicheaux, Administrator
**Web address:** www.etmc.org

| | | |
|---|---|---|
| **Owned, leased, sponsored:** | 15 hospitals | 1016 beds |
| **Contract–managed:** | 0 hospitals | 0 beds |
| **Totals:** | 15 hospitals | 1016 beds |

★● **0270:  EASTERN CONNECTICUT HEALTH NETWORK** (NP)
71 Haynes Street, Manchester, CT Zip 06040–4131; tel. 860/533–3400; Peter J. Karl, President and Chief Executive Officer
**(Centralized Physician/Insurance Health System)**

**CONNECTICUT:** MANCHESTER MEMORIAL HOSPITAL (O, 156 beds) 71 Haynes Street, Manchester, CT Zip 06040–4188; tel. 860/646–1222; Peter J. Karl, President and Chief Executive Officer
**Web address:** www.echn.org

ROCKVILLE GENERAL HOSPITAL (O, 47 beds) 31 Union Street, Vernon Rockville, CT Zip 06066–3160; tel. 860/872–0501; Peter J. Karl, President and Chief Executive Officer
**Web address:** www.echn.org

| | | |
|---|---|---|
| **Owned, leased, sponsored:** | 2 hospitals | 203 beds |
| **Contract–managed:** | 0 hospitals | 0 beds |
| **Totals:** | 2 hospitals | 203 beds |

★ **0555:  EASTERN MAINE HEALTHCARE SYSTEMS** (NP)
43 Whiting Hill Road, Brewer, ME Zip 04412; tel. 207/973–7045; M. Michelle Hood, President and Chief Executive Officer
**(Centralized Health System)**

**MAINE:** BLUE HILL MEMORIAL HOSPITAL (O, 25 beds) 57 Water Street, Blue Hill, ME Zip 04614–0823, Mailing Address: P.O. Box 1029, Zip 04614–1029; tel. 207/374–3400; Gregory E. Roraff, President and Chief Executive Officer
**Web address:** www.bhmh.org

CHARLES A. DEAN MEMORIAL HOSPITAL (O, 36 beds) 364 Pritham Avenue, Greenville, ME Zip 04441–1395, Mailing Address: P.O. Box 1129, Zip 04441–1129; tel. 207/695–5200; Geno Murray, President and Chief Executive Officer
**Web address:** www.cadean.org

EASTERN MAINE MEDICAL CENTER (O, 349 beds) 489 State Street, Bangor, ME Zip 04401–6674, Mailing Address: P.O. Box 404, Zip 04402–0404; tel. 207/973–7000; Deborah Carey Johnson, R.N., President and Chief Executive Officer
**Web address:** www.emh.org

INLAND HOSPITAL (O, 46 beds) 200 Kennedy Memorial Drive, Waterville, ME Zip 04901–4595; tel. 207/861–3000; John Dalton, President and Chief Executive Officer
**Web address:** www.inlandhospital.org

SEBASTICOOK VALLEY HEALTH (O, 25 beds) 447 North Main Street, Pittsfield, ME Zip 04967–1199; tel. 207/487–4000; Victoria Alexander–Lane, President and Chief Executive Officer
**Web address:** www.sebasticookvalleyhealth.org

THE ACADIA HOSPITAL (O, 72 beds) 268 Stillwater Avenue, Bangor, ME Zip 04401–3945, Mailing Address: P.O. Box 422, Zip 04402–0422; tel. 207/973–6100; Daniel B. Coffey, President and Chief Executive Officer
**Web address:** www.acadiahospital.org

THE AROOSTOOK MEDICAL CENTER (O, 122 beds) 140 Academy Street, Presque Isle, ME Zip 04769–3171, Mailing Address: P.O. Box 151, Zip 04769–0151; tel. 207/768–4000; Sylvia Getman, President and Chief Executive Officer
**Web address:** www.tamc.org

| Owned, leased, sponsored: | 7 hospitals | 675 beds |
|---|---|---|
| Contract–managed: | 0 hospitals | 0 beds |
| Totals: | 7 hospitals | 675 beds |

★**0256:  EMORY HEALTHCARE** (NP)
1440 Clifton Road N.E., Suite 145, Atlanta, GA Zip 30322–1102; tel. 404/778–5000; John T. Fox, Chief Executive Officer
**(Centralized Health System)**

**GEORGIA:** EMORY JOHNS CREEK HOSPITAL (O, 84 beds) 6325 Hospital Parkway, Johns Creek, GA Zip 30097; tel. 678/474–7000; Craig McCoy, Chief Executive Officer
**Web address:** www.emoryjohnscreek.com

EMORY UNIVERSITY HOSPITAL (O, 579 beds) 1364 Clifton Road N.E., Atlanta, GA Zip 30322–1102; tel. 404/712–2000; Robert J. Bachman, Chief Operating Officer
**Web address:** www.emoryhealthcare.org

EMORY UNIVERSITY HOSPITAL MIDTOWN (O, 469 beds) 550 Peachtree Street N.E., Atlanta, GA Zip 30308; tel. 404/686–4411; Dane C. Peterson, Chief Operating Officer
**Web address:** www.emoryhealthcare.org

WESLEY WOODS GERIATRIC HOSPITAL OF EMORY UNIVERSITY (O, 276 beds) 1821 Clifton Road N.E., Atlanta, GA Zip 30329–5102; tel. 404/728–6200; William Such, Chief Executive Officer
**Web address:** www.emoryhealthcare.org

WESLEY WOODS LONG TERM CARE HOSPITAL (O, 18 beds) 1821 Clifton Road N.E., 2nd Floor, Atlanta, GA Zip 30329; tel. 404/728–6200; William Such, Chief Executive Officer
**Web address:** www.emoryhealthcare.org

| Owned, leased, sponsored: | 5 hospitals | 1426 beds |
|---|---|---|
| Contract–managed: | 0 hospitals | 0 beds |
| Totals: | 5 hospitals | 1426 beds |

**0647:  ENCORE HEALTHCARE** (IO)
7150 Columbia Gateway Drove, Suite J., Columbia, MD Zip 21046–2974; tel. 443/539–2350; Tim Nicholson, Chief Executive Officer
**(Independent Hospital System)**

**OKLAHOMA:** SPECIALTY HOSPITAL OF MIDWEST CITY (O, 31 beds) 8210 National Avenue, Midwest City, OK Zip 73110; tel. 405/739–0800; Chad Lovett, Chief Executive Officer
**Web address:** www.specialtyhospitalmidwestcity.com/specialty_midwest/index.aspx

**TEXAS:** CORPUS CHRISTI SPECIALTY HOSPITAL (O, 31 beds) 1310 Third Street, Corpus Christi, TX Zip 78404–2208; tel. 361/888–4323; Judy Wolfe, Chief Executive Officer
**Web address:** www.encore–healthcare.com

MESA HILLS SPECIALTY HOSPITAL (O, 32 beds) 2311 North Oregon Street, El Paso, TX Zip 79902–3216; tel. 915/545–1823; William Balay, Jr., Chief Executive Officer
**Web address:** www.ihs–inc.com

PLANO SPECIALTY HOSPITAL (O, 43 beds) 1621 Coit Road, Plano, TX Zip 75075; tel. 972/758–5200; Jerry Amato, Chief Executive Officer
**Web address:** www.planospecialtyhospital.com

PLUM CREEK SPECIALTY HOSPITAL (O, 47 beds) 5601 Plum Creek Drive, Amarillo, TX Zip 79124–1801; tel. 806/351–1000; Billy Blasingame, Chief Executive Officer
**Web address:** www.specialtyhospital–plumcreek.net

| Owned, leased, sponsored: | 5 hospitals | 184 beds |
|---|---|---|
| Contract–managed: | 0 hospitals | 0 beds |
| Totals: | 5 hospitals | 184 beds |

**0525:  ERLANGER HEALTH SYSTEM** (NP)
975 East Third Street, Chattanooga, TN Zip 37403; tel. 423/778–7000; Charlesetta Woodard–Thompson, President and Chief Executive Officer
**(Independent Hospital System)**

**GEORGIA:** ERLANGER AT HUTCHESON (C, 185 beds) 100 Gross Crescent Circle, Fort Oglethorpe, GA Zip 30742–3669; tel. 706/858–2000; Roger Forgey, President and Chief Executive Officer
**Web address:** www.hutcheson.org

**TENNESSEE:** ERLANGER BLEDSOE HOSPITAL (C, 25 beds) 71 Wheeler Avenue, Pikeville, TN Zip 37367, Mailing Address: P.O. Box 699, Zip 37367–0699; tel. 423/447–2112; Stephanie Boynton, Administrator
**Web address:** www.erlanger.org

ERLANGER MEDICAL CENTER (O, 538 beds) 632 Morrison Springs Road, Chattanooga, TN Zip 37415; tel. 423/778–7000; Charlesetta Woodard–Thompson, President and Chief Executive Officer
**Web address:** www.erlanger.org

| Owned, leased, sponsored: | 1 hospital | 538 beds |
|---|---|---|
| Contract–managed: | 2 hospitals | 210 beds |
| Totals: | 3 hospitals | 748 beds |

**0382:  ERNEST HEALTH, INC.** (IO)
7770 Jefferson Street N.E., Suite 320, Albuquerque, NM Zip 87109; tel. 505/856–5300; Darby Brockette, Chief Executive Officer
**(Independent Hospital System)**

**ARIZONA:** MOUNTAIN VALLEY REGIONAL REHABILITATION HOSPITAL (O, 16 beds) 3700 North Windsong Drive, Prescott Valley, AZ Zip 86314; tel. 928/759–8800; Jennifer Roel, Chief Executive Officer
**Web address:** www.mvrrh.ernesthealth.com

**COLORADO:** NORTHERN COLORADO LONG TERM ACUTE HOSPITAL (O, 20 beds) 4401A Union Street, Johnstown, CO Zip 80534; tel. 970/619–3663; Joanne Fenton, MSN, FACHE, Chief Executive Officer
**Web address:** www.ncltah.ernesthealth.com/

NORTHERN COLORADO REHABILITATION HOSPITAL (O, 40 beds) 4401 Union Street, Johnstown, CO Zip 80534; tel. 970/619–3400; Sharon Scheller, Chief Executive Officer
**Web address:** www.ncrh.ernesthealth.com

**IDAHO:** NORTHERN IDAHO ADVANCED CARE HOSPITAL (O, 40 beds) 600 North Cecil Road, Post Falls, ID Zip 83854; tel. 208/262–2800; Richard M. Richards, Chief Executive Officer
**Web address:** www.niach.ernesthealth.com

SOUTHWEST IDAHO ADVANCED CARE HOSPITAL (O, 40 beds) Franklin Road and Allumbaugh Street, Boise, ID Zip 83706; tel. 208/376–5700; Nolan Hoffer, Chief Executive Officer
**Web address:** www.siach.ernesthealth.com/

**MONTANA:** ADVANCED CARE HOSPITAL OF MONTANA (O, 40 beds) 3528 Gabel Road, Billings, MT Zip 59102–7307; tel. 406/373–8000; Joseph McClure, Chief Executive Officer
**Web address:** www.achm.ernesthealth.com

**NEW MEXICO:** ADVANCED CARE HOSPITAL OF SOUTHERN NEW MEXICO (O, 40 beds) 4451 East Lohman Avenue, Las Cruces, NM Zip 88011; tel. 575/521–6600; Suzanne Quillen, R.N., Chief Executive Officer
**Web address:** www.achsnm.ernesthealth.com

REHABILITATION HOSPITAL OF SOUTHERN NEW MEXICO (O, 40 beds) 4441 East Lohman Avenue, Las Cruces, NM Zip 88011–8267; tel. 575/521–6400; Beverly Munoz, Chief Executive Officer
**Web address:** www.rhsnm.ernesthealth.com

**SOUTH CAROLINA:** GREENWOOD REGIONAL REHABILITATION HOSPITAL (O, 46 beds) 1530 Parkway, Greenwood, SC Zip 29646; tel. 864/330–9070; Timothy Kagle, Chief Executive Officer
**Web address:** www.grrh.ernesthealth.com

For explanation of codes following names, see page B2.
★ Indicates Type III membership in the American Hospital Association.

Section B

**TEXAS:** LAREDO SPECIALTY HOSPITAL (O, 60 beds) 2005 Bustamente Street, Laredo, TX Zip 78041–5470; tel. 956/753–5353; Mario Rodriguez, Chief Executive Officer
**Web address:** www.lsh.ernesthealth.com

MESQUITE REHABILITATION HOSPITAL (O, 20 beds) 1023 North Belt Line Road, Mesquite, TX Zip 75149–1788; tel. 972/216–2400; Brenda M. Antwine, Chief Executive Officer
**Web address:** www.mesquiterehab.ernesthealth.com

MESQUITE SPECIALTY HOSPITAL (O, 40 beds) 1024 North Galloway Avenue, Mesquite, TX Zip 75149–2434; tel. 972/216–2300; Brenda M. Antwine, Chief Executive Officer
**Web address:** www.msh.ernesthealth.com

NEW BRAUNFELS REGIONAL REHABILITATION HOSPITAL (O, 20 beds) 2041 Sundance Parkway, New Braunfels, TX Zip 78130–2779; tel. 830/625–6700; Jennifer Malatek, Chief Executive Officer
**Web address:** www.nbrrh.ernesthealth.com

SOUTH TEXAS REHABILITATION HOSPITAL (O, 40 beds) 425 East Alton Gloor Boulevard, Brownsville, TX Zip 78526; tel. 956/554–6000; Jessie Eason Smedley, Chief Executive Officer
**Web address:** www.strh.ernesthealth.com

**UTAH:** UTAH VALLEY SPECIALTY HOSPITAL (O, 40 beds) 306 West River Bend Lane, Provo, UT Zip 84604; tel. 801/226–8880; Marie Prothero, R.N., MSN, Chief Executive Officer
**Web address:** www.uvsh.ernesthealth.com

**WYOMING:** ELKHORN VALLEY REHABILITATION HOSPITAL (O, 40 beds) 5715 East 2nd Street, Casper, WY Zip 82609; tel. 307/265–0005; Michael Phillips, Chief Executive Officer
**Web address:** www.evrh.ernesthealth.com/

| | | |
|---|---|---|
| Owned, leased, sponsored: | 16 hospitals | 582 beds |
| Contract–managed: | 0 hospitals | 0 beds |
| Totals: | 16 hospitals | 582 beds |

**0396: ESSENTIA HEALTH** (NP)
502 East Second Street, Duluth, MN Zip 55805; tel. 218/786–8376; Peter E. Person, M.D., Chief Executive Officer
**(Moderately Centralized Health System)**

**IDAHO:** CLEARWATER VALLEY HOSPITAL AND CLINICS (O, 23 beds) 301 Cedar, Orofino, ID Zip 83544–9029; tel. 208/476–4555; Casey Meza, Chief Executive Officer
**Web address:** www.smh-cvhc.org

ST. LUKE'S JEROME FAMILY MEDICAL CENTER (O, 25 beds) 709 North Lincoln Street, Jerome, ID Zip 83338–1851, Mailing Address: P.O. Box 586, Zip 83338–0586; tel. 208/324–4301; James L. Angle, FACHE, Chief Executive Officer
**Web address:** www.stbenshospital.org

ST. MARY'S HOSPITAL (O, 28 beds) Lewiston and North Streets, Cottonwood, ID Zip 83522–9750, Mailing Address: P.O. Box 137, Zip 83522–0137; tel. 208/962–3251; Casey Meza, Chief Executive Officer
**Web address:** www.stmaryshospital.net

**MINNESOTA:** ESSENTIA HEALTH ADA (O, 14 beds) 201 9th Street West, Ada, MN Zip 56510–1243; tel. 218/784–5000; Ryan Hill, Interim Chief Executive Officer
**Web address:** www.essentiahealth.org

ESSENTIA HEALTH DULUTH (O, 154 beds) 502 East Second Street, Duluth, MN Zip 55805–1982; tel. 218/727–8762; Mike Metcalf, Chief Administrative Officer
**Web address:** www.smdcmedicalcenter.org

ESSENTIA HEALTH FOSSTON (O, 75 beds) 900 Hilligoss Boulevard S.E., Fosston, MN Zip 56542–1599; tel. 218/435–1133; Patricia Wangler, Chief Executive Officer
**Web address:** www.firstcare.org

ESSENTIA HEALTH NORTHERN PINES (O, 58 beds) 5211 Highway 110, Aurora, MN Zip 55705–1599; tel. 218/229–2211; Laura Ackman, Administrator
**Web address:** www.essentiahealth.org

ESSENTIA HEALTH SANDSTONE (O, 85 beds) 109 Court Avenue South, Sandstone, MN Zip 55072–5120; tel. 320/245–2212; Michael D. Hedrix, Interim Chief Executive Officer
**Web address:** www.pinemedicalcenter.org

ESSENTIA HEALTH ST. JOSEPH'S MEDICAL CENTER (O, 162 beds) 523 North Third Street, Brainerd, MN Zip 56401–3098; tel. 218/829–2861; Jani M. Wiebolt, President and Chief Executive Officer
**Web address:** www.sjmcmn.org

ESSENTIA HEALTH ST. MARY'S HOSPITAL – DETROIT LAKES (O, 58 beds) 1027 Washington Avenue, Detroit Lakes, MN Zip 56501–3598; tel. 218/847–5611; Peter Jacobson, President
**Web address:** www.trustedcareforlife.org

ESSENTIA HEALTH ST. MARY'S MEDICAL CENTER (O, 316 beds) 407 East Third Street, Duluth, MN Zip 55805–1984; tel. 218/786–4000; Daniel B. McGinty, Administrator
**Web address:** www.smdc.org

ESSENTIA HEALTH–HOLY TRINITY HOSPITAL (O, 65 beds) 115 West Second Street, Graceville, MN Zip 56240–0157, Mailing Address: P.O. Box 157, Zip 56240–0157; tel. 320/748–7223; Kevin Gish, Chief Executive Officer
**Web address:** www.essentiahealth.
org/HolyTrinityHospital/FindaClinic/Essentia–HealthHoly–Trinity–Hospital–96.aspx

MINNESOTA VALLEY HEALTH CENTER (O, 110 beds) 621 South Fourth Street, Le Sueur, MN Zip 56058–2298; tel. 507/665–3375; Patricia J. Townsdin–Woodruff, President and Chief Executive Officer
**Web address:** www.mvhc.org

**NORTH DAKOTA:** ESSENTIA HEALTH FARGO (O, 117 beds) 3000 32nd Avenue South, Fargo, ND Zip 58103; tel. 701/364–8000; Greg Glasner, M.D., Chief Executive Officer
**Web address:** www.essentiahealth.com

**WISCONSIN:** ESSENTIA HEALTH ST. MARY'S HOSPITAL OF SUPERIOR (O, 25 beds) 3500 Tower Avenue, Superior, WI Zip 54880–5395; tel. 715/395–5400; Mary Shaw, Chief Operating Officer
**Web address:** www.smdc.org

| | | |
|---|---|---|
| Owned, leased, sponsored: | 15 hospitals | 1315 beds |
| Contract–managed: | 0 hospitals | 0 beds |
| Totals: | 15 hospitals | 1315 beds |

**2395: EXCELA HEALTH** (NP)
532 West Pittsburgh Street, Greensburg, PA Zip 15601; tel. 724/832–5050; Robert Rogalski, Chief Executive Officer
**(Centralized Health System)**

**PENNSYLVANIA:** EXCELA FRICK HOSPITAL (O, 65 beds) 508 South Church Street, Mount Pleasant, PA Zip 15666–1790; tel. 724/547–1500; Ronald H. Ott, President
**Web address:** www.frickhospital.org

EXCELA HEALTH WESTMORELAND HOSPITAL (O, 359 beds) 532 West Pittsburgh Street, Greensburg, PA Zip 15601–2282; tel. 724/832–4000; Ronald H. Ott, President
**Web address:** www.excelahealth.org

EXCELA LATROBE AREA HOSPITAL (O, 153 beds) One Mellon Way, Latrobe, PA Zip 15650–1096; tel. 724/537–1000; Michael D. Busch, Executive Vice President and Chief Operating Officer
**Web address:** www.excelahealth.org

| | | |
|---|---|---|
| Owned, leased, sponsored: | 3 hospitals | 577 beds |
| Contract–managed: | 0 hospitals | 0 beds |
| Totals: | 3 hospitals | 577 beds |

**★0134: EXEMPLA HEALTHCARE, INC.** (NP)
2420 West 26th Avenue, Suite 100–D, Denver, CO Zip 80211; tel. 303/813–5000; Robert W. Ladenburger, President and Chief Executive Officer
**(Centralized Health System)**

**COLORADO:** EXEMPLA GOOD SAMARITAN MEDICAL CENTER (O, 192 beds) 200 Exempla Circle, Lafayette, CO Zip 80026; tel. 303/689–4000; David Hamm, President and Chief Executive Officer
**Web address:** www.exempla.org

EXEMPLA LUTHERAN MEDICAL CENTER (O, 449 beds) 8300 West 38th Avenue, Wheat Ridge, CO Zip 80033–6005; tel. 303/425–4500; Grant Wicklund, President and Chief Executive Officer
**Web address:** www.exempla.org

Section B

For explanation of codes following names, see page B2.
★ Indicates Type III membership in the American Hospital Association.

EXEMPLA SAINT JOSEPH HOSPITAL (C, 371 beds) 1835 Franklin Street, Denver, CO Zip 80218–1191; tel. 303/837–7111; Bain J. Farris, President and Chief Executive Officer
**Web address:** www.exempla.org

| Owned, leased, sponsored: | 2 hospitals | 641 beds |
|---|---|---|
| Contract–managed: | 1 hospital | 371 beds |
| Totals: | 3 hospitals | 1012 beds |

★**1325: FAIRVIEW HEALTH SERVICES** (NP)
2450 Riverside Avenue, Minneapolis, MN Zip 55454–1400; tel. 612/672–6141; Mark A. Eustis, President and Chief Executive Officer
**(Centralized Physician/Insurance Health System)**

**MINNESOTA:** FAIRVIEW LAKES HEALTH SERVICES (O, 47 beds) 5200 Fairview Boulevard, Wyoming, MN Zip 55092–8013; tel. 651/982–7000; Steven C. Housh, President
**Web address:** www.fairview.org/

FAIRVIEW NORTHLAND MEDICAL CENTER (O, 31 beds) 911 Northland Drive, Princeton, MN Zip 55371–2173; tel. 763/389–1313; John W. Herman, Chief Executive Officer
**Web address:** www.northland.fairview.org

FAIRVIEW RIDGES HOSPITAL (O, 165 beds) 201 East Nicollet Boulevard, Burnsville, MN Zip 55337–5799; tel. 952/892–2000; Beth Krehbiel, President and Chief Executive Officer
**Web address:** www.fairview.org

FAIRVIEW SOUTHDALE HOSPITAL (O, 335 beds) 6401 France Avenue South, Edina, MN Zip 55435–2199; tel. 952/924–5000; Bradley Beard, President
**Web address:** www.fairview.org

RANGE REGIONAL HEALTH SERVICES (O, 76 beds) 750 East 34th Street, Hibbing, MN Zip 55746–4600; tel. 218/262–4881; Debra K. Boardman, FACHE, President and Chief Executive Officer
**Web address:** www.range.fairview.org

UNIVERSITY OF MINNESOTA MEDICAL CENTER, FAIRVIEW (O, 814 beds) 2450 Riverside Avenue, Minneapolis, MN Zip 55454–1400; tel. 612/672–6000; Carolyn Wilson, President
**Web address:** www.fairview.org

| Owned, leased, sponsored: | 6 hospitals | 1468 beds |
|---|---|---|
| Contract–managed: | 0 hospitals | 0 beds |
| Totals: | 6 hospitals | 1468 beds |

**0814: FAITH REGIONAL HEALTH SERVICES** (NP)
2700 West Norfolk Avenue, Norfolk, NE Zip 68701–4438, Mailing Address: P.O. Box 869, Zip 68702–0869; tel. 402/644–7201; James J. Sinek, President and Chief Executive Officer

**NEBRASKA:** FAITH REGIONAL HEALTH SERVICES (O, 146 beds) 2700 West Norfolk Avenue, Norfolk, NE Zip 68701, Mailing Address: P.O. Box 869, Zip 68702–0869; tel. 402/644–7201; James J. Sinek, President and Chief Executive Officer
**Web address:** www.frhs.org

NIOBRARA VALLEY HOSPITAL (C, 20 beds) 401 South Fifth Street, Lynch, NE Zip 68746–0118, Mailing Address: P.O. Box 118, Zip 68746–0118; tel. 402/569–2451; Kelly Kalkowski, Chief Executive Officer
**Web address:** www.ci.lynch.ne.us/health.htm

TILDEN COMMUNITY HOSPITAL (C, 21 beds) 308 West Second Street, Tilden, NE Zip 68781–0340, Mailing Address: P.O. Box 340, Zip 68781–0340; tel. 402/368–5343; Lon Knievel, Chief Executive Officer
**Web address:** www.tildenhospital.org

WEST HOLT MEMORIAL HOSPITAL (C, 18 beds) 406 West Neely Street, Atkinson, NE Zip 68713–0200; tel. 402/925–2811; Michael F. Coyle, Chief Executive Officer
**Web address:** www.westholtmed.org

| Owned, leased, sponsored: | 1 hospital | 146 beds |
|---|---|---|
| Contract–managed: | 3 hospitals | 59 beds |
| Totals: | 4 hospitals | 205 beds |

**0397: FINGER LAKES HEALTH** (NP)
196 North Street, Geneva, NY Zip 14456; tel. 315/787–4000; Jose Acevedo, M.D., President and Chief Executive Officer
**(Independent Hospital System)**

**NEW YORK:** GENEVA GENERAL HOSPITAL (O, 132 beds) 196 North Street, Geneva, NY Zip 14456–1694; tel. 315/787–4000; Jose Acevedo, M.D., President and Chief Executive Officer
**Web address:** www.flhealth.org

SOLDIERS AND SAILORS MEMORIAL HOSPITAL OF YATES COUNTY (O, 186 beds) 418 North Main Street, Penn Yan, NY Zip 14527–1085; tel. 315/531–2000; Jose Acevedo, M.D., President and Chief Executive Officer
**Web address:** www.flhealth.org

| Owned, leased, sponsored: | 2 hospitals | 318 beds |
|---|---|---|
| Contract–managed: | 0 hospitals | 0 beds |
| Totals: | 2 hospitals | 318 beds |

★**0243: FIRSTHEALTH OF THE CAROLINAS** (NP)
155 Memorial Drive, Pinehurst, NC Zip 28374–8710, Mailing Address: P.O. Box 3000, Zip 28374–3000; tel. 910/715–1000; David J. Kilarski, Chief Executive Officer
**(Centralized Physician/Insurance Health System)**

**NORTH CAROLINA:** FIRSTHEALTH MONTGOMERY MEMORIAL HOSPITAL (O, 25 beds) 520 Allen Street, Troy, NC Zip 27371–2802, Mailing Address: P.O. Box 486, Zip 27371–0486; tel. 910/572–1301; Beth Walker, R.N., President
**Web address:** www.firsthealth.org

FIRSTHEALTH MOORE REGIONAL HOSPITAL (O, 379 beds) 155 Memorial Drive, Pinehurst, NC Zip 28374–8710, Mailing Address: P.O. Box 3000, Zip 28374–3000; tel. 910/715–1000; David J. Kilarski, Chief Executive Officer
**Web address:** www.firsthealth.org

FIRSTHEALTH RICHMOND MEMORIAL HOSPITAL (O, 91 beds) 925 Long Drive, Rockingham, NC Zip 28379–4815; tel. 910/417–3000; John J. Jackson, President
**Web address:** www.firsthealth.org

| Owned, leased, sponsored: | 3 hospitals | 495 beds |
|---|---|---|
| Contract–managed: | 0 hospitals | 0 beds |
| Totals: | 3 hospitals | 495 beds |

**0378: FIVE STAR QUALITY CARE** (IO)
400 Centre Street, Newton, MA Zip 02458–2076; tel. 617/796–8387; Bruce J. Mackey, Jr., President and Chief Executive Officer
**(Independent Hospital System)**

**MASSACHUSETTS:** BRAINTREE REHABILITATION HOSPITAL (O, 187 beds) 250 Pond Street, Braintree, MA Zip 02184–5351; tel. 781/348–2500; Randy Doherty, Administrator
**Web address:** www.braintreerehabhospital.com

NEW ENGLAND REHABILITATION HOSPITAL (O, 210 beds) Two Rehabilitation Way, Woburn, MA Zip 01801–6098; tel. 781/935–5050; Joel Rudin, Chief Executive Officer
**Web address:** www.newenglandrehab.com

| Owned, leased, sponsored: | 2 hospitals | 397 beds |
|---|---|---|
| Contract–managed: | 0 hospitals | 0 beds |
| Totals: | 2 hospitals | 397 beds |

**5345: FRANCISCAN ALLIANCE** (CC)
1515 Dragoon Trail, Mishawaka, IN Zip 46546–1290, Mailing Address: P.O. Box 1290, Zip 46546–1290; tel. 574/256–3935; Kevin D. Leahy, President and Chief Executive Officer
**(Moderately Centralized Health System)**

**ILLINOIS:** FRANCISCAN ST. JAMES HOSPITAL AND HEALTH CENTERS (O, 402 beds) 20201 South Crawford Avenue, Olympia Fields, IL Zip 60461–1080; tel. 708/747–4000; Seth C. R. Warren, President
**Web address:** www.stjameshhc.org

For explanation of codes following names, see page B2.
★ Indicates Type III membership in the American Hospital Association.

**B52** Health Care Systems, Networks and Alliances

© 2012 AHA Guide

**INDIANA:** FRANCISCAN PHYSICIANS HOSPITAL (O, 32 beds) 701 Superior Avenue, Munster, IN Zip 46321–4029; tel. 219/924–1300; Barbara M. Greene, President
**Web address:** www.heartlandmemorial.org

FRANCISCAN ST. ANTHONY HEALTH – CROWN POINT (O, 254 beds) 1201 South Main Street, Crown Point, IN Zip 46307–8483; tel. 219/738–2100; David Ruskowski, President
**Web address:** www.stanthonymedicalcenter.com

FRANCISCAN ST. ANTHONY HEALTH – MICHIGAN CITY (O, 171 beds) 301 West Homer Street, Michigan City, IN Zip 46360–4358; tel. 219/879–8511; James Callaghan, III, M.D., President
**Web address:** www.saintanthonymemorial.org

FRANCISCAN ST. ELIZABETH HEALTH – CRAWFORDSVILLE (O, 76 beds) 1710 Lafayette Road, Crawfordsville, IN Zip 47933–1099; tel. 765/362–2800; Thomas R. Peck, Chief Executive Officer
**Web address:** www.stclaremedical.org

FRANCISCAN ST. ELIZABETH HEALTH – LAFAYETTE CENTRAL (O, 302 beds) 1501 Hartford Street, Lafayette, IN Zip 47904–2134; tel. 765/423–6011; Terrance E. Wilson, President and Chief Executive Officer
**Web address:** www.ste.org

FRANCISCAN ST. FRANCIS HEALTH – BEECH GROVE (O, 206 beds) 1600 Albany Street, Beech Grove, IN Zip 46107–1593; tel. 317/787–3311; ,
**Web address:** www.stfrancishospitals.org

FRANCISCAN ST. FRANCIS HEALTH – INDIANAPOLIS (O, 234 beds) 8111 South Emerson Avenue, Indianapolis, IN Zip 46217; tel. 317/528–5000; Robert J. Brody, President and Chief Executive Officer
**Web address:** www.stfrancishospitals.org

FRANCISCAN ST. FRANCIS HEALTH – MOORESVILLE (O, 92 beds) 1201 Hadley Road, Mooresville, IN Zip 46158–1789; tel. 317/831–1160; Jared Stark, Executive Director
**Web address:** www.stfrancishospitals.org

FRANCISCAN ST. FRANCIS HEALTH–CARMEL (O, 6 beds) 12188B North Meridian Street, Carmel, IN Zip 46032; tel. 317/705–4500;

FRANCISCAN ST. MARGARET HEALTH – HAMMOND (O, 500 beds) 5454 Hohman Avenue, Hammond, IN Zip 46320–1999; tel. 219/933–2074; Thomas J. Gryzbek, President
**Web address:** www.smmhc.com

ST. ELIZABETH EAST (O, 140 beds) 1701 South Creasy Lane, Lafayette, IN Zip 47905–4972; tel. 765/502–4000; Terrance E. Wilson, President and Chief Executive Officer
**Web address:** www.ste.org

SURGICAL HOSPITAL OF MUNSTER (O, 9 beds) 7847 Calumet Avenue, Munster, IN Zip 46321; tel. 219/836–5102; Paul Skowron, Chief Executive Officer

| | | |
|---|---|---|
| Owned, leased, sponsored: | 13 hospitals | 2424 beds |
| Contract–managed: | 0 hospitals | 0 beds |
| Totals: | 13 hospitals | 2424 beds |

★1475:  **FRANCISCAN MISSIONARIES OF OUR LADY HEALTH SYSTEM, INC.** (CC)
4200 Essen Lane, Baton Rouge, LA Zip 70809; tel. 225/923–2701; John J. Finan, Jr., FACHE, President and Chief Executive Officer
**(Moderately Centralized Health System)**

**LOUISIANA:** ASSUMPTION COMMUNITY HOSPITAL (O, 6 beds) 135 Highway 402, Napoleonville, LA Zip 70390–2217; tel. 985/369–3600; Wayne M. Arboneaux, Chief Executive Officer
**Web address:** www.ololrmc.com

OUR LADY OF LOURDES REGIONAL MEDICAL CENTER (O, 218 beds) 611 St. Landry Street, Lafayette, LA Zip 70506–4627, Mailing Address: P.O. Box 4027, Zip 70502–4027; tel. 337/289–2000; William F. Barrow, II, President and Chief Executive Officer
**Web address:** www.lourdes.net

OUR LADY OF THE LAKE REGIONAL MEDICAL CENTER (O, 1049 beds) 5000 Hennessy Boulevard, Baton Rouge, LA Zip 70808–4375; tel. 225/765–6565; K. Scott Wester, FACHE, President and Chief Executive Officer
**Web address:** www.ololrmc.com

ST. ELIZABETH HOSPITAL (O, 48 beds) 1125 West Highway 30, Gonzales, LA Zip 70737–5004; tel. 225/647–5000; Dolores N. LeJeune, R.N., President and Chief Executive Officer
**Web address:** www.steh.com

ST. FRANCIS MEDICAL CENTER (O, 343 beds) 309 Jackson Street, Monroe, LA Zip 71201–7407, Mailing Address: P.O. Box 1901, Zip 71210–1901; tel. 318/966–4000; Louis H. Bremer, Jr., President and Chief Executive Officer
**Web address:** www.stfran.com

| | | |
|---|---|---|
| Owned, leased, sponsored: | 5 hospitals | 1664 beds |
| Contract–managed: | 0 hospitals | 0 beds |
| Totals: | 5 hospitals | 1664 beds |

★1455:  **FRANCISCAN SISTERS OF CHRISTIAN CHARITY SPONSORED MINISTRIES, INC.** (CC)
1415 South Rapids Road, Manitowoc, WI Zip 54220–9302; tel. 920/684–7071; Sister Laura J. Wolf, President
**(Moderately Centralized Health System)**

**NEBRASKA:** ST. FRANCIS MEMORIAL HOSPITAL (O, 92 beds) 430 North Monitor Street, West Point, NE Zip 68788–1555; tel. 402/372–2404; Ronald O. Briggs, FACHE, President and Chief Executive Officer
**Web address:** www.fcswp.org

**OHIO:** GENESIS HEALTHCARE SYSTEM (O, 358 beds) 2951 Maple Avenue, Zanesville, OH Zip 43701–2881; tel. 740/454–5000; Matthew J. Perry, President and Chief Executive Officer
**Web address:** www.genesishcs.org

**WISCONSIN:** HOLY FAMILY MEMORIAL MEDICAL CENTER (O, 62 beds) 2300 Western Avenue, Manitowoc, WI Zip 54220, Mailing Address: P.O. Box 1450, Zip 54221–1450; tel. 920/320–2011; Mark P. Herzog, President and Chief Executive Officer
**Web address:** www.hfmhealth.org

| | | |
|---|---|---|
| Owned, leased, sponsored: | 3 hospitals | 512 beds |
| Contract–managed: | 0 hospitals | 0 beds |
| Totals: | 3 hospitals | 512 beds |

★0271:  **FREEMAN HEALTH SYSTEM** (NP)
1102 West 32nd Street, Joplin, MO Zip 64804; tel. 417/347–1111; Paula F. Baker, President and Chief Executive Officer
**(Centralized Health System)**

**MISSOURI:** FREEMAN HOSPITAL WEST (O, 340 beds) 1102 West 32nd Street, Joplin, MO Zip 64804–3503; tel. 417/347–1111; Paula F. Baker, President and Chief Executive Officer
**Web address:** www.freemanhealth.com

FREEMAN NEOSHO HOSPITAL (O, 25 beds) 113 West Hickory Street, Neosho, MO Zip 64850–1705; tel. 417/455–4352; Daxton Holcomb, Chief Executive Officer
**Web address:** www.freemanhealth.com

| | | |
|---|---|---|
| Owned, leased, sponsored: | 2 hospitals | 365 beds |
| Contract–managed: | 0 hospitals | 0 beds |
| Totals: | 2 hospitals | 365 beds |

0182:  **FUNDAMENTAL LONG TERM CARE HOLDINGS, LLC** (IO)
930 Ridgebrook Road, Sparks Glencoe, MD Zip 21152; tel. 410/773–1000; W. Bradley Bennett, President and Chief Executive Officer
**(Independent Hospital System)**

**KANSAS:** SPECIALTY HOSPITAL OF MID–AMERICA (O, 104 beds) 6509 West 103rd Street, Overland Park, KS Zip 66212–1728; tel. 913/649–3701; Karen Leverich, Chief Executive Officer
**Web address:** www.thicare.com/SpecHospOfMidAmerica/

**NEVADA:** HARMON MEDICAL AND REHABILITATION HOSPITAL (O, 118 beds) 2170 East Harmon Avenue, Las Vegas, NV Zip 89119; tel. 702/794–0100; Bonnie Essex Hillegass, Chief Executive Officer

HORIZON SPECIALTY HOSPITAL (O, 53 beds) 640 Desert Lane, Las Vegas, NV Zip 89106; tel. 702/382–3155; Dave Tupper, Chief Executive Officer and Administrator

VEGAS VALLEY REHABILITATION HOSPITAL (O, 100 beds) 2945 Casa Vegas, Las Vegas, NV Zip 89109; tel. 702/735–7179; Maureen Davis, Administrator
**Web address:** www.fundltc.com

Section B

For explanation of codes following names, see page B2.
★ Indicates Type III membership in the American Hospital Association.

**NEW MEXICO:** SPECIALTY HOSPITAL OF ALBUQUERQUE (O, 24 beds) 235 Elm Street N.E., Albuquerque, NM Zip 87102; tel. 505/842–5550; William R. Fox, Chief Executive Officer

**TEXAS:** LLANO SPECIALTY HOSPITAL OF LUBBOCK (O, 30 beds) 1409 9th Street, Lubbock, TX Zip 79401–2601; tel. 806/767–9133; Dennis Fleenor, R.N., Chief Executive Officer
**Web address:** www.fundltc.com/Healthcare%20Facility% 20Locator/facility_page.aspx?locationID=190

TEXAS SPECIALTY HOSPITAL AT DALLAS (O, 62 beds) 7955 Harry Hines Boulevard, Dallas, TX Zip 75235–3395; tel. 214/637–0000; Glenna Carver, R.N., Chief Executive Officer
**Web address:** www.thicare.com

TEXAS SPECIALTY HOSPITAL AT HOUSTON (O, 25 beds) 6160 South Loop East, Houston, TX Zip 77087–1010; tel. 713/640–2400; Michael Higginbotham, Chief Executive Officer
**Web address:** www.thicare.com

TEXAS SPECIALTY HOSPITAL AT LUBBOCK (O, 37 beds) 4302 Princeton Street, Lubbock, TX Zip 79415–1304; tel. 806/723–8700; Deanna Graves, Chief Executive Officer

TEXAS SPECIALTY HOSPITAL AT WICHITA FALLS (O, 31 beds) 1103 Grace Street, Wichita Falls, TX Zip 76301–4414; tel. 940/720–6633; Delnita Bray, Administrator
**Web address:** www.thicare.com

| | | |
|---|---|---|
| Owned, leased, sponsored: | 10 hospitals | 584 beds |
| Contract–managed: | 0 hospitals | 0 beds |
| Totals: | 10 hospitals | 584 beds |

★**5570: GEISINGER HEALTH SYSTEM** (NP)
100 North Academy Avenue, Danville, PA Zip 17822; tel. 570/271–6211; Glenn Steele, Jr., M.D., Ph.D., President and Chief Executive Officer
**(Centralized Physician/Insurance Health System)**

**PENNSYLVANIA:** GEISINGER MEDICAL CENTER (O, 475 beds) 100 North Academy Avenue, Danville, PA Zip 17822–2201; tel. 570/271–6211; Thomas P. Sokola, Chief Administrative Officer
**Web address:** www.geisinger.org

GEISINGER WYOMING VALLEY MEDICAL CENTER (O, 242 beds) 1000 East Mountain Boulevard, Wilkes Barre, PA Zip 18711–0027; tel. 570/808–7300; John J. Buckley, Chief Administrative Officer
**Web address:** www.geisinger.org

GEISINGER–BLOOMSBURG HOSPITAL (O, 72 beds) 549 Fair Street, Bloomsburg, PA Zip 17815–1419; tel. 570/387–2100; Lissa Bryan–Smith, Chief Administrative Officer
**Web address:** www.bloomhealth.net

GEISINGER–COMMUNITY MEDICAL CENTER (O, 232 beds) 1800 Mulberry Street, Scranton, PA Zip 18510–2369; tel. 570/969–8000; Robert P. Steigmeyer, President and Chief Executive Officer
**Web address:** www.cmchealthsys.org

| | | |
|---|---|---|
| Owned, leased, sponsored: | 4 hospitals | 1021 beds |
| Contract–managed: | 0 hospitals | 0 beds |
| Totals: | 4 hospitals | 1021 beds |

★**0311: GENESIS HEALTH SYSTEM** (NP)
1227 East Rusholme Street, Davenport, IA Zip 52803–2498; tel. 563/421–1000; Douglas P. Cropper, President and Chief Executive Officer
**(Centralized Health System)**

**ILLINOIS:** GENESIS MEDICAL CENTER, ILLINI CAMPUS (O, 101 beds) 801 Illini Drive, Silvis, IL Zip 61282–1893; tel. 309/281–4000; Florence Spyrow, President
**Web address:** www.genesishealth.com

MERCER COUNTY HOSPITAL (C, 22 beds) 409 N.W. Ninth Avenue, Aledo, IL Zip 61231–1296; tel. 309/582–5301; Ted Rogalski, Chief Executive Officer
**Web address:** www.mercerhospital.org

**IOWA:** GENESIS MEDICAL CENTER, DEWITT (O, 86 beds) 1118 11th Street, De Witt, IA Zip 52742–1296; tel. 563/659–4200; Jeffrey M. Cooper, President
**Web address:** www.genesishealth.com

GENESIS MEDICAL CENTER–DAVENPORT (O, 380 beds) 1227 East Rusholme Street, Davenport, IA Zip 52803–2498; tel. 563/421–1000; Wayne A. Diewald, President
**Web address:** www.genesishealth.com

JACKSON COUNTY REGIONAL HEALTH CENTER (C, 25 beds) 700 West Grove Street, Maquoketa, IA Zip 52060–0910; tel. 563/652–2474; Curt Coleman, FACHE, Chief Executive Officer
**Web address:** www.jcrhc.org

| | | |
|---|---|---|
| Owned, leased, sponsored: | 3 hospitals | 567 beds |
| Contract–managed: | 2 hospitals | 47 beds |
| Totals: | 5 hospitals | 614 beds |

**0812: GEORGETOWN HOSPITAL SYSTEM** (NP)
606 Black River Road, Georgetown, SC Zip 29440–3304, Mailing Address: P.O. Box 421718, Zip 29442–4203; tel. 843/527–7000; Bruce P. Bailey, President and Chief Executive Officer
**(Independent Hospital System)**

**SOUTH CAROLINA:** GEORGETOWN MEMORIAL HOSPITAL (O, 136 beds) 606 Black River Road, Georgetown, SC Zip 29440–3368, Mailing Address: Drawer 421718, Zip 29442–1718; tel. 843/527–7000; Bruce P. Bailey, Chief Executive Officer
**Web address:** www.georgetownhospitalsystem.org

WACCAMAW COMMUNITY HOSPITAL (O, 169 beds) 4070 Highway 17 Bypass, Murrells Inlet, SC Zip 29576, Mailing Address: P.O. Drawer 3350, Zip 29576; tel. 843/652–1000; Gayle L. Resetar, Chief Operating Officer
**Web address:** www.gmhsc.com

| | | |
|---|---|---|
| Owned, leased, sponsored: | 2 hospitals | 305 beds |
| Contract–managed: | 0 hospitals | 0 beds |
| Totals: | 2 hospitals | 305 beds |

**0283: GILLIARD HEALTH SERVICES** (IO)
3091 Carter Hill Road, Montgomery, AL Zip 36111–1801; tel. 334/265–5009; William G. McKenzie, President, Chief Executive Officer and Chairman

**ALABAMA:** EVERGREEN MEDICAL CENTER (O, 44 beds) 101 Crestview Avenue, Evergreen, AL Zip 36401–0706, Mailing Address: P.O. Box 706, Zip 36401–0706; tel. 251/578–2480; William G. McKenzie, Interim Administrator
**Web address:** www.evergreenmedical.org

JACKSON MEDICAL CENTER (O, 26 beds) 220 Hospital Drive, Jackson, AL Zip 36545–2459, Mailing Address: P.O. Box 428, Zip 36545–0428; tel. 251/246–9021; Amy Gibson, Chief Executive Officer
**Web address:** www.jacksonmedicalcenter.org

TROY REGIONAL MEDICAL CENTER (O, 78 beds) 1330 Highway 231 South, Troy, AL Zip 36081–1224; tel. 334/670–5000; Teresa G. Grimes, Chief Executive Officer
**Web address:** www.troymedicalcenter.com

| | | |
|---|---|---|
| Owned, leased, sponsored: | 3 hospitals | 148 beds |
| Contract–managed: | 0 hospitals | 0 beds |
| Totals: | 3 hospitals | 148 beds |

**0654: GLOBALREHAB** (IO)
1420 West Mockingbird Lane, Suite 100, Dallas, TX Zip 75247–4931, Mailing Address: 1340 Empire Central Drive, Zip 75247–4022; tel. 214/879–7500; Hooman Sedighi, M.D., President and Chief Executive Officer
**(Independent Hospital System)**

**TEXAS:** GLOBALREHAB HOSPITAL – DALLAS (O, 42 beds) 1340 Empire Central Drive, Dallas, TX Zip 75247–4022; tel. 214/879–7300; Ellen Shankles, Chief Executive Officer
**Web address:** www.globalrehabhospitals.com

GLOBALREHAB HOSPITAL – FORT WORTH (O, 42 beds) 6601 Harris Parkway, Fort Worth, TX Zip 76132–6108; tel. 817/433–9600; Brigid Greenberg, Interim Chief Executive Officer
**Web address:** www.globalrehabhospitals.com

For explanation of codes following names, see page B2.
★ Indicates Type III membership in the American Hospital Association.

GLOBALREHAB HOSPITAL – SAN ANTONIO (O, 42 beds) 19126 Stonehue Road, San Antonio, TX Zip 78258–3490; tel. 210/482–3400; Travis Rich, Chief Executive Officer
**Web address:** www.globalrehabhospitals.com

| Owned, leased, sponsored: | 3 hospitals | 126 beds |
|---|---|---|
| Contract–managed: | 0 hospitals | 0 beds |
| **Totals:** | 3 hospitals | 126 beds |

---

## 0522: GOOD SHEPHERD HEALTH SYSTEM (NP)
700 East Marshall Avenue, Longview, TX Zip 75601–5580; tel. 903/315–2000; Edward D. Banos, President and Chief Executive Officer

**(Independent Hospital System)**

GOOD SHEPHERD MEDICAL CENTER (O, 399 beds) 700 East Marshall Avenue, Longview, TX Zip 75601–5571; tel. 903/315–2000; Edward D. Banos, President and Chief Executive Officer
**Web address:** www.gsmc.org

GOOD SHEPHERD MEDICAL CENTER–LINDEN (O, 25 beds) 404 North Kaufman Street, Linden, TX Zip 75563–5235; tel. 903/756–5561; Carla Roadcap, R.N., MSN, Chief Executive Officer
**Web address:** www.gsmclinden.org

GOOD SHEPHERD MEDICAL CENTER–MARSHALL (O, 142 beds) 811 South Washington Avenue, Marshall, TX Zip 75670–5336, Mailing Address: P.O. Box 1599, Zip 75671–1599; tel. 903/927–6000; Russell J. Collier, FACHE, President and Chief Executive Officer
**Web address:** www.gsmcmarshall.org

| Owned, leased, sponsored: | 3 hospitals | 566 beds |
|---|---|---|
| Contract–managed: | 0 hospitals | 0 beds |
| **Totals:** | 3 hospitals | 566 beds |

---

## 0648: GOOD SHEPHERD REHABILITATION NETWORK (IO)
850 South Fifth Street, Allentown, PA Zip 18103–3308; tel. 610/776–3100; Sally T. Gammon, FACHE, President and Chief Executive Officer

**(Independent Hospital System)**

**PENNSYLVANIA:** GOOD SHEPHERD PENN PARTNERS SPECIALTY HOSPITAL AT RITTENHOUSE (O, 38 beds) 1800 Lombard Street, Philadelphia, PA Zip 19146–1414; tel. 877/969–7342; Linda Dean, Chief Executive Officer
**Web address:** www.phillyrehab.com/longterm

GOOD SHEPHERD REHABILITATION HOSPITAL (O, 102 beds) 850 South 5th Street, Allentown, PA Zip 18103–3308; tel. 610/776–3299; Sally T. Gammon, FACHE, President and Chief Executive Officer
**Web address:** www.goodshepherdrehab.org

GOOD SHEPHERD SPECIALTY HOSPITAL (O, 32 beds) 2545 Schoenersville Road, 3rd Floor, Bethlehem, PA Zip 18017; tel. 484/884–5051; Lisa Marsilio, Vice President and Administrator
**Web address:** www.goodshepherdrehab.org

| Owned, leased, sponsored: | 3 hospitals | 172 beds |
|---|---|---|
| Contract–managed: | 0 hospitals | 0 beds |
| **Totals:** | 3 hospitals | 172 beds |

---

## ★1535: GREAT PLAINS HEALTH ALLIANCE, INC. (NP)
625 Third Street, Phillipsburg, KS Zip 67661–2138, Mailing Address: P.O. Box 366, Zip 67661–0366; tel. 785/543–2111; Roger S. John, President and Chief Executive Officer

**(Decentralized Health System)**

**KANSAS:** ASHLAND HEALTH CENTER (C, 45 beds) 709 Oak Street, Ashland, KS Zip 67831–0188, Mailing Address: P.O. Box 188, Zip 67831–0188; tel. 620/635–2241; Benjamin Anderson, Chief Executive Officer
**Web address:** www.ashlandhc.org

CHEYENNE COUNTY HOSPITAL (L, 16 beds) 210 West First Street, Saint Francis, KS Zip 67756–0547, Mailing Address: P.O. Box 547, Zip 67756–0547; tel. 785/332–2104; Leslie Lacy, Administrator
**Web address:** www.cheyennecountyhospital.com

COMANCHE COUNTY HOSPITAL (C, 12 beds) 202 South Frisco Street, Coldwater, KS Zip 67029, Mailing Address: HC 65, Box 8A, Zip 67029; tel. 620/582–2144; Nancy Zimmerman, R.N., Administrator
**Web address:** www.gpha.com

ELLINWOOD DISTRICT HOSPITAL (L, 25 beds) 605 North Main Street, Ellinwood, KS Zip 67526–1440; tel. 620/564–2548; Joyce Schulte, Chief Executive Officer
**Web address:** www.ellinwood.org

FREDONIA REGIONAL HOSPITAL (C, 34 beds) 1527 Madison Street, Fredonia, KS Zip 66736–1751, Mailing Address: P.O. Box 579, Zip 66736–0579; tel. 620/378–2121; Terry Deschaine, Chief Executive Officer
**Web address:** www.fredoniaregionalhospital.org

GRISELL MEMORIAL HOSPITAL DISTRICT ONE (C, 46 beds) 210 South Vermont Avenue, Ransom, KS Zip 67572; tel. 785/731–2231; Kristine Ochs, R.N., Administrator
**Web address:** www.grisellmemorialhospital.org

KIOWA COUNTY MEMORIAL HOSPITAL (L, 15 beds) 721 West Kansas Avenue, Greensburg, KS Zip 67054–1951; tel. 620/723–3341; Mary Sweet, Administrator
**Web address:** www.kcmh.net

LANE COUNTY HOSPITAL (C, 31 beds) 235 West Vine, Dighton, KS Zip 67839–0969, Mailing Address: P.O. Box 969, Zip 67839–0969; tel. 620/397–5321; Donna McGowan, Administrator
**Web address:** www.lchospital.com

MEDICINE LODGE MEMORIAL HOSPITAL (C, 25 beds) 710 North Walnut Street, Medicine Lodge, KS Zip 67104–1019; tel. 620/886–3771; Kevin A. White, Administrator
**Web address:** www.mlmh.net/

MINNEOLA DISTRICT HOSPITAL (C, 54 beds) 212 Main Street, Minneola, KS Zip 67865–0127, Mailing Address: P.O. Box 127, Zip 67865–0127; tel. 620/885–4264; Brian Roland, Administrator and Chief Executive Officer
**Web address:** www.minneolahealthcare.com

OSBORNE COUNTY MEMORIAL HOSPITAL (C, 25 beds) 424 West New Hampshire Street, Osborne, KS Zip 67473–0070, Mailing Address: P.O. Box 70, Zip 67473–0070; tel. 785/346–2121; Kiley Floyd, Administrator
**Web address:** www.ocmh.org

OTTAWA COUNTY HEALTH CENTER (L, 42 beds) 215 East Eighth, Minneapolis, KS Zip 67467–1999, Mailing Address: P.O. Box 290, Zip 67467–0290; tel. 785/392–2122; Joy Johnson, R.N., Interim Chief Executive Officer
**Web address:** www.ottawacountyhealthcenter.com

PHILLIPS COUNTY HOSPITAL (L, 25 beds) 1150 State Street, Phillipsburg, KS Zip 67661–1799, Mailing Address: P.O. Box 607, Zip 67661–0607; tel. 785/543–5226; David Engel, Chief Executive Officer
**Web address:** www.phillipshospital.org

RAWLINS COUNTY HEALTH CENTER (C, 24 beds) 707 Grant Street, Atwood, KS Zip 67730–4700, Mailing Address: P.O. Box 47, Zip 67730–4700; tel. 785/626–3211; Deanna Freeman, Administrator and Chief Executive Officer
**Web address:** www.rchc.us

REPUBLIC COUNTY HOSPITAL (L, 63 beds) 2420 G Street, Belleville, KS Zip 66935–2400; tel. 785/527–2254; Blaine K. Miller, Administrator
**Web address:** www.rphospital.org

SABETHA COMMUNITY HOSPITAL (L, 25 beds) 14th and Oregon Streets, Sabetha, KS Zip 66534–0229, Mailing Address: P.O. Box 229, Zip 66534–0229; tel. 785/284–2121; Lora Key, Chief Executive Officer
**Web address:** www.sabethahospital.com

SATANTA DISTRICT HOSPITAL (C, 57 beds) 401 South Cheyenne Street, Satanta, KS Zip 67870–0159, Mailing Address: P.O. Box 159, Zip 67870–0159; tel. 620/649–2761; Ron Baker, Administrator
**Web address:** www.satantahospital.org

SMITH COUNTY MEMORIAL HOSPITAL (L, 53 beds) 614 South Main Street, Smith Center, KS Zip 66967–0349; tel. 785/282–6845; Carolyn K. Hess, R.N., Administrator
**Web address:** www.gpha.com

TREGO COUNTY–LEMKE MEMORIAL HOSPITAL (C, 62 beds) 320 North 13th Street, Wakeeney, KS Zip 67672–2099; tel. 785/743–2182; Harold Courtois, Administrator and Chief Executive Officer
**Web address:** www.tclmh.org

---

For explanation of codes following names, see page B2.
★ Indicates Type III membership in the American Hospital Association.

**NEBRASKA:** HARLAN COUNTY HEALTH SYSTEM (C, 19 beds) 717 North Brown Street, Alma, NE Zip 68920–0836, Mailing Address: P.O. Box 836, Zip 68920–0836; tel. 308/928–2151; Jeffrey D. Shelton, Chief Executive Officer
**Web address:** www.harlancountyhealth.com

| Owned, leased, sponsored: | 8 hospitals | 264 beds |
| Contract–managed: | 12 hospitals | 434 beds |
| Totals: | 20 hospitals | 698 beds |

---

**★1555: GREENVILLE HOSPITAL SYSTEM** (NP)
701 Grove Road, Greenville, SC Zip 29605–5601; tel. 864/455–7000; Michael C. Riordan, President and Chief Executive Officer
**(Centralized Health System)**

**SOUTH CAROLINA:** GREENVILLE MEMORIAL HOSPITAL (O, 786 beds) 701 Grove Road, Greenville, SC Zip 29605–4295; tel. 864/455–7000; Paul F. Johnson, President
**Web address:** www.ghs.org

GREER MEMORIAL HOSPITAL (O, 70 beds) 830 South Bumcombe Road, Greer, SC Zip 29650–2400; tel. 864/848–8200; John F. Mansure, FACHE, President
**Web address:** www.ghs.org

HILLCREST MEMORIAL HOSPITAL (O, 43 beds) 729 S.E. Main Street, Simpsonville, SC Zip 29681–3280; tel. 864/454–6100; Eric Bour, M.D., President
**Web address:** www.ghs.org

PATEWOOD MEMORIAL HOSPITAL (O, 36 beds) 175 Patewood Drive, Greenville, SC Zip 29605; tel. 864/797–1000; Beverly J. Haines, R.N., Interim President
**Web address:** www.ghs.org/patewood

| Owned, leased, sponsored: | 4 hospitals | 935 beds |
| Contract–managed: | 0 hospitals | 0 beds |
| Totals: | 4 hospitals | 935 beds |

---

**★0675: GUTHRIE HEALTHCARE SYSTEM** (NP)
Guthrie Square, Sayre, PA Zip 18840; tel. 570/887–4312; Joseph A. Scopelliti, M.D., President and Chief Executive Officer
**(Moderately Centralized Health System)**

**NEW YORK:** CORNING HOSPITAL (O, 82 beds) 176 Denison Parkway East, Corning, NY Zip 14830–2899; tel. 607/937–7200; Shirley P. Magana, President and Chief Operating Officer
**Web address:** www.corninghospital.com

**PENNSYLVANIA:** ROBERT PACKER HOSPITAL (O, 238 beds) 1 Guthrie Square, Sayre, PA Zip 18840–1698; tel. 570/888–6666; Marie T. Droege, President
**Web address:** www.guthrie.org

TROY COMMUNITY HOSPITAL (O, 25 beds) 101 Elmira Street, Troy, PA Zip 16947–1271; tel. 570/297–2121; Staci Covey, R.N., MS, President
**Web address:** www.guthrie.org

| Owned, leased, sponsored: | 3 hospitals | 345 beds |
| Contract–managed: | 0 hospitals | 0 beds |
| Totals: | 3 hospitals | 345 beds |

---

**0409: HAMILTON HEALTH CARE SYSTEM, INC.** (NP)
1200 Memorial Drive, Dalton, GA Zip 30720–2529, Mailing Address: P.O. Box 1900, Zip 30722–1900; tel. 706/272–6000; Jeffrey D. Myers, President and Chief Executive Officer
**(Centralized Physician/Insurance Health System)**

**GEORGIA:** HAMILTON MEDICAL CENTER (O, 230 beds) 1200 Memorial Drive, Dalton, GA Zip 30720–2529, Mailing Address: P.O. Box 1168, Zip 30722–1168; tel. 706/272–6000; Jeffrey D. Myers, President and Chief Executive Officer
**Web address:** www.hamiltonhealth.com

MURRAY MEDICAL CENTER (O, 19 beds) 707 Old Dalton Ellijay Road, Chatsworth, GA Zip 30705–2060, Mailing Address: P.O. Box 1406, Zip 30705–1406; tel. 706/695–4564; James C. Hazel, FACHE, Chief Executive Officer
**Web address:** www.hamiltonhealth.com/

| Owned, leased, sponsored: | 2 hospitals | 249 beds |
| Contract–managed: | 0 hospitals | 0 beds |
| Totals: | 2 hospitals | 249 beds |

---

**0541: HARTFORD HEALTHCARE** (NP)
80 Seymour Street, Hartford, CT Zip 06102–8000, Mailing Address: P.O. Box 5037, Zip 06102–5037; Elliot T. Joseph, President and Chief Executive Officer
**(Moderately Centralized Health System)**

**CONNECTICUT:** HARTFORD HOSPITAL (O, 613 beds) 80 Seymour Street, Hartford, CT Zip 06102–5037, Mailing Address: P.O. Box 5037, Zip 06102–5037; tel. 860/545–5000; Jeffrey A. Flaks, President and Chief Executive Officer
**Web address:** www.harthosp.org

MIDSTATE MEDICAL CENTER (O, 134 beds) 435 Lewis Avenue, Meriden, CT Zip 06451–2101; tel. 203/694–8200; Lucille A. Janatka, President and Chief Executive Officer
**Web address:** www.midstatemedical.org

NATCHAUG HOSPITAL (O, 57 beds) 189 Storrs Road, Mansfield Center, CT Zip 06250–0260; tel. 860/456–1311; Stephen W. Larcen, Ph.D., President and Chief Executive Officer
**Web address:** www.natchaug.org

THE HOSPITAL OF CENTRAL CONNECTICUT (O, 249 beds) 100 Grand Street, New Britain, CT Zip 06052–2017, Mailing Address: P.O. Box 100, Zip 06050–0100; tel. 860/224–5011; Clarence J. Silvia, President and Chief Executive Officer
**Web address:** www.thocc.org

WINDHAM HOSPITAL (O, 79 beds) 112 Mansfield Avenue, Willimantic, CT Zip 06226–2040; tel. 860/456–9116; Stephen W. Larcen, Ph.D., President and Chief Executive Officer
**Web address:** www.windhamhospital.org

| Owned, leased, sponsored: | 5 hospitals | 1132 beds |
| Contract–managed: | 0 hospitals | 0 beds |
| Totals: | 5 hospitals | 1132 beds |

---

**0637: HAVEN BEHAVIORAL HEALTHCARE** (IO)
652 West Iris Drive, Nashville, TN Zip 37204–3191; tel. 615/250–9500; Vern Westrich, President and Chief Executive Officer
**(Independent Hospital System)**

**ARIZONA:** HAVEN SENIOR HORIZONS (O, 30 beds) 1201 South 7th Avenue, Suite 200, Phoenix, AZ Zip 85007–4076; tel. 623/236–2000; Kathy Shaw, Chief Executive Officer
**Web address:** www.havenbehavioral.com

**COLORADO:** HAVEN BEHAVIORAL SENIOR CARE OF NORTH DENVER (O, 40 beds) 8451 Pearl Street, Suite 100, Thornton, CO Zip 80229–4804; tel. 303/288–7807; Marc McComas, Executive Director
**Web address:** www.havenbehavioral.com/seniorcare/denver

HAVEN BEHAVIORAL WAR HEROES HOSPITAL (O, 20 beds) 1008 Minnequa Avenue, Suite 6100, Pueblo, CO Zip 81004–3733; tel. 719/546–6000; Carrin Harper, M.D., Chief Executive Officer

**PENNSYLVANIA:** HAVEN BEHAVIORAL HEALTH OF EASTERN PENNSYLVANIA (O, 48 beds) 145 North 6th Street, 3rd Floor, Reading, PA Zip 19601–3096; tel. 610/406–4340; John Baker, Interim Chief Executive Officer
**Web address:** www.havenbehavioralhospital.com

| Owned, leased, sponsored: | 4 hospitals | 138 beds |
| Contract–managed: | 0 hospitals | 0 beds |
| Totals: | 4 hospitals | 138 beds |

---

For explanation of codes following names, see page B2.
★ Indicates Type III membership in the American Hospital Association.

**★3555: HAWAII HEALTH SYSTEMS CORPORATION** (NP)
3675 Kilauea Avenue, Honolulu, HI Zip 96816; tel. 808/733–4151;
Bruce S. Anderson, Ph.D., President and Chief Executive Officer
**(Independent Hospital System)**

**HAWAII:** HALE HO'OLA HAMAKUA (O, 52 beds) 45–547 Plumeria Street,
Honokaa, HI Zip 96727–6902; tel. 808/775–7211; Cathy
Meyer–Uyehara, Administrator
**Web address:** www.hhsc.org

HILO MEDICAL CENTER (O, 276 beds) 1190 Waianuenue Avenue, Hilo, HI
Zip 96720–2095; tel. 808/932–3000; Howard N. Ainsley, Regional Chief
Executive Officer
**Web address:** www.hmc.hhsc.org

KAU HOSPITAL (O, 5 beds) 1 Kamani Street, Pahala, HI Zip 96777, Mailing
Address: P.O. Box 40, Zip 96777–0040; tel. 808/928–2050; Merilyn Harris,
Administrator
**Web address:** www.hhsc.org

KAUAI VETERANS MEMORIAL HOSPITAL (O, 45 beds) Waimea Canyon Road,
Waimea, HI Zip 96796, Mailing Address: P.O. Box 337, Zip 96796–0337;
tel. 808/338–9431; Jerry Walker, Interim Regional Chief Executive Officer
**Web address:** www.kvmh.hhsc.org

KOHALA HOSPITAL (O, 26 beds) 54–383 Hospital Road, Kohala, HI
Zip 96755, Mailing Address: P.O. Box 10, Kapaau, Zip 96755–0010;
tel. 808/889–6211; Eugene Amar, Jr., Administrator
**Web address:** www.koh.hhsc.org

KONA COMMUNITY HOSPITAL (O, 54 beds) 79–1019 Haukapila Street,
Kealakekua, HI Zip 96750–7920; tel. 808/322–9311; Jay E. Kreuzer,
FACHE, Chief Executive Officer
**Web address:** www.kch.hhsc.org

KULA HOSPITAL (O, 6 beds) 100 Keokea Place, Kula, HI Zip 96790–7450;
tel. 808/878–1221; Paul Harper, Interim Administrator
**Web address:** www.hhsc.org

LANAI COMMUNITY HOSPITAL (O, 14 beds) 628 Seventh Street, Lanai City, HI
Zip 96763–0650, Mailing Address: P.O. Box 630650, Zip 96763–0650;
tel. 808/565–8450; Paul Harper, Interim Administrator
**Web address:** www.lch.hhsc.org

LEAHI HOSPITAL (O, 188 beds) 3675 Kilauea Avenue, Honolulu, HI
Zip 96816–2398; tel. 808/733–8000; Vincent H. S. Lee, FACHE, Regional
Chief Executive Officer
**Web address:** www.hhsc.org

MALUHIA HOSPITAL (O, 146 beds) 1027 Hala Drive, Honolulu, HI Zip 96817;
tel. 808/832–5874; Sally T. Ishikawa, Administrator

MAUI MEMORIAL MEDICAL CENTER (O, 213 beds) 221 Mahalani Street,
Wailuku, HI Zip 96793–2581; tel. 808/244–9056; Wesley Lo, Regional Chief
Executive Officer
**Web address:** www.mmmc.hhsc.org

SAMUEL MAHELONA MEMORIAL HOSPITAL (O, 80 beds) 4800 Kawaihau
Road, Kapaa, HI Zip 96746–1998; tel. 808/822–4961; Jerry Walker, Interim
Regional Chief Executive Officer
**Web address:** www.smmh.hhsc.org

| Owned, leased, sponsored: | 12 hospitals | 1105 beds |
|---|---|---|
| Contract–managed: | 0 hospitals | 0 beds |
| Totals: | 12 hospitals | 1105 beds |

---

**0266: HAWAII PACIFIC HEALTH** (NP)
55 Merchant Street, Honolulu, HI Zip 96813; tel. 808/535–7414;
Charles A. Sted, Chief Executive Officer
**(Independent Hospital System)**

KAPIOLANI MEDICAL CENTER FOR WOMEN & CHILDREN (O, 225 beds) 1319
Punahou Street, Honolulu, HI Zip 96826–1032; tel. 808/983–6000; Raymond
Vara, Chief Executive Officer
**Web address:** www.kapiolani.org

PALI MOMI MEDICAL CENTER (O, 116 beds) 98–1079 Moanalua Road, Aiea,
HI Zip 96701–4713; tel. 808/486–6000; Raymond Vara, Chief Executive
Officer
**Web address:** www.kapiolani.org

STRAUB CLINIC & HOSPITAL (O, 107 beds) 888 South King Street, Honolulu,
HI Zip 96813–3009; tel. 808/522–4000; Raymond Vara, Chief Executive
Officer
**Web address:** www.straubhealth.org

WILCOX MEMORIAL HOSPITAL (O, 64 beds) 3–3420 Kuhio Highway, Lihue, HI
Zip 96766–1099; tel. 808/245–1100; Kathleen Clark, President and Chief
Executive Officer
**Web address:** www.wilcoxhealth.org

| Owned, leased, sponsored: | 4 hospitals | 512 beds |
|---|---|---|
| Contract–managed: | 0 hospitals | 0 beds |
| Totals: | 4 hospitals | 512 beds |

---

**★0048: HCA** (IO)
One Park Plaza, Nashville, TN Zip 37203–1548; tel. 615/344–9551;
Richard M. Bracken, Chairman and Chief Executive Officer
**(Decentralized Health System)**

**ALASKA:** ALASKA REGIONAL HOSPITAL (O, 132 beds) 2801 Debarr Road,
Anchorage, AK Zip 99508–2997, Mailing Address: P.O. Box 143889,
Zip 99514–3889; tel. 907/264–1754; Annie Holt, FACHE, Chief Executive
Officer
**Web address:** www.alaskaregional.com

**CALIFORNIA:** GOOD SAMARITAN HOSPITAL (O, 349 beds) 2425 Samaritan
Drive, San Jose, CA Zip 95124–3997, Mailing Address: P.O. Box 240002,
Zip 95154–2402; tel. 408/559–2011; Paul Beaupre, M.D., Chief
Executive Officer
**Web address:** www.goodsamsanjose.com

LOS ROBLES HOSPITAL AND MEDICAL CENTER (O, 273 beds) 215 West
Janss Road, Thousand Oaks, CA Zip 91360–1847; tel. 805/497–2727;
Gregory R. Angle, President and Chief Executive Officer
**Web address:** www.losrobleshospital.com

REGIONAL MEDICAL CENTER OF SAN JOSE (O, 193 beds) 225 North Jackson
Avenue, San Jose, CA Zip 95116–1691; tel. 408/259–5000; Michael T.
Johnson, Chief Executive Officer
**Web address:** www.regionalmedicalsanjose.com

RIVERSIDE COMMUNITY HOSPITAL (O, 373 beds) 4445 Magnolia Avenue,
Riverside, CA Zip 92501–4199, Mailing Address: P.O. Box 1669,
Zip 92502–1669; tel. 951/788–3000; Patrick D. Brilliant, President and
Chief Executive Officer
**Web address:** www.riversidecommunityhospital.com

WEST HILLS HOSPITAL AND MEDICAL CENTER (O, 293 beds) 7300 Medical
Center Drive, West Hills, CA Zip 91307–1910; tel. 818/676–4000; Beverly
Gilmore, President and Chief Executive Officer
**Web address:** www.westhillshospital.com

**COLORADO:** MEDICAL CENTER OF AURORA (O, 303 beds) 1501 South
Potomac Street, Aurora, CO Zip 80012–5499; tel. 303/695–2600; Bill
Voloch, Interim Chief Executive Officer
**Web address:** www.auroramed.com

NORTH SUBURBAN MEDICAL CENTER (O, 136 beds) 9191 Grant Street,
Thornton, CO Zip 80229–4341; tel. 303/451–7800; Jennifer Alderfer, Chief
Executive Officer
**Web address:** www.northsuburban.com

PRESBYTERIAN–ST. LUKE'S MEDICAL CENTER (O, 397 beds) 1719 East 19th
Avenue, Denver, CO Zip 80218–1281; tel. 303/839–6000; Madeleine
Roberson, Chief Executive Officer
**Web address:** www.pslmc.com

ROSE MEDICAL CENTER (O, 264 beds) 4567 East Ninth Avenue, Denver, CO
Zip 80220–3941; tel. 303/320–2121; Kenneth H. Feiler, Chief Executive
Officer
**Web address:** www.rosebabies.com

SKY RIDGE MEDICAL CENTER (O, 185 beds) 10101 Ridge Gate Parkway,
Lone Tree, CO Zip 80124; tel. 720/225–1000; Maureen Tarrant, Chief
Executive Officer
**Web address:** www.skyridgemedcenter.com

SPALDING REHABILITATION HOSPITAL (O, 40 beds) 900 Potomac Steet,
Aurora, CO Zip 80011–6716; tel. 303/367–1166; Cynthia Kreutz, Chief
Executive Officer
**Web address:** www.spaldingrehab.com

SWEDISH MEDICAL CENTER (O, 354 beds) 501 East Hampden Avenue,
Englewood, CO Zip 80113; tel. 303/788–5000; Mary M. White, Chief
Executive Officer
**Web address:** www.swedishhospital.com

For explanation of codes following names, see page B2.
★ Indicates Type III membership in the American Hospital Association.

**FLORIDA:** AVENTURA HOSPITAL AND MEDICAL CENTER (O, 359 beds) 20900 Biscayne Boulevard, Aventura, FL Zip 33180–1407; tel. 305/682–7000; Heather J. Rohan, Chief Executive Officer
**Web address:** www.aventurahospital.com

BLAKE MEDICAL CENTER (O, 294 beds) 2020 59th Street West, Bradenton, FL Zip 34209–4669; tel. 941/792–6611; Daniel J. Friedrich, III, Chief Executive Officer
**Web address:** www.blakemedicalcenter.com

BRANDON REGIONAL HOSPITAL (O, 359 beds) 119 Oakfield Drive, Brandon, FL Zip 33511–5799; tel. 813/681–5551; Bland Eng, Chief Executive Officer
**Web address:** www.brandonhospital.com

CAPITAL REGIONAL MEDICAL CENTER (O, 198 beds) 2626 Capital Medical Boulevard, Tallahassee, FL Zip 32308–4499; tel. 850/325–5000; Brian Cook, FACHE, Chief Executive Officer
**Web address:** www.capitalregionalmedicalcenter.com

CENTRAL FLORIDA REGIONAL HOSPITAL (O, 226 beds) 1401 West Seminole Boulevard, Sanford, FL Zip 32771–6764; tel. 407/321–4500; Wendy H. Brandon, Chief Executive Officer
**Web address:** www.centralfloridaregional.com

COLUMBIA HOSPITAL (O, 250 beds) 2201 45th Street, West Palm Beach, FL Zip 33407–2069; tel. 561/842–6141; Dana Oaks, Chief Executive Officer
**Web address:** www.columbiahospital.com

DOCTORS HOSPITAL OF SARASOTA (O, 168 beds) 5731 Bee Ridge Road, Sarasota, FL Zip 34233–5056; tel. 941/342–1100; Robert C. Meade, Chief Executive Officer
**Web address:** www.doctorsofsarasota.com

EDWARD WHITE HOSPITAL (O, 110 beds) 2323 Ninth Avenue North, Saint Petersburg, FL Zip 33713–6898, Mailing Address: P.O. Box 12018, Zip 33733–2018; tel. 727/323–1111; Richard S. Frank, Interim Chief Executive Officer
**Web address:** www.edwardwhitehospital.com

ENGLEWOOD COMMUNITY HOSPITAL (O, 100 beds) 700 Medical Boulevard, Englewood, FL Zip 34223–3978; tel. 941/475–6571; Thomas J. Rice, FACHE, President and Chief Executive Officer
**Web address:** www.englewoodcommunityhospital.com

FAWCETT MEMORIAL HOSPITAL (O, 238 beds) 21298 Olean Boulevard, Port Charlotte, FL Zip 33952–6765, Mailing Address: P.O. Box 494960, Punta Gorda, Zip 33949–4960; tel. 941/629–1181; Thomas J. Rice, FACHE, President and Chief Executive Officer
**Web address:** www.fawcetthospital.com

FORT WALTON BEACH MEDICAL CENTER (O, 257 beds) 1000 Mar–Walt Drive, Fort Walton Beach, FL Zip 32547–6795; tel. 850/862–1111; John A. Deardorff, Chief Executive Officer
**Web address:** www.fwbmc.com

GULF COAST MEDICAL CENTER (O, 176 beds) 449 West 23rd Street, Panama City, FL Zip 32405–4593, Mailing Address: P.O. Box 15309, Zip 32406–5309; tel. 850/769–8341; Carlton Ulmer, Chief Executive Officer
**Web address:** www.egulfcoastmedical.com

J. F. K. MEDICAL CENTER (O, 424 beds) 5301 South Congress Avenue, Atlantis, FL Zip 33462–1197; tel. 561/965–7300; Gina Melby, Chief Executive Officer
**Web address:** www.jfkmc.com

KENDALL REGIONAL MEDICAL CENTER (O, 300 beds) 11750 Bird Road, Miami, FL Zip 33175–3530; tel. 305/223–3000; Scott A. Cihak, Chief Executive Officer
**Web address:** www.kendallmed.com

LAKE CITY MEDICAL CENTER (O, 67 beds) 340 N.W. Commerce Drive, Lake City, FL Zip 32055–3718; tel. 386/719–9000; Mark Robinson, FACHE, Chief Executive Officer
**Web address:** www.lakecitymedical.com

LARGO MEDICAL CENTER (O, 243 beds) 201 14th Street S.W., Largo, FL Zip 33770–3133, Mailing Address: P.O. Box 2905, Zip 33779–2905; tel. 727/588–5200; Anthony M. Degina, President and Chief Executive Officer
**Web address:** www.largomedical.com

LAWNWOOD REGIONAL MEDICAL CENTER (O, 331 beds) 1700 South 23rd Street, Fort Pierce, FL Zip 34950–0188; tel. 772/461–4000; Rodney R. Smith, Chief Executive Officer
**Web address:** www.lawnwoodmed.com

MEDICAL CENTER OF TRINITY (O, 292 beds) 9330 State Road 54, Trinity, FL Zip 34655, Mailing Address: P.O. Box 996, New Port Richey, Zip 34656–0996; tel. 727/834–4900; Leigh Massengill, Chief Executive Officer
**Web address:** www.medicalcentertrinity.com

MEMORIAL HOSPITAL JACKSONVILLE (O, 425 beds) 3625 University Boulevard South, Jacksonville, FL Zip 32216–4240, Mailing Address: P.O. Box 16325, Zip 32245–6325; tel. 904/399–6111; James F. O'Loughlin, President and Chief Executive Officer
**Web address:** www.memorialhospitaljax.com

NORTH FLORIDA REGIONAL MEDICAL CENTER (O, 278 beds) 6500 Newberry Road, Gainesville, FL Zip 32605–4392, Mailing Address: P.O. Box 147006, Zip 32614–7006; tel. 352/333–4000; Ward Boston, III, Chief Executive Officer
**Web address:** www.nfrmc.com

NORTHSIDE HOSPITAL AND HEART INSTITUTE (O, 227 beds) 6000 49th Street North, Saint Petersburg, FL Zip 33709–2145; tel. 727/521–4411; Stephen J. Daugherty, Chief Executive Officer
**Web address:** www.northsidehospital.com

NORTHWEST MEDICAL CENTER (O, 215 beds) 2801 North State Road 7, Margate, FL Zip 33063; tel. 954/974–0400; Dianne Goldenberg, Chief Executive Officer
**Web address:** www.northwestmed.com

OAK HILL HOSPITAL (O, 214 beds) 11375 Cortez Boulevard, Brooksville, FL Zip 34613; tel. 352/596–6632; Mickey Smith, Chief Executive Officer
**Web address:** www.oakhillhospital.com

OCALA REGIONAL MEDICAL CENTER (O, 270 beds) 1431 S.W. First Avenue, Ocala, FL Zip 34474–4058, Mailing Address: P.O. Box 2200, Zip 34478–2200; tel. 352/401–1000; Randall McVay, Chief Executive Officer
**Web address:** www.ocalaregional.com

ORANGE PARK MEDICAL CENTER (O, 230 beds) 2001 Kingsley Avenue, Orange Park, FL Zip 32073–5156; tel. 904/276–8500; Thomas R. Pentz, President and Chief Executive Officer
**Web address:** www.opmedical.com

OSCEOLA REGIONAL MEDICAL CENTER (O, 235 beds) 700 West Oak Street, Kissimmee, FL Zip 34741–4996; tel. 407/846–2266; Kathryn Gillette, Chief Executive Officer
**Web address:** www.osceolaregional.com

PALMS WEST HOSPITAL (O, 166 beds) 13001 Southern Boulevard, Loxahatchee, FL Zip 33470–1150; tel. 561/798–3300; Eric Goldman, Chief Executive Officer
**Web address:** www.palmswesthospital.com

PLANTATION GENERAL HOSPITAL (O, 264 beds) 401 N.W. 42nd Avenue, Plantation, FL Zip 33317–2882; tel. 954/587–5010; Randy Gross, Chief Executive Officer
**Web address:** www.plantationgeneral.com

RAULERSON HOSPITAL (O, 100 beds) 1796 Highway 441 North, Okeechobee, FL Zip 34972–1918, Mailing Address: P.O. Box 1307, Zip 34973–1307; tel. 863/763–2151; Robert H. Lee, President
**Web address:** www.raulersonhospital.com

REGIONAL MEDICAL CENTER–BAYONET POINT (O, 280 beds) 14000 Fivay Road, Hudson, FL Zip 34667–7199; tel. 727/869–5400; Shayne George, Chief Executive Officer
**Web address:** www.rmchealth.com

SOUTH BAY HOSPITAL (O, 112 beds) 4016 Sun City Center Boulevard, Sun City Center, FL Zip 33573–5298; tel. 813/634–3301; Sharon L. Roush, Chief Executive Officer
**Web address:** www.southbayhospital.com

SPECIALTY HOSPITAL JACKSONVILLE (O, 62 beds) 4901 Richard Street, Jacksonville, FL Zip 32207–7328; tel. 904/737–3120; Barbara Walsh, Chief Executive Officer
**Web address:** www.specialtyhospitaljax.com

ST. LUCIE MEDICAL CENTER (O, 194 beds) 1800 S.E. Tiffany Avenue, Port St. Lucie, FL Zip 34952–7580; tel. 772/335–4000; Gary Cantrell, President and Chief Executive Officer
**Web address:** www.stluciemed.com

ST. PETERSBURG GENERAL HOSPITAL (O, 219 beds) 6500 38th Avenue North, Saint Petersburg, FL Zip 33710–1629; tel. 727/384–1414; Robert B. Conroy, Jr., Chief Executive Officer
**Web address:** www.stpetegeneral.com

For explanation of codes following names, see page B2.
★ Indicates Type III membership in the American Hospital Association.

TWIN CITIES HOSPITAL (O, 65 beds) 2190 Highway 85 North, Niceville, FL Zip 32578–1045; tel. 850/678–4131; David Whalen, Chief Executive Officer
**Web address:** www.tchealthcare.com

UNIVERSITY HOSPITAL AND MEDICAL CENTER (O, 317 beds) 7201 North University Drive, Tamarac, FL Zip 33321–2996; tel. 954/721–2200; Mark Rader, FACHE, Chief Executive Officer
**Web address:** www.uhmchealth.com

WEST FLORIDA HOSPITAL (O, 339 beds) 8383 North Davis Highway, Pensacola, FL Zip 32514–6088; tel. 850/494–4000; Brian Baumgardner, Chief Executive Officer
**Web address:** www.westfloridahospital.com

WESTSIDE REGIONAL MEDICAL CENTER (O, 224 beds) 8201 West Broward Boulevard, Plantation, FL Zip 33324–9937; tel. 954/473–6600; Lee B. Chaykin, Chief Executive Officer
**Web address:** www.westsideregional.com

**GEORGIA:** CARTERSVILLE MEDICAL CENTER (O, 80 beds) 960 Joe Frank Harris Parkway, Cartersville, GA Zip 30120–2129; tel. 770/382–1530; Keith Sandlin, Chief Executive Officer
**Web address:** www.cartersvillemedical.com

COLISEUM MEDICAL CENTERS (O, 227 beds) 350 Hospital Drive, Macon, GA Zip 31217–3871; tel. 478/765–7000; Charles Briscoe, Chief Executive Officer
**Web address:** www.coliseumhealthsystem.com

COLISEUM NORTHSIDE HOSPITAL (O, 103 beds) 400 Charter Boulevard, Macon, GA Zip 31210–4853, Mailing Address: P.O. Box 4627, Zip 31208–4627; tel. 478/757–8200; Mike Sherrod, Chief Executive Officer
**Web address:** www.coliseumhealthsystem.com

COLISEUM PSYCHIATRIC CENTER (O, 34 beds) 340 Hospital Drive, Macon, GA Zip 31217–8002; tel. 478/741–1355; James W. Eyler, FACHE, Chief Executive Officer
**Web address:** www.coliseumhealthsystem.com

DOCTORS HOSPITAL (O, 287 beds) 3651 Wheeler Road, Augusta, GA Zip 30909–6426; tel. 706/651–3232; Douglas Welch, Chief Executive Officer
**Web address:** www.doctors–hospital.net

EASTSIDE MEDICAL CENTER (O, 247 beds) 1700 Medical Way, Snellville, GA Zip 30078–2195; tel. 770/979–0200; Kimberly Ryan, Chief Executive Officer
**Web address:** www.eastsidemedical.com

FAIRVIEW PARK HOSPITAL (O, 168 beds) 200 Industrial Boulevard, Dublin, GA Zip 31021–2997, Mailing Address: P.O. Box 1408, Zip 31040–1408; tel. 478/275–2000; Donald R. Avery, FACHE, President and Chief Executive Officer
**Web address:** www.fairviewparkhospital.com

POLK MEDICAL CENTER (O, 18 beds) 424 North Main Street, Cedartown, GA Zip 30125–2698; tel. 770/748–2500; Kim Scoggins, Administrator
**Web address:** www.polkmedicalcenter.com

REDMOND REGIONAL MEDICAL CENTER (O, 230 beds) 501 Redmond Road, Rome, GA Zip 30165–7001, Mailing Address: P.O. Box 107001, Zip 30162–7001; tel. 706/291–0291; John Quinlivan, Chief Executive Officer
**Web address:** www.redmondregional.com

**IDAHO:** EASTERN IDAHO REGIONAL MEDICAL CENTER (O, 309 beds) 3100 Channing Way, Idaho Falls, ID Zip 83404–7533, Mailing Address: P.O. Box 2077, Zip 83403–2077; tel. 208/529–6111; Douglas Crabtree, Chief Executive Officer
**Web address:** www.eirmc.com

WEST VALLEY MEDICAL CENTER (O, 122 beds) 1717 Arlington, Caldwell, ID Zip 83605–4864; tel. 208/459–4641; Julie Taylor, Chief Executive Officer
**Web address:** www.westvalleymedctr.com

**INDIANA:** TERRE HAUTE REGIONAL HOSPITAL (O, 231 beds) 3901 South Seventh Street, Terre Haute, IN Zip 47802–5709; tel. 812/232–0021; Mary Ann Conroy, Chief Executive Officer
**Web address:** www.regionalhospital.com

**KANSAS:** ALLEN COUNTY HOSPITAL (O, 25 beds) 101 South First Street, Iola, KS Zip 66749–3505, Mailing Address: P.O. Box 540, Zip 66749–0540; tel. 620/365–1000; Cristina Rivera, Chief Executive Officer
**Web address:** www.allencountyhospital.com

MENORAH MEDICAL CENTER (O, 158 beds) 5721 West 119th Street, Overland Park, KS Zip 66209–3722; tel. 913/498–6000; Steven D. Wilkinson, President and Chief Executive Officer
**Web address:** www.menorahmedicalcenter.com

OVERLAND PARK REGIONAL MEDICAL CENTER (O, 276 beds) 10500 Quivira Road, Overland Park, KS Zip 66215–2306, Mailing Address: P.O. Box 15959, Zip 66215–5959; tel. 913/541–5000; Damond Boatwright, Chief Executive Officer
**Web address:** www.oprmc.com

WESLEY MEDICAL CENTER (O, 524 beds) 550 North Hillside, Wichita, KS Zip 67214–4976; tel. 316/962–2000; Hugh C. Tappan, President and Chief Executive Officer
**Web address:** www.wesleymc.com

**KENTUCKY:** FRANKFORT REGIONAL MEDICAL CENTER (O, 134 beds) 299 King's Daughters Drive, Frankfort, KY Zip 40601–4186; tel. 502/875–5240; Chip Peal, Chief Executive Officer
**Web address:** www.frankfortregional.com

GREENVIEW REGIONAL HOSPITAL (O, 167 beds) 1801 Ashley Circle, Bowling Green, KY Zip 42104–3362; tel. 270/793–1000; Mark A. Marsh, Chief Executive Officer
**Web address:** www.greenviewhospital.com

**LOUISIANA:** AMG SPECIALTY HOSPITAL–LAFAYETTE REGIONAL CAMPUS (O, 142 beds) 2810 Ambassador Caffery Parkway, Lafayette, LA Zip 70506–5906; tel. 337/981–2949; Kathy J. Bobbs, FACHE, Interim Chief Executive Officer
**Web address:** www.medicalcenterofacadiana.com

DAUTERIVE HOSPITAL (O, 103 beds) 600 North Lewis Street, New Iberia, LA Zip 70563; tel. 337/365–7311; Alan J. Fabian, Chief Executive Officer
**Web address:** www.dauterivehospital.com

LAKEVIEW REGIONAL MEDICAL CENTER (O, 172 beds) 95 Judge Tanner Boulevard, Covington, LA Zip 70433–7507; tel. 985/867–3800; Jason E. Cobb, FACHE, Chief Executive Officer
**Web address:** www.lakeviewregional.com

RAPIDES REGIONAL MEDICAL CENTER (O, 349 beds) 211 Fourth Street, Alexandria, LA Zip 71301; tel. 318/473–3000; David R. Williams, President and Chief Executive Officer
**Web address:** www.rapidesregional.com

TULANE MEDICAL CENTER (O, 327 beds) 1415 Tulane Avenue, New Orleans, LA Zip 70112–2600; tel. 504/988–5263; Robert Lynch, M.D., Chief Executive Officer
**Web address:** www.tuhc.com

TULANE–LAKESIDE HOSPITAL (O, 116 beds) 4700 South I. 10 Service Road West, Metairie, LA Zip 70001–1269; tel. 504/780–4200; Robert Lynch, M.D., Chief Executive Officer
**Web address:** www.tuhc.com

**MISSISSIPPI:** GARDEN PARK MEDICAL CENTER (O, 130 beds) 15200 Community Road, Gulfport, MS Zip 39503–3085, Mailing Address: P.O. Box 1240, Zip 39502–1240; tel. 228/575–7000; Brenda M. Waltz, FACHE, Chief Executive Officer
**Web address:** www.gpmedical.com

**MISSOURI:** BELTON REGIONAL MEDICAL CENTER (O, 38 beds) 17065 South 71 Highway, Belton, MO Zip 64012–4631; tel. 816/348–1200; Todd Krass, R.N., Chief Executive Officer
**Web address:** www.beltonregionalmedicalcenter.com

CENTERPOINT MEDICAL CENTER (O, 221 beds) 19600 East 39th Street, Independence, MO Zip 64057; tel. 816/698–7000; Carolyn W. Caldwell, President and Chief Executive Officer
**Web address:** www.centerpointmedical.com

LAFAYETTE REGIONAL HEALTH CENTER (O, 25 beds) 1500 State Street, Lexington, MO Zip 64067–1107; tel. 660/259–2203; Bret Kolman, CPA, Chief Executive Officer
**Web address:** www.lafayetteregionalhealthcenter.com

LEE'S SUMMIT MEDICAL CENTER (O, 64 beds) 2100 S.E. Blue Parkway, Lee's Summit, MO Zip 64063; tel. 816/282–5000; Jacqueline DeSouza, Chief Executive Officer
**Web address:** www.leessummitmedicalcenter.com

RESEARCH MEDICAL CENTER (O, 374 beds) 2316 East Meyer Boulevard, Kansas City, MO Zip 64132–1136; tel. 816/276–4000; Kevin J. Hicks, President and Chief Executive Officer
**Web address:** www.researchmedicalcenter.com

RESEARCH PSYCHIATRIC CENTER (O, 100 beds) 2323 East 63rd Street, Kansas City, MO Zip 64130–3462; tel. 816/444–8161; Richard Failla, Chief Executive Officer
**Web address:** www.researchpsychiatriccenter.com

For explanation of codes following names, see page B2.
★ Indicates Type III membership in the American Hospital Association.

**NEVADA:** MOUNTAINVIEW HOSPITAL (O, 235 beds) 3100 North Tenaya Way, Las Vegas, NV Zip 89128–0436; tel. 702/255–5000; William Wagnon, Chief Executive Officer
**Web address:** www.mountainview–hospital.com

SOUTHERN HILLS HOSPITAL AND MEDICAL CENTER (O, 134 beds) 9300 West Sunset Road, Las Vegas, NV Zip 89148; tel. 702/880–2100; Kimball Anderson, FACHE, Chief Executive Officer
**Web address:** www.southernhillshospital.com

SUNRISE HOSPITAL AND MEDICAL CENTER (O, 592 beds) 3186 Maryland Parkway, Las Vegas, NV Zip 89109–2306, Mailing Address: P.O. Box 98530, Zip 89193–8530; tel. 702/731–8000; Todd Sklamberg, President
**Web address:** www.sunrisehospital.com

**NEW HAMPSHIRE:** PARKLAND MEDICAL CENTER (O, 82 beds) One Parkland Drive, Derry, NH Zip 03038–2750; tel. 603/432–1500; Tina Marie Legere, Chief Executive Officer
**Web address:** www.parklandmedicalcenter.com

PORTSMOUTH REGIONAL HOSPITAL (O, 165 beds) 333 Borthwick Avenue, Portsmouth, NH Zip 03801–7004; tel. 603/436–5110; Anne Jamieson, FACHE, Chief Executive Officer
**Web address:** www.portsmouthhospital.com

**OKLAHOMA:** OU MEDICAL CENTER (O, 750 beds) 1200 Everett Drive, Oklahoma City, OK Zip 73104–5047, Mailing Address: P.O. Box 26307, Zip 73126–0307; tel. 405/271–3636; Cole C. Eslyn, FACHE, President and Chief Executive Officer
**Web address:** www.oumedcenter.com

**SOUTH CAROLINA:** COLLETON MEDICAL CENTER (O, 131 beds) 501 Robertson Boulevard, Walterboro, SC Zip 29488–5714; tel. 843/782–2000; Mitchell P. Mongell, FACHE, Chief Executive Officer
**Web address:** www.colletonmedical.com

GRAND STRAND REGIONAL MEDICAL CENTER (O, 221 beds) 809 82nd Parkway, Myrtle Beach, SC Zip 29572–1413; tel. 843/692–1000; Doug White, Chief Executive Officer
**Web address:** www.grandstrandmed.com

TRIDENT MEDICAL CENTER (O, 403 beds) 9330 Medical Plaza Drive, Charleston, SC Zip 29406–9195; tel. 843/797–7000; Todd Gallati, FACHE, President and Chief Executive Officer
**Web address:** www.tridenthealthsystem.com

**TENNESSEE:** HENDERSONVILLE MEDICAL CENTER (O, 81 beds) 355 New Shackle Island Road, Hendersonville, TN Zip 37075–2479; tel. 615/338–1000; Regina Bartlett, Chief Executive Officer
**Web address:** www.hendersonvillemedicalcenter.com

HORIZON MEDICAL CENTER (O, 130 beds) 111 Highway 70 East, Dickson, TN Zip 37055–2080; tel. 615/446–0446; John A. Marshall, Chief Executive Officer
**Web address:** www.horizonmedicalcenter.com

PARKRIDGE MEDICAL CENTER (O, 433 beds) 2333 McCallie Avenue, Chattanooga, TN Zip 37404–3258; tel. 423/698–6061; Darrell W. Moore, Chief Executive Officer
**Web address:** www.parkridgemedicalcenter.com

SKYLINE MADISON CAMPUS (O, 284 beds) 500 Hospital Drive, Madison, TN Zip 37115–5032; tel. 615/769–5000; Steve Otto, Chief Executive Officer
**Web address:** www.skylinemadison.com

SKYLINE MEDICAL CENTER (O, 295 beds) 3441 Dickerson Pike, Nashville, TN Zip 37207–2539; tel. 615/769–2000; Steve Otto, Chief Executive Officer
**Web address:** www.skylinemedicalcenter.com

SOUTHERN HILLS MEDICAL CENTER (O, 101 beds) 391 Wallace Road, Nashville, TN Zip 37211–4859; tel. 615/781–4000; Thomas H. Ozburn, Chief Executive Officer
**Web address:** www.southernhills.com

STONECREST MEDICAL CENTER (O, 101 beds) 200 StoneCrest Boulevard, Smyrna, TN Zip 37167–6810; tel. 615/768–2000; Mark E. Sims, Chief Executive Officer
**Web address:** www.stonecrestmedical.com

SUMMIT MEDICAL CENTER (O, 188 beds) 5655 Frist Boulevard, Hermitage, TN Zip 37076–2053; tel. 615/316–3000; Jeffrey T. Whitehorn, Chief Executive Officer
**Web address:** www.summitmedctr.com

TRISTAR ASHLAND CITY MEDICAL CENTER (O, 12 beds) 313 North Main Street, Ashland City, TN Zip 37015–1347; tel. 615/792–3030; Darrell White, R.N., Administrator
**Web address:** www.tristarcentennial.com

TRISTAR CENTENNIAL MEDICAL CENTER (O, 584 beds) 2300 Patterson Street, Nashville, TN Zip 37203–1528; tel. 615/342–1000; Thomas L. Herron, FACHE, Chief Executive Officer
**Web address:** www.tristarcentennial.com

**TEXAS:** BAYSHORE MEDICAL CENTER (O, 476 beds) 4000 Spencer Highway, Pasadena, TX Zip 77504–1294; tel. 713/359–2000; Jeffrey S. Holland, Chief Executive Officer
**Web address:** www.bayshoremedical.com

CLEAR LAKE REGIONAL MEDICAL CENTER (O, 655 beds) 500 Medical Center Boulevard, Webster, TX Zip 77598–4286; tel. 281/332–2511; Stephen K. Jones, Jr., FACHE, Chief Executive Officer
**Web address:** www.clearlakermc.com

CONROE REGIONAL MEDICAL CENTER (O, 292 beds) 504 Medical Boulevard, Conroe, TX Zip 77304, Mailing Address: P.O. Box 1538, Zip 77305–1538; tel. 936/539–1111; Jerry A. Nash, Chief Executive Officer
**Web address:** www.conroeregional.com

CORPUS CHRISTI MEDICAL CENTER (O, 453 beds) 3315 South Alameda Street, Corpus Christi, TX Zip 78411–1883, Mailing Address: P.O. Box 8991, Zip 78468–8991; tel. 361/761–1400; Jay Woodall, Chief Executive Officer
**Web address:** www.ccmedicalcenter.com

DENTON REGIONAL MEDICAL CENTER (O, 208 beds) 3535 South I–35 East, Denton, TX Zip 76210; tel. 940/384–3535; Caleb F. O'Rear, Chief Executive Officer
**Web address:** www.dentonregional.com

GREEN OAKS HOSPITAL (O, 106 beds) 7808 Clodus Fields Drive, Dallas, TX Zip 75251–2206; tel. 972/991–9504; Thomas M. Collins, President, Chairman and Chief Executive Officer
**Web address:** www.greenoakspsych.com

KINGWOOD MEDICAL CENTER (O, 248 beds) 22999 U.S. Highway 59 North, Kingwood, TX Zip 77339; tel. 281/348–8000; Melinda Stephenson, Chief Executive Officer
**Web address:** www.kingwoodmedical.com

LAS COLINAS MEDICAL CENTER (O, 90 beds) 6800 North MacArthur Boulevard, Irving, TX Zip 75039–2422; tel. 972/969–2000; Daniela Decell, Chief Executive Officer
**Web address:** www.lascolinasmedical.com

LAS PALMAS DEL SOL HEALTHCARE (O, 550 beds) 1801 North Oregon Street, El Paso, TX Zip 79902–3591; tel. 915/521–1200; Hank Hernandez, Chief Executive Officer
**Web address:** www.laspalmashealth.com

MEDICAL CENTER OF ARLINGTON (O, 297 beds) 3301 Matlock Road, Arlington, TX Zip 76015–2998; tel. 817/465–3241; Winston Borland, President and Chief Executive Officer
**Web address:** www.medicalcenterarlington.com

MEDICAL CENTER OF LEWISVILLE (O, 182 beds) 500 West Main, Lewisville, TX Zip 75057–3699; tel. 972/420–1000; Ashley McClellan, Chief Executive Officer
**Web address:** www.lewisvillemedical.com

MEDICAL CENTER OF MCKINNEY (O, 224 beds) 4500 Medical Center Drive, McKinney, TX Zip 75069–3499; tel. 972/547–8000; Ernest C. Lynch, III, Chief Executive Officer
**Web address:** www.medicalcenterofmckinney.com

MEDICAL CENTER OF PLANO (O, 306 beds) 3901 West 15th Street, Plano, TX Zip 75075–7799; tel. 972/596–6800; Troy Villarreal, Chief Executive Officer
**Web address:** www.medicalcenterplano.com

MEDICAL CITY DALLAS HOSPITAL (O, 592 beds) 7777 Forest Lane, Dallas, TX Zip 75230–2598; tel. 972/566–7000; Erol R. Akdamar, President and Chief Executive Officer
**Web address:** www.medicalcityhospital.com

METHODIST AMBULATORY SURGERY HOSPITAL (O, 23 beds) 9150 Huebner Road, Suite 100, San Antonio, TX Zip 78240–1545; tel. 210/575–5000; Elaine F. Morris, Administrator
**Web address:** www.mas.sahealth.com

METHODIST HOSPITAL (O, 1484 beds) 7700 Floyd Curl Drive, San Antonio, TX Zip 78229–3993; tel. 210/575–4000; Gay Nord, Chief Executive Officer
**Web address:** www.sahealth.com

METHODIST STONE OAK HOSPITAL (O, 134 beds) 1139 East Sonterra Boulevard, San Antonio, TX Zip 78258; tel. 210/638–2100; Dean M. Alexander, Chief Executive Officer
**Web address:** www.stoneoakhealth.com

---

For explanation of codes following names, see page B2.
★ Indicates Type III membership in the American Hospital Association.

NORTH HILLS HOSPITAL (O, 176 beds) 4401 Booth Calloway Road, North Richland Hills, TX Zip 76180–7399; tel. 817/255–1000; Randy Moresi, Chief Executive Officer
**Web address:** www.northhillshospital.com

PLAZA MEDICAL CENTER OF FORT WORTH (O, 219 beds) 900 Eighth Avenue, Fort Worth, TX Zip 76104–3986; tel. 817/336–2100; Clay Franklin, Chief Executive Officer
**Web address:** www.plazamedicalcenter.com

RIO GRANDE REGIONAL HOSPITAL (O, 320 beds) 101 East Ridge Road, McAllen, TX Zip 78503–1299; tel. 956/632–6000; Gregory A. Seiler, Chief Executive Officer
**Web address:** www.riohealth.com

ST. DAVID'S MEDICAL CENTER (O, 458 beds) 919 East 32nd Street, Austin, TX Zip 78705–2709, Mailing Address: P.O. Box 4039, Zip 78765–4039; tel. 512/476–7111; Donald H. Wilkerson, Chief Executive Officer
**Web address:** www.stdavids.com

ST. DAVID'S NORTH AUSTIN MEDICAL CENTER (O, 332 beds) 12221 North MoPac Expressway, Austin, TX Zip 78758–2496; tel. 512/901–1000; Allen Harrison, Chief Executive Officer
**Web address:** www.northaustin.com

ST. DAVID'S REHABILITATION CENTER (O, 64 beds) 1005 East 32nd Street, Austin, TX Zip 78705–2705, Mailing Address: P.O. Box 4270, Zip 78765–4270; tel. 512/544–5100; Diane Owens, Administrator
**Web address:** www.stdavids.com

ST. DAVID'S ROUND ROCK MEDICAL CENTER (O, 156 beds) 2400 Round Rock Avenue, Round Rock, TX Zip 78681–4097; tel. 512/341–1000; Deborah L. Ryle, Administrator and Chief Executive Officer
**Web address:** www.stdavids.com

ST. DAVID'S SOUTH AUSTIN MEDICAL CENTER (O, 222 beds) 901 West Ben White Boulevard, Austin, TX Zip 78704–6903; tel. 512/447–2211; Todd E. Steward, Chief Executive Officer
**Web address:** www.southaustinmc.com

TEXAS ORTHOPEDIC HOSPITAL (O, 49 beds) 7401 Main Street, Houston, TX Zip 77030–4509; tel. 713/799–8600; Trent Lind, Chief Executive Officer
**Web address:** www.texasorthopedic.com

THE WOMAN'S HOSPITAL OF TEXAS (O, 367 beds) 7600 Fannin Street, Houston, TX Zip 77054–1906; tel. 713/790–1234; Linda B. Russell, Chief Executive Officer
**Web address:** www.womanshospital.com

VALLEY REGIONAL MEDICAL CENTER (O, 214 beds) 100A Alton Gloor Boulevard, Brownsville, TX Zip 78526–3346, Mailing Address: P.O. Box 3710, Zip 78523–3710; tel. 956/350–7101; Susan Andrews, Chief Executive Officer
**Web address:** www.valleyregionalmedicalcenter.com

WEST HOUSTON MEDICAL CENTER (O, 227 beds) 12141 Richmond Avenue, Houston, TX Zip 77082–2499; tel. 281/558–3444; Todd Caliva, Chief Executive Officer
**Web address:** www.westhoustonmedical.com

**UTAH:** BRIGHAM CITY COMMUNITY HOSPITAL (O, 39 beds) 950 South Medical Drive, Brigham City, UT Zip 84302; tel. 435/734–9471; Richard Spuhler, Chief Executive Officer
**Web address:** www.brighamcityhospital.com

LAKEVIEW HOSPITAL (O, 116 beds) 630 East Medical Drive, Bountiful, UT Zip 84010–4996; tel. 801/299–2200; Rand Kerr, Chief Executive Officer
**Web address:** www.lakeviewhospital.com

MOUNTAIN VIEW HOSPITAL (O, 114 beds) 1000 East 100 North, Payson, UT Zip 84651–1690; tel. 801/465–7000; Kevin Johnson, Chief Executive Officer
**Web address:** www.mvhpayson.com

OGDEN REGIONAL MEDICAL CENTER (O, 167 beds) 5475 South 500 East, Ogden, UT Zip 84405–6978; tel. 801/479–2111; Mark B. Adams, Chief Executive Officer
**Web address:** www.ogdenregional.com

ST. MARK'S HOSPITAL (O, 317 beds) 1200 East 3900 South, Salt Lake City, UT Zip 84124–1390; tel. 801/268–7111; Steven B. Bateman, Chief Executive Officer
**Web address:** www.stmarkshospital.com

TIMPANOGOS REGIONAL HOSPITAL (O, 117 beds) 750 West 800 North, Orem, UT Zip 84059–3660; tel. 801/714–6000; Keith D. Tintle, Chief Executive Officer
**Web address:** www.timpanogosregionalhospital.com

**VIRGINIA:** CJW MEDICAL CENTER (O, 758 beds) 7101 Jahnke Road, Richmond, VA Zip 23225–4044; tel. 804/320–3911; Tim McManus, Interim Chief Executive Officer
**Web address:** www.cjwmedical.com

DOMINION HOSPITAL (O, 94 beds) 2960 Sleepy Hollow Road, Falls Church, VA Zip 22044–2030; tel. 703/536–2000; Suzanne B. Jackson, FACHE, Chief Executive Officer
**Web address:** www.dominionhospital.com

HENRICO DOCTORS' HOSPITAL (O, 488 beds) 1602 Skipwith Road, Richmond, VA Zip 23229–5205; tel. 804/289–4500; Patrick J. Farrell, Chief Executive Officer
**Web address:** www.henricodoctorshospital.com

JOHN RANDOLPH MEDICAL CENTER (O, 118 beds) 411 West Randolph Road, Hopewell, VA Zip 23860–2938; tel. 804/541–1600; Dia Nichols, Chief Executive Officer
**Web address:** www.johnrandolphmed.com

LEWIS–GALE MEDICAL CENTER (O, 521 beds) 1900 Electric Road, Salem, VA Zip 24153–7494; tel. 540/776–4000; Victor Giovanetti, President and Chief Executive Officer
**Web address:** www.lewis–gale.com

LEWISGALE HOSPITAL ALLEGHANY (O, 146 beds) One ARH Lane, Low Moor, VA Zip 24457, Mailing Address: P.O. Box 7, Zip 24457–0007; tel. 540/862–6011; Greg T. Madsen, Chief Executive Officer
**Web address:** www.alleghanyregional.com

LEWISGALE HOSPITAL AT PULASKI (O, 54 beds) 2400 Lee Highway, Pulaski, VA Zip 24301–0759, Mailing Address: P.O. Box 759, Zip 24301–0759; tel. 540/994–8100; Mark Nichols, FACHE, Chief Executive Officer
**Web address:** www.pch–va.com/

MONTGOMERY REGIONAL HOSPITAL (O, 103 beds) 3700 South Main Street, Blacksburg, VA Zip 24060–7081, Mailing Address: P.O. Box 90004, Zip 24062–9004; tel. 540/951–1111; Scott Hill, Chief Executive Officer
**Web address:** www.mrhospital.com

RESTON HOSPITAL CENTER (O, 187 beds) 1850 Town Center Parkway, Reston, VA Zip 20190–3219; tel. 703/689–9000; Tim McManus, President and Chief Executive Officer
**Web address:** www.restonhospital.com

SPOTSYLVANIA REGIONAL MEDICAL CENTER (O, 100 beds) 4600 Spotsylvania Parkway, Fredericksburg, VA Zip 22408; tel. 540/834–1500; Timothy C. Tobin, FACHE, President and Chief Executive Officer
**Web address:** www.spotsrmc.com

| | | |
|---|---|---|
| **Owned, leased, sponsored:** | 146 hospitals | 35106 beds |
| **Contract–managed:** | 0 hospitals | 0 beds |
| **Totals:** | 146 hospitals | 35106 beds |

---

**0328: HEALTH FIRST, INC.** (NP)
6450 U.S. Highway 1, Rockledge, FL Zip 32955; tel. 321/434–7000; Steven P. Johnson, Ph.D., President and Chief Executive Officer
**(Centralized Physician/Insurance Health System)**

**FLORIDA:** CAPE CANAVERAL HOSPITAL (O, 145 beds) 701 West Cocoa Beach Causeway, Cocoa Beach, FL Zip 32931–5595, Mailing Address: P.O. Box 320069, Zip 32932–0069; tel. 321/799–7111; Roy Wright, FACHE, President and Chief Executive Officer
**Web address:** www.health–first.org

HOLMES REGIONAL MEDICAL CENTER (O, 514 beds) 1350 South Hickory Street, Melbourne, FL Zip 32901–3276; tel. 321/434–7000; Judy Killebrew, President
**Web address:** www.health–first.org

PALM BAY HOSPITAL (O, 119 beds) 1425 Malabar Road N.E., Melbourne, FL Zip 32907; tel. 321/434–8000; Roy Wright, FACHE, President
**Web address:** www.health–first.org

VIERA HOSPITAL (O, 84 beds) 8745 North Wickham Road, Melbourne, FL Zip 32940–5997; tel. 321/434–9164; Christopher Kennedy, President
**Web address:** www.vierahospital.org

| | | |
|---|---|---|
| **Owned, leased, sponsored:** | 4 hospitals | 862 beds |
| **Contract–managed:** | 0 hospitals | 0 beds |
| **Totals:** | 4 hospitals | 862 beds |

Section B

## 1775: HEALTH MANAGEMENT ASSOCIATES (IO)
5811 Pelican Bay Boulevard, Suite 500, Naples, FL Zip 34108; tel. 239/598-3131; Gary D. Newsome, President and Chief Executive Officer
**(Decentralized Health System)**

**ALABAMA:** RIVERVIEW REGIONAL MEDICAL CENTER (O, 204 beds) 600 South Third Street, Gadsden, AL Zip 35901-5399, Mailing Address: P.O. Box 268, Zip 35902; tel. 256/543-5200; Lloyd F. Ford, Jr., Ph.D., FACHE, Chief Executive Officer
**Web address:** www.riverviewregional.com

STRINGFELLOW MEMORIAL HOSPITAL (L, 79 beds) 301 East 18th Street, Anniston, AL Zip 36207-0038, Mailing Address: P.O. Box 38, Zip 36207-0038; tel. 256/235-8900; John Gallagher, Chief Executive Officer
**Web address:** www.stringfellowhealth.com

**ARKANSAS:** SPARKS REGIONAL MEDICAL CENTER (O, 303 beds) 100 Towson Avenue, Fort Smith, AR Zip 72901-2632, Mailing Address: P.O. Box 17006, Zip 72917-7006; tel. 479/441-4000; Melody Trimble, Chief Executive Officer
**Web address:** www.sparks.org

SUMMIT MEDICAL CENTER (L, 103 beds) East Main and South 20th Streets, Van Buren, AR Zip 72956-5715, Mailing Address: P.O. Box 409, Zip 72957-0409; tel. 479/474-3401; Sue Conley, Chief Executive Officer
**Web address:** www.summitmedicalcenter.net

**FLORIDA:** BARTOW REGIONAL MEDICAL CENTER (O, 72 beds) 2200 Osprey Boulevard, Bartow, FL Zip 33830-3308, Mailing Address: P.O. Box 1050, Zip 33831-1050; tel. 863/533-8111; Troy DeDecker, Chief Executive Officer
**Web address:** www.bartowregional.com

BROOKSVILLE REGIONAL HOSPITAL (L, 91 beds) 17240 Cortez Boulevard, Brooksville, FL Zip 34601, Mailing Address: P.O. Box 37, Zip 34605-0037; tel. 352/796-5111; Kenneth R. Wicker, Chief Executive Officer
**Web address:** www.brooksvilleregionalhospital.org

CHARLOTTE REGIONAL MEDICAL CENTER (O, 208 beds) 809 East Marion Avenue, Punta Gorda, FL Zip 33950-3898, Mailing Address: P.O. Box 51-1328, Zip 33951-1328; tel. 941/639-3131; Jose F. Morillo, Chief Executive Officer
**Web address:** www.charlotteregional.com

HEART OF FLORIDA REGIONAL MEDICAL CENTER (O, 194 beds) 40100 Highway 27, Davenport, FL Zip 33837-5906; tel. 863/422-4971; Donnie Breeding, Chief Executive Officer
**Web address:** www.heartofflorida.com

HIGHLANDS REGIONAL MEDICAL CENTER (L, 126 beds) 3600 South Highlands Avenue, Sebring, FL Zip 33870-5495, Mailing Address: Drawer 2066, Zip 33871-2066; tel. 863/471-5800; Brian Hess, Chief Executive Officer
**Web address:** www.highlandsregional.com

LEHIGH REGIONAL MEDICAL CENTER (O, 88 beds) 1500 Lee Boulevard, Lehigh Acres, FL Zip 33936-4897; tel. 239/369-2101; Joanie Jeannette, MSN, Chief Executive Officer
**Web address:** www.lehighregional.com

LOWER KEYS MEDICAL CENTER (L, 90 beds) 5900 College Road, Key West, FL Zip 33040-4396, Mailing Address: P.O. Box 9107, Zip 33041-9107; tel. 305/294-5531; Nicki L. Will-Mowery, Ph.D., Chief Executive Officer
**Web address:** www.lkmc.com

PASCO REGIONAL MEDICAL CENTER (O, 120 beds) 13100 Fort King Road, Dade City, FL Zip 33525-5294; tel. 352/521-1100; Philip Minden, Chief Executive Officer
**Web address:** www.pascoregionalmc.com

PEACE RIVER REGIONAL MEDICAL CENTER (O, 190 beds) 2500 Harbor Boulevard, Port Charlotte, FL Zip 33952-5396; tel. 941/766-4122; Joseph T. Clancy, Chief Executive Officer
**Web address:** www.peaceriverregional.com

PHYSICIANS REGIONAL MEDICAL CENTER – PINE RIDGE (O, 70 beds) 6101 Pine Ridge Road, Naples, FL Zip 34119; tel. 239/348-4000; Geoffrey D. Moebius, Chief Executive Officer
**Web address:** www.physiciansregional.com

SANTA ROSA MEDICAL CENTER (L, 105 beds) 1450 Berryhill Road, Milton, FL Zip 32570-4028, Mailing Address: P.O. Box 648, Zip 32572-0648; tel. 850/626-7762; Phillip L. Wright, FACHE, Chief Executive Officer
**Web address:** www.santarosamedicalcenter.org

SEBASTIAN RIVER MEDICAL CENTER (O, 115 beds) 13695 North U.S. Highway 1, Sebastian, FL Zip 32958-3230, Mailing Address: Box 780838, Zip 32978-0838; tel. 772/589-3186; Steven Salyer, Chief Executive Officer
**Web address:** www.sebastianrivermedical.com

SEVEN RIVERS REGIONAL MEDICAL CENTER (O, 128 beds) 6201 North Suncoast Boulevard, Crystal River, FL Zip 34428-6712; tel. 352/795-6560; Joyce A. Brancato, Chief Executive Officer
**Web address:** www.srrmc.com

SHANDS LAKE SHORE (O, 85 beds) 368 N.E. Franklin Street, Lake City, FL Zip 32055-3047; tel. 386/292-8000; Rhonda Kay Sherrod, R.N., MSN, Administrator
**Web address:** www.shands.org

SHANDS LIVE OAK (O, 15 beds) 1100 S.W. 11th Street, Live Oak, FL Zip 32060-3608; tel. 386/362-0800; Ricardo Diaz, Chief Executive Officer
**Web address:** www.shands.org

SHANDS STARKE REGIONAL MEDICAL CENTER (O, 25 beds) 922 East Call Street, Starke, FL Zip 32091-3699; tel. 904/368-2300; Brent Burish, Chief Executive Officer
**Web address:** www.shands.org

SPRING HILL REGIONAL HOSPITAL (L, 75 beds) 10461 Quality Drive, Spring Hill, FL Zip 34609-9634; tel. 352/688-8200; Patrick Maloney, Interim Chief Executive Officer
**Web address:** www.springhillregionalhospital.org

ST. CLOUD REGIONAL MEDICAL CENTER (O, 84 beds) 2906 17th Street, Saint Cloud, FL Zip 34769-6099; tel. 407/892-2135; Lindell W. Orr, Interim Chief Executive Officer
**Web address:** www.stcloudregional.com

VENICE REGIONAL MEDICAL CENTER (O, 220 beds) 540 The Rialto, Venice, FL Zip 34285-2900; tel. 941/485-7711; Peter Wozniak, MS, R.N., Chief Executive Officer
**Web address:** www.veniceregional.com

WUESTHOFF MEDICAL CENTER – MELBOURNE (O, 115 beds) 250 North Wickham Road, Melbourne, FL Zip 32935; tel. 321/752-1200; Jeannette Skinner, R.N., FACHE, Chief Executive Officer
**Web address:** www.wuesthoff.org

WUESTHOFF MEDICAL CENTER – ROCKLEDGE (O, 291 beds) 110 Longwood Avenue, Rockledge, FL Zip 32955-2887, Mailing Address: P.O. Box 565002, Mail Stop 1, Zip 32956-5002; tel. 321/636-2211; Devon Hyde, Chief Operating Officer
**Web address:** www.wuesthoff.org

**GEORGIA:** BARROW REGIONAL MEDICAL CENTER (O, 56 beds) 316 North Broad Street, Winder, GA Zip 30680-2150, Mailing Address: P.O. Box 688, Zip 30680-0688; tel. 770/867-3400; Todd Dixon, R.N., Chief Executive Officer
**Web address:** www.barrowregional.com

EAST GEORGIA REGIONAL MEDICAL CENTER (O, 150 beds) 1499 Fair Road, Statesboro, GA Zip 30458, Mailing Address: P.O. Box 1048, Zip 30459-1048; tel. 912/486-1000; Robert F. Bigley, President and Chief Executive Officer
**Web address:** www.eastgeorgiaregional.com

WALTON REGIONAL MEDICAL CENTER (O, 115 beds) 330 Alcovy Street, Monroe, GA Zip 30655-2140, Mailing Address: P.O. Box 1346, Zip 30655-1346; tel. 770/267-8461; J. T. Barnhart, Chief Executive Officer
**Web address:** www.waltonregional.com

**KENTUCKY:** PAUL B. HALL REGIONAL MEDICAL CENTER (O, 72 beds) 625 James S. Trimble Boulevard, Paintsville, KY Zip 41240-0000; tel. 606/789-3511; Deborah Trimble, R.N., Chief Executive Officer
**Web address:** www.pbhrmc.com

**MISSISSIPPI:** BILOXI REGIONAL MEDICAL CENTER (L, 198 beds) 150 Reynoir Street, Biloxi, MS Zip 39530-4199, Mailing Address: P.O. Box 128, Zip 39533-0128; tel. 228/432-1571; Monte J. Bostwick, Chief Executive Officer
**Web address:** www.hmamississippi.com

CENTRAL MISSISSIPPI MEDICAL CENTER (L, 377 beds) 1850 Chadwick Drive, Jackson, MS Zip 39204-3479, Mailing Address: P.O. Box 59001, Zip 39204-9001; tel. 601/376-1000; Charlotte W. Dupre', Chief Executive Officer
**Web address:** www.centralmississippimedicalcenter.com

CROSSGATES RIVER OAKS HOSPITAL (L, 134 beds) 350 Crossgates Boulevard, Brandon, MS Zip 39042-2698; tel. 601/825-2811; J. Allen Tyra, Chief Executive Officer
**Web address:** www.crossgatesriveroaks.com

Section B

GILMORE MEMORIAL REGIONAL MEDICAL CENTER (O, 95 beds) 1105 Earl Frye Boulevard, Amory, MS Zip 38821–5500, Mailing Address: P.O. Box 459, Zip 38821–0459; tel. 662/256–7111; L. Dwayne Blaylock, Chief Executive Officer
**Web address:** www.gilmorehealth.com

MADISON RIVER OAKS MEDICAL CENTER (L, 67 beds) Highway 16 East, Canton, MS Zip 39046–8823, Mailing Address: P.O. Box 1607, Zip 39046–1607; tel. 601/859–1331; Glen Silverman, Chief Executive Officer
**Web address:** www.madisonriveroaks.com

NATCHEZ COMMUNITY HOSPITAL (O, 101 beds) 129 Jefferson Davis Boulevard, Natchez, MS Zip 39120–5100, Mailing Address: P.O. Box 1203, Zip 39121–1203; tel. 601/445–6200; Donald Rentfro, Chief Executive Officer
**Web address:** www.natchezcommunityhospital.com/default.aspx

NORTHWEST MISSISSIPPI REGIONAL MEDICAL CENTER (L, 195 beds) 1970 Hospital Drive, Clarksdale, MS Zip 38614–7204, Mailing Address: P.O. Box 1218, Zip 38614–1218; tel. 662/627–3211; Joan Strayham, R.N., Interim Chief Executive Officer
**Web address:** www.northwestregional.org

RIVER OAKS HOSPITAL (O, 158 beds) 1030 River Oaks Drive, Flowood, MS Zip 39232–9553, Mailing Address: P.O. Box 5100, Jackson, Zip 39296–5100; tel. 601/932–1030; Dennis R. Bruns, Chief Executive Officer
**Web address:** www.riveroakshosp.org

TRI–LAKES MEDICAL CENTER (O, 112 beds) 303 Medical Center Drive, Batesville, MS Zip 38606–8608; tel. 662/563–5611; Wes Sigler, Chief Executive Officer
**Web address:** www.trilakesmc.com

WOMAN'S HOSPITAL (O, 60 beds) 1026 North Flowood Drive, Flowood, MS Zip 39232–9532, Mailing Address: P.O. Box 4546, Jackson, Zip 39296–4546; tel. 601/932–1000; Sherry J. Pitts, Chief Executive Officer
**Web address:** www.womanshospitalms.com

**MISSOURI:** POPLAR BLUFF REGIONAL MEDICAL CENTER (O, 287 beds) 2620 North Westwood Boulevard, Poplar Bluff, MO Zip 63901–3396, Mailing Address: P.O. Box 88, Zip 63902–0088; tel. 573/686–5311; Charles L. Stewart, Chief Executive Officer
**Web address:** www.poplarbluffregional.com

TWIN RIVERS REGIONAL MEDICAL CENTER (O, 116 beds) 1301 First Street, Kennett, MO Zip 63857–2508, Mailing Address: P.O. Box 728, Zip 63857–0728; tel. 573/888–4522; Kenneth James, Chief Executive Officer
**Web address:** www.twinriversmedctr.com

**NORTH CAROLINA:** DAVIS REGIONAL MEDICAL CENTER (O, 131 beds) 218 Old Mocksville Road, Statesville, NC Zip 28625–1930, Mailing Address: P.O. Box 1823, Zip 28687–1823; tel. 704/873–0281; Vincent T. Cherry, Jr., Chief Executive Officer
**Web address:** www.davisregional.com

LAKE NORMAN REGIONAL MEDICAL CENTER (O, 103 beds) 171 Fairview Road, Mooresville, NC Zip 28117–9500, Mailing Address: P.O. Box 3250, Zip 28117–3250; tel. 704/660–4000; Greg Lowe, Chief Executive Officer
**Web address:** www.lnrmc.com

SANDHILLS REGIONAL MEDICAL CENTER (O, 64 beds) 1000 West Hamlet Avenue, Hamlet, NC Zip 28345–4522, Mailing Address: P.O. Box 1109, Zip 28345–1109; tel. 910/205–8000; Michael H. McNair, Chief Executive Officer
**Web address:** www.hma–corp.com

**OKLAHOMA:** INTEGRIS BLACKWELL REGIONAL HOSPITAL (O, 31 beds) 710 South 13th Street, Blackwell, OK Zip 74631–3700; tel. 580/363–2311; Julie M. McCormack, R.N., Administrator
**Web address:** www.integris–health.com

INTEGRIS CLINTON REGIONAL HOSPITAL (O, 49 beds) 100 North 30th Street, Clinton, OK Zip 73601–3117, Mailing Address: P.O. Box 1569, Zip 73601–1569; tel. 580/323–2363; Darcey O'Brien, Chief Executive Officer
**Web address:** www.integris–health.com

INTEGRIS MARSHALL COUNTY MEDICAL CENTER (O, 21 beds) 1 Hospital Drive, Madill, OK Zip 73446, Mailing Address: P.O. Box 827, Zip 73446–0827; tel. 580/795–3384; Matthew M. Lyden, Chief Executive Officer
**Web address:** www.integrismarshallcounty.com

INTEGRIS MAYES COUNTY MEDICAL CENTER (O, 39 beds) 111 North Bailey Street, Pryor, OK Zip 74361–4211, Mailing Address: P.O. Box 278, Zip 74362–0278; tel. 918/825–1600; Douglas K. Weaver, FACHE, President
**Web address:** www.integris–health.com

INTEGRIS SEMINOLE MEDICAL CENTER (O, 32 beds) 2401 Wrangler Boulevard, Seminole, OK Zip 74868–1917; tel. 405/303–4000; C. David Hill, President
**Web address:** www.hma.com

MEDICAL CENTER OF SOUTHEASTERN OKLAHOMA (O, 148 beds) 1800 University Boulevard, Durant, OK Zip 74701–3006, Mailing Address: P.O. Box 1207, Zip 74702–1207; tel. 580/924–3080; Patricia Dorris, Executive Director
**Web address:** www.mymcso.com

MIDWEST REGIONAL MEDICAL CENTER (L, 255 beds) 2825 Parklawn Drive, Midwest City, OK Zip 73110–4258; tel. 405/610–4411; Stan V. Holm, FACHE, Chief Executive Officer
**Web address:** www.midwestregional.com

**PENNSYLVANIA:** CARLISLE REGIONAL MEDICAL CENTER (O, 165 beds) 361 Alexander Spring Road, Carlisle, PA Zip 17015–6940; tel. 717/249–1212; John Kristel, Chief Executive Officer
**Web address:** www.carlislermc.com/default.aspx

HEART OF LANCASTER REGIONAL MEDICAL CENTER (O, 139 beds) 1500 Highlands Drive, Lititz, PA Zip 17543; tel. 717/625–5000; James Machado, Administrator
**Web address:** www.heartoflancaster.com

LANCASTER REGIONAL MEDICAL CENTER (O, 150 beds) 250 College Avenue, Lancaster, PA Zip 17603, Mailing Address: P.O. Box 3434, Zip 17604–3434; tel. 717/291–8211; Bob Moore, FACHE, Chief Executive Officer
**Web address:** www.lancasterregional.com

**SOUTH CAROLINA:** CAROLINA PINES REGIONAL MEDICAL CENTER (O, 99 beds) 1304 West Bobo Newsom Highway, Hartsville, SC Zip 29550–4710; tel. 843/339–2100; J. Timothy Browne, FACHE, Chief Executive Officer
**Web address:** www.cprmc.com

CHESTER REGIONAL MEDICAL CENTER (L, 136 beds) 1 Medical Park Drive, Chester, SC Zip 29706–9799; tel. 803/581–3151; Page H. Vaughan, Chief Executive Officer
**Web address:** www.chospital.org

**TENNESSEE:** HARTON REGIONAL MEDICAL CENTER (O, 104 beds) 1801 North Jackson Street, Tullahoma, TN Zip 37388–2201; tel. 931/393–3000; William R. Spray, Chief Executive Officer
**Web address:** www.hartonmedicalcenter.com

JAMESTOWN REGIONAL MEDICAL CENTER (O, 85 beds) 436 Central Avenue West, Jamestown, TN Zip 38556–3031, Mailing Address: P.O. Box 1500, Zip 38556–1500; tel. 931/879–8171; Kimberly L. Anthony, Chief Executive Officer
**Web address:** www.jamestownregional.org

JEFFERSON MEMORIAL HOSPITAL (L, 54 beds) 110 Hospital Drive, Jefferson City, TN Zip 37760–5281; tel. 865/471–2500; David V. Bunch, President
**Web address:** www.hma.com/content/jefferson–memorial–hospital

LAFOLLETTE MEDICAL CENTER (L, 164 beds) 923 East Central Avenue, La Follette, TN Zip 37766–3106, Mailing Address: P.O. Box 1301, Zip 37766–1301; tel. 423/907–1200; Mark Cain, Chief Executive Officer
**Web address:** www.hma.com/content/lafollette–medical–center

NEWPORT MEDICAL CENTER (O, 47 beds) 435 Second Street, Newport, TN Zip 37821–3799; tel. 423/625–2200; Spencer Thomas, Chief Executive Officer
**Web address:** www.hma.com/content/newport–medical–center

PHYSICIANS REGIONAL MEDICAL CENTER (O, 243 beds) 900 East Oak Hill Avenue, Knoxville, TN Zip 37917–4556; tel. 865/545–8000; Karen Metz, Chief Executive Officer
**Web address:** www.hma.com/content/physicians–regional–medical–center

TURKEY CREEK MEDICAL CENTER (O, 101 beds) 10820 Parkside Drive, Knoxville, TN Zip 37922–1956; tel. 865/218–7011; Lance W. Jones, Chief Executive Officer
**Web address:** www.hma.com/content/turkey–creek–medical–center

UNIVERSITY MEDICAL CENTER (O, 245 beds) 1411 Baddour Parkway, Lebanon, TN Zip 37087–2595; tel. 615/444–8262; Saad Ehtisham, R.N., FACHE, Chief Executive Officer
**Web address:** www.universitymedicalcenter.com

For explanation of codes following names, see page B2.
★ Indicates Type III membership in the American Hospital Association.

**TEXAS:** DALLAS REGIONAL MEDICAL CENTER (O, 85 beds) 1011 North Galloway Avenue, Mesquite, TX Zip 75149–2433; tel. 214/320–7000; Matthew T. Caldwell, Chief Executive Officer
**Web address:** www.dallasregionalmedicalcenter.com

**WASHINGTON:** TOPPENISH COMMUNITY HOSPITAL (O, 63 beds) 502 West Fourth Avenue, Toppenish, WA Zip 98948–0672, Mailing Address: P.O. Box 672, Zip 98948–0672; tel. 509/865–3105; Derrick Yu, Administrator
**Web address:** www.hma–corp.com

YAKIMA REGIONAL MEDICAL AND CARDIAC CENTER (O, 214 beds) 110 South Ninth Avenue, Yakima, WA Zip 98902–3397; tel. 509/575–5000; Richard H. Robinson, Chief Executive Officer
**Web address:** www.yakimaregional.net

**WEST VIRGINIA:** WILLIAMSON MEMORIAL HOSPITAL (O, 76 beds) 859 Alderson Street, Williamson, WV Zip 25661–3215, Mailing Address: P.O. Box 1980, Zip 25661–1980; tel. 304/235–2500; Todd C. Hubler, Chief Executive Officer
**Web address:** www.hmawmh.com

| | | |
|---|---|---|
| Owned, leased, sponsored: | 68 hospitals | 8532 beds |
| Contract–managed: | 0 hospitals | 0 beds |
| Totals: | 68 hospitals | 8532 beds |

---

**★0307: HEALTH QUEST SYSTEMS, INC.** (NP)
1351 Route 55, Lagrangeville, NY Zip 12540–5108; tel. 845/475–9500; Michael T. Weber, President and Chief Executive Officer
**(Moderately Centralized Health System)**

**NEW YORK:** NORTHERN DUTCHESS HOSPITAL (O, 68 beds) 6511 Springbrook Avenue, Rhinebeck, NY Zip 12572–5002, Mailing Address: P.O. Box 5002, Zip 12572–5002; tel. 845/876–3001; Denise George, R.N., President and Chief Executive Officer
**Web address:** www.health–quest.org/home_nd.cfm?id=9

PUTNAM HOSPITAL CENTER (O, 164 beds) 670 Stoneleigh Avenue, Carmel, NY Zip 10512–3997; tel. 845/279–5711; Maureen Zipparo, President and Chief Operating Officer
**Web address:** www.putnamhospital.org

VASSAR BROTHERS MEDICAL CENTER (O, 365 beds) 45 Reade Place, Poughkeepsie, NY Zip 12601–3947; tel. 845/454–8500; Janet L. Ready, President and Chief Operating Officer
**Web address:** www.health–quest.org

| | | |
|---|---|---|
| Owned, leased, sponsored: | 3 hospitals | 597 beds |
| Contract–managed: | 0 hospitals | 0 beds |
| Totals: | 3 hospitals | 597 beds |

---

**0534: HEALTHALLIANCE OF THE HUDSON VALLEY** (NP)
396 Broadway, Kingston, NY Zip 12401–4626; tel. 845/331–3131; David W. Lundquist, President and Chief Executive Officer
**(Independent Hospital System)**

BENEDICTINE HOSPITAL (O, 120 beds) 105 Marys Avenue, Kingston, NY Zip 12401–5894; tel. 845/338–2500; David W. Lundquist, President and Chief Executive Officer
**Web address:** www.benedictine.org

KINGSTON HOSPITAL (O, 150 beds) 396 Broadway, Kingston, NY Zip 12401–4692; tel. 845/331–3131; David W. Lundquist, President and Chief Executive Officer
**Web address:** www.kingstonregionalhealth.org

MARGARETVILLE HOSPITAL (O, 15 beds) 42084 State Highway 28, Margaretville, NY Zip 12455–2820; tel. 845/586–2631; Sandra A. Horan, Executive Director
**Web address:** www.margaretvillehospital.org

| | | |
|---|---|---|
| Owned, leased, sponsored: | 3 hospitals | 285 beds |
| Contract–managed: | 0 hospitals | 0 beds |
| Totals: | 3 hospitals | 285 beds |

---

**★2185: HEALTHEAST CARE SYSTEM** (NP)
559 Capitol Boulevard, 6–South, Saint Paul, MN Zip 55103–0000; tel. 651/232–2300; Kathryn G. Correia, President and Chief Executive Officer
**(Centralized Health System)**

**MINNESOTA:** HEALTHEAST BETHESDA HOSPITAL (O, 126 beds) 559 Capitol Boulevard, Saint Paul, MN Zip 55103–2101; tel. 651/232–2000; Catherine Barr, President
**Web address:** www.healtheast.org

ST. JOHN'S HOSPITAL (O, 192 beds) 1575 Beam Avenue, Saint Paul, MN Zip 55109–1126; tel. 651/232–7000; Scott L. North, FACHE, Chief Executive Officer
**Web address:** www.stjohnshospital–mn.org

ST. JOSEPH'S HOSPITAL (O, 232 beds) 45 West 10th Street, Saint Paul, MN Zip 55102–1053; tel. 651/232–3000; Scott L. North, FACHE, Chief Executive Officer
**Web address:** www.healtheast.org

WOODWINDS HEALTH CAMPUS (O, 86 beds) 1925 Woodwinds Drive, Woodbury, MN Zip 55125–4445; tel. 651/232–0228; Scott L. North, FACHE, Chief Executive Officer
**Web address:** www.woodwinds.org

| | | |
|---|---|---|
| Owned, leased, sponsored: | 4 hospitals | 636 beds |
| Contract–managed: | 0 hospitals | 0 beds |
| Totals: | 4 hospitals | 636 beds |

---

**0342: HEALTHPARTNERS** (NP)
8170 33rd Avenue South, Bloomington, MN Zip 55425–1514; tel. 952/883–7463; Mary K. Brainerd, President and Chief Executive Officer
**(Moderately Centralized Health System)**

LAKEVIEW HOSPITAL (O, 66 beds) 927 Churchill Street West, Stillwater, MN Zip 55082–5930; tel. 651/439–5330; Curt Geissler, President
**Web address:** www.lakeview.org

REGIONS HOSPITAL (O, 424 beds) 640 Jackson Street, Saint Paul, MN Zip 55101–2595; tel. 651/254–3456; Brock D. Nelson, President and Chief Executive Officer
**Web address:** www.regionshospital.com

**WISCONSIN:** WESTFIELDS HOSPITAL (O, 25 beds) 535 Hospital Road, New Richmond, WI Zip 54017–1495; tel. 715/243–2600; Steven Massey, President and Chief Executive Officer
**Web address:** www.westfieldshospital.com

| | | |
|---|---|---|
| Owned, leased, sponsored: | 3 hospitals | 515 beds |
| Contract–managed: | 0 hospitals | 0 beds |
| Totals: | 3 hospitals | 515 beds |

---

**★0023: HEALTHSOUTH CORPORATION** (IO)
3660 Grandview Parkway, Suite 200, Birmingham, AL Zip 35243; tel. 205/967–7116; Jay F. Grinney, President and Chief Executive Officer
**(Decentralized Health System)**

**ALABAMA:** HEALTHSOUTH LAKESHORE REHABILITATION HOSPITAL (O, 100 beds) 3800 Ridgeway Drive, Birmingham, AL Zip 35209–5599; tel. 205/868–2000; Terrence E. Brown, Chief Executive Officer
**Web address:** www.healthsouthlakeshorerehab.com

HEALTHSOUTH REHABILITATION HOSPITAL (O, 39 beds) 1736 East Main Street, Dothan, AL Zip 36301, Mailing Address: P.O. Box 6708, Zip 36302–6708; tel. 334/712–6333; Margaret A. Futch, Chief Executive Officer
**Web address:** www.healthsouthdothan.com

HEALTHSOUTH REHABILITATION HOSPITAL OF MONTGOMERY (O, 70 beds) 4465 Narrow Lane Road, Montgomery, AL Zip 36116–2900; tel. 334/284–7700; Linda Wade, Chief Executive Officer
**Web address:** www.healthsouthmontgomery.com

HEALTHSOUTH REHABILITATION HOSPITAL OF NORTH ALABAMA (O, 70 beds) 107 Governors Drive S.W., Huntsville, AL Zip 35801–4329; tel. 256/535–2300; Douglas H. Beverly, Chief Executive Officer
**Web address:** www.healthsouthhuntsville.com

---

For explanation of codes following names, see page B2.
★ Indicates Type III membership in the American Hospital Association.

HEALTHSOUTH REHABILITATION OF GADSDEN (O, 44 beds) 801 Goodyear Avenue, Gadsden, AL Zip 35903; tel. 256/439–5000; Michael W. Thompson, Chief Executive Officer
**Web address:** www.healthsouth.com

REGIONAL REHABILITATION HOSPITAL (O, 48 beds) 3715 Highway 280/431 North, Phenix City, AL Zip 36867; tel. 334/732–2200; Jill Jordan, Chief Executive Officer
**Web address:** www.regionalrehabhospital.com

**ARIZONA:** HEALTHSOUTH EAST VALLEY REHABILITATION HOSPITAL (O, 40 beds) 5652 East Baseline Road, Mesa, AZ Zip 85206–4713; tel. 480/567–0350; Timothy T. Poore, Chief Executive Officer
**Web address:** www.healthsoutheastvalley.com

HEALTHSOUTH REHABILITATION HOSPITAL OF SOUTHERN ARIZONA (O, 60 beds) 1921 West Hospital Drive, Tucson, AZ Zip 85704–7806; tel. 520/742–2800; Robin Conklin, R.N., InterimChief Executive Officer
**Web address:** www.healthsouthsouthernarizona.com

HEALTHSOUTH REHABILITATION INSTITUTE OF TUCSON (O, 80 beds) 2650 North Wyatt Drive, Tucson, AZ Zip 85712–6108; tel. 520/325–1300; Jeffrey Christensen, Chief Executive Officer
**Web address:** www.rehabinstituteoftucson.com

HEALTHSOUTH SCOTTSDALE REHABILITATION HOSPITAL (O, 60 beds) 9630 East Shea Boulevard, Scottsdale, AZ Zip 85260; tel. 480/551–5400; Richard Schulz, Chief Executive Officer
**Web address:** www.healthsouthscottsdale.com

HEALTHSOUTH VALLEY OF THE SUN REHABILITATION HOSPITAL (O, 75 beds) 13460 North 67th Avenue, Glendale, AZ Zip 85304–1042; tel. 623/878–8800; Beth Bacher, Chief Executive Officer
**Web address:** www.healthsouthvalleyofthesun.com

YUMA REHABILITATION HOSPITAL (O, 41 beds) 901 West 24th Street, Yuma, AZ Zip 85364; tel. 928/726–5000; Larry Barclift, Interim Chief Executive Officer
**Web address:** www.yumarehabhospital.com

**ARKANSAS:** HEALTHSOUTH REHABILITATION HOSPITAL (O, 60 beds) 153 East Monte Painter Drive, Fayetteville, AR Zip 72703–4002; tel. 479/444–2200; Jack C. Mitchell, FACHE, Chief Executive Officer
**Web address:** www.healthsouthfayetteville.com

HEALTHSOUTH REHABILITATION HOSPITAL OF FORT SMITH (O, 80 beds) 1401 South J Street, Fort Smith, AR Zip 72901–5155; tel. 479/785–3300; Ryan Cassedy, Chief Executive Officer
**Web address:** www.healthsouthfortsmith.com

HEALTHSOUTH REHABILITATION HOSPITAL OF JONESBORO (O, 67 beds) 1201 Fleming Avenue, Jonesboro, AR Zip 72401–4311, Mailing Address: P.O. Box 1680, Zip 72403–1680; tel. 870/932–0440; Donna Harris, Chief Executive Officer
**Web address:** www.healthsouthjonesboro.com

ST. VINCENT REHABILITATION HOSPITAL (O, 71 beds) 2201 Wildwood Avenue, Sherwood, AR Zip 72120–5074, Mailing Address: P.O. Box 6930, Zip 72124–6930; tel. 501/834–1800; Lee Frazier, FACHE, Chief Executive Officer
**Web address:** www.stvincenthealth.com/svrehabhospital/index.html

**CALIFORNIA:** HEALTHSOUTH BAKERSFIELD REHABILITATION HOSPITAL (O, 60 beds) 5001 Commerce Drive, Bakersfield, CA Zip 93309–0689; tel. 661/323–5500; Sandra Hegland, Chief Executive Officer
**Web address:** www.healthsouthbakersfield.com

HEALTHSOUTH TUSTIN REHABILITATION HOSPITAL (O, 48 beds) 14851 Yorba Street, Tustin, CA Zip 92780–2925; tel. 714/832–9200; Diana C. Hanyak, Chief Executive Officer
**Web address:** www.tustinrehab.com

**COLORADO:** HEALTHSOUTH REHABILITATION HOSPITAL OF COLORADO SPRINGS (O, 64 beds) 325 Parkside Drive, Colorado Springs, CO Zip 80910; tel. 719/630–8000; Stephen Schaefer, Chief Executive Officer
**Web address:** www.healthsouthcoloradosprings.com

**FLORIDA:** HEALTHSOUTH EMERALD COAST REHABILITATION HOSPITAL (O, 75 beds) 1847 Florida Avenue, Panama City, FL Zip 32405–4640; tel. 850/914–8600; Tony N. Bennett, Chief Executive Officer
**Web address:** www.healthsouthpanamacity.com

HEALTHSOUTH REHABILITATION HOSPITAL (O, 70 beds) 901 North Clearwater–Largo Road, Largo, FL Zip 33770–4126; tel. 727/586–2999; Donald D. Evans, Chief Executive Officer
**Web address:** www.healthsouthlargo.com

HEALTHSOUTH REHABILITATION HOSPITAL OF MIAMI (O, 60 beds) 20601 Old Cutler Road, Miami, FL Zip 33189–2400; tel. 305/251–3800; Elizabeth L. Izquierdo, CPA, Chief Executive Officer
**Web address:** www.healthsouthmiami.com

HEALTHSOUTH REHABILITATION HOSPITAL OF SARASOTA (O, 86 beds) 6400 Edgelake Drive, Sarasota, FL Zip 34240–8813; tel. 941/921–8600; Marcus Braz, Chief Executive Officer
**Web address:** www.healthsouthsarasota.com

HEALTHSOUTH REHABILITATION HOSPITAL OF SPRING HILL (O, 80 beds) 12440 Cortez Boulevard, Brooksville, FL Zip 34613–2628; tel. 352/592–4250; Lori Bedard, Chief Executive Officer
**Web address:** www.healthsouthspringhill.com

HEALTHSOUTH REHABILITATION HOSPITAL OF TALLAHASSEE (O, 76 beds) 1675 Riggins Road, Tallahassee, FL Zip 32308–5315; tel. 850/656–4800; Heath Phillips, Chief Executive Officer
**Web address:** www.healthsouthtallahassee.com

HEALTHSOUTH SEA PINES REHABILITATION HOSPITAL (O, 90 beds) 101 East Florida Avenue, Melbourne, FL Zip 32901–9966; tel. 321/984–4600; Denise B. McGrath, Chief Executive Officer
**Web address:** www.healthsouthseapines.com

HEALTHSOUTH SUNRISE REHABILITATION HOSPITAL (O, 126 beds) 4399 Nob Hill Road, Fort Lauderdale, FL Zip 33351–5899; tel. 954/749–0300; Kevin R. Conn, Chief Executive Officer
**Web address:** www.healthsouthsunrise.com

HEALTHSOUTH TREASURE COAST REHABILITATION HOSPITAL (O, 90 beds) 1600 37th Street, Vero Beach, FL Zip 32960–6549; tel. 772/778–2100; Kevin R. Conn, Interim Chief Executive Officer
**Web address:** www.healthsouthtreasurecoast.com

**ILLINOIS:** VAN MATRE HEALTHSOUTH REHABILITATION HOSPITAL (O, 50 beds) 950 South Mulford Road, Rockford, IL Zip 61108; tel. 815/381–8500; Ken Bowman, Chief Executive Officer
**Web address:** www.healthsouth.com

**INDIANA:** HEALTHSOUTH DEACONESS REHABILITATION HOSPITAL (O, 80 beds) 4100 Covert Avenue, Evansville, IN Zip 47714–5567, Mailing Address: P.O. Box 5349, Zip 47716–5349; tel. 812/476–9983; Barbara Butler, Chief Executive Officer
**Web address:** www.healthsouthdeaconess.com

**KANSAS:** KANSAS REHABILITATION HOSPITAL (O, 59 beds) 1504 S.W. Eighth Avenue, Topeka, KS Zip 66606–1632; tel. 785/235–6600; Marty Dernier, Chief Financial Officer and Administrator
**Web address:** www.kansasrehabhospital.com

MID–AMERICA REHABILITATION HOSPITAL (O, 98 beds) 5701 West 110th Street, Shawnee Mission, KS Zip 66211–2503; tel. 913/491–2400; Kristen De Hart, Chief Executive Officer
**Web address:** www.midamericarehabhospital.com

WESLEY REHABILITATION HOSPITAL (O, 65 beds) 8338 West 13th Street North, Wichita, KS Zip 67212–2984; tel. 316/729–9999; Bob Peck, Interim Chief Executive Officer
**Web address:** www.wesleyrehabhospital.com

**KENTUCKY:** HEALTHSOUTH LAKEVIEW REHABILITATION HOSPITAL (O, 40 beds) 134 Heartland Drive, Elizabethtown, KY Zip 42701–2778; tel. 270/769–3100; Lori Jarboe, Chief Executive Officer
**Web address:** www.healthsouthlakeview.com

HEALTHSOUTH NORTHERN KENTUCKY REHABILITATION HOSPITAL (O, 40 beds) 201 Medical Village Drive, Edgewood, KY Zip 41017–3407; tel. 859/341–2044; Richard R. Evens, Chief Executive Officer
**Web address:** www.healthsouthkentucky.com

**LOUISIANA:** HEALTHSOUTH REHABILITATION HOSPITAL OF ALEXANDRIA (O, 47 beds) 104 North Third Street, Alexandria, LA Zip 71301–8581; tel. 318/449–1370; William Bush, Chief Executive Officer
**Web address:** www.healthsouthalexandria.com

**MAINE:** NEW ENGLAND REHABILITATION HOSPITAL OF PORTLAND (O, 90 beds) 335 Brighton Avenue, Portland, ME Zip 04102–9735; tel. 207/775–4000; Jeanine Chesley, Chief Executive Officer
**Web address:** www.nerhp.org

**MARYLAND:** HEALTHSOUTH CHESAPEAKE REHABILITATION HOSPITAL (O, 54 beds) 220 Tilghman Road, Salisbury, MD Zip 21804–1921; tel. 410/546–4600; Steven Walas, Chief Executive Officer
**Web address:** www.healthsouthchesapeake.com

For explanation of codes following names, see page B2.
★ Indicates Type III membership in the American Hospital Association.

**MASSACHUSETTS:** FAIRLAWN REHABILITATION HOSPITAL (O, 110 beds) 189 May Street, Worcester, MA Zip 01602–4339; tel. 508/791–6351; R. David Richer, Chief Executive Officer
**Web address:** www.fairlawnrehab.org

HEALTHSOUTH REHABILITATION HOSPITAL OF WESTERN MASSACHUSETTS (O, 53 beds) 14 Chestnut Place, Ludlow, MA Zip 01056–3476; tel. 413/589–7581; Scott R. Keen, Chief Executive Officer
**Web address:** www.healthsouthrehab.org

**MISSOURI:** HOWARD A. RUSK REHABILITATION CENTER (O, 60 beds) 315 Business Loop 70 West, Columbia, MO Zip 65203–3248; tel. 573/817–2703; Bruce Eady, Chief Executive Officer
**Web address:** www.ruskrehab.com

THE REHABILITATION INSTITUTE OF ST. LOUIS (O, 96 beds) 4455 Duncan Avenue, Saint Louis, MO Zip 63110–1111; tel. 314/658–3800; Barbara Jacobsmeyer, Chief Executive Officer
**Web address:** www.rehabinstitutestl.com

**NEVADA:** HEALTHSOUTH DESERT CANYON REHABILITATION HOSPITAL (O, 50 beds) 9175 West Oquendo Road, Las Vegas, NV Zip 89148–1234; tel. 702/252–7342; Deanna Martin, MSN, Chief Executive Officer
**Web address:** www.healthsouthdesertcanyon.com

HEALTHSOUTH REHABILITATION HOSPITAL – HENDERSON (O, 70 beds) 10301 Jeffreys Street, Henderson, NV Zip 89052; tel. 702/939–9400; Robert Bollard, Interim Chief Executive Officer
**Web address:** www.hendersonrehabhospital.com

HEALTHSOUTH REHABILITATION HOSPITAL–LAS VEGAS (O, 79 beds) 1250 South Valley View Boulevard, Las Vegas, NV Zip 89102–1861; tel. 702/877–8898; Josh D. Luke, Ph.D., FACHE, Chief Executive Officer
**Web address:** www.healthsouthlasvegas.com

**NEW HAMPSHIRE:** HEALTHSOUTH REHABILITATION HOSPITAL (O, 50 beds) 254 Pleasant Street, Concord, NH Zip 03301–2508; tel. 603/226–9800; Catherine Devaney, Chief Executive Officer
**Web address:** www.healthsouthrehabconcordnh.com

**NEW JERSEY:** HEALTHSOUTH REHABILITATION HOSPITAL OF TOMS RIVER (O, 129 beds) 14 Hospital Drive, Toms River, NJ Zip 08755–6470; tel. 732/244–3100; Patricia Ostaszewski, MS, Chief Executive Officer
**Web address:** www.rehabnj.com/tomsriver

HEALTHSOUTH REHABILITATION HOSPITAL OF VINELAND (O, 40 beds) 1237 West Sherman Avenue, Vineland, NJ Zip 08360; tel. 856/696–7100; Tammy Feuer, Chief Executive Officer
**Web address:** www.rhsj.com

REHABILITATION HOSPITAL OF TINTON FALLS (O, 60 beds) 2 Centre Plaza, Tinton Falls, NJ Zip 07724; tel. 732/460–5320; Linda A. Savino, MS, Chief Executive Officer
**Web address:** www.rehabnj.com

**NEW MEXICO:** HEALTHSOUTH REHABILITATION HOSPITAL (O, 87 beds) 7000 Jefferson Street N.E., Albuquerque, NM Zip 87109–4313; tel. 505/344–9478; Sylvia K. Kelly, Chief Executive Officer
**Web address:** www.healthsouthnewmexico.com

**OHIO:** HEALTHSOUTH REHABILITATION HOSPITAL AT DRAKE (O, 40 beds) 151 West Galbraith Road, Cincinnati, OH Zip 45216–1015; tel. 513/418–5600; Mark S. Brodeur, FACHE, Chief Executive Officer
**Web address:** www.healthsouthatdrake.com

**PENNSYLVANIA:** GEISINGER HEALTHSOUTH REHABILITATION HOSPITAL (O, 42 beds) 2 Rehab Lane, Danville, PA Zip 17821; tel. 570/271–6733; Lorie Dillon, Chief Executive Officer
**Web address:** www.geisingerhealthsouth.com

HEALTHSOUTH HARMARVILLE REHABILITATION HOSPITAL (O, 202 beds) Guys Run Road, Pittsburgh, PA Zip 15238–0460, Mailing Address: P.O. Box 11460, Zip 15238–0460; tel. 412/828–1300; Kenneth J. Anthony, Chief Executive Officer
**Web address:** www.healthsouthharmarville.com

HEALTHSOUTH NITTANY VALLEY REHABILITATION HOSPITAL (O, 73 beds) 550 West College Avenue, Pleasant Gap, PA Zip 16823–7401; tel. 814/359–3421; Susan Hartman, Chief Executive Officer
**Web address:** www.nittanyvalleyrehab.com

HEALTHSOUTH READING REHABILITATION HOSPITAL (O, 60 beds) 1623 Morgantown Road, Reading, PA Zip 19607–9455; tel. 610/796–6000; Richard Kruczek, Chief Executive Officer
**Web address:** www.healthsouthreading.com

HEALTHSOUTH REHABILITATION HOSPITAL (O, 44 beds) 303 Camp Meeting Road, Sewickley, PA Zip 15143–8322; tel. 412/741–9500; Leah Laffey, MSN, R.N., Chief Executive Officer
**Web address:** www.healthsouthsewickley.com

HEALTHSOUTH REHABILITATION HOSPITAL OF ALTOONA (O, 70 beds) 2005 Valley View Boulevard, Altoona, PA Zip 16602–4598; tel. 814/944–3535; Scott Filler, Chief Executive Officer
**Web address:** www.healthsouthaltoona.com

HEALTHSOUTH REHABILITATION HOSPITAL OF ERIE (O, 100 beds) 143 East Second Street, Erie, PA Zip 16507–1501; tel. 814/878–1200; Lucretia Atti, Interim Chief Executive Officer
**Web address:** www.healthsoutherie.com

HEALTHSOUTH REHABILITATION HOSPITAL OF MECHANICSBURG (O, 75 beds) 175 Lancaster Boulevard, Mechanicsburg, PA Zip 17055–0736, Mailing Address: P.O. Box 2016, Zip 17055–2016; tel. 717/691–3700; Mark Freeburn, Chief Executive Officer
**Web address:** www.healthsouthpa.com

HEALTHSOUTH REHABILITATION HOSPITAL OF YORK (O, 90 beds) 1850 Normandie Drive, York, PA Zip 17408–1534; tel. 717/767–6941; Steven Alwine, Chief Executive Officer
**Web address:** www.healthsouthyork.com

**PUERTO RICO:** HEALTHSOUTH HOSPITAL OF MANATI (O, 40 beds) Carretera 2, Kilometro 47 7, Manati, PR Zip 00674; tel. 787/621–3800; Enrique A. Vicens–Rivera, Jr., J.D., Chief Executive Officer
**Web address:** http://healthsouth.com

HEALTHSOUTH REHABILITATION HOSPITAL (O, 32 beds) University Hospital, 3rd Floor, San Juan, PR Zip 00923, Mailing Address: P.O. Box 70344, Zip 00923; tel. 787/274–5100; Daniel Del Castillo, Chief Executive Officer
**Web address:** www.healthsouth.com

**SOUTH CAROLINA:** ANMED HEALTH REHABILITATION HOSPITAL (O, 45 beds) 1 Spring Back Way, Anderson, SC Zip 29621; tel. 864/716–2600; Michele M. Skripps, R.N., Administrator
**Web address:** www.anmedrehab.com

HEALTHSOUTH REHABILITATION HOSPITAL (O, 96 beds) 2935 Colonial Drive, Columbia, SC Zip 29203–6811; tel. 803/254–7777; James H. Rogers, FACHE, Regional Vice President
**Web address:** www.healthsouthcolumbia.com

HEALTHSOUTH REHABILITATION HOSPITAL (O, 88 beds) 900 East Cheves Street, Florence, SC Zip 29506–2704; tel. 843/679–9000; Thom King, Chief Executive Officer
**Web address:** www.healthsouthflorence.com

HEALTHSOUTH REHABILITATION HOSPITAL (O, 46 beds) 1795 Dr. Frank Gaston Boulevard, Rock Hill, SC Zip 29732; tel. 803/326–3500; Anthony W. Jackson, Chief Executive Officer
**Web address:** www.healthsouthrockhill.com

HEALTHSOUTH REHABILITATION HOSPITAL OF CHARLESTON (O, 46 beds) 9181 Medcom Street, Charleston, SC Zip 29406–9168; tel. 843/820–7777; Troy Powell, Chief Executive Officer
**Web address:** www.healthsouthcharleston.com

**TENNESSEE:** HEALTHSOUTH CANE CREEK REHABILITATION HOSPITAL (O, 40 beds) 180 Mt Pelia Road, Martin, TN Zip 38237–3812; tel. 731/587–4231; Eric Garrard, Chief Executive Officer
**Web address:** www.healthsouthcanecreek.com

HEALTHSOUTH CHATTANOOGA REHABILITATION HOSPITAL (O, 46 beds) 2412 McCallie Avenue, Chattanooga, TN Zip 37404–3398; tel. 423/698–0221; Scott Rowe, Chief Executive Officer
**Web address:** www.healthsouthchattanooga.com

HEALTHSOUTH REHABILITATION HOSPITAL (O, 50 beds) 113 Cassel Drive, Kingsport, TN Zip 37660–3775; tel. 423/246–7240; Susan Glenn, Chief Executive Officer
**Web address:** www.healthsouthkingsport.com

HEALTHSOUTH REHABILITATION HOSPITAL (O, 40 beds) 4100 Austin Peay Highway, Memphis, TN Zip 38128–2502; tel. 901/213–5400; Brad Kennedy, Chief Executive Officer
**Web address:** www.healthsouthnorthmemphis.com

HEALTHSOUTH REHABILITATION HOSPITAL OF MEMPHIS (O, 72 beds) 1282 Union Avenue, Memphis, TN Zip 38104–3414; tel. 901/722–2000; Michael L. Pierce, Chief Executive Officer
**Web address:** www.healthsouthmemphis.com

For explanation of codes following names, see page B2.
★ Indicates Type III membership in the American Hospital Association.

VANDERBILT STALLWORTH REHABILITATION HOSPITAL (O, 80 beds) 2201 Childrens Way, Nashville, TN Zip 37212–3165; tel. 615/320–7600; Susan Heath, Chief Executive Officer
**Web address:** www.vanderbiltstallworthrehab.com

**TEXAS:** HEALTHSOUTH PLANO REHABILITATION HOSPITAL (O, 65 beds) 2800 West 15th Street, Plano, TX Zip 75075–7526; tel. 972/612–9000; Jennifer Lynn Brewer, Chief Executive Officer
**Web address:** www.healthsouthplano.com

HEALTHSOUTH REHABILITATION HOSPITAL (O, 60 beds) 1212 West Lancaster Avenue, Fort Worth, TX Zip 76102–4510; tel. 817/870–2336; Trent Pierce, R.N., Chief Executive Officer
**Web address:** www.healthsouthfortworth.com

HEALTHSOUTH REHABILITATION HOSPITAL (O, 60 beds) 19002 McKay Drive, Humble, TX Zip 77338–5701; tel. 281/446–6148; Angela L. Simmons, Chief Executive Officer
**Web address:** www.healthsouthhumble.com

HEALTHSOUTH REHABILITATION HOSPITAL MIDLAND–ODESSA (O, 60 beds) 1800 Heritage Boulevard, Midland, TX Zip 79707–9750; tel. 432/520–1600; Christopher Wortham, Chief Executive Officer
**Web address:** www.healthsouthmidland.com

HEALTHSOUTH REHABILITATION HOSPITAL OF ARLINGTON (O, 65 beds) 3200 Matlock Road, Arlington, TX Zip 76015–2911; tel. 817/468–4000; Mark S. Deno, Chief Executive Officer
**Web address:** www.healthsoutharlington.com

HEALTHSOUTH REHABILITATION HOSPITAL OF AUSTIN (O, 55 beds) 1215 Red River Street, Austin, TX Zip 78701–1921; tel. 512/474–5700; Duke Saldivar, Chief Executive Officer
**Web address:** www.healthsouthaustin.com

HEALTHSOUTH REHABILITATION HOSPITAL OF BEAUMONT (O, 61 beds) 3340 Plaza 10 Boulevard, Beaumont, TX Zip 77707–2551; tel. 409/835–0835; H. J. Gaspard, Chief Executive Officer
**Web address:** www.healthsouthbeaumont.com

HEALTHSOUTH REHABILITATION HOSPITAL OF CYPRESS (O, 40 beds) 13031 Wortham Center Drive, Houston, TX Zip 77065–5662; tel. 832/280–2512; Sheila A. Kramer, Chief Executive Officer
**Web address:** www.healthsouthcypress.com

HEALTHSOUTH REHABILITATION HOSPITAL OF NORTH HOUSTON (O, 84 beds) 18550 I 45 South, Conroe, TX Zip 77384; tel. 281/364–2000; Krista Uselman, Chief Executive Officer
**Web address:** www.healthsouth.com

HEALTHSOUTH REHABILITATION HOSPITAL OF TEXARKANA (O, 60 beds) 515 West 12th Street, Texarkana, TX Zip 75501–4416; tel. 903/793–0088; Jerry Jasper, Chief Executive Officer
**Web address:** www.healthsouthtexarkana.com

HEALTHSOUTH REHABILITATION HOSPITAL–CITYVIEW (O, 62 beds) 6701 Oakmont Boulevard, Fort Worth, TX Zip 76132–2957; tel. 817/370–4700; Deborah Hopps, Chief Executive Officer
**Web address:** www.healthsouthcityview.com

HEALTHSOUTH REHABILITATION HOSPITAL–WICHITA FALLS (O, 63 beds) 3901 Armory Road, Wichita Falls, TX Zip 76302–2204; tel. 940/720–5700; Michael L. Bullitt, Chief Executive Officer
**Web address:** www.healthsouthwichitafalls.com

HEALTHSOUTH REHABILITATION INSTITUTE OF SAN ANTONIO (O, 96 beds) 9119 Cinnamon Hill, San Antonio, TX Zip 78240–5401; tel. 210/691–0737; Scott Butcher, Chief Executive Officer
**Web address:** www.hsriosa.com

HEALTHSOUTH SUGAR LAND REHABILITATION HOSPITAL (O, 50 beds) 1325 Highway 6, Sugar Land, TX Zip 77478; tel. 281/276–7574; Nicholas Hardin, Chief Executive Officer
**Web address:** www.healthsouthsugarland.com

TRINITY MOTHER FRANCES REHABILITATION HOSPITAL (O, 74 beds) 3131 Troup Highway, Tyler, TX Zip 75701–8352; tel. 903/510–7000; Sharla Anderson, Chief Executive Officer
**Web address:** www.tmfrehabhospital.com

**UTAH:** HEALTHSOUTH REHABILITATION HOSPITAL OF UTAH (O, 105 beds) 8074 South 1300 East, Sandy, UT Zip 84094–0743; tel. 801/561–3400; Philip Eaton, Chief Executive Officer
**Web address:** www.healthsouthutah.com

**VIRGINIA:** HEALTHSOUTH REHABILITATION HOSPITAL OF FREDERICKSBURG (O, 40 beds) 300 Park Hill Drive, Fredericksburg, VA Zip 22401–3387; tel. 540/368–7300; Donna Z. Phillips, M.D., Chief Executive Officer
**Web address:** www.fredericksburgrehabhospital.com

HEALTHSOUTH REHABILITATION HOSPITAL OF NORTHERN VIRGINIA (O, 40 beds) 24430 Millstream Drive, Aldie, VA Zip 20105–3098; tel. 703/957–2000; Christina Stover, Chief Executive Officer
**Web address:** www.healthsouthnorthernvirginia.com

HEALTHSOUTH REHABILITATION HOSPITAL OF PETERSBURG (O, 40 beds) 95 Pinehill Boulevard, Petersburg, VA Zip 23805–9233; tel. 804/504–8100; Scott Rotsted, Chief Executive Officer
**Web address:** www.healthsouthpetersburg.com

HEALTHSOUTH REHABILITATION HOSPITAL OF VIRGINIA (O, 40 beds) 5700 Fitzhugh Avenue, Richmond, VA Zip 23226–1877; tel. 804/288–5700; Jeff Ruskan, II, Chief Executive Officer
**Web address:** www.healthsouthrichmond.com

REHABILITATION HOSPITAL OF SOUTHWEST VIRGINIA (O, 25 beds) 103 North Street, Bristol, VA Zip 24201–3201; tel. 276/642–7900; Georgeanne Cole, Chief Executive Officer
**Web address:** www.rehabilitationhospitalswvirginia.com

UVA–HEALTHSOUTH REHABILITATION HOSPITAL (O, 50 beds) 515 Ray C. Hunt Drive, Charlottesville, VA Zip 22903; tel. 434/244–2000; Thomas J. Cook, Chief Executive Officer
**Web address:** www.uvahealthsouth.com

**WEST VIRGINIA:** HEALTHSOUTH HUNTINGTON REHABILITATION HOSPITAL (O, 52 beds) 6900 West Country Club Drive, Huntington, WV Zip 25705–2000; tel. 304/733–1060; Michael E. Zuliani, Chief Executive Officer
**Web address:** www.healthsouthhuntington.com

HEALTHSOUTH MOUNTAINVIEW REGIONAL REHABILITATION HOSPITAL (O, 80 beds) 1160 Van Voorhis Road, Morgantown, WV Zip 26505–3437; tel. 304/598–1100; Vickie Demers, Chief Executive Officer
**Web address:** www.healthsouthmountainview.com

HEALTHSOUTH SOUTHERN HILLS REHABILITATION HOSPITAL (O, 42 beds) 120 Twelfth Street, Princeton, WV Zip 24740–2312; tel. 304/487–8000; Deborah S. Guthrie, Chief Executive Officer
**Web address:** www.healthsouthsouthernhills.com

HEALTHSOUTH WESTERN HILLS REHABILITATION HOSPITAL (O, 50 beds) 3 Western Hills Drive, Parkersburg, WV Zip 26101–8122; tel. 304/420–1300; Alvin R. Lawson, JD, FACHE, Chief Executive Officer
**Web address:** www.healthsouthwesternhills.com

| | | |
|---|---|---|
| **Owned, leased, sponsored:** | 98 hospitals | 6473 beds |
| **Contract–managed:** | 0 hospitals | 0 beds |
| **Totals:** | 98 hospitals | 6473 beds |

---

★**0585: HEALTHTECH MANAGEMENT SERVICES** (IO)
405 Duke Drive, Suite 210, Franklin, TN Zip 37067; tel. 615/309–6053; Derek Morkel, Chief Executive Officer
**(Decentralized Health System)**

**ARIZONA:** COBRE VALLEY REGIONAL MEDICAL CENTER (C, 25 beds) 5880 South Hospital Drive, Globe, AZ Zip 85501–9454; tel. 928/425–3261; Neal Jensen, Chief Executive Officer
**Web address:** www.cvrmc.org

**CALIFORNIA:** PIONEERS MEMORIAL HEALTHCARE DISTRICT (C, 107 beds) 207 West Legion Road, Brawley, CA Zip 92227–7780; tel. 760/351–3333; Greg Moore, CPA, Interim Chief Executive Officer
**Web address:** www.pmhd.org

**GEORGIA:** UPSON REGIONAL MEDICAL CENTER (C, 115 beds) 801 West Gordon Street, Thomaston, GA Zip 30286–2831, Mailing Address: P.O. Box 1059, Zip 30286–1059; tel. 706/647–8111; David L. Castleberry, Chief Executive Officer
**Web address:** www.urmc.org

**ILLINOIS:** CARLINVILLE AREA HOSPITAL (C, 25 beds) 20733 North Broad Street, Carlinville, IL Zip 62626–1499; tel. 217/854–3141; Kenneth G. Reid, President and Chief Executive Officer
**Web address:** www.cahcare.com

HAMMOND–HENRY HOSPITAL (C, 79 beds) 600 North College Avenue, Geneseo, IL Zip 61254–1099; tel. 309/944–4625; Bradley Solberg, FACHE, Chief Executive Officer
**Web address:** www.hammondhenry.com

For explanation of codes following names, see page B2.
★ Indicates Type III membership in the American Hospital Association.

HILLSBORO AREA HOSPITAL (C, 25 beds) 1200 East Tremont Street, Hillsboro, IL Zip 62049–1900; tel. 217/532–6111; Rex H. Brown, Chief Executive Officer
**Web address:** www.hillsborohealth.org

**LOUISIANA:** DE SOTO REGIONAL HEALTH SYSTEM (C, 37 beds) 207 Jefferson Street, Mansfield, LA Zip 71052–2603, Mailing Address: P.O. Box 1636, Zip 71052–2603; tel. 318/871–3100; Douglas P. Efferson, FACHE, Chief Executive Officer
**Web address:** www.desotoregional.com

IBERIA MEDICAL CENTER (C, 83 beds) 2315 East Main Street, New Iberia, LA Zip 70560–4031, Mailing Address: P.O. Box 13338, Zip 70562–3338; tel. 337/364–0441; John A. Tucker, Chief Executive Officer
**Web address:** www.iberiamedicalcenter.com

**MONTANA:** BARRETT HOSPITAL & HEALTHCARE (C, 20 beds) 90 Highway 91 South, Dillon, MT Zip 59725–3597; tel. 406/683–3000; Ken Westman, Chief Executive Officer
**Web address:** www.barretthospital.org

**NEBRASKA:** TRI VALLEY HEALTH SYSTEM (C, 51 beds) 1305 West Highway 6 and 34, Cambridge, NE Zip 69022–0488, Mailing Address: P.O. Box 488, Zip 69022–0488; tel. 308/697–3329; Roger W. Steinkruger, Chief Executive Officer
**Web address:** www.trivalleyhealth.com

**NEW MEXICO:** UNION COUNTY GENERAL HOSPITAL (C, 21 beds) 300 Wilson Street, Clayton, NM Zip 88415–3321, Mailing Address: P.O. Box 489, Zip 88415–0489; tel. 575/374–2585; Donald Weidemann, Administrator
**Web address:** www.unioncountygeneral.com

**NEW YORK:** ADIRONDACK MEDICAL CENTER (C, 271 beds) 2233 State Route 86, Saranac Lake, NY Zip 12983, Mailing Address: P.O. Box 471, Zip 12983–0471; tel. 518/891–4141; Chandler M. Ralph, President and Chief Executive Officer
**Web address:** www.amccares.org

**OREGON:** BLUE MOUNTAIN HOSPITAL (C, 64 beds) 170 Ford Road, John Day, OR Zip 97845–2009; tel. 541/575–1311; Robert Houser, FACHE, Chief Executive Officer
**Web address:** www.bluemountainhospital.org

**WASHINGTON:** SUNNYSIDE COMMUNITY HOSPITAL (C, 25 beds) 1016 Tacoma Avenue, Sunnyside, WA Zip 98944–0719, Mailing Address: P.O. Box 719, Zip 98944–0719; tel. 509/837–1500; Robert L. Brendgard, Interim Chief Executive Officer
**Web address:** www.sunnysidehospital.com

**WISCONSIN:** GRANT REGIONAL HEALTH CENTER (C, 25 beds) 507 South Monroe Street, Lancaster, WI Zip 53813–2054; tel. 608/723–2143; Nicole Clapp, R.N., MSN, FACHE, President and Chief Executive Officer
**Web address:** www.grantregional.com

SOUTHWEST HEALTH CENTER (C, 119 beds) 1400 Eastside Road, Platteville, WI Zip 53818–9800; tel. 608/348–2331; Dan D. Rohrbach, President and Chief Executive Officer
**Web address:** www.southwesthealth.org

SPOONER HEALTH SYSTEM (C, 115 beds) 819 Ash Street, Spooner, WI Zip 54801–1299; tel. 715/635–2111; Michael Schafer, Chief Executive Officer and Administrator
**Web address:** www.spoonerhealthsystem.com

TOMAH MEMORIAL HOSPITAL (C, 25 beds) 321 Butts Avenue, Tomah, WI Zip 54660–1412; tel. 608/372–2181; Philip J. Stuart, Administrator and Chief Executive Officer
**Web address:** www.tomahhospital.org

**WYOMING:** HOT SPRINGS COUNTY MEMORIAL HOSPITAL (C, 25 beds) 150 East Arapahoe Street, Thermopolis, WY Zip 82443–2498; tel. 307/864–3121; Robin Roling, President and Chief Executive Officer
**Web address:** www.hscmh.org

POWELL VALLEY HEALTHCARE (C, 125 beds) 777 Avenue H, Powell, WY Zip 82435–2296; tel. 307/754–2267; Bill D. Patten, Chief Executive Officer
**Web address:** www.pvhc.org

| | | |
|---|---|---|
| Owned, leased, sponsored: | 0 hospitals | 0 beds |
| Contract–managed: | 20 hospitals | 1382 beds |
| Totals: | 20 hospitals | 1382 beds |

★**9505: HENRY FORD HEALTH SYSTEM** (NP)
One Ford Place, Detroit, MI Zip 48202–3450; tel. 313/876–8708; Nancy M. Schlichting, Chief Executive Officer
**(Centralized Health System)**

**MICHIGAN:** HENRY FORD HOSPITAL (O, 759 beds) 2799 West Grand Boulevard, Detroit, MI Zip 48202–2608; tel. 313/916–2600; John Popovich, M.D., President and Chief Executive Officer
**Web address:** www.henryfordhealth.org

HENRY FORD KINGSWOOD HOSPITAL (O, 100 beds) 10300 West Eight Mile Road, Ferndale, MI Zip 48220–2100; tel. 248/398–3200; C. Edward Coffey, M.D., Chief Executive Officer and Director Behavioral Health Services
**Web address:** www.henryford.com

HENRY FORD MACOMB HOSPITAL–WARREN CAMPUS (O, 122 beds) 13355 East Ten Mile Road, Warren, MI Zip 48089–2048; tel. 586/759–7300; Barbara Rossmann, President and Chief Executive Officer

HENRY FORD MACOMB HOSPITALS (O, 421 beds) 15855 19 Mile Road, Clinton Township, MI Zip 48038–6324; tel. 586/263–2300; Barbara Rossmann, President and Chief Executive Officer
**Web address:** www.henryfordmacomb.com

HENRY FORD WEST BLOOMFIELD HOSPITAL (O, 191 beds) 6777 West Maple Road, West Bloomfield, MI Zip 48322–3013; tel. 248/661–4100; Gerard van Grinsven, President and Chief Executive Officer
**Web address:** www.henryford.com

HENRY FORD WYANDOTTE HOSPITAL (O, 348 beds) 2333 Biddle Avenue, Wyandotte, MI Zip 48192–4668; tel. 734/246–6000; James J. Sexton, FACHE, President and Chief Executive Officer
**Web address:** www.henryfordhealth.org

| | | |
|---|---|---|
| Owned, leased, sponsored: | 6 hospitals | 1941 beds |
| Contract–managed: | 0 hospitals | 0 beds |
| Totals: | 6 hospitals | 1941 beds |

**0309: HERITAGE VALLEY HEALTH SYSTEM** (NP)
1000 Dutch Ridge Road, Beaver, PA Zip 15009–9727; tel. 724/773–2024; Norman F. Mitry, President and Chief Executive Officer
**(Independent Hospital System)**

**PENNSYLVANIA:** HERITAGE VALLEY BEAVER (O, 312 beds) 1000 Dutch Ridge Road, Beaver, PA Zip 15009–9727; tel. 724/728–7000; Norman F. Mitry, President and Chief Executive Officer
**Web address:** www.heritagevalley.org

SEWICKLEY VALLEY HOSPITAL, (A DIVISION OF VALLEY MEDICAL FACILITIES) (O, 171 beds) 720 Blackburn Road, Sewickley, PA Zip 15143–1459; tel. 412/741–6600; Norman F. Mitry, President and Chief Executive Officer
**Web address:** www.heritagevalley.org

| | | |
|---|---|---|
| Owned, leased, sponsored: | 2 hospitals | 483 beds |
| Contract–managed: | 0 hospitals | 0 beds |
| Totals: | 2 hospitals | 483 beds |

**0348: HMC/CAH CONSOLIDATED, INC.** (IO)
1100 Main Street, Suite 2350, Kansas City, MO Zip 64105–5186; tel. 816/474–7800; Lawrence J. Arthur, President
**(Independent Hospital System)**

**KANSAS:** HILLSBORO COMMUNITY HOSPITAL (O, 16 beds) 701 South Main Street, Hillsboro, KS Zip 67063–1595; tel. 620/947–3114; Marion Regier, Chief Executive Officer
**Web address:** www.hchks.com

HORTON COMMUNITY HOSPITAL (O, 25 beds) 240 West 18th Street, Horton, KS Zip 66439–1245; tel. 785/486–2642; Terry Nichols, Interim Chief Executive Officer

OSWEGO COMMUNITY HOSPITAL (O, 12 beds) 800 Barker Drive, Oswego, KS Zip 67356–9033; tel. 620/795–2921; Daniel Hiben, Chief Executive Officer
**Web address:** www.oswegocommunityhospital.com

**MISSOURI:** I–70 COMMUNITY HOSPITAL (O, 15 beds) 105 Hospital Drive, Sweet Springs, MO Zip 65351–2229; tel. 660/335–4700; Julie Davenport, Chief Executive Officer
**Web address:** www.i70medcenter.com

---

For explanation of codes following names, see page B2.
★ Indicates Type III membership in the American Hospital Association.

**NORTH CAROLINA:** WASHINGTON COUNTY HOSPITAL (O, 25 beds) 958 U.S. Highway 64 East, Plymouth, NC Zip 27962–9591; tel. 252/793–4135; Harley Smith, President
**Web address:** www.wchonline.com

YADKIN VALLEY COMMUNITY HOSPITAL (O, 22 beds) 624 West Main Street, Yadkinville, NC Zip 27055–7804, Mailing Address: P.O. Box 68, Zip 27055–0068; tel. 336/679–2041; Frederick L. Soule, Interim Chief Executive Officer
**Web address:** www.hmccah.com

**OKLAHOMA:** DRUMRIGHT REGIONAL HOSPITAL (O, 15 beds) 610 West Bypass, Drumright, OK Zip 74030–5957; tel. 918/382–2300; Darrel Morris, Chief Executive Officer
**Web address:** www.drumrighthospital.com

FAIRFAX COMMUNITY HOSPITAL (O, 15 beds) Taft Avenue and Highway 18, Fairfax, OK Zip 74637–4028, Mailing Address: P.O. Box 219, Zip 74637–0219; tel. 918/642–3291; Tina Steele, Chief Executive Officer and Chief Financial Officer
**Web address:** www.fairfaxmemorialhospital.com

HASKELL COUNTY COMMUNITY HOSPITAL (O, 32 beds) 401 Northwest H Street, Stigler, OK Zip 74462–1625, Mailing Address: P.O. Box 728, Zip 74462–0728; tel. 918/967–4682; Scott McIntyre, FACHE, Chief Executive Officer
**Web address:** www.hchs.otnnet.net

PRAGUE COMMUNITY HOSPITAL (O, 19 beds) 1322 Klabzuba Avenue, Prague, OK Zip 74864–9005, Mailing Address: P.O. Box S., Zip 74864–1090; tel. 405/567–4922; Joan Walters, R.N., MSN, Administrator
**Web address:** www.praguehospital.com

SEILING COMMUNITY HOSPITAL (O, 18 beds) Highway 60 N.E., Seiling, OK Zip 73663, Mailing Address: P.O. Box 720, Zip 73663–0720; tel. 580/922–7361; Larry Troxell, Chief Executive Officer

**TENNESSEE:** LAUDERDALE COMMUNITY HOSPITAL (O, 25 beds) 326 Asbury Avenue, Ripley, TN Zip 38063–9701; tel. 731/221–2200; Scott Tongate, Chief Executive Officer
**Web address:** www.lauderdalehospital.com/

| | | |
|---|---|---|
| **Owned, leased, sponsored:** | 12 hospitals | 239 beds |
| **Contract–managed:** | 0 hospitals | 0 beds |
| **Totals:** | 12 hospitals | 239 beds |

---

**★5355: HOSPITAL SISTERS HEALTH SYSTEM** (CC)
4936 LaVerna Road, Springfield, IL Zip 62707–9797, Mailing Address: P.O. Box 19456, Zip 62707; tel. 217/523–4747; Mary Starmann–Harrison, FACHE, President and Chief Executive Officer **(Decentralized Health System)**

**ILLINOIS:** ST. ANTHONY'S MEMORIAL HOSPITAL (O, 146 beds) 503 North Maple Street, Effingham, IL Zip 62401–2099; tel. 217/342–2121; Daniel J. Woods, President and Chief Executive Officer
**Web address:** www.stanthonyshospital.org

ST. ELIZABETH'S HOSPITAL (O, 260 beds) 211 South Third Street, Belleville, IL Zip 62220–1998; tel. 618/234–2120; Maryann Reese, R.N., FACHE, President and Chief Executive Officer
**Web address:** www.steliz.org

ST. FRANCIS HOSPITAL (O, 25 beds) 1215 Franciscan Drive, Litchfield, IL Zip 62056–1799, Mailing Address: P.O. Box 1215, Zip 62056–1215; tel. 217/324–2191; Daniel L. Perryman, President and Chief Executive Officer
**Web address:** www.stfrancis–litchfield.org

ST. JOHN'S HOSPITAL (O, 430 beds) 800 East Carpenter Street, Springfield, IL Zip 62769–0002; tel. 217/544–6464; Robert P. Ritz, Chief Executive Officer
**Web address:** www.st–johns.org

ST. JOSEPH'S HOSPITAL (O, 47 beds) 9515 Holy Cross Lane, Breese, IL Zip 62230–0099; tel. 618/526–4511; Mark D. Klosterman, FACHE, President and Chief Executive Officer
**Web address:** www.stjoebreese.com

ST. JOSEPH'S HOSPITAL (O, 25 beds) 1515 Main Street, Highland, IL Zip 62249–1656; tel. 618/654–7421; Peggy A. Sebastian, MSN, R.N., President and Chief Executive Officer
**Web address:** www.stjosephshighland.com

ST. MARY'S HOSPITAL (O, 220 beds) 1800 East Lake Shore Drive, Decatur, IL Zip 62521–3883; tel. 217/464–2966; Kevin F. Kast, President and Chief Executive Officer
**Web address:** www.stmarys–hospital.com

ST. MARY'S HOSPITAL (O, 98 beds) 111 Spring Street, Streator, IL Zip 61364–3399; tel. 815/673–2311; Brian E. Dietz, FACHE, Interim President and Chief Executive Officer
**Web address:** www.stmaryshospital.org

**WISCONSIN:** SACRED HEART HOSPITAL (O, 212 beds) 900 West Clairemont Avenue, Eau Claire, WI Zip 54701–6122; tel. 715/717–4121; Julie Manas, President and Chief Executive Officer
**Web address:** www.sacredhearthospital–ec.org

ST. JOSEPH'S HOSPITAL (O, 102 beds) 2661 County Highway I, Chippewa Falls, WI Zip 54729–1498; tel. 715/723–1811; Joan Coffman, President and Chief Executive Officer
**Web address:** www.stjoeschipfalls.com

ST. MARY'S HOSPITAL MEDICAL CENTER (O, 83 beds) 1726 Shawano Avenue, Green Bay, WI Zip 54303–3282; tel. 920/498–4200; Therese B. Pandl, President and Chief Executive Officer
**Web address:** www.stmgb.org

ST. NICHOLAS HOSPITAL (O, 78 beds) 3100 Superior Avenue, Sheboygan, WI Zip 53081; tel. 920/459–8300; Andrew Bagnall, Chief Executive Officer
**Web address:** www.stnicholashospital.org

ST. VINCENT HOSPITAL (O, 255 beds) 835 South Van Buren Street, Green Bay, WI Zip 54301–3526, Mailing Address: P.O. Box 13508, Zip 54307–3508; tel. 920/433–0111; Therese B. Pandl, President and Chief Executive Officer
**Web address:** www.stvgh.org

| | | |
|---|---|---|
| **Owned, leased, sponsored:** | 13 hospitals | 1981 beds |
| **Contract–managed:** | 0 hospitals | 0 beds |
| **Totals:** | 13 hospitals | 1981 beds |

---

**★0642: HOUSTON HEALTHCARE SYSTEM** (NP)
1601 Watson Boulevard, Warner Robins, GA Zip 31093–3431, Mailing Address: P.O. Box 2886, Zip 31099–2886; tel. 478/922–4281; Cary Martin, Chief Executive Officer **(Independent Hospital System)**

**GEORGIA:** HOUSTON MEDICAL CENTER (O, 237 beds) 1601 Watson Boulevard, Warner Robins, GA Zip 31093–3431, Mailing Address: P.O. Box 2886, Zip 31099–2886; tel. 478/922–4281; Cary Martin, Chief Executive Officer
**Web address:** www.hhc.org

PERRY HOSPITAL (O, 39 beds) 1120 Morningside Drive, Perry, GA Zip 31069–2906; tel. 478/987–3600; David Campbell, Administrator
**Web address:** www.hhc.org

| | | |
|---|---|---|
| **Owned, leased, sponsored:** | 2 hospitals | 276 beds |
| **Contract–managed:** | 0 hospitals | 0 beds |
| **Totals:** | 2 hospitals | 276 beds |

---

**0117: HUNTSVILLE HOSPITAL HEALTH SYSTEM** (NP)
101 Sivley Road S.W., Huntsville, AL Zip 35801–4421; tel. 265/256–1000; David S. Spillers, Chief Executive Officer

**ALABAMA:** HUNTSVILLE HOSPITAL (O, 834 beds) 101 Sivley Road, Huntsville, AL Zip 35801–4470; tel. 256/265–1000; David S. Spillers, Chief Executive Officer
**Web address:** www.huntsvillehospital.org

MADISON HOSPITAL (O, 60 beds) 8375 Highway 72 West, Madison, AL Zip 35758–9573; tel. 256/265–2012; Mary Lynne Wright, R.N., President
**Web address:** www.madisonalhospital.org/

| | | |
|---|---|---|
| **Owned, leased, sponsored:** | 2 hospitals | 894 beds |
| **Contract–managed:** | 0 hospitals | 0 beds |
| **Totals:** | 2 hospitals | 894 beds |

Section B

For explanation of codes following names, see page B2.
★ Indicates Type III membership in the American Hospital Association.

**0201: IASIS HEALTHCARE** (IO)
117 Seaboard Lane, Building E., Franklin, TN Zip 37067; tel. 615/844–2747; Carl Whitmer, President and Chief Executive Officer
**(Moderately Centralized Health System)**

**ARIZONA:** MOUNTAIN VISTA MEDICAL CENTER (O, 172 beds) 1301 South Crismon Road, Mesa, AZ Zip 85208; tel. 480/358–6100; Anthony Marinello, Chief Executive Officer
**Web address:** www.mvmedicalcenter.com

ST. LUKE'S BEHAVIORAL HEALTH CENTER (O, 85 beds) 1800 East Van Buren, Phoenix, AZ Zip 85006–3742; tel. 602/251–8546; Gregory L. Jahn, R.N., Chief Executive Officer
**Web address:** www.iasishealthcare.com

ST. LUKE'S MEDICAL CENTER (O, 225 beds) 1800 East Van Buren Street, Phoenix, AZ Zip 85006–3742; tel. 602/251–8100; Edward W. Myers, Chief Executive Officer
**Web address:** www.stlukesmedcenter.com

**COLORADO:** PIKES PEAK REGIONAL HOSPITAL (O, 15 beds) 16420 West Highway 24, Woodland Park, CO Zip 80863; tel. 719/687–9999; Dolores A. Horvath, Chief Executive Officer
**Web address:** www.pprmc.org

**FLORIDA:** MEMORIAL HOSPITAL OF TAMPA (O, 139 beds) 2901 Swann Avenue, Tampa, FL Zip 33609–4057; tel. 813/873–6400; John J. Mainieri, Chief Executive Officer
**Web address:** www.memorialhospitaltampa.com

PALMS OF PASADENA HOSPITAL (O, 307 beds) 1501 Pasadena Avenue South, Saint Petersburg, FL Zip 33707–3798; tel. 727/381–1000; Brian T. Flynn, Chief Executive Officer
**Web address:** www.palmspasadena.com

TOWN AND COUNTRY HOSPITAL (O, 200 beds) 6001 Webb Road, Tampa, FL Zip 33615–3291; tel. 813/888–7060; Dale Johns, Administrator
**Web address:** www.townandcountryhospital.com

**LOUISIANA:** GLENWOOD REGIONAL MEDICAL CENTER (O, 247 beds) 503 McMillan Road, West Monroe, LA Zip 71291–5327; tel. 318/329–4200; Ronald J. Elder, Chief Executive Officer
**Web address:** www.grmc.com

**NEVADA:** NORTH VISTA HOSPITAL (O, 198 beds) 1409 East Lake Mead Boulevard, North Las Vegas, NV Zip 89030–7197; tel. 702/649–7711; Richard L. Kilburn, Chief Executive Officer
**Web address:** www.northvistahospital.com

**TEXAS:** ODESSA REGIONAL MEDICAL CENTER (O, 194 beds) 520 East Sixth Street, Odessa, TX Zip 79761–4565, Mailing Address: P.O. Box 4859, Zip 79760–4859; tel. 432/582–8000; Stacey L. Gerig, Chief Executive Officer
**Web address:** www.odessaregionalmedicalcenter.com

SOUTHWEST GENERAL HOSPITAL (O, 265 beds) 7400 Barlite Boulevard, San Antonio, TX Zip 78224–1399; tel. 210/921–2000; Gregory Padilla, Chief Executive Officer
**Web address:** www.swgeneralhospital.com

ST. JOSEPH MEDICAL CENTER (O, 384 beds) 1401 St. Joseph Parkway, Houston, TX Zip 77002–8321; tel. 713/757–1000; Patrick J. Mathews, Chief Executive Officer and Chief Financial Officer
**Web address:** www.sjmctx.com

THE MEDICAL CENTER OF SOUTHEAST TEXAS (O, 185 beds) 2555 Jimmy Johnson Boulevard, Port Arthur, TX Zip 77640; tel. 409/724–7389; Matthew S. Roberts, Chief Executive Officer
**Web address:** www.medicalcentersetexas.com

WADLEY REGIONAL MEDICAL CENTER (O, 157 beds) 1000 Pine Street, Texarkana, TX Zip 75501–5170; tel. 903/798–8000; Thomas D. Gilbert, Chief Executive Officer
**Web address:** www.wadleyhealth.com

**UTAH:** DAVIS HOSPITAL AND MEDICAL CENTER (O, 200 beds) 1600 West Antelope Drive, Layton, UT Zip 84041–1142; tel. 801/807–1000; Michael E. Jensen, President and Chief Executive Officer
**Web address:** www.davishospital.com

JORDAN VALLEY MEDICAL CENTER (O, 183 beds) 3580 West 9000 South, West Jordan, UT Zip 84088–8811; tel. 801/561–8888; Bryanie W. Swilley, Jr., Chief Executive Officer
**Web address:** www.jordanvalleymc.com

PIONEER VALLEY HOSPITAL (O, 101 beds) 3460 South Pioneer Parkway, West Valley City, UT Zip 84120–2648; tel. 801/964–3100; Bryanie W. Swilley, Jr., Chief Executive Officer
**Web address:** www.pioneervalleyhospital.com

SALT LAKE REGIONAL MEDICAL CENTER (O, 132 beds) 1050 East South Temple, Salt Lake City, UT Zip 84102–1599; tel. 801/350–4111; Jeff Frandsen, Chief Executive Officer
**Web address:** www.saltlakeregional.com

| | | |
|---|---|---|
| Owned, leased, sponsored: | 18 hospitals | 3389 beds |
| Contract–managed: | 0 hospitals | 0 beds |
| **Totals:** | 18 hospitals | 3389 beds |

**★0231: INDIANA UNIVERSITY HEALTH** (NP)
340 West 10th Street, Suite 6100, Indianapolis, IN Zip 46202–3082, Mailing Address: P.O. Box 1367, Zip 46206–1367; tel. 317/962–5900; Daniel F. Evans, Jr., JD, President and Chief Executive Officer
**(Centralized Physician/Insurance Health System)**

**INDIANA:** INDIANA UNIVERSITY HEALTH ARNETT HOSPITAL (O, 141 beds) 5165 McCarty Lane, Lafayette, IN Zip 47905–8764, Mailing Address: P.O. Box 5545, Zip 47903–5545; tel. 765/448–8000; Alfonso W. Gatmaitan, Chief Executive Officer
**Web address:** www.iuhealth.org

INDIANA UNIVERSITY HEALTH BALL MEMORIAL HOSPITAL (O, 347 beds) 2401 University Avenue, Muncie, IN Zip 47303–3499; tel. 765/747–3111; Michael E. Haley, President and Chief Executive Officer
**Web address:** www.iuhealth.org

INDIANA UNIVERSITY HEALTH BEDFORD HOSPITAL (O, 25 beds) 2900 West 16th Street, Bedford, IN Zip 47421–3583; tel. 812/275–1200; Bradford W. Dykes, President and Chief Executive Officer
**Web address:** www.iuhealth.org

INDIANA UNIVERSITY HEALTH BLACKFORD HOSPITAL (O, 15 beds) 410 Pilgrim Boulevard, Hartford City, IN Zip 47348–1897; tel. 765/348–0300; Steven J. West, Chief Executive Officer
**Web address:** www.iuhealth.org

INDIANA UNIVERSITY HEALTH BLOOMINGTON HOSPITAL (O, 293 beds) 709 W. 1st Street, Bloomington, IN Zip 47402, Mailing Address: P.O. Box 1149, Zip 47402–1149; tel. 812/336–6821; Mark E. Moore, President and Chief Executive Officer
**Web address:** www.iuhealth.org

INDIANA UNIVERSITY HEALTH GOSHEN HOSPITAL (O, 122 beds) 200 High Park Avenue, Goshen, IN Zip 46526–4899, Mailing Address: P.O. Box 139, Zip 46527–0139; tel. 574/533–2141; James O. Dague, President and Chief Executive Officer
**Web address:** www.iuhealth.org

INDIANA UNIVERSITY HEALTH LA PORTE HOSPITAL (O, 204 beds) 1007 Lincolnway, La Porte, IN Zip 46350–3201, Mailing Address: P.O. Box 250, Zip 46352–0250; tel. 219/326–1234; G. Thor Thordarson, President and Chief Executive Officer
**Web address:** www.iuhealth.org

INDIANA UNIVERSITY HEALTH MORGAN HOSPITAL (O, 92 beds) 2209 John R. Wooden Drive, Martinsville, IN Zip 46151–1840, Mailing Address: P.O. Box 1717, Zip 46151–1717; tel. 765/342–8441; Doug Puckett, President and Chief Executive Officer
**Web address:** www.iuhealth.org/morgan/

INDIANA UNIVERSITY HEALTH NORTH HOSPITAL (O, 161 beds) 11700 North Meridian Avenue, Carmel, IN Zip 46032; tel. 317/688–2000; Jonathan R. Goble, FACHE, President and Chief Executive Officer
**Web address:** www.iuhealth.org

INDIANA UNIVERSITY HEALTH PAOLI HOSPITAL (O, 24 beds) 642 West Hospital Road, Paoli, IN Zip 47454–0499, Mailing Address: P.O. Box 499, Zip 47454–0499; tel. 812/723–2811; Larry Bailey, Chief Executive Officer
**Web address:** www.bhhs.org

INDIANA UNIVERSITY HEALTH STARKE HOSPITAL (O, 20 beds) 102 East Culver Road, Knox, IN Zip 46534–2299, Mailing Address: P.O. Box 339, Zip 46534–0339; tel. 574/772–6231; David W. Hyatt, Interim Chief Executive Officer
**Web address:** www.iuhealth.org

For explanation of codes following names, see page B2.
★ Indicates Type III membership in the American Hospital Association.

INDIANA UNIVERSITY HEALTH TIPTON HOSPITAL (O, 25 beds) 1000 South Main Street, Tipton, IN Zip 46072–9799; tel. 765/675–8500; Michael Harlowe, President and Chief Executive Officer
**Web address:** www.iuhealth.org

INDIANA UNIVERSITY HEALTH UNIVERSITY HOSPITAL (O, 1407 beds) 550 University Boulevard, Indianapolis, IN Zip 46202–5149, Mailing Address: P.O. Box 1367, Zip 46206–1367; tel. 317/962–2000; Daniel F. Evans, Jr., JD, President and Chief Executive Officer
**Web address:** www.iuhealth.org

INDIANA UNIVERSITY HEALTH WEST HOSPITAL (O, 127 beds) 1111 North Ronald Reagan Parkway, Avon, IN Zip 46123; tel. 317/217–3000; Matthew D. Bailey, FACHE, President and Chief Executive Officer
**Web address:** www.iuhealth.org

INDIANA UNIVERSITY HEALTH WHITE MEMORIAL HOSPITAL (O, 25 beds) 720 South Sixth Street, Monticello, IN Zip 47960–8182; tel. 574/583–7111; Stephanie Long, Chief Executive Officer
**Web address:** www.iuhealth.org/white–memorial

IU HEALTH SAXONY HOSPITAL (O, 42 beds) 13000 East 136th Street, Fishers, IN Zip 46037–9478; tel. 317/678–2000; Philip M. Dulberger, M.D., Chief Executive Officer

JAY COUNTY HOSPITAL (C, 35 beds) 500 West Votaw Street, Portland, IN Zip 47371–1322; tel. 260/726–7131; Joe Johnston, Chief Executive Officer
**Web address:** www.jaycountyhospital.com

| Owned, leased, sponsored: | 16 hospitals | 3070 beds |
|---|---|---|
| Contract–managed: | 1 hospital | 35 beds |
| **Totals:** | 17 hospitals | 3105 beds |

## 2025: INFIRMARY HEALTH SYSTEM (NP)
5 Mobile Infirmary Circle, Mobile, AL Zip 36607–3520; tel. 251/435–5500; D. Mark Nix, President and Chief Executive Officer

**ALABAMA:** INFIRMARY LONG TERM ACUTE CARE HOSPITAL (L, 191 beds) 5644 Girby Road, Mobile, AL Zip 36693–3320; tel. 251/660–5239; Susanne Marmande, Administrator
**Web address:** www.theinfirmary.com/

INFIRMARY WEST (L, 63 beds) 5600 Girby Road, Mobile, AL Zip 36693–3398; tel. 251/660–5120; Alan R. Whaley, Administrator
**Web address:** www.southalabama.edu/usakph/index.html

MOBILE INFIRMARY MEDICAL CENTER (O, 493 beds) 5 Mobile Infirmary Drive North, Mobile, AL Zip 36607–3513, Mailing Address: P.O. Box 2144, Zip 36652–2144; tel. 251/435–2400; Joe Strough, Administrator
**Web address:** www.mobileinfirmary.org

NORTH BALDWIN INFIRMARY (L, 35 beds) 1815 Hand Avenue, Bay Minette, AL Zip 36507–4110, Mailing Address: P.O. Box 1409, Zip 36507–1409; tel. 251/937–5521; Ormand P. Thompson, Administrator
**Web address:** www.mobileinfirmary.org

THOMAS HOSPITAL (L, 136 beds) 750 Morphy Avenue, Fairhope, AL Zip 36532–1812, Mailing Address: P.O. Drawer 929, Zip 36533–0929; tel. 251/928–2375; William J. McLaughlin, Administrator
**Web address:** www.thomashospital.com

| Owned, leased, sponsored: | 5 hospitals | 918 beds |
|---|---|---|
| Contract–managed: | 0 hospitals | 0 beds |
| **Totals:** | 5 hospitals | 918 beds |

## ★1305: INOVA HEALTH SYSTEM (NP)
8110 Gatehouse Road, Falls Church, VA Zip 22042; tel. 703/289–2069; J. Knox Singleton, President and Chief Executive Officer
**(Centralized Health System)**

**VIRGINIA:** INOVA ALEXANDRIA HOSPITAL (O, 334 beds) 4320 Seminary Road, Alexandria, VA Zip 22304–1594; tel. 703/504–3167; Christine Candio, Chief Executive Officer
**Web address:** www.inova.org

INOVA FAIR OAKS HOSPITAL (O, 196 beds) 3600 Joseph Siewick Drive, Fairfax, VA Zip 22033–1798; tel. 703/391–3600; John L. Fitzgerald, Chief Executive Officer
**Web address:** www.inova.org

INOVA FAIRFAX HOSPITAL (O, 927 beds) 3300 Gallows Road, Falls Church, VA Zip 22042–3300; tel. 703/776–4001; L. Reuven Pasternak, M.D., M.P.H., Chief Executive Officer
**Web address:** www.inova.org

INOVA LOUDOUN HOSPITAL (O, 290 beds) 44045 Riverside Parkway, Leesburg, VA Zip 20176–2799, Mailing Address: P.O. Box 6000, Zip 20177–0600; tel. 703/858–6000; Patrick Walters, Interim Chief Executive Officer
**Web address:** www.inova.org

INOVA MOUNT VERNON HOSPITAL (O, 237 beds) 2501 Parker's Lane, Alexandria, VA Zip 22306; tel. 703/664–7000; Barbara J. Doyle, R.N., MS, Senior Vice President and Chief Executive Officer
**Web address:** www.inova.org

| Owned, leased, sponsored: | 5 hospitals | 1984 beds |
|---|---|---|
| Contract–managed: | 0 hospitals | 0 beds |
| **Totals:** | 5 hospitals | 1984 beds |

## 0333: INTEGRATED HEALTHCARE (IO)
1301 North Tustin Avenue, Santa Ana, CA Zip 92705; tel. 714/953–3652; Kenneth K. Westbrook, President and Chief Executive Officer
**(Independent Hospital System)**

**CALIFORNIA:** CHAPMAN MEDICAL CENTER (O, 100 beds) 2601 East Chapman Avenue, Orange, CA Zip 92869–3206; tel. 714/633–0011; Don Kreitz, Chief Executive Officer
**Web address:** www.chapmanmedicalcenter.com

COASTAL COMMUNITIES HOSPITAL (O, 178 beds) 2701 South Bristol Street, Santa Ana, CA Zip 92704–6201; tel. 714/754–5454; Craig G. Myers, Chief Executive Officer
**Web address:** www.coastalcommhospital.com

WESTERN MEDICAL CENTER ANAHEIM (O, 188 beds) 1025 South Anaheim Boulevard, Anaheim, CA Zip 92805–5806; tel. 714/533–6220; Dennis M. Knox, Chief Executive Officer
**Web address:** www.westernmedanaheim.com

WESTERN MEDICAL CENTER–SANTA ANA (O, 282 beds) 1001 North Tustin Avenue, Santa Ana, CA Zip 92705–3577; tel. 714/835–3555; Daniel Brothman, Chief Executive Officer
**Web address:** www.westernmedicalcenter.com

| Owned, leased, sponsored: | 4 hospitals | 748 beds |
|---|---|---|
| Contract–managed: | 0 hospitals | 0 beds |
| **Totals:** | 4 hospitals | 748 beds |

## ★0305: INTEGRIS HEALTH (NP)
3366 N.W. Expressway, Suite 800, Oklahoma City, OK Zip 73112–9756; tel. 405/949–6066; Bruce Lawrence, President and Chief Executive Officer
**(Moderately Centralized Health System)**

**OKLAHOMA:** INTEGRIS BAPTIST MEDICAL CENTER (O, 569 beds) 3300 N.W. Expressway, Oklahoma City, OK Zip 73112–4418; tel. 405/949–3011; Chris Hammes, FACHE, President
**Web address:** www.integrisok.com

INTEGRIS BAPTIST REGIONAL HEALTH CENTER (O, 84 beds) 200 Second Street S.W., Miami, OK Zip 74354–6830, Mailing Address: P.O. Box 1207, Zip 74355–1207; tel. 918/542–6611; Joel A. Hart, FACHE, President
**Web address:** www.integris–health.com

INTEGRIS BASS BAPTIST HEALTH CENTER (O, 167 beds) 600 South Monroe Street, Enid, OK Zip 73701–7211, Mailing Address: P.O. Box 3168, Zip 73702–3168; tel. 580/233–2300; Jeffrey S. Tarrant, FACHE, President
**Web address:** www.integris–health.com

INTEGRIS BASS PAVILION (O, 24 beds) 401 South Third Street, Enid, OK Zip 73701–5737; tel. 580/249–4260; Jeffrey S. Tarrant, FACHE, President
**Web address:** www.integris–health.com/integris/en–us/locations/bass–enid

INTEGRIS CANADIAN VALLEY HOSPITAL (O, 75 beds) 1201 Health Center Parkway, Yukon, OK Zip 73099–6381; tel. 405/717–6800; Rex Van Meter, President
**Web address:** www.integris–health.com

For explanation of codes following names, see page B2.
★ Indicates Type III membership in the American Hospital Association.

INTEGRIS GROVE GENERAL HOSPITAL (O, 58 beds) 1001 East 18th Street, Grove, OK Zip 74344–2907; tel. 918/786–2243; Greg Martin, President
**Web address:** www.integris–health.com

INTEGRIS HEALTH EDMOND (O, 40 beds) 4801 Integris Parkway, Edmond, OK Zip 73034–8864; tel. 405/657–3000; Avilla Williams, MS, President
**Web address:** www.integrisok.com/edmond

INTEGRIS SOUTHWEST MEDICAL CENTER (O, 305 beds) 4401 South Western, Oklahoma City, OK Zip 73109–3441; tel. 405/636–7000; James D. Moore, FACHE, Chief Executive Officer
**Web address:** www.integris–health.com

| | | |
|---|---|---|
| Owned, leased, sponsored: | 8 hospitals | 1322 beds |
| Contract–managed: | 0 hospitals | 0 beds |
| Totals: | 8 hospitals | 1322 beds |

★**1815: INTERMOUNTAIN HEALTHCARE, INC** (NP)
36 South State Street, 22nd Floor, Salt Lake City, UT Zip 84111–1453; tel. 801/442–2000; Charles W. Sorenson, Jr., M.D., Chief Executive Officer
**(Centralized Physician/Insurance Health System)**

**IDAHO:** CASSIA REGIONAL MEDICAL CENTER (O, 25 beds) 1501 Hiland Avenue, Burley, ID Zip 83318–2648; tel. 208/678–4444; Rod Barton, Administrator
**Web address:** www.cassiaregional.org

**UTAH:** ALTA VIEW HOSPITAL (O, 71 beds) 9660 South 1300 East, Sandy, UT Zip 84094–3793; tel. 801/501–2600; Becky Kapp, Administrator
**Web address:** www.intermountainhealthcare.org

AMERICAN FORK HOSPITAL (O, 88 beds) 170 North 1100 East, American Fork, UT Zip 84003–2096; tel. 801/855–3300; Michael R. Olson, Administrator
**Web address:** www.intermountainhealthcare.org

BEAR RIVER VALLEY HOSPITAL (O, 14 beds) 905 North 1000 West, Tremonton, UT Zip 84337–2497; tel. 435/207–4500; Eric Packer, Administrator
**Web address:** www.ihc.com

DELTA COMMUNITY MEDICAL CENTER (O, 18 beds) 126 South White Sage Avenue, Delta, UT Zip 84624–8928; tel. 435/864–5591; James E. Beckstrand, Administrator
**Web address:** www.ihc.com

DIXIE REGIONAL MEDICAL CENTER (O, 261 beds) 1380 East Medical Center Drive, Saint George, UT Zip 84790; tel. 435/251–1000; Terri Kane, Administrator
**Web address:** www.intermountainhealthcare.org

FILLMORE COMMUNITY MEDICAL CENTER (O, 19 beds) 674 South Highway 99, Fillmore, UT Zip 84631–9701; tel. 435/743–5591; James E. Beckstrand, Administrator
**Web address:** www.ihc.com

GARFIELD MEMORIAL HOSPITAL AND CLINICS (C, 41 beds) 200 North 400 East, Panguitch, UT Zip 84759, Mailing Address: P.O. Box 389, Zip 84759–0389; tel. 435/676–8811; Alberto Vasquez, Administrator
**Web address:** www.ihc.com/xp/ihc/garfield

HEBER VALLEY MEDICAL CENTER (O, 19 beds) 1485 South Highway 40, Heber City, UT Zip 84032–3522; tel. 435/654–2500; Steve Anderson, Administrator
**Web address:** www.ihc.com

INTERMOUNTAIN MEDICAL CENTER (O, 452 beds) 5121 South Cottonwood Street, Murray, UT Zip 84157; tel. 801/507–7000; David Grauer, Administrator
**Web address:** www.intermountainhealthcare.org

LDS HOSPITAL (O, 236 beds) Eighth Avenue and C Street, Salt Lake City, UT Zip 84143–0001; tel. 801/408–1100; Jim Sheets, Administrator
**Web address:** www.intermountainhealthcare.org

LOGAN REGIONAL HOSPITAL (O, 135 beds) 1400 North 500 East, Logan, UT Zip 84341–2499; tel. 435/716–1000; Michael A. Clark, Administrator and Chief Executive Officer
**Web address:** www.loganregionalhospital.org

MCKAY–DEE HOSPITAL CENTER (O, 311 beds) 4401 Harrison Boulevard, Ogden, UT Zip 84403; tel. 801/387–2800; Timothy T. Pehrson, Chief Executive Officer
**Web address:** www.mckay–dee.org

OREM COMMUNITY HOSPITAL (O, 18 beds) 331 North 400 West, Orem, UT Zip 84057–1999; tel. 801/224–4080; Steven Badger, R.N., Administrator
**Web address:** www.intermountainhealthcare.org

PARK CITY MEDICAL CENTER (O, 26 beds) 900 Round Valley Drive, Park City, UT Zip 84060–7552; tel. 435/658–7000; Robert W. Allen, Chief Executive Officer
**Web address:** www.intermountainhealthcare.org

PRIMARY CHILDREN'S MEDICAL CENTER (O, 289 beds) 100 North Mario Capecchi Drive, Salt Lake City, UT Zip 84113–1100; tel. 801/662–1000; Katy Welkie, R.N., Administrator and Chief Executive Officer
**Web address:** www.intermountainhealthcare.org

RIVERTON HOSPITAL (O, 92 beds) 3741 West 12600 South, Riverton, UT Zip 84065–7215; tel. 801/285–4000; Blair Kent, Administrator
**Web address:** www.intermountainhealthcare.org/

SANPETE VALLEY HOSPITAL (O, 19 beds) 1100 South Medical Drive, Mount Pleasant, UT Zip 84647–2222; tel. 435/462–2441; Mark L. Allen, FACHE, Administrator
**Web address:** www.intermountainhealthcare.com

SEVIER VALLEY MEDICAL CENTER (O, 27 beds) 1000 North Main Street, Richfield, UT Zip 84701–1843; tel. 435/896–8271; Gary E. Beck, Administrator
**Web address:** www.intermountain.com

THE ORTHOPEDIC SPECIALTY HOSPITAL (O, 36 beds) 5848 South 300 East, Murray, UT Zip 84107; tel. 801/314–4100; Bryan Johnson, Administrator
**Web address:** www.intermountainhealthcare.org

UTAH VALLEY REGIONAL MEDICAL CENTER (O, 367 beds) 1034 North 500 West, Provo, UT Zip 84604–3337; tel. 801/357–7850; Steve Smoot, Administrator
**Web address:** www.utahvalleyregional.org

VALLEY VIEW MEDICAL CENTER (O, 48 beds) 1303 North Main Street, Cedar City, UT Zip 84720–3462; tel. 435/868–5000; Jason Wilson, Administrator
**Web address:** www.ihc.com

| | | |
|---|---|---|
| Owned, leased, sponsored: | 21 hospitals | 2571 beds |
| Contract–managed: | 1 hospital | 41 beds |
| Totals: | 22 hospitals | 2612 beds |

★**0061: IOWA HEALTH SYSTEM** (NP)
1776 West Lakes Parkway, Suite 400, Des Moines, IA Zip 50266; tel. 515/241–6161; William B. Leaver, President and Chief Executive Officer
**(Decentralized Health System)**

**ILLINOIS:** METHODIST MEDICAL CENTER OF ILLINOIS (O, 282 beds) 221 N.E. Glen Oak Avenue, Peoria, IL Zip 61636–4310; tel. 309/672–5522; Deborah R. Simon, R.N., President and Chief Executive Officer
**Web address:** www.mymethodist.net

TRINITY ROCK ISLAND (O, 317 beds) 2701 17th Street, Rock Island, IL Zip 61201–5393; tel. 309/779–5000; Richard A. Seidler, FACHE, President and Chief Executive Officer
**Web address:** www.trinityqc.com

**IOWA:** ALLEN MEMORIAL HOSPITAL (O, 201 beds) 1825 Logan Avenue, Waterloo, IA Zip 50703–1916; tel. 319/235–3941; Thomas Tibbitts, Interim Chief Executive Officer
**Web address:** www.allenhospital.org

BUENA VISTA REGIONAL MEDICAL CENTER (C, 35 beds) 1525 West Fifth Street, Storm Lake, IA Zip 50588–0309, Mailing Address: P.O. Box 309, Zip 50588–0309; tel. 712/732–4030; Steven Colerick, Chief Executive Officer
**Web address:** www.bvrmc.org

CLARKE COUNTY HOSPITAL (C, 25 beds) 800 South Fillmore Street, Osceola, IA Zip 50213–1619; tel. 641/342–2184; Brian G. Evans, FACHE, Chief Executive Officer
**Web address:** www.clarkehosp.org

COMMUNITY MEMORIAL HOSPITAL (C, 16 beds) 909 West First Street, Sumner, IA Zip 50674–1203, Mailing Address: P.O. Box 148, Zip 50674–0148; tel. 563/578–3275; Mary S. Wells, R.N., Chief Executive Officer
**Web address:** www.cmhsumner.org

For explanation of codes following names, see page B2.
★ Indicates Type III membership in the American Hospital Association.

FINLEY HOSPITAL (O, 119 beds) 350 North Grandview Avenue, Dubuque, IA Zip 52001–6392; tel. 563/582–1881; David R. Brandon, President and Chief Executive Officer
**Web address:** www.finleyhospital.org

GREATER REGIONAL MEDICAL CENTER (C, 25 beds) 1700 West Townline, Creston, IA Zip 50801–1099; tel. 641/782–7091; Monte Neitzel, Chief Executive Officer
**Web address:** www.greaterregional.org

GREENE COUNTY MEDICAL CENTER (C, 90 beds) 1000 West Lincolnway, Jefferson, IA Zip 50129–1697; tel. 515/386–2114; Carl P. Behne, Administrator and Chief Executive Officer
**Web address:** www.gcmchealth.com

GRUNDY COUNTY MEMORIAL HOSPITAL (C, 80 beds) 201 East J Avenue, Grundy Center, IA Zip 50638–2096; tel. 319/824–5421; Pamela K. Delagardelle, Chief Executive Officer
**Web address:** www.grundycountyhospital.com

GUTHRIE COUNTY HOSPITAL (C, 25 beds) 710 North 12th Street, Guthrie Center, IA Zip 50115–1544; tel. 641/332–2201; Gerald D. Neal, Chief Executive Officer and Administrator
**Web address:** www.guthriecountyhospital.org

GUTTENBERG MUNICIPAL HOSPITAL (C, 20 beds) 200 Main Street, Guttenberg, IA Zip 52052–0550, Mailing Address: P.O. Box 550, Zip 52052–0550; tel. 563/252–1121; Kimberley A. Gau, FACHE, Chief Executive Officer
**Web address:** www.guttenberghospital.org

HUMBOLDT COUNTY MEMORIAL HOSPITAL (C, 49 beds) 1000 North 15th Street, Humboldt, IA Zip 50548–1008; tel. 515/332–4200; James Atty, Chief Executive Officer
**Web address:** www.humboldthospital.org

IOWA LUTHERAN HOSPITAL (O, 187 beds) 700 East University Avenue, Des Moines, IA Zip 50316–2392; tel. 515/263–5612; Eric T. Crowell, President and Chief Executive Officer
**Web address:** www.iowahealth.org

IOWA METHODIST MEDICAL CENTER (O, 415 beds) 1200 Pleasant Street, Des Moines, IA Zip 50309–9976; tel. 515/241–6212; Eric T. Crowell, President and Chief Executive Officer
**Web address:** www.iowahealth.org

JONES REGIONAL MEDICAL CENTER (O, 22 beds) 1795 Highway 64 East, Anamosa, IA Zip 52205–2112; tel. 319/462–6131; Eric Briesemeister, Chief Executive Officer
**Web address:** www.jonesregional.org

LORING HOSPITAL (C, 25 beds) 211 Highland Avenue, Sac City, IA Zip 50583–0217; tel. 712/662–7105; Michael S. Ketcham, President and Chief Executive Officer
**Web address:** www.loringhospital.org

POCAHONTAS COMMUNITY HOSPITAL (C, 20 beds) 606 N.W. Seventh, Pocahontas, IA Zip 50574–1099; tel. 712/335–3501; James D. Roetman, President and Chief Executive Officer
**Web address:** www.pocahontashospital.org

ST. LUKE'S HOSPITAL (O, 363 beds) 1026 A Avenue N.E., Cedar Rapids, IA Zip 52402–3026, Mailing Address: P.O. Box 3026, Zip 52406–3026; tel. 319/369–7211; Theodore E. Townsend, FACHE, President and Chief Executive Officer
**Web address:** www.crstlukes.org

ST. LUKE'S REGIONAL MEDICAL CENTER (O, 160 beds) 2720 Stone Park Boulevard, Sioux City, IA Zip 51104–2000; tel. 712/279–3500; Peter W. Thoreen, FACHE, President and Chief Executive Officer
**Web address:** www.stlukes.org

TRINITY BETTENDORF (O, 59 beds) 4500 Utica Ridge Road, Bettendorf, IA Zip 52722–1626; tel. 563/742–5000; Richard A. Seidler, FACHE, President and Chief Executive Officer
**Web address:** www.trinityqc.com

TRINITY MUSCATINE (O, 56 beds) 1518 Mulberry Avenue, Muscatine, IA Zip 52761–3499; tel. 563/264–9100; James M. Hayes, Chief Executive Officer
**Web address:** www.trinitymuscatine.org

TRINITY REGIONAL MEDICAL CENTER (O, 132 beds) 802 Kenyon Road, Fort Dodge, IA Zip 50501–5795; tel. 515/573–3101; Susan K. Thompson, President and Chief Executive Officer
**Web address:** www.trmc.org

| Owned, leased, sponsored: | 12 hospitals | 2313 beds |
| Contract–managed: | 11 hospitals | 410 beds |
| **Totals:** | 23 hospitals | 2723 beds |

---

**★7775: JEFFERSON HEALTH SYSTEM** (NP)
259 Radnor–Chester Road, Suite 290, Radnor, PA Zip 19087–5288; tel. 610/225–6200; Joseph T. Sebastianelli, President and Chief Executive Officer
**(Moderately Centralized Health System)**

**PENNSYLVANIA:** MAGEE REHABILITATION HOSPITAL (O, 96 beds) 1513 Race Street, Philadelphia, PA Zip 19102–1177; tel. 215/587–3000; Jack A. Carroll, Ph.D., President and Chief Executive Officer
**Web address:** www.mageerehab.org

THOMAS JEFFERSON UNIVERSITY HOSPITAL (O, 930 beds) 211 S. 9th Street, Suite 300, Philadelphia, PA Zip 19107–5096; tel. 215/955–6000; David P. McQuaid, FACHE, President and Chief Operating Officer
**Web address:** www.jeffersonhospital.org

| Owned, leased, sponsored: | 2 hospitals | 1026 beds |
| Contract–managed: | 0 hospitals | 0 beds |
| **Totals:** | 2 hospitals | 1026 beds |

---

**★○0052: JEWISH HOSPITAL & ST. MARY'S HEALTHCARE** (NP)
200 Abraham Flexner Way, Louisville, KY Zip 40202–1886; tel. 502/587–4011; David Laird, President and Chief Executive Officer
**(Centralized Health System)**

**INDIANA:** SCOTT MEMORIAL HOSPITAL (C, 25 beds) 1415 North Gardner Street, Scottsburg, IN Zip 47170–0430, Mailing Address: Box 430, Zip 47170–0430; tel. 812/752–3456; Clifford D. Nay, Executive Director
**Web address:** www.scottmemorial.com

SOUTHERN INDIANA REHABILITATION HOSPITAL (O, 60 beds) 3104 Blackiston Boulevard, New Albany, IN Zip 47150–9579; tel. 812/941–8300; Randy L. Napier, President and Chief Executive Officer
**Web address:** www.sirh.org

**KENTUCKY:** FRAZIER REHAB INSTITUTE (O, 79 beds) 220 Abraham Flexner Way, Louisville, KY Zip 40202–1887; tel. 502/582–7400; Douglas Howell, Interim President and Chief Executive Officer
**Web address:** www.frazierrehab.org

JEWISH HOSPITAL (O, 462 beds) 200 Abraham Flexner Way, Louisville, KY Zip 40202–1886; tel. 502/587–4011; Douglas Howell, Interim President and Chief Executive Officer
**Web address:** www.jewishhospital.org

JEWISH HOSPITAL–SHELBYVILLE (O, 41 beds) 727 Hospital Drive, Shelbyville, KY Zip 40065–1699; tel. 502/647–4000; Michael L. Collins, President and Chief Executive Officer
**Web address:** www.jhsmh.org

OUR LADY OF PEACE (O, 261 beds) 2020 Newburg Road, Louisville, KY Zip 40205–1879; tel. 502/479–4500; Jennifer Nolan, President and Chief Executive Officer
**Web address:** www.hopehasaplace.org

STS. MARY & ELIZABETH HOSPITAL (O, 163 beds) 1850 Bluegrass Avenue, Louisville, KY Zip 40215–1199; tel. 502/361–6000; James Parobek, President
**Web address:** www.jhsmh.org

TAYLOR REGIONAL HOSPITAL (C, 90 beds) 1700 Old Lebanon Road, Campbellsville, KY Zip 42718–9600; tel. 270/465–3561; Jane Wheatley, Chief Executive Officer
**Web address:** www.trhosp.org

| Owned, leased, sponsored: | 6 hospitals | 1066 beds |
| Contract–managed: | 2 hospitals | 115 beds |
| **Totals:** | 8 hospitals | 1181 beds |

---

For explanation of codes following names, see page B2.
★ Indicates Type III membership in the American Hospital Association.

**★8855: JFK HEALTH SYSTEM** (NP)
80 James Street, 2nd Floor, Edison, NJ Zip 08820–3998;
tel. 732/321–7774; Raymond F. Fredericks, President and Chief
Executive Officer

**NEW JERSEY:** JFK JOHNSON REHABILITATION INSTITUTE (O, 92 beds) 65
James Street, Edison, NJ Zip 08818–3059; tel. 732/321–7050; Anthony
Cuzzola, Vice President Rehabilitation Services
**Web address:** www.solarishs.org

JFK MEDICAL CENTER (O, 441 beds) 65 James Street, Edison, NJ
Zip 08818–3059; tel. 732/321–7000; Raymond F. Fredericks, President and
CEO
**Web address:** www.jfkmc.org

| Owned, leased, sponsored: | 2 hospitals | 533 beds |
|---|---|---|
| Contract–managed: | 0 hospitals | 0 beds |
| Totals: | 2 hospitals | 533 beds |

**★0218: JOHN C. LINCOLN HEALTH NETWORK** (NP)
2500 West Utopia Road, Suite 100, Phoenix, AZ Zip 85027–4172;
tel. 623/434–6230; Rhonda Forsyth, President and Chief Executive
Officer
**(Independent Hospital System)**

**ARIZONA:** JOHN C. LINCOLN DEER VALLEY HOSPITAL (O, 204 beds) 19829
North 27th Avenue, Phoenix, AZ Zip 85027–4002; tel. 623/879–6100;
Bruce Pearson, FACHE, Executive Vice President and Chief Executive
Officer
**Web address:** www.jcl.com

JOHN C. LINCOLN NORTH MOUNTAIN HOSPITAL (O, 256 beds) 250 East
Dunlap Avenue, Phoenix, AZ Zip 85020–2446; tel. 602/943–2381; Bruce
Pearson, FACHE, Executive Vice President and Chief Executive Officer
**Web address:** www.jcl.com

| Owned, leased, sponsored: | 2 hospitals | 460 beds |
|---|---|---|
| Contract–managed: | 0 hospitals | 0 beds |
| Totals: | 2 hospitals | 460 beds |

**★0324: JOHN MUIR HEALTH** (NP)
1400 Treat Boulevard, Walnut Creek, CA Zip 94597–2142;
tel. 925/941–2100; Calvin K. Knight, President and Chief Executive
Officer
**(Centralized Health System)**

**CALIFORNIA:** JOHN MUIR BEHAVIORAL HEALTH CENTER (O, 70 beds) 2740
Grant Street, Concord, CA Zip 94520; tel. 925/674–4100; Elizabeth
Stallings, Chief Operating Officer
**Web address:** www.johnmuirhealth.com

JOHN MUIR MEDICAL CENTER, CONCORD (O, 182 beds) 2540 East Street,
Concord, CA Zip 94520; tel. 925/682–8200; Michael S. Thomas, President
and Chief Administrative Officer
**Web address:** www.johnmuirhealth.com

JOHN MUIR MEDICAL CENTER, WALNUT CREEK (O, 367 beds) 1601 Ygnacio
Valley Road, Walnut Creek, CA Zip 94598–3194; tel. 925/939–3000; Jane
Willemsen, Chief Administrative Officer
**Web address:** www.jmmdhs.com/index.php/jmmdhs_jmmc.html

| Owned, leased, sponsored: | 3 hospitals | 619 beds |
|---|---|---|
| Contract–managed: | 0 hospitals | 0 beds |
| Totals: | 3 hospitals | 619 beds |

**★1015: JOHNS HOPKINS HEALTH SYSTEM** (NP)
733 North Broadway, BRB 104, Baltimore, MD Zip 21205;
tel. 410/955–5000; Ronald R. Peterson, President
**(Centralized Physician/Insurance Health System)**

**DISTRICT OF COLUMBIA:** SIBLEY MEMORIAL HOSPITAL (O, 252 beds) 5255
Loughboro Road N.W., Washington, DC Zip 20016–2695;
tel. 202/537–4000; Richard O. Davis, Ph.D., President
**Web address:** www.sibley.org

**FLORIDA:** ALL CHILDREN'S HOSPITAL (O, 259 beds) 501 6th Avenue South,
Saint Petersburg, FL Zip 33701–4899; tel. 727/898–7451; Arnold T.
Stenberg, Jr., Executive Vice President and Chief Administrative Officer
**Web address:** www.allkids.org

**MARYLAND:** HOWARD COUNTY GENERAL HOSPITAL (O, 256 beds) 5755
Cedar Lane, Columbia, MD Zip 21044–2999; tel. 410/740–7890; Victor
A. Broccolino, President and Chief Executive Officer
**Web address:** www.hcgh.org

JOHNS HOPKINS BAYVIEW MEDICAL CENTER (O, 518 beds) 4940 Eastern
Avenue, Baltimore, MD Zip 21224–2780; tel. 410/550–0100; Richard G.
Bennett, M.D., President
**Web address:** www.hopkinsbayview.org

JOHNS HOPKINS HOSPITAL (O, 912 beds) 600 North Wolfe Street, Baltimore,
MD Zip 21287–2182; tel. 410/955–5000; Ronald R. Peterson, President
**Web address:** www.hopkinsmedicine.org

SUBURBAN HOSPITAL (O, 234 beds) 8600 Old Georgetown Road, Bethesda,
MD Zip 20814–1497; tel. 301/896–3100; Brian A. Gragnolati, FACHE,
President and Chief Executive Officer
**Web address:** www.suburbanhospital.org

| Owned, leased, sponsored: | 6 hospitals | 2431 beds |
|---|---|---|
| Contract–managed: | 0 hospitals | 0 beds |
| Totals: | 6 hospitals | 2431 beds |

**★2105: KAISER FOUNDATION HOSPITALS** (NP)
One Kaiser Plaza, Oakland, CA Zip 94612–3600;
tel. 510/271–5910; George C. Halvorson, Chairman and Chief
Executive Officer
**(Decentralized Health System)**

**CALIFORNIA:** ANAHEIM MEDICAL CENTER (O, 326 beds) 441 North Lakeview
Avenue, Anaheim, CA Zip 92807–3089; tel. 714/279–4000; Julie K.
Miller–Phipps, Senior Vice President and Executive Director
**Web address:** www.kp.org

ANTIOCH MEDICAL CENTER (O, 150 beds) 4501 Sand Creek Road, Antioch,
CA Zip 94531; tel. 925/813–6500; Tim F. Daly, Chief Operating Officer
**Web address:** www.kaiserpermanente.org

BALDWIN PARK MEDICAL CENTER (O, 254 beds) 1011 Baldwin Park
Boulevard, Baldwin Park, CA Zip 91706–5806; tel. 626/851–1011; Margaret
H. Pierce, Executive Director
**Web address:** www.kp.org

FONTANA MEDICAL CENTER (O, 390 beds) 9961 Sierra Avenue, Fontana, CA
Zip 92335–6720; tel. 909/427–5000; Greg Christian, Executive Director
**Web address:** www.kaiserpermanente.org

FRESNO MEDICAL CENTER (O, 169 beds) 7300 North Fresno Street, Fresno,
CA Zip 93720–2941; tel. 559/448–4500; Jeffrey A. Collins, Senior Vice
President and Area Manager
**Web address:** www.kaiserpermanente.org

HAYWARD MEDICAL CENTER (O, 208 beds) 27400 Hesperian Boulevard,
Hayward, CA Zip 94545–4235; tel. 510/784–4000; Colleen McKeown,
Senior Vice President and Area Manager
**Web address:** www.kaiserpermanente.org

KAISER PERMANENTE DOWNEY MEDICAL CENTER (O, 218 beds) 9333
Imperial Highway, Downey, CA Zip 90242–2812; tel. 562/657–9000; E. Jane
Finley, Senior Vice President and Executive Director
**Web address:** www.kaiserpermanente.org

LOS ANGELES MEDICAL CENTER (O, 464 beds) 4867 Sunset Boulevard, Los
Angeles, CA Zip 90027–5969; tel. 323/783–4011; Mark E. Costa, Executive
Director
**Web address:** www.kaiserpermanente.org

MANTECA MEDICAL CENTER (O, 146 beds) 1777 West Yosemite Avenue,
Manteca, CA Zip 95337–5187; tel. 209/825–3500; Corwin N. Harper, Senior
Vice President and Area Manager
**Web address:** www.kaiserpermanente.org

MORENO VALLEY COMMUNITY HOSPITAL (O, 72 beds) 27300 Iris Avenue,
Moreno Valley, CA Zip 92555–4800; tel. 951/243–0811; Corey A. Seale,
Administrator

OAKLAND MEDICAL CENTER (O, 341 beds) 280 West MacArthur Boulevard,
Oakland, CA Zip 94611–5693; tel. 510/752–1000; Nathaniel L. Oubre, Jr.,
Senior Vice President and Area Manager
**Web address:** www.kaiserpermanente.org

---

For explanation of codes following names, see page B2.
★ Indicates Type III membership in the American Hospital Association.

PANORAMA CITY MEDICAL CENTER (O, 218 beds) 13652 Cantara Street, Panorama City, CA Zip 91402–5497; tel. 818/375–2000; Dennis C. Benton, Administrator and Executive Director
**Web address:** www.kaiserpermanente.org

REDWOOD CITY MEDICAL CENTER (O, 213 beds) 1150 Veterans Boulevard, Redwood City, CA Zip 94063–2037; tel. 650/299–2000; Frank T. Beirne, Senior Vice President and Area Manager
**Web address:** www.kaiserpermanente.org

RIVERSIDE MEDICAL CENTER (O, 215 beds) 10800 Magnolia Avenue, Riverside, CA Zip 92505–3000; tel. 951/353–2000; Vita M. Willett, Administrator and Executive Director
**Web address:** www.kaiserpermanente.org

ROSEVILLE MEDICAL CENTER (O, 340 beds) 1600 Eureka Road, Roseville, CA Zip 95661–3027; tel. 916/784–4000; Edward S. Glavis, Senior Vice President and Area Manager
**Web address:** www.kp.org

SACRAMENTO MEDICAL CENTER (O, 287 beds) 2025 Morse Avenue, Sacramento, CA Zip 95825–2115; tel. 916/973–5000; Ronald Groepper, Senior Vice President and Area Manager
**Web address:** www.kp.org

SAN DIEGO MEDICAL CENTER (O, 392 beds) 4647 Zion Avenue, San Diego, CA Zip 92120–2507; tel. 619/528–5000; Mary Ann Barnes, Senior Vice President and Executive Director
**Web address:** www.kaiserpermanente.org

SAN FRANCISCO MEDICAL CENTER (O, 215 beds) 2200 O'Farrell Street, San Francisco, CA Zip 94115–3358; tel. 415/833–2000; Christine Robisch, Senior Vice President and Area Manager
**Web address:** www.kaiserpermanente.org

SAN JOSE MEDICAL CENTER (O, 217 beds) 250 Hospital Parkway, San Jose, CA Zip 95119–1199; tel. 408/972–7000; Irene Chavez, Senior Vice President and Area Manager
**Web address:** www.kaiserpermanente.org

SAN RAFAEL MEDICAL CENTER (O, 82 beds) 99 Montecillo Road, San Rafael, CA Zip 94903–3308; tel. 415/444–2000; Judy Coffey, Senior Vice President and Area Manager
**Web address:** www.kaiserpermanente.org

SANTA CLARA MEDICAL CENTER (O, 327 beds) 700 Lawrence Expressway, Santa Clara, CA Zip 95051–5173; tel. 408/851–1000; Christopher L. Boyd, Senior Vice President and Area Manager
**Web address:** www.kaiserpermanente.org

SANTA ROSA MEDICAL CENTER (O, 117 beds) 401 Bicentennial Way, Santa Rosa, CA Zip 95403–2192; tel. 707/571–4000; Judy Coffey, Senior Vice President and Area Manager
**Web address:** www.kaiserpermanente.org

SOUTH BAY MEDICAL CENTER (O, 235 beds) 25825 South Vermont Avenue, Harbor City, CA Zip 90710–3599; tel. 310/325–5111; Lesley A. Wille, Administrator and Executive Director
**Web address:** www.kaiserpermanente.org

SOUTH SACRAMENTO MEDICAL CENTER (O, 181 beds) 6600 Bruceville Road, Sacramento, CA Zip 95823–4671; tel. 916/688–2430; Patricia Rodriguez, Senior Vice President and Area Manager
**Web address:** www.kp.org

SOUTH SAN FRANCISCO MEDICAL CENTER (O, 120 beds) 1200 El Camino Real, South San Francisco, CA Zip 94080–3299; tel. 650/742–2000; Frank T. Beirne, Senior Vice President and Area Manager
**Web address:** www.kaiserpermanente.org

VACAVILLE MEDICAL CENTER (O, 64 beds) 1 Quality Drive, Vacaville, CA Zip 95688–9494; tel. 707/624–4000; Max Villalobos, Senior Vice President
**Web address:** www.kp.org

VALLEJO MEDICAL CENTER (O, 287 beds) 975 Sereno Drive, Vallejo, CA Zip 94589–2441; tel. 707/651–1000; Max Villalobos, Senior Vice President and Area Manager
**Web address:** www.kaiserpermanente.org

WALNUT CREEK MEDICAL CENTER (O, 233 beds) 1425 South Main Street, Walnut Creek, CA Zip 94596–5300; tel. 925/295–4000; Ginger Campbell, Senior Vice President and Area Manager
**Web address:** www.kaiserpermanente.org

WEST LOS ANGELES MEDICAL CENTER (O, 172 beds) 6041 Cadillac Avenue, Los Angeles, CA Zip 90034–1702; tel. 323/857–2201; Gloria C. Blackburn, Executive Director
**Web address:** www.kaiserpermanente.org

WOODLAND HILLS MEDICAL CENTER (O, 175 beds) 5601 DeSoto Avenue, Woodland Hills, CA Zip 91365–6701; tel. 818/719–2000; Catherine Casas, Executive Director
**Web address:** www.kaiserpermanente.org

**HAWAII:** KAISER PERMANENTE MEDICAL CENTER (O, 235 beds) 3288 Moanalua Road, Honolulu, HI Zip 96819–1469; tel. 808/432–0000; William F. Haug, FACHE, Administrator
**Web address:** www.kaiserpermanente.org

**OREGON:** SUNNYSIDE MEDICAL CENTER (O, 283 beds) 10180 S.E. Sunnyside Road, Clackamas, OR Zip 97015–9303; tel. 503/652–2880; Susan Mullaney, Administrator
**Web address:** www.kaiserpermanente.org

| | | |
|---|---|---|
| **Owned, leased, sponsored:** | 32 hospitals | 7346 beds |
| **Contract–managed:** | 0 hospitals | 0 beds |
| **Totals:** | 32 hospitals | 7346 beds |

---

**★0258: KETTERING HEALTH NETWORK** (NP)
3965 Southern Boulevard, Dayton, OH Zip 45429–1221; tel. 937/395–8150; Fred M. Manchur, President and Chief Executive Officer
**(Moderately Centralized Health System)**

**OHIO:** FORT HAMILTON HOSPITAL (O, 187 beds) 630 Eaton Avenue, Hamilton, OH Zip 45013–2770; tel. 513/867–2000; Jennifer Swenson, President
**Web address:** www.khnetwork.org/fort_hamilton

GRANDVIEW MEDICAL CENTER (O, 317 beds) 405 Grand Avenue, Dayton, OH Zip 45405–4796; tel. 937/226–3200; Richard Haas, FACHE, President
**Web address:** www.khnetwork.org

GREENE MEMORIAL HOSPITAL (O, 89 beds) 1141 North Monroe Drive, Xenia, OH Zip 45385–1600; tel. 937/352–2000; Terry M. Burns, President
**Web address:** www.greenehealth.org

KETTERING MEDICAL CENTER (O, 515 beds) 3535 Southern Boulevard, Kettering, OH Zip 45429; tel. 937/298–4331; Roy G. Chew, Ph.D., President
**Web address:** www.kmcnetwork.org

SOIN MEDICAL CENTER (O, 63 beds) 3535 Pentagon Boulevard, Beavercreek, OH Zip 45431; tel. 937/702–4000; Terry M. Burns, President
**Web address:** www.khnetwork.org/soin

SYCAMORE MEDICAL CENTER (O, 163 beds) 4000 Miamisburg–Centerville Road, Miamisburg, OH Zip 45342; tel. 937/866–0551; Mark T. Smith, JD, CPA, President
**Web address:** www.khnetwork.org

| | | |
|---|---|---|
| **Owned, leased, sponsored:** | 6 hospitals | 1334 beds |
| **Contract–managed:** | 0 hospitals | 0 beds |
| **Totals:** | 6 hospitals | 1334 beds |

---

**★0026: KINDRED HEALTHCARE** (IO)
680 South Fourth Street, Louisville, KY Zip 40202–2412; tel. 502/596–7300; Paul J. Diaz, President and Chief Executive Officer
**(Independent Hospital System)**

**ARIZONA:** KINDRED HOSPITAL ARIZONA–PHOENIX (O, 166 beds) 40 East Indianola Avenue, Phoenix, AZ Zip 85012–2059; tel. 602/280–7000; Rachelle Spencer, Administrator
**Web address:** www.khphoenix.com/

KINDRED HOSPITAL–TUCSON (O, 51 beds) 355 North Wilmot Road, Tucson, AZ Zip 85711–2635; tel. 520/584–4500; Heidi Miller, Chief Executive Officer
**Web address:** www.khtucson.com

**CALIFORNIA:** KINDRED HOSPITAL OF RIVERSIDE (O, 40 beds) 2224 Medical Center Drive, Perris, CA Zip 92571; tel. 951/436–3535; James Linhares, Administrator
**Web address:** www.khriverside.com

KINDRED HOSPITAL OF SOUTH BAY (O, 84 beds) 1246 West 155th Street, Gardena, CA Zip 90247–4011; tel. 310/323–5330; Kevin Chavez, Administrator
**Web address:** www.khsouthbay.com/

For explanation of codes following names, see page B2.
★ Indicates Type III membership in the American Hospital Association.

KINDRED HOSPITAL RANCHO (O, 55 beds) 10841 White Oak Avenue, Rancho Cucamonga, CA Zip 91730–3811; tel. 909/581–6400; Jody Knox, Administrator
**Web address:** www.khrancho.com

KINDRED HOSPITAL–BALDWIN PARK (C, 95 beds) 14148 East Francisquito Avenue, Baldwin Park, CA Zip 91706; tel. 626/388–2700; Swenda Moreh, Chief Executive Officer
**Web address:** www.khbaldwinpark.com

KINDRED HOSPITAL–BREA (O, 48 beds) 875 North Brea Boulevard, Brea, CA Zip 92821–2699; tel. 714/529–6842; Joyce Winters, R.N., MSN, Administrator
**Web address:** www.kindredhospitalbrea.com/

KINDRED HOSPITAL–LA MIRADA (O, 216 beds) 14900 East Imperial Highway, La Mirada, CA Zip 90638; tel. 562/944–1900; April Myers, Administrator
**Web address:** www.kindredlamirada.com/

KINDRED HOSPITAL–LOS ANGELES (O, 81 beds) 5525 West Slauson Avenue, Los Angeles, CA Zip 90056–1067; tel. 310/642–0325; Luke Tharasri, Administrator
**Web address:** www.kindredhospitalla.com/

KINDRED HOSPITAL–ONTARIO (O, 91 beds) 550 North Monterey Avenue, Ontario, CA Zip 91764–3399; tel. 909/391–0333; Robin Rapp, MS, R.N., Chief Executive Officer
**Web address:** www.khontario.com/

KINDRED HOSPITAL–SACRAMENTO (O, 37 beds) 330 Montrose Drive, Folsom, CA Zip 95630–2720; tel. 916/351–9151; Janet Biedron, R.N., Chief Executive Officer
**Web address:** www.kindredsacramento.com/

KINDRED HOSPITAL–SAN DIEGO (O, 70 beds) 1940 El Cajon Boulevard, San Diego, CA Zip 92104–1096; tel. 619/543–4500; Natalie Germuska, Chief Executive Officer
**Web address:** www.kindredsandiego.com

KINDRED HOSPITAL–SAN FRANCISCO BAY AREA (O, 99 beds) 2800 Benedict Drive, San Leandro, CA Zip 94577–6840; tel. 510/357–8300; Kelli Cole, Chief Executive Officer
**Web address:** www.kindredhospitalsfba.

KINDRED HOSPITAL–WESTMINSTER (O, 109 beds) 200 Hospital Circle, Westminster, CA Zip 92683–3910; tel. 714/893–4541; Adam Darvish, M.P.H., Chief Executive Officer
**Web address:** www.khwestminster.com/

**COLORADO:** KINDRED HOSPITAL–AURORA (O, 37 beds) 700 Potomac Street, Aurora, CO Zip 80012; tel. 720/857–8333; Linda A. W. McCaskill, Market Chief Executive Officer
**Web address:** www.khaurora.com/

KINDRED HOSPITAL–DENVER (O, 68 beds) 1920 High Street, Denver, CO Zip 80218–1213; tel. 303/320–5871; Linda A. W. McCaskill, Chief Executive Officer
**Web address:** www.kh–denver.com

**FLORIDA:** KINDRED HOSPITAL BAY AREA–TAMPA (O, 155 beds) 4555 South Manhattan Avenue, Tampa, FL Zip 33611–2397; tel. 813/839–6341; Julie Feasel, Chief Executive Officer
**Web address:** www.khtampa.com

KINDRED HOSPITAL MELBOURNE (O, 60 beds) 765 West Nasa Boulevard, Melbourne, FL Zip 32901–1815; tel. 321/733–5725; Angelica Cotshott, Chief Executive Officer
**Web address:** www.khmelbourne.com

KINDRED HOSPITAL NORTH FLORIDA (O, 80 beds) 801 Oak Street, Green Cove Springs, FL Zip 32043–4317; tel. 904/284–9230; Hoyt Ross, Chief Executive Officer
**Web address:** www.khnorthflorida.com

KINDRED HOSPITAL OCALA (O, 31 beds) 1500 S.W. 1st Avenue, Ocala, FL Zip 34474; tel. 352/369–0513; Marc Lemon, Administrator
**Web address:** www.kindredocala.com

KINDRED HOSPITAL SOUTH FLORIDA–FORT LAUDERDALE (O, 123 beds) 1516 East Las Olas Boulevard, Fort Lauderdale, FL Zip 33301–2399; tel. 954/764–8900; Theodore L. Welding, Administrator
**Web address:** www.khfortlauderdale.com/

KINDRED HOSPITAL SOUTH FLORIDA–HOLLYWOOD (O, 118 beds) 1859 Van Buren Street, Hollywood, FL Zip 33020–5127; tel. 954/920–9000; Christopher Clements, Administrator
**Web address:** www.khsfhollywood.com/

KINDRED HOSPITAL THE PALM BEACHES (O, 70 beds) 5555 West Blue Heron Boulevard, Riviera Beach, FL Zip 33418–7813; tel. 561/840–0754; Timothy Page, Chief Executive Officer
**Web address:** www.khthepalmbeaches.com/

KINDRED HOSPITAL–CENTRAL TAMPA (O, 102 beds) 4801 North Howard Avenue, Tampa, FL Zip 33603–1484; tel. 813/874–7575; Debra Plummer, Chief Executive Officer
**Web address:** www.kindredcentraltampa.com/

**GEORGIA:** KINDRED HOSPITAL ROME (O, 45 beds) 304 Turner McCall Boulevard, Rome, GA Zip 30162; tel. 706/378–6800; Susan M. Stovall, Chief Executive Officer
**Web address:** www.kindredrome.com

KINDRED HOSPITAL–ATLANTA (O, 70 beds) 705 Juniper Street N.E., Atlanta, GA Zip 30308; tel. 404/873–2871; Michael Schmitt, Chief Executive Officer
**Web address:** www.kindredatlanta.com/

**ILLINOIS:** KINDRED CHICAGO–CENTRAL HOSPITAL (O, 54 beds) 4058 West Melrose Street, Chicago, IL Zip 60641–4797; tel. 773/736–7000; Bruce Carey, Chief Executive Officer
**Web address:** www.khchicagocentral.com

KINDRED HOSPITAL CHICAGO–NORTHLAKE (O, 94 beds) 365 East North Avenue, Northlake, IL Zip 60164–2628; tel. 708/345–8100; Beverly Foster, Chief Executive Officer
**Web address:** www.kindrednorthlake.com/

KINDRED HOSPITAL PEORIA (O, 50 beds) 500 West Romeo B. Garrett Avenue, Peoria, IL Zip 61605; tel. 309/680–1500; Adam Novak, Chief Executive Officer
**Web address:** www.khpeoria.com/

KINDRED HOSPITAL SPRINGFIELD (O, 50 beds) 701 North Walnut Street, Springfield, IL Zip 62702–4913; tel. 217/528–1217; Sherry L. Hendricksen, R.N., MSN, Chief Executive Officer
**Web address:** www.kindredspringfield.com/

KINDRED HOSPITAL–SYCAMORE (O, 69 beds) 225 Edward Street, Sycamore, IL Zip 60178–2197; tel. 815/895–2144; Cindy Smith, Chief Executive Officer
**Web address:** www.kindredhospitalsyc.com/

**INDIANA:** KINDRED HOSPITAL INDIANAPOLIS SOUTH (O, 60 beds) 607 Greenwood Springs Drive, Greenwood, IN Zip 46143–1400; tel. 317/888–8155; Mona Euler, Chief Executive Officer
**Web address:** www.khindysouth.com/

KINDRED HOSPITAL NORTHWEST INDIANA (O, 70 beds) 5454 Hohman Avenue, 5th Floor, Hammond, IN Zip 46320; tel. 219/937–9900; Jeff Cellucci, Interim Chief Executive Officer
**Web address:** www.khnwindiana.com

KINDRED HOSPITAL OF NORTHERN INDIANA (O, 32 beds) 215 West Fourth Street, Suite 200, Mishawaka, IN Zip 46544–1917; tel. 574/252–2000; Christine T. Voorde, Chief Executive Officer
**Web address:** www.khnorthernindiana.com/

KINDRED HOSPITAL–INDIANAPOLIS (O, 59 beds) 1700 West 10th Street, Indianapolis, IN Zip 46222–3802; tel. 317/636–4400; Kristy Walden, R.N., Interim Administrator
**Web address:** www.kindredhospitalindy.com/

**KENTUCKY:** KINDRED HOSPITAL–LOUISVILLE (O, 164 beds) 1313 Saint Anthony Place, Louisville, KY Zip 40204–1740; tel. 502/587–7001; Michael L. Moody, Market Chief Executive Officer
**Web address:** www.kindredlouisville.com/

**LOUISIANA:** KINDRED HOSPITAL LAFAYETTE (O, 50 beds) 204 Energy Parkway, Lafayette, LA Zip 70508–3816; tel. 337/232–1905; Sharon Black, Chief Executive Officer
**Web address:** www.khlafayette.com

KINDRED HOSPITAL WEST–JEFFERSON (O, 56 beds) 1111 Medical Center Boulevard, Suite S–550, Marrero, LA Zip 70072; tel. 504/349–2470; Paul R. Newhouse, Chief Executive Officer
**Web address:** www.khwestjefferson.com/

KINDRED HOSPITAL–NEW ORLEANS (O, 80 beds) 3601 Coliseum Street, New Orleans, LA Zip 70115–3606; tel. 504/899–1555; Thomas G. Alexander, Chief Executive Officer
**Web address:** www.kindredhospitalnola.com

**MASSACHUSETTS:** KINDRED HOSPITAL BOSTON–NORTH SHORE (O, 50 beds) 15 King Street, Peabody, MA Zip 01960–4379; tel. 978/531–2900; Yolande Wilson, Chief Executive Officer
**Web address:** www.kindredbns.com

For explanation of codes following names, see page B2.
★ Indicates Type III membership in the American Hospital Association.

KINDRED HOSPITAL NORTHEAST–STOUGHTON (O, 170 beds) 909 Sumner Street, 1st Floor, Stoughton, MA Zip 02072; tel. 781/297–8200; Robert A. Gundersen, Market Chief Executive Officer
**Web address:** www.khstoughton.com

KINDRED HOSPITAL PARK VIEW (O, 202 beds) 1400 State Street, Springfield, MA Zip 01109–2550; tel. 413/726–6700; Jake Socha, Chief Executive Officer
**Web address:** www.khparkview.com/

KINDRED HOSPITAL–BOSTON (O, 59 beds) 1515 Commonwealth Avenue, Brighton, MA Zip 02135–3617; tel. 617/254–1100; Susan Downey, Chief Executive Officer
**Web address:** www.kindredbos.com/

**MICHIGAN:** KINDRED HOSPITAL DETROIT (O, 77 beds) 4777 East Outer Drive, Detroit, MI Zip 48234–3241; tel. 313/369–5800; Andrew G. Escamilla, MS, R.N., Chief Executive Officer
**Web address:** www.kindreddetroit.com/

**MISSOURI:** KINDRED HOSPITAL KANSAS CITY (O, 130 beds) 8701 Troost Avenue, Kansas City, MO Zip 64131–2767; tel. 816/995–2000; Aaron Anothayanontha, Chief Executive Officer
**Web address:** www.kindredhospitalkc.com

KINDRED HOSPITAL NORTHLAND (O, 35 beds) 500 Northwest 68th Street, Kansas City, MO Zip 64118; tel. 816/420–6300; Alexander Gill, Interim Chief Executive Officer
**Web address:** www.khnorthland.com

KINDRED HOSPITAL–ST. LOUIS (O, 98 beds) 4930 Lindell Boulevard, Saint Louis, MO Zip 63108–1510; tel. 314/361–8700; Stacy M. Howard, R.N., Chief Executive Officer
**Web address:** www.kindredstlouis.com/

ST. LUKE'S REHABILITATION HOSPITAL (O, 35 beds) 14709 Olive Boulevard, Chesterfield, MO Zip 63017–2221; tel. 314/317–5700; Della Abboud, Chief Executive Officer
**Web address:** www.khrehabstluke.com

**NEVADA:** KINDRED HOSPITAL LAS VEGAS–SAHARA (O, 238 beds) 5110 West Sahara Avenue, Las Vegas, NV Zip 89146–3406; tel. 702/871–1418; Christie Bond–Carafelli, Chief Executive Officer
**Web address:** www.kindredhospitalvs.com/

**NEW JERSEY:** KINDRED HOSPITAL–NEW JERSEY MORRIS COUNTY (O, 117 beds) 400 West Blackwell Street, Dover, NJ Zip 07801; tel. 973/537–3818; Wayne D. Blanchard, Chief Executive Officer
**Web address:** www.khmorriscounty.com/

**NEW MEXICO:** KINDRED HOSPITAL–ALBUQUERQUE (O, 61 beds) 700 High Street N.E., Albuquerque, NM Zip 87102–2565; tel. 505/242–4444; Michael R. Shaw, Chief Executive Officer
**Web address:** www.kindredalbuquerque.com/

**NORTH CAROLINA:** KINDRED HOSPITAL–GREENSBORO (O, 124 beds) 2401 Southside Boulevard, Greensboro, NC Zip 27406–3311; tel. 336/271–2800; Derek Murzyn, Chief Executive Officer
**Web address:** www.khgreensboro.com

**NORTH DAKOTA:** KINDRED HOSPITAL FARGO (O, 31 beds) 1720 University Drive South, Fargo, ND Zip 58103; tel. 701/241–9099; Custer Huseby, Chief Executive Officer
**Web address:** www.khfargo.com

KINDRED HOSPITAL–CENTRAL DAKOTAS (O, 41 beds) 1000 18th Street N.W., Mandan, ND Zip 58554; tel. 701/667–2000; April Bishop, Chief Executive Officer
**Web address:** www.khcentraldakotas.com

**OHIO:** KINDRED HOSPITAL CLEVELAND–GATEWAY (O, 153 beds) 2351 East 22nd Street, 7th Floor, Cleveland, OH Zip 44115; tel. 216/363–2671; Ian Cooper, Chief Executive Officer
**Web address:** www.kindredgateway.com

KINDRED HOSPITAL LIMA (O, 26 beds) 730 West Market Street, 6th Floor, Lima, OH Zip 45801; tel. 419/224–1888; Kris Karns, FACHE, Ph.D., Chief Executive Officer
**Web address:** www.khlima.com

KINDRED HOSPITAL OF CENTRAL OHIO (O, 33 beds) 335 Glessner Avenue, 5th Floor, Mansfield, OH Zip 44903; tel. 419/526–0777; Kris Karns, FACHE, Ph.D., Chief Executive Officer
**Web address:** www.khcentralohio.com/

KINDRED HOSPITAL–DAYTON (O, 67 beds) One Elizabeth Place, 5th Floor, Dayton, OH Zip 45408; tel. 937/222–5963; Lynn Schoen, Chief Executive Officer
**Web address:** www.khdayton.com

**OKLAHOMA:** KINDRED HOSPITAL TULSA (O, 60 beds) 3219 South 79th East Avenue, Tulsa, OK Zip 74145–1343; tel. 918/663–8183; Lee A. Simpson, Jr., Chief Executive Officer
**Web address:** www.khtulsa.com

KINDRED HOSPITAL– OKLAHOMA CITY (O, 93 beds) 1407 North Robinson Avenue, Oklahoma City, OK Zip 73103–4823; tel. 405/232–8000; Gayla Campbell, Chief Executive Officer
**Web address:** www.kindredoklahoma.com

**PENNSYLVANIA:** KINDRED HOSPITAL EASTON (O, 31 beds) 250 South 21st Street, 3rd Floor, Easton, PA Zip 18042; tel. 610/250–4724; Louise Cassidy, Chief Executive Officer
**Web address:** www.kheaston.com/

KINDRED HOSPITAL PITTSBURGH–NORTH SHORE (O, 111 beds) 1004 Arch Street, Pittsburgh, PA Zip 15212–5235; tel. 412/323–5800; Rodney B. Jones, Interim Administrator
**Web address:** www.kindrednorthshore.com/

KINDRED HOSPITAL SOUTH PHILADELPHIA (O, 58 beds) 1930 South Broad Street, Philadelphia, PA Zip 19145–2304; tel. 267/570–5200; Garrett Arneson, Chief Executive Officer
**Web address:** www.khsouthphilly.com

KINDRED HOSPITAL–DELAWARE COUNTY (O, 39 beds) 1500 Lansdowne Avenue, 6th Floor, Darby, PA Zip 19023; tel. 610/237–5780; Deborah Karn, Chief Executive Officer
**Web address:** www.kindreddelco.com/

KINDRED HOSPITAL–HERITAGE VALLEY (O, 35 beds) 1000 Dutch Ridge Road, Beaver, PA Zip 15009; tel. 724/773–8480; Rodney B. Jones, Administrator
**Web address:** www.kindredhospitalhv.com/

KINDRED HOSPITAL–PHILADELPHIA (O, 109 beds) 6129 Palmetto Street, Philadelphia, PA Zip 19111–5729; tel. 215/722–8555; Garrett Arneson, Interim Chief Executive Officer
**Web address:** www.kindredphila.com/

KINDRED HOSPITAL–PITTSBURGH (O, 63 beds) 7777 Steubenville Pike, Oakdale, PA Zip 15071–3409; tel. 412/494–5500; John T. Burton, Administrator
**Web address:** www.kindredhospitalpittsburgh.com/

KINDRED HOSPITAL–WYOMING VALLEY (O, 36 beds) 575 North River Street, 7th Floor, Wilkes Barre, PA Zip 18764–0999; tel. 570/552–7620; Sharon Yurkiewicz, Chief Executive Officer
**Web address:** www.kindredhospitalwv.com/

**SOUTH CAROLINA:** KINDRED HOSPITAL–CHARLESTON (O, 55 beds) 326 Calhoun Street, 3rd Floor, Charleston, SC Zip 29401; tel. 843/876–8670; Jennifer Sheets, R.N., Chief Executive Officer
**Web address:** www.khcharleston.com

**TENNESSEE:** KINDRED HOSPITAL–CHATTANOOGA (O, 44 beds) 709 Walnut Street, Chattanooga, TN Zip 37402–1916; tel. 423/266–7721; William J. Bryant, Chief Executive Officer
**Web address:** www.kindredchattanooga.com/

KINDRED HOSPITAL–NASHVILLE (O, 58 beds) 1412 County Hospital Road, Nashville, TN Zip 37218; tel. 615/687–2600; William P. Macri, Chief Executive Officer
**Web address:** www.khnashville.com/

**TEXAS:** CENTRAL TEXAS REHABILITATION HOSPITAL (O, 20 beds) 1201 West 38th Street, 8th Floor, Austin, TX Zip 78705–1006; tel. 512/406–6300; Peggy Barrett, R.N., Chief Executive Officer
**Web address:** www.khrehabcentraltexas.com/

KINDRED HOSPITAL DALLAS CENTRAL (O, 60 beds) 8050 Meadows Road, Dallas, TX Zip 75231; tel. 469/232–6500; Justin Smith, Interim Chief Executive Officer
**Web address:** www.khdallascentral.com/

KINDRED HOSPITAL EAST HOUSTON (O, 230 beds) 15101 East Freeway, Channelview, TX Zip 77530; tel. 832/200–5500; Angel Gradney, Chief Executive Officer
**Web address:** www.kheasthouston.com

KINDRED HOSPITAL EL PASO (O, 62 beds) 1740 Curie Drive, El Paso, TX Zip 79902; tel. 915/351–9044; Aleen D. Arabit, Chief Executive Officer
**Web address:** www.khelpaso.com

For explanation of codes following names, see page B2.
★ Indicates Type III membership in the American Hospital Association.

KINDRED HOSPITAL MIDTOWN (O, 40 beds) 105 Drew Avenue, Houston, TX Zip 77006; tel. 713/529–8922; James Poullard, Chief Executive Officer
**Web address:** www.khmidtown.com

KINDRED HOSPITAL NORTH HOUSTON (O, 288 beds) 7407 North Freeway, Houston, TX Zip 77076–1314; tel. 832/200–6000; Michael B. Davis, Chief Executive Officer
**Web address:** www.khnorthhouston.com

KINDRED HOSPITAL SUGAR LAND (O, 171 beds) 1550 First Colony Boulevard, Sugar Land, TX Zip 77479; tel. 281/275–6000; Lorene Perona, Chief Executive Officer
**Web address:** www.khsugarland.com

KINDRED HOSPITAL TARRANT COUNTY–ARLINGTON (O, 78 beds) 1000 North Cooper Street, Arlington, TX Zip 76011–5540; tel. 817/548–3400; Christina Richard, Administrator
**Web address:** www.kindredhospitalarl.com/

KINDRED HOSPITAL TARRANT COUNTY–FORT WORTH SOUTHWEST (O, 74 beds) 7800 Oakmont Boulevard, Fort Worth, TX Zip 76132–4299; tel. 817/346–0094; Anna Rojas, Chief Executive Officer
**Web address:** www.kindredhospitalfwsw.com/

KINDRED HOSPITAL VICTORIA (O, 23 beds) 506 East San Antonio Street, 3rd Floor, Victoria, TX Zip 77901–6060; tel. 361/575–1445; Tammy Barben, Chief Executive Officer
**Web address:** www.khvictoria.com

KINDRED HOSPITAL–AMARILLO (O, 72 beds) 7501 Wallace Boulevard, Amarillo, TX Zip 79124–2150; tel. 806/467–7000; Kay E. Peck, Ph.D., Chief Executive Officer
**Web address:** www.khamarillo.com/

KINDRED HOSPITAL–BAY AREA (O, 74 beds) 4801 East Sam Houston Parkway South, Pasadena, TX Zip 77505–3955; tel. 281/991–5463; Anne R. Leon, Administrator
**Web address:** www.khbayareahouston.com/

KINDRED HOSPITAL–CORPUS CHRISTI (O, 68 beds) 6226 Saratoga Boulevard, Corpus Christi, TX Zip 78414–3421; tel. 361/986–1600; Diana Schultz, Chief Executive Officer
**Web address:** www.khcorpuschristi.com/

KINDRED HOSPITAL–DALLAS (O, 100 beds) 9525 Greenville Avenue, Dallas, TX Zip 75243–4116; tel. 214/355–2600; Brenda Rowe, Chief Executive Officer
**Web address:** www.khdallas.com

KINDRED HOSPITAL–FORT WORTH (O, 67 beds) 815 Eighth Avenue, Fort Worth, TX Zip 76104; tel. 817/332–4812; Angela Harris, Chief Executive Officer
**Web address:** www.kindredfortworth.com/

KINDRED HOSPITAL–HOUSTON (O, 105 beds) 6441 Main Street, Houston, TX Zip 77030–1596; tel. 713/790–0500; Robert Stein, Chief Executive Officer
**Web address:** www.khhouston.com/

KINDRED HOSPITAL–HOUSTON NORTHWEST (O, 84 beds) 11297 Fallbrook Drive, Houston, TX Zip 77065–4292; tel. 281/897–8114; Mary Anne Craig, Chief Executive Officer
**Web address:** www.khhoustonnw.com/

KINDRED HOSPITAL–MANSFIELD (O, 55 beds) 1802 Highway 157 North, Mansfield, TX Zip 76063–9555; tel. 817/473–6101; Susan Schaetti, Administrator
**Web address:** www.kindredmansfield.com

KINDRED HOSPITAL–SAN ANTONIO (O, 59 beds) 3636 Medical Drive, San Antonio, TX Zip 78229–3184; tel. 210/616–0616; Katherine Eskew, Chief Executive Officer
**Web address:** www.khsanantonio.com/

KINDRED HOSPITAL–WHITE ROCK (O, 25 beds) 9440 Poppy Drive, 5th Floor, Dallas, TX Zip 75218; tel. 214/324–6562; Justin Smith, Administrator
**Web address:** www.khwhiterock.com/

KINDRED REHABILITATION HOSPITAL (O, 42 beds) 7200 West 9th Avenue, Amarillo, TX Zip 79106; tel. 806/468–2900; Kay E. Peck, Ph.D., Chief Executive Officer
**Web address:** www.khrehabamarillo.com/

KINDRED REHABILITATION HOSPITAL ARLINGTON (O, 24 beds) 2601 West Randol Mill Road, Arlington, TX Zip 76012; tel. 817/804–4400; Chetan Bhasin, Chief Executive Officer
**Web address:** www.khrehabarlington.com

KINDRED REHABILITATION HOSPITAL CLEAR LAKE (O, 60 beds) 655 East Medical Center Boulevard, Webster, TX Zip 77598–4328; tel. 281/286–1500; Dale R. Mulder, President and Chief Executive Officer
**Web address:** www.khrehabclearlake.com/

KINDRED REHABILITATION HOSPITAL NORTHEAST HOUSTON (O, 46 beds) 18839 McKay Road, Humble, TX Zip 77338; tel. 281/964–6600; Jeffrey Smith, Chief Executive Officer
**Web address:** www.khrehabnortheasthouston.com

**VIRGINIA:** KINDRED HOSPITAL RICHMOND (O, 60 beds) 2220 Edward Holland Drive, Richmond, VA Zip 23230–2519; tel. 804/678–7000; Greg Floyd, Chief Executive Officer
**Web address:** www.kindredrichmond.com/

**WASHINGTON:** KINDRED HOSPITAL SEATTLE–NORTHGATE (O, 42 beds) 10631 8th Avenue N.E., Seattle, WA Zip 98125–0716; tel. 206/364–2050; Lauren Suarez, Chief Executive Officer
**Web address:** www.kindredhospitalseattle.com/

**WISCONSIN:** KINDRED HOSPITAL–MILWAUKEE (O, 56 beds) 5017 South 110Th Street, Greenfield, WI Zip 53228–3131; tel. 414/427–8282; Linda Newberry-Ferguson, Chief Executive Officer
**Web address:** www.khmilwaukee.com/

| | | |
|---|---|---|
| Owned, leased, sponsored: | 97 hospitals | 7618 beds |
| Contract–managed: | 1 hospital | 95 beds |
| Totals: | 98 hospitals | 7713 beds |

**★0149: KISH HEALTH SYSTEM** (NP)
626 Bethany Road, De Kalb, IL Zip 60115–4939, Mailing Address: P.O. Box 707, DeKalb, Zip 60115–0707; tel. 815/756–1521; Kevin P. Poorten, President and Chief Executive Officer
**(Independent Hospital System)**

**ILLINOIS:** KISHWAUKEE COMMUNITY HOSPITAL (O, 94 beds) 1 Kish Hospital Drive, DeKalb, IL Zip 60115–9602, Mailing Address: P.O. Box 707, Zip 60115–0707; tel. 815/756–1521; Brad Copple, President
**Web address:** www.kishhospital.org

VALLEY WEST COMMUNITY HOSPITAL (O, 25 beds) 11 East Pleasant Avenue, Sandwich, IL Zip 60548–0901; tel. 815/786–8484; Brad Copple, President
**Web address:** www.vwch.org

| | | |
|---|---|---|
| Owned, leased, sponsored: | 2 hospitals | 119 beds |
| Contract–managed: | 0 hospitals | 0 beds |
| Totals: | 2 hospitals | 119 beds |

**0056: LAKELAND HEALTHCARE** (NP)
1234 Napier Avenue, Saint Joseph, MI Zip 49085–2158; tel. 269/983–8300; Loren Hamel, M.D., President and Chief Executive Officer
**(Centralized Health System)**

**MICHIGAN:** LAKELAND COMMUNITY HOSPITAL WATERVLIET (O, 38 beds) 400 Medical Park Drive, Watervliet, MI Zip 49098–9225; tel. 269/463–3111; Ray Cruse, Chief Executive Officer
**Web address:** www.communityhospitalwatervliet.com

LAKELAND REGIONAL MEDICAL CENTER–ST. JOSEPH (O, 250 beds) 1234 Napier Avenue, Saint Joseph, MI Zip 49085–2112; tel. 269/983–8300; Loren Hamel, M.D., President and Chief Executive Officer
**Web address:** www.lakelandhealth.org

LAKELAND SPECIALTY HOSPITAL–BERRIEN CENTER (O, 26 beds) 6418 Deans Hill Road, Berrien Center, MI Zip 49102–9750; tel. 269/473–3003; Loren Hamel, M.D., President and Chief Executive Officer
**Web address:** www.lakelandhealth.org

| | | |
|---|---|---|
| Owned, leased, sponsored: | 3 hospitals | 314 beds |
| Contract–managed: | 0 hospitals | 0 beds |
| Totals: | 3 hospitals | 314 beds |

**0393: LANDMARK HOSPITALS** (IO)
3255 Independence Street, Cape Girardeau, MO Zip 63701–4904; tel. 573/335–1091; William K. Kapp, III, M.D., President and Chief Executive Officer
**(Independent Hospital System)**

For explanation of codes following names, see page B2.
★ Indicates Type III membership in the American Hospital Association.

**GEORGIA:** LANDMARK HOSPITAL OF ATHENS (O, 42 beds) 775 Sunset Drive, Athens, GA Zip 30606–2211; tel. 706/425–1500; Tommy Jackson, Chief Executive Officer
**Web address:** www.landmarkhospitals.com

**MISSOURI:** LANDMARK HOSPITAL (O, 30 beds) 3255 Independence Street, Cape Girardeau, MO Zip 63701–4904; tel. 573/335–1091; Rodney Brown, Chief Executive Officer
**Web address:** www.landmarkhospitals.com

LANDMARK HOSPITAL OF COLUMBIA (O, 42 beds) 604 Old 63 North, Columbia, MO Zip 65201–6308; tel. 573/499–6600; Deborah Sabella, R.N., Chief Executive Officer
**Web address:** www.landmarkhospitals.com

LANDMARK HOSPITAL OF JOPLIN (O, 30 beds) 2040 West 32nd Street, Joplin, MO Zip 64804; tel. 417/627–1300; Dennis Nicely, Chief Executive Officer
**Web address:** www.landmarkhospitals.com

| Owned, leased, sponsored: | 4 hospitals | 144 beds |
| Contract–managed: | 0 hospitals | 0 beds |
| Totals: | 4 hospitals | 144 beds |

---

**0369: LEE MEMORIAL HEALTH SYSTEM** (NP)
2776 Cleveland Avenue, Fort Myers, FL Zip 33901, Mailing Address: P.O. Box 2218, Zip 33902–2218; tel. 239/343–2000; James R. Nathan, President and Chief Executive Officer
**(Centralized Health System)**

**FLORIDA:** CAPE CORAL HOSPITAL (O, 291 beds) 636 Del Prado Boulevard, Cape Coral, FL Zip 33990–2695; tel. 239/424–2000; James R. Nathan, President
**Web address:** www.leememorial.org

GULF COAST MEDICAL CENTER (O, 349 beds) 13681 Doctor's Way, Fort Myers, FL Zip 33912–4300; tel. 239/343–1000; James R. Nathan, President and Chief Executive Officer
**Web address:** www.leememorial.org

LEE MEMORIAL HOSPITAL (O, 835 beds) 2776 Cleveland Avenue, Fort Myers, FL Zip 33901–5855, Mailing Address: P.O. Box 2218, Zip 33902–2218; tel. 239/332–1111; James R. Nathan, President
**Web address:** www.leememorial.org

| Owned, leased, sponsored: | 3 hospitals | 1475 beds |
| Contract–managed: | 0 hospitals | 0 beds |
| Totals: | 3 hospitals | 1475 beds |

---

★**2755: LEGACY HEALTH** (NP)
1919 N.W. Lovejoy Street, Portland, OR Zip 97209–1503; tel. 503/415–5600; George J. Brown, M.D., President and Chief Executive Officer
**(Centralized Health System)**

**OREGON:** LEGACY EMANUEL HOSPITAL AND HEALTH CENTER (O, 406 beds) 2801 North Gantenbein Avenue, Portland, OR Zip 97227–1674; tel. 503/413–2200; Lori Morgan, M.D., Chief Administrative Officer
**Web address:** www.legacyhealth.org

LEGACY GOOD SAMARITAN HOSPITAL AND MEDICAL CENTER (O, 249 beds) 1015 N.W. 22nd Avenue, Portland, OR Zip 97210–3099; tel. 503/413–7711; Tony Melaragno, M.D., Chief Administrative Officer
**Web address:** www.legacyhealth.org

LEGACY MERIDIAN PARK HOSPITAL (O, 130 beds) 19300 S.W. 65th Avenue, Tualatin, OR Zip 97062–9741; tel. 503/692–1212; Allyson Anderson, Chief Administrative Officer
**Web address:** www.legacyhealth.org

LEGACY MOUNT HOOD MEDICAL CENTER (O, 90 beds) 24800 S.E. Stark, Gresham, OR Zip 97030–0154; tel. 503/667–1122; Gretchen Nichols, R.N., Chief Administrative Officer
**Web address:** www.legacyhealth.org

**WASHINGTON:** LEGACY SALMON CREEK MEDICAL CENTER (O, 194 beds) 2211 N.E. 139th Street, Vancouver, WA Zip 98686–2742; tel. 360/487–1000; Jonathan Avery, Chief Administrative Officer
**Web address:** www.legacyhealth.org

| Owned, leased, sponsored: | 5 hospitals | 1069 beds |
| Contract–managed: | 0 hospitals | 0 beds |
| Totals: | 5 hospitals | 1069 beds |

---

★**0370: LEHIGH VALLEY HEALTH NETWORK** (NP)
1200 South Cedar Crest Boulevard, Allentown, PA Zip 18103, Mailing Address: P.O. Box 689, Zip 18105–0689; tel. 610/402–8000; Ronald W. Swinfard, M.D., President and Chief Executive Officer
**(Centralized Health System)**

**PENNSYLVANIA:** LEHIGH VALLEY HOSPITAL (O, 783 beds) 1200 South Cedar Crest Boulevard, Allentown, PA Zip 18105–6248, Mailing Address: P.O. Box 689, Zip 18105–1556; tel. 610/402–8000; Ronald W. Swinfard, M.D., President and Chief Executive Officer
**Web address:** www.lvhhn.org

LEHIGH VALLEY HOSPITAL–MUHLENBERG (O, 168 beds) 2545 Schoenersville Road, Bethlehem, PA Zip 18017–7300; tel. 484/884–2201; Ronald W. Swinfard, M.D., President and Chief Executive Officer
**Web address:** www.lvhhn.org

| Owned, leased, sponsored: | 2 hospitals | 951 beds |
| Contract–managed: | 0 hospitals | 0 beds |
| Totals: | 2 hospitals | 951 beds |

---

**0632: LHC GROUP** (IO)
420 West Pinhook Road, Lafayette, LA Zip 70503–2131; tel. 337/223–1307; Keith G. Myers, Chairman and Chief Executive Officer

**LOUISIANA:** LOUISIANA EXTENDED CARE HOSPITAL OF LAFAYETTE (O, 42 beds) 1214 Coolidge Boulevard, 8th Floor, Lafayette, LA Zip 70503–2621; tel. 337/289–8180; Kevin Frank, Administrator
**Web address:** www.lhcgroup.com

LOUISIANA EXTENDED CARE HOSPITAL OF NATCHITOCHES (O, 21 beds) 501 Keyser Avenue, Natchitoches, LA Zip 71457; tel. 318/354–2044; Kermit Simmons, Administrator
**Web address:** www.lhcgroup.com

LOUISIANA EXTENDED CARE HOSPITAL WEST MONROE (O, 18 beds) 503 McMillan Road, 3rd Floor, West Monroe, LA Zip 71291; tel. 318/329–4300; Cleta Munholland, Administrator

OCHSNER EXTENDED CARE HOSPITAL OF KENNER (O, 34 beds) 180 West Esplanade Avenue, 5th Floor, Kenner, LA Zip 70065–2467; tel. 504/464–8590; Fritz Nelson, Administrator
**Web address:** www.lhcgroup.com/

| Owned, leased, sponsored: | 4 hospitals | 115 beds |
| Contract–managed: | 0 hospitals | 0 beds |
| Totals: | 4 hospitals | 115 beds |

---

★**0394: LHP HOSPITAL GROUP** (IO)
2800 North Dallas Parkway, Suite 200, Plano, TX Zip 75093–5994; tel. 866/465–9222; Daniel J. Moen, Chief Executive Officer
**(Independent Hospital System)**

**FLORIDA:** BAY MEDICAL CENTER (L, 273 beds) 615 North Bonita Avenue, Panama City, FL Zip 32401–3600, Mailing Address: P.O. Box 59515, Zip 32412–0515; tel. 850/769–1511; Steven M. Johnson, President and Chief Executive Officer
**Web address:** www.baymedical.org

**IDAHO:** PORTNEUF MEDICAL CENTER (O, 174 beds) 777 Hospital Way, Pocatello, ID Zip 83201–4004; tel. 208/239–1000; Norman F. Stephens, President and Chief Executive Officer
**Web address:** www.portmed.org

---

For explanation of codes following names, see page B2.
★ Indicates Type III membership in the American Hospital Association.

Section B

**TEXAS:** TEXAS HEALTH PRESBYTERIAN HOSPITAL–WNJ (O, 215 beds) 500 North Highland Avenue, Sherman, TX Zip 75092–7354; tel. 903/870–4611; Vance V. Reynolds, FACHE, CPA, Chief Executive Officer
**Web address:** www.wnj.org

| Owned, leased, sponsored: | 3 hospitals | 662 beds |
|---|---|---|
| Contract–managed: | 0 hospitals | 0 beds |
| Totals: | 3 hospitals | 662 beds |

★**0158:  LIFEBRIDGE HEALTH** (NP)
2401 West Belvedere Avenue, Baltimore, MD Zip 21215; tel. 410/601–5134; Warren A. Green, President and Chief Executive Officer
**(Centralized Health System)**

**MARYLAND:** LEVINDALE HEBREW GERIATRIC CENTER AND HOSPITAL (O, 443 beds) 2434 West Belvedere Avenue, Baltimore, MD Zip 21215–5299; tel. 410/466–8700; Aric Spitulnik, President and Chief Operating Officer
**Web address:** www.sinai-balt.com

NORTHWEST HOSPITAL (O, 230 beds) 5401 Old Court Road, Randallstown, MD Zip 21133–5185; tel. 410/521–2200; Brian M. White, President and Chief Operating Officer
**Web address:** www.lifebridgehealth.org

SINAI HOSPITAL OF BALTIMORE (O, 456 beds) 2401 West Belvedere Avenue, Baltimore, MD Zip 21215–5271; tel. 410/601–9000; Neil M. Meltzer, President and Chief Operating Officer
**Web address:** www.lifebridgehealth.org

| Owned, leased, sponsored: | 3 hospitals | 1129 beds |
|---|---|---|
| Contract–managed: | 0 hospitals | 0 beds |
| Totals: | 3 hospitals | 1129 beds |

★**0191:  LIFECARE MANAGEMENT SERVICES** (IO)
5340 Legacy Drive, Suite 150, Plano, TX Zip 75024; tel. 469/241–2100; Phillip B. Douglas, Chairman and Chief Executive Officer
**(Independent Hospital System)**

**COLORADO:** COLORADO ACUTE LONG TERM HOSPITAL (O, 63 beds) 1690 Meade Street, Denver, CO Zip 80204; tel. 303/264–6900; Terry W. Kepler, Administrator
**Web address:** www.lifecare–hospitals.com

**FLORIDA:** COMPLEX CARE HOSPITAL AT RIDGELAKE (O, 40 beds) 6150 Edgelake Drive, Sarasota, FL Zip 34240–8803; tel. 941/342–3000; Danny R. Edwards, Administrator
**Web address:** www.lifecare–hospitals.com/hospital.php?id=23

**IDAHO:** COMPLEX CARE HOSPITAL OF IDAHO (O, 60 beds) 2131 South Bonito Way, Meridian, ID Zip 83642–1659; tel. 877/801–2244; Colin O'Sullivan, Administrator
**Web address:** www.lifecare–hospitals.com

**LOUISIANA:** LIFECARE HOSPITALS OF SHREVEPORT (O, 119 beds) 9320 Linwood Avenue, Shreveport, LA Zip 71106–7003; tel. 318/688–8504; Keith Cox, Administrator
**Web address:** www.lifecare–hospitals.com

LIFECARE SPECIALTY HOSPITAL OF NORTH LOUISIANA (O, 90 beds) 1401 Ezell Street, Ruston, LA Zip 71270–7221; tel. 318/251–3126; Brent Martin, Chief Executive Officer
**Web address:** www.lifecare–hospitals.com/hospital.php?id=19

**NEVADA:** COMPLEX CARE HOSPITAL AT TENAYA (O, 70 beds) 2500 North Tenaya, Las Vegas, NV Zip 89128; tel. 702/562–2021; Timothy C. Deaton, Administrator
**Web address:** www.lifecare–hospitals.com

TAHOE PACIFIC HOSPITALS (O, 60 beds) 201 West Liberty Street, Suite 310, Reno, NV Zip 89501; tel. 775/355–5970; Colin O'Sullivan, Administrator
**Web address:** www.lifecare–hospitals.com

**NORTH CAROLINA:** LIFECARE HOSPITALS OF NORTH CAROLINA (O, 40 beds) 1051 Noell Lane, Rocky Mount, NC Zip 27804–1761; tel. 252/451–2300; Kevin S. Cooper, R.N., Administrator
**Web address:** www.lifecare–hospitals.com

**OHIO:** LIFECARE HOSPITAL OF DAYTON (O, 44 beds) 4000 Miamisburg–Centerville Road, Miamisburg, OH Zip 45342; tel. 937/384–8300; Russell Dean, Chief Executive Officer
**Web address:** www.lifecare–hospitals.com

**PENNSYLVANIA:** LIFECARE HOSPITALS OF CHESTER COUNTY (O, 39 beds) 400 East Marshall Street, West Chester, PA Zip 19380; tel. 484/826–0400; Rosalie Cox, Administrator
**Web address:** www.lifecare–hospitals.com

LIFECARE HOSPITALS OF MECHANICSBURG (O, 68 beds) 4950 Wilson Lane, Mechanicsburg, PA Zip 17055; tel. 717/697–7706; Nicholas Mezza, Chief Executive Officer
**Web address:** www.lifecare–hospitals.com/hospital.php?id=20

LIFECARE HOSPITALS OF PITTSBURGH (O, 236 beds) 225 Penn Avenue, Pittsburgh, PA Zip 15221–2148; tel. 412/247–2424; Richard Pletz, Administrator
**Web address:** www.lifecare–hospitals.com

LIFECARE HOSPITALS OF PITTSBURGH – MONROEVILLE (O, 87 beds) 2380 McGinley Road, Monroeville, PA Zip 15146–4400; tel. 412/856–2400; Richard Pletz, Administrator
**Web address:** www.lifecare–hospitals.com/hospital.php?id=8

**TEXAS:** LIFECARE HOSPITALS OF DALLAS (O, 60 beds) 6161 Harry Hines Boulevard, Suite 100, Dallas, TX Zip 75235–5369; tel. 214/525–6300; Jay Lindsey, Chief Executive Officer
**Web address:** www.lifecare–hospitals.com

LIFECARE HOSPITALS OF SAN ANTONIO (O, 62 beds) 8026 Floyd Curl Drive, San Antonio, TX Zip 78229–3915; tel. 210/690–7000; Randell G. Stokes, Administrator
**Web address:** www.lifecare–hospitals.com

LIFECARE HOSPITALS OF SOUTH TEXAS–NORTH MCALLEN (O, 94 beds) 5101 North Jackson, McAllen, TX Zip 78504; tel. 956/926–7000; Michelle Lozano, Adminstrator
**Web address:** www.lifecare–hospitals.com

**WISCONSIN:** LIFECARE HOSPITALS OF WISCONSIN (O, 35 beds) 2400 Golf Road, Pewaukee, WI Zip 53072; tel. 262/524–2600; Jevne Conover, Administrator
**Web address:** www.lifecare–hospitals.com

| Owned, leased, sponsored: | 17 hospitals | 1267 beds |
|---|---|---|
| Contract–managed: | 0 hospitals | 0 beds |
| Totals: | 17 hospitals | 1267 beds |

★**0180:  LIFEPOINT HOSPITALS, INC.** (IO)
103 Powell Court, Suite 200, Brentwood, TN Zip 37027; tel. 615/372–8500; William F. Carpenter, III, Chairman and Chief Executive Officer
**(Moderately Centralized Health System)**

**ALABAMA:** ANDALUSIA REGIONAL HOSPITAL (O, 87 beds) 849 South Three Notch Street, Andalusia, AL Zip 36420–5325, Mailing Address: P.O. Box 760, Zip 36420–0760; tel. 334/222–8466; Mark J. Dooley, Chief Executive Officer
**Web address:** www.andalusiaregionalhospital.com

LAKELAND COMMUNITY HOSPITAL (O, 42 beds) Highway 195 East, Haleyville, AL Zip 35565–9536, Mailing Address: P.O. Box 780, Zip 35565–0780; tel. 205/486–5213; James P. Jeansonne, Chief Executive Officer
**Web address:** www.lifepointhospitals.com

NORTHWEST MEDICAL CENTER (O, 76 beds) 1530 U.S. Highway 43, Winfield, AL Zip 35594–5056; tel. 205/487–7000; Chuck Spann, Chief Executive Officer
**Web address:** www.northwestmedcenter.com

RUSSELLVILLE HOSPITAL (O, 92 beds) 15155 Highway 43, Russellville, AL Zip 35653–1975, Mailing Address: P.O. Box 1089, Zip 35653–1089; tel. 256/332–1611; Christine R. Stewart, FACHE, Chief Executive Officer
**Web address:** www.russellvillehospital.com

VAUGHAN REGIONAL MEDICAL CENTER (O, 149 beds) 1015 Medical Center Parkway, Selma, AL Zip 36701–6352; tel. 334/418–4100; David R. Sirk, Chief Executive Officer
**Web address:** www.vaughanregional.com

For explanation of codes following names, see page B2.
★ Indicates Type III membership in the American Hospital Association.

Section B

**ARIZONA:** HAVASU REGIONAL MEDICAL CENTER (O, 138 beds) 101 Civic Center Lane, Lake Havasu City, AZ Zip 86403–5683; tel. 928/855–8185; Sandra C. Podley, Chief Executive Officer
**Web address:** www.havasuregional.com

VALLEY VIEW MEDICAL CENTER (O, 66 beds) 5330 South Highway 95, Fort Mohave, AZ Zip 86426; tel. 928/788–2273; Richard G. Carter, Chief Executive Officer
**Web address:** www.valleyviewmedicalcenter.net

**COLORADO:** COLORADO PLAINS MEDICAL CENTER (L, 50 beds) 1000 Lincoln Street, Fort Morgan, CO Zip 80701–3298; tel. 970/867–3391; Michael N. Patterson, Chief Executive Officer
**Web address:** www.coloradoplainsmedicalcenter.com

**FLORIDA:** PUTNAM COMMUNITY MEDICAL CENTER (O, 99 beds) Highway 20 West, Palatka, FL Zip 32177–8118, Mailing Address: P.O. Box 778, Zip 32178–0778; tel. 386/328–5711; Jerry Christine, Chief Executive Officer
**Web address:** www.pcmcfl.com

**GEORGIA:** ROCKDALE MEDICAL CENTER (O, 146 beds) 1412 Milstead Avenue N.E., Conyers, GA Zip 30012; tel. 770/918–3000; Deborah Armstrong, Chief Executive Officer
**Web address:** www.rockdalemedicalcenter.org

**KANSAS:** WESTERN PLAINS MEDICAL COMPLEX (O, 89 beds) 3001 Avenue A, Dodge City, KS Zip 67801–6508, Mailing Address: P.O. Box 1478, Zip 67801–1478; tel. 620/225–8400; Michael R. Burroughs, FACHE, Chief Executive Officer
**Web address:** www.westernplainsmc.com

**KENTUCKY:** BLUEGRASS COMMUNITY HOSPITAL (O, 25 beds) 360 Amsden Avenue, Versailles, KY Zip 40383–1286; tel. 859/873–3111; Tommy Haggard, Chief Executive Officer
**Web address:** www.bluegrasscommunityhospital.com

BOURBON COMMUNITY HOSPITAL (O, 58 beds) 9 Linville Drive, Paris, KY Zip 40361–2196; tel. 859/987–3600; Joseph G. Koch, Chief Executive Officer
**Web address:** www.bourbonhospital.com

CLARK REGIONAL MEDICAL CENTER (O, 100 beds) 175 Hospital Drive, Winchester, KY Zip 40391–9591; tel. 859/745–3500; Katherine S. Love, Chief Executive Officer
**Web address:** www.clarkregional.org

GEORGETOWN COMMUNITY HOSPITAL (O, 58 beds) 1140 Lexington Road, Georgetown, KY Zip 40324–9362; tel. 502/868–1100; Jerry C. Dooley, Chief Executive Officer
**Web address:** www.georgetowncommunityhospital.com

JACKSON PURCHASE MEDICAL CENTER (O, 106 beds) 1099 Medical Center Circle, Mayfield, KY Zip 42066–1179; tel. 270/251–4100; Fred L. Pelle, FACHE, Chief Executive Officer
**Web address:** www.jacksonpurchase.com

LAKE CUMBERLAND REGIONAL HOSPITAL (O, 295 beds) 305 Langdon Street, Somerset, KY Zip 42501–2750, Mailing Address: P.O. Box 620, Zip 42502–2750; tel. 606/679–7441; Mark T. Brenzel, Chief Executive Officer
**Web address:** www.lakecumberlandhospital.com

LOGAN MEMORIAL HOSPITAL (O, 52 beds) 1625 South Nashville Road, Russellville, KY Zip 42276–8834, Mailing Address: P.O. Box 10, Zip 42276–0010; tel. 270/726–4011; William Haugh, Chief Executive Officer
**Web address:** www.loganmemorial.com

MEADOWVIEW REGIONAL MEDICAL CENTER (O, 101 beds) 989 Medical Park Drive, Maysville, KY Zip 41056–8750; tel. 606/759–5311; Robert Parker, Chief Executive Officer
**Web address:** www.meadowviewregional.com

SPRING VIEW HOSPITAL (O, 60 beds) 320 Loretto Road, Lebanon, KY Zip 40033–1300; tel. 270/692–3161; Ruth A. McDaniel, Chief Executive Officer
**Web address:** www.springviewhospital.com

**LOUISIANA:** MERCY REGIONAL MEDICAL CENTER (O, 70 beds) 800 East Main Street, Ville Platte, LA Zip 70586, Mailing Address: P.O. Box 349, Zip 70586–0349; tel. 337/363–5684; Robert Alan Daugherty, Chief Executive Officer
**Web address:** www.mercyregionalmedicalcenter.com

MINDEN MEDICAL CENTER (O, 161 beds) 1 Medical Plaza, Minden, LA Zip 71055–3330, Mailing Address: P.O. Box 5003, Zip 71058–5003; tel. 318/377–2321; George E. French, III, FACHE, Chief Executive Officer
**Web address:** www.mindenmedicalcenter.com

RIVER PARISHES HOSPITAL (O, 106 beds) 500 Rue De Sante, La Place, LA Zip 70068–5418; tel. 985/652–7000; Gerald A. Fornoff, Interim Chief Executive Officer
**Web address:** www.riverparisheshospital.com

TECHE REGIONAL MEDICAL CENTER (L, 165 beds) 1125 Marguerite Street, Morgan City, LA Zip 70380–1855, Mailing Address: P.O. Box 2308, Zip 70381–2308; tel. 985/384–2200; James P. Frazier, III, Chief Executive Officer
**Web address:** www.techeregional.com

**MISSISSIPPI:** BOLIVAR MEDICAL CENTER (L, 127 beds) 901 East Sunflower Road, Cleveland, MS Zip 38732–9722, Mailing Address: P.O. Box 1380, Zip 38732–1380; tel. 662/846–0061; Scott M. Smith, Chief Executive Officer
**Web address:** www.bolivarmedical.com

**NEVADA:** NORTHEASTERN NEVADA REGIONAL HOSPITAL (O, 50 beds) 2001 Errecart Boulevard, Elko, NV Zip 89801–3499; tel. 775/738–5151; Gene Miller, Chief Executive Officer
**Web address:** www.nnrhospital.com

**NEW MEXICO:** LOS ALAMOS MEDICAL CENTER (O, 38 beds) 3917 West Road, Los Alamos, NM Zip 87544–2293; tel. 505/661–9500; Feliciano Jiron, Chief Executive Officer
**Web address:** www.losalamosmedicalcenter.com

MEMORIAL MEDICAL CENTER (L, 224 beds) 2450 South Telshor Boulevard, Las Cruces, NM Zip 88011–5076; tel. 575/522–8641; Paul F. Herzog, Chief Executive Officer
**Web address:** www.mmclc.org

**TENNESSEE:** ATHENS REGIONAL MEDICAL CENTER (O, 63 beds) 1114 West Madison Avenue, Athens, TN Zip 37303–4150, Mailing Address: P.O. Box 250, Zip 37371–0250; tel. 423/745–1411; John R. Workman, Chief Executive Officer
**Web address:** www.athensrmc.com

CROCKETT HOSPITAL (O, 90 beds) 1607 South Locust Avenue, Lawrenceburg, TN Zip 38464–4011, Mailing Address: P.O. Box 847, Zip 38464–0847; tel. 931/762–6571; Jeff Noblin, FACHE, Chief Executive Officer
**Web address:** www.crocketthospital.com

HILLSIDE HOSPITAL (O, 50 beds) 1265 East College Street, Pulaski, TN Zip 38478–4500; tel. 931/363–7531; Roxana J. Pool, R.N., M.P.H., Chief Executive Officer
**Web address:** www.hillsidehospital.com

LIVINGSTON REGIONAL HOSPITAL (O, 82 beds) 315 Oak Street, Livingston, TN Zip 38570, Mailing Address: P.O. Box 550, Zip 38570–0550; tel. 931/823–5611; Michael J. Meadows, Chief Executive Officer
**Web address:** www.livingstonhospital.com

RIVERVIEW REGIONAL MEDICAL CENTER NORTH (O, 63 beds) 158 Hospital Drive, Carthage, TN Zip 37030–1096; tel. 615/735–1560; Jimmy D. Stuart, Administrator
**Web address:** www.myriverviewmedical.com/

RIVERVIEW REGIONAL MEDICAL CENTER SOUTH (O, 25 beds) 130 Lebanon Highway, Carthage, TN Zip 37030–2955; tel. 615/735–9815; Jimmy D. Stuart, Administrator
**Web address:** www.myriverviewmedical.com

SOUTHERN TENNESSEE MEDICAL CENTER (O, 153 beds) 185 Hospital Road, Winchester, TN Zip 37398–2404; tel. 931/967–8200; J. Phillip Young, FACHE, Chief Executive Officer
**Web address:** www.southerntennessee.com

SUMNER REGIONAL MEDICAL CENTER (O, 145 beds) 555 Hartsville Pike, Gallatin, TN Zip 37066–2449, Mailing Address: P.O. Box 1558, Zip 37066–1558; tel. 615/452–4210; Mary Jo Lewis, FACHE, President and Chief Executive Officer
**Web address:** www.sumner.org

TROUSDALE MEDICAL CENTER (O, 25 beds) 500 Church Street, Hartsville, TN Zip 37074–1744; tel. 615/374–2221; William D. Mize, Interim Chief Executive Officer
**Web address:** www.trousdale.org

For explanation of codes following names, see page B2.
★ Indicates Type III membership in the American Hospital Association.

Section B

WOODS MEMORIAL HOSPITAL (O, 30 beds) 886 Highway 411 North, Etowah, TN Zip 37331–1912; tel. 423/263–3600; John R. Workman, Chief Executive Officer
**Web address:** www.woodshospital.org

**TEXAS:** ENNIS REGIONAL MEDICAL CENTER (L, 58 beds) 2201 West Lampasas Street, Ennis, TX Zip 75119–5644; tel. 972/875–0900; David Anderson, Chief Executive Officer
**Web address:** www.ennisregional.com

PALESTINE REGIONAL MEDICAL CENTER–EAST (O, 113 beds) 2900 South Loop 256, Palestine, TX Zip 75801–6958; tel. 903/731–1000; Alan E. George, Chief Executive Officer
**Web address:** www.palestineregional.com

PALESTINE REGIONAL REHABILITATION CENTER (O, 12 beds) 4000 South Loop 256, Palestine, TX Zip 75801–8467, Mailing Address: P.O. Box 4070, Zip 75802–4070; tel. 903/731–5100; Ronald Safford, Administrator
**Web address:** www.palestineregional.com

PARKVIEW REGIONAL HOSPITAL (L, 58 beds) 600 South Bonham, Mexia, TX Zip 76667–3608; tel. 254/562–0408; Kevin Zachary, Chief Executive Officer
**Web address:** www.parkviewregional.com

**UTAH:** ASHLEY REGIONAL MEDICAL CENTER (O, 39 beds) 150 West 100 North, Vernal, UT Zip 84078–2036; tel. 435/789–3342; Si Hutt, Chief Executive Officer
**Web address:** www.ashleyregional.com

CASTLEVIEW HOSPITAL (O, 57 beds) 300 North Hospital Drive, Price, UT Zip 84501–4200; tel. 435/637–4800; Mark Holyoak, Chief Executive Officer
**Web address:** www.castleviewhospital.net

**VIRGINIA:** CLINCH VALLEY MEDICAL CENTER (O, 111 beds) 6801 Governor G. C. Peery Highway, Richlands, VA Zip 24641–2194; tel. 276/596–6000; David B. Darden, Chief Executive Officer
**Web address:** www.clinchvalleymedicalcenter.com

DANVILLE REGIONAL MEDICAL CENTER (O, 151 beds) 142 South Main Street, Danville, VA Zip 24541–2922; tel. 434/799–2100; Eric Deaton, Chief Executive Officer
**Web address:** www.danvilleregional.org

MEMORIAL HOSPITAL (O, 220 beds) 320 Hospital Drive, Martinsville, VA Zip 24112–1981, Mailing Address: P.O. Box 4788, Zip 24115–4788; tel. 276/666–7200; Grady W. Philips, III, Chief Executive Officer
**Web address:** www.martinsvillehospital.com

WYTHE COUNTY COMMUNITY HOSPITAL (L, 90 beds) 600 West Ridge Road, Wytheville, VA Zip 24382–1099; tel. 276/228–0200; Timothy A. Bess, Chief Executive Officer
**Web address:** www.wcchcares.com

**WEST VIRGINIA:** LOGAN REGIONAL MEDICAL CENTER (O, 129 beds) 20 Hospital Drive, Logan, WV Zip 25601–3473; tel. 304/831–1101; John E. Walker, FACHE, Chief Executive Officer
**Web address:** www.loganregionalmedicalcenter.com

RALEIGH GENERAL HOSPITAL (O, 229 beds) 1710 Harper Road, Beckley, WV Zip 25801–3397; tel. 304/256–4100; Allen Peters, President and Chief Executive Officer
**Web address:** www.raleighgeneral.com

**WYOMING:** LANDER REGIONAL HOSPITAL (O, 89 beds) 1320 Bishop Randall Drive, Lander, WY Zip 82520–3996; tel. 307/332–4420; Ben Quinton, Chief Executive Officer
**Web address:** www.landerhospital.com

RIVERTON MEMORIAL HOSPITAL (O, 49 beds) 2100 West Sunset Drive, Riverton, WY Zip 82501–2274; tel. 307/856–4161; James Christian Smolik, Chief Executive Officer
**Web address:** www.riverton–hospital.com

| Owned, leased, sponsored: | 52 hospitals | 4961 beds |
|---|---|---|
| Contract–managed: | 0 hospitals | 0 beds |
| **Totals:** | 52 hospitals | 4961 beds |

---

**0060:  LIFESPAN CORPORATION** (NP)
167 Point Street, Providence, RI Zip 02903–4771;
tel. 401/444–3500
**(Moderately Centralized Health System)**

**RHODE ISLAND:** EMMA PENDLETON BRADLEY HOSPITAL (O, 51 beds) 1011 Veterans Memorial Parkway, East Providence, RI Zip 02915–5099; tel. 401/432–1000; Daniel J. Wall, President and Chief Executive Officer
**Web address:** www.lifespan.org

MIRIAM HOSPITAL (O, 247 beds) 164 Summit Avenue, Providence, RI Zip 02906–2895; tel. 401/793–2500; Arthur J. Sampson, FACHE, Executive Director
**Web address:** www.lifespan.org

NEWPORT HOSPITAL (O, 119 beds) 11 Friendship Street, Newport, RI Zip 02840–2299; tel. 401/846–6400; August B. Cordeiro, FACHE, President and Chief Executive Officer
**Web address:** www.newporthospital.org

RHODE ISLAND HOSPITAL (O, 672 beds) 593 Eddy Street, Providence, RI Zip 02903–4900; tel. 401/444–4000; Timothy J. Babineau, M.D., President and Chief Executive Officer
**Web address:** www.lifespan.org

| Owned, leased, sponsored: | 4 hospitals | 1089 beds |
|---|---|---|
| Contract–managed: | 0 hospitals | 0 beds |
| **Totals:** | 4 hospitals | 1089 beds |

---

**2175:  LOMA LINDA UNIVERSITY ADVENTIST HEALTH SCIENCES CENTER** (NP)
11175 Campus Street, Loma Linda, CA Zip 92354;
tel. 909/558–7572; Richard H. Hart, M.D., President and Chief Executive Officer
**(Moderately Centralized Health System)**

**CALIFORNIA:** LOMA LINDA UNIVERSITY BEHAVIORAL MEDICINE CENTER (O, 89 beds) 1710 Barton Road, Redlands, CA Zip 92373–5304; tel. 909/558–9200; Ruthita J. Fike, Chief Executive Officer
**Web address:** www.llu.edu

LOMA LINDA UNIVERSITY MEDICAL CENTER (O, 815 beds) 11234 Anderson Street, Loma Linda, CA Zip 92354–2870, Mailing Address: P.O. Box 2000, Zip 92354–0200; tel. 909/558–4000; Ruthita J. Fike, Chief Executive Officer
**Web address:** www.llumc.edu

LOMA LINDA UNIVERSITY MEDICAL CENTER–MURRIETA (O, 106 beds) 28062 Baxter Road, Murrieta, CA Zip 92563; tel. 951/290–4000; Richard L. Rawson, Chief Executive Officer
**Web address:** www.llumcmurrieta.org

| Owned, leased, sponsored: | 3 hospitals | 1010 beds |
|---|---|---|
| Contract–managed: | 0 hospitals | 0 beds |
| **Totals:** | 3 hospitals | 1010 beds |

---

**5755:  LOS ANGELES COUNTY–DEPARTMENT OF HEALTH SERVICES** (NP)
313 North Figueroa Street, Room 912, Los Angeles, CA Zip 90012–2691; tel. 213/240–8101; Mitchell H. Katz, M.D., Director
**(Independent Hospital System)**

LAC–HARBOR–UNIVERSITY OF CALIFORNIA AT LOS ANGELES MEDICAL CENTER (O, 350 beds) 1000 West Carson Street, Torrance, CA Zip 90502–2004; tel. 310/222–2345; Delvecchio Finley, Chief Executive Officer
**Web address:** www.humc.edu

LAC–OLIVE VIEW–UCLA MEDICAL CENTER (O, 238 beds) 14445 Olive View Drive, Sylmar, CA Zip 91342–1495; tel. 818/364–1555; Carolyn F. Rhee, Chief Executive Officer
**Web address:** www.ladhs.org

LAC/UNIVERSITY OF SOUTHERN CALIFORNIA MEDICAL CENTER (O, 633 beds) 1200 North State Street, Los Angeles, CA Zip 90033–1029; tel. 323/226–2622; Pete Delgado, Chief Executive Officer
**Web address:** www.lacusc.org

RANCHO LOS AMIGOS NATIONAL REHABILITATION CENTER (O, 207 beds) 7601 East Imperial Highway, Downey, CA Zip 90242–3496; tel. 562/401–7022; Jorge Orozco, Chief Executive Officer
**Web address:** www.rancho.org

For explanation of codes following names, see page B2.
★ Indicates Type III membership in the American Hospital Association.

| Owned, leased, sponsored: | 4 hospitals | 1428 beds |
|---|---|---|
| Contract–managed: | 0 hospitals | 0 beds |
| Totals: | 4 hospitals | 1428 beds |

## 0047: LOUISIANA STATE HOSPITALS (NP)
628 North 4th Street, Baton Rouge, LA Zip 70802–5342, Mailing Address: P.O. Box 629, Zip 70821–0628; tel. 225/342–9500; Shelby Price, Chief Executive Officer
**(Independent Hospital System)**

**LOUISIANA:** CENTRAL LOUISIANA STATE HOSPITAL (O, 128 beds) 242 West Shamrock Avenue, Pineville, LA Zip 71360, Mailing Address: P.O. Box 5031, Zip 71361–5031; tel. 318/484–6200; Wayne Hallford, Chief Executive Officer
**Web address:** www.dhh.la.gov/omh/inpatient–serv/clsh.htm

EASTERN LOUISIANA MENTAL HEALTH SYSTEM (O, 593 beds) 4502 Highway 951, Jackson, LA Zip 70748–5842, Mailing Address: P.O. Box 498, Zip 70748–0498; tel. 225/634–0100; Patricia Gonzales, Chief Executive Officer
**Web address:** www.dhh.louisiana.gov/offices/locations.asp?ID=62&Detail=126

SOUTHEAST LOUISIANA HOSPITAL (O, 153 beds) 23515 Highway 190, Mandeville, LA Zip 70448–5612, Mailing Address: P.O. Box 3850, Zip 70470–3850; tel. 985/626–6300; Richard Kramer, Interim Chief Executive Officer
**Web address:** www.selh.org

| Owned, leased, sponsored: | 3 hospitals | 874 beds |
|---|---|---|
| Contract–managed: | 0 hospitals | 0 beds |
| Totals: | 3 hospitals | 874 beds |

## ★0320: LRGHEALTHCARE (NP)
80 Highland Street, Laconia, NH Zip 03246–3298; tel. 603/524–3211; Thomas Clairmont, President
**(Independent Hospital System)**

**NEW HAMPSHIRE:** FRANKLIN REGIONAL HOSPITAL (O, 25 beds) 15 Aiken Avenue, Franklin, NH Zip 03235–1299; tel. 603/934–2060; Thomas Clairmont, President
**Web address:** www.lrgh.org

LAKES REGION GENERAL HOSPITAL (O, 104 beds) 80 Highland Street, Laconia, NH Zip 03246–3298; tel. 603/524–3211; Thomas Clairmont, President
**Web address:** www.lrgh.org

| Owned, leased, sponsored: | 2 hospitals | 129 beds |
|---|---|---|
| Contract–managed: | 0 hospitals | 0 beds |
| Totals: | 2 hospitals | 129 beds |

## 0715: LSU HEALTH CARE SERVICES DIVISION (NP)
Kirby Smith Hall, 1st Floor, MR, Room 151, Baton Rouge, LA Zip 70803, Mailing Address: P.O. Box 91308, Zip 70821–1308; tel. 225/922–0488; Roxane A. Townsend, M.D., Chief Executive Officer
**(Moderately Centralized Health System)**

**LOUISIANA:** EARL K. LONG MEDICAL CENTER (O, 103 beds) 5825 Airline Highway, Baton Rouge, LA Zip 70805–2498; tel. 225/358–1000; Roxane A. Townsend, M.D., Chief Executive Officer
**Web address:** www.lsuhsc.edu

INTERIM LSU PUBLIC HOSPITAL (O, 255 beds) 2021 Perdido Street, New Orleans, LA Zip 70112–1396; tel. 504/903–3000; Roxane A. Townsend, M.D., Chief Executive Officer
**Web address:** www.lsuhospitals.org/hospitals/mclno/mclno–directory.htm

LALLIE KEMP MEDICAL CENTER (O, 25 beds) 52579 Highway 51 South, Independence, LA Zip 70443–2231; tel. 985/878–9421; Sherre Pack–Hookfin, Administrator
**Web address:** www.lsuhospitals.org

LEONARD J. CHABERT MEDICAL CENTER (O, 87 beds) 1978 Industrial Boulevard, Houma, LA Zip 70363–7094; tel. 985/873–2200; Rhonda G. Green, Administrator
**Web address:** www.lsuhsc.edu/hcsd/ljc

LSU BOGALUSA MEDICAL CENTER (O, 74 beds) 433 Plaza Street, Bogalusa, LA Zip 70427–3793; tel. 985/730–6700; Kurt M. Scott, FACHE, Administrator
**Web address:** www.lsuhospitals.org

UNIVERSITY MEDICAL CENTER (O, 100 beds) 2390 West Congress Street, Lafayette, LA Zip 70506–4298, Mailing Address: P.O. Box 69300, Zip 70596–9300; tel. 337/261–6001; Lawrence T. Dorsey, Administrator
**Web address:** www.lsuhospitals.org

WALTER OLIN MOSS REGIONAL MEDICAL CENTER (O, 36 beds) 1000 Walters Street, Lake Charles, LA Zip 70607–4647; tel. 337/475–8100; Jimmy Pottorff, Interim Administrator
**Web address:** www.lsuhospitals.org/Hospitals/WOM/WOM.htm

| Owned, leased, sponsored: | 7 hospitals | 680 beds |
|---|---|---|
| Contract–managed: | 0 hospitals | 0 beds |
| Totals: | 7 hospitals | 680 beds |

## ★0340: MAIN LINE HEALTH (NP)
130 South Bryn Mawr Avenue, Bryn Mawr, PA Zip 19010; tel. 484/337–3000; John J. Lynch, III, FACHE, President and Chief Executive Officer
**(Moderately Centralized Health System)**

**PENNSYLVANIA:** BRYN MAWR HOSPITAL (O, 319 beds) 130 South Bryn Mawr Avenue, Bryn Mawr, PA Zip 19010–3160; tel. 484/337–3000; Andrea F. Gilbert, FACHE, President
**Web address:** www.brynmawrhospital.org

BRYN MAWR REHABILITATION HOSPITAL (O, 148 beds) 414 Paoli Pike, Malvern, PA Zip 19355–3300, Mailing Address: P.O. Box 3007, Zip 19355–0707; tel. 484/596–5400; Donna Phillips, President
**Web address:** www.brynmawrrehab.org

LANKENAU MEDICAL CENTER (O, 353 beds) 100 Lancaster Avenue West, Wynnewood, PA Zip 19096–3411; tel. 484/476–2000; Phillip D. Robinson, Chief Executive Officer
**Web address:** www.mainlinehealth.org

PAOLI HOSPITAL (O, 222 beds) 255 West Lancaster Avenue, Paoli, PA Zip 19301–1763; tel. 484/565–1000; Barbara J. Tachovsky, President
**Web address:** www.mainlinehealth.org

RIDDLE HOSPITAL (O, 209 beds) 1068 West Baltimore Pike, Media, PA Zip 19063–5177; tel. 484/227–9400; Gary L. Perecko, President
**Web address:** www.riddlehospital.org

| Owned, leased, sponsored: | 5 hospitals | 1251 beds |
|---|---|---|
| Contract–managed: | 0 hospitals | 0 beds |
| Totals: | 5 hospitals | 1251 beds |

## 0614: MAINEHEALTH (NP)
110 Free Street, Portland, ME Zip 04101–3537; William L. Caron, Jr., President
**(Moderately Centralized Health System)**

**MAINE:** MAINE MEDICAL CENTER (O, 637 beds) 22 Bramhall Street, Portland, ME Zip 04102–3175; tel. 207/662–0111; Richard W. Petersen, President and Chief Executive Officer
**Web address:** www.mmc.org

MILES MEMORIAL HOSPITAL (O, 38 beds) 35 Miles Street, Damariscotta, ME Zip 04543–9767; tel. 207/563–1234; James W. Donovan, President and Chief Executive Officer
**Web address:** www.lchcare.org

PEN BAY MEDICAL CENTER (O, 165 beds) 6 Glen Cove Drive, Rockport, ME Zip 04856–4240; tel. 207/596–8000; Wade C. Johnson, MS, FACHE, Chief Executive Officer
**Web address:** www.penbayhealthcare.org

SOUTHERN MAINE MEDICAL CENTER (O, 110 beds) One Medical Center Drive, Biddeford, ME Zip 04005–9496, Mailing Address: P.O. Box 626, Zip 04005–0626; tel. 207/283–7000; Edward J. McGeachey, President and Chief Executive Officer
**Web address:** www.smmc.org

SPRING HARBOR HOSPITAL (O, 88 beds) 123 Andover Road, Westbrook, ME Zip 04092–3850; tel. 207/761–2200; Dennis P. King, Chief Executive Officer
**Web address:** www.springharbor.org

For explanation of codes following names, see page B2.
★ Indicates Type III membership in the American Hospital Association.

ST. ANDREWS HOSPITAL AND HEALTHCARE CENTER (O, 73 beds) 6 St. Andrews Lane, Boothbay Harbor, ME Zip 04538–1732, Mailing Address: P.O. Box 417, Zip 04538–0417; tel. 207/633–2121; James W. Donovan, President and Chief Executive Officer
**Web address:** www.lincolncountyhealthcare.org

STEPHENS MEMORIAL HOSPITAL (O, 25 beds) 181 Main Street, Norway, ME Zip 04268–1297; tel. 207/743–5933; Timothy A. Churchill, President
**Web address:** www.wmhcc.com

WALDO COUNTY GENERAL HOSPITAL (O, 25 beds) 118 Northport Avenue, Belfast, ME Zip 04915–6072, Mailing Address: P.O. Box 287, Zip 04915–0287; tel. 207/338–2500; Mark A. Biscone, Executive Director
**Web address:** www.wchi.com

| | | |
|---|---|---|
| Owned, leased, sponsored: | 8 hospitals | 1161 beds |
| Contract–managed: | 0 hospitals | 0 beds |
| Totals: | 8 hospitals | 1161 beds |

★**5305: MARIAN HEALTH SYSTEM** (CC)
1923 South Utica Avenue, Tulsa, OK Zip 74104, Mailing Address: P.O. Box 4753, Zip 74159–0753; tel. 918/742–9988; Sister M. Therese Gottschalk, President
**(Moderately Centralized Health System)**

**MINNESOTA:** SAINT ELIZABETH'S MEDICAL CENTER (O, 168 beds) 1200 Grant Boulevard West, Wabasha, MN Zip 55981–1042; tel. 651/565–4531; Thomas Crowley, President and Chief Executive Officer
**Web address:** www.stelizabethswabasha.org

**OKLAHOMA:** JANE PHILLIPS MEDICAL CENTER (O, 140 beds) 3500 East Frank Phillips Boulevard, Bartlesville, OK Zip 74006–2411; tel. 918/333–7200; David R. Stire, President and Chief Executive Officer
**Web address:** www.jpmc.org

ST. JOHN BROKEN ARROW (S, 44 beds) 1000 West Boise Circle, Broken Arrow, OK Zip 74012–4900; tel. 918/994–8100; David L. Phillips, Chief Executive Officer
**Web address:** www.stjohnbrokenarrow.com

ST. JOHN MEDICAL CENTER (O, 547 beds) 1923 South Utica Avenue, Tulsa, OK Zip 74104–6502; tel. 918/744–2345; S. Charles Anderson, President and Chief Executive Officer
**Web address:** www.sjmc.org

ST. JOHN OWASSO (O, 36 beds) 12451 East 100th Street North, Owasso, OK Zip 74055–4600; tel. 918/274–5000; David L. Phillips, President and Chief Executive Officer
**Web address:** www.stjohnowasso.com

ST. JOHN SAPULPA (O, 25 beds) 519 South Division Street, Sapulpa, OK Zip 74066–4501, Mailing Address: P.O. Box 1368, Zip 74067–1368; tel. 918/224–4280; Valerie Round, Chief Executive Officer
**Web address:** www.sjmc.org

**WISCONSIN:** EAGLE RIVER MEMORIAL HOSPITAL (O, 9 beds) 201 Hospital Road, Eagle River, WI Zip 54521–8835; tel. 715/479–7411; Sheila Clough, President
**Web address:** www.ministryhealth.org

FLAMBEAU HOSPITAL (O, 25 beds) 98 Sherry Avenue, Park Falls, WI Zip 54552–1467, Mailing Address: P.O. Box 310, Zip 54552–0310; tel. 715/762–2484; David A. Grundstrom, Chief Administrative Officer
**Web address:** www.flambeauhospital.org

HOWARD YOUNG MEDICAL CENTER (O, 52 beds) 240 Maple Street, Woodruff, WI Zip 54568, Mailing Address: P.O. Box 470, Zip 54568–0470; tel. 715/356–8000; Sheila Clough, President
**Web address:** www.ministryhealth.org

MINISTRY DOOR COUNTY MEDICAL CENTER (O, 55 beds) 323 South 18th Avenue, Sturgeon Bay, WI Zip 54235–1495; tel. 920/743–5566; Gerald M. Worrick, President and Chief Executive Officer
**Web address:** www.dcmh.org

MINISTRY GOOD SAMARITAN HEALTH CENTER (O, 16 beds) 601 South Center Avenue, Merrill, WI Zip 54452–3404; tel. 715/536–5511; Kristine McGarigle, President
**Web address:** www.ministryhealth.org

MINISTRY SAINT MICHAEL'S HOSPITAL (O, 50 beds) 900 Illinois Avenue, Stevens Point, WI Zip 54481–3196; tel. 715/346–5000; Jeffrey L. Martin, President
**Web address:** www.ministryhealth.org/SMH/home.nws

OUR LADY OF VICTORY HOSPITAL (O, 7 beds) 1120 Pine Street, Stanley, WI Zip 54768–0220; tel. 715/644–5571; Cynthia Eichman, President
**Web address:** www.ministryhealth.org

SACRED HEART–ST. MARY'S HOSPITALS (O, 58 beds) 2251 North Shore Drive, Rhinelander, WI Zip 54501–3998; tel. 715/361–2000; Monica Hilt, President and Chief Operating Officer
**Web address:** www.ministryhealth.org

SAINT CLARE'S HOSPITAL (O, 60 beds) 3400 Ministry Parkway, Weston, WI Zip 54476; tel. 715/393–3000; Mary T. Krueger, President
**Web address:** www.ministryhealth.org

SAINT JOSEPH'S HOSPITAL (O, 319 beds) 611 St. Joseph Avenue, Marshfield, WI Zip 54449–1898; tel. 715/387–1713; Brian Kief, President and Chief Executive Officer
**Web address:** www.stjosephs–marshfield.org

| | | |
|---|---|---|
| Owned, leased, sponsored: | 16 hospitals | 1611 beds |
| Contract–managed: | 0 hospitals | 0 beds |
| Totals: | 16 hospitals | 1611 beds |

★**1975: MARSHALL HEALTH SYSTEM** (NP)
227 Britany Road, Guntersville, AL Zip 35976; tel. 256/894–6615; Gary R. Gore, Chief Executive Officer
**(Independent Hospital System)**

**ALABAMA:** MARSHALL MEDICAL CENTER NORTH (O, 90 beds) 8000 Alabama Highway 69, Guntersville, AL Zip 35976; tel. 256/753–8000; Cheryl M. Hays, FACHE, Administrator
**Web address:** www.mmcenters.com

MARSHALL MEDICAL CENTER SOUTH (O, 112 beds) U.S. Highway 431 North, Boaz, AL Zip 35957–0999, Mailing Address: P.O. Box 758, Zip 35957–0758; tel. 256/593–8310; John D. Anderson, FACHE, Administrator
**Web address:** www.mmcs.org

| | | |
|---|---|---|
| Owned, leased, sponsored: | 2 hospitals | 202 beds |
| Contract–managed: | 0 hospitals | 0 beds |
| Totals: | 2 hospitals | 202 beds |

★**0523: MARY WASHINGTON HEALTHCARE** (NP)
2300 Fall Hill Avenue, Suite 308, Fredericksburg, VA Zip 22401–3343; tel. 540/741–3100; Fred M. Rankin, III, President and Chief Executive Officer
**(Centralized Health System)**

**VIRGINIA:** MARY WASHINGTON HOSPITAL (O, 437 beds) 1001 Sam Perry Boulevard, Fredericksburg, VA Zip 22401–3354; tel. 540/741–1100; Fred M. Rankin, III, President and Chief Executive Officer
**Web address:** www.mwhc.com

STAFFORD HOSPITAL (O, 70 beds) 101 Hospital Center Boulevard, Stafford, VA Zip 22554–6200; tel. 540/741–9000; Fred M. Rankin, III, President and Chief Executive Officer
**Web address:** www.marywashingtonhealthcare.com

| | | |
|---|---|---|
| Owned, leased, sponsored: | 2 hospitals | 507 beds |
| Contract–managed: | 0 hospitals | 0 beds |
| Totals: | 2 hospitals | 507 beds |

**0013: MASSACHUSETTS DEPARTMENT OF MENTAL HEALTH** (NP)
25 Staniford Street, Boston, MA Zip 02114–2575; tel. 617/626–8123; Marcia Fowler, Commissioner

**MASSACHUSETTS:** DR. J. CORRIGAN MENTAL HEALTH CENTER (O, 16 beds) 49 Hillside Street, Fall River, MA Zip 02720–5266; tel. 508/235–7200; Steve Figueiredo, Director

TAUNTON STATE HOSPITAL (O, 185 beds) 60 Hodges Avenue Extension, Taunton, MA Zip 02780–3034, Mailing Address: PO Box 4007, Zip 02780–0997; tel. 508/977–3000; Roberta H. Guez, Chief Operating Officer

WORCESTER STATE HOSPITAL (O, 126 beds) 305 Belmont Street, Worcester, MA Zip 01604–1695; tel. 508/368–3300; Anthony Riccitelli, Chief Operating Officer

For explanation of codes following names, see page B2.
★ Indicates Type III membership in the American Hospital Association.

| | | |
|---|---|---|
| Owned, leased, sponsored: | 3 hospitals | 327 beds |
| Contract–managed: | 0 hospitals | 0 beds |
| Totals: | 3 hospitals | 327 beds |

**0280: MASSACHUSETTS DEPARTMENT OF PUBLIC HEALTH**
(NP)
250 Washington Street, Boston, MA Zip 02108–4619;
tel. 617/624–6000; John Auerbach, Commissioner
**(Independent Hospital System)**

LEMUEL SHATTUCK HOSPITAL (O, 260 beds) 170 Morton Street, Jamaica
Plain, MA Zip 02130–3735; tel. 617/522–8110; Paul Romary, Chief
Executive Officer
**Web address:** www.mass.gov/shattuckhospital.org

MASSACHUSETTS HOSPITAL SCHOOL (O, 93 beds) 3 Randolph Street,
Canton, MA Zip 02021–2397; tel. 781/828–2440; Katherine Ann Chmiel,
R.N., MS, Chief Executive Officer
**Web address:** www.mhsf.us/

TEWKSBURY HOSPITAL (O, 720 beds) 365 East Street, Tewksbury, MA
Zip 01876–1998; tel. 978/851–7321; Debra Tosti, Interim Chief Executive
Officer
**Web address:** www.state.ma.us/dph/hosp/th.htm

WESTERN MASSACHUSETTS HOSPITAL (O, 70 beds) 91 East Mountain Road,
Westfield, MA Zip 01085; tel. 413/562–4131; Derrick Tallman, Chief
Executive Officer
**Web address:** www.mass.gov/dph/hosp/wmh.htm

| | | |
|---|---|---|
| Owned, leased, sponsored: | 4 hospitals | 1143 beds |
| Contract–managed: | 0 hospitals | 0 beds |
| Totals: | 4 hospitals | 1143 beds |

**★1875: MAYO CLINIC HEALTH SYSTEM** (NP)
200 S.W. First Street, Rochester, MN Zip 55905–0002;
tel. 507/284–2511; John Noseworthy, M.D., President and Chief
Executive Officer
**(Moderately Centralized Health System)**

**ARIZONA:** MAYO CLINIC HOSPITAL (O, 244 beds) 5777 East Mayo Boulevard,
Phoenix, AZ Zip 85054–4502; tel. 480/515–6296; Ann M. Meyers, Chief
Executive Officer
**Web address:** www.mayoclinic.org/arizona/

**FLORIDA:** MAYO CLINIC JACKSONVILLE (O, 214 beds) 4500 San Pablo Road
South, Jacksonville, FL Zip 32224–1865; tel. 904/953–2000; Hilary G.
Mathews, MS, R.N., Administrator
**Web address:** www.mayoclinic.org

**GEORGIA:** MAYO CLINIC HEALTH SYSTEM IN WAYCROSS (O, 200 beds) 410
Darling Avenue, Waycross, GA Zip 31501–5246, Mailing Address: P.O.
Box 139, Zip 31502–0139; tel. 912/283–3030; Robert M. Trimm, Chief
Administrative Officer
**Web address:** www.satilla.org

**IOWA:** FLOYD COUNTY MEDICAL CENTER (C, 25 beds) 800 Eleventh Street,
Charles City, IA Zip 50616–3499; tel. 641/228–6830; Bill D. Faust,
Administrator
**Web address:** www.fcmc.us.com/

WINNESHIEK MEDICAL CENTER (C, 25 beds) 901 Montgomery Street,
Decorah, IA Zip 52101–2325; tel. 563/382–2911; Gretchen M. Dahlen,
FACHE, Chief Executive Officer
**Web address:** www.winmedical.org

**MINNESOTA:** MAYO CLINIC – METHODIST HOSPITAL (O, 335 beds) 201
West Center Street, Rochester, MN Zip 55902–3084;
tel. 507/266–7890; Lynn Frederick, Administrator
**Web address:** www.mayoclinic.org

MAYO CLINIC – SAINT MARYS HOSPITAL (O, 797 beds) 1216 Second Street
S.W., Rochester, MN Zip 55902–1970; tel. 507/255–5123; Lynn Frederick,
Administrator
**Web address:** www.mayoclinic.org

MAYO CLINIC HEALTH SYSTEM IN ALBERT LEA (O, 129 beds) 404 West
Fountain Street, Albert Lea, MN Zip 56007–2473; tel. 507/373–2384; Mark
Ciota, M.D., Chief Executive Officer
**Web address:** www.almedcenter.org

MAYO CLINIC HEALTH SYSTEM IN AUSTIN (O, 82 beds) 1000 First Drive
N.W., Austin, MN Zip 55912–2904; tel. 507/433–7351; David Agerter,
President and Chief Executive Officer
**Web address:** www.austinmedicalcenter.org

MAYO CLINIC HEALTH SYSTEM IN CANNON FALLS (O, 21 beds) 1116 West
Mill Street, Cannon Falls, MN Zip 55009–1898; tel. 507/263–4221; Thomas
J. Witt, M.D., President and Chief Executive Officer
**Web address:** www.cannonhealth.org/

MAYO CLINIC HEALTH SYSTEM IN FAIRMONT (O, 96 beds) 800 Medical
Center Drive, Fairmont, MN Zip 56031–0800; tel. 507/238–8100; Robert
Bartingale, Chief Administrative Officer
**Web address:** www.fairmontmedicalcenter.org

MAYO CLINIC HEALTH SYSTEM IN LAKE CITY (O, 108 beds) 500 West Grant
Street, Lake City, MN Zip 55041–1143; tel. 651/345–3321; Thomas J. Witt,
M.D., President and Chief Executive Officer
**Web address:** www.lakecitymedicalcenter.org

MAYO CLINIC HEALTH SYSTEM IN MANKATO (O, 166 beds) 1025 Marsh
Street, Mankato, MN Zip 56002–8673, Mailing Address: P.O. Box 8673,
Zip 56002–8673; tel. 507/625–4031; Gregory Kutcher, M.D., President and
Chief Executive Officer
**Web address:** www.isj–mhs.org

MAYO CLINIC HEALTH SYSTEM IN NEW PRAGUE (O, 25 beds) 301 Second
Street N.E., New Prague, MN Zip 56071–1799; tel. 952/758–4431; Mary J.
Klimp, Chief Administrative Officer
**Web address:** www.mayoclinichealthsystem.org/locations/new–prague

MAYO CLINIC HEALTH SYSTEM IN RED WING (O, 134 beds) 701 Fairview
Boulevard, Red Wing, MN Zip 55066–2848, Mailing Address: P.O. Box 95,
Zip 55066–0095; tel. 651/267–5000; Thomas J. Witt, M.D., President and
Chief Executive Officer
**Web address:** www.mayoclinichealthsystem.org/locations/red–wing

MAYO CLINIC HEALTH SYSTEM IN SAINT JAMES (O, 13 beds) 1101 Moulton
and Parsons Drive, Saint James, MN Zip 56081; tel. 507/375–3261; Ryan J.
Smith, Administrator
**Web address:** www.mayoclinichealthsystem.org/locations/st–james

MAYO CLINIC HEALTH SYSTEM IN SPRINGFIELD (O, 24 beds) 625 North
Jackson Avenue, Springfield, MN Zip 56087–1714, Mailing Address: P.O. Box
146, Zip 56087–0146; tel. 507/723–6201; Scott D. Thoreson, FACHE,
Administrator
**Web address:** www.smc–mhs.org

MAYO CLINIC HEALTH SYSTEM IN WASECA (O, 25 beds) 501 North State
Street, Waseca, MN Zip 56093–2811; tel. 507/835–1210; Jeffrey Carlson,
Chief Executive Officer
**Web address:** www.mayoclinichealthsystem.org

**WISCONSIN:** MAYO CLINIC HEALTH SYSTEM – CHIPPEWA VALLEY IN
BLOOMER (O, 55 beds) 1501 Thompson Street, Bloomer, WI
Zip 54724–1299; tel. 715/568–2000; Edward A. Wittrock, Vice President
Regional System
**Web address:** www.bloomermedicalcenter.org

MAYO CLINIC HEALTH SYSTEM – FRANCISCAN HEALTHCARE IN LA CROSSE
(O, 155 beds) 700 West Avenue South, La Crosse, WI Zip 54601–4783;
tel. 608/785–0940; Timothy J. Johnson, President and Chief Executive
Officer
**Web address:** www.franciscankemp.org

MAYO CLINIC HEALTH SYSTEM – FRANCISCAN HEALTHCARE IN SPARTA (O,
14 beds) 310 West Main Street, Sparta, WI Zip 54656–2171;
tel. 608/269–2132; Kimberly Hawthorne, Administrator
**Web address:** www.mayohealthsystem.com

MAYO CLINIC HEALTH SYSTEM – NORTHLAND IN BARRON (O, 45 beds) 1222
Woodland Avenue, Barron, WI Zip 54812–1798; tel. 715/537–3186; Maurita
Sullivan, Administrator
**Web address:** www.luthermidelfortnorthland.org

MAYO CLINIC HEALTH SYSTEM – OAKRIDGE IN OSSEO (O, 39 beds) 13025
Eighth Street, Osseo, WI Zip 54758–7673, Mailing Address: P.O. Box 70,
Zip 54758–0070; tel. 715/597–3121; Michael Ryan, Administrator
**Web address:** www.luthermidelfortoakridge.com

MAYO CLINIC HEALTH SYSTEM – RED CEDAR IN MENOMONIE (O, 25 beds)
2321 Stout Road, Menomonie, WI Zip 54751–2397; tel. 715/235–5531;
Steven Lindberg, Chief Administrative Officer
**Web address:** www.rcmc–mhs.org

For explanation of codes following names, see page B2.
★ Indicates Type III membership in the American Hospital Association.

MAYO CLINIC HEALTH SYSTEM IN EAU CLAIRE (O, 204 beds) 1221 Whipple Street, Eau Claire, WI Zip 54702–4105, Mailing Address: P.O. Box 5, Zip 54702–0005; tel. 715/838–3311; Randall L. Linton, M.D., President and Chief Executive Officer
**Web address:** www.mhs.mayo.edu

| | | |
|---|---|---|
| Owned, leased, sponsored: | 23 hospitals | 3150 beds |
| Contract–managed: | 2 hospitals | 50 beds |
| Totals: | 25 hospitals | 3200 beds |

---

**★0252: MCLAREN HEALTH CARE CORPORATION** (NP)
G3235 Beecher Road, Suite B., Flint, MI Zip 48532; tel. 810/342–1100; Philip A. Incarnati, President and Chief Executive Officer
**(Moderately Centralized Health System)**

**MICHIGAN:** MCLAREN BAY REGION (O, 338 beds) 1900 Columbus Avenue, Bay City, MI Zip 48708–6831; tel. 989/894–3000; Alice M. Gerard, President and Chief Executive Officer
**Web address:** www.bayregional.org

MCLAREN BAY SPECIAL CARE (O, 26 beds) 3250 East Midland Road, Suite 1, Bay City, MI Zip 48706–2835; tel. 989/667–6802; Cheryl A. Burzynski, President
**Web address:** www.bayspecialcare.org

MCLAREN CENTRAL MICHIGAN (O, 78 beds) 1221 South Drive, Mount Pleasant, MI Zip 48858–3234; tel. 989/772–6700; William P. Lawrence, President and Chief Executive Officer
**Web address:** www.cmch.org

MCLAREN FLINT (O, 336 beds) 401 South Ballenger Highway, Flint, MI Zip 48532–3685; tel. 810/342–2000; Donald C. Kooy, President and Chief Executive Officer
**Web address:** www.mclarenregional.org

MCLAREN GREATER LANSING (O, 318 beds) 401 West Greenlawn Avenue, Lansing, MI Zip 48910–2819; tel. 517/975–6000; Rick Wright, President and Chief Executive Officer
**Web address:** www.irmc.org

MCLAREN LAPEER REGION (O, 157 beds) 1375 North Main Street, Lapeer, MI Zip 48446–1350; tel. 810/667–5500; Barton Buxton, Ed.D., President and Chief Executive Officer
**Web address:** www.lapeerregional.org

MCLAREN MACOMB (O, 288 beds) 1000 Harrington Boulevard, Mount Clemens, MI Zip 48043–2920; tel. 586/493–8000; Mark S. O'Halla, President and Chief Executive Officer
**Web address:** www.mcrmc.org

MCLAREN NORTHERN MICHIGAN (O, 178 beds) 416 Connable Avenue, Petoskey, MI Zip 49770–2297; tel. 231/487–4000; Reezie DeVet, R.N., Ph.D., President and Chief Executive Officer
**Web address:** www.northernhealth.org

MCLAREN OAKLAND (O, 288 beds) 50 North Perry Street, Pontiac, MI Zip 48342–2253; tel. 248/338–5000; Clarence Sevillian, President and Chief Executive Officer
**Web address:** www.pohmedical.org

| | | |
|---|---|---|
| Owned, leased, sponsored: | 9 hospitals | 2007 beds |
| Contract–managed: | 0 hospitals | 0 beds |
| Totals: | 9 hospitals | 2007 beds |

---

**0391: MEDCENTRAL HEALTH SYSTEM** (NP)
335 Glessner Avenue, Mansfield, OH Zip 44903; tel. 419/526–8000; Joe Chamberlain, Interim Chief Executive Officer
**(Independent Hospital System)**

**OHIO:** MEDCENTRAL – MANSFIELD HOSPITAL (O, 268 beds) 335 Glessner Avenue, Mansfield, OH Zip 44903–2265; tel. 419/526–8000; James E. Meyer, President and Chief Executive Officer
**Web address:** www.medcentral.org

MEDCENTRAL – SHELBY HOSPITAL (O, 25 beds) 199 West Main Street, Shelby, OH Zip 44875–1490; tel. 419/342–5015; Ron Distl, Chief Executive Officer
**Web address:** www.medcentral.org/body.cfm?id=153

| | | |
|---|---|---|
| Owned, leased, sponsored: | 2 hospitals | 293 beds |
| Contract–managed: | 0 hospitals | 0 beds |
| Totals: | 2 hospitals | 293 beds |

---

**★0154: MEDSTAR HEALTH** (NP)
5565 Sterrett Place, 5th Floor, Columbia, MD Zip 21044; tel. 410/772–6500; Kenneth A. Samet, President and Chief Executive Officer
**(Decentralized Health System)**

**DISTRICT OF COLUMBIA:** MEDSTAR GEORGETOWN UNIVERSITY HOSPITAL (O, 406 beds) 3800 Reservoir Road N.W., Washington, DC Zip 20007–2197; tel. 202/444–2000; Richard L. Goldberg, M.D., President
**Web address:** www.georgetownuniversityhospital.org

MEDSTAR NATIONAL REHABILITATION NETWORK (O, 137 beds) 102 Irving Street N.W., Washington, DC Zip 20010–2949; tel. 202/877–1000; John D. Rockwood, President
**Web address:** www.medstarnrh.org

MEDSTAR WASHINGTON HOSPITAL CENTER (O, 799 beds) 110 Irving Street N.W., Washington, DC Zip 20010–2975; tel. 202/877–7000; John Sullivan, President
**Web address:** www.whcenter.org

**MARYLAND:** MEDSTAR FRANKLIN SQUARE MEDICAL CENTER (O, 368 beds) 9000 Franklin Square Drive, Baltimore, MD Zip 21237–2998; tel. 443/777–7000; Samuel E. Moskowitz, President
**Web address:** www.medstarfranklin.org

MEDSTAR GOOD SAMARITAN HOSPITAL (O, 310 beds) 5601 Loch Raven Boulevard, Baltimore, MD Zip 21239–2995; tel. 443/444–8000; Jeffrey A. Matton, President and Chief Executive Officer
**Web address:** www.goodsam–md.org

MEDSTAR HARBOR HOSPITAL (O, 187 beds) 3001 South Hanover Street, Baltimore, MD Zip 21225–1290; tel. 410/350–3200; Dennis W. Pullin, Chief Executive Officer
**Web address:** www.harborhospital.org

MEDSTAR MONTGOMERY MEDICAL CENTER (O, 158 beds) 18101 Prince Philip Drive, Olney, MD Zip 20832–1512; tel. 301/774–8882; Peter W. Monge, President
**Web address:** www.montgomerygeneral.com

MEDSTAR ST. MARY'S HOSPITAL (O, 115 beds) 25500 Point Lookout Road, Leonardtown, MD Zip 20650–0527, Mailing Address: P.O. Box 527, Zip 20650–0527; tel. 301/475–6001; Christine R. Wray, President
**Web address:** www.medstarstmarys.org

MEDSTAR UNION MEMORIAL HOSPITAL (O, 271 beds) 201 East University Parkway, Baltimore, MD Zip 21218–2895; tel. 410/554–2000; Bradley Chambers, President
**Web address:** www.unionmemorial.org

| | | |
|---|---|---|
| Owned, leased, sponsored: | 9 hospitals | 2751 beds |
| Contract–managed: | 0 hospitals | 0 beds |
| Totals: | 9 hospitals | 2751 beds |

---

**★0323: MEDWEST HEALTH SYSTEM** (NP)
68 Hospital Road, Sylva, NC Zip 28779; tel. 828/586–7000; Steve Heatherly, President
**(Independent Hospital System)**

**NORTH CAROLINA:** MEDWEST – HARRIS (O, 86 beds) 68 Hospital Road, Sylva, NC Zip 28779–2795; tel. 828/586–7000; J. Michael Poore, Chief Executive Officer
**Web address:** www.westcare.org

MEDWEST – HAYWOOD (O, 146 beds) 262 Leroy George Drive, Clyde, NC Zip 28721–9434; tel. 828/456–7311; John Young, Interim CEO
**Web address:** www.haymed.org

MEDWEST – SWAIN (O, 25 beds) 45 Plateau Street, Bryson City, NC Zip 28713–6784; tel. 828/488–2155; J. Michael Poore, Chief Executive Officer
**Web address:** www.westcare.org

---

For explanation of codes following names, see page B2.
★ Indicates Type III membership in the American Hospital Association.

| Owned, leased, sponsored: | 3 hospitals | 257 beds |
|---|---|---|
| Contract–managed: | 0 hospitals | 0 beds |
| **Totals:** | 3 hospitals | 257 beds |

★**0086:   MEMORIAL HEALTH SYSTEM** (NP)
701 North First Street, Springfield, IL Zip 62781–0001;
tel. 217/788–3000; Edgar J. Curtis, President and Chief Executive
Officer
**(Centralized Physician/Insurance Health System)**

**ILLINOIS:** ABRAHAM LINCOLN MEMORIAL HOSPITAL (O, 25 beds) 200
Stahlhut Drive, Lincoln, IL Zip 62656–2698; tel. 217/732–2161; Dolan
Dalpoas, President and Chief Executive Officer
**Web address:** www.almh.org

MEMORIAL MEDICAL CENTER (O, 471 beds) 701 North First Street,
Springfield, IL Zip 62781–0001; tel. 217/788–3000; Edgar J. Curtis,
President and Chief Executive Officer
**Web address:** www.memorialmedical.com

TAYLORVILLE MEMORIAL HOSPITAL (O, 45 beds) 201 East Pleasant Street,
Taylorville, IL Zip 62568–1597; tel. 217/824–3331; Daniel J. Raab,
President and Chief Executive Officer
**Web address:** www.taylorvillememorial.org

| Owned, leased, sponsored: | 3 hospitals | 541 beds |
|---|---|---|
| Contract–managed: | 0 hospitals | 0 beds |
| **Totals:** | 3 hospitals | 541 beds |

**0176:   MEMORIAL HEALTH SYSTEM OF EAST TEXAS** (NP)
1201 Frank Avenue, Lufkin, TX Zip 75904–3357;
tel. 936/634–8111; Gary N. Looper, President and Chief Executive
Officer
**(Moderately Centralized Health System)**

**TEXAS:** MEMORIAL ACUTE LONG TERM CARE HOSPITAL (O, 50 beds) 1201
Frank Street, 5th Floor, Lufkin, TX Zip 75904, Mailing Address: P.O. Box
1447, Zip 75901;

MEMORIAL MEDICAL CENTER – LIVINGSTON (O, 66 beds) 1717 Highway 59
Bypass, Livingston, TX Zip 77351–1257, Mailing Address: P.O. Box 1257,
Zip 77351–1257; tel. 936/329–8700; David LeMonte, Chief Executive
Officer
**Web address:** www.memorialhealth.org

MEMORIAL MEDICAL CENTER – LUFKIN (O, 217 beds) 1201 West Frank
Avenue, Lufkin, TX Zip 75904–3357, Mailing Address: P.O. Box 1447,
Zip 75902–1447; tel. 936/634–8111; Gary N. Looper, President and Chief
Executive Officer
**Web address:** www.memorialhealth.org

MEMORIAL MEDICAL CENTER – SAN AUGUSTINE (O, 18 beds) 511 East
Hospital Street, San Augustine, TX Zip 75972–2121, Mailing Address: P.O.
Box 658, Zip 75972–0658; tel. 936/275–3446; Darlene Williams, R.N.,
Administrator
**Web address:** www.memorialhealth.org

MEMORIAL SPECIALTY HOSPITAL (O, 26 beds) 1201 West Frank Avenue,
Lufkin, TX Zip 75904; tel. 936/639–7975; Leslie Leach, Administrator
**Web address:** www.memorialhealth.org

| Owned, leased, sponsored: | 5 hospitals | 377 beds |
|---|---|---|
| Contract–managed: | 0 hospitals | 0 beds |
| **Totals:** | 5 hospitals | 377 beds |

★**0083:   MEMORIAL HEALTHCARE SYSTEM** (NP)
3501 Johnson Street, Hollywood, FL Zip 33021–5421;
tel. 954/265–5805; Frank V. Sacco, FACHE, President and Chief
Executive Officer
**(Centralized Health System)**

**FLORIDA:** MEMORIAL HOSPITAL MIRAMAR (O, 178 beds) 1901 S.W. 172nd
Avenue, Miramar, FL Zip 33029; tel. 954/538–5000; Leah A. Carpenter,
Chief Executive Officer
**Web address:** www.mhs.net

MEMORIAL HOSPITAL PEMBROKE (L, 149 beds) 7800 Sheridan Street,
Pembroke Pines, FL Zip 33024–2536; tel. 954/883–8482; Chantal Leconte,
Chief Executive Officer
**Web address:** www.memorialpembroke.com/

MEMORIAL HOSPITAL WEST (O, 304 beds) 703 North Flamingo Road,
Pembroke Pines, FL Zip 33028–1014; tel. 954/436–5000; C. Kennon
Hetlage, FACHE, Chief Executive Officer and Administrator
**Web address:** www.mhs.net

MEMORIAL REGIONAL HOSPITAL (O, 713 beds) 3501 Johnson Street,
Hollywood, FL Zip 33021–5421; tel. 954/987–2000; Zeff Ross, FACHE,
Senior Vice President and Chief Executive Officer
**Web address:** www.mhs.net

MEMORIAL REGIONAL HOSPITAL SOUTH (O, 280 beds) 3600 Washington
Street, Hollywood, FL Zip 33021–8216; tel. 954/966–4500; Douglas Zaren,
FACHE, Administrator
**Web address:** www.memorialregionalsouth.com

| Owned, leased, sponsored: | 5 hospitals | 1624 beds |
|---|---|---|
| Contract–managed: | 0 hospitals | 0 beds |
| **Totals:** | 5 hospitals | 1624 beds |

★**2645:   MEMORIAL HERMANN HEALTHCARE SYSTEM** (NP)
929 Gessner, Suite 2700, Houston, TX Zip 77024;
tel. 713/242–2700; Daniel J. Wolterman, President and Chief
Executive Officer
**(Centralized Health System)**

**TEXAS:** MEMORIAL HERMANN – TEXAS MEDICAL CENTER (O, 868 beds)
6411 Fannin Street, Houston, TX Zip 77030–1501; tel. 713/704–4000;
Craig Cordola, Chief Executive Officer
**Web address:** www.mhhs.org

MEMORIAL HERMANN KATY HOSPITAL (O, 142 beds) 23900 Katy Freeway,
Katy, TX Zip 77494; tel. 281/644–7000; Brian S. Barbe, Chief Executive
Officer
**Web address:** www.memorialhermann.org

MEMORIAL HERMANN MEMORIAL CITY MEDICAL CENTER (L, 377 beds) 921
Gessner Road, Houston, TX Zip 77024–2501; tel. 713/242–3000; Keith N.
Alexander, Chief Executive Officer
**Web address:** www.memorialhermann.org

MEMORIAL HERMANN NORTHEAST (L, 227 beds) 18951 North Memorial
Drive, Humble, TX Zip 77338–4297; tel. 281/540–7700; Louis G. Smith, Jr.,
Chief Executive Officer
**Web address:** www.memorialhermann.org

MEMORIAL HERMANN NORTHWEST HOSPITAL (O, 1172 beds) 1635 North
Loop West, Houston, TX Zip 77008; tel. 713/867–3380; Gary Kerr, Chief
Executive Officer
**Web address:** www.mhbh.org

MEMORIAL HERMANN REHABILITATION HOSPITAL – KATY (O, 35 beds)
21720 Kingsland Boulevard, Katy, TX Zip 77450–2513; tel. 281/579–5555;
Noelle Lopez, Executive Director
**Web address:** www.memorialhermann.com

MEMORIAL HERMANN SUGAR LAND HOSPITAL (O, 77 beds) 17500 West
Grand Parkway South, Sugar Land, TX Zip 77479; tel. 281/725–5000; Jim
Brown, Chief Executive Officer
**Web address:** www.memorialhermann.org

TIRR MEMORIAL HERMANN (O, 119 beds) 1333 Moursund Street, Houston,
TX Zip 77030–3405; tel. 713/799–5000; Carl E. Josehart, Chief Executive
Officer
**Web address:** www.memorialhermann.org/locations/tirr.html

| Owned, leased, sponsored: | 8 hospitals | 3017 beds |
|---|---|---|
| Contract–managed: | 0 hospitals | 0 beds |
| **Totals:** | 8 hospitals | 3017 beds |

**0084:   MEMORIALCARE** (NP)
17360 Brookhurst Street, Fountain Valley, CA Zip 92708–3720,
Mailing Address: P.O. Box 1428, Long Beach, Zip 90801–1428;
tel. 714/377–2900; Barry S. Arbuckle, Ph.D., President and Chief
Executive Officer
**(Centralized Health System)**

For explanation of codes following names, see page B2.
★ Indicates Type III membership in the American Hospital Association.

Section B

**CALIFORNIA:** COMMUNITY HOSPITAL OF LONG BEACH (O, 148 beds) 1720 Termino Avenue, Long Beach, CA Zip 90804-2180; tel. 562/498-1000; Diana Hendel, PharmD, Chief Executive Officer
**Web address:** www.chlb.org

LONG BEACH MEMORIAL MEDICAL CENTER (O, 420 beds) 2801 Atlantic Avenue, Long Beach, CA Zip 90806-1737, Mailing Address: P.O. Box 1428, Zip 90801-1428; tel. 562/933-2000; Diana Hendel, PharmD, Chief Executive Officer
**Web address:** www.memorialcare.org/LongBeach

MILLER CHILDREN'S HOSPITAL (O, 383 beds) 2801 Atlantic Avenue, Long Beach, CA Zip 90806; tel. 562/933-5437; Diana Hendel, PharmD, Chief Executive Officer
**Web address:** www.memorialcare.org

ORANGE COAST MEMORIAL MEDICAL CENTER (O, 218 beds) 9920 Talbert Avenue, Fountain Valley, CA Zip 92708-5153; tel. 714/378-7000; Marcia Manker, Chief Executive Officer
**Web address:** www.memorialcare.org

SADDLEBACK MEMORIAL MEDICAL CENTER (O, 325 beds) 24451 Health Center Drive, Laguna Hills, CA Zip 92653-3689; tel. 949/837-4500; Steve Geidt, Chief Executive Officer
**Web address:** www.memorialcare.org

| | | |
|---|---|---|
| Owned, leased, sponsored: | 5 hospitals | 1494 beds |
| Contract-managed: | 0 hospitals | 0 beds |
| Totals: | 5 hospitals | 1494 beds |

---

**★5185: MERCY HEALTH** (CC)
14528 South Outer 40, Suite 100, Chesterfield, MO Zip 63017-5743; tel. 314/579-6100; Lynn Britton, President and Chief Executive Officer
**(Decentralized Health System)**

**ARKANSAS:** HOWARD MEMORIAL HOSPITAL (C, 20 beds) 130 Medical Circle, Nashville, AR Zip 71852-8606; tel. 870/845-4400; Debra J. Wright, R.N., Chief Executive Officer
**Web address:** www.howardmemorial.com

MERCY HOSPITAL BERRYVILLE (O, 25 beds) 214 Carter Street, Berryville, AR Zip 72616-4303; tel. 870/423-3355; Kristy Estrem, FACHE, President
**Web address:** www.mercy.net/berryvillear

MERCY HOSPITAL FORT SMITH (O, 374 beds) 7301 Rogers Avenue, Fort Smith, AR Zip 72903-4189, Mailing Address: P.O. Box 17000, Zip 72917-7000; tel. 479/314-6000; Ryan Gehrig, President
**Web address:** www.stedwardmercy.com

MERCY HOSPITAL HOT SPRINGS (O, 282 beds) 300 Werner Street, Hot Springs National Park, AR Zip 71913-9937, Mailing Address: P.O. Box 29001, Zip 71913-9001; tel. 501/622-1000; Timothy J. Johnsen, President and Chief Executive Officer
**Web address:** www.saintjosephs.com

MERCY HOSPITAL OZARK (O, 25 beds) 801 West River Street, Ozark, AR Zip 72949-3000; tel. 479/667-4138; Michael K. Smith, Regional Administator
**Web address:** www.gravettehospital.org

MERCY HOSPITAL PARIS (O, 16 beds) 500 East Academy, Paris, AR Zip 72855-4099; tel. 479/963-6101; Sharon Sorey, R.N., Regional Administrator
**Web address:** www.stedwardmercy.com

MERCY HOSPITAL ROGERS (O, 141 beds) 2710 Rife Medical Lane, Rogers, AR Zip 72758; tel. 479/338-8000; Scott Street, President and Chief Executive Officer
**Web address:** www.mercyhealthnwa.smhs.com

MERCY HOSPITAL WALDRON (O, 24 beds) 1341 West 6th Street, Waldron, AR Zip 72958-7001; tel. 479/637-4135; Steve Loveless, Regional Administrator
**Web address:** www.stedwardmercy.com

**KANSAS:** MERCY HOSPITAL COLUMBUS (O, 18 beds) 220 North Pennsylvania Street, Columbus, KS Zip 66725-1110; tel. 620/429-2545; Cindy Neely, Administrator
**Web address:** www.mercy.ne

MERCY HOSPITAL FORT SCOTT (O, 61 beds) 401 Woodland Hills Boulevard, Fort Scott, KS Zip 66701-8797; tel. 620/223-2200; Reta K. Baker, President
**Web address:** www.mercykansas.com

MERCY HOSPITAL INDEPENDENCE (O, 40 beds) 800 West Myrtle Street, Independence, KS Zip 67301-9980, Mailing Address: P.O. Box 388, Zip 67301-0388; tel. 620/331-2200; Eric Ammons, President and Chief Executive Officer
**Web address:** www.mercykansas.com

**MISSOURI:** MERCY HOSPITAL AURORA (O, 25 beds) 500 Porter Street, Aurora, MO Zip 65605-2365; tel. 417/678-2122; Douglas M. Stroemel, President
**Web address:** www.stjohns.com/aboutus/aurora.aspx

MERCY HOSPITAL CASSVILLE (O, 18 beds) 94 Main Street, Cassville, MO Zip 65625-1610; tel. 417/847-6000; Douglas M. Stroemel, President
**Web address:** www.southbarrycountyhospital.com

MERCY HOSPITAL JOPLIN (O, 341 beds) 2817 South St. John's Boulevard, Joplin, MO Zip 64804-1626; tel. 417/781-2727; Gary W. Pulsipher, President and Chief Executive Officer
**Web address:** www.stj.com

MERCY HOSPITAL LEBANON (O, 62 beds) 100 Hospital Drive, Lebanon, MO Zip 65536-9210; tel. 417/533-6100; Michael J. Gillen, FACHE, President
**Web address:** www.stjohnslebanon.com

MERCY HOSPITAL SPRINGFIELD (O, 613 beds) 1235 East Cherokee Street, Springfield, MO Zip 65804-2263; tel. 417/820-2000; Jon D. Swope, President and Chief Executive Officer
**Web address:** www.stjohns.com

MERCY HOSPITAL ST. LOUIS (O, 979 beds) 615 South New Ballas Road, Saint Louis, MO Zip 63141-8277; tel. 314/569-6000; Jeffrey A. Johnston, President
**Web address:** www.mercy.net/stlouismo

MERCY HOSPITAL WASHINGTON (O, 180 beds) 901 East Fifth Street, Washington, MO Zip 63090-3127; tel. 636/239-8000; Terri L. McLain, FACHE, President
**Web address:** www.mercy.net

MERCY MCCUNE-BROOKS HOSPITAL (L, 35 beds) 3125 Drive Russell Smith Way, Carthage, MO Zip 64836-7402; tel. 417/358-8121; Robert Y. Copeland, Jr., FACHE, Chief Executive Officer
**Web address:** www.mccune-brooks.org

MERCY REHABILITATION HOSPITAL (O, 68 beds) 14561 North Outer Forty Road, Chesterfield, MO Zip 63017; tel. 314/881-4000; Donna M. Flannery, Chief Executive Officer
**Web address:** www.stjohnsmercyrehab.com

MERCY ST. FRANCIS HOSPITAL (O, 20 beds) 100 West Highway 60, Mountain View, MO Zip 65548-7125; tel. 417/934-7000; Jonathan O. Wade, President and Chief Executive Officer
**Web address:** www.stjohns.com/aboutus/stfrancis.aspx

**OKLAHOMA:** ARBUCKLE MEMORIAL HOSPITAL (C, 10 beds) 2011 West Broadway Street, Sulphur, OK Zip 73086-4221; tel. 580/622-2161; Darin Farrell, Chief Executive Officer
**Web address:** www.arbucklehospital.com/

KINGFISHER REGIONAL HOSPITAL (C, 25 beds) 1000 Kingfisher Regional Hospital Drive, Kingfisher, OK Zip 73750-3528, Mailing Address: P.O. Box 59, Zip 73750-0059; tel. 405/375-3141; Nancy Schmid, Chief Executive Officer
**Web address:** www.kingfisherhospital.com

MERCY HEALTH LOVE COUNTY (C, 25 beds) 300 Wanda Street, Marietta, OK Zip 73448-1200; tel. 580/276-3347; Richard Barker, Administrator
**Web address:** www.mercyhealthlovecounty.com

MERCY HOSPITAL ARDMORE (O, 190 beds) 1011 14th Avenue N.W., Ardmore, OK Zip 73401-1828; tel. 580/223-5400; Mindy Burdick, FACHE, President
**Web address:** www.mercyok.net

MERCY HOSPITAL EL RENO (O, 48 beds) 2115 Parkview Drive, El Reno, OK Zip 73036-2199, Mailing Address: P.O. Box 129, Zip 73036-0129; tel. 405/262-2640; Doug Danker, Administrator
**Web address:** www.mercyok.net

MERCY HOSPITAL HEALDTON (L, 22 beds) 3462 Hospital Road, Healdton, OK Zip 73438, Mailing Address: P.O. Box 928, Zip 73438; tel. 580/229-0701; Jeremy A. Jones, Administrator
**Web address:** www.mercyok.com

MERCY HOSPITAL LOGAN COUNTY (O, 25 beds) Highway 33 West at Academy Road, Guthrie, OK Zip 73044-3700, Mailing Address: P.O. Box 1017, Zip 73044-1017; tel. 405/282-6700; Joshua Tucker, Chief Executive Officer
**Web address:** www.loganmedicalcenter.com

---

For explanation of codes following names, see page B2.
★ Indicates Type III membership in the American Hospital Association.

MERCY HOSPITAL OKLAHOMA CITY (O, 369 beds) 4300 West Memorial Road, Oklahoma City, OK Zip 73120–8362; tel. 405/755–1515; Jim Gebhart, Jr., FACHE, President
**Web address:** www.mercyok.net

MERCY HOSPITAL TISHOMINGO (O, 25 beds) 1000 South Byrd Street, Tishomingo, OK Zip 73460–3299; tel. 580/371–2327; Richard Barker, Interim Chief Executive Officer
**Web address:** www.mercy.net/

VALLEY VIEW REGIONAL HOSPITAL (C, 131 beds) 430 North Monta Vista, Ada, OK Zip 74820–4610; tel. 580/332–2323; W. Kent Rogers, Chief Executive Officer
**Web address:** www.valleyviewregional.com

| | | |
|---|---|---|
| **Owned, leased, sponsored:** | 26 hospitals | 4026 beds |
| **Contract–managed:** | 5 hospitals | 211 beds |
| **Totals:** | 31 hospitals | 4237 beds |

---

**0649: MERCY HEALTH SYSTEM** (NP)
1000 Mineral Point Avenue, Janesville, WI Zip 53548–2940, Mailing Address: P.O. Box 5003, Zip 53547–5003; tel. 608/756–6000; Javon R. Bea, President and Chief Executive Officer
**(Centralized Physician/Insurance Health System)**

**ILLINOIS:** MERCY HARVARD HOSPITAL (O, 54 beds) 901 Grant Street, Harvard, IL Zip 60033–1898, Mailing Address: P.O. Box 850, Zip 60033–0850; tel. 815/943–5431; Jennifer Hallatt, Chief Operating Officer
**Web address:** www.mercyhealthsystem.org

**WISCONSIN:** MERCY HOSPITAL AND TRAUMA CENTER (O, 148 beds) 1000 Mineral Point Avenue, Janesville, WI Zip 53547–2982, Mailing Address: P.O. Box 5003, Zip 53547–5003; tel. 608/756–6000; Javon R. Bea, President and Chief Executive Officer
**Web address:** www.mercyhealthsystem.org

MERCY WALWORTH HOSPITAL AND MEDICAL CENTER (O, 6 beds) N2950 State Road 67, Lake Geneva, WI Zip 53147; tel. 262/245–0535; Jennifer Hallatt, Administrator
**Web address:** www.mercyhealthsystem.org

| | | |
|---|---|---|
| **Owned, leased, sponsored:** | 3 hospitals | 208 beds |
| **Contract–managed:** | 0 hospitals | 0 beds |
| **Totals:** | 3 hospitals | 208 beds |

---

**★0257: MERIDIAN HEALTH** (NP)
1350 Campus Parkway, Neptune, NJ Zip 07753; tel. 732/751–7510; John K. Lloyd, President and Chief Executive Officer
**(Centralized Health System)**

**NEW JERSEY:** BAYSHORE COMMUNITY HOSPITAL (O, 142 beds) 727 North Beers Street, Holmdel, NJ Zip 07733–1598; tel. 732/739–5900; Anthony V. Cava, Executive Director
**Web address:** www.bchs.com

JERSEY SHORE UNIVERSITY MEDICAL CENTER (O, 540 beds) 1945 Route 33, Neptune, NJ Zip 07754–0397; tel. 732/775–5500; Steven G. Littleson, FACHE, President
**Web address:** www.meridianhealth.com

OCEAN MEDICAL CENTER (O, 265 beds) 425 Jack Martin Boulevard, Brick Township, NJ Zip 08724; tel. 732/840–2200; Dean Q. Lin, FACHE, President
**Web address:** www.meridianhealth.com

RIVERVIEW MEDICAL CENTER (O, 270 beds) 1 Riverview Plaza, Red Bank, NJ Zip 07701–9982; tel. 732/741–2700; Timothy J. Hogan, FACHE, President
**Web address:** www.riverviewmedicalcenter.com

SOUTHERN OCEAN MEDICAL CENTER (O, 176 beds) 1140 Route 72 West, Manahawkin, NJ Zip 08050–2499; tel. 609/978–8900; Joseph P. Coyle, President and Chief Executive Officer
**Web address:** www.soch.com

| | | |
|---|---|---|
| **Owned, leased, sponsored:** | 5 hospitals | 1393 beds |
| **Contract–managed:** | 0 hospitals | 0 beds |
| **Totals:** | 5 hospitals | 1393 beds |

---

**★2735: METHODIST HEALTH SYSTEM** (NP)
1441 North Beckley Avenue, Dallas, TX Zip 75203–1201, Mailing Address: P.O. Box 655999, Zip 75265–5999; tel. 214/947–8181; Stephen L. Mansfield, Ph.D., FACHE, President and Chief Executive Officer
**(Independent Hospital System)**

**TEXAS:** METHODIST CHARLTON MEDICAL CENTER (O, 258 beds) 3500 West Wheatland Road, Dallas, TX Zip 75237–3460, Mailing Address: P.O. Box 225357, Zip 75222–5357; tel. 214/947–7777; Jonathan S. Davis, FACHE, President
**Web address:** www.mhs.com

METHODIST DALLAS MEDICAL CENTER (O, 420 beds) 1441 North Beckley Avenue, Dallas, TX Zip 75203–1201, Mailing Address: P.O. Box 655999, Zip 75265–5999; tel. 214/947–8181; Laura Irvine, President
**Web address:** www.mhd.com

METHODIST HOSPITAL FOR SURGERY (O, 32 beds) 17101 North Dallas Parkway, Addison, TX Zip 75001–7103; tel. 469/248–3900; Chris Shoup, President
**Web address:** www.methodisthospitalforsurgery.com/

METHODIST MANSFIELD MEDICAL CENTER (O, 130 beds) 2700 East Broad Street, Mansfield, TX Zip 76063–5899; tel. 682/622–2000; John E. Phillips, FACHE, President and Chief Executive Officer
**Web address:** www.methodisthealthsystem.org

METHODIST MCKINNEY HOSPITAL (O, 23 beds) 8000 West Eldorado Parkway, McKinney, TX Zip 75070–5940; tel. 972/569–2700; Joseph Minissale, Interim President
**Web address:** www.methodistmckinneyhospital.com

METHODIST REHABILITATION HOSPITAL (O, 40 beds) 3020 West Wheatland Road, Dallas, TX Zip 75237–3537; tel. 972/708–8604; Barbara Mobley, Chief Executive Officer
**Web address:** www.methodist–rehab.com

METHODIST RICHARDSON MEDICAL CENTER (O, 147 beds) 401 West Campbell Road, Richardson, TX Zip 75080–3416; tel. 972/498–4000; E. Kenneth Hutchenrider, President
**Web address:** www.richardsonregional.com

| | | |
|---|---|---|
| **Owned, leased, sponsored:** | 7 hospitals | 1050 beds |
| **Contract–managed:** | 0 hospitals | 0 beds |
| **Totals:** | 7 hospitals | 1050 beds |

---

**9345: METHODIST LE BONHEUR HEALTHCARE** (CO)
1211 Union Avenue, Suite 700, Memphis, TN Zip 38104–6600; tel. 901/516–0543; Gary S. Shorb, President and Chief Executive Officer
**(Centralized Health System)**

**TENNESSEE:** METHODIST EXTENDED CARE HOSPITAL (O, 36 beds) 225 South Claybrook Street, Memphis, TN Zip 38104–3537; tel. 901/516–2152; Sandra Bailey–DeLeeuw, Administrator
**Web address:** www.methodisthealth.org

METHODIST HEALTHCARE MEMPHIS HOSPITALS (O, 1321 beds) 1265 Union Avenue, Memphis, TN Zip 38104; tel. 901/516–7000; Kevin M. Spiegel, FACHE, Chief Executive Officer
**Web address:** www.methodisthealth.org

METHODIST HEALTHCARE–FAYETTE HOSPITAL (O, 10 beds) 214 Lakeview Drive, Somerville, TN Zip 38068–9737; tel. 901/516–4000; David Crislip, Administrator
**Web address:** www.methodisthealth.org

| | | |
|---|---|---|
| **Owned, leased, sponsored:** | 3 hospitals | 1367 beds |
| **Contract–managed:** | 0 hospitals | 0 beds |
| **Totals:** | 3 hospitals | 1367 beds |

---

**0208: MID ATLANTIC HEALTH MANAGEMENT, INC.** (IO)
1220 Butterworth Court, Stevensville, MD Zip 21666–2504; tel. 410/643–3393; Harold A. McBee, Jr., President
**(Independent Hospital System)**

**WEST VIRGINIA:** POTOMAC VALLEY HOSPITAL (O, 25 beds) 100 Pin Oak Lane, Keyser, WV Zip 26726–2699; tel. 304/597–3500; Linda K. Shroyer, Administrator
**Web address:** www.potomacvalleyhospital.com

---

For explanation of codes following names, see page B2.
★ Indicates Type III membership in the American Hospital Association.

Section B

**WISCONSIN:** INDIANHEAD MEDICAL CENTER (O, 25 beds) 113 Fourth Avenue, Shell Lake, WI Zip 54871; Mailing Address: P.O. Box 300, Zip 54871–0300; tel. 715/468–7833; Paul Naglosky, Administrator
**Web address:** www.indianheadmedicalcenter.com

| Owned, leased, sponsored: | 2 hospitals | 50 beds |
| Contract–managed: | 0 hospitals | 0 beds |
| Totals: | 2 hospitals | 50 beds |

---

**★0001: MIDMICHIGAN HEALTH** (NP)
4000 Wellness Drive, Midland, MI Zip 48670–0001; tel. 989/839–3000; Richard M. Reynolds, President and Chief Executive Officer
**(Centralized Health System)**

**MICHIGAN:** MIDMICHIGAN MEDICAL CENTER–CLARE (O, 49 beds) 703 North Mcewan Street, Clare, MI Zip 48617–1440; tel. 989/802–5000; Raymond Stover, President
**Web address:** www.midmichigan.org

MIDMICHIGAN MEDICAL CENTER–GLADWIN (O, 25 beds) 515 South Quarter Street, Gladwin, MI Zip 48624–1959; tel. 989/426–9286; Raymond Stover, President and Chief Executive Officer
**Web address:** www.midmichigan.org

MIDMICHIGAN MEDICAL CENTER–GRATIOT (O, 136 beds) 300 East Warwick Drive, Alma, MI Zip 48801–1014; tel. 989/463–1101; Mark A. Santamaria, President
**Web address:** www.midmichigan.org/gratiot

MIDMICHIGAN MEDICAL CENTER–MIDLAND (O, 250 beds) 4000 Wellness Drive, Midland, MI Zip 48670–0001; tel. 989/839–3000; Gregory H. Rogers, President
**Web address:** www.midmichigan.org

| Owned, leased, sponsored: | 4 hospitals | 460 beds |
| Contract–managed: | 0 hospitals | 0 beds |
| Totals: | 4 hospitals | 460 beds |

---

**0368: MINNESOTA DEPARTMENT OF HUMAN SERVICES** (NP)
540 Cedar Street, Saint Paul, MN Zip 55164–0980, Mailing Address: P.O. Box 64980, Zip 55164–0980; tel. 651/431–2369; Michael Tessneer, Chief Executive Officer
**(Independent Hospital System)**

**MINNESOTA:** ANOKA–METROPOLITAN REGIONAL TREATMENT CENTER (O, 112 beds) 3301 Seventh Avenue, Anoka, MN Zip 55303–1119; tel. 763/712–4000; David Hartford, Administrator
**Web address:** www.health.state.mn.us

COMMUNITY BEHAVIORAL HEALTH HOSPITAL – ALEXANDRIA (O, 16 beds) 1610 8th Avenue East, Alexandria, MN Zip 55308; tel. 320/335–6201; John A. Cosco, Ph.D., FACHE, Administrator
**Web address:** www.health.state.mn.us

COMMUNITY BEHAVIORAL HEALTH HOSPITAL – ANNANDALE (O, 16 beds) 400 Annandale Boulevard, Annandale, MN Zip 55302–3141; tel. 651/259–3850; Pamela R. Bajari, R.N., Interim Administrator
**Web address:** www.health.state.mn.us

COMMUNITY BEHAVIORAL HEALTH HOSPITAL – BAXTER (O, 16 beds) 14241 Grand Oaks Drive, Baxter, MN Zip 56425; tel. 218/316–3101; Richard G. Slieter, Jr., Administrator

COMMUNITY BEHAVIORAL HEALTH HOSPITAL – BEMIDJI (O, 16 beds) 800 Bemidji Avenue North, Bemidji, MN Zip 56601–3054; tel. 218/308–2400; Theresa Vander Eyck, Administrator

COMMUNITY BEHAVIORAL HEALTH HOSPITAL – FERGUS FALLS (O, 16 beds) 1801 West Alcott Avenue, Fergus Falls, MN Zip 56538–0478, Mailing Address: P.O. Box 478, Zip 56538–0478; tel. 218/332–5001; Derrick A. Jones, Administrator

COMMUNITY BEHAVIORAL HEALTH HOSPITAL – ROCHESTER (O, 16 beds) 251 Wood Lake Drive S.E., Rochester, MN Zip 55904; tel. 507/206–2561; Mark S. Lancet, Administrator
**Web address:** www.health.state.mn.us

COMMUNITY BEHAVIORAL HEALTH HOSPITAL – ST. PETER (O, 16 beds) 2000 Klein Street, Saint Peter, MN Zip 56082–5800; tel. 507/933–5001; Carol Olson, Administrator
**Web address:** www.health.state.mn.us

COMMUNITY BEHAVIORAL HEALTH HOSPITAL – WADENA (O, 16 beds) 240 Shady Lane Drive, Wadena, MN Zip 56482, Mailing Address: P.O. Box 430, Zip 56482–0430; tel. 218/319–6001; Richard G. Slieter, Jr., Administrator

| Owned, leased, sponsored: | 9 hospitals | 240 beds |
| Contract–managed: | 0 hospitals | 0 beds |
| Totals: | 9 hospitals | 240 beds |

---

**★0143: MISSION HEALTH SYSTEM** (CO)
509 Biltmore Avenue, Asheville, NC Zip 28801; tel. 828/213–1111; Ronald A. Paulus, M.D., President and Chief Executive Officer
**(Moderately Centralized Health System)**

**NORTH CAROLINA:** ANGEL MEDICAL CENTER (C, 25 beds) 120 Riverview Street, Franklin, NC Zip 28734, Mailing Address: P.O. Box 1209, Zip 28744; tel. 828/524–8411; Martin Wadewitz, Interim Chief Executive Officer
**Web address:** www.angelmed.org

ASHEVILLE SPECIALTY HOSPITAL (O, 31 beds) 428 Biltmore Avenue, 4th Floor, Asheville, NC Zip 28801; tel. 828/213–5400; Robert C. Desotelle, President and Chief Executive Officer
**Web address:** www.ashevillespecialtyhospital.org

BLUE RIDGE REGIONAL HOSPITAL (O, 42 beds) 125 Hospital Drive, Spruce Pine, NC Zip 28777, Mailing Address: P.O. Box 9, Zip 28777; tel. 828/765–4201; Oscar K. Weinmeister, III, Chief Executive Officer
**Web address:** www.spchospital.org

MCDOWELL HOSPITAL (O, 49 beds) 430 Rankin Drive, Marion, NC Zip 28752–6568, Mailing Address: P.O. Box 730, Zip 28752–0730; tel. 828/659–5000; Lynn Ingram Boggs, President and Chief Executive Officer
**Web address:** www.mcdhospital.org

MISSION HOSPITAL (O, 744 beds) 509 Biltmore Avenue, Asheville, NC Zip 28801–4690; tel. 828/213–1111; Ronald A. Paulus, M.D., President and Chief Executive Officer
**Web address:** www.missionhospitals.org

TRANSYLVANIA REGIONAL HOSPITAL (C, 52 beds) 260 Hospital Drive, Brevard, NC Zip 28712–1116; tel. 828/884–9111; Robert J. Bednarek, President and Chief Executive Officer
**Web address:** www.trhospital.org

| Owned, leased, sponsored: | 4 hospitals | 866 beds |
| Contract–managed: | 2 hospitals | 77 beds |
| Totals: | 6 hospitals | 943 beds |

---

**★0336: MISSISSIPPI BAPTIST HEALTH SYSTEM** (NP)
1225 North State Street, Jackson, MS Zip 39202–2002; tel. 601/968–1000; Mark F. Slyter, FACHE, President and Chief Executive Officer
**(Independent Hospital System)**

**MISSISSIPPI:** BAPTIST MEDICAL CENTER LEAKE (O, 69 beds) 310 Ellis Street, Carthage, MS Zip 39051–3809, Mailing Address: P.O. Box 909, Zip 39051–0909; tel. 601/267–1100; Wayne Walters, Chief Executive Officer
**Web address:** www.leakemh.org

MISSISSIPPI BAPTIST MEDICAL CENTER (O, 638 beds) 1225 North State Street, Jackson, MS Zip 39202–2002; tel. 601/968–1000; Kerry R. Tirman, JD, FACHE, President
**Web address:** www.mbhs.org

MISSISSIPPI HOSPITAL FOR RESTORATIVE CARE (O, 25 beds) 1225 North State Street, Jackson, MS Zip 39202–2097, Mailing Address: P.O. Box 23695, Zip 39225–3695; tel. 601/968–1000; Bobbie K. Ware, R.N., FACHE, Chief Executive Officer and Chief Nursing Officer
**Web address:** www.mbhs.org

| Owned, leased, sponsored: | 3 hospitals | 732 beds |
| Contract–managed: | 0 hospitals | 0 beds |
| Totals: | 3 hospitals | 732 beds |

---

For explanation of codes following names, see page B2.
★ Indicates Type III membership in the American Hospital Association.

**2475: MISSISSIPPI COUNTY HOSPITAL SYSTEM** (NP)
1520 North Division Street, Blytheville, AR Zip 72315–1448, Mailing Address: Box 108, Zip 72316; Ralph E. Beaty, Chief Executive Officer
**(Independent Hospital System)**

**ARKANSAS:** GREAT RIVER MEDICAL CENTER (O, 73 beds) 1520 North Division Street, Blytheville, AR Zip 72315–1448, Mailing Address: P.O. Box 108, Zip 72316–0108; tel. 870/838–7300; Ralph E. Beaty, Chief Executive Officer

SOUTH MISSISSIPPI COUNTY REGIONAL MEDICAL CENTER (O, 25 beds) 611 West Lee Avenue, Osceola, AR Zip 72370–3001, Mailing Address: P.O. Box 607, Zip 72370–0607; tel. 870/563–7000; Ralph E. Beaty, Chief Executive Officer
**Web address:** www.mchealthsystem.com

| | | |
|---|---|---|
| Owned, leased, sponsored: | 2 hospitals | 98 beds |
| Contract–managed: | 0 hospitals | 0 beds |
| Totals: | 2 hospitals | 98 beds |

**0017: MISSISSIPPI STATE DEPARTMENT OF MENTAL HEALTH** (NP)
1101 Robert East Lee Building, 239 North Lamar Street, Jackson, MS Zip 39201–1101; tel. 601/359–1288; Edwin C. LeGrand, III, Executive Director
**(Independent Hospital System)**

**MISSISSIPPI:** EAST MISSISSIPPI STATE HOSPITAL (O, 327 beds) 4555 Highland Park Drive, Meridian, MS Zip 39307–5498, Mailing Address: Box 4128, West Station, Zip 39304–4128; tel. 601/482–6186; Charles Carlisle, Director
**Web address:** www.emsh.state.ms.us

MISSISSIPPI STATE HOSPITAL (O, 938 beds) 3550 Highway 468 West, Whitfield, MS Zip 39193, Mailing Address: P.O. Box 157–A, Zip 39193–0157; tel. 601/351–8000; James G. Chastain, FACHE, Director
**Web address:** www.msh.state.ms.us

NORTH MISSISSIPPI STATE HOSPITAL (O, 50 beds) 1937 Briar Ridge Road, Tupelo, MS Zip 38804; tel. 662/690–4200; Paul A. Callens, Ph.D., Director
**Web address:** www.nmsh.state.ms.us

SOUTH MISSISSIPPI STATE HOSPITAL (O, 50 beds) 823 Highway 589, Purvis, MS Zip 39475–4194; tel. 601/794–0100; Clint Ashley, Director
**Web address:** www.smsh.state.ms.us

| | | |
|---|---|---|
| Owned, leased, sponsored: | 4 hospitals | 1365 beds |
| Contract–managed: | 0 hospitals | 0 beds |
| Totals: | 4 hospitals | 1365 beds |

**1335: MORTON PLANT MEASE HEALTH CARE** (NP)
300 Pinellas Street, Clearwater, FL Zip 33756, Mailing Address: P.O. Box 210, Zip 33756–0210; tel. 727/462–7000; Glenn D. Waters, FACHE, President

**FLORIDA:** MEASE COUNTRYSIDE HOSPITAL (O, 100 beds) 3231 McMullen–Booth Road, Safety Harbor, FL Zip 34695–1098, Mailing Address: P.O. Box 1098, Zip 34695–1098; tel. 727/725–6222; Glenn D. Waters, FACHE, President
**Web address:** www.mpmhealth.com

MEASE HOSPITAL DUNEDIN (O, 258 beds) 601 Main Street, Dunedin, FL Zip 34698–5891, Mailing Address: P.O. Box 760, Zip 34697–0760; tel. 727/733–1111; Glenn D. Waters, FACHE, President and Chief Executive Officer
**Web address:** www.mpmhealth.com

MORTON PLANT HOSPITAL (O, 524 beds) 300 Pinellas Street, Clearwater, FL Zip 33756–3825, Mailing Address: P.O. Box 210, Zip 33757–0210; tel. 727/462–7000; Glenn D. Waters, FACHE, President
**Web address:** www.mortonplant.com

MORTON PLANT NORTH BAY HOSPITAL (O, 122 beds) 6600 Madison Street, New Port Richey, FL Zip 34652–1900; tel. 727/842–8468; Glenn D. Waters, FACHE, President
**Web address:** www.mpmhealth.com

MORTON PLANT REHABILITATION CENTER (O, 126 beds) 400 Corbett Street, Belleair, FL Zip 34640; tel. 813/462–7600; Linda A. Kirk, Administrator

| | | |
|---|---|---|
| Owned, leased, sponsored: | 5 hospitals | 1130 beds |
| Contract–managed: | 0 hospitals | 0 beds |
| Totals: | 5 hospitals | 1130 beds |

**0167: MOUNTAIN STATES HEALTH ALLIANCE** (NP)
400 North State of Franklin Road, Johnson City, TN Zip 37604–6035; tel. 423/431–1040; Dennis Vonderfecht, President and Chief Executive Officer
**(Centralized Health System)**

**TENNESSEE:** FRANKLIN WOODS COMMUNITY HOSPITAL (O, 114 beds) 300 MedTech Parkway, Johnson City, TN Zip 37604–2277; tel. 423/302–1000; Tony Benton, Chief Executive Officer
**Web address:** www.msha.com

INDIAN PATH MEDICAL CENTER (O, 189 beds) 2000 Brookside Drive, Kingsport, TN Zip 37660–4627; tel. 423/857–7000; Monty E. McLaurin, President and Chief Executive Officer
**Web address:** www.msha.com

JOHNSON CITY MEDICAL CENTER (O, 514 beds) 400 North State of Franklin Road, Johnson City, TN Zip 37604–6094; tel. 423/431–6111; David E. Nicely, Chief Executive Officer
**Web address:** www.msha.com

JOHNSON COUNTY COMMUNITY HOSPITAL (O, 2 beds) 1901 South Shady Street, Mountain City, TN Zip 37683–2271; tel. 423/727–1100; Lisa Heaton, Administrator and Chief Nursing Officer
**Web address:** www.msha.com

QUILLEN REHABILITATION HOSPITAL (O, 47 beds) 2511 Wesley Street, Johnson City, TN Zip 37601–1723; tel. 423/283–0700; Ann Fleming, Senior Vice President
**Web address:** www.msha.com

SYCAMORE SHOALS HOSPITAL (O, 79 beds) 1501 West Elk Avenue, Elizabethton, TN Zip 37643–2874; tel. 423/542–1300; Dwayne Taylor, Chief Executive Officer
**Web address:** www.msha.com

WOODRIDGE HOSPITAL (O, 84 beds) 403 State of Franklin Road, Johnson City, TN Zip 37604–6034; tel. 423/431–7060; Grace Pereira, Interim Chief Executive Officer
**Web address:** www.msha.com

**VIRGINIA:** DICKENSON COMMUNITY HOSPITAL (O, 2 beds) 312 Hospital Drive, Clintwood, VA Zip 24228, Mailing Address: P.O. Box 1440, Zip 24228–1440; tel. 276/926–0300; Mark T. Leonard, Chief Executive Officer
**Web address:** www.dchosp.com

JOHNSTON MEMORIAL HOSPITAL (O, 100 beds) 16000 Johnston Memorial Drive, Abingdon, VA Zip 24211; tel. 276/676–7000; Sean S. McMurray, FACHE, Vice President and Chief Executive Officer
**Web address:** www.jmh.org

NORTON COMMUNITY HOSPITAL (O, 40 beds) 100 15th Street N.W., Norton, VA Zip 24273–1616; tel. 276/679–9600; Mark T. Leonard, Chief Executive Officer
**Web address:** www.nchosp.org

RUSSELL COUNTY MEDICAL CENTER (O, 78 beds) 58 Carroll Street, Lebanon, VA Zip 24266, Mailing Address: P.O. Box 3600, Zip 24266–0200; tel. 276/883–8000; Edward C. Greene, Jr., Assistant Vice President and Administrator
**Web address:** www.rcmc.net

SMYTH COUNTY COMMUNITY HOSPITAL (O, 151 beds) 243 Medical Park Drive, Marion, VA Zip 24354, Mailing Address: P.O. Box 880, Zip 24354–0880; tel. 276/378–1000; Lindy P. White, President and Chief Executive Officer
**Web address:** www.msha.com/hospitals/smyth_county_community_hospital_l_marion_va.aspx

| | | |
|---|---|---|
| Owned, leased, sponsored: | 12 hospitals | 1400 beds |
| Contract–managed: | 0 hospitals | 0 beds |
| Totals: | 12 hospitals | 1400 beds |

For explanation of codes following names, see page B2.
★ Indicates Type III membership in the American Hospital Association.

**6555: MULTICARE HEALTH SYSTEM** (NP)
315 Martin Luther King Jr. Way, Tacoma, WA Zip 98415, Mailing Address: P.O. Box 5299, Zip 98415–0299; tel. 253/403–1000; Diane E. Cecchettini, R.N., President and Chief Executive Officer
**(Moderately Centralized Health System)**

**WASHINGTON:** MULTICARE GOOD SAMARITAN HOSPITAL (O, 256 beds) 407 14th Avenue S.E., Puyallup, WA Zip 98372–0118, Mailing Address: P.O. Box 1247, Zip 98371–1247; tel. 253/697–4000; Glenn Kasman, President and Chief Executive Officer
**Web address:** www.goodsamhealth.org

MULTICARE MARY BRIDGE CHILDREN'S HOSPITAL AND HEALTH CENTER (O, 72 beds) 317 Martin Luther King Jr. Way, Tacoma, WA Zip 98405–0299, Mailing Address: P.O. Box 5299, Zip 98415–0299; tel. 253/403–1400; Mady Murrey, R.N., Vice President and Administrator
**Web address:** www.multicare.org/marybridge

MULTICARE TACOMA GENERAL HOSPITAL (O, 420 beds) 315 Martin Luther King Jr. Way, Tacoma, WA Zip 98405–0299, Mailing Address: P.O. Box 5299, Zip 98415–0299; tel. 253/403–1000; Diane E. Cecchettini, R.N., President and Chief Executive Officer
**Web address:** www.multicare.org

| | | |
|---|---|---|
| Owned, leased, sponsored: | 3 hospitals | 748 beds |
| Contract–managed: | 0 hospitals | 0 beds |
| Totals: | 3 hospitals | 748 beds |

★**1465: MUNSON HEALTHCARE** (NP)
1105 Sixth Street, Traverse City, MI Zip 49684–2386; tel. 231/935–6703; Edwin Ness, President and Chief Executive Officer
**(Centralized Physician/Insurance Health System)**

**MICHIGAN:** KALKASKA MEMORIAL HEALTH CENTER (O, 96 beds) 419 South Coral Street, Kalkaska, MI Zip 49646–2503; tel. 231/258–7500; James D. Austin, FACHE, Administrator
**Web address:** www.munsonhealthcare.org

MUNSON MEDICAL CENTER (O, 391 beds) 1105 Sixth Street, Traverse City, MI Zip 49684–2345; tel. 231/935–5000; Edwin Ness, President and Chief Executive Officer
**Web address:** www.munsonhealthcare.org

PAUL OLIVER MEMORIAL HOSPITAL (O, 47 beds) 224 Park Avenue, Frankfort, MI Zip 49635–9658; tel. 231/352–2200; James D. Austin, FACHE, Administrator
**Web address:** www.munsonhealthcare.org

| | | |
|---|---|---|
| Owned, leased, sponsored: | 3 hospitals | 534 beds |
| Contract–managed: | 0 hospitals | 0 beds |
| Totals: | 3 hospitals | 534 beds |

**0261: NATIONAL SURGICAL HOSPITALS** (IO)
250 South Wacker Drive, Suite 500, Chicago, IL Zip 60606; tel. 312/627–8400; John G. Rex–Waller, Chief Executive Officer
**(Independent Hospital System)**

**ARIZONA:** ARIZONA SPINE AND JOINT HOSPITAL (O, 23 beds) 4620 East Baseline Road, Mesa, AZ Zip 85206; tel. 480/832–4770; Kristi McShay, Chief Executive Officer
**Web address:** www.azspineandjoint.com

**IDAHO:** NORTHWEST SPECIALTY HOSPITAL (O, 22 beds) 1593 East Polston Avenue, Post Falls, ID Zip 83854; tel. 208/262–2300; Ron Rock, Chief Executive Officer
**Web address:** www.northwestspecialtyhospital.com

**LOUISIANA:** LAFAYETTE SURGICAL SPECIALTY HOSPITAL (O, 20 beds) 1101 Kaliste Saloom Road, Lafayette, LA Zip 70508; tel. 337/769–4100; Buffy Domingue, Chief Executive Officer
**Web address:** www.lafayettesurgical.com

**MICHIGAN:** SOUTHEAST MICHIGAN SURGICAL HOSPITAL (O, 13 beds) 21230 Dequindre, Warren, MI Zip 48091–2287; tel. 586/427–1000; John Kolozsvary, Chief Executive Officer
**Web address:** www.nshinc.com

**NEW MEXICO:** PHYSICIANS MEDICAL CENTER OF SANTA FE HOSPITAL (O, 12 beds) 2990 Rodeo Park Drive East, Santa Fe, NM Zip 87505; tel. 505/428–5400; Lloyd Scarrow, Chief Executive Officer
**Web address:** www.pmchospital.com

**NORTH CAROLINA:** NORTH CAROLINA SPECIALTY HOSPITAL (O, 18 beds) 3916 Ben Franklin Boulevard, Durham, NC Zip 27704; tel. 919/956–9300; Randi L. Shults, Chief Executive Officer
**Web address:** www.ncspecialty.com

**TEXAS:** EL PASO SPECIALTY HOSPITAL (O, 27 beds) 1755 Curie Drive, El Paso, TX Zip 79902–2919; tel. 915/544–3636; James Wilcox, Chief Executive Officer
**Web address:** www.elpasospecialtyhospital.com

SOUTH TEXAS SPINE AND SURGICAL HOSPITAL (O, 30 beds) 18600 Hardy Oak Boulevard, San Antonio, TX Zip 78258; tel. 210/507–4090; Debbie Kelly, Chief Executive Officer
**Web address:** www.shst.net

SOUTH TEXAS SURGICAL HOSPITAL (O, 20 beds) 6130 Parkway Drive, Corpus Christi, TX Zip 78414–2455; tel. 361/993–2000; James Murphy, Chief Executive Officer
**Web address:** www.nshinc.com

SOUTHWEST SURGICAL HOSPITAL (O, 23 beds) 1612 Hurst Town Center Drive, Hurst, TX Zip 76054–6236; tel. 817/345–4100; Harold Stigler, Chief Executive Officer
**Web address:** www.swsurgery.com

**UTAH:** CACHE VALLEY SPECIALTY HOSPITAL (O, 15 beds) 2380 North 400 East, North Logan, UT Zip 84341; tel. 435/713–9700; John C. Worley, Jr., Chief Executive Officer
**Web address:** www.cvsh.com

**WISCONSIN:** OAKLEAF SURGICAL HOSPITAL (O, 13 beds) 3802 West Oakwood Mall Drive, Eau Claire, WI Zip 54701; tel. 715/831–8130; Anne Hargrave–Thomas, Chief Executive Officer
**Web address:** www.oakleafmedical.com

| | | |
|---|---|---|
| Owned, leased, sponsored: | 12 hospitals | 236 beds |
| Contract–managed: | 0 hospitals | 0 beds |
| Totals: | 12 hospitals | 236 beds |

★**9265: NEBRASKA METHODIST HEALTH SYSTEM, INC.** (CO)
8511 West Dodge Road, Omaha, NE Zip 68114; tel. 402/354–5411; John M. Fraser, President and Chief Executive Officer
**(Moderately Centralized Health System)**

**IOWA:** JENNIE EDMUNDSON HOSPITAL (O, 114 beds) 933 East Pierce Street, Council Bluffs, IA Zip 51503–4652, Mailing Address: P.O. Box 2C, Zip 51502–3002; tel. 712/396–6000; Steven P. Baumert, President and Chief Executive Officer
**Web address:** www.bestcare.org

**NEBRASKA:** NEBRASKA METHODIST HOSPITAL (O, 460 beds) 8303 Dodge Street, Omaha, NE Zip 68114–4108; tel. 402/354–4000; Stephen L. Goeser, FACHE, President and Chief Executive Officer
**Web address:** www.bestcare.org

| | | |
|---|---|---|
| Owned, leased, sponsored: | 2 hospitals | 574 beds |
| Contract–managed: | 0 hospitals | 0 beds |
| Totals: | 2 hospitals | 574 beds |

★**0213: NEW HANOVER REGIONAL MEDICAL CENTER** (NP)
2131 South 17th Street, Wilmington, NC Zip 28401–9000; tel. 910/343–7040; John K. Barto, Jr., President and Chief Executive Officer
**(Moderately Centralized Health System)**

**NORTH CAROLINA:** NEW HANOVER REGIONAL MEDICAL CENTER (O, 709 beds) 2131 South 17th Street, Wilmington, NC Zip 28401–7483, Mailing Address: P.O. Box 1990, Zip 28402–9000; tel. 910/343–7000; John K. Barto, Jr., President and Chief Executive Officer
**Web address:** www.nhhn.org

PENDER MEMORIAL HOSPITAL (C, 68 beds) 507 East Freemont Street, Burgaw, NC Zip 28425–5131; tel. 910/259–5451; Ruth Glaser, President
**Web address:** www.pendermemorial.org

For explanation of codes following names, see page B2.
★ Indicates Type III membership in the American Hospital Association.

| | | |
|---|---|---|
| Owned, leased, sponsored: | 1 hospital | 709 beds |
| Contract–managed: | 1 hospital | 68 beds |
| Totals: | 2 hospitals | 777 beds |

**★3075: NEW YORK CITY HEALTH AND HOSPITALS CORPORATION** (NP)
125 Worth Street, Room 514, New York, NY Zip 10013–4006;
tel. 212/788–3321; Alan D. Aviles, President
**(Decentralized Health System)**

**NEW YORK:** BELLEVUE HOSPITAL CENTER (O, 828 beds) 462 First Avenue, New York, NY Zip 10016–9198; tel. 212/562–4141; Lynda D. Curtis, Senior Vice President and Executive Director
**Web address:** www.nyc.gov/bellevue

COLER–GOLDWATER SPECIALTY HOSPITAL AND NURSING FACILITY (O, 2016 beds) One Main Street, New York, NY Zip 10044; tel. 212/318–8000; Robert Hughes, Executive Director
**Web address:** www.coler–goldwater.org

CONEY ISLAND HOSPITAL (O, 371 beds) 2601 Ocean Parkway, Brooklyn, NY Zip 11235–7795; tel. 718/616–3000; Arthur Wagner, Senior Vice President and Executive Director
**Web address:** www.ci.nyc.ny.us/html/hhc/html/coneyisland.html

ELMHURST HOSPITAL CENTER (O, 551 beds) 79–01 Broadway, Elmhurst, NY Zip 11373–1329; tel. 718/334–4000; Chris D. Constantino, Executive Director
**Web address:** www.elmhursthospitalcenter.org

GOUVERNEUR HOSPITAL (O, 196 beds) 227 Madison Street, New York, NY Zip 10002; tel. 212/238–7000; Gregory M. Kaladjian, Executive Director

HARLEM HOSPITAL CENTER (O, 272 beds) 506 Lenox Avenue, New York, NY Zip 10037–1894; tel. 212/939–1000; Denise C. Soares, R.N., Executive Director
**Web address:** www.nyc.gov/html/hhc/harlem

JACOBI MEDICAL CENTER (O, 457 beds) 1400 Pelham Parkway South, Bronx, NY Zip 10461–1197; tel. 718/918–5000; William P. Walsh, Senior Vice President and Executive Director
**Web address:** www.nyc.gov/html/hhc/jacobi/home.html

KINGS COUNTY HOSPITAL CENTER (O, 601 beds) 451 Clarkson Avenue, Brooklyn, NY Zip 11203–2097; tel. 718/245–3131; Antonio D. Martin, Senior Vice President and Executive Director
**Web address:** www.ci.nyc.ny.us/html/hhc/html/kings.html

LINCOLN MEDICAL AND MENTAL HEALTH CENTER (O, 335 beds) 234 East 149th Street, Bronx, NY Zip 10451–5504; tel. 718/579–5700; Iris Jimenez–Hernandez, Senior Vice President and Executive Director
**Web address:** www.nyc.gov/html/hhc/lincoln

METROPOLITAN HOSPITAL CENTER (O, 349 beds) 1901 First Avenue, New York, NY Zip 10029–7404; tel. 212/423–6262; Meryl Weinberg, Executive Director
**Web address:** www.nyc.gov/html/hhc/metropolitan.html

NORTH CENTRAL BRONX HOSPITAL (O, 213 beds) 3424 Kossuth Avenue, Bronx, NY Zip 10467–2489; tel. 718/519–3500; William P. Walsh, Director
**Web address:** www.ci.nyc.ny.us/html/hhc/html/northcentralbronx.html

QUEENS HOSPITAL CENTER (O, 303 beds) 82–68 164th Street, Jamaica, NY Zip 11432–1104; tel. 718/883–3000; Julius Wool, Executive Director
**Web address:** www.nyc.gov/html/hhc/qhc/html/home/home.shtml

SEA VIEW HOSPITAL REHABILITATION CENTER AND HOME (O, 304 beds) 460 Brielle Avenue, Staten Island, NY Zip 10314; tel. 212/390–8181; Jane M. Lyons, Executive Director

WOODHULL MEDICAL AND MENTAL HEALTH CENTER (O, 346 beds) 760 Broadway, Brooklyn, NY Zip 11206–5383; tel. 718/963–8000; George M. Proctor, Senior Vice President and Executive Director
**Web address:** www.nyc.gov/html/hhc

| | | |
|---|---|---|
| Owned, leased, sponsored: | 14 hospitals | 7142 beds |
| Contract–managed: | 0 hospitals | 0 beds |
| Totals: | 14 hospitals | 7142 beds |

**0142: NEW YORK PRESBYTERIAN HEALTHCARE SYSTEM** (NP)
177 Fort Washington Avenue, Room P123, New York, NY Zip 10032; tel. 212/746–3745; Steven J. Corwin, M.D., Chief Executive Officer
**(Moderately Centralized Health System)**

BROOKLYN HOSPITAL CENTER (S, 374 beds) 121 DeKalb Avenue, Brooklyn, NY Zip 11201–5425; tel. 718/250–8000; Richard B. Becker, M.D., President, Chief Executive Officer and Interim Chief Medical Officer
**Web address:** www.tbh.org

GRACIE SQUARE HOSPITAL (S, 157 beds) 420 East 76th Street, New York, NY Zip 10021–3104; tel. 212/988–4400; Frank Bruno, Chief Executive Officer
**Web address:** www.nygsh.org

HOSPITAL FOR SPECIAL SURGERY (S, 188 beds) 535 East 70th Street, New York, NY Zip 10021–4898; tel. 212/606–1000; Louis A. Shapiro, President and Chief Executive Officer
**Web address:** www.hss.edu

NEW YORK COMMUNITY HOSPITAL (S, 125 beds) 2525 Kings Highway, Brooklyn, NY Zip 11229–1798, Mailing Address: 2513 Avenue O, Zip 11210–5230; tel. 718/692–5300; Lin H. Mo, President and Chief Executive Officer
**Web address:** www.nych.com

NEW YORK HOSPITAL QUEENS (S, 519 beds) 56–45 Main Street, Flushing, NY Zip 11355–5000; tel. 718/670–1231; Stephen S. Mills, President and Chief Executive Officer
**Web address:** www.nyhq.org

NEW YORK METHODIST HOSPITAL (S, 591 beds) 506 Sixth Street, Brooklyn, NY Zip 11215–3609; tel. 718/780–3000; Mark J. Mundy, President and Chief Executive Officer
**Web address:** www.nym.org

NEW YORK WESTCHESTER SQUARE MEDICAL CENTER (S, 140 beds) 2475 Saint Raymonds Avenue, Bronx, NY Zip 10461–3124; tel. 718/430–7300; Alan Kopman, FACHE, President and Chief Executive Officer
**Web address:** www.nywsmc.org

NEW YORK–PRESBYTERIAN HOSPITAL (O, 2264 beds) 525 East 68th Street, New York, NY Zip 10065–4870; tel. 212/746–5454; Steven J. Corwin, M.D., Chief Executive Officer
**Web address:** www.nyp.org

NYACK HOSPITAL (S, 375 beds) 160 North Midland Avenue, Nyack, NY Zip 10960–1998; tel. 845/348–2000; David H. Freed, President and Chief Executive Officer
**Web address:** www.nyackhospital.org

| | | |
|---|---|---|
| Owned, leased, sponsored: | 9 hospitals | 4733 beds |
| Contract–managed: | 0 hospitals | 0 beds |
| Totals: | 9 hospitals | 4733 beds |

**0009: NEW YORK STATE OFFICE OF MENTAL HEALTH** (NP)
44 Holland Avenue, Albany, NY Zip 12229–3411; tel. 518/474–4403; Michael F. Hogan, Ph.D., Commissioner
**(Independent Hospital System)**

BRONX CHILDREN'S PSYCHIATRIC CENTER (O, 75 beds) 1000 Waters Place, Bronx, NY Zip 10461–2799; tel. 718/239–3600; June Dacosta, Acting Executive Director
**Web address:** www.omh.ny.gov

BRONX PSYCHIATRIC CENTER (O, 450 beds) 1500 Waters Place, Bronx, NY Zip 10461–2796; tel. 718/931–0600; Pamela Turner, Executive Director
**Web address:** www.omh.ny.gov

BROOKLYN CHILDREN'S PSYCHIATRIC CENTER (O, 36 beds) 1819 Bergen Street, Brooklyn, NY Zip 11233–4513; tel. 718/221–4500; Diane Aman, Acting Executive Director
**Web address:** www.omh.ny.gov

BUFFALO PSYCHIATRIC CENTER (O, 240 beds) 400 Forest Avenue, Buffalo, NY Zip 14213–1298; tel. 716/885–2261; Thomas Dodson, Executive Director
**Web address:** www.omh.ny.gov

CAPITAL DISTRICT PSYCHIATRIC CENTER (O, 200 beds) 75 New Scotland Avenue, Albany, NY Zip 12208–3474; tel. 518/447–9611; Lewis Campbell, Executive Director
**Web address:** www.omh.ny.gov/omhweb/facilities/cdpc/facility.htm

For explanation of codes following names, see page B2.
★ Indicates Type III membership in the American Hospital Association.

CENTRAL NEW YORK PSYCHIATRIC CENTER (O, 226 beds) Marcy, NY Zip 13403; tel. 315/765–3600; Maureen Bosco, Interim Executive Director
**Web address:** www.omh.ny.gov

CREEDMOOR PSYCHIATRIC CENTER (O, 380 beds) 79–25 Winchester Boulevard, Jamaica, NY Zip 11427–2199; tel. 718/264–3600; William A. Fisher, M.D., Executive Director
**Web address:** www.omh.ny.gov

ELMIRA PSYCHIATRIC CENTER (O, 100 beds) 100 Washington Street, Elmira, NY Zip 14901–2898; tel. 607/737–4739; Mark Stephany, Executive Director
**Web address:** www.omh.ny.gov/omhweb/facilities/elpc/facility.htm

GREATER BINGHAMTON HEALTH CENTER (O, 115 beds) 425 Robinson Street, Binghamton, NY Zip 13904–1735; tel. 607/724–1391; Margaret R. Dugan, Executive Director
**Web address:** www.omh.ny.gov/omhweb/facilities/bipc/facility.htm

KINGSBORO PSYCHIATRIC CENTER (O, 290 beds) 681 Clarkson Avenue, Brooklyn, NY Zip 11203–2125; tel. 718/221–7395; James McCummings, Executive Director
**Web address:** www.omh.ny.gov/omhweb/facilities/kbpc/facility/htm

MANHATTAN PSYCHIATRIC CENTER–WARD'S ISLAND (O, 745 beds) 600 East 125th Street, New York, NY Zip 10035–9998; tel. 646/672–6767; Stephen Rabinowitz, Executive Director
**Web address:** www.omh.ny.gov

MID–HUDSON FORENSIC PSYCHIATRIC CENTER (O, 268 beds) Route 17M, New Hampton, NY Zip 10958, Mailing Address: P.O. Box 158, Zip 10958–0158; tel. 845/374–8700; Peggi Healy, Executive Director
**Web address:** www.omh.ny.gov

MOHAWK VALLEY PSYCHIATRIC CENTER (O, 614 beds) 1400 Noyes Street, Utica, NY Zip 13502–3803; tel. 315/738–3800; Colleen A. Sawyer, R.N., MSN, Executive Director
**Web address:** www.omh.ny.gov/omhweb/facilities/mvpc/facility.htm

NEW YORK STATE PSYCHIATRIC INSTITUTE (O, 58 beds) 1051 Riverside Drive, New York, NY Zip 10032–1007; tel. 212/543–5000; Jeffrey A. Lieberman, M.D., Executive Director
**Web address:** www.nyspi.org

PILGRIM PSYCHIATRIC CENTER (O, 569 beds) 998 Crooked Hill Road, Brentwood, NY Zip 11717–1087; tel. 631/761–3500; Dean R. Weinstock, R.N., Executive Director
**Web address:** www.omh.ny.gov/omhweb/facilities/pgpc/facility.htm

QUEENS CHILDREN'S PSYCHIATRIC CENTER (O, 84 beds) 74–03 Commonwealth Boulevard, Jamaica, NY Zip 11426–1890; tel. 718/264–4506; June Dacosta, Acting Executive Director
**Web address:** www.omh.ny.gov

RICHARD H. HUTCHINGS PSYCHIATRIC CENTER (O, 131 beds) 620 Madison Street, Syracuse, NY Zip 13210–2319; tel. 315/426–3632; Colleen A. Sawyer, R.N., MSN, Executive Director
**Web address:** www.omh.ny.gov

ROCHESTER PSYCHIATRIC CENTER (O, 180 beds) 1111 Elmwood Avenue, Rochester, NY Zip 14620–3005; tel. 585/241–1200; Michael P. Zuber, Ph.D., Executive Director
**Web address:** www.omh.ny.gov/omhweb/facilities/ropc/facility.htm

ROCKLAND CHILDREN'S PSYCHIATRIC CENTER (O, 54 beds) 599 Convent Road, Orangeburg, NY Zip 10962; tel. 845/359–7400; Raul Silva, M.D., Executive Director
**Web address:** www.omh.ny.gov/

ROCKLAND PSYCHIATRIC CENTER (O, 525 beds) 140 Old Orangeburg Road, Orangeburg, NY Zip 10962–0071; tel. 845/359–1000; James H. Bopp, Executive Director
**Web address:** www.omh.ny.gov/

SAGAMORE CHILDREN'S PSYCHIATRIC CENTER (O, 69 beds) 197 Half Hollow Road, Dix Hills, NY Zip 11746–5861; tel. 631/370–1700; Tom McOlvin, Executive Director
**Web address:** www.omh.ny.gov

SOUTH BEACH PSYCHIATRIC CENTER (O, 340 beds) 777 Seaview Avenue, Staten Island, NY Zip 10305–3409; tel. 718/667–2300; Thomas Uttaro, Executive Director
**Web address:** www.omh.ny.gov

ST. LAWRENCE PSYCHIATRIC CENTER (O, 146 beds) 1 Chimney Point Drive, Ogdensburg, NY Zip 13669–2291; tel. 315/541–2001; Samua A. Bastien, IV, Ph.D., Executive Director
**Web address:** www.omh.ny.gov/omhweb/facilities/slpc/facility.htm

WESTERN NEW YORK CHILDREN'S PSYCHIATRIC CENTER (O, 46 beds) 1010 East and West Road, West Seneca, NY Zip 14224–3602; tel. 716/677–7000; Kathe Hayes, Executive Director
**Web address:** www.omh.ny.gov

| | | |
|---|---|---|
| Owned, leased, sponsored: | 24 hospitals | 5941 beds |
| Contract–managed: | 0 hospitals | 0 beds |
| **Totals:** | 24 hospitals | 5941 beds |

**0353: NEXUS HEALTH SYSTEMS** (IO)
One Riverway, Suite 600, Houston, TX Zip 77056; tel. 713/355–6111; John W. Cassidy, M.D., President, Chief Executive Officer and Chief Medical Officer
**(Independent Hospital System)**

**CALIFORNIA:** HEALTHBRIDGE CHILDRENS REHABILITATION HOSPITAL (O, 27 beds) 393 South Tustin Street, Orange, CA Zip 92868; tel. 714/289–2400; Ronell Myburgh, Administrator
**Web address:** www.nhsltd.com/HealthBridge–Orange/Default.htm

**TEXAS:** HEALTHBRIDGE CHILDREN'S HOSPITAL OF HOUSTON (O, 40 beds) 2929 Woodland Park Drive, Houston, TX Zip 77082; tel. 281/293–7774; Joseph Rafferty, Chief Executive Officer
**Web address:** www.healthbridgehouston.com/

NEXUS SPECIALTY HOSPITAL (O, 75 beds) 123 Vision Park Boulevard, Shenandoah, TX Zip 77384; tel. 281/364–0317; Erin Cassidy, Chief Executive Officer
**Web address:** www.nexusspecialty.com

| | | |
|---|---|---|
| Owned, leased, sponsored: | 3 hospitals | 142 beds |
| Contract–managed: | 0 hospitals | 0 beds |
| **Totals:** | 3 hospitals | 142 beds |

**0349: NOLAND HEALTH SERVICES, INC.** (NP)
600 Corporate Parkway, Suite 100, Birmingham, AL Zip 35242; tel. 205/783–8484; Gary M. Glasscock, President and Chief Executive Officer

**ALABAMA:** NOLAND HOSPITAL ANNISTON (O, 34 beds) 400 East 10th Street, 4th Floor, Anniston, AL Zip 36207; tel. 256/741–6141; Bob Notarianni, Administrator
**Web address:** www.nolandhealth.com

NOLAND HOSPITAL BIRMINGHAM (O, 23 beds) 50 Medical Park East Drive, 8th Floor, Birmingham, AL Zip 35235; tel. 205/808–5100; Thomas P. Harlan, Administrator
**Web address:** www.nolandhealth.com

NOLAND HOSPITAL DOTHAN (O, 30 beds) 1108 Ross Clark Circle, 4th Floor, Dothan, AL Zip 36302; tel. 334/699–4300; Kaye Burke, Administrator
**Web address:** www.nolandhealth.com

NOLAND HOSPITAL MONTGOMERY (O, 36 beds) 1725 Pine Street, 5 North, Montgomery, AL Zip 36106–1109; tel. 334/240–0532; John Heffner, Interim Administrator
**Web address:** www.nolandhealth.com

NOLAND HOSPITAL SHELBY (O, 52 beds) 1000 First Street North, 3rd Floor, Alabaster, AL Zip 35007–8703; tel. 205/620–8641; Laura S. Wills, Administrator
**Web address:** www.nolandhospitals.com/nhs.html

NOLAND HOSPITAL TUSCALOOSA (O, 27 beds) 809 University Boulevard E, 4th Floor, Tuscaloosa, AL Zip 35401; tel. 205/759–7241; Dale Jones, Administrator
**Web address:** www.nolandhealth.com

| | | |
|---|---|---|
| Owned, leased, sponsored: | 6 hospitals | 202 beds |
| Contract–managed: | 0 hospitals | 0 beds |
| **Totals:** | 6 hospitals | 202 beds |

★**0032: NORTH MISSISSIPPI HEALTH SERVICES, INC.** (NP)
830 South Gloster Street, Tupelo, MS Zip 38801–4996; tel. 662/377–3136; John R. Heer, President and Chief Executive Officer
**(Centralized Physician/Insurance Health System)**

For explanation of codes following names, see page B2.
★ Indicates Type III membership in the American Hospital Association.

NORTH MISSISSIPPI MEDICAL CENTER–HAMILTON (O, 36 beds) 1256 Military Street South, Hamilton, AL Zip 35570–5001; tel. 205/921–6200; Donald J. Jones, FACHE, Administrator
**Web address:** www.nmhs.net

**MISSISSIPPI:** CALHOUN HEALTH SERVICES (C, 150 beds) 140 Burke–Calhoun City Road, Calhoun City, MS Zip 38916–9690; tel. 662/628–6611; James P. Franklin, Administrator
**Web address:** www.nmhs.net/calhoun_city

NORTH MISSISSIPPI MEDICAL CENTER – TUPELO (O, 757 beds) 830 South Gloster Street, Tupelo, MS Zip 38801–4934; tel. 662/377–3000; Steve Altmiller, President and Chief Executive Officer
**Web address:** www.nmhs.net

NORTH MISSISSIPPI MEDICAL CENTER–EUPORA (O, 73 beds) 70 Medical Plaza, Eupora, MS Zip 39744–4018; tel. 662/258–6221; John R. Jones, Administrator
**Web address:** www.nmhs.net/eupora

NORTH MISSISSIPPI MEDICAL CENTER–IUKA (O, 48 beds) 1777 Curtis Drive, Iuka, MS Zip 38852–1001, Mailing Address: P.O. Box 860, Zip 38852–0860; tel. 662/423–6051; Fred A. Truesdale, Jr., Administrator
**Web address:** www.nmhs.net

NORTH MISSISSIPPI MEDICAL CENTER–PONTOTOC HOSPITAL AND NURSING HOME (L, 69 beds) 176 South Main Street, Pontotoc, MS Zip 38863–3311, Mailing Address: P.O. Box 790, Zip 38863–0790; tel. 662/488–7640; Fred B. Hood, FACHE, Administrator
**Web address:** www.nmhs.net

NORTH MISSISSIPPI MEDICAL CENTER–WEST POINT (O, 60 beds) 835 Medical Center Drive, West Point, MS Zip 39773–9320; tel. 662/495–2300; James W. Hahn, Administrator
**Web address:** www.nmhs.net/westpoint

| | | |
|---|---|---|
| Owned, leased, sponsored: | 6 hospitals | 1043 beds |
| Contract–managed: | 1 hospital | 150 beds |
| Totals: | 7 hospitals | 1193 beds |

**0867: NORTH OAKS HEALTH SYSTEM** (NP)
15790 Paul Vega MD Drive, Hammond, LA Zip 70403–1436, Mailing Address: P.O. Box 2668, Zip 70404; tel. 985/345–2700; James E. Cathey, Jr., Chief Executive Officer

**LOUISIANA:** NORTH OAKS MEDICAL CENTER (O, 255 beds) 15790 Paul Vega, M. D. Drive, Hammond, LA Zip 70403–1436, Mailing Address: PO Box 2668, Zip 70404–2668; tel. 985/345–2700; James E. Cathey, Jr., President and Chief Executive Officer
**Web address:** www.northoaks.org

NORTH OAKS REHABILITATION HOSPITAL (O, 27 beds) 1900 South Morrison Boulevard, Hammond, LA Zip 70403; tel. 504/230–5700; Sybil K. Paulson, R.N., Administrator
**Web address:** www.northoaks.org

| | | |
|---|---|---|
| Owned, leased, sponsored: | 2 hospitals | 282 beds |
| Contract–managed: | 0 hospitals | 0 beds |
| Totals: | 2 hospitals | 282 beds |

**★0062: NORTH SHORE–LONG ISLAND JEWISH HEALTH SYSTEM** (NP)
145 Community Drive, Great Neck, NY Zip 11021; tel. 516/465–8100; Michael J. Dowling, President and Chief Executive Officer
**(Centralized Health System)**

**NEW YORK:** FOREST HILLS HOSPITAL (O, 242 beds) 102–01 66th Road, Forest Hills, NY Zip 11375–2029; tel. 718/830–4000; Rita Mercieca, R.N., Executive Director
**Web address:** www.northshorelij.com

FRANKLIN HOSPITAL (O, 356 beds) 900 Franklin Avenue, Valley Stream, NY Zip 11580–2190; tel. 516/256–6000; Catherine Hottendorf, R.N., MS, Executive Director
**Web address:** www.northshorelij.com

GLEN COVE HOSPITAL (O, 265 beds) 101 St. Andrews Lane, Glen Cove, NY Zip 11542–2254; tel. 516/674–7300; Dennis Connors, Executive Director
**Web address:** www.northshorelij.com

HUNTINGTON HOSPITAL (O, 299 beds) 270 Park Avenue, Huntington, NY Zip 11743–2799; tel. 631/351–2200; Kevin F. Lawlor, President and Chief Executive Officer
**Web address:** www.hunthosp.org

LENOX HILL HOSPITAL (O, 539 beds) 100 East 77th Street, New York, NY Zip 10075–1850; tel. 212/434–2000; Frank J. Danza, Executive Director
**Web address:** www.lenoxhillhospital.org

LONG ISLAND JEWISH MEDICAL CENTER (O, 840 beds) 270–05 76th Avenue, New Hyde Park, NY Zip 11040–1496; tel. 718/470–7000; Chantal Weinhold, Executive Director
**Web address:** www.lij.edu

NORTH SHORE UNIVERSITY HOSPITAL (O, 804 beds) 300 Community Drive, Manhasset, NY Zip 11030–3816; tel. 516/562–0100; Susan Somerville, R.N., Executive Director
**Web address:** www.northshorelij.com

PLAINVIEW HOSPITAL (O, 204 beds) 888 Old Country Road, Plainview, NY Zip 11803–4978; tel. 516/719–3000; Michael Fener, Executive Director
**Web address:** www.northshorelij.com

SOUTHSIDE HOSPITAL (O, 300 beds) 301 East Main Street, Bay Shore, NY Zip 11706–8458; tel. 631/968–3000; ,
**Web address:** www.southsidehospital.org

STATEN ISLAND UNIVERSITY HOSPITAL (O, 663 beds) 475 Seaview Avenue, Staten Island, NY Zip 10305–3436; tel. 718/226–9000; Anthony C. Ferreri, President and Chief Executive Officer
**Web address:** www.siuh.edu

SYOSSET HOSPITAL (O, 75 beds) 221 Jericho Turnpike, Syosset, NY Zip 11791–4567; tel. 516/496–6400; Michael Fener, Executive Director
**Web address:** www.northshorelij.com

| | | |
|---|---|---|
| Owned, leased, sponsored: | 11 hospitals | 4587 beds |
| Contract–managed: | 0 hospitals | 0 beds |
| Totals: | 11 hospitals | 4587 beds |

**★0281: NORTHERN ARIZONA HEALTHCARE** (NP)
1200 North Beaver Street, Flagstaff, AZ Zip 86001; tel. 928/779–3366; William T. Bradel, President and Co–Chief Executive Officer
**(Moderately Centralized Health System)**

**ARIZONA:** FLAGSTAFF MEDICAL CENTER (O, 267 beds) 1200 North Beaver Street, Flagstaff, AZ Zip 86001–3198; tel. 928/779–3366; William T. Bradel, President
**Web address:** www.flagstaffmedicalcenter.com

VERDE VALLEY MEDICAL CENTER (O, 110 beds) 269 South Candy Lane, Cottonwood, AZ Zip 86326–4170; tel. 928/639–6000; James J. Bleicher, M.D., President and Chief Executive Officer
**Web address:** www.nahealth.com

| | | |
|---|---|---|
| Owned, leased, sponsored: | 2 hospitals | 377 beds |
| Contract–managed: | 0 hospitals | 0 beds |
| Totals: | 2 hospitals | 377 beds |

**★0470: NORTHSHORE UNIVERSITY HEALTHSYSTEM** (NP)
1301 Central Street, Evanston, IL Zip 60201–1613; tel. 847/570–2000; Mark R. Neaman, President and Chief Executive Officer
**(Moderately Centralized Health System)**

**ILLINOIS:** NORTHSHORE UNIVERSITY HEALTH SYSTEM EVANSTON HOSPITAL (O, 755 beds) 1301 Central Street, Evanston, IL Zip 60201–1613; tel. 847/570–2000; J. P. Gallagher, President
**Web address:** www.northshore.org

NORTHSHORE UNIVERSITY HEALTH SYSTEM SKOKIE HOSPITAL (O, 234 beds) 9600 Gross Point Road, Skokie, IL Zip 60076–1257; tel. 847/677–9600; Kristen Murtos, FACHE, President
**Web address:** www.northshore.org

| | | |
|---|---|---|
| Owned, leased, sponsored: | 2 hospitals | 989 beds |
| Contract–managed: | 0 hospitals | 0 beds |
| Totals: | 2 hospitals | 989 beds |

For explanation of codes following names, see page B2.
★ Indicates Type III membership in the American Hospital Association.

Section B

## 0410: NORTHSIDE HEALTHCARE SYSTEM (NP)
1000 Johnson Ferry Road N.E., Atlanta, GA Zip 30342–1611; tel. 404/851–8000; Robert Quattrocchi, President and Chief Executive Officer

**GEORGIA:** NORTHSIDE HOSPITAL (O, 571 beds) 1000 Johnson Ferry Road N.E., Atlanta, GA Zip 30342–1611; tel. 404/851–8000; Robert Quattrocchi, President and Chief Executive Officer
**Web address:** www.northside.com

NORTHSIDE HOSPITAL – CHEROKEE (O, 79 beds) 201 Hospital Road, Canton, GA Zip 30114–2408, Mailing Address: P.O. Box 906, Zip 30169; tel. 770/720–5100; William M. Hayes, Chief Executive Officer
**Web address:** www.northside.com

NORTHSIDE HOSPITAL FORSYTH (O, 187 beds) 1200 Northside Forsyth Drive, Cumming, GA Zip 30041–7659; tel. 770/844–3200; Lynn Jackson, Administrator
**Web address:** www.northside.com

| | | |
|---|---|---|
| Owned, leased, sponsored: | 3 hospitals | 837 beds |
| Contract–managed: | 0 hospitals | 0 beds |
| **Totals:** | 3 hospitals | 837 beds |

## ★0024: NORTHWESTERN MEMORIAL HEALTHCARE (NP)
251 East Huron Street, Chicago, IL Zip 60611; tel. 312/926–2000; Dean M. Harrison, President and Chief Executive Officer
**(Moderately Centralized Health System)**

**ILLINOIS:** NORTHWESTERN LAKE FOREST HOSPITAL (O, 205 beds) 660 North Westmoreland Road, Lake Forest, IL Zip 60045–1696; tel. 847/234–5600; Thomas J. McAfee, President
**Web address:** www.lfh.com

NORTHWESTERN MEMORIAL HOSPITAL (O, 868 beds) 251 East Huron Street, Chicago, IL Zip 60611–2908; tel. 312/926–2000; Dean M. Harrison, President and Chief Executive Officer
**Web address:** www.nmh.org

| | | |
|---|---|---|
| Owned, leased, sponsored: | 2 hospitals | 1073 beds |
| Contract–managed: | 0 hospitals | 0 beds |
| **Totals:** | 2 hospitals | 1073 beds |

## ★2285: NORTON HEALTHCARE (NP)
234 East Gray Street, Suite 225, Louisville, KY Zip 40202, Mailing Address: P.O. Box 35070, Zip 40232–5070; tel. 502/629–8000; Stephen Williams, President
**(Centralized Physician/Insurance Health System)**

**KENTUCKY:** KOSAIR CHILDREN'S HOSPITAL (O, 263 beds) 231 East Chestnut Street, Louisville, KY Zip 40202; tel. 502/629–6000; Thomas D. Kmetz, President
**Web address:** www.nortonhealthcare.org

NORTON AUDUBON HOSPITAL (O, 262 beds) One Audubon Plaza Drive, Louisville, KY Zip 40217–1397, Mailing Address: P.O. Box 17550, Zip 40217–0550; tel. 502/636–7111; Steven MacLauchlan, President
**Web address:** www.nortonhealthcare.org

NORTON BROWNSBORO HOSPITAL (O, 98 beds) 4960 Norton Healthcare Boulevard, Louisville, KY Zip 40141; tel. 502/446–8000; Doug Winkelhake, President
**Web address:** www.nortonhealthcare.org

NORTON HOSPITAL (O, 340 beds) 200 East Chestnut Street, Louisville, KY Zip 40202–1800, Mailing Address: P.O. Box 35070, Zip 40232–5070; tel. 502/629–8000; Kevin S. Wardell, President
**Web address:** www.nortonhealthcare.org

NORTON SUBURBAN HOSPITAL (O, 364 beds) 4001 Dutchmans Lane, Louisville, KY Zip 40207–4799; tel. 502/893–1000; Charlotte Ipsan, President
**Web address:** www.nortonhealthcare.com

| | | |
|---|---|---|
| Owned, leased, sponsored: | 5 hospitals | 1327 beds |
| Contract–managed: | 0 hospitals | 0 beds |
| **Totals:** | 5 hospitals | 1327 beds |

## ★0139: NOVANT HEALTH (NP)
2085 Frontis Plaza Boulevard, Winston–Salem, NC Zip 27103–3090; tel. 336/718–5600; Carl S. Armato, President and Chief Executive Officer
**(Moderately Centralized Health System)**

**NORTH CAROLINA:** BRUNSWICK NOVANT MEDICAL CENTER (O, 60 beds) 240 Hospital Drive N.E., Bolivia, NC Zip 28462; tel. 910/721–1000; Shelbourn Stevens, President
**Web address:** www.brunswicknovant.org

FORSYTH MEDICAL CENTER (O, 681 beds) 3333 Silas Creek Parkway, Winston–Salem, NC Zip 27103–3090; tel. 336/718–5000; Jeffery T. Lindsay, Chief Executive Officer
**Web address:** www.novanthealth.org

FRANKLIN REGIONAL MEDICAL CENTER (O, 70 beds) 100 Hospital Drive, Louisburg, NC Zip 27549–2256, Mailing Address: P.O. Box 609, Zip 27549–0609; tel. 919/497–8401; Jody Morris, President and Chief Executive Officer
**Web address:** www.franklinregional.org

MEDICAL PARK HOSPITAL (O, 22 beds) 1950 South Hawthorne Road, Winston–Salem, NC Zip 27103–3993; tel. 336/718–0600; Teresa Carter, Vice President and Chief Operating Officer
**Web address:** www.novanthealth.org

PRESBYTERIAN HOSPITAL (O, 582 beds) 200 Hawthorne Lane, Charlotte, NC Zip 28204–2528, Mailing Address: P.O. Box 33549, Zip 28233–3549; tel. 704/384–4000; Derrick Mark Billings, President
**Web address:** www.presbyterian.org

PRESBYTERIAN HOSPITAL HUNTERSVILLE (O, 60 beds) 10030 Gilead Road, Huntersville, NC Zip 28078, Mailing Address: P.O. Box 3508, Zip 28070–3508; tel. 704/316–4000; Tanya S. Blackmon, President
**Web address:** www.novanthealth.org

PRESBYTERIAN HOSPITAL MATTHEWS (O, 117 beds) 1500 Matthews Township Parkway, Matthews, NC Zip 28105–4656, Mailing Address: P.O. Box 3310, Zip 28106–3310; tel. 704/384–6500; Roland R. Bibeau, President
**Web address:** www.presbyterian.org

PRESBYTERIAN–ORTHOPAEDIC HOSPITAL (O, 80 beds) 1901 Randolph Road, Charlotte, NC Zip 28207–1195; tel. 704/316–2000; Mike Riley, Senior Vice President and Chief Operating Officer
**Web address:** www.novanthealth.org

ROWAN REGIONAL MEDICAL CENTER (O, 196 beds) 612 Mocksville Avenue, Salisbury, NC Zip 28144–2799; tel. 704/210–5000; Dari Caldwell, President
**Web address:** www.rowan.org

THOMASVILLE MEDICAL CENTER (O, 101 beds) 207 Old Lexington Road, Thomasville, NC Zip 27360–3428, Mailing Address: P.O. Box 789, Zip 27361–0789; tel. 336/472–2000; Kathie A. Johnson, R.N., MS, Ph.D., President and Chief Executive Officer
**Web address:** www.thomasvillemedicalcenter.org

**SOUTH CAROLINA:** UPSTATE CAROLINA MEDICAL CENTER (O, 125 beds) 1530 North Limestone Street, Gaffney, SC Zip 29340–4738; tel. 864/487–4271; Kimberly Taylor, Chief Operating Officer
**Web address:** www.upstatecarolina.org

**VIRGINIA:** PRINCE WILLIAM HOSPITAL (O, 168 beds) 8700 Sudley Road, Manassas, VA Zip 20110–4418, Mailing Address: P.O. Box 2610, Zip 20108–0867; tel. 703/369–8000; Melissa Robson, President
**Web address:** www.pwhs.org

| | | |
|---|---|---|
| Owned, leased, sponsored: | 12 hospitals | 2262 beds |
| Contract–managed: | 0 hospitals | 0 beds |
| **Totals:** | 12 hospitals | 2262 beds |

## ★1165: OAKWOOD HEALTHCARE, INC. (NP)
One Parklane Boulevard, Suite 1000E, Dearborn, MI Zip 48126; tel. 313/253–6050; Brian M. Connolly, President and Chief Executive Officer
**(Centralized Health System)**

**MICHIGAN:** OAKWOOD ANNAPOLIS HOSPITAL (O, 211 beds) 33155 Annapolis Street, Wayne, MI Zip 48184–2405; tel. 734/467–4000; Eric W. Widner, President
**Web address:** www.oakwood.org

For explanation of codes following names, see page B2.
★ Indicates Type III membership in the American Hospital Association.

© 2012 AHA Guide

OAKWOOD HERITAGE HOSPITAL (O, 183 beds) 10000 Telegraph Road, Taylor, MI Zip 48180–3330; tel. 313/295–5000; Michael Geheb, M.D., Division President
**Web address:** www.oakwood.org

OAKWOOD HOSPITAL & MEDICAL CENTER–DEARBORN (O, 553 beds) 18101 Oakwood Boulevard, Dearborn, MI Zip 48124–4089, Mailing Address: P.O. Box 2500, Zip 48123–2500; tel. 313/593–7000; Michael Geheb, M.D., Division President
**Web address:** www.oakwood.org

OAKWOOD SOUTHSHORE MEDICAL CENTER (O, 144 beds) 5450 Fort Street, Trenton, MI Zip 48183–4625; tel. 734/671–3800; Edith M. Hughes, President
**Web address:** www.oakwood.org

| Owned, leased, sponsored: | 4 hospitals | 1091 beds |
|---|---|---|
| Contract–managed: | 0 hospitals | 0 beds |
| Totals: | 4 hospitals | 1091 beds |

---

**0616: OCEANS HEALTHCARE** (IO)
2720 Rue de Jardin, Suite 100, Lake Charles, LA Zip 70605–4050; tel. 337/721–1900; Jason Reed, President and Chief Executive Officer

**LOUISIANA:** OCEANS BEHAVIORAL HOSPITAL OF ALEXANDRIA (O, 24 beds) 2621 North Bolton Avenue, Alexandria, LA Zip 71303–4506; tel. 318/448–8473; Gene Amons, Administrator
**Web address:** www.obha.info

OCEANS BEHAVIORAL HOSPITAL OF BATON ROUGE (O, 20 beds) 11135 Florida Boulevard, Baton Rouge, LA Zip 70815–2013; tel. 225/356–7030; Gene Amos, Administrator
**Web address:** www.obhbr.info/

OCEANS BEHAVIORAL HOSPITAL OF BROUSSARD (O, 38 beds) 418 Albertson Parkway, Broussard, LA Zip 70518; tel. 337/237–6444; Marlene Lucas, Administrator
**Web address:** www.obhb.info/

OCEANS BEHAVIORAL HOSPITAL OF DE RIDDER (O, 20 beds) 1420 Blankenship Drive, Deridder, LA Zip 70634–4604; tel. 337/460–9472; Ronald E. Hand, Administrator
**Web address:** www.obhd.info/

OCEANS BEHAVIORAL HOSPITAL OF GREATER NEW ORLEANS (O, 18 beds) 716 Village Road, Kenner, LA Zip 70065–2751; tel. 504/464–8895; Deborah Spier, Administrator
**Web address:** www.obhgno.info/

OCEANS BEHAVIORAL HOSPITAL OF KENTWOOD (O, 18 beds) 921 Avenue G., Kentwood, LA Zip 70444–2636; tel. 985/229–0717; Robert Pound, Administrator
**Web address:** www.obhk.info/

OCEANS BEHAVIORAL HOSPITAL OF LAKE CHARLES (O, 20 beds) 302 West Mcneese Street, Lake Charles, LA Zip 70605–5604; tel. 337/474–7581; Nicholas D. Guillory, MSN, Administrator
**Web address:** www.obhlc.info/

OCEANS BEHAVIORAL HOSPITAL OF OPELOUSAS (O, 20 beds) 1310 Heather Drive, Opelousas, LA Zip 70570–7714; tel. 337/948–8820; Remi Savoy, Administrator
**Web address:** www.obho.info/

OCEANS SPECIALTY HOSPITAL OF GRETNA (O, 27 beds) 535 Commerce Street, Suite B., Gretna, LA Zip 70056–7316; tel. 504/391–1500; Michael Rabalais, Chief Executive Officer
**Web address:** www.oshla.info

| Owned, leased, sponsored: | 9 hospitals | 205 beds |
|---|---|---|
| Contract–managed: | 0 hospitals | 0 beds |
| Totals: | 9 hospitals | 205 beds |

---

★**0359: OCHSNER HEALTH SYSTEM** (NP)
1514 Jefferson Highway, New Orleans, LA Zip 70121–2429; tel. 800/874–8984; Patrick J. Quinlan, M.D., Chief Executive Officer
**(Moderately Centralized Health System)**

OCHSNER BAPTIST MEDICAL CENTER (O, 55 beds) 2700 Napoleon Avenue, New Orleans, LA Zip 70115–6914; tel. 504/899–9311; Bradley R. Goodson, Chief Executive Officer
**Web address:** www.ochsner.org

OCHSNER MEDICAL CENTER (O, 771 beds) 1514 Jefferson Highway, New Orleans, LA Zip 70121–2429; tel. 504/842–3000; Michael Hulefeld, Chief Executive Officer
**Web address:** www.ochsner.org

OCHSNER MEDICAL CENTER – KENNER (O, 119 beds) 180 West Esplanade Avenue, Kenner, LA Zip 70065–6001; tel. 504/468–8600; Paolo Zambito, Chief Executive Officer
**Web address:** www.ochsner.org/locations/ochsner_health_center_kenner_w_esplanade_ave/

OCHSNER MEDICAL CENTER – NORTH SHORE (L, 110 beds) 100 Medical Center Drive, Slidell, LA Zip 70461–5520; tel. 985/646–5000; Polly J. Davenport, R.N., Chief Executive Officer
**Web address:** www.ochsner.org/locations/northshore

OCHSNER MEDICAL CENTER–BATON ROUGE (O, 115 beds) 17000 Medical Center Drive, Baton Rouge, LA Zip 70816–3224; tel. 225/752–2470; Eric McMillen, Interim Chief Executive Officer
**Web address:** www.ochsner.org/page.cfm?id=103

OCHSNER ST. ANNE GENERAL HOSPITAL (O, 35 beds) 4608 Highway 1, Raceland, LA Zip 70394–2623; tel. 985/537–6841; Milton D. Bourgeois, Jr., Chief Executive Officer
**Web address:** www.ochsnerstanne.org

| Owned, leased, sponsored: | 6 hospitals | 1205 beds |
|---|---|---|
| Contract–managed: | 0 hospitals | 0 beds |
| Totals: | 6 hospitals | 1205 beds |

---

**0388: OCONEE REGIONAL HEALTH SYSTEMS** (NP)
821 North Cobb Street, Milledgeville, GA Zip 31061; tel. 478/454–3505; Jean Aycock, President and Chief Executive Officer
**(Independent Hospital System)**

**GEORGIA:** JASPER MEMORIAL HOSPITAL (O, 67 beds) 898 College Street, Monticello, GA Zip 31064–1298; tel. 706/468–6411; Jan Gaston, Administrator
**Web address:** www.jaspermemorialhospital.org

OCONEE REGIONAL MEDICAL CENTER (O, 89 beds) 821 North Cobb Street, Milledgeville, GA Zip 31061–2351, Mailing Address: P.O. Box 690, Zip 31059–0690; tel. 478/454–3500; Jean Aycock, President and Chief Executive Officer
**Web address:** www.oconeeregional.com

| Owned, leased, sponsored: | 2 hospitals | 156 beds |
|---|---|---|
| Contract–managed: | 0 hospitals | 0 beds |
| Totals: | 2 hospitals | 156 beds |

---

**0537: OHIO DEPARTMENT OF MENTAL HEALTH** (NP)
30 East Broad Street, 8th Floor, Columbus, OH Zip 43215–3430; tel. 614/466–2297; Tracy Plouck, Director
**(Independent Hospital System)**

**OHIO:** APPALACHIAN BEHAVIORAL HEALTHCARE (O, 224 beds) 100 Hospital Drive, Athens, OH Zip 45701–2301; tel. 740/594–5000; Jane E. Krason, R.N., Chief Executive Officer
**Web address:** www.mh.state.oh.us

HEARTLAND BEHAVIORAL HEALTHCARE (O, 130 beds) 3000 Erie Street, Massillon, OH Zip 44646–7993, Mailing Address: P.O. Box 540, Zip 44648–0540; tel. 330/833–3135; James Ignelzi, Interim Chief Executive Officer
**Web address:** www.mh.state.oh.us/ibhs/bhos/hoh.html

NORTHCOAST BEHAVIORAL HEALTHCARE SYSTEM (O, 260 beds) 1756 Sagamore Road, Northfield, OH Zip 44067–1086; tel. 330/467–7131; David Celletti, Chief Executive Officer
**Web address:** www.mh.state.oh.us

NORTHWEST OHIO PSYCHIATRIC HOSPITAL (O, 24 beds) 930 Detroit Avenue, Toledo, OH Zip 43614–2701; tel. 419/381–1881; Mychail Scheramic, M.D., Chief Executive Officer
**Web address:** www.mh.state.oh.us/

Section B

For explanation of codes following names, see page B2.
★ Indicates Type III membership in the American Hospital Association.

SUMMIT BEHAVIORAL HEALTHCARE (O, 284 beds) 1101 Summit Road, Cincinnati, OH Zip 45237–2652; tel. 513/948–3600; Elizabeth Banks, Chief Executive Officer
**Web address:** www.mh.state.oh.us/

TWIN VALLEY BEHAVIORAL HEALTHCARE (O, 248 beds) 2200 West Broad Street, Columbus, OH Zip 43223–1295; tel. 614/752–0333; Karen Woods–Nyce, Chief Executive Officer
**Web address:** www.mh.state.oh.us/ibhs/bhos/tvbh.html

| | | |
|---|---|---|
| Owned, leased, sponsored: | 6 hospitals | 1170 beds |
| Contract–managed: | 0 hospitals | 0 beds |
| Totals: | 6 hospitals | 1170 beds |

---

**★0251:  OHIO STATE UNIVERSITY HEALTH SYSTEM** (NP)
370 West Ninth Avenue, Columbus, OH Zip 43210–1240; tel. 614/247–5555; Peter E. Geier, Chief Executive Officer
**(Centralized Health System)**

JAMES CANCER HOSPITAL AND SOLOVE RESEARCH INSTITUTE (O, 209 beds) 300 West Tenth Avenue, Columbus, OH Zip 43210–1240; tel. 614/293–3300; Michael Caligiuri, Chief Executive Officer
**Web address:** www.jamesline.com

OHIO STATE UNIVERSITY MEDICAL CENTER (O, 976 beds) 370 West 9th Avenue, Columbus, OH Zip 43210–1240; tel. 614/293–8000; Peter E. Geier, Chief Executive Officer
**Web address:** www.osumedcenter.edu

| | | |
|---|---|---|
| Owned, leased, sponsored: | 2 hospitals | 1185 beds |
| Contract–managed: | 0 hospitals | 0 beds |
| Totals: | 2 hospitals | 1185 beds |

---

**3315:  OHIO VALLEY HEALTH SERVICES AND EDUCATION CORPORATION** (NP)
2000 Eoff Street, Wheeling, WV Zip 26003; tel. 304/234–8383; Michael J. Caruso, President and Chief Executive Officer
**(Moderately Centralized Health System)**

EAST OHIO REGIONAL HOSPITAL (O, 172 beds) 90 North Fourth Street, Martins Ferry, OH Zip 43935–1648; tel. 740/633–1100; George G. Couch, FACHE, President and Chief Executive Officer
**Web address:** www.eorh–online.com

**WEST VIRGINIA:** OHIO VALLEY MEDICAL CENTER (O, 159 beds) 2000 Eoff Street, Wheeling, WV Zip 26003–3870; tel. 304/234–0123; Bernie Albertini, Chief Administrative Officer
**Web address:** www.ohiovalleymedicalcenter.com

| | | |
|---|---|---|
| Owned, leased, sponsored: | 2 hospitals | 331 beds |
| Contract–managed: | 0 hospitals | 0 beds |
| Totals: | 2 hospitals | 331 beds |

---

**★0162:  OHIOHEALTH** (NP)
180 East Broad Street, Columbus, OH Zip 43215; tel. 614/544–4455; David P. Blom, President and Chief Executive Officer
**(Centralized Physician/Insurance Health System)**

**OHIO:** DOCTORS HOSPITAL (O, 213 beds) 5100 West Broad Street, Columbus, OH Zip 43228–1607; tel. 614/544–1000; Michael L. Reichfield, President
**Web address:** www.ohiohealth.com

DOCTORS HOSPITAL NELSONVILLE (O, 25 beds) 1950 Mount Saint Mary Drive, Nelsonville, OH Zip 45764–1193; tel. 740/753–1931; LaMar L. Wyse, Chief Operating Officer
**Web address:** www.ohiohealth.com

DUBLIN METHODIST HOSPITAL (O, 92 beds) 7500 Hospital Drive, Dublin, OH Zip 43016; tel. 614/544–8000; Bruce P. Hagen, President
**Web address:** www.ohiohealth.com

GRADY MEMORIAL HOSPITAL (O, 61 beds) 561 West Central Avenue, Delaware, OH Zip 43015–1485; tel. 740/615–1000; Bruce P. Hagen, President
**Web address:** www.ohiohealth.com

GRANT MEDICAL CENTER (O, 392 beds) 111 South Grant Avenue, Columbus, OH Zip 43215–1898; tel. 614/566–9000; Vinson Yates, President
**Web address:** www.ohiohealth.com

HARDIN MEMORIAL HOSPITAL (O, 25 beds) 921 East Franklin Street, Kenton, OH Zip 43326–2099; tel. 419/673–0761; Mark R. Seckinger, Administrator and Chief Executive Officer
**Web address:** www.hardinmemorial.org

MORROW COUNTY HOSPITAL (C, 53 beds) 651 West Marion Road, Mount Gilead, OH Zip 43338–1027; tel. 419/946–5015; Christopher Truax, Chief Executive Officer
**Web address:** www.morrowcountyhospital.com

O'BLENESS MEMORIAL HOSPITAL (C, 132 beds) 55 Hospital Drive, Athens, OH Zip 45701–2302; tel. 740/593–5551; Greg Long, Chief Executive Officer
**Web address:** www.obleness.org

OHIOHEALTH MARION GENERAL HOSPITAL (O, 170 beds) 1000 McKinley Park Drive, Marion, OH Zip 43302–6397; tel. 740/383–8400; John W. Sanders, President
**Web address:** www.ohiohealth.com/mariongeneral

RIVERSIDE METHODIST HOSPITAL (O, 796 beds) 3535 Olentangy River Road, Columbus, OH Zip 43214–3998; tel. 614/566–5000; Stephen Markovich, M.D., President
**Web address:** www.ohiohealth.com

| | | |
|---|---|---|
| Owned, leased, sponsored: | 8 hospitals | 1774 beds |
| Contract–managed: | 2 hospitals | 185 beds |
| Totals: | 10 hospitals | 1959 beds |

---

**0018:  OKLAHOMA DEPARTMENT OF MENTAL HEALTH AND SUBSTANCE ABUSE SERVICES** (NP)
1200 N.E. 13th Street, Oklahoma City, OK Zip 73117, Mailing Address: P.O. Box 53277, Zip 73152–3277; tel. 405/522–3908; Terri White, Commissioner
**(Independent Hospital System)**

**OKLAHOMA:** GRIFFIN MEMORIAL HOSPITAL (O, 120 beds) 900 East Main Street, Norman, OK Zip 73071–5305, Mailing Address: P.O. Box 151, Zip 73070–0151; tel. 405/321–4880; Randy May, Executive Director
**Web address:** www.odmhsas.org

NORTHWEST CENTER FOR BEHAVIORAL HEALTH (O, 28 beds) 1222 Tenth Street, Fort Supply, OK Zip 73841–0001; tel. 580/766–2311; Trudy Hoffman, Executive Director
**Web address:** www.ncbhok.org/

OKLAHOMA FORENSIC CENTER (O, 200 beds) 24800 South 4420 Road, Vinita, OK Zip 74301, Mailing Address: P.O. Box 69, Zip 74301–0069; tel. 918/256–7841; William T. Burkett, Chief Executive Officer

| | | |
|---|---|---|
| Owned, leased, sponsored: | 3 hospitals | 348 beds |
| Contract–managed: | 0 hospitals | 0 beds |
| Totals: | 3 hospitals | 348 beds |

---

**3355:  ORLANDO HEALTH** (NP)
1414 Kuhl Avenue, Orlando, FL Zip 32806–2093; tel. 407/841–5111; Sherrie Sitarik, President and Chief Executive Officer
**(Moderately Centralized Health System)**

**FLORIDA:** HEALTH CENTRAL (O, 399 beds) 10000 West Colonial Drive, Ocoee, FL Zip 34761–3499; tel. 407/296–1000; Gregory P. Ohe, President and Chief Executive Officer
**Web address:** www.healthcentral.org

ORLANDO REGIONAL MEDICAL CENTER (O, 1491 beds) 1414 Kuhl Avenue, Orlando, FL Zip 32806–2093; tel. 407/841–5111; Shannon Elswick, President
**Web address:** www.orhs.org

ORLANDO REGIONAL SOUTH SEMINOLE HOSPITAL (O, 206 beds) 555 West State Road 434, Longwood, FL Zip 32750–4999; tel. 407/767–1200; Robert E. Snyder, Jr., President
**Web address:** www.orhs.org

SOUTH LAKE HOSPITAL (O, 122 beds) 1900 Don Wickham Drive, Clermont, FL Zip 34711–2787; tel. 352/394–4071; John Moore, Chief Executive fficer
**Web address:** www.southlakehospital.com

---

For explanation of codes following names, see page B2.
★ Indicates Type III membership in the American Hospital Association.

| | | |
|---|---|---|
| Owned, leased, sponsored: | 4 hospitals | 2218 beds |
| Contract–managed: | 0 hospitals | 0 beds |
| Totals: | 4 hospitals | 2218 beds |

★**5335:  OSF HEALTHCARE SYSTEM** (CC)
800 N.E. Glen Oak Avenue, Peoria, IL Zip 61603–3200;
tel. 309/655–2850; Kevin D. Schoeplein, President
**(Centralized Physician/Insurance Health System)**

**ILLINOIS:** OSF HOLY FAMILY MEDICAL CENTER (O, 23 beds) 1000 West
Harlem Avenue, Monmouth, IL Zip 61462–1099; tel. 309/734–3141;
Patricia A. Luker, Chief Executive Officer
**Web address:** www.osfholyfamily.org

OSF SAINT ANTHONY MEDICAL CENTER (O, 235 beds) 5666 East State
Street, Rockford, IL Zip 61108–2425; tel. 815/226–2000; David A. Schertz,
President and Chief Executive Officer
**Web address:** www.osfhealth.com

OSF SAINT FRANCIS MEDICAL CENTER (O, 574 beds) 530 N.E. Glen Oak
Avenue, Peoria, IL Zip 61637–0001; tel. 309/655–2000; Keith E. Steffen,
President and Chief Executive Officer
**Web address:** www.osfsaintfrancis.org

OSF SAINT JAMES – JOHN W. ALBRECHT MEDICAL CENTER (O, 42 beds)
2500 West Reynolds, Pontiac, IL Zip 61764–2194; tel. 815/842–2828;
David T. Ochs, President and Chief Executive Officer
**Web address:** www.osfsaintjames.org

OSF ST. JOSEPH MEDICAL CENTER (O, 149 beds) 2200 East Washington
Street, Bloomington, IL Zip 61701–4323; tel. 309/662–3311; Kenneth J.
Natzke, President and Chief Executive Officer
**Web address:** www.osfstjoseph.org

OSF ST. MARY MEDICAL CENTER (O, 90 beds) 3333 North Seminary Street,
Galesburg, IL Zip 61401–1299; tel. 309/344–3161; Richard S. Kowalski,
FACHE, President and Chief Executive Officer
**Web address:** www.osfstmary.org

SAINT CLARE HOME (O, 0 beds) 5533 North Galena Road, Peoria Heights, IL
Zip 61614–4499; tel. 309/682–5428; Candy Conover, Administrator

ST. ANTHONY'S CONTINUING CARE CENTER (O, 179 beds) 767 30th Street,
Rock Island, IL Zip 61201; Sister Mary Anthony Mazzaferri, Administrator

**MICHIGAN:** OSF ST. FRANCIS HOSPITAL (O, 48 beds) 3401 Ludington Street,
Escanaba, MI Zip 49829–1377; tel. 906/786–3311; Peter G. Jennings,
President and Chief Executive Officer
**Web address:** www.osfstfrancis.org

| | | |
|---|---|---|
| Owned, leased, sponsored: | 9 hospitals | 1340 beds |
| Contract–managed: | 0 hospitals | 0 beds |
| Totals: | 9 hospitals | 1340 beds |

**0367:  PACER HEALTH CORPORATION** (IO)
14100 Palmetto Frontage Road, Suite 110, Miami Lakes, FL
Zip 33016; tel. 305/828–7660; Rainier Gonzalez, Chairman and
Chief Executive Officer

**KENTUCKY:** KNOX COUNTY HOSPITAL (O, 25 beds) 80 Hospital Drive,
Barbourville, KY Zip 40906–1317, Mailing Address: P.O. Box 10,
Zip 40906–0160; tel. 606/546–4175; Craig Morgan, Chief Executive
Officer
**Web address:** www.knoxcohospital.com

**LOUISIANA:** CALCASIEU OAKS GERIATRIC PSYCHIATRIC HOSPITAL (O, 24
beds) 2837 Ernest Street, Lake Charles, LA Zip 70601;
tel. 337/439–8111; Charles Getwood, Assistant Chief Executive Officer

| | | |
|---|---|---|
| Owned, leased, sponsored: | 2 hospitals | 49 beds |
| Contract–managed: | 0 hospitals | 0 beds |
| Totals: | 2 hospitals | 49 beds |

**0435:  PACIFIC HEALTH CORPORATION** (IO)
14642 Newport Avenue, Suite 388, Tustin, CA Zip 92780;
tel. 714/619–9997; Georg J. Hopf, President and Chief Executive
Officer
**(Independent Hospital System)**

**CALIFORNIA:** ANAHEIM GENERAL HOSPITAL (O, 126 beds) 3350 West Ball
Road, Anaheim, CA Zip 92804–3799; tel. 714/827–6700; Michael O.
Choo, Interim Chief Executive Officer

BELLFLOWER MEDICAL CENTER (O, 110 beds) 9542 East Artesia Boulevard,
Bellflower, CA Zip 90706–6511; tel. 562/925–8355; Michael O. Choo,
President and Chief Executive Officer
**Web address:** www.bellflowermedicalctr.com

LOS ANGELES METROPOLITAN MEDICAL CENTER (O, 213 beds) 2231 South
Western Avenue, Los Angeles, CA Zip 90018–1302; tel. 323/730–7300; Ron
Stinnett, Chief Executive Officer
**Web address:** www.lammc.com

NEWPORT SPECIALTY HOSPITAL (O, 155 beds) 14662 Newport Avenue,
Tustin, CA Zip 92780–6064; tel. 714/838–9600; Peter Friedman, President
and Chief Executive Officer
**Web address:** www.newportspecialtyhospital.com/

| | | |
|---|---|---|
| Owned, leased, sponsored: | 4 hospitals | 604 beds |
| Contract–managed: | 0 hospitals | 0 beds |
| Totals: | 4 hospitals | 604 beds |

★**5235:  PALLOTTINE HEALTH SERVICES** (CC)
2900 First Avenue, Huntington, WV Zip 25702; tel. 304/526–1234;
Michael G. Sellards, Chief Executive Officer
**(Independent Hospital System)**

**WEST VIRGINIA:** ST. JOSEPH'S HOSPITAL OF BUCKHANNON (O, 69 beds) 1
Amalia Drive, Buckhannon, WV Zip 26201–2222; tel. 304/473–2000; Sue
E. Johnson–Phillippe, President and Chief Executive Officer
**Web address:** www.stj.net

ST. MARY'S MEDICAL CENTER (O, 375 beds) 2900 First Avenue, Huntington,
WV Zip 25702–1272; tel. 304/526–1234; Michael G. Sellards, President and
Chief Executive Officer
**Web address:** www.st-marys.org

| | | |
|---|---|---|
| Owned, leased, sponsored: | 2 hospitals | 444 beds |
| Contract–managed: | 0 hospitals | 0 beds |
| Totals: | 2 hospitals | 444 beds |

★**4155:  PALMETTO HEALTH** (NP)
1301 Taylor Street, Suite 9–A, Columbia, SC Zip 29201, Mailing
Address: P.O. Box 2266, Zip 29202–2266; tel. 803/296–2100;
Charles D. Beaman, Jr., Chief Executive Officer
**(Moderately Centralized Health System)**

**SOUTH CAROLINA:** BAPTIST EASLEY HOSPITAL (O, 89 beds) 200 Fleetwood
Drive, Easley, SC Zip 29640–2076, Mailing Address: P.O. Box 2129,
Zip 29641–2129; tel. 864/442–7200; Roddey E. Gettys, III, Chief
Executive Officer
**Web address:** www.palmettohealth.org

PALMETTO HEALTH BAPTIST (O, 451 beds) Taylor at Marion Street,
Columbia, SC Zip 29220–0001; tel. 803/296–5010; James M. Bridges,
Executive Vice President and Chief Operating Officer
**Web address:** www.palmettohealth.org

PALMETTO HEALTH RICHLAND (O, 669 beds) Five Richland Medical Park
Drive, Columbia, SC Zip 29203–6897; tel. 803/434–7000; Stan Hickson,
FACHE, Executive Vice President and Chief Operating Officer
**Web address:** www.palmettohealth.org

| | | |
|---|---|---|
| Owned, leased, sponsored: | 3 hospitals | 1209 beds |
| Contract–managed: | 0 hospitals | 0 beds |
| Totals: | 3 hospitals | 1209 beds |

★**7555:  PALOMAR HEALTH** (NP)
15255 Innovation Drive, San Diego, CA Zip 92128–3410;
tel. 858/675–5100; Michael H. Covert, FACHE, Chief Executive
Officer
**(Moderately Centralized Health System)**

**CALIFORNIA:** PALOMAR MEDICAL CENTER (O, 330 beds) 555 East Valley
Parkway, Escondido, CA Zip 92025–3084; tel. 760/739–3000; Gerald E.
Bracht, Chief Administrative Officer
**Web address:** www.pph.org

For explanation of codes following names, see page B2.
★ Indicates Type III membership in the American Hospital Association.

Section B

POMERADO HOSPITAL (O, 107 beds) 15615 Pomerado Road, Poway, CA Zip 92064–2460; tel. 858/613–4000; David A. Tam, M.D., FACHE, Chief Administrative Officer
**Web address:** www.pph.org

| | | |
|---|---|---|
| Owned, leased, sponsored: | 2 hospitals | 437 beds |
| Contract–managed: | 0 hospitals | 0 beds |
| Totals: | 2 hospitals | 437 beds |

★**1985:   PARK NICOLLET HEALTH SERVICES** (NP)
6500 Excelsior Boulevard, Saint Louis Park, MN Zip 55426–4702; tel. 952/993–5000; David Abelson, M.D., Chief Executive Officer
**(Independent Hospital System)**

**MINNESOTA:** GLENCOE REGIONAL HEALTH SERVICES (C, 135 beds) 1805 Hennepin Avenue North, Glencoe, MN Zip 55336–1416; tel. 320/864–3121; Jon D. Braband, FACHE, President and Chief Executive Officer
**Web address:** www.grhsonline.org

PARK NICOLLET METHODIST HOSPITAL (O, 426 beds) 6500 Excelsior Boulevard, Saint Louis Park, MN Zip 55426–4702; Minneapolis, tel. 952/993–5000; David Abelson, M.D., President and Chief Executive Officer
**Web address:** www.parknicollet.com

| | | |
|---|---|---|
| Owned, leased, sponsored: | 1 hospital | 426 beds |
| Contract–managed: | 1 hospital | 135 beds |
| Totals: | 2 hospitals | 561 beds |

★**0159:   PARKVIEW HEALTH** (NP)
10501 Corporate Drive, Fort Wayne, IN Zip 46845, Mailing Address: P.O. Box 5600, Zip 46895–5600; tel. 260/373–7001; Michael J. Packnett, President and Chief Executive Officer
**(Centralized Physician/Insurance Health System)**

**INDIANA:** PARKVIEW HOSPITAL (O, 620 beds) 2200 Randallia Drive, Fort Wayne, IN Zip 46805–4699; tel. 260/373–4000; Sue Ehinger, Ph.D., Executive Vice President and Chief Operating Officer
**Web address:** www.parkview.com

PARKVIEW HUNTINGTON HOSPITAL (O, 36 beds) 2001 Stults Road, Huntington, IN Zip 46750–3696; tel. 260/355–3000; Darlene Garrett, Chief Operating Officer
**Web address:** www.parkview.com

PARKVIEW LAGRANGE HOSPITAL (O, 25 beds) 207 North Townline Road, LaGrange, IN Zip 46761–1325; tel. 260/463–2143; Robert T. Myers, Chief Operating Officer
**Web address:** www.parkview.com

PARKVIEW NOBLE HOSPITAL (O, 31 beds) 401 Sawyer Road, Kendallville, IN Zip 46755–0728; tel. 260/347–8700; David C. Hunter, Chief Operating Officer
**Web address:** www.parkview.com

PARKVIEW ORTHO HOSPITAL (O, 30 beds) 11130 Parkview Circle Drive, Zip 46845–1735; tel. 260/672–5000; 5000 S Parkview Health, Fort Wayne, IN; Julie Fleck, Chief Operating Officer
**Web address:** www.parkview.com

PARKVIEW WHITLEY HOSPITAL (O, 97 beds) 1260 East State Road 205, Columbia City, IN Zip 46725–9492; tel. 260/248–9000; Scott F. Gabriel, Senior Vice President and Chief Operating Officer
**Web address:** www.parkview.com

| | | |
|---|---|---|
| Owned, leased, sponsored: | 5 hospitals | 839 beds |
| Contract–managed: | 0 hospitals | 0 beds |
| Totals: | 5 hospitals | 839 beds |

★**1785:   PARTNERS HEALTHCARE SYSTEM, INC.** (NP)
800 Boylston Street, Suite 1150, Boston, MA Zip 02199–8001; tel. 617/278–1004; Gary L. Gottlieb, M.D., President and Chief Executive Officer
**(Centralized Health System)**

**MASSACHUSETTS:** BRIGHAM AND WOMEN'S HOSPITAL (O, 779 beds) 75 Francis Street, Boston, MA Zip 02115–6110; tel. 617/732–5500; Elizabeth Nabel, M.D., President
**Web address:** www.brighamandwomens.org

FAULKNER HOSPITAL (O, 93 beds) 1153 Centre Street, Boston, MA Zip 02130–3400; tel. 617/983–7000; Elizabeth Nabel, M.D., President
**Web address:** www.faulknerhospital.org

MARTHA'S VINEYARD HOSPITAL (O, 25 beds) One Hospital Road, Oak Bluffs, MA Zip 02557, Mailing Address: P.O. Box 1477, Zip 02557–1477; tel. 508/693–0410; Timothy J. Walsh, Chief Executive Officer
**Web address:** www.marthasvineyardhospital.org

MASSACHUSETTS GENERAL HOSPITAL (O, 945 beds) 55 Fruit Street, Boston, MA Zip 02114–2696; tel. 617/726–2000; Peter L. Slavin, M.D., President
**Web address:** www.massgeneral.org

MCLEAN HOSPITAL (O, 177 beds) 115 Mill Street, Belmont, MA Zip 02478–9106; tel. 617/855–2000; Scott L. Rauch, M.D., President
**Web address:** www.mclean.harvard.edu

NANTUCKET COTTAGE HOSPITAL (O, 19 beds) 57 Prospect Street, Nantucket, MA Zip 02554–2799; tel. 508/825–8100; Margot Hartmann, M.D., Ph.D., President and Chief Executive Officer
**Web address:** www.nantuckethospital.org

NEWTON–WELLESLEY HOSPITAL (O, 232 beds) 2014 Washington Street, Newton Lower Falls, MA Zip 02462–1699; tel. 617/243–6000; Michael Jellinek, M.D., President
**Web address:** www.nwh.org

NORTH SHORE MEDICAL CENTER (O, 395 beds) 81 Highland Avenue, Salem, MA Zip 01970–2714; tel. 978/741–1200; Robert G. Norton, President and Chief Executive Officer
**Web address:** www.nsmc.partners.org

SPAULDING HOSPITAL FOR CONTINUING MEDICAL  CARE NORTH SHORE (O, 160 beds) 1 Dove Avenue, Salem, MA Zip 01970–2999; tel. 978/825–8900; Maureen Banks, R.N., MS, President
**Web address:** www.shaughnessy–kaplan.org

SPAULDING HOSPITAL FOR CONTINUING MEDICAL CARE CAMBRIDGE (O, 180 beds) 1575 Cambridge Street, Cambridge, MA Zip 02138–4308; tel. 617/876–4344; Maureen Banks, R.N., MS, President
**Web address:** www.spauldingrehab.org/OurLocations/HospitalCambridge

SPAULDING REHABILITATION HOSPITAL (O, 196 beds) 125 Nashua Street, Boston, MA Zip 02114–1198; tel. 617/573–7000; David E. Storto, President
**Web address:** www.spauldingrehab.org

SPAULDING REHABILITATION HOSPITAL CAPE COD (O, 60 beds) 311 Service Road, East Sandwich, MA Zip 02537–1370; tel. 508/833–4000; Maureen Banks, R.N., MS, President and Chief Executive Officer
**Web address:** www.rhci.org

| | | |
|---|---|---|
| Owned, leased, sponsored: | 12 hospitals | 3261 beds |
| Contract–managed: | 0 hospitals | 0 beds |
| Totals: | 12 hospitals | 3261 beds |

★**5415:   PEACEHEALTH** (CC)
14432 S.E. Eastgate Way, Suite 300, Bellevue, WA Zip 98007–6412; tel. 425/747–1711; Alan R. Yordy, President and Chief Mission Officer
**(Moderately Centralized Health System)**

**ALASKA:** PEACEHEALTH KETCHIKAN MEDICAL CENTER (L, 54 beds) 3100 Tongass Avenue, Ketchikan, AK Zip 99901–5746; tel. 907/225–5171; Patrick J. Branco, Chief Executive Officer
**Web address:** www.peacehealth.org

**OREGON:** COTTAGE GROVE COMMUNITY HOSPITAL (O, 14 beds) 1515 Village Drive, Cottage Grove, OR Zip 97424–9700; tel. 541/942–0511; MaryAnne McMurren, R.N., Administrator and Chief Executive Officer
**Web address:** www.peacehealth.org

PEACE HARBOR HOSPITAL (O, 21 beds) 400 Ninth Street, Florence, OR Zip 97439–7398; tel. 541/997–8412; Rick Yecny, Chief Executive Officer
**Web address:** www.peacehealth.org

SACRED HEART MEDICAL CENTER (O, 93 beds) 1255 Hilyard Street, Eugene, OR Zip 97401–3700, Mailing Address: P.O. Box 10905, Zip 97440–0905; tel. 541/686–7300; Thomas A. Reitinger, Interim Chief Executive Officer
**Web address:** www.peacehealth.org

For explanation of codes following names, see page B2.
★ Indicates Type III membership in the American Hospital Association.

SACRED HEART MEDICAL CENTER AT RIVERBEND (O, 388 beds) 3333 Riverbend Drive, Springfield, OR Zip 97477–8800; tel. 541/222–7300; John Hill, Chief Executive Officer
**Web address:** www.peacehealth.org

**WASHINGTON:** PEACEHEALTH SOUTHWEST MEDICAL CENTER (O, 450 beds) 400 N.E. Mother Joseph Place, Vancouver, WA Zip 98664–3200, Mailing Address: P.O. Box 1600, Zip 98668–1600; tel. 360/256–2000; Joseph M. Kortum, President and Chief Mission Officer
**Web address:** www.swmedicalcenter.org

PEACEHEALTH ST. JOHN MEDICAL CENTER (O, 202 beds) 1615 Delaware Street, Longview, WA Zip 98632–2310, Mailing Address: P.O. Box 3002, Zip 98632–3002; tel. 360/414–2000; Sy Johnson, Chief Executive Officer
**Web address:** www.peacehealth.org

PEACEHEALTH ST. JOSEPH MEDICAL CENTER (O, 253 beds) 2901 Squalicum Parkway, Bellingham, WA Zip 98225–1851; tel. 360/734–5400; Nancy Steiger, R.N., Chief Executive Officer and Chief Mission Officer
**Web address:** www.peacehealth.org

| | | |
|---|---|---|
| Owned, leased, sponsored: | 8 hospitals | 1475 beds |
| Contract–managed: | 0 hospitals | 0 beds |
| Totals: | 8 hospitals | 1475 beds |

---

★**0314: PHOEBE PUTNEY HEALTH SYSTEM** (NP)
417 Third Avenue, Albany, GA Zip 31702; tel. 229/312–1000; Joel Wernick, President and Chief Executive Officer
**(Centralized Health System)**

**GEORGIA:** PHOEBE NORTH (O, 102 beds) 2000 Palmyra Road, Albany, GA Zip 31702–1908, Mailing Address: P.O. Box 1908, Zip 31702–1908; tel. 229/434–2000; Hugh D. Wilson, Interim Chief Executive Officer
**Web address:** www.palmyramedicalcenters.com

PHOEBE PUTNEY MEMORIAL HOSPITAL (O, 440 beds) 417 Third Avenue, Albany, GA Zip 31701–1828, Mailing Address: P.O. Box 1828, Zip 31702–1828; tel. 229/883–1800; Joel Wernick, President and Chief Executive Officer
**Web address:** www.phoebeputney.com

PHOEBE SUMTER MEDICAL CENTER (O, 45 beds) 126 Highway 280 West, Americus, GA Zip 31719; tel. 229/924–6011; Keith J. Petersen, Chief Executive Officer
**Web address:** www.phoebesumter.org

PHOEBE WORTH MEDICAL CENTER (O, 25 beds) 807 South Isabella Street, Sylvester, GA Zip 31791–0545, Mailing Address: P.O. Box 545, Zip 31791–0545; tel. 229/776–6961; Kim Gilman, Chief Administrative Officer
**Web address:** www.phobeputney.com

| | | |
|---|---|---|
| Owned, leased, sponsored: | 4 hospitals | 612 beds |
| Contract–managed: | 0 hospitals | 0 beds |
| Totals: | 4 hospitals | 612 beds |

---

**0650: PHYSICIAN SYNERGY GROUP** (IO)
5605 North MacArthur Boulevard, Suite 310, Irving, TX Zip 75038–2617; tel. 214/350–7741; Corazon Ramirez, M.D., Chief Executive Officer
**(Independent Hospital System)**

**TEXAS:** DALLAS MEDICAL CENTER (O, 89 beds) Seven Medical Parkway, Dallas, TX Zip 75234, Mailing Address: P.O. Box 819094, Zip 75381–9094; tel. 972/247–1000; Raji Kumar, Chief Executive Officer
**Web address:** www.dallasmedcenter.com

PINE CREEK MEDICAL CENTER (O, 18 beds) 9032 Harry Hines Boulevard, Dallas, TX Zip 75235; tel. 214/231–2273; Corazon Ramirez, M.D., Chief Executive Officer
**Web address:** www.pinecreekmedicalcenter.com

| | | |
|---|---|---|
| Owned, leased, sponsored: | 2 hospitals | 107 beds |
| Contract–managed: | 0 hospitals | 0 beds |
| Totals: | 2 hospitals | 107 beds |

---

★**0043: PHYSICIANS FOR HEALTHY HOSPITALS** (IO)
1525 West Florida Avenue, Suite A., Hemet, CA Zip 92543; tel. 951/652–2811; Joel Bergenfeld, Chief Executive Officer

**CALIFORNIA:** HEMET VALLEY MEDICAL CENTER (O, 284 beds) 1117 East Devonshire Avenue, Hemet, CA Zip 92543–3083; tel. 951/652–2811; Joel Bergenfeld, Chief Executive Officer
**Web address:** www.valleyhealthsystem.com

MENIFEE VALLEY MEDICAL CENTER (O, 82 beds) 28400 McCall Boulevard, Sun City, CA Zip 92585–9537; tel. 951/679–8888; Joel Bergenfeld, Chief Executive Officer
**Web address:** www.valleyhealthsystem.com

| | | |
|---|---|---|
| Owned, leased, sponsored: | 2 hospitals | 366 beds |
| Contract–managed: | 0 hospitals | 0 beds |
| Totals: | 2 hospitals | 366 beds |

---

**0620: PHYSICIANS HOSPITAL SYSTEM** (IO)
1625 East Jefferson Boulevard, Mishawaka, IN Zip 46545–7103; tel. 574/255–1400; Cameron R. Gilbert, Ph.D., President and Chief Executive Officer
**(Independent Hospital System)**

**INDIANA:** DOCTOR'S HOSPITAL AND NEUROMUSCULAR CENTER (O, 20 beds) 411 South Whitlock Street, Bremen, IN Zip 46506, Mailing Address: P.O. Box 36, Zip 46506–0036; tel. 574/546–3830; DeWayne Long, Chief Executive Officer
**Web address:** www.physicianshospitalsystem.net

RIVERCREST SPECIALTY HOSPITAL (O, 30 beds) 1625 East Jefferson Boulevard, Mishawaka, IN Zip 46545; tel. 574/255–1400; Ronni Banks, Administrator
**Web address:** www.physicianshospitalsystem.net/

UNITY MEDICAL & SURGICAL HOSPITAL (O, 15 beds) 4455 Edison Lakes Parkway, Mishawaka, IN Zip 46545–1442; tel. 574/968–0867; John M. Day, Chief Executive Officer
**Web address:** www.physicianshospitalsystem.net

| | | |
|---|---|---|
| Owned, leased, sponsored: | 3 hospitals | 65 beds |
| Contract–managed: | 0 hospitals | 0 beds |
| Totals: | 3 hospitals | 65 beds |

---

★**0310: PIEDMONT HEALTHCARE** (NP)
1800 Howell Mill Road N.W., Suite 850, Atlanta, GA Zip 30318–2538; tel. 404/425–1314; R. Timothy Stack, FACHE, President and Chief Executive Officer
**(Independent Hospital System)**

**GEORGIA:** HENRY MEDICAL CENTER (L, 289 beds) 1133 Eagle's Landing Parkway, Stockbridge, GA Zip 30281–5099; tel. 678/604–1000; Charles F. Scott, President and Chief Executive Officer
**Web address:** www.henrymedical.com

PIEDMONT FAYETTE HOSPITAL (O, 148 beds) 1255 Highway 54 West, Fayetteville, GA Zip 30214; tel. 770/719–7000; W. Darrell Cutts, President and Chief Executive Officer
**Web address:** www.fayettehospital.org

PIEDMONT HOSPITAL (O, 481 beds) 1968 Peachtree Road N.W., Atlanta, GA Zip 30309–1231; tel. 404/605–5000; Leslie A. Donahue, President and Chief Executive Officer
**Web address:** www.piedmonthospital.org

PIEDMONT MOUNTAINSIDE HOSPITAL (O, 48 beds) 1266 Highway 515 South, Jasper, GA Zip 30143; tel. 706/692–2441; Mike Robertson, President and Chief Executive Officer
**Web address:** www.piedmontmountainsidehospital.org

PIEDMONT NEWNAN HOSPITAL (O, 143 beds) 60 Hospital Road, Newnan, GA Zip 30263–1210, Mailing Address: P.O. Box 997, Zip 30264–0997; tel. 770/253–1912; G. Michael Bass, President and Chief Executive Officer
**Web address:** www.piedmontnewnan.org

| | | |
|---|---|---|
| Owned, leased, sponsored: | 5 hospitals | 1109 beds |
| Contract–managed: | 0 hospitals | 0 beds |
| Totals: | 5 hospitals | 1109 beds |

Section B

**★0326: PIONEER HEALTH SERVICES** (IO)
110 Pioneer Way, Magee, MS Zip 39111, Mailing Address: P.O. Box 1100, Zip 39111; tel. 601/849–6440; Joseph S. McNulty, III, President and Chief Executive Officer
**(Independent Hospital System)**

PIONEER COMMUNITY HOSPITAL OF EARLY (L, 25 beds) 11740 Columbia Street, Blakely, GA Zip 39823–9604; tel. 229/723–4235; Adam Willmann, Administrator
**Web address:** www.pchearly.com

**MISSISSIPPI:** PIONEER COMMUNITY HOSPITAL OF ABERDEEN (O, 35 beds) 400 South Chestnut Street, Aberdeen, MS Zip 39730–3335, Mailing Address: P.O. Box 548, Zip 39730–0747; tel. 662/369–2455; John Tompkins, Administrator
**Web address:** www.pchaberdeen.com

PIONEER COMMUNITY HOSPITAL OF CHOCTAW (C, 20 beds) 311 West Cherry Street, Ackerman, MS Zip 39735–8708; tel. 662/285–6235; Sean Johnson, Chief Executive Officer
**Web address:** www.pchchoctaw.com

PIONEER COMMUNITY HOSPITAL OF NEWTON (O, 30 beds) 9421 Eastside Drive, Newton, MS Zip 39345–0299; tel. 601/683–2031; Mark Norman, Administrator
**Web address:** www.pchnewton.com

S. E. LACKEY MEMORIAL HOSPITAL (O, 55 beds) 330 Broad Street, Forest, MS Zip 39074–0428, Mailing Address: P.O. Box 428, Zip 39074–0428; tel. 601/469–4151; Donna Riser, Administrator
**Web address:** www.selackey.com

**NORTH CAROLINA:** PIONEER COMMUNITY HOSPITAL OF STOKES (L, 25 beds) 1570 Highway 8 and 89 North, Danbury, NC Zip 27016, Mailing Address: P.O. Box 10, Zip 27016–0010; tel. 336/593–2831; James R. White, Jr., Chief Executive Officer
**Web address:** www.pchstokes.com

**VIRGINIA:** PIONEER COMMUNITY HOSPITAL OF PATRICK COUNTY (O, 25 beds) 18688 Jeb Stuart Highway, Stuart, VA Zip 24171–1559; tel. 276/694–3151; Jeanette Filpi, Chief Executive Officer
**Web address:** www.phscorporate.com

| Owned, leased, sponsored: | 6 hospitals | 195 beds |
|---|---|---|
| Contract–managed: | 1 hospital | 20 beds |
| Totals: | 7 hospitals | 215 beds |

**0617: POST ACUTE MEDICAL, LLC** (IO)
3500 Market Street, Suite 202, Camp Hill, PA Zip 17011–4354; tel. 717/731–9660; Anthony F. Misitano, President and Chief Executive Officer

**LOUISIANA:** NORTHSHORE SPECIALTY HOSPITAL (O, 58 beds) 20050 Crestwood Boulevard, Covington, LA Zip 70433; tel. 985/875–7525; Douglas L. Johnson, FACHE, Chief Executive Officer
**Web address:** www.northshoreltach.com

**TEXAS:** WARM SPRINGS REHABILITATION HOSPITAL (O, 64 beds) 5101 Medical Drive, San Antonio, TX Zip 78229–6098; tel. 210/616–0100; Dennis Falck, Chief Executive Officer
**Web address:** www.warmsprings.org

WARM SPRINGS SPECIALTY HOSPITAL (O, 34 beds) 200 Memorial Drive, Luling, TX Zip 78648; tel. 830/875–8400; Jason Carter, Chief Executive Officer
**Web address:** www.warmsprings.org

WARM SPRINGS SPECIALTY HOSPITAL OF VICTORIA (O, 26 beds) 102 Medical Drive, Victoria, TX Zip 77904; tel. 361/576–6200; Brian Holt, Chief Executive Officer
**Web address:** www.warmsprings.org

| Owned, leased, sponsored: | 4 hospitals | 182 beds |
|---|---|---|
| Contract–managed: | 0 hospitals | 0 beds |
| Totals: | 4 hospitals | 182 beds |

**★0381: POUDRE VALLEY HEALTH SYSTEM** (NP)
2315 East Harmony Road, Suite 200, Fort Collins, CO Zip 80528; tel. 970/237–7001; Rulon F. Stacey, Ph.D., FACHE, President and Chief Executive Officer
**(Independent Hospital System)**

**COLORADO:** MEDICAL CENTER OF THE ROCKIES (O, 136 beds) 2500 Rocky Mountain Avenue, Loveland, CO Zip 80538; tel. 970/624–2500; George E. Hayes, FACHE, President and Chief Executive Officer
**Web address:** www.medctrrockies.org

POUDRE VALLEY HOSPITAL (O, 238 beds) 1024 South Lemay Avenue, Fort Collins, CO Zip 80524–3998; tel. 970/495–7000; Kevin L. Unger, FACHE, President and Chief Executive Officer
**Web address:** www.pvhs.org

| Owned, leased, sponsored: | 2 hospitals | 374 beds |
|---|---|---|
| Contract–managed: | 0 hospitals | 0 beds |
| Totals: | 2 hospitals | 374 beds |

**0240: PREFERRED MANAGEMENT CORPORATION** (IO)
120 West MacArthur, Suite 121, Shawnee, OK Zip 74804–2028; tel. 405/878–0202; Donald Freeman, President and Chief Executive Officer
**(Independent Hospital System)**

**TEXAS:** COLLINGSWORTH GENERAL HOSPITAL (L, 13 beds) 1013 15th Street, Wellington, TX Zip 79095–3703, Mailing Address: P.O. Box 1112, Zip 79095–1112; tel. 806/447–2521; Candy Powell, Administrator
**Web address:** www.collingsworthgeneral.net

CULBERSON HOSPITAL (L, 14 beds) Eisenhower–Farm Market Road 2185, Van Horn, TX Zip 79855, Mailing Address: P.O. Box 609, Zip 79855–0609; tel. 432/283–2760; Jared Chanski, Administrator
**Web address:** www.culbersonhospital.org

KIMBLE HOSPITAL (O, 15 beds) 2101 Main Street, Junction, TX Zip 76849–2101; tel. 325/446–3321; Steve Bowen, Chief Executive Officer
**Web address:** www.kimblehospital.org

PARMER MEDICAL CENTER (C, 15 beds) 1307 Cleveland Avenue, Friona, TX Zip 79035–1121; tel. 806/250–2754; B. Lance Gatlin, FACHE, Administrator
**Web address:** www.pcchtx.com

SABINE COUNTY HOSPITAL (L, 25 beds) Highway 83 West, Hemphill, TX Zip 75948, Mailing Address: P.O. Box 750, Zip 75948–0750; tel. 409/787–3300; Diana Taylor, Administrator
**Web address:** www.sabinecountyhospital.com/

SCHLEICHER COUNTY MEDICAL CENTER (L, 14 beds) 400 West Murchison, Eldorado, TX Zip 76936, Mailing Address: P.O. Box V., Zip 76936–1246; tel. 325/853–2507; Paul Burke, Administrator
**Web address:** www.scmc.us

| Owned, leased, sponsored: | 5 hospitals | 81 beds |
|---|---|---|
| Contract–managed: | 1 hospital | 15 beds |
| Totals: | 6 hospitals | 96 beds |

**★3505: PRESBYTERIAN HEALTHCARE SERVICES** (CO)
2501 Buena Vista Drive, S.E., Albuquerque, NM Zip 87106–4260, Mailing Address: P.O. Box 26666, Zip 87125–6666; tel. 505/841–1234; James H. Hinton, President and Chief Executive Officer
**(Centralized Physician/Insurance Health System)**

**NEW MEXICO:** COLFAX GENERAL HOSPITAL (C, 35 beds) 615 Prospect Avenue, Springer, NM Zip 87747, Mailing Address: P.O. Box 458, Zip 87747; tel. 505/483–2443; Bill Norris, Administrator

DR. DAN C. TRIGG MEMORIAL HOSPITAL (L, 17 beds) 301 East Miel De Luna Avenue, Tucumcari, NM Zip 88401–3810, Mailing Address: P.O. Box 608, Zip 88401–0608; tel. 575/461–7000; Lance C. Labine, Administrator
**Web address:** www.phs.org

ESPANOLA HOSPITAL (O, 80 beds) 1010 Spruce Street, Espanola, NM Zip 87532–2746; tel. 505/753–7111; Brenda Romero, Administrator
**Web address:** www.phs.org

LINCOLN COUNTY MEDICAL CENTER (L, 25 beds) 211 Sudderth Drive, Ruidoso, NM Zip 88345–6043, Mailing Address: P.O. Box 8000, Zip 88355–8000; tel. 575/257–8200; Alfred Santos, Administrator
**Web address:** www.phs.org

For explanation of codes following names, see page B2.
★ Indicates Type III membership in the American Hospital Association.

PLAINS REGIONAL MEDICAL CENTER (O, 106 beds) 2100 Martin Luther King Boulevard, Clovis, NM Zip 88101–9412, Mailing Address: P.O. Box 1688, Zip 88102–1688; tel. 575/769–2141; Hoyt Skabelund, Administrator
**Web address:** www.phs.org

PRESBYTERIAN HOSPITAL (O, 552 beds) 1100 Central Avenue S.E., Albuquerque, NM Zip 87106–4934, Mailing Address: P.O. Box 26666, Zip 87125–6666; tel. 505/841–1234; Clay Holderman, Interim Administrator
**Web address:** www.phs.org

PRESBYTERIAN KASEMAN HOSPITAL (O, 118 beds) 8300 Constitution Avenue N.E., Albuquerque, NM Zip 87110–7624, Mailing Address: P.O. Box 26666, Zip 87125–6666; tel. 505/291–2000; Doyle Boykin, R.N., MSN, Administrator
**Web address:** www.phs.org

SOCORRO GENERAL HOSPITAL (O, 24 beds) 1202 Highway 60 West, Socorro, NM Zip 87801, Mailing Address: P.O. Box 1009, Zip 87801–1009; tel. 505/835–1140; Bo Beames, Administrator
**Web address:** www.phs.org

| | | |
|---|---|---|
| Owned, leased, sponsored: | 7 hospitals | 922 beds |
| Contract–managed: | 1 hospital | 35 beds |
| Totals: | 8 hospitals | 957 beds |

---

★**0851: PRESENCE HEALTH** (CC)
7435 West Talcott Avenue, Chicago, IL Zip 60631; tel. 773/792–5150; Sandra B. Bruce, FACHE, President and Chief Executive Officer

**ILLINOIS:** HOLY FAMILY MEDICAL CENTER (O, 118 beds) 100 North River Road, Des Plaines, IL Zip 60016–1255; tel. 847/297–1800; Pamela Bell, R.N., Chief Executive Officer
**Web address:** www.reshealth.org

OUR LADY OF THE RESURRECTION MEDICAL CENTER (O, 279 beds) 5645 West Addison Street, Chicago, IL Zip 60634–4403; tel. 773/282–7000; Martin H. Judd, Executive Vice President and Chief Executive Officer
**Web address:** www.reshealthcare.org

OUR LADY OF THE RESURRECTION–LONG TERM CARE (O, 50 beds) 5645 West Addison Street, Chicago, IL Zip 60634;

PROVENA COVENANT MEDICAL CENTER (O, 181 beds) 1400 West Park Street, Urbana, IL Zip 61801–2396; tel. 217/337–2000; Michael L. Brown, President and Chief Executive Officer
**Web address:** www.provenacovenant.org

PROVENA MERCY MEDICAL CENTER (O, 124 beds) 1325 North Highland Avenue, Aurora, IL Zip 60506–1449; tel. 630/859–2222; Maureen A. Bryant, FACHE, President and Chief Executive Officer
**Web address:** www.provena.org/mercy/

PROVENA SAINT JOSEPH HOSPITAL (O, 119 beds) 77 North Airlite Street, Elgin, IL Zip 60123–4912; tel. 847/695–3200; Eugene J. McMahon, M.D., President and Chief Executive Officer
**Web address:** www.provena.org

PROVENA SAINT JOSEPH MEDICAL CENTER (O, 457 beds) 333 North Madison Street, Joliet, IL Zip 60435–6595; tel. 815/725–7133; Beth Hughes, President and Chief Executive Officer
**Web address:** www.provena.org/stjoes

PROVENA ST. MARY'S HOSPITAL (O, 143 beds) 500 West Court Street, Kankakee, IL Zip 60901–3661; tel. 815/937–2400; Amy LaFine, R.N., MSN, President and Chief Executive Officer
**Web address:** www.provena.org/stmarys/

PROVENA UNITED SAMARITANS MEDICAL CENTER (O, 127 beds) 812 North Logan, Danville, IL Zip 61832–3788; tel. 217/443–5000; Michael L. Brown, President and Chief Executive Officer
**Web address:** www.provena.org/usmc

RESURRECTION MEDICAL CENTER (O, 402 beds) 7435 West Talcott Avenue, Chicago, IL Zip 60631–3746; tel. 773/774–8000; John D. Baird, Chief Executive Officer
**Web address:** www.reshealthcare.org

RESURRECTION NURSING PAVILION (O, 295 beds) 1001 North Greenwood, Park Ridge, IL Zip 60068; Patricia Tiernan, Administrator

SAINT FRANCIS HOSPITAL (O, 244 beds) 355 Ridge Avenue, Evanston, IL Zip 60202–3399; tel. 847/316–4000; Jeffrey J. Murphy, Executive Vice President and Chief Executive Officer
**Web address:** www.reshealth.org

SAINT JOSEPH HOSPITAL (O, 327 beds) 2900 North Lake Shore Drive, Chicago, IL Zip 60657–6274; tel. 773/665–3000; Roberta Luskin–Hawk, M.D., Chief Executive Officer
**Web address:** www.reshealth.org

SAINTS MARY & ELIZABETH MEDICAL CENTER (O, 495 beds) 2233 West Division Street, Chicago, IL Zip 60622–3086; tel. 312/770–2000; Margaret McDermott, Chief Executive Officer
**Web address:** www.stmaryofnazareth.org

| | | |
|---|---|---|
| Owned, leased, sponsored: | 14 hospitals | 3361 beds |
| Contract–managed: | 0 hospitals | 0 beds |
| Totals: | 14 hospitals | 3361 beds |

---

**0357: PRIME HEALTHCARE SERVICES** (IO)
3300 East Guasti Road, Ontario, CA Zip 91761–8655; tel. 909/235–4400; Prem Reddy, M.D., Interim President and Chief Executive Officer
**(Independent Hospital System)**

**CALIFORNIA:** ALVARADO HOSPITAL (O, 121 beds) 6655 Alvarado Road, San Diego, CA Zip 92120–5208; tel. 619/287–3270; Robin Gomez, Administrator
**Web address:** www.alvaradohospital.com

CENTINELA HOSPITAL MEDICAL CENTER (O, 369 beds) 555 East Hardy Street, Inglewood, CA Zip 90301–4011, Mailing Address: P.O. Box 720, Zip 90312–6720; tel. 310/673–4660; Linda Bradley, Chief Executive Officer
**Web address:** www.centinelamed.com

CHINO VALLEY MEDICAL CENTER (O, 112 beds) 5451 Walnut Avenue, Chino, CA Zip 91710–2672; tel. 909/464–8600; Lex Reddy, Chief Executive Officer
**Web address:** www.cvmc.com

DESERT VALLEY HOSPITAL (O, 75 beds) 16850 Bear Valley Road, Victorville, CA Zip 92395; tel. 760/241–8000; Margaret R. Peterson, Ph.D., R.N., Chief Executive Officer
**Web address:** www.dvmc.com

ENCINO HOSPITAL MEDICAL CENTER (O, 151 beds) 16237 Ventura Boulevard, Encino, CA Zip 91436–2201; tel. 818/995–5000; Robert C. Bills, Chief Executive Officer
**Web address:** www.encinomed.com

GARDEN GROVE HOSPITAL AND MEDICAL CENTER (O, 74 beds) 12601 Garden Grove Boulevard, Garden Grove, CA Zip 92843–1908; tel. 714/537–5160; Virgis Narbutas, Chief Executive Officer
**Web address:** www.gardengrovehospital.com

HUNTINGTON BEACH HOSPITAL (O, 130 beds) 17772 Beach Boulevard, Huntington Beach, CA Zip 92647–6819; tel. 714/843–5000; Virgis Narbutas, Chief Executive Officer
**Web address:** www.hbhospital.com

LA PALMA INTERCOMMUNITY HOSPITAL (O, 141 beds) 7901 Walker Street, La Palma, CA Zip 90623–1722; tel. 714/670–7400; Virgis Narbutas, Chief Executive Officer
**Web address:** www.lapalmaintercommunityhospital.com

MONTCLAIR HOSPITAL MEDICAL CENTER (O, 102 beds) 5000 San Bernardino Street, Montclair, CA Zip 91763–2326; tel. 909/625–5411; Gregory Brentano, Chief Executive Officer
**Web address:** www.dhmcm.com

PARADISE VALLEY HOSPITAL (O, 205 beds) 2400 East Fourth Street, National City, CA Zip 91950–2099; tel. 619/470–4321; Luis Leon, Regional Chief Executive Officer
**Web address:** www.paradisevalleyhospital.org

SAN DIMAS COMMUNITY HOSPITAL (O, 64 beds) 1350 West Covina Boulevard, San Dimas, CA Zip 91773–3219; tel. 909/599–6811; Gregory Brentano, Chief Executive Officer
**Web address:** www.sandimashospital.com

SHASTA REGIONAL MEDICAL CENTER (O, 135 beds) 1100 Butte Street, Redding, CA Zip 96001–0853, Mailing Address: P.O. Box 496072, Zip 96049–6072; tel. 530/244–5400; Randall Hempling, Chief Executive Officer
**Web address:** www.shastaregional.com

SHERMAN OAKS HOSPITAL (O, 112 beds) 4929 Van Nuys Boulevard, Sherman Oaks, CA Zip 91403–1702; tel. 818/981–7111; Robert C. Bills, Chief Executive Officer
**Web address:** www.shermanoakshospital.com

For explanation of codes following names, see page B2.
★ Indicates Type III membership in the American Hospital Association.

Section B

VICTOR VALLEY COMMUNITY HOSPITAL (O, 115 beds) 15248 Eleventh Street, Victorville, CA Zip 92395; tel. 760/245–8691; Edward Matthews, Interim Chief Executive Officer
**Web address:** www.vvch.org

WEST ANAHEIM MEDICAL CENTER (O, 219 beds) 3033 West Orange Avenue, Anaheim, CA Zip 92804–3184; tel. 714/827–3000; Virgis Narbutas, Chief Executive Officer
**Web address:** www.westanaheimmedctr.com

**NEVADA:** SAINT MARY'S REGIONAL MEDICAL CENTER (O, 272 beds) 235 West Sixth Street, Reno, NV Zip 89503; tel. 775/770–3000; Helen Lidholm, Chief Executive Officer
**Web address:** www.saintmarysreno.com

**PENNSYLVANIA:** ROXBOROUGH MEMORIAL HOSPITAL (O, 137 beds) 5800 Ridge Avenue, Philadelphia, PA Zip 19128–1737; tel. 215/483–9900; Peter J. Adamo, Chief Executive Officer
**Web address:** www.roxboroughmemorial.com

**TEXAS:** HARLINGEN MEDICAL CENTER (O, 88 beds) 5501 South Expressway 77, Harlingen, TX Zip 78550; tel. 956/365–1000; Todd Mann, President and Chief Executive Officer
**Web address:** www.hmcrgv.com

PAMPA REGIONAL MEDICAL CENTER (O, 32 beds) One Medical Plaza, Pampa, TX Zip 79065; tel. 806/665–3721; Richard L. McConahy, Interim Chief Executive Officer
**Web address:** www.prmctx.com

| | | |
|---|---|---|
| Owned, leased, sponsored: | 19 hospitals | 2654 beds |
| Contract–managed: | 0 hospitals | 0 beds |
| Totals: | 19 hospitals | 2654 beds |

---

**★0153: PROHEALTH CARE, INC.** (NP)
N17 W24100 Riverwood Drive, Suite 130, Waukesha, WI Zip 53188; tel. 262/928–2242; Susan A. Edwards, President and Chief Executive Officer
**(Centralized Health System)**

**WISCONSIN:** OCONOMOWOC MEMORIAL HOSPITAL (O, 76 beds) 791 Summit Avenue, Oconomowoc, WI Zip 53066–3896; tel. 262/569–9400; John R. Robertstad, FACHE, President
**Web address:** www.oconomowocmemorial.org

REHABILITATION HOSPITAL OF WISCONSIN (O, 40 beds) 1625 Coldwater Creek Drive, Waukesha, WI Zip 53188–8028; tel. 262/521–8800; Anne E. Jurenec, Chief Executive Officer
**Web address:** www.rehabhospitalwi.com

WAUKESHA MEMORIAL HOSPITAL (O, 317 beds) 725 American Avenue, Waukesha, WI Zip 53188–5099; tel. 262/928–1000; John R. Robertstad, FACHE, President
**Web address:** www.waukeshamemorial.org

| | | |
|---|---|---|
| Owned, leased, sponsored: | 3 hospitals | 433 beds |
| Contract–managed: | 0 hospitals | 0 beds |
| Totals: | 3 hospitals | 433 beds |

---

**★0197: PROMEDICA HEALTH SYSTEM** (NP)
1801 Richards Road, Toledo, OH Zip 43607; tel. 419/469–3800; Randall D. Oostra, FACHE, President and Chief Executive Officer
**(Centralized Physician/Insurance Health System)**

**MICHIGAN:** PROMEDICA BIXBY HOSPITAL (O, 66 beds) 818 Riverside Avenue, Adrian, MI Zip 49221–1496; tel. 517/265–0900; Timothy Jakacki, President
**Web address:** www.promedica.org

PROMEDICA HERRICK HOSPITAL (O, 60 beds) 500 East Pottawatamie Street, Tecumseh, MI Zip 49286–2097; tel. 517/424–3000; Timothy Jakacki, President
**Web address:** www.promedica.org

**OHIO:** PROMEDICA BAY PARK HOSPITAL (O, 72 beds) 2801 Bay Park Drive, Oregon, OH Zip 43616; tel. 419/690–7900; Holly L. Bristoll, President
**Web address:** www.promedica.org

PROMEDICA DEFIANCE REGIONAL HOSPITAL (O, 35 beds) 1200 Ralston Avenue, Defiance, OH Zip 43512–1396; tel. 419/783–6955; Gary Cates, President and Chief Executive Officer
**Web address:** www.promedica.org

PROMEDICA FLOWER HOSPITAL (O, 218 beds) 5200 Harroun Road, Sylvania, OH Zip 43560–2196; tel. 419/824–1444; Alan Sattler, President
**Web address:** www.promedica.org

PROMEDICA FOSTORIA COMMUNITY HOSPITAL (O, 25 beds) 501 Van Buren Street, Fostoria, OH Zip 44830–0907, Mailing Address: P.O. Box 907, Zip 44830–0907; tel. 419/435–7734; Daniel Schwanke, President
**Web address:** www.promedica.org

PROMEDICA ST. LUKE'S HOSPITAL (O, 209 beds) 5901 Monclova Road, Maumee, OH Zip 43537–1899; tel. 419/893–5911; Daniel L. Wakeman, President
**Web address:** www.stlukeshospital.com

PROMEDICA TOLEDO HOSPITAL (O, 616 beds) 2142 North Cove Boulevard, Toledo, OH Zip 43606–3896; tel. 419/291–4000; Kevin C. Webb, Ph.D., President
**Web address:** www.promedica.org

| | | |
|---|---|---|
| Owned, leased, sponsored: | 8 hospitals | 1301 beds |
| Contract–managed: | 0 hospitals | 0 beds |
| Totals: | 8 hospitals | 1301 beds |

---

**0230: PROMISE HEALTHCARE** (IO)
999 Yamato Road, 3rd Floor, Boca Raton, FL Zip 33431; tel. 561/869–3100; Howard B. Koslow, President and Chief Executive Officer
**(Independent Hospital System)**

**ARIZONA:** PROMISE HOSPITAL OF PHOENIX (L, 40 beds) 433 East 6th Street, Mesa, AZ Zip 85203–7104; tel. 480/427–3000; Scott Floden, Chief Executive Officer
**Web address:** www.promise–phoenix.com

**CALIFORNIA:** PROMISE HOSPITAL OF EAST LOS ANGELES (L, 36 beds) 443 South Soto Street, Los Angeles, CA Zip 90033–4398; tel. 323/261–1181; Richard Luna, Chief Executive Officer
**Web address:** www.promiseeastla.com

PROMISE HOSPITAL OF EAST LOS ANGELES, SUBURBAN MEDICAL CENTER CAMPUS (L, 182 beds) 16453 South Colorado Avenue, Paramount, CA Zip 90723–5000; tel. 562/531–3110; Richard Luna, Chief Executive Officer
**Web address:** www.promiseeastla.com

PROMISE HOSPITAL OF SAN DIEGO (O, 100 beds) 5550 University Avenue, San Diego, CA Zip 92105–2307; tel. 619/582–3800; Roy Rodriguez, Chief Executive Officer
**Web address:** www.promisesandiego.com

**LOUISIANA:** PROMISE HOSPITAL BATON ROUGE (L, 50 beds) 5130 Mancuso Lane, Baton Rouge, LA Zip 70809–3583; tel. 225/621–1248; Richard Knowland, Area Chief Executive Officer
**Web address:** www.promisehealthcare.com

PROMISE HOSPITAL OF BATON ROUGE (O, 28 beds) 3600 Florida Boulevard, 4th Floor, Baton Rouge, LA Zip 70806; tel. 225/387–7770; Richard Knowland, Area Chief Executive Officer
**Web address:** www.promise–batonrouge.com

PROMISE HOSPITAL OF BATON ROUGE (O, 22 beds) 17000 Medical Center Drive, 3rd Floor, Baton Rouge, LA Zip 70816; tel. 225/236–5440; Richard Knowland, Area Chief Executive Officer
**Web address:** www.promise–batonrouge.com

PROMISE HOSPITAL OF BOSSIER CITY (O, 50 beds) 2525 Viking Drive, Bossier City, LA Zip 71111; tel. 318/841–2525; Rick Stockton, Chief Executive Officer
**Web address:** www.promise–bossiercity.com

PROMISE HOSPITAL OF LOUISIANA – SHREVEPORT CAMPUS (O, 146 beds) 1800 Irving Place, Shreveport, LA Zip 71101–4608; tel. 318/425–4096; Rick Stockton, Chief Executive Officer
**Web address:** www.promise–shreveport.com

PROMISE HOSPITAL OF MISS LOU (O, 40 beds) 209 Front Street, Vidalia, LA Zip 71373–2837; tel. 318/336–6500; Benny Costello, Chief Executive Officer
**Web address:** www.promise–misslou.com

---

For explanation of codes following names, see page B2.
★ Indicates Type III membership in the American Hospital Association.

**MISSISSIPPI:** PROMISE HOSPITAL OF VICKSBURG (L, 33 beds) 1111 North Frontage Road, 2nd Floor, Vicksburg, MS Zip 39180–5102; tel. 601/619–3526; Lee Huckaby, Chief Executive Officer
**Web address:** www.promise-vicksburg.com

**TEXAS:** PROMISE HOSPITAL OF SAN ANTONIO (L, 26 beds) 7400 Barlite Boulevard, 2nd Floor, San Antonio, TX Zip 78224; tel. 210/921–3550; Karen Pitcher, Vice President and Chief Executive Officer
**Web address:** www.promise-sanantonio.com

PROMISE SPECIALTY HOSPITAL OF SOUTHEAST TEXAS (O, 36 beds) 2600 Highway 365, Nederland, TX Zip 77627–6237; tel. 409/726–8700; Gayla Quillin, Administrator
**Web address:** www.promise-southeasttexas.com

**UTAH:** PROMISE SPECIALTY HOSPITAL OF SALT LAKE (O, 32 beds) 1050 East South Temple, 3rd Floor, Salt Lake City, UT Zip 84102; tel. 801/350–4110; Linda Hook, Chief Executive Officer
**Web address:** www.promise-saltlake.com

| | | |
|---|---|---|
| Owned, leased, sponsored: | 14 hospitals | 821 beds |
| Contract–managed: | 0 hospitals | 0 beds |
| Totals: | 14 hospitals | 821 beds |

★**0344: PROVIDENCE HEALTH & SERVICES** (CC)
1801 Lind Avenue S.W., 9016, Renton, WA Zip 98057–9016; tel. 425/525–3698; John F. Koster, M.D., President and Chief Executive Officer
**(Decentralized Health System)**

**ALASKA:** PROVIDENCE ALASKA MEDICAL CENTER (O, 371 beds) 3200 Providence Drive, Anchorage, AK Zip 99508–4615, Mailing Address: P.O. Box 196604, Zip 99519–6604; tel. 907/562–2211; Bruce Lamoureux, Vice President and Chief Executive Officer
**Web address:** www.providence.org/alaska/pamc/default.htm

PROVIDENCE KODIAK ISLAND MEDICAL CENTER (L, 25 beds) 1915 East Rezanof Drive, Kodiak, AK Zip 99615–6602; tel. 907/486–3281; Donald J. Rush, Chief Executive Officer
**Web address:** www.providence.org

PROVIDENCE SEWARD MEDICAL CENTER (L, 6 beds) 417 First Avenue, Seward, AK Zip 99664, Mailing Address: P.O. Box 365, Zip 99664–0365; tel. 907/224–5205; Christopher Bolton, Administrator
**Web address:** www.providence.org

PROVIDENCE VALDEZ MEDICAL CENTER (C, 21 beds) 911 Meals Avenue, Valdez, AK Zip 99686–0550, Mailing Address: P.O. Box 550, Zip 99686–0550; tel. 907/835–2249; Sean McCallister, Administrator
**Web address:** www.providence.org/alaska

**CALIFORNIA:** PROVIDENCE HOLY CROSS MEDICAL CENTER (O, 254 beds) 15031 Rinaldi Street, Mission Hills, CA Zip 91346–9600; tel. 818/365–8051; Larry Bowe, Chief Executive
**Web address:** www.providence.org/losangeles/facilities/providence_holy_cross/

PROVIDENCE LITTLE COMPANY OF MARY MEDICAL CENTER (O, 372 beds) 4101 Torrance Boulevard, Torrance, CA Zip 90503–4698; tel. 310/540–7676; Elizabeth Dunne, Chief Executive Officer
**Web address:** www.lcmweb.org

PROVIDENCE LITTLE COMPANY OF MARY MEDICAL CENTER SAN PEDRO (O, 327 beds) 1300 West Seventh Street, San Pedro, CA Zip 90732–3505; tel. 310/832–3311; Nancy Carlson, Chief Executive
**Web address:** www.https://california.providence.org/san-pedro

PROVIDENCE SAINT JOSEPH MEDICAL CENTER (O, 414 beds) 501 South Buena Vista Street, Burbank, CA Zip 91505–4866; tel. 818/843–5111; Kerry Carmody, Chief Executive Officer
**Web address:** www.providence.org

PROVIDENCE TARZANA MEDICAL CENTER (O, 245 beds) 18321 Clark Street, Tarzana, CA Zip 91356–3521; tel. 818/881–0800; Dale Surowitz, Chief Executive
**Web address:** www.providence.org/tarzana.com

**MONTANA:** COMMUNITY HOSPITAL OF ANACONDA (C, 87 beds) 401 West Pennsylvania Street, Anaconda, MT Zip 59711–1931; tel. 406/563–8500; Steve McNeece, Chief Executive Officer
**Web address:** www.communityhospitalofanaconda.org

ST. JOSEPH HOSPITAL (S, 22 beds) 6 Thirteenth Avenue East, Polson, MT Zip 59860–5316, Mailing Address: P.O. Box 1010, Zip 59860–1010; tel. 406/883–5377; James R. Kiser, II, Chief Executive Officer
**Web address:** www.saintjoes.org

ST. PATRICK HOSPITAL (S, 134 beds) 500 West Broadway, Missoula, MT Zip 59802–4096, Mailing Address: P.O. Box 4587, Zip 59806–4587; tel. 406/543–7271; Jeff Fee, Chief Executive Officer
**Web address:** www.saintpatrick.org

**OREGON:** PROVIDENCE HOOD RIVER MEMORIAL HOSPITAL (O, 25 beds) 811 13th Street, Hood River, OR Zip 97031–1204, Mailing Address: P.O. Box 149, Zip 97031–0149; tel. 541/386–3911; Edward E. Freysinger, Chief Executive Officer
**Web address:** www.providence.org/hoodriver

PROVIDENCE MEDFORD MEDICAL CENTER (O, 113 beds) 1111 Crater Lake Avenue, Medford, OR Zip 97504–6241; tel. 541/732–5000; Thomas S. Hanenburg, Chief Executive
**Web address:** www.providence.org

PROVIDENCE MILWAUKIE HOSPITAL (O, 64 beds) 10150 S.E. 32nd Avenue, Milwaukie, OR Zip 97222–6516; tel. 503/513–8300; Keith Hyde, Chief Executive Officer
**Web address:** www.providence.org

PROVIDENCE NEWBERG MEDICAL CENTER (O, 40 beds) 1001 Providence Drive, Newberg, OR Zip 97132–7485; tel. 503/537–1555; Alan C. Olive, Chief Executive Officer
**Web address:** www.phsor.org

PROVIDENCE PORTLAND MEDICAL CENTER (O, 412 beds) 4805 N.E. Glisan Street, Portland, OR Zip 97213–2967; tel. 503/215–5526; Theron Park, Chief Executive Officer
**Web address:** www.providence.org

PROVIDENCE SEASIDE HOSPITAL (L, 47 beds) 725 South Wahanna Road, Seaside, OR Zip 97138–7735; tel. 503/717–7000; Krista Farnham, Chief Executive
**Web address:** www.providence.org

PROVIDENCE ST. VINCENT MEDICAL CENTER (O, 552 beds) 9205 S.W. Barnes Road, Portland, OR Zip 97225–6661; tel. 503/216–1234; Janice Burger, Administrator
**Web address:** www.providence.org/portland/hospitals

PROVIDENCE WILLAMETTE FALLS MEDICAL CENTER (O, 89 beds) 1500 Division Street, Oregon City, OR Zip 97045–1597; tel. 503/656–1631; Russ Reinhard, Chief Executive
**Web address:** www.providence.org/pwfmc

**WASHINGTON:** PROVIDENCE CENTRALIA HOSPITAL (O, 100 beds) 914 South Scheuber Road, Centralia, WA Zip 98531–9027; tel. 360/736–2803; Cindy Mayo, Chief Executive
**Web address:** www.providence.org

PROVIDENCE HOLY FAMILY HOSPITAL (S, 182 beds) 5633 North Lidgerwood Street, Spokane, WA Zip 99208–1224; tel. 509/482–0111; Elaine Couture, R.N., Chief Executive Officer
**Web address:** www.providence.org

PROVIDENCE MOUNT CARMEL HOSPITAL (S, 25 beds) 982 East Columbia Avenue, Colville, WA Zip 99114–3352; tel. 509/685–5100; Robert D. Campbell, Jr., President and Chief Executive
**Web address:** www.mtcarmelhospital.org

PROVIDENCE REGIONAL MEDICAL CENTER EVERETT (O, 491 beds) 1321 Colby Avenue, Everett, WA Zip 98206–1147, Mailing Address: P.O. Box 1147, Zip 98206–1147; tel. 425/261–2000; David Brooks, Chief Executive Officer
**Web address:** www.providence.org

PROVIDENCE SACRED HEART MEDICAL CENTER & CHILDREN'S HOSPITAL (S, 628 beds) 101 West Eighth Avenue, Spokane, WA Zip 99204–2364, Mailing Address: P.O. Box 2555, Zip 99220–2555; tel. 509/474–3131; Elaine Couture, R.N., Chief Executive Officer
**Web address:** www.shmc.org

PROVIDENCE ST. JOSEPH'S HOSPITAL (S, 65 beds) 500 East Webster Street, Chewelah, WA Zip 99109–9523; tel. 509/935–8211; Robert D. Campbell, Jr., President and Chief Executive
**Web address:** www.sjhospital.org

PROVIDENCE ST. MARY MEDICAL CENTER (S, 76 beds) 401 West Poplar Street, Walla Walla, WA Zip 99362, Mailing Address: P.O. Box 1477, Zip 99362–0312; tel. 509/525–3320; Steven A. Burdick, Chief Executive Officer
**Web address:** www.smmc.com

For explanation of codes following names, see page B2.
★ Indicates Type III membership in the American Hospital Association.

PROVIDENCE ST. PETER HOSPITAL (O, 378 beds) 413 Lilly Road N.E., Olympia, WA Zip 98506–5166; tel. 360/491–9480; Medrice Coluccio, R.N., Chief Executive Officer
**Web address:** www.providence.org/swsa/facilities/st_peter_hospital

WHITMAN HOSPITAL AND MEDICAL CENTER (C, 25 beds) 1200 West Fairview Street, Colfax, WA Zip 99111–9579; tel. 509/397–3435; Deborah Glass, MS, R.N., Chief Executive Officer
**Web address:** www.whitmanhospital.com

| Owned, leased, sponsored: | 26 hospitals | 5457 beds |
|---|---|---|
| Contract–managed: | 3 hospitals | 133 beds |
| Totals: | 29 hospitals | 5590 beds |

★**0011:  PUERTO RICO DEPARTMENT OF HEALTH** (NP)
Building A – Medical Center, San Juan, PR Zip 00936, Mailing Address: Call Box 70184, Zip 00936; tel. 787/765–2929; Lorenzo Gonzalez Feliciano, M.D., Secretary of Health
**(Independent Hospital System)**

**PUERTO RICO:** CARDIOVASCULAR CENTER OF PUERTO RICO AND THE CARIBBEAN (O, 146 beds) Americo Miranda Centro Medico, San Juan, PR Zip 00936, Mailing Address: P.O. Box 366528, Zip 00936–6528; tel. 787/754–8500; Javier E. Malave Rosario, Executive Director
**Web address:** www.cardiovascular.gobierno.pr

HOSPITAL UNIVERSITARIO DR. RAMON RUIZ ARNAU (O, 102 beds) Avenue Laurel, Santa Juanita, Bayamon, PR Zip 00956; tel. 787/787–5151; Rafael Garcia Alvarez, Chief Executive Officer

UNIVERSITY HOSPITAL (O, 262 beds) Nineyas 869 Rio Piedras, San Juan, PR Zip 00922, Mailing Address: P.O. Box 2116, Zip 00922; tel. 787/754–0101; Jorge Matta Gonzalez, Executive Director

UNIVERSITY PEDIATRIC HOSPITAL (O, 145 beds) Barrio Monacenno, Carretera 22, Rio Piedras, PR Zip 00935, Mailing Address: P.O. Box 2129, San Juan, Zip 00922–2129; tel. 787/777–3535; Sylvia Mercado, Executive Director

| Owned, leased, sponsored: | 4 hospitals | 655 beds |
|---|---|---|
| Contract–managed: | 0 hospitals | 0 beds |
| Totals: | 4 hospitals | 655 beds |

★**0002:  QHR** (IO)
105 Continental Place, Brentwood, TN Zip 37027; tel. 800/233–1470; James L. Horrar, President and Chief Executive Officer
**(Decentralized Health System)**

**ALABAMA:** ELBA GENERAL HOSPITAL (C, 20 beds) 987 Drayton Street, Elba, AL Zip 36323–1494; tel. 334/897–2257; Ellen C. Briley, Administrator and Chief Executive Officer

**ALASKA:** BARTLETT REGIONAL HOSPITAL (C, 57 beds) 3260 Hospital Drive, Juneau, AK Zip 99801–7808; tel. 907/796–8900; John H. Vowell, Interim Chief Executive Officer
**Web address:** www.bartletthospital.org

**COLORADO:** ARKANSAS VALLEY REGIONAL MEDICAL CENTER (C, 163 beds) 1100 Carson Avenue, La Junta, CO Zip 81050–2799; tel. 719/383–6000; Lynn Crowell, Chief Executive Officer
**Web address:** www.avrmc.org

COMMUNITY HOSPITAL (C, 44 beds) 2021 North 12th Street, Grand Junction, CO Zip 81501–2999; tel. 970/242–0920; Chris Thomas, FACHE, President and Chief Executive Officer
**Web address:** www.yourcommunityhospital.com

MEMORIAL HOSPITAL (C, 25 beds) 750 Hospital Loop, Craig, CO Zip 81625–8750; tel. 970/824–9411; George A. Rohrich, Chief Executive Officer
**Web address:** www.thememorialhospital.com

MONTROSE MEMORIAL HOSPITAL (C, 69 beds) 800 South Third Street, Montrose, CO Zip 81401–4291; tel. 970/249–2211; David L. Hample, Chief Executive Officer
**Web address:** www.montrosehospital.com

MT. SAN RAFAEL HOSPITAL (C, 25 beds) 410 Benedicta Avenue, Trinidad, CO Zip 81082–2093; tel. 719/846–9213; James Robertson, Chief Executive Officer
**Web address:** www.msrhc.org

PARKVIEW MEDICAL CENTER (C, 370 beds) 400 West 16th Street, Pueblo, CO Zip 81003–2781; tel. 719/584–4000; Michael T. Baxter, Chief Executive Officer
**Web address:** www.parkviewmc.org

PIONEERS MEDICAL CENTER (C, 50 beds) 345 Cleveland Street, Meeker, CO Zip 81641–3238; tel. 970/878–5047; Kenneth Harman, Chief Executive Officer
**Web address:** www.pioneershospital.com

PROWERS MEDICAL CENTER (C, 25 beds) 401 Kendall Drive, Lamar, CO Zip 81052–3993; tel. 719/336–4343; Craig Loveless, Interim Chief Executive Officer
**Web address:** www.prowersmedical.com

**FLORIDA:** FISHERMEN'S HOSPITAL (C, 25 beds) 3301 Overseas Highway, Marathon, FL Zip 33050–0068; tel. 305/743–5533; Hal W. Leftwich, FACHE, Chief Executive Officer
**Web address:** www.fishermenshospital.com

HENDRY REGIONAL MEDICAL CENTER (C, 25 beds) 524 West Sagamore Avenue, Clewiston, FL Zip 33440–3094; tel. 863/983–9121; Lynn W. Beasley, FACHE, Chief Executive Officer
**Web address:** www.hendryregional.org

JACKSON HOSPITAL (C, 65 beds) 4250 Hospital Drive, Marianna, FL Zip 32446–1939, Mailing Address: P.O. Box 1608, Zip 32447–1608; tel. 850/526–2200; Larry Meese, Chief Executive Officer
**Web address:** www.jacksonhosp.com

**GEORGIA:** HABERSHAM MEDICAL CENTER (C, 137 beds) 541 Historic Highway 441, Demorest, GA Zip 30535–3118, Mailing Address: P.O. Box 37, Zip 30535–0037; tel. 706/754–2161; C. Richard Dwozan, Chief Executive Officer
**Web address:** www.hcmcmed.org

**IDAHO:** BENEWAH COMMUNITY HOSPITAL (C, 19 beds) 229 South Seventh Street, Saint Maries, ID Zip 83861–1803; tel. 208/245–5551; Brian Nall, Chief Executive Officer
**Web address:** www.bchmed.org

GRITMAN MEDICAL CENTER (C, 25 beds) 700 South Main Street, Moscow, ID Zip 83843–3047; tel. 208/882–4511; Kara Besst, President and Chief Executive Officer
**Web address:** www.gritman.org

STEELE MEMORIAL MEDICAL CENTER (C, 18 beds) 203 South Daisy Street, Salmon, ID Zip 83467–4109; tel. 208/756–5600; Jeff Hill, Chief Executive Officer
**Web address:** www.steelemh.org

**ILLINOIS:** CRAWFORD MEMORIAL HOSPITAL (C, 63 beds) 1000 North Allen Street, Robinson, IL Zip 62454–1167; tel. 618/544–3131; Donald E. Annis, Chief Executive Officer
**Web address:** www.crawfordmh.org

HOOPESTON REGIONAL HEALTH CENTER (C, 99 beds) 701 East Orange Street, Hoopeston, IL Zip 60942–1871; tel. 217/283–5531; Harry Brockus, Chief Executive Officer
**Web address:** www.hoopestonhospital.org

IROQUOIS MEMORIAL HOSPITAL AND RESIDENT HOME (C, 84 beds) 200 Fairman Avenue, Watseka, IL Zip 60970–1644; tel. 815/432–5841; Michael J. Stenger, Interim President and Chief Executive Officer
**Web address:** www.iroquoismemorial.com

LAWRENCE COUNTY MEMORIAL HOSPITAL (C, 25 beds) 2200 West State Street, Lawrenceville, IL Zip 62439–1853; tel. 618/943–1000; Doug Florkowski, Chief Executive Officer
**Web address:** www.lcmhosp.org

PEKIN HOSPITAL (C, 125 beds) 600 South 13th Street, Pekin, IL Zip 61554–5098; tel. 309/347–1151; Gary L. Jepson, Chief Executive Officer
**Web address:** www.pekinhospital.org

**INDIANA:** DAVIESS COMMUNITY HOSPITAL (C, 48 beds) 1314 East Walnut Street, Washington, IN Zip 47501–2198, Mailing Address: P.O. Box 760, Zip 47501–0760; tel. 812/254–2760; David Bixler, Chief Executive Officer
**Web address:** www.dchosp.org

SULLIVAN COUNTY COMMUNITY HOSPITAL (C, 25 beds) 2200 North Section Street, Sullivan, IN Zip 47882, Mailing Address: P.O. Box 10, Zip 47882–0010; tel. 812/268–4311; Michelle Sly-Smith, Chief Executive Officer
**Web address:** www.schosp.org

For explanation of codes following names, see page B2.
★ Indicates Type III membership in the American Hospital Association.

© 2012 AHA Guide

**IOWA:** BOONE COUNTY HOSPITAL (C, 25 beds) 1015 Union Street, Boone, IA Zip 50036–4821; tel. 515/432–3140; Joseph S. Smith, Chief Executive Officer
**Web address:** www.boonehospital.com

FORT MADISON COMMUNITY HOSPITAL (C, 50 beds) 5445 Avenue O, Fort Madison, IA Zip 52627–0174, Mailing Address: P.O. Box 174, Zip 52627–0174; tel. 319/372–6530; C. James Platt, Chief Executive Officer
**Web address:** www.fmchosp.com

**KANSAS:** COFFEYVILLE REGIONAL MEDICAL CENTER (C, 88 beds) 1400 West Fourth, Coffeyville, KS Zip 67337–0856; tel. 620/251–1200; John Smith, Chief Executive Officer
**Web address:** www.crmcinc.com

GREELEY COUNTY HEALTH SERVICES (C, 50 beds) 506 Third Street, Tribune, KS Zip 67879–0338, Mailing Address: P.O. Box 338, Zip 67879–0338; tel. 620/376–4221; Deborah Lehner, Administrator
**Web address:** www.phn.org

NEOSHO MEMORIAL REGIONAL MEDICAL CENTER (C, 25 beds) 629 South Plummer, Chanute, KS Zip 66720–0426, Mailing Address: P.O. Box 426, Zip 66720–0426; tel. 620/431–4000; Dennis Franks, FACHE, Chief Executive Officer
**Web address:** www.nmrmc.com

NEWMAN REGIONAL HEALTH (C, 59 beds) 1201 West 12th Avenue, Emporia, KS Zip 66801–2597; tel. 620/343–6800; John Rossfeld, Interim Chief Executive Officer
**Web address:** www.newmanrh.org

ST. LUKE HOSPITAL AND LIVING CENTER (C, 37 beds) 535 South Freeborn, Marion, KS Zip 66861–1299; tel. 620/382–2177; Jeremy Armstrong, FACHE, Chief Executive Officer
**Web address:** www.slhmarion.org

WILSON MEDICAL CENTER (C, 15 beds) 2600 Ottawa Road, Neodesha, KS Zip 66757–1817, Mailing Address: P.O. Box 360, Zip 66757–0360; tel. 620/325–2611; Dennis R. Shelby, Chief Executive Officer
**Web address:** www.wilsonmedical.org

**KENTUCKY:** CALDWELL MEDICAL CENTER (C, 25 beds) 100 Medical Center Drive, Princeton, KY Zip 42445–2430, Mailing Address: P.O. Box 410, Zip 42445–0410; tel. 270/365–0300; Charles D. Lovell, Jr., FACHE, President and Chief Executive Officer
**Web address:** www.caldwellhosp.org

FLEMING COUNTY HOSPITAL (C, 52 beds) 55 Foundation Drive, Flemingsburg, KY Zip 41041–9815, Mailing Address: P.O. Box 388, Zip 41041–0388; tel. 606/849–5000; David M. Faulkner, Chief Executive Officer
**Web address:** www.flemingcountyhospital.org

JENNIE STUART MEDICAL CENTER (C, 139 beds) 320 West 18th Street, Hopkinsville, KY Zip 42241–2400, Mailing Address: P.O. Box 2400, Zip 42241–2400; tel. 270/887–0100; Eric A. Lee, President and Chief Executive Officer
**Web address:** www.jsmc.org

MONROE COUNTY MEDICAL CENTER (C, 49 beds) 529 Capp Harlan Road, Tompkinsville, KY Zip 42167–1840; tel. 270/487–9231; Vicky McFall, Chief Executive Officer
**Web address:** www.mcmccares.com

OHIO COUNTY HOSPITAL (C, 25 beds) 1211 Main Street, Hartford, KY Zip 42347–1619; tel. 270/298–7411; Blaine Pieper, Chief Executive Officer
**Web address:** www.ohiocountyhospital.com

**LOUISIANA:** FRANKLIN FOUNDATION HOSPITAL (C, 22 beds) 1097 Northwest Boulevard, Franklin, LA Zip 70538–3724, Mailing Address: P.O. Box 577, Zip 70538–0577; tel. 337/828–0760; Parker Templeton, FACHE, Chief Executive Officer
**Web address:** www.franklinfoundation.org

OPELOUSAS GENERAL HEALTH SYSTEM (C, 201 beds) 539 East Prudhomme Street, Opelousas, LA Zip 70570, Mailing Address: P.O. Box 1389, Zip 70571–1389; tel. 337/948–3011; Gary I. Keller, President and Chief Executive Officer
**Web address:** www.opelousasgeneral.com

**MAINE:** CALAIS REGIONAL HOSPITAL (C, 25 beds) 24 Hospital Lane, Calais, ME Zip 04619–1398; tel. 207/454–7521; Michael K. Lally, Chief Executive Officer
**Web address:** www.calaishospital.com

CARY MEDICAL CENTER (C, 49 beds) 163 Van Buren Road, Suite 1, Caribou, ME Zip 04736–2599; tel. 207/498–3111; Kris A. Doody, R.N., Chief Executive Officer
**Web address:** www.carymedicalcenter.org

PENOBSCOT VALLEY HOSPITAL (C, 25 beds) 7 Transalpine Road, Lincoln, ME Zip 04457–0368, Mailing Address: P.O. Box 368, Zip 04457–0368; tel. 207/794–3321; David A. Shannon, Chief Executive Officer
**Web address:** www.pvhme.org

**MICHIGAN:** ALLEGAN GENERAL HOSPITAL (C, 25 beds) 555 Linn Street, Allegan, MI Zip 49010–1524; tel. 269/673–8424; Gerald J. Barbini, President and Chief Executive Officer
**Web address:** www.aghosp.org

HAYES GREEN BEACH MEMORIAL HOSPITAL (C, 25 beds) 321 East Harris Street, Charlotte, MI Zip 48813–1629; tel. 517/543–1050; Matthew Rush, President and Chief Executive Officer
**Web address:** www.hgbhealth.com

STURGIS HOSPITAL (C, 49 beds) 916 Myrtle Street, Sturgis, MI Zip 49091–2326; tel. 269/651–7824; Robert J. LaBarge, Chief Executive Officer
**Web address:** www.sturgishospital.com

THREE RIVERS HEALTH (C, 35 beds) 701 South Houthealth Parkway, Three Rivers, MI Zip 49093–8352; tel. 269/278–1145; William B. Russell, Chief Executive Officer
**Web address:** www.threerivershealth.org

**MINNESOTA:** RAINY LAKE MEDICAL CENTER (C, 25 beds) 1400 Highway 71, International Falls, MN Zip 56649–2189; tel. 218/283–4481; Bob Haley, Interim Chief Executive Officer
**Web address:** www.rainylakemedical.com

**MISSISSIPPI:** HANCOCK MEDICAL CENTER (C, 47 beds) 149 Drinkwater Boulevard, Bay Saint Louis, MS Zip 39521–2790, Mailing Address: P.O. Box 2790, Zip 39521–2790; tel. 228/467–8600; Robert A. Pascasio, FACHE, Chief Executive Officer
**Web address:** www.hmc.org

KING'S DAUGHTERS MEDICAL CENTER (C, 91 beds) 427 Highway 51 North, Brookhaven, MS Zip 39601–2600, Mailing Address: P.O. Box 948, Zip 39602–0948; tel. 601/833–6011; Alvin Hoover, FACHE, Chief Executive Officer
**Web address:** www.kdmc.org

TIPPAH COUNTY HOSPITAL (C, 85 beds) 1005 City Avenue North, Ripley, MS Zip 38663–0499, Mailing Address: P.O. Box 499, Zip 38663–0499; tel. 662/837–9221; Tom Hood, Administrator
**Web address:** www.tippahcounty.ripley.ms/hospital.html

**MISSOURI:** NEVADA REGIONAL MEDICAL CENTER (C, 71 beds) 800 South Ash Street, Nevada, MO Zip 64772–3223; tel. 417/667–3355; Judith K. Feuquay, Chief Executive Officer
**Web address:** www.nrmchealth.com

**MONTANA:** CENTRAL MONTANA MEDICAL CENTER (C, 90 beds) 408 Wendell Avenue, Lewistown, MT Zip 59457–2261; tel. 406/535–7711; Lee Rhodes, Chief Executive Officer
**Web address:** www.cmmccares.com

NORTH VALLEY HOSPITAL (C, 25 beds) 1600 Hospital Way, Whitefish, MT Zip 59937–7849; tel. 406/863–3500; Jason A. Spring, FACHE, Chief Executive Officer
**Web address:** www.nvhosp.org

**NEBRASKA:** PHELPS MEMORIAL HEALTH CENTER (C, 25 beds) 1215 Tibbals Street, Holdrege, NE Zip 68949–1255; tel. 308/995–2211; Mark Harrel, Chief Executive Officer
**Web address:** www.phelpsmemorial.com

**NEW MEXICO:** CIBOLA GENERAL HOSPITAL (C, 25 beds) 1016 East Roosevelt Avenue, Grants, NM Zip 87020–2118; tel. 505/287–4446; Michael Makosky, Chief Executive Officer
**Web address:** www.cibolahospital.com

GERALD CHAMPION REGIONAL MEDICAL CENTER (C, 86 beds) 2669 North Scenic Drive, Alamogordo, NM Zip 88310–8799; tel. 575/439–6100; Robert J. Heckert, Jr., Chief Executive Officer
**Web address:** www.gcrmc.org

HOLY CROSS HOSPITAL (C, 47 beds) 1397 Weimer Road, Taos, NM Zip 87571–6284; tel. 575/758–8883; Peter A. Hofstetter, Chief Executive Officer
**Web address:** www.taoshospital.org

For explanation of codes following names, see page B2.
★ Indicates Type III membership in the American Hospital Association.

**NORTH CAROLINA:** ALLEGHANY MEMORIAL HOSPITAL (C, 25 beds) 233 Doctors Street, Sparta, NC Zip 28675–0009, Mailing Address: P.O. Box 9, Zip 28675–0009; tel. 336/372–5511; James F. Heitzenrater, FACHE, Chief Executive Officer
**Web address:** www.amhsparta.org

ASHE MEMORIAL HOSPITAL (C, 85 beds) 200 Hospital Avenue, Jefferson, NC Zip 28640–9244; tel. 336/846–7101; R. D. Williams, Administrator and Chief Executive Officer
**Web address:** www.ashememorial.org

JOHNSTON HEALTH (C, 147 beds) 509 North Bright Leaf Boulevard, Smithfield, NC Zip 27577–1376, Mailing Address: P.O. Box 1376, Zip 27577–1376; tel. 919/934–8171; Charles W. Elliott, Jr., Chief Executive Officer
**Web address:** www.johnstonhealth.org

MOREHEAD MEMORIAL HOSPITAL (C, 214 beds) 117 East King's Highway, Eden, NC Zip 27288–5299; tel. 336/623–9711; Carl Martin, President and Chief Executive Officer
**Web address:** www.morehead.org

NORTHERN HOSPITAL OF SURRY COUNTY (C, 108 beds) 830 Rockford Street, Mount Airy, NC Zip 27030–5365, Mailing Address: P.O. Box 1101, Zip 27030–1101; tel. 336/719–7000; William B. James, Chief Executive Officer
**Web address:** www.northernhospital.com

RUTHERFORD REGIONAL MEDICAL CENTER (C, 116 beds) 288 South Ridgecrest Avenue, Rutherfordton, NC Zip 28139–3097; tel. 828/286–5000; Cindy D. Buck, Interim Chief Executive Officer
**Web address:** www.rutherfordhosp.org

**OHIO:** KNOX COMMUNITY HOSPITAL (C, 87 beds) 1330 Coshocton Road, Mount Vernon, OH Zip 43050–1495; tel. 740/393–9000; Bruce D. White, Chief Executive Officer
**Web address:** www.knoxcommhosp.org

MEMORIAL HOSPITAL (C, 71 beds) 715 South Taft Avenue, Fremont, OH Zip 43420–3200; tel. 419/332–7321; Wesley W. Oswald, Interim Chief Executive Officer
**Web address:** www.memorialhcs.org

WOOSTER COMMUNITY HOSPITAL (C, 150 beds) 1761 Beall Avenue, Wooster, OH Zip 44691–2342; tel. 330/263–8100; William E. Sheron, Chief Executive Officer
**Web address:** www.woosterhospital.org

**OKLAHOMA:** OKMULGEE MEMORIAL HOSPITAL (C, 36 beds) 1401 Morris Drive, Okmulgee, OK Zip 74447–6419, Mailing Address: P.O. Box 1038, Zip 74447–1038; tel. 918/756–4233; George N. Miller, Jr., Chief Executive Officer
**Web address:** www.okmulgeehospital.com

PERRY MEMORIAL HOSPITAL (C, 26 beds) 501 North 14th Street, Perry, OK Zip 73077–5099; tel. 580/336–3541; Terry W. Shambles, Interim Chief Executive Officer
**Web address:** www.pmh-ok.org

SHARE MEDICAL CENTER (C, 90 beds) 800 Share Drive, Alva, OK Zip 73717–3699, Mailing Address: P.O. Box 727, Zip 73717–0727; tel. 580/327–2800; Kandice K. Allen, R.N., Interim Chief Executive Officer
**Web address:** www.smcok.com

**PENNSYLVANIA:** CLARION HOSPITAL (C, 77 beds) One Hospital Drive, Clarion, PA Zip 16214–8501; tel. 814/226–9500; Byron Quinton, Chief Executive Officer
**Web address:** www.clarionhospital.org

J. C. BLAIR MEMORIAL HOSPITAL (C, 72 beds) 1225 Warm Springs Avenue, Huntingdon, PA Zip 16652–2398; tel. 814/643–2290; Lisa Mallon, Interim President and Chief Executive Officer
**Web address:** www.jcblair.org

JERSEY SHORE HOSPITAL (C, 25 beds) 1020 Thompson Street, Jersey Shore, PA Zip 17740–1794; tel. 570/398–0100; Carey W. Plummer, President and Chief Executive Officer
**Web address:** www.jsh.org

MEMORIAL HOSPITAL (C, 183 beds) One Hospital Drive, Towanda, PA Zip 18848–9702; tel. 570/265–2191; Gary A. Baker, President
**Web address:** www.memorialhospital.org

**SOUTH CAROLINA:** ABBEVILLE AREA MEDICAL CENTER (C, 25 beds) 420 Thomson Circle, Abbeville, SC Zip 29620–5656, Mailing Address: P.O. Box 887, Zip 29620–0887; tel. 864/366–5011; Richard D. Osmus, Chief Executive Officer
**Web address:** www.abbevilleareamc.com

NEWBERRY COUNTY MEMORIAL HOSPITAL (C, 32 beds) 2669 Kinard Street, Newberry, SC Zip 29108–0497, Mailing Address: P.O. Box 497, Zip 29108–0497; tel. 803/276–7570; Ronald J. Vigus, Chief Executive Officer
**Web address:** www.newberryhospital.org

REGIONAL MEDICAL CENTER (C, 286 beds) 3000 St. Matthews Road, Orangeburg, SC Zip 29118–1470; tel. 803/395–2200; Thomas C. Dandridge, FACHE, President and Chief Executive Officer
**Web address:** www.trmchealth.org

**SOUTH DAKOTA:** HURON REGIONAL MEDICAL CENTER (C, 25 beds) 172 Fourth Street S.E., Huron, SD Zip 57350–2590; tel. 605/353–6200; John L. Single, Chief Executive Officer
**Web address:** www.huronregional.org

**TENNESSEE:** LINCOLN COUNTY HEALTH SYSTEM (C, 353 beds) 106 Medical Center Boulevard, Fayetteville, TN Zip 37334–2684; tel. 931/438–1100; Jamie W. Guin, Jr., Chief Executive Officer
**Web address:** www.lchealthsystem.com

MACON COUNTY GENERAL HOSPITAL (C, 25 beds) 204 Medical Drive, Lafayette, TN Zip 37083–1799, Mailing Address: P.O. Box 378, Zip 37083–0378; tel. 615/666–2147; Dennis A. Wolford, FACHE, Executive Officer
**Web address:** www.mcgh.net

RHEA MEDICAL CENTER (C, 25 beds) 9400 Rhea County Highway, Dayton, TN Zip 37321–7922; tel. 423/775–1121; Kennedy L. Croom, Jr., Administrator and Chief Executive Officer
**Web address:** www.rheamedical.org

**TEXAS:** BRAZOSPORT REGIONAL HEALTH SYSTEM (C, 103 beds) 100 Medical Drive, Lake Jackson, TX Zip 77566–9983; tel. 979/297–4411; Daniel L. Buche, Chief Executive Officer
**Web address:** www.brhs.org

MATAGORDA REGIONAL MEDICAL CENTER (C, 58 beds) 104 7th Street, Bay City, TX Zip 77414–4853; tel. 979/245–6383; Steven L. Smith, Chief Executive Officer
**Web address:** www.matagordaregional.org

MEMORIAL HOSPITAL (C, 32 beds) 1110 Sarah Dewitt Drive, Gonzales, TX Zip 78629–2021, Mailing Address: P.O. Box 587, Zip 78629–0587; tel. 830/672–7581; Charles Norris, Chief Executive Officer
**Web address:** www.gonzaleshealthcare.com

**VERMONT:** NORTHWESTERN MEDICAL CENTER (C, 20 beds) 133 Fairfield Street, Saint Albans, VT Zip 05478–1726; tel. 802/524–5911; Jill Berry Bowen, President and Chief Executive Officer
**Web address:** www.northwesternmedicalcenter.org

**WASHINGTON:** KADLEC MEDICAL CENTER (C, 249 beds) 888 Swift Boulevard, Richland, WA Zip 99352–3514; tel. 509/946–4611; Rand J. Wortman, Chief Executive Officer
**Web address:** www.kadlecmed.org

**WISCONSIN:** AMERY REGIONAL MEDICAL CENTER (C, 35 beds) 265 Griffin Street East, Amery, WI Zip 54001–1439; tel. 715/268–8000; Michael Karuschak, Jr., Chief Executive Officer
**Web address:** www.amerymedicalcenter.org

**WYOMING:** MEMORIAL HOSPITAL OF CARBON COUNTY (C, 25 beds) 2221 West Elm Street, Rawlins, WY Zip 82301–0460, Mailing Address: P.O. Box 460, Zip 82301–0460; tel. 307/324–2221; Daniel E. Jessop, CPA, Chief Executive Officer
**Web address:** www.imhcc.com

WEST PARK HOSPITAL (C, 140 beds) 707 Sheridan Avenue, Cody, WY Zip 82414–3409; tel. 307/527–7501; Douglas A. McMillan, Administrator and Chief Executive Officer
**Web address:** www.westparkhospital.org

| Owned, leased, sponsored: | 0 hospitals | 0 beds |
|---|---|---|
| Contract–managed: | 88 hospitals | 6288 beds |
| **Totals:** | 88 hospitals | 6288 beds |

**★0040: QUEEN'S HEALTH SYSTEMS** (NP)
1301 Punchbowl Street, Honolulu, HI Zip 96813–2402; tel. 808/535–5448; Arthur A. Ushijima, President and Chief Executive Officer
**(Moderately Centralized Health System)**

For explanation of codes following names, see page B2.
★ Indicates Type III membership in the American Hospital Association.

**HAWAII:** MOLOKAI GENERAL HOSPITAL (O, 15 beds) Kaunakakai, HI Zip 96748–0408; tel. 808/553–5331; Janice Kalanihuia, President
**Web address:** www.queens.org

QUEEN'S MEDICAL CENTER (O, 495 beds) 1301 Punchbowl Street, Honolulu, HI Zip 96813–2499; tel. 808/538–9011; Arthur A. Ushijima, President
**Web address:** www.queens.org

| | | |
|---|---|---|
| **Owned, leased, sponsored:** | 2 hospitals | 510 beds |
| **Contract–managed:** | 0 hospitals | 0 beds |
| **Totals:** | 2 hospitals | 510 beds |

---

**★8495: REGIONAL HEALTH** (NP)
353 Fairmont Boulevard, Rapid City, SD Zip 57701, Mailing Address: P.O. Box 6000, Zip 57709–6000; tel. 605/719–1000; Charles E. Hart, M.D., MS, President and Chief Executive Officer
**(Moderately Centralized Health System)**

**SOUTH DAKOTA:** CUSTER REGIONAL HOSPITAL (L, 87 beds) 1039 Montgomery Street, Custer, SD Zip 57730–1397; tel. 605/673–2229; Veronica Schmidt, Chief Executive Officer
**Web address:** www.regionalhealth.com

LEAD–DEADWOOD REGIONAL HOSPITAL (O, 18 beds) 61 Charles Street, Deadwood, SD Zip 57732–1303; tel. 605/722–6101; Sherry Bea Smith, R.N., Chief Executive Officer and Chief Financial Officer
**Web address:** www.regionalhealth.com

PHILIP HEALTH SERVICES (C, 48 beds) 503 West Pine Street, Philip, SD Zip 57567, Mailing Address: P.O. Box 790, Zip 57567–0790; tel. 605/859–2511; Kent Olson, Administrator and Chief Executive Officer
**Web address:** www.rcrh.org/Facilities/Hospitals/HPPMemorial.asp

RAPID CITY REGIONAL HOSPITAL (O, 374 beds) 353 Fairmont Boulevard, Rapid City, SD Zip 57701–7393, Mailing Address: P.O. Box 6000, Zip 57709–6000; tel. 605/719–1000; Timothy H. Sughrue, Chief Executive Officer
**Web address:** www.rcrh.org

SPEARFISH REGIONAL HOSPITAL (O, 34 beds) 1440 North Main Street, Spearfish, SD Zip 57783–1504; tel. 605/644–4000; Larry W. Veitz, Chief Executive Officer
**Web address:** www.regionalhealth.com

STURGIS REGIONAL HOSPITAL (O, 109 beds) 949 Harmon Street, Sturgis, SD Zip 57785–2452; tel. 605/720–2400; Van D. Hyde, MS, Chief Executive Officer
**Web address:** www.rcrh.org/Facilities/Hospitals/SCHCC/Default.asp

**WYOMING:** CROOK COUNTY MEDICAL SERVICES DISTRICT (C, 48 beds) 713 Oak Street, Sundance, WY Zip 82729, Mailing Address: P.O. Box 517, Zip 82729–0517; tel. 307/283–3501; Jan VanBeek, Chief Executive Officer
**Web address:** www.crookcountymedical.com

WESTON COUNTY HEALTH SERVICES (C, 75 beds) 1124 Washington Boulevard, Newcastle, WY Zip 82701–2996; tel. 307/746–4491; Gary Bieganski, FACHE, Interim Chief Executive Officer
**Web address:** www.wchs–wy.org

| | | |
|---|---|---|
| **Owned, leased, sponsored:** | 5 hospitals | 622 beds |
| **Contract–managed:** | 3 hospitals | 171 beds |
| **Totals:** | 8 hospitals | 793 beds |

---

**0622: REGIONALCARE HOSPITAL PARTNERS** (IO)
103 Continental Place, Suite 200, Brentwood, TN Zip 37027–1087; tel. 615/844–9800; Martin S. Rash, Chairman and Chief Executive Officer
**(Moderately Centralized Health System)**

**ALABAMA:** ELIZA COFFEE MEMORIAL HOSPITAL (O, 278 beds) 205 Marengo Street, Florence, AL Zip 35630–6033, Mailing Address: P.O. Box 818, Zip 35631–0818; tel. 256/768–9191; Russell Pigg, Chief Executive Officer
**Web address:** www.chgroup.org

SHOALS HOSPITAL (O, 131 beds) 201 Avalon Avenue, Muscle Shoals, AL Zip 35661–2805, Mailing Address: P.O. Box 3359, Zip 35662–3359; tel. 256/386–1600; Ross Berry, Chief Executive Officer
**Web address:** www.chgroup.org

**CONNECTICUT:** SHARON HOSPITAL (O, 78 beds) 50 Hospital Hill Road, Sharon, CT Zip 06069–0789, Mailing Address: P.O. Box 789, Zip 06069–0789; tel. 860/364–4000; Kim Lumia, Chief Executive Officer
**Web address:** www.sharonhospital.com

**IOWA:** OTTUMWA REGIONAL HEALTH CENTER (O, 88 beds) 1001 Pennsylvania Avenue, Ottumwa, IA Zip 52501–2186; tel. 641/684–2300; Philip G. Dionne, Chief Executive Officer
**Web address:** www.orhc.com

**OHIO:** CLINTON MEMORIAL HOSPITAL (O, 85 beds) 610 West Main Street, Wilmington, OH Zip 45177–0600; tel. 937/382–6611; Michael C. Choo, M.D., Chief Executive Officer
**Web address:** www.cmhregional.com

**PENNSYLVANIA:** SOUTHWEST REGIONAL MEDICAL CENTER (O, 77 beds) 350 Bonar Avenue, Waynesburg, PA Zip 15370–1608; tel. 724/627–3101; Cynthia Cowie, Chief Executive Officer
**Web address:** www.sw–rmc.com

**TEXAS:** PARIS REGIONAL MEDICAL CENTER (O, 226 beds) 820 Clarksville Street, Paris, TX Zip 75460–9070; tel. 903/785–4521; Billy Porter, Chief Executive Officer
**Web address:** www.parisrmc.com

| | | |
|---|---|---|
| **Owned, leased, sponsored:** | 7 hospitals | 963 beds |
| **Contract–managed:** | 0 hospitals | 0 beds |
| **Totals:** | 7 hospitals | 963 beds |

---

**0411: RELIANT HEALTHCARE PARTNERS** (IO)
15851 Dallas Parkway, Suite 50, Addison, TX Zip 75001; tel. 972/308–8518; Emmett E. Moore, CPA, JD, Chief Executive Officer
**(Independent Hospital System)**

RELIANT REHABILITATION HOSPITAL ABILENE (O, 30 beds) 6401 Directors Parkway, Abilene, TX Zip 79606–5869; tel. 325/691–1600; Lisa M. Nelson, R.N., MS, Chief Executive Officer
**Web address:** www.reliantabilene.com

RELIANT REHABILITATION HOSPITAL CENTRAL TEXAS (O, 75 beds) 1400 Hester's Crossing, Round Rock, TX Zip 78681; tel. 512/244–4400; Abraham Sims, Interim Chief Executive Officer
**Web address:** www.reliantcentraltx.com/

RELIANT REHABILITATION HOSPITAL NORTH HOUSTON (O, 60 beds) 117 Vision Park Boulevard, Shenandoah, TX Zip 77384–3001; tel. 936/444–1700; Abraham Sims, Chief Executive Officer
**Web address:** www.reliantnorthhouston.com/

RELIANT REHABILITATION HOSPITAL NORTH TEXAS (O, 50 beds) 3351 Waterview Parkway, Richardson, TX Zip 75080; tel. 972/398–5700; Jim Ransom, Chief Executive Officer
**Web address:** www.relianthcp.com

| | | |
|---|---|---|
| **Owned, leased, sponsored:** | 4 hospitals | 215 beds |
| **Contract–managed:** | 0 hospitals | 0 beds |
| **Totals:** | 4 hospitals | 215 beds |

---

**0373: RENAISSANCE HEALTHCARE SYSTEMS** (IO)
14440 John F. Kennedy Boulevardd, Houston, TX Zip 77032; tel. 832/886–1900; Michael Smesney, Chief Executive Officer
**(Independent Hospital System)**

RENAISSANCE HOSPITAL (O, 28 beds) 5500 39th Street, Groves, TX Zip 77619–9805; tel. 409/962–5733; Eileen Nguyen, Administrator
**Web address:** www.renhealthcare.org

RENAISSANCE HOSPITAL TERRELL (L, 102 beds) 1551 Highway 34 South, Terrell, TX Zip 75160–4833; tel. 972/563–7611; Sean Astolfo, Administrator
**Web address:** www.terrell–hospital.com

SOUTH HAMPTON COMMUNITY HOSPITAL (O, 90 beds) 2929 South Hampton Road, Dallas, TX Zip 75224; tel. 214/623–4400; Steven Walker, Chief Executive Officer
**Web address:** www.shchospital.com

For explanation of codes following names, see page B2.
★ Indicates Type III membership in the American Hospital Association.

Section B

ST. ANTHONY'S HOSPITAL (O, 39 beds) 2807 Little York Road, Houston, TX Zip 77093–3495; tel. 713/697–7777; Jason B. Fisher, Chief Executive Officer
**Web address:** www.stanthonyshouston.com

| | | |
|---|---|---|
| Owned, leased, sponsored: | 4 hospitals | 259 beds |
| Contract–managed: | 0 hospitals | 0 beds |
| Totals: | 4 hospitals | 259 beds |

---

**★2625: RENOWN HEALTH** (NP)
1155 Mill Street, Reno, NV Zip 89502–1576; tel. 775/982–4100; James I. Miller, President and Chief Executive Officer
**(Centralized Health System)**

**NEVADA:** RENOWN REGIONAL MEDICAL CENTER (O, 654 beds) 1155 Mill Street, Reno, NV Zip 89502–1474; tel. 775/982–4100; Gregory E. Boyer, Chief Executive Officer
**Web address:** www.renown.org

RENOWN REHABILITATION HOSPITAL (O, 62 beds) 1495 Mill Street, Reno, NV Zip 89502–1449; tel. 775/982–3500; Blain Claypool, Chief Executive Officer
**Web address:** www.renown.org

RENOWN SOUTH MEADOWS MEDICAL CENTER (O, 76 beds) 10101 Double R Boulevard, Reno, NV Zip 89521; tel. 775/982–7000; Blain Claypool, Chief Executive Officer
**Web address:** www.renown.org

| | | |
|---|---|---|
| Owned, leased, sponsored: | 3 hospitals | 792 beds |
| Contract–managed: | 0 hospitals | 0 beds |
| Totals: | 3 hospitals | 792 beds |

---

**4810: RIVERSIDE HEALTH SYSTEM** (NP)
701 Town Center Drive, Suite 1000, Newport News, VA Zip 23606; tel. 757/534–7000; William B. Downey, President and Chief Executive Officer
**(Centralized Physician/Insurance Health System)**

**VIRGINIA:** HAMPTON ROADS SPECIALTY HOSPITAL (O, 25 beds) 245 Chesapeake Avenue, Newport News, VA Zip 23607–6038; tel. 757/534–5000; Courtney Detwiler, R.N., Administrator
**Web address:** www.hamptonroadsspecialtyhospital.com

RIVERSIDE BEHAVIORAL HEALTH CENTER (O, 79 beds) 2244 Executive Drive, Hampton, VA Zip 23666–2430; tel. 757/827–1001; Allan D. Erbe, Administrator
**Web address:** www.riversideonline.com

RIVERSIDE REGIONAL MEDICAL CENTER (O, 188 beds) 500 J. Clyde Morris Boulevard, Newport News, VA Zip 23601–1929; tel. 757/594–2000; Patrick Parcells, Senior Vice President and Administrator
**Web address:** www.riverside–online.com

RIVERSIDE REHABILITATION INSTITUTE (O, 30 beds) 245 Chesapeake Avenue, Newport News, VA Zip 23607–6038; tel. 757/928–8000; Edward Heckler, Administrator
**Web address:** www.riverside–online.com

RIVERSIDE SHORE MEMORIAL HOSPITAL (O, 48 beds) 9507 Hospital Avenue, Nassawadox, VA Zip 23413–1821, Mailing Address: P.O. Box 17, Zip 23413–0017; tel. 757/414–8000; Joseph P. Zager, Vice President and Administrator
**Web address:** www.shorehealthservices.org

RIVERSIDE TAPPAHANNOCK HOSPITAL (O, 17 beds) 618 Hospital Road, Tappahannock, VA Zip 22560–5000; tel. 804/443–3311; Elizabeth J. Martin, Vice President and Administrator
**Web address:** www.riverside–online.com

RIVERSIDE WALTER REED HOSPITAL (O, 30 beds) 7519 Hospital Drive, Gloucester, VA Zip 23061–4178, Mailing Address: P.O. Box 1130, Zip 23061–1130; tel. 804/693–8800; Megan K. Moore, Vice President and Administrator
**Web address:** www.riversideonline.com

| | | |
|---|---|---|
| Owned, leased, sponsored: | 7 hospitals | 417 beds |
| Contract–managed: | 0 hospitals | 0 beds |
| Totals: | 7 hospitals | 417 beds |

---

**0268: ROBERT WOOD JOHNSON HEALTH SYSTEM & NETWORK** (NP)
1 Robert Wood Johnson Place, New Brunswick, NJ Zip 08903–2601; tel. 732/828–3000; Stephen K. Jones, President and Chief Executive Officer
**(Moderately Centralized Health System)**

**NEW JERSEY:** CHILDREN'S SPECIALIZED HOSPITAL (O, 126 beds) 200 Somerset Street, New Brunswick, NJ Zip 08901; tel. 732/258–7000; Amy B. Mansue, President and Chief Executive Officer
**Web address:** www.childrens–specialized.org

ROBERT WOOD JOHNSON UNIVERSITY HOSPITAL (O, 610 beds) 1 Robert Wood Johnson Place, New Brunswick, NJ Zip 08903–2601; tel. 732/828–3000; Stephen K. Jones, President and Chief Executive Officer
**Web address:** www.rwjuh.edu

ROBERT WOOD JOHNSON UNIVERSITY HOSPITAL AT HAMILTON (O, 242 beds) One Hamilton Health Place, Hamilton, NJ Zip 08690–3599; tel. 609/586–7900; Anthony J. Cimino, President and Chief Executive Officer
**Web address:** www.rwjhamilton.org

ROBERT WOOD JOHNSON UNIVERSITY HOSPITAL RAHWAY (O, 163 beds) 865 Stone Street, Rahway, NJ Zip 07065–2797; tel. 732/381–4200; Kirk C. Tice, President and Chief Executive Officer
**Web address:** www.rwjuhr.com

| | | |
|---|---|---|
| Owned, leased, sponsored: | 4 hospitals | 1141 beds |
| Contract–managed: | 0 hospitals | 0 beds |
| Totals: | 4 hospitals | 1141 beds |

---

**0046: ROCHESTER GENERAL HEALTH SYSTEM** (NP)
1425 Portland Avenue, 5th Floor, Rochester, NY Zip 14621; tel. 585/922–4000; Mark C. Clement, President and Chief Executive Officer
**(Moderately Centralized Health System)**

**NEW YORK:** NEWARK–WAYNE COMMUNITY HOSPITAL (O, 270 beds) 1200 Driving Park Avenue, Newark, NY Zip 14513, Mailing Address: P.O. Box 111, Zip 14513–0111; tel. 315/332–2022; Mark F. Klyczek, President and Chief Executive Officer
**Web address:** www.rochestergeneral.org

ROCHESTER GENERAL HOSPITAL (O, 520 beds) 1425 Portland Avenue, Rochester, NY Zip 14621–3099; tel. 585/922–4000; Robert Nesselbush, President
**Web address:** www.rochestergeneral.org

| | | |
|---|---|---|
| Owned, leased, sponsored: | 2 hospitals | 790 beds |
| Contract–managed: | 0 hospitals | 0 beds |
| Totals: | 2 hospitals | 790 beds |

---

**★0109: RURAL HEALTH GROUP** (IO)
48 West 1500 North, Nephi, UT Zip 84648–1226; tel. 435/623–4924; Mark R. Stoddard, President and Chairman
**(Independent Hospital System)**

**NEVADA:** DESERT VIEW HOSPITAL (O, 25 beds) 360 South Lola Lane, Pahrump, NV Zip 89048; tel. 775/751–7500; Susan Davila, Administrator and Chief Executive Officer
**Web address:** www.desertviewhospital.com

**UTAH:** CENTRAL VALLEY MEDICAL CENTER (L, 25 beds) 48 West 1500 North, Nephi, UT Zip 84648; tel. 435/623–3000; Mark R. Stoddard, President
**Web address:** www.cvmed.net

| | | |
|---|---|---|
| Owned, leased, sponsored: | 2 hospitals | 50 beds |
| Contract–managed: | 0 hospitals | 0 beds |
| Totals: | 2 hospitals | 50 beds |

---

**★0220: RUSH HEALTH SYSTEMS** (NP)
1314 19th Avenue, Meridian, MS Zip 39301; tel. 601/483–0011; Wallace Strickland, President and Chief Executive Officer
**(Independent Hospital System)**

---

For explanation of codes following names, see page B2.
★ Indicates Type III membership in the American Hospital Association.

**MISSISSIPPI:** H. C. WATKINS MEMORIAL HOSPITAL (O, 25 beds) 605 South Archusa Avenue, Quitman, MS Zip 39355–2331; tel. 601/776–6925; Clinton Eaves, Administrator
**Web address:** www.rushhealthsystems.org/hcw/

JOHN C. STENNIS MEMORIAL HOSPITAL (O, 25 beds) 14365 Highway 16 West, De Kalb, MS Zip 39328–7974; tel. 769/486–1000; Jason Payne, Administrator
**Web address:** www.rushhealthsystems.org/stennis/

LAIRD HOSPITAL (O, 25 beds) 25117 Highway 15, Union, MS Zip 39365–9099; tel. 601/774–8214; Thomas G. Bartlett, III, M.D., Administrator
**Web address:** www.rushhealthsystems.org/laird/

RUSH FOUNDATION HOSPITAL (O, 182 beds) 1314 19th Avenue, Meridian, MS Zip 39301–4195; tel. 601/483–0011; Christopher Rush, Vice President and Administrator
**Web address:** www.rushhealthsystems.org

SCOTT REGIONAL HOSPITAL (O, 25 beds) 317 Highway 13 South, Morton, MS Zip 39117–3353, Mailing Address: P.O. Box 259, Zip 39117–0259; tel. 601/732–6301; Michael R. Edwards, Chief Executive Officer
**Web address:** www.rushhealthsystems.org

SPECIALTY HOSPITAL OF MERIDIAN (O, 49 beds) 1314 19th Avenue, Meridian, MS Zip 39301–4116; tel. 601/703–4211; Elizabeth C. Mitchell, Vice President and Administrator
**Web address:** www.rushhealthsystems.org

| | | |
|---|---|---|
| Owned, leased, sponsored: | 6 hospitals | 331 beds |
| Contract–managed: | 0 hospitals | 0 beds |
| Totals: | 6 hospitals | 331 beds |

---

**★3855: RUSH UNIVERSITY MEDICAL CENTER** (NP)
1653 West Congress Parkway, Chicago, IL Zip 60612–3864; tel. 312/942–5000; Larry J. Goodman, M.D., Chief Executive Officer
**(Moderately Centralized Health System)**

**ILLINOIS:** RUSH UNIVERSITY MEDICAL CENTER (O, 664 beds) 1653 West Congress Parkway, Chicago, IL Zip 60612–3833; tel. 312/942–5000; Peter W. Butler, President and Chief Operating Officer
**Web address:** www.rush.edu

RUSH–COPLEY MEDICAL CENTER (O, 210 beds) 2000 Ogden Avenue, Aurora, IL Zip 60504–7222; tel. 630/978–6200; Barry C. Finn, President and Chief Executive Officer
**Web address:** www.rushcopley.com

| | | |
|---|---|---|
| Owned, leased, sponsored: | 2 hospitals | 874 beds |
| Contract–managed: | 0 hospitals | 0 beds |
| Totals: | 2 hospitals | 874 beds |

---

**0351: SAINT CATHERINE HEALTHCARE, LLC** (IO)
101 Broad Street, Ashland, PA Zip 17921; tel. 570/875–2000; Daniel A. Colon, President and Chief Executive Officer

**INDIANA:** SAINT CATHERINE REGIONAL HOSPITAL (O, 64 beds) 2200 Market Street, Charlestown, IN Zip 47111–0009, Mailing Address: P.O. Box 9, Zip 47111–0009; tel. 812/256–3301; Daniel A. Colon, President and Chief Executive Officer
**Web address:** www.saintcatherinehospital.com

**PENNSYLVANIA:** SAINT CATHERINE MEDICAL CENTER FOUNTAIN SPRINGS (O, 79 beds) 101 Broad Street, Ashland, PA Zip 17921–2147; tel. 570/875–2000; Daniel A. Colon, President and Chief Executive Officer
**Web address:** www.stchc.com/scmcfs

| | | |
|---|---|---|
| Owned, leased, sponsored: | 2 hospitals | 143 beds |
| Contract–managed: | 0 hospitals | 0 beds |
| Totals: | 2 hospitals | 143 beds |

---

**★0318: SAINT FRANCIS CARE, INC.** (NP)
114 Woodland Street, Hartford, CT Zip 06105; tel. 860/714–5541; Christopher M. Dadlez, President and Chief Executive Officer
**(Independent Hospital System)**

**CONNECTICUT:** MOUNT SINAI REHABILITATION HOSPITAL (O, 30 beds) 490 Blue Hills Avenue, Hartford, CT Zip 06112; tel. 860/714–3500; Christopher M. Dadlez, President and Chief Executive Officer
**Web address:** www.stfranciscare.org

SAINT FRANCIS HOSPITAL AND MEDICAL CENTER (O, 569 beds) 114 Woodland Street, Hartford, CT Zip 06105–1208; tel. 860/714–4000; Christopher M. Dadlez, President and Chief Executive Officer
**Web address:** www.saintfranciscare.com

| | | |
|---|---|---|
| Owned, leased, sponsored: | 2 hospitals | 599 beds |
| Contract–managed: | 0 hospitals | 0 beds |
| Totals: | 2 hospitals | 599 beds |

---

**★0254: SAINT FRANCIS HEALTH SYSTEM** (NP)
6161 South Yale Avenue, Tulsa, OK Zip 74136–1902; tel. 918/494–8454; Jake Henry, Jr., President and Chief Executive Officer
**(Centralized Physician/Insurance Health System)**

**OKLAHOMA:** LAUREATE PSYCHIATRIC CLINIC AND HOSPITAL (O, 75 beds) 6655 South Yale Avenue, Tulsa, OK Zip 74136–3329; tel. 918/481–4000; William Schloss, Senior Vice President
**Web address:** www.laureate.com

SAINT FRANCIS HOSPITAL (O, 774 beds) 6161 South Yale Avenue, Tulsa, OK Zip 74136–1902; tel. 918/494–2200; Lynn A. Sund, R.N., MS, Senior Vice President, Administrator and Chief Nursing Executive
**Web address:** www.saintfrancis.com

SAINT FRANCIS HOSPITAL SOUTH (O, 60 beds) 10501 East 91St. Streeet, Tulsa, OK Zip 74133–5790; tel. 918/455–3535; David S. Weil, Senior Vice President and Administrator
**Web address:** www.sfh-ba.com

| | | |
|---|---|---|
| Owned, leased, sponsored: | 3 hospitals | 909 beds |
| Contract–managed: | 0 hospitals | 0 beds |
| Totals: | 3 hospitals | 909 beds |

---

**0120: SAINT LUKE'S HEALTH SYSTEM** (NP)
10920 Elm Avenue, Kansas City, MO Zip 64134–4108, Mailing Address: 4401 Wornall, Zip 64111; tel. 816/932–2000; Melinda Estes, M.D., President and Chief Executive Officer
**(Centralized Health System)**

**KANSAS:** ANDERSON COUNTY HOSPITAL (O, 41 beds) 421 South Maple, Garnett, KS Zip 66032–1334, Mailing Address: P.O. Box 309, Zip 66032–0309; tel. 785/448–3131; Dennis A. Hachenberg, FACHE, Chief Executive Officer
**Web address:** www.saint–lukes.org

CUSHING MEMORIAL HOSPITAL (O, 53 beds) 711 Marshall Street, Leavenworth, KS Zip 66048–3235; tel. 913/684–1100; N. Gary Wages, FACHE, Interim Chief Executive Officer
**Web address:** www.cushinghospital.org

SAINT LUKE'S SOUTH HOSPITAL (O, 110 beds) 12300 Metcalf Avenue, Overland Park, KS Zip 66213; tel. 913/317–7000; Kathy A. Howell, R.N., Chief Executive Officer
**Web address:** www.saint–lukes.org

**MISSOURI:** CRITTENTON CHILDREN'S CENTER (O, 54 beds) 10918 Elm Avenue, Kansas City, MO Zip 64134–4108; tel. 816/765–6600; Janine Hron, Chief Executive Officer
**Web address:** www.crittentonkc.org

HEDRICK MEDICAL CENTER (O, 25 beds) 100 Central Avenue, Chillicothe, MO Zip 64601–1554; tel. 660/646–1480; Matthew J. Wenzel, Chief Executive Officer
**Web address:** www.saintlukeshealthsystem.org

SAINT LUKE'S CANCER INSTITUTE (O, 9 beds) 4321 Washington, Medical Plaza III, Suite 5100, Kansas City, MO Zip 64111–3214; tel. 816/932–2823; Julie L. Quirin, FACHE, Chief Executive Officer
**Web address:** www.saint–lukes.org

SAINT LUKE'S EAST HOSPITAL (O, 125 beds) 100 Ne Saint Lukes Boulevard, Lee's Summit, MO Zip 64086–6000; tel. 816/347–5000; Ronald L. Baker, Chief Executive Officer
**Web address:** www.saint–lukes.org

For explanation of codes following names, see page B2.
★ Indicates Type III membership in the American Hospital Association.

SAINT LUKE'S HOSPITAL OF KANSAS CITY (O, 435 beds) 4401 Wornall Road, Kansas City, MO Zip 64111–3220; tel. 816/932–9886; Julie L. Quirin, FACHE, Chief Executive Officer
**Web address:** www.saint–lukes.org

SAINT LUKE'S NORTH HOSPITAL – BARRY ROAD (O, 137 beds) 5830 N.W. Barry Road, Kansas City, MO Zip 64154–2778; tel. 816/891–6000; Kevin T. Trimble, FACHE, President and Chief Executive Officer
**Web address:** www.saint–lukes.org

WRIGHT MEMORIAL HOSPITAL (O, 25 beds) 191 Iowa Boulevard, Trenton, MO Zip 64683–8343, Mailing Address: P.O. Box 628, Zip 64683–0628; tel. 660/358–5700; Gary W. Jordan, FACHE, Chief Executive Officer
**Web address:** www.saintlukeshealthsystem.org

| | | |
|---|---|---|
| Owned, leased, sponsored: | 10 hospitals | 1014 beds |
| Contract–managed: | 0 hospitals | 0 beds |
| Totals: | 10 hospitals | 1014 beds |

★**0264: SAINT VINCENT HEALTH SYSTEM** (CC)
232 West 25th Street, Erie, PA Zip 16544–0002; tel. 814/452–5000; Scott Whalen, Ph.D., FACHE, President and Chief Executive Officer
**(Moderately Centralized Health System)**

**NEW YORK:** WESTFIELD MEMORIAL HOSPITAL (O, 4 beds) 189 East Main Street, Westfield, NY Zip 14787–1195; tel. 716/326–4921; Scott Whalen, Ph.D., FACHE, President and Chief Executive Officer
**Web address:** www.wmhinc.org

**PENNSYLVANIA:** SAINT VINCENT HEALTH CENTER (O, 486 beds) 232 West 25th Street, Erie, PA Zip 16544–0002; tel. 814/452–5000; Scott Whalen, Ph.D., FACHE, President and Chief Executive Officer
**Web address:** www.svhs.org

| | | |
|---|---|---|
| Owned, leased, sponsored: | 2 hospitals | 490 beds |
| Contract–managed: | 0 hospitals | 0 beds |
| Totals: | 2 hospitals | 490 beds |

**0403: SALEM HEALTH** (NP)
890 Oak Street Building B. POB 14001, Salem, OR Zip 97309–5014; tel. 503/561–5200; Norman F. Gruber, President and Chief Executive Officer
**(Independent Hospital System)**

**OREGON:** SALEM HOSPITAL (O, 459 beds) 665 Winter Street S.E., Salem, OR Zip 97301–3959, Mailing Address: P.O. Box 14001, Zip 97309–5014; tel. 503/561–5200; Norman F. Gruber, President and Chief Executive Officer
**Web address:** www.salemhospital.org

WEST VALLEY HOSPITAL (O, 6 beds) 525 S.E. Washington Street, Dallas, OR Zip 97338–2899, Mailing Address: P.O. Box 378, Zip 97338–0378; tel. 503/623–8301; Robert C. Brannigan, Administrator
**Web address:** www.westvalleyhospital.org

| | | |
|---|---|---|
| Owned, leased, sponsored: | 2 hospitals | 465 beds |
| Contract–managed: | 0 hospitals | 0 beds |
| Totals: | 2 hospitals | 465 beds |

★**0186: SAMARITAN HEALTH SERVICES** (NP)
3600 N.W. Samaritan Drive, Corvallis, OR Zip 97330, Mailing Address: P.O. Box 1068, Zip 97339; tel. 541/768–5001; Larry A. Mullins, FACHE, President and Chief Executive Officer
**(Centralized Physician/Insurance Health System)**

GOOD SAMARITAN REGIONAL MEDICAL CENTER (O, 165 beds) 3600 N.W. Samaritan Drive, Corvallis, OR Zip 97330–3737, Mailing Address: P.O. Box 1068, Zip 97339–1068; tel. 541/768–5111; Steven W. Jasperson, Chief Executive Officer
**Web address:** www.samhealth.org

SAMARITAN ALBANY GENERAL HOSPITAL (O, 70 beds) 1046 West Sixth Avenue, Albany, OR Zip 97321–1999; tel. 541/812–4000; David G. Triebes, Chief Executive Officer
**Web address:** www.samhealth.org

SAMARITAN LEBANON COMMUNITY HOSPITAL (O, 25 beds) 525 North Santiam Highway, Lebanon, OR Zip 97355–4363, Mailing Address: P.O. Box 739, Zip 97355–0739; tel. 541/258–2101; Becky A. Pape, R.N., Chief Executive Officer
**Web address:** www.samhealth.org

SAMARITAN NORTH LINCOLN HOSPITAL (C, 25 beds) 3043 N.E. 28th Street, Lincoln City, OR Zip 97367–4523, Mailing Address: P.O. Box 767, Zip 97367–0767; tel. 541/994–3661; Marty Cahill, Chief Executive Officer
**Web address:** www.samhealth.org

SAMARITAN PACIFIC COMMUNITIES HOSPITAL (C, 25 beds) 930 S.W. Abbey Street, Newport, OR Zip 97365–4820, Mailing Address: P.O. Box 945, Zip 97365–4820; tel. 541/265–2244; David C. Bigelow, PharmD, Chief Executive Officer
**Web address:** www.samhealth.org

| | | |
|---|---|---|
| Owned, leased, sponsored: | 3 hospitals | 260 beds |
| Contract–managed: | 2 hospitals | 50 beds |
| Totals: | 5 hospitals | 310 beds |

★**0530: SANFORD HEALTH** (NP)
2301 East 60th Street North, Sioux Falls, SD Zip 57104–0589, Mailing Address: PO Box 5039, Zip 57117–5039; tel. 605/333–1000; Kelby K. Krabbenhoft, President and Chief Executive Officer
**(Decentralized Health System)**

**IOWA:** ORANGE CITY AREA HEALTH SYSTEM (C, 104 beds) 1000 Lincoln Circle S.E., Orange City, IA Zip 51041–1398; tel. 712/737–4984; Martin W. Guthmiller, Chief Executive Officer
**Web address:** www.ochealthsystem.org

SANFORD MEDICAL CENTER ROCK RAPIDS (L, 16 beds) 801 South Greene Street, Rock Rapids, IA Zip 51246–1998; tel. 712/472–2591; Tammy Loosbrock, Chief Executive Officer
**Web address:** www.sanfordmerrill.org

SANFORD SHELDON MEDICAL CENTER (O, 95 beds) 118 North Seventh Avenue, Sheldon, IA Zip 51201–1235, Mailing Address: P.O. Box 250, Zip 51201–0250; tel. 712/324–5041; Richard E. Nordahl, Chief Executive Officer
**Web address:** www.sanfordsheldon.org

**MINNESOTA:** ARNOLD MEMORIAL HEALTH CARE CENTER (L, 50 beds) 601 Louisiana Avenue, Adrian, MN Zip 56110–0279, Mailing Address: P.O. Box 279, Zip 56110–0279; tel. 507/483–2668; Michele Roban, Administrator

MAHNOMEN HEALTH CENTER (C, 18 beds) 414 West Jefferson Avenue, Mahnomen, MN Zip 56557–4912, Mailing Address: P.O. Box 396, Zip 56557–0396; tel. 218/935–2511; Susan K. Klassen, Chief Executive Officer and Administrator
**Web address:** www.mahnomenhealthcenter.com

MURRAY COUNTY MEDICAL CENTER (C, 18 beds) 2042 Juniper Avenue, Slayton, MN Zip 56172–1016; tel. 507/836–6111; Meldon L. Snow, Chief Executive Officer
**Web address:** www.murraycountymed.org

ORTONVILLE AREA HEALTH SERVICES (C, 89 beds) 450 Eastvold Avenue, Ortonville, MN Zip 56278–1133; tel. 320/839–2502; Richard M. Ash, Chief Executive Officer
**Web address:** www.oahs.us

PERHAM HEALTH (C, 19 beds) 1000 Coney Street West, Perham, MN Zip 56573–1199; tel. 218/347–4500; Chuck Hofius, Chief Executive Officer
**Web address:** www.perhamhealth.org

SANFORD BAGLEY MEDICAL CENTER (O, 95 beds) 203 Fourth Street N.W., Bagley, MN Zip 56621–8307; tel. 218/694–6501; Kirby Johnson, Administrator
**Web address:** www.clearwaterhealthservices.com

SANFORD BEMIDJI MEDICAL CENTER (O, 196 beds) 1300 Anne Street N.W., Bemidji, MN Zip 56601; tel. 218/751–5430; Paul A. Hanson, Chief Executive Officer
**Web address:** www.nchs.com

SANFORD JACKSON MEDICAL CENTER (L, 20 beds) 1430 North Highway, Jackson, MN Zip 56143–1098; tel. 507/847–2420; Mary J. Ruyter, Chief Executive Officer
**Web address:** www.sanfordjackson.org

For explanation of codes following names, see page B2.
★ Indicates Type III membership in the American Hospital Association.

**B112** Health Care Systems, Networks and Alliances

© 2012 AHA Guide

SANFORD LUVERNE MEDICAL CENTER (O, 25 beds) 1600 North Kniss Avenue, Luverne, MN Zip 56156–1067; tel. 507/283–2321; Tammy Loosbrock, Chief Executive Officer
**Web address:** www.sanfordluverne.org

SANFORD MEDICAL CENTER CANBY (L, 100 beds) 112 St. Olaf Avenue South, Canby, MN Zip 56220–1433; tel. 507/223–7277; Robert J. Salmon, Chief Executive Officer
**Web address:** www.sanfordcanby.org

SANFORD MEDICAL CENTER THIEF RIVER FALLS (O, 35 beds) 120 LaBree Avenue South, Thief River Falls, MN Zip 56701–2840; tel. 218/681–4240; Christine K. Harff, Chief Executive Officer
**Web address:** www.sanfordhealth.org

SANFORD TRACY MEDICAL CENTER (L, 25 beds) 251 Fifth Street East, Tracy, MN Zip 56175–1536; tel. 507/629–3200; Stacy Barstad, Chief Executive Officer
**Web address:** www.sanfordtracy.org

SANFORD WESTBROOK MEDICAL CENTER (L, 6 beds) 920 Bell Avenue, Westbrook, MN Zip 56183–0188, Mailing Address: P.O. Box 188, Zip 56183–0188; tel. 507/274–6121; Stacy Barstad, Chief Executive Officer
**Web address:** www.sanfordwestbrook.org

SANFORD WHEATON MEDICAL CENTER (O, 15 beds) 401 12th Street North, Wheaton, MN Zip 56296–1099; tel. 320/563–8226; JoAnn M. Foltz, R.N., Chief Executive Officer
**Web address:** www.wheatonhealthcare.org

SANFORD WORTHINGTON MEDICAL CENTER (O, 48 beds) 1018 Sixth Avenue, Worthington, MN Zip 56187–2202, Mailing Address: P.O. Box 997, Zip 56187–0997; tel. 507/372–2941; Michael Hammer, Chief Executive Officer

WINDOM AREA HOSPITAL (C, 25 beds) 2150 Hospital Drive, Windom, MN Zip 56101–0339, Mailing Address: P.O. Box 339, Zip 56101–0339; tel. 507/831–2400; Geraldine F. Burmeister, FACHE, Chief Executive Officer
**Web address:** www.windomareahospital.com

**NORTH DAKOTA:** HILLSBORO MEDICAL CENTER (C, 52 beds) 12 Third Street S.E., Hillsboro, ND Zip 58045, Mailing Address: P.O. Box 609, Zip 58045–0609; tel. 701/636–3200; Jac McTaggart, Chief Executive Officer
**Web address:** www.hillsboromedicalcenter.com

MEDCENTER ONE (O, 218 beds) 300 North Seventh Street, Bismarck, ND Zip 58501–4439, Mailing Address: P.O. Box 5525, Zip 58506–5525; tel. 701/323–6000; Craig Lambrecht, M.D., President and Chief Executive Officer
**Web address:** www.medcenterone.com

SANFORD MEDICAL CENTER FARGO (O, 456 beds) 801 Broadway North, Fargo, ND Zip 58122; tel. 701/234–2000; Dennis C. Millirons, FACHE, President
**Web address:** www.sanfordhealth.org

SANFORD MEDICAL CENTER MAYVILLE (O, 18 beds) 42 Sixth Avenue S.E., Mayville, ND Zip 58257–1598; tel. 701/786–3800; Roger Baier, Chief Executive Officer
**Web address:** www.unionhospital.com

SANFORD NORTHWOOD DEACONESS HEALTH CENTER (O, 73 beds) 4 North Park Street, Northwood, ND Zip 58267–0190, Mailing Address: P.O. Box 190, Zip 58267–0190; tel. 701/587–6060; Pete Antonson, Chief Executive Officer
**Web address:** www.ndhc.net

**SOUTH DAKOTA:** COMMUNITY MEMORIAL HOSPITAL (C, 16 beds) 809 Jackson Street, Burke, SD Zip 57523, Mailing Address: P.O. Box 319, Zip 57523–0319; tel. 605/775–2621; Jim Frank, Chief Executive Officer
**Web address:** www.sanfordhealth.org

PIONEER MEMORIAL HOSPITAL AND HEALTH SERVICES (C, 64 beds) 315 North Washington Street, Viborg, SD Zip 57070–2002, Mailing Address: P.O. Box 368, Zip 57070–0368; tel. 605/326–5161; Georgia C. Pokorney, Chief Executive Officer
**Web address:** www.pioneermemorial.org

SANFORD CANTON–INWOOD MEDICAL CENTER (O, 18 beds) 440 North Hiawatha Drive, Canton, SD Zip 57013–9404; tel. 605/987–2621; Eric C. Hilmoe, Chief Executive Officer
**Web address:** www.sanfordcantoninwood.org

SANFORD DEUEL COUNTY MEDICAL CENTER (L, 10 beds) 701 Third Avenue South, Clear Lake, SD Zip 57226–2016; tel. 605/874–2141; Robert J. Salmon, Chief Executive Officer
**Web address:** www.sanforddeuelcounty.org

SANFORD MEDICAL CENTER CHAMBERLAIN (O, 69 beds) 300 South Byron Boulevard, Chamberlain, SD Zip 57325–9741; tel. 605/234–5511; Maureen K. Cadwell, Chief Executive Officer
**Web address:** www.sanfordmiddakota.org

SANFORD MEDICAL CENTER WEBSTER (L, 20 beds) 1401 West 1st Street, Webster, SD Zip 57274–1816, Mailing Address: P.O. Box 489, Zip 57274–0489; tel. 605/345–3336; David Rogers, Chief Executive Officer
**Web address:** www.sanfordhealth.org

SANFORD UNIVERSITY OF SOUTH DAKOTA MEDICAL CENTER (O, 478 beds) 1305 West 18th Street, Sioux Falls, SD Zip 57105–0496, Mailing Address: P.O. Box 5039, Zip 57117–5039; tel. 605/333–1000; Charles O'Brien, M.D., President
**Web address:** www.sanfordhealth.org

SANFORD VERMILLION MEDICAL CENTER (L, 114 beds) 20 South Plum Street, Vermillion, SD Zip 57069–3346; tel. 605/624–2611; Timothy J. Tracy, Chief Executive Officer
**Web address:** www.sanfordvermillion.org

WINNER REGIONAL HEALTHCARE CENTER (C, 104 beds) 745 East Eighth Street, Winner, SD Zip 57580–2677; tel. 605/842–7100; John M. Osse, Interim Chief Executive Officer
**Web address:** www.winnerregional.org

| | | |
|---|---|---|
| **Owned, leased, sponsored:** | 23 hospitals | 2200 beds |
| **Contract–managed:** | 10 hospitals | 509 beds |
| **Totals:** | 33 hospitals | 2709 beds |

**0412: SCHUYLKILL HEALTH SYSTEM** (NP)
420 South Jackson Street, Pottsville, PA Zip 17901; tel. 570/621–5000; John E. Simodejka, President and Chief Executive Officer
**(Moderately Centralized Health System)**

**PENNSYLVANIA:** SCHUYLKILL MEDICAL CENTER – EAST NORWEGIAN STREET (O, 126 beds) 700 East Norwegian Street, Pottsville, PA Zip 17901–2710; tel. 570/621–4000; John E. Simodejka, President and Chief Executive Officer
**Web address:** www.schuylkillhealth.com

SCHUYLKILL MEDICAL CENTER – SOUTH JACKSON STREET (O, 191 beds) 420 South Jackson Street, Pottsville, PA Zip 17901–3625; tel. 570/621–5000; John E. Simodejka, President and Chief Executive Officer
**Web address:** www.schuylkillhealth.com

| | | |
|---|---|---|
| **Owned, leased, sponsored:** | 2 hospitals | 317 beds |
| **Contract–managed:** | 0 hospitals | 0 beds |
| **Totals:** | 2 hospitals | 317 beds |

★**0398: SCOTT & WHITE HEALTHCARE** (NP)
2401 South 31st Street, Temple, TX Zip 76508; tel. 254/724–2111; Robert W. Pryor, M.D., President and Chief Executive Officer
**(Centralized Physician/Insurance Health System)**

**TEXAS:** HILLCREST BAPTIST MEDICAL CENTER (C, 260 beds) 100 Hillcrest Medical Boulevard, Waco, TX Zip 76712–8897; tel. 254/202–2000; Glenn A. Robinson, Chief Executive Officer
**Web address:** www.hillcrest.net

SCOTT & WHITE HOSPITAL – BRENHAM (O, 60 beds) 700 Medical Parkway, Brenham, TX Zip 77833–5498; tel. 979/836–6173; John L. Simms, President and Chief Executive Officer
**Web address:** www.swbrenham.org

SCOTT & WHITE HOSPITAL – LLANO (O, 26 beds) 200 West Ollie Street, Llano, TX Zip 78643–2628; tel. 325/247–5040; Kevin Leeper, Chief Executive Officer
**Web address:** www.llanomemorial.org

SCOTT & WHITE HOSPITAL – TAYLOR (O, 23 beds) 305 Mallard Lane, Taylor, TX Zip 76574–1208; tel. 512/352–7611; Kevin E. Smith, Chief Operating Officer
**Web address:** www.swtaylor.org

**Section B**

For explanation of codes following names, see page B2.
★ Indicates Type III membership in the American Hospital Association.

SCOTT & WHITE HOSPITAL AT ROUND ROCK (O, 74 beds) 300 University Boulevard, Round Rock, TX Zip 78665–1032; tel. 512/509–0200; Ernest L. Bovio, Jr., Chief Executive Officer
**Web address:** www.scottandwhite.org

SCOTT AND WHITE CONTINUING CARE HOSPITAL (O, 50 beds) 546 North Kegley Road, Temple, TX Zip 76502; tel. 254/215–0900; Kimberly K. Langston, R.N., Executive Associate Director and Administrator
**Web address:** www.sw.org/location/temple-cch

SCOTT AND WHITE MEMORIAL HOSPITAL (O, 603 beds) 2401 South 31st Street, Temple, TX Zip 76508–0002; tel. 254/724–2111; Patricia M. Currie, FACHE, Chief Hospital Services
**Web address:** www.sw.org

| | | |
|---|---|---|
| Owned, leased, sponsored: | 6 hospitals | 836 beds |
| Contract–managed: | 1 hospital | 260 beds |
| Totals: | 7 hospitals | 1096 beds |

---

★0037: **SCOTTSDALE HEALTHCARE** (NP)
3621 Wells Fargo Avenue, Scottsdale, AZ Zip 85251–5607; tel. 480/882–4000; Thomas J. Sadvary, FACHE, President and Chief Executive Officer
**(Moderately Centralized Health System)**

ARIZONA: SCOTTSDALE HEALTHCARE SHEA MEDICAL CENTER (O, 409 beds) 9003 East Shea Boulevard, Scottsdale, AZ Zip 85260–6771; tel. 480/323–3000; Peggy J. Reiley, Ph.D., MS, R.N., Senior Vice President and Chief Clinical Officer
**Web address:** www.shc.org

SCOTTSDALE HEALTHCARE THOMPSON PEAK HOSPITAL (O, 64 beds) 7400 East Thompson Peak Parkway, Scottsdale, AZ Zip 85255; tel. 480/324–7000; Kimberly Post, R.N., Vice President and Administrator
**Web address:** www.shc.org

SCOTTSDALE HEALTHCARE–OSBORN MEDICAL CENTER (O, 347 beds) 7400 East Osborn Road, Scottsdale, AZ Zip 85251–6403; tel. 480/882–4000; Gary E. Baker, Senior Vice President and Administrator
**Web address:** www.shc.org

| | | |
|---|---|---|
| Owned, leased, sponsored: | 3 hospitals | 820 beds |
| Contract–managed: | 0 hospitals | 0 beds |
| Totals: | 3 hospitals | 820 beds |

---

★1505: **SCRIPPS HEALTH** (NP)
4275 Campus Point Court, San Diego, CA Zip 92121; tel. 858/678–6919; Chris D. Van Gorder, FACHE, President and Chief Executive Officer
**(Centralized Health System)**

CALIFORNIA: SCRIPPS GREEN HOSPITAL (O, 173 beds) 10666 North Torrey Pines Road, La Jolla, CA Zip 92037–1093; tel. 858/455–9100; Robin Brown, Senior Vice President and Chief Executive
**Web address:** www.scrippshealth.org

SCRIPPS MEMORIAL HOSPITAL–ENCINITAS (O, 158 beds) 354 Santa Fe Drive, Encinitas, CA Zip 92024–5182, Mailing Address: P.O. Box 230817, Zip 92023–0817; tel. 760/633–6501; Carl J. Etter, Senior Vice President and Chief Executive
**Web address:** www.scripps.org

SCRIPPS MEMORIAL HOSPITAL–LA JOLLA (O, 351 beds) 9888 Genesee Avenue, La Jolla, CA Zip 92037–1200, Mailing Address: P.O. Box 28, Zip 92038–0028; tel. 858/626–4123; Gary G. Fybel, Senior Vice President and Chief Executive
**Web address:** www.scrippshealth.org

SCRIPPS MERCY HOSPITAL (O, 439 beds) 4077 Fifth Avenue, San Diego, CA Zip 92103–2105; tel. 619/294–8111; Thomas A. Gammiere, Senior Vice President and Chief Executive
**Web address:** www.scrippshealth.org

| | | |
|---|---|---|
| Owned, leased, sponsored: | 4 hospitals | 1121 beds |
| Contract–managed: | 0 hospitals | 0 beds |
| Totals: | 4 hospitals | 1121 beds |

---

★0181: **SELECT MEDICAL CORPORATION** (IO)
4714 Gettysburg Road, Mechanicsburg, PA Zip 17055; tel. 717/972–1100; David S. Chernow, President and Chief Administrative Officer
**(Independent Hospital System)**

ALABAMA: SELECT SPECIALTY HOSPITAL–BIRMINGHAM (O, 38 beds) 800 Montclair Road, Birmingham, AL Zip 35213; tel. 205/599–4600; Andrea White, Chief Executive Officer
**Web address:** www.selectmedicalcorp.com

ARIZONA: SELECT SPECIALTY HOSPITAL–PHOENIX (O, 48 beds) 350 West Thomas Road, Phoenix, AZ Zip 85013; tel. 602/406–6802; Nancy L. Burton, Chief Executive Officer
**Web address:** www.selectmedicalcorp.com

SELECT SPECIALTY HOSPITAL–SCOTTSDALE (O, 62 beds) 7400 East Osborn Road, 3 West, Scottsdale, AZ Zip 85251–6432; tel. 480/882–4360; Nancy L. Burton, Chief Executive Officer
**Web address:** www.selectmedicalcorp.com

ARKANSAS: REGENCY HOSPITAL OF NORTHWEST ARKANSAS (O, 50 beds) 1125 North College, Fayetteville, AR Zip 72703; tel. 479/713–7000; Michael A. McLean, Chief Executive Officer
**Web address:** www.regencyhospital.com

SELECT SPECIALTY HOSPITAL–FORT SMITH (O, 34 beds) 1001 Towson Avenue, Fort Smith, AR Zip 72902–4921; tel. 479/441–3960; Cindy McLain, Chief Executive Officer
**Web address:** www.selectmedicalcorp.com

SELECT SPECIALTY HOSPITAL–LITTLE ROCK (O, 43 beds) 2 St. Vincent Circle, 6th Floor, Little Rock, AR Zip 72205; tel. 501/661–4198; Barry Ewy, Chief Executive Officer
**Web address:** www.selectmedicalcorp.com

COLORADO: SELECT LONG TERM CARE HOSPITAL – COLORADO SPRINGS (O, 30 beds) 6001 East Woodmen Road, 6th Floor, Colorado Springs, CO Zip 80923–2601; tel. 719/571–6000; James Elton, Chief Executive Officer
**Web address:** www.selectmedical.com

SELECT SPECIALTY HOSPITAL–DENVER (O, 65 beds) 1719 East 19th Avenue, 5th Floor, Denver, CO Zip 80218; tel. 303/563–3700; Deborah Dale, Chief Executive Officer
**Web address:** www.selectmedicalcorp.com

DELAWARE: SELECT SPECIALTY HOSPITAL–WILMINGTON (O, 35 beds) 7 Clayton Street, 5th Floor, Wilmington, DE Zip 19805; tel. 302/421–4545; H. Frank Schneider, Chief Executive Officer
**Web address:** www.selectmedicalcorp.com

FLORIDA: SELECT SPECIALTY HOSPITAL–GAINESVILLE (O, 44 beds) 2708 S.W. Archer Road, Gainesville, FL Zip 32608; tel. 352/337–3240; Russell A. Test, Chief Executive Officer
**Web address:** www.selectspecialtyhospitals.com

SELECT SPECIALTY HOSPITAL–MIAMI (O, 40 beds) 955 N.W. 3rd Street, Miami, FL Zip 33128; tel. 305/416–5700; Dionisio Bencomo, Chief Executive Officer
**Web address:** www.selectmedicalcorp.com

SELECT SPECIALTY HOSPITAL–ORLANDO (O, 75 beds) 2250 Bedford Road, Orlando, FL Zip 32803; tel. 407/303–7869; Nellie Castroman, Chief Executive Officer
**Web address:** www.selectmedicalcorp.com

SELECT SPECIALTY HOSPITAL–PALM BEACH (O, 60 beds) 3060 Melaleuca Lane, Lake Worth, FL Zip 33461; tel. 561/357–7200; Larry Melby, Chief Executive Officer
**Web address:** www.selectspecialtyhospitals.com

SELECT SPECIALTY HOSPITAL–PANAMA CITY (O, 30 beds) 615 North Bonita Avenue, 3rd Floor, Panama City, FL Zip 32401; tel. 850/767–3180; Debra R. Gibson, Chief Executive Officer
**Web address:** www.selectmedicalcorp.com

SELECT SPECIALTY HOSPITAL–PENSACOLA (O, 54 beds) 7000 Cobble Creek Drive, Pensacola, FL Zip 32504; tel. 850/473–4800; David Goodson, Chief Executive Officer
**Web address:** www.selectmedicalcorp.com

SELECT SPECIALTY HOSPITAL–TALLAHASSEE (O, 29 beds) 1554 Surgeons Drive, Tallahassee, FL Zip 32308; tel. 850/219–6800; Lora Davis, Chief Executive Officer
**Web address:** www.selectmedicalcorp.com

---

For explanation of codes following names, see page B2.
★ Indicates Type III membership in the American Hospital Association.

Section B

WEST GABLES REHABILITATION HOSPITAL (O, 60 beds) 2525 S.W. 75th Avenue, Miami, FL Zip 33155–2800; tel. 305/262–6800; Walter Concepcion, Chief Executive Officer
**Web address:** www.westgablesrehabhospital.com/

**GEORGIA:** REGENCY HOSPITAL OF CENTRAL GEORGIA (O, 34 beds) 535 Coliseum Drive, Macon, GA Zip 31217; tel. 478/803–7300; Michael S. Boggs, Chief Executive Officer
**Web address:** www.regencyhospital.com

REGENCY HOSPITAL OF SOUTH ATLANTA (O, 37 beds) 1170 Cleveland Avenue, 4th Floor, East Point, GA Zip 30344; tel. 404/466–6250; Alisa Jett, Chief Executive Officer
**Web address:** www.regencyhospital.com

SELECT SPECIALTY HOSPITAL–ATLANTA (O, 30 beds) 550 Peachtree Street N.E., Atlanta, GA Zip 30308; tel. 404/686–2270; Andrew Tatnall, Chief Executive Officer
**Web address:** www.selectmedical.com

SELECT SPECIALTY HOSPITAL–AUGUSTA (O, 80 beds) 1537 Walton Way, Augusta, GA Zip 30904; tel. 706/731–1169; David L. Mork, Jr., FACHE, Chief Executive Officer
**Web address:** www.selectmedical.com

SELECT SPECIALTY HOSPITAL–SAVANNAH (O, 36 beds) 5353 Reynolds Street, 4 South, Savannah, GA Zip 31405; tel. 912/819–7972; Coleen Zimmerman, Chief Executive Officer
**Web address:** www.selectmedicalcorp.com

**INDIANA:** REGENCY HOSPITAL OF NORTHWEST INDIANA (O, 25 beds) 4321 Fir Street, 4th Floor, East Chicago, IN Zip 46312; tel. 219/392–7790; Victor J. Galfano, FACHE, Chief Executive Officer
**Web address:** www.regencyhospital.com

SELECT SPECIALTY HOSPITAL–BEECH GROVE (O, 45 beds) 1600 Albany Street, Suite 200, Beech Grove, IN Zip 46107; tel. 317/783–8913; Cheryl G. Gentry, Chief Executive Officer
**Web address:** www.selectmedicalcorp.com

SELECT SPECIALTY HOSPITAL–EVANSVILLE (O, 60 beds) 400 S.E. 4th Street, Evansville, IN Zip 47713; tel. 812/421–2500; Tracy Conroy, Chief Executive Officer
**Web address:** www.selectmedicalcorp.com

SELECT SPECIALTY HOSPITAL–FORT WAYNE (O, 32 beds) 700 Broadway, 7th Floor, Fort Wayne, IN Zip 46802; tel. 260/425–3810; Lea Ann Klarner, Chief Executive Officer
**Web address:** www.selectmedicalcorp.com

**IOWA:** SELECT SPECIALTY HOSPITAL–QUAD CITIES (O, 50 beds) 1111 West Kimberly Road, Davenport, IA Zip 52806–5711; tel. 563/468–2000; Austin B. Cleveland, Chief Executive Officer
**Web address:** www.selectmedicalcorp.com

**KANSAS:** SELECT SPECIALTY HOSPITAL–KANSAS CITY (O, 40 beds) 8929 Parallel Parkway, 4th Floor, Kansas City, KS Zip 66112; tel. 913/596–7220; Matthew H. Blevins, Chief Executive Officer
**Web address:** www.selectmedicalcorp.com

SELECT SPECIALTY HOSPITAL–TOPEKA (O, 34 beds) 1700 S.W. Seventh Street, Suite 840, Topeka, KS Zip 66606–1660; tel. 785/295–5551; Jon W. Scott, Chief Executive Officer
**Web address:** www.selectmedical.com

SELECT SPECIALTY HOSPITAL–WICHITA (O, 58 beds) 929 North St. Francis Street, Wichita, KS Zip 67214; tel. 316/261–8303; Peggy Cliffe, Chief Executive Officer
**Web address:** www.selectmedicalcorp.com

**KENTUCKY:** SELECT SPECIALTY HOSPITAL–LEXINGTON (O, 41 beds) 310 South Limestone Street, 3rd Floor, Lexington, KY Zip 40508; tel. 859/226–7096; Mary Lou Guinle, FACHE, Chief Executive Officer
**Web address:** www.selectmedicalcorp.com

**LOUISIANA:** REGENCY HOSPITAL OF COVINGTON (O, 38 beds) 195 Highland Park Entrance, Covington, LA Zip 70433; tel. 985/867–3977; Keith Carruth, Chief Executive Officer
**Web address:** www.regencyhospital.com

**MICHIGAN:** GREAT LAKES SPECIALTY HOSPITAL–HACKLEY CAMPUS (O, 31 beds) 1700 Clinton Street, S2, Muskegon, MI Zip 49442–5502; tel. 231/728–5811; Brian Pangle, Chief Executive Officer
**Web address:** www.selectmedical.com

GREAT LAKES SPECIALTY HOSPITAL–OAK CAMPUS (O, 20 beds) 200 Jefferson Avenue S.E., 5th Floor, Grand Rapids, MI Zip 49503–4502; tel. 616/965–8701; Brian Pangle, Chief Executive Officer
**Web address:** www.selectmedicalcorp.com

SELECT SPECIALTY HOSPITAL–ANN ARBOR (O, 36 beds) 5301 East Huron River Drive, 5th Floor, Ypsilanti, MI Zip 48197–1051; tel. 734/712–0111; John O'Malley, FACHE, Chief Executive Officer
**Web address:** www.selectspecialtyhospitals.com

SELECT SPECIALTY HOSPITAL–BATTLE CREEK (O, 25 beds) 300 North Avenue, Battle Creek, MI Zip 49017–3307; tel. 269/964–9075; Gerrie Baarson, Chief Executive Officer
**Web address:** www.selectmedicalcorp.com

SELECT SPECIALTY HOSPITAL–DOWNRIVER (O, 40 beds) 10000 Telegraph Road, 2nd Floor, Taylor, MI Zip 48180–3330; tel. 313/375–7075; Robert Padalino, Chief Executive Officer
**Web address:** www.selectmedicalcorp.com

SELECT SPECIALTY HOSPITAL–FLINT (O, 26 beds) 401 South Ballenger Highway, 5th Floor, Flint, MI Zip 48532–3638; tel. 810/342–4500; Lorie Powell, Chief Executive Officer
**Web address:** www.selectmedicalcorp.com

SELECT SPECIALTY HOSPITAL–GROSSE POINTE (O, 30 beds) 468 Cadieux Road, Grosse Pointe Farms, MI Zip 48230–1507; tel. 313/473–6131; Miriam Deemer, Chief Executive Officer
**Web address:** www.selectmedicalcorp.com

SELECT SPECIALTY HOSPITAL–MACOMB COUNTY (O, 30 beds) 215 North Avenue, Mount Clemens, MI Zip 48043–1716; tel. 586/307–9000; Jon P. O'Malley, Chief Executive Officer
**Web address:** www.selectmedicalcorp.com

SELECT SPECIALTY HOSPITAL–NORTHWEST DETROIT (O, 36 beds) 6071 West Outer Drrive, Detroit, MI Zip 48235–2624; tel. 313/966–4747; Sandra Baumchen, Chief Executive Officer
**Web address:** www.selectmedicalcorp.com

SELECT SPECIALTY HOSPITAL–PONTIAC (O, 30 beds) 44405 Woodward Avenue, 8th Floor, Pontiac, MI Zip 48341–5023; tel. 248/452–5252; Peggy Kingston, Chief Executive Officer
**Web address:** www.https://www.selectmedicalcorp.com

SELECT SPECIALTY HOSPITAL–SAGINAW (O, 32 beds) 1447 North Harrison Street, Saginaw, MI Zip 48602–4727; tel. 989/583–4235; Dawn Frisbie, Chief Executive Officer
**Web address:** www.selectmedicalcorp.com

**MINNESOTA:** REGENCY HOSPITAL OF MINNEAPOLIS (O, 54 beds) 1300 Hidden Lakes Parkway, Golden Valley, MN Zip 55422–4299; tel. 763/588–2750; John Allen, Chief Executive Officer
**Web address:** www.regencyhospital.com

**MISSISSIPPI:** REGENCY HOSPITAL OF HATTIESBURG (O, 33 beds) 220 South 27th Avenue, Hattiesburg, MS Zip 39401; tel. 601/288–8510; Robert J. Trautman, Chief Executive Officer
**Web address:** www.regencyhospital.com/hattiesburg

REGENCY HOSPITAL OF JACKSON (O, 36 beds) 971 Lakeland Drive, Jackson, MS Zip 39216; tel. 601/364–6200; Michael L. Moore, Chief Executive Officer
**Web address:** www.regencyhospital.com

REGENCY HOSPITAL OF MERIDIAN (O, 40 beds) 1102 Constitution Avenue, 2nd Floor, Meridian, MS Zip 39301–4001; tel. 601/484–7900; Clifton Quinn, Chief Executive Officer
**Web address:** www.regencyhospital.com

SELECT SPECIALTY HOSPITAL–GULF COAST (O, 61 beds) 1520 Broad Avenue, Suite 300, Gulfport, MS Zip 39501; tel. 228/575–7500; John O'Keefe, Chief Executive Officer
**Web address:** www.selectmedicalcorp.com

SELECT SPECIALTY HOSPITAL–JACKSON (O, 53 beds) 5903 Ridgewood Road, Jackson, MS Zip 39211; tel. 601/899–3800; R. Shannon Canard, Chief Executive Officer
**Web address:** www.selectmedicalcorp.com

**MISSOURI:** SELECT SPECIALTY HOSPITAL–SPRINGFIELD (O, 44 beds) 1630 East Primrose Street, Springfield, MO Zip 65804; tel. 417/885–4700; Cynthia Whitten, R.N., Chief Executive Officer
**Web address:** www.selectspecialtyhospitals.com

SELECT SPECIALTY HOSPITAL–ST. LOUIS (O, 33 beds) 300 First Capitol Drive, Unit 1, Saint Charles, MO Zip 63301–2844; tel. 636/947–5010; Jordan Tenenbaum, Chief Executive Officer
**Web address:** www.selectmedicalcorp.com

For explanation of codes following names, see page B2.
★ Indicates Type III membership in the American Hospital Association.

**Section B**

**SELECT SPECIALTY HOSPITAL–WESTERN MISSOURI** (O, 34 beds) 2316 East Meyer Boulevard, 3 West, Kansas City, MO Zip 64132; tel. 816/276–3300; Matthew Paul Pearson, Chief Executive Officer
**Web address:** www.selectmedicalcorp.com

**NEBRASKA:** SELECT SPECIALTY HOSPITAL–OMAHA (O, 52 beds) 1870 South 75th Street, Omaha, NE Zip 68124–1700; tel. 402/361–5700; Thomas N. Theroult, Chief Executive Officer
**Web address:** www.selectmedicalcorp.com

**NEW JERSEY:** KESSLER INSTITUTE FOR REHABILITATION (O, 332 beds) 1199 Pleasant Valley Way, West Orange, NJ Zip 07052–1419; tel. 973/731–3600; Robert Brehm, Division President
**Web address:** www.kessler–rehab.com

**SELECT SPECIALTY HOSPITAL–NORTHEAST NEW JERSEY** (O, 59 beds) 96 Parkway, Rochelle Park, NJ Zip 07662; tel. 201/221–2358; Barbara E. Hannan, Chief Executive Officer
**Web address:** www.selectmedicalcorp.com

**NORTH CAROLINA:** SELECT SPECIALTY HOSPITAL–DURHAM (O, 30 beds) 3643 North Roxboro Road, 6th Floor, Durham, NC Zip 27704; tel. 919/470–9137; Robert F. Jernigan, Jr., Chief Executive Officer
**Web address:** www.selectmedicalcorp.com

**SELECT SPECIALTY HOSPITAL–GREENSBORO** (O, 30 beds) 1200 North Elm Street, 5th Floor, Greensboro, NC Zip 27401; tel. 336/832–8571; Deana Knight, Chief Executive Officer
**Web address:** www.selectmedicalcorp.com

**SELECT SPECIALTY HOSPITAL–WINSTON–SALEM** (O, 42 beds) 3333 Silas Creek Parkway, 6th Floor, Winston–Salem, NC Zip 27103; tel. 336/718–6300; Marion Reef, Chief Executive Officer
**Web address:** www.selectmedicalcorp.com

**OHIO:** REGENCY HOSPITAL CLEVELAND EAST (O, 44 beds) 4200 Interchange Corporate Center Road, Cleveland, OH Zip 44128–5631; tel. 216/910–3800; Barbara Wojtala, Chief Executive Officer
**Web address:** www.regencyhospital.com/

**REGENCY HOSPITAL OF CINCINNATI** (O, 31 beds) 311 Straight Street, Cincinnati, OH Zip 45219; tel. 513/559–5900; Angie Holden, Chief Executive Officer
**Web address:** www.regencyhospital.com

**REGENCY HOSPITAL OF COLUMBUS** (O, 43 beds) 1430 South High Street, Columbus, OH Zip 43207–1045; tel. 614/456–0300; Sara Poling, Chief Executive Officer
**Web address:** www.regencyhospital.com/

**REGENCY HOSPITAL OF TOLEDO** (O, 35 beds) 5220 Alexis Road, Sylvania, OH Zip 43560–2504; tel. 419/318–5700; Patrick J. Murtha, Chief Executive Officer
**Web address:** www.regencyhospital.com

**SELECT SPECIALTY HOSPITAL–AKRON** (O, 60 beds) 200 East Market Street, Akron, OH Zip 44308; tel. 330/761–7500; Kimberly A. Thomas, JD, MSN, R.N., Chief Executive Officer
**Web address:** www.selectmedicalcorp.com

**SELECT SPECIALTY HOSPITAL–CANTON** (O, 30 beds) 1320 Mercy Drive N.W., Canton, OH Zip 44708; tel. 330/489–8189; Dawne Wheeler, Chief Executive Officer
**Web address:** www.selectmedicalcorp.com

**SELECT SPECIALTY HOSPITAL–CINCINNATI** (O, 35 beds) 375 Dixmyth Avenue, Cincinnati, OH Zip 45220; tel. 513/872–4444; Salvatore Iweimrin, R.N., Chief Executive Officer
**Web address:** www.selectmedicalcorp.com

**SELECT SPECIALTY HOSPITAL–COLUMBUS** (O, 176 beds) 1087 Dennison Avenue, Columbus, OH Zip 43201; tel. 614/458–9000; Gene Cashman, Chief Executive Officer
**Web address:** www.selectmedicalcorp.com

**SELECT SPECIALTY HOSPITAL–YOUNGSTOWN** (O, 51 beds) 1044 Belmont Avenue, Youngstown, OH Zip 44501; tel. 330/480–2349; Sharon Noro, Chief Executive Officer
**Web address:** www.selectmedicalcorp.com

**SELECT SPECIALTY HOSPITAL–ZANESVILLE** (O, 35 beds) 800 Forest Avenue, 6th Floor, Zanesville, OH Zip 43701; tel. 740/588–7888; Linda Supplee, Chief Executive Officer
**Web address:** www.selectmedicalcorp.com

**OKLAHOMA:** SELECT SPECIALTY HOSPITAL–OKLAHOMA CITY (O, 72 beds) 3524 N.W. 56th Street, Oklahoma City, OK Zip 73112–4510; tel. 405/606–6700; Connie Strickland, Chief Executive Officer
**Web address:** www.selectmedicalcorp.com

**SELECT SPECIALTY HOSPITAL–TULSA MIDTOWN** (O, 56 beds) 1125 South Trenton Avenue, Tulsa, OK Zip 74104; tel. 918/579–7300; Linda Tiemens, Chief Executive Officer
**Web address:** www.selectmedicalcorp.com

**PENNSYLVANIA:** PENN STATE HERSHEY REHABILITATION HOSPITAL (O, 32 beds) 1135 Old West Chocolate Avenue, Hummelstown, PA Zip 17036; tel. 717/832–2600; Mary A. Zweifel, Chief Executive Officer
**Web address:** www.psh–rehab.com

**SELECT SPECIALTY HOSPITAL–CENTRAL PENNSYLVANIA** (O, 92 beds) 503 North 21st Street, 5th Floor, Camp Hill, PA Zip 17011; tel. 717/972–4575; Claudia Ann Eisenmann, Chief Executive Officer
**Web address:** www.selectmedicalcorp.com

**SELECT SPECIALTY HOSPITAL–DANVILLE** (O, 30 beds) 100 North Academy Avenue, 3rd Floor, Danville, PA Zip 17822–3050; tel. 570/214–9653; Brian Mann, Chief Executive Officer
**Web address:** www.selectmedicalcorp.com

**SELECT SPECIALTY HOSPITAL–ERIE** (O, 50 beds) 252 West 11th Street, Erie, PA Zip 16501; tel. 814/874–5300; Anne Frew, Chief Executive Officer
**Web address:** www.selectmedicalcorp.com

**SELECT SPECIALTY HOSPITAL–JOHNSTOWN** (O, 39 beds) 320 Main Street, Johnstown, PA Zip 15901; tel. 814/534–7300; Kelly Blake, Chief Executive Officer
**Web address:** www.selectmedicalcorp.com

**SELECT SPECIALTY HOSPITAL–LAUREL HIGHLANDS** (O, 40 beds) 121 West Second Street, Latrobe, PA Zip 15650; tel. 724/539–3230; Anthony Martino, Chief Executive Officer
**Web address:** www.selectmedicalcorp.com

**SELECT SPECIALTY HOSPITAL–MCKEESPORT** (O, 30 beds) 1500 Fifth Avenue, McKeesport, PA Zip 15132; tel. 412/664–2900; John St. Leger, Chief Executive Officer
**Web address:** www.selectmedicalcorp.com

**SELECT SPECIALTY HOSPITAL–PITTSBURGH/UPMC** (O, 32 beds) 200 Lothrop Street, E824, Pittsburgh, PA Zip 15213; tel. 412/586–9800; Anthony Martino, Interim Chief Executive Officer
**Web address:** www.selectmedicalcorp.com

**SOUTH CAROLINA:** REGENCY HOSPITAL OF FLORENCE (O, 40 beds) 121 East Cedar Street, Florence, SC Zip 29506; tel. 843/661–3499; Darrell Jones, Chief Executive Officer
**Web address:** www.regencyhospital.com

**REGENCY HOSPITAL OF GREENVILLE** (O, 32 beds) One St. Francis Drive, 4th Floor, Greenville, SC Zip 29601; tel. 864/255–1438; Stephanie James, Chief Executive Officer
**Web address:** www.regencyhospital.com

**SOUTH DAKOTA:** SELECT SPECIALTY HOSPITAL–SIOUX FALLS (O, 21 beds) 1325 South Cliff Avenue, Suite 3300, Sioux Falls, SD Zip 57105; tel. 605/322–3500; Carol Ulmer, Chief Executive Officer
**Web address:** www.selectmedicalcorp.com

**TENNESSEE:** SELECT SPECIALTY HOSPITAL–KNOXVILLE (O, 35 beds) 1901 Clinch Avenue, Suite 404, Knoxville, TN Zip 37916–2307; tel. 865/541–2615; Vanda Scott, Chief Executive Officer
**Web address:** www.selectmedicalcorp.com

**SELECT SPECIALTY HOSPITAL–MEMPHIS** (O, 38 beds) 5959 Park Avenue, 12th Floor, Memphis, TN Zip 38119–5200; tel. 901/765–1245; Mark A. Kelly, Chief Executive Officer
**Web address:** www.selectmedicalcorp.com

**SELECT SPECIALTY HOSPITAL–NASHVILLE** (O, 47 beds) 2000 Hayes Street, Nashville, TN Zip 37203–2318; tel. 615/284–4599; Michael McAlister, Chief Executive Officer
**Web address:** www.selectmedicalcorp.com

**SELECT SPECIALTY HOSPITAL–NORTH KNOXVILLE** (O, 33 beds) 900 East Oak Hill Avenue, Knoxville, TN Zip 37917; tel. 865/541–2615; Vanda Scott, Chief Executive Officer
**Web address:** www.selectmedicalcorp.com

**SELECT SPECIALTY HOSPITAL–TRICITIES** (O, 33 beds) One Medical Park Boulevard, 5th Floor, Bristol, TN Zip 37620–8964; tel. 423/844–5900; Megan Schmidt, Chief Executive Officer
**Web address:** www.selectmedicalcorp.com

For explanation of codes following names, see page B2.
★ Indicates Type III membership in the American Hospital Association.

**TEXAS:** REGENCY HOSPITAL OF FORT WORTH (O, 44 beds) 6801 Oakmont Boulevard, Fort Worth, TX Zip 76132–3918; tel. 817/840–2500; Brad Ervin, Chief Executive Officer
**Web address:** www.regencyhospital.com

REGENCY HOSPITAL OF ODESSA (O, 36 beds) 318 North Alleghaney, Suite 202, Odessa, TX Zip 79761; tel. 432/552–4000; Don Cubb, Chief Executive Officer
**Web address:** www.regencyhospital.com

SELECT REHABILITATION HOSPITAL OF DENTON (O, 44 beds) 2620 Scripture Street, Denton, TX Zip 76201; tel. 940/297–6500; Michele Powell, Chief Executive Officer
**Web address:** www.selectrehab–denton.com/

SELECT SPECIALTY HOSPITAL–DALLAS (O, 60 beds) 2329 West Parker Road, Carrollton, TX Zip 75010; tel. 469/892–1400; Curt L. Roberts, Chief Executive Officer
**Web address:** www.selectmedical.com

SELECT SPECIALTY HOSPITAL–HOUSTON (O, 277 beds) 1917 Ashland Street, Houston, TX Zip 77008–3994; tel. 713/861–6161; Jesse Ruiz, Chief Executive Officer
**Web address:** www.selectmedicalcorp.com

SELECT SPECIALTY HOSPITAL–LONGVIEW (O, 32 beds) 700 East Marshall Avenue, 1st Floor, Longview, TX Zip 75601; tel. 903/315–1111; Robert A. Turner, Chief Executive Officer
**Web address:** www.selectmedicalcorp.com

SELECT SPECIALTY HOSPITAL–MIDLAND (O, 29 beds) 4214 Andrews Highway, Suite 320, Midland, TX Zip 79703; tel. 432/522–3364; Connie K. Siffring, Chief Executive Officer
**Web address:** www.selectmedicalcorp.com

SELECT SPECIALTY HOSPITAL–SAN ANTONIO (O, 44 beds) 111 Dallas Street, 4th Floor, San Antonio, TX Zip 78205; tel. 210/297–7185; Sean Stricker, Chief Executive Officer
**Web address:** www.selectmedicalcorp.com

SELECT SPECIALTY HOSPITAL–SOUTH DALLAS (O, 100 beds) 800 Kirnwood Drive, De Soto, TX Zip 75115; tel. 972/780–6500; Jeff Jennings, Chief Executive Officer
**Web address:** www.selectmedicalcorp.com

**WEST VIRGINIA:** SELECT SPECIALTY HOSPITAL–CHARLESTON (O, 32 beds) 333 Laidley Street, Charleston, WV Zip 25322; tel. 304/720–7234; Frank Weber, Chief Executive Officer
**Web address:** www.selectmedical.com

**WISCONSIN:** SELECT SPECIALTY HOSPITAL–MADISON (O, 58 beds) 801 Braxton Place, Madison, WI Zip 53715; tel. 608/260–2703; Patrice L. Komoroski, Ph.D., R.N., Chief Executive Officer
**Web address:** www.selectmedicalcorp.com

SELECT SPECIALTY HOSPITAL–MILWAUKEE (O, 34 beds) 8901 West Lincoln Avenue, 6th Floor, Milwaukee, WI Zip 53227; tel. 414/328–7700; Richard Keddington, Chief Executive Officer
**Web address:** www.selectmedicalcorp.com

| Owned, leased, sponsored: | 98 hospitals | 4788 beds |
| Contract–managed: | 0 hospitals | 0 beds |
| Totals: | 98 hospitals | 4788 beds |

---

**★2565:  SENTARA HEALTHCARE** (NP)
6015 Poplar Hall Drive, Norfolk, VA Zip 23502–3819; tel. 757/455–7000; David L. Bernd, Chief Executive Officer
**(Centralized Health System)**

**VIRGINIA:** MARTHA JEFFERSON HOSPITAL (O, 139 beds) 500 Martha Jefferson Drive, Charlottesville, VA Zip 22911; tel. 434/654–7000; James E. Haden, President and Chief Executive Officer
**Web address:** www.marthajefferson.org

ROCKINGHAM MEMORIAL HOSPITAL (O, 238 beds) 2010 Health Campus Drive, Harrisonburg, VA Zip 22801–3293; tel. 540/433–4100; James D. Krauss, President and Chief Executive Officer
**Web address:** www.rmhonline.com

SENTARA CAREPLEX HOSPITAL (O, 182 beds) 3000 Coliseum Drive, Hampton, VA Zip 23666–5963; tel. 757/736–1000; Debra A. Flores, R.N., MS, President and Administrator
**Web address:** www.sentara.com

SENTARA LEIGH HOSPITAL (O, 238 beds) 830 Kempsville Road, Norfolk, VA Zip 23502–3920; tel. 757/261–6000; Teresa L. Edwards, Vice President and Administrator
**Web address:** www.sentara.com

SENTARA NORFOLK GENERAL HOSPITAL (O, 491 beds) 600 Gresham Drive, Norfolk, VA Zip 23507; tel. 757/388–3000; Mary L. Blunt, Corporate Vice President and Administrator
**Web address:** www.sentara.com

SENTARA NORTHERN VIRGINIA MEDICAL CENTER (O, 169 beds) 2300 Opitz Boulevard, Woodbridge, VA Zip 22191–3399; tel. 703/670–1313; Megan R. Perry, Vice President and Administrator
**Web address:** www.potomachospital.com

SENTARA OBICI HOSPITAL (O, 168 beds) 2800 Godwin Boulevard, Suffolk, VA Zip 23434–4323; tel. 757/934–4000; Kurt T. Hofelich, Vice President and Administrator
**Web address:** www.sentara.com

SENTARA PRINCESS ANNE HOSPITAL (O, 160 beds) 2025 Glenn Mitchell Drive, Virginia Beach, VA Zip 23456–0178; tel. 757/363–6100; Stephen D. Porter, President
**Web address:** www.sentara.com

SENTARA VIRGINIA BEACH GENERAL HOSPITAL (O, 234 beds) 1060 First Colonial Road, Virginia Beach, VA Zip 23454–3002; tel. 757/395–8000; Thomas B. Thames, M.D., Interim President
**Web address:** www.sentara.com

SENTARA WILLIAMSBURG REGIONAL MEDICAL CENTER (O, 145 beds) 100 Sentara Circle, Williamsburg, VA Zip 23188–5713; tel. 757/984–6000; Robert L. Graves, Vice President and Administrator
**Web address:** www.sentara.com

| Owned, leased, sponsored: | 10 hospitals | 2164 beds |
| Contract–managed: | 0 hospitals | 0 beds |
| Totals: | 10 hospitals | 2164 beds |

---

**★0111:  SHANDS HEALTHCARE** (NP)
1600 S.W. Archer Road, Gainesville, FL Zip 32610–0326; tel. 352/265–8929; Timothy M. Goldfarb, Chief Executive Officer
**(Moderately Centralized Health System)**

**FLORIDA:** SHANDS AT THE UNIVERSITY OF FLORIDA (O, 939 beds) 1600 S.W. Archer Road, Gainesville, FL Zip 32610–0326, Mailing Address: P.O. Box 100326, Zip 32610–0326; tel. 352/265–0111; Timothy M. Goldfarb, Chief Executive Officer
**Web address:** www.shands.org

SHANDS JACKSONVILLE MEDICAL CENTER (O, 620 beds) 655 West Eighth Street, Jacksonville, FL Zip 32209–6595; tel. 904/244–0411; James R. Burkhart, FACHE, President and Chief Executive Officer
**Web address:** www.shandsjacksonville.org

| Owned, leased, sponsored: | 2 hospitals | 1559 beds |
| Contract–managed: | 0 hospitals | 0 beds |
| Totals: | 2 hospitals | 1559 beds |

---

**★2065:  SHARP HEALTHCARE** (NP)
8695 Spectrum Center Boulevard, San Diego, CA Zip 92123–1489; tel. 858/499–4000; Michael Murphy, CPA, President and Chief Executive Officer
**(Centralized Health System)**

**CALIFORNIA:** SHARP CHULA VISTA MEDICAL CENTER (O, 343 beds) 751 Medical Center Court, Chula Vista, CA Zip 91911–6699, Mailing Address: P.O. Box 1297, Zip 91912–1297; tel. 619/482–5800; Pablo Velez, Chief Executive Officer
**Web address:** www.sharp.com

SHARP CORONADO HOSPITAL AND HEALTHCARE CENTER (L, 204 beds) 250 Prospect Place, Coronado, CA Zip 92118–1999; tel. 619/522–3600; Marcia K. Hall, Chief Executive Officer
**Web address:** www.sharp.com

SHARP GROSSMONT HOSPITAL (L, 521 beds) 5555 Grossmont Center Drive, La Mesa, CA Zip 91942–3019, Mailing Address: P.O. Box 158, Zip 91944–0158; tel. 619/740–6000; Michele T. Tarbet, R.N., Chief Executive Officer
**Web address:** www.sharp.com

**Section B**

For explanation of codes following names, see page B2.
★ Indicates Type III membership in the American Hospital Association.

SHARP MEMORIAL HOSPITAL (O, 400 beds) 7901 Frost Street, San Diego, CA Zip 92123–2701; tel. 858/939–3400; Tim Smith, Chief Executive Officer
**Web address:** www.sharp.com

SHARP MESA VISTA HOSPITAL (O, 149 beds) 7850 Vista Hill Avenue, San Diego, CA Zip 92123–2717; tel. 858/278–4110; Kathi Lencioni, Chief Executive Officer
**Web address:** www.sharp.com

| | | |
|---|---|---|
| Owned, leased, sponsored: | 5 hospitals | 1617 beds |
| Contract–managed: | 0 hospitals | 0 beds |
| Totals: | 5 hospitals | 1617 beds |

★**0304: SHORE HEALTH SYSTEM** (NP)
219 South Washington Street, Easton, MD Zip 21601; tel. 410/822–1000; Kenneth D. Kozel, FACHE, President and Chief Executive Officer
**(Centralized Health System)**

| | | |
|---|---|---|
| Owned, leased, sponsored: | 0 hospitals | 0 beds |
| Contract–managed: | 0 hospitals | 0 beds |
| Totals: | 0 hospitals | 0 beds |

**4125: SHRINERS HOSPITALS FOR CHILDREN** (NP)
2900 Rocky Point Drive, Tampa, FL Zip 33607–1435, Mailing Address: P.O. Box 31356, Zip 33631–3356; tel. 813/281–0300; Keith Gardner, Executive Vice President
**(Independent Hospital System)**

SHRINERS HOSPITALS FOR CHILDREN, LOS ANGELES (O, 30 beds) 3160 Geneva Street, Los Angeles, CA Zip 90020–1199; tel. 213/388–3151; Eugene Raynaud, Interim Chief Executive Officer and Administrator
**Web address:** www.shrinershospitals.org

SHRINERS HOSPITALS FOR CHILDREN, NORTHERN CALIFORNIA (O, 70 beds) 2425 Stockton Boulevard, Sacramento, CA Zip 95817–2215; tel. 916/453–2000; Margaret Bryan, Administrator
**Web address:** www.shrinershq.org

**FLORIDA:** SHRINERS HOSPITALS FOR CHILDREN, TAMPA (O, 25 beds) 12502 USF Pine Drive, Tampa, FL Zip 33612–9499; tel. 813/972–2250; Alice Reed Lanford, R.N., MSN, FACHE, Administrator
**Web address:** www.shrinershq.org

**HAWAII:** SHRINERS HOSPITALS FOR CHILDREN, HONOLULU (O, 16 beds) 1310 Punahou Street, Honolulu, HI Zip 96826–1099; tel. 808/941–4466; Stanley B. Berry, FACHE, Administrator
**Web address:** www.shrinershq.org

**ILLINOIS:** SHRINERS HOSPITALS FOR CHILDREN–CHICAGO (O, 36 beds) 2211 North Oak Park Avenue, Chicago, IL Zip 60707–3392; tel. 773/622–5400; Terry Wheat, R.N., Acting Administrator
**Web address:** www.shrinershospitals.org

**KENTUCKY:** SHRINERS HOSPITALS FOR CHILDREN–LEXINGTON (O, 50 beds) 1900 Richmond Road, Lexington, KY Zip 40502–1298; tel. 859/266–2101; Tony Lewgood, Administrator
**Web address:** www.shrinershq.com

**LOUISIANA:** SHRINERS HOSPITALS FOR CHILDREN, SHREVEPORT (O, 45 beds) 3100 Samford Avenue, Shreveport, LA Zip 71103–4289; tel. 318/222–5704; Garry Kim Green, FACHE, Administrator
**Web address:** www.shriners.com

**MASSACHUSETTS:** SHRINERS HOSPITALS FOR CHILDREN, SPRINGFIELD (O, 20 beds) 516 Carew Street, Springfield, MA Zip 01104–2396; tel. 413/787–2000; Charles Walczak, FACHE, Administrator
**Web address:** www.shrinershq.org

SHRINERS HOSPITALS FOR CHILDREN–BOSTON (O, 30 beds) 51 Blossom Street, Boston, MA Zip 02114–2601; tel. 617/722–3000; C. Thomas D'Esmond, FACHE, Administrator
**Web address:** www.shrinershospitals.org

**MINNESOTA:** SHRINERS HOSPITALS FOR CHILDREN, TWIN CITIES (O, 40 beds) 2025 East River Parkway, Minneapolis, MN Zip 55414–3696; tel. 612/596–6100; Charles C. Lobeck, Administrator
**Web address:** www.shrinershq.org

**MISSOURI:** SHRINERS HOSPITALS FOR CHILDREN, ST. LOUIS (O, 42 beds) 2001 South Lindbergh Boulevard, Saint Louis, MO Zip 63131–3597; tel. 314/432–3600; John Gloss, FACHE, Administrator
**Web address:** www.shrinershq.org

**OHIO:** SHRINERS HOSPITALS FOR CHILDREN, SHRINERS BURNS HOSPITAL, CINCINNATI (O, 30 beds) 3229 Burnet Avenue, Cincinnati, OH Zip 45229–3095; tel. 513/872–6000; Ronald R. Hitzler, Administrator
**Web address:** www.shrinershq.org

**OREGON:** SHRINERS HOSPITALS FOR CHILDREN, PORTLAND (O, 8 beds) 3101 S.W. Sam Jackson Park Road, Portland, OR Zip 97239; tel. 503/241–5090; J. Craig Patchin, Administrator
**Web address:** www.shcc.org

**PENNSYLVANIA:** SHRINERS HOSPITALS FOR CHILDREN, ERIE (O, 30 beds) 1645 West 8th Street, Erie, PA Zip 16505–5007; tel. 814/875–8700; Charles Walczak, FACHE, Administrator
**Web address:** www.shrinershq.org

SHRINERS HOSPITALS FOR CHILDREN, PHILADELPHIA (O, 39 beds) 3551 North Broad Street, Philadelphia, PA Zip 19140–4105; tel. 215/430–4000; Ernest N. Perilli, Administrator
**Web address:** www.shrinershq.org

**SOUTH CAROLINA:** SHRINERS HOSPITALS FOR CHILDREN, GREENVILLE (O, 24 beds) 950 West Faris Road, Greenville, SC Zip 29605–4277; tel. 864/271–3444; Randall R. Romberger, Administrator
**Web address:** www.shrinershospitalsforchildren.org

**TEXAS:** SHRINERS HOSPITALS FOR CHILDREN, GALVESTON BURNS HOSPITAL (O, 30 beds) 815 Market Street, Galveston, TX Zip 77550–2725; tel. 409/770–6600; David A. Ferrell, Chief Executive Officer
**Web address:** www.shrinershq.org

SHRINERS HOSPITALS FOR CHILDREN, HOUSTON (O, 40 beds) 6977 Main Street, Houston, TX Zip 77030–3701; tel. 713/797–1616; David A. Ferrell, Chief Executive Officer
**Web address:** www.shrinershospitals.org

**UTAH:** SHRINERS HOSPITALS FOR CHILDREN–INTERMOUNTAIN (O, 40 beds) Fairfax Road & Virginia Street, Salt Lake City, UT Zip 84103–4399; tel. 801/536–3500; Kevin Martin, R.N., M.P.H., Administrator
**Web address:** www.shriners.org

**WASHINGTON:** SHRINERS HOSPITALS FOR CHILDREN (O, 30 beds) 911 West Fifth Avenue, Spokane, WA Zip 99204, Mailing Address: P.O. Box 2472, Zip 99210–2472; tel. 509/455–7844; Eugene Raynaud, Administrator
**Web address:** www.shrinershospital.org

| | | |
|---|---|---|
| Owned, leased, sponsored: | 20 hospitals | 675 beds |
| Contract–managed: | 0 hospitals | 0 beds |
| Totals: | 20 hospitals | 675 beds |

●**0376: SIGNATURE HOSPITAL CORPORATION** (IO)
363 North Sam Houston Parkway East Suite 1700, Houston, TX Zip 77060–2424; tel. 281/598–9800; Steven G. Peterson, Chief Executive Officer
**(Independent Hospital System)**

**TEXAS:** GULF COAST MEDICAL CENTER (O, 59 beds) 10141 Highway 59, Wharton, TX Zip 77488–3004; tel. 979/282–6100; Martin R. Slack, Chief Executive Officer
**Web address:** www.gulfcoastmedical.com

| | | |
|---|---|---|
| Owned, leased, sponsored: | 1 hospital | 59 beds |
| Contract–managed: | 0 hospitals | 0 beds |
| Totals: | 1 hospital | 59 beds |

★**0284: SINAI HEALTH SYSTEM** (NP)
1500 South California Avenue, Chicago, IL Zip 60608–1729; tel. 773/542–2000; Alan H. Channing, President and Chief Executive Officer
**(Independent Hospital System)**

For explanation of codes following names, see page B2.
★ Indicates Type III membership in the American Hospital Association.
● Single hospital health care system

**ILLINOIS:** MOUNT SINAI HOSPITAL (O, 290 beds) California Avenue at 15th Street, Chicago, IL Zip 60608–1729; tel. 773/542–2000; Alan H. Channing, President and Chief Executive Officer
**Web address:** www.sinai.org

SCHWAB REHABILITATION HOSPITAL (O, 101 beds) 1401 South California Avenue, Chicago, IL Zip 60608–1858; tel. 773/522–2010; Alan H. Channing, President and Chief Executive Officer
**Web address:** www.schwabrehab.org

| Owned, leased, sponsored: | 2 hospitals | 391 beds |
|---|---|---|
| Contract–managed: | 0 hospitals | 0 beds |
| **Totals:** | 2 hospitals | 391 beds |

**5125: SISTERS OF CHARITY HEALTH SYSTEM** (CC)
2475 East 22nd Street, Cleveland, OH Zip 44115–3221; tel. 216/363–2797; Sister Judith Ann Karam, President and Chief Executive Officer
**(Moderately Centralized Health System)**

**OHIO:** MERCY MEDICAL CENTER (O, 337 beds) 1320 Mercy Drive N.W., Canton, OH Zip 44708–2641; tel. 330/489–1000; Thomas E. Cecconi, President and Chief Executive Officer
**Web address:** www.cantonmercy.org

ST. JOHN MEDICAL CENTER (O, 182 beds) 29000 Center Ridge Road, Westlake, OH Zip 44145–5293; tel. 440/835–8000; William A. Young, Jr., President and Chief Executive Officer
**Web address:** www.sjws.net

ST. VINCENT CHARITY MEDICAL CENTER (O, 203 beds) 2351 East 22nd Street, Cleveland, OH Zip 44115–3111; tel. 216/861–6200; David Perse, M.D., President
**Web address:** www.svch.net

**SOUTH CAROLINA:** PROVIDENCE HOSPITAL (O, 314 beds) 2435 Forest Drive, Columbia, SC Zip 29204–2098; tel. 803/865–4500; George A. Zara, President and Chief Executive Officer
**Web address:** www.provhosp.com

| Owned, leased, sponsored: | 4 hospitals | 1036 beds |
|---|---|---|
| Contract–managed: | 0 hospitals | 0 beds |
| **Totals:** | 4 hospitals | 1036 beds |

**★5095: SISTERS OF CHARITY OF LEAVENWORTH HEALTH SYSTEM** (CC)
2420 West 26th Avenue, Suite 100D, Denver, CO Zip 80211–5301; tel. 303/813–5180; Michael A. Slubowski, Chief Executive Officer
**(Moderately Centralized Health System)**

**CALIFORNIA:** SAINT JOHN'S HEALTH CENTER (O, 223 beds) 2121 Santa Monica Boulevard, Santa Monica, CA Zip 90404; tel. 310/829–5511; Lou Lazatin, President and Chief Executive Officer
**Web address:** www.newstjohns.org

**COLORADO:** ST. MARY'S HOSPITAL AND MEDICAL CENTER (O, 310 beds) 2635 North 7th Street, Grand Junction, CO Zip 81501–8209, Mailing Address: P.O. Box 1628, Zip 81502–1628; tel. 970/298–2273; Michael J. McBride, FACHE, President and Chief Executive Officer
**Web address:** www.stmarygj.com

**KANSAS:** PROVIDENCE MEDICAL CENTER (O, 196 beds) 8929 Parallel Parkway, Kansas City, KS Zip 66112–1636; tel. 913/596–4000; Randall G. Nyp, FACHE, President and Chief Executive Officer
**Web address:** www.providence–health.org

SAINT JOHN HOSPITAL (O, 56 beds) 3500 South Fourth Street, Leavenworth, KS Zip 66048–5043; tel. 913/680–6000; Randall G. Nyp, FACHE, President and Chief Executive Officer
**Web address:** www.providence–health.org/sjh

ST. FRANCIS HEALTH CENTER (O, 291 beds) 1700 S.W. 7th Street, Topeka, KS Zip 66606–1690; tel. 785/295–8000; Robert J. Erickson, Chief Executive Officer
**Web address:** www.stfrancistopeka.org

**MONTANA:** HOLY ROSARY HEALTHCARE (O, 90 beds) 2600 Wilson Street, Miles City, MT Zip 59301–5094; tel. 406/233–2600; Paul Lewis, Chief Executive Officer
**Web address:** www.holyrosaryhealthcare.org

ST. JAMES HEALTHCARE (O, 58 beds) 400 South Clark Street, Butte, MT Zip 59702–3300; tel. 406/723–2500; Charles T. Wright, President and Chief Executive Officer
**Web address:** www.stjameshealthcare.org

ST. VINCENT HEALTHCARE (O, 206 beds) 1233 North 30th Street, Billings, MT Zip 59101–0165, Mailing Address: P.O. Box 35200, Zip 59107–5200; tel. 406/237–7000; Jason Barker, Chief Executive Officer
**Web address:** www.svh–mt.org

| Owned, leased, sponsored: | 8 hospitals | 1430 beds |
|---|---|---|
| Contract–managed: | 0 hospitals | 0 beds |
| **Totals:** | 8 hospitals | 1430 beds |

**5805: SISTERS OF MARY OF THE PRESENTATION HEALTH SYSTEM** (CC)
1202 Page Drive S.W., Fargo, ND Zip 58103–2340, Mailing Address: P.O. Box 10007, Zip 58106–0007; tel. 701/237–9290; Aaron K. Alton, President and Chief Executive Officer
**(Independent Hospital System)**

**ILLINOIS:** ST. MARGARET'S HOSPITAL (O, 86 beds) 600 East First Street, Spring Valley, IL Zip 61362–2034; tel. 815/664–5311; Tim Muntz, President and Chief Executive Officer
**Web address:** www.aboutsmh.org

**NORTH DAKOTA:** PRESENTATION MEDICAL CENTER (O, 25 beds) 213 Second Avenue N.E., Rolla, ND Zip 58367–7153, Mailing Address: P.O. Box 759, Zip 58367–0759; tel. 701/477–3161; Michael Pfeifer, Chief Executive Officer
**Web address:** www.pmc–rolla.com

ST. ALOISIUS MEDICAL CENTER (O, 120 beds) 325 East Brewster Street, Harvey, ND Zip 58341–1653; tel. 701/324–4651; Rockford Zastoupil, President and Chief Executive Officer
**Web address:** www.staloisius.org

ST. ANDREW'S HEALTH CENTER (O, 25 beds) 316 Ohmer Street, Bottineau, ND Zip 58318–1018; tel. 701/228–9300; Jodi Atkinson, President and Chief Executive Officer
**Web address:** www.standrewshealth.com

| Owned, leased, sponsored: | 4 hospitals | 256 beds |
|---|---|---|
| Contract–managed: | 0 hospitals | 0 beds |
| **Totals:** | 4 hospitals | 256 beds |

**5955: SISTERS OF SAINT FRANCIS** (CC)
2500 Grant Boulevard, Syracuse, NY Zip 13208–1713; tel. 315/634–7000; Sister Marian Rose Mansius, Assistant General Minister
**(Independent Hospital System)**

**NEW YORK:** ST. ELIZABETH MEDICAL CENTER (S, 181 beds) 2209 Genesee Street, Utica, NY Zip 13501–5999; tel. 315/798–8100; Richard H. Ketcham, FACHE, President and Chief Executive Officer
**Web address:** www.stemc.org

ST. JOSEPH'S HOSPITAL HEALTH CENTER (S, 431 beds) 301 Prospect Avenue, Syracuse, NY Zip 13203–1807; tel. 315/448–5111; Kathryn H. Ruscitto, President
**Web address:** www.sjhsyr.org

| Owned, leased, sponsored: | 2 hospitals | 612 beds |
|---|---|---|
| Contract–managed: | 0 hospitals | 0 beds |
| **Totals:** | 2 hospitals | 612 beds |

**0629: SOLARA HEALTHCARE** (IO)
13455 Noel Road, Suite 1320, Dallas, TX Zip 75240–6702; tel. 469/621–6700; Michael Brohm, President and Chief Executive Officer
**(Independent Hospital System)**

**OKLAHOMA:** SOLARA HOSPITAL OF MUSKOGEE (O, 41 beds) 351 South 40th Street, Muskogee, OK Zip 74401–4916; tel. 918/682–6161; Craig Koele, Chief Executive Officer
**Web address:** www.solarahc.com

For explanation of codes following names, see page B2.
★ Indicates Type III membership in the American Hospital Association.

Section B

SOLARA HOSPITAL OF SHAWNEE (O, 34 beds) 1900 Gordon Cooper Drive, 2nd Floor, Shawnee, OK Zip 74801; tel. 405/395–5800; Michael E. Gerten, Chief Executive Officer
**Web address:** www.solarahc.com

**TEXAS:** SOLARA HOSPITAL CONROE (O, 41 beds) 1500 Grand Lake Drive, Conroe, TX Zip 77304; tel. 936/523–1800; Steve Hockert, Chief Executive Officer
**Web address:** www.solarahc.com/shcco.html

SOLARA HOSPITAL HARLINGEN (O, 82 beds) 508 Victoria Lane, Harlingen, TX Zip 78550–3225; tel. 956/425–9600; Paul E. Qualls, Jr., Chief Executive Officer
**Web address:** www.solarahc.com/shcha.html

SOLARA HOSPITAL MCALLEN (O, 78 beds) 301 West Expressway 83, McAllen, TX Zip 78503–3045; tel. 956/632–4880; Jack Boggess, Chief Executive Officer
**Web address:** www.solarahc.com/shcmc.html

| | | |
|---|---|---|
| Owned, leased, sponsored: | 5 hospitals | 276 beds |
| Contract–managed: | 0 hospitals | 0 beds |
| Totals: | 5 hospitals | 276 beds |

**0358:  SOUND SHORE HEALTH SYSTEM** (NP)
16 Guion Place, New Rochelle, NY Zip 10801–5500; tel. 914/632–5000; John R. Spicer, President and Chief Executive Officer
**(Centralized Physician/Insurance Health System)**

**NEW YORK:** MOUNT VERNON HOSPITAL (O, 132 beds) 12 North Seventh Avenue, Mount Vernon, NY Zip 10550–2098; tel. 914/664–8000; John R. Spicer, President and Chief Executive Officer
**Web address:** www.sshsw.org

SOUND SHORE MEDICAL CENTER OF WESTCHESTER (O, 356 beds) 16 Guion Place, New Rochelle, NY Zip 10801–5502; tel. 914/632–5000; John R. Spicer, President and Chief Executive Officer
**Web address:** www.sshsw.org

| | | |
|---|---|---|
| Owned, leased, sponsored: | 2 hospitals | 488 beds |
| Contract–managed: | 0 hospitals | 0 beds |
| Totals: | 2 hospitals | 488 beds |

**★0151:  SOUTH JERSEY HEALTHCARE** (NP)
2950 College Drive, Suite 1E, Vineland, NJ Zip 08360; tel. 856/641–8000; Chester B. Kaletkowski, President and Chief Executive Officer
**(Centralized Health System)**

**NEW JERSEY:** SOUTH JERSEY HEALTHCARE – ELMER HOSPITAL (O, 88 beds) 501 West Front Street, Elmer, NJ Zip 08318–1090; tel. 856/363–1000; Chester B. Kaletkowski, President and Chief Executive Officer
**Web address:** www.sjhealthcare.net

SOUTH JERSEY HEALTHCARE – REGIONAL MEDICAL CENTER (O, 325 beds) 1505 West Sherman Avenue, Vineland, NJ Zip 08360; tel. 856/641–8000; Chester B. Kaletkowski, President and Chief Executive Officer
**Web address:** www.sjhealthcare.net

| | | |
|---|---|---|
| Owned, leased, sponsored: | 2 hospitals | 413 beds |
| Contract–managed: | 0 hospitals | 0 beds |
| Totals: | 2 hospitals | 413 beds |

**★0253:  SOUTHEAST GEORGIA HEALTH SYSTEM** (NP)
2415 Parkwood Drive, Brunswick, GA Zip 31520–4252, Mailing Address: P.O. Box 1518, Zip 31521–1518; tel. 912/466–7000; Gary R. Colberg, FACHE, President and Chief Executive Officer

**GEORGIA:** SOUTHEAST GEORGIA HEALTH SYSTEM BRUNSWICK CAMPUS (O, 510 beds) 2415 Parkwood Drive, Brunswick, GA Zip 31520–4252, Mailing Address: P.O. Box 1518, Zip 31521–1518; tel. 912/466–7000; Gary R. Colberg, FACHE, President and Chief Executive Officer
**Web address:** www.sghs.org

SOUTHEAST GEORGIA HEALTH SYSTEM CAMDEN CAMPUS (O, 40 beds) 2000 Dan Proctor Drive, Saint Marys, GA Zip 31558–3810; tel. 912/576–6200; Howard W. Sepp, Jr., FACHE, Vice President and Administrator
**Web address:** www.sghs.org

| | | |
|---|---|---|
| Owned, leased, sponsored: | 2 hospitals | 550 beds |
| Contract–managed: | 0 hospitals | 0 beds |
| Totals: | 2 hospitals | 550 beds |

**★0628:  SOUTHEASTHEALTH** (NP)
1701 Lacey Street, Cape Girardeau, MO Zip 63701–5230; tel. 573/334–4822; Wayne Smith, President and Chief Executive Officer
**(Moderately Centralized Health System)**

**MISSOURI:** SOUTHEAST HEALTH CENTER OF RIPLEY COUNTY (L, 27 beds) 109 Plum Street, Doniphan, MO Zip 63935–1299; tel. 573/996–2141; Robert E. Garrison, Chief Executive Officer
**Web address:** www.rcmhospital.net

SOUTHEAST HOSPITAL (O, 227 beds) 1701 Lacey Street, Cape Girardeau, MO Zip 63701–5230; tel. 573/334–4822; Wayne Smith, Interim President and Chief Executive Officer
**Web address:** www.southeastmissourihospital.com

| | | |
|---|---|---|
| Owned, leased, sponsored: | 2 hospitals | 254 beds |
| Contract–managed: | 0 hospitals | 0 beds |
| Totals: | 2 hospitals | 254 beds |

**4175:  SOUTHERN ILLINOIS HOSPITAL SERVICES** (NP)
1239 East Main Street, Carbondale, IL Zip 62901, Mailing Address: P.O. Box 3988, Zip 62902–3988; tel. 618/457–5200; Rex P. Budde, President and Chief Executive Officer
**(Independent Hospital System)**

**ILLINOIS:** HERRIN HOSPITAL (O, 104 beds) 201 South 14th Street, Herrin, IL Zip 62948–3631; tel. 618/942–2171; Terence Farrell, Administrator
**Web address:** www.sih.net

MEMORIAL HOSPITAL OF CARBONDALE (O, 153 beds) 405 West Jackson Street, Carbondale, IL Zip 62901–1467, Mailing Address: P.O. Box 10000, Zip 62902–9000; tel. 618/549–0721; Bart Millstead, Administrator
**Web address:** www.sih.net

ST. JOSEPH MEMORIAL HOSPITAL (O, 25 beds) 2 South Hospital Drive, Murphysboro, IL Zip 62966–3333; tel. 618/684–3156; Scott Seaborn, Administrator
**Web address:** www.sih.net

| | | |
|---|---|---|
| Owned, leased, sponsored: | 3 hospitals | 282 beds |
| Contract–managed: | 0 hospitals | 0 beds |
| Totals: | 3 hospitals | 282 beds |

**0346:  SOUTHERN PLAINS MEDICAL GROUP** (IO)
3555 N.W. 58th Street, Suite 700, Oklahoma City, OK Zip 73112; tel. 405/917–0300; Thomas R. Rice, FACHE, President and Chief Operating Officer

**OKLAHOMA:** PHYSICIANS' HOSPITAL IN ANADARKO (O, 25 beds) 1002 Central Boulevard East, Anadarko, OK Zip 73005–4496; tel. 405/247–2551; Richard Carter, M.D., Chief Executive Officer

STROUD REGIONAL MEDICAL CENTER (O, 25 beds) Highway 66 West, Stroud, OK Zip 74079, Mailing Address: P.O. Box 530, Zip 74079–0530; tel. 918/968–3571; Regina Peters, Chief Executive Officer

| | | |
|---|---|---|
| Owned, leased, sponsored: | 2 hospitals | 50 beds |
| Contract–managed: | 0 hospitals | 0 beds |
| Totals: | 2 hospitals | 50 beds |

For explanation of codes following names, see page B2.
★ Indicates Type III membership in the American Hospital Association.

**0652: SOUTHWEST HEALTH SYSTEMS** (NP)

215 Marion Avenue, Mccomb, MS Zip 39648–2705, Mailing Address: P.O. Box 1307, Zip 39649–1307; tel. 601/249–5500; Norman M. Price, FACHE, Chief Executive Officer and Administrator

**(Independent Hospital System)**

**MISSISSIPPI:** LAWRENCE COUNTY HOSPITAL (O, 25 beds) Highway 84 East, Monticello, MS Zip 39654–0788, Mailing Address: P.O. Box 788, Zip 39654–0788; tel. 601/587–4051; Semmes Ross, Jr., Administrator
**Web address:** www.smrmc.com

SOUTHWEST MISSISSIPPI REGIONAL MEDICAL CENTER (O, 143 beds) 215 Marion Avenue, McComb, MS Zip 39648–2798, Mailing Address: P.O. Box 1307, Zip 39649–1307; tel. 601/249–5500; Norman M. Price, FACHE, Chief Executive Officer
**Web address:** www.smrmc.com

| | | |
|---|---|---|
| Owned, leased, sponsored: | 2 hospitals | 168 beds |
| Contract–managed: | 0 hospitals | 0 beds |
| Totals: | 2 hospitals | 168 beds |

**★1245: SPARROW HEALTH SYSTEM** (NP)

1215 East Michigan Avenue, Lansing, MI Zip 48912; tel. 517/364–1000; Dennis A. Swan, President and Chief Executive Officer

**(Centralized Health System)**

**MICHIGAN:** SPARROW CLINTON HOSPITAL (O, 25 beds) 805 South Oakland Street, Saint Johns, MI Zip 48879–2253; tel. 989/227–3400; Edward Bruun, President and Chief Executive Officer
**Web address:** www.clintonmemorial.org

SPARROW HOSPITAL (O, 638 beds) 1215 East Michigan Avenue, Lansing, MI Zip 48912–1811, Mailing Address: P.O. Box 30480, Zip 48909–7980; tel. 517/364–1000; Dennis A. Swan, President and Chief Executive Officer
**Web address:** www.sparrow.org

SPARROW IONIA HOSPITAL (O, 25 beds) 479 Lafayette Street, Ionia, MI Zip 48846–1834, Mailing Address: Box 1001, Zip 48846–1899; tel. 616/523–1400; William Roeser, President and Chief Executive Officer
**Web address:** www.ioniahospital.org

SPARROW SPECIALTY HOSPITAL (O, 36 beds) 1210 West Saginaw Street, Lansing, MI Zip 48915–1927, Mailing Address: P.O. Box 85201, Zip 48915; tel. 517/364–6800; Kira Carter–Robertson, Chief Executive Officer
**Web address:** www.sparrowspecialty.org

| | | |
|---|---|---|
| Owned, leased, sponsored: | 4 hospitals | 724 beds |
| Contract–managed: | 0 hospitals | 0 beds |
| Totals: | 4 hospitals | 724 beds |

**★4195: SPARTANBURG REGIONAL HEALTHCARE SYSTEM** (NP)

101 East Wood Street, Spartanburg, SC Zip 29303–3016; tel. 864/560–6000; Bruce Holstien, President and Chief Executive Officer

**(Centralized Health System)**

**SOUTH CAROLINA:** SPARTANBURG HOSPITAL FOR RESTORATIVE CARE (O, 91 beds) 389 Serpentine Drive, Spartanburg, SC Zip 29303–3026; tel. 864/560–3280; Anita M. Butler, Chief Executive Officer
**Web address:** www.srhs.com

SPARTANBURG REGIONAL MEDICAL CENTER (O, 539 beds) 101 East Wood Street, Spartanburg, SC Zip 29303–3016; tel. 864/560–6000; J. Philip Feisal, Senior Vice President Acute Care Hospitals
**Web address:** www.spartanburgregional.com

VILLAGE HOSPITAL (O, 34 beds) 250 Westmoreland Road, Greer, SC Zip 29651; tel. 864/530–6000; J. Philip Feisal, Chief Executive Officer
**Web address:** www.villageatpelham.com

| | | |
|---|---|---|
| Owned, leased, sponsored: | 3 hospitals | 664 beds |
| Contract–managed: | 0 hospitals | 0 beds |
| Totals: | 3 hospitals | 664 beds |

**0641: SPECIALTY HEALTHCARE, LLC** (IO)

305 West Harriet Street, Leesville, LA Zip 71446–4229; tel. 337/238–4449; Craig Ball, Chairman and Chief Executive Officer

**LOUISIANA:** SPECIALTY LONG TERM ACUTE CARE HOSPITAL OF HAMMOND (O, 20 beds) 42074 Veterans Avenue, Hammond, LA Zip 70403; tel. 985/902–8148; Charles Ball, Administrator
**Web address:** www.specialtyltchhammond.com

SPECIALTY REHABILITATION HOSPITAL (O, 12 beds) 1110 Ringgold Avenue Suite B., Coushatta, LA Zip 71019–9073; tel. 318/932–1770; Craig Ball, Chief Executive Officer
**Web address:** www.specialtyhealthcare.com

SPECIALTY REHABILITATION HOSPITAL OF LULING (O, 21 beds) 1125 Paul Maillard Road, Luling, LA Zip 70070–4351; tel. 985/785–5233; Lisa Miller, Administrator
**Web address:** www.specialtyrehabluling.com

| | | |
|---|---|---|
| Owned, leased, sponsored: | 3 hospitals | 53 beds |
| Contract–managed: | 0 hospitals | 0 beds |
| Totals: | 3 hospitals | 53 beds |

**0352: SPECIALTY HOSPITALS OF AMERICA, LLC** (IO)

155 Fleet Street, Portsmouth, NH Zip 03801; tel. 603/570–4888; Eric F. Rieseberg, President

**(Independent Hospital System)**

**DISTRICT OF COLUMBIA:** SPECIALTY HOSPITAL OF WASHINGTON (O, 177 beds) 700 Constitution Avenue N.E., Washington, DC Zip 20002–6058; tel. 202/546–5700; Susan P. Bailey, R.N., Chief Executive Officer
**Web address:** www.specialtyhospitalofwashington.com

SPECIALTY HOSPITAL OF WASHINGTON–HADLEY (O, 82 beds) 4601 Martin Luther King Jr. Avenue, S.W., Washington, DC Zip 20032–1199; tel. 202/574–5700; Peter Miller, FACHE, Chief Executive Officer

| | | |
|---|---|---|
| Owned, leased, sponsored: | 2 hospitals | 259 beds |
| Contract–managed: | 0 hospitals | 0 beds |
| Totals: | 2 hospitals | 259 beds |

**★0177: SPECTRUM HEALTH** (NP)

100 Michigan Street N.E., Grand Rapids, MI Zip 49503–2551; tel. 616/391–1774; Richard C. Breon, President and Chief Executive Officer

**(Moderately Centralized Health System)**

**MICHIGAN:** SPECTRUM HEALTH BUTTERWORTH HOSPITAL (O, 1066 beds) 100 Michigan Street N.E., Grand Rapids, MI Zip 49503–2560; tel. 616/774–7444; Matthew Van Vranken, President, Spectrum Health Hospital Group
**Web address:** www.spectrum–health.org

SPECTRUM HEALTH GERBER MEMORIAL (O, 40 beds) 212 South Sullivan Avenue, Fremont, MI Zip 49412–1548; tel. 231/924–3300; Randall Stasik, President and Chief Executive Officer
**Web address:** www.gerberhospital.org

SPECTRUM HEALTH REED CITY HOSPITAL (O, 74 beds) 300 North Patterson Road, Reed City, MI Zip 49677–0075, Mailing Address: P.O. Box 75, Zip 49677–0075; tel. 231/832–3271; Sam Daugherty, Ed.D., President
**Web address:** www.reedcity.spectrum–health.org

SPECTRUM HEALTH SPECIAL CARE HOSPITAL (O, 36 beds) 750 Fuller Avenue N.E., Grand Rapids, MI Zip 49503–1995; tel. 616/486–3000; Charles Tozer, Chief Executive Officer
**Web address:** www.spectrum–health.org

SPECTRUM HEALTH UNITED HOSPITAL (O, 117 beds) 615 South Bower Street, Greenville, MI Zip 48838–2614; tel. 616/754–4691; Christina Freese–Decker, President
**Web address:** www.spectrum–health.org/

| | | |
|---|---|---|
| Owned, leased, sponsored: | 5 hospitals | 1333 beds |
| Contract–managed: | 0 hospitals | 0 beds |
| Totals: | 5 hospitals | 1333 beds |

**Section B**

For explanation of codes following names, see page B2.
★ Indicates Type III membership in the American Hospital Association.

**★5455: SSM HEALTH CARE** (CC)
477 North Lindbergh Boulevard, Saint Louis, MO Zip 63141–7813;
tel. 314/994–7800; William P. Thompson, President and Chief
Executive Officer
**(Decentralized Health System)**

**ILLINOIS:** GOOD SAMARITAN REGIONAL HEALTH CENTER (O, 148 beds) 605
North 12th Street, Mount Vernon, IL Zip 62864–2899;
tel. 618/242–4600; Michael D. Warren, President
**Web address:** www.smgsi.com

ST. MARY'S HOSPITAL (O, 104 beds) 400 North Pleasant Avenue, Centralia,
IL Zip 62801–3091; tel. 618/436–8000; Bruce Merrell, FACHE, President
**Web address:** www.smgsi.com

**MISSOURI:** SSM CARDINAL GLENNON CHILDREN'S MEDICAL CENTER (O,
176 beds) 1465 South Grand Boulevard, Saint Louis, MO
Zip 63104–1095; tel. 314/577–5600; Sherlyn Hailstone, MSN, R.N.,
FACHE, President
**Web address:** www.cardinalglennon.com

SSM DEPAUL HEALTH CENTER (O, 476 beds) 12303 De Paul Drive,
Bridgeton, MO Zip 63044–2512; tel. 314/344–6000; Sean Hogan, President
**Web address:** www.ssmdepaul.com

SSM ST. CLARE HEALTH CENTER (O, 184 beds) 1015 Bowles Avenue,
Fenton, MO Zip 63026–2394; tel. 636/496–2000; R. William Hoefer, FACHE,
President
**Web address:** www.ssmstclare.com

SSM ST. JOSEPH HEALTH CENTER (O, 331 beds) 300 First Capitol Drive,
Saint Charles, MO Zip 63301–2844; tel. 636/947–5000; Gaspare Calvaruso,
President
**Web address:** www.ssmstjoseph.com

SSM ST. JOSEPH HOSPITAL WEST (O, 126 beds) 100 Medical Plaza, Lake
Saint Louis, MO Zip 63367–1366; tel. 636/625–5200; Lisle Wescott,
President
**Web address:** www.ssmstjoseph.com

SSM ST. MARY'S HEALTH CENTER (O, 374 beds) 6420 Clayton Road, Saint
Louis, MO Zip 63117–1811; tel. 314/768–8000; Kathleen R. Becker, M.P.H.,
JD, President
**Web address:** www.stmarys–stlouis.com

ST. FRANCIS HOSPITAL AND HEALTH SERVICES (O, 57 beds) 2016 South
Main Street, Maryville, MO Zip 64468–2655; tel. 660/562–2600; Gray Cox,
President
**Web address:** www.stfrancismaryville.com

ST. MARYS HEALTH CENTER (O, 139 beds) 100 St. Marys Medical Plaza,
Jefferson City, MO Zip 65101–1602; tel. 573/761–7000; R. Brent VanConia,
President
**Web address:** www.lethealingbegin.com

**OKLAHOMA:** ST. ANTHONY HOSPITAL (O, 499 beds) 1000 North Lee Street,
Oklahoma City, OK Zip 73102–1080, Mailing Address: P.O. Box 205,
Zip 73101–0205; tel. 405/272–7000; Joe Hodges, President
**Web address:** www.saintsok.com

ST. ANTHONY SHAWNEE HOSPITAL (O, 131 beds) 1102 West MacArthur
Street, Shawnee, OK Zip 74804–1744; tel. 405/273–2270; Charles E.
Skillings, President and Chief Executive Officer
**Web address:** www.stanthonyshawnee.com

**WISCONSIN:** ST. CLARE HOSPITAL AND HEALTH SERVICES (O, 54 beds) 707
14th Street, Baraboo, WI Zip 53913–1597; tel. 608/356–1400; Sandra
L. Anderson, President
**Web address:** www.stclare.com

ST. MARY'S HOSPITAL (O, 361 beds) 700 South Park Street, Madison, WI
Zip 53715–0450; tel. 608/251–6100; Frank D. Byrne, M.D., President
**Web address:** www.stmarysmadison.com

| | | |
|---|---|---|
| Owned, leased, sponsored: | 14 hospitals | 3160 beds |
| Contract–managed: | 0 hospitals | 0 beds |
| Totals: | 14 hospitals | 3160 beds |

---

**★0250: ST. CHARLES HEALTH SYSTEM, INC.** (NP)
2500 N.E. Neff Road, Bend, OR Zip 97701–6015;
tel. 541/382–4321; James A. Diegel, President and Chief Executive
Officer
**(Centralized Physician/Insurance Health System)**

**OREGON:** MOUNTAIN VIEW HOSPITAL DISTRICT (C, 25 beds) 470 N.E. A
Street, Madras, OR Zip 97741–1844; tel. 541/475–3882; Jeanine
Gentry, Chief Executive Officer
**Web address:** www.mvhd.org

PIONEER MEMORIAL HOSPITAL (L, 25 beds) 1201 N.E. Elm Street, Prineville,
OR Zip 97754–1206; tel. 541/447–6254; Robert Gomes, Chief Executive
Officer
**Web address:** www.stcharleshealthcare.org

ST. CHARLES MEDICAL CENTER – BEND (O, 261 beds) 2500 N.E. Neff Road,
Bend, OR Zip 97701–6015; tel. 541/382–4321; Jay Henry, Chief Executive
Officer
**Web address:** www.scmc.org

ST. CHARLES MEDICAL CENTER – REDMOND (O, 48 beds) 1253 N.W. Canal
Boulevard, Redmond, OR Zip 97756–1395; tel. 541/548–8131; Robert
Gomes, Chief Executive Officer
**Web address:** www.stcharleshealthcare.org

| | | |
|---|---|---|
| Owned, leased, sponsored: | 3 hospitals | 334 beds |
| Contract–managed: | 1 hospital | 25 beds |
| Totals: | 4 hospitals | 359 beds |

---

**0618: ST. ELIZABETH HEALTHCARE** (NP)
1 Medical Village Drive, Edgewood, KY Zip 41017–3403;
tel. 859/301–2370; John S. Dubis, FACHE, President and Chief
Executive Officer
**(Centralized Physician/Insurance Health System)**

**KENTUCKY:** ST. ELIZABETH EDGEWOOD (O, 510 beds) 1 Medical Village
Drive, Edgewood, KY Zip 41017–3403; tel. 859/301–2000; John S.
Dubis, FACHE, President and Chief Executive Officer
**Web address:** www.stelizabeth.com

ST. ELIZABETH FLORENCE (O, 170 beds) 4900 Houston Road, Florence, KY
Zip 41042–4824; tel. 859/212–5200; Chris Carle, Senior Vice President and
Chief Operating Officer
**Web address:** www.stelizabeth.com

ST. ELIZABETH FORT THOMAS (O, 194 beds) 85 North Grand Avenue, Fort
Thomas, KY Zip 41075–1796; tel. 859/572–3100; Thomas Saalfeld, Senior
Vice President and Chief Operating Officer
**Web address:** www.stelizabeth.com

ST. ELIZABETH GRANT (O, 16 beds) 238 Barnes Road, Williamstown, KY
Zip 41097–9460; tel. 859/824–8240; Paula Roe, Assistant Vice President
Operations
**Web address:** www.stelizabeth.com

| | | |
|---|---|---|
| Owned, leased, sponsored: | 4 hospitals | 890 beds |
| Contract–managed: | 0 hospitals | 0 beds |
| Totals: | 4 hospitals | 890 beds |

---

**★5425: ST. JOSEPH HEALTH** (CC)
500 South Main Street, Suite 1000, Orange, CA Zip 92868, Mailing
Address: P.O. Box 14132, Zip 92863–1532; tel. 714/347–7500;
Deborah A. Proctor, President and Chief Executive Officer
**(Moderately Centralized Health System)**

**CALIFORNIA:** MISSION HOSPITAL (O, 407 beds) 27700 Medical Center Road,
Mission Viejo, CA Zip 92691–6426; tel. 949/364–1400; Kenneth
McFarland, President and Chief Executive Officer
**Web address:** www.mission4health.com

PETALUMA VALLEY HOSPITAL (L, 29 beds) 400 North McDowell Boulevard,
Petaluma, CA Zip 94954–2369; tel. 707/778–1111; Kevin Klockenga,
President and Chief Executive Officer
**Web address:** www.stjosephhealth.org/petalumavalley

QUEEN OF THE VALLEY MEDICAL CENTER (O, 174 beds) 1000 Trancas
Street, Napa, CA Zip 94558–2906, Mailing Address: P.O. Box 2340,
Zip 94558–2340; tel. 707/252–4411; Walt Mickens, President and Chief
Executive Officer
**Web address:** www.thequeen.org

REDWOOD MEMORIAL HOSPITAL (O, 25 beds) 3300 Renner Drive, Fortuna,
CA Zip 95540–3198; tel. 707/725–3361; Joseph M. Mark, Chief Executive
Officer
**Web address:** www.stjosepheureka.org

For explanation of codes following names, see page B2.
★ Indicates Type III membership in the American Hospital Association.

SANTA ROSA MEMORIAL HOSPITAL (O, 272 beds) 1165 Montgomery Drive, Santa Rosa, CA Zip 95405–4897, Mailing Address: P.O. Box 522, Zip 95402–0522; tel. 707/546–3210; Kevin Klockenga, President and Chief Executive Officer
**Web address:** www.stjosephhealth.org

ST. JOSEPH HOSPITAL (O, 128 beds) 2700 Dolbeer Street, Eureka, CA Zip 95501–4799; tel. 707/445–8121; Joseph M. Mark, President and Chief Executive Officer
**Web address:** www.stjosepheureka.org

ST. JOSEPH HOSPITAL (O, 379 beds) 1100 West Stewart Drive, Orange, CA Zip 92863–5600, Mailing Address: P.O. Box 5600, Zip 92863–5600; tel. 714/633–9111; Steven C. Moreau, Chief Executive Officer
**Web address:** www.sjo.org

ST. JUDE MEDICAL CENTER (O, 384 beds) 101 East Valencia Mesa Drive, Fullerton, CA Zip 92835–3809; tel. 714/992–3000; Lee Penrose, President and Chief Executive Officer
**Web address:** www.stjudemedicalcenter.org

ST. MARY MEDICAL CENTER (O, 186 beds) 18300 Highway 18, Apple Valley, CA Zip 92307–2206, Mailing Address: P.O. Box 7025, Zip 92307–0725; tel. 760/242–2311; Alan H. Garrett, President and Chief Executive Officer
**Web address:** www.stmaryapplevalley.com/

| Owned, leased, sponsored: | 9 hospitals | 1984 beds |
|---|---|---|
| Contract–managed: | 0 hospitals | 0 beds |
| **Totals:** | 9 hospitals | 1984 beds |

---

★**0302:   ST. LUKE'S EPISCOPAL HEALTH SYSTEM** (NP)
6624 Fannin Street, Suite 1100, Houston, TX Zip 77030; tel. 832/355–7661; David J. Fine, Chief Executive Officer
**(Independent Hospital System)**

**TEXAS:** ST. LUKE'S EPISCOPAL HOSPITAL (O, 711 beds) 6720 Bertner Avenue, Houston, TX Zip 77030–2697, Mailing Address: P.O. Box 20269, Zip 77225–0269; tel. 832/355–1000; Margaret M. Van Bree, Dr.PH, Chief Executive Officer
**Web address:** www.stlukestexas.com

ST. LUKE'S HOSPITAL AT THE VINTAGE (O, 78 beds) 20171 Chasewood Park Drive, Houston, TX Zip 77070; tel. 832/534–5000; Francis X. Speidel, M.D., Chief Executive Officer
**Web address:** www.stlukesvintage.com/

ST. LUKE'S LAKESIDE HOSPITAL (O, 30 beds) 17400 St. Luke's Way, The Woodlands, TX Zip 77384; tel. 936/266–9000; Debra F. Sukin, Chief Executive Officer
**Web address:** www.stlukeslakeside.com/

ST. LUKE'S PATIENTS MEDICAL CENTER (O, 61 beds) 4600 East Sam Houston Parkway South, Pasadena, TX Zip 77505; tel. 713/948–7000; William Simmons, President and Chief Executive Officer
**Web address:** www.stlukestexas.com

ST. LUKE'S SUGAR LAND HOSPITAL (O, 84 beds) 1317 Lake Pointe Parkway, Sugar Land, TX Zip 77478; tel. 281/637–7000; Bryan J. Hargis, FACHE, Chief Executive Officer
**Web address:** www.stlukessugarland.com

ST. LUKE'S THE WOODLANDS HOSPITAL (O, 154 beds) 17200 St. Luke's Way, The Woodlands, TX Zip 77384; tel. 936/266–2000; Debra F. Sukin, Chief Executive Officer
**Web address:** www.stlukeswoodlands.com

| Owned, leased, sponsored: | 6 hospitals | 1118 beds |
|---|---|---|
| Contract–managed: | 0 hospitals | 0 beds |
| **Totals:** | 6 hospitals | 1118 beds |

---

★**0356:   ST. LUKE'S HEALTH SYSTEM** (NP)
420 West Idaho Street, Boise, ID Zip 83702; tel. 208/381–4200; David C. Pate, M.D., JD, President and Chief Executive Officer
**(Independent Hospital System)**

**IDAHO:** ELMORE MEDICAL CENTER (C, 57 beds) 895 North Sixth East Street, Mountain Home, ID Zip 83647–2207, Mailing Address: P.O. Box 1270, Zip 83647–1270; tel. 208/587–8401; Gregory L. Maurer, Administrator
**Web address:** www.elmoremedicalcenter.org

NORTH CANYON MEDICAL CENTER (C, 15 beds) 267 North Canyon Drive, Gooding, ID Zip 83330; tel. 208/934–4433; David Butler, Chief Executive Officer
**Web address:** www.goodinghospital.org

ST. LUKE'S MAGIC VALLEY MEDICAL CENTER (O, 201 beds) 801 Pole Line Road West, Twin Falls, ID Zip 83301, Mailing Address: P.O. Box 409, Zip 83303–0409; tel. 208/814–0000; James L. Angle, FACHE, Chief Executive Officer
**Web address:** www.stlukesonline.org

ST. LUKE'S MCCALL (O, 15 beds) 1000 State Street, McCall, ID Zip 83638–3704; tel. 208/634–2221; Michael A. Fenello, Chief Executive Officer
**Web address:** www.mccallhosp.org

ST. LUKE'S REGIONAL MEDICAL CENTER (O, 576 beds) 190 East Bannock Street, Boise, ID Zip 83712–6298; tel. 208/381–2222; Chris Roth, Chief Executive Officer
**Web address:** www.stlukesonline.org/boise

ST. LUKE'S WOOD RIVER MEDICAL CENTER (O, 25 beds) 100 Hospital Drive, Ketchum, ID Zip 83340, Mailing Address: P.O. Box 100, Zip 83340; tel. 208/727–8800; Cody Langbehn, Chief Executive Officer
**Web address:** www.slrmc.org

WEISER MEMORIAL HOSPITAL (C, 25 beds) 645 East Fifth Street, Weiser, ID Zip 83672–2202; tel. 208/549–0370; Tom Murphy, Chief Executive Officer
**Web address:** www.weisermemorialhospital.org

| Owned, leased, sponsored: | 4 hospitals | 817 beds |
|---|---|---|
| Contract–managed: | 3 hospitals | 97 beds |
| **Totals:** | 7 hospitals | 914 beds |

---

**0862:   ST. LUKE'S UNIVERSITY HEALTH NETWORK** (NP)
801 Ostrum Street, Bethlehem, PA Zip 18015–1000; tel. 610/954–4000; Richard A. Anderson, President and Chief Executive Officer

**NEW JERSEY:** ST. LUKE'S HOSPITAL – WARREN CAMPUS (O, 140 beds) 185 Roseberry Street, Phillipsburg, NJ Zip 08865–9955; tel. 908/859–6700; Thomas H. Litz, FACHE, President an Chief Executive Officer
**Web address:** www.warrenhospital.org

**PENNSYLVANIA:** ST. LUKE'S HOSPITAL – ANDERSON CAMPUS (O, 108 beds) 1872 Riverside Circle, Easton, PA Zip 18045–5669; tel. 484/503–3000; Edward Nawrocki, President
**Web address:** www.mystlukesonline.org

ST. LUKE'S HOSPITAL – MINERS CAMPUS (O, 92 beds) 360 West Ruddle Street, Coaldale, PA Zip 18218–1027; tel. 570/645–2131; William E. Moyer, President
**Web address:** www.slhn.org

ST. LUKE'S HOSPITAL – QUAKERTOWN CAMPUS (O, 57 beds) 1021 Park Avenue, Quakertown, PA Zip 18951–1573; tel. 215/538–4500; Edward Nawrocki, President
**Web address:** www.slhhn.org

ST. LUKE'S UNIVERSITY HOSPITAL – BETHLEHEM CAMPUS (O, 581 beds) 801 Ostrum Street, Bethlehem, PA Zip 18015–1065; tel. 610/954–4000; Richard A. Anderson, President and Chief Executive Officer
**Web address:** www.slhn–lehighvalley.org

| Owned, leased, sponsored: | 5 hospitals | 978 beds |
|---|---|---|
| Contract–managed: | 0 hospitals | 0 beds |
| **Totals:** | 5 hospitals | 978 beds |

---

**0156:   STANFORD HEALTH CARE** (NP)
300 Pasteur Drive, Palo Alto, CA Zip 94304–2299; tel. 650/723–4000; Amir Dan Rubin, President and Chief Executive Officer
**(Moderately Centralized Health System)**

**CALIFORNIA:** LUCILE SALTER PACKARD CHILDREN'S HOSPITAL AT STANFORD (O, 302 beds) 725 Welch Road, Palo Alto, CA Zip 94304–1601; tel. 650/497–8000; Christopher G. Dawes, President and Chief Executive Officer
**Web address:** www.lpch.org

For explanation of codes following names, see page B2.
★ Indicates Type III membership in the American Hospital Association.

Section B

STANFORD HOSPITAL AND CLINICS (O, 477 beds) 1520 Page Mill Road, Palo Alto, CA Zip 94304–1125; tel. 650/723–4000; Amir Dan Rubin, President and Chief Executive Officer
**Web address:** www.stanfordhospital.com/

| | | |
|---|---|---|
| Owned, leased, sponsored: | 2 hospitals | 779 beds |
| Contract–managed: | 0 hospitals | 0 beds |
| Totals: | 2 hospitals | 779 beds |

**0141: STEWARD HEALTH CARE SYSTEM, LLC** (IO)
500 Boylston Street, 5th Floor, Boston, MA Zip 02116–3740; tel. 617/419–4700; Ralph de la Torre, M.D., Chairman and Chief Executive Officer
**(Moderately Centralized Health System)**

**MASSACHUSETTS:** CARNEY HOSPITAL (O, 133 beds) 2100 Dorchester Avenue, Boston, MA Zip 02124–5615; tel. 617/296–4000; Margaret Hanson, R.N., Interim President
**Web address:** www.carneyhospital.org

GOOD SAMARITAN MEDICAL CENTER (O, 190 beds) 235 North Pearl Street, Brockton, MA Zip 02301–1794; tel. 508/427–3000; Jeffrey H. Liebman, President
**Web address:** www.stewardhealth.org/Good–Samaritan

HOLY FAMILY HOSPITAL AND MEDICAL CENTER (O, 239 beds) 70 East Street, Methuen, MA Zip 01844–4597; tel. 978/687–0151; Lester P. Schindel, President and Chief Executive Officer
**Web address:** www.stewardhealth.org/Holy–Family–Hospital

MERRIMACK VALLEY HOSPITAL (O, 90 beds) 140 Lincoln Avenue, Haverhill, MA Zip 01830–6798; tel. 978/374–2000; Michael F. Collins, Chief Executive Officer
**Web address:** www.merrimackvalleyhospital.com

MORTON HOSPITAL AND MEDICAL CENTER (O, 153 beds) 88 Washington Street, Taunton, MA Zip 02780–2465; tel. 508/828–7000; Michael J. Schwartz, Interim President
**Web address:** www.mortonhospital.org

NASHOBA VALLEY MEDICAL CENTER (O, 42 beds) 200 Groton Road, Ayer, MA Zip 01432–3300; tel. 978/784–9000; Steven P. Roach, Chief Executive Officer
**Web address:** www.nashobamed.com

NORWOOD HOSPITAL (O, 205 beds) 800 Washington Street, Norwood, MA Zip 02062–3487; tel. 781/769–4000; Emily L. Holliman, President
**Web address:** www.stewardhealth.org/Norwood–Hospital

QUINCY MEDICAL CENTER (O, 116 beds) 114 Whitwell Street, Quincy, MA Zip 02169–1899; tel. 617/773–6100; Daniel J. Knell, MSN, President
**Web address:** www.quincymc.org

SAINT ANNE'S HOSPITAL (O, 92 beds) 795 Middle Street, Fall River, MA Zip 02721–1798; tel. 508/674–5741; Craig A. Jesiolowski, FACHE, President
**Web address:** www.saintanneshospital.org

ST. ELIZABETH'S MEDICAL CENTER (O, 338 beds) 736 Cambridge Street, Brighton, MA Zip 02135–2997; tel. 617/789–3000; John Polanowicz, President
**Web address:** www.stewardhealth.org/St_Elizabeths

| | | |
|---|---|---|
| Owned, leased, sponsored: | 10 hospitals | 1598 beds |
| Contract–managed: | 0 hospitals | 0 beds |
| Totals: | 10 hospitals | 1598 beds |

**0858: STRATEGIC BEHAVIORAL HEALTH, LLC** (IO)
8295 Tournament Drive, Suite 201, Memphis, TN Zip 38125–8906; tel. 901/969–3100; Jim Shaheen, President

**COLORADO:** PEAK VIEW BEHAVIORAL HEALTH (O, 24 beds) 7353 Sisters Grove, Colorado Springs, CO Zip 80923–2615; tel. 719/444–8484; Gary Miller, Chief Executive Officer
**Web address:** www.strategicbh.com/peakview.html

**NEVADA:** MONTEVISTA HOSPITAL (O, 80 beds) 5900 West Rochelle Avenue, Las Vegas, NV Zip 89103–3327; tel. 702/364–1111; Robert E. Marshall, Chief Executive Officer
**Web address:** www.montevistahospital.com

RED ROCK BEHAVIORAL HOSPITAL (O, 21 beds) 5975 West Twain Avenue, Las Vegas, NV Zip 89103–1237; tel. 702/214–8099; Bob Mash, Chief Executive Officer
**Web address:** www.redrockhospital.com

| | | |
|---|---|---|
| Owned, leased, sponsored: | 3 hospitals | 125 beds |
| Contract–managed: | 0 hospitals | 0 beds |
| Totals: | 3 hospitals | 125 beds |

**0517: SUCCESS HEALTHCARE** (IO)
999 Yamato Road, 3rd Floor, Boca Raton, FL Zip 33431–4477; tel. 561/869–6300; Peter R. Baronoff, President and Chief Executive Officer
**(Independent Hospital System)**

**CALIFORNIA:** SILVER LAKE MEDICAL CENTER (O, 150 beds) 1711 West Temple Street, Los Angeles, CA Zip 90026–5421; tel. 213/989–6100; Steve Popkin, Chief Executive Officer
**Web address:** www.silverlakemc.com

**MISSOURI:** ST. ALEXIUS HOSPITAL – BROADWAY CAMPUS (O, 189 beds) 3933 South Broadway, Saint Louis, MO Zip 63118–4601; tel. 314/865–3333; Michael J. Motte, Chief Executive Officer
**Web address:** www.stalexiushospital.com

ST. ALEXIUS HOSPITAL – FOREST PARK CAMPUS (O, 178 beds) 6150 Oakland Avenue, Saint Louis, MO Zip 63139–3215; tel. 314/768–3000; Michael J. Motte, Chief Executive Officer
**Web address:** www.stalexiushospital.com

| | | |
|---|---|---|
| Owned, leased, sponsored: | 3 hospitals | 517 beds |
| Contract–managed: | 0 hospitals | 0 beds |
| Totals: | 3 hospitals | 517 beds |

**0399: SUMMA HEALTH SYSTEM** (NP)
525 East Market Street, Akron, OH Zip 44309–2090; tel. 330/375–3000; Thomas J. Strauss, President and Chief Executive Officer
**(Centralized Health System)**

**OHIO:** ROBINSON MEMORIAL HOSPITAL (O, 141 beds) 6847 North Chestnut Street, Ravenna, OH Zip 44266–1204, Mailing Address: P.O. Box 1204, Zip 44266–1204; tel. 330/297–0811; Stephen Colecchi, President and Chief Executive Officer
**Web address:** www.robinsonmemorial.org

SUMMA BARBERTON CITIZENS HOSPITAL (O, 212 beds) 155 Fifth Street N.E., Barberton, OH Zip 44203–3332; tel. 330/615–3000; Thomas DeBord, President
**Web address:** www.barbhosp.com

SUMMA HEALTH SYSTEM (O, 461 beds) 525 East Market Street, Akron, OH Zip 44309–2090; tel. 330/375–3000; Thomas J. Strauss, President and Chief Executive Officer
**Web address:** www.summahealth.org

SUMMA WADSWORTH–RITTMAN HOSPITAL (O, 62 beds) 195 Wadsworth Road, Wadsworth, OH Zip 44281–9505; tel. 330/331–1000; Thomas DeBord, President
**Web address:** www.wrhhs.org

SUMMA WESTERN RESERVE HOSPITAL (O, 105 beds) 1900 23rd Street, Cuyahoga Falls, OH Zip 44223–1499; tel. 330/971–7000; Robert Kent, D.O., President and Chief Executive Officer
**Web address:** www.westernreservehospital.org

| | | |
|---|---|---|
| Owned, leased, sponsored: | 5 hospitals | 981 beds |
| Contract–managed: | 0 hospitals | 0 beds |
| Totals: | 5 hospitals | 981 beds |

**★0189: SUMMIT HEALTH** (NP)
112 North Seventh Street, Chambersburg, PA Zip 17201; tel. 717/267–7138; Norman B. Epstein, FACHE, President and Chief Executive Officer
**(Independent Hospital System)**

For explanation of codes following names, see page B2.
★ Indicates Type III membership in the American Hospital Association.

**PENNSYLVANIA:** CHAMBERSBURG HOSPITAL (O, 240 beds) 112 North Seventh Street, Chambersburg, PA Zip 17201–1720; tel. 717/267–3000; Norman B. Epstein, FACHE, President
**Web address:** www.summithealth.org

WAYNESBORO HOSPITAL (O, 64 beds) 501 East Main Street, Waynesboro, PA Zip 17268–2394; tel. 717/765–4000; Melissa Dubrow, Interim Administrative Officer
**Web address:** www.summithealth.org

| | | |
|---|---|---|
| Owned, leased, sponsored: | 2 hospitals | 304 beds |
| Contract–managed: | 0 hospitals | 0 beds |
| Totals: | 2 hospitals | 304 beds |

**0237: SUNLINK HEALTH SYSTEMS** (IO)
900 Circle 75 Parkway, Suite 1120, Atlanta, GA Zip 30339; tel. 770/933–7000; Robert M. Thornton, Jr., Chief Executive Officer
**(Independent Hospital System)**

**GEORGIA:** CHESTATEE REGIONAL HOSPITAL (O, 49 beds) 227 Mountain Drive, Dahlonega, GA Zip 30533–1606; tel. 706/864–6136; Larry R. Jeter, Chief Executive Officer
**Web address:** www.chestateeregionalhospital.com

NORTH GEORGIA MEDICAL CENTER (O, 150 beds) 1362 South Main Street, Ellijay, GA Zip 30540–0346, Mailing Address: P.O. Box 2239, Zip 30540–0346; tel. 706/276–4741; Jeffrey Dunn, Chief Executive Officer
**Web address:** www.northgeorgiamedicalcenter.com

**MISSISSIPPI:** TRACE REGIONAL HOSPITAL (O, 61 beds) Highway 8 East, Houston, MS Zip 38851–9396, Mailing Address: P.O. Box 626, Zip 38851–0626; tel. 662/456–3700; Gary L. Staten, Chief Executive Officer
**Web address:** www.traceregional.com

**MISSOURI:** CALLAWAY COMMUNITY HOSPITAL (O, 31 beds) 10 South Hospital Drive, Fulton, MO Zip 65251–2510; tel. 573/642–3376; Allen D. AufderHeide, Chief Executive Officer
**Web address:** www.mycallaway.org

MISSOURI SOUTHERN HEALTHCARE (L, 45 beds) 1200 North One Mile Road, Dexter, MO Zip 63841–1000; tel. 573/624–5566; Amy Akers, Chief Executive Officer
**Web address:** www.msh–hospital.com

| | | |
|---|---|---|
| Owned, leased, sponsored: | 5 hospitals | 336 beds |
| Contract–managed: | 0 hospitals | 0 beds |
| Totals: | 5 hospitals | 336 beds |

**★0066: SUSQUEHANNA HEALTH SYSTEM** (NP)
700 High Street, Williamsport, PA Zip 17701–3109; tel. 570/321–1000; Steven P. Johnson, FACHE, President and Chief Executive Officer
**(Centralized Health System)**

**PENNSYLVANIA:** DIVINE PROVIDENCE HOSPITAL (O, 31 beds) 1100 Grampian Boulevard, Williamsport, PA Zip 17701–1995; tel. 570/326–8000; Robert E. Kane, Administrator and Chief Executive Officer
**Web address:** www.susquehannahealth.org

MUNCY VALLEY HOSPITAL (O, 156 beds) 215 East Water Street, Muncy, PA Zip 17756–8700; tel. 570/546–8282; Ronald J. Reynolds, President
**Web address:** www.susquehannahealth.org

WILLIAMSPORT REGIONAL MEDICAL CENTER (O, 224 beds) 700 High Street, Williamsport, PA Zip 17701–3109; tel. 570/321–1000; Neil G. Armstrong, FACHE, President

| | | |
|---|---|---|
| Owned, leased, sponsored: | 3 hospitals | 411 beds |
| Contract–managed: | 0 hospitals | 0 beds |
| Totals: | 3 hospitals | 411 beds |

**★8795: SUTTER HEALTH** (NP)
2200 River Plaza Drive, Sacramento, CA Zip 95833; tel. 916/733–8800; Patrick E. Fry, Chief Executive Officer
**(Decentralized Health System)**

**CALIFORNIA:** ALTA BATES SUMMIT MEDICAL CENTER (O, 527 beds) 2450 Ashby Avenue, Berkeley, CA Zip 94705–2067; tel. 510/204–4444; David Bradley, Chief Executive Officer
**Web address:** www.altabates.com

ALTA BATES SUMMIT MEDICAL CENTER – SUMMIT CAMPUS (O, 414 beds) 350 Hawthorne Avenue, Oakland, CA Zip 94609–3100; tel. 510/655–4000; David Bradley, Chief Executive Officer
**Web address:** www.altabatessummit.com

CALIFORNIA PACIFIC MEDICAL CENTER (O, 967 beds) 2333 Buchanan Street, San Francisco, CA Zip 94115–1925, Mailing Address: P.O. Box 7999, Zip 94120–7999; tel. 415/600–6000; Warren S. Browner, M.D., M.P.H., Chief Executive Officer
**Web address:** www.cpmc.org

EDEN MEDICAL CENTER (O, 271 beds) 20103 Lake Chabot Road, Castro Valley, CA Zip 94546–5341; tel. 510/537–1234; George Bischalaney, President and Chief Executive Officer
**Web address:** www.edenmedcenter.org

MEMORIAL HOSPITAL LOS BANOS (O, 46 beds) 520 West I Street, Los Banos, CA Zip 93635; tel. 209/826–0591; Richard S. Liszewski, Chief Executive Officer
**Web address:** www.memoriallosbanos.org/

MEMORIAL MEDICAL CENTER (O, 417 beds) 1700 Coffee Road, Modesto, CA Zip 95355–2869, Mailing Address: P.O. Box 942, Zip 95353–0942; tel. 209/526–4500; James E. Conforti, Chief Executive Officer
**Web address:** www.memorialmedicalcenter.org

MENLO PARK SURGICAL HOSPITAL (O, 16 beds) 570 Willow Road, Menlo Park, CA Zip 94025–2617; tel. 650/324–8500; Kathleen Palange, R.N., Chief Executive Officer
**Web address:** www.pamf.org/mpsh

MILLS–PENINSULA HEALTH SERVICES (O, 393 beds) 1501 Trousdale Drive, Burlingame, CA Zip 94010–3282; tel. 650/696–5400; Robert W. Merwin, Chief Executive Officer
**Web address:** www.mills–peninsula.org

NOVATO COMMUNITY HOSPITAL (O, 47 beds) 180 Rowland Way, Novato, CA Zip 94945–5009, Mailing Address: P.O. Box 1108, Zip 94948–1108; tel. 415/209–1300; Anne L. Hosfeld, Chief Administrative Officer
**Web address:** www.novatocommunity.sutterhealth.org

ST. LUKE'S HOSPITAL (O, 229 beds) 3555 Cesar Chavez Street, San Francisco, CA Zip 94110–4490; tel. 415/600–6000; Warren S. Browner, M.D., M.P.H., Chief Executive Officer
**Web address:** www.stlukes–sf.org

SUTTER AMADOR HOSPITAL (O, 42 beds) 200 Mission Boulevard, Jackson, CA Zip 95642–2132; tel. 209/223–7500; Anne Platt, Chief Executive Officer
**Web address:** www.sutteramador.org

SUTTER AUBURN FAITH HOSPITAL (O, 78 beds) 11815 Education Street, Auburn, CA Zip 95602–2410; tel. 530/888–4500; Mitchell J. Hanna, Chief Executive Officer
**Web address:** www.sutterhealth.org

SUTTER CENTER FOR PSYCHIATRY (O, 69 beds) 7700 Folsom Boulevard, Sacramento, CA Zip 95826–2608; tel. 916/386–3000; John W. Boyd, PsyD, Chief Administrative Officer
**Web address:** www.sutterpsychiatry.org

SUTTER COAST HOSPITAL (O, 59 beds) 800 East Washington Boulevard, Crescent City, CA Zip 95531–8359; tel. 707/464–8511; Eugene Suksi, Chief Executive Officer
**Web address:** www.sutterhealth.org

SUTTER DAVIS HOSPITAL (O, 48 beds) 2000 Sutter Place, Davis, CA Zip 95616–6201, Mailing Address: P.O. Box 1617, Zip 95617–1617; tel. 530/756–6440; Janet Wagner, R.N., Chief Executive Officer
**Web address:** www.sutterhealth.org

SUTTER DELTA MEDICAL CENTER (O, 136 beds) 3901 Lone Tree Way, Antioch, CA Zip 94509–6253; tel. 925/779–7200; Gary D. Rapaport, Chief Executive Officer
**Web address:** www.sutterdelta.org

SUTTER LAKESIDE HOSPITAL (O, 49 beds) 5176 Hill Road East, Lakeport, CA Zip 95453–6300; tel. 707/262–5000; Siri Nelson, Chief Administrative Officer
**Web address:** www.sutterlakeside.org

SUTTER MATERNITY AND SURGERY CENTER OF SANTA CRUZ (O, 30 beds) 2900 Chanticleer Avenue, Santa Cruz, CA Zip 95065–1816; tel. 831/477–2200; Richard Nichols, Administrator
**Web address:** www.suttermatsurg.org

For explanation of codes following names, see page B2.
★ Indicates Type III membership in the American Hospital Association.

Section B

SUTTER MEDICAL CENTER OF SANTA ROSA, CHANATE CAMPUS (O, 135 beds) 3325 Chanate Road, Santa Rosa, CA Zip 95404–1707; tel. 707/576–4000; Mike Purvis, Chief Administrative Officer
**Web address:** www.sutterhealth.org

SUTTER MEDICAL CENTER, SACRAMENTO (O, 654 beds) 5151 F Street, Sacramento, CA Zip 95819–3295; tel. 916/454–3333; Carrie Owen-Plietz, Chief Executive Officer
**Web address:** www.sutterhealth.org

SUTTER ROSEVILLE MEDICAL CENTER (O, 313 beds) One Medical Plaza, Roseville, CA Zip 95661–3037; tel. 916/781–1000; Patrick R. Brady, Chief Executive Officer
**Web address:** www.sutterroseville.org

SUTTER SOLANO MEDICAL CENTER (O, 102 beds) 300 Hospital Drive, Vallejo, CA Zip 94589–2517, Mailing Address: P.O. Box 3189, Zip 94590–0669; tel. 707/554–4444; Theresa Glubka, Chief Executive Officer
**Web address:** www.suttersolano.org

SUTTER TRACY COMMUNITY HOSPITAL (O, 82 beds) 1420 North Tracy Boulevard, Tracy, CA Zip 95376–3497; tel. 209/835–1500; David M. Thompson, Chief Executive Officer
**Web address:** www.suttertracy.org

**HAWAII:** KAHI MOHALA BEHAVIORAL HEALTH (O, 60 beds) 91–2301 Old Fort Weaver Road, Ewa Beach, HI Zip 96706–3602; tel. 808/671–8511; Leonard Licina, Chief Executive Officer
**Web address:** www.kahi.org

| Owned, leased, sponsored: | 24 hospitals | 5184 beds |
|---|---|---|
| Contract–managed: | 0 hospitals | 0 beds |
| Totals: | 24 hospitals | 5184 beds |

## 0871:  SWEDISH HEALTH SERVICES (NP)
747 Broadway, Seattle, WA Zip 98122; tel. 206/386–6000; Kevin Brown, Chief Executive

**WASHINGTON:** SWEDISH MEDICAL CENTER–CHERRY HILL CAMPUS (O, 198 beds) 500 17th Avenue, Seattle, WA Zip 98122–5711; tel. 206/320–2000; Rayburn Lewis, M.D., Executive
**Web address:** www.swedish.org

SWEDISH MEDICAL CENTER–FIRST HILL (O, 620 beds) 747 Broadway, Seattle, WA Zip 98122–4307; tel. 206/386–6000; Todd Strumwasser, M.D., Chief Executive
**Web address:** www.swedish.org

SWEDISH/EDMONDS (O, 161 beds) 21601 76th Avenue West, Edmonds, WA Zip 98026–7506; tel. 425/640–4000; David E. Jaffe, Chief Administrative Officer
**Web address:** www.swedish.org

SWEDISH/ISSAQUAH (O, 49 beds) 751 N.E. Blakely Drive, Issaquah, WA Zip 98029–6201; tel. 425/313–4000; Chuck Salmon, Chief Executive
**Web address:** www.swedish.org/issaquah

| Owned, leased, sponsored: | 4 hospitals | 1028 beds |
|---|---|---|
| Contract–managed: | 0 hospitals | 0 beds |
| Totals: | 4 hospitals | 1028 beds |

## ★5375:  SYLVANIA FRANCISCAN HEALTH (CC)
3231 Central Park West, Suite 106, Toledo, OH Zip 43617–3009; tel. 419/882–8373; James W. Pope, FACHE, President and Chief Executive Officer
**(Independent Hospital System)**

**OHIO:** PROVIDENCE CARE CENTER (S, 138 beds) 2025 Hayes Avenue, Sandusky, OH Zip 44870; Rick G. Ryan, Administrator and Chief Executive Officer

TRINITY HEALTH SYSTEM (S, 319 beds) 380 Summit Avenue, Steubenville, OH Zip 43952–2699; tel. 740/283–7000; Fred B. Brower, President and Chief Executive Officer
**Web address:** www.trinityhealth.com

TRINITY HOSPITAL TWIN CITY (S, 25 beds) 819 North First Street, Dennison, OH Zip 44621–1098; tel. 740/922–2800; Joseph J. Mitchell, President
**Web address:** www.twincityhospital.org

**TEXAS:** BURLESON ST. JOSEPH HEALTH CENTER (S, 25 beds) 1101 Woodson Drive, Caldwell, TX Zip 77836–1052, Mailing Address: P.O. Box 360, Zip 77836–0360; tel. 979/567–3245; John Hughson, Chief Executive Officer
**Web address:** www.st–joseph.org/

GRIMES ST. JOSEPH HEALTH CENTER (S, 18 beds) 210 South Judson Street, Navasota, TX Zip 77868–3704; tel. 936/825–6585; Dia Copeland, Administrator
**Web address:** www.st–joseph.org

MADISON ST. JOSEPH HEALTH CENTER (S, 25 beds) 100 West Cross Street, Madisonville, TX Zip 77864–0698, Mailing Address: Box 698, Zip 77864–0698; tel. 936/348–2631; Reed Edmundson, Administrator
**Web address:** www.st–joseph.org

ST. JOSEPH REGIONAL HEALTH CENTER (S, 238 beds) 2801 Franciscan Drive, Bryan, TX Zip 77802–2599; tel. 979/776–3777; Kathleen R. Krusie, Chief Executive Officer
**Web address:** www.st–joseph.org

| Owned, leased, sponsored: | 7 hospitals | 788 beds |
|---|---|---|
| Contract–managed: | 0 hospitals | 0 beds |
| Totals: | 7 hospitals | 788 beds |

## 0379:  TAHOE FOREST HEALTH SYSTEM (NP)
10121 Pine Avenue, Truckee, CA Zip 96161; tel. 530/587–6011; Robert A. Schapper, Chief Executive Officer

**CALIFORNIA:** TAHOE FOREST HOSPITAL DISTRICT (O, 25 beds) 10121 Pine Avenue, Truckee, CA Zip 96161–4856, Mailing Address: P.O. Box 759, Zip 96160–0759; tel. 530/587–6011; Robert A. Schapper, Chief Executive Officer
**Web address:** www.tfhd.com

**NEVADA:** INCLINE VILLAGE COMMUNITY HOSPITAL (O, 6 beds) 880 Alder Avenue, Incline Village, NV Zip 89450; tel. 775/833–4100; Judy Newland, R.N., Director
**Web address:** www.tfhd.com

| Owned, leased, sponsored: | 2 hospitals | 31 beds |
|---|---|---|
| Contract–managed: | 0 hospitals | 0 beds |
| Totals: | 2 hospitals | 31 beds |

## 0341:  TANNER HEALTH SYSTEM (NP)
705 Dixie Street, Carrollton, GA Zip 30117–3818; tel. 770/836–9580; Loy M. Howard, President and Chief Executive Officer

**GEORGIA:** HIGGINS GENERAL HOSPITAL (L, 25 beds) 200 Allen Memorial Drive, Bremen, GA Zip 30110–2012, Mailing Address: P.O. Box 655, Zip 30110–0655; tel. 770/537–5851; Michael Alexander, Administrator
**Web address:** www.tanner.org

TANNER MEDICAL CENTER (O, 176 beds) 705 Dixie Street, Carrollton, GA Zip 30117–3818; tel. 770/836–9666; Loy M. Howard, President and Chief Executive Officer
**Web address:** www.tanner.org

TANNER MEDICAL CENTER–VILLA RICA (O, 39 beds) 601 Dallas Road, Villa Rica, GA Zip 30180–1202, Mailing Address: P.O. Box 638, Zip 30180–0638; tel. 770/456–3100; Deborah Matthews, Administrator
**Web address:** www.tanner.org

| Owned, leased, sponsored: | 3 hospitals | 240 beds |
|---|---|---|
| Contract–managed: | 0 hospitals | 0 beds |
| Totals: | 3 hospitals | 240 beds |

## ★0169:  TEMPLE UNIVERSITY HEALTH SYSTEM (NP)
3509 North Broad Street, 9th Floor, Philadelphia, PA Zip 19140–4105; tel. 215/707–0900; Larry Kaiser, M.D., President and Chief Executive Officer
**(Moderately Centralized Health System)**

For explanation of codes following names, see page B2.
★ Indicates Type III membership in the American Hospital Association.

**PENNSYLVANIA:** FOX CHASE CANCER CENTER–AMERICAN ONCOLOGIC HOSPITAL (O, 65 beds) 333 Cottman Avenue, Philadelphia, PA Zip 19111; tel. 215/728–6900; Michael V. Seiden, President and Chief Executive Officer
**Web address:** www.fccc.edu

JEANES HOSPITAL (O, 176 beds) 7600 Central Avenue, Philadelphia, PA Zip 19111–2499; tel. 215/728–2000; Linda J. Grass, Executive Director and Chief Executive Officer
**Web address:** www.jeanes.com

TEMPLE UNIVERSITY HOSPITAL (O, 730 beds) 3401 North Broad Street, Philadelphia, PA Zip 19140–5192; tel. 215/707–2000; John N. Kastanis, FACHE, Interim Chief Executive Officer
**Web address:** www.tuh.templehealth.org/content/default.htm

| | | |
|---|---|---|
| Owned, leased, sponsored: | 3 hospitals | 971 beds |
| Contract–managed: | 0 hospitals | 0 beds |
| Totals: | 3 hospitals | 971 beds |

★0063:   **TENET HEALTHCARE CORPORATION** (IO)
1445 Ross Avenue, Suite 1400, Dallas, TX Zip 75202–2703, Mailing Address: P.O. Box 139036, Zip 75313–9036; tel. 469/893–2200; Trevor Fetter, President and Chief Executive Officer
**(Moderately Centralized Health System)**

**ALABAMA:** BROOKWOOD MEDICAL CENTER (O, 645 beds) 2010 Brookwood Medical Center Drive, Birmingham, AL Zip 35209–6875; tel. 205/877–1000; Garry L. Gause, President and Chief Executive Officer
**Web address:** www.brookwood–medical.com

**CALIFORNIA:** DESERT REGIONAL MEDICAL CENTER (L, 387 beds) 1150 North Indian Canyon Drive, Palm Springs, CA Zip 92262–4872, Mailing Address: P.O. Box 2739, Zip 92263–2739; tel. 760/323–6511; Karolee M. Sowle, R.N., MSN, FACHE, Chief Executive Officer
**Web address:** www.desertmedctr.com

DOCTORS HOSPITAL OF MANTECA (O, 73 beds) 1205 East North Street, Manteca, CA Zip 95336–4900; tel. 209/823–3111; Mark P. Lisa, FACHE, Chief Executive Officer
**Web address:** www.doctorsmanteca.com

DOCTORS MEDICAL CENTER (O, 441 beds) 1441 Florida Avenue, Modesto, CA Zip 95350–4418, Mailing Address: P.O. Box 4138, Zip 95352–4138; tel. 209/578–1211; Warren J. Kirk, Chief Executive Officer
**Web address:** www.dmc–modesto.com

FOUNTAIN VALLEY REGIONAL HOSPITAL AND MEDICAL CENTER (O, 400 beds) 17100 Euclid Street, Fountain Valley, CA Zip 92708–4043; tel. 714/966–7200; Debbie Walsh, MSN, Chief Executive Officer
**Web address:** www.fountainvalleyhospital.com

JOHN F. KENNEDY MEMORIAL HOSPITAL (O, 126 beds) 47111 Monroe Street, Indio, CA Zip 92201; tel. 760/347–6191; Daniel Bowers, Chief Executive Officer
**Web address:** www.jfkmemorialhosp.com

LAKEWOOD REGIONAL MEDICAL CENTER (O, 144 beds) 3700 East South Street, Lakewood, CA Zip 90712–1498, Mailing Address: P.O. Box 6070, Zip 90714–6070; tel. 562/531–2550; B. Joseph Badalian, President and Chief Executive Officer
**Web address:** www.lakewoodregional.com

LOS ALAMITOS MEDICAL CENTER (O, 120 beds) 3751 Katella Avenue, Los Alamitos, CA Zip 90720–3164; tel. 562/598–1311; Michele Finney, Chief Executive Officer
**Web address:** www.losalamitosmedctr.com

PLACENTIA–LINDA HOSPITAL (O, 114 beds) 1301 North Rose Drive, Placentia, CA Zip 92870–3899; tel. 714/993–2000; Kent G. Clayton, President and Chief Executive Officer
**Web address:** www.placentialinda.com

SAN RAMON REGIONAL MEDICAL CENTER (O, 123 beds) 6001 Norris Canyon Road, San Ramon, CA Zip 94583–5400; tel. 925/275–9200; Gary Sloan, Chief Executive Officer
**Web address:** www.sanramonmedctr.com

SIERRA VISTA REGIONAL MEDICAL CENTER (O, 164 beds) 1010 Murray Avenue, San Luis Obispo, CA Zip 93405–8800, Mailing Address: P.O. Box 1367, Zip 93406–1367; tel. 805/546–7600; Candace L. Markwith, Chief Executive Officer
**Web address:** www.sierravistaregional.com

TWIN CITIES COMMUNITY HOSPITAL (O, 122 beds) 1100 Las Tablas Road, Templeton, CA Zip 93465–9704; tel. 805/434–3500; Richard D. Lyons, Chief Executive Officer
**Web address:** www.twincitieshospital.com

**FLORIDA:** CORAL GABLES HOSPITAL (O, 256 beds) 3100 Douglas Road, Coral Gables, FL Zip 33134–6990; tel. 305/445–8461; Jay S. Miranda, Chief Executive Officer
**Web address:** www.coralgableshospital.com

DELRAY MEDICAL CENTER (O, 403 beds) 5352 Linton Boulevard, Delray Beach, FL Zip 33484–6580; tel. 561/498–4440; Mark Bryan, Chief Executive Officer
**Web address:** www.delraymedicalctr.com

FLORIDA MEDICAL CENTER (O, 459 beds) 5000 West Oakland Park Boulevard, Fort Lauderdale, FL Zip 33313–1585; tel. 954/735–6000; Ben A. Rodriguez, Chief Executive Officer
**Web address:** www.floridamedicalctr.com

GOOD SAMARITAN MEDICAL CENTER (O, 174 beds) 1309 North Flagler Drive, West Palm Beach, FL Zip 33401–3499; tel. 561/655–5511; Mark Nosacka, Chief Executive Officer
**Web address:** www.goodsamaritanmc.com

HIALEAH HOSPITAL (O, 378 beds) 651 East 25th Street, Hialeah, FL Zip 33013–3878; tel. 305/693–6100; Ralph A. Aleman, Chief Executive Officer
**Web address:** www.hialeahhosp.com

NORTH SHORE MEDICAL CENTER (O, 357 beds) 1100 N.W. 95th Street, Miami, FL Zip 33150–2098; tel. 305/835–6000; Manuel Linares, Chief Executive Officer
**Web address:** www.northshoremedical.com

PALM BEACH GARDENS MEDICAL CENTER (L, 199 beds) 3360 Burns Road, Palm Beach Gardens, FL Zip 33410–4304; tel. 561/622–1411; Michael Cowling, Chief Executive Officer
**Web address:** www.pbgmc.com

PALMETTO GENERAL HOSPITAL (O, 360 beds) 2001 West 68th Street, Hialeah, FL Zip 33016–1898; tel. 305/823–5000; Ana J. Mederos, Chief Executive Officer
**Web address:** www.palmettogeneral.com

ST. MARY'S MEDICAL CENTER (O, 463 beds) 901 45th Street, West Palm Beach, FL Zip 33407–2495; tel. 561/844–6300; Davide M. Carbone, FACHE, Chief Executive Officer
**Web address:** www.stmarysmc.com

WEST BOCA MEDICAL CENTER (O, 185 beds) 21644 State Road 7, Boca Raton, FL Zip 33428–1899; tel. 561/488–8000; Mitchell S. Feldman, Chief Executive Officer
**Web address:** www.westbocamedctr.com

**GEORGIA:** ATLANTA MEDICAL CENTER (O, 403 beds) 303 Parkway Drive N.E., Atlanta, GA Zip 30312–1212; tel. 404/265–4000; William T. Moore, Chief Executive Officer
**Web address:** www.atlantamedcenter.com

NORTH FULTON REGIONAL HOSPITAL (L, 196 beds) 3000 Hospital Boulevard, Roswell, GA Zip 30076–3899; tel. 770/751–2500; Deborah C. Keel, Chief Executive Officer
**Web address:** www.northfultonregional.com

SOUTH FULTON MEDICAL CENTER (O, 210 beds) 1170 Cleveland Avenue, Atlanta, GA Zip 30344–3665; tel. 404/466–1170; James Clements, Chief Executive Officer
**Web address:** www.southfultonmedicalcenter.com

SPALDING REGIONAL MEDICAL CENTER (O, 160 beds) 601 South Eighth Street, Griffin, GA Zip 30224–4294, Mailing Address: P.O. Drawer V, Zip 30224–1168; tel. 770/228–2721; John A. Quinn, Chief Executive Officer
**Web address:** www.spaldingregional.com

SYLVAN GROVE HOSPITAL (L, 23 beds) 1050 McDonough Road, Jackson, GA Zip 30233–1599; tel. 770/775–7861; Edward J. Whitehouse, Chief Executive Officer
**Web address:** www.sylvangrovehospital.com

**MISSOURI:** DES PERES HOSPITAL (O, 143 beds) 2345 Dougherty Ferry Road, Saint Louis, MO Zip 63122–3313; tel. 314/966–9100; John A. Grah, JD, FACHE, Chief Executive Officer
**Web address:** www.despereshospital.com

For explanation of codes following names, see page B2.
★ Indicates Type III membership in the American Hospital Association.

SAINT LOUIS UNIVERSITY HOSPITAL (O, 332 beds) 3635 Vista at Grand Boulevard, Saint Louis, MO Zip 63110–0250, Mailing Address: P.O. Box 15250, Zip 63110–0250; tel. 314/577–8000; Phillip E. Sowa, Chief Executive Officer
**Web address:** www.sluhospital.com

**NEBRASKA:** CREIGHTON UNIVERSITY MEDICAL CENTER (O, 223 beds) 601 North 30th Street, Omaha, NE Zip 68131–2197; tel. 402/449–4000; Gary Honts, Chief Executive Officer
**Web address:** www.saintjosephhospital.com

**NORTH CAROLINA:** CENTRAL CAROLINA HOSPITAL (O, 116 beds) 1135 Carthage Street, Sanford, NC Zip 27330–4111; tel. 919/774–2100; Doug Doris, Chief Executive Officer
**Web address:** www.centralcarolinahosp.com

FRYE REGIONAL MEDICAL CENTER (L, 306 beds) 420 North Center Street, Hickory, NC Zip 28601–5049; tel. 828/322–6070; Michael R. Blackburn, Chief Executive Officer
**Web address:** www.fryemedctr.com

**PENNSYLVANIA:** HAHNEMANN UNIVERSITY HOSPITAL (O, 496 beds) Broad and Vine Streets, Philadelphia, PA Zip 19102–1192; tel. 215/762–7000; Michael P. Halter, Chief Executive Officer
**Web address:** www.hahnemannhospital.com

ST. CHRISTOPHER'S HOSPITAL FOR CHILDREN (O, 181 beds) 3601 A. Street, Philadelphia, PA Zip 19134–1043; tel. 215/427–5000; Carolyn Jackson, Chief Executive Officer
**Web address:** www.stchristophershospital.com

**SOUTH CAROLINA:** COASTAL CAROLINA HOSPITAL (O, 41 beds) 1000 Medical Center Drive, Hardeeville, SC Zip 29927; tel. 843/784–8000; William J. Masterton, Chief Executive Officer
**Web address:** www.coastalhospital.com

EAST COOPER MEDICAL CENTER (O, 140 beds) 2000 Hospital Drive, Mount Pleasant, SC Zip 29464–3294; tel. 843/881–0100; Jason P. Alexander, FACHE, Chief Executive Officer
**Web address:** www.eastcoopermedctr.com

HILTON HEAD HOSPITAL (O, 93 beds) 25 Hospital Center Boulevard, Hilton Head Island, SC Zip 29926–2738; tel. 843/681–6122; Mark T. O'Neil, Jr., President and Chief Executive Officer
**Web address:** www.hiltonheadregional.com

PIEDMONT MEDICAL CENTER (O, 281 beds) 222 Herlong Avenue, Rock Hill, SC Zip 29732–1952; tel. 803/329–1234; Charles F. Miller, President and Chief Executive Officer
**Web address:** www.piedmontmedicalcenter.com

**TENNESSEE:** SAINT FRANCIS HOSPITAL (O, 511 beds) 5959 Park Avenue, Memphis, TN Zip 38119–5198, Mailing Address: P.O. Box 171808, Zip 38187–1808; tel. 901/765–1000; David L. Archer, Chief Executive Officer
**Web address:** www.saintfrancishosp.com

SAINT FRANCIS HOSPITAL–BARTLETT (O, 100 beds) 2986 Kate Bond Road, Bartlett, TN Zip 38133–4003; tel. 901/820–7000; Jeremy Clark, Chief Executive Officer
**Web address:** www.saintfrancisbartlett.com

**TEXAS:** CENTENNIAL MEDICAL CENTER (O, 118 beds) 12505 Lebanon Road, Frisco, TX Zip 75035–8298; tel. 972/963–3333; Joe D. Thomason, Chief Executive Officer
**Web address:** www.centennialmedcenter.com

CYPRESS FAIRBANKS MEDICAL CENTER (O, 181 beds) 10655 Steepletop Drive, Houston, TX Zip 77065–4297; tel. 281/890–4285; Terry J. Wheeler, Chief Executive Officer
**Web address:** www.cyfairhospital.com

DOCTORS HOSPITAL AT WHITE ROCK LAKE (O, 163 beds) 9440 Poppy Drive, Dallas, TX Zip 75218–3694; tel. 214/324–6100; G. Scott Manis, Chief Executive Officer
**Web address:** www.doctorshospitaldallas.com

HOUSTON NORTHWEST MEDICAL CENTER (O, 339 beds) 710 FM 1960 Road West, Houston, TX Zip 77090–3402; tel. 281/440–1000; Linda Mercier, R.N., MSN, Chief Executive Officer
**Web address:** www.hnmc.com

LAKE POINTE MEDICAL CENTER (O, 112 beds) 6800 Scenic Drive, Rowlett, TX Zip 75088–4552, Mailing Address: P.O. Box 1550, Zip 75030–1550; tel. 972/412–2273; J. Eric Evans, Chief Executive Officer
**Web address:** www.lakepointemedical.com

NACOGDOCHES MEDICAL CENTER (O, 109 beds) 4920 N.E. Stallings, Nacogdoches, TX Zip 75965–1200, Mailing Address: P.O. Box 631604, Zip 75963–1604; tel. 936/569–9481; Gary L. Stokes, Chief Executive Officer
**Web address:** www.nacmedicalcenter.com

PARK PLAZA HOSPITAL (O, 208 beds) 1313 Hermann Drive, Houston, TX Zip 77004–7092; tel. 713/527–5000; John Tressa, R.N., MSN, Chief Executive Officer
**Web address:** www.parkplazahospital.com

PLAZA SPECIALTY HOSPITAL (O, 56 beds) 1300 Binz, Houston, TX Zip 77004; tel. 713/285–1000; Steven Barr, R.N., MSN, Chief Executive Officer
**Web address:** www.plazaspecialtyhospital.com

PROVIDENCE MEMORIAL HOSPITAL (O, 359 beds) 2001 North Oregon Street, El Paso, TX Zip 79902–3368; tel. 915/577–6011; John Harris, Chief Executive Officer
**Web address:** www.sphn.com

SIERRA MEDICAL CENTER (O, 334 beds) 1625 Medical Center Drive, El Paso, TX Zip 79902–5044; tel. 915/747–4000; Edmundo Castaneda, Chief Executive Officer
**Web address:** www.sphn.com

SIERRA PROVIDENCE EAST MEDICAL CENTER (O, 110 beds) 2400 Trawood Drive, El Paso, TX Zip 79936; tel. 915/577–8000; Sally Hurt–Steffen, MSN, R.N., Chief Executive Officer
**Web address:** www.sphn.com

| | | |
|---|---|---|
| **Owned, leased, sponsored:** | 51 hospitals | 12137 beds |
| **Contract–managed:** | 0 hospitals | 0 beds |
| **Totals:** | 51 hospitals | 12137 beds |

---

**0020: TEXAS DEPARTMENT OF STATE HEALTH SERVICES** (NP)
1100 West 49th Street, Austin, TX Zip 78756–3199; tel. 512/458–7111; David L. Lakey, M.D., Commissioner
**(Independent Hospital System)**

AUSTIN STATE HOSPITAL (O, 314 beds) 4110 Guadalupe Street, Austin, TX Zip 78751–4296; tel. 512/452–0381; Carl Schock, Superintendent
**Web address:** www.mhmr.state.tx.us

BIG SPRING STATE HOSPITAL (O, 200 beds) 1901 North Highway 87, Big Spring, TX Zip 79720–0283; tel. 432/267–8216; Edward Moughon, Superintendent
**Web address:** www.dshs.state.tx.us/mhhospitals/BigSpringSH/default.shtm

EL PASO PSYCHIATRIC CENTER (O, 77 beds) 4615 Alameda Avenue, El Paso, TX Zip 79905–2702; tel. 915/532–2202; Zulema Carrillo, Chief Executive Officer

KERRVILLE STATE HOSPITAL (O, 202 beds) 721 Thompson Drive, Kerrville, TX Zip 78028–5154; tel. 830/896–2211; Jay Norwood, Acting Superintendent
**Web address:** www.dshs.state.tx.us/lmhospitals/kerrvillesh

NORTH TEXAS STATE HOSPITAL (O, 603 beds) Highway 70 Northwest, Vernon, TX Zip 76384, Mailing Address: P.O. Box 2231, Zip 76385–2231; tel. 940/552–9901; James E. Smith, Superintendent
**Web address:** www.mhmr.state.tx.us

RIO GRANDE STATE CENTER/SOUTH TEXAS HEALTH CARE SYSTEM (O, 128 beds) 1401 South Rangerville Road, Harlingen, TX Zip 78552–7638; tel. 956/364–8000; Sonia Hernandez–Keeble, Superintendent
**Web address:** www.dshs.state.tx.us/mhospital/riograndesc/default.shtm

RUSK STATE HOSPITAL (O, 290 beds) 805 North Dickinson, Rusk, TX Zip 75785, Mailing Address: P.O. Box 318, Zip 75785–0318; tel. 903/683–3421; Ted Debbs, Administrator
**Web address:** www.mhmr.state.tx.us

SAN ANTONIO STATE HOSPITAL (O, 302 beds) 6711 South New Braunfels, Suite 100, San Antonio, TX Zip 78223–3006; tel. 210/531–7711; Robert C. Arizpe, Superintendent
**Web address:** www.dshs.state.tx.us

TERRELL STATE HOSPITAL (O, 316 beds) 1200 East Brin Street, Terrell, TX Zip 75160–2938; tel. 972/524–6452; Joe Finch, PsyD, Superintendent
**Web address:** www.dshs.state.tx.us/mhhospitals/terrellsh

For explanation of codes following names, see page B2.
★ Indicates Type III membership in the American Hospital Association.

TEXAS CENTER FOR INFECTIOUS DISEASE (O, 75 beds) 2303 S.E. Military Drive, San Antonio, TX Zip 78223–3597; tel. 210/534–8857; James N. Elkins, FACHE, Director
**Web address:** www.dshs.state.tx.us/tcid

| Owned, leased, sponsored: | 10 hospitals | 2507 beds |
|---|---|---|
| Contract–managed: | 0 hospitals | 0 beds |
| Totals: | 10 hospitals | 2507 beds |

★**0129: TEXAS HEALTH RESOURCES** (NP)
612 East Lamar Boulevard, Suite 900, Arlington, TX Zip 76011; tel. 682/236–7900; Douglas D. Hawthorne, FACHE, Chief Executive Officer
**(Moderately Centralized Health System)**

TEXAS HEALTH ARLINGTON MEMORIAL HOSPITAL (O, 289 beds) 800 West Randol Mill Road, Arlington, TX Zip 76012–2503; tel. 817/548–6100; Kirk King, FACHE, President
**Web address:** www.arlingtonmemorial.org

TEXAS HEALTH HARRIS METHODIST HOSPITAL AZLE (O, 31 beds) 108 Denver Trail, Azle, TX Zip 76020–3614; tel. 817/444–8600; Bob S. Ellzey, FACHE, President
**Web address:** www.harrismethodisthospitals.org

TEXAS HEALTH HARRIS METHODIST HOSPITAL CLEBURNE (O, 85 beds) 201 Walls Drive, Cleburne, TX Zip 76033–4007; tel. 817/641–2551; Blake Kretz, President
**Web address:** www.texashealth.org

TEXAS HEALTH HARRIS METHODIST HOSPITAL FORT WORTH (O, 620 beds) 1301 Pennsylvania Avenue, Fort Worth, TX Zip 76104–2122; tel. 817/250–2000; Lillie Biggins, R.N., President
**Web address:** www.texashealth.org

TEXAS HEALTH HARRIS METHODIST HOSPITAL HURST–EULESS–BEDFORD (O, 259 beds) 1600 Hospital Parkway, Bedford, TX Zip 76022–6913, Mailing Address: P.O. Box 669, Zip 76095–0669; tel. 817/685–4000; Deborah Paganelli, President
**Web address:** www.texashealth.org

TEXAS HEALTH HARRIS METHODIST HOSPITAL SOUTHWEST FORT WORTH (O, 143 beds) 6100 Harris Parkway, Fort Worth, TX Zip 76132–4199; tel. 817/433–5000; Brett McClung, President
**Web address:** www.texashealth.org

TEXAS HEALTH HARRIS METHODIST HOSPITAL STEPHENVILLE (O, 54 beds) 411 North Belknap Street, Stephenville, TX Zip 76401–3415; tel. 254/965–1500; Christopher Leu, Chief Executive Officer
**Web address:** www.texashealth.org

TEXAS HEALTH PRESBYTERIAN HOSPITAL ALLEN (O, 73 beds) 1105 Central Expressway North, Allen, TX Zip 75013; tel. 972/747–1000; Sheila A. McKinney, President
**Web address:** www.texashealth.org

TEXAS HEALTH PRESBYTERIAN HOSPITAL DALLAS (O, 631 beds) 8200 Walnut Hill Lane, Dallas, TX Zip 75231–4402; tel. 214/345–6789; Britt Berrett, President and Chief Executive Officer
**Web address:** www.texashealth.org

TEXAS HEALTH PRESBYTERIAN HOSPITAL DENTON (O, 208 beds) 3000 I. 35 North, Denton, TX Zip 76201–3798; tel. 940/898–7000; Stan C. Morton, FACHE, President
**Web address:** www.dentonhospital.com

TEXAS HEALTH PRESBYTERIAN HOSPITAL KAUFMAN (O, 68 beds) 850 Ed Hall Drive, Kaufman, TX Zip 75142, Mailing Address: P.O. Box 1108, Zip 75142–1108; tel. 972/932–7200; Patsy Youngs, President
**Web address:** www.texashealth.org

TEXAS HEALTH PRESBYTERIAN HOSPITAL PLANO (O, 338 beds) 6200 West Parker Road, Plano, TX Zip 75093–7914; tel. 972/981–8000; Mike Evans, R.N., MS, President
**Web address:** www.texashealth.org

TEXAS HEALTH SPECIALTY HOSPITAL (O, 10 beds) 1301 Pennsylvania Avenue, 4th Floor, Fort Worth, TX Zip 76104–2190; tel. 817/250–5500; Susan Louise Baldwin, R.N., FACHE, President and Chief Nursing Officer
**Web address:** www.texashealth.org

| Owned, leased, sponsored: | 13 hospitals | 2809 beds |
|---|---|---|
| Contract–managed: | 0 hospitals | 0 beds |
| Totals: | 13 hospitals | 2809 beds |

★**7235: THE METHODIST HOSPITAL SYSTEM** (CO)
6565 Fannin Street, D–200, Houston, TX Zip 77030–2707; tel. 713/441–2221; Marc Boom, M.D., Chief Executive Officer
**(Centralized Health System)**

METHODIST SUGAR LAND HOSPITAL (O, 207 beds) 16655 S.W. Freeway, Sugar Land, TX Zip 77479–2343; tel. 281/274–7000; Christopher Siebenaler, Administrator and Chief Executive Officer
**Web address:** www.methodisthealth.com

METHODIST WEST HOUSTON HOSPITAL (O, 75 beds) 18500 Katy Freeway, Houston, TX Zip 77094–1110; tel. 832/522–1000; Wayne M. Voss, Chief Executive Officer
**Web address:** www.methodisthealth.com

METHODIST WILLOWBROOK HOSPITAL (O, 195 beds) 18220 Tomball Parkway, Houston, TX Zip 77070; tel. 281/477–1000; Beryl O. Ramsey, FACHE, Chief Executive Officer
**Web address:** www.methodisthealth.com

SAN JACINTO METHODIST HOSPITAL (O, 275 beds) 4401 Garth Road, Baytown, TX Zip 77521–2122; tel. 281/420–8600; Donna Gares, R.N., President and Chief Executive Officer
**Web address:** www.methodisthealth.com

THE METHODIST HOSPITAL (O, 884 beds) 6565 Fannin Street, Houston, TX Zip 77030–2707; tel. 713/790–3311; Roberta Schwartz, Executive Vice President
**Web address:** www.methodisthealth.com

| Owned, leased, sponsored: | 5 hospitals | 1636 beds |
|---|---|---|
| Contract–managed: | 0 hospitals | 0 beds |
| Totals: | 5 hospitals | 1636 beds |

**2445: THEDACARE, INC.** (NP)
122 East College Avenue, Appleton, WI Zip 54911, Mailing Address: P.O. Box 8025, Zip 54912; tel. 920/830–5880; Dean Gruner, M.D., President and Chief Executive Officer
**(Moderately Centralized Health System)**

**WISCONSIN:** APPLETON MEDICAL CENTER (O, 147 beds) 1818 North Meade Street, Appleton, WI Zip 54911–3496; tel. 920/731–4101; Kim Barnas, Senior Vice President
**Web address:** www.thedacare.org

NEW LONDON FAMILY MEDICAL CENTER (O, 25 beds) 1405 Mill Street, New London, WI Zip 54961–2155, Mailing Address: P.O. Box 307, Zip 54961–0307; tel. 920/531–2000; William Schmidt, President and Chief Executive Officer
**Web address:** www.thedacare.org

RIVERSIDE MEDICAL CENTER (O, 25 beds) 800 Riverside Drive, Waupaca, WI Zip 54981–1999; tel. 715/258–1000; Craig A. Kantos, Chief Executive Officer
**Web address:** www.riversidemedical.org

SHAWANO MEDICAL CENTER (O, 25 beds) 309 North Bartlette Street, Shawano, WI Zip 54166; tel. 715/526–2111; Dorothy Erdmann, Chief Executive Officer
**Web address:** www.shawanomed.org

THEDA CLARK MEDICAL CENTER (O, 147 beds) 130 Second Street, Neenah, WI Zip 54956–2883, Mailing Address: P.O. Box 2021, Zip 54957–2021; tel. 920/729–3100; Kim Barnas, Senior Vice President
**Web address:** www.thedacare.org

| Owned, leased, sponsored: | 5 hospitals | 369 beds |
|---|---|---|
| Contract–managed: | 0 hospitals | 0 beds |
| Totals: | 5 hospitals | 369 beds |

★**0643: THOMAS HEALTH SYSTEM, INC.** (NP)
4605 MacCorkle Avenue S.W., South Charleston, WV Zip 25309–1311; tel. 304/766–3600; Stephen P. Dexter, President and Chief Executive Officer
**(Moderately Centralized Health System)**

Section B

For explanation of codes following names, see page B2.
★ Indicates Type III membership in the American Hospital Association.

**WEST VIRGINIA:** SAINT FRANCIS HOSPITAL (O, 142 beds) 333 Laidley Street, Charleston, WV Zip 25301–1628, Mailing Address: P.O. Box 471, Zip 25322–0471; tel. 304/347–6500; Stephen P. Dexter, President and Chief Executive Officer
**Web address:** www.stfrancishospital.com

THOMAS MEMORIAL HOSPITAL (O, 241 beds) 4605 MacCorkle Avenue S.W., South Charleston, WV Zip 25309–1398; tel. 304/766–3600; Stephen P. Dexter, President and Chief Executive Officer
**Web address:** www.thomaswv.org

| | | |
|---|---|---|
| Owned, leased, sponsored: | 2 hospitals | 383 beds |
| Contract–managed: | 0 hospitals | 0 beds |
| Totals: | 2 hospitals | 383 beds |

---

**★0219: TRINITY HEALTH** (CC)
27870 Cabot Drive, Novi, MI Zip 48377; tel. 248/489–5004; Joseph R. Swedish, President and Chief Executive Officer
**(Decentralized Health System)**

**CALIFORNIA:** SAINT AGNES MEDICAL CENTER (O, 436 beds) 1303 East Herndon Avenue, Fresno, CA Zip 93720–3309; tel. 559/450–3000; Nancy Hollingsworth, R.N., MSN, President and Chief Executive Officer
**Web address:** www.samc.com

**IDAHO:** SAINT ALPHONSUS MEDICAL CENTER – NAMPA (S, 118 beds) 1512 12th Avenue Road, Nampa, ID Zip 83686–6008; tel. 208/463–5000; Karl Keeler, Chief Executive Officer
**Web address:** www.mercynampa.org

SAINT ALPHONSUS REGIONAL MEDICAL CENTER (O, 399 beds) 1055 North Curtis Road, Boise, ID Zip 83706–1370; tel. 208/367–2121; Sally E. Jeffcoat, President and Chief Executive Officer
**Web address:** www.saintalphonsus.org

**ILLINOIS:** GOTTLIEB MEMORIAL HOSPITAL (O, 268 beds) 701 West North Avenue, Melrose Park, IL Zip 60160–1692; tel. 708/681–3200; Patricia Cassidy, President
**Web address:** www.gottliebhospital.org

LOYOLA UNIVERSITY MEDICAL CENTER (O, 535 beds) 2160 South First Avenue, Maywood, IL Zip 60153–5585; tel. 708/216–9000; Patricia Cassidy, Interim President and Chief Executive Officer
**Web address:** www.loyolamedicine.org/Medical_Services/index.cfm

MERCY HOSPITAL AND MEDICAL CENTER (O, 291 beds) 2525 South Michigan Avenue, Chicago, IL Zip 60616–2477; tel. 312/567–2000; Sister Sheila Lyne, President and Chief Executive Officer
**Web address:** www.mercy–chicago.org

MORRISON COMMUNITY HOSPITAL (C, 60 beds) 303 North Jackson Street, Morrison, IL Zip 61270–3042; tel. 815/772–4003; Kent Jorgensen, Chief Executive Officer
**Web address:** www.morrisonhospital.com

**INDIANA:** SAINT JOSEPH REGIONAL MEDICAL CENTER (O, 258 beds) 5215 Holy Cross Parkway, Mishawaka, IN Zip 46545–1469; tel. 574/335–5000; Albert Gutierrez, FACHE, President and Chief Executive Officer
**Web address:** www.sjmed.com

SAINT JOSEPH REGIONAL MEDICAL CENTER–PLYMOUTH CAMPUS (O, 45 beds) 1915 Lake Avenue, Plymouth, IN Zip 46563–9905, Mailing Address: P.O. Box 670, Zip 46563–9905; tel. 574/936–3181; Lori Price, President
**Web address:** www.sjmed.com

**IOWA:** BAUM HARMON MERCY HOSPITAL (O, 13 beds) 255 North Welch Avenue, Primghar, IA Zip 51245–1034, Mailing Address: P.O. Box 528, Zip 51245–0528; tel. 712/957–2300; David Liebsack, Chief Executive Officer
**Web address:** www.baumharmon.org

CENTRAL COMMUNITY HOSPITAL (C, 16 beds) 901 Davidson Street N.W., Elkader, IA Zip 52043–9015; tel. 563/245–7000; Frances J. Zichal, Chief Executive Officer
**Web address:** www.centralcommunityhospital.com

ELLSWORTH MUNICIPAL HOSPITAL (C, 25 beds) 110 Rocksylvania Avenue, Iowa Falls, IA Zip 50126–2400; tel. 641/648–4631; Cherelle Montanye, Chief Executive Officer
**Web address:** www.emhia.com

FRANKLIN GENERAL HOSPITAL (C, 77 beds) 1720 Central Avenue East, Hampton, IA Zip 50441–1859; tel. 641/456–5000; Kim Price, Chief Executive Officer
**Web address:** www.franklingeneral.com

HANCOCK COUNTY MEMORIAL HOSPITAL (C, 25 beds) 532 First Street N.W., Britt, IA Zip 50423; tel. 641/843–5000; Vance Jackson, FACHE, Administrator and Chief Executive Officer
**Web address:** www.hancockmemhospital.com

HAWARDEN COMMUNITY HOSPITAL (C, 18 beds) 1111 11th Street, Hawarden, IA Zip 51023–1999; tel. 712/551–3100; Jayson Pullman, Chief Executive Officer
**Web address:** www.hawardencommunityhospital.org

KOSSUTH REGIONAL HEALTH CENTER (C, 22 beds) 1515 South Phillips Street, Algona, IA Zip 50511–3649; tel. 515/295–2451; Scott A. Curtis, Administrator and Chief Executive Officer
**Web address:** www.krhc.com

MERCY MEDICAL CENTER–CLINTON (O, 341 beds) 1410 North Fourth Street, Clinton, IA Zip 52732–2940; tel. 563/244–5555; Sean J. Williams, President and Chief Financial Officer
**Web address:** www.mercyclinton.com

MERCY MEDICAL CENTER–DUBUQUE (O, 272 beds) 250 Mercy Drive, Dubuque, IA Zip 52001–7360; tel. 563/589–8000; Russell M. Knight, President and Chief Executive Officer
**Web address:** www.mercydubuque.com

MERCY MEDICAL CENTER–DYERSVILLE (S, 25 beds) 1111 Third Street S.W., Dyersville, IA Zip 52040; tel. 563/875–7101; Russell M. Knight, President and Chief Executive Officer
**Web address:** www.mercydubuque.com/dyersville

MERCY MEDICAL CENTER–NEW HAMPTON (O, 18 beds) 308 North Maple Avenue, New Hampton, IA Zip 50659–1142; tel. 641/394–4121; Bruce E. Roesler, FACHE, President and Chief Executive Officer
**Web address:** www.mercynewhampton.com

MERCY MEDICAL CENTER–NORTH IOWA (O, 240 beds) 1000 Fourth Street S.W., Mason City, IA Zip 50401–2800; tel. 641/428–7000; Rod G. Schlader, Interim President and Chief Executive Officer
**Web address:** www.mercynorthiowa.com

MERCY MEDICAL CENTER–SIOUX CITY (O, 238 beds) 801 Fifth Street, Sioux City, IA Zip 51101–1326, Mailing Address: P.O. Box 3168, Zip 51102–3168; tel. 712/279–2010; Robert J. Peebles, President and Chief Executive Officer
**Web address:** www.mercysiouxcity.com

MITCHELL COUNTY REGIONAL HEALTH CENTER (C, 25 beds) 616 North Eighth Street, Osage, IA Zip 50461–1498; tel. 641/732–6000; Desiree Einsweiler, Interim Chief Executive Officer
**Web address:** www.mitchellcohospital–clinics.com

PALO ALTO COUNTY HEALTH SYSTEM (C, 47 beds) 3201 First Street, Emmetsburg, IA Zip 50536; tel. 712/852–5500; Vance Jackson, FACHE, Interim Administrator
**Web address:** www.pachs.com

REGIONAL HEALTH SERVICES OF HOWARD COUNTY (C, 20 beds) 235 Eighth Avenue West, Cresco, IA Zip 52136–1098; tel. 563/547–2101; Vance Jackson, FACHE, Interim Chief Executive Officer
**Web address:** www.rhshc.com

**MARYLAND:** HOLY CROSS HOSPITAL (O, 425 beds) 1500 Forest Glen Road, Silver Spring, MD Zip 20910–1487; tel. 301/754–7000; Kevin J. Sexton, President and Chief Executive Officer
**Web address:** www.holycrosshealth.org

**MICHIGAN:** CHELSEA COMMUNITY HOSPITAL (O, 102 beds) 775 South Main Street, Chelsea, MI Zip 48118–1383; tel. 734/475–1311; Nancy Kay Graebner, President and Chief Executive Officer
**Web address:** www.cch.org

MERCY HEALTH PARTNERS, HACKLEY CAMPUS (O, 213 beds) 1700 Clinton Street, Muskegon, MI Zip 49442–5502, Mailing Address: P.O. Box 3302, Zip 49443–3302; tel. 231/726–3511; Roger Spoelman, President and Chief Executive Officer
**Web address:** www.hackley.org

MERCY HEALTH PARTNERS, LAKESHORE CAMPUS (O, 24 beds) 72 South State Street, Shelby, MI Zip 49455–1299; tel. 231/861–2156; Jay Bryan, President and Chief Executive Officer
**Web address:** www.mercyhealthpartners.org

For explanation of codes following names, see page B2.
★ Indicates Type III membership in the American Hospital Association.

MERCY HEALTH PARTNERS, MERCY CAMPUS (O, 188 beds) 1500 East Sherman Boulevard, Muskegon, MI Zip 49444–1849; tel. 231/672–2000; Roger Spoelman, President and Chief Executive Officer
**Web address:** www.mghp.com

MERCY HOSPITAL CADILLAC (O, 65 beds) 400 Hobart Street, Cadillac, MI Zip 49601–2331; tel. 231/876–7200; John L. MacLeod, President and Chief Executive Officer
**Web address:** www.munsonhealthcare.org

MERCY HOSPITAL GRAYLING (O, 94 beds) 1100 East Michigan Avenue, Grayling, MI Zip 49738–1312; tel. 989/348–5461; Stephanie J. Riemer–Matuzak, Chief Executive Officer
**Web address:** www.mercygrayling.munsonhealthcare.org/

SAINT MARY'S HEALTH CARE (O, 344 beds) 200 Jefferson Avenue S.E., Grand Rapids, MI Zip 49503–4598; tel. 616/685–5000; Philip H. McCorkle, Jr., President and Chief Executive Officer
**Web address:** www.mercyhealthsaintmarys.org

ST. JOSEPH MERCY HOSPITAL (O, 530 beds) 5301 McAuley Drive, Ypsilanti, MI Zip 48197, Mailing Address: P.O. Box 995, Ann Arbor, Zip 48106–0995; tel. 734/712–3456; Robert F. Casalou, President and Chief Executive Officer
**Web address:** www.sjmercyhealth.org

ST. JOSEPH MERCY LIVINGSTON HOSPITAL (O, 55 beds) 620 Byron Road, Howell, MI Zip 48843–1093; tel. 517/545–6000; Robert F. Casalou, President and Chief Executive Officer
**Web address:** www.sjmh.com/who/mcphersn.shtml

ST. JOSEPH MERCY OAKLAND (O, 409 beds) 44405 Woodward Avenue, Pontiac, MI Zip 48341–5023; tel. 248/858–3000; Jack Weiner, President and Chief Executive Officer
**Web address:** www.stjoesoakland.com

ST. JOSEPH MERCY PORT HURON (O, 119 beds) 2601 Electric Avenue, Port Huron, MI Zip 48060–6518; tel. 810/985–1500; Rebecca Smith, Chief Executive Officer
**Web address:** www.mercyporthuron.com

ST. JOSEPH MERCY SALINE HOSPITAL (O, 0 beds) 400 West Russell Street, Saline, MI Zip 48176–1183; tel. 734/429–1500; Robert F. Casalou, President and Chief Executive Officer

ST. MARY MERCY HOSPITAL (O, 289 beds) 36475 West Five Mile Road, Livonia, MI Zip 48154–1988; tel. 734/655–4800; David A. Spivey, President and Chief Executive Officer
**Web address:** www.stmarymercy.org

**NEBRASKA:** OAKLAND MERCY HOSPITAL (O, 18 beds) 601 East Second Street, Oakland, NE Zip 68045–1400; tel. 402/685–5601; Roger W. Lenz, Interim Chief Executive Officer
**Web address:** www.oaklandhospital.org

PENDER COMMUNITY HOSPITAL (C, 67 beds) 100 Hospital Drive, Pender, NE Zip 68047–0100, Mailing Address: P.O. Box 100, Zip 68047–0100; tel. 402/385–3083; Richard Thomason, FACHE, Chief Executive Officer
**Web address:** www.pendercommunityhospital.com

**OHIO:** FAYETTE COUNTY MEMORIAL HOSPITAL (C, 25 beds) 1430 Columbus Avenue, Washington Court House, OH Zip 43160–1791; tel. 740/335–1210; Lyndon J. Christman, President and Chief Executive Officer
**Web address:** www.fcmh.org

MOUNT CARMEL (O, 729 beds) 793 West State Street, Columbus, OH Zip 43222–1551; tel. 614/234–5000; Claus von Zychlin, President and Chief Executive Officer
**Web address:** www.mountcarmelhealth.com

MOUNT CARMEL NEW ALBANY SURGICAL HOSPITAL (O, 60 beds) 7333 Smith's Mill Road, New Albany, OH Zip 43054; tel. 614/775–6600; Richard D'Enbeau, Chief Operating Officer
**Web address:** www.newalbanysurgicalhospital.com

MOUNT CARMEL ST. ANN'S (O, 250 beds) 500 South Cleveland Avenue, Westerville, OH Zip 43081–8998; tel. 614/898–4000; Claus von Zychlin, Executive Vice President and Chief Operating Officer
**Web address:** www.mountcarmelhealth.com

**OREGON:** SAINT ALPHONSUS MEDICAL CENTER – BAKER CITY (S, 65 beds) 3325 Pocahontas Road, Baker City, OR Zip 97814–1464; tel. 541/523–6461; H. Ray Gibbons, FACHE, Chief Executive Officer
**Web address:** www.stelizabethhealth.com

SAINT ALPHONSUS MEDICAL CENTER – ONTARIO (S, 49 beds) 351 S.W. Ninth Street, Ontario, OR Zip 97914–2693; tel. 541/881–7000; Richard L. Palagi, Chief Executive Officer
**Web address:** www.holyrosary–ontario.org

| Owned, leased, sponsored: | 35 hospitals | 7525 beds |
|---|---|---|
| Contract–managed: | 12 hospitals | 427 beds |
| **Totals:** | 47 hospitals | 7952 beds |

---

**0540: TRINITY MOTHER FRANCES HOSPITALS AND CLINICS** (NP)
910 East Houston, Tyler, TX Zip 75702–8369; tel. 903/593–8441; J. Lindsey Bradley, Jr., FACHE, President
**(Centralized Physician/Insurance Health System)**

**TEXAS:** MOTHER FRANCES HOSPITAL – JACKSONVILLE (O, 21 beds) 2026 South Jackson, Jacksonville, TX Zip 75766; tel. 903/541–4500; Thomas N. Cammack, Jr., Chief Administrative Officer
**Web address:** www.tmfhs.org

MOTHER FRANCES HOSPITAL – TYLER (O, 392 beds) 800 East Dawson Street, Tyler, TX Zip 75701–2036; tel. 903/593–8441; Laura Owen, Senior Vice President and Chief Executive Officer
**Web address:** www.tmfhs.org

MOTHER FRANCES HOSPITAL – WINNSBORO (O, 35 beds) 719 West Coke Road, Winnsboro, TX Zip 75494–0628, Mailing Address: P.O. Box 628, Zip 75494–0628; tel. 903/342–5227; Janet Coates, President and Chief Executive Officer
**Web address:** www.tmfhs.org

TYLER CONTINUECARE HOSPITAL AT MOTHER FRANCES (O, 51 beds) 800 East Dawson, 4th Floor, Tyler, TX Zip 75701; tel. 903/531–4080; Stephanie Hyde, Chief Executive Officer
**Web address:** www.continuecare.org

| Owned, leased, sponsored: | 4 hospitals | 499 beds |
|---|---|---|
| Contract–managed: | 0 hospitals | 0 beds |
| **Totals:** | 4 hospitals | 499 beds |

---

**★9255: TRUMAN MEDICAL CENTERS** (NP)
2301 Holmes Street, Kansas City, MO Zip 64108–2677; tel. 816/404–1000; John W. Bluford, President and Chief Executive Officer
**(Independent Hospital System)**

**MISSOURI:** TRUMAN MEDICAL CENTER–HOSPITAL HILL (O, 272 beds) 2301 Holmes Street, Kansas City, MO Zip 64108–2640; tel. 816/404–1000; John W. Bluford, President and Chief Executive Officer
**Web address:** www.trumed.org

TRUMAN MEDICAL CENTER–LAKEWOOD (O, 310 beds) 7900 Lee's Summit Road, Kansas City, MO Zip 64139–1236; tel. 816/404–7000; John W. Bluford, President and Chief Executive Officer
**Web address:** www.trumanmed.org

| Owned, leased, sponsored: | 2 hospitals | 582 beds |
|---|---|---|
| Contract–managed: | 0 hospitals | 0 beds |
| **Totals:** | 2 hospitals | 582 beds |

---

**0238: TY COBB HEALTHCARE SYSTEM, INC.** (NP)
461 Cook Street, Suite A., Royston, GA Zip 30662–4003; tel. 706/245–1832; Charles T. Adams, President and Chief Executive Officer
**(Independent Hospital System)**

**GEORGIA:** COBB MEMORIAL HOSPITAL (O, 186 beds) 521 Franklin Springs Street, Royston, GA Zip 30662–3909, Mailing Address: P.O. Box 589, Zip 30662–0589; tel. 706/245–5071; David H. Seagraves, Chief Executive Officer
**Web address:** www.tycobbhealthcare.org

HART COUNTY HOSPITAL (L, 120 beds) Gibson and Cade Streets, Hartwell, GA Zip 30643–0280, Mailing Address: P.O. Box 280, Zip 30643–0280; tel. 706/856–6100; Jerry R. Wise, Administrator and Vice President
**Web address:** www.tycobbhealthcare.org

| Owned, leased, sponsored: | 2 hospitals | 306 beds |
|---|---|---|
| Contract–managed: | 0 hospitals | 0 beds |
| **Totals:** | 2 hospitals | 306 beds |

**Section B**

For explanation of codes following names, see page B2.
★ Indicates Type III membership in the American Hospital Association.

## 9195:  U. S. INDIAN HEALTH SERVICE (FG)

801 Thompson Avenue, Rockville, MD Zip 20852;
tel. 301/443–1083; Yvette Roubideaux, M.D., M.P.H., Director
**(Independent Hospital System)**

**ARIZONA:** CHINLE COMPREHENSIVE HEALTH CARE FACILITY (O, 60 beds) Highway 191, Chinle, AZ Zip 86503, Mailing Address: P.O. Drawer PH, Zip 86503; tel. 928/674–7011; Ronald Tso, Chief Executive Officer
**Web address:** www.ihs.gov

FORT DEFIANCE INDIAN HEALTH SERVICE HOSPITAL (O, 39 beds) Fort Defiance, AZ Zip 86504; tel. 928/729–8014; Leland Leonard, M.D., Administrator
**Web address:** www.ihs.gov

HOPI HEALTH CARE CENTER (O, 6 beds) Keams Canyon, AZ Zip 86034; Polacca, tel. 928/737–6000; De Alva Honahnie, Chief Executive Officer
**Web address:** www.ihs.gov/index.asp

U. S. PUBLIC HEALTH SERVICE INDIAN HOSPITAL (O, 20 beds) 12033 Agency Road, Parker, AZ Zip 85344–7718; tel. 928/669–2137; Dee Hutchison, Acting Chief Executive Officer
**Web address:** www.ihs.gov

U. S. PUBLIC HEALTH SERVICE INDIAN HOSPITAL (O, 8 beds) San Carlos, AZ Zip 85550; tel. 928/475–2371; Nella J. Ben, Chief Executive Officer
**Web address:** www.ihs.gov

U. S. PUBLIC HEALTH SERVICE INDIAN HOSPITAL–SELLS (O, 12 beds) Sells, AZ Zip 85634; tel. 520/383–7251; Priscilla Whitethorne, Chief Executive Officer
**Web address:** www.ihs.gov

U. S. PUBLIC HEALTH SERVICE INDIAN HOSPITAL–WHITERIVER (O, 35 beds) 200 West Hospital Drive, Whiteriver, AZ Zip 85941–0860, Mailing Address: State Route 73, Box 860, Zip 85941–0860; tel. 928/338–4911; Michelle Martinez, Interim Chief Executive Officer
**Web address:** www.ihs.gov

U. S. PUBLIC HEALTH SERVICE PHOENIX INDIAN MEDICAL CENTER (O, 127 beds) 4212 North 16th Street, Phoenix, AZ Zip 85016–5389; tel. 602/263–1200; John Molina, Chief Executive Officer
**Web address:** www.ihs.gov

**MARYLAND:** NATIONAL INSTITUTES OF HEALTH CLINICAL CENTER (O, 161 beds) 9000 Rockville Pike, Building 10, Room 6–2551, Bethesda, MD Zip 20892–1504; tel. 301/496–4000; John I. Gallin, M.D., Director
**Web address:** www.clinicalcenter.nih.gov

**MINNESOTA:** U. S. PUBLIC HEALTH SERVICE INDIAN HOSPITAL (O, 11 beds) 7th Street & Grant Utley Avenue N.W., Cass Lake, MN Zip 56633, Mailing Address: Rural Route 3, Box 211, Zip 56633; tel. 218/335–3200; Norine Smith, Chief Executive Officer
**Web address:** www.ihs.gov

U.S. PUBLIC HEALTH SERVICE INDIAN HOSPITAL (O, 19 beds) Highway 1, Redlake, MN Zip 56671, Mailing Address: P.O. Box 497, Zip 56671–0497; tel. 218/679–3912; Mark Karzon, Chief Executive Officer
**Web address:** www.ihs.gov

**MONTANA:** CROW/NORTHERN CHEYENNE HOSPITAL (O, 24 beds) P.O. Box 9, Crow Agency, MT Zip 59022–0009; tel. 406/638–2626; Yvonne Misiaszek, Service Unit Director
**Web address:** www.ihs.
gov/facilitiesservices/areaoffices/billings/crow/index.asp

FORT BELKNAP U. S. PUBLIC HEALTH SERVICE INDIAN HOSPITAL (O, 6 beds) 669 Agency Main Street, Harlem, MT Zip 59526; tel. 406/353–3100; Steve Fox, Chief Executive Officer
**Web address:** www.ihs.gov

U. S. PUBLIC HEALTH SERVICE BLACKFEET COMMUNITY HOSPITAL (O, 25 beds) Saint Mary, MT Zip 59417–0760; Browning, tel. 406/338–6100; Timothy Davis, Interim Chief Executive Officer
**Web address:** www.phs.ihs.gov

**NEBRASKA:** U. S. PUBLIC HEALTH SERVICE INDIAN HOSPITAL (O, 30 beds) Highway 7577, Winnebago, NE Zip 68071; tel. 402/878–2231; Sheriann Moore, Service Unit Director
**Web address:** www.ihs.gov

**NEW MEXICO:** ACOMA–CANONCITO–LAGUNA HOSPITAL (O, 25 beds) 80B Veterans Boulevard, Acoma, NM Zip 87034, Mailing Address: P.O. Box 130, San Fidel, Zip 87049–0130; tel. 505/552–5300; William Thorne, Jr., Chief Executive Officer
**Web address:** www.ihs.gov/albuquerque/index.cfm?module=dsp_abq_acoma_canoncito_laguna

GALLUP INDIAN MEDICAL CENTER (O, 71 beds) 516 East Nizhoni Boulevard, Gallup, NM Zip 87301–5748, Mailing Address: P.O. Box 1337, Zip 87305–1337; tel. 505/722–1000; Bennie C. Yazzie, Interim Chief Executive Officer
**Web address:** www.ihs.
gov/facilitiesservices/areaoffices/navajo/naihs–hcc–gallup.asp

MESCALERO PUBLIC HEALTH SERVICE INDIAN HOSPITAL (O, 13 beds) Mescalero, NM Zip 88340; tel. 505/671–4441; Dorlynn Simmons, Chief Executive Officer
**Web address:** www.ihs.gov

NORTHERN NAVAJO MEDICAL CENTER (O, 62 beds) Shiprock, NM Zip 87420–0160; tel. 505/368–6001; Fannessa Comer, Chief Executive Officer
**Web address:** www.home.nnmc.ihs.gov/

PHS SANTA FE INDIAN HOSPITAL (O, 39 beds) 1700 Cerrillos Road, Santa Fe, NM Zip 87505–3554; tel. 505/988–9821; Robert J. Lyon, Chief Executive Officer
**Web address:** www.ihs.gov

U. S. PUBLIC HEALTH SERVICE INDIAN HOSPITAL (O, 12 beds) Crownpoint, NM Zip 87313; tel. 505/786–5291; Virgil Davis, Acting Chief Executive Officer
**Web address:** www.ihs.gov

U. S. PUBLIC HEALTH SERVICE INDIAN HOSPITAL (O, 32 beds) Route 301 North B. Street, Zuni, NM Zip 87327, Mailing Address: P.O. Box 467, Zip 87327–0467; tel. 505/782–4431; Jean Othole, Chief Executive Officer
**Web address:** www.ihs.gov

**NORTH DAKOTA:** PUBLIC HEALTH SERVICE INDIAN HOSPITAL – QUENTIN N. BURDICK MEMORIAL HEALTH FACILITY (O, 27 beds) 2 Blocks North of Highway 5, Belcourt, ND Zip 58316, Mailing Address: P.O. Box 160, Zip 58316–0160; tel. 701/477–6111; RoxAnne LaVallie–Unabia, Chief Executive Officer
**Web address:** www.ihs.gov

U. S. PUBLIC HEALTH SERVICE INDIAN HOSPITAL (O, 14 beds) N 10 North River Road, Fort Yates, ND Zip 58538, Mailing Address: P.O. Box J, Zip 58538; tel. 701/854–3831; Lisa Guardipee, Director
**Web address:** www.ihs.gov

**OKLAHOMA:** CLAREMORE INDIAN HOSPITAL (O, 46 beds) 101 South Moore Avenue, Claremore, OK Zip 74017–5091; tel. 918/342–6200; George Valliere, Chief Executive Officer
**Web address:** www.ihs.gov

LAWTON INDIAN HOSPITAL (O, 26 beds) 1515 Lawrie Tatum Road, Lawton, OK Zip 73507–3099; tel. 580/353–0350; Greg Ketcher, Administrator
**Web address:** www.ihs.gov

WILLIAM W. HASTINGS INDIAN HOSPITAL (O, 58 beds) 100 South Bliss Avenue, Tahlequah, OK Zip 74464–3399; tel. 918/458–3100; Charles Grim, D.D.S., Chief Executive Officer

**SOUTH DAKOTA:** INDIAN HEALTH SERVICE HOSPITAL (O, 5 beds) 3200 Canyon Lake Drive, Rapid City, SD Zip 57702–8197; tel. 605/355–2280; Helen Thompson, Interim Director
**Web address:** www.ihs.gov

U. S. PUBLIC HEALTH SERVICE INDIAN HOSPITAL (O, 11 beds) 317 Main Street, Eagle Butte, SD Zip 57625–1012, Mailing Address: P.O. Box 1012, Zip 57625–1012; tel. 605/964–7724; Charlene Red Thunder, Chief Executive Officer
**Web address:** www.ihs.gov

U. S. PUBLIC HEALTH SERVICE INDIAN HOSPITAL (O, 45 beds) East Highway 18, Pine Ridge, SD Zip 57770, Mailing Address: P.O. Box 1201, Zip 57770–1201; tel. 605/867–5131; William Pourier, Service Unit Director
**Web address:** www.ihs.gov

U. S. PUBLIC HEALTH SERVICE INDIAN HOSPITAL (O, 35 beds) Highway 18, Soldier Creek Road, Rosebud, SD Zip 57570; tel. 605/747–2231; Shelly Harris, Chief Executive Officer
**Web address:** www.ihs.gov

| | | |
|---|---|---|
| **Owned, leased, sponsored:** | 31 hospitals | 1104 beds |
| **Contract–managed:** | 0 hospitals | 0 beds |
| **Totals:** | 31 hospitals | 1104 beds |

## ★9105:  UAB HEALTH SYSTEM (NP)

500 22nd Street South, Suite 408, Birmingham, AL Zip 35233;
tel. 205/975–5362; William Ferniany, Ph.D., Chief Executive Officer
**(Moderately Centralized Health System)**

For explanation of codes following names, see page B2.
★ Indicates Type III membership in the American Hospital Association.

**ALABAMA:** MEDICAL WEST (O, 229 beds) 995 Ninth Avenue S.W., Bessemer, AL Zip 35022–4527; tel. 205/481–7000; Tom R. McDougal, Jr., President and Chief Executive Officer
**Web address:** www.uabmedicalwest.org

UNIVERSITY OF ALABAMA HOSPITAL (O, 1062 beds) 619 19th Street South, Birmingham, AL Zip 35249; tel. 205/934–4011; Michael Waldrum, M.D., Chief Executive Officer
**Web address:** www.health.uab.edu

| | | |
|---|---|---|
| Owned, leased, sponsored: | 2 hospitals | 1291 beds |
| Contract–managed: | 0 hospitals | 0 beds |
| Totals: | 2 hospitals | 1291 beds |

---

**★0082: UC HEALTH** (NP)
3200 Burnet Avenue, Cincinnati, OH Zip 45229; tel. 513/585–6000; James A. Kingsbury, President and Chief Executive Officer
**(Moderately Centralized Health System)**

**OHIO:** DRAKE CENTER (O, 269 beds) 151 West Galbraith Road, Cincinnati, OH Zip 45216–1015; tel. 513/418–2500; Debra C. Hampton, Ph.D., Vice President, Administration and Chief Nursing Officer
**Web address:** www.drakecenter.uchealth.com

UC HEALTH SURGICAL HOSPITAL (O, 8 beds) 7750 University Court, West Chester, OH Zip 45069; tel. 513/475–8300; Lesley Gilbertson, M.D., Executive and Medical Director
**Web address:** www.surgicalhospital.uchealth.com

UNIVERSITY HOSPITAL (O, 466 beds) 234 Goodman Street, Cincinnati, OH Zip 45219–2316; tel. 513/584–1000; W. Brian Gibler, M.D., President and Chief Executive Officer
**Web address:** www.universityhospital.uchealth.com

WEST CHESTER HOSPITAL (O, 126 beds) 7700 University Drive, West Chester, OH Zip 45069–2505; tel. 513/298–3000; Kevin Joseph, M.D., Chief Executive Officer
**Web address:** www.westchesterhospital.uchealth.com

| | | |
|---|---|---|
| Owned, leased, sponsored: | 4 hospitals | 869 beds |
| Contract–managed: | 0 hospitals | 0 beds |
| Totals: | 4 hospitals | 869 beds |

---

**0390: UK HEALTHCARE** (NP)
800 Rose Street, Lexington, KY Zip 40536–0293; tel. 859/323–5000; Michael Karpf, M.D., Executive Vice President Health Affairs
**(Independent Hospital System)**

**KENTUCKY:** UK HEALTHCARE GOOD SAMARITAN HOSPITAL (O, 158 beds) 310 South Limestone Street, Lexington, KY Zip 40508–3008; tel. 859/226–7000; Willem de Villiers, M.D., Chief Administrative Officer
**Web address:** www.ukhealthcare.uky.edu/samaritan

UNIVERSITY OF KENTUCKY ALBERT B. CHANDLER HOSPITAL (O, 524 beds) 800 Rose Street, N100, Lexington, KY Zip 40536–0293; tel. 859/323–5000; Richard P. Lofgren, M.D., Vice President Health Care Operations
**Web address:** www.ukhealthcare.uky.edu

| | | |
|---|---|---|
| Owned, leased, sponsored: | 2 hospitals | 682 beds |
| Contract–managed: | 0 hospitals | 0 beds |
| Totals: | 2 hospitals | 682 beds |

---

**★0224: UMASS MEMORIAL HEALTH CARE, INC.** (NP)
1 Biotech Park, Worcester, MA Zip 01605–2982; tel. 508/334–0100; John G. O'Brien, President and Chief Executive Officer
**(Moderately Centralized Health System)**

**MASSACHUSETTS:** CLINTON HOSPITAL (O, 41 beds) 201 Highland Street, Clinton, MA Zip 01510–1096; tel. 978/368–3000; Sheila Daly, President and Chief Executive Officer
**Web address:** www.clintonhospital.org

HEALTH ALLIANCE HOSPITALS (O, 83 beds) 60 Hospital Road, Leominster, MA Zip 01453–8004; tel. 978/466–2000; Patrick L. Muldoon, FACHE, President and Chief Executive Officer
**Web address:** www.healthalliance.com

UMASS MEMORIAL MEDICAL CENTER (O, 682 beds) 119 Belmont Street, Worcester, MA Zip 01605–2982; tel. 508/334–1000; John G. O'Brien, President and Chief Executive Officer
**Web address:** www.umassmemorial.org

UMASS MEMORIAL–MARLBOROUGH HOSPITAL (O, 67 beds) 157 Union Street, Marlborough, MA Zip 01752–1297; tel. 508/481–5000; Karen O. Moore, MS, R.N., President and Chief Executive Officer
**Web address:** www.marlboroughhospital.org

WING MEMORIAL HOSPITAL AND MEDICAL CENTERS (O, 74 beds) 40 Wright Street, Palmer, MA Zip 01069–1138; tel. 413/283–7651; Charles E. Cavagnaro, III, M.D., President and Chief Executive Officer
**Web address:** www.winghealth.org

| | | |
|---|---|---|
| Owned, leased, sponsored: | 5 hospitals | 947 beds |
| Contract–managed: | 0 hospitals | 0 beds |
| Totals: | 5 hospitals | 947 beds |

---

**0288: UNITED HEALTH SERVICES** (NP)
10–42 Mitchell Avenue, Binghamton, NY Zip 13903; tel. 607/762–2200; Matthew J. Salanger, President and Chief Executive Officer
**(Independent Hospital System)**

**NEW YORK:** CHENANGO MEMORIAL HOSPITAL (O, 138 beds) 179 North Broad Street, Norwich, NY Zip 13815–1097; tel. 607/337–4111; Drake M. Lamen, M.D., President and Chief Executive Officer
**Web address:** www.uhs.net/cmh

DELAWARE VALLEY HOSPITAL (O, 25 beds) 1 Titus Place, Walton, NY Zip 13856–1498; tel. 607/865–2100; Dru Cavanagh, R.N., Interim Chief Executive Officer
**Web address:** www.uhs.net

UNITED HEALTH SERVICES HOSPITALS–BINGHAMTON (O, 460 beds) 10–42 Mitchell Avenue, Binghamton, NY Zip 13903–1678; tel. 607/763–6000; Matthew J. Salanger, President and Chief Executive Officer
**Web address:** www.uhs.net

| | | |
|---|---|---|
| Owned, leased, sponsored: | 3 hospitals | 623 beds |
| Contract–managed: | 0 hospitals | 0 beds |
| Totals: | 3 hospitals | 623 beds |

---

**9605: UNITED MEDICAL CORPORATION** (IO)
603 Main Street, Windermere, FL Zip 34786–3548, Mailing Address: P.O. Box 1100, Zip 34786–1100; tel. 407/876–2200; Donald R. Dizney, Chairman and Chief Executive Officer

**PUERTO RICO:** HOSPITAL PAVIA–HATO REY (O, 180 beds) 435 Ponce De Leon Avenue, San Juan, PR Zip 00917–3428; tel. 787/754–0909; Astro Munoz, Chief Executive Officer
**Web address:** www.paviahealth.com

HOSPITAL PAVIA–SANTURCE (O, 215 beds) 1462 Asia Street, San Juan, PR Zip 00909–2143, Mailing Address: Box 11137, Santurce Station, Zip 00910–1137; tel. 787/727–6060; Jose Luis Rodriguez, Chief Executive Officer
**Web address:** www.paviahealth.com

HOSPITAL PEREA (O, 103 beds) 15 Basora Street, Mayaguez, PR Zip 00681, Mailing Address: P.O. Box 170, Zip 00681; tel. 787/834–0101; Marco Reyes Concepcion, Executive Director
**Web address:** www.paviahealth.com/perea_hospital.htm

SAN JORGE CHILDREN'S HOSPITAL (O, 125 beds) 252 San Jorge Street, Santurce, San Juan, PR Zip 00912–3310; tel. 787/727–1000; Domingo Cruz, Senior Vice President Operations
**Web address:** www.sanjorgechildrenshospital.com

| | | |
|---|---|---|
| Owned, leased, sponsored: | 4 hospitals | 623 beds |
| Contract–managed: | 0 hospitals | 0 beds |
| Totals: | 4 hospitals | 623 beds |

**Section B**

**0322:  UNITED SURGICAL PARTNERS INTERNATIONAL** (IO)
15305 Dallas Parkway, Suite 1600, Addison, TX Zip 75001–6491; tel. 972/713–3500; William H. Wilcox, President and Chief Executive Officer
**(Independent Hospital System)**

**ARIZONA:** ARIZONA ORTHOPEDIC SURGICAL HOSPITAL (O, 16 beds) 2905 West Warner Road, Chandler, AZ Zip 85224; tel. 480/603–9000; Duane Scholer, Chief Executive Officer
**Web address:** www.azosh.com

**OKLAHOMA:** OKLAHOMA CENTER FOR ORTHOPEDIC AND MULTI–SPECIALTY SURGERY (O, 10 beds) 8100 South Walker, Suite C., Oklahoma City, OK Zip 73139, Mailing Address: P.O. Box 890609, Zip 73189; tel. 405/602–6500; Teri Philbrick, Chief Executive Officer
**Web address:** www.okla–sc.com/

**TEXAS:** BAYLOR MEDICAL CENTER AT FRISCO (O, 68 beds) 5601 Warren Parkway, Frisco, TX Zip 75034; tel. 214/407–5000; William A. Keaton, Chief Executive Officer
**Web address:** www.bmcf.com

BAYLOR MEDICAL CENTER AT UPTOWN (O, 24 beds) 2727 East Lemmon Avenue, Dallas, TX Zip 75204–2895; tel. 214/443–3000; Matt Chance, Administrator
**Web address:** www.bmcuptown.com

IRVING COPPELL SURGICAL HOSPITAL (O, 12 beds) 400 West Interstate 635, Irving, TX Zip 75063; tel. 972/868–4000; Deonna Unell, Chief Executive Officer
**Web address:** www.ic–sh.com

SUGAR LAND SURGICAL HOSPITAL (O, 6 beds) 1211 Highway 6, Suite 70, Sugar Land, TX Zip 77478; tel. 281/243–1000; Daniel Smith, Interim Chief Executive Officer
**Web address:** www.sugarlandhospital.com

TOPS SURGICAL SPECIALTY HOSPITAL (O, 16 beds) 17080 Red Oak Drive, Houston, TX Zip 77090; tel. 281/539–2900; Samuel H. Rossmann, Chief Executive Officer
**Web address:** www.tops–hospital.com

| | | |
|---|---|---|
| **Owned, leased, sponsored:** | 7 hospitals | 152 beds |
| **Contract–managed:** | 0 hospitals | 0 beds |
| **Totals:** | 7 hospitals | 152 beds |

---

**9555:  UNIVERSAL HEALTH SERVICES, INC.** (IO)
367 South Gulph Road, King of Prussia, PA Zip 19406–0958, Mailing Address: P.O. Box 61558, Zip 19406–0958; tel. 610/768–3300; Alan B. Miller, President and Chief Executive Officer
**(Decentralized Health System)**

**ALABAMA:** HILL CREST BEHAVIORAL HEALTH SERVICES (O, 94 beds) 6869 Fifth Avenue South, Birmingham, AL Zip 35212–1866; tel. 205/833–9000; Steve McCabe, Chief Executive Officer
**Web address:** www.hillcrestbhs.com

LAUREL OAKS BEHAVIORAL HEALTH CENTER (O, 32 beds) 700 East Cottonwood Road, Dothan, AL Zip 36301; tel. 334/794–7373; Derek Johnson, Chief Executive Officer
**Web address:** www.laureloaksbhc.com

**ALASKA:** NORTH STAR BEHAVIORAL HEALTH SYSTEM (O, 200 beds) 2530 DeBarr Road, Anchorage, AK Zip 99508–2948; tel. 907/258–7575; Andrew Mayo, Chief Executive Officer and Managing Director
**Web address:** www.northstarbehavioral.com

**ARKANSAS:** PINNACLE POINTE HOSPITAL (O, 124 beds) 11501 Financial Center Parkway, Little Rock, AR Zip 72211–3715; tel. 501/223–3322; Lisa Evans, Chief Executive Officer
**Web address:** www.pinnaclepointehospital.com

RIVENDELL BEHAVIORAL HEALTH SERVICES OF ARKANSAS (O, 77 beds) 100 Rivendell Drive, Benton, AR Zip 72019–9100; tel. 501/316–1255; Duane Runyan, Chief Executive Officer and Managing Director
**Web address:** www.rivendellofarkansas.com

THE BRIDGEWAY (L, 103 beds) 21 Bridgeway Road, North Little Rock, AR Zip 72113–9516; tel. 501/771–1500; Barry Pipkin, Chief Executive Officer
**Web address:** www.thebridgeway.com

**CALIFORNIA:** BHC ALHAMBRA HOSPITAL (O, 85 beds) 4619 North Rosemead Boulevard, Rosemead, CA Zip 91770–1478, Mailing Address: P.O. Box 369, Zip 91770–0369; tel. 626/286–1191; Peggy Minnick, R.N., Chief Executive Officer
**Web address:** www.bhcalhambra.com

CANYON RIDGE HOSPITAL (O, 106 beds) 5353 G Street, Chino, CA Zip 91710–5250; tel. 909/590–3700; Jeff McDonald, Chief Executive Officer
**Web address:** www.canyonridgehospital.net

CORONA REGIONAL MEDICAL CENTER (O, 240 beds) 800 South Main Street, Corona, CA Zip 92882–3420; tel. 951/737–4343; Kevan Metcalfe, Chief Executive Officer
**Web address:** www.coronaregional.com

DEL AMO HOSPITAL (O, 70 beds) 23700 Camino Del Sol, Torrance, CA Zip 90505–5000; tel. 310/530–1151; Lisa K. Montes, Chief Executive Officer
**Web address:** www.delamohospital.com

FREMONT HOSPITAL (O, 96 beds) 39001 Sundale Drive, Fremont, CA Zip 94538–2005; tel. 510/796–1100; John C. Cooper, Chief Executive Officer
**Web address:** www.fremonthospital.com

HERITAGE OAKS HOSPITAL (O, 72 beds) 4250 Auburn Boulevard, Sacramento, CA Zip 95841–4164; tel. 916/489–3336; Chris Diamond, Chief Executive Officer
**Web address:** www.heritageoakshospital.com

INLAND VALLEY MEDICAL CENTER (L, 252 beds) 36485 Inland Valley Drive, Wildomar, CA Zip 92595–9700; tel. 951/677–1111; Kenneth I. Rivers, Chief Executive Officer
**Web address:** www.swhealthcaresystem.com

PALMDALE REGIONAL MEDICAL CENTER (O, 157 beds) 38600 Medical Center Drive, Palmdale, CA Zip 93551–4483; tel. 661/382–5000; Larry Coomes, Chief Executive Officer
**Web address:** www.palmdaleregional.com

RANCHO SPRINGS MEDICAL CENTER (O, 51 beds) 25500 Medical Center Drive, Murrieta, CA Zip 92562–5965; tel. 951/696–6000; Kenneth I. Rivers, Chief Executive Officer
**Web address:** www.swhcs.com

SIERRA VISTA HOSPITAL (O, 120 beds) 8001 Bruceville Road, Sacramento, CA Zip 95823–2329; tel. 916/288–0300; Mike Zauner, Chief Executive Officer

**COLORADO:** CEDAR SPRINGS BEHAVIORAL HEALTH SYSTEM (O, 110 beds) 2135 Southgate Road, Colorado Springs, CO Zip 80906–2693; tel. 719/633–4114; A. Elaine Crnkovic, Chief Executive Officer
**Web address:** www.cedarspringshospital.com

CENTENNIAL PEAKS HOSPITAL (O, 72 beds) 2255 South 88th Street, Louisville, CO Zip 80027–9716; tel. 303/673–9990; Elicia Bunch, Chief Executive Officer
**Web address:** www.centennialpeaks.com

HIGHLANDS BEHAVIORAL HEALTH SYSTEM (O, 86 beds) 8565 South Poplar Way, Littleton, CO Zip 80130; tel. 720/348–2800; David W. Morris, Chief Executive Officer
**Web address:** www.highlandsbhs.com

**DELAWARE:** DOVER BEHAVIORAL HEALTH SYSTEM (O, 52 beds) 725 Horsepond Road, Dover, DE Zip 19901; tel. 302/741–0140; William Weaver, Chief Executive Officer
**Web address:** www.doverbehavioral.com

ROCKFORD CENTER (O, 94 beds) 100 Rockford Drive, Newark, DE Zip 19713–2121; tel. 302/996–5480; John F. McKenna, Chief Executive Officer and Managing Director
**Web address:** www.rockfordcenter.com

**DISTRICT OF COLUMBIA:** GEORGE WASHINGTON UNIVERSITY HOSPITAL (O, 367 beds) 900 23rd Street N.W., Washington, DC Zip 20037–2377; tel. 202/715–4000; Barry A. Wolfman, Chief Executive Officer and Managing Director
**Web address:** www.gwhospital.com

**FLORIDA:** ATLANTIC SHORES HOSPITAL (O, 72 beds) 4545 North Federal Highway, Fort Lauderdale, FL Zip 33308–5274; tel. 954/771–2711; Manuel R. Llano, Chief Executive Officer
**Web address:** www.atlanticshoreshospital.com

For explanation of codes following names, see page B2.
★ Indicates Type III membership in the American Hospital Association.

CENTRAL FLORIDA BEHAVIORAL HOSPITAL (O, 120 beds) 6601 Central Florida Parkway, Orlando, FL Zip 32821–8064; tel. 407/370–0111; Vickie Lewis, Chief Executive Officer
**Web address:** www.centralfloridabehavioral.com

EMERALD COAST BEHAVIORAL HOSPITAL (O, 90 beds) 1940 Harrison Avenue, Panama City, FL Zip 32405–4542; tel. 850/763–0017; Tim Bedford, Chief Executive Officer
**Web address:** www.emeraldcoastbehavioral.com

FORT LAUDERDALE HOSPITAL (L, 100 beds) 1601 East Las Olas Boulevard, Fort Lauderdale, FL Zip 33301–2393; tel. 954/463–4321; Manuel R. Llano, Chief Executive Officer
**Web address:** www.fortlauderdalehospital.org

LAKEWOOD RANCH MEDICAL CENTER (O, 120 beds) 8330 Lakewood Ranch Boulevard, Bradenton, FL Zip 34202; tel. 941/782–2100; James D. Wilson, Chief Executive Officer
**Web address:** www.lakewoodranchmedicalcenter.com

MANATEE MEMORIAL HOSPITAL (O, 319 beds) 206 Second Street East, Bradenton, FL Zip 34208–1000; tel. 941/746–5111; Kevin DiLallo, Chief Executive Officer
**Web address:** www.manateememorial.com

MANATEE PALMS YOUTH SERVICES (O, 60 beds) 4480 51st Street West, Bradenton, FL Zip 34210; tel. 941/792–2222; George Shopland, Chief Executive Officer
**Web address:** www.mpys.com

RIVER POINT BEHAVIORAL HEALTH (O, 92 beds) 6300 Beach Boulevard, Jacksonville, FL Zip 32216–2782; tel. 904/724–9202; Gayle Eckerd, Chief Executive Officer
**Web address:** www.riverpointbehavioral.com

SANDYPINES (O, 80 beds) 11301 S.E. Tequesta Terrace, Tequesta, FL Zip 33469–8146; tel. 561/744–0211; John McCarthy, Chief Executive Officer

THE VINES (O, 90 beds) 3130 S.W. 27th Avenue, Ocala, FL Zip 34474; tel. 352/671–3130; Michael McDonald, Chief Executive Officer
**Web address:** www.tenbroeckocala.com

WEKIVA SPRINGS CENTER FOR WOMEN (O, 60 beds) 3947 Salisbury Road, Jacksonville, FL Zip 32216–6115; tel. 904/296–3533; Gayle Eckerd, Chief Executive Officer
**Web address:** www.wekivacenter.com

WELLINGTON REGIONAL MEDICAL CENTER (L, 108 beds) 10101 Forest Hill Boulevard, West Palm Beach, FL Zip 33414–6199; tel. 561/798–8500; Jerel T. Humphrey, Chief Executive Officer
**Web address:** www.wellingtonregional.com

WINDMOOR HEALTHCARE OF CLEARWATER (O, 120 beds) 11300 U.S. 19 North, Clearwater, FL Zip 33764; tel. 727/541–2646; Wendy Merson, Chief Executive Officer
**Web address:** www.windmoor–healthcare.com

**GEORGIA:** ANCHOR HOSPITAL (O, 111 beds) 5454 Yorktowne Drive, Atlanta, GA Zip 30349–5305; tel. 770/991–6044; Jennifer Morgan, Chief Executive Officer and Managing Director
**Web address:** www.anchorhospital.com

COASTAL HARBOR TREATMENT CENTER (O, 195 beds) 1150 Cornell Avenue, Savannah, GA Zip 31406–2797; tel. 912/354–3911; Ray Heckerman, Chief Executive Officer and Managing Director
**Web address:** www.coastalharbor.com

PEACHFORD BEHAVIORAL HEALTH SYSTEM (O, 224 beds) 2151 Peachford Road, Atlanta, GA Zip 30338–6599; tel. 770/455–3200; Matthew Crouch, Chief Executive Officer and Managing Director
**Web address:** www.peachfordhospital.com

SAINT SIMONS BY–THE–SEA HOSPITAL (O, 101 beds) 2927 Demere Road, Saint Simons Island, GA Zip 31522–1620; tel. 912/638–1999; Steve Glazier, Chief Executive Officer
**Web address:** www.ssbythesea.com

TURNING POINT HOSPITAL (O, 59 beds) 3015 Veterans Parkway South, Moultrie, GA Zip 31788–6705, Mailing Address: P.O. Box 1177, Zip 31776–1177; tel. 229/985–4815; Ben Marion, Chief Executive Officer and Managing Director
**Web address:** www.turningpointcare.com

**IDAHO:** INTERMOUNTAIN HOSPITAL (O, 140 beds) 303 North Allumbaugh Street, Boise, ID Zip 83704–9266; tel. 208/377–8400; Brent J. Bryson, Chief Executive Officer
**Web address:** www.intermountainhospital.com

**ILLINOIS:** HARTGROVE HOSPITAL (O, 128 beds) 5730 West Roosevelt Road, Chicago, IL Zip 60644; tel. 773/413–1700; Steven Airhart, Chief Executive Officer
**Web address:** www.uhsinc.com

LINCOLN PRAIRIE BEHAVIORAL HEALTH CENTER (O, 88 beds) 5230 South Sixth Street, Springfield, IL Zip 62703; tel. 217/585–1180; Mark Littrell, Chief Executive Officer
**Web address:** www.lincolnprairiebhc.com/

RIVEREDGE HOSPITAL (O, 224 beds) 8311 West Roosevelt Road, Forest Park, IL Zip 60130–2500; tel. 708/771–7000; Carey Carlock, Chief Executive Officer
**Web address:** www.riveredgehospital.com

STREAMWOOD BEHAVIORAL HEALTH CENTER (O, 177 beds) 1400 East Irving Park Road, Streamwood, IL Zip 60107–3203; tel. 630/837–9000; Roxane Harcourt, Chief Executive Officer
**Web address:** www.streamwoodhospital.com

THE PAVILION (O, 46 beds) 809 West Church Street, Champaign, IL Zip 61820–3399; tel. 217/373–1700; Joseph Sheehy, Chief Executive Officer and Managing Director
**Web address:** www.pavilionhospital.com

**INDIANA:** BLOOMINGTON MEADOWS HOSPITAL (O, 67 beds) 3600 North Prow Road, Bloomington, IN Zip 47404; tel. 812/331–8000; Jean Scallon, Chief Executive Officer
**Web address:** www.bloomingtonmeadows.com

MICHIANA BEHAVIORAL HEALTH CENTER (O, 76 beds) 1800 North Oak Drive, Plymouth, IN Zip 46563–3492; tel. 574/936–3784; Bryan W. Lett, Chief Executive Officer
**Web address:** www.michianabhc.com

VALLE VISTA HOSPITAL (O, 102 beds) 898 East Main Street, Greenwood, IN Zip 46143–1400; tel. 317/887–1348; Sherri R. Jewett, Chief Executive Officer
**Web address:** www.vallevistahospital.com

WELLSTONE REGIONAL HOSPITAL (O, 100 beds) 2700 Vissing Park Road, Jeffersonville, IN Zip 47130; tel. 812/284–8000; Thomas Stormanns, Chief Executive Officer
**Web address:** www.wellstonehospital.com

**KENTUCKY:** CUMBERLAND HALL HOSPITAL (O, 64 beds) 210 West 17th Street, Hopkinsville, KY Zip 42240–1912; tel. 270/886–1919; James Spruyt, Chief Executive Officer
**Web address:** www.cumberlandhallhospital.com

LINCOLN TRAIL BEHAVIORAL HEALTH SYSTEM (O, 67 beds) 3909 South Wilson Road, Radcliff, KY Zip 40160–9714, Mailing Address: P.O. Box 369, Zip 40159–0369; tel. 270/351–9444; Charles L. Webb, Jr., Administrator
**Web address:** www.lincolnbehavioral.com

RIDGE BEHAVIORAL HEALTH SYSTEM (O, 110 beds) 3050 Rio Dosa Drive, Lexington, KY Zip 40509–9990; tel. 859/269–2325; Nina W. Eisner, Chief Executive Officer and Managing Director
**Web address:** www.ridgebhs.com

RIVENDELL BEHAVIORAL HEALTH (O, 125 beds) 1035 Porter Pike, Bowling Green, KY Zip 42103; tel. 270/843–1199; Janice Richardson, Chief Executive Officer and Managing Director
**Web address:** www.rivendellbehavioral.com

THE BROOK AT DUPONT (O, 66 beds) 1405 Browns Lane, Louisville, KY Zip 40207; tel. 502/896–0495; Paul Andrews, Chief Executive Officer
**Web address:** www.thebrookhospitals.com/

THE BROOK HOSPITAL – KMI (O, 110 beds) 8521 Old Lagrange Road, Louisville, KY Zip 40223; tel. 502/426–6380; Paul Andrews, Chief Executive Officer
**Web address:** www.thebrookhospitals.com

**LOUISIANA:** BRENTWOOD HOSPITAL (O, 160 beds) 1006 Highland Avenue, Shreveport, LA Zip 71101–4103; tel. 318/678–7500; James Duff, Chief Executive Officer
**Web address:** www.brentwoodbehavioral.com

RIVER OAKS HOSPITAL (O, 126 beds) 1525 River Oaks Road West, New Orleans, LA Zip 70123–2162; tel. 504/734–1740; Evelyn Nolting, Chief Executive Officer and Managing Director
**Web address:** www.riveroakshospital.com

**MASSACHUSETTS:** ARBOUR H. R. I. HOSPITAL (O, 68 beds) 227 Babcock Street, Brookline, MA Zip 02146–6799; tel. 617/731–3200; Patrick Moallemian, Chief Executive Officer and Managing Director
**Web address:** www.arbourhealth.com

For explanation of codes following names, see page B2.
★ Indicates Type III membership in the American Hospital Association.

ARBOUR HOSPITAL (O, 118 beds) 49 Robinwood Avenue, Boston, MA Zip 02130–2156; tel. 617/522–4400; Joseph Murphy, Chief Executive Officer
**Web address:** www.arbourhealth.com

ARBOUR–FULLER HOSPITAL (O, 46 beds) 200 May Street, Attleboro, MA Zip 02703–5520; tel. 508/761–8500; Lisa Pappone, Chief Executive Officer
**Web address:** www.arbourhealth.com

PEMBROKE HOSPITAL (O, 80 beds) 199 Oak Street, Pembroke, MA Zip 02359–1953; tel. 781/829–7000; Thomas P. Hickey, Chief Executive Officer and Managing Director
**Web address:** www.arbourhealth.com/pembroke.htm

WESTWOOD LODGE HOSPITAL (O, 130 beds) 45 Clapboardtree Street, Westwood, MA Zip 02090–2930; tel. 781/762–7764; Gregory Brownstein, Chief Executive Officer
**Web address:** www.arbourhealth.com

**MICHIGAN:** FOREST VIEW PSYCHIATRIC HOSPITAL (O, 82 beds) 1055 Medical Park Drive S.E., Grand Rapids, MI Zip 49546–3607; tel. 616/942–9610; Andrew Hotaling, Chief Executive Officer
**Web address:** www.forestviewhospital.com

HAVENWYCK HOSPITAL (O, 242 beds) 1525 University Drive, Auburn Hills, MI Zip 48326–2673; tel. 248/373–9200; David C. Bell, Chief Executive Officer
**Web address:** www.havenwyckhospital.com

**MISSISSIPPI:** ALLIANCE HEALTH CENTER (O, 134 beds) 5000 Highway 39 North, Meridian, MS Zip 39301–1021; tel. 601/483–6211; William M. Patterson, Chief Executive Officer
**Web address:** www.alliancehealthcenter.com

BRENTWOOD BEHAVIORAL HEALTHCARE OF MISSISSIPPI (O, 105 beds) 3531 East Lakeland Drive, Jackson, MS Zip 39296–9794; tel. 601/936–2024; Michael J. Carney, Chief Executive Officer
**Web address:** www.brentwoodjackson.com

DIAMOND GROVE CENTER FOR CHILDREN AND ADOLESCENTS (O, 55 beds) 2311 Highway 15 South, Louisville, MS Zip 39339, Mailing Address: P.O. Box 848, Zip 39339; tel. 662/779–0119; Patrick R. Swoopes, Administrator
**Web address:** www.ccs.state.ms.us

PARKWOOD BEHAVIORAL HEALTH SYSTEM (O, 128 beds) 8135 Goodman Road, Olive Branch, MS Zip 38654–2103; tel. 662/895–4900; Ethan Permenter, Chief Executive Officer
**Web address:** www.parkwoodbhs.com

**MISSOURI:** HEARTLAND BEHAVIORAL HEALTH SERVICES (O, 37 beds) 1500 West Ashland Street, Nevada, MO Zip 64772–1710; tel. 417/667–2666; Alyson Wysong–Harder, Chief Executive Officer
**Web address:** www.heartlandbehavioral.com

TWO RIVERS BEHAVIORAL HEALTH SYSTEM (O, 105 beds) 5121 Raytown Road, Kansas City, MO Zip 64133–2141; tel. 816/382–6300; Scott Hullinger, Chief Executive Officer
**Web address:** www.tworivershospital.com

**NEVADA:** CENTENNIAL HILLS HOSPITAL MEDICAL CENTER (O, 171 beds) 6900 North Durango Drive, Las Vegas, NV Zip 89148; tel. 702/835–9700; Sajit Pullarkat, Chief Executive Officer and Managing Director
**Web address:** www.centennialhillshospital.com

DESERT SPRINGS HOSPITAL MEDICAL CENTER (O, 346 beds) 2075 East Flamingo Road, Las Vegas, NV Zip 89119–5121; tel. 702/733–8800; Samuel Kaufman, Chief Executive Officer and Managing Director
**Web address:** www.desertspringshospital.net

NORTHERN NEVADA MEDICAL CENTER (O, 80 beds) 2375 East Prater Way, Sparks, NV Zip 89434–9900; tel. 775/331–7000; Mark W. Crawford, Chief Executive Officer
**Web address:** www.nnmc.com

SPRING MOUNTAIN SAHARA (O, 30 beds) 5460 West Sahara, Las Vegas, NV Zip 89146; tel. 702/216–8900; Darryl S. Dubroca, Chief Executive Officer and Managing Director
**Web address:** www.springmountainsahara.com

SPRING MOUNTAIN TREATMENT CENTER (L, 82 beds) 7000 West Spring Mountain Road, Las Vegas, NV Zip 89117; tel. 702/873–2400; Darryl S. Dubroca, Chief Executive Officer and Managing Director
**Web address:** www.healthsouth.com

SPRING VALLEY HOSPITAL MEDICAL CENTER (O, 169 beds) 5400 South Rainbow Boulevard, Las Vegas, NV Zip 89118; tel. 702/853–3000; Leonard Freehof, Chief Executive Officer and Managing Director
**Web address:** www.springvalleyhospital.com

SUMMERLIN HOSPITAL MEDICAL CENTER (O, 148 beds) 657 Town Center Drive, Las Vegas, NV Zip 89144; tel. 702/233–7000; Robert S. Freymuller, Chief Executive Officer
**Web address:** www.summerlinhospital.org

VALLEY HOSPITAL MEDICAL CENTER (O, 365 beds) 620 Shadow Lane, Las Vegas, NV Zip 89106–4119; tel. 702/388–4000; Jay Finnegan, Chief Executive Officer
**Web address:** www.valleyhospital.net

WEST HILLS HOSPITAL (O, 95 beds) 1240 East Ninth Street, Reno, NV Zip 89512–2997, Mailing Address: P.O. Box 30012, Zip 89520–3012; tel. 775/323–0478; Steve Shell, Chief Executive Officer
**Web address:** www.westhillshospital.net

**NEW JERSEY:** HAMPTON BEHAVIORAL HEALTH CENTER (O, 110 beds) 650 Rancocas Road, Westampton Township, NJ Zip 08060–5613; Mount Holly, tel. 609/267–7000; Craig Hilton, Chief Executive Officer
**Web address:** www.hamptonhospital.com

SUMMIT OAKS HOSPITAL (O, 90 beds) 19 Prospect Street, Summit, NJ Zip 07902–0100; tel. 908/522–7000; James P. Gallagher, Chief Executive Officer
**Web address:** www.summitoakshospital.com/

**NEW MEXICO:** MESILLA VALLEY HOSPITAL (O, 126 beds) 3751 Del Rey Boulevard, Las Cruces, NM Zip 88012–8526; tel. 575/382–3500; Brian Hemmert, Chief Executive Officer
**Web address:** www.mesillavalleyhospital.com

PEAK BEHAVIORAL HEALTH SERVICES (O, 120 beds) 5065 McNutt Road, Santa Teresa, NM Zip 88008–9442; tel. 575/589–3000; Jacob Cuellar, M.D., Chief Executive Officer
**Web address:** www.peakbehavioral.com/

**NORTH CAROLINA:** BRYNN MARR HOSPITAL (O, 87 beds) 192 Village Drive, Jacksonville, NC Zip 28546–7299; tel. 910/577–1400; Jay Kortemeyer, Chief Executive Officer
**Web address:** www.brynnmarr.org

HOLLY HILL HOSPITAL (O, 152 beds) 3019 Falstaff Road, Raleigh, NC Zip 27610–1812; tel. 919/250–7000; Robert L. Turner, Ph.D., Chief Executive Officer
**Web address:** www.hollyhillhospital.com

OLD VINEYARD BEHAVIORAL HEALTH SERVICES (O, 102 beds) 3637 Old Vineyard Road, Winston–Salem, NC Zip 27104–4842; tel. 336/794–3550; Kevin Patton, Chief Executive Officer
**Web address:** www.oldvineyard.net

**NORTH DAKOTA:** PRAIRIE ST. JOHN'S (O, 89 beds) 510 4th Street South, Fargo, ND Zip 58103–1914; tel. 701/476–7200; Gregory LaFrancois, Chief Executive Officer
**Web address:** www.prairie–stjohns.com

**OHIO:** ARROWHEAD BEHAVIORAL HEALTH HOSPITAL (O, 42 beds) 1725 Timber Line Road, Maumee, OH Zip 43537–4015; tel. 419/891–9333; Elyssia Lowe–Narayan, Chief Executive Officer
**Web address:** www.arrowheadbehavioral.com

BELMONT PINES HOSPITAL (O, 46 beds) 615 Churchill–Hubbard Road, Youngstown, OH Zip 44505–1379; tel. 330/759–2700; George H. Perry, Ph.D., Chief Executive Officer
**Web address:** www.belmontpines.com

WINDSOR–LAURELWOOD CENTER FOR BEHAVIORAL MEDICINE (O, 152 beds) 35900 Euclid Avenue, Willoughby, OH Zip 44094–4648; tel. 440/953–3000; Daniel Aranda, Chief Executive Officer
**Web address:** www.windsorlaurelwood.com

**OKLAHOMA:** CEDAR RIDGE HOSPITAL (O, 116 beds) 6501 N.E. 50th Street, Oklahoma City, OK Zip 73141; tel. 405/605–6111; Kevan Finley, Chief Executive Officer
**Web address:** www.cedarridgebhs.com

SHADOW MOUNTAIN BEHAVIORAL HEALTH SYSTEM (O, 202 beds) 6262 South Sheridan Road, Tulsa, OK Zip 74133–4055; tel. 918/492–8200; Mike Kistler, Chief Executive Officer
**Web address:** www.shadowmountainbhs.com

ST. MARY'S REGIONAL MEDICAL CENTER (O, 163 beds) 305 South Fifth Street, Enid, OK Zip 73701–5899, Mailing Address: P.O. Box 232, Zip 73702–0232; tel. 580/233–6100; Stanley D. Tatum, FACHE, Chief Executive Officer
**Web address:** www.stmarysregional.com

For explanation of codes following names, see page B2.
★ Indicates Type III membership in the American Hospital Association.

**PENNSYLVANIA:** BROOKE GLEN BEHAVIORAL HOSPITAL (O, 146 beds) 7170 Lafayette Avenue, Fort Washington, PA Zip 19034–0209; tel. 215/641–5300; Neil Callahan, Chief Executive Officer
**Web address:** www.brookeglenbehavioral.com

CLARION PSYCHIATRIC CENTER (O, 74 beds) 2 Hospital Drive, Clarion, PA Zip 16214–8502; tel. 814/226–9545; Robert Scheffler, Chief Executive Officer
**Web address:** www.clarioncenter.com

FAIRMOUNT BEHAVIORAL HEALTH SYSTEM (O, 239 beds) 561 Fairthorne Avenue, Philadelphia, PA Zip 19128–2499; tel. 215/487–4000; Charles McLister, Chief Executive Officer
**Web address:** www.fairmountbhs.com

FOUNDATIONS BEHAVIORAL HEALTH (O, 102 beds) 833 East Butler Avenue, Doylestown, PA Zip 18901–2280; tel. 215/345–0444; Robert Weinhold, Chief Executive Officer
**Web address:** www.fbh.com

FRIENDS HOSPITAL (O, 219 beds) 4641 Roosevelt Boulevard, Philadelphia, PA Zip 19124–2343; tel. 215/831–4600; Geoff Botak, Chief Executive Officer
**Web address:** www.friendshospital.com

HORSHAM CLINIC (O, 138 beds) 722 East Butler Pike, Ambler, PA Zip 19002–2310; tel. 215/643–7800; Phyllis Weisfield, Chief Executive Officer and Managing Director
**Web address:** www.horshamclinic.com

MEADOWS PSYCHIATRIC CENTER (O, 101 beds) 132 The Meadows Drive, Centre Hall, PA Zip 16828–9231; tel. 814/364–2161; Thomas Kenny, Chief Executive Officer
**Web address:** www.themeadows.net

ROXBURY TREATMENT CENTER (O, 94 beds) 601 Roxbury Road, Shippensburg, PA Zip 17257–9302; tel. 800/648–4673; Geoff Botak, Chief Executive Officer
**Web address:** www.roxburyhospital.com

**PUERTO RICO:** FIRST HOSPITAL PANAMERICANO (O, 153 beds) State Road 787 KM 1 5, Cidra, PR Zip 00739, Mailing Address: P.O. Box 1400, Zip 00739; tel. 787/739–5555; Marta Rivera, Executive Director
**Web address:** www.hospitalpanamericano.com

**SOUTH CAROLINA:** AIKEN REGIONAL MEDICAL CENTERS (O, 256 beds) 302 University Parkway, Aiken, SC Zip 29801–2757; tel. 803/641–5000; Carlos Milanes, Chief Executive Officer and Managing Director
**Web address:** www.aikenregional.com

CAROLINA CENTER FOR BEHAVIORAL HEALTH (O, 112 beds) 2700 East Phillips Road, Greer, SC Zip 29650–4816; tel. 864/235–2335; John Willingham, Chief Executive Officer and Managing Director
**Web address:** www.thecarolinacenter.com

LIGHTHOUSE CARE CENTER OF CONWAY (O, 52 beds) 152 Waccamaw Medical Park Drive, Conway, SC Zip 29526–8901; tel. 843/347–8871; Thomas L. Ryba, Chief Executive Officer
**Web address:** www.lighthousecarecenterofconway.com/

PALMETTO LOWCOUNTRY BEHAVIORAL HEALTH (O, 112 beds) 2777 Speissegger Drive, Charleston, SC Zip 29405–8299; tel. 843/747–5830; Cherie Tolley, Chief Executive Officer
**Web address:** www.plbhs.com

THREE RIVERS BEHAVIORAL HEALTH (O, 98 beds) 2900 Sunset Boulevard, West Columbia, SC Zip 29169–3422; tel. 803/796–9911; Jeffrey Barnett, Chief Executive Officer
**Web address:** www.threeriversbehavioral.org

**TENNESSEE:** LAKESIDE BEHAVIORAL HEALTH SYSTEM (O, 311 beds) 2911 Brunswick Road, Memphis, TN Zip 38133–4199; tel. 901/377–4700; Shelley A. Nowak, Chief Executive Officer
**Web address:** www.lakesidebhs.com

ROLLING HILLS HOSPITAL (O, 80 beds) 2014 Quail Hollow Circle, Franklin, TN Zip 37067–5967; tel. 615/628–5700; Richard A. Bangert, Chief Executive Officer
**Web address:** www.rollinghillshospital.org/

**TEXAS:** AUSTIN LAKES HOSPITAL (O, 54 beds) 1025 East 32nd Street, Austin, TX Zip 78705–2714; tel. 512/544–5253; Ramona Key, Chief Executive Officer
**Web address:** www.austinlakeshospital.com

CORNERSTONE REGIONAL HOSPITAL (L, 14 beds) 2302 Cornerstone Boulevard, Edinburg, TX Zip 78539–8471; tel. 956/618–4444; Alma Medina, R.N., Chief Executive Officer
**Web address:** www.southtexashealthsystem.com/Facilities/Cornerstone–Regional–Hospital

CYPRESS CREEK HOSPITAL (O, 96 beds) 17750 Cali Drive, Houston, TX Zip 77090–2700; tel. 281/586–7600; Brian Brooker, Chief Executive Officer
**Web address:** www.cypresscreekhospital.com

DOCTORS HOSPITAL OF LAREDO (O, 183 beds) 10700 McPherson Road, Laredo, TX Zip 78045; tel. 956/523–2000; Elmo Lopez, Jr., Chief Executive Officer
**Web address:** www.doctorshosplaredo.com

FORT DUNCAN REGIONAL MEDICAL CENTER (O, 101 beds) 3333 North Foster Maldonado Boulevard, Eagle Pass, TX Zip 78852–5893; tel. 830/773–5321; Rene Lopez, Chief Executive Officer
**Web address:** www.fortduncanmedicalcenter.com

GLEN OAKS HOSPITAL (O, 54 beds) 301 Division Street, Greenville, TX Zip 75401–4101; tel. 903/454–6000; Joel Klein, Chief Executive Officer and Managing Director
**Web address:** www.glenoakshospital.com

HICKORY TRAIL HOSPITAL (O, 86 beds) 2000 Old Hickory Trail, Desoto, TX Zip 75115–2242; tel. 972/298–7323; Mercy Estevez, Chief Executive Officer
**Web address:** www.hickorytrail.com

KINGWOOD PINES HOSPITAL (O, 116 beds) 2001 Ladbrook Drive, Kingwood, TX Zip 77339; tel. 281/358–1495; James Burroughs, Chief Executive Officer
**Web address:** www.kingwoodpines.com

LAUREL RIDGE TREATMENT CENTER (O, 190 beds) 17720 Corporate Woods Drive, San Antonio, TX Zip 78259–3500; tel. 210/491–9400; Dan Thomas, Chief Executive Officer
**Web address:** www.laurelridgetc.com

MILLWOOD HOSPITAL (O, 122 beds) 1011 North Cooper Street, Arlington, TX Zip 76011–5517; tel. 817/261–3121; Jon C. O'Shaughnessy, Chief Executive Officer
**Web address:** www.millwoodhospital.com

NORTHWEST TEXAS HEALTHCARE SYSTEM (O, 426 beds) 1501 South Coulter Avenue, Amarillo, TX Zip 79106–1790, Mailing Address: P.O. Box 1110, Zip 79105–1110; tel. 806/354–1000; Sharon Oxendale, Interim Chief Executive Officer and Managing Director
**Web address:** www.nwtexashealthcare.com

RIVER CREST HOSPITAL (O, 80 beds) 1636 Hunters Glen Road, San Angelo, TX Zip 76901–5016; tel. 325/949–5722; Shelah Adams, Chief Executive Officer
**Web address:** www.rivercresthospital.com

SOUTH TEXAS HEALTH SYSTEM (O, 775 beds) 1102 West Trenton Road, Edinburg, TX Zip 78539–9105; tel. 956/388–6000; Linda Resendez, R.N., Chief Executive Officer
**Web address:** www.southtexashealthsystem.com

TEXAS NEUROREHAB CENTER (O, 47 beds) 1106 West Dittmar, Austin, TX Zip 78745–6388, Mailing Address: P.O. Box 150459, Zip 78715–0459; tel. 512/444–4835; Edgar E. Prettyman, PsyD, Chief Executive Officer
**Web address:** www.texasneurorehab.com

TEXOMA MEDICAL CENTER (O, 251 beds) 5016 U.S. Highway 75 S., Denison, TX Zip 75020–2035, Mailing Address: P.O. Box 890, Zip 75021–0890; tel. 903/416–4000; Ronald T. Seal, Chief Executive Officer
**Web address:** www.texomamedicalcenter.net

TIMBERLAWN MENTAL HEALTH SYSTEM (O, 144 beds) 4600 Samuell Boulevard, Dallas, TX Zip 75228–6800; tel. 214/381–7181; Craig Nuckles, Chief Executive Officer, Managing and Regional Vice President
**Web address:** www.timberlawn.com

WEST OAKS HOSPITAL (O, 144 beds) 6500 Hornwood Drive, Houston, TX Zip 77074–5095; tel. 713/995–0909; Tim C. Simmons, Chief Executive Officer
**Web address:** www.westoakshospital.com

**VIRGINIA:** CUMBERLAND HOSPITAL (O, 132 beds) 9407 Cumberland Road, New Kent, VA Zip 23124–0150; tel. 804/966–2242; Patrice Gay Brooks, Chief Executive Officer
**Web address:** www.cumberlandhospital.com

POPLAR SPRINGS HOSPITAL (O, 120 beds) 350 Poplar Drive, Petersburg, VA Zip 23805–9367; tel. 804/733–6874; Richard Clark, Chief Executive Officer
**Web address:** www.poplarsprings.com

Section B

For explanation of codes following names, see page B2.
★ Indicates Type III membership in the American Hospital Association.

VIRGINIA BEACH PSYCHIATRIC CENTER (O, 100 beds) 1100 First Colonial Road, Virginia Beach, VA Zip 23454; tel. 757/496–6000; Denise Webb, Administrator
**Web address:** www.absfirst.com

**WASHINGTON:** AUBURN REGIONAL MEDICAL CENTER (O, 120 beds) 202 North Division, Plaza One, Auburn, WA Zip 98001–4908; tel. 253/833–7711; Robert Dickens, Interim Chief Executive Officer
**Web address:** www.auburnregional.com

FAIRFAX HOSPITAL (O, 95 beds) 10200 N.E. 132nd Street, Kirkland, WA Zip 98034–2899; tel. 425/821–2000; Ron Escarda, Chief Executive Officer
**Web address:** www.fairfaxhospital.com

**WEST VIRGINIA:** RIVER PARK HOSPITAL (O, 147 beds) 1230 Sixth Avenue, Huntington, WV Zip 25701–2312, Mailing Address: P.O. Box 1875, Zip 25719–1875; tel. 304/526–9111; Terry A. Stephens, Chief Executive Officer
**Web address:** www.riverparkhospital.net

**WYOMING:** WYOMING BEHAVIORAL INSTITUTE (O, 124 beds) 2521 East 15th Street, Casper, WY Zip 82609–4126; tel. 307/237–7444; Joseph Gallagher, Chief Executive Officer
**Web address:** www.wbihelp.com

| | | |
|---|---|---|
| Owned, leased, sponsored: | 134 hospitals | 17178 beds |
| Contract–managed: | 0 hospitals | 0 beds |
| Totals: | 134 hospitals | 17178 beds |

---

**★0112: UNIVERSITY HOSPITALS** (NP)
11100 Euclid Avenue, Cleveland, OH Zip 44106–5000; tel. 216/844–1000; Thomas F. Zenty, III, President and Chief Executive Officer
**(Centralized Physician/Insurance Health System)**

**OHIO:** UNIVERSITY HOSPITALS AHUJA MEDICAL CENTER (O, 92 beds) 3999 Richmond Road, Beachwood, OH Zip 44122–6805; tel. 216/593–5500; Susan V. Juris, President
**Web address:** www.uhhospitals. org/ahuja/tabid/7051/uhahujamedicalcenter.aspx

UNIVERSITY HOSPITALS BEDFORD MEDICAL CENTER (O, 77 beds) 44 Blaine Avenue, Cleveland, OH Zip 44146–2709; tel. 440/735–3900; Laurie Delgado, President
**Web address:** www.uhbedford.org

UNIVERSITY HOSPITALS CASE MEDICAL CENTER (O, 777 beds) 11100 Euclid Avenue, Cleveland, OH Zip 44106–2602; tel. 216/844–1000; Fred C. Rothstein, M.D., President
**Web address:** www.UHhospitals.org

UNIVERSITY HOSPITALS CONNEAUT MEDICAL CENTER (O, 25 beds) 158 West Main Road, Conneaut, OH Zip 44030–2039; tel. 440/593–1131; Robert David, President and Chief Executive Officer
**Web address:** www.uhhospitals.org

UNIVERSITY HOSPITALS GEAUGA MEDICAL CENTER (O, 126 beds) 13207 Ravenna Road, Chardon, OH Zip 44024–7032; tel. 440/269–6000; M. Steven Jones, President
**Web address:** www.uhhospitals.org/geauga/

UNIVERSITY HOSPITALS GENEVA MEDICAL CENTER (O, 25 beds) 870 West Main Street, Geneva, OH Zip 44041–1295; tel. 440/466–1141; Robert David, President and Chief Executive Officer
**Web address:** www.uhhs.com

UNIVERSITY HOSPITALS RICHMOND MEDICAL CENTER (O, 60 beds) 27100 Chardon Road, Cleveland, OH Zip 44143–1116; tel. 440/585–6500; Laurie Delgado, President
**Web address:** www.uhrichmond.org

| | | |
|---|---|---|
| Owned, leased, sponsored: | 7 hospitals | 1182 beds |
| Contract–managed: | 0 hospitals | 0 beds |
| Totals: | 7 hospitals | 1182 beds |

---

**★6405: UNIVERSITY OF CALIFORNIA–SYSTEMWIDE ADMINISTRATION** (NP)
1111 Franklin Street, 11th Floor, Oakland, CA Zip 94607–5200; tel. 510/987–9071; John D. Stobo, M.D., Senior Vice President Health Sciences and Services
**(Moderately Centralized Health System)**

**CALIFORNIA:** RONALD REAGAN UNIVERSITY OF CALIFORNIA LOS ANGELES MEDICAL CENTER (O, 466 beds) 757 Westwood Plaza, Los Angeles, CA Zip 90095–8358; tel. 310/825–9111; David Feinberg, M.D., Chief Executive Officer
**Web address:** www.uclahealth.org

SANTA MONICA–UCLA MEDICAL CENTER AND ORTHOPAEDIC HOSPITAL (O, 316 beds) 1250 16th Street, Santa Monica, CA Zip 90404; tel. 310/319–4000; Posie Carpenter, R.N., MSN, Chief Administrative Officer
**Web address:** www.healthcare.ucla.edu

STEWART & LYNDA RESNICK NEUROPSYCHIATRIC HOSPITAL AT UCLA (O, 74 beds) 760 Westwood Plaza, Los Angeles, CA Zip 90095–8353; tel. 310/825–9989; Thomas Strouse, M.D., Medical Director
**Web address:** www.semel.ucla.edu/resnick

UC SAN DIEGO HEALTH SYSTEM (O, 530 beds) 200 West Arbor Drive, San Diego, CA Zip 92103–8970; tel. 619/543–6222; Paul S. Viviano, Chief Executive Officer
**Web address:** www.health.ucsd.edu

UCSF MEDICAL CENTER (O, 660 beds) 500 Parnassus Avenue, San Francisco, CA Zip 94143–0296, Mailing Address: 500 Parnassus Avenue, Box 0296, Zip 94143–0296; tel. 415/476–1000; Mark R. Laret, Chief Executive Officer
**Web address:** www.ucsfhealth.org

UNIVERSITY OF CALIFORNIA, DAVIS MEDICAL CENTER (O, 567 beds) 2315 Stockton Boulevard, Sacramento, CA Zip 95817–2282; tel. 916/734–2011; Ann Madden Rice, Chief Executive Officer
**Web address:** www.ucdmc.ucdavis.edu

UNIVERSITY OF CALIFORNIA, IRVINE HEALTHCARE (O, 363 beds) 101 The City Drive, Orange, CA Zip 92868–3298; tel. 714/456–6011; Terry A. Belmont, Chief Executive Officer
**Web address:** www.ucihealth.com

| | | |
|---|---|---|
| Owned, leased, sponsored: | 7 hospitals | 2976 beds |
| Contract–managed: | 0 hospitals | 0 beds |
| Totals: | 7 hospitals | 2976 beds |

---

**★0216: UNIVERSITY OF MARYLAND MEDICAL SYSTEM** (NP)
250 West Pratt Street, 24th Floor, Baltimore, MD Zip 21201–1595; tel. 410/328–8667; Robert A. Chrencik, President and Chief Executive Officer
**(Centralized Health System)**

**MARYLAND:** BALTIMORE WASHINGTON MEDICAL CENTER (O, 321 beds) 301 Hospital Drive, Glen Burnie, MD Zip 21061–5899; tel. 410/787–4000; Karen E. Olscamp, Chief Executive Officer
**Web address:** www.bwmc.umms.org

CHESTER RIVER HEALTH SYSTEM (O, 47 beds) 100 Brown Street, Chestertown, MD Zip 21620–1499; tel. 410/778–3300; James E. Ross, FACHE, President and Chief Executive Officer
**Web address:** www.chesterriverhealth.org

CIVISTA HEALTH (O, 124 beds) 5 Garrett Avenue, La Plata, MD Zip 20646–1070, Mailing Address: P.O. Box 1070, Zip 20646–1070; tel. 301/609–4000; Noel A. Cervino, President and Chief Executive Officer
**Web address:** www.civista.org

DORCHESTER GENERAL HOSPITAL (O, 44 beds) 300 Byrn Street, Cambridge, MD Zip 21613–1908; tel. 410/228–5511; Kenneth D. Kozel, FACHE, President and Chief Executive Officer
**Web address:** www.shorehealth.org

KERNAN ORTHOPAEDICS AND REHABILITATION (O, 104 beds) 2200 Kernan Drive, Baltimore, MD Zip 21207–6697; tel. 410/448–2500; Michael Jablonover, M.D., President and Chief Executive Officer
**Web address:** www.kernan.org

MARYLAND GENERAL HOSPITAL (O, 212 beds) 827 Linden Avenue, Baltimore, MD Zip 21201–4681; tel. 410/225–8000; Sylvia Smith Johnson, President and Chief Executive Officer
**Web address:** www.marylandgeneral.org

MEMORIAL HOSPITAL AT EASTON MARYLAND (O, 107 beds) 219 South Washington Street, Easton, MD Zip 21601–2996; tel. 410/822–1000; Kenneth D. Kozel, FACHE, President and Chief Executive Officer
**Web address:** www.shorehealth.org

---

For explanation of codes following names, see page B2.
★ Indicates Type III membership in the American Hospital Association.

MT. WASHINGTON PEDIATRIC HOSPITAL (O, 70 beds) 1708 West Rogers Avenue, Baltimore, MD Zip 21209–4537; tel. 410/578–8600; Sheldon J. Stein, President and Chief Executive Officer
**Web address:** www.mwph.org

UNIVERSITY OF MARYLAND MEDICAL CENTER (O, 819 beds) 22 South Greene Street, Baltimore, MD Zip 21201–1595; tel. 410/328–8667; Jeffrey A. Rivest, FACHE, President and Chief Executive Officer
**Web address:** www.umm.edu

| Owned, leased, sponsored: | 9 hospitals | 1848 beds |
| Contract–managed: | 0 hospitals | 0 beds |
| Totals: | 9 hospitals | 1848 beds |

---

**★0227: UNIVERSITY OF MISSOURI HEALTH CARE** (NP)
One Hospital Drive, DC 031, Columbia, MO Zip 65212–0001; tel. 573/884–8738; James H. Ross, Chief Executive Officer
**(Centralized Health System)**

**MISSOURI:** CAPITAL REGION MEDICAL CENTER (O, 114 beds) 1125 Madison Street, Jefferson City, MO Zip 65101–5200, Mailing Address: P.O. Box 1128, Zip 65102–1128; tel. 573/632–5000; Edward F. Farnsworth, FACHE, President
**Web address:** www.crmc.org

COOPER COUNTY MEMORIAL HOSPITAL (C, 32 beds) 17651 B Highway, Boonville, MO Zip 65233–2839, Mailing Address: P.O. Box 88, Zip 65233–0088; tel. 660/882–7461; Allen J. Waldo, FACHE, CPA, Chief Executive Officer
**Web address:** www.coopercmh.com

MISSOURI REHABILITATION CENTER (O, 79 beds) 600 North Main Street, Mount Vernon, MO Zip 65712–1004; tel. 417/466–3711; Steve Patterson, R.N., Executive Director
**Web address:** www.muhealth.org/~MOrehab

UNIVERSITY OF MISSOURI HOSPITALS AND CLINICS (O, 477 beds) One Hospital Drive, Columbia, MO Zip 65212–0001; tel. 573/882–4141; James H. Ross, Chief Executive Officer
**Web address:** www.muhealth.org

WOMEN'S AND CHILDREN'S HOSPITAL (O, 108 beds) 404 Keene Street, Columbia, MO Zip 65201–6626; tel. 573/875–9000; Keri Simon, Executive Director
**Web address:** www.muchildrenshospital.org

| Owned, leased, sponsored: | 4 hospitals | 778 beds |
| Contract–managed: | 1 hospital | 32 beds |
| Totals: | 5 hospitals | 810 beds |

---

**★0168: UNIVERSITY OF PENNSYLVANIA HEALTH SYSTEM** (NP)
3400 Civic Center Boulevard, Philadelphia, PA Zip 19104–5127; tel. 215/662–2203; Ralph W. Muller, President and Chief Executive Officer
**(Centralized Physician/Insurance Health System)**

**PENNSYLVANIA:** HOSPITAL OF THE UNIVERSITY OF PENNSYLVANIA (O, 782 beds) 3400 Spruce Street, Philadelphia, PA Zip 19104–4206; tel. 215/662–4000; Garry L. Scheib, Executive Director
**Web address:** www.pennhealth.com

PENN PRESBYTERIAN MEDICAL CENTER (O, 331 beds) 51 North 39th Street, Philadelphia, PA Zip 19104–2699; tel. 215/662–8000; Michele M. Volpe, Executive Director and Chief Executive Officer
**Web address:** www.pennmedicine.org/pmc/

PENNSYLVANIA HOSPITAL (O, 474 beds) 800 Spruce Street, Philadelphia, PA Zip 19107–6192; tel. 215/829–3000; R. Michael Buckley, M.D., Executive Director
**Web address:** www.pahosp.com

| Owned, leased, sponsored: | 3 hospitals | 1587 beds |
| Contract–managed: | 0 hospitals | 0 beds |
| Totals: | 3 hospitals | 1587 beds |

---

**★0223: UNIVERSITY OF ROCHESTER MEDICAL CENTER** (NP)
601 Elmwood Avenue, Rochester, NY Zip 14642–0002; tel. 585/275–2100; Steven I. Goldstein, General Director and Chief Executive Officer
**(Centralized Health System)**

**NEW YORK:** F. F. THOMPSON HOSPITAL (O, 267 beds) 350 Parrish Street, Canandaigua, NY Zip 14424–1731; tel. 585/396–6000; Michael Stapleton, R.N., MS, President and Chief Executive Officer
**Web address:** www.thompsonhealth.com

HIGHLAND HOSPITAL OF ROCHESTER (O, 261 beds) 1000 South Avenue, Rochester, NY Zip 14620–2733; tel. 585/473–2200; Steven I. Goldstein, President and Chief Executive Officer
**Web address:** www.stronghealth.com

STRONG MEMORIAL HOSPITAL OF THE UNIVERSITY OF ROCHESTER (O, 750 beds) 601 Elmwood Avenue, Rochester, NY Zip 14642–0002; tel. 585/275–2100; Steven I. Goldstein, President and Chief Executive Officer
**Web address:** www.urmc.rochester.edu

| Owned, leased, sponsored: | 3 hospitals | 1278 beds |
| Contract–managed: | 0 hospitals | 0 beds |
| Totals: | 3 hospitals | 1278 beds |

---

**★0057: UNIVERSITY OF SOUTH ALABAMA HOSPITALS** (NP)
2451 Fillingim Street, Mobile, AL Zip 36617–2238; tel. 251/471–7000; Stanley K. Hammack, Chief Executive Officer
**(Independent Hospital System)**

**ALABAMA:** UNIVERSITY OF SOUTH ALABAMA CHILDREN'S AND WOMEN'S HOSPITAL (O, 198 beds) 1700 Center Street, Mobile, AL Zip 36604–3301; tel. 251/415–1000; Owen Bailey, Administrator
**Web address:** www.usahealthsystem.com/usacwh

UNIVERSITY OF SOUTH ALABAMA MEDICAL CENTER (O, 114 beds) 2451 Fillingim Street, Mobile, AL Zip 36617–2293; tel. 251/471–7000; A. Elizabeth Anderson, Administrator
**Web address:** www.usahospitals.org

| Owned, leased, sponsored: | 2 hospitals | 312 beds |
| Contract–managed: | 0 hospitals | 0 beds |
| Totals: | 2 hospitals | 312 beds |

---

**★0033: UNIVERSITY OF TEXAS SYSTEM** (NP)
601 Colorado Street, Suite 205, Austin, TX Zip 78701–2982; tel. 512/499–4224; Kenneth Shine, M.D., Executive Vice Chancellor
**(Moderately Centralized Health System)**

**TEXAS:** UNIVERSITY OF TEXAS HARRIS COUNTY PSYCHIATRIC CENTER (O, 211 beds) 2800 South MacGregor Way, Houston, TX Zip 77021–1000, Mailing Address: P.O. Box 20249, Zip 77225–0249; tel. 713/741–5000; Jair C. Soares, M.D., Executive Director
**Web address:** www.uth.tmc.edu

UNIVERSITY OF TEXAS HEALTH SCIENCE CENTER AT TYLER (O, 116 beds) 11937 Highway 271, Tyler, TX Zip 75708–3154; tel. 903/877–7777; Kirk A. Calhoun, M.D., President
**Web address:** www.uthct.edu

UNIVERSITY OF TEXAS M.D. ANDERSON CANCER CENTER (O, 607 beds) 1515 Holcombe Boulevard, Box 91, Houston, TX Zip 77030–4095; tel. 713/792–2121; Ronald A. DePinho, M.D., President
**Web address:** www.mdanderson.org

UNIVERSITY OF TEXAS MEDICAL BRANCH HOSPITALS (O, 428 beds) 301 University Boulevard, Galveston, TX Zip 77555–0128; tel. 409/772–1011; Donna K. Sollenberger, Executive Vice President and Chief Executive Officer
**Web address:** www.utmb.edu

| Owned, leased, sponsored: | 4 hospitals | 1362 beds |
| Contract–managed: | 0 hospitals | 0 beds |
| Totals: | 4 hospitals | 1362 beds |

---

For explanation of codes following names, see page B2.
★ Indicates Type III membership in the American Hospital Association.

Section B

**0137: UPMC** (NP)
600 Grant Street, U.S. Steel Tower, Suite 6262, Pittsburgh, PA Zip 15219; tel. 412/647-4800; Jeffrey A. Romoff, President and Chief Executive Officer
**(Centralized Physician/Insurance Health System)**

**PENNSYLVANIA:** CHILDREN'S HOSPITAL OF PITTSBURGH OF UPMC (O, 296 beds) 4401 Penn Avenue, Pittsburgh, PA Zip 15224-1334; tel. 412/692-5325; Christopher Gessner, President
**Web address:** www.chp.edu

MAGEE-WOMENS HOSPITAL OF UPMC (O, 318 beds) 300 Halket Street, Pittsburgh, PA Zip 15213-3108; tel. 412/641-1000; Leslie C. Davis, President
**Web address:** www.magee.edu

UPMC BEDFORD MEMORIAL (O, 27 beds) 10455 Lincoln Highway, Everett, PA Zip 15537-7046; tel. 814/623-6161; Roger P. Winn, President
**Web address:** www.upmcbedfordmemorial.com

UPMC HAMOT (O, 387 beds) 201 State Street, Erie, PA Zip 16550-0002; tel. 814/877-6000; John T. Malone, President and Chief Executive Officer
**Web address:** www.hamot.org

UPMC HORIZON (O, 187 beds) 110 North Main Street, Greenville, PA Zip 16125-1726; tel. 724/588-2100; Donald R. Owrey, President
**Web address:** www.horizon.upmc.com

UPMC MCKEESPORT (O, 231 beds) 1500 Fifth Avenue, McKeesport, PA Zip 15132-2422; tel. 412/664-2000; Cynthia M. Dorundo, President
**Web address:** www.mckeesport.upmc.com

UPMC MERCY (O, 488 beds) 1400 Locust Street, Pittsburgh, PA Zip 15219-5166; tel. 412/232-8111; Will L. Cook, President
**Web address:** www.upmc.com/HospitalsFacilities/HFHome/Hospitals/Mercy/

UPMC NORTHWEST (O, 180 beds) 100 Fairfield Drive, Seneca, PA Zip 16346; tel. 814/676-7600; David Gibbons, President
**Web address:** www.northwest.upmc.com

UPMC PASSAVANT (O, 412 beds) 9100 Babcock Boulevard, Pittsburgh, PA Zip 15237-5815; tel. 412/367-6700; David T. Martin, President
**Web address:** www.upmc.edu/passavant

UPMC PRESBYTERIAN SHADYSIDE (O, 1763 beds) 200 Lothrop Street, Pittsburgh, PA Zip 15213-2585; tel. 412/647-2345; John Innocenti, Sr., President and Chief Executive Officer
**Web address:** www.upmc.edu

UPMC ST. MARGARET (O, 249 beds) 815 Freeport Road, Pittsburgh, PA Zip 15215-3301; tel. 412/784-4000; Teresa G. Petrick, President
**Web address:** www.stmargaret.upmc.com

| | | |
|---|---|---|
| Owned, leased, sponsored: | 11 hospitals | 4538 beds |
| Contract-managed: | 0 hospitals | 0 beds |
| Totals: | 11 hospitals | 4538 beds |

**0816: UPPER ALLEGHENY HEALTH SYSTEM** (NP)
130 South Union Street, Suite 300, Olean, NY Zip 14760-3676; tel. 716/375-6190; Timothy J. Finan, FACHE, President and Chief Executive Officer

**NEW YORK:** OLEAN GENERAL HOSPITAL (O, 186 beds) 515 Main Street, Olean, NY Zip 14760-1513; tel. 716/373-2600; Timothy J. Finan, FACHE, President and Chief Executive Officer
**Web address:** www.ogh.org

**PENNSYLVANIA:** BRADFORD REGIONAL MEDICAL CENTER (O, 182 beds) 116 Interstate Parkway, Bradford, PA Zip 16701-1036; tel. 814/368-4143; Timothy J. Finan, FACHE, President and Chief Executive Officer
**Web address:** www.brmc.com

| | | |
|---|---|---|
| Owned, leased, sponsored: | 2 hospitals | 368 beds |
| Contract-managed: | 0 hospitals | 0 beds |
| Totals: | 2 hospitals | 368 beds |

**0038: UPPER CHESAPEAKE HEALTH SYSTEM** (NP)
520 Upper Chesapeake Drive, Suite 405, Bel Air, MD Zip 21014-4324; tel. 443/643-3303; Lyle Ernest Sheldon, FACHE, President and Chief Executive Officer
**(Independent Hospital System)**

**MARYLAND:** HARFORD MEMORIAL HOSPITAL (O, 105 beds) 501 South Union Avenue, Havre De Grace, MD Zip 21078-3493; tel. 443/843-5000; Lyle Ernest Sheldon, FACHE, President and Chief Executive Officer
**Web address:** www.uchs.org

UPPER CHESAPEAKE MEDICAL CENTER (O, 175 beds) 500 Upper Chesapeake Drive, Bel Air, MD Zip 21014-4324; tel. 443/643-1000; Lyle Ernest Sheldon, FACHE, President and Chief Executive Officer
**Web address:** www.uchs.org

| | | |
|---|---|---|
| Owned, leased, sponsored: | 2 hospitals | 280 beds |
| Contract-managed: | 0 hospitals | 0 beds |
| Totals: | 2 hospitals | 280 beds |

**0868: USMD INC.** (IO)
6333 North State Highway 161 Suite 200, Irving, TX Zip 75038-2229; tel. 214/493-4000; Karen A. Fiducia, FACHE, President, Hospital Division

**TEXAS:** USMD HOSPITAL AT ARLINGTON (O, 34 beds) 801 West Interstate 20, Arlington, TX Zip 76017-5851; tel. 817/472-3400; Marcia Crim, R.N., MSN, Chief Executive Officer
**Web address:** www.usmdhospital.com

USMD HOSPITAL AT FORT WORTH (O, 8 beds) 5900 Dirks Road, Fort Worth, TX Zip 76132; tel. 817/433-9100; Stephanie Atkins-Guidry, Administrator
**Web address:** www.usmdfortworth.com/

| | | |
|---|---|---|
| Owned, leased, sponsored: | 2 hospitals | 42 beds |
| Contract-managed: | 0 hospitals | 0 beds |
| Totals: | 2 hospitals | 42 beds |

**0860: UVA HEALTH SYSTEM** (NP)
1215 Lee Street, Charlottesville, VA Zip 22908-0816; tel. 434/924-0211; R. Edward Howell, Vice President and Chief Executive Officer

**VIRGINIA:** TRANSITIONAL CARE HOSPITAL (O, 20 beds) 2965 Ivy Road (250 West), Charlottesville, VA Zip 22903-9330; tel. 434/924-7897; Michelle Hereford, Administrator
**Web address:** www.uvahealth.com/services/transitional-care-hospital

UNIVERSITY OF VIRGINIA MEDICAL CENTER (O, 570 beds) 1215 Lee Street, Charlottesville, VA Zip 22908-0001, Mailing Address: P.O. Box 800809, Zip 22908-0809; tel. 434/924-0211; R. Edward Howell, Vice President and Chief Executive Officer
**Web address:** www.healthsystem.virginia.edu

| | | |
|---|---|---|
| Owned, leased, sponsored: | 2 hospitals | 590 beds |
| Contract-managed: | 0 hospitals | 0 beds |
| Totals: | 2 hospitals | 590 beds |

**6415: UW MEDICINE** (NP)
4333 Brooklyn Avenue N.E., Seattle, WA Zip 98195, Mailing Address: P.O. Box 356350, Zip 98195-6350; tel. 206/543-7718; Paul G. Ramsey, Chief Executive Officer
**(Independent Hospital System)**

**WASHINGTON:** HARBORVIEW MEDICAL CENTER (O, 413 beds) 325 Ninth Avenue, Seattle, WA Zip 98104-2499, Mailing Address: P.O. Box 359717, Zip 98195-9717; tel. 206/744-3000; Eileen Whalen, R.N., Executive Director
**Web address:** www.uwmedicine.washington.edu/pages/default.aspx

NORTHWEST HOSPITAL & MEDICAL CENTER (O, 176 beds) 1550 North 115th Street, Seattle, WA Zip 98133-8401; tel. 206/364-0500; C. W. Schneider, President and Chief Executive Officer
**Web address:** www.nwhospital.org

UNIVERSITY OF WASHINGTON MEDICAL CENTER (O, 396 beds) 1959 N.E. Pacific Street, Seattle, WA Zip 98195-6151; tel. 206/598-3300; Stephen P. Zieniewicz, FACHE, Executive Director
**Web address:** www.uwmedicine.washington.edu/pages/default.aspx

VALLEY MEDICAL CENTER (O, 176 beds) 400 South 43rd Street, Renton, WA Zip 98055-5714; tel. 425/228-3450; Richard D. Roodman, Chief Executive Officer
**Web address:** www.valleymed.org

*For explanation of codes following names, see page B2.*
★ *Indicates Type III membership in the American Hospital Association.*

| Owned, leased, sponsored: | 4 hospitals | 1161 beds |
|---|---|---|
| Contract–managed: | 0 hospitals | 0 beds |
| Totals: | 4 hospitals | 1161 beds |

| Owned, leased, sponsored: | 1 hospital | 909 beds |
|---|---|---|
| Contract–managed: | 0 hospitals | 0 beds |
| Totals: | 1 hospital | 909 beds |

★**0386: VALLEY BAPTIST HEALTH SYSTEM** (NP)
2101 Pease Street, Harlingen, TX Zip 78550; tel. 956/389–1100;
Manuel Vela, President and Chief Executive Officer
**(Centralized Physician/Insurance Health System)**

**TEXAS:** VALLEY BAPTIST MEDICAL CENTER–BROWNSVILLE (O, 240 beds)
1040 West Jefferson Street, Brownsville, TX Zip 78520–5829, Mailing
Address: P.O. Box 3590, Zip 78523–3590; tel. 956/698–5400; Leslie
Bingham, Senior Vice President and Chief Executive Officer
**Web address:** www.valleybaptist.net/brownsville/

VALLEY BAPTIST MEDICAL CENTER–HARLINGEN (O, 416 beds) 2101 Pease
Street, Harlingen, TX Zip 78550–8307, Mailing Address: P.O. Drawer 2588,
Zip 78551–2588; tel. 956/389–1100; William D. Adams, Senior Vice
President and Chief Executive Officer
**Web address:** www.valleybaptist.net

| Owned, leased, sponsored: | 2 hospitals | 656 beds |
|---|---|---|
| Contract–managed: | 0 hospitals | 0 beds |
| Totals: | 2 hospitals | 656 beds |

★**0128: VALLEY HEALTH SYSTEM** (NP)
220 Campus Boulevard, Suite 310, Winchester, VA Zip 22601–2889,
Mailing Address: P.O. Box 3340, Zip 22604–1334;
tel. 540/536–8024; Mark H. Merrill, President
**(Moderately Centralized Health System)**

**VIRGINIA:** PAGE MEMORIAL HOSPITAL (O, 25 beds) 200 Memorial Drive,
Luray, VA Zip 22835–1005; tel. 540/743–4561; N. Travis Clark,
President
**Web address:** www.pagememorialhospital.org

SHENANDOAH MEMORIAL HOSPITAL (O, 18 beds) 759 South Main Street,
Woodstock, VA Zip 22664–1127; tel. 540/459–1100; Floyd Heater,
President
**Web address:** www.valleyhealthlink.com

WARREN MEMORIAL HOSPITAL (O, 166 beds) 1000 North Shenandoah
Avenue, Front Royal, VA Zip 22630–3598; tel. 540/636–0300; Patrick B.
Nolan, President and Chief Executive Officer
**Web address:** www.valleyhealthlink.com

WINCHESTER MEDICAL CENTER (O, 459 beds) 1840 Amherst Street,
Winchester, VA Zip 22601–2540, Mailing Address: P.O. Box 3340,
Zip 22604–3340; tel. 540/536–8000; Alfred E. Pilong, President and Chief
Executive Officer
**Web address:** www.valleyhealthlink.com

**WEST VIRGINIA:** HAMPSHIRE MEMORIAL HOSPITAL (O, 44 beds) 363 Sunrise
Boulevard, Romney, WV Zip 26757; tel. 304/822–4561; Neil R.
McLaughlin, R.N., Interim President
**Web address:** www.valleyhealthlink.com/hampshire

WAR MEMORIAL HOSPITAL (O, 41 beds) One Healthy Way, Berkeley Springs,
WV Zip 25411; tel. 304/258–1234; Neil R. McLaughlin, R.N., President
**Web address:** www.warmemorialhospital.com

| Owned, leased, sponsored: | 6 hospitals | 753 beds |
|---|---|---|
| Contract–managed: | 0 hospitals | 0 beds |
| Totals: | 6 hospitals | 753 beds |

● ★**0387: VANDERBILT HEALTHCARE** (NP)
1211 22nd Avenue South, Nashville, TN Zip 37232;
tel. 615/322–5000; Charles Wright Pinson, M.D., Deputy Vice
Chancellor for Health Affairs and Chief Executive Officer of Vanderbilt
Health System
**(Moderately Centralized Health System)**

**TENNESSEE:** VANDERBILT HOSPITAL AND CLINICS (O, 909 beds) 1211
22nd Avenue North, Nashville, TN Zip 37232–2102; tel. 615/322–5000;
David R. Posch, Chief Executive Officer
**Web address:** www.mc.vanderbilt.edu

**0193: VANGUARD HEALTH SYSTEM** (IO)
20 Burton Hills Boulevard, Suite 10, Nashville, TN Zip 37215;
tel. 615/665–6000; Charles N. Martin, Jr., Chairman and Chief
Executive Officer
**(Decentralized Health System)**

**ARIZONA:** ARROWHEAD HOSPITAL (O, 234 beds) 18701 North 67th Avenue,
Glendale, AZ Zip 85308–5722; tel. 623/561–1000; Frank L. Molinaro,
Chief Executive Officer
**Web address:** www.arrowheadhospital.com

MARYVALE HOSPITAL MEDICAL CENTER (O, 100 beds) 5102 West Campbell
Avenue, Phoenix, AZ Zip 85031–1799; tel. 623/848–5000; Crystal Hamilton,
R.N., Chief Executive Officer
**Web address:** www.maryvalehospital.com

PARADISE VALLEY HOSPITAL (O, 142 beds) 3929 East Bell Road, Phoenix,
AZ Zip 85032–2196; tel. 602/923–5000; Shawn G. Strash, Chief Executive
Officer
**Web address:** www.paradisevalleyhospital.com

PHOENIX BAPTIST HOSPITAL (O, 215 beds) 2000 West Bethany Home Road,
Phoenix, AZ Zip 85015–2443; tel. 602/249–0212; Wayne Gillis, Interim Chief
Executive Officer
**Web address:** www.phoenixbaptisthospital.com

WEST VALLEY HOSPITAL (O, 106 beds) 13677 West McDowell Road,
Goodyear, AZ Zip 85338; tel. 623/882–1500; Jo Adkins, Chief Executive
Officer
**Web address:** www.wvhospital.com

**ILLINOIS:** LOUIS A. WEISS MEMORIAL HOSPITAL (O, 184 beds) 4646 North
Marine Drive, Chicago, IL Zip 60640–1501; tel. 773/878–8700; Jeffrey
Steinberg, M.D., Chief Executive Officer
**Web address:** www.weisshospital.com

MACNEAL HOSPITAL (O, 373 beds) 3249 South Oak Park Avenue, Berwyn, IL
Zip 60402–0715; tel. 708/783–9100; Brian J. Lemon, Chief Executive
Officer
**Web address:** www.macneal.com

WEST SUBURBAN MEDICAL CENTER (O, 172 beds) 3 Erie Court, Oak Park, IL
Zip 60302–2599; tel. 708/383–6200; John J. Cleary, Chief Executive Officer
**Web address:** www.westsuburbanmc.com/Home.aspx

WESTLAKE HOSPITAL (O, 181 beds) 1225 Lake Street, Melrose Park, IL
Zip 60160–4000; tel. 708/681–3000; William A. Brown, FACHE, Chief
Executive Officer
**Web address:** www.wlhospital.com/Home.aspx

**MASSACHUSETTS:** METROWEST MEDICAL CENTER (O, 160 beds) 115
Lincoln Street, Framingham, MA Zip 01702–6342; tel. 508/383–1000;
Andrei Soran, Chief Executive Officer
**Web address:** www.mwmc.com

SAINT VINCENT HOSPITAL (O, 297 beds) 123 Summer Street, Worcester, MA
Zip 01608; tel. 508/363–5000; Erik G. Wexler, President and Chief
Executive Officer
**Web address:** www.stvincenthospital.com

**MICHIGAN:** CHILDREN'S HOSPITAL OF MICHIGAN (O, 222 beds) 3901
Beaubien Street, Detroit, MI Zip 48201–2119; tel. 313/745–5437;
Herman B. Gray, M.D., President
**Web address:** www.chmkids.org

DETROIT RECEIVING HOSPITAL/UNIVERSITY HEALTH CENTER (O, 268 beds)
4201 Saint Antoine Street, Detroit, MI Zip 48201–2153; tel. 313/745–3000;
Iris Taylor, Ph.D., R.N., President
**Web address:** www.dmc.org

HARPER UNIVERSITY HOSPITAL/HUTZEL WOMEN'S HOSPITAL (O, 535 beds)
3990 John R Street, Detroit, MI Zip 48201–2018; tel. 313/745–8040;
Thomas Malone, M.D., President
**Web address:** www.harperhospital.org

HURON VALLEY–SINAI HOSPITAL (O, 153 beds) 1 William Carls Drive,
Commerce Township, MI Zip 48382–2201; tel. 248/937–3300; Lynn M.
Torossian, President
**Web address:** www.hvsh.org

For explanation of codes following names, see page B2.
★ Indicates Type III membership in the American Hospital Association.
● Single hospital health care system

Section B

REHABILITATION INSTITUTE OF MICHIGAN (O, 74 beds) 261 Mack Boulevard, Detroit, MI Zip 48201–2495; tel. 313/745–1203; William H. Restum, Ph.D., President
**Web address:** www.rimrehab.org

SINAI–GRACE HOSPITAL (O, 337 beds) 6071 West Outer Drive, Detroit, MI Zip 48235–2679; tel. 313/966–3300; Reginald J. Eadie, M.D., President
**Web address:** www.sinaigrace.org

**TEXAS:** BAPTIST HEALTH SYSTEM (O, 1342 beds) 111 Dallas Street, San Antonio, TX Zip 78205–1230; tel. 210/297–7000; David S. Goldberg, President
**Web address:** www.baptisthealthsystem.com

| | | |
|---|---|---|
| Owned, leased, sponsored: | 18 hospitals | 5095 beds |
| Contract–managed: | 0 hospitals | 0 beds |
| Totals: | 18 hospitals | 5095 beds |

---

**5435: VIA CHRISTI HEALTH** (CC)
8200 East Thorn, Wichita, KS Zip 67226–2709; tel. 316/858–4900; Jeffrey Korsmo, President and Chief Executive Officer
**(Centralized Health System)**

**KANSAS:** KANSAS SURGERY AND RECOVERY CENTER (O, 32 beds) 2770 North Webb Road, Wichita, KS Zip 67226–8112; tel. 316/634–0090; Ely Bartal, M.D., Chief Executive Officer
**Web address:** www.ksrc.org

MERCY REGIONAL HEALTH CENTER (O, 111 beds) 1823 College Avenue, Manhattan, KS Zip 66502, Mailing Address: P.O. Box 1289, Zip 66505–1289; tel. 785/776–3322; John R. Broberg, FACHE, President and Chief Executive Officer
**Web address:** www.mercyregional.org

VIA CHRISTI HOSPITAL (O, 68 beds) 14800 West St. Teresa, Wichita, KS Zip 67235–9602; tel. 316/796–7000; Kevin Strecker, President
**Web address:** www.via–christi.org

VIA CHRISTI HOSPITAL (O, 111 beds) 1 Mt. Carmel Way, Pittsburg, KS Zip 66762–6643; tel. 620/232–0109; Randall R. Cason, FACHE, President and Chief Executive Officer
**Web address:** www.viachristi.org

VIA CHRISTI HOSPITALS WICHITA (O, 801 beds) 929 North St. Francis Street, Wichita, KS Zip 67214–3882; tel. 316/268–5000; Sherry Hausmann, President
**Web address:** www.via–christi.org

VIA CHRISTI REHABILITATION CENTER (O, 58 beds) 1151 North Rock Road, Wichita, KS Zip 67206–1262; tel. 316/634–3400; Cindy LaFleur, President
**Web address:** www.via–christi.org

| | | |
|---|---|---|
| Owned, leased, sponsored: | 6 hospitals | 1181 beds |
| Contract–managed: | 0 hospitals | 0 beds |
| Totals: | 6 hospitals | 1181 beds |

---

**0299: VIBRA HEALTHCARE** (IO)
4550 Lena Drive, Suite 225, Mechanicsburg, PA Zip 17055; tel. 717/591–5700; Brad Hollinger, Chairman and Chief Executive Officer
**(Independent Hospital System)**

**CALIFORNIA:** KENTFIELD REHABILITATION AND SPECIALTY HOSPITAL (O, 60 beds) 1125 Sir Francis Drake Boulevard, Kentfield, CA Zip 94904–1455; tel. 415/456–9680; Ann Gors, Chief Executive Officer
**Web address:** www.kentfieldrehab.com

NORTHERN CALIFORNIA REHABILITATION HOSPITAL (O, 88 beds) 2801 Eureka Way, Redding, CA Zip 96001; tel. 530/246–9000; Chris Jones, Chief Executive Officer
**Web address:** www.norcalrehab.com

ROBERT H. BALLARD REHABILITATION HOSPITAL (O, 60 beds) 1760 West 16th Street, San Bernardino, CA Zip 92411; tel. 909/473–1200; Edward C. Palacios, Chief Executive Officer
**Web address:** www.ballardhospital.com

SAN JOAQUIN VALLEY REHABILITATION HOSPITAL (O, 40 beds) 7173 North Sharon Avenue, Fresno, CA Zip 93720–3329; tel. 559/436–3600; Edward C. Palacios, Chief Executive Officer
**Web address:** www.sjvrehab.com

VIBRA HOSPITAL OF SAN DIEGO (O, 57 beds) 555 Washington Street, San Diego, CA Zip 92103; tel. 619/260–8300; Michael T. Phillips, FACHE, Chief Executive Officer
**Web address:** www.vhsandiego.com/

**COLORADO:** VIBRA HOSPITAL OF DENVER (O, 71 beds) 8451 Pearl Street, Thornton, CO Zip 80229–4804; tel. 303/288–3000; Dianne Chartier, R.N., Chief Executive Officer
**Web address:** www.vhdenver.com

**INDIANA:** VIBRA HOSPITAL OF FORT WAYNE (O, 50 beds) 2626 Fairfield Avenue, Fort Wayne, IN Zip 46807–1215; tel. 260/399–2900; Robert P. Gerick, Interim Chief Executive Officer
**Web address:** www.vhfortwayne.com

VIBRA HOSPITAL OF NORTHWESTERN INDIANA (O, 40 beds) 9509 Georgia Street, Crown Point, IN Zip 46307–6518; tel. 219/472–2200; Mark Senko, Chief Executive Officer
**Web address:** www.vhnwindiana.com/

**KENTUCKY:** SOUTHERN KENTUCKY REHABILITATION HOSPITAL (O, 60 beds) 1300 Campbell Lane, Bowling Green, KY Zip 42104–4162; tel. 270/782–6900; Stuart Locke, Interim Chief Executive Officer
**Web address:** www.skyrehab.com

**MASSACHUSETTS:** NEW BEDFORD REHABILITATION HOSPITAL (O, 90 beds) 4499 Acushnet Avenue, New Bedford, MA Zip 02745; tel. 508/995–6900; Edward B. Leary, Chief Executive Officer
**Web address:** www.newbedfordrehab.com

**MICHIGAN:** VIBRA HOSPITAL OF SOUTHEASTERN MICHIGAN (O, 140 beds) 26400 West Outer Drive, Lincoln Park, MI Zip 48146–2088; tel. 313/386–2000; Jonathan Cohee, Chief Executive Officer
**Web address:** www.vhsemichigan.com/

**NEW JERSEY:** MARLTON REHABILITATION HOSPITAL (O, 46 beds) 92 Brick Road, Marlton, NJ Zip 08053–2177; tel. 856/988–8778; Michael Long, MS, Chief Executive Officer
**Web address:** www.marltonrehab.com

**OHIO:** VIBRA HOSPITAL OF MAHONING VALLEY (O, 45 beds) 8049 South Avenue, Boardman, OH Zip 44512; tel. 330/726–5000; Mary Lou Sankovich, R.N., MSN, Chief Executive Officer and Chief Nursing Officer
**Web address:** www.mahoningvalleyhospital.com

**OREGON:** VIBRA SPECIALTY HOSPITAL OF PORTLAND (O, 60 beds) 10300 N.E. Hancock Street, Portland, OR Zip 97220; tel. 503/257–5500; Tina Key, Chief Executive Officer
**Web address:** www.vibrahealthcare.com

**TEXAS:** VIBRA SPECIALTY HOSPITAL OF DALLAS (O, 60 beds) 2700 Walker Way, Desoto, TX Zip 75115–2088; tel. 214/638–1500; Paul P. Hall, Jr., Chief Executive Officer and Chief Clinical Officer
**Web address:** www.vibrahealthcare.com

| | | |
|---|---|---|
| Owned, leased, sponsored: | 15 hospitals | 967 beds |
| Contract–managed: | 0 hospitals | 0 beds |
| Totals: | 15 hospitals | 967 beds |

---

**★0217: VIDANT HEALTH** (NP)
2100 Stantonsburg Road, Greenville, NC Zip 27834–2818, Mailing Address: P.O. Box 6028, Zip 27835–6028; tel. 252/847–4100; David C. Herman, M.D., Chief Executive Officer
**(Moderately Centralized Health System)**

**NORTH CAROLINA:** ALBEMARLE HEALTH (C, 140 beds) 1144 North Road Street, Elizabeth City, NC Zip 27909, Mailing Address: P.O. Box 1587, Zip 27906–1587; tel. 252/335–0531; Sharon M. Tanner, President
**Web address:** www.albemarlehealth.org

THE OUTER BANKS HOSPITAL (O, 61 beds) 4800 South Croatan Highway, Nags Head, NC Zip 27959–9704; tel. 252/449–4511; Ronald A. Sloan, FACHE, President
**Web address:** www.theouterbankshospital.com

VIDANT BEAUFORT HOSPITAL (L, 95 beds) 628 East 12th Street, Washington, NC Zip 27889–3409; tel. 252/975–4100; Harvey Case, President
**Web address:** www.beaufortregionalhealthsystem.org

---

For explanation of codes following names, see page B2.
★ Indicates Type III membership in the American Hospital Association.

VIDANT BERTIE HOSPITAL (L, 6 beds) 1403 South King Street, Windsor, NC Zip 27983–1726, Mailing Address: P.O. Box 40, Zip 27983–1726; tel. 252/794–6600; Jeffrey N. Sackrison, FACHE, President
**Web address:** www.vidanthealth.com

VIDANT CHOWAN HOSPITAL (L, 67 beds) 211 Virginia Road, Edenton, NC Zip 27932–0629, Mailing Address: P.O. Box 629, Zip 27932–0629; tel. 252/482–8451; Jeffrey N. Sackrison, FACHE, President
**Web address:** www.vidanthealth.com

VIDANT DUPLIN HOSPITAL (L, 74 beds) 401 North Main Street, Kenansville, NC Zip 28349–9989, Mailing Address: P.O. Box 278, Zip 28349–0278; tel. 910/296–0941; Jay Briley, Chief Executive Officer
**Web address:** www.vidanthealth.com

VIDANT EDGECOMBE HOSPITAL (O, 117 beds) 111 Hospital Drive, Tarboro, NC Zip 27886–2011; tel. 252/641–7700; Wendell H. Baker, Jr., President
**Web address:** www.VidantHealth.com

VIDANT MEDICAL CENTER (O, 847 beds) 2100 Stantonsburg Road, Greenville, NC Zip 27834, Mailing Address: P.O. Box 6028, Zip 27835–6028; tel. 252/847–4100; Steven Lawler, President
**Web address:** www.uhseast.com

VIDANT PUNGO HOSPITAL (O, 35 beds) 202 East Water Street, Belhaven, NC Zip 27810–9998; tel. 252/943–2111; Harvey Case, President
**Web address:** www.pungodistricthospital.org

VIDANT ROANOKE–CHOWAN HOSPITAL (L, 103 beds) 500 South Academy Street, Ahoskie, NC Zip 27910–3261, Mailing Address: P.O. Box 1385, Zip 27910–1385; tel. 252/209–3000; Susan S. Lassiter, President
**Web address:** www.vidanthealth.com

| | | |
|---|---|---|
| **Owned, leased, sponsored:** | 9 hospitals | 1405 beds |
| **Contract–managed:** | 1 hospital | 140 beds |
| **Totals:** | 10 hospitals | 1545 beds |

---

**0012: VIRGINIA DEPARTMENT OF MENTAL HEALTH** (NP)
1220 Bank Street, Richmond, VA Zip 23219, Mailing Address: P.O. Box 1797, Zip 23218–1797; tel. 804/786–3921; James S. Reinhard, M.D., Commissioner
**(Independent Hospital System)**

**VIRGINIA:** CATAWBA HOSPITAL (O, 110 beds) 5525 Catawba Hospital Drive, Catawba, VA Zip 24070–2115, Mailing Address: P.O. Box 200, Zip 24070–0200; tel. 540/375–4200; Walton F. Mitchell, III, Director
**Web address:** www.catawba.dmhmrsas.virginia.gov

CENTRAL STATE HOSPITAL (O, 277 beds) 26317 West Washington Street, Petersburg, VA Zip 23803, Mailing Address: P.O. Box 4030, Zip 23803–4030; tel. 804/524–7000; Charles M. Davis, M.D., Ph.D., Director
**Web address:** www.csh.dmhmrsas.virginia.gov

CENTRAL VIRGINIA TRAINING CENTER (O, 1112 beds) 210 East Colony Road, Madison Heights, VA Zip 24572–2005, Mailing Address: P.O. Box 1098, Lynchburg, Zip 24505–1098; tel. 434/947–6326; Denise D. Micheletti, R.N., Director
**Web address:** www.cvtc.dmhmrsas.virginia.gov/

COMMONWEALTH CENTER FOR CHILDREN AND ADOLESCENTS (O, 60 beds) 1355 Richmond Road, Staunton, VA Zip 24401–1091, Mailing Address: Box 4000, Zip 24402–4000; tel. 540/332–2100; William J. Tuell, MSN, Facility Director
**Web address:** www.ccca.dbhds.virginia.gov

EASTERN STATE HOSPITAL (O, 334 beds) 4601 Ironbound Road, Williamsburg, VA Zip 23188–2652; tel. 757/253–5161; John M. Favret, Director
**Web address:** www.esh.dmhmrsas.virginia.gov/

HIRAM W. DAVIS MEDICAL CENTER (O, 10 beds) 26317 West Washington Street, Petersburg, VA Zip 23803–2727, Mailing Address: P.O. Box 4030, Zip 23803–0030; tel. 804/524–7344; Bill Hawkins, Director

NORTHERN VIRGINIA MENTAL HEALTH INSTITUTE (O, 123 beds) 3302 Gallows Road, Falls Church, VA Zip 22042–3398; tel. 703/207–7110; R. Maxilimien del Rio, M.D., Facility Director
**Web address:** www.nvmhi.dmhmrsas.virginia.gov

PIEDMONT GERIATRIC HOSPITAL (O, 150 beds) 5001 East Patrick Henry Highway, Burkeville, VA Zip 23922–0427, Mailing Address: P.O. Box 427, Zip 23922–0427; tel. 434/767–4401; Stephen M. Herrick, Ph.D., Director
**Web address:** www.pgh.dmhmrsas.virginia.gov

SOUTHERN VIRGINIA MENTAL HEALTH INSTITUTE (O, 72 beds) 382 Taylor Drive, Danville, VA Zip 24541–4023; tel. 434/799–6220; David M. Lyon, Director
**Web address:** www.svmhi.dmhmrsas.virginia.gov

SOUTHWESTERN VIRGINIA MENTAL HEALTH INSTITUTE (O, 266 beds) 340 Bagley Circle, Marion, VA Zip 24354–3390; tel. 276/783–1200; Cynthia McClaskey, Ph.D., Director
**Web address:** www.swvmhi.dmhmrsas.virginia.gov/

WESTERN STATE HOSPITAL (O, 260 beds) 1301 Richmond Avenue, Staunton, VA Zip 24401, Mailing Address: P.O. Box 2500, Zip 24402–2500; tel. 540/332–8000; Jack W. Barber, M.D., Director
**Web address:** www.dbhds.virginia.gov

| | | |
|---|---|---|
| **Owned, leased, sponsored:** | 11 hospitals | 2774 beds |
| **Contract–managed:** | 0 hospitals | 0 beds |
| **Totals:** | 11 hospitals | 2774 beds |

---

**★6725: VIRTUA HEALTH** (NP)
50 Lake Center Executive Drive, Suite 401, Marlton, NJ Zip 08053; tel. 856/355–0010; Richard P. Miller, Chief Executive Officer
**(Moderately Centralized Health System)**

**NEW JERSEY:** VIRTUA BERLIN (O, 82 beds) 100 Townsend Avenue, Berlin, NJ Zip 08009–9035; tel. 856/322–3000; Gary L. Long, Chief Operating Officer
**Web address:** www.virtua.org

VIRTUA MARLTON (O, 192 beds) 90 Brick Road, Marlton, NJ Zip 08053–9697; tel. 856/355–6000; Gary L. Long, Chief Operating Officer
**Web address:** www.virtua.org

VIRTUA MEMORIAL (O, 312 beds) 175 Madison Avenue, Mount Holly, NJ Zip 08060–2099; tel. 609/267–0700; Stephen Kolesk, M.D., Vice President and Chief Operating Officer
**Web address:** www.virtua.org

VIRTUA VOORHEES (O, 398 beds) 100 Bowman Drive, Voorhees, NJ Zip 08043–9612; tel. 856/325–3000; Michael S. Kotzen, Vice President and Chief Operating Officer
**Web address:** www.virtua.org

| | | |
|---|---|---|
| **Owned, leased, sponsored:** | 4 hospitals | 984 beds |
| **Contract–managed:** | 0 hospitals | 0 beds |
| **Totals:** | 4 hospitals | 984 beds |

---

**★0221: WAKE FOREST BAPTIST HEALTH** (NP)
Medical Center Boulevard, Winston–Salem, NC Zip 27157; tel. 336/716–2011; John D. McConnell, M.D., Chief Executive Officer
**(Moderately Centralized Health System)**

**NORTH CAROLINA:** WAKE FOREST BAPTIST HEALTH–DAVIE HOSPITAL (O, 25 beds) 223 Hospital Street, Mocksville, NC Zip 27028–2038, Mailing Address: P.O. Box 1209, Zip 27028–1209; tel. 336/751–8100; Kevin Walsh, Administrator
**Web address:** www.daviehospital.org

WAKE FOREST BAPTIST HEALTH–LEXINGTON MEDICAL CENTER (O, 69 beds) 250 Hospital Drive, Lexington, NC Zip 27292–6728, Mailing Address: P.O. Box 1817, Zip 27293–1817; tel. 336/248–5161; Steven C. Snelgrove, Chief Executive Officer
**Web address:** www.lexingtonmemorial.com

WAKE FOREST BAPTIST MEDICAL CENTER (O, 853 beds) Medical Center Boulevard, Winston–Salem, NC Zip 27157–0001; tel. 336/716–2011; Sanjay K. Saha, Executive Vice President, Operations
**Web address:** www.wfubmc.edu

| | | |
|---|---|---|
| **Owned, leased, sponsored:** | 3 hospitals | 947 beds |
| **Contract–managed:** | 0 hospitals | 0 beds |
| **Totals:** | 3 hospitals | 947 beds |

---

**★6705: WAKEMED HEALTH & HOSPITALS** (NP)
3000 New Bern Avenue, Raleigh, NC Zip 27610; tel. 919/350–8000; William K. Atkinson, II, Ph.D., President and Chief Executive Officer
**(Moderately Centralized Health System)**

For explanation of codes following names, see page B2.
★ Indicates Type III membership in the American Hospital Association.

*Section B*

BETSY JOHNSON REGIONAL HOSPITAL (C, 89 beds) 800 Tilghman Drive, Dunn, NC Zip 28334–5599, Mailing Address: Drawer 1706, Zip 28335–1706; tel. 910/892–7161; Kenneth E. Bryan, President and Chief Executive Officer
**Web address:** www.bjrh.org

WAKEMED CARY HOSPITAL (O, 192 beds) 1900 Kildaire Farm Road, Cary, NC Zip 27518; tel. 919/350–2300; David C. Coulter, Senior Vice President and Chief Executive Officer
**Web address:** www.wakemed.org

WAKEMED RALEIGH CAMPUS (O, 647 beds) 3000 New Bern Avenue, Raleigh, NC Zip 27610–1295; tel. 919/350–8000; William K. Atkinson, II, Ph.D., President and Chief Executive Officer
**Web address:** www.wakemed.org

| Owned, leased, sponsored: | 2 hospitals | 839 beds |
|---|---|---|
| Contract–managed: | 1 hospital | 89 beds |
| **Totals:** | 3 hospitals | 928 beds |

★**0188:   WELLMONT HEALTH SYSTEM** (NP)
1905 American Way, Kingsport, TN Zip 37660–5882; tel. 423/230–8200; Margaret DeNarvaez, President and Chief Executive Officer
**(Moderately Centralized Health System)**

**TENNESSEE:** WELLMONT BRISTOL REGIONAL MEDICAL CENTER (O, 348 beds) 1 Medical Park Boulevard, Bristol, TN Zip 37620–7430; tel. 423/844–1121; Barton A. Hove, President
**Web address:** www.wellmont.org

WELLMONT HANCOCK COUNTY HOSPITAL (O, 10 beds) 1519 Main Street, Sneedville, TN Zip 37869–3657; tel. 423/733–5000; Fred L. Pelle, FACHE, President and Chief Executive Officer
**Web address:** www.wellmont.org/Hospitals/Hancock–County–Hospital.aspx

WELLMONT HAWKINS COUNTY MEMORIAL HOSPITAL (L, 50 beds) 851 Locust Street, Rogersville, TN Zip 37857–2407, Mailing Address: P.O. Box 130, Zip 37857–0130; tel. 423/921–7000; Greg Neal, President and Chief Executive Officer
**Web address:** www.wellmont.org

WELLMONT HOLSTON VALLEY MEDICAL CENTER (O, 345 beds) 130 West Ravine Street, Kingsport, TN Zip 37660, Mailing Address: P.O. Box 238, Zip 37662–0238; tel. 423/224–4000; Virginia Frank, President and Chief Executive Officer
**Web address:** www.wellmont.org

**VIRGINIA:** LEE REGIONAL MEDICAL CENTER (O, 58 beds) 1800 Combs Road, Pennington Gap, VA Zip 24277–1808, Mailing Address: P.O. Box 589, Zip 24277–0589; tel. 276/546–1440; Ron Prewitt, President
**Web address:** www.wellmont.org/Hospitals/Lee–Regional–Medical–Center.aspx

MOUNTAIN VIEW REGIONAL MEDICAL CENTER (O, 118 beds) 310 Third Street N.E., Norton, VA Zip 24273–1137; tel. 276/679–9100; David L. Brash, System Regional Vice President and President
**Web address:** www.wellmont.org

WELLMONT LONESOME PINE HOSPITAL (O, 60 beds) 1990 Holton Avenue East, Big Stone Gap, VA Zip 24219–3350; tel. 276/523–3111; David L. Brash, Interim President
**Web address:** www.wellmont.org

| Owned, leased, sponsored: | 7 hospitals | 989 beds |
|---|---|---|
| Contract–managed: | 0 hospitals | 0 beds |
| **Totals:** | 7 hospitals | 989 beds |

★**0068:   WELLSPAN HEALTH** (NP)
45 Monument Road, Suite 200, York, PA Zip 17403; tel. 717/851–2121; Bruce M. Bartels, President
**(Centralized Physician/Insurance Health System)**

**PENNSYLVANIA:** GETTYSBURG HOSPITAL (O, 76 beds) 147 Gettys Street, Gettysburg, PA Zip 17325–2534; tel. 717/334–2121; Jane E. Hyde, President
**Web address:** www.wellspan.org

YORK HOSPITAL (O, 549 beds) 1001 South George Street, York, PA Zip 17405–3645; tel. 717/851–2345; Keith Noll, President
**Web address:** www.wellspan.org

| Owned, leased, sponsored: | 2 hospitals | 625 beds |
|---|---|---|
| Contract–managed: | 0 hospitals | 0 beds |
| **Totals:** | 2 hospitals | 625 beds |

★**0995:   WELLSTAR HEALTH SYSTEM** (NP)
805 Sandy Plains Road, Marietta, GA Zip 30066; tel. 770/792–5012; Reynold J. Jennings, President and Chief Executive Officer
**(Centralized Health System)**

**GEORGIA:** WELLSTAR COBB HOSPITAL (O, 370 beds) 3950 Austell Road, Austell, GA Zip 30106–1121; tel. 770/732–4000; Kem Mullins, FACHE, Senior Vice President and Hospital President
**Web address:** www.wellstar.org

WELLSTAR DOUGLAS HOSPITAL (O, 102 beds) 8954 Hospital Drive, Douglasville, GA Zip 30134–2282; tel. 770/949–1500; Craig A. Owens, Senior Vice President and Administrator
**Web address:** www.wellstar.org

WELLSTAR KENNESTONE HOSPITAL (O, 580 beds) 677 Church Street, Marietta, GA Zip 30060–1148; tel. 770/793–5000; Candice Saunders, Senior Vice President and Administrator
**Web address:** www.wellstar.org

WELLSTAR PAULDING HOSPITAL (O, 216 beds) 600 West Memorial Drive, Dallas, GA Zip 30132–1335; tel. 770/445–4411; Mark Haney, Senior Vice President and Administrator
**Web address:** www.wellstar.org

WELLSTAR WINDY HILL HOSPITAL (O, 55 beds) 2540 Windy Hill Road, Marietta, GA Zip 30067–8632; tel. 770/644–1000; Lou Little, Senior Vice President and Administrator
**Web address:** www.wellstar.org

| Owned, leased, sponsored: | 5 hospitals | 1323 beds |
|---|---|---|
| Contract–managed: | 0 hospitals | 0 beds |
| **Totals:** | 5 hospitals | 1323 beds |

★**0199:   WEST PENN ALLEGHENY HEALTH SYSTEM** (NP)
30 Isabella Street, Suite 300, Pittsburgh, PA Zip 15212–5862; tel. 412/330–2403; Keith T. Ghezzi, M.D., Interim President and Chief Executive Officer
**(Moderately Centralized Health System)**

**PENNSYLVANIA:** ALLEGHENY GENERAL HOSPITAL (O, 366 beds) 320 East North Avenue, Pittsburgh, PA Zip 15212–4756; tel. 412/359–3131; Judith F. Zedreck, R.N., Interim Chief Executive Officer
**Web address:** www.wpahs.org

ALLEGHENY VALLEY HOSPITAL (O, 228 beds) 1301 Carlisle Street, Natrona Heights, PA Zip 15065–1152; tel. 724/224–5100; Ned Laubacher, President and Chief Executive Officer
**Web address:** www.wpahs.org

CANONSBURG GENERAL HOSPITAL (O, 60 beds) 100 Medical Boulevard, Canonsburg, PA Zip 15317–9762; tel. 724/745–6100; Terry Wiltrout, Chief Executive Officer
**Web address:** www.wpahs.org

FORBES REGIONAL HOSPITAL (O, 310 beds) 2570 Haymaker Road, Monroeville, PA Zip 15146–3513; tel. 412/858–2000; Reese Jackson, President and Chief Executive Officer
**Web address:** www.wpahs.org

WESTERN PENNSYLVANIA HOSPITAL (O, 439 beds) 4800 Friendship Avenue, Pittsburgh, PA Zip 15224–1722; tel. 412/578–5000; Duke Rupert, President and Chief Executive Officer
**Web address:** www.wpahs.org

| Owned, leased, sponsored: | 5 hospitals | 1403 beds |
|---|---|---|
| Contract–managed: | 0 hospitals | 0 beds |
| **Totals:** | 5 hospitals | 1403 beds |

★**0004:   WEST TENNESSEE HEALTHCARE** (NP)
620 Skyline Drive, Jackson, TN Zip 38301–3901; tel. 731/541–5000; Bobby Arnold, President and Chief Executive Officer
**(Centralized Health System)**

For explanation of codes following names, see page B2.
★ Indicates Type III membership in the American Hospital Association.

**TENNESSEE:** BOLIVAR GENERAL HOSPITAL (O, 21 beds) 650 Nuckolls Road, Bolivar, TN Zip 38008–1532, Mailing Address: P.O. Box 509, Zip 38008–0509; tel. 731/658–3100; Ruby Kirby, Administrator
**Web address:** www.wth.net

CAMDEN GENERAL HOSPITAL (O, 12 beds) 175 Hospital Drive, Camden, TN Zip 38320–1617; tel. 731/584–6135; Denny R. Smith, Administrator
**Web address:** www.wth.net

GIBSON GENERAL HOSPITAL (O, 32 beds) 200 Hospital Drive, Trenton, TN Zip 38382–3313; tel. 731/855–7900; Sherry Scruggs, Administrator
**Web address:** www.wth.net

HUMBOLDT GENERAL HOSPITAL (O, 30 beds) 3525 Chere Carol Road, Humboldt, TN Zip 38343–3699; tel. 731/784–2321; Sherry Scruggs, Administrator
**Web address:** www.wth.net

JACKSON–MADISON COUNTY GENERAL HOSPITAL (O, 619 beds) 620 Skyline Drive, Jackson, TN Zip 38301; tel. 731/541–5000; Bobby Arnold, President and Chief Executive Officer
**Web address:** www.wth.org

MILAN GENERAL HOSPITAL (O, 28 beds) 4039 Highland Street, Milan, TN Zip 38358–3483; tel. 731/686–1591; Sherry Scruggs, Administrator
**Web address:** www.wth.org

PATHWAYS OF TENNESSEE (O, 25 beds) 238 Summar Drive, Jackson, TN Zip 38301–3906; tel. 731/541–8200; Pam Henson, Executive Director
**Web address:** www.wth.net

| | | |
|---|---|---|
| Owned, leased, sponsored: | 7 hospitals | 767 beds |
| Contract–managed: | 0 hospitals | 0 beds |
| Totals: | 7 hospitals | 767 beds |

★**0119: WEST VIRGINIA UNITED HEALTH SYSTEM** (NP) 1000 Technology Drive, Suite 2320, Fairmont, WV Zip 26554; tel. 304/368–2700; J. Thomas Jones, President and Chief Executive Officer
**(Moderately Centralized Health System)**

**WEST VIRGINIA:** CAMDEN–CLARK MEDICAL CENTER (O, 435 beds) 800 Garfield Avenue, Parkersburg, WV Zip 26101–5378, Mailing Address: P.O. Box 718, Zip 26102–0718; tel. 304/424–2111; Michael A. King, FACHE, President and Chief Executive Officer
**Web address:** www.ccmh.org

CITY HOSPITAL (O, 171 beds) 2500 Hospital Drive, Martinsburg, WV Zip 25401–3402, Mailing Address: P.O. Box 1418, Zip 25402–1418; tel. 304/264–1000; Anthony Zelenka, Chief Administrative Officer
**Web address:** www.cityhospital.org

JEFFERSON MEMORIAL HOSPITAL (O, 25 beds) 300 South Preston Street, Ranson, WV Zip 25438–1699; tel. 304/728–1600; Christina D. Coad, Ph.D., Chief Administrative Officer
**Web address:** www.jeffmem.com

UNITED HOSPITAL CENTER (O, 264 beds) 327 Medical Park Drive, Bridgeport, WV Zip 26330–9006; tel. 681/342–1000; Bruce C. Carter, President
**Web address:** www.uhcwv.org

WEST VIRGINIA UNIVERSITY HOSPITALS (O, 509 beds) 1 Medical Center Drive, Morgantown, WV Zip 26506–4749; tel. 304/598–4000; Bruce McClymonds, President and Chief Executive Officer
**Web address:** www.health.wvu.edu

| | | |
|---|---|---|
| Owned, leased, sponsored: | 5 hospitals | 1404 beds |
| Contract–managed: | 0 hospitals | 0 beds |
| Totals: | 5 hospitals | 1404 beds |

★**0811: WESTERN CONNECTICUT HEALTHCARE, INC.** (NP) 24 Hospital Avenue, Danbury, CT Zip 06810–6099; tel. 203/739–7066; John M. Murphy, M.D., President
**(Moderately Centralized Health System)**

**CONNECTICUT:** DANBURY HOSPITAL (O, 354 beds) 24 Hospital Avenue, Danbury, CT Zip 06810–6099; tel. 203/739–7000; John M. Murphy, M.D., President and Chief Executive Officer
**Web address:** www.danburyhospital.org

NEW MILFORD HOSPITAL (O, 62 beds) 21 Elm Street, New Milford, CT Zip 06776–2993; tel. 860/355–2611; John M. Murphy, M.D., Executive Director and Senior Vice President
**Web address:** www.newmilfordhospital.org

| | | |
|---|---|---|
| Owned, leased, sponsored: | 2 hospitals | 416 beds |
| Contract–managed: | 0 hospitals | 0 beds |
| Totals: | 2 hospitals | 416 beds |

★**6745: WHEATON FRANCISCAN HEALTHCARE** (CC) 26W171 Roosevelt Road, Wheaton, IL Zip 60187–6078, Mailing Address: P.O. Box 667, Zip 60187–0667; tel. 630/909–6900; John D. Oliverio, President and Chief Executive Officer
**(Moderately Centralized Health System)**

**ILLINOIS:** MARIANJOY REHABILITATION HOSPITAL (O, 128 beds) 26 West 171 Roosevelt Road, Wheaton, IL Zip 60187–0795, Mailing Address: P.O. Box 795, Zip 60187–0795; tel. 630/909–8000; Kathleen C. Yosko, President and Chief Executive Officer
**Web address:** www.marianjoy.org

RUSH OAK PARK HOSPITAL (O, 114 beds) 520 South Maple Avenue, Oak Park, IL Zip 60304–1097; tel. 708/383–9300; Bruce M. Elegant, President and Chief Executive Officer
**Web address:** www.roph.org

**IOWA:** COVENANT MEDICAL CENTER (O, 243 beds) 3421 West Ninth Street, Waterloo, IA Zip 50702–5499; tel. 319/272–8000; Jack Dusenbery, President and Chief Executive Officer
**Web address:** www.wheatoniowa.org

MERCY HOSPITAL OF FRANCISCAN SISTERS (O, 64 beds) 201 Eighth Avenue S.E., Oelwein, IA Zip 50662–2447; tel. 319/283–6000; Terri Derflinger, Administrator
**Web address:** www.covhealth.com

SARTORI MEMORIAL HOSPITAL (O, 50 beds) 515 College Street, Cedar Falls, IA Zip 50613–2500; tel. 319/268–3000; Rose Fowler, MS, Administrator
**Web address:** www.wheatoniowa.org

**WISCONSIN:** MIDWEST ORTHOPEDIC SPECIALTY HOSPITAL (O, 16 beds) 10101 South 27th Street, 2nd Floor, Franklin, WI Zip 53132–7209; tel. 414/817–5800; Daniel Mattes, Chief Executive Officer
**Web address:** www.mymosh.com/

ST. ELIZABETH HOSPITAL (O, 206 beds) 1506 South Oneida Street, Appleton, WI Zip 54915–1397; tel. 920/738–2000; Travis Andersen, President
**Web address:** www.affinityhealth.org

UNITED HOSPITAL SYSTEM, ST. CATHERINE'S MEDICAL CENTER CAMPUS (O, 202 beds) 9555 76th Street, Pleasant Prairie, WI Zip 53158; tel. 262/656–2011; Richard O. Schmidt, Jr., President and Chief Executive Officer
**Web address:** www.uhsi.org

WHEATON FRANCISCAN HEALTHCARE – ALL SAINTS (O, 356 beds) 3801 Spring Street, Racine, WI Zip 53405–1690; tel. 262/687–4011; Kenneth R. Buser, President and Chief Executive Officer
**Web address:** www.allsaintshealth.com

WHEATON FRANCISCAN HEALTHCARE – ELMBROOK MEMORIAL (O, 100 beds) 19333 West North Avenue, Brookfield, WI Zip 53045–4198; tel. 262/785–2000; Debra K. Standridge, President
**Web address:** www.wfhealthcare.org

WHEATON FRANCISCAN HEALTHCARE – FRANKLIN (O, 19 beds) 10101 South 27th Street, Franklin, WI Zip 53132–7209; tel. 414/325–4700; Daniel Mattes, President
**Web address:** www.mywheaton.org/

WHEATON FRANCISCAN HEALTHCARE – ST. FRANCIS (S, 164 beds) 3237 South 16th Street, Milwaukee, WI Zip 53215–4592; tel. 414/647–5000; Daniel Mattes, President
**Web address:** www.mywheaton.org

WHEATON FRANCISCAN HEALTHCARE – ST. JOSEPH'S (O, 317 beds) 5000 West Chambers Street, Milwaukee, WI Zip 53210–9988; tel. 414/447–2000; Debra K. Standridge, President
**Web address:** www.whfc.org

For explanation of codes following names, see page B2.
★ Indicates Type III membership in the American Hospital Association.

WHEATON FRANCISCAN HEALTHCARE – THE WISCONSIN HEART HOSPITAL (O, 30 beds) 10000 West Bluemound Road, Wauwatosa, WI Zip 53226; tel. 414/778–7800; Debra K. Standridge, President
**Web address:** www.twhh.org

| Owned, leased, sponsored: | 14 hospitals | 2009 beds |
|---|---|---|
| Contract–managed: | 0 hospitals | 0 beds |
| **Totals:** | 14 hospitals | 2009 beds |

---

★**0468: WHITE RIVER HEALTH SYSTEM** (NP)
1710 Harrison Street, Batesville, AR Zip 72501–7303; tel. 870/262–1200; Gary Bebow, FACHE, Administrator and Chief Executive Officer
**(Moderately Centralized Health System)**

**ARKANSAS:** STONE COUNTY MEDICAL CENTER (O, 25 beds) 2106 East Main Street, Mountain View, AR Zip 72560, Mailing Address: P.O. Box 510, Zip 72560–0510; tel. 870/269–4361; Renie Taylor, Administrator
**Web address:** www.whiteriverhealthsystem.com

WHITE RIVER MEDICAL CENTER (O, 171 beds) 1710 Harrison Street, Batesville, AR Zip 72501–2197, Mailing Address: P.O. Box 2197, Zip 72503–2197; tel. 870/262–1200; Gary Bebow, FACHE, Administrator and Chief Executive Officer
**Web address:** www.whiteriverhealthsystem.com

| Owned, leased, sponsored: | 2 hospitals | 196 beds |
|---|---|---|
| Contract–managed: | 0 hospitals | 0 beds |
| **Totals:** | 2 hospitals | 196 beds |

---

**0646: WHITTIER HEALTH NETWORK** (IO)
25 Railroad Square, Haverhill, MA Zip 01832–5721; tel. 978/556–5858; Alfred L. Arcidi, M.D., President
**(Independent Hospital System)**

**MASSACHUSETTS:** WHITTIER REHABILITATION HOSPITAL (O, 74 beds) 150 Flanders Road, Westborough, MA Zip 01581; tel. 508/871–2000; Alfred J. Arcidi, M.D., Senior Vice President
**Web address:** www.whittierhealth.com

WHITTIER REHABILITATION HOSPITAL (O, 60 beds) 145 Ward Hill Avenue, Bradford, MA Zip 01835; tel. 978/372–8000; Alfred J. Arcidi, M.D., Senior Vice President
**Web address:** www.whittierhealth.com

| Owned, leased, sponsored: | 2 hospitals | 134 beds |
|---|---|---|
| Contract–managed: | 0 hospitals | 0 beds |
| **Totals:** | 2 hospitals | 134 beds |

---

**1945: WILLIS–KNIGHTON HEALTH SYSTEM** (NP)
2600 Greenwood Road, Shreveport, LA Zip 71130–2600; tel. 318/212–4000; James K. Elrod, FACHE, President and Chief Executive Officer
**(Centralized Physician/Insurance Health System)**

**LOUISIANA:** WILLIS–KNIGHTON MEDICAL CENTER (O, 902 beds) 2600 Greenwood Road, Shreveport, LA Zip 71103–2600, Mailing Address: P.O. Box 32600, Zip 71130–2600; tel. 318/212–4600; Jaf Fielder, Vice President and Administrator
**Web address:** www.wkhs.com

WK BOSSIER HEALTH CENTER (O, 134 beds) 2400 Hospital Drive, Bossier City, LA Zip 71111; tel. 318/212–7000; Clifford M. Broussard, FACHE, Administrator
**Web address:** www.wkhs.com/wkb/

| Owned, leased, sponsored: | 2 hospitals | 1036 beds |
|---|---|---|
| Contract–managed: | 0 hospitals | 0 beds |
| **Totals:** | 2 hospitals | 1036 beds |

---

★**0157: YALE NEW HAVEN HEALTH SYSTEM** (NP)
789 Howard Avenue, New Haven, CT Zip 06519; tel. 203/688–4608; Marna P. Borgstrom, President and Chief Executive Officer
**(Centralized Physician/Insurance Health System)**

**CONNECTICUT:** BRIDGEPORT HOSPITAL (O, 384 beds) 267 Grant Street, Bridgeport, CT Zip 06610–2805, Mailing Address: P.O. Box 5000, Zip 06610–5000; tel. 203/384–3000; William M. Jennings, President and Chief Executive Officer
**Web address:** www.bridgeporthospital.org

GREENWICH HOSPITAL (O, 184 beds) 5 Perryridge Road, Greenwich, CT Zip 06830–4697; tel. 203/863–3000; Frank A. Corvino, President and Chief Executive Officer
**Web address:** www.greenhosp.org

YALE–NEW HAVEN HOSPITAL (O, 962 beds) 20 York Street, New Haven, CT Zip 06510–3202; tel. 203/688–4242; Marna P. Borgstrom, President and Chief Executive Officer
**Web address:** www.ynhh.org

| Owned, leased, sponsored: | 3 hospitals | 1530 beds |
|---|---|---|
| Contract–managed: | 0 hospitals | 0 beds |
| **Totals:** | 3 hospitals | 1530 beds |

Section B

# Headquarters of Health Care Systems

## Geographically

### United States

#### ALABAMA

**Birmingham:** BAPTIST HEALTH SYSTEM 3201 4th Avenue South, Zip 35222–1723, Mailing Address: P.O. Box 830605, Zip 35283–0605; tel. 205/715–5319; M. Shane Spees, President and Chief Executive Officer, p. B18

BRADFORD HEALTH SERVICES 2101 Magnolia Avenue South, Suite 518, Zip 35205; tel. 205/251–7753; Jerry W. Crowder, President and Chief Executive Officer, p. B22

★ HEALTHSOUTH CORPORATION 3660 Grandview Parkway, Suite 200, Zip 35243; tel. 205/967–7116; Jay F. Grinney, President and Chief Executive Officer, p. B64

NOLAND HEALTH SERVICES, INC. 600 Corporate Parkway, Suite 100, Zip 35242; tel. 205/783–8484; Gary M. Glasscock, President and Chief Executive Officer, p. B94

★ UAB HEALTH SYSTEM 500 22nd Street South, Suite 408, Zip 35233; tel. 205/975–5362; William Ferniany, Ph.D., Chief Executive Officer, p. B132

**Guntersville:** ★ MARSHALL HEALTH SYSTEM 227 Britany Road, Zip 35976; tel. 256/894–6615; Gary R. Gore, Chief Executive Officer, p. B84

**Huntsville:** HUNTSVILLE HOSPITAL HEALTH SYSTEM 101 Sivley Road S.W., Zip 35801–4421; tel. 265/256–1000; David S. Spillers, Chief Executive Officer, p. B69

**Mobile:** INFIRMARY HEALTH SYSTEM 5 Mobile Infirmary Circle, Zip 36607–3520; tel. 251/435–5500; D. Mark Nix, President and Chief Executive Officer, p. B71

★ UNIVERSITY OF SOUTH ALABAMA HOSPITALS 2451 Fillingim Street, Zip 36617–2238; tel. 251/471–7000; Stanley K. Hammack, Chief Executive Officer, p. B139

**Montgomery:** ★ BAPTIST HEALTH 301 Brown Springs Road, Zip 36117; tel. 334/273–4400; W. Russell Tyner, President and Chief Executive Officer, p. B17

GILLIARD HEALTH SERVICES 3091 Carter Hill Road, Zip 36111–1801; tel. 334/265–5009; William G. McKenzie, President, Chief Executive Officer and Chairman, p. B54

**Tuscaloosa:** DCH HEALTH SYSTEM 809 University Boulevard East, Zip 35401; tel. 205/759–7111; Bryan N. Kindred, FACHE, President and Chief Executive Officer, p. B40

#### ARIZONA

**Flagstaff:** ★ NORTHERN ARIZONA HEALTHCARE 1200 North Beaver Street, Zip 86001; tel. 928/779–3366; William T. Bradel, President and Co–Chief Executive Officer, p. B95

**Phoenix:** ★ BANNER HEALTH 1441 North 12th Street, Zip 85006–2837, Mailing Address: P.O. Box 25489, Zip 85002–5489; tel. 602/747–4000; Peter S. Fine, FACHE, President and Chief Executive Officer, p. B16

★ JOHN C. LINCOLN HEALTH NETWORK 2500 West Utopia Road, Suite 100, Zip 85027–4172; tel. 623/434–6230; Rhonda Forsyth, President and Chief Executive Officer, p. B74

**Scottsdale:** ★ SCOTTSDALE HEALTHCARE 3621 Wells Fargo Avenue, Zip 85251–5607; tel. 480/882–4000; Thomas J. Sadvary, FACHE, President and Chief Executive Officer, p. B114

#### ARKANSAS

**Batesville:** ★ WHITE RIVER HEALTH SYSTEM 1710 Harrison Street, Zip 72501–7303; tel. 870/262–1200; Gary Bebow, FACHE, Administrator and Chief Executive Officer, p. B146

**Blytheville:** MISSISSIPPI COUNTY HOSPITAL SYSTEM 1520 North Division Street, Zip 72315–1448, Mailing Address: Box 108, Zip 72316; Ralph E. Beaty, Chief Executive Officer, p. B91

**Little Rock:** ★ BAPTIST HEALTH 9601 Interstate 630, Exit 7, Zip 72205–7299; tel. 501/202–2000; Russell D. Harrington, Jr., FACHE, President and Chief Executive Officer, p. B17

#### CALIFORNIA

**Alhambra:** AHMC & HEALTHCARE, INC. 55 South Raymond Avenue, Suite 105, Zip 91801–7100; tel. 626/457–9600; Jonathan Wu, M.D., President and Chairman, p. B7

**Corona:** AURORA BEHAVIORAL HEALTH CARE 4238 Green River Road, Zip 92882; tel. 951/549–8032; Soon K. Kim, M.D., President and Chief Executive Officer, p. B14

**Covina:** CITRUS VALLEY HEALTH PARTNERS 210 West San Bernardino Road, Zip 91723; tel. 626/331–7331; Robert H. Curry, President and Chief Executive Officer, p. B32

**El Segundo:** AVANTI HOSPITALS 222 North Sepulveda Boulevard, Suite 950, Zip 90245–5614; tel. 310/356–0550; John J. Ferrelli, Chief Operating Officer, p. B15

**Fountain Valley:** MEMORIALCARE 17360 Brookhurst Street, Zip 92708–3720, Mailing Address: P.O. Box 1428, Long Beach, Zip 90801–1428; tel. 714/377–2900; Barry S. Arbuckle, Ph.D., President and Chief Executive Officer, p. B87

**Fresno:** COMMUNITY MEDICAL CENTERS Fresno and Maddy Drive, Zip 93721, Mailing Address: P.O. Box 1232, Zip 93715–1232; tel. 559/459–6000; Tim A. Joslin, President and Chief Executive Officer, p. B37

**Hemet:** ★ PHYSICIANS FOR HEALTHY HOSPITALS 1525 West Florida Avenue, Suite A., Zip 92543; tel. 951/652–2811; Joel Bergenfeld, Chief Executive Officer, p. B101

**Loma Linda:** LOMA LINDA UNIVERSITY ADVENTIST HEALTH SCIENCES CENTER 11175 Campus Street, Zip 92354; tel. 909/558–7572; Richard H. Hart, M.D., President and Chief Executive Officer, p. B82

**Los Altos Hills:** ★ DAUGHTERS OF CHARITY HEALTH SYSTEM 26000 Altamont Road, Zip 94022; tel. 650/917–4500; Robert Issai, President and Chief Executive Officer, p. B40

**Los Angeles:** ALTA HEALTHCARE SYSTEM 10780 Santa Monica Boulevard, Suite 400, Zip 90025–7616; tel. 310/943–4500; David Topper, Chief Executive Officer, p. B9

LOS ANGELES COUNTY–DEPARTMENT OF HEALTH SERVICES 313 North Figueroa Street, Room 912, Zip 90012–2691; tel. 213/240–8101; Mitchell H. Katz, M.D., Director, p. B82

**Oakland:** ★ KAISER FOUNDATION HOSPITALS One Kaiser Plaza, Zip 94612–3600; tel. 510/271–5910; George C. Halvorson, Chairman and Chief Executive Officer, p. B74

★ UNIVERSITY OF CALIFORNIA–SYSTEMWIDE ADMINISTRATION 1111 Franklin Street, 11th Floor, Zip 94607–5200; tel. 510/987–9071; John D. Stobo, M.D., Senior Vice President Health Sciences and Services, p. B138

**Ontario:** PRIME HEALTHCARE SERVICES 3300 East Guasti Road, Zip 91761–8655; tel. 909/235–4400; Prem Reddy, M.D., Interim President and Chief Executive Officer, p. B103

**Orange:** ★ ST. JOSEPH HEALTH 500 South Main Street, Suite 1000, Zip 92868, Mailing Address: P.O. Box 14132, Zip 92863–1532; tel. 714/347–7500; Deborah A. Proctor, President and Chief Executive Officer, p. B122

**Palo Alto:** STANFORD HEALTH CARE 300 Pasteur Drive, Zip 94304–2299; tel. 650/723–4000; Amir Dan Rubin, President and Chief Executive Officer, p. B123

**Roseville:** ★ ADVENTIST HEALTH 2100 Douglas Boulevard, Zip 95661–3898, Mailing Address: P.O. Box 619002, Zip 95661–9002; tel. 916/781–2000; Robert G. Carmen, President, p. B4

**Sacramento:** ★ SUTTER HEALTH 2200 River Plaza Drive, Zip 95833; tel. 916/733–8800; Patrick E. Fry, Chief Executive Officer, p. B125

**San Diego:** PALOMAR HEALTH 15255 Innovation Drive, Zip 92128–3410; tel. 858/675–5100; Michael H. Covert, FACHE, Chief Executive Officer, p. B99

★ SCRIPPS HEALTH 4275 Campus Point Court, Zip 92121; tel. 858/678–6919; Chris D. Van Gorder, FACHE, President and Chief Executive Officer, p. B114

★ SHARP HEALTHCARE 8695 Spectrum Center Boulevard, Zip 92123–1489; tel. 858/499–4000; Michael Murphy, CPA, President and Chief Executive Officer, p. B117

**San Francisco:** ★ DIGNITY HEALTH 185 Berry Street, Suite 300, Zip 94107–1773; tel. 415/438–5500; Lloyd H. Dean, President and Chief Executive Officer, p. B46

**Santa Ana:** INTEGRATED HEALTHCARE 1301 North Tustin Avenue, Zip 92705; tel. 714/953–3652; Kenneth K. Westbrook, President and Chief Executive Officer, p. B71

**Santa Barbara:** ★ COTTAGE HEALTH SYSTEM Pueblo at Bath Streets, Zip 93105, Mailing Address: P.O. Box 689, Zip 93102–0689; tel. 805/569–7290; Ronald C. Werft, President and Chief Executive Officer, p. B39

**Santa Fe Springs:** COLLEGE HEALTH ENTERPRISES 11627 Telegraph Road, Suite 200, Zip 90670; tel. 562/923–9449; Barry J. Weiss, Chairman of the Board, p. B32

**Truckee:** TAHOE FOREST HEALTH SYSTEM 10121 Pine Avenue, Zip 96161; tel. 530/587–6011; Robert A. Schapper, Chief Executive Officer, p. B126

**Tustin:** PACIFIC HEALTH CORPORATION 14642 Newport Avenue, Suite 388, Zip 92780; tel. 714/619–9997; Georg J. Hopf, President and Chief Executive Officer, p. B99

**Walnut Creek:** ★ JOHN MUIR HEALTH 1400 Treat Boulevard, Zip 94597–2142; tel. 925/941–2100; Calvin K. Knight, President and Chief Executive Officer, p. B74

## COLORADO

**Denver:** ★ EXEMPLA HEALTHCARE, INC. 2420 West 26th Avenue, Suite 100–D, Zip 80211; tel. 303/813–5000; Robert W. Ladenburger, President and Chief Executive Officer, p. B51

★ SISTERS OF CHARITY OF LEAVENWORTH HEALTH SYSTEM 2420 West 26th Avenue, Suite 100D, Zip 80211–5301; tel. 303/813–5180; Michael A. Slubowski, Chief Executive Officer, p. B119

**Englewood:** ★ CATHOLIC HEALTH INITIATIVES 198 Inverness Drive West, Suite 800, Zip 80112–5202; tel. 303/298–9100; Kevin E. Lofton, FACHE, President and Chief Executive Officer, p. B27

**Fort Collins:** ★ POUDRE VALLEY HEALTH SYSTEM 2315 East Harmony Road, Suite 200, Zip 80528; tel. 970/237–7001; Rulon F. Stacey, Ph.D., FACHE, President and Chief Executive Officer, p. B102

## CONNECTICUT

**Danbury:** ★ WESTERN CONNECTICUT HEALTHCARE, INC. 24 Hospital Avenue, Zip 06810–6099; tel. 203/739–7066; John M. Murphy, M.D., President, p. B145

**Hartford:** CONNECTICUT DEPARTMENT OF MENTAL HEALTH AND ADDICTION SERVICES 410 Capitol Avenue, Zip 06106, Mailing Address: P.O. Box 341431, Zip 06134–1431; tel. 860/418–7000; Patricia Rehmer, Commissioner, p. B38

HARTFORD HEALTHCARE 80 Seymour Street, Zip 06102–8000, Mailing Address: P.O. Box 5037, Zip 06102–5037; Elliot T. Joseph, President and Chief Executive Officer, p. B56

★ SAINT FRANCIS CARE, INC. 114 Woodland Street, Zip 06105; tel. 860/714–5541; Christopher M. Dadlez, President and Chief Executive Officer, p. B111

**Manchester:** ★ EASTERN CONNECTICUT HEALTH NETWORK 71 Haynes Street, Zip 06040–4131; tel. 860/533–3400; Peter J. Karl, President and Chief Executive Officer, p. B49

**New Haven:** ★ YALE NEW HAVEN HEALTH SYSTEM 789 Howard Avenue, Zip 06519; tel. 203/688–4608; Marna P. Borgstrom, President and Chief Executive Officer, p. B146

## DELAWARE

**Wilmington:** ★ CHRISTIANA CARE HEALTH SYSTEM 501 West 14th Street, Zip 19801–1013, Mailing Address: P.O. Box 1668, Zip 19899; tel. 302/733–1000; Robert J. Laskowski, M.D., President and Chief Executive Officer, p. B31

## DISTRICT OF COLUMBIA

**Washington:** BUREAU OF MEDICINE AND SURGERY, DEPARTMENT OF THE NAVY 2300 East Street N.W., Zip 20372–5300; tel. 202/762–3701; Rear Admiral Matthew L. Nathan, Surgeon General, p. B23

DEPARTMENT OF THE AIR FORCE 1420 Pentagon, Room 4E1084, Zip 20330–1420; tel. 202/767–4765; Lieutenant General Charles B. Green, M.D., Surgeon General, p. B41

DEPARTMENT OF VETERANS AFFAIRS 810 Vermont Avenue N.W., Zip 20420; tel. 202/273–5781; Robert A. Petzel, M.D., Under Secretary for Health, p. B42

## FLORIDA

**Altamonte Springs:** ★ ADVENTIST HEALTH SYSTEM SUNBELT HEALTH CARE CORPORATION 900 Hope Way, Zip 32714–1502; tel. 407/357–1000; Donald L. Jernigan, Ph.D., President and Chief Executive Officer, p. B5

**Boca Raton:** PROMISE HEALTHCARE 999 Yamato Road, 3rd Floor, Zip 33431; tel. 561/869–3100; Howard B. Koslow, President and Chief Executive Officer, p. B104

SUCCESS HEALTHCARE 999 Yamato Road, 3rd Floor, Zip 33431–4477; tel. 561/869–6300; Peter R. Baronoff, President and Chief Executive Officer, p. B124

**Clearwater:** MORTON PLANT MEASE HEALTH CARE 300 Pinellas Street, Zip 33756, Mailing Address: P.O. Box 210, Zip 33756–0210; tel. 727/462–7000; Glenn D. Waters, FACHE, President, p. B91

**Coral Gables:** ★ BAPTIST HEALTH SOUTH FLORIDA 6855 Red Road, Suite 600, Zip 33143–3632; tel. 786/662–7111; Brian E. Keeley, President and Chief Executive Officer, p. B18

**Fort Lauderdale:** ★ BROWARD HEALTH 303 S.E. 17th Street, Zip 33316–2510; tel. 954/355–5100; Frank P. Nask, President and Chief Executive Officer, p. B23

**Fort Myers:** LEE MEMORIAL HEALTH SYSTEM 2776 Cleveland Avenue, Zip 33901, Mailing Address: P.O. Box 2218, Zip 33902–2218; tel. 239/343–2000; James R. Nathan, President and Chief Executive Officer, p. B79

**Gainesville:** ★ SHANDS HEALTHCARE 1600 S.W. Archer Road, Zip 32610–0326; tel. 352/265–8929; Timothy M. Goldfarb, Chief Executive Officer, p. B117

**Hollywood:** ★ MEMORIAL HEALTHCARE SYSTEM 3501 Johnson Street, Zip 33021–5421; tel. 954/265–5805; Frank V. Sacco, FACHE, President and Chief Executive Officer, p. B87

**Jacksonville:** ★ BAPTIST HEALTH 800 Prudential Drive, Zip 32207; tel. 904/202–4011; Hugh Greene, President and Chief Executive Officer, p. B17

**Leesburg:** CENTRAL FLORIDA HEALTH ALLIANCE 600 East Dixie Avenue, Zip 34748–5925; tel. 352/323–5762; Donald G. Henderson, FACHE, Chief Executive Officer, p. B30

**Miami Lakes:** PACER HEALTH CORPORATION 14100 Palmetto Frontage Road, Suite 110, Zip 33016; tel. 305/828–7660; Rainier Gonzalez, Chairman and Chief Executive Officer, p. B99

**Naples:** HEALTH MANAGEMENT ASSOCIATES 5811 Pelican Bay Boulevard, Suite 500, Zip 34108; tel. 239/598–3131; Gary D. Newsome, President and Chief Executive Officer, p. B62

**Orlando:** ORLANDO HEALTH 1414 Kuhl Avenue, Zip 32806–2093; tel. 407/841–5111; Sherrie Sitarik, President and Chief Executive Officer, p. B98

**Pensacola:** ★ BAPTIST HEALTH CARE CORPORATION 1717 North E Street, Suite 320, Zip 32501, Mailing Address: P.O. Box 17500, Zip 32522–7500; tel. 850/434–4011; Mark T. Faulkner, President, p. B18

**Rockledge:** HEALTH FIRST, INC. 6450 U.S. Highway 1, Zip 32955; tel. 321/434–7000; Steven P. Johnson, Ph.D., President and Chief Executive Officer, p. B61

WUESTHOFF HEALTH SYSTEM 110 Longwood Avenue, Zip 32955; tel. 321/636–2211; Steven P. Johnson, Chief Executive Officer, p. B136

**Tampa:** SHRINERS HOSPITALS FOR CHILDREN 2900 Rocky Point Drive, Zip 33607–1435, Mailing Address: P.O. Box 31356, Zip 33631–3356; tel. 813/281–0300; Keith Gardner, Executive Vice President, p. B118

**Windermere:** UNITED MEDICAL CORPORATION 603 Main Street, Zip 34786–3548, Mailing Address: P.O. Box 1100, Zip 34786–1100; tel. 407/876–2200; Donald R. Dizney, Chairman and Chief Executive Officer, p. B133

## GEORGIA

**Albany:** ★ PHOEBE PUTNEY HEALTH SYSTEM 417 Third Avenue, Zip 31702; tel. 229/312–1000; Joel Wernick, President and Chief Executive Officer, p. B101

**Atlanta:** ★ EMORY HEALTHCARE 1440 Clifton Road N.E., Suite 145, Zip 30322–1102; tel. 404/778–5000; John T. Fox, Chief Executive Officer, p. B50

NORTHSIDE HEALTHCARE SYSTEM 1000 Johnson Ferry Road N.E., Zip 30342–1611; tel. 404/851–8000; Robert Quattrocchi, President and Chief Executive Officer, p. B96

★ PIEDMONT HEALTHCARE 1800 Howell Mill Road N.W., Suite 850, Zip 30318–2538; tel. 404/425–1314; R. Timothy Stack, FACHE, President and Chief Executive Officer, p. B101

SUNLINK HEALTH SYSTEMS 900 Circle 75 Parkway, Suite 1120, Zip 30339; tel. 770/933–7000; Robert M. Thornton, Jr., Chief Executive Officer, p. B125

**Brunswick:** ★ SOUTHEAST GEORGIA HEALTH SYSTEM 2415 Parkwood Drive, Zip 31520–4252, Mailing Address: P.O. Box 1518, Zip 31521–1518; tel. 912/466–7000; Gary R. Colberg, FACHE, President and Chief Executive Officer, p. B120

**Carrollton:** TANNER HEALTH SYSTEM 705 Dixie Street, Zip 30117–3818; tel. 770/836–9580; Loy M. Howard, President and Chief Executive Officer, p. B126

**Columbus:** ★ COLUMBUS REGIONAL HEALTHCARE SYSTEM 707 Center Street, Suite 400, Zip 31901; tel. 706/660–6100; Charles A. Stark, FACHE, Chief Executive Officer, p. B32

**Dalton:** HAMILTON HEALTH CARE SYSTEM, INC. 1200 Memorial Drive, Zip 30720–2529, Mailing Address: P.O. Box 1900, Zip 30722–1900; tel. 706/272–6000; Jeffrey D. Myers, President and Chief Executive Officer, p. B56

**Decatur:** DEKALB REGIONAL HEALTH SYSTEM 2701 North Decatur Road, Zip 30033; tel. 404/501–1000; John Shelton, President and Chief Executive Officer, p. B41

**Marietta:** ★ WELLSTAR HEALTH SYSTEM 805 Sandy Plains Road, Zip 30066; tel. 770/792–5012; Reynold J. Jennings, President and Chief Executive Officer, p. B144

**Milledgeville:** OCONEE REGIONAL HEALTH SYSTEMS 821 North Cobb Street, Zip 31061; tel. 478/454–3505; Jean Aycock, President and Chief Executive Officer, p. B97

**Royston:** TY COBB HEALTHCARE SYSTEM, INC. 461 Cook Street, Suite A., Zip 30662–4003; tel. 706/245–1832; Charles T. Adams, President and Chief Executive Officer, p. B131

**Thomasville:** ★ ARCHBOLD MEDICAL CENTER 910 South Broad Street, Zip 31792–6113; tel. 229/228–2739; J. Perry Mustian, President, p. B10

**Warner Robins:** ★ HOUSTON HEALTHCARE SYSTEM 1601 Watson Boulevard, Zip 31093–3431, Mailing Address: P.O. Box 2886, Zip 31099–2886; tel. 478/922–4281; Cary Martin, Chief Executive Officer, p. B69

## HAWAII

**Honolulu:** ★ HAWAII HEALTH SYSTEMS CORPORATION 3675 Kilauea Avenue, Zip 96816; tel. 808/733–4151; Bruce S. Anderson, Ph.D., President and Chief Executive Officer, p. B57

HAWAII PACIFIC HEALTH 55 Merchant Street, Zip 96813; tel. 808/535–7414; Charles A. Sted, Chief Executive Officer, p. B57

★ QUEEN'S HEALTH SYSTEMS 1301 Punchbowl Street, Zip 96813–2402; tel. 808/535–5448; Arthur A. Ushijima, President and Chief Executive Officer, p. B108

## IDAHO

**Boise:** ★ ST. LUKE'S HEALTH SYSTEM 420 West Idaho Street, Zip 83702; tel. 208/381–4200; David C. Pate, M.D., JD, President and Chief Executive Officer, p. B123

## ILLINOIS

**Arlington Heights:** ALEXIAN BROTHERS HEALTH SYSTEM 3040 Salt Creek Lane, Zip 60005; tel. 847/463–8910; Mark A. Frey, President and Chief Executive Officer, p. B8

**Carbondale:** SOUTHERN ILLINOIS HOSPITAL SERVICES 1239 East Main Street, Zip 62901, Mailing Address: P.O. Box 3988, Zip 62902–3988; tel. 618/457–5200; Rex P. Budde, President and Chief Executive Officer, p. B120

**Chicago:** COOK COUNTY BUREAU OF HEALTH SERVICES 1900 West Polk Street, Suite 200, Zip 60612; tel. 312/864–6820; Ramanathan Raju, M.D., Chief Executive Officer, p. B38

NATIONAL SURGICAL HOSPITALS 250 South Wacker Drive, Suite 500, Zip 60606; tel. 312/627–8400; John G. Rex–Waller, Chief Executive Officer, p. B92

★ NORTHWESTERN MEMORIAL HEALTHCARE 251 East Huron Street, Zip 60611; tel. 312/926–2000; Dean M. Harrison, President and Chief Executive Officer, p. B96

★ PRESENCE HEALTH 7435 West Talcott Avenue, Zip 60631; tel. 773/792–5150; Sandra B. Bruce, FACHE, President and Chief Executive Officer, p. B103

★ RUSH UNIVERSITY MEDICAL CENTER 1653 West Congress Parkway, Zip 60612–3864; tel. 312/942–5000; Larry J. Goodman, M.D., Chief Executive Officer, p. B111

★ SINAI HEALTH SYSTEM 1500 South California Avenue, Zip 60608–1729; tel. 773/542–2000; Alan H. Channing, President and Chief Executive Officer, p. B118

**Crystal Lake:** ★ CENTEGRA HEALTH SYSTEM 385 Millennium Drive, Zip 60012; tel. 815/788–5800; Michael S. Eesley, Chief Executive Officer, p. B30

**De Kalb:** ★ KISH HEALTH SYSTEM 626 Bethany Road, Zip 60115–4939, Mailing Address: P.O. Box 707, DeKalb, Zip 60115–0707; tel. 815/756–1521; Kevin P. Poorten, President and Chief Executive Officer, p. B78

**Evanston:** ★ NORTHSHORE UNIVERSITY HEALTHSYSTEM 1301 Central Street, Zip 60201–1613; tel. 847/570–2000; Mark R. Neaman, President and Chief Executive Officer, p. B95

**Evergreen Park:** AMERICAN PROVINCE OF LITTLE COMPANY OF MARY SISTERS 9350 South California Avenue, Zip 60805–2595; tel. 708/229–5491; Sister Kathleen McIntyre, Province Leader, p. B9

**Maywood:** LOYOLA UNIVERSITY HEALTH SYSTEM 2160 South First Avenue, Zip 60153–5585; tel. 708/216–9000; Officer, Goldberg, President

**Oak Brook:** ★ ADVOCATE HEALTH CARE 2025 Windsor Drive, Zip 60523; tel. 630/990–5018; Jim H. Skogsbergh, President and Chief Executive Officer, p. B6

**Peoria:** ★ OSF HEALTHCARE SYSTEM 800 N.E. Glen Oak Avenue, Zip 61603–3200; tel. 309/655–2850; Kevin D. Schoeplein, President, p. B99

**Schaumburg:** CANCER TREATMENT CENTERS OF AMERICA 1336 Basswood Road, Zip 60173; tel. 847/342–7400; Stephen B. Bonner, President and Chief Executive Officer, p. B23

**Springfield:** DIVISION OF MENTAL HEALTH, DEPARTMENT OF HUMAN SERVICES 319 East Madison Street, S–3B, Zip 62701; tel. 217/785–6023; Lorrie Rickman Jones, Ph.D., Director, p. B48

★ HOSPITAL SISTERS HEALTH SYSTEM 4936 LaVerna Road, Zip 62707–9797, Mailing Address: P.O. Box 19456, Zip 62707; tel. 217/523–4747; Mary Starmann–Harrison, FACHE, President and Chief Executive Officer, p. B69

★ MEMORIAL HEALTH SYSTEM 701 North First Street, Zip 62781–0001; tel. 217/788–3000; Edgar J. Curtis, President and Chief Executive Officer, p. B87

**Wheaton:** ★ WHEATON FRANCISCAN HEALTHCARE 26W171 Roosevelt Road, Zip 60187–6078, Mailing Address: P.O. Box 667, Zip 60187–0667; tel. 630/909–6900; John D. Oliverio, President and Chief Executive Officer, p. B145

**Winfield:** ★ CADENCE HEALTH 25 North Winfield Road, Zip 60190; tel. 630/933–1600; Michael Vivoda, Chief Executive Officer, p. B23

## INDIANA

**Evansville:** ★ DEACONESS HEALTH SYSTEM 600 Mary Street, Zip 47747; tel. 812/450–5000; Linda E. White, President and Chief Executive Officer, p. B40

**Fort Wayne:** ★ PARKVIEW HEALTH 10501 Corporate Drive, Zip 46845, Mailing Address: P.O. Box 5600, Zip 46895–5600; tel. 260/373–7001; Michael J. Packnett, President and Chief Executive Officer, p. B100

**Hammond:** COMMUNITY HEALTHCARE SYSTEM 901 MacArthur Boulevard, Zip 46321–2959; tel. 219/836–1600; Donald Powers, Chairman, President and Chief Executive Officer, p. B37

**Indianapolis:** COMMUNITY HEALTH NETWORK 7330 Shadeland Station, Zip 46256–3957; tel. 317/355–1411; Bryan A. Mills, President and Chief Executive Officer, p. B33

★ INDIANA UNIVERSITY HEALTH 340 West 10th Street, Suite 6100, Zip 46202–3082, Mailing Address: P.O. Box 1367, Zip 46206–1367; tel. 317/962–5900; Daniel F. Evans, Jr., JD, President and Chief Executive Officer, p. B70

**Mishawaka:** FRANCISCAN ALLIANCE 1515 Dragoon Trail, Zip 46546–1290, Mailing Address: P.O. Box 1290, Zip 46546–1290; tel. 574/256–3935; Kevin D. Leahy, President and Chief Executive Officer, p. B52

PHYSICIANS HOSPITAL SYSTEM 1625 East Jefferson Boulevard, Zip 46545–7103; tel. 574/255–1400; Cameron R. Gilbert, Ph.D., President and Chief Executive Officer, p. B101

## IOWA

**Davenport:** ★ GENESIS HEALTH SYSTEM 1227 East Rusholme Street, Zip 52803–2498; tel. 563/421–1000; Douglas P. Cropper, President and Chief Executive Officer, p. B54

**Des Moines:** ★ IOWA HEALTH SYSTEM 1776 West Lakes Parkway, Suite 400, Zip 50266; tel. 515/241–6161; William B. Leaver, President and Chief Executive Officer, p. B72

## KANSAS

**Phillipsburg:** ★ GREAT PLAINS HEALTH ALLIANCE, INC. 625 Third Street, Zip 67661–2138, Mailing Address: P.O. Box 366, Zip 67661–0366; tel. 785/543–2111; Roger S. John, President and Chief Executive Officer, p. B55

**Wichita:** VIA CHRISTI HEALTH 8200 East Thorn, Zip 67226–2709; tel. 316/858–4900; Jeffrey Korsmo, President and Chief Executive Officer, p. B142

## KENTUCKY

**Bowling Green:** COMMONWEALTH HEALTH CORPORATION 800 Park Street, Zip 42101–2356; tel. 270/745–1500; Connie Smith, President and Chief Executive Officer, p. B33

**Edgewood:** ST. ELIZABETH HEALTHCARE 1 Medical Village Drive, Zip 41017–3403; tel. 859/301–2370; John S. Dubis, FACHE, President and Chief Executive Officer, p. B122

**Lexington:** APPALACHIAN REGIONAL HEALTHCARE, INC. 2285 Executive Drive, Suite 400, Zip 40505–4810, Mailing Address: P.O. Box 8086, Zip 40533–8086; tel. 859/226–2440; Jerry Haynes, President and Chief Executive Officer, p. B10

CARDINAL HILL HEALTHCARE SYSTEM 2050 Versailes Road, Zip 40504; tel. 859/254–5701; Gary Payne, President and Chief Executive Officer, p. B25

UK HEALTHCARE 800 Rose Street, Zip 40536–0293; tel. 859/323–5000; Michael Karpf, M.D., Executive Vice President Health Affairs, p. B133

**Louisville:** ALLIANT MANAGEMENT SERVICES 2650 Eastpoint Parkway, Suite 300, Zip 40223–5135; tel. 502/992–3525; Timothy L. Jarm, President and Chief Executive Officer, p. B8

★ BAPTIST HEALTHCARE SYSTEM 4007 Kresge Way, Zip 40207–4677; tel. 502/896–5000; Tommy J. Smith, President and Chief Executive Officer, p. B18

★ JEWISH HOSPITAL & ST. MARY'S HEALTHCARE 200 Abraham Flexner Way, Zip 40202–1886; tel. 502/587–4011; David Laird, President and Chief Executive Officer, p. B73

★ KINDRED HEALTHCARE 680 South Fourth Street, Zip 40202–2412; tel. 502/596–7300; Paul J. Diaz, President and Chief Executive Officer, p. B75

★ NORTON HEALTHCARE 234 East Gray Street, Suite 225, Zip 40202, Mailing Address: P.O. Box 35070, Zip 40232–5070; tel. 502/629–8000; Stephen Williams, President, p. B96

## LOUISIANA

**Baton Rouge:** ★ FRANCISCAN MISSIONARIES OF OUR LADY HEALTH SYSTEM, INC. 4200 Essen Lane, Zip 70809; tel. 225/923–2701; John J. Finan, Jr., FACHE, President and Chief Executive Officer, p. B53

LOUISIANA STATE HOSPITALS 628 North 4th Street, Zip 70802–5342, Mailing Address: P.O. Box 629, Zip 70821–0628; tel. 225/342–9500; Shelby Price, Chief Executive Officer, p. B83

LSU HEALTH CARE SERVICES DIVISION Kirby Smith Hall, 1st Floor, MR, Room 151, Zip 70803, Mailing Address: P.O. Box 91308, Zip 70821–1308; tel. 225/922–0488; Roxane A. Townsend, M.D., Chief Executive Officer, p. B83

**Benton:** CYPRESS HEALTH SYSTEMS 106 Preston Day Circle, Zip 71006; tel. 318/965–9914; Kim B. Bird, President and Chief Executive Officer, p. B40

**Hammond:** NORTH OAKS HEALTH SYSTEM 15790 Paul Vega MD Drive, Zip 70403–1436, Mailing Address: P.O. Box 2668, Zip 70404; tel. 985/345–2700; James E. Cathey, Jr., Chief Executive Officer, p. B95

**Lafayette:** AMG INTEGRATED HEALTHCARE MANAGEMENT 101 La Rue France, Suite 500, Zip 70508–3144; tel. 337/269–9828; August J. Rantz, III, Founder and Chief Executive Officer, p. B9

LHC GROUP 420 West Pinhook Road, Zip 70503–2131; tel. 337/223–1307; Keith G. Myers, Chairman and Chief Executive Officer, p. B79

**Lake Charles:** OCEANS HEALTHCARE 2720 Rue de Jardin, Suite 100, Zip 70605–4050; tel. 337/721–1900; Jason Reed, President and Chief Executive Officer, p. B97

**Leesville:** SPECIALTY HEALTHCARE, LLC 305 West Harriet Street, Zip 71446–4229; tel. 337/238–4449; Craig Ball, Chairman and Chief Executive Officer, p. B121

**New Orleans:** ★ OCHSNER HEALTH SYSTEM 1514 Jefferson Highway, Zip 70121–2429; tel. 800/874–8984; Patrick J. Quinlan, M.D., Chief Executive Officer, p. B97

**Shreveport:** ALLEGIANCE HEALTH MANAGEMENT 504 Texas Street, Suite 200, Zip 71101; tel. 318/226–8202; Rock Bordelon, President and Chief Executive Officer, p. B8

WILLIS–KNIGHTON HEALTH SYSTEM 2600 Greenwood Road, Zip 71130–2600; tel. 318/212–4000; James K. Elrod, FACHE, President and Chief Executive Officer, p. B146

## MAINE

**Brewer:** ★ EASTERN MAINE HEALTHCARE SYSTEMS 43 Whiting Hill Road, Zip 04412; tel. 207/973–7045; M. Michelle Hood, President and Chief Executive Officer, p. B49

**Portland:** MAINEHEALTH 110 Free Street, Zip 04101–3537; William L. Caron, Jr., President, p. B83

## MARYLAND

**Baltimore:** ★ JOHNS HOPKINS HEALTH SYSTEM 733 North Broadway, BRB 104, Zip 21205; tel. 410/955–5000; Ronald R. Peterson, President, p. B74

★ LIFEBRIDGE HEALTH 2401 West Belvedere Avenue, Zip 21215; tel. 410/601–5134; Warren A. Green, President and Chief Executive Officer, p. B80

★ UNIVERSITY OF MARYLAND MEDICAL SYSTEM 250 West Pratt Street, 24th Floor, Zip 21201–1595; tel. 410/328–8667; Robert A. Chrencik, President and Chief Executive Officer, p. B138

**Bel Air:** UPPER CHESAPEAKE HEALTH SYSTEM 520 Upper Chesapeake Drive, Suite 405, Zip 21014–4324; tel. 443/643–3303; Lyle Ernest Sheldon, FACHE, President and Chief Executive Officer, p. B140

**Cheverly:** DIMENSIONS HEALTHCARE SYSTEM 3001 Hospital Drive, 3rd Floor, Zip 20785; tel. 301/583–4000; Kenneth E. Glover, President and Chief Executive Officer, p. B47

**Columbia:** ENCORE HEALTHCARE 7150 Columbia Gateway Drove, Suite J., Zip 21046–2974; tel. 443/539–2350; Tim Nicholson, Chief Executive Officer, p. B50

★ MEDSTAR HEALTH 5565 Sterrett Place, 5th Floor, Zip 21044; tel. 410/772–6500; Kenneth A. Samet, President and Chief Executive Officer, p. B86

**Easton:** ★ SHORE HEALTH SYSTEM 219 South Washington Street, Zip 21601; tel. 410/822–1000; Kenneth D. Kozel, FACHE, President and Chief Executive Officer, p. B118

**Marriottsville:** ★ BON SECOURS HEALTH SYSTEM, INC. 1505 Marriottsville Road, Zip 21104–1399; tel. 410/442–5511; Richard Statuto, President and Chief Executive Officer, p. B22

**Rockville:** ★ ADVENTIST HEALTHCARE 1801 Research Boulevard, Suite 400, Zip 20850; tel. 301/315–3030; William G. Robertson, President and Chief Executive Officer, p. B6

U. S. INDIAN HEALTH SERVICE 801 Thompson Avenue, Zip 20852; tel. 301/443–1083; Yvette Roubideaux, M.D., M.P.H., Director, p. B132

**Sparks Glencoe:** FUNDAMENTAL LONG TERM CARE HOLDINGS, LLC 930 Ridgebrook Road, Zip 21152; tel. 410/773–1000; W. Bradley Bennett, President and Chief Executive Officer, p. B53

**Stevensville:** MID ATLANTIC HEALTH MANAGEMENT, INC. 1220 Butterworth Court, Zip 21666–2504; tel. 410/643–3393; Harold A. McBee, Jr., President, p. B89

## MASSACHUSETTS

**Boston:** MASSACHUSETTS DEPARTMENT OF MENTAL HEALTH 25 Staniford Street, Zip 02114–2575; tel. 617/626–8123; Marcia Fowler, Commissioner, p. B84

MASSACHUSETTS DEPARTMENT OF PUBLIC HEALTH 250 Washington Street, Zip 02108–4619; tel. 617/624–6000; John Auerbach, Commissioner, p. B85

★ PARTNERS HEALTHCARE SYSTEM, INC. 800 Boylston Street, Suite 1150, Zip 02199–8001; tel. 617/278–1004; Gary L. Gottlieb, M.D., President and Chief Executive Officer, p. B100

STEWARD HEALTH CARE SYSTEM, LLC 500 Boylston Street, 5th Floor, Zip 02116–3740; tel. 617/419–4700; Ralph de la Torre, M.D., Chairman and Chief Executive Officer, p. B124

**Haverhill:** WHITTIER HEALTH NETWORK 25 Railroad Square, Zip 01832–5721; tel. 978/556–5858; Alfred L. Arcidi, M.D., President, p. B146

**Hyannis:** ★ CAPE COD HEALTHCARE, INC. 88 Lewis Bay Road, Zip 02601–5210; tel. 508/862–5121; Michael K. Lauf, President and Chief Executive Officer, p. B24

**Newton:** FIVE STAR QUALITY CARE 400 Centre Street, Zip 02458–2076; tel. 617/796–8387; Bruce J. Mackey, Jr., President and Chief Executive Officer, p. B52

**Pittsfield:** ★ BERKSHIRE HEALTH SYSTEMS, INC. 725 North Street, Zip 01201–4124; tel. 413/447–2743; David E. Phelps, President and Chief Executive Officer, p. B21

**Springfield:** ★ BAYSTATE HEALTH, INC. 759 Chestnut Street, Zip 01199–0001; tel. 413/794–0000; Mark R. Tolosky, JD, FACHE, President and Chief Executive Officer, p. B20

**Tewksbury:** ★ COVENANT HEALTH SYSTEMS, INC. 100 Ames Pond Drive, Suite 102, Zip 01876–1293; tel. 978/654–6363; David R. Lincoln, President and Chief Executive Officer, p. B39

**Worcester:** ★ UMASS MEMORIAL HEALTH CARE, INC. 1 Biotech Park, Zip 01605–2982; tel. 508/334–0100; John G. O'Brien, President and Chief Executive Officer, p. B133

## MICHIGAN

**Dearborn:** ★ OAKWOOD HEALTHCARE, INC. One Parklane Boulevard, Suite 1000E, Zip 48126; tel. 313/253–6050; Brian M. Connolly, President and Chief Executive Officer, p. B96

**Detroit:** ★ DETROIT MEDICAL CENTER 3990 John R., Zip 48201; tel. 313/745–1250; Michael Duggan, Chief Executive Officer, p. B46

★ HENRY FORD HEALTH SYSTEM One Ford Place, Zip 48202–3450; tel. 313/876–8708; Nancy M. Schlichting, Chief Executive Officer, p. B68

**Flint:** ★ MCLAREN HEALTH CARE CORPORATION G3235 Beecher Road, Suite B., Zip 48532; tel. 810/342–1100; Philip A. Incarnati, President and Chief Executive Officer, p. B86

**Grand Rapids:** ★ SPECTRUM HEALTH 100 Michigan Street N.E., Zip 49503–2551; tel. 616/391–1774; Richard C. Breon, President and Chief Executive Officer, p. B121

**Kalamazoo:** ★ BRONSON HEALTHCARE GROUP, INC. 301 John Street, Zip 49007–5345; tel. 269/341–6000; Frank J. Sardone, President and Chief Executive Officer, p. B22

**Lansing:** ★ SPARROW HEALTH SYSTEM 1215 East Michigan Avenue, Zip 48912; tel. 517/364–1000; Dennis A. Swan, President and Chief Executive Officer, p. B121

**Midland:** ★ MIDMICHIGAN HEALTH 4000 Wellness Drive, Zip 48670–0001; tel. 989/839–3000; Richard M. Reynolds, President and Chief Executive Officer, p. B90

**Novi:** ★ TRINITY HEALTH 27870 Cabot Drive, Zip 48377; tel. 248/489–5004; Joseph R. Swedish, President and Chief Executive Officer, p. B130

**Port Huron:** ★ BLUE WATER HEALTH SERVICES CORPORATION 1221 Pine Grove Avenue, Zip 48061–5011; tel. 810/989–3717; Thomas D. DeFauw, FACHE, President and Chief Executive Officer, p. B22

**Royal Oak:** ★ BEAUMONT HEALTH SYSTEM 3711 West 13 Mile Road, Zip 48073–6767; tel. 248/898–5000; Gene Michalski, President and Chief Executive Officer, p. B20

**Saint Joseph:** LAKELAND HEALTHCARE 1234 Napier Avenue, Zip 49085–2158; tel. 269/983–8300; Loren Hamel, M.D., President and Chief Executive Officer, p. B78

**Traverse City:** ★ MUNSON HEALTHCARE 1105 Sixth Street, Zip 49684–2386; tel. 231/935–6703; Edwin Ness, President and Chief Executive Officer, p. B92

## MINNESOTA

**Bloomington:** HEALTHPARTNERS 8170 33rd Avenue South, Zip 55425–1514; tel. 952/883–7463; Mary K. Brainerd, President and Chief Executive Officer, p. B64

**Duluth:** ESSENTIA HEALTH 502 East Second Street, Zip 55805; tel. 218/786–8376; Peter E. Person, M.D., Chief Executive Officer, p. B51

**Minneapolis:** ★ ALLINA HEALTH 2925 Chicago Avenue, Zip 55407, Mailing Address: P.O. Box 43, Zip 55440; tel. 612/262–5000; Ken Paulus, President and Chief Executive Officer, p. B9

CHILDREN'S HOSPITALS AND CLINICS OF MINNESOTA 2525 Chicago Avenue South, Zip 55404; tel. 612/813–6100; Alan L. Goldbloom, M.D., President and Chief Executive Officer, p. B31

★ FAIRVIEW HEALTH SERVICES 2450 Riverside Avenue, Zip 55454–1400; tel. 612/672–6141; Mark A. Eustis, President and Chief Executive Officer, p. B52

**Rochester:** ★ MAYO CLINIC HEALTH SYSTEM 200 S.W. First Street, Zip 55905–0002; tel. 507/284–2511; John Noseworthy, M.D., President and Chief Executive Officer, p. B85

**Saint Cloud:** ★ CENTRACARE HEALTH SYSTEM 1406 Sixth Avenue North, Zip 56303; tel. 320/251–2700; Terence Pladson, M.D., President and Chief Executive Officer, p. B30

**Saint Louis Park:** ★ PARK NICOLLET HEALTH SERVICES 6500 Excelsior Boulevard, Zip 55426–4702; tel. 952/993–5000; David Abelson, M.D., Chief Executive Officer, p. B100

**Saint Paul:** ★ HEALTHEAST CARE SYSTEM 559 Capitol Boulevard, 6–South, Zip 55103–0000; tel. 651/232–2300; Kathryn G. Correia, President and Chief Executive Officer, p. B64

MINNESOTA DEPARTMENT OF HUMAN SERVICES 540 Cedar Street, Zip 55164–0980, Mailing Address: P.O. Box 64980, Zip 55164–0980; tel. 651/431–2369; Michael Tessneer, Chief Executive Officer, p. B90

## MISSISSIPPI

**Jackson:** ★ MISSISSIPPI BAPTIST HEALTH SYSTEM 1225 North State Street, Zip 39202–2002; tel. 601/968–1000; Mark F. Slyter, FACHE, President and Chief Executive Officer, p. B90

MISSISSIPPI STATE DEPARTMENT OF MENTAL HEALTH 1101 Robert East Lee Building, 239 North Lamar Street, Zip 39201–1101; tel. 601/359–1288; Edwin C. LeGrand, III, Executive Director, p. B91

**Magee:** ★ PIONEER HEALTH SERVICES 110 Pioneer Way, Zip 39111, Mailing Address: P.O. Box 1100, Zip 39111; tel. 601/849–6440; Joseph S. McNulty, III, President and Chief Executive Officer, p. B102

**Mccomb:** SOUTHWEST HEALTH SYSTEMS 215 Marion Avenue, Zip 39648–2705, Mailing Address: P.O. Box 1307, Zip 39649–1307; tel. 601/249–5500; Norman M. Price, FACHE, Chief Executive Officer and Administrator, p. B121

**Meridian:** ★ RUSH HEALTH SYSTEMS 1314 19th Avenue, Zip 39301; tel. 601/483–0011; Wallace Strickland, President and Chief Executive Officer, p. B110

**Tupelo:** ★ NORTH MISSISSIPPI HEALTH SERVICES, INC. 830 South Gloster Street, Zip 38801–4996; tel. 662/377–3136; John R. Heer, President and Chief Executive Officer, p. B94

## MISSOURI

**Cape Girardeau:** LANDMARK HOSPITALS 3255 Independence Street, Zip 63701–4904; tel. 573/335–1091; William K. Kapp, III, M.D., President and Chief Executive Officer, p. B78

★ SOUTHEASTHEALTH 1701 Lacey Street, Zip 63701–5230; tel. 573/334–4822; Wayne Smith, President and Chief Executive Officer, p. B120

**Chesterfield:** ★ MERCY HEALTH 14528 South Outer 40, Suite 100, Zip 63017–5743; tel. 314/579–6100; Lynn Britton, President and Chief Executive Officer, p. B88

**Columbia:** ★ UNIVERSITY OF MISSOURI HEALTH CARE One Hospital Drive, DC 031, Zip 65212–0001; tel. 573/884–8738; James H. Ross, Chief Executive Officer, p. B139

**Joplin:** ★ FREEMAN HEALTH SYSTEM 1102 West 32nd Street, Zip 64804; tel. 417/347–1111; Paula F. Baker, President and Chief Executive Officer, p. B53

**Kansas City:** HMC/CAH CONSOLIDATED, INC. 1100 Main Street, Suite 2350, Zip 64105–5186; tel. 816/474–7800; Lawrence J. Arthur, President, p. B68

SAINT LUKE'S HEALTH SYSTEM 10920 Elm Avenue, Zip 64134–4108, Mailing Address: 4401 Wornall, Zip 64111; tel. 816/932–2000; Melinda Estes, M.D., President and Chief Executive Officer, p. B111

★ TRUMAN MEDICAL CENTERS 2301 Holmes Street, Zip 64108–2677; tel. 816/404–1000; John W. Bluford, President and Chief Executive Officer, p. B131

**Saint Louis:** ★ ASCENSION HEALTH 4600 Edmundson Road, Zip 63134–3806; tel. 314/733–8000; Robert J. Henkel, FACHE, President and Chief Executive Officer, p. B11

★ BJC HEALTHCARE 4901 Forest Park Avenue, Suite 1200, Zip 63108–1401; tel. 314/747–9322; Steven H. Lipstein, President and Chief Executive Officer, p. B21

★ SSM HEALTH CARE 477 North Lindbergh Boulevard, Zip 63141–7813; tel. 314/994–7800; William P. Thompson, President and Chief Executive Officer, p. B122

**Springfield:** COXHEALTH 1423 North Jefferson Avenue, Zip 65802–1988; tel. 417/269–3108; Steven D. Edwards, President and Chief Executive Officer, p. B40

## MONTANA

**Great Falls:** BENEFIS HEALTH SYSTEM 1101 26th Street South, Zip 59405; tel. 406/455–5000; John H. Goodnow, Chief Executive Officer, p. B21

## NEBRASKA

**Lincoln:** ★ BRYANLGH HEALTH SYSTEM 1600 South 48th Street, Zip 68506; tel. 402/489–0200; Kimberly A. Russel, President and Chief Executive Officer, p. B23

**Norfolk:** FAITH REGIONAL HEALTH SERVICES 2700 West Norfolk Avenue, Zip 68701–4438, Mailing Address: P.O. Box 869, Zip 68702–0869; tel. 402/644–7201; James J. Sinek, President and Chief Executive Officer, p. B52

**Omaha:** ALEGENT HEALTH 12809 West Dodge Road, Zip 68154; tel. 402/343–4000; Richard A. Hachten, II, FACHE, President and Chief Executive Officer, p. B7

★ NEBRASKA METHODIST HEALTH SYSTEM, INC. 8511 West Dodge Road, Zip 68114; tel. 402/354–5411; John M. Fraser, President and Chief Executive Officer, p. B92

## NEVADA

**Reno:** ★ RENOWN HEALTH 1155 Mill Street, Zip 89502–1576; tel. 775/982–4100; James I. Miller, President and Chief Executive Officer, p. B110

## NEW HAMPSHIRE

**Laconia:** ★ LRGHEALTHCARE 80 Highland Street, Zip 03246–3298; tel. 603/524–3211; Thomas Clairmont, President, p. B83

**Portsmouth:** SPECIALTY HOSPITALS OF AMERICA, LLC 155 Fleet Street, Zip 03801; tel. 603/570–4888; Eric F. Rieseberg, President, p. B121

## NEW JERSEY

**Edison:** ★ JFK HEALTH SYSTEM 80 James Street, 2nd Floor, Zip 08820–3998; tel. 732/321–7774; Raymond F. Fredericks, President and Chief Executive Officer, p. B74

**Egg Harbor Township:** ★ ATLANTICARE 2500 English Creek Avenue, Building 500, Suite 501, Zip 08234; tel. 609/407–2309; David P. Tilton, President and Chief Executive Officer, p. B14

**Lakewood:** ACUTECARE HEALTH SYSTEM 500 River Avenue, Suite 150, Zip 08701–4743; tel. 732/364–0800; Daniel Czermak, Chairman and President, p. B4

**Marlton:** ★ VIRTUA HEALTH 50 Lake Center Executive Drive, Suite 401, Zip 08053; tel. 856/355–0010; Richard P. Miller, Chief Executive Officer, p. B143

**Morristown:** ★ ATLANTIC HEALTH 475 South Street, Zip 07962, Mailing Address: P.O. Box 1905, Zip 07962–1905; tel. 973/660–3270; Joseph A. Trunfio, Ph.D., President and Chief Executive Officer, p. B14

**Neptune:** ★ MERIDIAN HEALTH 1350 Campus Parkway, Zip 07753; tel. 732/751–7510; John K. Lloyd, President and Chief Executive Officer, p. B89

**New Brunswick:** ROBERT WOOD JOHNSON HEALTH SYSTEM & NETWORK 1 Robert Wood Johnson Place, Zip 08903–2601; tel. 732/828–3000; Stephen K. Jones, President and Chief Executive Officer, p. B110

**Trenton:** ★ CAPITAL HEALTH 750 Brunswick Avenue, Zip 08638–4174; tel. 609/394–6000; Al Maghazehe, Ph.D., FACHE, Chief Executive Officer, p. B24

DIVISION OF MENTAL HEALTH AND ADDICTION SERVICES, DEPARTMENT OF HUMAN SERVICES, STATE OF NEW JERSEY Capital Center, P.O. Box 727, Zip 08625–0727; tel. 609/777–0702; Lynn Kovich, Assistant Commissioner, p. B47

**Vineland:** ★ SOUTH JERSEY HEALTHCARE 2950 College Drive, Suite 1E, Zip 08360; tel. 856/641–8000; Chester B. Kaletkowski, President and Chief Executive Officer, p. B120

**West Orange:** ★ BARNABAS HEALTH 95 Old Short Hills Road, Zip 07052; tel. 973/322–4000; Barry Ostrowsky, President and Chief Executive Officer, p. B19

### NEW MEXICO

**Albuquerque:** ERNEST HEALTH, INC. 7770 Jefferson Street N.E., Suite 320, Zip 87109; tel. 505/856–5300; Darby Brockette, Chief Executive Officer, p. B50

★ PRESBYTERIAN HEALTHCARE SERVICES 2501 Buena Vista Drive, S.E., Zip 87106–4260, Mailing Address: P.O. Box 26666, Zip 87125–6666; tel. 505/841–1234; James H. Hinton, President and Chief Executive Officer, p. B102

### NEW YORK

**Albany:** NEW YORK STATE OFFICE OF MENTAL HEALTH 44 Holland Avenue, Zip 12229–3411; tel. 518/474–4403; Michael F. Hogan, Ph.D., Commissioner, p. B93

**Binghamton:** UNITED HEALTH SERVICES 10–42 Mitchell Avenue, Zip 13903; tel. 607/762–2200; Matthew J. Salanger, President and Chief Executive Officer, p. B133

**Buffalo:** ★ CATHOLIC HEALTH SYSTEM 2121 Main Street, Suite 300, Zip 14214; tel. 716/862–2410; Joseph D. McDonald, President and Chief Executive Officer, p. B29

**Cooperstown:** ★ BASSETT HEALTHCARE NETWORK 1 Atwell Road, Zip 13326–1301; tel. 607/547–3456; William F. Streck, M.D., President and Chief Executive Officer, p. B19

**Elmira:** ★ ARNOT HEALTH 600 Roe Avenue, Zip 14905–1629; tel. 607/737–4100; Anthony J. Cooper, FACHE, President and Chief Executive Officer, p. B11

**Geneva:** FINGER LAKES HEALTH 196 North Street, Zip 14456; tel. 315/787–4000; Jose Acevedo, M.D., President and Chief Executive Officer, p. B52

**Great Neck:** ★ NORTH SHORE–LONG ISLAND JEWISH HEALTH SYSTEM 145 Community Drive, Zip 11021; tel. 516/465–8100; Michael J. Dowling, President and Chief Executive Officer, p. B95

**Kingston:** HEALTHALLIANCE OF THE HUDSON VALLEY 396 Broadway, Zip 12401–4626; tel. 845/331–3131; David W. Lundquist, President and Chief Executive Officer, p. B64

**Lagrangeville:** ★ HEALTH QUEST SYSTEMS, INC. 1351 Route 55, Zip 12540–5108; tel. 845/475–9500; Michael T. Weber, President and Chief Executive Officer, p. B64

**New Rochelle:** SOUND SHORE HEALTH SYSTEM 16 Guion Place, Zip 10801–5500; tel. 914/632–5000; John R. Spicer, President and Chief Executive Officer, p. B120

**New York:** ASCEND HEALTH CORPORATION 32 East 57th Street, 17th Floor, Zip 10022–2513; Richard A. Kresch, M.D., President and Chief Executive Officer, p. B11

★ CONTINUUM HEALTH PARTNERS 555 West 57th Street, Zip 10019; tel. 212/523–8130; Stanley Brezenoff, President and Chief Executive Officer, p. B38

★ NEW YORK CITY HEALTH AND HOSPITALS CORPORATION 125 Worth Street, Room 514, Zip 10013–4006; tel. 212/788–3321; Alan D. Aviles, President, p. B93

NEW YORK PRESBYTERIAN HEALTHCARE SYSTEM 177 Fort Washington Avenue, Room P123, Zip 10032; tel. 212/746–3745; Steven J. Corwin, M.D., Chief Executive Officer, p. B93

**Olean:** UPPER ALLEGHENY HEALTH SYSTEM 130 South Union Street, Suite 300, Zip 14760–3676; tel. 716/375–6190; Timothy J. Finan, FACHE, President and Chief Executive Officer, p. B140

**Rochester:** ROCHESTER GENERAL HEALTH SYSTEM 1425 Portland Avenue, 5th Floor, Zip 14621; tel. 585/922–4000; Mark C. Clement, President and Chief Executive Officer, p. B110

★ UNIVERSITY OF ROCHESTER MEDICAL CENTER 601 Elmwood Avenue, Zip 14642–0002; tel. 585/275–2100; Steven I. Goldstein, General Director and Chief Executive Officer, p. B139

**Rockville Centre:** CATHOLIC HEALTH SERVICES OF LONG ISLAND 992 North Village Avenue, 1st Floor, Zip 11570; tel. 516/705–3700; Lawrence E. McManus, President and Chief Executive Officer, p. B29

**Syracuse:** SISTERS OF SAINT FRANCIS 2500 Grant Boulevard, Zip 13208–1713; tel. 315/634–7000; Sister Marian Rose Mansius, Assistant General Minister, p. B119

### NORTH CAROLINA

**Asheville:** ★ MISSION HEALTH SYSTEM 509 Biltmore Avenue, Zip 28801; tel. 828/213–1111; Ronald A. Paulus, M.D., President and Chief Executive Officer, p. B90

**Boone:** ★ APPALACHIAN REGIONAL HEALTHCARE SYSTEM 336 Deerfield Road, Zip 28607–5008, Mailing Address: P.O. Box 2600, Zip 28607–2600; tel. 828/262–4100; Richard G. Sparks, President and Chief Executive Officer, p. B10

**Charlotte:** ACUITYHEALTHCARE, LP 10200 Mallard Creek Road, Suite 300, Zip 28262–9705; tel. 877/228–4893; Edwin H. Cooper, Jr., MS, President and Chief Executive Officer, p. B4

★ CAROLINAS HEALTHCARE SYSTEM 1000 Blythe Boulevard, Zip 28203–5871, Mailing Address: P.O. Box 32861, Zip 28232–2861; tel. 704/355–2000; Michael C. Tarwater, Chief Executive Officer, p. B25

**Durham:** ★ DUKE UNIVERSITY HEALTH SYSTEM 201 Trent Drive, Zip 27710, Mailing Address: P.O. Box 3701, Zip 27710–3701; tel. 919/684–2255; Victor J. Dzau, M.D., President and Chief Executive Officer, p. B48

**Fayetteville:** CAPE FEAR VALLEY HEALTH SYSTEM 1638 Owen Drive, Zip 28304, Mailing Address: P.O. Box 2000, Zip 28302–2000; tel. 910/615–4000; Michael Nagowski, President and Chief Executive Officer, p. B24

**Greenville:** ★ VIDANT HEALTH 2100 Stantonsburg Road, Zip 27834–2818, Mailing Address: P.O. Box 6028, Zip 27835–6028; tel. 252/847–4100; David C. Herman, M.D., Chief Executive Officer, p. B142

**Pinehurst:** ★ FIRSTHEALTH OF THE CAROLINAS 155 Memorial Drive, Zip 28374–8710, Mailing Address: P.O. Box 3000, Zip 28374–3000; tel. 910/715–1000; David J. Kilarski, Chief Executive Officer, p. B52

**Raleigh:** ★ WAKEMED HEALTH & HOSPITALS 3000 New Bern Avenue, Zip 27610; tel. 919/350–8000; William K. Atkinson, II, Ph.D., President and Chief Executive Officer, p. B143

**Sylva:** ★ MEDWEST HEALTH SYSTEM 68 Hospital Road, Zip 28779; tel. 828/586–7000; Steve Heatherly, President, p. B86

**Wilmington:** ★ NEW HANOVER REGIONAL MEDICAL CENTER 2131 South 17th Street, Zip 28401–9000; tel. 910/343–7040; John K. Barto, Jr., President and Chief Executive Officer, p. B92

**Winston–Salem:** ★ NOVANT HEALTH 2085 Frontis Plaza Boulevard, Zip 27103–3090; tel. 336/718–5600; Carl S. Armato, President and Chief Executive Officer, p. B96

★ WAKE FOREST BAPTIST HEALTH Medical Center Boulevard, Zip 27157; tel. 336/716–2011; John D. McConnell, M.D., Chief Executive Officer, p. B143

### NORTH DAKOTA

**Bismarck:** BENEDICTINE SISTERS OF THE ANNUNCIATION 7520 University Drive, Zip 58504–9653; tel. 701/255–1520; Sister Susan Berger, Prioress, p. B20

**Fargo:** SISTERS OF MARY OF THE PRESENTATION HEALTH SYSTEM 1202 Page Drive S.W., Zip 58103–2340, Mailing Address: P.O. Box 10007, Zip 58106–0007; tel. 701/237–9290; Aaron K. Alton, President and Chief Executive Officer, p. B119

## OHIO

**Akron:** ★ AKRON GENERAL HEALTH SYSTEM 400 Wabash Avenue, Zip 44307–2433; tel. 330/344–6000; Thomas L. Stover, M.D., President and Chief Executive Officer, p. B7

SUMMA HEALTH SYSTEM 525 East Market Street, Zip 44309–2090; tel. 330/375–3000; Thomas J. Strauss, President and Chief Executive Officer, p. B124

**Canton:** AULTMAN HEALTH FOUNDATION 2600 Sixth Street S.W., Zip 44710–1702; Edward J. Roth, III, President and Chief Executive Officer, p. B14

**Cincinnati:** ★ CATHOLIC HEALTH PARTNERS 615 Elsinore Place, Zip 45202; tel. 513/639–2800; Michael D. Connelly, President and Chief Executive Officer, p. B28

★ UC HEALTH 3200 Burnet Avenue, Zip 45229; tel. 513/585–6000; James A. Kingsbury, President and Chief Executive Officer, p. B133

**Cleveland:** ★ CLEVELAND CLINIC HEALTH SYSTEM 9500 Euclid, Zip 44195–5108; tel. 216/444–2200; Delos Cosgrove, M.D., President and Chief Executive Officer, p. B32

SISTERS OF CHARITY HEALTH SYSTEM 2475 East 22nd Street, Zip 44115–3221; tel. 216/363–2797; Sister Judith Ann Karam, President and Chief Executive Officer, p. B119

★ UNIVERSITY HOSPITALS 11100 Euclid Avenue, Zip 44106–5000; tel. 216/844–1000; Thomas F. Zenty, III, President and Chief Executive Officer, p. B138

**Columbus:** OHIO DEPARTMENT OF MENTAL HEALTH 30 East Broad Street, 8th Floor, Zip 43215–3430; tel. 614/466–2297; Tracy Plouck, Director, p. B97

★ OHIO STATE UNIVERSITY HEALTH SYSTEM 370 West Ninth Avenue, Zip 43210–1240; tel. 614/247–5555; Peter E. Geier, Chief Executive Officer, p. B98

★ OHIOHEALTH 180 East Broad Street, Zip 43215; tel. 614/544–4455; David P. Blom, President and Chief Executive Officer, p. B98

**Dayton:** ★ KETTERING HEALTH NETWORK 3965 Southern Boulevard, Zip 45429–1221; tel. 937/395–8150; Fred M. Manchur, President and Chief Executive Officer, p. B75

**Findlay:** ★ BLANCHARD VALLEY HEALTH SYSTEM 1900 South Main Street, Zip 45840–1214; tel. 419/423–4500; Scott C. Malaney, President and Chief Executive Officer, p. B21

**Galion:** ★ AVITA HEALTH SYSTEM 269 Portland Way South, Zip 44833–2399; tel. 419/468–4841; Jerome Morasko, President and Chief Executive Officer, p. B16

**Mansfield:** MEDCENTRAL HEALTH SYSTEM 335 Glessner Avenue, Zip 44903; tel. 419/526–8000; Joe Chamberlain, Interim Chief Executive Officer, p. B86

**Toledo:** ★ PROMEDICA HEALTH SYSTEM 1801 Richards Road, Zip 43607; tel. 419/469–3800; Randall D. Oostra, FACHE, President and Chief Executive Officer, p. B104

★ SYLVANIA FRANCISCAN HEALTH 3231 Central Park West, Suite 106, Zip 43617–3009; tel. 419/882–8373; James W. Pope, FACHE, President and Chief Executive Officer, p. B126

## OKLAHOMA

**Oklahoma City:** ★ INTEGRIS HEALTH 3366 N.W. Expressway, Suite 800, Zip 73112–9756; tel. 405/949–6066; Bruce Lawrence, President and Chief Executive Officer, p. B71

OKLAHOMA DEPARTMENT OF MENTAL HEALTH AND SUBSTANCE ABUSE SERVICES 1200 N.E. 13th Street, Zip 73117, Mailing Address: P.O. Box 53277, Zip 73152–3277; tel. 405/522–3908; Terri White, Commissioner, p. B98

SOUTHERN PLAINS MEDICAL GROUP 3555 N.W. 58th Street, Suite 700, Zip 73112; tel. 405/917–0300; Thomas R. Rice, FACHE, President and Chief Operating Officer, p. B120

**Shawnee:** PREFERRED MANAGEMENT CORPORATION 120 West MacArthur, Suite 121, Zip 74804–2028; tel. 405/878–0202; Donald Freeman, President and Chief Executive Officer, p. B102

**Tulsa:** ★ MARIAN HEALTH SYSTEM 1923 South Utica Avenue, Zip 74104, Mailing Address: P.O. Box 4753, Zip 74159–0753; tel. 918/742–9988; Sister M. Therese Gottschalk, President, p. B84

★ SAINT FRANCIS HEALTH SYSTEM 6161 South Yale Avenue, Zip 74136–1902; tel. 918/494–8454; Jake Henry, Jr., President and Chief Executive Officer, p. B111

## OREGON

**Bend:** ★ ST. CHARLES HEALTH SYSTEM, INC. 2500 N.E. Neff Road, Zip 97701–6015; tel. 541/382–4321; James A. Diegel, President and Chief Executive Officer, p. B122

**Corvallis:** ★ SAMARITAN HEALTH SERVICES 3600 N.W. Samaritan Drive, Zip 97330, Mailing Address: P.O. Box 1068, Zip 97339; tel. 541/768–5001; Larry A. Mullins, FACHE, President and Chief Executive Officer, p. B112

**Medford:** ★ ASANTE HEALTH SYSTEM 2650 Siskiyou Boulevard, Suite 200, Zip 97504–8170; tel. 541/789–4100; Roy G. Vinyard, FACHE, President and Chief Executive Officer, p. B11

**Portland:** ★ LEGACY HEALTH 1919 N.W. Lovejoy Street, Zip 97209–1503; tel. 503/415–5600; George J. Brown, M.D., President and Chief Executive Officer, p. B79

**Salem:** SALEM HEALTH 890 Oak Street Building B. POB 14001, Zip 97309–5014; tel. 503/561–5200; Norman F. Gruber, President and Chief Executive Officer, p. B112

## PENNSYLVANIA

**Allentown:** GOOD SHEPHERD REHABILITATION NETWORK 850 South Fifth Street, Zip 18103–3308; tel. 610/776–3100; Sally T. Gammon, FACHE, President and Chief Executive Officer, p. B55

★ LEHIGH VALLEY HEALTH NETWORK 1200 South Cedar Crest Boulevard, Zip 18103, Mailing Address: P.O. Box 689, Zip 18105–0689; tel. 610/402–8000; Ronald W. Swinfard, M.D., President and Chief Executive Officer, p. B79

**Ashland:** SAINT CATHERINE HEALTHCARE, LLC 101 Broad Street, Zip 17921; tel. 570/875–2000; Daniel A. Colon, President and Chief Executive Officer, p. B111

**Beaver:** HERITAGE VALLEY HEALTH SYSTEM 1000 Dutch Ridge Road, Zip 15009–9727; tel. 724/773–2024; Norman F. Mitry, President and Chief Executive Officer, p. B68

**Bethlehem:** ST. LUKE'S UNIVERSITY HEALTH NETWORK 801 Ostrum Street, Zip 18015–1000; tel. 610/954–4000; Richard A. Anderson, President and Chief Executive Officer, p. B123

**Bryn Mawr:** ★ MAIN LINE HEALTH 130 South Bryn Mawr Avenue, Zip 19010; tel. 484/337–3000; John J. Lynch, III, FACHE, President and Chief Executive Officer, p. B83

**Camp Hill:** POST ACUTE MEDICAL, LLC 3500 Market Street, Suite 202, Zip 17011–4354; tel. 717/731–9660; Anthony F. Misitano, President and Chief Executive Officer, p. B102

**Chambersburg:** ★ SUMMIT HEALTH 112 North Seventh Street, Zip 17201; tel. 717/267–7138; Norman B. Epstein, FACHE, President and Chief Executive Officer, p. B124

**Danville:** ★ GEISINGER HEALTH SYSTEM 100 North Academy Avenue, Zip 17822; tel. 570/271–6211; Glenn Steele, Jr., M.D., Ph.D., President and Chief Executive Officer, p. B54

**Erie:** ★ SAINT VINCENT HEALTH SYSTEM 232 West 25th Street, Zip 16544–0002; tel. 814/452–5000; Scott Whalen, Ph.D., FACHE, President and Chief Executive Officer, p. B112

**Greensburg:** EXCELA HEALTH 532 West Pittsburgh Street, Zip 15601; tel. 724/832–5050; Robert Rogalski, Chief Executive Officer, p. B51

**Johnstown:** CONEMAUGH HEALTH SYSTEM 1086 Franklin Street, Zip 15905–4398; tel. 814/534–9000; Scott A. Becker, President and Chief Executive Officer, p. B38

**King of Prussia:** UNIVERSAL HEALTH SERVICES, INC. 367 South Gulph Road, Zip 19406–0958, Mailing Address: P.O. Box 61558, Zip 19406–0958; tel. 610/768–3300; Alan B. Miller, President and Chief Executive Officer, p. B134

**Lehighton:** BLUE MOUNTAIN HEALTH SYSTEM 211 North 12th Street, Zip 18235–1138; tel. 610/377–1300; Andrew E. Harris, President and Chief Executive Officer, p. B21

**Mechanicsburg:** ★ SELECT MEDICAL CORPORATION 4714 Gettysburg Road, Zip 17055; tel. 717/972–1100; David S. Chernow, President and Chief Administrative Officer, p. B114

VIBRA HEALTHCARE 4550 Lena Drive, Suite 225, Zip 17055; tel. 717/591–5700; Brad Hollinger, Chairman and Chief Executive Officer, p. B142

**Newtown Square:** ★ CATHOLIC HEALTH EAST 3805 West Chester Pike, Suite 100, Zip 19073; tel. 610/355–2000; Judith M. Persichilli, Chief Executive Officer, p. B26

**Philadelphia:** ALBERT EINSTEIN HEALTHCARE NETWORK 5501 Old York Road, Zip 19141–3098; tel. 215/456–7890; Barry R. Freedman, President and Chief Executive Officer, p. B7

★ TEMPLE UNIVERSITY HEALTH SYSTEM 3509 North Broad Street, 9th Floor, Zip 19140–4105; tel. 215/707–0900; Larry Kaiser, M.D., President and Chief Executive Officer, p. B126

★ UNIVERSITY OF PENNSYLVANIA HEALTH SYSTEM 3400 Civic Center Boulevard, Zip 19104–5127; tel. 215/662–2203; Ralph W. Muller, President and Chief Executive Officer, p. B139

**Pittsburgh:** UPMC 600 Grant Street, U.S. Steel Tower, Suite 6262, Zip 15219; tel. 412/647–4800; Jeffrey A. Romoff, President and Chief Executive Officer, p. B140

★ WEST PENN ALLEGHENY HEALTH SYSTEM 30 Isabella Street, Suite 300, Zip 15212–5862; tel. 412/330–2403; Keith T. Ghezzi, M.D., Interim President and Chief Executive Officer, p. B144

**Pottsville:** SCHUYLKILL HEALTH SYSTEM 420 South Jackson Street, Zip 17901; tel. 570/621–5000; John E. Simodejka, President and Chief Executive Officer, p. B113

**Radnor:** ★ JEFFERSON HEALTH SYSTEM 259 Radnor–Chester Road, Suite 290, Zip 19087–5288; tel. 610/225–6200; Joseph T. Sebastianelli, President and Chief Executive Officer, p. B73

**Sayre:** ★ GUTHRIE HEALTHCARE SYSTEM Guthrie Square, Zip 18840; tel. 570/887–4312; Joseph A. Scopelliti, M.D., President and Chief Executive Officer, p. B56

**Springfield:** ★ CROZER–KEYSTONE HEALTH SYSTEM 100 West Sproul Road, Zip 19064; tel. 610/338–8205; Joan K. Richards, President and Chief Executive Officer, p. B40

**Villanova:** DEVEREUX 444 Devereux Drive, Zip 19085, Mailing Address: P.O. Box 638, Zip 19085–0638; tel. 610/520–3000; Robert Q. Kreider, President and Chief Executive Officer, p. B46

**Williamsport:** ★ SUSQUEHANNA HEALTH SYSTEM 700 High Street, Zip 17701–3109; tel. 570/321–1000; Steven P. Johnson, FACHE, President and Chief Executive Officer, p. B125

**York:** ★ WELLSPAN HEALTH 45 Monument Road, Suite 200, Zip 17403; tel. 717/851–2121; Bruce M. Bartels, President, p. B144

## PUERTO RICO

**San Juan:** ★ PUERTO RICO DEPARTMENT OF HEALTH Building A – Medical Center, Zip 00936, Mailing Address: Call Box 70184, Zip 00936; tel. 787/765–2929; Lorenzo Gonzalez Feliciano, M.D., Secretary of Health, p. B106

## RHODE ISLAND

**Providence:** ★ CARE NEW ENGLAND HEALTH SYSTEM 45 Willard Avenue, Zip 02905–3218; tel. 401/453–7900; Dennis D. Keefe, President and Chief Executive Officer, p. B25

LIFESPAN CORPORATION 167 Point Street, Zip 02903–4771; tel. 401/444–3500; , p. B82

## SOUTH CAROLINA

**Anderson:** ANMED HEALTH 800 North Fant Street, Zip 29621–5793; tel. 864/512–1000; John A. Miller, Jr., FACHE, Chief Executive Officer, p. B10

**Columbia:** ★ PALMETTO HEALTH 1301 Taylor Street, Suite 9–A, Zip 29201, Mailing Address: P.O. Box 2266, Zip 29202–2266; tel. 803/296–2100; Charles D. Beaman, Jr., Chief Executive Officer, p. B99

**Georgetown:** GEORGETOWN HOSPITAL SYSTEM 606 Black River Road, Zip 29440–3304, Mailing Address: P.O. Box 421718, Zip 29442–4203; tel. 843/527–7000; Bruce P. Bailey, President and Chief Executive Officer, p. B54

**Greenville:** ★ GREENVILLE HOSPITAL SYSTEM 701 Grove Road, Zip 29605–5601; tel. 864/455–7000; Michael C. Riordan, President and Chief Executive Officer, p. B56

**Spartanburg:** ★ SPARTANBURG REGIONAL HEALTHCARE SYSTEM 101 East Wood Street, Zip 29303–3016; tel. 864/560–6000; Bruce Holstien, President and Chief Executive Officer, p. B121

## SOUTH DAKOTA

**Rapid City:** ★ REGIONAL HEALTH 353 Fairmont Boulevard, Zip 57701, Mailing Address: P.O. Box 6000, Zip 57709–6000; tel. 605/719–1000; Charles E. Hart, M.D., MS, President and Chief Executive Officer, p. B109

**Sioux Falls:** ★ AVERA HEALTH 3900 West Avera Drive, Suite 301, Zip 57108; tel. 605/322–4700; John T. Porter, President and Chief Executive Officer, p. B15

★ SANFORD HEALTH 2301 East 60th Street North, Zip 57104–0589, Mailing Address: PO Box 5039, Zip 57117–5039; tel. 605/333–1000; Kelby K. Krabbenhoft, President and Chief Executive Officer, p. B112

## TENNESSEE

**Brentwood:** CENTERRE HEALTHCARE 5250 Virginia Way, Suite 240, Zip 37027–7576; tel. 615/846–9508; Patrick A. Foster, President and Chief Executive Officer, p. B30

DUKE LIFEPOINT HEALTHCARE 103 Powell Court, Zip 37027–5079; Jeffrey G. Seraphine, FACHE, Division President, p. B48

★ LIFEPOINT HOSPITALS, INC. 103 Powell Court, Suite 200, Zip 37027; tel. 615/372–8500; William F. Carpenter, III, Chairman and Chief Executive Officer, p. B80

★ QHR 105 Continental Place, Zip 37027; tel. 800/233–1470; James L. Horrar, President and Chief Executive Officer, p. B106

REGIONALCARE HOSPITAL PARTNERS 103 Continental Place, Suite 200, Zip 37027–1087; tel. 615/844–9800; Martin S. Rash, Chairman and Chief Executive Officer, p. B109

**Chattanooga:** ERLANGER HEALTH SYSTEM 975 East Third Street, Zip 37403; tel. 423/778–7000; Charlesetta Woodard–Thompson, President and Chief Executive Officer, p. B50

**Franklin:** ACADIA HEALTHCARE COMPANY, INC. 830 Crescent Centre Drive, Suite 610, Zip 37067–7323; tel. 615/861–6000; Joey Jacobs, Chairman and Chief Executive Officer, p. B4

CAPELLA HEALTHCARE 501 Corporate Centre Drive, Suite 200, Zip 37067; tel. 615/764–3000; Daniel S. Slipkovich, Chief Executive Officer, p. B24

★ COMMUNITY HEALTH SYSTEMS, INC. 4000 Meridian Boulevard, Zip 37067–6325, Mailing Address: P.O. Box 689020, Zip 37068–9020; tel. 615/465–7000; Wayne T. Smith, Chairman, President and Chief Executive Officer, p. B33

★ HEALTHTECH MANAGEMENT SERVICES 405 Duke Drive, Suite 210, Zip 37067; tel. 615/309–6053; Derek Morkel, Chief Executive Officer, p. B67

IASIS HEALTHCARE 117 Seaboard Lane, Building E., Zip 37067; tel. 615/844–2747; Carl Whitmer, President and Chief Executive Officer, p. B70

**Jackson:** ★ WEST TENNESSEE HEALTHCARE 620 Skyline Drive, Zip 38301–3901; tel. 731/541–5000; Bobby Arnold, President and Chief Executive Officer, p. B144

**Johnson City:** MOUNTAIN STATES HEALTH ALLIANCE 400 North State of Franklin Road, Zip 37604–6035; tel. 423/431–1040; Dennis Vonderfecht, President and Chief Executive Officer, p. B91

**Kingsport:** ★ WELLMONT HEALTH SYSTEM 1905 American Way, Zip 37660–5882; tel. 423/230–8200; Margaret DeNarvaez, President and Chief Executive Officer, p. B144

**Knoxville:** ★ COVENANT HEALTH 100 Fort Sanders West Boulevard, Zip 37922; tel. 865/531–5555; Anthony Spezia, President and Chief Executive Officer, p. B39

**Memphis:** ★ BAPTIST MEMORIAL HEALTH CARE CORPORATION 350 North Humphreys Boulevard, Zip 38120–2177; tel. 901/227–5117; Stephen Curtis Reynolds, President and Chief Executive Officer, p. B19

METHODIST LE BONHEUR HEALTHCARE 1211 Union Avenue, Suite 700, Zip 38104–6600; tel. 901/516–0543; Gary S. Shorb, President and Chief Executive Officer, p. B89

STRATEGIC BEHAVIORAL HEALTH, LLC 8295 Tournament Drive, Suite 201, Zip 38125–8906; tel. 901/969–3100; Jim Shaheen, President, p. B124

**Nashville:** ★ ARDENT HEALTH SERVICES 1 Burton Hills Boulevard, Suite 250, Zip 37215; tel. 615/296–3000; David T. Vandewater, President and Chief Executive Officer, p. B10

BEHAVIORAL CENTERS OF AMERICA 3100 West End Avenue, Suite 1000, Zip 37203; tel. 615/463–3200; John E. Turner, President and Chief Executive Officer, p. B20

HAVEN BEHAVIORAL HEALTHCARE 652 West Iris Drive, Zip 37204–3191; tel. 615/250–9500; Vern Westrich, President and Chief Executive Officer, p. B56

★ HCA One Park Plaza, Zip 37203–1548; tel. 615/344–9551; Richard M. Bracken, Chairman and Chief Executive Officer, p. B57

★ VANDERBILT HEALTHCARE 1211 22nd Avenue South, Zip 37232; tel. 615/322–5000; Charles Wright Pinson, M.D., Deputy Vice Chancellor for Health Affairs and Chief Executive Officer of Vanderbilt Health System, p. B141

VANGUARD HEALTH SYSTEM 20 Burton Hills Boulevard, Suite 10, Zip 37215; tel. 615/665–6000; Charles N. Martin, Jr., Chairman and Chief Executive Officer, p. B141

## TEXAS

**Addison:** RELIANT HEALTHCARE PARTNERS 15851 Dallas Parkway, Suite 50, Zip 75001; tel. 972/308–8518; Emmett E. Moore, CPA, JD, Chief Executive Officer, p. B109

UNITED SURGICAL PARTNERS INTERNATIONAL 15305 Dallas Parkway, Suite 1600, Zip 75001–6491; tel. 972/713–3500; William H. Wilcox, President and Chief Executive Officer, p. B134

**Arlington:** ★ TEXAS HEALTH RESOURCES 612 East Lamar Boulevard, Suite 900, Zip 76011; tel. 682/236–7900; Douglas D. Hawthorne, FACHE, Chief Executive Officer, p. B129

**Austin:** TEXAS DEPARTMENT OF STATE HEALTH SERVICES 1100 West 49th Street, Zip 78756–3199; tel. 512/458–7111; David L. Lakey, M.D., Commissioner, p. B128

★ UNIVERSITY OF TEXAS SYSTEM 601 Colorado Street, Suite 205, Zip 78701–2982; tel. 512/499–4224; Kenneth Shine, M.D., Executive Vice Chancellor, p. B139

**Dallas:** ★ BAYLOR HEALTH CARE SYSTEM 3500 Gaston Avenue, Zip 75246; tel. 214/820–0111; Joel T. Allison, President and Chief Executive Officer, p. B20

CIRRUS HEALTH 9301 North Central Expressway, Suite 360, Zip 75231; tel. 214/217–0100; Timothy Parris, President and Chief Executive Officer, p. B32

CORNERSTONE HEALTHCARE GROUP 2200 Ross Avenue, suite 3060, Zip 75201–2708; tel. 469/621–6700; Harrison Price, Interim President and Chief Executive Officer, p. B38

GLOBALREHAB 1420 West Mockingbird Lane, Suite 100, Zip 75247–4931, Mailing Address: 1340 Empire Central Drive, Zip 75247–4022; tel. 214/879–7500; Hooman Sedighi, M.D., President and Chief Executive Officer, p. B54

★ METHODIST HEALTH SYSTEM 1441 North Beckley Avenue, Zip 75203–1201, Mailing Address: P.O. Box 655999, Zip 75265–5999; tel. 214/947–8181; Stephen L. Mansfield, Ph.D., FACHE, President and Chief Executive Officer, p. B89

SOLARA HEALTHCARE 13455 Noel Road, Suite 1320, Zip 75240–6702; tel. 469/621–6700; Michael Brohm, President and Chief Executive Officer, p. B119

★ TENET HEALTHCARE CORPORATION 1445 Ross Avenue, Suite 1400, Zip 75202–2703, Mailing Address: P.O. Box 139036, Zip 75313–9036; tel. 469/893–2200; Trevor Fetter, President and Chief Executive Officer, p. B127

**Harlingen:** ★ VALLEY BAPTIST HEALTH SYSTEM 2101 Pease Street, Zip 78550; tel. 956/389–1100; Manuel Vela, President and Chief Executive Officer, p. B141

**Houston:** ★ DUBUIS HEALTH SYSTEM 1700 West Loop South, Suite 1100A, Zip 77027–3007; tel. 713/277–2300; Stephen Mills, Chief Executive Officer, p. B48

DYNACQ HEALTHCARE, INC. 10304 Interstate 10 East, Suite 369, Zip 77029; tel. 713/367–2000; Chiu Moon Chan, Chairman, President and Chief Executive Officer, p. B49

★ MEMORIAL HERMANN HEALTHCARE SYSTEM 929 Gessner, Suite 2700, Zip 77024; tel. 713/242–2700; Daniel J. Wolterman, President and Chief Executive Officer, p. B87

NEXUS HEALTH SYSTEMS One Riverway, Suite 600, Zip 77056; tel. 713/355–6111; John W. Cassidy, M.D., President, Chief Executive Officer and Chief Medical Officer, p. B94

RENAISSANCE HEALTHCARE SYSTEMS 14440 John F. Kennedy Boulevardd, Zip 77032; tel. 832/886–1900; Michael Smesney, Chief Executive Officer, p. B109

SIGNATURE HOSPITAL CORPORATION 363 North Sam Houston Parkway East Suite 1700, Zip 77060–2424; tel. 281/598–9800; Steven G. Peterson, Chief Executive Officer, p. B118

★ ST. LUKE'S EPISCOPAL HEALTH SYSTEM 6624 Fannin Street, Suite 1100, Zip 77030; tel. 832/355–7661; David J. Fine, Chief Executive Officer, p. B123

★ THE METHODIST HOSPITAL SYSTEM 6565 Fannin Street, D–200, Zip 77030–2707; tel. 713/441–2221; Marc Boom, M.D., Chief Executive Officer, p. B129

**Irving:** ★ CHRISTUS HEALTH 6363 North Highway 161, Suite 450, Zip 75038; tel. 214/492–8500; Ernie W. Sadau, President and Chief Executive Officer, p. B31

PHYSICIAN SYNERGY GROUP 5605 North MacArthur Boulevard, Suite 310, Zip 75038–2617; tel. 214/350–7741; Corazon Ramirez, M.D., Chief Executive Officer, p. B101

USMD INC. 6333 North State Highway 161 Suite 200, Zip 75038–2229; tel. 214/493–4000; Karen A. Fiducia, FACHE, President, Hospital Division, p. B140

**Longview:** GOOD SHEPHERD HEALTH SYSTEM 700 East Marshall Avenue, Zip 75601–5580; tel. 903/315–2000; Edward D. Banos, President and Chief Executive Officer, p. B55

**Lubbock:** ★ COVENANT HEALTH SYSTEM 3615 19th Street, Zip 79410–1201; tel. 806/725–0447; Richard H. Parks, FACHE, President and Chief Executive Officer, p. B39

**Lufkin:** MEMORIAL HEALTH SYSTEM OF EAST TEXAS 1201 Frank Avenue, Zip 75904–3357; tel. 936/634–8111; Gary N. Looper, President and Chief Executive Officer, p. B87

**Plano:** ★ COMMUNITY HOSPITAL CORPORATION 5801 Tennyson Parkway, Suite 550, Zip 75024; tel. 972/943–6400; Michael D. Williams, President and Chief Executive Officer, p. B37

★ LHP HOSPITAL GROUP 2800 North Dallas Parkway, Suite 200, Zip 75093–5994; tel. 866/465–9222; Daniel J. Moen, Chief Executive Officer, p. B79

★ LIFECARE MANAGEMENT SERVICES 5340 Legacy Drive, Suite 150, Zip 75024; tel. 469/241–2100; Phillip B. Douglas, Chairman and Chief Executive Officer, p. B80

**San Antonio:** BAPTIST HEALTH SYSTEM 215 East Quincy, Suite 200, Zip 78216; tel. 210/297–1040; , p. B18

**Sherman:** CARRUS HOSPITALS 1810 West U.S. Highway 82, Zip 75092–7069; tel. 903/870–2600; Ronald E. Dorris, Chief Executive Officer, p. B26

**Temple:** ★ SCOTT & WHITE HEALTHCARE 2401 South 31st Street, Zip 76508; tel. 254/724–2111; Robert W. Pryor, M.D., President and Chief Executive Officer, p. B113

**Tyler:** ★ EAST TEXAS MEDICAL CENTER REGIONAL HEALTHCARE SYSTEM 1000 South Beckham Street, Zip 75701–1996, Mailing Address: P.O. Box 6400, Zip 75711–6400; tel. 903/535–6211; Elmer G. Ellis, FACHE, President and Chief Executive Officer, p. B49

TRINITY MOTHER FRANCES HOSPITALS AND CLINICS 910 East Houston, Zip 75702–8369; tel. 903/593–8441; J. Lindsey Bradley, Jr., FACHE, President, p. B131

## UTAH

**Nephi:** ★ RURAL HEALTH GROUP 48 West 1500 North, Zip 84648–1226; tel. 435/623–4924; Mark R. Stoddard, President and Chairman, p. B110

**Salt Lake City:** ★ INTERMOUNTAIN HEALTHCARE, INC 36 South State Street, 22nd Floor, Zip 84111–1453; tel. 801/442–2000; Charles W. Sorenson, Jr., M.D., Chief Executive Officer, p. B72

## VIRGINIA

**Charlottesville:** UVA HEALTH SYSTEM 1215 Lee Street, Zip 22908–0816; tel. 434/924–0211; R. Edward Howell, Vice President and Chief Executive Officer, p. B140

**Falls Church:** DEPARTMENT OF THE ARMY, OFFICE OF THE SURGEON GENERAL 5109 Leesburg Pike, Zip 22041; tel. 703/681–3000; Lieutenant General Eric B. Schoomaker, Surgeon General, p. B41

★ INOVA HEALTH SYSTEM 8110 Gatehouse Road, Zip 22042; tel. 703/289–2069; J. Knox Singleton, President and Chief Executive Officer, p. B71

**Fredericksburg:** ★ MARY WASHINGTON HEALTHCARE 2300 Fall Hill Avenue, Suite 308, Zip 22401–3343; tel. 540/741–3100; Fred M. Rankin, III, President and Chief Executive Officer, p. B84

**Lynchburg:** CENTRA HEALTH, INC. 1920 Atherholt Road, Zip 24501–1104; tel. 434/200–3000; W. Michael Bryant, President and Chief Executive Officer, p. B30

**Newport News:** RIVERSIDE HEALTH SYSTEM 701 Town Center Drive, Suite 1000, Zip 23606; tel. 757/534–7000; William B. Downey, President and Chief Executive Officer, p. B110

**Norfolk:** ★ SENTARA HEALTHCARE 6015 Poplar Hall Drive, Zip 23502–3819; tel. 757/455–7000; David L. Bernd, Chief Executive Officer, p. B117

**Richmond:** VIRGINIA DEPARTMENT OF MENTAL HEALTH 1220 Bank Street, Zip 23219, Mailing Address: P.O. Box 1797, Zip 23218–1797; tel. 804/786–3921; James S. Reinhard, M.D., Commissioner, p. B143

**Roanoke:** ★ CARILION CLINIC Belleview at Jefferson Street, Zip 24014, Mailing Address: P.O. Box 13727, Zip 24036–3727; tel. 540/981–7000; Nancy Howell Agee, President and Chief Executive Officer, p. B25

**Winchester:** ★ VALLEY HEALTH SYSTEM 220 Campus Boulevard, Suite 310, Zip 22601–2889, Mailing Address: P.O. Box 3340, Zip 22604–1334; tel. 540/536–8024; Mark H. Merrill, President, p. B141

## WASHINGTON

**Bellevue:** ★ PEACEHEALTH 14432 S.E. Eastgate Way, Suite 300, Zip 98007–6412; tel. 425/747–1711; Alan R. Yordy, President and Chief Mission Officer, p. B100

**Renton:** ★ PROVIDENCE HEALTH & SERVICES 1801 Lind Avenue S.W., 9016, Zip 98057–9016; tel. 425/525–3698; John F. Koster, M.D., President and Chief Executive Officer, p. B105

**Seattle:** SWEDISH HEALTH SERVICES 747 Broadway, Zip 98122; tel. 206/386–6000; Kevin Brown, Chief Executive, p. B126

UW MEDICINE 4333 Brooklyn Avenue N.E., Zip 98195, Mailing Address: P.O. Box 356350, Zip 98195–6350; tel. 206/543–7718; Paul G. Ramsey, Chief Executive Officer, p. B140

**Tacoma:** MULTICARE HEALTH SYSTEM 315 Martin Luther King Jr. Way, Zip 98415, Mailing Address: P.O. Box 5299, Zip 98415–0299; tel. 253/403–1000; Diane E. Cecchettini, R.N., President and Chief Executive Officer, p. B92

## WEST VIRGINIA

**Charleston:** ★ CHARLESTON AREA MEDICAL CENTER HEALTH SYSTEM, INC. 501 Morris Street, Zip 25301–1300, Mailing Address: P.O. Box 1547, Zip 25326–1547; tel. 304/388–5432; David L. Ramsey, President and Chief Executive Officer, p. B30

**Elkins:** ★ DAVIS HEALTH SYSTEM Reed Street and Gorman Avenue, Zip 26241, Mailing Address: P.O. Box 1697, Zip 26241–1697; tel. 304/636–3300; Mark Doak, President and Chief Executive Officer, p. B40

**Fairmont:** ★ WEST VIRGINIA UNITED HEALTH SYSTEM 1000 Technology Drive, Suite 2320, Zip 26554; tel. 304/368–2700; J. Thomas Jones, President and Chief Executive Officer, p. B145

**Huntington:** ★ PALLOTTINE HEALTH SERVICES 2900 First Avenue, Zip 25702; tel. 304/526–1234; Michael G. Sellards, Chief Executive Officer, p. B99

**South Charleston:** ★ THOMAS HEALTH SYSTEM, INC. 4605 MacCorkle Avenue S.W., Zip 25309–1311; tel. 304/766–3600; Stephen P. Dexter, President and Chief Executive Officer, p. B129

**Wheeling:** OHIO VALLEY HEALTH SERVICES AND EDUCATION CORPORATION 2000 Eoff Street, Zip 26003; tel. 304/234–8383; Michael J. Caruso, President and Chief Executive Officer, p. B98

## WISCONSIN

**Appleton:** THEDACARE, INC. 122 East College Avenue, Zip 54911, Mailing Address: P.O. Box 8025, Zip 54912; tel. 920/830–5880; Dean Gruner, M.D., President and Chief Executive Officer, p. B129

**Janesville:** MERCY HEALTH SYSTEM 1000 Mineral Point Avenue, Zip 53548–2940, Mailing Address: P.O. Box 5003, Zip 53547–5003; tel. 608/756–6000; Javon R. Bea, President and Chief Executive Officer, p. B89

**Manitowoc:** ★ FRANCISCAN SISTERS OF CHRISTIAN CHARITY SPONSORED MINISTRIES, INC. 1415 South Rapids Road, Zip 54220–9302; tel. 920/684–7071; Sister Laura J. Wolf, President, p. B53

**Milwaukee:** ★ AURORA HEALTH CARE 3000 West Montana, Zip 53215–3268, Mailing Address: P.O. Box 341880, Zip 53234–1880; tel. 414/647–3000; Nick Turkal, M.D., President and Chief Executive Officer, p. B15

CHILDREN'S HOSPITAL AND HEALTH SYSTEM 9000 West Wisconsin Avenue, Zip 53226–4810, Mailing Address: P.O. Box 1997, Zip 53201–1997; tel. 414/226–2000; Peggy N. Troy, President and Chief Executive Officer, p. B31

**Waukesha:** ★ PROHEALTH CARE, INC. N17 W24100 Riverwood Drive, Suite 130, Zip 53188; tel. 262/928–2242; Susan A. Edwards, President and Chief Executive Officer, p. B104

**Wausau:** ASPIRUS, INC. 425 Pine Ridge Boulevard, Zip 54401–4123; tel. 715/847–2118; Duane L. Erwin, President and Chief Executive Officer, p. B14

# Networks and their Hospitals

## ALASKA

**PEACEHEALTH KETCHIKAN MEDICAL CENTER**
**3100 Tongass Avenue, Ketchikan, AK 99901–5746; tel. 907/225–5171; Patrick J. Branco, Chief Executive Officer**

PEACEHEALTH KETCHIKAN MEDICAL CENTER, 3100 Tongass Avenue, Ketchikan, AK, Zip 99901–5746; tel. 907/225–5171; Patrick J. Branco, Chief Executive Officer

## ARIZONA

**NORTHERN ARIZONA HEALTHCARE**
**1200 North Beaver Street, Flagstaff, AZ 86001; tel. 928/779–3366; William T. Bradel, President and Co–Chief Executive Officer; James J. Breidel, Co–President**

FLAGSTAFF MEDICAL CENTER, 1200 North Beaver Street, Flagstaff, AZ, Zip 86001–3198; tel. 928/779–3366; William T. Bradel, President
VERDE VALLEY MEDICAL CENTER, 269 South Candy Lane, Cottonwood, AZ, Zip 86326–4170; tel. 928/639–6000; James J. Bleicher, M.D., President and Chief Executive Officer

## CALIFORNIA

**NORTHERN CALIFORNIA NETWORK**
**821 South St. Helena Highway Suite 208, St. Helena, CA 95661–3804; tel. 707/967–7515; Terry Newmyer, President and Chief Executive Officer**

FRANK R. HOWARD MEMORIAL HOSPITAL, One Madrone Street, Willits, CA, Zip 95490–4225; tel. 707/459–6801; Rick Bockmann, Chief Executive Officer
ST. HELENA HOSPITAL, 10 Woodland Road, Saint Helena, CA, Zip 94574; tel. 707/963–3611; Terry Newmyer, President and Chief Executive Officer
ST. HELENA HOSPITAL CLEARLAKE, 15630 18th Avenue, Clearlake, CA, Zip 95422–9339, Mailing Address: P.O. Box 6720, Zip 95422–6720; tel. 707/994–6486; Terry Newmyer, President and Chief Executive Officer
ST. HELENA HOSPITAL–CENTER FOR BEHAVIORAL HEALTH, 525 Oregon Street, Vallejo, CA, Zip 94590–3201; tel. 707/648–2200; Terry Newmyer, President and Chief Executive Officer
UKIAH VALLEY MEDICAL CENTER, 275 Hospital Drive, Ukiah, CA, Zip 95482–4531; tel. 707/462–3111; Gwen Matthews, R.N., MSN, Chief Executive Officer

**PROVIDENCE HEALTH AND SERVICES – SOUTHERN CALIFORNIA**
**501 South Buena Vista Street, Burbank, CA 91505–4809; tel. 818/843–5111; Kerry Carmody, Interim Chief Executive Officer**

PROVIDENCE HOLY CROSS MEDICAL CENTER, 15031 Rinaldi Street, Mission Hills, CA, Zip 91346–9600; tel. 818/365–8051; Larry Bowe, Chief Executive
PROVIDENCE LITTLE COMPANY OF MARY MEDICAL CENTER, 4101 Torrance Boulevard, Torrance, CA, Zip 90503–4698; tel. 310/540–7676; Elizabeth Dunne, Chief Executive Officer
PROVIDENCE LITTLE COMPANY OF MARY MEDICAL CENTER SAN PEDRO, 1300 West Seventh Street, San Pedro, CA, Zip 90732–3505; tel. 310/832–3311; Nancy Carlson, Chief Executive
PROVIDENCE SAINT JOSEPH MEDICAL CENTER, 501 South Buena Vista Street, Burbank, CA, Zip 91505–4866; tel. 818/843–5111; Kerry Carmody, Chief Executive Officer
PROVIDENCE TARZANA MEDICAL CENTER, 18321 Clark Street, Tarzana, CA, Zip 91356–3521; tel. 818/881–0800; Dale Surowitz, Chief Executive

## COLORADO

**CENTURA HEALTH**
**188 Inverness Drive West, Suite 500, Englewood, CO 80112–5204; tel. 303/290–6500; Gary Campbell, Chief Executive Officer**

AVISTA ADVENTIST HOSPITAL, 100 Health Park Drive, Louisville, CO, Zip 80027–9583; tel. 303/673–1000; John Sackett, Chief Executive Officer
LITTLETON ADVENTIST HOSPITAL, 7700 South Broadway Street, Littleton, CO, Zip 80122–2628; tel. 303/730–8900; Morre Dean, Interim Chief Executive Officer
PARKER ADVENTIST HOSPITAL, 9395 Crown Crest Boulevard, Parker, CO, Zip 80138; tel. 303/269–4000; Morre Dean, Chief Executive Officer
PENROSE–ST. FRANCIS HEALTH SERVICES, 2222 North Nevada Avenue, Colorado Springs, CO, Zip 80907–6799, Mailing Address: P.O. Box 7021, Zip 80933–7021; tel. 719/776–5000; Margaret D. Sabin, President and Chief Executive Officer
PORTER ADVENTIST HOSPITAL, 2525 South Downing Street, Denver, CO, Zip 80210–5876; tel. 303/778–1955; Randall L. Haffner, Ph.D., Chief Executive Officer

ST. ANTHONY HOSPITAL, 11600 West Second Place, Lakewood, CO, Zip 80228–1527; tel. 720/321–0000; Jeffrey Brickman, FACHE, President and Chief Executive Officer
ST. ANTHONY NORTH HOSPITAL, 2551 West 84th Avenue, Westminster, CO, Zip 80031; tel. 303/426–2151; Carole Peet, R.N., MSN, President and Chief Executive Officer
ST. ANTHONY SUMMIT MEDICAL CENTER, 340 Peak One Drive, Frisco, CO, Zip 80443, Mailing Address: P.O. Box 738, Zip 80443–0738; tel. 970/668–3300; Paul J. Chodkowski, Chief Executive Officer
ST. MARY–CORWIN MEDICAL CENTER, 1008 Minnequa Avenue, Pueblo, CO, Zip 81004–3798; tel. 719/557–4000; Robert Ryder, Chief Executive Officer
ST. THOMAS MORE HOSPITAL, 1338 Phay Avenue, Canon City, CO, Zip 81212–2221; tel. 719/285–2000; Robert Ryder, Chief Executive Officer

**COMMUNITY HEALTH PROVIDERS ORGANIZATION**
**2021 North 12th Street, Grand Junction, CO 81501–2980; tel. 970/256–6200; Chris Thomas, FACHE, President and Chief Executive Officer**

COMMUNITY HOSPITAL, 2021 North 12th Street, Grand Junction, CO, Zip 81501–2999; tel. 970/242–0920; Chris Thomas, FACHE, President and Chief Executive Officer

**HCA HEALTHONE, LLC**
**4900 South Monaco Street, Suite 380, Denver, CO 80237–3487; tel. 303/788–2500; Sylvia Young, President**

MEDICAL CENTER OF AURORA, 1501 South Potomac Street, Aurora, CO, Zip 80012–5499; tel. 303/695–2600; Bill Voloch, Interim Chief Executive Officer
NORTH SUBURBAN MEDICAL CENTER, 9191 Grant Street, Thornton, CO, Zip 80229–4341; tel. 303/451–7800; Jennifer Alderfer, Chief Executive Officer
PRESBYTERIAN–ST. LUKE'S MEDICAL CENTER, 1719 East 19th Avenue, Denver, CO, Zip 80218–1281; tel. 303/839–6000; Madeleine Roberson, Chief Executive Officer
ROSE MEDICAL CENTER, 4567 East Ninth Avenue, Denver, CO, Zip 80220–3941; tel. 303/320–2121; Kenneth H. Feiler, Chief Executive Officer
SKY RIDGE MEDICAL CENTER, 10101 Ridge Gate Parkway, Lone Tree, CO, Zip 80124; tel. 720/225–1000; Maureen Tarrant, Chief Executive Officer
SPALDING REHABILITATION HOSPITAL, 900 Potomac Steet, Aurora, CO, Zip 80011–6716; tel. 303/367–1166; Cynthia Kreutz, Chief Executive Officer
SWEDISH MEDICAL CENTER, 501 East Hampden Avenue, Englewood, CO, Zip 80113; tel. 303/788–5000; Mary M. White, Chief Executive Officer

**UNIVERSITY OF COLORADO HEALTH**
**12605 East 16th Avenue, Aurora, CO 80045–2545; tel. 720/848–0000; Rulon F. Stacey, Ph.D., FACHE, Chief Executive Officer**

MEDICAL CENTER OF THE ROCKIES, 2500 Rocky Mountain Avenue, Loveland, CO, Zip 80538; tel. 970/624–2500; George E. Hayes, FACHE, President and Chief Executive Officer
POUDRE VALLEY HOSPITAL, 1024 South Lemay Avenue, Fort Collins, CO, Zip 80524–3998; tel. 970/495–7000; Kevin L. Unger, FACHE, President and Chief Executive Officer
UNIVERSITY OF COLORADO HOSPITAL, 12605 East 16th Avenue, Aurora, CO, Zip 80045–2545; tel. 720/848–0000; Bruce Schroffel, President and Chief Executive Officer

## CONNECTICUT

**EASTERN CONNECTICUT HEALTH NETWORK**
**71 Haynes Street, Manchester, CT 06040–4131; tel. 860/533–3400; Peter J. Karl, President and Chief Executive Officer**

MANCHESTER MEMORIAL HOSPITAL, 71 Haynes Street, Manchester, CT, Zip 06040–4188; tel. 860/646–1222; Peter J. Karl, President and Chief Executive Officer
ROCKVILLE GENERAL HOSPITAL, 31 Union Street, Vernon Rockville, CT, Zip 06066–3160; tel. 860/872–0501; Peter J. Karl, President and Chief Executive Officer

## FLORIDA

**BAYCARE HEALTH SYSTEM**
**16255 Bay Vista Drive, Clearwater, FL 33760–3127; tel. 877/692–2922; Stephen R. Mason, President and Chief Executive Officer**

BAYCARE ALLIANT HOSPITAL, 601 Main Street, Dunedin, FL, Zip 34698–5848; tel. 727/736–9999; Jacqueline Arocho, Administrator
MEASE COUNTRYSIDE HOSPITAL, 3231 McMullen–Booth Road, Safety Harbor, FL, Zip 34695–1098, Mailing Address: P.O. Box 1098, Zip 34695–1098; tel. 727/725–6222; Glenn D. Waters, FACHE, President

MEASE HOSPITAL DUNEDIN, 601 Main Street, Dunedin, FL, Zip 34698–5891, Mailing Address: P.O. Box 760, Zip 34697–0760; tel. 727/733–1111; Glenn D. Waters, FACHE, President and Chief Executive Officer

MORTON PLANT HOSPITAL, 300 Pinellas Street, Clearwater, FL, Zip 33756–3825, Mailing Address: P.O. Box 210, Zip 33757–0210; tel. 727/462–7000; Glenn D. Waters, FACHE, President

MORTON PLANT NORTH BAY HOSPITAL, 6600 Madison Street, New Port Richey, FL, Zip 34652–1900; tel. 727/842–8468; Glenn D. Waters, FACHE, President

SOUTH FLORIDA BAPTIST HOSPITAL, 301 North Alexander Street, Plant City, FL, Zip 33563–9058, Mailing Address: Drawer H, Zip 33564–9058; tel. 813/757–1200; Isaac Mallah, President and Chief Executive Officer

ST. ANTHONY'S HOSPITAL, 1200 Seventh Avenue North, Saint Petersburg, FL, Zip 33705–1388, Mailing Address: P.O. Box 12588, Zip 33733–2588; tel. 727/825–1100; William G. Ulbricht, President

ST. JOSEPH'S HOSPITAL, 3001 West Martin Luther King Boulevard, Tampa, FL, Zip 33607–6387, Mailing Address: P.O. Box 4227, Zip 33677–4227; tel. 813/870–4000; Isaac Mallah, President and Chief Executive Officer

### HEALTH MANAGEMENT ASSOCIATES
**5811 Pelican Bay Boulevard, Suite 500, Naples, FL 34108; tel. 239/598–3131; Gary D. Newsome, President and Chief Executive Officer**

CHESTER REGIONAL MEDICAL CENTER, 1 Medical Park Drive, Chester, SC, Zip 29706–9799; tel. 803/581–3151; Page H. Vaughan, Chief Executive Officer

## GEORGIA

### EMORY HEALTHCARE
**1440 Clifton Road N.E., Suite 145, Atlanta, GA 30322–1102; tel. 404/778–5000; John T. Fox, Chief Executive Officer**

EMORY UNIVERSITY HOSPITAL, 1364 Clifton Road N.E., Atlanta, GA, Zip 30322–1102; tel. 404/712–2000; Robert J. Bachman, Chief Operating Officer

EMORY UNIVERSITY HOSPITAL MIDTOWN, 550 Peachtree Street N.E., Atlanta, GA, Zip 30308; tel. 404/686–4411; Dane C. Peterson, Chief Operating Officer

WESLEY WOODS GERIATRIC HOSPITAL OF EMORY UNIVERSITY, 1821 Clifton Road N.E., Atlanta, GA, Zip 30329–5102; tel. 404/728–6200; William Such, Chief Executive Officer

### FIRST MEDICAL NETWORK
**1899 Powers Ferry Road S.E., Suite 400, Atlanta, GA 30339; tel. 678/742–9100; Gary Hutchins, Chief Executive Officer**

APPLING HEALTHCARE SYSTEM, 163 East Tollison Street, Baxley, GA, Zip 31513–2898; tel. 912/367–9841; Dale Spell, Chief Executive Officer

ATHENS REGIONAL MEDICAL CENTER, 1199 Prince Avenue, Athens, GA, Zip 30606–2793; tel. 706/475–7000; James G. Thaw, President and Chief Executive Officer

BROOKS COUNTY HOSPITAL, 903 North Court Street, Quitman, GA, Zip 31643–1315, Mailing Address: P.O. Box 5000, Zip 31643–5000; tel. 229/263–4171; Kenneth D. Rhudy, Chief Executive Officer

CANDLER HOSPITAL, 5353 Reynolds Street, Savannah, GA, Zip 31405–6013; tel. 912/819–6000; Paul P. Hinchey, President and Chief Executive Officer

CRISP REGIONAL HOSPITAL, 902 North Seventh Street, Cordele, GA, Zip 31015–5007; tel. 229/276–3100; Steven Gautney, Chief Executive Officer

EASTSIDE MEDICAL CENTER, 1700 Medical Way, Snellville, GA, Zip 30078–2195; tel. 770/979–0200; Kimberly Ryan, Chief Executive Officer

EFFINGHAM HOSPITAL, 459 Highway 119 South, Springfield, GA, Zip 31329–3021, Mailing Address: P.O. Box 386, Zip 31329–0386; tel. 912/754–6451; Norma J. Morgan, Chief Executive Officer

ELBERT MEMORIAL HOSPITAL, 4 Medical Drive, Elberton, GA, Zip 30635–1897; tel. 706/283–3151; James Yarborough, FACHE, Interim Chief Executive Officer

EMORY UNIVERSITY HOSPITAL, 1364 Clifton Road N.E., Atlanta, GA, Zip 30322–1102; tel. 404/712–2000; Robert J. Bachman, Chief Operating Officer

EMORY UNIVERSITY HOSPITAL MIDTOWN, 550 Peachtree Street N.E., Atlanta, GA, Zip 30308; tel. 404/686–4411; Dane C. Peterson, Chief Operating Officer

EMORY–ADVENTIST HOSPITAL, 3949 South Cobb Drive S.E., Smyrna, GA, Zip 30080–6300; tel. 770/434–0710; Dennis Kiley, President

FAIRVIEW PARK HOSPITAL, 200 Industrial Boulevard, Dublin, GA, Zip 31021–2997, Mailing Address: P.O. Box 1408, Zip 31040–1408; tel. 478/275–2000; Donald R. Avery, FACHE, President and Chief Executive Officer

FLOYD MEDICAL CENTER, 304 Turner McCall Boulevard, Rome, GA, Zip 30165–2734, Mailing Address: P.O. Box 233, Zip 30162–0233; tel. 706/509–5000; Kurt Stuenkel, FACHE, President and Chief Executive Officer

GEORGIA HEALTH SCIENCES MEDICAL CENTER, 1120 15th Street, Augusta, GA, Zip 30912–5000; tel. 706/721–0211; David S. Hefner, President and Chief Executive Officer

GRADY GENERAL HOSPITAL, 1155 Fifth Street S.E., Cairo, GA, Zip 39828–0360, Mailing Address: P.O. Box 360, Zip 39828–0360; tel. 229/377–1150; LaDon Toole, Chief Operating Officer and Administrator

HABERSHAM MEDICAL CENTER, 541 Historic Highway 441, Demorest, GA, Zip 30535–3118, Mailing Address: P.O. Box 37, Zip 30535–0037; tel. 706/754–2161; C. Richard Dwozan, Chief Executive Officer

HIGGINS GENERAL HOSPITAL, 200 Allen Memorial Drive, Bremen, GA, Zip 30110–2012, Mailing Address: P.O. Box 655, Zip 30110–0655; tel. 770/537–5851; Michael Alexander, Administrator

HOUSTON MEDICAL CENTER, 1601 Watson Boulevard, Warner Robins, GA, Zip 31093–3431, Mailing Address: P.O. Box 2886, Zip 31099–2886; tel. 478/922–4281; Cary Martin, Chief Executive Officer

JOHN D. ARCHBOLD MEMORIAL HOSPITAL, 915 Gordon Avenue, Thomasville, GA, Zip 31792–6614, Mailing Address: P.O. Box 1018, Zip 31799–1018; tel. 229/228–2000; J. Perry Mustian, President and Chief Executive Officer

LIBERTY REGIONAL MEDICAL CENTER, 462 Elma G. Miles Parkway, Hinesville, GA, Zip 31313–4000, Mailing Address: P.O. Box 919, Zip 31310–0919; tel. 912/369–9400; H. Scott Kroell, Jr., Chief Executive Officer

LOUIS SMITH MEMORIAL HOSPITAL, 116 West Thigpen Avenue, Lakeland, GA, Zip 31635–1099; tel. 229/482–3110; Neil W. Ginty, Administrator

MEDICAL CENTER OF CENTRAL GEORGIA, 777 Hemlock Street, Macon, GA, Zip 31201–2155; tel. 478/633–1000; A. Donald Faulk, Jr., FACHE, President

MITCHELL COUNTY HOSPITAL, 90 East Stephens Street, Camilla, GA, Zip 31730–1836, Mailing Address: P.O. Box 639, Zip 31730–0639; tel. 229/336–5284; Mark E. Kimball, Administrator

NEWTON MEDICAL CENTER, 5126 Hospital Drive, Covington, GA, Zip 30014–2567; tel. 770/786–7053; James F. Weadick, Administrator and Chief Executive Officer

NORTHSIDE HOSPITAL, 1000 Johnson Ferry Road N.E., Atlanta, GA, Zip 30342–1611; tel. 404/851–8000; Robert Quattrocchi, President and Chief Executive Officer

OCONEE REGIONAL MEDICAL CENTER, 821 North Cobb Street, Milledgeville, GA, Zip 31061–2351, Mailing Address: P.O. Box 690, Zip 31059–0690; tel. 478/454–3500; Jean Aycock, President and Chief Executive Officer

PHOEBE NORTH, 2000 Palmyra Road, Albany, GA, Zip 31702–1908, Mailing Address: P.O. Box 1908, Zip 31702–1908; tel. 229/434–2000; Hugh D. Wilson, Interim Chief Executive Officer

PIONEER COMMUNITY HOSPITAL OF EARLY, 11740 Columbia Street, Blakely, GA, Zip 39823–9604; tel. 229/723–4235; Adam Willmann, Administrator

SOUTH GEORGIA MEDICAL CENTER, 2501 North Patterson Street, Valdosta, GA, Zip 31602–1735, Mailing Address: P.O. Box 1727, Zip 31603–1727; tel. 229/333–1000; Randy Sauls, Chief Executive Officer and Administrator

SOUTHEAST GEORGIA HEALTH SYSTEM BRUNSWICK CAMPUS, 2415 Parkwood Drive, Brunswick, GA, Zip 31520–4252, Mailing Address: P.O. Box 1518, Zip 31521–1518; tel. 912/466–7000; Gary R. Colberg, FACHE, President and Chief Executive Officer

SOUTHEAST GEORGIA HEALTH SYSTEM CAMDEN CAMPUS, 2000 Dan Proctor Drive, Saint Marys, GA, Zip 31558–3810; tel. 912/576–6200; Howard W. Sepp, Jr., FACHE, Vice President and Administrator

SOUTHERN REGIONAL MEDICAL CENTER, 11 Upper Riverdale Road S.W., Riverdale, GA, Zip 30274–2615; tel. 770/991–8000; Stephen W. Mahan, President and Chief Executive Officer

SPALDING REGIONAL MEDICAL CENTER, 601 South Eighth Street, Griffin, GA, Zip 30224–4294, Mailing Address: P.O. Drawer V, Zip 30224–1168; tel. 770/228–2721; John A. Quinn, Chief Executive Officer

TANNER MEDICAL CENTER, 705 Dixie Street, Carrollton, GA, Zip 30117–3818; tel. 770/836–9666; Loy M. Howard, President and Chief Executive Officer

TANNER MEDICAL CENTER–VILLA RICA, 601 Dallas Road, Villa Rica, GA, Zip 30180–1202, Mailing Address: P.O. Box 638, Zip 30180–0638; tel. 770/456–3100; Deborah Matthews, Administrator

THE MEDICAL CENTER, 710 Center Street, Columbus, GA, Zip 31901–1527, Mailing Address: P.O. Box 951, Zip 31902–0951; tel. 706/571–1000; Ryan Chandler, President and Chief Executive Officer

TIFT REGIONAL MEDICAL CENTER, 901 East 18th Street, Tifton, GA, Zip 31794–3648, Mailing Address: Drawer 747, Zip 31793–0747; tel. 229/382–7120; William T. Richardson, President and Chief Executive Officer

UPSON REGIONAL MEDICAL CENTER, 801 West Gordon Street, Thomaston, GA, Zip 30286–2831, Mailing Address: P.O. Box 1059, Zip 30286–1059; tel. 706/647–8111; David L. Castleberry, Chief Executive Officer

WALTON REGIONAL MEDICAL CENTER, 330 Alcovy Street, Monroe, GA, Zip 30655–2101, Mailing Address: P.O. Box 1346, Zip 30655–1346; tel. 770/267–8461; J. T. Barnhart, Chief Executive Officer

WEST GEORGIA HEALTH, 1514 Vernon Road, La Grange, GA, Zip 30240–4199; tel. 706/882–1411; Gerald N. Fulks, President and Chief Executive Officer

### ST. JOSEPH'S/CANDLER HEALTH SYSTEM, INC.
**5353 Reynolds Street, Savannah, GA 31405–6015; tel. 912/819–6000; Paul P. Hinchey, President and Chief Executive Officer**

APPLING HEALTHCARE SYSTEM, 163 East Tollison Street, Baxley, GA, Zip 31513–2898; tel. 912/367–9841; Dale Spell, Chief Executive Officer

CANDLER HOSPITAL, 5353 Reynolds Street, Savannah, GA, Zip 31405–6013; tel. 912/819–6000; Paul P. Hinchey, President and Chief Executive Officer

EFFINGHAM HOSPITAL, 459 Highway 119 South, Springfield, GA, Zip 31329–3021, Mailing Address: P.O. Box 386, Zip 31329–0386; tel. 912/754–6451; Norma J. Morgan, Chief Executive Officer

EMORY UNIVERSITY HOSPITAL, 1364 Clifton Road N.E., Atlanta, GA, Zip 30322–1102; tel. 404/712–2000; Robert J. Bachman, Chief Operating Officer

LIBERTY REGIONAL MEDICAL CENTER, 462 Elma G. Miles Parkway, Hinesville, GA, Zip 31313–4000, Mailing Address: P.O. Box 919, Zip 31310–0919; tel. 912/369–9400; H. Scott Kroell, Jr., Chief Executive Officer

MEADOWS REGIONAL MEDICAL CENTER, 1703 Meadows Lane, Vidalia, GA, Zip 30474–8915, Mailing Address: P.O. Box 1048, Zip 30475–1048; tel. 912/535–5555; Alan Kent, Chief Executive Officer

ST. JOSEPH'S HOSPITAL, 11705 Mercy Boulevard, Savannah, GA, Zip 31419–1791; tel. 912/819–4100; Paul P. Hinchey, President and Chief Executive Officer

WILLINGWAY HOSPITAL, 311 Jones Mill Road, Statesboro, GA, Zip 30458–4765; tel. 912/764–6236; Jimmy Mooney, Chief Executive Officer

## IDAHO

**HOSPITAL COOPERATIVE**
**850 East Young Street, Pocatello, ID 83201–5736; tel. 208/239–2162; Jon Smith, Executive Director**

BEAR LAKE MEMORIAL HOSPITAL, 164 South Fifth Street, Montpelier, ID, Zip 83254–1597; tel. 208/847–1630; Rodney D. Jacobson, Administrator

BINGHAM MEMORIAL HOSPITAL, 98 Poplar Street, Blackfoot, ID, Zip 83221–1799; tel. 208/785–4100; Louis D. Kraml, FACHE, Chief Executive Officer

CARIBOU MEMORIAL HOSPITAL AND LIVING CENTER, 300 South Third West, Soda Springs, ID, Zip 83276–1598; tel. 208/547–3341; John L. Hoopes, Chief Executive Officer

FRANKLIN COUNTY MEDICAL CENTER, 44 North First East Street, Preston, ID, Zip 83263–1399; tel. 208/852–0137; Michael G. Andrus, Administrator and Chief Executive Officer

LOST RIVERS DISTRICT HOSPITAL, 551 Highland Drive, Arco, ID, Mailing Address: P.O. Box 145, Zip 83213–0145; tel. 208/527–8206; Kim Dahlman, Administrator

MADISON MEMORIAL HOSPITAL, 450 East Main Street, Rexburg, ID, Zip 83440–2048, Mailing Address: P.O. Box 310, Zip 83440–0310; tel. 208/359–6900; Rachel Gonzales, MSN, R.N., Chief Executive Officer

MINIDOKA MEMORIAL HOSPITAL, 1224 Eighth Street, Rupert, ID, Zip 83350–1599; tel. 208/436–0481; Carl Hanson, Administrator

ONEIDA COUNTY HOSPITAL, 150 North 200 West, Malad City, ID, Zip 83252–0126, Mailing Address: Box 126, Zip 83252–0126; tel. 208/766–2231; Todd V. Winder, Administrator and Chief Executive Officer

PORTNEUF MEDICAL CENTER, 777 Hospital Way, Pocatello, ID, Zip 83201–4004; tel. 208/239–1000; Norman F. Stephens, President and Chief Executive Officer

POWER COUNTY HOSPITAL DISTRICT, 510 Roosevelt Road, American Falls, ID, Zip 83211–0420, Mailing Address: P.O. Box 420, Zip 83211–0420; tel. 208/226–3200; Dallas Clinger, Administrator

ST. LUKE'S JEROME FAMILY MEDICAL CENTER, 709 North Lincoln Street, Jerome, ID, Zip 83338–1851, Mailing Address: P.O. Box 586, Zip 83338–0586; tel. 208/324–4301; James L. Angle, FACHE, Chief Executive Officer

STAR VALLEY MEDICAL CENTER, 901 Adams Street, Afton, WY, Zip 83110–0579, Mailing Address: P.O. Box 579, Zip 83110–0579; tel. 307/885–5800; Don Herbert, Interim Chief Executive Officer

STEELE MEMORIAL MEDICAL CENTER, 203 South Daisy Street, Salmon, ID, Zip 83467–4109; tel. 208/756–5600; Jeff Hill, Chief Executive Officer

TETON VALLEY HOSPITAL AND SURGICENTER, 120 East Howard Street, Driggs, ID, Zip 83422–5112; tel. 208/354–2383; Virgil Boss, Chief Executive Officer

**NORTH IDAHO HEALTH NETWORK**
**1250 West Ironwood Drive, Suite 201, Coeur D'Alene, ID 83814–2681; tel. 208/666–3212; Richard McMaster, Executive Director**

BENEWAH COMMUNITY HOSPITAL, 229 South Seventh Street, Saint Maries, ID, Zip 83861–1803; tel. 208/245–5551; Brian Nall, Chief Executive Officer

BONNER GENERAL HOSPITAL, 520 North Third Avenue, Sandpoint, ID, Zip 83864–0877, Mailing Address: Box 1448, Zip 83864–0877; tel. 208/263–1441; Sheryl Rickard, Chief Executive Officer

BOUNDARY COMMUNITY HOSPITAL, 6640 Kaniksu Street, Bonners Ferry, ID, Zip 83805–7532; tel. 208/267–3141; Craig A. Johnson, Chief Executive Officer and Chief Financial Officer

KOOTENAI MEDICAL CENTER, 2003 Kootenai Health Way, Coeur D'Alene, ID, Zip 83814–2677; tel. 208/666–2000; Jon Ness, Chief Executive Officer

SHOSHONE MEDICAL CENTER, 25 Jacobs Gulch, Kellogg, ID, Zip 83837–2096; tel. 208/784–1221; Gary Moore, Chief Executive Officer

**SOUTHWEST IDAHO COMMUNITY HEALTH NETWORK**
**PO Box 607, Boise, ID 83701–0607; tel. 208/381–1571; Stephen R. Stoddard, FACHE, Executive Director**

CASCADE MEDICAL CENTER, 402 Old State Highway, Cascade, ID, Zip 83611, Mailing Address: P.O. Box 1330, Zip 83611–1330; tel. 208/382–4242; William C. Behnke, Jr., Administrator

ELKS REHAB HOSPITAL, 600 North Robbins Road, Boise, ID, Zip 83702–4597, Mailing Address: P.O. Box 1100, Zip 83701–1100; tel. 208/489–4444; Joseph P. Caroselli, Chief Executive Officer

ELMORE MEDICAL CENTER, 895 North Sixth East Street, Mountain Home, ID, Zip 83647–2207, Mailing Address: P.O. Box 1270, Zip 83647–1270; tel. 208/587–8401; Gregory L. Maurer, Administrator

NORTH CANYON MEDICAL CENTER, 267 North Canyon Drive, Gooding, ID, Zip 83330; tel. 208/934–4433; David Butler, Chief Executive Officer

ST. LUKE'S JEROME FAMILY MEDICAL CENTER, 709 North Lincoln Street, Jerome, ID, Zip 83338–1851, Mailing Address: P.O. Box 586, Zip 83338–0586; tel. 208/324–4301; James L. Angle, FACHE, Chief Executive Officer

ST. LUKE'S MAGIC VALLEY MEDICAL CENTER, 801 Pole Line Road West, Twin Falls, ID, Zip 83301, Mailing Address: P.O. Box 409, Zip 83303–0409; tel. 208/814–0000; James L. Angle, FACHE, Chief Executive Officer

ST. LUKE'S MCCALL, 1000 State Street, McCall, ID, Zip 83638–3704; tel. 208/634–2221; Michael A. Fenello, Chief Executive Officer

ST. LUKE'S REGIONAL MEDICAL CENTER, 190 East Bannock Street, Boise, ID, Zip 83712–6298; tel. 208/381–2222; Chris Roth, Chief Executive Officer

ST. LUKE'S WOOD RIVER MEDICAL CENTER, 100 Hospital Drive, Ketchum, ID, Zip 83340, Mailing Address: P.O. Box 100, Zip 83340; tel. 208/727–8800; Cody Langbehn, Chief Executive Officer

SYRINGA HOSPITAL AND CLINICS, 607 West Main Street, Grangeville, ID, Zip 83530–1396; tel. 208/983–1700; Joseph Cladouhos, Chief Executive Officer

WALTER KNOX MEMORIAL HOSPITAL, 1202 East Locust Street, Emmett, ID, Zip 83617–2715; tel. 208/365–3561; John N. Olson, Chief Executive Officer

WEISER MEMORIAL HOSPITAL, 645 East Fifth Street, Weiser, ID, Zip 83672–2202; tel. 208/549–0370; Tom Murphy, Chief Executive Officer

## ILLINOIS

**FELICIAN SERVICES, INC.**
**3800 West Peterson Avenue, Chicago, IL 60659–3116; tel. 773/463–3806; Sister Mary Clarette Stryzewski, President and Chief Executive Officer**

ST. MARY'S HOSPITAL, 400 North Pleasant Avenue, Centralia, IL, Zip 62801–3091; tel. 618/436–8000; Bruce Merrell, FACHE, President

WHEATON FRANCISCAN HEALTHCARE – ST. FRANCIS, 3237 South 16th Street, Milwaukee, WI, Zip 53215–4592; tel. 414/647–5000; Daniel Mattes, President

**SWEDISHAMERICAN HEALTH SYSTEM**
**1401 East State Street, Rockford, IL 61104–2227; tel. 815/489–4400; William R. Gorski, M.D., President and Chief Executive Officer**

## INDIANA

**ST. VINCENT HEALTH**
**2001 West 86Th Street, Indianapolis, IN 46260–1902; tel. 317/338–8455; Vincent C. Caponi, FACHE, Chief Executive Officer**

SAINT JOHN'S HEALTH SYSTEM, 2015 Jackson Street, Anderson, IN, Zip 46016–4339; tel. 765/649–2511; Thomas J. VanOsdol, President

ST. JOSEPH HOSPITAL AND HEALTH CENTER, 1907 West Sycamore Street, Kokomo, IN, Zip 46901–4197, Mailing Address: P.O. Box 9010, Zip 46904–9010; tel. 765/452–5611; Kathlene A. Young, MS, FACHE, President and Chief Executive Officer

ST. VINCENT CARMEL HOSPITAL, 13500 North Meridian Street, Carmel, IN, Zip 46032; tel. 317/582–7000; Michael D. Chittenden, President

ST. VINCENT CLAY HOSPITAL, 1206 East National Avenue, Brazil, IN, Zip 47834–2797, Mailing Address: P.O. Box 489, Zip 47834–0489; tel. 812/442–2500; Jerry Laue, Administrator

ST. VINCENT FRANKFORT HOSPITAL, 1300 South Jackson Street, Frankfort, IN, Zip 46041–3394, Mailing Address: P.O. Box 669, Zip 46041–0669; tel. 765/656–3000; Thomas Crawford, Administrator

ST. VINCENT INDIANAPOLIS HOSPITAL, 2001 West 86th Street, Indianapolis, IN, Zip 46260–1991, Mailing Address: P.O. Box 40970, Zip 46240–0970; tel. 317/338–2345; Kyle De Fur, FACHE, President

ST. VINCENT JENNINGS HOSPITAL, 301 Henry Street, North Vernon, IN, Zip 47265–1097; tel. 812/352–4200; Carl W. Risk, II, Administrator

ST. VINCENT MERCY HOSPITAL, 1331 South A Street, Elwood, IN, Zip 46036–1942; tel. 765/552–4600; Deborah Y. Rasper, FACHE, Administrator

ST. VINCENT RANDOLPH HOSPITAL, 473 Greenville Avenue, Winchester, IN, Zip 47394–2235, Mailing Address: P.O. Box 407, Zip 47394–0407; tel. 765/584–0004; Francis G. Albarano, Administrator

ST. VINCENT SETON SPECIALTY HOSPITAL, 1501 Hartford Street, Lafayette, IN, Zip 47904; tel. 765/236–8900; Peter H. Alexander, Administrator

ST. VINCENT WILLIAMSPORT HOSPITAL, 412 North Monroe Street, Williamsport, IN, Zip 47993–0215; tel. 765/762–4000; Jane Craigin, Chief Executive Officer

**SUBURBAN HEALTH ORGANIZATION**
**2780 Waterfront Parkway East Drive, Suite 300, Indianapolis, IN 46214; tel. 317/692–5222; Julie M. Carmichael, President**

COMMUNITY WESTVIEW HOSPITAL, 3630 Guion Road, Indianapolis, IN, Zip 46222–1699; tel. 317/924–6661; Jon P. Anderson, CPA, Chief Executive Officer

HANCOCK REGIONAL HOSPITAL, 801 North State Street, Greenfield, IN, Zip 46140–1270, Mailing Address: P.O. Box 827, Zip 46140–0827; tel. 317/462–5544; Robert C. Keen, Ph.D., FACHE, President and Chief Executive Officer

HENDRICKS REGIONAL HEALTH, 1000 East Main Street, Danville, IN, Zip 46122–0409, Mailing Address: P.O. Box 409, Zip 46122–0409; tel. 317/745–4451; Dennis W. Dawes, FACHE, President

HENRY COUNTY HOSPITAL, 1000 North 16th Street, New Castle, IN, Zip 47362–4319, Mailing Address: P.O. Box 490, Zip 47362–0490; tel. 765/521–0890; Paul Janssen, President and Chief Executive Officer

INDIANA UNIVERSITY HEALTH MORGAN HOSPITAL, 2209 John R. Wooden Drive, Martinsville, IN, Zip 46151–1840, Mailing Address: P.O. Box 1717, Zip 46151–1717; tel. 765/342–8441; Doug Puckett, President and Chief Executive Officer

RIVERVIEW HOSPITAL, 395 Westfield Road, Noblesville, IN, Zip 46060–1425, Mailing Address: P.O. Box 220, Zip 46061–0220; tel. 317/773–0760; Patricia K. Fox, President and Chief Executive Officer

WITHAM MEMORIAL HOSPITAL, 2605 North Lebanon Street, Lebanon, IN, Zip 46052, Mailing Address: P.O. Box 1200, Zip 46052–3005; tel. 765/485–8000; Raymond V. Ingham, M.D., Ph.D., President and Chief Executive Officer

## IOWA

**GENESIS HEALTH SYSTEM**
**1227 East Rusholme Street, Davenport, IA 52803–2498; tel. 563/421–1000; Douglas P. Cropper, President and Chief Executive Officer**

GENESIS MEDICAL CENTER, DEWITT, 1118 11th Street, De Witt, IA, Zip 52742–1296; tel. 563/659–4200; Jeffrey M. Cooper, President

GENESIS MEDICAL CENTER, ILLINI CAMPUS, 801 Illini Drive, Silvis, IL, Zip 61282–1893; tel. 309/281–4000; Florence Spyrow, President

GENESIS MEDICAL CENTER–DAVENPORT, 1227 East Rusholme Street, Davenport, IA, Zip 52803–2498; tel. 563/421–1000; Wayne A. Diewald, President

**MERCY HEALTH NETWORK – CENTRAL IOWA**
**1111 6th Avenue, Des Moines, IA 50314–2611; tel. 515/247–3121; Sara Drobnich, Senior Vice President**

ADAIR COUNTY MEMORIAL HOSPITAL, 609 S.E. Kent Street, Greenfield, IA, Zip 50849–9454; tel. 641/743–2123; Angela Mortoza, Administrator

AUDUBON COUNTY MEMORIAL HOSPITAL, 515 Pacific Street, Audubon, IA, Zip 50025–1052; tel. 712/563–2611; Thomas G. Smith, Administrator and Chief Executive Officer

CLARINDA REGIONAL HEALTH CENTER, 823 South 17th Street, Clarinda, IA, Zip 51632, Mailing Address: P.O. Box 217, Zip 51632–0217; tel. 712/542–2176; Christopher R. Stipe, FACHE, Chief Executive Officer

DALLAS COUNTY HOSPITAL, 610 10th Street, Perry, IA, Zip 50220–2221; tel. 515/465–3547; Matt Wille, Chief Executive Officer

DAVIS COUNTY HOSPITAL, 509 North Madison Street, Bloomfield, IA, Zip 52537–1271; tel. 641/664–2145; Deborah L. Herzberg, R.N., MS, FACHE, Chief Executive Officer

DECATUR COUNTY HOSPITAL, 1405 N.W. Church Street, Leon, IA, Zip 50144–1299; tel. 641/446–4871; Lynn Milnes, Chief Executive Officer

GRINNELL REGIONAL MEDICAL CENTER, 210 Fourth Avenue, Grinnell, IA, Zip 50112–1833; tel. 641/236–7511; Todd C. Linden, President and Chief Executive Officer

MADISON COUNTY HEALTH CARE SYSTEM, 300 Hutchings Street, Winterset, IA, Zip 50273–2109; tel. 515/462–2373; Marcia Hendricks, R.N., Chief Executive Officer

MANNING REGIONAL HEALTHCARE CENTER, 410 Main Street, Manning, IA, Zip 51455–1093; tel. 712/655–2072; John O'Brien, Chief Executive Officer

MERCY MEDICAL CENTER–CENTERVILLE, 1 St. Joseph's Drive, Centerville, IA, Zip 52544–8055; tel. 641/437–4111; Clinton J. Christianson, FACHE, President and Chief Executive Officer

MERCY MEDICAL CENTER–DES MOINES, 1111 6th Avenue, Des Moines, IA, Zip 50314–2611; tel. 515/247–3121; David H. Vellinga, FACHE, President and Chief Executive Officer

MONROE COUNTY HOSPITAL, 6580 165th Street, Albia, IA, Zip 52531–8793; tel. 641/932–2134; Gregory A. Paris, FACHE, Chief Executive Officer

RINGGOLD COUNTY HOSPITAL, 504 North Cleveland Street, Mount Ayr, IA, Zip 50854–2201; tel. 641/464–3226; Gordon W. Winkler, Administrator and Chief Executive Officer

STEWART MEMORIAL COMMUNITY HOSPITAL, 1301 West Main, Lake City, IA, Zip 51449–1585; tel. 712/464–3171; Leah Marxen, Administrator and Chief Executive Officer

STORY COUNTY MEDICAL CENTER, 640 South 19th Street, Nevada, IA, Zip 50201–2266; tel. 515/382–2111; Todd Willert, Administrator

VAN DIEST MEDICAL CENTER, 2350 Hospital Drive, Webster City, IA, Zip 50595–2824, Mailing Address: P.O. Box 430, Zip 50595–0430; tel. 515/832–9400; Palmer Schneider, Administrator

WAYNE COUNTY HOSPITAL, 417 South East Street, Corydon, IA, Zip 50060–1860, Mailing Address: P.O. Box 305, Zip 50060–0305; tel. 641/872–2260; Daren Relph, Chief Executive Officer

**MERCY HEALTH NETWORK – NORTH IOWA**
**1000 4th Street S.W., Mason City, IA 50401–2800; tel. 641/428–7000; Rod G. Schlader, Interim Chief Executive Officer**

ELLSWORTH MUNICIPAL HOSPITAL, 110 Rocksylvania Avenue, Iowa Falls, IA, Zip 50126–2400; tel. 641/648–4631; Cherelle Montanye, Chief Executive Officer

FRANKLIN GENERAL HOSPITAL, 1720 Central Avenue East, Hampton, IA, Zip 50441–1859; tel. 641/456–5000; Kim Price, Chief Executive Officer

HANCOCK COUNTY MEMORIAL HOSPITAL, 532 First Street N.W., Britt, IA, Zip 50423; tel. 641/843–5000; Vance Jackson, FACHE, Administrator and Chief Executive Officer

IOWA SPECIALTY HOSPITAL–BELMOND, 403 First Street S.E., Belmond, IA, Zip 50421–1201; tel. 641/444–3223; Nancy Gabrielson, Administrator and Chief Executive Officer

KOSSUTH REGIONAL HEALTH CENTER, 1515 South Phillips Street, Algona, IA, Zip 50511–3649; tel. 515/295–2451; Scott A. Curtis, Administrator and Chief Executive Officer

MERCY MEDICAL CENTER–NEW HAMPTON, 308 North Maple Avenue, New Hampton, IA, Zip 50659–1142; tel. 641/394–4121; Bruce E. Roesler, FACHE, President and Chief Executive Officer

MERCY MEDICAL CENTER–NORTH IOWA, 1000 Fourth Street S.W., Mason City, IA, Zip 50401–2800; tel. 641/428–7000; Rod G. Schlader, Interim President and Chief Executive Officer

MITCHELL COUNTY REGIONAL HEALTH CENTER, 616 North Eighth Street, Osage, IA, Zip 50461–1498; tel. 641/732–6000; Desiree Einsweiler, Interim Chief Executive Officer

PALO ALTO COUNTY HEALTH SYSTEM, 3201 First Street, Emmetsburg, IA, Zip 50536; tel. 712/852–5500; Vance Jackson, FACHE, Interim Administrator

REGIONAL HEALTH SERVICES OF HOWARD COUNTY, 235 Eighth Avenue West, Cresco, IA, Zip 52136–1098; tel. 563/547–2101; Vance Jackson, FACHE, Interim Chief Executive Officer

## KANSAS

**HAYS MEDICAL CENTER**
**2220 Canterbury Drive, Hays, KS 67601–2370; tel. 785/623–2300; John H. Jeter, M.D., President and Chief Executive Officer**

CHEYENNE COUNTY HOSPITAL, 210 West First Street, Saint Francis, KS, Zip 67756–0547, Mailing Address: P.O. Box 547, Zip 67756–0547; tel. 785/332–2104; Leslie Lacy, Administrator

CITIZENS MEDICAL CENTER, 100 East College Drive, Colby, KS, Zip 67701–3799; tel. 785/462–7511; Kevan Trenkle, Chief Executive Officer

CLARA BARTON HOSPITAL, 250 West Ninth Street, Hoisington, KS, Zip 67544–1706; tel. 620/653–2114; Curt Colson, President and Chief Executive Officer

EDWARDS COUNTY HOSPITAL AND HEALTHCARE CENTER, 620 West Eighth Street, Kinsley, KS, Zip 67547–2329, Mailing Address: P.O. Box 99, Zip 67547–0099; tel. 620/659–3621; Robert Krickbaum, Chief Executive Officer

GOVE COUNTY MEDICAL CENTER, 520 West Fifth Street, Quinter, KS, Zip 67752–0129, Mailing Address: P.O. Box 129, Zip 67752–0129; tel. 785/754–3341; Richard Q. Bergling, Chief Executive Officer

GRAHAM COUNTY HOSPITAL, 304 West Prout Street, Hill City, KS, Zip 67642–1435; tel. 785/421–2121; Melissa Atkins, CPA, Chief Executive Officer

GRISELL MEMORIAL HOSPITAL DISTRICT ONE, 210 South Vermont Avenue, Ransom, KS, Zip 67572; tel. 785/731–2231; Kristine Ochs, R.N., Administrator

LANE COUNTY HOSPITAL, 235 West Vine, Dighton, KS, Zip 67839–0969, Mailing Address: P.O. Box 969, Zip 67839–0969; tel. 620/397–5321; Donna McGowan, Administrator

LOGAN COUNTY HOSPITAL, 211 Cherry Street, Oakley, KS, Zip 67748–1201; tel. 785/672–3211; Darcy Howard, Chief Executive Officer and Chief Financial Officer

MINNEOLA DISTRICT HOSPITAL, 212 Main Street, Minneola, KS, Zip 67865–0127, Mailing Address: P.O. Box 127, Zip 67865–0127; tel. 620/885–4264; Brian Roland, Administrator and Chief Executive Officer

NESS COUNTY HOSPITAL, 312 Custer Street, Ness City, KS, Zip 67560–1654; tel. 785/798–2291; Curt Thomas, Administrator

NORTON COUNTY HOSPITAL, 102 East Holme, Norton, KS, Zip 67654–0250, Mailing Address: P.O. Box 250, Zip 67654–0250; tel. 785/877–3351; Richard Miller, Administrator and Chief Executive Officer

PHILLIPS COUNTY HOSPITAL, 1150 State Street, Phillipsburg, KS, Zip 67661–1799, Mailing Address: P.O. Box 607, Zip 67661–0607; tel. 785/543–5226; David Engel, Chief Executive Officer

RAWLINS COUNTY HEALTH CENTER, 707 Grant Street, Atwood, KS, Zip 67730–4700, Mailing Address: P.O. Box 47, Zip 67730–4700; tel. 785/626–3211; Deanna Freeman, Administrator and Chief Executive Officer

ROOKS COUNTY HEALTH CENTER, 1210 North Washington Street, Plainville, KS, Zip 67663–1632, Mailing Address: P.O. Box 389, Zip 67663–0389; tel. 785/434–4553; Michael Sinclair, Chief Executive Officer

RUSH COUNTY MEMORIAL HOSPITAL, 801 Locust Street, La Crosse, KS, Zip 67548–9673, Mailing Address: P.O. Box 520, Zip 67548–0520; tel. 785/222–2545; Jonathan Owens, Chief Executive Officer

RUSSELL REGIONAL HOSPITAL, 200 South Main Street, Russell, KS, Zip 67665–2997; tel. 785/483–3131; Shelley Boden, Administrator and Chief Executive Officer

SCOTT COUNTY HOSPITAL, 310 East Third Street, Scott City, KS, Zip 67871–1203; tel. 620/872–5811; Mark Burnett, President and Chief Executive Officer

SHERIDAN COUNTY HEALTH COMPLEX, 826 18th Street, Hoxie, KS, Zip 67740–0167, Mailing Address: P.O. Box 167, Zip 67740–0167; tel. 785/675–3281; Steven L. Granzow, Chief Executive Officer

SMITH COUNTY MEMORIAL HOSPITAL, 614 South Main Street, Smith Center, KS, Zip 66967–0349; tel. 785/282–6845; Carolyn K. Hess, R.N., Administrator

TREGO COUNTY–LEMKE MEMORIAL HOSPITAL, 320 North 13th Street, Wakeeney, KS, Zip 67672–2099; tel. 785/743–2182; Harold Courtois, Administrator and Chief Executive Officer

**HEALTH INNOVATIONS NETWORK OF KANSAS**
**1500 S.W. 10th Avenue, Topeka, KS 66604–1301; tel. 785/354–6137; Kristi Grosser, Network Operations Director**

CLAY COUNTY MEDICAL CENTER, 617 Liberty Street, Clay Center, KS, Zip 67432–0512, Mailing Address: P.O. Box 512, Zip 67432–0512; tel. 785/632–2144; Ron Bender, Chief Executive Officer

COFFEY COUNTY HOSPITAL, 801 North Fourth Street, Burlington, KS, Zip 66839–0189, Mailing Address: P.O. Box 189, Zip 66839–0189; tel. 620/364–2121; Karen Smith, Interim Chief Executive Officer

COMMUNITY HEALTH CARE SYSTEM, 120 West Eighth Street, Onaga, KS, Zip 66521–0120; tel. 785/889–4272; Greg Unruh, Chief Executive Officer

COMMUNITY MEMORIAL HEALTHCARE, 708 North 18th Street, Marysville, KS, Zip 66508–1338; tel. 785/562–2311; Curtis R. Hawkinson, Chief Executive Officer

F. W. HUSTON MEDICAL CENTER, 408 Delaware Street, Winchester, KS, Zip 66097–4003; tel. 913/774–4340; LaMont Cook, Administrator

GEARY COMMUNITY HOSPITAL, 1102 St. Mary's Road, Junction City, KS, Zip 66441–4196, Mailing Address: P.O. Box 490, Zip 66441–0490; tel. 785/238–4131; David K. Bradley, FACHE, Chief Executive Officer

HERINGTON MUNICIPAL HOSPITAL, 100 East Helen Street, Herington, KS, Zip 67449–1606; tel. 785/258–2207; Michael J. Ryan, Chief Executive Officer

HIAWATHA COMMUNITY HOSPITAL, 300 Utah Street, Hiawatha, KS, Zip 66434–2314; tel. 785/742–2131; John Moore, Administrator

HOLTON COMMUNITY HOSPITAL, 1110 Columbine Drive, Holton, KS, Zip 66436–1545; tel. 785/364–2116; Carrie L. Saia, R.N., Interim Chief Executive Officer

HORTON COMMUNITY HOSPITAL, 240 West 18th Street, Horton, KS, Zip 66439–1245; tel. 785/486–2642; Terry Nichols, Interim Chief Executive Officer

KANSAS REHABILITATION HOSPITAL, 1504 S.W. Eighth Avenue, Topeka, KS, Zip 66606–1632; tel. 785/235–6600; Marty Dernier, Chief Financial Officer and Administrator

MORRIS COUNTY HOSPITAL, 600 North Washington Street, Council Grove, KS, Zip 66846–1422; tel. 620/767–6811; James H. Reagan, Jr., Ph.D., Chief Executive Officer

NEMAHA VALLEY COMMUNITY HOSPITAL, 1600 Community Drive, Seneca, KS, Zip 66538–9739; tel. 785/336–6181; Stan Regehr, President and Chief Executive Officer

SABETHA COMMUNITY HOSPITAL, 14th and Oregon Streets, Sabetha, KS, Zip 66534–0229, Mailing Address: P.O. Box 229, Zip 66534–0229; tel. 785/284–2121; Lora Key, Chief Executive Officer

STORMONT-VAIL HEALTHCARE, 1500 S.W. Tenth Avenue, Topeka, KS, Zip 66604–1353; tel. 785/354–6000; Randall Peterson, President and Chief Executive Officer

WASHINGTON COUNTY HOSPITAL, 304 East Third Street, Washington, KS, Zip 66968–2033; tel. 785/325–2211; Doyle L. McKimmy, FACHE, Chief Executive Officer

**MED-OP, INC.**
**205 East 7th Street, Hays, KS 67601–4907; tel. 785/621–4510; David Brittain, Executive Director**

CITIZENS MEDICAL CENTER, 100 East College Drive, Colby, KS, Zip 67701–3799; tel. 785/462–7511; Kevan Trenkle, Chief Executive Officer

CLARA BARTON HOSPITAL, 250 West Ninth Street, Hoisington, KS, Zip 67544–1706; tel. 620/653–2114; Curt Colson, President and Chief Executive Officer

GOODLAND REGIONAL MEDICAL CENTER, 220 West Second Street, Goodland, KS, Zip 67735–1602; tel. 785/890–3625; Jay P. Jolly, Chief Executive Officer

GOVE COUNTY MEDICAL CENTER, 520 West Fifth Street, Quinter, KS, Zip 67752–0129, Mailing Address: P.O. Box 129, Zip 67752–0129; tel. 785/754–3341; Richard Q. Bergling, Chief Executive Officer

GRAHAM COUNTY HOSPITAL, 304 West Prout Street, Hill City, KS, Zip 67642–1435; tel. 785/421–2121; Melissa Atkins, CPA, Chief Executive Officer

HAYS MEDICAL CENTER, 2220 Canterbury Drive, Hays, KS, Zip 67601–2370, Mailing Address: P.O. Box 8100, Zip 67601–8100; tel. 785/623–5000; John H. Jeter, M.D., President and Chief Executive Officer

LOGAN COUNTY HOSPITAL, 211 Cherry Street, Oakley, KS, Zip 67748–1201; tel. 785/672–3211; Darcy Howard, Chief Executive Officer and Chief Financial Officer

MERCY HOSPITAL AND TRAUMA CENTER, 1000 Mineral Point Avenue, Janesville, WI, Zip 53547–2982, Mailing Address: P.O. Box 5003, Zip 53547–5003; tel. 608/756–6000; Javon R. Bea, President and Chief Executive Officer

NESS COUNTY HOSPITAL, 312 Custer Street, Ness City, KS, Zip 67560–1654; tel. 785/798–2291; Curt Thomas, Administrator

NORTON COUNTY HOSPITAL, 102 East Holme, Norton, KS, Zip 67654–0250, Mailing Address: P.O. Box 250, Zip 67654–0250; tel. 785/877–3351; Richard Miller, Administrator and Chief Executive Officer

RICE COUNTY DISTRICT HOSPITAL, 619 South Clark Street, Lyons, KS, Zip 67554–0828, Mailing Address: P.O. Box 828, Zip 67554–0828; tel. 620/257–5173; George M. Stover, Chief Executive Officer

ROOKS COUNTY HEALTH CENTER, 1210 North Washington Street, Plainville, KS, Zip 67663–1632, Mailing Address: P.O. Box 389, Zip 67663–0389; tel. 785/434–4553; Michael Sinclair, Chief Executive Officer

RUSH COUNTY MEMORIAL HOSPITAL, 801 Locust Street, La Crosse, KS, Zip 67548–9673, Mailing Address: P.O. Box 520, Zip 67548–0520; tel. 785/222–2545; Jonathan Owens, Chief Executive Officer

RUSSELL REGIONAL HOSPITAL, 200 South Main Street, Russell, KS, Zip 67665–2997; tel. 785/483–3131; Shelley Boden, Administrator and Chief Executive Officer

SCOTT COUNTY HOSPITAL, 310 East Third Street, Scott City, KS, Zip 67871–1203; tel. 620/872–5811; Mark Burnett, President and Chief Executive Officer

SHERIDAN COUNTY HEALTH COMPLEX, 826 18th Street, Hoxie, KS, Zip 67740–0167, Mailing Address: P.O. Box 167, Zip 67740–0167; tel. 785/675–3281; Steven L. Granzow, Chief Executive Officer

STAFFORD COUNTY HOSPITAL, 502 South Buckeye Street, Stafford, KS, Zip 67578–2035, Mailing Address: P.O. Box 190, Zip 67578–0190; tel. 620/234–5221; Todd Taylor, Chief Executive Officer

**NEK CENTER FOR HEALTH & WELLNESS**
**240 West 18th Street, Horton, KS 66439–1245; tel. 785/486–2642; Terry Nichols, Chief Executive Officer**

COMMUNITY HEALTH CARE SYSTEM, 120 West Eighth Street, Onaga, KS, Zip 66521–0120; tel. 785/889–4272; Greg Unruh, Chief Executive Officer

COMMUNITY MEMORIAL HEALTHCARE, 708 North 18th Street, Marysville, KS, Zip 66508–1338; tel. 785/562–2311; Curtis R. Hawkinson, Chief Executive Officer

GEARY COMMUNITY HOSPITAL, 1102 St. Mary's Road, Junction City, KS, Zip 66441–4196, Mailing Address: P.O. Box 490, Zip 66441–0490; tel. 785/238–4131; David K. Bradley, FACHE, Chief Executive Officer

HOLTON COMMUNITY HOSPITAL, 1110 Columbine Drive, Holton, KS, Zip 66436–1545; tel. 785/364–2116; Carrie L. Saia, R.N., Interim Chief Executive Officer

HORTON COMMUNITY HOSPITAL, 240 West 18th Street, Horton, KS, Zip 66439–1245; tel. 785/486–2642; Terry Nichols, Interim Chief Executive Officer

MERCY REGIONAL HEALTH CENTER, 1823 College Avenue, Manhattan, KS, Zip 66502, Mailing Address: P.O. Box 1289, Zip 66505–1289; tel. 785/776–3322; John R. Broberg, FACHE, President and Chief Executive Officer

MORRIS COUNTY HOSPITAL, 600 North Washington Street, Council Grove, KS, Zip 66846–1422; tel. 620/767–6811; James H. Reagan, Jr., Ph.D., Chief Executive Officer

NEMAHA VALLEY COMMUNITY HOSPITAL, 1600 Community Drive, Seneca, KS, Zip 66538–9739; tel. 785/336–6181; Stan Regehr, President and Chief Executive Officer

ST. FRANCIS HEALTH CENTER, 1700 S.W. 7th Street, Topeka, KS, Zip 66606–1690; tel. 785/295–8000; Robert J. Erickson, Chief Executive Officer

WAMEGO CITY HOSPITAL, 711 Genn Drive, Wamego, KS, Zip 66547–1179; tel. 785/456–2295; Shannan Flach, Chief Executive Officer

**PIONEER HEALTH NETWORK, INC.**
**310 East Walnut Street, Suite 210, Garden City, KS 67846–5565; tel. 620/276–6100; Mary Adam, Executive Director**

BOB WILSON MEMORIAL GRANT COUNTY HOSPITAL, 415 North Main Street, Ulysses, KS, Zip 67880–2133; tel. 620/356–1266; Arthur H. Frable, Chief Executive Officer

CITIZENS MEDICAL CENTER, 100 East College Drive, Colby, KS, Zip 67701–3799; tel. 785/462–7511; Kevan Trenkle, Chief Executive Officer

EDWARDS COUNTY HOSPITAL AND HEALTHCARE CENTER, 620 West Eighth Street, Kinsley, KS, Zip 67547–2329, Mailing Address: P.O. Box 99, Zip 67547–0099; tel. 620/659–3621; Robert Krickbaum, Chief Executive Officer

GREELEY COUNTY HEALTH SERVICES, 506 Third Street, Tribune, KS, Zip 67879–0338, Mailing Address: P.O. Box 338, Zip 67879–0338; tel. 620/376–4221; Deborah Lehner, Administrator

HAMILTON COUNTY HOSPITAL, East Avenue G & Huser Street, Syracuse, KS, Zip 67878–0948, Mailing Address: P.O. Box 948, Zip 67878–0948; tel. 620/384–7461; Jeremy Clingenpeel, Administrator and Chief Executive Officer

HODGEMAN COUNTY HEALTH CENTER, 809 Bramley Street, Jetmore, KS, Zip 67854–9320, Mailing Address: P.O. Box 310, Zip 67854–0310; tel. 620/357–8361; Teresa L. Deuel, Chief Executive Officer

KEARNY COUNTY HOSPITAL, 500 Thorpe Street, Lakin, KS, Zip 67860; tel. 620/355–7111; John Loebl, Chief Executive Officer

LANE COUNTY HOSPITAL, 235 West Vine, Dighton, KS, Zip 67839–0969, Mailing Address: P.O. Box 969, Zip 67839–0969; tel. 620/397–5321; Donna McGowan, Administrator

MEADE DISTRICT HOSPITAL, 510 East Carthage Street, Meade, KS, Zip 67864–0820, Mailing Address: P.O. Box 820, Zip 67864–0820; tel. 620/873–2141; Michael P. Thomas, Administrator

MORTON COUNTY HEALTH SYSTEM, 445 Hilltop Street, Elkhart, KS, Zip 67950–0937, Mailing Address: P.O. Box 937, Zip 67950–0937; tel. 620/697–2141; Leonard Hernandez, Chief Executive Officer

SATANTA DISTRICT HOSPITAL, 401 South Cheyenne Street, Satanta, KS, Zip 67870–0159, Mailing Address: P.O. Box 159, Zip 67870–0159; tel. 620/649–2761; Ron Baker, Administrator

SCOTT COUNTY HOSPITAL, 310 East Third Street, Scott City, KS, Zip 67871–1203; tel. 620/872–5811; Mark Burnett, President and Chief Executive Officer

SOUTHWEST MEDICAL CENTER, 315 West 15th Street, Liberal, KS, Zip 67901–1340, Mailing Address: Box 1340, Zip 67905–1340; tel. 620/624–1651; Bill Ermann, Interim Chief Executive Officer

ST. CATHERINE HOSPITAL, 401 East Spuce Street, Garden City, KS, Zip 67846–5679; tel. 620/272–2561; Scott J. Taylor, President and Chief Executive Officer

STANTON COUNTY HOSPITAL, 404 North Chestnut Street, Johnson, KS, Zip 67855–0779, Mailing Address: P.O. Box 779, Zip 67855–0779; tel. 620/492–6250; Jay Tusten, Chief Executive Officer

STEVENS COUNTY HOSPITAL, 1006 South Jackson Street, Hugoton, KS, Zip 67951–2842, Mailing Address: P.O. Box 10, Zip 67951–0010; tel. 620/544–8511; Linda Stalcup, Chief Executive Officer

WICHITA COUNTY HEALTH CENTER, 211 East Earl Street, Leoti, KS, Zip 67861–9620; tel. 620/375–2233; Victoria J. Hahn, Administrator and Chief Executive Officer

**SUNFLOWER HEALTH NETWORK**
**139 North Penn Avenue, Salina, KS 67401–3044; tel. 785/452–6102; Heather Fuller, Executive Director**

CLAY COUNTY MEDICAL CENTER, 617 Liberty Street, Clay Center, KS, Zip 67432–0512, Mailing Address: P.O. Box 512, Zip 67432–0512; tel. 785/632–2144; Ron Bender, Chief Executive Officer

CLOUD COUNTY HEALTH CENTER, 1100 Highland Drive, Concordia, KS, Zip 66901–3923; tel. 785/243–1234; James E. Wahlmeier, President and Chief Executive Officer

ELLSWORTH COUNTY MEDICAL CENTER, 1604 Aylward Street, Ellsworth, KS, Zip 67439–0087, Mailing Address: P.O. Box 87, Zip 67439–0087; tel. 785/472–3111; Roger A. Masse, FACHE, Chief Executive Officer

HERINGTON MUNICIPAL HOSPITAL, 100 East Helen Street, Herington, KS, Zip 67449–1606; tel. 785/258–2207; Michael J. Ryan, Chief Executive Officer

HILLSBORO COMMUNITY HOSPITAL, 701 South Main Street, Hillsboro, KS, Zip 67063–1595; tel. 620/947–3114; Marion Regier, Chief Executive Officer

JEWELL COUNTY HOSPITAL, 100 Crestvue Avenue, Mankato, KS, Zip 66956–2407, Mailing Address: P.O. Box 327, Zip 66956–0327; tel. 785/378–3137; Doyle L. McKimmy, FACHE, Chief Executive Officer

LINCOLN COUNTY HOSPITAL, 624 North Second Street, Lincoln, KS, Zip 67455–1738, Mailing Address: P.O. Box 406, Zip 67455–0406; tel. 785/524–4403; Greg R. McNeil, Chief Executive Officer

LINDSBORG COMMUNITY HOSPITAL, 605 West Lincoln Street, Lindsborg, KS, Zip 67456–2328; tel. 785/227–3308; Larry VanDerWege, Administrator and Chief Executive Officer

MCPHERSON HOSPITAL, 1000 Hospital Drive, McPherson, KS, Zip 67460–2321; tel. 620/241–2250; Robert Monical, President and Chief Executive Officer

MEMORIAL HEALTH SYSTEM, 511 N.E. Tenth Street, Abilene, KS, Zip 67410–2153; tel. 785/263–2100; Mark A. Miller, FACHE, Chief Executive Officer

MITCHELL COUNTY HOSPITAL HEALTH SYSTEMS, 400 West Eighth, Beloit, KS, Zip 67420–1605, Mailing Address: P.O. Box 399, Zip 67420–0399; tel. 785/738–2266; David Dick, Chief Executive Officer

OSBORNE COUNTY MEMORIAL HOSPITAL, 424 West New Hampshire Street, Osborne, KS, Zip 67473–0070, Mailing Address: P.O. Box 70, Zip 67473–0070; tel. 785/346–2121; Kiley Floyd, Administrator

OTTAWA COUNTY HEALTH CENTER, 215 East Eighth, Minneapolis, KS, Zip 67467–1999, Mailing Address: P.O. Box 290, Zip 67467–0290; tel. 785/392–2122; Joy Johnson, R.N., Interim Chief Executive Officer

REPUBLIC COUNTY HOSPITAL, 2420 G Street, Belleville, KS, Zip 66935–2400; tel. 785/527–2254; Blaine K. Miller, Administrator

SALINA REGIONAL HEALTH CENTER, 400 South Santa Fe Avenue, Salina, KS, Zip 67401–4198, Mailing Address: P.O. Box 5080, Zip 67402–5080; tel. 785/452–7000; Micheal Terry, President and Chief Executive Officer

SMITH COUNTY MEMORIAL HOSPITAL, 614 South Main Street, Smith Center, KS, Zip 66967–0349; tel. 785/282–6845; Carolyn K. Hess, R.N., Administrator

## KENTUCKY

**COMMONWEALTH HEALTH CORPORATION**
**800 Park Street, Bowling Green, KY 42101–2356; tel. 270/745–1500; Connie Smith, President and Chief Executive Officer**

COMMONWEALTH REGIONAL SPECIALTY HOSPITAL, 250 Park Drive, 6th Floor, Bowling Green, KY, Zip 42101, Mailing Address: P.O. Box 90010, Zip 42101; tel. 270/796–6200; Emily Howard Martin, Administrator

MEDICAL CENTER AT BOWLING GREEN, 250 Park Street, Bowling Green, KY, Zip 42101–1795, Mailing Address: P.O. Box 90010, Zip 42102–9010; tel. 270/745–1000; Connie Smith, Chief Executive Officer

MEDICAL CENTER AT FRANKLIN, 1100 Brookhaven Road, Franklin, KY, Zip 42134–2746; tel. 270/598–4800; Clara M. Sumner, Senior Vice President and Chief Executive Officer

MEDICAL CENTER AT SCOTTSVILLE, 456 Burnley Road, Scottsville, KY, Zip 42164–6355; tel. 270/622–2800; Eric Hagan, R.N., Vice President

**COMMUNITY CARE NETWORK**
**110 A. Second Street, Henderson, KY 42420; tel. 619/278–2273; Roberta Alexander, Director**

CALDWELL MEDICAL CENTER, 100 Medical Center Drive, Princeton, KY, Zip 42445–2430, Mailing Address: P.O. Box 410, Zip 42445–0410; tel. 270/365–0300; Charles D. Lovell, Jr., FACHE, President and Chief Executive Officer

CRITTENDEN COUNTY HOSPITAL, 520 West Gum Street, Marion, KY, Zip 42064–6201, Mailing Address: P.O. Box 386, Zip 42064–0386; tel. 270/965–5281; Jim Christensen, Chief Executive Officer

JENNIE STUART MEDICAL CENTER, 320 West 18th Street, Hopkinsville, KY, Zip 42241–2400, Mailing Address: P.O. Box 2400, Zip 42241–2400; tel. 270/887–0100; Eric A. Lee, President and Chief Executive Officer

LIVINGSTON HOSPITAL AND HEALTHCARE SERVICES, 131 Hospital Drive, Salem, KY, Zip 42078–8043; tel. 270/988–2299; Mark A. Edwards, Chief Executive Officer

MEDICAL CENTER AT FRANKLIN, 1100 Brookhaven Road, Franklin, KY, Zip 42134–2746; tel. 270/598–4800; Clara M. Sumner, Senior Vice President and Chief Executive Officer

METHODIST HOSPITAL, 1305 North Elm Street, Henderson, KY, Zip 42420–2775, Mailing Address: P.O. Box 48, Zip 42420–0048; tel. 270/827–7700; Bruce D. Begley, Executive Director

METHODIST HOSPITAL UNION COUNTY, 4604 Highway 60 West, Morganfield, KY, Zip 42437–9570; tel. 270/389–5000; Patrick Donahue, Administrator

MURRAY–CALLOWAY COUNTY HOSPITAL, 803 Poplar Street, Murray, KY, Zip 42071–2432; tel. 270/762–1100; Colonel Jerome Penner, Chief Executive Officer

REGIONAL MEDICAL CENTER OF HOPKINS COUNTY, 900 Hospital Drive, Madisonville, KY, Zip 42431–1694; tel. 270/825–5100; E. Berton Whitaker, FACHE, Chief Executive Officer

STS. MARY & ELIZABETH HOSPITAL, 1850 Bluegrass Avenue, Louisville, KY, Zip 40215–1199; tel. 502/361–6000; James Parobek, President

**ST. ELIZABETH EDGEWOOD**
**1 Medical Village Drive, Edgewood, KY 41017–3403; tel. 859/301–2000; John S. Dubis, FACHE, President and Chief Executive Officer**

ST. ELIZABETH GRANT, 238 Barnes Road, Williamstown, KY, Zip 41097–9460; tel. 859/824–8240; Paula Roe, Assistant Vice President Operations

## MAINE

**BLUE HILL MEMORIAL HOSPITAL**
**57 Water Street, Blue Hill, ME 04614–0823; tel. 207/374–3400; Gregory E. Roraff, President and Chief Executive Officer**

BLUE HILL MEMORIAL HOSPITAL, 57 Water Street, Blue Hill, ME, Zip 04614–0823, Mailing Address: P.O. Box 1029, Zip 04614–1029; tel. 207/374–3400; Gregory E. Roraff, President and Chief Executive Officer

**MAINE NETWORK FOR HEALTH**
Key Plaza, 23 Water Street, Bangor, ME 04401; tel. 207/942–2844;
Stephen A. Ryan, President and Chief Executive Officer

BLUE HILL MEMORIAL HOSPITAL, 57 Water Street, Blue Hill, ME,
Zip 04614–0823, Mailing Address: P.O. Box 1029, Zip 04614–1029;
tel. 207/374–3400; Gregory E. Roraff, President and Chief Executive Officer

CHARLES A. DEAN MEMORIAL HOSPITAL, 364 Pritham Avenue, Greenville, ME,
Zip 04441–1395, Mailing Address: P.O. Box 1129, Zip 04441–1129;
tel. 207/695–5200; Geno Murray, President and Chief Executive Officer

EASTERN MAINE MEDICAL CENTER, 489 State Street, Bangor, ME,
Zip 04401–6674, Mailing Address: P.O. Box 404, Zip 04402–0404;
tel. 207/973–7000; Deborah Carey Johnson, R.N., President and Chief
Executive Officer

HOULTON REGIONAL HOSPITAL, 20 Hartford Street, Houlton, ME,
Zip 04730–9998; tel. 207/532–9471; Thomas J. Moakler, Chief Executive
Officer

INLAND HOSPITAL, 200 Kennedy Memorial Drive, Waterville, ME,
Zip 04901–4595; tel. 207/861–3000; John Dalton, President and Chief
Executive Officer

MILLINOCKET REGIONAL HOSPITAL, 200 Somerset Street, Millinocket, ME,
Zip 04462–1298; tel. 207/723–5161; Marie E. Vienneau, R.N., Chief
Executive Officer

MOUNT DESERT ISLAND HOSPITAL, 10 Wayman Lane, Bar Harbor, ME,
Zip 04609–0008, Mailing Address: P.O. Box 8, Zip 04609–0008;
tel. 207/288–5081; Arthur J. Blank, President and Chief Executive Officer

NORTHERN MAINE MEDICAL CENTER, 194 East Main Street, Fort Kent, ME,
Zip 04743–1497; tel. 207/834–3155; Peter Sirois, Interim Chief Executive
Officer

SEBASTICOOK VALLEY HEALTH, 447 North Main Street, Pittsfield, ME,
Zip 04967–1199; tel. 207/487–4000; Victoria Alexander–Lane, President
and Chief Executive Officer

THE ACADIA HOSPITAL, 268 Stillwater Avenue, Bangor, ME, Zip 04401–3945,
Mailing Address: P.O. Box 422, Zip 04402–0422; tel. 207/973–6100;
Daniel B. Coffey, President and Chief Executive Officer

THE AROOSTOOK MEDICAL CENTER, 140 Academy Street, Presque Isle, ME,
Zip 04769–3171, Mailing Address: P.O. Box 151, Zip 04769–0151;
tel. 207/768–4000; Sylvia Getman, President and Chief Executive Officer

## MASSACHUSETTS

**LAHEY CLINIC MEDICAL CENTER**
41 Mall Road, Burlington, MA 01803–4136; tel. 781/744–5796; David
M. Barrett, M.D.

LAHEY CLINIC HOSPITAL, 41 Mall Road, Burlington, MA, Zip 01805–0001;
tel. 781/744–5100; Howard R. Grant, JD, M.D., President and Chief
Executive Officer

**NORTHEAST HEALTH SYSTEM**
85 Herrick Street, Beverly, MA 01915–1790; tel. 978/922–3000;
Kenneth Hanover, President and Chief Executive Officer

BEVERLY HOSPITAL, 85 Herrick Street, Beverly, MA, Zip 01915–1777;
tel. 978/922–3000; Kenneth Hanover, President and Chief Executive Officer

## MICHIGAN

**GENESYS HEALTH SYSTEM**
1 Genesys Parkway, Grand Blanc, MI 48439–8065; tel. 810/606–5000;
Christine Gleason, Director of Marketing

GENESYS REGIONAL MEDICAL CENTER, One Genesys Parkway, Grand Blanc, MI,
Zip 48439–8066; tel. 810/606–5000; Elizabeth Aderholdt, President

**HOSPITAL NETWORK VENTURES, LLC**
6212 American Avenue, Portage, MI 49002; tel. 269/329–3200;
Gregory L. Hedegore, President and Chief Executive Officer

ALLEGAN GENERAL HOSPITAL, 555 Linn Street, Allegan, MI, Zip 49010–1524;
tel. 269/673–8424; Gerald J. Barbini, President and Chief Executive Officer

BRONSON METHODIST HOSPITAL, 601 John Street, Kalamazoo, MI,
Zip 49007–5346; tel. 269/341–6000; Frank J. Sardone, President and
Chief Executive Officer

OAKLAWN HOSPITAL, 200 North Madison Street, Marshall, MI, Zip 49068–1199;
tel. 269/781–4271; Rob Covert, President and Chief Executive Officer

PENNOCK HOSPITAL, 1009 West Green Street, Hastings, MI, Zip 49058–1790;
tel. 269/945–3451; Sheryl Lewis Blake, FACHE, Chief Executive Officer

STURGIS HOSPITAL, 916 Myrtle Street, Sturgis, MI, Zip 49091–2326;
tel. 269/651–7824; Robert J. LaBarge, Chief Executive Officer

**LAKELAND REGIONAL HEALTH SYSTEM**
1234 Napier Avenue, Saint Joseph, MI 49085–2112;
tel. 269/983–8300; Loren Hamel, M.D., President and Chief Executive
Officer

LAKELAND REGIONAL MEDICAL CENTER–ST. JOSEPH, 1234 Napier Avenue, Saint
Joseph, MI, Zip 49085–2112; tel. 269/983–8300; Loren Hamel, M.D.,
President and Chief Executive Officer

**ST. JOHN PROVIDENCE HEALTH SYSTEM**
28000 Dequindre Drive, Warren, MI 48092; tel. 586/753–1259;
Patricia A. Maryland, Dr.PH, President and Chief Executive Officer; Jean
Meyer, Executive Vice President, President Acute Care Operations

BRIGHTON CENTER FOR RECOVERY, 12851 Grand River Road, Brighton, MI,
Zip 48116–8506; tel. 810/227–1211; Ken Van Elsander, Director

PROVIDENCE HOSPITAL, 16001 West Nine Mile Road, Southfield, MI,
Zip 48075–4818, Mailing Address: P.O. Box 2043, Zip 48037–2043;
tel. 248/424–3000; Michael Wiemann, M.D., President

ST. JOHN HOSPITAL AND MEDICAL CENTER, 22101 Moross Road, Detroit, MI,
Zip 48236–2172; tel. 313/343–4000; Frank W. Poma, Interim President

ST. JOHN MACOMB–OAKLAND HOSPITAL, MACOMB CENTER, 11800 East Twelve
Mile Road, Warren, MI, Zip 48093–3494; tel. 586/573–5000; Terry
Hamilton, President

ST. JOHN MACOMB–OAKLAND HOSPITAL, OAKLAND CENTER, 27351 Dequindre,
Madison Heights, MI, Zip 48071–3499; tel. 248/967–7000; Diane M.
Radloff, President and Chief Executive Officer

ST. JOHN RIVER DISTRICT HOSPITAL, 4100 River Road, East China, MI,
Zip 48054–2909; tel. 810/329–7111; Frank W. Poma, President

**UPPER PENINSULA HEALTH CARE NETWORK (UPHCN)**
228 West Washington Street, Marquette, MI 49855–4330;
tel. 906/225–3146; Dennis Smith, Chief Executive Officer

ASPIRUS GRAND VIEW HOSPITAL, N10561 Grand View Lane, Ironwood, MI,
Zip 49938–9622; tel. 906/932–2525; Carol Goffnett, Chief Executive
Officer

ASPIRUS KEWEENAW HOSPITAL, 205 Osceola Street, Laurium, MI,
Zip 49913–2134; tel. 906/337–6500; Charles Nelson, Chief Executive
Officer

ASPIRUS ONTONAGON HOSPITAL, 601 South Seventh Street, Ontonagon, MI,
Zip 49953–1448; tel. 906/884–8000; Michael Hauswirth, Chief Operating
Officer

BARAGA COUNTY MEMORIAL HOSPITAL, 18341 U.S. Highway 41, L'Anse, MI,
Zip 49946–8024; tel. 906/524–3300; Tim E. Zwickey, Chief Executive
Officer

BELL HOSPITAL, 901 Lakeshore Drive, Ishpeming, MI, Zip 49849–1367;
tel. 906/486–4431; Barbara Larson, Interim Chief Executive Officer

DICKINSON COUNTY HEALTHCARE SYSTEM, 1721 South Stephenson Avenue,
Iron Mountain, MI, Zip 49801–3637; tel. 906/774–1313; John Schon,
Administrator and Chief Executive Officer

HELEN NEWBERRY JOY HOSPITAL, 502 West Harrie Street, Newberry, MI,
Zip 49868–1209; tel. 906/293–9200; Scott Pillion, Chief Executive Officer

MACKINAC STRAITS HEALTH SYSTEM, 1140 North State Street, Saint Ignace, MI,
Zip 49781–1013; tel. 906/643–8585; Rodney M. Nelson, Chief Executive
Officer

MARQUETTE GENERAL HEALTH SYSTEM, 580 West College Avenue, Marquette,
MI, Zip 49855–2705; tel. 906/228–9440; A. Gary Muller, FACHE, President
and Chief Executive Officer

MUNISING MEMORIAL HOSPITAL, 1500 Sand Point Road, Munising, MI,
Zip 49862–1406; tel. 906/387–4110; Kevin P. Calhoun, Chief Executive
Officer

OSF ST. FRANCIS HOSPITAL, 3401 Ludington Street, Escanaba, MI,
Zip 49829–1377; tel. 906/786–3311; Peter G. Jennings, President and
Chief Executive Officer

PORTAGE HEALTH, 500 Campus Drive, Hancock, MI, Zip 49930–1569;
tel. 906/483–1000; James Bogan, FACHE, President and Chief Executive
Officer

SCHOOLCRAFT MEMORIAL HOSPITAL, 500 Main Street, Manistique, MI,
Zip 49854–1522; tel. 906/341–3200; George H. Montgomery, Chief
Executive Officer

WAR MEMORIAL HOSPITAL, 500 Osborn Boulevard, Sault Sainte Marie, MI,
Zip 49783–1822; tel. 906/635–4460; David B. Jahn, President and Chief
Executive Officer

## MISSOURI

**MERCY HEALTH EAST**
615 South New Ballas Road, Saint Louis, MO 63141–8221;
tel. 314/364–3000; Donn Sorensen, President, East Region

MERCY HOSPITAL ST. LOUIS, 615 South New Ballas Road, Saint Louis, MO,
Zip 63141–8277; tel. 314/569–6000; Jeffrey A. Johnston, President

MERCY HOSPITAL WASHINGTON, 901 East Fifth Street, Washington, MO,
Zip 63090–3127; tel. 636/239–8000; Terri L. McLain, FACHE, President

## MONTANA

**MONTANA HEALTH NETWORK**
11 South 7th Street, Suite 241, Miles City, MT 59301;
tel. 406/234–1420; Janet Bastian, Chief Executive Officer

BEARTOOTH BILLINGS CLINIC, 2525 North Broadway, Red Lodge, MT,
Zip 59068, Mailing Address: P.O. Box 590, Zip 59068–0590;
tel. 406/446–2345; Kelley Evans, Chief Executive Officer

Section B

BILLINGS CLINIC, 2800 10th Avenue North, Billings, MT, Zip 59101, Mailing Address: P.O. Box 37000, Zip 59107-7000; tel. 406/657-4000; Nicholas Wolter, M.D., President and Chief Executive Officer

CENTRAL MONTANA MEDICAL CENTER, 408 Wendell Avenue, Lewistown, MT, Zip 59457-2261; tel. 406/535-7711; Lee Rhodes, Chief Executive Officer; David M. Faulkner, Co-Acting Chief Executive Officer

DANIELS MEMORIAL HEALTHCARE CENTER, 105 Fifth Avenue East, Scobey, MT, Zip 59263, Mailing Address: P.O. Box 400, Zip 59263-0400; tel. 406/487-2296; David Hubbard, Chief Executive Officer

FALLON MEDICAL COMPLEX, 202 South 4th Street West, Baker, MT, Zip 59313-0820, Mailing Address: P.O. Box 820, Zip 59313-0820; tel. 406/778-3331; David Espeland, Chief Executive Officer

FRANCES MAHON DEACONESS HOSPITAL, 621 Third Street South, Glasgow, MT, Zip 59230-2699; tel. 406/228-3500; Randall G. Holom, Chief Executive Officer

GLENDIVE MEDICAL CENTER, 202 Prospect Drive, Glendive, MT, Zip 59330-1999; tel. 406/345-3306; Scott A. Duke, Chief Executive Officer

HOLY ROSARY HEALTHCARE, 2600 Wilson Street, Miles City, MT, Zip 59301-5094; tel. 406/233-2600; Paul Lewis, Chief Executive Officer

MCCONE COUNTY HEALTH CENTER, 605 Sullivan Avenue, Circle, MT, Zip 59215, Mailing Address: P.O. Box 48, Zip 59215-0048; tel. 406/485-3381; Nancy Rosaaen, Chief Executive Officer

PHILLIPS COUNTY HOSPITAL, 417 South Fourth East, Malta, MT, Zip 59538, Mailing Address: P.O. Box 640, Zip 59538-0640; tel. 406/654-1100; Ward C. VanWichen, Chief Executive Officer

ROOSEVELT MEDICAL CENTER, 818 Second Avenue East, Culbertson, MT, Zip 59218, Mailing Address: P.O. Box 419, Zip 59218-0419; tel. 406/787-6401; Audrey Stromberg, Administrator

ROUNDUP MEMORIAL HEALTHCARE, 1202 Third Street West, Roundup, MT, Zip 59072-1816, Mailing Address: P.O. Box 40, Zip 59072-0040; tel. 406/323-2301; Bradley Howell, Chief Executive Officer

SHERIDAN MEMORIAL HOSPITAL, 440 West Laurel Avenue, Plentywood, MT, Zip 59254-1596; tel. 406/765-1420; Sandra Christensen, Chief Executive Officer

SIDNEY HEALTH CENTER, 216 14th Avenue S.W., Sidney, MT, Zip 59270-3586; tel. 406/488-2100; Richard Haraldson, Chief Executive Officer

STILLWATER COMMUNITY HOSPITAL, 44 West Fourth Avenue North, Columbus, MT, Zip 59019-0959, Mailing Address: P.O. Box 959, Zip 59019-0959; tel. 406/322-5316; Tim Russell, Administrator

## NEBRASKA

### ALEGENT HEALTH
**12809 West Dodge Road, Omaha, NE 68154; tel. 402/343-4000; Richard A. Hachten II, FACHE, President and Chief Executive Officer**

ALEGENT HEALTH MERCY HOSPITAL, 603 Rosary Drive, Corning, IA, Zip 50841-1685; tel. 641/322-3121; Debra Goldsmith, Chief Executive Officer

ALEGENT HEALTH-BERGAN MERCY MEDICAL CENTER, 7500 Mercy Road, Omaha, NE, Zip 68124-2319; tel. 402/398-6060; Marie E. Knedler, R.N., Vice President and Chief Operating Officer

ALEGENT HEALTH-COMMUNITY MEMORIAL HOSPITAL, 631 North Eighth Street, Missouri Valley, IA, Zip 51555-1199; tel. 712/642-2784; Robert A. Valentine, Regional Administrator

ALEGENT HEALTH-IMMANUEL MEDICAL CENTER, 6901 North 72nd Street, Omaha, NE, Zip 68122-1799; tel. 402/572-2121; Ann Schumacher, MSN, R.N., Vice President and Chief Operating Officer

ALEGENT HEALTH-MEMORIAL HOSPITAL, 104 West 17th Street, Schuyler, NE, Zip 68661-1396; tel. 402/352-2441; Connie Peters, R.N., Operations Leader and Regional Health Administrator

ALEGENT HEALTH-MERCY HOSPITAL, 800 Mercy Drive, Council Bluffs, IA, Zip 51503-3128, Mailing Address: P.O. Box 1C, Zip 51502-3001; tel. 712/328-5000; Marie E. Knedler, R.N., Vice President and Chief Operating Officer

ALEGENT HEALTH-MIDLANDS HOSPITAL, 11111 South 84th Street, Papillion, NE, Zip 68046-4122; tel. 402/593-3000; Kevin J. Nokels, FACHE, Vice President and Chief Operating Officer

### BLUE RIVER VALLEY HEALTH NETWORK
**2222 North Lincoln Avenue, York, NE 68467-1030; tel. 402/362-0445; Charles K. Schulz, President**

ANNIE JEFFREY MEMORIAL COUNTY HEALTH CENTER, 531 Beebe Street, Osceola, NE, Zip 68651, Mailing Address: P.O. Box 428, Zip 68651-0428; tel. 402/747-2031; Joseph W. Lohrman, Chief Executive Officer

BOONE COUNTY HEALTH CENTER, 723 West Fairview Street, Albion, NE, Zip 68620-1725, Mailing Address: P.O. Box 151, Zip 68620-0151; tel. 402/395-2191; Victor N. Lee, FACHE, President and Chief Executive Officer

BRODSTONE MEMORIAL HOSPITAL, 520 East Tenth Street, Superior, NE, Zip 68978-1225, Mailing Address: P.O. Box 187, Zip 68978-0187; tel. 402/879-3281; John E. Keelan, Administrator and Chief Executive Officer

BUTLER COUNTY HEALTH CARE CENTER, 372 South Ninth Street, David City, NE, Zip 68632-2116; tel. 402/367-1200; Donald T. Naiberk, Administrator

COMMUNITY MEMORIAL HOSPITAL, 1579 Midland Street, Syracuse, NE, Zip 68446-9732, Mailing Address: P.O. Box N, Zip 68446-0518; tel. 402/269-2011; Michael Harvey, Chief Executive Officer

CRETE AREA MEDICAL CENTER, 2910 Betten Drive, Crete, NE, Zip 68333-0220, Mailing Address: P.O. Box 220, Zip 68333-0220; tel. 402/826-2102; Carol Friesen, Chief Executive Officer

FILLMORE COUNTY HOSPITAL, 1900 F Street, Geneva, NE, Zip 68361-1325, Mailing Address: P.O. Box 193, Zip 68361-0193; tel. 402/759-3167; Paul Utemark, Chief Executive Officer

HENDERSON HEALTH CARE SERVICES, 1621 Front Street, Henderson, NE, Zip 68371; tel. 402/723-4512; Cheryl Brown, Administrator

HOWARD COUNTY MEDICAL CENTER, 1113 Sherman Street, Saint Paul, NE, Zip 68873-1536, Mailing Address: P.O. Box 406, Zip 68873-0406; tel. 308/754-4421; Arlan D. Johnson, Chief Executive Officer

JEFFERSON COMMUNITY HEALTH CENTER, 2200 H Street, Fairbury, NE, Zip 68352-1119, Mailing Address: P.O. Box 277, Zip 68352-0277; tel. 402/729-3351; William L. Welch, FACHE, Chief Executive Officer

JOHNSON COUNTY HOSPITAL, 202 High Street, Tecumseh, NE, Zip 68450-0599, Mailing Address: P.O. Box 599, Zip 68450-0599; tel. 402/335-3361; Diane Newman, Administrator

LITZENBERG MEMORIAL COUNTY HOSPITAL, 1715 26th Street, Central City, NE, Zip 68826-9620; tel. 308/946-3015; Tad M. Hunt, MS, Chief Executive Officer

MEMORIAL COMMUNITY HEALTH, 1423 Seventh Street, Aurora, NE, Zip 68818-1197; tel. 402/694-3171; Diane R. Keller, Chief Executive Officer

MEMORIAL HEALTH CARE SYSTEMS, 300 North Columbia Avenue, Seward, NE, Zip 68434-9907; tel. 402/643-2971; Roger J. Reamer, Chief Executive Officer

THAYER COUNTY HEALTH SERVICES, 120 Park Avenue, Hebron, NE, Zip 68370-2019, Mailing Address: P.O. Box 49, Zip 68370-0049; tel. 402/768-6041; Joyce Beck, Administrator

VALLEY COUNTY HEALTH SYSTEM, 2707 L. Street, Ord, NE, Zip 68862-1675; tel. 308/728-4200; Ashley Woodward, Interim Chief Executive Officer

WARREN MEMORIAL HOSPITAL, 905 Second Street, Friend, NE, Zip 68359-1133; tel. 402/947-2541; John W. Wilson, Chief Executive Officer

YORK GENERAL HOSPITAL, 2222 North Lincoln Avenue, York, NE, Zip 68467-1095; tel. 402/362-6671; Charles K. Schulz, Chief Executive Officer

### CENTRAL NEBRASKA PRIMARY
**1518 J. Street, Ord, NE 68862-1439; tel. 308/728-3011; Victoria Bauer, Executive Director**

VALLEY COUNTY HEALTH SYSTEM, 2707 L. Street, Ord, NE, Zip 68862-1675; tel. 308/728-4200; Ashley Woodward, Interim Chief Executive Officer

### NORTHEAST HEALTH SERVICES
**PO Box 186, Creighton, NE 68729-0186; tel. 402/358-5700; Jeff Lingerfelt, Chief Executive Officer**

ALEGENT HEALTH PLAINVIEW HOSPITAL, 704 North Third Street, Plainview, NE, Zip 68769, Mailing Address: P.O. Box 489, Zip 68769-0489; tel. 402/582-4245; Richard B. Gamel, Administrator

AVERA CREIGHTON HOSPITAL, 1503 Main Street, Creighton, NE, Zip 68729-0186, Mailing Address: P.O. Box 186, Zip 68729-0186; tel. 402/358-5700; Mark Schulte, Chief Executive Officer

OSMOND GENERAL HOSPITAL, 402 North Maple Street, Osmond, NE, Zip 68765-0429, Mailing Address: P.O. Box 429, Zip 68765-0429; tel. 402/748-3393; Celine M. Mlady, Chief Executive Officer

### REGIONAL CARE, INC.
**905 West 27th Street, Scottsbluff, NE 69361-1545; tel. 308/635-2260; Steve Hetzel, President**

BOX BUTTE GENERAL HOSPITAL, 2101 Box Butte Avenue, Alliance, NE, Zip 69301-0810, Mailing Address: P.O. Box 810, Zip 69301-0810; tel. 308/762-6660; Dan Griess, Chief Executive Officer

CHADRON COMMUNITY HOSPITAL AND HEALTH SERVICES, 825 Centennial Drive, Chadron, NE, Zip 69337-9400; tel. 308/432-5586; Harold L. Krueger, Jr., Chief Executive Officer

GARDEN COUNTY HEALTH SERVICES, 1100 West Second Street, Oshkosh, NE, Zip 69154; tel. 308/772-3283; Jimmie W. Hansel, Chief Executive Officer

GORDON MEMORIAL HOSPITAL, 300 East Eighth Street, Gordon, NE, Zip 69343-1123; tel. 308/282-0401; James LeBrun, Chief Executive Officer

KIMBALL HEALTH SERVICES, 505 South Burg Street, Kimball, NE, Zip 69145-1398; tel. 308/235-1952; Ken Hunter, R.N., Chief Executive Officer

MORRILL COUNTY COMMUNITY HOSPITAL, 1313 S Street, Bridgeport, NE, Zip 69336-0579, Mailing Address: P.O. Box 579, Zip 69336-0579; tel. 308/262-1616; Robin Stuart, Interim Administrator

REGIONAL WEST MEDICAL CENTER, 4021 Avenue B, Scottsbluff, NE, Zip 69361-4695; tel. 308/635-3711; Todd Sorensen, M.D., Chief Executive Officer

## NEW HAMPSHIRE

**CARING COMMUNITY NETWORK OF THE TWIN RIVERS**
**c/o First Health, 841 Central Street, Franklin, NH 03235-2026;**
**tel. 603/934-0177; Rick Silverberg, Managing Director**

FRANKLIN REGIONAL HOSPITAL, 15 Aiken Avenue, Franklin, NH, Zip 03235-1299;
tel. 603/934-2060; Thomas Clairmont, President

## NEW JERSEY

**ATLANTICARE**
**2500 English Creek Avenue, Building 500, Suite 501, Egg Harbor**
**Township, NJ 08234; tel. 609/407-2309; David P. Tilton, President and**
**Chief Executive Officer**

ATLANTICARE REGIONAL MEDICAL CENTER, 1925 Pacific Avenue, Atlantic City,
NJ, Zip 08401-6713; tel. 609/441-8994; Lori Herndon, President and Chief
Executive Officer

**QUALCARE, INC.**
**242 Old New Brunswick Road, Piscataway, NJ 08854-3754;**
**tel. 732/562-2800; Jerry Eisenberg, Network Contact**

CAPITAL HEALTH MEDICAL CENTER–HOPEWELL, 1 Capital Way, Pennington, NJ,
Zip 8534; tel. 609/303-4000; Al Maghazehe, Ph.D., FACHE, Chief Executive
Officer

CHILTON HOSPITAL, 97 West Parkway, Pompton Plains, NJ, Zip 07444-1696;
tel. 973/831-5000; Deborah Zastocki, R.N., FACHE, President and Chief
Executive Officer

CHRIST HOSPITAL, 176 Palisade Avenue, Jersey City, NJ, Zip 07306-1196,
Mailing Address: P.O. Box J-1, Zip 07306-1196; tel. 201/795-8200; Peter
A. Kelly, President and Chief Executive Officer

CLARA MAASS MEDICAL CENTER, One Clara Maass Drive, Belleville, NJ,
Zip 07109-3557; tel. 973/450-2000; Mary Ellen Clyne, Ph.D., President
and Chief Executive Officer

DEBORAH HEART AND LUNG CENTER, 200 Trenton Road, Browns Mills, NJ,
Zip 08015-1799; tel. 609/893-6611; Joseph P. Chirichella, President and
Chief Executive Officer

ENGLEWOOD HOSPITAL AND MEDICAL CENTER, 350 Engle Street, Englewood,
NJ, Zip 07631-1898; tel. 201/894-3000; Douglas A. Duchak, President
and Chief Executive Officer

HACKETTSTOWN REGIONAL MEDICAL CENTER, 651 Willow Grove Street,
Hackettstown, NJ, Zip 07840-1792; tel. 908/852-5100; Jason C. Coe,
President and Chief Executive Officer

JFK MEDICAL CENTER, 65 James Street, Edison, NJ, Zip 08818-3059;
tel. 732/321-7000; Raymond F. Fredericks, President and CEO

MEMORIAL HOSPITAL OF SALEM COUNTY, 310 Woodstown Road, Salem, NJ,
Zip 08079-2080; tel. 856/935-1000; Richard Grogan, Chief Executive
Officer

OCEAN MEDICAL CENTER, 425 Jack Martin Boulevard, Brick Township, NJ,
Zip 8724; tel. 732/840-2200; Dean Q. Lin, FACHE, President

PIEDMONT MOUNTAINSIDE HOSPITAL, 1266 Highway 515 South, Jasper, GA,
Zip 30143; tel. 706/692-2441; Mike Robertson, President and Chief
Executive Officer

RARITAN BAY MEDICAL CENTER, 530 New Brunswick Avenue, Perth Amboy, NJ,
Zip 8861; tel. 732/442-3700; Michael R. D'Agnes, President and Chief
Executive Officer

RIVERVIEW MEDICAL CENTER, 1 Riverview Plaza, Red Bank, NJ, Zip 07701-9982;
tel. 732/741-2700; Timothy J. Hogan, FACHE, President

ROBERT WOOD JOHNSON UNIVERSITY HOSPITAL, 1 Robert Wood Johnson Place,
New Brunswick, NJ, Zip 08903-2601; tel. 732/828-3000; Stephen K.
Jones, President and Chief Executive Officer

SAINT MICHAEL'S MEDICAL CENTER, 111 Central Avenue, Newark, NJ,
Zip 07102-2094; tel. 973/877-5549; David A. Ricci, President and Chief
Executive Officer

SOUTH JERSEY HEALTHCARE – REGIONAL MEDICAL CENTER, 1505 West
Sherman Avenue, Vineland, NJ, Zip 8360; tel. 856/641-8000; Chester B.
Kaletkowski, President and Chief Executive Officer

ST. MARY'S HOSPITAL, 350 Boulevard, Passaic, NJ, Zip 7055;
tel. 973/365-4300; Michael J. Sniffen, FACHE, President and Chief
Executive Officer

UNIVERSITY MEDICAL CENTER OF PRINCETON AT PLAINSBORO, One Plainsboro
Road, Plainsboro, NJ, Zip 8536; tel. 609/853-7100; Mark T. Jones,
President

UNIVERSITY OF MEDICINE AND DENTISTRY OF NEW JERSEY–UNIVERSITY
HOSPITAL, 150 Bergen Street, Newark, NJ, Zip 07103-2496;
tel. 973/972-4300; James R. Gonzalez, Acting President and Chief
Executive Officer

VIRTUA BERLIN, 100 Townsend Avenue, Berlin, NJ, Zip 08009-9035;
tel. 856/322-3000; Gary L. Long, Chief Operating Officer

VIRTUA MARLTON, 90 Brick Road, Marlton, NJ, Zip 08053-9697;
tel. 856/355-6000; Gary L. Long, Chief Operating Officer

## NEW YORK

**ALLEGANY WESTERN STEUBEN RURAL HEALTH NETWORK, INC.**
**85 North Main Street, Suite 4, Wellsville, NY 14895-1254;**
**tel. 585/593-5223; Carrie Whitwood, Executive Director**

JONES MEMORIAL HOSPITAL, 191 North Main Street, Wellsville, NY,
Zip 14895-1197, Mailing Address: P.O. Box 72, Zip 14895-0072;
tel. 585/593-1100; Eva Benedict, President and Chief Executive Officer

ST. JAMES MERCY HEALTH SYSTEM, 411 Canisteo Street, Hornell, NY,
Zip 14843-2197; tel. 607/324-8000; Mary E. LaRowe, FACHE, President
and Chief Executive Officer

**ARNOT HEALTH**
**600 Roe Avenue, Elmira, NY 14905-1629; tel. 607/737-4100; Anthony**
**J. Cooper, FACHE, President**

ARNOT OGDEN MEDICAL CENTER, 600 Roe Avenue, Elmira, NY,
Zip 14905-1629; tel. 607/737-4100; H. Fred Farley, R.N., Ph.D., FACHE,
President and Chief Operating Officer

IRA DAVENPORT MEMORIAL HOSPITAL, 7571 State Route 54, Bath, NY,
Zip 14810-9590; tel. 607/776-8500; James B. Watson, Chief Executive
Officer

**BASSETT HEALTHCARE NETWORK**
**1 Atwell Road, Cooperstown, NY 13326-1301; tel. 607/547-3456;**
**William F. Streck, M.D., President and Chief Executive Officer**

AURELIA OSBORN FOX MEMORIAL HOSPITAL, 1 Norton Avenue, Oneonta, NY,
Zip 13820-2629; tel. 607/432-2000; John R. Remillard, President

BASSETT MEDICAL CENTER, One Atwell Road, Cooperstown, NY,
Zip 13326-1394; tel. 607/547-3100; William F. Streck, M.D., President
and Chief Executive Officer

COBLESKILL REGIONAL HOSPITAL, 178 Grandview Drive, Cobleskill, NY,
Zip 12043-5144; tel. 518/254-3456; Eric H. Stein, FACHE, President and
Chief Executive Officer

LITTLE FALLS HOSPITAL, 140 Burwell Street, Little Falls, NY, Zip 13365-1725;
tel. 315/823-1000; Michael L. Ogden, President and Chief Executive Officer

O'CONNOR HOSPITAL, 460 Andes Road, State Route 28, Delhi, NY, Zip 13753;
tel. 607/746-0300; Daniel M. Ayres, Chief Executive Officer

**LAKE ERIE REGIONAL HEALTH SYSTEM OF NEW YORK**
**529 Central Avenue, Dunkirk, NY 14048-2514; tel. 716/366-1111;**
**Jonathan I. Lawrence, President and Chief Executive Officer**

BROOKS MEMORIAL HOSPITAL, 529 Central Avenue, Dunkirk, NY,
Zip 14048-2599; tel. 716/366-1111; Jonathan I. Lawrence, President and
Chief Executive Officer

LAKE SHORE HEALTH CARE CENTER, 845 Route 5 and 20, Irving, NY,
Zip 14081-9716; tel. 716/951-7000; Louis J. Frascella, President and
Chief Executive Officer

**MOHAWK VALLEY NETWORK, INC.**
**1710 Burrstone Road, New Hartford, NY 13413-1002;**
**tel. 315/624-6001; Scott H. Perra, President and Chief Executive**
**Officer**

FAXTON–ST. LUKE'S HEALTHCARE, 1656 Champlin Avenue, Utica, NY,
Zip 13502-4830, Mailing Address: P.O. Box 479, Zip 13503-0479;
tel. 315/624-6000; Scott H. Perra, President and Chief Executive Officer

**MOUNT SINAI NYU HEALTH NETWORK**
**One Gustave L. Levy Place, New York, NY 10029; tel. 212/659-8888;**
**Kenneth Davis, M.D., President and Chief Executive Officer**

COMMUNITY HOSPITAL AT DOBBS FERRY, 128 Ashford Avenue, Dobbs Ferry, NY,
Zip 10522-1896; tel. 914/693-0700; Ronald Corti, President and Chief
Executive Officer

ELMHURST HOSPITAL CENTER, 79-01 Broadway, Elmhurst, NY,
Zip 11373-1329; tel. 718/334-4000; Chris D. Constantino, Executive
Director

ENGLEWOOD HOSPITAL AND MEDICAL CENTER, 350 Engle Street, Englewood,
NJ, Zip 07631-1898; tel. 201/894-3000; Douglas A. Duchak, President
and Chief Executive Officer

LIBERTYHEALTH–JERSEY CITY MEDICAL CENTER, 355 Grand Street, Jersey City,
NJ, Zip 7302; tel. 201/915-2000; Joseph F. Scott, FACHE, President and
Chief Executive Officer

LUTHERAN MEDICAL CENTER, 150 55th Street, Brooklyn, NY, Zip 11220-2559;
tel. 718/630-7000; Wendy Z. Goldstein, President and Chief Executive
Officer

MEADOWLANDS HOSPITAL MEDICAL CENTER, 55 Meadowlands Parkway,
Secaucus, NJ, Zip 07094-1580; tel. 201/392-3100; Lynn McVey, President
and Chief Executive Officer

MORRISTOWN MEDICAL CENTER, 100 Madison Avenue, Morristown, NJ,
Zip 07962-1956; tel. 973/971-5000; David J. Shulkin, M.D., President and
Chief Executive Officer

MOUNT SINAI HOSPITAL, One Gustave L. Levy Place, New York, NY,
Zip 10029-6574; tel. 212/241-6500; Wayne Keathley, M.P.H., President
and Chief Operating Officer

OVERLOOK MEDICAL CENTER, 99 Beauvoir Avenue, Summit, NJ,
Zip 07902-0220; tel. 908/522-2000; Alan R. Lieber, President

PHELPS MEMORIAL HOSPITAL CENTER, 701 North Broadway, Sleepy Hollow, NY,
Zip 10591-1020; tel. 914/366-3000; Keith F. Safian, President and Chief
Executive Officer

QUEENS HOSPITAL CENTER, 82-68 164th Street, Jamaica, NY,
Zip 11432-1104; tel. 718/883-3000; Julius Wool, Executive Director

Section B

ST. JOHN'S RIVERSIDE HOSPITAL, 967 North Broadway, Yonkers, NY, Zip 10701–1399; tel. 914/964–4444; James Foy, President and Chief Executive Officer

ST. JOSEPH'S REGIONAL MEDICAL CENTER, 703 Main Street, Paterson, NJ, Zip 07503–2691; tel. 973/754–2000; William A. McDonald, President and Chief Executive Officer

ST. LUKE'S CORNWALL HOSPITAL, 70 Dubois Street, Newburgh, NY, Zip 12550–4851; tel. 845/561–4400; Allan E. Atzrott, FACHE, President and Chief Executive Officer

THE MOUNT SINAI HOSPITAL OF QUEENS, 25–10 30th Avenue, Long Island City, NY, Zip 11102–2448; tel. 718/932–1000; Caryn A. Schwab, Executive Director

VASSAR BROTHERS MEDICAL CENTER, 45 Reade Place, Poughkeepsie, NY, Zip 12601–3947; tel. 845/454–8500; Janet L. Ready, President and Chief Operating Officer

VETERANS AFFAIRS MEDICAL CENTER, 130 West Kingsbridge Road, Bronx, NY, Zip 10468–3992; tel. 718/584–9000; Maryann Musumeci, Director

**NORTHEAST HEALTH**
**2212 Burdett Avenue, Troy, NY 12180–2475; tel. 518/274–3382; James K. Reed, M.D., President and Chief Executive Officer**

ALBANY MEMORIAL HOSPITAL, 600 Northern Boulevard, Albany, NY, Zip 12204–1083; tel. 518/471–3221; Steven P. Boyle, Executive Vice President

SAMARITAN HOSPITAL, 2215 Burdett Avenue, Troy, NY, Zip 12180–2475; tel. 518/271–3300; Norman E. Dascher, Jr., Chief Executive Officer

SUNNYVIEW REHABILITATION HOSPITAL, 1270 Belmont Avenue, Schenectady, NY, Zip 12308–2104; tel. 518/382–4500; Edward Eisenman, Chief Executive Officer

**NORTHERN NY RURAL HEALTH CARE ALLIANCE**
**800 Starbuck Avenue, Suite A–5, Watertown, NY 13601; tel. 315/755–2500; Patricia Bishop, Executive Director**

CARTHAGE AREA HOSPITAL, 1001 West Street, Carthage, NY, Zip 13619–9703; tel. 315/493–1000; Adel Amir, Interim Chief Executive Officer

RIVER HOSPITAL, 4 Fuller Street, Alexandria Bay, NY, Zip 13607–1316; tel. 315/482–2511; Ben Moore, III, President and Chief Executive Officer

SAMARITAN MEDICAL CENTER, 830 Washington Street, Watertown, NY, Zip 13601–4034; tel. 315/785–4000; Thomas H. Carman, President and Chief Executive Officer

**RURAL HEALTH NETWORK OF OSWEGO COUNTY**
**10 George Street, Oswego, NY 13126; tel. 315/342–0827; Danielle Wert, Coordinator**

OSWEGO HOSPITAL, 110 West Sixth Street, Oswego, NY, Zip 13126–9985; tel. 315/349–5511; Ann C. Gilpin, President and Chief Executive Officer

**STELLARIS HEALTH**
**1 North Greenwich Road, Armonk, NY 10504–2311; tel. 914/273–5454; Arthur Nizza, President and Chief Executive Officer**

LAWRENCE HOSPITAL CENTER, 55 Palmer Avenue, Bronxville, NY, Zip 10708–3403; tel. 914/787–1000; Edward M. Dinan, President and Chief Executive Officer

NORTHERN WESTCHESTER HOSPITAL, 400 East Main Street, Mount Kisco, NY, Zip 10549–3477; tel. 914/666–1200; Joel Seligman, President and Chief Executive Officer

PHELPS MEMORIAL HOSPITAL CENTER, 701 North Broadway, Sleepy Hollow, NY, Zip 10591–1020; tel. 914/366–3000; Keith F. Safian, President and Chief Executive Officer

WHITE PLAINS HOSPITAL CENTER, 41 East Post Road, White Plains, NY, Zip 10601–4699; tel. 914/681–0600; Jon B. Schandler, President and Chief Executive Officer

# NORTH CAROLINA

**COASTAL CAROLINAS HEALTH ALLIANCE**
**5305–D Wrightsville Avenue, Wilmington, NC 28403; tel. 910/332–8012; Yvonne Hughes, Executive Director**

CAPE FEAR VALLEY – BLADEN COUNTY HOSPITAL, 501 South Poplar Street, Elizabethtown, NC, Zip 28337–0398, Mailing Address: P.O. Box 398, Zip 28337–0398; tel. 910/862–5100; Cameron Highsmith, Chief Executive Officer

COLUMBUS REGIONAL HEALTHCARE SYSTEM, 500 Jefferson Street, Whiteville, NC, Zip 28472–9987; tel. 910/642–8011; Henry Hawthorne, III, President and Chief Executive Officer

J. ARTHUR DOSHER MEMORIAL HOSPITAL, 924 North Howe Street, Southport, NC, Zip 28461–3099; tel. 910/457–3800; Edgar Haywood, III, Chief Executive Officer

MCLEOD LORIS HEALTHCARE, 3655 Mitchell Street, Box 690001, Loris, SC, Zip 29569–9601; tel. 843/716–7000; Edward D. Tinsley, III, Chief Executive Officer

MCLEOD REGIONAL MEDICAL CENTER, 555 East Cheves Street, Florence, SC, Zip 29502–2617, Mailing Address: P.O. Box 100551, Zip 29502–0551; tel. 843/777–2000; Robert L. Colones, President and Chief Executive Officer

NEW HANOVER REGIONAL MEDICAL CENTER, 2131 South 17th Street, Wilmington, NC, Zip 28401–7483, Mailing Address: P.O. Box 1990, Zip 28402–9000; tel. 910/343–7000; John K. Barto, Jr., President and Chief Executive Officer

PENDER MEMORIAL HOSPITAL, 507 East Freemont Street, Burgaw, NC, Zip 28425–5131; tel. 910/259–5451; Ruth Glaser, President

SAMPSON REGIONAL MEDICAL CENTER, 607 Beaman Street, Clinton, NC, Zip 28328–2697, Mailing Address: P.O. Box 260, Zip 28329–0260; tel. 910/592–8511; David J. Masterson, Chief Executive Officer

SCOTLAND HEALTH CARE SYSTEM, 500 Lauchwood Drive, Laurinburg, NC, Zip 28352–5599; tel. 910/291–7000; Gregory C. Wood, Chief Executive Officer

SOUTHEASTERN REGIONAL MEDICAL CENTER, 300 West 27th Street, Lumberton, NC, Zip 28358–3017, Mailing Address: P.O. Box 1408, Zip 28359–1408; tel. 910/671–5000; Joann Anderson, President and Chief Executive Officer

VIDANT DUPLIN HOSPITAL, 401 North Main Street, Kenansville, NC, Zip 28349–9989, Mailing Address: P.O. Box 278, Zip 28349–0278; tel. 910/296–0941; Jay Briley, Chief Executive Officer

VIDANT MEDICAL CENTER, 2100 Stantonsburg Road, Greenville, NC, Zip 27834, Mailing Address: P.O. Box 6028, Zip 27835–6028; tel. 252/847–4100; Steven Lawler, President

**MISSION HEALTH SYSTEM**
**509 Biltmore Avenue, Asheville, NC 28801; tel. 828/213–1111; Ronald A. Paulus, M.D., President and Chief Executive Officer**

BLUE RIDGE REGIONAL HOSPITAL, 125 Hospital Drive, Spruce Pine, NC, Zip 28777, Mailing Address: P.O. Box 9, Zip 28777; tel. 828/765–4201; Oscar K. Weinmeister, III, Chief Executive Officer

MCDOWELL HOSPITAL, 430 Rankin Drive, Marion, NC, Zip 28752–6568, Mailing Address: P.O. Box 730, Zip 28752–0730; tel. 828/659–5000; Lynn Ingram Boggs, President and Chief Executive Officer

MISSION HOSPITAL, 509 Biltmore Avenue, Asheville, NC, Zip 28801–4690; tel. 828/213–1111; Ronald A. Paulus, M.D., President and Chief Executive Officer

**WNC HEALTH NETWORK, INC.**
**1200 Ridgefield Boulevard Suite 200, Asheville, NC 28806–2280; tel. 828/667–8220; Janice M. Lato, President and Chief Executive Officer**

ALAMANCE REGIONAL MEDICAL CENTER, 1240 Huffman Mill Road, Burlington, NC, Zip 27216–0202, Mailing Address: P.O. Box 202, Zip 27216–0202; tel. 336/538–7000; John G. Currin, Jr., President

ANGEL MEDICAL CENTER, 120 Riverview Street, Franklin, NC, Zip 28734, Mailing Address: P.O. Box 1209, Zip 28744; tel. 828/524–8411; Martin Wadewitz, Interim Chief Executive Officer

ASHEVILLE SPECIALTY HOSPITAL, 428 Biltmore Avenue, 4th Floor, Asheville, NC, Zip 28801; tel. 828/213–5400; Robert C. Desotelle, President and Chief Executive Officer

BLOUNT MEMORIAL HOSPITAL, 907 East Lamar Alexander Parkway, Maryville, TN, Zip 37804–5016; tel. 865/983–7211; Don Heinemann, Administrator and Chief Executive Officer

BLOWING ROCK HOSPITAL, 418 Chestnut Street, Blowing Rock, NC, Zip 28605–0148, Mailing Address: P.O. Box 148, Zip 28605–0148; tel. 828/295–3136; Timothy R. Ford, Chief Executive Officer

BLUE RIDGE REGIONAL HOSPITAL, 125 Hospital Drive, Spruce Pine, NC, Zip 28777, Mailing Address: P.O. Box 9, Zip 28777; tel. 828/765–4201; Oscar K. Weinmeister, III, Chief Executive Officer

BUCHANAN GENERAL HOSPITAL, 1535 Slate Creek Road, Grundy, VA, Zip 24614–6974; tel. 276/935–1000; Robert D. Ruchti, R.N., Interim Chief Executive Officer

CALDWELL MEMORIAL HOSPITAL, 321 Mulberry Street S.W., Lenoir, NC, Zip 28645–5720, Mailing Address: P.O. Box 1890, Zip 28645–1890; tel. 828/757–5100; Laura J. Easton, R.N., President and Chief Executive Officer

CAPE FEAR VALLEY – BLADEN COUNTY HOSPITAL, 501 South Poplar Street, Elizabethtown, NC, Zip 28337–0398, Mailing Address: P.O. Box 398, Zip 28337–0398; tel. 910/862–5100; Cameron Highsmith, Chief Executive Officer

CAPE FEAR VALLEY MEDICAL CENTER, 1638 Owen Drive, Fayetteville, NC, Zip 28304–3431, Mailing Address: P.O. Box 2000, Zip 28302–2000; tel. 910/615–4000; Michael Nagowski, President and Chief Executive Officer

CAREPARTNERS HEALTH SERVICES, 68 Sweeten Creek Road, Asheville, NC, Zip 28803–1599, Mailing Address: P.O. Box 5779, Zip 28813–5779; tel. 828/277–4800; Tracy Buchanan, Chief Executive Officer

CARTERET GENERAL HOSPITAL, 3500 Arendell Street, Morehead City, NC, Zip 28557–1619, Mailing Address: P.O. Box 1619, Zip 28557–1619; tel. 252/808–6000; Richard A. Brvenik, FACHE, President

CATAWBA VALLEY MEDICAL CENTER, 810 Fairgrove Church Road S.E., Hickory, NC, Zip 28602–9643; tel. 828/326–3000; J. Anthony Rose, President and Chief Executive Officer

CHARLES A. CANNON MEMORIAL HOSPITAL, 434 Hospital Drive, Linville, NC, Zip 28646, Mailing Address: P.O. Box 767, Zip 28646; tel. 828/737–7000; Carmen Lacey, MSN, R.N., President

CHARLES GEORGE VETERANS AFFAIRS MEDICAL CENTER, 1100 Tunnel Road, Asheville, NC, Zip 28805–2087; tel. 828/298–7911; Cynthia Breyfogle, Director

CHEROKEE INDIAN HOSPITAL, 1 Hospital Road, Cherokee, NC, Zip 28719, Mailing Address: 1 Hospital Drive, Zip 28719; tel. 828/497–9163; Casey Cooper, Chief Executive Officer

COMMUNITY MEMORIAL HEALTHCENTER, 125 Buena Vista Circle, South Hill, VA, Zip 23970–0090, Mailing Address: P.O. Box 90, Zip 23970–0090; tel. 434/447–3151; W. Scott Burnette, President and Chief Executive Officer

CONWAY MEDICAL CENTER, 300 Singleton Ridge Road, Conway, SC, Zip 29526–9175, Mailing Address: P.O. Box 829, Zip 29528–0829; tel. 843/347–7111; Philip A. Clayton, President and Chief Executive Officer

CUMBERLAND MEDICAL CENTER, 421 South Main Street, Crossville, TN, Zip 38555–5031; tel. 931/484–9511; Barry Wagner, D.O., President and Chief Executive Officer

DICKENSON COMMUNITY HOSPITAL, 312 Hospital Drive, Clintwood, VA, Zip 24228, Mailing Address: P.O. Box 1440, Zip 24228–1440; tel. 276/926–0300; Mark T. Leonard, Chief Executive Officer

FIRSTHEALTH MONTGOMERY MEMORIAL HOSPITAL, 520 Allen Street, Troy, NC, Zip 27371–2802, Mailing Address: P.O. Box 486, Zip 27371–0486; tel. 910/572–1301; Beth Walker, R.N., President

FIRSTHEALTH MOORE REGIONAL HOSPITAL, 155 Memorial Drive, Pinehurst, NC, Zip 28374–8710, Mailing Address: P.O. Box 3000, Zip 28374–3000; tel. 910/715–1000; David J. Kilarski, Chief Executive Officer

FIRSTHEALTH RICHMOND MEMORIAL HOSPITAL, 925 Long Drive, Rockingham, NC, Zip 28379–4815; tel. 910/417–3000; John J. Jackson, President

FRANKLIN WOODS COMMUNITY HOSPITAL, 300 MedTech Parkway, Johnson City, TN, Zip 37604–2277; tel. 423/302–1000; Tony Benton, Chief Executive Officer

GRANVILLE HEALTH SYSTEM, 1010 College Street, Oxford, NC, Zip 27565–2507, Mailing Address: P.O. Box 947, Zip 27565–0947; tel. 919/690–3000; L. Lee Isley, Chief Executive Officer

HALIFAX REGIONAL MEDICAL CENTER, 250 Smith Church Road, Roanoke Rapids, NC, Zip 27870, Mailing Address: P.O. Box 1089, Zip 27870; tel. 252/535–8011; William Mahone, V, President and Chief Executive Officer

HIGHLANDS–CASHIERS HOSPITAL, 190 Hospital Drive, Highlands, NC, Zip 28741–7600, Mailing Address: P.O. Drawer 190, Zip 28741–0190; tel. 828/526–1200; Craig B. James, Chief Executive Officer

INDIAN PATH MEDICAL CENTER, 2000 Brookside Drive, Kingsport, TN, Zip 37660–4627; tel. 423/857–7000; Monty E. McLaurin, President and Chief Executive Officer

IREDELL MEMORIAL HOSPITAL, 557 Brookdale Drive, Statesville, NC, Zip 28677–1828, Mailing Address: P.O. Box 1828, Zip 28687–1828; tel. 704/873–5661; Ed Rush, President and Chief Executive Officer

JOHNSON CITY MEDICAL CENTER, 400 North State of Franklin Road, Johnson City, TN, Zip 37604–6094; tel. 423/431–6111; David E. Nicely, Chief Executive Officer

JOHNSON COUNTY COMMUNITY HOSPITAL, 1901 South Shady Street, Mountain City, TN, Zip 37683–2271; tel. 423/727–1100; Lisa Heaton, Administrator and Chief Nursing Officer

JOHNSTON MEMORIAL HOSPITAL, 16000 Johnston Memorial Drive, Abingdon, VA, Zip 24211; tel. 276/676–7000; Sean S. McMurray, FACHE, Vice President and Chief Executive Officer

LAUGHLIN MEMORIAL HOSPITAL, 1420 Tusculum Boulevard, Greeneville, TN, Zip 37745–5825; tel. 423/787–5000; Charles H. Whitfield, Jr., President and Chief Executive Officer

LENOIR MEMORIAL HOSPITAL, 100 Airport Road, Kinston, NC, Zip 28501–1634, Mailing Address: P.O. Box 1678, Zip 28503–1678; tel. 252/522–7000; Gary E. Black, President and Chief Executive Officer

LEXINGTON MEDICAL CENTER, 2720 Sunset Boulevard, West Columbia, SC, Zip 29169–4816; tel. 803/791–2000; Michael J. Biediger, FACHE, President and Chief Executive Officer

MARGARET R. PARDEE MEMORIAL HOSPITAL, 800 North Justice Street, Hendersonville, NC, Zip 28791; tel. 828/696–1000; James M. Kirby, II, Chief Executive Officer

MCDOWELL HOSPITAL, 430 Rankin Drive, Marion, NC, Zip 28752–6568, Mailing Address: P.O. Box 730, Zip 28752–0730; tel. 828/659–5000; Lynn Ingram Boggs, President and Chief Executive Officer

MCLEOD REGIONAL MEDICAL CENTER, 555 East Cheves Street, Florence, SC, Zip 29502–2617, Mailing Address: P.O. Box 100551, Zip 29502–0551; tel. 843/777–2000; Robert L. Colones, President and Chief Executive Officer

MEDWEST – HARRIS, 68 Hospital Road, Sylva, NC, Zip 28779–2795; tel. 828/586–7000; J. Michael Poore, Chief Executive Officer

MEDWEST – HAYWOOD, 262 Leroy George Drive, Clyde, NC, Zip 28721–9434; tel. 828/456–7311; John Young, Interim CEO

MEDWEST – SWAIN, 45 Plateau Street, Bryson City, NC, Zip 28713–6784; tel. 828/488–2155; J. Michael Poore, Chief Executive Officer

MISSION HOSPITAL, 509 Biltmore Avenue, Asheville, NC, Zip 28801–4690; tel. 828/213–1111; Ronald A. Paulus, M.D., President and Chief Executive Officer

MURPHY MEDICAL CENTER, 3990 U.S. Highway 64 East Alt, Murphy, NC, Zip 28906–7917; tel. 828/837–8161; Michael Stevenson, Administrator

NORTON COMMUNITY HOSPITAL, 100 15th Street N.W., Norton, VA, Zip 24273–1616; tel. 276/679–9600; Mark T. Leonard, Chief Executive Officer

OCONEE MEDICAL CENTER, 298 Memorial Drive, Seneca, SC, Zip 29672–9499; tel. 864/882–3351; Jeanne L. Ward, Ed.D., R.N., President and Chief Executive Officer

PARK RIDGE HEALTH, 100 Hospital Drive, Hendersonville, NC, Zip 28792–5272; tel. 828/684–8501; Jimm Bunch, President and Chief Executive Officer

QUILLEN REHABILITATION HOSPITAL, 2511 Wesley Street, Johnson City, TN, Zip 37601–1723; tel. 423/283–0700; Ann Fleming, Senior Vice President

RANDOLPH HOSPITAL, 364 White Oak Street, Asheboro, NC, Zip 27203–5400, Mailing Address: P.O. Box 1048, Zip 27204–1048; tel. 336/625–5151; Steve E. Eblin, Chief Executive Officer

RUSSELL COUNTY MEDICAL CENTER, 58 Carroll Street, Lebanon, VA, Zip 24266, Mailing Address: P.O. Box 3600, Zip 24266–0200; tel. 276/883–8000; Edward C. Greene, Jr., Assistant Vice President and Administrator

RUTHERFORD REGIONAL MEDICAL CENTER, 288 South Ridgecrest Avenue, Rutherfordton, NC, Zip 28139–3097; tel. 828/286–5000; Cindy D. Buck, Interim Chief Executive Officer

SELF REGIONAL HEALTHCARE, 1325 Spring Street, Greenwood, SC, Zip 29646–3860; tel. 864/725–4111; James A. Pfeiffer, FACHE, President and Chief Executive Officer

SMYTH COUNTY COMMUNITY HOSPITAL, 243 Medical Park Drive, Marion, VA, Zip 24354, Mailing Address: P.O. Box 880, Zip 24354–0880; tel. 276/378–1000; Lindy P. White, President and Chief Executive Officer

SOUTHEASTERN REGIONAL MEDICAL CENTER, 300 West 27th Street, Lumberton, NC, Zip 28358–3017, Mailing Address: P.O. Box 1408, Zip 28359–1408; tel. 910/671–5000; Joann Anderson, President and Chief Executive Officer

SPARTANBURG REGIONAL MEDICAL CENTER, 101 East Wood Street, Spartanburg, SC, Zip 29303–3016; tel. 864/560–6000; J. Philip Feisal, Senior Vice President Acute Care Hospitals

ST. LUKE'S HOSPITAL, 101 Hospital Drive, Columbus, NC, Zip 28722–9473; tel. 828/894–3311; Kenneth A. Shull, FACHE, Chief Executive Officer

SYCAMORE SHOALS HOSPITAL, 1501 West Elk Avenue, Elizabethton, TN, Zip 37643–2874; tel. 423/542–1300; Dwayne Taylor, Chief Executive Officer

THE UNIVERSITY OF TENNESSEE MEDICAL CENTER, 1924 Alcoa Highway, Box 81, Knoxville, TN, Zip 37920–6900; tel. 865/305–9000; Joseph Landsman, President and Chief Executive Officer

TRANSYLVANIA REGIONAL HOSPITAL, 260 Hospital Drive, Brevard, NC, Zip 28712–1116; tel. 828/884–9111; Robert J. Bednarek, President and Chief Executive Officer

TWIN COUNTY REGIONAL HOSPITAL, 200 Hospital Drive, Galax, VA, Zip 24333–2283; tel. 276/236–8181; Jon D. Applebaum, President and Chief Executive Officer

UNICOI COUNTY MEMORIAL HOSPITAL, 100 Greenway Circle, Erwin, TN, Zip 37650–2196, Mailing Address: P.O. Box 802, Zip 37650–0802; tel. 423/743–3141; Jim S. Pate, President and Chief Executive Officer

WATAUGA MEDICAL CENTER, 336 Deerfield Road, Boone, NC, Zip 28607–5008, Mailing Address: P.O. Box 2600, Zip 28607–2600; tel. 828/262–4100; Chuck Mantooth, President

WAYNE MEMORIAL HOSPITAL, 2700 Wayne Memorial Drive, Goldsboro, NC, Zip 27534, Mailing Address: P.O. Box 8001, Zip 27533; tel. 919/736–1110; J. William Paugh, President and Chief Executive Officer

WILSON MEDICAL CENTER, 1705 Tarboro Street, S.W., Wilson, NC, Zip 27893–3428; tel. 252/399–8040; Richard E. Hudson, FACHE, President and Chief Executive Officer

WOODRIDGE HOSPITAL, 403 State of Franklin Road, Johnson City, TN, Zip 37604–6034; tel. 423/431–7060; Grace Pereira, Interim Chief Executive Officer

## NORTH DAKOTA

### MEDCENTER ONE
**300 North Seventh Street, Bismarck, ND 58501–4439; tel. 701/323–6000; Craig Lambrecht, M.D., President and Chief Executive Officer**

MEDCENTER ONE, 300 North Seventh Street, Bismarck, ND, Zip 58501–4439, Mailing Address: P.O. Box 5525, Zip 58506–5525; tel. 701/323–6000; Craig Lambrecht, M.D., President and Chief Executive Officer

## OHIO

### CLEVELAND HEALTH NETWORK
**6000 West Creek Road, Suite 20, Independence, OH 44131–2139; tel. 216/986–1100; Fred M. DeGrandis, President**

AKRON CHILDREN'S HOSPITAL, One Perkins Square, Akron, OH, Zip 44308–1062; tel. 330/543–1000; William H. Considine, President

ASHTABULA COUNTY MEDICAL CENTER, 2420 Lake Avenue, Ashtabula, OH, Zip 44004–4954; tel. 440/997–2262; Michael J. Habowski, President and Chief Executive Officer

CLEVELAND CLINIC CHILDREN'S HOSPITAL FOR REHABILITATION, 2801 Martin Luther King Jr. Drive, Cleveland, OH, Zip 44104–3865; tel. 216/448–6400; Michael J. McHugh, M.D., Medical Director

Section B

CLEVELAND CLINIC FOUNDATION, 9500 Euclid Avenue, Cleveland, OH, Zip 44195–5108; tel. 216/444–2200; Delos Cosgrove, M.D., President and Chief Executive Officer

EMH ELYRIA MEDICAL CENTER, 630 East River Street, Elyria, OH, Zip 44035–5902; tel. 440/329–7500; Donald S. Sheldon, M.D., President and Chief Executive Officer

EUCLID HOSPITAL, 18901 Lake Shore Boulevard, Euclid, OH, Zip 44119–1090; tel. 216/531–9000; Mark Froimson, President

FAIRVIEW HOSPITAL, 18101 Lorain Avenue, Cleveland, OH, Zip 44111–5656; tel. 216/476–7000; Janice Murphy, President

FIRELANDS REGIONAL HEALTH SYSTEM, 1111 Hayes Avenue, Sandusky, OH, Zip 44870; tel. 419/557–7400; Martin Tursky, President and Chief Executive Officer

FISHER–TITUS MEDICAL CENTER, 272 Benedict Avenue, Norwalk, OH, Zip 44857–2374; tel. 419/668–8101; Patrick J. Martin, President and Chief Executive Officer

HILLCREST HOSPITAL, 6780 Mayfield Road, Cleveland, OH, Zip 44124–2202; tel. 440/312–4500; Jeffrey A. Leimgruber, President

LAKEWOOD HOSPITAL, 14519 Detroit Avenue, Lakewood, OH, Zip 44107–4383; tel. 216/521–4200; Robert Weil, M.D., President

LUTHERAN HOSPITAL, 1730 West 25th Street, Cleveland, OH, Zip 44113–3170; tel. 216/696–4300; Brian Donley, M.D., President

MARYMOUNT HOSPITAL, 12300 McCracken Road, Garfield Heights, OH, Zip 44125–2975; tel. 216/581–0500; Joanne Zeroske, President and Chief Executive Officer

METROHEALTH MEDICAL CENTER, 2500 MetroHealth Drive, Cleveland, OH, Zip 44109–1998; tel. 216/778–7800; Mark J. Moran, President and Chief Executive Officer

PARMA COMMUNITY GENERAL HOSPITAL, 7007 Powers Boulevard, Parma, OH, Zip 44129–5495; tel. 440/743–3000; Terrence G. Deis, President and Chief Executive Officer

ST. ELIZABETH HEALTH CENTER, 1044 Belmont Avenue, Youngstown, OH, Zip 44504–1096, Mailing Address: P.O. Box 1790, Zip 44501–1790; tel. 330/746–7211; Robert W. Shroder, President and Chief Executive Officer

ST. JOSEPH HEALTH CENTER, 667 Eastland Avenue S.E., Warren, OH, Zip 44484–4531; tel. 330/841–4000; John Finizio, President

SUMMA BARBERTON CITIZENS HOSPITAL, 155 Fifth Street N.E., Barberton, OH, Zip 44203–3332; tel. 330/615–3000; Thomas DeBord, President

SUMMA HEALTH SYSTEM, 525 East Market Street, Akron, OH, Zip 44309–2090; tel. 330/375–3000; Thomas J. Strauss, President and Chief Executive Officer

SUMMA WADSWORTH–RITTMAN HOSPITAL, 195 Wadsworth Road, Wadsworth, OH, Zip 44281–9505; tel. 330/331–1000; Thomas DeBord, President

SUMMA WESTERN RESERVE HOSPITAL, 1900 23rd Street, Cuyahoga Falls, OH, Zip 44223–1499; tel. 330/971–7000; Robert Kent, D.O., President and Chief Executive Officer

**COMPREHENSIVE HEALTHCARE OF OHIO, INC.**
**630 East River Street, Elyria, OH 44035–5902; tel. 440/329–7700; Donald S. Sheldon, M.D., President and Chief Executive Officer**

EMH ELYRIA MEDICAL CENTER, 630 East River Street, Elyria, OH, Zip 44035–5902; tel. 440/329–7500; Donald S. Sheldon, M.D., President and Chief Executive Officer

**LAKE HEALTH**
**7590 Auburn Road, Concord Township, OH 44077–3472; tel. 440/375–8100; Cynthia Moore–Hardy, President and Chief Executive Officer**

LAKE HEALTH, 7590 Auburn Road, Concord Township, OH, Zip 44077–3472; tel. 440/375–8100; Cynthia Moore–Hardy, President and Chief Executive Officer

**MERCY HEALTH PARTNERS – SOUTHWEST OHIO**
**4600 McAuley Place, Cincinnati, OH 45242; tel. 513/981–6000; James May, President and Chief Executive Officer**

MERCY HEALTH – FAIRFIELD HOSPITAL, 3000 Mack Road, Fairfield, OH, Zip 45014; tel. 513/870–7000; Thomas S. Urban, Market Leader and President

MERCY HOSPITAL ANDERSON, 7500 State Road, Cincinnati, OH, Zip 45255–2492; tel. 513/624–4500; Patricia A. Schroer, President and Chief Executive Officer

MERCY HOSPITAL CLERMONT, 3000 Hospital Drive, Batavia, OH, Zip 45103–1921; tel. 513/732–8200; Gayle M. Heintzelman, President and Chief Executive Officer

MERCY HOSPITAL MOUNT AIRY, 2446 Kipling Avenue, Cincinnati, OH, Zip 45239–6650; tel. 513/853–5000; Michael R. Stephens, President and Market Leader

MERCY HOSPITAL WESTERN HILLS, 3131 Queen City Avenue, Cincinnati, OH, Zip 45238–2396; tel. 513/389–5000; Michael R. Stephens, President and Market Leader

**OHIO STATE HEALTH NETWORK**
**660 Ackerman Road, Suite 601F, Columbus, OH 43202–4500; tel. 614/293–3785; Joann Ort, Executive Director**

BARNESVILLE HOSPITAL, 639 West Main Street, Barnesville, OH, Zip 43713–0309, Mailing Address: P.O. Box 309, Zip 43713–0309; tel. 740/425–3941; Richard L. Doan, FACHE, Chief Executive Officer

MADISON COUNTY HOSPITAL, 210 North Main Street, London, OH, Zip 43140–1115; tel. 740/845–7000; Fred L. Kolb, Chief Executive Officer

MARY RUTAN HOSPITAL, 205 Palmer Avenue, Bellefontaine, OH, Zip 43311–2281; tel. 937/592–4015; Mandy C. Goble, President and Chief Executive Officer

MERCER COUNTY JOINT TOWNSHIP COMMUNITY HOSPITAL, 800 West Main Street, Coldwater, OH, Zip 45828–1698; tel. 419/678–2341; Paula J. Detterman, FACHE, Chief Executive Officer

OHIO STATE UNIVERSITY MEDICAL CENTER, 370 West 9th Avenue, Columbus, OH, Zip 43210–1240; tel. 614/293–8000; Peter E. Geier, Chief Executive Officer

TRINITY HOSPITAL TWIN CITY, 819 North First Street, Dennison, OH, Zip 44621–1098; tel. 740/922–2800; Joseph J. Mitchell, President

WYANDOT MEMORIAL HOSPITAL, 885 North Sandusky Avenue, Upper Sandusky, OH, Zip 43351–1098; tel. 419/294–4991; Joseph A. D'Ettorre, Chief Executive Officer

**PREMIER HEALTH PARTNERS**
**40 West Fourth Street, Suite M–20, Dayton, OH 45402; tel. 937/208–2000; James R. Pancoast, President and Chief Executive Officer**

ATRIUM MEDICAL CENTER, One Medical Center Drive, Middletown, OH, Zip 45005–1066; tel. 513/424–2111; Carol Turner, President and Chief Executive Officer

GOOD SAMARITAN HOSPITAL, 2222 Philadelphia Drive, Dayton, OH, Zip 45406–1813; tel. 937/734–2612; Eloise Broner, President and Chief Executive Officer

MIAMI VALLEY HOSPITAL, One Wyoming Street, Dayton, OH, Zip 45409–2793; tel. 937/208–8000; Bobbie Gerhart, President and Chief Executive Officer

UPPER VALLEY MEDICAL CENTER, 3130 North County Road 25A, Troy, OH, Zip 45373–1309; tel. 937/440–4000; Thomas Parker, Chief Executive Officer

**TRIHEALTH**
**619 Oak Street, Cincinnati, OH 45206; tel. 513/569–6507; John S. Prout, President and Chief Executive Officer**

BETHESDA NORTH HOSPITAL, 10500 Montgomery Road, Cincinnati, OH, Zip 45242–4402; tel. 513/865–1111; Sher McClanahan, Chief Operating Officer

GOOD SAMARITAN HOSPITAL, 375 Dixmyth Avenue, Cincinnati, OH, Zip 45220–2489; tel. 513/862–1400; David Dornheggen, Chief Operating Officer

**WEST CENTRAL OHIO REGIONAL HEALTHCARE ALLIANCE, LLC**
**2615 Fort Amanda Road, Lima, OH 45804–3704; tel. 419/226–9085; Robin Johnson, Executive Director**

JOINT TOWNSHIP DISTRICT MEMORIAL HOSPITAL, 200 St. Clair Street, Saint Marys, OH, Zip 45885–2400; tel. 419/394–3335; Kevin W. Harlan, President

MARY RUTAN HOSPITAL, 205 Palmer Avenue, Bellefontaine, OH, Zip 43311–2281; tel. 937/592–4015; Mandy C. Goble, President and Chief Executive Officer

MERCER COUNTY JOINT TOWNSHIP COMMUNITY HOSPITAL, 800 West Main Street, Coldwater, OH, Zip 45828–1698; tel. 419/678–2341; Paula J. Detterman, FACHE, Chief Executive Officer

ST. RITA'S MEDICAL CENTER, 730 West Market Street, Lima, OH, Zip 45801–4670; tel. 419/227–3361; Robert O. Baxter, President

VAN WERT COUNTY HOSPITAL, 1250 South Washington Street, Van Wert, OH, Zip 45891–2599; tel. 419/238–2390; Mark J. Minick, President and Chief Executive Officer

# OKLAHOMA

**MERCY HEALTH SYSTEM OF OKLAHOMA**
**4300 West Memorial Road, Oklahoma City, OK 73120–8304; tel. 405/752–3756; Diane Smalley, President and Chief Executive Officer**

ARBUCKLE MEMORIAL HOSPITAL, 2011 West Broadway Street, Sulphur, OK, Zip 73086–4221; tel. 580/622–2161; Darin Farrell, Chief Executive Officer

KINGFISHER REGIONAL HOSPITAL, 1000 Kingfisher Regional Hospital Drive, Kingfisher, OK, Zip 73750–3528, Mailing Address: P.O. Box 59, Zip 73750–0059; tel. 405/375–3141; Nancy Schmid, Chief Executive Officer

MERCY HEALTH LOVE COUNTY, 300 Wanda Street, Marietta, OK, Zip 73448–1200; tel. 580/276–3347; Richard Barker, Administrator

MERCY HOSPITAL ARDMORE, 1011 14th Avenue N.W., Ardmore, OK, Zip 73401–1828; tel. 580/223–5400; Mindy Burdick, FACHE, President

MERCY HOSPITAL EL RENO, 2115 Parkview Drive, El Reno, OK, Zip 73036–2199, Mailing Address: P.O. Box 129, Zip 73036–0129; tel. 405/262–2640; Doug Danker, Administrator

MERCY HOSPITAL HEALDTON, 3462 Hospital Road, Healdton, OK, Zip 73438, Mailing Address: P.O. Box 928, Zip 73438; tel. 580/229-0701; Jeremy A. Jones, Administrator

MERCY HOSPITAL OKLAHOMA CITY, 4300 West Memorial Road, Oklahoma City, OK, Zip 73120-8362; tel. 405/755-1515; Jim Gebhart, Jr., FACHE, President

MERCY HOSPITAL TISHOMINGO, 1000 South Byrd Street, Tishomingo, OK, Zip 73460-3299; tel. 580/371-2327; Richard Barker, Interim Chief Executive Officer

OKLAHOMA HEART HOSPITAL, 4050 West Memorial Road, Oklahoma City, OK, Zip 73120; tel. 405/608-3200; John Harvey, M.D., President and Chief Executive Officer

VALLEY VIEW REGIONAL HOSPITAL, 430 North Monta Vista, Ada, OK, Zip 74820-4610; tel. 580/332-2323; W. Kent Rogers, Chief Executive Officer

## OREGON

### HEALTH FUTURE, LLC
**916 Town Centre Drive, Medford, OR 97504-6100; tel. 541/772-3062; Chris Chang-Howitz, Chief Executive Officer**

ASANTE HEALTH SYSTEM, 2650 Siskiyou Boulevard, Suite 200, Medford, OR, Zip 97504-8170; Roy G. Vinyard, President and Chief Executive Officer

ASHLAND COMMUNITY HOSPITAL, 280 Maple Street, Ashland, OR, Zip 97520-1593; tel. 541/201-4000; Mark E. Marchetti, President and Chief Executive Officer

BAY AREA HOSPITAL, 1775 Thompson Road, Coos Bay, OR, Zip 97420-2198; tel. 541/269-8111; Paul Janke, FACHE, President and Chief Executive Officer

MID-COLUMBIA MEDICAL CENTER, 1700 East 19th Street, The Dalles, OR, Zip 97058-3316; tel. 541/296-1111; Duane Francis, President and Chief Executive Officer

OHSU HOSPITAL, 3181 S.W. Sam Jackson Park Road, Portland, OR, Zip 97201-3098; tel. 503/494-8311; Peter F. Rapp, Vice President and Executive Director

PIONEER MEMORIAL HOSPITAL, 1201 N.E. Elm Street, Prineville, OR, Zip 97754-1206; tel. 541/447-6254; Robert Gomes, Chief Executive Officer

SKY LAKES MEDICAL CENTER, 2865 Daggett Avenue, Klamath Falls, OR, Zip 97601-1180; tel. 541/882-6311; Paul R. Stewart, President and Chief Executive Officer

ST. CHARLES MEDICAL CENTER - BEND, 2500 N.E. Neff Road, Bend, OR, Zip 97701-6015; tel. 541/382-4321; Jay Henry, Chief Executive Officer

ST. CHARLES MEDICAL CENTER - REDMOND, 1253 N.W. Canal Boulevard, Redmond, OR, Zip 97756-1395; tel. 541/548-8131; Robert Gomes, Chief Executive Officer

## PENNSYLVANIA

### COMMONWEALTH HEALTH
**575 North River Street, Wilkes Barre, PA 18764-0999; tel. 570/829-8111; Cornelio R. Catena, Chief Executive Officer**

BERWICK HOSPITAL CENTER, 701 East 16th Street, Berwick, PA, Zip 18603-2397; tel. 570/759-5000; Ronald R. Beer, Chief Executive Officer

FIRST HOSPITAL WYOMING VALLEY, 562 Wyoming Avenue, Wilkes-Barre, PA, Zip 18704-3721; tel. 570/552-3900; Mark Schor, Chief Executive Officer

MID-VALLEY HOSPITAL, 1400 Main Street, Peckville, PA, Zip 18452-2009; tel. 570/383-5500; Ann Marie Stevens, Chief Executive Officer

MOSES TAYLOR HOSPITAL, 700 Quincy Avenue, Scranton, PA, Zip 18510-1724; tel. 570/340-2100; Justin Davis, Chief Executive Officer

REGIONAL HOSPITAL OF SCRANTON, 746 Jefferson Avenue, Scranton, PA, Zip 18510-1624; tel. 570/348-7100; Brooks Turkel, Chief Executive Officer

SPECIAL CARE HOSPITAL, 128 West Washington Street, Nanticoke, PA, Zip 18634-3113; tel. 570/735-5000; Robert D. Williams, Chief Executive Officer

TYLER MEMORIAL HOSPITAL, 880 State Road 6 West, Tunkhannock, PA, Zip 18657-6149; tel. 570/836-2161; Denise S. Gieski, MS, Chief Executive Officer

WILKES-BARRE GENERAL HOSPITAL, 575 North River Street, Wilkes-Barre, PA, Zip 18764-0001; tel. 570/829-8111; Cornelio R. Catena, President and Chief Executive Officer

### LAUREL HEALTH SYSTEM
**22 Walnut Street, Wellsboro, PA 16901; tel. 570/724-0500; Ronald J. Butler, President and Chief Executive Officer**

SOLDIERS AND SAILORS MEMORIAL HOSPITAL, 32-36 Central Avenue, Wellsboro, PA, Zip 16901-1899; tel. 570/724-1631; Jan E. Fisher, President and Chief Executive Officer

### PENN HIGHLANDS HEALTHCARE
**100 Hospital Avenue, Du Bois, PA 15801-1440; tel. 814/371-2200; David J. McConnell, Chief Executive Officer**

BROOKVILLE HOSPITAL, 100 Hospital Road, Brookville, PA, Zip 15825-1367; tel. 814/849-2312; Rose Campbell, R.N., President

CLEARFIELD HOSPITAL, 809 Turnpike Avenue, Clearfield, PA, Zip 16830-1232, Mailing Address: P.O. Box 992, Zip 16830-0992; tel. 814/765-5341; Gary Macioce, President and Chief Executive Officer

DUBOIS REGIONAL MEDICAL CENTER, 100 Hospital Avenue, Du Bois, PA, Zip 15801-1440, Mailing Address: P.O. Box 447, Zip 15801-0447; tel. 814/371-2200; John Sutika, President

### SAINT VINCENT HEALTH SYSTEM
**232 West 25th Street, Erie, PA 16544-0002; tel. 814/452-5000; Scott Whalen, Ph.D., FACHE, President and Chief Executive Officer**

SAINT VINCENT HEALTH CENTER, 232 West 25th Street, Erie, PA, Zip 16544-0002; tel. 814/452-5000; Scott Whalen, Ph.D., FACHE, President and Chief Executive Officer

WESTFIELD MEMORIAL HOSPITAL, 189 East Main Street, Westfield, NY, Zip 14787-1195; tel. 716/326-4921; Scott Whalen, Ph.D., FACHE, President and Chief Executive Officer

### VANTAGE HEALTHCARE NETWORK, INC.
**18282 Technology Drive, Suite 202, Meadville, PA 16335; tel. 814/337-0000; David Petrarca, Director Retail Operations**

BRADFORD REGIONAL MEDICAL CENTER, 116 Interstate Parkway, Bradford, PA, Zip 16701-1036; tel. 814/368-4143; Timothy J. Finan, FACHE, President and Chief Executive Officer

BROOKVILLE HOSPITAL, 100 Hospital Road, Brookville, PA, Zip 15825-1367; tel. 814/849-2312; Rose Campbell, R.N., President

CLARION HOSPITAL, One Hospital Drive, Clarion, PA, Zip 16214-8501; tel. 814/226-9500; Byron Quinton, Chief Executive Officer

ELK REGIONAL HEALTH CENTER, 763 Johnsonburg Road, Saint Marys, PA, Zip 15857-3498; tel. 814/788-8000; Gregory P. Bauer, President and Chief Executive Officer

JAMESON HOSPITAL, 1211 Wilmington Avenue, New Castle, PA, Zip 16105-2516; tel. 724/658-9001; Douglas Danko, President and Chief Executive Officer

KANE COMMUNITY HOSPITAL, 4372 Route 6, Kane, PA, Zip 16735-3060; tel. 814/837-8585; J. Gary Rhodes, FACHE, Chief Executive Officer

MEADVILLE MEDICAL CENTER, 751 Liberty Street, Meadville, PA, Zip 16335-2559; tel. 814/333-5000; Philip Pandolph, Chief Executive Officer

PUNXSUTAWNEY AREA HOSPITAL, 81 Hillcrest Drive, Punxsutawney, PA, Zip 15767-2616; tel. 814/938-1800; Daniel D. Blough, Jr., Chief Executive Officer

TITUSVILLE AREA HOSPITAL, 406 West Oak Street, Titusville, PA, Zip 16354-1404; tel. 814/827-1851; Anthony J. Nasralla, FACHE, President and Chief Executive Officer

UPMC BEDFORD MEMORIAL, 10455 Lincoln Highway, Everett, PA, Zip 15537-7046; tel. 814/623-6161; Roger P. Winn, President

UPMC HAMOT, 201 State Street, Erie, PA, Zip 16550-0002; tel. 814/877-6000; John T. Malone, President and Chief Executive Officer

UPMC MCKEESPORT, 1500 Fifth Avenue, McKeesport, PA, Zip 15132-2422; tel. 412/664-2000; Cynthia M. Dorundo, President

UPMC NORTHWEST, 100 Fairfield Drive, Seneca, PA, Zip 16346; tel. 814/676-7600; David Gibbons, President

UPMC PASSAVANT, 9100 Babcock Boulevard, Pittsburgh, PA, Zip 15237-5815; tel. 412/367-6700; David T. Martin, President

UPMC ST. MARGARET, 815 Freeport Road, Pittsburgh, PA, Zip 15215-3301; tel. 412/784-4000; Teresa G. Petrick, President

WARREN GENERAL HOSPITAL, Two Crescent Park West, Warren, PA, Zip 16365-0068, Mailing Address: P.O. Box 68, Zip 16365-0068; tel. 814/723-4973; John P. Papalia, FACHE, Chief Executive Officer

## SOUTH DAKOTA

### REGIONAL HEALTH
**353 Fairmont Boulevard, Rapid City, SD 57701; tel. 605/719-1000; Charles E. Hart, M.D., MS, President and Chief Executive Officer**

CUSTER REGIONAL HOSPITAL, 1039 Montgomery Street, Custer, SD, Zip 57730-1397; tel. 605/673-2229; Veronica Schmidt, Chief Executive Officer

LEAD-DEADWOOD REGIONAL HOSPITAL, 61 Charles Street, Deadwood, SD, Zip 57732-1303; tel. 605/722-6101; Sherry Bea Smith, R.N., Chief Executive Officer and Chief Financial Officer

PHILIP HEALTH SERVICES, 503 West Pine Street, Philip, SD, Zip 57567, Mailing Address: P.O. Box 790, Zip 57567-0790; tel. 605/859-2511; Kent Olson, Administrator and Chief Executive Officer

RAPID CITY REGIONAL HOSPITAL, 353 Fairmont Boulevard, Rapid City, SD, Zip 57701-7393, Mailing Address: P.O. Box 6000, Zip 57709-6000; tel. 605/719-1000; Timothy H. Sughrue, Chief Executive Officer

SAME DAY SURGERY CENTER, 651 Cathedral Drive, Rapid City, SD, Zip 57701; tel. 605/719-5000; Doris Fritts, R.N., Executive Director

SPEARFISH REGIONAL HOSPITAL, 1440 North Main Street, Spearfish, SD, Zip 57783-1504; tel. 605/644-4000; Larry W. Veitz, Chief Executive Officer

SPEARFISH REGIONAL SURGERY CENTER, 1316 North 10th Street, Spearfish, SD, Zip 57783; tel. 605/642-3113; Michael DeLano, Administrator

STURGIS REGIONAL HOSPITAL, 949 Harmon Street, Sturgis, SD, Zip 57785-2452; tel. 605/720-2400; Van D. Hyde, MS, Chief Executive Officer

WESTON COUNTY HEALTH SERVICES, 1124 Washington Boulevard, Newcastle, WY, Zip 82701-2996; tel. 307/746-4491; Gary Bieganski, FACHE, Interim Chief Executive Officer


## TEXAS

### HEALTHCARE PARTNERS OF EAST TEXAS, INC.
**426 North Center Street, Longview, TX 75601-6403; tel. 903/238-8845; Mark Hobgood, Executive Director**

ALLEGIANCE SPECIALTY HOSPITAL OF KILGORE, 1612 South Henderson Boulevard, Kilgore, TX, Zip 75662-3594; tel. 903/984-3505; Sherry Bustin, Chief Executive Officer

ATLANTA MEMORIAL HOSPITAL, 1007 South William Street, Atlanta, TX, Zip 75551-3245; tel. 903/799-3000; Deborah Robison, R.N., Interim Chief Executive Officer

CHRISTUS ST. MICHAEL HEALTH SYSTEM, 2600 St. Michael Drive, Texarkana, TX, Zip 75503-2372; tel. 903/614-1000; Chris Karam, President and Chief Executive Officer

COZBY-GERMANY HOSPITAL, 707 North Waldrip Street, Grand Saline, TX, Zip 75140-1555; tel. 903/962-4242; Patty Vasquez, Administrator

DUBUIS HOSPITAL OF TEXARKANA, 2400 St. Michael Drive, 2nd Floor, Texarkana, TX, Zip 75503-2372; tel. 903/614-7600; Holly Powell, Administrator

EAST TEXAS MEDICAL CENTER ATHENS, 2000 South Palestine Street, Athens, TX, Zip 75751-5610; tel. 903/676-1000; Patrick L. Wallace, Administrator

EAST TEXAS MEDICAL CENTER CARTHAGE, 409 Cottage Road, Carthage, TX, Zip 75633-1466, Mailing Address: P.O. Box 549, Zip 75633-0549; tel. 903/693-3841; Gary Mikeal Hudson, Administrator

EAST TEXAS MEDICAL CENTER CLARKSVILLE, 3000 West Main Street, Clarksville, TX, Zip 75426, Mailing Address: P.O. Box 1270, Zip 75426-1270; tel. 903/427-6400; John S. Hart, Administrator

EAST TEXAS MEDICAL CENTER CROCKETT, 1100 Loop 304 East, Crockett, TX, Zip 75835-1810; tel. 936/546-3862; Terry Cutler, Administrator and Chief Operating Officer

EAST TEXAS MEDICAL CENTER FAIRFIELD, 125 Newman Street, Fairfield, TX, Zip 75840-1499; tel. 903/389-2121; Ruth Cook, Administrator

EAST TEXAS MEDICAL CENTER HENDERSON, 300 Wilson Street, Henderson, TX, Zip 75652-5956; tel. 903/657-7541; Mark Leitner, Chief Executive Officer

EAST TEXAS MEDICAL CENTER JACKSONVILLE, 501 South Ragsdale Street, Jacksonville, TX, Zip 75766-2413; tel. 903/541-5000; Jack R. Endres, Administrator

EAST TEXAS MEDICAL CENTER PITTSBURG, 2701 Highway 271 North, Pittsburg, TX, Zip 75686-1032; tel. 903/946-5000; W. Perry Henderson, Administrator

EAST TEXAS MEDICAL CENTER REHABILITATION CENTER, 701 Olympic Plaza Circle, Tyler, TX, Zip 75701-1996; tel. 903/596-3000; Eddie L. Howard, Vice President and Chief Operating Officer

EAST TEXAS MEDICAL CENTER TRINITY, 317 Prospect Drive, Trinity, TX, Zip 75862, Mailing Address: P.O. Box 3169, Zip 75862; tel. 936/744-1100; Brett Kirkham, Administrator

EAST TEXAS MEDICAL CENTER TYLER, 1000 South Beckham Street, Tyler, TX, Zip 75701-1996, Mailing Address: Box 6400, Zip 75711-6400; tel. 903/597-0351; Robert B. Evans, Administrator and Chief Executive Officer

EAST TEXAS MEDICAL CENTER-MOUNT VERNON, 500 Highway 37 South, Mount Vernon, TX, Zip 75457-3602, Mailing Address: P.O. Box 477, Zip 75457-0477; tel. 903/537-8000; David Bailey, Administrator

EAST TEXAS MEDICAL CENTER-QUITMAN, 117 Winnsboro Street, Quitman, TX, Zip 75783-2144, Mailing Address: P.O. Box 1000, Zip 75783-1000; tel. 903/763-6300; Warren Robicheaux, Administrator

GOOD SHEPHERD MEDICAL CENTER, 700 East Marshall Avenue, Longview, TX, Zip 75601-5571; tel. 903/315-2000; Edward D. Banos, President and Chief Executive Officer

GOOD SHEPHERD MEDICAL CENTER-LINDEN, 404 North Kaufman Street, Linden, TX, Zip 75563-5235; tel. 903/756-5561; Carla Roadcap, R.N., MSN, Chief Executive Officer

GOOD SHEPHERD MEDICAL CENTER-MARSHALL, 811 South Washington Avenue, Marshall, TX, Zip 75670-5336, Mailing Address: P.O. Box 1599, Zip 75671-1599; tel. 903/927-6000; Russell J. Collier, FACHE, President and Chief Executive Officer

HOPKINS COUNTY MEMORIAL HOSPITAL, 115 Airport Road, Sulphur Springs, TX, Zip 75482-0115; tel. 903/885-7671; Michael McAndrew, Chief Executive Officer

HOWARD MEMORIAL HOSPITAL, 130 Medical Circle, Nashville, AR, Zip 71852-8606; tel. 870/845-4400; Debra J. Wright, R.N., Chief Executive Officer

HUNTSVILLE MEMORIAL HOSPITAL, 110 Memorial Hospital Drive, Huntsville, TX, Zip 77340-4362, Mailing Address: P.O. Box 4001, Zip 77342-4001; tel. 936/291-3411; Sally I. Nelson, Chief Executive Officer

LITTLE RIVER MEMORIAL HOSPITAL, 451 West Locke Street, Ashdown, AR, Zip 71822-3398; tel. 870/898-5011; David Deaton, Administrator and Chief Executive Officer

MAGNOLIA REGIONAL MEDICAL CENTER, 101 Hospital Drive, Magnolia, AR, Zip 71753-2416, Mailing Address: P.O. Box 629, Zip 71754-0629; tel. 870/235-3000; Margaret M. West, MS, Chief Executive Officer

MCCURTAIN MEMORIAL HOSPITAL, 1301 Lincoln Road, Idabel, OK, Zip 74745-7341; tel. 580/286-7623; Bristol Messer, Chief Executive Officer

MEMORIAL MEDICAL CENTER – LIVINGSTON, 1717 Highway 59 Bypass, Livingston, TX, Zip 77351-1257, Mailing Address: P.O. Box 1257, Zip 77351-1257; tel. 936/329-8700; David LeMonte, Chief Executive Officer

MEMORIAL MEDICAL CENTER – LUFKIN, 1201 West Frank Avenue, Lufkin, TX, Zip 75904-3357, Mailing Address: P.O. Box 1447, Zip 75902-1447; tel. 936/634-8111; Gary N. Looper, President and Chief Executive Officer

MEMORIAL MEDICAL CENTER – SAN AUGUSTINE, 511 East Hospital Street, San Augustine, TX, Zip 75972-2121, Mailing Address: P.O. Box 658, Zip 75972-0658; tel. 936/275-3446; Darlene Williams, R.N., Administrator

NACOGDOCHES MEMORIAL HOSPITAL, 1204 North Mound Street, Nacogdoches, TX, Zip 75961-4061; tel. 936/564-4611; Tim Hayward, Administrator

PALESTINE REGIONAL MEDICAL CENTER-EAST, 2900 South Loop 256, Palestine, TX, Zip 75801-6958; tel. 903/731-1000; Alan E. George, Chief Executive Officer

PARIS REGIONAL MEDICAL CENTER, 820 Clarksville Street, Paris, TX, Zip 75460-9070; tel. 903/785-4521; Billy Porter, Chief Executive Officer

SABINE COUNTY HOSPITAL, Highway 83 West, Hemphill, TX, Zip 75948, Mailing Address: P.O. Box 750, Zip 75948-0750; tel. 409/787-3300; Diana Taylor, Administrator

SHELBY REGIONAL MEDICAL CENTER, 602 Hurst Street, Center, TX, Zip 75935-3414, Mailing Address: P.O. Box 1749, Zip 75935-1749; tel. 936/598-2781; Tariq Mahmood, Chief Executive Officer

TITUS REGIONAL MEDICAL CENTER, 2001 North Jefferson Avenue, Mount Pleasant, TX, Zip 75455-2398; tel. 903/577-6000; Ronald D. Davis, Chief Executive Officer

TYLER COUNTY HOSPITAL, 1100 West Bluff Street, Woodville, TX, Zip 75979-4799, Mailing Address: P.O. Box 549, Zip 75979-0549; tel. 409/283-8141; Sandra Gayle Wright, R.N., Ed.D., Chief Executive Officer

### REGIONAL HEALTHCARE ALLIANCE
**530 South Beckham Avenue, Tyler, TX 75702-8310; tel. 903/531-4449; John Webb, President**

ALLEGIANCE SPECIALTY HOSPITAL OF KILGORE, 1612 South Henderson Boulevard, Kilgore, TX, Zip 75662-3594; tel. 903/984-3505; Sherry Bustin, Chief Executive Officer

ATLANTA MEMORIAL HOSPITAL, 1007 South William Street, Atlanta, TX, Zip 75551-3245; tel. 903/799-3000; Deborah Robison, R.N., Interim Chief Executive Officer

BAYLOR UNIVERSITY MEDICAL CENTER, 3500 Gaston Avenue, Dallas, TX, Zip 75246-2088; tel. 214/820-0111; John B. McWhorter, III, President

CHILDREN'S MEDICAL CENTER OF DALLAS, 1935 Medical District Drive, Dallas, TX, Zip 75235-7794; tel. 214/456-7000; Christopher J. Durovich, President and Chief Executive Officer

COZBY-GERMANY HOSPITAL, 707 North Waldrip Street, Grand Saline, TX, Zip 75140-1555; tel. 903/962-4242; Patty Vasquez, Administrator

EAST TEXAS MEDICAL CENTER HENDERSON, 300 Wilson Street, Henderson, TX, Zip 75652-5956; tel. 903/657-7541; Mark Leitner, Chief Executive Officer

GOOD SHEPHERD MEDICAL CENTER, 700 East Marshall Avenue, Longview, TX, Zip 75601-5571; tel. 903/315-2000; Edward D. Banos, President and Chief Executive Officer

GOOD SHEPHERD MEDICAL CENTER-LINDEN, 404 North Kaufman Street, Linden, TX, Zip 75563-5235; tel. 903/756-5561; Carla Roadcap, R.N., MSN, Chief Executive Officer

HOPKINS COUNTY MEMORIAL HOSPITAL, 115 Airport Road, Sulphur Springs, TX, Zip 75482-0115; tel. 903/885-7671; Michael McAndrew, Chief Executive Officer

MOTHER FRANCES HOSPITAL – JACKSONVILLE, 2026 South Jackson, Jacksonville, TX, Zip 75766; tel. 903/541-4500; Thomas N. Cammack, Jr., Chief Administrative Officer

MOTHER FRANCES HOSPITAL – TYLER, 800 East Dawson Street, Tyler, TX, Zip 75701-2036; tel. 903/593-8441; Laura Owen, Senior Vice President and Chief Executive Officer

NACOGDOCHES MEDICAL CENTER, 4920 N.E. Stallings, Nacogdoches, TX, Zip 75965-1200, Mailing Address: P.O. Box 631604, Zip 75963-1604; tel. 936/569-9481; Gary L. Stokes, Chief Executive Officer

PALESTINE REGIONAL MEDICAL CENTER-EAST, 2900 South Loop 256, Palestine, TX, Zip 75801-6958; tel. 903/731-1000; Alan E. George, Chief Executive Officer

PARIS REGIONAL MEDICAL CENTER, 820 Clarksville Street, Paris, TX, Zip 75460-9070; tel. 903/785-4521; Billy Porter, Chief Executive Officer

TITUS REGIONAL MEDICAL CENTER, 2001 North Jefferson Avenue, Mount Pleasant, TX, Zip 75455-2398; tel. 903/577-6000; Ronald D. Davis, Chief Executive Officer

TRINITY MOTHER FRANCES REHABILITATION HOSPITAL, 3131 Troup Highway, Tyler, TX, Zip 75701–8352; tel. 903/510–7000; Sharla Anderson, Chief Executive Officer

TYLER CONTINUECARE HOSPITAL AT MOTHER FRANCES, 800 East Dawson, 4th Floor, Tyler, TX, Zip 75701; tel. 903/531–4080; Stephanie Hyde, Chief Executive Officer

UNIVERSITY OF TEXAS HEALTH SCIENCE CENTER AT TYLER, 11937 Highway 271, Tyler, TX, Zip 75708–3154; tel. 903/877–7777; Kirk A. Calhoun, M.D., President

### ST. DAVID'S HEALTH NETWORK
**98 San Jacinto Boulevard, Austin, TX 78701–4082; tel. 512/708–9700; C. David Huffstutler, President and Chief Executive Officer**

AUSTIN LAKES HOSPITAL, 1025 East 32nd Street, Austin, TX, Zip 78705–2714; tel. 512/544–5253; Ramona Key, Chief Executive Officer

ST. DAVID'S MEDICAL CENTER, 919 East 32nd Street, Austin, TX, Zip 78705–2709, Mailing Address: P.O. Box 4039, Zip 78765–4039; tel. 512/476–7111; Donald H. Wilkerson, Chief Executive Officer

ST. DAVID'S NORTH AUSTIN MEDICAL CENTER, 12221 North MoPac Expressway, Austin, TX, Zip 78758–2496; tel. 512/901–1000; Allen Harrison, Chief Executive Officer

ST. DAVID'S REHABILITATION CENTER, 1005 East 32nd Street, Austin, TX, Zip 78705–2705, Mailing Address: P.O. Box 4270, Zip 78765–4270; tel. 512/544–5100; Diane Owens, Administrator

ST. DAVID'S ROUND ROCK MEDICAL CENTER, 2400 Round Rock Avenue, Round Rock, TX, Zip 78681–4097; tel. 512/341–1000; Deborah L. Ryle, Administrator and Chief Executive Officer

ST. DAVID'S SOUTH AUSTIN MEDICAL CENTER, 901 West Ben White Boulevard, Austin, TX, Zip 78704–6903; tel. 512/447–2211; Todd E. Steward, Chief Executive Officer

## VIRGINIA

### CENTRAL VIRGINIA HEALTH NETWORK
**2201 West Broad Street, Suite 202, Richmond, VA 23220–2022; tel. 804/359–4500; Michael Matthews, Chief Executive Officer**

BON SECOURS MARYVIEW MEDICAL CENTER, 3636 High Street, Portsmouth, VA, Zip 23707–3270; tel. 757/398–2200; Joseph M. Oddis, Chief Executive Officer

BON SECOURS MEMORIAL REGIONAL MEDICAL CENTER, 8260 Atlee Road, Mechanicsville, VA, Zip 23116–1844; tel. 804/764–6000; Michael Robinson, Chief Executive Officer

BON SECOURS ST. FRANCIS MEDICAL CENTER, 13710 St. Francis Boulevard, Midlothian, VA, Zip 23114–3267; tel. 804/594–7300; Mark M. Gordon, Executive Vice President

BON SECOURS ST. MARY'S HOSPITAL, 5801 Bremo Road, Richmond, VA, Zip 23226–1907; tel. 804/285–2011; Toni R. Ardabell, R.N., Chief Executive Officer

BON SECOURS–DEPAUL MEDICAL CENTER, 150 Kingsley Lane, Norfolk, VA, Zip 23505–4650; tel. 757/889–5000; John E. Barrett, III, Chief Executive Officer

BON SECOURS–RICHMOND COMMUNITY HOSPITAL, 1500 North 28th Street, Richmond, VA, Zip 23223–5396, Mailing Address: P.O. Box 27184, Zip 23261–7184; tel. 804/225–1700; Michael Robinson, Executive Vice President and Administrator

CENTRA SOUTHSIDE COMMUNITY HOSPITAL, 800 Oak Street, Farmville, VA, Zip 23901–1199; tel. 434/392–8811; E. W. Tibbs, President and Chief Executive Officer

COMMUNITY MEMORIAL HEALTHCENTER, 125 Buena Vista Circle, South Hill, VA, Zip 23970–0090, Mailing Address: P.O. Box 90, Zip 23970–0090; tel. 434/447–3151; W. Scott Burnette, President and Chief Executive Officer

MARY IMMACULATE HOSPITAL, 2 Bernardine Drive, Newport News, VA, Zip 23602–4499; tel. 757/886–6000; Patricia L. Robertson, Executive Vice President

RAPPAHANNOCK GENERAL HOSPITAL, 101 Harris Drive, Kilmarnock, VA, Zip 22482, Mailing Address: P.O. Box 1449, Zip 22482–1449; tel. 804/435–8000; James M. Holmes, Jr., President and Chief Executive Officer

SHELTERING ARMS REHABILITATION HOSPITAL, 8254 Atlee Road, Mechanicsville, VA, Zip 23116–1844; tel. 804/764–7055; James E. Sok, FACHE, President and Chief Executive Officer

UNIVERSITY OF VIRGINIA MEDICAL CENTER, 1215 Lee Street, Charlottesville, VA, Zip 22908–0001, Mailing Address: P.O. Box 800809, Zip 22908–0809; tel. 434/924–0211; R. Edward Howell, Vice President and Chief Executive Officer

### VIRGINIA HEALTH NETWORK
**7400 Beaufont Springs Drive, Suite 505, Richmond, VA 23225–5521; tel. 804/320–3837; James Brittain, President**

AUGUSTA HEALTH, 78 Medical Center Drive, Fishersville, VA, Zip 22939–2332, Mailing Address: P.O. Box 1000, Zip 22939–1000; tel. 540/932–4000; Mary N. Mannix, FACHE, President and Chief Executive Officer

BATH COMMUNITY HOSPITAL, 83 Park Drive, Hot Springs, VA, Zip 24445, Mailing Address: P.O. Box Z, Zip 24445–0750; tel. 540/839–7000; Deborah Lipes, R.N., Chief Executive Officer

BEDFORD MEMORIAL HOSPITAL, 1613 Oakwood Street, Bedford, VA, Zip 24523–0688, Mailing Address: P.O. Box 688, Zip 24523–0688; tel. 540/586–2441; Patti Jurkus, President and Chief Executive Officer

BON SECOURS MARYVIEW MEDICAL CENTER, 3636 High Street, Portsmouth, VA, Zip 23707–3270; tel. 757/398–2200; Joseph M. Oddis, Chief Executive Officer

BON SECOURS MEMORIAL REGIONAL MEDICAL CENTER, 8260 Atlee Road, Mechanicsville, VA, Zip 23116–1844; tel. 804/764–6000; Michael Robinson, Chief Executive Officer

BON SECOURS ST. FRANCIS MEDICAL CENTER, 13710 St. Francis Boulevard, Midlothian, VA, Zip 23114–3267; tel. 804/594–7300; Mark M. Gordon, Executive Vice President

BON SECOURS ST. MARY'S HOSPITAL, 5801 Bremo Road, Richmond, VA, Zip 23226–1907; tel. 804/285–2011; Toni R. Ardabell, R.N., Chief Executive Officer

BON SECOURS–DEPAUL MEDICAL CENTER, 150 Kingsley Lane, Norfolk, VA, Zip 23505–4650; tel. 757/889–5000; John E. Barrett, III, Chief Executive Officer

BON SECOURS–RICHMOND COMMUNITY HOSPITAL, 1500 North 28th Street, Richmond, VA, Zip 23223–5396, Mailing Address: P.O. Box 27184, Zip 23261–7184; tel. 804/225–1700; Michael Robinson, Executive Vice President and Administrator

BUCHANAN GENERAL HOSPITAL, 1535 Slate Creek Road, Grundy, VA, Zip 24614–6974; tel. 276/935–1000; Robert D. Ruchti, R.N., Interim Chief Executive Officer

CARILION FRANKLIN MEMORIAL HOSPITAL, 180 Floyd Avenue, Rocky Mount, VA, Zip 24151–1389; tel. 540/483–5277; William D. Jacobsen, Chief Executive Officer

CARILION GILES COMMUNITY HOSPITAL, 159 Hartley Way, Pearisburg, VA, Zip 24134–2471; tel. 540/921–6000; James E. Tyler, Vice President and Administrator

CARILION MEDICAL CENTER, Belleview at Jefferson Street, Roanoke, VA, Zip 24014, Mailing Address: P.O. Box 13367, Zip 24033–3367; tel. 540/981–7000; Nancy Howell Agee, President and Chief Executive Officer

CARILION NEW RIVER VALLEY MEDICAL CENTER, 2900 Lamb Circle, Christiansburg, VA, Zip 24073–5041, Mailing Address: P.O. Box 5, Radford, Zip 24143–0005; tel. 540/731–2000; John S. Piatkowski, M.D., President and Chief Executive Officer

CARILION STONEWALL JACKSON HOSPITAL, 1 Health Circle, Lexington, VA, Zip 24450–2492; tel. 540/458–3300; Charles E. Carr, Chief Executive Officer

CARILION TAZEWELL COMMUNITY HOSPITAL, 141 Ben Bolt Avenue, Tazewell, VA, Zip 24651–9700; tel. 276/988–8700; John S. Piatkowski, M.D., Chief Executive Officer

CENTRA SOUTHSIDE COMMUNITY HOSPITAL, 800 Oak Street, Farmville, VA, Zip 23901–1199; tel. 434/392–8811; E. W. Tibbs, President and Chief Executive Officer

CHESAPEAKE REGIONAL MEDICAL CENTER, 736 Battlefield Boulevard North, Chesapeake, VA, Zip 23320–4941, Mailing Address: P.O. Box 2028, Zip 23327–2028; tel. 757/312–8121; Wynn L. Dixon, Jr., Chief Executive Officer

CHILDREN'S HOSPITAL OF RICHMOND, 2924 Brook Road, Richmond, VA, Zip 23220–1298; tel. 804/321–7474; Leslie G. Wyatt, Senior Vice President Children's Services and Executive Director

CHILDREN'S HOSPITAL OF THE KING'S DAUGHTERS, 601 Children's Lane, Norfolk, VA, Zip 23507–1910; tel. 757/668–7000; James D. Dahling, President and Chief Executive Officer

CJW MEDICAL CENTER, 7101 Jahnke Road, Richmond, VA, Zip 23225–4044; tel. 804/320–3911; Tim McManus, Interim Chief Executive Officer

CLINCH VALLEY MEDICAL CENTER, 6801 Governor G. C. Peery Highway, Richlands, VA, Zip 24641–2194; tel. 276/596–6000; David B. Darden, Chief Executive Officer

COMMUNITY MEMORIAL HEALTHCENTER, 125 Buena Vista Circle, South Hill, VA, Zip 23970–0090, Mailing Address: P.O. Box 90, Zip 23970–0090; tel. 434/447–3151; W. Scott Burnette, President and Chief Executive Officer

CULPEPER REGIONAL HOSPITAL, 501 Sunset Lane, Culpeper, VA, Zip 22701–3917, Mailing Address: P.O. Box 592, Zip 22701–0592; tel. 540/829–4100; H. Lee Kirk, Jr., President and Chief Executive Officer

DOMINION HOSPITAL, 2960 Sleepy Hollow Road, Falls Church, VA, Zip 22044–2030; tel. 703/536–2000; Suzanne B. Jackson, FACHE, Chief Executive Officer

FAUQUIER HOSPITAL, 500 Hospital Drive, Warrenton, VA, Zip 20186–3099; tel. 540/316–5000; Rodger H. Baker, President and Chief Executive Officer

HEALTHSOUTH REHABILITATION HOSPITAL OF VIRGINIA, 5700 Fitzhugh Avenue, Richmond, VA, Zip 23226–1877; tel. 804/288–5700; Jeff Ruskan, II, Chief Executive Officer

HENRICO DOCTORS' HOSPITAL, 1602 Skipwith Road, Richmond, VA, Zip 23229–5205; tel. 804/289–4500; Patrick J. Farrell, Chief Executive Officer

INOVA ALEXANDRIA HOSPITAL, 4320 Seminary Road, Alexandria, VA, Zip 22304–1594; tel. 703/504–3167; Christine Candio, Chief Executive Officer

INOVA FAIR OAKS HOSPITAL, 3600 Joseph Siewick Drive, Fairfax, VA, Zip 22033–1798; tel. 703/391–3600; John L. Fitzgerald, Chief Executive Officer

INOVA FAIRFAX HOSPITAL, 3300 Gallows Road, Falls Church, VA, Zip 22042–2300; tel. 703/776–4001; L. Reuven Pasternak, M.D., M.P.H., Chief Executive Officer

INOVA LOUDOUN HOSPITAL, 44045 Riverside Parkway, Leesburg, VA, Zip 20176–2799, Mailing Address: P.O. Box 6000, Zip 20177–0600; tel. 703/858–6000; Patrick Walters, Interim Chief Executive Officer

INOVA MOUNT VERNON HOSPITAL, 2501 Parker's Lane, Alexandria, VA, Zip 22306; tel. 703/664–7000; Barbara J. Doyle, R.N., MS, Senior Vice President and Chief Executive Officer

JOHN RANDOLPH MEDICAL CENTER, 411 West Randolph Road, Hopewell, VA, Zip 23860–2938; tel. 804/541–1600; Dia Nichols, Chief Executive Officer

JOHNSTON MEMORIAL HOSPITAL, 16000 Johnston Memorial Drive, Abingdon, VA, Zip 24211; tel. 276/676–7000; Sean S. McMurray, FACHE, Vice President and Chief Executive Officer

LEWISGALE HOSPITAL ALLEGHANY, One ARH Lane, Low Moor, VA, Zip 24457, Mailing Address: P.O. Box 7, Zip 24457–0007; tel. 540/862–6011; Greg T. Madsen, Chief Executive Officer

LEWISGALE HOSPITAL AT PULASKI, 2400 Lee Highway, Pulaski, VA, Zip 24301–0759, Mailing Address: P.O. Box 759, Zip 24301–0759; tel. 540/994–8100; Mark Nichols, FACHE, Chief Executive Officer

MARTHA JEFFERSON HOSPITAL, 500 Martha Jefferson Drive, Charlottesville, VA, Zip 22911; tel. 434/654–7000; James E. Haden, President and Chief Executive Officer

MARY IMMACULATE HOSPITAL, 2 Bernardine Drive, Newport News, VA, Zip 23602–4499; tel. 757/886–6000; Patricia L. Robertson, Executive Vice President

MARY WASHINGTON HOSPITAL, 1001 Sam Perry Boulevard, Fredericksburg, VA, Zip 22401–3354; tel. 540/741–1100; Fred M. Rankin, III, President and Chief Executive Officer

MEMORIAL HOSPITAL, 320 Hospital Drive, Martinsville, VA, Zip 24112–1981, Mailing Address: P.O. Box 4788, Zip 24115–4788; tel. 276/666–7200; Grady W. Philips, III, Chief Executive Officer

MOUNTAIN VIEW REGIONAL MEDICAL CENTER, 310 Third Street N.E., Norton, VA, Zip 24273–1137; tel. 276/679–9100; David L. Brash, System Regional Vice President and President

NORTHERN HOSPITAL OF SURRY COUNTY, 830 Rockford Street, Mount Airy, NC, Zip 27030–5365, Mailing Address: P.O. Box 1101, Zip 27030–1101; tel. 336/719–7000; William B. James, Chief Executive Officer

PIONEER COMMUNITY HOSPITAL OF PATRICK COUNTY, 18688 Jeb Stuart Highway, Stuart, VA, Zip 24171–1559; tel. 276/694–3151; Jeanette Filpi, Chief Executive Officer

PRINCE WILLIAM HOSPITAL, 8700 Sudley Road, Manassas, VA, Zip 20110–4418, Mailing Address: P.O. Box 2610, Zip 20108–0867; tel. 703/369–8000; Melissa Robson, President

RAPPAHANNOCK GENERAL HOSPITAL, 101 Harris Drive, Kilmarnock, VA, Zip 22482, Mailing Address: P.O. Box 1449, Zip 22482–1449; tel. 804/435–8000; James M. Holmes, Jr., President and Chief Executive Officer

RESTON HOSPITAL CENTER, 1850 Town Center Parkway, Reston, VA, Zip 20190–3219; tel. 703/689–9000; Tim McManus, President and Chief Executive Officer

RIVERSIDE BEHAVIORAL HEALTH CENTER, 2244 Executive Drive, Hampton, VA, Zip 23666–2430; tel. 757/827–1001; Allan D. Erbe, Administrator

RIVERSIDE REGIONAL MEDICAL CENTER, 500 J. Clyde Morris Boulevard, Newport News, VA, Zip 23601–1929; tel. 757/594–2000; Patrick Parcells, Senior Vice President and Administrator

RIVERSIDE REHABILITATION INSTITUTE, 245 Chesapeake Avenue, Newport News, VA, Zip 23607–6038; tel. 757/928–8000; Edward Heckler, Administrator

RIVERSIDE SHORE MEMORIAL HOSPITAL, 9507 Hospital Avenue, Nassawadox, VA, Zip 23413–1821, Mailing Address: P.O. Box 17, Zip 23413–0017; tel. 757/414–8000; Joseph P. Zager, Vice President and Administrator

RIVERSIDE TAPPAHANNOCK HOSPITAL, 618 Hospital Road, Tappahannock, VA, Zip 22560–5000; tel. 804/443–3311; Elizabeth J. Martin, Vice President and Administrator

RIVERSIDE WALTER REED HOSPITAL, 7519 Hospital Drive, Gloucester, VA, Zip 23061–4178, Mailing Address: P.O. Box 1130, Zip 23061–1130; tel. 804/693–8800; Megan K. Moore, Vice President and Administrator

RUSSELL COUNTY MEDICAL CENTER, 58 Carroll Street, Lebanon, VA, Zip 24266, Mailing Address: P.O. Box 3600, Zip 24266–0200; tel. 276/883–8000; Edward C. Greene, Jr., Assistant Vice President and Administrator

SENTARA CAREPLEX HOSPITAL, 3000 Coliseum Drive, Hampton, VA, Zip 23666–5963; tel. 757/736–1000; Debra A. Flores, R.N., MS, President and Administrator

SENTARA LEIGH HOSPITAL, 830 Kempsville Road, Norfolk, VA, Zip 23502–3920; tel. 757/261–6000; Teresa L. Edwards, Vice President and Administrator

SENTARA NORFOLK GENERAL HOSPITAL, 600 Gresham Drive, Norfolk, VA, Zip 23507; tel. 757/388–3000; Mary L. Blunt, Corporate Vice President and Administrator

SENTARA NORTHERN VIRGINIA MEDICAL CENTER, 2300 Opitz Boulevard, Woodbridge, VA, Zip 22191–3399; tel. 703/670–1313; Megan R. Perry, Vice President and Administrator

SENTARA OBICI HOSPITAL, 2800 Godwin Boulevard, Suffolk, VA, Zip 23434–4323; tel. 757/934–4000; Kurt T. Hofelich, Vice President and Administrator

SENTARA PRINCESS ANNE HOSPITAL, 2025 Glenn Mitchell Drive, Virginia Beach, VA, Zip 23456–0178; tel. 757/363–6100; Stephen D. Porter, President

SENTARA VIRGINIA BEACH GENERAL HOSPITAL, 1060 First Colonial Road, Virginia Beach, VA, Zip 23454–3002; tel. 757/395–8000; Thomas B. Thames, M.D., Interim President

SENTARA WILLIAMSBURG REGIONAL MEDICAL CENTER, 100 Sentara Circle, Williamsburg, VA, Zip 23188–5713; tel. 757/984–6000; Robert L. Graves, Vice President and Administrator

SHELTERING ARMS REHABILITATION HOSPITAL, 8254 Atlee Road, Mechanicsville, VA, Zip 23116–1844; tel. 804/764–7055; James E. Sok, FACHE, President and Chief Executive Officer

SMYTH COUNTY COMMUNITY HOSPITAL, 243 Medical Park Drive, Marion, VA, Zip 24354, Mailing Address: P.O. Box 880, Zip 24354–0880; tel. 276/378–1000; Lindy P. White, President and Chief Executive Officer

SOUTHAMPTON MEMORIAL HOSPITAL, 100 Fairview Drive, Franklin, VA, Zip 23851–1206, Mailing Address: P.O. Box 817, Zip 23851–0817; tel. 757/569–6100; Phil A. Wright, II, Chief Executive Officer

SOUTHERN VIRGINIA REGIONAL MEDICAL CENTER, 727 North Main Street, Emporia, VA, Zip 23847–1274; tel. 434/348–4400; Britton Phelps, Chief Executive Officer

SOUTHSIDE REGIONAL MEDICAL CENTER, 200 Medical Park Boulevard, Petersburg, VA, Zip 23805; tel. 804/765–5000; Michael Yungmann, Chief Executive Officer

TWIN COUNTY REGIONAL HOSPITAL, 200 Hospital Drive, Galax, VA, Zip 24333–2283; tel. 276/236–8181; Jon D. Applebaum, President and Chief Executive Officer

UNIVERSITY OF VIRGINIA MEDICAL CENTER, 1215 Lee Street, Charlottesville, VA, Zip 22908–0001, Mailing Address: P.O. Box 800809, Zip 22908–0809; tel. 434/924–0211; R. Edward Howell, Vice President and Chief Executive Officer

UVA–HEALTHSOUTH REHABILITATION HOSPITAL, 515 Ray C. Hunt Drive, Charlottesville, VA, Zip 22903; tel. 434/244–2000; Thomas J. Cook, Chief Executive Officer

VCU HEALTH SYSTEM, 1250 East Marshall Street, Richmond, VA, Zip 23219, Mailing Address: P.O. Box 980510, Zip 23298–0510; tel. 804/828–9000; John Duval, Chief Executive Officer

VIRGINIA HOSPITAL CENTER – ARLINGTON, 1701 North George Mason Drive, Arlington, VA, Zip 22205–3698; tel. 703/558–5000; James B. Cole, Chief Executive Officer

WYTHE COUNTY COMMUNITY HOSPITAL, 600 West Ridge Road, Wytheville, VA, Zip 24382–1099; tel. 276/228–0200; Timothy A. Bess, Chief Executive Officer

## WASHINGTON

### GROUP HEALTH COOPERATIVE
**320 Westlake Avenue North, Suite 100, Seattle, WA 98109–5233; tel. 206/448–5083; Scott Armstrong, Chief Executive Officer**

CASCADE VALLEY HOSPITAL AND CLINICS, 330 South Stillaguamish Avenue, Arlington, WA, Zip 98223–1642; tel. 360/435–2133; W. Clark Jones, Administrator

DAYTON GENERAL HOSPITAL, 1012 South Third Street, Dayton, WA, Zip 99328–1696; tel. 509/382–2531; Charles A. Button, Chief Executive Officer

DEACONESS MEDICAL CENTER, 800 West Fifth Avenue, Spokane, WA, Zip 99204–2803, Mailing Address: P.O. Box 248, Zip 99210–0248; tel. 509/458–5800; William L. Gilbert, Chief Executive Officer

GROUP HEALTH COOPERATIVE CENTRAL HOSPITAL, 201 16th Avenue East, Seattle, WA, Zip 98112; tel. 206/326–6300; Jane Hutcheson, Administrator

HARRISON MEDICAL CENTER, 2520 Cherry Avenue, Bremerton, WA, Zip 98310–4229; tel. 360/377–3911; Scott W. Bosch, President and Chief Executive Officer

ISLAND HOSPITAL, 1211 24th Street, Anacortes, WA, Zip 98221–2590; tel. 360/299–1300; Vincent Oliver, Administrator

KADLEC MEDICAL CENTER, 888 Swift Boulevard, Richland, WA, Zip 99352–3514; tel. 509/946–4611; Rand J. Wortman, Chief Executive Officer

KENNEWICK GENERAL HOSPITAL, 900 South Auburn Street, Kennewick, WA, Zip 99336–6128, Mailing Address: P.O. Box 6128, Zip 99336–0128; tel. 509/586–6111; Glen Marshall, Chief Executive Officer

KITTITAS VALLEY COMMUNITY HOSPITAL, 603 South Chestnut Street, Ellensburg, WA, Zip 98926–3875; tel. 509/962–7302; Paul E. Nurick, Chief Executive Officer

KOOTENAI MEDICAL CENTER, 2003 Kootenai Health Way, Coeur D'Alene, ID, Zip 83814–2677; tel. 208/666–2000; Jon Ness, Chief Executive Officer

LOURDES MEDICAL CENTER, 520 North Fourth Avenue, Pasco, WA, Zip 99301–2568, Mailing Address: P.O. Box 2568, Zip 99302–2568; tel. 509/547–7704; John Serle, President and Chief Executive Officer

MULTICARE MARY BRIDGE CHILDREN'S HOSPITAL AND HEALTH CENTER, 317 Martin Luther King Jr. Way, Tacoma, WA, Zip 98405–0299, Mailing Address: P.O. Box 5299, Zip 98415–0299; tel. 253/403–1400; Mady Murrey, R.N., Vice President and Administrator

NORTHWEST SPECIALTY HOSPITAL, 1593 East Polston Avenue, Post Falls, ID, Zip 83854; tel. 208/262–2300; Ron Rock, Chief Executive Officer

OVERLAKE HOSPITAL MEDICAL CENTER, 1035 116th Avenue N.E., Bellevue, WA, Zip 98004–4604; tel. 425/688–5000; Craig L. Hendrickson, President and Chief Executive Officer

PEACEHEALTH ST. JOSEPH MEDICAL CENTER, 2901 Squalicum Parkway, Bellingham, WA, Zip 98225–1851; tel. 360/734–5400; Nancy Steiger, R.N., Chief Executive Officer and Chief Mission Officer

PROSSER MEMORIAL HOSPITAL, 723 Memorial Street, Prosser, WA, Zip 99350–1593; tel. 509/786–2222; Julie Petersen, Chief Executive Officer

PROVIDENCE CENTRALIA HOSPITAL, 914 South Scheuber Road, Centralia, WA, Zip 98531–9027; tel. 360/736–2803; Cindy Mayo, Chief Executive

PROVIDENCE HOLY FAMILY HOSPITAL, 5633 North Lidgerwood Street, Spokane, WA, Zip 99208–1224; tel. 509/482–0111; Elaine Couture, R.N., Chief Executive Officer

PROVIDENCE REGIONAL MEDICAL CENTER EVERETT, 1321 Colby Avenue, Everett, WA, Zip 98206–1147, Mailing Address: P.O. Box 1147, Zip 98206–1147; tel. 425/261–2000; David Brooks, Chief Executive Officer

PROVIDENCE SACRED HEART MEDICAL CENTER & CHILDREN'S HOSPITAL, 101 West Eighth Avenue, Spokane, WA, Zip 99204–2364, Mailing Address: P.O. Box 2555, Zip 99220–2555; tel. 509/474–3131; Elaine Couture, R.N., Chief Executive Officer

PROVIDENCE ST. MARY MEDICAL CENTER, 401 West Poplar Street, Walla Walla, WA, Zip 99362, Mailing Address: P.O. Box 1477, Zip 99362–0312; tel. 509/525–3320; Steven A. Burdick, Chief Executive Officer

PULLMAN REGIONAL HOSPITAL, 835 S.E. Bishop Boulevard, Pullman, WA, Zip 99163–5512; tel. 509/332–2541; Scott K. Adams, Chief Executive Officer

SEATTLE CHILDREN'S HOSPITAL, 4800 Sand Point Way N.E., Seattle, WA, Zip 98105–3901, Mailing Address: P.O. Box 5371, Zip 98145–5005; tel. 206/987–2000; Thomas N. Hansen, M.D., Chief Executive Officer

SKAGIT VALLEY HOSPITAL, 1415 East Kincaid Street, Mount Vernon, WA, Zip 98273, Mailing Address: P.O. Box 1376, Zip 98273–1376; tel. 360/424–4111; Gregg A. Davidson, FACHE, Chief Executive Officer

ST. FRANCIS HOSPITAL, 34515 Ninth Avenue South, Federal Way, WA, Zip 98003–6799; tel. 253/944–8100; Anthony McLean, President

ST. JOSEPH MEDICAL CENTER, 1717 South J Street, Tacoma, WA, Zip 98405–3004, Mailing Address: P.O. Box 2197, Zip 98401–2197; tel. 253/426–4101; Syd Bersante, President

SUNNYSIDE COMMUNITY HOSPITAL, 1016 Tacoma Avenue, Sunnyside, WA, Zip 98944–0719, Mailing Address: P.O. Box 719, Zip 98944–0719; tel. 509/837–1500; Robert L. Brendgard, Interim Chief Executive Officer

TOPPENISH COMMUNITY HOSPITAL, 502 West Fourth Avenue, Toppenish, WA, Zip 98948–0672, Mailing Address: P.O. Box 672, Zip 98948–0672; tel. 509/865–3105; Derrick Yu, Administrator

UNITED GENERAL HOSPITAL, 2000 Hospital Drive, Sedro Woolley, WA, Zip 98284–4327; tel. 360/856–6021; Gregory C. Reed, FACHE, Chief Executive Officer

VALLEY HOSPITAL AND MEDICAL CENTER, 12606 East Mission Avenue, Spokane Valley, WA, Zip 99216–1090; tel. 509/924–6650; Dennis Barts, Chief Executive Officer

VIRGINIA MASON MEDICAL CENTER, 1100 Ninth Avenue, Seattle, WA, Zip 98101–2756, Mailing Address: P.O. Box 900, Zip 98111–0900; tel. 206/223–6600; Gary Kaplan, M.D., Chairman and Chief Executive Officer

WALLA WALLA GENERAL HOSPITAL, 1025 South Second Avenue, Walla Walla, WA, Zip 99362–1398, Mailing Address: P.O. Box 1398, Zip 99362–0309; tel. 509/525–0480; Monty E. Knittel, President and Chief Executive Officer

WHIDBEY GENERAL HOSPITAL, 101 North Main Street, Coupeville, WA, Zip 98239–3413; tel. 360/678–5151; Tom Tomasino, Administrator and Chief Executive Officer

WHITMAN HOSPITAL AND MEDICAL CENTER, 1200 West Fairview Street, Colfax, WA, Zip 99111–9579; tel. 509/397–3435; Deborah Glass, MS, R.N., Chief Executive Officer

YAKIMA REGIONAL MEDICAL AND CARDIAC CENTER, 110 South Ninth Avenue, Yakima, WA, Zip 98902–3397; tel. 509/575–5000; Richard H. Robinson, Chief Executive Officer

YAKIMA VALLEY MEMORIAL HOSPITAL, 2811 Tieton Drive, Yakima, WA, Zip 98902–3761; tel. 509/575–8000; Richard W. Linneweh, Jr., President and Chief Executive Officer

**LINCOLN COUNTY HEALTH DEPARTMENT**
**90 Nichols Street, Davenport, WA 99122–9729; tel. 509/725–1001; Ed Dzedzy, Public Health Administration**

LINCOLN HOSPITAL, 10 Nichols Street, Davenport, WA, Zip 99122–9729; tel. 509/725–7101; Thomas J. Martin, Chief Executive Officer

ODESSA MEMORIAL HEALTHCARE CENTER, 502 East Amende Drive, Odessa, WA, Zip 99159–0368, Mailing Address: P.O. Box 368, Zip 99159–0368; tel. 509/982–2611; Gary L. DelForge, Administrator

## WEST VIRGINIA

**HEALTH PARTNERS NETWORK, INC.**
**1000 Technology Drive, Suite 2320, Fairmont, WV 26554–8834; tel. 304/368–2740; William G. MacLean, Executive Director**

BROADDUS HOSPITAL, 1 Healthcare Drive, Philippi, WV, Zip 26416–1051, Mailing Address: P.O. Box 930, Zip 26416–1051; tel. 304/457–1760; Jeffrey A. Powelson, Chief Executive Officer

CAMDEN–CLARK MEDICAL CENTER, 800 Garfield Avenue, Parkersburg, WV, Zip 26101–5378, Mailing Address: P.O. Box 718, Zip 26102–0718; tel. 304/424–2111; Michael A. King, FACHE, President and Chief Executive Officer

CITY HOSPITAL, 2500 Hospital Drive, Martinsburg, WV, Zip 25401–3402, Mailing Address: P.O. Box 1418, Zip 25402–1418; tel. 304/264–1000; Anthony Zelenka, Chief Administrative Officer

DAVIS MEMORIAL HOSPITAL, Gorman Avenue and Reed Street, Elkins, WV, Zip 26241, Mailing Address: P.O. Box 1484, Zip 26241–1484; tel. 304/636–3300; Mark Doak, President and Chief Executive Officer

FAIRMONT GENERAL HOSPITAL, 1325 Locust Avenue, Fairmont, WV, Zip 26554–1435; tel. 304/367–7100; Robert C. Marquardt, FACHE, President and Chief Executive Officer

GRAFTON CITY HOSPITAL, 500 Market Street, Grafton, WV, Zip 26354–1187; tel. 304/265–0400; Patrick Shaw, Chief Executive Officer

HEALTHSOUTH HUNTINGTON REHABILITATION HOSPITAL, 6900 West Country Club Drive, Huntington, WV, Zip 25705–2000; tel. 304/733–1060; Michael E. Zuliani, Chief Executive Officer

HEALTHSOUTH MOUNTAINVIEW REGIONAL REHABILITATION HOSPITAL, 1160 Van Voorhis Road, Morgantown, WV, Zip 26505–3437; tel. 304/598–1100; Vickie Demers, Chief Executive Officer

HEALTHSOUTH WESTERN HILLS REHABILITATION HOSPITAL, 3 Western Hills Drive, Parkersburg, WV, Zip 26101–8122; tel. 304/420–1300; Alvin R. Lawson, JD, FACHE, Chief Executive Officer

JEFFERSON MEMORIAL HOSPITAL, 300 South Preston Street, Ranson, WV, Zip 25438–1699; tel. 304/728–1600; Christina D. Coad, Ph.D., Chief Administrative Officer

MINNIE HAMILTON HEALTHCARE CENTER, 186 Hospital Drive, Grantsville, WV, Zip 26147; tel. 304/354–9244; Steve Whited, Chief Executive Officer

ST. JOSEPH'S HOSPITAL OF BUCKHANNON, 1 Amalia Drive, Buckhannon, WV, Zip 26201–2222; tel. 304/473–2000; Sue E. Johnson–Phillippe, President and Chief Executive Officer

STONEWALL JACKSON MEMORIAL HOSPITAL, 230 Hospital Plaza, Weston, WV, Zip 26452–8558; tel. 304/269–8000; Avah Stalnaker, Chief Executive Officer

UNITED HOSPITAL CENTER, 327 Medical Park Drive, Bridgeport, WV, Zip 26330–9006; tel. 681/342–1000; Bruce C. Carter, President

WEST VIRGINIA UNIVERSITY HOSPITALS, 1 Medical Center Drive, Morgantown, WV, Zip 26506–4749; tel. 304/598–4000; Bruce McClymonds, President and Chief Executive Officer

**PARTNERS IN HEALTH NETWORK, INC.**
**405 Capitol Street, Suite 505, Charleston, WV 25301–1783; tel. 304/388–7385; Robert D. Whitler, Executive Director**

BOONE MEMORIAL HOSPITAL, 701 Madison Avenue, Madison, WV, Zip 25130–1699; tel. 304/369–1230; Tommy H. Mullins, Administrator

BRAXTON COUNTY MEMORIAL HOSPITAL, 100 Hoylman Drive, Gassaway, WV, Zip 26624–9320; tel. 304/364–5156; Ben Vincent, FACHE, Chief Executive Officer

CAMC TEAYS VALLEY HOSPITAL, 1400 Hospital Drive, Hurricane, WV, Zip 25526–9202; tel. 304/757–1700; Randall H. Hodges, President and Chief Executive Officer

CHARLESTON AREA MEDICAL CENTER, 501 Morris Street, Charleston, WV, Zip 25301–1300, Mailing Address: P.O. Box 1547, Zip 25326–1547; tel. 304/388–5432; David L. Ramsey, President and Chief Executive Officer

EYE AND EAR CLINIC OF CHARLESTON, 1306 Kanawha Boulevard East, Charleston, WV, Zip 25301–3001, Mailing Address: P.O. Box 2271, Zip 25328–2271; tel. 304/343–4371; Christina Arvon, Administrator and Chief Executive Officer

HIGHLAND HOSPITAL, 300 56th Street S.E., Charleston, WV, Zip 25304–2361, Mailing Address: P.O. Box 4107, Zip 25364–4107; tel. 304/926–1600; David M. McWatters, III, President and Chief Executive Officer

JACKSON GENERAL HOSPITAL, 122 Pinnell Street, Ripley, WV, Zip 25271–9101, Mailing Address: P.O. Box 720, Zip 25271–0720; tel. 304/372–2731; Stephanie McCoy, President and Chief Executive Officer

MINNIE HAMILTON HEALTHCARE CENTER, 186 Hospital Drive, Grantsville, WV, Zip 26147; tel. 304/354–9244; Steve Whited, Chief Executive Officer

MONTGOMERY GENERAL HOSPITAL, 401 Sixth Avenue, Montgomery, WV, Zip 25136–0270, Mailing Address: P.O. Box 270, Zip 25136–0270; tel. 304/442–5151; Vickie Gay, Chief Executive Officer

POCAHONTAS MEMORIAL HOSPITAL, Buckeye, WV, Zip 24924; tel. 304/799–7400; Barbara Lay, Chief Executive Officer

ROANE GENERAL HOSPITAL, 200 Hospital Drive, Spencer, WV, Zip 25276–1060; tel. 304/927–4444; Douglas E. Bentz, Chief Executive Officer

STONEWALL JACKSON MEMORIAL HOSPITAL, 230 Hospital Plaza, Weston, WV, Zip 26452–8558; tel. 304/269–8000; Avah Stalnaker, Chief Executive Officer

SUMMERSVILLE REGIONAL MEDICAL CENTER, 400 Fairview Heights Road, Summersville, WV, Zip 26651–0400; tel. 304/872–2891; Deborah A. Hill, R.N., FACHE, Chief Executive Officer

WEBSTER COUNTY MEMORIAL HOSPITAL, 324 Miller Mountain Drive, Webster Springs, WV, Zip 26288–1087, Mailing Address: P.O. Box 312, Zip 26288–0312; tel. 304/847–5682; Annette M. Keenan, Chief Executive Officer

## WISCONSIN

### AFFINITY HEALTH SYSTEM
**1570 Midway Place, Menasha, WI 54952–1165; tel. 920/720–1713; Daniel Neufelder, President and Chief Executive Officer**

CALUMET MEDICAL CENTER, 614 Memorial Drive, Chilton, WI, Zip 53014–1597; tel. 920/849–2386; Timothy Richman, President

MERCY MEDICAL CENTER, 500 South Oakwood Road, Oshkosh, WI, Zip 54904–7944, Mailing Address: P.O. Box 3370, Zip 54903–3370; tel. 920/223–2000; William Calhoun, President

ST. ELIZABETH HOSPITAL, 1506 South Oneida Street, Appleton, WI, Zip 54915–1397; tel. 920/738–2000; Travis Andersen, President

### ASPIRUS, INC.
**425 Pine Ridge Boulevard, Wausau, WI 54401–4123; tel. 715/847–2118; Duane L. Erwin, President and Chief Executive Officer**

ASPIRUS GRAND VIEW HOSPITAL, N10561 Grand View Lane, Ironwood, MI, Zip 49938–9622; tel. 906/932–2525; Carol Goffnett, Chief Executive Officer

ASPIRUS KEWEENAW HOSPITAL, 205 Osceola Street, Laurium, MI, Zip 49913–2134; tel. 906/337–6500; Charles Nelson, Chief Executive Officer

ASPIRUS ONTONAGON HOSPITAL, 601 South Seventh Street, Ontonagon, MI, Zip 49953–1448; tel. 906/884–8000; Michael Hauswirth, Chief Operating Officer

ASPIRUS WAUSAU HOSPITAL, 333 Pine Ridge Boulevard, Wausau, WI, Zip 54401–4187; tel. 715/847–2121; Diane Postler–Slattery, Ph.D., President and Chief Operating Officer

LANGLADE MEMORIAL HOSPITAL, 112 East Fifth Avenue, Antigo, WI, Zip 54409–2796; tel. 715/623–2331; David R. Schneider, Executive Director

MEMORIAL HEALTH CENTER, 135 South Gibson Street, Medford, WI, Zip 54451–1696; tel. 715/748–8100; Gregory A. Olson, President and Chief Executive Officer

### COLUMBIA ST. MARY'S
**2025 East Newport Avenue, Milwaukee, WI 53211–2906; tel. 414/961–3300; Mark R. Taylor, FACHE, President and Chief Executive Officer**

COLUMBIA ST. MARY'S HOSPITAL MILWAUKEE, 2301 North Lake Drive, Milwaukee, WI, Zip 53211–4508; tel. 414/291–1000; Mark R. Taylor, FACHE, President and Chief Executive Officer

COLUMBIA ST. MARY'S OZAUKEE HOSPITAL, 13111 North Port Washington Road, Mequon, WI, Zip 53097–2416; tel. 262/243–7300; Deborah G. Friberg, President

SACRED HEART REHABILITATION INSTITUTE, 2025 East Newport Avenue, Milwaukee, WI, Zip 53211–2906; tel. 414/298–6700; Deborah G. Friberg, President

### COMMUNITY HEALTH NETWORK, INC.
**225 Memorial Drive, Berlin, WI 54923–1243; tel. 920/361–5580; John Feeney, President and Chief Executive Officer**

BERLIN MEMORIAL HOSPITAL, 225 Memorial Drive, Berlin, WI, Zip 54923–1295; tel. 920/361–1313; John Feeney, President and Chief Executive Officer

WILD ROSE COMMUNITY MEMORIAL HOSPITAL, 601 Grove Avenue, Wild Rose, WI, Zip 54984, Mailing Address: P.O. Box 243, Zip 54984–0243; tel. 920/622–3257; Donald Caves, President

### GUNDERSON LUTHERAN HEALTH SYSTEM
**1900 South Avenue, La Crosse, WI 54601–5467; tel. 608/782–7300; Jeffrey E. Thompson, M.D., Chief Executive Officer**

GUNDERSEN LUTHERAN MEDICAL CENTER, 1900 South Avenue, La Crosse, WI, Zip 54601–9980; tel. 608/782–7300; Jeffrey E. Thompson, M.D., Chief Executive Officer

PALMER LUTHERAN HEALTH CENTER, 112 Jefferson Street, West Union, IA, Zip 52175–1022; tel. 563/422–3811; Debrah Chensvold, FACHE, President and Chief Executive Officer

TRI–COUNTY MEMORIAL HOSPITAL, 18601 Lincoln Street, Whitehall, WI, Zip 54773–8605; tel. 715/538–4361; Brian Theiler, President and Chief Executive Officer

### MERCY ALLIANCE, INC.
**1000 Mineral Point Avenue, Janesville, WI 53548–2940; tel. 608/756–6000; Javon R. Bea, President and Chief Executive Officer**

MERCY HARVARD HOSPITAL, 901 Grant Street, Harvard, IL, Zip 60033–1898, Mailing Address: P.O. Box 850, Zip 60033–0850; tel. 815/943–5431; Jennifer Hallatt, Chief Operating Officer

MERCY HOSPITAL AND TRAUMA CENTER, 1000 Mineral Point Avenue, Janesville, WI, Zip 53547–2982, Mailing Address: P.O. Box 5003, Zip 53547–5003; tel. 608/756–6000; Javon R. Bea, President and Chief Executive Officer

MERCY WALWORTH HOSPITAL AND MEDICAL CENTER, N2950 State Road 67, Lake Geneva, WI, Zip 53147; tel. 262/245–0535; Jennifer Hallatt, Administrator

### MINISTRY HEALTH CARE
**11925 West Lake Park Drive, Milwaukee, WI 53224–3002; tel. 414/359–1060; Nicholas Desien, President and Chief Executive Officer**

CALUMET MEDICAL CENTER, 614 Memorial Drive, Chilton, WI, Zip 53014–1597; tel. 920/849–2386; Timothy Richman, President

EAGLE RIVER MEMORIAL HOSPITAL, 201 Hospital Road, Eagle River, WI, Zip 54521–8835; tel. 715/479–7411; Sheila Clough, President

FLAMBEAU HOSPITAL, 98 Sherry Avenue, Park Falls, WI, Zip 54552–1467, Mailing Address: P.O. Box 310, Zip 54552–0310; tel. 715/762–2484; David A. Grundstrom, Chief Administrative Officer

HOWARD YOUNG MEDICAL CENTER, 240 Maple Street, Woodruff, WI, Zip 54568, Mailing Address: P.O. Box 470, Zip 54568–0470; tel. 715/356–8000; Sheila Clough, President

MERCY MEDICAL CENTER, 500 South Oakwood Road, Oshkosh, WI, Zip 54904–7944, Mailing Address: P.O. Box 3370, Zip 54903–3370; tel. 920/223–2000; William Calhoun, President

MINISTRY DOOR COUNTY MEDICAL CENTER, 323 South 18th Avenue, Sturgeon Bay, WI, Zip 54235–1495; tel. 920/743–5566; Gerald M. Worrick, President and Chief Executive Officer

MINISTRY GOOD SAMARITAN HEALTH CENTER, 601 South Center Avenue, Merrill, WI, Zip 54452–3404; tel. 715/536–5511; Kristine McGarigle, President

MINISTRY SAINT MICHAEL'S HOSPITAL, 900 Illinois Avenue, Stevens Point, WI, Zip 54481–3196; tel. 715/346–5000; Jeffrey L. Martin, President

OUR LADY OF VICTORY HOSPITAL, 1120 Pine Street, Stanley, WI, Zip 54768–0220; tel. 715/644–5571; Cynthia Eichman, President

SACRED HEART HOSPITAL, 401 West Mohawk Drive, Tomahawk, WI, Zip 54487; tel. 715/453–7700; Monica Hilt, President

SACRED HEART–ST. MARY'S HOSPITALS, 2251 North Shore Drive, Rhinelander, WI, Zip 54501–3998; tel. 715/361–2000; Monica Hilt, President and Chief Operating Officer

SAINT CLARE'S HOSPITAL, 3400 Ministry Parkway, Weston, WI, Zip 54476; tel. 715/393–3000; Mary T. Krueger, President

SAINT ELIZABETH'S MEDICAL CENTER, 1200 Grant Boulevard West, Wabasha, MN, Zip 55981–1042; tel. 651/565–4531; Thomas Crowley, President and Chief Executive Officer

SAINT JOSEPH'S HOSPITAL, 611 St. Joseph Avenue, Marshfield, WI, Zip 54449–1898; tel. 715/387–1713; Brian Kief, President and Chief Executive Officer

ST. ELIZABETH HOSPITAL, 1506 South Oneida Street, Appleton, WI, Zip 54915–1397; tel. 920/738–2000; Travis Andersen, President

### WHEATON FRANCISCAN HEALTHCARE
**400 West River Woods Parkway, Glendale, WI 53212–1060; tel. 414/465–3000; John D. Oliverio, President and Chief Executive Officer**

WHEATON FRANCISCAN HEALTHCARE – ALL SAINTS, 3801 Spring Street, Racine, WI, Zip 53405–1690; tel. 262/687–4011; Kenneth R. Buser, President and Chief Executive Officer

WHEATON FRANCISCAN HEALTHCARE – ELMBROOK MEMORIAL, 19333 West North Avenue, Brookfield, WI, Zip 53045–4198; tel. 262/785–2000; Debra K. Standridge, President

WHEATON FRANCISCAN HEALTHCARE – ST. FRANCIS, 3237 South 16th Street, Milwaukee, WI, Zip 53215–4592; tel. 414/647–5000; Daniel Mattes, President

WHEATON FRANCISCAN HEALTHCARE – ST. JOSEPH'S, 5000 West Chambers Street, Milwaukee, WI, Zip 53210–9988; tel. 414/447–2000; Debra K. Standridge, President

WHEATON FRANCISCAN HEALTHCARE – THE WISCONSIN HEART HOSPITAL, 10000 West Bluemound Road, Wauwatosa, WI, Zip 53226; tel. 414/778–7800; Debra K. Standridge, President

# Alliances

**ALLIANCE OF INDEPENDENT ACADEMIC MEDICAL CENTERS**
233 East Erie Street, Ste 306, Chicago, IL Zip 60611; tel. 312/988–7572; Nancie Noie Thompson, Executive Director

## ARIZONA
**Phoenix**
Member
Maricopa Integrated Health System
St. Joseph's Hospital and Medical Center

**Scottsdale**
Member
Scottsdale Healthcare

## CONNECTICUT
**Hartford**
Member
Mount Sinai Rehabilitation Hospital
Saint Francis Hospital and Medical Center

## DELAWARE
**Wilmington**
Member
Christiana Care Health System

## DISTRICT OF COLUMBIA
**Washington**
Member
Medstar National Rehabilitation Network
Medstar Washington Hospital Center

## FLORIDA
**Miami Beach**
Member
Mount Sinai Medical Center

**Orlando**
Member
Florida Hospital
Orlando Regional Medical Center

## ILLINOIS
**Chicago**
Member
Advocate Illinois Masonic Medical Center

**Oak Lawn**
Member
Advocate Christ Medical Center

**Park Ridge**
Member
Advocate Lutheran General Hospital

**Peoria**
Member
OSF Saint Francis Medical Center

## IOWA
**Des Moines**
Member
Iowa Health System

## KENTUCKY
**Louisville**
Member
Norton Healthcare

## LOUISIANA
**New Orleans**
Member
Ochsner Health System

## MAINE
**Portland**
Member
Maine Medical Center

## MARYLAND
**Baltimore**
Sinai Hospital of Baltimore
Member
Medstar Franklin Square Medical Center
Medstar Good Samaritan Hospital
Medstar Harbor Hospital
Medstar Union Memorial Hospital

**Bethesda**
Member
National Institutes of Health Clinical Center

**Columbia**
Member
MedStar Health

## MASSACHUSETTS
**Burlington**
Member
Lahey Clinic Hospital

**Pittsfield**
Member
Berkshire Medical Center

**Springfield**
Member
Baystate Health, Inc.

## MICHIGAN
**Detroit**
Member
Henry Ford Health System

**Grand Rapids**
Member
Spectrum Health

**Royal Oak**
Member
Beaumont Hospital – Royal Oak

## MINNESOTA
**Bloomington**
Member
HealthPartners

## MISSOURI
**Saint Louis**
Member
Mercy Hospital St. Louis

## NEW JERSEY
**Livingston**
Member
Saint Barnabas Medical Center

**Long Branch**
Member
Monmouth Medical Center

**Morristown**
Member
Morristown Medical Center

**Newark**
Member
Newark Beth Israel Medical Center

**Summit**
Member
Overlook Medical Center

## NEW YORK
**Brooklyn**
Member
Maimonides Medical Center

**Mineola**
Member
Winthrop–University Hospital

## NORTH CAROLINA
**Charlotte**
Member
Carolinas Medical Center

## OHIO
**Akron**
Member
Akron General Medical Center

**Cincinnati**
Member
TriHealth

**Columbus**
Member
Grant Medical Center
Riverside Methodist Hospital

## PENNSYLVANIA
**Bethlehem**
Member
St. Luke's University Hospital – Bethlehem Campus

**Danville**
Member
Geisinger Medical Center

**Gettysburg**
Member
Gettysburg Hospital

**Philadelphia**
Member
Einstein Medical Center Philadelphia

**Sayre**
Member
Robert Packer Hospital

**West Reading**
Member
Reading Hospital and Medical Center

**Wilkes Barre**
Member
Geisinger Wyoming Valley Medical Center

**York**
Member
York Hospital

## SOUTH DAKOTA
**Sioux Falls**
Member
Sanford Health

## TEXAS
**Dallas**
Member
Baylor Health Care System
Parkland Health & Hospital System

**Fort Worth**
Member
JPS Health Network

## WASHINGTON
**Seattle**
Member
Virginia Mason Medical Center

## WISCONSIN
**Milwaukee**
Member
Aurora Sinai Medical Center
Aurora St. Luke's Medical Center

**CATHOLIC CEO HEALTHCARE CONNECTION**
3333 Warrenville Rd, Ste 200, Lisle, IL Zip 60532; tel. 630/799–8315; Roger N. Butler, Executive Director

## CALIFORNIA
**Orange**
Member
St. Joseph Health

**San Francisco**
Member
Dignity Health

## COLORADO
**Denver**
Shareholder
Sisters of Charity of Leavenworth Health System

**Englewood**
Member
Catholic Health Initiatives

## ILLINOIS
**Springfield**
Member
Hospital Sisters Health System

**Wheaton**
Member
Wheaton Franciscan Healthcare

## KANSAS

**Wichita**
Member
  Via Christi Health

## LOUISIANA

**Baton Rouge**
Member
  Franciscan Missionaries of Our Lady Health System, Inc.

## MARYLAND

**Marriottsville**
Member
  Bon Secours Health System, Inc.

## MASSACHUSETTS

**Tewksbury**
Member
  Covenant Health Systems, Inc.

## MICHIGAN

**Novi**
Member
  Trinity Health

## MISSOURI

**Chesterfield**
Member
  Mercy Health

**Saint Louis**
Member
  Ascension Health

## OHIO

**Cincinnati**
Member
  Catholic Health Partners

**Toledo**
Member
  Sylvania Franciscan Health

## PENNSYLVANIA

**Newtown Square**
Member
  Catholic Health East

## SOUTH DAKOTA

**Sioux Falls**
Member
  Avera Health

## TEXAS

**Irving**
Member
  CHRISTUS Health

## WASHINGTON

**Bellevue**
Member
  PeaceHealth

**Renton**
Member
  Providence Health & Services

## WISCONSIN

**Manitowoc**
Member
  Franciscan Sisters of Christian Charity Sponsored Ministries, Inc.

## COMMUNITY HEALTH COLLABORATIVE, LLC

630 East River Street, Elyria, OH
Zip 44035–5902; tel. 440/329–7500;
Frank L. Lordeman, President and Chief
Executive Officer

## OHIO

**Elyria**
Member
  EMH Elyria Medical Center

**Middleburg Heights**
Member
  Southwest General Health Center

**Parma**
Member
  Parma Community General Hospital

## HOSPITAL NETWORK VENTURES, LLC

6212 American Avenue, Portage, MI
Zip 49002; tel. 269/329–3200; Gregory
L. Hedegore, President and Chief
Executive Officer

## MICHIGAN

**Allegan**
Networks
  Allegan General Hospital
Partner
  Allegan General Hospital

**Big Rapids**
Partner
  Mecosta County Medical Center

**Charlotte**
Partner
  Hayes Green Beach Memorial Hospital

**Chelsea**
Partner
  Chelsea Community Hospital

**Coldwater**
Partner
  Community Health Center of Branch County

**Hastings**
Networks
  Pennock Hospital
Partner
  Pennock Hospital

**Kalamazoo**
Member
  Bronson Methodist Hospital
Networks
  Bronson Methodist Hospital
Partner
  Bronson Healthcare Group, Inc.

**Marlette**
Partner
  Marlette Regional Hospital

**Marshall**
Networks
  Oaklawn Hospital
Partner
  Oaklawn Hospital

**Owosso**
Partner
  Memorial Healthcare

**Paw Paw**
Member
  Bronson LakeView Hospital

**Saint Joseph**
Partner
  Lakeland Healthcare

**South Haven**
Member
  South Haven Health System

**Sturgis**
Networks
  Sturgis Hospital
Partner
  Sturgis Hospital

**Vicksburg**
Member
  Bronson Vicksburg Hospital

**Watervliet**
Partner
  Lakeland Community Hospital Watervliet

## MEDI–SOTA, INC.

1280 Locust Street Suite 16, Dawson,
MN Zip 56232–2375;
tel. 320/769–2269; Deb Ranallo,
Executive Director

## MINNESOTA

**Appleton**
Member
  Appleton Area Health Services
Networks
  Appleton Area Health Services

**Arlington**
Member
  Sibley Medical Center
Networks
  Sibley Medical Center

**Benson**
Member
  Swift County–Benson Hospital
Networks
  Swift County–Benson Hospital

**Canby**
Member
  Sanford Medical Center Canby
Networks
  Sanford Medical Center Canby

**Dawson**
Member
  Johnson Memorial Health Services
Networks
  Johnson Memorial Health Services

**Elbow Lake**
Networks
  Prairie Ridge Hospital and Health Services

**Glencoe**
Member
  Glencoe Regional Health Services
Networks
  Glencoe Regional Health Services

**Glenwood**
Member
  Glacial Ridge Health System
Networks
  Glacial Ridge Health System

**Graceville**
Member
  Essentia Health–Holy Trinity Hospital
Networks
  Essentia Health–Holy Trinity Hospital

**Granite Falls**
Member
  Granite Falls Municipal Hospital and Manor
Networks
  Granite Falls Municipal Hospital and Manor

**Hendricks**
Member
  Hendricks Community Hospital
Networks
  Hendricks Community Hospital

**Litchfield**
Member
  Meeker Memorial Hospital
Networks
  Meeker Memorial Hospital

**Long Prairie**
Networks
  CentraCare Health System – Long Prairie

**Madelia**
Member
  Madelia Community Hospital
Networks
  Madelia Community Hospital

**Mahnomen**
Member
  Mahnomen Health Center
Networks
  Mahnomen Health Center

**Marshall**
Member
  Avera Marshall Regional Medical Center
Networks
  Avera Marshall Regional Medical Center

**Montevideo**
Member
  Chippewa County–Montevideo Hospital
Networks
  Chippewa County–Montevideo Hospital

**Olivia**
Member
  RC Hospital and Clinics
Networks
  RC Hospital and Clinics

**Ortonville**
Member
  Ortonville Area Health Services
Networks
  Ortonville Area Health Services

**Paynesville**
Member
  Paynesville Area Health Care System
Networks
  Paynesville Area Health Care System

**Perham**
Member
  Perham Health
Networks
  Perham Health

**Pipestone**
Member
  Pipestone County Medical Center Avera
Networks
  Pipestone County Medical Center Avera

**Redwood Falls**
Member
  Redwood Area Hospital
Networks
  Redwood Area Hospital

**Saint Peter**
Member
  River's Edge Hospital and Clinic
Networks
  River's Edge Hospital and Clinic

**Slayton**
Member
  Murray County Medical Center
Networks
  Murray County Medical Center

**Sleepy Eye**
Member
  Sleepy Eye Medical Center
Networks
  Sleepy Eye Medical Center

**Tracy**
Member
  Sanford Tracy Medical Center
Networks
  Sanford Tracy Medical Center

**Tyler**
Member
  Tyler Healthcare Center Avera
Networks
  Tyler Healthcare Center Avera

**Wadena**
Member
  Tri–County Hospital
Networks
  Tri–County Hospital

**Willmar**
Member
  Rice Memorial Hospital
Networks
  Rice Memorial Hospital

**Windom**
Member
  Windom Area Hospital
Networks
  Windom Area Hospital

**SOUTH DAKOTA**

**Watertown**
Member
  Prairie Lakes Healthcare System

## NORTH REGION HEALTH ALLIANCE
120 East Bridge Avenue, Warren, MN
Zip 56762; tel. 218/745–5343; Jon E.
Linnell, Chief Executive Officer

**MINNESOTA**

**Ada**
Member
  Essentia Health Ada

**Bagley**
Member
  Sanford Bagley Medical Center

**Baudette**
Member
  LakeWood Health Center

**Crookston**
Member
  RiverView Health

**Fosston**
Member
  Essentia Health Fosston

**Hallock**
Member
  Kittson Memorial Healthcare Center

**Roseau**
Member
  LifeCare Medical Center

**Thief River Falls**
Member
  Sanford Medical Center Thief River Falls

**Warren**
Member
  North Valley Health Center

## NORTH DAKOTA

**Cavalier**
Member
  Pembina County Memorial Hospital and Wedgewood
    Manor

**Cooperstown**
Member
  Cooperstown Medical Center

**Devils Lake**
Member
  Mercy Hospital

**Grafton**
Member
  Unity Medical Center

**Grand Forks**
Member
  Altru Health System

**Hillsboro**
Member
  Hillsboro Medical Center

**Langdon**
Member
  Cavalier County Memorial Hospital

**Mayville**
Member
  Sanford Medical Center Mayville

**McVille**
Member
  Nelson County Health System

**Northwood**
Member
  Sanford Northwood Deaconess Health Center

**Park River**
Member
  First Care Health Center

## NORTHWEST KANSAS HEALTH ALLIANCE
2220 Canterbury Drive, Hays, KS
Zip 67601–2370; tel. 785/623–2300

**KANSAS**

**Atwood**
  Rawlins County Health Center

**Colby**
  Citizens Medical Center

**Dighton**
  Lane County Hospital

**Greensburg**
  Kiowa County Memorial Hospital

**Hill City**
  Graham County Hospital

**Hoisington**
  Clara Barton Hospital

**Hoxie**
  Sheridan County Health Complex

**Kinsley**
  Edwards County Hospital and Healthcare Center

**La Crosse**
  Rush County Memorial Hospital

**Larned**
  Pawnee Valley Community Hospital

**Minneola**
  Minneola District Hospital

**Ness City**
  Ness County Hospital

**Norton**
  Norton County Hospital

**Oakley**
  Logan County Hospital

**Phillipsburg**
  Phillips County Hospital

**Plainville**
  Rooks County Health Center

**Quinter**
  Gove County Medical Center

**Ransom**
  Grisell Memorial Hospital District One

**Russell**
  Russell Regional Hospital

**Saint Francis**
  Cheyenne County Hospital

**Scott City**
  Scott County Hospital

**Smith Center**
  Smith County Memorial Hospital

**Wakeeney**
  Trego County–Lemke Memorial Hospital

## PENNANT HEALTH ALLIANCE
2122 Health Drive SW Suite 100,
Wyoming, MI Zip 49519–9698;
tel. 616/252–6800; Michael D. Faas,
Chief Executive Officer

**MICHIGAN**

**Ann Arbor**
Member
  University of Michigan Hospitals and Health Centers

**Battle Creek**
Member
  Bronson Battle Creek

**Cadillac**
Member
  Mercy Hospital Cadillac

**Grand Rapids**
Member
  Saint Mary's Health Care

**Grayling**
Member
  Mercy Hospital Grayling

**Muskegon**
Member
  Mercy Health Partners, Hackley Campus
  Mercy Health Partners, Mercy Campus

**Novi**
Member
  Trinity Health

**Shelby**
Member
  Mercy Health Partners, Lakeshore Campus

**Wyoming**
Member
  Metro Health Hospital

## PREMIER, INC.
13034 Ballantyne Corporate Place,
Charlotte, NC Zip 28277–1498;
tel. 704/816–5353; Susan DeVore,
President and Chief Executive Officer

**ALABAMA**

**Dothan**
Owner
  Southeast Alabama Medical Center

**Opelika**
Owner
  East Alabama Medical Center

## ALASKA

**Fairbanks**
Member
   Fairbanks Memorial Hospital

**Ketchikan**
Member
   PeaceHealth Ketchikan Medical Center

## ARIZONA

**Chandler**
   Chandler Regional Medical Center

**Gilbert**
   Mercy Gilbert Medical Center

**Glendale**
   Banner Thunderbird Medical Center

**Mesa**
   Banner Desert Medical Center
   Banner Heart Hospital
Member
   Banner Baywood Medical Center

**Page**
   Page Hospital

**Phoenix**
   Banner Estrella Medical Center
   Banner Good Samaritan Medical Center
   St. Joseph's Hospital and Medical Center
Owner
   Banner Health

**Scottsdale**
   Banner Behavioral Health Hospital – Scottsdale

**Sun City**
   Banner Boswell Medical Center

**Sun City West**

   Banner Del E. Webb Medical Center

## ARKANSAS

**Pine Bluff**
Owner
   Jefferson Regional Medical Center

## CALIFORNIA

**Arroyo Grande**
Member
   Arroyo Grande Community Hospital

**Bakersfield**
   Bakersfield Memorial Hospital
   Mercy Hospitals of Bakersfield
Member
   San Joaquin Community Hospital

**Camarillo**
   St. John's Pleasant Valley Hospital

**Carmichael**
   Mercy San Juan Medical Center

**Chula Vista**
Member
   Sharp Chula Vista Medical Center

**Clearlake**
Member
   St. Helena Hospital Clearlake

**Coronado**
Member
   Sharp Coronado Hospital and Healthcare Center

**Daly City**
   Seton Medical Center

**Folsom**
   Mercy Hospital of Folsom

**Gilroy**
   Saint Louise Regional Hospital

**Glendale**
Member
   Glendale Adventist Medical Center
   Glendale Memorial Hospital and Health Center

**Grass Valley**
   Sierra Nevada Memorial Hospital

**Hanford**
   Central Valley General Hospital
Member
   Hanford Community Medical Center

**La Mesa**
Member
   Sharp Grossmont Hospital

**Long Beach**
   St. Mary Medical Center

**Los Altos Hills**
   Daughters of Charity Health System

**Los Angeles**
   St. Vincent Medical Center
Member
   California Hospital Medical Center
   White Memorial Medical Center

**Lynwood**
   St. Francis Medical Center

**Merced**
   Mercy Medical Center Merced

**Moss Beach**
   Seton Medical Center Coastside

**Mount Shasta**
   Mercy Medical Center Mount Shasta

**Northridge**
Member
   Northridge Hospital Medical Center–Roscoe Boulevard
     Campus

**Oakdale**
   Oak Valley Hospital District

**Oceanside**
   Tri–City Medical Center

**Orange**
Owner
   St. Joseph Health

**Oxnard**
   St. John's Regional Medical Center

**Paradise**
Member
   Feather River Hospital

**Rancho Mirage**
Owner
   Eisenhower Medical Center

**Red Bluff**
   St. Elizabeth Community Hospital

**Redding**
   Mercy Medical Center Redding

**Redwood City**
   Sequoia Hospital

**Roseville**
Owner
   Adventist Health

**Sacramento**
   Mercy General Hospital
   Methodist Hospital of Sacramento

**Saint Helena**
Member
   St. Helena Hospital

**San Andreas**
   Mark Twain St. Joseph's Hospital

**San Bernardino**
   Community Hospital of San Bernardino
   St. Bernardine Medical Center

**San Diego**
Member
   Sharp Memorial Hospital
Owner
   Palomar Health
   Sharp HealthCare

**San Francisco**
   Saint Francis Memorial Hospital
   St. Mary's Medical Center
Owner
   Dignity Health

**San Gabriel**
Member
   San Gabriel Valley Medical Center

**San Jose**
   O'Connor Hospital

**San Luis Obispo**
Member
   French Hospital Medical Center

**Santa Cruz**
   Dominican Hospital

**Santa Maria**
   Marian Medical Center

**Simi Valley**
Member
   Simi Valley Hospital and Health Care Services

**Sonora**
Member
   Sonora Regional Medical Center

**Stockton**
   St. Joseph's Behavioral Health Center
   St. Joseph's Medical Center

**Susanville**
Member
   Banner Lassen Medical Center

**Ukiah**
Member
   Ukiah Valley Medical Center

**Vallejo**
Member
   St. Helena Hospital–Center for Behavioral Health

**Willits**
Member
   Frank R. Howard Memorial Hospital

**Woodland**
   Woodland Healthcare

## COLORADO

**Brush**
Member
   East Morgan County Hospital

**Denver**
   Porter Adventist Hospital

**Greeley**
Member
   North Colorado Medical Center

**Littleton**
   Littleton Adventist Hospital

**Louisville**
   Avista Adventist Hospital

**Loveland**
Member
   McKee Medical Center

**Parker**
   Parker Adventist Hospital

**Sterling**
Member
   Sterling Regional MedCenter

## CONNECTICUT

**Hartford**
Owner
   Saint Francis Hospital and Medical Center

**New Haven**
Member
   Hospital of Saint Raphael

**Waterbury**
   Saint Mary's Hospital

## DELAWARE

**Dover**
Owner
   Bayhealth Medical Center

**Lewes**
Owner
   Beebe Medical Center

**Wilmington**
Member
   Alfred I. duPont Hospital for Children

## DISTRICT OF COLUMBIA

**Washington**
Owner
   Sibley Memorial Hospital

## FLORIDA

**Altamonte Springs**
Owner
   Adventist Health System Sunbelt Health Care
     Corporation

**Clearwater**
   Morton Plant Hospital

**Coral Gables**
   Baptist Health South Florida, Doctors Hospital
Owner
   Baptist Health South Florida

**Coral Springs**
Member
   Broward Health Coral Springs

**Daytona Beach**
Member
  Florida Hospital Memorial Medical Center

**Deerfield Beach**
Member
  Broward Health North

**DeLand**
Member
  Florida Hospital DeLand

**Dunedin**
Member
  Mease Hospital Dunedin

**Fernandina Beach**
Member
  Baptist Medical Center Nassau

**Fort Lauderdale**
Member
  Broward Health Imperial Point
  Broward Health Medical Center
Owner
  Broward Health

**Hollywood**
Member
  Memorial Regional Hospital

**Homestead**
Member
  Baptist Health South Florida, Homestead Hospital

**Jacksonville**
  Baptist Health
  Baptist Medical Center

**Jacksonville Beach**
Member
  Baptist Medical Center Beaches

**Miami**
Member
  Baptist Health South Florida, Baptist Hospital of Miami
  Baptist Health South Florida, South Miami Hospital

**Miami Beach**
Owner
  Mount Sinai Medical Center

**Miramar**
  Memorial Hospital Miramar

**Naples**
Owner
  NCH Downtown Naples Hospital

**New Port Richey**
Member
  Morton Plant North Bay Hospital

**Orange City**
Member
  Florida Hospital Fish Memorial

**Orlando**
Member
  Florida Hospital

**Palm Coast**
Member
  Florida Hospital–Flagler

**Pembroke Pines**
Member
  Memorial Hospital Pembroke
  Memorial Hospital West

**Plant City**
Member
  South Florida Baptist Hospital

**Safety Harbor**
Member
  Mease Countryside Hospital

**Saint Petersburg**
Member
  Bayfront Medical Center
  St. Anthony's Hospital

**Sebring**
Member
  Florida Hospital Heartland Medical Center

**Tampa**
Member
  H. Lee Moffitt Cancer Center and Research Institute
  St. Joseph's Hospital

**Tavares**
Member
  Florida Hospital Waterman

**Tavernier**
Member
  Baptist Health South Florida, Mariners Hospital

**Vero Beach**
Owner
  Indian River Medical Center

**Wauchula**
  Florida Hospital Wauchula

**Weston**
Member
  Cleveland Clinic Florida

**Winter Haven**
Owner
  Winter Haven Hospital

**Zephyrhills**
Member
  Florida Hospital Zephyrhills

## GEORGIA
**Brunswick**
  Southeast Georgia Health System
Member
  Southeast Georgia Health System Brunswick Campus

**Calhoun**
Member
  Gordon Hospital

**Columbus**
Owner
  St. Francis Hospital

**Fort Oglethorpe**
Owner
  Erlanger at Hutcheson

**La Grange**
Owner
  West Georgia Health

**Saint Marys**
Member
  Southeast Georgia Health System Camden Campus

**Savannah**
Owner
  Candler Hospital
  Memorial Health

**Smyrna**
Member
  Emory–Adventist Hospital

## HAWAII
**Honolulu**
Owner
  Kuakini Medical Center

**Kailua**
  Castle Medical Center

**Kamuela**
  North Hawaii Community Hospital

## IDAHO
**Coeur D'Alene**
  Kootenai Medical Center

**Moscow**
Member
  Gritman Medical Center

**Post Falls**
  Northwest Specialty Hospital

## ILLINOIS
**Arlington Heights**
  Alexian Brothers Health System

**Centralia**
Member
  St. Mary's Hospital

**Chicago**
  Presence Health
  Saint Joseph Hospital
  Saints Mary & Elizabeth Medical Center
  Schwab Rehabilitation Hospital
  Sinai Health System
Member
  Our Lady of the Resurrection Medical Center
  Resurrection Medical Center
Owner
  Mercy Hospital and Medical Center
  Mount Sinai Hospital

**Des Plaines**
  Holy Family Medical Center

**Elk Grove Village**
Member
  Alexian Brothers Medical Center

**Evanston**
  Saint Francis Hospital

**Glendale Heights**
  Adventist GlenOaks Hospital

**Hinsdale**
Member
  Adventist Hinsdale Hospital

**Hoffman Estates**
  Alexian Brothers Behavioral Health Hospital
  St. Alexius Medical Center

**La Grange**
  Adventist La Grange Memorial Hospital

**Melrose Park**
Member
  Gottlieb Memorial Hospital

**Mount Vernon**
Member
  Good Samaritan Regional Health Center

**Urbana**
Owner
  Carle Foundation Hospital

**Winfield**
Owner
  Central DuPage Hospital

## INDIANA
**Gary**
Owner
  Methodist Hospitals

**Princeton**
Member
  Gibson General Hospital

## IOWA
**Ames**
Member
  Mary Greeley Medical Center

**Charles City**
Member
  Floyd County Medical Center

**Corning**
Member
  Alegent Health Mercy Hospital

**Council Bluffs**
Member
  Alegent Health–Mercy Hospital

**Davenport**
Member
  Genesis Medical Center–Davenport

**De Witt**
Member
  Genesis Medical Center, DeWitt

**Estherville**
Member
  Avera Holy Family Hospital

**Fairfield**
Member
  Jefferson County Health Center

**Iowa City**
Member
  Mercy Iowa City

**Le Mars**
  Floyd Valley Hospital

**Manchester**
Member
  Regional Medical Center

**Maquoketa**
Member
  Jackson County Regional Health Center

**Marshalltown**
Member
  Marshalltown Medical & Surgical Center

**Missouri Valley**
Owner
  Alegent Health–Community Memorial Hospital

**Mount Pleasant**
  Henry County Health Center

**Newton**
Member
Skiff Medical Center

**Oskaloosa**
Member
Mahaska Health Partnership

**Ottumwa**
Member
Ottumwa Regional Health Center

**Pella**
Member
Pella Regional Health Center

**Rock Valley**
Member
Hegg Memorial Health Center Avera

**Sibley**
Member
Osceola Community Hospital

**Sioux Center**
Sioux Center Community Hospital and Health Center Avera

**West Burlington**
Member
Great River Medical Center

## KENTUCKY

**Ashland**
King's Daughters Medical Center
Our Lady of Bellefonte Hospital

**Bowling Green**
Commonwealth Regional Specialty Hospital

**Corbin**
Member
Baptist Regional Medical Center

**Danville**
Ephraim McDowell Regional Medical Center

**Edgewood**
St. Elizabeth Edgewood

**Elizabethtown**
Member
Hardin Memorial Hospital

**Glasgow**
Owner
T. J. Samson Community Hospital

**Henderson**
Owner
Methodist Hospital

**Irvine**
Member
Marcum and Wallace Memorial Hospital

**La Grange**
Member
Baptist Hospital Northeast

**Lexington**
Member
Central Baptist Hospital

**Louisville**
Norton Audubon Hospital
Norton Brownsboro Hospital
Norton Suburban Hospital

Norton Hospital
Member
Baptist Hospital East
University of Louisville Hospital
Owner
Baptist Healthcare System
Norton Healthcare

**Madisonville**
Regional Medical Center of Hopkins County

**Manchester**
Member
Manchester Memorial Hospital

**Murray**
Owner
Murray–Calloway County Hospital

**Paducah**
Member
Lourdes Hospital
Western Baptist Hospital

**Salem**
Member
Livingston Hospital and Healthcare Services

## LOUISIANA

**Baton Rouge**
Baton Rouge General Medical Center
Member
Woman's Hospital

**Columbia**
Caldwell Memorial Hospital

**Hammond**
Member
North Oaks Medical Center

**Houma**
Owner
Terrebonne General Medical Center

**Lafayette**
Owner
Lafayette General Medical Center

**Marrero**
Owner
West Jefferson Medical Center

**New Orleans**
Owner
Touro Infirmary

**West Monroe**
Owner
Glenwood Regional Medical Center

**Zachary**
Lane Regional Medical Center

## MAINE

**Bangor**
St. Joseph Hospital

## MARYLAND

**Annapolis**
Owner
Anne Arundel Medical Center

**Baltimore**
Greater Baltimore Medical Center
Member
Bon Secours Baltimore Health System
Mercy Medical Center
Sinai Hospital of Baltimore

**Bethesda**
Owner
Suburban Hospital

**Columbia**
Owner
Howard County General Hospital

**Elkton**
Owner
Union Hospital

**Frederick**
Owner
Frederick Memorial Hospital

**Hagerstown**
Owner
Meritus Medical Center

**La Plata**
Civista Health

**Lanham**
Owner
Doctors Community Hospital

**Marriottsville**
Owner
Bon Secours Health System, Inc.

**Olney**
Owner
Medstar Montgomery Medical Center

**Randallstown**
Member
Northwest Hospital

**Rockville**
Adventist Behavioral Health Rockville
Adventist Rehabilitation Hospital of Maryland
Member
Shady Grove Adventist Hospital
Owner
Adventist HealthCare

**Salisbury**
Owner
Peninsula Regional Health System

**Takoma Park**
Member
Washington Adventist Hospital

**Westminster**
Owner
Carroll Hospital Center

## MASSACHUSETTS

**Andover**
Yankee Alliance

**Attleboro**
Member
Sturdy Memorial Hospital

**Boston**
Member
Beth Israel Deaconess Medical Center
Boston Medical Center

**Brockton**
Member
Signature Healthcare Brockton Hospital

**Cambridge**
Member
Spaulding Hospital for Continuing Medical Care Cambridge

**Fall River**
Owner
Southcoast Hospitals Group

**Great Barrington**
Member
Fairview Hospital

**Greenfield**
Member
Baystate Franklin Medical Center

**Lowell**
Member
Saints Medical Center

**North Adams**
North Adams Regional Hospital

**Pittsfield**
Member
Berkshire Medical Center

**Springfield**
Member
Baystate Medical Center
Owner
Baystate Health, Inc.

**Ware**
Member
Baystate Mary Lane Hospital

**Winchester**
Member
Winchester Hospital

## MICHIGAN

**Bay City**
McLaren Bay Region

**Detroit**
Member
Henry Ford Hospital
Owner
Henry Ford Health System

**Ferndale**
Henry Ford Kingswood Hospital

**Flint**
McLaren Health Care Corporation
Owner
McLaren Flint

**Grosse Pointe**
Member
Beaumont Hospital Grosse Pointe

**Lansing**
Member
McLaren Greater Lansing
Owner
Sparrow Hospital

**Lapeer**
Member
McLaren Lapeer Region

**Rochester**
Member
   Crittenton Hospital Medical Center

**Warren**
Member
   Henry Ford Macomb Hospital–Warren Campus

**Wyandotte**
Member
   Henry Ford Wyandotte Hospital

## MINNESOTA

**Burnsville**
Member
   Fairview Ridges Hospital

**Edina**
Member
   Fairview Southdale Hospital

**Fairmont**
Member
   Mayo Clinic Health System in Fairmont

**Glencoe**
Member
   Glencoe Regional Health Services

**Hibbing**
Member
   Range Regional Health Services

**Marshall**
   Avera Marshall Regional Medical Center

**Minneapolis**
Member
   University of Minnesota Medical Center, Fairview
Owner
   Fairview Health Services

**Pipestone**
Member
   Pipestone County Medical Center Avera

**Princeton**
Member
   Fairview Northland Medical Center

**Red Wing**
Member
   Mayo Clinic Health System in Red Wing

**Saint Louis Park**
   Park Nicollet Methodist Hospital
Member
   Park Nicollet Health Services

**Tyler**
Member
   Tyler Healthcare Center Avera

**Wyoming**
Member
   Fairview Lakes Health Services

## MISSISSIPPI

**Grenada**
Owner
   Grenada Lake Medical Center

**Jackson**
   Mississippi Baptist Health System
   Mississippi Hospital for Restorative Care
Owner
   Mississippi Baptist Medical Center
   University Hospitals and Health System, University of
   Mississippi Medical Center

**Laurel**
Owner
   South Central Regional Medical Center

**Meridian**
   Specialty Hospital of Meridian
Member
   Rush Foundation Hospital
Owner
   Rush Health Systems

**Picayune**
Member
   Highland Community Hospital

## MISSOURI

**Bridgeton**
   SSM DePaul Health Center

**Fenton**
Member
   SSM St. Clare Health Center

**Jefferson City**
Member
   St. Marys Health Center

**Lake Saint Louis**
Member
   SSM St. Joseph Hospital West

**Maryville**
Member
   St. Francis Hospital and Health Services

**Saint Charles**
Member
   SSM St. Joseph Health Center

**Saint Louis**
Member
   SSM Cardinal Glennon Children's Medical Center
   SSM St. Mary's Health Center
Owner
   SSM Health Care

## NEBRASKA

**Blair**
   Memorial Community Hospital and Health System

**O'Neill**
Member
   Avera St. Anthony's Hospital

**Ogallala**
Member
   Ogallala Community Hospital

**Omaha**
   Alegent Health
   Alegent Health–Lakeside Hospital
Owner
   Alegent Health–Bergan Mercy Medical Center
   Alegent Health–Immanuel Medical Center

**Papillion**
Owner
   Alegent Health–Midlands Hospital

**Schuyler**
Owner
   Alegent Health–Memorial Hospital

## NEVADA

**Fallon**
Member
   Banner Churchill Community Hospital

**Henderson**
   St. Rose Dominican Hospitals – Rose de Lima
   Campus
   St. Rose Dominican Hospitals – Siena Campus

## NEW HAMPSHIRE

**Manchester**
Member
   Catholic Medical Center
   Elliot Hospital

**Nashua**
Member
   St. Joseph Hospital

## NEW JERSEY

**Hackettstown**
Member
   Hackettstown Regional Medical Center

**Secaucus**
Member
   Meadowlands Hospital Medical Center

## NEW MEXICO

**Albuquerque**
Member
   Presbyterian Hospital
   Presbyterian Kaseman Hospital
Owner
   Presbyterian Healthcare Services

**Clovis**
Member
   Plains Regional Medical Center

**Espanola**
Member
   Espanola Hospital

**Ruidoso**
Member
   Lincoln County Medical Center

**Socorro**
Member
   Socorro General Hospital

**Tucumcari**
Member
   Dr. Dan C. Trigg Memorial Hospital

## NEW YORK

**Albany**
Member
   Albany Medical Center

**Batavia**
Member
   United Memorial Medical Center

**Bath**
Member
   Ira Davenport Memorial Hospital

**Brockport**
Member
   Lakeside Memorial Hospital

**Bronx**
   St. Barnabas Hospital

**Buffalo**
Member
   BryLin Hospitals

**Canandaigua**
Member
   F. F. Thompson Hospital

**Carthage**
   Carthage Area Hospital

**Clifton Springs**
Member
   Clifton Springs Hospital and Clinic

**Corning**
Member
   Corning Hospital

**Dansville**
Member
   Nicholas H. Noyes Memorial Hospital

**Elizabethtown**
Member
   Elizabethtown Community Hospital

**Elmira**
Member
   Arnot Ogden Medical Center
   St. Joseph's Hospital

**Geneva**
   Geneva General Hospital

**Glens Falls**
Member
   Glens Falls Hospital

**Hornell**
Member
   St. James Mercy Health System

**Medina**
Member
   Medina Memorial Hospital

**Montour Falls**
Member
   Schuyler Hospital

**Newark**
   Newark–Wayne Community Hospital

**Olean**
   Olean General Hospital

**Penn Yan**
Member
   Soldiers and Sailors Memorial Hospital of Yates
   County

**Plattsburgh**
Member
   Champlain Valley Physicians Hospital Medical Center

**Port Jervis**
   Bon Secours Community Hospital

**Rochester**
   Highland Hospital of Rochester
   Rochester Psychiatric Center
   Strong Memorial Hospital of the University of
   Rochester
   Unity Hospital
Member
   Rochester General Hospital
Owner
   Rochester General Health System

**Suffern**
Good Samaritan Hospital

**Syracuse**
Member
Upstate University Hospital

**Troy**
Member
Samaritan Hospital

**Warwick**
St. Anthony Community Hospital

**Wellsville**
Jones Memorial Hospital

**NORTH CAROLINA**

**Albemarle**
Owner
Stanly Regional Medical Center

**Asheboro**
Owner
Randolph Hospital

**Asheville**
Owner
Mission Hospital

**Boone**
Owner
Watauga Medical Center

**Bryson City**
Member
MedWest – Swain

**Burlington**
Owner
Alamance Regional Medical Center

**Clyde**
Owner
MedWest – Haywood

**Fayetteville**
Cape Fear Valley Medical Center

**Gastonia**
Owner
Gaston Memorial Hospital

**Goldsboro**
Owner
Wayne Memorial Hospital

**Hendersonville**
Member
Park Ridge Health
Owner
Margaret R. Pardee Memorial Hospital

**Hickory**
Owner
Catawba Valley Medical Center

**Kinston**
Owner
Lenoir Memorial Hospital

**Lumberton**
Owner
Southeastern Regional Medical Center

**Pinehurst**
FirstHealth of the Carolinas
Owner
FirstHealth Moore Regional Hospital

**Roanoke Rapids**
Owner
Halifax Regional Medical Center

**Rockingham**
FirstHealth Richmond Memorial Hospital

**Statesville**
Owner
Iredell Memorial Hospital

**Sylva**
MedWest Health System
Owner
MedWest – Harris

**Troy**
Owner
FirstHealth Montgomery Memorial Hospital

**Wilmington**
Owner
New Hanover Regional Medical Center

**Wilson**
Owner
Wilson Medical Center

**OHIO**

**Akron**
Owner
Summa Health System

**Amherst**
Specialty Hospital of Lorain

**Batavia**
Member
Mercy Hospital Clermont

**Cincinnati**
Mercy Hospital Mount Airy
Mercy Hospital Western Hills
Member
Mercy Hospital Anderson
Owner
Bethesda North Hospital
Catholic Health Partners
Good Samaritan Hospital

**Cleveland**
Cleveland Clinic Health System
Metrohealth Center for Skilled Nursing Care
Member
Cleveland Clinic Children's Hospital for Rehabilitation
Fairview Hospital
Lutheran Hospital
MetroHealth Medical Center
Owner
Cleveland Clinic Foundation
Hillcrest Hospital

**Dayton**
Grandview Medical Center
Kettering Health Network

**Defiance**
Mercy Hospital of Defiance

**Elyria**
Member
EMH Elyria Medical Center

**Euclid**
Member
Euclid Hospital

**Fairfield**
Mercy Health – Fairfield Hospital

**Garfield Heights**
Member
Marymount Hospital

**Kettering**
Kettering Medical Center

**Lakewood**
Member
Lakewood Hospital

**Lima**
Institute for Orthopaedic Surgery
Member
St. Rita's Medical Center

**Lorain**
Member
Mercy Regional Medical Center

**Miamisburg**
Sycamore Medical Center

**Oberlin**
Member
Mercy Allen Hospital

**Oregon**
Member
Mercy St. Charles Hospital

**Parma**
Member
Parma Community General Hospital

**Springfield**
Springfield Regional Medical Center

**Tiffin**
Member
Mercy Tiffin Hospital

**Toledo**
Mercy St. Anne Hospital
Member
Mercy St. Vincent Medical Center

**Urbana**
Member
Mercy Memorial Hospital

**Warren**
Member
St. Joseph Health Center

**Warrensville Heights**
Owner
South Pointe Hospital

**Willard**
Member
Mercy Willard Hospital

**Youngstown**
Member
St. Elizabeth Health Center

**OKLAHOMA**

**Oklahoma City**
Member
St. Anthony Hospital

**Tulsa**
Member
Laureate Psychiatric Clinic and Hospital
Owner
Saint Francis Hospital

**OREGON**

**Cottage Grove**
Cottage Grove Community Hospital

**Eugene**
Member
Sacred Heart Medical Center

**Florence**
Member
Peace Harbor Hospital

**Medford**
Providence Medford Medical Center

**Portland**
Member
Adventist Medical Center

**Salem**
Member
Salem Hospital

**Tillamook**
Member
Tillamook County General Hospital

**PENNSYLVANIA**

**Bethlehem**
Owner
St. Luke's University Hospital – Bethlehem Campus

**Bryn Mawr**
Member
Bryn Mawr Hospital

**Canonsburg**
Canonsburg General Hospital

**Corry**
Member
Corry Memorial Hospital

**Danville**
Member
Geisinger Health System
Geisinger Medical Center

**Du Bois**
DuBois Regional Medical Center

**Ellwood City**
Ellwood City Hospital

**Erie**
Member
Millcreek Community Hospital
Saint Vincent Health Center

**Greensburg**
Excela Health
Excela Health Westmoreland Hospital

**Greenville**
UPMC Horizon

**Kane**
Member
Kane Community Hospital

**Kittanning**
ACMH Hospital

**Latrobe**
Excela Latrobe Area Hospital

**Malvern**
Member
  Bryn Mawr Rehabilitation Hospital

**Meadville**
Member
  Meadville Medical Center

**Monroeville**
Member
  Forbes Regional Hospital

**Mount Pleasant**
  Excela Frick Hospital

**Nanticoke**
Member
  Special Care Hospital

**Natrona Heights**
  Allegheny Valley Hospital

**Paoli**
Member
  Paoli Hospital

**Philadelphia**
  Aria Health
  Magee Rehabilitation Hospital
Member
  Einstein Medical Center Philadelphia
  Thomas Jefferson University Hospital

**Pittsburgh**
  Allegheny General Hospital
  West Penn Allegheny Health System
Owner
  Western Pennsylvania Hospital

**Radnor**
Owner
  Jefferson Health System

**Scranton**
Member
  Regional Hospital of Scranton

**Seneca**
  UPMC Northwest

**Titusville**
Member
  Titusville Area Hospital

**Warren**
Owner
  Warren General Hospital

**Wilkes Barre**
Member
  Geisinger Wyoming Valley Medical Center

**Wynnewood**
Member
  Lankenau Medical Center

## SOUTH CAROLINA
**Anderson**
Owner
  AnMed Health Medical Center

**Columbia**
  Palmetto Health Baptist
Member
  Palmetto Health Richland
Owner
  Palmetto Health

**Conway**
Owner
  Conway Medical Center

**Easley**
  Baptist Easley Hospital

**Florence**
Owner
  McLeod Regional Medical Center

**Greenville**
  Bon Secours St. Francis Health System
Member
  Greenville Memorial Hospital
Owner
  Greenville Hospital System

**Greenwood**
Owner
  Self Regional Healthcare

**Greer**
Member
  Greer Memorial Hospital

**Spartanburg**
Owner
  Spartanburg Regional Medical Center

**West Columbia**
Owner
  Lexington Medical Center

## SOUTH DAKOTA
**Aberdeen**
Member
  Avera St. Luke's Hospital

**Britton**
Member
  Marshall County Healthcare Center Avera

**Dell Rapids**
Member
  Avera Dells Area Hospital

**Eureka**
Member
  Eureka Community Health Services Avera

**Flandreau**
Member
  Avera Flandreau Hospital

**Gregory**
Member
  Avera Gregory Hospital

**Milbank**
Member
  Milbank Area Hospital Avera

**Miller**
Member
  Avera Hand County Memorial Hospital & Clinic

**Mitchell**
Member
  Avera Queen of Peace Hospital

**Parkston**
Member
  Avera St. Benedict Hospital

**Platte**
Member
  Platte Health Center Avera

**Rapid City**
Owner
  Rapid City Regional Hospital

**Scotland**
Member
  Landmann–Jungman Memorial Hospital Avera

**Sioux Falls**
Member
  Avera McKennan Hospital and University Health Center
Owner
  Avera Health

**Tyndall**
Member
  St. Michael's Hospital Avera

**Wagner**
Member
  Wagner Community Memorial Hospital Avera

**Wessington Springs**
Member
  Avera Weskota Memorial Hospital

**Yankton**
Member
  Avera Sacred Heart Hospital

## TENNESSEE
**Elizabethton**
  Sycamore Shoals Hospital
**Etowah**
Member
  Woods Memorial Hospital

**Greeneville**
Member
  Takoma Regional Hospital

**Jefferson City**
Member
  Jefferson Memorial Hospital

**Jellico**
Member
  Jellico Community Hospital

**Johnson City**
  Franklin Woods Community Hospital
  Quillen Rehabilitation Hospital
  Woodridge Hospital
Member
  Johnson City Medical Center
Owner
  Mountain States Health Alliance

**Kingsport**
  Indian Path Medical Center

**Knoxville**
  Turkey Creek Medical Center
Member
  Physicians Regional Medical Center

**La Follette**
Member
  LaFollette Medical Center

**Madison**
  Skyline Madison Campus

**Maryville**
Owner
  Blount Memorial Hospital

**Memphis**
  Methodist Extended Care Hospital
Member
  Methodist Healthcare Memphis Hospitals
  Methodist Le Bonheur Healthcare

**Mountain City**
  Johnson County Community Hospital

**Nashville**
Owner
  Vanderbilt Hospital and Clinics

**Newport**
Member
  Newport Medical Center

**Somerville**
Owner
  Methodist Healthcare–Fayette Hospital

**Tazewell**
Member
  Claiborne County Hospital

## TEXAS
**Abilene**
Owner
  Hendrick Health System

**Allen**
  Texas Health Presbyterian Hospital Allen

**Arlington**
  Texas Health Arlington Memorial Hospital
  Texas Health Resources

**Azle**
Member
  Texas Health Harris Methodist Hospital Azle

**Bedford**
Member
  Texas Health Harris Methodist Hospital
    Hurst–Euless–Bedford

**Cleburne**
Member
  Texas Health Harris Methodist Hospital Cleburne

**Dallas**
  University of Texas Southwestern Medical Center
Member
  Methodist Charlton Medical Center
  Methodist Dallas Medical Center
  Texas Health Presbyterian Hospital Dallas
Owner
  Methodist Health System

**Denison**
Owner
  Texoma Medical Center

**El Paso**
Owner
  University Medical Center of El Paso

**Fort Worth**
  Texas Health Specialty Hospital
Member
  Huguley Memorial Medical Center
  Texas Health Harris Methodist Hospital Fort Worth
  Texas Health Harris Methodist Hospital Southwest
    Fort Worth

Section B

**Henderson**
Member
East Texas Medical Center Henderson

**Houston**
Harris County Hospital District
St. Luke's Episcopal Health System
Member
The Methodist Hospital
Owner
St. Luke's Episcopal Hospital
The Methodist Hospital System
University of Texas M.D. Anderson Cancer Center

**Kaufman**
Member
Texas Health Presbyterian Hospital Kaufman

**Killeen**
Member
Metroplex Adventist Hospital

**Lampasas**
Rollins–Brook Community Hospital

**Livingston**
Member
Memorial Medical Center – Livingston

**Lubbock**
Owner
University Medical Center

**Lufkin**
Memorial Specialty Hospital
Owner
Memorial Medical Center – Lufkin

**Nacogdoches**
Owner
Nacogdoches Memorial Hospital

**Plano**
Member
Texas Health Presbyterian Hospital Plano

**San Augustine**
Member
Memorial Medical Center – San Augustine

**San Marcos**
Member
Central Texas Medical Center

**Stephenville**
Member
Texas Health Harris Methodist Hospital Stephenville

**The Woodlands**
St. Luke's The Woodlands Hospital

**Weslaco**
Owner
Knapp Medical Center

**Winnsboro**
Member
Mother Frances Hospital – Winnsboro

**VIRGINIA**
**Abingdon**
Owner
Johnston Memorial Hospital

**Bedford**
Member
Bedford Memorial Hospital

**Chesapeake**
Owner
Chesapeake Regional Medical Center

**Christiansburg**
Member
Carilion New River Valley Medical Center

**Front Royal**
Member
Warren Memorial Hospital

**Galax**
Owner
Twin County Regional Hospital

**Lexington**
Member
Carilion Stonewall Jackson Hospital

**Marion**
Owner
Smyth County Community Hospital

**Mechanicsville**
Member
Bon Secours Memorial Regional Medical Center

**Midlothian**
Bon Secours St. Francis Medical Center

**Newport News**
Member
Mary Immaculate Hospital

**Norfolk**
Member
Bon Secours–DePaul Medical Center

**Pearisburg**
Member
Carilion Giles Community Hospital

**Portsmouth**
Member
Bon Secours Maryview Medical Center

**Richmond**
Member
Bon Secours St. Mary's Hospital
Bon Secours–Richmond Community Hospital

**Roanoke**
Member
Carilion Medical Center
Owner
Carilion Clinic

**Rocky Mount**
Member
Carilion Franklin Memorial Hospital

**South Hill**
Owner
Community Memorial Healthcenter

**Suffolk**
Owner
Sentara Obici Hospital

**Tazewell**
Member
Carilion Tazewell Community Hospital

**Winchester**
Member
Winchester Medical Center
Owner
Valley Health System

**Woodstock**
Member
Shenandoah Memorial Hospital

**WASHINGTON**
**Anacortes**
Island Hospital
**Arlington**
Cascade Valley Hospital and Clinics
**Bellevue**
Member
Overlake Hospital Medical Center
Owner
PeaceHealth
**Bellingham**
Member
PeaceHealth St. Joseph Medical Center
**Bremerton**
Harrison Medical Center
**Burien**
Member
Highline Medical Center
**Centralia**
Member
Providence Centralia Hospital
**Chelan**
Member
Lake Chelan Community Hospital
**Clarkston**
Member
Tri–State Memorial Hospital
**Colfax**
Member
Whitman Hospital and Medical Center
**Coupeville**
Member
Whidbey General Hospital

**Davenport**
Member
Lincoln Hospital
**Dayton**
Dayton General Hospital
**Edmonds**
Member
Swedish/Edmonds
**Ellensburg**
Kittitas Valley Community Hospital
**Ephrata**
Member
Columbia Basin Hospital
**Everett**
Member
Providence Regional Medical Center Everett
**Federal Way**
St. Francis Hospital
**Grand Coulee**
Member
Coulee Medical Center
**Kennewick**
Kennewick General Hospital
**Lakewood**
St. Clare Hospital
**Longview**
Member
PeaceHealth St. John Medical Center
**Medical Lake**
Eastern State Hospital
**Moses Lake**
Member
Samaritan Healthcare
**Mount Vernon**
Skagit Valley Hospital
**Newport**
Member
Newport Hospital and Health Services
**Odessa**
Member
Odessa Memorial Healthcare Center
**Olympia**
Member
Providence St. Peter Hospital
**Othello**
Member
Othello Community Hospital
**Pasco**
Lourdes Medical Center
**Prosser**
Member
Prosser Memorial Hospital
**Pullman**
Member
Pullman Regional Hospital
**Quincy**
Member
Quincy Valley Medical Center
**Renton**
Member
Valley Medical Center
**Republic**
Member
Ferry County Memorial Hospital
**Richland**
Member
Kadlec Medical Center
**Ritzville**
Member
East Adams Rural Hospital
**Seattle**
Virginia Mason Medical Center
**Sedro Woolley**
United General Hospital
**Spokane**
Member
Providence Holy Family Hospital
Providence Sacred Heart Medical Center & Children's
Hospital

**Spokane Valley**
Member
Valley Hospital and Medical Center

**Sunnyside**
Sunnyside Community Hospital

**Tacoma**
MultiCare Mary Bridge Children's Hospital and Health Center
St. Joseph Medical Center

**Tonasket**
Member
North Valley Hospital

**Toppenish**
Member
Toppenish Community Hospital

**Vancouver**
Member
PeaceHealth Southwest Medical Center

**Walla Walla**
Member
Providence St. Mary Medical Center
Walla Walla General Hospital

**Yakima**
Yakima Valley Memorial Hospital

**WEST VIRGINIA**

**Berkeley Springs**
Member
War Memorial Hospital

**Bluefield**
Owner
Bluefield Regional Medical Center

**Bridgeport**
Member
United Hospital Center

**Buckhannon**
Member
St. Joseph's Hospital of Buckhannon

**Elkins**
Owner
Davis Memorial Hospital

**Fairmont**
Owner
West Virginia United Health System

**Huntington**
Cabell Huntington Hospital
Owner
St. Mary's Medical Center

**Martinsburg**
Member
City Hospital

**Morgantown**
West Virginia University Hospitals
Owner
Monongalia General Hospital

**Parkersburg**
Owner
Camden–Clark Medical Center

**Point Pleasant**
Owner
Pleasant Valley Hospital

**Ranson**
Member
Jefferson Memorial Hospital

**South Charleston**
Owner
Thomas Memorial Hospital

**Weirton**
Owner
Weirton Medical Center

**WISCONSIN**

**Baraboo**
Member
St. Clare Hospital and Health Services

**Boscobel**
Boscobel Area Health Care

**Burlington**
Member
Aurora Memorial Hospital of Burlington

**Durand**
Member
Chippewa Valley Hospital and Oakview Care Center

**Elkhorn**
Member
Aurora Lakeland Medical Center

**Green Bay**
Aurora BayCare Medical Center

**Hartford**
Member
Aurora Medical Center of Washington County

**Kenosha**
Aurora Medical Center

**Madison**
Member
St. Mary's Hospital

**Milwaukee**
Member
Aurora Sinai Medical Center
Aurora St. Luke's Medical Center
Owner
Aurora Health Care

**Oshkosh**
Aurora Medical Center of Oshkosh

**Sheboygan**
Member
Aurora Sheboygan Memorial Medical Center

**Two Rivers**
Member
Aurora Medical Center – Manitowoc County

**Wauwatosa**
Aurora Psychiatric Hospital

**West Allis**
Member
Aurora West Allis Medical Center

**WYOMING**

**Torrington**
Member
Community Hospital

**Wheatland**
Platte County Memorial Hospital

**Worland**
Member
Washakie Medical Center

## SYNERNET, INC.
222 St John Street, Portland, ME
Zip 04102; tel. 207/771–3456; Gerry Vicenzi, President and Chief Executive Officer

**MAINE**

**Bangor**
Affiliate
St. Joseph Hospital

**Bar Harbor**
Affiliate
Mount Desert Island Hospital

**Biddeford**
Affiliate
Southern Maine Medical Center

**Boothbay Harbor**
Owner
St. Andrews Hospital and Healthcare Center

**Brunswick**
Affiliate
Mid Coast Hospital

**Damariscotta**
Owner
Miles Memorial Hospital

**Farmington**
Owner
Franklin Memorial Hospital

**Fort Kent**
Affiliate
Northern Maine Medical Center

**Norway**
Owner
Stephens Memorial Hospital

**Portland**
Owner
Maine Medical Center
New England Rehabilitation Hospital of Portland

**Rockport**
Affiliate
Pen Bay Medical Center

**Sanford**
Owner
Henrietta D. Goodall Hospital

**Skowhegan**
Affiliate
Redington–Fairview General Hospital

**Waterville**
Affiliate
MaineGeneral Medical Center–Waterville Campus

**Westbrook**
Owner
Spring Harbor Hospital

## THE NEW JERSEY COUNCIL OF TEACHING HOSPITALS
154 West State Street, Trenton, NJ
Zip 08608; tel. 609/656–9600; J. Richard Goldstein M.D., President

**NEW JERSEY**

**Camden**
Member
Cooper Health System

**Hamilton**
Member
Robert Wood Johnson University Hospital at Hamilton

**Morristown**
Member
Atlantic Health

**Neptune**
Member
Meridian Health

**New Brunswick**
Member
Robert Wood Johnson University Hospital

**Newark**
Member
University of Medicine and Dentistry of New Jersey–University Hospital

**Paterson**
Member
St. Joseph's Regional Medical Center

**Phillipsburg**
Member
St. Luke's Hospital – Warren Campus

**Somerville**
Member
Somerset Medical Center

## UNIVERSITY HEALTHSYSTEM CONSORTIUM, INC.
155 North Wacker Drive, Chicago, IL
Zip 60606–1787; tel. 630/954–1700; Irene M. Thompson, President and Chief Executive Officer

**ALABAMA**

**Birmingham**
Member
University of Alabama Hospital

**Mobile**
Affiliate
Infirmary West
Member
University of South Alabama Medical Center

**ARIZONA**

**Douglas**
Member
Southeast Arizona Medical Center

**Phoenix**
Member
Maricopa Integrated Health System
Mayo Clinic Hospital

Section B

**Tucson**
Member
  University of Arizona Medical Center – University
    Campus

## ARKANSAS
**Little Rock**
Member
  UAMS Medical Center

## CALIFORNIA
**Colton**
Member
  Arrowhead Regional Medical Center

**Downey**
Affiliate
  Rancho Los Amigos National Rehabilitation Center

**French Camp**
Member
  San Joaquin General Hospital

**Joshua Tree**
Member
  Hi–Desert Medical Center

**Los Angeles**
Member
  Cedars–Sinai Medical Center
  LAC/University of Southern California Medical Center
  Ronald Reagan University of California Los Angeles
    Medical Center

**Martinez**
Affiliate
  Contra Costa Regional Medical Center

**Moreno Valley**
Member
  Riverside County Regional Medical Center

**Orange**
Member
  University of California, Irvine Healthcare

**Palo Alto**
Member
  Lucile Salter Packard Children's Hospital at Stanford
  Stanford Hospital and Clinics

**Sacramento**
Member
  University of California, Davis Medical Center

**San Diego**
Member
  UC San Diego Health System

**San Francisco**
Member
  Laguna Honda Hospital and Rehabilitation Center
  San Francisco General Hospital Medical Center
  UCSF Medical Center

**San Jose**
Affiliate
  Santa Clara Valley Medical Center

**Santa Monica**
Affiliate
  Santa Monica–UCLA Medical Center and Orthopaedic
    Hospital

**Sylmar**
Affiliate
  LAC–Olive View–UCLA Medical Center

**Torrance**
Member
  LAC–Harbor–University of California at Los Angeles
    Medical Center

**Valencia**
Affiliate
  Henry Mayo Newhall Memorial Hospital

## COLORADO
**Aurora**
Member
  University of Colorado Hospital

**Denver**
Affiliate
  National Jewish Health
Member
  Denver Health Medical Center

## CONNECTICUT
**Bridgeport**
Member
  Bridgeport Hospital

**Farmington**
Member
  University of Connecticut Health Center, John
    Dempsey Hospital

**Greenwich**
Member
  Greenwich Hospital

**New Haven**
Member
  Yale–New Haven Hospital

## DISTRICT OF COLUMBIA
**Washington**
Member
  Howard University Hospital
  Medstar Georgetown University Hospital

## FLORIDA
**Gainesville**
Member
  Shands at the University of Florida

**Jacksonville**
Owner
  Shands Jacksonville Medical Center

**Lake City**
Affiliate
  Shands Lake Shore

**Live Oak**
Affiliate
  Shands Live Oak

**Miami**
Member
  Jackson Health System

**Starke**
Affiliate
  Shands Starke Regional Medical Center

**Tampa**
Member
  Tampa General Hospital

## GEORGIA
**Atlanta**
Member
  Emory University Hospital
  Emory University Hospital Midtown
  Grady Memorial Hospital
  Wesley Woods Geriatric Hospital of Emory University

**Augusta**
Member
  Georgia Health Sciences Medical Center

## ILLINOIS
**Chicago**
Affiliate
  Louis A. Weiss Memorial Hospital
Member
  John H. Stroger Jr. Hospital of Cook County
  La Rabida Children's Hospital
  Northwestern Memorial Hospital
  Provident Hospital of Cook County
  Rush University Medical Center
  University of Chicago Medical Center
  University of Illinois Hospital & Health Sciences
    System

**Hinsdale**
Member
  R M L Specialty Hospital

**Maywood**
Member
  Loyola University Medical Center

**Oak Forest**
Member
  Oak Forest Health Center of Cook County

**Oak Park**
Member
  Rush Oak Park Hospital

**Skokie**
Member
  NorthShore University Health System Skokie Hospital

## INDIANA
**Indianapolis**
Member
  Indiana University Health University Hospital
  Wishard Health Services

## IOWA
**Iowa City**
Member
  University of Iowa Hospitals and Clinics

## KANSAS
**Kansas City**
Member
  The University of Kansas Hospital

## KENTUCKY
**Cynthiana**
Member
  Harrison Memorial Hospital

**Lexington**
Member
  University of Kentucky Albert B. Chandler Hospital

**Louisville**
Member
  University of Louisville Hospital

**Morehead**
Member
  St. Claire Regional Medical Center

**Mount Vernon**
Member
  Rockcastle Regional Hospital and Respiratory Care
    Center

**Richmond**
Member
  Pattie A. Clay Regional Medical Center

## LOUISIANA
**Baton Rouge**
Member
  Earl K. Long Medical Center

**Bogalusa**
Member
  LSU Bogalusa Medical Center

**Houma**
Member
  Leonard J. Chabert Medical Center

**Independence**
Member
  Lallie Kemp Medical Center

**Lafayette**
Member
  University Medical Center

**Lake Charles**
Member
  Walter Olin Moss Regional Medical Center

**New Orleans**
Member
  Interim LSU Public Hospital

**Pineville**
Member
  Huey P. Long Medical Center

**Shreveport**
Member
  LSU Medical Center–University Hospital

**Winnsboro**
Member
  Franklin Medical Center

## MAINE
**Portland**
Member
  Maine Medical Center

## MARYLAND
**Baltimore**
Affiliate
  Kernan Orthopaedics and Rehabilitation
Member
  Johns Hopkins Bayview Medical Center
  Johns Hopkins Hospital
  Maryland General Hospital
  Mt. Washington Pediatric Hospital
  University of Maryland Medical Center

**Cambridge**
Member
  Dorchester General Hospital

**Easton**
Member
  Memorial Hospital at Easton Maryland

**Glen Burnie**
Member
  Baltimore Washington Medical Center

## MASSACHUSETTS

**Boston**
  Dana–Farber Cancer Institute
Member
  Boston Medical Center
  Brigham and Women's Hospital
  Carney Hospital
  Faulkner Hospital
  Massachusetts General Hospital
  Tufts Medical Center

**Brighton**
Member
  St. Elizabeth's Medical Center

**Brockton**
Member
  Good Samaritan Medical Center

**Cambridge**
Member
  Cambridge Health Alliance

**Clinton**
Affiliate
  Clinton Hospital

**Fall River**
Member
  Saint Anne's Hospital

**Marlborough**
Affiliate
  UMass Memorial–Marlborough Hospital

**Methuen**
Member
  Holy Family Hospital and Medical Center

**Newton Lower Falls**
Member
  Newton–Wellesley Hospital

**Norwood**
Member
  Norwood Hospital

**Salem**
Member
  North Shore Medical Center

**Springfield**
Member
  Baystate Medical Center

**Ware**
Member
  Baystate Mary Lane Hospital

## MICHIGAN

**Ann Arbor**
Member
  University of Michigan Hospitals and Health Centers

**Flint**
Member
  Hurley Medical Center

## MINNESOTA

**Burnsville**
Member
  Fairview Ridges Hospital

**Edina**
Member
  Fairview Southdale Hospital

**Hibbing**
Member
  Range Regional Health Services

**Minneapolis**
Affiliate
  Hennepin County Medical Center
Member
  University of Minnesota Medical Center, Fairview

**Rochester**
Member
  Mayo Clinic – Methodist Hospital
  Mayo Clinic – Saint Marys Hospital

**Saint Paul**
Member
  Regions Hospital

## MISSISSIPPI

**Jackson**
Member
  University Hospitals and Health System, University of Mississippi Medical Center

## MISSOURI

**Boonville**
Member
  Cooper County Memorial Hospital

**Columbia**
Member
  University of Missouri Health Care
  University of Missouri Hospitals and Clinics
  Women's and Children's Hospital

**Hermann**
Member
  Hermann Area District Hospital

**Jefferson City**
Member
  Capital Region Medical Center

**Kansas City**
Member
  Truman Medical Center–Hospital Hill
  Truman Medical Center–Lakewood

**Milan**
Member
  Sullivan County Memorial Hospital

**Saint Louis**
Member
  Barnes–Jewish Hospital

## NEBRASKA

**O'Neill**
Member
  Avera St. Anthony's Hospital

**Omaha**
Member
  Nebraska Medical Center

## NEVADA

**Las Vegas**
Affiliate
  University Medical Center

## NEW JERSEY

**Hamilton**
Member
  Robert Wood Johnson University Hospital at Hamilton

**Morristown**
Member
  Morristown Medical Center

**New Brunswick**
Member
  Robert Wood Johnson University Hospital

**Newark**
Member
  University of Medicine and Dentistry of New Jersey–University Hospital

**Rahway**
Member
  Robert Wood Johnson University Hospital Rahway

**Summit**
Member
  Overlook Medical Center

## NEW MEXICO

**Albuquerque**
Member
  University of New Mexico Hospitals

## NEW YORK

**Albany**
Member
  Albany Medical Center

**Brooklyn**
Member
  Kings County Hospital Center
  SUNY Downstate Medical Center University Hospital of Brooklyn

**Elmhurst**
Member
  Elmhurst Hospital Center

**Greenport**
Member
  Eastern Long Island Hospital

**New York**
Member
  Bellevue Hospital Center
  Mount Sinai Hospital
  New York–Presbyterian Hospital

**Riverhead**
Member
  Peconic Bay Medical Center

**Rochester**
Member
  Highland Hospital of Rochester
  Strong Memorial Hospital of the University of Rochester

**Stony Brook**
Member
  Stony Brook University Medical Center

**Syracuse**
Member
  Upstate University Hospital

## NORTH CAROLINA

**Ahoskie**
Affiliate
  Vidant Roanoke–Chowan Hospital

**Chapel Hill**
Member
  University of North Carolina Hospitals

**Danbury**
Member
  Pioneer Community Hospital of Stokes

**Durham**
Member
  Duke University Hospital
  Durham Regional Hospital

**Edenton**
Member
  Vidant Chowan Hospital

**Greenville**
Member
  Vidant Medical Center

**Mocksville**
Member
  Wake Forest Baptist Health–Davie Hospital

**Raleigh**
Member
  Duke Raleigh Hospital

**Tarboro**
Member
  Vidant Edgecombe Hospital

**Windsor**
Affiliate
  Vidant Bertie Hospital

**Winston–Salem**
Member
  Old Vineyard Behavioral Health Services
  Wake Forest Baptist Medical Center

**Yadkinville**
Member
  Yadkin Valley Community Hospital

## OHIO

**Barnesville**
Member
  Barnesville Hospital

**Bellefontaine**
Member
  Mary Rutan Hospital

**Bucyrus**
Member
  Bucyrus Community Hospital

**Canton**
Member
  Mercy Medical Center

**Chardon**
Affiliate
  University Hospitals Geauga Medical Center

Section B

**Cincinnati**
Member
   Cincinnati Children's Hospital Medical Center
   University Hospital

**Cleveland**
Affiliate
   University Hospitals Bedford Medical Center
Member
   St. Vincent Charity Medical Center
   University Hospitals Case Medical Center
   University Hospitals Richmond Medical Center

**Coldwater**
Member
   Mercer County Joint Township Community Hospital

**Columbus**
Member
   Ohio State University Medical Center

**Conneaut**
Affiliate
   University Hospitals Conneaut Medical Center

**Dennison**
Member
   Trinity Hospital Twin City

**Geneva**
Affiliate
   University Hospitals Geneva Medical Center

**London**
Member
   Madison County Hospital

**Middleburg Heights**
Member
   Southwest General Health Center

**Toledo**
Member
   The University of Toledo Medical Center

**Upper Sandusky**
Member
   Wyandot Memorial Hospital

**Waverly**
Affiliate
   Pike Community Hospital

**Westlake**
Member
   St. John Medical Center

**Willoughby**
Affiliate
   Windsor–Laurelwood Center for Behavioral Medicine

**OREGON**

**Grants Pass**
Member
   Three Rivers Medical Center

**Medford**
Member
   Asante Health System
   Rogue Valley Medical Center

**Portland**
Member
   OHSU Hospital

**PENNSYLVANIA**

**Allentown**
Member
   Lehigh Valley Hospital

**Bryn Mawr**
Member
   Bryn Mawr Hospital

**Media**
Member
   Riddle Hospital

**Paoli**
Member
   Paoli Hospital

**Philadelphia**
Affiliate
   Friends Hospital
   Penn Presbyterian Medical Center
   Thomas Jefferson University Hospital
Member
   Hospital of the University of Pennsylvania
   Pennsylvania Hospital

**Phoenixville**
Affiliate
   Phoenixville Hospital

**Pittsburgh**
Member
   UPMC Presbyterian Shadyside

**Wynnewood**
Member
   Lankenau Medical Center

**RHODE ISLAND**

**Westerly**
Member
   Westerly Hospital

**SOUTH CAROLINA**

**Charleston**
Member
   MUSC Medical Center of Medical University of South
   Carolina

**Greenville**
Member
   Greenville Hospital System

**TENNESSEE**

**Knoxville**
Member
   The University of Tennessee Medical Center

**Nashville**
Member
   Vanderbilt Hospital and Clinics

**TEXAS**

**Baytown**
Member
   San Jacinto Methodist Hospital

**Dallas**
Member
   Parkland Health & Hospital System
   University of Texas Southwestern Medical Center

**Galveston**
Member
   University of Texas Medical Branch Hospitals

**Houston**
Member
   Memorial Hermann – Texas Medical Center
   Methodist Willowbrook Hospital
   St. Luke's Episcopal Hospital
   The Methodist Hospital

**Sugar Land**
Member
   Methodist Sugar Land Hospital

**The Woodlands**
Member
   St. Luke's The Woodlands Hospital

**Tyler**
Affiliate
   University of Texas Health Science Center at Tyler

**UTAH**

**Moab**
Member
   Moab Regional Hospital

**Monticello**
Member
   San Juan Hospital

**Salt Lake City**
Member
.   University of Utah Health Care – Hospital and Clinics

**VERMONT**

**Burlington**
Member
   Fletcher Allen Health Care

**VIRGINIA**

**Charlottesville**
Member
   University of Virginia Medical Center

**Richmond**
Member
   VCU Health System

**WASHINGTON**

**Seattle**
Member
   Harborview Medical Center
   University of Washington Medical Center

**WEST VIRGINIA**

**Martinsburg**
Member
   City Hospital

**Morgantown**
Member
   West Virginia University Hospitals

**Ranson**
Member
   Jefferson Memorial Hospital

**WISCONSIN**

**Antigo**
Affiliate
   Langlade Memorial Hospital

**Friendship**
Member
   Moundview Memorial Hospital & Clinics

**Hudson**
Member
   Hudson Hospital

**Madison**
Member
   University of Wisconsin Hospital and Clinics

**Medford**
Affiliate
   Memorial Health Center

**Merrill**
Affiliate
   Ministry Good Samaritan Health Center

**Milwaukee**
Member
   Froedtert Memorial Lutheran Hospital

**New Richmond**
Member
   Westfields Hospital

**Wausau**
Affiliate
   Aspirus Wausau Hospital

**Wisconsin Rapids**
Member
   Riverview Hospital Association

## VANTAGE HEALTHCARE NETWORK, INC.
18282 Technology Drive, Suite 202,
Meadville, PA Zip 16335;
tel. 814/337–0000; David Petrarca,
Director Retail Operations

## VHA, INC.
901 New York Avenue NW, Suite 510
East Tower, Washington, DC
Zip 20001–4436; tel. 972/830–0253;
Curtis W. Nonomaque, President and
Chief Executive Officer

**ALABAMA**

**Alabaster**
   Shelby Baptist Medical Center

**Anniston**
Partner
   Northeast Alabama Regional Medical Center

**Athens**
Partner
   Athens–Limestone Hospital

**Atmore**
   Atmore Community Hospital

**Birmingham**
   Princeton Baptist Medical Center
Shareholder
   Baptist Health System

**Boaz**
   Marshall Medical Center South

**Brewton**
   D. W. McMillan Memorial Hospital

**Carrollton**
   Pickens County Medical Center

**Chatom**
   Washington County Hospital and Nursing Home

**Decatur**
Decatur General Hospital
**Fairhope**
Thomas Hospital
**Fayette**
Fayette Medical Center
**Fort Payne**
DeKalb Regional Medical Center
**Grove Hill**
Grove Hill Memorial Hospital
**Guntersville**
Marshall Medical Center North
Partner
Marshall Health System
**Hamilton**
North Mississippi Medical Center–Hamilton
**Huntsville**
Huntsville Hospital
**Jasper**
Walker Baptist Medical Center
**Montgomery**
Baptist Medical Center East
Shareholder
Baptist Medical Center South
**Moulton**
Lawrence Medical Center
**Northport**
Northport Medical Center
**Opp**
Mizell Memorial Hospital
**Ozark**
Dale Medical Center
**Prattville**
Prattville Baptist Hospital
**Scottsboro**
Partner
Highlands Medical Center
**Sylacauga**
Coosa Valley Medical Center
**Talladega**
Citizens Baptist Medical Center
**Tuscaloosa**
DCH Regional Medical Center
Partner
DCH Health System
**Union Springs**
Bullock County Hospital

## ALASKA
**Anchorage**
Providence Alaska Medical Center
**Cordova**
Cordova Community Medical Center
**Kodiak**
Providence Kodiak Island Medical Center
**Seward**
Providence Seward Medical Center
**Valdez**
Providence Valdez Medical Center
**Wrangell**
Wrangell Medical Center

## ARIZONA
**Bisbee**
Copper Queen Community Hospital
**Phoenix**
Mayo Clinic Hospital
**Safford**
Mt. Graham Regional Medical Center
**Scottsdale**
Scottsdale Healthcare Shea Medical Center
Scottsdale Healthcare Thompson Peak Hospital
Unit_of
Scottsdale Healthcare–Osborn Medical Center
**Tucson**
TMC Healthcare

## ARKANSAS
**Arkadelphia**
Baptist Health Medical Center–Arkadelphia
**Booneville**
Booneville Community Hospital
**Clinton**
Ozark Health Medical Center

**Conway**
Partner
Conway Regional Medical Center
**Fayetteville**
Partner
Washington Regional Medical Center
**Heber Springs**
Baptist Health Medical Center–Heber Springs
**Jonesboro**
NEA Baptist Memorial Hospital
Partner
St. Bernards Medical Center
**Little Rock**
Baptist Health Medical Center–Little Rock
Shareholder
Baptist Health
**North Little Rock**
Baptist Health Medical Center – North Little Rock
**Paragould**
Partner
Arkansas Methodist Medical Center
**Piggott**
Piggott Community Hospital
**Searcy**
White County Medical Center
**Stuttgart**
Baptist Health Medical Center–Stuttgart
**Walnut Ridge**
Lawrence Memorial Hospital
**West Memphis**
Crittenden Regional Hospital
**Wynne**
CrossRidge Community Hospital

## CALIFORNIA
**Alameda**
Alameda Hospital
**Antioch**
Sutter Delta Medical Center
**Arcadia**
Methodist Hospital of Southern California
**Auburn**
Sutter Auburn Faith Hospital
**Berkeley**
Alta Bates Medical Center–Herrick Campus
Alta Bates Summit Medical Center
**Burbank**
Providence Saint Joseph Medical Center
**Burlingame**
Mills–Peninsula Health Services
**Castro Valley**
Eden Medical Center
**Clovis**
Clovis Community Medical Center
**Concord**
John Muir Medical Center, Concord
**Covina**
Citrus Valley Health Partners
Citrus Valley Medical Center–Inter-Community Campus
**Crescent City**
Sutter Coast Hospital
**Davis**
Sutter Davis Hospital
**El Centro**
El Centro Regional Medical Center
**Encinitas**
Scripps Memorial Hospital–Encinitas
**Escondido**
Palomar Medical Center
**Fresno**
Community Regional Medical Center
Fresno Heart and Surgical Hospital
Shareholder
Community Medical Centers
**Glendora**
Foothill Presbyterian Hospital
**Greenbrae**
Marin General Hospital
**Jackson**
Sutter Amador Hospital

**La Jolla**
Scripps Green Hospital
Shareholder
Scripps Memorial Hospital–La Jolla
**Lakeport**
Sutter Lakeside Hospital
**Lancaster**
Partner
Antelope Valley Hospital
**Los Angeles**
Shareholder
Cedars–Sinai Medical Center
**Mariposa**
John C. Fremont Healthcare District
**Menlo Park**
Menlo Park Surgical Hospital
**Mission Hills**
Providence Holy Cross Medical Center
**Modesto**
Partner
Memorial Medical Center
**Monterey**
Community Hospital of the Monterey Peninsula
**Novato**
Novato Community Hospital
**Oakland**
Alta Bates Summit Medical Center – Summit Campus
**Pasadena**
Huntington Memorial Hospital
**Pleasanton**
ValleyCare Medical Center
**Pomona**
Partner
Pomona Valley Hospital Medical Center
**Poway**
Pomerado Hospital
**Roseville**
Sutter Roseville Medical Center
**Sacramento**
Sutter Medical Center, Sacramento
Shareholder
Sutter Health
**San Diego**
Palomar Health
Scripps Health
Scripps Mercy Hospital
**San Francisco**
California Pacific Medical Center–Davies Campus
Chinese Hospital
St. Luke's Hospital
Shareholder
California Pacific Medical Center
**San Pedro**
Providence Little Company of Mary Medical Center San Pedro
**Santa Barbara**
Cottage Health System
Goleta Valley Cottage Hospital
Partner
Santa Barbara Cottage Hospital
**Santa Cruz**
Sutter Maternity and Surgery Center of Santa Cruz
**Santa Rosa**
Sutter Medical Center of Santa Rosa, Chanate Campus
**Solvang**
Santa Ynez Valley Cottage Hospital
**Tarzana**
Providence Tarzana Medical Center
**Torrance**
Providence Little Company of Mary Medical Center
Partner
Torrance Memorial Medical Center
**Tracy**
Sutter Tracy Community Hospital
**Turlock**
Partner
Emanuel Medical Center
**Vallejo**
Sutter Solano Medical Center

Section B

**Walnut Creek**
John Muir Health
John Muir Medical Center, Walnut Creek
**West Covina**
Citrus Valley Medical Center–Queen of the Valley
Campus
**Whittier**
Partner
Presbyterian Intercommunity Hospital

## COLORADO

**Alamosa**
Partner
San Luis Valley Regional Medical Center

**Aspen**
Partner
Aspen Valley Hospital District

**Boulder**
Partner
Boulder Community Hospital

**Colorado Springs**
Partner
Memorial Health System

**Denver**
Exempla Healthcare, Inc.
Exempla Saint Joseph Hospital

**Englewood**
Craig Hospital

**Estes Park**
Estes Park Medical Center

**Fort Collins**
Poudre Valley Hospital

**Gunnison**
Partner
Gunnison Valley Hospital

**Haxtun**
Haxtun Hospital District

**Kremmling**
Kremmling Memorial Hospital

**La Jara**
Conejos County Hospital

**Lafayette**
Exempla Good Samaritan Medical Center

**Longmont**
Partner
Longmont United Hospital

**Loveland**
Medical Center of the Rockies

**Steamboat Springs**
Partner
Yampa Valley Medical Center

**Vail**
Shareholder
Vail Valley Medical Center

**Wheat Ridge**
Shareholder
Exempla Lutheran Medical Center

**Yuma**
Yuma District Hospital

## CONNECTICUT

**Bridgeport**
Bridgeport Hospital

**Danbury**
Partner
Danbury Hospital

**Greenwich**
Partner
Greenwich Hospital

**Hartford**
Connecticut Children's Medical Center
Shareholder
Hartford Hospital

**Manchester**
Eastern Connecticut Health Network
Manchester Memorial Hospital

**Meriden**
Partner
MidState Medical Center

**Middletown**
Partner
Middlesex Hospital

**New Haven**
Yale New Haven Health System
Yale–New Haven Hospital

**New Milford**
New Milford Hospital

**Norwalk**
Norwalk Hospital

**Putnam**
Day Kimball Hospital

**Stamford**
Partner
Stamford Hospital

**Torrington**
Partner
The Charlotte Hungerford Hospital

**Vernon Rockville**
Rockville General Hospital

**Wallingford**
Gaylord Hospital

**Willimantic**
Windham Hospital

## DISTRICT OF COLUMBIA

**Washington**
Medstar Georgetown University Hospital
Medstar Washington Hospital Center

## FLORIDA

**Apalachicola**
George E. Weems Memorial Hospital

**Boca Raton**
Partner
Boca Raton Regional Hospital

**Boynton Beach**
Partner
Bethesda Memorial Hospital

**Cape Coral**
Cape Coral Hospital

**Clermont**
South Lake Hospital

**Cocoa Beach**
Cape Canaveral Hospital

**Daytona Beach**
Shareholder
Halifax Health Medical Center of Daytona Beach

**Fort Myers**
Gulf Coast Medical Center
Partner
Lee Memorial Hospital

**Gulf Breeze**
Gulf Breeze Hospital

**Inverness**
Partner
Citrus Memorial Health System

**Jacksonville**
Mayo Clinic Jacksonville

**Jay**
Jay Hospital

**Lakeland**
Shareholder
Lakeland Regional Medical Center

**Leesburg**
Leesburg Regional Medical Center

**Longwood**
Orlando Regional South Seminole Hospital

**Melbourne**
Circles of Care
Palm Bay Hospital
Shareholder
Holmes Regional Medical Center

**New Smyrna Beach**
Bert Fish Medical Center

**Ocala**
Partner
Munroe Regional Medical Center

**Ocoee**
Health Central

**Orlando**
Orlando Regional Medical Center
Shareholder
Orlando Health

**Panama City**
Bay Medical Center

**Pensacola**
Baptist Hospital
Shareholder
Baptist Health Care Corporation

**Rockledge**
Health First, Inc.

**Stuart**
Martin Health System

**Tallahassee**
Shareholder
Tallahassee Memorial HealthCare

**Tampa**
Florida Hospital–Carrollwood
Partner
Florida Hospital Tampa

**Tarpon Springs**
Florida Hospital North Pinellas

**Titusville**
Partner
Parrish Medical Center

## GEORGIA

**Albany**
Phoebe Putney Health System
Partner
Phoebe Putney Memorial Hospital

**Americus**
Phoebe Sumter Medical Center

**Athens**
Partner
Athens Regional Medical Center

**Atlanta**
Partner
Northside Hospital

**Augusta**
University Health Care System

**Austell**
WellStar Cobb Hospital

**Blakely**
Pioneer Community Hospital of Early

**Brunswick**
Southeast Georgia Health System
Southeast Georgia Health System Brunswick Campus

**Cairo**
Grady General Hospital

**Camilla**
Mitchell County Hospital

**Canton**
Northside Hospital – Cherokee

**Chatsworth**
Murray Medical Center

**Cochran**
Bleckley Memorial Hospital

**Columbus**
Columbus Regional Healthcare System
Columbus Specialty Hospital
Doctors Hospital of Columbus
Hughston Hospital
Partner
The Medical Center

**Cordele**
Crisp Regional Hospital

**Cumming**
Northside Hospital Forsyth

**Cuthbert**
Southwest Georgia Regional Medical Center

**Dallas**
WellStar Paulding Hospital

**Dalton**
Partner
Hamilton Medical Center

**Decatur**
DeKalb Medical at Downtown Decatur
Partner
DeKalb Medical at North Decatur

**Douglas**
Coffee Regional Medical Center

**Douglasville**
WellStar Douglas Hospital

**Fitzgerald**
Dorminy Medical Center

**Gainesville**
Northeast Georgia Medical Center
**Hawkinsville**
Taylor Regional Hospital
**Homerville**
Clinch Memorial Hospital
**Lakeland**
Louis Smith Memorial Hospital
**Lawrenceville**
Partner
Gwinnett Hospital System
**Lithonia**
DeKalb Medical at Hillandale
**Macon**
Partner
Medical Center of Central Georgia
**Marietta**
WellStar Health System
WellStar Windy Hill Hospital
Partner
WellStar Kennestone Hospital
**Moultrie**
Colquitt Regional Medical Center
**Perry**
Perry Hospital
**Quitman**
Brooks County Hospital
**Riverdale**
Partner
Southern Regional Medical Center
**Rome**
Kindred Hospital Rome
Partner
Floyd Medical Center
**Saint Marys**
Southeast Georgia Health System Camden Campus
**Sylvester**
Phoebe Worth Medical Center
**Thomasville**
Partner
Archbold Medical Center
John D. Archbold Memorial Hospital
**Tifton**
Tift Regional Medical Center
**Valdosta**
Partner
South Georgia Medical Center
**Warner Robins**
Houston Medical Center
**Waycross**
Mayo Clinic Health System in Waycross

**HAWAII**
**Honolulu**
Queen's Health Systems
Queen's Medical Center
**Kaunakakai**
Molokai General Hospital
**Wahiawa**
Wahiawa General Hospital

**IDAHO**
**American Falls**
Power County Hospital District
**Arco**
Lost Rivers District Hospital
**Blackfoot**
Bingham Memorial Hospital
**Boise**
Elks Rehab Hospital
St. Luke's Health System
Shareholder
St. Luke's Regional Medical Center
**Bonners Ferry**
Boundary Community Hospital
**Cascade**
Cascade Medical Center
**Coeur D'Alene**
Kootenai Medical Center
**Emmett**
Walter Knox Memorial Hospital

**Gooding**
North Canyon Medical Center
**Grangeville**
Syringa Hospital and Clinics
**Jerome**
St. Luke's Jerome Family Medical Center
**Ketchum**
St. Luke's Wood River Medical Center
**Malad City**
Oneida County Hospital
**McCall**
St. Luke's McCall
**Montpelier**
Bear Lake Memorial Hospital
**Mountain Home**
Elmore Medical Center
**Orofino**
Clearwater Valley Hospital and Clinics
**Preston**
Franklin County Medical Center
**Rupert**
Minidoka Memorial Hospital
**Sandpoint**
Partner
Bonner General Hospital
**Twin Falls**
Partner
St. Luke's Magic Valley Medical Center
**Weiser**
Weiser Memorial Hospital

**ILLINOIS**
**Alton**
Alton Memorial Hospital
**Belleville**
Partner
Memorial Hospital
**Canton**
Graham Hospital
**Carbondale**
Memorial Hospital of Carbondale
Partner
Southern Illinois Hospital Services
**Chester**
Memorial Hospital
**Chicago**
Partner
Swedish Covenant Hospital
**De Kalb**
Kish Health System
**Decatur**
Decatur Memorial Hospital
**DeKalb**
Partner
Kishwaukee Community Hospital
**Elgin**
Partner
Sherman Hospital
**Elmhurst**
Partner
Elmhurst Memorial Hospital
**Eureka**
Advocate Eureka Hospital
**Evanston**
NorthShore University Health System Evanston Hospital
**Evergreen Park**
Partner
Little Company of Mary Hospital and Health Care Centers
**Flora**
Clay County Hospital
**Freeport**
Partner
FHN Memorial Hospital
**Geneseo**
Hammond–Henry Hospital
**Geneva**
Delnor Hospital
**Greenville**
Greenville Regional Hospital

**Herrin**
Herrin Hospital
**Jacksonville**
Partner
Passavant Area Hospital
**Jerseyville**
Jersey Community Hospital
**Lake Forest**
Partner
Northwestern Lake Forest Hospital
**Lincoln**
Abraham Lincoln Memorial Hospital
**Macomb**
Partner
McDonough District Hospital
**Maryville**
Partner
Anderson Hospital
**Mattoon**
Sarah Bush Lincoln Health Center
**Mendota**
Mendota Community Hospital
**Monticello**
Kirby Medical Center
**Murphysboro**
St. Joseph Memorial Hospital
**Naperville**
Edward Hospital
**New Lenox**
Partner
Silver Cross Hospital
**Normal**
Partner
Advocate BroMenn Medical Center
**Peoria**
Partner
Proctor Hospital
**Pittsfield**
Illini Community Hospital
**Quincy**
Partner
Blessing Hospital
**Rockford**
SwedishAmerican Hospital
**Rushville**
Sarah D. Culbertson Memorial Hospital
**Salem**
Salem Township Hospital
**Sandwich**
Valley West Community Hospital
**Shelbyville**
Shelby Memorial Hospital
**Skokie**
NorthShore University Health System Skokie Hospital
**Springfield**
Memorial Health System
Shareholder
Memorial Medical Center
**Taylorville**
Taylorville Memorial Hospital

**INDIANA**
**Anderson**
Community Hospital of Anderson and Madison County
**Avon**
Indiana University Health West Hospital
**Batesville**
Margaret Mary Community Hospital
**Bedford**
Indiana University Health Bedford Hospital
**Bloomington**
Partner
Indiana University Health Bloomington Hospital
**Bremen**
Community Hospital of Bremen
Doctor's Hospital and Neuromuscular Center
**Carmel**
Indiana University Health North Hospital
**Clinton**
Union Hospital Clinton

**Columbia City**
Parkview Whitley Hospital
**Columbus**
Partner
Columbus Regional Hospital
**Danville**
Partner
Hendricks Regional Health
**Elkhart**
Partner
Elkhart General Healthcare System
**Evansville**
Deaconess Health System
Shareholder
Deaconess Hospital
**Fort Wayne**
Parkview Health
Partner
Parkview Hospital
**Franklin**
Johnson Memorial Hospital
**Goshen**
Indiana University Health Goshen Hospital
**Greenfield**
Hancock Regional Hospital
**Hartford City**
Indiana University Health Blackford Hospital
**Huntington**
Parkview Huntington Hospital
**Indianapolis**
Community Health Network
Community Hospital East
Community Hospital North
Community Hospital South
Community Westview Hospital
Indiana Heart Hospital
Indiana University Health Methodist Hospital
Shareholder
Indiana University Health University Hospital
**Kendallville**
Parkview Noble Hospital
**Knox**
Indiana University Health Starke Hospital
**Kokomo**
Partner
Community Howard Regional Hospital
**La Porte**
Partner
Indiana University Health La Porte Hospital
**Lafayette**
Franciscan St. Elizabeth Health – Lafayette Central
Indiana University Health Arnett Hospital
**LaGrange**
Parkview LaGrange Hospital
**Madison**
Partner
King's Daughters' Hospital and Health Services
**Marion**
Partner
Marion General Hospital
**Martinsville**
Indiana University Health Morgan Hospital
**Muncie**
Shareholder
Indiana University Health Ball Memorial Hospital
**New Albany**
Partner
Floyd Memorial Hospital and Health Services
**New Castle**
Henry County Hospital
**Noblesville**
Partner
Riverview Hospital
**Paoli**
Indiana University Health Paoli Hospital
**Portland**
Jay County Hospital
**Richmond**
Partner
Reid Hospital and Health Care Services

**Seymour**
Schneck Medical Center
**Shelbyville**
Major Hospital
**South Bend**
Healthwin Hospital
Madison Center and Hospital
Memorial Hospital of South Bend
**Terre Haute**
Partner
Union Hospital
**Tipton**
Indiana University Health Tipton Hospital
**Vincennes**
Partner
Good Samaritan Hospital
**IOWA**
**Atlantic**
Shareholder
Cass County Memorial Hospital
**Council Bluffs**
Shareholder
Jennie Edmundson Hospital
**Decorah**
Winneshiek Medical Center
**Hamburg**
George C Grape Community Hospital
**Harlan**
Partner
Myrtue Medical Center
**Keokuk**
Shareholder
Keokuk Area Hospital
**Le Mars**
Partner
Floyd Valley Hospital
**Muscatine**
Trinity Muscatine
**Onawa**
Partner
Burgess Health Center
**Orange City**
Orange City Area Health System
**Red Oak**
Shareholder
Montgomery County Memorial Hospital
**Rock Rapids**
Sanford Medical Center Rock Rapids
**Sheldon**
Sanford Sheldon Medical Center
**Sioux City**
Shareholder
St. Luke's Regional Medical Center
**West Union**
Palmer Lutheran Health Center
**KANSAS**
**Abilene**
Memorial Health System
**Anthony**
Anthony Medical Center
**Atchison**
Shareholder
Atchison Hospital
**Atwood**
Rawlins County Health Center
**Belleville**
Republic County Hospital
**Beloit**
Mitchell County Hospital Health Systems
**Clay Center**
Clay County Medical Center
**Colby**
Shareholder
Citizens Medical Center
**Coldwater**
Comanche County Hospital
**Concordia**
Cloud County Health Center
**Dighton**
Lane County Hospital

**El Dorado**
Susan B. Allen Memorial Hospital
**Ellinwood**
Ellinwood District Hospital
**Ellsworth**
Ellsworth County Medical Center
**Fredonia**
Fredonia Regional Hospital
**Garnett**
Anderson County Hospital
**Goodland**
Goodland Regional Medical Center
**Greensburg**
Kiowa County Memorial Hospital
**Hays**
Shareholder
Hays Medical Center
**Herington**
Herington Municipal Hospital
**Hiawatha**
Partner
Hiawatha Community Hospital
**Hill City**
Graham County Hospital
**Hoisington**
Clara Barton Hospital
**Hoxie**
Sheridan County Health Complex
**Junction City**
Geary Community Hospital
**La Crosse**
Rush County Memorial Hospital
**Lawrence**
Lawrence Memorial Hospital
**Leavenworth**
Cushing Memorial Hospital
**Leoti**
Wichita County Health Center
**Liberal**
Shareholder
Southwest Medical Center
**Lincoln**
Lincoln County Hospital
**Lindsborg**
Lindsborg Community Hospital
**Lyons**
Rice County District Hospital
**Mankato**
Jewell County Hospital
**McPherson**
McPherson Hospital
**Medicine Lodge**
Medicine Lodge Memorial Hospital
**Minneapolis**
Ottawa County Health Center
**Minneola**
Minneola District Hospital
**Ness City**
Ness County Hospital
**Norton**
Norton County Hospital
**Oakley**
Logan County Hospital
**Osborne**
Osborne County Memorial Hospital
**Overland Park**
Saint Luke's South Hospital
**Parsons**
Partner
Labette Health
**Phillipsburg**
Phillips County Hospital
Shareholder
Great Plains Health Alliance, Inc.
**Plainville**
Rooks County Health Center
**Pratt**
Shareholder
Pratt Regional Medical Center
**Quinter**
Gove County Medical Center

**Ransom**
Grisell Memorial Hospital District One
**Russell**
Russell Regional Hospital
**Sabetha**
Sabetha Community Hospital
**Saint Francis**
Cheyenne County Hospital
**Salina**
Salina Surgical Hospital
Partner
Salina Regional Health Center
**Satanta**
Satanta District Hospital
**Scott City**
Scott County Hospital
**Smith Center**
Smith County Memorial Hospital
**Stafford**
Stafford County Hospital
**Topeka**
Shareholder
Stormont–Vail HealthCare
**Wakeeney**
Trego County–Lemke Memorial Hospital

## KENTUCKY
**Pikeville**
Pikeville Medical Center

## LOUISIANA
**Amite**
Hood Memorial Hospital
**Baton Rouge**
Franciscan Missionaries of Our Lady Health System, Inc.
Ochsner Medical Center–Baton Rouge
Member
Our Lady of the Lake Regional Medical Center
Partner
Woman's Hospital
**Bossier City**
WK Bossier Health Center
**Bunkie**
Bunkie General Hospital
**Church Point**
Acadia–St. Landry Hospital
**Columbia**
Citizens Medical Center
**Covington**
Partner
St. Tammany Parish Hospital
**Crowley**
Partner
American Legion Hospital
**De Ridder**
Partner
Beauregard Memorial Hospital
**Ferriday**
Riverland Medical Center
**Gonzales**
St. Elizabeth Hospital
**Greensburg**
St. Helena Parish Hospital
**Jennings**
Jennings American Legion Hospital
**Kenner**
Ochsner Medical Center – Kenner
**Lafayette**
Partner
Our Lady of Lourdes Regional Medical Center
**Lake Charles**
Partner
Lake Charles Memorial Hospital
**Mansfield**
De Soto Regional Health System
**Monroe**
Partner
St. Francis Medical Center
**Napoleonville**
Assumption Community Hospital
**Natchitoches**
Natchitoches Regional Medical Center

**New Iberia**
Iberia Medical Center
**New Orleans**
Ochsner Baptist Medical Center
Shareholder
Ochsner Medical Center
**Oak Grove**
West Carroll Memorial Hospital
**Raceland**
Ochsner St. Anne General Hospital
**Shreveport**
Willis–Knighton Health System
Shareholder
Willis–Knighton Medical Center
**Springhill**
Springhill Medical Center
**Sulphur**
Partner
West Calcasieu Cameron Hospital
**Vivian**
North Caddo Medical Center

## MAINE
**Augusta**
MaineGeneral Medical Center–Augusta Campus
**Bangor**
Eastern Maine Medical Center
The Acadia Hospital
**Bar Harbor**
Mount Desert Island Hospital
**Belfast**
Waldo County General Hospital
**Biddeford**
Shareholder
Southern Maine Medical Center
**Blue Hill**
Blue Hill Memorial Hospital
**Boothbay Harbor**
St. Andrews Hospital and Healthcare Center
**Brewer**
Partner
Eastern Maine Healthcare Systems
**Bridgton**
Bridgton Hospital
**Brunswick**
Mid Coast Hospital
**Damariscotta**
Miles Memorial Hospital
**Dover–Foxcroft**
Mayo Regional Hospital
**Ellsworth**
Maine Coast Memorial Hospital
**Greenville**
Charles A. Dean Memorial Hospital
**Houlton**
Houlton Regional Hospital
**Machias**
Down East Community Hospital
**Millinocket**
Unit_of
Millinocket Regional Hospital
**Norway**
Stephens Memorial Hospital
**Pittsfield**
Sebasticook Valley Health
**Portland**
Shareholder
Maine Medical Center
**Presque Isle**
The Aroostook Medical Center
**Rockport**
Pen Bay Medical Center
**Skowhegan**
Redington–Fairview General Hospital
**Waterville**
Inland Hospital
Shareholder
MaineGeneral Medical Center–Waterville Campus
**Westbrook**
Spring Harbor Hospital
**York**
York Hospital

## MARYLAND
**Baltimore**
Medstar Franklin Square Medical Center
Medstar Good Samaritan Hospital
Medstar Harbor Hospital
Medstar Union Memorial Hospital
**Bel Air**
Upper Chesapeake Medical Center
Partner
Upper Chesapeake Health System
**Columbia**
MedStar Health
**Havre De Grace**
Harford Memorial Hospital
**Leonardtown**
Medstar St. Mary's Hospital
**Olney**
Medstar Montgomery Medical Center
**Prince Frederick**
Calvert Memorial Hospital

## MASSACHUSETTS
**Belmont**
McLean Hospital
**Beverly**
Northeast Health System
Partner
Beverly Hospital
**Boston**
Brigham and Women's Hospital
Dana–Farber Cancer Institute
Faulkner Hospital
Massachusetts General Hospital
Spaulding Rehabilitation Hospital
Partner
Massachusetts Eye and Ear Infirmary
Shareholder
Partners HealthCare System, Inc.
**Burlington**
Partner
Lahey Clinic Hospital
**Cambridge**
Spaulding Hospital for Continuing Medical Care Cambridge
Partner
Mount Auburn Hospital
**Concord**
Partner
Emerson Hospital
**East Sandwich**
Spaulding Rehabilitation Hospital Cape Cod
**Falmouth**
Falmouth Hospital
**Gardner**
Partner
Heywood Hospital
**Hyannis**
Cape Cod Healthcare, Inc.
Partner
Cape Cod Hospital
**Lawrence**
Owner
Lawrence General Hospital
**Lowell**
Partner
Lowell General Hospital
**Melrose**
Hallmark Health System
Partner
Melrose–Wakefield Hospital
**Nantucket**
Nantucket Cottage Hospital
**Newton Lower Falls**
Newton–Wellesley Hospital
**Northampton**
Cooley Dickinson Hospital
**Oak Bluffs**
Martha's Vineyard Hospital
**Salem**
North Shore Medical Center
Spaulding Hospital for Continuing Medical Care North Shore

Section B

**South Weymouth**
Partner
   South Shore Hospital

**Southbridge**
Partner
   Harrington Memorial Hospital

## MICHIGAN

**Adrian**
   ProMedica Bixby Hospital

**Allegan**
   Allegan General Hospital

**Alpena**
   Alpena Regional Medical Center

**Bad Axe**
   Huron Medical Center

**Big Rapids**
   Mecosta County Medical Center

**Cass City**
   Hills & Dales General Hospital

**Coldwater**
   Community Health Center of Branch County

**Dearborn**
Member
   Oakwood Healthcare, Inc.
Partner
   Oakwood Hospital & Medical Center–Dearborn

**Detroit**
   St. John Detroit Riverview Center
Partner
   St. John Hospital and Medical Center

**East China**
   St. John River District Hospital

**Fremont**
   Spectrum Health Gerber Memorial

**Grand Haven**
   North Ottawa Community Hospital

**Grand Rapids**
   Mary Free Bed Rehabilitation Hospital
   Spectrum Health
   Spectrum Health Butterworth Hospital

**Greenville**
   Spectrum Health United Hospital

**Hastings**
   Pennock Hospital

**Holland**
Partner
   Holland Hospital

**Jackson**
   Allegiance Health

**Kalamazoo**
Partner
   Bronson Healthcare Group, Inc.
   Bronson Methodist Hospital

**Laurium**
   Aspirus Keweenaw Hospital

**Ludington**
   Memorial Medical Center of West Michigan

**Madison Heights**
   St. John Macomb–Oakland Hospital, Oakland Center

**Marquette**
   Marquette General Health System

**Marshall**
   Oaklawn Hospital

**Monroe**
Partner
   Mercy Memorial Hospital System

**Ontonagon**
   Aspirus Ontonagon Hospital

**Owosso**
Partner
   Memorial Healthcare

**Paw Paw**
   Bronson LakeView Hospital

**Petoskey**
   McLaren Northern Michigan

**Port Huron**
   Port Huron Hospital
Partner
   Blue Water Health Services Corporation

**Reed City**
   Spectrum Health Reed City Hospital

**Royal Oak**
Shareholder
   Beaumont Hospital – Royal Oak

**Saginaw**
   Covenant Medical Center

**Saint Ignace**
   Mackinac Straits Health System

**Saint Joseph**
   Lakeland Healthcare
   Lakeland Regional Medical Center–St. Joseph

**Shelby**
   Mercy Health Partners, Lakeshore Campus

**South Haven**
   South Haven Health System

**Taylor**
   Oakwood Heritage Hospital

**Tecumseh**
   ProMedica Herrick Hospital

**Trenton**
   Oakwood Southshore Medical Center

**Troy**
   Beaumont Hospital – Troy

**Vicksburg**
   Bronson Vicksburg Hospital

**Warren**
   St. John Macomb–Oakland Hospital, Macomb Center

**Wayne**
   Oakwood Annapolis Hospital

**West Branch**
Partner
   West Branch Regional Medical Center

**Wyoming**
   Metro Health Hospital

**Zeeland**
   Spectrum Health Zeeland Community Hospital

## MINNESOTA

**Ada**
   Essentia Health Ada

**Albert Lea**
   Mayo Clinic Health System in Albert Lea

**Arlington**
   Sibley Medical Center

**Austin**
   Mayo Clinic Health System in Austin

**Bemidji**
Partner
   Sanford Bemidji Medical Center

**Benson**
   Swift County–Benson Hospital

**Blue Earth**
   United Hospital District

**Brainerd**
   Essentia Health St. Joseph's Medical Center

**Buffalo**
   Buffalo Hospital

**Cambridge**
   Cambridge Medical Center

**Canby**
   Sanford Medical Center Canby

**Cannon Falls**
   Mayo Clinic Health System in Cannon Falls

**Coon Rapids**
   Mercy Hospital

**Detroit Lakes**
   Essentia Health St. Mary's Hospital – Detroit Lakes

**Duluth**
   Essentia Health
   Essentia Health Duluth
   Essentia Health St. Mary's Medical Center
Partner
   St. Luke's Hospital

**Fairmont**
   Mayo Clinic Health System in Fairmont

**Fergus Falls**
Partner
   Lake Region Healthcare Corporation

**Fosston**
   Essentia Health Fosston

**Fridley**
   Unity Hospital

**Graceville**
   Essentia Health–Holy Trinity Hospital

**Grand Rapids**
   Grand Itasca Clinic and Hospital

**Hallock**
   Kittson Memorial Healthcare Center

**Hutchinson**
   Hutchinson Area Health Care

**Jackson**
   Sanford Jackson Medical Center

**Lake City**
   Mayo Clinic Health System in Lake City

**Le Sueur**
   Minnesota Valley Health Center

**Long Prairie**
   CentraCare Health System – Long Prairie

**Luverne**
   Sanford Luverne Medical Center

**Madelia**
   Madelia Community Hospital

**Mahnomen**
   Mahnomen Health Center

**Mankato**
Partner
   Mayo Clinic Health System in Mankato

**Maple Grove**
   Maple Grove Hospital

**Melrose**
   CentraCare Health System – Melrose

**Minneapolis**
   Abbott Northwestern Hospital
Shareholder
   Allina Health

**Morris**
   Stevens Community Medical Center

**New Ulm**
   New Ulm Medical Center

**Ortonville**
   Ortonville Area Health Services

**Owatonna**
   Owatonna Hospital

**Paynesville**
   Paynesville Area Health Care System

**Perham**
   Perham Health

**Redwood Falls**
   Redwood Area Hospital

**Robbinsdale**
   North Memorial Health Care

**Rochester**
   Mayo Clinic – Methodist Hospital
   Mayo Clinic – Saint Marys Hospital
   Mayo Clinic Health System

**Roseau**
   LifeCare Medical Center

**Saint Cloud**
   CentraCare Health System
Partner
   St. Cloud Hospital

**Saint James**
   Mayo Clinic Health System in Saint James

**Saint Paul**
   HealthEast Bethesda Hospital
   St. John's Hospital
   St. Joseph's Hospital
   United Hospital
Shareholder
   HealthEast Care System

**Saint Peter**
   River's Edge Hospital and Clinic

**Sandstone**
   Essentia Health Sandstone

**Shakopee**
   St. Francis Regional Medical Center

**Slayton**
   Murray County Medical Center

**Springfield**
   Mayo Clinic Health System in Springfield

**Thief River Falls**
   Sanford Medical Center Thief River Falls

**Tracy**
   Sanford Tracy Medical Center

**Waconia**
Partner
Ridgeview Medical Center

**Warren**
North Valley Health Center

**Waseca**
Mayo Clinic Health System in Waseca

**Westbrook**
Sanford Westbrook Medical Center

**Willmar**
Partner
Rice Memorial Hospital

**Windom**
Windom Area Hospital

**Woodbury**
Woodwinds Health Campus

**Worthington**
Sanford Worthington Medical Center

## MISSISSIPPI

**Batesville**
Tri–Lakes Medical Center

**Booneville**
Baptist Memorial Hospital–Booneville

**Calhoun City**
Calhoun Health Services

**Columbus**
Baptist Memorial Hospital–Golden Triangle

**Corinth**
Magnolia Regional Health Center

**Eupora**
North Mississippi Medical Center–Eupora

**Greenville**
Delta Regional Medical Center

**Greenwood**
Partner
Greenwood Leflore Hospital

**Gulfport**
Partner
Memorial Hospital at Gulfport

**Hattiesburg**
Partner
Forrest General Hospital

**Jackson**
Partner
St. Dominic–Jackson Memorial Hospital

**McComb**
Partner
Southwest Mississippi Regional Medical Center

**Meridian**
Partner
Anderson Regional Medical Center

**Monticello**
Lawrence County Hospital

**New Albany**
Baptist Memorial Hospital–Union County

**Oxford**
Baptist Memorial Hospital–North Mississippi

**Pascagoula**
Singing River Health System

**Picayune**
Highland Community Hospital

**Pontotoc**
North Mississippi Medical Center–Pontotoc Hospital
and Nursing Home

**Southaven**
Baptist Memorial Hospital–Desoto

**Starkville**
OCH Regional Medical Center

**Tupelo**
North Mississippi Health Services, Inc.
North Mississippi Medical Center – Tupelo

**Tylertown**
Walthall County General Hospital

**West Point**
North Mississippi Medical Center–West Point

## MISSOURI

**Bolivar**
Partner
Citizens Memorial Hospital

**Bonne Terre**
Parkland Health Center–Bonne Terre

**Branson**
Partner
Skaggs Regional Medical Center

**Brookfield**
General John J. Pershing Memorial Hospital

**Cameron**
Partner
Cameron Regional Medical Center

**Cape Girardeau**
Landmark Hospital
Partner
Saint Francis Medical Center

**Carthage**
Partner
Mercy McCune–Brooks Hospital

**Chillicothe**
Hedrick Medical Center

**Clinton**
Golden Valley Memorial Healthcare

**Columbia**
Boone Hospital Center

**Crystal City**
Jefferson Regional Medical Center

**Farmington**
Parkland Health Center

**Joplin**
Freeman Health System
Freeman Hospital East

**Kansas City**
Crittenton Children's Center
Saint Luke's North Hospital – Barry Road
Shareholder
Saint Luke's Health System
Saint Luke's Hospital of Kansas City

**Lamar**
Barton County Memorial Hospital

**Lee's Summit**
Saint Luke's East Hospital

**Liberty**
Partner
Liberty Hospital

**Macon**
Samaritan Memorial Hospital

**Marshall**
Fitzgibbon Hospital

**Monett**
Cox Monett

**Neosho**
Freeman Neosho Hospital

**Potosi**
Washington County Memorial Hospital

**Saint Louis**
Barnes–Jewish Hospital
Barnes–Jewish West County Hospital
Christian Hospital
Missouri Baptist Medical Center
St. Louis Children's Hospital
Shareholder
BJC HealthCare

**Saint Peters**
Barnes–Jewish St. Peters Hospital

**Salem**
Salem Memorial District Hospital

**Sikeston**
Missouri Delta Medical Center

**Springfield**
CoxHealth
Lester E. Cox Medical Center North
Shareholder
Lester E. Cox Medical Centers

**Ste Genevieve**
Ste. Genevieve County Memorial Hospital

**Sullivan**
Missouri Baptist Sullivan Hospital

**Trenton**
Wright Memorial Hospital

**Warrensburg**
Western Missouri Medical Center

## MONTANA

**Anaconda**
Community Hospital of Anaconda

**Big Timber**
Pioneer Medical Center

**Billings**
Partner
Billings Clinic

**Bozeman**
Partner
Bozeman Deaconess Hospital

**Columbus**
Unit_of
Stillwater Community Hospital

**Fort Benton**
Missouri River Medical Center

**Glasgow**
Frances Mahon Deaconess Hospital

**Glendive**
Partner
Glendive Medical Center

**Great Falls**
Benefis Hospitals

**Hamilton**
Partner
Marcus Daly Memorial Hospital

**Helena**
Partner
St. Peter's Hospital

**Kalispell**
The HealthCenter

**Livingston**
Livingston Memorial Hospital

**Missoula**
St. Patrick Hospital
Partner
Community Medical Center

**Plains**
Clark Fork Valley Hospital

**Polson**
St. Joseph Hospital

**Red Lodge**
Beartooth Billings Clinic

**Ronan**
Partner
St. Luke Community Hospital

**Scobey**
Daniels Memorial Healthcare Center

**Sidney**
Partner
Sidney Health Center

## NEBRASKA

**Alliance**
Box Butte General Hospital

**Alma**
Harlan County Health System

**Atkinson**
West Holt Memorial Hospital

**Beatrice**
Partner
Beatrice Community Hospital and Health Center

**Bridgeport**
Morrill County Community Hospital

**Broken Bow**
Jennie M. Melham Memorial Medical Center

**Columbus**
Partner
Columbus Community Hospital

**Crete**
Crete Area Medical Center

**Falls City**
Community Medical Center

**Franklin**
Franklin County Memorial Hospital

**Gordon**
Gordon Memorial Hospital

**Hastings**
Partner
Mary Lanning Healthcare

**Lexington**
Partner
   Lexington Regional Health Center

**Lincoln**
   BryanLGH Health System
   BryanLGH Medical Center
Partner
   Madonna Rehabilitation Hospital

**Lynch**
   Niobrara Valley Hospital

**McCook**
Partner
   Community Hospital

**Minden**
   Kearney County Health Services

**Neligh**
   Antelope Memorial Hospital

**Norfolk**
Partner
   Faith Regional Health Services

**Omaha**
   Nebraska Methodist Health System, Inc.
Shareholder
   Nebraska Methodist Hospital

**Ord**
   Valley County Health System

**Oshkosh**
   Garden County Health Services

**Osmond**
   Osmond General Hospital

**Plainview**
   Alegent Health Plainview Hospital

**Scottsbluff**
Partner
   Regional West Medical Center

**Tilden**
   Tilden Community Hospital

**York**
Partner
   York General Hospital

## NEW HAMPSHIRE

**Claremont**
   Valley Regional Hospital

**Colebrook**
   Upper Connecticut Valley Hospital

**Dover**
Partner
   Wentworth–Douglass Hospital

**Keene**
Partner
   Cheshire Medical Center

**Lancaster**
   Weeks Medical Center

**Lebanon**
   Alice Peck Day Memorial Hospital
   Dartmouth–Hitchcock Medical Center

**Nashua**
Partner
   Southern New Hampshire Medical Center

**New London**
   New London Hospital

**Peterborough**
   Monadnock Community Hospital

**Rochester**
Partner
   Frisbie Memorial Hospital

**Woodsville**
   Cottage Hospital

## NEW JERSEY

**Atlantic City**
   AtlantiCare Regional Medical Center

**Edison**
   JFK Health System
   JFK Medical Center

**Egg Harbor Township**
   AtlantiCare

**Elmer**
   South Jersey Healthcare – Elmer Hospital

**Flemington**
Partner
   Hunterdon Medical Center

**Newton**
Partner
   Newton Medical Center

**Pennington**
   Capital Health Medical Center–Hopewell

**Phillipsburg**
Partner
   St. Luke's Hospital – Warren Campus

**Pomona**
   Bacharach Institute for Rehabilitation

**Pompton Plains**
Partner
   Chilton Hospital

**Ridgewood**
   Valley Hospital

**Somers Point**
Partner
   Shore Medical Center

**Trenton**
   Capital Health
   Capital Health Regional Medical Center

**Vineland**
   South Jersey Healthcare
   South Jersey Healthcare – Regional Medical Center

**Woodbury**
Partner
   Underwood–Memorial Hospital

## NEW MEXICO

**Artesia**
   Artesia General Hospital

**Farmington**
Partner
   San Juan Regional Medical Center

**Gallup**
Partner
   Rehoboth McKinley Christian Health Care Services

## NEW YORK

**Binghamton**
Shareholder
   United Health Services Hospitals–Binghamton

**Bronx**
   New York Westchester Square Medical Center

**Bronxville**
   Lawrence Hospital Center

**Brooklyn**
   New York Community Hospital
   New York Methodist Hospital
   Wyckoff Heights Medical Center

**Buffalo**
   Erie County Medical Center
   Roswell Park Cancer Institute

**Cobleskill**
Partner
   Cobleskill Regional Hospital

**Cooperstown**
Partner
   Bassett Medical Center

**Corning**
   Corning Hospital

**Elmira**
   St. Joseph's Hospital

**Flushing**
   New York Hospital Queens

**Geneva**
   Finger Lakes Health
Partner
   Geneva General Hospital

**Hamilton**
   Community Memorial Hospital

**Ithaca**
Partner
   Cayuga Medical Center at Ithaca

**Jamestown**
   Woman's Christian Association Hospital

**Little Falls**
   Little Falls Hospital

**Malone**
   Alice Hyde Medical Center

**Mineola**
   Winthrop–University Hospital

**Mount Kisco**
Partner
   Northern Westchester Hospital

**New York**
   New York–Presbyterian Hospital
Shareholder
   New York–Presbyterian/Columbia University Medical Center

**Norwich**
   Chenango Memorial Hospital

**Nyack**
   Nyack Hospital

**Ogdensburg**
   Claxton–Hepburn Medical Center

**Penn Yan**
   Soldiers and Sailors Memorial Hospital of Yates County

**Rochester**
   Strong Memorial Hospital of the University of Rochester
   Unity Hospital
   University of Rochester Medical Center
Partner
   Highland Hospital of Rochester

**Sleepy Hollow**
   Phelps Memorial Hospital Center

**Syracuse**
Partner
   Crouse Hospital

**Utica**
   Faxton–St. Luke's Healthcare

**Walton**
   Delaware Valley Hospital

**White Plains**
Partner
   White Plains Hospital Center

## NORTH CAROLINA

**Ahoskie**
   Vidant Roanoke–Chowan Hospital

**Bolivia**
   Brunswick Novant Medical Center

**Cary**
   WakeMed Cary Hospital

**Charlotte**
   Carolinas Medical Center
   Carolinas Medical Center–Mercy
   Presbyterian Hospital
   Presbyterian–Orthopaedic Hospital
Shareholder
   Carolinas HealthCare System

**Clinton**
   Sampson Regional Medical Center

**Concord**
Shareholder
   Carolinas Medical Center–NorthEast

**Dunn**
   Betsy Johnson Regional Hospital

**Edenton**
   Vidant Chowan Hospital

**Greensboro**
   Cone Health

**Greenville**
Shareholder
   Vidant Medical Center

**High Point**
Shareholder
   High Point Regional Health System

**Huntersville**
   Presbyterian Hospital Huntersville

**Kenansville**
   Vidant Duplin Hospital

**Lexington**
   Wake Forest Baptist Health–Lexington Medical Center

**Lincolnton**
   Carolinas Medical Center–Lincoln

**Louisburg**
   Franklin Regional Medical Center

**Matthews**
   Presbyterian Hospital Matthews

**Monroe**
   Carolinas Medical Center–Union

**Nags Head**
The Outer Banks Hospital
**Raleigh**
WakeMed Health & Hospitals
Partner
WakeMed Raleigh Campus
**Rocky Mount**
Partner
Nash Health Care Systems
**Salisbury**
Partner
Rowan Regional Medical Center
**Tarboro**
Vidant Edgecombe Hospital
**Thomasville**
Partner
Thomasville Medical Center
**Windsor**
Vidant Bertie Hospital
**Winston–Salem**
Forsyth Medical Center
Medical Park Hospital
Novant Health

**NORTH DAKOTA**

**Bismarck**
Partner
Medcenter One
**Fargo**
Essentia Health Fargo
Sanford Medical Center Fargo
**Grafton**
Unity Medical Center
**Grand Forks**
Partner
Altru Health System
**Hillsboro**
Hillsboro Medical Center
**Jamestown**
Partner
Jamestown Regional Medical Center
**Kenmare**
Kenmare Community Hospital
**Mayville**
Sanford Medical Center Mayville
**McVille**
Nelson County Health System
**Minot**
Trinity Health

**OHIO**

**Akron**
Akron General Health System
Shareholder
Akron General Medical Center
**Ashland**
Samaritan Regional Health System
**Athens**
O'Bleness Memorial Hospital
**Bellaire**
Belmont Community Hospital
**Bowling Green**
Wood County Hospital
**Cambridge**
Partner
Southeastern Ohio Regional Medical Center
**Cincinnati**
UC Health
Shareholder
Christ Hospital
**Cleveland**
University Hospitals Case Medical Center
**Columbus**
Doctors Hospital
Grant Medical Center
Riverside Methodist Hospital
Member
OhioHealth
**Concord Township**
Partner
Lake Health
**Cuyahoga Falls**
Edwin Shaw Rehab

**Dayton**
Miami Valley Hospital
Partner
Good Samaritan Hospital
**Defiance**
ProMedica Defiance Regional Hospital
**Delaware**
Grady Memorial Hospital
**Dover**
Partner
Union Hospital
**Dublin**
Dublin Methodist Hospital
**Findlay**
Blanchard Valley Hospital
**Fostoria**
ProMedica Fostoria Community Hospital
**Fremont**
Partner
Memorial Hospital
**Galion**
Galion Community Hospital
**Georgetown**
Southwest Regional Medical Center
**Greenville**
Wayne Hospital
**Kenton**
Hardin Memorial Hospital
**Lima**
Partner
Lima Memorial Health System
**Lodi**
Lodi Community Hospital
**Logan**
Hocking Valley Community Hospital
**Mansfield**
MedCentral – Mansfield Hospital
**Marion**
OhioHealth Marion General Hospital
**Maumee**
Partner
ProMedica St. Luke's Hospital
**Middletown**
Partner
Atrium Medical Center
**Mount Gilead**
Morrow County Hospital
**Nelsonville**
Doctors Hospital Nelsonville
**Newark**
Partner
Licking Memorial Hospital
**Norwalk**
Fisher–Titus Medical Center
**Oregon**
ProMedica Bay Park Hospital
**Oxford**
McCullough–Hyde Memorial Hospital
**Portsmouth**
Southern Ohio Medical Center
**Shelby**
MedCentral – Shelby Hospital
**Sidney**
Wilson Memorial Hospital
**Steubenville**
Partner
Trinity Health System
**Sylvania**
ProMedica Flower Hospital
**Toledo**
ProMedica Health System
Shareholder
ProMedica Toledo Hospital
**Troy**
Partner
Upper Valley Medical Center
**Warren**
Hillside Rehabilitation Hospital
**Wauseon**
Fulton County Health Center

**Youngstown**
Northside Medical Center
**Zanesville**
Partner
Genesis HealthCare System

**OKLAHOMA**

**Ada**
Partner
Valley View Regional Hospital
**Altus**
Partner
Jackson County Memorial Hospital
**Blackwell**
Integris Blackwell Regional Hospital
**Carnegie**
Carnegie Tri–County Municipal Hospital
**Chickasha**
Partner
Grady Memorial Hospital
**Clinton**
Integris Clinton Regional Hospital
**Duncan**
Partner
Duncan Regional Hospital
**El Reno**
Mercy Hospital El Reno
**Elk City**
Great Plains Regional Medical Center
**Enid**
Integris Bass Baptist Health Center
Integris Bass Pavilion
**Frederick**
Memorial Hospital and Physician Group
**Grove**
Integris Grove General Hospital
**Guymon**
Partner
Memorial Hospital of Texas County
**Hobart**
Elkview General Hospital
**Lawton**
Partner
Comanche County Memorial Hospital
**Madill**
Integris Marshall County Medical Center
**McAlester**
Partner
McAlester Regional Health Center
**Miami**
Integris Baptist Regional Health Center
**Norman**
Norman Regional Health System
**Oklahoma City**
Integris Baptist Medical Center
INTEGRIS Health
Integris Southwest Medical Center
**Pryor**
Integris Mayes County Medical Center
**Purcell**
Purcell Municipal Hospital
**Seminole**
Integris Seminole Medical Center
**Shawnee**
St. Anthony Shawnee Hospital
**Stillwater**
Partner
Stillwater Medical Center
**Tahlequah**
Tahlequah City Hospital
**Waurika**
Jefferson County Hospital
**Yukon**
INTEGRIS Canadian Valley Hospital

**OREGON**

**Hillsboro**
Partner
Tuality Healthcare
**Hood River**
Providence Hood River Memorial Hospital

**Medford**
Providence Medford Medical Center

**Milwaukie**
Providence Milwaukie Hospital

**Newberg**
Providence Newberg Medical Center

**Oregon City**
Providence Willamette Falls Medical Center

**Portland**
Providence Portland Medical Center
Providence St. Vincent Medical Center

**Seaside**
Providence Seaside Hospital

**Silverton**
Silverton Hospital

## PENNSYLVANIA

**Abington**
Partner
Abington Memorial Hospital

**Allentown**
Shareholder
Lehigh Valley Hospital

**Bethlehem**
Lehigh Valley Hospital–Muhlenberg

**Brookville**
Brookville Hospital

**Butler**
Partner
Butler Health System

**Chambersburg**
Chambersburg Hospital
Summit Health

**Clearfield**
Clearfield Hospital

**Coudersport**
Charles Cole Memorial Hospital

**Drexel Hill**
Delaware County Memorial Hospital

**Du Bois**
DuBois Regional Medical Center

**East Stroudsburg**
Pocono Medical Center

**Ephrata**
Partner
Ephrata Community Hospital

**Erie**
Shareholder
UPMC Hamot

**Gettysburg**
Gettysburg Hospital

**Hanover**
Hanover Hospital

**Harrisburg**
Community Hospital
Pinnacle Health System

**Hastings**
Miners Medical Center

**Indiana**
Indiana Regional Medical Center

**Jefferson Hills**
Jefferson Regional Medical Center

**Johnstown**
Conemaugh Health System
Memorial Medical Center

**Kane**
Kane Community Hospital

**Kittanning**
ACMH Hospital

**Lancaster**
Partner
Lancaster General Health

**Lebanon**
The Good Samaritan Hospital

**Lehighton**
Blue Mountain Health System
Gnaden Huetten Memorial Hospital

**Mc Connellsburg**
Fulton County Medical Center

**Meadowbrook**
Holy Redeemer Hospital and Medical Center

**Meyersdale**
Meyersdale Medical Center

**Monongahela**
Monongahela Valley Hospital

**New Castle**
Jameson Hospital

**Norristown**
Partner
Montgomery Hospital Medical Center

**Palmerton**
Palmerton Hospital

**Philadelphia**
Hospital of the University of Pennsylvania
Penn Presbyterian Medical Center
University of Pennsylvania Health System
Shareholder
Pennsylvania Hospital

**Pittsburgh**
Partner
St. Clair Memorial Hospital

**Punxsutawney**
Punxsutawney Area Hospital

**Renovo**
Bucktail Medical Center

**Roaring Spring**
Nason Hospital

**Saint Marys**
Elk Regional Health Center

**Sayre**
Robert Packer Hospital
Shareholder
Guthrie Healthcare System

**Scranton**
Partner
Geisinger–Community Medical Center

**Sellersville**
Partner
Grand View Hospital

**Sharon**
Partner
Sharon Regional Health System

**Springfield**
Crozer–Keystone Health System

**State College**
Mount Nittany Medical Center

**Troy**
Troy Community Hospital

**Tyrone**
Tyrone Hospital

**Uniontown**
Partner
Uniontown Hospital

**Upland**
Crozer–Chester Medical Center

**Waynesboro**
Waynesboro Hospital

**Wellsboro**
Soldiers and Sailors Memorial Hospital

**West Chester**
Partner
Chester County Hospital

**West Reading**
Reading Hospital and Medical Center

**Williamsport**
Divine Providence Hospital
Partner
Susquehanna Health System

**Windber**
Windber Medical Center

**York**
Partner
WellSpan Health
Shareholder
York Hospital

## RHODE ISLAND

**East Providence**
Emma Pendleton Bradley Hospital

**Newport**
Newport Hospital

**Pawtucket**
Memorial Hospital of Rhode Island

**Providence**
Butler Hospital
Care New England Health System
Miriam Hospital
Women & Infants Hospital of Rhode Island
Shareholder
Lifespan Corporation
Rhode Island Hospital

**Warwick**
Kent County Memorial Hospital

**Westerly**
Westerly Hospital

## SOUTH CAROLINA

**Gaffney**
Upstate Carolina Medical Center

## SOUTH DAKOTA

**Armour**
Douglas County Memorial Hospital

**Burke**
Community Memorial Hospital

**Canton**
Sanford Canton–Inwood Medical Center

**Chamberlain**
Sanford Medical Center Chamberlain

**Clear Lake**
Sanford Deuel County Medical Center

**Sioux Falls**
Sanford Health
Shareholder
Sanford University of South Dakota Medical Center

**Vermillion**
Sanford Vermillion Medical Center

**Viborg**
Pioneer Memorial Hospital and Health Services

**Watertown**
Prairie Lakes Healthcare System

**Webster**
Sanford Medical Center Webster

**Winner**
Winner Regional Healthcare Center

## TENNESSEE

**Bolivar**
Bolivar General Hospital

**Camden**
Camden General Hospital

**Chattanooga**
Erlanger Health System
Erlanger North Hospital

**Collierville**
Baptist Memorial Hospital–Collierville

**Columbia**
Partner
Maury Regional Hospital

**Covington**
Baptist Memorial Hospital–Tipton

**Franklin**
Williamson Medical Center

**Harriman**
Roane Medical Center

**Humboldt**
Humboldt General Hospital

**Huntingdon**
Baptist Memorial Hospital–Huntingdon

**Jackson**
Shareholder
Jackson–Madison County General Hospital

**Knoxville**
Covenant Health
East Tennessee Children's Hospital
Fort Sanders Regional Medical Center
Parkwest Medical Center

**Lenoir City**
Fort Loudoun Medical Center

**Lewisburg**
Marshall Medical Center

**Louisville**
Peninsula Hospital

**Memphis**
Baptist Memorial Health Care Corporation
Baptist Memorial Hospital for Women

Baptist Memorial Hospital – Memphis

**Milan**
Milan General Hospital

**Oak Ridge**
Partner
Methodist Medical Center of Oak Ridge

**Paris**
Henry County Medical Center

**Parsons**
Decatur County General Hospital

**Pikeville**
Erlanger Bledsoe Hospital

**Ripley**
Lauderdale Community Hospital

**Savannah**
Hardin Medical Center

**Sevierville**
LeConte Medical Center

**Trenton**
Gibson General Hospital

**Union City**
Baptist Memorial Hospital–Union City

**Waynesboro**
Wayne Medical Center

## TEXAS

**Amarillo**
Partner
Baptist St. Anthony Health System

**Andrews**
Permian Regional Medical Center

**Atlanta**
Atlanta Memorial Hospital

**Beaumont**
Baptist Hospitals of Southeast Texas

**Bellville**
Bellville General Hospital

**Caldwell**
Burleson St. Joseph Health Center

**Dallas**
Baylor Jack and Jane Hamilton Heart and Vascular Hospital
Baylor Specialty Hospital
Baylor University Medical Center
Children's Medical Center of Dallas
Methodist Health System
Shareholder
Baylor Health Care System

**Decatur**
Wise Regional Health System

**Del Rio**
Val Verde Regional Medical Center

**Electra**
Electra Memorial Hospital

**Floresville**
Connally Medical Center

**Fort Worth**
Shareholder
Baylor All Saints Medical Center at Fort Worth

**Garland**
Baylor Medical Center at Garland

**Gatesville**
Coryell Memorial Hospital

**Grapevine**
Partner
Baylor Regional Medical Center at Grapevine

**Houston**
Memorial Hermann – Texas Medical Center
Memorial Hermann Healthcare System
Memorial Hermann Northwest Hospital

**Humble**
Memorial Hermann Northeast

**Huntsville**
Huntsville Memorial Hospital

**Irving**
Partner
Baylor Medical Center at Irving

**Jacksonville**
Mother Frances Hospital – Jacksonville

**Katy**
Memorial Hermann Katy Hospital

**Levelland**
Covenant Hospital–Levelland

**Linden**
Good Shepherd Medical Center–Linden

**Longview**
Partner
Good Shepherd Medical Center

**Lubbock**
Covenant Children's Hospital
Covenant Medical Center
Covenant Medical Center–Lakeside
Shareholder
Covenant Health System

**Madisonville**
Madison St. Joseph Health Center

**Marshall**
Partner
Good Shepherd Medical Center–Marshall

**Midland**
Midland Memorial Hospital
Partner
Midland Memorial Hospital

**Navasota**
Grimes St. Joseph Health Center

**Odessa**
Medical Center Health System

**Orange**
Baptist Orange Hospital

**Pearsall**
Frio Regional Hospital

**Plainview**
Covenant Hospital Plainview

**Plano**
Baylor Regional Medical Center at Plano
Community Hospital Corporation
The Heart Hospital Baylor Plano

**Port Lavaca**
Memorial Medical Center

**Richardson**
Partner
Methodist Richardson Medical Center

**Rockdale**
Little River Medical Center

**Round Rock**
Scott & White Hospital at Round Rock

**San Angelo**
Shannon Medical Center

**Sherman**
Partner
Texas Health Presbyterian Hospital–WNJ

**Sugar Land**
Memorial Hermann Sugar Land Hospital

**Sulphur Springs**
Hopkins County Memorial Hospital

**Sweeny**
Sweeny Community Hospital

**Temple**
Scott and White Memorial Hospital

**Tomball**
Tomball Regional Medical Center

**Tyler**
Partner
Mother Frances Hospital – Tyler

**Waco**
Partner
Hillcrest Baptist Medical Center

**Waxahachie**
Baylor Medical Center at Waxahachie

**Wichita Falls**
Partner
United Regional Health Care System
United Regional Health Care System–Eighth Street Campus

**Winnie**
Winnie Community Hospital

**Yoakum**
Yoakum Community Hospital

## VERMONT

**Bennington**
Southwestern Vermont Medical Center

**Berlin**
Partner
Central Vermont Medical Center

**Morrisville**
Copley Hospital

**Newport**
North Country Hospital and Health Center

**Rutland**
Partner
Rutland Regional Medical Center

**Saint Johnsbury**
Northeastern Vermont Regional Hospital

**Windsor**
Mt. Ascutney Hospital and Health Center

## VIRGIN ISLANDS

**Saint Thomas**
Schneider Regional Medical Center

## VIRGINIA

**Charlottesville**
Partner
Martha Jefferson Hospital

**Farmville**
Centra Southside Community Hospital

**Fredericksburg**
Mary Washington Hospital

**Hampton**
Sentara CarePlex Hospital

**Harrisonburg**
Partner
Rockingham Memorial Hospital

**Lynchburg**
Centra Lynchburg General Hospital

**Manassas**
Prince William Hospital

**Norfolk**
Hospital for Extended Recovery
Sentara Leigh Hospital
Sentara Norfolk General Hospital
Shareholder
Sentara Healthcare

**Suffolk**
Sentara Obici Hospital

**Virginia Beach**
Sentara Princess Anne Hospital
Sentara Virginia Beach General Hospital

**Williamsburg**
Sentara Williamsburg Regional Medical Center

**Woodbridge**
Sentara Northern Virginia Medical Center

## WASHINGTON

**Aberdeen**
Grays Harbor Community Hospital

**Centralia**
Providence Centralia Hospital

**Chewelah**
Providence St. Joseph's Hospital

**Colfax**
Whitman Hospital and Medical Center

**Colville**
Providence Mount Carmel Hospital

**Everett**
Providence Regional Medical Center Everett

**Morton**
Morton General Hospital

**Olympia**
Providence St. Peter Hospital

**Puyallup**
MultiCare Good Samaritan Hospital

**Renton**
Providence Health & Services

**Seattle**
Swedish Medical Center–Cherry Hill Campus

**Spokane**
Providence Holy Family Hospital

**Tacoma**
MultiCare Tacoma General Hospital
Shareholder
MultiCare Health System

**Vancouver**
PeaceHealth Southwest Medical Center

**Walla Walla**
Providence St. Mary Medical Center

**Wenatchee**
Central Washington Hospital

**Yakima**
Partner
Yakima Valley Memorial Hospital

## WEST VIRGINIA

**Charleston**
Charleston Area Medical Center
Women and Children's Hospital
Shareholder
Charleston Area Medical Center Health System, Inc.

**Gassaway**
Braxton County Memorial Hospital

**Glen Dale**
Partner
Reynolds Memorial Hospital

**Madison**
Boone Memorial Hospital

**Montgomery**
Montgomery General Hospital

**Princeton**
Partner
Princeton Community Hospital

**Ripley**
Jackson General Hospital

**Spencer**
Roane General Hospital

**Wheeling**
Partner
Wheeling Hospital

## WISCONSIN

**Antigo**
Langlade Memorial Hospital

**Appleton**
Appleton Medical Center
Shareholder
ThedaCare, Inc.

**Barron**
Mayo Clinic Health System – Northland in Barron

**Beaver Dam**
Partner
Beaver Dam Community Hospitals

**Beloit**
Partner
Beloit Health System

**Bloomer**
Mayo Clinic Health System – Chippewa Valley in
Bloomer

**Eau Claire**
Partner
Mayo Clinic Health System in Eau Claire

**Green Bay**
Partner
Bellin Memorial Hospital

**La Crosse**
Mayo Clinic Health System – Franciscan Healthcare in
La Crosse
Shareholder
Gundersen Lutheran Medical Center

**Madison**
Shareholder
Meriter Hospital

**Marinette**
Bay Area Medical Center

**Medford**
Memorial Health Center

**Menomonee Falls**
Partner
Community Memorial Hospital

**Menomonie**
Mayo Clinic Health System – Red Cedar in Menomonie

**Milwaukee**
Partner
Froedtert Memorial Lutheran Hospital

**Neenah**
Theda Clark Medical Center

**Neillsville**
Memorial Medical Center – Neillsville

**New London**
New London Family Medical Center

**Oconomowoc**
Oconomowoc Memorial Hospital

**Oconto**
Oconto Hospital & Medical Center

**Osseo**
Mayo Clinic Health System – Oakridge in Osseo

**River Falls**
River Falls Area Hospital

**Sparta**
Mayo Clinic Health System – Franciscan Healthcare in
Sparta

**Superior**
Essentia Health St. Mary's Hospital of Superior

**Watertown**
Partner
Watertown Regional Medical Center

**Waukesha**
ProHealth Care, Inc.
Waukesha Memorial Hospital

**Waupaca**
Riverside Medical Center

**Wausau**
Aspirus Wausau Hospital

**West Bend**
Owner
St. Joseph's Community Hospital of West Bend

**Whitehall**
Tri–County Memorial Hospital

**Wisconsin Rapids**
Riverview Hospital Association

## WYOMING

**Buffalo**
Johnson County Healthcare Center

**Casper**
Partner
Wyoming Medical Center

**Cheyenne**
Partner
Cheyenne Regional Medical Center

**Douglas**
Memorial Hospital of Converse County

**Gillette**
Campbell County Memorial Hospital

**Jackson**
St. John's Medical Center and Living Center

**Kemmerer**
South Lincoln Medical Center

**Laramie**
Partner
Ivinson Memorial Hospital

**Lovell**
North Big Horn Hospital District

**Lusk**
Niobrara Health and Life Center

**Rawlins**
Memorial Hospital of Carbon County

**Sheridan**
Sheridan Memorial Hospital

# YANKEE ALLIANCE
138 River Road, Andover, MA
Zip 01810–1083; tel. 978/470–2000; R.
Paul O'Neill, President

## CONNECTICUT

**New Haven**
Member
Hospital of Saint Raphael

**New London**
Member
Lawrence & Memorial Hospital

**Stafford Springs**
Member
Johnson Memorial Hospital

## MAINE

**Bangor**
Member
St. Joseph Hospital

**Lewiston**
Member
St. Mary's Regional Medical Center

**Sanford**
Member
Henrietta D. Goodall Hospital

## MASSACHUSETTS

**Attleboro**
Member
Sturdy Memorial Hospital

**Boston**
Member
Boston Medical Center
New England Baptist Hospital
Tufts Medical Center

**Brockton**
Member
Signature Healthcare Brockton Hospital

**Cambridge**
Member
Spaulding Hospital for Continuing Medical Care
Cambridge

**Fall River**
Member
Charlton Memorial Hospital
Southcoast Hospitals Group

**Great Barrington**
Member
Fairview Hospital

**Lowell**
Member
Saints Medical Center

**New Bedford**
Member
St. Luke's Hospital

**Newburyport**
Member
Anna Jaques Hospital

**North Adams**
Member
North Adams Regional Hospital

**Oak Bluffs**
Member
Martha's Vineyard Hospital

**Pittsfield**
Member
Berkshire Health Systems, Inc.
Berkshire Medical Center

**Quincy**
Member
Quincy Medical Center

**Stoughton**
Member
New England Sinai Hospital and Rehabilitation Center

**Wareham**
Member
Tobey Hospital

**Winchester**
Member
Winchester Hospital

## NEW HAMPSHIRE

**Exeter**
Member
Exeter Hospital

**Manchester**
Member
Catholic Medical Center
Elliot Hospital

**Nashua**
Member
St. Joseph Hospital

**North Conway**
Member
Memorial Hospital

## NEW YORK

**Albany**
Member
Albany Medical Center

**Batavia**
Member
    United Memorial Medical Center

**Elizabethtown**
Member
    Elizabethtown Community Hospital

**Glens Falls**
Member
    Glens Falls Hospital

**Gloversville**
Member
    Nathan Littauer Hospital and Nursing Home

**Plattsburgh**
Member
    Champlain Valley Physicians Hospital Medical Center

**Troy**
Member
    Samaritan Hospital

**RHODE ISLAND**
**Providence**
Member
    Roger Williams Medical Center

**Wakefield**
Member
    South County Hospital

**Woonsocket**
Member
    Landmark Medical Center

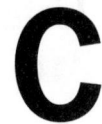

†List supplied by The Joint Commission

Section C

*This section of AHA Guide was compiled to provide a directory of information useful to the health care field.*

## National and International Organizations

The national and international lists include many types of voluntary organizations concerned with matters of interest to the health care field. The organizational information includes address, telephone number, FAX number, and the primary contact. The information was obtained directly from the organizations.

Organizations are searchable by state, then city within state, and "kind of organization."

We present these organization listings simply as a convenient directory. Inclusion or omission of any organization's name indicates neither approval nor disapproval by Health Forum LLC, an American Hospital Association company.

## United States Government Agencies

National agencies concerned with health–related matters are listed by the major department of government under which the different functions fall.

## State and Local Organizations and Agencies

The lists of organizations in states, associated areas, and provinces include Blue Cross and Blue Shield plans, group purchasing organizations, hospital associations and councils, quality improvement organizations, and regional health information organizations.

There are many active local organizations that do not fall within these categories. Contact the hospital association of the state or province for information about such additional groups. The hospital association and councils listed have offices with full-time executives.

The selected state and provincial government agencies include the state department of health, facility licensure, medical and nursing licensure, and managed care organization licensure.

## Other Providers

A list of Freestanding Ambulatory Surgery Centers is provided.

Lists of The Joint Commission Accredited Long Term Care Organizations and Joint Commission Accredited Behavioral Health Organizations are provided for your information.

These lists are provided simply as a convenient reference. Inclusion or omission of any organization's name indicates neither approval or disapproval by Health Forum L.L.C.

## A

**AARP,** 601 E Street NW, Washington, DC 20049; tel. 202/434–2277; FAX. 888/836–3985; Addison Barry Rand, Chief Executive Officer

**Academic Pediatric Association,** 6728 Old McLean Village Drive, McLean, VA 22101; tel. 703/556–9222; FAX. 703/556–8729; Marge Degnon, Executive Director

**AcademyHealth,** 1150 17th Street NW, Suite 600, Washington, DC 20036; tel. 202/292–6700; FAX. 202/292–6800; Lisa Simpson, MB, BCh, MPH, FAAP, President and Chief Executive Officer

**Accreditation Association for Ambulatory Health Care,** 5250 Old Orchard Rd., Suite 200, Skokie, IL 60077; tel. 847/853–6060; FAX. 847/853–9028; John E. Burke, Ph. D., Executive Director

**Accreditation Council for Graduate Medical Education, ACGME,** 515 N. State Street, Suite 2000, Chicago, IL 60654; tel. 312/755–5000; FAX. 312/755–7498; Thomas J. Nasca, MD, MACP, Chief Executive Officer

**Accreditation Council for Pharmacy Education, ACPE,** 135 S. LaSalle Street, Suite 4100, Chicago, IL 60603–4810; tel. 312/664–3575; FAX. 312/664–4652; Peter H. Vlasses, Pharm. D., BCPS, FCCP, Executive Director

**Acute Long Term Hospital Association,** 1667 K Street, NW, Suite 1050, Washington, DC 20006; tel. 202/266–9800; William Walters, Chief Executive Officer

**Advanced Medical Technology Association,** 701 Pennsylvania Avenue, NW, Suite 800, Washington, DC 20004; tel. 202/783–8700; FAX. 202/783–8750; Stephen J. Ubl, President and Chief Executive Officer

**Aerospace Medical Association,** 320 South Henry Street, Alexandria, VA 22314–3579; tel. 703/739–2240; FAX. 703/739–9652; Jeffrey C. Sventek, MS, CASP, Executive Director

**Alcoholics Anonymous World Services, Inc.,** PO Box 459, New York, NY 10163; tel. 212/870–3400; FAX. 202/870–3003

**Alexander Graham Bell Association for the Deaf & Hard of Hearing,** 3417 Volta Place, NW, Washington, DC 20007; tel. 202/204–4683; FAX. 202/337–5087; Garrett W. Yates, Acting Development Director

**Allergy Associates,** 2004 Grand Avenue, Baldwin, NY 11510; tel. 516/223–7656; FAX. 516/223–0583; Joe D' Amore, MD, President

**Alliance for Children & Families,** 11700 West Lake Park Drive, Milwaukee, WI 53224; tel. 414/359–1040; FAX. 414/359–1074; Susan N. Greyfus, President and Chief Executive Officer

**Alzheimer's Association, (Alzheimer's Disease and Related Disorders Association, Inc.),** 225 North Michigan Avenue, Suite 1700, Chicago, IL 60601; tel. 312/335–8700; FAX. 312/335–1110; Cyndy Cordell, Healthcare Professional Services

**America's Blood Centers,** 725 15th Street, NW, Suite 700, Washington, DC 20005–2109; tel. 202/393–5725; FAX. 202/393–1282; Jim MacPherson, Chief Executive Officer

**America's Health Insurance Plans,** 601 Pennsylvania Ave NW, South Bldg, Suite 500, Washington, DC 20004; tel. 202/778–3200; FAX. 202/778–8486; Charles W. Stellar, Executive Vice President

**American Academy for Cerebral Palsy and Developmental Medicine,** 555 E. Wells Street, Suite 1100, Milwaukee, WI 53202; tel. 414/918–3014; FAX. 414/276–2146; Tracy Burr, Executive Director

**American Academy of Allergy, Asthma and Immunology,** 555 East Wells Street, Suite 1100, Milwaukee, WI 53202; tel. 414/272–6071; FAX. 414/272–6070; Kay Whalen, Executive Director

**American Academy of Child and Adolescent Psychiatry,** 3615 Wisconsin Avenue, NW, Washington, DC 20016; tel. 202/966–7300; FAX. 202/966–2891; Virginia Q. Anthony, Executive Director

**American Academy of Dental Practice Administration,** 1063 Whippoorwill Lane, Palatine, IL 60067; tel. 847/934–4404; Kathleen Uebel, Executive Director

**American Academy of Dermatology,** 930 East Woodfield Road, Schaumburg, IL 60173; tel. 847/330–0230; FAX. 847/330–0050; Robert S. Bolan, PhD, Interim Executive Director

**American Academy of Family Physicians,** 11400 Tomahawk Creek Parkway, Leawood, KS 66211; tel. 913/906–6000; FAX. 913/906–6083

**American Academy of Medical Administrators,** 701 Lee Street, Suite 600, Des Plaines, IL 60016; tel. 847/759–8601; FAX. 847/759–8602; Renee Schleicher, CAE, President and Chief Executive Officer

**American Academy of Neurology,** 201 Chicago Avenue South, Minneapolis, MN 55415; tel. 612/928–6100; FAX. 612/454–2744; Catherine M. Rydell, CAE, Executive Director

**American Academy of Ophthalmology,** 655 Beach Street, P.O. Box 7424, San Francisco, CA 94120; tel. 415/561–8500; FAX. 415/561–8533; David W. Parke, II, Executive Vice President and Chief Executive Officer

**American Academy of Optometry,** 2909 Fairgreen Street, Orlando, FL 32803; tel. 3217103937; FAX. 4108939890; Lois Schoenbrun, CAE, FAAO Executive Director

**American Academy of Oral Medicine,** 23607 Highway 99, Suite 2C, Edmonds, WA 98020–9516; tel. 425/778–6162; FAX. 425/771–9588; Nick Senzee, Executive Director

**American Academy of Orthopaedic Surgeons,** 6300 North River Road, Rosemont, IL 60018–4262; tel. 847/823–7186; FAX. 847/823–8125; Karen L. Hackett, FACHE, CAE, Chief Executive Officer

**American Academy of Otolaryngic Allergy,** 1990 M. Street, NW, Suite 680, Washington, DC 20036; tel. 202/955–5010; FAX. 202/955–5016; Jami Lucas, Executive Director

**American Academy of Otolaryngology-Head and Neck Surgery, Inc.,** 1650 Diagonal Road, Alexandria, VA 22314; tel. 703/836–4444; FAX. 703/683–5100; David R. Nielsen, MD, FACS, Chief Executive Officer and Executive Vice President

**American Academy of Pain Management,** 13947 Mono Way, Suite A, Sonora, CA 95370–2807; tel. 209/533–9744; FAX. 209/533–9750; Kathryn A. Padgett, PhD, Executive Director

**American Academy of Pediatrics,** 141 Northwest Point Boulevard, Elk Grove Village, IL 60007–1098; tel. 847/434–4000; FAX. 847/434–8000; Errol R. Alden MD., Executive Director and Chief Executive Officer

**American Academy of Physical Medicine and Rehabilitation,** 9700 West Bryn Mawr Avenue, Suite 200, Rosemont, IL 60018–5701; tel. 847/737–6000; FAX. 847/737–6001; Thomas E. Stautzenbach, CAE, Executive Director

**American Academy of Physician Assistants,** 2318 Mill Road, Suite 1300, Alexandria, VA 22314; tel. 703/836–2272; FAX. 703/684–1924; James G. Potter, CAE, Executive Vice President and Interim Chief Executive Officer

**American Academy of Psychoanalysis And Dynamic Psychiatry,** One Regency Drive, PO Box 30, Bloomfield, CT 06002; tel. 888/691–8281; FAX. 860/286–0787; Jacquelyn T. Coleman, CAE, Executive Director

**American Aging Association, The Sally Balin Medical Center,** 110 Chesley Drive, Media, PA 19063; tel. 610/627–2626; FAX. 610/565–9747; Arthur K. Balin, MD, PhD., FACP

**American Ambulance Association,** 8400 Westpark Drive, Second Floor, McLean, VA 22102; tel. 703/610–9018; FAX. 703/610–0210; Maria Bianchi, Executive Vice President

**American Art Therapy Association, Inc.,** 11160 - C1 South Lakes Drive, Suite 813, Reston, VA 20191; tel. 703/212–2238; Peg Dunn-Snow, PhD, ATR-BC, President

**American Assembly for Men In Nursing,** PO Box 130220, Birmingham, AL 35213; tel. 205/956–0146; FAX. 205/956–0149; Byron McCain, Executive Director

**American Association for Clinical Chemistry, Inc. (AACC),** 1850 K Street, NW, Washington, DC 20006; tel. 202/857–0717; FAX. 202/877–5093; Richard Flaherty, Executive Vice President

**American Association for Dental Research,** 1619 Duke Street, Alexandria, VA 22314–3406; tel. 703/548–0066; FAX. 703/548–1883; Christopher Fox, Executive Director

**American Association for Health Education,** 1900 Association Drive, Reston, VA 20191; tel. 703/476–3400; FAX. 703/476–9527; Malcolm Goldsmith, Executive Director

**American Association For Homecare,** 2011 Crystal Drive, Suite 725, Arlington, VA 22202–3709; tel. 703/836–6263; FAX. 703/836–6730; Michael Reinemer, Vice President

**American Association for Laboratory Animal Science, AALAS,** 9190 Crestwyn Hills Drive, Memphis, TN 38125; tel. 901/754–8620; FAX. 901/753–0046; Ann T. Turner, PhD, CAE, Executive Director

**American Association for Respiratory Care,** 9425 N. MacArthur, Suite 100, Irving, TX 75063; tel. 972/243–2272; FAX. 972/484–2720

**American Association for the Advancement of Science,** 1200 New York Avenue, NW, Washington, DC 20005; tel. 202/326–6640; FAX. 202/371–9526; Alan Leshner, Chief Executive Officer

**American Association for the Surgery of Trauma,** 633 N. Saint Clair Street, Suite 2600, Chicago, IL 60611; tel. 800/789–4006; FAX. 312/202–5064; Sharon Gautschy, Executive Director

**American Association of Ambulatory Surgery Centers,** 1012 Cameron Street, Alexandria, VA 22314; tel. 703/836–8808; FAX. 703/549–0976; Kathy Bryant, President

**American Association of Anatomists,** 9650 Rockville Pike, Bethesda, MD 20814; tel. 301/634–7910; FAX. 301/634–7965; Andrea Pendleton

**American Association of Bioanalysts,** 906 Olive, Suite 1200, St. Louis, MO 63101–1448; tel. 314/241–1445; FAX. 314/241–1449; Mark S. Birenbaum, PhD, Administrator

**American Association of Certified Orthoptists,** Greater Baltimore Medical Center, 6569 North Charles Street, Baltimore, MD 21204; tel. 734/764–7558; FAX. 734/763–7114; Cheryl McCarus, CO, COMT, OSA, President

**American Association of Colleges of Nursing,** One DuPont Circle, NW, Suite 530, Washington, DC 20036; tel. 202/463–6930; FAX. 202/785–8320; Geraldine Bednash, PhD, RN FAAN, Chief Executive Officer and Executive Director

**American Association of Colleges of Osteopathic Medicine,** 5550 Friendship Boulevard, Suite 310, Chevy Chase, MD 20815–7231; tel. 301/968–4100; FAX. 301/968–4101; Stephen C. Shannon, DO, MPH, President and Chief Executive Officer

**American Association of Colleges of Pharmacy,** 1727 King Street, Floor 2, Alexandria, VA 22314–2700; tel. 703/739–2330; FAX. 703/836–8982; Lucinda Maine, PhD, Executive Vice President

**American Association of Colleges of Podiatric Medicine,** 15850 Crabbs Branch Way, Suite 320, Rockville, MD 20855–2622; tel. 301/948–9760; FAX. 301/948–1928; Moraith G. North, Executive Director

**American Association of Critical-Care Nurses,** 101 Columbia, Aliso Viejo, CA 92656–1491; tel. 949/362–2000; FAX. 949/362–2020; Wanda L. Johansson, RN, MN, Chief Executive Officer

**American Association of Dental Consultants, Inc.,** 10032 Wind Hill Drive, Greenville, IN 47124; tel. 812/923–2600; FAX. 812/923–2900; Judy Salisbury, Executive Director

**American Association of Endodontists,** 211 East Chicago Avenue, Suite 1100, Chicago, IL 60611–2691; tel. 312/266–7255; FAX. 312/266–9867; Trina Anderson, Executive Assistant to the Executive Director

**American Association of Healthcare Administrative Management,** 11240 Waples Mill Road, Suite 200, Fairfax, VA 22030; tel. 703/281–4043; FAX. 703/359–7562; Sharon Galler, Executive Director

**American Association of Healthcare Consultants,** 5938 N. Drake Avenue, Chicago, IL 60659; tel. 888/350–2242; FAX. 773/463–3552; Linda Campbell, CAE, Executive Director

**American Association of Kidney Patients,** 2701 North Rocky Point Drive, Suite 150, Tampa, FL 33607; tel. 800/749–2257; FAX. 813/636–8122; Karen E. Ryals, Executive Director

**American Association of Medical Assistants,** 20 North Wacker Drive, Suite 1575, Chicago, IL 60606; tel. 312/899–1500; FAX. 312/899–1259; Donald A. Balasa, JD, MBA, Executive Director, Legal Counsel

**American Association of Nurse Anesthetists,** 222 South Prospect Avenue, Park Ridge, IL 60068–4001; tel. 847/692–7050; FAX. 847/685–4501; Wanda O. Wilson, CRNA, PhD, Executive Director

**American Association of Occupational Health Nurses, Inc.,** 7794 Grow Drive, Pensacola, FL 32514; tel. 770/455–7757; FAX. 770/455–7271; Ann R. Cox, CAE, Executive Director

**American Association of Oral and Maxillofacial Surgeons,** 9700 West Bryn Mawr Avenue, Rosemont, IL 60018–5701; tel. 847/678–6200; FAX. 847/678–6286; Robert C. Rinaldi, PhD, Executive Director

**American Association of Orthodontists,** 401 North Lindbergh Boulevard, St. Louis, MO 63141–7816; tel. 314/993–1700; FAX. 314/997–1745; Chris P. Vranas, Executive Director

**American Association of Pastoral Counselors,** 9504A Lee Highway, Fairfax, VA 22031–2303; tel. 703/385–6967; FAX. 703/352–7725; Douglas M. Ronsheim, D.Min, Executive Director

**American Association of Physicists in Medicine,** One Physics Ellipse, College Park, MD 20740–3846; tel. 301/209–3350; FAX. 301/209–0862; Angela R. Keyser, Executive Director

**American Association of Plastic Surgeons,** 500 Cummings Center, Suite 4550, Beverly, MA 01915; tel. 978/927–8330; FAX. 978/524–0461; Aurelie Alger, JD, Executive Director

**American Association of Poison Control Centers,** 515 King Street, Suite 510, Alexandria, VA 22314; tel. 703/894–1858; FAX. 703/683–2812; Debbie Carr, Executive Director

**American Association of Psychiatric Technicians, Inc., A.A.P.T.,** 1220 S Street, Suite 100, Sacramento, CA 95814–7138; tel. 800/391–7589; FAX. 916/329–9145; Debi Loger, Executive Director

**American Association of Public Health Dentistry,** 3085 Stevenson Drive, Suite 200, Springfield, IL 62703; tel. 217/529–6941; FAX. 217/529–9120; Pamela T. Tolson, CAE, Executive Director

**American Association on Intellectual and Developmental Disabilities (AAIDD),** 501 Third Street, NW, Suite 200, Washington, DC 20001–2760; tel. 202/387–1968; FAX. 202/387–2193; Margaret A. Nygren, Executive Director & Chief Executive Officer

**American Baptist Homes and Caring Ministries,** PO Box 851 (National Ministries), Valley Forge, PA 19482–0851; tel. 610/768–2051; Laura Miraz, Liaison

**American Board of Allergy and Immunology,** 111 S. Independence Mall East, Suite 701, Philadelphia, PA 19106–3699; tel. 215/592–9466; FAX. 215/592–9411; Stephen I. Wasserman, MD, President

**American Board of Cardiovascular Medicine and Credentialing,** PO Box 3395, Riverview, FL 33568; tel. 813/394–4968; Jonni Cooper, BSN, MBA, PhD, FACCN-III, Chief Executive Officer

**American Board of Cardiovascular Perfusion,** 207 North 25th Avenue, Hattiesburg, MS 39401; tel. 601/582–2227; FAX. 601/582–2271; Beth A. Richmond, PhD, Stephen Oshrin, PhD, Executive Co-Directors

**American Board of Colon and Rectal Surgery,** 20600 Eureka Road, Suite 600, Taylor, MI 48180; tel. 734/282–9400; FAX. 734/282–9402; David J. Schoetz, MD, Executive Director

**American Board of Dermatology, Inc.,** Henry Ford Health System, One Ford Place, Detroit, MI 48202–3450; tel. 313/874–1088; FAX. 313/872–3221; Antoinette F. Hood, MD, Executive Director

**American Board of Emergency Medicine,** 3000 Coolidge Road, East Lansing, MI 48823; tel. 517/332–4800; FAX. 517/332–2234; Earl J. Reisdorff, MD, Executive Director

**American Board of Family Medicine, Inc.,** 1648 McGrathiana Parkway, Suite 550, Lexington, KY 40511–1247; tel. 859/269–5626; FAX. 859/335–7501; James Puffer, MD, President and Chief Executive Officer

**American Board of Internal Medicine,** 510 Walnut Street, Suite 1700, Philadelphia, PA 19106–3699; tel. 215/446–3500; FAX. 215/446–3473; Christine K. Cassel, MD, President

**American Board of Medical Specialties,** 222 N LaSalle St, Suite 1500, Chicago, IL 60601; tel. 312/436–2600; FAX. 312/436–2700; Lori Boukas, Communications Director

**American Board of Neurological Surgery,** 245 Amity Road #208, Woodbridge, CT 06525; tel. 713/441–6015; FAX. 713/794–0207; Mary Louise Spencer, Executive Director

**American Board of Nuclear Medicine,** 4555 Forest Park Blvd, Suite 119, St. Louis, MO 63108; tel. 314/367–2225; Henry D. Royal, MD, Executive Director

**American Board of Ophthalmology,** 111 Presidential Boulevard, Suite 241, Bala Cynwyd, PA 19004; tel. 610/664–1175; FAX. 610/664–6503; John G. Clarkson, MD, Executive Director

**American Board of Oral and Maxillofacial Surgery,** 625 North Michigan Avenue, Suite 1820, Chicago, IL 60611; tel. 312/642–0070; FAX. 312/642–8584; Cheryl E. Mounts, Executive Secretary

**American Board of Orthopedic Surgery, Inc.,** 400 Silver Cedar Court, Chapel Hill, NC 27514; tel. 919/929–7103; FAX. 919/942–8988; Shepard R. Hurwitz, MD, Executive Director

**American Board of Pathology,** One Urban Centre, 4830 West Kennedy Boulevard, Suite 690, Tampa, FL 33622–5915; tel. 813/286–2444; FAX. 813/289–5279; Rebecca L. Johnson, MD, Executive Vice President

**American Board of Pediatrics, Inc.,** 111 Silver Cedar Court, Chapel Hill, NC 27514; tel. 919/929–0461; FAX. 919/929–9255; James A. Stockman, III, MD, President

**American Board of Physical Medicine and Rehabilitation,** 3015 Allegro Park Lane SW, Rochester, MN 55902; tel. 507/282–1776; FAX. 507/282–9242; Anthony M. Tarvestad, JD, Executive Director

**American Board of Podiatric Surgery,** 445 Fillmore Street, San Francisco, CA 94117–3404; tel. 415/553–7800; FAX. 415/553–7801; James A. Lamb, Executive Director

**American Board of Preventive Medicine, Inc.,** 111 West Jackson Boulevard, Suite 1110, Chicago, IL 60604; tel. 312/939–2276; FAX. 312/939–2218; William W. Greaves, MD, MSPH, Executive Director

**American Board of Prosthodontics,** PO Box 271894, West Hartford, CT 06127–1894; tel. 860/679–2649; FAX. 860/206–1169; Thomas D. Taylor, DDS, MSD, Executive Director

**American Board of Psychiatry and Neurology, Inc.,** 2150 E. Lake Cook Road, Suite 900, Buffalo Grove, IL 60089; tel. 847/229–6500; FAX. 847/229–6600; Larry Faulkner, MD, Executive Vice President

**American Board of Quality Assurance and Utilization Review Physicians, Inc., ABQAURP,** 6640 Congress St, New Port Richey, FL 34653; tel. 800/998–6030; FAX. 727/569–0195; Arthur I. Broder, MD, Chairman

**American Board of Radiology,** 5441 E. Williams Blvd, Suite 200, Tucson, AZ 85711; tel. 520/790–2900; FAX. 520/790–3200; Gary J. Becker, MD, Executive Director

**American Board of Surgery, Inc.,** 1617 John F. Kennedy Boulevard, Suite 860, Philadelphia, PA 19103; tel. 215/568–4000; FAX. 215/563–5718; Frank R. Lewis, MD, Executive Director

**American Board of Thoracic Surgery,** 633 N. Street Clair Street, Suite 2320, Chicago, IL 60611; tel. 312/202–5900; FAX. 312/202–5960; William A. Baumgartner, MD, Executive Director

**American Broncho-Esophagological Association, Office of the Secretary,** Stanford University School of Medicine, Division of Pediatric Otolaryngology, Stanford, CA 94305–5739; tel. 650/725–6500; FAX. 650/725–8502; Peter Koltai, MD, Secretary

**American Burn Association,** 311 South Wacker Drive, Suite 4150, Chicago, IL 60606; tel. 312/642–9260; FAX. 312/642–9130; John Krichbaum, JD, Executive Director

**American Cancer Society,** 250 Williams Street NW, Suite 600, Atlanta, GA 30303; tel. 800/227–2345; Otis Brawley, MD, Chief Medical Officer

**American Center for the Alexander Technique, Inc.,** 39 W. 14th Street, #507, New York, NY 10011; tel. 212/633–2229; FAX. 212/633–2239; Jane Tomkiewicz, Executive Director

**American Chiropractic Association,** 1701 Clarendon Boulevard, Arlington, VA 22209; tel. 703/276–8800; FAX. 703/243–2593; Janet Ridgely, Acting Executive Vice President

**American Cleft Palate-Craniofacial Association,** 1504 E. Franklin Street, Suite 102, Chapel Hill, NC 27514; tel. 919/933–9044; FAX. 919/933–9604; Nancy C. Smythe, Executive Director

**American College Health Association,** 1362 Mellon Road, Suite 180, Hanover, MD 21076; tel. 410/859–1500; FAX. 410/859–1510; Doyle E. Randol, MS, Executive Director

**American College of Allergy, Asthma and Immunology,** 85 West Algonquin Road, Suite 550, Arlington Heights, IL 60005; tel. 847/427–1200; FAX. 847/427–1294; Rick Slawny, Executive Director

**American College of Apothecaries,** PO Box 341266, Bartlett, TN 38184; tel. 901/383–8119; FAX. 901/383–8882; D. C. Huffman, Jr., PhD, Executive Vice President

**American College of Cardiology,** 2400 N Street, NW, Washington, DC 20037; tel. 202/375–6180; FAX. 202/375–6819; Jack Lewin, MD, Chief Executive Officer

**American College of Cardiovascular Nurses, Inc.,** PO Box 3395, Riverview, FL 33568; tel. 813/394–4968; Jonni Cooper, BSN, MBA, PhD, FACCN-III, Chief Executive Officer

**American College of Chest Physicians,** 3300 Dundee Road, Northbrook, IL 60062; tel. 847/498–8300; FAX. 847/498–8318; Paul A. Markowski, CAE

**American College of Dentists,** 839J Quince Orchard Boulevard, Gaithersburg, MD 20878–1614; tel. 301/977–3223; FAX. 301/977–3330; Stephen A. Ralls, DDS

**American College of Emergency Physicians,** PO Box 619911, Dallas, TX 75261–9911; tel. 972/550–0911; FAX. 972/580–2816; Dean Wilikerson, Executive Director

**American College of Foot and Ankle Surgeons,** 8725 W. Higgins Rd, Suite 555, Chicago, IL 60631; tel. 773/693–9300; FAX. 773/693–9304; J.C. Mahaffey, CAE, Executive Director

**American College of Gastroenterology,** 6400 Goldsboro Road, Suite 200, Bethesda, MD 20817; tel. 3012639000; FAX. 7039314520; Thomas F. Fise, Executive Director

**American College of Healthcare Executives,** One North Franklin, Suite 1700, Chicago, IL 60606–3491; tel. 312/424–2800; FAX. 312/424–0023; Thomas C. Dolan, PhD, FACHE, CAE, President and Chief Executive Officer

**American College of Mohs Surgery,** 555 E. Wells, Suite 1100, Milwaukee, WI 53202–3823; tel. 414/347–1103; FAX. 414/276–2146; Kim Schardin, CAE, Executive Director

**American College of Nurse-Midwives,** Silver Spring Metro Plaza, 8403 Colesville Rd, Ste.1550, Silver Spring, MD 20910–6374; tel. 240/485–1800; FAX. 240/485–1818; Lorrie Kline Kaplan, Executive Director

**American College of Obstetricians and Gynecologists,** 409 12th Street, SW, Washington, DC 20090–6920; tel. 202/638–5577; FAX. 202/484–5107; Ralph W. Hale, MD, Executive Vice President

**American College of Occupational and Environmental Medicine, (Includes Occupational & Environmental Health Foundation and The Occupational Physicians Scholarship Fund),** 25 Northwest Point Blvd, Suite 700, Elk Grove Village, IL 60007; tel. 847/818–1800; FAX. 847/818–9266; Barry S. Eisenberg, CAE., Executive Director

**American College of Physician Executives,** 400 N. Ashley Drive, Suite 400, Tampa, FL 33602; tel. 813/287–2000; FAX. 813/287–8993; Peter Angood, MD, Chief Executive Officer

**American College of Physicians,** 190 North Independence Mall West, Philadelphia, PA 19106–1572; tel. 215/351–2600; FAX. 215/351–2829; John Tooker, MD, MBA, FACP, Executive VP, Chief Executive Officer

**American College of Preventive Medicine,** 455 Massachusetts Avenue NW, Suite 200, Washington, DC 20001; tel. 202/466–2044; FAX. 202/466–2662; Mike Barry, Executive Director

**American College of Radiology,** 1891 Preston White Drive, Reston, VA 20191–4397; tel. 703/648–8900; FAX. 703/648–9176; Harvey L. Neiman, MD, Executive Director

**American College of Rheumatology,** 2200 Lake Boulevard NE, Suite 250, Atlanta, GA 30319; tel. 404/633–3777; FAX. 404/633–1870; Helen Anne Richards, Director of Membership

**American College of Sports Medicine,** PO Box 1440, Indianapolis, IN 46206–1440; tel. 317/637–9200; FAX. 317/634–7817; James R. Whitehead, Executive Vice President

**American College of Surgeons,** 633 N. Saint Clair Street, Chicago, IL 60611; tel. 312/202–5000; FAX. 312/202–5001; David B. Hoyt, MD, FACS, Executive Director

**American Congress of Rehabilitation Medicine,** 11654 Plaza America Drive #535, Reston, VA 20190–4700; tel. 317/471–8760; FAX. 866/692–1619; Jon W. Lindbergh, MBA, CAE, Chief Executive Officer

**American Dental Assistants Association,** 35 E. Wacker Driver, Suite 1730, Chicago, IL 60601; tel. 312/541–1550; FAX. 312/541–1496; Lawrence H. Sepin, Executive Director

**American Dental Association,** 211 East Chicago Avenue, Chicago, IL 60611; tel. 312/440–2500; Kathleen T. O'Loughlin, DMD, MPH, Executive Director

**American Dental Education Association,** 1400 K. Street NW, Suite 1100, Washington, DC 20005; tel. 202/289–7201; FAX. 202/289–7204; Richard Valachovic, Executive Director

**American Dental Society of Anesthesiology, Inc.,** 211 East Chicago Avenue, Suite 780, Chicago, IL 60611; tel. 312/664–8270; FAX. 312/224–8624; R. Knight Charlton, Executive Director

**American Diabetes Association, Inc.,** 1701 N. Beauregard Street, Alexandria, VA 22311; tel. 703/549–1500; FAX. 703/836–7439; Larry Hausner, Chief Executive Officer

**American Federation for Aging Research,** 55 West 39th Street, 16th Floor, New York, NY 10018; tel. 212/703–9977; FAX. 212/997–0330; Stephanie Lederman, Director

**American Foundation for the Blind, Inc.,** 11 Penn Plaza, Suite 300, New York, NY 10001; tel. 212/502–7600; FAX. 212/502–7770; Liz Greco - Rocks, Vice President, Communications

**American Group Psychotherapy Association, Inc.,** 25 East 21st Street, Sixth Floor, New York, NY 10010; tel. 212/477–2677; FAX. 212/979–6627; Marsha S. Block, CAE, Chief Executive Officer

**American Head and Neck Society,** 11300 W. Olympic Blvd #600, Los Angles, CA 90064; tel. 310/437–0559; FAX. 310/437–0585; Christina Kasendorf, Executive Director

**American Headache Society,** 19 Mantua Road, Mt. Royal, NJ 08061; tel. 856/423–0043; FAX. 856/423–0082; Linda McGillicuddy, Executive Director

**American Health Care Association,** 1201 L Street, NW, Washington, DC 20005; tel. 202/842–4444; FAX. 202/842–3860; Mark Parkinson, President and Chief Executive Officer

**American Health Information Management Association (AHIMA),** 233 North Michigan Avenue, 21st Floor, Chicago, IL 60601–5800; tel. 312/233–1100; FAX. 312/233–1090; Alan F. Dowling PhD, Chief Executive Officer

**American Health Lawyers Association,** 1620 Eye Street NW, Washington, DC 20006–4010; tel. 202/833–1100; FAX. 202/833–1105; Peter M. Leibold, Esq, Executive Vice President and Chief Executive Officer

**American Health Planning Association,** 7245 Arlington Boulevard, Suite 300, Falls Church, VA 22042; tel. 703/573–3103; FAX. 703/573–3103; Dean Montgomery, Director

**American Healthcare Radiology Administrators,** 490 - B Boston, Post Road, Suite 101, Sudbury, MA 01776; tel. 978/443–7591; FAX. 978/443–8046; Mary S. Reitter, Executive Director

**American Heart Association, Inc.,** 7272 Greenville Avenue, Dallas, TX 75231; tel. 214/706–1574; FAX. 214/373–9818; Rose Marie Robertson, MD, FAHA, Chief Science Officer

**American Hospital Association,** 325 Seventh Street, NW, Suite 700, Washington, DC 20004; tel. 202/626–2363; Richard Umbdenstock, President and Chief Executive Officer

**American Hospital Association,** 155 N. Wacker Drive, Suite 400, Chicago, IL 60606; tel. 312/422–3000; Richard Umbdenstock, President and Chief Executive Officer

**American Hospital Association, Washington Office,** 325 Seventh Street, NW, Suite 700, Washington, DC 20004; tel. 202/638–1100; FAX. 202/626–2355; Rick Pollack, Executive Vice President

**American International Health Alliance,** 1250 Eye Street, NW, Suite 350, Washington, DC 20005; tel. 202/789–1136; FAX. 202/789–1277; James P. Smith, Executive Director

**American Laryngological Association, Office of the Secretary,** Vanderbilt University Medical Center, Department of Otolaryngology, Nashville, TN 37212–8783; tel. 615/343–0429; FAX. 615/322–9102; C. Gaelyn Garrett, MD, Scretary

**American Library Association,** 50 East Huron Street, Chicago, IL 60611; tel. 312/280–5063; FAX. 312/280–5270; Cynthia Vivian, Director

**American Lung Association,** 1301 Pennsylvania Avenue, NW, Washington, DC 20004–1725; tel. 202/785–3355; FAX. 202/452–1805; Charles D. Connor, President & Chief Executive Officer

**American Lung Association in Ohio,** 4050 Executive Park Drive, Suite 405, Cincinnati, OH 45241; tel. 513/985–3990; FAX. 513/985–3995; Gale Steitz, Program Director

**American Medical Association,** 515 North State Street, Chicago, IL 60610; tel. 312/464–5000; FAX. 312/464–4184

**American Medical Association Alliance,** 515 North State Street, 9th Floor, Chicago, IL 60610; tel. 312/464–4470; FAX. 312/464–5020; Hazel J. Lewis, Executive Director

**American Medical Group Association,** 1422 Duke Street, Alexandria, VA 22314–3403; tel. 703/838–0033; FAX. 703/548–1890; Donald W. Fisher, PhD, President and Chief Executive Officer

**American Medical Student Association/Foundation,** 1902 Association Drive, Reston, VA 20191; tel. 703/620–6600; FAX. 703/620–5873; Carol Williams-Nickelson, PsyD, Executive Director

**American Medical Technologists,** 10700 W. Higgins Road, Suite 150, Rosemont, IL 60018; tel. 847/823–5169; FAX. 847/823–0458; Christopher Damon, Executive Director

**American Medical Women's Association,** 100 North 20th Street, 4th Floor, Philadelphia, PA 19103; tel. 866/564–2483; FAX. 215/564–2175; Gina Marinilli, Associate Director

**American Medical Writers Association,** 30 West Gude Drive #525, Rockville, MD 20850; tel. 204/238–0940; FAX. 301/294–9006; Mark Rosal, Member Services Coordinator

**American Music Therapy Association,** 8455 Colesville Road, Suite 1000, Silver Spring, MD 20910; tel. 301/589–3300; FAX. 301/589–5175; Andrea Farbman, Ed.D., Executive Director

**American National Standards Institute,** 25 West 43rd Street, Fourth Floor, New York, NY 10036; tel. 212/642–4900; FAX. 212/398–0023; S. Joe Bhatia, President and Chief Executive Officer

**American Nephrology Nurses' Association,** East Holly Avenue, PO Box 56, Pitman, NJ 08071; tel. 856/256–2320; FAX. 856/589–7463

**American Neurological Association,** 5841 Cedar Lake Road, Suite 204, Minneapolis, MN 55416; tel. 952/545–6208; FAX. 952/545–6073; JoAnn Taie, Associate Executive Director

**American Occupational Therapy Association, Inc.,** 4720 Montgomery Lane, P.O. Box 31220, Bethesda, MD 20814–1220; tel. 301/652–2682; FAX. 301/652–7711; Frederick P. Somers, Executive Director

**American Ontological Society, Inc.,** 3096 Riverdale Rd., The Villages, FL 32162; tel. 352/751–0932; FAX. 352/751–0696; Shirley Gossard, Administrator

**American Ophthalmological Society,** PO Box 193940, San Francisco, CA 94119–3940; tel. 415/561–8578; FAX. 415/561–8531; Thomas J. Liesegang, MD, Executive Vice President

**American Optometric Association,** 243 North Lindbergh Boulevard, St. Louis, MO 63141; tel. 314/991–4100; FAX. 314/991–4101; Barry J. Barresi, OD, PhD, Executive Director

**American Organization of Nurse Executives (AONE),** 325 Seventh Street, NW, Suite 700, Washington, DC 20004; tel. 202/626–2240; FAX. 202/638–5499; Pamela A. Thompson, MS, RN, CENP, FAAN, Chief Executive Officer, and AHA Senior Vice President for Nursing

**American Orthopsychiatric Association,** Department of Psychology, Box 871104, Tempe, AZ 85287–1104; tel. 480/965–0380; FAX. 480/965–8544; Nicole Bruno, Director

**American Orthoptic Council,** 3914 Nakoma Road, Madison, WI 53711; tel. 608/233–5383; FAX. 608/263–4247; Leslie France, CO, Administrator

**American Osteopathic Association,** 142 East Ontario Street, Chicago, IL 60611; tel. 312/202–8003; FAX. 312/202–8303; John B. Crosby, JD, Executive Director

**American Parkinson Disease Association, Inc.,** 135 Parkinson Avenue, Parkinson Plaza, Staten Island, NY 10305; tel. 800/223–2732; FAX. 718/981–4399; G. Maestrone, DVM, Scientific and Medical Affairs Director

**American Pediatric Society, Inc.,** 3400 Research Forest Drive, Suite B7, The Woodlands, TX 77381; tel. 281/419–0052; FAX. 281/419–0082; Kathy Cannon, Associate Executive Director

**American Pharmacists Association,** 2215 Constitution Avenue NW, Washington, DC 20037; tel. 202/628–4410; FAX. 202/783–2351; Thomas E. Menighan, MBA, Executive Vice President/Chief Executive Officer

**American Physical Therapy Association,** 1111 North Fairfax Street, Alexandria, VA 22314–1488; tel. 703/684–2782; FAX. 703/684–7343; John D. Barnes, Chief Executive Officer

**American Physiological Society,** 9650 Rockville Pike, Bethesda, MD 20814–3991; tel. 301/634–7118; FAX. 301/634–7241; Martin Frank, PhD, Executive Director

**American Podiatric Medical Association,** 9312 Old Georgetown Road, Bethesda, MD 20814–1698; tel. 301/571–9200; FAX. 301/530–2752; Glenn B. Gastwirth, DPM, Executive Director

**American Psychiatric Association,** 1000 Wilson Boulevard, Suite 1825, Arlington, VA 22209; tel. 703/907–7300; FAX. 703/907–1086; James H. Scully Jr., MD, Medical Director and Chief Executive Officer

**American Psychoanalytic Association,** 309 East 49th Street, New York, NY 10017; tel. 212/752–0450; FAX. 212/593–0571; Dean K. Stein, Executive Director

**American Psychological Association,** 750 First Street, NE, Washington, DC 20002–4242; tel. 202/336–5800; FAX. 202/336–5797; Katherine Nordal, PhD, Executive Director For Professional Practice

**Section C**

**American Psychosomatic Society,** 6728 Old McLean Village Drive, McLean, VA 22101–3906; tel. 703/556–9222; FAX. 703/556–8729; George K. Degnon, Executive Director

**American Public Health Association,** 800 I Street, NW, Washington, DC 20001–3710; tel. 202/777–2742; FAX. 202/777–2534; Georges C. Benjamin, MD, FACP, FACEP(E), Executive Director

**American Public Human Services Association,** 1133 Nineteenth Street, NW, Suite 400, Washington, DC 20036; tel. 202/682–0100; FAX. 202/289–6555; Amy Plotnick, Publications Manager

**American Red Cross,** National Headquarters, 2025 E. Street, NW, Washington, DC 20006; tel. 202/303–5214; Pam Denning, Manager, Public Inquiry

**American Registry of Medical Assistants,** 61 Union Street, Ste. 5, Westfield, MA 01085–2476; tel. 413/562–7336; FAX. 413/562–9021; Annette H. Heyman, RMA, Director

**American Registry of Radiologic Technologists,** 1255 Northland Drive, St. Paul, MN 55120; tel. 651/687–0048; Jerry B. Reid, PhD, Executive Director

**American Rhinologic Society,** PO Box 495, Warwick, NY 10990; tel. 845/988–1631; FAX. 845/986–1527; Wendi Perez, Administrator/ Executive Director

**American Roentgen Ray Society,** 44211 Slate Stone Court, Leesburg, VA 20176; tel. 703/729–3353; FAX. 703/729–4839; Susan Brown Cappitelli, Executive Director

**American School Health Association,** 4340 East West Highway, Suite 403, Bethesda, MD 20814; tel. 301/652–8072; FAX. 301/652–8077; Stephen Conley, Executive Director

**American Society for Adolescent Psychiatry,** PO Box 570218, Dallas, TX 75357–0218; tel. 972/613–0985; FAX. 972/613–5532; Frances M. Roton, Executive Director

**American Society for Biochemistry and Molecular Biology, Inc.,** 9650 Rockville Pike, Bethesda, MD 20814–3996; tel. 301/634–7145; FAX. 301/634–7126; Charles C. Hancock, Executive Officer

**American Society for Clinical Laboratory Science,** 2025 M Street, NW, Suite 800, Washington, DC 20036; tel. 202/367–1174; FAX. 202/367–2174; Elissa Passiment, Executive Vice President

**American Society for Clinical Pathology, (Includes Board of Certification),** 33 W. Monroe Street, Suite 1600, Chicago, IL 60603; tel. 312/541–4999; FAX. 312/541–4767; E. Blair Holladay, PhD, SCT (ASCP), Executive Vice President

**American Society for Clinical Pharmacology and Therapeutics,** 528 North Washington Street, Alexandria, VA 22314; tel. 703/836–6981; FAX. 703/836–5223; Sharon J. Swan, CAE, Executive Director

**American Society for Cytotechnology,** 1500 Sunday Drive, Suite 102, Raleigh, NC 27607; tel. 800/948–3947; FAX. 919/787–4916; Beth Denny, Executive Director

**American Society for Healthcare Engineering (ASHE),** 155 N. Wacker Drive, Suite 400, Chicago, IL 60606–1725; tel. 312/422–3800; FAX. 312/422–4571; Dale Woodin, CHFM, FASHE, Executive Director

**American Society for Healthcare Human Resources Administration (ASHHRA),** 155 N. Wacker Drive, Suite 400, Chicago, IL 60606; tel. 312/422–3720; FAX. 312/422–4577; Stephanie Drake, MBA, Executive Director

**American Society for Healthcare Risk Management (ASHRM),** 155 N. Wacker Drive, Suite 400, Chicago, IL 60606; tel. 312/422–3980; FAX. 312/422–4580; Kim Hoarle, MBA, CAE, Executive Director

**American Society for Investigative Pathology,** 9650 Rockville Pike, Bethesda, MD 20814–3993; tel. 301/634–7130; FAX. 301/634–7990; Mark E. Sobel, MD, Ph.D, Executive Director

**American Society for Laser Medicine and Surgery, Inc.,** 2100 Stewart Avenue, Suite 240, Wausau, WI 54401; tel. 715/845–9283; FAX. 715/848–2493; Elizabeth Tanzi, MD, Secretary

**American Society for Microbiology,** 1752 North Street, NW, Washington, DC 20036; tel. 202/924–9265; FAX. 202/942–9333; Michael I. Goldberg, PhD, Executive Director

**American Society for Pharmacology and Experimental Therapeutics,** 9650 Rockville Pike, Bethesda, MD 20814–3995; tel. 301/634–7060; FAX. 301/634–7061; Christine K. Carrico, PhD, Executive Officer

**American Society for Public Administration,** 1301 Pennsylvania Avenue, NW, Suite 840, Washington, DC 20004; tel. 202/393–7878; FAX. 202/638–4952; Antoinette Samuel, CAE

**American Society for Radiation Oncology,** 8280 Willow Oaks Corporate Drive, Suite 500, Fairfax, VA 22031; tel. 703/502–1550; FAX. 703/502–7852; Laura I. Thevenot, Chief Executive Officer

**American Society for Reproductive Medicine,** 1209 Montgomery Highway, Birmingham, AL 35216–2809; tel. 205/978–5000; FAX. 205/293–5201; Robert W. Rebar, MD, Executive Director

**American Society for the Advancement of Anesthesia and Sedation in Dentistry,** Six East Union Avenue, PO Box 551, Bound Brook, NJ 08805; tel. 732/469–9050; FAX. 732/271–1985; David Crystal, DDS, Executive Secretary

**American Society of Anesthesiologists,** 520 North Northwest Highway, Park Ridge, IL 60068; tel. 847/825–5586; FAX. 847/825–2085; John A. Thorner, JD, CAE, Executive Vice President

**American Society of Colon and Rectal Surgeons,** 85 West Algonquin Road, Suite 550, Arlington Heights, IL 60005; tel. 847/290–9184; FAX. 847/290–9203; James Slawny, Executive Director

**American Society of Consultant Pharmacists,** 1321 Duke Street, Alexandria, VA 22314–3563; tel. 703/739–1300; FAX. 703/739–1321; Vera Jackson, PhD, Executive Director and Chief Executive Officer

**American Society of Cytopathology,** 100 West 10th Street, Suite 605, Wilmington, DE 19801; tel. 302/543–6583; FAX. 302/543–6597; Elizabeth A. Jenkins, Executive Director

**American Society of Health-System Pharmacists,** 7272 Wisconsin Avenue, Bethesda, MD 20814; tel. 301/664–8794; FAX. 301/664–8877; Paul Abramowitz, Chief Executive Officer and Executive Vice President

**American Society of Law, Medicine & Ethics,** 765 Commonwealth Avenue, Suite 1634, Boston, MA 02215; tel. 617/262–4990; FAX. 617/437–7596; Edward Hutchinson, Executive Director

**American Society of Neuroimaging,** 5841 Cedar Lake Road, Suite 204, Minneapolis, MN 55416; tel. 952/545–6291; FAX. 952/545–6073; Shannon Wild, Associate Executive Director

**American Society of Plastic Surgeons,** 444 East Algonquin Road, Arlington Heights, IL 60005; tel. 847/228–9900; FAX. 847/228–9131; Paul Pomerantz, CAE, Executive Vice President

**American Society of Radiologic Technologists,** 15000 Central Avenue, SE, Albuquerque, NM 87123–3909; tel. 505/298–4500; FAX. 505/298–5063; Ceela McElveny, Chief Communications and Membership Officer

**American Speech-Language-Hearing Association,** 2200 Research Boulevard, Rockville, MD 20850–3289; tel. 301/296–5700; FAX. 301/296–8580

**American Surgical Association,** 500 Cummings Center, Suite 4550, Beverly, MA 01915; tel. 978/927–8330; FAX. 978/524–8890; Jon Blackstone, Executive Director

**American Thoracic Society,** 61 Broadway, New York, NY 10006–2755; tel. 212/315–6444; FAX. 212/315–8630; Stephen C. Crane, PhD, MPH, Executive Director

**American Trauma Society,** 201 Park Washington Court, Falls Church, VA 22046; tel. 800/556–7890; FAX. 703/241–5603; Harry Teter, Executive Director

**American Urological Association, Inc.,** 1000 Corporate Boulevard, Linthicum, MD 21090; tel. 410/689–3700; Michael Sheppard, Executive Director

**amfAR, The Foundation for AIDS Research,** 120 Wall Street, 13th Floor, New York, NY 10005–3902; tel. 212/806–1600; FAX. 212/806–1601; Rachel Carr, Assistant Coordinator, Public Information

**AORN, Association of periOperative Registered Nurses,** 2170 South Parker Road, Suite 400, Denver, CO 80231–5711; tel. 303/755–6300; FAX. 303/750–2927; Linda Groah, RN, MSN, CNOR, FAAN, Executive Director and Chief Executive Officer

**Arthritis Foundation,** 1330 West Peachtree Street, Suite 100, Atlanta, GA 30309; tel. 404/872–7100; FAX. 404/965–7712; John H. Klippel, MD, President and Chief Executive Officer

**ASET - The Neurodiagnostic Society,** 402 East Bannister Road, Suite A, Kansas City, MO 64131; tel. 816/931–1120; FAX. 816/931–1145; Arlen Reimnitz, Executive Director

**Association for Applied Psychophysiology and Biofeedback,** 10200 West 44th Avenue, Suite 304, Wheat Ridge, CO 80033; tel. 303/422–8436; FAX. 303/422–8894; David Stumph, Executive Director

**Association for Clinical Pastoral Education, Inc.,** 1549 Clairmont Road, Suite 103, Decatur, GA 30033; tel. 404/320–1472; FAX. 404/320–0849; Teresa E. Snorton, Executive Director

**Association for Community Health Improvement (ACHI),** 155 N. Wacker Drive, Suite 400, Chicago, IL 60606; tel. 312/422–2193; FAX. 312/422–4522; Michael Bilton, Executive Director

**Association for Healthcare Administrative Professionals (AHCAP),** 455 S. Fourth Street, Suite 650, Louisville, KY 40202; tel. 8883200808; FAX. 5025893602; Monica Harper, Executive Director

**Association for Healthcare Foodservice, AHF,** 455 S. Fourth Street, Suite 650, Louisville, KY 40202; tel. 888/528–9552; FAX. 502/589–3602; Billye Potts, Executive Vice President

**Association for Healthcare Philanthropy,** 313 Park Avenue, Suite 400, Falls Church, VA 22046; tel. 703/532–6243; FAX. 703/532–7170

**Association for Healthcare Resource & Materials Management (AHRMM),** 155 N. Wacker Drive, Suite 400, Chicago, IL 60606; tel. 312/422–3840; FAX. 312/422–4573; Deborah L. Sprindzunas, Executive Director

**Association for Healthcare Volunteer Resource Professionals (AHVRP),** 155 N. Wacker Drive, Suite 400, Chicago, IL 60606; tel. 312/422–3939; FAX. 312/278–0884; Joan M. Miller, MHA, Executive Director

**Association for Hospital Medical Education,** 109 Brush Creek Road, Irwin, PA 15642; tel. 724/864–7321; FAX. 724/864–6153; Kimball Mohn, Executive Director

**Association for Professionals in Infection Control and Epidemiology,** 1275 K Street, NW, Suite 1000, Washington, DC 20005; tel. 202/789–1890; FAX. 202/789–1899; Kathy L. Warye, Chief Executive Officer

**Association for the Advancement of Automotive Medicine (AAAM),** PO Box 4176, Barrington, IL 60146; tel. 847/844–3880; FAX. 847/844–3884; Irene Herzau, Executive Director

**Association for the Healthcare Environment (AHE),** 155 N. Wacker Drive, Suite 400, Chicago, IL 60606; tel. 312/422–3860; FAX. 312/422–4578; Patti Costello, Executive Director

**Association of American Medical Colleges,** 2450 N Street, NW, Washington, DC 20037–1127; tel. 202/828–0400; FAX. 202/828–1125; Darrell G. Kirch, MD, President and Chief Executive Officer

**Association of American Physicians and Surgeons, Inc.,** 1601 North Tucson Boulevard, Suite Nine, Tucson, AZ 85716; tel. 520/327–4885; FAX. 520/325–4230; Jane M. Orient, MD, Executive Director

**Association of American Veterinary Medical Colleges,** 1101 Vermont Ave, NW, Suite 301, Washington, DC 20005; tel. 202/371–9195; FAX. 202/842–0773; Dr. Michael Chaddock, Deputy Director

**Association of Community Cancer Centers,** 11600 Nebel Street, Suite 201, Rockville, MD 20852–2557; tel. 301/984–9496; FAX. 301/770–1949; Christian Downs, JD, MHA, Executive Director

**Association of Environmental Health Academic Programs,** 8620 Roosevelt Way NE, Suite A, Seattle, WA 98115; tel. 206/522-5272; FAX. 206/985-9805; Yalonda Sinde, Executive Director

**Association of Healthcare Administrative Professionals, AHCAP,** 455 S. Fourth Street, Suite 650, Louisville, KY 40202; tel. 502/574-9040; FAX. 502/589-3602; Monica Harper, Executive Director

**Association of Nutrition and Foodservice Professionals,** 406 Surrey Woods Drive, St. Charles, IL 60174; tel. 630/587-6336; FAX. 630/587-6308; William St. John, President

**Association of Occupational & Environmental Clinics,** 1010 Vermont Avenue, NW # 513, Washington, DC 20005; tel. 202/347-4976; Katherine Kirkland, Dr PH, MPH, Executive Director

**Association of Professional Chaplains,** 1701 East Woodfield Road, Suite 400, Schaumburg, IL 60173; tel. 847/240-1014; FAX. 847/240-1015; Patricia F. Appelhans, JD, Executive Director

**Association of Public Health Laboratories,** 8515 Georgia Avenue, Suite 700, Silver Spring, MD 20910; tel. 240/485-2745; FAX. 240/485-2700; Scott J. Becker, MS, Executive Director

**Association of Schools of Allied Health Professions,** 4400 Jennifer Street, NW, Suite 333, Washington, DC 20015; tel. 202/237-6481; FAX. 202/237-6485; Thomas W. Elwood, Dr. PH, Executive Director

**Association of Schools of Public Health,** 1900 M Street, NW, Suite 710, Washington, DC 20036; tel. 202/296-1099; FAX. 202/296-1252; Harrison C. Spencer, MD, MPH, President and Chief Executive Officer

**Association of Specialized and Cooperative Library Agencies,** 50 East Huron Street, Chicago, IL 60611; tel. 312/280-4398; FAX. 312/280-5273; Susan Hornung, Executive Director

**Association of State and Territorial Health Officials,** 2231 Crystal Drive, Suite 450, Arlington, VA 22202; tel. 202/371-9090; FAX. 571/527-3189; Paul E. Jarris, MD, MBA, Executive Director

**Association of Surgical Technologists, Inc.,** 6 West Dry Creek Circle, Suite 200, Littleton, CO 80120; tel. 303/694-9130; FAX. 303/694-9169; William J. Teutsch, CAE, Chief Executive Officer

**Association of University Programs in Health Administration,** 2000 14th Street, N., Suite 780, Arlington, VA 22201; tel. 703/894-0940; FAX. 703/894-0941; Lydia Middleton, MBA, CAE, President and Chief Executive Officer

**Asthma and Allergy Foundation of America,** 8201 Corporate Drive, Suite 1000, Landover, MD 20785; tel. 800-7-ASTHMA; FAX. 202/466-8940; William McLin, M.Ed., President and Chief Executive Officer

**At Large of the AHA,** 155 N. Wacker Drive, Suite 400, Chicago, IL 60606; tel. 312/422-3700; FAX. 312/278-0882; Elizabeth Summy, Vice President

# B

**Bereavement and Advance Care Planning Services, Gundersen Lutheran Medical Foundation, Inc.,** 1900 South Avenue-Alex, La Crosse, WI 54601; tel. 608/775-4747; FAX. 608/775-5137; Rana Limbo, Director

**Bioethics Research Library, Georgetown University,** 102 Healy Hall, 37th and O Streets, NW, Washington, DC 20057; tel. 202/687-3885; FAX. 202/687-6770; Doris Goldstein, MLS, MA, Director of Library and Information Services

**Biological Stain Commission,** University of Rochester Medical Center, Department Pathology and Lab Medicine, Rochester, NY 14642-0001; tel. 585/275-2751; FAX. 585/442-8993; Chad Ragan, Laboratory Operations

**Birth Defect Research for Children,** 976 Lake Baldwin Lane, Suite 104, Orlando, FL 32814; tel. 407/895-0802; Betty Mekdeci, Executive Director

**Blinded Veterans Association,** 477 H Street, NW, Washington, DC 20001; tel. 202/371-8880; FAX. 202/371-8258; Thomas H. Miller, Executive Director

**Blue Cross and Blue Shield Association,** 225 N. Michigan Avenue, Chicago, IL 60601-7680; tel. 312/297-6000; Scott P. Serota, President and Chief Executive Officer

**Brady Center to Prevent Gun Violence,** 1225 Eye Street, NW, Suite 1100, Washington, DC 20005; tel. 202/289-7319; FAX. 202/408-1851; Paul Helmke, President

# C

**California Distance Learning Health Network,** 9245 Sky Park Court, Suite 100, San Diego, CA 92123; tel. 619/594-3364; Violet Macias-Reynolds, MS, M.Ed, Executive Director

**CARE Program, (Community Action for a Renewed Environment Program),** EPA, Washington, DC 20460; tel. 877/227-3909; FAX. 202/343-2395; Dennis O'Connor, Senior Policy Advisor

**CARF International,** 6951 East Southpoint, Tucson, AZ 85756; tel. 866/888-1122; FAX. 202/587-5009; Christine MacDonell, Managing Director

**Catholic Health Association of the United States,** 1875 Eye Street NW, Suite 1000, Washington, DC 20006; tel. 202/296-3993; FAX. 202/296-3997; Sr. Carol Keehan, DC, President and Chief Executive Officer

**Catholic Medical Association,** 29 Bala Avenue, Suite 205, Bala Cynwyd, PA 19004; tel. 484/270-8002; FAX. 866/666-2319; John Brehany, PhD, STL, Executive Director

**Center for Health Administration Studies, University of Chicago,** 969 East 60th Street, Chicago, IL 60637; tel. 773/702-7104; FAX. 773/702-7222; Jeanne Marsh, PhD., Director

**Center for Healthcare Governance (CHG),** 155 N. Wacker Drive, Suite 400, Chicago, IL 60606; tel. 888/540-6111; FAX. 312/278-0868; John R. Combes, MD, President and Chief Operating Officer

**Center for Healthy Aging, c/o National Council on Aging,** 1901 L Street, NW, 4th Floor, Washington, DC 20036; tel. 202/479-1200; FAX. 202/479-0735; Nancy Whitelaw, PhD, Director, Center for Healthy Aging

**Central Surgical Association, University of Chicago,** 5841 S. Maryland m/c 5094, Chicago, IL 60637; tel. 913/402-7102; FAX. 913/273-1116; Nonie Lowry, Meeting Coordinator

**Children's Eye Foundation,** 1631 Lancaster Drive, #200, Grapevine, TX 76051; tel. 817/301-2641; FAX. 817/329-5532; Thomas Rogers, Executive Director

**Children's Hospital Association,** 401 Wythe Street, Alexandria, VA 22314; tel. 703/684-1355; FAX. 703/684-1589; Mark Wietecha, President and Chief Executive Officer

**Christian Record Services, Inc.,** 4444 South 52nd Street, Lincoln, NE 68516; tel. 402/488-0981; FAX. 402/488-1902; Matthew Orian, Treasurer

**College of American Pathologists,** 325 Waukegan Road, Northfield, IL 60093-2750; tel. 847/832-7000; FAX. 847/832-8000; Charles Roussel, Chief Executive Officer

**Community Anti-Drug Coalitions of America,** 625 Slaters Lane, Suite 300, Alexandria, VA 22314; tel. 800/542-2322; FAX. 703/706-0565; Arthur T. Dean, Chairman and Chief Executive Officer

**Community Health Accreditation Program,** 1275 K Street NW, Suite 800, Washington, DC 20005; tel. 202/862-3413; FAX. 202/862-3419; Terry A. Duncombe, President and Chief Executive Officer

**Consortium of African American Public Health Programs (CAAPHP), Florida A&M University,** College of Pharmacy and Pharmaceutical Sciences, Institute of Public Health, Atlanta, GA 30310-1495; tel. 850/599-8655; FAX. 850/599-8830; Cynthia M. Harris, PhD, DABT, Director and Professor

**Cooley's Anemia Foundation, Inc.,** 330 Seventh Avenue, Suite 200, New York, NY 10001; tel. 212/279-8090; FAX. 212/279-5999; Gina Cioffi, National Executive Director

**Corporate Angel Network, Inc. (CAN),** Westchester County Airport, One Loop Road, White Plains, NY 10604; tel. 914/328-1313; FAX. 914/328-3938; Judith Runyan, Patient Advocate

**Council of Medical Specialty Societies,** 35 E. Wacker Drive, Suite 850, Chicago, IL 60601; tel. 312/224-2535; FAX. 312/644-8557; Norman B. Kahn, Jr., MD, EVP, and Chief Executive Officer

**Council on Education for Public Health,** 800 Eye Street, NW, Suite 202, Washington, DC 20001-3710; tel. 202/789-1050; FAX. 202/789-1895; Laura Rasar King, Executive Director

**Crohn's & Colitis Foundation of America, Inc.,** 386 Park Avenue, S., 17th Floor, New York, NY 10016-8804; tel. 800/932-2423; FAX. 212/779-4098; Richard J. Geswell, President

**Cystic Fibrosis Foundation,** 6931 Arlington Road, Bethesda, MD 20814; tel. 301/951-4422; FAX. 301/951-6378; Robert J. Beall, PhD, President and Chief Executive Officer

# D

**Damien Dutton Society for Leprosy Aid, Inc.,** 616 Bedford Avenue, Bellmore, NY 11710; tel. 516/221-5829; FAX. 516/221-5909; Elizabeth Campbell, Vice President

**Depression and Bipolar Support Alliance,** 730 North Franklin Street, Suite 501, Chicago, IL 60654-7225; tel. 800/826-3632; FAX. 312/642-7243; Allen Doederlein, President

**Dysautonomia Foundation, Inc.,** 315 W. 39th Street, Suite 701, New York, NY 10018; tel. 212/279-1066; FAX. 212/279-2066; David Brenner, Executive Director

# E

**Easter Seals, Inc.,** 233 South Wacker Drive, Suite 2400, Chicago, IL 60606; tel. 800/221-6827; FAX. 312/726-1494; Rosemary Garza, Information & Referral

**ECRI Institute,** 5200 Butler Pike, Plymouth Meeting, PA 19462; tel. 610/825-6000; FAX. 610/834-1275; Jeffrey C. Lerner, PhD, President and Chief Executive Officer

**Educational Commission for Foreign Medical Graduates,** 3624 Market Street, 4th Floor, Philadelphia, PA 19104-2685; tel. 215/823-2101; Emmanuel G. Cassimatis, MD, President and Chief Executive Officer

**Ehlers-Danlos National Foundation,** PO Box 13157, Richmond, VA 23225; tel. 804/276-9940; FAX. 804/276-9940; Susan L. Stephenson, Patient Advocate

**Emergency Nurses Association,** 915 Lee Street, Des Plaines, IL 60016; tel. 800/900-9659; FAX. 847/460-4006

**Epilepsy Foundation,** 8301 Professional Place-East, Landover, MD 20785; tel. 301/459-3700; FAX. 301/577-2684; Richard P. Denness, Chief Executive Officer

**Epilepsy Foundation of Connecticut,** 386 Main Street, Middletown, CT 06457; tel. 860/346-1924; FAX. 860/346-1928; Linda Wallace, Executive Director

# F

**Federated Ambulatory Surgery Association,** 1012 Cameron Street, Alexandria, VA 22314; tel. 703/836-8808; FAX. 703/549-0976; Kathy Bryant, Executive Director

Section C

**Federation of American Hospitals,** 750 9th Street, NW, Suite 600, Washington, DC 20001; tel. 202/624–1500; FAX. 202/737–6462; Chip Kahn, President

**Federation of State Medical Boards of the United States, Inc.,** 400 Fuller Wiser Rd, Suite 300, Euless, TX 76039; tel. 817/868–4000; FAX. 817/868–4097; Humayun J. Chaudhry, DO, FACP President and Chief Executive Officer

**Financial Accounting Standards Board,** 401 Merritt 7, P.O. Box 5116, Norwalk, CT 06856–5116; tel. 203/847–0700; FAX. 203/849–9714

**Frontline Healthcare Workers Safety Foundation, Ltd.,** Three Dunwoody Park, Suite 103, Atlanta, GA 30338; tel. 678/781–5241; FAX. 678/781–5242; Jennifer Elin Cole, MSW, Associate Director

# G

**Gerontological Society of America,** 1220 L Street, NW, Suite 901, Washington, DC 20005–4018; tel. 202/842–1275; FAX. 202/842–1150; James Appleby, Executive Director

**Great Plains Health Alliance, Inc.,** 625 Third Street, Box 366, Phillipsburg, KS 67661; tel. 785/543–2111; FAX. 785/543–5098; Roger S. John, President and Chief Executive Officer

**Guide Dog Users, Inc.,** 14311 Astrodome Drive, Silver Spring, MD 20906–2245; tel. 866/799–8436; FAX. 301/871–7591; Jane Sheehan, Office Manager

# H

**Health Industry Distributors Association,** 310 Montgomery Street, Alexandria, VA 22314–1516; tel. 703/549–4432; FAX. 703/549–6495; Matthew J. Rowan, President and Chief Executive Officer

**Health Research and Educational Trust (HRET),** 155 N. Wacker Drive, Suite 400, Chicago, IL 60606; tel. 312/422–2600; FAX. 312/422–4568; Maulik Joshi, President

**Healthcare Financial Management Association,** Two Westbrook Corporate Center, Suite 700, Westchester, IL 60154; tel. 708/531–9600; FAX. 708/531–0032; Richard L. Clarke, DHA, FHFMA, President and Chief Executive Officer

**Healthcare Information and Management Systems Society (HIMSS),** 230 East Ohio Street, Suite 500, Chicago, IL 60611–3201; tel. 312/664–4467; FAX. 312/664–6143; H. Stephen Lieber, President, Chief Executive Officer

**HEAR Center,** 301 East Del Mar Boulevard, Pasadena, CA 91101; tel. 626/796–2016; FAX. 626/796–2320; Ellen Simon, Executive Director

**Huntington's Disease Society of America, Inc.,** 505 Eighth Avenue, Suite 902, New York, NY 10018; tel. 800/345–4372; FAX. 212/239–3430; Louise Vetter, National Executive Director and Chief Executive Officer

# I

**iKeepSafe Internet Safety Coalition,** 4301 N. Fairfax Drive, Suite 190, Arlington, VA 22203; tel. 703/717–9066; FAX. 202/737–4097; Marsali S. Hancock, President

**Infusion Nurses Society,** 315 Norwood Park South, Norwood, MA 02062; tel. 781/440–9408; FAX. 781/440–9409; Mary Alexander, Chief Executive Officer

**Institute for Diversity in Health Management (IFD),** 155 N. Wacker Drive, Suite 400, Chicago, IL 60606; tel. 312/422–2630; FAX. 312/278–0893; Frederick D. Hobby, President and Chief Executive Officer

**Institute of Medicine,** 500 Fifth Street, NW, Washington, DC 20001; tel. 202/334–2352; FAX. 202/334–1412; Harvey V. Fineberg, MD, PhD, President

**Institute of Medicine of The National Academies,** 500 Fifth Street NW, Washington, DC 20001–2721; tel. 202/334–2000; FAX. 202/334–3851; Harvey V. Fineberg, President, Institute of Medicine

**Institutes for the Achievement of Human Potential,** 8801 Stenton Avenue, Wyndmoor, PA 19038; tel. 215/233–2050; FAX. 215/233–3940; Leland Green, Medical Director

**International Childbirth Education Association, Inc.,** 1500 Sunday Drive, Suite 102, Raleigh, NC 27607; tel. 919/863–9487; FAX. 919/787–4916

**International College of Surgeons/United States Section,** 1516 North Lake Shore Drive, Chicago, IL 60610–1694; tel. 312/787–6274; FAX. 312/787–9289; Maggie Kearney, Meeting and Publications Manager

**International Council for Health, Physical Education, Recreation, Sport and Dance,** 1900 Association Drive, Reston, VA 20191; tel. 703/476–3486; FAX. 703/476–9527; Dr. Dong Ja Yang, President

# L

**Leading Age,** 2519 Connecticut Avenue, NW, Washington, DC 20008–1520; tel. 202/783–2242; FAX. 202/783–2255; William L. Minnix, Jr., D. Min., President and Chief Executive Officer

**Lupus Foundation of America, Inc.,** 2000 L Street, NW, Suite 410, Washington, DC 20036; tel. 202/349–1155; FAX. 202/349–1156; Dawn Isherwood, Health Educator

# M

**March of Dimes Foundation,** 1275 Mamaroneck Avenue, White Plains, NY 10605; tel. 914/428–7100; FAX. 914/428–8203; Jennifer L. Howse, PhD, President

**Marriott Memorial Heart Foundation, International,** PO Box 3395, Riverview, FL 33568; tel. 623/204–4848; Jonni Cooper, BSN, MBA, PhD, FACCN-III, Chief Executive Officer

**Medical Fitness Association (MFA),** 1905 Huguenot Road, Suite 203, Richmond, VA 23235; tel. 804/897–5701; FAX. 804/897–5704; Ken Germano, Executive Director

**Medical Library Association,** 65 East Wacker Place, Suite 1900, Chicago, IL 60601–7298; tel. 312/419–9094; FAX. 312/419–8950; Carla J. Funk, Executive Director

**MedicAlert Foundation,** 2323 Colorado Avenue, Turlock, CA 95382; tel. 800/432–5378; FAX. 209/669–2495; Ramesh Srinvasan, SVP Marketing

**Men's Health Network,** PO Box 75972, Washington, DC 20013; tel. 202/543–6461; FAX. 202/543–2727; Ana Fadich, MPH, CHES, Director, Programs and Outreach

**Mental Health America, (formerly known as the National Mental Health Association),** 2000 N. Beauregard Street, 6th Floor, Alexandria, VA 22311; tel. 703/684–7722; FAX. 703/684–5968; David L. Shern, PhD, President and Chief Executive Officer

**MGMA-ACMPE,** 104 Inverness Terrace, E., Englewood, CO 80112–5306; tel. 877/275–6462; FAX. 303/784–6108; Susan L. Turney, MD, MS, FACP, FACMPE, President and Chief Executive Officer

**Midwives Alliance of North America,** 611 Pennsylvania Avenue SE, # 1700, Washington, DC 20003–4303; tel. 8889236262; Geradine Simkins, President

**Muscular Dystrophy Association,** 3300 East Sunrise Drive, Tucson, AZ 85718; tel. 520/529–2000; FAX. 520/529–5300; Valerie A. Cwik, MD, Interim President and Medical Director

# N

**National Academy of Sciences, Division on Earth and Life Studies,** 500 Fifth Street, NW, Keck 654, Washington, DC 20001; tel. 202/334–2500; FAX. 202/334–3362; Warren R. Muir, PhD, Executive Director

**National Accreditation Council for Agencies for, Blind and Low Vision Services (NAC),** 7017 Pearl Road, Middleburg Hts., OH 44130; tel. 440/545–1601; FAX. 423/875–3135; William A. Robinson, III, CPA, Executive Director

**National Accrediting Agency for Clinical Laboratory Sciences,** 5600 N. River Road, Suite 720, Rosemont, IL 60018; tel. 773/714–8880; FAX. 773/714–8886; Dianne M. Cearlock, Chief Executive Officer

**National Alliance for Hispanic Health,** 1501 16th Street NW, Washington, DC 20036; tel. 202/387–5000; FAX. 202/797–4353; Mr. Adolph Falcón, Senior Vice President

**National Alliance for the Mentally Ill (NAMI),** 3803 N. Fairfax Drive, Ste 100, Arlington, VA 22203; tel. 703/524–7600; FAX. 703/524–9094; Michael J. Fitzpatrick, MSW, Executive Director

**National Assembly on School-Based Health Care,** 1010 Vermont Avenue, NW, Suite 600, Washington, DC 20005; tel. 202/638–5872; FAX. 202/638–5879; Linda Juszczak, President

**National Association for Home Care & Hospice,** 228 Seventh Street, SE, Washington, DC 20003; tel. 202/547–7424; FAX. 202/547–3540; Val J. Halamandaris, President

**National Association for Practical Nurse Education and Service,** Mail Processing, 1940 Duke Street, Alexandria, VA 22314; tel. 703/933–1003; FAX. 703/940–4089; Helen Larsen, JD, Executive Director

**National Association Medical Staff Services,** 2025 M Street, NW, Suite 800, Washington, DC 20036; tel. 202/367–1196; FAX. 202/367–2196; Megan Cohen, Executive Director

**National Association of Boards of Pharmacy,** 1600 Feehanville Drive, Mt. Prospect, IL 60056; tel. 847/391–4406; FAX. 847/391–4502; Carmen A. Catizone, MS, R.Ph., D.Ph., Executive Director/Secretary

**National Association of County and City Health Officials,** 1100 17th Street, NW, 7th Floor, Washington, DC 20036; tel. 202/783–5550; FAX. 202/783–1583

**National Association of Dental Assistants,** 900 South Washington Street, Suite G13, Falls Church, VA 22046; tel. 703/237–8616; FAX. 703/533–1153; S. Young, Director

**National Association of Dental Laboratories, (Includes National Board for Certification in Dental Laboratory Technology),** 325 John Knox Rd, #L 103, Tallahassee, FL 32303; tel. 800/950–1150; FAX. 850/222–0053; Bennett Napier, CAE, Co-Executive Director

**National Association of Health Services Executives,** 1050 Connecticut Avenue, NW, 10th Floor, Washington, DC 20036; tel. 202/772–1030; FAX. 202/772–1072; Beverly Glover, Association Manager

**National Association of Psychiatric Health Systems,** 900 17th Street NW, Suite 420, Washington, DC 20006–2507; tel. 202/393–6700; FAX. 202/783–6041; Mark J. Covall, President and Chief Executive Officer

**National Association of Social Workers,** 750 First Street, NE, Suite 700, Washington, DC 20002; tel. 202/336–8200; FAX. 202/336–8313; Elizabeth Clark, PhD, ACSW, MPH, Executive Director

Section C

**National Association of State Mental Health Program Directors,** 66 Canal Center Plaza, Suite 302, Alexandria, VA 22314; tel. 703/739–9333; FAX. 703/548–9517; Robert W. Glover, PhD, Executive Director

**National Board for Respiratory Care, NBRC Executive Office,** 18000 W 105th Street, Olathe, KS 66061–7543; tel. 913/895–4900; FAX. 913/895–4650; Gary A. Smith, Executive Director

**National Board of Anesthesiology, Inc,** 11817 Summit, Kansas, MO 64114; tel. 785/842–7067; FAX. 816/836–8953; R. Scott Richart, JD, Executive Director

**National Board of Medical Examiners,** 3750 Market Street, Philadelphia, PA 19104; tel. 215/590–9500; FAX. 215/590–9430; Donald E. Melnick, MD, President

**National Board of Public Health Examiners,** 1900 M Street NW #710, Washington, DC 20036; tel. 866/514–7569; Molly M. Eggleston, Executive Director

**National Council of State Boards of Nursing,** 111 E. Wacker Drive, Suite 2900, Chicago, IL 60601; tel. 312/525–3600; FAX. 312/279–1032; Kathy Apple, Chief Executive Officer

**National Council on Aging, Inc., NCOA Headquarters,** 1901 L Street, NW, 4th Floor, Washington, DC 20024; tel. 202/479–1200; FAX. 202/479–0735; James P. Firman, Ed.D., President and Chief Executive Officer

**National Council on Alcoholism and Drug Dependence, Inc., NCADD,** 217 Broadway, Suite 712, New York, NY 10007; tel. 212/269–7797; FAX. 212/269–7510; Robert J. Lindsey, M.Ed., CEAP President and Chief Executive Officer

**National Council on Radiation Protection and Measurements,** 7910 Woodmont Avenue, Suite 400, Bethesda, MD 20814; tel. 301/657–2652; FAX. 301/907–8768; David A. Schauer, Executive Director

**National Dental Association,** 3517 16th Street, NW, Washington, DC 20010; tel. 202/588–1697; FAX. 202/588–1244; Robert S. Johns, Executive Director

**National Environmental Health Association,** 720 South Colorado Boulevard, North Tower, Suite 1000-N, Denver, CO 80246–1926; tel. 303/756–9090; FAX. 303/691–9490; Nelson Fabian, Executive Director

**National Federation of Licensed Practical Nurses,** 111 West Main Street, #100, Garner, NC 27529; tel. 919/779–0046; FAX. 919/779–5642; Charlene Barbour, Executive Director

**National Fire Protection Association,** PO Box 9101, One Batterymarck Park, Quincy, MA 02269–9101; tel. 617/770–3000; FAX. 617/770–7110; Richard P. Bielen, PE Director of Fire Protection Systems Engineering

**National Gaucher Foundation,** 2227 Idlewood Road, Suite 6, Tucker, GA 30084; tel. 800/504–3189; FAX. 770/934–2911; Rhonda Buyers, Executive Director and Chief Executive Officer

**National Headache Foundation,** 820 N. Orleans, Suite 217, Chicago, IL 60610–3132; tel. 888/643–5552; FAX. 312/640–9049; Robert Dalton, Executive Director

**National Health Council, Inc.,** 1730 M Street, NW, Suite 500, Washington, DC 20036; tel. 202/785–3910; FAX. 202/785–5923; Myrl Weinberg, CAE, President

**National Hemophilia Foundation,** 116 West 32nd Street, 11th Floor, New York, NY 10001; tel. 212/328–3700; FAX. 212/328–3799; Val Bias, Chief Executive Officer

**National Institute for Jewish Hospice, Central Telephone Network,** PO Box 48025, Los Angeles, CA 90048; tel. 800/446–4448; FAX. 516/791–6999; Shirley Lamm, Executive Director

**National Institute for Occupational Safety and Health,** 395 E Street, SW, Suite 9200, Washington, DC 20201; tel. 202/245–0625; John Howard, MD, Director

**National Kidney Foundation,** 30 East 33rd Street, New York, NY 10016; tel. 800/622–9010; FAX. 212/779–0068; John Davis, Chief Executive Officer

**National League for Nursing, NLN,** 61 Broadway, 33rd Floor, New York, NY 10006; tel. 212/363–5555; FAX. 212/812–0391; Beverly Malone, PhD, RN, FAAN, Chief Executive Officer

**National Multiple Sclerosis Society,** 733 Third Avenue, New York, NY 10017; tel. 212/986–3240; FAX. 212/986–7981; Joyce Nelson, President & Chief Executive Officer

**National Organization for Rare Disorders,** 55 Kenosia Avenue, PO Box 1968, Danbury, CT 06813–1968; tel. 203/744–0100; FAX. 203/798–2291; Names Peter L. Saltonstal, President and Chief Executive Officer

**National Parkinson Foundation, Inc.,** 1501 Northwest Ninth Avenue, Miami, FL 33136–1494; tel. 800/327–4545; FAX. 305/243–5540; Pamela Olmo, Vice President, Finance and Administration

**National Perinatal Association,** 457 State Street, Binghampton, NY 13901; tel. 888/971–3295; FAX. 607/772–0468; Mary Anne Laffin, CNM, FACNM, President

**National Registry of Emergency Medical Technicians,** 6610 Busch Boulevard, PO Box 29233, Columbus, OH 43229; tel. 614/888–4484; FAX. 614/888–8920; William E. Brown, Jr., Executive Director

**National Rehabilitation Association, (Includes Nine National Divisions and 58 Affiliate Chapters),** 633 South Washington Street, Alexandria, VA 22314; tel. 703/836–0850; FAX. 703/836–0848; Linda R. Winslow, Executive Director

**National Resident Matching Program,** 2121 K Street, NW, Washington, DC 20037–1127; tel. 202/828–0676; FAX. 202/828–4797; Mona M. Signer, Executive Director

**National Rural Health Association,** 1108 K. Street NW, 2nd Floor, Washington, DC 20005; tel. 202/639–0550; FAX. 202/639–0559; Alan Morgan, Chief Executive Officer

**National Safety Council,** 1121 Spring Lake Drive, Itasca, IL 60143–3201; tel. 800/621–7619; FAX. 630/285–0797; Customer Service Department

**National Stroke Association,** 9707 E Easter Lane, Building B, Centennial, CO 80112; tel. 303/754–0924; FAX. 303/649–1328; Teran Nash, Customer Relations Coordinator

**National Student Nurses' Association, Inc.,** 45 Main Street, Suite 606, Brooklyn, NY 11201; tel. 718/210–0705; FAX. 718/797–1186; Diane J. Mancino, Ed.D., RN, CAE, Executive Director

**National Tay-Sachs and Allied Diseases Association,** 2001 Beacon Street, Suite 204, Brighton, MA 02135; tel. 800/906–8723; FAX. 617/277–0134; Susan R. Kahn, Executive Director

**National Women's Health Network,** 1413 K Street NW, Fourth Floor, Washington, DC 20005; tel. 202/682–2640; FAX. 202/682–2648; Cynthia Pearson, Executive Director

**New England Gerontological Association,** One Cutts Road, Durham, NH 03824–3102; tel. 603/868–5757; Eugene E. Tillock, Ed.D., Executive Director

**New York State Nurses Association, NYSNA,** 11 Cornell Road, Latham, NY 12110; tel. 518/782–9400; FAX. 518/782–9530; Julie Pinkham, Interim Executive Director

**NSF International,** 789 Dixboro Road, PO Box 130140, Ann Arbor, MI 48113–0140; tel. 734/769–8010; FAX. 313/769–0109

## O

**Office of Radiation and Indoor Air, Environmental Protection Agency,** 1200 Pennsylvania Avenue, NW, Mail Code 6601J, Washington, DC 20460; tel. 202/343–9213; Dennis O'Connor, Senior Policy Advisor

**Osteogenesis Imperfecta Foundation, Inc.,** 804 West Diamond Avenue, Suite 210, Gaithersburg, MD 20878; tel. 301/947–0083; FAX. 301/947–0456; Tracy Smith Hart, Chief Executive Officer

## P

**Pan American Health Organization, Pan American Sanitary Bureau, Regional Office of the World Health Organization,** 525 23rd Street, NW, Washington, DC 20037; tel. 202/974–3000; FAX. 202/974–3663; Dr. Mirta Roses Periago, Director

**Parkinson's Disease Foundation, Inc, (Formerly United Parkinson Foundation),** 1359 Broadway, Suite 1509, New York, NY 10018; tel. 800/457–6676; FAX. 212/923–4778; Rasnahia Cororreal, Director of Administration

**Partnership for Food Safety Education,** 2345 Crystal Drive, Suite 800, Arlington, VA 22202; tel. 202/220–0651; FAX. 202/220–0873; Shelley Feist, Executive Director

**Partnership for Prevention,** 1015 18th Street NW, Suite 300, Washington, DC 20036; tel. 202/833–0009; FAX. 202/833–0113; Jud Richland, MPH, President and Chief Executive Officer

**Physician Executive Leadership Center,** 3403 West Fletcher Avenue, Tampa, FL 33618–2813; tel. 813/963–1800; Jennifer R. Grebenschikoff, Executive Vice President

**Pilot Dogs, Inc.,** 625 West Town Street, Columbus, OH 43215; tel. 614/221–6367; FAX. 614/221–1577; J. Jay Gray, Executive Director

**Practice Greenhealth,** 12355 Sunrise Valley Drive, Suite 680, Reston, VA 20191; tel. 888/688–3332; FAX. 866/379–8705; Anna Gilmore Hall, RN, MS, CAE, Executive Director

**Prevent Blindness America,** 211 W. Wacker Drive, Suite 1700, Chicago, IL 60606; tel. 800/331–2020; FAX. 312/363–6052; Hugh Parry, President and Chief Executive Officer

**Public Health Foundation,** 1300 L Street NW, Suite 800, Washington, DC 20005–4208; tel. 202/218–4400; FAX. 202/218–4409; Sue Madden, Deputy Executive Director

**Public Relations Society of America,** 33 Maiden Lane 11th Floor, New York, NY 10038–5150; tel. 212/460–1400; FAX. 212/995–0757; Catherine A. Bolton, Executive Director and Chief Operating Officer

## R

**Radiological Society of North America, Inc.,** 820 Jorie Boulevard, Oak Brook, IL 60523–2251; tel. 630/571–2670; FAX. 630/571–7837; Jennifer Divelbiss, Director of Marketing

**Recording for the Blind and Dyslexic,** 20 Roszel Road, Princeton, NJ 08540; tel. 866/732–3585; FAX. 609/520–7990; Richard O. Scribner, President

**Renal Physicians Association,** 1700 Rockville Pike, Suite 220, Rockville, MD 20852; tel. 301/468–3515; FAX. 301/468–3511; Dale Singer, MHA, Executive Director

**Robert Wood Johnson Foundation,** PO Box 2316, Route One and College Road East, Princeton, NJ 08543–2316; tel. 877/843–7953; FAX. 609/927–7582; Lydia Ryba, Manager, Office of Proposal Management

## S

**Safe Kids Worldwide,** 1301 Pennsylvania Avenue, NW, Suite 1000, Washington, DC 20004; tel. 202/662–0600; FAX. 202/393–2072; Kate Carr, President and Chief Executive Officer

**Shriners Hospitals for Children,** PO Box 31356, Tampa, FL 33631–3356; tel. 813/281–8111; FAX. 813/281–8174; Keith A. Gardner, Interim Executive Vice President

Section C

**SNMTS, Society of Nuclear Medicine Technologist Section,** 1850 Samuel Morse Drive, Reston, VA 20190; tel. 703/708–9000; FAX. 703/708–9015; Nikki Wenzel-Lamb, MBA, Administrator and Director of Leadership Services

**Society for Academic Emergency Medicine,** 2340 S. River Road, Suite 200, Des Plaines, IL 60018; tel. 847/813–9823; FAX. 847/813–5450; Ronald S. Moen, Interim Executive Director

**Society for Adolescent Health and Medicine (SAHM),** 111 Deer Lake Road, Suite 100, Deefield, IL 60015; tel. 847/753–5226; FAX. 847/480–9282; Debbie Trueblood, Executive Director

**Society for Healthcare Consumer Advocacy (SHCA),** 155 N. Wacker Drive, Suite 400, Chicago, IL 60606; tel. 312/422–3700; FAX. 312/278–0881; Elizabeth Summy, Vice President

**Society for Healthcare Strategy and Market Development (SHSMD),** 155 N. Wacker Drive, Suite 400, Chicago, IL 60606; tel. 312/422–3888; FAX. 312/278–0883; Lauren A. Barnett, Executive Director

**Society for Occupational and Environmental Health,** 6728 Old McLean Village Drive, McLean, VA 22101; tel. 703/556–9222; FAX. 703/556–8729; Connie MacKay, Account Manager

**Society for Pediatric Pathology,** 3643 Walton Way Extension, Augusta, GA 30909; tel. 706/364–3375; FAX. 706/733–8033; Kerry Crockett, Director of Operations and Meetings

**Society for Social Work Leadership in Health Care (SSWLHC),** 100 North 20th Street, Suite 400, Philadelphia, PA 19103; tel. 866/237–9542; FAX. 215/564–2175; Kyle Fernley, Account Manager

**Society of Cardiac Monitoring, Inc.,** PO Box 3395, Riverview, FL 33568; tel. 623/204–4848; Jonni Cooper, BSN, MBA, PhD, Chief Executive Officer

**Society of Chest Pain Centers,** 6161 Riverside Drive, Dublin, OH 43017; tel. 614/442–5950; FAX. 614/442–5953; Wilbert D. Mick, Chief Executive Officer

**Society of Critical Care Medicine,** 500 Midway Drive, Mount Prospect, IL 60056; tel. 847/827–6869; FAX. 847/827–6886; David J. Martin, CAE, Chief Executive Officer and EVP

**Society of Neurological Surgeons,** 3303 SW Bond Avenue, Portland, OR 97239; tel. 503/494–7978; Kim J. Burchiel, MD, FACS, Secretary

**Society of University Otolaryngologists-Head and Neck Surgeons,** USC School of Medicine, Department of Otolaryngology, Los Angeles, CA 90033; tel. 323/226–7315; FAX. 323/226–2780; Donna Hoffman, M.A., Executive Director

**Special Care Dentistry Association,** 401 N. Michigan Avenue, 2nd Floor, Chicago, IL 60611; tel. 312/527–6764; FAX. 312/673–6663; Kaye Englebrecht

**Spina Bifida Association,** 4590 MacArthur Boulevard, NW, Suite 250, Washington, DC 20007; tel. 800/621–3141; FAX. 202/944–3295; Cindy Brownstein, President and Chief Executive Officer

**Susan G. Komen Breast Cancer Foundation,** 5005 LBJ Freeway, Suite 250, Dallas, TX 75244; tel. 800/465–6636; Kimberly Simpson, Chief Operating Officer

# T

**The Academy of Nutrition and Dietetics,** 120 South Riverside Plaza, Suite 2000, Chicago, IL 60606–6995; tel. 312/899–0040; FAX. 312/899–4765; Patricia M. Babjak, Chief Executive Officer

**The American Association of Immunologists, Inc.,** 9650 Rockville Pike, Bethesda, MD 20814; tel. 301/634–7178; FAX. 301/634–7887; M. Michele Hogan, PhD, Executive Director

**The American Board of Anesthesiology, Inc.,** 4208 Six Forks Road, Suite 900, Raleigh, NC 27609–5735; tel. 919/745–2200; FAX. 919/745–2201; Mary E. Post, MBA, CAE, Executive Director, Administrative Affairs

**The American Board of Disability Analysts (ABDA),** Belle Meade Office Park, 4525 Harding Road, Nashville, TN 37205; tel. 615/327–2984; FAX. 615/327–9235; Alexander Horowitz, MD, Executive Officer Emeritus

**The American Board of Obstetrics and Gynecology, Inc.,** 2915 Vine Street, Dallas, TX 75204; tel. 214/871–1619; FAX. 214/871–1943; Larry Gilstrap, MD, Executive Director

**The American Board of Pediatric Dentistry,** 325 E. Washington Street, Suite 208, Iowa City, IA 52240–3960; tel. 319/341–8488; FAX. 319/341–9499; Jeffrey A. Dean, Executive Director

**The American Board of Plastic Surgery, Inc.,** Seven Penn Center, Suite 400, 1635 Market Street, Philadelphia, PA 19103–2204; tel. 215/587–9322; FAX. 215/587–9622; Terry M. Cullison, RN, MSN, Administrator

**The American Board of Urology, Inc.,** 600 Peter Jefferson Pkwy, Suite 150, Charlottesville, VA 22911; tel. 434/979–0059; FAX. 434/979–0266; Gerald H. Jordan, MD, Executive Secretary

**The American Orthopaedic Association,** 6300 North River Road, Suite 505, Rosemont, IL 60018–4263; tel. 847/318–7330; FAX. 847/318–7339; Kristin Olds Glavin, Executive Director

**The Arc of the United States,** 1825 K Street NW, Suite 1200, Washington, DC 20006; tel. 202/534–3700; FAX. 202/534–3731; Peter V. Berns, Chief Executive Officer

**The Association for Research in Vision and Ophthalmology,** 1801 Rockville Pike, Ste 400, Rockville, MD 20852–5622; tel. 240/221–2900; FAX. 240/221–0370; Iris M. Rush, CAE, Interim Executive Director

**The Association of Medical Illustrators,** 201 E Main Street, Suite 1405, Lexington, KY 40507; tel. 866/393–4264; FAX. 859/514–9166; Melanie Bowzer, Executive Director

**The Association of Women's Health, Obstetric and Neonatal Nurses,** 2000 L. Street, NW, Suite 740, Washington, DC 20036; tel. 202/261–2400; FAX. 202/728–0575; Karen Peddicord, RNC, PhD, Chief Executive Officer

**The Christopher and Dana Reeve Foundation, Paralysis Resource Center,** Short Hills Plaza, 636 Morris Turnpike, Suite #3A, Short Hills, NJ 07078–7503; tel. 800/539–7309; Angela Cantillon, Associate Director-Operations

**The Duke Endowment,** 100 North Tryon Street, Suite 3500, Charlotte, NC 28202; tel. 704/376–0291; FAX. 704/376–9336; Mary L. Piepenbring, Vice President

**The Endocrine Society,** 8401 Connecticut Avenue, Suite 900, Chevy Chase, MD 20815; tel. 301/941–0200; FAX. 301/941–0259; Janet Kreizman, Deputy Executive Director & Chief Policy Officer

**The Foundation Fighting Blindness, Inc.,** 7168 Columbia Gateway Drive, Suite 100, Columbia, MD 21046; tel. 410/423–0600; FAX. 410/872–0438; William T. Schmidt, Chief Executive Officer

**The Foundation for Ichthyosis and Related Skin Types, Inc. (FIRST),** 2616 N. Broad Street, Colmar, PA 18915; tel. 215/997–9400; FAX. 215/997–9403; Jean Pickford, Executive Director

**The Histochemical Society,** 9650 Rockville Pike, Bethesda, MD 20814; tel. 301/634–7026; FAX. 301/634–7099; W.L. Stahl, PhD, Executive Director

**The International Dyslexia Association,** 40 York Road, 4th Floor, Baltimore, MD 21204; tel. 410/296–0232; FAX. 410/321–5069; Kristi Bowman, Director of Development

**The Joint Commission,** One Renaissance Boulevard, Oakbrook Terrace, IL 60181; tel. 630/792–5650; FAX. 630/792–4650; Mark R. Chassin, MD, MPP, MPH, President

**The Leukemia & Lymphoma Society,** 1311 Mamaroneck Avenue, White Plains, NY 10650; tel. 914/949–5213; FAX. 914/949–6691; John E. Walter, President and Chief Executive Officer

**The Mended Hearts, Inc.,** 8150 N. Central Expy., M2075, Dallas, TX 75206; tel. 214/390–3265; FAX. 214/295–9552; Karen Caruth, Executive Director

**The National Commission for Health Education Credentialing, Inc.,** 1541 Alta Drive, Suite 303, Whitehall, PA 18052–5642; tel. 484/223–0770; FAX. 800/813–0727; Linda Lysoby, MS, MCHES, CAE, Executive Director

**The Seeing Eye, Inc.,** PO Box 375, Morristown, NJ 07963–0375; tel. 973/539–4425; FAX. 973/539–0922; Jim Kutsch, President

**The Southwestern Surgical Congress,** 5019 W 147th St, Leawood, KS 66224; tel. 913/402–7102; FAX. 913/273–9940; James A. Edney, MD, Executive Director

**The Vision Council,** 225 Reinekers Lane, Suite 700, Alexandria, VA 22314; tel. 703/548–4560; FAX. 703/548–4580; Ed Greene, Chief Executive Officer

# U

**UCLA Medical Center, Neurosurgery,** Box 956901, Los Angeles, CA 90095–6901; tel. 301/267–9449; FAX. 310/825–7245; Neil A. Martin, MD

**United Cerebral Palsy Associations, Inc.,** 1660 L Street, NW, Suite 700, Washington, DC 20036; tel. 800/872–5827; FAX. 202/776–0414; Stephen Bennett, President and Chief Executive Officer

**United Methodist Association of Health and Welfare Ministries,** 2800 W Main Street, Tupelo, MS 38801–3027; tel. 662/269–2955; FAX. 662/269–2956; Stephen L. Vinson, President and Chief Executive Officer

**United Way of America,** 701 North Fairfax Street, Alexandria, VA 22314–2045; tel. 703/836–7100; FAX. 703/683–7846; Brian A. Gallagher, President and Chief Executive Officer

**USP, United States Pharmacopeia,** 12601 Twinbrook Parkway, Rockville, MD 20852; tel. 301/816–8368; FAX. 301/816–8511; Arline M. Bilbo, Director, Member and Professional Relations

# W

**Western Orthopedic Association,** 154-A W. Foothill Boulevard, # 107, Upland, CA 91786; tel. 866/962–1388; FAX. 410/494–0515; Chuck Freitag, Executive Director

**Wound, Ostomy and Continence Nursing Certification Board (WOCNCB),** 555 E. Wells Street, Suite 1100, Milwaukee, WI 53202; tel. 888/496–2622; FAX. 414/276–2146; Tracy Burr, Executive Director

Section C

## ARGENTINA

**Camara Argentina De Empresas De Salud, (Argentina Hospital Association),** Tucuman 1668, 2 Piso, C.P. 1050, Buenos Aires; tel. 541143725915; FAX. 541143723229; Norberto Larroca-President

## AUSTRALIA

**Australian Healthcare Association,** Unit 2, 1 Napier Close, Deakin, ACT 2600; tel. 1261620780; FAX. 1261620779; Prue Power, Executive Director

## CANADA

**Canadian Blood Services, Head Office,** 1800 Alta Vista Drive, Ottawa, ON K1G 4J5; tel. 613/739–2300; FAX. 613/731–1411; Dr. Graham D. Sher, CEO

**Canadian Healthcare Association,** 17 York Street, Ottawa, ON K1N 9J6; tel. 613/241–8005; FAX. 613/241–5055; Pamela C. Fralick, MA, President and CEO

**Canadian Medical Engineering Consultants,** 594 Bush Street, Belfountain, ON L7K 0E8; tel. 519/927–3286; FAX. 519/927–9440; A. M. Dolan, President

**Canadian Orthopaedic Association,** 4150 Street Catherine Street West, Suite 360, Westmount, PQ; tel. 514/874–9003; FAX. 514/874–0464; Douglas C. Thomson, CEO

**Canadian Public Health Association,** 1565 Carling Avenue, Suite 300, Ottawa, ON K1Z 8R1; tel. 613/725–3769; FAX. 613/725–9826; Debra Lynkowski, Chief Executive Officer

**Canadian Society of Hospital Pharmacists,** 30 Concourse Gate, Unit 3, Ottawa, ON K2E7V7; tel. 613/736–9733; FAX. 613/736–5660

**Catholic Health Association of Canada,** Annex C, Saint-Vincent Hospital, 60 Cambridge Street North, Ottawa, ON K14 7A5; tel. 613/562–6262; FAX. 613/782–2857; James Roche, President

**The Canadian Medical Association,** 1867 Alta Vista Drive, Ottawa, ON K1G 3Y60G8; tel. 613/731–4552; FAX. 613/731–7314; Paul-Emile Cloutier, Secretary General and CEO

## COSTA RICA

**Asociacion Costarricense De Hospitales, (Costa Rica Hospital Association),** Apartado 267-1005, Barrio Mexico San Jose Costa Rica, Costa Rica; tel. 506/221–4919; FAX. 506/255–0363; Dr. Kenneth Gonzalez Arias, Presidente

## ENGLAND

**British Medical Association (BMA),** BMA House, Tavistock Square, London, WCIH 9JP; tel. 02073874499; FAX. 02073836400; Mr. Tony Bourne, Chief Executive and Secretary

## FRANCE

**Federation Hospitaliere De France, (France Hospital Association),** 1 bis, Rue Cabanis, Paris, 75014; tel. Gerard Vincent, Delegue General

**International Hospital Federation,** Immeuble JB SAY, 13 Chemin du Levant, Ferney Voltaire; tel. 334/50–42600; FAX. 334/504–2601; Jose Carlos de Souza Abrahao, President

**World Medical Association,** 13, ch. du Levant, CIB - Bâtiment A, Voltaire; tel. 33450407575; FAX. 33450405937; Dr. Otmar Kloiber, Secretary General

## GERMANY

**Deutsche Krankenhausgesellschaft, (German Hospital Federation),** Wegelystrabe 3, D - 10623, Berlin; tel. +4930398040; FAX. 493039087307; Georg Baum, Chief Executive

## HUNGARY

**Magyar Korhazszovetseg, (Hungarian Hospital Association),** 1113 Budapest, Ibrahim u. 19., Hungary; Dr. Zoltan Ajkay, President

## INDIA

**Indian Hospital Association,** B-401 Sarita Vihar, New Delhi, 110044; FAX. 91–11–694126; Dr. P.Ghez, Secretary General

## INDONESIA

**Indonesian Hospital Association,** Jl. Boulevard Artha Gading Blok, A-7A No. 28, Jakarta, Utara, 14240; tel. 214/–5845303; FAX. 214/458–7832; Muki Reksoprodjo

## ITALY

**Federazione Italiana delle Aziende Sanitarie e Ospedaliere (FIASO), (Italy Hospital Association),** Corso Vi Horis Emmanuele II n. 24, Roma, 00186; Dott. Francesco Ripa di Meana, Presidente

## KOREA

**Korean Hospital Association,** (Mapo Hyun Dai Building), 35-1 Mapo-Dong, Seoul; tel. 822/718–7521; FAX. 822/718–7522; (International Cooperation Officer)

## MEXICO

**Asociacion Mexicana De Hospitales AC, (Mexico Hospital Association),** Queretaro 210, Mexico City, 06700; tel. 55740135; FAX. 55841882; LIC. Francisco Spindola Salazar, Manager

## MONGOLIA

**Mongolian Hospital Association,** PO Box 48/54, Enkhtaivan Street 13b, Ulaanbaatar, 210648; tel. 976/999–9020; FAX. 976/999–6070; Jambaljav Lkhamsuren, MD, President

## PANAMA

**Asociacion Panamena De Hospitales Privados, (Panama Hospital Association),** Apartado 07503, Panama, Panama; tel. 507/269–0615; FAX. 507/966–4223; Rodrigo A. Moreno, President

## PERU

**Association Private Clinics of Peru,** Av. Dos De Mayo 1502 Of. 202, San Isidro, Lima; tel. 511/441–9546; FAX. 511/441–9546; Clodoaldo Barreda Dominguez, Administrator

## PHILIPPINES

**Philippine Hospital Association,** 14 Kamias Road, Quezon City-1, Metro Minila, 01102; tel. 632/992–7674; FAX. 632/921–2219

## SOUTH AFRICA

**Provincial Administration, Health Services Branch,** P.O. Box 227, South Africa, 9300; tel. 0514081107; FAX. 0514081058; Dr. S. Kabane

**South Africa Department of Health,** Room 725, Hallmark Building, Pretoria; Dr. Thabo Sibeko, Director - Hospital Services

## SWITZERLAND

**H+ Die Spitaeler der Schweiz, (Swiss Hospital Association),** Lorrainestrasse 4 A, Bern; M. Bernhart Wegmuller, Director

**World Federation of Public Health Associations,** c/o Institute for Social and Preventative Medicine, University of Geneva, CMU, Geneva, 4 CH-1211; Bettina Borisch, MD, PBH, FRCPath, Director of the Office of the Secretariat

**World Health Organization,** Avenue Appia 20, 1211 Geneva 27, Geneva; tel. 412/279–12111; FAX. 412/2791–3111; Dr. Margaret Chan, Director-General

## THE NETHERLANDS

**International Council on Social Welfare,** C/O MOVISIE - Netherlands Centre for Social Development, 3501 DC, Utrecht, 20002; Denys Correll, Executive Director

## THE UNITED STATES

**International Association of Healthcare Central Service Materiel Management,** 213 W. Institute Place, Suite 307, Chicago, IL 60610; tel. 312/440–0078; FAX. 312/440–9474; Betty Hanna, Executive Director

**Rehabilitation International,** 25 East 21st Street, New York, NY 10010; tel. 212/420–1500; FAX. 212/505–0871; Venus Ilagan, Secretary General

# U. S. GOVERNMENT AGENCIES

*The following information is based on data available as of May 2012.*
*For more information about U.S. government agencies, consult the* U.S. Government Manual. *Additional assistance may be obtained by contacting the American Hospital Association's Washington office, 325 Seventh Street, NW, Washington, DC 20004.*

**Executive Office of the President, The White House**
1600 Pennsylvania Avenue NW
Washington, DC 20500
202/456-1414
Barack H. Obama, President of the United States
http://www.whitehouse.gov

**Office of the Vice President of the United States**
The White House
1600 Pennsylvania Avenue NW
Washington, DC 20501
202/456-1414
Joseph R. Biden, Vice President of the United States
http://www.whitehouse.gov/administration/vice-president-biden

**Centers for Disease Control and Prevention**
1600 Clifton Road
Atlanta, GA 30333
404/639-3311
Dr. Thomas Frieden, MD, MPH, Director
http://www.cdc.gov

**Centers for Medicare & Medicaid Services**
7500 Security Blvd
Baltimore, MD 21244
877/267-2323
http://www.cms.gov

**Council of Economic Advisors**
Eisenhower Executive Office Building
Washington, DC 20502
202/395-5109
http://www.whitehouse.gov/administration/eop/cea/

**Council on Environmental Quality**
722 Jackson Place NW
Washington, DC 20503
202/395-5750
Nancy Sutley, Chair
http://www.whitehouse.gov/administration/eop/ceq

**Department of Agriculture**
1400 Independence Avenue SW
Washington, DC 20250
202/720-3631
Thomas J. Vilsack, Secretary of Agriculture
http://www.usda.gov

**Department of Commerce**
1401 Constitution Avenue NW
Washington, DC 20230
202/482-2000
http://www.commerce.gov

**Department of Defense**
Office of the Secretary
The Pentagon
Washington, DC 20301-1400
703/545-6700
http://www.defenselink.mil

**Department of Education**
400 Maryland Avenue SW
Washington, DC 20202
800/872-5327
Arne Duncan, Secretary of Education
http://www.ed.gov

**Department of Energy**
1000 Independence Avenue SW
Washington, DC 20585
202/586-5000
Steven Chu, Secretary of Energy
http://www.energy.gov

**Department of Health and Human Services**
200 Independence Avenue SW
Washington, DC 20201
877/696-6775
Kathleen Sebelius, Secretary of Health and Human Services
http://www.hhs.gov

**Department of Justice**
950 Pennsylvania Ave NW
Washington, DC 20530-0001
202/514-2000
Eric H. Holder, Jr., The Attorney General
http://www.usdoj.gov

**Department of Labor**
Frances Perkins Building
200 Constitution Avenue NW
Washington, DC 20210
202/693-6000
Hilda L. Solis, Labor Secretary
http://www.dol.gov

**Department of State**
2201 C Street NW
Washington, DC 20520
202/647-4000
Hilary Rodham Clinton, Secretary of State
http://www.state.gov

**Department of the Air Force**
1670 Air Force Pentagon
Washington, DC 20330-1670
703/695-9664
Michael B. Donley, Secretary of the Air Force
http://www.af.mil/main/welcome.asp

**Department of the ARMY**
1400 Defense Pentagon
Washington, DC 20301-1400
703/695-4311
John McHugh, Secretary of the ARMY
http://www.army.mil

**Department of the NAVY**
2000 Navy Pentagon
Washington, DC 20350-2000
703/545-6700
Ray Mabus, Secretary of the NAVY
http://www.navy.mil

**Department of the Treasury**
1500 Pennsylvania NW
Washington, DC 20220
202/622-2000
Timothy F. Geithner, Secretary of the Treasury
http://www.treasury.gov

**Department of Veterans Affairs**
810 Vermont Avenue NW
Washington, DC 20420
202/273-5400
www.va.gov

**Drug Enforcement Administration**
8701 Morrissette Drive
Springfield, VA 22102
202/307-1000
Michele Leonhart, Administrator
http://www.justice.gov/dea/index.htm

**Environmental Protection Agency**
Ariel Rios Building
1200 Pennsylvania Avenue NW
Washington, DC 20460
202/564-4700
Lisa P. Jackson, Administrator
http://www.epa.gov

**Equal Employment Opportunity Commission**
131 M Street NE
Washington, DC 20507
202/663-4191
Jacqueline Berrien, Chair
www.eeoc.gov

**Food and Drug Administration**
10903 New Hampshire Ave
Silver Spring, MD 20903
888/463-6332
http://www.fda.gov

**Health Resources and Services Administration**
5600 Fishers Lane
Room 14-71
Rockville, MD 20857
301/443-2216
Mary K. Wakefield, PhD, RN, Administrator
http://www.hrsa.gov

**Office of Management and Budget**
725 17th Street NW
Washington, DC 20503
202/395-3080
http://www.whitehouse.gov/omb/

**Office of National Drug Control Policy**
750 17th Street NW
Washington, DC 20503
202/395-6700
http://www.whitehousedrugpolicy.gov

**Social Security Administration, Office of Public Inquiries**
Windsor Park Building
6401 Security Blvd.
Baltimore, MD 21235
800/772-1213
www.ssa.gov

**Substance Abuse and Mental Health Services Administration**
One Choke Cherry Road
Rockville, MD 20857
240/276-2000
www.samhsa.gov

# Blue Cross–Blue Shield Plans

*The following listing is based on information provided by the agencies themselves and the Blue Cross and Blue Shield Association. Inclusion or omission of any organization's name indicates neither approval nor disapproval by Health Forum LLC, an American Hospital Association Company.*

## United States

**ALABAMA: Blue Cross and Blue Shield of Alabama,** 450 Riverchase Parkway, East, Birmingham, AL 35244; tel. 205/220–2100; Terry D. Kellogg, President and CEO

**ALASKA: Premera Blue Cross Blue Shield of Alaska,** 2550 Denali Street, Suite 1404, Anchorage, AK 99503; tel. 907/258–5065 (See Washington-Premera Blue Cross for additional information)

**ARIZONA: Blue Cross Blue Shield of Arizona,** 2444 West Las Palmaritas Drive, Phoenix, AZ 85021-4872; tel. 602/864–4100; Richard L. Boals, President and CEO

**ARKANSAS: Arkansas Blue Cross and Blue Shield,** 601 Gaines Street, Little Rock, AR 72201; tel. 501/378–2000; P. Mark White, President and CEO

**CALIFORNIA: Blue Cross of California,** 21555 Oxnard Street, Woodland Hills, CA 91367; tel. 818/234–5548 (See Indiana- WellPoint, Inc. for additional information)
**Blue Shield of California,** 50 Beale Street, San Francisco, CA 94105; tel. 415/229–5000; Bruce G. Bodaken, Chairman, President and CEO

**COLORADO: Anthem Blue Cross and Blue Shield,** 700 Broadway, Denver, CO 80273; tel. 303/831–2131 (See Indiana- WellPoint, Inc. for additional information)

**CONNECTICUT: Anthem Blue Cross and Blue Shield,** 370 Bassett Road, North Haven, CT 06473; tel. 203/239–4911 (See Indiana- WellPoint, Inc. for additional information)

**DELAWARE: Highmark Blue Cross Blue Shield of Delaware, Inc.,** 800 Delaware Avenue, Suite 900, Wilmington, DE 19801-1368; tel. 302/421–3000; (see Pennsylvania- Highmark, Inc. for additional information)

**DISTRICT OF COLUMBIA: CareFirst BlueCross BlueShield,** Washington, DC (See Maryland-CareFirst BlueCross BlueShield for additional information)

**FLORIDA: Blue Cross and Blue Shield of Florida,** 4800 Deerwood Campus Parkway, Jacksonville, FL 32246-8273; tel. 904/791–6111; Robert I. Lufrano, MD, Chairman, CEO and President

**GEORGIA: Blue Cross and Blue Shield of Georgia,** Capital City Plaza, 3350 Peachtree Rd NE, Atlanta, GA 30326; tel. 404/842–8000 (See Indiana-WellPoint, Inc. for additional information)

**HAWAII: Blue Cross and Blue Shield of Hawaii, (Hawaii Medical Service Association),** 818 Keeaumoku Street, Honolulu, HI 96814; tel. 808/948–6111; Robert P. Hiam, President and CEO

**IDAHO: Blue Cross of Idaho Health Service,** 3000 East Pine Avenue, Meridian, ID 83642-5995; tel. 208/345–4550; Ray Flachbart, President and CEO
**Regence BlueShield of Idaho,** 1602 21st Avenue, Lewiston, ID 83501; tel. 208/746–2671; Scott D. Kreiling, President

**ILLINOIS: Health Care Service Corporation, (Blue Cross and Blue Shield Plans in Illinois, New Mexico, Oklahoma and Texas),** 300 East Randolph Street, Chicago, IL 60601-5099; tel. 312/653–6000; Patricia A. Hemingway-Hall, President and Chief Executive Officer

**INDIANA: WellPoint, Inc.,** 120 Monument Circle, Indianapolis, IN 46204; tel. 317/488–6000; Angela F. Braly, Chair, President and Chief Executive Officer

**IOWA: Wellmark Blue Cross and Blue Shield of Iowa,** 1331 Grand Avenue, Des Moines, IA 50309; tel. 515/376–4500; John D. Forsyth, Chairman and CEO

**KANSAS: Blue Cross and Blue Shield of Kansas,** 1133 SW Topeka Boulevard, Topeka, KS 66629-0001; tel. 785/291–7000; Andrew C. Corbin, President and CEO

**KENTUCKY: Anthem Blue Cross and Blue Shield,** 13550 Triton Park Boulevard, Louisville, KY 40223; tel. 502/889–2000 (See Indiana- WellPoint, Inc. for additional information)

**LOUISIANA: Blue Cross and Blue Shield of Louisiana,** 5525 Reitz Avenue, Baton Rouge, LA 70809-3802; tel. 225/295–3307; Michael H. Reitz, President and CEO

**MAINE: Anthem Blue Cross and Blue Shield,** 2 Gannett Drive, South Portland, ME 04106-6911; tel. 207/822–7000 (See Indiana- WellPoint, Inc. for additional information)

**MARYLAND: CareFirst BlueCross BlueShield,** 1501 S. Clinton Street, Suite 700, Baltimore, MD 21224; tel. 410/581–3000; Chester E. Burrell, President and CEO

**MASSACHUSETTS: Blue Cross and Blue Shield of Massachusetts, Inc.,** Landmark Center, 401 Park Drive, Boston, MA 02215; tel. 617/246–5000; Andrew Dreyfus, President and CEO

**MICHIGAN: Blue Cross Blue Shield of Michigan,** 600 East Lafayette Boulevard, Detroit, MI 48226-2998; tel. 313/225–9000; Daniel J. Loepp, President and CEO

**MINNESOTA: Blue Cross and Blue Shield of Minnesota,** 3535 Blue Cross Road, Eagan, MN 55122; tel. 651/662–8000; Patrick J. Geraghty, President and CEO

**MISSISSIPPI: Blue Cross & Blue Shield of Mississippi,** 3545 Lakeland Drive, Jackson, MS 39232-9799; tel. 601/932–3704; M. Carol Pigott, President and CEO

**MISSOURI: Anthem Blue Cross and Blue Shield,** 1831 Chestnut Street, St. Louis, MO 63103; tel. 314/923–4444 (See Indiana- WellPoint, Inc. for additional information)
**Blue Cross and Blue Shield of Kansas City,** 2301 Main Street, Kansas City, MO 64108; tel. 816/395–2222; David R. Gentile, President and Chief Executive Officer

**MONTANA: Blue Cross and Blue Shield of Montana,** 560 North Park Avenue, Helena, MT 59601; tel. 406/437–5000; Michael E. Frank, President and Chief Executive Officer

**NEBRASKA: Blue Cross and Blue Shield of Nebraska,** 1919 Aksarben Drive, Omaha, NE 68106; tel. 402/982–7000; Steven S. Martin, President and CEO

**NEVADA: Anthem Blue Cross and Blue Shield,** 9133 W. Russell Road, Las Vegas, NV 89148; tel. 702/586–6100 (See Indiana- WellPoint, Inc. for additional information)

**NEW HAMPSHIRE: Anthem Blue Cross and Blue Shield,** 3000 Goffs Falls Rd, Manchester, NH 03111; tel. 603/695–7000 (See Indiana- WellPoint, Inc. for additional information)

**NEW JERSEY: Horizon Blue Cross and Blue Shield of New Jersey, Inc.,** 3 Penn Plaza East, Newark, NJ 07105; tel. 973/466–4000; Robert A. Marino, President and CEO

**NEW MEXICO: Blue Cross and Blue Shield of New Mexico,** 5701 Balloon Fiesta Parkway NE, Albuquerque, NM 87113; tel. 505/291–3500 (See Illinois- Health Care Service Corporation for additional information)

**NEW YORK: Empire Blue Cross and Blue Shield,** 165 Broadway, New York, NY 10006; tel. 212/476–1000 (See Indiana- WellPoint, Inc. for additional information)

**Excellus BlueCross BlueShield,** 165 Court Street, Rochester, NY 14647; tel. 585/454–1700; David H. Klein, President and CEO
**HealthNow New York Inc., d/b/a BlueCross BlueShield of Western New York and BlueShield of Northeastern New York,** 257 W. Genesee Street, Buffalo, NY 14202; tel. 716/887–6900; Alphonso O'Neil-White, President and CEO

**NORTH CAROLINA: Blue Cross and Blue Shield of North Carolina,** 5901 Chapel Hill Road, Durham, NC 27707; tel. 800/446–8053; J. Bradley Wilson, President and CEO

**NORTH DAKOTA: Blue Cross Blue Shield of North Dakota,** 4510 13th Avenue South, Fargo, ND 58121-0001; tel. 701/282–1100; Paul von Ebers, President and CEO

**OHIO: Anthem Blue Cross and Blue Shield,** 4361 Irwin Simpson Rd., Mason, OH 45040; tel. 513/872–8100 (See Indiana- WellPoint, Inc. for additional information)

**OKLAHOMA: Blue Cross and Blue Shield of Oklahoma,** 1400 S. Boston Avenue, Tulsa, OK 74119; tel. 918/560–3500 (See Illinois- Health Care Service Corporation for additional information)

**OREGON: The Regence Group, Regence BlueCross BlueShield of Oregon,** 100 SW Market Street, Portland, OR 97201; tel. 503/225–5221; Mark B. Ganz, President and CEO

**PENNSYLVANIA: Blue Cross of Northeastern Pennsylvania,** 19 North Main Street, Wilkes-Barre, PA 18711; tel. 570/200–4300; Denise S. Cesare, President and CEO
**Capital BlueCross,** 2500 Elmerton Avenue, Harrisburg, PA 17177-9799; tel. 717/541–7000; William Lehr, Jr., Chairman and CEO
**Highmark, Inc.,** 120 Fifth Avenue, Pittsburgh, PA 15222-3099; tel. 412/544–7000; Kenneth R. Melani, MD, President and CEO
**Independence Blue Cross,** 1901 Market Street, Philadelphia, PA 19103; tel. 215/241–2400; Daniel J. Hilferty, President and CEO

**RHODE ISLAND: Blue Cross & Blue Shield of Rhode Island,** 500 Exchange Street, Providence, RI 02903-2699; tel. 401/459–1000; James E. Purcell, President and Chief Executive Officer

**SOUTH CAROLINA: Blue Cross and Blue Shield of South Carolina,** I-20 East at Alpine Road, Columbia, SC 29219; tel. 803/788–3860; David S. Pankau, President and CEO

**SOUTH DAKOTA: Wellmark Blue Cross and Blue Shield of South Dakota,** 1601 West Madison Street, Sioux Falls, SD 57104; tel. 605/373–7200 (See Iowa- Wellmark Blue Cross and Blue Shield for additional information)

**TENNESSEE: BlueCross BlueShield of Tennessee, Inc.,** 1 Cameron Hill Circle, Chattanooga, TN 37402; tel. 423/535–5600; Vicky B. Gregg, Chief Executive Officer

**TEXAS: Blue Cross and Blue Shield of Texas,** 1001 E. Lookout Drive, Richardson, TX 75082; tel. 972/766–6900 (See Illinois- Health Care Service Corporation for additional information)

**UTAH: Regence BlueCross BlueShield of Utah,** 2890 E. Cottonwood Parkway, Salt Lake City, UT 84121; tel. 801/333–2000 (See Oregon- The Regence Group for additional information)

**VERMONT: Blue Cross and Blue Shield of Vermont,** Mailing Address: PO Box 186, Montpelier, VT 05601-0186; tel. 802/223–6131; Don C. George, President and CEO

**VIRGINIA: Anthem Blue Cross and Blue Shield,** 2015 Staples Mill Road, Richmond, VA 23230; tel. 804/354–7000 (See Indiana- WellPoint, Inc. for additional information)

**WASHINGTON: Premera Blue Cross,** 7001 220th Street SW Bldg. 3, Mountlake Terrace, WA 98043-2124; tel. 425/918–4000; H. R. Brereton Barlow, President and CEO

**Regence Blue Shield,** 1800 Ninth Avenue, Seattle, WA 98101; tel. 206/464–3600 (See Oregon- The Regence Group for additional information)

**WEST VIRGINIA: Highmark Blue Cross Blue Shield West Virginia,** 700 Market Square, Parkersburg, WV 26101; tel. 304/424–7700 (See Pennsylvania-Highmark, Inc. for additional information)

**WISCONSIN: Anthem Blue Cross and Blue Shield,** 6775 W. Washington Street, Milwaukee, WI 53214; tel. 414/459–5000 (See Indiana- WellPoint, Inc. for additional information)

**WYOMING: Blue Cross and Blue Shield of Wyoming,** 4000 House Avenue, Cheyenne, WY 82001-2266; tel. 307/634–1393; Tim J. Crilly, President and CEO

# U.S. Associated Areas

**PUERTO RICO: Triple-S Management Corporation,** 1441 F.D. Roosevelt Avenue, San Juan, PR 00920; tel. 787/749–4949; Ramon M. Ruiz-Comas, CPA, President and CEO

Section C

# Group Purchasing Organizations

*The following list of Group Purchasing Organizations is derived from the AHA Annual Survey of Hospitals and the organizations themselves. It reflects Group Purchasing Organizations serving hospitals. Inclusion or omission of any organization's name indicates neither approval nor disapproval by Health Forum LLC, an American Hospital Association company.*

## A

**Advantage Healthcare Net**, 2100 South Columbia Road, Suite 104, Grand Forks, ND 58201; tel. 800/548-2744; FAX. 701/772-0984; F. Wade Johnson, Vice President and Chief Operating Officer; www.advantage-healthcare.net

**Advantage/Amerinet**
see Advantage Healthcare Net

**Adventist Health**, 2100 Douglas Boulevard, Roseville, CA 95661; tel. 916/781-2000; Lowell Church, Vice President, Material Management; www.adventisthealth.org

**Adventist Premier**
see Premier Inc.

**Affiliated Materiel Services**, 931 Union Street, P. O. Box 940, Bangor, ME 04401; tel. 800/648-2727; Scott Oxley, Senior Vice President, Support Services; www.bigbluea.com/dynamic_div.aspx?id=85952

**Alegent NPG/Health Link Premier**
see Prairie Health Ventures

**All Health**
see Amerinet, Inc.

**Allegiance Health**, 205 North East Avenue, Jackson, MI 49201-1789; tel. 517/788-4800; www.allegiancehealth.org

**Allegiance Health Care Corporation**
see Cardinal Health, Inc.

**Alliant Purchasing, LLC**
see Alliant-HAS

**Alliant-HAS**, 2650 Eastpoint Parkway, Suite 320, Louisville, KY 40223; tel. 800/446-8760; FAX. 502/992-3526; Joe Broyles, President; www.alliant-has.com

**Altus Management LLC**, 840 Aero Drive, Suite 150, Cheektowaga, NY 14225; tel. 716/633-0563; Kevin Connor, Chief Executive Officer

**Amerinet, Inc.**, 2060 Craigshire Road, St. Louis, MO 63146; tel. 800/388-2638; Todd C. Ebert, President and Chief Executive Officer; www.amerinet-gpo.com

**Amerinet/Shared Health**
see Shared Health Services Corporation

**AmeriPath, Inc.**; www.ameripath.com

**AmerisourceBergen Corporation**, P.O. Box 959, Valley Forge, PA 19482; tel. 610/727-7000; Steven H. Collis, President and Chief Executive Officer; www.amerisourcebergen.com

**ArchCare**, 205 Lexington Avenue, 3rd Floor, New York, NY 10016; tel. 646/633-4700; Terence Gallagher, Vice President, Supply Chain; www.archcare.org

**Ascension Health**
see Resource and Supply Management Group, LLC

**Ascension Health/Consorta**
see Resource and Supply Management Group, LLC

**Associated Purchasing Services**, 7015 College Boulevard, Suite 150, Overland Park, KS 66211; tel. 913/327-8730; FAX. 913/327-7210; Dennis George, Chief Executive Officer; www.apskc.org

**Avera PACE**, 3900 West Avera Drive, Suite 200, Sioux Falls, SD 57108; tel. 800/657-8059; FAX. 605/322-4666; Steve Statz, Senior Vice President of Business Development; www.averapace.com

## B

**Banner Health System**
see Banner Support Services, Corporate Supply Chain Management

**Banner Support Services, Corporate Supply Chain Management**, 7300 West Detroit Street, Chandler, AZ 85226; tel. 602/685-5391; FAX. 602/685-5065; Richard Hahn, Director, Materials Management; www.bannerhealth.com

**Baptist Health Care Services**
see VHA, Inc.

**Baycare Purchasing Partners, LLC**, 8731 Florida Mining Boulevard, Tampa, FL 33634

**BJC Healthcare**
see Novation LLC

**Boone Hospital Center**, 1600 East Broadway, Columbia, MO 65201-5844; tel. 573/815-8000; FAX. 573/815-2638; Daniel J. Rothery, President; www.boone.org

**Borschow Hospital & Medical Supplies, Inc.**, Centro Internacional de Distribucion, Edificio # 10 Carr, 869 KM 4.2, Guaynabo, PR 00965; tel. 800/981-2301; FAX. 787/625-4395; Debbie Weitzman, Senior Vice President and General Manager; www.borschow.com/default.aspx?LN=EN

**Briggs Healthcare**, 7300 Westown Parkway, Suite 100, West Des Moines, IA 50266; tel. 800/247-2343; FAX. 800/222-1996; www.briggscorp.com

**Broadlane Group**
see MedAssets, Inc.

**Broadlane/MedAssets**
see MedAssets, Inc.

**Buffalo Hospital Supply Co., Inc.**, 4039 Genesee Street, Buffalo, NY 14225; tel. 716/626-9400; FAX. 716/626-4307; Michael J. Burke, Chief Executive Officer; www.buffalohospital.com

**Burrows Company**
see Owens & Minor, Inc.

**BuyPower**
see MedAssets, Inc.

## C

**California Department of General Services**, Ziggurat Building, 707 Third Street, West Sacramento, CA 95605; tel. 916/376-5000; Fred Klass, Director; www.dgs.ca.gov/Default.aspx?alias=www.dgs.ca.gov/dgs

**CALTC Purchasing Group**
see Connecticut Alliance for Long Term Care

**Capella Healthcare**, 501 Corporate Centre Drive, Suite 200, Franklin, TN 37067; tel. 615/764-3000; Brian K. Hitchcock, Vice President, Materiel Resource Operations; www.capellahealth.com

**Cardinal Health Pharmacy Distributor**
see Cardinal Health, Inc.

**Cardinal Health, Inc.**, 7000 Cardinal Place, Dublin, OH 43017; tel. 614/757-5000; George S. Barrett, Chairman and Chief Executive Officer; www.cardinalhealth.com

**Cardinal Industries**
see Cardinal Health, Inc.

**Care New England**
see VHA, Inc.

**Carilion Clinic**, P.O. Box 13367, Roanoke, VA 24033; tel. 800/422-8482; Nancy Howell Agee, President and Chief Executive Officer; www.carilionclinic.org

**Carolinas Shares Services**, P.O. Box 35126, Charlotte, NC 28235; tel. 704/512-7271; FAX. 704/512-7037; James Olsen, Senior Vice President and Chief Operating Officer; www.carolinassharedservices.org

**Catholic Health East**, 3805 West Chester Pike, Suite 100, Newtown Square, PA 19073; tel. 610/355-2092; Florence Doyle, Vice President, Supply Chain; www.che.org/services/materiels.php

**Catholic Health Initiatives**
see HealthTrust Purchasing Group

**Catholic Health Service-Long Island**
see Catholic Health Services of Long Island

**Catholic Health Services of Long Island**, 992 North Village Avenue, Rockville Centre, NY 11570; tel. 516/705-3700; Lawrence E. McManus, President and Chief Executive Officer; www.chsli.org

**Catholic Materials Management Alliance**
see HealthTrust Purchasing Group

**Central Atlantic Health Network, LLC**
see VHA, Inc.

**CHAMPS Healthcare**, 1226 Huron Road East, Cleveland, OH 44115; tel. 216/696-6900; FAX. 216/696-1875; Bob Stein, Vice President, Business Development; champshealthcare.com/en/GroupPurchasing.aspx

**CHCA**
see Child Health Corporation of America

**Child Health Corporation of America**, 6803 West 64th Street, Shawnee Mission, KS 66202; tel. 913/262-1436; FAX. 913/262-1575; Tim Rezash, Group Vice President, GPS; www.chca.com

**Children's Hospital Corporation of America**
see Child Health Corporation of America

**Christus Health**
see MedAssets, Inc.

**CHS**
see HealthTrust Purchasing Group

**Claflin Company**, 455 Warwick Industrial Drive, Warwick, RI 02886; tel. 800/343-7776; FAX. 401/739-4360; Ted Almon, President and Chief Executive Officer; www.claflin.com

**Clarian Health**
see IU Health Supply Chain Operations

**CoalesCo, Inc.**, 19 South Sea Winds Lane, Ponte Vedra Beach, FL 32082; tel. 904/543-8799; Robert P. Bissell, President and Chief Executive Officer; www.coalescoinc.com

**Coalition of Health Services**
see HealthShare/THA

**Coastal Cooperative of New Jersey, LLC**, 1350 Campus Parkway, Wall, NJ 07753; tel. 732/751-3404; www.coastalcoop.com

**Colonial Regional Alliance, LLC**, 10715 Downsville Pike, Suite 102, Hagerstown, MD 21740; tel. 240/313-9960; Stephen Carpenter, Executive Director; www.colonialregional.com

**Commonwealth of Massachusetts, Executive Office for Administration and Finance**, State House, Room 373, Boston, MA; tel. 617/727-2040; FAX. 617/727-2779; Jay Gonzalez, Executive Secretary; www.mass.gov/anf

**Community Health Systems**
see HealthTrust Purchasing Group

**Connecticut Alliance for Long Term Care**, 705-A New Britain Avenue, Hartford, CT 06106; tel. 860/547-0531; FAX. 860/953-6741; Marilyn Burlenski, President and Chief Executive Officer; www.caltc.org

**Consolidated Supply Chain Services, LLC**, 780 Commonwealth Drive, Suite 201, Warrendale, PA 15086; Gary R. Metcalfe, Chief Executive Officer

**Consorta, Inc.**
see HealthTrust Purchasing Group

**Cooperative Services of Florida**, 401 Leonard Boulevard North, Lehigh Acres, FL 33971; tel. 239/303–0606; FAX. 203/303–0754; Robert Simpson, President and Chief Executive Officer; www.csofl.com

**Corporate Express, Inc.**
see Staples Advantage

**Covenant Health**, 3615 19th Street, Lubbock, TX 79410; tel. 806/725–0000; Richard H. Parks, FACHE, President and Chief Executive Officer; www.covenanthealth.org

**CRC Health Group**, 20400 Stevens Creek Boulevard, 6th floor', Cupertino, CA 95014; tel. 877/272–8668; FAX. 408/367–0030; R. Andrew Eckert, Chief Executive Officer; www.crchealth.com

# D

**Defense Logistics Agency**, Andrew T. McNamara Building, 8725 John J. Kingman Road, Fort Belvoir, VA 22060-6221; tel. 703/767–5200; Vice Admiral Mark D. Harnitchek, SC, USN, Director; www.dla.mil

**DeKroyft-Metz & Co., Inc.**, 201 N.E. Adams Street, Peoria, IL 61602; tel. 800/322–3568; FAX. 309/673–4775; Gary Haluska, President; www.dekroyftmetz.com

**Delcrest Medical Services**, 100 Commerce Drive, Ivyland, PA 18974; tel. 800/672–8400; FAX. 215/675–1128; www.delcrest.com/index.html

**Department of Veterans Affairs**
see VA listings

**Direct Supply, Inc.**, 6767 North Industrial Road, Milwaukee, WI 53223; tel. 800/634–7328; Bob Hillis, Chief Executive Officer; www.directsupply.com

**Directs.com**
see Direct Supply, Inc.

**Distribution Cooperative, Inc.**, 5356 East Ponce de Leon Avenue, Suite 100, Stone Mountain, GA 30083; tel. 770/496–5900; Roy Gilleland, Chief Executive Officer

**Distribution Operations Center, LLC**, 9225 Polaris Lane, NE, Suite D, Olympia, WA 98516-7155; tel. 360/486–5620; docnw.com

**DSSI, LLC**, 40 Oak Hollow Street, Suite 225, Southfield, MI 48033; tel. 248/208–8375; Bhagwan P. Thacker, President and Chief Executive Officer; www.directsourcing.com

# E

**East Texas Medical Center Regional Healthcare System**, 1000 South Beckham Avenue, Tyler, TX 75701; tel. 903/597–0351; Elmer G. Ellis, President and Chief Executive Officer; www.etmc.org

**Eastern Maine Healthcare Systems**
see Northeast Purchasing Coalition LLC

# F

**Fairview Purchasing Network**, 400 Stinson Boulevard., N.E., Minneapolis, MN 55413; tel. 612/672–4409; FAX. 612/672–4440; Chris Hanson, Manager; www.fairview.org/About/PurchasingNetwork/index.htm

**Federal Strategic Sourcing Initiative**, 2200 Crystal Drive, Suite 11104, Arlington, VA 22202-3713; tel. 703/785–3013; Michel Kareis; www.gsa.gov/fssi

**FirstChoice Cooperative**, 4815 Troup Highway, Tyler, TX 75703; tel. 800/250–3457; Freddie Sanchez, Chairman; www.fccoop.org

**FSSI**
see Federal Strategic Sourcing Initiative

# G

**General Medical**
see McKesson Corporation

**General Services Commission**
see Texas Facilities Commission

**Genesis Health Alliance**, 3700 Washington Avenue, Evansville, IN 47750; tel. 812/485–4000; J. D. LeClere, Executive Director; www.stmarys.org/genesis

**Genesis Health System**, 1227 East Rusholme Street, Davenport, IA 52803; tel. 563/421–1000; Doug Cropper, President and Chief Executive Officer

**Genesis Purchasing Alliance**
see Genesis Health Alliance

**GHS for Premier**
see Genesis Health System

**GNYHA Services, Inc.**, 555 West 57th Street, New York, NY 10019; tel. 212/246–7100; FAX. 212/262–6350; Lee H. Perlman, President; www.gnyha.org/276/Default.aspx

**Government Services Administration**
see United States General Services Administration

**Greater New York Hospital Association**
see GNYHA Services, Inc.

**Grogan's Healthcare Supply**, 1016 South Broadway at Virginia Avenue, Lexington, KY 40504; tel. 800/365–1020; FAX. 859/254–6666; Alan Grogan, President and Chief Executive Officer; www.grogans.com

**GSA & Consolidated**
see United States General Services Administration

**GSA Contract**
see United States General Services Administration

**Gulf South Medical Supply**, 4345 Southpoint Boulevard, Jacksonville, FL 32216; tel. 800/347–2456; FAX. 800/827–2002; Gary A. Corless, President and Chief Executive Officer; www.pssworldmedical.com/gs

# H

**Hartford Hospital**, 80 Seymour Street, Hartford, CT 06102; tel. 860/545–5000; FAX. 860/545–5066; Jeffrey A. Flaks, President and Chief Executive Officer; www.harthosp.org/default.aspx

**HCA Health Trust Purchasing**
see HealthTrust Purchasing Group

**HCA Supply Chain**
see Parallon Business Solutions

**HCSA Healthcare Service Corp.**
see MedAssets, Inc.

**HCSC**
see Hospital Central Services Inc. and Affiliates

**Health Affiliated Services**, Century Plaza II, 2 Village Drive, Abilene, TX 79606; tel. 800/487–4274; Nancy Bander, Executive Director/National Accounts Manager; www.healthaffiliated.com

**Health Care Coalition of Texas**
see Healthcare Coalition of Texas

**Health Enterprises Cooperative**
see Health Enterprises of Iowa

**Health Enterprises of Iowa**, 5825 Dry Creek Lane, N.E., Cedar Rapids, IA 52402; tel. 319/368–3619; FAX. 319/368–3626; Jon S. Sewell, President and Chief Executive Officer; www.healthenterprises.org

**Health Future, LLC**, 916 Town Centre Drive, Medford, OR 97504; tel. 800/452–2558; Chris Chang-Howitz, Chief Executive Officer; www.healthfuture.org

**Health Purchasing Group**
see HealthTrust Purchasing Group

**Health Services Corporation of America**
see MedAssets, Inc.

**Healthcare Coalition of Texas**, 7160 Dallas Parkway, Suite 600, Plano, TX 75024; tel. 469/366–2100; FAX. 469/366–2101; Geoff Brenner, President and Chief Executive Officer; www.hcotx.com

**Healthcare Purchasing Alliance, Inc.**, 1417 Kuhl Avenue, Suite 100, Orlando, FL 32806; tel. 321/841–4724; FAX. 321/843–4724; Rosaline Parson, Corporate Director; https://hpainc.orlandohealth.com/about

**Healthcare Purchasing Partners**
see Novation LLC

**Healthcare Purchasing Partners International**
see Novation LLC

**HealthGroup of Alabama, Huntsville Hospital**, 101 Sivley Road, Huntsville, AL 35801; tel. 256/265–1000; David Spillers, Chief Executive Officer; www.huntsvillehospital.org/services/hga

**HealthShare/THA**, P.O. Box 679010, Austin, TX 78767-9010; tel. 512/465–1070; FAX. 512/692–2709; Jim Dixon, President and Chief Executive Officer; www.healthshare-tha.com

**HealthSouth Supply Chain Operations**
see MedAssets, Inc.

**HealthTech Management Services**, 405 Duke Drive, Suite 210, Franklin, TN 37067; tel. 800/228–0647; Derek Morkel, President and Chief Executive Officer; www.ht-llc.com

**HealthTrust Purchasing Group**, 155 Franklin Road, Suite 400, Brentwood, TN 37027; tel. 615/344–3000; Jim Fitzgerald, President and Chief Executive Officer; www.healthtrustcorp.com

**HEc**
see Health Enterprises of Iowa

**Hendrick Health Affiliated/Premier**
see Health Affiliated Services

**Henry Schein, Inc.**, 135 Duryea Road, Melville, NY 11747; tel. 631/843–5500; Stanley M. Bergman, Chairman and Chief Executive Officer; www.henryschein.com/Default.aspx

**HGA**
see HealthGroup of Alabama

**HHS/Amerinet**
see Amerinet, Inc.

**Hospital Central Services Inc. & Affiliates**, 2171 28th Street, S.W., Allentown, PA 18103; tel. 800/444–4272; FAX. 610/791–2919; J. Michael Lee, DBA, FACHE, President and Chief Executive Officer; www.hcsc.org

**Hospital Purchasing Service**, 3275 North M-37 Highway, P.O. Box 247, Middleville, MI 49333-0247; tel. 800/632–4572; FAX. 269/795–9788; Tom LaPres, President and Chief Executive Officer; www.hpsnet.com

**HPG**
see HealthTrust Purchasing Group

**HPPI**
see Novation LLC

**HPS**
see Hospital Purchasing Service

**HPSI**, 1 Ada, Suite 150, Irvine, CA 92618; tel. 800/223–4774; David Lindahl, Managing Director, Sales and Marketing; www.hpsionline.com

**HSCA**
see MedAssets, Inc.

**HSS**
see Amerinet, Inc.

**Huntsville Hospital**
see HealthGroup of Alabama

## I

**IHS Consolidate/Contracting**
see Iowa Health System

**IHS Contracting**
see Iowa Health System

**Illinois Department of Central Management Services**, JRTC, 100 West Randolph, Chicago, IL 60601-3219; tel. 312/814-2141; Malcolm Weems, Acting Director; www.cms.illinois.gov

**Illinois Purchasing Collaborative**
see IPC Group Purchasing

**Indiana University Health**
see IU Health Supply Chain Operations

**Innovatix, LLC**, 555 West 57th Street, 12th floor, New York, NY 10019; tel. 888/258-3273; FAX. 646/638-2641; John P. Sganga, FACHE, President and Chief Executive Officer; www.innovatix.com

**Integrated Services of Iowa Health**
see Iowa Health System

**Intermountain Healthcare Supply Chain Organization**, 36 South State Street, Salt Lake City, UT 84111; tel. 801/442-3615; Charles W. Sorenson, MD, President and Chief Executive Officer; www.intermountainhealthcare.org

**Intermountain Healthcare/Amerinet**
see Intermountain Healthcare Supply Chain Organization

**Iowa Health System**, 1200 Pleasant Street, Des Moines, IA 50309; tel. 515/241-6161; Bill Leaver, President and Chief Executive Officer; www.ihs.org

**IPC Group Purchasing**, 1151 East Warrenville Road, Naperville, IL 60563; tel. 630/276-5400; Patrick Sonin, Managing Executive; www.ipcgrouppurchasing.com

**Iroquois Healthcare Alliance**
see United Iroquois Shared Services, Inc.

**IU Health Supply Chain Operations**, 340 West 10th Street, Suite 6100, Indianapolis, IN 46202-3082; tel. 317/962-3556; Daniel F. Evans, Jr., President and Chief Executive Officer; iuhealth.org/about-iu-health/vendor-relations

## J

**J & B Medical Supply Co., Inc.**, 50496 West Pontiac Trail, Wixom, MI 48393; tel. 800/980-0047; Mary E. Shaya, President

**Jewish Hospital & St. Mary's HealthCare**, 200 Abraham Flexner Way, Louisville, KY 40202; tel. 800/333-2230; Sandra French, Vice President, Supply Chain; www.jhsmh.org

**JHHU**
see Johns Hopkins Health System

**JHSMH Regional Service Center**
see Jewish Hospital & St. Mary's HealthCare

**Johns Hopkins Health System**, 733 North Broadway, BRB 104, Baltimore, MD 21205; tel. 410/955-5000; Ronald R. Peterson, President; www.hopkinsmedicine.org

## K

**Kaiser National Purchasing Organization**
see Kaiser Permanente

**Kaiser Permanente**, One Kaiser Plaza, Oakland, CA 94612-3600; tel. 510/271-5860; George C. Halvorson, Chairman and Chief Executive Officer; www.kaiserpermanente.org

**Kaiser Permanente National Purchasing Program**
see Kaiser Permanente

**Kansas Department of Administration, Office of Business Improvement, Procurement and Contracts**, 900 S.W. Jackson, Room 651, Topeka, KS; tel. 785/296-2376; FAX. 785/296-2376; Marsha Stafford; www.da.ks.gov/purch

**Kreisers, Inc.**, 2200 West 46th Street, Sioux Falls, SD 57105; tel. 800/843-7948; FAX. 800/336-1175; David Larson; https://www.kreisers.com/cart/index.php

## L

**Lake Erie Health Alliance**
see Lake Erie Regional Cooperative

**Lake Erie Regional Cooperative**, 2142 North Cove Boulevard, Toledo, OH 43606; tel. 800/471-3110; Kathleen Krueger, President; www.lercnet.org

**LeeSar, Inc.**, 401 Leonard Boulevard North, Lehigh Acres, FL 33971; tel. 239/303-0606; FAX. 239/303-0046; Bob Simpson, President and Chief Executive Officer; www.leesar.com

**LEHA**
see Lake Erie Regional Cooperative

**Louisiana Division of Administration, Office of State Purchasing & Travel**, 1201 North Third Street, Suite 7-210, Baton Rouge, LA 70802; tel. 800/354-9548; FAX. 225/342-8688; Denise Lea, State Purchasing Director; www.doa.louisiana.gov/osp/osp.htm

**Louisiana Office of Purchasing**
see Louisiana Division of Administration

## M

**MaineHealth**
see Synernet, Inc.

**Mayo Clinic Health System**, 200 First Street, S.W., Rochester, MN 55905; tel. 507/284-2511; John Noseworthy, MD, President and Chief Executive Officer; mayoclinichealthsystem.org

**McKesson Corporation**, One Post Street, San Francisco, CA 94104; tel. 415/983-8300; John H. Hammergren, Chairman, President and Chief Executive Officer; www.mckesson.com

**Med-Op, Inc.**, 205 East 7th Street, Suite 133, Hays, KS 67601; tel. 785/621-4510; FAX. 785/621-4511; David Brittain, Executive Director; www.medopinc.com

**MedAssets, Inc.**, 100 North Point Center East, Suite 200, Alpharetta, GA 30022; tel. 678/323-2500; John A. Bardis, Chairman, President and Chief Executive Officer; www.medassets.com

**Medcenter Direct**, 3350 Peachtree Road, N.E., Suite 1610, Atlanta, GA 30326; tel. 404/233-2563

**Medi-Sota**, 1280 Locust Street, Suite 16, Dawson, MN 56232; tel. 320/769-2269; FAX. 320/769-2298; Deb Ranallo, Director; medi-sota.org/main

**Medline Industries, Inc.**, One Medline Place, Mundelein, IL 600690; tel. 800/633-5463; FAX. 800/351-1512; Andy Mills, President; www.medline.com

**Mercy Health Network**, 1111 Sixth Avenue, Suite 201, Des Moines, IA 50314; tel. 515/643-5300; FAX. 515/643-5350; David Vellinga, Chief Executive Officer; www.mercyhealthnetwork.com

**Mercy Health Network - North Iowa**
see Mercy Health Network

**Mercy Hospital Medical Center**
see Mercy Health Network

**Mercy ROi**
see ROi

**MHA Ventures, Inc.**, 1720 Ninth Avenue, Helena, MT 59601; tel. 406/442-1911; FAX. 406/443-3894; Dick Brown, President and Chief Executive Officer; www.mtha.org/ventures1.htm

**Mid-America Service Solutions**
see VHA, Inc. - Mid-America

**Midland Medical Supply Company**, 4850 Old Cheney Road, Lincoln, NE 68516; tel. 402/423-8877; FAX. 402/423-2931; Al Borchardt; www.midmed.com/index.asp

**Midsouth Healthcare Network**
see VA MidSouth Healthcare Network - VISN 9

**Minnesota MultiState Contracting Alliance for Pharmacy, (MMCAP)**, 50 Sherburne Avenue, Room 112, St. Paul, MN 55155; tel. 651/201-2420; FAX. 651/297-3996; Alan Dahlgren, Managing Director; www.mmcap.org

**Missouri Office of Administration Division of Purchasing & Materials Management**, Harry S Truman Building, 301 West High Street, Jefferson City, MO 65101; tel. 573/751-2387; FAX. 573/526-9815; James Miluski, CPPO, Director; www.oa.mo.gov/purch

**MMCAP**
see Minnesota Multi-State Contracting Alliance for Pharmacy

**Mohawk Hospital Equipment, Inc.**, 335 Columbia Street, Utica, NY 13502; tel. 800/962-5660; FAX. 315/797-0365; Thomas J. Spellman, President; www.mohawkhospital.com/index.php

**Morris & Dickson Co., L.L.C.**, 410 Kay Lane, Shreveport, LA 71115; tel. 800/388-3833; FAX. 318/798-6007; www.morrisdickson.com

**MSS**
see VHA, Inc., - Mid-America Service Solutions LLC

## N

**National Acquisition Center**
see United States Department of Veterans Affairs National Acquisition Center

**Navigator Group Purchasing, Inc.**, 1000 Corporate Centre Drive, Suite 100, Franklin, TN 37067; tel. 615/771-0800; FAX. 615/771-0064; John Markes, Chief Operating Officer; www.navigatorgpo.com

**Nebraska Purchasing Group, LLC**
see Prairie Health Ventures

**Nevada Healthcare Cooperative**, 1000 Ryland Street, Suite 403, Reno, NV 89502; tel. 775/982-4100; Gary Michealree, President

**New England Alliance for Health**, One Medical Center Drive, Lebanon, NH 03756; tel. 603/650-5340; Stephen LeBlanc, Executive Director; www.neahllc.org

**New Jersey Hospital Association, Group Purchasing Services**, 760 Alexander Road, P.O. Box 1, Princeton, NJ 08543-0001; tel. 972/910-6676; Susan Revell; www.njha.com/hbs/GroupPurchasingServices.aspx

**New York City Health & Hospitals Corporation**, 346 Broadway, 5th floor West, New York, NY 10013; tel. 212/442-3933; Richard Olah, Acting Senior Director; www.nyc.gov/html/hhc/html/contracting/contracting.shtml

**New York Hospital Association**
see GNYHA Services, Inc.

**New York State Office of Mental Health**, 44 Holland Avenue, Albany, NY 12229; tel. 518/474-4403; FAX. 518/474-2149; Michael F. Hogan, Ph.D., Commissioner; www.omh.state.ny.us

**North Carolina Department of Administration, Division of Purchase & Contract**, 116 W. Jones Street, 4th Floor, Raleigh, NC 27603-8002; tel. 919/807-4500; William Sam Byassee, State Purchasing Officer; www.pandc.nc.gov/index.htm

**North Shore-Long Island Jewish Health System**, 145 Community Drive, Great Neck, NY 11021; tel. 516/465-8100; Michael J. Dowling, President and Chief Executive Officer; www.northshorelij.com/NSLIJ/NSLIJ+HomePage

**Northeast Purchasing Coalition LLC**; Paul Benyo, Supply Network Director

**Northern Michigan Supply Alliance, LLC**, 2651 Aero Park Drive, Traverse City, MI 49686; tel. 231/935-8233; FAX. 231/947-2436; Mark Deponio, President; www.nmsa-mi.org

**Section C**

**Northwest Ohio Shared Services**, 3231 Central Park West Drive, Suite 200, Toledo, OH 43617; tel. 419/843–8880; FAX. 419/843–8886; John Pilewski, Vice President; www.hcno.org/noss/noss.html

**Novation - Upper Midwest**
see VHA, Inc. - Upper Midwest

**Novation - VHA OK/AR**
see VHA, Inc. - Oklahoma/Arkansas

**Novation LLC**, 125 East John Carpenter Freeway, Suite 1400, Irving, TX 75062; tel. 888/766–8283; Jody Hatcher, President and Chief Executive Officer; www.Novationco.com

**Novation West Coast**
see VHA, Inc. - West Coast

**Novation/AROK**
see VHA, Inc. - Oklahoma/Arkansas

**Novation/VHA**
see Novation LLC

**NPG**
see Prairie Health Ventures

**NSLIJ**
see North Shore-Long Island Jewish Health System

**NYC Health and Hospital**
see New York City Health & Hospitals Corporation

**NYS Office of Mental Health**
see New York State Office of Mental Health

## O

**Ohio State Health Network**, 370 West 9th Avenue, Columbus, OH 43210-1240; tel. 888/722–6746; FAX. 614/293–3768; Joann Ort, Executive Director; www.oshn.org

**Ohio State Office of Procurement Services**, 4200 Surface Road, Columbus, OH 43228-1395; tel. 614/466–5090; Gretchen Adkins, State Chief Procurement Officer; procure.ohio.gov/proc/index.asp

**OUHSC**
see University of Oklahoma, Purchasing Department

**Our Lady of the Lake Regional Medical Center**, 5000 Hennessey Boulevard, Baton Rouge, LA 70808; tel. 225/765–6565; K. Scott Wester, FACHE, President and Chief Executive Officer; www.ololrmc.com/default.cfm

**Owens & Minor, Inc.**, 9120 Lockwood Blvd., Mechanicsville, VA 23116; tel. 804/723–7000; FAX. 804/723–7100; Craig R. Smith President and Chief Executive Officer; www.owens-minor.com

## P

**Pace Premier**
see Avera PACE

**Parallon Business Solutions**, 6640 Carothers Parkway, Franklin, TN 37067; tel. 615/807–8000; Michael O'Boyle, President and Chief Executive Officer; parallon.net/index.html

**Partners Cooperative, Inc.**, 3625 Cumberland Boulevard, S.E., Suite 1425, Atlanta, GA 30339; tel. 678/842–7300; FAX. 678/842–7329; www.pcgpo.org

**Partners Healthcare, Materials Management**, 529 Main Street, Charlestown, MA 02129; tel. 617/726–2142; www.partners.org/About/Vendor-Information/Default.aspx

**PCGPO**
see Partners Cooperative, Inc.

**PeaceHealth Oregon Region**
see Premier Inc.

**Physician Sales & Services**, 4345 Southpoint Boulevard, Jacksonville, FL 32216; tel. 904/332–3000; Gary A. Corless, President and Chief Executive Officer; www.pssd.com

**PR1ME**, 6820 Deerpath Road, Elkridge, MD 21075; tel. 800/899–2199; Amy Ginsberg, Senior Client Manager; www.pr1me.org

**PR1ME MedAssets**
see PR1ME

**Prairie Health Ventures**, 421 South 9th Street, Suite 102, Lincoln, NE 68508-2245; tel. 800/409–4990; FAX. 402/476–7422; Dave Christensen, Chief Executive Officer; www.phvne.com

**Premier Inc.**, 13034 Ballantyne Corporate Place, Charlotte, NC 28277; tel. 877/777–1552; John Biggers, Senior Vice President, Group Purchasing; www.premierinc.com

**Premier/Adventist West**
see Premier Inc.

**Premier/Alegent NPG**
see Prairie Health Ventures

**Premier/Baptist Healthcare**
see Premier Inc.

**Premier/Health Enterprises Cooperative**
see Health Enterprises of Iowa

**Premier/Norton Purchasing**
see Alliant-HAS

**Premier/Seagate**
see Seagate Alliance, LLC

**Premier/SSM Health Care**
see SSM Health Care System

**Presbyterian Healthcare Services**
see Owens & Minor, Inc.

**Professional Health Services, Inc.**, 83 South Eagle Road, Havertown, PA 19083; tel. 800/833–3005; Michael Kleinman, President; phsmobile.com/default.aspx

**Professional Hospital Supply**, 42500 Winchester Road, Temecula, CA 92590; tel. 951/296–2600; FAX. 951/296–2624; Jenise Luttgens, Chief Executive Officer; www.phsyes.com

**Providence Health & Services**, 1801 Lind Avenue, S.W., Suite 9016, Renton, WA 98057; tel. 425/525–3355; John Koster, MD, President and Chief Executive Officer; www2.providence.org/Pages/default.aspx

**Provista**, 220 East Las Colinas Boulevard, Irving, TX 75039; tel. 888/538–4662; Dan Thomas, President; www.provistaco.com

**Provista/Novation**
see Provista

## Q

**Quorum Health Resources**
see HealthTrust Purchasing Group

## R

**Rapid City Regional Hospital**
see Regional Health

**Regional Health**, 353 Fairmont Boulevard, Rapid City, SD 57701; tel. 605/719–1000; Charles E. Hart, MD, MS, President and Chief Executive Officer; www.regionalhealth.com

**Regional Service Center**
see Jewish Hospital & St. Mary's HealthCare

**Resource and Supply Management Group, LLC**, 4600 Edmundson Road, St. Louis, MO 63134; tel. 314/733–8000; Scott Caldwell, Senior Vice President and Chief Supply Chain Officer; www.ascensionhealth.org

**Resource Optimization & InNovation, LLC**
see ROi

**ROi**, 645 Maryville Centre Drive, Suite 200, St. Louis, MO 63141; tel. 314/364–6400; Gene Kirtser, President and Chief Executive Officer; www.roiscs.com

**Rural Health Alliance**
see Medi-Sota

## S

**Sanford Health**, 1305 West 18th Street, P.O. Box 5039, Sioux Falls, SD 57117-5039; tel. 605/333–1000; Kelby K. Krabbenhoft, President and Chief Executive Officer; www.sanfordhealth.org

**SCM Alliance, Inc.**
see CoalesCo, Inc.

**Seagate Alliance, LLC**, 3445 Winton Place, Suite 222, Rochester, NY 14623-2950; tel. 888/732–4282; FAX. 585/273–8189; Diane H. Ashley, President and Chief Executive Officer; www.seagatealliance.com

**Seneca Medical**, 85 Shaffer Park Drive, P.O. Box 399, Tiffin, OH 44883; tel. 800/447–0225; FAX. 419/447–7201; Roger Benz, President; www.senecamedical.com/wps/portal/aboutUs

**ServiShare**, 100 East Grand Avenue, Suite 100, Des Moines, IA 50309-1835; tel. 800/240–1046; FAX. 515/283–9366; Dennis White, Senior Vice President, ServiShare; www.ihaonline.org/servishare/servishare2.shtml

**Shared Health**
see Shared Health Services Corporation

**Shared Health Services Corporation**, 2635 Hemstock Street, La Crosse, WI 54603; tel. 800/637–4445; FAX. 608/781–4412; Wade E. Turner, Executive Director; www.shsc-gpo.com

**Sisters of Mercy Health System**
see ROi

**Spectrum Health**
see VHA, Inc.

**SSM Health Care of Wisconsin**, 2901 Landmark Place, Suite 300, Madison, WI 53713; tel. 608/258–6120; Steven M. Barney, Interim Regional President, Chief Executive Officer; www.ssmhcwi.com/pages/default.aspx

**SSM Health Care System**, 477 North Lindbergh Boulevard, St. Louis, MO 63141; tel. 314/994–7800; FAX. 314/994–7900; William P. Thompson, President and Chief Executive Officer; www.ssmhc.com/internet/home/ssmcorp.nsf

**St. John's Health System**
see ROi

**St. Mary's Medical Center**, 2900 First Avenue, Huntington, WV 25702; tel. 304/526–1234; Michael G. Sellards, President and Chief Executive Officer; www.st-marys.org

**St. Patrick Healthcare/Novation**
see Providence Health & Services

**St. Vincent Health**, Resource and Supply Management Group, LLC

**Staples Advantage**, 500 Staples Drive, Framingham, MA; tel. 877/826–7755; Joseph G. Goody, President, Staples North American Delivery; www.staplesadvantage.com

**State of Ohio/State Purchasing**
see Ohio State Office of Procurement Services

**Sutter Health**, 2200 River Plaza Drive, Sacramento, CA 95833; tel. 916/733–8800; Patrick Fry, President and Chief Executive Officer

**Synernet, Inc.**, 222 St. John Street, Suite 329, Portland, ME 04102; tel. 800/545–0042; Gerry Vicenzi, President and Chief Executive Officer; www.synernet.net

## T

**TBPC**
see Texas Facilities Commission

**Tenet/Broadlane**
see MedAssets, Inc.

**Texas Building & Procurement Commission**
see Texas Facilities Commission

**Texas Facilities Commission**, 1711 San Jacinto, Austin, TX 78701; tel. 512/463–3446; Terry Keel, Executive Director; www.tfc.state.tx.us

**Texas Health Resources**, Supply Chain Management Office, 612 East Lamar Boulevard, Arlington, TX 76011; tel. 682/236–7517

**Texas Procurement**
see Texas Facilities Commission

**Texas Purchasing Coalition**, 7160 Dallas Parkway, Suite 600, Plano, TX 75024; tel. 469/366–2100; FAX. 469/366–2101; Geoff Brenner, President; www.texaspurchasingcoalition.com/content/home/?id=1390

**Tidewater Group Purchasing**
see Navigator Group Purchasing, Inc.

**Trinity Health**
see HealthTrust Purchasing Group

# U

**U.P. Health Care Network**
see Upper Peninsula Health Care Network

**U.S. Army Medical Command**
see Unites States Army Medical Department, Medical Research and Materiel Command

**UHC**, 155 North Wacker Drive, Chicago, IL 60606; tel. 312/775–4100; Jake Groenewold, Senior Vice President, Supply Chain; www.uhc.edu

**UHS Consortium**
see UHC

**United Healthcare Shared Services**
see United Iroquois Shared Services, Inc.

**United Iroquois Shared Services, Inc.**, 5740 Commons Park, East Syracuse, NY 13057; tel. 315/410–6476; FAX. 315/445–2293; Terry A. Field, Manager, Supply Chain Strategies; www.iroquois.org/Index.aspx?ID=4

**United States Army Medical Department, Medical Research and Materiel Command, MCMR-PA**, 504 Scott Street, Fort Detrick, MD 21702-5012; tel. 301/619–2736; Major General James Gilman, MD, Commanding General; https://mrmc.amedd.army.mil/index.cfm?pageid=medical_materiel.overview

**United States Department of Veterans Affairs National Acquisition Center**, P. O. Box 76, Building 37, 1st Avenue, Hines, IL 60141; tel. 708/786–5157; FAX. 708/786–5148; Craig Robinson, Associate Deputy Assistant Secretary; www1.va.gov/oamm/nac/index.htm

**United States General Services Administration**, One Constitution Square, 1275 First Street, N.E., Washington, DC 20417; tel. 866/606–8220; Daniel M. Tangherlini, Acting Administrator; www.gsa.gov

**University HealthSystem Consortium (UHC)/ Novation**
see UHC

**University Hospital Consortium**
see UHC

**University of Iowa, Accounts Payable, Purchasing and Travel Department**, 202 Plaza Centre One, Iowa City, IA 52242; tel. 319/335–0115; FAX. 319/335–2443; Deborah Zumbach, Senior Associate Director - Business Services and Director of Purchasing; www.uiowa.edu/purchasing

**University of Oklahoma Health Sciences Center**
see University of Oklahoma, Purchasing Department

**University of Oklahoma, Purchasing Department**, 2750 Venture Drive, Norman, OK 73069-8279; tel. 405/325–2811; FAX. 405/329–8394; Jan Duke, Interim Associate Director - Purchasing/Property Control; www.ou.edu/purchasing/index.html

**University of Pittsburgh**
see UPMC Supply Chain Management

**UPMC Supply Chain Management**, 200 Lothrop Street, Pittsburgh, PA 15213-2582; tel. 800/533–8762; Jeffrey A. Romoff, President and Chief Executive Officer; www.upmc.com/services/supplychainmanagement

**Upper Peninsula Health Care Network**, 228 West Washington Street, Suite 2, Marquette, MI 49855; tel. 906/225–3146; FAX. 902/225–7868; Dennis H. Smith, Executive Director; www.uphcn.org

# V

**VA Desert Pacific Healthcare Network - VISN 22**, 300 Oceangate, Suite 700, Long Beach, CA 90802; tel. 562/826–5963; FAX. 562/826–5987; Stan Johnson, Network Director; www.desertpacific.va.gov

**VA Great Lakes Health Care System - VISN 12**, Four Westbrook Corporate Tower, 11301 West Cermak Road, Westchester, IL 60154; tel. 708/492–3900; FAX. 708/492–3948; Jeffrey A. Murawsky, MD, Network Director; www.visn12.va.gov

**VA Health Care Upstate New York - VISN 2**, 113 Holland Avenue, Building 67, Albany, NY 12208; tel. 518/626–7327; David J. West, MSHA, FACHE, Network Director; www.visn2.va.gov

**VA Healthcare - VISN 4**, 323 North Shore Drive, Suite 400, Pittsburgh, PA 15212; tel. 412/822–3316; FAX. 412/822–3275; Michael E. Moreland, FACHE, Network Director; www.visn4.va.gov

**VA Healthcare System of Ohio - VISN 10**; www.visn10.va.gov

**VA Heartland Network - VISN 15**, 1201 Walnut Street, Suite 800, Kansas City, MO 64106; tel. 816/701–3000; James R. Floyd, Director; www.visn15.va.gov

**VA Mid-Atlantic Health Care Network - VISN 6**, 300 West Morgan Street, Suite 700, Durham, NC 27701; tel. 919/956–5541; FAX. 919/956–7152; Daniel F. Hoffmann, FACHE, Network Director; www.visn6.va.gov

**VA MidSouth Healthcare Network - VISN 9**, 1801 West End Avenue, Suite 600, Nashville, TN 37203; tel. 615/695–2200; FAX. 615/695–2210; John Dandridge, Jr., Network Director; www.visn9.va.gov/about/index.asp

**VA New England Healthcare System - VISN 1**, 200 Springs Road, Building #61, Bedford, MA 01730; tel. 781/687–4821; FAX. 781/687–3470; Michael F. Mayo-Smith, MD, MPH; www.newengland.va.gov

**VA NY/NJ Veterans Healthcare Network - VISN 3**, 130 West Kingsbridge Road, Bronx, NY 10468; tel. 718/584–9000; FAX. 718/579–1671; Michael A. Sabo, FACHE, Network Director; www.nynj.va.gov

**VA Southeast Network - VISN 7**, 3700 Crestwood Parkway, Suite 500, Duluth, GA 30096; tel. 678/924–5700; FAX. 678/924–5757; James Clark, Interim Network Director; www.southeast.va.gov

**VA System**
see United States Department of Veterans Affairs National Acquisition Center

**Vector Amerinet**
see Amerinet, Inc.

**Veterans Integrated Services Network (VISN)**
see VA listings

**VHA Inc.**, 220 Las Colinas Boulevard East, Irving, TX 75039; tel. 800/842–5146; Curt Nonomaque, President and Chief Executive Officer; https://www.vha.com/Pages/default.aspx

**VHA, Inc. - Central**, 8900 Keystone Crossing, Suite 480, Indianapolis, IN 46240; tel. 317/818–8000; https://www.vha.com/AboutVHA/Offices/Central/Pages/Default.aspx

**VHA, Inc. - Central Atlantic**, 521 East Morehead Street, Suite 300, Charlotte, NC 28202; tel. 704/377–7140; https://www.vha.com/AboutVHA/Offices/CentralAtlantic/Pages/Default.aspx

**VHA, Inc. - East Coat**, 8 Neshaminy Interplex, Suite 115, Trevose, PA 19053; tel. 215/245–4888; https://www.vha.com/AboutVHA/Offices/EastCoast/Pages/Default.aspx

**VHA, Inc. - Gulf States, Inc.**, 8940 Bluebonnet Boulevard, Suite 200, Baton Rouge, LA 70810; tel. 225/761–1568; FAX. 225/761–1582; https://www.vha.com/AboutVHA/Offices/GulfStates/Pages/Default.aspx

**VHA, Inc. - Mid-America**, 7415 West 130th Street, Suite 200, Overland Park, KS 66213; https://www.vha.com/AboutVHA/Offices/MidAmerica/Pages/Default.aspx

**VHA, Inc. - Mid-America Service Solutions LLC**; https://www.vha.com/AboutVHA/Offices/MidAmerica/Pages/MidAmericaServiceSolutions.aspx

**VHA, Inc. - Midwest**
see VHA, Inc. - Mid-America

**VHA, Inc. - Mountain States**, 1401 17th Street, Suite 850, Denver, CO 80202; tel. 303/308–4100; https://www.vha.com/AboutVHA/Offices/MountainStates/Pages/Default.aspx

**VHA, Inc. - New England**, 350 Granite Street, Suite 2304, Braintree, MA 02184; tel. 781/794–6500; FAX. 781/794–6529; https://www.vha.com/AboutVHA/Offices/NewEngland/Pages/Default.aspx

**VHA, Inc. - North Central**
see VHA, Inc. - Upper Midwest

**VHA, Inc. - Oklahoma/Arkansas**, 4013 Northwest Expressway Street, Oklahoma City, OK 73116; https://www.vha.com/AboutVHA/Offices/OKAR/Pages/Default.aspx

**VHA, Inc. - Pennsylvania**, 415 Holiday Drive, Pittsburgh, PA 15220; tel. 412/922–9124; FAX. 412/922–9345; https://www.vha.com/AboutVHA/Offices/Pennsylvania/Pages/Default.aspx

**VHA, Inc. - Southeast**, 4211 West Boy Scout Boulevard, Suite 750, Tampa, FL 33607; tel. 813/350–8300; FAX. 813/350–8383; https://www.vha.com/AboutVHA/Offices/Southeast/Pages/Default.aspx

**VHA, Inc. - Southwest**
see Healthcare Coalition of Texas

**VHA, Inc. - Texas**
see Healthcare Coalition of Texas

**VHA, Inc. - Tri-State**
see VHA, Inc. - Central

**VHA, Inc. - Upper Midwest**, 7601 France Avenue South, Suite 500, Edina, MN 55435; tel. 952/837–4700; https://www.vha.com/AboutVHA/Offices/UpperMidwest/Pages/Default.aspx

**VHA, Inc. - West Coast**, 880 Apollo Street, Suite 300, El Segundo, CA 90245; tel. 888/619–1900; https://www.vha.com/AboutVHA/Offices/WestCoast/Pages/Default.aspx

**VHA/Novation**
see VHA, Inc.

**Via Christi Health**
see MedAssets, Inc.

**Voluntary Hospitals of America**
see VHA Inc.

# W

**West Virginia Department of Health and Human Resources**, One Davis Square, Suite 100 East, Charlestown, WV 25301; tel. 304/558–0684; FAX. 304/558–1130; Michael J. Lewis, MD, Ph.D., Cabinet Secretary; www.wvdhhr.org

**Western New York Purchasing Alliance**
see Altus Management LLC

**Western States Contracting Alliance**
see WSCA/NASPO

**Westnet, Inc.**, 30 North Street, Canton, MA 02021; tel. 781/828–7772; FAX. 781/828–2011; Gordon O. Thompson, President; www.westnetmed.com/Default.aspx

**Wisconsin Valley Health Network, LLC**, 3000 Westhill Drive, Suite 300, Wausau, WI 54401; tel. 715/847–2999; FAX. 715/847–2813; Michael J. Murphy, Executive Director

**WNC Health Network**, 1200 Ridgefield Boulevard, Suite 200, Asheville, NC 28806; tel. 877/667–8220; FAX. 828/667–8228; Janice Lato, President and Chief Executive Officer; www.wnchn.org

**WNCHN**
see WNC Health Network

**WSCA/NASPO**, 201 East Main Street, Suite 1405, Lexington, KY 40507; tel. 859/514–9159; FAX. 859/514–9166; Lee Ann Pope, WSCA Program Director; www.aboutwsca.org

# Y

**Yale New Haven Health System**, 789 Howard Avenue, New Haven, CT 06519; tel. 203/688–4242; Marna P. Borgstrom, President and Chief Executive Officer; www.yalenewhavenhealth.org

**Yankee Alliance**, 138 River Road, Andover, MA 01810-1083; tel. 978/470–2000; FAX. 978/681–6100; James W. Oliver, President and Chief Executive Officer; www.yankeealliance.com

Section C

# Hospital Associations

*The following list of state and metropolitan hospital associations is derived from the American Hospital Association. For additional information visit the American Hospital Association website: www.aha.org.*

## United States

**ALABAMA: Alabama Hospital Association,** 500 North East Boulevard, Montgomery, AL 36117; tel. 334/272–8781; FAX. 334/270–9527; J. Michael Horsley, President and Chief Executive Officer

**ALASKA: Alaska State Hospital and Nursing Home Association,** 1049 W. Fifth Avenue, Suite 100, Anchorage, AK 99501; tel. 907/646–1444; FAX. 907/646–3964; Karen Perdue, President and Chief Executive Officer

**ARIZONA: Arizona Hospital and Healthcare Association,** 2800 North Central Avenue, Suite 1450, Phoenix, AZ 85004; tel. 602/445–4300; FAX. 602/445–4299; Laurie Liles, President and Chief Executive Officer

**ARKANSAS: Arkansas Hospital Association,** 419 Natural Resources Drive, Little Rock, AR 72205-1539; tel. 501/224–7878; FAX. 501/224–0519; Robert "Bo" Ryall, President and Chief Executive Officer

**CALIFORNIA: California Hospital Association,** 1215 K Street, Suite 800, Sacramento, CA 95814; tel. 916/552–7547; FAX. 916/552–7680; C. Duane Dauner, President and Chief Executive Officer

**Hospital Association of San Diego and Imperial Counties,** 5575 Ruffin Road, Suite 225, San Diego, CA 92123; tel. 858/614–0200; FAX. 858/614–0201; Steven A. Escoboza, President and Chief Executive Officer

**Hospital Association of Southern California,** 515 South Figueroa Street, Suite 1300, Los Angeles, CA 90071-3322; tel. 213/538–0700; FAX. 213/629–4272; James D. Barber, President and Chief Executive Officer

**Hospital Council of Northern and Central California,** 1215 K Street, Suite 730, Sacramento, CA 95814; tel. 916/552–7608; FAX. 916/554–2216; Arthur A. Sponseller, President and Chief Executive Officer

**COLORADO: Colorado Hospital Association,** 7335 East Orchard Road, Greenwood Village, CO 80111; tel. 720/489–1630; FAX. 720/489–9400; Steven Summer, President and Chief Executive Officer

**CONNECTICUT: Connecticut Hospital Association,** 110 Barnes Road, PO Box 90, Wallingford, CT 06492-0090; tel. 203/265–7611; FAX. 203/269–7713; Jennifer Jackson, President and Chief Executive Officer

**DELAWARE: Delaware Healthcare Association,** 1280 South Governors Avenue, Dover, DE 19904-4802; tel. 302/674–2853; FAX. 302/734–2731; Wayne A. Smith, President and Chief Executive Officer

**DISTRICT OF COLUMBIA: District of Columbia Hospital Association,** 1152 15th Street, NW, Suite 900, Washington, DC 20005-1723; tel. 202/682–1581; FAX. 202/371–8151; Robert A. Malson, President

**FLORIDA: Florida Hospital Association,** 306 East College Avenue, Tallahassee, FL 32301; tel. 850/222–9800; FAX. 850/561–6230; Bruce Rueben, President

**South Florida Hospital and Healthcare Association, Inc,** 6030 Hollywood Boulevard, Suite 140, Hollywood, FL 33024; tel. 954/964–1660; FAX. 954/962–1260; Linda S. Quick, President

**GEORGIA: Georgia Hospital Association (GHA),** 1675 Terrell Mill Road, Marietta, GA 30067; tel. 770/249–4500; FAX. 770/955–5801; Joseph A. Parker, President

**HAWAII: Healthcare Association of Hawaii,** 707 Richards Street, PH2, Honolulu, HI 96813; tel. 808/521–8961; FAX. 808/599–2879; George W. Greene, President and Chief Executive Officer

**IDAHO: Idaho Hospital Association,** 615 N. Seventh Street, Boise, ID 83701-1278; tel. 208/338–5100; FAX. 208/338–7800; Steven A. Millard, President

**ILLINOIS: Illinois Hospital Association,** 1151 East Warrenville Road, P.O. Box 3015, Naperville, IL 60566-7015; tel. 630/276–5400; FAX. 630/276–5431; Maryjane Wurth, President and Chief Executive Officer

**Metropolitan Chicago Healthcare Council,** 222 South Riverside Plaza, 19th Floor, Chicago, IL 60606; tel. 312/906–6000; FAX. 312/506–4900; Kevin Scanlan, President and Chief Executive Officer

**INDIANA: Indiana Hospital Association,** 1 American Square, Suite 1900, Indianapolis, IN 46282; tel. 317/633–4870; FAX. 317/633–4875; Douglas J. Leonard, FACHE, President

**IOWA: Iowa Hospital Association,** 100 East Grand Avenue, Suite 100, Des Moines, IA 50309-1835; tel. 515/288–1955; FAX. 515/283–9366; Kirk Norris, President

**KANSAS: Kansas Hospital Association,** 215 SE 8th Street, Topeka, KS 66603; tel. 785/233–7436; FAX. 785/233–6955; Tom Bell, President and Chief Executive Officer

**Health Alliance of MidAmerica,** 7015 College Boulevard, Suite 150, Overland Park, KS 66211; tel. 913/327–7200; FAX. 913/327–7210; Michael R. Dunaway, President

**KENTUCKY: Kentucky Hospital Association,** 2501 Nelson Miller Parkway, P.O. Box 436629, Louisville, KY 40253-6629; tel. 502/426–6220; FAX. 502/426–6226; Michael T. Rust, President

**Healthservices Council of Metropolitan Louisville,** 2501 Nelson Miller Parkway, Louisville, KY 40223; tel. 502/426–6220; FAX. 502/426–6226; Nancy Galvagni, Executive Director

**LOUISIANA: Louisiana Hospital Association,** 9521 Brookline Avenue, Baton Rouge, LA 70809-1431; tel. 225/928–0026; FAX. 225/923–1004; John Matessino, President and Chief Executive Officer

**Metropolitan Hospital Council of New Orleans,** 2450 Severn Avenue, Suite 210, Metairie, LA 70001; tel. 504/837–1171; FAX. 504/837–1174; Paul Salles, President

**MAINE: Maine Hospital Association,** 33 Fuller Road, Augusta, ME 04330; tel. 207/622–4794; FAX. 207/622–3073; Steven R. Michaud, President

**MARYLAND: Maryland Hospital Association,** 6820 Deerpath Road, Elkridge, MD 21075-6234; tel. 410/379–6200; FAX. 410/379–8239; Carmela Coyle, President and Chief Executive Officer

**Healthcare Council of the National Capital Area,** 8201 Corporate Drive, Suite 250, Landover, MD 20785-2229; tel. 301/731–4700; FAX. 301/731–8286; Joseph P. Burns, President and Chief Executive Officer

**MASSACHUSETTS: Massachusetts Hospital Association,** Five New England Executive Park, Burlington, MA 01803; tel. 781/262–6001; FAX. 781/272–1524; Lynn Nicholas, FACHE, President and Chief Executive Officer

**MICHIGAN: Michigan Health & Hospital Association,** 6215 West Street Joseph Highway, Lansing, MI 48917; tel. 517/323–3443; FAX. 517/323–0946; Spencer C. Johnson, President

**Hospital Council of East Central Michigan,** 315 Mullholland Street, Bay City, MI 48708; tel. 989/891–8810; FAX. 989/891–8161; Elizabeth S. Schnettler, President

**North Central Council of Michigan Health and Hospital Association,** 616 Petoskey Street, Suite 208, Petoskey, MI 49770-2779; tel. 231/439–9812; FAX. 231/439–9813; Elizabeth Gertz, Executive Director

**Upper Peninsula Hospital Council,** 6215 West Street Joseph Highway, Lansing, MI 48917; tel. 517/323–3443; FAX. 517/323–0946; Clark R. Ballard, President

**MINNESOTA: Minnesota Hospital Association,** 2550 University Avenue W, Suite 350S, St. Paul, MN 55114-1900; tel. 651/641–1121; FAX. 651/659–1477; Lawrence J. Massa, President and Chief Executive Officer

**MISSISSIPPI: Mississippi Hospital Association,** 116 Woodgreen Crossing, PO Box 1909, Madison, MS 39130; tel. 800/289–8884; FAX. 601/368–3200; Sam W. Cameron, President and Chief Executive Officer

**MISSOURI: Missouri Hospital Association,** PO Box 60, Jefferson City, MO 65102-0060; tel. 573/893–3700; FAX. 573/893–2809; Herb Kuhn, President and Chief Executive Officer

**MONTANA: MHA...An Association of Montana Health Care Providers,** 1720 Ninth Avenue, PO Box 5119, Helena, MT 59601; tel. 406/442–1911; FAX. 406/443–3894; Dick Brown, President and Chief Executive Officer

**NEBRASKA: Nebraska Hospital Association,** 3255 Salt Creek Circle, Suite 100, Lincoln, NE 68504; tel. 402/742–8140; FAX. 402/742–8191; Laura J. Redoutey, FACHE, President

**NEVADA: Nevada Hospital Association,** 5250 Neil Road, Suite 302, Reno, NV 89502; tel. 775/827–0184; FAX. 775/827–0190; Bill M. Welch, President and Chief Executive Officer

**NEW HAMPSHIRE: New Hampshire Hospital Association, Foundation for Healthy Communities,** 125 Airport Road, Concord, NH 03301-7300; tel. 603/225–0900; FAX. 603/225–4346; Stephen Ahnen, President

**NEW JERSEY: New Jersey Hospital Association,** PO Box 1, 760 Alexander Road, Princeton, NJ 08543-0001; tel. 609/275–4000; FAX. 609/452–8097; Elizabeth A. Ryan, Esq., President and Chief Executive Officer

**Hospital Alliance of New Jersey,** 150 West State Street, Trenton, NJ 08608; tel. 609/989–8200; FAX. 609/989–7768; Suzanne Ianni, President & Chief Executive Officer

**NEW MEXICO: New Mexico Hospital Association,** 7471 Pan American Freeway NE, Albuquerque, NM 87109; tel. 505/343–0010; FAX. 505/343–0012; Jeff Dye, President and Chief Executive Officer

**NEW YORK: Healthcare Association of New York State,** One Empire Drive, Rensselaer, NY 12144; tel. 518/431–7600; FAX. 518/431–7915; Daniel Sisto, President

**Greater New York Hospital Association,** 555 West 57 Street, 15th Floor, New York, NY 10019; tel. 212/246–7100; FAX. 212/262–6350; Kenneth E. Raske, President

**Iroquois Healthcare Alliance,** 17 Executive Park Drive, Clifton Park, NY 12065; tel. 518/383–5060; FAX. 518/383–2616; Gary J. Fitzgerald, President

**Nassau-Suffolk Hospital Council, Inc,** 1383 Veterans Memorial Highway, Suite 26, Hauppauge, NY 11788; tel. 631/435–3000; FAX. 631/435–2343; Wendy Darwell, Vice President and Chief Operating Officer

**New York City Health & Hospitals Corporation,** 125 Worth Street, New York, NY 10013; tel. 212/788–3321; FAX. 212/788–0040; Alan D. Aviles, President

**Northern Metropolitan Hospital Association,** 400 Stony Brook Court, Newburgh, NY 12550; tel. 845/562–7520; FAX. 845/562–0187; Kevin W. Dahill, President and Chief Executive officer

**Rochester Regional Healthcare Association,** 3445 Winton Place, Suite 222, Rochester, NY 14623; tel. 585/273–8180; FAX. 585/475–0266; Diane H. Ashley, President and Chief Executive Officer

**Western New York Healthcare Association,** 1876 Niagara Falls Boulevard, Tonawanda, NY 14150-6439; tel. 716/695–0843; FAX. 716/695–0073; John E. Bartimole, President

**NORTH CAROLINA: North Carolina Hospital Association,** PO Box 4449, Cary, NC 27519-4449; tel. 919/677–2400; FAX. 919/677–4200; William A. Pully, President

**NORTH DAKOTA: North Dakota Hospital Association,** 1622 E. Interstate Avenue, PO Box 7340, Bismarck, ND 58507; tel. 701/224–9732; FAX. 701/224–9529; Jerry E. Jurena, President

**OHIO: Ohio Hospital Association,** 155 East Broad Street, Floor 15, Columbus, OH 43215; tel. 614/221–7614; FAX. 614/221–4771; Michael D. Abrams, President and Chief Executive Officer

**Akron Regional Hospital Association,** 3200 West Market Street, Suite 200, Akron, OH 44333; tel. 330/873–1500; FAX. 330/873–1501; Sarah Metzger

**Central Ohio Hospital Council,** 155 East Broad Street, 23rd Floor, Columbus, OH 43215; tel. 614/358–2710; FAX. 614/358–2725; Jeff Klingler, President & Chief Executive Officer

**Greater Cincinnati Health Council,** 2100 Sherman Avenue, Suite 100, Cincinnati, OH 45212-2775; tel. 513/531–0200; FAX. 513/531–0278; Colleen K. O'Toole, President

**Greater Dayton Area Hospital Association,** 2 Riverplace, Suite 400, Dayton, OH 45405; tel. 937/228–1000; FAX. 937/228–1035; Bryan J. Bucklew, President and Chief Executive Officer

**Hospital Council of Northwest Ohio,** 3231 Central Park West Drive, Suite 200, Toledo, OH 43617; tel. 419/842–0800; FAX. 419/843–8889; W. Scott Fry, President and Chief Executive Officer

**The Center for Health Affairs,** 1226 Huron Road East, Cleveland, OH 44115; tel. 216/696–6900; FAX. 216/696–1875; William T. (Bill) Ryan, President and Chief Executive Officer

**OKLAHOMA: Oklahoma Hospital Association,** 4000 Lincoln Boulevard, Oklahoma City, OK 73105; tel. 405/427–9537; FAX. 405/424–4507; Craig W. Jones, President

**OREGON: Oregon Association of Hospitals and Health Systems,** 4000 Kruse Way Place, Building 2, Suite 100, Lake Oswego, OR 97035-2543; tel. 503/636–2204; FAX. 503/636–8310; Andy Davidson, President and Chief Executive Officer

**PENNSYLVANIA: The Hospital & Healthsystem Association of Pennsylvania,** 4750 Lindle Road, P.O. Box 8600, Harrisburg, PA 17105-8600; tel. 717/564–9200; FAX. 717/561–5334; Carolyn F. Scanlan, President and Chief Executive Officer

**Hospital Council of Western Pennsylvania,** 500 Commonwealth Drive, Warrendale, PA 15086; tel. 724/772–7206; FAX. 724/772–8339; A.J. Harper, President

**The Delaware Valley Healthcare Council of HAP,** 1835 Market Street, 10th Floor, Suite 1050, Philadelphia, PA 19103; tel. 215/563–2229; FAX. 215/563–2442; Carolyn F. Scanlon, President and Chief Executive Officer

**RHODE ISLAND: Hospital Association of Rhode Island,** 100 Midway Road, Suite 21, Cranston, RI 02920; tel. 401/946–7887; FAX. 401/946–8188; Edward Quinlan, President

**SOUTH CAROLINA: South Carolina Hospital Association,** 1000 Center Point Road, Columbia, SC 29210-5802; tel. 803/796–3080; FAX. 803/796–2938; Thorton Kirby, President

**SOUTH DAKOTA: South Dakota Association of Healthcare Organizations (SDAHO),** 3708 West Brooks Place, Sioux Falls, SD 57106; tel. 605/361–2281; FAX. 605/361–5175; David R. Hewett, President and Chief Executive Officer

**TENNESSEE: Tennessee Hospital Association,** 500 Interstate Boulevard, South, Nashville, TN 37210; tel. 615/256–8240; FAX. 615/242–4803; Craig A. Becker, President

**TEXAS: Texas Hospital Association,** P.O. Box 679010, Austin, TX 78768-9010; tel. 512/465–1000; FAX. 512/465–1090; Dan Stultz, President and Chief Executive Officer, MD, FACP, FACHE

**Dallas-Fort Worth Hospital Council,** 250 Decker Drive, Irving, TX 75062; tel. 972/719–4900; FAX. 972/719–4009; W. Stephen Love, President and Chief Executive Officer

**UTAH: UHA, Utah Hospital Association,** 2180 South 1300 East, Suite 440, Salt Lake City, UT 84106-2843; tel. 801/486–9915; FAX. 801/486–0882; Rod L. Betit, President and Chief Executive Officer

**VERMONT: Vermont Association of Hospitals and Health Systems,** 148 Main Street, Montpelier, VT 05602; tel. 802/223–3461; FAX. 802/223–0364; Beatrice Grause, President and Chief Executive Officer

**VIRGINIA: Virginia Hospital & Healthcare Association,** 4200 Inslake Drive, Glen Allen, VA 23060; tel. 804/965–1227; FAX. 804/965–0475; Laurens Sartoris, President

**WASHINGTON: Washington State Hospital Association,** 300 Elliott Avenue West, Suite 300, Seattle, WA 98119-4118; tel. 206/281–7211; FAX. 206/283–6122; C. Scott Bond, President and Chief Executive Officer

**WEST VIRGINIA: West Virginia Hospital Association,** 100 Association Drive, Charleston, WV 25311-1571; tel. 304/344–9744; FAX. 304/414–0210; Joseph M. Letnaunchyn, President and Chief Executive Officer

**WISCONSIN: Wisconsin Hospital Association,** 5510 Research Park Drive, P.O.Box 259038, Madison, WI 53725-9038; tel. 608/274–1820; FAX. 608/274–8554; Stephen Brenton, President

**WYOMING: Wyoming Hospital Association,** 2005 Warren Avenue, Cheyenne, WY 82001; tel. 307/632–9344; FAX. 307/632–9347; Dan Perdue, President

# U.S. Associated Areas

**PUERTO RICO: Puerto Rico Hospital Association,** Villa Nevarez Professional Center, Suite 101, San Juan, PR 00927; tel. 787/764–0290; FAX. 787/753–9748; Ruby Rodriguez, Vice President

# Canada

**NOVA SCOTIA: Health Association Nova Scotia,** Bedford Professional Centre, Two Dartmouth Road, Bedford, NS B4A-2K7; tel. 902/832–8500; FAX. 902/832–8505; Mary Lee, President and Chief Executive Officer

**ONTARIO: Catholic Health Alliance of Canada,** Annex C, Saint-Vincent Hospital, 60 Cambridge Street North, Ottawa, ON K1R-7A5; tel. 613/562–6262; FAX. 613/782–2857; James Roche, Executive Director

**Ontario Hospital Association,** 200 Front Street, West, Suite 2800, Toronto, ON M5V-3L1; tel. 416/205–1300; FAX. 416/205–1301; Susan Britton, President and Chief Executive Officer

**PRINCE EDWARD ISLAND: Health Association of PEI, Inc.,** 10 Pownal Street, Charlottetown, PEI C1A-3V6; tel. 902/368–3901; FAX. 902/368–3231; Ken Ezeard, Executive Director

**SASKATCHEWAN: Saskatchewan Association of Health Organizations,** 800-2002 Victoria Avenue, Regina, SK S4P-0R7; tel. 306/347–5500; FAX. 306/525–1960; Dale Markewich, Interim President and Chief Executive Officer

# Quality Improvement Organizations

*The following list of QIOs was obtained from the agencies themselves and the Centers for Medicare and Medicaid Services, Quality Improvement Organization programs.*

## United States

**ALABAMA: Alabama Quality Assurance Foundation,** Two Perimeter Park, S., Suite 200 West, Birmingham, AL 35243-2337; tel. 205/970–1600; FAX. 205/970–1616; Susan B. Holmes, Chief Financial Officer

**ALASKA: Mountain-Pacific Quality Health-Alaska QIO,** 4241 B Street, Suite 303, Anchorage, AK 99503; tel. 907/561–3202; FAX. 907/561–3204; Sharon C. Scudder, Office Director

**ARIZONA: Health Services Advisory Group, Inc.,** 3133 E. Camelback, Suite 300, Phoenix, AZ 85016; tel. 602/801–6600; FAX. 602/241–0757; Mary Ellen Dalton, Chief Executive officer

**ARKANSAS: Arkansas Foundation for Medical Care, Inc.,** 1020 W 4th Street, Suite 300, Little Rock, AR 72201; tel. 501/212–8660; FAX. 501/375–1201; Janna Williams, Director, Communications

**CALIFORNIA: Health Services Advisory Group of California,** 700 N. Brand Boulevard, Suite 370, Glendale, CA 91203; tel. 818/409–9229; FAX. 818/409–0835; Rick Potter, CPA, MBA, CHCA, Chief Executive Officer

**COLORADO: Colorado Foundation for Medical Care,** 23 Inverness Way East, Suite 100, Englewood, CO 80112; tel. 303/695–3300; FAX. 303/659–3350; Arja Pl. Adair, Jr., President and Chief Executive Officer

**CONNECTICUT: Qualidigm,** 1111 Cromwell Avenue, Suite 201, Rocky Hill, CT 06067; tel. 860/632–2008; FAX. 860/632–5865; Marcia K. Petrillo, Chief Executive Officer

**DELAWARE: Quality Insights of Delaware,** Baynard Building Suite 100, 3411 Silverside Rd, Wilmington, DE 19810-4812; tel. 302/478–3600; FAX. 302/478–3873; Les DelPizzo, Chief Operating Officer

**DISTRICT OF COLUMBIA: Delmarva Foundation of the District of Columbia,** 2175 K Street, NW, Suite 250, Washington, DC 20037; tel. 800/937–3362; FAX. 201/293–9650; Thomas Jackson, MBA, Chief Executive Officer

**FLORIDA: FMQAI,** 5201 W. Kennedy Boulevard, Suite 900, Tampa, FL 33609; tel. 813/354–9111; FAX. 813/354–1319; Tony Freedman, Chief Executive Officer

**GEORGIA: Georgia Medical Care Foundation,** 1455 Lincoln Parkway, Suite 800, Atlanta, GA 30346; tel. 404/982–0411; FAX. 404/982–7584; Dennis White, Chief Executive Officer

**HAWAII: Mountain-Pacific Quality Health Foundation - Hawaii,** 1360 South Beretania Street, Suite 501, Honolulu, HI 96814; tel. 808/545–2550; FAX. 808/440–6030; Dee Dee Nelson, Director of Hawaii Office

**IDAHO: Qualis Health,** 720 Park Boulevard, Suite 120, Boise, ID 83712-7756; tel. 208/343–4617; FAX. 208/343–4705; Linda Rowe, MS, Director, Idaho Care Transitions and Patient Safety

**ILLINOIS: Telligen,** 711 Jorie Blvd, Suite 301, Oak Brook, IL 60523-4425; tel. 630/928–5800; FAX. 630/928–5865; Jeff Chungath, Chief Executive Officer

**INDIANA: Health Care Excel, Incorporated,** 2629 Waterfront Parkway East Drive, Suite 150, Indianapolis, IN 46214; tel. 317/347–4500; FAX. 317/347–4567; Joy Casterton, Chief Executive Officer

**IOWA: Telligen,** 1776 West Lakes Parkway, West Des Moines, IA 50266; tel. 515/223–2900; FAX. 515/222–2407; Jeff Chungath, Chief Executive Officer

**KANSAS: The Kansas Foundation for Medical Care, Inc.,** 2947 Southwest Wanamaker Drive, Topeka, KS 66614; tel. 785/273–2552; FAX. 785/273–0737; Kenneth Mishler, President and Chief Executive Officer

**KENTUCKY: Health Care Excel of Kentucky Incorporated,** 1941 Bishop Lane, Suite 400, Louisville, KY 40218; tel. 502/454–5112; FAX. 502/454–5113; Joy Casterton, Chief Executive Officer

**LOUISIANA: eQHealth Solutions,** 8591 United Plaza Blvd, Suite 270, Baton Rouge, LA 70809; tel. 225/248–7003; FAX. 225/923–0957; Gary Curtis, Chief Executive Officer

**MARYLAND: Delmarva Foundation for Medical Care, Inc.,** 9240 Centreville Road, Easton, MD 21601; tel. 410/822–0697; FAX. 410/763–6250; Thomas Jackson, MBA, Chief Executive Officer

**MASSACHUSETTS: Masspro,** 245 Winter Street, Waltham, MA 02451-1231; tel. 781/890–0011; FAX. 781/487–0083; Laura Moore, MPA, President and Chief Executive Officer

**MICHIGAN: MPRO,** 22670 Haggerty Rd, Suite 100, Farmington Hills, MI 48335-2611; tel. 248/465–7300; FAX. 248/465–7428; Robert J. Yellan, President and Chief Executive Officer

**MINNESOTA: Stratis Health,** 2901 Metro Drive, Suite 400, Bloomington, MN 55425; tel. 952/854–3306; FAX. 952/853–8503; Jennifer Lundblad, PhD, MBA, Chief Executive Officer

**MISSISSIPPI: Information & Quality Healthcare,** Renaissance Place, 385B Highland Colony Parkway, Suite 504, Ridgeland, MS 39157; tel. 601/957–1575; FAX. 601/956–1713; James McIlwain, MD, President

**MISSOURI: Primaris,** 200 N. Keene Street, Suite 101, Columbia, MO 65201; tel. 573/817–8300; FAX. 573/777–9039; Richard A. Royer, Chief Executive Officer

**MONTANA: Mountain-Pacific Quality Health Foundation,** 3404 Cooney Drive, Helena, MT 59602; tel. 406/457–5812; FAX. 406/513–1920; Liz Campbell, Director, Corporate Affairs

**NEBRASKA: CIMRO of Nebraska,** 1230 O Street, Suite 120, Lincoln, NE 68508; tel. 402/476–1399; FAX. 402/476–1335; Janet Dooley, Director of Medicare Operations

**NEVADA: HealthInsight,** 6830 W Oquendo Road, Suite 102, Las Vegas, NV 89118; tel. 702/385–9933; FAX. 702/385–4586; Marc Bennett, MA, President and Chief Executive Officer

**NEW HAMPSHIRE: Northeast Health Care Quality Foundation (ME, NH, VT),** 15 Old Rollinsford Road, Suite 302, Dover, NH 03820-2830; tel. 603/749–1641; FAX. 603/749–1195; Robert A. Aurilio, FACHE, Chief Executive Officer

**NEW JERSEY: Healthcare Quality Strategies, Inc.,** 557 Cranbury Road, Suite 21, East Brunswick, NJ 08816; tel. 732/238–5570; FAX. 732/432–5647; Mary Jane Brubaker, Chief Operating Officer

**NEW MEXICO: HealthInsight New Mexico,** 5801 Osuna RD NE, Suite 200, Albuquerque, NM 87109; tel. 505/998–9898; FAX. 505/998–9899; Richard Kozoll, MD, MPH, President, Board of Directors

**NEW YORK: IPRO,** 1979 Marcus Avenue, Lake Success, NY 11042-1002; tel. 516/326–7767; FAX. 516/328–2310; Theodore O. Will, Chief Executive Officer

**NORTH CAROLINA: Carolinas Center for Medical Excellence,** 100 Regency Forest Drive, Suite 200, Cary, NC 27518-8598; tel. 919/461–5501; FAX. 919/461–5701; Charles Riddick, Chief Executive Officer

**NORTH DAKOTA: North Dakota Health Care Review Inc. (NDHCRI),** 3520 North Broadway, Minot, ND 58703; tel. 701/852–4231; FAX. 701/857–9755; Barbara Groutt, Chief Executive Officer

**OHIO: Ohio KePRO, Inc.,** Rock Run Center, 5700 Lombardo Center Drive, Seven Hills, OH 44131; tel. 216/447–9604; FAX. 216/447–7925; Rita Bowling, RN, BSN, MBA, CPHQ, Project Director

**OKLAHOMA: Oklahoma Foundation for Medical Quality,** 14000 Quail Springs Parkway, Suite 400, Oklahoma City, OK 73134; tel. 405/840–2891; FAX. 405/840–1343; Gregg Koehn, CPA, President and Chief Executive Officer

**OREGON: Acumentra Health,** 2020 SW Fourth Avenue, Suite 520, Portland, OR 97201-4960; tel. 503/279–0100; FAX. 503/279–0190; Jon Mitchell, FACHE, President and Chief Executive Officer

**PENNSYLVANIA: Quality Insights of Pennsylvania,** Commerce Court, 2601 Market Place Street, Suite 320, Harrisburg, PA 17110; tel. 717/671–5425; FAX. 717/671–5970; John C. Wiesendanger, Chief Executive Officer

**RHODE ISLAND: Healthcentric Advisors, formerly Quality Partners of Rhode Island,** 235 Promenade Street, Suite 500, Providence, RI 02908; tel. 401/528–3200; FAX. 401/528–3210; H. John Keimig, MHA, FACHE, President and Chief Executive Officer

**SOUTH CAROLINA: The Carolinas Center for Medical Excellence,** 246 Stoneridge Dr, Suite 200, Columbia, SC 29210; tel. 803/212–7500; FAX. 803/212–7600; Melinda Postal, Director of Communications

**SOUTH DAKOTA: South Dakota Foundation for Medical Care,** 2600 West 49th Street, Suite 300, Sioux Falls, SD 57105; tel. 605/336–3505; FAX. 605/373–0580; Mark Hoven, Chief Executive Officer

**TENNESSEE: Qsource,** 3340 Players Club Pkwy, Suite300, Memphis, TN 38125; tel. 800/528–2655; FAX. 901/273–2695

**TEXAS: TMF, Health Quality Institute,** Bridgepoint 1, Suite 300, 5918 West Courtyard Drive, Austin, TX 78730-5036; tel. 512/329–6610; FAX. 512/327–7159; Tom Manley, Chief Executive Officer

**UTAH: HealthInsight,** 756 East Winchester Street, Suite 200, Salt Lake City, UT 84107; tel. 801/892–0155; FAX. 801/892–0160; Marc Bennett, President and Chief Executive Officer

**VIRGINIA: VHQC,** 9830 Mayland Drive, Suite J, Richmond, VA 23233; tel. 804/289–5320; FAX. 804/289–5324; Donald A. Glozer, MHA, CHE, President and Chief Executive Officer

**WASHINGTON: Qualis Health,** 10700 Meridian Avenue, N., Suite 100, Seattle, WA 98133-9075; tel. 206/364–9700; FAX. 206/368–2419; Jonathan Sugarman, MD, MPH, President and Chief Executive Officer

**WEST VIRGINIA: West Virginia Medical Institute, Inc.,** 3001 Chesterfield Avenue, Charleston, WV 25304; tel. 304/346–9864; FAX. 304/346–9863; John Wiesendanger, MHA, Chief Executive Officer

**WISCONSIN: MetaStar, Inc.,** 2909 Landmark Place, Madison, WI 53713; tel. 608/274–1940; FAX. 608/274–5008; Greg E. Simmons, President and Chief Executive Officer

**WYOMING: Mountain-Pacific Quality Health Foundation - Wyoming,** 145 S. Durbin, Ste 105, Casper, WY 82601; tel. 877/810–6248; FAX. 307/472–1791; Deborah Fleming, Wyoming Director

## U.S. Associated Areas

**PUERTO RICO: Quality Improvement Professional Research Organization,** View Plaza Torre I, Suite 412, San Juan, PR 00918-1696; tel. 787/641–1240; FAX. 787/641–1248; Jose Robles, Chief Executive Officer

**VIRGIN ISLANDS: Virgin Islands Medical Institute, Inc.,** 1AD Estate Diamond Ruby, PO Box 5989, Christiansted, VI 00823-5989; tel. 340/712–2400; FAX. 340/712–2449; M. "Rikki" Nelthropp, Chief Executive Officer

# Regional Health Information Organizations

*The following list of Regional Health Information Organizations (RHIOs) is based on information provided by the agencies themselves. There are many local organizations that are not included. Inclusion or omission of any organization's name indicates neither approval nor disapproval by Health Forum, LLC, an American Hospital Association company.*

## United States

**ALABAMA: Montgomery Area Community Wellness Coalition,** 3060 Mobile Highway, Montgomery, AL 36108; tel. 334/293–6502; FAX. 334/293–6674; Cynthia Bisbee, PhD; www.wellness-coalition.org

**ALASKA: Alaska eHealth Network,** PMB 1143, 2440 E Tudor Road, Anchorage, AK 99507; tel. 907/770–2626; FAX. 907/770–1413; Rebecca Madison, Executive Director; www.ak-ehealth.com

**ARIZONA: Arizona Health-e Connection,** 3877 N. 7th Street, Suite 130, Phoenix, AZ 85014; tel. 602/688–7200; FAX. 602/264–8823; Melissa Rutala, Chief Executive Officer; www.azhec.org

**ARKANSAS: HITArkansas, Arkansas Foundation for Medical Care,** 1020 West 4th Street, Suite 420, Little Rock, AR 72201; tel. 501/212–8616; FAX. 501/212–8689; Johnathan Fuchs, FACHE, Chief Operating Officer; www.hitarkansas.com

**CALIFORNIA: California eHealth Collaborative,** 1966 Tice Valley Boulevard #144, Walnut Creek, CA 94595; tel. 415/260–6277; Lori Hack, MBA, Chief Executive Officer; caehc.org

**COLORADO: CORHIO, Colorado Regional Health Information Organization,** 3773 North Cherry Creek Drive, Suite 615, Denver, CO 80209; tel. 720/285–3200; FAX. 720/285–3205; Phyllis Albritton, Executive Director; www.corhio.org

**CONNECTICUT: eHealth Connecticut,** 1111 Cromwell Avenue, Building 201, Rocky Hill, CT 06067; tel. 860/240–5600; FAX. 860/278–2400; Scott Cleary, Program Manager; www.ehealthconnecticut.org

**DELAWARE: Delaware Health Information Network,** 107 Wolf Creek Boulevard, Suite 2, Dover, DE 19901; tel. 302/678–0220; FAX. 302/645–0398; Dr. Jan Lee, Executive Director; www.dhin.org

**FLORIDA: Big Bend Regional Healthcare Information Organization (BBRHIO),** 3411 Capital Medical Boulevard, Tallahassee, FL 32308; tel. 850/702–0365; Allen Byington, Executive Director; www.bigbendhealth.com
**Central Florida RHIO,** 4401 Vineland Rd., Suite A-10, Orlando, FL 32811; tel. 407/425–9500; FAX. 407/425–9559; Michael Kovner, Project Director; www.centralfloridarhio.org
**Florida Health Information Network, Agency for Health Care Administration,** 2727 Mahan Drive, Tallahassee, FL 32308; tel. 850/922–7036; FAX. 850/414–7831; Christine Nye, Director; www.fhin.net
**Health Network of the Palm Beaches, Inc.,** 3540 Forest Hill Blvd, Suite 101, West Palm Beach, FL 33406; tel. 561/433–3940; FAX. 561/433–2385; www.pbccha.org
**North East Florida Regional Health Organization, Inc.,** 6484 Ft. Caroline Road, Jacksonville, FL 32277; tel. 904/731–0221; Mark Renfro, Administrator; www.nefrho.org
**SunCoast RHIO,** 5020 Clark Road, #127, Sarasota, FL 34233; tel. 941/426–6093; Lee S. Gross, MD, President; www.suncoastrhio.org

**GEORGIA: GA Health Information Exchange,** 2 Peachtree Street, Atlanta, GA 30303; tel. 404/656–7282; FAX. 770/344–4035; Archie Banks, Director Office of Information Technology and Transparency; www.dch.georgia.gov

**HAWAII: Hawaii Health Information Corp. (HHIC),** 733 Bishop Street, Suite 1870, Makai Tower, Honolulu, HI 96813-4002; tel. 808/534–0288; FAX. 808/534–0292; Deborah Higashi, Operations Manager; www.hhic.org

**IDAHO: Idaho Health Data Exchange,** 450 W. State Street, PO Box 6978, Boise, ID 83707; tel. 208/332–7253; FAX. 208/332–7217; Scott Carrell, Interim Executive Director; www.idahohde.org

**ILLINOIS: Illinois Office of Health Information Technology,** 100 W. Randolph Street, 2-201, Chicago, IL 60601; tel. 312/793–0063; Laura Zaremba, Director/State HIT Coordinator; www.hie.illinois.gov

**INDIANA: Indiana Health Information Exchange,** 846 N. Senate Avenue, Suite 110, Indianapolis, IN 46202; tel. 317/644–1750; FAX. 317/644–1751; Harold Apple, President and Chief Executive Officer; www.ihie.org

**IOWA: Iowa e-Health, Iowa Department of Public Health,** Lucas Building, 321 E. 12th Street, Des Moines, IA 50319; tel. 515/281–4236; FAX. 515/281–4958; Kim Norby, Executive Director; www.iowaehealth.org

**KANSAS: Kansas E-Health Advisory Council, Kansas Department of Health and Environment,** Room 540, Curtis State Office Building, Topeka, KS 66612; tel. 785/296–0461; FAX. 785/296–4813; Rod Bremby, Program Director; www.kdheks.gov

**LOUISIANA: Louisiana Health Care Quality Forum,** 8550 United Plaza Blvd, Suite 500, Baton Rouge, LA 70809; tel. 225/334–9299; FAX. 225/334–9847; Nadine Robin, HIT Program Manager; www.lhcqf.org

**MAINE: HealthInfoNet,** 125 Presumpscot Street, Portland, ME 04103; tel. 207/541–9250; FAX. 207/541–9258; Devore Culver, Executive Director and Chief Executive Officer; www.hinfonet.org

**MASSACHUSETTS: Massachusetts Health Data Consortium,** 460 Totten Pond Rd., Suite 690, Waltham, MA 02451; tel. 781/419–7800; FAX. 781/795–0155; Ray Campbell, Executive Director and Chief Executive Officer; www.mahealthdata.org

**MINNESOTA: MN eHealth Initiative, Minnesota Department of Health,** 85 E. Seventh Place, Suite 200, St. Paul, MN 55164; tel. 651/201–4856; FAX. 651/201–3830; Bob B. Johnsno, Senior Planner; www.health.state.mn.us/e-health

**MONTANA: HealthShare Montana,** 2475 Village Lane, Suite 302, Billings, MT 59102; tel. 406/794–0170; FAX. 406/791–0170; Brad Putnam, Interim Administrator; www.healthsharemontana.org

**NEBRASKA: eHealth Council, Nebraska Information Technology Commission,** 501 S. 14th Street, P.O. Box 95045, Lincoln, NE 68509-5045; tel. 402/471–3560; Anne Byers, Project Manager; www.nitc.nebraska.gov/eHc

**NEVADA: HealthInsight,** 6830 W. Oquendo Road, Suite 102, Las Vegas, NV 89118; tel. 702/385–9933; FAX. 702/385–4586; Marc Bennett, President and Chief Executive Officer; www.healthinsight.org

**NEW HAMPSHIRE: NH Citizen's Health Initiative,** 501 South Street, 2nd Floor, Bow, NH 03304; tel. 603/573–3373; Jeanne Ryer, Executive Director; www.steppingupnh.org; www.citizenshealthinitiative.org

**NEW JERSEY: New Jersey Health Information Technology Commission, New Jersey Department of Health & Senior Services,** PO Box 360, Trenton, NJ 08625-0360; tel. 609/292–9382; Emmanouil Skoufos, PhD, Executive Director; www.state.nj.us/health/bc/hitc.shtml

**NEW MEXICO: New Mexico Health Information Collaborative (NMHIC),** 2309 Renard Place SE, Suite 103, Albuquerque, NM 87106; tel. 505/938–9904; FAX. 505/938–9940; Jeff Blair, MBA, Director of Health Informatics; www.nmhic.org

**NEW YORK: Healthcare Information Xchange of New York (HIXNY),** 15 Cornell Road, Latham, NY 12110; tel. 518/783–0518; FAX. 518/785–3101; Mark McKinney, Chief Executive Officer; www.hixny.org

**NORTH CAROLINA: NC Healthcare Information and Communications Alliance, Inc. (NCHICA),** 3200 NC Highway 54, Cape Fear Building, Suite 200, Research Triangle Park, NC 27709-3048; tel. 919/558–9258; FAX. 919/558–2198; Holt Anderson, Executive Director; www.nchica.org

**NORTH DAKOTA: North Dakota Health Information Technology,** 600 E. Boulevard Avenue, Dept. 112, Bismark, ND 58505-0100; tel. 701/328–1991; FAX. 701/328–1991; Sheldon H. Wolf, Director; www.healthit.nd.gov

**OHIO: Ohio Health Information Technology, Health Policy Institute of Ohio,** 37 W. Broad Street, Suite 350, Columbus, OH 43215; tel. 614/224–4950; FAX. 614/224–2205; William Hayes, President; www.healthpolicyohio.org/ohhit

**OREGON: Oregon Health Information Technology Oversight Council (HITOC),** Oregon Health Policy and Research, 1225 Ferry Street SE, Salem, OR 97301; tel. 503/373–7859; FAX. 503/378–5511; Carol Robinson, Director; www.oregon.gov/OHPPR/HITOC/index.shtml

**PENNSYLVANIA: Pennsylvania eHealth Initiative,** c/o The Hospital & Healthsystem Association of Pennsylvania, 4750 Lindle Road, Harrisburg, PA 17105; tel. 717/561–5338; FAX. 717/561–5216; Chris Cavanaugh, PAeHI Executive Director; www.paehi.org

**RHODE ISLAND: Rhode Island Health Information Exchange, Rhode Island Quality Institute,** 235 Promenade Street, Suite 600, Providence, RI 02908; tel. 401/276–9141; FAX. 401/276–9144; Laura Adams, Chief Executive Officer; www.riqi.org

**SOUTH DAKOTA: South Dakota e-Health Collaborative, South Dakota Department of Health,** 600 East Capitol Avenue, Pierre, SD 57501; tel. 605/773–3361; Kevin DeWald, State Health IT Coordinator; www.ehealth.dsu.edu

**TENNESSEE: Office of eHealth Initiatives,** 310 Great Circle Road, Fourth floor, east wing, Nashville, TN 37243; tel. 615/507–6406; FAX. 615/532–2849; Will Rice, Director; www.tn.gov/ehealth

**TEXAS: Greater Houston Health Information Exchange,** 1310 Prairie Street, Suite 1080, Houston, TX 77002; Kay Carr, President and Chief Executive Officer; www.ghhie.org
**miRHIO, Southeast Texas Health System,** PO Box 947, Goliad, TX 77963-0947; tel. 361/645–1762; FAX. 361/645–1743; Shannon Calhoun, Executive Director; www.mirhio.com
**Statewide Health Coordinating Council, Texas State Health Plan, Department of State Health Services,** 1100 W. 49th Street, M-660, PO Box 149347, MC 1898, Austin, TX 78714-9347; tel. 512/776–3548; FAX. 512/776–7344; Bobby D. Schmidt, M.Ed., Project Director; www.dshs.state.tx.us/chs/shcc

**UTAH: Utah Health Information Network,** 151 E. 5600 South, Suite 320, Murray, UT 84107; tel. 801/466–7705; FAX. 801/466–7169; Teresa L. Rivera, Chief Operating Officer; www.uhin.com

**VERMONT: Vermont Information Technology Leaders (VITL),** 144 Main Street, Suite 1, Montpelier, VT 05602; tel. 802/233–4100; FAX. 802/223–4100; David Cochran, MD, President; www.vitl.net

**VIRGINIA: Office of Health Information Technology,** Patrick Henry Building, 1111 East Broad Street, Richmond, VA 23219; tel. 804/371–0828; Kim Barnes, Director of Health IT; www.healthitcouncil.vi.virginia.gov

**WASHINGTON: Washington State Health Care Authority,** 626 8th Avenue SE, Olympia, WA 98504-2710; tel. 360/725–0859; Annette Burgin, WA HCA Project Assistant; www.hca.wa.gov/hit

**WEST VIRGINIA: WV Health Information Network (WVHIN), State designated HIE,** 100 Dee Drive, Charleston, WV 25311; tel. 304/558–4503; FAX. 304/558–2734; Phil Weikle, Chief Operations Officer; www.wvhin.org

**WISCONSIN: Wisconsin Statewide Health Information Network (WISHIN),** PO Box 259038, Madison, WI 53725; tel. 608/274–1820; FAX. 608/274–8554; Joseph Kachelski, Chief Executive Officer; www.wishin.org

**WYOMING: Wyoming Health Information Organization (WyHIO),** 109 E. 17th Street, Cheyenne, WY 82001; tel. 307/432–4025; Larry Biggio, Executive Director; www.wyhio.org

**Section C**

*The following list includes state departments of health and welfare, and their subagencies. The information was obtained directly from the agencies.*

## United States

### ALABAMA
The Honorable Robert Bentley, Governor, 334/242-7100

**Facility Licensure Agencies**

**Alabama Department of Public Health, Division of Licensure and Certification,** 201 Monroe Street, Suite 600, Montgomery, AL 36130-3017; tel. 334/206-5175; FAX. 334/206-5219; Walter T. Geary, MD, Bureau Director and Medical Director

**Health Agencies**

**Department of Public Health,** The RSA Tower, Suite 1552, PO Box 303017, Montgomery, AL 36130-3017; tel. 334/206-5200; FAX. 334/206-2008; Donald E. Williamson, MD, State Health Officer

**State Health Planning and Development Agency,** 100 North Union Street, Suite 870, Montgomery, AL 36103-3025; tel. 334/242-4103; FAX. 334/242-4113; Alva Lambert, Executive Director

**Managed Care Agencies**

**Department of Insurance,** 201 Monroe Street, Suite 1700, Montgomery, AL 36130-3351; tel. 334/269-3550; FAX. 334/241-4192; Jim Ridling, Commissioner

**Medical & Nursing Licensure Agencies**

**Alabama Board of Nursing,** 770 Washington Avenue, Suite 250, RSA Plaza, Montgomery, AL 36104; tel. 800/656-5318; FAX. 334/293-5201; N. Genell Lee, RN, MSN, JD, Executive Officer

**Alabama State Board of Medical Examiners,** 848 Washington Avenue, PO Box 946, Montgomery, AL 36101-0946; tel. 334/242-4116; FAX. 334/242-4155; Larry D. Dixon, Executive Director

### ALASKA
The Honorable Sean Parnell, Governor, 907/465-3500

**Facility Licensure Agencies**

**Facilities Section, Department of Health and Social Services,** PO Box 110650, Juneau, AK 99811-0650; tel. 907/465-1870; FAX. 907/465-2607; Jennifer Klein, Section Chief

**Health Agencies**

**Department of Health and Social Services,** 350 Main Street, Room 404, PO Box 110601, Juneau, AK 99811-0601; tel. 907/465-3030; FAX. 907/465-3068; William J. Steur, Commissioner

**Managed Care Agencies**

**Alaska Division of Insurance,** 333 Willoughby, Ninth Floor, State Office Building, Juneau, AK 99811-0805; tel. 907/465-2515; FAX. 907/465-3422; Linda Hall, Director

**Medical & Nursing Licensure Agencies**

**Alaska Board of Nursing, Division of Corporations, Business, and Professional Licensing,** 550 W. Seventh Avenue, Suite 1500, Anchorage, AK 99501; tel. 907/269-8161; FAX. 907/269-8196; Nancy Sanders, Executive Administrator

**Alaska State Board of Medical Examiners,** 550 W. Seventh Avenue, Suite 1500, Anchorage, AK 99501; tel. 907/269-8163; FAX. 907/269-8196; Debora J. Stovern, Executive Administrator

### ARIZONA
The Honorable Janice K. Brewer, Governor, 602/542-4331

**Facility Licensure Agencies**

**Arizona Department of Health Services, Medical Facilities Licensing Office,** 150 N. 18th Avenue, Suite 450, Phoenix, AZ 85007; tel. 602/364-3064; FAX. 602/364-4808; Alan Oppenheim, Assistant Director

**Health Agencies**

**Arizona Department of Health Services,** 150 N. 18th Ave, Suite 500, Phoenix, AZ 85007; tel. 602/542-1027; FAX. 602/542-1062; Will Humble, Interim Director

**Managed Care Agencies**

**Arizona Department of Insurance,** 2910 North 44th Street, Suite 210, Phoenix, AZ 85018-7269; tel. 602/364-2393; FAX. 602/364-2175; Christina Urias, Director of Insurance

**Medical & Nursing Licensure Agencies**

**Arizona Board of Osteopathic Examiners in Medicine and Surgery,** 9535 E. Doubletree Ranch Road, Suite 200, Scottsdale, AZ 85258; tel. 480/657-7703; FAX. 480/657-7715; Jenna Jones, Executive Director

**Arizona Department of Health Services, Division of Licensing Services,** 150 N 18th Avenue, Suite 400 - Receptionist, Phoenix, AZ 85007; tel. 602/364-3031; FAX. 602/364-4764; Colby Dower, Assistant Director

**Arizona Medical Board,** 9545 E. Doubletree Ranch Road, Scottsdale, AZ 85258; tel. 480/551-2791; FAX. 480/551-2828; Lisa S. Wynn, Executive Director

**Arizona State Board of Nursing,** 4747 N. Seventh Street, Suite 200, Phoenix, AZ 85014-3653; tel. 602/771-7800; FAX. 602/771-7888; Joey Ridenour, RN, MN, FAAN, Executive Director

### ARKANSAS
The Honorable Mike Beebe, Governor, 501/682-2345

**Facility Licensure Agencies**

**Health Facility Services, Arkansas Department of Health,** 5800 West 10th Street, Suite 400, Little Rock, AR 72204-1704; tel. 501/661-2201; FAX. 501/661-2165; Connie Melton, Section Chief

**Health Agencies**

**Arkansas Department of Health,** 4815 West Markham, Little Rock, AR 72205; tel. 501/661-2000; FAX. 501/661-2388; Paul K. Halverson, DrPH, Director and State Health Officer

**Managed Care Agencies**

**Arkansas Insurance Department,** 1200 West Third Street, Little Rock, AR 72201-1904; tel. 501/371-2600; FAX. 501/371-2618; Jay Bradford, Insurance Commissioner

**Medical & Nursing Licensure Agencies**

**Arkansas State Board of Nursing,** University Tower Building, 1123 South University Avenue, Little Rock, AR 72204; tel. 501/686-2700; FAX. 501/686-2714; Sue A. Tedford, ASBN Executive Director

**Arkansas State Medical Board,** 1401 W. Capitol, Suite 340, Little Rock, AR 72201; tel. 501/296-1802; FAX. 501/603-3555; Trent P. Pierce, MD, Chairman

### CALIFORNIA
The Honorable Edmund Brown, Jr., Governor, 916/445-2841

**Facility Licensure Agencies**

**Department of Public Health - Center for Health Care Quality, Licensing and Certification Program,** 1615 Capitol Avenue, MS 0512, PO Box 997413, Sacramento, CA 95899-7377; tel. 916/324-6630; FAX. 916/324-4820; Debby Rogers, RN, MS, PAEA, Deputy Director

**Health Agencies**

**California Department of Public Health,** PO Box 997377, MS 0500, Sacramento, CA 95899-7377; tel. 916/558-1700; FAX. 916/558-1762; Dr. Ron Chapman, Director

**Department of Health Care Services,** PO Box 997413, MS 0000, Sacramento, CA 95899-7413; tel. 916/440-7400; Toby Douglas, Director

**Healthcare Workforce Development Division,** 400 R Street, Room 330, Sacramento, CA 95811; tel. 916/326-3700; FAX. 916/322-2588; Lupe Alonzo-Diaz, MPA, Acting Deputy Director

**Managed Care Agencies**

**Department of Managed Health Care,** 980 Ninth St, Suite 500, Sacramento, CA 95814; tel. 888/466-2219; FAX. 916/255-5241; Brent Barnhart, Director

**Ombudsman's Office, California Department of Insurance,** 300 Capitol Mall, Suite 1600, Sacramento, CA 95814; tel. 916/492-3545; Dave Jones, Insurance Commissioner

**Medical & Nursing Licensure Agencies**

**Board of Vocational Nursing and Psychiatric Technicians,** 2535 Capitol Oaks Drive, Suite 205, Sacramento, CA 95833; tel. 916/263-7800; FAX. 916/263-7859; Teresa Bello-Jones, JD, MSN, RN, Executive Officer

**California Board of Registered Nursing,** 1747 N. Market Boulevard, Suite 150, Sacramento, CA 95834-1924; tel. 916/322-3350; FAX. 916/574-7700; Louise Bailey, M.Ed, RN, Executive Director

**Medical Board of California,** 2005 Evergreen Street, Suite 1200, Sacramento, CA 95815; tel. 916/263-2382; FAX. 916/263-2387; Linda K. Whitney, Executive Director

### COLORADO
The Honorable John Hickenlooper, Governor, 303/866-2471

**Facility Licensure Agencies**

**Health Facilities Division, Colorado Department of Public Health and Environment,** 4300 Cherry Creek Drive South, Building A, Second Floor, Denver, CO 80246-1530; tel. 303/692-2800; FAX. 303/753-6214; Howard Roitman, Director

**Health Agencies**

**Colorado Department of Public Health and Environment, Business Office,** 4300 Cherry Creek Drive, S., Denver, CO 80246-1530; tel. 303/692-2016; FAX. 303/751-3043; Christopher E. Urbina, Executive Director and Chief Medical Officer

**Managed Care Agencies**

**Department of Regulatory Agencies, Colorado Division of Insurance,** 1560 Broadway, Suite 850, Denver, CO 80202; tel. 303/894-7499; FAX. 303/894-7455; Jim Riesberg, Commissioner

**Medical & Nursing Licensure Agencies**

**Colorado Medical Board,** 1560 Broadway, Suite 1350, Denver, CO 80202-5140; tel. 303/894-7690; FAX. 303/894-7692; Marschall S. Smith, Program Director

**Colorado State Board of Nursing Department of Regulatory Agencies,** 1560 Broadway, Suite 1350, Denver, CO 80202; tel. 303/894-2430; FAX. 303/894-7693; Kenneth Julien, Program Director

**Department of Regulatory Agencies,** 1560 Broadway, Suite 1550, Denver, CO 80202; tel. 303/894-7855; FAX. 303/894-7885; Barbara Kelley, Executive Director

### CONNECTICUT
The Honorable Dan Malloy, Governor, 800/406-1527

**Facility Licensure Agencies**

**Department of Public Health, Healthcare Quality and Safety Branch,** 410 Capitol Avenue, MS 12HCS, P.O. Box 340308, Hartford, CT 06134-0308; tel. 860/509-7406; FAX. 860/509-7539; Wendy Furniss, RNC, MS, Branch Chief

**Health Agencies**

**Department of Public Health,** 410 Capitol Avenue, Mail Stop 12APP, Hartford, CT 06134-0308; tel. 860/509-7590; FAX. 860/707-1931; Jennifer Filippone, Chief Practitioner, Licensing and Investigations

**Managed Care Agencies**

**State of Connecticut, Insurance Department, Life & Health Division,** PO Box 816, 153 Market St., Hartford, CT 06142-0816; tel. 860/297-3857; FAX. 860/297-3941; Mary Ellen Breault, Director

**Medical & Nursing Licensure Agencies**

**Connecticut Board of Examiners for Nursing, Department of Public Health,** 410 Capitol Avenue, MS #13PHO, PO Box 340308, Hartford, CT 06134-0308; tel. 860/509-7624; FAX. 860/509-7553; Janice Wojick, Board Liaison

**Connecticut Department of Public Health,** 410 Capitol Avenue, MS #12 APP, PO Box 340308, Hartford, CT 06134-0308; tel. 860/509-7590; FAX. 860/509-8457; Jewel Mullen, MD, Commissioner

## DELAWARE
The Honorable Jack Markell, Governor, 302/744–4101

**Facility Licensure Agencies**
Department of Health and Social Services - Division of Public Health, Office of Health Facilities Licensing and Certification, 258 Chapman Road, Suite 101, Chopin Building, Newark, DE 19702; tel. 302/283–7220; FAX. 302/283–7221; Roseann Sapp, Office Manager

**Health Agencies**
Delaware Health and Social Services, 1901 North DuPont Highway, Main Administration Building, New Castle, DE 19720; tel. 302/255–9040; FAX. 302/255–4429; Rita M. Landgraf, Cabinet Secretary
Division of Public Health, Jesse Cooper Building, 417 Federal Street, Dover, DE 19901; tel. 302/744–4700; FAX. 302/739–6659; Karyl Thomas Rattay, MD, MS, FAAP, FACPM, Director

**Managed Care Agencies**
Delaware Department of Insurance, Consumer Department, 841 Silver Lake Boulevard, Dover, DE 19904; tel. 302/674–7300; FAX. 302/739–6278; Karen Weldin-Stewart, Commissioner

**Medical & Nursing Licensure Agencies**
Delaware Board of Medical Practice Delaware Division of Professional Regulation, Cannon Building, 861 Silver Lake Boulevard, Suite 203, Dover, DE 19904; tel. 302/744–4500; FAX. 302/739–2711; James L. Collins, Director
Delaware Board of Nursing, 861 Silver Lake Boulevard, Suite 203, Dover, DE 19904; tel. 302/744–4500; FAX. 302/739–2712; Pamela C. Zickafoose, Ed.D., MSN, RN, Executive Director

## DISTRICT OF COLUMBIA
Governor Switchboard, 202/624–5300

**Facility Licensure Agencies**
District of Columbia Department of Health, Health Regulation Licensing Administration, 899 N Capitol Street, NE, Washington, DC 20002; tel. 202/442–5955; FAX. 202/442–4795; Mohammad N. Akhter, MD, Director

**Health Agencies**
Department of Health, Government of the District of Columbia, 899 North Capitol Street NE, Washington, DC 20002; tel. 202/442–5955; FAX. 202/442–4795; Mohammad N. Akhter, Acting Director

**Managed Care Agencies**
District of Columbia Department of Insurance, Securities and Banking, Union Center Plaza, 810 First Street NE, Washington, DC 20002; tel. 202/727–8000; FAX. 202/535–1196; William P. White, Commissioner

**Medical & Nursing Licensure Agencies**
DC Board of Nursing, Department of Health, 899 North Capitol Street, NE, First Floor, Washington, DC 20002; tel. 202/724–8800; FAX. 202/724–8677; Karen Skinner, Executive Director
District of Columbia Board of Medicine, 899 North Capital Street NE, 2nd Floor, Washington, DC 20002; tel. 202/724–8800; FAX. 202/724–8677; Jacqueline Watson, MD, Executive Director

## FLORIDA
The Honorable Rick Scott, Governor, 850/488–2272

**Facility Licensure Agencies**
Agency for Health Care Administration, Bureau of Health Facility Regulation, Hospital and Outpatient Services Unit, 2727 Mahan Drive, Mail Stop 31, Tallahassee, FL 32308; tel. 850/412–4549; FAX. 850/922–4351; Laura MacLafferty, Unit Manager

**Health Agencies**
Department of Health, State Surgeon General, 4052 Bald Cypress Way, Bin #A00, Tallahassee, FL 32399-1701; tel. 850/245–4321; FAX. 850/922–9453

**Managed Care Agencies**
Office of Insurance Regulation, 200 East Gaines Street, Tallahassee, FL 32399; tel. 850/413–3140; FAX. 850/488–3334; Kevin M. McCarty, Commissioner

**Medical & Nursing Licensure Agencies**
Department of Health Florida Board of Nursing, 4052 Bald Cypress Way, Bin C-02, Tallahassee, FL 32399-3252; tel. 850/245–4125; FAX. 850/245–4172; Joe Baker, Jr., Executive Director

Florida Board of Medicine, 4052 Bald Cypress Way, Bin #C03, Tallahassee, FL 32399-3253; tel. 850/245–4131; FAX. 850/488–0596; Joy A. Tootte, JD, Executive Board Director
Florida Board of Osteopathic Medicine, 4052 Bald Cypress Way, Bin #C-06, Tallahassee, FL 32399-3256; tel. 850/245–4161; FAX. 850/921–6184; Christy Robinson, Program Operations Administrator

## GEORGIA
The Honorable Nathan Deal, Governor, 404/656–1776

**Facility Licensure Agencies**
Department of Community Health, Healthcare Facility Regulation Division, Two Peachtree Street, NW, Room 31-447, Atlanta, GA 30303-3142; tel. 404/657–5550; FAX. 404/657–8934; Carol Zafiratos, Program Director

**Health Agencies**
Department of Public Health, 2 Peachtree Street, NW, Suite 15-470, Atlanta, GA 30303-3682; tel. 404/657–2700; FAX. 404/657–2715; Brenda Fitzgerald, MD, Director

**Managed Care Agencies**
Office of Commissioner of Insurance, State of Georgia, Two Martin Luther King, Jr. Drive, Suite 604, West Tower, Atlanta, GA 30334; tel. 404/656–2085; FAX. 770/408–5931; Thomas F. Carswell, FLMI, Assistant Director, Division of Insurance

**Medical & Nursing Licensure Agencies**
Georgia Board of Nursing, 237 Coliseum Drive, Macon, GA 31217-3858; tel. 478/207–2440; FAX. 877/371–5712; Jim Cleghorn, Executive Director
Georgia Composite Medical Board, Two Peachtree Street, NW, 36th Floor, Atlanta, GA 30303; tel. 404/656–3913; FAX. 404/656–9723; LaSharn Hughes, MBA, Executive Director

## HAWAII
The Honorable Neil Abercrombie, Governor, 808/586–0034

**Facility Licensure Agencies**
Hawaii State Department of Health, Office Health Care Assurance, 601 Kamokila Blvd, Room 395, Kapolei, HI 96707; tel. 808/692–7420; FAX. 808/692–7447; Keith Ridley, Chief

**Health Agencies**
Hawaii Department of Health, PO Box 3378, 1250 Punchbowl Street, Honolulu, HI 96801; tel. 808/586–4401; FAX. 808/586–4368; Loretta J. Fuddy, ACSW, MPH, Director
Hawaii State Health Planning and Development Agency, 1177 Alakea Street, Suite 402, Honolulu, HI 96813; tel. 808/587–0788; FAX. 808/587–0783; Romala Sue Radcliffe, Administrator

**Managed Care Agencies**
State of Hawaii Department of Labor and Industrial Relations, Disability Compensation Division, PO Box 3769, 830 Punchbowl St., Honolulu, HI 96812; tel. 808/586–9151; FAX. 808/586–9219; Walter B. Kawamura, Administrator

**Medical & Nursing Licensure Agencies**
Hawaii Board of Nursing, Professional and Vocational Licensing Division, PO Box 3469, Honolulu, HI 96801; tel. 808/586–3000; Lee Ann Teshima, Executive Officer
Hawaii Medical Board, Department of Commerce and Consumer Affairs, 335 Merchant Street, Room 301, Honolulu, HI 96801; tel. 808/586–3000; Constance Cabral, Executive Officer

## IDAHO
The Honorable C.L. "Butch" Otter, Governor, 208/334–2100

**Facility Licensure Agencies**
Bureau of Facility Standards, Department of Health and Welfare, PO Box 83720, 3232 Elder Street, Boise, ID 83720; tel. 208/334–6626; FAX. 208/364–1888; Sylvia Creswell, Co-Supervisor NLTC

**Health Agencies**
Department of Health and Welfare, Division of Public Health, 450 West State, Fourth Floor, PO Box 83720, Boise, ID 83720-0036; tel. 208/334–6996; FAX. 208/334–6581; Jane Smith, Administrator

**Managed Care Agencies**
Idaho Department of Insurance, 700 West State Street, Third Floor, P.O. Box 83720, Boise, ID 83720-0042; tel. 208/334–4250; FAX. 208/334–4398; Joan Krosch, Health Care Policy and Program Specialist

**Medical & Nursing Licensure Agencies**
Idaho State Board of Medicine, PO Box 83720, Boise, ID 83720-0058; tel. 208/327–7000; FAX. 208/327–7005; Nancy Kerr, Executive Director
Idaho State Board of Nursing, 280 North 8th Street, Suite 210, PO Box 83720, Boise, ID 83720-0061; tel. 208/334–3110; FAX. 208/334–3262; Sandra Evans, MAEd., RN Executive Director

## ILLINOIS
The Honorable Pat Quinn, Governor, 217/782–6830

**Facility Licensure Agencies**
Division of Health Care Facilities and Programs, Illinois Department of Public Health, 525 West Jefferson Street, Fourth Floor, Springfield, IL 62761-0001; tel. 217/782–7412; FAX. 217/782–0382; William A. Bell, Division Chief

**Health Agencies**
Illinois Department of Public Health, 535 West Jefferson Street, Springfield, IL 62761; tel. 217/782–4977; FAX. 217/557–3497; Damon T. Arnold, MD, MPH, Director

**Managed Care Agencies**
Illinois Department of Insurance, 320 West Washington Street, Springfield, IL 62767-0001; tel. 217/782–4515; FAX. 217/782–5020; Andrew Boron, Director

**Medical & Nursing Licensure Agencies**
Illinois Department of Financial & Professional Regulation, James R. Thompson Center, 100 West Randolph Street, Chicago, IL 60601; tel. 312/814–2715; FAX. 312/814–5392; Michele Bromberg, MSN, APN, BC, Nursing Coordinator
Illinois Department of Financial and Professional Regulation, Division of Professional Regulation, 320 West Washington Street, Third Floor, Springfield, IL 62786; tel. 217/785–0800; FAX. 217/782–7645; Jay Stewart, Director

## INDIANA
The Honorable Mitch Daniels, Governor, 317/232–4567

**Facility Licensure Agencies**
Division of Acute Care, Indiana State Department of Health, Two North Meridian Street, Suite 4A, Indianapolis, IN 46204; tel. 317/233–7472; FAX. 317/233–7157; Randy Snyder, Program Director

**Health Agencies**
Indiana State Department of Health, Two North Meridian Street, Indianapolis, IN 46204; tel. 317/233–1325; FAX. 317/233–7157; Gregory N. Larson, MD, Commissioner

**Managed Care Agencies**
Indiana Department of Insurance Company Compliance Division, 311 West Washington Street, Suite 300, Indianapolis, IN 46204; tel. 317/232–2385; FAX. 317/232–5251; Logan P. Harrison, Chief Deputy Commissioner

**Medical & Nursing Licensure Agencies**
Indiana Professional Licensing Agency, Medical Licensing Board of Indiana, 402 West Washington, Room W072, Indianapolis, IN 46204; tel. 317/234–2060; FAX. 317/233–4236; Kristen Kelley, Director
Indiana State Board of Nursing, Indiana Professional Licensing Agency, 402 West Washington, Room W072, Indianapolis, IN 46204; tel. 317/234–2043; FAX. 317/233–4236; Elizabeth Kiefner Crawford, Board Director

## IOWA
The Honorable Terry Branstad, Governor, 515/281–5211

**Facility Licensure Agencies**
Iowa Department of Inspections and Appeals, Health Facilities Division, Lucas State Office Building, 321 East 12th Street, Des Moines, IA 50319-0083; tel. 515/281–4115; FAX. 515/242–5022; Mary Spracklin, Bureau Chief

**Health Agencies**
Iowa Department of Public Health, Lucas State Office Building, 321 E. 12th Street, Des Moines, IA 50319-0075; tel. 515/281–8474; FAX. 515/281–4958; Mariannette Miller-Meeks, MD

**Managed Care Agencies**

**Iowa Department of Commerce, Insurance Division**, 330 Maple, Des Moines, IA 50319-0065; tel. 515/281–5705; FAX. 515/281–3059; Susan E. Voss, Commissioner

**Medical & Nursing Licensure Agencies**

**Iowa Board of Medicine**, 400 SW 8th Street, Suite C, Des Moines, IA 50309-4686; tel. 515/281–5171; FAX. 515/242–5908; Mark Bowden, Executive Director

**Iowa Board of Nursing**, 400 SW 8th Street, Suite B, Des Moines, IA 50309; tel. 515/281–3255; FAX. 515/281–4825; Lorinda K. Inman, RN, MSN, Executive Director

**KANSAS**

**The Honorable Sam Brownback, Governor, 785/296–3232**

**Facility Licensure Agencies**

**Kansas Department of Health and Environment, Bureau of Child Care & Health Facilities**, 1000 Southwest Jackson, Suite 200, Topeka, KS 66612-1365; tel. 785/296–0131; FAX. 785/291–3419; Charles Moore, Director of Medical Facilities and Support

**Health Agencies**

**Kansas Department of Health and Environment**, Curtis Building, 1000 SW Jackson, Topeka, KS 66612-1368; tel. 785/296–0461; FAX. 785/368–6368; Robert Moser, MD, Secretary, Kansas Health and Environment

**Managed Care Agencies**

**Kansas Insurance Department**, 420 Southwest Ninth Street, Topeka, KS 66612; tel. 785/296–7850; FAX. 785/296–2537; Jay Rogers, Accident and Health Policy Examiner

**Medical & Nursing Licensure Agencies**

**Kansas State Board of Healing Arts**, 800 SW Jackson, Lower Level-Suite A, Topeka, KS 66612; tel. 785/296–7413; FAX. 785/296–0852; Kathleen Selzler Lippert, Executive Director

**Kansas State Board of Nursing**, Landon State Office Building, 900 SW Jackson, Topeka, KS 66612-1230; tel. 785/296–4929; FAX. 785/296–3929; Mary Blubaugh MSN, RN, Executive Administrator

**KENTUCKY**

**The Honorable Stephen L. Beshear, Governor, 502/564–2611**

**Facility Licensure Agencies**

**Office of Inspector General, Division of Healthcare**, Cabinet for Health and Family Services, 275 East Main Street, 5E-A, Frankfort, KY 40621; tel. 502/564–7963; FAX. 502/564–6546; Connie Payne, Director

**Health Agencies**

**Department for Public Health, Cabinet for Health & Family Services**, 275 East Main Street, Mail Stop HS1WA, Frankfort, KY 40621; tel. 502/564–3970; FAX. 502/564–9377; Audrey Tayse Haynes, Commissioner

**Managed Care Agencies**

**Department of Insurance, Health and Life Division**, 215 West Main Street, PO Box 517, Frankfort, KY 40601; tel. 502/564–6088; FAX. 502/564–2728; William J. Nold, Director

**Medical & Nursing Licensure Agencies**

**Kentucky Board of Medical Licensure**, 310 Whittington Parkway, Suite 1B, Louisville, KY 40222; tel. 502/429–7150; FAX. 502/429–7158; Preston P. Nunnelley, MD, President

**Kentucky Board of Nursing**, 312 Whittington Parkway, Suite 300, Louisville, KY 40222-2042; tel. 502/429–3300; FAX. 502/429–3311; Charlotte F. Beason, Executive Director

**LOUISIANA**

**The Honorable Bobby Jindal, Governor, 225/342–7015**

**Facility Licensure Agencies**

**Department of Health and Hospitals, Bureau of Health Services, Ambulatory Surgery Centers**, 602 N. Fifth Street, 2nd Floor, Baton Rouge, LA 70802; tel. 225/342–9348; FAX. 225/342–0157; Hedra Dubea, RN, Program Manager, Ambulatory Surgery Centers

**Department of Health and Hospitals, Bureau of Health Services, Health Standards**, 602 N. Fifth Street, 2nd Floor, Baton Rouge, LA 70821-3767; tel. 225/342–6446; FAX. 225/342–0157; Lori Guillory, Hospital Program Manager

**Health Agencies**

**Louisiana Department of Health and Hospitals**, 628 North 4th Street, Baton Rouge, LA 70802; tel. 225/342–9500; FAX. 225/342–5568; Bruce Greenstein, Secretary

**Managed Care Agencies**

**Louisiana Department of Insurance**, 1702 North Third Street, Baton Rouge, LA 70802; tel. 225/342–0800; FAX. 225/342–7401; Mike Boutwell, Asst. Commissioner, Licensing & Compliance

**Medical & Nursing Licensure Agencies**

**Louisiana State Board of Medical Examiners**, 630 Camp Street, New Orleans, LA 70130; tel. 504/568–6820; FAX. 504/568–5754; Robert L. Marier, MD., Executive Director

**Louisiana State Board of Nursing**, 17373 Perkins Road, Baton Rouge, LA 70810; tel. 225/755–7500; FAX. 225/755–7580; Barbara L. Morvant, MN, RN, Executive Director

**Louisiana State Board of Practical Nurse Examiners**, 3421 N. Causeway Boulevard, Suite 505, Metairie, LA 70002; tel. 504/838–5791; FAX. 504/838–5279; Claire Glaviano, BSN, MN, RN, Executive Director

**MAINE**

**The Honorable Paul LePage, Governor, 207/287–3531**

**Facility Licensure Agencies**

**Division of Licensing and Regulatory Services, Department of Health and Human Services**, 41 Anthony Avenue, 11 State House Station, Augusta, ME 04333; tel. 207/287–9300; FAX. 207/287–5807; Kenneth Albert, RN, Esq., Director

**Health Agencies**

**Department of Health and Human Services**, 11 State House Station, Augusta, ME 04333-0011; tel. 207/287–4223; FAX. 207/287–3005; Mary C. Mayhew, Commissioner

**Managed Care Agencies**

**Department of Professional and Financial Regulation, Bureau of Insurance**, #34 State House Station, Augusta, ME 04333-0334; tel. 207/624–8494; FAX. 207/624–8599; Glenn Griswold, Director, Consumer Health Care Division

**Medical & Nursing Licensure Agencies**

**Maine Board of Licensure in Medicine**, 161 Capitol Street, 137 State House Station, Augusta, ME 04333-0137; tel. 207/287–3601; FAX. 207/287–6590; Randal C. Manning, Executive Director

**Maine Board of Osteopathic Licensure**, 142 State House Station, 161 Capitol Street, Augusta, ME 04333-0142; tel. 207/287–2480; FAX. 207/287–3015; Susan E. Strout, Executive Secretary

**Maine State Board of Nursing**, 161 Capitol Street, 158 State House Station, Augusta, ME 04333-0158; tel. 207/287–1133; FAX. 207/287–1149; Myra A. Broadway, JD, MS, RN, Executive Director

**MARYLAND**

**The Honorable Martin O'Malley, Governor, 410/974–3901**

**Facility Licensure Agencies**

**Maryland Department of Health and Mental Hygiene, Freestanding Ambulatory Surgery Centers and Hospices**, Spring Grove Hospital Center, 55 Wade Avenue, Cantonville, MD 21288; tel. 410/402–8040; FAX. 410/402–8441; Barbara Fagan, Manager and Coordinator

**Maryland Office of Health Care Quality, Department of Health & Mental Hygiene**, Spring Grove Hospital Center, 55 Wade Avenue, Cantonville, MD 21228; tel. 410/402–8002; FAX. 410/402–8218; Nancy Grimm, Director

**Health Agencies**

**Department of Health and Mental Hygiene**, 201 West Preston Street, Baltimore, MD 21201; tel. 410/767–6500; FAX. 410/767–6489; Joshua M. Sharfstein, MD, Secretary

**Managed Care Agencies**

**Maryland Insurance Administration, Life & Health Complaints and Investigations**, 200 Street Paul Place, Suite 2700, Baltimore, MD 21202; tel. 410/468–2244; FAX. 410/468–2260; Brenda Wilson

**Medical & Nursing Licensure Agencies**

**Maryland Board of Nursing**, 4140 Patterson Avenue, Baltimore, MD 21215-2254; tel. 410/585–1900; FAX. 410/358–3530; Patricia A. Noble, MSN, RN, Executive Director

**Maryland Board of Physicians**, 4201 Patterson Avenue, 4th Floor, PO Box 2571, Baltimore, MD 21215-0095; tel. 800/492–6836; FAX. 410/358–2252; C. Irving Pinder, Jr., Executive Director

**MASSACHUSETTS**

**The Honorable Deval Patrick, Governor, 617/725–4000**

**Facility Licensure Agencies**

**Massachusetts Department of Public Health, Bureau of Health Care Safety and Quality**, 99 Chauncy Street, 11th Floor, Boston, MA 02111; tel. 617/753–8000; FAX. 617/753–8125; Madeleine Biondolillo, Bureau Director

**Health Agencies**

**Massachusetts Department of Public Health**, 250 Washington Street, 6th Floor, Boston, MA 02108; tel. 617/624–6000; FAX. 617/624–5185; John Auerbach, Commissioner

**Managed Care Agencies**

**Commonwealth of Massachusetts, Division of Insurance**, 1000 Washington St, Suite 810, Boston, MA 02118-2208; tel. 617/521–7794; FAX. 617/521–7575; Joseph G. Murphy, Commissioner

**Medical & Nursing Licensure Agencies**

**Commonwealth of Massachusetts, Board of Registration in Medicine**, 200 Harvard Mill Square, Suite 330, Wakefield, MA 01880; tel. 781/876–8200; FAX. 781/876–8383; Dr. Stan Riley, Executive Director

**MICHIGAN**

**The Honorable Rick Snyder, Governor, 517/373–3400**

**Facility Licensure Agencies**

**Division of Licensing and Certification, Michigan Department of Licensing and Regulatory Affairs, Bureau of Health Systems**, PO Box 30664, 611 West Ottawa, Lansing, MI 48909; tel. 517/241–4160; FAX. 517/241–3354; Larry Horvath

**Health Agencies**

**Michigan Department of Community Health, Public Health Administration**, 201 Townsend Street, Lansing, MI 48913; tel. 517/335–8024; FAX. 517/335–9032; Jean Chabut, Deputy Director for Public Health

**Managed Care Agencies**

**Department of Licensing and Regulatory Affairs**, PO Box 30220, 611 West Ottawa, Lansing, MI 48909-7979; tel. 517/373–0220; FAX. 517/335–4978; R. Kevin Clinton, Commissioner

**Medical & Nursing Licensure Agencies**

**Michigan Board of Medicine**, 611 West Ottawa Street, First Floor, Lansing, MI 48909; tel. 517/335–0918; FAX. 517/241–2895; Rae Ramsdell, Director, Bureau of Health Professions

**Michigan Board of Nursing, Bureau of Health Professions**, 611 West Ottawa Street, First Floor, Lansing, MI 48909; tel. 517/335–0918; FAX. 517/373–2179; Joseph Campbell, Director of Health Licensing Division

**Michigan Board of Osteopathic Medicine and Surgery**, 611 West Ottawa Street, First Floor, PO Box 30670, Lansing, MI 48909; tel. 517/335–0918; FAX. 517/373–2179; Joseph Campbell, Director of Health Licensing Division

**MINNESOTA**

**The Honorable Mark Dayton, Governor, 651/201–3400**

**Facility Licensure Agencies**

**Minnesota Department of Health, Compliance Monitoring Division**, Licensing and Certification Program, PO Box 64900, St. Paul, MN 55164-0900; tel. 651/201–4100; FAX. 651/215–9697; Mary Absolon, Program Manager

**Health Agencies**

**Minnesota Department of Health**, 625 Robert Street N, P.O. Box 64975, St. Paul, MN 55164-0975; tel. 651/201–5000; Edward Ehlinger, MD, Commissioner

**Managed Care Agencies**

**Minnesota Department of Health, Managed Care Systems**, PO Box 64882, 85 E. Seventh Place, St. Paul, MN 55164-0882; tel. 651/201–5166; FAX. 651/201–5186; Irene Goldman, Manager

**Medical & Nursing Licensure Agencies**

**Minnesota Board of Medical Practice**, 2829 University Avenue, SE, Suite 500, Minneapolis, MN 55414-3246; tel. 612/617–2149; FAX. 612/617–2166; Robert A. Leach, Executive Director

**Minnesota Board of Nursing,** 2829 University Avenue SE, Suite 200, Minneapolis, MN 55414-3253; tel. 612/617–2270; FAX. 612/617–2190; Shirley A. Brekken, RN, MS, Executive Director

## MISSISSIPPI
The Honorable Phil Bryant, Governor, 601/359–3150

**Facility Licensure Agencies**

**Bureau of Health Facilities Licensure and Certification, Mississippi State Department of Health,** PO Box 1700, 143 B Lefleur's Square, Jackson, MS 39215; tel. 601/364–1100; FAX. 601/364–5054; Marilynn Winborne, Director

**Health Agencies**

**Mississippi State Department of Health, Office of Health Policy and Planning,** 570 East Woodrow Wilson, P.O. Box 1700, Jackson, MS 39215-1700; tel. 601/576–7874; FAX. 601/576–7530; Donald E. Eicher, III, Director

**Managed Care Agencies**

**Mississippi Department of Insurance,** PO Box 79, 501 North West Street, Jackson, MS 39205; tel. 601/359–3577; FAX. 601/359–2474; Josel Jones, Special Assistant Attorney General

**Medical & Nursing Licensure Agencies**

**Mississippi Board of Nursing,** 1080 River Oaks Drive, Suite A 100, Flowood, MS 39232; tel. 601/987–4188; FAX. 601/664–9303; Melinda E. Rush, DSN, FNP, Executive Director

**Mississippi State Board of Medical Licensure,** 1867 Crane Ridge Drive, Suite 200-B, Jackson, MS 39216; tel. 601/987–3079; FAX. 601/987–4159; H. Vann Craig, MD, Executive Director

## MISSOURI
The Honorable Jeremiah W. (Jay) Nixon, Governor, 573/751–3222

**Facility Licensure Agencies**

**Bureau of Home Care and Rehabilitative Standards,** PO Box 570, Jefferson City, MO 65018; tel. 573/751–6336; FAX. 573/751–6315; Lisa Coots, RN, Administrator

**Bureau of Hospital Standards, Missouri Department of Health and Senior Services,** PO Box 570, Jefferson City, MO 65102; tel. 573/751–6303; FAX. 573/526–3621; Donya Lowrie, Bureau Chief

**Health Agencies**

**Department of Health and Senior Services,** PO Box 570, 920 Wildwood, Jefferson City, MO 65102; tel. 573/751–6001; FAX. 573/751–6041; Margaret T. Donnelly, Director

**Managed Care Agencies**

**Department of Insurance, Division of Market Regulation, Life and Healthcare Section,** PO Box 690, Jefferson City, MO 65102; tel. 573/526–4106; FAX. 573/526–6075; Molly White, Insurance Regulatory Manager

**Medical & Nursing Licensure Agencies**

**Missouri State Board of Nursing,** 3605 Missouri Boulevard, PO Box 656, Jefferson City, MO 65102; tel. 573/751–0681; FAX. 573/751–0075; Lori Scheidt, Executive Director

**Missouri State Board of Registration for the Healing Arts,** 3605 Missouri Boulevard, PO Box 4, Jefferson City, MO 65102; tel. 573/751–0098; FAX. 573/751–3166; Tina Steinman, Executive Director

## MONTANA
The Honorable Brian Schweitzer, Governor, 406/444–3111

**Facility Licensure Agencies**

**Quality Assurance Division, Department of Public Health and Human Services,** 2401 Colonial Drive, Second Floor, P.O. Box 202953, Helena, MT 59620-2953; tel. 406/444–2037; FAX. 406/444–1742; Jeff Buska, Administrator

**Health Agencies**

**Montana Department of Public Health and Human Services,** 111 North Sanders, P.O. Box 4210, Helena, MT 59604; tel. 406/444–5622; FAX. 406/444–1970; Anna Whiting Sorrell, Director

**Managed Care Agencies**

**Montana State Auditor, Insurance Department,** 840 Helena Avenue, Helena, MT 59601; tel. 406/444–2040; FAX. 406/444–3497; Steve Matthews, Chief Financial Examiner

**Medical & Nursing Licensure Agencies**

**Montana Board of Medical Examiners,** 301 S. Park Avenue, 4th Floor, PO Box 200513, Helena, MT 59620-0513; tel. 406/841–2360; FAX. 406/841–2305; Ian Marquand, Executive Director

**Montana State Board of Nursing,** 301 S. Park Avenue, 4th Floor, PO Box 200513, Helena, MT 59620-0513; tel. 406/841–2340; FAX. 406/841–2305; Cynthia Gustafson, Executive Director

## NEBRASKA
The Honorable Dave Heineman, Governor, 402/471–2244

**Facility Licensure Agencies**

**Nebraska Department of Health and Human Services, Division of Public Health - Licensure Unit,** 301 Centennial Mall South, Third Floor, Lincoln, NE 68509-4986; tel. 402/471–2115; FAX. 402/471–3577; Helen L. Meeks, Licensure Unit Administrator

**Health Agencies**

**Nebraska Department of Health and Human Services,** 301 Centennial Mall, South., PO Box 95026, Lincoln, NE 68509-5026; tel. 402/471–3121; FAX. 402/471–9449; Kerry T. Winterer, Chief Executive Officer

**Managed Care Agencies**

**Nebraska Department of Insurance, Life & Health Division,** 941 O Street, Suite 400, Lincoln, NE 68508-3639; tel. 402/471–2201; FAX. 402/471–4610; Bruce Ramge, Director

**Medical & Nursing Licensure Agencies**

**Licensure Unit, Department of Health and Human Services,** 301 Centennial Mall, South, PO Box 94986, Lincoln, NE 68509-4986; tel. 402/471–4963; FAX. 402/471–3577; Helen Meeks, Administrator

**Nebraska Board of Medicine and Surgery, Licensure Unit,** 301 Centennial Mall, S., PO Box 94986, Lincoln, NE 68509-4986; tel. 402/471–2118; FAX. 402/471–8614; Becky Wisell, Executive Director

**Office of Community Health Development,** 301 Centennial Mall, South, PO Box 95026, Lincoln, NE 68509; tel. 402/471–2353; FAX. 402/471–8259; David Palm, PhD, Administrator

## NEVADA
The Honorable Brian Sandoval, Governor, 775/684–5670

**Facility Licensure Agencies**

**Bureau of Health Care Quality and Compliance, Nevada Health Division,** 727 Fairview Drive, Suite E, Carson City, NV 89701-5493; tel. 775/687–4475; FAX. 775/687–6588; Laura Hale, Bureau Chief

**Health Agencies**

**Department of Health and Human Services,** 4126 Technology Way, Suite 100, Carson City, NV 89706-2009; tel. 775/684–4000; FAX. 775/684–4010; Michael J. Willden, Director

**Nevada Division of Health,** 4150 Technology Way, Suite 300, Carson City, NV 89706; tel. 775/684–4200; FAX. 775/684–4211; Richard Whitley, Administrator

**Managed Care Agencies**

**Nevada Division of Insurance,** 1818 E. College Pkwy, Suite 103, Carson City, NV 89706; tel. 775/687–0700; FAX. 775/687–0787; Scott J. Kipper, Insurance Commissioner

**Medical & Nursing Licensure Agencies**

**Nevada State Board of Medical Examiners, Licensing,** PO Box 7238, 1105 Terminal Way, Reno, NV 89502-2144; tel. 775/688–2559; FAX. 775/688–2321; Lynnette L. Daniels, Chief of Licensing

**Nevada State Board of Nursing,** 5011 Meadowood Mall Way, Suite 300, Reno, NV 89502; tel. 775/687–7700; FAX. 775/687–7707; Debra Scott, Executive Director

**Nevada State Board of Osteopathic Medicine,** 901 American Pacific Dr, Unit 180, Henderson, NV 89014; tel. 702/732–2147; FAX. 702/732–2079; Barbara Longo, Deputy Executive Director

## NEW HAMPSHIRE
The Honorable John Lynch, Governor, 603/271–2121

**Facility Licensure Agencies**

**Bureau of Health Facilities Administration, Office of Operations Support, Licensure and Regulation,** 129 Pleasant Street, Concord, NH 03301; tel. 603/271–9011; FAX. 603/271–4968; Michael Fleming, Bureau Chief

**Health Facilities Administration - Licensing,** 129 Pleasant Street, Concord, NH 03256; tel. 603/271–9305; FAX. 603/271–4968; Rodney Bascom, Chief of HFA-Licensing

**Health Agencies**

**Office of Health Services Planning and Review,** 29 Hazen Drive, Concord, NH 03301-6527; tel. 603/271–4606; FAX. 603/271–4141; Cindy Carrier, Managing Analyst

**Managed Care Agencies**

**Department of Health and Human Services, Division of Public Health Services,** 29 Hazen Drive, Concord, NH 03301-6521; tel. 603/271–4501; FAX. 603/271–4827; Dr. José T. Montero, Director

**Medical & Nursing Licensure Agencies**

**New Hampshire Board of Medicine,** Two Industrial Park Drive #8, Concord, NH 03301; tel. 603/271–1203; FAX. 603/271–6702; Penny Taylor, Administrator

**NH Board of Nursing,** 21 S. Fruit Street, Suite 16, Concord, NH 03301-2431; tel. 603/271–2323; FAX. 603/271–6605; Denise M. Nies

## NEW JERSEY
The Honorable Christopher Christie, Governor, 609/292–6000

**Facility Licensure Agencies**

**New Jersey Department of Health and Senior Services, Certificate of Need and Healthcare Facility Licensure,** PO Box 358, Trenton, NJ 08625-0358; tel. 609/292–8773; FAX. 609/292–3780; John A. Calabria, Director

**Health Agencies**

**New Jersey Department of Health and Senior Services, Office of the Commissioner,** PO Box 360, Trenton, NJ 08625-0360; tel. 609/292–7837; FAX. 609/292–0053; Mary O'Dowd, State Commissioner of Health and Senior Services

**Managed Care Agencies**

**Division of Medical Assistance and Health Services, Office of Managed Health Care,** PO Box 712, Trenton, NJ 08625-0712; tel. 609/588–2705; FAX. 609/588–6290; Karen Brodsky, Chief of Managed Care Contracting

**Medical & Nursing Licensure Agencies**

**New Jersey Board of Nursing,** 124 Halsey St, PO Box 45010, Newark, NJ 07101; tel. 973/504–6430; FAX. 973/648–3481; George Hebert, RN, MA, Executive Director

**New Jersey State Board of Medical Examiners,** PO Box 183, Trenton, NJ 08625-0183; tel. 609/826–7100; FAX. 609/826–7117; William V. Roeder, JD, Executive Director

## NEW MEXICO
The Honorable Susana Martinez, Governor, 505/476–2200

**Facility Licensure Agencies**

**New Mexico Department of Health, Health Facility Licensing and Certification Bureau,** 2040 S. Pacheco Street, 2nd Floor, Room 413, Santa Fe, NM 87505; tel. 505/476–9025; FAX. 505/476–9026; Judy Parks, Acting Director

**Health Agencies**

**New Mexico Department of Health,** 1190 S. Street Francis Drive, PO Box 26110, Santa Fe, NM 87502-6110; tel. 505/827–2613; FAX. 505/827–2530; Mary Altenberg, MPH, Bureau Chief

**Managed Care Agencies**

**Public Regulation Commission, Insurance Division,** PO Box 1269, 1120 Paseo de Peralta, Santa Fe, NM 87504-1269; tel. 505/827–4297; FAX. 505/476–0326; John G. Franchini, Superintendent of Insurance

**Medical & Nursing Licensure Agencies**

**New Mexico Board of Osteopathic Medical Examiners,** 2550 Cerrillos Rd., Second Floor, Santa Fe, NM 87505; tel. 505/476–4622; FAX. 505/476–4665; Santos R. Molano, Licensing Administrator

**New Mexico Medical Board,** 2055 S. Pacheco, Building 400, Santa Fe, NM 87505; tel. 505/476–2220; FAX. 505/476–7237; Lynn S. Hart, Executive Director

**Section C**

**State of New Mexico Board of Nursing,** 6301 Indian School NE, Suite 710, Albuquerque, NM 87110; tel. 505/841–8340; FAX. 505/841–8347; Nancy Darbro, PhD, APRN, RN, CNS, Executive Director

### NEW YORK
**The Honorable Andrew Cuomo, Governor, 518/474–7516**

**Facility Licensure Agencies**

**Center for Health Care Quality & Surveillance, New York State Department of Health,** Office of Long Term Care, 875 Central Ave., Albany, NY 12206; tel. 518/402–5673; FAX. 518/408–1636; Mark L. Kissinger, Director

**Division of Certification and Surveillance,** 855 Central Ave, Albany, NY 12206; tel. 518/402–1004; FAX. 518/402–1010; Mary Ellen Hennessy, Director

**New York State Department of Health, Office of Health Systems Management,** Corning Tower, Empire State Plaza, Albany, NY 12237; tel. 518/474–7028; FAX. 518/486–2564; Lora K. Lefebvre, Deputy Director

**Health Agencies**

**New York State Department of Health,** Empire State Plaza, Corning Tower, Room 1495, Albany, NY 12237; tel. 518/474–2011; FAX. 518/474–5450; Nirav R. Shah, MD, Commissioner of Health

**Managed Care Agencies**

**NYS DOH, Bureau of Managed Care Certification and Surveillance,** Room 1911 Corning Tower, Empire State Plaza, Albany, NY 12237; tel. 518/474–5515; FAX. 518/473–3583; Nina Daratsos, Director

**Medical & Nursing Licensure Agencies**

**New York State Board for Nursing NY State Education Department, Office of the Professions,** 89 Washington Avenue, Albany, NY 12234-1000; tel. 518/474–3817; FAX. 518/474–3706; Suzanne Sullivan, RN, Executive Secretary

**New York State Board of Medicine,** 89 Washington Avenue, West Wing, Third Floor, Albany, NY 12234; tel. 518/474–3817; FAX. 518/486–4846; Walter Ramos, Executive Secretary

**New York State Education Department, Office of the Professions,** State Education Building, 2nd Floor, Albany, NY 12234; tel. 518/474–3817; FAX. 518/474–1449; Susan Naccarato, Acting Director of Professional Licensing

### NORTH CAROLINA
**The Honorable Beverly Perdue, Governor, 919/733–4240**

**Facility Licensure Agencies**

**Department of Health and Human Services, Division of Health Service Regulation,** 2712 Mail Service Center, 1205 Umstead Drive, Raleigh, NC 27699; tel. 919/855–4620; FAX. 919/715–8476; Azzie Y. Conley, Chief, Acute and Home Care Licensure and Certification

**Health Agencies**

**NC Department of Health and Human Services,** 2001 Mail Service Center, Raleigh, NC 27699-2001; tel. 919/855–4800; FAX. 919/715–4645; Amanda Parks

**Managed Care Agencies**

**North Carolina Department of Insurance, Financial Evaluation Division,** 1203 Mail Service Center, 430 N. Salisbury Street, Raleigh, NC 27699-1203; tel. 919/733–2205; FAX. 919/733–2206; Jackie Obusek, Assistant Chief Financial Analyst

**Medical & Nursing Licensure Agencies**

**North Carolina Board of Nursing,** PO Box 2129, 4516 Lake Boone Trail, Raleigh, NC 27602-2129; tel. 919/782–3211; FAX. 919/781–9461; Julia L. George, RN, MSN, FRE, Executive Director

**North Carolina Medical Board,** 1203 Front Street, Raleigh, NC 27609; tel. 919/326–1100; FAX. 919/326–1130; David Henderson, Executive Director

### NORTH DAKOTA
**The Honorable Jack Dalrymple, Governor, 701/328–2200**

**Facility Licensure Agencies**

**North Dakota Department of Health, Division of Health Facilities,** 600 East Boulevard Avenue, Department 301, Bismarck, ND 58505-0200; tel. 701/328–2352; FAX. 701/328–1890; Darleen Bartz, PhD, Chief - Health Resources Section

**Health Agencies**

**State Department of Health,** 600 East Boulevard Avenue, Bismarck, ND 58505-0200; tel. 701/328–2372; FAX. 701/328–4727; Londa Rodahl, Administrative Assistant

**Managed Care Agencies**

**North Dakota Insurance Department,** 600 East Boulevard Avenue, Department 401, Bismarck, ND 58505-0320; tel. 701/328–2440; FAX. 701/328–4880; Adam Hamm, Commissioner

**Medical & Nursing Licensure Agencies**

**North Dakota Board of Nursing,** 919 South Seventh Street, Suite 504, Bismarck, ND 58504-5881; tel. 701/328–9777; FAX. 701/328–9785; Constance Kalanek, PhD, RN, Executive Director

**North Dakota State Board of Medical Examiners,** 418 East Broadway Avenue, Suite 12, Bismarck, ND 58501; tel. 701/328–6500; FAX. 701/328–6505; Duane Houdek, JD, Executive Secretary

### OHIO
**The Honorable John Kasich, Governor, 614/466–3555**

**Facility Licensure Agencies**

**Division of Quality Assurance, Ohio Department of Health,** 246 North High Street, Columbus, OH 43215; tel. 614/466–7857; FAX. 614/644–0208; Rebecca Maust, Chief, Division of Quality Assurance

**Health Agencies**

**Ohio Department of Health,** 246 North High Street, Columbus, OH 43215; tel. 614/466–3543; FAX. 614/644–0085; Theodore E. Wymyslo, MD, Director

**Managed Care Agencies**

**The Ohio Department of Insurance,** 50 W. Town Street, Third Floor, Suite 300, Columbus, OH 43215; tel. 614/644–2661; FAX. 614/728–5238; William Preston, Chief, Life and Health Division

**Medical & Nursing Licensure Agencies**

**Ohio Board of Nursing,** 17 South High Street, Suite 400, Columbus, OH 43215-7410; tel. 614/466–3947; FAX. 614/466–0388; Betsy J. Houchen, JD, RN, MS, Executive Director

**State Medical Board of Ohio,** 30 E. Broad Street, Third Floor, Columbus, OH 43215-6127; tel. 614/466–3934; FAX. 614/728–5946; Richard A. Whitehouse, Esq., Executive Director

### OKLAHOMA
**The Honorable Mary Fallin, Governor, 405/521–2342**

**Facility Licensure Agencies**

**Oklahoma State Department of Health, Protective Health Services, Medical Facilities Service,** 1000 Northeast 10th Street, Oklahoma City, OK 73117-1299; tel. 405/271–6576; FAX. 405/271–1308; Tom Welin, Chief of Medical Facilities Services

**Health Agencies**

**State Department of Health,** 1000 Northeast 10th St, Room 1114, Oklahoma City, OK 73117-1299; tel. 405/271–6576; FAX. 405/271–1308; Tom Welin, Chief, Medical Facilities

**Managed Care Agencies**

**Oklahoma State Department of Health, Managed Care Systems - Health Resources Development Service,** 1000 Northeast 10th Street, Room 1011, Oklahoma City, OK 73117-1299; tel. 405/271–6868; FAX. 405/271–7360; John W. Judge, Jr.

**Medical & Nursing Licensure Agencies**

**Oklahoma Board of Nursing,** 2915 N. Classen Boulevard, Suite 524, Oklahoma City, OK 73106; tel. 405/962–1800; FAX. 405/962–1821; Kimberly Glazier, M.Ed., RN, Executive Director

**Oklahoma State Board of Medical Licensure and Supervision,** 101 NE 51st Street, PO Box 18256, Oklahoma City, OK 73154-0256; tel. 405/962–1400; FAX. 405/962–1499; Lyle Kelsey, MBA, CMBE, Executive Director

**Oklahoma State Board of Osteopathic Examiners,** 4848 North Lincoln Boulevard, Suite 100, Oklahoma City, OK 73105-3321; tel. 405/528–8625; FAX. 405/557–0653; Deborah J. Bruce, Executive Director

### OREGON
**The Honorable John Kitzhaber, Governor, 503/373–1027**

**Facility Licensure Agencies**

**Health Care Regulation and Quality Improvement,** 800 Northeast Oregon Street, Suite 305, Portland, OR 97232; tel. 971/673–0540; FAX. 971/673–0556; Dana Selover, MD MPH

**Health Agencies**

**Oregon Health Authority-Public Health Division, Health Care Regulation and Quality Improvement,** 800 NE Oregon Street, Suite 305, Portland, OR 97232; tel. 971/673–0540; FAX. 971/673–0556; Dana Selover, Section Manager

**Managed Care Agencies**

**Department of Consumer and Business Services, Insurance Division,** PO Box 14480, 350 Winter Street NE, Salem, OR 97309-0405; tel. 503/947–7980; FAX. 503/378–4351; Patrick Allen, Commissioner

**Medical & Nursing Licensure Agencies**

**Oregon Medical Board,** 1500 SW First Avenue, Suite 620, Portland, OR 97201-5847; tel. 971/673–2700; FAX. 971/673–2670; Kathleen Haley, JD, Executive Director

**Oregon State Board of Nursing,** 17938 SW Upper Boones Ferry Road, Portland, OR 97224-7012; tel. 971/673–0685; FAX. 971/673–0684; Holly Mercer, Executive Director

### PENNSYLVANIA
**The Honorable Tom Corbett, Governor, 717/787–2500**

**Facility Licensure Agencies**

**Bureau of Facility Licensure and Certification,** 625 Forster Street, Room 932, Harrisburg, PA 17120; tel. 717/787–8015; FAX. 717/705–7298; Ann Chronister, Bureau Director

**Department of Health, Division of Home Health,** 132 Kline Plaza, Suite A, Harrisburg, PA 17104; tel. 717/783–1379; FAX. 717/772–0232; Linda Chamberlain, MS, BSN, RN, Division Director

**Division of Acute and Ambulatory Care, Pennsylvania Department of Health,** Health & Welfare Building, Room 532, Harrisburg, PA 17120; tel. 717/783–8980; FAX. 717/705–6663; Joanne Salsgiver, Director

**Health Agencies**

**Pennsylvania Department of Health,** Health and Welfare Building, Suite 802, Harrisburg, PA 17120; tel. 877/724–3258; FAX. 717/787–0191; Eli N. Avila, MD, JD, MPH, FCLM, Secretary

**Managed Care Agencies**

**Pennsylvania Insurance Department, Office of Corporate and Financial Regulation,** Company Licensing Division, 1345 Strawberry Square, Harrisburg, PA 17120; tel. 717/787–2317; FAX. 717/787–8557; Robert E. Brackbill, Chief of Company Licensing Division

**Medical & Nursing Licensure Agencies**

**Pennsylvania Department of Health, Quality Assurance,** 625 Forster Street, Eighth Floor West, Harrisburg, PA 17120; tel. 717/783–1078; FAX. 717/525–5506; Miranda Kerstetter, Executive Secretary

**Pennsylvania State Board of Medicine,** PO Box 2649, Harrisburg, PA 17105-2649; tel. 717/783–1400; FAX. 717/787–7769; Tammy Dougherty, Administrator

**Pennsylvania State Board of Nursing,** PO Box 2649, Harrisburg, PA 17105-2649; tel. 717/783–7142; FAX. 717/783–0822; Laurette Keiser, Executive Secretary

**Pennsylvania State Board of Osteopathic Medicine,** PO Box 2649, Harrisburg, PA 17105-2649; tel. 717/783–4858; FAX. 717/787–7769; Tammy Dougherty, Administrator

### RHODE ISLAND
**The Honorable Lincoln Chafee, Governor, 401/222–2080**

**Facility Licensure Agencies**

**Rhode Island Department of Health, Division of Facilities Regulation,** Three Capitol Hill, Room 306, Providence, RI 02908-5097; tel. 401/222–2566; FAX. 401/222–3999; Raymond Rusin, Chief of Facilities Regulation

**Health Agencies**

**Department of Health,** Three Capitol Hill, Providence, RI 02908-5097; tel. 401/222–5960; FAX. 401/277–6548; Leonard Green, Deputy Director

**Managed Care Agencies**

**Department of Business Regulation, Insurance Regulation Division,** 1511 Pontiac Avenue, Cranston, RI 02920; tel. 401/462–9520; FAX. 401/462–9602; Paul McGreevy, Director

**Medical & Nursing Licensure Agencies**

**Division of Professional Regulation, Rhode Island Department of Health,** Three Capitol Hill, Suite 104, Providence, RI 02908-5097; tel. 401/222-2827; FAX. 401/222-1272; Michael Simoli, Supervisor

**Rhode Island Board of Medical Licensure & Discipline,** Three Capitol Hill, Room 205, Providence, RI 02908-5097; tel. 401/222-3855; FAX. 401/222-2158; James McDonald, MD, Chief Admistrative Officer

**Rhode Island Board of Nurse Registration and Nursing Education,** 3 Capitol Hill, Room 105, Providence, RI 02908-5097; tel. 401/222-5700; FAX. 401/222-3352

**SOUTH CAROLINA**
**The Honorable Nikki Haley, Governor,** 803/734-2100

**Facility Licensure Agencies**

**SC Department of Health & Environmental Control, Division of Health Licensing,** 2600 Bull Street, Columbia, SC 29201; tel. 803/545-4370; FAX. 803/545-4212; Gwendolyn C. Thopmson, Director

**Health Agencies**

**Department of Health and Human Services,** 1801 Main Street, P.O. Box 8206, Columbia, SC 29202-8206; tel. 888/549-0820; FAX. 803/255-8235; Anthony E. Keck, Director

**Managed Care Agencies**

**South Carolina Department of Insurance, Financial Regulation & Solvency Services,** 1201 Main Street Street, Suite 1000, Capitol Center, Columbia, SC 29201; tel. 803/737-6199; FAX. 803/737-6232; Lee Hill, Financial Analyst

**Medical & Nursing Licensure Agencies**

**Department of Labor, Licensing and Regulation, State Board of Nursing for South Carolina,** PO Box 12367, 110 Centerview Drive, Columbia, SC 29211-2367; tel. 803/896-4550; FAX. 803/896-4515; Nancy Murphy, Administrator

**South Carolina Board of Medical Examiners,** Synergy Business Park, Kingstree Building, 110 Centerview Drive, Columbia, SC 29211; tel. 803/896-4500; FAX. 803/896-4515; Bruce Duke, Administrator

**SOUTH DAKOTA**
**The Honorable Dennis Daugaard, Governor,** 605/773-3212

**Facility Licensure Agencies**

**Office of Health Care Facilities Licensure and Certification, State Department of Health,** 615 E. Fourth Street, Pierre, SD 57501-1700; tel. 605/773-3356; FAX. 605/773-6667; Bob Stahl, Administrator

**Health Agencies**

**South Dakota Department of Health,** 600 East Capitol, Pierre, SD 57501-2536; tel. 605/773-3361; FAX. 605/773-5683; Doneen B. Hollingsworth, Secretary of Health

**Managed Care Agencies**

**Division of Insurance,** 445 E. Capitol Avenue, Pierre, SD 57501; tel. 605/773-3563; FAX. 605/773-5369; Melissa Klemann, Senior Policy Analyst

**Medical & Nursing Licensure Agencies**

**South Dakota Board of Medical and Osteopathic Examiners,** 101 N. Main Avenue, Suite 301, Sioux Falls, SD 57104; tel. 605/367-7781; FAX. 605/367-7786; Margaret B. Hansen, PA-C, MPAS, Executive Director

**South Dakota Board of Nursing,** 4305 South Louise Avenue, Suite 201, Sioux Falls, SD 57106; tel. 605/362-2760; FAX. 605/362-2768; Gloria Damgaard, RN, MS, Executive Director

**TENNESSEE**
**The Honorable Bill Haslam, Governor,** 615/741-2001

**Facility Licensure Agencies**

**Board for Licensing Health Care Facilities,** 227 French Landing Drive, Metro Center, Nashville, TN 37243; tel. 615/741-7221; FAX. 615/253-1535; Ann Rutherford Reed, RN, BSN, MBA, Director of Licensure

**Health Agencies**

**Department of Health,** Cordell Hull Building, 3rd Floor, 425 Fifth Avenue, N., Nashville, TN 37243; tel. 615/741-3111; FAX. 615/741-2491; John J. Dreyzehner, MD, MPH, FACOEM, Commissioner

**Managed Care Agencies**

**Department of Commerce and Insurance, Insurance Division,** 500 James Robertson Parkway, Nashville, TN 37243-1135; tel. 615/741-1670; FAX. 615/532-2788; Mark Jaquish, Insurance Analysis Director

**Medical & Nursing Licensure Agencies**

**Department of Health Bureau of Health Licensure and Regulation,** 220 Athens Way, Suite 104, Nashville, TN 37243; tel. 615/741-8404; FAX. 615/741-5542; Michelle J. Long, JD, Assistant Commissioner

**Tennessee Board of Medical Examiners,** 227 French Landing, Suite 300, Heritage Place Metro Center, Nashville, TN 37243; tel. 800/778-4123; FAX. 615/253-4484; Mitchell Mutter, MD, President

**Tennessee Board of Nursing,** 227 French Landing Suite 300, Heritage Place Metro Center, Nashville, TN 37243; tel. 800/778-4123; FAX. 615/741-7899; Elizabeth J. Lund, MSN, RN, Executive Director

**Tennessee Medical Laboratory Board,** 227 French Landing, Suite 300, Nashville, TN 37247; tel. 615/532-5128; FAX. 615/741-7698; Lynda S. England, Director

**Tennessee State Board of Osteopathic Examination, Office of Licensing Health Care Professionals,** 227 French Landing, Heritage Place Metro Center #300, Nashville, TN 37243; tel. 800/778-4123; FAX. 615/253-4484; Jill Robinson, DO, President

**TEXAS**
**The Honorable Rick Perry, Governor,** 512/463-2000

**Facility Licensure Agencies**

**Texas Department of Aging and Disability Services,** 701 W. 51st Street, PO Box 149030, Austin, TX 78714-9030; tel. 512/438-3011; FAX. 512/438-2738; Chris Taylor, Commissioner

**Texas Department of State Health Services, Facility Licensing Group,** Mail Code: 2835, P.O. Box 149347, Austin, TX 78714-9347; tel. 512/834-6648; FAX. 512/834-4514; Ellen Cooper, MSW, RN, MSN, Manager

**Health Agencies**

**Texas Department of State Health Services,** 1100 West 49th Street, Austin, TX 78756; tel. 512/776-7363; FAX. 512/776-7477; David L. Lakey, MD, Commissioner

**Managed Care Agencies**

**Texas Department of Insurance,** Mail Code 103-6A, P.O. Box 149104, Austin, TX 78714-9104; tel. 512/322-4266; FAX. 512/490-1013; Debra Diaz-Lara, Director

**Medical & Nursing Licensure Agencies**

**Texas Board of Nursing,** 333 Guadalupe, Suite 3-460, Austin, TX 78701; tel. 512/305-7400; FAX. 512/305-7401; Katherine A. Thomas, MN, RN, FAAN, Executive Director

**Texas State Board of Medical Examiners,** 333 Guadalupe, Tower Three, Suite 610, PO Box 2018, Austin, TX 78768-2018; tel. 512/305-7010; FAX. 512/305-7008; Mari Robinson, JD, Executive Director

**UTAH**
**The Honorable Gary R. Herbert, Governor,** 801/538-1000

**Facility Licensure Agencies**

**Utah Department of Health, Health Facility Licensing and Medicare Certification,** PO Box 144103, 288 North 1460 West, Salt Lake City, UT 84114-4103; tel. 801/538-6158; FAX. 801/538-6163; Joel Hoffman, Director

**Health Agencies**

**Utah Department of Health,** PO Box 141000, Salt Lake City, UT 84114-1000; tel. 801/538-6111; FAX. 801/538-6306; W. David Patton, Executive Director

**Managed Care Agencies**

**Utah Insurance Department,** State Office Building, Room 3110, Salt Lake City, UT 84114-6901; tel. 801/538-3803; FAX. 801/538-3829; Jilane Whitby, Information Specialist

**Medical & Nursing Licensure Agencies**

**Utah Physicians Licensing Board, Division of Occupational and Professional Licensure,** Heber M. Wells Building, First Floor, 160 East 300 South, Salt Lake City, UT 84114-6741; tel. 801/530-6621; FAX. 801/530-6511; Noel Taxin, Bureau Manager

**Utah State Board of Nursing,** 160 East 300 South, Box 146741, Salt Lake City, UT 84114-6741; tel. 801/530-6628; FAX. 801/530-6511; Laura Poe, Executive Administrator

**VERMONT**
**The Honorable Peter Shumlin, Governor,** 802/828-3333

**Facility Licensure Agencies**

**Hospice and Palliative Care, Council of Vermont,** 10 Main Street, Montpelier, VT 05602; tel. 802/229-0579; FAX. 802/223-6218; Virginia L. Fry, Executive Director

**Medical Practice Board, Vermont Department of Health,** 108 Cherry Street, PO Box 70, Burlington, VT 05402; tel. 802/657-4220; FAX. 802/657-4227; David Herlihy, Director

**Health Agencies**

**Vermont Department of Health,** 108 Cherry Street, P.O. Box 70, Burlington, VT 05402; tel. 802/863-7280; FAX. 802/951-1275; Harry L. Chen, MD, Commissioner

**Managed Care Agencies**

**Green Mountain Care Board,** 89 Main Street, 3rd Floor, Montpelier, VT 05620; tel. 802/828-2177

**Medical & Nursing Licensure Agencies**

**Licensing and Protection,** Ladd Hall, 103 South Main Street, Waterbury, VT 05671-2306; tel. 802/241-2345; FAX. 802/241-2358; Frances Keeler, Director

**Vermont Board of Nursing,** National Life Building, North Fl 2, Montpelier, VT 05620-3402; tel. 802/828-2396; FAX. 802/828-2484; Linda Davidson, MS, APRN, Executive Director

**Vermont Board of Osteopathic Physicians and Surgeons, Office of Professional Regulation,** National Life Building, North Fl 2, Montpelier, VT 05620-3402; tel. 802/828-2373; FAX. 802/828-2465; Kristy Pirie, Licensing Board Specialist

**Vermont Department of Disabilities Aging and Independent Living, Division of Licensing and Protection,** Ladd Hall, 103 South Main Street, Waterbury, VT 05671-2306; tel. 802/871-3317; FAX. 802/871-3318; Frances L. Keeler, RN, MSN, DBA, Director

**VIRGINIA**
**The Honorable Bob McDonnell, Governor,** 804/786-2211

**Facility Licensure Agencies**

**Office of Licensure and Certification, Virginia Department of Health,** 9960 Mayland Drive, Suite 401, Richmond, VA 23233; tel. 804/367-2102; FAX. 804/527-4502; Erik Bodin, Acting Director

**Health Agencies**

**Virginia Department of Health,** PO Box 2448, Richmond, VA 23218; tel. 804/864-7001; FAX. 804/864-7022; Karen Remley, MD, MBA, State Health Commissioner

**Virginia Department of Health, Division of Certificate of Public Need,** 9960 Mayland Drive, Suite 401, Richmond, VA 23233; tel. 804/367-2126; FAX. 804/527-4501; Erik O. Bodin, III, Director

**Managed Care Agencies**

**State Corporation Commission, Bureau of Insurance,** PO Box 1157, 1300 East Main St., Richmond, VA 23218; tel. 804/371-9741; FAX. 804/371-9511; Connie Doung, Senior Financial Analyst

**Medical & Nursing Licensure Agencies**

**Virginia Board of Medicine,** Perimeter Center, 9960 Mayland Drive, Richmond, VA 23233-1463; tel. 804/367-4600; FAX. 804/527-4426; William L. Harp, MD, Executive Director

**Virginia Board of Nursing,** Perimeter Center, 9960 Mayland Drive, Henrico, VA 23233-1463; tel. 804/367-4515; FAX. 804/527-4455; Jay P. Douglas, RN, MSM, CSAC, Executive Director

**WASHINGTON**
**The Honorable Chris Gregoire, Governor,** 360/902-4111

**Facility Licensure Agencies**

**Credentialing, Washington Department of Health,** PO Box 47877, 310 Israel Rd., SE, Olympia, WA 98504-7852; tel. 360/236-4900; FAX. 360/236-4909; Diane Young, Credentialing Manager

**State Department of Health, Investigations and Inspections Office,** PO Box 47874, Olympia, WA 98504-7874; tel. 360/236-2920; FAX. 360/586-0123; Linda Foss, Executive Manager of Clinical Care Facilities

**Section C**

**Health Agencies**

**Washington State Department of Health,** PO Box 47890, Olympia, WA 98504-7890; tel. 360/236–4501; FAX. 360/586–7424; Mary Selecky, Secretary of Health

**Managed Care Agencies**

**Office of the Insurance Commissioner, Rates & Forms, Healthcare, Life, Disability,** PO Box 40255, Olympia, WA 98504-0255; tel. 360/725–7111; FAX. 360/586–0759; Janis LaFlash, Manager, Health and Disability

**Medical & Nursing Licensure Agencies**

**Health Systems Quality Assurance, Department of Health,** 111 Israel Road, SE, Mail Stop 47850, Tumwater, WA 98501; tel. 360/236–4600; FAX. 360/236–4626; Karen Jensen, Assistant Secretary

**Washington State Board of Osteopathic Medicine and Surgery, Department of Health,** 310 Israel Rd., SE, PO Box 47852, Olympia, WA 98504-7852; tel. 360/236–4700; FAX. 360/236–2901; Erin Obenland, Program Manager

**Washington State Department of Health, Medical Quality Assurance Commission,** PO Box 47866, Olympia, WA 98504-7866; tel. 360/236–2750; FAX. 360/236–2795; Julie Kitten

**Washington State Nursing Care Quality Assurance Commission, Department of Health,** Point Plaza East, 310 Israel Rd. SE, Olympia, WA 98504-7864; tel. 360/236–4700; FAX. 360/236–4818; Paula Meyer, RN, MSN, Executive Director

**WEST VIRGINIA**
**The Honorable Earl Ray Tomblin, Governor, 304/558–2000**

**Facility Licensure Agencies**

**Office of Health Facility Licensure and Certification, West Virginia Division of Health,** 408 Leon Sullivan Way, Charleston, WV 25301-3718; tel. 304/558–0050; FAX. 304/558–2515; Anita Barnhouse, Program Manager II

**Health Agencies**

**Department of Health and Human Resources,** One Davis Square, Suite 100-East, Charleston, WV 25301; tel. 304/558–0684; FAX. 304/558–1130; Michael Lewis, Cabinet Secretary

**West Virginia Health Care Authority,** 100 Dee Drive, Charleston, WV 25311-1600; tel. 304/558–7000; FAX. 304/558–7001; James L. Pitrolo, Chair

**Managed Care Agencies**

**West Virginia Offices of the Insurance Commissioner,** PO Box 50540, 1124 Smith Street, Charleston, WV 25301; tel. 304/558–3354; FAX. 304/558–3869; Jason Butcher, Director of Communications

**Medical & Nursing Licensure Agencies**

**Office of Chief Medical Examiner,** 619 Virginia Street West, Charleston, WV 25302; tel. 304/558–6920; FAX. 304/558–7886; James A. Kaplan, MD, Chief Medical Examiner

**West Virginia Board of Examiners for Registered Professional Nurses,** 101 Dee Drive, Suite 102, Charleston, WV 25311-1620; tel. 304/558–3596; FAX. 304/558–3666; Laura S. Rhodes, RN, MSN, Executive Director

**West Virginia Board of Osteopathic Medicine,** 405 Capitol Street, Suite 402, Charleston, WV 25301; tel. 304/558–6095; FAX. 304/558–6096; Diana Shepard, Executive Director

**West Virginia State Board of Examiners for Licensed Practical Nurses,** 101 Dee Drive, Suite 100, Charleston, WV 25311; tel. 304/558–3572; FAX. 304/558–4367; Lanette Anderson, MSN, JD, RN, Executive Director

**WISCONSIN**
**The Honorable Scott Walker, Governor, 608/266–1212**

**Facility Licensure Agencies**

**Division of Quality Assurance, Department of Health Services,** One West Wilson Street, PO Box 2969, Madison, WI 53701-2969; tel. 608/267–7185; FAX. 608/267–0352; Otis Woods, Administrator

**Health Agencies**

**Department of Health Services,** PO Box 7850, Madison, WI 53707-7850; tel. 608/266–9622; FAX. 608/266–7882; Dennis G. Smith

**Managed Care Agencies**

**Office of the Commissioner of Insurance,** 125 S. Webster Street, P.O. Box 7873, Madison, WI 53707-7873; tel. 608/266–3585; FAX. 608/266–9935; Theodore Nickel, Commissioner

**Medical & Nursing Licensure Agencies**

**Wisconsin Department of Saftey and Professional Services,** 1400 East Washington Avenue, Room 178, PO Box 8935, Madison, WI 53708-8935; tel. 608/266–2112; FAX. 608/267–3816; Dan Williams, Director, Bureau of Health Services Professions

**Wisconsin Medical Examining Board,** 1400 East Washington Avenue, PO Box 8935, Madison, WI 53708; tel. 608/261–2378; FAX. 608/267–3816; Tom Ryan, Executive Director

**WYOMING**
**The Honorable Matthew Mead, Governor, 307/777–7434**

**Facility Licensure Agencies**

**Wyoming Department of Health, Healthcare Licensing and Surveys,** 6101 Yellowstone Road, Suite 186C, Cheyenne, WY 82002; tel. 307/777–7123; FAX. 307/777–7127; Ron Pearson, State Survey Agency Director

**Health Agencies**

**Department of Health,** 401 Hathaway Building, Cheyenne, WY 82002; tel. 307/777–7656; FAX. 307/777–7439; Thomas O. Forslund, Director

**Managed Care Agencies**

**State of Wyoming Department of Insurance,** 106 E. Sixth Avenue, Cheyenne, WY 82002; tel. 307/777–7401; FAX. 307/777–2446; Ken Vines, Commissioner

**Medical & Nursing Licensure Agencies**

**Wyoming Board of Medicine,** 320 West 25th Street, Suite 200, Cheyenne, WY 82002; tel. 307/778–7053; FAX. 307/778–2069; Deborah Gillette, Licensing Manager

**Wyoming State Board of Nursing,** 1810 Pioneer Avenue, Cheyenne, WY 82002; tel. 307/777–7601; FAX. 307/777–3519; Mary Kay Goetter, PhD, RNC, NEA-BC

# U.S. Associated Areas

**GUAM**
**Health Agencies**

**Department of Public Health and Social Services,** 123 Chalan Kareta, Mangilao, GU 96913-6304; tel. 671/735–7173; FAX. 671/734–5910; James W. Gillan, Director, DPHSS

**Managed Care Agencies**

**Department of Public Health and Social Services, Government of Guam,** 123 Chalan Kareta Route 10, Mangilao, GU 96923; tel. 671/735–7102; FAX. 671/734–5910; J. Peter Roberto, ACSW, Director

**Medical & Nursing Licensure Agencies**

**Guam Board of Medical Examiners, Health Professional Licensing Office,** 651 Legacy Square Commerical Complex, Rte. 10, Suite 9, Mangilao, GU 96913; tel. 671/735–7406; FAX. 671/735–7413; MaryLou Loualhati, Acting Administrator

**Guam Board of Nurse Examiners Department of Public Health and Social Services,** 123 Chalan Kareta, South Route 10, Mangilao, GU 96913-6304; tel. 671/733–7408; FAX. 671/477–4733; Margaret Guerrero

**PUERTO RICO**
**Facility Licensure Agencies**

**Department of Health Commonwealth of Puerto Rico, Departamento de Salud,** Box 70184, Calle Maga, Edifico E altos, San Juan, PR 00936-0184; tel. 787/274–7676; FAX. 787/250–6547; Jaime Rivera Dueno, MD, Secretary of Health

**Health Agencies**

**Puerto Rico Department of Health,** Building A - Medical Center, Call Box 70184, San Juan, PR 00936-8184; tel. 787/274–6822; FAX. 787/767–8341; Rosa Perez-Perdomo, MD, MPH, PhD, Secretary of Health

**Managed Care Agencies**

**Office of the Commissioner of Insurance,** B5 Calle Tabonuco, Suite 216, PMB 356, Guaynabo, PR 00968-3029; tel. 787/304–8686; FAX. 787/273–6365; Ana Lopez, Chief Deputy Commisioner

**Medical & Nursing Licensure Agencies**

**Junta de Licenciatmiento y Disciplina Medica,** PO Box 13969, San Juan, PR 00908; tel. 787/999–8989; Ernesto Caballero del Valle, Executive Director

**Puerto Rico Board of Medical Examiners,** PO Box 13969, San Juan, PR 00908; tel. 787/999–8989; FAX. 787/792–4436; Ernesto Caballero del Valle, Executive Director

**VIRGIN ISLANDS**
**Health Agencies**

**Virgin Islands Department of Health,** Charles Harwood Complex, 3500 Richmond Est, St. Croix, VI 00820-4370; tel. 340/773–6551; FAX. 340/773–1376; Fern Clark, MPH, Acting Commissioner of Health

# Canada

**ALBERTA**
**Medical & Nursing Licensure Agencies**

**College of Physicians & Surgeons of Alberta,** Suite 2700, 10020 100th Street, NW, Edmonton, AB T5J 0N3; tel. 7804234764; FAX. 7804200651; Dr. Trevor Theman, Registrar

**MANITOBA**
**Health Agencies**

**Department of Health,** 302 Legislative Building, 450 Broadway, Winnipeg, MB R3C 0V8; tel. 204/945–3731; FAX. 204/945–0441; Honourable Theresa Oswald, Minister

**Medical & Nursing Licensure Agencies**

**College of Physicians and Surgeons of Manitoba,** 1000-1661 Portage Avenue, Winnipeg, MB R3J 3T7; tel. 2047744344; FAX. 2047740750; William D.B. Pope, MD, Registrar

**NEW BRUNSWICK**
**Medical & Nursing Licensure Agencies**

**College of Physicians and Surgeons of New Brunswick,** One Hampton Road, Suite 300, Rothesay, NB E2E 5K8; tel. 5068495050; FAX. 5068495069; Dr. Ed Schollenberg, Registrar

**NEWFOUNDLAND**
**Health Agencies**

**Department of Health and Community Services,** Confederation Building (West Block), P.O. Box 8700, St. John's, NF A1B 4J6; tel. 709/729–3124; FAX. 709/729–0121; Susan Sullivan, Minister, Health and Community Services

**NOVA SCOTIA**
**Health Agencies**

**Department of Health and Wellness,** PO Box 488, Halifax, NS B3J 2R8; tel. 902/424–3377; FAX. 902/424–0559; Maureen MacDonald, Minister of Health & Wellness

**Medical & Nursing Licensure Agencies**

**College of Physicians and Surgeons of Nova Scotia, Office of the Registrar,** Suite 5005, 7071 Bayers Road, Halifax, NS B3L 2C2; tel. 9024225823; FAX. 9024225035; Gus Grant, MD, Registrar and Chief Executive Officer

**PRINCE EDWARD ISLAND**
**Medical & Nursing Licensure Agencies**

**College of Physicians and Surgeons of Prince Edward Island,** 14 Paramount Drive, Charlottetown, PE C1E 0C7; tel. 9025663861; FAX. 9025663986; C. Moyse, MD, Registrar

**QUEBEC**
**Health Agencies**

**Ministry of Health and Social Services,** Ministere de la Sante et des Services Sociaux, Quebec, PQ G1S 2M1; tel. 418/644–4545; Yves Bolduc, Minister

**SASKATCHEWAN**
**Health Agencies**

**Ministry of Health,** 3475 Albert Street, Third Floor, Regina, SK S4S 6X6; tel. 306/787–3696; FAX. 306/787–8310; Minister, The Hon. Don McMorris

**Medical & Nursing Licensure Agencies**

**College of Physicians and Surgeons of Saskatchewan,** 500 321A 21st Street, E., Saskatoon, SK S7K 0C1; tel. 3062447355; FAX. 3062440090; Karen Shaw, MD, Registrar

*The following list of freestanding ambulatory surgery centers was developed with the assistance of state government agencies and the individual facilities listed.*

*The AHA Guide contains two types of ambulatory surgery center listings; those that are hospital based and those that are freestanding. Hospital based ambulatory surgery centers are listed in section A of the AHA Guide and are identified by Facility Code F8 and F70.*

*We present this list simply as a convenient directory. Inclusion or omission of any organization's name indicates neither approval nor disapproval by Health Forum LLC, an American Hospital Association company.*

## United States

### ALABAMA
**Baptist Surgery Center,** 2035 East South Boulevard, Montgomery, AL 36111-0000; tel. 334/286-3180; FAX. 334/286-3381; Kay Catliffe, Nurse Manager

**Birmingham Surgery Center, Inc.,** 2621 19th Street, South, Homewood, AL 35209; tel. 205/271-8200; Kathy Houton, RN, Administrator

**Dothan Surgery Center,** 1450 Ross Clark Circle, SE, Suite 4, Dothan, AL 36301; tel. 334/793-3442; FAX. 334/793-3318; W. Berry Sowell, Chief Executive Officer and Administrator

**Florence Surgery Center, L.P.,** 103 Helton Court, Florence, AL 35630; tel. 256/760-0672; FAX. 256/766-4547; Jennifer Lathram, Administrator

**Gadsden Surgery Center,** 418 South Fifth Street, Gadsden, AL 35901; tel. 256/543-1253; FAX. 256/543-1260; Harriet Willoughby, Administrator

**Huntsville Endoscopy Center, Inc.,** 119 Longwood Drive, Huntsville, AL 35801; tel. 256/533-6488; FAX. 256/533-6495; Dalia Biggerstaff, RN, Clinical Director

**Montgomery Eye Surgery Center,** 2752 Zelda Road, Montgomery, AL 36106; tel. 334/270-9677; FAX. 334/213-0622; Deborah Cauthen, Administrator

**Montgomery Surgical Center,** 470 Taylor Road, Montgomery, AL 36117; tel. 334/284-9600; FAX. 334/284-4233; Linda Westhoff, Interim Administrator

**Outpatient Services East, Inc.,** 52 Medical Park Drive, E., Suite 401, Birmingham, AL 35235; tel. 205/838-3888; FAX. 205/314-2469; H. Alan Perry, President, Chairman of the Board

**The Kirklin Clinic,** 2000 Sixth Avenue, S., Birmingham, AL 35233; tel. 205/801-8000; Reid F. Jones, EVP and Sr. VP for Ambulatory Services

**The Surgery Center of Huntsville,** 721 Madison Street, Huntsville, AL 35801; tel. 256/533-4888; FAX. 256/532-9510; William Sammons, Chief Executive Officer

**Tuscaloosa Endoscopy Center,** 100 Rice Mine Road, N, Suite E, Tuscaloosa, AL 35406; tel. 205/345-0010; FAX. 205/752-1175; A. B. Reddy, MD, Medical Director

**Tuscaloosa Surgical Center,** 1400 McFarland Boulevard, N., Tuscaloosa, AL 35406; tel. 205/345-5500; Jeff Hayes, Administrator

### ALASKA
**Alaska Women's Health P.C.,** 4115 Lake Otis Parkway, Anchorage, AK 99508; tel. 907/563-7228; FAX. 907/563-6278; Carol Mitchell-Springer, President

**Geneva Woods Surgical Center,** 3730 Rhone Circle, Suite 100, Anchorage, AK 99508; tel. 907/562-4764; FAX. 907/561-8519; Barbara Cope, Administrator

**Pacific Cataract & Laser Institute,** 1600 "A" Street, Suite 200, Anchorage, AK 99501; tel. 907/272-2423; FAX. 907/272-2428

### ARIZONA
**Adobe Surgery Center,** 2585 North Wyatt Drive, Tucson, AZ 85712; tel. 520/721-2728; FAX. 520/720-0719; Sam E. Moussa, MD, Administrator

**Arizona Outpatient Surgery Center,** 6245 N. 16th Street, Phoenix, AZ 85016; tel. 602/274-1705; FAX. 602/253-4273

**Arizona Surgical Arts, Inc.,** 1245 North Wilmot Road, Tucson, AZ 85712; tel. 520/296-7550; FAX. 520/722-6937; Robert M. Dryden, MD

**Banner Canyon Springs Surgery Center,** 2940 E. Banner Gateway Drive, #100, Gilbert, AZ 85234; tel. 480/641-9292; Christine Casto, RN, Administrator

**Barnet Dulaney Perkin Eye Center,** 4800 N 22nd Street, Phoenix, AZ 85016; tel. 602/508-4721; FAX. 602/759-1336; Imelda Kelly, Director of Nursing

**CIGNA Healthplan of Arizona, Outpatient Surgery,** 755 East McDowell Road, Phoenix, AZ 85006; tel. 602/271-3020; Katie Rousey, RN Manager

**Cochise Eye and Laser, PC,** 2445 East Wilcox Drive, Sierra Vista, AZ 85635; tel. 520/458-8131; FAX. 520/458-0422; Sheree H. Christian, Administrator

**Cottonwood Day Surgery Center, Inc.,** 55 South Sixth Street, Cottonwood, AZ 86326; tel. 928/634-5118; FAX. 928/634-8522; Linda Davis, Administrator

**Desert Mountain Surgicenter,** 895 S. Dobson Rd., Ste 1, Chandler, AZ 85224-5721; tel. 480/899-3737; FAX. 480/899-6262; David M. Creech, MD

**Desert Samaritan Surgicenter,** 1500 South Dobson Road, Suite 101, Mesa, AZ 85202; tel. 602/835-3590; FAX. 480/835-8774; Brenda Mastopietro, Administrator

**Eye Institute at Boswell,** 10541 West Thunderbird Boulevard, Sun City, AZ 85351; tel. 602/933-3402; FAX. 602/972-5014; Jan Zellmann, Administrator

**Fifty-Ninth Avenue Surgical Facility, Ltd.,** 8608 North 59th Avenue, Glendale, AZ 85302; tel. 623/934-3211; FAX. 623/930-1891; Mark Gorman, Administrator

**Fishkind and Bakewell Eye Care and Surgery Center,** 5599 North Oracle Road, Tucson, AZ 85704; tel. 520/293-6740; FAX. 520/293-6771; Kathleen A. Brown, Surgery Center Supervisor

**Flagstaff Foot Doctors,** 421 North Humphries Street, Flagstaff, AZ 86001; tel. 928/774-4191; FAX. 888/464-1135; Anthony Rosales, MD, President

**Good Samaritan Surgicenter,** 1111 B East McDowell Road, Phoenix, AZ 85006; tel. 602/239-2776; FAX. 602/239-5352; Brenda Mastopietro, Administrator

**Havasu Foot and Ankle Surgi-Center,** 90 Riviera Drive, Lake Havasu, AZ 86403; tel. 928/855-7800; FAX. 928/855-5392; Robert Novack, DPM, Director

**Hodges Eye Care & Surgery Center,** 1502 North Tucson Boulevard, Tucson, AZ 85716; tel. 520/326-4321; FAX. 520/326-4736; Dr. Timothy L. Hodges, MD

**Kokopelli Eye Care, P.C.,** 2820 North Glassford Hill Road, Suite 101, Prescott Valley, AZ 86314; tel. 928/775-5606; FAX. 928/772-4999

**Kokopelli Eye Care, P.C.,** 412 Whipple Street, Prescott, AZ 86301; tel. 928/771-9000; FAX. 928/771-9460

**Metro Surgery Center, L.P.,** 3131 West Peoria Avenue, Phoenix, AZ 85029; tel. 602/375-1083; FAX. 602/789-6833; Diane Elmore, Administrator

**Outpatient Surgical Care, Ltd.,** 1530 West Glendale, Suite 105, Phoenix, AZ 85021; tel. 602/995-3395; FAX. 602/995-1853; Raymond Zimmerman, MD, Medical Director

**Phoenix Eye Surgical Center, LLC,** 5133 North Central Avenue, Suite 100, Phoenix, AZ 85012; tel. 602/279-2434; FAX. 602/279-6475; Sharon Stulstao, Administrator

**Physicians Surgery Center of Tempe, LLC,** 1940 East Southern Avenue, Tempe, AZ 85282; tel. 480/820-7101; FAX. 480/820-9291; Susan Vitort, Administrator

**Prescott Outpatient Surgery Center, LLP,** 815 Ainsworth Drive, Prescott, AZ 86301; tel. 602/778-9770; Derron DeRouin, Administrative Director

**Prescott Urocenter, Ltd.,** 811 Ainsworth, Suite 101, Prescott, AZ 86301; tel. 928/771-5282; FAX. 928/771-5283; Jo Clark, Billing

**Scottsdale Eye Surgery Center, P.C.,** 3320 North Miller Road, Scottsdale, AZ 85251; tel. 480/429-0700; FAX. 480/429-1700; Joyce Schweikert, Administrator

**Southwester Eye Center,** 2005 Injo, Suite 102, Lake Havasu City, AZ 86403-5874; tel. 928/505-3696; FAX. 928/505-6129; Gary Dillon, Director, Contract Services

**Southwestern Eye Center,** 2610 E. University Drive, Mesa, AZ 85213; tel. 480/892-8400; FAX. 480/892-9533; Gary Dillon, Director, Contract Services

**Southwestern Eye Center,** 1919 Florence Avenue, Kingman, AZ 86401; tel. 928/753-5454; FAX. 928/753-7790; Richard Hinton, Administrator

**Southwestern Eye Center,** 3321 E. Bell Road, Suite B12, Phoenix, AZ 85032-2755; tel. 602/787-9100; FAX. 602/787-9101; Gary Dillon, Director, Contract Services

**Southwestern Eye Center,** 3003 Highway 95 Ste 63, Bullhead City, AZ 86442-7860; tel. 928/763-7555; FAX. 928/763-7565; Gary Dillon, Director, Contract Services

**Southwestern Eye Center,** 270 S. Candy Lane, Cottonwood, AZ 86326-4164; tel. 928/634-4202; FAX. 928/634-5693; Gary Dillon, Director, Contract Services

**Southwestern Eye Center,** 2650 E. Show Low Lake Rd, Suite 2, Show Low, AZ 85901-7955; tel. 928/537-4240; FAX. 928/537-3892; Gary Dillon, Director, Contract Services

**Southwestern Eye Center,** 1600 Willow Creek Rd., Prescott, AZ 86301-1108; tel. 928/776-7477; FAX. 928/776-0693; Gary Dillon, Director, Contract Services

**Southwestern Eye Center,** 2242 W. 16th Street, Safford, AZ 85546-4081; tel. 928/428-0068; FAX. 928/428-0713; Gary Dillon, Director, Contract Services

**Southwestern Eye Center,** 1055 S. Stapley Drive, Mesa, AZ 85204-5013; tel. 480/833-9100; FAX. 480/833-6000; Gary Dillon, Director, Contract Services

**Southwestern Eye Center,** 10615 W. Thunderbird Bldg., A100, Sun City, AZ 85351-3018; tel. 623/977-9600; FAX. 623/977-9602; Gary Dillon, Director, Contract Services

**Southwestern Eye Center,** 75 Colonia De Salud A-100, Sierra Vista, AZ 85635-2487; tel. 520/459-6860; FAX. 520/459-6858; Gary Dillon, Director, Contract Services

**Southwestern Eye Center,** 2149 W. 24th Street, Yuma, AZ 85364-6163; tel. 928/726-4120; FAX. 928/341-0315; Gary Dillon, Director, Contract Services

**Southwestern Eye Center-Casa Grande,** 560 N. Camino Mercado, Suite 1, Casa Grande, AZ 85222; tel. 520/426-9224; FAX. 520/426-1554; Ellen Lopez, RN, Director of Surgical Services

**Southwestern Eye Surgicenter-Nogales,** 1815 North Mastick Way, Nogales, AZ 85621; tel. 520/761-3533; FAX. 520/281-1950; Gary Dillon, Director, Contract Services

**Summit Surgery & Recovery Care Center,** 1485 N. Turquoise Drive, #100, Flagstaff, AZ 86001; tel. 928/214-3211; FAX. 928/214-3219; Jantina Wilson, Administrator

**Sun City Endoscopy Center, Inc.,** 13203 North 103rd Avenue, Suite C 3, Sun City, AZ 85351; tel. 623/972-5083; FAX. 623/523-0505; Jagdish Patel, MD

**Surgery Center of Peoria,** 13260 North 94th Drive, Suite 200, Peoria, AZ 85381; tel. 623/933-2900; FAX. 623/933-0017; Kolette Al-Jamal, Administrator

**Surgi-Care,** 5115 North Central Avenue, Phoenix, AZ 85012; tel. 602/264-1818; FAX. 602/264-2172; Ellison F. Herro, MD, Administrator

**Swagel Wootton Eye Center,** 220 South 63rd Street, Mesa, AZ 85206; tel. 602/641–3937; FAX. 602/924–5096; S. Joyce Graham

**T.A.S.I. Surgery Center,** 5585 North Oracle Road, Suite B, Tucson, AZ 85704; tel. 520/293–7077; FAX. 520/293–7561; John A. Pierce, MD, Medical Director

**Tempe New Day Surgery Center LP,** 2000 East Southern Avenue, Suite 106, Tempe, AZ 85282; tel. 480/838–9313; FAX. 480/491–8802; John L. Titus, President

**The PAIN MDS ASC,** 2525 W Carefree Hwy, Suite 134, Phoenix, AZ 85085; tel. 623/580–4357; FAX. 623/580–5249; Linda Davis, Administrator

**Thunderbird Samaritan Surgicenter,** 5555 B West Thunderbird Road, Glendale, AZ 85306-4622; tel. 602/588–5475; FAX. 602/588–5472; Diane Elmore, RN, Administrator

**Valley Outpatient Surgery Center,** 160 West University Drive #1, Mesa, AZ 85201; tel. 602/835–7373; FAX. 602/969–7981; Craig R. Cassidy, DO, President

**Vital Sight P.C., dba Eye Institute of Southern Arizona,** 5632 East Fifth Street, Tucson, AZ 85711; tel. 520/790–8888; FAX. 520/790–1427; Mary Lou Lara, Administrator

**Warner Park Surgery Center,** 604 West Warner Road, Building A, Chandler, AZ 85225; tel. 480/899–2571; FAX. 480/899–4263; Dale Holmes

**White Mountain Ambulatory Surgery Center,** 2650 East Show Low Lake Road, Suite Two, Show Low, AZ 85901; tel. 908/537–4240; William J. Waldo

## ARKANSAS

**Arkansas Endoscopy Center, P.A.,** 9501 Baptist Health Drive, Suite 100, Little Rock, AR 72205; tel. 501/224–9100; FAX. 501/224–0420; Ronald D. Hardin, MD

**Arkansas Surgery and Endoscopy Center,** 4800 Hazel Street, Pine Bluff, AR 71603; tel. 870/536–4800; FAX. 870/534–5535; Syed Samad, MD, FACP, FACG

**Arkansas Surgery Center,** 10 Hospital Circle, Batesville, AR 72501; tel. 870/793–4040; FAX. 870/793–5649; Ronald L. Lowery, MD, Administrator

**Boozman-Hof Eye Surgery and Laser Center, LLC,** 3737 West Walnut Street, P.O. Box 1353, Rogers, AR 72757-1353; tel. 501/246–1751; FAX. 501/631–2702; Donna R. Acord, Director

**Doctors Surgery Center PA,** 303 West Polk Ave, Suite B, West Memphis, AR 72301; tel. 870/732–2100; Lois Meyers, RN

**Endoscopy Center of Hot Springs,** 151 McGowan Court, Hot Springs, AR 71913; tel. 501/623–4101; FAX. 501/623–0103; Barbara Hulsey, Administrator

**H. Lewis Pearson Eye Institute,** 3211 Surger Hill Road, Texarkana, AR 71854-9265; tel. 501/772–4440; FAX. 501/772–7190; James Loomis, Comptroller

**James Trice, M.D., P.A., dba Digestive Disease Center,** 7005 South Hazel Street, Pine Bluff, AR 71603; tel. 870/536–3070; FAX. 870/536–3171; Louis Trice, Administrator

**Little Rock Surgery Center,** 8820 Knoedl Court, Little Rock, AR 72205; tel. 501/224–6767; FAX. 501/224–8203; Kim Hamma, RN, Administrator

**Lowery Medical/Surgical Eye Center, P.A.,** 105 Central Avenue, Searcy, AR 72143; tel. 501/268–7154; FAX. 501/268–9071; Robert D. Lowery, MD, Administrator

**North Hills Gastroenterology Endoscopy Center, Inc.,** 3344 North Futrall Drive, Fayetteville, AR 72703; tel. 501/582–7280; FAX. 510/582–7279; William C. Martin, MD

**Novamed Surgery Center of Jonesboro, dba Eye Surgery Center of Arkansas,** 601 East Matthews, Jonesboro, AR 72401; tel. 870/935–6396; FAX. 870/935–4063; Tracy Gholson, Director

**Ozark Eye Center,** 360 Highway Five North, Mountain Home, AR 72653; tel. 870/425–2277; Cheryl Pearman, Administrator

**Physicians' Surgery Center of Fayetteville,** 3873 North Parkview Drive, Suite One, Fayetteville, AR 72703; tel. 479/527–0050; FAX. 479/582–1338; Russ Greene RN Administrator

**South Arkansas Surgery Center,** 4310 South Mulberry, Pine Bluff, AR 71603; tel. 870/535–5719; FAX. 870/536–1963; Heather Walters, Business Manager

**The Gastro-Intestinal Center,** 405 North University, Little Rock, AR 72205; tel. 501/663–1074; FAX. 501/663–0906; Brett Kirkman, Administrator

## CALIFORNIA

**Advanced Surgery Center,** 5771 North Fresno Street, Suite 101, Fresno, CA 93710; tel. 559/448–9900; FAX. 559/448–9546; B. David Singh MD, Administrator

**Aestheticare Outpatient Surgery Center,** 30260 Rancho Viejo Road, San Juan Capistrano, CA 92675; tel. 949/661–1700; FAX. 949/661–4321; Ronald E. Moser, MD

**Alliance Surgery Center,** 20377 Acacia Street, Suite 120, Newport Beach, CA 92660; tel. 949/870–3602; Naomi Hadden, Chief Financial Officer

**Ambulatory Surgical Center of Southern California, Gastroenterology Diagnostic Center,** 880 South Atlantic Boulevard G-10, Monterey Park, CA 91754; tel. 626/293–8851; FAX. 626/293–1606; Zelman Weingaren, MD

**Ambulatory Surgical Center of Zeiter Eye,** 117 North San Joaquin Street, Stockton, CA 95202; tel. 209/466-5566; FAX. 209/466–0535; Erin McCarthy, Office Manager

**Ambulatory Surgical Center, Inc.,** 14400 Bear Valley Road, Suite 201, Victorville, CA 92392; tel. 760/951–5162; FAX. 818/985–0055; Garey L. Weber, DPM, Administrator

**Antelope Valley Surgery Center,** 44301 North Lorimer Avenue, Lancaster, CA 93534; tel. 661/940–1112; FAX. 661/940–6856; Justina Geeter, Business Office Manager

**Arlington Podiatry Surgery Center,** 7310 Magnolia Avenue, Riverside, CA 92504; tel. 951/354–8787; FAX. 951/354–0350; James A. De Silva, Administrator

**Bakersfield Endoscopy Center,** 1408 Commercial Way, Bakersfield, CA 93309; tel. 661/327–4455; FAX. 661/633–5484; Ramesh Gupta, MD, Medical Director

**Ballas Outpatient Surgery Center,** 9320 Willowgrove Ave Ste L, Santee, CA 92071-2991; Raymond Mangrich, Administrator

**Bascom Surgery Center,** 3803 S. Bascom Avenue, Suite 106, Campbell, CA 95008; tel. 408/369–9535; FAX. 408/369–9106

**Bedford Surgery Center,** 100 UCLA Medical Plaza, Suite 310, Los Angeles, CA 90024-6999; tel. 310/777–8820; FAX. 310/777–8890; Patricia Adams, RN,PHD, Director of Nursing

**Beverly Hills Sunset Surgery Center, Inc.,** 9201 Sunset Boulevard, Suite 405, Los Angeles, CA 90069; tel. 310/887–1730; FAX. 310/887–1734; Sue Kim, Nursing Administrator

**Bolsa Outpatient Surgery Center,** 10362 Bolsa Avenue, Suite 100, Westminster, CA 92683; tel. 714/775–5690; FAX. 714/775–7405; Van Kychuong, MD, Medical Director

**Brockton Surgery Center,** 6958 Brockton Avenue, Riverside, CA 92506-3832; tel. 951/788–4400; Michael N. Durrant, DPM, MPH

**Camden Surgery Center of Beverly Hills,** 414 North Camden Drive, Suite 800, Beverly Hills, CA 90210; tel. 310/859–3991; FAX. 310/859–7126; Yvette L. Lee Administrator

**Campus Surgery Center, LP,** 901 Campus Drive, Suite 102, Daly City, CA 94015; tel. 650/991–2000; FAX. 650/755–8638

**Center for Surgery of Encinitas,** 477 North El Camino Real, Suite C-100, Encinitas, CA 92024; tel. 760/942–8800; FAX. 760/942–0106; Chris Clinton, RN, CASC Administrator

**Crown Valley Surgicenter,** 26921 Crown Valley Parkway, Suite 110, Mission Viejo, CA 92691; tel. 949/348–7252; FAX. 949/348–7246; Maurice Chammas, MD, Administrator

**Cypress Outpatient Surgical Center, Inc.,** 1665 Dominican Way, Suite 120, Santa Cruz, CA 95065; tel. 831/476–6943; FAX. 831/476–1473; Nicole Gonzalez Administrator

**Digestive Disease Center,** 24411 Health Center Drive, Suite 450, Laguna Hills, CA 92653; tel. 949/586–9386; FAX. 949/586–0864; Robert Dyer, Medical Director

**E N T Facial Surgery Center,** 1351 East Spruce, Fresno, CA 93720; tel. 559/432–3724; FAX. 559/432–8579; JoAnn LoForti, RN, MS, Division of Nursing

**El Mirador Surgical Center,** 1180 North Indian Canyon Drive, Suite 110, Palm Springs, CA 92262; tel. 760/416–4600; FAX. 760/416–4668; David Wiche, Director

**Endoscopy Center of Chula Vista,** 681 Third Avenue, Suite B, Chula Vista, CA 91910; tel. 619/425–2150; FAX. 619/425–2848; Robert Penner, MD, Administrator

**Endoscopy Center of Southern California,** 2336 Santa Monica Boulevard, Suite 204, Santa Monica, CA 90404; tel. 310/453–4477; FAX. 310/453–4811; Richard F. Corlin MD

**Endoscopy Center of the Central Coast,** 77 Casa Street, Suite 106, San Luis Obis, CA 93405; tel. 805/541–1021; FAX. 805/541–3142; Sue McMillan, Nurse Manager

**Escondido Surgery Center,** 343 East Second Avenue, Escondido, CA 92025; tel. 760/480–6606; FAX. 760/480–6671; L. Richard Greenstein, MD, Medical Director

**Eye Center of Northern California,** 6500 Fairmount Avenue, Suite Two, El Cerrito, CA 94530; tel. 510/525–2600; FAX. 510/524–1887; William Ellis

**Eye Life Institute,** 6283 Clark Road, Suite 11, Paradise, CA 95969; tel. 530/877–2020; FAX. 530/877–4641; Almary Hivale, RN, Director of ASC

**Eye Surgery Center of Southern California, Inc./ Med. Group, dba Tri-City Surgery Center,** 2023 West Vista Way, Suite E, Vista, CA 92083; tel. 760/941–8152; FAX. 760/941–8967; Daniel Lee, DDS, Medical Director

**Eye Surgery Center of the Desert,** 39700 Bob Hope Drive, Suite 111, Rancho Mirage, CA 92270; tel. 760/340–3937; FAX. 760/773–3823; Timothy D. Milauskas, Administrator

**Feather River Surgery Center,** 370 Del Norte Avenue, Yuba City, CA 95991; tel. 530/751–4800; FAX. 530/751–4884; Ann Perry, Administrator

**Foothill Ambulatory Surgery Center,** 1030 East Foothill Boulevard, Suite 101B, Upland, CA 91786; tel. 909/981–5859; FAX. 909/981–8293; Natee Poopat, MD, Office Director

**Fremont Surgery Center,** 2675 Stevenson Boulevard-South, Fremont, CA 94538; tel. 510/793–4987; FAX. 510/793–5084; Debi Ford, RN, Director of Nursing

**GastroDiagnostics, A Medical Group,** 1140 West La Veta, Suite 550, Orange, CA 92868; tel. 714/835–3636; FAX. 714/835–5567; Stephanie Quinn, Administrator

**Glendale Eye Surgery Center,** 607 North Central, Suite 103, Glendale, CA 91203; tel. 818/956–1010; FAX. 818/543–6083; Richard Weise, MD

**Golden Triangle Surgicenter,** 25405 Hancock Avenue, Suite 103, Murrieta, CA 92562; tel. 909/698–4670; FAX. 909/698–4675; Ella Stockstill, Administrator

**Greater Sacramento Surgery Center,** 2288 Auburn Boulevard, Suite 201, Sacramento, CA 95821; tel. 916/929–7229; FAX. 916/929–2590; Susan Brunone, MHS, Administrator

**Grossmont Plaza Surgery Center,** 5525 Grossmont Center Drive, La Mesa, CA 91942; tel. 619/644–4561; Chris Ekern, Manager

**Halcyon Laser and Surgery Center, Inc.,** 303 South Halcyon Road, Arroyo Grande, CA 93420; tel. 805/489–8254; FAX. 805/474–1997; Michelle Mele, Administrator

**HealthSouth Arcadia Outpatient Surgery, Inc.,** 614 West Duarte Road, Arcadia, CA 91007; tel. 626/445–4714; FAX. 626/445–1701; Sara Lamm, Administrator

**HealthSouth Forest Surgery Center,** 2110 Forest Avenue, San Jose, CA 95128; tel. 408/297–3432; FAX. 408/298–3338; Camille Magamon RN

**HealthSouth Grossmont Surgery Center,** 8881 Fletcher Parkway, Suite 100, La Mesa, CA 91942; tel. 619/698–0930; FAX. 619/698–3093; Administrator

**HealthSouth North Coast Surgery Center,** 3903 Waring Road, Oceanside, CA 92056; tel. 760/940–0997; FAX. 760/940–0407; Donna Danley, Administrator

**HealthSouth Surgery Center,** 75 Scripts Drive, Sacramento, CA 95825; tel. 916/929–9431; FAX. 916/929–0132; Deanne Conner, Administrator

**HealthSouth Surgery Center-Scripps,** 75 Scripps Drive, Sacramento, CA 95825; tel. 916/929–9431; FAX. 916/929–0132; Jodean Lake, Administrator

**Hemet Endoscopy Center,** 1003 East Florida Avenue, Suite 104, Hemet, CA 92543; tel. 951/652–2252; FAX. 951/925–9252; Milan S. Chakrabarty, MD

**Hemet Healthcare Surgicenter,** 301 North San Jacinto Avenue, Hemet, CA 92543; tel. 909/765–1717; FAX. 909/765–1716; Josh Hoffner, Business Office Manager

**High Desert Endoscopy,** 18523 Corwin Road, Suite H2, Apple Valley, CA 92307; tel. 760/242–3000; FAX. 760/242–1802; Raman S. Poola, MD, Administrator

**Hope Square Surgical Center,** 39700 Bob Hope Drive, Suite 301, Rancho Mirage, CA 92270; tel. 760/346-7696; FAX. 760/776-1069; BJ Clarke, RN, MPA, Administrator

**Huntington Outpatient Surgery Center,** 797 South Fair Oaks Avenue, Pasadena, CA 91105; tel. 626/535-2434; FAX. 626/535-2430; Robin Waldvogel, Medical Director

**Inland Endoscopy Center, Inc., dba Mountain View Surgery Center,** 10408 Industrial Circle, Redlands, CA 92374; tel. 909/796-7803; FAX. 909/796-0614; Khushal Stanisai

**Inland Surgery Center,** 1620 Laurel Avenue, Redlands, CA 92373; tel. 909/793-4701; FAX. 909/792-6397; Jacquelin Belcher, Facility Administrator

**Inland Surgery Center,** 3053 W. Stetson Ave, Hemet, CA 92545; tel. 951/652-4343; FAX. 951/658-3953; Barratt Phillips MD.

**Irvine Multi-Specialty Surgical Care,** 4900 Barranca Parkway, Suite 104, Irvine, CA 92604-8603; tel. 949/726-0677; FAX. 949/726-0678; Lauren Parrott, BS, Administrator

**Kaiser Ambulatory Surgical Center,** 2025 Morse Avenue, Sacramento, CA 95825; tel. 916/973-7786; FAX. 916/973-5530; Brian J. Brosnahan, RN, BSN, ASU Manager

**Kaiser Ambulatory Surgical Center,** 10725 International Drive, Rancho Cordov, CA 95670; tel. 916/631-2000; FAX. 916/631-2013; Steven Metzger, RN, Manager

**La Jolla Endoscopy Center,** 9850 Genesee Avenue, Suite 980, La Jolla, CA 92037; tel. 858/453-7525; FAX. 858/453-5753; Dr. David Roseman

**La Veta Surgical Center, an Affiliate of SCA,** 725 West La Veta, Suite 270, Orange, CA 92868; tel. 714/744-0900; FAX. 714/744-0283; Kelly Ruiz, Administrator

**Laser Surgery Center, Ltd.,** 2021 Ygnacio Valley Road, Building H-102, Walnut Creek, CA 94598; tel. 925/944-9400; FAX. 925/947-2160; Michele McKinley, Administrator

**Lassen Surgery Center,** 103 Fair Drive, PO Box 1150, Susanville, CA 96130; tel. 530/257-7772; FAX. 530/257-2939; Kim Sibert, Medical Staff Coordinator

**Lodi Outpatient Surgical Center,** 521 South Ham Lane, Suite F, Lodi, CA 95242; tel. 209/333-0905; FAX. 209/333-0219; Marklin E. Brown, Administrator, CASC

**Loma Linda Ambulatory Surgical Center, Podiatry Corp,** 11332 Mountain View Avenue, Suite A, Loma Linda, CA 92354; tel. 909/796-3707; FAX. 909/796-3709; Mariam Amiri, DPM, Administrator

**Los Altos Surgery Center,** 795 Altos Oaks Drive, Los Altos, CA 94024; tel. 650/209-1100; Harry Mittelman, MD

**Los Gatos Surgical Center,** 15195 National Avenue, Suite 100, Los Gatos, CA 95032; tel. 408/356-0454; FAX. 408/358-3924; David Hokeness, Administrator

**M/S Surgery Center, LLC,** 3510 Martin Luther King Boulevard, Lynwood, CA 90262; tel. 310/635-7550; FAX. 310/603-8749; John H. Shammas, MD, Medical Director

**Marin Ophthalmic Surgery Center,** 901 E Street, Suite 270, San Rafael, CA 94901; tel. 415/454-2112; FAX. 415/454-6542; Vicki Wininger, RN Clinical Director

**Martel Eye Institute, LLC,** 11216 Trinity River, Rancho Cordova, CA 95670; tel. 916/631-7868; FAX. 916/631-3788; Joseph Martel, MD

**Medical Arts Ambulatory Surgery Center,** 205 South West Street, Suite B, Visalia, CA 93291; tel. 209/625-9601; FAX. 209/625-3124; Thomas F. Mitts, MD, Administrator

**Medical Plaza Orthopedic Surgery Center,** 1301 20th Street, Suite 140, Santa Monica, CA 90404; tel. 310/315-0333; FAX. 310/315-0341; Trish Fowler, Director Surgical Services

**Merced Ambulatory Endoscopy Center,** 750 West Olive Avenue, Suite 107A, Merced, CA 95348; tel. 209/384-3116; FAX. 209/384-0878; Vijaya Tangella, Administrator

**Mission Ambulatory Surgicenter,** 26730 Crown Valley Parkway, First Floor, Mission Viejo, CA 92691; tel. 949/364-2201; FAX. 949/364-5372; Mary Parker, Administrator

**Mission Valley Surgery Center,** 39263 Mission Boulevard, Fremont, CA 94539; tel. 510/796-4500; FAX. 510/796-4573; Sarb S. Hundal, MD

**Modesto Surgery Center, Inc.,** 400 East Orangeburg Avenue, Suite One, Modesto, CA 95350; tel. 209/526-3000; FAX. 209/526-3133; Dr. Greg Tesluk, Administrator

**Monterey Peninsula Surgery Center, LLC,** 966 Cass Street, Suite 210, Monterey, CA 93940; tel. 831/372-2169; FAX. 408/372-6323; David J. Ogimachi, Administrator

**Napa Surgery Center,** 3444 Valle Verde Drive, Napa, CA 94558; tel. 707/252-9669; FAX. 707/257-3328; Eric Grigsby, MD, Owner

**Newport Beach Orange Coast Endoscopy Center,** 1525 Superior Avenue, Suite 114, Newport Beach, CA 92663; tel. 949/646-6999; FAX. 949/646-9699; Donald Abraham

**Newport Surgery Institute,** 360 San Miguel Drive, Suite 406, Newport Beach, CA 92660; tel. 949/759-0995; Suzanne Tavenner, Office Manager

**North Anaheim Surgicenter,** 1154 North Euclid, Anaheim, CA 92801; tel. 714/635-6272; FAX. 714/635-0943; Jeanette Rasmussen, Administrator

**North Bay Eye Associates, Inc., Ambulatory Surgery Center,** 380 Tesconi Court, Santa Rosa, CA 95401; tel. 707/544-3375; FAX. 707/544-0808; William H. Bartlett, Medical Director

**North Texas Surgi-Center,** PO Box 713150, Santee, CA 76302; tel. 940/767-7273; FAX. 940/723-9059; Barbara Dawson, Administrator

**Optima Ophthalmic Medical Associates, Inc.,** 1237 B Street, Hayward, CA 94541-2977; tel. 510/886-3937; FAX. 510/886-6304; Kelly Best, Office Manager

**Orange County Institute of Gastroenterology and Endoscopy,** 26732 Crown Valley Parkway, Suite 241, Mission Viejo, CA 92691; tel. 949/364-2611; FAX. 949/364-0226; Dina Moatazedi, Office Manager

**Out-Patient Surgery Center,** 17762 Beach Boulevard, Huntington Beach, CA 92647; tel. 714/842-1426; FAX. 714/849-3737; Patricia Galdamez, RN, DON

**Pacific Eye Institute,** 555 North 13th Avenue, Upland, CA 91786; tel. 909/982-8846; FAX. 909/982-4007; Robert Fabricant, MD, FACS, Medical Director

**Pacific Hills Surgery Center, LLC,** 24022 Calle De La Plata, Suite 180, Laguna Hills, CA 92653; tel. 949/458-3551; FAX. 949/951-9478; Kristi Morse, RN, Nurse Manager, Compliance

**Pacific Surgicenter, Inc.,** 1301 20th Street, Suite 470, Santa Monica, CA 90404; tel. 310/315-0222; FAX. 310/828-8852; Randi Ogilvie- Manager

**Petaluma Surgicenter,** 1400 Professional Drive, Suite 102, Petaluma, CA 94954; tel. 707/763-9325; FAX. 707/769-0751; Ronald M. La Vigna, DPM Manager

**Physicians Plaza Surgical Center,** 6000 Physicians Boulevard, Bakersfield, CA 93301; tel. 661/322-4744; FAX. 661/322-2938; Terri Waller, Administrator

**Plastic and Reconstructive Surgery Center,** 1387 Santa Rita Road, Pleasanton, CA 94566; tel. 925/462-3700; FAX. 510/462-4681; Ronald Iverson, Administrator

**Podiatric Surgery Center,** 255 North Gilbert, Suite B, Hemet, CA 92543; tel. 909/925-2186; FAX. 909/925-4947; Robert Drake, DPM, Administrator

**Premiere Surgery Center, Inc.,** 700 West El Norte Parkway, Escondido, CA 92026; tel. 760/738-7830; FAX. 760/738-7834; R. K. Massengill, MD, President

**Providence Ambulatory Surgical Center,** 1310 West Stewart Drive, Suite 310, Orange, CA 92668; tel. 714/771-6363; FAX. 714/771-0754; Harrell E. Robinson, MD, President

**Providence Holy Cross Surgery Center,** 11550 Indian Hills Road, Suite 160, Mission Hills, CA 91345; tel. 818/256-2100; FAX. 818/256-2156; Dale Bowman, Administrator

**Redlands Dental Surgery Center,** 1180 Nevada Street, Suite 100, Redlands, CA 92374; tel. 909/335-0474; FAX. 909/335-0477; Russell O. Seheult, DDS

**Richburg Valley Eye Institute Ambulatory Surgical Center,** 1680 East Herndon Avenue, Fresno, CA 93720; tel. 209/432-4200; FAX. 209/432-0147; Frederick Richburg, MD, Administrator

**Riverside Medical Clinic Surgery Center,** 7160 Brockton Avenue, Riverside, CA 92506; tel. 951/782-3801; FAX. 951/328-9742; Anette Nunn, RN, VP, Clinical Operations

**Sacramento Eye Surgicenter,** 3150 J Street, Sacramento, CA 95816; tel. 916/444-7052; FAX. 916/446-1145; Yvonne Jones, ASC Director

**Sacramento Midtown Endoscopy Center,** 3941 J Street, Suite 460, Sacramento, CA 95819; tel. 916/733-6940; FAX. 916/733-6934; Gautam Gandhi, MD

**Saddleback Eye Center,** 23161 Moulton Parkway, Laguna Hills, CA 92653; tel. 949/951-4641; FAX. 949/951-4601; Linda Riley, Administrator

**Saddleback Valley Outpatient Surgery,** 24302 Paseo De Valencia, Laguna Hills, CA 92653; tel. 949/472-0244; FAX. 949/472-0380; Brian Fitzgerald, Administrator

**Salinas Surgery Center,** 955-A Blanco Circle, Salinas, CA 93901; tel. 831/753-5800; FAX. 831/753-5808; Christine Gallagher, Executive Director

**San Francisco Surgi Center,** 1635 Divisidero Street, Suite 200, San Francisco, CA 94115; tel. 415/346-1218; FAX. 415/346-2930; Judith Mulligan, Administrator

**San Gabriel Valley Surgical Center,** 1250 South Sunset Avenue, Suite 100, West Covina, CA 91790; tel. 626/960-6623; FAX. 626/962-4341; Susan Raub, Administrator

**San Joaquin Laser Surgery Center,** 1805 North California Street, # 101A, Stockton, CA 95204; tel. 209/948-3241; FAX. 209/948-8009; Susan Ford, Administrator

**San Leandro Surgery Center,** 15035 East 14th Street, San Leandro, CA 94578; tel. 510/276-2800; FAX. 510/276-2890; Sheila L. Cook, Executive Director

**Sani Eye Surgery Center,** 1315 Las Tablas Road, Templeton, CA 93465; tel. 805/434-2533; FAX. 805/434-3037; Karim Rasheed, MD, Director

**Santa Cruz Surgery Center,** 3003 Paul Sweet Road, Santa Cruz, CA 95065; tel. 408/462-5512; FAX. 408/462-2451; Mary Ann Dunlap, RN

**Sequoia Surgery Center, LLC,** 842 South Akers Street, Visalia, CA 93277; tel. 559/740-4094; FAX. 559/740-4100; Renda Liden, CASC, Administrator

**Shepard Surgical Center,** 1418 East Main Street, Suite 110, Santa Maria, CA 93454-4806; tel. 805/614-7005; FAX. 805/614-7006; Dennis D. Shepard, MD

**Sierra Surgery Center Inc.,** 6153 North Thesta, Fresno, CA 93710; tel. 559/432-2757; FAX. 559/432-3556; John F. Burnett, MD, Owner and President

**Silicon Valley Surgery Center, LP,** 14601 S. Bascom Avenue, Suite 100, Los Gatos, CA 95032; tel. 408/402-0663; FAX. 408/402-7055

**Sonora Eye Surgery Center,** 940 Sylva Lane, Suite G, Sonora, CA 95370; tel. 209/532-2020; FAX. 209/532-1687; Desiree Torres, RN, Surgery Administrator

**South Coast Laser Center,** 3420 Bristol Street, Suite 701, Costa Mesa, CA 92626; tel. 714/957-0272; FAX. 714/641-2020; Marc R. Rose, MD, Medical Director

**Southern California Surgery Center,** 7305 Pacific Boulevard, Huntington Pa, CA 90255; tel. 323/584-8222; FAX. 323/584-8606; Ruth Huezo, Administrator

**Southland Endoscopy Center,** 949 East Calhoun Place, Suite B, Hemet, CA 92543; tel. 909/929-1177; FAX. 909/765-9111; Sreenivasa R. Nakka, MD, FACP

**Southwest Surgical Center, Health South,** 201 New Stine Road, Suite 130, Bakersfield, CA 93309; tel. 661/396-8900; FAX. 661/397-2929; Linda Bloomquist, Administrator

**St. Joseph Surgery and Laser Center, Inc., dba St. Mary and Joseph Surgery and Laser Center, Inc.,** 436 South Glassell Street, Orange, CA 92866; tel. 714/633-9566; FAX. 714/633-5193; Kathleen Ruper, Administrator

**Starpoint Health Foundation,** PO Box 7459, Newport Beach, CA 92658-7459; tel. 949/705-5100; FAX. 949/985-0055; Eric D. Friedlander, Chief Executive Officer

**Surgecenter of Palo Alto,** 795 El Camino Real, Palo Alto, CA 94301; tel. 650/324-1832; FAX. 650/330-4520; Margo Mynderse-Isola, Chief Executive Officer

**Surgery Center of San Buena Ventura,** 3525 Loma Vista Road, Suite B, Ventura, CA 93003; tel. 805/641-6434; FAX. 805/641-6437; Chris Behm, Administrator

**Surgery Center of Santa Monica,** 2121 Wilshire Boulevard, Suite 201, Santa Monica, CA 90403; tel. 310/264-7300; FAX. 310/828-8626

**Section C**

**Surgitek Outpatient Center, Inc.,** 460 North Greenfield Avenue, Suite Eight, Hanford, CA 93230; tel. 559/582-0238; FAX. 559/582-9341; Wiley Elick, Owner, Administrator

**Sutter Alhambra Surgery Center,** 1201 Alhambra Boulevard, Suite 110, Sacramento, CA 95816; tel. 916/733-8222; FAX. 916/733-8224; Ken Schwam, Administrator

**Sutter Auburn Surgery Center,** 3123 Professional Drive, Suite 100, Auburn, CA 95603; tel. 530/888-8899; FAX. 530/888-1464; Richard Lewis, Administrator

**Sutter North Procedure Center,** 550 B Street, Yuba City, CA 95991; tel. 530/749-3653; FAX. 530/749-3493; Deborah Smith, Ancillary Services Director

**The Center for Endoscopy,** 3921 Waring Road, Suite B, Oceanside, CA 92056; tel. 760/940-6300; FAX. 760/940-8074; Barbara Bockover, RN, Administrator

**The Centre for Plastic Surgery,** 1869 N Waterman Avenue, San Bernardino, CA 92404; tel. 909/883-8686; FAX. 909/881-6537; David Nguyen, MD

**The Endoscopy Center,** 870 Shasta Street, Suite 200, Yuba City, CA 95991; tel. 530/671-3636; Floyd V. Burton, MD

**The Endoscopy Center of the South Bay,** 23560 Madison Street, Suite 114, Torrance, CA 90505; tel. 310/325-6331; FAX. 310/325-6335; Jerome Cohen MD, Medical Director

**The Eye Surgery Center (Colton),** 1900 East Washington Street, Colton, CA 92324; tel. 909/825-8002; FAX. 909/424-1662; Melissa Goins, RN, Director

**The Eye Surgery Center of Northern California,** 5959 Greenback Lane Suite 310, Citrus Height, CA 95621; tel. 916/723-7400; FAX. 916/723-4449; Scott George, Clinic Director

**The Montebello Surgery Center,** 229 East Beverly Boulevard, Montebello, CA 90640; tel. 323/728-7998; FAX. 323/728-5041; Millie Kelly, Administrator

**The Palos Verdes Ambulatory Surgery Medical Center,** 3400 West Lomita Boulevard, Suite 307A, Torrance, CA 90505; tel. 310/539-5888; FAX. 310/517-9916; Christine Petti, MD, Medical Director

**The Plastic Surgery Center,** 95 Scripps Drive, Sacramento, CA 95825; tel. 916/929-1833; FAX. 916/929-6730; Marlin Schriock, Administrator

**The San Luis Obispo Surgery Center,** 1304 Ella Street, Suite C, San Luis Obis, CA 93401; tel. 805/544-7874; FAX. 866/384-2036; Judy Shapazian, RN, Administrator

**The Surgery Center of Alta Bates Summit Medical Center,** 3875 Telegraph Avenue, Oakland, CA 94609; tel. 510/547-2244; FAX. 510/653-5242; Kim D'Ambrosia, Administrator

**The Surgery Center Of Riverside, Inc.,** 8990 Garfield, Suite One, Riverside, CA 92503; tel. 951/785-5421; FAX. 951/785-0130

**The Surgery Center of Santa Rosa,** 1111 Sonoma Avenue, Lower Level, Santa Rosa, CA 95405; tel. 707/578-4100; FAX. 707/578-7997; Ken Alban, Administrator

**Third Street Surgery Center,** 420 East Third Street, Suite 110, Los Angeles, CA 90013; tel. 213/617-9194; FAX. 213/617-0605; Tomoko Okuda, RN, Clinical Coordinator

**Time Surgical Facility,** 720 North Tustin Avenue, Suite 202, Santa Ana, CA 92705; tel. 714/972-1811; FAX. 714/972-0986; Tracey Mora, RN, Nurse Manager

**Torrance Surgicenter,** 22410 Hawthorne Boulevard, Suite Three, Torrance, CA 90505; tel. 310/373-2238; FAX. 310/373-8238; Gary Barnes, Administrator

**Truxtun Surgery Center, Inc.,** 4260 Truxtun Avenue, Suite 120, Bakersfield, CA 93309; tel. 661/327-3636; Mary Moeder, AOM

**Twin Cities Surgicenter, Inc.,** 812 Fourth Street, Suite A, Marysville, CA 95901; tel. 530/741-3937; FAX. 530/743-0427; Karen M. Wasilenko, CASC Administrator

**University Ambulatory Surgery Center,** 8929 University Center Lane, Suite 103, San Diego, CA 92122; tel. 858/554-0220; FAX. 858/554-0458; Eileen Smith, Administrator

**Upland Outpatient Surgical Center, Inc.,** 1330 San Bernardino Road #F, Upland, CA 91786; tel. 909/981-8755; FAX. 909/981-9462; Brian Olson, Administrator

**Valencia Outpatient Surgical Center Partners, L.P., dba Valencia Surgical Center,** 24355 Lyons Avenue, Suite 120, Santa Clarita, CA 91321; tel. 661/255-6644; FAX. 661/255-7653; Pat Monolias, RN, Director of Nursing

**Valley Endoscopy Center,** 18425 Burbank Boulevard, Suite 525, Tarzana, CA 91356; tel. 818/708-6050; FAX. 818/708-6055; Christine Scoggins, RN, Clinical Director

**Ventura Out-Patient Surgery, Inc.,** 3555 Loma Vista Road, Suite 204, Ventura, CA 93003; tel. 805/653-5460; FAX. 805/653-1470; Brian D. Brantner, MD

**Washington Outpatient Surgery Center,** 2299 Mowry Avenue, First Floor, Fremont, CA 94538; tel. 510/791-5374; FAX. 510/790-8916; Dr. Jeffery Stuart, Medical Director

**Waverley Surgery Center, LP,** 400 Forest Avenue, Palo Alto, CA 94301; tel. 650/324-0600; FAX. 650/269-1620

**West Hills Surgical Center,** 7240 Medical Center Drive, West Hills, CA 91307; tel. 818/226-9151; FAX. 818/226-0947

**Westlake Eye Surgery Center,** 2900 Townsgate Road, Suite 201, Westlake Village, CA 91361; tel. 805/496-6789; FAX. 805/494-8392; John Darin, MD, Medical Director

**Zeiter Eye Surgical Center, Inc.,** 1801 E. March Lane, Suite C360, Stockton, CA 95210; tel. 209/337-2020; FAX. 209/337-2021; Theresa Slaton, RN, Surgical Administrator

## COLORADO

**Avista Surgery Center,** 2525 Fourth Street, Lower Level, Boulder, CO 80304; tel. 303/443-3672; John Sackett, Administrator

**Boulder Medical Center, P C,** 2750 Broadway, Boulder, CO 80304; tel. 303/440-3000; Mr. Bradford McKane, Chief Executive Officer

**Centennial Medical Plaza,** 14200 East Arapahoe Road, Centennial, CO 80112; tel. 303/699-3000; FAX. 303/699-3152; Mary Beth Savory, Director of Operations

**Centrum Surgical Center,** 8200 East Belleview, Suite 300, East Tower, Greenwood Village, CO 80111; tel. 303/290-0600; FAX. 303/290-6359; Ken Kolb, Administrator

**Choice Surgicare,** 1300 S. Potomac Street, #122, Aurora, CO 80012; tel. 720/748-6400; FAX. 720/748-6401; Tina Sherman, Administrator

**Colorado Center for Reproductive Medicine,** 10290 Ridgegate Circle, Lone Tree, CO 80124-5331; tel. 303/788-8300; FAX. 303/788-8310; Dr. William Schoolcraft, Administrator

**Colorado Outpatient Eye Surgical Center,** 2480 South Downing, Suite G-20, Denver, CO 80210; tel. 303/777-7303; FAX. 303/282-0266; Diane Nelson, RN, ASC Administrator

**Colorado Springs Eye Surgery Center,** 2920 North Cascade Avenue, Colorado Springs, CO 80907; tel. 719/636-5054; FAX. 719/520-3576; Dr. Robert Foerster, Medical Director

**Colorado Springs Health Partners Ambulatory Surgery Unit,** 209 South Nevada Avenue, Colorado Springs, CO 80903; tel. 719/475-7700; FAX. 719/538-2999; Ms. Joan Compton, VP Operations

**Colorado Springs Surgery Center An Affiliate of SCA,** 1615 Medical Center Point, Colorado Springs, CO 80907; tel. 719/635-7740; FAX. 719/635-7750; Jenny (Jen) Knellinger, Administrator

**Day Surgery of Grand Junction, Inc.,** 1000 Wellington Avenue, Grand Junction, CO 81501; tel. 970/245-5989; FAX. 970/243-9023; Karen Higuera, RN, Surgery Center Administrator

**Denver Eye Surgery Center, Inc.,** 13772 Denver West Parkway, Building 55, Suite 120, Lakewood, CO 80401; tel. 303/273-8770; FAX. 303/273-8775

**Denver Midtown Surgery Center,** 1919 East 18th Avenue, Denver, CO 80206; tel. 303/322-3993; FAX. 303/322-7329; Lisa Cross, Administrator

**Dishler Laser Institute,** 8400 East Prentice Avenue, Suite 1200, Greenwood Village, CO 80111; tel. 303/793-3000; FAX. 303/793-3008; Jon Dishler, MD, President

**Durango Surgicenter, LLC,** 316 Sawyer Drive, Durango, CO 81303; tel. 970/259-3818; FAX. 970/259-9553; D.J. Winder, MD, Administrator

**Eye Center of Northern Colorado Surgery Center,** 1725 E. Prospect Avenue, Fort Collins, CO 80525; tel. 970/221-2222; FAX. 970/221-2223; Carol Wittmer, Administrator

**Eye Surgery Center of Colorado, P.C.,** 8403 Bryant Street, Westminster, CO 80031; tel. 303/426-4810; FAX. 303/426-8708; William G. Self, Jr., MD, Administrator

**Foot Surgery Center of Northern Colorado,** 1355 Riverside Avenue, #B, Fort Collins, CO 80524; tel. 970/484-4620; FAX. 970/407-1194; Linda Kunkel, RN, Nurse Administrator

**Kaiser Permanente Ambulatory Surgery Center,** 2045 Franklin Street, Denver, CO 80205; tel. 303/764-4444; Elizabeth Reimann

**Littleton Day Surgery Center,** 8381 South Park Lane, Littleton, CO 80120; tel. 303/795-2244; FAX. 303/795-5965; Cindy Richardson, RN, BS, CLNC, Clinical Director/Administrator

**North Denver Endoscopy Center.,** 10001 North Washington, Thornton, CO 80229; tel. 303/252-0083; FAX. 303/252-9095; Craig J. Bakken, Administrator

**Orthopaedic & Spine Center of the Rockies Ambulatory Surgery Center,** 2500 East Prospect Road, Fort Collins, CO 80525; tel. 970/493-0010; FAX. 970/419-7151; Yvonne Boechmer, RN, BSN, CASC, Director of Surgical Operations

**Park Meadows Outpatient Surgery,** 7430 Park Meadows Drive #300, Lone Tree, CO 80124; tel. 303/706-1100; FAX. 303/790-7322; Charlene A. Sherwood, Administrator

**Peak One Surgery Center, LLC,** 350 Peak One Drive, P.O. Box 4460, Frisco, CO 80443; tel. 970/668-1458; FAX. 970/668-6677; Lisa Austin, Administrator

**Pikes Peak Endoscopy & Surgery Center,** 1699 Medical Center Pt., Colorado Springs, CO 80907; tel. 719/632-7101; FAX. 719/632-4468; Tricia Tappan, Chief Executive Officer

**Pueblo Surgery Center,** 25 Montebello Road, Pueblo, CO 81001; tel. 719/544-1600; FAX. 719/544-2599; Jennifer Arellano, Administrator

**South Denver Endoscopy Center, Inc.,** 499 East Hampden Avenue, Suite 430, Englewood, CO 80110; tel. 303/874-0350; Dr. Dan Hruza, Medical Director

**Surgery Center of Fort Collins,** 1100 East Prospect Road, Fort Collins, CO 80525; tel. 970/494-4800; FAX. 970/493-2380; Ross Alexander, Administrator

**U.S. Air Force Academy Clinic,** 4102 Pinion Drive, USAF Academy, CO 80840-4000; tel. 719/333-5660; FAX. 719/333-5670; Colonel Kenneth K. Knight

## CONNECTICUT

**Connecticut Foot Surgery Center,** 318 New Haven Avenue, Milford, CT 06460; tel. 203/882-0065; FAX. 203/882-0248; Martin Pressman, DPM, Administrator

**HealthSouth Surgery Center of Hartford,** 100 Retreat Avenue, Hartford, CT 06106; tel. 860/549-9970; FAX. 860/247-4121; Theresa Klimczyk, Administrative Director

**Stamford Surgical Center,** 32 Strawberry Hill Court, Stamford, CT 06902; tel. 203/276-6196; FAX. 203/276-4921; Patrice Kelly, Executive Director of Perioperative Services

## DELAWARE

**Bayview Endoscopy Center, Inc.,** 1539 Savannah Road, Lewes, DE 19958; tel. 302/644-0455; FAX. 302/645-5214; Harry J. Anagnostakos, DO, President

**Cataract and Laser Center, LLC,** 4102 Ogletown/Stanton Road, Suite 1, Newark, DE 19713; tel. 302/454-8802; FAX. 302/454-8801; Alexandra Meyer, Center Administrator

**Central Delaware Endoscopy Unit,** 644 South Queen Street, Suite 105, Dover, DE 19904; tel. 302/677-1617; FAX. 302/677-1669; William M. Kaplan, MD, Medical Director

**Limestone Medical Center, Inc.,** 1941 Limestone Road, Suite 113, Wilmington, DE 19808; tel. 302/633-9873; FAX. 302/992-0563; Thomas E. Mulhern, MBA, CASC Executive Director

## DISTRICT OF COLUMBIA

**Center for Ambulatory Surgery, Inc.,** 1145 19th Street, NW, Suite 850, Washington, DC 20036; tel. 202/223-9040; FAX. 202/223-9047; William Heron, MD, Medical Director

**Planned Parenthood of Metropolitan Washington, D.C.,** 1108 16th Street, NW, Washington, DC 20036; tel. 202/347-8512; FAX. 202/347-0281; Takina Wilson, Director of Patient Services

**Premier Surgery Center of D.C.,** 6323 Georgia Avenue, NW, Suite 200, Washington, DC 20011; tel. 202/291-0126; FAX. 202/291-0126; Lenora Hollaway, RN, Administrative Director

**The Endoscopy Center of Washington, DC, L.P.,** 2021 K Street, NW, Suite T-115, Washington, DC 20006; tel. 202/775-8692; FAX. 202/463-1165; Debra Jay RN, Center Director

## FLORIDA

**Aker-Kasten Eye Center,** 1445 Northwest Boca Raton Boulevard, Boca Raton, FL 33432; tel. 561/338-7722; FAX. 561/338-7785; Kim Harrington, Administrator

**All Saints Surgery Center,** 11377 Cortez Boulevard, Brooksville, FL 34613; tel. 352/597-3060; FAX. 352/597-3077; Julie Curky, RN, Administrator and Clinical Director

**Alpha Ambulatory Surgery, Inc.,** 2160 Capital Circle, NE, Tallahassee, FL 32308; tel. 850/385-0033; FAX. 850/422-0201; Juanita Legree, RN, Administrator

**Ambulatory Surgery Center,** 4500 East Fletcher Avenue, Tampa, FL 33613; tel. 813/977-8550; FAX. 813/977-7941; Edward J. Tennant, CASC, Administrator

**Ambulatory Surgery Center of Brevard,** 719 East New Haven Avenue, Melbourne, FL 32901; tel. 321/726-4106; FAX. 321/728-3001; Norm Gagnon, General Manager

**Ambulatory Surgical Care,** 1045 North Courtenay Parkway, Merritt Island, FL 32953; tel. 321/452-4448; FAX. 321/452-4533; Robyn Allard, RN, Administrator

**Atlantic Surgery Center,** 541 Health Boulevard, Daytona Beach, FL 32114; tel. 386/239-0021; FAX. 386/248-8226; Shirley A. Hines, RN, CASC, Administrator

**Atlantic Surgery Center,** 1707 South 25th Street, Fort Pierce, FL 34947; tel. 772/464-8900; FAX. 561/464-1104; Michele Weinberg, Business Office Manager

**Atlantic Surgical Center, Inc.,** 150 Southwest 12th Avenue, Suite 450, Pompano Beach, FL 33069; tel. 954/941-3369; FAX. 954/941-8470; Andrew Byers, Administrator

**Barkley Surgicenter,** 63 Barkley Circle, Suite 104, Fort Myers, FL 33907; tel. 239/275-8452; FAX. 239/275-1969; Kerri Gantt LHRM, CMM, Administrative Director

**Bayfront Same Day Surgery Center, LLC,** 603 Seventh Street South, St. Petersburg, FL 33701; tel. 727/553-7906; FAX. 727/553-7880; Jatin Motiwal, Executive Director

**Belleair Surgery Center,** 1130 Ponce de Leon Boulevard, Clearwater, FL 33756; tel. 727/581-4800; FAX. 813/585-0319; Ed Callahan, Administrator

**Beraja Healthcare Corp.,** 2550 Douglas Road, Coral Gables, FL 33134; tel. 305/443-7070; FAX. 305/357-1701; Margarita Caffe, RN, DON

**Bethesda Outpatient Surgery Center, LLC,** 10301 Hagen Ranch Road, Suite 520, Boynton Beach, FL 33437; tel. 561/374-5550; FAX. 561/374-9977; Maddie Linder, RN, Director of Surgical Services

**Boynton Beach ASC, LLC,** 1717-1799 Woolbright Road, Boynton Beach, FL 33426; tel. 516/737-8031; FAX. 561/736-5062; Lily Lee, Administrator

**Brandon Surgery Center,** 711 South Parsons, Brandon, FL 33511; tel. 813/654-7771; FAX. 813/654-3347; Edward J. Tennant, CASC, Administrator and Chief Executive Officer

**Brevard Surgery Center,** 665 Apollo Boulevard, Melbourne, FL 32901; tel. 321/984-3200; FAX. 321/984-0032; Gary R. Hardey, MBA, Administrator

**Cape Surgery Center,** 1941 Waldemere Street, Sarasota, FL 34239-3555; tel. 941/917-1900; FAX. 941/917-2356; Sharon Tolhurst, RN, MBA, Administrator

**Center for Digestive Health and Pain Management,** 12700 Creekside Lane, Suite 202, P.O. Box 33906, Fort Myers, FL 33919; tel. 941/489-4454; FAX. 941/489-2114; Vivian DiCarlo, RN, Nursing Director

**Center for Special Surgery,** 4650 Fourth Street, N., St. Petersburg, FL 33703; tel. 727/527-1919; FAX. 727/527-0714; Jan Silinsky, Administrator

**Central Florida Eye Institute,** 3133 Southwest 32nd Avenue, Ocala, FL 34474; tel. 352/237-8400; FAX. 352/237-7190; Thomas L. Croley, MD

**Citrus Endoscopy and Surgery Center,** 6412 West Gulf to Lake Highway, Crystal River, FL 34429; tel. 352/563-0223; FAX. 352/563-2961

**Citrus Surgery Center,** 110 North Lecanto Highway, Lecanto, FL 34461; tel. 352/527-1825; FAX. 352/527-1827; Richard Rice, Facility Administrator

**Clearwater Endoscopy Center,** 401 Corbett Street, Suite 220, Clearwater, FL 33756; tel. 727/443-0100; FAX. 727/461-4893; Nancy Wheeling RN, LHRM Administrator

**Collier Surgery Center,** 800 Goodlette Road, N., Suite 120, Naples, FL 34104; tel. 239/262-5757; FAX. 239/262-6073; David W. Douglas, Administrator

**Coral View Surgery Center,** 8390 West Flager, Suite 216, Miami, FL 33144; tel. 305/226-5574; Ruben Paradela, Chief Executive Officer

**Cortez Foot Surgery Center, PA,** 1800 Cortez Road W, Suite B, Bradenton, FL 34207; tel. 941/758-4608; FAX. 941/758-4438; Connie Belculfine, Administrator

**Countryside Surgery Center,** 3291 North McMullen Booth Road, Clearwater, FL 33761; tel. 727/725-5800; FAX. 727/797-4002; Diana Procuniar, Administrator

**Dermatologic and Cosmetic Surgery Center, L.C.,** 2668 Swamp Cabbage Court, Fort Myers, FL 33901; tel. 239/936-1145; FAX. 239/275-5074; Charles Eby, MD

**Doctors Surgery Center,** 921 North Main Street, Kissimmee, FL 34744; tel. 407/933-7800; FAX. 407/933-0564; Deloris Hillman, Administrator

**Emerald Coast Surgery Center,** 995 Northwest Mar Walt Drive, Fort Walton Beach, FL 32547; tel. 850/863-7887; FAX. 850/863-4955; Karen Payne, Administrator

**Endoscopy Center of Ocala, Inc.,** 1901 SE 18th Avenue, #400, Ocala, FL 34471; tel. 352/732-8905; FAX. 352/732-2661; Bill Emerson, Administrator

**Endoscopy Center of Sarasota,** 1435 Osprey Avenue, Suite 100, Sarasota, FL 34239; tel. 941/366-4475; FAX. 941/366-4390; Pam Copeland, RN, Administrator

**Eye Care and Surgery Center of Ft. Lauderdale,** 2540 Northeast Ninth Street, Ft. Lauderdale, FL 33304; tel. 954/561-3533; FAX. 954/565-9706; Jane M. Beatly, Administrator

**Eye Surgery and Laser Center,** 4120 Del Prado Boulevard, Cape Coral, FL 33904; tel. 239/542-4068; FAX. 239/542-0704; Latosha Underwood, RN, BSN, Risk Manager Designee

**Eye Surgery and Laser Center, LLC,** 409 Avenue K, SE, Winter Haven, FL 33880; tel. 863/299-8574; FAX. 863/294-8305; Eileen D. Beltramba, RN, BS, Center Director

**Eye Surgicenter,** 2521 Northwest 41st Street, Gainesville, FL 32606; tel. 352/377-7733; FAX. 352/377-9577; William A. Newsome, MD

**Florida Eye Clinic Ambulatory Surgical Center,** 160 Boston Avenue, Altamonte Springs, FL 32701; tel. 407/834-7776; FAX. 407/834-2478; Scott Bridgeman, Chief Executive Officer

**Florida Eye Institute Surgicenter, LLC,** 2750 Indian River Boulevard, Vero Beach, FL 32960; tel. 772/569-9500; FAX. 772/569-9507; Lyn M. Lane, Administrator

**Florida Medical Clinic Special Procedures Center,** 38135 Market Square, Zephyrhills, FL 33542; tel. 813/780-8266; FAX. 813/715-4150; Melissa LoParco, RN, Manager

**Florida Surgery Center,** 180 Boston Avenue, Altamonte Springs, FL 32701; tel. 407/830-0573; FAX. 407/830-4373; Patricia Rustin, Administrator

**Foundation for Advanced Eye Care,** 3737 N. Pine Island Rd, Sunrise, FL 33351; tel. 954/572-5888; Wayne Bizer, DO Medical Director

**Gaskins Eye Care and Surgery Center,** 2335 Ninth Street, N., Suite 304, Naples, FL 34103; tel. 239/263-7750; William Darrell Gaskins, MD

**Gulf Coast Surgery Center,** 411 Second Street, E., Bradenton, FL 34208; tel. 941/746-1121; FAX. 941/746-7816; Carlene Bailey, RN, Administrator

**Gulfcoast Surgery Center,** 12132 Cortez Boulevard, Brooksville, FL 34613; tel. 352/596-0744; Fawzi Soliman, MD

**HealthPark Surgery Center,** 1283 Jacaranda Boulevard, Venice, FL 34292; tel. 941/497-5660; FAX. 941/492-3942; Kermit Knight, CASC Administrator

**HealthSouth Orlando Center for Outpatient Surgery,** 1405 South Orange Avenue, Suite 400, Orlando, FL 32806; tel. 407/426-8331; FAX. 407/425-9582

**Hillmoor Eye Surgery Center, LLC dba One Day Surgery,** 1715 Southeast Tiffany Avenue, Port St. Lucie, FL 34952; tel. 772/335-7005; FAX. 772/335-3394; Diane DelRosario, Administrator

**Holiday Surgery Center,** 1109 U.S. Highway 19, Suite B, Holiday, FL 34691; tel. 727/934-5705; FAX. 727/937-3756; David Wall, Practice Administrator

**Jacksonville Surgery Center,** 7021 A.C. Skinner Parkway, Jacksonville, FL 32256; tel. 904/281-0021; FAX. 904/281-0988; Katherine Anderson, RN, BSN, Administrtor

**Jupiter Eye Center, LLC,** 102 Coastal Way, Jupiter, FL 33477; tel. 561/747-1111; FAX. 560/747-6682; Tom M. Coffman, MD, Medical Director

**Kissimmee Surgery Center,** 2275 North Central Avenue, Kissimmee, FL 34741; tel. 407/870-0573; FAX. 407/870-1859; Mark Aanonson, Administrator

**Lake Surgery and Endoscopy Center,** 8100 Country Road 44 LEG A, Leesburg, FL 34788; tel. 352/323-1995; FAX. 352/326-9990; Ismail A. Ismail, RPH, Chief Financial Officer

**Lee County Center for Foot and Ankle Surgery, Inc.,** 12734 Kenwood Lane, Suite 44, Fort Myers, FL 33907; tel. 941/936-2454; FAX. 941/936-1974; Sandra Desai, DPM

**Martin Memorial SurgiCenter,** 509 Riverside Drive, Suite 100, Stuart, FL 34994; tel. 772/223-5920; FAX. 772/288-5820

**Mayo Clinic Jacksonville Ambulatory Surgery Center for G.I.,** 4500 San Pablo Road, Jacksonville, FL 32224; tel. 904/223-2000; Patricia Sayles, ASC for GI Coordinator

**Medical Development Corporation of Pasco County,** 7315 Hudson Avenue, Hudson, FL 34667; tel. 727/868-9563; FAX. 727/863-6914; Dawn M. Ernst, Director, Nursing

**Melbourne Surgery Center,** 1340 Medical Park Drive, Suite 101, Melbourne, FL 32901; tel. 321/729-9493; FAX. 321/768-6043; Brian Rye, Administrator

**Merritt Island Surgery Center,** 220 North Sykes Creek Parkway, Suite 101, Merritt Island, FL 32953; tel. 321/459-0015; FAX. 321/459-2291; Cynthia Johnson, Administrator

**Miami Eye Center,** 619 Northwest 12th Avenue, Miami, FL 33136; tel. 305/326-0260; FAX. 305/326-1907; Edward C. Gelber, MD, FACS

**Mid Florida Surgery Center,** 17564 West Highway 441, Mt. Dora, FL 32757; tel. 352/735-4100; FAX. 352/735-2444; Patsy Lentz, RN, Administrative Director

**Montgomery Eye Center,** 700 Neapolitan Way, Naples, FL 34103; tel. 239/261-8383; FAX. 239/261-8443; Jay E. Montgomery, Administrator

**Mullis Eye Institute, Inc.,** 1600 Jenks Avenue, Panama City, FL 32405; tel. 904/763-6666; FAX. 904/763-6665; Colette Smith, RN, Director

**Naples Day Surgery North,** 11161 Health Park Boulevard, Naples, FL 34110; tel. 239/598-3111; FAX. 239/598-1707; Thomas C. Buckley, Executive Director

**New Port Richey Surgery Center,** 5415 Gulf Drive, New Port Richey, FL 34652; tel. 727/848-0446; FAX. 727/842-3166; Sandra McFarland, RN, Administrator

**Newgate Surgery Center, Inc.,** 5200 Tamiami Trail, Suite 202, Naples, FL 34103; tel. 239/263-6766; FAX. 239/263-3320; Dr. R. Crane

**North County Surgicenter,** 4000 Burns Road, Palm Beach Gardens, FL 33410; tel. 561/626-6446; FAX. 561/626-7244; Brenna Fazio, Business Manager

**North Florida Surgery Center,** 256 Professional Glen, Lake City, FL 32025; tel. 386/758-8937; FAX. 386/755-2169; Kathy Lovelace, Administrator

**North Florida Surgical Pavilion,** 6705 Northwest 10th Place, Gainesville, FL 32605; tel. 352/333-4555; FAX. 352/333-4569; Susan Roland, Administrative Director

**North Tampa Outpatient Surgical Facility,** 5329 Primrose Lake Circle, Tampa, FL 33647; tel. 813/463-9762; Becky Furniss, Administrator

**Northwest Florida Surgery Center,** 767 Airport Road, Panama City, FL 32405; tel. 850/747-0400; FAX. 850/913-9744; Ron Samuelian, Chief Executive Officer

**Novamed Surgery Center of Sebring,** 3601 South Highlands Avenue, Sebring, FL 33870; tel. 863/382-7500; FAX. 863/385-7332; Dana G. Cowart, ASC Director

**Oakwater Surgical Center, Inc.,** 3885 Oakwater Circle, Suite B, Orlando, FL 32806; tel. 407/438-9533; FAX. 407/438-9542; Carol Terry, RN

**Orange Park Surgery Center,** 2050 Professional Center Drive, Orange Park, FL 32073; tel. 904/272-2550; FAX. 904/272-7911; Michele K. Cook, RN, Administrator

**Outpatient Surgical Services, Ltd.,** 301 Northwest 82nd Avenue, Plantation, FL 33324; tel. 954/693-8600; FAX. 954/424-1966; Wayne C. Jones, FACHE, Administrator

**Palm Beach Eye Clinic,** 130 Butler Street, West Palm Beach, FL 33407; tel. 561/832-6113; FAX. 561/833-3003; Andre J. Golino, MD

**Section C**

**Palm Beach Lakes Surgery Center,** 2047 Palm Beach Lakes Boulevard, West Palm Beach, FL 33409; tel. 561/296-1330; FAX. 561/296-1350; Jonathan Cutler DPM, Manager

**Parkside Surgery Center,** 2731 Park Street, Jacksonville, FL 32205; tel. 904/389-1077; FAX. 904/338-9016; David Manning, Administrator

**Physician's Surgical Care Center,** 2056 Aloma Avenue, Winter Park, FL 32792; tel. 407/647-5100; FAX. 407/647-1966

**Physicians Ambulatory Surgery Center,** 300 Clyde Morris Boulevard, Suite B, Ormond Beach, FL 32174; tel. 386/672-1080; FAX. 386/672-8628; Joel M. Wilder, RN, Administrator

**Physicians Surgery Center, Ltd., dba Lee Island Coast Surgery Center,** 4035 Evans Avenue, Fort Myers, FL 33901; tel. 941/939-7375; FAX. 941/275-5248; Michael Pankey, RN, Administrator

**Port Orange Endoscopy & Surgery Center,** 1185 Dunlawton Avenue, Suite 100, Port Orange, FL 32127; tel. 386/672-0017; FAX. 386/672-6732; Susan K. Amon, RN, DON LHCRM

**Rand Surgical Pavilion Corp.,** Five West Sample Road, Deerfield Beach, FL 33064; tel. 954/782-1700; FAX. 954/782-7490; Deborah Rand, Administrator

**Reed Centre for Ambulatory Urological Surgery,** 1111 Kane Concourse, Suite 311, Bay Harbor, FL 33154; tel. 305/865-2000

**Same Day Surgicenter of Orlando,** 88 West Kaley Street, Orlando, FL 32806; tel. 407/423-0573; FAX. 407/841-3872; Bob Bashore, Administrator

**Samuel Wells Surgicenter, Inc.,** 3599 University Boulevard, S., Suite 604, Jacksonville, FL 32216; tel. 904/399-0905; FAX. 904/346-0757; Faye T. Evans, Risk Manager

**Seven Springs Surgery Center, Inc.,** 2024 Seven Springs Boulevard, New Port Richey, FL 34655; tel. 727/376-7000; FAX. 727/375-8944; Kathleen M. Geiger, RN, Surgery Director

**Southwest Florida Endoscopy Center,** 5050 Mason Corbin Court, Ft. Myers, FL 33907; tel. 239/275-6678; FAX. 239/275-5216; Jansi Prabakaran, MD, Administrator

**Southwest Florida Institute of Ambulatory Surgery,** 3700 Central Avenue, Suite Two, Ft. Myers, FL 33901; tel. 239/275-0665; FAX. 239/275-0503; Susan Hanzevack, Executive Director

**Specialty Surgery Of Ocala, LLC,** 3201 Southwest 34th Street, Ocala, FL 34474; tel. 352/237-6162; FAX. 352/509-9409; DeeDee Burroughs, RN, LHRM, Nurse Administrator

**St. Augustine Endoscopy Center,** 212 Southpark Circle, East, St. Augustine, FL 32086; tel. 904/824-6108; FAX. 904/823-9613; Santiago A. Rosado, MD, FACP, FACG, President

**St. Lucy's Outpatient Surgery Center,** 21275 Olean Boulevard, Port Charlotte, FL 33952; tel. 941/625-1325; FAX. 941/255-6985; Barb Vivas, RN, DON, Clinical Administrator

**St. Luke's Outpatient Surgery Center - Satellite,** 4500 San Pablo Road, Jacksonville, FL 32224; tel. 904/953-0100; FAX. 904/953-0019; Carla Pats, Manager

**St. Luke's Surgical Center,** 43309 U.S. Highway 19, N., Tarpon Spring, FL 34689; tel. 727/938-2020; FAX. 727/938-5606; Gustavo Gamero, MD, Medical Director

**Suncoast Eye Center, Eye Surgery Institute,** 14003 Lakeshore Boulevard, Hudson, FL 34667; tel. 727/868-9442; FAX. 727/862-6210; Lawrence A. Seigel, MD, PA, Medical Director

**Suncoast Medical Clinic, LLC,** 601 Seventh Street, S., St. Petersburg, FL 33701; tel. 727/894-1818; FAX. 727/824-7177; David Bailey, Executive Director

**Surgery Center at Coral Springs,** 967 University Drive, Coral Springs, FL 33071; tel. 954/341-5553; FAX. 954/344-7054; Jeff Rosenberg, Administrator

**Surgery Center at St. Andrews, Inc.,** 1350 East Venice Avenue, Venice, FL 34285; tel. 941/484-2030; FAX. 941/484-2010; Carol Carr, Administrator

**Surgery Center of North Florida, Inc.,** 6520 Northwest Ninth Boulevard, Gainsville, FL 32615; tel. 352/331-7987; FAX. 352/331-2787; Joy Ingram, Administrator

**Surgery Center of Stuart,** 2096 Southeast Ocean Boulevard, Stuart, FL 34996; tel. 772/223-0174; FAX. 772/223-0946; Barbara Tidwell, Administrator

**Surgical Licensed Ward, dba Underwood Surgery Center,** 110 West Underwood Street, Suite B, Orlando, FL 32806; tel. 407/648-9151; FAX. 407/426-7017; Doug Oakley, Administrator

**Surgical Park Center, Ltd.,** 9100 Southwest 87th Avenue, Miami, FL 33176; tel. 305/271-9100; FAX. 305/598-5509; Lionel Lima

**Surgicare Center, Inc.,** 4101 Evans Avenue, Ft. Myers, FL 33901; tel. 239/939-3456; FAX. 239/939-1164; Sharon A. Sileno, Director of Nursing

**Tallahassee Endoscopy Center,** 2400 Miccosukee Road, Tallahassee, FL 32308; tel. 850/877-2105; FAX. 850/942-1761; Noel Withers, Administrator

**Tallahassee Outpatient Surgery Center, Inc.,** 3334 Capital Medical Boulevard, Suite 500, Tallahassee, FL 32308; tel. 904/877-4688; FAX. 904/877-0368; Judi Cleckner RN, Administrator

**Tallahassee Single Day Surgery,** 1661 Phillips Road, Tallahassee, FL 32308; tel. 850/878-5165; FAX. 850/942-5545; Elizabeth Trikardos, Director of Nursing

**Tampa Bay Surgery Center,** 11811 North Dale Mabry Hwy, Tampa, FL 33618; tel. 813/961-8500; FAX. 813/265-2564; Jay L. Rosen, MD, Chief Executive Officer

**Tampa Bay Surgery Center,** 2727 MLK Blvd, Tampa, FL 33607; tel. 813/961-8500; FAX. 813/265-2564; Jay L. Rosen, MD, Chief Executive Officer

**Tampa Eye Surgery Center,** 4302 North Gomez, Tampa, FL 33607; tel. 813/870-6330; FAX. 813/871-3956; Beverly Martin, Administrator

**Tampa Outpatient Surgical Facility,** 5013 North Armenia Avenue, Tampa, FL 33603; tel. 813/875-0562; FAX. 813/871-5236; Christina McDonald, Administrator

**The Aesthetic Plastic Surgery Center,** 135 San Marco Drive, Venice, FL 34285; tel. 941/484-6836; FAX. 941/484-9690; Linda Martin, Administrative Director

**The Endoscopy Center,** 4810 North Davis Highway, Pensacola, FL 32503; tel. 850/474-8988; FAX. 850/478-9903; Steve Dunn, Administrator

**The Endoscopy Center, Inc.,** 5101 Southwest 8th Street, Miami, FL 33134; tel. 305/461-1881; FAX. 305/445-2406; Carla Guerrero, Administration

**The Eye Associates Surgery Center,** 6002 Pointe West Boulevard, Bradenton, FL 34209; tel. 941/792-2020; FAX. 941/792-2832; Pamela Morgan, RN, ASC Director

**The Gastrointestinal Center of Hialeah, Inc.,** 135 West 49th Street, Hialeah, FL 33012; tel. 305/825-1487; FAX. 305/825-9731; Maria T. Pineda, Administrator

**The Ocala Eye Surgery Center,** 3330 Southwest 33rd Road, Ocala, FL 34474; tel. 352/873-9311; FAX. 352/873-9652; Ann Hotaling, Director

**The Sarasota Ophthalmology, ASC, LLC, dba Center for Advanced Eye Surgery,** 3920 Bee Ridge Road Building F, Suite C, Sarasota, FL 34233; tel. 941/925-0000; FAX. 941/927-2726; Darice Downs, RN, LHRM,Center Director

**The Sheridan Surgery Center,** 95 Bulldog Boulevard, Suite 104, Melbourne, FL 32901; tel. 321/952-9800; FAX. 321/952-7889; Anne Latorra, Director

**The Surgery Center of Coral Gables, LLC,** 1097 SW Le Jeune Road, Miami, FL 33134; tel. 305/461-1300; Laura Lilburn, RN, CNOR, Center Director

**Total Surgery Center,** 130 Tamiami Trail, Suite 210, Naples, FL 34102; tel. 239/434-4118; FAX. 239/434-6343; Mary Boedeker, Administrator

**Treasure Coast Center for Surgery,** 1411 East Ocean Boulevard, Stuart, FL 34996; tel. 772/286-8028; FAX. 772/283-6628; Andrea Day, Business Office Manager

**University Surgical Center,** 7251 University Boulevard, Suite 100, Winter Park, FL 32792; tel. 407/677-0066; FAX. 407/677-4199; Laura Hofma Butrick, MBA, RHIA, CASC, Administrator

**Urological Ambulatory Surgery Center, Inc.,** 1812 North Mills Avenue, Orlando, FL 32803; tel. 407/992-2640; FAX. 407/897-2290; William Hamiger, Administrator

**Venture Ambulatory Surgery Center,** 16853 Northeast Second Avenue, Suite 400, North Miami Beach, FL 33162; tel. 305/652-2999; FAX. 305/652-8156; Lali Perez, RN, BSN, Center Director

**Vero Eye Center,** 70 Royal Palm Pointe, Vero Beach, FL 32960; tel. 772/569-6600; FAX. 772/569-5341; E.S. Branigan, III, MD

**Volusia Endoscopy & Surgery Center, Inc.,** 550 Memorial Circle, Suite G, Ormond Beach, FL 32174; tel. 386/672-0017; FAX. 386/672-6732; Susan K. Amon, RN, DON LHCRM

**Waterside Ambulatory Surgical Center, Inc.,** 2001 North Flagler Drive, West Palm Beach, FL 33407; tel. 561/659-6543; FAX. 561/659-3533; Lisa Bolognini, Administrative Director

## GEORGIA

**Advanced Aesthetics Plastic Surgery Center,** 874 Lanier Avenue West, One Prestige Park, Fayetteville, GA 30124; tel. 770/461-4000; FAX. 770/603-7064; Paul D. Feldman, President

**Advanced Surgery Center of Georgia,** 220 Hospital Road, Canton, GA 30114; tel. 770/479-2202; FAX. 770/479-6666; Marguerite Cammarata, Administrator

**Aesthetic Laser & Surgery Facility,** 416 Gordon Avenue, Thomasville, GA 31792-6644; tel. 229/228-7200; FAX. 229/228-5193; G. Courtney Houston, MD, Medical Director

**Aestheticare Surgicenter, P.C.,** 975 Johnson Ferry Road, Suite 160, Atlanta, GA 30342; tel. 404/303-7542; FAX. 404/531-0649; Sharon A. Pesselato, Director

**Affinity Outpatient Services,** 2224 US Highway 41 North, Tifton, GA 31794; tel. 912/391-4299; FAX. 912/391-4291; Barry L. Cutts, Administrator

**Albany Surgery Center, LLP,** 531 Seventh Avenue, Albany, GA 31701; tel. 229/883-3535; FAX. 229/883-3783; Stephen M. Wilder, DPM, Medical Director

**Ambulatory Foot and Leg Surgical Center,** 1650 Mulkey Road, Austell, GA 30106; tel. 770/941-3633; FAX. 770/944-9038; Douglas Elleby, DPM, Chief Executive Officer

**Ambulatory Laser and Surgery Center,** 425 Forest Parkway, Suite 103, Forest Park, GA 30297-2135; tel. 404/363-1087; FAX. 404/363-9951; Dr. Paul A. Colon, Medical Director

**Athens Plastic Surgery Center,** 2325 Prince Avenue, Athens, GA 30606; tel. 706/546-0280; FAX. 404/548-0258; Stephen B. Lober, MD, Administrator

**Atlanta Aesthetic Surgery Center, LLC,** 4200 Northside Parkway, Building Eight, Atlanta, GA 30327; tel. 404/233-3833; FAX. 404/233-8447; Debbie Clotfelter, Administrator

**Atlanta Center for Women's Choice, Inc.,** 1874 Piedmont Ave NE, Ste 585 E, Atlanta, GA 30324; tel. 404/892-8608; FAX. 404/892-8143; Toni P. Hawkins, Administrator

**Atlanta Endoscopy Center, Ltd.,** 2665 North Decatur Road, Suite 545, Decatur, GA 30033; tel. 404/297-5000; FAX. 404/296-9890; Kevin Mussared RN Clinical Coordinator

**Atlanta Gastroenterology Associates,** 301 Philip Blvd, Suite A, Lawrenceville, GA 30046; tel. 770/822-5560; Diane Wilkins, Office Manager

**Atlanta Outpatient Peachtree Dunwoody Center,** 5505 Peachtree-Dunwoody Road, Suite 150, Atlanta, GA 30342; tel. 404/847-0893; FAX. 404/843-8664; Kim Ashe, Chief Executive Officer, Director

**Atlanta Women's Medical Center, Inc.,** 235 West Wieuca Road, Atlanta, GA 30342; tel. 404/257-0057; FAX. 404/257-1245; Golda Melnik, Administrator

**Augusta Plastic Surgery Center, Inc.,** 1348 Walton Way, Suite 6300, Augusta, GA 30901-2772; tel. 706/724-5611; FAX. 706/724-5435

**Augusta Surgical Center,** 915 Russell Street, Augusta, GA 30904-4115; tel. 706/738-4925; FAX. 706/738-7224; Jeff Simless, Administrator

**Brunswick Endoscopy Center,** 3217 4th Street, Brunswick, GA 31520-3759; tel. 912/267-1802; FAX. 912/267-0061; Rita Warren, Administrator

**Center for Plastic Surgery, Inc.,** 365 East Paces Ferry Road, Atlanta, GA 30305; tel. 404/814-0868; FAX. 404/814-0869; Dr. Vincent Zubowicz, Medical Director

**Clayton Outpatient Surgical Center, Inc.,** 6911 Tara Boulevard, Jonesboro, GA 30236; tel. 770/477-9535; FAX. 770/471-7826; Renee Grimsley, Administrator

**Cobb Foot and Leg Surgery Center,** 792 Church Street, Suite 102, Marietta, GA 30060; tel. 770/422-9864; FAX. 770/984-0303; Glyn Lewis, Administrator

**Coliseum Same Day Surgery,** 340 Hospital Drive, P.O. Box 6154, Macon, GA 31208; tel. 912/742-1403; FAX. 912/742-1671; Lenore Sell, Administrator

**Columbus Women's Health Organization, Inc.,** 3850 Rosemont Drive, Columbus, GA 31901; tel. 706/323-8363

**DeKalb Gastroenterology Associates II, LLC, dba DeKalb Endoscopy Center,** 2675 North Decatur Road, Suite 506, Decatur, GA 30033; tel. 404/299-1679; FAX. 404/508-7558; Mark A. Stern, MD

**Dennis Surgery Center, Inc.,** 3193 Howell Mill Road, Suite 215, Atlanta, GA 30327; tel. 404/355-1312; FAX. 404/352-2798; Valerie Garrett, Administrator

**Dunwoody Outpatient Surgicenter, Inc.,** 4553 North Shallowford Road, Suite 60C, Atlanta, GA 30338; tel. 770/455-1983; FAX. 770/457-2823; Janet Davies, Administrator

**Endoscopy Center of Columbus, LLC,** 1130 Talbotton Road, Columbus, GA 31904-8745; tel. 706/641-6900; FAX. 706/327-0757; Jean Patterson, RN, Administrator

**Endoscopy Center of Southeast Georgia, Inc.,** 200 Maple Drive, P.O. Box 1367, Vidalia, GA 30474; tel. 912/538-1003; FAX. 912/537-9843; Dixie Calhoun, RN, Administrator

**Evans Surgery Center,** 635 Ronald Reagan Drive, Evans, GA 30809; tel. 706/868-3110; FAX. 706/868-3156; Sharon Gelinas, Administrator

**Feminist Women's Health Center,** 1924 Cliff Valley Way, Atlanta, GA 30329; tel. 404/728-7900; FAX. 404/728-7907; Erin Mabile, Clinical Director

**G.I. Endoscopy Center,** 6555 Professional Place, Suite B, Riverdale, GA 30274; tel. 770/692-0100; FAX. 770/692-6190; Aruna Prakash, BSc, Administrator

**Gainesville Surgery Center,** 1945 Beverly Road, Gainesville, GA 30501-2034; tel. 770/287-1500; Karen Fankhauser, Administrator

**Georgia Surgical Centers - South,** 541 Forest Parkway, Suite 14, Forest Park, GA 30297-6110; tel. 404/366-5652; Trudy Hunley, Administrator

**Gwinnett Endoscopy Center,** 301 Philip Blvd, NW, Suite B, Lawrenceville, GA 30046; tel. 770/682-7220; FAX. 770/338-0510; Kerry H. King, MD, Medical Director

**HealthSouth Surgery Center of Atlanta,** 1140 Hammond Drive, Building F, Suite 6100, Atlanta, GA 30328; tel. 770/551-9944; FAX. 770/551-8826; Mary Hardwick, Administrator

**HealthSouth Surgery Center of Gwinnett,** 2131 Fountain Drive, Snellville, GA 30078; tel. 770/979-8200; FAX. 770/979-1327; Holly Kouts, Administrator

**Kramer Professional Building,** 215 Clairemont Avenue, Decatur, GA 30030; tel. 404/373-2529; FAX. 404/373-1655; Jerald N. Kramer, DPM, President

**Marietta Surgical Center,** 780 Canton Road, Suite 100, Marietta, GA 30060; tel. 770/422-1579; FAX. 770/428-4861; Faith Wheeler, RNCNOR, QA and Risk Manager

**Medical Eye Associates, Inc.,** 1429 Oglethorpe Street, Macon, GA 31201; tel. 478/743-7061; FAX. 478/743-6296; Diane Vaughn, Practice Manager

**Midtown Urology Surgical Center,** 128 North Avenue, NE, Suite 100, Atlanta, GA 30308; tel. 404/881-0966; FAX. 404/874-5902; Jenelle E. Foote, MD, Medical Director

**North Atlanta Head and Neck Surgery Center, LLC,** 980 Johnson Ferry Road, Northside Doctors Centre, Atlanta, GA 30342; tel. 404/843-9171; FAX. 404/250-1881; Pradeep K. Snha, MD, PhD

**North Georgia Endoscopy Center, Inc.,** 320 Hospital Road, Canton, GA 30114; tel. 770/479-5535; FAX. 770/479-8821; Kevin V. Kellogg, Administrator

**North Georgia Outpatient Surgery Center,** 795 Red Bud Road, Calhoun, GA 30701; tel. 706/629-1852; FAX. 706/629-8004; Herbert E. Kosmahl, President

**North Oak Ambulatory Surgery Center, LLC,** 2718 North Oak Street, Valdosta, GA 31602; tel. 229/242-3668; FAX. 229/253-8666; T.E. Pitts, DPM

**Northeast Endoscopy Center, LLC,** 721 Wellness Way, Suite 110, Lawrenceville, GA 30045; tel. 770/995-7989; FAX. 770/339-8646; Betsy Roberts, Practice Manager

**Northeast Georgia Plastic Surgery Center,** 1296 Sims Street, Gainesville, GA 30501; tel. 770/534-1856; FAX. 770/531-0355; Sam Richwine, Medical Director

**Northlake Endoscopy Center,** 1459 Montreal Road, Suite 204, Tucker, GA 30084; tel. 770/939-4721; FAX. 770/939-1187; Ellen Burney, Administrator

**Northside Foot and Ankle Outpatient Surgical Center,** 3415 Holcomb Bridge Road, Norcross, GA 30092; tel. 770/449-1122; FAX. 770/242-8709; Steven T. Arminio, DPM, Administrator

**Northside Women's Clinic, Inc.,** 3543 Chamblee-Dunwoody Road, Atlanta, GA 30341; tel. 770/455-4210; FAX. 770/451-9529; James W. Gay, MD, Administrator

**Outpatient Center for Foot Surgery, Inc.,** 730 South Eighth Street, Suite B, Griffin, GA 30224; tel. 770/228-6644; FAX. 770/228-5769; Mark Henson, Administrator

**Paces Plastic Surgery Center, Inc.,** 3200 Downwood Circle, Suite 640, Atlanta, GA 30327; tel. 404/351-0051; FAX. 404/351-0632; Delene Graham, Office Manager

**Planned Parenthood of Reproductive Health Services,** 1289 Broad Street, Augusta, GA 30911; tel. 706/724-5557; FAX. 706/724-5293; Vanetta D. King, Center Manager

**Pulliam Ambulatory Surgical Center,** 4167 Hospital Drive, P.O. Box 469, Covington, GA 30015; tel. 770/786-1234; M.M. Pulliam, PC, Medical Director

**Resurgens Surgical Center,** 5671 Peachtree Dunwoody Road, Suite 800, Atlanta, GA 30342; tel. 404/531-8532; Leslie Mattson, RN Administrator

**Savannah Foot And Ankle Surgery Center,** 310 Eisenhower Drive, Savannah, GA 31406; tel. 912/356-8440; FAX. 912/356-8439; Kay J. West, Administrator

**Savannah Medical Clinic,** 120 East 34th Street, Savannah, GA 31401; tel. 912/236-1603; FAX. 912/236-1605; William Knorr, MD, Administrator

**Savannah Plastic Surgicenter,** 7208 Hodgson Memorial, Savannah, GA 31406; tel. 912/351-5050; FAX. 912/351-5051; Scott W. Vann MD

**Statesboro Ambulatory Surgery Center,** 95 Bel-Air Drive, Statesboro, GA 30461-6879; tel. 912/489-6519; FAX. 912/764-7882; Luane L. Jordan, RN

**The Emory Clinic Ambulatory Surgery Center,** 1365 Clifton Road, NE, Atlanta, GA 30322; tel. 404/778-5000; W. Mike Mason, Administrator

**The Foot Surgery Center,** 2520 Windy Hill Road, Suite 105, Marietta, GA 30067; tel. 770/952-0868; FAX. 770/952-4833; Donna L. Cowan, Nurse Administrator

**The Rome Surgery Center,** 16 John Maddox Drive, Rome, GA 30165; tel. 706/802-3727; FAX. 706/802-3883; Neal Jochimsen, Administrator

**The Surgery Center, LLC,** 2548 Weems Rd, Columbus, GA 31909-6248; tel. 706/323-8803; FAX. 706/323-9101; Sharon Johnson, Administrator

**Tifton Endoscopy Center, Inc.,** 1111 E. 20th Street, Tifton, GA 31794-3668; tel. 229/382-9338; FAX. 229/382-4282; Linda Ingram, RN, Nursing Administrator

**Village Podiatry,** 1350 Upper Hembree Road, Suite 100, Roswell, GA 30076; tel. 770/663-8011; FAX. 770/754-9820; Dr. Mitch Hilsen, Administrator

## HAWAII

**Aloha Surgical Center,** 239 Hoohana Street, Kahului, HI 96732; tel. 808/893-0578; FAX. 808/893-0580; Russell T. Stodd, MD, Medical Director

**Big Island Endoscopy Center, LLC,** 64-5188 Kinohou Street, Kamuela, HI 96743; tel. 808/887-0600; FAX. 808/887-6699; Aulii Delenia, Administrator

**Cataract and Vision Center of Hawaii,** 1712 Liliha Street, Suite 400, Honolulu, HI 96817; tel. 808/524-1010; FAX. 808/531-1030; Worldster Lee, MD, Director

**Hawaii Endoscopy Center, LLC,** 2226 Liliha Street, Suite 307, Honolulu, HI 96817; tel. 808/531-5828; FAX. 808/531-5819; Linda Oshiro, Administrator

**Hawaiian Eye Surgicenter,** 606 Kilani Avenue, Wahiawa, HI 96786; tel. 808/621-8448; FAX. 808/621-3177; Christopher M. Tortora, MD, Surgeon, Director

**Hilo Community Surgery Center,** 82 Pu'uhonu Place, Suite 100, Hilo, HI 96720; tel. 808/969-9669; FAX. 808/969-9608; Allan S. Takase, MD, Administrator

**Kaiser Honolulu Clinic,** 1010 Pensacola Street, Honolulu, HI 96814; tel. 808/545-2950; FAX. 808/597-2249; Jonathan Ganz, Administrator

**Kaiser Wailuku Clinic,** 80 Mahalani Street, Wailuku, HI 96793; tel. 808/243-6112; FAX. 808/243-6609; Martha Turner, Director

**Surgicare of Hawaii, an affiliate of S.C.A.,** 550 South Beretania Street, Suite 700, Honolulu, HI 96813; tel. 808/528-0211; FAX. 808/526-0651; Kare Klungreseter, Administrator

**The Endoscopy Center,** 134 Puuhonu Way, Hilo, HI 96720; tel. 808/935-1956; FAX. 808/935-7657; Jody Montell, Administrator

**The Surgical Suites, LLC,** 1100 Ward Avenue, Suite 1001, Honolulu, HI 96814; tel. 808/531-0127; FAX. 808/531-0455; Carlos Omphroy, MD, President

## IDAHO

**Addison Surgery Center,** 191 Addison Avenue, Twin Falls, ID 83301; tel. 208/734-5993; FAX. 208/734-5993; David A. Blackmer, DPM, President

**Boise Gastroenterology Associates, P.A., Idaho Endoscopy Center,** 6259 W. Emerald Street, Boise, ID 83704; tel. 208/489-1900; FAX. 208/375-5286; Robb F. Gibson, MD, President

**Coeur D'Alene Foot and Ankle Surgery Center,** 101 Ironwood Drive, Suite 131, Coeur D'Alene, ID 83814; tel. 208/666-0814; Stephen A. Isham, DPM, Chief Executive Officer

**Coeur D'Alene Surgery Center,** 2121 Ironwood Center Drive, Coeur D'Alene, ID 83814; tel. 208/765-9059; FAX. 208/664-9998; Peter C. Jones, MD, President

**Emerald Surgical Center,** 811 North Liberty, Boise, ID 83704; tel. 208/323-4522; FAX. 208/321-9585; Camille Miley, Nurse Director

**Idaho Ambucare Center, Inc.,** 4400 Flamingo Avenue, Nampa, ID 83686; tel. 208/288-4750; FAX. 208/288-4765; Gary Botimer, Administrator

**Idaho Eye Surgicenter,** 2025 East 17th Street, Idaho Falls, ID 83404; tel. 208/524-2025; FAX. 208/529-1924; Bradley P. Garnder, MD

**Idaho Falls Surgical Center,** 1945 East 17th Street, Idaho Falls, ID 83404; tel. 208/529-1945; FAX. 208/529-1961; Steven V. Klippert, MD, Chief Executive Officer

**Idaho Foot Surgery Center,** 1540 Elk Creek Drive, Idaho Falls, ID 83401; tel. 208/529-8393; FAX. 208/529-8078; Bruce G. Tolman, DPM, Facility Director

**Jefferson Day Surgery Center,** 220 West Jefferson, Boise, ID 83702; tel. 208/343-3802; FAX. 208/343-9161; William Stano, President

**Millennium Surgery Center,** 1828 S. Millenium Way, Suite 100, Meridian, ID 83642; tel. 208/381-0262; FAX. 208/429-8575; Shane Ricks, Administrator

**North Idaho Cataract and Laser Center, Inc.,** 1814 Lincoln Way, Coeur D'Alene, ID 83814; tel. 208/667-2531; FAX. 208/765-9385; Karen Sines, Administrator

**Pacific Cataract and Laser Institute,** 2822 South Vista Avenue, Boise, ID 83705; tel. 208/385-7576; FAX. 208/385-0050; Lisa Brady, Site Manager

**St. Luke's Clinic, Gastroenterology,** 775 Pole Line Rd West, Suite 203, Twin Falls, ID 83301; tel. 208/732-3030; FAX. 208/733-8970; Karen R. Butler, Clinical Manager

**Surgicare Center of Idaho, LLC,** 360 East Mallard Drive, Suite 125, Boise, ID 83706; tel. 208/336-8700; FAX. 208/426-0902; Mark Hollingshead, Medical Director

## ILLINOIS

**25 East Same Day Surgery,** 25 East Washington, Suite 300, Chicago, IL 60602; tel. 312/726-3329; FAX. 312/726-3823; Kimberly Zidonis, RN, Administrator

**Aanchor Health Center, Ltd.,** 1186 Roosevelt Rd., Glen Ellyn, IL 60137; tel. 630/495-4400; FAX. 630/629-5892; Aimee Dillard, Assistant Administrator

**Able Health Center, Ltd.,** 1640 Arlington Heights Road, Suite 110, Arlington Heights, IL 60004; tel. 847/255-7400; FAX. 847/398-4585

**Access Health Center, Ltd.,** 1700 75th Street, Downers Grove, IL 60516; tel. 630/964-0000; FAX. 630/964-0047; Jenny Mitchell, Administrator

**ACU Health Center, Ltd.,** 736 N. York Rd., Hinsdale, IL 60521; tel. 630/794-0645; FAX. 630/794-0169; Vera Schmidt, Chief of Operations

**Advantage Health Care, Ltd.,** 203 E. Irving Park Rd, Wood Dale, IL 60191; tel. 630/595-1515; FAX. 630/595-9907; Aimee Dillard, Assistant Administrator

**Ambulatory Surgicenter of Downers Grove, Ltd.,** 4333 Main Street, Downers Grove, IL 60515; tel. 630/322-9451; FAX. 630/322-9455; Inga Ferdkoff, MD, Administrator

**Bel-Clair Ambulatory Surgical Treatment Center,** 325 West Lincoln, Belleville, IL 62220; tel. 618/235-2299; FAX. 618/235-2556; David Horace, Administrator

**Belleville Surgical Center,** 28 North 64th Street, Belleville, IL 62223; tel. 618/398-5705; FAX. 618/398-5764; Diana Geoghegan, Administrator

**Belmont & Harlem Surgery Center,** 3101 North Harlem Avenue, Chicago, IL 60634; tel. 773/889-2000; FAX. 773/745-5522; Sandra Ankebrant, Executive Director

**Carle Surgicenter,** 1702 South Mattis Avenue, Champaign, IL 61821; tel. 217/326-2030; Administrator

**Children's Pediatric Specialty Services In Westchester,** 2301 Enterprise Drive, Westchester, IL 60154; tel. 708/836-4800; FAX. 708/836-4805; Kristen DiCicco, Administrator

**Community Health and Emergency Services,** 13245 Kessler Road, P.O. Box 233, Cairo, IL 62914; tel. 618/734-4400; FAX. 618/734-9046; Frederick L. Bernstein, Chief Executive Officer

**Dimensions Medical Center, Ltd.,** 1455 East Golf Road, Suite 108, Des Plaines, IL 60016; tel. 847/390-9300; FAX. 847/390-0001; Vera Schmidt, Administrator

**Dreyer Ambulatory Surgery Center,** 1221 North Highland Avenue, Aurora, IL 60506; tel. 630/264-8400; FAX. 630/264-8402; Brad Hlavacek, RN, BSN, MBA, Administrative Director

**Eastland Medical Plaza SurgiCenter, LLC,** 1505 Eastland Drive, Suite 180, Bloomington, IL 61701; tel. 309/662-2500; FAX. 309/662-7143; Brenda Cyrulik, Manager

**Edwardsville Ambulatory Surgical Center, LLC,** 12, Ginger Creek Parkway, Glen Carbon, IL 62034; tel. 618/656-8200; FAX. 618/656-8204; Michelle Looney, Director of Operations

**Elmwood Park Same Day Surgery Center,** 1614 North Harlem Avenue, Elmwood Park, IL 60607; tel. 708/452-5000; FAX. 708/452-5588; Mark Mayo, Administrator

**Foot and Ankle Surgical Center, Ltd.,** 1455 Golf Road, Suite 131, Des Plaines, IL 60016; tel. 847/390-7666; Lowell S. Weil, DPM, FACHS, Medical Director

**Forestview Medical Center, Ltd.,** 2750 S. River Road, Des Plaines, IL 60018; tel. 847/375-1000; FAX. 847/827-5977; Nancy Nelson, Administrator

**Fullerton Kimball Medical & Surgical Center,** 3412 West Fullerton Avenue, Chicago, IL 60647; tel. 773/235-8000; FAX. 773/235-7018; Renlin Xia, MD, Medical Director

**Golf Surgical Center,** 8901 Golf Road, Des Plaines, IL 60016; tel. 847/299-2273; FAX. 847/299-2297; Nicholas Lylizos, MD, Executive Director

**Hawthorn Surgery Center,** 1900 Hollister Drive, Suite 100, Libertyville, IL 60048; tel. 847/367-8100; FAX. 847/367-8335; Dr. Gary Rippberger, Administrator

**Hinsdale Surgical Center, LLC,** 908 North Elm Street, Suite 401, Hinsdale, IL 60521; tel. 630/325-5035; FAX. 630/325-5134; Shirley E. Zemansky, RN, Executive Director

**Hope Clinic for Women, Ltd.,** 1602 21st Street, Granite City, IL 62040; tel. 618/451-5722; FAX. 615/451-9092; Sally Burgess, MBA, Executive Director

**Illinois Eye Surgeons Cataract Surgery,** 3990 North Illinois Street, Belleville, IL 62221; tel. 618/235-3100; Nancy Mueth, Administrator

**Loyola Ambulatory Surgery Center at Oakbrook,** One South 224 Summit Avenue, Suite 201, Oakbrook Terrace, IL 60181; tel. 630/916-7088; Geoff Abbott, Administrator

**Michigan Avenue Center for Health, Ltd.,** 2415 S. Michigan Avenue, Chicago, IL 60616; tel. 312/328-1200; FAX. 312/328-1240; Aimee Dillard, Assistant Administrator

**Midwest Center for Day Surgery,** 3811 Highland Avenue, Downers Grove, IL 60515; tel. 630/852-9300; FAX. 630/852-7773; Ronald P. Ladniak, Administrator

**Midwest Eye Center, S.C.,** 1700 East West Road, Calumet City, IL 60409; tel. 708/891-3330; FAX. 708/891-0904; Afzal Ahmad, MD, Medical Director

**Naperville Surgical Centre,** 1263 Rickert Drive, Naperville, IL 60540; tel. 630/305-3300; FAX. 630/305-3301; Ronald P. Ladniak

**North Shore Endoscopy Center,** 101 South Waukegan Road, Suite 980, Lake Bluff, IL 60044; tel. 847/604-8700; FAX. 847/604-8711; Everett P. Kirch, MD, Administrator

**North Shore Surgicenter,** 3725 West Touhy Avenue, Lincolnwood, IL 60712-2603; tel. 847/324-7770; FAX. 847/324-7762; Gary Rippberger, MD, Administrator

**Northwest Community Day Surgery Center,** 675 West Kirchoff Road, Arlington Heights, IL 60005; tel. 874/618-7004; FAX. 874/618-7069; Roxanne Matias, Director

**Northwest Surgicare,** 1100 West Central Road, Arlington Heights, IL 60005; tel. 847/259-3080; FAX. 847/259-3190; Karolynn Welu-Kuecker, RN, Administrator

**Nova Med Eye Surgery Center of Maryville, LLC,** 12 Maryville Professional Park Drive, Maryville, IL 62062; tel. 618/288-7483; Sarah Davis, Administrator

**Novamed Center for Reconstructive Surgery- Oak Lawn,** 6311 West 95th Street, Oak Lawn, IL 60453; tel. 708/499-3355; FAX. 708/425-5654; Carmen Hollimon, Administrator

**Novamed Surgery Center of Chicago - Northshore,** 3034 West Peterson Avenue, Chicago, IL 60659; tel. 773/973-7432; FAX. 773/973-4134

**NovaMed Surgery Center River Forest, LLC,** 7427 Lake Street, River Forest, IL 60305; tel. 708/488-1300; FAX. 708/771-7321; Kelly Spillane, RN, ASC Director

**Oak Brook Surgical Centre, Inc.,** 2425 West 22nd Street, Suite 101, Oak Brook, IL 60523; tel. 630/990-2212; FAX. 630/990-3130; Ali Nili, Chief Operating Officer

**Oak Park Eye Center, SC,** 7638 W North Avenue, Elmwood Park, IL 60707; tel. 708/452-4257; FAX. 708/452-4283; Manuel Santiago, MD, Administrator

**Palos Surgicenter,** 7340 West College Drive, Palos Heights, IL 60463; tel. 708/361-3233; FAX. 708/361-4876; Thomas Holecek, Administrator

**Peoria Ambulatory Surgery Center,** 4909 North Glen Park Place, Peoria, IL 61614; tel. 309/691-9069; FAX. 309/690-9005; Cynthia J. Leisinger, MBA,CASC, Director of Surgical Services

**Peoria Day Surgery Center,** 7309 North Knoxville, Peoria, IL 61614; tel. 309/692-9210; FAX. 309/693-6472; Rita Hancock, Administrator

**Physicians' Surgery Center,** 2601 West Main Street, Carbondale, IL 62901; tel. 618/351-7300; FAX. 618/457-7890; Stephen Renfro, Administrator

**Physicians' Surgical Center, LLC,** 311 West Lincoln Suite 300, Belleville, IL 62220; tel. 618/233-7077; FAX. 618/233-2814; Bev LeMaster, RN, Nurse Manager

**Planned Parenthood of East Central Illinois,** 302 East Stoughton Street, Champaign, IL 61820; tel. 217/359-8022; FAX. 217/359-2683; Robin Beach, Vice President and Chief Operating Officer

**Premier Dermatology,** 2051 Plainfield Road, Crest Hill, IL 60403; tel. 815/741-4343; FAX. 815/741-8660; Rose Przenieslo, Practice Manager

**Quad City Ambulatory Surgery Center,** 520 Valley View Drive, Suite 300, Moline, IL 61265; tel. 309/762-1952; FAX. 309/762-3642; Gloria Catlett, RN, Manager

**Regionai Surgicenter, Ltd.,** 545 Valley View Drive, Moline, IL 61265; tel. 309/762-5560; FAX. 309/762-7351; Jennifer Swanson, Administrator

**River North Same Day Surgery,** One East Erie, Suite 300, Chicago, IL 60611; tel. 312/649-3939; FAX. 312/649-5747; Jonette Marino, RN, MBA, Administrator

**Rockford Ambulatory Surgery Center,** 1016 Featherstone Drive, Rockford, IL 61107; tel. 815/226-3300; FAX. 815/226-9990; Dr. Steven Gunderson, Chief Executive Officer and Medical Director

**Rockford Endoscopy Center,** 401 Roxbury Road, Rockford, IL 61107; tel. 815/397-7340; FAX. 815/397-7388; Nancy Garry, Administrator

**Rogers Park One Day Surgery Center,** 7616 North Paulina, Chicago, IL 60626; tel. 773/761-0500; FAX. 773/761-1355; Mira Pekic, Credentialing Dept. Manager

**Southwestern Medical Center, LLC, dba Magna Surgical Center,** 9831 South Western Avenue, Chicago, IL 60643; tel. 773/445-9696; FAX. 773/445-9590; Michelle Lipscomb, Assistant Administrator

**Springfield Clinic Ambulatory Surgery and Endoscopy Center,** 1025 South Seventh Street, Springfield, IL 62794-9248; tel. 217/528-7541; FAX. 217/527-8956; Ginny Timke

**Surgery Center of Southern Illinois,** PO Box 1729, 806 N. Treas, Marion, IL 62959; tel. 618/993-2113; FAX. 618/993-2041; Linda Bickers, RN, Administrator

**Surgicare Center, Inc.,** 333 Dixie Highway, Chicago Heights, IL 60411; tel. 708/754-4890; FAX. 708/709-6242; Dolores Stam, RN - Supervisor

**Surgicore, Inc.,** 10547 South Ewing Avenue, Chicago, IL 60617; tel. 773/221-1690; FAX. 773/221-1675; Michael A. Wood, DPM, Medical Director

**The Center for Orthopedic Medicine, LLC, dba The Center For Outpatient Medicine,** 2502-B East Empire Street, Bloomington, IL 61704; tel. 309/662-6120; FAX. 309/661-0060; Sarah Gardner, Business Director

**The Center for Surgery,** 475 East Diehl Road, Naperville, IL 60563-1253; tel. 630/505-7733; FAX. 630/505-0656; Eric Myers, Administrator

**The Surgery Center of Centralia,** 1045 Martin Luther King Jr. Drive, Centralia, IL 62801; tel. 618/532-3110; FAX. 618/532-7226; Mark Murfin, MD, Medical Director

**Valley Ambulatory Surgery Center and Valley Medical Inn,** 2210 Dean Street, St. Charles, IL 60175; tel. 630/584-9800; FAX. 630/584-9805; Deborah Lee Crook, RN, Administrator

**Women's Aid Clinic,** 4751 West Touhy Avenue, Lincolnwood, IL 60712-2212; tel. 847/676-2428; Iris Schneider

## INDIANA

**Aesthetic Surgery Center,** 13590 N. Meridian, Carmel, IN 46032; tel. 317/846-0846; FAX. 317/846-0722; William H. Beeson, MD, Medical Director

**Broadwest Specialty Surgical Center, LLC,** 315 West 89th Avenue, Merrillville, IN 46410-2904; tel. 219/757-5275; FAX. 219/757-5290; Angela Leach, Business Administrator

**Central Indiana Surgery Center,** 9002 North Meridian, Lower Level, Indianapolis, IN 46260; tel. 317/848-1763; FAX. 317/848-1895; Francis Price, Jr., MD, Medical Director

**Columbus Surgery Center,** 940 North Marr Road, Suite B, Columbus, IN 47201; tel. 812/372-1370; FAX. 812/373-9526; Marcy Ross, RN, Director

**Digestive Health Center,** 1120 AAA Way, Suite A, Carmel, IN 46032-3210; tel. 317/848-5494; FAX. 317/575-0392; Daniel J. Stout, MD, President

**Evansville Surgery Center,** 520 Mary Street, Evansville, IN 47710; tel. 812/433-3166; FAX. 812/433-3176; Cathy Head RN, BS, MHA, CASA Administrator

**Eye Specialists Surgery Centers, LLC,** 200 North Tillotson Avenue, Muncie, IN 47304-3988; tel. 765/286-8888; FAX. 765/747-7962; Rita Singh, MD, Chief Executive Officer

**Foot and Ankle Surgery Center, Inc.,** 8651 Township Line Road, Indianapolis, IN 46260-1578; tel. 317/334-0232; FAX. 317/334-0268; Anthony E. Miller, DPM, Owner

**Fort Wayne Ambulatory Surgery Center,** 321 East Wayne Street, Ft. Wayne, IN 46802-2713; tel. 260/422-5976; FAX. 260/969-1041; Nicole Johnson, OR Supervisor

**Fort Wayne Cardiology Outpatient Catheterization Laboratory,** 1819 Carew Street, Fort Wayne, IN 46805; tel. 260/481-4896; FAX. 260/481-4814; Douglas W. Martin, RN, MBA, Director of Clinical Operations

**Franciscan Physicians Hospital,** 701 Superior Avenue, Munster, IN 46321; tel. 219/924-1300; FAX. 219/922-4810; Barb Greene, President

**Gastrointestinal Endoscopy Center,** 801 Street Mary's Drive, Suite 110 West, Evansville, IN 47714; tel. 812/477-6103; FAX. 812/477-4897; Butch Moors, CPA, Administrator

**Grand Park Surgical Center,** 1479 East 84th Place, Merrillville, IN 46410; tel. 219/738-2828; FAX. 219/756-3349; Chris Macarthy, Administrator

**Grossnickle Eye Surgery Center, Inc.,** 2251 DuBois Drive, Warsaw, IN 46580-3292; tel. 574/269-3777; FAX. 574/371-4697; Diana Ostrom, RN, Administrator

**IMA Endoscopy Surgicenter, P.C.,** 8895 Broadway, Merrillville, IN 46410; tel. 219/736-4660; FAX. 219/736-4663; Dawn Bailey, Administrator

**Indiana Endoscopy Center,** 1801 North Senate, Suite 410, Indianapolis, IN 46202; tel. 317/962-5660; FAX. 317/963-5255; David B. Thomas, Medical Director

**Indiana Eye Clinic,** 30 North Emerson Avenue, Greenwood, IN 46143-9760; tel. 317/881-3937; FAX. 317/887-4008; Ken Dyar, RN, BSN, MBA, Executive Director

**Indiana Surgery Center,** 1550 East County Line Road, Suite 100, Indianapolis, IN 46227; tel. 317/621-7600; FAX. 317/621-7606; Peggy Davidson, Administrator

**Indiana Surgery Center - North,** 8040 Clearvista Parkway, Suite 150, Indianapolis, IN 46256; tel. 317/621-2000; FAX. 317/621-2050; Shannon Arrendale, RN, MBA, Executive Director

**Indianapolis Endoscopy Center,** 8315 E. 56th Street, Suite 100, Indianapolis, IN 46216; tel. 317/621-2232; FAX. 317/621-3232; Kathy Anderson, Executive Director

**Meridian Plastic Surgery Center,** 170 West 106th Street, Indianapolis, IN 46290-1004; tel. 317/575–0336; FAX. 317/571–8667; Joann Jones, RN, Director

**Michiana Endoscopy Center, LLC,** 53830 Generation Drive, South Bend, IN 46635; tel. 574/271–0893; FAX. 574/271–1285; David Mark, MD, Chief Executive Officer

**Munster Same Day Surgery Center,** 761 Forty Fifth Avenue, Suite 116, Munster, IN 46321; tel. 219/924–3090; FAX. 219/924–2160; Georgia Tsiongas, Administrator

**North Meridian Surgery Center,** 13225 N. Meridian Street, Carmel, IN 46032; tel. 317/574–5400; FAX. 317/575–0173; Julie Berzins, Director and Chief Executive Officer

**Northeast Indiana Endoscopy Center,** 7900 West Jefferson Boulevard, Suite 200, Fort Wayne, IN 46804; tel. 206/969–7181; FAX. 260/969–7182; Jerry Steele, Administrator

**Oakview Surgical Center, Inc.,** 120 E. 18th Street, Rochester, IN 46975; tel. 574/224–7500; FAX. 574/223–3057; Laurence C. Rogers, DPM, Administrator

**Outpatient Surgery Center of Indiana, LLP,** 711 Gardner Drive, Marion, IN 46952; tel. 317/664–2000; FAX. 317/668–6797; Dixie Hewitt, RN, Director

**Premier Surgery Center,** 11141 Parkview Plaza Drive, Suite 200, Fort Wayne, IN 46845-1714; tel. 260/266–9070; FAX. 260/266–9071; Nora Bass, NP, MSN, MBA, Senior Vice President Surgery Services

**Riverpointe Surgery Center,** 500 Arcade Avenue, Suite 100, Elkhart, IN 46514-2459; tel. 574/522–9505; FAX. 574/296–6484; John Cloyd, PhD, Executive Director

**Sagamore Surgical Services, Inc.,** 2320 Concord Road, Suite B, Lafayette, IN 47909; tel. 765/474–7854; FAX. 765/474–1317; Carol Blanar, Administrator

**South Bend Clinic Surgicenter,** 211 North Eddy Street, P.O. Box 1755, South Bend, IN 46634-4061; tel. 574/237–9366; FAX. 574/237–9363; Paul J. Meyer, Executive Director

**Southern Indiana Surgery Center,** 2800 Rex Grossman Boulevard, Bloomington, IN 47403; tel. 812/333–8969; FAX. 812/335–2309; Laura Baugh, RN, CNOR Clinical Manager, Administrative Director

**Surgery Center of Merrillville, LLC,** 8514 Broadway, Merrillville, IN 46410; tel. 219/756–5010; FAX. 219/736–5106; Tina Jackson, Director

**Surgery ONE,** 5052 North Clinton, Fort Wayne, IN 46825-5822; tel. 219/482–5194; FAX. 219/482–5686; Debra McCarter, Director

**Surgical Care Center, Inc.,** 8103 Clearvista Parkway, Indianapolis, IN 46256-4600; tel. 317/842–5173; FAX. 317/570–7429; Janelle Gray, RN, Director

**Surgical Center of New Albany,** 2201 Green Valley Road, New Albany, IN 47150-4648; tel. 812/949–1223; FAX. 812/945–4765; Tamara E. Jones, BSN, Administrator

**Surgicare,** 2907 McIntire Drive, Suite C, Bloomington, IN 47403; tel. 812/339–8000; FAX. 812/339–2524; Rhonda Jacobs, RN, Administrator

**Surgicare of Jeffersonville,** 1305 Wall Street, Suite 101, Jeffersonville, IN 47130-3898; tel. 812/288–9674; FAX. 812/283–6955; Marsha Parker, Administrator

**The Endoscopy Center at St. Francis,** 8051 South Emerson, Suite 150, Indianapolis, IN 46237; tel. 317/865–2955; FAX. 317/865–2952; James Turner, Chief Executive Officer

**The Indiana Hand to Shoulder Center,** 8501 Harcourt Road, P.O. Box 80434, Indianapolis, IN 46260-0434; tel. 317/875–9105; FAX. 317/872–1423; Valeria M. Wareham, DON, Chief Operating Officer

**Valley Cataract and Laser Institute, Inc., dba Valley Surgery Center,** 220 East Virginia, Evansville, IN 47711; tel. 812/435–1600; FAX. 812/435–1603; Lisa J. Gossman-Werner, Facility Administrator

**Whitewater Surgery Center,** 1900 Chester Boulevard, Richmond, IN 47374; tel. 765/966–1776; FAX. 765/962–1191; Mary Pordifio, RN, Nurse Manager

**Williams Eye Surgery Center,** 6836 Hohman Avenue, Hammond, IN 46324; tel. 219/937–5063; FAX. 219/937–5068; Renee Peters, Administrator

## IOWA

**Iowa Digestive Disease Center, Iowa Endoscopy Center,** 1378 NW124th Street, Suite 100, Clive, IA 50325; tel. 515/288–6097; FAX. 515/288–0384; Veryl Kroon, Chief Executive Officer

**Jones Eye Clinic,** 4405 Hamilton Boulevard, Sioux City, IA 51104-1140; tel. 712/239–3937; FAX. 712/239–4946; Charles E. Jones, MD, Medical Director

**Mississippi Valley Surgery Center, L.C.,** 3400 Dexter Court, Suite 200, Davenport, IA 52807; tel. 563/344–6600; FAX. 563/344–6699; John B. Dooley, Administrator

**Spencer Surgery and Laser Center, LLC,** 1721 West 18th Street, P.O. Box 420, Spencer, IA 51301; tel. 712/580–3278; FAX. 712/580–3279; Dennis D. Gordy, MD, Administrator

**Spring Park Surgery Center, LLC,** 3319 Spring Street, Suite 202-A, Davenport, IA 52807; tel. 563/355–6236; FAX. 563/359–6347; William Rosen, Medical Director

**Surgery Center of Des Moines,** 717 Lyon Street, Des Moines, IA 50312; tel. 515/266–3140; FAX. 515/266–3073; Michael Peabody, Administrator and Chief Executive Officer

## KANSAS

**Cotton-O'Neil Clinic Endoscopy Center,** 720 SW Lane St, Topeka, KS 66606-1539; tel. 785/270–4800; FAX. 785/270–4801; Mark Davis, Director

**Emporia Ambulatory Surgery Center,** 2528 West 15th Avenue, Emporia, KS 66801-6102; tel. 602/343–2233; J. E. Bosiljevac, MD, Administrator

**Endoscopic Services, P.A.,** 1431 South Bluffview Street, Suite 215, Wichita, KS 67218-3000; tel. 316/687–0234; FAX. 316/687–0360; Jace Hyder, MD

**Endoscopy and Surgery Center of Topeka, L.P.,** 2200 Southwest Sixth Avenue, Suite 103, Topeka, KS 66606-1707; tel. 913/354–1254; FAX. 913/354–1255; Ashraf M. Sufi, MD, Medical Director

**Eye Surgical Center,** 1100 North Topeka Street, Wichita, KS 67214-2810; tel. 316/263–6273; FAX. 316/263–5568; David A. Kingrey, Medical Director

**Hutchinson Clinic Ambulatory Surgery Center,** 2205 North Waldron, Hutchinson, KS 67502; tel. 620/728–2700; FAX. 620/728–2728; Mary Wood, Director

**Newton Surgery Center,** 800 Medical Center Drive, Newton, KS 67114-3761; tel. 316/283–4400; FAX. 316/283–6606; Joyce Hartner RN, BA, CNOR Director

**Surgicare of Wichita, Inc.,** 810 North Lorraine, Wichita, KS 67214-4841; tel. 316/685–2207; FAX. 316/685–2861; Tracie Johanek, RN, Administrator

**Team Vision Surgery Center East,** 6100 East Central Street, Suite Six, Wichita, KS 67208-4237; tel. 316/681–2020; FAX. 316/684–4939; Patricia Kusnerus, Administrator

**Team Vision Surgery Center West,** 834 North Socora, Suite One, Wichita, KS 67212-3238; tel. 316/681–2020; FAX. 316/684–4939; Patricia Kusnerus, Administrator

**Via Christi Surgery Center,** 1947 Founders' Circle, Wichita, KS 67206; tel. 316/613–4607; FAX. 316/613–4725; Penny Freeman, RN, BSN, CNOR, Manager

## KENTUCKY

**Ambulatory Surgery Center,** 2831 Lone Oak Road, Paducah, KY 42003; tel. 270/554–8373; FAX. 270/554–8987; Laxmaiah Manchikanti, MD

**Asethetic Plastic Surgery Institute of Louisville, LLC, dba Louisville Surgery Center,** 444 S. First Street, Suite 201, Louisville, KY 40202; tel. 502/238–2861; FAX. 502/238–2897; Amy McKiernan, Director of Nursing

**Baptist-Physicians' Surgery Center,** 1720 Nicholasville Rd, Suite 101, Lexington, KY 40503; tel. 859/260–7000; FAX. 859/260–7010; Robert Ramey, Administrator

**Bluegrass Surgery & Laser Center,** 1400 Poplar Level Road, Suite 1, Louisville, KY 40217; tel. 502/637–4800; FAX. 502/637–1550; Don E. Lenz, RN, Administrator

**Center For Surgical Care,** 7575 U.S. 42, Florence, KY 41042; tel. 606/283–6050; FAX. 606/283–6060; Jenny Brallier, RN, Director

**Commonwealth Eye Surgery Center,** 2353 Alexandria Drive, Suite 350, Lexington, KY 40504; tel. 859/224–2655; Jenny Lackey, Administrator

**Cumberland Valley Surgical Center,** 275 Hwy 770, Corbin, KY 40729; tel. 606/526–7874; FAX. 606/526–7836; Kim Turner, Business Director

**Dermatology Associates Of KY, PSC,** 250 Fountain Court, Lexington, KY 40509; tel. 859/263–4444; Joy Hayes, Administrator

**Dupont Surgery Center,** 4004 Dupont Circle, Louisville, KY 40207; tel. 502/896–6428; FAX. 502/893–5270; Sherry Oeswein, Administrator

**E.M.W. Women's Surgical Center,** 138 West Market Street, Louisville, KY 40202; tel. 502/589–2124; FAX. 502/589–1588; Anne Ahola, Executive Director

**Eyecare Network, Ltd.,** 1360 Medical Park Dr, Maysville, KY 41056; tel. 606/759–5341; Bryan Prater, Administrator

**Healthsouth Lexington Surgery Center,** 1451 Harrodsburg Rd, Suite 102, Lexington, KY 40504; tel. 859/276–2525; Dianna Bennett, Administrator

**Healthsouth Louisville Surgery Center,** 614 E Chestnut St, Louisville, KY 40202; tel. 502/589–9488; Vanessa McDermott, Administrator

**Jewish Hospital Medical Center East,** 3920 Dutchman's Lane, Louisville, KY 40207; tel. 502/259–6003; FAX. 502/259–6111; Shelley Neal, Administrator

**Kentucky Surgery Center,** 240 Fountain Court, Lexington, KY 40509; tel. 859/278–1460; FAX. 859/514–5107; Glenda Staterly, RN, Administrative Director

**Lake Cumberland Surgery Center,** 301 Langdon Street, Somerset, KY 42501; tel. 606/678–9688; FAX. 606/679–7479; Michael Everett, Administrative Director

**Lexington Clinic, PSC, dba Lexington Clinic Ambulatory Surgery Center,** 1221 South Broadway, Lexington, KY 40504; tel. 859/258–4600; FAX. 859/258–4664; Ashley Karathanasis, ASC Administrator

**Louisville Endoscopy Center,** 1400 Poplar Level Road, Suite 2, Louisville, KY 40217; tel. 502/636–2003; FAX. 502/636–4032; Rosemary Gentry, RN, BSN, CGRN, Center Director

**Louisville Surgery Center,** 614 East Chestnut Street, Louisville, KY 40202; tel. 502/589–9488; FAX. 502/589–9928; Vanessa McDermott, Administrator

**Mangat-KUY-Holzapfel Plastic Surgery Center,** 133 Barnwood Drive, Edgewood, KY 41017; tel. 859/331–9600; FAX. 859/578–3321; Linda Robinson, Administrator

**McPeak Surgery Center,** 108 Bravo Boulevard, Glasgow, KY 42141; tel. 270/651–2181; FAX. 270/651–2183; Sheila Dishman, Administrator

**Muhlenberg Surgery Center,** 1008 Medical Center Dr, Suite B, Powderly, KY 42367; tel. 270/338–9929; FAX. 270/338–9282; Susan Hust, Administrator

**Patient First Digestive Disease Center,** 340 Thomas More Parkway, Suite 160B, Crestview, KY 41017; tel. 859/331–6466; FAX. 859/331–1932; Gail Hynko, Site Manager

**Somerset Surgery Center,** 30 Medpark Drive, Somerset, KY 42503-2797; tel. 606/679–9322; FAX. 606/678–2666; Kathy Turner, Administrator

**Stone Road Surgery Center,** 280 Pasadena Dr, Lexington, KY 40503; tel. 859/278–1316; Heather C. Wright, Administrator

**Surgical Center of Elizabethtown,** 108 Financial Drive, Elizabethtown, KY 42701; tel. 270/737–5200; FAX. 270/737–2422; Robin Boles, Administrator

**Surgicare Lourdes Ambulatory Surgery Center,** 225 Medical Center Drive, Suite 105, Paducah, KY 42003; tel. 270/441–4500; FAX. 270/441–4577; Nancy Edwards, Director

**The Pain Treatment Center Inc. dba Stone Road Surgery Center,** 280 Pasadena Drive, Lexington, KY 40503; tel. 859/278–1316; FAX. 859/276–3847; Healther C. Wright, Chief Executive Officer

**Tri-State Digestive Disorder Center Ambulatory Surgery Center,** 425 Centre View Blvd, Crestview Hills, KY 41017; tel. 859/341–3575; FAX. 859/341–5701; Ross McHenry, MD

## LOUISIANA

**Acadiana Surgery Center, Inc.,** 2309 East Main Street, Suite 102, New Iberia, LA 70560; tel. 337/364–9680; FAX. 337/364–9689; Dana W. Stokes, RN. Director of Nurses

**Alexandria Laser and Surgery Center,** 4100 Parliament Drive, Alexandria, LA 71303; tel. 318/487–8342; FAX. 318/487–9942; Martina Anders, RN., Center Director

**Ambulatory Eye Surgery Center of Louisiana,** 3900 Veterans Boulevard, Suite 100, Metairie, LA 70002; tel. 504/455–1550; FAX. 504/455–2011; Judy Dufrechou RN, Director

**Brass Surgery Center,** 5328 Didesse Drive, Baton Rouge, LA 70808; tel. 225/766–1718; FAX. 225/766–1225; Derald W. Smith, Administrator

**Colonnade Endoscopy Center,** 555 Dr. Michael DeBakey Drive, Suite 102, Lake Charles, LA 70601; tel. 337/439–6226; FAX. 337/436–6223; Nellie Rideaux, Administrative Assistant

Health Organizations, Agencies, and Providers **C41**

**Foot Surgery Center of Shreveport,** 9308 Mansfield Road, Suite 300, Shreveport, LA 71118; tel. 318/686–9622; Richard Havens, DPM, Administrator

**Greater New Orleans Surgery Center,** 3434 Houma Boulevard, Suite 300, Metairie, LA 70006; tel. 504/454–2017; FAX. 530/869–5348; Penny A. Nichols, Administrator

**Houma Outpatient Surgery Center, Ltd.,** 3717 Houma Boulevard, Suite 300, Metairie, LA 70006; tel. 504/456–1515; FAX. 504/454–3810; Landon Tucker, Administrator

**Houma Surgi Center, Inc.,** 1020 School Street, Houma, LA 70360; tel. 985/868–4320; FAX. 985/868–3617; Pat Hitt, RN Assistant Administrator

**LaHaye Eye and Ambulatory Surgical Center,** 4313 I-49 S. Service Rd., Opelousas, LA 70570; tel. 337/942–2024; FAX. 337/948–8869; Bridget Ray, Administrator

**LaHaye Total Eye Care,** 201 Rue Iberville, Suite 800, Lafayette, LA 70508; tel. 337/235–2149; FAX. 337/231–4012; Bridget Ray

**Lake Charles Medical-Surgical Clinic,** 501 Dr. Michael DeBakey Drive, Lake Charles, LA 70601; tel. 337/433–8400; FAX. 337/433–7350; Karen Guillory, RN, Administrator

**Laser and Surgery Center of Acadiana,** 514 Street Landry Street, Lafayette, LA 70506; tel. 337/234–2020; FAX. 318/234–8230; Jackie Ipson, Office Manager

**Louisiana Endoscopy Center, Inc.,** 9103 Jefferson Highway, Baton Rouge, LA 70809; tel. 225/927–0970; FAX. 225/706–0160; Albert Hart, IV, Administrator

**LSU Eye Surgery Center,** 2020 Gravier Street, Suite B, New Orleans, LA 70112; tel. 504/412–1590; FAX. 504/472–1268; W. L. Blackwell, Chief Executive Officer

**Magnolia Surgical Facility,** 3939 Houma Boulevard, Suite 216, Metairie, LA 70006; tel. 504/455–7771; FAX. 504/885–5063; Melissa Johnson, Administrator, Medical Director

**MGA-GI Diagnostic and Therapeutic Center,** 1111 Medical Center Boulevard, Suite 450, Marrero, LA 70072; tel. 504/349–6310; FAX. 504/349–6444; Thomas D. McCaffery, Jr., President

**MGA-GI Diagnostic and Therapeutic Center,** 2633 Napoleon Avenue, Suite 707, New Orleans, LA 70115; tel. 504/896–8680; FAX. 504/896–8699; Thomas D. McCaffery, Jr., President

**Ochsner Outpatient Surgery Center,** 103 Medical Center Drive, Slidell, LA 70461; tel. 985/646–4466; FAX. 985/646–5699; Allison F. Maestri, RN

**Omega Hospital, LLC,** 2525 Severn Avenue, Metairie, LA 70001; tel. 504/832–4200; FAX. 504/832–4209; Deborah Scnenck, Administrator

**Outpatient Eye Surgery Center,** 4324 Veterans Boulevard #101, Metairie, LA 70006; tel. 504/455–4046; FAX. 504/455–9890; Cheryl Crouse, RN, Administrator

**Shreveport Endoscopy Center, AMC,** 3217 Mabel Street, PO Box 37045, Shreveport, LA 71133-7045; tel. 318/631–0072; FAX. 318/631–9688; Linda Ray, Administrator

**Shreveport Surgery Center,** 745 Olive Street, Suite 100, Shreveport, LA 71104; tel. 318/227–1163; FAX. 318/227–0413; Mary Jones, Administrator

**Surgery Center, Inc.,** 1101 South College Road, Suite 100, Lafayette, LA 70503; tel. 337/233–8603; FAX. 337/234–0341; Russell J. Arceneaux, Administrator

**Surginet Outpatient Surgery, LLC,** 101 La Rue France, Suite 400, Lafayette, LA 70508; tel. 318/269–9828; FAX. 318/269–9823; Millissa R. Coco, Administrator

**Thibodaux Laser & Surgery Center, LLC,** 1101 Audubon Avenue, Suite S-Four, Thibodaux, LA 70301; tel. 985/447–7258; FAX. 985/448–1521; Nate Graff, Administrator

**Urology Specialty and Surgery Center,** 234 Dr. Michael DeBakey Drive, Lake Charles, LA 70601; tel. 337/433–5282; FAX. 337/433–1159; Shari Davis, Administrator

**West Monroe Endoscopy Center,** 102 Thomas Road, Suite 506, West Monroe, LA 71291; tel. 318/388–8878; FAX. 318/388–8870; J.B. Duke McHugh, MD

## MAINE

**Acadia Medical Arts Ambulatory Surgical Suite,** 404 State Street, Bangor, ME 04401; tel. 207/990–0928; FAX. 207/945–4354; Paulette Blue, RN, Administrator

**Eyecare Medical Group,** 53 Sewall Street, Portland, ME 04102; tel. 207/828–2020; FAX. 207/773–7034; Clement Berry, Chief Executive Officer

**Maine Eye Center, P.A.,** 15 Lowell Street, Portland, ME 04102; tel. 207/774–8277; FAX. 207/871–1415; Curtis M. Libby, MD, Director

**Northern Maine Ambulatory Endoscopy Center,** 11 Martin Street, P.O. Box 748, Presque Isle, ME 04769-0151; tel. 207/764–2482; FAX. 207/764–1569; Devin McHalten, Administrator

**OA Centers for Orthopaedics,** 33 Sewall Street, Portland, ME 04102; tel. 207/828–2100; FAX. 207/828–2190; Linda M. Ruterbories, ASU Director

**Vision Care of Maine-Ardostook, LLC,** 173 Academy Street, Presque Isle, ME 04769; tel. 207/764–0376; FAX. 207/764–7612; Craig W. Young, MD, Director

## MARYLAND

**Ambulatory Endoscopy Center of Maryland, Inc.,** 7350 Van Dusen Road, Suite 230, Laurel, MD 20707; tel. 301/498–5500; FAX. 301/604–5956; Kim Wilson RN, Center Director

**Ambulatory Plastic Surgery Center Associates, CHTD,** 15245 Shady Grove Road, Suite 155, Rockville, MD 20850; tel. 301/738–9137; FAX. 301/738–7920; Mary Vincent, Office Manager

**Anne Arundel Gastroenterology Associates,** Bestgate Medical Clinic, 820 Bestgate Road, Annapolis, MD 21401; tel. 410/224–2116; Gary M. Evans, Administrator

**Baltimore Ambulatory Center for Endoscopy,** 19 Fontana Lane, Suite 104, Rosedale, MD 21237; tel. 410/574–7776; FAX. 410/574–9038; Dr. J. Khan, Medical Director

**Baltimore Podiatry Group,** 5205 East Drive, Suite I, Arbutus, MD 21227; tel. 410/247–5333; Neil Scheffler, DPM, President

**Baltimore Washington Eye Center,** 200 Hospital Drive, Suite 600, Glen Burnie, MD 21061; tel. 410/766–3937; FAX. 410/766–2904; Katie Guglietta, RN, ASC Coordinator

**Bayside Surgical Center, Inc.,** 8023 Ritchie Highway, Pasadena, MD 21122; tel. 410/761–4190; FAX. 410/761–0265; Sheila Freeze, Office Manager

**Beitler, Samuel D., DPM Ambulatory Surgery Center, Glen Burnie Podiatric Surgery Center,** 795 Aquahart Road, Suite 125, Glen Burnie, MD 21061; tel. 410/768–0702; FAX. 410/768–0649; Samuel D. Beitler, DPM

**Bel Air Ambulatory Surgical Center, LLC,** 2007 Rock Spring Road, Lower Level, Forest Hill, MD 21050; tel. 410/879–2474; FAX. 410/879–8194; Karen Carey, RN, Administrator

**Belcrest Surgery Center,** 6505 Belcrest Road, Suite One, Hyattsville, MD 20782; tel. 301/699–5900; FAX. 301/699–9297; Mark H. Sugar, DPM, Director

**Bethesda Ambulatory Surgical Center,** 5620 Shields Drive, Bethesda, MD 20817; tel. 301/530–4181; FAX. 301/530–4373; John Lydon, DPM, Administrator

**Bethesda Surgery Center, LLC,** 10215 Fernwood Road, Suite 412, Bethesda, MD 20817; tel. 301/530–6100; FAX. 301/530–6104; Janet Scanlon

**Center for Oral & Maxillofacial Surgery,** 1212 York Road, Suite A201, Lutherville, MD 21093; tel. 410/337–7755; FAX. 410/337–7922; Laurie Kolmer, Office Manager

**Chesapeake Ambulatory Surgery Center, LLC,** 8028 Governor Ritchie Highway, Suite 100, Pasadena, MD 21122; tel. 410/768–5800; FAX. 410/768–5806; Ira J. Gottlieb, DPM, Owner, Administrator

**Chesapeake Plastic Surgery,** 134 Holiday Court, Ste 305, Annapolis, MD 21401; tel. 410/646–3226; FAX. 443/949–7508; Haven Barlow, MD, Director

**Cumberland Valley Surgical Center, LLC,** 1110 Professional Court, Hagerstown, MD 21740; tel. 240/420–5559; Stacey Taylor, RN, BSN, Administrator, CASC

**De Leonibus and Palmer, LLC, ASC, MedSurg Foot Center,** 2086 Generals Highway, Suite 101, Annapolis, MD 21401; tel. 410/266–7666; FAX. 410/266–7703; John DeLeonibus, DPM, Owner

**Dimensions Surgery Center,** 14999 Health Center Drive, Ste 103, Bowie, MD 20716; tel. 301/809–2000; FAX. 301/464–3572; Joan McHale, Director of Operations

**Drs. Liss & Mirkin PA T-A Foot & Ankle Associates dba Foot and Ankle Associates, dba Kensington Surgery Center,** 10901 Connecticut Avenue, Suite 200 B, Kensington, MD 20895; tel. 301/949–2000; FAX. 301/949–2002; Dr. Gene Mirkin

**Dulaney Eye Institute,** 901 Dulaney Valley Road, Suite 220, Towson, MD 21204; tel. 410/583–1000; FAX. 410/583–4718; Andrea Hyatt, CASC, Administrator

**Dundalk Ambulatory Surgery Center,** 1123 Merritt Boulevard, Baltimore, MD 21222; tel. 410/282–6666; FAX. 410/282–0357; Pam Green, Office Manager

**Ellicott City Ambulatory Surgery Center,** 2850 North Ridge Road, Ellicott City, MD 21043; tel. 410/461–1600; FAX. 410/750–7615; Maureen Hartley, Administrator

**Eye Surgery Center of Ophthalmology Associates, LLC,** 10755 Falls Road, Suite 110B, Lutherville, MD 21093; tel. 410/583–2811; FAX. 410/583–2814; Lynne Young, Administrator

**Facial Plastic Surgicenter, Ltd.,** 1838 Greene Tree Road, Baltimore, MD 21208; tel. 410/486–3400; FAX. 410/486–0092; Ira D. Papel, MD, President

**Flaum, Martin/Rockville Ambulatory Surgical Center, LLC,** 50 West Edmonston Drive, Suite 306, Rockville, MD 20852; tel. 301/340–8666; FAX. 301/340–7448; Martin C. Flaum, Owner

**Foot Care Associates Ambulatory Care Center at Joppa Foot Care,** 2316 East Joppa Road, Baltimore, MD 21234; tel. 410/882–5100

**Four Corners Ambulatory Surgical Center, LLC, Dr. Gary A. Lieberman, PA,** 10101 Lorain Avenue, Silver Spring, MD 20901; tel. 301/681–8400; FAX. 301/681–3339; Gayle Rickert, Administrator

**Frederick Surgical Center,** 45 Thomas Johnson Drive, Ste 202, Frederick, MD 21702; tel. 301/694–3400; FAX. 301/694–3620; Tracey Tylicki, RN, BSN, Administrator and Director of Surgical Services

**Giardina and Glubo, P.A.,** 4660 Wilkens Avenue, Baltimore, MD 21229; tel. 410/242–7066; FAX. 410/242–4126; Eileen Giardina, RN

**Gynemed Surgi-Center,** 17 Fontana Lane, Suite 201, Baltimore, MD 21237; tel. 410/686–8220; FAX. 410/391–0943; David O'Neil, MD

**Harford County Ambulatory Surgery Center,** 1952-A Pulaski Highway, Edgewood, MD 21040; tel. 410/538–7000; FAX. 410/679–4291; Ms. Kim Merrill, RN, BN, Nurse Administrator

**Harford Endoscopy Center, LLC,** Two North Avenue, Suite 102, Belair, MD 21014; tel. 410/838–6345; FAX. 410/838–1595; Sherry Adkins, Center Director

**Johns Hopkins Plastic Surgery Associates,** JHOC 8, 601 North Caroline Street, Baltimore, MD 21287; tel. 410/955–6897; FAX. 410/614–4333; Dawn Lichtenberg

**Kaiser-Permanente-Kensington,** 10810 Connecticut Avenue, Kensington, MD 20895; tel. 301/929–7275; FAX. 301/929–7577; Wanda McCulley, RN, Administrator

**Lake Forest Ambulatory Surgical Center,** 702 Russell Avenue, Gaithersburg, MD 20877; tel. 301/948–3668; FAX. 301/926–7787; Fatimah, Office Manager

**Laser Surgery Center, Inc.,** 484A Ritchie Highway, Severna Park, MD 21146; tel. 410/544–4600; FAX. 410/544–0997; Barbara Stein, Office Manager

**Laurel Foot and Ankle Surgery Center Inc.,** 14440 Cherry Lane Court, Suite 104, Laurel, MD 20707; tel. 301/953–3668; Dr. Frank Smith, Administrator

**Maple Springs Ambulatory Surgery Center,** 10810 Darnstown Road, Suite 101, Gaithersburg, MD 20878; tel. 301/762–3338; FAX. 301/762–1585; Dr. Stuart Snyder, PA, President

**Maryland Endoscopy Center, LLC,** 100 West Road, Suite 115, Towson, MD 21204; tel. 410/494–0144; FAX. 410/494–0147; Irma Haak, RN, Center Director

**Maryland Urology Surgicenters, LLC,** 6830 Hospital Drive, Suite 204, Baltimore, MD 21237; tel. 410/391–6131; FAX. 410/391–6144; Dr. William Dowling, Head Doctor

**Metropolitan Ambulatory Urologic Institute LLC,** 7759 Belle Point Drive, Greenbelt, MD 20770; tel. 301/474–5583; FAX. 301/474–5742; Bernie Schwartz, Manager

**Michetti, Michael, Dr. of District Heights,** 6400 Marlboro Pike, District Heights., MD 20747; tel. 301/736–6900

**Mid Shore Surgical Eye Center,** 8420 Ocean Gateway, Suite One, Easton, MD 21601; tel. 410/822-0424; FAX. 410/822-2283; Cheryl Schmitt, RN

**Montgomery Endoscopy Center P.A., Montgomery Gastroenterology P.A.,** 12012 Veirs Mill Road, Silver Spring, MD 20906; tel. 301/942-3550; FAX. 301/933-3621; Sindu Stephen, MD, ASC Director

**Montgomery Surgical Center,** 46 West Gude Drive, Rockville, MD 20850; tel. 301/424-6901; FAX. 301/294-7847; Patti Hartsfield, Administrator

**Moulsdale, Murphy, Siegelbaum and Lerner,** 7505 Osler Drive, Suite 508, Towson, MD 21204; tel. 410/296-0166; FAX. 410/828-7275

**North Arundel Plastic Surgery Specialists,** 489 Ritchie Highway, Building C, 2nd Floor, Severna Park, MD 21146; tel. 410/841-5355; FAX. 410/841-6589; Ajia S. Markland, Administrator

**Parris-Castoro Eye & Laser Center,** 620 Boulton Street, Bel Air, MD 21014; tel. 410/399-8427; FAX. 410/399-8427; Mary Ripley, RN, Nurse Manager

**Plastic Surgery Specialists,** 2448 Holly Avenue, Suite 400, Annapolis, MD 21401; tel. 410/841-5355; FAX. 410/841-6589; Amanada Freeland, Adminstrator

**Plaza Ambulatory Surgical Center,** 6506 Reisterstown Road, Suite 501, Baltimore, MD 21215; tel. 410/764-7044; FAX. 410/764-8637; Dr. Brian Kashan, Administrator

**Podiatry Associates, P.A.,** One North Main Street, Bel Air, MD 21014; tel. 410/879-1212; FAX. 410/893-1081

**Podiatry Associates, P.A.,** 6569 North Charles Street, Suite 702, Towson, MD 21204; tel. 410/828-5420; FAX. 410/828-1663; Stan Book, Billing Manager

**Podiatry Associates, P.A., Charter Professional Center,** 10700 Charter Drive, Suite 300, Columbia, MD 21044; tel. 410/730-0970; FAX. 410/730-0161; Dr. Boyd, Capello, Ritter, Podiatrist

**Prince George's Multi-Specialty Surgery Centre, Inc.,** 8700 Central Avenue, Suite 106, Landover, MD 20785; tel. 301/499-3338; FAX. 301/499-1266; John Bubser, Administrator

**River Reach Outpatient Surgery Center,** 790 Governor Ritchie Highway, Suite E-35, Severna Park, MD 21146; tel. 410/544-2487; FAX. 410/544-1872; Pat Hofmeier, Administrator

**Riverside Ambulatory Surgery Center,** 560 Riverside Drive, Suite A-101, Salisbury, MD 21801; tel. 410/749-0121; FAX. 410/749-6807; Patricia Timmons, PMAC, Administrator

**Robinwood Surgery Center, LLC,** 11110 Medical Campus Road, Suite 200, Hagerstown, MD 21742; tel. 301/714-4300; FAX. 301/714-4324; Donna Trueax, Director

**Saint Mary's Multispecialty Surgery Center, Inc.,** Route 235 and Chancellors Run Road, Suite 15, PO Box 1310, California, MD 20619; tel. 301/862-3338; FAX. 301/862-3335; Douglas H. Hallgren, Administrator

**Spector, Adam, DPM, Ambulatory Surgery Center,** 2730 University Boulevard W., Suite 1000, Wheaton, MD 20902; tel. 301/949-3668; FAX. 301/949-8833; Adam Spector, DPM, Administrator

**Suburban Endoscopy Center, LLC,** 10215 Fernwood Road, Suite 260, Bethesda, MD 20817; tel. 301/530-2800; FAX. 301/530-9560

**Summit Ambulatory Surgery Center, Ambulatory Surgery Center,** 1001 Pine Heights Avenue, Suite 104, Baltimore, MD 21229; tel. 410/644-0929; Narang Ashok, Administrator

**SurgiCenter of Baltimore, LLP,** 23 Crossroads Drive, Suite 100, Owings Mills, MD 21117; tel. 410/356-0300; FAX. 410/356-7507; Rosemary L. Lambie, RN, Administrator

**The Adult and Pediatric Urology Surgery Center of MD,** 3455 Wilkens Avenue, Suite 100, Baltimore, MD 21229; tel. 410/646-0330; FAX. 410/644-6182; Bridget Mastrounni, Practice Administrator

**The Ambulatory Urosurgical Center,** 401 East Jefferson Street, Suite 105, Rockville, MD 20850; tel. 301/309-8219; FAX. 301/309-9370; Bernadette Noel, RN, Administrative Director

**The ASC at Waugh Chapel,** 2401 Brandermill Blvd, Suite 340, Gambrills, MD 21054; tel. 410/451-3206; FAX. 410/451-3207; Lance Caffiero, Administrator and Owner

**The Endoscopy Center,** 7402 York Road, Suite 101, Towson, MD 21204; tel. 410/494-0156; FAX. 410/828-1706; Barry Gendason, General Manager

**The Friendship Ambulatory Surgery Center, PC,** 5550 Friendship Boulevard, Suite 270, Chevy Chase, MD 20815; tel. 301/215-7347; FAX. 301/215-7345; Anthony Ruffin, Administrator

**Total Foot Care Surgery Center, Inc.,** 7525 Greenway Center Drive, Suite 112, Greenbelt, MD 20770; tel. 301/345-4087; FAX. 301/345-0482; Kathi Reinhart, Office Manager

**Waldorf Endoscopy Center,** 11340 Pembroke Square, Suite 202, Waldorf, MD 20603; tel. 301/638-5354; FAX. 301/843-5184; Center Director

**Western Maryland Eye Surgical Center,** 1003 West Seventh Street, Suite 400, Frederick, MD 21701; tel. 301/662-3721; FAX. 301/698-8164

## MASSACHUSETTS

**Andover Surgery Center, LP,** 138 Haverhill Street, Andover, MA 01810; tel. 508/475-2880; FAX. 508/475-9562; Nancy Aucoin, Executive Director

**Boston Center for Ambulatory Surgery, Inc.,** 170 Commonwealth Avenue, Boston, MA 02116; tel. 617/267-0710; FAX. 617/236-8704; Philip J. Gaven, MBA, Administrator

**Boston Eye Surgery & Laser Center, P.C.,** 50 Stanford Street, Boston, MA 02114; tel. 617/723-2015; FAX. 617/723-7787; Sheila M. Harney, Business Manager

**Boston University Eye Assoc., Inc.,** 90 New State Highway, Raynham, MA 02767; tel. 508/822-8839; FAX. 508/880-3616; Judith A. Orsie, RNBSN, Director of Surgical Services

**Cataract and Laser Center West, LLC,** 171 Interstate Drive, West Springfield, MA 01089; tel. 413/737-5500; FAX. 413/732-3514; C. Michael Duca, Administrator

**Cataract and Laser Center, Inc.,** 333 Elm Street, Dedham, MA 02026; tel. 781/326-3800; FAX. 728/326-2120; John Dunne, Administrator

**HealthSouth Maple Surgery Center,** 298 Carew Street, Springfield, MA 01104; tel. 413/739-9668; FAX. 413/781-3652; Kathleen S. Loomis, RN, Facility Administrator

**New England Eye Surgery Center,** 696 Main Street, Weymouth, MA 02190; tel. 617/331-3820; FAX. 617/331-1076; Kenneth Camerota

**Northeast Ambulatory Center,** Three Woodland Road, Suite 321, Stoneham, MA 02180; tel. 781/665-5233; FAX. 781/662-4878; Anil Kumar MD, Medical Director

**Plymouth Laser and Surgical Center,** 40 Industrial Park Road, Plymouth, MA 02360; tel. 508/746-8600; FAX. 508/747-0824; Kathleen Murphy, Administrator

**Same Day SurgiClinic,** 272 Stanley Street, Fall River, MA 02720; tel. 508/672-2290; FAX. 508/679-3766; Steven Pimental, Administrator

**Surgery Center of Waltham,** 130 2nd Avenue, Waltham, MA 02451; tel. 781/434-6400; FAX. 781/434-6593; Sharon Edwards, Chief Operating Officer

**The Cosmetic Surgery Center,** 68 Camp Street, Hyannis, MA 02601; tel. 508/775-7026; FAX. 508/771-0499; Maryanne Savage, RN

**Worcester Surgical Center, Inc.,** 300 Grove Street, Worcester, MA 01650; tel. 508/754-0700; FAX. 508/831-9989; Andy H. Poritz, MD, Professional Services Director

## MICHIGAN

**Balian Eye Center,** 432 West University Drive, Rochester, MI 48307; tel. 248/651-6122; FAX. 248/651-4825; E. Mike Raphtis, MD

**Centre for Plastic Surgery,** 426 Michigan Street, NE, Suite 300, Grand Rapids, MI 49503; tel. 616/454-1256; FAX. 616/454-0308; Patty Bakker, Administrator

**East Michigan Surgery Center,** 701 South Ballenger, Flint, MI 48532; tel. 810/238-3603; FAX. 810/767-5194; Destiny Hahn, Administrator

**Eastside Endoscopy Center,** 28963 Little Mack, Suite 103, St. Clair Shores, MI 48081; tel. 586/447-5110; FAX. 586/774-6091; Beth Miller, Administrator

**Eastside Endoscopy Center,** 17700 23 Mile Road, Macomb Township, MI 48044; tel. 586/416-7501; FAX. 586/416-7506; Beth Miller, Administrator

**Endoscopy and Surgery Center at Woodbridge Hills,** 7901 Angling Road, Portage, MI 49024; tel. 269/324-8406; FAX. 269/324-8476; Renee Langeland, Administrator

**Health Care Midwest Surgery Center,** 125 West Walnut, Kalamazoo, MI 49007; tel. 616/343-1381; Gregor W. Blix, MD, Medical Director

**Hemorrhoid Clinics of America,** 22000 Greenfield Road, Oak Park, MI 48237; tel. 248/967-4140; FAX. 248/967-0745; Max Ali, MD, President

**Henry Ford Medical Center,** 6777 West Maple Road, West Bloomfield, MI 48322; tel. 248/661-4100; FAX. 248/661-6494; Sally Bertonia, Administrative Manager

**Henry Ford Medical Center-Lakeside Ambulatory Surgery,** 14500 Hall Road, Sterling Heights, MI 48313; tel. 586/247-2680; FAX. 586/247-2682; Peter Tate, Administrator

**John Michael Garrett, MD,** 1301 Carpenter Avenue, Iron Mountain, MI 49801; tel. 906/774-1404; FAX. 906/774-8132; Susan Brunnette, RN, ASC Supervisor

**Lakeshore Eye Surgery Center,** 21711 Greater Mack Avenue, St. Clair Shores, MI 48080; tel. 586/774-4080; FAX. 586/541-3399; Mariann Pomaville, Center Director

**Lansing Surgery Center,** 1707 Lake Lansing Road, Lansing, MI 48912; tel. 517/708-3333; FAX. 517/267-0430; Richard Smith, Chief Executive Officer

**M.D. Surgicenter,** 375 Barclay Circle, Rochester Hill, MI 48307; tel. 248/852-3636; FAX. 248/852-3631; David Boberg, Administrator

**Michigan Center for Outpatient Ocular Surgery,** 33080 Utica Road, P.O. Box 26010, Fraser, MI 48026; tel. 810/296-7250; FAX. 810/296-0276; Norbert P. Czajkowski, MD, Director

**Midwest Health Center,** 5050 Schaefer Avenue, Dearborn, MI 48126; tel. 313/581-5500; FAX. 313/581-6013; Mark B. Saffer, MD, President and Chief Executive Officer

**North Oakland ASC, LLC,** 1305 North Oakland Boulevard, Waterford, MI 48327; tel. 248/666-5552; FAX. 248/666-5508; Bonnie Kalous, Charge Nurse

**Oakland Surgi Center, Inc.,** 2820 Crooks Road, Suite 200, Rochester Hills, MI 48309; tel. 248/852-7484; FAX. 248/852-4279; Shela Matthews, CMM, Administrator

**Planned Parenthood Mid and South Michigan,** 3100 Professional Drive, P.O. Box 3673, Ann Arbor, MI 48106-3673; tel. 734/973-0710; FAX. 734/973-0595; Danielle Terry

**Planned Parenthood of South Central Michigan,** 4201 West Michigan Avenue, Kalamazoo, MI 49006-5833; tel. 269/372-1205; FAX. 269/372-1279; Amy Steward, MSN, FNP, Associate Medical Director

**Southgate Surgery Center,** 14050 Dix-Toledo Road, Southgate, MI 48195; tel. 734/281-0100; FAX. 734/281-7447; Linda Phillips, RN, Administrator

**Spectrum Health Surgical Center,** 1000 East Paris SE, Suite 100, Grand Rapids, MI 49546; tel. 616/285-1822; FAX. 616/285-1820; Deb Williams, Nurse Manager

**St. John Surgery Center,** 21000 12 Mile Road, St. Clair Shores, MI 48081; tel. 810/447-5015; FAX. 810/447-5012; Cheri Dendy, Administrator

**St. Mary's Ambulatory Care Center,** 4599 Towne Centre, Saginaw, MI 48604; tel. 517/797-3000; FAX. 517/797-3010; Lori Jurgens, Director

**Superior Endoscopy Center/U P Digestive Disease Associates, P.C.,** 1414 West Fair Avenue, Suite 135, Marquette, MI 49855; tel. 906/226-6025; FAX. 906/226-5366; Kristine Gorsalitz, RN, Director of Nursing

**Surgery Center of Michigan,** 44650 Delco Boulevard, Sterling Heights, MI 48313; tel. 586/254-3391; FAX. 586/254-3344; Jay Novetsky, MD, Medical Director

**Surgical Care Center of Michigan,** 750 East Beltline, NE, Grand Rapids, MI 49525; tel. 616/940-3600; FAX. 616/954-0216; Kris Kilgore, RN, BSN, Administrative Director

**The Berry Surgery Center,** 28500 Orchard Lake Road, Suite100, Farmington Hills, MI 48334; tel. 248/851-6767; FAX. 248/851-2077; Aaron Betel, Medical Director

## MINNESOTA

**Centennial Lakes Surgery Center,** 7373 France Avenue, S., Suite 404, Edina, MN 55435; tel. 952/832-9360; FAX. 952/832-5079; Pamela Spohn, Administrator

**Children's - Minnetonka,** 6050 Clearwater Drive, Minnetonka, MN 55343; tel. 612/930-8600; FAX. 612/930-8650; Ann Huhn, Business Manager

**DL Surgery Center,** 125 Frazee Street East, Detroit Lakes, MN 56501; tel. 218/844-2372; Abigail Ring, MD, President

**Landmark Surgery Center,** 17 West Exchange Street, Suite 222, St. Paul, MN 55102; tel. 651/968-5468; FAX. 651/968-5493; Beckie Hines, Site Supervisor

**Midwest Surgery Centers,** 2080 Woodwinds Drive, Woodbury, MN 55125; tel. 651/642-1106; FAX. 651/642-9837; H. Joseph Drannen, Administrator

**Section C**

**WestHealth, Inc.,** 2855 Campus Drive, Plymouth, MN 55441; tel. 763/577–7000; Sue Durkin, Director, Clinical Operations

**Willmar Surgery Center,** 1320 South First Street, Willmar, MN 56201; tel. 320/235–6506; FAX. 320/235–7069; Harley Pakola, Medical Director

## MISSISSIPPI

**Better Living Clinic Endoscopy Center,** 3000 Halls Ferry Road, Vicksburg, MS 39180; tel. 601/638–9800; FAX. 601/638–9808; Barbara Neal, Office Manager

**Cedar Lake Surgery Center,** 1720 B Medical Park Drive, Biloxi, MS 39532; tel. 228/702–2000; FAX. 228/702–2019; Michael T. Gossman, Administrator

**Columbus Endoscopy Center, Inc.,** 600 Leigh Drive, Columbus, MS 39705; tel. 662/327–7525; FAX. 662/243–2252; Justin Oswalt, Administrator

**East Mississippi Endoscopic Center, LLC,** 1926 23rd Ave, Meridian, MS 39302; tel. 601/485–1131; FAX. 601/485–1336; Crystal Bowler, Director

**Endoscopy Center of North Mississippi,** 1206 Office Park Drive, Oxford, MS 38655; tel. 662/234–9888; FAX. 662/234–9872; Roger Franck, Administrator

**ENT and Facial Plastic Surgery, PA, dba Head & Neck Surgery Center, LLC,** 107 Millsaps Drive, P.O. Box 17829, Hattiesburg, MS 39402; tel. 601/268–5131; FAX. 601/268–5138; Jean Lincoln, Business Manager

**Eye Surgical Center of Mississippi, LLC,** 1053 River Oaks Drive, Flowood, MS 39232; tel. 601/969–1430; FAX. 601/709–2117; Dr. Brannon Aden, Administrator

**Gastrointestinal Association Endoscopy,** 1405 North State Street, Third Floor, Jackson, MS 39205; tel. 601/354–1234; FAX. 601/352–4882; Diane Winsner, Administrator

**Gulf Coast Outpatient Surgery Center,** 2781 C T Switzer Sr Drive, Suite 101, Biloxi, MS 39531; tel. 228/594–2900; FAX. 228/594–2901; Diane Farris, Administrator

**Gulf South Surgery Center,** 1206 31st Avenue, P.O. Box 1778, Gulfport, MS 39501; tel. 228/864–0008; FAX. 228/864–0742; Warren Hiatt, Jr., MD, President

**Gulfport Surgery Center,** 1300 Broad Ave, Gulfport, MS 39501; tel. 228/575–2200; FAX. 228/575–2249; William Hertzog, Administrator

**Jackson Eye Institute & ASC,** 2500 Lakeland Drive, Suite B, Flowood, MS 39208; tel. 601/933–1197; FAX. 601/939–6823; Dr. James Bruce, Administrator

**Laurel Surgery and Endoscopy Center, LLC,** 1710 West 12th Street, Laurel, MS 39440; tel. 601/369–2021; FAX. 601/369–2022; Meredith Baker, Administrator

**Lowery A. Woodall Outpatient Surgery Facility,** 105 South 28th Avenue, Hattiesburg, MS 39401; tel. 601/579–3400; FAX. 601/264–2025; Ed Curtis, Administrator

**MAE Physicians Surgery Center, LLC,** 1190 North State Street, Suite 102, Jackson, MS 39202; tel. 601/968–1790; FAX. 601/292–4531; Carla Glaze, Administrator

**Magnolia Regional Health Center Surgery Center,** 401 Alcorn Drive, Corinth, MS 38834; tel. 662/293–2000; FAX. 662/287–3562; Angela Jackson, Administrator

**Meridian Surgery Center,** 2100 13 Street, Meridian, MS 39301; tel. 601/485–4443; FAX. 601/485–9060; Debbi Funck, Administrator

**Mississippi Coast Endoscopy & ASC,** 2406 Catalpa Ave, Pascagoula, MS 39567; tel. 228/696–0818; FAX. 228/696–0893; Mary Lynn, Administrator

**Mississippi Surgical Center,** 1421 North State Street, Suite 101, Jackson, MS 39202; tel. 601/353–8000; FAX. 601/948–2507; Judy Gray, Administrator

**New Gulf Coast Surgery Center, LLC,** 3882 Bienville Blvd, Ocean Springs, MS 39564; tel. 228/872–6290; FAX. 228/818–5538; Donna Griggs, CNO, Administrator

**North Mississippi Ambulatory Surgery Center, LLC,** 589 Garfield, Tupelo, MS 38801; tel. 662/377–4700; FAX. 662/377–3101; Scott Edwards, Administrator

**Ocean Springs Surgical & Endoscopy Center,** 3301 Bienville Blvd, Ocean Springs, MS 39564; tel. 228/872–8854; FAX. 228/872–0265; Mary Lynn, Administrator

**Oxford Surgery Center,** 499 Azalea Drive, Oxford, MS 38655; tel. 662/234–7979; FAX. 662/234–7079; Margaret Tatum, Administrator

**Pain Treatment Center, LLC,** 106 Asbury Circle, Hattiesburg, MS 39402; tel. 601/268–8698; FAX. 601/296–3049; Tracey Oden, Administrator

**Southern Eye Center of Excellence,** 1420 South 28th Avenue, Hattiesburg, MS 39402; tel. 601/264–3937; FAX. 601/264–5930; Lynn McMahan, MD, Medical Director

**Surgicare of Jackson,** 760 Lakeland Drive, Jackson, MS 39216; tel. 601/362–8700; FAX. 601/362–6349; Dawn Thomas, Administrator

## MISSOURI

**Auburn Surgery Center, Inc.,** 300 South Mount Auburn Road, Suite 200, Cape Girardeau, MO 63703; tel. 573/332–7881; FAX. 573/332–7176; Lanna Kelley, Administrator

**Cataract and Glaucoma Outpatient Surgicenter,** 7220 Watson Road, St. Louis, MO 63119; tel. 314/352–5500; Stanley C. Becker, MD

**CMMP Surgical Center,** 1705 Christy Drive, Suite 100, Jefferson City, MO 65101; tel. 573/635–7022; FAX. 573/635–7029; Angela R. Erosenko, Administrator

**Creekwood Surgery Center,** 211 Northeast 54th Street, Suite 100, Kansas City, MO 64118; tel. 816/455–4214; FAX. 816/455–4216; Nancy Sturgeon, Administrator

**Creve Coeur Surgery Center, LLC, dba City Place Surgery Center, LLC,** 845 N. New Ballas Ct., Suite 100, Creve Coeur, MO 63141; tel. 314/872–7100; FAX. 314/872–9176; Carolyn Hollowood, Administrator, RN,BSN,CASC

**Doctors' Park Surgery, Inc.,** 30 Doctors' Park, Cape Girardeau, MO 63703; tel. 573/334–9606; FAX. 573/334–9608; Darin Roberts, Chief Executive Officer/Administrator

**Eye Surgery Center-The Cliffs,** 4801 Cliff Avenue, Suite 101, Independence, MO 64055; tel. 816/478–4400; FAX. 816/478–8240; Jacki Wyrick, RN, BSN, Direct of Nursing

**NovaMed Eye Surgery Center of North County, dba Cataract Surgery Center,** 900 North Highway 67 (Lindbergh), Florissant, MO 63031; tel. 314/838–0321; FAX. 314/838–6532; Karen L. Bell, RN, ASC Director

**Saint Luke's -- G.I. Diagnostics, Inc.,** 4321 Washington, Suite 5700, Kansas City, MO 64111; tel. 816/561–2000; FAX. 816/931–7559; Craig B. Reeves, Administrator

**South County Surgical Center, LLC,** 12345 West Bend Drive, Suite 201, St. Louis, MO 63128; tel. 314/722–2530; FAX. 314/525–0198; Ellen Kluesner, Administrator

**Surgery Center of St. Joseph,** 3201 Ashland Avenue, Suite C & D, St. Joseph, MO 64506; tel. 816/279–0079; FAX. 816/364–1100; Brenda Wilzbach, Administrator

**Surgicenter of Kansas City, LLC,** 1800 East Meyer Boulevard, Kansas City, MO 64132; tel. 816/523–0100; FAX. 816/995–3190; Rita Gooding, Administrator

**The Endoscopy Center,** 3800 South Whitney, Independence, MO 64055; tel. 816/478–4887; FAX. 816/478–7140; Jean Hansen, MBA, FACMPE, Chief Executive Officer

**The Endoscopy Center,** 5330 North Oak Traffic Way #100, Kansas City, MO 64118; tel. 816/478–4887; FAX. 816/478–7140; Jean Hansen, MBA, FACMPE, Chief Executive Officer

**The Endoscopy Center,** 9601 NE 79th Street, Kansas City, MO 64158; tel. 816/478–4887; FAX. 816/478–7140; Jean Thompson, MBA, FACMPE, Chief Executive Officer

**The Endoscopy Center,** 5330 N. Oak Trafficway, Kansas City, MO 64118; tel. 816/478–4887; FAX. 816/478–7140; Jean Hansen, MBA, FACMPE, Chief Executive Officer

**The Endoscopy Center,** 9601 NE 79th Street, Kansas City, MO 64158; tel. 816/478–4887; FAX. 816/478–7140; Jean Hansen, MBA, FACMPE, Chief Executive Officer

**The Endoscopy Center II,** 5330 North Oak Trafficway, Suite 100, Kansas City, MO 64118; tel. 816/478–4887; FAX. 816/478–7140; Jean Thompson, Chief Executive Officer

**The Tobin Eye Institute,** 3902 Sherman Avenue, St. Joseph, MO 64506; tel. 816/279–1363; FAX. 816/233–8936; Lindsey Williams, RN, Director of Nursing and Operations

**Tri-County Surgery Center, LP,** 1111 East Sixth Street, Washington, MO 63090; tel. 636/239–1766; FAX. 636/239–2964; Candy Garofalo, Administrator

## MONTANA

**Billings Cataract and Laser Surgicenter,** 1221 North 26th Street, Billings, MT 59101; tel. 406/252–5681; FAX. 406/252–5025; Brenda Emerick, Business Manager

**Northern Rockies Surgery Center,** 940 North 30th Street, Billings, MT 59101; tel. 406/248–7186; FAX. 406/248–6889; Debbie Howe, RN, MSN, Administrator

**Same Day Surgery Center, LLC,** 300 North Wilson, Suite 600F, Bozeman, MT 59715; tel. 406/586–1956; Suellen Bradley, Clinical Director

**The Eye Surgicenter,** 2475 Village Lane, Suite 202, Billings, MT 59102; tel. 406/252–6608; FAX. 406/252–6600; Cheri Salthe, Office Manager

## NEBRASKA

**Aesthetic Surgical Images, P.C.,** 8900 West Dodge Road, Omaha, NE 68114; tel. 402/390–0100; FAX. 402/390–2711; Rita Petersen, Administrator

**Bergan Mercy Surgery Center, Health Inventures,** 7500 Mercy Road, Suite 4300, Omaha, NE 68124; tel. 402/398–5665; FAX. 402/398–6606; Leslie Voigt

**Lincoln Eye and Laser Institute,** 1500 South 48th Street, Suite 610, Lincoln, NE 68506; tel. 402/483–4448; FAX. 402/483–4750; Rhonda Assmus, Manager

**Lincoln Surgical Center,** 1710 South 70th, Suite 200, Lincoln, NE 68506; tel. 402/484–9090; FAX. 402/483–0476; Robin Linnafelter, Chief Executive Officer

**Omaha Ambulatory Surgery Center,** 825 North 90th Street, Omaha, NE 68114; tel. 402/397–1180; FAX. 402/408–1783; Jake Cook, Director

**Omega Surgery Center, LLC,** 1500 S. 48th Street, Suite 612, Lincoln, NE 68506; tel. 402/483–4448; FAX. 402/483–4750; Ann Perl, RN, ASC Administrator

**Omega Surgery Centers, LLC,** 11606 Nicholas Street, Suite 200, Omaha, NE 68154; tel. 402/493–2020; FAX. 402/431–8569; Ann Perl, RN, ASC Administrator

**The Urology Center, P.C.,** 111 1/2 South 90th Street, Omaha, NE 68114; tel. 402/397–9800; Laura Forehead, Administrator

## NEVADA

**Associated Foot Health Group,** 1300 E Plumb Ln Ste A, Reno, NV 89502; tel. 702/829–8066; FAX. 702/829–8069; Dr. Frank M. Davis, Jr., Administrator

**Carson Endoscopy Center,** 1385 Vista Lane, Carson City, NV 89703; tel. 775/884–4567; FAX. 775/884–4569; Autumn Uyechi, Director of Center Operations

**Digestive Disease Center,** 2136 East Desert Inn Road, Suite B, Las Vegas, NV 89109; tel. 702/734–0075; FAX. 702/734–3912; Osama Haikal, MD, Administrator

**Digestive Health Center,** 5250 Kietzke Lane, Reno, NV 89511; tel. 775/829–8855; FAX. 775/770–2717; Laura Kennedy, RN, Center Director

**Ford Center for Foot Surgery,** 2321 Pyramid Way, Sparks, NV 89431; tel. 702/331–1919; FAX. 702/331–2008; Dr. L. Bruce Ford, Administrator

**Las Vegas Surgicare, Ltd.,** 870 South Rancho Drive, Las Vegas, NV 89106; tel. 702/870–2090; FAX. 702/870–5468; Tony Burns, Administrator

**Shepherd Eye Surgicenter,** 3575 Pecos McLeod, Las Vegas, NV 89121; tel. 702/731–2088; FAX. 702/734–7836; Christina Kennelley, Administrator

**Sierra Center for Foot Surgery,** 1801 North Carson, Suite B, Carson City, NV 89701; tel. 775/882–1441; FAX. 775/882–6844; Dr. Jeffrey Bean, DPM, Administrator

**SMA Surgery Center,** 2450 West Charleston, Las Vegas, NV 89102; tel. 702/877–8660; FAX. 702/877–5180; Steve Evans, MD, Medical Director

## NEW HAMPSHIRE

**Bedford Ambulatory Surgical Center,** 11 Washington Place, Bedford, NH 03110; tel. 603/622–3670; FAX. 603/626–9750; Laurie T. Roderiques, CRNFA, Nurse Director

**Dartmouth Ambulatory Surgery Center,** 100 Hitchcock Way, Manchester, NH 03104; tel. 603/695–1800; FAX. 603/629–1730; Sean E. Hunt, MD, Medical Director, ASC

**Dr. O'Connell's Pain Care Centers, Inc.,** Pinewood Medical Center, 255 Route 108, Somersworth, NH 03878; tel. 603/692–3166; FAX. 603/692–3168; Tom Barnes, Administrator

**Dunning Street Ambulatory Care Center,** Seven Dunning Street, Claremont, NH 03743; tel. 603/543–3501; Ruth Ticknor, Administrator

Section C

**Elliot One Day Surgery Center,** One Elliot Way, Manchester, NH 03103; tel. 603/663–5932; FAX. 603/626–4300; William J. Oifederico, MHA, Administrative Director

**Nashua Eye Surgery Center, Inc.,** Five Coliseum Avenue, Nashua, NH 03063; tel. 603/882–9800; FAX. 603/882–0556; Paul O'Leary, Administrator

**Orthopaedic Surgery Center,** 264 Pleasant Street, Concord, NH 03301; tel. 603/228–7211; FAX. 603/228–7192; Donna Quinn, Administrator

**Salem Surgery Center,** 32 Stiles Road, Salem, NH 03079; tel. 603/898–3610; FAX. 603/890–3313; Cynthia C. Fortune, Director

**NEW JERSEY**

**Advanced Gastroenterology of Bergen County, PA, AGBC Endoscopy Center,** 140 Sylvan Avenue, Suite 101A/101B, Englewood Cliffs, NJ 07632-2554; tel. 201/945–6564; FAX. 201/461–9038; Michael Gailie, Practice Administrator

**Arthur W. Perry, M.D., FACS Plastic Surgery Center,** 3055 Route 27, Franklin Park, NJ 08823; tel. 732/422–9600; Arthur W. Perry, MD, Director

**Atlantic Surgery Center, LLC,** 279 Third Avenue, Suite 105, Long Branch, NJ 07740; tel. 732/222–7373; FAX. 732/571–9212; Daniel B. Goldberg, MD, President

**Atrium Surgery Center, Inc.,** 195 Route 46, Suite 202, Mine Hill, NJ 07803; tel. 973/989–5185; FAX. 973/328–4097; Jennifer Rand, RN, CNOR, Director of Nursing

**Bergen-Passaic Cataract Surgery and Laser Center, Inc.,** 18-01 Pollitt Drive, Ste 1A, Fair Lawn, NJ 07410-2815; tel. 201/794–8444; FAX. 201/794–1615; Caroline B. Ivanovski-Hauser, Project Manager

**Berkeley Heights Eye Group, PA, Summit Eye Group,** 369 Springfield Avenue, Berkeley Heights, NJ 07922; tel. 908/464–4600; FAX. 908/464–4737; Elizabeth Way, RN, Administrator

**Campus Eye Group Ambulatory Surgery Center, Inc.,** 1700 Whitehorse Hamilton Square Road, Suite A, Hamilton, NJ 08690; tel. 609/587–2020; FAX. 609/588–9545; Denise Agness, OD, Office Manager

**Center for Special Surgery,** 104 Lincoln Avenue, Hawthorne, NJ 07506; tel. 973/427–6800; FAX. 973/427–9602; John Tauber, Business Administrator

**Clifton Surgery Center,** 1117 Route 46 East Suite 303, Clifton, NJ 07013; tel. 973/779–7210; FAX. 973/779–7387; Ramon Silen, MD, President and Medical Director

**East Brunswick Surgery Center, dba University Surgi Center,** 561 Cranbury Road, East Brunswick, NJ 08816; tel. 732/390–4300; FAX. 732/390–0556; Paula Zuckerman, Clinical Director

**Endo-Surgi Center,** 1201 Morris Avenue, Union, NJ 07083; tel. 908/686–0066; FAX. 908/686–5388; Sharon DeMato, Administrator

**Endo-Surgi Center of Old Bridge,** 42 Throckmorton Lane, Old Bridge, NJ 08857; tel. 732/679–8808; Sharon DeMato, Executive Director

**Endo/Surgical Center of North Jersey,** 999 Clifton Avenue, Clifton, NJ 07013; tel. 973/777–3938; FAX. 973/591–0178; Ellen Tummillo RN, CGRN, Director of Nursing

**Englewood Endoscopic Associates,** 420 Grand Avenue, Suite 101, Englewood, NJ 07631; tel. 201/569–7044; FAX. 201/569–1999; Carmen Rivera, Office Manager

**Essex Surgical, LLC,** 776 Northfield Avenue, West Orange, NJ 07052; tel. 973/324–2300; FAX. 973/324–1421; George C. Peck, Jr., MD

**Eye Institute of Essex Surgeye Center,** 50 Newark Avenue, Belleville, NJ 07109; tel. 973/751–6060; FAX. 973/450–1464; Eileen Beltramba, Administrator

**Eye Physician of Sussex County Surgical Center,** 183 High Street, Newton, NJ 07860; tel. 973/383–6345; FAX. 973/383–0032; Patricia Fowler, RN

**Eye Surgery Princeton,** 419 North Harrison Street, Princeton, NJ 08540; tel. 609/921–9437; FAX. 609/921–0277; Richard H. Wong, MD, Medical Director

**Gastroenterology Diagnosis Northern New Jersey,** 205 Browertown Road, Suite 102, West Paterson, NJ 07424; tel. 973/890–4780; FAX. 973/890–1097; Ann Kalafsky, RN, Administrative Director

**Hand Surgery and Rehabilitation Center of New Jersey, P.A.,** 5000 Sagemore Drive, Suite 106, Marlton, NJ 08053; tel. 856/983–4263; FAX. 856/983–3894; Sheila McAteer, RN, BSN, Administrator of Surgical Center

**Hunterdon Center for Surgery, LLC T/A Surgery Today,** 121 Highway 31, Suite 1300, Flemington, NJ 08822; tel. 908/806–7017; FAX. 908/806–2838; Saleha Faruqi, MD, Medical Director

**James Street Surgical Suite,** 261 James Street, Suite 3E, Morristown, NJ 07960; tel. 973/267–7181; FAX. 973/267–3656; Patricia D'Amico, RN, Director of Nursing

**Mediplex Surgery Center,** 98 James Street, Suite 108, Edison, NJ 08820-3998; tel. 732/632–1600; FAX. 732/632–1678; Janet Kovacs, Director

**Mid Atlantic Eye Center,** 70 East Front Street, Red Bank, NJ 07701; tel. 732/741–0858; FAX. 732/219–0180; Walter J. Kahn, MD

**Northern New Jersey Eye Institute,** 71 Second Street, South Orange, NJ 07079; tel. 973/763–2203; FAX. 973/763–5207; Shirley Vitale, Practice Administrator

**Northwest Jersey Ambulatory Surgery Center,** 350 Sparta Avenue, Building A, Sparta, NJ 07871; tel. 973/729–8580; FAX. 973/729–2344; D. Crowley, RN, MSN, ASC Supervisor

**Ocean Surgical Pavilion, Inc.,** 1907 Highway 35, Suite Nine, Oakhurst, NJ 07755; tel. 732/517–8885; FAX. 732/517–0304; Barbara DeMaria, RN, CNOR, Center Director

**Pavonia Surgery Center, PC,** 600 Pavonia Avenue, Fourth Floor, Jersey City, NJ 07306; tel. 201/216–1700; FAX. 201/216–1800; William H. Constad, MD, President

**Penn Cardiology at Willingboro,** 200 Campbell Drive, Suite 115, Willingboro, NJ 08046; tel. 609/871–7070; FAX. 609/835–4510; Constance G. Matarese, Senior Practice Manager

**Physicians of Monmouth, LLC,** 733 North Beers Street, Holmdel, NJ 07733; tel. 732/739–0707; FAX. 732/739–8533; Renee Sharkey, RN, Surgical Coordinator

**Princeton Orthopaedic Associates, P.A.,** 727 State Road, Princeton, NJ 08540; tel. 609/924–8131; FAX. 609/924–8532; William G. Hyncik, Jr., Executive Director

**Retina Consultants Surgery Center,** 39 Sycamore Avenue, Little Silver, NJ 07739; tel. 732/530–7730; FAX. 732/530–3837

**Ridgedale Surgery Center,** 14 Ridgedale Avenue, Suite 120, Cedar Knolls, NJ 07927; tel. 973/605–5151; FAX. 973/605–1208; Diana Ruccio, Office Manager

**Ridgewood Ambulatory Surgery Center,** 1200 Ridgewood Avenue, Ridgewood, NJ 07450; tel. 201/444–9002; FAX. 201/612–8114; Kristine Williams, RN

**Saddle Brook Surgicenter, Inc.,** 289 Market Street, Saddle Brook, NJ 07663; tel. 201/843–4444; FAX. 201/368–2817; Dr. Ronald Sollitto, President and Chief Executive Officer

**Seashore Ambulatory Surgery Center,** 1907 New Road, Northfield, NJ 08225; tel. 609/645–8884; FAX. 609/645–9780; Kathleen Clark, Administrator

**Somerset Eye Institute, P.C.,** 562 Easton Avenue, Somerset, NJ 08873; tel. 732/828–5900; FAX. 732/828–3327; Lois Laudati, Manager of Professional Services

**Somerset Surgical Center, PA,** 1081 Route 22 West, Suite 201, Bridgewater, NJ 08807; tel. 908/575–0020; FAX. 908/575–1515; Joan McKibben, Administrator

**South Jersey Endoscopy Center,** 26 East Red Bank Avenue, Woodbury, NJ 08096; tel. 856/848–4464; FAX. 856/848–8706; Barbara Fargnoli, Billing Manager

**South Jersey Surgicenter,** 2835 South Delsea Drive, Vineland, NJ 08360; tel. 856/696–0020; FAX. 856/205–0300; Susy Olmeda, Administrative Coordinator

**Summit Surgical Center, LLC,** 200 Bowman Drive, Suite D-160, Voorhees, NJ 08043; tel. 856/247–7800; FAX. 856/325–5858; Barbara Diomede, Interim Administrator

**Surgery Center of Cherry Hill,** 408 Route 70 East, Cherry Hill, NJ 08034; tel. 856/354–1600; FAX. 856/429–7555; Deborah M. O'Donnell, RN, Administrator

**Surgical Center of South Jersey, an SCA affiliate,** 130 Gaither Drive, Suite 160, Mount Laurel, NJ 08054; tel. 856/722–7000; FAX. 856/722–8962; Eleanor O. Peschko, Administrator

**Surgicare of Central Jersey, Inc.,** 40 Stirling Road, Watchung, NJ 07060; tel. 908/769–8000; FAX. 908/769–4139; Linda Kollar, Executive Director

**Surgicare Surgical Associates of Fair Lawn, LLC,** 1501 Broadway, Route 4 West, Suite One and Three, Fairlawn, NJ 07410; tel. 201/703–8487; FAX. 201/791–6585; John H. Hajjar, MD, Member

**Teaneck Gastroenterology and Endoscopy Center,** 1086 Teaneck Road, Suite Three B, Teaneck, NJ 07666; tel. 201/837–9636; FAX. 201/837–9544; Mia D. Oliver, Manager

**The Endoscopy Center of Red Bank,** 365 Broad Street, Red Bank, NJ 07701; tel. 732/842–4294; FAX. 732/842–3854; Donna D. Spring, Director of Operations

**The New Jersey Eye Center,** 1 North Washington Avenue, Bergenfield, NJ 07621; tel. 201/384–7333; FAX. 201/384–9915; James Dello Russo, OD

**The Surgical Center at South Jersey Eye Physicians, P.A.,** 509 South Lenola Road, Suite 11B, Moorestown, NJ 08057; tel. 856/234–0258; FAX. 609/727–0064; Elizabeth Hanley, RN

**NEW MEXICO**

**Alamogordo Eye Clinic and Surgical Center,** 1124 10th Street, Alamogordo, NM 88310; tel. 505/434–1200; FAX. 505/437–3947; Cindy Buttram, RN

**HealthSouth Albuquerque Surgery Center,** 1720 Wyoming Boulevard, NE, Albuquerque, NM 87112; tel. 505/292–9200; FAX. 505/292–1398; Terry Sanchez, Administrator

**Northside Presbyterian,** PO Box 26666, 5901 Harper Drive, NE, Albuquerque, NM 87125; tel. 505/291–2114; FAX. 505/291–2983; Karin Vantiunen

**The Endoscopy Center of Santa Fe,** 1650 Hospital Drive, Suite 900, Santa Fe, NM 87505; tel. 505/988–3373; FAX. 505/984–1858; Betsy Libowitz, RN, Center Director

**NEW YORK**

**Ambulatory Surgery Center of Brooklyn,** 313 43rd Street, Brooklyn, NY 11232; tel. 718/369–1900; FAX. 718/965–4157; Frank A. Mazzagatti, PhD, Vice President of Operations and Administrator

**Ambulatory Surgery Center of Greater New York, LLC,** 1101 Pelham Parkway, N., Bronx, NY 10469; tel. 718/515–3500; Joanne McLaughlin, RN, MHA, Administrator

**Boulevard Surgical Center,** 46-04 31st Avenue, Long Island C, NY 11103; tel. 718/545–5050; FAX. 718/545–0032; Linda M. Smith, RN, Consultant

**Brook Plaza Ambulatory Surgical Center,** 1901 Utica Avenue, Brooklyn, NY 11234; tel. 718/629–5590; FAX. 347/587–4770; Steven Ackerman, Chief Executive Officer

**Brooklyn Eye Surgery Center, LLC,** 1301 Avenue J, Brooklyn, NY 11230; tel. 718/688–3937; FAX. 718/692–4456; Jay Raifman, Administrator

**Buffalo Ambulatory Surgery Center,** 3095 Harlem Road, Cheektowaga, NY 14225; tel. 716/896–3815; FAX. 716/896–3015; Dorothy L. Zimdahl, RN, BS, CNOR, CASC, Administrator

**Central New York Eye Center,** 22 Green Street, Poughkeepsie, NY 12601; tel. 845/471–3720; FAX. 845/471–9516; Kim M. Quick, RN, CRNO, COE

**Day-Op Center of Long Island, Inc.,** 110 Willis Avenue, Mineola, NY 11501; tel. 516/294–0030; FAX. 516/294–0228; Juliette LaRegina, Administrator

**Fifth Avenue Surgery Center,** 1049 Fifth Avenue, New York, NY 10028; tel. 212/772–6667; FAX. 212/988–8018; Charles J. Raab, Chief Executive Officer

**Garden City SurgiCenter.,** 400 Endo Boulevard, Garden City, NY 11530; tel. 516/832–8504; FAX. 516/228–9429; Kelly Fitzpatrick, Administrator

**Harrison Center Outpatient Surgery,** 5700 Genesee Street, Suite 11, Camillus, NY 13031; tel. 315/701–9378; FAX. 315/701–0871; Margaret M. Alteri, Administrator and Chief Executive Officer

**Harrison Center Outpatient Surgery, dba Holdings, LLC,** 550 Harrison Street, Suite 230, Syracuse, NY 13202; tel. 315/472–4424; FAX. 315/475–8056; Margaret M. Alteri, Administrator and Chief Executive Officer

**Kingston Ambulatory Surgical Center, LLC,** 40 Hurley Avenue, Suite 13, Kingston, NY 12401; tel. 845/338–4777; FAX. 845/339–7339; Kathleen Keily, Administrator

**Lattimore Community Surgicenter,** 125 Lattimore Road, Rochester, NY 14620; tel. 585/473–9000; FAX. 585/697–3519; Peter G. Varlan, Administrator

**North Shore Surgi Center, Inc.,** 989 West Jericho Turnpike, Smithtown, NY 11787; tel. 631/864–7100; FAX. 631/864–7129; Michael Guarino, Administrator

**Queens Surgi-Center,** 83-40 Woodhaven Boulevard, Glendale, NY 11385; tel. 718/849–8700; FAX. 718/849–6523; Adce Abadir, Administrator

**Section C**

**The Mackool Eye Institute,** 31-27 41st Street, Astoria, NY 11103; tel. 718/728–3400; FAX. 718/721–7562

**Westfall Surgery Center, LLP,** 1065 Senator Keating Boulevard, Rochester, NY 14618; tel. 585/256–1330; FAX. 585/256–3823; Gary J. Scott, Administrative Director

## NORTH CAROLINA

**Asheboro Endoscopy Center,** 700 Sunset Avenue, PO Box 4830, Asheboro, NC 27203; tel. 336/625–0305; FAX. 336/625–9941; Vickie Whitaker, RN, Clinical Director

**Blue Ridge Day Surgery Center,** 2308 Wesvill Court, Raleigh, NC 27607; tel. 919/781–4311; FAX. 919/781–0625; Kathy Leibl Administrator

**Caromont Specialty Surgery,** 2511 Court Drive, Gastonia, NC 28054; tel. 704/671–5600; FAX. 704/671–5650; Lisa Lineberger, Manager

**Carteret Surgery Center,** 3714 Guardian Avenue, Morehead City, NC 28557; tel. 252/247–0314; FAX. 252/247–2031; Kim Blaine, Business Manager

**Chapel Hill Surgical Center,** 109 Conner Drive, Suite 1201, Chapel Hill, NC 27514; tel. 919/968–0611; FAX. 919/967–8637; Gary S. Berger, MD, President

**Charlotte Surgery Center,** 2825 Randolph Road, Charlotte, NC 28211; tel. 704/377–1647; FAX. 704/358–8267; Connie M. Wilson, Administrator

**Cleveland Ambulatory Services,** 1100 North Lafayette Street, Shelby, NC 28150; tel. 704/482–1331; FAX. 704/482–4833; John Reynolds, MD, Administrator

**Craven Surgery Center,** 630 McCarthy Blvd, P.O. Box 12446, New Bern, NC 28561; tel. 252/633–2000; FAX. 252/633–9045; Joseph Hageman, RN, Executive Director

**Eye Surgery and Laser Clinic,** 500 Lake Concord Road, NE, Concord, NC 28025; tel. 704/782–1127; FAX. 704/782–1207; Administrator

**Eye Surgery Center of Shelby,** 1622 East Marion Street, Shelby, NC 28150; tel. 704/482–2020; FAX. 704/482–7707; Frank T. Hannah, MD, Medical Director

**Fayetteville Ambulatory Surgery Center,** 1781 Metromedical Drive, Fayetteville, NC 28304; tel. 910/323–1647; FAX. 910/323–4142; John T. Henley, Jr., MD, Medical Director

**Goldsboro Endoscopy Center, Inc.,** 2705 Medical Office Place, Goldsboro, NC 27534; tel. 919/580–9111; FAX. 919/580–0988; Venkata C. Motaparthy, MD, Chief Executive Officer

**HealthSouth Surgery Center of Hickory, L.P.,** PO Box 3529, Hickory, NC 28503-3528; Kevin Deal, RN, Administrator

**High Point Surgery Center,** 600 Lindsay Street, P.O. Box 2476, High Point, NC 27261; tel. 336/878–6068; FAX. 336/878–6111; Joan D. White, Administrative Director

**Iredell Head, Neck and Ear Ambulatory Surgery Center, Inc.,** 707 Bryant Street, Statesville, NC 28677; tel. 704/873–5224; FAX. 704/873–5984; Angie Kerr, Office Manager

**Iredell Surgical Center,** 1720 Davie Avenue, Statesville, NC 28677; tel. 704/871–0081; FAX. 704/871–0086; Glenda Tallent, MBA, Administrator

**Plastic Surgery Center of North Carolina, Inc.,** 2901 Maplewood Avenue, Winston-Salem, NC 27103; tel. 336/768–6210; FAX. 336/768–6236; Melba Edwards, Administrator

**Raleigh Plastic Surgery Center, Inc.,** 1112 Dresser Court, Raleigh, NC 27609; tel. 919/872–2616; FAX. 919/872–2771; Nancy Nicoll O'Neil, Administrator

**Regional Medical Services Surgery Center,** 5200 North Croatan Highway, Kitty Hawk, NC 27949; tel. 252/261–9000; FAX. 919/261–4329; Yvonne Burdick, Executive Director

**Southern Eye Associates, P.A., Ophthalmic Surgery Center,** 2801 Blue Ridge Road, Suite 200, Raleigh, NC 27607; tel. 919/571–0081; Kathryn O'Neill, Director of Clinical Services

**Surgical Eye Center,** 3312 Battleground Avenue, Greensboro, NC 27410; tel. 336/282–8330; FAX. 336/282–2625; Trudy Wester, Center Director

**SurgiCare of Jacksonville,** 166 Memorial Court, Jacksonville, NC 28546; tel. 910/353–9565; FAX. 919/353–5497; Takey Crist, Medical Director

**Vidant SurgiCenter,** 102 Bethesda Drive, Greenville, NC 27834; tel. 252/847–7700; FAX. 252/847–7784; Stephen W. Tripp, RPh, President

**WHA Medical Clinic, PLLC,** 1202 Medical Center Drive, Wilmington, NC 28401; tel. 910/341–3433; Diane A. Atkinson, Executive Director

**Wilmington SurgCare,** 1801 South 17th Street, Wilmington, NC 28401; tel. 910/763–4555; FAX. 910/332–8920; James Shafer, Facility Administrator

## NORTH DAKOTA

**Bismarck Surgical Associates,** 600 N. 9th Street, Bismarck, ND 58501; tel. 701/221–2299; FAX. 701/323–3370; Scott Osadchuk, Director

**Dakota Surgery & Laser Center,** 430 E. Sweet Avenue, Bismarck, ND 58504; tel. 701/222–4900; FAX. 701/222–4999; Charles R. Volk, Administrator

**Day Surgery-Wahpeton,** 275 South 11th Street, Wahpeton, ND 58075; tel. 701/642–2000; FAX. 701/671–4106; Kevin Gish, Administrator

**FM Endoscopy Center,** 4344 20th Ave SW, Fargo, ND 58103; tel. 701/371–5094; Rodney Ludwig, Administrator

**Great Plains Clinic Surgery Center,** 33 Ninth Street, W., Dickinson, ND 58601; tel. 701/483–6017; FAX. 701/483–5018; Mark Grove, Administrator

**Innovis Health,** 1702 S. University Drive, Fargo, ND 58103; tel. 701/364–8900; FAX. 701/364–8990; Dennis Furman, Chief Operating Officer

**Institute For Lower Back Care,** 4344 20th Ave SW, Fargo, ND 58103; tel. 701/297–0817; Panjin Sivanna, MD, Administrator

**Institute for Special Surgery,** 2301 25th Street, Fargo, ND 58103; tel. 702/271–1045; FAX. 702/271–1044; Timothy Haugen, Administrator

**Lamb Plastic Surgery Center,** 1507 S University Dr, Fargo, ND 58103; tel. 701/237–9592; Donald Lamb, MD, Administrator

**Laser and Surgery Center,** 4344 20th Ave S, Fargo, ND 58103; tel. 701/277–7200; Steve Bagan, MD, Administrator

**Mid Dakota Clinic Surgicenter,** 401 N 9th Street, Bismarck, ND 58501; tel. 701/530–6010; FAX. 701/530–5996; Marlene Sapa, Nursing Manager, Administrator

**North Dakota Surgery Center,** 3035 Demers Avenue, Grand Forks, ND 58201; tel. 701/775–3151; FAX. 701/775–3153; Ross J. Gonitzke, Administrator

**Northern Plains Surgery Center,** 44 4th St S, Fargo, ND 58103; tel. 701/232–9200; Sarah Ouse, RN, ASC Coordinator

**St. Alexius Same Day Surgery Center,** 810 East Rosser, Bismarck, ND 58501; tel. 701/530–5000; Sandy Gerving, Director

**Trinity Community Clinic-Western Dakota,** 1102 Main, Williston, ND 58801; tel. 701/572–7711; FAX. 701/572–2283; Mary E. Banta, Administrator

**Trinity Health-MA Same Day Surgery,** 400 E Burdick Expwy, Suite 400, Minot, ND 58702; tel. 701/857–7000; Renda Wilson, Administrator

## OHIO

**Amend Center for Eye Surgery,** 5939 Colerain Avenue, Cincinnati, OH 45239; tel. 513/923–3900; FAX. 513/923–3012

**Bloomberg Eye Center,** 1651 West Main Street, Newark, OH 43055; tel. 740/522–3937; FAX. 740/522–0063; Judy Mackey, Director of Corp. Services

**Central Ohio Endoscopy Center, LLC, Dublin Center,** 6670 Perimeter Drive, Suite 200, Dublin, OH 43016; tel. 614/754–5500; FAX. 614/707–4204; Debbie Sauls, RN, Nurse Manager

**Central Ohio Endoscopy Center, LLC, East Center,** 85 McNaughten Road, Suite 320, Columbus, OH 43213; tel. 614/754–5500; FAX. 614/864–2062; Debbie Sauls, RN, Nurse Manager

**Central Ohio Endoscopy Center, LLC, North Center,** 3800 Olentangy River Road, Columbus, OH 43214; tel. 614/754–5500; FAX. 614/754–5501; Debbie Sauls, RN, Nurse Manager

**Central Ohio Endoscopy Center, LLC, West Center,** 815 W. Broad Street, Suite 220, Columbus, OH 43222; tel. 614/754–5500; FAX. 614/707–4204; Debbie Sauls, RN, Nurse Manager

**Cincinnati Eye Institute and Ambulatory Surgery Center,** 1945 CEI Drive, Cincinnati, OH 45242; tel. 513/984–5133; FAX. 513/984–4240; Clyde Bell, President

**Cincinnati Foot Clinic, Inc.,** 8111 Cheviot Road, Cincinnati, OH 45247; tel. 513/385–6946; Robert Hayman, MD, President

**Columbus Eye Surgery Center,** 5965 East Broad Street, Suite 460, Columbus, OH 43213; tel. 614/751–4080; FAX. 614/751–4092; Janie Norman, RN, Center Director

**Consultants in Gastroenterology, Inc.,** 5900 Landerbrook Drive, Suite 195, Mayfield Heights, OH 44124; tel. 440/461–3596; FAX. 440/460–0130; Karen Wahl, Manager

**Consultants in Gastroenterology, Inc.,** 7530 Fredle Drive, Concord, OH 44077; tel. 440/386–2250; FAX. 440/386–2251; Karen Wahl, Administrator

**Crystal Clinic Surgery Center,** 3975 Embassy Parkway, Suite 202, Akron, OH 44313; tel. 330/668–4085; FAX. 330/668–2624; Katherine L. McNeal, RN, Administrator

**Digestivecare Endoscopy Unit,** 75 Sylvania Drive, Beavercreek, OH 45440; tel. 937/320–5050; FAX. 937/320–5060; Craig Penno, Administrator

**Endoscopy Center of Dayton Ltd.,** 4200 Indian Ripple Road, Beavercreek, OH 45440; tel. 937/427–2078; FAX. 937/427–9081; Jennette Papalios, RN, Nurse Manager

**Endoscopy Center West,** 3654 Werk Road, Cincinnati, OH 45248; tel. 513/451–6001; FAX. 513/451–7310; Angela Tiemann, Administrator

**Eye Institute of Northwestern Ohio, Inc.,** 3509 Briarfield Blvd, Maumee, OH 43537; tel. 419/865–3866; FAX. 419/865–3451; Carol R. Kollarits, MD, President

**Facial Surgery Center,** 1130 Congress Avenue, Glendale, OH 45246; tel. 513/772–2442; FAX. 513/772–2844; Joseph J. Moravec, MD, Medical Director

**Fairview Hospital Surgery Center,** 850 Columbia Road, Westlake, OH 44145; tel. 216/808–4000; FAX. 216/808–4010; Michelle Padden, RN, Administrator

**Firas Atassi, M.D. Outpatient Surgery Center,** 34500 Center Ridge Road, North Ridgeville, OH 33039; tel. 216/327–2414

**Gastroenterology Associates, Inc.,** 4665 Belpar Street, NW, PO Box 36329, Canton, OH 44735; tel. 330/493–1480; FAX. 330/493–6805; Erin Garner, RN, Endoscopy Nurse Manager

**Gastroenterology Specialists, Inc.,** 2726 Fulton Drive, NW, Canton, OH 44718; tel. 330/455–5011; FAX. 330/588–7127; Connie M. Kowalski, RN

**Kunesh Eye Surgery Center,** 2601 Far Hills Avenue, Dayton, OH 45419-1665; tel. 937/298–1093; FAX. 937/298–6344; Lucy Helmers, Administrator

**Midwest Eye Surgery Center,** 4452 Eastgate Boulevard, Suite 305, Cincinnati, OH 45245; tel. 513/752–5700; FAX. 513/752–5716; Holly Schwab, RN, Surgery Manager

**North Coast Endoscopy, Inc.,** 9500 Mentor Avenue, Suite 380, Mentor, OH 44060; tel. 440/352–9400; FAX. 440/352–9407; Ahmad Ascha, MD

**North Shore Endoscopy Center,** 850 Columbia Road, Suite 200, Westlake, OH 44145; tel. 440/808–1212; FAX. 440/808–0321; Christine St.George-Gray, RN, BSN, Operations Manager

**Ohio Eye Associates, Eye Surgery & Laser Center,** 466 South Trimble Road, Mansfield, OH 44906; tel. 419/756–8000; FAX. 419/756–7100; Thomas F. Marquardt, Administrator

**Optivue Vision,** 2740 Navarre Avenue, Oregon, OH 43616; tel. 419/697–3616; FAX. 419/697–3655; Karen R. Hess, RN, LMT, OR Manager

**Parkway Surgery Center, Ltd.,** 3500 Executive Parkway, Toledo, OH 43606; tel. 419/531–8349; FAX. 419/531–6833; Richard I. Tapper, MD, Medical Executive Director

**Sidney Foot and Ankle Center,** 1000 Michigan, Sidney, OH 45365; tel. 937/492–1211; FAX. 937/492–6557; Norma Polasky, Administrative Director

**Surgery Alliance Ltd.,** 975 Sawburg Avenue, Alliance, OH 44601; tel. 330/821–7997; FAX. 330/821–7295; Hazel Thomas, Administrator

**Taylor Station Surgery Center,** 275 Taylor Station Road, Columbus, OH 43213; tel. 614/751–4466; FAX. 614/751–4474; Julie Bernard, Director

**The Endoscopy Center,** 3439 Granite Circle, Toledo, OH 43617; tel. 419/843–7993; FAX. 419/841–7789; Alice Horner, RN Nurse Manager

**The Surgery Center,** 19250 East Bagley Road, Middleburg Heights, OH 44130; tel. 440/826–3240; FAX. 440/826–3250; Barb Draves, CASC, Administrator

**Tippecanoe Endoscopy, Inc.,** 1210 Boardman Canfield Road, Youngstown, OH 44512; tel. 330/726–0132; FAX. 330/726–2571; Mary Amorn, RN, Administrator

**Toledo Clinic, Inc.,** 4235 Secor Road, Toledo, OH 43623; tel. 419/479–5650; FAX. 419/479–3982; Scott Porterfield, Administrator

**Tri-State Centers, For Sight Surgery Center,** 8044 Montgomery Road, Suite 155, Cincinnati, OH 45236; tel. 513/791–7967; FAX. 513/791–1473; Jo Slocum RN, BSN, Administrator

**University Suburban Health Center, Wright Surgery Center Department,** 1611 South Green Road, Suite 124, South Euclid, OH 44121; tel. 216/382-1868; FAX. 216/382-0584; Thomas Stellato, MD, Medical Director

**Western Reserve Surgery Center,** 1930 State Route 59, Kent, OH 44240; tel. 330/677-3292; FAX. 330/677-3624; Laurie Simon, Administrator

**Zeeba Ambulatory Surgery Center,** 29017 Cedar Road, Lyndhurst, OH 44124; tel. 440/460-8000; FAX. 440/460-4225; Franklin Keathley, Administrator

**OKLAHOMA**

**Ambulatory Surgery Associates,** 6160 South Yale Avenue, Tulsa, OK 74136; tel. 918/495-2625; FAX. 918/497-3259; Kathy Helberg, RN, Director

**Central Oklahoma Ambulatory Surgical Center, Inc.,** 3301 Northwest 63rd Street, Oklahoma City, OK 73116; tel. 405/842-9732; FAX. 405/842-9771; W. Edward Dalton, MD, Administrator

**Eastern Oklahoma Surgery Center, LLC,** 5020 East 68th Street, Tulsa, OK 74136; tel. 918/492-1539; FAX. 918/494-8683; Linda Taylor, RN Supervisor

**Great Plains Ambulatory Surgery Center,** 5404 West Lee Boulevard, Suite 100, Lawton, OK 73505; tel. 580/536-7533; FAX. 580/536-7535; Richard Wedig, Administrator

**Heritage Eye Surgicenter of Oklahoma,** 6922 South Western, Oklahoma City, OK 73139; tel. 405/636-1508; FAX. 405/636-1239; Edward D. Glinski, DO, MBA, Administrator

**McGee Eye Surgery Center,** 1000 North Lincoln, Suite 150, Oklahoma City, OK 73104; tel. 405/232-8696; FAX. 405/235-4023; Glenda Woodside, Administrator

**Medical Plaza Endoscopy Unit,** 1125 North Porter, Suite 304, Norman, OK 73071; tel. 405/360-2799; FAX. 405/447-0321; Philip C. Bird, MD

**Oklahoma Surgicare,** 4317 W. Memorial Road, Oklahoma City, OK 73134; tel. 405/755-6240; FAX. 405/752-1819; Lindie Slater, Administrator

**Orthopedic Associates Ambulatory Surgery Center, Inc.,** 3301 Northwest 50th Street, Oklahoma City, OK 73112; tel. 405/947-5610; FAX. 405/948-5166; Carolyn Moles, RN, Director

**Outpatient Surgical Center of Ponca City,** 400 Fairview, Suite 50, Ponca City, OK 74601; tel. 580/762-0695; FAX. 580/765-9406; Steffi Cowan, Operations Manager

**Physicians Surgical Center,** 805 East Robinson, Norman, OK 73071-6610; tel. 405/364-9789; FAX. 405/366-8081; Sandra Vaughn, RN, Administrator

**Southern Oklahoma Surgical Center, Inc.,** 2412 North Commerce, Ardmore, OK 73401; tel. 580/226-5000; FAX. 580/226-5035; Christy Morris, RN, BSN, Administrator

**Southern Plains Medical Center, Inc.,** 2222 Iowa Avenue, PO Box 1069, Chickasha, OK 73023; tel. 405/224-8111; FAX. 405/222-5359; Steven Browning, Administrator

**Southwest Ambulatory Surgery Center, LLC,** 8125 South Walker Avenue, Oklahoma City, OK 73139; tel. 405/631-1015; FAX. 405/631-1050; Anthony L. Cruse, DO, Medical Director

**Surgery Center of South Oklahoma City,** 100 Southeast 59th Street, Oklahoma City, OK 73109; tel. 405/634-9300; FAX. 405/634-8300; Larry Smith, Administrator

**Tower Day Surgery,** 1044 Southwest 44th Street, Suite 100, Oklahoma City, OK 73109; tel. 405/636-1701; FAX. 405/636-4314; Marie Smith, RN, Director of Nursing

**Triad Eye Medical Clinic and Cataract Institute,** 6140 South Memorial, Tulsa, OK 74133; tel. 918/252-2020; FAX. 918/252-7466; Marc L. Abel, DO, Medical Director

**OREGON**

**Aesthetic Breast and Cosmetic Surgery Center,** 10201 Southeast Main, Suite 20, Portland, OR 97216; tel. 503/253-3458; FAX. 503/253-0856; Ronald V. DeMars, MD, Administrator

**Center for Cosmetic and Plastic Surgery,** 1353 East McAndrews Road, Medford, OR 97504; tel. 541/770-6776; FAX. 541/770-5791; Robert M. Jensen, MD, Administrator

**Eye Surgery Center,** 1408 E. Barnett Road, Medford, OR 97504-8279; tel. 541/779-2020; FAX. 541/770-6838; Loren R. Barrus, MD, Administrator

**Eye Surgery Institute,** 813 SW Highland Avenue, Redmond, OR 97756; tel. 541/548-7170; FAX. 541/548-3842; Sara Edwards, Administrator

**Futures Outpatient Surgical Center, Inc.,** 1849 Northwest Kearney, Suite 302, Portland, OR 97209; tel. 503/553-3653; FAX. 503/224-0722; Bryce E. Potter, MD, Principal

**Lovejoy Surgicenter, Inc.,** 933 Northwest 25th Avenue, Portland, OR 97210; tel. 503/221-1870; FAX. 503/221-1488; Kayla Reich, Administrator

**McKenzie Surgery Center,** 940 Country Club Road, Eugene, OR 97401; tel. 541/344-2600; FAX. 541/344-3317; Lynn M. Stapes, RN, Administrator

**North Bend Medical Center, Inc.,** 1900 Woodland Drive, Coos Bay, OR 97420; tel. 541/267-5151; FAX. 541/266-4501; J. Peter Johnson, Chief Executive Officer

**Ontario Surgery Center,** 251 SW 19th Street, Ontario, OR 97914; tel. 541/889-3198; FAX. 541/889-3904; Jeffrey C. Pitts, MD, Administrator

**Oregon Eye Surgery Center, Inc.,** 1550 Oak Street, Suite 8, Eugene, OR 97401; tel. 541/683-8771; FAX. 541/434-0995; Virginia Pecora, RN, Administrator

**The Oregon Clinic Portland Gastroenterology ASC,** 1111 NE 99th Street, Suite 302, Portland, OR 97220; tel. 503/963-2707; FAX. 503/963-2802; David Neale, Administrator

**The Portland Clinic Surgical Center,** 800 Southwest 13th Avenue, Portland, OR 97205; tel. 503/221-0161; FAX. 503/221-4451; J. Michael Schwab, Chief Executive Officer

**Westside Surgery Center,** 13240 Southwest Pacific Highway, Suite 200, Tigard, OR 97223; tel. 503/639-6571; FAX. 503/624-6037; Julie Solso, RN, ASC Director

**Willamette Valley Eye SurgiCenter,** 2001 Commercial Street, SE, Salem, OR 97302; tel. 503/363-1500; FAX. 503/588-2028; Gordon Miller, MD, Administrator

**PENNSYLVANIA**

**Abington Surgical Center,** 2701 Blair Mill Road, Suite 35, Willow Grove, PA 19090; tel. 215/443-8505; FAX. 215/957-0565; Stanley E. Grissinger, MBA, CHE, Executive Director

**Aestique Ambulatory Surgical Center,** One Aesthetic Way, Greensburg, PA 15601; tel. 724/832-7555; FAX. 724/832-7568; Theodore A. Lazzaro, MD, Medical Director

**Delaware Valley Laser Surgery Institute, (Nevyas Eye Associates),** Two Bala Plaza, Pl 33, Bala Cynwd, PA 19004; tel. 215/668-2847; FAX. 215/668-1509; Herbert J. Nevyas, MD, Medical Director

**Dermatologic SurgiCenter,** 1200 Locust Street, Philadelphia, PA 19107; tel. 215/546-3666; FAX. 215/546-6060; Anthony V. Benedetto, DO, FACP, Medical Director

**Dermatologic SurgiCenter,** 2221 Garrett Rd., Drexel Hill, PA 19026; tel. 610/623-5885; FAX. 610/623-7276; Anthony V. Benedetto, DO, FACP, Medical Director

**Digestive Disease Institute,** 899 Poplar Church Road, Camp Hill, PA 17011; tel. 717/763-1239; FAX. 717/763-9854; Iris Garman, Administrator

**Fairgrounds Surgical Center,** 400 North 17th Street, Suite 300, Allentown, PA 18104; tel. 610/821-2020; FAX. 610/821-2016; Darlene G. Hinkle and Debi Baker, Co-Administrative Directors

**Fort Washington Surgery Center,** 467 Pennsylvania Avenue, Fort Washington, PA 19034; tel. 215/628-4300; FAX. 215/628-4253; Charles Pappas, MD

**Kremer Eye Center,** 200 Mall Boulevard, King of Prussia, PA 19406; tel. 610/337-1580; FAX. 610/337-3184; Carol Hughes, RN

**Lebanon Outpatient Surgical Center, L.P.,** 830 Tuck Street, Lebanon, PA 17042; tel. 717/228-1620; FAX. 717/228-1642; Anita Gingrich Fuhrman, RN, BS, CASC, Director

**Mt. Lebanon Surgical Center,** Professional Office Building, 1050 Bower Hill Road, Suite 102, Pittsburgh, PA 15243; tel. 412/563-6808; FAX. 412/563-6857; Cynthia Fabus, Manager

**Mt. Pleasant Surgery Center,** 200 Bessemer Road, Mt. Pleasant, PA 15666; tel. 724/547-5432; FAX. 724/547-2435; Brian Konieczny, Administrative Director

**NEI Ambulatory Surgery Center Inc., PC,** 204 Mifflin Avenue, Scranton, PA 18503; tel. 570/340-8090; FAX. 570/342-3136; Mary Ann Labas, RN, Director of Nursing

**Northwood Surgery Center,** 3729 Easton-Nazareth Highway, Easton, PA 18045; tel. 610/559-7110; FAX. 610/559-7317; Chitu Patel, Administrator

**Ophthalmology Laser and Surgery Center, Inc.,** 92 Tuscarora Street, Harrisburg, PA 17104; tel. 717/233-2020; FAX. 717/233-0825

**Paoli Surgery Center,** One Industrial Boulevard, Paoli, PA 19301; tel. 610/408-0822; FAX. 610/408-9933; Caryl Berlin, Facility Manager

**Pennsylvania Eye Surgery Center,** 4100 Linglestown Road, Harrisburg, PA 17112; tel. 717/657-2020; FAX. 717/657-2071; Jill Stileler, RN, Director, Surgical Services

**Pocono Ambulatory Surgery Center,** One Storm Street, Stroudsburg, PA 18360; tel. 570/421-4978; Mary P. Hayden RN, BS, CASC, Administrative Director

**Shadyside Surgi-Center, Inc.,** 5727 Centre Avenue, Pittsburgh, PA 15206; tel. 412/363-6626; FAX. 412/363-7008; Susan M. Katch, RN, Director

**Southwestern Ambulatory Surgery Center,** 500 Lewis Run Road, Suite 202, Pittsburgh, PA 15122; tel. 412/469-6964; FAX. 412/469-6948; Pamela Wrobleski, CRNA, MPM, CASC Administrator

**Southwestern Pennsylvania Eye Surgery Center,** 750 East Beau Street, Washington, PA 15301; tel. 412/228-7477; FAX. 412/228-6271; Mary Roth, RN, Clinical Director

**Surgical Center of York,** 1750 Fifth Avenue, P.O. Box 290, York, PA 17405; tel. 717/843-7613; FAX. 717/849-5662; Pam Neiderer, Clinical Services Manager

**The Surgery Center of Chester County, Suite 100,** 460 Creamery Way, Oaklands Corporate Center, Exton, PA 19341-2533; tel. 610/594-8900; FAX. 610/594-8907; Dean Daringer, MBA, Administrator

**The SurgiCenter at Ligonier,** 221 West Main Street, Ligonier, PA 15658; tel. 724/238-9573; FAX. 724/238-4709; Kim Kenney-Ciarimboli, Ambulatory Services Director

**UPMC Monroeville Surgery Center,** 125 Daugherty Drive, Monroeville, PA 15146-2749; tel. 412/374-9385; FAX. 412/374-9490; Carol Fiske Boumbouras, CMSC, Administrative Assistant, Medical Staff Manager

**Valley Surgery Center,** 1130 Highway 315, Wilkes-Barre, PA 18702; tel. 570/821-2830; FAX. 570/823-7921; Patricia Williams, Administrator

**West Shore Endoscopy Center,** 423 North 21st Street, Camp Hill, PA 17011; tel. 717/975-2430; FAX. 717/730-2158; Lisa Scichitano, RN, BSN, Administrator

**Wills Surgery Center of Bucks County,** 401 North York Road, Warminster, PA 18974; tel. 215/443-3022; FAX. 215/443-5859; Patricia Cobb, RN, Administrator

**Zitelli & Brodland, Ambulatory Surgery Facility,** 5200 Centre Avenue, Suite 303, Pittsburgh, PA 15232; tel. 412/681-9400; FAX. 412/681-5240; John A. Zitelli, MD

**RHODE ISLAND**

**Bayside Endoscopy Center, LLC,** 33 Staniford Street, Providence, RI 02905; tel. 401/274-1810; FAX. 401/273-9689; Kathryn Abiri, RN, MSN, Administrator

**Ocean State Endoscopy,** 148 West River Street, Providence, RI 02904; tel. 401/274-1260; Rose Morton, MD, Administrator

**St. James Surgery Center,** 444 Quaker Lane, Warwick, RI 02886; tel. 401/384-6537; FAX. 401/384-6541; Paul S. Koch, MD, Medical Director

**Women's Medical Center,** 1725 Broad Street, Cranston, RI 02905; tel. 401/467-9111; FAX. 401/461-1390; Nancy Ganem, Administrator

**SOUTH CAROLINA**

**Ambulatory Eye Surgery and Laser Center, Inc.,** 9297 Medical Plaza Drive, Charleston, SC 29406; tel. 803/572-2888; Margaret A. Thompson

**AnMed Health Medicus Surgery Center, LLC,** 107 Professional Court, P.O. Box 1886, Anderson, SC 29622-1886; tel. 864/225-1933; FAX. 864/716-7965; Angela Kay, RN, Administrator

**Bay Microsurgical Unit, Inc.,** 1200 Highmarket Street, Georgetown, SC 29440; tel. 843/546-8421; FAX. 843/546-1173; Janet Spring, Director of Nursing

**Bearwood Ambulatory Surgery Center,** 3031 Highway 81, N., Anderson, SC 29621; tel. 864/226-7371; FAX. 864/226-8367; Meryle Martin, Office Manager

**Charleston Plastic Surgery Center, Inc.,** 261 Calhoun Street, Suite 200, Charleston, SC 29401; tel. 843/722-1985; FAX. 843/722-4840; Linda Crosby, Office Manager

**Columbia Gastrointestinal Endoscopy Center,** 2739 Laurel Street, Suite One-B, Columbia, SC 29240; tel. 803/254-9588; FAX. 803/931-8085; Cindy Sease, RN, Administrator

**Columbia Surgery Center, Inc.,** 238 Shuler RD, Columbia, SC 29212-8048; tel. 803/732-6180; FAX. 803/732-6563; Vickie H. Ott, Administrator

Section C

**Cross Creek Surgery Center of Greenville Hospital System,** Nine Doctors Drive, Crosscreek Medical Park, Greenville, SC 29605; tel. 803/455-8400; Barbara Callahan, Administrator

**Greenville Endoscopy Center,** 317 Street Francis Drive, Suite 150, Greenville, SC 29601; tel. 864/232-7338; FAX. 864/240-8140; Rebecca K. Swoyer, Administrator

**Greenville Endoscopy Center,** 200 Patewood Drive, Ste 100B, Greenville, SC 29615; tel. 864/232-7338; FAX. 864/240-8140; Rebecca K. Swoyer, Administrator

**Greenville Surgery Center,** Five Memorial Medical Court, Greenville, SC 29605; tel. 864/295-3067; FAX. 864/295-3096; Angela Kay, Administrator

**HealthSouth Surgery Center of Charleston,** 2690 Lake Park Drive, North Charles, SC 29406; tel. 803/764-0992; FAX. 803/764-3187; Rosina Feagin, RN, MSN, Administrator

**Roper West Ashley Surgery Center,** 325 Folly Rd, Ste 200, Charleston, SC 29412-2507; tel. 843/763-3763; FAX. 843/763-3721; Maria I. Sample, Administrator

**Spartanburg Urology Surgicenter, L.P.,** 391 Serpentine Drive, Suite 200, Spartanburg, SC 29303; tel. 864/585-2002; FAX. 864/585-3300; Rick Sizemore, RN, Administrator

**Upstate Surgery Center, LLC,** 10 Enterprise Boulevard, Suite 109, Greenville, SC 29615; tel. 864/458-7141; FAX. 864/676-9116; Geoffrey Hibbert, Interim Director

## SOUTH DAKOTA

**Avera Medical Group - Pierre,** 100 Mac Lane, Pierre, SD 57501; tel. 605/945-5210; FAX. 605/945-5084; Lynne Kurth, RN, Administrator

**Black Hills Regional Eye Surgery Center,** 2800 Third Street, Rapid City, SD 57701-7394; tel. 605/341-2000; FAX. 605/341-0278; Richard B. Hanafin, Executive Director

**Mallard Pointe Surgical Center,** 1201 Mickelson Drive, Watertown, SD 57201-7100; tel. 605/882-4743; FAX. 605/882-6064; Mary Petersen, Administrative Director

## TENNESSEE

**Bristol Surgery Center,** 350 Blountville Highway, Suite 108, Bristol, TN 37620; tel. 423/844-6120; FAX. 423/844-6119; Karen Williams,GCHC,MPH,NHA,CHES Administrator

**Cataract Surgery Center,** 825 Ridge Lake Blvd, Suite 200, Memphis, TN 38120-9411; tel. 901/360-8081; FAX. 901/368-3822

**Chattanooga Surgery Center,** 400 North Holtzclaw Avenue, Chattanooga, TN 37404; tel. 423/698-6871; FAX. 423/622-8993; K.D. Ratchford, Administrator

**Clarksville Endoscopy Center,** 132 Hillcrest Drive, Clarksville, TN 37043; tel. 931/552-0180; FAX. 931/572-0915; Deborah Glassell, Clinical Director

**D D C Surgery Center,** Nine Physicians Drive, Jackson, TN 38305; tel. 731/661-0086; FAX. 731/661-9783; Kelly Joyce, Clinical Director

**East Memphis Surgery Center,** 80 Humphreys Center Drive, Suite 101, Memphis, TN 38120; tel. 901/747-3233; FAX. 901/747-3230; Cathy Gilland, RN, Facility Administrator

**Endoscopy Center of Kingsport, dba Sullivan Digestive Center,** 2204 Pavilion Drive, Kingsport, TN 37660; tel. 423/392-6100; FAX. 423/392-6159; Penny Lloyd, Administrator

**Eye Surgery Center of East Tennessee,** 1124 Weisgarber Road, Suite 110, Knoxville, TN 37909; tel. 865/588-1037; FAX. 865/909-9104; Mary Beth Solocinski, RN, Center Director

**Eye Surgery Center of Middle Tennessee,** Parkview Tower, Suite 900, 210 25th Avenue, N., Nashville, TN 37203; tel. 615/327-2244; FAX. 615/327-9254; Stephen J. Molnar, Jr., Executive Administrator

**Fort Sanders West Outpatient Surgery Center, LLC,** 210 Fort Sanders West Boulevard, Knoxville, TN 37922; tel. 865/531-5200; FAX. 865/531-5770; Erma Morgan, Director

**Germantown Ambulatory Surgical Center, Inc.,** 7499 Poplar Pike, Germantown, TN 38138; tel. 901/755-6465

**HealthSouth Nashville Surgery Center,** 1717 Patterson Street, Nashville, TN 37203; tel. 615/329-1888; FAX. 615/329-0179; Lori Seymore, Administrator

**Knoxville Center for Reproductive Health,** 1547 West Clinch Avenue, Knoxville, TN 37916; tel. 865/637-3861; FAX. 865/637-0222; Kim Denison, Director

**Lebanon HMA Surgical Center,** 1414 Baddour Parkway, Lebanon, TN 37087; tel. 615/453-8252; FAX. 615/444-8994; Sylvia Black, Clinical Director

**LeBonheur East Surgery Center, L.P.,** 786 Estate Place, Memphis, TN 38120; tel. 901/287-4100; FAX. 901/287-4140; Sherrye Crone, Administrative Director, Carol Langston, Asst. Director

**Lisa Ross Birth & Women's Center, Inc., Maternity Center of East Tennessee (formerly),** 1925-B Ailor Avenue, Knoxville, TN 37921; tel. 865/524-4422; FAX. 865/523-3687; Linda Cole, CNM Executive Director

**Mays & Schnapp Pain Clinic and Rehabilitation Center,** 55 Humphreys Center Drive, Suite 200, Memphis, TN 38120; tel. 901/747-0040; FAX. 901/747-0042; Victoria Saunders, Practice Administrator

**Memphis Center for Reproductive Health,** 1462 Poplar Avenue, Memphis, TN 38104; tel. 901/274-3550; FAX. 901/274-3551; Rebecca L. Terrell, Executive Director

**Memphis Eye and Cataract Ambulatory Surgery Center,** 6485 Poplar Avenue, Memphis, TN 38119; tel. 901/767-3937; FAX. 901/767-1695

**Memphis Gastroenterology Endoscopy Center,** 8000 Wolf River Blvd, #200, Germantown, TN 38138-1727; tel. 901/747-3630; FAX. 901/747-4039; Sylvia Hawkins, RN, Compliance Manager

**Memphis Regional Gamma Knife Center,** 1211 Union Ave, Ste 220, Memphis, TN 38104; tel. 901/726-6444; FAX. 901/726-6145; Betsy Smith, Administrator

**Memphis Surgery Center,** 1044 Cresthaven Road, Memphis, TN 38119; tel. 901/682-1516; FAX. 901/682-1545; Cathy Gilland, RN, BS, Facility Administrator

**Mid-State Endoscopy Center,** 2010 Church Street, Suite 420, Nashville, TN 37203; tel. 615/329-2141; FAX. 615/321-0522; Allan H. Bailey, MD, Medical Director

**Nashville Endoscopy Center,** 300 20th N, Eighth Floor, Nashville, TN 37203; tel. 615/284-1335; FAX. 615/284-1316; Gregory A. Winston, Administrator

**Nashville Gastrointestinal Endoscopy Center,** 4230 Harding Road, Suite 309, Nashville, TN 37205; tel. 615/383-0165; FAX. 615/292-4657; Ron E. Pruitt, MD

**Northridge Surgery Center,** 647 Myatt Drive, Madison, TN 37115; tel. 615/868-8942; FAX. 615/860-3820; Tim Shannon, Administrator

**Oral Facial Surgery Center,** 322 22nd Avenue, N., Nashville, TN 37203; tel. 615/321-6160; FAX. 615/327-9612; Ronda Landers, Administrator

**Planned Parenthood - Greater Memphis Region,** 2430 Poplar Avenue, Suite 100, Memphis, TN 38112; tel. 901/725-1717; FAX. 901/274-4790; Ellen Ruby - Markie, Chief Executive Officer

**Ridge Lake Ambulatory Surgery Center,** 825 Ridge Lake Boulevard, Memphis, TN 38119; tel. 901/685-2200; Jana Jones, ASC Administrator

**Shea Ear Clinic,** 6133 Poplar Pike, Memphis, TN 38119; tel. 901/761-9720; FAX. 901/763-4400; John J. Shea Jr., MD, Medical Director

**Southern Endoscopy Center,** 330 Wallace Road, Suite 103, Nashville, TN 37211; tel. 615/832-5530; FAX. 615/832-5713; Robert W. Herring, Jr., MD, Medical Director

**St. Thomas Medical Group Endoscopy Center,** 4230 Harding Road, Suite 400, Nashville, TN 37205; tel. 615/297-2700; Jeff May RN, Center Director

**Surgery Center of Clarksville,** 121 Hillcrest Drive, Clarksville, TN 37043; tel. 931/552-9992; FAX. 931/648-1816; Angela Farmer, Administrator

**Surgical Services, P.C.,** 604 South Main Street, Sweetwater, TN 37874; tel. 423/337-4508; FAX. 423/337-4588

**Surgicenter Of Murfreesboro Medical Clinic, P.A.,** 1272 Garrison Drive, Murfreesboro, TN 37129; tel. 615/867-8160; FAX. 615/876-7876; Sandy Gordon, Coordinator

**Tennessee Endoscopy Center,** 1706 East Lamar Alexander Parkway, Maryville, TN 37804; tel. 615/983-0073; FAX. 615/984-1731; Craig Jarvis, MD, Administrator

**The Cookeville Surgery Center,** 100 West Fourth Street, Suite 100, Cookeville, TN 38501; tel. 931/526-8115; FAX. 931/526-7619; Jeanie McGinnis, RN Administrator

**The Endoscopy Center of Centennial, L.P.,** 2400 Patterson Street, Suite 515, Nashville, TN 37203; tel. 615/327-2111; FAX. 615/327-9292; Donna Crumley, RN, BS, MBA, Endoscopy Administrator

**The Eye Surgery Center of Oak Ridge,** 90 Vermont Avenue, Oak Ridge, TN 37830; tel. 865/482-8894; FAX. 865/481-8349; Regina Harkleroad, Director of Nursing

**Urology Surgery Center, L.P.,** 2801 Charlotte Avenue, Nashville, TN 37209; tel. 615/250-9202; FAX. 615/250-9251; Mary Ellen, Danielson, RN, CNOR, CASC, Director

**Volunteer Women's Medical Clinic,** 313 Concord Street, Knoxville, TN 37919; tel. 865/522-5173; FAX. 865/522-9907; Elizabeth Fraley-Dumas, Clinical Director

**Wesberry Surgery Center,** 2900 South Perkins Road, Memphis, TN 38118-3237; tel. 901/362-3100; FAX. 901/362-3372; Jesse Wesberry, Jr., MD, President

**Wesley Ophthalmic Plastic Surgery Center,** 1800 Church Street, Suite 100, Nashville, TN 37203; tel. 615/329-3624; Janie Stucker, RN, Director

## TEXAS

**Abilene Cataract and Refractive Surgery Center,** 2120 Antilley Road, Abilene, TX 79606; tel. 325/695-2020; FAX. 325/695-2326; Paul B. Thames MD Medical Director

**Abilene Endoscopy Center,** 1249 Ambler Avenue, Abilene, TX 79601; tel. 325/677-2626; FAX. 325/677-6835; Steve Johnson, MD, Medical Director

**Amarillo Cataract and Eye Surgery Center, Inc.,** 7310 Fleming Avenue, Amarillo, TX 79106; tel. 806/354-8891; FAX. 806/354-2591; Carol A. Pearson, Director

**Ambulatory Urological Surgery Center, Inc.,** 1149 Ambler, Abilene, TX 79601; tel. 915/676-3557; FAX. 915/673-2143; Angela X. Young, RN, Manager

**American Surgery Centers of South Texas, LTD,** 7810 Louis Pasteur, Suite 100, San Antonio, TX 78229; tel. 210/692-0218; FAX. 210/692-7980; Letty Herrera, Administrator

**Arlington Day Surgery Center,** 918 North Davis Street, Arlington, TX 76012; tel. 817/860-9933; FAX. 817/860-2314; Dan Chambers, Administrator

**Bailey Square Surgical Center, Ltd.,** 1111 West 34th Street, Austin, TX 78705; tel. 512/454-6753; FAX. 512/454-4314; Randy Humphrey, Administrator

**Bay Area Endoscopy Center,** 444 FM 1959, Suite B, Houston, TX 77034; tel. 281/481-9400; FAX. 281/481-9490; N.S. Bala, Medical Director

**Bay Area Surgicare Center,** 502 Medical Center Boulevard, Webster, TX 77598; tel. 281/332-2433; FAX. 281/332-0619; Carol Simons, Administrator

**Baylor SurgiCare,** 3920 Worth Street, Dallas, TX 75246; tel. 214/820-2581; FAX. 214/820-7484; Robin Shaw, Administrative Director

**Baylor Surgicare at Valley View,** 5744 LBJ Freeway, Suite 200, Dallas, TX 75240; tel. 972/490-4333; FAX. 972/991-1649; Gina Schilthuis, RN, Administrator

**Brazosport Eye Institute,** 103 Parking Way, P.O. Box 369, Lake Jackson, TX 77566; tel. 979/297-2961; FAX. 979/297-2395; Frank J. Grady, MD, PhD, FACS, Director

**Coastal Bend Ambulatory Surgical Center,** 900 Morgan, Corpus Christ, TX 78404; tel. 361/888-4288; FAX. 361/888-4786; Barbara VandenBout, Administrator

**Columbia Physicians DaySurgery Center,** 3930 Crutcher Street, Dallas, TX 75246; tel. 214/827-0760; FAX. 214/827-0944; Robin Shaw, RN, Administrator

**Conroe Surgery Center,** 1501 River Pointe Drive, Suite 200, Conroe, TX 77304; tel. 936/760-3443; FAX. 936/760-1322; Kathy Schutz, RN, BSN, CASC, Facility Administrator

**Covenant Surgicenter, Ltd.,** 2301 Quaker Avenue, Lubbock, TX 79410; tel. 806/725-8801; FAX. 806/725-8820; Elizabeth Hawronsky, Director

**Crystal Outpatient Surgery Center, Inc.,** 215 Oak Drive, S., Suite J, Lake Jackson, TX 77566; tel. 409/299-6118; FAX. 409/299-1007; R. Scott Yarish, MD, Administrator

**Cy-Fair Surgery Center,** 11250 Fallbrook Drive, Houston, TX 77065; tel. 713/955-7194; FAX. 713/890-0895; Sonja Christmas, Administrator

**Dallas DaySurgery of Texas North, Ltd.,** 9101 North Central Expressway, Suite 650, Dallas, TX 75231; tel. 214/821-8613; FAX. 214/821-4958; Elizabeth Toony, RN, BSN, CASC, Administrator

**Dallas Ophthalmology Center, Inc.,** 4633 North Central Expressway, Suite 310, Dallas, TX 75205; tel. 214/520-7600; FAX. 214/528-6522; Susan Points, RN, Administrator

**DeHaven Surgical Center,** 1424 East Front Street, Tyler, TX 75702; tel. 903/595-4144; FAX. 903/595-0236; Terri McDougal, RN, Administrator

**Doctors' Surgery Center, Inc.,** 5300 North Street, Nacogdoches, TX 75965; tel. 936/569–8278; FAX. 936/569–0275; Robert P. Lehmann, MD, Director

**East El Paso Surgery Center,** 7835 Corral Drive, El Paso, TX 79915; tel. 915/595–3353; FAX. 915/595–6796; Laura Ice, Administrator

**East Side Surgery Center, Inc.,** 10918 East Freeway, Houston, TX 77029; tel. 713/451–4299; FAX. 713/451–4383; Vicky Mizell, Administrator

**East Texas Eye Associates Surgery Center,** 1306 Frank Avenue, Lufkin, TX 75904; tel. 409/634–8381; Jo Ann O'Neill, COT, Administrator

**El Paso Institute of Eye Surgery, Inc.,** 1717 North Brown Street, Building #3, El Paso, TX 79902; tel. 915/544–0526; FAX. 915/544–2877; Esther A. Calderon, Administrator

**Elm Place Ambulatory Surgical Center,** 2217 South Danville Drive, Abilene, TX 79605; tel. 325/695–0600; FAX. 325/695–3908; Rebecca Laird, RN

**Endoscopy Center of Dallas, Ambulatory Endoscopy Clinic of Dallas,** 6390 LBJ Freeway, Suite 200, Dallas, TX 75240; tel. 972/934–3691; FAX. 972/934–3694; Jeane Suggs, Administrator

**Facial Plastic and Cosmetic Surgery Center,** 6300 Humana Plaza, Suite 475, Abilene, TX 79606; tel. 915/695–3630; FAX. 915/695–3633; Howard A. Tobin, MD, FACS, Medical Director

**Fort Worth Endoscopy Center,** 900 W. Magnolia Street, Suite 101, Fort Worth, TX 76104; tel. 817/332–6500; Jenny Hunter, Administrator

**Forth Worth Surgery Center,** 2001 West Rosedale, Fort Worth, TX 76104; tel. 817/877–4777; David Yodge, Administrator

**Foundation Surgery Center of Dickinson,** 3810 Hughes Court, Dickinson, TX 77539; tel. 713/337–7001; FAX. 713/337–7091; Theresa Mitcham, Administrator Assistant

**Gastroenterology Consultants Outpatient Surgical Center,** 8214 Wurzbach, San Antonio, TX 78229; tel. 210/614–1234; FAX. 210/614–7749; Robert Rosso, Chief Executive Officer

**Good Shepard Ambulatory Surgical Center, Ltd.,** 703 East Marshall Avenue, Suite 2000, Longview, TX 75601-5563; tel. 903/315–5300; FAX. 903/315–5301; Marion Benson, VP and Executive Director

**Gramercy Outpatient Surgery Center, Ltd.,** 2727 Gramercy, Houston, TX 77025; tel. 713/660–6900; FAX. 713/660–0704; Walter W. Topp, III, Administrator

**Greenville Surgery Center,** 7150 Greenville Avenue, Suite 200, Dallas, TX 75231; tel. 214/891–0466; FAX. 214/739–4702; Christine Locke, Administrator

**Heart of Texas Outpatient Cataract Center,** 100 South Park Drive, Brownwood, TX 76801; tel. 325/643–3561; Larry Smith, CRNA, Administrator

**Heritage Surgery Center,** 1501 Redbud Boulevard, McKinney, TX 75069; tel. 972/548–0771; FAX. 972/562–2300; Rudolf Churner, MD, Administrator

**Howerton Surgical Center,** 2610 I.H. 35 South, Austin, TX 78704-5703; tel. 512/443–9715; FAX. 512/443–9845; Michael D. Laney, CMPE, COE

**Key Whitman Surgery Center,** 2801 Lemmon Avenue, Suite 400, Dallas, TX 75204; tel. 214/754–0000; FAX. 214/754–0079; Jeffrey Whitman, MD

**Knapp Medical Center ASC,** 1402 East Sixth Street, Weslaco, TX 78596; tel. 956/968–6155; FAX. 956/968–8291; Paul Giles, Administrator

**Las Colinas Surgery Center,** 4255 North Macarthur Boulevard, Irving, TX 75038; tel. 214/257–0144; FAX. 214/258–0436; Michael Scott, Administrator

**Lufkin Endoscopy Center,** 317 Gaslight Boulevard, Lufkin, TX 75904; tel. 936/634–3713; FAX. 936/634–8136; Bhagvan R. Malladi, MD, Administrator

**Medical City Dallas Ambulatory Surgery Center,** 7777 Forest Lane, Suite C-150, Dallas, TX 75230; tel. 972/566–6171; FAX. 972/566–2502; Vickie Roberts, Administrator

**Metroplex Ambulatory Surgical Center,** 2717 Osler Drive, Suite 102, Grand Prairie, TX 75051; tel. 972/647–6272; FAX. 972/660–1822; Glenda Daniels, RN, Director

**Metroplex Surgicare Partners, Ltd., dba Baylor Surgicare at Bedford,** 1600 Central Drive, Suite 180, Bedford, TX 76022; tel. 817/571–1999; FAX. 817/571–1220; Brandon Shows, Administrator

**Mid-Town Surgical Center, LLP,** 2105 Jackson Street, Suite 200, Houston, TX 77003; tel. 713/571–8141; FAX. 713/571–8184; Louis Varela, MD

**North Carrier Surgicenter,** 517 North Carrier Parkway, Suite A, Grand Prairie, TX 75050-5494; tel. 972/264–0533; FAX. 972/262–5974; Abraham F. Syrquin, MD, Medical Director

**North Dallas Surgicare,** 375 Municipal Drive, Suite 214, Richardson, TX 75080; tel. 214/918–9400; FAX. 214/918–9749; Houston Landry, Administrator

**Northeast Texas Surgical Center,** 1902 Moores Ln, Suite B, Texarkana, TX 75503; tel. 903/792–2108; FAX. 903/792–0606; Penny Howard, RN, Administrator

**Park Central Surgical Center,** 12200 Park Central Drive, Third Floor, Dallas, TX 75251; tel. 972/661–0505; FAX. 972/661–5511; Molly Paulose, Administrator

**Physicians SurgiCenter of Houston True Results,** 7515 South Main Street, Suite 800, Houston, TX 77030; tel. 713/799–9990; FAX. 713/796–1142; Sean Bayette, MBA, MHA, Administrator

**Plano Ambulatory Surgery Associates, L.P., dba Surgery Center of Plano,** 1620 Coit Road, Plano, TX 75075-7799; tel. 972/519–1100; DeWayne Hodges, Administrator

**Plaza Day Surgery,** 909 Ninth Avenue, Fort Worth, TX 76104-3986; tel. 817/339–2300; FAX. 817/339–2329; Gina Basham, RN, Administrator

**Port Arthur Day Surgery Center,** 2555 Jimmy Johnson Boulevard, Port Arthur, TX 77640-2007; tel. 409/983–6144; Vicki Clark, Administrative Director

**Premier Ambulatory Surgery of Austin, dba South Austin Surgery Center,** 4207 James Casey, Suite 203, Austin, TX 78745; tel. 512/440–7894; FAX. 512/440–1932; Tammy Smittle, RN, CASC, Administrator

**Q Plus Outpatient Surgery Center,** 2507 Medical Row, Suite 101, Grand Prairie, TX 75051; tel. 972/647–8520; FAX. 972/336–0488; James L. Grace Administrator

**Renaissance Northeast Surgery Center,** 1475 FM 1960 East Bypass, Humble, TX 77338; tel. 281/446–4053; Julie McKase-Martin, Administrator

**Rio Grande Surgery Center,** 1809 South Cynthia, McAllen, TX 78503; tel. 956/618–4402; FAX. 956/618–4174; Jill Finke, CNOR Administrator

**San Antonio Digestive Disease Endoscopy Center,** 1804 Northeast Loop 410, Suite 101, San Antonio, TX 78217; tel. 210/828–8400; FAX. 210/804–4454; Kathy Favela, RN, Clinical Director

**San Antonio Gastroenterology Endoscopy Center,** 520 Euclid Avenue, San Antonio, TX 78212; tel. 210/271–0606; FAX. 210/271–0180; Ernesto Guerra, MD

**San Antonio Surgery Center, Inc., dba The Center for Special Surgery,** 21 Spurs Lane, Sub-Level 100, San Antonio, TX 78240; tel. 210/614–0187; FAX. 210/692–7757; Hong Nguyen, Administrator

**Southwest Endoscopy & Surgery Center,** 701 East Rendon Crowley Rd., Burleson, TX 76028; tel. 817/568–5188; FAX. 817/568–1568; J. Leslie Hill

**Surgery Center of Texas,** 155 East Loop 338, Suite 500, Odessa, TX 79762; tel. 432/367–3906; FAX. 432/367–3895; Libby Palma, Administrator

**SurgEyeCare, Inc.,** 5421 La Sierra Drive, Dallas, TX 75231; tel. 214/361–1443; FAX. 214/691–3299; Sandra J. Yankee, Administrator

**Surgical and Diagnostic Center, LP.,** 729 Bedford Euless Road West, Suite 100, Hurst, TX 76053; tel. 817/282–1001; FAX. 817/282–4040; Bart Steele, Administrator

**Surgical Center of El Paso,** 1815 North Stanton, El Paso, TX 79902; tel. 915/533–8412; FAX. 915/542–0367; Raymond Sainz, Administrator

**Texarkana Surgery Center,** 5404 Summerhill Road, Texarkana, TX 75503; tel. 903/793–4872; FAX. 903/794–6300; Kimble Hatridge, Administrator

**Texoma Outpatient Surgery Center, Inc.,** 1712 Eleventh Street, Wichita Falls, TX 76301; tel. 940/723–2499; FAX. 940/923–2497; Tracy Youngblood, Administrator

**The Cataract Center of East Texas, dba Novamed Surgery Center of Tyler,** 802 Turtle Creek Drive, Tyler, TX 75701; tel. 903/595–4333; FAX. 903/535–9845; S. Stephens, RN, Clinical Administrator

**The Center for Sight, P.A.,** 2 Medical Center Boulevard, Lufkin, TX 75904-3175; tel. 936/634–8434; FAX. 936/639–2581; Richard J. Ruckman, MD

**The Endoscopy Center of Southeast Texas,** 950 North 14th Street,#200, Beaumont, TX 77702; tel. 409/833–5555; FAX. 409/833–9911; JoAnn Hughes, RNBC, Center Director

**The Ocular Surgery Center, Inc.,** 1100 North Main Avenue, San Antonio, TX 78212; tel. 210/222–2154; FAX. 512/222–0706; Jane Wilson, Administrator

**The Surgery Center of Mesquite,** 2690 North Galloway Avenue, Mesquite, TX 75150; tel. 972/279–8100; FAX. 972/279–3300; Susan Erickson, Administrator

**The Surgery Center of the Woodlands,** 1441 Woodstead Court, Suite 100, The Woodlands, TX 77380; tel. 281/363–0058; FAX. 281/363–0450; Susan Olis, Administrator

**Urological Surgery Center of Fort Worth,** 418 South Henderson, Fort Worth, TX 76104; tel. 817/870–9165; FAX. 817/335–5421; Charles Bamberger, MD

**Valley Endoscopy Center, LLP,** 3101 South 77 Sunshine Strip, Suite B, Harlingen, TX 78550; tel. 956/421–2324; FAX. 956/421–5791; Susan R. Gonzalez, Center Director

**Vista Surgical Center West,** 2500 Fondren, Suite 350, Houston, TX 77063; tel. 713/782–8279; FAX. 713/782–3139; Diana Hastings, RN, CNOR - Clinical Director

**West Houston Surgicare,** 970 Campbell Road, Houston, TX 77024-2804; tel. 713/461–3547; FAX. 713/722–8921; Charles Mattea, Administrator

**Wilson Surgicenter,** 4315 28th Street, Lubbock, TX 79410; tel. 806/792–2104; Bill W. Wilson, MD, Chief Executive Officer

### UTAH

**Central Utah Surgical Center,** 1067 North 500 West, Provo, UT 84604; tel. 801/374–0354; FAX. 801/717–2364; Jill Andrews, RN, BSN, CNOR, Administrator

**Institute of Facial and Cosmetic Surgery,** 5929 Fashion Boulevard, Salt Lake City, UT 84107; tel. 801/261–3637; FAX. 801/261–4096; Dr. Brent D. Kennedy, Director

**Salt Lake Endoscopy Center,** 24 South 1100 East, Salt Lake City, UT 84102; tel. 801/355–2987; FAX. 801/531–9704; Cher Struck, Office Manager

**Salt Lake Surgical Center,** 617 East 3900 South, Salt Lake City, UT 84107; tel. 801/261–3141; FAX. 801/268–2599; Robyn Archer, Administrator

**St. George Surgical Center,** 676 South Bluff Street, St. George, UT 84770; tel. 435/673–8080; FAX. 435/673–0096; Kelly Kendall, Administrator

**St. Mark's Outpatient Surgery Center,** 1250 East 3900 South, Suite 100, Salt Lake City, UT 84124; tel. 801/262–0358; FAX. 801/262–0901; Diana McPherson, MBA, CASC, Administrator

**The SurgiCare Center of Utah,** 755 East 3900 South, Salt Lake City, UT 84107; tel. 801/266–2283; FAX. 801/268–6151; Helen Sikes, Administrator

**Wasatch Endoscopy,** 1220 East 3900 South, Suite 1B, Salt Lake City, UT 84124; tel. 801/281–3657; FAX. 801/281–4258; Jeri Fowles, Administrator

**Wasatch Surgery Center,** 555 South Foothill Boulevard, Salt Lake City, UT 84112; tel. 801/581–7782; FAX. 801/581–8962; Karen Ipson, Administrator, Manager

### VIRGINIA

**Blue Ridge Surgery Center,** 1802 Braeburn Drive, Salem, VA 24153; tel. 540/772–3601; FAX. 540/725–4543; Kay D'Ardenne, Administrator

**Cataract and Refractive Surgery Center, LLC,** 2010 Bremo Road, Suite 132, Richmond, VA 23226; tel. 804/673–5272; FAX. 804/673–5279; Patricia Lampman, Director

**Fredericksburg Ambulatory Surgery Center,** 1201 Sam Perry Boulevard, Suite 101, Fredericksburg, VA 22401; tel. 540/741–7000; FAX. 540/899–6893; Jeane Bullock, Administrator

**Kaiser Permanente Falls Church Ambulatory Surgery Center,** 201 North Washington Street, Falls Church, VA 22046; tel. 703/531–1623; FAX. 703/536–1400; Eileen Field, Director, ASC

**Lakeview Medical Center, Inc.,** 2000 Meade Parkway, Suffolk, VA 23424; tel. 757/934–9433; FAX. 757/934–9497; Laura E. Joyner, Chief Operations Officer

**Parham Surgery Center,** 7640 E Parham Road, Henrico, VA 23294; tel. 804/285–4763; FAX. 804/288–8946; Sandra W. Pearson, Administrator

**Piedmont Day Surgery Center, Inc.,** 1040 Main Street, P.O. Box 1360, Danville, VA 24543-1360; tel. 434/792–1433; FAX. 434/797–2807; Joseph Carbone, MD, President

Section C

**Riverside Hampton Surgery Center,** 850 Enterprise Parkway, Suite 1000, Hampton, VA 23666-6255; tel. 757/251-7700; FAX. 757/251-7799; Sheila Rilee, RN, Administrator

**Surgi Center of Central Virginia, Inc.,** 12 Chatham Heights Rd, Fredericksburg, VA 22405; tel. 703/371-5349; FAX. 703/373-1745; William A. Keeney, Facility Administrator

**Surgi-Center of Winchester, Inc.,** 1860 Amherst Street, PO Box 2660, Winchester, VA 22604; tel. 540/536-8934; FAX. 540/536-8936; David J. Kliewer, MD, Medical Director

**Urosurgical Center of Richmond,** 9105 Stony Point Dr, Richmond, VA 23235; tel. 804/330-9105; FAX. 804/560-0914; Terry W. Coffey, Administrator

**Urosurgical Center of Richmond-North,** 8228 Meadowbridge Road, Mechanicsville, VA 23116; tel. 804/730-5023; FAX. 804/746-4015; Terry W. Coffey, Administrator

**Virginia Ambulatory Surgery, Inc.,** 337-15th Street, SW, Charlottesville, VA 22903; tel. 434/951-4600; FAX. 434/817-8465; Gerry Dobrasz, Administrator

**Virginia Beach Ambulatory Surgery Center,** 1700 Will-o-Wisp Drive, Virginia Beach, VA 23454; tel. 757/496-6400; FAX. 757/496-3137; Martha R. Colen, Administrator

**Virginia Eye Institute/Eye Surgeons of Richmond, Inc.,** 400 Westhampton Station, Richmond, VA 23226; tel. 804/287-4244; FAX. 804/287-4207; Jane Broadbent, Marketing and Communications Director

**Woodburn Surgery Center,** 3289 Woodburn Road, Suite 100, Annandale, VA 22003; tel. 703/207-7520; Jolene Tornabeni, Senior Vice President, Administrator

**WASHINGTON**

**Allure Laser Center,** 625 4th Avenue, Suite 301, Kirkland, WA 98033; tel. 425/216-7200; FAX. 425/216-7272; Janet Jordan, Administrator

**Auburn Outpatient Surgery Center,** 1427 Jefferson Avenue, Suite 101, Enumclaw, WA 98022; tel. 360/825-4466; FAX. 360/825-2064; Nancy A. Becker, DO, Medical Director

**Bel-Red Ambulatory Surgical Facility,** 1260 116th Avenue, NE, #110, Bellevue, WA 98004; tel. 425/455-7225; FAX. 425/455-0045; Jan Zemplenyi, MD, Director

**Cascade Medical Group PS, Inc.,** 111 S. 13th Street, Mount Vernon, WA 98274; tel. 360/336-2178; FAX. 360/336-1674; Alex O'Dell, Business Administrator

**Cascade Valley Arlington Surgery Center,** 875 Wesley Street, Suite 160, Arlington, WA 98223; tel. 360/435-6969; FAX. 360/435-1068; Jola Barnett, Assistant Administrator

**Edmonds Surgery Center,** 21229 84th Avenue W., Edmonds, WA 98026; tel. 206/775-1505; FAX. 206/775-9078; Mark A. Kuzel, DPM, F.A.C.F.S

**Evergreen Endoscopy Center,** 11800 NE 128th Street, Suite 100, Kirkland, WA 98034; tel. 425/899-4500; FAX. 425/899-4510; Darlene Buckley, RN, Endoscopy Unit Supervisor

**Evergreen Eye Center,** 34719 Sixth Avenue South, Federal Way, WA 98003; tel. 800/340-3595; FAX. 206/212-2194; Richard A. Boudreau, Administrator

**Eye Surgery Center Northwest,** 842 South Cowley, Suite 3, Spokane, WA 99202; tel. 509/747-6358; FAX. 509/321-5020; Michael H. Cunningham, MD, President

**First Hill Surgery Center,** 515 Minor Avenue, Suite 130, Seattle, WA 98104; tel. 206/682-6103; FAX. 206/682-3511; Debbie Perdue, Director

**Foot Care Associates Ambulatory Surgery Center,** 16146 Cleveland Street, Redmond, WA 98052; tel. 425/885-7004; Dr. Brunsman, Medical Director

**GH TASC,** 209 Martin Luther King Jr. Way, Tacoma, WA 98405; tel. 253/596-3590; Nancy Sowers, RN, MBA, CNOR, Manager

**Good Samaritan Surgery Center,** 1322 Third Street SE, Suite 100, Puyallup, WA 98372; tel. 253/697-5700; FAX. 253/697-4120; William Rinker, MD, Medical Director

**Minor & James Medical, PLLC,** 515 Minor Avenue, Suite 200, Seattle, WA 98104; tel. 206/386-9500; FAX. 206/576-3807; Patricia Creed, RN, ASC Manager

**Moses Lake Clinic ASC,** 840 E. Hill Avenue, Moses Lake, WA 98837; tel. 509/764-6400; FAX. 509/764-6434; David Olson, Administrator

**North Kitsap Ambulatory Surgical Center Inc., dba Pacific Surgery Center,** 20669 Bond Road, NE, Suite 200, Poulsbo, WA 98370; tel. 360/779-6527; FAX. 360/697-2743; Susan Simons, RN, BSN, CASC, Administrator

**Northwest Center for Plastic and Reconstructive Surgery,** 16259 Sylvester Road, SW, Suite 302, Seattle, WA 98166; tel. 206/241-5400; FAX. 206/241-8591; Sindi Miller, Office Manager

**Northwest Gastroenterology, dba Northwest Endoscopy,** 2930 Squalicum Parkway, Suite 202, Bellingham, WA 98225; tel. 360/734-1420; FAX. 360/734-8748; Sandra Vander Yacht, Manager

**Northwest Nasal Sinus Center,** 1200 Northgate Way, Seattle, WA 98133; tel. 206/525-2525; FAX. 206/525-0346; Rick Fischer, Business Administrator

**Northwest Nasal Sinus Center,** 3100 Carillon Point, Kirkland, WA 98033; tel. 425/576-1700; FAX. 425/827-7725; Rick Fischer, Business Administrator

**Northwest Surgery Center,** 1920 100th Street, SE, Everett, WA 98208; tel. 425/316-3700; FAX. 425/316-6881; Chris Vance, President

**Northwest Surgery Center, Inc.,** West 123 Francis, Spokane, WA 99205; tel. 509/483-9363; FAX. 509/483-0355; Douglas P. Romney

**Olympic Plastic Surgery Suite,** 2600 Cherry Avenue, Suite 201, Bremerton, WA 98310; tel. 360/415-0762; Suzanne Fletcher, Administrator

**Pacific Cataract and Laser Institute,** 2517 Northeast Kresky, Chehalis, WA 98532; tel. 206/748-8632; FAX. 360/748-4007; Debbie Eldredge, Vice President and Chief Operating Officer

**Pacific Cataract and Laser Institute,** 10500 Northeast Eighth Street, Suite 1650, Bellevue, WA 98004-4332; tel. 425/462-7664; FAX. 425/462-6429; Maynard Pohl, OD, Clinical Director

**Pacific Cataract and Laser Institute,** 8200 West Grandridge, Kennewick, WA 99336; FAX. 360/748-4007; Debbie Eldredge, Vice President and Chief Operating Officer

**Pacific NW Facial Plastic Ambulatory Surgery Center,** 600 Broadway, Suite 280, Seattle, WA 98122; tel. 206/386-3550; FAX. 206/386-3553; Sherry Gizewski, Practice Manager

**Parkway Surgical Center,** 2940 Squalicum Parkway, Suite 204, Bellingham, WA 98225; tel. 206/676-8350; FAX. 206/676-8351; Orville Vandergriend, MD, Administrator

**PeaceHealth St. Joseph Medical Center, PeaceHealth Medical Group,** 4545 Cordata Parkway, Bellingham, WA 98226; tel. 360/738-2200; FAX. 360/752-5681; Debra L. Taylor, Dir Operations Specialty SVS

**Phillip C. Kierney, M.D., Cosmetic and Plastic Surgery,** 105 27th Avenue, SE, Puyallup, WA 98374; tel. 253/848-8110; FAX. 253/845-3561; P. Kierney, Owner

**Physicians Eye Surgical Center,** 3930 Hoyt Avenue, Everett, WA 98201; tel. 206/259-2020; Ms. Mello Johnson, Administrator

**Premier Orthopedic Group Surgery Center,** 21600 Highway 99, Suite 150, Edmonds, WA 98026; tel. 425/774-2636; FAX. 425/774-2688; Marilyn Degan, Director

**Rockwood Clinic, dba Gastrointestinal Endoscopy Unit,** 400 East 5th Avenue, Spokane, WA 99202; tel. 509/838-2531; FAX. 509/755-6580; Craig Whiting, MD, Administrator

**Seattle Endoscopy Center,** 11027 Meridian Avenue, N., Suite 100, Seattle, WA 98133; tel. 206/365-4492; FAX. 206/368-3456; Mary Beth Philips, BSN, RN, CGRN, Manager

**Seattle Hand Surgery Group, P.C.,** 600 Broadway, Suite 440, Seattle, WA 98122; tel. 206/292-6252; FAX. 206/292-7893

**Seattle Plastic Surgery Center,** 600 Broadway, Suite 320, Seattle, WA 98122; tel. 206/324-1120; FAX. 206/720-0800; Gail Boren, Manager

**Seattle Surgery Center, Columbus Pavilion,** 900 Terry Avenue, Third Floor, Seattle, WA 98104-1240; tel. 206/382-1021; FAX. 206/332-9369; Jim Sapienza, FACHE, Chief Executive Officer

**Sequim Same Day Surgery,** 777 North Fifth Avenue, Sequim, WA 98382; tel. 360/582-2632; FAX. 360/582-2631; Tammy Paolini, Operational Manager

**South Hill Ambulatory Surgical Center,** South 3028 Grand Boulevard, Spokane, WA 99203; tel. 509/747-0279; FAX. 509/747-3220; Borys Markewych

**Spokane Digestive Disease Center, P.S.,** 105 West Eighth Avenue, Suite 6010, Spokane, WA 99204-2341; tel. 509/838-5950; FAX. 509/838-5961; Michelle Avenger, RN, CGRN, Director

**Spokane Surgery Center,** North 1120 Pines Road, Spokane, WA 99206; tel. 509/928-1990; FAX. 509/928-2933; Stewart P. Brim, DPM

**Surgery Center Of Spokane,** 205 N. University #4, Spokane, WA 99206; tel. 509/922-3199; Dr. Jacqueline Borbol

**Tacoma Ambulatory Surgery Center,** 1112 Sixth Avenue, Suite 100, Tacoma, WA 98405; tel. 253/272-3916; FAX. 253/627-1713; Deborah Gist, Clinical Director

**Tacoma Endoscopy Center,** 1112 Sixth Avenue, Suite 200, Tacoma, WA 98405; tel. 253/272-8664; FAX. 253/627-7880; John G. Carrougher, MD, Medical Director

**The Eastside Endoscopy Center, LLC, A Physicians Endoscopy Partnered Facility,** 1135 116th Ave NE Suite 570, Bellevue, WA 98004-3049; tel. 425/451-7335; FAX. 425/451-1226; Michelle Steele, CGRN, Nurse Administrator

**The Plastic SurgiCentre, Inc.,** 535 South Pine Street, Spokane, WA 99202; tel. 509/623-2160; FAX. 509/623-1135; Vern Myrick, RN, Nurse Manager

**The Polyclinic, Inc.,** 1145 Broadway, Seattle, WA 98122; tel. 206/329-1760

**Virginia Mason-Issaquah,** 100 Northeast Gilman Boulevard, Issaquah, WA 98027; tel. 425/557-8000; Bobbie Eatmon, Director Ambulatory Services

**Washington Centre for Reproductive Medicine, ASC,** 1370 116th Avenue, NE, Suite 202, Bellevue, WA 98004; tel. 425/462-6100; FAX. 425/635-0742; Dr. James Kustin, Medical Director

**Washington Orthopedic Center, Inc., PS,** 1900 Cooks Hill Road, Centralia, WA 98531; tel. 360/736-2889; Dondi Sahlinger, OR Manager

**Whidbey SurgiCare,** PO Box 11782, Suite A Two, Olympia, WA 98508-1782; tel. 360/679-3117; FAX. 360/679-3118; Stephen T. Miller, DPM, Medical Director

**WEST VIRGINIA**

**Anwar Eye Center,** 1500 Lafayette Avenue, Moundsville, WV 26041; tel. 304/845-0908; FAX. 304/845-1250; M. F. Anwar, MD

**Cabell Huntington Surgery Center,** 1201 Hal Greer Boulevard, Huntington, WV 25701; tel. 304/523-1885; FAX. 304/523-8942; Lexa Woodyard, Administrator

**Day Surgery Center,** Chesterfield Medical Plaza, 2335 Chesterfield Ave. #400, Charleston, WV 25304; tel. 304/925-9300; FAX. 304/925-2924; Olivia Price, Administrator

**Greenbrier Clinic Surgery Center, Inc.,** 320 W. Main Street, White Sulphur Spring, WV 24986; tel. 304/536-4870; FAX. 304/536-1125; William N. Cunningham, MD, Medical Director

**Jerry N. Black, M.D., Surgical Suite,** 10 Amalia Drive, Suite 3C, Buckhannon, WV 26201; tel. 304/472-2100; FAX. 304/472-2118; Jerry N. Black, MD, Medical Director

**Kanawha Valley Surgi-Center,** 4803 MacCorkle Avenue, SE, Charleston, WV 25304; tel. 304/925-6390; FAX. 304/925-7931; Gorli Harish, MD, Medical Director

**Surgical Eye Center of Morgantown,** 1299 Pineview Drive, Morgantown, WV 26505; tel. 304/598-5755; Heather Huffman, Administrator

**Tri State Surgical Center, LLC,** 1006 Tavern Road, Martinsburg, WV 25401; tel. 304/267-0556; Stacey Ferguson, Administrator

**WISCONSIN**

**BayCare Surgery Center,** 2253 West Mason, P.O. Box 33227, Green Bay, WI 54303-0102; tel. 920/592-9100; FAX. 920/497-8056; Tammy Krueger, Executive Director

**Green Bay Surgical Center, Ltd.,** 704 South Webster Avenue, Ste 301, Green Bay, WI 54301; tel. 920/432-7433; FAX. 920/432-6003

**Menomonee Falls Ambulatory Surgery Center,** W180 N8045 Town Hall Road, Menomonee Falls, WI 53051; tel. 262/250-0950; FAX. 262/250-0955; Dianne Wallace, Executive Director

**North Shore Surgical Center,** 7007 North Range Line Road, Milwaukee, WI 53209; tel. 414/352-3341; FAX. 414/247-4588; Helen Kowalski, Executive Director

**Northwest Surgery Center,** 2300 North Mayfair Road, Suite 295, Wauwatosa, WI 53226; tel. 414/257-3322; FAX. 414/257-3364; Gail Wuestoff, Administrator

**Riverview Surgery Center,** 616 North Washington Street, Janesville, WI 53545; tel. 608/758-7300; FAX. 608/758-1050; Lynn Jenkins, Director

**St. Mary's Dean Ventures Surgery Centers,** PO Box 259630, Madison, WI 53725-9630; tel. 608/259–3510; FAX. 608/255–1272; Jonathan Lewis, Vice President

**Surgicenter of Greater Milwaukee,** 3223 South 103rd Street, Milwaukee, WI 53227; tel. 414/328–5800; FAX. 414/328–5805; Denise Augustin, Executive Director

**Surgicenter of Racine, Ltd.,** 5802 Washington Avenue, Racine, WI 53406; tel. 262/886–9100; FAX. 262/886–9130; Dennis J. Kontra, Administrator

**Wauwatosa Surgery Center,** 10900 West Potter Road, Wauwatosa, WI 53226-3424; tel. 414/774–9227; FAX. 414/774–0957; Cathy Logue, Administrator

**WYOMING**

**Wyoming Outpatient Services,** 5050 Powderhouse Road, Cheyenne, WY 82009; tel. 307/634–1311; FAX. 307/432–7550; Jan VanAlyn, LPN, Manager

**Yellowstone Surgery Center, LLC,** 5201 Yellowstone Road, Cheyenne, WY 82009; tel. 307/635–7070; FAX. 307/632–9920; Deborah Wright, Office Administrator

# U.S. Associated Areas

**PUERTO RICO**

**ASC Espanola Clinic,** Box 490, La Quinta, Mayaguez, PR 00681; tel. 787/832–2094

**Clinica de Cirugia Ambulatoria de Puerto Rico,** Box 3748, Mayaguez, PR 00681; tel. 787/833–4400; FAX. 787/265–6621; Roberto Ruiz, Administrator

**Damas Hospital,** Edificio Parra Office 201, Ponce, PR 00717-1320; tel. 787/840–8686; FAX. 787/841–0387; Mr. Enrique Vicens, MHSA

**Instituto Cirugia Plastica Del Oeste,** 165 Este Mendez Vigo Street, Mayaguez, PR 00680; tel. 787/833–3248; FAX. 787/831–4400; Oscar Vargas, MD, Medical Director

**Instituto Quirurgico De Un Dia - Dr. Pila,** PO Box 331910, Ponce, PR 00733-1910; tel. 787/848–5600; FAX. 787/841–1085; Mrs. Joselyn Irizarry RN, Supervisor

**OJOS, Eye Surgery Specialists of P.R.LLC,** Hipodromo Street 809, Santurce, PR 00909; tel. 787/721–8330; FAX. 787/722–3222; Maria Delos A. Tirado, Administrator

**San Juan Health Centre Ambulatory Clinic,** 150 De Diego Avenue, Badorioty Corner, San Juan, PR 00907; tel. 787/977–7575; FAX. 787/977–7587; Pedro Rivera-Archilla, Executive Director

Section C

# Joint Commission Accredited Freestanding Long–Term Care Organizations

*The accredited freestanding long–term care organizations listed have been accredited as of April, 2012 by The Joint Commission on Accreditation of Healthcare Organizations by decision of the Accreditation Committee of the Board of Commissioners.*

*The organizations listed here have been found to be in compliance with the Joint Commission standards for long–term care organizations, as found in the Comprehensive Accreditation Manual for the Long–Term Care Organizations.*

*Please refer to section A of the AHA Guide for information on hospitals with Long–Term Care services. These hospitals are identified by Facility Code 127. In section A, those hospitals identified by Approval Code 1 are Joint Commission accredited.*

*We present this list simply as a convenient directory. Inclusion or omission of any organization's name indicates neither approval nor disapproval by Health Forum LLC, an American Hospital Association company.*

## United States

### ALABAMA

**Central Alabama Veterans Health Care System,** 215 Perry Hill Road, Montgomery, AL 36109; tel. 334/272–4670

**Marion Regional Medical Center, Inc.,** 1256 Military Street South, Hamilton, AL 35570; tel. 205/921–6200

**Tuscaloosa VA Medical Center,** 3701 Loop Road East, Tuscaloosa, AL 35404; tel. 205/554–2000

### ARIZONA

**CareMeridian-Phoenix,** 5301 E. Thomas Avenue, Phoenix, AZ 85018; tel. 602/687–1100

**Citadel Care Center,** 5121 East Broadway Road, Mesa, AZ 85206; tel. 480/832–5555

**Desert Cove Nursing Center,** 1750 West Frye Road, Chandler, AZ 85224; tel. 480/899–0641

**Glendale Care Center,** 4704 West Diana Avenue, Glendale, AZ 85302; tel. 623/247–3949

**Heritage Health Care Center,** 1300 South Street, Globe, AZ 85501; tel. 928/425–3118

**La Canada Care Center,** 7970 North LaCanada Drive, Tucson, AZ 85704; tel. 520/797–1191

**Las Fuentes Care Center,** 1045 Scott Drive, Prescott, AZ 86301; tel. 928/778–9603

**Life Care Center of North Glendale,** 13620 North 55th Avenue, Glendale, AZ 85304; tel. 602/843–8433

**Life Care Center of Paradise Valley,** 4065 East Bell Road, Phoenix, AZ 85032; tel. 602/867–0212

**Life Care Center of Scottsdale,** 9494 East Becker Lane, Scottsdale, AZ 85260; tel. 480/860–6396

**Life Care Center of Sierra Vista,** 2305 East Wilcox Drive, Sierra Vista, AZ 85635; tel. 520/458–1050

**Life Care Center of South Mountain,** 8008 South Jesse Owens Parkway, Phoenix, AZ 85040; tel. 602/243–2780

**Life Care Center of Tucson,** 6211 North LaCholla Boulevard, Tucson, AZ 85741; tel. 520/575–0900

**Life Care Center of Yuma,** 2450 South 19th Avenue, Yuma, AZ 85364; tel. 928/344–0425

**Mi Casa Nursing Center,** 330 S. Pinnule Circle, Mesa, AZ 85206; tel. 480/981–0687

**Mountain View Care Center,** 1313 West Magee Road, Tucson, AZ 85704; tel. 520/797–2600

**Northern Arizona VA Health Care System,** 500 Highway 89 North, Prescott, AZ 86313; tel. 928/445–4860

**Payson Care Center,** 107 East Lone Pine Drive, Payson, AZ 85541; tel. 928/474–6896

**Phoenix VA Health Care System,** 650 East Indian School Road, Phoenix, AZ 85012-1892; tel. 602/277–5551

**Scottsdale Heritage Court,** 3339 N. Drinkwater Blvd, Scottsdale, AZ 85251; tel. 480/949–5400

**Southern Arizona VA Health Care System,** 3601 South Sixth Avenue, Tucson, AZ 85723; tel. 520/629–1821

**Sun Grove Village Care Center,** 20625 N. Lake Pleasant Road, Peoria, AZ 85382; tel. 623/566–0642

### ARKANSAS

**Central Arkansas Veterans Healthcare System,** 4300 West Seventh Street (00/LR), Little Rock, AR 72205; tel. 501/257–5314

### CALIFORNIA

**Bel Tooren Villa Convalescent Hospital,** 16910 Woodruff Avenue, Bellflower, CA 90706; tel. 562/867–1761

**CareMeridian,** 18792 East 17th Street, Santa Ana, CA 92705; tel. 949/263–6630

**CareMeridian,** 18-A Journey, Suite 200, Aliso Viejo, CA 92656; tel. 949/263–6630

**CareMeridian-Artesia,** 17724 Gridley Road, Artesia, CA 90701; tel. 562/865–0806

**CareMeridian-Cowan Heights,** 10631 Cowan Heights Drive, Santa Ana, CA 92705; tel. 714/731–7263

**CareMeridian-Elk Grove,** 7601 Jacinto Road, Elk Grove, CA 95758; tel. 916/688–3830

**CareMeridian-Escondido,** 2960 Bernardo Avenue, Escondido, CA 92029; tel. 760/739–8255

**CareMeridian-Fairfax,** 2390 Sir Francis Drake Boulevard, Fairfax, CA 94930; tel. 415/256–8007

**CareMeridian-Garden Grove,** 12461 Springdale Street, Garden Grove, CA 92845; tel. 949/263–6630

**CareMeridian-Granite Bay,** 7150 Sierra Ponds Lane, Granite Bay, CA 95746; tel. 916/772–2990

**CareMeridian-La Habra Heights,** 102 E. Avocado Crest Road, La Habra Heights, CA 90631; tel. 562/691–2486

**CareMeridian-Northridge,** 10318 Laramie Street, Chatsworth, CA 91311; tel. 818/882–5204

**CareMeridian-Oxnard,** 1540 Teal Club Road, Oxnard, CA 93030; tel. 805/382–1921

**CareMeridian-San Martin,** 11500 Center Avenue, San Martin, CA 95046; tel. 408/686–0758

**CareMeridian-Santiago Canyon,** 17722 Santiago Canyon Road, Silverado, CA 92676; tel. 714/649–0533

**CareMeridian-Weber,** 2020 N. Weber Avenue, Fresno, CA 93705; tel. 559/264–0535

**CHW Dominican Hospital,** 1555 Soquel Drive, Santa Cruz, CA 95065; tel. 831/462–7700

**East Los Angeles Doctors Hospital,** 4060 East Whittier Boulevard, Los Angeles, CA 90023; tel. 323/268–5514

**Fallbrook Hospital Corporation,** 624 East Elder Street, Fallbrook, CA 92028-3099; tel. 760/728–1191

**Goleta Valley Cottage Hospital,** PO Box 6306, Santa Barbara, CA 93160-6306; tel. 805/967–3411

**Hemet Valley Medical Center,** 1117 East Devonshire Avenue, Hemet, CA 92543; tel. 951/652–2811

**Hi Desert Medical Center,** 6601 White Feather Road, Joshua Tree, CA 92252; tel. 760/366–6260

**Hollenbeck Palms,** 573 South Boyle Avenue, Los Angeles, CA 90033; tel. 323/263–6195

**Imperial Convalescent Center,** 11926 La Mirada Boulevard, La Mirada, CA 90638; tel. 562/943–7156

**La Habra Convalescent Hospital,** 1233 West La Habra Boulevard, La Habra, CA 90631; tel. 562/691–0781

**Lake Forest Nursing Center,** 25652 Old Trabuco Road, Lake Forest, CA 92630; tel. 949/380–9380

**Life Care Center of Escondido,** 1980 Felicita Road, Escondido, CA 92025; tel. 760/741–6109

**Life Care Center of Menifee,** 27600 Encanto Drive, Menifee, CA 92586; tel. 951/679–6858

**Life Care Center of Vista,** 304 North Melrose Drive, Vista, CA 92083; tel. 760/724–8222

**Los Robles Hospital and Medical Center,** 215 West Janss Road, Thousand Oaks, CA 91360; tel. 805/370–4421

**Marian Medical Center,** 1400 East Church Street, Santa Maria, CA 93454; tel. 805/739–3000

**Metropolitan State Hospital,** 11401 South Bloomfield Avenue, Norwalk, CA 90650; tel. 562/863–7011

**Mills-Peninsula Health Services,** 1501 Trousdale Drive, Burlingame, CA 94010; tel. 650/696–5270

**Mirada Hills Rehabilitation and Convalescent Hospital,** 12200 La Mirada Boulevard, La Mirada, CA 90638; tel. 562/947–8691

**North Walk Villa Convalescent Hospital,** 12350 Rosecrans Avenue, Norwalk, CA 90650; tel. 562/921–6624

**Oak Valley District Hospital,** 350 S. Oak Avenue, Oakdale, CA 95361; tel. 209/847–3011

**Orangegrove Rehabilitation Hospital,** 12332 Garden Grove Boulevard, Garden Grove, CA 92843; tel. 714/534–1041

**Pacifica Nursing and Rehabilitation Center,** 385 Esplanade Avenue, Pacifica, CA 94044; tel. 650/993–5576

**Rady Children's Hospital San Diego,** 3020 Children's Way, MC 5069, San Diego, CA 92123-4282; tel. 858/576–1700

**Reche Canyon Rehabilitation and Health Care Center,** 1350 Reche Canyon Road, Colton, CA 92324; tel. 909/370–4411

**Rimrock Villa Convalescent Hospital,** 27555 Rimrock Road, Barstow, CA 92311; tel. 760/252–2515

**San Francisco General Hospital and Trauma Center,** 1001 Potrero Avenue, Bldg 20, Room 2300, San Francisco, CA 94110; tel. 415/206–3455

**San Francisco VA Medical Center,** 4150 Clement Street, San Francisco, CA 94121; tel. 415/750–2014

**Seton Medical Center,** 1900 Sullivan Avenue, Daly City, CA 94015; tel. 650/992–4000

**Totally Kids Specialty Healthcare,** 1720 Mountain View Avenue, Loma Linda, CA 92354; tel. 909/796–6915

**VA Central California Health Care System,** 2615 East Clinton Avenue, Fresno, CA 93703; tel. 559/225–6100

**VA Greater Los Angeles Healthcare System,** 11301 Wilshire Boulevard, Los Angeles, CA 90073; tel. 310/268–3132

**VA Loma Linda Healthcare System,** 11201 Benton Street, Loma Linda, CA 92357; tel. 909/583–6002

**VA Long Beach Health Care System,** 5901 East Seventh Street, Long Beach, CA 90822; tel. 562/826–5400

**VA Northern California Health Care System,** 10535 Hospital Way, Mather, CA 95655; tel. 925/372–2010

**VA Palo Alto Health Care System,** 3801 Miranda Avenue, Palo Alto, CA 94304; tel. 650/493–5000

**VA San Diego Health Care System,** 3350 La Jolla Village Drive, San Diego, CA 92161; tel. 858/552–8585

### COLORADO

**Berkley Medical Investors, LLC,** 735 South Locust Street, Denver, CO 80224; tel. 303/320–4377

**Briarwood Health Care Center,** 1440 Vine Street, Denver, CO 80206; tel. 303/399–0350

**Canon Lodge Care Center,** 905 Harding Avenue, Canon City, CO 81212; tel. 719/275–4106

**Columbine Manor Care Center,** 530 W 16th Street, Salida, CO 81201; tel. 719/539–6112

**Evergreen Nursing Home,** 1991 Carroll Avenue, Alamosa, CO 81101; tel. 719/589–4951

**Garden Terrace Alzheimer's Center of Excellence,** 1600 South Potomac Street, Aurora, CO 80012; tel. 303/750–8418

**Grand Junction Veterans Affairs Medical Center,** 2121 North Avenue, Grand Junction, CO 81501; tel. 970/242–0731

**Hallmark Nursing Center,** 3701 West Radcliff Avenue, Denver, CO 80236; tel. 303/794–6484

**Heritage Park Care Center,** 1200 Village Road, Carbondale, CO 81623; tel. 970/963–1500

**Life Care Center of Aurora,** 14101 East Evans Avenue, Aurora, CO 80014; tel. 303/751–2000

**Life Care Center of Colorado Springs,** 2490 International Circle, Colorado Springs, CO 80910; tel. 719/630-8888

**Life Care Center of Evergreen,** 2987 Bergen Peak Drive, Evergreen, CO 80439; tel. 303/674-4500

**Life Care Center of Greeley,** 4800 25th Street, Greeley, CO 80634; tel. 970/330-6400

**Life Care Center of Littleton,** 1500 W. Mineral Avenue, Littleton, CO 80120; tel. 303/795-7300

**Life Care Center of Longmont,** 2451 Pratt Street, Longmont, CO 80501; tel. 303/776-5000

**Life Care Center of Pueblo,** 2118 Chatalet Lane, Pueblo, CO 81005; tel. 719/564-2000

**Life Care Center of Westminster,** 7751 Zenobia Court, Westminster, CO 80030; tel. 303/412-9121

**San Luis Care Center,** 240 Craft Drive, Alamosa, CO 81101; tel. 719/589-9081

**University Park Care Center,** 945 Desert Flower Boulevard, Pueblo, CO 81001; tel. 719/545-5321

**VA Eastern Colorado Healthcare System,** 1055 Clermont Street, Denver, CO 80220; tel. 303/399-8020

**Valley View Villa,** 815 Fremont Avenue, Fort Morgan, CO 80701; tel. 970/867-8261

**Villa Manor Care Center,** 7950 W. Mississippi Avenue, Lakewood, CO 80226; tel. 303/986-4511

**Western Hills Health Care Center,** 1625 Carr Street, Lakewood, CO 80214; tel. 303/232-6881

## CONNECTICUT

**VA Connecticut Healthcare System,** 950 Campbell Avenue, West Haven, CT 06516; tel. 203/932-5711

**Woodlake at Tolland (ECHN Eldercare Services),** 26 Shenipsit Lake Road, Tolland, CT 06084; tel. 860/872-2999

**Yale Health,** 55 Lock Street, New Haven, CT 06520; tel. 203/432-4096

## DELAWARE

**VA Medical Center,** 1601 Kirkwood Highway, Wilmington, DE 19805; tel. 302/994-2511

## DISTRICT OF COLUMBIA

**VA Medical Center,** 50 Irving Street, Northwest, Washington, DC 20422; tel. 202/745-8000

## FLORIDA

**Bay Pines VA Healthcare System,** 10000 Bay Pines Boulevard, Bay Pines, FL 33744; tel. 727/398-6611

**Bon Secours Maria Manor Nursing & Rehabilitation Center,** 10300 4th Street North, Saint Petersburg, FL 33716; tel. 727/576-1025

**Darcy Hall of Life Care,** 2170 Palm Beach Lakes Boulevard, West Palm Beach, FL 33409; tel. 561/683-3333

**Florida Institute for Neurologic Rehabilitation, Inc,** 1962 Vandolah Road, Wauchula, FL 33873; tel. 863/773-2857

**Jackson Plaza Nursing and Rehabilitation Center,** 1861 Northwest 8th Avenue, Miami, FL 33136; tel. 305/347-3380

**James A. Haley Veterans' Hospital,** 13000 Bruce B. Downs Boulevard, Tampa, FL 33612; tel. 813/972-2000

**Lakeside Health Center,** 2501 Australian Avenue, West Palm Beach, FL 33407; tel. 561/655-7780

**Life Care Center of Altamonte Springs,** 989 Orienta Avenue, Altamonte Springs, FL 32701; tel. 407/831-3446

**Life Care Center of Citrus County,** 3325 Jerwayne Lane, Lecanto, FL 34461; tel. 352/746-4434

**Life Care Center of Estero,** 3850 Williams Road, Estero, FL 33928; tel. 239/495-4000

**Life Care Center of Hilliard,** 3756 W. 3rd Street, Hilliard, FL 32046; tel. 904/845-3988

**Life Care Center of Inverrary,** 4300 Rock Island Road, Lauderhill, FL 33319; tel. 954/485-6144

**Life Care Center of Jacksonville,** 4813 Lenoir Avenue, Jacksonville, FL 32216; tel. 904/332-4546

**Life Care Center of Melbourne,** 606 East Sheridan Road, Melbourne, FL 32901; tel. 321/727-0984

**Life Care Center of New Port Richey,** 7400 Trouble Creek Road, New Port Richey, FL 34653; tel. 727/375-2999

**Life Care Center of Ocala,** 2800 Southwest 41st Street, Ocala, FL 34474; tel. 352/873-7570

**Life Care Center of Orange Park,** 2145 Kingsely Avenue, Orange Park, FL 32073; tel. 904/272-2424

**Life Care Center of Orlando,** 3211 Rouse Road, Orlando, FL 32817; tel. 407/281-1070

**Life Care Center of Palm Bay,** 175 Villa Nueva Avenue, Palm Bay, FL 32907; tel. 321/952-1818

**Life Care Center of Pensacola,** 3291 East Olive Road, Pensacola, FL 32507; tel. 850/494-2327

**Life Care Center of Port St. Lucie,** 3720 SE Jennings Road, Port Saint Lucie, FL 34952; tel. 772/398-8080

**Life Care Center of Punta Gorda,** 450 Shreve Street, Punta Gorda, FL 33950; tel. 941/639-8771

**Life Care Center of Sarasota,** 8104 Tuttle Avenue, Sarasota, FL 34243; tel. 941/360-6411

**Life Care Center of Wells Crossing,** 355 Crossing Boulevard, Orange Park, FL 32073; tel. 904/264-1950

**Life Care Center of Winter Haven,** 1510 Cypress Gardens Boulevard, Winter Haven, FL 33884; tel. 863/318-8646

**Miami VA Healthcare System,** 1201 NW 16th Street, Miami, FL 33125; tel. 305/575-7000

**North Florida/South Georgia Veterans Health System,** 1601 Southwest Archer Road, Gainesville, FL 32608-1197; tel. 352/376-1611

**Orlando VA Medical Center,** 5201 Raymond Street, Orlando, FL 32803; tel. 407/629-1599

**St. Anne's Nursing Center,** 11855 Quail Roost Drive, Miami, FL 33177; tel. 305/252-4000

**St. Catherine's Rehabilitation Hospital/Villa Maria Nursing Center,** 1050 NE 125th Street, Miami, FL 33161; tel. 305/891-8850

**St. John's Rehabilitation Hospital and Nursing Center,** 3075 Northwest 35th Avenue, Lauderdale Lakes, FL 33311; tel. 954/739-6233

**The Gardens Court,** 3803 PGA Boulevard, Palm Beach Gardens, FL 33410; tel. 561/626-1125

**VA Medical Center-West Palm Beach, Florida,** 7305 N. Military Trail, West Palm Beach, FL 33410-6400; tel. 561/422-8600

## GEORGIA

**Camellia Gardens of Life Care,** 804 South Broad Street, Thomasville, GA 31792; tel. 229/226-0076

**Charlie Norwood VA Medical Center,** 1 Freedom Way, Augusta, GA 30904; tel. 706/733-0188

**Emanuel Medical Center,** 117 Kite Road, Swainsboro, GA 30401; tel. 478/289-1100

**Georgia War Veterans Home,** 2249 Vinson Highway, Milledgeville, GA 31061; tel. 478/445-4516

**Georgia War Veterans Nursing Home,** 1101 15th Street, Augusta, GA 30901; tel. 706/721-2531

**Gwinnett Medical Center,** 1000 Medical Center Boulevard, Lawrenceville, GA 30046; tel. 678/312-4321

**Life Care Center of Gwinnett,** 3850 Safehaven Drive, Lawrenceville, GA 30044; tel. 770/923-0005

**Life Care Center of Lawrenceville,** 210 Collins Industrial Way, Lawrenceville, GA 30043; tel. 678/442-0777

**Sadie G. Mays Health and Rehabilitation Center,** 1821 Anderson Avenue, NW, Atlanta, GA 30314; tel. 404/794-2477

**VA Medical Center-Atlanta,** 1670 Clairmont Road, Decatur, GA 30033; tel. 404/728-7601

**VA Medical Center-Carl Vinson,** 1826 Veterans Boulevard, Dublin, GA 31021; tel. 478/277-2701

## HAWAII

**Hale Anuenue Restorative Care Center,** 1333 Waianuenue Avenue, Hilo, HI 96720; tel. 808/961-6644

**Ka Punawai Ola,** 91-575 Farrington Highway, Kapolei, HI 96707; tel. 808/674-9262

**Life Care Center of Hilo,** 944 West Kawailani Street, Hilo, HI 96720; tel. 808/959-9151

**Life Care Center of Kona,** 78-6957 Kamehameha III Road, Kailua Kona, HI 96740; tel. 808/322-2790

**VA Pacific Islands Health Care System,** 459 Patterson Road, Honolulu, HI 96819-1522; tel. 808/433-0100

## IDAHO

**Boise VA Medical Center,** 500 West Fort Street, Boise, ID 83702-4598; tel. 208/422-1100

**Bridgeview Estates,** 1828 Bridgeview Boulevard, Twin Falls, ID 83301; tel. 208/736-3933

**Life Care Center of Boise,** 808 North Curtis Road, Boise, ID 83706; tel. 208/376-5273

**Life Care Center of Coeur d'Alene,** 500 West Aqua Avenue, Coeur D Alene, ID 83815; tel. 208/762-1122

**Life Care Center of Idaho Falls,** 2725 East 17th Street, Idaho Falls, ID 83406; tel. 208/529-4567

**Life Care Center of Lewiston,** 325 Warner Drive, Lewiston, ID 83501; tel. 208/798-8500

**Life Care Center of Post Falls,** 460 N Garden Plaza, Post Falls, ID 83854; tel. 208/755-9522

**Life Care Center of Sandpoint,** 1125 North Division Street, Sandpoint, ID 83864; tel. 208/265-9299

**Life Care Center of Treasure Valley,** 502 North Kimball Place, Boise, ID 83704; tel. 208/377-1900

**Life Care Center of Valley View,** 1130 N Allumbaugh Street, Boise, ID 83704; tel. 208/854-8500

## ILLINOIS

**Anna Hospital Corporation,** 517 North Main, Anna, IL 62906; tel. 618/833-4511

**Edward Hines Jr. VA Hospital,** 5000 South 5th Avenue, Hines, IL 60141-5000; tel. 708/202-5652

**James A. Lovell Federal Health Care Center,** 3001 Green Bay Road, North Chicago, IL 60064; tel. 224/610-3700

**Jesse Brown VA Medical Center,** 820 South Damen Avenue, Chicago, IL 60612; tel. 312/569-6101

**MacNeal Hospital,** 3249 South Oak Park Avenue, Berwyn, IL 60402; tel. 708/783-9100

**Mercy Harvard Hospital,** 901 Grant Street, Harvard, IL 60033; tel. 815/943-5431

**Northwestern Lake Forest Hospital,** 660 North Westmoreland Road, Lake Forest, IL 60045; tel. 847/234-5600

**Red Bud Regional Hospital, LLC,** 325 Spring Street, Red Bud, IL 62278; tel. 618/282-3831

**Sherman West Court,** 1950 Larkin Avenue, Elgin, IL 60123; tel. 847/742-7070

**VA Medical Center,** 2401 West Main Street, Marion, IL 62959; tel. 618/997-5311

**VA-Illiana Health Care System,** 1900 East Main Street, Danville, IL 61832; tel. 217/554-3000

**Washington County Hospital,** 705 South Grand Avenue, Nashville, IL 62263; tel. 618/327-8236

## INDIANA

**Gibson General Hospital, Inc.,** 1808 Sherman Drive, Princeton, IN 47670; tel. 812/385-9221

**Green Valley Care Center,** 3118 Green Valley Road, New Albany, IN 47150; tel. 812/945-2341

**Hammond Whiting Care Center,** 1000 114th Street, Whiting, IN 46394; tel. 219/659-2770

**Heritage Healthcare,** 3401 Soldiers Home Road, West Lafayette, IN 47906; tel. 765/463-1541

**Life Care Center of Fort Wayne,** 1649 Spy Run Avenue, Fort Wayne, IN 46805; tel. 260/422-8520

**Life Care Center of LaGrange,** 0770 N 075 E, Lagrange, IN 46761; tel. 260/463-7445

**Life Care Center of Michigan City,** 802 US Highway 20 East, Michigan City, IN 46360; tel. 219/872-7251

**Life Care Center of Rochester,** 827 West 13th Street, Rochester, IN 46975; tel. 574/223-4331

**Life Care Center of Valparaiso,** 3405 Campbell Road, Valparaiso, IN 46385; tel. 219/462-1023

**Life Care Center of Willows,** 1000 Elizabeth Street, Valparaiso, IN 46383; tel. 219/464-4858

**Mitchell Manor,** 24 Teke Burton Drive, Mitchell, IN 47446; tel. 812/849-2221

**Parkview Care Center,** 2819 North Saint Joseph Avenue, Evansville, IN 47712; tel. 812/424-2941

**Rensselaer Care Center,** 1309 East Grace Street, Rensselaer, IN 47978; tel. 219/866-4181

**The Lane House,** 1000 Lane Avenue, Crawfordsville, IN 47933; tel. 765/362-0007

**The Woodlands,** 3820 W Jackson Street, Muncie, IN 47304; tel. 765/289-3451

**VA Northern Indiana Health Care System,** 2121 Lake Avenue, Fort Wayne, IN 46805; tel. 260/460-1310

**Westside Village Nursing Center,** 8616 W. 10th Street, Indianapolis, IN 46234; tel. 317/209-2800

## IOWA

**VA Central Iowa Health Care System,** 3600 30th Street, Des Moines, IA 50310-5774; tel. 515/699-5850

## KANSAS

**Garden Terrace at Overland Park,** 7541 Switzer Road, Overland Park, KS 66214; tel. 913/631-2273

**Life Care Center of Andover,** 621 West 21st Street, Andover, KS 67002; tel. 316/733-1349

**Life Care Center of Burlington,** 601 Cross Street, Burlington, KS 66839; tel. 620/364-2117

**Life Care Center of Kansas City,** 3231 N. 61st Street, Kansas City, KS 66104; tel. 913/299-1770

**Life Care Center of Osawatomie,** 1615 Parker Street - Box 159, Osawatomie, KS 66064; tel. 913/755-4165

**Life Care Center of Seneca,** 512 Community Drive, Seneca, KS 66538; tel. 785/336-3528

**Life Care Center of Wichita,** 622 North Edgemoor, Wichita, KS 67208; tel. 316/686-5100

**Robert J. Dole VA Medical Center,** 5500 East Kellogg, Wichita, KS 67218; tel. 316/651-3601

**VA Eastern Kansas Health Care System,** 2200 SW Gage, Topeka, KS 66622; tel. 785/350-3111

## KENTUCKY

**Appalachian Regional Healthcare,** 260 Hospital Drive, South Williamson, KY 41503; tel. 606/237-1700

Section C

**Bureau of Prisons - FMC Lexington,** 3301 Leestown Road, Lexington, KY 40511-8799; tel. 859/255-6812

**Highlandspring of Ft. Thomas,** 960 Highland Avenue, Fort Thomas, KY 41075; tel. 859/572-0660

**Laurel Creek Health Care Center,** 1033 North Highway 11, Manchester, KY 40962; tel. 606/598-6163

**Life Care Center of Bardstown,** 120 Life Care Way, Bardstown, KY 40004; tel. 502/348-4220

**Life Care Center of LaCenter,** 252 W. 5th Street, La Center, KY 42056; tel. 270/665-5681

**Life Care Center of Morehead,** 933 North Tolliver Road, Morehead, KY 40351; tel. 606/784-7518

**Mountain View Health Care,** 945 West Russell Street, Elkhorn City, KY 41522; tel. 606/754-4134

**Murray-Calloway County Hospital,** 803 Poplar Street, Murray, KY 42071-2432; tel. 270/762-1102

**Parkview Nursing and Rehabilitation Center,** 544 Lone Oak Road, Paducah, KY 42003; tel. 270/443-6543

**Rockcastle Regional Hospital and Respiratory Care Center,** 145 Newcomb Avenue P.O. Box 1310, Mount Vernon, KY 40456; tel. 606/256-2195

**The Medical Center,** 250 Park Street, Bowling Green, KY 42102; tel. 270/745-1000

**VA Medical Center,** 1101 Veterans Drive, Lexington, KY 40502-2236; tel. 859/233-4511

**Villaspring Healthcare Center,** 630 Viox Drive, Erlanger, KY 41018; tel. 859/727-6700

### LOUISIANA

**Lane Regional Medical Center,** 6300 Main Street, Zachary, LA 70791; tel. 225/658-4303

**Trinity Neurologic Rehabilitation Center, LLC,** 1400 Lindberg Drive, Slidell, LA 70458; tel. 985/641-4985

**VA Medical Center,** PO Box 69004, Alexandria, LA 71306; tel. 318/473-0010

### MAINE

**VA Maine Healthcare System,** 1 Va Center, Augusta, ME 04330; tel. 207/623-8411

### MARYLAND

**Levindale Hebrew Geriatric Center and Hospital,** 2434 West Belvedere Avenue, Baltimore, MD 21215; tel. 410/466-8700

**VA Maryland Health Care System,** 10 North Greene Street, Baltimore, MD 21201; tel. 410/605-7000

**Western Maryland Hospital Center,** 1500 Pennsylvania Avenue, Hagerstown, MD 21742-3194; tel. 301/745-4200

### MASSACHUSETTS

**Cedar Hill Health Care Center,** 49 Thomas Patten Drive, Randolph, MA 02368; tel. 781/961-1160

**Chelsea Jewish Nursing Home,** 17 Lafayette Avenue, Chelsea, MA 02150; tel. 617/884-6766

**Deutsches Altenheim Inc.,** 2222 Centre Street, West Roxbury, MA 02132; tel. 617/325-1230

**Edith Nourse Rogers Memorial Veterans Hospital,** 200 Springs Road, Bedford, MA 01730; tel. 781/687-3080

**Federal Bureau of Prisons Federal Medical Center Devens,** PO Box 880, Ayer, MA 01432; tel. 978/796-1443

**Golden Living Center Cohasset,** 1 Chief Justice Cushing Hwy, Cohasset, MA 02025; tel. 781/383-9060

**Golden Living-Oak Hill Rehabilitation and Nursing Center,** 76 North Street, Middleboro, MA 02346; tel. 508/947-4774

**JML Care Center, Inc.,** 184 Ter Heun Drive, Falmouth, MA 02540-2503; tel. 508/457-4621

**Life Care Center of Acton,** One Great Road, Acton, MA 01720; tel. 978/263-9101

**Life Care Center of Auburn,** 14 Masonic Circle, Auburn, MA 01501; tel. 508/832-4800

**Life Care Center of Leominster,** 370 West Street, Leominster, MA 01453; tel. 978/537-0771

**Life Care Center of Nashoba Valley,** 191 Foster Street, Littleton, MA 01460; tel. 978/486-3512

**Life Care Center of Plymouth,** 94 Obery Street, Plymouth, MA 02360; tel. 508/747-9800

**Life Care Center of Raynham,** 546 South Street East, Raynham, MA 02767; tel. 508/821-5700

**Life Care Center of Stoneham,** 25 Woodland Road, Stoneham, MA 02180; tel. 781/662-2545

**Life Care Center of the North Shore,** 111 Birch Street, Lynn, MA 01902; tel. 781/592-9667

**Life Care Center of the South Shore,** 309 Driftway, Scituate, MA 02066; tel. 781/545-1370

**Life Care Center of West Bridgewater,** 765 West Center Street, West Bridgewater, MA 02379; tel. 508/580-4400

**Life Care Center of Wilbraham,** 2399 Boston Road, Wilbraham, MA 01095; tel. 413/596-3111

**Meadow Green Nursing and Rehabilitation Center,** 45 Woburn Street, Waltham, MA 02452; tel. 781/894-9530

**Park Avenue Nursing and Rehabilitation Center,** 146 Park Avenue, Arlington, MA 02476-5896; tel. 781/648-9530

**Seacoast Nursing and Rehabilitation Center,** 292 Washington Street, Gloucester, MA 01930; tel. 978/283-0300

**Sippican Healthcare Center,** 15 Mill Street, Marion, MA 02738; tel. 508/748-3830

**Soldiers' Home in Holyoke,** 110 Cherry Street, Holyoke, MA 01040; tel. 413/532-9475

**Soldiers' Home in Massachusetts,** 91 Crest Ave, Chelsea, MA 02150; tel. 617/884-5660

**The Highlands,** 335 Nichols Road, Fitchburg, MA 01420; tel. 978/343-4411

**The Oaks Nursing Center,** 4525 Acushnet Avenue, New Bedford, MA 02745; tel. 508/998-7807

**VA Boston Healthcare System,** 1400 VFW Parkway, West Roxbury, MA 02132; tel. 617/323-7700

**VA Central Western Massachusetts Healthcare System,** 421 North Main Street, Leeds, MA 01053-9764; tel. 413/584-4040

### MICHIGAN

**Aleda E. Lutz VA Medical Center,** 1500 Weiss Street, Saginaw, MI 48602; tel. 989/497-2500

**Battle Creek VA Medical Center,** 5500 Armstrong Road, Battle Creek, MI 49037; tel. 269/966-5600

**John D. Dingell VA Medical Center,** 4646 John R, Detroit, MI 48201; tel. 313/576-1000

**Life Care Center of Plainwell,** 320 Brigham Street, Plainwell, MI 49080; tel. 269/688-9805

**Oscar G. Johnson VA Medical Center,** 325 East H Street, Iron Mountain, MI 49801; tel. 906/774-3300

**Rivergate Health Care Center,** 14041 Pennsylvania Road, Riverview, MI 48192; tel. 734/284-7200

**Rivergate Terrace,** 14141 Pennsylvania Road, Riverview, MI 48193; tel. 734/284-8000

**Special Tree NeuroCare Center,** 39000 Chase Road, Romulus, MI 48174; tel. 734/893-1044

**VA Ann Arbor Healthcare System,** 2215 Fuller Road, Ann Arbor, MI 48105; tel. 734/769-7100

### MINNESOTA

**Bureau of Prisons - FMC Rochester,** PO Box 4600, Rochester, MN 55903; tel. 507/287-0674

**St. Cloud VA Health Care System,** 4801 Veterans Drive, Saint Cloud, MN 56303; tel. 320/255-6480

**VA Health Care System-Minneapolis,** One Veterans Drive, Minneapolis, MN 55417; tel. 612/725-2000

### MISSISSIPPI

**Mississippi State Hospital,** 3550 Highway 468 West, Whitfield, MS 39193; tel. 601/351-8000

**North Mississippi Medical Center, Inc.,** 830 South Gloster Street, Tupelo, MS 38801; tel. 662/377-3837

**Pontotoc Health Services, Inc.,** 176 S. Main Street, Pontotoc, MS 38863; tel. 662/488-7670

**VA Gulf Coast Veterans Health Care System,** 400 Veterans Avenue, Biloxi, MS 39531; tel. 228/523-5000

**VA Medical Center-G. V. (Sonny) Montgomery,** 1500 East Woodrow Wilson Avenue, Jackson, MS 39216; tel. 601/364-1201

**Webster Health Services, Inc.,** 70 Medical Plaza, Eupora, MS 39744; tel. 662/258-6221

### MISSOURI

**Barnes-Jewish Hospital,** 216 South Kingshighway Boulevard, Mailstop 90-31-640, Saint Louis, MO 63108; tel. 314/747-3000

**Bravo Care of Northbrook, Inc.,** 11701 Borman Drive, Suite 315, Saint Louis, MO 63146; tel. 314/994-9070

**Excelsior Springs City Hospital,** 1700 Rainbow Boulevard, Excelsior Springs, MO 64024; tel. 816/630-6091

**Harry S. Truman Memorial Veterans' Hospital,** 800 Hospital Drive, Columbia, MO 65201; tel. 573/814-6000

**John J. Pershing VA Medical Center,** 1500 North Westwood Boulevard, Poplar Bluff, MO 63901; tel. 573/686-4151

**Life Care Center of Bridgeton,** 12145 Bridge Square Drive, Bridgeton, MO 63044; tel. 314/298-7444

**Life Care Center of Brookfield,** 315 Hunt Street, Brookfield, MO 64628; tel. 660/258-3367

**Life Care Center of Cape Girardeau,** 2852 Independence Street, Cape Girardeau, MO 63703; tel. 573/335-2086

**Life Care Center of Carrollton,** 300 Life Care Lane, Carrollton, MO 64633; tel. 660/542-0155

**Life Care Center of Grandview,** 6301 East 125th Street, Grandview, MO 64030; tel. 816/765-7714

**Life Care Center of Saint Louis,** 3520 Chouteau Avenue, Saint Louis, MO 63129; tel. 314/771-2100

**Life Care Center of Sullivan,** 875 Dunsford Drive, Sullivan, MO 63080; tel. 573/468-3128

**Life Care Center of Waynesville,** 700 Birch Lane, Waynesville, MO 65583; tel. 573/774-6456

**Northwood Hills Care Center LLC,** 800 N. Arthur Street, Humansville, MO 65674; tel. 417/754-2208

**The Westchester House,** 550 White Road, Chesterfield, MO 63017; tel. 314/469-1200

**U.S. Medical Center for Federal Prisoners,** 1900 West Sunshine Street, Springfield, MO 65807; tel. 417/862-7041

**VA Medical Center,** 915 North Grand Boulevard, Saint Louis, MO 63106; tel. 314/289-7020

### MONTANA

**VA Montana Healthcare System,** 3687 Veterans Drive, Fort Harrison, MT 59636-1500; tel. 406/447-7900

### NEBRASKA

**Life Care Center of Elkhorn,** 20275 Hopper Street, Elkhorn, NE 68022; tel. 402/289-2572

**Life Care Center of Omaha,** 6032 Ville De Sante Drive, Omaha, NE 68104; tel. 402/571-6770

**VA Nebraska-Western Iowa Health Care System,** 4101 Woolworth Avenue, Omaha, NE 68105; tel. 402/449-0600

### NEVADA

**CareMeridian-Las Vegas,** 7690 Carmen Boulevard, Las Vegas, NV 89128; tel. 702/255-7399

**Life Care Center of Las Vegas,** 6151 Vegas Drive, Las Vegas, NV 89108; tel. 702/648-4900

**Life Care Center of Paradise Valley,** 2325 East Harmon, Las Vegas, NV 89119; tel. 702/798-7990

**Life Care Center of Reno,** 445 Holcomb Ranch Lane, Reno, NV 89511; tel. 775/851-0123

**VA Sierra Nevada Health Care System,** 975 Kirman Avenue, Reno, NV 89502-2597; tel. 775/786-7200

### NEW HAMPSHIRE

**VA Medical Center,** 718 Smyth Road, Manchester, NH 03104-4098; tel. 603/624-4366

### NEW JERSEY

**Bergen Regional Medical Center,** 230 East Ridgewood Avenue, Paramus, NJ 07652; tel. 201/967-4000

**Camden County Health Services Center,** 425 Woodbury Turnersville Road, Blackwood, NJ 08012; tel. 856/374-6500

**Gateway Care Center, LLC,** 139 Grant Avenue, Eatontown, NJ 07724; tel. 732/542-4700

**Robert Wood Johnson University Hospital at Rahway,** 865 Stone Street, Rahway, NJ 07065; tel. 732/499-6050

**St. Lawrence Rehabilitation Center,** 2381 Lawrenceville Road, Lawrenceville, NJ 08648; tel. 609/896-9500

**VA New Jersey Health Care System,** 385 Tremont Avenue, Director's Office (00), East Orange, NJ 07018; tel. 973/676-1000

### NEW MEXICO

**Deming Hospital Corporation,** 900 W Ash Street, Deming, NM 88030; tel. 575/546-5800

**Life Care Center of Farmington,** 1101 West Murray Drive, Farmington, NM 87401; tel. 505/326-1600

**New Mexico Behavioral Health Institute at Las Vegas,** 3695 Hot Springs Boulevard, Las Vegas, NM 87701; tel. 505/454-2404

**New Mexico VA Health Care System,** 1501 San Pedro Drive SE, Albuquerque, NM 87108; tel. 505/265-1711

### NEW YORK

**Casa Promesa, Residential Health Care Facility, Inc.,** 308 East 175th Street, Bronx, NY 10457; tel. 718/960-7600

**Coler-Goldwater Specialty Hospital and Nursing Facility-Coler Campus,** 900 Main Street, New York, NY 10044-0052; tel. 212/848-6318

**Coler-Goldwater Specialty Hospital and Nursing Facility-Goldwater Campus,** 1 Main Street, New York, NY 10044; tel. 212/318-4361

**Dr. Susan Smith McKinney Nursing/Rehabilitation Center,** 594 Albany Avenue, Brooklyn, NY 11203; tel. 718/245-7170

**Gouverneur Skilled Nursing Facility,** 227 Madison Street, New York, NY 10002; tel. 212/238-7800

**Helen Hayes Hospital,** 51-55 Route 9, West, West Haverstraw, NY 10993; tel. 845/786-4000

**James J Peters Bronx VA Medical Center,** 130 West Kingsbridge Road, Bronx, NY 10468; tel. 718/584–9000

**Long Beach Medical Center,** 455 East Bay Drive, Long Beach, NY 11561; tel. 516/897–1208

**Orleans Community Health,** 200 Ohio Street, Medina, NY 14103; tel. 585/798–2000

**Providence Rest,** 3304 Waterbury Avenue, Bronx, NY 10465; tel. 718/931–3000

**Samuel S. Stratton VA Medical Center,** 113 Holland Avenue, Albany, NY 12208; tel. 518/626–5000

**Sea View Hospital Rehabilitation Center and Home,** 460 Brielle Avenue, Staten Island, NY 10314; tel. 718/317–3000

**Upstate New York VA Health Care Network at Canandaigua,** 400 Fort Hill Avenue, Canandaigua, NY 14424; tel. 585/394–2000

**VA Healthcare Network Upstate New York at Bath,** 76 Veterans Avenue, Bath, NY 14810; tel. 607/664–4722

**VA Healthcare Network Upstate New York at Syracuse,** 800 Irving Avenue, Syracuse, NY 13210; tel. 315/425–4400

**VA Hudson Valley Health Care System,** 2094 Albany Post Road, Route 9A, Montrose, NY 10548; tel. 914/737–4400

**VA Medical Center Northport,** 79 Middleville Road, Northport, NY 11768; tel. 631/261–4400

**VA New York Harbor Health Care System,** 800 Poly Place, Brooklyn, NY 11209; tel. 718/630–3521

**VA Western New York Health Care System,** 3495 Bailey Avenue, Buffalo, NY 14215; tel. 716/862–8529

**NORTH CAROLINA**

**Carolinas Medical Center - Union,** 600 Hospital Drive, Monroe, NC 28112; tel. 704/283–3100

**Charles George VA Medical Center at Asheville,** 1100 Tunnel Road, Asheville, NC 28805; tel. 828/298–7911

**Life Care Center of Banner Elk,** 185 Norwood Hollow Road, Banner Elk, NC 28604; tel. 828/898–5136

**Life Care Center of Hendersonville,** 400 Thompson Street, Hendersonville, NC 28792; tel. 828/697–4348

**Person Memorial Hospital,** 615 Ridge Road, Roxboro, NC 27573; tel. 336/599–2121

**Sampson Regional Medical Center,** 607 Beaman Street, Clinton, NC 28329; tel. 910/592–8511

**Southeastern Regional Medical Center,** 300 West 27th Street, Lumberton, NC 28358; tel. 910/671–5860

**United Veteran Services of North Carolina,** 214 Cochran Avenue, Fayetteville, NC 28301; tel. 910/482–4131

**VA Medical Center,** 2300 Ramsey Street, Fayetteville, NC 28301; tel. 910/822–7091

**VA Medical Center,** 508 Fulton Street, Durham, NC 27705; tel. 919/286–0411

**W. G. (Bill) Hefner VA Medical Center,** 1601 Brenner Avenue, Salisbury, NC 28144; tel. 704/638–9000

**NORTH DAKOTA**

**Fargo VA Health Care System,** 2101 Elm Street North, Fargo, ND 58102; tel. 701/239–3241

**OHIO**

**DaySpring of Miami Valley Health Care Center and Rehabilitation,** 8001 Dayton-Springfield Road, Fairborn, OH 45324; tel. 937/864–5800

**Department of Veterans Affairs Medical Center, Dayton, Ohio,** 4100 West 3rd Street, Dayton, OH 45428; tel. 937/268–6511

**Eastgatespring Health Care Center and Rehabilitation,** 4400 Gleneste Withamsville Rd, Cincinnati, OH 45245; tel. 513/752–3710

**Franciscan Care Center of Sylvania,** 4111 North Holland Sylvania Road, Toledo, OH 43623; tel. 419/882–6582

**Heritagespring Health Care and Rehabilitation Center,** 7235 Heritagespring Drive, West Chester, OH 45069; tel. 513/759–5777

**Hillspring Healthcare & Rehabilitation Center,** 325 East Central Avenue Route 73, Springboro, OH 45066; tel. 937/748–1100

**Lakewood Hospital Association,** 14519 Detroit Avenue, Lakewood, OH 44107; tel. 216/521–4200

**Life Care Center of Elyria,** 1212 South Abbe Road, Elyria, OH 44035; tel. 440/365–5200

**Life Care Center of Medina,** 2400 Columbia Road, Medina, OH 44256; tel. 330/483–3131

**Life Care Center of Westlake,** 26520 Center Ridge Road, Westlake, OH 44145; tel. 440/871–3030

**Louis Stokes, Cleveland VA Medical Center,** 10701 East Boulevard, Cleveland, OH 44106; tel. 216/231–3456

**Mayfair Village Nursing Care Center,** 3000 Bethel Road, Columbus, OH 43220; tel. 614/889–6320

**Parma Community General Hospital,** 7007 Powers Boulevard, Parma, OH 44129; tel. 440/743–3000

**Providence Care Center,** 2025 Hayes Avenue, Sandusky, OH 44870; tel. 419/627–2273

**Rosary Care Center,** 6832 Convent Boulevard, Sylvania, OH 43560; tel. 419/824–3600

**Shawneespring Health Care and Rehabilitation Center,** 10111 Simonson Road, Harrison, OH 45030; tel. 513/367–7780

**St. Leonard Health Care Center,** 8100 Clyo Road, Centerville, OH 45458; tel. 937/433–0480

**The Ohio Eastern Star Health Care Center,** 1451 Gambier Road, Mount Vernon, OH 43050; tel. 740/397–1706

**VA Healthcare System of Ohio-Cincinnati Campus,** 3200 Vine Street, Cincinnati, OH 45220; tel. 513/861–3100

**VA Medical Center-Chillicothe,** 17273 State Route 104, Chillicothe, OH 45601; tel. 740/773–1141

**OKLAHOMA**

**Department of Veterans Affairs Medical Center,** 921 Northeast 13th Street, Oklahoma City, OK 73104; tel. 405/456–3312

**OREGON**

**Life Care Center of Coos Bay,** 2890 Ocean Boulevard, Coos Bay, OR 97420; tel. 541/267–5433

**Life Care Center of McMinnville,** 1309 East 27th Street, McMinnville, OR 97128; tel. 503/472–4678

**Life Care Center Valley West Health Care Center,** 2300 Warren Street, Eugene, OR 97405; tel. 541/686–2828

**Portland VA Medical Center,** 3710 SW US Veterans Hospital Road, Portland, OR 97239; tel. 503/273–5267

**VA Roseburg Health Care System,** 913 NW Garden Valley Boulevard, Roseburg, OR 97471; tel. 541/440–1000

**PENNSYLVANIA**

**Albert Einstein Medical Center,** 5501 Old York Road, Philadelphia, PA 19141; tel. 215/456–7890

**Barclay Friends,** 700 North Franklin Street, West Chester, PA 19380; tel. 610/696–5211

**Berwick Hospital Center,** 701 East 16th Street, Berwick, PA 18603; tel. 570/759–5000

**Erie VA Medical Center,** 135 East 38th Street, Erie, PA 16504; tel. 814/868–8661

**Fellowship Community,** 3000 Fellowship Drive, Whitehall, PA 18052; tel. 610/799–3000

**Gnaden Huetten Memorial Hospital,** 211 North 12th Street, Lehighton, PA 18235-1195; tel. 610/377–1300

**Good Shepherd Rehabilitation Hospital,** 850 S. Fifth Street, Allentown, PA 18103-3295; tel. 610/776–3133

**Hickory House Nursing Home,** 3120 Horseshoe Pike, Honey Brook, PA 19344; tel. 610/273–2915

**Lebanon VA Medical Center,** 1700 South Lincoln Avenue, Lebanon, PA 17042; tel. 717/272–6621

**Philadelphia VA Medical Center,** University and Woodland Avenues, Philadelphia, PA 19104; tel. 215/823–5857

**St. Luke's Hospital Miners Campus,** 360 West Ruddle Street, Coaldale, PA 18218-0067; tel. 570/645–8229

**VA Butler Healthcare,** 325 New Castle Road, Butler, PA 16001-2480; tel. 724/287–4781

**VA Medical Center,** 1400 Black Horse Hill Road, Coatesville, PA 19320-2097; tel. 610/384–7711

**VA Medical Center Wilkes-Barre,** 1111 East End Boulevard, Wilkes Barre, PA 18711; tel. 570/821–7204

**VA Medical Center-James E. Van Zandt,** 2907 Pleasant Valley Boulevard, Altoona, PA 16602-4377; tel. 814/943–8164

**VA Pittsburgh Health Care System,** University Drive, Pittsburgh, PA 15240; tel. 412/360–1858

**RHODE ISLAND**

**Cherry Hill Manor,** 2 Cherry Hill Road, Johnston, RI 02919; tel. 401/231–3102

**Evergreen House Health Center,** One Evergreen Drive, East Providence, RI 02914; tel. 401/438–3250

**Roger Williams Medical Center,** 825 Chalkstone Avenue, Providence, RI 02908; tel. 401/456–2043

**SOUTH CAROLINA**

**Life Care Center of Charleston,** 2600 Elms Plantation Boulevard, North Charleston, SC 29406; tel. 843/764–3500

**Life Care Center of Columbia,** 2514 Faraway Drive, Columbia, SC 29223; tel. 803/865–1999

**Life Care Center of Hilton Head,** 120 Lamotte Drive, Hilton Head Island, SC 29926; tel. 843/681–6006

**Marion Regional Hospital,** 1115 N. Main Street, Marion, SC 29571; tel. 843/431–2000

**Pepper Hill Nursing and Rehabilitation Center,** 3525 Augustus Road, Aiken, SC 29802-3188; tel. 803/642–8376

**Ralph H. Johnson VA Medical Center,** 109 Bee Street, Charleston, SC 29401-5799; tel. 843/577–5011

**William Jennings Bryan Dorn VA Medical Center,** 6439 Garners Ferry Road, Columbia, SC 29209; tel. 803/776–4000

**SOUTH DAKOTA**

**Sioux Falls VA Health Care System,** PO Box 5046, Sioux Falls, SD 57117; tel. 605/336–3230

**VA Black Hills Health Care System-Fort Meade-Hot Springs, SD,** 113 Comanche Road, Fort Meade, SD 57741; tel. 605/720–7170

**TENNESSEE**

**Hardin Medical Center,** 935 Wayne Road, Savannah, TN 38372; tel. 731/926–8121

**Hickman Community Health Care Services,** 135 East Swan Street, Centerville, TN 37033; tel. 931/729–4271

**Life Care Center of Athens,** 1234 Frye Street, Athens, TN 37371; tel. 423/754–8181

**Life Care Center of Centerville,** 112 Old Dickson Road, Centerville, TN 37033; tel. 931/729–4236

**Life Care Center of Cleveland,** 3530 Keith Street NW, Cleveland, TN 37312; tel. 423/476–3254

**Life Care Center of Collegedale,** 9210 Apison Pike, Collegedale, TN 37363; tel. 423/396–2182

**Life Care Center of Columbia,** 841 W. James Campbell Boulevard, Columbia, TN 38401; tel. 931/388–5035

**Life Care Center of Copper Basin,** 166 Industrial Drive, Ducktown, TN 37326; tel. 423/496–3245

**Life Care Center of East Ridge,** 1500 Fincher Avenue, East Ridge, TN 37412; tel. 423/894–1254

**Life Care Center of Elizabethton,** 1641 Hwy 19E Bypass, Elizabethton, TN 37643; tel. 423/542–4133

**Life Care Center of Gray,** 791 Old Gray Station Road, Gray, TN 37615; tel. 423/477–7146

**Life Care Center of Greeneville,** 725 Crum Street, Greeneville, TN 37743; tel. 423/639–8131

**Life Care Center of Jefferson City,** 336 W Old Andrew Johnson Hwy, Jefferson City, TN 37760; tel. 865/475–6097

**Life Care Center of Morgan County,** 419 South Kingston Street, Wartburg, TN 37887; tel. 423/346–6691

**Life Care Center of Morristown,** 501 West Economy Road, Morristown, TN 37814; tel. 423/581–5435

**Life Care Center of Red Bank,** 1020 Runyan Drive, Chattanooga, TN 37405; tel. 423/473–5553

**Life Care Center of Sparta,** 508 Mose Drive, Sparta, TN 38583; tel. 931/738–9430

**Life Care Center of Tullahoma,** 1715 No. Jackson Street, Tullahoma, TN 37388; tel. 931/455–8557

**Lynchburg Nursing Center,** 40 Nursing Home Road, Lynchburg, TN 37352; tel. 931/759–6000

**Milford Medical Investors, LP,** 105 Rowland Avenue, Bruceton, TN 38317; tel. 731/586–2061

**Ridgeview Terrace of Life Care,** Route 2 Coffey Lane, Rutledge, TN 37861; tel. 865/828–5295

**The Heritage Center,** 1026 McFarland Street, Morristown, TN 37814; tel. 423/581–5100

**VA Medical Center-James H. Quillen,** PO Box 4000, Mountain Home, TN 37684; tel. 423/926–1171

**VA Tennessee Valley Health Care System,** 1310 24th Avenue South, Nashville, TN 37212-2637; tel. 615/327–4751

**TEXAS**

**Alameda Oaks Nursing Center,** 1101 South Alameda, Corpus Christi, TX 78404; tel. 361/882–2711

**Amarillo VA Health Care System,** 6010 Amarillo Boulevard, West, Amarillo, TX 79106; tel. 806/355–9703

**Central Texas Veterans Health Care System,** 1901 Veterans Memorial Drive, Temple, TX 76504; tel. 254/743–2306

**Garden Terrace Alzheimer's Center of Excellence,** 7500 Oakmont Boulevard, Fort Worth, TX 76132; tel. 817/346–8080

**Garden Terrace Alzheimer's Center of Excellence,** 7887 Cambridge Street, Houston, TX 77054; tel. 713/796–2777

**Life Care Center of Haltom,** 2936 Markum Drive, Haltom City, TX 76117; tel. 817/831–0545

**Life Care Center of Plano,** 3800 West Park Boulevard, Plano, TX 75075; tel. 972/612–1700

Section C

**Michael E. DeBakey VA Medical Center,** 2002 Holcombe Boulevard, Houston, TX 77030; tel. 713/794–7100

**North Texas VA Health Care System,** 4500 South Lancaster Road, Dallas, TX 75216; tel. 202/329–8673

**Renaissance Park Multi-Care Center,** 4252 Bryant Irvin Road, Fort Worth, TX 76109; tel. 817/738–2975

**South Texas Veterans Health Care System,** 7400 Merton Minter Boulevard, San Antonio, TX 78229-4404; tel. 210/617–5205

**The Vosswood Nursing Center,** 815 South Voss Road, Houston, TX 77057; tel. 713/827–0883

**West Texas VA Health Care System,** 300 Veterans Boulevard, Big Spring, TX 79720; tel. 432/263–7361

**Wooldridge Place Nursing Center,** 7352 Wooldridge Road, Corpus Christi, TX 78414; tel. 361/991–9633

**UTAH**

**Garden Terrace Alzheimer's Center of Excellence,** 1201 East 4500 South, Salt Lake City, UT 84117; tel. 801/261–3664

**Life Care Center of Bountiful,** 460 West 2600 South, Bountiful, UT 84010; tel. 801/295–3135

**VIRGINIA**

**Life Care Center of New Market,** 315 East Lee Highway, New Market, VA 22844; tel. 540/740–8041

**Salem VA Medical Center,** 1970 Roanoke Boulevard, Salem, VA 24153; tel. 540/982–2463

**Southampton Memorial Hospital,** 100 Fairview Drive, Franklin, VA 23851; tel. 757/569–6100

**VA Medical Center-Hampton,** 100 Emancipation Drive, Hampton, VA 23667; tel. 757/722–9961

**VA Medical Center-Hunter Holmes McGuire,** 1201 Broad Rock Boulevard, Richmond, VA 23249; tel. 804/675–5756

**WASHINGTON**

**Alderwood Manor,** 3600 East Hartson Avenue, Spokane, WA 99202; tel. 509/535–2071

**Cascade Park Care Center,** 801 SE Park Crest Avenue, Vancouver, WA 98683; tel. 360/260–2200

**Cottesmore of Life Care,** 2909 14th Avenue NW, Gig Harbor, WA 98335; tel. 253/851–5433

**Garden Terrace Alzheimers Center of Excellence,** 491 S 338th Street, Federal Way, WA 98003; tel. 253/661–2226

**Hallmark Manor,** 32300 1st Avenue South, Federal Way, WA 98003; tel. 253/874–3580

**Life Care Center of Federal Way,** 1045 S. 308th Street, Federal Way, WA 98003; tel. 253/946–2273

**Life Care Center of Kennewick,** 1508 W. Seventh Avenue, Kennewick, WA 99336; tel. 509/586–9185

**Life Care Center of Kirkland,** 10101 Northeast 120th Street, Kirkland, WA 98034; tel. 425/823–2323

**Life Care Center of Mount Vernon,** 2120 East Division Street, Mount Vernon, WA 98274; tel. 360/424–4258

**Life Care Center of Port Orchard,** 2031 Pottery Avenue, Port Orchard, WA 98366; tel. 360/876–8035

**Life Care Center of Port Townsend,** 751 Kearney Street, Port Townsend, WA 98368; tel. 360/385–3555

**Life Care Center of Puyallup,** 511 10th Avenue SE, Puyallup, WA 98372; tel. 253/845–7566

**Life Care Center of Richland,** 44 Goethals Drive, Richland, WA 99352; tel. 509/943–1117

**Life Care Center of San Juan Island,** 660 Spring Street, Friday Harbor, WA 98250; tel. 360/378–2117

**Life Care Center of Skagit Valley,** 1462 West SR 20, Sedro Woolley, WA 98284; tel. 360/856–6867

**Life Care Center of West Seattle,** 4700 SW Admiral Way, Seattle, WA 98116; tel. 206/935–2480

**Marysville Care Center,** 1821 Grove Street, Marysville, WA 98270; tel. 360/659–3926

**Ritzville Medical Investors, Inc.,** 506 South Jackson Street, Ritzville, WA 99169; tel. 509/659–1600

**VA Medical Center,** North 4815 Assembly Street, Spokane, WA 99205; tel. 509/434–7000

**VA Puget Sound Health Care System,** 1660 South Columbian Way (S-002-QI), Seattle, WA 98108-1597; tel. 206/764–2731

**WEST VIRGINIA**

**VA Medical Center,** 200 Veterans Avenue, Beckley, WV 25801; tel. 304/255–2121

**VA Medical Center,** 510 Butler Avenue, Martinsburg, WV 25405; tel. 304/263–0811

**VA Medical Center-Louis A. Johnson,** 1 Medical Center Drive, Clarksburg, WV 26301; tel. 304/623–3461

**WISCONSIN**

**Clement J. Zablocki VA Medical Center,** 5000 West National Avenue, Milwaukee, WI 53295-1000; tel. 414/384–2000

**Divine Savior Healthcare, Inc.,** 2817 New Pinery Road, Portage, WI 53901; tel. 608/742–4131

**VA Medical Center-Great Lakes Health Care System,** 500 East Veterans Street, Tomah, WI 54660; tel. 608/372–1777

**WYOMING**

**Life Care Center of Casper,** 4041 South Poplar Street, Casper, WY 82601; tel. 307/266–0000

**Life Care Center of Cheyenne,** 1330 Prairie Avenue, Cheyenne, WY 82009; tel. 307/778–8997

**Sheridan VA Medical Center,** 1898 Fort Road, Sheridan, WY 82801; tel. 307/675–3530

**St. John's Medical Center,** 625 E. Broadway, Jackson, WY 83001; tel. 307/733–3636

**VA Medical Center,** 2360 East Pershing Boulevard, Cheyenne, WY 82001; tel. 307/778–7550

**Westview Health Care Center,** 1990 West Loucks, Sheridan, WY 82801; tel. 307/672–9789

# U.S. Associated Areas

**PUERTO RICO**

**VA Caribbean Healthcare System,** 10 Casia Street, San Juan, PR 00921-3201; tel. 787/641–7582

# Joint Commission Accredited Freestanding Behavioral Health Care Organizations

*The accredited freestanding mental health care organizations listed have been accredited as of April, 2012 by The Joint Commission by decision of the Accreditation Committee of the Board of Commissioners.*

*The organizations listed here have been found to be in compliance with the Joint Commissions standards for Accreditation Manual for Mental Health, Chemical Dependency, and Mental Retardation/Development Disabilities Services.*

*Please refer to section A of the AHA Guide for information on hospitals with inpatient and/or outpatient services. These hospitals are identified by Facility Codes F99, F100, F101, F102, F103, F104, F105, F106. In section A, those hospitals identified by Approval Code 1 are Joint Commission accredited.*

*We present this list simply as a convenient directory. Inclusion or omission of any organization's name indicates neither approval nor disapproval by Health Forum LLC, an American Hospital Association company.*

## United States

### ALABAMA

*A Center for Eating Disorders, P.O. Box 55901, Birmingham, AL 35255; tel. 205/933–0041

Alabama Clinical Schools, Inc., P.O. Box 100968, Birmingham, AL 35210; tel. 205/836–9923

AltaPointe Health Systems, Inc., 5750-A Southland Drive, Mobile, AL 36693; tel. 251/450–5901

*Birmingham Health Care, P.O. Box 11523, Birmingham, AL 35202; tel. 205/212–5600

*Bradford Health Services-Huntsville Lodge, 1600 Browns Ferry Road, Madison, AL 35758; tel. 256/461–7272

*Bradford Health Services-Warrior, PO Box 129, Warrior, AL 35180; tel. 205/647–1945

*Brookwood Medical Center, 2010 Brookwood Medical Center Drive, Birmingham, AL 35209; tel. 205/877–1000

*Central Alabama Veterans Health Care System, 215 Perry Hill Road, Montgomery, AL 36109; tel. 334/272–4670

*Fox Army Health Center US Army Medical Department Activity, 4100 Goss Road, Huntsville, AL 35809-7000; tel. 256/955–8888

*Franklin Primary Health Center, Inc., 1303 Dr. Martin Luther King Jr. Avenue, Mobile, AL 36603; tel. 251/434–8188

Glenwood, Inc., 150 Glenwood Lane, Birmingham, AL 35242; tel. 205/969–2880

Hill Crest Behavioral Health Services, 6869 Fifth Avenue South, Birmingham, AL 35212; tel. 205/833–9000

Laurel Oaks Behavioral Health Center, 700 East Cottonwood Road, Dothan, AL 36301; tel. 334/794–7373

*Lyster Army Health Clinic, 301 Andrews Avenue, Fort Rucker, AL 36362-5333; tel. 334/255–7609

Magnolia Creek Treatment Center for Eating Disorders, 645 Crenshaw Road, Columbiana, AL 35051; tel. 205/678–4373

Mountain View Hospital, PO Box 8406, Gadsden, AL 35902-8406; tel. 256/546–9265

Pathway, Inc., P.O. Box 311206, Enterprise, AL 36331; tel. 334/894–5591

*The University of Alabama Hospital at Birmingham, 1802 6th Avenue South, Birmingham, AL 35294; tel. 205/934–4444

*Tuscaloosa VA Medical Center, 3701 Loop Road East, Tuscaloosa, AL 35404; tel. 205/554–2000

*VA Medical Center, 700 19th Street South, Birmingham, AL 35233; tel. 205/933–8101

### ALASKA

Alaska Children's Services Inc., 4600 Abbott Road, Anchorage, AK 99507-4314; tel. 907/346–2101

*Alaska VA Healthcare System and Regional Office, 1201 N. Muldoon Road, Anchorage, AK 99504; tel. 907/257–5400

Boys and Girls Home of Alaska, Inc., 3101 Lathrop Street, Fairbanks, AK 99701; tel. 907/459–4700

*Bristol Bay Area Health Corporation, PO Box 130, Dillingham, AK 99576; tel. 907/842–5201

North Star Behavioral Health, 2530 DeBarr Road, Anchorage, AK 99508-2948; tel. 907/258–7575

Providence Adolescent Residential Treatment Program, 3400 East 20th, Anchorage, AK 99508; tel. 907/272–2148

*Yukon Kuskokwim Delta Regional Hospital, PO Box 287, Bethel, AK 99559; tel. 907/543–6300

### ARIZONA

A New Leaf, Inc., 868 East University Drive, Mesa, AZ 85203; tel. 480/969–4024

ANASAZI Foundation, 1424 S. Stapley Drive, Mesa, AZ 85204; tel. 480/892–7403

*Aurora Behavioral Health System, 6015 W Peoria Ave, Glendale, AZ 85302; tel. 623/344–4400

*Chandler Valley Hope, PO Box 1839, Chandler, AZ 85244-1839; tel. 602/899–3335

*Community Counseling Centers, Inc., 105 North Fifth Avenue, Holbrook, AZ 86025; tel. 928/524–6701

Crisis Response Network of Southern Arizona, 2802 E. District Street, Tucson, AZ 85714; tel. 602/427–4600

*Desert Visions Youth Wellness Center, PO Box 458, Sacaton, AZ 85247; tel. 520/562–4205

Devereux/Arizona-Richard L. Raskin Treatment Network, 11000 N Scottsdale Rd, Ste 260, Scottsdale, AZ 85254; tel. 480/998–2920

*Helping Associates, Inc., 1901 North Trekell Road, Ste A, Casa Grande, AZ 85122; tel. 520/836–1029

*Horizon Human Services, Inc., 210 East Cottonwood Lane, Casa Grande, AZ 85122; tel. 520/836–1688

*Little Colorado Behavioral Health Centers, Post Office Box 579, Saint Johns, AZ 85936; tel. 928/337–4301

*Main Street Diagnostics, LLC, 636 N. Main Street, Cottonwood, AZ 86326; tel. 928/639–4440

Mingus Mountain Estate Residential Center, Inc., PO Box 26485, Prescott Valley, AZ 86312; tel. 602/335–2000

*Mohave Mental Health Clinic, Inc., 1743 Sycamore Avenue, Kingman, AZ 86409; tel. 928/757–8111

Northern Arizona VA Health Care System, 500 Highway 89 North, Prescott, AZ 86313; tel. 928/445–4860

Parc Place, 2190 North Grace Boulevard, Chandler, AZ 85225; tel. 480/917–9301

*Phoenix VA Health Care System, 650 East Indian School Road, Phoenix, AZ 85012-1892; tel. 602/277–5551

*Pinal Hispanic Council, 712 North Main Street, Eloy, AZ 85131; tel. 520/466–7765

*Raymond W. Bliss Army Health Center, 2240 E. Winrow Avenue, Fort Huachuca, AZ 85613-7079; tel. 520/533–9026

Recovery Innovations, Inc., 2701 N. 16th Street, Suite 316, Phoenix, AZ 85006; tel. 602/650–1212

Remuda Ranch, One East Apache Street, Wickenburg, AZ 85390; tel. 928/684–3913

Rosewood Ranch L.P., 36075 South Rincon Road, Wickenburg, AZ 85390; tel. 928/684–9594

*Sierra Tucson, Inc., 39580 S. Lago del Oro Parkway, Tucson, AZ 85739; tel. 520/624–4000

Southern Arizona Mental Health Corporation, 2502 North Dodge Boulevard, Suite 190, Tucson, AZ 85716; tel. 520/617–0043

*Southern Arizona VA Health Care System, 3601 South Sixth Avenue, Tucson, AZ 85723; tel. 520/629–1821

*St. Luke's Behavioral Hospital, LP, 1800 East Van Buren, Phoenix, AZ 85006; tel. 602/251–8808

*The Guidance Center, Inc., 2187 North Vickey Street, Flagstaff, AZ 86004; tel. 928/527–1899

The Meadows of Wickenburg, Inc., 1655 North Tegner, Wickenburg, AZ 85390; tel. 928/684–3926

The New Foundation, 1200 North 77th Street, Scottsdale, AZ 85257; tel. 480/945–3302

*The River Sources Treatment, 950 N. Arizola Road Suite 3, Casa Grande, AZ 85122; tel. 520/381–2531

*The Sundance Center, 12816 E. Turquoise Avenue, Scottsdale, AZ 85259; tel. 480/773–7329

Touchstone Behavioral Health, 15648 N. 35th Ave, Phoenix, AZ 85053; tel. 623/930–8705

UBH of Phoenix LLC, 3550 East Pinchot, Phoenix, AZ 85018; tel. 940/320–8994

Urgent Psychiatric Center, 903 North 2nd Street, Phoenix, AZ 85004-1906; tel. 602/416–7600

*Verde Valley Guidance Clinic, Inc., 8 East Cottonwood Street, Cottonwood, AZ 86326; tel. 928/634–2236

*West Yavapai Guidance Clinic, 505 South Cortez Street, Prescott, AZ 86303; tel. 928/445–5211

Youth Development Institute, 1830 East Roosevelt Street, Phoenix, AZ 85006; tel. 602/256–5300

### ARKANSAS

Amicare of Arkansas, 4253 Crossover Road, Fayetteville, AR 72703; tel. 479/587–1408

Arkansas State Hospital, 305 South Palm Street, Little Rock, AR 72205; tel. 501/686–9000

BHC Pinnacle Pointe Hospital, Inc., 11501 Financial Centre Parkway, Little Rock, AR 72211; tel. 501/223–3322

*Central Arkansas Veterans Healthcare System, 4300 West Seventh Street (00/LR), Little Rock, AR 72205; tel. 501/257–5314

Community Counseling Services, Inc., 125 Dons Way, Hot Springs National Park, AR 71913; tel. 501/624–7111

Cornerstone Community Counseling Corporation, 106 East Third Street, Imboden, AR 72434; tel. 870/869–1500

Counseling and Education Center, Inc., 406 Pecan Street, Helena, AR 72342; tel. 870/338–8447

Delta Counseling Associates, Inc., 790 Roberts Drive, Monticello, AR 71655; tel. 870/367–9732

Delta Family Health and Fitness Center for Children, Inc., 815 East Street Louis Street, Hamburg, AR 71646; tel. 870/853–4224

Families, Inc. of Arkansas, 1815 Pleasant Grove Road, Jonesboro, AR 72401; tel. 870/933–6886

Habilitation Centers, Inc., PO Box 727, Fordyce, AR 71742; tel. 870/352–8203

Hometown Behavioral Health Services of Arkansas, Inc., PO Box 299, Hoxie, AR 72433; tel. 870/886–1333

Hope Behavioral Health Care, P.O. Box 176, Cherokee Village, AR 72525; tel. 870/257–3336

Inspiration Day Treatment, Inc., 1014 Autumn Road Suite 4, Little Rock, AR 72211; tel. 501/221–1941

*Life Strategies Counseling, Inc., 1217 Stone Street, Jonesboro, AR 72401; tel. 870/972–1268

Life Strategies of Arkansas, LLC, 703 Calvin Avery, West Memphis, AR 72301; tel. 870/732–1878

Living Hope Southeast, LLC, 100 South University, Suite 401, Little Rock, AR 72205; tel. 501/663–5473

Maxus, Inc., 1033 Old Burr Road, Warm Springs, AR 72478; tel. 870/647–1400

NeuroRestorative Timber Ridge, PO Box 208, Benton, AR 72018; tel. 501/594–5211

---

*Indicates organization is a Joint Commission accredited Chemical Dependency organization.

Section C

*Ozark Guidance Center, Inc., PO Box 6430, Springdale, AR 72766-6430; tel. 479/750-2020

Rivendell Behavioral Health Services of Arkansas, 100 Rivendell Drive, Benton, AR 72019; tel. 501/316-1255

Texarkana Behavioral Associates, L.C., 10301 Mayo Drive, Barling, AR 72923; tel. 479/494-5700

Texarkana Behavioral Associates, L.C., 4253 Crossover Road, Fayetteville, AR 72703; tel. 479/521-5731

*The BridgeWay, Inc., 21 BridgeWay Road, North Little Rock, AR 72113; tel. 501/771-1500

The Centers for Youth and Families, P.O. Box 251970, Little Rock, AR 72225-1970; tel. 501/666-8686

The Logan Centers, Inc., 70 CR 7010, Wynne, AR 72396; tel. 870/494-4600

Trinity Behavioral Health Care System, Inc., 1033 Old Burr Road, Warm Springs, AR 72478; tel. 870/647-1400

United Methodist Behavioral Hospital, 1601 Murphy Drive, Maumelle, AR 72113; tel. 501/803-3388

*United Methodist Children's Home, Inc., PO Box 56050, Little Rock, AR 72215; tel. 501/661-0720

*University of Arkansas for Medical Sciences, 4301 W. Markham, Little Rock, AR 72205; tel. 501/526-8100

*Veterans Health Care System of the Ozarks, 1100 North College Avenue, Fayetteville, AR 72703; tel. 479/444-5000

Woodridge Behavioral Care, 603 Kittle Road, Forrest City, AR 72335; tel. 870/633-3200

Youth Home, Inc., 20400 Colonel Glenn Road, Little Rock, AR 72210-5323; tel. 501/821-5500

CALIFORNIA

*Action Family Counseling, Inc., 26893 Bouquet Canyon Road, Suite C-134, Santa Clarita, CA 91350; tel. 661/297-6644

*Adolescent Growth, Inc., 6323 Zindell Avenue, Commerce, CA 90040; tel. 323/948-9998

Alameda County Medical Center, 1411 E. 31 Street, Oakland, CA 94602; tel. 510/437-4943

AltaMed Health Services Corporation, 500 Citadel Drive Suite 490, Los Angeles, CA 90040; tel. 323/889-7307

*Alvarado Parkway Institute Behavioral Health System, 7050 Parkway Drive, La Mesa, CA 91942; tel. 619/465-4411

*Associates in Counseling and Mediation, 265 S. Anita Drive - Suite 117, Orange, CA 92868; tel. 714/978-1090

*Aurora Behavioral Health Care/ San Diego, 11878 Avenue of Industry, San Diego, CA 92128; tel. 858/487-3200

*Aurora Behavioral Health Care/Las Encinas Hospital, 2900 East Del Mar Boulevard, Pasadena, CA 91107; tel. 626/795-9901

*Aurora Charter Oak-Los Angeles, L.L.C., 1161 East Covina Boulevard, Covina, CA 91724; tel. 626/966-1632

Berkeley Addiction Treatment Services, Inc., 2975 Sacramento Street, Berkeley, CA 94702; tel. 510/644-0200

*Betty Ford Center, 39000 Bob Hope Drive, Rancho Mirage, CA 92270; tel. 760/773-4100

*BHC Alhambra Hospital, 4619 North Rosemead Boulevard, Rosemead, CA 91770; tel. 626/286-1191

*BHC Fremont Hospital, 39001 Sundale Drive, Fremont, CA 94538; tel. 510/796-1100

BHC Heritage Oaks Hospital, 4250 Auburn Boulevard, Sacramento, CA 95841; tel. 916/489-3336

*BHC Sierra Vista Hospital, 8001 Bruceville Road, Sacramento, CA 95823; tel. 916/288-0300

California Institution for Women, P.O. Box 6000, Corona, CA 92878-6000; tel. 909/597-1771

*Casa Palmera Care Center, Inc., 14750 El Camino Real, Del Mar, CA 92014; tel. 858/481-4411

Cedars-Sinai Medical Center, 8700 Beverly Blvd, Los Angeles, CA 90048; tel. 310/423-5191

*Clinica Sierra Vista, PO BOX 1559, Bakersfield, CA 93302-1559; tel. 661/635-3050

College Hospital, 10802 College Place, Cerritos, CA 90703; tel. 562/924-9581

College Hospital Costa Mesa, 301 Victoria Street, Costa Mesa, CA 92627; tel. 949/642-2734

Community Hospital of San Bernardino, 1805 Medical Center Drive, San Bernardino, CA 92411-1288; tel. 909/887-6333

*Cornerstone of Southern California, 13682 Yorba Street, Tustin, CA 92780; tel. 714/730-5399

Corona Regional Medical Center, 800 South Main Street, Corona, CA 92882; tel. 951/737-4343

Del Amo Hospital, 23700 Camino Del Sol, Torrance, CA 90505; tel. 310/530-1151

Discovery Practice Management, Inc., 4281 Katella Ave, Suite 111, Los Alamitos, CA 90720; tel. 714/981-0700

*Dual Diagnosis Treatment Center, Inc., 209 Avenida Fabricante, San Clemente, CA 92672; tel. 949/369-1300

*El Camino Hospital, 2500 Grant Ave, Mountain View, CA 94040; tel. 650/940-7000

*Glendale Adventist Medical Center, 1509 Wilson Terrace, Glendale, CA 91206; tel. 818/409-8258

*Good Samaritan Hospital, 901 Olive Drive, Bakersfield, CA 93308; tel. 661/215-7500

*Good Samaritan Hospital, LP, 2425 Samaritan Drive, San Jose, CA 95124; tel. 408/559-2011

HAART-Hayward, 20094 Mission Boulevard, Hayward, CA 94541; tel. 510/727-9755

HAART-Oakland, 10850 MacArthur Boulevard Suite 200, Oakland, CA 94605; tel. 510/875-2300

Hathaway-Sycamores Child and Family Services, 210 South De Lacey Avenue, Suite 110, Pasadena, CA 91105; tel. 626/395-7100

*Huntington Memorial Hospital, PO Box 7013, Pasadena, CA 91109-7013; tel. 626/397-5555

ICE-San Diego, P O Box 439020, San Ysidro, CA 92143; tel. 619/710-8339

*Impact Drug and Alcohol Treatment Center, PO Box 93607, Pasadena, CA 91103; tel. 626/798-0884

*John Muir Behavioral Health, 2740 Grant Street, Concord, CA 94520; tel. 925/674-4100

Kaiser Foundation Hospital-Los Angeles Medical Center, 4733 Sunset Boulevard, Los Angeles, CA 90027; tel. 323/783-8101

La Palma Intercommunity Hospital, 7901 Walker Street, La Palma, CA 90623; tel. 714/670-7400

Langley Porter Psychiatric Hospital and Clinics-UCSF, 401 Parnassus Avenue, HOS 0984, San Francisco, CA 94143-0984; tel. 415/476-7000

*Loma Linda University Behavioral Medicine Center, 1710 Barton Road, Redlands, CA 92373; tel. 909/558-9204

Marin General Hospital, 250 Bon Air Road, Greenbrae, CA 94904; tel. 415/925-7000

*Mission Hospital Regional Medical Center, 27700 Medical Center Road, Mission Viejo, CA 92691; tel. 949/365-2248

Monte Nido Residential Center, Inc., 514 Live Oak Circle, Calabasas, CA 91302; tel. 310/457-9958

Northridge Hospital Medical Center, 18300 Roscoe Boulevard, Northridge, CA 91328; tel. 818/885-5321

Oak Grove Insutute Foundation, Inc., 24275 Jefferson Avenue, Murrieta, CA 92562; tel. 951/677-5599

Opioid Replacement Treatment Prog., Department of Veterans Affairs, 525 21st Street, Oakland, CA 94612; tel. 510/587-3434

Opioid Treatment Programs Los Angeles Ambulatory Care Center, 11301 Wilshire Boulevard Bldg.500, Rm.6404, Los Angeles, CA 90073; tel. 310/268-3132

*Optimum Performance Institute, 3080 Eucalyptus Hill Road, Santa Barbara, CA 93108; tel. 818/610-3956

Our Children's Keeper Child & Family Services, P.O. Box 276372, Sacramento, CA 95827; tel. 916/486-1737

*Pacifica Recovery Services, P O Box 2041, Upland, CA 91785; tel. 909/447-5081

Palomar Medical Center, 555 East Valley Parkway, Escondido, CA 92025; tel. 760/739-3104

*Passages, 241 Market Street, Port Hueneme, CA 93041; tel. 805/283-4737

Prime Healthcare Paradise Valley, LLC, 2400 East Fourth Street, National City, CA 91950-2099; tel. 619/470-4115

Puente de Vida, P.O. Box 86020, San Diego, CA 92138; tel. 858/452-3915

*R House, Inc., P.O. Box 2587, Santa Rosa, CA 95405; tel. 707/571-2215

Redlands Community Hospital, 350 Terracina Boulevard, Redlands, CA 92373; tel. 909/335-5500

River Oak Center for Children, 5030 El Camino Avenue, Carmichael, CA 95608; tel. 916/609-5100

*Riverside Center for Behavioral Medicine, 5900 Brockton Avenue, Riverside, CA 92506; tel. 951/275-8400

Saint Francis Memorial Hospital, 900 Hyde Street, San Francisco, CA 94109; tel. 415/353-6000

San Fernando Community Hospital, 14850 Roscoe Boulevard, Panorama City, CA 91402; tel. 818/904-3685

*San Francisco VA Medical Center, 4150 Clement Street, San Francisco, CA 94121; tel. 415/750-2014

*Santa Barbara Cottage Hospital, PO Box 689, Santa Barbara, CA 93102; tel. 805/569-7404

Santa Rosa Memorial Hospital, 1165 Montgomery Drive, Santa Rosa, CA 95405; tel. 707/522-1520

Scripps Mercy Hospital, 4077 Fifth Avenue- MER 1, San Diego, CA 92103; tel. 619/294-8111

Seneca Family of Agencies, 2275 Arlington Drive, San Leandro, CA 94578; tel. 510/317-1444

Sepulveda CA VAH Opioid Treatment Program, 11301 Wilshire Boulevard Bldg.500, Rm.6404, Los Angeles, CA 90073; tel. 310/268-3132

*Sharp McDonald Center, 7850 Vista Hill Avenue, San Diego, CA 92123; tel. 858/637-6920

Silver Lake Medical Center, 1711 W. Temple Street, Los Angeles, CA 90026; tel. 213/989-6100

*Soba Living, LLC dba Malibu Recovery Center, 22669 Pacific Coast Highway, Malibu, CA 90265; tel. 310/924-2053

*Spencer Recovery Centers, Inc., PO Box 118, Monrovia, CA 91017; tel. 949/376-3705

St. Helena Hospital Center for Behavioral Health, 525 Oregon Street, Vallejo, CA 94590; tel. 707/648-2200

*St. Joseph Hospital, 1100 West Stewart Drive, Orange, CA 92863-5600; tel. 714/771-8000

St. Mary Medical Center, 1050 Linden Avenue, Long Beach, CA 90813; tel. 562/491-9000

St. Mary's Medical Center, 450 Stanyan Street, San Francisco, CA 94117; tel. 415/668-1000

Stewart & Lynda Resnick Neuropsychiatric Hospital at UCLA, 150 Medical Plaza 4230C, MC 746330, Los Angeles, CA 90095; tel. 310/267-9092

Summit Eating Disorders and Outreach Program, 3610 American River Drive, Suite 140, Sacramento, CA 95864; tel. 916/574-1000

*Sutter East Bay Hospitals, 2450 Ashby Avenue, Berkeley, CA 94705; tel. 510/204-2606

Sutter Medical Center, Sacramento, 2801 L Street, Sacramento, CA 95816; tel. 916/454-2222

*Tarzana Treatment Centers, Inc., 18646 Oxnard Street, Tarzana, CA 91356; tel. 818/654-3815

Tessie Cleveland Community Services Corporation, 8019 S COMPTON AVENUE, Los Angeles, CA 90001; tel. 323/586-7333

*The Discovery House Residential Treatment, 847 Barton Ave, Camarillo, CA 93010; tel. 805/228-2826

The Huntington Beach Hospital, 17772 Beach Boulevard, Huntington Beach, CA 92647; tel. 714/843-5000

*Therapeutic Solutions, 3255 Esplanade, Chico, CA 95973; tel. 530/899-3150

*Twin Town Corporation, 4388 E. Katella Ave, Los Alamitos, CA 90720; tel. 562/594-8844

*VA Central California Health Care System, 2615 East Clinton Avenue, Fresno, CA 93703; tel. 559/225-6100

*VA Greater Los Angeles Healthcare System, 11301 Wilshire Boulevard, Los Angeles, CA 90073; tel. 310/268-3132

*VA Loma Linda Healthcare System, 11201 Benton Street, Loma Linda, CA 92357; tel. 909/583-6002

*VA Long Beach Health Care System, 5901 East Seventh Street, Long Beach, CA 90822; tel. 562/826-5400

*VA Northern California Health Care System, 10535 Hospital Way, Mather, CA 95655; tel. 925/372-2010

*VA Palo Alto Health Care System, 3801 Miranda Avenue, Palo Alto, CA 94304; tel. 650/493-5000

*VA San Diego Healthcare System, 3350 La Jolla Village Drive, San Diego, CA 92161; tel. 858/552-8585

Vista Del Mar Child and Family Services, 3200 Motor Avenue, Los Angeles, CA 90034; tel. 310/836-1223

West Anaheim Medical Center, 3033 West Orange Avenue, Anaheim, CA 92804; tel. 714/229-4000

West Los Angeles Drug Treatment Services, 11301 Wilshire Blvd, Bldg.500, Rm.6404, Los Angeles, CA 90073; tel. 310/268-3132

*West Oakland Health Council, 700 Adeline Street, Oakland, CA 94607; tel. 510/835-9610

---

*Indicates organization is a Joint Commission accredited Chemical Dependency organization.

**Western Medical Center Anaheim,** 1025 S. Anaheim Boulevard, Anaheim, CA 92805-0880; tel. 714/533-6220

**Westside Community Mental Health, Inc.,** 1301 Pierce Street, San Francisco, CA 94115; tel. 415/563-8200

**COLORADO**

*Adolescent and Family Institute of Colorado, Inc.,** 10001 West 32nd Avenue, Wheat Ridge, CO 80033; tel. 303/238-1231

*AspenPointe Behavioral Health Services,** 525 N. Cascade Avenue, Suite 100, Colorado Springs, CO 80903; tel. 719/572-6100

*Cedar Springs Hospital, Inc.,** 2135 Southgate Road, Colorado Springs, CO 80906; tel. 719/633-4114

**Children's Hospital Colorado,** 13123 East 16th Avenue, Aurora, CO 80045; tel. 720/777-1234

**Colorado Boys Ranch Foundation,** PO Box 681, La Junta, CO 81050; tel. 719/384-5981

**Comprehensive Addiction Treatment Services,** 2222 East 18Th Ave, Unit C, Denver, CO 80206; tel. 303/394-2714

**Denver Health and Hospital Authority,** 777 Bannock Street, Denver, CO 80204; tel. 303/436-5690

**Devereux Cleo Wallace,** 8405 Church Ranch Blvd, Westminster, CO 80021; tel. 303/466-7391

**Eating Disorder Center of Denver,** 950 S. Cherry Suite 1010, Denver, CO 80246; tel. 303/771-0861

**Eating Recovery Center, LLC,** 1830 Franklin Street Suite 500, Denver, CO 80218; tel. 303/825-8584

**El Pueblo Boys' & Girls' Ranch, Inc.,** One El Pueblo Ranch Way, Pueblo, CO 81006; tel. 719/544-7496

**Forest Heights Lodge,** PO Box 789, Evergreen, CO 80437-0789; tel. 303/674-6681

*Grand Junction Veterans Affairs Medical Center,** 2121 North Avenue, Grand Junction, CO 81501; tel. 970/242-0731

**North Colorado Medical Center,** 1801 16th Street, Greeley, CO 80631; tel. 970/352-4121

*Parker Valley Hope,** PO Box 670, Parker, CO 80134; tel. 303/841-7857

*Parkview Medical Center,** Medical Staff Services 400 West 16th Street Ste 245, Pueblo, CO 81003; tel. 719/584-4000

*Porter Adventist Hospital,** 2525 South Downing Street, Denver, CO 80210; tel. 303/778-1955

*Poudre Valley Hospital,** 1024 South Lemay Avenue, Fort Collins, CO 80524-3998; tel. 970/495-7000

**Southern Peaks Regional Treatment Center,** 700 Four Mile Parkway, Canon City, CO 81212; tel. 719/276-7511

*University of Colorado Hospital Authority,** 12401 E. 17th Avenue, F417, Aurora, CO 80045; tel. 720/848-7800

*VA Eastern Colorado Healthcare System,** 1055 Clermont St, Denver, CO 80220; tel. 303/399-8020

**VCPHCS X, LLC dba The Boulder Clinic, Inc.,** 1317 Spruce Street, Boulder, CO 80302; tel. 303/245-0123

**VCPHCS XI, LLC dba North Denver Behavioral Health Center,** 7290 Samuel Drive, Ste 110, Denver, CO 80221; tel. 303/487-7776

**VCPHCS XII, LLC dba Downtown Denver Behavioral Health Center,** 1337 Delaware Street, First Floor, Denver, CO 80204; tel. 303/629-5293

**CONNECTICUT**

**Blue Hills Substance Abuse Services,** 500 Vine Street, Hartford, CT 06112-1639; tel. 860/666-7665

**Bridgeport Hospital,** 267 Grant Street, Bridgeport, CT 06610; tel. 203/384-3000

*Bristol Hospital, Inc.,** PO Box 977, Bristol, CT 06011-0977; tel. 860/585-3222

**Capitol Region Mental Health Center,** 500 Vine Street, Hartford, CT 06112; tel. 860/297-0903

*Community Health Resources, Inc.,** 995 Day Hill Road, Windsor, CT 06095; tel. 860/731-5522

**Community Health Resources: CPAS Division,** 391 Pomfret Street, Putnam, CT 06260; tel. 860/646-3888

*Community Mental Health Affiliates, Inc.,** 270 John Downey Drive, New Britain, CT 06051; tel. 860/826-1358

*Community Renewal Team,** 555 Windsor Street, Hartford, CT 06120; tel. 860/560-5784

*Connecticut Mental Health Center,** 34 Park Street, New Haven, CT 06519; tel. 203/974-7300

*Connecticut Valley Hospital,** PO Box 351, Middletown, CT 06457-7023; tel. 860/262-5887

*Cornell Scott-Hill Health Corporation,** 400 Columbus Avenue, New Haven, CT 06519; tel. 203/503-3000

*Hartford Community Mental Health Center, Inc.,** One Main Street, Hartford, CT 06106; tel. 860/727-8703

*Hartford Hospital,** 80 Seymour Street, Hartford, CT 06102-5037; tel. 860/545-2100

*Hospital of Saint Raphael,** 1450 Chapel Street, New Haven, CT 06511; tel. 203/789-3000

**InterCommunity, Inc.,** 281 Main Street, East Hartford, CT 06118; tel. 860/569-5900

**John Dempsey Hospital/Univ of Connecticut Health Center,** 263 Farmington Avenue, Farmington, CT 06030-3802; tel. 860/679-2233

**Klingberg Family Centers, Inc.,** 370 Linwood Street, New Britain, CT 06052; tel. 860/224-9113

**Lawrence & Memorial Hospital,** 365 Montauk Avenue, New London, CT 06320; tel. 860/442-0711

**Manchester Memorial Hospital,** 71 Haynes Street, Manchester, CT 06040; tel. 860/533-3432

**Middlesex Hospital,** 28 Crescent Street, Middletown, CT 06457; tel. 860/358-6000

*Natchaug Hospital, Inc.,** 189 Storrs Road, Mansfield Center, CT 06250; tel. 860/456-1311

**New Era Rehabilitation Center,** 3851 Main Street, 2nd floor, Bridgeport, CT 06606; tel. 203/372-3333

*Perception Programs, Inc.,** PO Box 407, Willimantic, CT 06226; tel. 860/450-7122

**River Valley Services,** PO Box 351, Middletown, CT 06457; tel. 860/262-5200

*Rushford Center, Inc.,** 883 Paddock Avenue, Meriden, CT 06450; tel. 203/235-1792

**Saint Francis Hospital & Medical Center-8 West Unit,** 500 Blue Hills Avenue, Hartford, CT 06112; tel. 860/714-2333

*Saint Mary's Hospital, Inc.,** 56 Franklin Street, Waterbury, CT 06706; tel. 203/709-6000

*Silver Hill Hospital,** 208 Valley Road, New Canaan, CT 06840; tel. 203/801-2297

**South Central Rehabilitation Center,** 232 Cedar Street, New Haven, CT 06519; tel. 203/503-3356

*Southwest Community Health Center, Inc.,** 968 Fairfield Avenue, Bridgeport, CT 06605; tel. 203/332-3506

**Southwest Connecticut Mental Health System,** 97 Middle Street, Bridgeport, CT 06604; tel. 203/579-7368

**St. Vincent's Medical Center,** 2800 Main Street, Bridgeport, CT 06606; tel. 203/576-5473

**State of CT DMHAS-Southeastern Mental Health Authority,** 401 West Thames Street, Bldg. 301, Norwich, CT 06360; tel. 860/859-4674

*Stonington Behavioral Health, Inc.,** 75 Swantown Hill Road, North Stonington, CT 06359; tel. 860/535-1010

**The Charlotte Hungerford Hospital,** PO Box 988, Torrington, CT 06790; tel. 860/496-6666

*The Children's Center of Hamden, Inc.,** 1400 Whitney Avenue, Hamden, CT 06517; tel. 203/248-2116

*The Danbury Hospital,** 24 Hospital Avenue, Danbury, CT 06810; tel. 203/739-7000

*The Hospital of Central Connecticut,** PO Box 100, New Britain, CT 06050-0100; tel. 860/224-5666

*The Waterbury Hospital,** 64 Robbins Street, Waterbury, CT 06721; tel. 203/573-6000

**The Wellspring Foundation, Inc.,** 21 Arch Bridge Road, Bethlehem, CT 06751; tel. 203/266-8000

*The Wheeler Clinic,** 91 Northwest Drive, Plainville, CT 06062; tel. 860/793-3500

*United Services, Inc.,** Post Office Box 839, Dayville, CT 06241; tel. 860/774-2020

*VA Connecticut Healthcare System,** 950 Campbell Avenue, West Haven, CT 06516; tel. 203/932-5711

**Western Connecticut Mental Health Network,** 55 West Main Street, Suite 410, Waterbury, CT 06702; tel. 203/805-6400

**Yale Health,** P.O. Box 208237, New Haven, CT 06520; tel. 203/432-4096

**Yale-New Haven Hospital,** 20 York Street, New Haven, CT 06510-3203; tel. 203/688-4242

**DELAWARE**

*Brandywine Counseling & Community Services,** 2500 West Fourth Street, Wilmington, DE 19805; tel. 302/472-0381

**Brandywine Counseling & Community Services, South Chapel,** 24 Brookhill Drive, Newark, DE 19702; tel. 302/454-3020

**Brandywine Counseling & Community Services, Lancaster,** 2713 Lancaster Avenue, Wilmington, DE 19805; tel. 302/656-2347

**Christiana Care-Christiana Hospital,** PO Box 6001, Newark, DE 19718; tel. 302/733-1274

**Delaware Guidance Services for Children and Youth, Inc.,** 1213 Delaware Avenue, Wilmington, DE 19806; tel. 302/652-3948

*Dover Behavioral Health System,** 725 Horsepond Road, Dover, DE 19901; tel. 302/747-1198

*Gateway Foundation Delaware City Treatment Center,** P.O. Box 547, Delaware City, DE 19706; tel. 312/663-1130

**Meadow Wood Behavioral Health System,** 575 South DuPont Highway, New Castle, DE 19720; tel. 302/328-3330

**Rockford Center,** 100 Rockford Drive, Newark, DE 19713; tel. 302/996-5480

*SODAT-Delaware, Inc.,** 625 N. Orange Street, Wilmington, DE 19801; tel. 302/656-4044

*Thresholds, Inc.,** 20505 DuPont Boulevard, Suite 1, Georgetown, DE 19947; tel. 302/856-1835

**VA Medical Center,** 1601 Kirkwood Highway, Wilmington, DE 19805; tel. 302/994-2511

**DISTRICT OF COLUMBIA**

**McClendon Center,** 1313 New York Avenue, NW, Washington, DC 20005; tel. 202/737-6191

**The Episcopal Center for Children,** 5901 Utah Avenue, NW, Washington, DC 20015-1616; tel. 202/363-1333

*The Psychiatric Institute of Washington,** 4228 Wisconsin Avenue, Northwest, Washington, DC 20016; tel. 202/885-5600

*VA Medical Center,** 50 Irving Street, Northwest, Washington, DC 20422; tel. 202/745-8000

**Walter Reed Army Medical Center,** 6900 Georgia Avenue, Northwest, Washington, DC 20307-5001; tel. 202/782-3501

*Washington Hospital Center,** 110 Irving Street, Northwest, Washington, DC 20010; tel. 202/877-7000

**FLORIDA**

*ALPHA Community Mental Health Center,** 7811 SW 24th Street # 137, Miami, FL 33155; tel. 305/264-3225

*Alpha Health Care Clinic, Inc.,** 1990 NE 163rd Street Suite 102, North Miami Beach, FL 33162; tel. 305/945-9906

**Alternate Family Care, Inc.,** 10001 W Oakland Park Blvd, Suite 200, Sunrise, FL 33351; tel. 954/746-5200

*Alternative Treatment International, Inc.,** 2919 Northfield Drive, Tarpon Springs, FL 34688; tel. 727/796-3719

*Ambrosia of the Palm Beaches,** 2626 Lake Drive, Singer Island, FL 33404; tel. 561/721-8800

*Ambrosia Treatment Center,** 546 NW University Boulevard, Suite 103, Port Saint Lucie, FL 34986; tel. 772/323-2099

*Apalachee Center, Inc.,** 2634-J Capital Circle NE, Tallahassee, FL 32308; tel. 850/523-3333

*Atlantic Shores Hospital,** 4545 North Federal Highway, Fort Lauderdale, FL 33308; tel. 954/771-2711

*Avanti Wellness Center,** 3574 US 1 South Suite 113, Saint Augustine, FL 32086-6467; tel. 904/824-7597

*Bay Pines VA Healthcare System,** 10000 Bay Pines Boulevard, Bay Pines, FL 33744; tel. 727/398-6611

*Bayview Center for Mental Health, Inc.,** 700 SE 3rd Avenue, Suite 100, Fort Lauderdale, FL 33316; tel. 954/414-8700

*Beachcomber Rehab, Inc.,** 4493 North Ocean Boulevard, Delray Beach, FL 33483; tel. 561/276-6226

*Behavioral Health of the Palm Beaches, Inc.,** 3153 Canada Court, Lake Worth, FL 33461; tel. 561/615-6664

**Behavioral Support Services, Inc.,** 315 N. Lakemont Avenue, Suite B, Winter Park, FL 32792; tel. 407/831-6412

**Biscayne Milieu Health Center, Inc.,** 13499 Biscayne Boulevard Suite 101, Miami, FL 33181; tel. 305/948-9000

*Broward Addiction Recovery Division,** 1011 SW 2nd Court, Fort Lauderdale, FL 33312; tel. 954/357-4860

**Broward Center for Mental Health, PA.,** 3127 West Hallandale Beach Boulevard Suite 115, Hallandale, FL 33009; tel. 754/816-3071

---

*Indicates organization is a Joint Commission accredited Chemical Dependency organization.

Section C

*Center for Alcohol & Drug Studies, Inc., 2976 S. Military Trail, Ste 1, West Palm Beach, FL 33415; tel. 561/963-4371

Central Florida Treatment Center-Ft. Pierce Clinic, 1302 Lawnwood Circle, Suite B, Fort Pierce, FL 34950; tel. 772/468-6800

CFSATC, Inc., 1800 West Colonial Drive, Orlando, FL 32804; tel. 407/843-0041

CFSATC, Inc. Cocoa, 7 North Cocoa Boulevard, Cocoa, FL 32922; tel. 321/631-4578

CFSATC, Inc. Lake Worth, Inc., 3155 Lake Worth Road Suite #2, Lake Worth, FL 33461; tel. 561/439-8440

CFSATC, Inc. Palm Bay, 2198 Harris Avenue, Palm Bay, FL 32905; tel. 321/951-9750

*Circles of Care, Inc., 400 East Sheridan Road, Melbourne, FL 32901-3184; tel. 321/984-4900

Citrus Health Network, Inc., 4175 West 20th Avenue, Hialeah, FL 33012; tel. 305/424-3100

*Coastal Behavioral Healthcare, Inc., 1565 State Street, Sarasota, FL 34236; tel. 941/927-8900

Coastal Mental Health Services, Inc., 1745 Travertine Terrace, Sanford, FL 32771; tel. 800/614-4124

Columbia Hospital, 2201 45th Street, West Palm Beach, FL 33407; tel. 561/863-3104

*Community Health of South Florida, Inc., 10300 SW 216 Street, Miami, FL 33190; tel. 305/252-4853

Comprehensive Psychiatric Center, 9735 East Fern Street, Miami, FL 33157; tel. 305/238-5121

Comprehensive Psychiatric Center Central, 4790 N. W. 7th Street Suite #101 & 102, Miami, FL 33126; tel. 305/529-5810

Comprehensive Psychiatric Center North, 240 Northwest 183rd Street, Miami, FL 33169; tel. 305/651-2332

*Dade Family Counseling Community Mental Health Center, 4343 West Flagler Street Suite 100, Miami, FL 33134; tel. 305/774-9570

*David Lawrence Center, 6075 Bathey Lane, Naples, FL 34116; tel. 239/455-8500

*Destination Hope, Inc., 6555 NW 9th Avenue Suite 214, Fort Lauderdale, FL 33309; tel. 954/771-2091

Fair Oaks Pavilion at Delray Medical Center, 5352 Linton Boulevard, Delray Beach, FL 33484; tel. 561/495-3278

*Fairwinds Treatment Center, 1569 S Fort Harrison Avenue, Clearwater, FL 33756; tel. 727/449-0300

*Family Resource Center of South Florida, Inc., 155 South Miami Avenue 4th Fl, Miami, FL 33130-1617; tel. 305/374-6006

*Florida Center for Recovery, 3451 West Midway Road, Fort Pierce, FL 34981; tel. 772/460-2777

Florida Hospital Zephyrhills, 7050 Gall Boulevard, Zephyrhills, FL 33541; tel. 813/788-0411

Florida Institute for Neurologic Rehabilitation, Inc., PO Box 1348, Wauchula, FL 33873; tel. 863/773-2857

*Focus Healthcare of Florida, 5960 Southwest 106th Avenue, Cooper City, FL 33328; tel. 954/680-2700

*Fort Lauderdale Hospital Management, LLC, 1601 East Las Olas Boulevard, Fort Lauderdale, FL 33301; tel. 954/463-4321

Fort Lauderdale Hospital-Opioid Treatment Programs, 1601 East Las Olas Blvd, Fort Lauderdale, FL 33301; tel. 954/463-4321

Future Care Solution, Inc., 3911 SW 67 Ave, Miami, FL 33155; tel. 305/740-6960

*G&G Holistic Addiction Treatment, Inc., 1590 NE 162nd Street Suite 200, North Miami Beach, FL 33162; tel. 305/945-8384

Geo Care, Inc. / Treasure Coast Forensic Treatment Center, 96 SW Allapattah Road, Indiantown, FL 34956; tel. 772/597-9400

Gulf Coast Treatment Center, 1015 Mar Walt Drive, Fort Walton Beach, FL 32547; tel. 850/863-4160

Halifax Health, PO Box 2830, Daytona Beach, FL 32120-9718; tel. 386/425-4773

*Hanley Center, 933 45th Street, West Palm Beach, FL 33407-2374; tel. 561/841-1000

*HealthCare Connection of Tampa, Inc., 825 West Linebaugh Avenue, Tampa, FL 33612; tel. 813/931-5560

*Hendry Glades Mental Health Clinic, Inc., 601 West Alverdez Avenue, Clewiston, FL 33440; tel. 863/983-1423

Hollywood Pavilion, LLC, 1201 North 37th Avenue, Hollywood, FL 33021; tel. 954/962-1355

Homestead Behavioral Health Clinic, 654 NE 9th Place, Homestead, FL 33030; tel. 305/248-3488

*Jackson Memorial Hospital, 1611 Northwest 12th Avenue, Miami, FL 33136-1094; tel. 305/585-1111

*Jackson North Community Mental Health Center, 20201 NW 37th Ave, Opa Locka, FL 33056; tel. 786/466-2700

*James A. Haley Veterans' Hospital, 13000 Bruce B. Downs Boulevard, Tampa, FL 33612; tel. 813/972-2000

*Jessie Trice Community Health Center, Inc., 700 S. Royal Poinciana Blvd, Suite 300, Miami, FL 33166; tel. 305/805-1700

*John's Place, Inc., 315 SE 11th Street, Fort Lauderdale, FL 33316; tel. 954/463-9590

La Amistad Behavioral Health Services, 1650 Park Avenue North, Maitland, FL 32751; tel. 407/647-0660

La Amistad Residential Treatment Center, LLC, 6601 Central Florida Parkway, Orlando, FL 32821; tel. 407/370-0111

Lakeside Behavioral Healthcare, Inc., 1800 Mercy Dr, Orlando, FL 32808; tel. 407/667-1666

*Lakeview Health Systems, LLC, 1900 Corporate Square Blvd, Jacksonville, FL 32216; tel. 904/727-6455

Larkin Community Hospital, Inc., 7031 Southwest 62nd Avenue, South Miami, FL 33143; tel. 305/284-7700

Lee Memorial Health System Behavioral Health Services, 12550 New Brittany Blvd, Ste 200, 201, Fort Myers, FL 33907; tel. 239/936-1114

Lehigh HMA LLC, 1500 Lee Boulevard, Lehigh Acres, FL 33936; tel. 239/368-4503

*Manatee Glens, PO Box 9478, Bradenton, FL 34206-9478; tel. 941/782-4299

Manatee Palms Group Homes, 4480 51st Street West, Bradenton, FL 34210; tel. 941/792-2222

Mental Health Care, Inc., 5707 North 22nd Street, Tampa, FL 33610; tel. 813/272-2244

*Miami VA Healthcare System, 1201 NW 16th Street, Miami, FL 33125; tel. 305/575-7000

Milestones In Recovery, Inc., 2525 Embassy Lake Drive, Suite 8, Cooper City, FL 33328; tel. 954/272-0806

Miracle Mile Community Mental Health Center, 955 NW 3rd Street, Suite 105, Miami, FL 33128; tel. 305/324-9494

Multicultural Community Mental Health Center, 2721 Poinsettia Avenue, West Palm Beach, FL 33407; tel. 561/653-6292

National Deaf Academy, LLC, 19650 US Highway 441, Mount Dora, FL 32757; tel. 352/735-9500

New Directions Community Mental Health Center, 28870 South Dixie Highway, Homestead, FL 33030; tel. 305/247-4009

*New Era Health Center, Inc., 9600 Southwest 8th Street Suite 1, Miami, FL 33174; tel. 305/559-8838

*New Horizons Community Mental Health Center, Inc., 1469 NW 36th Street 2nd Floor, Miami, FL 33142; tel. 305/637-7258

*North Florida/South Georgia Veterans Health System, 1601 Southwest Archer Road, Gainesville, FL 32608-1197; tel. 352/376-1611

Northside Mental Health Center, 12512 Bruce B. Downs Boulevard, Tampa, FL 33612-9209; tel. 813/977-8700

Nueva America, Inc., 2682 SW 87th Avenue, Miami, FL 33165; tel. 305/480-5680

Oliver-Pyatt Centers, Inc., 6150 SW 76 Street, Miami, FL 33143; tel. 305/663-1738

*Orlando VA Medical Center, 5201 Raymond Street, Orlando, FL 32803; tel. 407/629-1599

*Palm Partners, LLC, 816 Palm Trail, Delray Beach, FL 33483; tel. 561/819-3009

Parent's Information and Resource Center, Inc., 817 N. Dixie Highway, Pompano Beach, FL 33060; tel. 954/785-8285

*PB Institute Partners Limited Partnership, 1017 N. Olive Avenue, West Palm Beach, FL 33401; tel. 800/433-5098

*Peace River Center for Personal Development, Inc., P.O. Box 1559, Bartow, FL 33831-1559; tel. 863/519-0575

Personal Enrichment through Mental Health Services, Inc., 11254 58th Street North, Pinellas Park, FL 33782; tel. 727/545-6477

Phoenix Clinic, 2212 SW 60th Terrace, Miramar, FL 33023; tel. 954/491-2133

*Professional Training Association Corporation, 321 Northlake Blvd Suite 102, North Palm Beach, FL 33408; tel. 561/494-0866

*RBHS & MHRC & MHCJ, PO Box 19249, Jacksonville, FL 32245-9249; tel. 904/743-1883

Recapturing the Vision International, 9780 E Indigo Street Suite 302, Palmetto Bay, FL 33157; tel. 305/232-6003

*Recovery First, Inc., 4110 Davie Road Extension, Hollywood, FL 33024; tel. 954/981-4545

Reflections Wellness Center of Broward, Inc., 6848 Stirling Road, Hollywood, FL 33024; tel. 954/362-0104

*River Point Behavioral Health, PO Box 17128, Jacksonville, FL 32245-7128; tel. 904/724-9202

Santa Rosa Medical Center, 6002 Berryhill Road, Milton, FL 32570; tel. 850/626-5102

*Serenity Now CMHC, 2724 N. Australia Avenue Building 1, West Palm Beach, FL 33407; tel. 561/381-7707

South County Mental Health Center, Inc., 16158 South Military Trail, Delray Beach, FL 33484; tel. 561/637-1000

SP Behavioral, LLC, 11301 SE Tequesta Terrace, Tequesta, FL 33469; tel. 561/744-0211

*Springbrook Hospital, 7007 Grove Road, Brooksville, FL 34609; tel. 352/596-4306

*Stepping Stone Center for Recovery, 2701 Gateway Drive, Pompano Beach, FL 33069; tel. 954/489-2588

Stepping Stone Center for Recovery-Opioid Treatment Programs, 8889 Corporate Square Court, Jacksonville, FL 32216; tel. 954/489-2580

Suncoast Mental Health Center, Inc., 2814 S. US Hwy 1 Suite D - 4, Fort Pierce, FL 34982; tel. 772/489-4726

*Sunrise Detoxification Center, LLC, 3185 Boutwell Road, Lake Worth, FL 33461; tel. 561/533-0074

*The Centers, 5664 SW 60th Ave, Ocala, FL 34474; tel. 352/291-5456

*The Centre for Women, Inc., 305 South Hyde Park Avenue, Tampa, FL 33606; tel. 813/251-8437

The Devereux Foundation, Inc., 5850 T. G. Lee Blvd, Suite 400, Orlando, FL 32822; tel. 407/362-9210

*The Hazelden Foundation, 950 Sixth Avenue North, Naples, FL 34102; tel. 651/213-4150

*The Jerome Golden Center for Behavioral Health, Inc., 1041 45th Street, West Palm Beach, FL 33407; tel. 561/383-8000

*The Recovery Place, Inc., 3100 E. Commercial Boulevard, Fort Lauderdale, FL 33308; tel. 954/200-8308

The Renfrew Center of Florida, 7700 Renfrew Lane, Coconut Creek, FL 33073; tel. 215/482-5353

*The Treatment Center of the Palm Beaches, LLC, 4905 Lantana Road, Lake Worth, FL 33463; tel. 561/253-6790

*The Village South, Inc., 3050 Biscayne Boulevard, Miami, FL 33137; tel. 305/573-3784

*The Vines Hospital, 3130 SW 27th Avenue, Ocala, FL 34471; tel. 352/671-3130

*The Watershed Treatment Programs, 200 Congress Park Drive, #100, Delray Beach, FL 33445; tel. 561/361-6608

*The Willough at Naples, 9001 Tamiami Trail East, Naples, FL 34113; tel. 239/775-4500

*Transitions Recovery Program, 1928 Northeast 154th Street, Miami, FL 33162; tel. 305/949-9001

*Treatment Alternatives, 7000 North Federal Hwy, Boca Raton, FL 33487; tel. 561/637-4766

*Treatment Resources of Margate, Inc., 5100 Coconut Creek Parkway, Margate, FL 33063; tel. 954/917-3334

*Treatment Solutions of South Florida, Inc., 6278 N. Federal Hwy. PMB 392, Fort Lauderdale, FL 33308; tel. 954/627-6157

*Turning Point of Tampa, Inc., 6227 Sheldon Road, Tampa, FL 33615; tel. 813/882-3003

*Tykes & Teens, 3577 SW Corporate Parkway, Palm City, FL 34990; tel. 772/220-3439

*Unity Recovery Center, Inc., 11900 SE Federal Hwy Suite 212, Hobe Sound, FL 33455; tel. 772/546-3455

University Behavioral, LLC, 2500 Discovery Drive, Orlando, FL 32826; tel. 407/281-7000

*VA Medical Center-West Palm Beach, Florida, 7305 N. Military Trail, West Palm Beach, FL 33410-6400; tel. 561/422-8600

Volunteers of America of Florida, Inc., 1205 East 8th Avenue, Tampa, FL 33605; tel. 813/282-1525

*Wekiva Springs Center, LLC, 3947 Salisbury Road, Jacksonville, FL 32216; tel. 904/296-3533

*Indicates organization is a Joint Commission accredited Chemical Dependency organization.

*Windmoor Healthcare of Clearwater, Inc., 11300 US 19 North, Clearwater, FL 33764; tel. 727/541-2646

## GEORGIA

*Acadia Riverwoods, 223 Medical Center Drive, Riverdale, GA 30274; tel. 770/991-8500

Central State Hospital, 620 Broad St, Milledgeville, GA 31062; tel. 478/445-4128

Chanan Foundation, Inc., 6470 Cedar Mountain Road, Douglasville, GA 30134; tel. 678/715-8891

*Charlie Norwood VA Medical Center, 1 Freedom Way, Augusta, GA 30904; tel. 706/733-0188

*Coastal Harbor Treatment Center, 1150 Cornell Avenue, Savannah, GA 31406; tel. 912/354-3911

*Coliseum Psychiatric Center, LLC, 340 Hospital Drive, Macon, GA 31217-8002; tel. 478/741-1355

Cord of Three Counseling Services, 206 Screven Avenue, Waycross, GA 31501; tel. 912/288-7480

Devereux Georgia Treatment Network, 1291 Stanley Road, Kennesaw, GA 30152-4359; tel. 770/427-0147

DM & ADR, Inc., 1710 Commerce Road, Athens, GA 30607; tel. 706/552-0688

East Central Regional Hospital, 100 Myrtle Blvd, Gracewood, GA 30812; tel. 706/790-2030

East Georgia Regional Medical Center, P.O. Box 1048, Statesboro, GA 30458; tel. 912/486-1000

*Families Matter Counseling and Psychological Services, 747 Lauren Parkway, Stone Mountain, GA 30083; tel. 404/602-0182

*Fulton County Department of BHDD, 99 Jesse Hill Jr Dr Suite 408, Atlanta, GA 30303; tel. 404/730-1202

*Georgia Pines Community Service Board, 1102 Smith Avenue Suite K, Thomasville, GA 31799; tel. 229/225-4335

Georgia Regional Hospital at Atlanta, PO Box 37047, Decatur, GA 30034-0407; tel. 404/243-2100

*Georgia Regional Hospital at Savannah, 1915 Eisenhower Drive, Savannah, GA 31406; tel. 912/356-2011

Grady Memorial Hospital Corporation, 80 Jesse Hill, Jr., Drive, SE, Atlanta, GA 30303; tel. 404/616-4252

Hopes of Honorable Youth, LLC, 130 W. Wieuca Suite 204 B, Atlanta, GA 30342; tel. 404/797-7126

KidsPeace National Centers of Georgia, Inc., 101 KidsPeace Drive, Bowdon, GA 30108; tel. 770/437-7200

Laurel Heights Hospital, 934 Briarcliff Road, Northeast, Atlanta, GA 30306; tel. 404/888-7860

Macon Behavioral Health System, 3500 Riverside Drive, Macon, GA 31210; tel. 478/477-3829

*Martin Army Community Hospital, 7950 Martin Loop, Fort Benning, GA 31905-5637; tel. 706/544-4762

*Metro Atlanta Recovery Residences, Inc., PO Box 48349, Atlanta, GA 30342; tel. 678/805-5100

Mind, Body & Soul, LLC, 2221 Peachtree Road, Suite X16, Atlanta, GA 30309; tel. 678/793-6488

Murphy Harpst Children's Centers, Inc., 740 Fletcher Street, Cedartown, GA 30125; tel. 770/748-1500

*Northside Hospital, Inc., 1000 Johnson Ferry Road, Atlanta, GA 30342-1611; tel. 404/851-8000

*Ogeechee Behavioral Health Services, PO Box 1259, Swainsboro, GA 30401; tel. 478/289-2522

*Peachford Behavioral Health System of Atlanta, 2151 Peachford Road, Atlanta, GA 30338; tel. 770/455-3200

*Ridgeview Institute, 3995 South Cobb Drive, Smyrna, GA 30080; tel. 770/434-4567

Skyland Trail, 1961 North Druid Hills Road, Atlanta, GA 30329; tel. 404/315-8333

Southside Behavioral Lifestyle Enrichment Center, 2685 Metropolitan Parkway, Suite C, Atlanta, GA 30315; tel. 404/627-1385

*Southside Medical Center, Inc., 1046 Ridge Avenue, Atlanta, GA 30315; tel. 404/688-1350

*Southwestern State Hospital, PO Box 1378, Thomasville, GA 31799-1378; tel. 229/227-3020

*St. Francis Hospital, Inc., PO Box 7000, Columbus, GA 31908-7000; tel. 706/596-4000

*Talbott Recovery Campus, 5448 Yorktowne Drive, Atlanta, GA 30349; tel. 770/994-0185

Tanner Medical Center / Villa Rica, 601 Dallas Highway, Villa Rica, GA 30180; tel. 770/456-3000

Tanner Medical Center, Inc., 705 Dixie Street, Carrollton, GA 30117; tel. 770/836-9580

*Turning Point Hospital, PO Box 1177, Moultrie, GA 31776; tel. 229/985-4815

*UHS of Anchor, LP, 5454 Yorktowne Drive, Atlanta, GA 30349; tel. 770/991-6044

*VA Medical Center-Atlanta, 1670 Clairmont Road, Decatur, GA 30033; tel. 404/728-7601

*VA Medical Center-Carl Vinson, 1826 Veterans Boulevard, Dublin, GA 31021; tel. 478/277-2701

*WellStar Cobb Hospital, 805 Sandy Plains Road, Marietta, GA 30066; tel. 770/732-4000

West Central Georgia Regional Hospital, PO Box 12435, Columbus, GA 31917-2435; tel. 706/568-5203

*Willingway Hospital, 311 Jones Mill Road, Statesboro, GA 30458; tel. 912/764-6236

*Winn Army Community Hospital, 1061 Harmon Avenue, Fort Stewart, GA 31314-5674; tel. 912/435-6911

## HAWAII

Benchmark Behavioral Health Systems-Pearl City, P.O Box 1196, Pearl City, HI 96782; tel. 808/454-1411

Hawaii State Hospital, 45 710 Keaahala Road, Kaneohe, HI 96744; tel. 808/247-2191

*Naval Health Clinic Hawaii, 480 Central Avenue, Pearl Harbor, HI 96860-4908; tel. 808/471-3025

Sutter Health Pacific, 91-2301 Old Fort Weaver Road, Ewa Beach, HI 96706; tel. 808/671-8511

The Queen's Medical Center, 1301 Punchbowl Street, Honolulu, HI 96813; tel. 808/538-9011

*VA Pacific Islands Health Care System, 459 Patterson Road, Honolulu, HI 96819-1522; tel. 808/433-0100

## IDAHO

*Boise VA Medical Center, 500 West Fort Street, Boise, ID 83702-4598; tel. 208/422-1100

Eastern Idaho Health Services, PO Box 2077, Idaho Falls, ID 83404; tel. 208/529-6210

*Kootenai Health, 2003 Kootenai Health Way, Coeur D Alene, ID 83814; tel. 208/666-2000

Project Patch, PO Box 450, Garden Valley, ID 83622; tel. 360/690-8495

## ILLINOIS

*Adventist Hinsdale Hospital, 120 North Oak Street, Hinsdale, IL 60521; tel. 630/856-6001

*Advocate Addiction Treatment Program, 701 Lee Street, Suite 800, Des Plaines, IL 60016; tel. 847/795-3900

*Advocate Christ Medical Center, 4440 West 95th Street, Oak Lawn, IL 60453; tel. 708/684-8000

*Advocate Illinois Masonic Medical Center, 836 West Wellington Avenue, Chicago, IL 60657; tel. 773/975-1600

Advocate Lutheran General Hospital, 1775 Dempster Street, Park Ridge, IL 60068; tel. 847/723-2210

*Alexian Brothers Behavioral Health Hospital, 1650 Moon Lake Boulevard, Hoffman Estates, IL 60169; tel. 847/882-1600

Alexian Brothers Center for Mental Health, 3436 N. Kennicott Avenue, Arlington Heights, IL 60004; tel. 847/952-7460

Allendale Association, PO Box 1088, Lake Villa, IL 60046; tel. 847/356-2351

*Aunt Martha's Youth Service Center, Inc., 19990 Governors Highway, Olympia Fields, IL 60461; tel. 708/747-7100

*Aurora Chicago Lakeshore Hospital, 4840 North Marine Drive, Chicago, IL 60640; tel. 773/878-9700

Beacon Therapeutic Diagnostic and Treatment Center, 1912 West 103rd Street, Chicago, IL 60643; tel. 773/298-1243

*Ben Gordon Center, 12 Health Services Drive, Dekalb, IL 60115; tel. 815/756-4875

CAP of Downers Grove, 4954 South Main Street, Downers Grove, IL 60515; tel. 630/810-0186

*Centegra Hospital Woodstock, 385 Millennium Drive, Crystal Lake, IL 60012; tel. 815/759-4689

Center for Addictive Problems, 609 North Wells Street, Chicago, IL 60654; tel. 312/266-0404

Center on Deafness, 3444 Dundee Road, Northbrook, IL 60062; tel. 847/559-0110

*Central DuPage Hospital, 25 North Winfield Road, Winfield, IL 60190; tel. 630/933-1600

Central Illinois Center for the Treatment of Addictions, 3420 N Rochelle, Peoria, IL 61604; tel. 309/671-8005

*Chestnut Health Systems, 1003 Martin Luther King Drive, Bloomington, IL 61701; tel. 309/827-6026

Coles County Mental Health Association, Inc., 750 Broadway Avenue East, Mattoon, IL 61938; tel. 217/238-5700

*Community Counseling Centers of Chicago, 4740 North Clark Street, Chicago, IL 60640; tel. 773/765-0810

*Comprehensive Behavioral Health Center of St. Clair County, 505 South 8th Street, East Saint Louis, IL 62201; tel. 618/482-7330

*Counseling Center of Lake View, 3225 North Sheffield Avenue, Chicago, IL 60657; tel. 773/549-5886

DuPage County Health Department/ Mental Health Services, 111 North County Farm Road, Wheaton, IL 60187; tel. 630/682-7400

*DuPage Interventions, 11 S 250 Route 83, Hinsdale, IL 60521; tel. 630/325-5050

Ecker Center for Mental Health, 1845 Grandstand Place, Elgin, IL 60123; tel. 847/695-0484

*Edward Hines Jr. VA Hospital, 5000 South 5th Avenue, Hines, IL 60141-5000; tel. 708/202-5652

*Elmhurst Memorial Hospital, 155 East Brush Hill Road, Elmhurst, IL 60126; tel. 331/221-1000

Family Alliance, Inc., 2028 N. Seminary Avenue, Woodstock, IL 60098; tel. 815/338-3590

Family Guidance Centers at Triangle Center-Methadone, 2525 E Oakton, Arlington Heights, IL 60005; tel. 217/544-9858

Family Guidance Centers, Inc., 310 West Chicago Avenue, Chicago, IL 60654; tel. 312/943-6545

Family Guidance Centers, Inc., 484 Lee Street, Des Plaines, IL 60016; tel. 847/827-7517

Family Guidance Centers, Inc., 751 Aurora Avenue, Aurora, IL 60505; tel. 630/801-0017

*Family Service and Community Mental Health Center/McHenry, 4100 Veterans Parkway, McHenry, IL 60050; tel. 815/385-6400

FHN Family Counseling Center, 421 W. Exchange Street, Freeport, IL 61032; tel. 815/599-7337

Garfield Counseling Center, Inc., 4132 West Madison, Chicago, IL 60624; tel. 773/533-0433

*Gateway Foundation, Inc., 55 East Jackson Blvd, Suite 1500, Chicago, IL 60604; tel. 312/663-1130

Hartgrove Hospital, 5730 W. Roosevelt. Road, Chicago, IL 60644; tel. 773/413-1700

*Heartland Human Services, PO Box 1047, Effingham, IL 62401; tel. 217/347-7179

*Human Service Center, PO Box 1346, Peoria, IL 61654-1346; tel. 309/671-8005

*Insight Psychological Centers, 333 North Michigan Avenue, Suite 1900, Chicago, IL 60601; tel. 312/540-9955

Jackson Park Hospital and Medical Center, 7531 South Stony Island Avenue, Chicago, IL 60649; tel. 773/947-7500

*James A. Lovell Federal Health Care Center, 3001 Green Bay Road, North Chicago, IL 60064; tel. 224/610-3700

*Jesse Brown VA Medical Center, 820 South Damen Avenue, Chicago, IL 60612; tel. 312/569-6101

Kenneth Young Center, 1001 Rohlwing Road, Elk Grove Village, IL 60007; tel. 847/524-8800

*Lake County Health Department / Behavioral Health Services, 3010 Grand Avenue, Waukegan, IL 60085; tel. 847/377-8299

*Leyden Family Service and Mental Health Center, 10001 West Grand Avenue, Franklin Park, IL 60131; tel. 847/451-0330

*Little Company of Mary Hospital & Health Care Centers, 2800 West 95th Street, Evergreen Park, IL 60805; tel. 708/422-6200

*Maryville Academy Scott Nolan Center, 555 Wilson Lane, Des Plaines, IL 60016; tel. 847/768-5430

Memorial Medical Center, 701 North First Street, Springfield, IL 62781-0001; tel. 217/788-3000

Mental Health and Deafness Resources, Inc., 614 Anthony Trail, Northbrook, IL 60062; tel. 847/509-8260

*Naperville Psychiatric Venture dba Linden Oaks Hospital, 801 South Washington, Naperville, IL 60566-7060; tel. 630/305-5500

*Near North Health Service Corporation, 1276 North Clybourn Avenue, Chicago, IL 60610; tel. 312/337-1073

*North Central Behavioral Health Systems, Inc., PO Box 1488, La Salle, IL 61301; tel. 815/223-0160

*NorthShore University HealthSystem, 1301 Central Street, Suite 300, Evanston, IL 60201; tel. 847/570-5005

*Northwest Community Hospital Youth Center, 901 Kirchoff Road, Arlington Heights, IL 60005; tel. 847/618-1000

---

*Indicates organization is a Joint Commission accredited Chemical Dependency organization.

*Palos Community Hospital, 12251 South 80th Avenue, Palos Heights, IL 60463; tel. 708/923-4000

PEER Services, Inc., 906 Davis Street, Evanston, IL 60201; tel. 847/492-1778

*Pioneer Center for Human Services/Youth Service Bureau, 101 South Jefferson Street, Woodstock, IL 60098; tel. 815/338-7360

*ProCare Centers, 1820 South 25th Avenue, Broadview, IL 60153; tel. 708/338-3806

*Provena Mercy Medical Center, 1325 North Highland Avenue, Aurora, IL 60506; tel. 630/859-2222

*Remedies Renewing Lives, 516 Green Street, Rockford, IL 61102; tel. 815/966-1285

Riveredge Hospital, 8311 West Roosevelt Road, Forest Park, IL 60130; tel. 708/771-7000

*Riverside Medical Center, 350 North Wall Street, Kankakee, IL 60901; tel. 815/933-1671

Rosecrance, Inc., 1021 N. Mulford Road, Rockford, IL 61107; tel. 815/387-5600

Rush University Medical Center, 1653 West Congress Parkway, Chicago, IL 60612; tel. 312/942-5000

Sequel Schools, LLC, 1150 North River Road, 100 Quigley Bldg., Des Plaines, IL 60016; tel. 847/391-8000

*Sinnissippi Centers, Inc., 325 Illinois Route 2, Dixon, IL 61021; tel. 815/284-6611

*Southeastern Illinois Counseling Centers, Inc., Drawer M, Olney, IL 62450; tel. 618/395-4306

*Southwood Interventions, 5701 South Wood, Chicago, IL 60636; tel. 773/737-4600

St. Mary's Hospital, 400 North Pleasant Avenue, Centralia, IL 62801; tel. 618/436-6519

Streamwood Behavioral Healthcare System, 1400 East Irving Park Road, Streamwood, IL 60107; tel. 630/837-9000

*Tazwood Mental Health Center, Inc., 3248 Vandever Avenue, Pekin, IL 61554; tel. 309/347-5579

*The Child, Adolescent and Family Recovery Center, LLC, 900 North Shore Drive Suite 140, Lake Bluff, IL 60044; tel. 847/457-6730

*The Pavilion Foundation, 809 West Church Street, Champaign, IL 61820; tel. 217/373-1700

*The South Suburban Council on Alcoholism and Substance Abuse, 1909 Cheker Square, Hazel Crest, IL 60429; tel. 708/647-3333

*The Women's Treatment Center, 140 N. Ashland Avenue, Chicago, IL 60607; tel. 312/850-0050

*Timberline Knolls, 40 Timberline Drive, Lemont, IL 60439; tel. 630/257-9600

*VA Medical Center, 2401 West Main Street, Marion, IL 62959; tel. 618/997-5311

*VA-Illiana Health Care System, 1900 East Main Street, Danville, IL 61832; tel. 217/554-3000

Waukegan IL Hospital Company, LLC, 2615 Washington Street, Waukegan, IL 60085; tel. 847/249-3900

Westlake Hospital-Opioid Treatment Programs, 1225 W. Lake Street, Melrose Park, IL 60160; tel. 708/938-4000

*Woodridge Interventions, 2221 64th Street, Woodridge, IL 60517; tel. 630/968-6477

## INDIANA

Adult and Child Mental Health Center, Inc., 222 E. Ohio Street Suite 600, Indianapolis, IN 46204; tel. 317/882-5122

*Aspire Indiana, 9516 East 148th Street, Noblesville, IN 46060; tel. 317/587-0500

*Bloomington Meadows Hospital, 3600 North Prow Road, Bloomington, IN 47404; tel. 812/331-8000

Columbus Hospital LLC, 2223 Poshard Drive, Columbus, IN 47203; tel. 812/376-1711

*Community Hospital East, 1500 North Ritter Avenue, Indianapolis, IN 46219; tel. 317/355-5520

Crossroad Child & Family Services, Inc., 2525 Lake Avenue, Fort Wayne, IN 46805-5457; tel. 260/484-4153

*Cummins Behavioral Health Systems, Inc., 6655 East US 36, Avon, IN 46123; tel. 317/272-3330

Elder Alternative Adult Day Services, 2236 E 10TH ST, Indianapolis, IN 46201-2006; tel. 317/633-3104

Evansville Psychiatric Children's Center, 3300 East Morgan Avenue, Evansville, IN 47715; tel. 812/477-6436

*Fairbanks Hospital, Inc., 8102 Clearvista Parkway, Indianapolis, IN 46256-4698; tel. 317/849-8222

*Family & Children's Center. Counseling & Development Services, 315 W. Jefferson, South Bend, IN 46601; tel. 574/968-9660

*Four County Comprehensive Mental Health, Inc., 1015 Michigan Avenue, Logansport, IN 46947; tel. 574/722-5151

*Good Samaritan Hospital, 520 South Seventh Street, Vincennes, IN 47591; tel. 812/885-3334

*Grant-Blackford Mental Health, Inc., 505 Wabash Avenue, Marion, IN 46952; tel. 765/662-3971

*Howard Regional Health System, PO Box 9011, Kokomo, IN 46904; tel. 765/453-8547

*LifeSpring, Inc., 460 Spring Street, Jeffersonville, IN 47130; tel. 812/280-0280

Logansport State Hospital, 1098 South State Road 25, Logansport, IN 46947; tel. 574/722-4141

Madison State Hospital, 711 Green Road, Madison, IN 47250; tel. 812/265-2611

*Meridian Services, Corporation, 240 North Tillotson Avenue, Muncie, IN 47304; tel. 765/288-1928

Michiana Behavioral Health Center, 1800 North Oak Drive, Plymouth, IN 46563; tel. 574/936-3784

*Oaklawn Psychiatric Center, Inc., PO Box 809 330 Lakeview Drive, Goshen, IN 46527-0809; tel. 574/533-1234

Options Treatment Center, 5602 Caito Drive, Indianapolis, IN 46226; tel. 317/544-4340

Person First Consulting, Inc, 6002 Morning Dove Drive, Indianapolis, IN 46228; tel. 317/750-0222

Persons Centered Value Partners, LLC, 4459 Peggy Hollow Road, Shoals, IN 47581; tel. 812/936-3543

Premier Care of Indiana, Inc., 317 S. Norton Avenue, Marion, IN 46952; tel. 765/664-0101

R.T.C. Resource Acquisition Corporation, 1404 South State, Indianapolis, IN 46203; tel. 317/783-4003

*Regional Mental Health Center, 8555 Taft Street, Merrillville, IN 46410-6199; tel. 219/769-4005

Resolute Acquisition Corporation, 320 North Tibbs, Indianapolis, IN 46222; tel. 317/630-5215

Riverview Adult Day Center, 2715 E Jackson Blvd, Elkhart, IN 46516-5053; tel. 574/293-6886

*Saint John's Health System, 2015 Jackson Street, Anderson, IN 46016; tel. 765/646-8373

Samlind of Indiana, Inc., 33149 State Road 2, New Carlisle, IN 46552; tel. 574/654-8700

*Southwestern Behavioral Healthcare, Inc., 415 Mulberry Street, Evansville, IN 47713-1298; tel. 812/436-4231

Starline Community Services, Inc., 2201 N. Division St, Mishawaka, IN 46545; tel. 574/323-8707

*Tara Treatment Center, Inc., 6231 South US 31, Franklin, IN 46131; tel. 812/526-2611

The Children's Campus, Inc., 1411 Lincoln Way West, Mishawaka, IN 46544-1690; tel. 574/259-5666

The Midwest Center for Youth and Families, PO Box 669, Kouts, IN 46347; tel. 219/766-2999

*The Otis R. Bowen Center for Human Services, Inc., PO Box 497, Warsaw, IN 46581-0497; tel. 574/267-7169

*VA Medical Center-Richard L. Roudebush VAMC, 1481 West 10th Street, Indianapolis, IN 46202; tel. 317/988-2121

*VA Northern Indiana Health Care System, 2121 Lake Avenue, Fort Wayne, IN 46805; tel. 260/460-1310

*Valle Vista Hospital, LLC, 898 East Main Street, Greenwood, IN 46143; tel. 317/887-1348

*Wabash Valley Alliance, Inc., 2900 North River Road, West Lafayette, IN 47906; tel. 765/464-0401

*Wellstone Regional Hospital Acquisition, LLC, 2700 Vissing Park Road, Jeffersonville, IN 47130; tel. 812/284-8000

Willowglen Academy-Indiana, Inc., 308 East 21st Avenue, Gary, IN 46407; tel. 219/886-1320

Wishard Health Services, 1001 W 10th Street, Indianapolis, IN 46202; tel. 317/655-2255

*Wishard Health Services, 1001 West Tenth Street, Indianapolis, IN 46202; tel. 317/639-6671

## IOWA

*Alegent Health Mercy Hospital, PO Box 1C, Council Bluffs, IA 51503; tel. 712/328-5000

Boys and Girls Home and Family Services, Inc., 2101 Court Street, Sioux City, IA 51104; tel. 712/293-4700

*Broadlawns Medical Center, 1801 Hickman Road, Des Moines, IA 50314; tel. 515/282-2200

Clarinda Youth Corporation, 1820 North 16th Street, Clarinda, IA 51632; tel. 712/542-3103

Hillcrest Family Services, 2005 Asbury Road, Dubuque, IA 52001; tel. 563/583-7357

*Iowa City VA Health Care System, 601 Highway 6 West, Iowa City, IA 52246; tel. 319/338-0581

Mental Health Institute, 2277 Iowa Avenue, Independence, IA 50644; tel. 319/334-2583

*Mercy Medical Center, 1111 6th Avenue, Des Moines, IA 50314; tel. 515/247-3121

*Orchard Place, 925 Porter Avenue, Des Moines, IA 50315; tel. 515/285-6781

Special Needs Services, P.O. Box 4117, Waterloo, IA 50704; tel. 319/277-3966

*St. Luke's Methodist Hospital, 1026 A Avenue Northeast, Cedar Rapids, IA 52402; tel. 319/369-7211

*The University of Iowa Hospitals and Clinics, 200 Hawkins Drive, Iowa City, IA 52242; tel. 319/384-5897

*VA Central Iowa Health Care System, 3600 30th Street, Des Moines, IA 50310-5774; tel. 515/699-5850

Woodward Academy, 1251 334th Street, Woodward, IA 50276; tel. 515/438-3481

## KANSAS

*Atchison Valley Hope, PO Box 312, Atchison, KS 66002; tel. 913/367-1618

Haskell Health Center, 2415 Massachusetts, Lawrence, KS 66046; tel. 785/843-4890

Kansas City Metro Methadone Program, MS 4015, 3901 Rainbow Boulevard, Kansas City, KS 66160-7341; tel. 913/588-6493

KVC Behavioral HealthCare, Inc., 21350 West 153rd Street, Olathe, KS 66061; tel. 913/322-4900

*Marillac Center Inc., 8000 W. 127th Street, Overland Park, KS 66213; tel. 816/508-3300

*Moundridge Valley Hope, P.O. Box 956, Moundridge, KS 67107; tel. 620/345-4673

*Munson Army Health Center, Building 343 - 550 Pope Avenue, Fort Leavenworth, KS 66027-2332; tel. 913/684-6420

*Norton Valley Hope, PO Box 510, Norton, KS 67654; tel. 785/877-5101

*Prairie View, Inc., PO Box 467, Newton, KS 67114; tel. 316/284-6400

*Robert J. Dole VA Medical Center, 5500 East Kellogg, Wichita, KS 67218; tel. 316/651-3601

*Saint Francis Community Services, Inc., 509 East Elm Street, Salina, KS 67401; tel. 785/825-0541

Sequel of Kansas, LLC, 2050 West 11th Street, Wichita, KS 67203; tel. 316/267-5710

*United Methodist Youthville, Inc., 4505 E 47th Street South, Wichita, KS 67210; tel. 316/529-9100

*VA Eastern Kansas Health Care System, 2200 SW Gage, Topeka, KS 66622; tel. 785/350-3111

VCPHCS XIV, LLC dba Bridge Way Recovery, 6331 West 110th ST, Overland Park, KS 66211; tel. 936/524-2140

## KENTUCKY

*Blanchfield Army Community Hospital, MCXD-DCMCC 650 Joe Drive, Fort Campbell, KY 42223-5349; tel. 270/798-8512

*Bluegrass Regional Mental Health-Mental Retardation Board, 1351 Newtown Pike, Bldg 1, Lexington, KY 40511-1277; tel. 859/253-1686

*Cumberland River Regional MH/MR Board, Inc., PO Box 568, Corbin, KY 40702; tel. 606/528-7010

*Ireland Army Community Hospital, 851 Ireland Ave, Fort Knox, KY 40121-5520; tel. 502/624-0251

*Jewish Hospital & St. Mary's HealthCare, Inc., 200 Abraham Flexner Way, Louisville, KY 40202-1886; tel. 502/587-4011

KVC Behavioral HealthCare Kentucky, Inc., 900 Beasley Street, #120, Lexington, KY 40509; tel. 859/254-1035

*Lincoln Trail Behavioral Health System, PO Box 369, Radcliff, KY 40160; tel. 270/351-9444

*NorthKey Community Care, PO Box 2680, Covington, KY 41012; tel. 859/578-3233

*Recovery Works Drug & Alcohol Rehabilitation Center, 3107 Cincinnati Road, Georgetown, KY 40324; tel. 502/570-9313

*Seven Counties Services, Inc., 101 West Muhammad Ali Blvd, Louisville, KY 40202; tel. 502/589-8600

Spectrum Care Academy, Inc., PO Box 911, Columbia, KY 42728; tel. 270/384-6444

Sunrise Children's Services, P.O. Box 1429, Mount Washington, KY 40047-1429; tel. 502/538-1000

*Indicates organization is a Joint Commission accredited Chemical Dependency organization.

Section C

**\*The Brook Hospital-Dupont,** 1405 Browns Lane, Louisville, KY 40207; tel. 502/426-0495

**\*The Brook Hospital-KMI,** 8521 LaGrange Road, Louisville, KY 40242; tel. 502/426-6380

**\*VA Medical Center,** 1101 Veterans Drive, Lexington, KY 40502-2236; tel. 859/233-4511

**\*VA Medical Center,** 800 Zorn Avenue, Louisville, KY 40206; tel. 502/287-4000

**LOUISIANA**

**Acadia Vermilion Hospital,** 2520 North University Avenue, Lafayette, LA 70507; tel. 337/234-5614

**Acceptable Health Services, LLC,** 5640 Rad Blvd, Ste 740, New Orleans, LA 70126; tel. 504/245-2440

**\*Brentwood Acquisition-Shreveport, Inc.,** 1006 Highland Avenue, Shreveport, LA 71101; tel. 318/678-7500

**Community Care Hospital,** 1421 General Taylor Street, New Orleans, LA 70115; tel. 504/899-2500

**Crossroads Regional Hospital,** 44 Versailles Blvd, Alexandria, LA 71303; tel. 318/445-5111

**DRD New Orleans Medical Clinic,** 417 S. Johnson Street, New Orleans, LA 70112; tel. 504/524-7205

**Eastern Louisiana Mental Health System,** PO Box 498, Jackson, LA 70748-0498; tel. 225/634-0216

**Ekems Healthcare, Inc.,** 8470 Morrison Road suite A, New Orleans, LA 70127; tel. 504/248-1581

**Leesville Rehabilitation Hospital,** 900 South Sixth Street, Leesville, LA 71446; tel. 337/392-8118

**Liberty HealthCare Systems, LLC,** 4673 Eugene Ware Blvd, Bastrop, LA 71220; tel. 318/281-2448

**Minden Medical Center,** P.O. Box 5003, Minden, LA 71058-5003; tel. 318/377-2321

**Natchitoches Regional Medical Center,** PO Box 2009, Natchitoches, LA 71457; tel. 318/214-4200

**Oceans Behavioral Hospital of Greater New Orleans,** 716 Village Road, Kenner, LA 70065; tel. 504/464-8895

**Oceans Behavioral Hospital of Lafayette,** 420 Albertson Parkway, Broussard, LA 70518; tel. 337/839-9008

**\*Overton Brooks VA Medical Center,** 510 East Stoner Avenue, Shreveport, LA 71101-4295; tel. 318/221-8411

**Positive Choices Counseling Services, Inc.,** P.O. Box 614, Vidalia, LA 71373; tel. 318/336-4700

**Provision Rehab LLC.,** 6 Bienville Square South Drive, Natchitoches, LA 71457; tel. 318/238-4030

**River Oaks, Inc.,** 1525 River Oaks Road West, New Orleans, LA 70123; tel. 504/734-1740

**Seaside Health System,** 615 E. Worthy Road, Gonzales, LA 70737; tel. 225/238-3043

**Southeast Louisiana Veterans Healthcare System,** P.O. Box 61011, New Orleans, LA 70161-1011; tel. 504/565-4836

**Success Counseling Services-North,** 1504 Barksdale Boulevard, Bossier City, LA 71111; tel. 318/222-4299

**\*VA Medical Center,** PO Box 69004, Alexandria, LA 71306; tel. 318/473-0010

**VCPHCS V, LLC d.b.a, New Orleans Narcotic Treatment Program,** 1141 Whitney Avenue Building 4, Gretna, LA 70056; tel. 504/347-1120

**VCPHCS VI, LLC d.b.a. Lake Charles Substance Abuse Clinic,** 2829 4th Ave, Suite 200, Lake Charles, LA 70601; tel. 337/433-8281

**MAINE**

**Acadia Hospital-Narcotic Treatment Program,** PO Box 422, Bangor, ME 04402-0422; tel. 207/973-6100

**Cap Quality Care, Inc.,** 1 Delta Drive, Suite A, Westbrook, ME 04092; tel. 207/856-7227

**Cary Medical Center,** 163 Van Buren Road, Caribou, ME 04736; tel. 207/498-3111

**Maine Medical Center,** 22 Bramhall Street, Portland, ME 04102; tel. 207/662-0111

**MaineGeneral Medical Center,** 149 North Street, ME, 04901,, Waterville, ME 04901; tel. 207/872-1000

**Mercy Recovery Center,** 40 Park Road, Westbrook, ME 04092; tel. 207/857-8085

**Riverview Psychiatric Center,** 11 State House Station, Augusta, ME 04333-0011; tel. 207/624-4683

**\*St. Mary's Regional Medical Center,** PO Box 291, Campus Avenue, Lewiston, ME 04243-0291; tel. 207/777-8100

**\*The Acadia Hospital,** PO Box 422, Bangor, ME 04402-0422; tel. 207/973-6100

**\*VA Maine Healthcare System,** 1 Va Center, Augusta, ME 04330; tel. 207/623-8411

**MARYLAND**

**Addiction Treatment Services of Hopkins Bayview,** 5200 Eastern Avenue, MFL-6-E, Baltimore, MD 21224; tel. 410/550-0004

**Adventist Behavioral Health Eastern Shore,** 821 Fieldcrest Road, Cambridge, MD 21613; tel. 410/221-0288

**\*Adventist Health Care, Inc.,** 14901 Broschart Road, Rockville, MD 20850; tel. 301/251-4500

**\*Ashley, Inc.,** 800 Tydings Lane, Havre De Grace, MD 21078; tel. 410/273-6600

**Awakenings,** 2 West Aylesbury Road, Timonium, MD 21093; tel. 410/561-9591

**\*Baltimore Behavioral Health, Inc.,** 1001 W Pratt Street/201 S. Arlington, Baltimore, MD 21223; tel. 410/962-7180

**Behavioral Pharmacology Research Unit,** 5510 Nathan Shock Drive, Baltimore, MD 21224; tel. 410/550-0035

**\*Bon Secours Hospital Baltimore, Inc.,** 2000 West Baltimore Street, Baltimore, MD 21223; tel. 410/362-3011

**Bon Secours New Hope Treatment Center,** 2401 West Baltimore Street, Baltimore, MD 21223; tel. 410/945-7706

**Brook Lane Health Services,** PO Box 1945, Hagerstown, MD 21742-1945; tel. 301/733-0330

**Calvert Memorial Hospital,** 100 Hospital Road, Prince Frederick, MD 20678; tel. 410/535-4000

**\*Carroll Hospital Center, Inc.,** 200 Memorial Avenue, Westminster, MD 21157; tel. 410/871-6523

**Catholic Charities Child and Family Services,** 2300 Dulaney Valley Road, Timonium, MD 21093; tel. 410/252-4700

**Center for Addiction Medicine,** 827 Linden Avenue, Baltimore, MD 21201; tel. 410/225-8240

**\*Chase Brexton Health Services, Inc.,** 1001 Cathedral Street, Baltimore, MD 21201; tel. 410/837-2050

**\*Crossroads Center of Frederick,** 203 Broadway Street Suite A, Frederick, MD 21701; tel. 301/696-1950

**Daybreak Rehabilitation Center,** 2490 Giles Road, Baltimore, MD 21225; tel. 410/396-1646

**Eastern Shore Hospital Center,** PO Box 800, Cambridge, MD 21613; tel. 410/221-2527

**\*Family Health Centers of Baltimore, Inc.,** 631 Cherry Hill Road, Baltimore, MD 21225; tel. 410/354-2000

**\*Fort Meade USA MEDDAC,** 2480 Llewellyn Avenue, Fort George G Meade, MD 20755-5129; tel. 301/677-8171

**Frederick County Health Department /Substance Abuse Services,** 300-B Scholl's Lane, Frederick, MD 21701; tel. 301/600-1775

**Glass Substance Abuse Program, Inc.,** 821 North Eutaw Street, Baltimore, MD 21202; tel. 410/225-9185

**\*Health Care for the Homeless, Inc.,** 421 Fallsway, Baltimore, MD 21202; tel. 410/837-5533

**Hope Health Systems, Inc.,** 6707 Whitestone Road, Ste 106, Woodlawn, MD 21207; tel. 410/265-8737

**House of the Good Shepherd of the City of Baltimore,** 4100 Maple Avenue, Baltimore, MD 21227; tel. 410/247-2770

**\*Hudson Health Services, Inc.,** PO Box 1096, Salisbury, MD 21802-1096; tel. 410/219-9000

**John L. Gildner Regional Institute for Children & Adolescents,** 15000 Broschart Road, Rockville, MD 20850; tel. 301/251-6800

**\*Johns Hopkins Bayview Medical Center,** 4940 Eastern Avenue, Baltimore, MD 21224-2780; tel. 410/550-0120

**Laurel Regional Hospital,** 7300 Van Dusen Road, Laurel, MD 20707; tel. 301/497-7984

**Levindale Hebrew Geriatric Center and Hospital,** 2434 West Belvedere Avenue, Baltimore, MD 21215; tel. 410/466-8700

**Maple Shade Youth & Family Services, Inc.,** 23704 Ocean Gateway, Mardela Springs, MD 21837; tel. 410/742-7400

**\*Maryland Treatment Centers, Inc.,** PO Box 136, Emmitsburg, MD 21727; tel. 301/447-2361

**MBA Southeast Baltimore County,** 8860 Citation Road Suite B, Essex, MD 21221; tel. 410/486-2500

**MBA-Cherry Hill,** 2490 Giles Road, Baltimore, MD 21225; tel. 410/225-9185

**MedStar St. Mary's Hospital,** PO Box 527, Leonardtown, MD 20650; tel. 301/475-8981

**\*Meritus Medical Center,** 11116 Medical Campus Road, Hagerstown, MD 21742; tel. 301/790-8000

**Methadone for Business Achievers (MBA),** 821 North Eutaw Street, Baltimore, MD 21201; tel. 410/225-9185

**Methadone for Business Achievers-Timonium,** 2 West Aylesbury Road, Timonium, MD 21093; tel. 410/561-9591

**\*Mid-Atlantic Treatment Services,** 2100 North Charles Street, Baltimore, MD 21218; tel. 410/752-0505

**\*Montgomery General Hospital,** 18101 Prince Philip Drive, Olney, MD 20832; tel. 301/774-8770

**\*National Naval Medical Center,** 8901 Wisconsin Avenue, Bethesda, MD 20889-5600; tel. 301/319-4618

**\*Naval Health Clinic Annapolis,** 250 Wood Road, Annapolis, MD 21402-5050; tel. 410/293-1330

**\*Naval Health Clinic, Patuxent River,** 47149 Buse Road, Building 1370, Patuxent River, MD 20670-5370; tel. 301/342-1418

**\*Pathways,** 2620 Riva Road, Annapolis, MD 21401; tel. 410/573-5400

**\*People's Community Health Center, Inc.,** 2524 Kirk Avenue, Baltimore, MD 21218; tel. 410/467-6040

**\*Prince George's County Health Department,** 1701 McCormick Drive, Suite 230, Largo, MD 20774; tel. 301/883-7903

**Reflective Treatment Center,** 301 N Gay Street, Baltimore, MD 21202; tel. 410/752-3500

**Regional Institute for Children and Adolescents-Baltimore,** 605 South Chapel Gate Lane, Baltimore, MD 21229; tel. 410/368-7800

**Saint Luke Institute,** 8901 New Hampshire Avenue, Silver Spring, MD 20903; tel. 301/445-7970

**Sheppard Pratt Health System, Inc.,** PO Box 6815, Baltimore, MD 21285-6815; tel. 410/938-4281

**Sinai Hospital Addictions Recovery Program,** 2401 West Belvedere Avenue, Baltimore, MD 21215; tel. 410/601-5355

**Spring Grove Hospital Center,** 55 Wade Avenue, Catonsville, MD 21228; tel. 410/402-6000

**Springfield Hospital Center,** 6655 Sykesville Road, Sykesville, MD 21784; tel. 410/970-7000

**\*The Johns Hopkins Hospital,** 600 North Wolfe Street, Baltimore, MD 21287; tel. 410/955-5000

**The Union Memorial Hospital,** 201 East University Parkway, Baltimore, MD 21218; tel. 410/554-2000

**Thomas B. Finan Center,** PO Box 1722 Country Club Road, Cumberland, MD 21501-1722; tel. 301/777-2405

**\*Tuerk House, Inc.,** 730 Ashburton Street, Baltimore, MD 21216-6116; tel. 410/233-0684

**\*University of Maryland Medical Center,** 22 South Greene Street, Baltimore, MD 21201-1595; tel. 410/328-6027

**\*VA Maryland Health Care System,** 10 North Greene Street, Baltimore, MD 21201; tel. 410/605-7000

**Wicomico County Health Department,** 108 East Main Street, Salisbury, MD 21801; tel. 410/742-3784

**Woodbourne Center, Inc.,** 1301 Woodbourne Avenue, Baltimore, MD 21239; tel. 410/433-1000

**\*Worcester County Health Department,** PO Box 249, Snow Hill, MD 21863; tel. 410/632-1100

**MASSACHUSETTS**

**Academic & Behavioral Clinic,** P.O. Box 190789, Roxbury, MA 02119; tel. 617/822-0829

**\*AdCare Hospital of Worcester, Inc.,** 107 Lincoln Street, Worcester, MA 01605-2499; tel. 508/799-9000

**Arbour Hospital Inc.,** 49 Robinwood Avenue, Jamaica Plain, MA 02130; tel. 617/522-4400

**Arbour-Fuller Hospital,** 200 May Street, South Attleboro, MA 02703; tel. 508/761-8500

**Arbour-HRI Hospital,** 227 Babcock Street, Brookline, MA 02446; tel. 617/731-3200

**Austen Riggs Center,** 25 Main Street, Stockbridge, MA 01262-0962; tel. 413/298-5511

**Baldpate Hospital,** 83 Baldpate Road, Georgetown, MA 01833; tel. 978/352-2131

**Baystate Franklin Medical Center,** 164 High Street, Greenfield, MA 01301; tel. 413/773-0211

**Baystate Medical Center,** 759 Chestnut Street, Springfield, MA 01199; tel. 413/794-5960

**\*Berkshire Medical Center,** 725 North Street, Pittsfield, MA 01201; tel. 413/447-2464

---

\*Indicates organization is a Joint Commission accredited Chemical Dependency organization.

**\*Bournewood Hospital,** 300 South Street, Chestnut Hill, MA 02467; tel. 617/469–0300

**Bridgewater State Hospital,** 20 Administration Road, Bridgewater, MA 02324; tel. 508/279–4500

**Brockton Multi Service Center,** 165 Quincy Street, Brockton, MA 02302; tel. 508/897–2000

**Cambridge Eating Disorder Center,** 3 Bow Street, Cambridge, MA 02138; tel. 617/547–2255

**Cape Cod and Islands Community Mental Health Center,** 830 County Road, Pocasset, MA 02559; tel. 508/564–9600

**Centerpoint,** PO Box 374, Tewksbury, MA 01876; tel. 978/858–3776

**Cohannet Academy,** 60 Hodges Avenue - Goss 3, Taunton, MA 02780; tel. 508/977–3730

**Counseling & Assessment Clinic of Worcester, LLC,** 38 Front Street, 5th Floor, Worcester, MA 01608; tel. 508/756–5400

**\*Dimock Community Foundation, Inc.,** 45 Dimock Street, Roxbury, MA 02119; tel. 617/442–8800

**Dimock Community Foundation, Inc.-Opioid Treatment Programs,** 55 Dimock Street, Roxbury, MA 02119; tel. 617/442–8800

**Doctor Franklin Perkins School,** 971 Main Street, Lancaster, MA 01523; tel. 978/365–7376

**Dr. John C. Corrigan Mental Health Center,** 49 Hillside Street, Fall River, MA 02720; tel. 508/235–7200

**Dr. Solomon Carter Fuller Mental Health Center,** 85 E. Newton Street, Boston, MA 02118; tel. 917/626–8861

**\*Edith Nourse Rogers Memorial Veterans Hospital,** 200 Springs Road, Bedford, MA 01730; tel. 781/687–3080

**Federal Bureau of Prisons Federal Medical Center Devens,** PO Box 880, Ayer, MA 01432; tel. 978/796–1443

**\*Fenway Community Health Center, Inc.,** 1340 Boylston Street, Boston, MA 02215; tel. 617/267–0900

**Franciscan Hospital for Children, Inc.,** 30 Warren Street, Boston, MA 02135-3680; tel. 617/254–3800

**\*Gosnold, Inc.,** 200 Ter Heun Drive, Falmouth, MA 02540; tel. 508/540–6550

**\*High Point Treatment Center, Inc.,** 100 North Front Street 3rd Fl, New Bedford, MA 02740; tel. 774/628–1095

**High Point Treatment Center, Inc.,** 1233 State Road, Plymouth, MA 02360-5133; tel. 508/224–7701

**High Point Treatment Center-Opioid Treatment Programs,** 10 Meadowbrook Road, Brockton, MA 02301; tel. 508/742–4400

**Hillcrest Educational Centers, Inc.,** 788 South Street, Pittsfield, MA 01201; tel. 413/499–7924

**Justice Resource Institute Behavioral Health Centers,** 380 Massachusetts Ave, Acton, MA 01720; tel. 978/264–3500

**Justice Resource Institute--The Meadowridge Schools,** 56-58 Framingham Road, Marlborough, MA 01752; tel. 617/450–0500

**LAMOUR By Design Inc.,** 4244 Diauto Drive, Randolph, MA 02368; tel. 781/885–7252

**Laurel Hill Inn, Ltd.,** PO Box 368, Medford, MA 02155-0004; tel. 781/396–1116

**\*Lowell Community Health Center,** 586 Merrimack Street, Lowell, MA 01854; tel. 978/937–9700

**\*Lynn Community Health Center,** PO Box 526, Lynn, MA 01903; tel. 781/596–2502

**\*McLean Hospital,** 115 Mill Street, Belmont, MA 02478; tel. 617/855–3450

**\*Mercy Hospital,** 271 Carew Street, Springfield, MA 01104; tel. 413/748–9000

**Mercy Medical Center Inpatient Detox Program,** 1233 Main Street, Holyoke, MA 01040; tel. 413/539–2950

**Mercy Medical Center-MMTP,** 227 Mill Street, Springfield, MA 01102; tel. 413/539–2400

**MetroWest Medical Center,** 115 Lincoln Street, Framingham, MA 01702; tel. 508/383–1000

**NFI Massachusetts(Northeastern Family Institute),** PO Box 732, Westborough, MA 01581; tel. 978/774–0774

**North End Community Health Committee, Inc.,** 332 Hanover Street, Boston, MA 02113; tel. 617/643–8000

**\*Northeast Hospital Corporation,** 85 Herrick Street, Beverly, MA 01915-1777; tel. 978/922–3000

**Osiris Family Institute, LLC,** 184 Dudley Street Suite 107 LL, Roxbury, MA 02119; tel. 617/442–2002

**Priority Professional Care, LLC,** 1613 Blue Hill Ave Suite 302, Mattapan, MA 02126; tel. 857/598–4774

**Pyramid Builders Associates,** 1960 Washington Street, Boston, MA 02118; tel. 617/516–0280

**SSTAR,** 1010 South Main Street, Fall River, MA 02721; tel. 508/235–5010

**SSTAR DETOX,** 386 Stanley Street, Fall River, MA 02720; tel. 508/324–3500

**Steward Saint Anne's Hospital,** 795 Middle Street, Fall River, MA 02721-1798; tel. 508/674–5600

**The Three Rivers Treatment Program,** 26 Ridgewood Terrace, Springfield, MA 01105; tel. 413/733–4032

**The Whitney Academy, Inc.,** PO Box 619, East Freetown, MA 02717; tel. 508/763–3737

**University of Massachusetts Medical School, Transitions IRTP,** 305 Belmont Street, 7th Flr C, Worcester, MA 01604; tel. 508/856–1439

**\*VA Boston Healthcare System,** 1400 VFW Parkway, West Roxbury, MA 02132; tel. 617/323–7700

**Walden Behavioral Care,** 9 Hope Avenue, Waltham, MA 02453; tel. 781/647–6767

**Westwood Pembroke Health System,** 45 Clapboardtree Street, Westwood, MA 02090; tel. 781/762–7764

**Whittier Pavilion,** 76 Summer Street, Haverhill, MA 01830; tel. 978/373–8222

**Wild Acre Inns, Inc.,** 108 Pleasant Street, Arlington, MA 02476; tel. 781/643–0643

## MICHIGAN

**\*ACAC, Inc.,** 3949 Sparks Drive SE Suite 103, Grand Rapids, MI 49546; tel. 616/957–5850

**\*Access Behavioral Healthcare, LLC,** 42189 E. Ann Arbor Road, Plymouth, MI 48170; tel. 734/453–5603

**\*Aleda E. Lutz VA Medical Center,** 1500 Weiss Street, Saginaw, MI 48602; tel. 989/497–2500

**\*Apex Behavioral Health, PLLC,** 1547 S. Wayne Rd., Westland, MI 48186; tel. 734/729–3133

**\*Apex Behavioral Health-Dearborn,** 6 Parklane Blvd, Ste 695, Dearborn, MI 48126; tel. 313/271–8170

**\*Apex Downriver Behavioral Health,** 19366 Allen Road, Ste C, Brownstown, MI 48183; tel. 734/479–0949

**\*Arbor Circle Corporation,** 1115 Ball Avenue, Grand Rapids, MI 49505; tel. 616/456–7775

**\*Battle Creek VA Medical Center,** 5500 Armstrong Road, Battle Creek, MI 49037; tel. 269/966–5600

**\*Bay Mills Indian Community,** 12124 West Lake Shore Drive, Brimley, MI 49715; tel. 906/248–5526

**Beacon Specialized Living Services, Inc.,** 555 Railroad Street P.O. 69, Bangor, MI 49013; tel. 269/427–8400

**\*Brighton Hospital,** 12851 Grand River Road, Brighton, MI 48116; tel. 810/227–1211

**C.W. Enterprises LLC,** 50630 Chesterfield Road, Chesterfield, MI 48051; tel. 586/949–7680

**\*Catholic Services of Macomb, Inc.,** 15945 Canal Road, Clinton Township, MI 48038; tel. 586/416–2300

**\*Community Care Services,** 26184 West Outer Drive, Lincoln Park, MI 48146; tel. 313/389–7525

**Community Mental Health for Central Michigan,** 301 South Crapo, Suite 100, Mount Pleasant, MI 48858; tel. 989/772–5938

**Delta Family Clinic South,** 6195 Miller Road, Suite A, Swartz Creek, MI 48473; tel. 810/630–1152

**Forest View Psychiatric Hospital,** 1055 Medical Park Drive SE, Grand Rapids, MI 49546; tel. 616/942–9610

**Genesys Practice Partners, Inc.,** 8435 Holly Road, Grand Blanc, MI 48439; tel. 810/424–2400

**\*Growth Works Incorporated,** PO Box 6115, Plymouth, MI 48170-6115; tel. 734/455–4095

**\*Harbor Oaks Hospital,** 35031 23 Mile Road, New Baltimore, MI 48047; tel. 586/725–5777

**Havenwyck Hospital,** 1525 University Drive, Auburn Hills, MI 48326; tel. 248/373–9200

**\*Hegira Programs, Inc.,** 8623 N Wayne Road, Suite 200, Westland, MI 48185; tel. 734/458–4601

**\*Henry Ford Macomb Hospital,** 15855 Nineteen Mile Road, Clinton Township, MI 48038; tel. 586/263–2700

**\*Horizon Treatment Services, LLC,** 17515 W. 9 Mile Rd., Suite 720, Southfield, MI 48075; tel. 248/423–1728

**Huron Valley Consultation Center, Inc.,** 2750 South State Street, Ann Arbor, MI 48104; tel. 734/662–6300

**Integro, LLC,** 1200 N West Avenue, Suite 300, Jackson, MI 49202; tel. 517/789–1234

**\*Ionia County Substance Abuse,** 175 E. Adams, Ionia, MI 48846; tel. 616/527–5341

**\*John D. Dingell VA Medical Center,** 4646 John R, Detroit, MI 48201; tel. 313/576–1000

**\*Jump Start Consulting, LLC dba Inner Door Center,** 317 East Eleven Mile Road, Royal Oak, MI 48067; tel. 248/336–2868

**\*Karalee & Associates, P.C.,** 1308 South Main Street, Plymouth, MI 48170; tel. 734/451–3440

**Kingswood Hospital,** 10300 West Eight Mile Road, Ferndale, MI 48220; tel. 313/874–6260

**Lakeside Academy,** 3921 Oakland Drive, Kalamazoo, MI 49008; tel. 269/381–4760

**\*Latino Family Services, Inc.,** 3815 West Fort Street, Detroit, MI 48216; tel. 313/841–7380

**Lenawee Community Mental Health Authority,** 1040 S. Winter Street, Suite#1022, Adrian, MI 49221; tel. 517/263–8905

**Livingston County Community Mental Health Authority,** 2280 East Grand River, Howell, MI 48843; tel. 517/546–4126

**\*McLaren Regional Medical Center,** 401 South Ballenger Highway, Flint, MI 48532; tel. 810/342–2000

**\*Meridian Professional Psychological Consultants, PC,** 5031 Park Lake Road, East Lansing, MI 48823; tel. 517/332–0811

**Metro East Substance Abuse Treatment Corporation,** PO Box 13408, Detroit, MI 48213; tel. 313/371–0055

**Michigan Access Center, Inc.,** 2722 East Michigan Avenue Suite 104, Lansing, MI 48912; tel. 517/332–9000

**\*Michigan Behavior Medicine,** 2525 Crooks Rd suite100, Troy, MI 48084; tel. 248/740–9360

**\*Michigan Psychiatric & Behavioral Associates, P.C.,** 690 South Trumbull Street, Bay City, MI 48708; tel. 989/922–4900

**Monroe Community Mental Health Authority,** P.O. Box 726, Monroe, MI 48161-0726; tel. 734/243–7340

**Nardin Park Recovery Center,** 9605 Grand River, Detroit, MI 48204; tel. 313/834–5930

**New Center Community Services,** 2051 West Grand Boulevard, Detroit, MI 48208; tel. 313/961–3200

**\*Oakland Psychological Clinic, P.C.,** 2550 South Telegraph Road Suite 250, Bloomfield Hills, MI 48302; tel. 248/322–0003

**Oakwood Heritage Hospital,** 10000 Telegraph Road, Taylor, MI 48180; tel. 313/295–5000

**Opioid Treatment Program-John D. Dingell VA Medical Center,** 4646 John R. Street, Detroit, MI 48201; tel. 313/576–4314

**\*Oscar G. Johnson VA Medical Center,** 325 East H Street, Iron Mountain, MI 49801; tel. 906/774–3300

**Rainbow Center of Michigan (Monroe),** 14733 South Telegraph Road, Monroe, MI 48161; tel. 734/243–8707

**Rainbow Center of Michigan, Inc.,** 20724 Eureka Road, Taylor, MI 48180; tel. 734/759–0510

**Rainbow Center of Michigan, Inc.,** P O Box 725098, Berkley, MI 48072; tel. 313/865–1580

**\*Recovery Pathways, LLC,** 717 E. Midland Street, Bay City, MI 48706; tel. 989/928–3566

**\*Redford Counseling Center,** 25945 West Seven Mile Road, Redford, MI 48240; tel. 313/535–6560

**\*River's Bend, P.C.,** 800 Stephenson Highway, Suite 250, Troy, MI 48083; tel. 248/585–3239

**Rose Hill Center, Inc.,** 5130 Rose Hill Boulevard, Holly, MI 48442; tel. 248/634–5530

**Safehaus, Inc.,** 21056 Dean Street, Warren, MI 48091; tel. 586/806–4678

**Saint Mary's Health Care,** 200 Jefferson Avenue Southeast, Grand Rapids, MI 49503; tel. 616/685–5000

**St. John Providence Macomb-Oakland Hospital,** 11800 East Twelve Mile Road, Warren, MI 48093; tel. 586/573–5443

**\*St. Joseph Mercy Hospital,** 5301 E Huron River Drive PO Box 995, Ann Arbor, MI 48106-0995; tel. 734/712–3456

**Star Center, Inc.,** 13575 Lesure, Detroit, MI 48227; tel. 313/493–4410

**\*Sterling Area Health Center,** PO Box 740, Sterling, MI 48659; tel. 989/654–2491

**Summit Pointe,** 140 West Michigan Avenue, Battle Creek, MI 49017; tel. 269/966–1460

**Sunshine Treatment Institute,** P.O. Box 690, Southfield, MI 48037; tel. 313/368–4800

**Taylor Psychological Clinic, PC,** 1172 Robert T Longway Blvd, Flint, MI 48503; tel. 810/232–8466

---

*Indicates organization is a Joint Commission accredited Chemical Dependency organization.

Section C

**TBCI, PC,** 1059 Owendale, Troy, MI 48083; tel. 248/526-0110

*****The Guidance Center,** 13101 Allen Road, Southgate, MI 48195; tel. 734/785-7700

**The Montcalm Center for Behavioral Health,** 611 North State Street, Stanton, MI 48888; tel. 989/831-7520

*****The Salvation Army Turning Point Programs,** 72 Sheldon Boulevard, SE, Grand Rapids, MI 49503; tel. 616/742-0351

*****The University of Michigan Hospitals and Health Centers,** 2101 Commonwealth, Suite A, Ann Arbor, MI 48105; tel. 734/647-2478

**Ultimate Solutions,** 29240 Buckingham, Suite 11, Livonia, MI 48154; tel. 734/513-2800

*****VA Ann Arbor Healthcare System,** 2215 Fuller Road, Ann Arbor, MI 48105; tel. 734/769-7100

*****WA Foote Memorial Hospital,** 205 North East Avenue, Jackson, MI 49201; tel. 517/788-4800

*****Washtenaw County Community Supports and Treatment Services,** 2140 East Ellsworth Road, Ann Arbor, MI 48108; tel. 734/544-3000

### MINNESOTA

**Abbott Northwestern Hospital,** 800 East 28th Street, Minneapolis, MN 55407; tel. 612/863-4875

**Andrew Residence,** 1215 South 9th Street, Minneapolis, MN 55404; tel. 612/333-0111

**Anoka-Metro Regional Treatment Center,** 3301 7th Avenue North, Anoka, MN 55303; tel. 651/431-5000

**Bureau of Prisons-FMC Rochester,** PO Box 4600, Rochester, MN 55903; tel. 507/287-0674

**Child and Adolescent Behavioral Health Services,** 1701 Technology Drive, Willmar, MN 56201; tel. 218/330-7406

*****Community Addiction Recovery Enterprise,** 3301 Seventh Avenue North, Anoka, MN 55303; tel. 651/431-5020

**Community Addiction Recovery Enterprise-Willmar Opioid Treatment Programs,** 1801 Technology Drive Northeast, Willmar, MN 56201; tel. 320/231-5356

*****Hazelden Foundation, Recovery Services Division,** PO Box 11, Center City, MN 55012; tel. 612/257-4200

**Hennepin Faculty Associates,** 600 Shapiro Building 914 South Eighth Street, Minneapolis, MN 55404; tel. 612/347-5000

**Hennepin Faculty Associates Addiction Medicine Program,** 914 South Eighth Street Suite 131, Minneapolis, MN 55404; tel. 612/347-7600

**Hennepin Healthcare System, Inc.,** 701 Park Avenue, Minneapolis, MN 55415; tel. 612/873-2338

*****Mayo Clinic Health System in Albert Lea,** 404 West Fountain Street, Albert Lea, MN 56007; tel. 507/373-2384

**Mercy Hospital,** 4050 Coon Rapids Boulevard, Coon Rapids, MN 55433; tel. 763/236-6000

**Minnesota Security Hospital,** 100 Freeman Drive, Saint Peter, MN 56082; tel. 507/985-3128

**Minnesota Specialty Health Systems-Brainerd,** 11615 State Avenue, Brainerd, MN 56401; tel. 218/828-6123

**Minnesota Specialty Health Systems-Wadena,** 240 Shady Lane Drive, Wadena, MN 56482; tel. 218/319-6001

**Minnesota Specialty Health Systems-Willmar,** 1208 Olena Avenue SE, Willmar, MN 56201; tel. 320/235-0018

*****New Beginnings at Waverly, LLC,** 109 North Shore Drive, Waverly, MN 55390-9743; tel. 763/658-5800

**Park Nicollet Health Services,** PO Box 650, Minneapolis, MN 55440; tel. 952/993-5000

**PrairieCare,** 12915 63rd Avenue North, Maple Grove, MN 55369; tel. 952/838-5800

*****Saint Cloud Hospital,** 1406 Sixth Avenue North, Saint Cloud, MN 56303; tel. 320/251-2700

*****SMDC Medical Center,** 502 East Second Street, Duluth, MN 55805; tel. 218/727-8762

*****St. Cloud VA Health Care System,** 4801 Veterans Drive, Saint Cloud, MN 56303; tel. 320/255-6480

**St. Joseph's Hospital Chemical Dependency Unit,** 45 W. 10th Street, Saint Paul, MN 55102; tel. 651/232-3256

**United Hospital,** 333 North Smith Avenue, Saint Paul, MN 55102; tel. 651/241-8802

*****University of Minnesota Medical Center, Fairview,** 2450 Riverside Avenue, Minneapolis, MN 55455; tel. 612/273-3000

*****VA Health Care System-Minneapolis,** One Veterans Drive, Minneapolis, MN 55417; tel. 612/725-2000

**Veterans Affairs Medical Center Outpatient Methadone Program,** One Veterans Drive, Minneapolis, MN 55417; tel. 612/725-2228

### MISSISSIPPI

**Adams County Correctional Center,** 20 Hobo Forks Rd, Natchez, MS 39120; tel. 601/304-2500

**Bolivar Medical Center,** PO Box 1380, Cleveland, MS 38732-1380; tel. 662/846-2534

**Brentwood Behavioral Healthcare of Mississippi, LLC,** 3531 Lakeland Drive, Flowood, MS 39232; tel. 601/936-2024

*****CARES Center, Inc. and Mississippi Children's Home Society,** 1900 North West Street, Jackson, MS 39202; tel. 601/352-7784

**Central Mississippi Medical Center,** PO Box 59001, Jackson, MS 39204; tel. 601/376-1000

*****COPAC, Inc.,** 3949 Highway 43 North, Brandon, MS 39047; tel. 601/829-2500

**Crossgates River Oaks Hospital,** 350 Crossgates Boulevard, Brandon, MS 39042; tel. 601/825-2811

*****Delta Regional Medical Center,** PO Box 5247, Greenville, MS 38704-5247; tel. 662/378-3783

**Diamond Grove Center for Children and Adolescents,** PO Box 848, Louisville, MS 39339; tel. 662/779-0119

**Millcreek of Pontotoc,** PO Box 619, Pontotoc, MS 38863; tel. 662/488-8878

*****Mississippi State Hospital,** PO Box 157-A, Whitfield, MS 39193-0157; tel. 601/351-8000

**Natchez Community Hospital,** PO Box 1203, Natchez, MS 39121; tel. 601/445-6205

**Northwest Mississippi Regional Medical Center,** PO Box 1218, Clarksdale, MS 38614; tel. 662/624-3401

*****Parkwood Behavioral Health System,** 8135 Goodman Road, Olive Branch, MS 38654; tel. 662/895-4900

**PSI Crossings,** 5000 Highway 39 North, Meridian, MS 39301; tel. 601/483-5452

**Rehabilitation Centers, Inc.,** PO Box 1160, Magee, MS 39111; tel. 601/849-4221

*****Specialized Treatment Facility,** 14426 James Bond Road, Gulfport, MS 39503; tel. 228/328-6000

*****VA Gulf Coast Veterans Health Care System,** 400 Veterans Avenue, Biloxi, MS 39531; tel. 228/523-5000

*****VA Medical Center-G. V. (Sonny) Montgomery,** 1500 East Woodrow Wilson Avenue, Jackson, MS 39216; tel. 601/364-1201

### MISSOURI

*****Alternative Behavioral Care,** 255 Spenser Road, Suite 101, Saint Peters, MO 63376; tel. 636/477-6111

**Barnes-Jewish Hospital,** 216 South Kingshighway Boulevard, Mailstop 90-31-640, Saint Louis, MO 63108; tel. 314/747-3000

**BJC Behavioral Health,** 1430 Olive Street - Suite 400, Saint Louis, MO 63103; tel. 314/206-3712

*****Boonville Valley Hope,** 1415 Ashley Road, Boonville, MO 65233; tel. 660/882-6547

**Center for Behavioral Medicine,** 1000 East 24th Street, Kansas City, MO 64108-2620; tel. 816/512-7000

*****CenterPointe Hospital,** 4801 Weldon Spring Parkway, Saint Charles, MO 63304; tel. 636/441-7300

*****Centrec Care, Inc.,** 1224 Fern Ridge Parkway, Suite 305, Saint Louis, MO 63141; tel. 314/205-8068

**Change Academy Lake of the Ozarks (CALO),** 130 Calo Lane, Lake Ozark, MO 65049; tel. 573/365-2221

**Child Advocacy Services Center, Inc.,** 2 East 59th Street, Kansas City, MO 64113-2116; tel. 816/363-1898

*****Christian Hospital Northeast-Northwest,** 11133 Dunn Road, Saint Louis, MO 63136; tel. 314/653-5616

**Columbia Treatment Clinic,** 1301 Vandiver Suite Y, Columbia, MO 65202; tel. 573/449-8338

**Cottonwood Residential Treatment Center,** 1025 N. Sprigg, Cape Girardeau, MO 63701; tel. 573/290-5888

*****Crittenton,** 10918 Elm Avenue, Kansas City, MO 64134-4199; tel. 816/765-6600

**DRD Kansas City Medical Clinic,** 723 East 18th Street, Kansas City, MO 64108; tel. 816/283-3877

**DRD Springfield Medical Clinic,** 404 East Battlefield Street, Springfield, MO 65807; tel. 417/865-8045

**Epworth Children & Family Services,** 110 North Elm Avenue, Saint Louis, MO 63119; tel. 314/961-5718

**Fulton State Hospital,** 600 East Fifth Street, Fulton, MO 65251-1798; tel. 573/592-4100

**Great Circle,** PO Box 189, Saint James, MO 65559; tel. 573/265-3251

*****Harry S. Truman Memorial Veterans' Hospital,** 800 Hospital Drive, Columbia, MO 65201; tel. 573/814-6000

**Hawthorn Children's Psychiatric Hospital,** 1901 Pennsylvania Avenue, Saint Louis, MO 63133; tel. 314/512-7800

**Heartland Behavioral Health Services,** 1500 West Ashland, Nevada, MO 64772; tel. 417/667-2666

*****Kansas City Veterans Affairs Medical Center,** 4801 Linwood Boulevard, Kansas City, MO 64128; tel. 816/861-4700

**Lakeland Regional Hospital,** 440 South Market Avenue, Springfield, MO 65806; tel. 417/865-5581

**McCallum Place Eating Disorders Treatment,** 231 W. Lockwood Avenue Suite 201, Saint Louis, MO 63119; tel. 314/968-1900

*****Northland Family Counseling Center, Inc.,** 429 East US Highway 69, Kansas City, MO 64119-3118; tel. 816/452-8777

**Ozarks Medical Center,** PO Box 1100, West Plains, MO 65775; tel. 417/256-9111

*****Provident, Inc.,** 2650 Olive Street., Saint Louis, MO 63103; tel. 314/371-6500

*****Research Psychiatric Center,** 2323 East 63rd Street, Kansas City, MO 64130; tel. 816/444-8161

*****Signature Behavioral Healthcare,** 763 South New Ballas Road, Suite 300, Saint Louis, MO 63141; tel. 816/795-1445

**Southeast Missouri Mental Health Center,** 1010 West Columbia Street, Farmington, MO 63640-2997; tel. 573/218-6792

*****SSM DePaul Health Center,** 12303 DePaul Drive, Bridgeton, MO 63044-2588; tel. 314/344-6000

**SSM Health Care-St. Louis,** 6420 Clayton Road, Richmond Heights, MO 63117; tel. 314/768-8000

**SSM St. Joseph Health Center,** 300 First Capitol Drive, Saint Charles, MO 63301; tel. 636/947-5000

*****St. Anthony's Medical Center,** 10010 Kennerly Road, Saint Louis, MO 63128; tel. 314/525-1000

**St. Louis Psychiatric Rehabilitation Center,** 5300 Arsenal Street, Saint Louis, MO 63139; tel. 314/877-6500

*****Swope Health Services,** 3801 Blue Parkway, Kansas City, MO 64130; tel. 816/922-3166

**The Salvation Army Children's Shelter,** 101 W Linwood, Kansas City, MO 64111; tel. 816/285-2480

*****Truman Medical Center,** 2301 Holmes Street, Kansas City, MO 64108; tel. 816/404-0905

**Two Rivers Psychiatric Hospital,** 5121 Raytown Road, Kansas City, MO 64133; tel. 816/356-5688

**U.S. Medical Center for Federal Prisoners,** 1900 West Sunshine Street, Springfield, MO 65807; tel. 417/862-7041

*****VA Medical Center,** 915 North Grand Boulevard, Saint Louis, MO 63106; tel. 314/289-7020

**VCPHCS XV, LLC dba Joplin Treatment Clinic,** P.O Box 4692, Joplin, MO 64803; tel. 214/365-6111

**Woodridge of Missouri, LLC,** PO Box 4067, Waynesville, MO 65583; tel. 573/774-5353

### MONTANA

**Acadia Montana,** 55 Basin Creek Road, Butte, MT 59701; tel. 406/494-4183

**Billings Clinic,** PO Box 37000, Billings, MT 59107-3700; tel. 406/657-4000

**Intermountain Children's Home,** 500 South Lamborn, Helena, MT 59601; tel. 406/442-7920

**Montana Academy,** 9705 Lost Prairie Road, Marion, MT 59925; tel. 406/858-2339

*****Rocky Mountain Treatment Center,** 920 Fourth Avenue North, Great Falls, MT 59401; tel. 406/727-8832

**Shodair Children's Hospital,** PO Box 5539, Helena, MT 59604; tel. 406/444-7500

*****VA Montana Healthcare System,** 3687 Veterans Drive, Fort Harrison, MT 59636-1500; tel. 406/447-7900

### NEBRASKA

*****Alegent Health Immanuel Medical Center,** 6901 North 72nd Street, Omaha, NE 68122; tel. 402/572-2291

---

*Indicates organization is a Joint Commission accredited Chemical Dependency organization.

**Section C**

*Behavioral Health Specialists, Inc., 900 W Norfolk Avenue, Ste 200, Norfolk, NE 68701; tel. 402/370-3140

*Blue Valley Behavioral Health, Inc., 1123 North 9th Street, Beatrice, NE 68310; tel. 402/228-3386

Boys Town National Research Hospital, 555 North 30th Street, Omaha, NE 68131; tel. 402/498-6525

*BryanLGH Medical Center, 1600 South 48th Street, Lincoln, NE 68506; tel. 402/489-0200

Epworth Village, Inc., PO Box 503, York, NE 68467-0503; tel. 402/362-3353

*Hastings Regional Center, PO Box 579, Hastings, NE 68902-0579; tel. 402/462-1971

Lincoln Lancaster County Child Guidance Center, 2444 'O' Street, Lincoln, NE 68510; tel. 402/475-7666

Lincoln Regional Center, PO Box 94949, Lincoln, NE 68509-4949; tel. 402/471-4444

*O'Neill Valley Hope, 1421 North 10th Street, Oneill, NE 68763; tel. 402/336-3747

OMNI Behavioral Health, 5115 F Street, Omaha, NE 68117; tel. 402/397-9866

*VA Nebraska-Western Iowa Health Care System, 4101 Woolworth Avenue, Omaha, NE 68105; tel. 402/449-0600

**NEVADA**

*Community Counseling Center, Carson City, 205 South Pratt Avenue, Carson City, NV 89701; tel. 775/882-3945

Desert Willow Treatment Center, 6171 W Charleston Boulevard, Building #17, Las Vegas, NV 89146; tel. 702/486-8900

*Las Vegas Recovery Center, 3371 N. Buffalo Drive, Las Vegas, NV 89129; tel. 702/515-1374

*Montevista Hospital, 5900 West Rochelle Avenue, Las Vegas, NV 89103-3327; tel. 702/364-1111

*New Frontier Treatment Center, PO Box 1240, Fallon, NV 89407; tel. 775/423-1412

Northern Nevada Adult Mental Health Services, 480 Galletti Way, Sparks, NV 89431; tel. 775/688-2001

*Seven Hills Behavioral Institute, Inc., 3021 W. Horizon Ridge Parkway, Henderson, NV 89052; tel. 702/646-5000

Southern Nevada Adult Mental Health Services, 6161 West Charleston Boulevard, Las Vegas, NV 89146; tel. 702/486-4400

Spring Mountain Treatment Center, 7000 Spring Mountain Road, Las Vegas, NV 89117; tel. 702/873-2400

*VA Sierra Nevada Health Care System, 975 Kirman Avenue, Reno, NV 89502-2597; tel. 775/786-7200

*VA Southern Nevada Healthcare System, PO Box 360001, North Las Vegas, NV 89036; tel. 702/636-3000

Willow Springs Center, 690 Edison Way, Reno, NV 89502; tel. 775/858-4515

**NEW HAMPSHIRE**

Community Council of Nashua, NH, 7 Prospect Street, Nashua, NH 03060; tel. 603/889-6147

Lakeview NeuroRehabilitation Center, 244 Highwatch Road, Effingham, NH 03882; tel. 603/539-7451

NFI North, Inc., 40 Park Lane, Contoocook, NH 03229; tel. 603/746-7550

**NEW JERSEY**

AtlantiCare Behavioral Health, 2511 Fire Road, Unit B10 Bellevue Commons, Egg Harbor Township, NJ 08234; tel. 609/645-7600

AtlantiCare Regional Medical Center, 1925 Pacific Avenue, Atlantic City, NJ 08401; tel. 609/407-2309

Bancroft Rehabilitation Services, 425 Kings Highway East, Haddonfield, NJ 08033; tel. 856/429-5637

*Bayonne Community Mental Health Center, 601 Broadway, Bayonne, NJ 07002; tel. 201/339-9200

*Bergen Regional Medical Center, 230 East Ridgewood Avenue, Paramus, NJ 07652; tel. 201/967-4000

*Bonnie Brae, 3415 Valley Road, P. O. Box 825, Liberty Corner, NJ 07938-0825; tel. 908/647-0800

*Cape Counseling Services, 1129 Route 9, Cape May Court House, NJ 08210; tel. 609/778-6100

*Care Plus NJ, Inc., 610 Valley Health Plaza, Paramus, NJ 07652; tel. 201/265-8200

*Carrier Clinic, PO Box 147, Belle Mead, NJ 08502-0147; tel. 908/281-1000

*Catholic Charities-Diocese of Metuchen, 319 Maple Street, Perth Amboy, NJ 08861; tel. 732/324-8200

Christian Health Care Center, 301 Sicomac Avenue, Wyckoff, NJ 07481; tel. 201/848-5200

*CPC Behavioral Healthcare, Inc., 10 Industrial Way East, Eatontown, NJ 07724; tel. 732/935-2220

*East Orange General Hospital, 300 Central Avenue, East Orange, NJ 07018; tel. 973/672-8400

*GenPsych of South Carolina, LLC, 981 Route 22 West, Bridgewater, NJ 08807; tel. 908/526-8370

Hampton Behavioral Health Center, 650 Rancocas Rd, Westampton, NJ 08060; tel. 609/267-7000

*High Focus Centers, 47 Maple Street, Suite 401, Summit, NJ 07901; tel. 908/363-1023

*Hoboken University Medical Center, 308 Willow Avenue, Hoboken, NJ 07030; tel. 201/418-1000

*Hunterdon Medical Center, 2100 Wescott Drive, Flemington, NJ 08822; tel. 908/788-6151

*Jersey City Medical Center, 355 Grand Street, Jersey City, NJ 07302; tel. 201/915-2000

*Jersey Shore University Medical Center, 1945 Route 33, Neptune, NJ 07754-0397; tel. 732/776-4900

*Kennedy University Hospital, 1099 White Horse Road, Voorhees, NJ 08043; tel. 856/566-5200

Khaleidoscope Health Care, Inc., Jones and Associates-111 Wayne Street, Jersey City, NJ 07302; tel. 201/451-5425

Merit Mountainside dba Mountainside Hospital, 1 Bay Avenue, Montclair, NJ 07042; tel. 973/429-6000

Monmouth Medical Center, 300 Second Avenue, Long Branch, NJ 07740; tel. 732/222-5200

*Morristown Medical Center, 100 Madison Avenue, Morristown, NJ 07962-1956; tel. 973/971-5450

Newark Beth Israel Medical Center, 201 Lyons Avenue, Newark, NJ 07112; tel. 973/926-7000

Newton Medical Center, 175 High Street, Newton, NJ 07860; tel. 973/383-2121

*North Hudson Community Action Corporation, 800-31st Street, Union City, NJ 07087; tel. 201/866-2727

*Overlook Medical Center, PO Box 220, Summit, NJ 07902-0220; tel. 908/522-4912

*Princeton HealthCare System, 253 Witherspoon Street, Princeton, NJ 08540; tel. 609/497-4000

Raritan Bay Medical Center-Methadone Program, 530 New Brunswick Avenue, Perth Amboy, NJ 08861; tel. 732/442-3700

*Recovery Services of New Jersey, Inc., 5034 Atlantic Avenue, Mays Landing, NJ 08330; tel. 609/625-4900

Richard Hall Community Mental Health Center, 500 North Bridge Street, Bridgewater, NJ 08807; tel. 908/725-2800

Riverview Medical Center, One Riverview Plaza, Red Bank, NJ 07701; tel. 732/741-2700

Saint Barnabas Behavioral Health Center, Inc., 1691 US Highway 9, CN 2025, Toms River, NJ 08754; tel. 732/914-1688

*Saint Clare's Health System, 25 Pocono Road, Denville, NJ 07834; tel. 973/983-2233

Saint Peter's Healthcare System, PO Box 591, New Brunswick, NJ 08903-0591; tel. 732/745-8555

Sequel of New Jersey-Capital Academy, 1770 Mt Ephraim Avenue, Haddon Township, NJ 08104; tel. 856/635-0200

Somerset Medical Center, 110 Rehill Avenue, Somerville, NJ 08876-2598; tel. 908/685-2200

South Jersey Drug Treatment, PO Box 867, Bridgeton, NJ 08302; tel. 856/455-5441

St. Francis Medical Center, 601 Hamilton Avenue, Trenton, NJ 08629; tel. 609/599-5000

St. Mary's Hospital, 350 Boulevard, Passaic, NJ 07055; tel. 973/365-4300

*Summit Oaks Hospital, 19 Prospect Street, Summit, NJ 07901; tel. 908/522-7000

*The Lester A. Drenk Behavioral Health Center, Inc., 1289 Route 38 West, Suite 203, Hainesport, NJ 08036; tel. 609/267-5656

*Trinitas Regional Medical Center, 225 Williamson Street, Elizabeth, NJ 07207; tel. 908/994-5754

UMDNJ-University Behavioral HealthCare, PO Box 1392, Piscataway, NJ 08855-1392; tel. 732/235-5500

Underwood-Memorial Hospital, 509 North Broad Street, Woodbury, NJ 08097; tel. 856/845-0100

*VA New Jersey Health Care System, 385 Tremont Avenue, Director's Office (00), East Orange, NJ 07018; tel. 973/676-1000

Virtua Health, Inc., 401 Route 73 North, 50 Lake Center Drive, Suite 402, Marlton, NJ 08053; tel. 856/355-0029

VisionQuest-New Jersey, P.O. Box 370, New Lisbon, NJ 08064; tel. 609/894-4856

Willowglen Academy New Jersey, Inc., 8 Wilson Drive, Sparta, NJ 07871; tel. 973/579-3700

*Youth Consultation Service, 284 Broadway, Newark, NJ 07104; tel. 973/482-8411

**NEW MEXICO**

E L Rocky Mountain Management & Services, LLC, 712 Rencher, Clovis, NM 88101; tel. 505/762-6091

*Mesilla Valley Hospital, 3751 Del Rey Boulevard, Las Cruces, NM 88012; tel. 575/382-3500

New Mexico Behavioral Health Institute at Las Vegas, 3695 Hot Springs Boulevard, Las Vegas, NM 87701; tel. 505/454-2404

*New Mexico VA Health Care System, 1501 San Pedro Drive SE, Albuquerque, NM 87108; tel. 505/265-1711

Peak Behavioral Health Services, LLC, 5045 McNutt Road, Santa Teresa, NM 88008; tel. 575/589-3000

*Presbyterian Medical Services, 1422 Paseo de Peralta, Santa Fe, NM 87504-2267; tel. 505/982-5565

Sequel of New Mexico, LLC, 5400 Gibson Blvd, Albuquerque, NM 87108; tel. 505/924-6330

Sequoyah Adolescent Treatment Center, 3405 W Pan American Freeway NE, Albuquerque, NM 87107; tel. 505/222-0375

*University of New Mexico Health Sciences Center, 2211 Lomas Blvd NE, Albuquerque, NM 87106; tel. 505/272-2111

Youth and Family Centered Services of New Mexico, Inc., 5310 Sequoia NW, Albuquerque, NM 87120; tel. 505/836-7330

**NEW YORK**

*A.R.E.B.A.-Casriel, Inc., 500 West 57th Street, New York, NY 10019; tel. 212/376-1810

Acute Chemical Dependency Detox Unit-Kings County, 410 Winthrop Street, Brooklyn, NY 11203; tel. 718/245-3901

*Arms Acres, Inc., 75 Seminary Hill Road, Carmel, NY 10512; tel. 845/225-3400

Astor Services for Children & Families, PO Box 5005, Rhinebeck, NY 12572-5005; tel. 845/871-1000

August Aichhorn R.T.F., 23 West 106th Street, New York, NY 10025; tel. 212/316-9353

Baker Victory Services, Inc., 780 Ridge Road, Lackawanna, NY 14218; tel. 716/828-9515

*Bellevue Hospital Center, 462 First Avenue, New York, NY 10016; tel. 212/562-3718

*Benedictine Hospital, 105 Mary's Avenue, Kingston, NY 12401; tel. 845/338-2500

Beth Israel Medical Center MMTP-Avenue A Clinic, 26 Avenue A, New York, NY 10009; tel. 212/420-2078

Beth Israel Medical Center MMTP-Cumberland Clinic, 100 Flatbush Avenue, Brooklyn, NY 11217; tel. 718/237-9600

Beth Israel Medical Center MMTP-Gouverneur Clinic, 109-11 Delancey Street, New York, NY 10002; tel. 212/420-2086

Beth Israel Medical Center MMTP-Harlem, 103 East 125th Street, New York, NY 10035; tel. 212/774-3260

Beth Israel Medical Center MMTP-Harlem Clinic 1, First Avenue @ 16th Street, New York, NY 10003; tel. 212/774-3210

Beth Israel Medical Center MMTP-Marie Nyswander Clinic, 160 Water Street, New York, NY 10038; tel. 212/774-3258

Beth Israel Medical Center MMTP-St Vincent's, 201 West 13th Street, New York, NY 10011; tel. 212/420-2015

Beth Israel Medical Center MMTP-Vincent P Dole, 25 - 12th Street, Brooklyn, NY 11215; tel. 718/965-7900

Bon Secours Community Hospital-Opioid Treatment Programs, 160 East Main Street, Port Jervis, NY 12771; tel. 845/858-7000

Bronx Children's Psychiatric Center, 1000 Waters Place, Bronx, NY 10461-2799; tel. 718/239-3621

Bronx Psychiatric Center, 1500 Waters Place, Bronx, NY 10461; tel. 718/862-3300

---

*Indicates organization is a Joint Commission accredited Chemical Dependency organization.

Section C

**Bronx Veterans Administration Medical Center Substance Abuse,** 130 W Kingsbridge Rd, Ward 5B, Bronx, NY 10468; tel. 718/584-9000

*****Bronx-Lebanon Hospital Center,** 1650 Grand Concourse, Bronx, NY 10457; tel. 718/590-1800

**Bronx-Lebanon Hospital Center-MMTP,** 1650 Selwyn Avenue Suite 3A, Bronx, NY 10457; tel. 718/960-1075

**Brooklyn Children's Center,** 1819 Bergen Street, Brooklyn, NY 11233; tel. 718/221-4500

**Buffalo Psychiatric Center,** 400 Forest Avenue, Buffalo, NY 14213; tel. 716/885-2261

**Canton-Potsdam Hospital-Opioid Treatment Program,** 50 Leroy Street, Potsdam, NY 13676; tel. 315/265-3300

**Carnegie Hill Institute,** 116 East 92nd Street, New York, NY 10128; tel. 212/289-7166

**Central New York Psychiatric Center,** PO Box 300, Marcy, NY 13403-0300; tel. 315/765-3660

*****Coney Island Hospital,** 2601 Ocean Parkway, Brooklyn, NY 11235; tel. 718/616-3000

*****Conifer Park, Inc.,** 79 Glenridge Road, Glenville, NY 12302; tel. 518/399-6446

**Creedmoor Psychiatric Center,** 79-25 Winchester Boulevard, Queens Village, NY 11427; tel. 718/264-3607

**Crouse Hospital Methadone Maintenance Treatment Program,** 410 South Crouse Avenue, Syracuse, NY 13210; tel. 315/470-8300

**Drug Treatment & Education Cen North Shore Univ Hospital,** 400 Community Drive, Manhasset, NY 11030; tel. 516/562-3010

**Ellis Medicine Ellis Hospital,** 1101 Nott Street, Schenectady, NY 12308; tel. 518/243-4000

*****Elmhurst Hospital Center,** 79-01 Broadway, Elmhurst, NY 11373; tel. 718/334-4000

**Elmira Psychiatric Center,** 100 Washington Street, Elmira, NY 14901-2898; tel. 607/737-4739

**Erie County Medical Center,** 462 Grider Street, Buffalo, NY 14215; tel. 716/898-3000

**Flushing Hospital Medical Center / Chemical Dependency Unit,** 45th Avenue at Parsons Blvd, Flushing, NY 11355; tel. 718/670-5918

*****Fort Drum Ambulatory Health Care,** 11050 Mt. Belvedere Boulevard, Fort Drum, NY 13602-5004; tel. 315/772-7817

**Four Winds, Inc.,** 800 Cross River Road, Katonah, NY 10536; tel. 914/763-8151

**Four Winds-Saratoga,** 30 Crescent Avenue, Saratoga Springs, NY 12866; tel. 518/584-3600

*****Glens Falls Hospital,** 100 Park Street, Glens Falls, NY 12801; tel. 518/926-1000

**Good Samaritan Hospital-Opioid Treatment Programs,** 255 Lafayette Avenue, Suffern, NY 10901; tel. 845/368-5220

**Gracie Square Hospital-Opioid Treatment Programs,** 420 East 76th Street, New York, NY 10021; tel. 212/434-5322

**Greater Binghamton Health Center,** 425 Robinson Street, Binghamton, NY 13904; tel. 607/773-4082

**Greater Hudson Valley Family Health Center-Opioid Treatment Programs,** 3 Commerical Place, Newburgh, NY 12550; tel. 845/220-2146

*****Harlem Hospital Center,** 506 Lenox Avenue, New York, NY 10037-1802; tel. 212/939-1340

*****Hudson River HealthCare, Inc.,** 1037 Main Street, Peekskill, NY 10566; tel. 914/734-8800

**Hudson Valley Hospital Center MMTP,** 1980 Crompond Road, Cortlandt Manor, NY 10567; tel. 914/737-6117

**Hutchings Psychiatric Center,** 620 Madison Street, Syracuse, NY 13210; tel. 315/426-3600

*****Interfaith Medical Center,** 1545 Atlantic Avenue, Brooklyn, NY 11213; tel. 718/613-4001

**Jacobi Medical Center Chemical Dependence/ Medically Detox,** 1400 Pelham Parkway, Bronx, NY 10461; tel. 718/918-5322

*****John T. Mather Memorial Hospital,** 75 North Country Road, Port Jefferson, NY 11777-2190; tel. 631/473-1320

*****Keller Army Community Hospital,** 900 Washington Road, West Point, NY 10996; tel. 845/938-3305

*****Kings County Hospital Center,** 451 Clarkson Avenue, Brooklyn, NY 11203; tel. 718/245-5315

**Long Beach Medical Center Chemical Dependency Unit,** 455 East Bay Drive, Long Beach, NY 11561; tel. 516/897-1000

**Long Beach Medical Center MMTP,** 450 East Bay Drive, Long Beach, NY 11561; tel. 516/897-1330

*****Long Island Center for Recovery, Inc.,** 320 West Montauk Highway, Hampton Bays, NY 11946; tel. 631/728-3100

*****Long Island Jewish Medical Center,** 270-05 76th Avenue, New Hyde Park, NY 11040; tel. 516/470-7000

**Long Island Jewish Medical Center-MMTP,** 75-59 263rd Street, Glen Oaks, NY 11004; tel. 718/470-8285

**Loyola Recovery Foundation, Inc.,** 1159 Pittsford-Victor Road, Pittsford, NY 14534; tel. 585/203-1005

**Loyola Recovery Foundation, Inc.,** 76 Veterans Ave, Bath, NY 14810; tel. 585/205-1005

**Lutheran Medical Center (Acute Care Addiction Program),** 150 55th Street, Brooklyn, NY 11220; tel. 718/630-7300

**Maimonides Medical Center,** 4802 Tenth Avenue, Brooklyn, NY 11219-2916; tel. 718/283-6000

**Manhattan Psychiatric Center,** 600 East 125th Street - Ward's Island, New York, NY 10035; tel. 646/672-6000

**Medically Managed Inpatient Detoxification,** 2 Park Avenue, Yonkers, NY 10703; tel. 914/964-7383

**Methadone Treatment Program,** 648 Albany Avenue, Brooklyn, NY 11203; tel. 718/245-3901

**Metropolitan Correctional Center-New York / Opioid Treatment Programs,** 150 Park Row, New York, NY 10007; tel. 646/836-6300

*****Metropolitan Hospital Center,** 1901 First Avenue, New York, NY 10029; tel. 212/423-6501

**Mohawk Valley Psychiatric Center,** 1400 Noyes Street, Utica, NY 13502; tel. 315/738-3800

**Montefiore Medical Center-SATP,** 111 East 210th Street, Bronx, NY 10467; tel. 718/920-2001

**Montefiore Medical Center-SATP-Opioid Treatment Programs-Unit III,** 2005 Jerome Avenue, 1st Floor, Bronx, NY 10467; tel. 718/583-0600

**Narco Freedom Inc. MMTP,** 2910 Grand Concourse, Bronx, NY 10455; tel. 718/292-2240

**Narco Freedom, Inc.-Bridge Plaza MMTP,** 37-18 34th Street, Long Island City, NY 11101; tel. 718/292-2240

**Nassau County Department Methadone Maintenance Treatment Program,** NUMC, 2201 Hempstead Turnpike Building K, East Meadow, NY 11554; tel. 516/572-5906

**Nassau Health Care Corporation,** 2201 Hempstead Turnpike, East Meadow, NY 11554; tel. 516/572-4876

**New York State Psychiatric Institute,** 1051 Riverside Drive, New York, NY 10032; tel. 212/543-5000

*****New York-Presbyterian Hospital,** 525 East 68th Street, Box 437, New York, NY 10065; tel. 212/746-5454

**North Central Bronx Hospital,** 3424 Kossuth Avenue, Bronx, NY 10467; tel. 718/519-3500

*****North Shore University Hospital at Glen Cove,** 101 Saint Andrews Lane, Glen Cove, NY 11542; tel. 516/674-7580

**Oswego Hospital,** 110 West Sixth Street, Oswego, NY 13126; tel. 315/349-5566

**Pathways, Sisters of Charity Hospital,** 158 Holden Street, Buffalo, NY 14214; tel. 716/862-1000

*****Phelps Memorial Hospital Center,** 701 North Broadway, Sleepy Hollow, NY 10591; tel. 914/366-1000

**Pilgrim Psychiatric Center,** 998 Crooked Hill Road, West Brentwood, NY 11717; tel. 631/761-3500

**PROMESA Methadone Treatment Program,** 1776 Clay Ave, Bronx, NY 10457; tel. 718/960-7601

**Quannacut at Eastern Long Island Hospital,** 201 Manor Place, Greenport, NY 11944; tel. 631/477-1000

**Queens Children's Psychiatric Center,** 74-03 Commonwealth Boulevard, Bellerose, NY 11426; tel. 718/264-4600

*****Queens Hospital Center,** 82-68 164th Street, Jamaica, NY 11432; tel. 718/883-2351

*****Richmond Medical Center,** 355 Bard Avenue, Staten Island, NY 10310; tel. 718/818-1234

*****Rochester General Hospital,** 1425 Portland Avenue, Rochester, NY 14621; tel. 585/922-4000

**Rochester Mental Health Center,** 490 East Ridge Road, Rochester, NY 14621; tel. 585/922-2500

**Rochester Pathways, Sisters of Charity Hospital,** 435 East Henrietta Road, Rochester, NY 14607; tel. 585/424-6580

**Rockland Children's Psychiatric Center,** 2 First Avenue, Orangeburg, NY 10962; tel. 845/680-4040

**Rockland Psychiatric Center,** 140 Old Orangeburg Road, Orangeburg, NY 10962; tel. 845/359-1000

**Sagamore Children's Psychiatric Center,** 197 Half Hollow Road, Dix Hills, NY 11746; tel. 631/370-1701

**Saint Joseph's Hospital, Yonkers,** 275 North St, Harrison, NY 10528; tel. 718/485-3400

**Saint Vincent's Hospital White Plains OTC,** 77 East Post Road, White Plains, NY 10601; tel. 914/286-2820

*****Samuel S. Stratton VA Medical Center,** 113 Holland Avenue, Albany, NY 12208; tel. 518/626-5000

**SBH Chemical Dependence Methadone Substance Abuse Treatment,** 4535-39 Third Avenue, Bronx, NY 10457; tel. 718/960-6170

**SBH Chemical Dependence-Medically Managed,** 183rd Street and Third Avenue, Bronx, NY 10457; tel. 718/960-6170

*****Seafield Center, Inc.,** 7 Seafield Lane, Westhampton Beach, NY 11978; tel. 631/288-1122

**Sound Shore Medical Center of Westchester,** 16 Guion Place, New Rochelle, NY 10802; tel. 914/632-5000

**South Beach Psychiatric Center,** 777 Seaview Avenue, Staten Island, NY 10305; tel. 718/667-2300

**South Nassau Communities Hospital,** 1 Healthy Way, Oceanside, NY 11572; tel. 516/632-3999

*****St. Barnabas Hospital,** 4422 Third Avenue, Bronx, NY 10457; tel. 718/960-6108

*****St. James Mercy Hospital,** 411 Canisteo Street, Hornell, NY 14843; tel. 607/324-8703

*****St. John's Episcopal Hospital-South Shore,** 327 Beach 19th Street, Far Rockaway, NY 11691; tel. 718/869-7000

**St. Johns Riverside Hospital MMTP,** 2 Park Avenue, Yonkers, NY 10703; tel. 914/964-4000

*****St. Joseph's Hospital,** 127 South Broadway, Yonkers, NY 10701; tel. 914/378-7839

**St. Joseph's Hospital Yonkers,** 147-18 Archer Avenue, Jamaica, NY 11435; tel. 718/291-1888

**St. Joseph's Hospital-MMTP,** 8 Guion Street, 1st Floor, Yonkers, NY 10701; tel. 914/378-7000

*****St. Joseph's Villa of Rochester,** 3300 Dewey Avenue, Rochester, NY 14616; tel. 585/865-1550

**St. Lawrence Psychiatric Center,** One Chimney Point Drive, Ogdensburg, NY 13669; tel. 315/541-2279

*****St. Luke's-Roosevelt Hospital Center,** 1000 10th Avenue, New York, NY 10019; tel. 212/523-4000

**St. Luke's-Roosevelt Hospital Center - Clark 6,** 1111 Amsterdam Ave, New York, NY 10025; tel. 212/523-4000

*****St. Mary's Hospital,** 427 Guy Park Avenue, Amsterdam, NY 12010; tel. 518/770-7592

**St. Vincent's Hospital, Westchester MMTP Clinic I,** 275 North Street, Harrison, NY 10528; tel. 718/953-2302

**Staten Island Univ Hospital Inpatient Chemical Dependency Detox Unit,** 375 Seguine Avenue, Staten Island, NY 10309; tel. 718/226-6939

*****Staten Island University Hospital,** 475 Seaview Avenue, Staten Island, NY 10305; tel. 718/226-9000

**Stony Brook University Hospital Medical Center,** Nicolls Road, Stony Brook, NY 11794-8503; tel. 631/444-1956

**Stony Lodge Hospital, Inc.,** PO Box 1250, Briarcliff Manor, NY 10510; tel. 914/941-7400

*****Strong Memorial Hospital,** 601 Elmwood Avenue, Rochester, NY 14642; tel. 585/275-2644

**Stuyvesant Square Chemical Dependency Outpatient Detox,** 1-9 Nathan Perlman Place, New York, NY 10003; tel. 212/420-4220

**Suffolk County Department of Health Services, Huntington MMTP,** PO Box 6100, Building C-928, North County Complex, Hauppauge, NY 11788; tel. 631/854-4400

**Suffolk County Department of Health-East End Clinic,** 300 Center Drive, Riverhead, NY 11901; tel. 631/852-2680

**Suffolk County Department of Health-Hauppauge Clinic,** 200 Wireless Blvd, Hauppauge, NY 11788; tel. 631/853-7373

**Suffolk County Department of Health-North County Complex,** PO Box 6100, Bldg 151, North County Complex, Hauppauge, NY 11788; tel. 631/853-6410

**Summit Park Hospital,** 50 Sanitorium Road, Pomona, NY 10970; tel. 845/364-2700

*****Syracuse Community Health Center, Inc.,** 819 South Salina Street, Syracuse, NY 13202; tel. 315/476-7921

*Indicates organization is a Joint Commission accredited Chemical Dependency organization.

**The Brooklyn Hospital Center Parkside Drug Detox Program,** 121 DeKalb Avenue, Brooklyn, NY 11201; tel. 718/250–8005

**The Children's Home RTF, Inc.,** 638 Squirrel Hill Road, Chenango Forks, NY 13746; tel. 607/656–9004

**The Family Foundation School,** 431 Chapel Hill Road, Hancock, NY 13783; tel. 845/887–5213

**The Guidance Center Chemical Dependency Treatment Center,** 70 Grand Street, New Rochelle, NY 10801; tel. 914/636–4440

**The House of the Good Shepherd,** 1550 Champlin Avenue, Utica, NY 13502; tel. 315/235–7600

*****The Institute for Family Health,** 16 East 16th Street, New York, NY 10003; tel. 212/633–0800

**The Kingston Hospital Methadone Treatment Program,** 2 Barbarossa Lane, Kingston, NY 12401; tel. 845/943–6022

*****The Long Island Home,** 400 Sunrise Highway, Amityville, NY 11701; tel. 631/264–4000

*****The Mount Sinai Medical Center,** One Gustave L. Levy Place, Box 1051, New York, NY 10029-6574; tel. 212/241–5719

*****The Mount Vernon Hospital,** 12 North Seventh Avenue, Mount Vernon, NY 10550; tel. 914/361–6278

**The Mount Vernon Hospital Methadone Maintenance Program,** 3 South 6th Avenue, 3rd Floor, Mount Vernon, NY 10550; tel. 914/361–6000

**United Health Services Hospitals,** 33-57 Harrison Street, Johnson City, NY 13790; tel. 607/763–6130

*****Upstate New York VA Health Care Network at Canandaigua,** 400 Fort Hill Avenue, Canandaigua, NY 14424; tel. 585/394–2000

*****VA Healthcare Network Upstate New York at Bath,** 76 Veterans Avenue, Bath, NY 14810; tel. 607/664–4722

*****VA Healthcare Network Upstate New York at Syracuse,** 800 Irving Avenue, Syracuse, NY 13210; tel. 315/425–4400

*****VA Hudson Valley Health Care System,** 2094 Albany Post Road, Route 9A, Montrose, NY 10548; tel. 914/737–4400

*****VA Medical Center Northport,** 79 Middleville Road, Northport, NY 11768; tel. 631/261–4400

*****VA New York Harbor Health Care System,** 800 Poly Place, Brooklyn, NY 11209; tel. 718/630–3521

**VA New York Harbor Healthcare System-Opioid Treatment Programs,** 437 West 16th Street, New York, NY 10011; tel. 212/462–4461

*****VA Western New York Health Care System,** 3495 Bailey Avenue, Buffalo, NY 14215; tel. 716/862–8529

*****West Midtown Medical Group,** 505 Eighth Avenue, 4th Floor, New York, NY 10018; tel. 212/736–5900

**Westchester Medical Center,** 100 Woods Road, Taylor Pavilion, Valhalla, NY 10595; tel. 914/493–7000

**Western New York Children's Psychiatric Center,** 1010 East and West Road, West Seneca, NY 14224; tel. 716/677–7000

**Whitney M. Young, Jr. MMTP,** 10 Dewitt Street, Albany, NY 12207; tel. 518/463–3882

**Woodhull Medical and Mental Health Center,** 760 Broadway, Brooklyn, NY 11206; tel. 718/963–8101

**NORTH CAROLINA**

**A Caring Home, Inc.,** 8616 Nations Ford Road, Charlotte, NC 28217-5126; tel. 704/525–2840

**Alexander Youth Network,** PO Box 220632, Charlotte, NC 28222-9979; tel. 704/366–8712

**Allegiance Community Care, LLC,** 604 Calavaras Ln, Knightdale, NC 27545; tel. 919/264–7517

*****AssistedCare Management Group, Inc.,** 1003 Old Waterford Way, Suite 2C, Leland, NC 28451; tel. 910/332–2346

**Autumn Halls of Unaka,** 14949 Joe Brown Hwy, Murphy, NC 28906; tel. 828/835–8103

**Behavioral Enrichment Services, Inc.,** 10130 Mallard Creek Rd Ste 300, Charlotte, NC 28262; tel. 704/968–1864

**Bethesda Care dba Keston Care,** 11312 US 15/ 501 N, Chatham Crossing, Suite 400, Chapel Hill, NC 27517; tel. 919/967–0507

**Blessed Alms,** P.O. Box 16527, Greensboro, NC 27416; tel. 336/997–0971

**Brynn Marr Hospital,** 192 Village Drive, Jacksonville, NC 28546; tel. 910/577–1400

**Canaan Care Home, Inc.,** 2804 Stirrup Court, Wake Forest, NC 27587; tel. 919/274–0596

**Carelink Solutions, Inc.,** P. O. Box 3137, Asheboro, NC 27204; tel. 336/327–2088

**Caring Hands and Supplementary Enrichment Education, LLC,** 3209 Guess Road, Durham, NC 27705; tel. 919/479–6806

**Caring Touch Home Health Care, LLC,** 799 James Lynn Drive, Pembroke, NC 28372; tel. 910/521–9175

**Carolina Comprehensive Services, LLC,** 312 West Millbrook Rd Suite 137, Raleigh, NC 27609; tel. 919/847–0550

*****Carolinas Medical Center,** PO Box 32861, Charlotte, NC 28232; tel. 704/355–7359

*****Carter's Circle of Care, Inc.,** 2031 Martin Luther King Jr. Dr, Ste, E,D,, Greensboro, NC 27406; tel. 336/271–5817

**Champion Healthcare Services, Inc.,** 4428 Louisburg Road Suite 105, Raleigh, NC 27616; tel. 919/522–9896

*****Charles George VA Medical Center at Asheville,** 1100 Tunnel Road, Asheville, NC 28805; tel. 828/298–7911

**Community Treatment Alternatives, Inc.,** 2750 E. W.T. Harris Blvd, Ste 102, Charlotte, NC 28213; tel. 704/323–9266

*****Connections BWB Incorporated,** 8430 University Executive Park Drive Suite 655, Charlotte, NC 28262; tel. 704/596–5553

**Continuum Care Services, Inc.,** P.O. Box 6331, Concord, NC 28027; tel. 704/784–0753

**Crystal E. Nickerson dba Choice Behavioral Health & Consultation,** 2302 West Meadowview Road, Suite 228, Greensboro, NC 27407; tel. 336/617–0764

**Davis Regional Medical Center,** PO Box 1823, Statesville, NC 28687; tel. 704/873–0281

**Eagle Healthcare Services, Inc.,** 4428 Louisburg Road, Suite 109, Raleigh, NC 27604; tel. 919/872–7686

**Enterpro STC Services dba Carolina Care Health Services,** 1100 South Mint Street, Charlotte, NC 28203; tel. 704/379–1850

**Extended Reach Day Treatment,** 2716 Custer Avenue, Fayetteville, NC 28312; tel. 910/484–0095

*****Fellowship Hall, Inc.,** PO Box 13890, Greensboro, NC 27415; tel. 336/621–3381

**First Genesis Group Home, Inc.,** 1903 Delmar Drive, Greensboro, NC 27406; tel. 336/274–4447

**Good Deeds,** 381 Northwoods Drive, Raeford, NC 28376; tel. 910/848–2273

**Good Kids Therapeutic Resources,** 200 Wilson St, Williamston, NC 27892; tel. 919/491–3299

**Grandfather Home for Children,** P. O. Box 98, Banner Elk, NC 28604; tel. 828/898–5465

**Greater Image Healthcare Corporation,** 609 Murchison Road, Fayetteville, NC 28301; tel. 910/527–8466

**Healthcare Solutions Network of North Carolina,** 170 Old Naples Rd., Hendersonville, NC 28792; tel. 828/684–4228

**I Innovations, Inc.,** 176 Sandollar Court, Sanford, NC 27332; tel. 919/770–2457

**Jabez Management, LLC,** P.O. Box 1404, Reidsville, NC 27323-1404; tel. 336/361–9579

**JMJ Enterprise LLC dba Fresh Start Home for Children,** 2020 Textile Drive, Greensboro, NC 27405; tel. 336/271–6982

*****Julian F. Keith Alcohol and Drug Abuse Treatment Center,** 201 Tabernacle Road, Black Mountain, NC 28711; tel. 828/257–6200

**KidsPeace National Centers of North America, Inc.,** 3109 Poplarwood Court, Suite 310, Raleigh, NC 27604; tel. 919/872–6447

**Leading Into New Communities, Inc.,** 907 Castle Street, Wilmington, NC 28401; tel. 910/762–4635

**McLaurin Vocational Training Center, Inc.,** 10 North Bridges Street, Hamlet, NC 28345; tel. 910/582–0934

**Midstate Health Systems, Inc.,** 3721 Legion Rd, Hope Mills, NC 28348; tel. 910/484–3717

**Miss Daisy's Gentlemen of Future,** P.O. Box 1991, Wilson, NC 27894-1991; tel. 252/363–5446

*****Naval Hospital Camp Lejeune,** 100 Brewster Boulevard, Camp Lejeune, NC 28547-2538; tel. 910/450–4007

**New Beginning Youth Facility,** 525 Greenbriar Farm Trl, Siler City, NC 27344; tel. 336/302–0801

**New Beginnings Resources,** 175 Northpoint Avenue, Suite 109, High Point, NC 27264; tel. 336/457–9034

**New Directions Group Care Management,** PO Box 1442, Whiteville, NC 28472; tel. 910/640–1737

**Noir Enterprises, llc,** PO Box 1794, Arden, NC 28704; tel. 828/654–9452

**Old Vineyard Behavioral Health Services,** 3637 Old Vineyard Road, Winston Salem, NC 27104-4842; tel. 336/794–3550

**Patterson Home, Inc.,** p.o.box 64013, Fayetteville, NC 28306; tel. 910/527–8427

**Phoenix Supported Living, Inc.,** 2996 NC 69 S # 6, Hayesville, NC 28904; tel. 828/389–1795

**Positive Outlook Services, LLC,** P.O. Box 2121, Henderson, NC 27536; tel. 252/492–9410

**Quality Home Care Services, Inc,** 3552 Beatties Ford Road, Charlotte, NC 28216; tel. 704/394–8968

**Recovery Innovations of North Carolina,** 300 Parkview Drive West, Henderson, NC 27536; tel. 252/438–4145

**Reintegration Targeting, Inc.,** 2210 North Tyron Street Suite A, Charlotte, NC 28206-2772; tel. 704/334–2600

**Residential Services, Inc.,** 111 Providence Road, Chapel Hill, NC 27514; tel. 919/942–7391

*****Robeson Health Care Corporation,** 60 Commerce Drive, Pembroke, NC 28372; tel. 910/521–2900

**SBH-Wilmington, LLC,** 2050 Mercantile Drive, Leland, NC 28451; tel. 910/371–2500

**Spigner Management Systems, Inc.,** 601 Mann Street, Fayetteville, NC 28301; tel. 910/864–1807

**The Circle of Courage Support Services, LLC,** 3806 Park Avenue, South A, Wilmington, NC 28403; tel. 910/338–0001

**The Renfrew of North Carolina,** 6633 Fairview Road, Charlotte, NC 28210; tel. 704/366–1264

**Timber Ridge Treatment Center,** P O Box 259, Gold Hill, NC 28071; tel. 704/279–1199

**Total Care & Concern, Inc.,** 1428 Orchard Lake Drive, Charlotte, NC 28270; tel. 704/321–1635

*****Tri-County Community Health Council, Inc.,** PO Box 227, Newton Grove, NC 28366; tel. 910/567–6194

**Unique Home Care, Inc.,** P.O. Box 835, Jefferson, NC 28640; tel. 336/246–6991

**United Health Rehabilitation Services, LLC,** 1314 Headquarters Drive, Greensboro, NC 27405; tel. 336/271–6800

*****Unity Healing Center,** PO Box c-201, Cherokee, NC 28719; tel. 828/497–3958

**Unity Home Care, Inc.,** 211 Fairway Drive Suite A, Fayetteville, NC 28305; tel. 910/864–1799

*****VA Medical Center,** 2300 Ramsey Street, Fayetteville, NC 28301; tel. 910/822–7091

*****VA Medical Center,** 508 Fulton Street, Durham, NC 27705; tel. 919/286–0411

**VIRTUE, Inc.,** POB 35492, Charlotte, NC 28235; tel. 704/568–1490

**VisionOne Health Services, Inc.,** 4822 Albemarle Road, Ste 112A, Charlotte, NC 28205; tel. 704/323–7617

*****W & B Health Care, Inc.,** P.O. Box 168, Red Springs, NC 28377; tel. 910/843–1997

*****W. G. (Bill) Hefner VA Medical Center,** 1601 Brenner Avenue, Salisbury, NC 28144; tel. 704/638–9000

*****Walter B. Jones Alcohol & Drug Abuse Treatment Center,** 2577 W. 5th Street, Greenville, NC 27834; tel. 252/830–3426

**Well Care LLC,** 2715 Ashton Drive, Suite 200, Wilmington, NC 28412; tel. 910/452–1555

**Wellness Solution Center,** 1100 North Miami Blvd Suite 601, Durham, NC 27703; tel. 919/682–6909

**Whitaker PRTF,** 1003 12th Street, Butner, NC 27509; tel. 919/575–7927

*****Wilmington Treatment Center, Inc.,** 2520 Troy Drive, Wilmington, NC 28401; tel. 910/762–2727

*****Womack Army Medical Center,** Bldg # 4-2817, Reilly Road, Fort Bragg, NC 28310; tel. 910/907–8917

**NORTH DAKOTA**

**Altru Health System,** P.O. Box 6002, Grand Forks, ND 58206-6002; tel. 701/780–5000

*****Center for Solutions PC,** 7448 68th Avenue NE, Cando, ND 58324; tel. 701/968–2568

*****Fargo VA Health Care System,** 2101 Elm Street North, Fargo, ND 58102; tel. 701/239–3241

*****North Dakota State Hospital,** 2605 Circle Drive, Jamestown, ND 58401-6905; tel. 701/253–3964

*****Prairie St. John's,** PO Box 2027, Fargo, ND 58107-2027; tel. 701/476–7200

**Saint Alexius Medical Center,** 900 East Broadway, Bismarck, ND 58502; tel. 701/530–7600

---

*Indicates organization is a Joint Commission accredited Chemical Dependency organization.

© 2012 AHA Guide

Section C

*Sanford Medical Center Fargo, 801 Broadway North, Fargo, ND 58122; tel. 701/234-2000

*Trinity Health, PO Box 5020, Minot, ND 58702-5020; tel. 701/857-5000

**OHIO**

*Abraxas Counseling Center, 899 East Broad Street, Columbus, OH 43205; tel. 614/220-8655

Access Ohio, 99 N Brice Rd Suite 360, Columbus, OH 43213; tel. 614/225-0400

Akron Children's Hospital, One Perkins Square, Akron, OH 44308-1082; tel. 330/543-1000

*Akron-Urban Minority Alcoholism Drug Abuse Outreach, 665 W Market Street, Akron, OH 44303; tel. 330/379-3467

Appalachian Behavioral Healthcare, 100 Hospital Drive, Athens, OH 45701; tel. 740/594-5000

Applewood Centers, Inc., 2525 East 22nd St, Cleveland, OH 44115-3266; tel. 216/696-5800

*Beech Brook, 3737 Lander Road, Cleveland, OH 44124; tel. 216/831-2255

*Behavioral Connections of Wood County, Inc., Post Office Box 29, Bowling Green, OH 43402; tel. 419/352-5387

*Bellefaire Jewish Children's Bureau, 22001 Fairmount Boulevard, Shaker Heights, OH 44118; tel. 216/932-2800

Belmont Pines Hospital, 615 Churchhill-Hubbard Road, Youngstown, OH 44505; tel. 330/759-2700

BHC Fox Run Hospital, 67670 Traco Drive, Saint Clairsville, OH 43950; tel. 740/695-2131

*Center for Chemical Addictions Treatment, 830 Ezzard Charles Drive, Cincinnati, OH 45214; tel. 513/381-6672

*Chalmers P. Wylie Ambulatory Care Center, 420 North James Road, Columbus, OH 43219; tel. 614/257-5200

Child Guidance & Family Solutions, 312 Locust Street, Akron, OH 44302; tel. 330/762-0591

Cincinnati Children's Hospital Medical Center, 3333 Burnet Avenue, Cincinnati, OH 45229-3039; tel. 513/636-3333

Cleveland Clinic, 9500 Euclid Avenue HS1-04, Cleveland, OH 44195; tel. 216/444-2200

Cleveland Clinic Children's Hospital for Rehabilitation, 2801 Martin Luther King, Jr. Drive, Cleveland, OH 44104; tel. 216/448-6400

Community Behavioral Health Center, 3355 Richmond Road, 225-A, Beachwood, OH 44122; tel. 216/831-1494

*Community Behavioral Health, Inc., 520 Eaton Ave, Hamilton, OH 45013; tel. 513/785-4784

*Community Counseling Center of Ashtabula County, 2801 C Court, Ashtabula, OH 44004; tel. 440/998-4210

*Community Health Center, 725 East Market Street, Akron, OH 44305; tel. 330/434-4141

Comprehensive Psychiatry Group, Inc., 955 Windham Court, Youngstown, OH 44512; tel. 330/726-9570

*Cornell Abraxas, 2775 State Route 39, Shelby, OH 44875; tel. 419/747-3322

*Craig and Frances Lindner Center of HOPE, 4075 Old Western Row Road, Mason, OH 45040; tel. 513/536-4673

*Crisis Intervention and Recovery Center, Inc., 832 McKinley Avenue NW, Canton, OH 44703; tel. 330/452-9812

*Department of Veterans Affairs Medical Center-Dayton, 4100 West 3rd Street, Dayton, OH 45428; tel. 937/268-6511

Far West Center, 29133 Health Campus Drive, Westlake, OH 44145; tel. 440/835-6212

*Glenbeigh, PO Box 298, Rock Creek, OH 44084-0298; tel. 440/563-3400

*Interval Brotherhood Homes, Inc., 3445 South Main Street, Akron, OH 44319; tel. 330/644-4095

Lake Health, 7590 Auburn Road, Painesville, OH 44077; tel. 440/375-8100

Lifessentials Counseling, 131 N Ludlow Street, Suite 1212, Dayton, OH 45402; tel. 937/222-5496

*Lorain County Alcohol and Drug Abuse Services, Inc., 2115 W PARK DR, Lorain, OH 44053-1138; tel. 440/282-4777

*Louis Stokes, Cleveland VA Medical Center, 10701 East Boulevard, Cleveland, OH 44106; tel. 216/231-3456

Marymount Hospital, 12300 McCracken Road, Garfield Heights, OH 44125; tel. 216/581-0500

Maumee Valley Guidance Center, 211 Biede Avenue, Defiance, OH 43512; tel. 419/782-8856

*Mental Health Services for Clark and Madison Counties, Inc., 1345 Fountain Boulevard, Springfield, OH 45504; tel. 937/399-9500

*Nationwide Children's Hospital, Inc., 700 Children's Drive, Columbus, OH 43205; tel. 614/722-5950

*Neil Kennedy Recovery Clinic, 2151 Rush Boulevard, Youngstown, OH 44507; tel. 330/744-1181

New Albany Home Health Solutions, LLC, 4401 Oaks Shadow Drive, New Albany, OH 43054; tel. 614/557-1145

*New Directions, Inc., 30800 Chagrin Boulevard, Cleveland, OH 44124; tel. 216/591-0324

Northcoast Behavioral Healthcare, 1756 Sagamore Road, Northfield, OH 44067; tel. 330/467-7131

*Northland/The Ridge, 50 W. Technecenter Drive Suite B5, Milford, OH 45150; tel. 513/753-9964

Ohio Hospital for Psychiatry, 880 Greenlawn Avenue, Columbus, OH 43223; tel. 614/449-9664

Opiate Substitution Services-SUDEP, CVAMC, 3200 Vine Street, Cincinnati, OH 45220; tel. 513/861-3100

Phoenix Rising Behaviorall Healthcare And Recovery, Inc., 4974 Higbee ave, suite 209, Canton, OH 44718; tel. 330/493-4553

Pomegranate Health Systems of Central Ohio, 765 Pierce Drive, Columbus, OH 43223; tel. 614/223-1650

Portage Path Behavioral Health, 340 South Broadway, Akron, OH 44308; tel. 330/253-3100

*Promedica Toledo Hospital, 2142 North Cove Boulevard, Toledo, OH 43606; tel. 419/291-7460

PsyCare, Inc., 2980 Belmont Avenue, Youngstown, OH 44505; tel. 330/759-2310

*Rakesh Ranjan MD and Associates, Inc, 12300 McCraken Road, Suite 137, Garfield Heights, OH 44105; tel. 216/587-6727

*Ravenwood Mental Health Center, 12557 Ravenwood Drive, Chardon, OH 44024; tel. 440/285-3568

*Rescue Incorporated, 3350 Collingwood Boulevard, Toledo, OH 43610; tel. 419/255-9585

Rocking Horse Children's Health Center, 651 S. Limestone Street, Springfield, OH 45505; tel. 937/324-1111

Shaker Clinic, LLC, 20600 Chagrin Boulevard Suite 620, Shaker Heights, OH 44122; tel. 216/751-4762

*Southeast, Inc., 16 West Long Street, Columbus, OH 43215; tel. 614/225-0980

*Southwest General Health Center, 18697 East Bagley Road, Middleburg Heights, OH 44130; tel. 440/816-8469

Specialty Care Counseling Services, Ltd, 2000 East Market Street, Warren, OH 44483; tel. 330/399-1221

*St. Vincent Charity Medical Center, 2351 East 22nd Street, Cleveland, OH 44115; tel. 216/861-6200

*Stella Maris, Inc., 1320 Washington Avenue, Cleveland, OH 44113; tel. 216/781-0550

*The Buckeye Ranch, Inc., 5665 Hoover Road, Grove City, OH 43123; tel. 614/875-2371

*The Crossroads Center, 311 Martin Luther King Drive, Cincinnati, OH 45220; tel. 513/475-5300

The MetroHealth System, 2500 MetroHealth Drive, Cleveland, OH 44109-1998; tel. 216/778-7800

*The Ohio State University Hospital, 452 W. 10th Ave, RHH 1255, Columbus, OH 43210; tel. 614/293-9700

The University of Toledo Medical Center, 3000 Arlington Avenue, Toledo, OH 43614; tel. 419/383-3407

*The Woods at Parkside, 349 Olde Ridenour Road, Columbus, OH 43230; tel. 614/471-2552

Twin Valley Behavioral Healthcare, 2200 West Broad Street, Columbus, OH 43223; tel. 614/752-0333

*Unison Behavioral Health Group, PO Box 10015, Toledo, OH 43699-0015; tel. 419/242-9577

*VA Healthcare System of Ohio-Cincinnati Campus, 3200 Vine Street, Cincinnati, OH 45220; tel. 513/861-3100

*VA Medical Center-Chillicothe, 17273 State Route 104, Chillicothe, OH 45601; tel. 740/773-1141

Visiting Nurse Association Healthcare Partners of Ohio, 2500 East 22nd Street, Cleveland, OH 44115; tel. 216/931-1300

*Windsor Laurelwood Center for Behavioral Medicine, 35900 Euclid Avenue, Willoughby, OH 44094; tel. 440/953-3000

*Wood County Children's Services Association, PO Box 738, Bowling Green, OH 43402; tel. 419/352-7588

Zepf Center, 6605 West Central Avenue, Toledo, OH 43617; tel. 419/841-7701

**OKLAHOMA**

*Advantage Community Resources LLC, 11032 Quail Creek Road, Suite # 175, Oklahoma City, OK 73120; tel. 405/206-0177

AHS Hillcrest Medical Center, LLC, 1120 South Utica Avenue, Tulsa, OK 74104-4090; tel. 918/579-1000

Alliance of Tulsa, Inc., 5214 E. 71st Street Suite 1400, Tulsa, OK 74136; tel. 918/747-0155

*Alpha II, Inc., 1608 N. Main Street, Tonkawa, OK 74653; tel. 580/628-2539

BetterLife Counseling Services, Inc., 9700 South Pennsylvania Avenue, Oklahoma City, OK 73159; tel. 405/735-9732

*Broadway House, Inc, 221 Second Avenue NW, Ardmore, OK 73401; tel. 580/226-3252

*Brookhaven Hospital, 201 South Garnett Road, Tulsa, OK 74128-1800; tel. 918/438-4257

Carl Albert Community Mental Health Center, PO Box 579, McAlester, OK 74502; tel. 918/426-7800

Cedar Ridge, 6501 NE 50th Street, Oklahoma City, OK 73141; tel. 405/605-6111

Central Oklahoma Family Medical Center, Inc., P.O. Box 358, Konawa, OK 74849; tel. 580/925-3286

Child & Family Wellness Center, 355004 E 750 Rd, Cushing, OK 74023; tel. 918/225-0750

*Children's Recovery Center of Oklahoma, 320 12th Avenue Northeast, Norman, OK 73071; tel. 405/364-9004

Choices Institute, 529 N. Grand, Enid, OK 73701; tel. 580/234-8880

Core Life Counseling Center, LLC, P.O. Box 3013, Enid, OK 73703; tel. 580/237-3432

*Cornerstone Clinical Services, Inc., 1919 West Elk Avenue, Duncan, OK 73533; tel. 580/595-7000

*Cushing Valley Hope, PO Box 472, Cushing, OK 74023-0472; tel. 918/225-1736

Daybreak Family Services, 1516 S. Boston Avenue Suite 1, Tulsa, OK 74119; tel. 918/561-6000

*Department of Veterans Affairs Medical Center, 921 Northeast 13th Street, Oklahoma City, OK 73104; tel. 405/456-3312

Discovery Uttuwah LLC, 118 So. Main, Wagoner, OK 74467; tel. 918/485-1573

Duncan Regional Hospital, Inc., 1407 Whisenant Drive, Duncan, OK 73533; tel. 580/252-5300

Family Options, 2914 Epperly Drive, Del City, OK 73115; tel. 405/604-9790

*Health Concepts Family Services Outpatient Behavioral Health, 1843 SE 15th Street, Tulsa, OK 74104; tel. 918/872-6135

Health Network, LLC, 1366 Southeast Washington Boulevard, Suite A, Bartlesville, OK 74006; tel. 918/333-0222

IMPACT (University of Oklahoma-Tulsa), 4502 E. 41st Street Room 2G07, Tulsa, OK 74135; tel. 918/660-3150

Improving Lives Counseling Services, Inc., 6216 S. Lewis Avenue, Suite 180, Tulsa, OK 74136; tel. 918/812-6010

Integrated Comprehensive Health Care (ICHC), LLC, 4801 N Classen BLVD, Oklahoma City, OK 73118; tel. 405/843-7300

*INTEGRIS Baptist Medical Center, 3300 NW Expressway, Oklahoma City, OK 73112-4481; tel. 405/949-4069

*Jack C. Montgomery VA Medical Center, 1011 Honor Heights Drive, Muskogee, OK 74401; tel. 918/577-3000

Jennifer M Smith MCP, LPC, PLC, 3910 W. 6th Ave, Stillwater, OK 74074; tel. 918/978-1109

*Jim Taliaferro Community Mental Health Center, 602 SW 38th st, Lawton, OK 73505; tel. 580/248-5780

Land Of Hope, 57523 Moccasin Trail Road, Prague, OK 74864; tel. 405/567-0054

*Laureate Psychiatric Clinic and Hospital, 6655 South Yale Avenue, Tulsa, OK 74136; tel. 918/481-4000

Lifeworks Counseling Solutions, LLC, 311 West Main Street, Canton, OK 73724; tel. 580/515-1010

Medical Center of Southeastern Oklahoma, PO Box 1207, Durant, OK 74701; tel. 580/924-3080

Next Step Counseling, 1301 Martin Luther King Avenue, Suite 101, Oklahoma City, OK 73117; tel. 405/476-8412

Norman Counseling Clinic, 2416 Tee Circle, Norman, OK 73069; tel. 405/809-2004

**Section C**

**Norman Regional Health System,** PO Box 1308, Norman, OK 73070-1308; tel. 405/307-1000

**\*Northwest Center for Behavioral Health (NCBH),** 1222 10th Street, Suite 211, Woodward, OK 73801; tel. 580/256-8615

**Oklahoma Counseling Services, Inc.,** 3100 S. Elm Place, Suite B, Broken Arrow, OK 74012; tel. 918/286-2535

**Oklahoma Forensic Center,** PO Box 69, Vinita, OK 74301-0069; tel. 918/256-7841

**Oklahoma Play Therapy Counseling Center,** 502 W. Randolph, Enid, OK 73701; tel. 580/484-5683

**Parkside, Inc.,** 1620 East 12th Street, Tulsa, OK 74120; tel. 918/582-2131

**Pennington Creek Lifehouse,** 801 E Main, Tishomingo, OK 73460; tel. 580/310-4164

**Positive Changes,** 744 SE 25th Street, Oklahoma City, OK 73129; tel. 405/636-1463

**Professional Counseling Solutions, PLLC,** 1500 North Main, Frederick, OK 73542; tel. 580/335-3320

**Promise Family Center, PLLC,** 5350 South Western Suite 305, Oklahoma City, OK 73109; tel. 405/431-0232

**Sequel of Oklahoma, LLC,** 3301 North Martin Luther King Avenue, Oklahoma City, OK 73111; tel. 405/548-1280

**Solutions for Life Counseling Services,** 309 W. Cherokee, Enid, OK 73701; tel. 580/234-4700

**Southeastern Psychiatric Services,** P.O. Box 1589, McAlester, OK 74502; tel. 918/423-3700

**SouthWest Counseling Services, PLLC,** 703 Frisco Avenue, Clinton, OK 73601; tel. 580/323-9100

**Southwest Foster Care Of Oklahoma,** 4801 North Classen Blvd Suite 135, Oklahoma City, OK 73118; tel. 405/848-0011

**Southwest Oklahoma Counseling,** P.O. Box 691, Clinton, OK 73601; tel. 580/323-9800

**\*St. Anthony Hospital,** 1000 North Lee Street, Oklahoma City, OK 73101; tel. 405/272-7000

**Substance Abuse Treatment Center, OKC VAMC,** 921 NE 13th St, Bldg 1, Oklahoma City, OK 73104; tel. 405/456-3312

**Tulsa Center for Behavioral Health,** 2323 South Harvard, Tulsa, OK 74114; tel. 918/293-2140

**Universal Health Services, Inc.,** 6262 South Sheridan Road, Tulsa, OK 74133; tel. 918/492-8200

**VCPHCS IV, LLC dba BHG Oklahoma City Clinic (Opioid Treatment Programs),** 5401 SW 29th, Oklahoma City, OK 73128; tel. 405/681-2003

**Willow Crest Hospital, Inc.,** 130 A Street South West, Miami, OK 74354; tel. 918/542-1836

**\*YCO, Inc.,** P.O.Box 95207, Oklahoma City, OK 73143; tel. 405/917-5677

**OREGON**

**Catherine Freer Wilderness Therapy Programs,** PO Box 1064, Albany, OR 97321; tel. 541/926-7252

**CODA, Inc.,** 1027 E. Burnside, Portland, OR 97214-1328; tel. 503/239-8400

**\*Hazelden Foundation,** 1901 Esther Street, Newberg, OR 97132; tel. 503/554-4300

**Kerr Youth and Family Services,** 722 Northeast 162nd Avenue, Portland, OR 97230; tel. 503/255-4205

**Northwest Behavioral Healthcare Services,** 18000 Southeast Webster Road, Gladstone, OR 97027; tel. 503/722-4470

**Northwest Human Services,** 681 Center Street, NE, Salem, OR 97301; tel. 503/588-5828

**Oregon State Hospital,** 2600 Center Street, NE, Salem, OR 97301-2682; tel. 503/945-2870

**\*Portland VA Medical Center,** 3710 SW US Veteran's Hospital RD, PO Box 1034, (P3OTP), Portland, OR 97207; tel. 503/273-5267

**\*Providence Portland Medical Center,** 4805 Northeast Glisan Street, Portland, OR 97213; tel. 503/215-2349

**\*Providence St. Vincent Medical Center,** 9205 Southwest Barnes Road, Portland, OR 97225; tel. 503/216-1234

**Rainrock Treatment Center,** 1863 Pioneer Parkway East Suite 304, Springfield, OR 97477; tel. 541/896-9300

**\*Serenity Lane,** 2133 Centennial Plaza, Eugene, OR 97401; tel. 541/284-8611

**Southern Oregon Adolescent Study and Treatment Center,** 715 SW Ramsey Avenue, Grants Pass, OR 97527; tel. 541/956-4943

**Trillium Family Services,** 3415 SE Powell Blvd, Portland, OR 97202; tel. 503/234-9591

**\*UBH of Oregon,** 10300 SW Eastridge Street, Portland, OR 97225; tel. 503/944-5000

**\*VA Roseburg Healthcare System,** 913 NW Garden Valley Boulevard, Roseburg, OR 97471; tel. 541/440-1000

**\*VA Southern Oregon Rehabilitation Center and Clinics,** 8495 Crater Lake Highway, White City, OR 97503; tel. 541/826-2111

**Youth Villages-ChristieCare of Oregon,** PO Box 368, Marylhurst, OR 97036; tel. 503/635-3416

**PENNSYLVANIA**

**Abraxas Academy,** 1000 Academy Drive, Morgantown, PA 19543; tel. 610/913-8000

**\*Abraxas I,** PO Box 59, Marienville, PA 16239; tel. 814/927-6615

**\*Abraxas, a GEO Group Company,** 429 West 6th Street, Erie, PA 16507; tel. 814/459-0618

**\*Adelphoi Village, Inc.,** 1119 Village Way, Latrobe, PA 15650; tel. 724/520-1111

**Albert Einstein Medical Center,** 5501 Old York Road, Philadelphia, PA 19141; tel. 215/456-7890

**Associates in Counseling and Child Guidance,** 272 East Connelly Boulevard, Sharon, PA 16146; tel. 724/983-1381

**Beacon Light Behavioral Health Systems,** 800 East Main Street, Bradford, PA 16701; tel. 814/362-5250

**Belmont Center for Comprehensive Treatment,** 4200 Monument Road, Philadelphia, PA 19131; tel. 215/877-2000

**Bethesda Children's Home,** 15667 State Highway 86, Meadville, PA 16335; tel. 814/724-7510

**Bryn Mawr Hospital,** 130 South Bryn Mawr Avenue, Bryn Mawr, PA 19010; tel. 484/337-3000

**Bustleton Mental Health Institute, Inc.,** 1701 Grant Avenue, Philadelphia, PA 19115-3160; tel. 215/464-3838

**Child Guidance Resource Centers,** 2000 Old West Chester Pike, Havertown, PA 19083; tel. 484/454-8700

**Children's Aid Home Programs of Somerset County, Inc.,** PO Box 1195, Somerset, PA 15501; tel. 814/443-1637

**Children's BehavioralHealth, Inc.,** 203 College Park Plaza, Johnstown, PA 15904; tel. 814/262-0768

**Children's Service Center of Wyoming Valley, Inc.,** 335 South Franklin Street, Wilkes Barre, PA 18702; tel. 570/825-6425

**Choices Program of Wyoming Valley,** 307 Laird Street, Plains, PA 18705; tel. 570/552-3700

**CHOR Youth & Family Services, Inc.,** 1010 Centre Avenue, Reading, PA 19601-1498; tel. 610/478-8266

**\*Clear Brook, Inc.,** 1003 Wyoming Avenue, Forty Fort, PA 18704; tel. 570/288-6692

**\*Corecare Behavioral Health Management, Inc.,** 111 North 49th Street, Philadelphia, PA 19139; tel. 215/471-2600

**Crozer Chester Medical Center-Community Hospital of Chester,** One Medical Center Boulevard, Chester, PA 19013; tel. 610/447-2000

**Devereux Children's Behavioral Health Services,** 655 Sugartown Road, PO Box 297, Malvern, PA 19355-0297; tel. 484/595-6733

**Diversified Treatment Alternatives, Inc.,** 148 Fairfield Road, Lewisburg, PA 17837; tel. 570/523-3457

**\*Eagleville Hospital,** 100 Eagleville Road, PO Box 45, Eagleville, PA 19408-0045; tel. 610/539-6000

**EIHAB Human Services, Inc.,** 1200 SR 92 South, Tunkhannock, PA 18657; tel. 570/388-6155

**\*Erie VA Medical Center,** 135 East 38th Street, Erie, PA 16504; tel. 814/868-8661

**\*Fairmount Behavioral Health System,** 561 Fairthorne Avenue, Philadelphia, PA 19128; tel. 215/487-4000

**Foundations Medical Services,** 124 Hollywood Drive Bantam Commons Bld 2, Butler, PA 16001; tel. 724/431-2006

**\*Friends Behavioral Health System, LP,** 4641 Roosevelt Boulevard, Philadelphia, PA 19124-2399; tel. 215/831-4600

**\*Gateway Rehabilitation Center / Genesis Division,** 311 Rouser Road, Moon Township, PA 15108; tel. 412/604-8900

**Geisinger Medical Center,** 100 North Academy Avenue, Danville, PA 17822; tel. 570/271-6211

**Glade Run Lutheran Services,** PO Box 70, Zelienople, PA 16063-0070; tel. 724/452-4453

**\*Greater Philadelphia Health Action, Inc. (GPHA),** 432 North 6th Street, Philadelphia, PA 19123; tel. 215/925-2400

**\*Greenbriar Treatment Center,** 800 Manor Drive, Washington, PA 15301; tel. 724/225-9700

**Hoffman Homes, Inc.,** PO Box 4777, Gettysburg, PA 17325; tel. 717/359-7148

**\*Holcomb Behavioral Health Systems,** 835 Springdale Drive Suite 100, Exton, PA 19341; tel. 610/363-1488

**Holy Spirit Hospital,** 503 North 21st Street, Camp Hill, PA 17011-2288; tel. 717/763-2100

**Kensington Hospital Outpatient Treatment Program,** 136 West Diamond Street, Philadelphia, PA 19122; tel. 215/426-8100

**KidsPeace National Centers, Inc/KidsPeace Children's Hospital,** 4085 Independence Drive, Schnecksville, PA 18078; tel. 610/799-8000

**Kirkbride Center,** 111 North 49th Street, Philadelphia, PA 19139; tel. 215/471-2600

**\*Lebanon VA Medical Center,** 1700 South Lincoln Avenue, Lebanon, PA 17042; tel. 717/272-6621

**Lehigh Valley Hospital,** PO Box 689, Cedar Crest & I-78, Allentown, PA 18105-1556; tel. 610/402-8000

**Lehigh Valley Hospital-Muhlenberg,** 2545 Schoenersville Road, Bethlehem, PA 18017-7384; tel. 484/884-2200

**\*Live Well Services, Inc.,** 203 Floral Vale Blvd, Yardley, PA 19067; tel. 215/968-7600

**\*Livengrin Foundation, Inc.,** 4833 Hulmeville Road, Bensalem, PA 19020-3099; tel. 215/638-5200

**\*Marworth,** PO Box 36, Waverly, PA 18471; tel. 570/563-1112

**Mercy Catholic Medical Center/Mercy Hospital of Philadelphia,** 501 South 54th Street, Philadelphia, PA 19143; tel. 215/748-9300

**\*Mirmont Treatment Center,** 100 Yearsley Mill Road, Media, PA 19063-5593; tel. 484/227-1400

**Montgomery County Emergency Service, Inc.,** 50 Beech Drive, Norristown, PA 19403-5421; tel. 610/279-6100

**Narcotic Addict Rehabilitation Program of Thomas Jefferson University,** 1020 South 21st St (NE Corner of 21st & Washington Ave, Philadelphia, PA 19146; tel. 215/735-5979

**NATP of Western Psychiatric Institute & Clinic of UPMC P-S,** 6714 Kelly Street, Pittsburgh, PA 15208; tel. 412/624-1000

**New Vitae, Inc. Partial Hospital Program and Outpatient Clinic,** 16 South Main Street, Quakertown, PA 18951; tel. 215/538-3403

**Nulton Diagnostic and Treatment Center, PC,** 214 College Park Plaza, Johnstown, PA 15904; tel. 814/262-0025

**Pamela Ralph MD PC, Inc.,** 1489 Baltimore Pike, Springfield, PA 19064; tel. 484/472-7430

**Paoletta Counseling Services,** 456 N Pitt Street, Mercer, PA 16137; tel. 724/662-7202

**Paoli Hospital,** 255 W. Lancaster Avenue, Paoli, PA 19301; tel. 610/648-1000

**Pennsylvania Hospital,** 800 Spruce Street, Philadelphia, PA 19107; tel. 215/829-6511

**Pennsylvania Psychiatric Institute,** 2501 Third Street, Harrisburg, PA 17110; tel. 717/782-4734

**Perseus House, Inc.,** 1511 Peach Street, Erie, PA 16501; tel. 814/480-5900

**\*Philadelphia VA Medical Center,** University and Woodland Avenues, Philadelphia, PA 19104; tel. 215/823-5857

**Philhaven,** PO Box 550, Mount Gretna, PA 17064; tel. 717/273-8871

**Presbyterian Children's Village Services,** 452 South Roberts Road, Bryn Mawr, PA 19010; tel. 610/525-5400

**Progressive Medical Specialists, Inc.,** 2453 West Pike Road, Houston, PA 15342; tel. 724/873-5655

**Progressive Medical Specialists, Inc.,** 2900 Smallman Street, Pittsburgh, PA 15201; tel. 412/391-6384

**Psychiatric Care Systems, PC,** 110 Hidden Valley Road, McMurray, PA 15317; tel. 724/941-4070

**Pyramid Healthcare Inc., Dolminis Methadone Clinic,** 2 Sellers Drive, Altoona, PA 16601; tel. 814/940-0407

**\*Pyramid Healthcare, Inc.,** P.O. Box 967, Duncansville, PA 16635; tel. 814/940-0407

**Pyramid Healthcare, Inc.-York, Opioid Treatment Programs,** 104 Davies Drive, York, PA 17402; tel. 717/840-2300

**RHH Medical Center, Inc.,** 1005 Old State Rt.119, Hunker, PA 15639; tel. 724/696-9600

**RHJ Medical Center, Inc., Vandergrift, LLC,** 2994 River Road, Vandergrift, PA 15690; tel. 724/842-0357

**\*Roxbury Treatment Center,** 601 Roxbury Road, Shippensburg, PA 17257; tel. 717/532-4217

---

\*Indicates organization is a Joint Commission accredited Chemical Dependency organization.